P9-DHY-898

Williams
Hematology

NOTICE

Medicine is an ever-changing science. As new research and clinical experience broaden our knowledge, changes in treatment and drug therapy are required. The authors and the publisher of this work have checked with sources believed to be reliable in their efforts to provide information that is complete and generally in accord with the standards accepted at the time of publication. However, in view of the possibility of human error or changes in medical sciences, neither the authors nor the publisher nor any other party who has been involved in the preparation or publication of this work warrants that the information contained herein is in every respect accurate or complete, and they disclaim all responsibility for any errors or omissions or for the results obtained from use of the information contained in this work. Readers are encouraged to confirm the information contained herein with other sources. For example and in particular, readers are advised to check the product information sheet included in the package of each drug they plan to administer to be certain that the information contained in this work is accurate and that changes have not been made in the recommended dose or in the contraindications for administration. This recommendation is of particular importance in connection with new or infrequently used drugs.

Williams Hematology

Eighth Edition

Kenneth Kaushansky, MD
Helen M. Ranney Professor and Chair
Department of Medicine
University of California, San Diego
La Jolla, California

Marshall A. Lichtman, MD
Professor of Medicine and of Biochemistry and Biophysics
University of Rochester Medical Center
Rochester, New York

Ernest Beutler, MD*
Professor and Chairman
Department of Molecular and Experimental Medicine
The Scripps Research Institute
La Jolla, California
Senior Consultant
Division of Hematology Oncology
Scripps Clinic Medical Group, Inc.
Clinical Professor of Medicine
University of California, San Diego
La Jolla, California

Thomas J. Kipps, MD, PhD
Evelyn and Edwin Tasch Chair in Cancer Research
Professor of Medicine
Division of Hematology/Oncology
Deputy Director for Research Operations
Moores UCSD Cancer Center
University of California, San Diego
La Jolla, California

Uri Seligsohn, MD
Professor and Director
Amalia Biron Research Institute of Thrombosis and Hemostasis
Department of Hematology
Chaim Sheba Medical Center
Tel-Hashomer and Sackler Faculty of Medicine
Tel Aviv University
Tel Aviv, Israel

*Deceased (5 October 2008)

Josef T. Prchal, MD
Professor of Medicine, Pathology, and Genetics
Hematology Division
University of Utah
Salt Lake City, Utah
Department of Pathophysiology
First Faculty of Medicine
Charles University in Prague
Czech Republic

Mc Graw Hill Medical

New York Chicago San Francisco Lisbon London Madrid Mexico City
Milan New Delhi San Juan Seoul Singapore Sydney Toronto

The McGraw·Hill Companies

Williams HEMATOLOGY, Eighth Edition

Copyright © 2010, by The McGraw-Hill Companies, Inc. All rights reserved. Printed in China. Except as permitted under the United States Copyright Act of 1976, no part of this publication may be reproduced or distributed in any form or by any means, or stored in a data base or retrieval system, without the prior written permission of the publisher.

1 2 3 4 5 6 7 8 9 0 CTP/CTP 14 13 12 11 10

Set ISBN 978-0-07-162151-9; MHID 0-07-162151-2
Book ISBN 978-0-07-162144-1 MHID 0-07-162144-X
CD ISBN 978-0-07-162145-8; MHID 0-07-162145-8

This book was set in Minion Pro by Silverchair Science + Communications, Inc.
The editors were James Shanahan and Harriet Lebowitz.
The production supervisor was Sherri Souffrance.
Production services were provided by Sylvia Rebert of Progressive Publishing Alternatives.
The designer was Alan Barnett.
The cover designer was Margaret Webster-Shapiro.
China Translation & Printing Services, Ltd., was printer and binder.

This book is printed on acid-free paper.

Library of Congress Cataloging-in-Publication Data

Williams hematology / editors, Kenneth Kaushansky ... [et al.]. — 8th ed.
p. ; cm.
Other title: Hematology
Rev. ed. of: Williams hematology / editors, Marshall A. Lichtman ... [et al.]. 7th ed. c2006.
Includes bibliographical references and index.
Summary: "A comprehensive textbook outlining all facets of hematology"—Provided by publisher.
ISBN-13: 978-0-07-162151-9 (set : alk. paper)
ISBN-10: 0-07-162151-2 (set : alk. paper)
ISBN-13: 978-0-07-162144-1 (alk. paper)
ISBN-10: 0-07-162144-X (alk. paper)
1. Blood—Diseases. 2. Hematology. I. Kaushansky, Kenneth. II. Williams, William J. (William Joseph), 1926– III. Title: Hematology.
[DNLM: 1. Hematologic Diseases. WH 100 W721 2011]
RC633.H43 2011
616.1'5—dc22

2010001715

McGraw-Hill books are available at special quantity discounts to use as premiums and sales promotions, or for use in corporate training programs. To contact a representative please e-mail us at bulksales@mcgraw-hill.com.

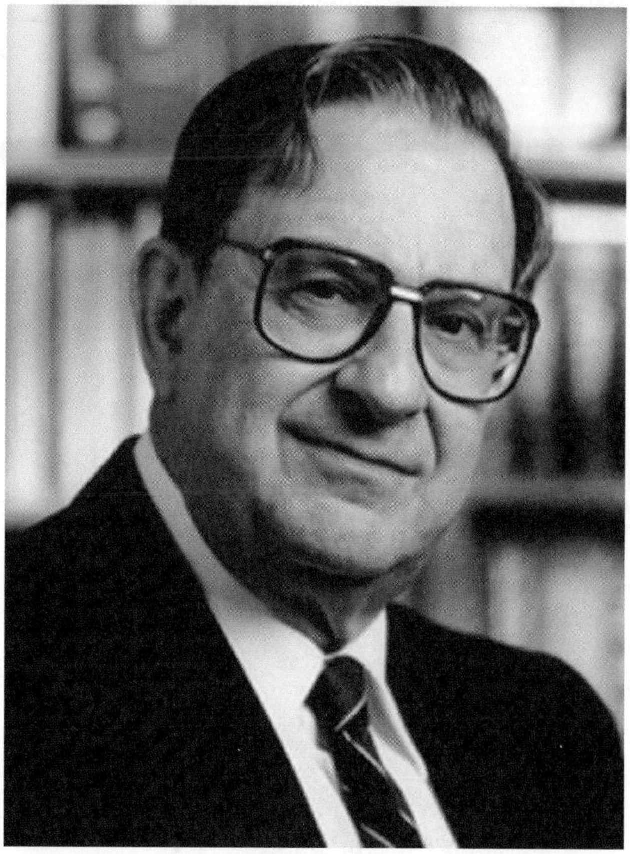

Ernest Beutler, MD
1928–2008

This 8th edition of *Williams Hematology* is dedicated to Ernest Beutler,
committed physician, extraordinary scientist, stimulating educator,
gifted administrator, dear friend, valued colleague,
and one of the founding editors of *Hematology*.

CONTENTS

PART VII

Neutrophils, Eosinophils, Basophils, and Mast Cells

PART VIII

Monocytes and Macrophages

PART IX

Lymphocytes and Plasma Cells

PART X

Neoplastic Myeloid Diseases

PART XIII

Transfusion Medicine

CONTRIBUTORS

Charles S. Abrams, MD [122]
Professor of Medicine
Division of Hematology-Oncology
University of Pennsylvania School of Medicine
Philadelphia, Pennsylvania

Archana M. Agarwal, MD [44]
Department of Pathology, University of Utah
Salt Lake City, Utah

Neeraj Agarwal, MD [49]
Assistant Professor of Medicine
Department of Internal Medicine
University of Utah
Salt Lake City, Utah

Doru T. Alexandrescu, MD [123]
Department of Medicine
Division of Dermatology
University of California, San Diego
VA San Diego Health Care System
San Diego, California

Carl E. Allen, MD, PhD [72]
Texas Children's Cancer Center/Hematology
Baylor College of Medicine
Houston, Texas

Elias Anaissie, MD [109]
Myeloma Institute for Research and Therapy
University of Arkansas for Medical Sciences
Little Rock, Arkansas

Karl E. Anderson, MD, FACP [57]
Professor, Departments of Preventative Medicine and Community Health, Internal Medicine, and Pharmacology and Toxicology
University of Texas Medical Branch
Galveston, Texas

Edgardo Angtuaco [109]
Myeloma Institute for Research and Therapy
University of Arkansas for Medical Sciences
Little Rock, Arkansas

Daniel A. Arber, MD [63]
Director of Clinical Hematology
Clinical Laboratories
Stanford University Medical Center
Stanford, California

Kelty R. Baker, MD [50]
Clinical Assistant Professor
Baylor College of Medicine
Houston, Texas

Bart Barlogie, MD, PhD [109]
Myeloma Institute for Research and Therapy
University of Arkansas for Medical Sciences
Little Rock, Arkansas

Jeffery Barnes [20]
Massachusetts General Hospital Cancer Center
Boston, Massachusetts

Twyla Bartel [109]
Myeloma Institute for Research and Therapy
University of Arkansas for Medical Sciences
Little Rock, Arkansas

Philip A. Beer, MD [87]
Department of Haematology
University of Cambridge
Cambridge Institute for Medical Research
Cambridge, United Kingdom

Joel S. Bennett, MD [122]
Professor of Medicine and Pharmacology
Division of Hematology-Oncology
University of Pennsylvania School of Medicine
Philadelphia, Pennsylvania

Carolina Berger, MD [24]
Fred Hutchinson Cancer Research Center
Seattle, Washington

Robert F. Betts, MD [84]
University of Rochester Medical Center
Rochester, New York

Bruce Beutler, MD [18]
Professor and Chairman
Department of Genetics
The Scripps Research Institute
La Jolla, California

Ernest Beutler, MD [1, 9, 30, 32, 42]*
Professor and Chairman
Department of Molecular and Experimental Medicine
The Scripps Research Institute
La Jolla, California
Senior Consultant
Division of Hematology Oncology
Scripps Clinic Medical Group, Inc.
Clinical Professor of Medicine
University of California, San Diego
La Jolla, California

Lisa Beutler [22]
Genome Sciences
University of Washington
Seattle, Washington

Steven Beutler, MD [22]
Redlands Community Hospital
Redlands, California

*Deceased (5 October 2008)

Neil Blumberg, MD [138, 140]
Professor and Director, Clinical Laboratories and Transfusion Medicine
Department of Pathology and Laboratory Medicine
University of Rochester
Rochester, New York

Niels Borregaard, MD, PhD [66]
Professor of Internal Medicine and Hematology
Department of Hematology
Copenhagen, Denmark

Laurence A. Boxer, MD [66]
Henry and Mala Dorfman Professorship of Pediatric Hematology/Oncology
Professor of Pediatric Hematology/Oncology
University of Michigan
Ann Arbor, Michigan

Michael Boyiadzis [100]
Division of Hematology-Oncology
University of Pittsburgh Cancer Institute
University of Pittsburgh School of Medicine
Pittsburgh, Pennsylvania

H. Elizabeth Broome [74, 107]
Clinical Professor of Medicine
University of California, San Diego
Department of Pathology
Moores Cancer Center
La Jolla, California

Brian S. Bull, MD [29, 51]
Professor and Chair
Department of Pathology and Human Anatomy
Loma Linda University Medical Center
Loma Linda, California

Joel N. Buxbaum, MD [110]
The Scripps Research Institute
La Jolla, California

Jamie Caro, MD [36, 55]
Professor of Medicine
Department of Medicine
Thomas Jefferson University
Cardeza Foundation for Hematologic Research
Philadelphia, Pennsylvania

Dennis A. Carson, MD [13]
Professor of Medicine
Director, Moores CSD Cancer Center
La Jolla, California

Januario E. Castro, MD [27]
Associate Professor of Medicine
University of California, San Diego
Moores Cancer Center
La Jolla, California

Bruce A. Chabner, MD [20]
Massachusetts General Hospital Cancer Center
Boston, Massachusetts

Junmei Chen [119]
Research Scientist
Puget Sound Blood Center
Seattle, Washington

James Cleary [20]
Massachusetts General Hospital Cancer Center
Boston, Massachusetts

Barry S. Coller, M.D. [114, 121]
Professor
Laboratory of Blood and Vascular Medicine
Physician-in-Chief
Vice President for Medical Affairs
Hospital Medical Affairs
The Rockefeller University
New York, New York

Myra Coppage [138]
Department of Pathology and Laboratory Medicine
University of Rochester
Rochester, New York

Gay M. Crooks, MB, BS, FRACP [76]
Professor of Medicine
Department of Pathology and Laboratory Medicine
David Geffen School of Medicine
University of California, Los Angeles
Los Angeles, California

Mark Crowther, MD, MSC, FRCPC [23]
Professor of Medicine and Pathology and Molecular Medicine
McMaster University
Hamilton, Ontario, Canada

David C. Dale, MD [65]
Professor of Medicine
Department of Medicine
University of Washington
Seattle, Washington

Nam H. Dang, MD, PhD [106]
Department of Hematologic Malignancies
Nevada Cancer Institute
Las Vegas, Nevada

Philip G. De Groot, PhD [129]
Department of Clinical Chemistry and Hematology
University Medical Center Utrecht
Utrecht, The Netherlands

Jean Delaunay, MD, PhD [39]
Professor of Genetics
INSERUM U 779
Secteur Paul-Broca
78 rue du Général-Leclerc
Hôpital de Bicêtre
94275 Le Kremlin-Bicêtre
France

Philippe de Moerloose, MD [126]
Haemostasis Unit
University Hospital of Geneva and University of Geneva Faculty of Medicine
Geneva, Switzerland

Madhav Dhodapkar, MD [19]
Bunker Professor of Medicine
Chief, Section of Hematology
Yale University
New Haven, Connecticut

Reyhan Diz-Kucukkaya, MD [119]
Associate Professor
Department of Internal Medicine
Division of Hematology
Istanbul University
Istanbul Faculty of Medicine
Istanbul, Turkey

Steven D. Douglas, MD [67]
Professor and Associate Chair Pediatrics
Chief Section of Immunology and Director of Clinical Immunology Laboratories
Children's Hospital of Philadelphia
Philadelphia, Pennsylvania

Ann M. Dvorak, MD [63]
Director, Electron Microscopy Unit
Senior Pathologist, Professor of Pathology
Department of Pathology
Beth Israel Deaconess Medical Center
Harvard Medical School
Boston, Massachusetts

Deborah Elstein, PhD [73]
Gaucher Clinic
Shaare Zedek Medical Center
Jerusalem, Israel

Joshua Epstein, DSC [109]
Myeloma Institute for Research and Therapy
University of Arkansas for Medical Sciences
Little Rock, Arkansas

William B. Ershler, MD [8]
Senior Investigator
Deputy Clinical Director
Intramural Research Program
National Institute on Aging
National Institute of Health
Baltimore, Maryland

Miguel A. Escobar, MD [124]
Associate Professor of Medicine and Pediatrics
Division of Hematology
University of Texas Health Science Center at Houston
Houston, Texas

Kenneth A. Foon, MD [97, 100]
Nevada Cancer Institute
Department of Hematological Malignancies
Las Vegas, Nevada

Charles W. Francis, MD [23]
Hematology/Oncology Division
University of Rochester Medical Center
Rochester, New York

Deborah L. French, PhD [121]
Assistant Professor
Department of Medicine
Mount Sinai School of Medicine
New York, New York

Jonathan W. Friedberg, MD [104]
Chief, Hematology/Oncology Division
James P. Wilmot Cancer Center
Associate Professor of Medicine
University of Rochester Medical Center
Rochester, New York

Patrick G. Gallagher, MD [45]
Professor
Department of Pediatrics and Genetics
Yale University School of Medicine
New Haven, Connecticut

Stephen J. Galli, MD [63]
Mary Hewitt Loveless, MD, Professor
Professor of Pathology and Microbiology and Immunology
Chair, Department of Pathology
Stanford University School of Medicine
Stanford University Medical Center
Stanford, California

Richard L. Gallo, MD, PhD [123]
Department of Medicine
Division of Dermatology
University of California, San Diego
VA San Diego Health Care System
San Diego, California

Tomas Ganz, MD, PhD [37]
Departments of Medicine and Pathology, David Geffen School of Medicine
University of California, Los Angeles
Los Angeles, California

Randy D. Gascoyne, MD, FRCPC [98]
Clinical Professor of Pathology
Research Director, Centre for Lymphoid Cancers
Departments of Pathology and Advanced Therapeutics British Columbia Cancer Agency, the BC Centre Research Center and University of British Columbia
Vancouver, BC, Canada

Amy Geddis, MD, PhD [119]
Associate Professor
Department of Pediatrics
Division of Hematology/Oncology
Univeristy of California School of Medicine
University of California
San Diego, California

Larisa J. Geskin, MD, FAAD [105]
Director, Cutaneous Oncology Center
University of Pittsburgh Medical Center
Pittsburgh, Pennsylvania

David Ginsburg, MD [127]
Professor, Department of Internal Medicine and Human Genetics
Investigator, Howard Hughes Medical Institute
University of Michigan
Ann Arbor, Michigan

Lucy A. Godley, MD, PhD [11]
Section of Hematology/Oncology
Department of Medicine and the Center Research Center
University of Chicago
Chicago, Illinois

Oscar B. Goodman Jr. [106]
Departments of Clinical Oncology
Nevada Cancer Institute
Las Vegas, Nevada

Siamon Gordon, MD, ChB, PhD [68, 69]
Sir William Dunn School of Pathology
University of Oxford
Oxford, United Kingdom

Roberta A. Gottlieb, MD [12]
San Diego State University
San Diego, California

Anthony R. Green, PhD, FRCP, FRCPath, FMedSci [87]
Professor
Department of Haematology
University of Cambridge
Cambridge Institute for Medical Research
Cambridge, United Kingdom

Ralph Green, MD, PhD, FRCPath [41, 43]
Professor of Pathology and Medicine
University of California Medical Center
Sacramento, California

Xylina T. Gregg, MD [38]
Utah Cancer Specialists
Salt Lake City, Utah

John H. Griffin, PhD [116]
Professor
Department of Molecular and Experimental Medicine
The Scripps Research Institute
La Jolla, California

Katherine A. Hajjar, MD [117, 136]
Brine Family Professor and Chair
Department of Cell and Developmental Biology
Weill Cornell Medical College
Professor of Pediatrics
New York Presbyterian Hospital
New York, New York

Paul C. Herrmann, MD, PhD [29, 51]
Associate Professor
Department of Pathology and Human Anatomy
Loma Linda University Medical Center
Loma Linda, California

Maureane Hoffman, MD, PhD [115]
Professor of Pathology
Duke University Medical Center and Durham Veterans Affairs Medical Center
Durham, North Carolina

Sandra J. Horning, MD [99]
Emeritus Professor of Medicine/Oncology
Stanford University Medical Center
Sr. VP, Global Head, Clinical Hematology/Oncology
Genentech, Inc.
Stanford Cancer Center
Stanford, California

Russell D. Hull, MD [134]
Professor
Department of Medicine
University of Calgary
Active Staff
Department of Internal Medicine
Foothills Hospital
Calgary, Alberta, Canada

Joseph E. Italiano Jr., PhD [114]
Assistant Professor of Medicine
Brigham and Women's Hospital
Harvard Medical School
Boston, Massachusetts

Daniel R. Jacobson, MD [110]
A Boston Health Care System
Boston, Massachusetts

Jill M. Johnsen, MD [127]
Assistant Member, Research Division
Puget Sound Blood Center
Assistant Professor, Division of Hematology
Department of Medicine
University of Washington
Seattle, Washington

Lynn B. Jorde, PhD [10]
H. A. and Edna Benning Presidential Professor
Department of Human Genetics
University of Utah School of Medicine
Salt Lake City, Utah

Marshall E. Kadin, MD [96]
Associate Professor of Pathology, Harvard Medical School
Professor of Dermatology
Boston University School of Medicine
Director, Cutaneous Lymphoma Program
Providence, Rhode Island

Kenneth Kaushansky, MD [14, 16, 113, 118, 120]
Helen M. Ranney Professor and Chair
Department of Medicine
University of California, San Diego
La Jolla, California

Armand Keating, MD [28]
Princess Margaret Hospital
Institute of Biomaterials and Biomedical Engineering
Department of Medicine
University of Toronto
Toronto, Ontario, Canada

Nigel S. Key, MB, FRCP [124]
Harold R. Roberts Distinguished Professor of Medicine
Division of Hematology/Oncology
Department of Medicine
University of North Carolina
Chapel Hill, North Carolina

Thomas J. Kipps, MD, PhD [5, 15, 27, 75, 77, 78, 80, 81, 92, 94]
Evelyn and Edwin Tasch Chair in Cancer Research
Professor of Medicine
Division of Hematology/Oncology
Deputy Director for Research Operations
Moores UCSD Cancer Center
University of California, San Diego
La Jolla, California

Mark J. Koury, MD [4]
Vanderbilt University Medical Center
Nashville, Tennessee

Abdullah Kutlar, MD [48]
Professor of Medicine
Georgia Sickle Cell Center
Medical College of Georgia
Sickle Cell Center
Augusta, Georgia

Larry W. Kwak, MD, PhD [25]
Chairman, Department of Lymphoma and Myeloma
Justin Distinguished Chair in Leukemia Research
Associate Director, Center for Cancer Immunology Research
Division of Cancer Medicine
The University of Texas M. D. Anderson Cancer Center
Houston, Texas

Robert A. Kyle, MD [112]
Consultant
Division of Hematology
Mayo Clinic
Professor of Medicine
Laboratory of Medicine and Pathology
Mayo Clinic, College of Medicine
Rochester, Minnesota

Andrew Lane [20]
Dana-Farber Cancer Institute
Boston, Massachusetts

Lewis L. Lanier, PhD [79]
Professor
Department of Microbiology and Immunology
University of California, San Francisco
San Francisco, California

Michelle M. Le Beau, PhD [11]
Section of Hematology/Oncology
Department of Medicine and the Center Research Center
University of Chicago
Chicago, Illinois

Norma B. Lerner, MD, MPH [140]
St. Christopher's Hospital for Children
Philadelphia, Pennsylvania

Marcel Levi, MD, PhD [130]
Department of Medicine/Vascular Medicine
Academic Medical Center
University of Amsterdam
Amsterdam, The Netherlands

Marshall A. Lichtman, MD [1, 4, 34, 52, 64, 70, 71, 85, 88, 89, 90, 91, 97, 108]
Professor of Medicine and of Biochemistry and Biophysics
University of Rochester Medical Center
Rochester, New York

Jane L. Liesveld, MD [88, 89, 90]
James P. Wilmot Cancer Center
University of Rochester Medical Center
Rochester, New York

Ton Lisman, PhD [129]
Associate Professor of Experimental Surgery
Surgical Research Laboratory and Section of Hepatobiliary Surgery and Liver Transplantation
Department of Surgery
University Medical Center, Groningen
Groningen, The Netherlands

John S. (Pete) Lollar III, MD [128]
Aflac Cancer Center and Blood Disorders Services
Department of Pediatrics
Emory University
Emory Children's Center
Atlanta, Georgia

Dan L. Longo, MD [8]
Senior Investigator
Scientific Director
Intramural Research Program
National Institute on Aging
National Institute of Health
Baltimore, Maryland

Jose A. Lopez, MD [119]
Professor of Medicine and Molecular and Human Genetics
Scientific Director, Thrombosis Research Section
Vice Chairman of Medicine for Research
Baylor College of Medicine
Houston, Texas

Thomas P. Loughran, MD [96]
Director, Penn State Hershey Cancer Institute
Professor of Medicine
Penn State College of Medicine
Hershey, Pennsylvania

Robert Lowsky, MD [21]
Stanford University
Division of Blood and Marrow Transplantation
Stanford, California

Naomi L.C. Luban, MD [54]
Professor, Pediatrics and Pathology
George Washington University Medical Center
Division Chief, Laboratory Medicine
Director, Transfusion Medicine/Donor Center
Children's National Medical Center
Washington, D.C.

Aaron Lubetsky, MD [131]
Institute of Thrombosis and Hemostasis and National Hemophilia Center
Sheba Medical Center
Tel Hashomer, Israel

Aaron J. Marcus, MD [117]
Professor of Medicine and of Pathology and Laboratory Medicine
Weill Cornell Medical College
Chief of Hematology-Oncology
VA New York Harbor Healthcare System
New York, New York

Kenneth L. McClain, MD, PhD [72]
Professor of Pediatrics
Texas Children's Cancer Center/Hematology
Baylor College of Medicine
Houston, Texas

Jeffery McCullough, MD [139]
Professor
Department of Laboratory Medicine and Pathology
Director, Division of Laboratory Medicine and Section of Transfusion Medicine
University of Minnesota Medical School
Minneapolis, Minnesota

Janice McFarland, MD [138]
Blood Center of Southeast Wisconsin
Milwaukee, Wisconsin

Peter W. McLaughlin, MD [102]
Department of Lymphoma/Myeloma
University of Texas
Houston, Texas

Bruce C. McLeod, MD [26]
Rush University Medical Center
Chicago, Illinois

Giampaolo Merlini [111]
Director, Center for Research and Treatment of Systematic Amyloidoses
University Hospital Policlinico San Matteo
Professor, Department of Medicine
University of Pavia
Pavia, Italy

Dean D. Metcalfe, MD [63]
Chief, Laboratory of Allergic Diseases
NAID/National Institute of Health
Bethesda, Maryland

Martha P. Mims, MD, PhD [7]
Associate Professor, Department of Medicine
Section Chief, Section of Hematology/Oncology
Baylor College of Medicine
Houston, Texas

Constantine Mitsiades [20]
Dana-Farber Cancer Institute
Boston, Massachusetts

Joel Moake, MD [50]
Senior Research Scientist and Associate Director
Biomedical Engineering Laboratory
Rice University
Houston, Texas

Emile R. Mohler III, MD [135]
Director, Vascular Medicine
Director, Vascular Diagnostic Center
Division of Cardiovascular Medicine
University of Pennsylvania School of Medicine
Director, Vascular Medicine Program
Presbyterian Medical Center
Philadelphia, Pennsylvania

Dougald M. Monroe III, PhD [115]
Professor of Medicine
Division of Hematology
University of North Carolina
School of Medicine
Chapel Hill, North Carolina

William A. Muller, MD, PhD [117]
Magerstadt Professor and Chairman
Department of Pathology
Feinberg School of Medicine
Northwestern University
Chicago, Illinois

Mike Murphy [141]
Professor of Blood Transfusion Medicine University of Oxford
Consultant Haematologist, National Blood Service and Oxford Radcliffe Hospitals
Oxford, United Kingdom

Bijay Nair [109]
Myeloma Institute for Research and Therapy
University of Arkansas for Medical Sciences
Little Rock, Arkansas

Kavita Natarajan, MBBS [48]
Assistant Professor of Medicine
Medical College of Georgia
Division of Hematology/Oncology
Augusta, Georgia

Sattva S. Neelapu, MD [25]
Department of Lymphoma and Myeloma
Division of Center Medicine
The University of Texas M. D. Anderson Cancer Center
Houston, Texas

Marguerite Neerman-Arbez, PhD [126]
Department of Genetic Medicine and Development
University of Geneva Faculty of Medicine
Geneva, Switzerland

Robert S. Negrin, MD [21]
Stanford University
Stanford, California

Luigi D. Notarangelo, MD [82]
Division of Immunology
Children's Hospital
Harvard Medical School
Boston, Massachusetts

Hans D. Ochs, MD [82]
Professor of Pediatrics
Jeffrey Modell Chair of Pediatric Immunology Research
Division of Immunology
Seattle Children's Research Hospital
Department of Pediatrics
University of Washington
Seattle, Washington

Ubaldo Martinez Outschoorn, MD [36, 55]
Assistant Professor
Department of Medical Oncology
Cardeza Foundation for Hematologic Research
Thomas Jefferson University
Philadelphia, Pennsylvania

Charles H. Packman, MD [53]
Clinical Professor of Medicine
University of North Carolina School of Medicine
Chapel Hill, North Carolina
Chief, Hematology-Oncology Section
Department of Internal Medicine and Blumenthal Cancer Center
Carolinas Medical Center
Charlotte, North Carolina

James Palis, MD [6]
Department of Pediatrics
University of Rochester Medical Center
Rochester, New York

Charles J. Parker, MD [40]
Professor of Medicine
Division of Hematology and Bone Marrow Transplantation
University of Utah School of Medicine
Salt Lake City, Utah

Archibald S. Perkins, MD [104]
Professor
Department of Pathology and Lab Medicine
University of Rochester Medical Center
Rochester, New York

John D. Phillips, PhD [57]
Associate Professor of Medicine
Division of Hematology
University of Utah School of Medicine
Salt Lake City, Utah

Graham F. Pineo, MD [134]
Professor of Medicine
Department of Medicine and Oncology
University of Calgary
Department of Medicine
Foothills Hospital
Calgary, Alberta, Canada

Annette Pluddemann [68, 69]
Department of Primary Health Care
University of Oxford
Oxford, United Kingdom

Mortimer Poncz, MD [133]
Professor of Pediatrics
University of Pennsylvania School of Medicine
Children's Hospital of Philadelphia
Philadelphia, Pennsylvania

Prem Ponka, MD [58]
Professor of Physiology and Medicine
Lady Davis Institute
McGill University
Montreal, Quebec, Canada

Jaroslav F. Prchal, MD [86]
Associate Professor of Medicine and Oncology
McGill University
St. Mary's Hospital
Montreal, Quebec, Canada

Josef T. Prchal, MD [7, 31, 33, 38, 44, 49, 56, 58, 86]
Professor of Medicine, Pathology, and Genetics
Division of Hematology
University of Utah
Salt Lake City, Utah
Department of Pathophysiology
First Faculty of Medicine
Charles University
Prague, Czech Republic

Oliver W. Press, MD, PhD [101]
Member, Fred Hutchinson Cancer Research Center
Professor of Medicine/Oncology
University of Washington
Director of Hematology/Hematologic Malignancies
Seattle Cancer Care Alliance
Seattle, Washington

Ching-Hon Pui, MD [93]
Chair
American Cancer Society
Professor, Department of Oncology
St. Jude Children's Research Hospital
Professor of Pediatrics
University of Tennessee Health Science Center
Memphis, Tennessee

Jayashree Ramasethu, MD, FAAP [54]
Associate Professor of Clinical Pediatrics
Director, Neonatal Perinatal Medicine Fellowship Program
Georgetown University Hospital
Division of Neonatology
Washington, D.C.

Jacob H. Rand, M.D. [132]
Professor of Pathology and Medicine
Director of Hematology Laboratory
Montefiore Medical Center
The University Hospital for the Albert Einstein College of Medicine
Bronx, New York

A. Koneti Rao, MD [121]
Assistant Professor of Pathology and Laboratory Medicine
Assistant Director, Transfusion Medicine/Blood Bank
Strong Memorial Hospital
University of Rochester Medical Center
Rochester, New York

Gary E. Raskob, PhD [134]
Dean, College of Public Health
Professor, Epidemiology and Medicine
The University of Oklahoma Health Science Center
Oklahoma City, Oklahoma

Majed A. Refaai, MD [140]
Department of Pathology and Laboratory Medicine
University of Rochester Medical Center
Rochester, New York

Erin Gourley Reid, MD [83]
Associate Professor of Medicine
Vice Chair, Lymphoma Working Group
AIDS Malignancy Consortium
University of California, San Diego
Moores Cancer Center
La Jolla, California

Marion E. Reid, PhD [137]
New York Blood Center
New York, New York

Paul Richardson, MD [20]
Dana-Farber Cancer Institute
Boston, Massachusetts

Stanley R. Riddell, MD [24]
Fred Hutchinson Cancer Research Center
Seattle, Washington

Harold R. Roberts, MD [115, 124]
Sarah Graham Kenan Distinguished Professor of Medicine and Pathology
Division of Hematology/Oncology
Department of Medicine
University of North Carolina School of Medicine
Chapel Hill, North Carolina
Department of Pathology
Duke University School of Medicine
Durham, North Carolina

Jorge E. Romaguera, MD [102]
Professor
Department of Lymphoma Myeloma
The University of Texas M. D. Anderson Cancer Center
Houston, Texas

Jia Ruan, MD, PhD [136]
Assistant Professor of Medicine
Department of Medicine
Weill Cornell Medical College
Assistant Attending Physician
New York Presbyterian Hospital
New York, New York

Daniel H. Ryan, MD [2, 3]
University of Rochester Medical Center
Rochester, New York

J. Evan Sadler, MD, PhD [133]
Professor and Director
Division of Hematology
Department of Medicine
Washington University School of Medicine
St. Louis, Missouri

Ophira Salomon, MD [125]
Amalia Biron Research Institute of Thrombosis and Hemostasis
Department of Hematology
Sheba Medical Center
Tel Hashomer and Sackler Faculty of Medicine
Tel Aviv University
Tel Aviv, Israel

Vaishali Sanchorawala, MD [110]
Associate Professor of Medicine
Amyloid Research and Treatment Program and Sections of Hematology-Oncology
Boston University School of Medicine and Boston Medical Center
Boston, Massachusetts

Alan Saven, MD [95]
Head, Division of Hematology/Oncology
Scripps Clinic Medical Group
La Jolla, California

Andrew I. Schafer, MD [135]
Frank Wister Thomas Professor of Medicine
Chairman, Department of Medicine
University of Pennsylvania School of Medicine
Philadelphia, Pennsylvania

Mathias Schmid, MD [13]
Assistant Professor
University Hospital Ulm
Ulm, Germany

David C. Seldin, MD, PhD [110]
Chief, Hematology-Oncology Section and Director
Amyloid Treatment and Research Program
Boston University School of Medicine and Boston Medical Center
Boston, Massachusetts

George B. Segel, MD [6, 34]
Department of Pediatrics
University of Rochester Medical Center
Rochester, New York

Uri Seligsohn, MD [118, 125, 130, 131]
Professor of Hematology and Director
Amalia Biron Research Institute of Thrombosis and Hemostasis
Sheba Medical Center
Tel-Hashomer and Sackler Faculty of Medicine
Tel Aviv University
Tel Aviv, Israel

Sanford J. Shattil, MD [122]
Professor and Chief, Division of Hematology-Oncology
Department of Medicine
University of California, San Diego
Adjunct Professor of Molecular and Experimental Medicine
The Scripps Research Institute
La Jolla, California

John Shaughnessy, PhD [109]
Myeloma Institute for Research and Therapy
University of Arkansas for Medical Sciences
Little Rock, Arkansas

Darren Sigal, MD [95]
Division of Hematology/Oncology
Scripps Clinic Medical Group
La Jolla, California

Brian F. Skinnider, MD [98]
Department of Pathology
British Columbia Cancer Agency and University of British Columbia
Vancouver, British Columbia, Canada

C. Wayne Smith, MD [59, 60, 61]
Professor and Head, Section of Leukocyte Biology
Department of Pediatrics
Baylor College of Medicine
Houston, Texas

Susan S. Smyth, MD, PhD [114]
Research Assistant Professor of Medicine
Carolina Center for Cardiovascular Biology
Center for Thrombosis and Hemostasis
University of North Carolina School of Medicine
Chapel Hill, North Carolina

Ralph M. Steinman, MD [19]
Henry G. Kunkle Professor
Head, Laboratory of Cellular Physiology and Immunology
Rockefeller University
New York, New York

David Stroncek [138]
Department of Transfusion Medicine
National Institutes of Health
Bethesda, Maryland

Ayalew Tefferi, MD [91]
Mayo Clinic
Rochester, Minnesota

Tim M. Townes, PhD [48]
Professor and Chair
Department of Biochemistry and Molecular Genetics
University of Alabama at Birmingham
Birmingham, Alabama

Steven P. Treon [111]
Director, Bing Center for Waldenstrom's Macroglobulinemia
Dana-Farber Cancer Institute
Associate Professor, Harvard Medical School
Boston, Massachusetts

Giorgio Trinchieri, MD [79]
Director, Cancer and Inflammation Program
Chief, Laboratory of Experimental Immunology
Center for Cancer Research, NCI, NIH
Frederick, Maryland

Florin Tuluc, MD, PhD [67]
Research Assistant Professor of Pediatrics
University of Pennsylvania School of Medicine
Joseph Stokes Jr. Research Institute
The Children's Hospital of Philadelphia
Philadelphia, Pennsylvania

Frits van Rhee, MD, PhD, MRCP (UK), FRCPath [109]
Professor of Medicine
Director of Clinical Research
Myeloma Institute for Research and Therapy
University of Arkansas for Medical Sciences
Little Rock, Arkansas

Wouter W. van Solinge, PhD [46]
Professor of Laboratory Medicine
Head of Department
Medical Director Division Laboratories and Pharmacy
Department of Clinical Chemistry and Haematology
University Medical Center Utrecht
Utrecht, The Netherlands

Richard van Wijk, PhD [46]
Associate Professor
Department of Clinical Chemistry and Haematology
University Medical Center Utrecht
Utrecht, The Netherlands

Ralph Vassallo Jr., MD [141]
Medical Director
American Red Cross Services
Penn-Jersey Region
Philadelphia, Pennsylvania

Dietlind L. Wahner-Roedler, MD [112]
Consultant
Division of General Internal Medicine
Mayo Clinic
Associate Professor of Medicine
Mayo Clinic College of Medicine
Mayo Clinic
Rochester, Minnesota

Huan-You Wang, MD, PhD [92]
Associate Clinical Professor of Pathology
Co-Director of Hematopathology
Department of Pathology
University of California, San Diego
La Jolla, California

Peter A. Ward, MD [17]
Department of Pathology
University of Michigan Medical School
Ann Arbor, Michigan

Andrew J. Wardlaw, MD, PhD [62]
Institute for Lung Health
Department of Infection
Immunity and Inflammation
Leicester University Medical School
Leicester, United Kingdom

Jeffery S. Warren, MD [17]
Department of Pathology
University of Michigan Medical School
Ann Arbor, Michigan

Sir David J. Weatherall, MD [47]
Professor
Weatherall Institute of Molecular Medicine
John Radcliffe Hospital
Headington, Oxford, United Kingdom

Sidney Whiteheart, PhD [114]
Professor
Molecular and Cellular Biochemistry
University of Kentucky College of Medicine
Lexington, Kentucky

Shmuel Yaccoby [109]
Myeloma Institute for Research and Therapy
University of Arkansas for Medical Sciences
Little Rock, Arkansas

Neal S. Young, MD [35]
Hematology Branch
National Heart, Lung, and Blood
National Institutes of Health
Bethesda, Maryland

Ari Zimran, MD [73]
Gaucher Clinic
Shaare Zedek Medical Center
Jerusalem, Israel

Ariella Zivelin, PhD [125]
Laboratory Manager
Institute of Thrombosis and Hemostasis
Sheba Medical Center
Tel Hashomer, Israel

Emanuele Zucca, MD [103]
IOSI-Oncology Institute of Southern Switzerland
Ospedale San Giovanni
Bellinzona, Switzerland

PREFACE

The rate of growth in our understanding of diseases of blood cells and coagulation proteins provides a challenge for the editors of a comprehensive textbook of hematology. The sequencing of individual genomes and the acquisition of knowledge in proteomics, metabolomics, and all the other burgeoning "-omics" fields as applied to hematologic disorders have accelerated the understanding of the pathogenesis of the diseases of our interest. The rate at which basic knowledge in molecular and cell biology and molecular immunology has been translated into improved diagnostic and therapeutic methods is equally impressive. Specific molecular targets for therapy in a myriad of hematological disorders have become reality, and it is not hyperbole to state that hematology has become the poster child for the rational design of therapeutics throughout all of medicine.

This edition of *Williams Hematology* includes many changes, we believe, for the better. Each chapter has been extensively revised or rewritten to provide the most current information available. Two new chapters have been added, Chapter 10 entitled Epigenetics and Genomics, to reflect the growing importance of this basic science in hematology, and Chapter 28 entitled Principles of Multipotential Cell Therapy for Tissue Replacement. In addition, several chapters have been divided, most notably the single chapter on non-Hodgkin lymphoma has been split into its constituent diseases, and the chapters on erythrocytosis and thrombocytosis have been divided into the myeloproliferative and reactive forms, to reflect our growing understanding of the pathophysiology of these disorders and more targeted approaches to their therapy. Recognizing that at the heart of hematology is blood and marrow cell morphology, we have incorporated most of the collection of 274 images that appeared in a separate section of color plates in the 7th edition (as well as additional images) into the relevant topics in each chapter, allowing far easier access to highly informative illustrations and cellular morphology.

Apropos the age of information, the new edition of *Williams Hematology* is also available online, as part of the popular www.accessmedicine.com website. With direct links to a comprehensive drug therapy database and to other important medical texts, including *Harrison's Principles of Internal Medicine* and *Goodman and Gilman's The Pharmacological Basis of Therapeutics*, *Williams Hematology Online* is part of a powerful resource covering all disciplines within medical education and practice. The online edition of *Williams Hematology* also includes PubMed links to journal articles cited in the references in our new edition.

For the first time, a CD accompanies the *Williams Hematology* book. The CD features a large selection of morphologies, illustrations, and drawings, from this new edition of *Williams Hematology*; these can be easily transported into PowerPoint™ format for use in lectures and presentations.

Finally, the *Williams Manual of Hematology* will once again be revised. The convenient *Manual* features the most clinically salient content from the parent text, and is perfect for use in time-restricted clinical situations. The *Manual* will be available for iPhone™ and other mobile formats.

The readers of the 8th edition of *Williams Hematology* will note the passing of a legend in hematology, Dr. Ernest Beutler. Ernie was a founding editor and the lead editor of *Hematology* for the 5th and 6th editions, continued to contribute as an editor for the 7th edition, and passed away in October 2008, while the 8th edition's revised and new chapters were being compiled. Ernie's thumbprint continues to permeate the 8th edition, including F1 and F2 generations of the Beutler pedigree, and it is to Ernie that we dedicate this edition.

The production of this book required the timely cooperation of 191 contributors. We are grateful for their work in providing this comprehensive and up-to-date text. Despite the growth of both basic and clinical knowledge and the passion that each of our contributors brings to the topic of their chapter, we have been able to maintain the text in a single volume through scrupulous attention to chapter length.

Each editor has had expert administrative assistance in the management of the manuscripts for which they were primarily responsible. We thank Carolina Bump in La Jolla, California; Susan Madden in Salt Lake City, Utah; and Orly Katz in Tel Aviv, Israel, for their very helpful participation in the production of the book. Special thanks go to Susan Daley in Rochester, New York, and Monica Gudea in La Jolla, California, who were responsible for coordinating the management of 141 chapters, including many new figures and tables, and managing other administrative matters, a challenging task that Ms. Daley and Ms. Gudea performed with skill and good humor. The editors also acknowledge the interest and support of our colleagues from McGraw-Hill, including James F. Shanahan, Editor-in-Chief, Internal Medicine; Harriet Lebowitz, Senior Project Development Editor for *Williams Hematology*; and Sylvia Rebert, Project Manager for *Williams Hematology.*

Kenneth Kaushansky
Marshall A. Lichtman
Thomas J. Kipps
Uri Seligsohn
Josef T. Prchal

PART I

Clinical Evaluation of the Patient

CHAPTER 1

INITIAL APPROACH TO THE PATIENT: HISTORY AND PHYSICAL EXAMINATION

Marshall A. Lichtman and Ernest Beutler

SUMMARY

The care of a patient with a suspected hematologic abnormality begins with a systematic attempt to determine the nature of the illness by eliciting an in-depth medical history and performing a physical examination. The physician should identify the patient's symptoms systematically and obtain as much relevant information as possible about their origin and evolution and about the general health of the patient by appropriate questions designed to explore the patient's recent and remote experience. Reviewing previous records may add important data for understanding the onset or progression of illness. Hereditary and environmental factors should be carefully sought and evaluated. The use of drugs and medications, nutritional patterns, and sexual behavior should be considered. The physician follows the medical history with a physical examination to obtain evidence for tissue and organ abnormalities that can be accessed through bedside observation to permit a careful search for signs of the illnesses suggested by the history. Skin changes and hepatic, splenic, or lymph nodal enlargement are a few findings that may be of considerable help in pointing toward a diagnosis. Additional history is obtained during the physical examination, as findings suggest an additional or alternative consideration. Thus, the history and physical examination should be considered as a unit, providing the basic information with which further diagnostic information is integrated: blood and marrow studies and imaging studies and biopsies.

Primary hematologic diseases are common in the aggregate, but hematologic manifestations secondary to other diseases occur even more frequently. For example, the signs and symptoms of anemia and the presence of enlarged lymph nodes are common clinical findings that may be related to a hematologic disease but occur frequently as secondary manifestations of disorders not considered primarily hematologic. A wide variety of diseases may produce signs or symptoms of hematologic illness. Thus, in patients with a connective tissue disease, all the signs and symptoms of anemia may be elicited and lymphadenopathy may be notable, but additional findings are usually present that indicate primary involvement of some system besides the hematopoietic (marrow) or lymphopoietic (lymph nodes or other lymphatic sites). In this discussion, emphasis is placed on the clinical findings resulting from either primary hematologic disease or the complications of hematologic disorders so as to avoid presenting an extensive catalog of signs and symptoms encountered in general clinical medicine.

In each discussion of specific diseases in subsequent chapters, the signs and symptoms that accompany the particular disorder are presented, and the clinical findings are covered in detail. In this chapter a more general systematic approach is taken.

Acronyms and abbreviations that appear in this chapter include: HELLP syndrome, hemolytic anemia, elevated liver enzymes, and low platelet count; Ig, immunoglobulin; IL, interleukin; POEMS, polyneuropathy, organomegaly, endocrinopathy, monoclonal gammopathy, and skin changes; PS, performance status.

THE HEMATOLOGY CONSULTATION

Table 1–1 lists the major abnormalities that result in the evaluation of the patient by the hematologist. The signs indicated in Table 1–1 may reflect a primary or secondary hematologic problem. For example, immature granulocytes in the blood may be signs of myeloid diseases such as myelogenous leukemia, or, depending on the frequency of these cells and the level of immaturity, the dislodgment of cells resulting from bone marrow metastases of a carcinoma. Nucleated red cells in the blood may reflect the breakdown in the marrow–blood interface seen in primary myelofibrosis or the hypoxia of congestive heart failure. Certain disorders have a propensity for secondary hematologic abnormalities; renal, liver, and connective tissue diseases are prominent among such abnormalities. Chronic alcoholism, nutritional fetishes, use of certain medications may be causal factors in blood cell or coagulation protein disorders. Pregnant women and persons of older age are prone to certain hematologic disorders: anemia, thrombocytopenia, or disseminated coagulation in the former case, and hematologic malignancies and pernicious anemia in the latter. The history and physical examination can provide vital clues to the possible diagnosis and also to the rationale choice of laboratory tests.

THE HISTORY

In today's technology- and procedure-driven medical environment, the importance of carefully gathering information from patient inquiry and examination is at risk of losing its primacy. The history (and physical examination) remains the vital starting point for the evaluation of any clinical problem.[1–3]

GENERAL SYMPTOMS AND SIGNS

Performance status (PS) is used to establish semiquantitatively the extent of a patient's disability. This status is important in evaluating patient comparability in clinical trials, in determining the likely tolerance to cytotoxic therapy, and in evaluating the effects of therapy. A well-founded set of criteria for measuring performance status is presented in Table 1–2.[4] An abbreviated version sometimes is used, as proposed by the Eastern Cooperative Oncology Group (Table 1–3).[5]

Weight loss is a frequent accompaniment of many serious diseases, including primary hematologic entities, but it is not a prominent accompaniment of most hematologic disease. Many "wasting" diseases, such as disseminated carcinoma and tuberculosis, cause anemia, and pronounced emaciation should suggest one of these diseases rather than anemia as the primary disorder.

Fever is a common early manifestation of the aggressive lymphomas or acute leukemias as a result of pyrogenic cytokines (e.g., interleukin (IL)-1, IL-6, IL-8 and others) released as a reflection of the disease itself. After chemotherapy-induced cytopenias or in the face of accompanying immunodeficiency, infection is usually the cause of fever. In patients with "fever of unknown origin," lymphoma, particularly Hodgkin lymphoma, should be considered. Occasionally, primary myelofibrosis, acute leukemia, advanced myelodysplastic syndrome, and other lymphomas may also cause fever. In rare patients with severe pernicious anemia or hemolytic anemia, fever may be present. *Chills* may accompany severe hemolytic processes and the bacteremia that may complicate the immunocompromised or neutropenic patient. *Night sweats* suggest the presence of low-grade fever and may occur in patients with lymphoma or leukemia.

Fatigue, malaise, and *lassitude* are such common accompaniments of both physical and emotional disorders that their evaluation is complex

TABLE 1–1. Findings That May Lead to a Hematology Consultation

Decreased hemoglobin concentration (anemia)
Increased hemoglobin concentration (polycythemia)
Elevated serum ferritin level
Accelerated sedimentation rate
Leukopenia or neutropenia
Immature granulocytes or nucleated red cells in the blood
Pancytopenia
Granulocytosis: neutrophilia, eosinophilia, basophilia, or mastocytosis
Monocytosis
Lymphocytosis
Lymphadenopathy
Splenomegaly
Hypergammaglobulinemia: monoclonal or polyclonal
Purpura
Thrombocytopenia
Thrombocytosis
Exaggerated bleeding: spontaneous or trauma related
Prolonged partial thromboplastin or prothrombin coagulation times
Venous thromboembolism
Thrombophilia
Obstetrical adverse events (e.g., recurrent fetal loss, stillbirth, and HELLP* syndrome)

*Hemolytic anemia, elevated liver enzymes, and low platelet count.

and often difficult. In patients with serious disease, these symptoms may be readily explained by fever, muscle wasting, or other associated findings. Patients with moderate or severe anemia frequently complain of fatigue, malaise, or lassitude and these symptoms may accompany the hematologic malignancies. Fatigue or lassitude may occur also with iron deficiency even in the absence of sufficient anemia to account for the symptom. In slowly developing chronic anemias, the patient may not recognize reduced exercise tolerance, or other loss of physical capabilities except in retrospect, after a remission has been induced by appropriate therapy. Anemia may be responsible for more symptoms than has been traditionally recognized, as suggested by the remarkable improvement in quality of life of most uremic patients treated with erythropoietin.

Weakness may accompany anemia or the wasting of malignant processes, in which cases it is manifest as a general loss of strength or reduced capacity for exercise. The weakness may be localized as a result of neurologic complications of hematologic disease. In vitamin B_{12} deficiency (e.g., pernicious anemia), there may be weakness of the lower extremities, accompanied by numbness, tingling, and unsteadiness of gait. Peripheral neuropathy also occurs with monoclonal immunoglobulinemias. Weakness of one or more extremities in patients with leukemia, myeloma, or lymphoma may signify central or peripheral nervous system invasion or compression as a result of vertebral collapse, a paraneoplastic syndrome (e.g. encephalitis), or brain or meningeal involvement. Myopathy secondary to malignancy occurs with the hematologic malignancies and is usually manifest as weakness of proximal muscle groups. Foot drop or wrist drop may occur in lead poisoning, amyloidosis, systemic autoimmune diseases, or as a complication of vincristine therapy. Paralysis may occur in acute intermittent porphyria.

TABLE 1–2. Criteria of Performance Status (Karnovsky Scale)[4]

Able to carry on normal activity; no special care is needed.	
100%	Normal; no complaints, no evidence of disease
90%	Able to carry on normal activity; minor signs or symptoms of disease
80%	Normal activity with effort; some signs or symptoms of disease
Unable to work; able to live at home, care for most personal needs; a varying amount of assistance is needed.	
70%	Cares for self; unable to carry on normal activity or to do active work
60%	Requires occasional assistance but is able to care for most personal needs
50%	Requires considerable assistance and frequent medical care
Unable to care for self; requires equivalent of institutional or hospital care; disease may be progressing rapidly.	
40%	Disabled; requires special care and assistance
30%	Severely disabled; hospitalization is indicated though death not imminent
20%	Very sick; hospitalization necessary; active supportive treatment necessary
10%	Moribund; fatal processes progressing rapidly
0%	Dead

SPECIFIC SYMPTOMS OR SIGNS

Nervous System

Headache may be the result of a number of causes related to hematologic diseases. Anemia or polycythemia may cause mild to severe headache. Invasion or compression of the brain by leukemia or lymphoma, or opportunistic infection of the central nervous system by *Cryptococcus* or *Mycobacterium* species, may also cause headache in patients with hematologic malignancies. Hemorrhage into the brain or subarachnoid space in patients with thrombocytopenia or other bleeding disorders may cause sudden, severe headache.

TABLE 1–3. Eastern Cooperative Oncology Group Performance Status[5]

Grade	Activity
0	Fully active, able to carry on all predisease performance without restriction
1	Restricted in physically strenuous activity but ambulatory and able to carry out work of a light or sedentary nature, e.g., light housework, office work
2	Ambulatory and capable of all self-care but unable to carry out any work activities; up and about more than 50% of waking hours
3	Capable of only limited self-care, confined to bed or chair more than 50% of waking hours
4	Completely disabled; cannot carry on any self-care; totally confined to bed or chair
5	Dead

Paresthesias may occur because of peripheral neuropathy in pernicious anemia or secondary to hematologic malignancy or amyloidosis. They may also result from therapy with vincristine.

Confusion may accompany malignant or infectious processes involving the brain, sometimes as a result of the accompanying fever. Confusion may also occur with severe anemia, hypercalcemia (e.g., myeloma), or high-dose glucocorticoid therapy. Confusion or apparent senility may be a manifestation of pernicious anemia. Frank psychosis may develop in acute intermittent porphyria or with high-dose glucocorticoid therapy.

Impairment of consciousness may be a result of increased intracranial pressure secondary to hemorrhage or leukemia or lymphoma in the central nervous system. It may also accompany severe anemia, polycythemia, hyperviscosity secondary, usually, to an immunoglobulin (Ig)M monoclonal protein (uncommonly IgA or IgG) in the plasma, or a leukemic hyperleukocytosis syndrome, especially in chronic myelogenous leukemia.

Eyes

Conjunctival plethora is a feature of polycythemia and pallor a result of anemia. Occasionally blindness may result from retinal hemorrhages secondary to severe anemia and thrombocytopenia or blurred vision resulting from severe hyperviscosity resulting from macroglobulinemia or extreme hyperleukocytosis of leukemia. Partial or complete visual loss can stem from retinal vein or artery thrombosis. Diplopia or disturbances of ocular movement may occur with orbital tumors or paralysis of the third, fourth, or sixth cranial nerves because of compression by tumor, especially extranodal lymphoma, extramedullary myeloma, or myeloid (granulocytic) sarcoma.

Ears

Vertigo, tinnitus, and "roaring" in the ears may occur with marked anemia, polycythemia, hyperleukocytic leukemia, or macroglobulinemia-induced hyperviscosity. Ménière disease was first described in a patient with acute leukemia and inner ear hemorrhage.

Nasopharynx, Oropharynx, and Oral Cavity

Epistaxis may occur in patients with thrombocytopenia, acquired or inherited platelet function disorders and von Willebrand disease. *Anosmia* or *olfactory hallucinations* occur in pernicious anemia. The nasopharynx may be invaded by a granulocytic sarcoma or extranodal lymphoma; the symptoms are dependent on the structures invaded. The paranasal sinuses may be involved by opportunistic organisms, such as fungus in patients with severe, prolonged neutropenia. *Pain or tingling in the tongue* occurs in pernicious anemia and may accompany severe iron deficiency or vitamin deficiencies. *Macroglossia* occurs in amyloidosis. *Bleeding gums* may occur with bleeding disorders. Infiltration of the gingiva with leukemic cells occurs notably in acute monocytic leukemia. *Ulceration* of the tongue or oral mucosa may be severe in the acute leukemias or in patients with severe neutropenia. *Dryness of the mouth* may be caused by hypercalcemia, secondary, for example, to myeloma. *Dysphagia* may be seen in patients with severe mucous membrane atrophy associated with chronic iron-deficiency anemia.

Neck

Painless swelling in the neck is characteristic of lymphoma but may be caused by a number of other diseases as well. Occasionally, the enlarged lymph nodes of lymphomas may be tender or painful because of secondary infection or rapid growth. Painful or tender lymphadenopathy is usually associated with inflammatory reactions, such as infectious mononucleosis or suppurative adenitis. *Diffuse swelling* of the neck and face may occur with obstruction of the superior vena cava due to lymphomatous compression.

Chest and Heart

Both *dyspnea* and *palpitations*, usually on effort but occasionally at rest, may occur because of anemia or pulmonary embolism. *Congestive heart failure* may supervene, and *angina pectoris* may become manifest in anemic patients. The impact of anemia on the circulatory system depends in part on the rapidity with which it develops, and chronic anemia may become severe without producing major symptoms; with severe acute blood loss, the patient may develop shock with a nearly normal hemoglobin level, prior to compensatory hemodilution. *Cough* may result from enlarged mediastinal nodes compressing the trachea or bronchi. *Chest pain* may arise from involvement of the ribs or sternum with lymphoma or multiple myeloma, nerve-root invasion or compression, or herpes zoster; the pain of herpes zoster usually precedes the skin lesions by several days. Chest pain with inspiration suggests a pulmonary infarct, as does *hemoptysis*. *Tenderness of the sternum* may be quite pronounced in chronic myelogenous or acute leukemia, and occasionally in primary myelofibrosis, or if intramedullary lymphoma or myeloma proliferation is explosive.

Gastrointestinal System

Dysphagia has already been mentioned under "Nasopharynx, Oropharynx, and Oral Cavity." *Anorexia* frequently occurs but usually has no specific diagnostic significance. Hypercalcemia and azotemia cause anorexia, nausea, and vomiting. A variety of ill-defined gastrointestinal complaints grouped under the heading "indigestion" may occur with hematologic diseases. *Abdominal fullness, premature satiety, belching,* or *discomfort* may occur because of a greatly enlarged spleen, but such splenomegaly may also be entirely asymptomatic. *Abdominal pain* may arise from intestinal obstruction by lymphoma, retroperitoneal bleeding, lead poisoning, ileus secondary to therapy with the *Vinca* alkaloids, acute hemolysis, allergic purpura, the abdominal crises of sickle cell disease, or acute intermittent porphyria. *Diarrhea* may occur in pernicious anemia. It also may be prominent in the various forms of intestinal malabsorption, although significant malabsorption may occur without diarrhea. In small-bowel malabsorption, steatorrhea may be a notable feature. Malabsorption may be a manifestation of small-bowel lymphoma. *Gastrointestinal bleeding* related to thrombocytopenia or other bleeding disorder may be occult but often is manifest as *hematemesis* or *melena*. *Hematochezia* can occur if a bleeding disorder is associated with a colonic lesion. *Constipation* may occur in the patient with hypercalcemia or in one receiving treatment with the *Vinca* alkaloids.

Genitourinary and Reproductive Systems

Impotence or *bladder dysfunction* may occur with spinal cord or peripheral nerve damage due to one of the hematologic malignancies or with pernicious anemia. Priapism may occur in hyperleukocytic leukemia, essential thrombocythemia, or sickle cell disease. *Hematuria* may be a manifestation of hemophilia A or B. *Red urine* may also occur with intravascular hemolysis (hemoglobinuria), myoglobinuria, or porphyrinuria. Injection of anthracycline drugs or ingestion of drugs such as phenazopyridine (Pyridium) regularly causes the urine to turn red. The use of deferoxamine mesylate (Desferal) may result in a rust color of the urine. Beeturia, a benign, possibly genetic trait, affecting approximately 4 percent of individuals, causes pinkish-red urine (and feces) as a result of exaggerated excretion of the beetroot pigments betacyanins. *Amenorrhea* may also be induced by certain drugs, such as antimetabolites or alkylating agents. *Menorrhagia* is a common cause of iron deficiency, and care must be taken to obtain an accurate history of the extent of menstrual blood loss. Semiquantification can be obtained from estimates of the number of days of heavy bleeding (usually <3), the number of days of any bleeding (usually <7), number of tampons or pads used (requirement for double pads suggests excessive bleeding), degree of blood soaking, and clots formed, and inquiries such as, "Have you experienced a gush of blood when a tampon is removed?" However, an objective distinction between menorrhagia (loss of more than 80 mL blood per period) and normal blood loss can best be made by a visual assessment technique using pictorial charts of towels or tampons.[6] Menorrhagia may occur in patients with bleeding disorders.

Back and Extremities

Back pain may accompany acute hemolytic reactions or be a result of involvement of bone or the nervous system in acute leukemia or aggressive lymphoma. It is one of the most common manifestations of myeloma.

Arthritis or *arthralgia* may occur with gout secondary to increased uric acid production in patients with hematologic malignancies, especially acute lymphocytic leukemia in childhood, myelofibrosis, myelodysplastic syndrome, and hemolytic anemia. They also occur in the plasma cell dyscrasias, acute leukemias, and sickle cell disease without evidence of gout, and in allergic purpura. Arthritis may accompany hemochromatosis, although the association has not been carefully established. In the latter case the arthritis starts typically in the small joints of the hand (second and third metacarpal joints), and episodes of acute synovitis may be related to deposition of calcium pyrophosphate dehydrate crystals. Hemarthroses in patients with severe bleeding disorders cause marked joint pain. Autoimmune diseases may present as anemia and/or thrombocytopenia, and arthritis appears as a later manifestation. *Shoulder pain* on the left may be a result of infarction of the spleen and on the right of gall bladder disease associated with chronic hemolytic anemia such as hereditary spherocytosis. *Bone pain* may occur with bone involvement by the hematologic malignancies; it is common in the congenital hemolytic anemias, such as sickle cell anemia, and may occur in myelofibrosis. In patients with Hodgkin lymphoma, ingestion of alcohol may induce pain at the site of any lesion, including those in bone. *Edema* of the lower extremities, sometimes unilateral, may occur because of obstruction to veins or lymphatics by lymphomatous masses or from deep venous thrombosis. The latter can also cause edema of the upper extremities.

Skin

Skin manifestations of hematologic disease may be of great importance; they include changes in texture or color, itching, and the presence of specific or nonspecific lesions. The skin in iron-deficient patients may become dry, the hair dry and fine, and the nails brittle. In hypothyroidism, which may cause anemia, the skin is dry, coarse, and scaly. *Jaundice* may be apparent with pernicious anemia or congenital or acquired hemolytic anemia. The skin of patients with pernicious anemia is said to be "lemon yellow" because of the simultaneous appearance of jaundice and pallor. Jaundice may also occur in patients with hematologic malignancies, especially lymphomas, as a result of liver involvement or biliary tract obstruction. *Pallor* is a common accompaniment of anemia, although some severely anemic patients may not appear pale. Erythromelalgia may be a troublesome complication of polycythemia vera. Patchy plaques or widespread *erythroderma* occur in cutaneous T-cell lymphoma (especially Sézary syndrome) and in some cases of chronic lymphocytic leukemia or lymphocytic lymphoma. The skin is often involved, sometimes severely, in graft-versus-host disease following marrow transplantation. Patients with hemochromatosis may have bronze or grayish pigmentation of the skin. *Cyanosis* occurs with methemoglobinemia, either hereditary or acquired; sulfhemoglobinemia; abnormal hemoglobins with low oxygen affinity; and primary and secondary polycythemia. Cyanosis of the ears or the fingertips may occur after exposure to cold in individuals with cryoglobulins or cold agglutinins.

Itching may occur in the absence of any visible skin lesions in Hodgkin lymphoma and may be extreme. Mycosis fungoides or other lymphomas with skin involvement may also present as itching. A significant number of patients with polycythemia vera will complain of itching after bathing.

Petechiae and *ecchymoses* are most often seen in the extremities in patients with thrombocytopenia, nonthrombocytopenic purpura, or acquired or inherited platelet function abnormalities and von Willebrand disease. Unless secondary to trauma, these lesions usually are painless; the lesions of psychogenic purpura and erythema nodosum are painful. *Easy bruising* is a common complaint, especially among women, and when no other hemorrhagic symptoms are present, usually no abnormalities are found after detailed study. This symptom may, however, indicate a mild hereditary bleeding disorder, such as von Willebrand disease or one of the platelet disorders.

Infiltrative lesions may occur in the leukemias (leukemia cutis) and lymphomas (lymphoma cutis) and are sometimes the presenting complaint. Monocytic leukemia has a higher frequency of skin infiltration than other forms of leukemia. *Necrotic lesions* may occur with intravascular coagulation, purpura fulminans, and warfarin-induced skin necrosis, or rarely with exposure to cold in patients with circulating cryoproteins or cold agglutinins.

Leg ulcers are a common complaint in sickle cell anemia and occur rarely in other hereditary anemias.

■ DRUGS AND CHEMICALS

Drugs

Drug therapy, either self-prescribed or ordered by a physician, is extremely common in our society. Drugs often induce or aggravate hematologic disease, and it is therefore essential that a careful history of drug ingestion, including beneficial and adverse reactions, should be obtained from all patients. Drugs taken regularly often become a part of the patient's way of life and are often forgotten or are not recognized as "drugs." Agents such as aspirin, laxatives, tranquilizers, medicinal iron, vitamins, other nutritional supplements, and sedatives belong to this category. Furthermore, drugs may be ingested in unrecognized form, such as antibiotics in food or quinine in tonic water. Specific, persistent questioning, often on several occasions, may be necessary before a complete history of drug use is obtained. It is very important to obtain detailed information on alcohol consumption from every patient. The four "CAGE" questions—about **c**utting down, being **a**nnoyed by criticism, having **g**uilt feelings, and needing an **e**ye-opener—provide an effective approach to the history of alcohol use. Patients should also be asked about the use of recreational drugs. The use of "alternative medicines" and herbal medicines is common, and many patients will not consider these medications or may actively withhold information about their use. Nonjudgmental questioning may be successful in identifying agents in this category that the patient is taking. Some patients equate the term "drugs," as opposed to "medicines," with illicit drugs. Establishing that the examiner is interested in all forms of ingestants—prescribed drugs, self-remedies, alternative remedies, etcetera—is important to ensure getting the information required.

Chemicals

In addition to drugs, most people are exposed regularly to a variety of chemicals in the environment, some of which may be potentially harmful agents in hematologic disease. Similarly, occupational exposure to chemicals must be considered. When a toxin is suspected, the patient's daily activities and environment must be carefully reviewed, since significant exposure to toxic chemicals may occur incidentally.

VACCINATION

Vaccinations can exacerbate immune thrombocytopenia.

NUTRITION

Children who are breast-fed without iron supplementation may develop iron-deficiency anemia. Nutritional information can be useful in deducing the possible role of dietary deficiency in anemia. The avoidance of certain food groups, as might be the case with vegans, or the ingestion of uncooked fish can be clues to the pathogenesis of megaloblastic anemia.

FAMILY HISTORY

A carefully obtained family history may be of great importance in the study of patients with hematologic disease (see Chap. 9). In the case of hemolytic disorders, questions should be asked regarding jaundice, anemia, and gallstones in relatives. In patients with disorders of hemostasis or venous thrombosis, particular attention must be given to bleeding manifestations or venous thromboembolism in family members. In the case of autosomal recessive disorders such as pyruvate kinase deficiency, the parents are usually not affected, but a similar clinical syndrome may have occurred in siblings. It is particularly important to inquire about siblings who may have died in infancy, as these may be forgotten, especially by older patients. When sex-linked inheritance is suspected, it is necessary to inquire about symptoms in the maternal grandfather, maternal uncles, male siblings, and nephews. In patients with disorders with dominant inheritance, such as hereditary spherocytosis, one may expect to find that one of the parents and possibly siblings and children of the patient have stigmata of the disease. Ethnic background may be important in the consideration of certain diseases such as α- and β-thalassemia, sickle cell anemia, glucose-6-phosphate dehydrogenase deficiency, hemoglobin E, and other inherited disorders that are prevalent in specific geographic areas, such as the Mediterranean basin or Southeast Asia.

SEXUAL HISTORY

Because of the frequency of infections with the human immunodeficiency viruses, it is important to ascertain the sexual behavior of the patient, especially risk factors for transmission of HIV.

PREVENTIVE HEMATOLOGY

Ideally, the physician's goal is to prevent illness, and opportunities exist for hematologists to prevent the development of hematologic disorders. These opportunities include identification of individual genetic risk factors and avoidance of situations that may make a latent disorder manifest. Prophylactic therapy, as for example in avoiding venous stasis in patients heterozygous for protein C deficiency or administering prophylactic heparin at the time of major surgery, is a more immediate aspect of prevention because it depends on the physician's intervention. Hematologists may also prevent disease by reinforcing community medicine efforts. Examples include fostering the elimination of sources of environmental lead that may result in childhood anemia and fostering the careful regulation of environmental toxins, such as benzene, organochlorine and organophosphate pesticides, and phenoxyherbicides that may increase the risk of lymphohematopoietic malignancies. Prenatal diagnosis can provide information to families as to whether a fetus is affected with a hematologic disorder.

PHYSICAL EXAMINATION

A detailed physical examination should be performed on every patient, with sufficient attention paid to all systems to obtain a full evaluation of the general health of the individual. Certain body areas are especially pertinent to hematologic disease and therefore deserve special attention. These are the skin, eyes, tongue, lymph nodes, skeleton, spleen and liver, and nervous system.

SKIN

Pallor and Flushing

The color of the skin is a result of the pigment contained therein and to the blood flowing through the skin capillaries. The component of skin color related to the blood may be a useful guide to anemia or polycythemia, as pallor may result when the hemoglobin level is reduced, and redness when the hemoglobin level is increased. The amount of pigment in the skin modifies skin color and can mislead the clinician, as in individuals with pallor due to decreased pigment, or make skin color useless as a guide because of the intense pigmentation present.

Alterations in blood flow and in hemoglobin content may change skin color; this too can mislead the clinician. Thus emotion may cause either pallor or blushing. Exposure of the skin to cold or heat may similarly cause pallor or blushing. Chronic exposure to wind or sun may lead to permanent redness of the skin, and chronic ingestion of alcohol to a flushed face. The degree of erythema of the skin can be evaluated by pressing the thumb firmly against the skin, as on the forehead, so that the capillaries are emptied, and then comparing the color of the compressed spot with the surrounding skin immediately after the thumb is removed.

The mucous membranes and nail beds are usually more reliable guides to anemia or polycythemia than the skin. The conjunctivae and gums may be inflamed, however, and therefore not reflect the hemoglobin level, or the gums may appear pale because of pressure from the lips. The gums and the nail beds may also be pigmented and the capillaries correspondingly obscured. In some individuals, the color of the capillaries does not become fully visible through the nails unless pressure is applied to the fingertip, either laterally or on the end of the nail.

The palmar creases are useful guides to the hemoglobin level and appear pink in the fully opened hand unless the hemoglobin is 7 g/dL or less. Liver disease may induce flushing of the thenar and hypothenar eminences of the palm, even in patients with anemia.

Cyanosis

The detection of cyanosis, like the detection of pallor, may be made difficult by skin pigmentation. Cyanosis is a function of the total amount of reduced hemoglobin, methemoglobin, or sulfhemoglobin present. The minimum amounts of these pigments that cause detectable cyanosis are approximately 5 g/dL blood of reduced hemoglobin, 1.5 to 2.0 g/dL of methemoglobin, and 0.5 g/dL of sulfhemoglobin.

Jaundice

Jaundice may be observed in the skin of individuals who are not otherwise deeply pigmented or in the sclerae or the mucous membranes. The patient should be examined in daylight rather than under incandescent or fluorescent light, because the yellow color of the latter masks the yellow color of the patient. Jaundice is a result of actual staining of the skin by bile pigment, and bilirubin glucuronide (direct-reacting or conjugated bilirubin) stains the skin more readily than the unconjugated form. Jaundice of the skin may not be visible if the bilirubin level is below 2 to 3 mg/dL. Yellow pigmentation of the skin may also occur with carotenemia, especially in young children.

Petechiae and Ecchymoses

Petechiae are small (1 to 2 mm), round, red or brown lesions resulting from hemorrhage into the skin and are present primarily in areas with high venous pressure, such as the lower extremities. These lesions do not blanch on pressure, and this can be demonstrated most readily by compressing the skin with a glass microscope slide or magnifying lens. Petechiae may occasionally be elevated slightly, that is, palpable; this finding suggests vasculitis. Ecchymoses may be of various sizes and shapes and may be red, purple, blue, or yellowish green, depending on the intensity of the skin hemorrhage and its age. They may be flat or elevated; some are painful and tender. The lesions of hereditary hemorrhagic telangiectasia are small, flat, nonpulsatile, and violaceous. They blanch with pressure.

Excoriation

Itching may be intense in some hematologic disorders such as Hodgkin lymphoma, even in the absence of skin lesions. Excoriation of the skin from scratching is the only physical manifestation of this severe symptom.

Leg Ulcers

Open ulcers or scars from healed ulcers are often found in the region of the internal or external malleoli in patients with sickle cell anemia, and, rarely, in other hereditary anemias.

Nails

Detection of pallor or rubor by examining the nails was discussed earlier. The fingernails in chronic, severe iron-deficiency anemia may be ridged longitudinally and flattened or concave rather than convex. The latter change is referred to as *koilonychia* and is uncommon in present practice.

Eyes

Jaundice, pallor, or *plethora* may be detected from examination of the eyes. Jaundice is usually more readily detected in the sclerae than in the skin. Ophthalmoscopic examination is also essential in patients with hematologic disease. *Retinal hemorrhages* and *exudates* occur in patients with severe anemia and thrombocytopenia. These hemorrhages are usually the typical "flame-shaped" hemorrhages, but they may be quite large and elevate the retina so that they may appear as a darkly colored tumor. Round hemorrhages with white centers are also often seen. *Dilatation of the veins* may be seen in polycythemia; in patients with macroglobulinemia, the veins are engorged and segmented, resembling link sausages.

Mouth

Pallor of the mucosa has already been discussed. *Ulceration* of the oral mucosa occurs commonly in neutropenic patients. In leukemia there may also be infiltration of the gums with swelling, redness, and bleeding. *Bleeding* from the mucosa may occur with a hemorrhagic disease. A dark line of lead sulfide may be deposited in the gums at the base of the teeth in lead poisoning. The *tongue* may be completely smooth in pernicious anemia and iron-deficiency anemia. Patients with an upper dental prosthesis may also have papillary atrophy, presumably on a mechanical basis. The tongue may be smooth and red in patients with nutritional deficiencies. This may be accompanied by fissuring at the corners of the mouth, but fissuring may also be due to ill-fitting dentures. An enlarged tongue, abnormally firm to palpation, may indicate the presence of primary amyloidosis.

Lymph Nodes

Lymph nodes are widely distributed in the body, and in disease any node or group of nodes may be involved. The major concern on physical examination is the detection of enlarged or tender nodes in the cervical, supraclavicular, axillary, epitrochlear, inguinal, or iliofemoral regions. Under normal conditions in adults, the only readily palpable lymph nodes are in the inguinal region, where several firm nodes 0.5 to 2.0 cm long are normally attached to the dense fascia below the inguinal ligament and in the femoral triangle. In children, multiple small (0.5 to 1.0 cm) nodes may be palpated in the cervical region as well. Supraclavicular nodes may sometimes be palpable only when the patient performs the Valsalva maneuver.

Enlarged lymph nodes are ordinarily detected in the superficial areas by palpation, although they are sometimes large enough to be seen. Palpation should be gentle and is best performed with a circular motion of the fingertips, using slowly increasing pressure. Tender lymph nodes usually indicate an inflammatory etiology, although rapidly proliferative lymphoma may be tender to palpation.

Nodes too deep to palpate may be detected by specific imaging procedures, including computerized tomography, magnetic resonance imaging, ultrasound studies, gallium scintography, and positron emission tomography.[7,8]

Chest

Increased rib or sternal tenderness is an important physical sign often ignored. Increased bone pain may be generalized, as in leukemia, or spotty, as in plasma cell myeloma or in metastatic tumors. The superficial surfaces of all bones should be examined thoroughly by applying intermittent firm pressure with the fingertips to locate potential areas of disease.

Spleen

The normal adult spleen is usually not palpable on physical examination but occasionally the tip may be felt.[9] Palpability of the normal spleen may be related to body habitus, but there is disagreement on this point. Percussion, palpation, or a combination of these two methods may detect enlarged spleens.[10] Some enlarged spleens may be visible by protrusion of the abdominal wall.

The normal spleen weighs approximately 150 g and lies in the peritoneal cavity against the diaphragm and the posterolateral abdominal wall at the level of the lower three ribs. As it enlarges it remains close to the abdominal wall, while the lower pole moves downward, anteriorly, and to the right. Spleens enlarged only 40 percent above normal may be palpable, but significant splenic enlargement may occur and the organ still not be felt on physical examination. A good but imperfect correlation has been reported between spleen size estimated from radioisotope scanning or ultrasonography and spleen weight determined after splenectomy or at autopsy.[11] Although it is common to fail to palpate an enlarged spleen on physical examination, palpation of a normal-sized spleen is unusual, and therefore a palpable spleen is usually a significant physical finding.

An enlarged spleen lies just beneath the abdominal wall and can be identified by its movement during respiration. The splenic notch may be evident if the organ is moderately enlarged. During the examination the patient lies in a relaxed, supine position. The examiner, standing on the patient's right, lightly palpates the left upper abdomen with the right hand while exerting pressure forward with the palm of the left hand placed over the lower ribs posterolaterally. This action permits the spleen to descend and be felt by the examiner's fingers. If nothing is felt, the palpation should

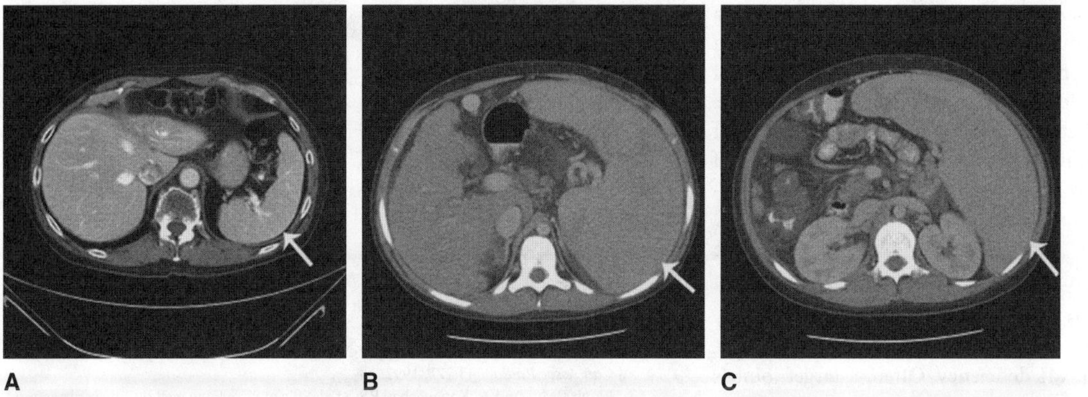

FIGURE 1–1. A three-way composite of abdominal computerized tomography. **A.** Normal spleen size. **B.** Enlarged spleen. **C.** Massively enlarged spleen at the level of mid-kidney. Normally the spleen would either not be visualized or only a small lower pole would be evident at the latter level. (*White arrow* in the three images mark edge of splenic silhouette.) *(Images kindly provided by Deborah Rubens, MD, The University of Rochester Medical Center.)*

be performed repeatedly, moving the examining hand approximately 2 cm toward the inguinal ligament each time. It is often advantageous to carry out the examination initially with the patient lying on the right side with left knee flexed and to repeat it with the patient supine.

It is not always possible to be sure that a left upper quadrant mass is spleen; masses in the stomach, colon, kidney, or pancreas may mimic splenomegaly on physical examination. When there is uncertainty regarding the nature of a mass in the left upper quadrant, imaging procedures will usually permit accurate diagnosis.[11–13] Figure 1–1 is an example of splenic enlargement as seen by computerized tomography of the abdomen and Figure 1–2 as seen by ultrasonography.

Liver

Palpation of the edge of the liver in the right upper quadrant of the abdomen is commonly used to detect hepatic enlargement, although the inaccuracies of this method have been demonstrated. It is necessary to determine both the upper and lower borders of the liver by percussion in order to properly assess liver size.[14,15] The normal liver may be palpable as much as 4 to 5 cm below the right costal margin but is usually not palpable in the epigastrium. The height of liver dullness is best measured in a specific line 8, 10, or 12 cm to the right of the midline. Techniques should be standardized so that serial measurements can be made. The vertical span of the normal liver determined in this manner will range approximately 10 cm in an average-size man and approximately 2 cm smaller in a woman. Because of variations introduced by technique, each physician should determine the normal area of liver dullness by his or her own procedure. Correlation of radioisotope imaging data with results from routine physical examinations indicates that often a liver of normal size is considered enlarged on physical examination and an enlarged liver is considered normal. Ultrasonography and computed tomography measurements are useful in determining size and demonstrating localized infiltrative lesions.[16–18]

Nervous System

A thorough evaluation of neurologic function is necessary in many patients with hematologic disease. Vitamin B_{12} deficiency impairs cerebral, olfactory, spinal cord, and peripheral nerve function, and severe chronic deficiency may lead to irreversible neurologic degeneration. Leukemic meningitis is often manifested by headache, visual impairment, or cranial nerve dysfunction. Tumor growth in the brain or spinal

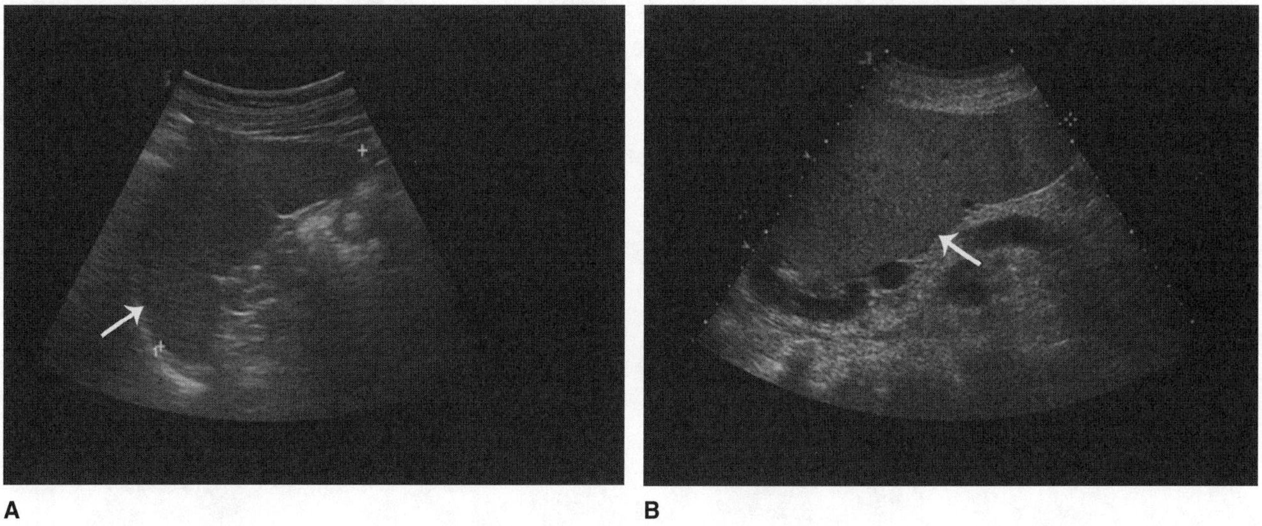

FIGURE 1–2. A two-way composite of ultrasonographic examination for spleen size. Patient's head is to the left side of the longitudinal image. **A.** Image of echo indicating normal spleen size with cranial to caudal longitudinal dimension of 10.3 cm. **B.** Image of echo indicating enlarged spleen with cranial to caudal longitudinal dimension of 16.2 cm. (*White arrows* mark edge of splenic silhouette.) The normal spleen is usually less than 13 cm in length, but the examiner has to consider other dimensions in assessing spleen size (volume). *(Images kindly provided by Deborah Rubens, MD, The University of Rochester Medical Center.)*

cord compression may be caused by malignant lymphoma or plasma cell myeloma. A variety of neurologic abnormalities may develop in patients with leukemias, lymphomas, and myeloma as a consequence of tumor infiltration, bleeding, infection, or a paraneoplastic syndrome. Essential monoclonal gammopathy is associated with several types of sensory and motor neuropathies. Polyneuropathy is a feature of POEMS, a syndrome marked by polyneuropathy, organomegaly, endocrinopathy, monoclonal gammopathy, and skin changes.

Joints

Deformities of the knees, elbows, ankles, shoulders, wrists, or hips may be the result of repeated hemorrhage in patients with hemophilia A, hemophilia B, or severe factor VII deficiency. Often, a target joint is prominently affected.

REFERENCES

1. Bickley LS, Szilagyi PG: *Bates Guide to Physical Examination and History Taking,* 9th ed. Lippincott Williams & Wilkins, Philadelphia, 2007.
2. Sackett DL: A primer on the precision and accuracy of the clinical examination. *JAMA* 267:2638, 1992.
3. Williams ME: *Geriatric Physical Diagnosis: A Guide to Observation and Assessment.* McFarland & Company, Jefferson, NC, 2008.
4. Mor V, Laliberte L, Morris JN, Wiemann M: The Karnovsky performance status scale: An examination of its reliability and validity in a research setting. *Cancer* 53:2002, 1984.
5. Oken MM, Creech RH, Tormey DC, et al: Toxicity and response criteria of the Eastern Cooperative Oncology Group. *Am J Clin Oncol* 5:649, 1982.
6. Janssen CAH, Scholten PC, Heintz APM: A simple visual assessment technique to discriminate between menorrhagia and normal menstrual blood loss. *Obstet Gynecol* 85:977, 1995.
7. Grubnic S, Vinnicombe SJ, Norman AR, Husband JE: MR evaluation of normal retroperitoneal and pelvic lymph nodes. *Clin Radiol* 57:193, 2002.
8. Atula TS, Varpula MJ, Kurki TJI, et al: Assessment of cervical lymph node status in head and neck cancer patients: Palpation, computed tomography and low-field magnetic resonance imaging compared with ultrasound-guided fine needle aspiration cytology. *Eur J Radiol* 25:152, 1997.
9. Arkles LB, Gill GD, Nolan MP: A palpable spleen is not necessarily enlarged or pathological. *Med J Aust* 145:15, 1986.
10. Barkun AN, Camus M, Green L, et al: The bedside assessment of splenic enlargement. *Am J Med* 91:512, 1991.
11. Downey MT: Estimation of splenic weight from ultrasonographic measurements. *Can Assoc Radiol J* 43:273, 1992.
12. Lamb PM, Lund A, Kanagasbay RR, et al: Spleen size: How well do linear ultrasound measurements correlate with three-dimensional CT volume assessments? *Br J Radiol* 75:573, 2002.
13. Halpern S, Coel M, Ashburn W, et al: Correlation of liver and spleen size: Determinations by nuclear medicine studies and physical examination. *Arch Intern Med* 134:123, 1974.
14. Castell DO, O'Brien KD, Muench H, Chalmers TC: Estimation of liver size by percussion in normal individuals. *Ann Intern Med* 70:1183, 1969.
15. Tucker WN, Saab S, Rickman LS, Mathews WC: The scratch test is unreliable for detecting the liver edge. *J Clin Gastroenterol* 25:410, 1997.
16. Bennett WF, Dova JG: Review of hepatic imaging and a problem-oriented approach to liver masses. *Hepatology* 12:761, 1990.
17. Barloon TJ, Brown BP, Abu-Yousef MM, et al: Teaching physical examination of the adult liver with the use of real-time sonography. *Acad Radiol* 5:101, 1998.
18. Elstein D, Hadas-Halpern I, Azuri Y, et al: Accuracy of ultrasonography in assessing spleen and liver. *J Ultrasound Med* 16:209, 1997.

CHAPTER 2
EXAMINATION OF BLOOD CELLS

Daniel H. Ryan

SUMMARY

Examination of the blood cell counts and their appearance on a blood film is central to the diagnosis of blood cell diseases and can give important information about numerous other degenerative, inflammatory, and neoplastic diseases that are reflected in quantitative or qualitative changes of blood cells. Examples are the anemia accompanying chronic renal disease, chronic inflammation, or iron deficiency, the presence of malarial parasites in red cells, the eosinophilia of parasitic infection, the decrease in platelets resulting from immune thrombocytopenia, and other key findings on a blood examination that reflect numerous disease states. By careful examination of the blood, an experienced observer can diagnose all types of leukemia and closely related diseases. In few other disciplines can a physician make a specific diagnosis with easily accessible tissue samples and methods that can be used in a physician's office. Today, blood examination is conducted almost exclusively in diagnostic laboratories, but the results can be provided to the clinician within a few hours of drawing the sample. Assessment of the concentration of red cells, reticulocytes, leukocytes, specific leukocyte types, and platelets; morphology of red cells, white cells, and platelets; identification of intracellular parasites, malignant cells, and marrow precursors (e.g., nucleated red cells) provides a large amount of information from the "complete blood count," quickly and accurately.

The blood is examined so as to answer these questions: Is the marrow producing appropriate numbers of mature cells in the major hematopoietic lineages? Is the development of each hematopoietic lineage qualitatively normal? Quantitative measures available from automated cell counters are reliable and provide a rapid and cost-effective way to screen for major disturbances of hematopoiesis or abnormalities that reflect nonhematopoietic diseases, such as inflammatory, degenerative, or neoplastic states. Light microscopic observation of the blood film is essential to confirm certain quantitative results and to investigate qualitatively abnormal differentiation of the hematopoietic lineages. Based on examination of the blood, the physician is directed toward a more focused assessment of marrow function or to systemic disorders that secondarily involve the hematopoietic system.

The complete blood count is a necessary part of the diagnostic evaluation in a broad variety of clinical conditions. Similarly, the leukocyte differential count and examination of the blood film, in spite of limitations as a screening test for occult disease,[1] is important in initial consideration of the differential diagnosis in most ill patients. Although quantitative and morphologic examination of the cells of the blood are considered separately in this chapter, the distinction between these two is not absolute, and measures once considered "qualitative" become quantitative as technology advances.

Acronyms and abbreviations that appear in the chapter include: CHr, reticulocyte-specific hemoglobin content; EDTA, ethylenediaminetetraacetic acid; fl, femtoliter; Hct, hematocrit; Ig, immunoglobulin; MCH, mean cell hemoglobin; MCHC, mean cell hemoglobin concentration; MCV, mean cell volume; MCVr, mean cell volume of reticulocytes; MPV, mean platelet volume; NHANES, National Health and Nutrition Examination Survey; NK, natural killer; PDW, platelet volume distribution width; RBC, red blood cell; RDW, red cell distribution width; RET-He, reticulocyte-specific hemoglobin content.

QUANTITATIVE MEASURES OF CELLS IN THE BLOOD

Automated blood cell analysis is the cornerstone of the modern hematology laboratory, allowing rapid, cost-effective, and accurate analysis of the cells of the blood, including many new parameters with diagnostic utility. The morphologic and functional complexity of blood cells is significant, so that definitive interpretation in some cases requires direct microscopic examination of a stained blood film by a trained observer. However, it is possible to use automated techniques to analyze and report on the majority of samples and to use defined criteria to select those that need further review. Depending on workload and space considerations, laboratories may choose to link automated hematology analyzers with automated blood film preparation and automated image analyzers to facilitate manual morphologic review of cells by traditional light microscopy or online review of digitized images. The newer automated analyzers are capable of providing accurate digitized images of normal and abnormal cells identified on a stained slide, obviating much of the manual effort involved in searching for cells.[2] These instruments may be able to categorize the cells, provisionally, but final cell classification and examination of the blood film by microscopy by a technologist or physician is required.

The characteristics of various automated hematology analyzer systems have been reviewed.[3] A detailed description of individual instruments is beyond the scope of this chapter, but the general principles employed by state-of-the-art instrumentation are summarized below. The major analytical challenges are the frequency of the different cell types, which vary over many orders of magnitude, from red cells (millions per μL) to basophils (dozens per μL), and the complexity of the structure of normal and abnormal blood cells. Over the past several decades, instruments have become increasingly sophisticated with the use of multiple parameters to produce more precise results in the great majority of patient samples. In a typical automated hematology analyzer, the blood sample is aspirated and separated into different fluidic streams. The streams are mixed with various buffers that accomplish specific purposes in the analysis, for instance, using differential lysis to separate all or subsets of leukocytes, reagents to measure hemoglobin or detect myeloperoxidase containing leukocytes, and various fluorescent dyes. Measurements of each fluidic stream are made in flow as the sample passes through a series of detectors in what are essentially modified flow cytometers (see Chap. 3). Commonly used principles include light scatter at various angles, electrical impedance and conductivity, and fluorescence, and light absorption of cells stained in flow. Light scatter yields information about cell size (using scatter at low-incident angles), and nuclear lobulation and cytoplasmic granularity (using high-angle light scatter), with polarization of the scattered light as an additional parameter. If red cells are converted to spherocytes by the buffer solution to eliminate the variability of cell shape, light scatter at different angles can provide information about hemoglobin content, as well as size of individual red cells. Cell size is also estimated by measuring change in electrical resistance, which is proportional to cell size as cells enter a narrow orifice through which a direct current is maintained, the original Coulter principle, named for Wallace Coulter who developed the electronic particle counter.[4] Both methods provide a cell

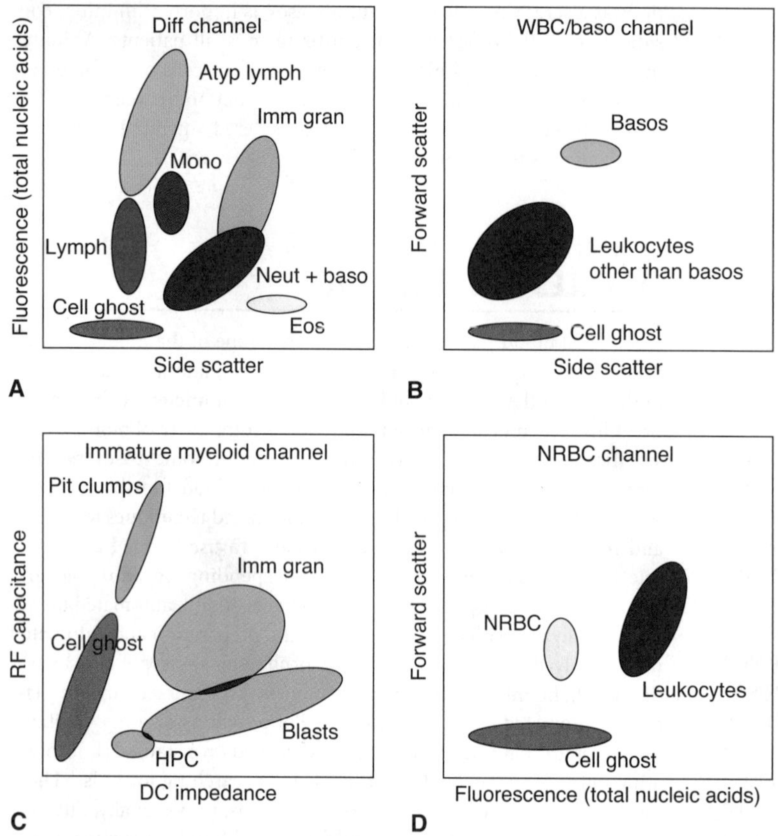

FIGURE 2–1. Schematic of multiparameter cell discrimination in an automated hematology analyzer. The Sysmex XE-2100 is used as an example, in which leukocytes are discriminated by **(A)** DNA/RNA fluorescence using a polymethine dye versus high angle (side) light scatter in lysed blood (abnormal cell types in light shading); **(B)** side scatter versus low angle (forward) light scatter after acidic lysis in a separate aliquot that preserves basophil structure; and **(C)** direct current (DC) impedance versus radio frequency (RF) capacitance of cells subjected to a lysis reagent that relatively preserves immature cells with lower membrane lipid content. Nucleated red blood cells (NRBC) are distinguished **(D)** in a lysed sample stained with nucleic acid dye where leukocyte nuclei have detectably higher DNA/RNA content than red cell nuclei. Atyp Lymph, atypical lymphocytes; Baso, basophils; Blasts, blast cells; Diff Channel, differential count channel; Eos, eosinophils; HPC, hematopoietic progenitor cells; Imm Gran, immature granulocytes; Lymph, lymphocytes; Mono, monocytes; Neut + Baso, neutrophils + basophils; Plt Clumps, platelet clumps; WBC, white blood cells.

count with a prespecified volume of blood analyzed. Radiofrequency capacitance measurement yields additional intracellular structural information that complements the direct current measurement, which relates to cell size. Differential lysis with detergents of varying strength or pH is used to separate certain leukocyte types, such as basophils and immature granulocytic cells from the major normal blood cell types. In addition, nucleic-acid-binding fluorescent dyes incorporated into the lysis buffer measure total RNA plus DNA in the cells and are used in some analyzers to help differentiate leukocyte types. Fluorescence measurements after staining with RNA binding dyes are commonly used for reticulocyte counting as well as defining newer parameters of reticulocyte and platelet level of maturity. Light absorption is the principle used for hemoglobin measurement and in some instruments for identifying peroxidase-positive granulocytes. An individual instrument can use a combination of techniques to improve the accuracy and precision of the analysis (Fig. 2–1). Complex algorithms are invoked to determine whether the distribution of variables for a specific result or for the specimen as a whole fit sufficiently within a known variable space so that the results can be reported with high confidence, or whether the specimen should be "flagged" for further analysis (Fig. 2–2). These instruments have replaced a great deal of laborious manual work, but also demand increasing interpretive skills on the part of laboratory technologists.

RED CELLS

Most automated blood cell counters measure the number of red cells, the mean red cell volume (MCV), and hemoglobin concentration. The other red cell parameters, including the hematocrit, mean cell hemoglobin (MCH), and mean cell hemoglobin concentration (MCHC) are derived from these primary measurements.

Measurement of the Red Cell Count and Hematocrit

In electronic instruments, the hematocrit (Hct; proportional volume of blood occupied by erythrocytes) is calculated from the product of direct measurements of the erythrocyte count and the MCV (Hct [μL/100 μL] = RBC [$\times 10^{-6}/\mu$L] $\times$ MCV [fl]/10). Falsely elevated MCV and decreased red cell counts can be observed when red cell autoantibodies are present and retain binding capability at room temperature (cold agglutinins and some cases of autoimmune hemolytic anemia).[5] This causes red cells to clump and affects the accuracy of both red blood cell (RBC) count and MCV, as well as the resultant hematocrit. MCV, and hence measured hematocrit, can increase up to 5 percent after 24 hours of storage at room temperature.[6]

The hematocrit may also be determined by subjecting the blood to sufficient centrifugal force to pack the cells while minimizing trapped extracellular fluid.[7] This approach was traditionally done in capillary tubes filled with blood and centrifuged at very high speed in a small tabletop centrifuge, and the technique was referred to as the "microhematocrit." Although the hematocrit is the volume (mL) of red cells per volume (100 mL) of blood, it is usually expressed as a percent. Before standardized methods for hemoglobin quantification were available, the hematocrit was the simplest and most accurate method for determining the volume of red cells in blood and by inference the hemoglobin. However, this is a manual procedure not well adapted to routine processing in a high-volume clinical laboratory, and is affected by varying amounts of plasma trapped between red cells in the packed cell volume,[8] typically about 2 to 3 percent of the packed volume.[9] The hematocrit from polycythemic samples (hematocrit greater than 55 mL/dL, i.e., 55%) or blood containing abnormal erythrocytes (sickle cells, thalassemic red cells, iron-deficient red cells, spherocytes, macrocytes) are increased because of enhanced plasma trapping that generally is caused by increased red cell rigidity.[9,10] Therefore, although automated hematocrit values are adjusted to be equivalent to spun hematocrit for normal samples, in abnormal samples, the spun hematocrit may be spuriously elevated (up to 6% in microcytosis).[11] The hemoglobin determination now is preferred to the hematocrit, because it is measured directly and is the best indicator of the oxygen-carrying capacity of the blood.

Measurement of Hemoglobin

Hemoglobin is intensely colored, and this property has been used in methods for estimating its concentration in blood. Erythrocytes contain a mixture of hemoglobin, oxyhemoglobin, carboxyhemoglobin, methemoglobin, and minor amounts of other forms of hemoglobin. To

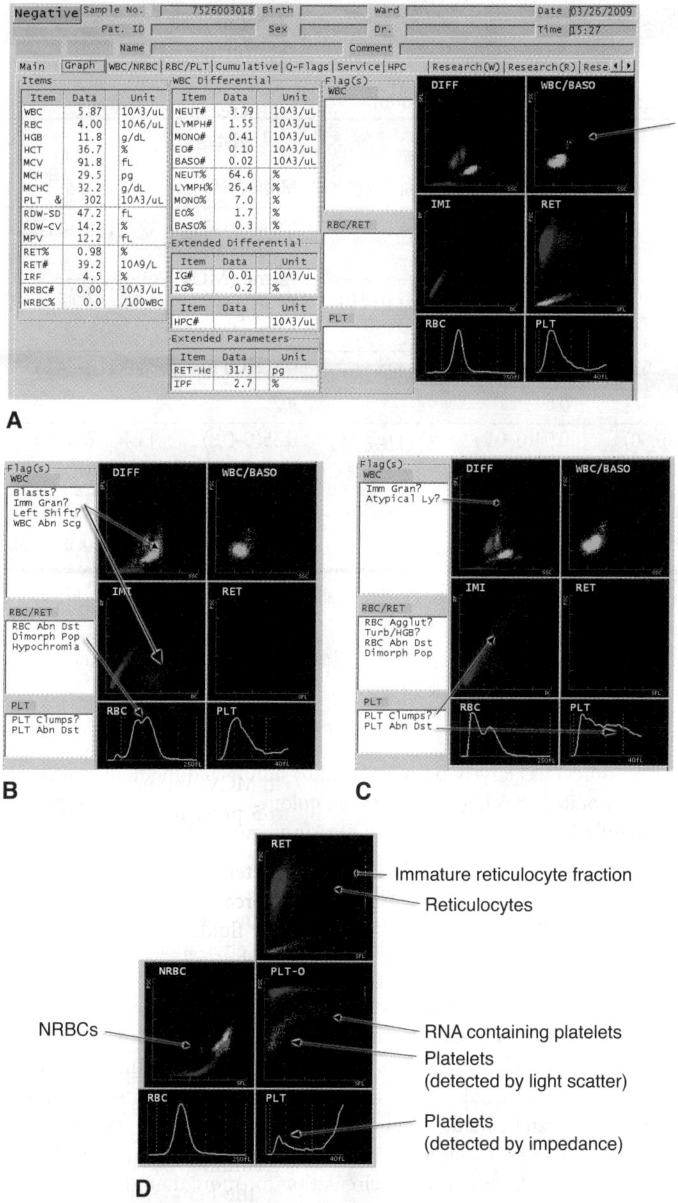

FIGURE 2–2. Examples of how samples containing various abnormal findings are flagged for manual review. **A.** Normal sample showing how the major variables and results are displayed. **B.** Immature granulocytes appearing on the DIFF (leukocyte differential count) and IMI (immature myeloid) histograms, as well as a dimorphic red cell population. **C.** Multiple flags, including cells in the area of atypical lymphocytes, and platelet clumps with abnormal platelet volume distribution. **D.** Appearance of nucleated red blood cells (NRBCs), reticulocytes, and reticulated platelets on a different set of parameters. This figure is not intended as a comprehensive illustration of the technical details, but serves to demonstrate that differential lysing reactions coupled with multiparameter light-scatter, impedance, capacitance, and fluorescence measurements are used to analyze blood cells in current high-throughput instruments.

determine hemoglobin concentration in the blood, red cells are lysed and hemoglobin variants are converted to the stable compound cyanmethemoglobin for quantification by absorption at 540 nm.[12] All forms of hemoglobin are readily converted to cyanmethemoglobin except sulfhemoglobin, which is rarely present in significant amounts. In automated blood cell counters, hemoglobin is usually measured by a modified cyanmethemoglobin or an alternate lauryl sulphate method. Hemoglobin measurement is accurate and preferable to the hematocrit for the diagnosis of anemia. In practice, the major interference with this measurement is chylomicronemia, but newer instruments identify and minimize this interference.

The hemoglobin level varies with age (Table 2–1). Chap. 6 discusses changes in hemoglobin in the neonatal period. After the first week or two of extrauterine life, the hemoglobin falls from levels of approximately 17 g/dL to levels of approximately 12 g/dL by 2 months of age. Thereafter, the levels remain relatively constant throughout the first year of life. Any child with a hemoglobin level below 11 g/dL should be considered anemic.[13] Chap. 8 discusses changes in hemoglobin levels in older persons.

Size and Hemoglobin Content of Erythrocytes (Red Cell Indices)

The size and hemoglobin content of erythrocytes (red cell indices) have traditionally been used to assist in the differential diagnosis of anemia.[14] In current practice, the most useful parameter is the MCV.[15]

Automated blood counters measure the MCV directly by either electrical impedance or light scatter measurements of individual red cells. The MCV has been used to guide the diagnostic workup in patients with anemia, for example testing patients with microcytic anemia for iron deficiency or thalassemia,[16] and those with macrocytic anemia for folate or vitamin B_{12} deficiency.[17] This approach has practical value, but also limitations[18]; for instance, MCV may be normal in some older patients with pernicious anemia,[19] or in advanced pernicious anemia with severe red cell fragmentation.[20] One-third of older patients have an elevated MCV without an evident cause.[21] Mathematical manipulations of the red cell indices take advantage of the trend toward higher red cell count, lower red cell distribution width (RDW), MCH, and MCV in thalassemia trait versus iron-deficiency anemia to assist in the differential diagnosis of these disorders,[22] but their usefulness has been questioned.[23] Although more definitive tests are preferred when available, the MCV, MCH, and formulas using these parameters may be useful in screening of high-prevalence populations where laboratory resources are limited.[24]

The other red cell indices have little independent value in clinical decision making. The MCH, the amount of hemoglobin per red cell, is calculated by the formula:

$$\text{MCH(pg/cell)} = \text{hemoglobin (g/dL)/red cell count } (\times 10^6 \text{ cells}/\mu\text{L}) \times 10$$

The MCH increases or decreases in parallel with the MCV and generally provides little additional diagnostic information. The MCHC, the concentration of hemoglobin per unit red cell volume, is calculated by the formula:

$$\text{MCHC (g/dL of red cells)} = \text{hemoglobin (g/dL)/hematocrit (mL/100 dL)} \times 100$$

The range of the MCHC measurement in most automated instruments is limited by technical factors,[25] and is primarily useful for quality control purposes, such as detecting sample turbidity.

These red cell indices are average quantities and therefore may not detect abnormalities in blood with mixed-cell populations. In situations such as sideroblastic anemia, recently transfused patients, patients with severe pernicious anemia with red cell fragmentation, and folate plus iron deficiency, both large and small red cells are present, diminishing

TABLE 2–1. Reference Ranges for Leukocyte Count, Differential Count, and Hemoglobin Concentration in Children*

	Leukocytes	Neutrophils							Hemoglobin
Age	Total (×10³/μL)	Total	Band	Segmented	Eosinophils	Basophils	Lymphocytes	Monocytes	g/dL Blood
12 mo	11.4(6.0–17.5)	3.5(1.5–8.5)	0.35(0–1.0)	3.2(1.0–8.5)	0.30(0.05–0.70)	0.05(0–0.20)	7.0(4.0–10.5)	0.55(0.05–1.1)	12.6(11.1–14.1)
		31	*3.1*	*28*	*2.6*	*0.4*	*61*	*4.8*	
4 yr	9.1(5.5–15.5)	3.8(1.5–8.5)	0.27(0–1.0)	3.5(1.5–7.5)	0.25(0.02–0.65)	0.05(0–0.2)	4.5(2.0–8.0)	0.45(0–0.8)	12.7(11.2–14.3)
		42	*3.0*	*39*	*2.8*	*0.6*	*50*	*5.0*	
6 yr	8.5(5.0–14.5)	4.3(1.5–8.0)	0.25(0–1.0)	4.0(1.5–7.0)	0.23(0–0.65)	0.05(0–0.2)	3.5(1.5–7.0)	0.40(0–0.8)	13.0(11.4–14.5)
		51	*3.0*	*48*	*2.7*	*0.6*	*42*	*4.7*	
10 yr	8.1(4.5–13.5)	4.4(1.8–8.0)	0.24(0–1.0)	4.2(1.8–7.0)	0.20(0–0.60)	0.04(0–0.2)	3.1(1.5–6.5)	0.35(0–0.8)	13.4(11.8–15.0)
		54	*3.0*	*51*	*2.4*	*0.5*	*38*	*4.3*	
21 yr	7.4(4.5–11.0)	4.4(1.8–7.7)	0.22(0–0.7)	4.2(1.8–7.0)	0.20(0–0.45)	0.04(0–0.2)	2.5(1.0–4.8)	0.30(0–0.8)	M: 15.5(13.5–17.5)
		59	*3.0*	*56*	*2.7*	*0.5*	*34*	*4.0*	F: 13.8(12.0–15.6)

*The means and ranges are in thousands of cells per mL. This table is provided as a guide. Normal ranges should be validated by the clinical laboratory for the specific methods in use. The number in *italic* is mean percentage of total leukocytes.

For leukocyte and differential count, see Altman PL, Dittmer DS (eds): *Blood and Other Body Fluids*. Federation of American Societies for Experimental Biology, Washington, DC, 1961. By permission.

For hemoglobin concentration, see Rudolph AM, Hoffman JI (eds): *Pediatrics*, 18th ed, pp 1011, 1012. Appleton and Lange, Norwalk, CT, 1987.

the value of the MCV measurement. In these cases, RDW would be expected to increase, as this parameter measures the variation in red cell size and is a quantitative expression of anisocytosis. An elevated RDW may be an early sign of iron-deficiency anemia[26] and although proposed as an aid in distinguishing iron deficiency from other causes of microcytic anemia,[27] such as thalassemia, the RDW is not sufficiently specific to obviate the need for more focused tests.[28] The RDW can be used in the laboratory as a flag to select those samples that should have manual review of blood films for red cell morphology. Quantitative measurement of fragmented red cells is available on two analyzers, and this parameter can sensitively detect fragmented cells as seen in macro- and microangiopathies, although specificity is low[29] because the detection principle is by size and cell content, not shape. The RDW has been repeatedly associated with risk of cardiovascular disease in various settings,[30–33] and is elevated in a variety of chronic disorders.[34,35] These associations may indicate RDW as a surrogate marker of inflammation (through inflammation-associated erythroid maturation impairment),[30] but this remains to be proven.

A number of disorders, such as immune and hereditary spherocytosis (Chaps. 45 and 53), hemoglobin C disease (Chap. 48), elliptocytosis (Chap. 45), inherited granule abnormalities (Chap. 66), and malaria and other parasitic diseases (Chap. 52), may not be reliably detected by the various flagging strategies on automated analyzers, and morphologic findings such as basophilic stippling (Chap. 29), toxic granulation (Chap. 59), siderocytes (Chap. 29), and pathologic rouleaux formation (Chap. 111) are only detectable by microscopic examination of the blood film.

Reticulocyte Enumeration

The reticulocyte is a newly released anucleate red cell that enters the blood with residual detectable amounts of RNA (Chaps. 29 and 31). The number of reticulocytes in a volume of blood permits an estimate of marrow erythrocyte production and is thus useful in evaluating the pathogenesis of anemia by distinguishing inadequate production from accelerated destruction (hemolysis; Chap. 31). The manual method for enumerating reticulocytes by placing a sample of blood in a tube containing new methylene blue and preparing a blood film to enumerate the proportion of cells that show blue beaded precipitates (residual chains of ribosomes) has largely been replaced by automated methods, which are incorporated into high-volume hematology analyzers. Reticulocytes are identified by direct fluorescence measurement after staining with RNA-binding dyes (thiazole orange, polymethine dyes, CD4K530, auramine O, coriphosphine O) or light scatter measurements to detect staining with nonfluorescent RNA-binding dyes (new methylene blue, oxazine 750).[36] Various proprietary combinations of light scatter and other parameters are used to minimize interferences such as nucleated red cells, nuclear remnants (Howell-Jolly bodies), malaria parasites, or platelet clumps.

Automated reticulocyte counts are typically reported in absolute numbers (reticulocytes per μL or per L of blood), obviating the need to correct for a reduced red cell count (anemia), if present. An additional correction can be made to consider the effect of elevated erythropoietin levels secondary to anemia, which results in premature release of reticulocytes, which persist in the circulation for more than the usual 1 day and correspondingly inflate estimates of marrow reticulocyte production based on the reticulocyte count (see Chap. 31). The correlation between manual and automated methods of reticulocyte enumeration is good, but reference ranges differ slightly among the methods,[37] given the different dyes and conditions used and the continuous nature of the variables separating reticulocytes from mature red cells.

Reticulocyte Indices

The ability of new automated analyzers to measure parameters specifically in reticulocytes on a cell-by-cell basis opens up the possibility of reticulocyte-specific indices. The theoretical advantage is that acute changes in red cell function would be detected more rapidly and reliably in the reticulocyte fraction as opposed to the total red cell population.

Estimates of reticulocyte-specific hemoglobin content (CHr and RET-He,[38] which are comparable[39]) by light scatter measurements of reticulocytes are closely related to adequacy of iron availability to erythroid precursors, and have been described as diagnostically useful in detecting functional iron deficiency in complex clinical settings, such as chronic inflammation[40] and chronic renal disease,[39,41] and are recommended by the National Kidney Foundation for the latter purpose.[42] The increase in serum ferritin as an acute phase reactant combined with the physiologic variation of serum iron and iron-binding capacity limits the value of conventional parameters in these settings. The CHr may be a better predictor of marrow iron stores than traditional serum iron parameters in nonmacrocytic patients,[43] and is a more sensitive predictor of iron deficiency than hemoglobin for screening infants[44] and adolescents[45] for iron deficiency. Mean cell volume of reticulocytes (MCVr) is available on several instruments but is less well studied. This parameter responds as expected to iron and vitamin B_{12} or folate therapy of the respective nutritional anemias, and also reflects erythropoietin effect. These reticulocyte parameters have the advantage of ready access in the context of an automated blood count, but the CHr and RET-He are limited by availability on only two instruments, and the MCVr is not a standardized parameter across instruments.

Many hematology analyzers now report some quantitative measure of reticulocyte RNA content. Increase in the immature (highest RNA content) reticulocyte fraction is an early sign of marrow recovery from the conditioning regimens of stem cell transplantation,[46] cancer chemotherapy, or treatment for nutritional anemias, usually preceding the rise in total reticulocyte count. It has been used as a marker of ineffective erythropoiesis, distinguishing macrocytosis caused by megaloblastic anemia or myelodysplasia from other causes,[47] and as a predictor of insufficient stem cell mobilization for transplantation.[48] A limitation at present is that the methods lack standardization and reference ranges for these parameters are instrument dependent.[49]

LEUKOCYTES

Leukocyte Count

Leukocyte counts are performed by automated cell counters on blood samples appropriately diluted with a solution that lyses the erythrocytes (e.g., an acid or a detergent), but preserves leukocyte integrity. Manual counting of leukocytes is used only when the instrument reports a potential interference or the count is beyond instrument linearity limits. Manual counts are subject to much greater technical variation than automated counts because of technical and statistical factors. Automated leukocyte counts may be falsely elevated as a result of cryoglobulins or cryofibrinogen,[50,50a] clumped platelets or fibrin from an inadequately anticoagulated or mixed sample, ethylenediaminetetraacetic acid (EDTA)-induced platelet aggregation,[51] nucleated red blood cells, or nonlysed red cells, and falsely decreased because of EDTA-induced neutrophil aggregation.[52] This potential interference is very instrument dependent, and current analyzers use a variety of algorithms to minimize their effect and flag those rare samples in which accurate automated analysis cannot be performed. With respect to nucleated red cells, high-end analyzers routinely and accurately quantify these cells with detection limits of 1 to 2 nucleated red cells per 100 leukocytes.[53] Nucleated red cells are normally present in small numbers in neonatal blood, and are increased in a variety of hematopoietic disorders and conditions of severe hematopoietic stress (see Chap. 44).

Leukocyte Differential

Leukocytes in the blood serve different functions and arise from different hematopoietic lineages, so it is important to evaluate each of the major leukocyte types separately. Modern automated instruments use multiple parameters to identify and enumerate the five major morphologic leukocyte types in blood: neutrophils, basophils, eosinophils, lymphocytes, and monocytes, as well as indicate the possible presence of immature or abnormal forms. Absolute neutrophil counts are accurately performed,[54] but "band" neutrophils cannot be identified as such by automated analyzers, although they will usually trigger a manual review flag if present in increased numbers. Quantification of immature granulocytes available on one analyzer (Sysmex XE 2100) compares well with microscopic methods,[55] but this is not a widely available or standardized parameter. This analyzer also detects a population enriched in hematopoietic progenitor cells that may allow rapid identification of samples with either very few or adequate numbers of CD34+ cells.[56] Current high-throughput instruments can perform an accurate automated "five-part" differential count with a false-positive rate of less than 15 percent in samples from a medical center patient population.[6] Small numbers of abnormal cells can escape detection by either automated or manual methods. The false-negative rate for detection of abnormal cells varies from 1 to 20 percent, depending on the instrument and the detection limit desired (1 to 5% abnormal cells).[57–59] Lymphoma cells and reactive lymphocytes are the most difficult for both automated instruments and the human observer to identify. If one needs to search for infrequent abnormal cells or evaluate leukocyte morphology, there is still no substitute for microscopic examination of a properly stained blood film by a trained observer, although manual evaluation of atypical lymphocytes can be influenced by prior knowledge of automated instrument flags.[60] The variability of morphologic quantification of band neutrophils is so high that some have advocated ceasing quantitative reporting of band cells.[61] In spite of instrumentation that permits automated analysis of a majority of clinical samples, the test is still quite labor-intensive relative to other high-volume laboratory tests, and its value as a cause-finding tool in screening of asymptomatic patients has been questioned.[62]

The normal differential leukocyte count varies with age. As described in detail in Chap. 6, polymorphonuclear neutrophils are predominant in the first few days after birth, but thereafter lymphocytes account for the majority of leukocytes. This pattern persists up to approximately 4 to 5 years of age, when the polymorphonuclear leukocyte again becomes the predominant cell and remains so throughout the rest of childhood and adult life. Chapter 8 discusses the leukocyte count in older persons. The leukocyte count may decrease slightly in older subjects because of a fall in the lymphocyte count with age. The reference range for neutrophil counts is lower in Americans of African descent, and in African, Afro-Caribbean, and some Middle Eastern populations than in persons of European descent.[63,64]

PLATELETS

Platelet Count

Platelets are usually counted electronically by enumerating particles in the unlysed sample within a specified volume window (e.g., 2–20 fl), where volume may be measured by electrical impedance or light scatter.[65] The platelet count was more difficult to automate than the red cell count because of the small size, tendency to aggregate, and potential overlap of platelets with more numerous smaller red cells and cellular debris. Current instruments typically construct a platelet volume histogram based on platelet size within a reliably measured platelet volume window and mathematically extrapolate this histogram to account for platelets whose size overlaps with debris (smaller) or small red cells (larger). This works because platelet volumes in health or disease follow a log-normal distribution.[66] Some analyzers compare platelet counts determined by different methods (e.g., impedance, light scatter or fluorescence) to improve accuracy, especially useful for low platelet counts. Based on analysis of volume distribution histograms of platelets and red cells and comparison of optical and impedance-based platelet counts, suspect samples are flagged for microscopic review. Automated platelet counting by current instrumentation is accurate and far more precise than manual methods.[67] However, very low platelet counts in the range of $10 \times 10^3/\mu L$ still present some difficulties, with most modern analyzers overestimating by 10 to 30 percent in comparison to international standardized methods using monoclonal antibodies.[68]

Causes of falsely decreased platelet counts include incomplete anticoagulation of the sample (sometimes accompanied by small clots in the specimen or fibrin strands on the stained film), and platelet clumping or "satellitism" (adherence of platelets to neutrophils), caused by nonpathogenic antibodies recognizing platelet adhesion molecule epitopes exposed as a result of chelation of divalent cations in the anticoagulated sample.[65,69] The latter condition occurs in approximately 0.1 percent of hospitalized patients.[70] Platelet counting under these conditions is difficult, but can be approached by collecting blood in citrate[70] or estimating platelet count from a freshly prepared fingerstick blood film (a method which also typically shows small platelet clumps but avoids chelation of calcium). Classical causes of falsely elevated platelet count include severe microcytosis, cryoglobulins, and leukocyte fragmentation.[65] Infrequently, it may be necessary to confirm automated results by a microscopic (phase contrast) platelet count or platelet estimate from the blood film, bearing in mind that these methods are imprecise.

The mean platelet volume (MPV) has been proposed as a useful clinical tool in the differential diagnosis of thrombocytopenias,[71] and is associated with cardiovascular risk, stroke, and metabolic disease.[72–74] Increased MPV may be related in a complex way to thrombopoietic stimuli that affect megakaryocyte ploidy,[75] and not platelet age per se.[76] However, in spite of the association of increased platelet size on blood films with consumptive thrombocytopenias, platelet size is a difficult parameter to accurately quantify and use diagnostically because of a wide physiologic variation of the MPV in normal subjects (e.g.) Mediterranean macrothrombocytopenia[77]) and susceptibility of anticoagulated platelets to time-dependent swelling *in vitro*.[78] Healthy subjects demonstrate an inverse correlation between platelet count and MPV, such that the platelet mass is relatively stable across the wide range of normal platelet counts. Mediterranean macrothrombocytopenia, prevalent in those of Greek and Italian origin, is an expression of this wide normal variation. There is a strong linkage of MPV to three genetic loci in a genome-wide association study.[79] A platelet volume distribution width (PDW) can be calculated just as the RDW, and is correlated with platelet count and MPV.[80] This measurement has yet to find a clinical use.

Newly released platelets contain RNA, as do newly released red cells, and are functionally more active. The number of platelets with high RNA content (sometimes termed reticulated platelets or immature platelet fraction, measured with RNA-binding fluorescent dyes) is a marker of marrow megakaryocytopoiesis and has been proposed as a way of differentiating decreased production of platelets from circulatory destruction or removal as a cause of thrombocytopenia, in an analogous fashion to the use of the reticulocyte count. The percentage of reticulated platelets is increased in destructive thrombocytopenias, but remains within the reference range in hypoproductive states.[81] Reticulated platelet number or RNA content correlates with imminent platelet recovery after chemotherapy.[82,83] Clinical application of this parameter has been limited by lack of standardization and availability on routine automated instruments, although this is changing with the addition of the immature platelet fraction as a stable and reproducible parameter to the high-end Sysmex instrument.[84]

REFERENCE RANGES

The use of reference ranges for quantitative hematology measurements deserves some additional comment. The physiologic variation of certain blood cell counts is notably higher than usually found in blood chemistry analytes. This is presumably a reflection of the adaptive responsiveness of the marrow and other tissues to cytokine and hormonal signaling. For instance, the leukocyte and differential counts are affected by stress, diurnal variation, tobacco smoking, and ethnic origin. With increasing globalization of clinical research and therapy, ethnic characterization of populations used for reference ranges is critical to data interpretation of clinical studies.[85] Platelet count and MPV are typically inversely related in normal individuals, and also show substantial ethnic variation.[86] The platelet and absolute neutrophil counts are lower in individuals of African ethnic origin.[64] American men and women of African descent have lower hemoglobin concentrations than do men and women of European descent, a difference that is reduced by half, but still significant, when subjects with iron deficiency, thalassemia, sickle trait, and renal disease are excluded.[87] Important clinical consequences may result from these differences, for instance, reduced neutrophil counts in Americans of African descent result in lower-dose intensity of treatment in early stage breast cancer, which may be related to survival outcome disparities.[88] Beutler and West[87] summarize the situation well: "The problem cannot be solved by simply establishing different ranges for different ethnic groups, especially since all represent some degree of admixture. Thus, it is basically information that the physician must possess that becomes one of the many factors that we designate as clinical judgment." With these caveats in mind, reference ranges for children, and African American, Hispanic, and white adults are presented in Tables 2–1 and 2–2. As with all laboratory parameters, clinical interpretation of patient results should be based on laboratory specific reference ranges. Therefore, these tables are not presented to guide interpretation of specific laboratory results, but to indicate the challenges facing laboratories and physicians in constructing and interpreting reference ranges of even standard and traditional assays.

Note the variation in reference ranges obtained from different studies. The major variability is likely population selection, especially the degree to which chronic illness or asymptomatic iron deficiency are excluded, and physiologic factors, such as diurnal variation, are considered. For example, the Wakeman study[89] exclusively used early morning samples, hence the upper limit of leukocyte count is lower because of diurnal physiologic variation. The National Health and Nutritional Examination Surveys (NHANES) III national database has the advantage of being a very large broad nationwide sampling, which as used by Cheng and colleagues[90] excluded any subjects with history of smoking, alcohol consumption, contraceptive use, and a variety of chronic diseases (60% of the tested subjects were excluded). However, those with asymptomatic iron deficiency were not excluded, so hemoglobins tend to be lower than in studies that may have been weighted toward groups of individuals in which undiagnosed iron deficiency and other asymptomatic disorders are less common. α- and β-thalassemia trait are also quite common in healthy individuals of certain ethnic groups, and inclusion of subjects with these disorders will also affect reference ranges. When subjects with low transferrin saturation, low ferritin, and high creatinine, sedimentation rate, or C-reactive protein measurements were excluded in analysis of the NHANES III and Kaiser-Scripps subjects ages 20 to 59, lower limits of hemoglobin were determined to be 13.7 g/dL (white men), 12.2 g/dL (white women), 12.9 g/dL (African American men), and 11.5 g/dL (African American women).[91] Such considerations also affect determination of the upper (97.5th percentile) limit of normal hematocrit and hemoglobin in relation to a possible diagnosis of polycythemia, where one has to carefully weigh the likelihood that a "normal-range" study has adequately excluded iron-deficient subjects.[92,93] Biomedical parameters are also subject to historical trends, such as the observed improvement in hemoglobin levels in the post–folic-acid-fortification era.[94]

Finally, when one observes significant changes in reference ranges based on age (e.g., glomerular filtration rate, lipid parameters, hemoglobin), there is the question of whether this is physiologic or a result of increased prevalence of undiagnosed occult disease. Most hematologic variables show more stability within an individual than between individuals, illustrating one reason for the lack of sensitivity and specificity of any test "cutoff," which is typically designed for a population rather than

TABLE 2–2. Published Reference Ranges for Key Blood Variables

	NORIP[98]	Wakeman[89]	Cheng[90]*			Bain[64]	
Date	2003	2004	1994	1994	1994	1996	1996
Ethnicity	Nordic	United Kingdom	U.S. European descent	U.S. African descent	U.S. Mexican descent	U.K. European descent	U.K. African descent
No.	1800	250	3125	1712	1735		
Hgb (g/dL) (M)	13.4–17.0	13.7–17.2	13.2–16.9	12.0–16.2	13.1–16.7		
(F)	11.7–15.3	12.0–15.2	10.7–15.1	10.2–14.4	11.4–15.0		
Hct (%) (M)	40–50	40–50	39–50	36–48	39–50		
(F)	35–46	37–46	34–45	32–43	33–45		
MCV (fl)	82–98	83–98 (M)	79–97 (M)	75–97 (M)	83–96 (M)		
		85–98 (F)	77–97 (F)	75–97 (F)	81–98 (F)		
WBC (×10⁹/L)	3.5–8.8	3.6–9.2	4.1–11.7 (M)	3.5–9.5 (M)	4.6–10.6 (M)	3.6–9.2 (M)	2.8–7.2 (M)
			4.3–12.0 (F)	3.4–10.5 (F)	4.3–11.3 (F)	3.5–10.8 (F)	3.2–7.8 (F)
Neutrophils (×10⁹/L)		1.7–6.2	2.7–8.1 (M)	1.5–7.4 (M)	2.2–6.6 (M)	1.7–6.1 (M)	0.9–4.2 (M)
			2.5–6.9 (F)	1.5–8.4 (F)	2.5–7.9 (F)	1.7–7.5 (F)	1.3–4.2 (F)
Lymphocytes (×10⁹/L)		1.0–3.4	1.1–3.7 (M)	1.1–3.6 (M)	1.3–3.4 (M)	1.0–2.9 (M)	1.0–3.2 (M)
			1.2–3.7 (F)	1.3–3.9 (F)	1.3–3.9 (F)	1.0–3.5 (F)	1.1–3.6 (F)
Monocytes (×10⁹/L)		0.2–0.8	0.13–0.86 (M)	0.11–0.72 (M)	0.14–0.70 (M)	0.18–0.62 (M)	0.15–0.58 (M)
			0.11–0.78 (F)	0.12–0.83 (F)	0.12–0.79 (F)	0.14–0.61 (F)	0.15–0.39 (F)
Platelets (×10⁹/L) (M)	145–348	140–320	161–385	161–381	166–388	143–332	115–290
(F)	165–387	180–380	178–434	178–452	171–411	169–358	125–342

F, female; Hgb, hemoglobin; Hct, hematocrit; M, male; MCV, mean cell; NORIP, Nordic Reference Interval Project; U.K., United Kingdom volume; U.S., United States volume; WBC, white blood cell count.

*Ranges calculated from adult (>18 years) data, assuming equal contribution of subjects from each of multiple adult age groups, derived from the National Health and Nutrition Examination Survey (NHANES) III.

NOTE: This table is provided as a guide. Normal ranges should be validated by the clinical laboratory for the specific methods in use.

for an individual person. A study of repeated analyses of blood variables from older subjects[95] graphically demonstrates this phenomenon. Some normal subjects have a normal steady-state platelet count between 170,000 and 200,000/μL, whereas others have one between 280,000 and 310,000/μL (Fig. 2–3). For the latter group, a progressive fall in platelet count because of marrow failure may not be detected as quickly as the former group. The same observations are shown for absolute neutrophil count, hemoglobin, and MCV, among others. This normal variation may be genetically influenced as shown for the MCV.[96]

MORPHOLOGIC EXAMINATION OF THE BLOOD

Microscopic examination of the blood spread on a glass slide or coverslip yields useful information regarding all the cells of the blood. The process of preparing a thin blood film causes mechanical trauma to the cells. Also, the cells flatten on the glass during drying, and the fixation and staining involve exposure to methanol and water. Some artifacts are inevitably introduced, but these can be minimized by good technique. The optimal part of the stained blood film to use for morphologic examination of the blood cells should be sufficiently thin that only a few erythrocytes in a ×100 magnification field touch each other, but not so thin that no red cells are touching. Figure 2–4 is a composite image taken from the optimal portion of the film showing the five major leukocyte types, normal red cells, and platelets. Selection of a portion of the blood film for analysis that is too thick or too thin for proper morphologic evaluation is by far the most common error in blood film interpretation. For example, leukemic blasts may appear dense and rounded and lose their characteristic features when viewed in the thick part of the film. For specific purposes, the thick portion or side and "feathered" edges of the film are of interest (for instance, to detect microfilariae and malarial parasites or to search for large abnormal cells and platelet clumps).

The blood film is first scanned at low magnification (×200) to confirm reasonably even distribution of leukocytes and to check for abnormally large or immature cells in the side and feathered edges of the film. The feathered edge is examined for platelet clumps. Abnormal cells, red cell aggregation or rouleaux, background bluish staining consistent with paraproteinemia, and parasites are all findings that can be suggested by medium magnification examination (×400). The optimal portion of the film is then examined at high magnification (×1000, oil immersion) to systematically assess the size, shape, and morphology of the major cell lineages.

■ RED CELL MORPHOLOGY

Normal erythrocytes on dried films are nearly uniform in size, with a normal distribution of about a mean diameter of 7.2 to 7.9 μm. The

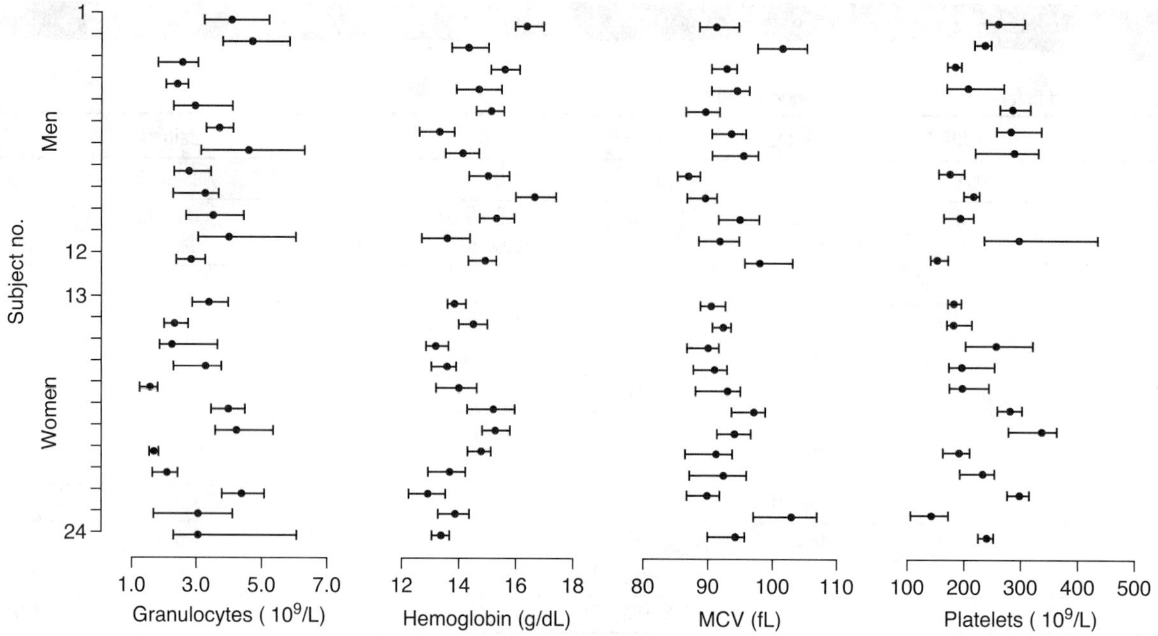

FIGURE 2–3. Absolute neutrophil count, hemoglobin, mean cell volume (MCV), and platelet count determined repeatedly by automated hematology analyzer on 24 healthy elderly subjects. Fasting (7–9 AM) blood samples were obtained 9 to 10 times at 14-day intervals from seated elderly subjects with minimal stasis by the same phlebotomist and performed in duplicate on the morning specimen collection. Subjects had no chronic medical conditions requiring therapy and were not taking drugs. The mean and range for each patient is shown separately for each assay. This is an illustration of the relatively narrow range within which most variables are maintained in an individual, whereas there are striking differences in both mean and variance between subjects. Reference ranges need to encompass at least 95% of values from all healthy individuals, placing limits on diagnostic sensitivity in detecting progressive decrease or a dysregulated change in a hematologic variable, previously maintained in a homeostatic range. *(Adapted from Fraser CG, Wilkinson SP, Neville RG, et al,[95] with permission.)*

normal-sized erythrocyte is about the diameter of the nucleus of a small lymphocyte (Chap. 29). The MCV is a more sensitive measure of red cell volume than the red cell diameter. However, an experienced observer should be able to recognize abnormalities in average red cell size when the MCV is significantly elevated or decreased. *Anisocytosis* is the term that describes variation in erythrocyte size (Chap. 29), and is the morphologic correlate of the RDW. The *macrocyte*, a red cell larger than normal (Chap. 29), may be seen in a number of disease states, for example, in folic acid or vitamin B_{12} deficiency. Cells are considered to be macrocytes if they are well hemoglobinized and their diameters exceed 9 μm. Early ("shift" or "stress") *reticulocytes* (i.e., those with the most residual RNA) appear in stained films as large, bluish cells, referred to as *polychromatophilic* cells (Chap. 31). These cells roughly correspond to those quantified by automated analyzers as the immature reticulocyte fraction. *Microcyte*, meaning a red cell smaller than normal (Chap. 42), is the term used to describe a cell less than 6 μm in diameter.

The normal erythrocyte on a blood film is circular with central pallor. *Poikilocytosis* is a term used to describe variations in the shape of erythrocytes (Chap. 29). The predominant appearance of a specific abnormality in red cell shape can be an important diagnostic clue in patients with anemia. Erythrocytes with evenly spaced spikes (echinocytes or crenated cells [Chap. 29]) can be an artifact caused by prolonged storage, or may reflect metabolic erythrocyte abnormalities.

The normal erythrocyte appears as a disc with a rim of hemoglobin and a clear central area. The central pallor normally occupies less than one-half the diameter of the cells. Increased central pallor *(hypochromia)* is associated with disorders characterized by diminished hemoglobin synthesis, such as iron deficiency (Chap. 42). Evaluation of red cell hemoglobin content, as well as red cell size, is dependent on examining the proper part of the blood film. Cells at the far "feathered edge" will always be large and lack central pallor, whereas cells in the thick part of the film will look small and rounded and will also lack central pallor. A sharp refractile border demarcating the central area of pallor is an artifact secondary to inadequate drying of the film before staining (because of high humidity; more common in anemic samples). *Spherocytes* are more densely stained and appear smaller because of their rounded shape; they show decreased or absent central pallor (Chap. 29). The hemoglobin may appear to be abnormally distributed in erythrocytes, particularly in a form of cell in which there is a spot or disc of hemoglobin in the center surrounded by a clear area which is, in turn, surrounded by a rim of hemoglobin at the outer edge of the cell, giving the appearance of a target—a *target cell* (Chap. 29). This is in reality a cup-shaped cell that is distorted as it is flattened on the glass slide. These cells are typically found in disorders of hemoglobin synthesis (e.g., thalassemia), liver disease, and postsplenectomy where the cell-surface-to-cell-volume ratio is high. Figure 2–5 illustrates some common red cell morphologic abnormalities and associated diseases (see Chap. 29).

Erythrocytes are usually distributed evenly throughout the blood film. In some cases the cells become aligned in overlapping stacks, referred to as rouleaux (Chap. 111), resembling overlapping rows of coins. Such rouleaux formation is normal in the thicker part of the film; when found in the optimal viewing portion of the film (pathologic rouleaux), it may be a result of the presence of an increase in immunoglobulin (Ig), especially IgM, and suggests the diagnosis of macroglobulinemia. Occasionally, high concentrations of IgA or IgG in patients with myeloma may produce pathologic rouleaux, as a manifestation of myeloma.

Chap. 29 describes the inclusions that may be observed in erythrocytes on films stained with Wright or Giemsa stain. Nucleated red cells are not normally observed in blood films but may be found in newborns, particularly if physiologically stressed, and in a variety of disorders, including

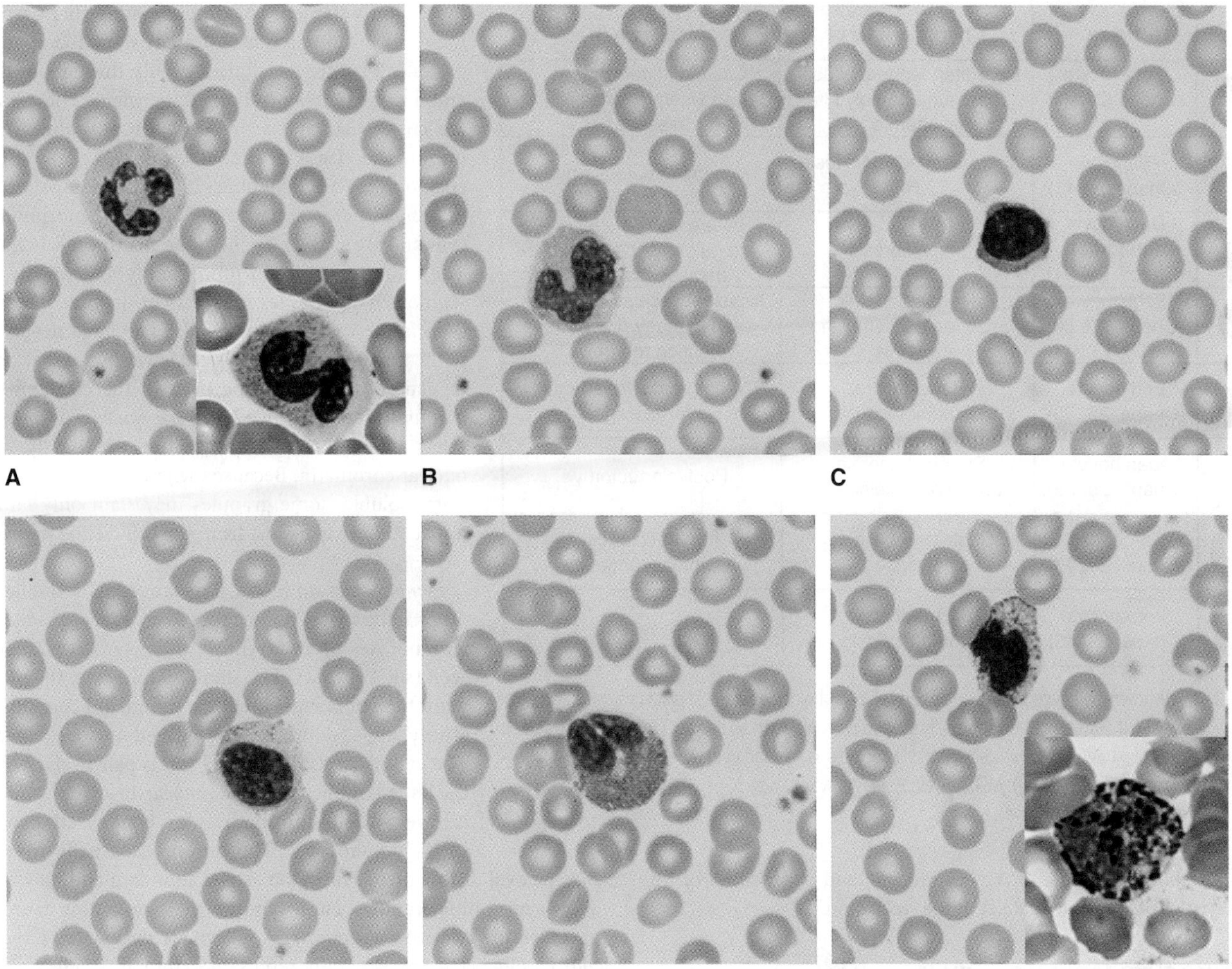

A B C D E F

FIGURE 2–4. Images from a normal blood film showing major leukocyte types. The red cells are normocytic (normal size) and normochromic (normal hemoglobin content) with normal shape. The scattered platelets are normal in frequency and morphology. **A.** A platelet caught sitting in the biconcavity of the red cell in the preparation of the blood film. This normal finding should not be mistaken for a red cell inclusion. Images are taken from the optimal portion of the blood film for morphologic analysis. Image shows a **(A)** segmented (polymorphonuclear) neutrophil and in the inset a band neutrophil; **(B)** monocyte; **(C)** small lymphocyte; **(D)** large granular lymphocyte, note larger size than lymphocyte in **(C)** and increased amount of cytoplasm containing scattered eosinophilic granules; and **(E)** eosinophil. Virtually all normal blood eosinophils are bilobed and filled with relatively large (compared to the neutrophil) eosinophilic granules. **F.** Basophil and in inset a basophil that was less degranulated during film preparation, showing relatively large basophilic granules. The eosinophilic and basophilic granules are readily resolvable by light microscopy (×1000), whereas the neutrophilic granule is not resolvable but they in the aggregate impart a faint tan coloration to the neutrophil cytoplasm, quite distinctly different from the blue-gray cytoplasmic coloring of the monocyte and lymphocyte.

hypoxic states (congestive heart failure), severe hemolytic anemia, primary myelofibrosis, and infiltrative disease of the marrow (Chap. 44).

■ PLATELET MORPHOLOGY

Platelets appear in normal stained blood film as small blue or colorless bodies with red or purple granules (see Fig. 2–4). Normal platelets average about 1 to 2 μm in diameter, but show wide variation in shape, from round to elongated, cigar-shaped forms. A rough estimate of the platelet count can be made by observation of the stained blood film. If the platelet count is normal, approximately 8 to 15 platelets (individually or in small clumps) should be visible in each oil-immersion (×1000) field. There should be 1 platelet present for approximately every 20 erythrocytes. This is a valuable check when the automated platelet count is in question or an unexpected result is obtained.

In improperly prepared films, platelets may form large aggregates in some areas and appear to be diminished or absent in others. The occurrence of giant platelets or platelet masses may indicate a myeloproliferative disorder or improper collection of the blood specimen. The latter circumstance can occur when venipuncture technique is faulty and platelets become activated before the blood sample is thoroughly mixed with anticoagulant. These platelet masses are apparent typically in the thin "feathered edge" of the film. This maldistribution may create a mistaken impression of thrombocytopenia if the aggregates are not detected. Platelet clumping throughout the blood film, or platelet "satellitism" (adherence of platelets to neutrophils), may be a result of platelet agglutinins, as previously discussed (Fig. 2–6).

A platelet will occasionally overlie an erythrocyte, where it may be mistaken for an inclusion body or a parasite. The differentiation depends on the observation of a halo around the platelet, determination

	Name	Characteristic of	Also seen in
	Spherocyte (Chaps. 29, 45, 53)	Hereditary spherocytosis, immune hemolytic anemia	Clostridial perfringens septicemia, Wilson disease
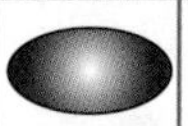	Elliptocyte (Chaps. 29,45)	Hereditary elliptocytosis (HE)	Iron deficiency, megaloblastic anemia, thalassemia, myelofibrosis, MDS
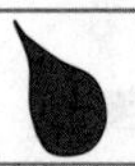	Dacryocyte (teardrop) (Chaps. 29, 91)	Myelofibrosis	Severe iron deficiency, megaloblastic anemia, thalassemia, MDS
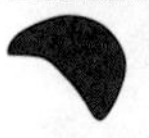	Schistocyte (Chaps. 29, 50, 130, 133)	Microangiopathic, mechanical hemolytic anemia	Occasional schistocytes are seen in many disorders affecting red cells.
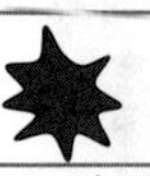	Echinocyte (Chaps. 29, 36)	Renal failure, malnutrition	Common *in vitro* artifact after storage
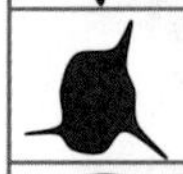	Acanthocyte (Chaps. 29, 55)	Spur cell anemia, abetalipoproteinemia	Postsplenectomy
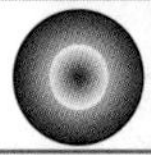	Target cell (Chaps. 29, 47)	Cholestasis, Hgb C disease	Iron deficiency, thalassemia
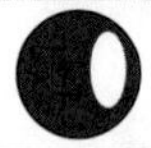	Stomatocyte (Chaps. 29, 45)	Hereditary stomatocytosis	Alcoholism

FIGURE 2–5. Disorders associated with certain red cell morphologic changes. *Poikilocytosis* is a general term used to indicate the presence of abnormally shaped red cells, such as dacryocytes (teardrop-shaped red cells), schistocytes (fragmented red cells), and elliptocytes, as is found in the most extreme form in hereditary pyropoikilocytosis (Chap. 45). MDS, myelodysplastic syndromes.

that it lies above the plane of the erythrocyte, and observation of the characteristics of a normal platelet in the "inclusion."

LEUKOCYTE MORPHOLOGY

The distribution of leukocytes on glass slides is not uniform, and the larger cells, such as monocytes and segmented neutrophils, tend to be concentrated on the edges and thin end of the blood film. The cells that are normally found in blood are polymorphonuclear leukocytes of the neutrophilic, eosinophilic, and basophilic types; lymphocytes; and monocytes, with smaller numbers of eosinophils and basophils (see Fig. 2–4). *Neutrophils* are round cells ranging from 10 to 14 μm in diameter on a blood film. The nucleus is lobulated, with two to four lobes connected by a thin chromatin thread. The defining feature of the segmented neutrophil is the round lobes with condensed chromatin, because the chromatin thread may overlie the nucleus and not be visible. The chromatin stains purple and is coarse and arranged in clumps. The nucleus of 1 to 16 percent of the neutrophils from females may have an appendage that is shaped like a drumstick and is attached to one lobe by a strand of chromatin. The cytoplasm is clear and contains many small, tan to pink granules distributed evenly throughout the cell, although they may not be apparent when they lie over the nucleus.

Bands are identical in appearance to mature polymorphonuclear leukocytes except that the nucleus is not segmented but is sausage-shaped or U-shaped (see Fig. 2–4). It may have incipient segmentation, as evidenced by beginning constrictions but not sufficient to be categorized as a segmented neutrophil. The nuclear chromatin is slightly less condensed than the mature neutrophil (Chap. 59).

Eosinophils are on the average slightly larger than neutrophils (Chap. 62). The nucleus usually has two lobes (see Fig. 2–4). The chromatin pattern is the same as that in the neutrophil, but the nucleus tends to be more lightly stained. The differentiating characteristic of these cells is the presence of many refractile, orange-red granules that are distributed evenly throughout the cell and may be visible overlying the nucleus. These granules are larger than those in the neutrophil and are more uniform in size. Occasionally, some of the granules in eosinophils stain light blue rather than orange-red.

Basophils are similar to the other polymorphonuclear cells and are slightly smaller than neutrophils (Chap. 63). The nucleus may stain more faintly and usually is less segmented and has less distinct chromatin condensation than is the case in neutrophils. The large deeply basophilic granules of basophils are fewer in number and less regular in size and shape than in the eosinophil. The granules are visible overlying the nucleus and, in some cells, almost completely obscure the lightly stained nuclear chromatin. Because the granular constituents are water soluble, some granules may stain only faintly or not at all or may be lost from the cell during preparation (see Fig. 2–4).

Lymphocytes on blood films are usually smaller than other leukocytes, about 10 μm in diameter, but large lymphocytes up to 20 μm in diameter occasionally are seen (see Fig. 2–4). The small lymphocyte, the predominant type in normal blood, is round and contains a relatively large, round, densely stained nucleus (Chap. 74). The cytoplasm is scanty and stains pale to dark blue. In the large lymphocytes, the nuclear-to-cytoplasmic ratio is lower and the chromatin is less condensed than in the small lymphocytes. The nucleus is usually round but may be oval or indented. The cytoplasm is abundant and may contain a few azurophilic granules. Large lymphocytes containing azurophilic granules and relatively abundant cytoplasm are designated *large granular lymphocytes*, and generally represent cytotoxic T cells or natural killer (NK) cells (Chap. 96). *Reactive lymphocytes*, as seen in viral infections caused by Epstein-Barr virus, cytomegalovirus, adenovirus, or other organisms, are large with indented nuclei and abundant blue cytoplasm (Chap. 84). Nuclear chromatin condensation is variable, and nucleoli may be evident. A low nuclear-to-cytoplasmic ratio and greater degree of chromatin condensation distinguishes these reactive T lymphocytes from neoplastic cells.

Monocytes are the largest normal cells in the blood, usually measuring from 15 to 22 μm in diameter (see Fig. 2–4). The nucleus is of various shapes—round, kidney-shape, oval, or lobular—and frequently appears to be folded (Chap. 67). The chromatin is arranged in fine strands with sharply defined margins. The cytoplasm is light gray, contains variable numbers of fine lilac or purple granules, and is frequently vacuolated, especially in films made from blood anticoagulated with EDTA. The gray (as opposed to blue) color of monocyte cytoplasm is a result of fine granules (staining pink) seen on the background of RNA-containing cytoplasm (staining blue), and helps to distinguish between monocytes and reactive lymphocytes. The monocyte nuclear chromatin contains a fine, string-like structure as opposed to the smudgy-appearing clumps of the lymphoid chromatin. Nuclear shape and cytoplasmic vacuolization are less reliable distinguishing features between monocytic and lymphoid cells.

LEUKOCYTE INCLUSIONS

Leukocytes may contain abnormal inclusions as a result of genetic or acquired disorders.

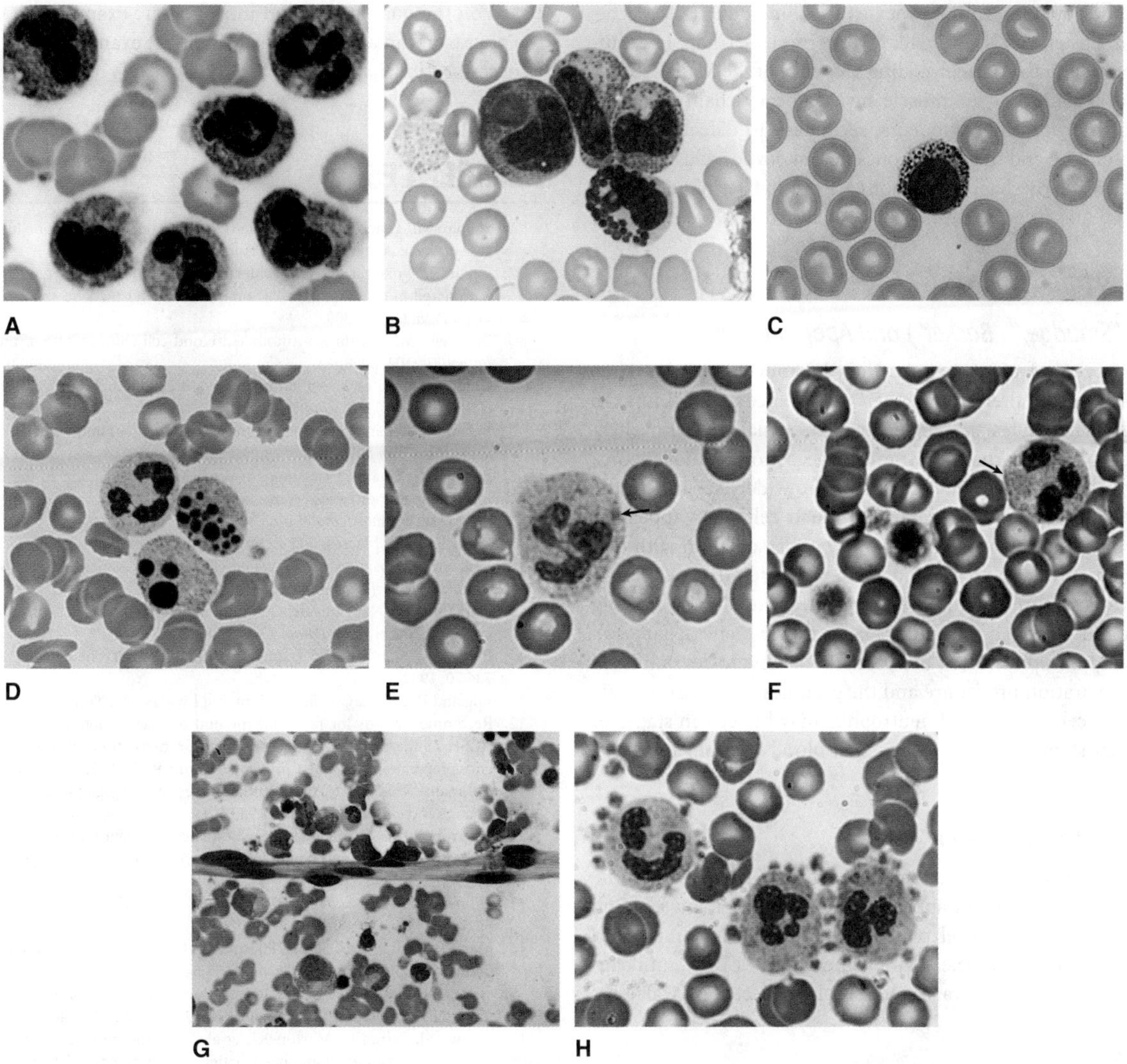

FIGURE 2–6. Blood films. **A.** Toxic granules in neutrophils. In inflammatory states the neutrophil may develop overt purplish granules as shown in this example of reactive neutrophilia. **B.** Chédiak-Higashi disease. Note the giant eosinophilic granule in the monocyte and the numerous enlarged granules in the lymphocyte (see Chap. 66). **C.** Hurler syndrome. Note characteristic prominent dense cytoplasmic inclusions in the mononuclear cell. These inclusions are accumulations of glycosaminoglycans resulting from a deficiency of α-L-iduronidase in leukocytes and other tissues. **D.** Examples of apoptosis of two neutrophils in normal anticoagulated blood during standing at room temperature. Nuclear condensation and fragmentation are evident. A normal neutrophil is also present. **E.** Döhle bodies. These RNA remnants of rough endoplasmic reticulum appear as blue rod-shaped structures (*arrow* points to one) in neutrophils involved in inflammatory reactions. **F.** May-Hegglin disease. The large blue-gray inclusions (*arrow*) represent precipitates of nonmuscle myosin heavy chain type IIA. Note also the two macrothrombocytes (the size of red cells) characteristic of this disorder (see Chap. 114). The neutrophil inclusions stain with fluorescent antibodies to nonmuscle myosin heavy chain type IIA. **G.** Marrow film. A strand of endothelial cells derived from vascular tissue caught on the biopsy needle. Individual endothelial cells may be found, rarely in a blood film. **H.** Platelet satellitism. Three neutrophils surrounded by adherent platelets. This blood film was prepared from an EDTA-anticoagulated sample. *(Used with permission from* Lichtman's Atlas of Hematology, *www.accessmedicine.com.)*

Abnormal Granules

In patients with conditions associated with a systemic inflammatory reaction, neutrophil granules may appear larger than normal and stain more darkly, often assuming a dark blue-black color. This has been called *toxic granulation* (see Fig. 2–6). These granules can be confused with the larger granules of basophils. In *mucopolysaccharidoses*, coarse, dark granules may be found in the neutrophils, and large azurophilic granules are often found in some lymphocytes and monocytes (see Fig. 2–6). Huge misshapen granules are found in the polymorphonuclear leukocytes, and giant azurophilic granules are present in the lymphocytes of patients exhibiting the *Chédiak-Higashi* anomaly (see Fig. 2–6; Chap. 66). *Auer rods* are sharply outlined, red-staining rods found in the cytoplasm in blast cells, and occasionally in more mature leukemic cells, in the blood of some patients with acute myelogenous leukemia (Chap. 89).

Abnormal Neutrophil Inclusions

Light blue round or oval *Döhle bodies,* about 1 to 2 μm in diameter, may be seen in the cytoplasm of neutrophils of patients with infections, burns, and other inflammatory states (see Fig. 2–6). The blue staining is caused by RNA of the rough-surfaced endoplasmic reticulum contained in Döhle bodies.[97] These bodies are thought to be a reflection of accelerated maturation of neutrophils with residual endoplasmic reticulum from the promyelocyte stage. They usually occur in circumstances in which toxic granulation may be present. *May-Hegglin* anomaly is one of several MYH9 disorders, autosomal dominant macrothrombocytopenias, with leukocyte inclusion bodies (also Fechtner, Sebastian, Epstein, and Alport-like syndromes; see Chap. 114) Single-point mutation in the protein-coding sequence of the *MYH9* results in disordered assembly of nonmuscle myosin heavy-chain type IIA. This leads to macrothrombocytopenia, secondary to defective megakaryocyte maturation and fragmentation. The leukocytic inclusions, pale blue-stained, irregularly shaped inclusions are precipitates of nonmuscle myosin heavy chains (see Fig. 2–6). Neutrophil function is normal.

LEUKOCYTE ARTIFACTS

Damaged ("Smudge," "Basket") and Apoptotic Cells

During the process of preparing the film, leukocytes may be damaged, with consequent alteration in their appearance and staining. In some damaged leukocytes the nucleus appears enlarged, with alteration of the chromatin so that the strands appear more homogeneous, stain with a distinct reddish hue, and are more widely separated; the cytoplasm may or may not appear intact. Such cells may appear to have a large blue nucleolus. There is no specific association with disease other than chronic lymphocytic leukemia, where the neoplastic lymphocytes are ruptured by the shearing forces generated in making a blood film and damaged ("smudge") cells are frequent (Chap. 94). Eosinophils and basophils often are partially or largely degranulated by the film preparation procedure and the granules may be seen scattered beside the cell. Occasional neutrophils may be seen in stages of apoptosis when standing in anticoagulated blood at room temperature (see Fig. 2–6).

Radial Nuclear Segmentation

This refers to abnormal segmentation of the nuclei of leukocytes on the blood film, in which the lobes appear to radiate from a single point, giving a cloverleaf or cartwheel picture. This change is common in cytocentrifuged preparations (i.e., from a body fluid), EDTA anticoagulated blood after excessive storage, and samples collected in oxalate.

Vacuolization

Vacuoles may develop in the nucleus and cytoplasm of leukocytes, especially monocytes and neutrophils, with prolonged storage in EDTA anticoagulated blood. Vacuoles may be associated with swelling of the nuclei and loss of granules from the cytoplasm. In blood films prepared without anticoagulation, vacuoles in neutrophils suggest sepsis.

Endothelial Cells

If the blood film is prepared from the first drop of blood issuing from the microsampling wound, endothelial cells may be present singly, in clumps, or as strings of attached cells (see Fig. 2–6). These cells en face may simulate the appearance of abnormal cells and may be misinterpreted as blasts or metastatic tumor cells.

THE NEED FOR EXAMINATION OF THE BLOOD FILM

The quantitative determinations discussed earlier in this chapter describe the blood in sufficient detail that the physician will often recognize the need for further laboratory and clinical workup. Quantitative analysis of the blood may suggest certain diseases involving erythrocytes, leukocytes, and/or platelets that should be confirmed by examination of a stained blood film. In many cases, examination of the blood film will be prompted by flags detected in automated analysis. Based on the quantitative and morphologic examination of the blood, the physician can assess the need for direct examination of the marrow, as described in Chap. 3.

REFERENCES

1. Shapiro MF, Hatch RL, Greenfield S: Cost containment and labor-intensive tests. The case of the leukocyte differential count. *JAMA* 252:231, 1984.
2. Ceelie H, Dinkelaar RB, van Gelder W: Examination of peripheral blood films using automated microscopy; evaluation of Diffmaster Octavia and Cellavision DM96. *J Clin Pathol* 60:72, 2007.
3. Buttarello M, Plebani M: Automated blood cell counts: State of the art. *Am J Clin Pathol* 130:104, 2008.
4. Coulter WH: High speed automatic blood cell counter and cell size analyzer. *Proc Natl Elect Conf* 12:1034, 1956.
5. Bessman JD, Banks D: Spurious macrocytosis, a common clue to erythrocyte cold agglutinins. *Am J Clin Pathol* 74:797, 1980.
6. Bourner G, Dhaliwal J, Sumner J: Performance evaluation of the latest fully automated hematology analyzers in a large, commercial laboratory setting: A 4-way, side-by-side study. *Lab Hematol* 11:285, 2005.
7. Wintrobe MM: Macroscopic examination of the blood. *Am J Med Sci* 185:58, 1933.
8. England JM, Walford DM, Waters DA: Re-assessment of the reliability of the haematocrit. *Br J Haematol* 23:247, 1972.
9. Fairbanks VF: Nonequivalence of automated and manual hematocrit and erythrocyte indices. *Am J Clin Pathol* 73:55, 1980.
10. Pearson TC, Guthrie DL: Trapped plasma in the microhematocrit. *Am J Clin Pathol* 78:770, 1982.
11. England JM: *Blood Cell Sizing*. Churchill Livingstone, New York, 1991.
12. Recommendations for reference method for haemoglobinometry in human blood (ICSH standard 1986) and specifications for international haemiglobincyanide reference preparation (3rd ed). *Clin Lab Haematol* 9:73, 1987.
13. Dallman PR, Siimes MA: Percentile curves for hemoglobin and red cell volume in infancy and childhood. *J Pediatr* 94:26, 1979.
14. Wintrobe MM: Anemia: Classification and treatment on the basis of differences in the average volume and hemoglobin content of the red corpuscles. *Arch Intern Med* 54:256, 1934.
15. Hillman RS: After sixty years: The MCV is still alive and well. *J Gen Intern Med* 5:264, 1990.
16. Mach-Pascual S, Darbellay R, Pilotto PA, et al: Investigation of microcytosis: A comprehensive approach. *Eur J Haematol* 57:54, 1996.
17. Griner PF, Oranburg PR: Predictive values of erythrocyte indices for tests of iron, folic acid, and vitamin B_{12} deficiency. *Am J Clin Pathol* 70:748, 1978.
18. Seward SJ, Safran C, Marton KI, et al: Does the mean corpuscular volume help physicians evaluate hospitalized patients with anemia? *J Gen Intern Med* 5:187, 1990.
19. Carmel R: Pernicious anemia. The expected findings of very low serum cobalamin levels, anemia, and macrocytosis are often lacking. *Arch Intern Med* 148:1712, 1988.
20. Sekhar J, Stabler SP: Life-threatening megaloblastic pancytopenia with normal mean cell volume: Case series. *Eur J Intern Med* 18:548, 2007.
21. Mahmoud MY, Lugon M, Anderson CC: Unexplained macrocytosis in elderly patients. *Age Ageing* 25:310, 1996.
22. Eldibany MM, Totonchi KF, Joseph NJ, et al: Usefulness of certain red blood cell indices in diagnosing and differentiating thalassemia trait from iron-deficiency anemia. *Am J Clin Pathol* 111:676, 1999.
23. Lafferty JD, Crowther MA, Ali MA, et al: The evaluation of various mathematical RBC indices and their efficacy in discriminating between thalassemic and non-thalassemic microcytosis. *Am J Clin Pathol* 106:201, 1996.
24. Rathod DA, Kaur A, Patel V, et al: Usefulness of cell counter-based parameters and formulas in detection of beta-thalassemia trait in areas of high prevalence. *Am J Clin Pathol* 128:585, 2007.
25. Rose MS: Epitaph for the M.C.H.C. *Br Med J* 4:169, 1971.
26. McClure S, Custer E, Bessman JD: Improved detection of early iron deficiency in nonanemic subjects. *JAMA* 253:1021, 1985.
27. Bessman JD, Gilmer PR Jr, Gardner FH: Improved classification of anemias by MCV and RDW. *Am J Clin Pathol* 80:322, 1983.
28. Flynn MM, Reppun TS, Bhagavan NV: Limitations of red blood cell distribution width (RDW) in evaluation of microcytosis. *Am J Clin Pathol* 85:445, 1986.
29. Lesesve JF, Salignac S, Alla F, et al: Comparative evaluation of schistocyte counting by an automated method and by microscopic determination. *Am J Clin Pathol* 121:739, 2004.
30. Tonelli M, Sacks F, Arnold M, et al: Relation between red blood cell distribution width and cardiovascular event rate in people with coronary disease. *Circulation* 117:163, 2008.
31. Ani C, Ovbiagele B: Elevated red blood cell distribution width predicts mortality in persons with known stroke. *J Neurol Sci* 277:103, 2009.

32. Cavusoglu E, Chopra V, Gupta A, et al: Relation between red blood cell distribution width (RDW) and all-cause mortality at two years in an unselected population referred for coronary angiography. *Int J Cardiol* 2009.
33. Felker GM, Allen LA, Pocock SJ, et al: Red cell distribution width as a novel prognostic marker in heart failure: Data from the CHARM Program and the Duke Databank. *J Am Coll Cardiol* 50:40, 2007.
34. Cakal B, Akoz AG, Ustundag Y, et al: Red cell distribution width for assessment of activity of inflammatory bowel disease. *Dig Dis Sci* 54:842, 2009.
35. Lippi G, Targher G, Montagnana M, et al: Relationship between red blood cell distribution width and kidney function tests in a large cohort of unselected outpatients. *Scand J Clin Lab Invest* 68:745, 2008.
36. Riley RS, Ben-Ezra JM, Tidwell A, et al: Reticulocyte analysis by flow cytometry and other techniques. *Hematol Oncol Clin North Am* 16:373, 2002.
37. Buttarello M, Bulian P, Farina G, et al: Flow cytometric reticulocyte counting. Parallel evaluation of five fully automated analyzers: An NCCLS-ICSH approach. *Am J Clin Pathol* 115:100, 2001.
38. Buttarello M, Temporin V, Ceravolo R, et al: The new reticulocyte parameter (RET-Y) of the Sysmex XE 2100: Its use in the diagnosis and monitoring of posttreatment sideropenic anemia. *Am J Clin Pathol* 121:489, 2004.
39. Brugnara C, Schiller B, Moran J: Reticulocyte hemoglobin equivalent (Ret He) and assessment of iron-deficient states. *Clin Lab Haematol* 28:303, 2006.
40. Thomas L, Franck S, Messinger M, et al: Reticulocyte hemoglobin measurement—Comparison of two methods in the diagnosis of iron-restricted erythropoiesis. *Clin Chem Lab Med* 43:1193, 2005.
41. Tsuchiya K, Saito M, Okano-Sugiyama H, et al: Monitoring the content of reticulocyte hemoglobin (CHr) as the progression of anemia in nondialysis chronic renal failure (CRF) patients. *Ren Fail* 27:59, 2005.
42. Group AiCKDW. KDOQI clinical practice guidelines and clinical practice recommendations for anemia in chronic kidney disease. *Am J Kidney Dis* 47(5 Suppl 3):S11, 2006.
43. Mast AE, Blinder MA, Lu Q, et al: Clinical utility of the reticulocyte hemoglobin content in the diagnosis of iron deficiency. *Blood* 99:1489, 2002.
44. Ullrich C, Wu A, Armsby C, et al: Screening healthy infants for iron deficiency using reticulocyte hemoglobin content. *JAMA* 294:924, 2005.
45. Stoffman N, Brugnara C, Woods ER: An algorithm using reticulocyte hemoglobin content (CHr) measurement in screening adolescents for iron deficiency. *J Adolesc Health* 36:529, 2005.
46. Noronha JF, De Souza CA, Vigorito AC, et al: Immature reticulocytes as an early predictor of engraftment in autologous and allogeneic bone marrow transplantation. *Clin Lab Haematol* 25:47, 2003.
47. Torres Gomez A, Casano J, Sanchez J, et al: Utility of reticulocyte maturation parameters in the differential diagnosis of macrocytic anemias. *Clin Lab Haematol* 25:283, 2003.
48. Dunlop LC, Cohen J, Harvey M, et al: The immature reticulocyte fraction: A negative predictor of the harvesting of CD34 cells for autologous peripheral blood stem cell transplantation. *Clin Lab Haematol* 28:245, 2006.
49. Buttarello M, Bulian P, Farina G, et al: Five fully automated methods for performing immature reticulocyte fraction: Comparison in diagnosis of bone marrow aplasia. *Am J Clin Pathol* 117:871, 2002.
50. Gulliani GL, Hyun BH, Gagaldon H: Falsely elevated automated leukocyte count on cryoglobulinemic and/or cryofibrinogenic blood samples. *Lab Med* 8:14, 1977.
50a. Taft EG, Grossman J, Abraham GN, et al: Pseudoleukocytosis due to cryoprotein crystals. *Am J Clin Pathol* 60:669, 1973.
51. Lombarts AJ, de Kieviet W: Recognition and prevention of pseudothrombocytopenia and concomitant pseudoleukocytosis. *Am J Clin Pathol* 89:534, 1988.
52. Zandecki M, Genevieve F, Gerard J, et al: Spurious counts and spurious results on haematology analysers: A review. Part II: White blood cells, red blood cells, haemoglobin, red cell indices and reticulocytes. *Int J Lab Hematol* 29:21, 2007.
53. Gulati G, Behling E, Kocher W, et al: An evaluation of the performance of Sysmex XE-2100 in enumerating nucleated red cells in peripheral blood. *Arch Pathol Lab Med* 131:1077, 2007.
54. Hijiya N, Onciu M, Howard SC, et al: Utility of automated counting to determine absolute neutrophil counts and absolute phagocyte counts for pediatric cancer treatment protocols. *Cancer* 101:2681, 2004.
55. Field D, Taube E, Heumann S: Performance evaluation of the immature granulocyte parameter on the Sysmex XE-2100 automated hematology analyzer. *Lab Hematol* 12:11, 2006.
56. Letestu R, Marzac C, Audat F, et al: Use of hematopoietic progenitor cell count on the Sysmex XE-2100 for peripheral blood stem cell harvest monitoring. *Leuk Lymphoma* 48:89, 2007.
57. Thalhammer-Scherrer R, Knobl P, Korninger L, et al: Automated five-part white blood cell differential counts. Efficiency of software-generated white blood cell suspect flags of the hematology analyzers Sysmex SE-9000, Sysmex NE-8000, and Coulter STKS: *Arch Pathol Lab Med* 121:573, 1997.
58. Ruzicka K, Veitl M, Thalhammer-Scherrer R, et al: The new hematology analyzer Sysmex XE-2100: Performance evaluation of a novel white blood cell differential technology. *Arch Pathol Lab Med* 125:391, 2001.
59. Aulesa C, Pastor I, Naranjo D, et al: Application of receiver operating characteristics curve (ROC) analysis when definitive and suspect morphologic flags appear in the new Coulter LH 750 analyzer. *Lab Hematol* 10:14, 2004.
60. van der Meer W, Scott CS, de Keijzer MH: Automated flagging influences the inconsistency and bias of band cell and atypical lymphocyte morphological differentials. *Clin Chem Lab Med* 42:371, 2004.
61. van der Meer W, van Gelder W, de Keijzer R, et al: Does the band cell survive the 21st century? *Eur J Haematol* 76:251, 2006.
62. Atwater S, Corash L: Advances in leukocyte differential and peripheral blood stem cell enumeration. *Curr Opin Hematol* 3:71, 1996.
63. Reed WW, Diehl LF: Leukopenia, neutropenia, and reduced hemoglobin levels in healthy American blacks. *Arch Intern Med* 151:501, 1991.
64. Bain BJ: Ethnic and sex differences in the total and differential white cell count and platelet count. *J Clin Pathol* 49:664, 1996.
65. Zandecki M, Genevieve F, Gerard J, et al: Spurious counts and spurious results on haematology analysers: A review. Part I: Platelets. *Int J Lab Hematol* 29:4, 2007.
66. Paulus JM: Platelet size in man. *Blood* 46:321, 1975.
67. Lawrence JB, Yomtovian RA, Dillman C, et al: Reliability of automated platelet counts: Comparison with manual method and utility for prediction of clinical bleeding. *Am J Hematol* 48:244, 1995.
68. Segal HC, Briggs C, Kunka S, et al: Accuracy of platelet counting haematology analysers in severe thrombocytopenia and potential impact on platelet transfusion. *Br J Haematol* 128:520, 2005.
69. Fiorin F, Steffan A, Pradella P, et al: IgG platelet antibodies in EDTA-dependent pseudothrombocytopenia bind to platelet membrane glycoprotein IIb. *Am J Clin Pathol* 110:178, 1998.
70. Bartels PC, Schoorl M, Lombarts AJ: Screening for EDTA-dependent deviations in platelet counts and abnormalities in platelet distribution histograms in pseudothrombocytopenia. *Scand J Clin Lab Invest* 57:629, 1997.
71. Levin J, Bessman JD: The inverse relation between platelet volume and platelet number. Abnormalities in hematologic disease and evidence that platelet size does not correlate with platelet age. *J Lab Clin Med* 101:295, 1983.
72. Huczek Z, Kochman J, Filipiak KJ, et al: Mean platelet volume on admission predicts impaired reperfusion and long-term mortality in acute myocardial infarction treated with primary percutaneous coronary intervention. *J Am Coll Cardiol* 46:284, 2005.
73. Muscari A, De Pascalis S, Cenni A, et al: Determinants of mean platelet volume (MPV) in an elderly population: Relevance of body fat, blood glucose and ischaemic electrocardiographic changes. *Thromb Haemost* 99:1079, 2008.
74. Tavil Y, Sen N, Yazici HU, et al: Mean platelet volume in patients with metabolic syndrome and its relationship with coronary artery disease. *Thromb Res* 120:245, 2007.
75. Bessman JD: The relation of megakaryocyte ploidy to platelet volume. *Am J Hematol* 16:161, 1984.
76. Thompson CB, Love DG, Quinn PG, et al: Platelet size does not correlate with platelet age. *Blood* 62:487, 1983.
77. Behrens WE: Mediterranean macrothrombocytopenia. *Blood* 46:199, 1975.
78. O'Malley T, Ludlam CA, Fox KA, et al: Measurement of platelet volume using a variety of different anticoagulant and antiplatelet mixtures. *Blood Coagul Fibrinolysis* 7:431, 1996.
79. Meisinger C, Prokisch H, Gieger C, et al: A genome-wide association study identifies three loci associated with mean platelet volume. *Am J Hum Genet* 84:66, 2009.
80. Osselaer JC, Jamart J, Scheiff JM: Platelet distribution width for differential diagnosis of thrombocytosis. *Clin Chem* 43:1072, 1997.
81. Kurata Y, Hayashi S, Kiyoi T, et al: Diagnostic value of tests for reticulated platelets, plasma glycocalicin, and thrombopoietin levels for discriminating between hyperdestructive and hypoplastic thrombocytopenia. *Am J Clin Pathol* 115:656, 2001.
82. Chaoui D, Chakroun T, Robert F, et al: Reticulated platelets: A reliable measure to reduce prophylactic platelet transfusions after intensive chemotherapy. *Transfusion* 45:766, 2005.
83. Wang C, Smith BR, Ault KA, et al: Reticulated platelets predict platelet count recovery following chemotherapy. *Transfusion* 42:368, 2002.
84. Briggs C, Kunka S, Hart D, et al: Assessment of an immature platelet fraction (IPF) in peripheral thrombocytopenia. *Br J Haematol* 126:93, 2004.
85. Eller LA, Eller MA, Ouma B, et al: Reference intervals in healthy adult Ugandan blood donors and their impact on conducting international vaccine trials. *PLoS ONE* 3:e3919, 2008.
86. Peng L, Yang J, Lu X, et al: Effects of biological variations on platelet count in healthy subjects in China. *Thromb Haemost* 91:367, 2004.
87. Beutler E, West C: Hematologic differences between African-Americans and whites: The roles of iron deficiency and alpha-thalassemia on hemoglobin levels and mean corpuscular volume. *Blood* 106:740, 2005.
88. Hershman D, Weinberg M, Rosner Z, et al: Ethnic neutropenia and treatment delay in African American women undergoing chemotherapy for early-stage breast cancer. *J Natl Cancer Inst* 95:1545, 2003.
89. Wakeman L, Al-Ismail S, Benton A, et al: Robust, routine haematology reference ranges for healthy adults. *Int J Lab Hematol* 29:279, 2007.
90. Cheng CK, Chan J, Cembrowski GS, et al: Complete blood count reference interval diagrams derived from NHANES III: Stratification by age, sex, and race. *Lab Hematol* 10:42, 2004.
91. Beutler E, Waalen J: The definition of anemia: What is the lower limit of normal of the blood hemoglobin concentration? *Blood* 107:1747, 2006.

92. Fairbanks VF, Tefferi A: Normal ranges for packed cell volume and hemoglobin concentration in adults: Relevance to "apparent polycythemia." *Eur J Haematol* 65:285, 2000.
93. Pearson TC: Correspondence: Normal ranges for packed cell volume and hemoglobin concentration in adults: Relevance to "apparent polycythemia." *Eur J Haematol* 67:56, 2001.
94. Ganji V, Kafai MR: Hemoglobin and hematocrit values are higher and prevalence of anemia is lower in the post-folic acid fortification period than in the pre-folic acid fortification period in US adults. *Am J Clin Nutr* 89:363, 2009.
95. Fraser CG, Wilkinson SP, Neville RG, et al: Biologic variation of common hematologic laboratory quantities in the elderly. *Am J Clin Pathol* 92:465, 1989.
96. Lin JP, O'Donnell CJ, Jin L, et al: Evidence for linkage of red blood cell size and count: Genome-wide scans in the Framingham Heart Study. *Am J Hematol* 82:605, 2007.
97. Jenis EH, Takeuchi A, Dillon DE, et al: The May-Hegglin anomaly: Ultrastructure of the granulocytic inclusion. *Am J Clin Pathol* 55:187, 1971.
98. Gerdes U, Johnsson JJ, Kairisto V, et al: Nordic Reference Interval Project. www.furst.no/norip/, 2003.

CHAPTER 3
EXAMINATION OF THE MARROW

Daniel H. Ryan

SUMMARY

Microscopic examination of the marrow is a mainstay of hematologic diagnosis. Even with the advent of specialized biochemical and molecular assays that capitalize on advances in our understanding of the cell biology of hematopoiesis, the primary diagnosis of hematologic malignancies and many nonneoplastic hematologic disorders relies upon examination of the cells in the marrow. An aspirate and biopsy of the marrow can be obtained with minimal risk and only minor discomfort and are quickly and easily processed for examination. The marrow should be examined when the clinical history, blood cell counts, blood film, or laboratory test results suggest the possibility of a primary or secondary hematologic disorder for which morphologic analysis or special studies of the marrow would aid in the diagnosis. Leukopenia, thrombocytopenia, bicytopenia, or tricytopenia nearly always require a marrow examination for diagnosis. Nonhemolytic anemia that is not readily diagnosed as iron deficiency, thalassemia, vitamin B_{12} deficiency, folate deficiency, or another type of anemia defined by blood cell examination and supporting laboratory tests often requires a marrow examination. Abnormal cells in the blood, such as nucleated red cells, white cell precursors, abnormal lymphocytes not explained by concurrent infection, and blast cells, usually require a marrow examination. In addition to determining the cellularity and morphology of precursor cells or the presence of nonhematopoietic cells, the study provides marrow cells for immunophenotyping by cell flow analysis, for cytogenetic studies, and in special cases for marrow cell culture. Granulomatous and storage diseases may be uncovered in the marrow, and the marrow can be used to culture fastidious organisms such as fungi and mycobacteria. Searching for extranodal spread of lymphoma (staging) is another important use of the marrow examination.

HISTORY OF THE MARROW EXAMINATION

The first recorded examinations of marrow in living patients occurred in the first decades of the 20th century, first using the tibia as a source and then open biopsies. Neither technique led to routine examination of the marrow because in the former case the tibia usually was hypocellular in adults and in the latter case because of the invasiveness of an open procedure and the discomfort and risk of infection and bleeding.[1] In 1923, Arinkin, who was working in Leningrad, devised the marrow aspiration technique,[2] which was the prototype for our current aspiration procedure. Thirty years passed before the suggestion that the pelvis might be preferable to the sternum gained hold, and another 10 years passed before a practical marrow biopsy instrument was put to use.[1] Regular use of the posterior iliac crest for aspiration and biopsy and regular use of biopsy to complement aspiration did not occur until the 1970s, when staging of lymphoma made biopsy a frequent procedure and new simpler biopsy instruments became readily available.

Acronyms and abbreviations that appear in this chapter include: CD, cluster of differentiation; DMSO, dimethylsulfoxide; EDTA, ethylenediaminetetraacetic acid; FISH, fluorescence *in situ* hybridization; GPI, glycosylphosphatidylinositol; MDS, myelodysplastic syndrome; M:E, myeloid:erythroid cell ratio; PCR, polymerase chain reaction.

INDICATIONS FOR MARROW ASPIRATE OR BIOPSY

The International Council for Standardization in Hematology has published guidelines for marrow aspirate and biopsy to promote consistency in performance and reporting.[3] Although marrow aspiration and biopsy techniques are safe, they should be performed with a clear idea as to how the results will help distinguish the differential diagnoses under consideration or provide follow-up of treatment.[4–6] In many hematologic disorders, such as most cases of iron deficiency anemia, thalassemia, and acquired and inherited hemolytic anemia, examination of the blood and specialized laboratory tests may suffice to make the diagnosis without the need for a marrow examination.

When examination of the marrow is indicated, the decision as to whether an aspirate only or an aspirate plus biopsy is desired should be made. Aspiration is always attempted because of the superior morphology offered by examination of the aspirate smear. However, a marrow biopsy is superior to the aspirate in quantifying marrow cellularity and diagnosing infiltrative diseases of the marrow and should be performed when these conditions are part of the differential diagnosis.[7–11] In low-grade lymphoma, the marrow frequently is involved at the time of diagnosis, and this involvement is most sensitively detected by marrow biopsy.[12] Marrow biopsy is useful for diagnosing and following the course of disorders that are commonly associated with reticulin fibrosis, such as megakaryoblastic leukemia, hairy cell leukemia, and the chronic myeloproliferative disorders.[13,14] In myelodysplastic syndromes, marrow biopsy is useful for evaluating abnormal localization of immature precursor cells and abnormal megakaryocytes.[14] Marrow necrosis and gelatinous transformation are more readily detected in marrow sections than in aspirate films. The marrow aspirate may be useful in the severely anemic patient with suspected megaloblastic anemia as a result of vitamin B_{12} or folic acid deficiency. Marrow aspirate alone may be appropriate in some clinical settings where the diagnostic question is very targeted, such as diagnosis of childhood immune thrombocytopenia purpura or surveillance followup of leukemia patients in apparent remission.

Depending on the diagnostic question, availability of material, and expected frequency of the abnormal cells, an appropriate selection of specialized diagnostic methods may be needed to support the clinical diagnosis. Morphology of marrow cells is still the gold standard for diagnosis of hematologic malignancy and allows construction of a good differential diagnosis for nonmalignant disorders. Immunocytochemistry provides excellent phenotype–morphology correlation on an individual cell basis, but is limited to epitopes that resist fixation and/or drying. Flow cytometry allows study of almost any surface or intracellular protein, with the added ability to detect important quantitative changes in cellular proteins and simultaneous determination of multiple proteins within the same cell. However, flow cytometry requires that cells be viable and dissociated from tissue. Gene expression arrays allow analysis of complex patterns of RNA expression by sophisticated mathematical algorithms to detect diagnostic patterns based on the broadest range of cellular gene products, but with relatively less ability to study small subpopulations. Attempts at clinical validation of gene expression data are significant and ongoing. Classic metaphase cytogenetics, fluorescence *in situ* hybridization (FISH), and reverse transcriptase polymerase chain reaction (PCR) each assesses the underlying oncogenetic mechanisms involved in hematopoietic malignancies. In the order given, these techniques are characterized by increasing ability to detect rare malignant cells but increasingly limited sequences of DNA queried.

■ MARROW ASPIRATION TECHNIQUE

At birth, all bones contain hematopoietic marrow. Fat cells begin to replace hemopoietic marrow in the extremities in the fifth to seventh year. By adulthood, the hemopoietic marrow is limited to the axial skeleton and the proximal portions of the extremities (see Chaps. 4 and 8). Chapter 4 discusses the structure and function of the marrow and the distribution of marrow in the skeleton. Fatty marrow appears yellow, whereas hematopoietic marrow is red. Red marrow contains fat, however, and fat droplets are visible grossly in aspirated marrow specimens. Histologically, yellow marrow consists almost entirely of fat cells and supporting connective tissue. Red marrow contains an abundance of hemopoietic cells, fat cells, and connective tissue. The marrow fills the spaces between the trabeculae of bone in the marrow cavity. Marrow is soft and friable and can be readily aspirated or biopsied with a needle.

The posterior iliac crest (Fig. 3–1) is the preferred site for marrow aspiration and biopsy. In adults, the sternum and the anterior iliac crest also can be used (Fig. 3–2). The sternum should be used for aspiration

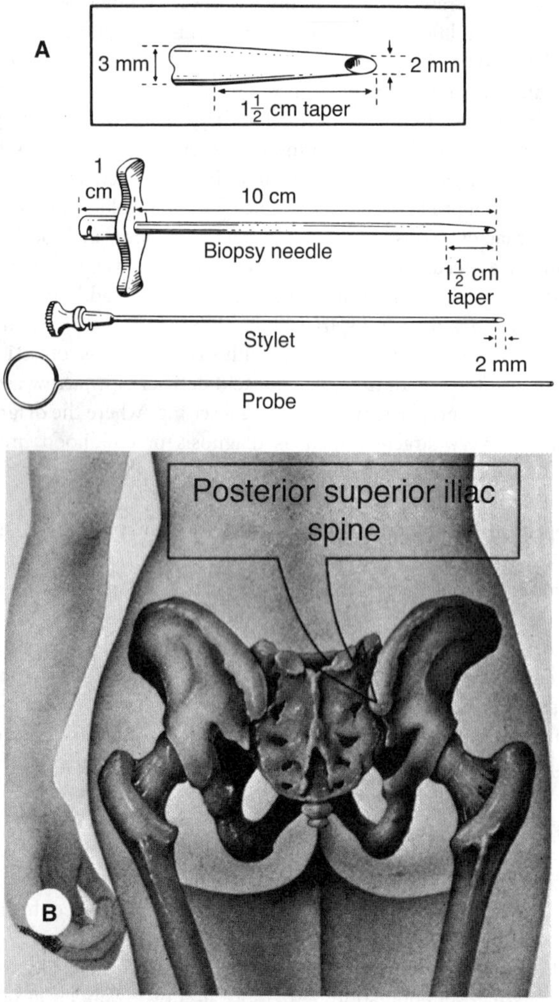

FIGURE 3–1. A. Jamshidi biopsy instrument. *(From Jamshidi K, Swaim WR,[22] with permission.)* **B.** Site of marrow biopsy. *(From Ellis LD, Jensen WN, Westerman MP,[7] with permission.)*

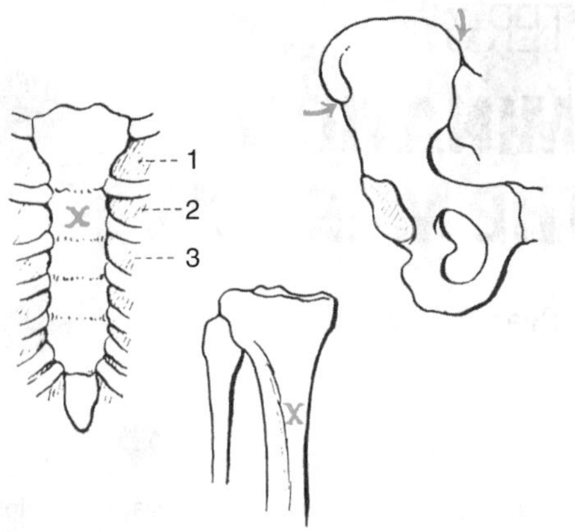

FIGURE 3–2. Sites used for marrow aspiration. *(Modified from Schwartz SO, Hartz WH Jr, Robbins JH,* Hematology in Practice, *part 1, p 36. McGraw-Hill, New York, 1961.)*

only. The anterior iliac crest is less preferred than the posterior crest in adults because of the crest's thick cortical bone. The anteromedial surface of the tibia is an option for infants younger than 1 year old (particularly newborns), but the posterior iliac crest is still the preferred site. The spinous processes of the vertebrae, the ribs, or other marrow-containing bones are rarely used. Serious adverse outcomes after marrow aspiration or biopsy are rare, less than 0.05 percent. In this study one direct fatality, and three episodes of prolonged but not permanent disability were observed in nearly 55,000 bone marrow biopsies.[15] Morbidity most frequently involved hemorrhage, which were associated more with platelet function impairment than thrombocytopenia or coagulation factor defects.[15] Infection and reactions to anesthetic agents are other infrequent complications. Penetration of the bone with damage to the underlying structures is possible with all marrow aspirations, but the hazard is greatest in sternal aspirations because the sternum at the second interspace is only approximately 1 cm thick in adults. To prevent this, a guard should be in place on the needle when a sternal aspirate is done.

For either a marrow biopsy or aspiration, sedation minimizes anxiety and pain,[16] particularly in children,[17,18] where propofol administered under carefully controlled conditions is frequently used. Midazolam (Versed) is a popular choice for conscious sedation.[19] However, the sedation must be performed with proper monitoring to minimize risk.[20] Marrow biopsies and aspirations for staging purposes often can be performed while the patient is under anesthesia for other procedures. Several different types of needles, most of which are satisfactory, are available for marrow aspiration.[4] For adults, an 18-gauge needle is sufficiently large to permit aspiration of adequate specimens; larger needles are unnecessary. The patient is prone or in the left or right lateral decubitus position. Sterile precautions must be observed. The skin over the puncture site is shaved if necessary and cleansed with a disinfectant solution. The skin, subcutaneous tissues, and periosteum are infiltrated with a local anesthetic solution, such as 1 percent lidocaine. Adequate infiltration of the anesthetic at the periosteal surface is important, but no more than 20 mL of 1 percent lidocaine should be used in an adult.[21] Adequate anesthesia can be achieved with much less lidocaine in virtually all cases. An air gun can be used to anesthetize the skin surface prior to application of anesthetic to the periosteal surface by injection. After the anesthesia has taken effect, usually in 3 to 5 minutes, the marrow needle is inserted through the skin, subcutaneous tissue, and cortex of the bone using a slight twisting motion. In obese patients, the length of the needle must be sufficient to reach the iliac crest. The stylet should be locked into place on the hub of the needle to prevent plugging of the needle with tissue prior to needle entry into the marrow cavity. Penetration of the cortex can be sensed by a slight, rapid forward movement accompanied by a sudden increase in the ease of advancing the needle. The stylet of the needle is removed promptly, the hub is attached to a 10- or 20-mL syringe, and approximately 0.5 to 1.5 mL of fluid is aspirated. The actual aspiration of the marrow causes a transient painful sensation for most patients. If additional specimen volume is required, another syringe is fitted on the marrow needle, the syringe and needle is rotated and an adjacent area is entered and marrow is aspirated. The stylet may be reinserted and the marrow needle slightly repositioned between aspirations. When aspiration is complete, the stylet is reinserted and the needle immediately removed from the bone. Pressure is applied to the skin over the aspiration site for at least 5 minutes to minimize bruising at the site. In a thrombocytopenic patient, firm pressure should be applied for at least 10 to 15 minutes. The bloody fluid that is aspirated contains light-colored particles of marrow approximately 0.5 to 1 mm in diameter. They often are readily visible in the syringe but may not be detected until the syringe contents are discharged on glass slides for film preparation.

If nothing enters the syringe when aspiration is performed, the needle was not properly placed in the marrow cavity. The needle can be cautiously advanced 1 to 2 mm after reinsertion of the stylet and aspiration attempted again. Perhaps as a more desired alternative, the needle can be removed from the bone and reinserted in a nearby site in the anesthetized area. The thickness of the bone must be considered when the needle is being adjusted in the bone. Occasionally the needle must be rotated on its longitudinal axis, or in a larger orbit, in order to loosen the marrow mechanically before the marrow can be aspirated. If a small amount of blood has been aspirated, a new needle should be used because of the probability of clotting of the aspirate when it finally is obtained. Aspiration with a 50-mL syringe may succeed if use of a smaller syringe failed. Leukemic marrow may be so densely packed in the bone as to resist all attempts at aspiration, in which case biopsy is necessary. Fibrotic marrow may be impossible to aspirate. The most common cause of failure to obtain marrow is faulty positioning of the needle, and a second attempt at aspiration usually succeeds.

■ NEEDLE BIOPSY TECHNIQUE

Needle biopsy usually is performed with the Jamshidi needle,[22] using the same preparation as described above in "Marrow Aspiration Technique." The Jamshidi instrument (see Fig. 3–1) consists of a cylindrical needle with constant bore, except for a concentrically tapered distal portion ending in a sharp, beveled cutting tip. The stylet fits precisely inside the opening at the tapered tip, interlocks at the hub of the needle, and extends 1 to 2 mm beyond the end of the needle. An 11-gauge needle is most commonly used in the United States. After the skin and the periosteum of the biopsy site are anesthetized, a 3-mm incision is made in the skin. The needle, with obturator in place, is inserted into the skin incision and through the subcutaneous tissue to the cortex of the bone. The needle is directed toward the posterior iliac spine and advanced with a twisting motion. Penetration of the cortex is sensed by a decreased resistance to forward movement of the needle. The obturator is removed, and the needle is slowly advanced with reciprocal clockwise–counterclockwise twisting motions around the long axis. After sufficient penetration of the bone (up to approximately 3 cm), the needle is rotated several times on its axis and withdrawn approximately 2 to 3 mm. Some needles now come with a "trap" that snares the biopsy so that the needle can be directly removed. The needle is reinserted to the original depth at a slightly different angle, taking care not to bend the needle, and rotated several times to free the specimen from attachments in the marrow cavity. The needle is slowly withdrawn, with the same twisting motion used during insertion. The core of marrow inside the needle is removed by inserting the probe through the cutting tip and extruding the specimen through the hub of the needle. The smaller size of the cutting aperture relative to the bore of the shaft of the Jamshidi instrument yields a specimen that fits loosely inside the needle and therefore is less subject to compression, distortion, or fragmentation. The technique reliably produces good-quality biopsy specimens. Marrow biopsy should be performed before marrow aspiration is attempted (or in a slightly different site on the iliac crest) to avoid hemorrhage and distorted marrow architecture in the biopsy core. With the availability of the biopsy needles described in this section, open (surgical) biopsies rarely are necessary but may be performed, for example, for diagnosis of deeply situated bone lesions or at the time of a surgical procedure performed for related indications (e.g., staging).

PREPARATION OF MARROW SPECIMENS FOR STUDY

Several types of preparations can be made from the marrow aspirate to maximize use of the diagnostic material. Most important is the *direct film*, which is made immediately from a drop of marrow suspension from the unmanipulated aspirate. This preparation is the best for evaluating cellular morphology and differential counts of the marrow. The *particle film* is best for estimating marrow cellularity and megakaryocyte abundance, but morphology is obscured in the thicker parts of the film. A *concentrate film*, which is prepared from a concentrate of nucleated cells (marrow buffy coat) achieved by centrifugation of a small volume of anticoagulated marrow, is useful for detecting low-abundance cells, such as megakaryocytes and metastatic tumor, or hematopoietic precursors or lymphoma or leukemia cells when the marrow is hypocellular. The relative proportions of cell lineages are not maintained in the concentrate film preparation (often erythroid precursors are relatively enriched). In addition, this preparation is subject to anticoagulant-induced changes in nuclear morphology or cytoplasmic vacuolization. The *touch imprint* from the biopsy is important for evaluating cellular morphology in the case of a "dry tap,"[23] and provides cytologic detail of cells that may not appear in the aspirate specimen.[24]

■ MARROW FILMS

After aspiration, approximately 0.5 mL of marrow is placed on a glass slide; the rest is mixed into a tube containing ethylenediaminetetraacetic acid (EDTA) solution. The marrow specimen is examined to ensure the presence of "spicules" or particles of marrow containing bony or fatty pieces, indicating successful aspiration of the marrow cavity. Direct marrow films are immediately prepared by transferring drops of the unanticoagulated marrow pool to fresh slides and making push films with coverslips. Sufficient films should be made for special stains. Heparinization of the aspirate is not necessary if the operator works rapidly and should be avoided because heparinization may introduce artifacts.

A useful technique is preparing a thick film of marrow by discharging a drop or two of the aspirate on a slide, covering the aspirate with a second slide, gently pressing the slides together to express most of the blood into a gauze sponge, and then pulling the slides apart longitudinally. Such preparations may contain an increased number of broken cells if too much pressure is applied, but they provide a large number of particles from which marrow cellularity can be estimated and which are useful for estimating the amount of hemosiderin present.

The EDTA-anticoagulated sample may be centrifuged (1500 g for 10 minutes) in a Wintrobe tube to concentrate the cellular elements of the marrow. After centrifugation, the fatty layer and plasma are removed, and the "buffy coat" is mixed with an equal amount of plasma. Multiple films of this preparation are made. These films can be air dried, labeled, and retained as unstained preparations in case special stains are required.

TOUCH PREPARATIONS

After a biopsy specimen is obtained using the Jamshidi needle, the specimen should be extruded through the hub of the needle and then gently rolled across a glass slide (using an applicator stick to move the specimen) before it is placed in fixative, taking care to avoid crushing. The touch preparations are allowed to dry and are stained in the same manner as films.

SPECIAL STUDIES

It is essential to formulate the diagnostic question before performing a marrow aspiration to ensure an adequate sample is obtained for all the special studies that may be needed to make the correct diagnosis. A sterile anticoagulated sample containing viable unfixed cells in single-cell suspension is the best substrate for nearly all special studies of a marrow sample that likely will be required. Specifically, flow cytometry, is best performed on EDTA- or heparin-anticoagulated aspirate specimens, which are stable for at least 24 hours at room temperature. For cytogenetic or cell culture analysis, heparin-anticoagulated marrow should be added to tissue culture medium and analyzed as soon as possible to maintain optimal cell viability. Cytogenetic samples are generally not adversely affected by overnight incubation.[25] In cases where the marrow aspirate is dry, a duplicate biopsy specimen can be disaggregated to produce a cell suspension for morphology, flow cytometry, and cytogenetic studies.[26]

For molecular analysis of fresh specimens, sample storage should be minimized, and storage at 4°C is preferable. EDTA is the preferred anticoagulant because heparin can interfere with some molecular assays. DNA is relatively stable, but RNA has a variable half-life in an intact cell and is degraded rapidly (on the order of seconds to minutes) in a cell lysate by ubiquitous ribonucleases. Sample storage prior to RNA isolation should be minimized.[27] Collection tubes have been designed for stabilization of RNA, but for maximal RNA recovery, samples should be transported to the laboratory immediately, where cell suspensions (typically buffy coat or mononuclear cell preparations) will be prepared and nucleic acids extracted under conditions that inhibit ribonucleases. DNA and messenger RNA can be extracted and analyzed from paraffin-embedded tissue sections[28,29] and dried stained films,[30] but degradation is significant, and its impact is proportional to the length of sequence required.

Archival storage of marrow specimens is important in light of advances in molecular diagnosis that may necessitate validation studies using samples of known origin or testing of diagnostic material from a patient now in remission. Isolated DNA or RNA can be stored for long periods at –70°C, whereas viable, intact cells can be reliably preserved only by controlled rate freezing in dimethylsulfoxide (DMSO) and storage in liquid nitrogen.

HISTOLOGIC SECTIONS

A variety of techniques for preparing aspirated material for histologic study have been advocated. All of the techniques are designed to collect a sufficient number of marrow particles in a small volume so that adequate sections can be prepared. This goal can be accomplished by discharging the marrow aspirate onto a glass slide, allowing the particles to settle for a few seconds, and then gently tilting the slide so that the excess blood runs off. The particles then are pushed together with an applicator stick, and the remaining blood is allowed to clot. The clot is promptly fixed, typically in buffered formalin,[31] for tissue processing and sectioning. An alternative method using filtration of the anticoagulated aspirate specimen has been described.[32]

The core marrow biopsy specimen is processed for histologic examination typically by fixation in neutral buffered formalin, followed by decalcification and embedding in paraffin. B5 fixative is usually avoided to limit environmental exposure to mercury, although zinc-based substitutes are available. Decalcification can be accomplished with acid reagents or EDTA, the latter of which provides better preservation of nucleic acid and protein antigens, but is slower. Sections of high quality cut at 3 μm and stained with hematoxylin and eosin or with Giemsa are satisfactory for routine work. Refinements in fixation and embedding techniques have enabled use of most immunologic markers in decalcified paraffin-embedded marrow biopsy specimens.[32] Fixation in neutral-buffered formalin and embedding without decalcification in plastic have the advantage of superior morphology[33] and suitability for most immunochemical procedures[34] if methylmethacrylate is used rather than glycomethacrylate, but the method is technically more demanding and expensive.[35]

MORPHOLOGIC INTERPRETATION OF MARROW PREPARATIONS

OVERVIEW

The Wright-Giemsa–stained direct marrow aspirate film should be examined as quickly as possible to provide a preliminary assessment of the marrow morphology and allow setup of specialized testing based on this preliminary evaluation while the sample is fresh. Final interpretation of the marrow biopsy and aspirate should be integrated with results from the clinical history, blood film, cell counts, laboratory data, cell marker studies, and molecular or cytogenetic data. No other histologic specimen exists in which a state-of-the-art interpretation is dependent on such an array of supportive data. This situation results from the wealth of basic biologic information gained from *in vitro* studies of blood cells, which has been translated into useful diagnostic tests. The challenge for the hematopathologist and hematologist is to understand the advantages and limitations of each diagnostic approach so that results can be reconciled and placed into perspective.

ADEQUACY OF THE MARROW SAMPLE

The first question in interpreting the marrow is whether the sample is adequate for diagnosis. At the time of the procedure, the presence of marrow particles in the aspirate is the best indicator that the needle entered the medullary cavity and marrow was successfully withdrawn. Marrow particles are bony with a glistening appearance caused by fat in the particles. Specimens containing cortical bone, muscle, or other tissue with little or no medullary bone are inadequate for marrow interpretation but may provide other information. Samples with extensive crush artifact or hemorrhage also are inadequate, underscoring the importance of proper technique in obtaining a useful sample. An unspoken assumption is that the piece of marrow provided for diagnostic evaluation is representative of the marrow as a whole. Based on reproducibility of bilateral biopsies, this more likely is true in leukemia and myeloma than in lymphoma and metastatic tumor.[36] A biopsy specimen should contain at least a 0.5-cm length of marrow cavity. However, for detection of lymphoma or metastatic tumor, current recommendations suggest a biopsy length of 1.6 to 2.0 cm,[37] with examination of two to four deeper sections to maximize sensitivity.[38] A significant proportion of biopsies obtained in routine practice may fall short of this recommended length.[39]

The marrow cavity was entered if the aspirate contains marrow particles or hematopoietic precursors (e.g., megakaryocytes, nucleated red cells) not found in the blood film. However, this finding does not ensure the specimen is adequate for diagnosis, because the amount of marrow actually aspirated can vary significantly in disease states.[40] Also, some cell types, notably fibroblasts and metastatic tumor cells, are not as readily removed from the marrow space by aspiration as are normal precursors. Lack of particles or precursor cells does not prove the marrow cavity was not entered, because marrow packed with leukemic cells or infiltrated with fibroblasts may yield few cells ("dry tap").[23] Marrow aspirations resulting in a dry tap usually are a consequence of significant pathology (only 7% show normal histology on biopsy[23]) and indicate the need to examine a biopsy specimen.

MARROW CELLULARITY

The "gold standard" for overall marrow cellularity is examination of an adequate marrow biopsy specimen.[41,42] The normal cellularity (percentage of marrow space occupied by hematopoietic cells as opposed to fatty and nonhematopoietic tissue of iliac crest marrow decreases from a mean of 80 percent in early childhood to 50 percent by age 30 years, with further decreases after age 70 years.[43] Consequently, marrow cellularity should be evaluated with reference to normal individuals of the same age as the patient.[44] The normal range of iliac crest marrow cellularity is broader than expected.[43] When evaluating cellularity, consider that the marrow spaces directly adjacent to cortical bone frequently are fatty and are not representative of the cellularity of the deeper marrow spaces.[45]

Cellularity assessment by examination of the direct marrow aspirate film is more difficult because of loss of histologic structure and mixture with blood. The aspirate may suggest the marrow is more hypocellular than indicated by the biopsy.[42] Marrow particles (seen in the direct film or a particle preparation) are the best indicators of cellularity. These particles are like "mini-biopsies" and contain sufficient hematopoietic and fatty elements to give some idea of marrow cellularity. Cellularity estimates based on careful examination of particles in the aspirate preparation agree well with cellularity estimated from the marrow biopsy.[44]

The degree of dilution of marrow aspirate specimens with blood during the aspiration is variable and may affect interpretation of marrow cellularity. Adult marrows with greater than 30 percent lymphocytes plus monocytes likely are substantially admixed with blood, as shown by cytokinetic studies of paired marrow aspirate and biopsy preparations.[46] Radiolabeled erythrocytes and serum albumin have been used to estimate the admixture of nucleated cells from blood with those from marrow in sternal marrow aspirates.[40] In patients with hematologic disease, from 6 to 93 percent of the nucleated cells were derived from the blood.[40] The greatest admixture was observed in patients with leukemia. Substantial dilution with blood may occur in aspirates that were difficult to obtain or when multiple draws were taken from the same puncture site. Based on cell markers and progenitor assays, the first 1.0 mL of marrow aspirated from healthy donors was only 8 percent contaminated with blood nucleated cells. In contrast, subsequent aspirates obtained for marrow harvesting were 20 percent contaminated with nucleated blood cells.[47] The bulk volume of the "marrow" aspirate (i.e., plasma, red cells) is almost completely derived from blood, even if the nucleated cells are mostly marrow derived.[47] Assessment of marrow cellularity by measuring the "buffy coat" observed after centrifugation of the aspirate specimen is unreliable.[42]

Cellularity of individual lineages is best assessed by examination of the biopsy specimen. Erythroid cells typically are arranged in clusters, whereas megakaryocytes are scattered throughout the biopsy. Erythroid and megakaryocytic cellularity is best appreciated at low power. In the aspirate, a myeloid-to-erythroid (M:E) ratio frequently is calculated to give some impression of the relative cellularity of these two major lineages. As a rule of thumb, the M:E ratio normally should be between 2:1 and 4:1 (Table 3–1 lists the normal ranges in men and women). The relative proportions of cell types should be assessed only on the direct marrow film, biopsy imprint, or particle preparation, not a concentrate film, which has been manipulated by centrifugation. A decreased M:E ratio can be interpreted as either myeloid hypocellularity or erythroid hyperplasia, depending on the overall marrow cellularity. Automated hematology instruments offer the possibility of performing automated marrow erythroid and myeloid cell counts.[48] Megakaryocyte numbers can be assessed from the direct marrow aspirate film, where at least five megakaryocytes should be present in the optimal portion of the film. In the particle preparation, most large particles should contain one or more megakaryocytes. Megakaryocyte number varies markedly in direct marrow aspirate films of normal subjects[49] (Table 3–1) and depends on the degree of admixture of the specimen with blood. Megakaryocytes are enriched at the feathered edge of concentrate films.

INFILTRATIVE DISEASES OF THE MARROW

Malignant Neoplasms

Metastatic nonhematopoietic tumor in the marrow biopsy is characterized by disruption of the marrow architecture with groups of cytologically abnormal cells. Assessment of the tissue of origin is primarily based on morphology, clinical history, and immunocytochemical staining. The tendency of carcinoma cells to form tightly adherent clusters frequently is helpful in recognizing these neoplasms (Chap. 44). The clumps can appear on the marrow aspirate, but the aspirate is less sensitive than the biopsy for detecting metastatic tumor. Tumor clumps may occur infrequently in the aspirate, often appearing only on side or feathered edges of the film, or only in the concentrate preparation. These tumor clumps must be distinguished from clumps of damaged hematopoietic cells, which commonly appear in aspirate preparations, especially the concentrate film. The distinction is best accomplished by examining cells at the periphery of the clumps to determine if the cells show the morphology of hematopoietic precursors or are cytologically atypical cells. Isolated nonhematopoietic tumor cells are seen infrequently in aspirate preparations, even when tumor is obvious in the biopsy, because of the adherent nature of most nonhematopoietic tumors. Examination of multiple films may be necessary to find isolated tumor cell clumps.[50] Metastatic carcinoma cells can be identified by immunocytochemical staining for epithelial markers, such as cytokeratins, markers not found on hematopoietic cells (Chap. 44). The presence of such cells in node-negative breast cancer conveys a negative prognostic risk,[51] although full-blown metastatic disease does not always occur. Molecular evidence suggests that tumor cells in breast cancer may disseminate with far less advanced genomic mutations than previously thought, and that the tumor cells acquire genomic aberrations typical of metastatic cells thereafter.[52] This finding may explain the variable clinical outcome of micrometastatic disease.

Myeloma[53] and lymphomas[12] are more reliably detected on the biopsy preparation, where the typical aggregation pattern of abnormal lymphoid cells can be appreciated. Abnormal lymphoid aggregates should be distinguished from lymphoid aggregates found in reactive conditions or in older patients.[54] Neoplastic aggregates are more likely show cytologic atypia and monomorphous cellular population, and they often are adjacent to bony trabeculae, but the distinction can be difficult in some cases. The cellular morphology often can be better appreciated on the marrow aspirate, but the key histologic features are lost. Lymphoma cells do not form the tight clusters seen in nonhematopoietic

TABLE 3–1. Normal Values for Marrow Differential Cell Count at Different Ages (Percent of Cells)

	Rosse et al[68]: Infants Tibial Marrow			Glaser et al[85]: Subjects Aged 1–20 Years Sternal Marrow, 1 mL Aspirated	Bain[49]: Subjects Aged 21–56 Years Iliac Marrow, 0.1–0.2 mL Aspirated Men (n = 30), Women (n = 20)
Type of Cell	<1 month (n = 57)	1 month (n = 7)	18 months (n = 19)		
Myeloblast	–	–	–	1.2 (0–3)	1.4 (0–3.0)
Promyelocyte	0.79 ± 0.91	0.76 ± 0.65	0.64 ± 0.59	1.8 (0–4)	7.8 (3.2–12.4)
Myelocyte	3.95 ± 2.93	2.50 ± 1.48	2.49 ± 1.39	16.5 (8–25)	
Neutrophilic					7.6 (3.7–10.0)
Eosinophilic					1.3 (0–2.8)
Basophilic					
Metamyelocyte	19.37 ± 4.84	11.34 ± 3.59	12.42 ± 4.15	23 (14–34)	4.1 (2.3–5.9)
Band form	28.89 ± 7.56	14.10 ± 4.63	14.20 ± 5.63	–	**
Segmented					
Neutrophil	7.37 ± 4.64	3.64 ± 2.97	6.31 ± 3.91	12.9 (4.5–29)	Men: 32.1 (21.9–42.3); women: 37.4 (28.8–4.9)
Eosinophil	2.70 ± 1.27	2.61 ± 1.40	2.70 ± 2.16	–	2.2 (0.3–4.2)
Basophil	0.12 ± 0.20	0.07 ± 0.16	0.10 ± 0.12		0.1 (0–0.4)
Lymphocyte	14.42 ± 5.54	47.05 ± 9.24	43.55 ± 8.56	16 (5–36)	13.1 (6.0–20.0)
Monocyte	0.88 ± 0.85	1.01 ± 0.89	2.12 ± 1.59	–	1.3 (0–2.6)
Plasma cell	0.00 ± 0.02	0.02 ± 0.06	0.06 ± 0.08	–	0.6 (0–1.2)
Proerythroblast	0.02 ± 0.06	0.10 ± 0.14	0.08 ± 0.13	0.5 (0–1.5)	
Erythroblast					Men: 28.1 (16.2–40.1)§; women: 22.5 (13.0–32.0)§
Basophilic	0.24 ± 0.25	0.34 ± 0.33	0.50 ± 0.34	1.7 (0–5)	
Polychromatophilic	13.06 ± 6.78	6.90 ± 4.45	6.97 ± 3.56	18 (5–34)	
Orthochromatic	0.09 ± 0.73	0.54 ± 1.88	0.44 ± 0.49	2.7 (0–8)	
Megakaryocyte	0.06 ± 0.15	0.05 ± 0.09	0.07 ± 0.12	–	31 (6–77)‡
Macrophage					0.4 (0–1.3)
Others					¶
Transitional cells*	1.18 ± 1.13	1.95 ± 0.94	1.99 ± 1.00	–	
Broken cell	5.79 ± 2.78	5.50 ± 2.46	5.05 ± 2.15	–	
M/E ratio	4.4	4.4	4.8	2.9 (1–5)	Men: 2.1 (1.1–4.1); women: 2.8 (1.6–5.2)

*Immature lymphoid cells.

**Bands included in segmented neutrophil count.

§All erythroblast forms (basophilic, polychromatophilic, orthochromatic) grouped together.

‡Number of megakaryocytes near the advancing edge of the film (mean, range).

¶Osteoclasts noted in 8 of 50 subjects, osteoblasts in 5 of 50, no mast cells observed.

tumors on the marrow aspirate film. In hairy cell leukemia (Chap. 95), the hematopoietic cells are sufficiently adherent to each other and the marrow matrix with variably increased collagen matrix that the aspirate specimen is often markedly hypocellular (dry tap), whereas biopsy specimens show extensive infiltration with hairy cells. Special studies, such as *in situ* hybridization for κ versus λ light-chain messenger RNA[55] or immunohistochemistry/flow cytometry to determine cell lineage and demonstrate surface light-chain restriction, may be necessary to distinguish a reactive process from malignant lymphoma or plasma cell myeloma. Detection of clonal immunoglobulin gene rearrangements by PCR amplification of messenger RNA transcripts may be used for this purpose, but clinical interpretation of the results can be problematic, and morphology remains the standard in evaluating marrow involvement by lymphoma.[56]

Fibrosis

Marrow fibrosis typically is recognizable only on a marrow biopsy specimen; the aspirate merely shows reduced or absent recovery of hematopoietic cells. Early stages of fibrosis are characterized by increased stainable marrow reticulin fibers (see Chap. 91). Fibrosis may

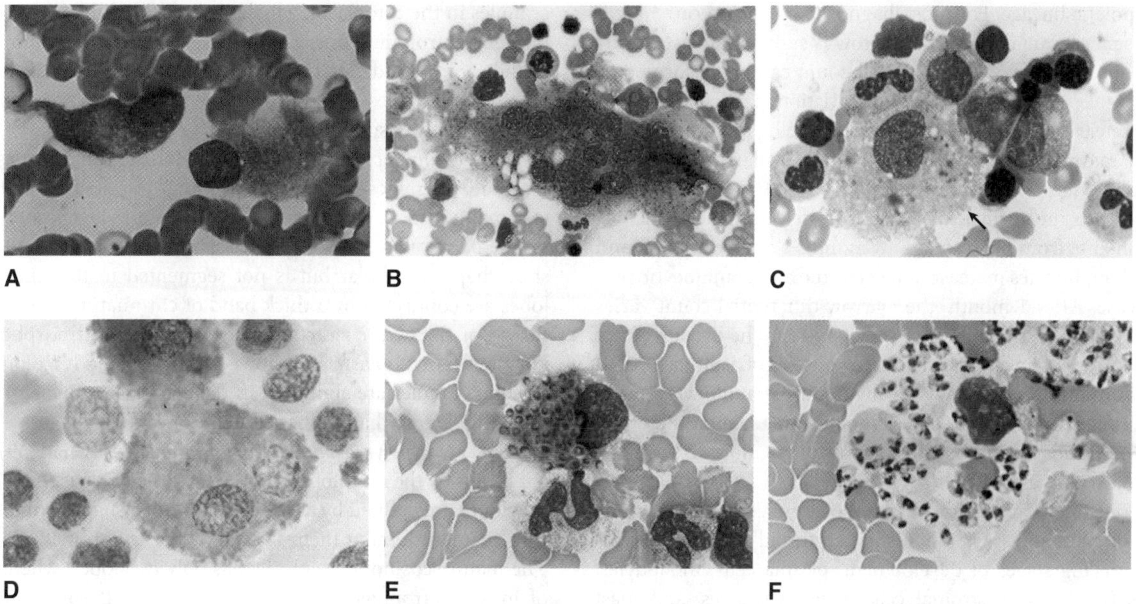

FIGURE 3–3. Marrow findings. **A.** Two osteoblasts are in this field. Elongated ovoid cells with nucleus at extreme end, a morphology which characteristically looks like the nucleus is falling out of the cell. A clear area is apparent spaced at an interval from the nucleus. **B.** Osteoclast. Multinucleated giant cell. The nuclei are characteristically scattered throughout the cell, appearing separate. **C.** Macrophage (*arrow*), relatively large cell with circular nucleus and abundant cytoplasm. Ingested debris and few vacuoles. **D.** Macrophage (two). Prussian blue stain. Relatively large cell with circular nuclei. One binucleate. Each macrophage is full of iron as indicated by blue reaction product of stain. **E.** Macrophage engorged with *Histoplasma capsulatum.* **F.** Macrophage engorged with amastigote forms of *Leishmania donovani*. *(Used with permission from* Lichtman's Atlas of Hematology. *www.accessmedicine.com.)*

accompany either primary hematopoietic disorders (e.g., myelofibrosis) or infiltrative diseases such as metastatic tumor.

Storage Diseases

Storage disorders, such as Gaucher and Niemann-Pick diseases (see Chap. 73), are characterized by abnormal macrophages containing stored material in various forms.[57] These cells can be appreciated on both the biopsy and aspirate specimens. In the latter preparation, they typically are more common in the feathered edge of the films. Reactive cells, such as the histiocytes with "sea-blue" inclusion granules (see Chap. 73) or pseudo-Gaucher cells associated with chronic myelogenous leukemia (see Chap. 90),[57] can resemble the cells seen in storage disorders.

■ INFECTIONS

Infectious organisms with an intracellular location, such as *Leishmania,*[58] *Histoplasma*, and *Toxoplasma,*[59] can be visualized in monocytic cells by morphologic examination of the marrow (Fig. 3–3). Identification of mycobacterial organisms in the marrow by acid-fast staining lacks sensitivity but allows early diagnosis in one-third of cases with HIV-related *Mycobacterium avium* complex infection.[60] Microscopic examination and culture of the marrow are the most sensitive diagnostic tests for disseminated leishmaniasis, a troublesome problem in HIV-infected patients exposed to this organism.[61] Marrow morphology also is a sensitive diagnostic tool for detecting disseminated histoplasmosis in patients with AIDS.[62] However, marrow culture has a low diagnostic yield in the workup of fever of unknown origin in nonimmunosuppressed patients.[63]

The presence of marrow granulomas, recognizable only on biopsy specimens, necessitates examination by special stains for fungal and mycobacterial organisms, but the differential diagnosis is extensive.[57,64]

■ NECROSIS AND GELATINOUS TRANSFORMATION

Marrow necrosis may occur in a variety of disorders, particularly sickle cell disease and neoplastic processes involving the marrow.[65] Aspirates of necrotic marrow stained with polychrome stains contain cells with indistinct margins and smudged basophilic nuclei surrounded by acidophilic material. Marrow sections stained with hematoxylin and eosin show loss of normal marrow architecture, indistinct cellular margins, and a background of amorphous eosinophilic material. Patients with severe weight loss may develop *gelatinous transformation* of the marrow, characterized by amorphous extracellular material (proteoglycans), fat atrophy, and marrow hypoplasia.[66] The findings of gelatinous transformation are reversible.[67]

MORPHOLOGIC DIFFERENTIATION OF HEMATOPOIETIC LINEAGES

■ OVERVIEW

Marrow aspirate films should be examined under low-power magnification to assess the relative amounts of fat and hemopoietic cells in particles and the number of megakaryocytes, plasma cells, and mast cells present. Low-power examination also permits detection of osteoclasts or osteoblasts, groups of malignant cells, Gaucher cells, lymphoid follicles, and granulomas. The entire film should be examined, including the particles, and higher magnification should be used to study any abnormalities discovered. Similarly, biopsy sections are examined at low power to assess adequacy, overall cellularity, presence of infiltrative disease, and cellularity of the major hematopoietic lineages.

After the low-power survey, the films should be examined at higher power and under oil-immersion magnification to determine the various hemopoietic cell types present and assess adequacy of differentiation in each hematopoietic lineage. For most diagnostic questions, careful and systematic visual examination of the marrow is sufficient to assess differentiation, but a marrow differential cell count can be performed to quantify the status of hematopoietic differentiation, particularly in the granulocytic lineages. Because a large variety of cell types normally are present in the marrow and their distribution is irregular, accurate marrow differential count requires examination of 300 to 500 nucleated cells. Table 3–1 lists the normal values for these determinations, including data for infants from birth to age 18 months.[68] Between birth and age 1 month, lymphocytes increase and erythroid and granulocytic precursors decrease. After 1 month, the marrow differential count varies little to age 18 months, the duration of the study.[68] The proportion of segmented neutrophils increases with large volumes of aspirate, probably because of dilution of marrow cells by mature granulocytes in the blood.[69] The range of normal for all cell types is broad, and differential counts and M:E ratios should be considered rough guides to the character of the marrow as a whole.

Morphologically recognizable cells in the normal marrow include mature granulocytes and their precursors, erythroid precursors, lymphocytes in varying stages of development, plasma cells, monocytes, macrophages (histiocytes), stromal cells, megakaryocytes, and mast cells. Typically only the later stages of differentiation, in which progenitors become fully committed to a given lineage, are morphologically recognizable. Progenitors of all lineages typically are unremarkable cells without distinctive morphologic attributes. The next stage of maturation, in which precursor cells take on identifiable morphologic features, can be identified in marrow samples and provide essential evidence for diagnosis of many hematologic diseases.

The characteristics of each cell type are briefly described, and the nomenclature is discussed. Further details of the morphology of these cells are discussed in the relevant specific chapters of this book (see Chap. 29 for discussion of erythrocyte precursors; Chap. 59 for granulocyte precursors; Chap. 67 for monocytes; and Chap. 74 for lymphocytes and plasma cells).

GRANULOCYTES

The term *granulocytes* refers to the precursors and mature forms of leukocytes characterized by neutrophilic, eosinophilic, or basophilic granules in their cytoplasm in the more mature stages of development. This series sometimes is referred to as the *myeloid series*. The overall trend is a gradual decrease in nuclear size and enhanced clumping of nuclear chromatin as cells lose proliferative capacity, while granules of varying types progressively appear in the cytoplasm.

The *myeloblast* (Chap. 59) is round and large, approximately 14 to 18 μm in diameter on a dried film. The nucleus occupies most of the cell. The nuclear chromatin is very fine, and two to five nucleoli are present. The cytoplasm is basophilic but less so than the cytoplasm of the erythroid series. No granules are present.

The *promyelocyte* (Chap. 59) is larger than the myeloblast. The chromatin pattern is coarser than that of the myeloblast, but nucleoli usually are present. The cytoplasm is basophilic with a clear Golgi area and is characterized by a small number of prominent, large red granules—the primary, nonspecific, or azurophilic granules. In the marrow, the granules usually mark the cell as a granulocyte precursor, although similar-appearing granules (with different enzymatic composition) may occur in large lymphocytes.

The *myelocyte* (Chap. 59) is slightly smaller than the promyelocyte. The myelocyte is the most mature mitotic cell in the myeloid lineage. Its nucleus is round or oval and often eccentrically located. The chromatin pattern is coarser than that of the promyelocyte, and nucleoli usually are not visible. The defining feature is the presence of specific granules in the cytoplasm, which identify the cell lineage. The granules may be neutrophilic (fine, variable size, lilac color), eosinophilic (larger, round, orange–red), or basophilic (larger still, irregular in size, deep blue). The granules first appear in the perinuclear area. The cytoplasm is only slightly basophilic.

The *metamyelocyte* (Chap. 59) is about the same size as the myelocyte and resembles it closely, except that the nucleus is indented, the chromatin is more coarse, and the cytoplasm is less basophilic.

The *band cell* (Chap. 59) is characterized by a nucleus that is horseshoe shape or lobular but is not segmented in that the rudimentary lobes are connected by a thick band of chromatin rather than the thin thread or filament characterizing the mature polymorphonuclear leukocyte. The cytoplasm is yellowish–pink or nearly colorless. Lineage specific granules are abundant in the cytoplasm. Nuclear chromatin is dense but less so than in the segmented granulocyte.

Segmented (polymorphonuclear) granulocytes (Chap. 59) differ from band cells by the multilobed character of the nucleus. At least two separate lobes are defined by a complete rounded shape, whether or not the thin filament joining them is seen. Nuclear chromatin is very dense. The mature eosinophil typically has only two lobes, whereas the nuclei of most neutrophils have two to four lobes. Basophil nuclei may be obscured by the abundant basophilic granules.

MONOCYTES

Monocytes in normal marrow are identical morphologically to those in the blood. Promonocytes (Chap. 67) have more delicate chromatin, visible nucleoli, often a few fine granules, and somewhat more basophilic cytoplasm.

MACROPHAGES (HISTIOCYTES)

The term histiocyte is an obsolete synonym for macrophage. When identifying these cells in the marrow the term macrophage is used. Diseases of macrophages were termed histiocytic disorders and because that term is still in common use by hematopathologists, the term "histiocyte" lives on when discussing diseases of macrophages. These cells are derived from monocytes but are larger, reaching 20 to 30 μm in the longest dimension (Chap. 67). The nucleus is oval with delicate reticular chromatin and one or two small nucleoli. The cytoplasm ranges from blue-gray to pale and colorless, and often contains phagocytosed cells, degenerating cell debris, and vacuoles. Normally, intact red cells are rarely visible inside marrow macrophages. However, uncontrolled activation of these cells leads to a "hemophagocytic syndrome" in which macrophages phagocytize red cells, erythroblasts, other leukocytes, and platelets. This phenomenon is associated with a variety of neoplastic, viral, and reactive conditions (see Chap. 72).[70]

ERYTHROID CELLS

During erythroid differentiation, the nucleus progressively becomes smaller and nuclear chromatin more condensed, as the cell's proliferative capacity decreases. The cytoplasm gradually loses the bluish color imparted by RNA, which is replaced by the pink-staining hemoglobin. Cells in the erythroid series are termed *erythroblasts* (previously the term "normoblast" was used to distinguish the normal sequence from the sequence observed in megaloblastic anemia). These stages are arbitrary divisions within a continuum of differentiation. Chap. 29 provides more detailed descriptions of normal red cell precursors.

The *proerythroblast* (Chap. 29) is a large, round cell measuring from 15 to 20 μm in diameter. The nucleus occupies most of the cell. The chromatin is present in a fine reticular or stippled pattern but is usually more densely stained than the chromatin of the myeloblast. Nucleoli are present and often are bluish. The cytoplasm typically is more basophilic than the myeloblast.

The *basophilic erythroblast* (Chap. 29) is smaller than the proerythroblast, and the nucleus occupies less of the cell. The chromatin pattern is stippled, and the small, condensed masses of chromatin are sharply defined and separated by pale parachromatin. The cytoplasm is deeply basophilic.

The *polychromatophilic erythroblast* (Chap. 29) is smaller than the basophilic erythroblast. The nucleus occupies even less of the cell, and the chromatin pattern is more condensed, with larger masses of chromatin sharply defined by pale parachromatin. The cytoplasm is gray or grayish-pink because of the increasing amounts of hemoglobin.

The *orthochromatic erythroblast* (Chap. 29) is only slightly larger than the mature erythrocyte. The nucleus is small and pyknotic. The cytoplasm is red, like that of the mature erythrocyte.

The *erythrocyte* (Chap. 29) is the mature anucleate red cell. *Polychromatophilic erythrocytes* are mature anucleate red cells that are just released from the marrow (corresponding to early reticulocytes) and still have sufficient residual RNA to impart a slight grayish tinge to the cytoplasm (Chap. 31). The gray color of the cytoplasm results from a combination of cytoplasmic RNA and hemoglobin.

■ EVALUATION OF IRON STORES

Marrow examination often should include evaluation of the iron stores, especially if the patient is anemic. The examination is accomplished by staining a marrow film or section by the Prussian blue technique. Because decalcification of marrow biopsy specimens results in decreased recovery of stainable iron,[71] a nondecalcified specimen or aspirate should be stained when evaluating iron stores in the differential diagnosis of anemia. Marrow macrophages (seen best in the aspirate particle preparation) are evaluated for storage iron (see Fig. 3–3), and erythroblasts (best evaluated in the direct film or concentrate) are examined for the presence of iron granules in the cytoplasm (sideroblasts). Late erythroblasts are readily identified by their small size and the size, shape, and chromatin pattern of the nucleus. The proportion of late erythroblasts that contain one or more Prussian blue granules is extremely variable (3–69%) in normal subjects.[49] Abnormal sideroblasts are characterized by increased number (>5) of iron granules arranged in a ring around the nucleus, reflecting accumulation of iron in mitochondria (Chaps. 58 and 88).

■ MEGAKARYOCYTES

Chapter 113 discusses the megakaryocyte in detail. Megakaryocytes are large cells (30–150 μm) with darkly stained, irregularly lobed nuclei (Chap. 113). The cytoplasm is blue "cotton candy" textured, and the more mature cells contain many red granules. About half the megakaryocytes should have platelets adjacent to their periphery.

■ LYMPHOCYTES

In normal marrow, lymphocytes similar to those found in the blood occur in variable numbers, depending on the degree of blood contamination of the marrow (see Chap 74). Immature lymphoid cells with a very high nuclear to cytoplasmic ratio and moderately dense but finely distributed chromatin often are seen in marrow aspirates of children. The immature lymphoid cells may cause diagnostic difficulty in some clinical settings, such as the "rebound" lymphocytosis that occurs after cessation of maintenance chemotherapy for acute lymphoblastic leukemia.[72] These lymphocytes mostly represent varying stages of B-cell precursor development.[73] Mature lymphocytes and the smaller numbers of immature lymphoid forms prominent in infant marrows diminish in number with age.

■ PLASMA CELLS

Normal plasma cells vary in size but usually are 12 to 16 μm in diameter when spread on a slide. They are round or oval. The nucleus is small, round, eccentrically placed, and stained densely purple. The chromatin is coarse and clumped. Nucleoli are not visible. The cytoplasm is deep blue, often with a paranuclear clear zone (Chap. 74). Binucleate forms may be found in normal marrow.

■ OTHER CELL TYPES

Mast cells are readily recognized by their content of dark-blue granules, which usually completely fill the cytoplasm and may obscure the nucleus (Chap. 63). The cells are round or spindle shaped and often are located deep in the particles, frequently lying along blood vessels. The nucleus often is not visible but when seen is round or oval with a vesicular chromatin pattern.

Osteoclasts and *osteoblasts* are uncommon, but can be seen in hypocellular marrow or marrow obtained from children and from adults with hyperparathyroidism or osteoblastic reactions to tumors. Osteoclasts are large cells and may be larger than 100 μm in diameter (see Fig. 3–3). They superficially resemble megakaryocytes but contain multiple separated nuclei that have a moderately fine chromatin pattern with nucleoli. The cytoplasm varies from slightly basophilic to intensely acidophilic because of the content of acidophilic granules. Osteoclasts may contain coarse basophilic debris.

Osteoblasts usually are oval cells up to 30 μm in the longest diameter (see Fig. 3–3). They often occur in groups. The nucleus usually is quite eccentric and may seem to be spilling out of the cell. The chromatin pattern is uniform, and one to three nucleoli are present. The cytoplasm is light blue and may contain a few red granules. Osteoblasts may be mistaken for plasma cells. In osteoblasts, the pale centrosomal region of the cytoplasm is separated from the nucleus, in contrast to that of the plasma cell, in which the centrosomal region directly abuts the nucleus.

PRINCIPLES OF FLOW CYTOMETRY INTERPRETATION

Immunophenotyping is complementary to morphology in the contemporary practice of marrow cell identification. Flow cytometers use similar principles to the automated hematology analyzers discussed in Chap. 2, with the notable difference that fluorescence-labeled monoclonal antibodies directed toward cluster of differentiation (CD) antigens (described in detail in Chap. 15) are used to aid in the specific diagnosis of hematologic malignancies. As described in the World Health Organization classification of hematologic malignancies,[74] immunophenotypic data (expression of cell surface, intracytoplasmic, and nuclear antigens) is a key determinant of diagnosis and classification of hematopoietic malignancies. The principle of immunophenotyping is similar to RNA expression analysis, which differs primarily by way of the enormous quantity of data obtained when the entire transcriptome, rather than selected RNA products (proteins), are analyzed, necessitating advanced data analysis techniques. Both methods are attempting to cluster neoplastic cell populations by virtue of differential patterns of gene or protein expression. Only the basic principles of flow cytometry analysis are described in this chapter, so that the reader has the basis for understanding the phenotypic characteristics associated with the hematopoietic disorders described in greater detail in other chapters of this book.

METHODOLOGY

Flow cytometers are automated hematology analyzers that use principles of light scatter and fluorescence to define cellular populations in which to analyze expression of proteins identified by fluorescent tagged antibodies. Direct current impedance, radio frequency capacitance, and absorption measurements are typically not employed. A single-cell suspension is aspirated into a laminar flow of isotonic diluent that passes in front of one or more laser beams. Light scatter and fluorescence data are collected using specific photomultiplier tubes with appropriate filtration to collect scattered light (same wavelength as the incident laser light) or fluorescence emitted light (at a longer wavelength determined by the dye used). Multiple detectors with different filtration coupled with single or multiple lasers are used to collect highly multiplexed data. For instance, four colors can be analyzed at once with a single laser provided all four can be excited at one incident wavelength, and the Stokes shift (difference between exciting wavelength and fluorescence emitted wavelength) is substantially different for each dye used. As with automated hematology analyzers, light scatter information is collected at a low angle (correlates with cell size) and 90-degree angle (correlates with cellular granularity and nuclear complexity; see Chap. 2, Fig. 2–1). The latter measurement is especially useful in separating developing myeloid progenitors, monocytes, and mature granulocytes from lymphoid cells and blasts.

Immunophenotyping can be achieved by using monoclonal antibodies specific to certain cell surface proteins, most of which have CD designations that are periodically updated by international workshops (see Chap. 15). A primary requirement for flow cytometry analysis is that cells must be viable and in single-cell suspension prior to staining,[75] which is why this method is used largely for hematopoietic malignancies and immunologic disorders and not for analysis of solid tumors. This consideration also explains differences in results between flow cytometry and morphologic or immunohistochemical observations when samples with highly adherent neoplastic cells are analyzed. For instance, in multiple myeloma or large cell lymphoma the proportion of abnormal plasma cells or lymphoma cells observed by flow cytometry is typically lower, sometimes much lower or undetectable, than that shown in a marrow biopsy. In a well-equipped and appropriately staffed clinical laboratory, preliminary information often can be provided within 3 to 4 hours after the initial sample collection, thereby facilitating institution of appropriate therapy (e.g., in the case of newly diagnosed acute leukemias).

Four-color marker analysis is the current clinical standard of practice, but six-color analysis will be widely used in the next few years. For research immunology and hematologic research, simultaneous analysis of 14 or more markers is possible. At present, routine use of that many simultaneously measured markers is not necessary for clinical diagnosis. Most markers are analyzed as cell surface proteins by directly adding conjugated antibodies to cell suspension, followed by washing and lysis of red cells.[75] Assessment of intracytoplasmic and nuclear-associated proteins is accomplished by first fixing cells in suspension and adding the relevant antibodies in conjunction with a membrane permeabilizing agent. Some of the more important and lineage-specific markers (CD3 in precursor T cells; CD79a and CD22 in B cells; myeloperoxidase in granulocyte lineage; cyclin D1 in mantle cell lymphoma; terminal deoxynucleotidyl transferase in precursor lymphocytic lymphoma/leukemia) are intracytoplasmic or intranuclear. Fluorescence and light scatter data are stored electronically as list mode data files that can be archived on compact disk or digital video disk and later reanalyzed using appropriate software.

GATING STRATEGIES

In heterogeneous specimens such as marrow, in which the relevant clinical population (such as blasts) may be a minor population overall, a strategy for specifically identifying the population(s) of interest is necessary. As discussed in Chap. 2, this is accomplished for blood cells by very complex cluster analysis using multiple parameters. Because the flow cytometer has a much more sophisticated analytical capability at the back end with the fluorescent markers, the front end selection of cells doesn't need to be as definitive, but should broadly include the cells of interest and exclude most nonrelevant cells. This process, referred to as *gating*, is typically accomplished by a combination of CD45 (common leukocyte antigen) and 90-degree light scatter (side scatter). As shown in Figure 3–4, lymphocytes, monocytes, myeloid precursors, and blast cells can be reasonably distinguished in marrow using this method. It is important to exclude monocytes, which express high affinity Fc receptors that nonspecifically bind antibodies and may cause false-positive fluorescence signals. Individual lineages, such as eosinophils, basophils, and neutrophils, or stages of neutrophilic maturation, are not distinguished as automated hematology analyzers do for blood, but this is not necessary for the diagnostic questions asked by flow cytometric immunophenotyping. Identification of as few as 1 percent blast cells permits immunophenotypic evaluation of this population if desired. For samples with low cell viability, gating strategies based on light scatter and/or vital exclusion dyes such as 7α-actinomycin-D to limit analysis to the viable cell population only may be used.[75] Identification of CD45-negative metastatic tumor by flow cytometry using epithelial associated antigens is limited by the difficulty in bringing these adherent cells into single-cell suspension. Immunocytochemistry of a marrow biopsy specimen is the preferred method for phenotyping solid tumors (and Hodgkin lymphoma) and is also complementary to flow cytometry in diagnosis of lymphoid infiltrates.

DETERMINING THE IMMUNOPHENOTYPE OF AN ABNORMAL POPULATION

Typically, the diagnostic question involves characterizing an expanded blast population or detection and analysis of a monoclonal lymphoid population (see Fig. 3–4). These determinations can be achieved by examining lineage-specific or maturation stage-specific markers. For instance, in marrow, immature cell populations can be identified by expression of antigens such as CD34 and terminal deoxynucleotidyl transferase. In some instances, the stage of differentiation can be determined using combinations of markers that are expressed only during certain phases of differentiation (e.g., dual expression of CD4 and CD8 in an immature T-precursor population). Stage-specific phenotypes are sometimes valuable clues to clinically relevant diagnoses, such as the characteristic lack of human leukocyte antigen-D related (HLA-DR) expression in promyelocytic leukemia, a phenotype that mimics the normal loss of this antigen in promyelocytes. Among lymphoid leukemia/lymphomas, chronic lymphocytic leukemia/small cell lymphoma, mantle cell lymphoma, hairy cell leukemia, and B- or T-precursor lymphoblastic leukemia, among others, have distinctive immunophenotypes. This method also may allow identification of aberrant phenotype combinations not seen in normal samples, thereby providing indirect evidence of malignancy. For example, coexpression of high levels of CD56 on a strongly

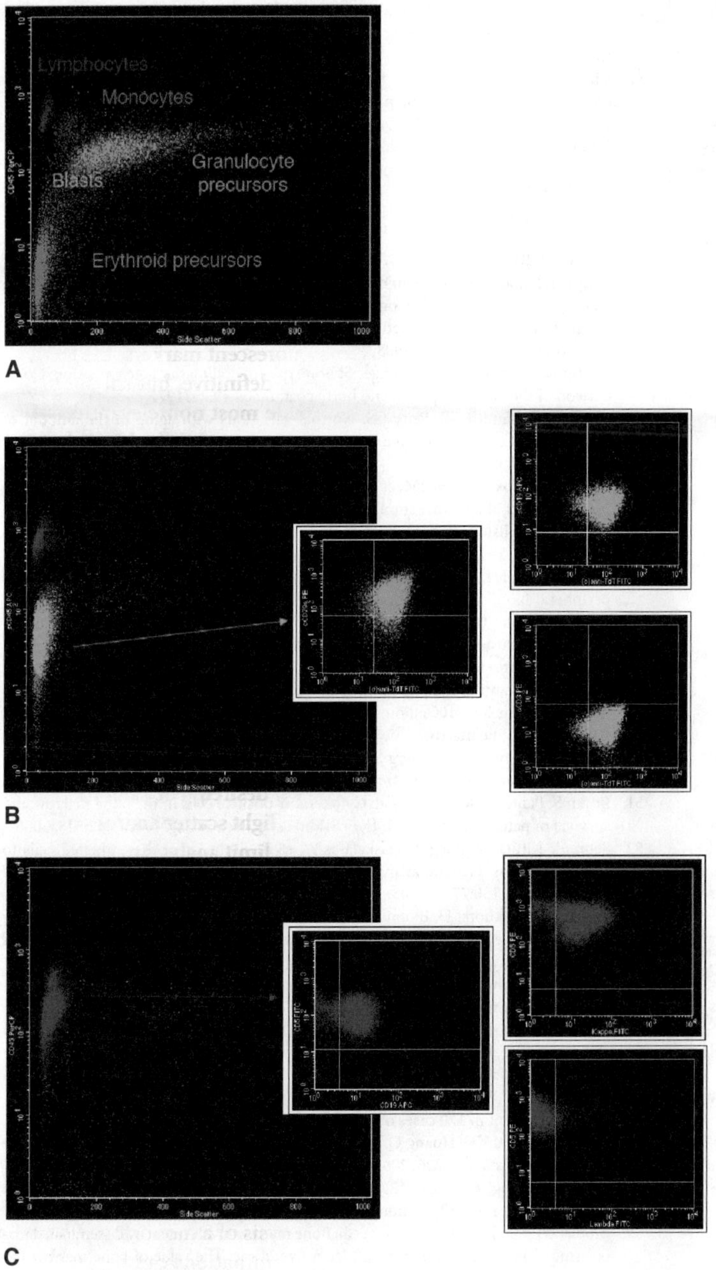

FIGURE 3–4. Flow cytometry examples: **A.** Normal marrow showing CD45 versus side scatter, which identifies major cell populations as indicated. **B.** Acute lymphoid leukemia, in which an expanded blast population is evident in the CD45 versus side scatter histogram (shown in green). Those cells with dim CD45 and negative side scatter (green) are then gated, so that expression of cell markers on this population only can be analyzed, as shown in the three histograms to the right, where the population is shown to be CD19+/CD79a+ (B cell), terminal deoxynucleotidyl transferase (TdT)+ (immature lymphoid), and CD3− (not T cell), hence B-precursor lymphoblastic leukemia. **C.** Chronic lymphocytic leukemia (CLL), in which an expanded lymphocyte population is evident on the CD45 versus side scatter histogram (shown in red), with coexpression of CD5 and CD19 (consistent with CLL), and expression of only surface immunoglobulin light-chain κ isotype on the CD5+ cells, showing that the population is monoclonal.

CD38+ plasma cells is an atypical phenotype suggestive of myeloma, and loss of the pan–T-cell marker CD7 on an otherwise mature-appearing T cell may suggest T-cell lymphoma. Coexpression of lymphoid- and myeloid-associated markers or immature- and mature-stage-specific markers is associated with leukemia, and has been used to detect minimal residual disease. The latter determination is useful in prediction of outcome in acute myeloid and lymphoid leukemias,[76,77] and myeloma,[78] and in considering the next step in therapy. Detection of minimal residual disease should involve carefully defined marker combinations that are tested in normal marrow to determine the upper limit of normal expression and have been shown to be diagnostically useful in clinical trials. Expression intensity is a frequent clue to diagnosis; for example, the weak surface immunoglobulin and weak CD20 expression in chronic lymphocytic leukemia. In some samples, loss of expected light scatter features may provide diagnostic hints. Loss of 90-degree light scatter in myeloid populations often correlates with the hypogranularity of neutrophils that can be seen in myelodysplasia. Increased forward-angle light scatter (an indicator of cell size) may be seen in some blast cell populations, large cell lymphomas, and metastatic tumors of nonhematopoietic origin. In reporting flow cytometry immunophenotyping results, the summary immunophenotype of the relevant population(s) should be described, rather than simply a listing of the percentage of cells positive for each marker, with subpopulations noted as observed.

OTHER COMMON FLOW CYTOMETRY APPLICATIONS

Immunophenotyping of granulocyte precursors has been used to demonstrate abnormal granulocyte maturation in myelodysplastic syndrome (MDS).[79] Although it is not clear that this approach improves upon the sensitivity or specificity of a morphologic diagnosis, poorer clinical outcome of MDS patients with more highly abnormal phenotypes in MDS may be predicted.[80] Clonality of immunoglobulin-expressing B-cell malignancies involving marrow (e.g., chronic lymphocytic leukemia and lymphoplasmacytic lymphoma) can be determined by simultaneous assessment of surface κ and λ immunoglobulin light-chain expression.[81] Cytoplasmic κ and λ identification can also be useful in establishing the clonality of plasma cell neoplasm in marrow. Technical considerations are important to minimize nonspecific binding of serum monoclonal immunoglobulins to the surface of lymphocytes in the performance of these applications.

Flow cytometry is used to enumerate CD34+ progenitors when evaluating the adequacy of blood stem cell collections (Chaps. 21 and 26).[82] Lymphocyte subset quantitation is diagnostically important in acquired and congenital immunodeficiency states. Diagnosis of paroxysmal nocturnal hemoglobinuria (Chap. 40) by flow cytometry has involved measuring expression of several glycophosphatidylinositol-linked proteins in different cell lineages in blood, providing a more sensitive detection method than traditional *in vitro* assays.[83] A new assay using FLAER (fluorescently labeled inactive variant of the protein aerolysin), which binds to glycosylphosphatidylinositol (GPI) anchors, detects GPI-linked protein expression in multiple cell lineages sufficiently sensitive to detect a <1 percent of paroxysmal nocturnal hemoglobinuria cells in the clone.[84]

REFERENCES

1. Arinkin M: Die intravital Untersuchungsmethodik des Knockenmarks. Folia Haematol (Frankf) 38:233,1929, reproduced in Lichtman MA, Spivak JL, Boxer LA, Shattil SJ, Henderson ES, editors, *Hematology: Landmark papers of the Twentieth Century*. English translation, p 824. Academic Press, New York, 2000.

2. Custer RP, Ahlfeldt FE: Studies on the structure and function of bone marrow. II: Variations in cellularity in various bones with advancing years of life and their relative response to stimuli. *J Lab Clin Med* 17:960, 1932.
3. Lee SH, Erber WN, Porwit A, et al: ICSH guidelines for the standardization of bone marrow specimens and reports. *Int J Lab Hematol* 30:349, 2008.
4. Riley RS, Hogan TF, Pavot DR, et al: A pathologist's perspective on bone marrow aspiration and biopsy: I: Performing a bone marrow examination. *J Clin Lab Anal* 18:70, 2004.
5. Bain B: Bone marrow trephine biopsy. *J Clin Pathol* 54:737, 2001.
6. Bain B: Bone marrow aspiration. *J Clin Pathol* 54:657, 2001.
7. Ellis LD, Jensen WN, Westerman MP: Needle biopsy of bone marrow: An experience with 1,445 biopsies. *Arch Intern Med* 114:213, 1964.
8. Sabharwal BD, Malhotra V, Aruna S, et al: Comparative evaluation of bone marrow aspirate particle smears, imprints and biopsy sections. *J Postgrad Med* 36:194, 1990.
9. Bearden JD, Ratkin GA, Coltman CA: Comparison of the diagnostic value of bone marrow biopsy and bone marrow aspiration in neoplastic disease. *J Clin Pathol* 27:738, 1974.
10. Pasquale D, Chikkappa G: Comparative evaluation of bone marrow aspirate particle smears, biopsy imprints, and biopsy sections. *Am J Hematol* 22:381, 1986.
11. Kidd PG, Saminathan T, Drachtman RA, et al: Comparison of the cellularity and presence of residual leukemia in bone marrow aspirate and biopsy specimens in pediatric patients with acute lymphoblastic leukemia (ALL) at day 7–14 of chemotherapy. *Med Pediatr Oncol* 29:541, 1997.
12. Montserrat E, Villamor N, Reverter JC, et al: Bone marrow assessment in B-cell chronic lymphocytic leukaemia: Aspirate or biopsy? A comparative study in 258 patients. *Br J Haematol* 93:111, 1996.
13. Winfield DA, Polacarz SU: Bone marrow histology 3: Value of bone marrow core biopsies in acute leukemia, myelodysplastic syndromes, and chronic myeloid leukemia. *J Clin Pathol* 45:855, 1992.
14. Bartl R, Frisch B, Wilmanns W: Potential of bone marrow biopsy in chronic myeloproliferative disorders (MPD). *Eur J Haematol* 50:41, 1993.
15. Bain BJ: Bone marrow biopsy morbidity and mortality. *Br J Haematol* 121:949, 2003.
16. Dunlop TJ, Deen C, Lind S, et al: Use of combined oral narcotic and benzodiazepine for control of pain associated with bone marrow examination. *South Med J* 92:477, 1999.
17. Hertzog J, Dalton H, Anderson B: Prospective evaluation of propofol anesthesia in the pediatric intensive care unit for elective oncology procedures in ambulatory and hospitalized children. *Pediatrics* 106:742, 2000.
18. Holdsworth M, Raisch D, Winter S: Pain and distress from bone marrow aspirations and lumbar punctures. *Ann Pharmacother* 37:17, 2003.
19. Cheuk DK, Wong WH, Ma E, et al: Use of midazolam and ketamine as sedation for children undergoing minor operative procedures. *Support Care Cancer* 13:1001, 2005.
20. Reeves ST, Havidich JE, Tobin DP: Conscious sedation of children with propofol is anything but conscious. *Pediatrics* 114:e74, 2004.
21. Cannell H: Evidence for safety margins of lignocaine local anaesthetics for peri-oral use. *Br Dent J* 181:243, 1996.
22. Jamshidi K, Swaim WR: Bone marrow biopsy with unaltered architecture: A new biopsy device. *J Lab Clin Med* 77:335, 1971.
23. Humphries J: Dry tap bone marrow aspiration: Clinical significance. *Am J Hematol* 35:247, 1990.
24. James L, Stass S, Schumacher H: Value of imprint preparation of bone marrow biopsies in hematologic diagnosis. *Cancer* 46:173, 1980.
25. Tomkins DJ, Scheid EE: Effect of sample holding, cryopreservation, and storage on the human lymphocyte cytogenetic test. *Am J Ind Med* 9:385, 1986.
26. Novotny JR, Schmucker U, Staats B, et al: Failed or inadequate bone marrow aspiration: A fast, simple and cost-effective method to produce a cell suspension from a core biopsy specimen. *Clin Lab Haematol* 27:33, 2005.
27. Breit S, Nees M, Schaefer U, et al: Impact of pre-analytical handling on bone marrow mRNA gene expression. *Br J Haematol* 126:231, 2004.
28. Wickham C, Boyce M, Joyner MV: Amplification of PCR products in excess of 600 base pairs using DNA extracted from decalcified, paraffin wax embedded bone marrow trephine biopsies. *Mol Pathol* 53:19, 2000.
29. Bock O, Lehmann U, Kreipe H: Quantitative intra-individual monitoring of BCR-ABL transcript levels in archival bone marrow trephines of patients with chronic myeloid leukemia. *J Mol Diagn* 5:54, 2003.
30. Akoury DA, Seo JJ, James CD, et al: RT-PCR detection of mRNA recovered from archival glass slide smears. *Mod Pathol* 6:195, 1993.
31. Lillie RD, Fullmer HM: *Histopathologic Technic and Practical Histochemistry,* 4th ed, p 54. McGraw-Hill, New York, 1976.
32. Hyun BH, Stevenson AJ, Hanau CA: Fundamentals of bone marrow examination. *Hematol Oncol Clin North Am* 8:651, 1994.
33. Moosavi H, Lichtman MA, Donnelly JA, et al: Plastic-embedded human marrow biopsy specimens: Improved histochemical methods. *Arch Pathol Lab Med* 105:269, 1981.
34. Blythe D, Hand NM, Jackson P, et al: Use of methyl methacrylate resin for embedding bone marrow trephine biopsy specimens. *J Clin Pathol* 50:45, 1997.
35. Brown DC, Gatter KC: The bone marrow trephine biopsy. A review of normal histology. *Histopathology* 22:411, 1992.
36. Wang J, Wiess L, Chang K, et al: Diagnostic utility of bilateral bone marrow examination: Significance of morphologic and ancillary technique study in malignancy. *Cancer* 94:1522, 2002.
37. Cheson B, Horning S, Coiffier B, et al: Report of an international workshop to standardize response criteria for non-Hodgkin's lymphomas. NCI Sponsored International Working Group. *J Clin Oncol* 17:1244, 1999.
38. Campbell JK, Matthews JP, Seymour JF, et al: Optimum trephine length in the assessment of bone marrow involvement in patients with diffuse large cell lymphoma. *Ann Oncol* 14:273, 2003.
39. Bishop PW, McNally K, Harris M: Audit of bone marrow trephines. *J Clin Pathol* 45:1105, 1992.
40. Holdrinet RSG, Egmond J, Wessels JMC, et al: A method for quantification of peripheral blood admixture in bone marrow aspirates. *Exp Hematol* 8:103, 1980.
41. Ozkaynak MF, Scribano P, Gomperts E, et al: Comparative evaluation of the bone marrow by the volumetric method, particle smears, and biopsies in pediatric disorders. *Am J Hematol* 29:144, 1988.
42. Gruppo RA, Lampkin BC, Granger S: Bone marrow cellularity determination: Comparison of the biopsy, aspirate, and buffy coat. *Blood* 49:29, 1977.
43. Hartsock RJ, Smith EB, Petty CS: Normal variations with aging of the amount of hemopoietic tissue in bone marrow from the anterior iliac crest. *Am J Clin Pathol* 43:326, 1965.
44. Tuzuner N, Cox C, Rowe JM, et al: Bone marrow cellularity in myeloid stem cell disorders: Impact of age correction. *Leuk Res* 18:559, 1994.
45. Wilkins BS: Histology of normal haemopoiesis: Bone Marrow histology I. *J Clin Pathol* 45:645, 1992.
46. Abrahamsen JF, Lund-Johansen F, Laerum OD, et al: Flow cytometric assessment of peripheral blood contamination and proliferative activity of human bone marrow cell populations. *Cytometry* 19:77, 1995.
47. Batinic D, Marusic M, Pavletic Z, et al: Relationship between differing volumes of bone marrow aspirates and their cellular composition. *Bone Marrow Transplant* 6:103, 1990.
48. Mori Y, Mizukami T, Hamaguchi Y, et al: Automation of bone marrow aspirate examination using the XE-2100 automated hematology analyzer. *Cytometry* 58B:25, 2004.
49. Bain BJ: The bone marrow aspirate of healthy subjects. *Br J Haematol* 94:206, 1996.
50. Atac B, Lawrence C, Goldberg S: Metastatic tumor: The complementary role of the marrow aspirate and biopsy. *Am J Med Sci* 302:211, 1991.
51. Braun S, Pantel K, Müller P, et al: Cytokeratin-positive cells in the bone marrow and survival of patients with stage I, II, or III breast cancer. *N Engl J Med* 342:525, 2000.
52. Schmidt-Kittler O, Ragg T, Daskalakis A, et al: From latent disseminated cells to overt metastasis: Genetic analysis of systemic breast cancer progression. *Proc Natl Acad Sci U S A* 100:7737, 2003.
53. Terpstra W, Lokhorst H, Blomjous F: Comparison of plasma cell infiltration in bone marrow biopsies and aspirates in patients with multiple myeloma. *Br J Haematol* 82:46, 1992.
54. Navone R, Valpreda M, Pich A: Lymphoid nodules and nodular lymphoid hyperplasia in bone marrow biopsies. *Acta Haematol* 74:19, 1985.
55. Erber WN, Asbahr HD, Phelps PN: In situ hybridization of immunoglobulin light chain mRNA on bone marrow trephines using biotinylated probes and the APAAP method. *Pathology* 25:63, 1993.
56. Kang Y, Park C, Seo E, et al: Polymerase chain reaction-based diagnosis of bone marrow involvement in 170 cases of non-Hodgkin lymphoma. *Cancer* 94:3073, 2002.
57. Chang KL, Gaal KK, Huang Q, et al: Histiocytic lesions involving the bone marrow. *Semin Diagn Pathol* 20:226, 2003.
58. Magill AJ, Grogl M, Gasser RA, Jr, et al: Visceral infection caused by Leishmania tropica in veterans of Operation Desert Storm. *N Engl J Med* 328:1383, 1993.
59. Brouland JP, Audouin J, Hofman P, et al: Bone marrow involvement by disseminated toxoplasmosis in acquired immunodeficiency syndrome: The value of bone marrow trephine biopsy and immunohistochemistry for the diagnosis. *Hum Pathol* 27:302, 1996.
60. Hussong J, Peterson LR, Warren JR, et al: Detecting disseminated Mycobacterium avium complex infections in HIV-positive patients. The usefulness of bone marrow trephine biopsy specimens, aspirate cultures, and blood cultures. *Am J Clin Pathol* 110:806, 1998.
61. Agostoni C, Dorigoni N, Malfitano A, et al: Mediterranean leishmaniasis in HIV-infected patients: Epidemiological, clinical, and diagnostic features of 22 cases. *Infection* 26:93, 1998.
62. Neubauer MA, Bodensteiner DC: Disseminated histoplasmosis in patients with AIDS. *South Med J* 85:1166, 1992.
63. Mourad O, Palda V, Detsky AS: A comprehensive evidence-based approach to fever of unknown origin. *Arch Intern Med* 163:545, 2003.
64. Eid A, Carion W, Nystrom JS: Differential diagnoses of bone marrow granuloma. *West J Med* 164:510, 1996.
65. Norgard MJ, Carpenter JTJ, Conrad ME: Bone marrow necrosis and degeneration. *Arch Intern Med* 139:905, 1979.
66. Seaman JP, Kjeldsberg CR, Linker A: Gelatinous transformation of the bone marrow. *Hum Pathol* 9:685, 1978.
67. Tavassoli M, Eastlund DT, Yam LT, et al: Gelatinous transformation of bone marrow in prolonged self-induced starvation. *Scand J Haematol* 16:311, 1976.
68. Rosse C, Krauner MJ, Dillon TL, et al: Bone marrow cell populations of normal infants: The predominance of lymphocytes. *J Lab Clin Med* 89:1225, 1977.
69. Dresch C, Faille A, Poirier O, et al: The cellular composition of the granulocyte series in the normal human bone marrow according to the volume of the sample. *J Clin Pathol* 27:106, 1974.

70. Janka G, Imashuku S, Elinder G, et al: Infection- and malignancy-associated hemophagocytic syndromes. Secondary hemophagocytic lymphohistiocytosis. *Hematol Oncol Clin North Am* 12:435, 1998.
71. DePalma L: The effect of decalcification and choice of fixative on histiocytic iron in bone marrow core biopsies. *Biotech Histochem* 71:57, 1996.
72. Pritchard-Jones K, Toogood IR, Rice MS: The significance of an M2 bone marrow at cessation of chemotherapy in childhood acute lymphoblastic leukemia. *Am J Pediatr Hematol Oncol* 10:292, 1988.
73. Longacre TA, Foucar K, Crago S, et al: Hematogones: A multiparameter analysis of bone marrow precursor cells. *Blood* 73:543, 1989.
74. Jaffe ES, Harris NL, Stein H: *Tumours of Haematopoietic and Lymphoid Tissues (World Health Organization Classification of Tumours)*. International Agency for Research on Cancer, Lyon, France, 2008.
75. Stelzer GT, Marti G, Hurley A, et al: U.S.-Canadian Consensus recommendations on the immunophenotypic analysis of hematologic neoplasia by flow cytometry: Standardization and validation of laboratory procedures. *Cytometry* 30:214, 1997.
76. Campana D: Status of minimal residual disease testing in childhood haematological malignancies. *Br J Haematol* 143:481, 2008.
77. Freeman SD, Jovanovic JV, Grimwade D: Development of minimal residual disease-directed therapy in acute myeloid leukemia. *Semin Oncol* 35:388, 2008.
78. Paiva B, Vidriales MB, Cervero J, et al: Multiparameter flow cytometric remission is the most relevant prognostic factor for multiple myeloma patients who undergo autologous stem cell transplantation. *Blood* 112:4017, 2008.
79. Loken MR, van de Loosdrecht A, Ogata K, et al: Flow cytometry in myelodysplastic syndromes: Report from a working conference. *Leuk Res* 32:5, 2008.
80. Scott BL, Wells DA, Loken MR, et al: Validation of a flow cytometric scoring system as a prognostic indicator for posttransplantation outcome in patients with myelodysplastic syndrome. *Blood* 112:2681, 2008.
81. Kawano-Yamamoto C, Muroi K, Izumi T, et al: Two-color flow cytometry with a CD19 gate for the evaluation of bone marrow involvement of B-cell lymphoma. *Leuk Lymphoma* 43:2133, 2002.
82. Sutherland DR, Anderson L, Keeney M, et al: The ISHAGE guidelines for CD34+ cell determination by flow cytometry. International Society of Hematotherapy and Graft Engineering. *J Hematother* 5:213, 1996.
83. Krauss JS: Laboratory diagnosis of paroxysmal nocturnal hemoglobinuria. *Ann Clin Lab Sci* 33:401, 2003.
84. Brodsky RA, Mukhina GL, Li S, et al: Improved detection and characterization of paroxysmal nocturnal hemoglobinuria using fluorescent aerolysin. *Am J Clin Pathol* 114:459, 2000.
85. Glaser K, Limarzi LR, Poncher HG: Cellular composition of the bone marrow in normal infants and children. *Pediatrics* 6:789, 1950.

[illegible] tolerance [illegible]
[illegible] 1998.
[illegible] Hazardous [illegible]
[illegible] Commission [illegible]
[illegible] Industrial [illegible]
[illegible] Cincinnati, Ohio [illegible]
[illegible] Association [illegible]
[illegible]
[illegible]
[illegible]
[illegible]
[illegible]
[illegible]
[illegible]
[illegible]
[illegible]

PART II

The Organization of the Lymphohematopoietic Tissues

CHAPTER 4

STRUCTURE OF THE MARROW AND THE HEMATOPOIETIC MICROENVIRONMENT

Mark J. Koury and Marshall A. Lichtman*

SUMMARY

The marrow, located in the medullary cavity of bone, is the sole site of effective hematopoiesis in humans. The marrow produces approximately six billion cells per kilogram of body weight per day. Hematopoietically active (red) marrow regresses after birth until late adolescence, after which it is focused in the lower skull, vertebrae, shoulder and pelvic girdles, ribs, and sternum. Fat cells replace hematopoietic cells in the bones of the hands, feet, legs, and arms (yellow marrow). Fat occupies approximately 50 percent of the space of red marrow in the adult. Further fatty metamorphosis continues slowly with aging. In very old individuals, a gelatinous transformation of fat to a mucoid material may occur (white marrow). Yellow marrow can revert to hematopoietically active marrow if prolonged demand is present, as in chronic hemolytic anemia. Hematopoiesis can be expanded by increasing the volume of red marrow (expanding proliferating populations) and decreasing the development (transit) time from progenitor to mature cell.

The marrow stroma consists principally of a network of sinuses that originate at the endosteum from cortical capillaries and terminate in collecting vessels that enter the systemic venous circulation. The trilaminar sinus wall is composed of endothelial cells; an underdeveloped, thin basement membrane; and adventitial reticular cells that are fibroblasts capable of transforming into adipocytes. The endothelium and reticular cells are sources of hematopoietic cytokines. Hematopoiesis occurs in the intersinus spaces and is controlled by a complex array of stimulatory and inhibitory cytokines, cell–cell contacts, and the effects of extracellular matrix components on proximate cells. In this unique environment, lymphohematopoietic stem cells differentiate into all the blood cell lineages. Mature cells are produced and released to maintain steady-state blood cell levels. The system also can respond to meet increased demands for additional cells as a result of blood loss, hemolysis, inflammation, immune cytopenias, and other causes. Stem cells can leave and reenter marrow as part of their normal circulation. Their extramedullary circulation can be increased by exogenous cytokines and chemokines.

The evolutionary factors that led to confinement of hematopoiesis to the medullary cavity of bone are not fully understood. Two relationships that may underlie this requirement for proximity are the biochemical and receptor contributions of osteoblasts to hematopoiesis and the homing of hematopoietic stem cells to endosteum.

Acronyms and abbreviations that appear in this chapter include: IIICS, type III connecting segment; AGM, aorta-gonad-mesonephros; ALCAM, activated leukocyte adhesion molecule; bFGF, basic fibroblast growth factor; BFU-E, burst-forming unit–erythroid; BMP, bone morphogenetic protein; CAR, CXCL 12-abundant reticular cells; CD, cluster of differentiation; CFU-E, colony forming unit–erythroid; CFU-S, colony forming unit–spleen; CLA, cutaneous lymphocyte antigen; EC, endothelial cell; ECM, extracellular matrix protein; ELAM, endothelial leukocyte adhesion molecule; FN, fibronectin; GAG, glycosaminoglycan; G-CSF, granulocyte colony-stimulating factor; G-CSF-R, granulocyte colony-stimulating factor receptor; GlyCAM, glycosylation-dependent cell adhesion molecule; GM-CSF, granulocyte-macrophage colony-stimulating factor; HCA, hematopoietic cell antigen; HCAM, homing cell adhesion molecule; HGF, hepatocyte growth factor; HLA, human leukocyte antigen; HPP-CFC, high proliferative potential–colony forming cell; HSA, heat-stable antigen; IAP, integrin-associated protein; ICAM, intercellular adhesion molecule; iC3b, inactive complement 3b complex; IHH, Indian hedgehog family of proteins; IL, interleukin; LFA, lymphocyte function antigen; LPAM, lymphocyte Peyer patch-specific adhesion molecule; MAdCAM, mucosal addressin cell adhesion molecule; M-CSF, macrophage colony-stimulating factor; MGC-24, multiglycosylated core of 24 kDa; MIP, macrophage inflammatory protein; MMP, matrix metalloproteinase; NF-κB, nuclear factor κB; NFAT, nuclear factor of activated T cells; NK, natural killer; ODF, osteoclast differentiation and activation factor; OPG, osteoprotegerin; PCLP, podocalyxin; PDGF, platelet-derived growth factor; PECAM, platelet endothelial cell adhesion molecule; PRR2, poliovirus receptor-related–2 protein; PSGL, P-selectin glycoprotein ligand; RANTES, regulated on activation, normal T-cell expressed, presumed secreted; RTC, receptor tyrosine kinase; SDF, stromal cell-derived factor; SHP-1, Src homology 2 domain-bearing protein tyrosine phosphatase-1; sLe, sialyl Lewis; SP, side population; TGF-β, transforming growth factor-beta; TPO, thrombopoietin; TSP, thrombospondin; VAP, vascular adhesion protein; VCAM, vascular cell adhesion molecule; VEGF, vascular endothelial growth factor; VLA, very-late antigen; VNR, vitronectin receptor.

*Camille N. Abboud was an author of the chapter in the last edition and some material from that edition has been retained.

HISTORY AND GENERAL CONSIDERATIONS

The marrow, one of the largest organs in the human body, is the principal site for blood cell formation. In the normal adult, daily marrow production amounts to approximately 2.5 billion red cells, 2.5 billion platelets, and 1 billion granulocytes per kilogram of body weight. The rate of production adjusts to actual needs and can vary from nearly zero to many times normal.[1] Until the late 19th century, blood cell formation was thought to be the prerogative of the lymph nodes or the liver and spleen. In 1868, Neuman[2] and Bizzozero[3] independently observed nucleated blood cells in material squeezed from the ribs of human cadavers and proposed that the marrow is the major source of blood cells.[4] The first *in vivo* marrow biopsy probably was done in 1876 by Mosler,[5] who used a regular wood drill to obtain marrow particles from a patient with leukemia. Studies by Arinkin[6] in 1929 established marrow aspiration as a safe, easy, and useful technique (see Chap. 3).

Kinetic studies of marrow cells, using radioisotopes and *in vitro* cultures, have shown that cell lineages consist of maturing end cells with a finite functional life span. The cells are capable of limited proliferation before they reach full maturation and do not have the capacity for self-renewal. On the other hand, sustained cellular production depends on pools of primordial cells capable of both differentiation and self-replication.[7] The most primitive pool consists of pluripotential lymphohematopoietic stem cells (HSCs) with the capacity for continuous self-renewal. The more mature pools consist of differentiated unipotential progenitor cells, with their maturation restricted to single cell lineages and no capacity for self-renewal (see Chap. 16). The proliferative activity of these pools involves humoral feedback from peripheral target tissues[8] and cell–cell and cell–matrix interactions within the microenvironment of the marrow.[9] The marrow stroma provides a unique structural and chemical environment (niches) that supports the survival, differentiation, and proliferation of pluripotential HSCs. Primitive hematopoietic stem cell interactive niches[10] have been identified at the structural and molecular[11] levels and are dynamically controlled by bone morphogenetic proteins (BMPs)[12] and factors regulating intramedullary osteoblastic cells.[13] Early stem cells can be identified and isolated using a unique array of surface antigen-receptor expressions (CD34+/–, Thy-1lo, KIT+, CD38–, CD33–, vascular endothelial [VE]-cadherin+, KDR/FLK1+, FLK2–/FLT3–, CD133+/–)[14–19] and have a unique molecular signature.[20,21] Isolated cell populations enriched in HSC can be quantified using *in vitro* long-term progenitor assays and surrogate *in vivo* repopulating assays in severely immunodeficient mice and xenogeneic animal models (see Chap. 16).

SITES OF HEMATOPOIESIS

EMBRYOGENESIS AND EARLY STEM CELL DEVELOPMENT

As shown in Figure 4–1, the marrow is the last in a series of anatomical sites of hematopoiesis that change several times during embryonic and fetal development.[22–25] The earliest hematopoietic cells develop in the blood islands of the extraembryonic yolk sac during late gastrulation and form the primitive hematopoietic system. This primitive hematopoiesis is transient lasting from the appearance of the blood islands on embryonic days 7.5 in mice and day 19 in humans through the final cellular divisions in the circulating embryonic blood on day 13 in mice and week 6 in humans.[25,26] The large majority of primitive blood cells produced are erythrocytes that enucleate after release into the circulation, and their hemoglobin contains the embryonic α- and β-globin chains. However, primitive hematopoietic cells also give rise to primitive macrophages and megakaryocytes. Overlapping with this transient primitive hematopoiesis is definitive hematopoiesis that gives rise to all of the blood cell types found in the adult (see Chap. 6).

Transplantation experiments in hematopoietically ablated mice have demonstrated that definitive hematopoietic cells arise on days 8.5 to 11.5 in mice and weeks 4 to 6 in humans in three different embryonic locations: the yolk sac blood islands, the anterior portion of the aorta-gonad-mesonephros (AGM) region, and the allantoic portion of the developing placenta.[23–25] Although the HSC pool expands greatly in the placenta compared to the yolk sac and the AGM region, HSCs from all three sites migrate through the blood circulation to the fetal liver where they seed themselves and mature into all of the cellular elements of the blood.[22–25] The HSCs do not differentiate in the yolk sac, AGM, and placenta, but they do function in the fetal liver, which is the main site of hematopoiesis during mid-gestation. As in primitive hematopoiesis, erythrocytes are the predominant cell produced in definitive hematopoiesis. Definitive erythrocytes are smaller than the primitive erythrocytes, and their hemoglobin contains the fetal and adult globin chains. In the last third of gestation, the HSCs and early hematopoietic progenitor cells migrate from the fetal liver through the circulation seeding the spleen and marrow. During the last third of gestation, fetal liver hematopoiesis declines steadily as the spleen and marrow become the major hematopoietic sites. By the time of birth, marrow is the major hematopoietic site in humans, while the spleen remains a prominent but decreasing site in the mouse (see Chap. 6).

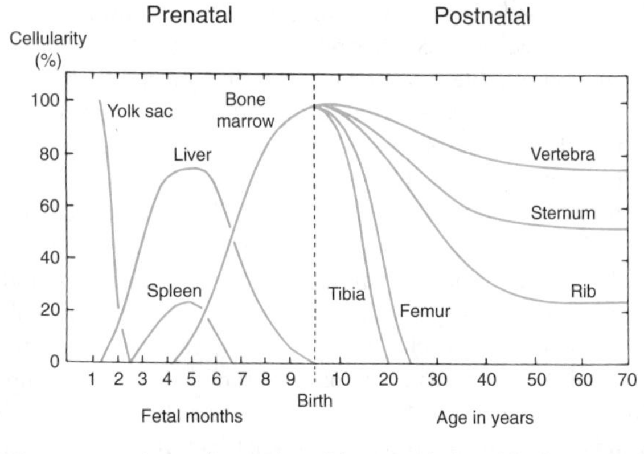

FIGURE 4–1. Expansion and recession of hematopoietic activity in extramedullary and medullary sites. For details regarding the nature of yolk sac and hepatic hematopoiesis, see "Sites of Hematopoiesis: Embryogenesis and Early Stem Cell Development." Chap. 6 provides a more comprehensive treatment of this topic (see Fig. 6–1).

In each of the three sites where HSCs are generated, visceral endoderm is in close proximity to the mesoderm that is been formed by gastrulation. This proximity is important in that the endoderm appears to induce both endothelial and blood cell development in the adjacent mesoderm through secretion of Indian hedgehog (IHH), member of the hedgehog family of proteins.[27] IHH, in turn, upregulates the expression of BMP-4 in the developing mesodermal cells.[27] BMP-4 upregulation is important for the development of both the endothelial cells that form blood vessels and the HSCs located within these vessels.[27,28] Developing endothelial cells and hematopoietic cells in the vessels formed by these endothelial cells are found in each site of primitive and definitive hematopoiesis. The close association of these two cell types in the developing embryo has led to the proposal for their having a common precursor, the hemangioblast.[29–31] A very limited number of hemangioblasts was demonstrated to arise in mice in the posterior region of the primitive streak during the mid-streak through neural stages of gastrulation.[32] The hemangioblasts migrate from this area to the sites of vessel and hematopoietic cell generation. In addition to BMP-4, other important proteins involved in the development of the hemangioblasts are the vascular endothelial growth factor receptor KDR/Flk-1, the transcription factor TAL1, and its binding partner LMO2.[29–31]

In the generation of definitive hematopoietic cells, it is possible that the hemangioblasts give rise to the HSCs directly or that they give rise to specialized endothelial cells, the hemogenic endothelium, which, in turn, produces the HSCs.[31,33] The differentiation of HSCs from hemangioblasts or hemogenic endothelium require the signaling protein Notch1 and the transcription factors GATA-2, MYB, and Runx1.[29–31,34,35] The mechanisms of this earliest expansion of HSC is not well-defined, but two factors that also play roles later, KIT ligand/stem cell factor (SCF) and interleukin-3 (IL-3), are important in the embryo. BMP-4, in addition to its role in the induction of hematopoietic and endothelial differentiation, increases proliferative and self-renewal of HSCs,[27,28] as it differentially upregulates c-KIT/stem cell factor (SCF) receptor in the HSCs, but not in adjacent endothelial cells.[36] Expansion of the earliest definitive HSC is also mediated by Notch signaling as it induces the Runx1 transcription factor[34,35] and one of its targets, the IL-3 gene.[37]

STEM CELL AND MESENCHYMAL CELL PLASTICITY

Primitive stem cells obtained from human fetal liver or marrow reconstitute all lymphohematopoietic-derived cells and part of the stromal microenvironment in *in vivo* repopulation assays.[38] These observations are consistent with the early derivation of hematopoietic, vascular, and stromal cells from a CD34-negative, KDR/Flk-1-positive, multipotential mesenchymal stem cell.[15–17,39] Identification of AC133-positive, CD34-negative, CD7-negative HSCs[40] and demonstration of endothelial precursors in AC133-positive progenitor cells[41] underscore the crosstalk between hematopoiesis and angiogenesis signaling pathways and establish the functional role of hemangioblasts in ontogeny.[42–45] As early fetal hematopoiesis is established, the yolk sac vascular networks remain active sites of progenitor production and hematopoiesis.[25] Long-term reconstituting HSCs express two members of the ATP-binding cassette genes (ABCG-2 and P-glycoprotein), allowing the efflux of mitochondrial vital dyes such as Hoechst 33342 and rhodamine 123 and their isolation by multiparameter flow cytometry based on their low side scatter (side population [SP] cells).[46–49] Enrichment of the SP population for HSC has been achieved in both adult marrow[50] and fetal liver[51] populations by using the signaling lymphocyte and activation markers (SLAMs) to select cells with the specific phenotype (CD150+, CD244–, CD48–). Nearly half of the individual cells in the CD150+CD244–CD48– population provide long-term hematopoietic reconstitution in irradiated mice.[50]

Early HSCs have been found in skeletal tissue[52] and in brain-derived neural cells,[53] indicating the widespread tissue distribution of these pluripotential cells. Heterogeneity in SP and non-SP marrow-derived progenitor cells within muscle shows SP cells are incorporated into endothelial structures during vasculogenesis, whereas non-SP cells differentiate into smooth muscle.[54] These findings confirm the intimate overlap of HSC and hemangioblast activity,[29–31,44] while showing that resident marrow-derived mesenchymal stem cell progenitors can differentiate into nonhematopoietic tissue cell types.[54] Derivation of hematopoietic cells from adult tissue (muscle, liver) has been attributed to resident marrow-derived stem cells in these tissues.[55,56] Tissue (muscle, neural, hepatic)-committed stem cells have been detected in CD34+, AC133+, CXCR4+ marrow cell populations, providing an explanation for the cells' ability to be mobilized after growth factor administration and to participate in distal organ regeneration.[57] There is a role for adult marrow-derived mesenchymal stem cells in the repair and regeneration of nonmarrow organs, including cardiac and smooth muscle, liver, and brain.[58,59] However, these marrow-derived mesenchymal stem cells function mainly by providing a microenvironment through various cytokines that induce cell growth and stimulate vascularization or by fusing with local cells, rather than any significant transdifferentiation into specific differentiated cells of the organ undergoing repair (see Chap. 16).[58,59]

■ HISTOGENESIS

Stroma and Hematopoietic Tissue

Cavities within bone occur in the human being at about the fifth fetal month and soon become the exclusive site for granulocytic and megakaryocytic proliferation. Erythropoietic activity at the time is confined to the liver. The microenvironment in the marrow becomes supportive of erythroblasts only toward the end of the last trimester (see Fig. 4–1). The formation of the marrow cavities in the developing mouse bones appear at a relatively later time in the prenatal life of mice than humans, but it involves an IHH-regulated,[60] synchronized maturation of osteoblast progenitors arising from mesenchymal stem cells and osteoclast progenitors arising from HSCs in the areas of mineralized cartilage of the fetal bones.[61] As these respective progenitors differentiate *in situ* they acquire the phenotype of osteoblasts with expression of osteopontin, osteonectin, bone sialoprotein and M-CSF and of osteoclasts with expression of tartrate-resistant acid phosphatase (TRAP), calcitonin receptors, and c-FMS (M-CSF receptor).[61] In the human, marrow hematopoiesis begins at the 11th week of gestation in specialized mesodermal structures termed primary logettes.[62] The logettes are composed of mesenchymal cells and fibers that surround a central artery and protrude into the venous sinuses of the developing marrow cavities. The myeloid and erythroid hematopoietic cells that populate the logettes are derived not from HSCs but rather from later-committed progenitors.[62] Just after birth the HSCs are found in the marrow, and hematopoiesis is evident throughout the marrow cavity.

Adipose Tissue

By the fourth year of life, a significant number of fat cells have appeared in the diaphysis of the human long bones.[63] These cells slowly replace hematopoietic elements and expand centripetally until, at approximately age 18 years, hematopoietic marrow is found only in the vertebrae, ribs, skull, pelvis, and proximal epiphyses of the femora and humeri. Direct measurements of the volume of bone cavities reveal bone cavity volume increases from 1.4 percent of body weight at birth to 4.8 percent in the adult,[63] whereas blood volume decreases from 8 percent of body weight in the newborn to approximately 7 percent in the adult.[64] Expansion of marrow space continues throughout life, resulting in a further gradual increase in the amount of fatty tissue in all bone cavities, especially in the long bones.[65,66] The preference of hematopoietic tissue for centrally located bones has been ascribed to higher central tissue temperature with greater vascularity.[67] However, because complete reactivation of fatty marrow can occur in experimental animals in which hematopoietic expansion is induced, other factors (cytokines, hormonal signals) must be involved.[68–71]

MARROW STRUCTURE

■ VASCULATURE

The blood supply to the marrow comes from two major sources. The nutrient artery, the principal source, penetrates the cortex through the nutrient canal. In the marrow cavity, the nutrient artery bifurcates into ascending and descending central or medullary arteries from which radial branches travel to the inner face of the cortex. After repenetrating the endosteum, the radial vessels diminish in caliber to structures of capillary size that course within the canalicular system of the cortex. Here arterial blood from the nutrient artery mixes with blood that enters the cortical capillary system from the periosteal capillaries derived from muscular arteries.[72] After reentering the marrow cavity, the cortical capillaries form a sinusoidal network (Fig. 4–2). Hematopoietic cells are located in the intersinusoidal tissue spaces. Some arteries have specialized, thin-walled segments that arise abruptly as continuations of

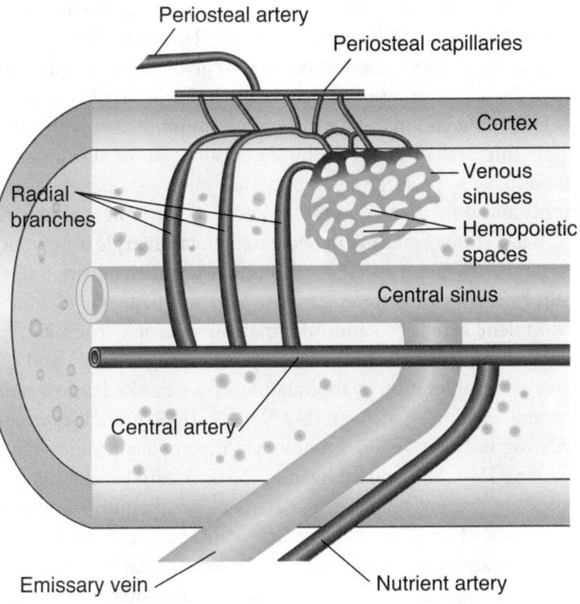

FIGURE 4–2. Schematic of the marrow circulation (see "Marrow Structure" for further explanation).

arteries with walls of normal thickness.[73] These vessels give off nearly perpendicular branches analogous to the arterial branching observed in the spleen and kidney, permitting volume compensation for changes in intramedullary pressure. In the marrow cavity, blood flows through a highly branching network of medullary sinuses. These sinuses collect into a large central sinus from which the blood enters the systemic venous circulation through emissary veins.

Vascular networks consisting of cells expressing CD31, CD34, and CD105 (endoglin) but lacking intercellular adhesion molecule (ICAM)-1, ICAM-2, ICAM-3, or endothelial leukocyte adhesion molecule (ELAM)-1 (E-selectin) can form within the stroma of long-term marrow cultures. These findings underscore the intimate relationship of blood vessels to hematopoietic activity.[74] A study of early hematopoiesis of human marrow from long bones (ages 6–28 weeks) has shown an absence of CD34-positive hematopoietic progenitors before onset of hematopoiesis, a predominance of CD68-positive cells mediating chondrolysis, and CD34-positive endothelial cells developing into specific vascular structures organized by endothelial cells and myoid cells.[75] Vascular endothelial growth factor (VEGF) receptors found on CD34-positive cells[17] and AGM primitive stem cells underscore the common ontogeny.[30,32] Subsets of CD34-positive cells expressing the AC133 antigen and the human VEGF receptor-2 define the functional endothelial precursor phenotype.[76] Endothelial progenitors residing in the CD34+, CD11b+ subsets are capable of producing and binding angiopoietins,[77] and fibronectin enhances VEGF-induced CD34 cell differentiation into endothelial cells.[78]

INNERVATION

Myelinated and nonmyelinated nerve fibers are present in periarterial sheaths in marrow,[79] where they are believed to regulate arterial vessel tone. Nerve terminals are distributed between layers of periarterial adventitial cells or localize next to arterial smooth muscle cells.[80] Nonmyelinated fibers terminate in the hematopoietic spaces, implying that neurohumors elaborated from free-nerve terminals affect hematopoiesis. Intimate cell–cell communication between sympathetic nerve cells and structural elements within the marrow sinuses occurs at less than 5 percent of nerve terminals that terminate within the hematopoietic parenchyma or on sinus walls. This anatomical unit, termed a *neuroreticular complex*, consists of efferent (autonomic) nerves and marrow stromal cells connected by gap junctions.[80] The marrow is supplied by sensory and autonomic innovation seen by glyoxylic acid-induced fluorescence histochemistry of catecholaminergic nerve fibers and nerve fibers exhibiting cholinacetyltransferase immunoreactivity.[81] Bone also is highly innervated, as shown by the localization of substance P and neurokinin-1 receptors.[82] Osteoblasts and osteoclasts express glutamate receptors and transporters, as underscored by the bone loss induced by sciatic neurectomy resulting in decreased glutaminergic innervation.[83]

Nerve growth factor receptor antibody reacts with adventitial reticular cells.[84] Tachykinins have demonstrated stimulatory and inhibitory hematopoietic activities within the marrow microenvironment.[85] Substance P stimulates primitive hematopoietic progenitors[86] and CD34-positive cell proliferation by modulating stromal cell release of stem cell factor and cytokines such as IL-1,[85] IL-3, IL-6, granulocyte colony-stimulating factor (G-CSF), granulocyte-macrophage colony-stimulating factor (GM-CSF), and kit ligand.[87] Neurokinin-1 receptors for substance P are present on marrow vascular endothelium[88] and regulate blood flow and angiogenesis.[89] Mice with specific denervation have decreased marrow cellularity with increased circulating hematopoietic progenitors.[90] The sympathetic nervous system controls circadian fluctuations in circulating HSC numbers though its affect on the expression of the chemokine CXCL12 stromal-derived factor (SDF) 1α in the marrow.[91] Studies in mice with defective myelinization and mice treated with adrenergic antagonists or agonists indicate that the adrenergic nervous system in the marrow also regulates mobilization of HSCs by G-CSF.[92] Adrenergic neurotransmission in response to G-CSF suppresses osteoblast function, decreases release of CXCL12 from bone, and increases the circulating HSCs.[92]

SINUS ARCHITECTURE AND CELLULAR ORGANIZATION

In mammals, hematopoiesis occurs in the extravascular spaces between marrow sinuses. The sinus wall is composed of a luminal layer of endothelial cells and an abluminal coat of adventitial reticular cells, which forms an incomplete outer lining (Fig. 4–3). A thin, interrupted basement lamina is present between the cell layers. The endothelial cells and adventitial reticular cells provide a vascular/perivascular niche that is separate from the endosteal niche provided by the bone cells of the endosteum and from the stromal cells: adipocytes, macrophages, and lymphocytes.

Endothelial Cells

Endothelial cells are broad flat cells that completely cover the inner surface of the sinus.[93] They form the major barrier and control the system for chemicals and particles entering and leaving the hematopoietic spaces, with overlapping or interdigitating unions permitting volume expansion.[94] The endothelium of marrow sinusoids is actively endocytic and contains clathrin-coated pits, clathrin-coated vesicles, lysosomes, phagosomes, transfer tubules, and diaphragmed fenestrae.[95,96] Particles are endocytosed by endothelial cells primarily through clathrin-coated pits.[97] Such endocytic features are in accordance with studies demonstrating colony-stimulating factor receptors on endothelial cells[98] and their shared antigenic determinants with macrophages.[99,100] Marrow endothelial cells express von Willebrand factor antigen,[101] type IV collagen, and laminin.[102] They also constitutively express adhesion molecules: ICAM-3,[103] vascular cell adhesion molecule (VCAM)-1, and E-selectin.[104] The distribution of sialic acid and other carbohydrates on the luminal surface of marrow sinus endothelium is discontinued at diaphragmed fenestrae and coated pits, suggesting such sugars play a role in endothelial membrane function and cellular interactions.[97] *In vivo*, the conditional deletion in endothelial cells of gp130, the common receptor component for several cytokines including IL-6, leads to a hypocellular marrow as mice age.[105] The loss of gp130 from marrow endothelial cells affects the progenitor cell populations rather than the HSC leading to a lethal anemia, with normal platelets and a leukocytosis.[104] Marrow microvascular endothelium can be isolated using *Ulex europaeus* lectin[106] and CD34 monoclonal antibodies.[107]

Marrow endothelial cells via direct cell–cell contacts and secreted peptides uniquely influence osteoprogenitor cell differentiation[108,109] and regulate hematopoiesis by elaborating cytokines such as IL-5,[110] negative regulators thymosin β_4, AcSDKP,[111] and transforming growth factor-beta (TGF-β) antagonists such as B-type natriuretic peptide.[112] Reciprocal regulation of CD34 expression and adhesion molecules by vascular endothelial cells exposed to inflammatory stimuli such as IL-1, interferon-γ, and tumor necrosis factor-alpha (TNF-α) is observed.[113] Receptors for the complement component C1q are upregulated on marrow microvascular endothelium by inflammatory cytokines.[114] Endothelial cells regulate cellular trafficking into and out of the marrow sinusoidal spaces by altering their permeability and reorganizing their cytoskeleton by ICAM-3, by VE-cadherin–mediated cell–cell contacts,[103,115] and via specialized heparin sulfate proteoglycans,[116] CXCL12 bound to surface proteoglycans,[117] and other chemokines/chemokine receptors[118,119] such as fractalkine, a membrane-bound

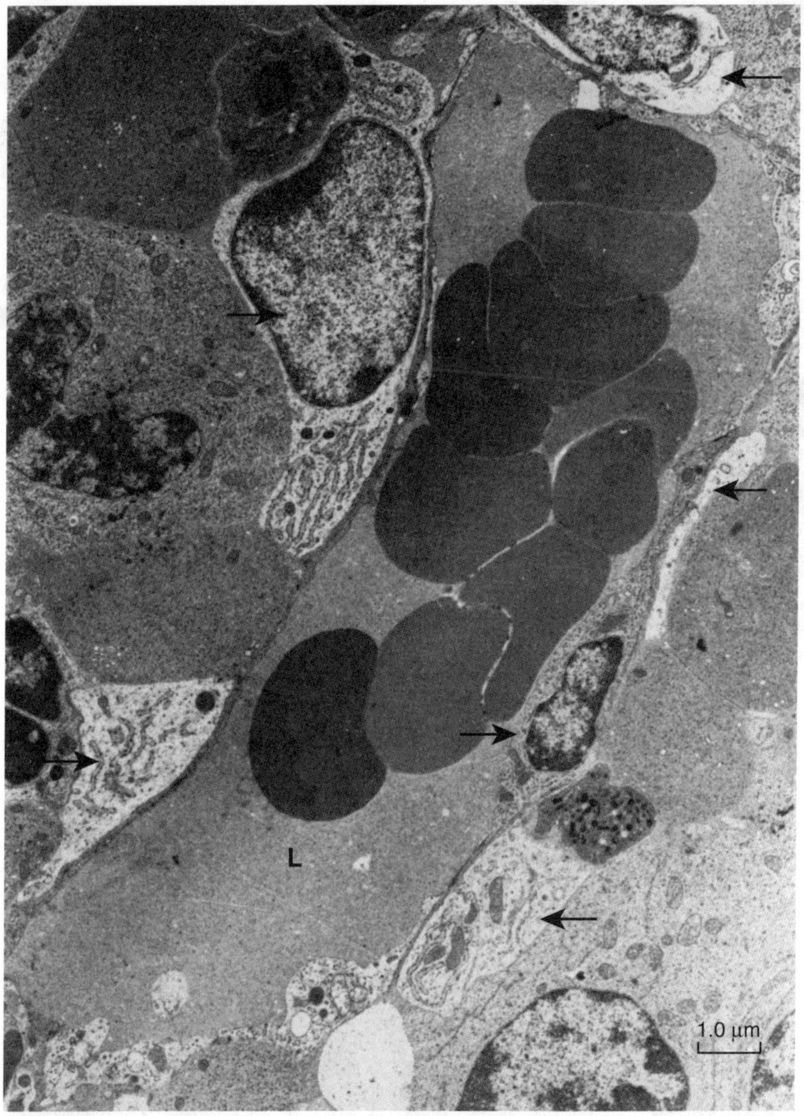

FIGURE 4–3. Transmission electron micrograph of a mouse marrow sinus. The *small arrow* in the sinus lumen (*L*) indicates the perikaryon of an endothelial cell. Several endothelial cell junctions are present along the circumference of the sinus endothelial wall. Thus, the wall is composed of the cytoplasm of endothelial cells that overlap or interdigitate. Two adventitial reticular cell bodies are identified by *arrows* at the top and upper left of the sinus. The cytoplasm of the adventitial reticular cells is discontinuous as it is followed around the sinus. Three cytoplasmic processes of adventitial reticular cells are indicated by *arrows*. Other, smaller processes of reticular cell cytoplasm are found upon close inspection of the sinus periphery and the hematopoietic spaces. The scattered rough endoplasmic reticulum and dense bodies are characteristic of the reticular cell cytoplasm. *(From Lichtman MA,[79] with permission.)*

chemokine with a mucin stalk expressed in activated vascular beds.[120] Marrow sinusoidal endothelium specifically expresses sialylated CD22 ligands, which are homing receptors for recirculating B lymphocytes.[121]

Adventitial Reticular Cells

The abluminal or adventitial surface of the vascular sinus is composed of reticular cells.[93,122,123] The reticular cell bodies are contiguous with the sinus, forming part of its adventitial coat (see Fig. 4–3). Their extensive branching cytoplasmic processes envelop the outer wall of the sinus to form an adventitial sheath. The sheath is interrupted and is estimated to cover approximately two-thirds of the abluminal surface area of sinuses. The reticular cells synthesize reticular (argentophilic) fibers that, with their cytoplasmic processes, extend into the hematopoietic compartments and form a meshwork on which hematopoietic cells rest (Figs. 4–4 and 4–5). The cell bodies, their broad processes, and their fibers constitute the reticulum of the marrow.

Adventitial reticular cells have a high concentration of alkaline phosphatase in their membranes, express CD10, CD13, and class I human leukocyte antigen (HLA) antigens,[135] react with the 6/19 and STRO-1 monoclonal antibodies,[124,125] and express all neurotrophin receptors including the low affinity nerve growth factor receptor (p75LNGFR) and the Trk receptors (TrkA, TrkB, and TrkC),[126] even though nerve growth factor is not a growth factor for STRO-1–derived stromal cells.[127] These adventitial reticular cells can differentiate along the smooth muscle pathway and contain α smooth-muscle actin, vimentin, laminin, fibronectin, and collagens I, III, and IV.[128,129] Unlike embryonic fibroblasts,[130] adventitial reticular cells usually are CD34-negative.[94,128,131] Stromal cells display cell–cell contacts via connexin-43 gap junctions, which are critical for normal hematopoiesis.[132,133] These gap junctions are localized to areas of adherence of stromal cells and hematopoietic cells in marrow recovering from cytotoxic injury.[134] The importance of direct cell–cell communication between progenitors and stromal cells remains unclear, because the hematopoietic capacity of connexin-43 wild-type and knockout fetal liver cells does not differ on wild-type stroma.[135] Marrow-derived stromal cell lines display heterogeneity at the molecular level (expression of cytokines such as SCF, thrombopoietin [TPO], and FLT3 ligand or differentiation regulatory genes such as human Jagged-1) and at the functional level (cobblestone formation, CD34+ cell proliferation), with variable expression of ICAM-1, VCAM-1, and collagens I, III, and IV.[136]

A population of reticular cells that express high amounts of CXCL12, termed CXCL12-abundant reticular (CAR) cells, are the major producers of CXCL12 in the marrow.[137] The majority of CAR cells are in close association with the sinusoidal endothelial cells but some are also associated with the endosteum. The CXCL12 produced by CAR cells is required for the normal development of HSC,[137] various differentiation stages of B-lymphocytes[138] and the plasmacytoid dendritic cells[139] that are all found in close physical association with CAR cells.

More specialized contractile reticular "barrier cells" have been described in mouse spleen and marrow after hematopoietic stress, such as malarial infection or administration of IL-1.[140] Barrier cells increase in number and seem to enclose developing hematopoietic progenitors in these animals. The cells may regulate the release of precursors into the circulation.[140] Human counterparts of barrier cells are α smooth-muscle–positive cells that appear in culture after 2 weeks and are represented by myoid cells lining sinuses at the abluminal side of endothelial cells in marrow biopsies.[128] These cells also have been described in fetal marrow and are increased in areas of active marrow proliferation after inflammation.[140]

Adipocytes

Adipocytes in marrow develop by lipogenesis in fibroblast-like cells, most likely the adventitial reticular cells (Fig. 4–6). Reticular cells in mouse and human marrow can undergo transformation to fat cells *in vitro* and can revert into fibroblasts in culture by lipolysis.[93,141] Marrow fat cells are relatively resistant to lipolysis during starvation. Their

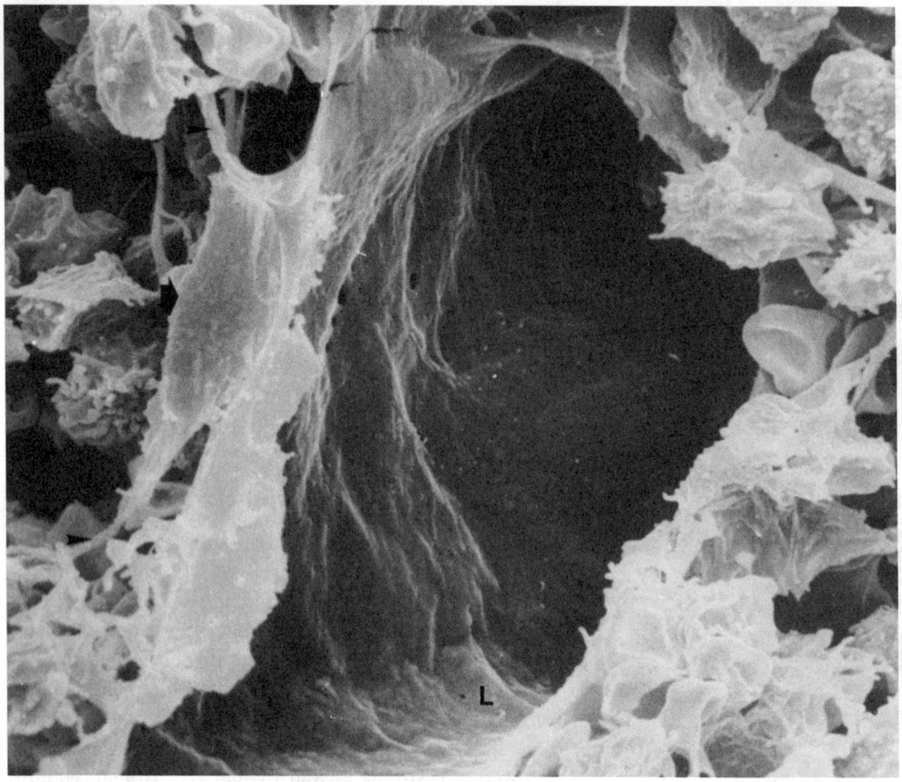

FIGURE 4–4. Scanning electron micrograph of rat marrow sinus. The floor of the lumen (*L*) is indicated. The *arrow on the left* indicates the cell body of an adventitial reticular cell, which is just beneath the endothelial cell layer. Reticular cell processes can be seen coursing between the sinus wall and the hematopoietic compartment (*small arrows*). *(From Lichtman MA,[79] with permission.)*

proportion of saturated fatty acids is lower than in other fat deposits, but their composition depends on whether they are located in red, hematopoietically active, or yellow, hematopoietically inactive, marrow.[141] Adipocytes express leptin, osteocalcin, and increased prolactin receptors during differentiation, thereby promoting hematopoiesis and influencing osteogenesis.[142–144] Adipocyte maturation *in vitro* is inhibited by stromal-derived cytokines such as IL-1 and IL-11.[145,146] Marrow brown fat[141] is a source of leptin[147] and an adipocyte-derived hormone adiponectin,[148] which inhibit preadipocyte differentiation and B lymphopoiesis while supporting myeloid hematopoietic progenitor growth *in vitro*.[149,150] This stromal-mediated inhibition of B-cell lymphopoiesis is mediated by activation of cyclooxygenase pathways and prostaglandin release.[151] Adiponectin, which is present at a low level in obesity, has antiangiogenic properties and induces apoptosis of endothelial cells.[152] Adipocyte differentiation by marrow stromal cells is modulated in a dose-dependent fashion by TGF-β[153] and bone morphogenetic proteins.[154,155] Other hormonal signaling pathways, such as the peroxisome proliferator-activated receptor gamma 2 (PPARγ2),[156] growth hormone,[157] 1,25-dihydroxy-vitamin $D_3(1,25(OH)_2D_3)$,[158] and estrogens,[159] also influence adipocyte differentiation, supporting the reciprocal regulation of osteogenesis and adipogenesis in the marrow microenvironment.[160]

Stromal Cells

Stromal cells obtained from animal or human marrow can be studied in cultures.[161] They presumably are derived from fibroblasts. They have unique phenotypic and functional characteristics that allow them to nurture hematopoietic development in highly specialized microenvironmental niches.[162] These cells express nerve growth factor receptor, VCAM-1, tenascin, endoglin, and collagens IV and VI, but they do not express intercellular adhesion molecules.[163] Unlike marrow fibroblasts, marrow stromal cells fail to upregulate collagenase when exposed to IL-1.[164] Stromal cells and cell lines differ in their capacities to support the growth of myeloid,[165,166] pro-B,[167,168] and T-cell precursors.[169] This hematopoietic nurturing function of stromal cells parallels growth factor expression such as FLT3 ligand,[170] KIT ligand,[171] TPO,[172] LIF,[173] IL-6 and soluble IL-6 receptor,[174,175] IL-7,[176] insulin-like growth factor I,[177] early acting growth-arrest-specific gene-6 (a ligand for the Axl, Sky, and Mer families of tyrosine kinases),[178] and chemokines.[179] Other interactions that regulate hematopoietic

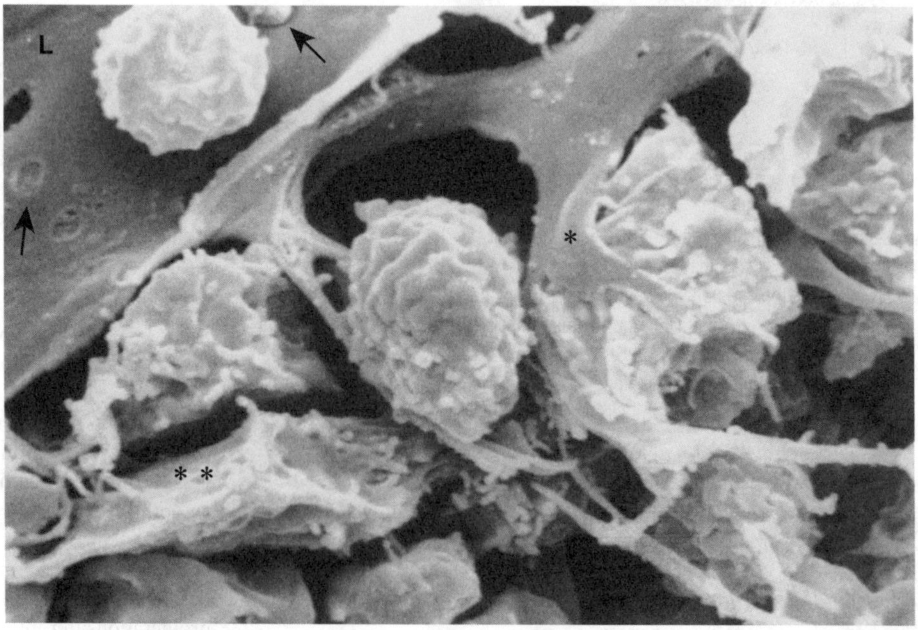

FIGURE 4–5. Scanning electron micrograph of rat femoral marrow sinus. The lumen (*L*) of an exposed sinus that has been cut open is indicated. The *single asterisk* indicates the process of an adventitial reticular cell and the intimate contact it makes with a hematopoietic cell. To the left of this process are adventitial reticular cell fibers, which form a scaffold for hematopoietic cells. The *double asterisk* identifies a portion of a reticular cell. The hole in the sinus floor is an artifact of preparation or a migration channel bereft of the emigrating cell. Empty spaces between cells and fibers are artifacts of preparation. The *arrow to the left* points to thin-walled fenestrae in the endothelial cytoplasm. The *arrow to the right* identifies the portion of a reticulocyte that may be penetrating the sinus wall, early in egress (see Fig. 4–8A).

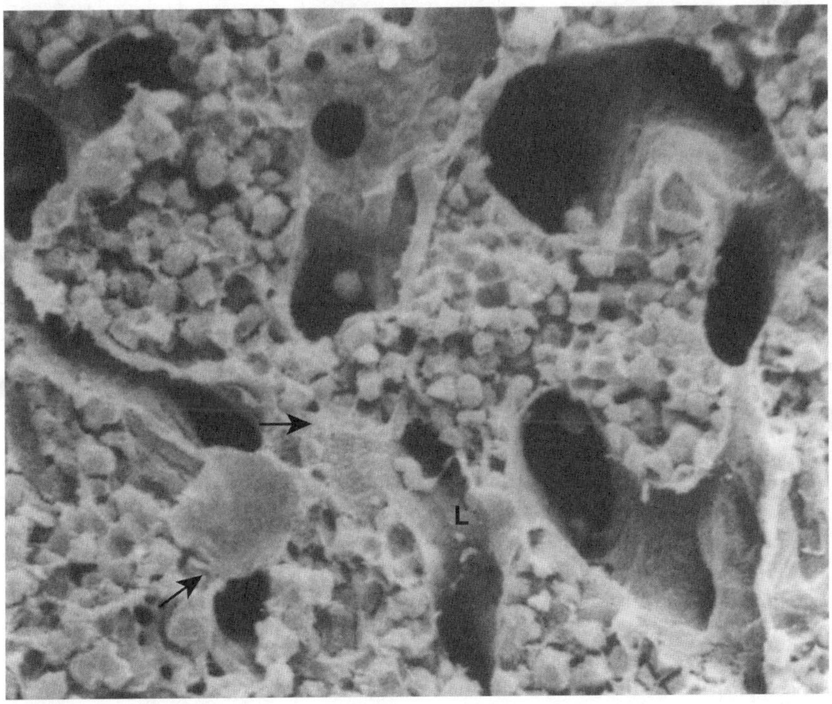

FIGURE 4–6. Scanning electron micrograph of rat femoral marrow. Several sinuses and the intervening hematopoietic cords are evident. The exposed lumen (*L*) of one branching sinus is indicated. The sinus, just above the *L*, contains a bean-shaped proplatelet with an attenuated strand connected to a separating smaller proplatelet fragment. Smaller proplatelet fragments are below the *L*. The *short horizontal arrow* points to the cytoplasm of a transected megakaryocyte. The *lower arrow* points to a fat cell. The rat femoral marrow contains a modest number of fat cells. Spaces in the hematopoietic cords are artifacts resulting from transecting the femur. *(From Lichtman MA,[79] with permission.)*

cell survival and differentiation are mediated by cell–cell contact via negative regulators of hematopoiesis such as TGF-β, which downregulates *c-KIT* expression[180]; the Notch/Jagged pathway, which inhibits myeloid differentiation[181]; specific receptors (e.g., WNT protein family[182] or angiogenins such as neuropilin-1[183]); and adhesion molecules (MUC18, CD164, hematopoietic cell antigen [HCA]) on stromal cells and hematopoietic CD34-positive cells.[184–186] Stromal cells produce nerve growth factor[187] and express neuronal markers[188] and brain natriuretic peptide, a potent vasodilator. These functions underscore their versatile differentiating capacity and crucial role in repair mechanisms.[189] Human stromal cells and cell lines *in vitro* activate CD14+ monocytes to secrete osteopontin (a matrix-associated glycoprotein important for T-cell activation)[190] and chemokines (CXCL1/growth-related oncogene [GROα], and CXCL7/neutrophil-activating protein [NAP]-2).[191] Osteopontin, in turn, downregulates Notch-1 gene expression in CD34+ cells,[191] modifying Notch-1/Jagged-1 signaling and their capacity to expand and differentiate.[192] The stromal cell-derived membrane protein mKirre (a mammalian homologue of the genkirre of *Drosophila melanogaster*) encodes a type Ia membrane protein that is cleaved by metalloproteinases and supports via its extracellular domain HSCs in a murine stromal cell line (OP9).[193] Another example of cellular interactions between adipocytes and stromal cells involves a transmembrane protein with epidermal growth factor-like repeat motifs dlk (delta-like)[194] that inhibits stromal cell adipogenesis and promotes cobblestone-area colony formation, bypassing the IL-7 requirement for B lymphopoiesis. This function implies the complexity and redundancy of microenvironmental signals regulating hematopoiesis.[195,196]

Bone Cells

Osteoblasts, osteoclasts, and elongated flat cells with a spindle-shaped nucleus form the marrow endosteal lining.[197] Resting endosteal cells express vimentin, tenascin, α smooth-muscle actin, osteocalcin, CD51, and CD56. They do not react with antibodies to CD3, CD15, CD20, CD34, CD45, CD68, or CD117.[198] Enriched CD56-positive, CD45-negative, CD34-negative endosteal cells grown in the presence of cytokines (insulin growth factor I, basic fibroblast growth factor [bFGF], kit ligand, IL-3, GM-CSF) do not give rise to hematopoietic cells, which suggests they are not totipotent mesenchymal stem cells in these culture conditions.[198] Cultured human bone cells have high levels of the integrins $\alpha_1\beta_1$, $\alpha_3\beta_1$, $\alpha_5\beta_1$, and $\alpha_v\beta_5$.[199] Endosteal cells are a rich source of stem cells (using the *in vivo* colony-forming unit–spleen [CFU-S] assay; see Chap. 16)[200] and provide a homing niche for newly transplanted early HSC expressing hyaluronic acid.[201] Mesenchymal stem cells positive for the STRO-1 antibody can differentiate into adipocyte, chondrocytic, and osteogenic cells.[202–204] Similar osteogenic potential is found in STRO-1–positive vascular pericytes.[205] Mesenchymal stem cell to osteogenic differentiation is associated with loss of the activated leukocyte adhesion molecule (CD166).[206]

Osteoblasts

Osteoblasts have three major functions: formation of new bone by regulating the secretion of the bone matrix proteins, regulation of bone resorption via osteoclast activity, and regulation of the hematopoietic environment mainly by their secretion of cytokines that affect HSC. Hematopoietic cells and osteoblasts are derived from a common marrow progenitor after marrow transplantation.[207] Bone-forming osteoblast progenitor cells, like stromal precursors, reside in the CD34-negative, STRO-1–positive nonadherent marrow cell population.[208,209] The differentiation of mesenchymal cells into either osteoblasts or adipocytes is related to the relative activities of Rux2 and PPARγ, respectively.[210] With aging, the sensitivity to PPARγ appears to increase, contributing to the increase in adipose tissue in the marrow found with older age.[210] BMP-2,[211] bFGF,[212] hepatocyte growth factor (HGF),[213] parathyroid hormone[13] and endothelin-1[214] promote osteoblast growth, whereas TGF-β[215] and osterix[216] affect their differentiation.[208,215] Osteoblasts expand early hematopoietic progenitor survival in long-term cultures and secrete hematopoietic growth factors such as macrophage colony-stimulating factor (M-CSF), G-CSF, GM-CSF, IL-1, and IL-6.[217,218] Osteoblasts also produce various cytokines such as hematopoietic cell-cycle inhibitory factors TGF-β,[219] osteopontin,[220] and CXCL12,[13,92] as well as cell-cycle stimulatory factor Dickkopf-1,[221] which may contribute to their intimate role in stem cell regulation within the marrow microenvironment. These cells can be transplanted in nonablated mice[222] and facilitate engraftment of purified allogeneic HSC, which is in keeping with their ability to support hematopoiesis.[223] Subcapsular renal explants of bone can form a suitable hematopoietic microenvironment for early stem cells, underscoring the potential for osteoblasts to nurture hematopoiesis.[224] Direct cell–cell communication has been shown in marrow and in osteoblastic cell networks,[225] indicating a potential regulatory role for these anatomical gap junctions in hematopoiesis.[132,133] *In vivo*, the size of stem cell niches increases after osteoblastic expansion and Notch activation in transgenic models.[12,13]

In another model, intramedullary hematopoiesis and stem cell numbers are severely diminished following *in vivo* ablation of osteoblasts,[226] underscoring the importance of this cell type to the marrow hematopoietic inductive microenvironment.[227]

Osteoclasts

Mature osteoclasts are multinucleated giant cells derived from fusion of progenitor cells of the monocyte/macrophage lineage of the HSC.[228] The mature osteoclasts resorb and remodel bone, regulate osteoblast activity, and help control the HSC entry into and exit from the marrow.[221,229,230] The osteoclasts have motile and resorptive phases. They require the Wiskott-Aldrich syndrome protein during clustering and fusion of actin-based adhesion structures named *podosomes*.[231] Podosomes are involved in the formation of specific structures termed *sealing zones* in which actin rings surround an area of ruffled plasma membrane at the face of the endosteal bone. Within these sealing zones the osteoclasts secrete hydrochloric acid and digestive enzymes that resorb bone. Osteoclasts also can be derived from pro-B cells, as shown by Pax-5 knockout mice, which have increased osteoclasts and severe osteopenia.[232] When osteoclast activity or number are reduced or eliminated in mice through null mutations or homologous recombination, the marrow cavities fail to form resulting in osteopetrosis. From analyses of various osteopetrotic mice, proteins required for osteoclast differentiation were identified. These proteins include the macrophage transcription factor PU.1; the secreted and surface displayed cytokine M-CSF of stromal cells and its receptor c-FMS on osteoclasts; the transcription factor c-FOS; the osteoblast and stromal cell surface protein receptor activator of NF-κB ligand (RANKL); its osteoclast receptor RANK, the signaling transducer tumor necrosis factor (TNF) receptor-associated factor 6 (TRAF 6); the downstream transcription factor NF-κB, and nuclear factor of activated T cells (NFAT).[230,233,234] Other osteopetrotic mice strains have deficiency of proteins required for the bone resorption function of osteoclasts. These proteins include the β_3 component of the $\alpha_v\beta_3$ (vitronectin receptor) required for binding of the osteoclast sealing zone to bone; c-Src signaling protein; the proton transporting H^+ adenosine triphosphatase (ATPase) and chloride channel protein required for HCl secretion; and the secreted osteoclast proteins cathepsin K, matrix metalloproteinases, and TRAP that digest the bone matrix.[229,230,234]

Osteoblast/stromal cells regulate differentiation of osteoclasts through intimate cell–cell contacts. They are found in direct apposition to osteoclasts with coated pit formation, suggesting accumulation of receptor–ligand complexes in endocytic vesicles.[235,236] In areas of active bone remodeling, osteoblasts and osteoclasts are separated from the rest of the marrow in bone-remodeling compartments that are covered with a flat monolayer of cells with osteoblast markers.[237] The recruitment of the osteoblasts and osteoclasts appears to be through capillaries associated with the remodeling compartment.[238] A major regulatory mechanism by which osteoblasts and osteoclasts interact is the RANK/RANKL/osteoprotegerin (OPG) system of signaling.[238] Osteoclast differentiation and maturation require the signaling cascade from RANK on the cell surface through TRAF 6, NF-κB, and NFAT.[235] Osteoblasts and their progenitor cells display RANKL on their surfaces, and binding of RANKL to the RANK on the osteoclasts and their progenitors promotes differentiation and activation of the osteoclasts. Osteoblasts also secrete OPG, a decoy receptor for RANKL, which inactivates RANKL by binding to the active site of RANKL, thereby preventing its binding to RANK. As a result, osteoclastic activity is decreased when OPG concentrations are high and increased when they are low.[239] Another signaling mechanism by which osteoclasts and osteoblasts reciprocally regulate the differentiation and activities of each other is the ephrinB2-EphB4 signaling system.[240] Osteoclasts express ephrinB2 on their surfaces while the osteoblasts express EphB4, a member of the receptor tyrosine kinase (RTK) family, that is the receptor for ephrinB2. Binding of ephrinB2-EphB4 results in bidirectional signaling in which osteoclast differentiation is decreased though suppression of the c-FOS–NFATc1 activity, whereas osteoblast differentiation is increased by EphB4 signaling.[240]

Osteoclasts produce HGF and express c-Met, the HGF receptor, implying a paracrine and autocrine regulatory pathway between them and adjoining osteoblasts.[213,241] Similarly, blocking expression of cadherin-6 interferes with heterotypic interactions between osteoclasts and stromal cells, impairing their ability to support osteoclast formation.[242] CD9, a tetraspanin transmembrane adhesion protein on stromal cells,[243] influences myelopoiesis in long-term marrow cultures.[244] Inhibition of stromal cell CD9-mediated signaling by a blocking antibody reduces osteoclast differentiation factor transcription, leading to reduced osteoclastogenesis.[245] Macrophage-stimulating protein, a HGF-like protein, signals through the stem cell-derived tyrosine kinase, a member of the HGF receptor family. It also stimulates osteoclast bone-resorbing activity by enhanced cytoskeletal reorganization without affecting proliferation of osteoclast precursors.[246,247] Osteoclast differentiation is influenced by monocytes expressing ADAM-8 (CD156), a protein of the disintegrin and metalloproteinase family,[248] and eosinophil chemotactic factor-L (ECFL),[249] characterizing complex cell–cell, cell adhesion protein, stromal cell cytokine, and chemokine signals within the marrow microenvironment.

■ MACROPHAGES, LYMPHOCYTES, AND PLASMA CELLS

Macrophages, including monocyte-derived, antigen-presenting dendritic cells, and lymphocytes, including T, natural killer (NK), B, and plasma cells, arise from the HSC and form part of the marrow microenvironment through growth factor production (IL-3, CCL3) and cell–cell interactions with developing progenitors.[79,93,250–253] *In vivo*, lymphocytes and macrophages concentrate around arterial vessels, near the center of the hematopoietic cords. Macrophages[254] and lymphocytes[255] are an integral part of the adherent monolayer found in long-term lymphohematopoietic cultures. Mature T and B lymphocytes and plasma cells are found near foci of granulopoiesis in the adherent layers of long-term cultures in humans.[256] Marrow stroma can support thymocyte differentiation,[257] and an early T-cell progenitor maturation pathway occurs in the marrow.[258] Stromal cells facilitate the maturation of NK cells,[259] an effect likely mediated by stromal-derived FLT3 ligand and IL-15.[260] Within the marrow, both NK cells and CD8+ memory T cells require the coordinated expression of secreted IL-15 and surface IL-15 receptors by other marrow cells for their survival and development.[261] Marrow stroma regulates B lymphopoiesis by different stromal cell niches and homing receptors (VCAM-1) and by production of cytokines such as FLT3 ligand, KIT ligand, IL-7, and TGF-β.[262–264] Mature B and T lymphocytes in the marrow are in contact with a specific set of monocyte-derived, antigen-presenting dendritic cells that are clustered around the blood vessels.[265] These dendritic cells produce macrophage migration-inhibition factor, a cytokine required for survival of mature B lymphocytes that have matured in secondary lymphoid organs and re-circulated to the marrow.[265]

A marrow niche that controls B lymphopoiesis has been reported.[266] In this niche, the stromal cells expressing VCAM-1 and CXCL12, which have direct contact with the HSC, are also in contact with the earliest progenitors the B-cell lineage, the prepro-B cells. The next stage of differentiation, the pro-B cells, is not found near the CXCL12-producing cells, but instead have contact with the marrow stromal cells that produce IL-7. The subsequent stage, the pre-B cell phase, is not in contact with either the IL-7- or CXCL12-producing cells. The stages after the pre-B cell occur after the cells enter the blood and seed the lymphoid follicles of the secondary lymphoid organs, mainly spleen and lymph nodes. From these lymphoid organs, the cells then reenter the blood as B lymphocytes or immature plasma cells. The immature plasma cells that have differentiated in the spleen and will become the long-lived plasma cells home to the marrow, where they are located in contact with CXCL12-producing stromal cells. A negative feedback is completed as the mature plasma cells compete with the prepro-B cells for sites on the CXCL12-producing stromal cells or directly induce apoptosis of the prepro-B cells.[267] In addition, to its role as site of early T-lymphocyte development, the marrow acts a secondary organ for the proliferation of mature CD8 and CD4 memory T lymphocytes. Although no specific organized structure or niche has been found for these T lymphocytes, they can represent up to 4 percent of nucleated cells in the marrow that they reenter by migrating through the sinusoidal endothelium from the blood.[268]

Stromal cells elaborate and respond to protein growth factors, such as platelet-derived growth factor (PDGF).[269] PDGF upregulates M-CSF secretion by stromal cells, establishing a paracrine stimulatory loop between the two cell types.[270] Addition of PDGF to macrophages expressing PDGF receptors upregulates IL-1 secretion and thereby activates primitive hematopoietic cells.[271] Macrophages also modulate the structure and composition of the extracellular matrix and its fibronectin content.[272] Marrow macrophage phenotype[273] is regulated by adjoining stromal cell–accessory cell–derived colony-stimulating factors and cytokines,[274] such as M-CSF upregulation of $\alpha_4\beta_1$- and $\alpha_5\beta_1$-integrin expression[275] and FLT3 ligand-promoting macrophage outgrowth with B-cell–associated antigens.[276]

Macrophages are an integral component of the local microenvironment and regulate hematopoiesis via a complex array of dual-acting stem cell stimulatory and inhibitory factors, such as IL-1, CCL3, TNF-α, and TGF-β.[277–281] Stromal cells and accessory cells are needed for optimum hematopoietic cell development.[282] Signals regulating the pluripotential HSCs are not entirely defined but require intimate cell–cell contact for signaling through cytokine–chemokine receptors, integrin receptors, alone or together with heparan sulfate or chondroitin sulfate-containing glycoproteins. This regulatory paradigm is underscored by several studies: (1) A neutralizing antibody to c-KIT, although able to abrogate myelopoiesis in stromal–stem cell cocultures, did not affect stem cell survival.[283] (2) Stromal-cell-derived BMPs (BMP-2, BMP-4, BMP-7) regulate the proliferation and differentiation of CD34-positive, CD38-negative, lineage-negative cells, with high amounts of BMP-2 and BMP-7 inhibiting proliferation and maintaining repopulating capacity, whereas BMP-4 at higher concentrations extends the survival of these repopulating cells *ex vivo*.[284] (3) Several adhesion receptors of the sialomucin family mediate inhibitory signals to limit stem cell expansion or differentiation.[285] (4) Direct contact of enriched CD34-positive, lineage-negative cells and stroma induces a soluble factor that increases primitive hematopoietic cell production.[286]

EXTRACELLULAR MATRIX

Mesenchymal cells forming the cellular stroma in marrow are active in laying down a rich carpet of extracellular matrix proteins (ECMs),[287] such as proteoglycans or glycosaminoglycans (GAGs),[287,288] fibronectin,[287,289] tenascin,[287,290] collagen,[287,290] laminin,[290] hemonectin,[291] and thrombospondin (TSP).[287,292] Localizing signals are provided by stromal–ECM hematopoietic cell adhesive interactions,[293,294] in concert with chemokines[295] and cytokines, bound to heparin-like structures in the GAGs.[296] The binding of specific cytokines may enhance the activity of a cytokine if the GAG-binding site does not interfere with the site that binds the cytokine receptor, whereas GAG-binding sites that overlap or interfere with a cytokine receptor-binding site can inhibit the cytokine function.[297] These interactions form specialized niches that may facilitate lymphocytic (B and T) or lineage-specific development along the erythroid, myeloid, or megakaryocytic pathways.[298,299] Other functions of these niches include stem cell survival[300] and quiescence.[298,301] Table 4–1 lists the cytokines that are presented on the surface of stromal cells and matrix-binding chemokines and cytokines.[296,302–314] Sl/Sl[d] mice that have a deficient hematopoietic microenvironment as a result of a deficiency in KIT ligand[315] processing or membrane presentation are anemic and have altered extracellular matrix composition.[316]

TABLE 4–1. Cell Membrane Presentation and Matrix Association of Cytokines and Chemokines

Cell Membrane	Matrix Association
Chemokine	*Chemokine*
Fractalkine	RANTES, PF-4, IP-10, IL-8
	Macrophage inflammatory proteins (MIP-1α, MIP-1β)
	CXCL12/stromal cell-derived growth factor-1 (SDF-1α, SDF-1β)
	Monocyte chemoattractant protein-1 (MCP-1)
Cytokine	*Cytokine*
c-KIT ligand	Granulocyte-macrophage colony-stimulating factor
Tumor necrosis factor alpha (TNF-α)	Interferon gamma (IFN-γ)
Interleukin-1 (IL-1)	Leukemia inhibitory factor (LIF)
Macrophage colony-stimulating factor (M-CSF)	Interleukins (IL-1α, IL-1β, IL-2, IL-3, IL-4, IL-5, IL-6, IL-7, IL-12)
	Basic fibroblast growth factor (bFGF)
Transforming growth factor alpha (TGF-α)	Hepatocyte growth factor (HGF)
	Transforming growth factor beta (TGF-β; binding to endoglin and heparan sulfate)

IP-10, interferon-inducible protein 10; PF-4, platelet factor 4; RANTES, regulated upon activation normal T-cell expressed and secreted.

In long-term marrow cultures, collagen, fibronectin, and laminin are secreted early, and extracellular deposition of these proteins coincides with active hematopoiesis.[316] Antibodies to GM-CSF stain adipocyte membranes.[317] Cultures actively generating granulocyte-macrophage precursors produce M-CSF, GM-CSF, and, to a lesser extent, KIT ligand and G-CSF within the adherent layer.[318] GM-CSF, G-CSF, and bFGF are detected on the surface of endothelial cells and fibroblasts. GM-CSF localizes to the extracellular matrix, as shown by double labeling of heparan sulfate proteoglycans and GM-CSF.[319] Negative regulators such as TGF-β exert their effects early on long-term marrow cultures by limiting megakaryocyte progenitor and stem cell expansion.[320]

Proteoglycans

Proteoglycans are polyanionic macromolecules (heparan sulfate, dermatan, chondroitin sulfate, hyaluronic acid) that are distributed on the surface of adventitial reticular cells and within the extracellular matrix.[287,321] Heparan sulfate is the main cell-surface GAG in long-term marrow cultures, and chondroitin sulfate is the major secreted species.[316,322] D-xylosides, which stimulate artificial sulfated GAG synthesis, increase chondroitin sulfate synthesis and hematopoietic cell production.[322] Hyaluronic acid and chondroitin sulfate-containing proteoglycans are prominent in the adherent and nonadherent compartments of long-term marrow cultures.[321] Heparin-containing and heparan sulfate-containing proteoglycans interact with laminin and type IV collagen[323] and may play a role in cell–cell interactions, cytokine presentation, and cell differentiation.[324–327] They also mediate progenitor cell binding to stroma and other extracellular matrix molecules such as fibronectin.[328–332]

Another important lymphocyte–progenitor cell–associated proteoglycan, CD44, uses hyaluronate as a ligand and promotes stromal adhesive interactions.[255,333] A binding site for lymphocyte CD44 on the carboxy-terminal heparin-binding domain of fibronectin is present,[334] and neutralizing antibodies to CD44 inhibit hematopoiesis in long-term marrow cultures.[335] Cytokines (GM-CSF, IL-3, KIT ligand) rapidly induce CD44 expression and increase CD44-mediated adhesion of CD34-positive hematopoietic progenitors to hyaluronan.[336] Chondroitin sulfates A and B mediate monocyte and B-cell activation via a CD44-dependent pathway.[337] Hyaluronate, the CD44 ligand, enhances hematopoiesis by releasing IL-1 (CD44-dependent) and IL-6 (CD44-independent pathway), supporting the important role of this proteoglycan receptor in hematopoiesis.[338]

Heparan sulfate mediates IL-7–dependent lymphopoiesis[311] and modulates hematopoiesis and stromal cell–matrix remodeling[339] by anchoring HGF[312,340] and bFGF.[339,341,342] Marrow stromal cell-surface heparan sulfate-containing proteoglycans consist mainly of syndecan-3, syndecan-4, and glypican-1. The major extracellular matrix-associated form is perlecan.[343] Syndecan-3 is expressed in marrow stromal cells as a variant form with a core protein of 50 to 55 kDa, suggesting syndecan-3 plays a role in hematopoiesis.[343] Perlecan promotes bFGF receptor binding and mitogenesis and can bind GM-CSF.[337,344] Heparan sulfate expression is induced on the cell surface in early erythroid differentiation of multipotential HSC.[345] Glypican-4, another member of this family, is found on marrow stromal cells and progenitor cells.[346] Syndecan-1 expression in B lymphoid cells is reduced by IL-6, which implies similar regulatory pathways in other cell types.[347] Biglycan, a matrix glycoprotein SC1, with homology to osteonectin, and the molecule SIM selectively increase IL-7–dependent proliferation of B cells.[348] Interactions of B cells with other components of the immune system are mediated by syndecan-4, which facilitates the formation of dendritic processes[349] and regulates focal adhesion, stress fiber formation, and cell migration.[350] Together, these observations underscore the major contribution of proteoglycans in the formation of specialized microenvironmental niches to promote lineage-specific hematopoiesis.

Fibronectin

Fibronectin localizes at sites of attachment of hematopoietic cells and marrow stromal cells *in vitro*,[289,351] and at sites of interaction between these cells and developing granulocytes or monocytes.[352] Early erythroid progenitors attach to the cell-binding domain of fibronectin.[353,354] This association can be inhibited by blocking antibodies to the fibronectin integrin receptors $\alpha_5\beta_1$ and $\alpha_4\beta_1$.[355] Adhesion of hematopoietic progenitor cells to stroma is partly mediated by fibronectin.[328,356] This binding can be enhanced by protein kinase C activators such as phorbol esters, suggesting the involvement of integrin receptors in the process.[357–359] The alternatively spliced form of fibronectin (type III connecting segment [IIICS]) is expressed uniquely within the marrow microenvironment[359] and associates with the $\alpha_4\beta_1$-integrin receptor on HSC.[360] Additional IIICS fibronectin variants have been detected in marrow stroma, providing for a fine control using messenger RNA splicing of progenitor–stem cell interactions.[361] Fibronectin adhesion to peptide domains, such as the CS1 domain (which activates α_4 integrins) or stromal cells, has dual effects of stimulation and inhibition of hematopoietic progenitor growth.[362–365]

The integrins very-late antigen (VLA)-4 and -5 ($\alpha4\beta1$ and $\alpha5\beta1$) and CD44 cooperate to promote fibronectin adhesive interactions.[362,366–368] Cytokines such as IL-3, KIT ligand, and TPO augment the magnitude of fibronectin-mediated hematopoietic progenitor cell adhesion and migration.[369–372] Fibronectin facilitates maturation of CD34-positive progenitor-derived dendritic cells[373] and is involved in adhesion of mature cells, including megakaryocytes,[374,375] mast cells,[376] chemokine-activated T lymphocytes,[377] eosinophils,[378] and neutrophils.[379] Fibronectin is required for expression of gelatinase in macrophages[380] and regulates cytokine release by M-CSF–activated macrophages[381] and chondrocytes.[382] These interactions of fibronectin and its integrin counterreceptors on hematopoietic cells are associated with activation of the sodium–hydrogen exchanger and result in improved cell survival or stimulation.[383]

Tenascin

Tenascin is an extracellular matrix glycoprotein family consisting of three members: tenascin-C, tenascin-R (restrictin), and tenascin-X.[290,384] Tenascin-C is expressed on the surface of stromal cells in the marrow. Like fibronectin and collagen III, tenascin-C is found in the microenvironment surrounding maturing hematopoietic cells.[287,385] In a long-term marrow culture system (Whitlock-Witte), thiol 2-mercaptoethanol induced expression of tenascin-C and improved lymphoid-lineage differentiation.[386] Glucocorticoids, on the other hand, promote myeloid differentiation in long-term marrow cultures and downregulate tenascin expression.[387] Tenascin-C has distinct functional domains that promote hematopoietic cell adhesion to stroma or extracellular matrix proteins or mediate a strong mitogenic signal to marrow mononuclear cells.[388] In tenascin-C–deficient mutant mice, the colony-forming capacity of marrow is markedly decreased.[389] Long-term marrow cultures from these tenascin-deficient animals result in decreased progenitor cell output.[389] Addition of tenascin-C to these cultures restores hematopoietic cell production.[389] Mutant tenascin-C–deficient animals also display decreased fibronectin in their marrow, suggesting a possible mechanistic interaction between tenascin-C and fibronectin in the marrow microenvironment.[390] These studies underscore the important role of extracellular matrix proteins such as fibronectin and tenascin-C in hematopoiesis.

Collagen

Collagen types I and III are associated with microvascular walls, whereas collagen type IV is confined to basal lamina beneath endothelial cells.[100,216,391] Marrow-derived capillary networks grow in collagen gel cultures,[392] and inhibition of collagen synthesis reduces hematopoiesis *in vitro*,[393] highlighting the importance of the underlying matrix in reconstituting an intact hematopoietic microenvironment.[394] Erythroid and granulocytic progenitors adhere to collagen type I *in vitro*,[395] and a low-molecular-weight collagen has been described in lithium-stimulated marrow cultures,[396] emphasizing the effects of induction on matrix composition and stromal support of hematopoiesis.[397] Marrow-derived fibroblasts and stromal cells synthesize collagens I, III, IV, V, and VI.[398] Collagen VI is a strong cytoadhesive component of the marrow microenvironment. Collagen VI binds von Willebrand factor.[399] Collagen type XIV, another fibril-associated collagen, promotes hematopoietic cell adhesion of myeloid and lymphoid cell lines.[400] Collagen-induced, intracellular calcium-mediated signaling events occur in megakaryocytes (see Chap. 113).[401] *In situ* immunolocalization of ECMs in murine marrow showed that collagen types I and IV and fibronectin localize to the endosteum.[402]

The distinct spatial distribution of these matrix proteins indicates their role in the preferential homing of engrafted HSC to marrow.[201]

Laminin

Laminin is a multidomain glycoprotein with mitogenic and adhesive sites. It is a major component of the extracellular matrix and basement membranes.[316,403] Because laminin interacts with collagen type IV and basement membrane components such as proteoglycans and entactin,[404] it can regulate leukocyte chemotaxis.[405,406] Similarly, CD34-positive granulocytic progenitors,[407] mature monocytes,[408] and neutrophils[409] adhere to laminin. Its role within the cytomatrix may be to strengthen adhesive interactions with $\alpha_5\beta_1$ (VLA-5) and $\alpha_6\beta_1$ (VLA-6) on hematopoietic cells.[410] Laminin, in combination with fibronectin *in vitro*, can expand both HSCs and several more differentiated progenitors.[411] Laminins are composed of α, β, and γ polypeptides. Laminin-1 ($\alpha_1\beta_1\gamma_1$) is not expressed in marrow, which expresses laminin-2 ($\alpha_2\beta_1\gamma_1$), laminin-8 ($\alpha_4\beta_1\gamma_1$), and laminin-10 ($\alpha_5\beta_1\gamma_1$).[412] Stromal cells in cultures and cytokine-expanded CD34-positive cells also express laminin β_2, which is found in the pericellular space in marrow and intracellularly in megakaryocytes.[413,414] Laminin-γ_2 chain expression is unique to marrow-derived stromal cells. It colocalizes with α smooth-muscle actin in marrow and is not expressed in endothelial cells or megakaryocytes.[415]

Integrins $\alpha_6\beta_1$ and $\alpha_6\beta_4$ are receptors for laminin-10/11 and laminin-8.[416] Laminin-10/11 ($\alpha_5\beta_1\gamma_1/\gamma_5\beta_2\gamma_1$) and fibronectin bind CD34-positive and CD34-positive CD38-negative progenitors, whereas laminin-8 ($\alpha_4\beta_1\gamma_1$) and laminin-10/11 facilitate CXCL12–stimulated transmigration of CD34-positive cells.[416] In mouse repopulation studies, specific antibodies that block the α_6 components of these laminin receptors decreased the homing of HSCs and of colony-forming unit–granulocyte-macrophage (CFU-GM).[417] Furthermore, when combined with antibodies to the α_4 component of integrins, they synergized in decreasing the homing of the short-term, multipotent repopulating cells. In contrast to this role of these integrin receptors in the homing of HSC, a 67-kDa, nonintegrin laminin receptor is appears to be upregulated in HSCs following G-CSF stimulation and plays a significant role in the mobilization.[418] This 67-kDa, nonintegrin receptor for laminin, also found on erythroid progenitor and precursor cells, has a role in the homing of burst-forming unit–erythroid (BFU-E), progenitors that circulate in the blood and to the marrow.[419] $\alpha_6\beta_1$ mediates mast cell adhesion to laminin,[420] whereas the Lutheran blood group glycoproteins on the late-stage erythroid cells serve as receptors for the α_5 integrin component of laminins.[421] Laminin promotes the M-CSF–dependent proliferation of marrow-derived macrophages and macrophage cell lines. This effect is partially mediated via an α_6-integrin subunit.[422]

Thrombospondin

The thrombospondins (TSPs) are a small family of secreted matricellular glycoproteins that modulate cell function by altering cell–matrix interactions.[423] Thrombospondin-1 (TSP1) is a 450-kDa multifunctional extracellular matrix protein, initially identified in platelet α granules. TSP1 has domains that interact with collagen and fibronectin and may participate in stem cell lodgement.[424] Receptors on hematopoietic and nonhematopoietic cells can interact with TSP, including CD36[425] and the CLA-1 protein of the CD36/LIMP II gene family.[426] Perlecan mediates the binding of TSP to endothelial cells.[427] The TSP receptor CD36 is expressed during erythroid (CFU-E [colony-forming unit–erythroid] stage) and megakaryocytic maturation.[428] TSP binds to matrix heparan sulfates[233] and inhibits *in vitro* megakaryopoiesis via CD36.[429] Mature megakaryocytes require thrombospondin-2 (TSP2) for normal hemostasis, as shown in mice lacking TSP2.[430] TSP2 is a matrix-associated protein necessary for the release of functionally competent platelets by megakaryocytes. TSP2 is taken up in an integrin-dependent manner from the marrow milieu, illustrating another important function of this matricellular protein.[430] TSP has a stimulatory effect on NK cells by activating latent TGF-β.[431,432] All-*trans*-retinoic acid-induced granulocytic differentiation of HL-60 cells is associated with increased TSP secretion. The process is delayed by a blocking anti-TSP antibody.[433] TSP decreases the proliferation and promotes the differentiation of HL-60 cells; these effects are not mediated by latent TGF-β activation.[433] A 140-kDa fragment of TSP1 binds bFGF, and TSP1 acts as a scavenger for matrix-associated angiogenic factors (fibroblast growth factor [FGF]2, VEGF, HGF), underscoring its antiangiogenic properties.[434,435] Endothelial cell TSP expression is inhibited by proangiogenic inflammatory cytokines such as IL-1 and TNF-α.[436] TSP stimulates matrix metalloproteinase-9 activity in endothelial cells[437] and is chemotactic to monocytes[438] and neutrophil-like HL-60 cells.[439]

Vitronectin

Vitronectin, also known as *serum-spreading factor*, is a 75-kDa protein present in plasma, platelets, and connective tissue.[282] Vitronectin, a major cytoadhesive glycoprotein, binds to the specific integrin $\alpha_v\beta_3$ receptor (CD51) on fibroblasts, endothelial cells, mature hematopoietic cells,[440] including platelets and megakaryocytes,[441] mast cells,[442] and bone cells[443] such as osteoblasts and osteoclasts.[444,445] The vitronectin receptor CD51($\alpha_V\beta_3$) cooperates with c-FMS in osteoclast differentiation[446] and contributes to cell fusion and bone resorption in osteoclasts stimulated by TGF-β.[447] The integrin $\alpha_V\beta_3$ is expressed on monocyte-macrophages and neutrophils and mediates their transendothelial migration.[448,449] Metargidin (ADAM-15) is a type I transmembrane glycoprotein that binds the $\alpha_v\beta_3$ receptor on a monocytic cell line.[450] It uses integrin receptor, $\alpha_5\beta_1$, to mediate adhesion of a lymphoid cell line, indicating the complexity of cell adhesive interactions in different hematopoietic cells. The vitronectin receptor cooperates with TSP and CD36 in the recognition and phagocytosis of apoptotic cells by neutrophils, macrophages, and dendritic cells.[451–453] Vitronectin and the platelet-derived GAG serglycin augment megakaryocyte proplatelet formation.[454,455] Soluble vitronectin inhibits bFGF-mediated endothelial cell adhesion by interfering with its interaction with the $\alpha_v\beta_3$ receptor.[456] Cytotoxic T lymphocytes,[457] γ/δ-lymphocytes,[458] and NK cells[459] utilize the integrin $\alpha_V\beta_3$ as a costimulatory molecule mediating activation signals and cell proliferation. The TSP receptor integrin-associated protein CD47 and the integrin $\alpha_V\beta_3$ mediate monocyte activation and cytokine release after interacting with soluble CD23.[460] Hence, vitronectin appears to contribute mainly to terminal megakaryocyte maturation and platelet formation, while exerting a major role in apoptotic cell clearance, cellular activation, and trafficking to areas of inflammation, bone remodeling, and angiogenesis.

Other Matrix Proteins

Osteopontin, a glycoprotein produced by osteoblasts and hematopoietic cells in the marrow, binds to fibronectin and collagen.[461] Osteopontin can bind numerous integrins and CD44, and its binding through β_1-integrin results in suppression of proliferation and maintenance of quiescence in HSCs.[461] Conversely, the same osteopontin-β_1-integrin pathway induces proliferation in erythroblasts.[462] Osteopontin also plays a role in the development of NK cells[463,464] and T lymphocytes.[461] The fibulins are proteins secreted by the stromal cells of marrow, including osteoblasts and endothelial cells.[465,466] The metalloproteinase-resistant fibulin-1 accumulates in the extracellular matrix where it binds to a specific site on fibronectin.[465,466] Through this interaction with fibronectin, fibulin-1 disrupts HSC binding to fibronectin resulting in their decreased proliferation and differentiation.[466] Thus, fibulin-1 can act as a negative regulator that can maintain the quiescence of HSCs in the marrow. Hemonectin, a 60-kDa glycoprotein that is closely related to fetuin, mediates the attachment of granulocytes in the marrow[291] through its galactose and mannose residues.[432] Hemonectin and its receptor have not been characterized, making its existence and role in the marrow hematopoietic microenvironment unclear.

HEMATOPOIETIC CELL ORGANIZATION

Erythroblasts

The hematopoietic cells lie in cords or wedges between the vascular sinuses. BFU-Es, the earliest progenitor cells committed solely to erythroid differentiation, are not erythropoietin (EPO)-dependent, whereas CFU-Es and their immediate progeny, proerythroblasts, depend upon EPO to prevent apoptosis. EPO, the major regulator of erythropoiesis, has tightly controlled production rates by the kidneys in response to hypoxia, which, in turn, is regulated by numbers of circulating red blood cells.[467] Proerythroblasts differentiate into basophilic, polychromatophilic, and orthochromatic erythroblasts that have progressive accumulations of hemoglobin, reductions in cell size, and condensations of nuclear chromatin (see Chap. 29). In a process that requires an actin-based constriction ring like that involved in cytokinesis,[468] erythroblast-macrophage protein (EMP),[469] Rac guanosine triphosphatases,[470] and histone deacetylation,[471] orthochromatic erythroblasts enucleate and become reticulocytes that are released into the circulation. The irregularly shaped, motile nascent reticulocytes are near the sinuses, which they enter by transit through the sinus endothelial cells.[472]

Erythroid differentiation occurs within the erythroblastic islands (EBIs),[473] which consist of a central stromal macrophage surrounded by developing erythroid cells (see Chap. 29, Fig. 29–1).[474] EBIs are increased in patients with hemolytic anemias and decreased in hypertransfused mice.[475] EBIs with more mature erythroblasts appear nearer the sinusoids of the marrow.[476] In EBIs reconstructed *in vitro*, erythroblasts can dissociate from the macrophages as they mature,[477,478] suggesting that increased maturity of the erythroblasts near the sinusoids represents migration of the erythroblasts rather than the island. The central macrophage sends out extensive slender membranous processes that envelop each erythroblast and may phagocytize defective erythroblasts and extruded nuclei.[479] The extruded nuclei display phosphatidylserine on their plasma membranes that leads to rapid phagocytosis by the central macrophage.[480] Phagocytosis of extruded nuclei with recycling of the DNA components is essential in that deoxyribonuclease II-deficient mice die from an underproduction anemia with fetal liver macrophages filled with extruded erythroid nuclei.[481]

At least five cell-surface protein pairs contribute to adherence between macrophages and erythroblasts in erythroblastic islands.[473] These binding pairs are (1) VCAM-1 on macrophages and $\alpha_4\beta_1$ integrin (VLA-4) on erythroblasts; (2) α_V component of integrins on macrophages and ICAM-4 on erythroblasts; (3) erythroblast-macrophage protein (EMP), on both erythroblasts and macrophages that mediates a homophilic reaction; (4) CD169/Siglec 1 on macrophages and sialated glycoproteins on erythroblasts; and (5) hemoglobin-haptoglobin receptor (CD163) on macrophages and an unknown binding partner on erythroblasts.

Contact with macrophages in erythroblastic islands, increases the proliferation of erythroid cells without affecting their survival or differentiation.[478] Chemical depletion of macrophages prevents the erythropoietic response of mice to blood loss.[482] Several surface proteins or secreted products of macrophages have been demonstrated to stimulate erythroid cell proliferation, including KIT ligand,[483,484] ephrin-2,[485] and BMP-4.[486] In addition to these potential enhancers of erythroid cell proliferation, a series of negative regulators of erythroid cell growth have also been identified in the macrophages and erythroblasts that compose the EBIs. These negative regulators act mostly in pathologic situations and include the inflammatory cytokines TNF-α, TGF-β, TNF-related apoptosis-inducing ligand (TRAIL), and receptor-binding cancer antigen of SiSo cells.[473] A proposed negative regulation acting between early stage erythroid progenitors that express on their surface the apoptosis regulator FAS and the late-stage erythroblasts displaying FAS ligand[487] may be active within the EBIs.

Megakaryocytes

Megakaryocytes lie directly outside the vascular wall[488] in normal and myeloproliferative diseases (see Chap. 113).[489] Such discrete spatial structural distribution may be determined by specific adhesive interactions and the provision of specific growth factors for a given cell lineage.[490–492] In thrombopoiesis, HSC in the subcortical regions of the hematopoietic cords generate megakaryocytic progenitors that proliferate and differentiate with the acquisition of polyploidy and development of pronounced branched extensions, the proplatelets. Expression of the transcription factors GATA-1 and its binding partner, friend of GATA (FOG), play an important role in the differentiation of a common erythroid/megakaryocytic progenitor cell from a common granulocyte/macrophage progenitor.[493,494] Subsequent differentiation of the megakaryocytic lineage from the erythroid lineage involves the NF-E2 and TEL transcription factors.[493] TPO, the major regulator of megakaryocyte development acts in concert with several synergistic cytokines including IL-11, KIT ligand, IL-6, and leukemia inhibitory factor.[493,494] TPO levels are inversely related to megakaryocyte and platelet numbers as a result of a simple feedback loop in which a relatively constant TPO production by various tissues is balanced by TPO catabolism through binding to its receptor c-MPL on megakaryocytes and platelets.[494]

During their differentiation, megakaryocytic progenitors and megakaryocytes migrate toward the venous sinuses. Each stage of this migration requires platelet endothelial adhesion molecule (PECAM)-1[495,496] and, at the later stages, sinus endothelial cell production of CXCL12.[497,498] The intimate relation of megakaryocyte to sinus endothelium is explained by their expression of CXCR4, the receptor for CXCL12, which, in concert with TPO or FGF-4, increases megakaryocyte progenitor adhesion to the endothelial cells of the marrow venous sinus.[499] The adhesion appears to be regulated by VCAM-1 expression on megakaryocytic cells and enhances the survival and differentiation of the megakaryocytes.[499] In the proplatelets of the mature megakaryocytes, a microtubule sliding mechanism allows their elongation as well as helping redistribute cytoplasmic platelet granules to bulbous formations at their distal ends.[493] The proplatelets can be separated from the megakaryocyte in the marrow, but their fate is not certain, and they may not give rise to platelets.[500] However, the megakaryocyte extends many of the proplatelets through the adjacent sinus endothelial cells where the shear force of the blood flow breaks off individual platelets and some proplatelets themselves, which later fragment in the circulation.[500]

Granulocytes

Stem cells and granulocytic progenitor cells are concentrated in the subcortical regions of the hematopoietic cords (see Chap. 16).[501] Differentiation of the common granulocyte/macrophage progenitor from the common erythroid/megakaryocytic progenitor is regulated by the expression of multiple transcription factors. PU.1 expression promotes the development of the granulocyte/macrophage progenitor phenotype and antagonizes the activity of the GATA-1/FOG transcription factor that promotes erythroid/megakaryocytic progenitor differentiation.[502] The myeloid commitment of the common granulocyte/macrophage progenitor is reinforced by the CCAAT/enhancer-binding protein α (C/EBPα), which promotes myeloid differentiation while suppressing the lymphoid transcription factor Pax5.[502,503] The further expression of C/EBPα is associated with granulocytic differentiation, whereas increased PU.1 activity is associated with monocytic differentiation.[503] The progression of myeloid differentiation beyond the promyelocyte stage, including the formation of secondary and tertiary granules, requires both C/EBP and the GFI-1 transcription factors.[503,504] GFI-1 also antagonizes the activity of the Egr-1 and Egr-2 transcription factors that are associated with monocytic differentiation.[503] The timing of expression and relative ratios of C/EBPα and GATA-2 transcription factors regulate differentiation of the common granulocyte progenitor, a cell that can become a neutrophil, eosinophil, basophil, or mast cell.[505] Increased C/EBPα at this stage promotes a differentiation pathway toward neutrophils and eosinophils, whereas increased GATA-2 promotes differentiation toward basophils and mast cells.[505] Those cells differentiating along the neutrophil/eosinophil pathway will follow a terminal neutrophil path when only C/EBPα is expressed, and a terminal eosinophil path when both C/EBPα and GATA-2 are expressed. Those cells differentiating along the basophil/mast cell pathway will follow a terminal mast cell path when only GATA-2 is expressed, and a terminal basophil path when both GATA-2 and C/EBPα are expressed.

A group of related hematopoietic growth factors support granulocytic progenitor and precursor viability and proliferation and in some cases the mobilization of these cells and their mature progeny from the marrow. These growth factors include KIT ligand, GM-CSF, M-CSF, G-CSF, IL-6, IL-3, and IL-5. They are produced in sites of inflammation in peripheral tissues although some such as KIT ligand and M-CSF are normally expressed by the marrow stroma. Two hematopoietic growth factors have specific lineage targets for the late stage granulocytic cells, IL-5 for eosinophil progenitors and G-CSF for the neutrophilic progenitors. IL-5 is a hematopoietic cytokine produced mainly by the T-helper type 2 (Th2) lymphocytes in response to allergens (see Chap. 62).[506,507] The eosinophilic progenitor cells display a IL-5α receptor protein that when associated with the common β receptor, binds IL-5, leading to the survival and proliferation of the eosinophilic progenitor cells.[506] Mature eosinophils have survival and chemotactic responses to IL-5 that mediates their entry into the circulation and accumulation in sites of allergic inflammation.[507] Despite GM-CSF, G-CSF, IL-3, and IL-6 all stimulating granulopoiesis *in vivo*, only the lack of G-CSF results in marked but incomplete neutropenia, making it the likely regulator of normal circulating granulocyte numbers.[508] Under normal steady-state conditions, 1 to 2 percent of neutrophils circulate transiently in the blood, while the majority remain in the marrow unless mobilized by inflammation in other areas of the body.

Models of G-CSF regulation of granulopoiesis and circulating neutrophils under normal conditions and during increased production of inflammation have been proposed.[509,510] Newly formed neutrophils have low expression of CXCR4 and can exit the marrow by migration through the sinusoidal endothelial cells. As they normally age in the circulation they express more CXCR4 and are attracted back to the marrow by its stromal production of CXCL12, the CXCR4 ligand.[509] After reentering the marrow, the senescent neutrophils undergo apoptosis and are phagocytosed by macrophages that, in turn, produce G-CSF that stimulates granulopoiesis.[509] With inflammation, cells in the site of inflammation produce both G-CSF and chemokines, including KC chemokine (CXCL1), and macrophage inhibitory protein-2 (MIP-2; CXCL2). The secreted G-CSF acts on the marrow mobilizing neutrophils by its ability to reduce both marrow CXCL12 production and the neutrophil CXCR4 expression. G-CSF, however, does not recruit the neutrophils to the site of inflammation from the blood.[509] By their chemotactic properties, CXCL1 and CXCL2 also induce rapid mobilization from the marrow into the blood and to the site of inflammation.[509] Another model involves a similar migration of neutrophils from the marrow that depends on G-CSF downregulating CXCL12 production and neutrophil CXCR4 expression, but the feedback that decreases G-CSF occurs in the peripheral tissues.[510] In this model, macrophages that phagocytose apoptotic neutrophils in the peripheral tissues decrease IL-23 production which decreases IL-17 production by a subset of T lymphocytes that, in turn, results in decreased G-CSF in the marrow.

THREE-DIMENSIONAL ORGANIZATION

Computer-assisted three-dimensional reconstruction analysis of human marrow confirms the megakaryocyte apposition against the sinus wall and the position of granulocytic cells along the wall of the central arteriole.[511] Erythropoietic cells located mainly around the sinus wall form a continuous network or cord instead of separate "islands." On this basis, the unitary structure of marrow has been defined as a hematopoietic cord with a central arteriole and surrounded by sinuses.[511] A similar structure termed a hematon serves as a multicellular functional unit of marrow and contains adipocytes, stromal elements, macrophages, and HSC in a compact spheroid.[512]

CELL ADHESION AND HOMING

After their initial migration from the yolk sac, AGM, or placenta to the marrow, the HSCs are located in specific sites in the marrow through interactions with other types of cells and with matrix proteins. HSCs do not remain permanently in the marrow because at any one time a small percentage exit the marrow through the venous sinusoids and enter the blood where they circulate briefly.[513,514] In addition to the HSCs, the more differentiated progenitor cells, such as the short-term repopulating cells and the primitive BFU-Es, can circulate prior to homing to specific sites in the marrow. When circulating, the HSCs can either reenter the marrow or they can enter other organs. After entering the interstitium of a peripheral organ, the HSCs can give rise to myeloid progeny and/or they enter the lymphatic drainage of the organ and circulate through lymphatic vessels and thoracic duct before reentering the blood.[515] HSCs have multiple adhesion and cytokine receptors that allow them to attach to cellular and matrix components within the marrow sinusoidal spaces.[355,357–360] Such attachment facilitates their homing and lodgment in the marrow and provide the close cell–cell contacts required for cell survival and regulated steady-state proliferation,[511] as shown by the membrane-bound KIT ligand in regulating the lodgment of stem cells within the endosteal marrow region.[516]

Most of the various lineages of differentiated cells also have marrow release followed by a circulatory phase and eventual homing of some of the cells to the marrow. In some cell types, the circulating cells will differentiate further in peripheral organs such as B lymphocytes in the lymph nodes or spleen and T lymphocytes in the thymus. After a period of residence in these secondary lymphoid organs, some lymphocytes travel through the lymph and blood, homing to the marrow, where they become functioning mature cells, such as plasma cells and CD4 and CD8 mature T lymphocytes.[266–268] Mature and band forms of neutrophils exit the marrow, circulate in the blood and, if not recruited to a site of inflammation, home as senescent cells to the marrow by the CXCL12/CXCR4 mechanism described in the section above, Granulocytes.[509] Senescent erythrocytes are also removed from circulation through a mechanism that involves binding surface ICAM-4 to integrin $\alpha_L\beta_2$ (leukocyte function-associated antigen [LFA]-1) on macrophages found in the spleen and marrow.[517] Mature leukocytes that participate in inflammatory reactions, such as the lymphocytes, monocytes/macrophages, and eosinophils, exit the circulation in areas of infection, allergic reactions, or injury. Table 4–2 lists the adhesive receptors and their ligands, present on hematopoietic stem progenitor cells, and components of the hematopoietic microenvironment, but receptor–ligand interactions that regulate the trafficking of mature leukocytes are not included exhaustively.[518,519]

INTEGRINS

Members of the integrin family are divalent cation-requiring heterodimeric proteins (18 α subunits and 8 β subunits). Integrins mediate important cellular functions, including embryonic development, cell differentiation, and adhesive interactions between hematopoietic cells and inflammatory cells and surrounding vascular and stromal microenvironment.[359,520,521] They are subdivided based on the β-chain composition. Table 4–2 indicates that α-chains can associate with more than one β-chain subunit. The principal integrin receptors of the β_1 subgroup involved in HSC's endothelial and stromal interactions are $\alpha_4\beta_1$ (VLA-4), $\alpha_5\beta_1$ (VLA-5), and $\alpha_L\beta_2$ (LFA-1) of the β_2 subgroup. $\alpha_4\beta_1$-based stromal adhesion events regulate erythropoiesis in the stages after EPO dependence.[522] This receptor also stimulates granulopoiesis over established marrow stromal cells in cooperation with PECAM-1 (CD31), an immunoglobulin superfamily member.[523] The high expression of VLA-4 in granulocytic precursor cells and newly formed granulocytes has an important role in their adherence to VCAM-1 in the marrow, whereas the downregulation of $\alpha_4\beta_1$ in the more mature neutrophils works in concert with the CXCL12 and CXCR4 mechanism for their release into the blood.[524] The $\alpha_4\beta_1$ integrin on B lymphocytes are important for interactions with the VCAM-1 on the stromal cells in the B lymphocyte niche, both in the early B lymphocyte development prior to migration out of the marrow and the later development of immature plasma cells that have reentered the marrow.[266] An acquired defect in stromal function, characterized by a deficiency in VCAM-1 and IL-7 expression,[525–527] accounts for the delayed B lymphoid reconstitution seen after marrow transplantation. During thrombopoiesis, CXCL12 induces VCAM-1 in the marrow sinusoid endothelial cells[499] that mediates the binding of the megakaryocytes to the endothelium.[490] Integrin $\alpha_4\beta_7$ and its counterreceptor mucosal addressin cell adhesion molecule (MAdCAM)-1, like the integrin $\alpha_4\beta_1$/VCAM-1 receptor,[528] contribute equally to the homing of HSC to the marrow.[529]

Integrins are signaling molecules. After engaging their ligands, or subsequent to activation by monoclonal antibodies, multiple events (tyrosine phosphorylation of focal adhesion kinase, paxillin, and ERK-2) are triggered (outside–in signaling), culminating with Ras activation.[530–534] Integrin receptor cross-talk[535] with other adhesive receptor members, such as the immunoglobulin superfamily (NK cell–T cell [$\alpha_1\beta_2$/DYNAM-1], CD34-positive–endothelial cell PECAM-1,[536–539] or selectins[540]), also results from outside–in signaling events that regulate receptor-binding affinity[541,542] and mediates inhibitory signals for erythroid, myeloid, and lymphoid progenitor growth.[543–547] Integrin binding to their counterreceptors, such as $\alpha_4\beta_1$/VCAM-1 or $\alpha_4\beta_1$/FN, in early CD34-positive progenitors enhances their viability and preserves their long-term repopulating ability.[548] In studies of isolated SP cells, high expression of the vitronectin receptor $\alpha_v\beta_3$ (CD51/CD61) was associated with quiescence and long-term repopulating ability.[549] Conversely, expression of the α_2 integrin was associated with only short-term repopulating capacity.[550]

IMMUNOGLOBULIN SUPERFAMILY

The immunoglobulin superfamily[293] designates a group of molecules containing one or more amino acid repeats also found in immunoglobulins and includes PECAM-1 (CD31), ICAM-3/R (CD50) and ICAM-1 (CD54), LFA-3 (CD58), ICAM-2 (CD102), VCAM-1 (CD106), c-KIT (CD117), and LW/ICAM-4 (CD242) (see Table 4–2).[551–569] VCAM-1 is upregulated by inflammatory cytokines (IL-4, IL-13).[566,567] Immunoglobulin-like adhesion molecules also include NCAM, a neural cell-adhesion molecule that binds lymphocytes but not hematopoietic progenitors; Thy-1, a stem cell antigen major histocompatibility complex classes I and II; and CD2, CD4, and CD8 (see Table 4–2).[327] LW/ICAM-4 on erythroblasts binds the α_V component of integrins on macrophages in erythroblastic islands,[473] whereas the function of Lutheran red blood cell antigen, Lu/B-CAM (CD239), is unknown.[569] Lu/B-CAM binds laminin and is expressed late in erythroblast differentiation, suggesting a role in enucleation or reticulocyte entry into the sinusoid.[569] The sialic acid-binding immunoglobulin (Ig)-like lectins (siglecs) are a family of surface proteins found on lymphocytes and myeloid cells that bind sialic acid residues of glycoproteins.[570] Some siglecs are evolutionarily conserved, such as siglec-1 (sialoadhesin), which is highly expressed on macrophages including the central macrophages of erythroblastic islands, and CD22, a coreceptor on B lymphocytes. The remaining siglecs, which are phylogenetically evolving rapidly, include CD33, which is expressed in lymphocytes and in all stages of myeloid cells where it is a commonly used marker for acute myeloid leukemia.

LECTINS (SELECTINS)

Homing of stem cells requires lectin receptors with galactosyl and mannosyl specificities.[571,572] The selectins are a family of adhesion molecules, each containing type C lectin structures.[573] The leukocyte selectin (L-selectin, CD62L) is expressed on hematopoietic stem-progenitors[574] and mediates adhesive interactions with other receptors (addressins), such as the CD34 sialomucin present on specialized endothelium, using sialylated fucosyl-glucoconjugates (see Table 4–2). The CD34 receptor on stem cells, however, does not bind L-selectin,[574] as a putative L-selectin ligand yet to be defined exists on these cells. The selectin family also contains CD62E, an E-selectin constitutively expressed on marrow sinusoidal endothelium that regulates transmigration of leukocytes and CD34-positive stem cell homing. The third member of this family is P-selectin, which is found on platelets. P-selectin can bind HSC using a mucin receptor, CD162 also known as the P-selectin glycoprotein ligand (PSGL)-1, which binds to all three selectins (see Table 4–2). These proteins are responsible for leukocyte rolling over endothelial surfaces and tethering, thereby allowing integrin-mediated firm adhesion to the endothelium and mediating cellular homing events using specialized high endothelial venule lymphocyte homing sites.[573,575–578] In addition to their role in HSC homing in the marrow, E-selectin and P-selectin can promote either growth inhibition in HSC and apoptosis of late-stage myeloid progenitors while promoting the expansion (P-selectin) or differentiation (E-selectin) of short-term repopulating cells.[579]

SIALOMUCINS

Three members of the CD34 family—CD34, podocalyxin, and endoglycan—are expressed on vascular endothelium, HSCs, and various hematopoietic cell lineages.[578] When expressed on lymphoid high endothelial venules, these sialomucins are receptors for L-selectin, but their different glycosylation in hematopoietic cells prevents L-selectin binding and results in their reducing nonspecific adhesion and potentially enhancing mobility.[578] Although its function has not been determined, endomucin is another CD34-like sialomucin expressed in endothelium and in HSCs.[580] In T lymphocytes, where it affects mobility, CD43 (leukosialin)[581] acts in concert with PSGL-1 and binds both P-selectin and E-selectin.[582] CD43 in neutrophils can be adhesive when binding E-selectin on endothelial cells, but it is antiadhesive in most instances.[582] CD43 can regulate hematopoietic progenitor survival.[583] CD162 (PSGL-1), a sialomucin that binds all three selectins, is important in leukocyte trafficking and stem cell homing.[573,575–578] CD164 (endolyn), another sialomucin receptor displayed on HSCs, forms a

TABLE 4–2. Hematopoietic and Microenvironment Adhesion Receptors and Their Ligands

Receptor Subgroups	Receptor	Cellular Distribution	Ligand
Integrins			
β_1 subgroup (CD29)	CD49d, $\alpha_4\beta_1$ (VLA-4)	CD34+ cells (erythroid, and lymphomyeloid progenitors)	VCAM-1 (CD106), FN, TSP
	CD49e, $\alpha_5\beta_1$ (VLA-5)	CD34+ cells, bone cells	FN, laminin
	CD49f, $\alpha_6\beta_1$ (VLA-6)	Rare CD34+ cells, monocytes	Collagen, laminin
β_2 subgroup (CD18)	CD11a/CD18, $\alpha_L\beta_2$ (LFA-1)	CD34+ cell subsets, not on repopulating stem cells	ICAM-1, ICAM-2, ICAM-3, DYNAM-1
	CD11b/CD18, $\alpha_M\beta_2$ (Mac-1)	CD34+ subsets, monocytes	ICAM-1, ICAM-2, iC3b, fibrinogen
β_3 subgroup	Vβ_3 (VNR)	Megakaryocytes, osteoclast	FN, TSP, CD31
β_7 subgroup	$\alpha_4\beta_7$ (LPAM-1)	Lymphoid and myeloid progenitor cells, mature myeloid cells	MAdCAM-1, VCAM-1, FN
Immunoglobulins			
	CD31 (PECAM-1)	ECs, CD34+ cells, monocytes	CD31 homophilic adhesion, $\alpha_V\beta_3$ (VNR), CD38
	CD50 (ICAM-3, ICAM-R)	CD34+ cells, monocytes	$\alpha_L\beta_2$ (LFA-1), CD11d/CD18 ($\alpha_D\beta_2$)
	CD54 (ICAM-1)	CD34+ cells, stroma, activated ECs	$\alpha_L\beta_2$ (LFA-1), $\alpha_M\beta_2$ (Mac-1)
	CD58 (LFA-3)	CD34+ progenitors, stroma, ECs	CD2
	CD102 (ICAM-2)	ECs, monocytes	$\alpha_L\beta_2$ (LFA-1)
	CD106 (VCAM-1)	Stroma, activated ECs	$\alpha_4\beta_1$ (VLA-4), $\alpha_4\beta_7$ (LPAM-1)
	CD117 (*c-KIT*)	CD34+ progenitors	Membrane KIT ligand
	CD242 (ICAM-4)	Erythroid cells	α_V-integrins
	PRR2 (related to CD155, the poliovirus receptor)	CD34+, CD33+, CD41+, myelomonocytic cells, megakaryocytic cells, ECs	PRR2 homophilic adhesion
Lectins			
	CD62L (L-selectin)	Stroma, CD34+ cells	GlyCAM-1, MAdCAM-1, CD162, CD34, sLe^x, PCLP1
	CD62E (E-selectin)	Activated ECs, (marrow ECs express CD62E constitutively)	CD15, sLe^a, CD162, CLA, sLe^x
	CD62P (P-selectin)	Activated ECs	CD162, sLe^x, CD24 (HSA)
Sialomucins			
	CD34	CD34+ cells, endothelial cells	Selectins, other ligands?
	CD43	CD34+, monocytes, NK cells	CD54 (ICAM-1)
	CD162 (PSGL-1)	CD34+ cells, endothelial cells	CD62L, CD62E, CD62P
	CD164 (MGC-24v)	CD34+ cells, stroma, monocytes	Unknown
	CD166 (HCA, ALCAM)	CD34+ cells, stromal cells, ECs	CD6, CD166
Hyaladherin			
	CD44	CD34+ cells, broad distribution	Hyaluronan, bFGF, HGF
Other			
	CD38	CD34+ subsets, early T and B cells, plasma cells, thymocytes	CD31, hyaluronan
	CD144 (VE-cadherin)	CFU-E, stromal cells, ECs	E-cadherin
	CD157 (BST-1)	Stroma, T and B cells, myeloid cells	Unknown

ALCAM, activated leukocyte adhesion molecule; bFGF, basic fibroblast growth factor; CD, cluster designation; CFU-E, colony forming unit–erythroid; CLA, cutaneous lymphocyte antigen; EC, endothelial cell; FN, fibronectin; GlyCAM, glycosylation-dependent cell adhesion molecule; HCA, hematopoietic cell antigen; HGF, hepatocyte growth factor; HSA, heat-stable antigen; ICAM, intercellular adhesion molecule; iC3b, inactive complement 3b complex; LFA, lymphocyte function antigen; LPAM, lymphocyte Peyer patch-specific adhesion molecule; MAdCAM, mucosal addressin cell adhesion molecule; MGC-24, multiglycosylated core of 24 kDa; PCLP, podocalyxin-like protein; PECAM, platelet/endothelial cell adhesion molecule; PRR2, poliovirus receptor-related protein2; PSGL-P, selectin glycoprotein ligand; sLe, sialyl Lewis; TSP, thrombospondin; VLA, very-late antigen; VCAM, vascular cell adhesion molecule; VNR, vitronectin receptor.

complex with CXCR4, VLA-4, and VLA-5 on the leading edge of migrating HSCs after exposure to fibronectin-bound CXCL12, indicating a role for CD164 in the homing of HSCs.[584] CD166 (HCA, activated leukocyte adhesion molecule [ALCAM]) forms homodimers (CD166) and heterodimers with CD6.[585,586]

HYALADHERINS

The fifth subgroup listed in Table 4–2 is the cartilage-related proteoglycan, CD44, also known as the *lymphocyte homing cell adhesion molecule* (HCAM). This adhesion receptor, which binds the hyaluronic acid in the marrow matrix and can be a receptor for E-selectin, is expressed on neutrophils, lymphocytes, erythroblasts, and HSC.[573,575,576] CD44 displayed on HSCs facilitates their homing and adhesion to marrow and plays a role in their mobilization in response to G-CSF.[573,575,576,587] Studies with CD44-deficient mice show no defects in HSC homing and growth, and no decrease in hematopoiesis,[588] suggesting that another hyaladherin receptor may compensate for the absence of CD44. The other hyaladherin receptor on HSC is the receptor for hyaluron-mediated mobility (CD168/RHAMM),[573,576,588] which does provide hyaluronic acid binding by neutrophils under inflammatory conditions in CD44 deficiency.[589] Thus, CD44 and CD168/RHAMM may provide redundant hyaluronic acid binding in HSC.

OTHER ADHESION MOLECULES

CD38 is a newly recognized adhesion receptor that binds the CD31 receptor and matrix hyaluronan. It is expressed on early T and B cells and subsets of CD34-positive hematopoietic progenitors.[590,591] Cadherins are large molecules involved in cell–cell junctions and vascular integrity. CD144 (E-cadherin) is expressed on CD34-positive progenitors, marrow stroma, and endothelial cells, thereby providing another pathway for stem cell lodgement.[592] Downregulation of VE-cadherin is associated with cross-linking of VCAM-1, resulting in enhanced transendothelial migration of CD34-positive cells in response to CXCL12.[115] Although N-cadherin expression by both HSC and osteoblasts has been proposed to play a role in their interactions,[12] experimental results in mice did not find any evidence for such a role.[593] The stromal adhesion receptor BST-1 (CD157) is an adenosine diphosphate-ribosyl cyclase with similarity to CD38. CD157 is expressed on marrow stroma, T and B cells, and myeloid cells. It promotes pre–B-cell adhesion and growth.[594–597]

CELLULAR HOMING

Mechanisms of tissue homing by circulating cells have been revealed by studies of leukocytes that home to areas of inflammation as well as lymphocytes homing to secondary lymphoid organs via the specialized high endothelial venules (HEVs). A sequence of specific events by which leukocytes adhere to and migrate through the endothelium begins with tethering of the leukocytes to the luminal surface of the endothelial cells.[598] P-selectin and E-selectin are upregulated in response to various inflammatory cytokines on the endothelial cell surface, where they bind their respective counterreceptors PSGL-1 and CD44 on leukocytes.[573,577] In the secondary lymphoid organs, the tethering is mediated by L-selectin on the naïve lymphocytes that bind peripheral node addressins such as MAdCAM-1, podocalyxin, CD34, and endomucin.[573,577,599] Tethering results in rolling of the leukocytes along the endothelial surface. Interactions of VLA-4 and $\alpha_4\beta_7$ integrin on the surface of lymphocytes with their respective ligands VCAM-1 and MAdCAM-1 on HEVs may also mediate rolling.[573,599] The rolling of neutrophils is slowed further by PSGL-1 and L-selectin activation of other adhesion molecules that include the β_2 integrins $\alpha_L\beta_2$ (LFA-1) and $\alpha_M\beta_2$ (Mac-1).[577,599,600] These β_2 integrins, in turn, bind ICAM-1 on endothelial cells. The rolling leukocytes also receive signals through surface G-protein-coupled receptors that bind chemokines in the heparan sulfate proteoglycans on the endothelial cells.[577,599,600]

The interaction of PSGL-1, L-selectin, integrins, and G-protein-coupled receptors with their endothelial ligands leads to cytoskeletal changes with arrest of rolling and adhesion to the endothelium. The adherent leukocytes undergo a rapid diapedesis, with migration either through or between the endothelial cells into the abluminal interstitium. At the interface with the adherent leukocyte, ICAM-1 and VCAM-1 in the endothelial cell are concentrated in a cup-like, caveolin-rich structure that internalizes ICAM-1.[600–602] This caveolin-rich structure is linked to the endothelial cell cytoskeleton through vimentin. The internalization of the ICAM caveolae leads to the formation of a channel through the cell to the abluminal surface. When leukocytes follow a paracellular route through the endothelium, they require the coordinated activity of multiple adhesion proteins. These include PECAM-1, CD99, JAM proteins, and VE-cadherin, each of which mediates homophilic interactions at intercellular junctions between endothelial cells, and ICAM-2.[600–602] Although the roles of these proteins is uncertain, antibody inhibition and knockout mice demonstrate that they are necessary for the unidirectional migration of the leukocyte through the endothelium. PECAM-1, CD99, and JAM-C are expressed on leukocytes and may be involved in homophilic interactions between the migrating leukocyte and the endothelial junction. LFA-1 and Mac-1 on leukocytes can bind and interact with ICAM-2 and JAM-A on endothelium, whereas leukocyte VLA-4 can interact with endothelial JAM-B.

The driving force for the migration and homing of leukocytes is the expression of chemoattractants at the site of inflammation or areas of constitutive production, such as the secondary lymphoid organs or the marrow. Bacterial peptides, complement components, and cytokines are produced in inflammatory sites. More than 40 different but structurally related chemotactic cytokines (chemokines) can be produced by leukocytes in inflammatory sites.[603,604] Chemokines accumulate on cell surfaces or in extracellular matrices through their binding to glycosaminoglycans (GAGs).[603–605] Concentrations and chemotactic activities of each cytokine are related to production rate, binding affinities to GAGs, presence of decoy chemokines that can compete with chemotactic activity, and modulation by metalloproteinases that enhance or diminish activities of substrate chemokines.[603,605]

Based on the location of one or two cysteine residues in the amino terminus, chemokines are divided into four subfamilies.[295,603–605] One large subfamily comprises the CXC ligand (CXCL) chemokines (e.g., platelet factor 4, IL-8, melanocyte growth-stimulating activity/GROα, neutrophil activating protein-2, granulocyte chemotactic protein-2), which mediate neutrophil migration and activation. The other large subfamily comprises the CC ligand (CCL) chemokines (e.g., CCL3 [MIP-1α], CCL4 [MIP-1β], [CCL5] RANTES [regulated on activation, normal T-cell expressed, presumed secreted], MCP-1 through MCP-5), which mediate mostly monocyte and in some cases lymphocyte chemotaxis. A chemokine with CXXXCL structure is fractalkine, an endothelial transmembrane mucin–chemokine hybrid molecule that mediates the rapid capture, firm adhesion, and activation under physiologic flow of circulating monocytes, resting or IL-2–activated CD8 lymphocytes, and NK cells.[606] The cytokines TNF-α and IL-1 upregulate fractalkine, in keeping with the need to recruit effector cells rapidly at sites of inflammation.[605] The chemokines receptors on the surface of leukocytes are coupled to G proteins that initiate signaling for chemotaxis upon chemokine ligand binding.[603,604] The chemokine receptors for the two large subfamilies bind those members such that CXCLs bind CXCRs and CCLs bind CCRs. However, within these two subfamilies is significant redundancy and promiscuity in chemokine-receptor binding. Table 4–3 gives a detailed listing of chemokine receptors and the cellular targets and ligands interacting with each receptor subgroup.[603,604]

TABLE 4–3. Chemokine Receptors, Interacting Chemokine Ligands, and Cellular Specificity

Receptors	Receptor Expression	Chemokine Ligands
CXCR1	Neutrophils, monocytes	CXCL2 (GROβ), CXCL3 (GROγ), CXCL5 (ENA78), CXCL6 (GCP-2), CXCL8 (IL-8)
CXCR2	Neutrophils, IL-5–primed Eos, monocytes	CXCL1,2,3 (GROα/β/γ), CXCL5 (ENA78), CXCL6, CXCL7 (NAP-2), CXCL8(IL-8),
CXCR3	Activated memory and naïve T cells, NK cells; T (preferentially Th1) cells, B cells	CXCL9 (MIG), CXCL10 (IP-10), CXCL11 (I-TAC)
CXCR4	Neutrophils, monocytes, megakaryocytes, CD34+ and pre–B-cell precursors, resting and activated T cells, DCs	CXCL12 (SDF-1α, SDF-1β)
CXCR5	B lymphocytes, T lymphocytes	CXCL13 (BCA-1/BLC)
CXCR6	T lymphocytes	CXCL16 (SR-PSOX)
CXCR7	B lymphocyte, T lymphocytes, Basos, monocytes, NK cells	CXCL11 (I-TAC), CXCL12 (SDF-1α)
CX3CR1	Monocytes, DCs, CD34+ cells, NK cells; in nodal tissues activated T helper lymphocytes, activated B cells, and follicular DCs	CX3CL1 (fractalkine/neurotactin)
XCR1	Resting T cells, NK cells	XCL1 (lymphotactin/SCM-1α/ATAC), XCL2 (SCM-1β)
CCR1	Monocytes, Eos, basophils, activated Neu and T cells, CD34+ cells, immature DCs	CCL3 (MIP-1α), CCL5 (RANTES), CCL7 (MCP-3), CCL8 (MCP-2), CCL13 (MCP-4), CCL22 (MDC), CCL23 (MPIF-1)
	Monocytes, T cells (not Neu, Eos, or B cells)	CCL14 (HCC-1), CCL15 (HCC-2/MIP-5), CCL16 (HCC-4/LEC)
CCR2	Monocytes, basophils, DCs, T cells, activated memory CD4 T cells, NK cells	CCL2(MCP-1), CCL7 (MCP-3), CCL8 (MCP-2), CCL13 (MCP-4)
CCR3	Eos, thymocytes, basophils, DCs, activated memory CD4 T cells	CCL5 (RANTES), CCL7 (MCP-3), CCL8 (MCP-2), CCL11 (Eotaxin-1), CCL13 (MCP-4), CCL15 (HCC-2/MIP-5), CCL24 (Eotaxin-2/MPIF-2), CCL26 (Eotaxin-3)
CCR4	Activated T cells, immature DCs	CCL17 (TARC)
	Monocyte-derived DCs, activated NK cells	CCL22 (MDC)
	Thymocytes (CD3+, CD4+, $CD8^{low}$)	CCL22 (MDC)
CCR5	Monocytes, activated memory CD4 T cells	CCL5 (RANTES), CCL8 (MCP-2), CCL13 (MCP-4), CCL14 (HCC-1)
	Immature DCs, CD34+ cells, NK cells	CCL3 (MIP-1α), CCL4 (MIP-1β)
	Human thymocytes	CCL4 (MIP-1β)
CCR6	T cells, CD34+– derived dendritic cells	CCL20 (MIP-3α/LARC/exodus-1)
CCR7	Activated T (naïve and memory T cells) > B lymphocytes, NK cells subsets, CD34+ macrophage progenitors, mature DCs	CCL19 (MIP-3β/ELC/exodus-3), CCL21 (SLC/exodus-2/6Ckine) [6Ckine inactive on B cells]
CCR8	Monocytes, T (Th2) cells, NK cells	CCL1 (I309), CCL17 (TARC)
CCR9	Thymocytes (CD4+/CD8+, CD4+/CD8–), activated macrophages	CCL25 (TECK)
CCR10	Skin-homing memory T cells, CD4/CD8 cells	CCL26 (Eotaxin-3), CCL27 (CTACK/ILC/ESkine), CCL28 (MEC)
CCR1 and CCR3	Neutrophils, monocytes, lymphocytes	CCL15 (HCC-2/MIP-5)
Not known	Resting T cells	CCL18 (DC-CK1/PARC)
CCR3/CCR10	Memory lymphocytes, Eos, IgA plasmablasts	CCL28 (MEC)

6Ckine, chemokine with 6 cysteines; ATAC, activation-induced, chemokine-related molecule; Baso, basophil; BCA, B-cell attracting chemokine; BLC, B cell homing chemokine that activates Burkitt lymphoma receptor 1 (BLR1); CTACK, cutaneous T cell-attracting chemokine; DC, dendritic cell; ELC, EBI1-ligand chemokine; ENA, epithelial neutrophil activating protein; EOS, eosinophil; ESkine, embryonal stem cell chemokine; GCP, granulocyte chemotactic protein; GRO, growth related oncogene; HCC, human C-C-chemokine; IL-8 is also chemotactic for a specific subset of (CD3+, CD8+, CD56+, CD26–) T cells; IP, Interferon-inducible protein; I-TAC, interferon-inducible T-cell α chemoattractant; LARC, liver and activation-regulated chemokine; LEC, liver-expressed chemokine; MCP, monocyte chemoattractant protein; MDC, macrophage-derived chemokine, MDC is chemotactic to eosinophils, in a CCR3- and CCR4-independent manner; MEC, mucosae-associated epithelial chemokine; MIG, monokine induced by interferon-γ, MIP, macrophage inflammatory protein; MPIF, myeloid progenitor inhibitory factor; NAP, neutrophil activating peptide; NK, natural killer; PARC, pulmonary and activation-regulated chemokine; RANTES, regulated on activation, normal T-cell expressed and secreted; SCM, single-C motif; SDF, stromal cell-derived factor; SLC, secondary lymphoid-tissue chemokine, also known as exodus-2 and 6Ckine; SR-PSOX, scavenger receptor for phosphatylserine and oxidized lipoprotein; TARC, thymus and activation-regulated chemokine; TECK, thymus-expressed chemokine.

A major exception to this redundant and promiscuous chemokine-receptor interaction is the specific binding of CXCL12/SDF-1α to its receptor CXCR4, which is associated with homeostatic maintenance of cell populations, including the HSCs and their progeny in the marrow.[604,607] Although CXCL12 can bind one other chemokine receptor (CXCR7),[604,607] mouse knockout experiments show that absence CXCR4 or CXCL12 is lethal in the embryonic period.[604] CXCL12 is produced by the bone, endothelial, perivascular reticular cells and some hematopoietic cells in the marrow, and its receptor CXCR4 is expressed on various hematopoietic and mature blood cells.[575,576,607,608] CXCL12 and CXCR4 are involved in the trafficking of HSCs, committed progenitor cells, and mature cells, including neutrophils, dendritic cells, NK cells, and T and B lymphocytes.[508,509,603,607,608] The cellular specificity of the homing, localization, and mobilization that are driven by CXCL12 and CXCR4 are regulated by additional chemokines, adhesion proteins, and metalloproteinases associated with specific hematopoietic cell types and/or the organs to which they home, in which they reside, and from which they are mobilized.[607,608] In the case of HSCs homing from the peripheral tissues through which they migrate, their initial entry into the lymphatic vessels is driven by the lipid chemoattractant sphingosine-1-phosphate (S-1-P).[515] HSC display S-1-P receptors that respond to high levels in the lymph compared to the peripheral tissues where S-1-P is degraded.

For the HSC and the marrow, multiple experiments using inhibitors and antibodies with stem cell transplantation in mice and humans, parabiotic experiments with mice, and transplantation of human HSC into immunocompromised mice (e.g, NOD/SCID strains) have contributed to an understanding of some interactions of these multiple factors that influence HSC within the marrow. Two adhesion mechanisms that play major roles in CXCL12-mediated HSC homing to marrow are the binding and activation of $\alpha_4\beta_1$ integrin and selectin ligands, particularly PSGL-1,[575,576] on HSC to their respective receptors, VCAM-1, and P- and E-selectins on the marrow sinusoidal endothelium.[528,576,609] Although $\alpha_4\beta_1$ integrin appears to be the major integrin on HSC involved in the first step of homing, other integrins have been implicated as having supporting roles including $\alpha_5\beta_1$, $\alpha_4\beta_7$, and $\alpha_6\beta_1$ or $\alpha_6\beta_4$ integrin that bind to fibronectin, MAdCAM-1, and laminins in the marrow.[417,576] The E-selectin ligands appear to cooperate with the α_4 integrins rather than the P-selectin ligands in HSC homing.[576] Similarly, a coordinated action between CXCR4 that has bound CXCL12 and the CD44 isoform on HSC,[610] or another hyaladherin such as RHAMM,[588] may provide a source of adhesion for HSC to hyaluronic acid on marrow endothelial cells in the homing process.[576] In cord blood cells enriched for HSC, the colocalization and cooperative activity of the endolyn with CXCR4, $\alpha_4\beta_1$, and $\alpha_5\beta_1$ integrin appears to enhance HSC homing to the marrow in response to CXCL12.[584] CXCR4 has also been colocalized in lipid rafts on HSC with Rac 1, a member of the receptor-associated RhoGTPases.[611] The RhoGTPases have two members, Rac-2 and RhoH, that are hematopoietic specific and that with other more widely expressed members such as Rac-1, Cdc42, and Rho A, are downstream effectors of CXCR4, β_1-integrin, and KIT signaling in HSC.[612] The various RhoGTPases modulate actin polymerization and lead to cytoskeletal changes that are required for the survival, proliferation, homing, and mobilization of HSC and their progeny.[612] In the homing of HSC, the RhoGTPase-mediated signaling provided by the coordinated action of CXCR4, β_1 integrins, and CD44 leads to the rolling, arrest, and transmigration of the marrow sinus endothelial cells.

Once the HSCs have migrated across the sinusoidal endothelial cells, they migrate further within the marrow in response to CXCL12. Using fluorescent SLAM-labeled markers for the identification of HSC in murine transplantation experiments, the homing of HSC in the marrow cavity is associated with reticular cells that express the highest amounts of CAR cells in the marrow.[137] The majority of CAR cells are in the perivascular areas[137] to which the HSCs home.[50] Another factor that may contribute to perivascular homing, especially after stress like lethal irradiation, is the ability of the marrow sinusoidal endothelial cells that express CXCR4 to bind circulating CXCL12 and transport it into the perivascular areas of the marrow.[608,613] A second area in marrow to which of HSC home is the endosteal niche because of the proximity of these endosteal areas to the perivascular areas,[613] as well as the abundant CXCL12 production by osteoblasts and osteoclasts.[221,612] The remaining 25 percent of HSCs home to other locations in the marrow.[50,613] Thus, two HSC niches are recognized in marrow—perivascular and endosteal—with HSCs in the perivascular areas are more likely to proliferate, differentiate, and mobilize into the blood than HSCs in the endosteal areas.[221,613–616]

In the marrow, multiple mechanisms act to stabilize and reinforce the lodgement of HSC, that is, to maintain the HSC in niches. One prominent mechanism is the binding of KIT ligand, either secreted in and adherent to the marrow matrix or displayed on stromal cells, to its receptor c-KIT on HSC. The absence of either c-KIT or KIT ligand results in embryonic failure of hematopoiesis due to impaired homing of HSC to the fetal liver where KIT ligand acts cooperatively with CXCL12 as a chemoattractant and to impaired retention of HSC in marrow[617] where c-KIT upregulates HSC expression of integrins $\alpha_4\beta_1$ and $\alpha_5\beta_1$.[618] The β_1 integrins of the HSC also bind osteopontin, which, in turn, is bound to other matrix proteins, such as fibronectin and collagen. Similarly, CD44 on HSC binds to hyaluronic acid, fibronectin, and collagen the marrow matrix.[220] Two receptors on HSC that contribute specifically to endosteal niche retention are the calcium-sensing receptor,[619] which is needed for effective binding to collagen, and the Tie family receptor kinases,[620] specifically Tie-2 receptor,[621] which mediates HSC integrin binding to fibronectin after engaging its ligand, angiopoitein-1, that is expressed by osteoblasts. Marrow SP cells enriched with long-term repopulating quiescent HSC have high expression of β_3-integrin, most likely as the vitronectin receptor $\alpha_V\beta_3$, suggesting another integrin–matrix protein interaction that helps with HSC retention.[622] One mechanism of retention in the endosteal niche is the long-term maintenance of HSC by TPO produced by adjacent osteoblasts.[623,624] The binding of TPO by its receptor induces HSC quiescence, whereas the absence of TPO leads to active cell cycling and to a protracted and progressive depletion of HSCs.[623,624]

CELL PROLIFERATION AND MATURATION

Irrespective of their location during the post-natal period, HSC undergo continued self-renewal divisions, but at 3 to 4 weeks of age in mice (corresponding to 2–4 years in humans), they switch to their characteristic cell-cycle quiescence found in adult HSC.[625] This switch appears to be an intrinsic event that also decreases the myeloid differentiation potential of the HSCs.[625] In the adult marrow, specifically in the endosteal niche, HSCs have multiple stimuli that induce cell-cycle quiescence. These stimuli include high concentrations of CXCL12 and its binding by CXCR4[607,608]; low concentrations of CD34, podocalyxin, and endoglycan[578]; TPO binding by MPL[623,624]; variable binding to matrix proteins such as osteopontin, fibronectin, and fibulin, depending upon angiopoetin-1/Tie-2, and KIT ligand/c-KIT activities.[461,618,621] Compared to HSCs located outside the endosteal niche, HSCs that are tightly adherent to the endosteum have greater proliferative potential, marrow homing, and long-term reconstitution capacity.[626]

In murine transplantation studies, cell-cycle status is significant because HSCs in G_0/G_1 phases have high rates of engraftment and long-term reconstitution, whereas those in S, G_2, or M phases provide minimal engraftment or long-term reconstitution.[625,627,628] In long-term labeling with bromodeoxyuridine (BrdU), murine HSC with the lin–Sca+KIT+CD150+CD48–CD34– phenotype, representing both classical and SLAM HSC markers, have the greatest reconstitution capacity and are located in both endosteal and central areas of the marrow.[629] These HSC are extremely quiescent with an estimated division rate of only four or five times over the life of the adult mouse. However, the large majority of them can enter cell cycle and are mobilized within a day or two of stressful stimuli, including G-CSF or 5-fluorouracil (5-FU) administration.[629] But after they home and reestablish their marrow residence, almost all resume their deep quiescence, indicating that the long-term reconstituting HSC provide a large reserve of HSC that are ready to respond, but only do so under situations of stress.[629]

External stimuli promote cell cycling by inducing one or more of the three D-cyclin family members.[627,630] In G_1 phase, the D1, D2, and D3 cyclins in complexes with two cyclin-dependent kinases, cdk-4 and cdk-6, phosphorylate the retinoblastoma protein (pRB) and related repressors of the E2F transcription factors that promote the entry into S phase from G_1.[627,630] Although cellular proliferation of early multipotent progenitors, the short-term repopulating cells and the colony-forming unit–granulocyte-erythroid-monocyte-macrophages, have relatively low rates of proliferation, they are greatly increased compared to the very infrequent cell divisions of HSC. The D cyclins and cdk-4 and cdk-6 kinases are important in these early progenitor cells because murine knockouts that lack either all three D cyclins[631] or lack both cdk-4 and cdk-6 kinases[632] have specific, lethal hematopoietic failures at the fetal liver stage of definitive hematopoiesis. In both of these knockout models, the HSC populations have little or no loss of numbers, but the multipotent progenitors are severely reduced, indicating these cell cycle regulators are required for the process that commits the HSC to increased proliferation during differentiation.[631,632]

As they divide, multipotent progenitors have progressively restricted lineage potential, which is regulated by various transcription factors as described above in the sections on the individual cell types in the marrow. The single-lineage progenitors further increase the percentages of their populations in active cell cycle so that by the later stages of CFU-E, CFC-G, and the more mature hematopoietic precursor cell development, the majority are in the S, G_2, and M phases.[627] The two potential sources of extracellular stimuli that increase the hematopoietic cell division are soluble hematopoietic cytokines and local interactions of the progenitors with other cells and matrix in the marrow. Hematopoietic cytokines include those produced either in remote organs, such as EPO, or those produced in a wide variety of organs including the marrow, such as TPO, GM-CSF, and G-CSF.[633] These latter hematopoietic cytokines have multiple effects on their target progenitor cells, including the promotion of survival, maturation, and migration, that are important for the increased production and recruitment of the mature cells to sites of inflammation.[633] Among the cytokines, M-CSF has been shown to be mitogenic, that is, promote progression from G_1 to S phase, in macrophages and their precursors.[634] The signaling from FMS, the M-CSF receptor, that leads to the S-phase progression, is mediated by both cyclin D1 and the transcription factor MYC.[635] Among the various cellular interactions of late progenitors and precursors, attachment to central macrophages of erythroblastic islands has been demonstrated to promote G_1 to S phase progression in erythroid progenitors/precursors.[478] This mitogenic effect of macrophage-erythroid cell interaction is unrelated to the antiapoptotic effect of EPO on the erythroid cells during these stages of erythroid differentiation.[478]

Mature hematopoietic cells cease their cell division prior to their release from the marrow, but the mechanisms that signal the cessation of division in hematopoietic cells as they mature are uncertain. Among the potential mediators of this cessation are Rb and several intracellular inhibitors of the cyclin-dependent kinases, specifically the INK4 proteins (p15, p16, p18, p19) that inhibit cdk-4 and cdk-6 and the CIP/KIP family of cdk-2 inhibitors (p21, p27, and p57).[627] Rb knockout mice have a lethal anemia during fetal liver hematopoiesis that is associated with persistent progression through cell cycle, but the erythroblast apoptosis appears to be related to failure of mitochondrial biogenesis.[628] Understanding activity of the of $p16^{INK4a}$ in regulating cell cycle is complicated by its potential role in senescence and apoptosis of HSC.[636] Although p21 and p27 proteins have been proposed as having roles in the TGF-β–induced HSC quiescence and in the increased proliferation of later progenitor stages, cdk-2 knockout mice do not have impaired hematopoiesis,[637] indicating that other cell-cycle mediators are required for the cessation of proliferation that accompanies terminal differentiation.

Apoptosis is the major regulator of cellular populations in the marrow. Because of the exponential expansion of cells in a proliferating population, cell death has a dramatic effect on the numbers of cells in subsequent generations.[638] Thus, the regulation of hematopoietic cell populations by apoptosis provides a mechanism for dramatic and prompt changes in blood cell production. During various stages of their differentiations, hematopoietic cells depend upon specific hematopoietic cytokines to prevent apoptosis.[633,638] A wide range of sensitivities to the hematopoietic cytokines among the dependent cells, as has been demonstrated for erythroid cells and EPO,[639] results in differential survival that allows for a graded response. Experiments in knockout mice have identified specific proteins in the Bcl-2 family as principal regulators of the intrinsic or mitochondrial apoptosis pathway in the homeostasis of the hematopoietic cells populations in the marrow.[640,641] Antiapoptotic members of the Bcl-2 family (Bcl-2, Bcl-X_L, Mcl-1, and A1) stabilize the mitochondrial membranes by preventing mitochondrial depolarization by the pore-forming family members, Bax and Bak.[640,641] The antiapoptotic members are also opposed by the proapoptotic, regulatory family members that consist of the BH3-only domain, such as Bim, Bid, Nix, and Puma.

In HSC and multipotent progenitors, Mcl-1 is required to prevent apoptosis, and KIT ligand stimulation increases the Mcl-1 expression.[642] In the later stages of single-lineage progenitors, Mcl-1 continues to be required for survival of neutrophil, and B and T lymphocytes, but it is antagonized by the expression of Bim and Puma in these progenitors, providing a means to eliminate specific cells, such as the autoreactive B and T lymphocytes.[640,641] A1 is required for normal neutrophil survival.[643] In the erythroid lineage, Bcl-X_L is required to prevent apoptosis at the late erythroblast stage,[644] and the proapoptotic Nix protein is also expressed.[645] The sequential proapoptotic and antiapoptotic stimuli that regulate erythropoiesis demonstrate overlapping and cooperative interactions that affect erythroid cell homeostasis by both survival and differentiation. Following moderate blood loss, an increased percentage of HSC enter cell cycle and self-renewal.[646] In the BFU-E through CFU-E stages, KIT ligand and glucocorticoids act in concert to upregulate proliferation according to the erythropoietic requirements.[647] However, because CFU-E depends upon EPO, KIT ligand and EPO act together, enhancing the proliferation and survival, respectively, of CFU-E.[648] EPO prevents apoptosis of CFU-E through basophilic erythroblast stages by a mechanism other than upregulating the antiapoptotic Bcl-X_L, but its upregulation of Bcl-X_L prevents the apoptosis of the late-stage hemoglobin-producing erythroblasts.[644] Expression of proapoptotic Nix in very late erythroblasts and reticulocytes plays a major role in targeting mitochondria for nontoxic elimination by autophagy.[649,650]

Various mathematical models have been constructed to explain the production rates for each cell type during homeostasis and during

TABLE 4–4. Normal Precursor Cell Kinetics

	Marrow		
Cell Type	Number (cells/kg)	Transit Time (days)	Production Rate (cells/kg/day)
I. Red cells			
Erythroblasts	5.3×10^9	~5.0	3.0×10^9
Reticulocytes	8.2×10^9	2.8	3.0×10^9
II. Megakaryocytes	15.0×10^6	~7.0	2.0×10^6
III. Granulocytes			
Proliferation pool	2.1×10^9	~5.0	0.85×10^9
Postmitotic pool	5.6×10^9	6.6	0.85×10^9

SOURCE: Finch CA, Harker LA, Cook JD,[651] with permission.

periods of increased and decreased production. A model of homeostatic human marrow has been based upon marrow films and sections relating differential counts of marrow samples to their content of injected radioactive iron. A number of assumptions and approximations are made,[651] but the summary data (Table 4–4) agree well with many other observations on the cellular content and kinetics of normal marrows. Under pathologic conditions such as infection, inflammation, or hematopoietic dysplasia, the proliferation and differentiation of hematopoietic progenitors may be affected by microbial products, cytokines, and cellular interactions that do not have a role in normal hematopoietic development. Infections, for example, can lead to increased myelopoiesis without the involvement of the hematopoietic cytokines. HSC and their myeloid and lymphoid progeny have a multiple toll-like receptors (TLRs) which bind specific bacterial or viral molecules.[652,653] The activation of TLRs leads to increased myelopoietic proliferation and differentiation, especially of the monocyte/macrophage lineage, and differentiation of lymphoid cells toward the dendritic cell phenotype.[652,654] Although increased hematopoietic cytokines are produced by TLR activation, a direct response to TLR activation in hematopoietic cells changes the prevalent myeloid transcription factor from C/EBPα, which mediates homeostasis by hematopoietic cytokines, to C/EBPβ, which mediates the emergency responses to TLR activation.[655] In response to the activation of TLRs, mature neutrophils have decreased apoptosis as a result of increased Mcl-1 and decreased Bad activity.[653] An alternative path to apoptosis in hematopoietic cells is the activation of specific death-domain receptors for the ligands such as FAS ligand, TNFα, and TRAIL. Although these ligands are most commonly associated with pathologic states where they may play a role in the anemias of chronic disease, they have also been proposed to have a regulatory role in normal erythropoiesis.[656]

CELLULAR RELEASE

Cell migration from the marrow occurs between adventitial cells and through endothelial cell channels that develop at the time of cell transit. Electron micrographs of leukocytes partially translocated across endothelium indicate that marked deformation of these cells occurs as they penetrate the cytoplasm of the endothelial cell and enter the sinus lumen (Fig. 4–7).[657] As with reticulocytes, egress occurs adjacent to junctions of endothelial cells.[479] The nucleus of the granulocyte, usually segmented, does not require as marked a deformation to traverse the migration pore as do the nuclei of monocytes and lymphocytes.[657] This transendothelial migration is likely to be related to leukocyte migration from the blood and into areas of inflammation described in the section on adhesion and homing because the marrow sinusoidal endothelial cells constitutively express adhesion proteins that are upregulated in inflammation, including VCAM-1, ICAM-1, and E- and P-selectin.[509] The immature granulocytes in marrow are anchored to adventitial reticular cells through lectin-like adhesion molecules. Gradual loss of these molecules (e.g., shedding of L-selectin) during maturation or after activation could permit movement toward the sinus wall.[658] Transient changes in surface glycoproteins (upregulation of α-2,6-sialylation of CD11b and CD18) of maturing marrow myeloid cells lead to decreased stromal and fibronectin adhesion and may favor contact with endothelium and cell egress.[659] The complement component C5a and G-CSF administration recruit neutrophils by altering integrins (low CD11a with G-CSF) and decreased L-selectin expression (with both agents).[660,661] Similar findings obtained in mice lacking two or all three selectins underscore the essential role of selectins in neutrophil recruitment.[662]

A number of releasing factors have been implicated in the initiation of marrow granulocyte egress, including G-CSF,[663,664] GM-CSF,[665] the $C3_e$ component of complement,[666] zymosan-activated plasma-containing complement fragments,[667] glucocorticoid hormones,[668] androgenic steroids,[669] and endotoxin.[670] Neutrophils residing in the marrow venous sinusoids are rapidly released into the circulation by IL-8.[671] In a rat model in which releasing factors can be given through the femoral artery and neutrophils collected from the femoral vein, chemokines CXCL2 (MIP-2) and CXCL1 (KC) that are produced at sites of inflammation will induce rapid, selective neutrophil migration from the marrow compartment into the blood.[672,673] Blocking or inhibiting the α_4-integrin component, β_2-integrin component, or the sheddase that catalyzes the shedding of L-selectin on migrating HSC indicates that the interaction of the highly expressed VLA-4 on neutrophils with VCAM-1 on the sinusoidal endothelial cells is required for transendothelial migration, whereas shedding of L-selectin has no effect and β_2-integrin binding helps retain the neutrophils in the marrow.[672] Blocking the neutrophil enzyme matrix metalloproteinase-9 (MMP-9) had no effect on the chemokine-induced neutrophil migration.[673] CXCL2 and CXCL1-induced migration is synergistic with the rapid, selective neutrophil migration from the marrow induced by G-CSF,[674] which is mediated by interrupting the interaction of CXCL12 in the marrow and CXC4R on neutrophils.[675] In a similar hind-leg model in guinea pigs, IL-5 and eotaxin, both of which are produced in sites of allergic inflammation, induce the rapid, selective migration of eosinophils from the marrow to blood with a synergistic effect when both are administered.[676] CCL11(eotaxin) alone induces the migration of both eosinophil progenitor cells and mature eosinophils.[676] The route of migration is transendothelial, and blocking experiments demonstrate that β_2-integrin binding enhances eosinophil migration from the marrow to the blood, whereas α_4-integrin binding helps retain eosinophils in the marrow.[677] Prostaglandin D_2 (PDG_2) is produced by mast cells in sites of allergic inflammation, and it induces rapid, selective migration of eosinophils from the marrow to the blood in the guinea pig model.[678] The eosinophils respond via two PDG_2 receptors, chemoattractant receptor-homologous molecule on Th2 (CRHTH2) and D-type prostanoid (DP) receptors.[678]

Releasing factors for reticulocytes have been more difficult to identify. Adventitial reticular cell cytoplasm is a barrier to the reticulocytes on the abluminal surface of the endothelium.[679] Phlebotomy, phenylhydrazine-induced hemolytic anemia, and EPO result in marked reduction of the adventitial cell cover of the sinus, a process that is thought to facilitate cell egress through the endothelium.[680] To leave the marrow, the reticulocyte depends on a pressure gradient across the membrane to drive it through

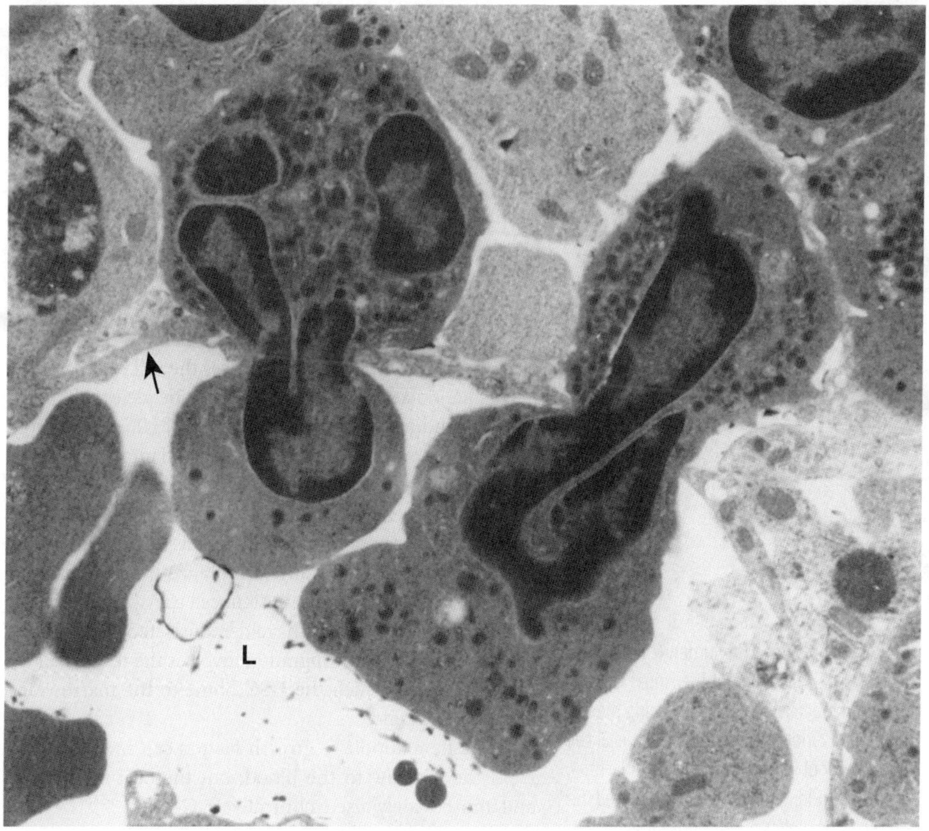

FIGURE 4–7. Transmission electron micrograph of mouse femoral marrow. The lumen (*L*) of a sinus is indicated. Endothelial cell cytoplasm separates the sinus lumen from the hematopoietic spaces (*arrow*). Two neutrophils are evident traversing the sinus wall. Note deformation of the cell producing a narrow waist where the cell passes through endothelium. The luminal portion of the migrating cells is granule-poor. The remainder of the cytoplasm is granule-rich, possibly reflecting gel-sol transformation during pseudopod formation.

the pore (Fig. 4–8).[679,680] The pressures within the marrow sinuses are pulsatile, and pressures sufficient to cause egress may be transient.[681] All of these estimations are based on a passive release mechanism, in part because mature reticulocytes are not motile and although very deformable compared to older reticulocytes,[682] making active migration by nascent reticulocytes through the endothelial cells improbable.

Platelet release is initiated by megakaryocyte cytoplasm invaginating the abluminal surface of the marrow sinus endothelial cell until a pore is made (Fig. 4–9). Cytoplasm flows through this pore into the marrow sinus and eventually is separated from the body of the megakaryocyte, resulting in a multiplatelet fragment or proplatelet (Fig. 4–10).[488] The proplatelets often are string bean–shaped structures and are found in the marrow sinus lumen.[493] The shear force of blood flow in the sinus fragments some proplatelets into single platelets.[454,455,500] Megakaryocyte nuclei are left in marrow after platelet release and are phagocytized and degraded there.[683]

Occasional immature granulocytes and megakaryocyte nuclei or whole megakaryocytes are present in cell concentrates of normal blood.[684] Nucleated red cells rarely escape from the marrow under normal conditions. The absence of circulating erythroblasts may relate to the spleen's capacity to sequester and enucleate circulating

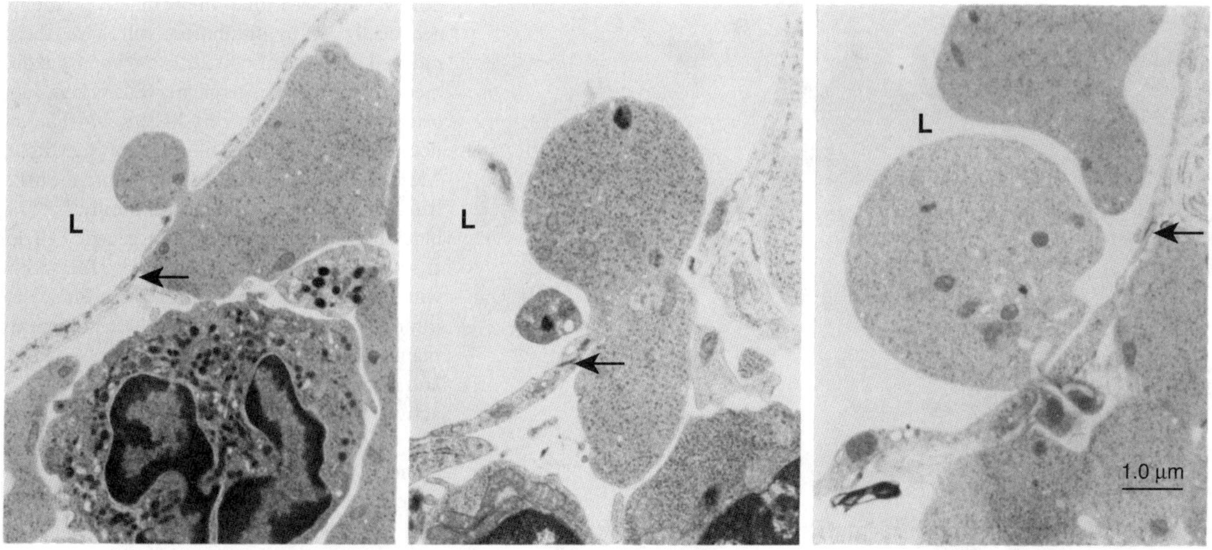

FIGURE 4–8. Transmission electron micrograph of mouse femoral marrow. Composite of reticulocytes in egress. **A.** Small protrusion of marrow reticulocyte into sinus lumen (*L*). **B.** Reticulocyte in egress, with approximately half the cell in the sinus lumen. **C.** Reticulocyte virtually in the sinus. Egress occurs through a migration pore that is parajunctional in position (*arrows* point to endothelial cell junctions). *(From Lichtman MA, Waugh RE,[479] with permission.)*

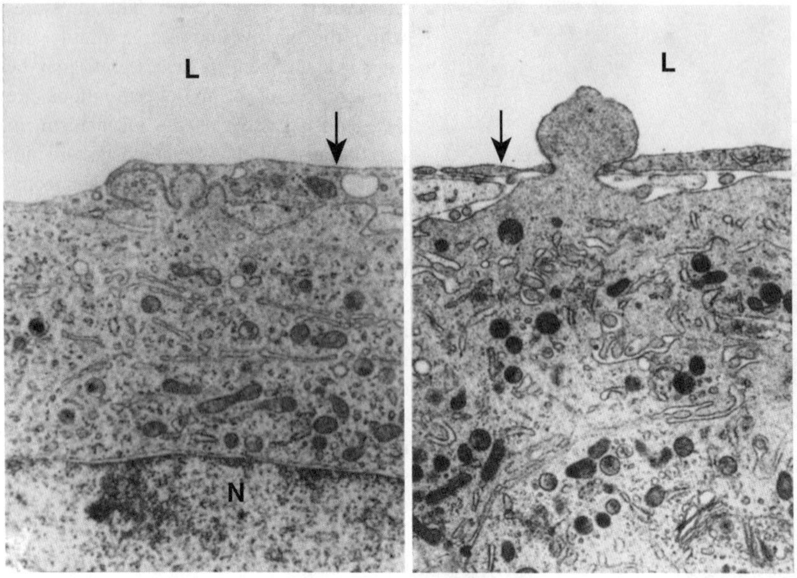

FIGURE 4–9. Transmission electron micrograph of mouse femoral marrow. **A.** The lumen (*L*) of a marrow sinus is indicated. The *arrow* points to the thin endothelial cytoplasmic lining of the sinus. The nucleus of a megakaryocyte (*N*) is indicated, with the cytoplasm of the megakaryocyte invaginating the endothelial cell cytoplasm in three places below the lumen. **B.** The arrow indicates the thin endothelial cell cytoplasmic lining of the sinus. The endothelium is attenuated to a double membrane in two places. A small process of megakaryocyte cytoplasm has formed a pore in the endothelial cell and has entered the sinus lumen (*L*). Cytoplasm flows through such pores and delivers proplatelets to the sinus lumen.

erythroblasts. The late myelocytes and metamyelocytes have the capacity to move, respond to chemoattractants, and deform, albeit less well than the mature neutrophils, and thus occasionally exit marrow by normal mechanisms. Invasion of marrow by neoplastic cells or replacement of marrow by fibrous tissue is associated with an increased prevalence of immature cells in the circulation. Damage to the architecture of marrow with a breakdown of the integrity of sinus walls may allow cells to enter the circulation less discriminately. Tumor cells elaborate chemoattractive cytokines (chemokines), which explains their ability to facilitate cell egress from marrow.[685]

Under homeostatic conditions, the migration of HSC from marrow into the blood is a rare but steady process.[514,515,629] With the stress of chemotherapeutic agents or pharmacologic doses of G-CSF administration, many HSCs are recruited into active cell cycle,[629] and they migrate into the blood before homing again to the marrow.[514] The stress of moderate blood loss also increases the cell cycling of the HSC, but those cycling HSC cannot be detected in the blood,[646] indicating that the migration of HSC in response to stress is very likely related to the inflammatory/injury component of the stress. This relationship between inflammation/injury and HSC migration has been used experimentally to understand the mechanisms of HSC migration into the blood and clinically to mobilize the HSC into the blood for collection for use in stem cell transplantation. Not surprisingly, these studies have demonstrated that much of the regulation of HSC migration involves the reversal of the mechanisms by which the HSC home to the marrow and develop quiescence.

Many hematopoietic growth factors can mobilize HSC from the marrow to the blood, but the best understood and most widely used clinically is G-CSF.[576,686–688] Like the other growth factors, the G-CSF mobilization of HSC requires several days for maximal effect. A major determinant in the both homing to and migration from the marrow is the interaction of CXCR4 on HSC and its ligand CXCL12 in the marrow. G-CSF induces stem cell mobilization by decreasing CXCL12.[689] Inhibitor studies originally identified the mechanism as the degradation of CXCL12 by neutrophil-associated enzymes such as neutrophil elastase, cathepsin G, and MMP-9 or the HSC enzyme CD26/dipeptidylpepetidase.[576,607,686,689] Later studies, however, showed that mice that lack the proteases genetically or by inhibition still have the G-CSF–induced decrease of CXCL12,[690,691] and the decrease is mediated by the adrenergic nervous system suppressing osteoblast production of CXCL12.[91,92] The successful development of small blockers of CXCR4, such as AMD-3100, has provided a more rapid means to mobilize HSC that could be used clinically.[687,688] Similarly, blocking α_4-integrin binding or genetic deletion of the α_4-integrin component leads to HSC mobilization within 1 or 2 days under both homeostatic or G-CSF–induced conditions.[576,616] This effect appears to be mainly mediated through disruption of VLA-4 activity and is further enhanced by interfering with the binding activity of other adhesion mediators such as the β_2-integrins or E-selectin whose blocking has no effect alone.[576,616,687,692] Some of these β_2-integrin synergistic effects may be indirect through the action on other cells.[576,693] The results of interfering with two other adhesion mediators of HSC homing, CD44 and KIT ligand, are unclear in that blocking experiments using antibodies to CD44 or administration of soluble KIT ligand induced HSC mobilization while genetic deficiencies of CD44 or c-KIT leads to decreased G-CSF mobilization.[576,687,688] Two chemokine ligands of the

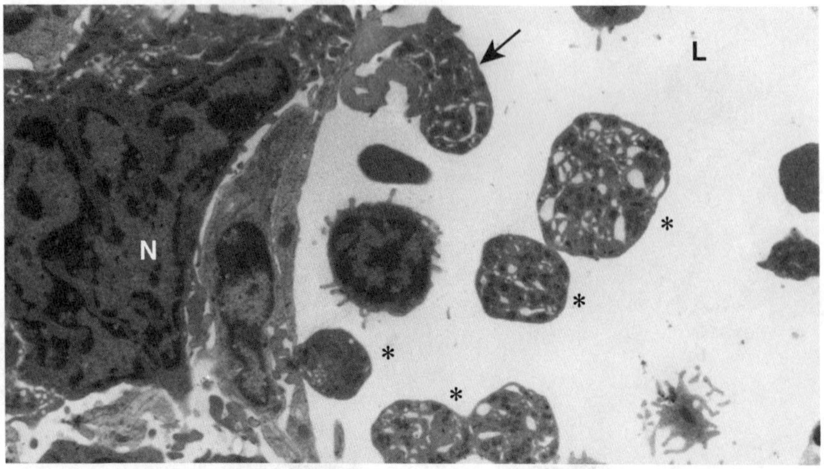

FIGURE 4–10. Transmission electron micrograph of mouse femoral marrow. The marrow sinus lumen (*L*) and a megakaryocyte nucleus (*N*) virtually denuded of cytoplasm are indicated. The megakaryocyte nucleus abuts the nucleus of an adventitial reticular cell; the latter is separated from the lumen by the very thin endothelial cell cytoplasm. A portion of residual megakaryocyte cytoplasm (proplatelet) can be seen streaming into the lumen (*arrow*). The lumen contains several proplatelets (*asterisks*). Compare the size of the proplatelets to that of lymphocyte in the sinus. The bean-shaped, three-dimensional appearance of the proplatelets can be seen in the scanning micrograph shown in Figure 4–6.

CXCR2 receptor, IL-8 and GRO-β (KC in mice), will induce HSC mobilization within minutes to hours and can synergize with G-CSF, but their action is more complex in that it is mediated through neutrophils and their enzymes including MMP-9.[607,687,688,694]

REFERENCES

1. Testa NG, Molineux G: *Haemopoiesis: A Practical Approach*. IRL Press, New York, 1993.
2. Neuman E: Ueber die Bedeutung des Knochenmarks für die Blutbildung. *Cbl Med Wiss* 6:689, 1868.
3. Bizzozero G: Sulla fungione ematopoietica del midollo delle ossa. *Gazz Med Ital-Lomb* 46, 1868.
4. Neuman E: Du Role de la möelle des os dans la formation du sang. *C R Acad Sci (Paris)* 68:1112, 1869.
5. Mosler F: Klinische Symptome und Therapie der medullalären Leukemi. *Berl Klin Wochenschr* 13:233, 1876.
6. Arinkin MJ: Die intravitale Untersuchungsmetodik des Knochenmarks. *Folia Haematol Int Mag Klin Morphol Blutforsch (Leipzig)* 38:233, 1929.
7. Lajtha LG: The common ancestral cell, in *Blood Pure and Eloquent*, edited by MM Wintrobe, p 81. McGraw-Hill, New York, 1980.
8. Erslev AJ: Feedback circuits in the control of stem cell differentiation. *Am J Pathol* 65:629, 1971.
9. Trentin JJ: Determination of bone marrow stem cell differentiation by stroma hemopoietic inductive microenvironment (HIM). *Am J Pathol* 65:621, 1971.
10. Lemischka IR, Moore KA: Stem cells: Interactive niches. *Nature* 425:778, 2003.
11. Hackney JA, Charbord P, Brunk BP, et al: A molecular profile of a hematopoietic stem cell niche. *Proc Natl Acad Sci U S A* 99:13061, 2002.
12. Zhang J, Niu C, Ye L, et al: Identification of the haematopoietic stem cell niche and control of the niche size. *Nature* 425:836, 2003.
13. Calvi LM, Adams GB, Weibrecht KW, et al: Osteoblastic cells regulate the haematopoietic stem cell niche. *Nature* 425:841, 2003.
14. Weissman IL, Anderson DJ, Gage F: Stem and progenitor cells: Origins, phenotypes, lineage commitments, and transdifferentiations. *Annu Rev Cell Dev Biol* 17:387, 2001.
15. Dao MA, Arevalo J, Nolta JA: Reversibility of CD34 expression on human hematopoietic stem cells that retain the capacity for secondary reconstitution. *Blood* 101:112, 2003.
16. Kuci S, Wessels JT, Buhring HJ, et al: Identification of a novel class of human adherent CD34-stem cells that give rise to SCID-repopulating cells. *Blood* 101:869, 2003.
17. Ziegler BL, Valtieri M, Almeida-Porada G, et al: KDR receptor: A key marker defining hematopoietic stem cells. *Science* 285:1553, 1999.
18. Christensen JL, Weissman IL: Flk-2 is a marker in hematopoietic stem cell differentiation: A simple method to isolate long-term stem cells. *Proc Natl Acad Sci U S A* 98:14541, 2001.
19. Bhatia M: AC133 expression in human stem cells. *Leukemia* 15:1686, 2001.
20. Steidl U, Krovenwett R, Rohr UP, et al: Gene expression profiling identifies significant differences between the molecular phenotypes of bone marrow-derived and circulating human CD34+ hematopoietic stem cells. *Blood* 99:2037, 2002.
21. Ivanova NB, Dimos JT, Schaniel C, et al: A stem cell molecular signature. *Science* 298:601, 2002.
22. Baron MH: Embryonic origins of mammalian hematopoiesis. *Exp Hematol* 31:1160, 2003.
23. Mikkola HK, Gekas C, Orkin SH, Dieterlen-Lievre F: Placenta as a site for hematopoietic stem cell development. *Exp Hematol* 33:1048, 2005.
24. Dieterlen-Lièvre F: Emergence of haematopoietic stem cells during development. *C R Biol* 330:504, 2007.
25. McGrath K, Palis J: Ontogeny of erythropoiesis in the mammalian embryo. *Curr Top Dev Biol* 82:1, 2008.
26. Migliaccio G, Migliaccio AR, Petti S, et al: Human embryonic hemopoiesis. Kinetics of progenitors and precursors underlying the yolk sac—Liver transition. *J Clin Invest* 78:51, 1986.
27. Snyder A, Fraser ST, Baron MH: Bone morphogenetic proteins in vertebrate hematopoietic development. *J Cell Biochem* 93:224, 2004.
28. Durand C, Robin C, Bollerot K, et al: Embryonic stromal clones reveal developmental regulators of definitive hematopoietic stem cells. *Proc Natl Acad Sci U S A* 104:20838, 2007.
29. Nishikawa SI: A complex linkage in the developmental pathway of endothelial and hematopoietic cells. *Curr Opin Cell Biol* 13:673, 2001.
30. Park C, Ma YD, Choi K: Evidence for the hemangioblast. *Exp Hematol* 33:965, 2005.
31. Jaffredo T, Nottingham W, Liddiard K, et al: From hemangioblast to hematopoietic stem cell: An endothelial connection? *Exp Hematol* 33:1029, 2005.
32. Huber TL, Kouskoff V, Fehling HJ, et al: Haemangioblast commitment is initiated in the primitive streak of the mouse embryo. *Nature* 432:625, 2004.
33. Zovein AC, Hofmann JJ, Lynch M, et al: Fate tracing reveals the endothelial origin of hematopoietic stem cells. *Cell Stem Cell* 3:625, 2008.
34. Burns CE, Traver D, Mayhall E, et al: Hematopoietic stem cell fate is established by the Notch-Runx pathway. *Genes Dev* 19:2331, 2005.
35. Nakagawa M, Ichikawa M, Kumano K, et al: AML1/Runx1 rescues Notch1-null mutation-induced deficiency of para-aortic splanchnopleural hematopoiesis. *Blood* 108:3329, 2006.
36. Marshall CJ, Sinclair JC, Thrasher AJ, Kinnon C: Bone morphogenetic protein 4 modulates c-Kit expression and differentiation potential in murine embryonic aorta-gonad-mesonephros haematopoiesis *in vitro*. *Br J Haematol* 139:321, 2007.
37. Robin C, Ottersbach K, Durand C, et al: An unexpected role for IL-3 in the embryonic development of hematopoietic stem cells. *Dev Cell* 11:171, 2006.
38. Almeida-Porada GD, Hoffman R, Manalo P, et al: Detection of human cells in human/sheep chimeric lambs with in vitro human stroma-forming potential. *Exp Hematol* 24:482, 1996.
39. Zanjani ED, Almeida-Porada G, Livingston AG, et al: Reversible expression of CD34 by adult human bone marrow long-term engrafting hematopoietic stem cells. *Exp Hematol* 31:406, 2003.
40. Gallacher L, Murdoch B, Wu DM, et al: Isolation and characterization of human CD34(−)Lin(−) and CD34(+)Lin(−) hematopoietic stem cells using cell surface markers AC133 and CD7. *Blood* 95:2813, 2000.
41. Gehling UM, Ergun S, Schumacher U, et al: *In vitro* differentiation of endothelial cells from AC133-positive progenitor cells. *Blood* 95:3106, 2000.
42. Takakura N, Watanabe T, Suenobu S, et al: A role for hematopoietic stem cells in promoting angiogenesis. *Cell* 102:199, 2000.
43. Wang L, Li L, Shojaei F, et al: Endothelial and hematopoietic cell fate of human embryonic stem cells originates from primitive endothelium with hemangioblastic properties. *Immunity* 21:31, 2004.
44. Cogle CR, Wainman DA, Jorgensen ML, et al: Adult human hematopoietic cells provide functional hemangioblast activity. *Blood* 103:133, 2004.
45. Bailey AS, Jiang S, Afentoulis M, et al: Transplanted adult hematopoietic stems cells differentiate into functional endothelial cells. *Blood* 103:13, 2004.
46. Nadin BM, Goodell MA, Hirschi KK: Phenotype and hematopoietic potential of side population cells throughout embryonic development. *Blood* 102:2436, 2003.
47. Scharenberg CW, Harkey MA, Tork-Storb B: The ABCG2 transporter is an efficient Hoechst 33342 efflux pump and is preferentially expressed by immature human progenitors. *Blood* 99:507, 2002.
48. Pearce DJ, Ridler CM, Simpson C, Bonnet D: Multiparameter analysis of murine bone marrow side population cells. *Blood* 103:2541, 2004.
49. Eaker SS, Hawley TS, Ramezani A, Hawley RG: Detection and enrichment of hematopoietic stem cells by side population phenotype. *Methods Mol Biol* 263:161, 2004.
50. Kiel MJ, Yilmaz OH, Iwashita T, et al: SLAM family receptors distinguish hematopoietic stem and progenitor cells and reveal endothelial niches for stem cells. *Cell* 121:1109, 2005.
51. Kim I, He S, Yilmaz OH, et al: Enhanced purification of fetal liver hematopoietic stem cells using SLAM family receptors. *Blood* 108:737, 2006.
52. Jackson KA, Mi T, Goodell MA: Hematopoietic potential of stem cells isolated from murine skeletal muscle. *Proc Natl Acad Sci U S A* 96:14482, 1999.
53. Bjornson CR, Rietze RL, Reynolds BA, et al: Turning brain into blood: A hematopoietic fate adopted by adult neural stem cells *in vivo*. *Science* 283:534, 1999.
54. Majka SM, Jackson KA, Kienstra KA, et al: Distinct progenitor populations in skeletal muscle are bone marrow derived and exhibit different cell fates during vascular regeneration. *J Clin Invest* 111:71, 2003.
55. Geiger H, True JM, Grimes B, et al: Analysis of the hematopoietic potential of muscle-derived cells in mice. *Blood* 100:721, 2002.
56. Issarachai S, Priestley GV, Nakamoto B, Papayannopoulou T: Cells with hemopoietic potential residing in muscle are itinerant bone marrow-derived cells. *Exp Hematol* 30:366, 2002.
57. Ratajczak MZ, Kucia M, Reca R, et al: Stem cell plasticity revisited: CXCR4-positive cells expressing mRNA for early muscle, liver and neural cells "hide out" in the bone marrow. *Leukemia* 18:29, 2004.
58. Zipori D: The stem state: Mesenchymal plasticity as a paradigm. *Curr Stem Cell Res Ther* 1:95, 2006.
59. Phinney DG, Prockop DJ: Concise review: Mesenchymal stem/multipotent stromal cells: The state of transdifferentiation and modes of tissue repair—Current views. *Stem Cells* 25:2896, 2007.
60. Colnot C, de la Fuente L, Huang S, et al: Indian hedgehog synchronizes skeletal angiogenesis and perichondrial maturation with cartilage development. *Development* 132:1057, 2005.
61. Cecchini MG, Hofstetter W, Halasy J, et al: Role of CSF-1 in bone and bone marrow development. *Mol Reprod Dev* 46:75, 1997.
62. Tavian M, Péault B: The changing cellular environments of hematopoiesis in human development in utero. *Exp Hematol* 33:1062, 2005.
63. Custer RP, Ahlfeldt FE: Studies on the structure and function of the bone marrow. *J Lab Clin Med* 17:960, 1932.
64. Gregersen MI, Rawson RA: Blood volume. *Physiol Rev* 39:307, 1969.
65. Christy M: Active marrow distribution as a function of age in humans. *Phys Med Biol* 26:389, 1981.
66. Babyn PS, Ranson M, McCarvelle ME: Normal bone marrow signal characteristics and fatty conversion. *Med Clin North Am* 6:473, 1998.
67. Huggins C, Blocksom BH Jr: Changes in outlying bone marrow accompanying a local increase in temperature within physiologic limits. *J Exp Med* 64:253, 1936.
68. Maniatis A, Tavassoli M, Crosby WH: Factors affecting the conversion of yellow to red marrow. *Blood* 37:581, 1971.

69. Crosby WH: Experience with injured and implanted bone marrow: Relation of function to structure, in *Hemopoietic Cellular Proliferation*, edited by F Stohlman Jr, p 87. Grune & Stratton, New York, 1970.
70. Ji X, Chen D, Xu C, et al: Patterns of gene expression associated with BMP-2-induced osteoblast and adipocyte differentiation of mesenchymal progenitor cell 3T3-F442A. *J Bone Miner Metab* 18:132, 2000.
71. Martin RB, Chow BD, Lucas PA: Bone marrow fat content in relation to bone remodeling and serum chemistry in intact and ovariectomized dogs. *Calcif Tissue Int* 46:189, 1990.
72. Brookes M: *The Blood Supply of Bone*. Butterworth, London, 1971.
73. Tavassoli M: Arterial structure of the bone marrow in rabbits with special reference to thin walled arteries. *Acta Anat (Basel)* 90:608, 1974.
74. Wilkins BS, Jones DB: Vascular networks within the stroma of human long-term bone marrow cultures. *J Pathol* 177:295, 1995.
75. Charbord P, Tavian M, Humeau L, Peault B: Early ontogeny of the human marrow from long bones: An immunohistochemical study of hematopoiesis and its microenvironment. *Blood* 87:4109, 1996.
76. Peichev M, Naiyer AJ, Pereira D, et al: Expression of VEGFR-2 and AC133 by circulating human CD34(+) cells identifies a population of functional endothelial precursors. *Blood* 95:952, 2000.
77. Hildebrand P, Cirulli V, Prinsen RC, et al: The role of angiopoietins in the development of endothelial cells from cord blood CD34+ progenitors. *Blood* 104:2010, 2004.
78. Wijelath ES, Rahman S, Murray J, et al: Fibronectin promotes VEGF-induced CD34 cell differentiation into endothelial cells. *J Vasc Surg* 39:655, 2004.
79. Lichtman MA: The ultrastructure of the hemopoietic environment of the marrow: A review. *Exp Hematol* 9:391, 1981.
80. Yamazaki K, Allen TD: Ultrastructural morphometric study of efferent nerve terminals on murine bone marrow stromal cells, and the recognition of a novel anatomical unit: The "neuro-reticular complex." *Am J Anat* 187:261, 1990.
81. Artico M, Bosco S, Cavallotti C, et al: Noradrenergic and cholinergic innervation of the bone marrow. *Int J Mol Med* 10:77, 2002.
82. Goto T, Yamaza T, Kido MA, et al: Light and electron microscopy study of the distribution of axon containing substance-P and the localization of neurokinin-1 receptor in bone. *Cell Tissue Res* 293:87, 1998.
83. Chenu C: Glutaminergic innervation in bone. *Microsc Res Tech* 58:70, 2002.
84. Cattoretti G, Schiro R, Orazi A, et al: Bone marrow stroma in humans: Anti-nerve growth factor receptor antibodies selectively stain reticular cells *in vivo* and *in vitro*. *Blood* 81:1726, 1993.
85. Rameshwar P, Gascon P: Substance P (SP) mediates production of stem cell factor and interleukin-1 in bone marrow stroma: Potential autoregulatory role for these cytokines in SP receptor expression and induction. *Blood* 86:482, 1995.
86. Rameshwar P, Zhu G, Donelly RJ, et al: The dynamics of bone marrow stromal cells in the proliferation of multipotent hematopoietic progenitors by substance P: An understanding of the effects of a neurotransmitter on the differentiating hematopoietic stem cell. *J Neuroimmunol* 121:22, 2001.
87. Hiramoto M, Aizawa S, Iwase O, et al: Stimulatory effects of substance P on CD34 positive cell proliferation and differentiation in vitro are mediated by the modulation of stromal cell function. *Int J Mol Med* 1:347, 1998.
88. Greeno EW, Mantyh P, Vercellotti GM, Moldow CF: Functional neurokin 1 receptors for substance P are expressed by human vascular endothelium. *J Exp Med* 177:1269, 1993.
89. Pelletier L, Angonin R, Regnard J, et al: Human bone marrow angiogenesis: In vitro modulation by substance P and neurokinin A. *Br J Haematol* 119:1083, 2002.
90. Afan AM, Broome CS, Nicholls SE, et al: Bone marrow innervation regulates cellular retention in the murine haematopoietic system. *Br J Haematol* 98:569, 1997.
91. Méndez-Ferrer S, Lucas D, Battista M, Frenette PS: Haematopoietic stem cell release is regulated by circadian oscillations. *Nature* 452:442, 2008.
92. Katayama Y, Battista M, Kao WM, et al: Signals from the sympathetic nervous system regulate hematopoietic stem cell egress from bone marrow. *Cell* 124:407, 2006.
93. Abboud CN, Liesveld JL, Lichtman MA: The architecture of marrow and its role in hematopoietic cell lodgement, in *The Hematopoietic Microenvironment*, edited by MW Long, MS Wicha, p 2. Johns Hopkins University Press, Baltimore, MD, 1993.
94. Tavassoli M, Shaklai M: Absence of tight junctions in endothelium of marrow sinuses: Possible significance for marrow cell egress. *Br J Haematol* 41:303, 1979.
95. Bankston PW, DeBruyn PPH: The permeability to carbon of the sinusoidal lining cells of the embryonic rat liver and rat bone marrow. *Am J Anat* 141:281, 1974.
96. Lichtman MA, Packman CH, Constine LS: Molecular and cellular traffic across the marrow sinus wall, in *Blood Cell Formation: The Role of Hemopoietic Microenvironment*, edited by M. Tavassoli, p 87. Humana Press, Clifton, NJ, 1989.
97. Kataoka M, Tavassoli M: Identification of lectin-like substances recognizing galactosyl residues of glycoconjugates on the plasma membrane of marrow sinus endothelium. *Blood* 65:1163, 1985.
98. Bussolino F, Colotta F, Bocchietto E, et al: Recent developments in the cell biology of granulocyte-macrophage colony-stimulating factor and granulocyte colony-stimulating factor: Activities on endothelial cells. *Int J Clin Lab Res* 23:8, 1993.
99. Koch AE, Burrows JC, Domer PH, et al: Monoclonal antibodies defining shared human macrophage-endothelial antigens. *Pathobiology* 60:59, 1992.
100. Penn PE, Jiang D-Z, Fei R-G, et al: Dissecting the hematopoietic microenvironment: IX. Further characterization of murine bone marrow stromal cells. *Blood* 81:1205, 1993.
101. Hasthorpe S, Bogdanovski M, Rogerson J, Radley JM: Characterization of endothelial cells in murine long-term marrow culture: Implication for hemopoietic regulation. *Exp Hematol* 20:386, 1992.
102. Perkins S, Fleischman RA: Stromal cell progeny of murine bone marrow fibroblast colony-forming units are clonal endothelial-like cells that express collagen IV and laminin. *Blood* 75:620, 1990.
103. van Buul JD, Mul FP, Van der Schoot CE, Hordijk PL: ICAM-3 activation modulates cell-cell contacts of human bone marrow endothelial cells. *J Vasc Res* 41:28, 2004.
104. Schweitzer KM, Drager AM, Van der Valk P, et al: Constitutive expression of E-selectin and vascular cell adhesion molecule-1 on endothelial cells of hematopoietic tissues. *Am J Pathol* 148:165, 1996.
105. Yao L, Yokota T, Xia L, et al: Bone marrow dysfunction in mice lacking the cytokine receptor gp130 in endothelial cells. *Blood* 106:4093, 2005.
106. Masek LC, Sweetenham JW, Whitehouse JMA, Schumacher U: Immuno-, lectin-, and enzyme-histochemical characterization of human bone marrow endothelium. *Exp Hematol* 22:1203, 1994.
107. Rafii S, Shapiro F, Rimarachin J, et al: Isolation and characterization of human bone marrow microvascular endothelial cells: Hematopoietic progenitor adhesion. *Blood* 84:10, 1994.
108. Villars F, Guillotin B, Amedee T, et al: Effect of HUVEC on human osteoprogenitor cell differentiation needs heterotypic gap junction communication. *Am J Physiol Cell Physiol* 282:C775, 2002.
109. Guillotin B, Bourget C, Remy-Zolgadri M, et al: Human primary endothelial cells stimulate human osteoprogenitor cell differentiation. *Cell Physiol Biochem* 14:325, 2004.
110. Mohle R, Salemi P, Moore MA, Rafii S: Expression of interleukin-5 by human bone marrow microvascular endothelial cells: Implications for the regulation of eosinophilopoiesis *in vivo*. *Br J Haematol* 99:732, 1997.
111. Huang WQ, Wang QR: Bone marrow endothelial cells secrete thymosin beta4 and AcSDKP. *Exp Hematol* 29:12, 2001.
112. Bordenave L, Georges A, Bareille R, et al: Human bone marrow endothelial cells: A new identified source of B-type natriuretic peptide. *Peptides* 23:935, 2002.
113. Delia D, Lampugnani MG, Resnati M, et al: CD34 expression is regulated reciprocally with adhesion molecules in vascular cells *in vitro*. *Blood* 81:1001, 1993.
114. Guo WX, Ghebrehiwet B, Weksler B, et al: Up-regulation of endothelial cell binding proteins/receptors for complement component C1q by inflammatory cytokines. *J Lab Clin Med* 133:541, 1999.
115. van Buul JD, Voermans C, Van den Berg V, et al: Migration of human hematopoietic progenitor cells across bone marrow endothelium is regulated by vascular endothelial cadherin. *J Immunol* 168:588, 2002.
116. Netelenbos T, Van den Born J, Kessler FL, et al: In vitro model for hematopoietic progenitor cell homing reveals endothelial heparan sulfate proteoglycans as direct adhesive ligands. *J Leukoc Biol* 74:1035, 2003.
117. Netelenbos T, Van den Born J, Kessler FL, et al: Proteoglycans on bone marrow endothelial cells bind and present SDF-1 towards hematopoietic progenitor cells. *Leukemia* 17:175, 2003.
118. Hillyer P, Mordelet E, Flynn G, Male D: Chemokines, chemokine receptors and adhesion molecules on different human endothelia: Discriminating the tissue-specific functions that affect leucocyte migration. *Clin Exp Immunol* 134:431, 2003.
119. Yun HJ, Jo DY: Production of stromal cell-derived factor-1 (SDF-1), and expression of CXCR4 in human bone marrow endothelial cells. *J Korean Med Sci* 18:679, 2003.
120. Imai T, Hieshima K, Haskell C, et al: Identification and molecular characterization of fractalkine receptor CX3CR1 which mediates both leukocyte migration and adhesion. *Cell* 91:521, 1997.
121. Nitschke L, Floyd H, Ferguson DJ, Crocker PR: Identification of CD22 ligands on bone marrow sinusoidal endothelium implicated in CD22-dependent homing of recirculating B cells. *J Exp Med* 189:1513, 1999.
122. Weiss L, Chen L-T: The organization of hemopoietic cords and vascular sinuses in bone marrow. *Blood Cells* 1:617, 1975.
123. Leblond PF, Chamberlain JK, Weed RI: Scanning electron microscopy of erythropoietin-stimulated bone marrow. *Blood Cells* 1:639, 1975.
124. Abboud CN, Duerst RE, Frantz CN, et al: Lysis of human fibroblast colony-forming cells and endothelial cells by monoclonal antibody (6–19) and complement. *Blood* 68:1196, 1986.
125. Simmons PJ, Torok-Storb B: Identification of stromal cell precursors in human bone marrow by a novel monoclonal antibody, STRO-1. *Blood* 78:55, 1991.
126. Labouyrie E, Dubus P, Groppi A, et al: Expression of neurotrophins and their receptors in human bone marrow. *Am J Pathol* 154:405, 1999.
127. Gronthos S, Simmons PJ: The growth factor requirements of STRO-1-positive human bone marrow stromal precursors under serum-deprived conditions in vitro. *Blood* 85:929, 1995.
128. Galmiche MC, Koteliansky VE, Briere J, et al: Stromal cells from human long-term marrow cultures are mesenchymal cells that differentiate following a vascular smooth muscle differentiation pathway. *Blood* 82:66, 1993.
129. Dennis JE, Charbord P: Origin and differentiation of human and murine stroma. *Stem Cells* 20:205, 2002.
130. Brown J, Greaves MF, Molgaard HV: The gene encoding the stem cell antigen, CD34 is conserved in mouse and expressed in haemopoietic progenitor cell lines, brain, and embryonic fibroblasts. *Int Immunol* 3:175, 1991.
131. Simmons PJ, Torok-Storb B: CD34 expression by stromal precursors in normal adult bone marrow. *Blood* 78:2848, 1991.

132. Dorshkind K, Green L, Godwin A, Fletcher WH: Connexin-43-type gap junctions mediate communication between bone marrow stromal cells. *Blood* 82:38, 1993.
133. Montecino RE, Leathers H, Dorshkind K: Expression of connexin 43(Gx43) is critical for normal hematopoiesis. *Blood* 96:917, 2000.
134. Durig J, Rosenthal C, Halfmeyer K, et al: Intercellular communication between bone marrow stromal cell and CD34+ haematopoietic progenitor cells is mediated by connexin 43-type gap junctions. *Br J Haematol* 111:416, 2000.
135. Rosendaal M, Jopling C: Hematopoietic capacity of connexin43 wild-type and knock-out fetal liver cells not different on wild-type stroma. *Blood* 101:2996, 2003.
136. Torok-Storb B, Iwata M, Graf L, et al: Dissecting the marrow micro-environment. *Ann N Y Acad Sci* 872:164, 1999.
137. Sugiyama T, Kohara H, Noda M, Nagasawa T: Maintenance of the hematopoietic stem cell pool by CXCL12-CXCR4 chemokine signaling in bone marrow stromal cell niches. *Immunity* 25:977, 2006.
138. Nagasawa T: The chemokine CXCL12 and regulation of HSC and B lymphocyte development in the bone marrow niche. *Adv Exp Med Biol* 602:69, 2007.
139. Kohara H, Omatsu Y, Sugiyama T, et al: Development of plasmacytoid dendritic cells in bone marrow stromal cell niches requires CXCL12-CXCR4 chemokine signaling. *Blood* 110:4153, 2007.
140. Weiss L, Geduldig U: Barrier cells: Stromal regulation of hematopoiesis and blood cell release in normal and stressed murine bone marrow. *Blood* 78:975, 1991.
141. Tavassoli M: Fatty evolution of marrow and the role of adipose tissue in hematopoiesis, in *Handbook of the Hemopoietic Microenvironment*, edited by M Tavassoli, p 157. Humana Press, Clifton, NJ, 1989.
142. Laharrague P, Larrouy D, Fontanilles AM, et al: High expression of leptin by human bone marrow adipocytes in primary cultures. *FASEB J* 12:747, 1998.
143. Benayahu D, Shamay A, Wientroub S: Osteocalcin (BGP), gene expression, and protein production by marrow stromal adipocytes. *Biochem Biophys Res Commun* 13:442, 1997.
144. McAveny KM, Gimble JM, Yu-Lee L: Prolactin receptor expression during adipocyte differentiation of bone marrow stroma. *Endocrinology* 137:5723, 1996.
145. Delikat S, Harris RJ, Galvani DW: IL-1 beta inhibits adipocyte formation in human long-term bone marrow culture. *Exp Hematol* 21:31, 1993.
146. Keller DC, Du XX, Srour EF, et al: Interleukin-11 inhibits adipogenesis and stimulates myelopoiesis in human long-term marrow cultures. *Blood* 82:1428, 1993.
147. Fantuzzi G, Fraggioni R: Leptin in the regulation of immunity, inflammation, and hematopoiesis. *J Leukoc Biol* 68:437, 2000.
148. Yokota T, Meka CS, Kouro T, et al: Adiponectin, a fat cell product, influences the earliest lymphocyte precursors in bone marrow cultures by activation of the cyclooxygenase-prostaglandin pathway in stromal cells. *J Immunol* 171:5091, 2003.
149. Thomas T, Gori F, Khosla S, et al: Leptin acts on human marrow stromal cells to enhance differentiation to osteoblasts and to inhibit differentiation to adipocytes. *Endocrinology* 140:1630, 1999.
150. Yokota T, Meka CS, Medina KL, et al: Paracrine regulation of fat cell formation in bone marrow cultures via adiponectin and prostaglandins. *J Clin Invest* 109:1303, 2002.
151. Yokota T, Meka CS, Kouro T, et al: Adiponectin, a fat cell product, influences the earliest lymphocyte precursors in bone marrow cultures by activation of the cyclooxygenase-prostaglandin pathway in stromal cells. *J Immunol* 171:5091, 2003.
152. Brakenhielm E, Veitonmaki N, Cao R, et al: Adiponectin-induced antiangiogenesis and antitumor activity involve caspase-mediated endothelial cell apoptosis. *Proc Natl Acad Sci U S A* 101:2476, 2004.
153. Zhou S, Eid K, Glowacki J: Cooperation between TGF-beta and Wnt pathways during chondrocyte and adipocyte differentiation of human marrow stromal cells. *J Bone Miner Res* 19:463, 2004.
154. Gimble JM, Morgan C, Kelly K, et al: Bone morphogenetic proteins inhibit adipocyte differentiation by bone marrow stromal cells. *J Cell Biochem* 58:393, 1995.
155. Chen TL, Shen WJ, Kraemer FB: Human BMP-7/OP-1 induces the growth and differentiation of adipocytes and osteoblasts in bone marrow stromal cell cultures. *J Cell Biochem* 82:187, 2001.
156. Li X, Cui Q, Kao C, et al: Lovastatin inhibits adipogenic and stimulates osteogenic differentiation by suppressing PPARgamma2 and increasing Cbfa1/Runx2 expression in bone marrow mesenchymal cell cultures. *Bone* 33:652, 2003.
157. Gevers EF, Loveridge N, Robinson IC: Bone marrow adipocytes: A neglected target tissue for growth hormone. *Endocrinology* 143:4065, 2002.
158. Duque G, Macoritto M, Kremer R: 1, 25(OH)2D3 inhibits bone marrow adipogenesis in senescence accelerated mice (SAM-P/6) by decreasing the expression of peroxisome proliferators-activated receptor gamma 2 (PPARgamma2). *Exp Gerontol* 39:333, 2004.
159. Okazaki R, Inoue D, Shibata M, et al: Estrogen promotes early osteoblast differentiation and inhibits adipocyte differentiation in mouse bone marrow stromal cell lines that express estrogen receptor (ER) alpha or beta. *Endocrinology* 143:2349, 2002.
160. Nuttal ME, Gimble JM: Controlling the balance between osteoblasto-genesis and adipogenesis and the consequent therapeutic implications. *Curr Opin Pharmacol* 4:290, 2004.
161. Lichtman MA: The relationship of stromal cells to hemopoietic cells in marrow, in *Long-Term Bone Marrow Culture*, edited by DG Wright, JS Greenberger, p 3. Liss, New York, 1984.
162. Seshi B, Kumar S, Sellers D: Human bone marrow stromal cell: Coexpression of markers specific for multiple mesenchymal cell lineages. *Blood Cells Mol Dis* 26:234, 2000.
163. Wilkins BS, Jones DB: Immunophenotypic characterization of stromal cells in aspirated human bone marrow samples. *Exp Hematol* 26:1061, 1998.
164. Takahashi GW, Moran D, Andrews DF III, Singer JW: Differential expression of collagenase by human fibroblasts and bone marrow stromal cells. *Leukemia* 8:305, 1994.
165. Liesveld JL, Abboud CN, Duerst RE, et al: Characterization of human marrow stromal cells: Role in progenitor cell binding and granulopoiesis. *Blood* 73:1794, 1989.
166. Li J, Sensebe L, Herve P, Charbord P: Nontransformed colony-derived stromal cell lines from normal human marrows: III. The maintenance of hematopoiesis from CD34+ cell populations. *Exp Hematol* 25:582, 1997.
167. Osmond DG, Kim N, Manoukina R, et al: Dynamics and localization of early B-lymphocyte precursor cells (pro-B cells) in the bone marrow of SCID mice. *Blood* 79:1695, 1992.
168. Moreau I, Duvert V, Caux C, et al: Myofibroblastic stromal cells isolated from human bone marrow induce the proliferation of both early myeloid and B lymphoid cells. *Blood* 82:2396, 1993.
169. Tamir M, Eren R, Globerson A, et al: Selective accumulation of lymphocyte precursor cells mediated by stromal cells of hemopoietic origin. *Exp Hematol* 18:332, 1990.
170. Lisovsky M, Braun SE, Ge Y, et al: Flt3-ligand production by human bone marrow stromal cells. *Leukemia* 10:1012, 1996.
171. Besmer P: Kit-ligand-stem cell factor, in *Colony-Stimulating Factors: Molecular and Cellular Biology*, edited by JM Garland, PJ Quesenberry, DJ Hilton, p 369. Marcel Dekker, New York, 1997.
172. Guerriero A, Worford L, Holland HK, et al: Thrombopoietin is synthesized by bone marrow stromal cells. *Blood* 90:3444, 1997.
173. Waring PM: Leukemia inhibitory factor, in *Colony-Stimulating Factors: Molecular and Cellular Biology*, edited by JM Garland, PJ Quesenberry, DJ Hilton, p 467. Marcel Dekker, New York, 1997.
174. Rodriguez Mdel C, Bernad A, Aracil M: Interleukin-6 deficiency affects bone marrow stromal precursors, resulting in defective hematopoietic support. *Blood* 103:3349, 2004.
175. Ueda T, Tsuji K, Yoshino H, et al: Expansion of human NOD/SCID repopulating cells by stem cell factor, Flk2/Flt3 ligand, thrombopoietin, Il-6, and soluble Il-6 receptor. *J Clin Invest* 105:1013, 2000.
176. Iwata M, Graf L, Awaya N, Torok-Storb B: Functional interleukin-7 receptors (IL-7Rs) are expressed by marrow stromal cells: Binding of IL-7 increases levels of IL-6, mRNA and secreted protein. *Blood* 100:1318, 2002.
177. Abboud SL, Bethel CR, Aron DC: Secretion of insulinlike growth factor I and insulinlike growth factor-binding proteins by murine bone marrow stromal cells. *J Clin Invest* 88:470, 1991.
178. Dormady SP, Zhang X-M, Basch RS: Hematopoietic progenitor cells grow on 3T3 fibroblast monolayers that overexpress growth arrest-specific gene-6 (GAS6). *Proc Natl Acad Sci U S A* 97:12260, 2000.
179. Hidalgo A, Sanz-Rodriguez F, Rodriguez-Fernandez JL, et al: Chemokine stromal cell-derived factor-1alpha modulates VLA-4 integrin-dependent adhesion to fibronectin and VCAM-1 on bone marrow hematopoietic progenitor cells. *Exp Hematol* 29:345, 2001.
180. Heberlein C, Friel J, Laker C, et al: Downregulation of c-kit (stem cell factor receptor) in transformed hematopoietic precursor cells by stroma cells. *Blood* 93:554, 1999.
181. Walker L, Lynch M, Silverman S, et al: The Notch/Jagged pathway inhibits proliferation of human hematopoietic progenitors in vitro. *Stem Cells* 17:162, 1999.
182. Van Den Berg DJ, Sharma AK, Bruno E, Hoffman R: Role of members of the Wnt gene family in human hematopoiesis. *Blood* 92:89, 1998.
183. Tordjman R, Ortega N, Coulombel L, et al: Neuropilin-1 is expressed on bone marrow stromal cells: A novel interaction with hematopoietic cells? *Blood* 94:2301, 1999.
184. Filshie RJ, Zannettino AC, Makrynikola V, et al: MUC18, a member of the immunoglobulin superfamily, is expressed on bone marrow fibroblasts and a subset of hematological malignancies. *Leukemia* 12:414, 1998.
185. Zannettino ACW, Buhring H-J, Niutta S, et al: The sialomucin CD164 (MCG-24v) is an adhesive glycoprotein expressed by human hematopoietic progenitors and bone marrow stromal cells that serves as a potent negative regulator of hematopoiesis. *Blood* 92:2613, 1998.
186. Cortes F, Deschaseaux F, Uchida N, et al: HCA, an immunoglobulin-like adhesion molecule present on the earliest human hematopoietic precursor cells, is also expressed by stromal cells in blood-forming tissues. *Blood* 93:826, 1999.
187. Garcia R, Agular J, Alberti E, et al: Bone marrow stromal cells produce nerve growth factor and glial cell line–derived neurotrophic factors. *Biochem Biophys Res Commun* 316:753, 2004.
188. Padovan CS, Jahn K, Birnbaum T, et al: Expression of neuronal markers in differentiated marrow stromal cells and CD133+ stem-like cells. *Cell Transplant* 12:839, 2003.
189. Song S, Kamath S, Mosquera D, et al: Expression of brain natriuretic peptide by human bone marrow stromal cells. *Exp Neurol* 185:191, 2004.
190. Denhardt DT, Noda M, O'Regan AW, et al: Osteopontin as a means to cope with environmental insults: Regulation of inflammation, tissue remodeling, and cell survival. *J Clin Invest* 107:1055, 2001.
191. Iwata M, Awaya N, Graf L, et al: Human marrow stromal cells activate monocytes to secrete osteopontin, which down-regulates Notch 1 gene expression in CD34+ cells. *Blood* 103:4496, 2004.
192. Kumano K, Chiba S, Kunisato A, et al: Notch1, but not Notch2, is essential for generating hematopoietic stem cells from endothelial cells. *Immunity* 18:699, 2003.

193. Ueno H, Sakita-Ishikawa M, Morikawa Y, et al: A stromal cell-derived membrane protein that supports hematopoietic stem cells. *Nat Immunol* 4:457, 2003.
194. Moore KA, Pytowski B, Witte L, et al: Hematopoietic activity of a stromal cell transmembrane protein containing epidermal growth factor-like repeat motifs. *Proc Natl Acad Sci U S A* 94:4011, 1997.
195. Bauer SR, Ruiz-Hildalgo MJ, Rudikoff EK, et al: Modulated expression of the epidermal growth factor-like homeotic protein dlk influences stromal-cell-pre-B-cell interactions, stromal cell adipogenesis, and preB-cell interleukin-7 requirements. *Mol Cell Biol* 18:5247, 1998.
196. Ohno N, Izawaa A, Hattori M, et al: Dlk inhibits stem cell factor-induced colony formation of murine hematopoietic progenitors. Hes-1 independent effects. *Stem Cells* 19:7109, 2001.
197. Miller SC, De Saint-Georges L, Bowman BM, Jee WS: Bone lining cells: Structure and function. *Scanning Microsc* 3:953, 1989.
198. Sillaber C, Walchshofer S, Mosberger I, et al: Immunophenotypic characterization of human bone marrow endosteal cells. *Tissue Antigens* 53:559, 1999.
199. Saito T, Albelda SM, Brighton CT: Identification of integrin receptors on cultured human bone cells. *J Orthop Res* 12:384, 1994.
200. Gong J: Endosteal marrow: A rich source of hematopoietic stem cells. *Science* 199:1443, 1978.
201. Nilsson SK, Haylock DN, Johnston HM, et al: Hyaluronan is synthesized by primitive hemopoietic cells, participates in their lodgement at the endosteum following transplantation, and is involved in the regulation of their proliferation and differentiation in vitro. *Blood* 101:856, 2003.
202. Park SR, Oreffo RO, Triffitt JT: Interconversion potential of cloned human marrow adipocytes in vitro. *Bone* 24:549, 1999.
203. Pittenger MF, Mackay AM, Beck SC, et al: Multilineage potential of adult human mesenchymal stem cells. *Science* 284:143, 1999.
204. Oyajobi BO, Lomri A, Hott M, Marie PJ: Isolation and characterization of human clonogenic osteoblast progenitors immunoselected from fetal bone marrow stroma using STRO-1 monoclonal antibody. *J Bone Miner Res* 14:351, 1999.
205. Doherty MJ, Ashton BA, Walsh S, et al: Vascular pericytes express osteogenic potential *in vitro* and *in vivo*. *J Bone Miner Res* 13:828, 1999.
206. Bruder SP, Ricalton NS, Boynton RE, et al: Mesenchymal stem cell surface antigen SB-10 corresponds to activated leukocyte cell adhesion molecule and is involved in osteogenic differentiation. *J Bone Miner Res* 13:655, 1998.
207. Dominici M, Pritchard C, Garlits JE, et al: Hematopoietic cells and osteoblasts are derived from a common marrow progenitor after bone marrow transplantation. *Proc Natl Acad Sci U S A* 101:11761, 2004.
208. Long MW, Robinson JA, Ashcraft EA, Mann KG: Regulation of human bone marrow-derived osteoprogenitor cells by osteogenic growth factors. *J Clin Invest* 95:881, 1995.
209. Gronthos S, Zannettino AC, Graves SE, et al: Differential cell surface expression of the STRO-1 and alkaline phosphatase antigens on discrete developmental stages in primary cultures of human bone cells. *J Bone Miner Res* 14:47, 1999.
210. Moerman EJ, Teng K, Lipschitz DA, Lecka-Czernik B: Aging activates adipogenic and suppresses osteogenic programs in mesenchymal marrow stroma/stem cells: The role of PPAR-gamma2 transcription factor and TGF-beta/BMP signaling pathways. *Aging Cell* 3:379, 2004.
211. Hanada K, Dennis JE, Caplan AI: Stimulatory effects of basic fibroblast growth factor and bone morphogenetic protein-2 on osteogenic differentiation of rat bone marrow-derived mesenchymal stem cells. *J Bone Miner Res* 12:1606, 1997.
212. Blanquaert F, Delany AM, Canalis E: Fibroblast growth factor-2 induces hepatocyte growth factor/scatter factor expression in osteoblasts. *Endocrinology* 140:1069, 1999.
213. Grano M, Galimi F, Zambonin G, et al: Hepatocyte growth factor is a coupling factor for osteoclasts and osteoblasts *in vitro*. *Proc Natl Acad Sci U S A* 93:7644, 1996.
214. Yin JJ, Mohammad KS, Kakonen SM, et al: A causal role for endothelin-1 in the pathogenesis of osteoblastic bone metastases. *Proc Natl Acad Sci U S A* 100:10954, 2003.
215. Erlebacher A, Filvaroff EH, Ye J-Q, Derynck R: Osteoblastic responses to TGF-β during bone remodeling. *Mol Biol Cell* 9:1903, 1998.
216. Nakashima K, Zhou X, Kunkel G, et al: The novel zinc finger-containing transcription factor osterix is required for osteoblast differentiation and bone formation. *Cell* 108:17, 2002.
217. Taichman RS, Emerson SG: The role of osteoblasts in the hematopoietic microenvironment. *Stem Cells* 16:7, 1998.
218. Ahmed N, Khokher MA, Hassan HT: Cytokine-induced expansion of human CD34+ stem/progenitor and CD34+CD41+ early megakaryocytic marrow cells cultured on normal osteoblasts. *Stem Cells* 17:92, 1999.
219. Gehron Robey P, Young MF, Flanders KC, et al: Osteoblasts synthesize and respond to transforming growth factor-type β (TGF-beta) *in vitro*. *J Cell Biol* 105:457, 1987.
220. Haylock DN, Nilsson SK: Osteopontin: A bridge between bone and blood. *Br J Haematol* 134:467, 2006.
221. Frisch BJ, Porter RL, Calvi LM: Hematopoietic niche and bone meet. *Curr Opin Support Palliat Care* 2:211, 2008.
222. Nilsson SK, Dooner MS, Weier HU, et al: Cells capable of bone production engraft from whole bone marrow transplants in nonablated mice. *J Exp Med* 189:729, 1999.
223. El-Badri NS, Wang B-Y, Cherry, Good RA: Osteoblasts promote engraftment of allogeneic hematopoietic stem cells. *Exp Hematol* 26:110, 1998.
224. Gurevitch O, Fabian I: Ability of the hemopoietic microenvironment in the induced bone to maintain the proliferative potential of early hemopoietic precursors. *Stem Cells* 11:56, 1993.
225. Civitelli R, Beyer EC, Warlow PM, et al: Connexin43 mediates direct intercellular communication in human osteoblastic cell networks. *J Clin Invest* 91:1888, 1993.
226. Visnjic D, Kalajzic Z, Rowe DW, et al: Hematopoiesis is severely altered in mice with an induced osteoblast deficiency. *Blood* 103, 3258, 2004.
227. Zhu J, Emerson SG: A new bone to pick: Osteoblasts and the haematopoietic stem-cell niche. *Bioessays* 26:595, 2004.
228. Matayoshi A, Brown C, DiPersio JF, et al: Human blood-mobilized hematopoietic precursors differentiate into osteoclasts in the absence of stromal cells. *Proc Natl Acad Sci U S A* 93:10785, 1996.
229. Edwards CM, Mundy GR: Eph receptors and ephrin signaling pathways: a role in bone homeostasis. *Int J Med Sci* 5:263, 2008.
230. Askmyr MK, Fasth A, Richter J: Towards a better understanding and new therapeutics of osteopetrosis. *Br J Haematol* 140:597, 2008.
231. Calle Y, Jones GE, Jagger C, et al: WASp deficiency in mice results in failure to form osteoclast sealing zones and defects in bone resorption. *Blood* 103:3552, 2004.
232. Horowitz MC, Lorenzo JA: The origins of osteoclasts. *Curr Opin Rheumatol* 16:464, 2004.
233. Dai X-M, Zong X-H, Sylvestre V, Stanley R: Incomplete restoration of colony-stimulating factor 1 (CSF-1) function in CSF-1-deficient *Csf1^{op}/Csf1^{op}* mice by transgenic expression of cell surface CSF-1. *Blood* 103:1114, 2004.
234. Asagiri M, Takayanagi H: The molecular understanding of osteoclast differentiation. *Bone* 40:251, 2007.
235. Udagawa N, Takahashi N, Yasuda H, et al: Osteoprotegerin produced by osteoblasts is an important regulator of osteoclast development and function. *Endocrinology* 141:3478, 2000.
236. Domon T, Yamazaki Y, Fukui A, et al: Ultrastructural study of cell-cell interaction between osteoclasts osteoblasts/stroma cells in vitro. *Ann Anat* 184:221, 2002.
237. Andersen TL, Sondergaard TE, Skorzynska KE, et al: A physical mechanism for coupling bone resorption and formation in adult human bone. *Am J Pathol* 174:239, 2009.
238. Takahashi N, Udagawa N, Suda T: A new member of tumor necrosis factor ligand family, ODF/OPGL/TRANCE/RANKL, regulates osteoclast differentiation and function. *Biochem Biophys Res Commun* 256:449, 1999.
239. Shalhoub V, Faust J, Boyle WJ, et al: Osteoprotegerin and osteoprotegerin ligand effects on osteoclast formation from human peripheral blood mononuclear cell precursors. *J Cell Biochem* 72:251, 1999.
240. Zhao C, Irie N, Takada Y, et al: Bidirectional ephrinB2-EphB4 signaling controls bone homeostasis. *Cell Metab* 4:111, 2006.
241. Jimi E, Nakamura I, Amano H, et al: Osteoblast function is activated by osteoblastic cells through a mechanism involving cell-to-cell contact. *Endocrinology* 137:2187, 1996.
242. Mbalaviele G, Nishimura R, Myoi A, et al: Cadherin-6 mediates the heterotypic interactions between the hemopoietic osteoclast cell lineage and stromal cells in a murine model of osteoclast differentiation. *J Cell Biol* 141:1467, 1998.
243. Hayashi S, Miyake K, Kincade PW: The CD9 molecule on stromal cells. *Leuk Lymphoma* 38:265, 2000.
244. Oritani K, Wu X, Medina K, et al: Antibody ligation of CD9 modifies production of myeloid cells in long-term cultures. *Blood* 87:2252, 1996.
245. Tanio Y, Yamazaki H, Kunisada T, et al: CD9 molecule expressed on stromal cells is involved in osteoclastogenesis. *Exp Hematol* 27:853, 1999.
246. Iwama A, Yamaguchi N, Suda T: STK/RON receptor tyrosine kinase mediates both apoptotic and growth signals via the multifunctional docking site conserved in the HGF receptor family. *EMBO J* 15:5866, 1996.
247. Kurihara N, Tatsumi J, Arai F, et al: Macrophage-stimulating protein (MSP) and its receptor, RON, stimulate human osteoclast activity but not proliferation: Effect of MSP distinct from that of hepatocyte growth factor. *Exp Hematol* 26:1080, 1998.
248. Choi SJ, Han JH, Roodman GD: ADAM8: A novel osteoclast stimulating factor. *J Bone Miner Res* 16:814, 2001.
249. Oba Y, Chung HY, Choi SJ, Roodman GD: Eosinophil chemotactic factor-L (ECF-L): A novel osteoclast stimulating factor. *J Bone Miner Res* 18:1332, 2003.
250. Quesenberry PJ, Crittenden RB, Lowry P, et al: *In vitro* and *in vivo* studies of stromal niches. *Blood Cells* 20:97, 1994.
251. Gibson FM, Scopes J, Daly S, et al: IL-3 is produced by normal stroma in long-term bone marrow cultures. *Br J Haematol* 90:518, 1995.
252. Verfaillie CM, Catanzarro PM, Li WN: Macrophage inflammatory protein 1 alpha, interleukin-3, and diffusible marrow stromal factors maintain human hematopoietic stem cells for at least eight weeks *in vitro*. *J Exp Med* 179:643, 1994.
253. Crocker PR, Morris L, Gordon S: Novel cell surface adhesion receptors involved in interactions between stromal macrophages and haematopoietic cells. *J Cell Sci* 9(Suppl):185, 1988.
254. Wang QR, Wolf NS: Dissecting the hematopoietic microenvironment: VIII. Clonal isolation and identification of cell types in murine CFU-F colonies by limiting dilution. *Exp Hematol* 18:355, 1990.
255. Kincade PW: Cell interaction molecules and cytokines which participate in B lymphopoiesis. *Baillieres Clin Haematol* 5:575, 1992.
256. Berneman ZN, Chen ZZ, Van Bockstaele D, et al: The nature of the adherent hemopoietic cells in human long-term bone marrow cultures (HLTBMCs): Presence of lymphocytes and plasma cells next to the myelomonocytic population. *Leukemia* 9:648, 1989.
257. Tong J, Kishi H, Matsuda T, Muraguchi A: A bone marrow-derived stroma line, ST2 can support the differentiation of fetal thymocytes from CD4+ CD8+ double negative to the CD4+ CD8+ double positive differentiation stage *in vitro*. *Immunology* 97:672, 1999.

258. Dejbakhsh-Jones S, Strober S: Identification of an early T cell progenitor for a pathway of T cell maturation in the bone marrow. *Proc Natl Acad Sci U S A* 96:14493, 1999.
259. Tsuji JM, Pollack SB: Maturation of murine natural killer precursor cells in the absence of exogenous cytokines requires contact with bone marrow stroma. *Nat Immunol* 14:44, 1995.
260. Yu H, Fehniger TA, Fuschsuber P, et al: Flt3 ligand promotes the generation of a distinct CD34(+) human natural killer cell progenitor that responds to interleukin-15. *Blood* 92:3647, 1998.
261. Burkett PR, Koka R, Chien M, et al: Coordinate expression and trans presentation of interleukin (IL)-15Ralpha and IL-15 supports natural killer cell and memory CD8+ T cell homeostasis. *J Exp Med* 200:825, 2004.
262. Kurosaka D, LeBien TW, Priby JAR: Comparative studies of different stromal cell microenvironments in support of human B-cell development. *Exp Hematol* 27:1271, 1999.
263. Funk PE, Stephan RP, Witte PL: Vascular adhesion molecule-1-positive reticular cells express interleukin-7 and stem cell factor in the bone marrow. *Blood* 86:2661, 1995.
264. Tang J, Nuccie BL, Ritterman I, et al: TGF-beta down-regulates stromal IL-7 secretion and inhibits proliferation of human B cell precursors. *J Immunol* 159:117, 1997.
265. Sapoznikov A, Pewzner-Jung Y, Kalchenko V, et al: Perivascular clusters of dendritic cells provide critical survival signals to B cells in bone marrow niches. *Nat Immunol* 9:388, 2008.
266. Tokoyoda K, Egawa T, Sugiyama T, et al: Cellular niches controlling B lymphocyte behavior within bone marrow during development. *Immunity* 20:707, 2004.
267. Fairfax KA, Kallies A, Nutt SL, Tarlinton DM: Plasma cell development: From B-cell subsets to long-term survival niches. *Semin Immunol* 20:49, 2008.
268. Di Rosa F, Pabst R: The bone marrow: A nest for migratory memory T cells. *Trends Immunol* 26:360, 2005.
269. Abboud SL: A bone marrow stromal cell line is a source and target for platelet-derived growth factor. *Blood* 81:2547, 1993.
270. Abboud SL, Pinzani M: Peptide growth factors stimulate macrophage colony-stimulating factor in murine stromal cells. *Blood* 78:103, 1991.
271. Yan XQ, Brady G, Iscove NN: Platelet-derived growth factor (PDGF) activates primitive hematopoietic precursors (pre-CFCmulti) by upregulating IL-1 in PDGF receptor-expressing macrophages. *J Immunol* 150:2440, 1993.
272. Lerat H, Lissitzky JC, Singer JW, et al: Role of stromal cells and macrophages in fibronectin biosynthesis and matrix assembly in human long-term marrow cultures. *Blood* 82:1480, 1993.
273. Baldus SE, Wickenhauser C, Stefanovic A, et al: Enrichment of human bone marrow mononuclear phagocytes and characterization of macrophage subpopulations by immunoenzymatic double staining. *Histochem J* 30:285, 1998.
274. Wijffels JF, De Rover Z, Kraal G, Beelen RH: Macrophage phenotype regulation by colony-stimulating factors at bone marrow level. *J Leukoc Biol* 53:249, 1993.
275. Shima M, Teitelbaum SL, Holers VM, et al: Macrophage-colony-stimulating factor regulates expression of the integrins alpha 4, beta 1 and alpha 5, beta 1 by murine marrow macrophages. *Proc Natl Acad Sci U S A* 92:5179, 1995.
276. Dannaeus K, Johannisson A, Nilsson K, Jonsson JI: Flt3 ligand induces the outgrowth of Mac-1+ B22+ mouse bone marrow progenitor cells restricted to macrophage differentiation that coexpress early B cell-associated genes. *Exp Hematol* 27:1646, 1999.
277. Wright EC, Pragnell IB: Stem cell proliferation inhibitors. *Baillieres Clin Haematol* 5:723, 1992.
278. Su S, Mukaida N, Wang J, et al: Inhibition of immature progenitor cell proliferation by 1macrophage inflammatory protein-1 alpha by interacting mainly with a C-C chemokine receptor, CCR1. *Blood* 90:605, 1997.
279. Jacobsen SEW, Ruscetti FW, Dubois CM, Keller JR: Tumor necrosis factor α directly and indirectly regulates hematopoietic progenitor cell proliferation: Role of colony-stimulating factor receptor modulation. *J Exp Med* 175:1759, 1992.
280. Dufour C, Corcione A, Svahn J, et al: TNF-alpha and IFN-gamma are overexpressed in the bone marrow of Fanconi anemia patients and TNF-alpha suppresses erythropoiesis in vitro. *Blood* 102:2053, 2003.
281. Rogers JA, Berman JW: A tumor necrosis factor-responsive long-term-culture-initiating cell is associated with the stromal layer of mouse long-term bone marrow cultures. *Proc Natl Acad Sci U S A* 90:5777, 1993.
282. Knospe WH, Husseini SG, Zipori D, Fried W: Hematopoiesis on cellulose ester membranes: XIII. A combination of cloned stromal cells is needed to establish a hematopoietic microenvironment supportive of trilineal hematopoiesis. *Exp Hematol* 21:257, 1993.
283. Winerman JP, Nishikawa S, Muller-Sieburg CE: Maintenance of high levels of pluripotent hematopoietic stem cells *in vitro*: Effect of stromal cells and c-kit. *Blood* 81:365, 1993.
284. Bhatia M, Bonnet D, Wu D, et al: Bone morphogenetic proteins regulate the developmental program of human hematopoietic stem cells. *J Exp Med* 189:1139, 1999.
285. Simmons PJ, Zannettino A, Gronthos S, Leavesley D: Potential adhesion mechanisms for localization of haemopoietic progenitors to bone marrow stroma. *Leuk Lymphoma* 12:353, 1994.
286. Koller MR, Oxender M, Jensen TC, et al: Direct contact between CD34+ lin− cells and stroma induces a soluble activity that specifically increases primitive hematopoietic cell production. *Exp Hematol* 27:734, 1999.
287. Klein G: The extracellular matrix of the hematopoietic microenvironment. *Experientia* 51:914, 1995.
288. Singer JW, Keating A, Wright TN: The human haemopoietic microenvironment, in *Recent Advances in Haematology*, edited by AV Hoff-brand, p 1. Churchill Livingstone, London, 1985.
289. Bentley SA, Tralka TS: Fibronectin-mediated attachment of hematopoietic cells to stromal elements in continuous bone marrow culture. *Exp Hematol* 11:129, 1983.
290. Postlethwaite A, Kang AH: Fibroblasts and matrix proteins, in *Inflammation Basic Principles and Clinical Correlates*, 3rd ed, edited by JI Gallin, R Snyderman, p 227. Lippincott Williams & Wilkins, Philadelphia, 1999.
291. Campbell AD, Long MW, Wicha MS: Haemonectin: A bone marrow adhesion protein specific for cells of granulocytic lineage. *Nature* 329:445, 1987.
292. Lawler J: The structural and functional properties of thrombospondin. *Blood* 67:1197, 1986.
293. Simmons PJ, Levesque JP, Zannettino AC: Adhesion molecules in haemopoiesis. *Baillieres Clin Haematol* 10:485, 1997.
294. Verfaille CM: Adhesion receptors as regulators of the hematopoietic process. *Blood* 92:2609, 1998.
295. Broxmeyer HE, Kim CH: Regulation of hematopoiesis in a sea of chemokine family members with a plethora of redundant activities. *Exp Hematol* 27:1113, 1999.
296. Gordon MY: Extracellular matrix- and membrane-bound cytokines, in *Colony-Stimulating Factors: Molecular and Cellular Biology*, edited by JM Garland, PJ Quesenberry, DJ Hilton, p 133. Marcel Dekker, New York, 1997.
297. Coombe DR: Biological implications of glycosaminoglycan interactions with haemopoietic cytokines. *Immunol Cell Biol* 86:598, 2008.
298. Long MW: Hematopoietic microenvironments, in *Colony-Stimulating Factors: Molecular and Cellular Biology*, edited by JM Garland, PJ Quesenberry, DJ Hilton, p 117. Marcel Dekker, New York, 1997.
299. Oritani K, Kanakura Y, Aoyama K, et al: Matrix glycoprotein SC1/ECM2 augments B lymphopoiesis. *Blood* 90:3404, 1997.
300. Koller MR, Oxender M, Jensen TC, et al: Direct contact between CD34+ lin− cells and stroma induces a soluble activity that specifically increases primitive hematopoietic cell production. *Exp Hematol* 27:734, 1999.
301. Varnum-Finney B, Purton LE, Yu M, et al: The Notch ligand, Jagged-1 influences the development of primitive hematopoietic precursor cells. *Blood* 91:4084, 1998.
302. Hoogewerf AJ, Kuschert GS, Proudfoot AE, et al: Glycosaminoglycans mediate cell surface oligomerization of chemokines. *Biochemistry* 36:13570, 1997.
303. Luster AD, Greenberg SM, Leder P: The IP-10 chemokine binds to a specific cell surface heparan sulfate site shared with platelet factor 4 and inhibits endothelial cell proliferation. *J Exp Med* 182:219, 1995.
304. Tanaka T, Adams DH, Hubscher S, et al: T-cell adhesion induced by proteoglycan immobilized cytokine MIP-1β. *Nature* 361:78, 1993.
305. Chakravarty L, Rogers L, Quach T, et al: Lysine 58 and histidine 66, at the C-terminal alpha-helix of monocyte chemoattractant protein-1, are essential for glycosaminoglycan binding. *J Biol Chem* 273:29641, 1998.
306. Spillman D, Witt D, Lindahl U: Defining the interleukin-8-binding domain of heparan sulfate. *J Biol Chem* 273:15487, 1998.
307. Koopman W, Ediriwickrema C, Krangel MS: Structure and function of the glycosaminoglycan binding site of chemokine macrophage-inflammatory protein-1 beta. *J Immunol* 163:2120, 1999.
308. Amara A, Lorthioir O, Valenzuela A, et al: Stromal cell derived factor-1 alpha associates with heparan sulfates through the first beta-strand of the chemokine. *J Biol Chem* 274:23916, 1999.
309. Wolff EA, Greenfield B, Taub DD, et al: Generation of artificial proteoglycans containing glycosaminoglycan-modified CD44. Demonstration of the interaction between rantes and chondroitin sulfate. *J Biol Chem* 274:2518, 1999.
310. Lipscombe RJ, Nakhoul AM, Sanderson CJ, Coombe DR: Interleukin-5 binds to heparin/heparan sulfate. A model for an interaction with extracellular matrix. *J Leukoc Biol* 63:342, 1998.
311. Borghesi LA, Yamashita Y, Kincade PW: Heparan sulfate proteogly-cans mediate interleukin-7-dependent B lymphopoiesis. *Blood* 93:140, 1999.
312. Lyon M, Deakin JA, Nakamura T, Gallagher JT: Interaction of hepatocyte growth factor with heparan sulfate. Elucidation of major heparan sulfate structural determinants. *J Biol Chem* 269:11216, 1994.
313. Kiefer MC, Stephans JC, Crawford K, et al: Ligand-affinity cloning and structure of a cell surface heparan sulfate proteoglycan that binds basic fibroblast growth factor. *Proc Natl Acad Sci U S A* 87:6985, 1990.
314. Robledo MM, Ursa MA, Sanchez-Madrid F, Teixido J: Associations between TGF-beta1 receptors in human bone marrow stromal cells. *Br J Haematol* 102:804, 1998.
315. Kapur R, Cooper R, Xiao X, et al: The presence of novel amino acids in the cytoplasmic domain of stem cell factor results in hematopoietic defects in the *Steel*^{17H} mice. *Blood* 94:1915, 1999.
316. Gay RE, Prince CW, Zuckerman KS, Gay S: The collagenous hemopoietic microenvironment, in *Handbook of the Hemopoietic Microenvironment*, edited by M Tavassoli, p 369. Humana Press, Clifton, NJ, 1989.
317. De Wynter E, Allen T, Coutinho L, et al: Localization of granulocytic macrophage colony-stimulating factor in human long-term bone marrow cultures. Biological and immunocytochemical characterization. *J Cell Sci* 106:761, 1993.
318. Deschaseaux ML, Herve P, Charbord P: The detection of colony-stimulating factors and steel factor in adherent layers of human long-term marrow cultures using reverse-transcriptase polymerase chain reaction. *Leukemia* 8:513, 1994.

319. Liu J, De Wynter E, Testa NG, et al: Immunoelectron microscopic localization of growth factors and other markers of human long-term bone marrow cultures. *Chin Med Sci J* 11:129, 1996.
320. Waegell WO, Higley HR, Kincade PW, Dasch JR: Growth acceleration and stem cell expansion in Dexter-type cultures by neutralization of TGF-beta. *Exp Hematol* 22:1051, 1994.
321. Wight TN, Kinsella MG, Keating A, Singer JW: Proteoglycans in human long-term bone marrow cultures: Biochemical and ultrastructural analyses. *Blood* 67:1333, 1986.
322. Allen TD, Dexter TM, Simmons PJ: Marrow biology and stem cells, in *Colony Stimulating Factors, Molecular and Cellular Biology, Immunology Series*, vol 49, edited by TM Dexter, JM Garland, NG Testa, p 1. Marcel Dekker, New York, 1990.
323. Yurchenco PD, Schittny JC: Molecular architecture of basement membranes. *FASEB J* 4:1577, 1990.
324. Keating A, Gordon MY: Hierarchical organization of hematopoietic microenvironments: Role of proteoglycans. *Leukemia* 2:766, 1988.
325. Gordon MY, Riley GP, Clarke D: Heparan sulfate is necessary for adhesive interactions between human early hemopoietic progenitor cells and the extracellular matrix of the marrow microenvironment. *Leukemia* 2:804, 1988.
326. Uhlman DL, Luikart SD: The role of proteoglycans in the adhesion and differentiation of hematopoietic cells, in *The Hematopoietic Microenvironment*, edited by MW Long, MS Wicha, p 232. Johns Hopkins University Press, Baltimore, MD, 1993.
327. Bruno E, Luikart SD, Long MW, Hoffman R: Marrow-derived heparan sulfate proteoglycan mediates the adhesion of hematopoietic progenitor cells to cytokines. *Exp Hematol* 23:1212, 1995.
328. Minguell JJ, Hardy C, Tavassoli M: Membrane-associated chondroitin sulfate proteoglycan and fibronectin mediate the binding of hemopoietic progenitor cells to stromal cells. *Exp Cell Res* 201:200, 1992.
329. Han ZC, Bellucci S, Shen ZX, et al: Glycosaminoglycans enhance megakaryopoiesis by modifying the activities of hematopoietic growth regulators. *J Cell Physiol* 168:97, 1996.
330. Gordon MY, Lewis JL, Marley SB, et al: Stromal cells negatively regulate primitive haematopoietic progenitor cell activation via a phosphatidylinositol-anchored cell adhesion/signaling mechanism. *Br J Haematol* 96:647, 1997.
321. Gupta P, Oegema TR Jr, Brazil JJ, et al: Structurally specific heparan sulfates support primitive human hematopoiesis by formation of a multimolecular stem cell niche. *Blood* 92:4641, 1998.
332. Da Prato I, Valentini P, Testi R, et al: Differential activity of glycosaminoglycans on colony-forming cells from cord blood. Preliminary results. *Leuk Res* 23:1015, 1999.
333. Lewinsohn DM, Nagler A, Ginzton N, et al: Hematopoietic progenitor cell expression of the H-CAM (CD44) homing-associated adhesion molecule. *Blood* 75:589, 1990.
334. Jalkanen S, Jalkanen M: Lymphocyte CD44 binds the COOH-terminal heparin-binding domain of fibronectin. *J Cell Biol* 116:817, 1992.
335. Miyake K, Medina KL, Mayashi S-I, et al: Monoclonal antibodies to Pgp-1/CD44 block lympho-hemopoiesis in long-term bone marrow cultures. *J Exp Med* 171:477, 1990.
336. Legras S, Levesque JP, Charrad R, et al: CD44-mediated adhesiveness of human hematopoietic progenitors to hyaluronan is modulated by cytokines. *Blood* 89:1905, 1997.
337. Rachmilewitz J, Tykocinski ML: Differential effects of chondroitin sulfates A and B on monocyte and B cell activation: Evidence for B-cell activation via a CD44-dependent pathway. *Blood* 92:223, 1998.
338. Khaldoyanidi S, Moll J, Karakhanova S, et al: Hyaluronate-enhanced hematopoiesis: Two different receptors trigger the release of interleukin-1β and interleukin-6 from bone marrow macrophages. *Blood* 94:940, 1999.
339. Sternberg D, Peled A, Shezen E, et al: Control of stroma-dependent hematopoiesis by basic fibroblast growth factor: Stromal phenotypic plasticity and modified myelopoietic functions. *Cytokines Mol Ther* 2:29, 1996.
340. Weimar IS, Miranda N, Muller EJ, et al: Hepatocyte growth factor/scatter factor (HGF/SF) is produced by bone marrow stromal cells and promotes proliferation, adhesion and survival of human hematopoietic progenitor cells (CD34+). *Exp Hematol* 26:885, 1998.
341. Pivak-Kroizman T, Lemmon MA, Dikic I, et al: Heparin-induced oligomerization of FGF molecules is responsible for FGF receptor dimerization, activation, and cell proliferation. *Cell* 79:1015, 1994.
342. Ratajczak MZ, Ratajczak J, Slorska M, et al: Effect of basic (FGF-2) and acidic (FGF-1) fibroblast growth factors on early haematopoietic cell development. *Br J Haematol* 93:772, 1996.
343. Schofield KP, Gallagher JT, David G: Expression of proteoglycan core proteins in human bone marrow stroma. *Biochem J* 343:663, 1999.
344. Klein G, Conzelmann S, Beck S, et al: Perlecan in human bone marrow: A growth-factor-presenting, but anti-adhesive, extracellular matrix component for hematopoietic cells. *Matrix Biol* 14:457, 1995.
345. Drzeniek Z, Stoocker G, Siebertz B, et al: Heparan sulfate proteoglycan expression is induced during early erythroid differentiation of multipotential hematopoietic stem cells. *Blood* 93:2884, 1999.
346. Siebertz B, Stocker G, Drzeniek Z, et al: Expression of glypican-4 in haematopoietic-progenitor and bone-marrow-stromal cells. *Biochem J* 344:937, 1999.
347. Sneed TB, Stanley DJ, Young LA, Sanderson RD: Interleukin-6 regulates expression of the syndecan-1 proteoglycan on B lymphoid cells. *Cell Immunol* 153:456, 1994.
348. Oritani K, Kincade PW: Identification of stromal cell products that interact with pre-B cells. *J Cell Biol* 134:771, 1996.
349. Yamashita Y, Oritani K, Miyoshi EK, et al: Syndecan-4 is expressed by B lineage lymphocytes and can transmit a signal for formation of dendritic processes. *J Immunol* 162:5940, 1999.
350. Longley RL, Woods A, Fleetwood A, et al: Control of morphology, cytoskeleton and migration by syndecan-4. *J Cell Sci* 112:3421, 1999.
351. Zukerman KS, Wicha MS: Extracellular matrix production by the adherent cells of long-term murine bone marrow cultures. *Blood* 61:540, 1983.
352. Sorrel JM: Ultrastructural localization of fibronectin in bone marrow of the embryonic chick and its relationship to granulopoiesis. *Cell Tissue Res* 252:565, 1988.
353. Tsai S, Patel V, Beaumont E, et al: Differential binding of erythroid and myeloid progenitors to fibroblasts and fibronectin. *Blood* 69:1587, 1987.
354. Vuillet-Gaugler MH, Breton-Gorius J, Vainchenker W, et al: Loss of attachment to fibronectin with terminal human erythroid differentiation. *Blood* 75:865, 1990.
355. Rosemblatt M, Vuillet-Gaugler MH, Leroy C, Coulombel L: Coexpression of two fibronectin receptors, VLA-4, and VLA-5 by immature human erythroblastic precursor cells. *J Clin Invest* 87:6, 1991.
356. Liesveld JL, Winslow J, Kempski MC, et al: Adhesive interactions of normal and leukemic human CD34+ myeloid progenitors: Role of marrow stroma, fibroblasts and cytomatrix components. *Exp Hematol* 19:63, 1991.
357. Kerst JM, Sanders JB, Slaper Cortenbach IC, et al: Alpha 4, beta 1 and alpha 5, beta 1 are differentially expressed during myelopoiesis and mediate the adherence of human CD34+ cells to fibronectin in an activation-dependent way. *Blood* 81:344, 1993.
358. Ryan DH, Nuccie BL, Abboud CN, Winslow JM: Vascular cell adhesion molecule-1 and the integrin VLA-4 mediate adhesion of human B cell precursors to cultured bone marrow adherent cells. *J Clin Invest* 88:995, 1991.
359. Hynes RO: Integrins: Versatility, modulation, and signaling in cell adhesion. *Cell* 69:11, 1992.
360. Williams DA, Rios M, Stephens C, Patel VP: Fibronectin and VLA-4 in haematopoietic stem cell-microenvironment interactions. *Nature* 352:438, 1991.
361. Schofield KP, Humphries MJ: Identification of fibronectin IIICS variants in human bone marrow stroma. *Blood* 93:410, 1999.
362. Verfaillie CM, Benis A, Iida J, et al: Adhesion of committed human hematopoietic progenitors to synthetic peptides from the C-terminal heparin-binding domain of fibronectin: Cooperation between the integrin alpha 4, beta 1 and the CD44 adhesion receptor. *Blood* 84:1802, 1994.
363. Hassan HT, Sadovinkova EY, Drize NJ, et al: Fibronectin increases both non-adherent cells and CFU-GM while collagen increases adherent cells in human normal long-term bone marrow cultures. *Haematologia (Budap)* 28:77, 1997.
364. Yokota T, Oritani K, Mitsui H, et al: Growth-supporting activities of fibronectin on hematopoietic stem/progenitor cells *in vitro* and *in vivo*: Structural requirements for fibronectin activities of CS1 and cell-binding domains. *Blood* 91:3263, 1998.
365. Hurley RW, McCarthy JB, Verfaillie CM: Direct adhesion to bone marrow stroma via fibronectin receptors inhibits hematopoietic progenitor proliferation. *J Clin Invest* 96:511, 1995.
366. Goltry KL, Patel VP: Specific domains of fibronectin mediate adhesion and migration of early murine erythroid progenitors. *Blood* 90:138, 1997.
367. Van der Loo JC, Xiao X, McMillin D, et al: VLA-5 is expressed by mouse and human long-term repopulating hematopoietic cells and mediates adhesion to extracellular matrix protein fibronectin. *J Clin Invest* 102:1051, 1998.
368. Robledo MM, Sanz-Rodrigues F, Hidalgo A, Teixido J: Differential use of very late antigen-4 and -5 integrins by hematopoietic precursors and myeloma cells to adhere to transforming growth factor-beta-1-treated bone marrow stroma. *J Biol Chem* 273:12056, 1998.
369. Schofield KP, Rushton G, Humphries MJ, et al: Influence of interleukin-3 and other growth factors on alpha$_4$beta$_1$ integrin-mediated adhesion and migration of human hematopoietic progenitor cells. *Blood* 90:1858, 1997.
370. Levesque JP, Haylock DN, Simmons PJ: Cytokine regulation of proliferation and cell adhesion are correlated events in human CD34+ hemopoietic progenitors. *Blood* 88:1168, 1996.
371. Cui L, Ramsfjell V, Borge OJ, et al: Thrombopoietin promotes adhesion of primitive human hemopoietic cells to fibronectin and vascular cell adhesion molecule-1: Role of activation of very late antigen (VLA)-4 and VLA-5. *J Immunol* 159:1961, 1997.
372. Schofield KP, Humphries MJ, De Wynter E, et al: The effect of $\alpha_4\beta_1$-integrin binding sequences of fibronectin on growth of cells from human hematopoietic progenitors. *Blood* 91:3230, 1998.
373. Staquet MJ, Jacquet C, Dezutter-Dambuyant C, Schmitt D: Fibronectin upregulates in vitro generation of dendritic Langerhans cells from human cord blood CD34+ progenitors. *J Invest Dermatol* 109:738, 1997.
374. Berthier R, Jacquier-Sarlin M, Schweitzer A, et al: Adhesion of mature polypoid megakaryocytes to fibronectin is mediated by beta 1 integrins and leads to cell damage. *Exp Cell Res* 242:315, 1998.
375. Schick PK, Wojenski CM, He X, et al: Integrins involved in the adhesion of megakaryocytes to fibronectin and fibrinogen. *Blood* 92:2650, 1998.
376. Krugger-Krasagakes S, Grutzkau A, Krasagakis K, et al: Adhesion of human mast cells to extracellular matrix provides a co-stimulatory signal for cytokine production. *Immunology* 98:253, 1999.
377. Lloyd AR, Oppenheim JJ, Kelvin DJ, Taub DD: Chemokines regulate T cell adherence to recombinant adhesion molecules and extracellular matrix proteins. *J Immunol* 156:932, 1996.

378. Higashimoto I, Chihara J, Kawabata M, et al: Adhesion to fibronectin regulates expression of intercellular adhesion molecule-1 on eosinophilic cells. *Int Arch Allergy Immunol* 120(Suppl 1):34, 1999.
379. Xu X, Hakansson L: Simultaneous analysis of eosinophil and neutrophil adhesion to plasma and tissue fibronectin, fibrinogen, and albumin. *J Immunol Methods* 226:93, 1999.
380. Xie B, Laouar A, Huberman E: Fibronectin-mediated cell adhesion is required for induction of 92-kDa type IV collagenase/gelatinase (MMP-9) gene expression during macrophage differentiation. The signaling role of protein kinase C-beta. *J Biol Chem* 273:11576, 1998.
381. Kremlev SG, Chapoval AI, Evans R: Cytokine release by macrophages after interacting with CSF-1 and extracellular matrix proteins: Characteristics of a mouse model of inflammatory responses *in vitro*. *Cell Immunol* 185:59, 1998.
382. Yonezawa I, Kato K, Yagita H, et al: VLA-5-mediated interactions with fibronectin induces cytokine production by human chondrocytes. *Biochem Biophys Res Commun* 219:261, 1996.
383. Rich IN, Brackmann I, Worthington-White D, Dewey MJ: Activation of sodium/hydrogen exchanger via the fibronectin-integrin pathway results in hematopoietic stimulation. *J Cell Physiol* 177:109, 1998.
384. Klein G, Beck S, Muller CA: Tenascin is a cytoadhesive extracellular matrix component of the human hematopoietic microenvironment. *J Cell Biol* 123:1027, 1993.
385. Chiquet-Ehrismann R, Matsuoka Y, Hofer U, et al: Tenascin variants: Differential binding to fibronectin and distinct distribution in cell cultures and tissues. *Cell Regul* 2:927, 1991.
386. Sakai T, Ohta M, Kawakatsu H, et al: Tenascin-C induction in Whitlock-Witte culture: A relevant role of the thiol moiety in lymphoid-lineage differentiation. *Exp Cell Res* 217:395, 1995.
387. Ekblom M, Fassler R, Tomasini-Johansson B, et al: Downregulation of tenascin expression by glucocorticoids in bone marrow stromal cells and in fibroblasts. *J Cell Biol* 123:1037, 1993.
388. Seiffert M, Beck SC, Schermutzki F, et al: Mitogenic and adhesive effects of tenascin-C on human hematopoietic cells are mediated by various functional domains. *Matrix Biol* 17:47, 1998.
389. Ohta M, Sakai T, Saga Y, et al: Suppression of hematopoietic activity in tenascin-C-deficient mice. *Blood* 91:4074, 1998.
390. Mackie EJ, Tucker RP: The tenascin-C knockout revisited. *J Cell Sci* 112:3847, 1999.
391. Bentley SA: Collagen synthesis by bone marrow stromal cells: A quantitative study. *Br J Haematol* 50:491, 1982.
392. Mori M, Sadahira Y, Kawasaki S, et al: Formation of capillary networks from bone marrow cultured in collagen gel. *Cell Struct Funct* 14:393, 1989.
393. Zukerman KS, Rhodes RK, Goodrum DD, et al: Inhibition of collagen deposition in the extracellular matrix prevents the establishment of a stroma supportive of hematopoiesis in long-term murine bone marrow cultures. *J Clin Invest* 75:970, 1985.
394. Zukerman KS, Prince CW, Gay S: The hemopoietic extracellular matrix, in *Handbook of the Hemopoietic Microenvironment*, edited by M Tavassoli, p 399. Humana Press, Clifton, NJ, 1989.
395. Koenigsmann M, Griffin JD, DiCarlo J, Cannistra SA: Myeloid and erythroid progenitor cells from normal bone marrow adhere to collagen type I. *Blood* 79:657, 1992.
396. Waterhouse EJ, Quesenberry PJ, Balian G: Collagen synthesis by murine bone marrow cell culture. *J Cell Physiol* 127:397, 1987.
397. Charbord P, Tamayo E, Saeland S, et al: Granulocyte-macrophage colony-stimulating factor (GM-CSF) in human long-term bone marrow cultures: Endogenous production in the adherent layer and effect on exogenous GM-CSF on granulomonopoiesis. *Blood* 78:1230, 1991.
398. Chichester CO, Fernández M, Minguel JJ: Extracellular matrix gene expression by human bone marrow stroma and by marrow fibroblasts. *Cell Adhes Commun* 1:93, 1993.
399. Klein G, Muller CA, Tillet E, et al: Collagen type VI in the human bone marrow microenvironment: A strong cytoadhesive component. *Blood* 86:1740, 1995.
400. Klein G, Kibler C, Schermutzki F, et al: Cell binding properties of collagen type XIV for human hematopoietic cells. *Matrix Biol* 16:307, 1998.
401. Briddon SJ, Melford SK, Turner M, et al: Collagen mediates changes in intracellular calcium in primary mouse megakaryocytes through syk-dependent and -independent pathways. *Blood* 93:3847, 1999.
402. Nilsson SK, Debatis ME, Dooner MS, et al: Immunofluorescence characterization of key extracellular matrix proteins in murine bone marrow in situ. *J Histochem Cytochem* 46:371, 1998.
403. Kleinman HK, Weeks BS: Laminin: Structure, function and receptors. *Curr Opin Cell Biol* 1:964, 1989.
404. Senior RM, Gresham HD, Griffin GL, et al: Entactin stimulates neutrophil adhesion and chemotaxis through interactions between its Arg-GlyAsp (RGD) domain and the leukocyte response integrin. *J Clin Invest* 90:2251, 1992.
405. Bryant G, Rao CN, Brentani M, et al: A role for the laminin receptor in leukocyte chemotaxis. *J Leukoc Biol* 41:220, 1987.
406. Lundgren-Akerlund E, Olofsson AM, Berger E, Arfors KE: CD11b/CD18-dependent polymorphonuclear leucocyte interaction with matrix proteins in adhesion and migration. *Scand J Immunol* 37:569, 1993.
407. Liesveld JL, Ryan DH, Kempski MC, et al: Quantitation of the binding of human CD34 positive myeloid progenitors to marrow stroma fibroblasts, and components of the extracellular matrix, in *Hematopoiesis, UCLA Symposia on Molecular and Cellular Biology New Series*, edited by SC Clark, DW Golde, p 157. Wiley-Liss, New York, 1990.
408. Tobias JW, Bern MM, Netland PA, Zetter BR: Monocyte adhesion to subendothelial components. *Blood* 69:1265, 1987.
409. Bohnsack JF, Akiyama SK, Damsky CH, et al: Human neutrophil adherence to laminin in vitro: Evidence for a distinct neutrophil integrin receptor for laminin. *J Exp Med* 171:1221, 1990.
410. Bohnsack JF: CD11/CD18-independent neutrophil adherence to laminin is mediated by the integrin VLA-6. *Blood* 79:1545, 1992.
411. Sagar BM, Rentala S, Gopal PN, et al: Fibronectin and laminin enhance engraftibility of cultured hematopoietic stem cells. *Biochem Biophys Res Commun* 350:1000, 2006.
412. Gu Y, Sorokin L, Durbeej M, et al: Characterization of bone marrow laminins and identification of α_5-containing laminins as adhesive proteins for multipotent hematopoietic FDCP-mix cells. *Blood* 93:2533, 1999.
413. Monturi N, Selleri C, Risitano AM, et al: Expression of the 67-kDa laminin receptor in acute myeloid leukemia cells mediates adhesion to laminin and is frequently associated with monocytic differentiation. *Clin Cancer Res* 5:1465, 1999.
414. Vogel W, Kanz L, Brugger W, et al: Expression of laminin β_2 chain in normal human bone marrow. *Blood* 94:1143, 1999.
415. Siler U, Roussell P, Muller CA, Klein G: Laminin gamma$_2$ chain is a stromal cell marker of the human bone marrow microenvironment. *Br J Haematol* 119:212, 2002.
416. Gu Y-C, Kortesmaa J, Tryggvason K, et al: Laminin isoform-specific promotion of adhesion and migration of human bone marrow progenitor cells. *Blood* 101:877, 2003.
417. Qian H, Tryggvason K, Jacobsen SE, Ekblom M: Contribution of alpha$_6$ integrins to hematopoietic stem and progenitor cell homing to bone marrow and collaboration with alpha4 integrins. *Blood* 107:3503, 2006.
418. Selleri C, Ragno P, Ricci P, et al: The metastasis-associated 67-kDa laminin receptor is involved in G-CSF-induced hematopoietic stem cell mobilization. *Blood* 108:2476, 2006.
419. Bonig H, Chang KH, Nakamoto B, Papayannopoulou T: The p67 laminin receptor identifies human erythroid progenitor and precursor cells and is functionally important for their bone marrow lodgment. *Blood* 108:1230, 2006.
420. Fehlner-Gardiner C, Uniyal S, Von Ballestrem C, et al: Integrin VLA-6 (alpha 6, beta 1) mediates adhesion of mouse bone marrow-derived mast cells to laminin. *Allergy* 51:650, 1996.
421. El-Nemer W, Gane P, Colin Y, et al: The Lutheran blood group glycoproteins, the erythroid receptors for laminin, are adhesion molecules. *J Biol Chem* 273:16686, 1998.
422. Ohki K, Kohashi O: Laminin promotes proliferation of bone marrow-derived macrophages and macrophage cell lines. *Cell Struct Funct* 19:63, 1994.
423. Bornstein P: Thrombospondins as matricellular modulators of cell function. *J Clin Invest* 107:929, 2001.
424. Long MW, Dixit VM: Thrombospondin functions as a cytoadhesion molecule for human hematopoietic progenitor cells. *Blood* 75:2311, 1990.
425. Li WX, Howard RJ, Leung LL: Identification of SVTCG in thrombospondin as the conformation-dependent, high affinity binding site for its receptor, CD36. *J Biol Chem* 268:16179, 1993.
426. Calvo D, Vega MA: Identification, primary structure, and distribution of CLA-1, a novel member of the CD36/LIMPII gene family. *J Biol Chem* 268:18929, 1993.
427. Vischer P, Feitsma K, Schon P, Volker W: Perlecan is responsible for thrombospondin 1 binding on the surface of cultured porcine endothelial cells. *Eur J Cell Biol* 73:332, 1997.
428. Nakahata T, Okumura N: Cell surface antigen expression in human erythroid progenitors: Erythroid and megakaryocytic markers. *Leuk Lymphoma* 13:401, 1994.
429. Yang M, Li K, Ng MH, et al: Thrombospondin-1 inhibits in vitro megakaryocytopoiesis via CD36. *Thromb Res* 109:47, 2003.
430. Kyriakides TR, Rojnuckarin P, Reidy MA, et al: Megakaryocytes require thrombospondin-2 for normal platelet formation and function. *Blood* 101:3915, 2003.
431. Pierson BA, Gupta K, Hu WS, Miller JS: Human natural killer cell expansion is regulated by thrombospondin-mediated activation of transforming growth factor-beta 1 and independent accessory cell-derived contact and soluble factors. *Blood* 87:180, 1996.
432. Crawford SE, Stellmach V, Murphy-Ullrich JE, et al: Thrombospondin-1 is a major activator of TGF-beta 1 *in vivo*. *Cell* 93:1159, 1998.
433. Touhami M, Fauvel-Lafeve F, Da Silva N, et al: Induction of thrombospondin-1 by all-*trans* retinoic acid modulates growth and differentiation of HL-60 myeloid leukemia cells. *Leukemia* 11:2137, 1997.
434. Taraboletti G, Belotti D, Borsotti P, et al: The 140-kilodalton antiangiogenic fragment of thrombospondin-1 binds to basic fibroblast growth factor. *Cell Growth Differ* 8:471, 1997.
435. Margosio B, Marchetti D, Vergani V, et al: Thrombospondin 1 as a scavenger for matrix-associated fibroblast growth factor 2. *Blood* 102:4399, 2003.
436. Loganadane LD, Berge N, Legrand C, Fauvel-Lafeve F: Endothelial cell proliferation regulated by cytokines modulates thrombospondin-1 secretion into the subendothelium. *Cytokine* 9:740, 1997.
437. Qian X, Wang TN, Rothman VL, et al: Thrombospondin-1 modulates angiogenesis in vitro by up-regulation of matrix metalloproteinase-9 in endothelial cells. *Exp Cell Res* 235:403, 1997.

438. Mansfield PJ, Suchard SJ: Thrombospondin promotes both chemotaxis and haptotaxis of human peripheral blood monocytes. *J Immunol* 153:4219, 1994.
439. Mansfield PJ, Suchard SJ: Thrombospondin promotes both chemotaxis and haptotaxis in neutrophil-like HL-60 cells. *J Immunol* 150:1959, 1993.
440. Horton MA: The alpha$_v$beta$_3$ integrin "vitronectin receptor." *Int J Biochem Cell Biol* 29:721, 1997.
441. Poujol C, Nurden AT, Nurden P: Ultrastructural analysis of the distribution of vitronectin receptor (alpha v beta 3) in human platelets and megakaryocytes reveals an intracellular pool and labeling of the alpha-granule membrane. *Br J Haematol* 96:823, 1997.
442. Shimizu Y, Irani AM, Brown EJ, et al: Human mast cells derived from fetal liver cells cultured with stem cell factor express a functional CD51/ CD61 (alpha$_v$beta$_3$) integrin. *Blood* 86:930, 1995.
443. Hughes DE, Salter DM, Dedhar S, Simpson R: Integrin expression in human bone. *J Bone Miner Res* 8:527, 1993.
444. Mbalaviele G, Jaiswal N, Meng A, et al: Human mesenchymal stem cells promote human osteoclast differentiation from CD34+ bone marrow hematopoietic progenitors. *Endocrinology* 140:3736, 1999.
445. Boissy P, Machuca I, Pfaff M, et al: Aggregation of mononucleated precursors triggers cell surface expression of alpha$_v$beta$_3$ integrin, essential to formation of osteoclast-like multinucleated cells. *J Cell Sci* 111:2563, 1998.
446. Faccio R, Takeshita S, Zallone A, et al: C-Fms and the $\alpha_v\beta_3$ integrin collaborate during osteoclast differentiation. *J Clin Invest* 111:749, 2003.
447. Chin SL, Johnson SA, Quinn J, et al: A role for alpha V integrin subunit in TGF-beta-stimulated osteoclastogenesis. *Biochem Biophys Res Commun* 307:1051, 2003.
448. Weerasinghe D, McHugh KP, Ross FP, et al: A role for the alpha$_v$beta$_3$ integrin in the transmigration of monocytes. *J Cell Biol* 142:595, 1998.
449. Rainger GE, Buckley CD, Simmons DL, Nash GB: Neutrophils sense flow-generated stress and direct their migration through alpha$_v$beta$_3$ integrin. *Am J Physiol* 276:H858, 1999.
450. Nath D, Slocombe PM, Stephens PE, et al: Interactions of metargidin (ADAM-15) with alpha$_v$beta$_3$ and alpha$_5$beta$_1$ integrins on different haemopoietic cells. *J Cell Sci* 112:579, 1999.
451. Savill J, Hogg N, Ren Y, Haslett C: Thrombospondin cooperates with CD36 and the vitronectin receptor in macrophage recognition of neutrophils undergoing apoptosis. *J Clin Invest* 90:1513, 1992.
452. Fadok VA, Warner ML, Bratton DL, Henson PM: CD36 is required for phagocytosis of apoptotic cells by human macrophages that use either a phosphatidylserine receptor or the vitronectin receptor (alpha$_v$beta$_3$). *J Immunol* 161:6250, 1998.
453. Rubartelli A, Poggi A, Zocchi MR: The selective engulfment of apoptotic bodies by dendritic cells is mediated by the alpha$_{(v)}$beta$_3$ integrin and requires intracellular calcium and extracellular calcium. *Eur J Immunol* 27:1893, 1997.
454. Hunt P, Hokom MM, Hornkohl A, et al: The effect of platelet-derived glycosaminoglycan serglycin on in vitro proplatelet-like process formation. *Exp Hematol* 21:1295, 1993.
455. Leven RM: Differential regulation of integrin-mediated proplatelet formation and megakaryocyte spreading. *J Cell Physiol* 163:597, 1995.
456. Rusnati M, Tanghetti E, Dell'Era P, et al: Alpha$_v$beta$_3$ integrin mediates the cell-adhesive capacity and biological activity of basic fibroblast growth factor (FGF-2) in cultured endothelial cells. *Mol Cell Biol* 8:2449, 1997.
457. Ybarrondo B, O'Rouke AM, McCarthy JB, Mescher MF: Cytotoxic T lymphocyte interaction with fibronectin and vitronectin: Activated adhesion and cosignalling. *Immunology* 91:186, 1997.
458. Roberts K, Yokoyama WM, Kehn PJ, Shevach EM: The vitronectin receptor serves as an accessory molecule for the activation of a subset of gamma/delta T cells. *J Exp Med* 173:231, 1991.
459. Rabinowich H, Lin WC, Amoscato A, et al: Expression of vitronectin receptor on human NK cells and its role in protein phosphorylation, cytokine production, and cell proliferation. *J Immunol* 154:1124, 1995.
460. Hermann P, Armant M, Brown E, et al: The vitronectin receptor and its associated CD47 molecule mediates proinflammatory cytokine synthesis in human monocytes by interactions with soluble CD23. *J Cell Biol* 144:767, 1999.
461. Stier S, Ko Y, Forkert R, et al: Osteopontin is a hematopoietic stem cell niche component that negatively regulates stem cell pool size. *J Exp Med* 201:1781, 2005.
462. Kang JA, Zhou Y, Weis TL, et al: Osteopontin regulates actin cytoskeleton and contributes to cell proliferation in primary erythroblasts. *J Biol Chem* 283:6997, 2008.
463. Chung JW, Kim MS, Piao ZH, et al: Osteopontin promotes the development of natural killer cells from hematopoietic stem cells. *Stem Cells* 26:2114, 2008.
464. Diao H, Iwabuchi K, Li L, et al. Osteopontin regulates development and function of invariant natural killer T cells. *Proc Natl Acad Sci U S A* 105:15884, 2008.
465. Gu YC, Nilsson K, Eng H, Ekblom M: Association of extracellular matrix proteins fibulin-1 and fibulin-2 with fibronectin in bone marrow stroma. *Br J Haematol* 109:305, 2000.
466. Hergeth SP, Aicher WK, Essl M, et al: Characterization and functional analysis of osteoblast-derived fibulins in the human hematopoietic stem cell niche. *Exp Hematol* 36:1022, 2008.
467. Koury MJ: Erythropoietin: The story of hypoxia and a finely regulated hematopoietic hormone. *Exp Hematol* 33:1263, 2005.
468. Koury ST, Koury MJ, Bondurant MC: Cytoskeletal distribution and function during the maturation and enucleation of mammalian erythroblasts. *J Cell Biol* 109:3005, 1989.
469. Soni S, Bala S, Gwynn B, et al: Absence of erythroblast macrophage protein (Emp) leads to failure of erythroblast nuclear extrusion. *J Biol Chem* 281:20181, 2006.
470. Ji P, Jayapal SR, Lodish HF: Enucleation of cultured mouse fetal erythroblasts requires Rac GTPases and mDia2. *Nat Cell Biol* 10:314, 2008.
471. Popova EY, Krauss SW, Short SA, et al: Chromatin condensation in terminally differentiating mouse erythroblasts does not involve special architectural proteins but depends on histone deacetylation. *Chromosome Res* 17: 47, 2009.
472. Wilson JG, Tavassoli M: Microenvironmental factors involved in the establishment of erythropoiesis in bone marrow. *Ann N Y Acad Sci* 718:271, 1994.
473. Chasis JA, Mohandas N: Erythroblastic islands: Niches for erythropoiesis. *Blood* 112:470, 2008.
474. Bessis M: L'ilot èrythroblastique, unitè fonctionelle de le moelle osseuse. *Rev Hematol* 13:8, 1958.
475. Le Charpentier Y, Prenant M: Isoloment de l'ilot erythroblastique: Etude en microscopie optique et electronique a balayage. *Nouv Rev Fr Hematol* 15:119, 1975.
476. Yokoyama T, Etoh T, Kitagawa H, et al: Migration of erythroblastic islands toward the sinusoid as erythroid maturation proceeds in rat bone marrow. *J Vet Med Sci* 65:449, 2003.
477. Spike BT, Dibling BC, Macleod KF: Hypoxic stress underlies defects in erythroblast islands in the Rb-null mouse. *Blood* 110:2173, 2007.
478. Rhodes MM, Kopsombut P, Bondurant MC, et al: Adherence to macrophages in erythroblastic islands enhances erythroblast proliferation and increases erythrocyte production by a different mechanism than erythropoietin. *Blood* 111:1700, 2008.
479. Lichtman MA, Waugh RE: Red cell egress from the marrow: Ultrastructural and biophysical aspects, in *Regulation of Erythropoiesis*, edited by ED Zanjani, M Tavassoli, J Ascencao, p 15. PMA Literary & Film Management, Great Neck, NY, 1989.
480. Yoshida H, Kawane K, Koike M, et al: Phosphatidylserine-dependent engulfment by macrophages of nuclei from erythroid precursor cells. *Nature* 437:754, 2005.
481. Kawane K, Fukuyama H, Kondoh G, et al: Requirement of DNase II for definitive erythropoiesis in the mouse fetal liver. *Science* 292:1546, 2001.
482. Sadahira Y, Yasuda T, Yoshino T, et al: Impaired splenic erythropoiesis in phlebotomized mice injected with CL2MDP-liposome: An experimental model for studying the role of stromal macrophages in erythropoiesis. *J Leukoc Biol* 68:464, 2000.
483. Wu H, Klingmuller U, Acurio A, et al: Functional interaction of erythropoietin and stem cell factor receptors is essential for erythroid colony formation. *Proc Natl Acad Sci U S A* 94:1806, 1997.
484. Muta K, Krantz SB, Bondurant MC, Dai CH: Stem cell factor retards differentiation of normal human erythroid progenitor cells while stimulating proliferation. *Blood* 86:572, 1995.
485. Suenobu S, Takakura N, Inada T, et al: A role of EphB4 receptor and its ligand, ephrin-B2 in erythropoiesis. *Biochem Biophys Res Commun* 293:1124, 2002.
486. Lenox LE, Perry JM, Paulson RF: BMP4 and Madh5 regulate the erythroid response to acute anemia. *Blood* 105:2741, 2005.
487. De Maria R, Testa U, Luchetti L, et al: Apoptotic role of Fas/Fas ligand system in the regulation of erythropoiesis. *Blood* 93:796, 1999.
488. Lichtman MA, Chamberlain JK, Simon W, et al: Parasinusoidal location of megakaryocytes in marrow: A determinant of platelet release. *Am J Hematol* 4:303, 1978.
489. Thiele J, Galle R, Sander C, Fischer R: Interactions between megakaryocytes and sinus wall: An ultrastructural study of bone marrow tissue in primary (essential) thrombocythemia. *J Submicrosc Cytol Pathol* 23:595, 1991.
490. Avraham H, Cowley S, Chi SY, et al: Characterization of adhesive interactions between human endothelial cells and megakaryocytes. *J Clin Invest* 91:2378, 1993.
491. Zweegman S, Veenhof MA, Huijgens PC, et al: Regulation of megakaryopoiesis in an in vitro stroma model: Preferential adhesion of megakaryocytic progenitors and subsequent inhibition of maturation. *Exp Hematol* 28:401, 2000.
492. Yang M, Li K, Lam AC, et al: Platelet-derived growth factor enhances granulopoiesis via bone marrow stromal cells. *Int J Hematol* 73:327, 2001.
493. Battinelli EM, Hartwig JH, Italiano JE Jr: Delivering new insight into the biology of megakaryopoiesis and thrombopoiesis. *Curr Opin Hematol* 14:419, 2007.
494. Kaushansky K: Historical review: Megakaryopoiesis and thrombopoiesis. *Blood* 111:981, 2008.
495. Dhanjal TS, Pendaries C, Ross EA, et al: A novel role for PECAM-1 in megakaryocytokinesis and recovery of platelet counts in thrombocytopenic mice. *Blood* 109:4237, 2007.
496. Wu Y, Welte T, Michaud M, Madri JA: PECAM-1: A multifaceted regulator of megakaryocytopoiesis. *Blood* 110:851, 2007.
497. Riviere C, Subra F, Cohen-Solal K, et al: Phenotypic and functional evidence for the expression of CXCR4 receptor during megakaryopoiesis. *Blood* 93:1511, 1999.
498. Hamada T, Mohle R, Hesselgesser J, et al: Transendothelial migration of megakaryocytes in response to stromal cell-derived factor 1 (SDF-1) enhances platelet formation. *J Exp Med* 188:539, 1998.
499. Avecilla ST, Hattori K, Heissig B, et al: Chemokine-mediated interaction of hematopoietic progenitors with the bone marrow vascular niche is required for thrombopoiesis. *Nat Med* 10:64, 2004.
500. Junt T, Schulze H, Chen Z, et al: Dynamic visualization of thrombopoiesis within bone marrow. *Science* 317:1767, 2007.
501. Lambertsen RH, Weiss L: A model of intramedullary hemopoietic microenvironments based on stereologic study of the distribution of endoclonal colonies. *Blood* 63:287, 1984.

502. Rosmarin AG, Yang Z, Resendes KK: Transcriptional regulation in myelopoiesis: Hematopoietic fate choice, myeloid differentiation, and leukemogenesis. *Exp Hematol* 33:131, 2005.
503. Hock H, Orkin SH: Zinc-finger transcription factor Gfi-1: Versatile regulator of lymphocytes, neutrophils and hematopoietic stem cells. *Curr Opin Hematol* 13:1, 2006.
504. Friedman AD: Transcriptional control of granulocyte and monocyte development. *Oncogene* 26:6816, 2007.
505. Iwasaki H, Akashi K: Myeloid lineage commitment from the hematopoietic stem cell. *Immunity* 26:726, 2007.
506. Mori Y, Iwasaki H, Kohno K, et al: Identification of the human eosinophil lineage-committed progenitor: Revision of phenotypic definition of the human common myeloid progenitor. *J Exp Med* 206:183, 2009.
507. Rosenberg HF, Phipps S, Foster PS: Eosinophil trafficking in allergy and asthma. *J Allergy Clin Immunol* 119:1303, 2007.
508. Christopher MJ, Link DC: Regulation of neutrophil homeostasis. *Curr Opin Hematol* 14:3, 2007.
509. Furze RC, Rankin SM: Neutrophil mobilization and clearance in the bone marrow. *Immunology* 125:281, 2008.
510. Stark MA, Huo Y, Burcin TL, et al: Phagocytosis of apoptotic neutrophils regulates granulopoiesis via IL-23 and IL-17. *Immunity* 22:285, 2005.
511. Naito K, Tamahashi N, Chiba T, et al: The microvasculature of the human bone marrow correlated with the distribution of hematopoietic cells: A computer-assisted three-dimensional reconstruction study. *Tohoku J Exp Med* 166:439, 1992.
512. Blazsek I, Misset JL, Benavides M, et al: Hematon, a multicellular functional unit in normal human bone marrow: Structural organization, hemopoietic activity, and its relationship to myelodysplasia and myeloid leukemias. *Exp Hematol* 18:259, 1990.
513. Wright DE, Wagers AJ, Gulati AP, et al: Physiological migration of hematopoietic stem and progenitor cells. *Science* 294:1933, 2001.
514. Abkowitz JL, Robinson AE, Kale S, et al: Mobilization of hematopoietic stem cells during homeostasis and after cytokine exposure. *Blood* 102:1249, 2003.
515. Massberg S, Schaerli P, Knezevic-Maramica I, et al: Immunosurveillance by hematopoietic progenitor cells trafficking through blood, lymph, and peripheral tissues. *Cell* 131:994, 2007.
516. Driessen RL, Johnston HM, Nilsson SK: Membrane bound stem cell factor is a key regulator in the initial lodgement of stem cells within the endosteal marrow region. *Exp Hematol* 31:1284, 2003.
517. Ihanus E, Uotila LM, Toivanen A: Red-cell ICAM-4 is a ligand for the monocyte/macrophage integrin CD11c/CD18: Characterization of the binding sites on ICAM-4. *Blood* 109:802, 2007.
518. Kishimoto TK, Baldwin ET, Anderson DC: The role of β_2 integrins in inflammation, in *Inflammation Basic Principles and Clinical Correlates*, 3rd ed, edited by JI Gallin, R Snyderman, p 537. Lippincott Williams & Wilkins, Philadelphia, 1999.
519. Lasky LA: Selectin-carbohydrate interactions and the initiation of the inflammatory response. *Annu Rev Biochem* 64:113, 1995.
520. Hynes RO: Integrins: Bidirectional, allosteric signaling machines. *Cell* 110:673, 2002.
521. Takada Y, Ye X, Simon S: The integrins. *Genome Biol* 8:215, 2007.
522. Eshghi S, Vogelezang MG, Hynes RO, et al: Alpha4beta1 integrin and erythropoietin mediate temporally distinct steps in erythropoiesis: Integrins in red cell development. *J Cell Biol* 177:871, 2007.
523. Iguchi A, Okuyama R, Koguma M, et al: Selective stimulation of granulopoiesis in vitro by established bone marrow stromal cells. *Cell Struct Funct* 22:357, 1997.
524. Petty JM, Lenox CC, Weiss DJ, et al: Crosstalk between CXCR4/stromal derived factor-1 and VLA-4/VCAM-1 pathways regulates neutrophil retention in the bone marrow. *J Immunol* 182:604, 2009.
525. Dittel BN, LeBien TW: Reduced expression of vascular cell adhesion molecule-1 on bone marrow stromal cells isolated from marrow transplant recipients correlates with a reduced capacity to support human B lymphopoiesis in vitro. *Blood* 86:2833, 1995.
526. Funk PE, Stephan RP, Witte PL: Vascular cell adhesion molecule 1-positive reticular cells express interleukin-7 and stem cell factor in the bone marrow. *Blood* 86:2661, 1995.
527. Galotto M, Berisso G, Delfino L, et al: Stromal damage as a consequence of high-dose chemo/radiotherapy in bone marrow transplant recipients. *Exp Hematol* 27:1460, 1999.
528. Priestley GV, Ulyanova T, Papayannopoulou T: Sustained alterations in biodistribution of stem/progenitor cells in Tie2Cre+ alpha4(f/f) mice are hematopoietic cell autonomous. *Blood* 109:109, 2007.
529. Katayama Y, Hildalgo A, Peired A, Frenette PS: $\alpha_4\beta_7$ and its counter-receptor MAdCAM-1 contribute to hematopoietic progenitor recruitment into bone marrow following transplantation. *Blood* 104:2020, 2004.
530. Aplin AE, Howe A, Alahari SK, Juliano RL: Signal transduction and signal modulation by cell adhesion receptors: The role of integrins, cadherins, immunoglobulin-cell adhesion molecules and selectins. *Pharmacol Rev* 50:197, 1998.
531. Jarvis LJ, Maguire JE, LeBien TW: Contact between human bone marrow stromal cells and B lymphocytes enhances very late antigen-4/vascular cell adhesion molecule-1-independent tyrosine phosphorylation of focal adhesion kinase, paxillin, and ERK-2 in stromal cells. *Blood* 90:1626, 1997.
532. Shibayama H, Anzai N, Braun SE, et al: H-Ras is involved in the inside-out signaling pathway of interleukin-3-induced integrin activation. *Blood* 93:1540, 1999.
533. Levesque JP, Simmons PJ: Cytoskeleton and integrin-mediated adhesion signaling in human CD34+ hemopoietic progenitor cells. *Exp Hematol* 27:579, 1999.
534. Arai A, Nosaka Y, Kohsaka H, et al: CrkL activates integrin-mediated hematopoietic cell adhesion through the guanine nucleotide exchange factor C3G. *Blood* 93:3713, 1999.
535. Porter JC, Hogg N: Integrin cross talk: Activation of lymphocyte function-associated antigen-1 on human T cells alters $alpha_4beta_1$- and $alpha_5beta_1$-mediated function. *J Cell Biol* 138:1437, 1997.
536. Shibuya A, Campbell D, Hannum C, et al: DYNAM-1, a novel adhesion molecule involved in the cytolytic function of T lymphocytes. *Immunity* 4:573, 1996.
537. Shibuya K, Lanier LL, Phillips JH, et al: Physical and functional association of LFA-1 with DYNAM-1 adhesion molecule. *Immunity* 11:615, 1999.
538. Rodriguez-Fernandez JL, Gomez M, Luque A, et al: The interaction of activated integrin lymphocyte function-associated antigen 1 with ligand intercellular adhesion molecule 1 induces activation and redistribution of focal adhesion kinase and proline-rich tyrosine kinase 2 in T lymphocytes. *Mol Biol Cell* 10:1891, 1999.
539. Leavesley DI, Oliver JM, Swart BW, et al: Signals from platelet/endothelial cell adhesion molecule enhance the adhesive activity of the very late antigen-4 integrin of human CD34+ hematopoietic progenitor cells. *J Immunol* 153:4673, 1994.
540. Vestweber D, Blanks JE: Mechanisms that regulate the function of the selectins and their ligands. *Physiol Rev* 79:181, 1999.
541. Oostendorp RA, Dormer P: VLA-4-mediated interactions between normal human hematopoietic progenitors and stromal cells. *Leuk Lymphoma* 24:423, 1997.
542. Gotoh A, Ritchie A, Takahira H, Broxmeyer HE: Thrombopoietin and erythropoietin activate inside-out signaling of integrin and enhance adhesion to immobilized fibronectin in human growth-factor-dependent hematopoietic cells. *Ann Hematol* 75:207, 1997.
543. Liesveld JL, Winslow JM, Frediani KE, et al: Expression of integrins and examination of their adhesive function in normal and leukemic hematopoietic cells. *Blood* 81:112, 1993.
544. Ryan DH, Nuccie BL, Abboud CN: Inhibition of human bone marrow lymphoid progenitor colonies by antibodies to VLA integrins. *J Immunol* 149:3759, 1992.
545. Sugahara H, Kanakura Y, Furitsu T, et al: Induction of programmed cell death in human hematopoietic cell lines by fibronectin via its interaction with very late antigen 5. *J Exp Med* 179:1757, 1994.
546. Hurley RW, McCarthy JB, Wayner EA, Verfaillie CM: Monoclonal antibody crosslinking of the alpha 4 beta 1 integrin inhibits committed clonogenic hematopoietic progenitor proliferation. *Exp Hematol* 25:321, 1997.
547. Oostendorp RA, Spitzer E, Reisbach G, Dormer P: Antibodies to the beta 1-integrin chain, CD44, or ICAM-3 stimulate adhesion of blast colony-forming cells and may inhibit their growth. *Exp Hematol* 25:345, 1997.
548. Dao MA, Nolta JA: Cytokine and integrin stimulation synergize to promote higher levels of GATA-2, c-myb, and CD34 protein in primary human hematopoietic progenitors from bone marrow. *Blood* 109:2373, 2007.
549. Umemoto T, Yamato M, Shiratsuchi Y, et al: Expression of Integrin beta3 is correlated to the properties of quiescent hemopoietic stem cells possessing the side population phenotype. *J Immunol.* 177:7733, 2006.
550. Wagers AJ, Weissman IL: Differential expression of alpha2 integrin separates long-term and short-term reconstituting Lin-/loThy1.1(lo)c-kit+ Sca-1+ hematopoietic stem cells. *Stem Cells* 24:1087, 2006.
551. Petri B, Bixel MG: Molecular events during leukocyte diapedesis. *FEBS J* 273:4399, 2006.
552. Woodfin A, Voisin MB, Nourshargh S: PECAM-1: A multi-functional molecule in inflammation and vascular biology. *Arterioscler Thromb Vasc Biol* 27:2514, 2007.
553. Arkin S, Naprstek B, Guarini L, et al: Expression of intercellular adhesion molecule-1 (CD54) on hematopoietic progenitors. *Blood* 77:948, 1991.
554. Gunji Y, Nakamura M, Hagiwara T, et al: Expression and function of adhesion molecules on human hematopoietic stem cells: CD34+ LFA-1(neg) cells are more primitive than CD34+ LFA-1+ cells. *Blood* 80:429, 1992.
555. Makgoba MW, Sanders ME, Ginther Luce GE, et al: ICAM-1, a ligand for LFA-1-dependent adhesion of B, T, and myeloid cells. *Nature* 331:86, 1988.
556. Rao SG, Chitnis VS, Deora A, et al: An ICAM-1-like cell adhesion molecule is responsible for CD34-positive haemopoietic stem cells adhesion to bone-marrow stroma. *Cell Biol Int* 20:255, 1996.
557. Staunton DE, Dustin ML, Springer TA: Functional cloning of ICAM-2, a cell adhesion ligand for LFA-1, homologous to ICAM-1. *Nature* 339:61, 1989.
558. Fawcett J, Holness CLL, Needham LA, et al: Molecular cloning of ICAM-3, a third ligand for LFA-1, constitutively expressed on resting leukocytes. *Nature* 360:481, 1992.
559. Campanero MR, Sanchez-Mateos P, del Pozo MA, Sanchez-Madrid F: ICAM-3 regulates lymphocyte morphology and integrin-mediated T cell interactions with endothelial cell and extracellular matrix ligands. *J Cell Biol* 127:867, 1994.
560. Wang JH, Smolyar A, Tan K, et al: Structure of a heterophilic adhesion complex between the human CD2 and CD58 (LFA-3) counterreceptors. *Cell* 97:791, 1999.
561. Nielsen M, Gerwien J, Geisler C, et al: MHC class II ligation induces CD58 (LFA-3)-mediated adhesion in human T cells. *Exp Clin Immunogenet* 15:61, 1998.
562. LeGuiner S, Le Drean E, Labarriere N, et al: LFA-3 co-stimulates cytokine secretion by cytotoxic T lymphocytes by providing a TCR-independent activation signal. *Eur J Immunol* 28:1322, 1998.
563. Itzhaky D, Raz N, Hollander N: The glycosylphosphatidylinositol-anchored form and the transmembrane form of CD58 associate with protein kinases. *J Immunol* 60:4361, 1998.

564. Kirby AC, Cahen P, Porter SR, Olsen I: LFA-3 (CD58) mediates T lymphocyte adhesion in chronic inflammatory infiltrates. *Scand J Immunol* 50:469, 1999.
565. De Waele M, Renmans W, Jochmans K, et al: Different expression of adhesion molecules on CD34+ cells in AML and B lineage ALL and their normal bone marrow counterparts. *Eur J Haematol* 63:192, 1999.
566. McCarty JM, Yee EK, Deisher TA, et al: Interleukin-4 induces endothelial vascular cell adhesion molecule-1 (VCAM-1) by an NF-kappa b-independent mechanism. *FEBS Lett* 372:194, 1995.
567. Bochner BS, Klunk DA, Sterbinsky SA, et al: IL-13 selectively induces vascular cell adhesion molecule-1 expression in human endothelial cells. *J Immunol* 154:799, 1995.
568. Kinashi T, Springer TA: Regulation of cell-matrix adhesion by receptor tyrosine kinases. *Leuk Lymphoma* 18:203, 1995.
569. Toivanen A, Ihanus E, Mattila M, et al: Importance of molecular studies on major blood groups—intercellular adhesion molecule-4, a blood group antigen involved in multiple cellular interactions. *Biochim Biophys Acta* 1780:456, 2008.
570. Crocker PR, Redelinghuys P: Siglecs as positive and negative regulators of the immune system. *Biochem Soc Trans* 36:1467, 2008.
571. Aizawa S, Tavassoli M: *In vitro* homing of hemopoietic stem cells mediated by a recognition system with galactosyl and mannosyl specificities. *Proc Natl Acad Sci U S A* 84:4485, 1987.
572. Tavassoli M, Hardy CL: Molecular basis of homing of intravenously transplanted stem cells. *Blood* 76:1059, 1990.
573. Sperandio M: Selectins and glycosyltransferases in leukocyte rolling *in vivo*. *FEBS J* 273:4377, 2006.
574. Sackstein R: Expression of an L-selectin ligand on hematopoietic progenitor cells. *Acta Haematol* 97:22, 1997.
575. Chute JP: Stem cell homing. *Curr Opin Hematol* 13:399, 2006.
576. Méndez-Ferrer S, Frenette PS: Hematopoietic stem cell trafficking: Regulated adhesion and attraction to bone marrow microenvironment. *Ann N Y Acad Sci* 1116:392, 2007.
577. Zarbock A, Ley K: Neutrophil adhesion and activation under flow. *Microcirculation* 16:31, 2009.
578. Nielsen JS, McNagny KM: Novel functions of the CD34 family. *J Cell Sci* 121:3683, 2008.
579. Eto T, Winkler I, Purton LE, Lévesque JP: Contrasting effects of P-selectin and E-selectin on the differentiation of murine hematopoietic progenitor cells. *Exp Hematol* 33:232, 2005.
580. Matsubara A, Iwama A, Yamazaki S, et al: Endomucin, a CD34-like sialomucin, marks hematopoietic stem cells throughout development. *J Exp Med* 202:1483, 2005.
581. Stockton BM, Cheng G, Manjunath N, et al: Negative regulation of T cell homing by CD43. *Immunity* 8:373, 1998.
582. Matsumoto M, Shigeta A, Miyasaka M, Hirata T: CD43 plays both antiadhesive and proadhesive roles in neutrophil rolling in a context-dependent manner. *J Immunol* 181:3628, 2008.
583. Bazil V, Brandt J, Chen S, et al: A monoclonal antibody recognizing CD43 (leukosialin) initiates apoptosis of human hematopoietic progenitor cells but not stem cells. *Blood* 87:1272, 1996.
584. Forde S, Tye BJ, Newey SE, et al: Endolyn (CD164) modulates the CXCL12-mediated migration of umbilical cord blood CD133+ cells. *Blood* 109:1825, 2007.
585. Bowen MA, Aruffo A: Adhesion molecules, their receptors, and their regulation: Analysis of CD6-activated leukocyte cell-adhesion molecule (ALCAM/CD166) interactions. *Transplant Proc* 31:795, 1999.
586. Ohneda O, Ohneda K, Arai F, et al: ALCAM (CD166): Its role in hematopoietic and endothelial development. *Blood* 98:2134, 2001.
587. Nervi B, Link DC, DiPersio JF: Cytokines and hematopoietic stem cell mobilization. *J Cell Biochem* 99:690, 2006.
588. Oostendorp RA, Ghaffari S, Eaves CJ: Kinetics of in vivo homing and recruitment into cycle of hematopoietic cells are organ-specific but CD44-independent. *Bone Marrow Transplant* 26:559, 2000.
589. Nedvetzki S, Gonen E, Assayag N, et al: RHAMM, a receptor for hyaluronan-mediated motility, compensates for CD44 in inflamed CD44-knockout mice: A different interpretation of redundancy. *Proc Natl Acad Sci U S A* 101:18081, 2004.
590. Funaro A, Malavasi F: Human CD38, a surface receptor, an enzyme, an adhesion molecule and not a simple marker. *J Biol Regul Homeost Agents* 13:54, 1999.
591. Hoenstein AL, Stokinger H, Imhof BA, Malavasi F: CD38 binding to human myeloid cells is mediated by mouse and human CD31. *Biochem J* 330:1129, 1998.
592. Turel KR, Rao SG: Expression of the cell adhesion molecule E-cadherin by the human bone marrow stromal cells and its probable role in CD34(+) stem cell adhesion. *Cell Biol Int* 22:641, 1998.
593. Kiel MJ, Acar M, Radice GL, Morrison SJ: Hematopoietic stem cells do not depend on N-cadherin to regulate their maintenance. *Cell Stem Cell* 4:170, 2009.
594. Hirata Y, Kimura N, Sato K, et al: ADP ribosyl cyclase activity of a novel bone marrow stromal cell surface molecule, BST-1. *FEBS Lett* 356:244, 1994.
595. Kaisho T, Ishikawa J, Oritani K, et al: BST-1, a surface molecule of bone marrow stromal cell lines that facilitates pre-B-cell growth. *Proc Natl Acad Sci U S A* 91:5325, 1994.
596. Vicari AP, Bean AG, Slotnik A: A role for BP-3/BST-1 antigen in early T cell development. *Int Immunol* 8:183, 1996.
597. Okuyama Y, Ishihara K, Kimura N, et al: Human BST-1 expressed on myeloid cells functions as a receptor molecule. *Biochem Biophys Res Commun* 228:838, 1996.
598. Springer TA: Traffic signals for lymphocyte recirculation and leukocyte emigration: The multistep paradigm. *Cell* 76:301, 1994.
599. Pals ST, de Gorter DJ, Spaargaren M: Lymphoma dissemination: The other face of lymphocyte homing. *Blood* 110:3102, 2007.
600. Petri B, Bixel MG: Molecular events during leukocyte diapedesis. *FEBS J* 273:4399, 2006.
601. Hordijk PL: Endothelial signalling events during leukocyte transmigration. *FEBS J* 273:4408, 2006.
602. Garrido-Urbani S, Bradfield PF, Lee BP, Imhof BA: Vascular and epithelial junctions: A barrier for leucocyte migration. *Biochem Soc Trans* 36:203, 2008.
603. Pease JE, Williams TJ: The attraction of chemokines as a target for specific anti-inflammatory therapy. *Br J Pharmacol* 147(Suppl 1):S212, 2006.
604. Watt SM, Forde SP: The central role of the chemokine receptor, CXCR4, in haemopoietic stem cell transplantation: Will CXCR4 antagonists contribute to the treatment of blood disorders? *Vox Sang* 94:18, 2008.
605. Bacon KB, Greaves DR, Dairaghi DJ, Schall TJ: The expanding universe of C, CX3C and CC chemokines, in *The Cytokine Handbook*, 3rd ed, edited by AW Thompson, p 753. Academic Press, San Diego, 1998.
606. Fong AM, Robinson LA, Steeber DA, et al: Fractalkine and CX3CR1 mediate a novel mechanism of leukocyte capture, firm adhesion, and activation under physiologic flow. *J Exp Med* 188:1413, 1998.
607. Broxmeyer HE: Chemokines in hematopoiesis. *Curr Opin Hematol* 15:49, 2008.
608. Dar A, Kollet O, Lapidot T: Mutual, reciprocal SDF-1/CXCR4 interactions between hematopoietic and bone marrow stromal cells regulate human stem cell migration and development in NOD/SCID chimeric mice. *Exp Hematol* 34:967, 2006.
609. Scott LM, Priestley GV, Papayannopoulou T: Deletion of alpha4 integrin from adult hematopoietic cells reveals roles in homeostasis, regeneration, and homing. *Mol Cell Biol* 23:9349, 2003.
610. Avigdor A, Goichberg P, Shivtiel S, et al: CD44 and hyaluronic acid cooperate with SDF-1 in the trafficking of human CD34+ stem/progenitor cells to the bone marrow. *Blood* 103:2981, 2004.
611. Wysoczynski M, Reca R, Ratajczak J, et al: Incorporation of CXCR4 into membrane lipid rafts primes homing-related responses of hematopoietic stem/progenitor cells to an SDF-1 gradient. *Blood* 10:40, 2005.
612. Williams DA, Zheng Y, Cancelas JA: Rho GTPases and regulation of hematopoietic stem cell localization. *Methods Enzymol* 439:365, 2008.
613. Kiel MJ, Morrison SJ: Uncertainty in the niches that maintain haematopoietic stem cells. *Nat Rev Immunol* 8:290, 2008.
614. Yin T, Li L: The stem cell niches in bone. *J Clin Invest* 116:1195, 2006.
615. Laird DJ, von Andrian UH, Wagers AJ: Stem cell trafficking in tissue development, growth, and disease. *Cell* 132:612, 2008.
616. Papayannopoulou T, Scadden DT: Stem-cell ecology and stem cells in motion. *Blood* 111:3923, 2008.
617. Czechowicz A, Kraft D, Weissman IL, Bhattacharya D: Efficient transplantation via antibody-based clearance of hematopoietic stem cell niches. *Science* 318:1296, 2007.
618. Levesque JP, Leavesley DI, Niutta S, et al: Cytokines increase human hemopoietic cell adhesiveness by activation of very late antigen (VLA)-4 and VLA-5 integrins. *J Exp Med* 181:1805, 1995.
619. Adams GB, Chabner KT, Alley IR, et al: Stem cell engraftment at the endosteal niche is specified by the calcium-sensing receptor. *Nature* 439:599, 2006.
620. Puri MC, Bernstein A: Requirement for the TIE family of receptor tyrosine kinases in adult but not fetal hematopoiesis. *Proc Natl Acad Sci U S A* 100:12753, 2003.
621. Arai F, Hirao A, Ohmura M, et al: Tie2/angiopoietin-1 signaling regulates hematopoietic stem cell quiescence in the bone marrow niche. *Cell* 118:149, 2004.
622. Umemoto T, Yamato M, Shiratsuchi Y, et al: Expression of Integrin beta3 is correlated to the properties of quiescent hemopoietic stem cells possessing the side population phenotype. *J Immunol.* 177:7733, 2006.
623. Qian H, Buza-Vidas N, Hyland CD, et al: Critical role of thrombopoietin in maintaining adult quiescent hematopoietic stem cells. *Cell Stem Cell* 1:671, 2007.
624. Yoshihara H, Arai F, Hosokawa K, et al: Thrombopoietin/MPL signaling regulates hematopoietic stem cell quiescence and interaction with the osteoblastic niche. *Cell Stem Cell* 1:685, 2007.
625. Bowie MB, Kent DG, Dykstra B, et al: Identification of a new intrinsically timed developmental checkpoint that reprograms key hematopoietic stem cell properties. *Proc Natl Acad Sci U S A* 104:5878, 2007.
626. Haylock DN, Williams B, Johnston HM, et al: Hemopoietic stem cells with higher hemopoietic potential reside at the bone marrow endosteum. *Stem Cells* 25:1062, 2007.
627. Steinman RA: Cell cycle regulators and hematopoiesis. *Oncogene* 21:3403, 2002.
628. Walkley CR, Sankaran VG, Orkin SH: Rb and hematopoiesis: Stem cells to anemia. *Cell Div* 3:13, 2008.
629. Wilson A, Laurenti E, Oser G, et al: Hematopoietic stem cells reversibly switch from dormancy to self-renewal during homeostasis and repair. *Cell* 135:1118, 2008.
630. Sherr CJ, Roberts JM: Living with or without cyclins and cyclin-dependent kinases. *Genes Dev* 18:2699, 2004.
631. Kozar K, Ciemerych MA, Rebel VI, et al: Mouse development and cell proliferation in the absence of D-cyclins. *Cell* 118:477, 2004.

632. Malumbres M, Sotillo R, Santamaría D, et al: Mammalian cells cycle without the D-type cyclin-dependent kinases Cdk4 and Cdk6. *Cell* 118(4):493, 2004.
633. Metcalf D: Hematopoietic cytokines. *Blood* 111:485, 2008.
634. Tushinski RJ, Stanley ER: The regulation of mononuclear phagocyte entry into S phase by the colony stimulating factor CSF-1. *J Cell Physiol* 122:221, 1985.
635. Roussel MF, Theodoras AM, Pagano M, Sherr CJ: Rescue of defective mitogenic signaling by D-type cyclins. *Proc Natl Acad Sci U S A* 92:6837, 1995.
636. Oguro H, Iwama A: Life and death in hematopoietic stem cells. *Curr Opin Immunol* 19:503, 2007.
637. Berthet C, Rodriguez-Galan MC, Hodge DL, et al: Hematopoiesis and thymic apoptosis are not affected by the loss of Cdk2. *Mol Cell Biol* 27:5079, 2007.
638. Koury MJ: Programmed cell death (apoptosis) in hematopoiesis. *Exp Hematol* 20:391, 1992.
639. Kelley LL, Koury MJ, Bondurant MC: Survival or death of individual proerythroblasts results from differing erythropoietin sensitivities: A mechanism for controlled rates of erythrocyte production. *Blood* 82:2340, 1993.
640. Opferman JT: Life and death during hematopoietic differentiation. *Curr Opin Immunol* 19:497, 2007.
641. Reed JC: Bcl-2-family proteins and hematologic malignancies: History and future prospects. *Blood* 111:3322, 2008.
642. Opferman JT, Iwasaki H, Ong CC, et al: Obligate role of anti-apoptotic MCL-1 in the survival of hematopoietic stem cells. *Science* 307:1101, 2005.
643. Hamasaki A, Sendo F, Nakayama K, et al: Accelerated neutrophil apoptosis in mice lacking A1-a, a subtype of the bcl-2-related A1 gene. *J Exp Med* 188:1985, 1998.
644. Rhodes MM, Kopsombut P, Bondurant MC, et al: Bcl-x(L) prevents apoptosis of late-stage erythroblasts but does not mediate the antiapoptotic effect of erythropoietin. *Blood* 106:1857, 2005.
645. Aerbajinai W, Giattina M, Lee YT, et al: The proapoptotic factor Nix is coexpressed with Bcl-xL during terminal erythroid differentiation. *Blood* 102:712, 2003.
646. Cheshier SH, Prohaska SS, Weissman IL: The effect of bleeding on hematopoietic stem cell cycling and self-renewal. *Stem Cells Dev* 16:707, 2007.
647. von Lindern M, Schmidt U, Beug H: Control of erythropoiesis by erythropoietin and stem cell factor: A novel role for Bruton's tyrosine kinase. *Cell Cycle* 3:876, 2004.
648. Muta K, Krantz SB, Bondurant MC, et al: Distinct roles of erythropoietin, insulin-like growth factor I, and stem cell factor in the development of erythroid progenitor cells. *J Clin Invest* 94:34, 1994.
649. Schweers RL, Zhang J, Randall MS, et al: NIX is required for programmed mitochondrial clearance during reticulocyte maturation. *Proc Natl Acad Sci U S A* 104:19500, 2007.
650. Sandoval H, Thiagarajan P, Dasgupta SK, et al: Essential role for Nix in autophagic maturation of erythroid cells. *Nature* 454:232, 2008.
651. Finch CA, Harker LA, Cook JD: Kinetics of the formed elements of human blood. *Blood* 50:699, 1977.
652. Nagai Y, Garrett KP, Ohta S, et al: Toll-like receptors on hematopoietic progenitor cells stimulate innate immune system replenishment. *Immunity* 24:801, 2006.
653. McGettrick AF, O'Neill LA: Toll-like receptors: Key activators of leucocytes and regulator of haematopoiesis. *Br J Haematol* 139:185, 2007.
654. Sioud M, Fløisand Y, Forfang L, Lund-Johansen F: Signaling through toll-like receptor 7/8 induces the differentiation of human bone marrow CD34+ progenitor cells along the myeloid lineage. *J Mol Biol* 364:945, 2006.
655. Hirai H, Zhang P, Dayaram T, et al: C/EBPbeta is required for "emergency" granulopoiesis. *Nat Immunol* 7:732, 2006.
656. Testa U: Apoptotic mechanisms in the control of erythropoiesis. *Leukemia* 18:1176, 2004.
657. Lichtman MA, Chamberlain JK, Santillo PA: Factors thought to contribute to the regulation of egress of cells from marrow, in *The Year in Hematology 1978,* edited by R Silber, J LoBue, A Gordon, p 243. Plenum Press, New York, 1978.
658. Van Eeden SF, Miyagashima R, Haley L, Hogg JC: A possible role for L-selectin in the release of polymorphonuclear leukocytes from bone marrow. *Am J Physiol* 272:H1717, 1997.
659. Le Marer N, Skacel PO: Up-regulation of alpha2,6 sialylation during myeloid maturation: A potential role in myeloid cell release from the bone marrow. *J Cell Physiol* 179:315, 1999.
660. Jagels MA, Chambers JD, Arfors KE, Hugli TE: C5a- and tumor necrosis factor-alpha-induced leukocytosis occurs independently of beta 2 integrins and L-selectin: Differential effects on neutrophil adhesion molecule expression *in vivo*. *Blood* 85:2900, 1995.
661. Stroncek DF, Kaszcz W, Herr GP, et al: Expression of neutrophil antigens after 10 days of granulocyte-colony-stimulating factor. *Transfusion* 38:663, 1998.
662. Jung U, Ley K: Mice lacking two or all three selectins demonstrate overlapping and distinct functions for each selectin. *J Immunol* 162:6755, 1999.
663. Yong KL: Granulocyte colony-stimulating factor (G-CSF) increases neutrophil migration across vascular endothelium independent of an effect on adhesion: Comparison with granulocyte-macrophage colony-stimulating factor (GM-CSF). *Br J Haematol* 94:40, 1996.
664. Ulich TR, Del Castillo J, Souza L: Kinetics and mechanisms of recombinant human granulocyte-colony stimulating factor-induced neutrophilia. *Am J Pathol* 133:630, 1988.
665. DiPersio JF, Abboud CN: Activation of neutrophils by granulocyte-macrophage colony-stimulating factor, in *Granulocyte Responses to Cytokines: Basic and Clinical Research, Immunology Series*, vol 57, edited by RG Coffey, p 457. Marcel Dekker, New York, 1992.
666. Ghebrehiwet B, Muller-Eberhard HJ: C3e: An acidic fragment of human C3 with leukocytosis-inducing activity. *J Immunol* 123:616, 1979.
667. Kubo H, Graham L, Doyle NA, et al: Complement fragment-induced release of neutrophils from bone marrow and sequestration within pulmonary capillaries in rabbits. *Blood* 92:283, 1998.
668. Deinard AS, Page AR: A study of steroid-induced granulocytosis. *Br J Haematol* 28:333, 1974.
669. Vogel MJ, Yankee RA, Kimball HR, et al: The effect of etiocholanolone on granulocyte kinetics. *Blood* 30:474, 1967.
670. Cybulsky MI, McCoumb DJ, Movat HZ: Neutrophil leukocyte emigration induced by endotoxin: Mediator roles of interleukin-1 and tumor necrosis factor alpha. *J Immunol* 140:3144, 1988.
671. Terashima T, English D, Hogg JC, Van Eeden SF: Release of polymorphonuclear leukocytes from the bone marrow by interleukin-8. *Blood* 92:1062, 1998.
672. Burdon PC, Martin C, Rankin SM: The CXC chemokine MIP-2 stimulates neutrophil mobilization from the rat bone marrow in a CD49d-dependent manner. *Blood* 105:2543, 2005.
673. Burdon PC, Martin C, Rankin SM: Migration across the sinusoidal endothelium regulates neutrophil mobilization in response to ELR + CXC chemokines. *Br J Haematol* 142:100, 2008.
674. Wengner AM, Pitchford SC, Furze RC, Rankin SM: The coordinated action of G-CSF and ELR + CXC chemokines in neutrophil mobilization during acute inflammation. *Blood* 111:42, 2008.
675. Suratt BT, Petty JM, Young SK, et al: Role of the CXCR4/SDF-1 chemokine axis in circulating neutrophil homeostasis. *Blood* 104:565, 2004..
676. Palframan RT, Collins PD, Williams TJ, Rankin SM: Eotaxin induces a rapid release of eosinophils and their progenitors from the bone marrow. *Blood* 91:2240, 1998.
677. Palframan RT, Collins PD, Severs NJ, et al: Mechanisms of acute eosinophil mobilization from the bone marrow stimulated by interleukin 5: The role of specific adhesion molecules and phosphatidylinositol 3-kinase. *J Exp Med* 188:1621, 1998.
678. Schratl P, Royer JF, Kostenis E, et al: The role of the prostaglandin D2 receptor, DP, in eosinophil trafficking. *J Immunol* 179:4792, 2007.
679. Chamberlain JK, Weiss L, Weed RI: Bone marrow sinus cell packing: A determinant of cell release. *Blood* 46:91, 1975.
680. Waugh RE, Sassi M: An *in vitro* model of erythroid egress in bone marrow. *Blood* 68:250, 1986.
681. Dabrowski A, Szygula Z, Miszta H: Do changes in bone marrow pressure contribute to the egress of cells from the bone marrow? *Acta Physiol Pol* 32:729, 1981.
682. Chasis JA, Prenant M, Leung A, Mohandas N: Membrane assembly and remodeling during reticulocyte maturation. *Blood* 74:1112, 1989.
683. Radley JM, Haller CJ: Fate of senescent megakaryocytes in bone marrow. *Br J Haematol* 53:277, 1983.
684. Efrati P, Rozenszajn L: The morphology of buffy coats in normal human adults. *Blood* 16:1012, 1960.
685. Mantovani A, Vecchi A, Sozzani S, et al: Tumors as a paradigm for the *in vivo* role of chemokines in leukocyte recruitment, in *Chemokines and Cancer, Contemporary Cancer Research*, edited by BJ Rollins, p 35. Humana Press, Totowa, NJ, 1999.
686. Papayannopoulou T: Current mechanistic scenarios in hematopoietic stem/progenitor cell mobilization. *Blood* 103:1580, 2004.
687. Nervi B, Link DC, DiPersio JF: Cytokines and hematopoietic stem cell mobilization. *J Cell Biochem* 99:690, 2006.
688. Pelus LM: Peripheral blood stem cell mobilization: New regimens, new cells, where do we stand. *Curr Opin Hematol* 15:285, 2008.
689. Petit I, Szyper-Kravitz M, Nagler A, et al: G-CSF induces stem cell mobilization by decreasing bone marrow SDF-1 and up-regulating CXCR4. *Nat Immunol* 3:687, 2002.
690. Levesque J-P, Liu F, Simmons PJ, et al: Characterization of hematopoietic progenitor mobilization in protease-deficient mice. *Blood* 104:65, 2004.
691. Semerad CL, Christopher MJ, Liu F, et al: G-CSF potently inhibits osteoblast activity and CXCL12 mRNA expression in the bone marrow. *Blood* 106:3020, 2005.
692. Papayannopoulou T, Priestley GV, Nakamoto B, et al: Synergistic mobilization of hemopoietic progenitor cells using concurrent beta1 and beta2 integrin blockade or beta2-deficient mice. *Blood* 97:1282, 2001.
693. Velders GA, Pruijt JF, Verzaal P, et al: Enhancement of G-CSF-induced stem cell mobilization by antibodies against the beta 2 integrins LFA-1 and Mac-1. *Blood* 100:327, 2002.
694. Pruijt JFM, Verzaal P, Van Ros R, et al: Neutrophils are indispensable for hematopoietic stem cell mobilization by interleukin-8 in mice. *Proc Natl Acad Sci U S A* 99:6228, 2002.

CHAPTER 5
THE ORGANIZATION AND STRUCTURE OF LYMPHOID TISSUES

Thomas J. Kipps

SUMMARY

The lymphoid tissues can be divided into primary and secondary lymphoid organs. Primary lymphoid tissues are sites where lymphocytes develop from progenitor cells into functional and mature lymphocytes. The major primary lymphoid tissue is the marrow, the site where all lymphocyte progenitor cells reside and initially differentiate. This organ is discussed in Chap. 4. The other primary lymphoid tissue is the thymus, the site where progenitor cells from the marrow differentiate into mature thymus-derived (T) cells. Secondary lymphoid tissues are sites where lymphocytes interact with each other and nonlymphoid cells to generate immune responses to antigens. These include the spleen, lymph nodes, and mucosa-associated lymphoid tissues (MALT). The structure of these tissues provides insight into how the immune system discriminates between self-antigens and foreign antigens and develops the capacity to orchestrate a variety of specific and nonspecific defenses against invading pathogens.

THE THYMUS

The thymus is the site for development of thymic-derived lymphocytes, or T cells. In this organ, developing T cells, called thymocytes, differentiate from lymphoid stem cells derived from the marrow into functional, mature T cells.[1] It is here that T cells acquire their repertoire of specific antigen receptors to cope with the antigenic challenges received throughout one's life span. Once they have completed their maturation, the T cells leave the thymus and circulate in the blood and through secondary lymphoid tissues.

THYMIC ANATOMY

The thymus is located in the superior mediastinum, overlying, in order, the left brachiocephalic (or innominate) vein, the innominate artery, the left common carotid artery, and the trachea. It overlaps the upper limit of the pericardial sac below and extends into the neck beneath the upper anterior ribs. It receives its blood supply from the internal thoracic arteries. Venous blood from the thymus drains into the brachiocephalic and internal thoracic veins, which communicate above with the inferior thyroid veins.

Acronyms and abbreviations that appear in this chapter include: *AIRE*, autoimmune regulatory gene; APECED, autoimmune polyendocrinopathy-candidiasis-ectodermal dystrophy; C, capsule; CT, computed tomography; GALT, gastrointestinal-associated lymphoid tissue; LN, lymphatic nodule; MALT, mucosa-associated lymphoid tissues; MHC, major histocompatibility complex; PALS, periarteriolar lymphoid sheath; PGA syndrome, polyglandular autoimmune syndrome; T, thymus-derived; TCR, T-cell receptor.

Arising from the third and fourth brachial pouches as an epithelial organ populated by lymphoid cells and endoderm-derived thymic epithelial cells, the thymus develops at about the eighth week of gestation.[2] The thymus increases in size through fetal and postnatal life and remains ample into puberty,[3] when it weighs approximately 40 g. Thereafter, the size progressively decreases with aging as a consequence of thymic involution (see Chap. 8, Fig. 8–1).[4]

The volume of the thymus can be estimated by sonography. In one study of 149 healthy term infants within 1 week of birth, there was a significant correlation between the estimated thymic volume and the weight of the infant.[5] However, no correlation was apparent between the estimated thymic volume and the infant's sex, length, or gestational age. Also, there was no apparent correlation between estimated volume and the proportions of CD4+ T cells or CD8+ T cells found in the blood. The estimated thymic volume of healthy infants increases from birth to 4 and 8 months of age and then decreases.[3] Most of the individual variation at 4 and 10 months of age appears to correlate with breast-feeding status, body size, and, to a lesser extent, illness. Breast-fed infants at 4 months of age have significantly larger estimated thymic volumes than do age-matched formula-fed infants with similar thymic volumes at birth.[6]

THYMIC STRUCTURE

A longitudinal fissure divides the thymus into two asymmetrical lobes, a larger right and a smaller left, that are derived from the right and left brachial pouches, respectively. These two developmentally separate parts of the thymus are easily separated from each other by blunt dissection.

Each lobe of the thymus is divided into multiple lobules by fibrous septa (Fig. 5–1). Each lobule consists of an outer cortex and an inner medulla. The cortex contains dense collections of thymocytes that appear as lymphocytes of slightly variable size with scattered, rare mitoses. The lighter-staining medulla is more sparsely populated with cells. It contains loosely arranged mature thymocytes and characteristic tightly packed whorls of squamous-appearing epithelial cells, called *thymic* or *Hassall corpuscles* (Fig. 5–2). These appear to be remnants of degenerating cells and are rich in high-molecular-weight cytokeratins.

The thymus contains several other important cell types in addition to thymocytes. There are several types of specialized epithelial cells within the thymus.[7] The three main categories of thymic epithelial cells are the medullary epithelial cells, which are organized into clusters, the cortical epithelial cells, which form an epithelial network, and the epithelial cells of the outer cortex. The epithelial cells in the cortex and medulla often have a stellate shape, display desmosomal connections to one another, and may function as nurse cells to developing thymocytes. In addition, the thymus contains marrow-derived antigen-presenting cells, primarily interdigitating dendritic cells and macrophages, particularly at the corticomedullary junction.

After puberty, thymic involution begins within the cortex. This region may disappear completely with aging, while medullary remnants persist throughout life. Glucocorticoids also may induce atrophy of the cortex secondary to glucocorticoid-induced apoptosis of cortical thymocytes.[8] This also may be seen in conditions that are associated with increases in circulating glucocorticoid hormones, for example, pregnancy or stress.[9,10]

THYMIC IMMUNE FUNCTION

The thymus is the site of T-cell development. The importance of the thymus is underscored by patients with DiGeorge syndrome, or chromosome 22q11.2 deletion syndrome, who lack the genes required for

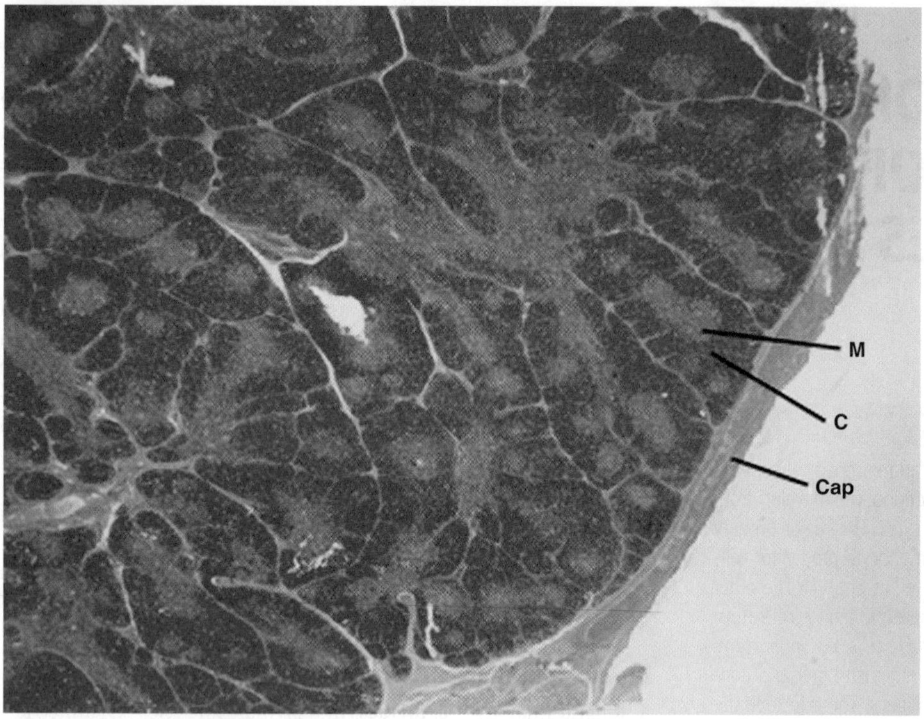

FIGURE 5–1. Normal human infant thymus. The thymus is surrounded by dense connective tissue capsule (*Cap*). It is organized into adjacent lobules separated by capsular connective tissue extensions or trabeculae. The lobules each have a dense cortex (*C*) and a lighter staining medulla (*M*). The medulla is a continuous tissue surrounded by the cortex that extends throughout the thymus, which cannot be appreciated in a single section. *(Reproduced from* Lichtman's Atlas of Hematology, *www.accessmedicine.com, with permission.)*

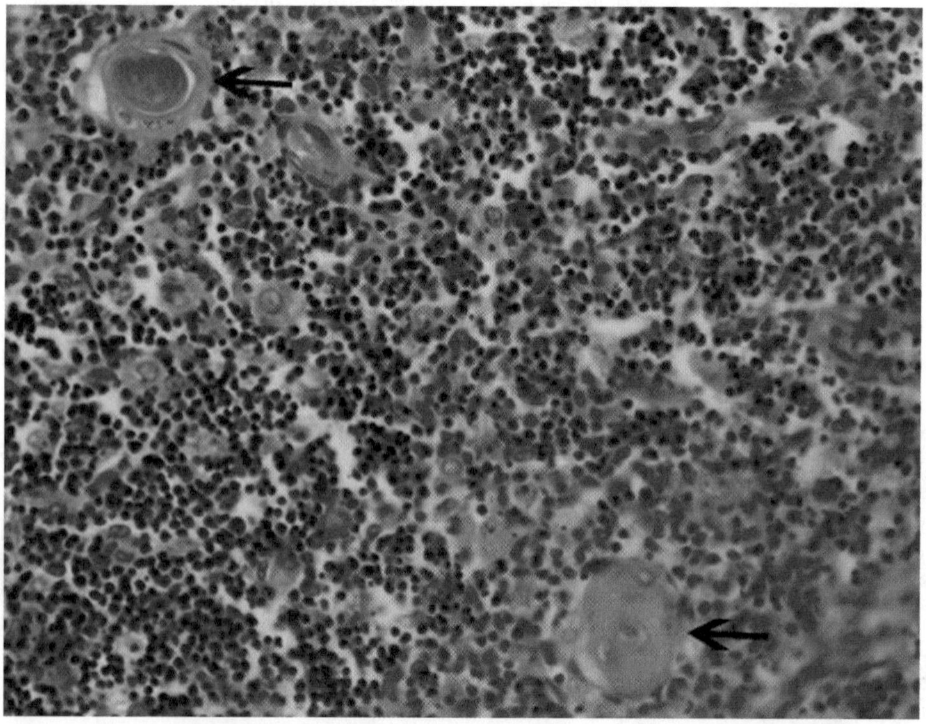

FIGURE 5–2. Normal human infant thymus. Higher magnification. Medulla. The *arrows* indicate thymic corpuscles (synonymous with Hassall corpuscles). They are composed of tightly packed, concentrically arranged, type IV endothelioreticular cells with flattened nuclei. The central mass is composed of keratinized cells. In addition to thymic corpuscles and the mass of small densely stained T lymphocytes, the medulla contains scattered, larger, type V epithelioreticular cells with their light nuclei, dark nucleolus, and eosinophilic cytoplasm, evident on this section. *(Reproduced from* Lichtman's Atlas of Hematology, *www.accessmedicine.com, with permission.)*

thymic development.[11] These patients do not develop T cells and hence have profound immune deficiency.

Prothymocytes originate in the marrow and migrate to the thymus, where they mature into T cells (see Chaps. 76 and 78). Maturation of T cells is accompanied by the sequential acquisition by thymocytes of the various T-cell markers (Fig. 5–3).[12] Terminal deoxynucleotidyl transferase is found in prothymocytes and immature thymocytes but is absent in mature T cells.

Pre-T cells enter the cortex via small blood vessels and are double negative for CD4 and CD8 antigens.[1] One of the earliest identifiable T-cell membrane antigens is CD2. As the thymocytes proliferate and differentiate in the cortex, they acquire CD4 and CD8 antigens. They subsequently acquire the CD3 antigen and the T-cell receptor for antigen as they migrate toward the medulla.

Positive and negative selection of maturing T cells takes place in the thymus.[13] Double-positive (CD4+ and CD8+) thymocytes undergo an initial positive selection step that is mediated exclusively by thymic cortical epithelium.[14] Thymocytes that have T-cell receptors (TCRs) capable of interacting with the major histocompatibility complex (MHC) molecules expressed by thymic cortical epithelial cells undergo expansion, whereas thymocytes with defective TCR undergo apoptosis.[15–17] In the cortex, the thymocytes are induced to expressed the chemokine receptor CCR7, which directs their migration to CCL19– and CCL21–producing cells in the thymic medulla.[18] As these positively selected cells migrate toward the medulla, they experience negative selection through their interaction with thymic medullary epithelial cells, which express the autoimmune regulatory gene (*AIRE*). *AIRE* encodes a transcriptional regulator that promotes ectopic expression of a large repertoire of transcripts encoding proteins that ordinarily are restricted to differentiated organs residing in the periphery.[19] This allows the thymic medullary epithelial cells to express many different self-antigens, which are presented to developing thymocytes. Those thymocytes that have TCR that react too vigorously with the MHC molecules of the medullary epithelium will undergo apoptosis.[16] Most of the developing thymocytes are destroyed. In this way, only those T cells that have the appropriate level of low affinity for self-MHC molecules will reach the final maturation stages and be allowed to exit the thymus.

Patients with the rare disease *autoimmune polyendocrinopathy-candidiasis-ectodermal*

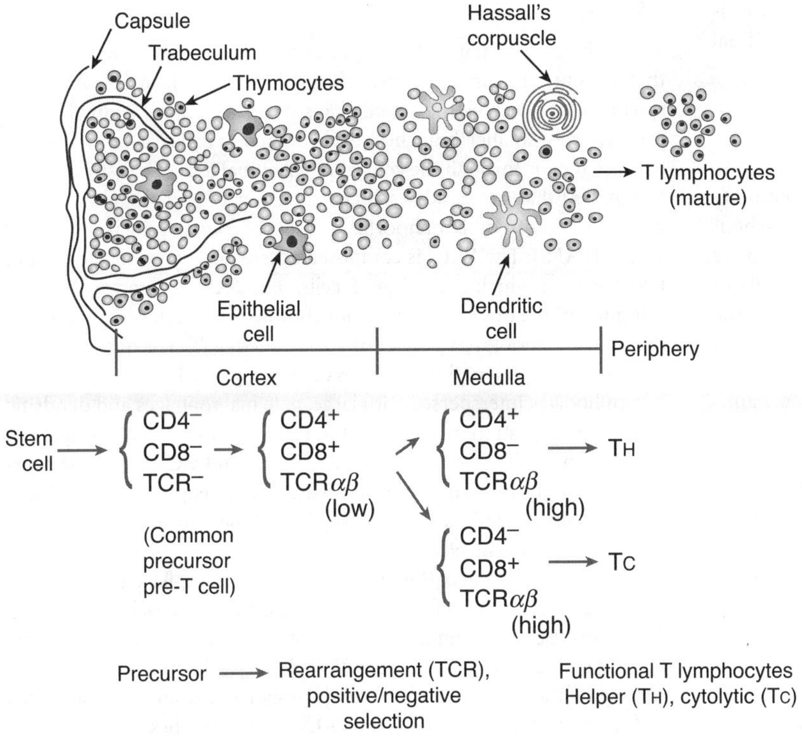

FIGURE 5–3. Structure of the thymus. The top half of the figure provides a cross section of a thymic lobule, indicating the outer cortex (*left*), inner medulla (*center*), and periphery (*far right*). The *arrows* indicate various structures and cell types. As thymocytes mature, they migrate from the cortex toward the medullary region and acquire phenotypic features that are outlined at the bottom of the figure, as described in the text (see Chap. 76).

dystrophy (APECED) or *polyglandular autoimmune* (PGA) syndrome type I (PGA I) underscore the importance of negative selection of thymocytes by thymic medullary epithelial cells. APECED, or PGA I, is characterized by chronic mucocutaneous candidiasis, hypoparathyroidism, and adrenal insufficiency, but most patients also have a number of other autoimmune manifestations, including thyroiditis, type 1 diabetes, ovarian failure, alopecia, and/or hepatitis.[20] These patients have genetic defects in *AIRE*,[21] which precludes their thymic epithelial cells from expressing the large variety of tissue differentiation self-antigens required for the negative selection of self-reactive thymocytes and the generation of central T-cell tolerance.[19,22]

The selected thymocytes enter the thymic medulla, where they further mature and differentiate to become positive for either CD4 or CD8 and acquire the capacity for future helper or cytolytic functions, respectively.[1] Here they also may interact with scattered B cells during their final stages of thymic education (see Chaps. 19, 76, and 78). A small percentage of the lymphocytes produced in the thymus finally exit the medulla via efferent lymphatics as mature, naïve T cells.

THE SPLEEN

The spleen is a secondary lymphoid organ. Secondary lymphoid tissues provide an environment in which the cells of the immune system can interact with antigen and with one another to develop an immune response to antigen. The spleen is a major site of immune response to bloodborne antigens. In addition, the splenic red pulp contains macrophages that are responsible for clearing the blood of unwanted foreign substances and senescent erythrocytes, even in the absence of specific immunity. Thus, it acts as a filter for the blood.

■ SPLENIC ANATOMY

The spleen is located within the peritoneum in the left upper quadrant of the abdomen between the fundus of the stomach and the diaphragm. It receives its blood supply from the systemic circulation via the splenic artery, which branches off the celiac trunk, and the left gastroepiploic artery.[23] The blood returning from the spleen drains into the portal circulation via the splenic vein. Therefore, the spleen can become congested with blood and increase in size when there is portal vein hypertension (see Chap. 55).

Approximately 10 percent of individuals have one or more accessory spleens. Accessory spleens are usually 1 cm in diameter and resemble lymph nodes. However, they usually are covered with peritoneum, as is the spleen itself. Accessory spleens typically lie along the course of the splenic artery or its gastroepiploic branch, but they may be elsewhere.[24] The commonest location is near the hilus of the spleen, but approximately 1 in 6 accessory spleens can be found embedded in the tail of the pancreas, where they may be occasionally mistaken for a pancreatic mass lesion.[25]

The average weight of the spleen in the adult human is 135 g (range: 100–250 g). However, when emptied of blood it weighs only approximately 80 g. On autopsy of 539 subjects with normal spleens, there was a positive correlation between the spleen weight and both the degree of acute splenic congestion and the subject's height and weight, but not with the subject's sex or age.[26]

The splenic volume can be estimated by computed tomography (CT) of the abdomen.[27] In one study, the splenic volume was calculated from the linear and the maximal cross-sectional area measurements of the spleen, using the following formula: splenic volume = 30 cm^3 + 0.58 (the product of the width, length, and thickness of the spleen measured in centimeters).[28] Using this formula, the mean value of the calculated splenic volume for 47 normal subjects was 214.6 cm^3, with a range of 107.2 to 314.5 cm^3. The calculated splenic volume did not appear to vary significantly with the subject's age, gender, height, weight, body mass index, or the diameter of the first lumbar vertebra, the latter being considered representative of body habitus on CT.

The splenic volume also can be estimated by sonography, which provides good correlation with volumes measured by helical abdominal CT or actual volume displaced by the excised organ (see Fig. 1–1). In one study of 50 patients, the linear measurement by sonography that correlated most closely with CT volume was the spleen width measured on a longitudinal section with the patient in the right lateral decubitus position (correlation coefficient [r] = 0.89, $p < 0.001$). There was also good correlation between splenic length measured in the right lateral decubitus position and CT volume ($r = 0.86$, $p < 0.001$). In another study of 32 normal spleens from adult corpses, the ultrasonogram measurements of maximal height, width, and breadth of the spleen were compared with the actual volume displaced by the excised organ.[29] The mean actual splenic volume was approximately 148 cm^3 (±81 cm^3 SD), whereas mean splenic volume estimated from ultrasonography was 284 cm^3 (±168 cm^3 SD). Despite the differences between the actual and estimated volumes, these investigators did find a roughly linear correlation between actual splenic volume and the estimated splenic volume measured by ultrasound (see Fig. 1–2). However, there may be operator-to-operator variation in measurement of the estimated splenic volume, making the use of sonography in longitudinal studies technically demanding.

SPLENIC STRUCTURE

The spleen has an open circulation, which lacks endothelial continuity from artery to vein. When isolated spleens are perfused in washout studies, erythrocytes that appear in the splenic vein appear to be flushed out from three compartments. The red cells that are flushed out first come from a compartment that presumably is formed by the splenic vessels. The erythrocytes that are flushed out next come from a second compartment, where they presumably are loosely held within the filtration beds. The erythrocytes that are flushed out last presumably were adherent to cells of the filtration beds. Although 90 percent of the blood flow passes through the splenic vessels, only approximately 10 percent of the total splenic red cells are found within this first compartment. The second compartment is perfused by 9 percent of the total inflow yet contains 70 percent of the splenic red cells. The last compartment is perfused by only 1 percent of the inflow but contains 20 percent of the splenic red cells.

These compartments reflect the anatomy of the spleen and its stroma. The stroma is composed of branched, fibroblast-like cells called reticular cells. These cells produce slender collagen fibers, the reticular fibers, which are rich in type III collagen. The reticular cells and fibers form a meshwork, or reticulum, which filters the blood. Three major types of filtration beds can be distinguished by their structure and content: the white pulp, the marginal zone, and the red pulp.

White Pulp

The white pulp contains the lymphocytes and other mononuclear cells that surround the arterioles branching off the splenic artery. After the splenic artery pierces the splenic capsule at the hilum, it divides into progressively smaller branches. Each branch is called a central artery because it runs through the central longitudinal axis of a distinctive filtration bed that surrounds each central artery (Fig. 5–4). This is composed of a cuff of lymphocytes called the periarteriolar lymphoid sheath (PALS). The PALS is composed mostly of T lymphocytes, about two-thirds of which are CD4+ T cells. The PALS around white pulp arterioles of the human spleen is not continuous.[30] Indeed, segments of the central arterioles might not be surrounded by T cells in areas where they run through lymphoid follicles containing pale kernels of activated B lymphocytes interspersed with large, pale macrophages and dendritic cells.[1] The migration of T cells to the PALS is governed by stromal cell production of chemokines, primarily CCL19 and CCL21, which interact with the chemokine receptor CCR7 that is expressed by naïve T cells.[31] Stromal production of these chemokines can be stimulated by certain cytokines, such as lymphotoxin.[32]

On gross inspection of the surface of a freshly cut spleen, these follicles appear as white dots referred to as malpighian corpuscles (Fig. 5–5). These corpuscles contain a germinal center and have the same anatomic features and functions as secondary follicles in the lymph node. Branches coming off the central artery deliver disproportionate amounts of plasma and lymphocytes to the rim of the PALS (Fig. 5–6). These branches tend to run at acute angles, leading to a selective loss of plasma from the blood, a phenomenon referred to as skimming. After becoming relatively depleted of plasma, the arterioles then carry high-hematocrit blood into the filtration beds of the red pulp and marginal zone. As a result, the red pulp and marginal zone beds contain relatively high concentrations of red cells.

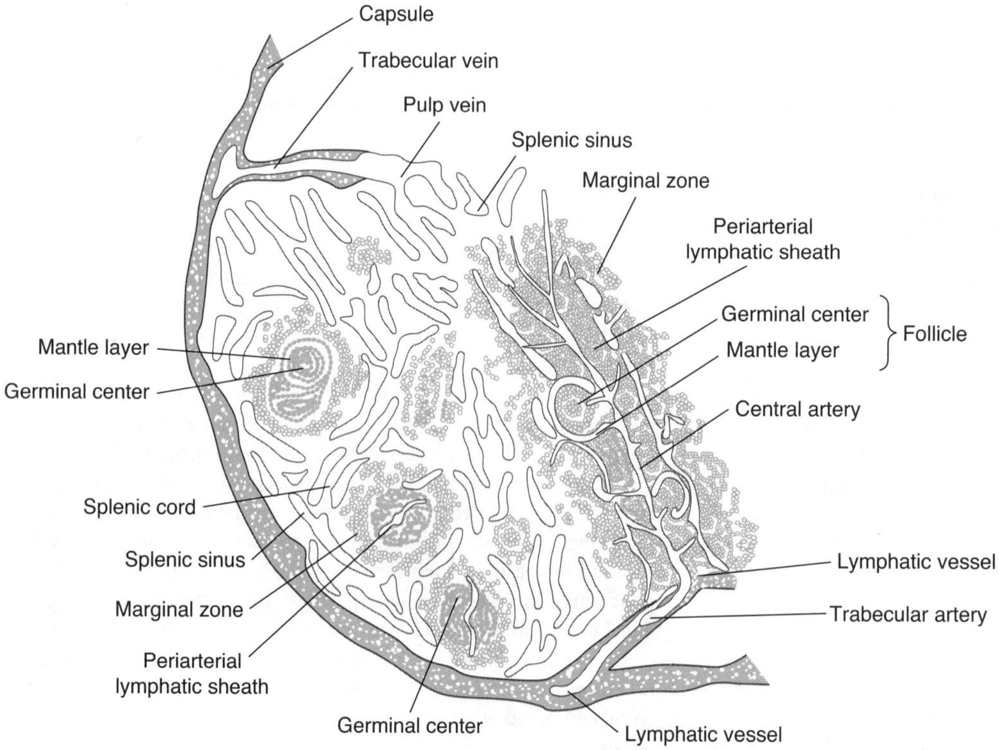

FIGURE 5–4. Structure of the spleen. A branch of the splenic artery enters the pulp and becomes a central artery. Surrounding the central artery is a periarterial lymphoid sheath (PALS). At the circumference of the PALS is the marginal zone, which generally separates the white pulp of the PALS from the red pulp. Follicles of B cells with occasional germinal centers (malpighian corpuscles) are located at the outer margins of the PALS for the depicted central artery and the PALS of central arteries that are in a different plane from that of the figure.

The Marginal Zone

The marginal zone surrounds the PALS and follicles. It is composed of a reticulum, which forms a finely meshed filtration bed, serving as a vestibule for much of the blood that flows through the spleen. The marginal zone surrounds the white pulp and merges insensibly into the red pulp. It contains more lymphocytes than the red pulp. These are primarily memory B cells and CD4+ T cells that appear especially well equipped for rapid antibody immune responses to bloodborne antigens.[33–35] However, like the red pulp, the marginal zone may become congested and remove damaged and senescent red cells and parasites.

The Red Pulp

The red pulp of the spleen is composed of a reticular meshwork, called the splenic cords of Billroth, and splenic sinuses.[36] This region predominantly contains erythrocytes but has large numbers of

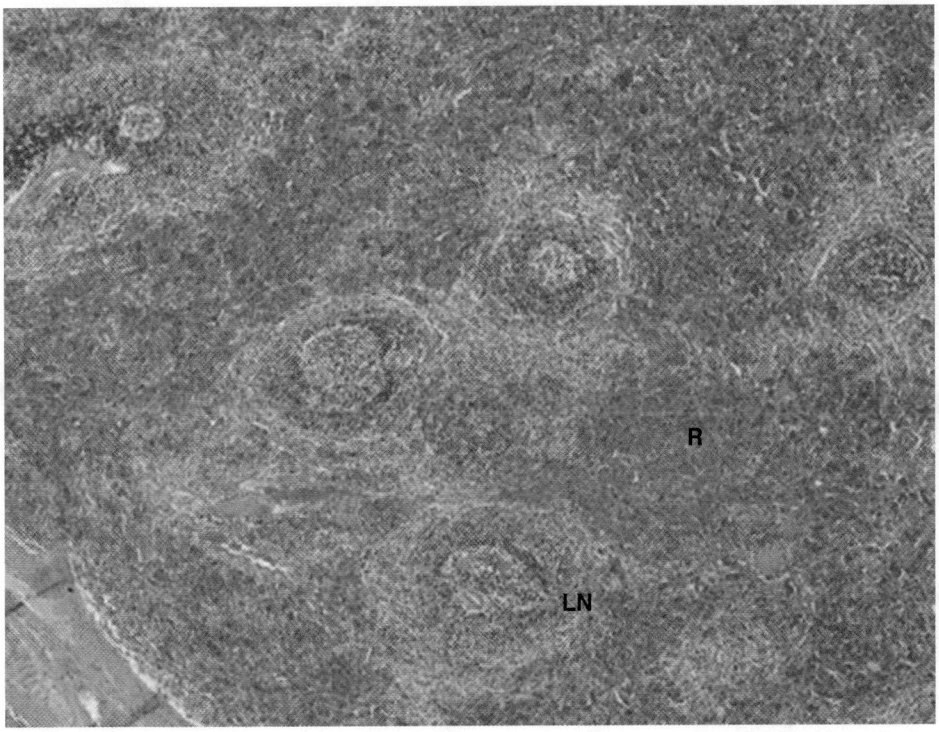

FIGURE 5–5. Normal human spleen. The splenic tissue is composed of red and white pulp. The red pulp (*R*), shown here as masses of red cells, is imparted a red color in living tissue as a result of the natural color of hemoglobin in red cells and in stained sections as a result of the intensified red (eosinophilic) stain taken up by hemoglobin. The red pulp contains venous sinuses separated by cords of red cells (cords of Billroth), which cannot be seen in a light micrograph. The white pulp is composed of spherical aggregates of lymphocytes (lymphatic nodule [*LN*]) with a lighter staining germinal center and an outer, relatively thin, darker stained marginal zone, which separates white pulp from red pulp. Thick-walled central arteries are usually evident penetrating the white pulp. The central artery is cut obliquely in the white pulp at the upper left. Two arteries are seen penetrating the nodule in the center-left of the field and a single artery penetrating the white pulp in the lower-center of the field. The central artery is often seen in the lymphatic nodule in an eccentric position. Other nodules do not show a vessel in this plane of section. *(Reproduced from* Lichtman's Atlas of Hematology, *www.accessmedicine.com, with permission.)*

macrophages and dendritic cells. There are relatively few lymphocytes and plasma cells in this area.

As the central arteries branch and decrease in size, the PALS also branches and decreases in diameter to but a few cells surrounding the arteriole. The small arteriole finally emerges from its sheath and then terminates in either the marginal zone or the red pulp. Here these vessels are suspended and anchored by adventitial reticular cells in the periarterial beds. They often terminate abruptly as arteriolar capillaries or as vessels with a trumpet-like flare with widened slits called interendothelial slits. The blood flows through these slits into filtration beds composed of large-meshed loculi that open to one another.

The blood in the red pulp and marginal zone drains into venous sinuses that form anastomosing, blind-ending vessels. These venous sinuses actually are specialized postcapillary venules. The endothelial cells are shaped as tapered rods that are stiffened by basal, longitudinal, intermediate cytoskeletal filaments and contractile filaments of actin and myosin. These intracellular contractile filaments can shorten the vein, causing the endothelium to buckle and form interendothelial gaps, favoring transmural passage.

The endothelial cells are attached to a basement membrane. Although this appears to be fashioned of fibers, the basement membrane actually is an extracellular membranous wall with large, regular defects that expose considerable basal endothelial surface. This includes the interendothelial slits through which blood may flow from the filtration bed and into the vein. Ordinarily the interendothelial slits are narrow or even closed unless forced apart by cells in transmural transit or by endothelial contraction.

Splenic arterioles terminate at varied distances from the walls of venous vessels. Blood flowing from arterioles that terminate at the venous vessel wall may flow directly into the splenic vein. However, blood flowing from arterioles that terminate at a distance from a vein must traffic through the spleen. In so doing, the blood either may pass quickly through a nonsinusal venous aperture or slowly through sinusoidal interendothelial slits and the fibroblast stroma.

The fibroblast stroma contains reticular cells and myofibroblast cells, which are also called barrier cells. The latter may fuse with each other to form a syncytial membrane that connects the arterial terminals with venous interendothelial slits or apertures. Like other myofibroblasts, these cells contain actin and myosin and may contract, thereby approximating splenic arterial and venous vessels with one another. Thus, the fibroblast stroma may affect the relative proportion of blood that flows through the stroma or the sinusal interendothelial slits. Such redistribution might occur during periods of acute physiologic stress, allow for increased expulsion of red cells from the spleen, and account for some of the increase in hematocrit observed during strenuous exercise.[37]

■ SPLENIC FUNCTION

Red Cell Clearance

Mixed within the stroma of the red pulp and marginal zone are monocytes and macrophages. As the blood passes through the stroma, monocytes may be held on the stroma, where the microenvironment is conducive to their maturation into macrophages and large, dendritic, lysosome-rich phagocytes. These cells may assist the reticular cells in mechanical filtration. More important, these cells have phagocytic activity that allows them to ingest imperfect erythrocytes, store platelets, and remove infectious agents, such as plasmodia, from the circulation.[38] In addition, these cells have nonphagocytic functions, such as the presentation of antigens to T cells or the elaboration of certain cytokines.

Collectively, the anatomy of the spleen allows the marginal zone and red pulp to cull defective erythrocytes. As the blood passes slowly through the sinusal interendothelial slits and the fibroblast stroma, the erythrocytes must undergo alterations in shape to squeeze through the mechanical barrier generated by this filtration compartment. Normal red cells that are supple may pass through readily because the interendothelial slits can open to about 0.5 μm. However, blood cells containing large, rigid inclusions, such as plasmodium-containing erythrocytes, are delayed or sequestered.[39]

Splenic macrophages residing within these filtration beds also can sequester erythrocytes that are coated with antibody. Polymorphisms of Fcγ-RII (CD32) or Fcγ-RIII (CD16) that affect immunoglobulin (Ig) G binding *in vitro* can alter the efficiency of clearance of antibody-coated red cells *in vivo*.[40]

When these filtration beds sequester imperfect red cells, the blood pools inside the spleen, causing stasis and congestion. This stimulates

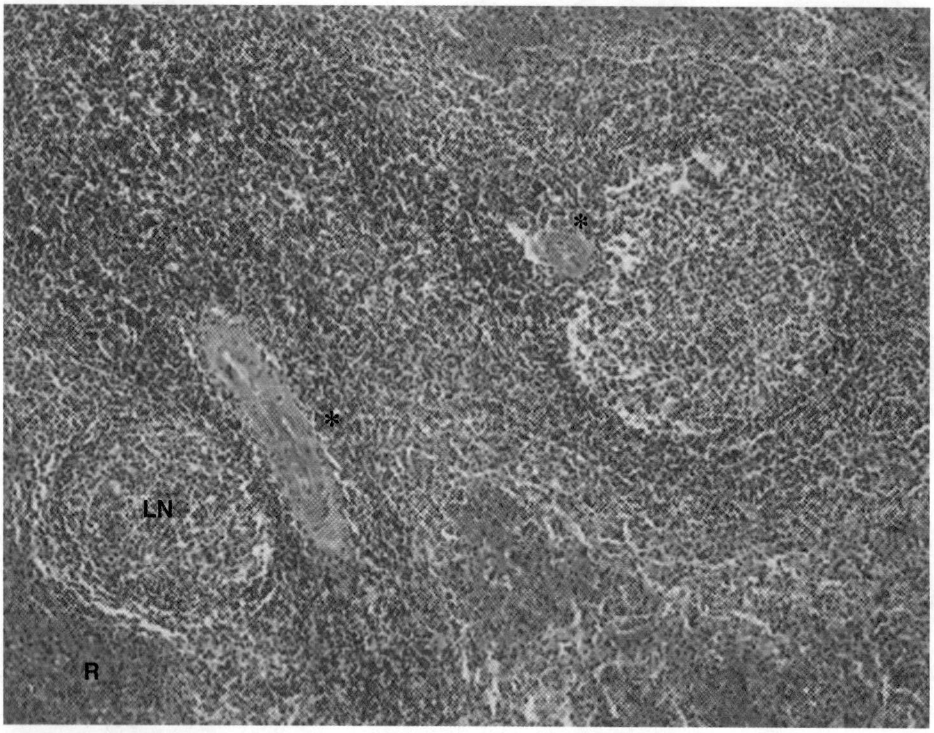

FIGURE 5–6. Normal human spleen (higher magnification of white pulp). The white pulp is composed of spherical aggregates of lymphocytes (lymphatic nodules [*LN*]) with a lighter staining germinal center and an outer, relatively thin, darker stained marginal zone, which separates white pulp from red pulp. The lymphatic nodules largely consist of B lymphocytes. Thick-walled central arteries are usually evident penetrating the white pulp, often in an eccentric position as shown here. The T-cell–rich PALS surrounds the central artery, which is cut longitudinally in the lymphatic nodule at the left. A single central artery penetrating the lymphatic nodule in the upper-right part of the field is in a characteristically eccentric position. *(Reproduced from* Lichtman's Atlas of Hematology, *www.accessmedicine.com, with permission.)*

sphincter-like contraction of the distal vein, resulting in proximal plasma transudation that produces a viscous luminal mass of high-hematocrit blood. During episodes of enhanced red cell sequestration, as occur during malarial crises or hemolytic episodes in a small proportion of patients with sickle cell disease, the splenic volume and weight may increase 10- to 20-fold (see Chap. 48).[41] Although the white pulp may enlarge, particularly in germinal centers, the marginal zones and red pulp become greatly widened with pooled erythrocytes and macrophages in this setting.

Regulation of Blood Volume

The spleen also can play a role in modulating blood volume. Release of high-hematocrit blood through splenic contraction occurs in response to activation of the baroreflex, which also may be activated during conditions of decreased blood pressure and cardiac output.[42,43] On the other hand, physiologic agents such as atrial natriuretic peptide, nitric oxide, and adrenomedullin can induce fluid extravasation from the splenic circulation into lymphatic reservoirs.[44] Excessive splenic extravasation can contribute to the inability to maintain adequate intravascular volume during septic shock. There also is evidence that the splenic afferent and renal sympathetic nerves play a role in maintaining renal microvascular tone.[44] This splenorenal reflex can influence blood pressure and, during septic shock, help promote renal sodium and water reabsorption and release of the vasoconstrictor angiotensin II. On the other hand, in portal hypertension, the splenorenal reflex can promote renal sodium and water retention and possibly play a role in the hemodynamic complications of portal hypertension through neurohormonal modulation of the mesenteric vascular bed.

Splenic Immune Function

The spleen and its responses to antigens are similar to those of lymph nodes, the major difference being that the spleen is the major site of immune responses to bloodborne antigens, while lymph nodes are involved in responses to antigens in the lymph.[36] Antigens and lymphocytes enter the spleen through the vascular sinuses, because the spleen lacks high endothelial venules. Upon entry, the lymphocytes home to the white pulp. T cells, which express the chemokine receptor CCR7,[45] migrate to the PALS in response to CCL19 and CCL21, and B cells, which express CXCR5, migrate to the lymphoid nodules in response to CXCL13.[31] Dendritic cells also express CCR7 and hence migrate to the same area as do naïve T cells. T and B cells migrate within these compartments for about 5 and 7 hours, respectively. In the absence of an immune response, these cells migrate through a reticulum arranged around the circumference of the central artery.

Upon immune activation in response to antigen, the lymphocytes may remain in the spleen to sustain a primary or secondary immune response. Activation of B cells is initiated in the marginal zones that are adjacent to CD4+ T cells in the PALS. Activated B cells then migrate into germinal centers or into the red pulp.[46] Lymphoid nodules appear and expand by recruiting lymphocytes from the blood and the peripheral zone of the follicles, termed the mantle zone. These cells then proliferate and differentiate in the center of a lymphoid nodule, forming a germinal center.[47] In their path from the marginal zone to the follicles, B cells pass into the PALS, where they remain in contact with T lymphocytes for a few hours, allowing ample time for T- and B-cell interaction in response to antigens. If they are not recruited in an immune response to antigen, both T and B lymphocytes exit the spleen via deep efferent lymphatics, not the splenic veins.

These efferent lymphatics are not distinguished as separate structures within the PALS, being quite thin-walled and often packed with efferent lymphocytes. However, they are important in moving nonreactive lymphocytes out of the spleen and in producing high-hematocrit pulp blood. After leaving the spleen, the efferent lymphocytes become the afferent lymphatics of the perisplenic mesenteric lymph nodes or empty into the thoracic duct. This duct empties into the left subclavian vein, thus returning the lymphocytes to the venous circulation.

LYMPH NODES

The lymphoid nodes are secondary lymphoid tissues. They form part of a network that filters antigens from the interstitial tissue fluid and lymph during its passage from the periphery to the thoracic duct. Thus, the lymph nodes are the primary sites of immune response to tissue antigens.

LYMPH NODE ANATOMY

The lymph nodes are round or kidney-shaped clusters of mononuclear cells that normally are less than 1 cm in diameter (Fig. 5–7). A collagenous capsule surrounds a typical lymph node and has an indentation called the hilus where blood vessels enter and leave.

Lymph nodes typically are present at the branches of the lymphatic vessels and form part of the extensive network of lymphatic channels that extends throughout the body. Several afferent lymphatic channels that drain lymph from regional tissues into the lymph node perforate the capsule of each lymph node. The lymph draining from the node leaves through one efferent lymphatic vessel at the hilus. The lymph from the node, in turn, empties into efferent lymphatic vessels that eventually drain into larger lymphatic channels leading eventually to the thoracic duct. The thoracic duct in turns drains into the left subclavian vein, thus returning lymph into the systemic circulation.

Clusters of lymph nodes are placed strategically in areas that drain various superficial and deep regions of the body, such as the neck, axillae, groin, mediastinum, and abdominal cavity. The lymph nodes that receive lymph that drains from the skin, termed somatic nodes, are superficial. The lymph nodes that receive their lymph from the mucosal surface of the respiratory, digestive, or genitourinary tract, termed visceral nodes, are usually deep within body cavities.

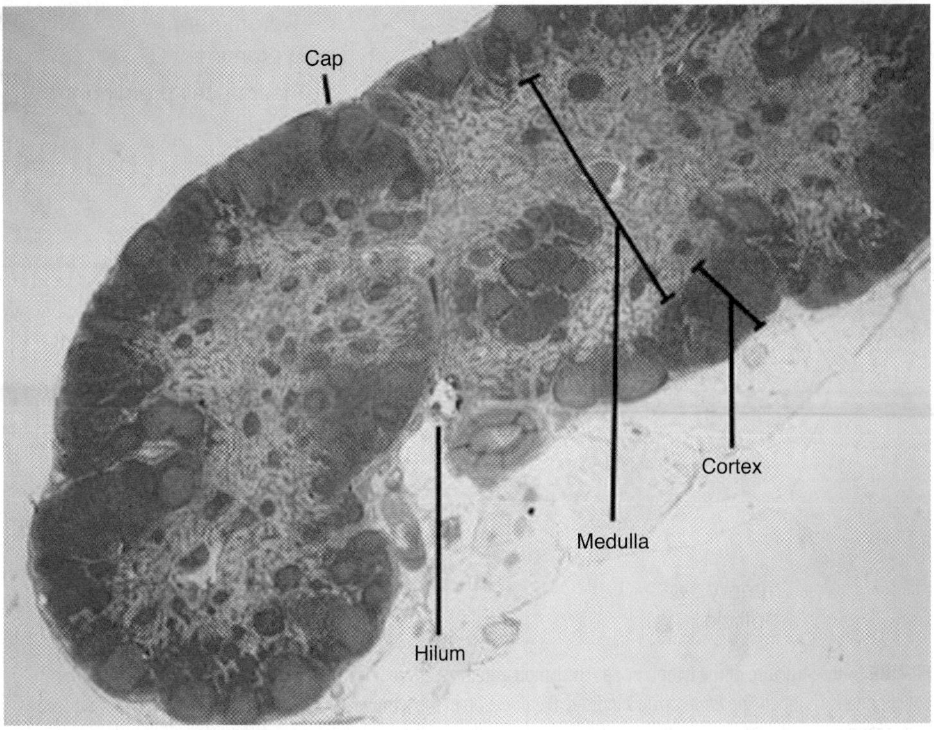

FIGURE 5–7. Normal human lymph node. Low power. Capsule (*Cap*) is a thin connective tissue covering. Below the capsule is the subcapsular sinus. Lymphatics penetrate the capsule and enter the subcapsular sinus. The cortex is composed of adjacent lymphatic nodules, usually with fine connective tissue trabecula extending from the capsule separating the nodules. The nodule has a germinal center that stains lighter than the outer mantle zone because of the proliferating medium-sized and large lymphocytes with less dense staining properties. The medulla is composed of interconnecting medullary cords composed of lymphocytes and interspersed light staining channels, the medullary sinuses. Lymph flows from the subcapsular sinus down the trabecular sinuses and into the medullary sinuses and exits the node via efferent lymphatics at the hilum. *(Reproduced from* Lichtman's Atlas of Hematology, *www.accessmedicine.com, with permission.)*

LYMPH NODE STRUCTURE

Beneath the collagenous capsule is the subcapsular sinus, into which the afferent lymphatic channels drain (Fig. 5–8). This sinus is lined with phagocytic cells. Fibrous trabeculae radiate from the medulla adjacent to the hilus of the node to the subcapsular sinus, thus breaking the node into several follicles, called cortical follicles. These trabeculae, together with the capsule and a network of reticulin fibers, support the various cellular components of the node and serve as the scaffolding for lymphatic spaces, namely, the subcapsular and cortical sinuses. These lymphatic spaces are continuous with medullary sinuses and the solitary efferent lymphatic channel exiting the hilus.

Each cortical follicle contains dense collections of small, mature, recirculating lymphocytes. These consist of a B-cell area (cortex), a T-cell area (paracortex), and a central medulla with cellular cords that contain T cells, B cells, plasma cells, and macrophages.[1] Some follicles contain lightly staining areas of 1- to 2-mm in diameter, called germinal centers. Germinal centers are the specialized sites for the generation of memory B cells and antibody affinity maturation via the process of immunoglobulin variable-region somatic hypermutation.[48] Follicles without germinal centers are called primary follicles, and those with germinal centers are called secondary follicles. Primary lymphoid follicles contain nodules that consist predominantly of small, mature, recirculating B lymphocytes.

Within 1 week after antigenic stimulation, secondary follicles develop a germinal center, which contains proliferating B cells and macrophages.[49,50] The small, nonreactive B cells are apparently forced to the periphery of the follicle, where they form a dense follicular mantle. The B cells within the germinal center, on the other hand, are highly activated, typically forming blasts that have abundant cytoplasm and round, cleaved, or convoluted shapes. Follicular dendritic cells also are found within the germinal centers. These cells can trap and retain antigens for months, possibly in the form of immune complexes.[51] The germinal centers of the secondary follicle may gradually regress after the antigenic stimulus is eliminated.

Surrounding the lymphoid follicles of the superficial cortex are sheets of lymphocytes that extend to the deep cortex, the paracortex, that blend into medullary cords of cells. The paracortical zones are formed mostly of T cells. The ratio of T cells to B cells in these zones is approximately 3:1. The medulla, however, contains scattered B cells, dendritic cells, macrophages, and, during an immune response, plasma cells. The superficial cortex and medulla of the lymph nodes are the thymic-independent areas, while the deep cortex is particularly enriched with T cells, forming an area that sometimes is referred to as the thymic-dependent area. The major T-cell population found within the lymph node consists of CD4+ T cells. The scattering of CD4+ T cells in the follicles, and in more prominent numbers in the interfollicular zones, reveals the proximity of CD4+ T and B cells important for T-B cooperation during proliferation and maturation of antigen-stimulated B cells.[52]

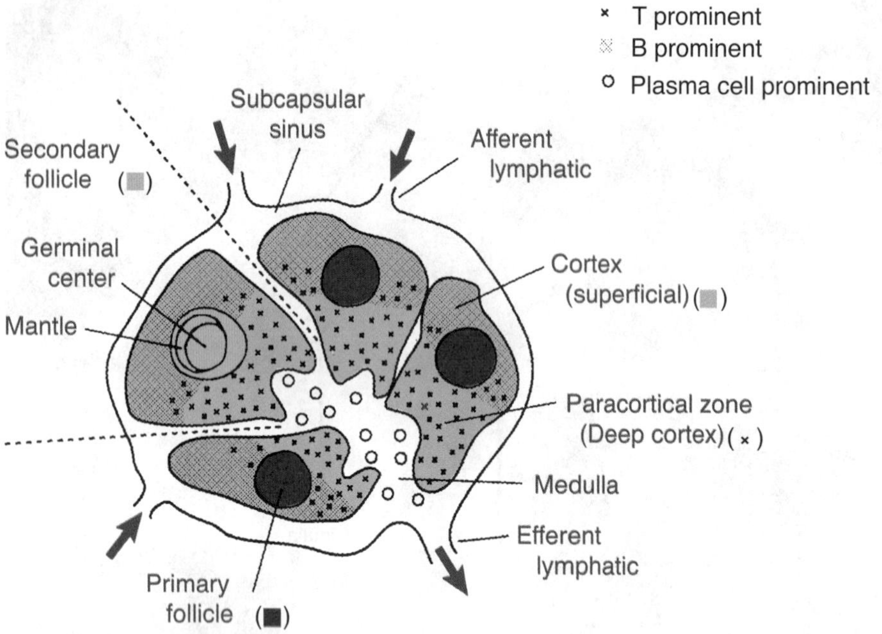

FIGURE 5–8. Structure of the lymph node. The lymph enters via afferent lymphatic channels and exits via the efferent lymphatic channel. The *large arrows* indicate the direction of the lymphatic flow into and out of the lymph node. The legend shows the symbols used for the T-cell zone (*x*) and the B-cell zone (*shade*) of each follicle. The follicle in the lower left part of the node contains a primary follicle lacking a germinal center. The follicle immediately above this follicle contains a germinal center. Thus, the entire follicle delineated by the dashed lines is a secondary follicle. The cortex, paracortical area, and medulla are also shown.

Lymphocytes primarily enter lymphatic tissues from the blood by migrating across the tall, active endothelium of specialized postcapillary venules called high endothelial venules.[53] Cellular adhesion molecules and various chemokines are responsible for the pattern of lymphocyte trafficking and determine the associations among stromal (e.g., reticular and endothelial) and parenchymal (e.g., T and B lymphocytes, dendritic cells, and macrophages) cells in the lymphoid tissues.[48,54]

■ LYMPH NODE FUNCTION

The lymph node is the site where different types of lymphocytes, macrophages, and dendritic cells can interact with one another to generate an immune response to antigens carried within the lymph. As the lymph passes across the nodes from afferent to efferent lymphatic vessels, particulate antigens are removed by the phagocytic cells and transported into the lymphoid tissue of the lymph node.[1] Abnormal cells within the lymph, such as neoplastic cells, also can be trapped within the lymph node.

Within the lymph node, antigen is presented to T cells as processed peptides by MHC molecules of antigen-presenting cells (see Chap. 78). Various T-cell subsets comprise a network of interactive cells. CD4+ and CD8+ cell-mediated contacts, as well as T-cell–derived soluble factors, induce and regulate the immune response (see Chap. 19). T-cell recognition is mediated by the TCR for antigen (see Chap. 78). Which T cells are activated is determined by the specificity of the TCRs, the structure of MHC molecules, and the nature of antigen-presenting cells, including the dendritic reticular cells, macrophages, and B cells.

However, along with TCR recognition of processed antigen presented in the MHC of the antigen-presenting cell, adequate T-cell activation requires second signals, or costimulation, delivered through accessory molecules, such as CD28 on T cells (see Chap. 78).[55] Without these second signals, the T cells may become anergic, or specifically nonresponsive to antigen stimulation.[56] This specific suppression is thought to play an important regulatory role in the maintenance of self-tolerance.[57,58]

T-cell recognition of specific antigen may induce release of soluble factors, such as the interleukins, that can activate T cells, B cells, and/or monocytes.[59] Also, the activated T cells express surface molecules, such as CD40-ligand (CD154), that also can activate B cells, dendritic cells, or macrophages.[60,61]

The T-dependent immune response includes the formation of early germinal centers within days after antigen exposure. There is a mixture of B cells and activated CD4+ T cells in the lymphoid follicles. T-B cooperation involves the accessory B-cell antigen CD40 and the CD154 antigen expressed on activated T cells (see Chap. 19). Activated B cells become blasts and comprise the largest numbers of cells in the early germinal center.[49] Subsequently, B-cell blasts give rise to smaller B cells, the centrocytes. B cells undergo affinity maturation within the germinal center. During this process, the genes encoding the surface immunoglobulin of B cells undergo high rates of mutation, called somatic hypermutation.[47,62] B cells that express immunoglobulin with little or no affinity for antigen undergo apoptosis.[63] The resulting cellular debris is tingible, or capable of being stained, and is found prominently within macrophages specifically designated tingible body macrophages. On the other hand, B cells expressing surface immunoglobulin with high affinity for antigen are selected to proliferate and differentiate to memory B cells or plasma cells.[48] As well as promoting activation of B cells, CD4+ T cells, and CD8+ T cells, the T-cell limb of the primary immune response may generate circulating CD4+ and CD8+ memory T cells.[64,65]

Following release of specific antibody, antigen–antibody complexes may form and become sequestered on the surface of follicular dendritic cells within the germinal centers. These antigen–antibody complexes produce a coating of small, bead-like, immune complex-coated bodies called *iccosomes*. Iccosomes may be presented to CD4+ T cells by B cells and dendritic cells. Iccosomes also appear to assist in anamnestic recall of high levels of antibody following reentry of antigen in the host.[66] T- and B-cell memory functions and self-tolerance depend upon persistence of antigen.[67]

PERIPHERAL LYMPHOID TISSUES

■ MUCOSA-ASSOCIATED LYMPHOID TISSUES

The mucosa-associated lymphoid tissues (MALT) are diffusely organized aggregates of lymphocytes that protect the respiratory and gastrointestinal epithelium.[68] The lymphoid aggregates associated with the respiratory epithelium are sometimes referred to as the bronchial-associated lymphoid tissue. The lymphoid aggregates associated with the intestinal epithelium are sometimes referred to as the gut-associated lymphoid tissue (GALT). Lymphocytes in the GALT are located in three main regions: within the epithelial layer, scattered through the lamina propria, and clustered in organized collections in the lamina propria. The latter includes the tonsils, adenoids, appendix, and specialized

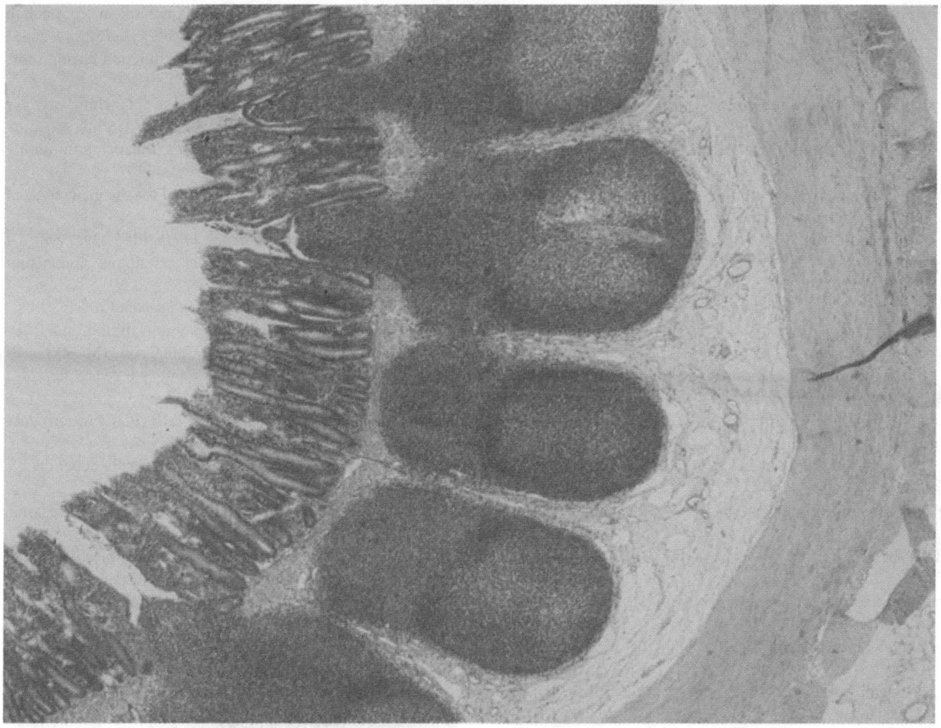

FIGURE 5–9. A cross section of human terminal ileum. The columnar epithelium is organized into villi. A series of lymphatic nodules in the mucosa extending from the lamina propria to the submucosa is part of the gastrointestinal-associated lymphoid tissue (GALT). In the ileum, this highly organized lymphatic tissue is referred to as Peyer patches. They each contain a germinal center. The GALT is a subset of the mucosa-associated lymphatic tissue. Scattered lymphatic nodules may also be seen in the mucosa of other parts of the small bowel and colon but they are usually isolated single nodules. *(Reproduced from* Lichtman's Atlas of Hematology, *www.accessmedicine.com, with permission.)*

structures called Peyer patches found in the ileum (Fig. 5–9). Most of intraepithelial lymphocytes are CD8+ T cells, 10 percent of which express the γ/δ form of the TCR (see Chap. 78). On the other hand, the intestinal lamina propria contains a mixed population of cells, including activated CD4-positive T cells. Similar to the lymphoid follicles of the spleen and lymph nodes, the mucosal follicles in the lamina propria contain mostly B cells, which sometimes are organized into germinal centers.

Solitary lymph nodules with follicular and germinal center structures occur in the mucosa and submucosa of the respiratory tract, the gastrointestinal tract (particularly within the ileum), the urinary tract, and the vagina. Microfolds overlying specialized epithelial cells in the gut transport antigenic material by pinocytosis, with potential subsequent activation of the immune response. During states of chronic inflammation, lymphoid nodules may form as a localized center of lymphocytes with marked follicular activity. The Waldeyer ring of pharyngeal lymphoid tissues and Peyer patches in the ileum contain prominent aggregated nodular lymphoid tissue. No capsule or efferent or afferent lymphatic vessels are present in these accessory lymphoid tissues.

The MALT are rich in plasma cells and eosinophils. The plasma cells are a source of secretory immunoglobulin that is transferred into the lumina of the bronchi and gastrointestinal tract. The majority of plasma cells in the mucosa of the bronchi and gut contain IgA.[69] IgA is released from the plasma cell and then combines with a secretory piece synthesized within the mucosal epithelium to become secretory IgA (see Chap. 77). Secretory IgA then is secreted across the microvilli of mucosal epithelium into the lumen, where it may prevent colonization of mucosal membranes by pathogens. Lymphoid nodules along mucosa-lined tracts serve as precursors of IgA-producing cells. These nodules form a barrier against many microorganisms and antigens.[70]

Peyer Patches

Peyer patches are the most important and highly organized of the gut-associated lymphoid tissues.[68] They are found in the lamina propria of the ileum (near the ileocolonic junction) and consist of up to 50 or more lymphoid nodules covered by a single layer of columnar epithelium (see Fig. 5–9). They are well developed in youth and regress with age. Antigens from the intestinal epithelium are collected by specialized epithelial cells called M cells, allowing for generation of specific immune responses against intestinal pathogens.[71] Peyer patches are the sites at which B cells differentiate, in response to these antigens, into the plasma cells found within the intestine.[72]

Tonsils

The tonsils are the major component of the Waldeyer ring of pharyngeal lymphoid tissues. They are covered by variable epithelial surfaces that have deep, branching depressions called crypts. Fused lymphatic nodules lie adjacent to the crypts, and germinal centers are prominent. A pseudocapsule of condensed connective tissue surrounds the tonsils, and septae within the structures form lobulations. Together with the other lymphoid tissues of the Waldeyer ring, the tonsils provide the initial barrier to pathogens entering the oral pharynx.

REFERENCES

1. Crivellato E, Vacca A, Ribatti D: Setting the stage: An anatomist's view of the immune system. *Trends Immunol* 25:210, 2004.
2. Blackburn CC, Manley NR: Developing a new paradigm for thymus organogenesis. *Nat Rev Immunol* 4:278, 2004.
3. Hasselbalch H, Jeppesen DL, Ersbrøll AK, et al: Thymus size evaluated by sonography. A longitudinal study on infants during the first year of life. *Acta Radiol* 38:222, 1997.
4. Linton PJ, Dorshkind K: Age-related changes in lymphocyte development and function. *Nat Immunol* 5:133, 2004.
5. Hasselbalch H, Jeppesen DL, Ersbøll AK, et al: Sonographic measurement of thymic size in healthy neonates. Relation to clinical variables. *Acta Radiol* 38:95, 1997.
6. Hasselbalch H, Jeppesen DL, Engelmann MD, et al: Decreased thymus size in formula-fed infants compared with breastfed infants. *Acta Paediatr* 85:1029, 1996.
7. Rezzani R, Bonomini F, Rodella LF: Histochemical and molecular overview of the thymus as site for T-cells development. *Prog Histochem Cytochem* 43:73, 2008.
8. Cifone MG, Migliorati G, Parroni R, et al: Dexamethasone-induced thymocyte apoptosis: Apoptotic signal involves the sequential activation of phosphoinositide-specific phospholipase C, acidic sphingomyelinase, and caspases. *Blood* 93:2282, 1999.
9. Rijhsinghani AG, Thompson K, Bhatia SK, Waldschmidt TJ: Estrogen blocks early T cell development in the thymus. *Am J Reprod Immunol* 36:269, 1996.
10. Ayala A, Herdon CD, Lehman DL, et al: Differential induction of apoptosis in lymphoid tissues during sepsis: Variation in onset, frequency, and the nature of the mediators. *Blood* 87:4261, 1996.
11. Sullivan KE: Chromosome 22q11.2 deletion syndrome: DiGeorge syndrome/velocardiofacial syndrome. *Immunol Allergy Clin North Am* 28:353, 2008.

12. Hale LP: Histologic and molecular assessment of human thymus. *Ann Diagn Pathol* 8:50, 2004.
13. Starr TK, Jameson SC, Hogquist KA: Positive and negative selection of T cells. *Annu Rev Immunol* 21:139, 2003.
14. Laufer TM, Glimcher LH, Lo D: Using thymus anatomy to dissect T cell repertoire selection. *Semin Immunol* 11:65, 1999.
15. Blackman M, Kappler J, Marrack P: The role of the T cell receptor in positive and negative selection of developing T cells. *Science* 248:1335, 1990.
16. Müller-Hermelink HK, Wilisch A, Schultz A, Marx A: Characterization of the human thymic microenvironment: Lymphoepithelial interaction in normal thymus and thymoma. *Arch Histol Cytol* 60:9, 1997.
17. Nikolich-Zugich J, Slifka MK, Messaoudi I: The many important facets of T-cell repertoire diversity. *Nat Rev Immunol* 4:123, 2004.
18. Kwan J, Killeen N: CCR7 directs the migration of thymocytes into the thymic medulla. *J Immunol* 172:3999, 2004.
19. Mathis D, Benoist C: Aire. *Annu Rev Immunol* 27:287, 2009.
20. Betterle C, Greggio NA, Volpato M: Clinical review 93: Autoimmune polyglandular syndrome type 1. *J Clin Endocrinol Metab* 83:1049, 1998.
21. Vogel A, Strassburg CP, Obermayer-Straub P, et al: The genetic background of autoimmune polyendocrinopathy-candidiasis-ectodermal dystrophy and its autoimmune disease components. *J Mol Med* 80:201, 2002.
22. Mathis D, Benoist C: Back to central tolerance. *Immunity* 20:509, 2004.
23. Romero-Torres R: The true splenic blood supply and its surgical applications. *Hepatogastroenterology* 45:885, 1998.
24. Paul R, Bielmeier J, Breul J, et al: [Accessory spleen of the spermatic cord]. *Urologe A* 36:262, 1997.
25. Lauffer JM, Baer HU, Maurer CA, et al: Intrapancreatic accessory spleen. A rare cause of a pancreatic mass. *Int J Pancreatol* 25:65, 1999.
26. Sprogøe-Jakobsen S, Sprogøe-Jakobsen U: The weight of the normal spleen. *Forensic Sci Int* 88:215, 1997.
27. Watanabe Y, Todani T, Noda T, Yamamoto S: Standard splenic volume in children and young adults measured from CT images. *Surg Today* 27:726, 1997.
28. Prassopoulos P, Daskalogiannaki M, Raissaki M, et al: Determination of normal splenic volume on computed tomography in relation to age, gender and body habitus. *Eur Radiol* 7:246, 1997.
29. Rodrigues Junior AJ, Rodrigues CJ, Germano MA, et al: Sonographic assessment of normal spleen volume. *Clin Anat* 8:252, 1995.
30. Steiniger B, Ruttinger L, Barth PJ: The three-dimensional structure of human splenic white pulp compartments. *J Histochem Cytochem* 51:655, 2003.
31. Müller G, Höpken UE, Lipp M: The impact of CCR7 and CXCR5 on lymphoid organ development and systemic immunity. *Immunol Rev* 195:117, 2003.
32. Schneider K, Potter KG, Ware CF: Lymphotoxin and LIGHT signaling pathways and target genes. *Immunol Rev* 202:49, 2004.
33. Mebius RE, Nolte MA, Kraal G: Development and function of the splenic marginal zone. *Crit Rev Immunol* 24:449, 2004.
34. Steiniger B, Timphus EM, Barth PJ: The splenic marginal zone in humans and rodents: An enigmatic compartment and its inhabitants. *Histochem Cell Biol* 126:641, 2006.
35. Weill JC, Weller S, Reynaud CA: Human marginal zone B cells. *Annu Rev Immunol* 27:267, 2009.
36. Kraus MD: Splenic histology and histopathology: An update. *Semin Diagn Pathol* 20:84, 2003.
37. Stewart IB, McKenzie DC: The human spleen during physiological stress. *Sports Med* 32:361, 2002.
38. Chotivanich K, Udomsangpetch R, McGready R, et al: Central role of the spleen in malaria parasite clearance. *J Infect Dis* 185:1538, 2002.
39. Suwanarusk R, Cooke BM, Dondorp AM, et al: The deformability of red blood cells parasitized by *Plasmodium falciparum* and *P. vivax*. *J Infect Dis* 189:190, 2004.
40. Kumpel BM, De Haas M, Koene HR, et al: Clearance of red cells by monoclonal G3 anti-D *in vivo* is affected by the VF polymorphism of Fcgamma RIIIa (CD16). *Clin Exp Immunol* 132:81, 2003.
41. Smith NC, Fell A, Good MF: The immune response to asexual blood stages of malaria parasites. *Chem Immunol* 70:144, 1998.
42. Bakovic D, Eterovic D, Saratlija-Novakovic Z, et al: Effect of human splenic contraction on variation in circulating blood cell counts. *Clin Exp Pharmacol Physiol* 32:944, 2005.
43. Palada I, Eterovic D, Obad A, et al: Spleen and cardiovascular function during short apneas in divers. *J Appl Physiol* 103:1958, 2007.
44. Hamza SM, Kaufman S: Role of spleen in integrated control of splanchnic vascular tone: Physiology and pathophysiology. *Can J Physiol Pharmacol* 87:1, 2009.
45. Forster R, Davalos-Misslitz AC, Rot A: CCR7 and its ligands: Balancing immunity and tolerance. *Nat Rev Immunol* 8:362, 2008.
46. Rizzo LV, Secord EA, Tsiagbe VK, et al: Components essential for the generation of germinal centers. *Dev Immunol* 6:325, 1998.
47. Hollowood K, Goodlad JR: Germinal centre cell kinetics. *J Pathol* 185:229, 1998.
48. Klein U, Dalla-Favera R: Germinal centres: Role in B-cell physiology and malignancy. *Nat Rev Immunol* 8:22, 2008.
49. Tarlinton D: Germinal centers: Form and function. *Curr Opin Immunol* 10:245, 1998.
50. Dunn-Walters DK, Isaacson PG, Spencer J: Analysis of mutations in immunoglobulin heavy chain variable region genes of microdissected marginal zone (MGZ) B cells suggests that the MGZ of human spleen is a reservoir of memory B cells. *J Exp Med* 182:559, 1995.
51. Burton GF, Masuda A, Heath SL, et al: Follicular dendritic cells (FDC) in retroviral infection: Host/pathogen perspectives. *Immunol Rev* 156:185, 1997.
52. Gulbranson-Judge A, Casamayor-Palleja M, MacLennan IC: Mutually dependent T and B cell responses in germinal centers. *Ann N Y Acad Sci* 815:199, 1997.
53. Butcher EC, Williams M, Youngman K, et al: Lymphocyte trafficking and regional immunity. *Adv Immunol* 72:209, 1999.
54. Warnock RA, Askari S, Butcher EC, von Andrian UH: Molecular mechanisms of lymphocyte homing to peripheral lymph nodes. *J Exp Med* 187:205, 1998.
55. Greenfield EA, Nguyen KA, Kuchroo VK: CD28/B7 costimulation: A review. *Crit Rev Immunol* 18:389, 1998.
56. Schwartz RH: T cell anergy. *Annu Rev Immunol* 21:305, 2003.
57. Van Parijs L, Abbas AK: Homeostasis and self-tolerance in the immune system: Turning lymphocytes off. *Science* 280:243, 1998.
58. Malvey EN, Telander DG, Vanasek TL, Mueller DL: The role of clonal anergy in the avoidance of autoimmunity: Inactivation of autocrine growth without loss of effector function. *Immunol Rev* 165:301, 1998.
59. Seder RA, Gazzinelli RT: Cytokines are critical in linking the innate and adaptive immune responses to bacterial, fungal, and parasitic infection. *Adv Intern Med* 44:353, 1999.
60. Ranheim EA, Kipps TJ: Activated T cells induce expression of B7/BB1 on normal or leukemic B cells through a CD40-dependent signal. *J Exp Med* 177:925, 1993.
61. Grewal IS, Flavell RA: CD40 and CD154 in cell-mediated immunity. *Annu Rev Immunol* 16:111, 1998.
62. Vora KA, Ravetch JV, Manser T: Insights into the mechanisms of antibody-affinity maturation and the generation of the memory B-cell compartment using genetically altered mice. *Dev Immunol* 6:305, 1998.
63. Liu YJ, de Bouteiller O, Fugier-Vivier I: Mechanisms of selection and differentiation in germinal centers. *Curr Opin Immunol* 9:256, 1997.
64. Doherty PC, Topham DJ, Tripp RA: Establishment and persistence of virus-specific CD4+ and CD8+ T cell memory. *Immunol Rev* 150:23, 1996.
65. Callan MF, Annels N, Steven N, et al: T cell selection during the evolution of CD8+ T cell memory in vivo. *Eur J Immunol* 28:4382, 1998.
66. Liu YJ, Grouard G, de Bouteiller O, Banchereau J: Follicular dendritic cells and germinal centers. *Int Rev Cytol* 166:139, 1996.
67. Freitas AA, Rocha B: Peripheral T cell survival. *Curr Opin Immunol* 11:152, 1999.
68. MacDonald TT: The mucosal immune system. *Parasite Immunol* 25:235, 2003.
69. Macpherson AJ, McCoy KD, Johansen FE, Brandtzaeg P: The immune geography of A induction and function. *Mucosal Immunol* 1:11, 2008.
70. Mason KL, Huffnagle GB, Noverr MC, Kao JY: Overview of gut immunology. *Adv Exp Med Biol* 635:1, 2008.
71. Clark MA, Jepson MA: Intestinal M cells and their role in bacterial infection. *Int J Med Microbiol* 293:17, 2003.
72. Dunn-Walters DK, Isaacson PG, Spencer J: Sequence analysis of human V_H genes indicates that ileal lamina propria plasma cells are derived from Peyer's patches. *Eur J Immunol* 27:463, 1997.

PART III

Epochal Hematology

CHAPTER 6
HEMATOLOGY OF THE FETUS AND NEWBORN

James Palis and George B. Segel

SUMMARY

During embryogenesis, hematopoiesis occurs in spatially and temporally distinct sites, including the extraembryonic yolk sac, the fetal liver, and the preterm marrow. The development of primitive erythroblasts in the yolk sac is critical for embryonic survival. Primitive erythroblasts differentiate within the vascular network rather than in the extravascular space and circulate as nucleated cells. Although it is widely assumed that primitive red cells remain nucleated throughout their life span, it is likely that many ultimately enucleate upon terminal differentiation. After 7 weeks' gestation, hematopoietic progenitors are no longer detected in the yolk sac. The liver serves as the primary source of red cells from the 9th to the 24th week of gestation. Like primitive erythropoiesis in the yolk sac, definitive erythropoiesis in the fetal liver is necessary for continued survival of the embryo. In contrast to the yolk sac, where hematopoiesis is restricted to maturing primitive erythroid, macrophage, and megakaryocytic cells, hematopoiesis in the fetal liver consists of definitive erythroid, megakaryocyte, and multiple myeloid, as well as lymphoid lineages. Hematopoietic cells are first seen in the marrow of the 10- to 11-week embryo, and they remain confined to the diaphyseal regions of long bones until 15 weeks' gestation. Lymphopoiesis is present in the lymph plexuses and the thymus beginning at 9 weeks' gestation. Yolk sac stem cells were first thought to seed the liver and eventually the marrow. However, later experiments in avian and amphibian embryos indicate that the hematopoietic stem cells that seed the marrow arise within the body of the embryo proper rather than from the yolk sac. The aorta-gonad-mesonephros (AGM) region generates hematopoietic stem cells that seed the liver and the marrow to provide lifelong hematopoiesis. Hgb Gower-1 ($\zeta_2\varepsilon_2$) is the major hemoglobin in embryos younger than 5 weeks. Hgb F ($\alpha_2\gamma_2$) is the major hemoglobin of fetal life. The fetal hemoglobin concentration in blood decreases after birth by approximately 3 percent per week and is generally less than 2 to 3 percent of the total hemoglobin by 6 months of age. The mean hemoglobin level in cord blood at term is 16.8 g/dL, with 95 percent of the values falling between 13.7 and 20.1 g/dL. The red cells of the newborn are macrocytic, with a mean corpuscular volume (MCV) in excess of 110 fl/cell. The red cell, hemoglobin, and hematocrit values decrease only slightly during the first week, but decline more rapidly in the following 5 to 8 weeks, producing the physiologic anemia of the newborn. The absolute number of neutrophils in the blood of term and premature infants is usually greater than that found in older children. Segmented neutrophils are the predominant leukocytes in the first few days after birth. As their number decreases, the lymphocyte becomes the most numerous cell and remains so during the first 4 postnatal years. Phagocytosis of bacteria and latex granules by neutrophils from premature and term infants is normal. Bactericidal activity varies according to the conditions of testing and the clinical status of the neonates. The platelet counts in term and preterm infants are between 150 and 400 × 10^9/L (150,000 to 400,000/μL), comparable to adult values. The absolute number of lymphocytes in the newborn is equivalent to that in older children, with lower values in premature infants at birth. The absolute number of CD3+ and CD4+ (helper/inducer phenotype) T-cell subsets in blood of newborns is significantly higher than in adults. Humoral (B-cell) immunity also develops early in gestation, but it is not fully active until after birth. In the newborn, approximately 15 percent of lymphocytes have immunoglobulin on their surface, with all immunoglobulin (Ig) isotypes represented. The term newborn has reduced mean plasma levels (<60% of adult levels) of factors II, IX, X, XI, and XII, prekallikrein, and high-molecular-weight kininogen. In contrast, the plasma concentration of factor VIII is similar and von Willebrand factor is increased compared to older children and adults.

Acronyms and abbreviations that appear in this chapter include: ADP, adenosine diphosphate; AGM, aorta-gonad-mesonephros; ATP, adenosine triphosphate; ATPase, adenosine triphosphatase; BFU-E, burst-forming unit–erythroid; BPG, bisphosphoglycerate; BPI, bacterial permeability-increasing protein; cAMP, cyclic adenosine monophosphate; CFU-E, colony-forming unit–erythroid; CFU-GEMM, colony-forming unit–granulocyte-erythroid-monocyte-macrophage; CFU-GM, colony-forming unit–granulocyte-monocyte; CFU-Meg, colony-forming unit–megakaryocyte; G-CSF, granulocyte colony-stimulating factor; GM-CSF, granulocyte-monocyte colony-stimulating factor; IL, interleukin; MCV, mean corpuscular volume; NADPH, nicotinamide adenine dinucleotide phosphate (reduced form); NBT, nitroblue tetrazolium; NK, natural killer; RDW, red cell distribution width; SIDS, sudden infant death syndrome; TNF, tumor necrosis factor; TPO, thrombopoietin.

FETAL HEMATOLYMPHOPOIESIS

PRODUCTION OF EMBRYONIC AND FETAL HEMATOPOIETIC CELLS

During embryogenesis, hematopoiesis occurs in spatially and temporally distinct sites, including the extraembryonic yolk sac, the fetal liver, the thymus, and the preterm marrow. The origin of hematopoietic cells is closely tied to gastrulation, the formation of mesoderm cells, and to the emergence of the endothelial lineage. Hematopoiesis is first established soon after implantation of the blastocyst, with the appearance of primitive erythroid cells in blood islands of the yolk sac beginning at day 18 of gestation.[1] The spatial and temporal association of embryonic red cells and endothelial cells in these blood islands suggests that the transient erythromyeloid potential of the yolk sac arises from hemangioblast precursors that also contain endothelial potential.[2] This concept is supported by *in vitro* studies of human embryonic stem cells cultured as embryoid bodies.[3,4] It now appears likely that hematopoietic stem cells containing erythromyeloid and lymphoid potential subsequently arise from intraembryonic vasculature, particularly the aorta (Fig. 6–1). These hematopoietic stem cells provide for fetal and long-term postnatal blood cell production. The ontogeny of the hematopoietic system remains a topic of active research using mammalian and several nonmammalian model systems.

Yolk Sac Hematopoiesis

"Primitive" red cells derived from the yolk sac constitute a distinct transient erythroid lineage that differs from "definitive" red cells that subsequently mature in the fetal liver and marrow. The development of primitive erythroblasts is critical for embryonic survival. In the mouse, targeted disruption of the transcription factors SCL (TAL1), LM02 (RBTN2), and GATA-1 each abrogates primitive erythropoiesis in the yolk sac and leads to early embryonic death.[5–7] In the human, primitive erythroblasts begin to enter the embryo proper at days 21 to 22 of gestation with the onset of cardiac contractions[8] and circulate until approximately 12 weeks of gestation. Yolk sac erythroblasts have several characteristics that distinguish them from their later definitive counterparts. Primitive erythroblasts circulate as nucleated cells, accumulating embryonic hemoglobins and completing terminal differentiation within the vascular network.[9] Because of their

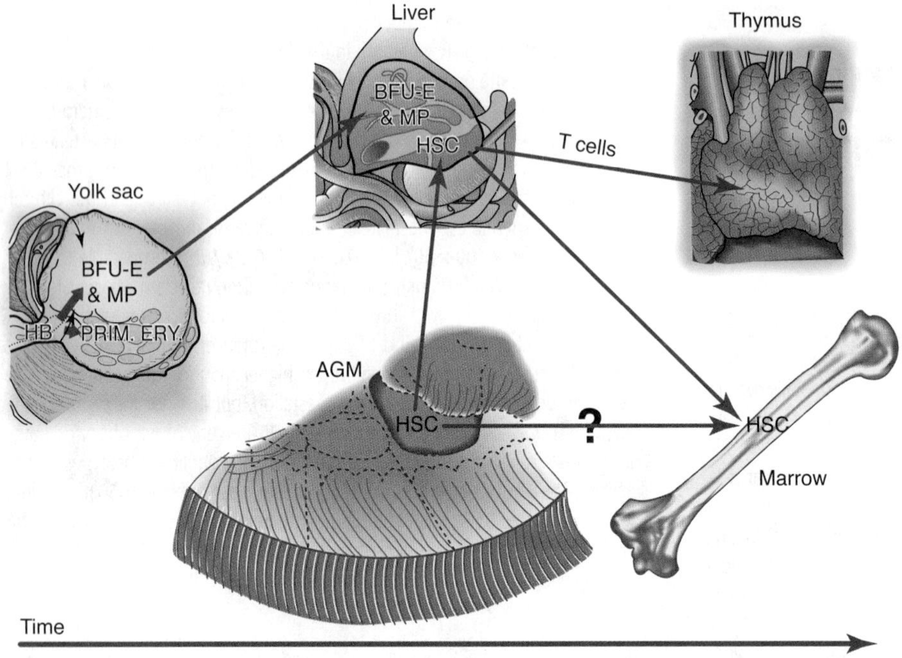

FIGURE 6–1. Hypothetical model of human hematopoietic ontogeny based on amphibian, avian, murine, and human developmental data. The yolk sac provides two transient populations of committed progenitors that are thought to arise from a mesoderm-derived hemangioblast (HB) precursor. The first wave of progenitors produces primitive erythroblasts (PRIM. ERY.) (see text). The second wave produces burst-forming unit–erythroid (BFU-E) and several myeloid progenitors (MP) that seed the liver. Long-term hematopoietic stem cells (HSC) arise later in the aorta-gonad-mesonephros (AGM) region that subsequently populate the liver and ultimately the marrow to generate the full panoply of definitive hematopoiesis. The HSC from liver also provide naïve lymphoid cells to the thymus, and T-lineage maturation occurs there.

extremely large size, with an estimated mean corpuscular volume (MCV) of >400 fl/cell, yolk sac erythroblasts have been termed "megaloblasts." Although it is widely assumed that primitive red cells remain nucleated throughout their life span, it is likely that many if not all, like their murine counterparts, ultimately enucleate upon terminal differentiation.[10–12]

In the mouse, primitive red cells are derived from a transient population of primitive erythroid progenitors that is confined to the yolk sac.[13] Ultrastructural examination of the human yolk sac reveals the presence, not only of primitive erythroblasts, but also of macrophage cells and megakaryocytes.[11] These findings are consistent with hematopoietic progenitor studies in the mouse embryo suggesting that primitive hematopoiesis in the yolk sac includes the primitive erythroid, macrophage, and megakaryocyte lineages.[13,14]

The initial wave of primitive erythroid progenitors is followed by a second wave of yolk sac–derived definitive erythroid progenitors, termed burst forming units–erythroid (BFU-E). BFU-E are present in the human yolk sac as early as 4 weeks' gestation and are found in the fetal liver by 5 weeks' gestation.[15] These findings suggest that the fetal liver is initially seeded by hematopoietic progenitors derived from the yolk sac (see Fig. 6–1).[16] Erythroid and nonerythroid progenitors are evident also in the nonliver regions of the embryo proper.[17] After 7 weeks' gestation, hematopoietic progenitors are no longer detected in the yolk sac.[18]

Hepatic Hematopoiesis

The liver serves as the primary source of red cells from the 9th to the 24th weeks of gestation. Between 7 and 15 weeks' gestation, 60 percent of the liver cells are hematopoietic.[19] Erythroid cells differentiate in close physical association with macrophages and extrude their nuclei prior to entering the bloodstream. These fetal-liver-derived definitive "macrocytes" are smaller than yolk sac–derived primitive megaloblasts and contain one-third the amount of hemoglobin. Differentiation of murine erythroid cells in the fetal liver is critically dependent on erythropoietin signaling through its receptor and the Janus kinase 2 (JAK2).[20,21] Fetal-liver-derived erythroid progenitors will differentiate *in vitro* with erythropoietin alone, in contrast to adult-marrow-derived BFU-E which requires erythropoietin plus interleukin (IL)-3.[22,23] Erythropoietin transcripts are present during the first trimester in the liver.[15] The liver remains the primary site of erythropoietin transcription throughout fetal life.[24] Erythropoietin transcripts also are present in the developing human kidney as early as 17 weeks' gestation and increase after 30 weeks.[24] Like primitive erythropoiesis in the yolk sac, definitive erythropoiesis in the fetal liver is necessary for continued survival of the embryo. Targeted disruption of the c-myb transcription factor in the mouse blocks fetal liver erythropoiesis and leads to fetal death.[25] This mutation does not affect primitive erythropoiesis, indicating fundamental differences in the transcriptional regulation of these distinct forms of erythropoiesis.

In contrast to the yolk sac, where hematopoiesis is restricted to erythromyeloid lineages, hematopoiesis in the fetal liver eventually will consist of definitive erythroid, megakaryocyte, multiple myeloid, as well as lymphoid, lineages. Megakaryocytes are present in the liver by 6 weeks' gestation. Platelets are first evident in the circulation at 8 to 9 weeks' gestation.[19] Granulopoiesis is present in the liver parenchyma as early as 7 weeks' gestation and small numbers of circulating leukocytes are present at the 11th week of gestation. Despite the low number and immature appearance of hepatic neutrophils, the fetal liver contains abundant hematopoietic progenitor cells, including the multipotential colony-forming unit–granulocyte-erythroid-monocyte-macrophage (CFU-GEMM) and colony-forming unit–granulocyte-monocyte (CFU-GM).[26] CFU-GM growth depends upon several cytokines, including granulocyte colony-stimulating factor (G-CSF), granulocyte-monocyte colony-stimulating factor (GM-CSF), and interleukins.[27] When compared to adult marrow-derived myeloid progenitors, these fetal-liver-derived myeloid progenitors have a similar dose–response *in vitro* to G-CSF.[28] G-CSF is expressed by hepatocytes at 14 weeks' gestation.[29]

Lymphopoiesis

Lymphopoiesis is present in the lymph plexuses and the thymus beginning at 9 weeks' gestation.[19] B cells with surface immunoglobulin (Ig)M are present in the liver, and circulating lymphocytes also are seen at 9 weeks' gestation. T lymphocytes are found only rarely before 12 weeks' gestation.[30] Lymphocyte subpopulations are detected by 13 weeks' gestation in fetal liver.[31] Absolute numbers of major lymphoid subsets in 20- to 26-week-old fetuses, as defined by the antigens CD2, CD3, CD4, CD8, CD16, CD19, and CD20 (see Chap. 15 for functional significance of these phenotypes), are similar to those in newborns (see "Neonatal Lymphopoiesis" below).[32,33]

Marrow Hematopoiesis

Hematopoietic cells are first seen in the marrow of the 10- to 11-week embryo,[1] and they remain confined to the diaphyseal regions of long bones until 15 weeks' gestation.[34] Initially there are approximately equal numbers of myeloid and erythroid cells in the fetal marrow. However, myeloid cells predominate by 12 weeks' gestation, and the myeloid-to-erythroid ratio approaches the adult level of 3:1 by 21 weeks' gestation.[19] Macrophage cells in the fetal marrow, but not in the fetal liver, express the lipopolysaccharide receptor CD14.[29] The marrow becomes the major site of hematopoiesis after the 24th week of gestation and remains so throughout the remainder of fetal life.

■ ONTOGENY OF HEMATOPOIETIC STEM CELLS

The reconstitution of the entire hematopoietic system by transplantation with cord blood indicates that hematopoietic stem cells are circulating in the bloodstream at birth.[35] The immunologic reconstitution of an immunodeficient human fetus with fetal-liver-derived cells also indicates that hematopoietic stem cells exist in the later fetal liver.[36] It was first postulated that hematopoietic stem cells originate independently in each hematopoietic site (yolk sac, liver, and marrow) of the embryo.[37] However, experiments in the mammalian embryo indicate that the liver rudiment, like the marrow, is seeded by exogenous hematopoietic cells.[38,39] It was initially thought that the liver, and eventually the marrow, were seeded by yolk sac–derived stem cells.[40] However, experiments in avian and amphibian embryos indicate that the hematopoietic stem cells that ultimately provide for adult hematopoiesis arise within the body of the embryo proper rather than from the yolk sac.[41,42] Subsequent investigations in the mouse embryo indicate that stem cells capable of engrafting myeloablated adult recipients originate in the aorta-gonad-mesonephros (AGM) region of the embryo proper.[43] This correlates anatomically with the transient appearance of clusters of CD34+ blood cells closely associated with the ventral wall of the aorta in several mammalian species, including the 5 weeks' gestation human embryo.[44,45] These findings suggest that hematopoietic stem cells arise from "hemogenic" aortic endothelium and then seed the liver and eventually the marrow to provide lifelong hematopoiesis (see Fig. 6–1). Studies in the murine embryo suggest that the placenta also serves as a site of hematopoietic stem cell origin and expansion.[46] It is not known if the placenta serves similar functions during human development. The underlying relationship of the transient erythromyeloid hematopoiesis derived from the yolk sac to long-term hematopoietic stem cell–derived intraembryonic hematopoiesis remains unclear.

■ SYNTHESIS OF FETAL HEMOGLOBINS

Human hemoglobin (Hgb) is a tetramer composed of two α-type and two β-type globin chains (Table 6–1). The α-globin gene cluster is located on chromosome 16 and contains the ζ gene 5′ to the pair of α-globin genes. The β-globin gene cluster is located on chromosome 11 and contains five globin genes oriented 5′ to 3′ as ε-γ^A-γ^G-δ-β.[47] During embryogenesis the genes on both chromosomes are activated sequentially from the 5′ to the 3′ end. This globin "switching" is related not only to the relative positions of the globin genes within their respective chromosomal clusters, but also to interacting upstream "locus control regions."[48]

Hgb Gower-1 ($\zeta_2\varepsilon_2$) is the major hemoglobin in embryos younger than 5 weeks' gestation (see Table 6–1).[49] Hgb Gower-2 ($\alpha_2\varepsilon_2$) has been found in embryos with a gestational age as young as 4 weeks and is absent in embryos older than 13 weeks.[50] Hgb Portland ($\zeta_2\gamma_2$) is found in young embryos, but persists in infants with homozygous α-thalassemia. Synthesis of the ζ and ε chains decreases as those of the α and γ chains increase

TABLE 6–1. Embryonic Hemoglobins

Hemoglobin	Chain Composition	Primary Site	Appearance
Gower-1	$\zeta_2\varepsilon_2$	Yolk sac	<5–6 weeks
Gower-2	$\alpha_2\varepsilon_2$	Yolk sac	4–13 weeks
Portland	$\zeta_2\gamma_2$	Yolk sac	4–13 weeks
Fetal (F)	$\alpha_2\gamma_2$	Liver	Early, 53–95% at term
Adult (A)	$\alpha_2\beta_2$	Marrow	9 weeks, 5–45% at term

(Fig. 6–2). The ζ-to-α-globin switch precedes the ε-to-γ-globin switch as the liver replaces the yolk sac as the main site of erythropoiesis.[9,51]

Hgb F ($\alpha_2\gamma_2$) is the major hemoglobin of fetal life[52] (see Fig. 6–2). Synthesis of Hgb A can be demonstrated in fetuses as young as 9 weeks' gestation.[53,54] In fetuses of 9 to 21 weeks' gestation, the amount of Hgb A ($\alpha_2\beta_2$) rises from 4 to 13 percent of the total hemoglobin.[54] These levels of Hgb A have enabled the antenatal diagnosis of β-thalassemia using globin-chain synthesis. After 34 to 36 weeks' gestation the percentage of Hgb A rises, whereas that of Hgb F decreases (see Fig. 6–2). The mean synthesis of Hgb F in term infants was 59.0 ± 10 percent (1 SD) of total hemoglobin synthesis as assessed by ^{14}C-leucine uptake.[55] The amount of Hgb F in blood varies in term infants from 53 to 95 per cent of total hemoglobin.[56,57]

The fetal hemoglobin concentration in blood decreases after birth by approximately 3 percent per week and is generally less than 2 to 3 percent of the total hemoglobin by 6 months of age. This rate of decrease in Hgb F production is closely related to the gestational age of the infant and is not affected by the changes in environment and oxygen tension that occur at the time of birth.[58] Hgb A_2 ($\alpha_2\delta_2$) has not been detected in fetuses. Normal adult levels of Hgb A_2 are achieved by 4 months of age.[59] Increased proportions of Hgb F at birth have been reported in infants who are small for gestational age, who have experienced chronic intrauterine hypoxia, who have trisomy 13, or who have died from sudden infant death syndrome (SIDS).[60–64] Decreased levels of Hgb F at birth are found in trisomy 21.[65]

■ FETAL BLOOD

The cellular composition of fetal blood changes markedly during the second and third trimesters. The mean hemoglobin in fetuses progressively increases from 9.0 ± 2.8 g/dL at age 10 weeks to 16.5 ± 4.0 g/dL at age 39 weeks.[66] There is a concomitant decrease in the MCV of fetal red cells from a mean of 134 fl/cell at 18 weeks' gestation to 118 fl/cell at 30 weeks' gestation.[67] The total white blood cell count averages 2×10^9/L between 10 and 17 weeks of gestation,[31] and increases during the middle trimester to between 4 and 4.5×10^9/L, with an 80 to 85 percent preponderance of lymphocytes and 5 to 10 percent neutrophils.[67] The percentage of circulating nucleated red cells decreases from a mean of 12 percent at 18 weeks to 4 percent at 30 weeks.[67] The platelet count remains greater than 150,000/μL from 15 weeks' gestation to term.[67,68]

Large numbers of committed hematopoietic progenitors circulate in the fetal blood. Blood samples obtained by fetoscopy at 12 to 19 weeks' gestation reveal a mean of 20,450 BFU-E/mL and 12,490 CFU-GM/mL.[69] This is in striking contrast to adult blood, which contains many fewer erythroid progenitors and 30 to 250 CFU-GM/mL.[70] Most (70 to 80%) circulating hematopoietic progenitors at 26 to 28 weeks' gestation are cycling.[70] In contrast, adult-marrow-derived progenitors in the bloodstream are relatively quiescent with only 0 to 5 percent cycling.

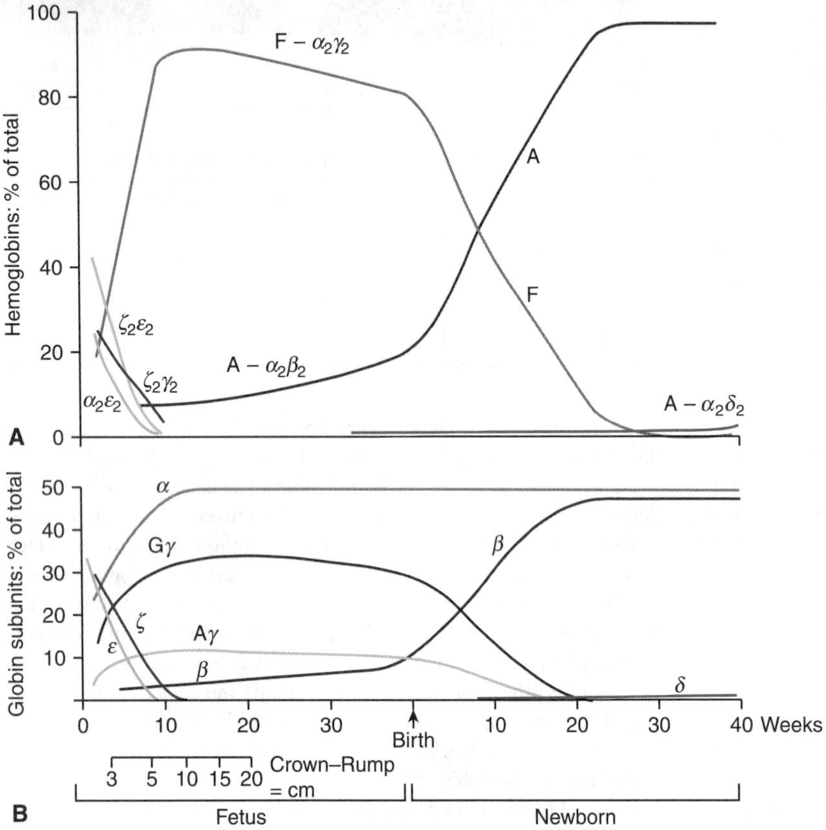

FIGURE 6–2. Changes in hemoglobin tetramers **(A)** and in globin subunits **(B)** during human development from embryo to early infancy. *(Reproduced from Bunn HF, Forget BG:* Hemoglobin: Molecular, Genetic and Clinical Aspects, *p 68. WB Saunders, Philadelphia, 1986, with permission.)*

NEONATAL HEMATOPOIESIS

NEONATAL ERYTHROPOIESIS AND RED CELLS

Hemoglobin, Hematocrit, and Indices

The mean hemoglobin level in cord blood at term is 16.8 g/dL, with 95 percent of the values falling between 13.7 and 20.1 g/dL.[71] This variation reflects perinatal events, particularly asphyxia,[72] and also the amount of blood transferred from the placenta to the infant after delivery. Early cord clamping appears to heighten the occurrence of anemia at 2 months and to impair cardiopulmonary adaptation.[73] Delay of cord clamping may increase the blood volume and red cell mass of the infant by as much as 55 percent.[74,75] This results in fewer transfusions and fewer days requiring oxygen and ventilation in preterm infants.[73] The mean total blood volume after birth is 86 mL/kg for the term infant and 89 mL/kg for the premature infant.[76] The blood volume per kilogram decreases over the ensuing weeks, reaching a mean value of about 65 mL/kg by 3 to 4 months of age.

Normally the hemoglobin and hematocrit values rise in the first several hours after birth because of the movement of plasma from the intravascular to the extravascular space.[77] A venous hemoglobin concentration of less than 14 g/dL in a term infant and/or a fall in hemoglobin or hematocrit level in the first postnatal day are abnormal. Table 6–2 shows the normal red cell values from capillary blood samples for term infants in the first 12 weeks after birth.[78] Capillary hematocrit values in newborns are higher than those in simultaneous venous samples, particularly during the first postnatal days, and the capillary-to-venous ratio is approximately 1.1:1.[79] This difference reflects circulatory factors and is greater in preterm and sick infants.

The red cells of the newborn are macrocytic, with an MCV in excess of 110 fl/cell. The MCV begins to fall after the first week, reaching adult values by the ninth week (see Table 6–2).[78,80] The blood film from a newborn infant shows macrocytic normochromic cells, polychromasia, and a few nucleated red blood cells. Even in healthy infants there may be mild anisopoikilocytosis.[81] Three to 5 percent of the red cells may be fragments, target cells, or distorted. By 3 to 5 days after birth, nucleated red blood cells are not found normally in the blood of term or premature infants, but they may be present in markedly elevated numbers in the presence of hemolysis or hypoxic stress. As expected from these findings, the red cell distribution width (RDW) is markedly elevated in the newborn period.[82]

There are significant numbers of circulating progenitor cells in cord blood.[83–86] Cord blood BFU-E and colony-forming unit–erythroid (CFU-E) differentiate more rapidly than their adult counterparts.[87] Furthermore, the proportion of cord blood hematopoietic progenitors in the mitotic cycle is approximately 50 percent, intermediate between the proportions found in fetal and adult progenitor cells.[70,85]

In several,[88,89] but not all,[90] studies premature infants at birth had lower hemoglobin levels, higher reticulocyte counts, and higher nucleated red cell counts than did the term infants. The reticulocyte counts of premature infants are inversely proportional to their gestational age, with a mean of 8 percent reticulocytes evident at 32 weeks' gestation and 4 to 5 percent at term.[91] Infants who are small for their gestational ages have higher red cell counts, hematocrit levels, and hemoglobin concentrations as compared with infants whose size is appropriate for their gestational age.[89,92]

Erythropoietin and Physiologic Anemia of the Newborn Erythropoietin is the primary regulator of erythropoiesis. Although erythropoietin is present in cord blood, it falls to undetectable levels after birth in healthy infants.[93] Subsequently, the reticulocyte count falls to less than 1 percent by the sixth day after birth.[78,94] The red cell, hemoglobin, and hematocrit values decrease only slightly during the first week, but decline more rapidly in the following 5 to 8 weeks (see Table 6–2),[78] producing the physiologic anemia of the newborn. The lowest hemoglobin values in the term infant occur at approximately 2 months of age.[80] When the hemoglobin concentration falls below 11 g/dL, erythropoietic activity begins to increase. Erythropoietin can be measured after the 60th postnatal day,[95] corresponding to the recovery from physiologic anemia. If there is sufficient stimulus, such as hemolytic anemia or cyanotic heart disease, the newborn infant is able to produce erythropoietin prior to the 60th postnatal day.[93]

The fall in hemoglobin level is more pronounced in the premature infant. In one study of premature infants the mean hemoglobin level at 2 months was 9.4 g/dL, with a 95 percent range of 7.2 to 11.7 g/dL.[96] In healthy premature infants erythropoietin becomes detectable when the hemoglobin level falls to approximately 12 g/dL. In infants with a lower percentage of Hgb F (as from transfusion) and consequently better oxygen delivery, erythropoietin does not rise until the hemoglobin falls to approximately 9.5 g/dL.[97] The mean values for iron-sufficient premature infants reached those of term infants by 4 months for red cell count, 5 months for hemoglobin

TABLE 6–2. Red Cell Values for Term Infants during the First 12 Weeks after Birth*

Age	Hbg, g/dL ± SD	RBC × 10^{12}/L ± SD	Hematocrit, % ± SD	MCV, fl ± SD	MCHC, g/dL ± SD	Reticulocytes, % ± SD
Days						
1	19.3 ± 2.2	5.14 ± 0.7	61 ± 7.4	119 ± 9.4	31.6 ± 1.9	3.2 ± 1.4
2	19.0 ± 1.9	5.15 ± 0.8	60 ± 6.4	115 ± 7.0	31.6 ± 1.4	3.2 ± 1.3
3	18.8 ± 2.0	5.11 ± 0.7	62 ± 9.3	116 ± 5.3	31.1 ± 2.8	2.8 ± 1.7
4	18.6 ± 2.1	5.00 ± 0.6	57 ± 8.1	114 ± 7.5	32.6 ± 1.5	1.8 ± 1.1
5	17.6 ± 1.1	4.97 ± 0.4	57 ± 7.3	114 ± 8.9	30.9 ± 2.2	1.2 ± 0.2
6	17.4 ± 2.2	5.00 ± 0.7	54 ± 7.2	113 ± 10.0	32.2 ± 1.6	0.6 ± 0.2
7	17.9 ± 2.5	4.86 ± 0.6	56 ± 9.4	118 ± 11.2	32.0 ± 1.6	0.5 ± 0.4
Weeks						
1–2	17.3 ± 2.3	4.80 ± 0.8	54 ± 8.3	112 ± 19.0	32.1 ± 2.9	0.5 ± 0.3
2–3	15.6 ± 2.6	4.20 ± 0.6	46 ± 7.3	111 ± 8.2	33.9 ± 1.9	0.8 ± 0.6
3–4	14.2 ± 2.1	4.00 ± 0.6	43 ± 5.7	105 ± 7.5	33.5 ± 1.6	0.6 ± 0.3
4–5	12.7 ± 1.6	3.60 ± 0.4	36 ± 4.8	101 ± 8.1	34.9 ± 1.6	0.9 ± 0.8
5–6	11.9 ± 1.5	3.55 ± 0.2	36 ± 6.2	102 ± 10.2	34.1 ± 2.9	1.0 ± 0.7
6–7	12.0 ± 1.5	3.40 ± 0.4	36 ± 4.8	105 ± 12.0	33.8 ± 2.3	1.2 ± 0.7
7–8	11.1 ± 1.1	3.40 ± 0.4	33 ± 3.7	100 ± 13.0	33.7 ± 2.6	1.5 ± 0.7
8–9	10.7 ± 0.9	3.40 ± 0.5	31 ± 2.5	93 ± 12.0	34.1 ± 2.2	1.8 ± 1.0
9–10	11.2 ± 0.9	3.60 ± 0.3	32 ± 2.7	91 ± 9.3	34.3 ± 2.9	1.2 ± 0.6
10–11	11.4 ± 0.9	3.70 ± 0.4	34 ± 2.1	91 ± 7.7	33.2 ± 2.4	1.2 ± 0.7
11–12	11.3 ± 0.9	3.70 ± 0.3	33 ± 3.3	88 ± 7.9	34.8 ± 2.2	0.7 ± 0.3

MCHC, mean corpuscular hemoglobin concentration; MCV, mean corpuscular volume; RBC, red blood cell.

*Capillary blood samples. The RBC count and MCV measurements were made on an electronic counter.

SOURCE: Adapted from Matoth Y, Zaizor R, Varsano I.[78]

level, and 6 months for mean corpuscular volume and mean corpuscular hemoglobin.[96]

Blood Viscosity The viscosity of blood increases logarithmically in relation to the hematocrit.[98,99] Hyperviscosity was found in 5 percent of infants,[100] and in 18 percent of infants who were small for gestational age.[101] Newborn infants with hematocrit values of greater than 65 to 70 percent may become symptomatic because of increased viscosity.[102] In one study of infants with documented hyperviscosity and a mean hematocrit greater than 65 percent, 38 percent had symptoms of irritability, hypotonia, tremors, or poor suck reflex.[103] Partial plasma exchange transfusion reduced blood viscosity, improved cerebral blood flow, and relieved the symptoms. However, cerebral blood flow was normal in the asymptomatic infants with hyperviscosity, and there consequently was no benefit from exchange transfusion.[103] Studies of neurodevelopmental status do not show any clear long-term benefits for the use of partial exchange transfusions in asymptomatic neonates.[104]

Red Cell Antigens The blood group antigens on neonatal red cells differ from those of the older child and adult. The i antigen is expressed strongly, whereas the I antigen and the A and B antigens are expressed only weakly on neonatal red cells. The i antigen is a straight-chain carbohydrate that is replaced by the branched-chain derivative, I antigen, as a result of the developmental acquisition of a glycosyltransferase.[105] By 1 year of age the i antigen is undetectable, and the ABH antigens increase to adult levels by age 3 years. The ABH, Kell, Duffy, and Vel antigens can be detected on the cells of the fetus in the first trimester and are present at birth.[106] The Lu^a and Lu^b antigens also are detectable on fetal red cells and are more weakly expressed at birth, increasing to adult levels by age 15 years.[106] The Xg antigen is variably expressed in the fetus and is weaker on newborn than on adult red cells. Moreover, particularly poor expression of Xg has been noted in newborns with trisomy 13, 18, and 21.[106] The Lewis group (Le^a/Le^b) antigens are adsorbed on the red cell membrane and become detectable within 1 to 2 weeks after birth as the receptor sites develop. Anti-A and anti-B isohemagglutinins develop during the first 6 postnatal months, reaching adult levels by 2 years of age.

Red Cell Life Span The life span of the red cells in the newborn infant is shorter than that of red cells in the adult. The average of several studies of mean half-life of newborn red cells is 60 to 80 days.[107] The reasons for this shortened survival are unclear, but the known susceptibility to oxidant injury of newborn red cells may be a contributing factor.

Iron and Transferrin The serum iron level in cord blood of the normal infant is elevated compared to maternal levels. The mean value is about 150 ± 40 mcg/dL (1 SD).[108] Infants on an iron-supplemented diet have a median serum iron level of 125 mcg/dL at 1 month of age and of approximately 75 mcg/dL at 6 months of age. The total iron-binding capacity rises throughout the first year. The median transferrin saturation falls from almost 65 percent at 2 weeks to 25 percent at 1 year, and saturations as low as 10 percent may be observed in the absence of iron deficiency.[109] The mean serum ferritin levels in iron-sufficient infants are high at birth, 160 mcg/L, rise further during the first month, and then fall to a mean of 30 mcg/L by 1 year of age.[110] The amount of stainable iron in the marrow at birth is small but increases in both term and premature infants during the first weeks after birth. Stainable marrow iron begins to decrease after 2 months and is gone by 4 to 6 months in term infants and earlier in premature infants.[111] Iron is preferentially allocated to erythropoiesis if the availability of iron is limited.[112] This makes the availability of adequate iron particularly important to avoid iron lack in the brain, heart, and skeletal muscle.

Red Cell Functions

Oxygen Delivery The oxygen affinity of cord blood is greater than that of maternal blood, because the affinity of Hgb F for 2,3-bisphosphoglycerate (2,3-BPG) is less than that of Hgb A.[113] Levels of 2,3-BPG are lower in newborn red cells than in adult cells and even more decreased in the red cells of premature infants,[114] and this low 2,3-BPG level further heightens the oxygen affinity of newborn red cells. Consequently, the red cell oxygen equilibrium curve of the newborn is shifted to the left of that of the adult (Fig. 6–3). The mean partial pressure of oxygen at which hemoglobin is 50 percent saturated with oxygen at 1 day of age in term infants is 19.4 ± 1.8 torr, as compared with the normal adult value of 27.0 ± 1.1 torr.[115] This results in a decrease in the oxygen released at the tissue level, as shown in Figure 6–3. As the partial pressure of oxygen (P_{O2}) falls from 90 torr in arterial to 40 torr in the venous blood, 3.0 mL/dL of oxygen are released from newborn blood, whereas 4.5 mL/dL are released from adult Hgb A-containing blood. The shift to the left of the oxygen equilibrium curve is even more pronounced in the premature infant, requiring a larger fall in P_{O2} to release an equivalent amount of oxygen. After birth the oxygen equilibrium curve shifts gradually to the right, reaching the position of the adult curve by 6 months of age. The position of the curve in the premature infant correlates with gestational age rather than with postnatal age,[115] and its shift to the adult position is more gradual.

Metabolism Many differences have been found between the metabolism of the red cells of newborn infants and that of adults.[116,117] Some of the differences may be explained by the younger mean cell age in the newborn, but others seem to be properties of the fetal cell. The glucose consumption in newborn red cells is lower than that in adult red cells.[118] Elevated levels of glucose phosphate isomerase, glyceraldehyde-3-phosphate dehydrogenase, phosphoglycerate kinase, and enolase beyond those explainable by the young cell age have been found in neonatal cells.[114,119] The level of phosphofructokinase is low in red cells of term and premature infants.[114,119,120] The pentose phosphate shunt is active in red cells of term and premature infants,[121] but glutathione instability leads to a heightened susceptibility to oxidant injury. The result of oxidant stress is depletion of adenosine triphosphate (ATP) and adenine nucleotides leading to iron release, denaturing of membrane proteins, and hemoglobin and membrane peroxidation.[122] The levels of ATP and adenosine diphosphate (ADP) are higher in the red cells of term and preterm infants,[120] but may merely reflect the younger age of the erythrocyte population. Finally, lower-than-adult activities have been found for several other red cell enzymes, including cytochrome B_5 reductase[123] and glutathione peroxidase.[124]

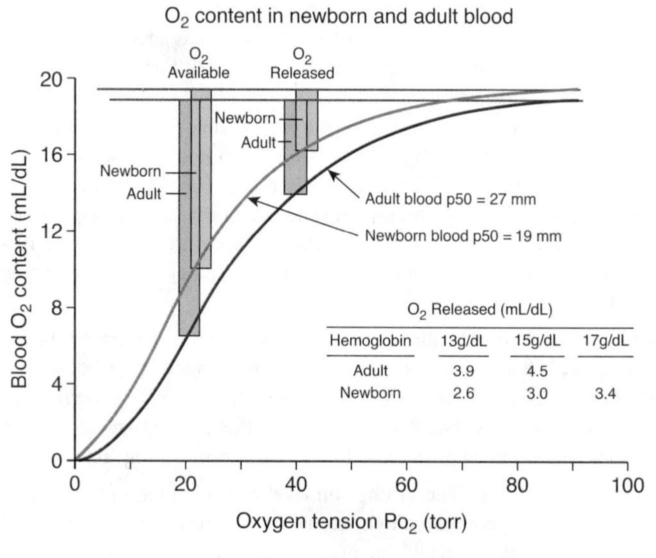

FIGURE 6–3. The oxygen equilibrium curves are based on the assumption that the Hgb concentration is 15 g/dL and that there is full O_2 saturation of Hgb at a partial pressure of arterial oxygen (Pao_2) of 100 torr. The O_2 released is the difference in O_2 content between a Pao_2 of 90 torr and the mixed venous Pao_2 of 40 torr. The O_2 available is the difference in O_2 content between a Pao_2 of 90 torr and a mixed venous Pao_2 of 20 torr. This is the maximum O_2 available without evoking compensatory mechanisms such as increased cardiac output.

Membrane The membrane of the newborn red cell also is different from that of the adult red cell. Ouabain-sensitive adenosine triphosphatase (ATPase) is decreased,[125] and active potassium influx is significantly less in neonatal red cells.[126] Newborn cells are more sensitive to osmotic hemolysis and to oxidant injury than are adult cells. Newborn red cell membranes have higher total lipid, phospholipid, and cholesterol per cell than adult red cells.[127,128] The patterns of phospholipid and phospholipid fatty acid composition also differ from those in adult red cells. Red cells of newborns have the same pattern of membrane proteins on polyacrylamide gel electrophoresis[129] and the same rate of mobility in an electric field[130] as do red cells from adults. After trypsin treatment of newborn and adult cells, however, there is a difference in electrophoretic mobility, indicating that the surface trypsin-resistant proteins are different.[130] The relationship of the metabolic and membrane alterations in neonatal red cells to their shorter life span is not clear.

WHITE CELLS

Granulocytopoiesis and Monocytopoiesis

Colony-Stimulating Factors and Granulomonopoiesis The absolute number of neutrophils in the blood of term and premature infants usually is greater than that found in older children (Table 6–3).[131] The neutrophil count tends to be lower in the premature than in the term infant, and the proportion of myelocytes and band neutrophils is higher.[132] Serum and urinary colony-stimulating activity are elevated during the period of neutrophilia.[133] When granulopoiesis was studied in cord blood, blood, and marrow of infants, the macrophage colony-forming unit was predominant despite the clinical neutrophilia, and this pattern was not altered by different sources of colony-stimulating factors.[134,135] The endogenous cytokines produced by mononuclear cells from cord or systemic venous blood support the growth of neutrophil colonies in assays using marrow from adults.[134] However, there is diminished GM-CSF, G-CSF, and IL-3 production in stimulated newborn compared to adult mononuclear cells,[136–138] which may limit the response to bacterial infection in the newborn. Furthermore, preterm infants have a reduced neutrophil storage pool and a restricted capacity to increase their progenitor proliferation, and their neutrophil count may fall precipitously with neonatal bacterial infection.[139] Dysregulation as well as diminished capacity of neonatal granulopoiesis may impair the neonatal response to infection.[140] Smaller numbers of CFU-GM colonies were observed in the blood of sick infants, who also have diminished endogenous production of colony-stimulating factors in culture.[135] The clinical use of cytokines to treat neonatal sepsis remains controversial,[141]

TABLE 6–3. The White Cell Count and the Differential Count during the First 2 Weeks after Birth*

Age	Leukocytes	Neutrophils			Eosinophils	Basophils	Lymphocytes	Monocytes
		Total	Segmented	Bands				
Birth								
Mean	18.0	11.0	9.4	1.6	0.40	0.10	5.5	1.05
Range	9.0–30.0	6.0–26.0	–	–	0.02–0.85	0–0.64	2.0–11.0	0.4–3.1
Mean %	–	61	52	9	2.2	0.6	31	5.8
7 days								
Mean	12.2	5.5	4.7	0.83	0.50	0.05	5.0	1.1
Range	5.0–21.0	1.5–10.0	–	–	0.07–1.1	0–0.25	2.0–17.0	0.3–2.7
Mean %	–	45	39	6	4.1	0.4	41	9.1
14 days								
Mean	11.4	4.5	3.9	0.63	0.35	0.05	5.5	1.0
Range	5.0–20.0	1.0–9.5	–	–	0.07–1.0	0–0.23	2.0–17.0	0.2–2.4
Mean %	–	40	34	5.5	3.1	0.4	48	8.8

*All white cell counts are expressed as cells × 10^9/L.

SOURCE: Modified from Altman PL, Dittmer DS,[131] and from Dallman PR: *Pediatrics*, 16th edition, edited by AM Rudolph, HL Barnett, AH Einhorn. Appleton-Century-Crofts, New York, 1977.

but circulating neutrophils are increased in preterm infants treated with recombinant G-CSF, and the infants' length of stay in the neonatal intensive care unit is shortened.[142]

White Cell and Differential Counts Table 6–3 gives the values for the white cell and differential counts during the first 2 weeks after birth. The absolute number of segmented neutrophils rises in both term and premature infants in the first 24 hours.[143] In term infants, the mean value increases from 8 × 10^9/L (8000/μL) to a peak of 13 × 10^9/L (13,000/μL) and then falls to 4 × 10^9/L (4000/μL) by 72 hours of age, remaining at this level through the following 7 days. In the premature infant, the mean values for neutrophils are 5 × 10^9/L (5000/μL) at birth, 8 × 10^9/L (8000/μL) at 12 hours, and 4 × 10^9/L (4000/μL) at 72 hours. The mean count then falls gradually to 2.5 × 10^9/L (2500/μL) by the 28th postnatal day. The level after the first 72 hours is very stable for an individual infant, whether term or premature. Immature forms, including an occasional promyelocyte and blast cell, may be seen in the blood of healthy infants in the first few days after birth and are more frequent in premature infants than in term infants.[143] Segmented granulocytes are the predominant cells in the first few days after birth. As their number decreases, the lymphocyte becomes the most numerous cell and remains so during the first 4 years of life. An absolute eosinophil count of greater than 0.7 × 10^9/L (700/μL) was found in 76 percent of premature infants at 2 to 3 weeks of age. The onset of the eosinophilia coincided with the establishment of steady weight gain in the infants.[144] It is increased by the use of total parenteral nutrition, endotracheal intubation, and blood transfusions.

Phagocyte Functions

Bacterial infections are a major cause of morbidity and mortality in the newborn period.[145] The infections frequently are caused by organisms of low virulence in normal children and adults, including *Staphylococcus*, Lancefield group B β-hemolytic streptococci, *Pseudomonas*, and other Gram-negative bacilli. Cellular defense mechanisms and humoral immunity of the newborn differ from those found later in life, and these undoubtedly contribute to the unusual susceptibility to infection noted in the neonatal period.[145]

Opsonins and Complement Engulfment and destruction of bacteria by neutrophils depend on opsonic activity of the plasma and on chemotaxis, phagocytosis, and the bacteriocidal capacity of the leukocyte. The serum factors necessary for optimal phagocytosis (opsonins) include the immunoglobulins and complement components. In term infants, opsonic activity is normal for *Staphylococcus aureus*,[146,147] but it is low for yeast[148] and *Escherichia coli*.[147] Diminished opsonic antibody is associated with group B streptococcal infection and represents one risk factor for neonatal infection.[149]

In premature infants, opsonic activity is low for *S. aureus* and *Serratia marcescens*,[146] but is normal for *Pseudomonas aeruginosa*.[150] When serum concentrations of fibronectin and IgG subclasses C3 and C4 were measured at birth, 1 month, 3 months, and 6 months, early gestational age was correlated with lower initial levels.[151] The decreased opsonic activity for some organisms in premature infants has been attributed to diminished IgG levels, because additional IgG will correct the opsonic defect both *in vivo* and *in vitro*.[146] The added IgG improves bacterial opsonization by serum of premature infants in part because complement consumption and deposition of C3 on the bacterial surface are augmented.[152,153]

Complement components appear in fetal blood before 20 weeks' gestation and increase markedly during the third trimester. However, in many newborns both the classical and alternative complement pathways are decreased in activity and in levels of individual components.[154] The mean level of C3, the first common component of the two pathways of complement activation, is approximately 65 percent of that in normal adults.[155–157] There is no transplacental transfer of this protein, and levels in infants are lower than those in their mothers.[155] Total serum hemolytic complement (CH_{50}) and alternative pathway activity (PH_{50}) in newborns are lower than in adults, as are mean levels of C1q, C2–C9, properdin, and factors B, I, and H.[156–158] In general, the mean levels in full-term infants are greater than 50 percent of those in normal adult controls and may be somewhat less in premature infants. There is considerable overlap, however, between levels in infants and in controls. A functional deficiency in the alternative pathway has been detected in infants.[159]

Fibronectin mediates more efficient interactions between phagocytes and infectious agents. Fibronectin, a 450-kDa glycoprotein found in plasma and in the intercellular matrix, promotes the attachment of staphylococci to neutrophils[160] and enhances opsonic activity of antibodies against group B streptococci.[161] Because both these bacteria are common pathogens for neonates, the deficiency in fibronectin observed in neonates[162] may further compromise opsonic capacity and hence bactericidal activity in the neonate.

The administration of intravenous IgG may be useful in the treatment or prophylaxis of infection in preterm infants based on the reduced placental transfer of maternal antibody and the restricted endogenous synthesis of IgG.[163] IgG administered to septic neonates appears to enhance serum opsonic capacity as well as to increase the quantity of circulating neutrophils.[164] In premature neonates, added IgG heightens granulocyte phagocytosis.[165] Intravenous IgG has been reported to effectively treat infected premature neonates, but these reports involved small numbers of subjects.[166,167] The clinical efficacy of IgG prophylaxis against neonatal pathogens is not firmly established.[168–170] New IgG preparations with consistent, adequate levels of antibodies directed against neonatal pathogens can be achieved by selection of sera with high levels of functional antibodies,[171] or potentially by the addition of monoclonal antibodies, and these may prove more effective.

Chemotaxis Chemotactic function of leukocytes is low in neonates, whereas random motility is normal.[172–174] Neonatal serum does not generate as much chemotactic factor as does adult serum, even after the addition of purified C3. The defect in chemotaxis may be related to decreased granulocyte deformability and impaired capping of cell surface receptors.[175] The role of observed cyclic adenosine monophosphate (cAMP) and membrane potential alterations in the defective chemotaxis is not clear.[175] The ability of neutrophils to roll along the blood vessel endothelium also is impaired in neonates. Diminished upregulation and surface migration of β_2 integrins and fewer L-selectin receptors reduce the ability of neonatal neutrophils to interact with adhesion molecules on the endothelium.[139]

The densities of the C3bi receptor (CD11b/CD18) and of the low-affinity receptor for immunoglobulin, FcRIII (CD16), are decreased on neutrophils of premature infants, whereas term infants' cells show a lesser impairment.[176–179] The deficient upregulation of C3bi correlates with decreased adherence and chemotaxis by neonatal neutrophils.[180] Low FcRIII is associated with impaired chemotaxis of neonatal neutrophils,[181] although decreased FcRIII might also be responsible for subtle defects in adherence and subsequent phagocytosis of opsonized[171] and unopsonized[182] organisms by neutrophils.

Phagocytic and Bactericidal Activity Phagocytosis of bacteria and latex granules by neutrophils from premature and term infants is normal.[146,150,183,184] Bactericidal activity varies according to the conditions of testing and the clinical status of the neonates. The intracellular killing of *S. aureus* and *S. marcescens* in cells from most term and low-birth-weight infants is normal,[146,185] as is that of *E. coli* in term infants.[147] Similar studies have shown defective bactericidal activity against *S. aureus* in some infants in the first 12 hours after birth,[183] *P. aeruginosa* in cells from premature infants,[150] and *Candida albicans* in granulocytes from term and premature infants.[186] With bacteria-to-neutrophil ratios of 1:1, newborn cells kill *S. aureus* and *E. coli* as effectively as controls; however, at the higher ratio of 100:1, killing and oxidative responses as measured by chemiluminescence are markedly depressed, although phagocytosis is normal.[184] Depressed activity also has been found in cells from newborns who have had clinical stress, either from infection or other disorders, shown both as decreased chemiluminescence and impaired bactericidal activity against *S. aureus*, *E. coli*, and group B streptococci.[187–189] The decreased granulocyte function shown in these studies also is found in liquid culture, where neutrophils from newborns do not survive as long as those from adults, perhaps because of decreased resistance to autoxidation.[188] Although superoxide dismutase levels are normal and superoxide production is normal or increased in neutrophils from newborns, glutathione peroxidase and catalase levels are decreased.[189,190] The relationship of these *in vitro* cellular defects to bacterial infections in the newborn is still not clear.

Antimicrobial proteins and peptides are present in neutrophil cytoplasmic granules. Bacterial permeability-increasing protein (BPI), located in the primary granules, is markedly lower in newborns, particularly preterm newborns.[191,192] BPI is an antimicrobial protein that binds and neutralizes endotoxin. Other granule components, such as myeloperoxidase (bacterial killing) and defensins (antimicrobial proteins), are not diminished.

Monocytes from newborn infants have normal nitroblue tetrazolium (NBT) reduction,[193] normal antibody-dependent cellular cytotoxicity,[194] and normal *in vitro* killing of *S. aureus* and *E. coli*.[195] However, they are slower than monocytes from adults in phagocytosis of polystyrene spheres,[196] and they have reduced ATP production.[197] Furthermore, chemotaxis to serum-derived factors is decreased, as is monocyte appearance in skin windows.[198] These functional aspects may contribute to the observed susceptibility of newborns to a variety of infectious agents.

Cytokine Effects on Neonatal Phagocytic Function There is a complex interaction between cytokines produced by lymphocytes and macrophages, and the activation status of neutrophils during infection. There is decreased production of interferon-γ by neonatal leukocytes.[199,200] Interferon-γ causes the upregulation of the C3bi receptor and induces the surface expression of the high-affinity immunoglobulin receptor FcRI (CD64)[201] on neutrophils. C3bi is required for adherence and efficient chemotaxis by neutrophils. Low levels of this receptor also impair complement-mediated phagocytosis and oxidative metabolism. FcRI also mediates oxidative responses, and appears on neutrophils of adults during infection. The diminished production of G-CSF and GM-CSF by neonatal mononuclear cells[136–138] may not only limit progenitor colony growth, but may also impair neonatal neutrophil functions, including chemotaxis, superoxide production, and C3bi expression, which are enhanced by these factors.[202,203] Tumor necrosis factor (TNF)-α and IL-4, cytokines that modulate neutrophil functions, also may be produced at lower levels in neonates.[204]

THROMBOPOIESIS AND PLATELETS

The platelet counts in term and preterm infants are between 150 and 400×10^9/L (150,000 to 400,000/μL), comparable to adult values.[205,206] Thrombocytopenia of fewer than 100×10^9/L (100,000/μL) may occur in high-risk infants with respiratory distress or sepsis,[207] small-for-date infants,[208] and newborns with trisomy syndromes.[209] Even normal newborns are unable to regulate thrombopoiesis and myelopoiesis in a wholly effective manner.[210] Although committed megakaryocyte progenitors (colony-forming unit–megakaryocyte [CFU-Meg]) are increased in the marrow and cord blood of newborns, they are less able to produce adequate numbers of platelets when severely stressed. Reduced levels of G-CSF, GM-CSF, and IL-3 may play a role in the impaired response.[211] Thrombopoietin (TPO) is a major regulator of platelet production in adults. TPO transcripts have been detected as early as 6 weeks postconception and the primary source of TPO in the fetus and neonate is thought to be the liver.[212] Serum TPO levels are higher in preterm and term neonates compared to adults. However, thrombocytopenic newborns do not increase serum TPO levels as robustly as thrombocytopenic adults, which may contribute to the high incidence of thrombocytopenia seen in sick infants.[212]

Platelet Functions

Bleeding Time and Closure Time The expected inverse relationship between the platelet count and bleeding time has been described in term and preterm newborns.[213] However, the bleeding time often is longer than would be predicted by the platelet count because of sepsis or respiratory distress resulting in impaired platelet function, aggravating the effects of thrombocytopenia.

The bleeding time reflects platelet function and capillary integrity, as well as the platelet count, and traditionally has been used to assess these parameters. However, there are technical difficulties in applying a technique for measuring bleeding time to neonates or preterm infants because of the need for venous occlusion of the forearm, where the test normally is performed, and for a minimal incision to avoid scarring of the skin. Bleeding times were measured using an automatic device to minimize trauma in normal neonates, with venous occlusion of 20 torr for infants who weigh less than 1000 g, 25 torr for those who weigh 1000 to 2000 g, and 30 torr for those who weigh more than 2000 g. In 82 observations, 97 percent of the measurements were below 3.5 minutes, which was suggested as the upper limit for normal in these infants.[214] A similar upper limit (200 seconds) for the bleeding time of normal infants has been obtained using an automated device and vertical incisions.[215] Generally, newborn infants have shorter bleeding times than do children and adults, which may reflect their higher hematocrit, increased concentration of von Willebrand factor, and higher proportion of high-molecular-weight multimers of von Willebrand factor.[216] Children have longer bleeding times than either adults or newborns,[217] and the upper limit measured with an automated pediatric device may be as high as 13 minutes before age 10 years, compared to an upper limit of 7 minutes in adults measured with the same device.[217]

The bleeding times in newborns may be prolonged for a variety of reasons, including neonatal infection and respiratory distress syndrome, which do not necessarily result in thrombocytopenia.[218] Platelets from healthy newborns are relatively deficient in phospholipid metabolism, granule secretion, and aggregation,[219] but there is heightened platelet adhesion because of increased large von Willebrand multimers. The result of these differences is shortened bleeding and closure times in normal neonates (see below).

The use of indomethacin for treatment of patent ductus arteriosus in preterm infants has been questioned because this agent interferes with prostaglandin metabolism and the production of thromboxane A_2, an important initiator of platelet aggregation. Although bleeding times are prolonged from a normal 3.5 minutes to approximately 9 minutes in indomethacin-treated patients,[220] indomethacin did not result in an increase in periventricular or intraventricular hemorrhage in preterm infants treated for patent ductus arteriosus.

The closure time to assess platelet function may replace the bleeding time, particularly for neonates and young children in whom bleeding times are difficult to perform and interpret. The closure time is measured using the PFA-100 system (Dade-Behring Inc., Deerfield, IL) and employs a fine capillary attached to membranes containing collagen-epinephrine and collagen-ADP, combinations of agents that activate platelets. An anticoagulated (3.2% sodium citrate) blood sample is passed through the capillary, and the time to occlusion of the membrane with each agent is measured as the closure time. Newborn infants have closure times that are shorter than those of adults, likely related to their higher hematocrits, increased von Willebrand multimers and hence ristocetin cofactor, and higher leukocyte counts.[221–223] The normal adult value for collagen-epinephrine closure time is less than 164 seconds, and for collagen-ADP closure time is less than 116 seconds. However, each laboratory must determine its own normal range for these tests.

Platelet Aggregation and Metabolism A variety of differences have been described in the platelet function of neonates. These include decreased ADP release, platelet factor 3 activity, platelet adhesiveness, and platelet aggregation in response to ADP, epinephrine, collagen, or thrombin.[224,225] These defects result from intrinsic differences in neonatal compared to adult platelets.[226] Paradoxically, these insufficiencies have little effect on the bleeding time of neonates. The *in vitro* findings do not appear related to a significant defect in prostaglandin synthesis or to storage pool deficiency of adenine nucleotides.[224] Furthermore, electron micrographs of neonatal platelets do not differ from those of platelets from normal adults.[227] This leaves unexplained the *in vitro* observations in neonatal platelets, which may be related to platelet membrane immaturity. These *in vitro* abnormalities may aggravate the impairment in platelet function and the predisposition to bleeding that results from neonatal diseases, particularly respiratory distress syndrome and sepsis.

Maternal aspirin ingestion also results in abnormalities in platelet aggregation in the newborn in response to collagen.[228,229] However, aspirin has been studied extensively in patients with preeclampsia, and there is no significant bleeding in the fetus or newborn.[230,231]

Newborn infants commonly have petechiae, particularly on the head, neck, and shoulders, after vertex deliveries. They are presumably caused by trauma associated with passage through the birth canal and disappear within a few days. Petechiae usually are not present in infants delivered by cesarean section.

Platelet Antigens and Glycoproteins The glycoprotein complex GPIIb/IIIa represents approximately 15 percent of platelet surface protein and exhibits two allelic forms, Pl^{A1} and Pl^{A2}.[232] The Pl^{A1} antigen can be identified on fetal platelets by 16 weeks' gestation.[233] Pl^{A1} antigen is observed in a higher percentage of fetuses between 18 and 26 weeks' gestation than in adults. Approximately 2 percent of the population in the United States of European descent is homozygous for Pl^{A2} and hence they are Pl^{A1}-negative. The complete expression of the Pl^{A1} antigen during early gestation likely permits sensitization in women who are Pl^{A1}-negative even during their first pregnancy.[233] The membrane glycoprotein GPIb, as well as the GPIIb/IIIa complex, is expressed by 18 weeks of gestation.[233] The difference between Pl^{A1} and Pl^{A2} is a leucine 33–proline 33 amino acid polymorphism in glycoprotein IIIA.[232] Prenatal diagnosis of the glycoprotein genotype using DNA from amniocytes and the polymerase chain reaction can establish the potential for neonatal alloimmune thrombocytopenia[234] as well as the diagnosis of Glanzmann thrombasthenia. Rarely, other fetal platelet antigens such as Pl^{E2}, $DUZO^a$, Ko^a, and Bak^a have caused maternal sensitization and neonatal alloimmune thrombocytopenia.[235] The gestational ages for expression of these antigens have not been defined but are sufficiently early to permit sensitization.

NEONATAL LYMPHOPOIESIS

T-Lymphocyte Functions—Cellular Immunity

The absolute number of lymphocytes in the newborn is equivalent to that in older children, ages 6 months to 2 years, with lower values in premature infants at birth. Thymus-derived cells (T cells) develop early in gestation.[236] Tables 6–4 and 6–5 show the various lymphocyte subsets

TABLE 6–4. Blood Lymphocyte Subsets: Infants Age 1 to 3 Days

	Median (10th–90th percentile range)	
Lymphocyte Subsets	Infants (1–3 Days)	Adults
Lymphocytes × 10^9/L	3.1 × 10^9/L (3.1–6.8)	—
CD3+ % of lymphocytes	83% (72–90)	77 (69–84)
Count × 10^9/L	3.7 (2.6–5.8)	—
CD3–/CD19+ % of lymphocytes	14% (6–22)	14 (8–18)
Count × 10^9/L	0.58 (0.23–1.2)	—
NK (CD3–/CD16+ or CD56+) % of lymphocytes	4% (2–8)	11 (6–17)
Count × 10^9/L	0.2 (0.06–0.38)	—
CD3+/CD4+ % of lymphocytes	63% (52–72)	46 (37–55)
Count × 10^9/L	2.7 (2.0–4.4)	—
CD3+/CD8+ % of lymphocytes	23% (16–29)	28 (20–34)
Count × 10^9/L	1.1 (0.55–1.9)	—

SOURCE: Data from O'Gorman MRG, Millard DD, Lowder JN, et al.[237]

in infants and children.[237,238] The absolute number of CD3+ and CD4+ (helper/inducer phenotype) T-cell subsets in blood of newborns is higher than in adults.[239] This is a result of an increased total lymphocyte count in neonates (and older children) as compared with adults.[240] The percentages of major lymphoid subsets (CD2, CD3, CD4, CD8, CD19) and natural killer (NK) cells are not markedly different in neonates, children, and adults when measured by flow cytometry methods.[241,242] However, functional defects are present in the NK cell population.[242] Furthermore, the responses of T-helper type 1 (Th1 cell-mediated immunity) and T-helper type 2 (Th2-assisted humoral immunity) differ in newborns and adults in response to various antigens such as vaccines, infectious agents, and environmental antigens.[243] The numbers of T and B lymphocytes are sustained or increased during the first 2 postnatal months.[244] There is a trend toward increased CD4 and decreased CD8 lymphocytes in newborns and children, resulting in an increased CD4:CD8 ratio.[245,246] In spite of this, T-cell suppressor activity may be increased in newborns.[247] Most responses of the cellular immunity system, such as antigen recognition and binding, antibody-dependent cytotoxicity, and graft-versus-host reactivity are present in the newborn,[247] although some are decreased in comparison with adults.[248] The *in vitro* response to phytohemagglutinin of cord blood lymphocytes is increased,[249,250] but the response of the newborn to 2,4-dinitrofluoro-benzene, a potent inducer of delayed hypersensitivity, is not as consistent as that seen in older children.[251] Impaired T-cell production of interferon-γ and other lymphokines may be related to immature macrophage rather than to T-lymphocyte function, because intercellular cooperation is a requisite for these processes.[252] Furthermore, cord blood T lymphocytes form a functional IL-2 receptor complex and have normal IL-2 receptors, but they do not upregulate interferon-γ in response to IL-2.[253]

B-Lymphocyte Functions–Humoral Immunity

Humoral (B-cell) immunity also develops early in gestation,[236] but it is not fully active until after birth. In the newborn, approximately 15

TABLE 6–5. Blood Lymphocyte Subsets: Infants and Children to Age 18 Years

Lymphocyte Subsets	0–3 months	3–6 months	6–12 months	1–2 years	2–6 years	6–12 years	12–18 years
WBC × 10^9/L	10.60 (7.20–18.00)	9.20 (6.70–14.00)	9.10 (6.40–13.00)	8.80 (6.40–12.00)	7.10 (5.20–11.00)	6.50 (4.40–9.50)	6.00 (4.40–8.10)
Lymphocytes × 10^9/L	5.40 (3.40–7.60)	6.30 (3.90–9.00)	5.90 (3.40–9.00)	5.50 (3.60–8.90)	3.60 (2.30–5.40)	2.70 (1.90–3.70)	2.20 (1.40–3.30)
CD3+							
% of lymphocytes	73% (53–84)	66% (51–77)	65% (49–76)	65% (53–75)	66% (56–75)	69% (60–76)	73% (56–84)
Count × 10^9/L	3.68 (2.50–5.50)	3.75 (2.50–5.60)	3.93 (1.90–5.90)	3.55 (2.10–6.20)	2.39 (1.40–3.70)	1.82 (1.20–2.60)	1.48 (1.00–2.20)
CD19+							
% of lymphocytes	15% (06–32)	25% (11–41)	24% (14–37)	25% (16–35)	21% (14–33)	18% (13–27)	14% (06–23)
Count × 10^9/L	0.73 (0.30–2.00)	1.55 (0.43–3.00)	1.52 (0.61–2.60)	1.31 (0.72–2.60)	0.75 (0.39–1.40)	0.48 (0.27–0.86)	0.30 (0.11–0.57)
CD16+/CD56+							
% of lymphocytes	8% (04–18)	6% (03–14)	7% (03–15)	7% (03–15)	9% (04–17)	9% (04–17)	9% (03–22)
Count × 10^9/L	0.42 (0.17–1.10)	0.42 (0.17–0.83)	0.40 (0.16–0.95)	0.36 (0.18–0.92)	0.30 (0.13–0.72)	0.23 (0.10–0.48)	0.19 (0.07–0.48)
CD4+							
% of lymphocytes	52% (35–64)	46% (35–56)	46% (31–56)	41% (32–51)	38% (28–47)	37% (31–47)	41% (31–52)
Count × 10^9/L	2.61 (1.60–4.00)	2.85 (1.80–4.00)	2.67 (1.40–4.30)	2.16 (1.30–3.40)	1.38 (0.07–2.20)	0.98 (0.65–1.50)	0.84 (0.53–1.30)
CD8+							
% of lymphocytes	18% (12–28)	16% (12–23)	17% (12–24)	20% (14–30)	23% (16–30)	25% (18–35)	26% (18–35)
Count × 10^9/L	0.98 (0.56–1.70)	1.05 (0.59–1.60)	1.04 (0.50–1.70)	1.04 (0.62–2.00)	0.84 (0.49–1.30)	0.68 (0.37–1.10)	0.53 (0.33–0.92)

SOURCE: Data from Shearer WT, Rosenblatt HM, Gelman RS, et al.[238]

percent of lymphocytes have immunoglobulin on their surface, with all Ig isotypes represented.[254] A percentage of these cells are CD5+ B cells (B-1 cells), which produce polyreactive autoantibodies whose function is yet unclear.[255] The proportion of CD5+ B cells is markedly higher in the fetus compared to adults. The percentages of B cells expressing specific immunoglobulin isotypes are not related to the plasma levels of those isotypes. Variation in antibody response to specific antigens relates to the interaction of macrophages, T cells, and B cells. B lymphocytes are well represented in newborns, but T-lymphocyte-independent B-lymphocyte responses are limited during the first year.[256] T-lymphocyte-dependent B-lymphocyte antibody production matures much earlier.[256]

Fetal lymphocytes synthesize little immunoglobulin, presumably because of the sheltered environment *in utero*. Animals kept germ-free after birth have few plasma cells and markedly decreased production of immunoglobulins.[257] IgG levels of term infants are similar to maternal levels because of transplacental transfer.[258] IgM, IgD, and IgE do not cross the placenta,[258,259] and the levels of these immunoglobulins and of IgA are low or not detectable at birth. Breast feeding provides some transfer of antibodies, particularly secretory IgA, lysozyme, and lactoferrin. Large numbers of lymphocytes and monocytes (10^6 cells/mL) are found in colostrum and milk during the first 2 months postpartum.[260] These may provide local gastrointestinal protection against infection,[261,262] and there is some evidence for absorption of immunoglobulin and transfer of tuberculin sensitivity to the infant.

Although the newborn infant can produce specific IgG antibody,[263] only small amounts of IgG are usually produced by the fetus. IgG levels in premature infants are reduced in relation to gestational age because of the low placental transport early in pregnancy.[264–266] The ability of the fetus to produce IgM and IgA with appropriate stimuli is indicated by the presence of these antibodies in many newborn infants who have had prenatal infections[267] and by the presence of IgM isohemagglutinins in more than half of term newborn infants.[268] In human newborns and in fetal animals, the IgM response is predominant, and the appearance of IgG after exposure to specific antigens is delayed. These differences from the adult may relate to functional immaturity of B and T lymphocytes,[269–271] to increased activity of suppressor T cells,[258,269] and perhaps to altered macrophage function.[272]

Newborns also may have relative splenic hypofunction, suggested by the large number of "pocked" red cells seen in the blood films of neonates, particularly premature infants. These "pocks" represent residual intraerythrocyte inclusions, which remain because of monocyte and macrophage hypofunction.[273,274]

COAGULATION IN THE NEONATE

Plasma Coagulation Factors

When the term newborn is compared to older children and adults, several differences in the coagulation and fibrinolytic systems are described.[275–280] A comprehensive evaluation of the developmental changes in the levels of clotting factors and coagulation tests in preterm and term infants has been published.[281,282] The term newborn has reduced mean plasma levels (<60% of adult levels) of factors II, IX, X, XI, XII, prekallikrein, and high-molecular-weight kininogen (Table 6–6). This is not a result of impaired messenger ribonucleic acid (mRNA) expression, at least in the case of factors II and X.[283] In contrast, the plasma concentration of factor VIII is similar and von Willebrand factor is increased compared to that of older children and adults. In spite of the lower levels of factors, the functional tests (prothrombin and partial thromboplastin times) are only slightly prolonged compared to adult normal values (Table 6–6). Although different coagulation factors show different postnatal patterns of maturation, near-adult values are achieved for most components by 6 months of age.[278]

Factors II (prothrombin), VII, IX, and X require vitamin K for the final γ-glutamyl carboxylation step in their synthesis.[284] These factors decrease during the first 3 to 4 days after birth. This fall may be lessened by administration of vitamin K,[285] effectively preventing classic, early occurring (first few days after birth) hemorrhagic disease of the newborn. Inactive prothrombin molecules have been found in the plasma of some newborns, but they disappear after administration of vitamin K.[286] Early occurring hemorrhagic disease is most often associated with maternal administration of medications such as phenytoin (Dilantin)[287] and warfarin,[288] which reduce the vitamin K-dependent factors. In rare cases, no contributing factor is found.

A hemorrhagic diathesis also may occur later, 2 to 12 weeks after birth, as a result of lack of vitamin K, and is called *late hemorrhagic disease of the newborn* or *acquired prothrombin complex deficiency*.[289,290] The etiology of the vitamin K lack is unclear but may result from poor dietary intake, particularly related to breast feeding, alterations in liver function with cholestasis and decreased vitamin K absorption, or a toxic or infectious impairment of hepatic utilization.[289] Unfortunately, intracranial hemorrhage frequently is the presenting event in this condition. This problem can be prevented by parenteral or oral vitamin K, but the preferred route of administration remains controversial.[291] The parenteral route may result rarely in neuromuscular complications,[292] and an association of intramuscular vitamin K prophylaxis and cancer in infancy was suggested but not substantiated. Oral administration, however, appears less reliable and may require repeated doses.[289] The current recommendation of the American Academy of Pediatrics suggests that vitamin K_1, 0.5 to 1 mg, be administered intramuscularly at birth.[293] Even the lower (0.5 mg) parenteral dose may be excessive for preterm (<32 weeks' gestation) infants, although no toxic effects have been reported as a result of very high plasma values.[294] Recent data suggest that 0.2 mg vitamin K may be appropriate prophylaxis for infants delivered at fewer than 32 weeks' gestation, but additional oral supplementation is needed when feeding is established.[295] A mixed micellar vitamin K_1 preparation is particularly well absorbed and may permit prophylaxis with a single oral dose,[296] but the efficacy and safety of oral prophylaxis require further study.

Table 6–6 shows the values for coagulation factors in healthy 30- to 36-weeks' gestation premature infants. More prominent decreases in factors IX, XI, and XII are noted, which tend to prolong the partial thromboplastin time. Table 6–6 also shows the values for coagulation factors in 28- to 31-weeks' gestation infants. All of the coagulation factors are lower at earlier gestational ages.

There are no significant differences in mean prothrombin time determinations between 30- and 36-weeks' gestation premature and full-term infants who have not received vitamin K.[297] Premature infants given vitamin K have a longer mean prothrombin time than do term infants similarly treated. In some small infants there is no improvement in prothrombin time or levels of prothrombin, and factors VII and X after the intramuscular administration of vitamin K.[285,298] These results suggest a greater degree of "immaturity" of the liver in the small infants.

Bleeding and Thrombosis

Significant bleeding occurs more often in low-birth-weight infants than in term newborn infants. Increased capillary fragility is frequently found in premature infants in the first 2 days after birth and

TABLE 6–6. Reference Values for Coagulation Tests in Preterm and Full-Term Infants*

	Preterm 28–31-Week Infants	Preterm 30–36-Week Infants			Full-Term Infants			
Coagulation Test	Day 1	Day 1	Day 30	Day 180	Day 1	Day 30	Day 180	Adults
PT(s)	15.4 (14.6–16.9)	13.0 (10.6–16.2)	11.8 (10.0–13.6)	12.5 (10.0–15.0)	13.0 (10.1–15.9)	11.8 (10.0–14.3)	12.3 (10.7–13.9)	12.4 (10.8–13.9)
INR		1.0 (0.61–1.70)	0.79 (0.53–1.11)	0.91 (0.53–1.48)	1.00 (0.53–1.62)	0.79 (0.53–1.26)	0.88 (0.61–1.17)	0.89 (0.64–1.17)
APTT(s)	108(80.0–168)	53.6(27.5–79.4)	44.7(26.9–62.5)	37.5(27.2–53.5)	42.9(31.3–54.5)	40.4(32.0–55.2)	35.5(28.1–42.9)	33.5(26.6–40.3)
TCT(s)	24.8 (19.2–30.4)	24.4 (18.8–29.9)	25.2 (18.9–31.5)	23.5 (19.0–28.3)	24.3 (19.4–29.2)	25.5 (19.8–31.2)	25.0 (19.7–30.3)	
Fibrinogen (g/L)	2.56 (1.60–5.50)	2.43 (1.50–3.73)	2.54 (1.50–4.14)	2.28 (1.50–3.60)	2.83 (1.67–3.99)	2.70 (1.62–3.78)	2.51 (1.50–3.87)	2.78 (1.56–4.00)
II(U/mL)	0.31(0.19–0.54)	0.45(0.20–0.77)	0.57(0.36–0.95)	0.87(0.51–1.23)	0.48(0.26–0.70)	0.68(0.34–1.02)	0.88(0.60–1.16)	1.08(0.70–1.46)
V (U/mL)	0.65(0.43–0.80)	0.88(0.41–1.44)	1.02(0.48–1.56)	1.02(0.58–1.46)	0.72(0.34–1.08)	0.98(0.62–1.34)	0.91(0.55–1.27)	1.06(0.62–1.50)
VII (U/mL)	0.37(0.24–0.76)	0.67(0.21–1.13)	0.83(0.21–1.45)	0.99(0.47–1.51)	0.66(0.28–1.04)	0.90(0.42–1.38)	0.87(0.47–1.27)	1.05(0.67–1.43)
VIII (U/mL)	0.79(0.37–1.26)	1.11(0.50–2.13)	1.11(0.50–1.99)	0.99(0.50–1.87)	1.00(0.50–1.78)	0.91(0.50–1.57)	0.73(0.50–1.09)	0.99(0.50–1.49)
vWF (U/mL)	1.41(0.83–2.23)	1.36(0.78–2.10)	1.36(0.66–2.16)	0.98(0.54–1.58)	1.53(0.50–2.87)	1.28(0.50–2.46)	1.07(0.50–1.97)	0.92(0.50–1.58)
IX (U/mL)	0.18(0.17–0.20)	0.35(0.19–0.65)	0.44(0.13–0.80)	0.81(0.50–1.20)	0.53(0.15–0.91)	0.51(0.21–0.81)	0.86(0.36–1.36)	1.09(0.55–1.63)
X (U/mL)	0.36(0.25–0.64)	0.41(0.11–0.71)	0.56(0.20–0.92)	0.77(0.35–1.19)	0.40(0.12–0.68)	0.59(0.31–0.87)	0.78(0.38–1.18)	1.06(0.70–1.52)
XI (U/mL)	0.23(0.11–0.33)	0.30(0.08–0.52)	0.43(0.15–0.71)	0.78(0.46–1.10)	0.38(0.10–0.66)	0.53(0.27–0.79)	0.86(0.49–1.34)	0.97(0.67–1.27)
XII (U/mL)	0.25(0.05–0.35)	0.38(0.10–0.66)	0.43(0.11–0.75)	0.82(0.22–1.42)	0.53(0.13–0.93)	0.49(0.17–0.81)	0.77(0.39–1.15)	1.08(0.52–1.64)
PK (U/mL)	0.26(0.15–0.32)	0.33(0.09–0.57)	0.59(0.31–0.87)	0.78(0.40–1.16)	0.37(0.18–0.69)	0.57(0.23–0.91)	0.86(0.56–1.16)	1.12(0.62–1.62)
HK (U/mL)	0.32(0.19–0.52)	0.49(0.09–0.89)	0.64(0.16–1.12)	0.83(0.41–1.25)	0.54(0.06–1.02)	0.77(0.33–1.21)	0.82(0.36–1.28)	0.92(0.50–1.36)
XIIIa (U/mL)		0.70(0.32–1.08)	0.99(0.51–1.47)	1.13(0.65–1.61)	0.79(0.27–1.31)	0.93(0.39–1.47)	1.04(0.46–1.62)	1.05(0.55–1.55)
XIIIb (U/mL)		0.81(0.35–1.27)	1.07(0.57–1.57)	1.15(0.67–1.63)	0.76(0.30–1.22)	1.11(0.39–1.73)	1.10(0.50–1.70)	0.97(0.57–1.37)

APTT, activated partial thromboplastin time; HK, high-molecular-weight kininogen; INR, international normalized ratio; PK, prekallikrein; PT, prothrombin time; TCT, thrombin clotting time; vWF, von Willebrand factor.

*All factors except fibrinogen are expressed as units per milliliter (U/mL), where pooled plasma contains 1.0 U/mL. All values are expressed as the mean of 40 to 77 samples for each population. The range of values encompassing 95% of the population is shown in parentheses.

SOURCE: Modified from Andrew M, Paes B, Milner B, et al,[278] and Andrew M, Paes B, Johnston M,[281] with permission.

TABLE 6–7. Reference Values for Inhibitors of Coagulation in Preterm and Full-Term Infants*

Inhibitor Levels	Day 1	Day 30	Day 180	Day 1	Day 30	Day 180	Adults
AT (U/mL)	0.38 (0.14–0.62)	0.59 (0.37–0.81)	0.90 (0.52–1.28)	0.63 (0.39–0.87)	0.78 (0.48–1.08)	1.04 (0.84–1.24)	1.05 (0.79–1.31)
α_2M (U/mL)	1.10 (0.56–1.82)	1.38 (0.72–2.04)	2.09 (1.10–3.21)	1.39 (0.95–1.83)	1.50 (1.06–1.94)	1.91 (1.49–2.33)	0.86 (0.52–1.20)
C_1E-INH (U/mL)	0.65 (0.31–0.99)	0.74 (0.40–1.24)	1.40 (0.96–2.04)	0.72 (0.36–1.08)	0.89 (0.47–1.31)	1.41 (0.89–1.93)	1.01 (0.71–1.31)
α_1AT (U/mL)	0.90 (0.36–1.44)	0.76 (0.38–1.12)	0.82 (0.48–1.16)	0.93 (0.49–1.37)	0.62 (0.36–0.88)	0.77 (0.47–1.07)	0.93 (0.55–1.31)
HCII (U/mL)	0.32 (0.10–0.60)	0.43 (0.15–0.71)	0.89 (0.45–1.40)	0.43 (0.10–0.93)	0.47 (0.10–0.87)	1.20 (0.50–1.90)	0.96 (0.66–1.26)
Protein C (U/mL)	0.28 (0.12–0.44)	0.37 (0.15–0.59)	0.57 (0.31–0.83)	0.35 (0.17–0.53)	0.43 (0.21–0.65)	0.59 (0.37–0.81)	0.96 (0.64–1.28)
Protein S (U/mL)	0.26 (0.14–0.38)	0.56 (0.22–0.90)	0.82 (0.44–1.20)	0.36 (0.12–0.60)	0.63 (0.33–0.93)	0.87 (0.55–1.19)	0.92 (0.60–1.24)

α_1AT, α_1-antitrypsin; α_2M, α_2-macroglobulin; AT, antithrombin; C_1 esterase inhibitor; C_1E-INH, HCII, heparin cofactor II.

*All values are expressed in units per milliliter (U/mL) where pooled plasma contains 1.0 U/mL. All values are expressed as the mean of 40 to 75 samples for each population. The range of values encompassing 95% of the population is shown in parentheses.

SOURCE: Modified from Andrew M, Paes B, Milner B, et al,[278] and Andrew M, Paes B, Johnston M,[281] with permission.

is not associated with thrombocytopenia.[285] Bleeding under the scalp or in other superficial areas may be caused by trauma at birth coupled with increased capillary fragility. The more serious disorders of periventricular–intraventricular hemorrhage and pulmonary hemorrhage probably are not caused by coagulation disorders, although such disorders may increase the bleeding.[299] Hypoxia seems to affect the clotting status of low-birth-weight infants.[300] Many infants with markedly abnormal prothrombin times have had hypoxia during delivery or shortly thereafter.[295] Cardiovascular collapse seen with episodes of cardiac arrest or with profound shock may cause disseminated intravascular coagulation and generalized bleeding. In many sick premature infants, a combination of shock, sepsis, liver immaturity, hypoxia, and other factors may contribute to the pathogenesis of coagulation abnormalities.

Arterial and venous thromboses are relatively frequent in newborns as compared to other age groups, but greater than 90 percent of arterial and greater than 80 percent of venous clots are related to catheters. Spontaneous thromboses are much less common, and most involve the renal veins or, rarely, the pulmonary vasculature.[301] Relative hypercoagulability in the newborn could result from a difference in the vascular endothelium, activation of the coagulation cascade, diminished coagulation inhibitor activity, or a defect in fibrinolysis. Inhibitors of coagulation include antithrombin, heparin cofactor II, protein C, and protein S.[282,302] The levels of proteins C and S, which are vitamin K-dependent, as well as antithrombin and heparin cofactor II, are low in the newborn; they are in a range associated with thrombotic episodes in adults with inherited deficiencies.[302] In addition, the presence of factor V Leiden may occur in as many as 6 percent of newborns.[303] This produces resistance to the action of protein C and may heighten the susceptibility to thrombosis. Hyperprothrombinemia caused by the 20210A allele prothrombin gene may affect 1 percent of the population,[304] but the elevated prothrombin level predisposing to thrombosis occurs in older patients.[305] The combined deficiency of these anticoagulant proteins may further intensify the thrombotic risk. However, the precise role of these inhibitors of coagulation in newborn hypercoagulability is uncertain because a proportionate decrease in vitamin K-dependent procoagulant factors (II, VII, IX, X) also is present, and an additional inhibitor, α_2-macroglobulin, is increased. Table 6–7 shows the values for plasma inhibitors of coagulation in premature and term infants.

HEMATOLOGIC EFFECTS OF MATERNAL DRUGS ON THE FETUS AND NEWBORN

Hemostatic Effects

A number of maternally administered pharmacologic agents have been implicated in hematologic abnormalities of the fetus or newborn (Table 6–8). Maternal aspirin ingestion results in impaired platelet aggregation but does not foster neonatal bleeding. Other agents taken by the mother, including diazoxide and thiazides, might be associated with neonatal thrombocytopenia.[306–308]

The newborn's plasma coagulation factors may be depressed by maternal warfarin ingestion.[288] This drug is best avoided during pregnancy because it is teratogenic (first trimester) and may cause growth retardation of the fetus as well as bleeding.[288] In contrast, heparin does not cross the placenta, and maternal treatment with heparin appears to be safe for the fetus.[309]

Phenytoin (Dilantin) and/or phenobarbital also may reduce the newborn's vitamin K-dependent factors, possibly by microsomal enzyme induction, which enhances their degradation.[287] Furthermore, phenytoin may depress the platelet count as a result of prenatal exposure[310] and cause teratogenic effects, for example, the fetal hydantoin syndrome.[311] The decision to use this agent during pregnancy should reflect an assessment of the need for this specific drug, and also the risk of maternal seizures to the fetus and mother versus the potential side effects of treatment. Newborns of mothers taking rifampin and isoniazid also may have depressed vitamin K-dependent factors.[312]

Hyperbilirubinemia and Kernicterus

Nitrofurantoin and nalidixic acid may cause oxidant injury to the red cell membrane and hemoglobin.[313,314] If there is glucose-6-phosphate dehydrogenase deficiency, or if reduced glutathione is diminished, as in newborn red cells, these drugs have the potential to induce hemolysis and heighten neonatal hyperbilirubinemia. Although this problem has not been documented by transplacental transfer of nitrofurantoin or nalidixic acid, hemolysis has occurred in glucose-6-phosphate dehydrogenase-deficient infants who acquired the drugs from breast milk.[314,315] Alternatively, sulfonamides may cause displacement of bilirubin bound to albumin and heighten the risk of kernicterus.[316] Salicylates, phenylbutazone, and naproxen may have a similar effect at very high plasma concentrations.[316] Ideally, all these medications should be

TABLE 6–8. Hematologic Effects of Maternal Drugs on the Fetus and Newborn

Drug	Effect	Certainty*	Mechanism	Reference
Antiretroviral agents in combination	Decreased hemoglobin	Established	Unknown—only seen with combination of zidovudine, lamivudine + nelfinavir	317
Aspirin	Bleeding; kernicterus	Established; potential	Interference with platelet function	122, 224, 228
			Displacement of bilirubin from albumin	316
Diazoxide	Bleeding	Questionable	Thrombocytopenia	306
Nalidixic acid	Hyperbilirubinemia	Potential	Oxidant damage to hemoglobin	314
Nitrofurantoin	Hyperbilirubinemia	Potential	Oxidant damage to hemoglobin	313, 315
Phenytoin (Dilantin/ phenobarbital)	Bleeding	Suspected	Depletion of vitamin K-dependent coagulation factors by hepatic enzyme induction and factor degradation	287
Rifampin/isoniazid	Bleeding	Suspected	Depletion of vitamin K-dependent coagulation factors	312
Sulfonamides	Kernicterus	Established	Displacement of bilirubin from albumin	316
Thiazides	Bleeding	Suspected	Thrombocytopenia	307, 308
Warfarin (Coumadin)	Bleeding	Established	Known depletion of vitamin K-dependent coagulation factors by blocking carboxylation	287, 288

*Certainty reflects the level of confidence in the data, assigned in increasing order from potential through questionable, suspected, and established.

SOURCE: Based on Miller RK, Kellogg CR, Saltzman RA.[306]

avoided during pregnancy unless their indication outweighs the potential risk to the fetus and newborn.

REFERENCES

1. Bloom W, Bartelmez GW: Hematopoiesis in young human embryos. *Am J Anat* 67:21, 1940.
2. Huber TL, Kouskoff V, Fehling HJ, et al: Haemangioblast commitment is initiated in the primitive streak of the mouse embryo. *Nature* 432:625, 2004.
3. Zambidis ET, Peault B, Park TS, et al: Hematopoietic differentiation of human embryonic stem cells progresses through sequential hematoendothelial, primitive, and definitive stages resembling human yolk sac development. *Blood* 106:860, 2005.
4. Kennedy M, D'Souza SL, Lynch-Kattman, et al: Development of the hemangioblast defines the onset of hematopoiesis in human ES cell differentiation cultures. *Development* 109:2679, 2007.
5. Shivdasani RA, Mayer EL, Orkin SH: Absence of blood formation in mice lacking T-cell leukemia oncoprotein tal-1/SCL. *Nature* 373:432, 1995.
6. Warren AJ, Colledge WH, Carlton MBL, et al: The oncogenic cysteine-rich LIM domain protein is essential for erythroid development. *Cell* 78:45, 1994.
7. Fujiwara Y, Browne CP, Cuniff K, Goff SC, Orkin SH: Arrested development of embryonic red cell precursors in mouse embryos lacking transcription factor GATA-1. *Proc Natl Acad Sci U S A* 93:12355, 1996.
8. Tavian M, Hallais M-F, Peault B: Emergence of intraembryonic hematopoietic precursors in the pre-liver human embryo. *Development* 126:793, 1999.
9. Peschle C, Mavilio F, Care A, et al: Haemoglobin switching in human embryos: Asynchrony of zeta→alpha and epsilon→gamma-globin switches in primitive and definite erythropoietic lineage. *Nature* 313:235, 1985.
10. Knoll W: Blut und blutbildende organe menschlicher embryonen. *Denkschriften der Schweizerischen Naturforschenden Gesellschaft* 64:1, 1927.
11. Fukuda T: Fetal hemopoiesis. I. Electron microscopic studies on human yolk sac hemopoiesis. *Virchows Arch B Cell Pathol* 14:197, 1973.
12. Kingsley PD, Malik J, Fantauzzo KA, Palis J: Yolk sac derived primitive erythroblasts enucleate during mammalian embryogenesis. *Blood* 104:19, 2004.
13. Palis J, Robertson S, Kennedy M, Wall C, Keller G: Development of erythroid and myeloid progenitors in the yolk sac and embryo proper of the mouse. *Development* 126:5073, 1999.
14. Tober J, Koniski A, McGrath KE, et al: The megakaryocyte lineage originates from hemangioblast precursors and is an integral component both of primitive and definitive hematopoiesis. *Blood* 109:1433, 2007.
15. Migliaccio G, Migliaccio AR, Petti S, et al: Human embryonic hemopoiesis. Kinetics of progenitors and precursors underlying the yolk sac–liver transition. *J Clin Invest* 78:51, 1986.
16. Tavian M, Peault B: Embryonic development of the human hematopoietic system. *Int J Dev Biol* 49:243, 2005.
17. Huyhn A, Dommergues M, Izac B, et al: Characterization of hematopoietic progenitors from human yolk sacs and embryos. *Blood* 86:4474, 1995.
18. Dommergues M, Aubeny E, Dumez Y, et al: Hematopoiesis in the human yolk sac: Quantitation of erythroid and granulopoietic progenitors between 3.5 and 8 weeks of development. *Bone Marrow Transplant* 9:23, 1992.
19. Keleman E, Calvo W, Fliedner TM: *Atlas of Human Hemopoietic Development*. Springer-Verlag, Berlin, 1979.
20. Lin C-S, Lim S-K, D'Agati V, Constantini F: Differential effects of an erythropoietin receptor gene disruption on primitive and definitive erythropoiesis. *Genes Dev* 10:154, 1996.
21. Neubauer H, Cumano A, Muller M, et al: Jak2 deficiency defines an essential developmental checkpoint in definitive hematopoiesis. *Cell* 93:397, 1998.
22. Valtieri M, Gabbianelli M, Pelosi E, et al: Erythropoietin alone induces erythroid burst formation by human embryonic but not adult BFU-E in unicellular serum-free culture. *Blood* 74:460, 1989.
23. Emerson SG, Shanti T, Ferrara JL, Greenstein JL: Developmental regulation of erythropoiesis by hematopoietic growth factors: Analysis on populations of BFU-E from bone marrow, peripheral blood, and fetal liver. *Blood* 74:49, 1989.
24. Dame C, Fahnenstich H, Feitag P, et al: Erythropoietin mRNA expression in human fetal and neonatal tissue. *Blood* 92:3218, 1998.
25. Mucenski ML, McLain K, Kier AB, et al: A functional c-myb gene is required for normal murine fetal hepatic hematopoiesis. *Cell* 65:677, 1991.
26. Hann IM, Bodger MP, Hoffbrand AV: Development of pluripotent hematopoietic progenitor cells in the human fetus. *Blood* 62:118, 1983.
27. Nicola NA, Metcalf D: Specificity of action of colony-stimulating factors in the differentiation of granulocytes and macrophages. *CIBA Found Symp* 118:7, 1986.
28. Ohls RK, Li Y, Abdel-Mageed A, et al: Neutrophil pool sizes and granulocyte colony-stimulating factor production in human mid-trimester fetuses. *Pediatr Res* 37:806, 1995.
29. Slayton WB, Juul SE, Calhoun DA, et al: Hematopoiesis in the liver and marrow of human fetuses at 5 to 16 weeks postconception: quantitative assessment of macrophage and neutrophil populations. *Pediatr Res* 43:774, 1998.
30. Pahal GS, Jauniaux E, Kinnon C, et al: Normal development of human hematopoiesis between eight and seventeen weeks' gestation. *Am J Obstet Gynecol* 183:1029, 2000.
31. Gupta S, Pahwa R, O'Reilly R, et al: Ontogeny of lymphocyte subpopulation in human fetal liver. *Proc Natl Acad Sci U S A* 73:919, 1976.
32. Rainaut M, Pagniez M, Hercend T, et al: Characterization of mononuclear cell subpopulations in normal fetal peripheral blood. *Hum Immunol* 18:331, 1987.
33. Hann IM, Gibson BES, Letsky EA: *Fetal and Neonatal Hematology*. Baillaire Tindale, Philadelphia, 1991.
34. Charbord P, Tavian M, Humeau L, Peault B: Early ontogeny of the human marrow from long bones: An immunohistochemical study of hematopoiesis and its microenvironment. *Blood* 87:4109, 1996.

35. Cairo MS, Wagner JE: Placental and/or umbilical cord blood: An alternative source of hematopoietic stem cells for transplantation. *Blood* 90:4665, 1997.
36. Touraine JL, Raudrant D, Laplace S: Transplantation of hemopoietic cells from the fetal liver to treat patients with congenital diseases postnatally or prenatally. *Transplant Proc* 29:712, 1997.
37. Maximow AA: Relation of blood cells to connective tissues and endothelium. *Physiol Rev* IV(4):532, 1924.
38. Houssaint E: Differentiation of the mouse hepatic primordium. II. Extrinsic origin of the haemopoietic cell line. *Cell Differ* 10:243, 1981.
39. Cudennec CA, Thiery J-P, Le Douarin N-M: *In vitro* induction of adult erythropoiesis in early mouse yolk sac. *Proc Natl Acad Sci U S A* 78:2412, 1981.
40. Moore MAS, Owen JJT: Stem-cell migration in developing myeloid and lymphoid systems. *Lancet* i:658, 1967.
41. Dieterlen-Lievre F: On the origin of hematopoietic stem cells in the avian embryo: An experimental approach. *J Embryol Exp Morphol* 33:607, 1975.
42. Carpenter KL, Turpen JB: Experimental studies on hemopoiesis in the pronephros of *Rana pipiens*. *Differentiation* 14:167, 1979.
43. Muller AM, Medvinsky A, Strouboulis J, et al: Development of hematopoietic stem cell activity in the mouse embryo. *Immunity* 1:291, 1994.
44. Smith RA, Glomski CA: "Hemogenic endothelium" of the embryonic aorta: Does it exist? *Dev Comp Immunol* 6:359, 1982.
45. Tavian M, Coulombel L, Luton D, et al: Aorta-associated CD-34+ hematopoietic cells in the early human embryo. *Blood* 87:67, 1996.
46. Gekas C, Dieterlen-Lièvre F, Orkin SH, Mikkola HK: The placenta is a niche for hematopoietic stem cells. *Dev Cell* 8:297, 2005.
47. Proudfoot NJ, Shander MH, Manley JL, et al: Structure and in vitro transcription of human globin genes. *Science* 209:1329, 1980.
48. Grosveld F, Van Assendelft GB, Greaves DR, Kolias B: Position independent, high-level expression of the human globin gene in transgenic mice. *Cell* 51:975, 1987.
49. Hecht F, Motulsky AG, Lemire RJ, et al: Predominance of hemoglobin Gower 1 in early human embryonic development. *Science* 152:91, 1966.
50. Huehns ER, Dance N, Beaven GH, et al: Human embryonic hemoglobins. *Cold Spring Harb Symp Quant Biol* 29:327, 1964.
51. Gale RE, Clegg JB, Huehns ER: Human embryonic haemoglobins Gower 1 and Gower 2. *Nature* 280:162, 1979.
52. Pataryas HA, Stomatoyannopoulos G: Hemoglobins in human fetuses: Evidence of adult hemoglobin production after the 11th gestational week. *Blood* 39:688, 1972.
53. Thomas ED, Lochte HL Jr, Greenough WB III, et al: *In vitro* synthesis of foetal and adult haemoglobin by foetal haematopoietic tissues. *Nature* 185:396, 1960.
54. Kazazian HH, Woodhead AP: Hemoglobin A synthesis in the developing fetus. *N Engl J Med* 289:58, 1973.
55. Bard H: The effect of placental insufficiency on fetal and adult hemoglobin synthesis. *Am J Obstet Gynecol* 120:67, 1974.
56. Kirschbaum T: Fetal hemoglobin content of cord blood determined by column chromatography. *Am J Obstet Gynecol* 84:1375, 1962.
57. Armstrong D, Schroeder WA, Fenninger W: A comparison of the percentage of fetal hemoglobin in human umbilical cord blood as determined by chromatography and by alkali denaturation. *Blood* 22:554, 1963.
58. Bard H: Postnatal fetal and adult hemoglobin synthesis in early preterm newborn infants. *J Clin Invest* 60:1789, 1973.
59. Metaxotou-Mavromati AD, Antonopoulou HK, Laskari SA, et al: Developmental changes in hemoglobin F levels during the first two years of life in normal and heterozygous -thalassemia infants. *Pediatrics* 69:734, 1982.
60. Bard H, Makowski EL, Meschia G, et al: The relative rates of synthesis of hemoglobins A and F in red cells of newborn infants. *Pediatrics* 45:766, 1970.
61. Bromberg YN, Abrahamov A, Salzberger M: The effect of maternal anoxemia on the foetal haemoglobin of the newborn. *J Obstet Gynaecol Br Commonw* 63:875, 1956.
62. Huehns ER, Hecht F, Keil JV, et al: Developmental hemoglobin anomalies in a chromosomal triplication. *Proc Natl Acad Sci U S A* 51:89, 1964.
63. Lee CSN, Boyer SH, Bowen P, et al: The D1 trisomy syndrome: Three subjects with unequally advancing development. *Johns Hopkins Med J* 118:374, 1966.
64. Giulian GG, Gilbert EF, Moss RL: Elevated fetal hemoglobin levels in sudden infant death syndrome. *N Engl J Med* 316:1122, 1987.
65. Wilson MG, Schroeder WA, Graves DA: Postnatal change of hemoglobins F and A2 in infants with Down's syndrome (G trisomy). *Pediatrics* 42:349, 1968.
66. Brown MS: Fetal and neonatal erythropoieses, in *Developmental and Neonatal Hematology*, edited by JA Stockman, III, C Pochedly, p 39. Raven Press, New York, 1988.
67. Forestier F, Daffos F, Galacteros F, et al: Haematological values of 163 normal fetuses between 18 and 30 weeks of gestation. *Pediatr Res* 20:342, 1986.
68. Millar DS, Davis LR, Rodich CH, et al: Normal blood cell values in the early midtrimester fetus. *Prenat Diagn* 5:367, 1985.
69. Linch DC, Knott LJ, Rodech CH, et al: Studies of circulating hemopoietic progenitor cells in human fetal blood. *Blood* 59:976, 1982.
70. Christensen RD: Hematopoiesis in the fetus and neonate. *Pediatr Res* 26:531, 1989.
71. Marks J, Gairdner D, Roscoe JD: Blood formation in infancy. III. Cord blood. *Arch Dis Child* 30:117, 1955.
72. Linderkamp O, Versmold HT, Messow-Zahn K, et al: The effect of intrapartum and intra-uterine asphyxia on placental transfusion in premature and full-term infants. *Eur J Pediatr* 127:91, 1978.
73. Mercer JS: Current best evidence: A review of the literature on umbilical cord clamping. *J Midwifery Womens Health* 46:402, 2001.
74. Yao AC, Hirvensalo M, Lind J: Placental transfusion rate and uterine contraction. *Lancet* 1:380, 1968.
75. Usher R, Shepard M, Lind J, et al: The blood volume of the newborn and placental transfusion. *Acta Paediatr* 52:497, 1963.
76. Bratteby LE: Studies on erythro-kinetics in infancy. XI. The change in circulating red cell volume during the first five months of life. *Acta Paediatr Scand* 57:215, 1968.
77. McCue CM, Garner FB, Hurt WG, et al: Placental transfusion. *J Pediatr* 72:15, 1968.
78. Matoth Y, Zaizor R, Varsano I: Postnatal changes in some red cell parameters. *Acta Paediatr Scand* 60:317, 1971.
79. Linderkamp O, Versmold HT, Strohhacker I, et al: Capillary-venous hematocrit differences in newborn infants. *Eur J Pediatr* 127:9, 1977.
80. Saarinen UM, Simmes MA: Developmental changes in red blood cell counts and indices of infants after exclusion of iron deficiency by laboratory criteria and continuous iron supplementation. *J Pediatr* 92:412, 1978.
81. Zipursky A, Brown E, Palko J, et al: The erythrocyte differential count in newborn infants. *Am J Pediatr Hematol Oncol* 5:45, 1983.
82. Alter BP, Goldberg JD, Berkowitz RL: Red cell size heterogeneity during ontogeny. *Am J Pediatr Hematol Oncol* 10:279, 1988.
83. Shannon KM, Naylor GS, Torkildson JC, et al: Circulating erythroid progenitors in the anemia of prematurity. *N Engl J Med* 317:728, 1987.
84. Linch DC, Knott LJ, Rodeck CH, Huehns ER: Studies of circulating hemopoietic progenitor cells in human fetal blood. *Blood* 59:976, 1983.
85. Christensen RD: Circulating pluripotent hematopoietic progenitor cells in neonates. *J Pediatr* 11:622, 1987.
86. Clapp DW, Baley JE, Gerson SL: Gestational age dependent changes in circulating hematopoietic stem cells in newborn infants. *J Lab Clin Med* 113:422, 1989.
87. Holbrook SR, Christensen RD, Rothstein G: Erythroid colonies derived from fetal blood display different growth patterns from those derived from adult marrow. *Pediatr Res* 24:605, 1988.
88. Burman D, Morris AF: Cord hemoglobin in low birth weight infants. *Arch Dis Child* 49:382, 1974.
89. Meberg A: Haemoglobin concentrations and erythropoietin levels in appropriate and small for gestational age infants. *Scand J Haematol* 24:162, 1980.
90. Zaizov R, Matoth Y: Red cell values on the first postnatal day during the last 16 weeks of gestation. *Am J Hematol* 1:275, 1976.
91. Lockridge S, Pass R, Cassidy G: Reticulocyte counts in intrauterine growth retardation. *Pediatrics* 47:919, 1971.
92. Humbert JR, Abelson H, Hathaway WE, et al: Polycythemia in small for gestational age infants. *J Pediatr* 75:1812, 1969.
93. Halvorsen S, Finne PH: Erythropoietin production in the human fetus and newborn. *Ann N Y Acad Sci* 149:576, 1968.
94. Seip M: The reticulocyte level and the erythrocyte production judged from reticulocyte studies in newborn infants during the first week of life. *Acta Paediatr Scand* 44:355, 1955.
95. Mann DL, Sites ML, Donati RM, et al: Erythropoietic stimulating activity during the first ninety days of life. *Proc Soc Exp Biol Med* 118: 212, 1965.
96. Lundstrom U, Simmes MA: Red blood cell values in low-birth-weight infants: Ages at which values become equivalent to those of term infants. *J Pediatr* 96:1040, 1980.
97. Stockman JA III, Garcia JF, Oski FA: The anemia of prematurity: Factors governing the erythropoietin response. *N Engl J Med* 296:647, 1977.
98. MackIntosh TF, Walker CHM: Blood viscosity in the newborn. *Arch Dis Child* 48:547, 1973.
99. Bergqvist G: Viscosity of the blood in the newborn infant. *Acta Paediatr Scand* 63:858, 1974.
100. Wirth FH, Goldberg WR, Lubchenco L: Neonatal hyperviscosity. I. Incidence. *Pediatrics* 63:833, 1979.
101. Hakanson DO, Oh W: Hyperviscosity in the small-for-gestational age infant. *Biol Neonate* 37:190, 1980.
102. Ramamurthy RS, Berlanga M: Postnatal alteration in hematocrit and viscosity in normal and polycythemic infants. *J Pediatr* 110:929, 1987.
103. Bada HS, Korones SB, Pourcyrous M, et al: Asymptomatic syndrome of polycythemic hyperviscosity: Effect of partial plasma exchange transfusion. *J Pediatr* 120:579, 1992.
104. Sarkar S, Rosenkrantz TS: Neonatal polycythemia and hyperviscosity. *Semin Fetal Neonatal Med* 13:248, 2008.
105. Bierhuizen MF, Mattei MG, Fukuda M: Expression of the developmental I antigen by a cloned human cDNA encoding a member of a beta-1,6-N-acetylglucosaminyltransferase gene family. *Genes Dev* 7:468, 1993.
106. Race RR, Sanger R: *Blood Groups in Man*, 6th ed. Blackwell Scientific, London, 1975.
107. Pearson HA: Life-span of the fetal red blood cell. *J Pediatr* 70:166, 1967.
108. Weipple G, Pantlitschko M, Bauer P, et al: Normal values and distribution of serum iron in cord blood. *Clin Chim Acta* 44:147, 1973.
109. Saarinen UM, Siimes MA: Developmental changes in serum iron, total iron-binding capacity, and transferrin saturation in infancy. *J Pediatr* 91:875, 1977.
110. Saarinen UM, Siimes MA: Serum ferritin in assessment of iron nutrition in healthy infants. *Acta Paediatr Scand* 67:745, 1978.
111. Seip M, Halvorsen S: Erythrocyte production and iron stores in premature infants during the first months of life. The anemia of prematurity—Etiology, pathogenesis, iron requirement. *Acta Paediatr Scand* 45:600, 1956.

112. Rao R, Georgieff MK: Perinatal aspects of iron metabolism. *Acta Paediatr Suppl* 91:124, 2002.
113. Bauer C, Ludwig I, Ludwig M: Different effects of 2,3-diphosphoglycerate and adenosine triphosphate on oxygen affinity of adult and fetal hemoglobin. *Life Sci* 7:1339, 1968.
114. Oski FA: Red cell metabolism in the newborn infant. V. Glycolytic intermediates and glycolytic enzymes. *Pediatrics* 44:84, 1969.
115. Oski FA, Delivoria-Papadopoulos M: The red cell, 2,3-diphosphoglycerate, and tissue oxygen release. *J Pediatr* 77:941, 1970.
116. Zipursky A: The erythrocytes of the newborn infant. *Semin Hematol* 2:167, 1965.
117. Oski FA, Komazawa M: Metabolism of the erythrocytes of the newborn infant. *Semin Hematol* 12:209, 1975.
118. Oski FA, Smith CA: Red cell metabolism in the premature infant. III. Apparent inappropriate glucose consumption for cell age. *Pediatrics* 41:473, 1968.
119. Konrad PN, Valentine WN, Paglia DE: Enzymatic activities and glutathione content of erythrocytes in the newborn: comparison with red cells of older normal subjects and those with comparable reticulocytosis. *Acta Haematol* 48:193, 1972.
120. Gross RT, Schroeder EAR, Brounstein SA: Energy metabolism in the erythrocytes of premature infants compared to full term newborn infants and adults. *Blood* 21:755, 1963.
121. Oski FA: Red cell metabolism in the premature infant. II. The pentose phosphate pathway. *Pediatrics* 39:689, 1967.
122. Bracci R, Perrone S, Buonocore G: Oxidant injury in neonatal erythrocytes during the neonatal period. *Acta Paediatr Suppl* 91:130, 2002.
123. Ross JD: Deficient activity of DPNH-dependent methemoglobin diaphorase in cord blood erythrocytes. *Blood* 21:51, 1963.
124. Gross RT, Bracci R, Rudolph N, et al: Hydrogen peroxide toxicity and detoxification in erythrocytes of newborn infants. *Blood* 29:481, 1967.
125. Whaun JM, Oski FA: Red cell stromal adenosine triphosphatase (ATPase) of newborn infants. *Pediatr Res* 3:105, 1969.
126. Blum SF, Oski FA: Red cell metabolism in the newborn infant. IV. Transmembrane potassium flux. *Pediatrics* 43:396, 1969.
127. Crowley J, Ways P, Jones JW: Human fetal erythrocyte and plasma lipids. *J Clin Invest* 44:989, 1965.
128. Neerhout RC: Erythrocyte lipids in the neonate. *Pediatr Res* 2:172, 1968.
129. Shapiro DL, Pasqualini P: Erythrocyte membrane proteins of premature and full-term infants. *Pediatr Res* 12:176, 1978.
130. Kosztolanyi G, Jobst K: Electrokinetic analysis of the fetal erythrocyte membrane after trypsin digestion. *Pediatr Res* 14:138, 1980.
131. Altman PL, Dittmer DS: *Blood and Other Body Fluids.* Federation of American Societies for Experimental Biology, Washington, DC, 1961.
132. Coulombel L, Dehan M, Tchernia G, et al: The number of polymorphonuclear leukocytes in relation to gestational age in the newborn. *Acta Paediatr Scand* 68:709, 1979.
133. Laver J, Duncan E, Abboud M, et al: High levels of granulocyte and granulocyte-macrophage colony-stimulating factors in cord blood of normal full-term neonates. *J Pediatr* 116:627, 1990.
134. Ijima H, Suda T, Miura Y: Predominance of macrophage-colony formation in human cord blood. *Exp Hematol* 10:234, 1982.
135. Prindull G, Ben-Ishay Z, Gabriel M, et al: A comparison of spontaneous and CSF added CFU-GM colony formation in healthy, sick and hypotrophic pre-term infants. *Blut* 45:167, 1982.
136. Satwani P, Morris E, van de Ven C, et al: Dysregulation of expression of immunoregulatory and cytokine genes and its association with the immaturity in neonatal phagocytic and cellular immunity. *Biol Neonate* 88:214, 2005.
137. English BK, Hammond WP, Lewis DB, et al: Decreased granulocyte-macrophage colony-stimulating factor production by human neonatal blood mononuclear cells and T cells. *Pediatr Res* 31:211, 1992.
138. Cairo MS, Suen Y, Knoppel E, et al: Decreased G-CSF and IL-3 production and gene expression from mononuclear cells of newborn infants. *Pediatr Res* 31:574, 1992.
139. Carr R: Neutrophil production and function in newborn infants. *Br J Haematol* 110:18, 2000.
140. Rosenthal J, Cairo MS: The role of cytokines in modulating neonatal myelopoiesis and host defense. *Cytokines Mol Ther* 1:165, 1995.
141. Banerjea MC, Speer CP: The current role of colony-stimulating factors in prevention and treatment of neonatal sepsis. *Semin Neonatol* 7:335, 2002.
142. Kucukoduk S, Sezer T, Yildiran A, et al: Randomized, double- blinded, placebo-controlled trial of early administration of recombinant human granulocyte colony-stimulating factor to non-neutropenic preterm newborns between 33 and 36 weeks with presumed sepsis. *Scand J Infect Dis* 34:893, 2002.
143. Xanthou M: Leucocyte blood picture in healthy full-term and premature babies during neonatal period. *Arch Dis Child* 45:242, 1970.
144. Gibson EL, Vaucher Y, Corrigan JJ Jr: Eosinophilia in premature infants. Relationship to weight gain. *J Pediatr* 95:99, 1979.
145. Koenig JM and Yoder MC: Neonatal neutrophils: The good, the bad and the ugly. *Clin Perinatol* 31:39, 2004.
146. Forman ML, Stiehm ER: Impaired opsonic activity but normal phagocytosis in low-birth-weight infants. *N Engl J Med* 281:926, 1969.
147. Dossett JH, Williams RC Jr, Quie PG: Studies on interaction of bacteria, serum factors and polymorphonuclear leukocytes in mothers and newborns. *Pediatrics* 44:49, 1969.
148. Miller ME: Phagocytosis in the newborn infant: Humoral and cellular factors. *J Pediatr* 74:255, 1969.
149. Hill HR, Shigeoka AO, Pincus S, Christensen RD: Intravenous IgG in combination with other modalities in the treatment of neonatal infection. *Pediatr Infect Dis* 5:180, 1986.
150. Cocchi P, Marianelli L: Phagocytosis and intracellular killing of *Pseudomonas aeruginosa* in premature infants. *Helv Paediatr Acta* 22:110, 1967.
151. Drossou V, Kanakoudi F, Diamanti E, et al: Concentrations of main serum opsonins in early infancy. *Arch Dis Child* 72:F172, 1995.
152. Yang KD, Bathras JM, Shigeoka AO, et al: Mechanisms of bacterial opsonization by immune globulin intravenous correlation of complement consumption with opsonic activity and protective efficacy. *J Infect Dis* 159:701, 1989.
153. Shaio MF, Yang KD, Bohnsack JF, Hill HR: Effect of immune globulin intravenous on opsonization of bacteria by classic and alternative complement pathways in premature serum. *Pediatr Res* 25:634, 1989.
154. Hill H: Host defenses in the neonate: prospects for enhancement. *Semin Perinatol* 9:2, 1985.
155. Propp RP, Alper CA: C3 synthesis in the human fetus and lack of transplacental passage. *Science* 162:672, 1968.
156. Johnston RB Jr, Altenburger KM, Atkinson AW Jr, et al: Complement in the newborn infant. *Pediatrics* 64:781, 1979.
157. Strunk RC, Fenton LJ, Gaines JA: Alternative pathway of complement activation in full term and premature infants. *Pediatr Res* 13:641, 1979.
158. Davis CA, Vallota EH, Forristal J: Serum complement levels in infancy: Age related changes. *Pediatr Res* 13:1043, 1979.
159. Mills EL, Bjorksten B, Quie PG: Deficient alternative complement pathway activity in newborn sera. *Pediatr Res* 13:1341, 1979.
160. Proctor RA, Prendergast E, Mosher DF: Fibronectin mediates attachment of *Staphylococcus aureus* to human neutrophils. *Blood* 59:681, 1982.
161. Hill HR, Shigeoka AO, Augustine NH, et al: Fibronectin enhances the opsonic and protective activity of monoclonal and polyclonal antibody against group B streptococci. *J Exp Med* 159:1618, 1984.
162. Harris MC, Levitt J, Douglas SD, et al: Effect of fibronectin on adherence of neutrophils from newborn infants. *J Clin Microbiol* 21:243, 1985.
163. Hill HR, Shigeoka AO, Gonzales LA, Christensen RD: Intravenous immune globulin use in newborns. *J Allergy Clin Immunol* 84:617, 1989.
164. Christensen RD, Brown MS, Hall DC, et al: Effect on neutrophil kinetics and serum opsonic capacity of intravenous administration of immune globulin to neonates with clinical signs of early-onset sepsis. *J Pediatr* 118:606, 1991.
165. Fujiwara T, Taniuchi S, Hattori K, et al: Effect of immunoglobulin therapy on phagocytosis by polymorphonuclear leucocytes in whole blood of neonates. *Clin Exp Immunol* 107:435, 1997.
166. Weisman LE, Stoll BJ, Kueser TJ, et al: Intravenous immune globulin therapy for early-onset sepsis in premature neonates. *J Pediatr* 121:434, 1992.
167. Schreiber JR, Berger M: Intravenous immune globulin therapy for sepsis in premature neonates. *J Pediatr* 121:401, 1992.
168. Baker CJ, Melish ME, Hall RT, et al: Intravenous immune globulin for the prevention of nosocomial infection in low-birth-weight infants. *N Engl J Med* 327:213, 1992.
169. Fanaroff A, Wright E, Korones S, Wright L: A controlled trial of prophylactic intravenous immunoglobulin to reduce nosocomial infections in VLBW infants. *Pediatr Res* 31:202A, 1992.
170. Suri M, Harrison L, Van de Ven C, et al: Immunotherapy in the prophylaxis of neonatal sepsis. *Curr Opin Pediatr* 15:155, 2003.
171. Fischer GW, Weisman LE, Hemming VG: Directed immune globulin for the prevention or treatment of neonatal group B streptococcal infections: A review. *Clin Immunol Immunopathol* 62:S92, 1992.
172. Miller ME: Chemotactic function in the neonate. Humoral and cellular aspects. *Pediatr Res* 5:487, 1971.
173. Klei RB, Fischer TJ, Gard SE, et al: Decreased mononuclear and polymorphonuclear chemotaxis in human newborns, infants, and young children. *Pediatrics* 60:467, 1977.
174. Tono-oka T, Nakayama M, Uehara H, et al: Characteristics of impaired chemotactic function in cord blood leukocytes. *Pediatr Res* 13:148, 1979.
175. Hill HR, Augustine NH, Newton JA, et al: Correction of a developmental defect in neutrophil activation and movement. *Am J Pathol* 128:307, 1987.
176. Bruce MC, Baley JE, Medvik KA, et al: Impaired surface membrane expression of C3bi but not C3b receptors on neonatal neutrophils. *Pediatr Res* 21:306, 1987.
177. Anderson DC, Freeman KLB, Heerdt B, et al: Abnormal stimulated adherence of neonatal granulocytes: Impaired induction of surface MAC-1 by chemotactic factors or secretagogues. *Blood* 70:740, 1987.
178. Smith JB, Campbell DE, Ludomirsky A, et al: Expression of the complement receptors CR1 and CR3 and the type III Pc-gamma receptor on neutrophils from newborn infants and from fetuses with Rh disease. *Pediatr Res* 28:120, 1990.
179. Carr R, Davies JM: Abnormal PcRIII expression by neutrophils from very preterm neonates. *Blood* 76:607, 1990.
180. Anderson DC, Rothlein R, Marlin SD, et al: Impaired transendothelial migration by neonatal neutrophils: Abnormalities of Mac-1(CD11b/CD18)-dependent adherence reactions. *Blood* 76:2613, 1990.
181. Masuda K, Kinoshita Y, Kobayashi Y: Heterogeneity of Fc expression in chemotaxis and adherence of neonatal neutrophils. *Pediatr Res* 25:6, 1989.

182. Tosi MF, Berger M: Functional differences between the 40 kDa and 50 kDa IgG Fc receptors on human neutrophils revealed by elastase treatment and antireceptor antibodies. *J Immunol* 141:2097, 1988.
183. Coen R, Grush O, Kander E: Studies of bactericidal activity and metabolism of the leukocyte in full-term neonates. *J Pediatr* 78:400, 1969.
184. Mills EL, Thompson T, Bjorksten B, et al: The chemiluminescence response and bactericidal activity of polymorphonuclear neutrophils from newborns and their mothers. *Pediatrics* 63:429, 1979.
185. Park BH, Holmes B, Good RA: Metabolic activities in leukocytes of newborn infants. *J Pediatr* 76:237, 1970.
186. Xanthou M, Valassi-Adam E, Kintronidou E, et al: Phagocytosis and killing ability of *Candida albicans* by blood leucocytes of healthy term and preterm babies. *Arch Dis Child* 50:72, 1975.
187. Shigeoka AO, Charette RP, Wyman ML, et al: Defective oxidative metabolic responses of neutrophils from stressed neonates. *J Pediatr* 98:392, 1981.
188. Strauss RG, Snyder EL: Neutrophils from human infants exhibit decreased viability. *Pediatr Res* 15:794, 1981.
189. Strauss RG, Snyder EL, Wallace PO, et al: Oxygen-detoxifying enzymes in neutrophils of infants and their mothers. *J Lab Clin Med* 95:897, 1980.
190. Yamazaki M, Matsuoka T, Yasui K, et al: Increased production of superoxide anion by neonatal polymorphonuclear leukocytes stimulated with a chemotactic peptide. *Am J Hematol* 27:169, 1988.
191. Levy O: Impaired innate immunity at birth: deficiency of bacteriocidal/permeability-increasing protein (BPI) in the neutrophils of newborns. *Pediatr Res* 51:667, 2002.
192. Neupponen I, Turunen R, Nevalainen T, et al: Extracellular release of bactericidal/permeability increasing protein in newborn infants. *Pediatr Res* 51:670, 2002.
193. Kretschmer RR, Papierniak CK, Stewardson-Krieger P, et al: Quantitative nitroblue tetrazolium reduction by normal newborn monocytes. *J Pediatr* 91:306, 1977.
194. Milgrom H, Shore SL: Assessment of monocyte function in the normal newborn infant by antibody-dependent cellular cytotoxicity. *J Pediatr* 91:612, 1977.
195. Orlowski JP, Sieger L, Anthony BF: Bactericidal capacity of monocytes of newborn infants. *J Pediatr* 89:797, 1976.
196. Schuit KE, Powell DA: Phagocytic dysfunction in monocytes of normal newborn infants. *Pediatrics* 65:501, 1980.
197. Das M, Henderson T, Feig SA: Neonatal mononuclear cell metabolism: Further evidence for diminished monocyte function in the neonate. *Pediatr Res* 13:632, 1979.
198. Mills EL: Mononuclear phagocytes in the newborn: Their relation to the state of relative immunodeficiency. *Am J Pediatr Hematol Oncol* 5:189, 1983.
199. Bryson YJ, Winter HS, Gard SE, et al: Deficiency of immune interferon production by leukocytes of normal newborns. *Cell Immunol* 55:191, 1987.
200. Frenkel L, Bryson YJ: Ontogeny of phytohemagglutinin-induced gamma interferon by leukocytes of healthy infants and children: Evidence for decreased production in infants younger than 2 months of age. *J Pediatr* 111:97, 1987.
201. Perussia B, Dayton ET, Lazarus R, et al: Immune interferon induces the receptor for monomeric IgG on human monocytic and myeloid cells. *J Exp Med* 158:1092, 1983.
202. Cairo MS: Review of G-CSF and GM-CSF effects on neonatal neutrophil kinetics. *Am J Pediatr Hematol Oncol* 11:238, 1989.
203. Cairo MS, VandeVen C, Toy C, et al: GM-CSF primes and modulates neonatal PMN motility: Up-regulation of C3bi (Mol) expression with alteration in PMN adherence and aggregation. *Am J Pediatr Hematol Oncol* 13:249, 1991.
204. Sautois B, Fillet G, Beguin Y: Comparative cytokine production by in vitro stimulated mononucleated cells from cord blood and adult blood. *Exp Hematol* 25:103, 1997.
205. Fogel BJ, Arais D, Kung F: Platelet counts in healthy premature infants. *J Pediatr* 73:108, 1968.
206. Sell EJ, Corrigan JJ: Platelet counts, fibrinogen concentrations and factor V and factor VIII levels in healthy infants according to gestational age. *J Pediatr* 82:1028, 1973.
207. Mehta P, Vasa R, Neumann L, Karpatkin M: Thrombocytopenia in the high-risk infant. *J Pediatr* 97:791, 1980.
208. Meberg A, Halvorsen S, Orstavik I: Transitory thrombocytopenia in small-for-dates infants, possibly related to maternal smoking. *Lancet* 2:303, 1977.
209. Thuring W, Tonz O: Neonatale thrombozytenwere be: Kindern mit Down-Syndrom und anderen autosomalen trisomien. *Helv Paediatr Acta* 34:545, 1979.
210. Cairo, MS: The regulation of hematopoietic growth factor production from cord mononuclear cells and its effect on newborn rat hematopoiesis. *J Hematother* 2:217, 1993.
211. Suen Y, Chang M, Lee SM, et al: Regulation of interleukin-11 protein and mRNA expression in neonatal and adult fibroblasts and endothelial cells. *Blood* 84:4125, 1994.
212. Murray NA, Watts TL, Roberts IAG: Thrombopoietin in the fetus and neonate. *Early Hum Dev* 59:1, 2000.
213. Feusner JH: Normal and abnormal bleeding times in neonates and young children utilizing a fully standardized template technic. *Am J Clin Pathol* 74:73, 1980.
214. Rennie JM, Gibson T, Cooke RWI: Micromethod for bleeding time in the newborn. *Arch Dis Child* 60:51, 1985.
215. Andrew M, Paes B, Bowker J, Vegh P: Evaluation of an automated bleeding time device in the newborn. *Am J Hematol* 35:275, 1990.
216. Weinstein MJ, Blanchard R, Moake JL, et al: Fetal and neonatal von Willebrand factor (vWF) is unusually large and similar to the vWF in patients with thrombotic thrombocytopenic purpura. *Br J Haematol* 72:68, 1989.
217. Andrew M, Vegh P, Johnston M, et al: Maturation of the hemostatic system during childhood. *Blood* 80:1998, 1992.
218. Andrew M, Castle V, Saigal S, et al: Clinical impact of neonatal thrombocytopenia. *J Pediatr* 110:457, 1987.
219. Israels SJ, Rand ML, Michelson AD: Neonatal platelet function [review]. *Semin Thromb Hemost* 29:363, 2003.
220. Corazza MS, Davis RF, Merritt TA, et al: Prolonged bleeding time in preterm infants receiving indomethacin for patent ductus arteriosus. *J Pediatr* 105:292, 1984.
221. Israels SJ, Cheang T, McMillan-Ward EM, et al: Evaluation of primary hemostasis in neonates with a new in vitro platelet function analyzer. *J Pediatr* 138:116, 2001.
222. Knofler R, Weissbach G, Kuhlisch E: Platelet function tests in childhood. Measuring aggregation and release reaction in whole blood. *Semin Thromb Hemost* 24:513, 1998.
223. Saxonhouse MA, Sola MC: Platelet function in term and preterm neonates. *Clin Perinatol* 31:15, 2004.
224. Stuart MJ: Platelet function in the neonate. *Am J Pediatr Hematol Oncol* 1:227, 1979.
225. Israels SJ, Daniels M, McMillan EM: Deficient collagen-induced activation in the newborn platelet. *Pediatr Res* 27:337, 1990.
226. Rajasekhar D, Kestin AS, Bednarek FJ, et al: Neonatal platelets are less reactive than adult platelets to physiological agonists in whole blood. *Thromb Haemost* 72:957, 1994.
227. Ts'ao C, Green D, Schultz K: Function and ultrastructure of platelets of neonates; enhanced ristocetin aggregation of neonatal platelets. *Br J Haematol* 32:225, 1976.
228. Blieyer WA, Breckenridge RT: Studies on the detection of adverse drug reactions in the newborn. II. The effects of prenatal aspirin on newborn hemostasis. *JAMA* 213:2049, 1970.
229. Corby DG, Schulman I: The effects of antenatal drug administration on aggregation of platelets of newborn infants. *J Pediatr* 79:307, 1971.
230. Hauth JC, Goldenberg RL, Parker CR Jr, et al: Low-dose aspirin: Lack of association with an increase in abruptio placentae or perinatal mortality. *Obstet Gynecol* 85:1055, 1995.
231. Sibai BM, Caritis SN, Thom E, et al: Low-dose aspirin in nulliparous women: Safety of continuous epidural block and correlation between bleeding time and maternal-neonatal bleeding complications. National Institute of Child Health and Human Developmental Maternal–Fetal Medicine Network. *Am J Obstet Gynecol* 172:1553, 1995.
232. Newman PJ, Derbes RS, Aster RH: The human platelet alloantigens, PLA1 and PLA2, are associated with a leucine 33/proline 33 amino acid polymorphism in membrane glycoprotein IIIa, and are distinguishable by DNA typing. *J Clin Invest* 83:1778, 1989.
233. Gruel Y, Boizard B, Daffos F, et al: Determination of platelet antigens and glycoproteins in the human fetus. *Blood* 68:488, 1986.
234. McFarland JG, Aster RH, Bussel JB, et al: Prenatal diagnosis of neonatal alloimmune thrombocytopenia using allele-specific oligonucleotide probes. *Blood* 78:2276, 1991.
235. Shulman NR, Jordan JV Jr: Platelet immunology, in *Hemostasis and Thrombosis: Basic Principles and Clinical Practice*, 2nd ed, edited by RW Colman, J Hirsh, VJ Marder, EW Salzman, pp 476–483. JB Lippincott, Philadelphia, 1987.
236. Pabst HF: Ontogeny of the immune response as a basis of childhood diseases. *J Pediatr* 97:519, 1980.
237. O'Gorman MRG, Millard DD, Lowder JN, et al: Lymphocyte subpopulations in 1–3 day old infants. *Cytometry* 34:235 1998.
238. Shearer WT, Rosenblatt HM, Gelman RS, et al: Lymphocyte subsets in healthy children from birth through 18 years of age: The Pediatric AIDS Clinical Trials Group P1009 Study. *J Allergy Clin Immunol* 112:973, 2003.
239. De Waele M, Foulon W, Renmans W, et al: Hematologic values and lymphocyte subsets in fetal blood. *Am J Clin Pathol* 89:742, 1988.
240. Hicks MJ, Jones JF, Minnich LL, et al: Age-related changes in T- and B-lymphocyte subpopulations in the peripheral blood. *Arch Pathol Lab Med* 107:518, 1983.
241. Kotylo PA, Baenzinger JC, Yoder MC, et al: Rapid analysis of lymphocyte subsets in cord blood. *Am J Clin Pathol* 93:263, 1990.
242. Kohl S: Human neonatal natural killer cell cytotoxicity function. *Pediatr Infect Dis J* 18:635, 1999.
243. Adkins B. Neonatal T cell function. *J Pediatr Gastroenterol Nutr* 40:S5, 2005.
244. Comans-Bitter WM, de Groot R, van den Beemd R, et al: Immunophenotyping of blood lymphocytes in childhood. Reference values for lymphocyte subpopulations. *J Pediatr* 130:388, 1997.
245. Slukvin II, Chernishov VP: Two-color flow cytometric analysis of natural killer and cytotoxic T-lymphocyte subsets in peripheral blood of normal human neonates. *Biol Neonate* 61:156, 1992.
246. Neubert R, Delgado I, Abraham K, et al: Evaluation of the age-dependent development of lymphocyte surface receptors in children. *Life Sci* 62:1099, 1998.
247. Miller ME: Immune-inflammatory response in the human neonate. *Am J Pediatr Hematol Oncol* 3:199, 1981.
248. Stiehm ER, Winter HS, Bryson YF: Cellular (T cell) immunity in the human newborn. *Pediatrics* 64:814, 1979.
249. Carr MC, Stites DP, Fudenberg HH: Cellular immune aspects of the human fetal-maternal relationship. I. In vitro response of cord blood lymphocytes to phytohemagglutinin. *Cell Immunol* 5:21, 1972.
250. Papiernick M: Comparison of human foetal with child blood lymphocytic kinetics. *Biol Neonate* 19:163, 1971.

251. Uhr JW, Dancis J, Newmann CG: Delayed-type hypersensitivity in premature neonatal humans. *Nature* 187:1130, 1960.
252. Blaese RM, Poplack DG, Muchmore AV: The mononuclear phagocyte system: Role in expression of immunocompetence in neonatal and adult life. *Pediatrics* 64(Suppl):829, 1979.
253. Von Freeden U, Zessack N, Van Valen F, Burdach S: Defective interferon gamma production in neonatal T cells is independent of interleukin-2 receptor binding. *Pediatr Res* 30:270, 1991.
254. Sterm CMM: Changes in lymphocytes subpopulations in the blood of healthy and sick newborn infants. *Pediatr Res* 13:792, 1979.
255. Raveche ES: Possible immunoregulatory role for CD5+ B cells. *Clin Immunol Immunopathol* 56:135, 1990.
256. Wilson CB, Kollmann TR: Induction of antigen specific immunity in human neonates and infants [review]. *Nestle Nutr Workshop Ser Pediatr Program* 61:183 2008.
257. Gustafsson BE, Laurell CB: Gamma globulin production in germ free rats after bacterial contamination. *J Exp Med* 110:675, 1959.
258. Gitlin D: The differentiation and maturation of specific immune mechanisms. *Acta Paediatr Scand* 172(Suppl):60, 1967.
259. Stiehm ER: Fetal defense mechanisms. *Am J Dis Child* 129:438, 1975.
260. Goldman AS, Garza C, Nichols BL, Goldblum RM: Immunological factors in human milk during the first year of lactation. *J Pediatr* 100:563, 1982.
261. Goldman AS, Ham Pong AJ, Goldblum RM: Host defenses: Development and maternal contributions. *Adv Pediatr* 32:71, 1985.
262. Newburg DS, Walker WA: Protection of the neonate by the innate immune system of developing gut and of human milk. *Pediatr Res* 61:2 2007.
263. Rothberg RM: Immunoglobulin and specific antibody synthesis during the first weeks of life of premature infants. *J Pediatr* 75:391, 1969.
264. Harworth JC, Norris M, Dilling L: A study of the immunoglobulins in premature infants. *Arch Dis Child* 40:243, 1965.
265. Thom H, McKay E, Gray DWG: Protein concentrations in the umbilical cord plasma of premature and mature infants. *Clin Sci* 33:433, 1967.
266. Yeung CY, Hoffs JR: Serum gamma-G-globulin levels in normal, premature, postmature, and "small-for-dates" newborn babies. *Lancet* 1:1167, 1968.
267. Sever JH: Immunological responses to perinatal responses to perinatal infections. *J Pediatr* 75:1111, 1969.
268. Thomaidis T, Agathopoulos A, Matsaniotis N: Natural isohemagglutinin production by the fetus. *J Pediatr* 74:39, 1969.
269. Morito T, Bankhurst AD, Williams RC Jr: Studies of human cord blood and adult lymphocyte interactions with in vitro immunoglobulin production. *J Clin Invest* 64:990, 1979.
270. Miyagawa Y, Sugita K, Komiyama A, et al: Delayed in vitro immunoglobulin production by cord lymphocytes. *Pediatrics* 65:497, 1980.
271. Ferguson AC, Cheung SC: Modulation of immunoglobulin M and G synthesis by monocytes and T lymphocytes in the newborn infant. *J Pediatr* 98:385, 1981.
272. Blaese RM, Poplack DG, Muchmore AV: The mononuclear phagocyte system: role in expression of immunocompetence in neonatal and adult life. *Pediatrics* 64:829, 1977.
273. Holroyde CP, Oski FA, Gardner FH: The "pocked" erythrocyte. *N Engl J Med* 281:516, 1969.
274. Freedman RM, Johnston D, Mahoney MJ, et al: Development of splenic reticuloendothelial function in neonates. *J Pediatr* 96:466, 1980.
275. Gross SJ, Stuart MJ: Hemostasis in the premature infant. *Clin Perinatol* 4:259, 1977.
276. Barnard DR, Hathaway WE: Neonatal thrombosis. *Am J Pediatr Hematol Oncol* 1:235, 1979.
277. Bleyer WA, Hakami N, Shepard TH: The development of hemostasis in the human fetus and newborn infant. *J Pediatr* 79:838, 1971.
278. Andrew M, Paes B, Milner B, et al: Development of the human coagulation system in the full-term infant. *Blood* 70:165, 1987.
279. Andrew M, Paes B, Milner R, et al: Development of the human coagulation system in the healthy premature infant. *Blood* 72:1651, 1988.
280. Corrigan JJ Jr: Neonatal thrombosis and the thrombolytic system: Pathophysiology and therapy. *Am J Pediatr Hematol Oncol* 10:83, 1988.
281. Andrew M, Paes B, Johnston M: Development of the hemostatic system in the neonate and young infant. *Am J Pediatr Hematol Oncol* 12:95, 1990.
282. Andrew M: The relevance of developmental hemostasis to hemorrhagic disorders of newborns. *Semin Perinatol* 21:70, 1997.
283. Karpatkin M, Lee M, Cohen L, et al: Synthesis of coagulation proteins in the fetus and neonate. *J Pediatr Hematol Oncol* 22:276, 2000.
284. Furie B, Furie BC: Molecular basis of gamma-carboxylation. Role of the propeptide in the vitamin K-dependent proteins. *Ann N Y Acad Sci* 614:1, 1991.
285. Aballi AJ, deLamerens S: Coagulation changes in the neonatal period and in early infancy. *Pediatr Clin North Am* 9:785, 1962.
286. Muntean W, Petek W, Rosanelli K, et al: Immunologic studies of prothrombin in newborns. *Pediatr Res* 13:1262, 1979.
287. Lane PA, Hathaway WE: Vitamin K in infancy. *J Pediatr* 106:351, 1985.
288. Stevenson RE, Burton OM, Ferlauto GJ, et al: Hazards of oral anticoagulants during pregnancy. *JAMA* 243:1549, 1980.
289. Shearer MJ: Annotation: Vitamin K and vitamin K-dependent proteins. *Br J Haematol* 75:156, 1990.
290. von Kries R, Hanawa Y: Neonatal vitamin K prophylaxis. Report of Scientific and Standardization Subcommittee on Perinatal Haemostasis. *Thromb Haemost* 69:293, 1993.
291. Sutor AH, Gobel U, Kries RV, et al: Vitamin K prophylaxis in the newborn. *Blut* 60:275, 1990.
292. Hathaway WE, Isarangkura PB, Mahasandana C, et al: Comparison of oral and parenteral vitamin K prophylaxis for prevention of late hemorrhagic disease of the newborn. *J Pediatr* 119:461, 1991.
293. Blackmon L, Batton DG, Bell EF, et al: Controversies concerning vitamin K and the newborn. American Academy of Pediatrics Policy Statement. *Pediatrics* 112:191, 2003.
294. Costakos DT, Porte M: Did "controversies concerning vitamin K and the newborn" cover all the controversies? *Pediatrics* 113:1466, 2004.
295. Clarke P, Mitchell SJ, Wynn R, et al: Vitamin K prophylaxis for preterm infants: A randomized, controlled trial of three regimens. *Pediatrics* 118:1657, 2006.
296. Amadee-Manesme O, Labert WE, Alagille D, De Leenheer AP: Pharmacokinetics and safety of a new solution of vitamin K_1 (20) in children with cholestasis. *J Pediatr Gastroenterol Nutr* 14:160, 1996.
297. Aballi AJ: The action of vitamin K in the neonatal period. *South Med J* 58:48, 1965.
298. Gray OP, Ackerman A, Fraser AJ: Intracranial haemorrhage and clotting in low birth weight infants. *Lancet* 1:543, 1968.
299. Volpe JJ: Neonatal intraventricular hemorrhage. *N Engl J Med* 304:886, 1981.
300. Appleyard WJ, Cottom DG: Effect of asphyxia on Thrombotest values in low birth-weight infants. *Arch Dis Child* 45:705, 1970.
301. Schmidt B, Zipursky A: Thrombotic disease in newborn infants. *Clin Perinatol* 2:461, 1984.
302. Rodgers GM, Shuman MA: Congenital thrombotic disorders. *Am J Hematol* 21:419, 1986.
303. Sifontes MT, Nuss R, Hunger SP, et al: Correlation between the functional assay for activated protein C resistance and factor V Leiden in the neonate. *Pediatr Res* 42:776, 1997.
304. Leroyer C, Mercier B, Oger E, et al: Prevalence of 20210 A allele of the prothrombin gene in venous thromboembolism patients. *Thromb Haemost* 80:49, 1998.
305. Poort SR, Rosendaal FR, Reitsma PH, Bertina RM: A common genetic variation in the 3′-untranslated region of the prothrombin gene is associated with elevated plasma prothrombin levels and an increase in venous thrombosis. *Blood* 88:3698, 1996.
306. Miller RK, Kellogg CR, Saltzman RA: Reproductive and perinatal toxicology, in *Handbook of Toxicology*, edited by TJ Haley, WO Berndt, pp 195–309. Hemisphere Publishing, Washington, DC, 1987.
307. Gray MJ: Use and abuse of thiazides in pregnancy. *Clin Obstet Gynecol* 11:568, 1968.
308. Leikin SL: Thiazide and neonatal thrombocytopenia. *N Engl J Med* 271:161, 1964.
309. Ginsberg JS, Kowalchuk G, Hirsh J, Brill-Edwards P, Burrows R: Heparin therapy during pregnancy. *Arch Intern Med* 149:2233, 1989.
310. Page TE, Hoyme HE, Markarian M, et al: Neonatal hemorrhage secondary to thrombocytopenia: An occasional effect of prenatal hydantoin exposure. *Birth Defects Orig Artic Ser* 18:47, 1982.
311. Hanson JW, Buehler BA: Fetal hydantoin syndrome: Current status. *J Pediatr* 101:816, 1982.
312. Eggermont E, Logghe N, van de Casseye W, et al: Haemorrhagic disease of the newborn in the offspring of rifampin and isoniazid treated mothers. *Acta Paediatr Belg* 29:87, 1976.
313. Powell RD, DeGowin RL, Alving AS, et al: Nitrofurantoin-induced hemolysis. *J Lab Clin Med* 62:1002, 1963.
314. Belton EM, Jones RV: Haemolytic anaemia due to nalidixic acid. *Lancet* 2:691, 1965.
315. Varsano I, Fischl J, Tikvah P, et al: The excretion of orally ingested nitrofurantoin in human milk. *J Pediatr* 82:886, 1973.
316. Brodersen R: Prevention of kernicterus, based on recent progress in bilirubin chemistry. *Acta Paediatr* 66:625, 1977.
317. El Beitune P, Duarte G: Antiretroviral agents during pregnancy: Consequences on hematologic parameters in HIV-exposed, uninfected newborn infants. *Eur J Obstet Gynecol Reprod Biol* 128:59, 2006.

CHAPTER 7
HEMATOLOGY DURING PREGNANCY

Martha P. Mims and Josef T. Prchal

SUMMARY

Normal pregnancy involves many changes in maternal physiology including alterations in hematologic parameters. These changes include expansion in maternal blood and plasma volume. The increase in plasma volume is relatively larger than the increase in red cell mass resulting in a decrease in hemoglobin concentration. An increase in the levels of some plasma proteins alters the balance of coagulation and fibrinolysis. Worldwide, the predominant cause of anemia in pregnancy is iron deficiency. Fetal requirements for iron are met despite maternal deficiency, but maternal iron deficiency has a number of adverse consequences including an increased frequency of preterm delivery and low-birth-weight infants. Bleeding disorders in pregnancy are a common reason for hematologic consultation and evoke concern for both the mother and child. Life-threatening bleeding caused by disseminated intravascular coagulation is seen with some complications unique to pregnancy, including placental abruption, retained dead fetus, and amniotic fluid embolism. Von Willebrand disease is the commonest inherited bleeding disorder, but because of increases in factor VIII level and von Willebrand factor (VWF) during pregnancy, excessive bleeding at delivery is rarely a problem. Factor levels fall rapidly postpartum, and serious hemorrhage can occur during this period. Carriers of hemophilia A and B should be monitored during pregnancy to determine if factor levels will be adequate for delivery at term. Caution should be exercised at delivery and during the first few days of life with offspring of hemophilia carriers until hemophilia testing is completed and the infant's status is known. Acquired hemophilia as a result of factor VIII autoantibodies is rare, but can occur during pregnancy or the puerperium. Thrombocytopenia is not uncommon in pregnancy, and its causes include several conditions that are unique to pregnancy, such as preeclampsia. Idiopathic thrombocytopenic purpura (ITP) is common, it is often exacerbated in pregnancy, and is managed conservatively if possible; close followup of newborns of mothers with ITP is essential. HELLP (hemolysis, elevated liver enzymes, and low platelet count) syndrome and TTP (thrombotic thrombocytopenic purpura)/HUS (hemolytic uremic syndrome) are also seen in pregnancy and the puerperium. HELLP syndrome is managed with delivery if possible, whereas TTP requires plasma exchange. Inherited and acquired prothrombotic conditions can be exacerbated by pregnancy and can result in adverse reproductive outcomes as well as venous thromboembolism. The strongest evidence for an association between a thrombophilia and recurrent fetal loss exists for antiphospholipid antibody syndrome; however, evidence is mounting for a connection between inherited thrombophilias and the severity of some complications of pregnancy. These thrombophilias increase the risk of venous thromboembolism in pregnancy and the puerperium. Treatment of hematologic malignancies in pregnancy can present a difficult dilemma both in terms of staging studies and management. In many cases of Hodgkin lymphoma, treatment can be delayed safely until after delivery. In aggressive lymphomas and acute leukemias however rapid initiation of chemotherapy is often necessary to save the life of the mother. In general, the teratogenic effects of chemotherapy are greatest in the first trimester; however, care must be taken in later trimesters to avoid cytopenias of both mother and fetus at delivery. Hemorrhagic and thrombotic complications associated with pregnancy in females with essential thrombocythemia and polycythemia vera present a unique challenge due to the lack of controlled trials in these situations.

Acronyms and abbreviations that appear in this chapter include: DDAVP, desmopressin acetate, a synthetic analogue of the pituitary hormone vasopressin; DIC, disseminated intravascular coagulation; DVT, deep vein thrombosis; ESR, erythrocyte sedimentation rate; ET, essential thrombocythemia; HELLP, hemolysis, elevated liver enzymes, low platelets syndrome; ITP, idiopathic thrombocytopenic purpura; PV, polycythemia vera; TTP, thrombotic thrombocytopenic purpura; VTE, venous thromboembolism; VWD, von Willebrand disease; VWF, von Willebrand factor.

BLOOD VOLUME, ERYTHROPOIETIN LEVEL, AND HEMOGLOBIN CONCENTRATION

Maternal blood volume increases by an average of 40 to 50 percent above the nonpregnant level.[1] Plasma volume begins to rise early in pregnancy, with most of the escalation taking place in the second trimester and prior to week 32 of gestation.[2] Red cell mass increases significantly beginning in the second trimester and continues to expand throughout pregnancy, but to a lesser extent than plasma volume.[2] Erythropoietin levels increase throughout pregnancy, reaching approximately 150 percent of their prepregnancy levels at term.[3,4] The overall effect of these changes in most women is a slight drop in hemoglobin concentration, which is most pronounced at the end of the second trimester and slowly improves approaching term.

■ PLATELET AND WHITE CELL COUNTS

The effect of pregnancy on maternal platelet count is somewhat more controversial; some studies demonstrate a mild decline in platelet count over the course of gestation,[5] whereas others do not.[6] In general, white cell counts rise during pregnancy with the occasional appearance of myelocytes or metamyelocytes in the blood.[7] During labor and the early puerperium, there is a rise in the leukocyte count. Leukocytosis appears to be linearly related to the duration of labor.[8]

■ PLASMA PROTEINS

The levels of some plasma proteins also increase during pregnancy. In particular, C-reactive protein concentration is higher in pregnant women and rises even further during labor.[9] Erythrocyte sedimentation rate (ESR) rises during pregnancy, and is affected by both hemoglobin concentration and gestational age.[10] The rise in ESR during pregnancy, in large part a result of an increase in levels of plasma globulins and fibrinogen, makes its use as a marker of inflammation difficult. The levels of many of the procoagulant factors increase during pregnancy whereas activity of the fibrinolytic system diminishes in preparation for the hemostatic challenge of delivery. Plasma levels of von Willebrand factor (VWF), fibrinogen, and factors VII, VIII, and X all increase markedly, whereas factors II, V, IX, and XII are essentially unchanged and factor XIII declines.[11] Levels of protein C and antithrombin remain stable throughout pregnancy whereas total and free protein S fall with increasing gestational age.[12] Fibrinolysis is also impaired by increases in plasminogen activator inhibitors I and II, the latter a product of the placenta.[13]

ANEMIA IN PREGNANCY

■ IRON DEFICIENCY

Worldwide the contribution of anemia to maternal and fetal morbidity and mortality is well recognized; in some parts of Africa, more than 75 percent of pregnant women are anemic, and there is a significant correlation between maternal mortality and anemia.[14] Iron deficiency may protect against placental malaria, but epidemiologic studies have not been conducted to verify this supposition.[15] In pregnant women, anemia is defined as a hemoglobin concentration of less than 11 g/dL in the first and third trimesters, and less than 10.5 g/dL in the second trimester.[15] In both the industrialized and the developing world, iron-deficiency anemia (see Chap. 42) is the commonest cause of anemia.[16] On average approximately 1 g of iron is required during a normal pregnancy; 300 mg of iron are required by the fetus and the placenta, whereas expansion of the maternal red blood cell mass requires 500 mg, and 200 mg are lost via excretion.[17] These requirements exceed the iron storage of most young women and in general cannot be met by the diet. Even in cases of maternal iron deficiency, the fetal requirements for iron are always met; thus there is no correlation between the hemoglobin of the fetus and that of the mother.[18]

Iron-deficiency anemia during the first two trimesters of pregnancy is associated with a twofold increased risk for preterm delivery and a threefold increased risk for delivery of a low-birth-weight infant.[19] However, a large randomized trial comparing routine iron prophylaxis in pregnancy versus iron supplementation given only as needed demonstrated no significant differences in adverse maternal or fetal outcomes.[20] As in nonpregnant individuals, iron-deficiency anemia can generally be diagnosed using laboratory values such as serum ferritin, and transferrin saturation levels (see Chap. 42). *Pica*, the ingestion of nonnutritive substances, is said to be more common among iron-deficient pregnant women than among other populations with iron deficiency. Ice, clay or dirt, and starch are the most frequent substances ingested (see Chap. 42); to some extent, however, the choice appears to be cultural and much more widespread than most practitioners realize.[21]

FOLATE AND VITAMIN B_{12} DEFICIENCY

Apart from iron deficiency, folate deficiency is the next most frequent nutritional deficiency leading to anemia in pregnant women. In the United States, where foodstuffs are supplemented with folate and the level of awareness of the association between folate deficiency and neural tube defects in the embryo is high, folate deficiency is relatively unusual. Folate requirements in pregnancy are roughly twice those in the nonpregnant state (800 mcg/day vs. 400 mcg/day), and if diet is insufficient may exceed the body's stores of folate (5–10 mg) relatively quickly.[22] Anemia related to folate deficiency most often presents in the third trimester and responds to folate supplementation with reticulocytosis within 24 to 72 hours.[16] Reports of severe pancytopenia and even states resembling the HELLP (hemolysis, elevated liver enzymes, and low platelet count) syndrome as a result of folate deficiency in pregnancy have appeared in the literature.[23,24] Despite these case reports, a review of 21 trials measuring the effect of folate supplementation on biochemical and hematologic parameters and pregnancy outcome (excluding neural tube defects) revealed improvement in low hemoglobin level in late pregnancy, but had no measurable effect on any substantive measures of pregnancy outcome (see Chap. 41).[25]

Vitamin B_{12} deficiency during pregnancy is rare, in part because deficiency of this vitamin leads to infertility. Serum cobalamin levels are known to fall during pregnancy.[26] A shift from the serum to tissue stores is proposed to account for the drop in serum B_{12} levels. However, values less than 180 pmol/L usually are not observed in healthy women, and these low-normal levels are not accompanied by increased levels of methylmalonic acid, an indicator of cellular deficiency (see Chap. 41).[27]

RED CELL APLASIA

A rare cause of anemia in pregnancy is pure red cell aplasia (see Chap. 35). In pure red cell aplasia, anemia tends to occur early in pregnancy and often resolves within weeks of delivery. The pathogenic mechanism leading to red cell aplasia does not appear to be transferred to the fetus, but does tend to recur in subsequent pregnancies.[28,29] Conservative treatment, if feasible, is probably best until delivery; successful prenatal treatments with glucocorticoids and with intravenous immunoglobulin have been reported.[30,31]

BLEEDING DISORDERS AND CAUSES OF THROMBOCYTOPENIA

Bleeding disorders in pregnancy require consideration of maternal bleeding and hemorrhagic complications in the newborn. Data on the fetus is often lacking, and the practitioner must base decisions on past experience and the mother's previous reproductive history.

DISSEMINATED INTRAVASCULAR COAGULATION

Life-threatening bleeding is seen with some pregnancy-unique complications resulting in disseminated intravascular coagulation (DIC) stemming from placental abruption, a retained dead fetus, and amniotic fluid embolism (see Chap. 130). Although amniotic fluid embolism is a significant cause of maternal death in developed countries, the mortality decreased from 86 percent in 1979 to less than 30 percent in 1994 and 1995, perhaps from a better supportive therapy.[32] Amniotic fluid embolism is heralded by maternal vascular collapse with dyspnea, hypotension, and cardiac arrhythmias followed by DIC that is manifested by oozing from intravenous lines, hematuria, hemoptysis, and excessive uterine bleeding. Atypical presentations have also been reported in which there is rapid deterioration of the fetus followed by maternal respiratory and cardiovascular deterioration postpartum with development of DIC.[33]

In amniotic fluid embolism, DIC is thought to arise from the procoagulant properties of amniotic fluid containing vernix, caseosa, and fetal squamous epithelial cells in the pulmonary circulation followed by a secondary fibrinolytic response.[34] Treatment is not significantly different than in other cases of DIC with bleeding (see Chap. 130); however, there are some reports of successful management with uterine artery embolization.[35]

Placental abruption has also led to development of DIC, and the spectrum of hemostatic failure is broad and appears to be related to the degree of placental separation.[36] Volume resuscitation, delivery of the fetus, and infusion of blood products to correct the maternal coagulation defect are indicated. Regional anesthesia is contraindicated because of the risk of bleeding in the epidural space and of the pooling of blood in the lower limb vascular bed, which could worsen hypovolemia.[36] Fetal trophoblast cells have distinct properties which may activate coagulation including expression of tissue factor, suppression of fibrinolysis, and exposure of anionic phospholipids.[38] Finally, intrauterine fetal death can also lead to DIC. Thromboplastic substances, and specifically tissue factor released from dead fetal tissues into the maternal circulation are thought to trigger DIC; however, this is not usually detectable by laboratory tests until 3 or 4 weeks after fetal demise. Overt DIC is present in approximately 50 percent of women who retain a dead fetus for 5 weeks or longer.[37]

VON WILLEBRAND DISEASE

Although von Willebrand disease (VWD) is transmitted in an autosomal dominant fashion, women appear to be disproportionately affected with bleeding symptoms; primarily menorrhagia and postpartum hemorrhage (see Chap. 127). In normal women and in types 1 and 2 (but not type 3) VWD patients, levels of factor VIII and VWF rise during pregnancy, with the most pronounced increase in the third trimester.[38] As a result, prophylactic administration of VWF-containing factor concentrates at delivery is often unnecessary in type 1 and type 2 VWD patients; however, the risk of postpartum hemorrhage is significant (13–29%) as levels fall rapidly after birth.[39] Thus in type 1 patients, factor VIII levels should be tested not only late in the third trimester, but also for 1 to 2 weeks postpartum. These patients should be monitored for increases in menstrual blood flow for at least 1 month. Risk of bleeding appears to be minimal when factor VIII levels are greater than 40 U/dL. There are several reports of severe thrombocytopenia developing late in pregnancy in patients with type 2B VWD[40,41] and at least one of these patients developed a pulmonary embolus while receiving cryoprecipitate for postpartum hemorrhage. Despite the possible risk of thrombosis, these patients may require treatment with plasma-derived VWF-containing concentrates at delivery or postpartum if there is abnormal bleeding, and with platelets if thrombocytopenic bleeding is not controlled with infusion of VWF concentrate. Type 3 VWD patients require infusion of a plasma-derived VWF-containing concentrate at delivery, typically 40 to 80 IU/kg, followed by doses of 20 to 40 IU/kg daily for a week then tapered over the next few weeks.[42] Use of desmopressin acetate (DDAVP) antepartum is controversial because of the theoretical risk of vasoconstriction and placental insufficiency and the risk of maternal hyponatremia. Guidelines for management of VWD at delivery and during the puerperium have been published and are also reviewed in Chap. 127.[45,46]

COAGULATION FACTOR DEFICIENCIES

Carriers of hemophilia A and B generally have factor levels approximately 50 percent of normal; however, a wide range of values have been reported as a result of random inactivation of the X chromosome (see Chaps. 9 and 124).[47] Ideally, carriers are identified before pregnancy when prenatal counseling can be offered. Baseline factor levels should be tested at the first visit during pregnancy and again in the third trimester, but it should be noted that factor IX levels generally do not rise during the course of the pregnancy.[43] The sex of the fetus should be determined to guide the obstetrician at delivery. Cranial hemorrhage is the commonest site of bleeding in newborns with severe hemophilia and has the highest potential for long-term serious sequelae. Risk factors for cranial hemorrhage include prolonged labor and use of instruments during delivery.[49] To protect a potentially affected or known hemophiliac fetus, vacuum extraction should be avoided at delivery and forceps should be used only with caution. All intramuscular injections should be withheld from the newborn until hemophilia testing is completed. Testing should be done on cord blood to avoid potential bleeding or bruising after a blood draw.[44] The mother's factor level should be followed for a few days after delivery and menstrual bleeding should be monitored to ensure adequate hemostasis.

There is also an association between pregnancy and acquired hemophilia caused by factor VIII autoantibodies (see Chap. 128). This condition usually appears 1 to 4 months postpartum, but emerges during pregnancy in up to 14 percent of patients.[45] In general, the Bethesda titer of the inhibitor is low and in most cases the inhibitor disappears spontaneously. Inhibitors can recur in subsequent pregnancies.[46]

Rarely, pregnant women with factor deficiencies other than factors VIII and IX may be identified. The most important of these to recognize is deficiency of factor XIII, which is associated with habitual hemorrhagic abortions and postpartum hemorrhage. In rare pregnancies reaching term, bleeding complications, including intracranial hemorrhage in the infant, have been observed.[47,48] Treatment of this deficiency with fresh-frozen plasma, cryoprecipitate, or plasma-derived factor XIII concentrates prevents abortion in women, although there are no controlled studies.[49] Most authorities recommend more frequent prophylactic therapy during pregnancy (every 3 weeks vs. every 5–6 weeks) with booster doses during labor or before cesarean section to ensure a level of 5 percent or greater.[50]

THROMBOCYTOPENIA

Thrombocytopenia in pregnancy is relatively common, with up to 5 percent of all pregnant women exhibiting asymptomatic thrombocytopenia.[51] Many of the causes of thrombocytopenia in pregnancy are identical to those seen in the nonpregnant state, with some predisposing to bleeding whereas others predispose to clotting. However, there are several conditions leading to thrombocytopenia that are unique to pregnancy, including gestational thrombocytopenia, preeclampsia/HELLP syndrome/eclampsia, and acute fatty liver of pregnancy.

Gestational and Immune Thrombocytopenia

Gestational thrombocytopenia and idiopathic thrombocytopenic purpura (ITP) are best discussed together as they can be difficult to differentiate and in fact may be two extremes of a spectrum of disease. In general, gestational thrombocytopenia is asymptomatic and is said to occur later in pregnancy and be less severe than ITP. Most sources suggest that gestational thrombocytopenia occurs in the second and third trimesters, with platelet counts rarely falling below 70,000/μL.[52] Gestational thrombocytopenia can sometimes be diagnosed with certainty only after delivery; usually there is no past history of low platelets, except perhaps with previous pregnancies, the platelet count returns to normal after delivery, and there is no association with fetal thrombocytopenia. It is not clear whether or not gestational thrombocytopenia is a variant of immune-mediated platelet destruction (see Chap. 119). [52]

In contrast to gestational thrombocytopenia, ITP can occur at any point in pregnancy and the fall in platelet count can be severe. Diagnosis is essentially the same as it would be in any patient in that alternative causes of thrombocytopenia must be ruled out. As in other cases, treatment of ITP in pregnancy must take into account the severity of the thrombocytopenia and the presence or absence of symptoms. In general, platelet counts less than 10,000/μL require treatment regardless of the trimester; platelet counts of 30,000 to 50,000/μL without bleeding require no treatment, and platelet counts of 10,000 to 30,000/μL in later trimesters or in the presence of bleeding require treatment. Although glucocorticoid and intravenous immunoglobulin are safe in pregnancy, it should be recognized that they may have no effect on fetal counts and should only be used to treat the mother.[53] Splenectomy for ITP in pregnancy is best done in the second trimester if platelet counts are extremely low and unresponsive to treatment.[52] One small study evaluated the safety of anti-D antibodies during pregnancy; all 10 of the women studied achieved a platelet count greater than 30,000/μL, but larger studies are needed before this intervention can be recommended.[60] Similarly, there are case reports of rituximab administration for treatment of refractory ITP in pregnancy; at least one report demonstrated transient inhibition of neonatal B-lymphocyte development.[61] Maternal platelet counts of greater than 50,000/μL usually are safe for both vaginal and cesarean delivery. In terms of predicting fetal platelet count, it should be noted that less than 5 percent of babies born to mothers with ITP have platelet counts less than 20,000/μL, although there does seem to be some correlation between very severely depressed maternal platelet count and thrombocytopenia in the newborn.[54] No clear recommendations can be given for measuring fetal platelet count prior to or at delivery as measurements are fraught with error; however, if the fetal platelet count is known to be less than 20,000/μL, cesarean section is probably reasonable. Newborns of mothers with ITP should be monitored for 5 to 7 days after delivery to ensure that the platelet count does not drop (see Chap. 54).

Eclampsia and HELLP Syndrome

The spectrum of hypertensive disorders of pregnancy ranging from preeclampsia to severe preeclampsia and HELLP syndrome to eclampsia (see Chap. 50) may also result in thrombocytopenia, although thrombosis is more of an issue than is bleeding. There is some debate in the literature as to whether thrombocytopenia can be diagnosed in preeclampsia without HELLP syndrome; however, data from one large study[51] demonstrate that approximately 15 percent of cases of preeclampsia are complicated by thrombocytopenia. In general, the symptoms of preeclampsia, including hematologic manifestations, resolve with delivery; however, in a small proportion of cases they persist, worsen, or even develop immediately postpartum. When symptoms persist postpartum, the differentiation from thrombotic thrombocytopenic purpura (TTP)/hemolytic uremic syndrome becomes more difficult. Some data suggest that maternal recovery from the HELLP syndrome is accelerated by administration of intravenous dexamethasone[55]; however, a meta-analysis demonstrated no clear advantage to the use of glucocorticoids in terms of maternal or perinatal morbidity or mortality.[56] Observation or treatment of HELLP with glucocorticoids alone postpartum should probably not persist beyond the third postpartum day. If the patient is not clearly improving, plasma exchange should be initiated as one would do for TTP.[57,58] Although not associated with hypertension, acute fatty liver of pregnancy is another rare disorder that can present in the third trimester with severe liver dysfunction, but thrombocytopenia, if present, is generally mild and does not require treatment (see Chaps. 50, 119, and 130).

■ THROMBOPHILIA

Fetal Loss and Complications

Pregnancy is a prothrombotic state. Inherited prothrombotic conditions contribute to 50 percent of the cases of venous thromboembolism and pulmonary embolism, as well as to stroke in pregnancy and the puerperium. Evidence is mounting that hereditary thrombophilias (see Chap. 131) may also predispose to fetal loss through placental vascular disorders. The best evidence for an association between a thrombophilia, albeit acquired, and recurrent fetal loss exists for antiphospholipid antibody syndrome in which the association between the antibodies and pregnancy loss has been recognized for more than 20 years.[59] As many as 20 percent of women with recurrent fetal loss have antiphospholipid antibodies,[60] and studies show that without treatment up to 90 percent will experience fetal loss.[61] One study suggests that poor pregnancy outcomes occur more frequently in primary antiphospholipid syndrome when patients have more than one positive laboratory test (lupus anticoagulant, immunoglobulin [Ig] G/IgM anticardiolipin, IgG/IgM antihuman β_2-glycoprotein I antibodies).[70] In a randomized controlled trial including 90 women with a history of recurrent miscarriage associated with phospholipid antibodies (or antiphospholipid antibodies), lupus anticoagulant, and cardiolipin antibodies (or anticardiolipin antibodies), the rate of livebirths with low-dose aspirin (75 mg/day) and unfractionated heparin (5000 U subcutaneously twice per day) was 71 percent (32 of 45 pregnancies) and 42 percent (19 of 45 pregnancies) with low-dose aspirin alone (odds ratio, 3.37 [95% confidence interval: 1.40–8.10]).[62]

Although an association between inherited thrombophilias and pregnancy loss has been elusive and there are inconsistencies between studies, there does appear to be an association between factor V Leiden and recurrent fetal loss.[63,64] Less-convincing data exist for prothrombin 20210A, but there is no clear association with homozygous methylene tetrahydrofolate reductase C677T polymorphism (hyperhomocysteinemia).[65] Published trials examining the use of low-molecular-weight heparins or aspirin to prevent adverse pregnancy outcomes in women with inherited thrombophilias have been criticized for lack of an untreated control group.[75–77] Pregnancy outcomes from a large ongoing trial conducted with a no-treatment control have yet to be published.[78] Studies evaluating a role for inherited thrombophilias in preeclampsia and intrauterine growth retardation indicate that these factors may not be causative, but may contribute to disease severity.[66,67]

Thromboembolic Events

Risk Factors Estimates place the relative risk of arterial and venous thromboembolism (VTE) in pregnant women (see Chaps. 134 and 135) at two to six times that of nonpregnant women.[11,68] Factors specific to pregnancy that increase the risk of VTE include obstruction of venous return by the gravid uterus, acquired prothrombotic changes in hemostatic proteins, and venous atonia caused by hormonal factors.[69] Additional risk factors include cesarean section (especially emergency), obesity, and increasing age. Approximately 80 percent of deep vein thromboses in pregnancy occur in the iliofemoral veins on the left, probably as a consequence of compression of the left iliac vein by the right iliac and ovarian arteries.[70,71] Rates of VTE immediately postpartum are difficult to assess as many occur after the patient is discharged; however, some studies suggest that postpartum rates may be even higher than antepartum rates.[72,73] Inherited thrombophilia (Chap. 131) plays a role in VTE in pregnancy. The highest rates occur with inherited antithrombin deficiency where it has been estimated that in the absence of anticoagulation, 32 to 44 percent of patients will experience thromboembolism.[72] In a large retrospective study of more than 70,000 pregnancies,[74] the risk of VTE in pregnancy was estimated at approximately 1 in 437 for carriers of factor V Leiden, 1 in 113 for protein C deficiency, and 1 in 2.8 for type I antithrombin deficiency. Based on results from other studies, the risk for carriers of protein S deficiency appears to be similar to that for protein C deficiency, and risk for carriers of the prothrombin 20210A gene mutation is similar to or lower than that of factor V Leiden carriers.[75–77]

Diagnostic Methods Diagnosis of VTE in pregnancy is complicated both because the presenting complaints—leg edema, back pain, and chest pain—are common in pregnancy, and because radiologic studies used to make the diagnosis in nonpregnant individuals are relatively contraindicated in pregnant women. Compression ultrasonography is the initial test of choice in pregnant women. If this test is nondiagnostic, several other tests may be considered. If pulmonary embolus is suspected, lung ventilation perfusion scanning, which gives relatively low-dose radiation, may be used. Magnetic resonance imaging or magnetic resonance venography are also informative if available. Measurement of D-dimers is a useful adjunct in nonpregnant patients to rule out VTE (D-dimers are sensitive, but not specific, for VTE). However, D-dimer levels rise over the course of normal pregnancy[78,79] and with several complications of pregnancy, including preterm labor, hypertension, and placental abruption,[80] and thus may not be useful in excluding VTE.

Prophylaxis Prophylaxis for VTE is a controversial issue as only a few prospective studies have been done to assess the risk of use.[81,82] There is general agreement, however, that because of its teratogenic potential, warfarin should not be used during pregnancy and that low-molecular-weight heparins are the anticoagulant of choice because they do not cross the placenta and have a lower risk of osteoporosis and heparin-induced thrombocytopenia.[83] Most experts agree that women with low risk, including those with no prior history of VTE and a confirmed hypercoagulable state or with a single prior VTE associated with a transient risk factor, can be managed with careful surveillance during pregnancy (except for patients with antithrombin deficiency and antiphospholipid syndrome who should receive prophylactic doses of low-molecular-weight heparin or unfractionated heparin during pregnancy). Postpartum risk increases somewhat, and anticoagulation should be continued for 6 to 8 weeks. Newer recommendations suggest that women with thrombophilia, but no prior VTE, should receive postpartum anticoagulation. Treatment of patients with a single previous thromboembolism and a hypercoagulable state not on warfarin at conception is more controversial. Some recommend careful clinical surveillance, whereas others counsel use of prophylactic low-molecular-weight heparins antepartum; postpartum most experts recommend 6 to 8 weeks of prophylaxis for all patients in this category. Patients with two or more episodes of VTE should be treated throughout pregnancy and the puerperium.[84–88] Treatment of VTE in pregnancy should be with full-dose low-molecular-weight heparin. Ideally, women on treatment doses of heparin have elective induction of labor. Heparin is usually discontinued 24 hours prior to induction; however, women deemed to be at very high risk of recurrent VTE can then receive IV heparin up to 4 to 6 hours prior to delivery.[86,87] Great care should be taken with epidural anesthesia, and it should be avoided if there is any question of a significant anticoagulant effect. Heparins and warfarin are safe postpartum, even when breast-feeding.[89]

TREATMENT OF HEMATOLOGIC MALIGNANCIES IN PREGNANCY

Although not common, leukemias and lymphomas do occur in pregnancy and present problems with proper diagnosis, staging, and treatment (see Chaps. 89, 90, 93, 99, 100, and 104). The literature suggests that the incidence of Hodgkin lymphoma is 1:1000 to 1:6000 pregnancies, whereas the incidence of non-Hodgkin lymphoma is manyfold lower.[90] Leukemia in pregnancy is uncommon.

HODGKIN LYMPHOMA

A review of the literature suggests that neither the histology nor the outcome of patients who present during pregnancy is worse than that of other patients.[91] Diagnosis, usually by biopsy of a lymph node, is usually not problematic, but staging can be difficult. Posterior–anterior chest films with abdominal shielding and marrow biopsy (in the presence of B symptoms, leukopenia, or thrombocytopenia) should be done and present little risk to the fetus. Laboratory studies, including blood counts, liver functions tests, and ESR, should be done, but care should be taken in interpreting the alkaline phosphatase and ESR measurements, which both rise during the course of a normal pregnancy. Evaluation for the presence of abdominopelvic disease is difficult because computed tomography imaging is contraindicated in pregnant women. Abdominal ultrasonograms are safe, but provide limited information. If necessary, magnetic resonance imaging scans can probably be done safely in pregnancy; however, this is rarely necessary. The toxicities of treatment and the risks of delaying treatment until later in pregnancy or postpartum need to be considered carefully in each case. Fetal risks of chemotherapy are greatest in the first trimester during the period of organogenesis, with folate antagonists and antimetabolites carrying the largest risk.[92] Despite the changes in physiology that occur during pregnancy, there is no evidence that dosing should be changed. If chemotherapy is indicated, it should be delayed until the second trimester; however, single-agent vinblastine has been given in the first trimester with a low incidence of fetal abnormalities.[93] Treatment should be timed so that there is the maximum amount of time possible between the last dose of chemotherapy and delivery to avoid cytopenias in either the mother or the fetus. In some cases, radiotherapy may be a feasible alternative in the second and third trimesters of pregnancy. Of 16 patients who received radiotherapy for supradiaphragmatic Hodgkin lymphoma (clinical stages IA and IIA) during pregnancy, 11 received full mantle irradiation, and all patients had lead shielding of the uterus.[94] All 16 pregnancies were carried to completion with full-term deliveries of normal infants. However, a review of the records of 382 women treated with radiotherapy for Hodgkin lymphoma suggests that the risk of breast cancer after radiation therapy is nearly sevenfold greater with irradiation around the time of pregnancy.[95] Additional studies are needed to confirm these findings, but this potential risk should be borne in mind by the clinician when making therapeutic decisions. Relapse of Hodgkin lymphoma usually occurs within the first 2 years following treatment, and patients are counseled to avoid pregnancy during this period. Vigilance for second cancers in these patients is also advised as is monitoring for hypothyroidism in those who receive radiation therapy, especially during subsequent pregnancies when hypothyroidism could have profound maternal and fetal effects.

NON-HODGKIN LYMPHOMA

As compared with Hodgkin lymphoma, other lymphomas are less frequent in pregnancy, tend to present with a higher stage disease, and have a poorer prognosis.[96] Burkitt or Burkitt-like lymphoma can involve the breasts of young pregnant or lactating women and typically behaves aggressively.[97,98] In patients with high-grade lymphomas, chemotherapy often cannot be delayed and difficult decisions must be made. However, in one report of 16 pregnant patients who received aggressive chemotherapy for non-Hodgkin lymphoma during their pregnancies, all survived to delivery.[99] Half of the 16 patients received chemotherapy in their first trimester and all 16 delivered healthy infants despite episodes of myelosuppression during the pregnancies. In a subsequent report, the health of 84 children born to mothers who received chemotherapy for hematologic malignancies during pregnancy revealed no abnormalities in physical or cognitive development and no increase in cancers at a median followup of 18.7 years.[100] Rituximab in pregnancy, both as a single agent and in combination with chemotherapy, has not been associated with abnormalities of the newborn when given in the first, second, or third trimester[115]; however, there is one report of prolonged lymphopenia in a neonate whose mother received rituximab in pregnancy.[101,102]

ACUTE LEUKEMIA

Leukemia is distinctly uncommon in pregnancy; estimates derived from studies beginning in the 1950s place the incidence at about 1:75,000 pregnancies (Chaps. 89 and 93).[103,104] Acute leukemias make up nearly 90 percent of the total, followed by chronic myeloid leukemia, which comprises an additional 10 percent; chronic lymphocytic leukemia is extremely rare.[105] The acute leukemias require urgent treatment, and while pregnancy itself does not alter the course of the leukemia, the outcome is much worse if treatment is delayed.[106] A summary of data on 96 pregnant women reported in the literature from 1983 to 1995 who were treated with cytotoxic chemotherapy for leukemias (most of which were acute) revealed that most patients received regimens that included multiple drugs and were not different from those given to nonpregnant patients.[107] Nearly one-third of patients were treated in the first trimester of pregnancy. Among the 96 pregnancies, there were 2 maternal deaths, 2 children were stillborn, 2 therapeutic abortions were performed, 1 child had chromosomal abnormalities, and 8 had congenital defects. Seven of the eight children born with congenital defects were born to mothers who had been treated in the first trimester. It was not possible to identify a drug (or drugs) that was most likely responsible for adverse outcomes. Treatment in the first trimester carries a high risk of fetal anomaly or miscarriage. Case reports of treatment of acute promyelocytic leukemia in pregnancy with all-*trans*-retinoic acid[108–110] suggest that it may be safe after the first trimester.

Arsenic trioxide is not recommended for use at any stage of pregnancy because of its high potential for embryotoxicity.[124] For patients who require chemotherapy postpartum, breast-feeding is not recommended so as to avoid exposure of the newborn to cytotoxic drugs in the breast milk.[111] Patients with chronic myeloid leukemia have been successfully treated in pregnancy with interferon-α, hydroxyurea, leukapheresis, and even busulfan.[112–114] A review of 125 women treated with imatinib mesylate during pregnancy revealed that most pregnancies had successful outcomes; however, 12 infants had abnormalities, 3 of which involved complex malformations.[115]

ESSENTIAL THROMBOCYTHEMIA

The management of pregnant patients with essential thrombocythemia (ET) is a challenge because thrombosis is the main complication of ET (see Chap. 87) and is accentuated by the prothrombotic state of pregnancy. In addition, of all the myeloproliferative disorders, ET has the highest proportion of affected females of child-bearing age. One study reviewed 155 pregnancies in 86 women with ET, and only 59 percent of these pregnancies resulted in a live neonate.[116] First-trimester abortion was seen in 31 percent of pregnancies, the main cause being placental infarction. Maternal thrombotic or hemorrhagic complications were infrequent, but were more common than in normal pregnancy. Pregnancy did not appear to adversely affect the course and prognosis of ET.

A meta-analysis claimed to reveal a benefit for aspirin treatment, while the benefit of heparin prophylaxis has not been established, but may have a role in selected cases.[117] If cytoreductive therapy becomes necessary, interferon-α is the drug of choice. A similar incidence of ET pregnancy complications was reported in a series from the Mayo clinic.[118] Another large single institution study of 68 young ET patients demonstrated that for both polycythemia vera (PV) and ET, most thromboses in young patients occurred at the time of diagnosis and also suggested, but did not prove, the benefit of aspirin.[119] The most detailed analysis was published by the Italian Society of Hematology in its guidelines.[117] The Society's report analyzed pooled outcome data from 461 pregnancies in women with ET. The mean age of the pregnant patients was 29 years, and the mean platelet count at the beginning of pregnancy was 1000×10^9/L, which declined to 400×10^9/L in the second trimester. This decrease in the platelet count during pregnancy documented for the first time the anecdotal observation that some women with ET spontaneously normalize their platelet count during their pregnancy (the authors of this chapter have rarely observed this phenomenon; however, in one of their ET patients a spontaneous, but transient, ET remission occurred in the first pregnancy, but not in the following pregnancy). The Italian study found that 44 percent of pregnancies were unsuccessful in women with ET, a figure that is threefold higher than in the general population. Among the 461 pregnancies there were 13 pre- or postpartum significant bleeding events. The median duration of gestation was 38 weeks because of abortions and preterm deliveries. Cesarean section was necessary in 15 percent of the patients. The platelet count at the beginning of pregnancy did not predict pregnancy outcome. Placental infarctions were reported in 18 pregnancies and these were associated with intrauterine fetal growth retardation (11 pregnancies). Placental abruption was reported in 3.6 percent of ET pregnancies compared to 1 percent in the non-ET population. Preeclampsia was seen at a rate equal to that seen in non-ET pregnancies. Postpartum thrombotic episodes were reported in 5.2 percent of the pregnancies and included venous thrombosis, pulmonary embolism, sagittal sinus thrombosis, transient ischemic attacks, and Budd-Chiari syndrome (rates for all problems were significantly higher than in non-ET pregnancies). The impact of therapy was difficult to evaluate because management of ET pregnancies was heterogeneous; no specific therapy for ET was given in 48 percent of the pregnancies. Aspirin therapy at doses ranging from 75 mg to 500 mg per day was used in 106 pregnancies, low-molecular-weight heparin (pre-/postpartum) was used in 26, interferon-α was used in 19 pregnancies, and a handful of patients had various chemotherapies and radioactive phosphorus. When the outcome of the ET pregnancies was reviewed, 74 percent of patients treated with aspirin during pregnancy had successful pregnancies, whereas 55 percent of the patients not receiving aspirin had successful pregnancies. Based on the detailed analyses of all variables, this panel of experts felt that there was no direct evidence of the efficacy of aspirin in pregnant ET women, but that "it seems possible that aspirin increases the rate of successful pregnancies." The panel also recommended that ET patients with a thrombotic episode (peripheral or placental) during pregnancy should receive low-molecular-weight heparin at therapeutic doses and oral anticoagulant therapy (prothrombin time international normalized ratio 2–3) for at least 6 weeks postpartum. Longer periods of anticoagulation were recommended for patients with familial thrombophilia. Pregnant women deemed candidates for platelet-lowering therapy (a history of major thrombosis, or of major bleeding, platelet count greater than 1000×10^9/L, familial thrombophilia or cardiovascular risk factors) were recommended to receive interferon. The Italian panel also recommended avoidance of anagrelide in pregnancy because of uncertainty about its teratogenic potential; however, several normal infants have been born to women who inadvertently took this drug during pregnancy (FDA documents submitted by the manufacturer). Although the risk of congenital anomalies among infants of women treated with hydroxyurea during pregnancy was thought to be substantial, of 15 infants born to women treated with hydroxyurea at conception and/or during pregnancy, no malformations were observed, and only one stillbirth was reported in a woman who also had eclampsia. At least one publication has identified the presence of the *JAK2* V617F mutation as a risk factor for pregnancy complications; however, to date there is no consensus on whether to manage these patients differently.[134]

POLYCYTHEMIA VERA

Although there is significant overlap in the clinical features of PV and ET, there are some noteworthy differences (see Chap. 86). In PV, the number of reported pregnancies is low because most PV patients are past child-bearing age, and comorbid conditions are more frequent. One authoritative review suggests maintaining the hemoglobin below 45 percent[120] in pregnancy and another recommends using interferon-α when myelosuppression is indicated.[121] Another noted authority in PV recommends that the hemoglobin be kept lower than 35 percent in pregnancy.[122] However, because of a dearth of data and controlled studies, optimal management of PV pregnancies is poorly defined and agreed upon protocols are not available. None of the available information allows definite therapeutic recommendations; however, some authorities recommend that at a minimum, all pregnant patients with PV be treated with low-dose aspirin.[138]

HEMOGLOBINOPATHIES

■ SICKLE SYNDROMES

Although pregnancy in patients with sickle cell trait is typically uneventful, these patients probably have an increased risk for urinary tract infection.[123] Earlier studies suggested an increased risk for preeclampsia in patients with sickle cell trait, but a large study demonstrated that sickle cell trait is not an independent risk factor for preeclampsia (see Chap. 48).[124]

Patients with sickle cell anemia should receive at least 1 mg of folate per day; however, they should not receive iron supplementation until a ferritin level is checked and iron deficiency is documented.[125] Because of the risk of fetal malformation, hydroxyurea should be discontinued at least 3 months before pregnancy. However, successful outcomes have been reported in sickle cell disease patients who were exposed to the drug while pregnant.[126] Women with sickle cell anemia and their fetuses have an increased risk of complications during pregnancy. In a retrospective review of 127 deliveries of women with sickle cell disease,[127] nearly 50 percent of women with hemoglobin SS experienced pain crises during pregnancy. As compared with deliveries among women with hemoglobin AA, deliveries among women with sickle cell disease were at increased risk for intrauterine growth restriction, low birth weight, prematurity, and preterm labor. In general, these risks were lower for patients with SC disease than with SS disease. More than half of the patients with SS disease in this study had received a blood transfusion during pregnancy. The issue of prophylactic versus need-based transfusion in sickle cell patients is controversial. The single randomized study to address this issue demonstrated no difference in perinatal outcome between the offspring of mothers with sickle cell disease who were assigned to treatment with prophylactic transfusions and those who were not.[128]

Although the incidence of cesarean section in sickle cell patients is reported to be as high as 36 percent,[129] delivery can generally be accomplished vaginally. Most experts recommend avoiding induction of labor as this can lead to sickle crisis.[130] Epidural anesthesia is reported to be safe and to decrease the risk of peripartum painful crises.[131]

THALASSEMIA SYNDROMES

■ β-THALASSEMIA SYNDROMES

Preconception evaluation of patients with β-thalassemia syndromes is recommended and should include assessment of transfusion needs, chelation therapy, body iron status and organ function, and the presence of antibodies to red cell antigens.[132] Patients with β-thalassemia minor generally tolerate pregnancy well; however, doses of at least 4 mg of folate per day are recommended in the preconception period and the first trimester as there is some data to suggest an increased risk of neural tube defects in their offspring.[133] Transfusion and iron chelation therapy has improved both life expectancy and fertility in patients with β-thalassemia intermedia and major, and successful pregnancies have been reported in both disorders.[134] During pregnancy, regular transfusions are recommended to keep the hemoglobin level at 10 mg/dL.[135] Iron-chelation therapy with deferoxamine in pregnancy is controversial and most authorities recommend a hiatus during pregnancy; however, no fetal abnormalities have been reported in pregnancies in which it was continued (see Chap. 47).[136]

■ α-THALASSEMIA SYNDROMES

Patients with the silent carrier state or α-thalassemia trait have no increase in pregnancy complications; however, identification of patients with heterozygous α-thalassemia trait is important in assessing the risk of having a fetus that has hemoglobin H or hemoglobin Bart. Although women with hemoglobin H are generally able to have successful pregnancies, the chronic anemia often worsens, requiring blood transfusion. Patients with hemoglobin H are sensitive to oxidizing compounds and medications, which should be borne in mind, particularly during pregnancy (see Chap. 47).

REFERENCES

1. Pritchard JA: Changes in the blood volume during pregnancy and delivery. *Anesthesiology* 26:393, 1965.
2. Scott DE: Anemia in pregnancy. *Obstet Gynecol Annu* 1:219, 1972.
3. Harstad TW, Mason RA, Cox SM: Serum erythropoietin quantitation in pregnancy using an enzyme-linked immunoassay. *Am J Perinatol* 9:233, 1992.
4. McMullin MF, White R, Lappin T, et al: Haemoglobin during pregnancy: Relationship to erythropoietin and haematinic status. *Eur J Haematol* 71:44, 2003.
5. Pitkin RM, Witte DL: Platelet and leukocyte counts in pregnancy. *JAMA* 242:2696, 1979.
6. van Buul EJA SE, Johnsman HW, et al: Haematological and biochemical profile of uncomplicated pregnancy in nulliparous women: A longitudinal study. *Neth J Med* 46:73, 1995.
7. England JM, Bain BJ: Total and differential leucocyte count. *Br J Haematol* 33:1, 1976.
8. Acker DB, Johnson MP, Sachs BP, et al: The leukocyte count in labor. *Am J Obstet Gynecol* 153:737, 1985.
9. Watts DH, Krohn MA, Wener MH, et al: C-reactive protein in normal pregnancy. *Obstet Gynecol* 77:176, 1991.
10. van den Broe NR, Letsky EA: Pregnancy and the erythrocyte sedimentation rate. *BJOG* 108:1164, 2001.
11. Greer IA: Thrombosis in pregnancy: Maternal and fetal issues. *Lancet* 353:1258, 1999.
12. Clark P, Brennand J, Conkie JA, et al: Activated protein C sensitivity, protein C, protein S and coagulation in normal pregnancy. *Thromb Haemost* 79:1166, 1998.
13. Halligan A BJ, Sheppard B, et al: Haemostatic, fibrinolytic and endothelial variables in normal pregnancies and pre-eclampsia. *Br J Obstet Gynaecol* 101:448, 1992.
14. Brabin BJ, Hakimi M, Pelletier D: An analysis of anemia and pregnancy-related maternal mortality. *J Nutr* 131:604S, 2001.
15. CDC criteria for anemia in children and childbearing-aged women. *MMWR Morb Mortal Wkly Rep* 38:400, 1989.
16. Sifakis S, Pharmakides G: Anemia in pregnancy. *Ann N Y Acad Sci* 900:125, 2000.
17. FAO/WHO: *Joint Expert Consultation Report: Requirements of Vitamin A, Iron, Folate, and Vitamin B12.* FAO Food and Nutrition Series 23. FAO, Rome, 1988.
18. Harthoorn-Lasthuizen EJ, Lindemans J, Langenhuijsen MM: Does iron-deficient erythropoiesis in pregnancy influence fetal iron supply? *Acta Obstet Gynecol Scand* 80:392, 2001.
19. Scholl TO, Hediger ML, Fischer RL, et al: Anemia vs iron deficiency: Increased risk of preterm delivery in a prospective study. *Am J Clin Nutr* 55:985, 1992.
20. Hemminki E, Rimpela U: A randomized comparison of routine versus selective iron supplementation during pregnancy. *J Am Coll Nutr* 10:3, 1991.
21. Horner RD, Lackey CJ, Kolasa K, et al: Pica practices of pregnant women. *J Am Diet Assoc* 91:34, 1991.
22. Shojania AM: Folic acid and vitamin B12 deficiency in pregnancy and in the neonatal period. *Clin Perinatol* 11:433, 1984.
23. Van de Velde A, Van Droogenbroeck J, Tjalma W, et al: Folate and Vitamin B(12) deficiency presenting as pancytopenia in pregnancy: A case report and review of the literature. *Eur J Obstet Gynecol Reprod Biol* 100:251, 2002.
24. Walker SP, Wein P, Ihle BU: Severe folate deficiency masquerading as the syndrome of hemolysis, elevated liver enzymes, and low platelets. *Obstet Gynecol* 90:655, 1997.
25. Mahomed K: Folate supplementation in pregnancy. *Cochrane Database Syst Rev* CD000183, 2000.
26. Bruinse HW, van den Berg H: Changes of some vitamin levels during and after normal pregnancy. *Eur J Obstet Gynecol Reprod Biol* 61:31, 1995.
27. Frenkel EP, Yardley DA: Clinical and laboratory features and sequelae of deficiency of folic acid (folate) and vitamin B12 (cobalamin) in pregnancy and gynecology. *Hematol Oncol Clin North Am* 14:1079, 2000.
28. Aggio MC, Zunini C: Reversible pure red-cell aplasia in pregnancy. *N Engl J Med* 297:221, 1977.
29. Baker RI, Manoharan A, de Luca E, et al: Pure red cell aplasia of pregnancy: A distinct clinical entity. *Br J Haematol* 85:619, 1993.
30. Makino Y, Nagano M, Tamura K, et al: Pregnancy complicated with pure red cell aplasia: A case report. *J Perinat Med* 31:530, 2003.
31. Mant MJ: Chronic idiopathic pure red cell aplasia: Successful treatment during pregnancy and durable response to intravenous immunoglobulin. *J Intern Med* 236:593, 1994.
32. Tuffnell DJ: Amniotic fluid embolism. *Curr Opin Obstet Gynecol* 15:119, 2003.
33. Awad IT, Shorten GD: Amniotic fluid embolism and isolated coagulopathy: Atypical presentation of amniotic fluid embolism. *Eur J Anaesthesiol* 18:410, 2001.
34. Bick RL: Syndromes of disseminated intravascular coagulation in obstetrics, pregnancy, and gynecology. Objective criteria for diagnosis and management. *Hematol Oncol Clin North Am* 14:999, 2000.
35. Goldszmidt E, Davies S: Two cases of hemorrhage secondary to amniotic fluid embolus managed with uterine artery embolization. *Can J Anaesth* 50:917, 2003.
36. Letsky EA: Disseminated intravascular coagulation. *Best Pract Res Clin Obstet Gynaecol* 15:623, 2001.
37. Romero R, Copel JA, Hobbins JC: Intrauterine fetal demise and hemostatic failure: The fetal death syndrome. *Clin Obstet Gynecol* 28:24, 1985.
38. Conti M, Mari D, Conti E, et al: Pregnancy in women with different types of von Willebrand disease. *Obstet Gynecol* 68:282, 1986.
39. Batlle J, Noya MS, Giangrande P, et al: Advances in the therapy of von Willebrand disease. *Haemophilia* 8:301, 2002.
40. Mathew P, Greist A, Maahs JA, et al: Type 2B vWD: The varied clinical manifestations in two kindreds. *Haemophilia* 9:137, 2003.

41. Rick ME, Williams SB, Sacher RA, et al: Thrombocytopenia associated with pregnancy in a patient with type IIB von Willebrand's disease. *Blood* 69:786, 1987.
42. Foster PA: The reproductive health of women with von Willebrand Disease unresponsive to DDAVP: Results of an international survey. On behalf of the Subcommittee on von Willebrand Factor of the Scientific and Standardization Committee of the ISTH. *Thromb Haemost* 74:784, 1995.
43. Briet E, Reisner HM, Blatt PM: Factor IX levels during pregnancy in a women with hemophilia B. *Haemostasis* 11:87, 1982.
44. Giangrande PL: Management of pregnancy in carriers of haemophilia. *Haemophilia* 4:779, 1998.
45. Michiels JJ, Hamulyak K, Nieuwenhuis HK, et al: Acquired haemophilia A in women postpartum: Management of bleeding episodes and natural history of the factor VIII inhibitor. *Eur J Haematol* 59:105, 1997.
46. Solymoss S: Postpartum acquired factor VIII inhibitors: Results of a survey. *Am J Hematol* 59:1, 1998.
47. Kobayashi T, Terao T, Kojima T, et al: Congenital factor XIII deficiency with treatment of factor XIII concentrate and normal vaginal delivery. *Gynecol Obstet Invest* 29:235, 1990.
48. Rodeghiero F, Castaman GC, Di Bona E, et al: Successful pregnancy in a woman with congenital factor XIII deficiency treated with substitutive therapy. Report of a second case. *Blut* 55:45, 1987.
49. Burrows RF, Ray JG, Burrows EA: Bleeding risk and reproductive capacity among patients with factor XIII deficiency: A case presentation and review of the literature. *Obstet Gynecol Surv* 55:103, 2000.
50. Anwar R, Miloszewski KJ: Factor XIII deficiency. *Br J Haematol* 107:468, 1999.
51. Burrows RF, Kelton JG: Fetal thrombocytopenia and its relation to maternal thrombocytopenia. *N Engl J Med* 329:1463, 1993.
52. George JN, Woolf SH, Raskob GE, et al: Idiopathic thrombocytopenic purpura: A practice guideline developed by explicit methods for the American Society of Hematology. *Blood* 88:3, 1996.
53. Kaplan C, Daffos F, Forestier F, et al: Fetal platelet counts in thrombocytopenic pregnancy. *Lancet* 336:979, 1990.
54. Valat AS, Caulier MT, Devos P, et al: Relationships between severe neonatal thrombocytopenia and maternal characteristics in pregnancies associated with autoimmune thrombocytopenia. *Br J Haematol* 103:397, 1998.
55. Martin JN Jr, Perry KG Jr, Blake PG, et al: Better maternal outcomes are achieved with dexamethasone therapy for postpartum HELLP (hemolysis, elevated liver enzymes, and thrombocytopenia) syndrome. *Am J Obstet Gynecol* 177:1011, 1997.
56. Matchaba P, Moodley J: Corticosteroids for HELLP syndrome in pregnancy. *Cochrane Database Syst Rev* CD002076, 2004.
57. Martin JN Jr, Blake PG, Perry KG Jr, et al: The natural history of HELLP syndrome: Patterns of disease progression and regression. *Am J Obstet Gynecol* 164:1500, 1991.
58. Martin JN Jr, Files JC, Blake PG, et al: Postpartum plasma exchange for atypical preeclampsia-eclampsia as HELLP (hemolysis, elevated liver enzymes, and low platelets) syndrome. *Am J Obstet Gynecol* 172:1107, 1995.
59. Rouget JP, Goudemand J, Ducloux G, et al: [Circulating anticoagulant, recurrent abortions and venous thrombosis: A new entity or a pre-lupus syndrome? 2 cases]. *Ann Med Interne (Paris)* 134:111, 1983.
60. Kutteh WH: Antiphospholipid antibodies and reproduction. *J Reprod Immunol* 35:151, 1997.
61. Rai RS, Clifford K, Cohen H, et al: High prospective fetal loss rate in untreated pregnancies of women with recurrent miscarriage and antiphospholipid antibodies. *Hum Reprod* 10:3301, 1995.
62. Rai R, Cohen H, Dave M, et al: Randomised controlled trial of aspirin and aspirin plus heparin in pregnant women with recurrent miscarriage associated with phospholipid antibodies (or antiphospholipid antibodies). *BMJ* 314:253, 1997.
63. Martinelli I, Taioli E, Cetin I, et al: Mutations in coagulation factors in women with unexplained late fetal loss. *N Engl J Med* 343:1015, 2000.
64. Ridker PM, Miletich JP, Buring JE, et al: Factor V Leiden mutation as a risk factor for recurrent pregnancy loss. *Ann Intern Med* 128:1000, 1998.
65. Rey E, Kahn SR, David M, et al: Thrombophilic disorders and fetal loss: A meta-analysis. *Lancet* 361:901, 2003.
66. Greer IA: Thrombophilia: Implications for pregnancy outcome. *Thromb Res* 109:73, 2003.
67. Morrison ER, Miedzybrodzka ZH, Campbell DM, et al: Prothrombotic genotypes are not associated with pre-eclampsia and gestational hypertension: Results from a large population-based study and systematic review. *Thromb Haemost* 87:779, 2002.
68. Gerhardt A, Scharf RE, Beckmann MW, et al: Prothrombin and factor V mutations in women with a history of thrombosis during pregnancy and the puerperium. *N Engl J Med* 342:374, 2000.
69. Macklon NS, Greer IA, Bowman AW: An ultrasound study of gestational and postural changes in the deep venous system of the leg in pregnancy. *Br J Obstet Gynaecol* 104:191, 1997.
70. Cockett FB, Thomas ML: The iliac compression syndrome. *Br J Surg* 52:816, 1965.
71. Ginsberg JS, Brill-Edwards P, Burrows RF, et al: Venous thrombosis during pregnancy: Leg and trimester of presentation. *Thromb Haemost* 67:519, 1992.
72. Conard J, Horellou MH, Van Dreden P, et al: Thrombosis and pregnancy in congenital deficiencies in AT III, protein C or protein S: Study of 78 women. *Thromb Haemost* 63:319, 1990.
73. Pabinger I, Schneider B: Thrombotic risk in hereditary anti-thrombin III, protein C or protein S deficiency. *Arterioscler Thromb Vasc Biol* 16:742, 1996.
74. McColl MD, Ramsay JE, Tait RC, et al: Risk factors for pregnancy associated venous thromboembolism. *Thromb Haemost* 78:1183, 1997.
75. De Stefano V, Leone G, Mastrangelo S, et al: Thrombosis during pregnancy and surgery in patients with congenital deficiency of antithrombin III, protein C, protein S. *Thromb Haemost* 71:799, 1994.
76. Grandone E, Margaglione M, Colaizzo D, et al: Genetic susceptibility to pregnancy-related venous thromboembolism: Roles of factor V Leiden, prothrombin G20210A, and methylenetetrahydrofolate reductase C677T mutations. *Am J Obstet Gynecol* 179:1324, 1998.
77. Martinelli I, De Stefano V, Taioli E, et al: Inherited thrombophilia and first venous thromboembolism during pregnancy and puerperium. *Thromb Haemost* 87:791, 2002.
78. Chabloz P, Reber G, Boehlen F, et al: TAFI antigen and D-dimer levels during normal pregnancy and at delivery. *Br J Haematol* 115:150, 2001.
79. Paniccia R, Prisco D, Bandinelli B, et al: Plasma and serum levels of D-dimer and their correlations with other hemostatic parameters in pregnancy. *Thromb Res* 105: 257, 2002.
80. Kobayashi T, Tokunaga N, Sugimura M, et al: Coagulation/fibrinolysis disorder in patients with severe preeclampsia. *Semin Thromb Hemost* 25:451, 1999.
81. Brill-Edwards P, Ginsberg JS, Gent M, et al: Safety of withholding heparin in pregnant women with a history of venous thromboembolism. Recurrence of Clot in This Pregnancy Study Group. *N Engl J Med* 343:1439, 2000.
82. Pabinger I, Grafenhofer H, Kyrle PA, et al: Temporary increase in the risk for recurrence during pregnancy in women with a history of venous thromboembolism. *Blood* 100:1060, 2002.
83. Ageno W, Crotti S, Turpie AG: The safety of antithrombotic therapy during pregnancy. *Expert Opin Drug Saf* 3:113, 2004.
84. Bauer KA: Management of thrombophilia. *J Thromb Haemost* 1:1429, 2003.
85. Bowles L, Cohen H: Inherited thrombophilias and anticoagulation in pregnancy. *Best Pract Res Clin Obstet Gynaecol* 17:471, 2003.
86. Ginsberg JS, Bates SM: Management of venous thromboembolism during pregnancy. *J Thromb Haemost* 1:1435, 2003.
87. Kearon C, Crowther M, Hirsh J: Management of patients with hereditary hypercoagulable disorders. *Annu Rev Med* 51:169, 2000.
88. Schafer AI, Levine MN, Konkle BA, et al: Thrombotic disorders: Diagnosis and treatment. *Hematology Am Soc Hematol Educ Program* 520, 2003.
89. Clark SL, Porter TF, West FG: Coumarin derivatives and breast-feeding. *Obstet Gynecol* 95:938, 2000.
90. Ward FT, Weiss RB: Lymphoma and pregnancy. *Semin Oncol* 16:397, 1989.
91. Lishner M, Zemlickis D, Sutcliffe SB, et al: Non-Hodgkin's lymphoma and pregnancy. *Leuk Lymphoma* 14:411, 1994.
92. Doll DC, Ringenberg QS, Yarbro JW: Antineoplastic agents and pregnancy. *Semin Oncol* 16:337, 1989.
93. Nisce LZ, Tome MA, He S, et al: Management of coexisting Hodgkin's disease and pregnancy. *Am J Clin Oncol* 9:146, 1986.
94. Woo SY, Fuller LM, Cundiff JH, et al: Radiotherapy during pregnancy for clinical stages IA-IIA Hodgkin's disease. *Int J Radiat Oncol Biol Phys* 23:407, 1992.
95. Chen J, Lee RJ, Tsodikov A, et al: Does radiotherapy around the time of pregnancy for Hodgkin's disease modify the risk of breast cancer? *Int J Radiat Oncol Biol Phys* 58:1474, 2004.
96. Gelb AB, van de Rijn M, Warnke RA, et al: Pregnancy-associated lymphomas. A clinicopathologic study. *Cancer* 78:304, 1996.
97. Bobrow LG, Richards MA, Happerfield LC, et al: Breast lymphomas: A clinicopathologic review. *Hum Pathol* 24:274, 1993.
98. Brogi E, Harris NL: Lymphomas of the breast: Pathology and clinical behavior. *Semin Oncol* 26:357, 1999.
99. Aviles A, Diaz-Maqueo JC, Talavera A, et al: Growth and development of children of mothers treated with chemotherapy during pregnancy: Current status of 43 children. *Am J Hematol* 36:243, 1991.
100. Aviles A, Neri N: Hematological malignancies and pregnancy: A final report of 84 children who received chemotherapy *in utero*. *Clin Lymphoma* 2:173, 2001.
101. Herold M, Schnohr S, Bittrich H: Efficacy and safety of a combined rituximab chemotherapy during pregnancy. *J Clin Oncol* 19:3439, 2001.
102. Kimby E, Sverrisdottir A, Elinder G: Safety of rituximab therapy during the first trimester of pregnancy: A case history. *Eur J Haematol* 72:292, 2004.
103. Catanzarite VA, Ferguson JE, 2nd: Acute leukemia and pregnancy: A review of management and outcome, 1972–1982. *Obstet Gynecol Surv* 39:663, 1984.
104. Yahia C, Hyman GA, Phillips LL: Acute leukemia and pregnancy. *Obstet Gynecol Surv* 13:1, 1958.
105. Pavlidis NA: Coexistence of pregnancy and malignancy. *Oncologist* 7:279, 2002.
106. Kawamura S, Yoshiike M, Shimoyama T, et al: Management of acute leukemia during pregnancy: From the results of a nationwide questionnaire survey and literature survey. *Tohoku J Exp Med* 174:167, 1994.
107. Ebert U, Loffler H, Kirch W: Cytotoxic therapy and pregnancy. *Pharmacol Ther* 74:207, 1997.
108. Delgado-Lamas JL, Garces-Ruiz OM: Malignancy: Case report: Acute promyelocytic leukemia in late pregnancy. Successful treatment with all-*trans*-retinoic acid (ATRA) and chemotherapy. *Hematology* 4:415, 2000.
109. Giagounidis AA, Beckmann MW, Giagounidis AS, et al: Acute promyelocytic leukemia and pregnancy. *Eur J Haematol* 64:267, 2000.

110. Lipovsky MM, Biesma DH, Christiaens GC, et al: Successful treatment of acute promyelocytic leukaemia with all-*trans*-retinoic-acid during late pregnancy. *Br J Haematol* 94:699, 1996.
111. Pejovic T, Schwartz PE: Leukemias. *Clin Obstet Gynecol* 45:866, 2002.
112. Baer MR, Ozer H, Foon KA: Interferon-alpha therapy during pregnancy in chronic myelogenous leukaemia and hairy cell leukaemia. *Br J Haematol* 81:167, 1992.
113. Bazarbashi MS, Smith MR, Karanes C, et al: Successful management of Ph chromosome chronic myelogenous leukemia with leukapheresis during pregnancy. *Am J Hematol* 38:235, 1991.
114. Delmer A, Rio B, Bauduer F, et al: Pregnancy during myelosuppressive treatment for chronic myelogenous leukemia. *Br J Haematol* 82:783, 1992.
115. Gleevec package insert. Novartis Pharmaceuticals, East Hanover, NJ, 2001.
116. Griesshammer M, Grunewald M, Michiels JJ: Acquired thrombophilia in pregnancy: Essential thrombocythemia. *Semin Thromb Hemost* 29:205, 2003.
117. Barbui T, Barosi G, Grossi A, et al: Practice guidelines for the therapy of essential thrombocythemia. A statement from the Italian Society of Hematology, the Italian Society of Experimental Hematology and the Italian Group for Bone Marrow Transplantation. *Haematologica* 89:215, 2004.
118. Elliott MA, Tefferi A: Thrombocythaemia and pregnancy. *Best Pract Res Clin Haematol* 16:227, 2003.
119. Randi ML, Rossi C, Fabris F, et al: Essential thrombocythemia in young adults: Major thrombotic complications and complications during pregnancy—A follow-up study in 68 patients. *Clin Appl Thromb Hemost* 6:31, 2000.
120. Griesshammer M, Bergmann L, Pearson T: Fertility, pregnancy and the management of myeloproliferative disorders. *Baillieres Clin Haematol* 11:859, 1998.
121. Silver RT: Interferon alfa: Effects of long-term treatment for polycythemia vera. *Semin Hematol* 34:40, 1997.
122. Spivak JL: Polycythemia vera: Myths, mechanisms, and management. *Blood* 100:4272, 2002.
123. Pastore LM, Savitz DA, Thorp JM Jr: Predictors of urinary tract infection at the first prenatal visit. *Epidemiology* 10:282, 1999.
124. Stamilio DM, Sehdev HM, Macones GA: Pregnant women with the sickle cell trait are not at increased risk for developing preeclampsia. *Am J Perinatol* 20:41, 2003.
125. Thinkhamrop J, Apiwantanakul S, Lumbiganon P, et al: Iron status in anemic pregnant women. *J Obstet Gynaecol Res* 29:160, 2003.
126. Diav-Citrin O, Hunnisett L, Sher GD, et al: Hydroxyurea use during pregnancy: A case report in sickle cell disease and review of the literature. *Am J Hematol* 60:148, 1999.
127. Sun PM, Wilburn W, Raynor BD, et al: Sickle cell disease in pregnancy: Twenty years of experience at Grady Memorial Hospital, Atlanta, Georgia. *Am J Obstet Gynecol* 184:1127, 2001.
128. Koshy M, Burd L, Wallace D, et al: Prophylactic red-cell transfusions in pregnant patients with sickle cell disease. A randomized cooperative study. *N Engl J Med* 319:1447, 1988.
129. Koshy M, Burd L: Management of pregnancy in sickle cell syndromes. *Hematol Oncol Clin North Am* 5:585, 1991.
130. Rappaport VJ, Velazquez M, Williams K: Hemoglobinopathies in pregnancy. *Obstet Gynecol Clin North Am* 31:287, 2004.
131. Finer P, Blair J, Rowe P: Epidural analgesia in the management of labor pain and sickle cell crisis—A case report. *Anesthesiology* 68:799, 1988.
132. Aessopos A, Karabatsos F, Farmakis D, et al: Pregnancy in patients with well-treated beta-thalassemia: Outcome for mothers and newborn infants. *Am J Obstet Gynecol* 180:360, 1999.
133. Ibba RM, Zoppi MA, Floris M, et al: Neural tube defects in the offspring of thalassemia carriers. *Fetal Diagn Ther* 18:5, 2003.
134. Tamakoudis P, Tsatalas C, Mamopoulos M, et al: Transfusion-dependent homozygous beta-thalassemia major: Successful pregnancy in five cases. *Eur J Obstet Gynecol Reprod Biol* 74:1997.
135. Kumar RM, Rizk DE, Khuranna A: Beta-thalassemia major and successful pregnancy. *J Reprod Med* 42:294, 1997.
136. Singer ST, Vichinsky EP: Deferoxamine treatment during pregnancy: Is it harmful? *Am J Hematol* 60:24, 1999.

CHAPTER 8
HEMATOLOGY IN OLDER PERSONS

William B. Ershler and Dan L. Longo

SUMMARY

Those who are older than the age of 75 years comprise a rapidly growing segment of the population. Marrow, like other organs, undergoes characteristic changes with advancing age, and many of these changes are evident by standard examination. For example, within the marrow space, hematopoietic cells occupy approximately one-half the volume at mid-life, with adipose tissue making up the difference. Yet, in the absence of disease, blood counts are generally maintained within a range established as normal for younger individuals. This is possible because hematopoietic stem cells increase in number with age and are of sufficient functional capacity to respond to homeostatic signals. Older people are more likely to have chronic diseases that may produce additional stress on marrow reserve. Anemia, for example, is present in just over 10 percent of community-dwelling individuals older than the age of 65 years, and for those residing in nursing homes, the prevalence is closer to 50 percent. One distinction between anemia in older people compared with younger people is that for approximately one-third of older anemic patients, a specific cause for the anemia cannot be determined. This "unexplained anemia" is likely the result of multiple factors, including inappropriately low erythropoietin response, inflammatory cytokines, androgen deficiency, and to some extent, early myelodysplasia. Platelet and neutrophil changes with age have been incompletely characterized but are likely to be subtle and of little clinical consequence. There is a well-characterized, age-associated involution of the thymus gland that precedes the histologic changes within the marrow, and marrow-derived T- and B-cell precursors are affected. Older people have fewer naïve, reactive T cells and an increase in relatively inert memory T cells. Thus, the capacity to react to new antigenic challenges is reduced and there is an increased susceptibility to certain infections and vaccines. Also evident are deficient regulatory functions, which may explain the observed increase in autoantibody, paraprotein, and inflammatory cytokines in those of advanced age. In the absence of disease, however, these alterations are of little consequence. In the presence of chronic debilitating disease, they are likely to become more pronounced and as such, contribute to an exaggerated decline in overall function. Similar conclusions can be drawn regarding dysregulated inflammatory pathways and coagulation. In balance, advancing age is associated with a procoagulant profile that may be of clinical importance in the presence of underlying atherosclerotic vascular disease.

Abbreviations and acronyms used in this chapter include: EPSE, Established Populations for the Epidemiological Study of the Elderly; HSC, hematopoietic stem cells; IADL, independent activities of daily living; IL, interleukin; LIF, leukemia inhibitory factor; NHANES, National Health and Nutrition Examination Survey; OSM, oncostatin M; PAI-1, plasminogen-activator inhibitor-I; TAFI, thrombin-activatable fibrinolysis inhibitor; TCR, T-cell receptor; TF, tissue factor; TGF-β, transforming growth factor-beta; Th, T-helper lymphocytes; TNF-α, tumor necrosis factor-alpha; t-PA, tissue-type plasminogen activator; WHO, World Health Organization.

Over the next several decades, the percentage of the population older than the age of 65 years will nearly double.[1] In anticipation, an increased research effort is being made to better understand the basic biology of aging and the mechanisms whereby individuals become susceptible to disease.[2] This chapter presents a current appraisal of our understanding of aging followed by a more detailed description of age-associated changes in hematopoiesis and their clinical consequences.

A PRIMER ON AGING

A central dogma in gerontology is that aging is not a disease. One common feature of aging is that for any variable that can be measured, the range of values among normal individuals in an aging population is much wider than the range of normal among younger individuals. Although functional declines that accompany normal aging have been well characterized,[3] in general these are of insufficient magnitude to account for symptoms or be mistaken for disease. For example, that kidney function declines with age is well recognized,[4] and, in fact, has proven to be a useful biologic marker of aging. Yet, clinical consequences of this change in renal function, in the absence of a disease or the exposure to an exogenous nephrotoxic agent, do not occur commonly. Similarly, the marrow changes with age. Marrow stem cells increase in number and proliferative capacity, yet the *in vitro* proliferative potential of progenitor and cells is less.[5–7] Although clinically significant cytopenias do not occur in the absence of disease, mild to moderate anemia that has not been fully characterized occurs with increasing frequency, especially in the frail elderly. Furthermore, in frail individuals even a mild reduction in hemoglobin level is associated with untoward clinical outcomes.[8,9]

Certain immune functions decrease with age,[10,11] but these may be of only marginal clinical significance. For example, whether the laboratory-observed declines in immune function contribute to a heightened susceptibility to infection is a subject of debate, but data support an association of age-associated qualitative change in lymphocyte function and susceptibility to reactivation of tuberculosis[12,13] or herpes zoster[14,15] and diminished response to influenza vaccine.[16–19] The immune decline, however, is not considered of sufficient magnitude or duration to account for the increased incidence of cancer in older people,[20] although this remains a point of contention.[21] Similarly, autoantibody and monoclonal gammopathies appear with increasing frequency with advancing age, but these have been considered a marker of an acquired dysregulation of humoral immunity but unlikely to be of clinical importance.[22]

THEORIES OF AGING

Providing a rational, unifying explanation for the aging process has been the subject of a great number of theoretical expositions. Yet, no single proposal suffices to account for the complexities observed (Table 8–1).

Genetic Effects

That genetic controls are involved seems obvious when one considers that life span is highly species specific. For example, mice generally live approximately 30 months and humans approximately 90 years. However, the aging phenomenon is not necessarily a direct consequence of primary DNA sequence. For example, mice and bats have 0.25 percent difference in their primary DNA sequence but bats live for 25 years, 10 times longer than mice. Thus, regulation of gene expression seems likely to be the major source of species longevity differences.

Although within a species there is considerable variation in longevity, this variability is much less within inbred strains or among monozygotic

TABLE 8–1. Theories of Aging

Intrinsic-stochastic	Somatic mutation[29,30]
	Intrinsic mutagenesis[34]
	Impaired DNA repair[35]
	Error catastrophe[37]
Extrinsic-stochastic	Ionizing radiation[29,30,32,37]
	Free radical[42,43]
Genetically determined	Neuroendocrine[240]
	Immune[56]

twins, when compared to dizygotic twins or nontwin siblings. Also, various genetically determined syndromes have remarkable (albeit incomplete) features of accelerated aging. These include Hutchison-Guilford (early onset progeria), Werner (adult-onset progeria), and Down syndromes.[23] Although no progeria syndrome manifests a complete phenotype of advanced age, the identification of the genes responsible for these particular syndromes is beginning to pay dividends by providing clues to the molecular mechanisms involved in the aging process. For example, Werner syndrome is now known to be caused by mutations in a single gene on chromosome 8 that encodes a protein containing a helicase-like domain.[24,25] Similarly, a mutation in the lamin A (*LMNA*) gene localized to chromosome 1 has been demonstrated to be the cause of the Hutchison-Guilford syndrome.[26] The future functional characterization of these specific proteins will, no doubt, increase our level of understanding of the aging process.

Examination of aging in yeast has also been informative with regard to the genetic controls of aging. These single-cell organisms follow the replicative limits of mammalian cells and it has been observed that "life span" is related to silencing large chromosomal regions. Mutations in these silencing genes lead to increased longevity.[27] Thus, if there are certain genes that regulate normal aging, or at least are associated with the development of an aged phenotype, it stands to reason that acquired damage to those genes might influence the rate of aging.

Over the years several theories have been proposed that relate to this supposition. In general, they hypothesize a random or stochastic accumulation of damage, either to DNA or protein that leads eventually to dysfunctional cells, cell death, and subsequent organ dysfunction and ultimately death. Prominent among these is the *somatic mutation* theory,[28] which predicts that genetic damage from background radiation, for example, accumulates and produces mutations that ultimately result in functional decline. A variety of refinements have been suggested to this theory invoking the importance of mutational interactions,[29] transposable elements,[30] and changes in DNA methylation status.[31]

Intrinsic Mutagenesis Theory

A related hypothesis is Burnet's *theory of intrinsic mutagenesis*[32] which proposes that spontaneous or endogenous mutations occur at different rates in different species and that this accounts for the variability observed in life span. Closely related to this notion is the *DNA repair* theory.[33] Initially there was great excitement about this idea as it was found that long-lived animals had demonstrably more active DNA repair mechanisms than shorter-lived species.[33] However, longitudinal studies within a species have not revealed a consistent decline in repair mechanisms with age. This, of course, does not rule out the possibility that repair of certain specific and critical DNA lesions is altered with advancing age. We now understand that there are multiple DNA repair mechanisms including base excision repair, transcription-coupled repair, and even mitochondrial DNA repair mechanisms. Disorders involving one or a subset of repair mechanisms could lead to accumulation of DNA damage and dysfunction.

Error Catastrophe Theory

In yet another intrinsic/stochastic model, the theory of *error catastrophe* proposed by Orgel,[34] it is suggested that random errors in protein synthesis occur and when the proteins involved are those responsible for DNA or RNA synthesis, there is resultant DNA damage and the consequences thereof to daughter cells. Although this model has appeal, there has been no reported evidence for impaired or inaccurate protein synthesis machinery with advancing age. However, a candidate protein that may eventually be shown to be so affected is telomerase. This critical enzyme is necessary for maintaining telomere length and cell replicative potential. *In vitro* cellular senescence is associated with diminished telomerase activity,[35] but whether this relates to aging of the organism as a whole remains controversial.[36]

Posttranslational Effects

Evidence that exogenous factors are involved in the acquisition of age-associated damage to DNA and protein is derived from a number of observations, many of which are circumstantial or correlative, but nonetheless provocative. It now appears that the accumulation of abnormal protein within senescent cells, as predicted by the *error catastrophe* theory, actually reflects posttranslational events, such as glycation or oxidation-resultant crosslinking. There is theoretic appeal to the concept that key proteins, such as collagen or other extracellular matrix proteins and DNA become dysfunctional with age as a result of the impairment produced by these crosslinks.[37–39]

Glycation One mechanism producing crosslinks is called glycation, the nonenzymatic reaction of glucose with the amino groups of proteins. Presumably, glycation would occur more readily in the presence of higher serum levels of glucose; consequently, this theory fits well with the observed, age-associated dysregulation of glucose metabolism and prevalent hyperglycemia in geriatric populations. Of course, these findings also point out the theory's deficiency as a unifying mechanism, as there is no question that individuals with well-maintained glucose levels throughout their life span are still subject to the acquired changes typical of aging.

Free Radical Hypothesis

Another mechanism held responsible for crosslinking is the damage produced by free radicals, and this forms the basis of the *free radical hypothesis* initially promoted by Harman.[40,41] This theory offers that aging is the result of DNA and protein damage (e.g., mutagenesis or crosslinking) by atoms or molecules that contain unpaired electrons (free radicals). These highly reactive species are produced as byproducts of a variety of metabolic processes and are normally inhibited by intrinsic cellular antioxidant defense mechanisms. Nitrate-based free radicals are also generated by *in vivo* processes and another set of nitrogen free-radical scavenging mechanisms are in place. If free radical generation increases with age, or the defense mechanisms that scavenge free radicals (e.g., glutathione) or repair free radical damage decline, the accumulated free radical damage may account for altered DNA and protein function. Evidence to support this widely held notion is incomplete. It is known that free radical generation in mammals correlates inversely with longevity[42] and, similarly, the level of free radical inhibiting enzymes, such as superoxide dismutase were higher in those species with longer life spans.[42] However, efforts at enhancing antioxidant mechanisms with dietary vitamin E have resulted in only a modest enhancement of median survival in mice and no affect on maximum lifespan.[43–45]

Much attention has been focused on mitochondrial function in the context of free radical damage because the bulk of oxidative metabolism and the production of reactive oxygen species occur in these organelles. Although mitochondrial DNA codes for antioxidant enzymes in addition to enzymes involved in energy production, it is currently believed that energy production declines with age, as a result of mitochondrial DNA damage by those reactive products. Indeed, mitochondrial damage increases with age in experimental models[46–48] and the shortened survival of knockout mice deficient in mitochondrial antioxidant enzymes has supported the potential importance of this mechanism.[49]

The most compelling data to date in support of the free radical hypothesis come from the experiments of Orr and Sohal in which transgenic *Drosophila* producing enhanced levels of superoxide dismutase and catalase had a maximum survival 33 percent greater than controls.[26] Furthermore, it is known that flies produce high levels of free radicals associated with their impressive metabolic requirements, and that survival is enhanced dramatically when the ability to fly is experimentally hindered.[44] However, the generalizability of these findings has been questioned. It has been noted that transgenic mice overexpressing free radical scavenging enzymes have produced very modest effects on life span.[50] Thus, the conclusion that augmentation of free radical scavenging mechanisms increases longevity in mammalian species is not established.

Neuroendocrine Theory

From a different perspective, very good evidence implicates a nonrandom, perhaps genetically regulated, endogenous mechanism involved in aging. For example, the theory of *neuroendocrine effects* suggests that the decrements in neuronal and associated hormonal function are central to aging. It has been suggested that age-associated decline of hypothalamic–pituitary–adrenal axis function results in a physiologic cascade leading ultimately to the "frail" phenotype. This hypothesis is appealing because it is well established that this neuroendocrine axis regulates much of development and also the involution of ovarian and testicular function. Furthermore, age-associated declines in growth hormone and related factors,[51] dehydroepiandrosterone,[52] and secondary sex steroids[53] are implicated in age-associated impairments, including a reduction in lean body mass and bone density. Furthermore, pharmacologic reconstitution using these or related hormones has met with some success at reversing age-associated functional decline.[54,55]

Immunologic Theory

Similarly, it has been argued that involution of the thymus gland and subsequent decline in immune function (see "Marrow and Thymus: Anatomical Changes" on the next page) is a key regulator of aging.[56] The argument is based upon the observation that the decline in immune function occurs in all mammalian species, but occurs later in those with longer survival.[57] Furthermore, dietary restriction is associated with maintained thymic mass and measurable immune function as well as prolonged survival, suggesting an association of a decline in immunity with primary aging processes.

The possibility is highlighted by the observation that differences in maximum survival of different mouse strains is associated with specific alleles in the major histocompatibility complex, which, in turn, code for immunologic determinants.[58] This hypothesis, although not without its appeal, is not widely accepted as a major explanation for aging. Perhaps this relates to the fact that biologic aging is a universal phenomenon and certain features are held in common, even in organisms with primitive or no immune function. (The same could also be said for the neuroendocrine theory.) It is obvious that the immune system is of great importance in minimizing the chance of early death, particularly from infectious diseases. However, immunologic reconstitution of middle-aged or old animals has not been shown to prolong survival.[59]

LIFE SPAN: MEDIAN AND MAXIMUM SURVIVAL

From the perspective of those who study aging, an important distinction is made between median (life expectancy) and maximum life span. Over the past century, a dramatic increase in median survival has been mostly attributable to modern sanitation and refrigeration, as well as public health measures, including vaccination and antibiotics.[60] Early deaths have been diminished and more individuals are reaching old age. In the United States today, expected survival from birth is approximately 80 years.[61] Median survival is what concerns public health officials and healthcare providers. In contrast, maximum survival is the focus of those gerontologists interested in the biology of aging and longevity.

The oldest human being alive today is approximately 120 years old. It is intriguing that the oldest age limit has remained stable, unchanged by the public health initiatives mentioned above. In the laboratory, limits on age have been established for a variety of species. *Drosophila*, free of predators, disease, or flyswatters, can live 30 days, whereas C57BL/6 mice in a laboratory environment and allowed to eat a healthy diet *ad libitum*, may survive 40 months. Unlike health-related interventions in humans, certain experimental interventions in lower species have been associated with a prolongation of maximum survival. In *Drosophila*, for example, transgenic offspring producing extra copies of the free radical scavenging enzymes superoxide dismutase and catalase survive approximately 33 percent longer than controls.[62] In nutritional intervention studies involving lower species, controlled restriction of dietary intake (dietary restriction) has become a common experimental paradigm exploited in the investigation of primary processes of aging and maximum survival.[63,64]

DIETARY RESTRICTION

Dietary restriction typically involves a reduction of 30 to 40 percent in caloric intake with careful attention to the provision of adequate amounts of essential nutrients. It is associated with both a delay in the acquisition of age-related diseases (including cancer) and a reduction in the rate of achieving certain established biomarkers of aging (i.e., a retardation in primary aging). The critical questions remain: What is the mechanism of the dietary restriction effect, and will it be applicable to higher species? With regard to the latter, there are now comprehensive and interactive studies within the United States in which dietary restriction is being examined in nonhuman primates[65,66] and human studies are also under way.[67,68] Although it appears that the calorie-restricted monkeys in these studies are assuming a more youthful phenotype in a variety of physiologic measures,[65,69,70] it remains too early to predict whether maximum survival will be affected.

CELLULAR VERSUS ORGANISMAL AGING

After a finite number of divisions, normal somatic cells invariably enter a state of irreversibly arrested growth, a process termed *replicative senescence*.[71] It has been proposed that escape from the regulators of senescence is what oncologists term *malignant transformation*. However, the role of replicative senescence as an explanation of organismal aging remains the subject of vigorous debate. The controversy relates, in part, to the fact that certain organisms (e.g., *Drosophila, Caenorhabditis elegans*) undergo an aging process, yet all of their adult cells are postreplicative.

What is clear is that the loss of proliferative capacity of human cells in culture is intrinsic to the cells and not dependent on either environmental factors or culture conditions.[71] Unless transformation occurs,

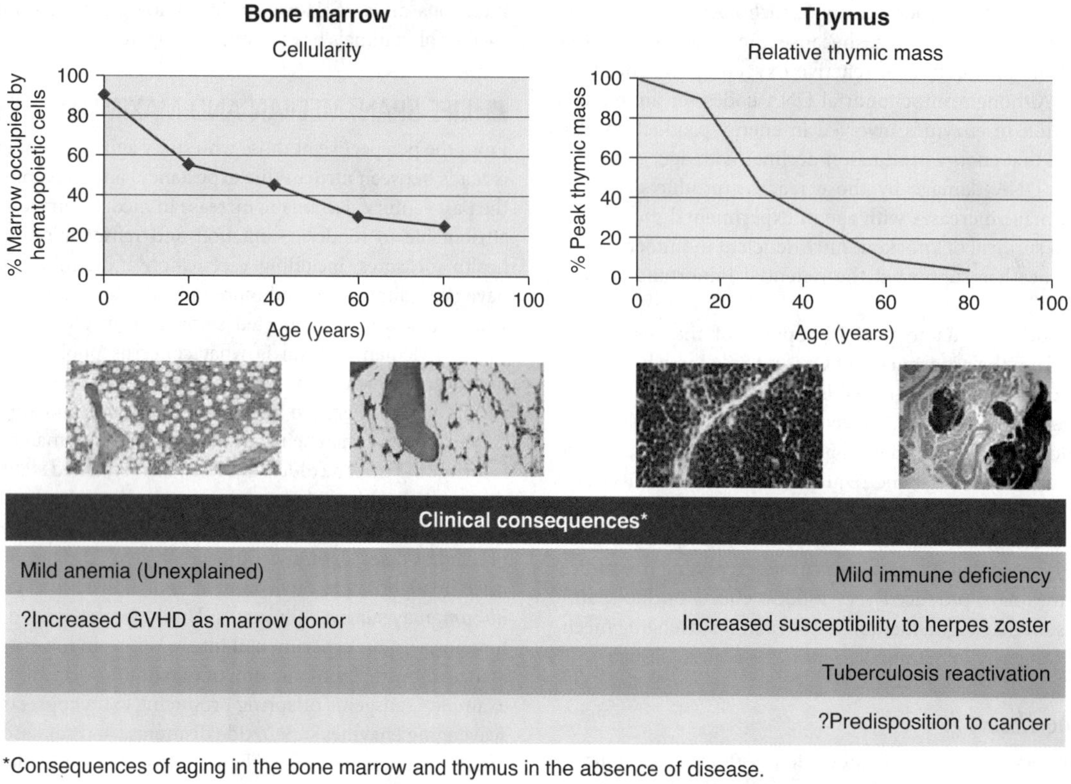

FIGURE 8–1. Aging of marrow and thymus. Marrow cellularity declines from birth in a manner comparably to thymic mass. This is reflected histologically by the increased presence of fat. The clinical consequences of these age-associated changes, in the absence of disease, are a mild anemia and immune deficiency. The latter is reflected by an increased predisposition to certain infections (e.g., herpes zoster or reactivation of latent tuberculosis) and possibly to the increased predisposition to cancer. GVHD, graft-versus-host disease.

cells age with each successive division. The number of divisions turns out to be more important than the actual amount of time passed. Thus, cells held in a quiescent state for months, when allowed back into a proliferative environment, will continue approximately the same number of divisions as those that were allowed to proliferate without a quiescent period.[72] The question remains whether this *in vitro* phenomenon is relevant to animal aging.[72] Although when various species are compared, replicative potential is directly and significantly related to life span,[73] within an organism there is great variability in proliferative capacity from tissue to tissue and organ to organ. Thus, age-associated changes in the marrow or gut might relate to replicative senescence, whereas in muscle or brain other processes most certainly are involved.

AGING AND HEMATOPOIESIS

Aging is a universal phenomenon that affects all normal cells, tissues, organ systems, and organisms. Accordingly, the marrow undergoes changes with age. Age-related hematologic changes are reflected by a decline in marrow cellularity, an increased risk of myeloproliferative diseases[74] and anemia,[75–77] and a declining adaptive immunity.[78,79]

MARROW AND THYMUS: ANATOMIC CHANGES

The percentage of marrow space occupied by the hematopoietic tissue declines from 90 percent at birth to a level of approximately 50 percent at age 30 years and 30 percent at age 70 years.[80,81] A similar change occurs in the thymus, where involution begins at an earlier age and is reflected anatomically by a reduction in lymphoid mass with an increase in fat[82] and functionally by a steady decrease in the production of naïve T cells[59,83] (Fig. 8–1). Fat infiltration into the marrow and thymus results in a diminished volume of hematopoietic tissue.

Although age-related change in the marrow is well described, the exact mechanisms that regulate these changes remains speculative. For example, it remains unclear whether the age-associated expansion of marrow fat is a cause or an effect of aging and whether the changes seen in marrow and histologically similar changes within the thymus are intrinsically related. Because of the intricate association of hematologic and immune functions and these common histologic patterns of change with age, both changes in blood and innate immunity are discussed below.

Marrow: Stem Cells

The ontogeny of hematopoietic stem cells (HSC) is the focus of much attention. In fetal development the manufacture of blood occurs in various organs but after birth this function is subsumed by the marrow (see Chaps. 4 and 6). Current evidence identifies early hematopoietic cells both in the extraembryonic yolk sac as well as an intraembryonic site within the ventral wall of dorsal aorta–gonad–mesonephros.[84] At approximately 5 to 6 weeks of gestation, progenitors derived from the yolk sac colonize the fetal liver and become the major source for blood cells for the remainder of intrauterine life.[85] At around 7 weeks of gestation, hematopoietic cells also colonize the spleen[85] and multipotent progenitor cells are seen in the fetal circulation by the end of 12 to 14 weeks of gestation.[86] At around 8 to 9 weeks of gestation, while hematopoiesis within the yolk sac per se is becoming extinct, T-cell production starts in the thymus.[87] T-cell precursors derived from the fetal liver colonize the thymus and undergo maturation and differentiation.[88–90] Hematopoietic cells first appear in the medullary cavities of bone at around 14 weeks of gestation[91] and by birth the marrow has become the primary site of hematopoiesis.

Unlike the commonly held notion that stem cell compartments diminish either in number or function with age ultimately resulting in an inability to meet homeostatic demands, age-related HSC changes appear to be an exception, at least for murine species in which this question has been most directly addressed. Early work demonstrated that marrow serially transplanted could reconstitute hematopoietic function for an estimated 15 to 20 life spans.[92] Furthermore, the capacity for old marrow to reconstitute proved superior to that of young.[93] Subsequently, a number of investigators using a variety of techniques have concluded that HSC frequency in old mice is approximately twice that found in young.[94–97] Some evidence suggests that the intrinsic function of HSC changes somewhat with age, most notably in a shift in lineage potential from lymphoid to myeloid development. This may contribute to an observed relative increase in neutrophils and decrease in lymphocytes in the blood of older people.[98]

Marrow also serves as one of the organs of the immune system. B-lymphocyte maturation begins within the marrow where precursor cells acquire surface immunoglobulin. Marrow-derived T-lymphocyte precursors are reduced in number with advancing age.[79] Thus, to some extent the decline in immune function with age is a consequence of marrow aging.

Marrow during Adult Life

The most apparent change seen in the marrow with aging is decreased cellularity.[80] Under normal circumstances, the marrow is the only site of hematopoiesis. Extramedullary hematopoiesis may occur in the liver, spleen, and lymph nodes in pathologic states when the marrow compensatory mechanisms are outstripped. Until puberty the entire skeleton remains hematopoietically active but by age 18 years only the vertebrae, ribs, sternum, skull, pelvis, proximal epiphyseal regions of humerus, and femur remain active sites of blood production, with other medullary sites replaced with fatty tissue. By age 40 years, the marrow in sternum, ribs, pelvis, and vertebrae is composed of equal amounts of hematopoietic tissue and fat, and cellularity declines gradually thereafter. By age 65 years, marrow cellularity has been estimated to be approximately 30 percent[80,81] with a corresponding increase in marrow fat. Age-associated imbalanced bone remodeling and osteoporosis results in decreased trabecular bone, which itself may contribute to diminished hematopoiesis.[99] The presence of marrow fat correlates with the occurrence and severity of osteoporosis, both of which are evident with aging.[100] Several age-related qualitative changes have been identified in hematopoietic cells, including skewed X-chromosome inactivation, telomere shortening,[101–103] accumulation of mitochondrial DNA mutations,[104,105] and micronuclei formation,[106] any of which could result in cellular dysfunction. Furthermore, growth hormone production declines with age and this, too, is linked with deposition of fat within the marrow.[107] Administration of growth hormone to old rats reduces marrow fat and increases hematopoietic tissue.[108]

Blood Cell Changes with Age

Red Blood Cells Anemia is a significant health problem in the elderly because of both a high prevalence and significant associated morbidity, including reduced quality of life, clinical depression, falls, functional impairment, slower walking speed, reduced grip strength, loss of mobility, worsening comorbidities, and mortality.[109,110]

In older men and women, anemia defined using the World Health Organization (WHO) criteria of hemoglobin levels less than 13 g/dL for men and 12 g/dL for women[111] is associated with an increase in mortality.[112–117] The WHO criteria do not take into account inherent ethnic variations particularly with respect to Americans of African descent who have lower levels of hemoglobin without significant adverse outcomes.[118,119] In a study that analyzed 1018 Americans of African descent and 1583 Americans of European descent, adults ages 71 to 82 years, anemia defined by the WHO criteria was associated with increased mortality in the latter but not the former.[118,119] The reasons for these ethnic differences are undefined. However, the difference is one of degree. In general, the impact of anemia on functional status and mortality in Americans of African descent becomes apparent at hemoglobin levels about 1 g/dL lower than in those of European descent. The issue of establishing criteria for the diagnosis of anemia is relevant in the context of age, as well. Older women, for example, have better physical performance and function at hemoglobin values between 13 and 15 g/dL than at 12 to 12.9 g/dL,[120] suggesting that a cutoff level of 12 g/dL is too low. Nevertheless, the WHO definition remains the standard used in most current epidemiologic surveys and many clinical laboratories.

Prevalence of Anemia The third National Health and Nutrition Examination Survey (NHANES III) database, a nationally representative sample of community-dwelling persons, was used to determined age- and sex-specific prevalence rates of anemia in the total U.S. population.[121] For those older than the age of 65 years, by WHO criteria, approximately 11 percent were anemic (Table 8–2). The prevalence of anemia was lowest (1.5%) among males between 17 and 49 years of age and highest (26.1%) in males older than age 85 years. Among those age 65 years and older, the prevalence rate was notably higher in Americans of African descent as compared to Americans of European or Hispanic descent. Prevalence rates of anemia in the elderly vary in community-dwelling and institutionalized populations. Anemia is more common among frail elderly. In the nursing home, for example, anemia prevalence approaches 50 percent or higher.[122–125]

Unexplained Anemia Hematologists are usually successful in uncovering the cause of anemia in young and middle-aged adults. However, in older populations, a specific explanation cannot be defined by routine evaluation in approximately one-third of anemic patients (see Table 8–2).

TABLE 8–2. Prevalence of Anemia in the Elderly Using the WHO* Criteria

Study	Age (Years)	Population	Prevalence (%)
Guralnik, Eisenstaedt, Ferrucci, et al (2004)[121]	≥65	Community-dwelling elderly Americans	10.6
Ferrucci, Guralnik, Bandinelli, et al (2007)[241]	>70	Community-dwelling elderly Italian	11
Denny, Kuchibhatla, Cohen (2006)[242]	≥71	Community-dwelling	24
Joosten, Pelemans, Hiele, et al (1992)[243]	≥65	Hospitalized	24†
Artz, Fergusson, Drinka, et al (2004)[122]	Most ≥65	Nursing-home	48
Robinson, Artz, Culleton, et al (2007)[125]	≥65	Nursing-home	59.6

*World Health Organization anemia criteria: hemoglobin <13 g/dL for adult men and <12 g/dL for adult women.

†In this study, anemia defined as hemoglobin <11.5 g/dL.

Typically, this anemia is mild (hemoglobin concentration in the 10–12 g/dL range), normocytic, and hypoproliferative (relatively low absolute reticulocyte count). It has been postulated that the cause relates to a number of factors, including declining testosterone level,[126] occult inflammation,[127] impaired renal function with inappropriately low serum erythropoietin,[128] and occult myelodysplasia.[129] Likely, unexplained anemia represents an amalgam of these and perhaps other factors, such as shortened red cell survival, refractoriness of the erythroid precursors to erythropoietin stimulation, and/or the presence of as yet undiagnosed illness.

Serum Erythropoietin Data on erythropoietin levels in nonanemic older persons are inconsistent. Some suggest that nonanemic older persons have higher erythropoietin levels compared to younger adults,[130–132] but other studies fail to confirm these findings.[10–12] One longitudinal analysis demonstrated that serum erythropoietin levels rose gradually in healthy individuals who maintained normal hemoglobin levels but the rise was not observed in those who developed diabetes or hypertension during the evaluation period.[133] An explanation for the rise in serum erythropoietin with age has not been established, but in theory, it could be the result of age-associated shortened red cell survival or reduced sensitivity of erythroid progenitor cells to the erythropoietin signal. Studies in older subjects are ongoing to define the basis for the increasing need for erythropoietin to maintain normal levels of red cells.

White Blood Cells Although no significant change is seen in the blood leukocyte count or differential count with normal aging,[134,135] among those who acquire features of frailty, an increased neutrophil count may be observed.[98,136] Furthermore, several qualitative neutrophil defects have been described. For example, a decreased respiratory burst response to soluble signals,[134] defective phagocytosis,[135] and impaired neutrophil migration to sites of stress[137] have been described in accordance with advanced age. Although the exact cause for these functional changes has not been clarified, it may be associated with an age-related alteration in actin cytoskeleton and receptor expression in leukocytes.[138] A mild decrease in the blood lymphocyte count is first noticeable in the fourth decade with a gradually progressive decrease thereafter throughout the remainder of the life span.[139] Qualitative alterations in T-lymphocyte function in the elderly have also been demonstrated,[140] as discussed in Aging and Immunity, below.

Platelets At present, knowledge about the influence of age on platelet counts has been limited to cross-sectional data derived from selected populations. From those data, no or very limited changes in platelet number are noted with age.[141–144] To date, a longitudinal data set describing alterations in platelet number with advancing age has not been produced nor are there conclusive studies describing age-associated changes in platelet function.

COAGULANT AND ANTICOAGULANT FACTORS

Plasma Factor Concentrations

A number of proteins critical to clot formation and fibrinolysis change in characteristic ways with advancing age.[145–147] Plasma concentrations of factor VII coagulant activity and antigen,[145–149] and factor VIIIC,[132,147,150] as well as von Willebrand factor,[132,150] fibrinogen,[132,147,149,151] fibrinopeptide A,[132,147,148] and tissue plasminogen activator antigen[132,152–154] increase with age (see Chaps. 115, 116, and 136 for general discussions of coagulation proteins and their regulation). In healthy centenarians, levels of activated factor VII, activation peptides of prothrombin, factors IX and X, and thrombin–antithrombin complex concentration were increased, which are signs of higher-than-expected coagulation enzyme activity.[147] Age-associated increases in levels of protein C occur in both sexes. Aging is also associated with increasing levels of free protein S.[145] In contrast, antithrombin III tends to decrease with age in males and increases with age in females following menopause.[155] Higher D-dimer and plasmin–antiplasmin complexes indicate an accompanying increase in fibrinolytic activity.[147,156] In contrast, plasma tissue-type plasminogen activator (t-PA) inhibitor levels increase with increasing age, as do levels of thrombin-activatable fibrinolysis inhibitor (TAFI) in women[157] and its proenzyme form, procarboxypeptidase U, in both sexes (see Chap. 136 for a general discussion of fibrinolysis).[158] These latter findings are suggestive of a possible age-dependent compromise in fibrinolytic activity.[159] Thus, procoagulant and, in some studies, fibrinolytic activities appear to be increased in older subjects by both *in vitro*[147,160,161] and *in vivo* studies.[162,163] Older patients may show an exaggerated anticoagulant response to warfarin.[164]

Aging as a Prothrombotic State

Activation of the coagulation system and increase in procoagulant markers have been associated with the pathogenesis of atherosclerosis.[165,166] However, procoagulant markers, most notably D-dimer,[167] fibrinogen, and factor VIII,[168] also increase with advancing age, and may, in fact, correlate better with aging than with cardiovascular disease. The Established Populations for the Epidemiological Study of the Elderly (EPESE) cohort, examined 1729 participants age 70 years and older, and showed that increasing age was associated with high D-dimer levels.[165,166] For example, 23 percent of the participants ages 90 to 99 years had high D-dimer levels (>600 mcg/L) compared to 13 percent in the 80 to 89 years age group and 7 percent in the 70 to 79 years age group.[156] Fibrinogen concentrations in healthy subjects ages 19 to 96 years were significantly higher in participants older than the age of 60 years when compared to younger subjects.[169] An examination of healthy individuals across the life span found that fibrinogen levels increased by 25 mg/dL per decade of life and that levels as high as 320 mg/dL were found in more than 80 percent of people older than 65 years of age.[170] Other markers of activated coagulation, such as plasminogen-activation inhibitor-1 (PAI-1) and factor VIII increase with age.[150,171,172] Thus, aging is associated with markers of activated coagulation. In this context, it is notable that the incidence of venous thrombosis and pulmonary emboli increases dramatically in geriatric populations.[173,174] Bleeding complications from anticoagulation therapy are also increased in older patients. No interventional study has identified an at-risk population of normal subjects without prior thrombosis in whom prophylactic anticoagulation is of value.

Coagulation and Functional Decline

The EPESE study demonstrated that increases in D-dimer and interleukin-6 (IL-6) were related to increases in both morbidity and mortality.[156] In fact, the correlation for adverse outcomes was stronger with D-dimer than IL-6.[175] In this, and other studies,[176–178] D-dimer and other markers of activated coagulation were associated with limitation in a wide variety of functional domains including independent activities of daily living (IADL), lower-extremity function, and performance on cognitive testing. The age-associated changes in coagulation markers occur earlier than other aging biomarkers, and hence it has been argued that they could be early predictors of those elderly at increased risk for functional decline.[179]

This age-associated risk association of coagulation factors has also been reproduced in animals. For example, when stress associated with physical restraint was compared in old versus young C57BL/6J mice, significantly increased expression of PAI-1 messenger RNA (mRNA) was noted in almost all the tissues in older mice.[180] Similar results were seen for expression of tissue factor (TF) mRNA in older mice.[180] In both these experimental models an increase in microthrombi was noted, with clots distributed through multiple organ systems in the older mice.

In humans, both the presence of depression and/or psychological stress are associated with increased coagulation[181–183] and decreased fibrinolytic activity.[184] In elderly subjects without cardiovascular disease, physical exhaustion, a characteristic frequently used to distinguish frail from nonfrail individuals, was associated with significant increases in both inflammatory and coagulation factors as assessed by fibrinogen, C-reactive protein, and white cell levels.[181] The frail and prefrail subjects from the Cardiovascular Health Study had significantly higher levels of fibrinogen, factor VIII, and D-dimer levels as compared to the nonfrail group. The association with frailty persisted even after adjusting for the presence of cardiovascular disease and diabetes.[185] Frailty is also associated with increased risk of venous thromboembolism when compared to nonfrail individuals of the same age, especially in association with increased factor VIII levels.[186]

AGING AND IMMUNITY

Whether related to primary processes of aging or not, the thymus gland undergoes a very characteristic pattern of involution beginning well in advance of other phenotypic changes attributed to aging. Among the consequences are a decreased generation of naïve T lymphocytes.[187] Despite this, the total lymphocyte count does not decline greatly because circulating T cells are capable of expanding to fill the T-cell niche in the absence of generation of new T cells. However, when they do so, the repertoire for antigen recognition becomes less comprehensive. Thymic involution may result from an aging T-cell progenitor population,[188] a consequence of defects in rearrangement of T-cell receptor β genes,[189,190] loss of self-peptide expressing thymic epithelium,[191] and/or because of the loss of thymic trophic cytokines.[192] Thymic epithelial cells produce a variety of colony-stimulating factors and hematopoietic cytokines such as IL-1, IL-3, IL-6, IL-7, transforming growth factor-β, oncostatin M (OSM), and leukemia inhibitory factor (LIF)[193–195] which influence the complex process of T-cell production. It is proposed that thymic atrophy and decreased thymopoiesis is an active process and mediated by the upregulation of thymosuppressive cytokines (LIF, IL-6 and OSM), which results in the altered peripheral T-lymphocyte function with aging (see Chaps. 76 and 78 for general discussions of T-lymphocyte biology).[196]

There is a notable shift in the overall blood T-cell population toward lymphocytes with memory T-cell markers[197] and many of these are thought to have attained replicative senescence.[198] With the decreasing numbers of naïve T cells in the periphery and increasing memory T cells reaching senescence, elderly persons have difficulties responding to old and new antigens and demonstrate impaired reactions to vaccinations. The decreased efficacy of vaccines may also be a result of alterations in antigen presentation with age. Within the T-helper cell fraction there is a shift to the T-helper type 2 (Th2) subset and away from Th1,[199] thereby influencing cytokine production and overall immune response.

In addition to the anatomic changes within marrow and thymus, similar age-associated morphologic changes within the paracortical and medullary zones of secondary lymphoid tissues (spleen and lymph nodes) occur, including a decline in the paracortical and medullary zones and increased deposition of fat within the germinal centers.[200,201] It remains unclear to what extent these changes contribute to the overall change in immune function with age.

A wide range of lymphocyte functional changes have been described in the context of aging; however, cataloging these would be beyond the scope of this chapter. Such changes are detailed in several excellent reviews.[11,202–205] Briefly stated, there is a shift in the T-cell population toward memory T cells,[197] which attain replicative senescence in response to repeated antigen exposures.[198] With the relative and absolute decrease in numbers of naïve T cells in the periphery and the accumulation of functionally diminished memory senescent T cells, primary and secondary immune responses are reduced in elderly persons.

Coincident with the age-related changes in lymphocyte function is the increase in levels of circulating proinflammatory cytokines, measurable in some, even in the absence of definable inflammatory disease. IL-6 is the prototype in this regard. In young adults expression of IL-6 is tightly regulated, and serum levels are usually unmeasurable or very low in the absence of inflammatory conditions. Animal studies reveal an increased production of IL-6[206,207] from peripheral mononuclear cells and lymphoid cells after stimulation with lipopolysaccharide or other mitogens. Similarly, in humans serum IL-6 levels increase significantly with age.[208–212] Other inflammatory proteins, including tumor necrosis factor (TNF)-α and C-reactive protein are also seen at higher levels in the elderly.[213–215] Visceral adipose tissue from older mice express greater levels of both IL-6 and TNF-α mRNA than younger mice[216] and thus, some of the age-associated rise in IL-6 may be the consequence of those metabolic shifts mentioned above.

CLINICAL CONSEQUENCES

MARROW AGING

Although a number of measurable changes occur in the marrow, not the least of which is a dramatic reduction in cellularity, apparent compensatory stem cell changes allow the sustenance of normal or near normal blood counts throughout the life span. From allogeneic hematopoietic stem cell transplant experience, when marrow is donated from a 65-year-old person to an human leukocyte antigen-matched younger recipient, the transferred marrow supports hematopoiesis for the life of the recipient, although allogeneic marrow from older donors has a greater chance of being associated with graft-versus-host disease.[217]

UNEXPLAINED ANEMIA

To the extent that marrow contains continuously repopulating cell lines, it is remarkable that changes attributable to aging alone (i.e., in the absence of disease) are subtle. Nonetheless unexplained anemia accounts for up to one-third of cases of anemia in older patients and its frequency increases with advancing age.[218]

The anemia is most commonly mild, with hemoglobin levels approximately 1 g/dL lower than the WHO standard. The red cells are typically of normal size and examination of the blood film reveals no evidence for intravascular destruction or morphologic features suggestive of myelodysplasia. Although inflammatory cytokine levels may be elevated, the intensity of inflammation is insufficient to produce increased levels of hepcidin; thus, the anemia has a distinct pathogenesis from the anemia of chronic disease. Because unexplained anemia is typically mild, it is likely to be overlooked. In one population-based cohort that included elderly patients with even more significant anemia, the medical records of affected individuals did not mention anemia as a problem in 75 percent of the cases.[112] However, this casual acceptance of lower hemoglobin levels in older populations might not be advisable.[109] Not only can a decline in important functional measures be related to mild anemia,[113,219–222] but longitudinal studies demonstrate increased mortality among individuals with even mild anemia.[115,120,223] Furthermore, a retrospective cohort study of Veterans Administration National Surgical Quality Improvement database indicated that of 310,311 subjects age 65 years and older who underwent noncardiac surgery, the 30-day mortality and cardiac event rates increased by 1.6 percent for each 1 percent change in hematocrit below the level of 39 percent.[216] Thus, although in younger individuals mild anemia may be well tolerated, in many older individuals it is associated with important negative consequences. That stated, it remains to be established whether the correction of anemia for those with unexplained anemia will result in improved quality of life, physical function, or survival.

In elderly patients with unexplained anemia, the presence of macrocytosis, thrombocytopenia, neutropenia, splenomegaly; or unexplained constitutional symptoms of fever, chills, or weight loss; or symptoms of early satiety or bone pain should prompt consideration of an evaluation to consider megaloblastic anemia, myelodysplasia, or other relevant causes of marrow malfunction, most of which occur with increasing frequency with advancing age.

IMMUNE SENESCENCE

The complex alterations in immune function with age have been briefly presented above and in more detail elsewhere.[202–205] The described changes may explain an age-associated predisposition to certain infections (herpes zoster, tuberculosis reactivation) and perhaps a failure to mount a sufficient vaccine response (e.g., to influenza hemagglutinin).[224–228] The more profound immune deficiency commonly observed in older people most often reflects the debilitating effects of concurrent diseases, most of which occur more commonly with age, and side effects of the medicines used to manage those diseases.

INFLAMMATION AND COAGULATION DYSREGULATION AND FRAILTY

Presumably on the basis of chronic inflammatory stimuli, there is an age-associated activation of coagulation[174] and fibrinolytic[229] pathways that favor thrombus formation. Fibrinogen levels are typically high with more than 80 percent of those age 65 years and older having levels above 320 mg/dL.[169] Similarly an analysis of D-dimer levels in the EPESE, including 1727 community elderly, revealed an age-associated increase, and this correlated with declining overall physical function.[156] Furthermore, when combining D-dimer and IL-6 levels, it was discovered that those individuals who had elevations of both were at greatest

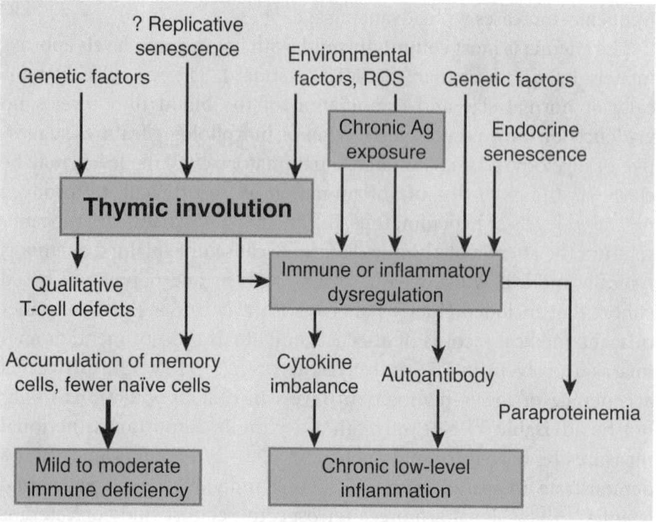

FIGURE 8–2. Immunity and aging. A variety of factors are associated with thymic involution, the consequence of which is a mild to moderate immune deficiency. Dysregulated inflammatory pathways are also observed with advancing age, and these may be of greater clinical importance. Ag, antigen; ROS, reactive oxygen species.

risk for mortality over a 4-year interval.[175] In the Cardiovascular Health Study, which included relatively healthy elderly, higher fibrinogen and factor VIII levels were associated with a greater risk for cardiovascular disease and mortality, even after adjustment for other cardiovascular risk factors.[174,230] Summarizing what has now become a robust literature, higher IL-6, TNF-α, D-dimer, and C-reactive protein have each been associated with negative physiologic consequences, including reduced lower-extremity muscle mass and strength,[231,232] cognitive decline,[233] insulin resistance,[234] subclinical and clinical cardiovascular disease,[235,236] renal insufficiency,[237] loss of bone mineral density,[238] depression,[239] anemia,[127] dementia,[177] and mortality.[231] As a result, a general consensus has emerged that activated inflammatory mediators are, at least in part, contributing to the physiology of aging, and to the extent that these pathways are dysregulated, important functional outcomes are impaired (Fig. 8–2).

REFERENCES

1. Kinsella K, Velkoff VA: *An Aging World*. Vol. Series P95/01–1. US Government Printing Office, US Census Bureau, Washington, DC, 2001.
2. Walston J, Hadley EC, Ferrucci L, et al: Research agenda for frailty in older adults: Toward a better understanding of physiology and etiology: Summary from the American Geriatrics Society/National Institute on Aging Research conference on frailty in older adults. *J Am Geriatr Soc* 54:991, 2006.
3. Shock NW, Gueulich RC, Andres R: *Normal human aging: The Baltimore Longitudinal Study of Aging*. NIH U.S. Public Health Service, Washington, DC. Publication No. 84–2450. 1984.
4. Lindeman RD: Overview: Renal physiology and pathophysiology of aging. *Am J Kidney Dis* 16:275, 1990.
5. Gazit R, Weissman IL, Rossi DJ: Hematopoietic stem cells and the aging hematopoietic system. *Semin Hematol* 45:218, 2008.
6. Rossi DJ, Bryder D, Zahn JM, et al: Cell intrinsic alterations underlie hematopoietic stem cell aging. *Proc Natl Acad Sci U S A* 102:9194, 2005.
7. Sudo K, Ema H, Morita Y, Nakauchi H: Age-associated characteristics of murine hematopoietic stem cells. *J Exp Med* 192:1273, 2000.
8. Artz AS: Anemia and the frail elderly. *Semin Hematol* 45:261, 2008.
9. Chaves PHM: Functional outcomes of anemia in older adults. *Semin Hematol* 45:255, 2008.
10. Pawelec G, Larbi A: Immunity and ageing in man: Annual review 2006/2007. *Exp Gerontol* 43:34, 2008.
11. Longo DL: Immunology of aging, in *Fundamental Immunology*, 5th ed, edited by WE Paul, p 1043. Lippicott, Williams and Wilkins, Philadelphia, 2003.
12. Dubrow EL: Reactivation of tuberculosis: A problem of aging. *J Am Geriatr Soc* 24:481, 1976.
13. Nagami PH, Yoshikawa TT: Tuberculosis in the geriatric patient. *J Am Geriatr Soc* 31:356, 1983.
14. Arvin A: Aging, immunity, and the varicella-zoster virus. *N Engl J Med* 352:2266, 2005.
15. Schmader K: Herpes zoster in older adults. *Clin Infect Dis* 32:1481, 2001.
16. Arden NH, Patriarca PA, Kendal A: Experiences in the use and efficacy of inactivated influenza vaccine in the nursing home. *Options for the Control of Influenza*, edited by AP Kendal, PA Patriarca, p 155. Alan Liss, New York, 1986.
17. Deng Y, Jing Y, Campbell AE, Gravenstein S: Age-related impaired type 1 T cell responses to influenza: Reduced activation ex vivo, decreased expansion in CTL culture in vitro, and blunted response to influenza vaccination in vivo in the elderly. *J Immunol* 172:3437, 2004.
18. Hilleman MR: Realities and enigmas of human viral influenza: Pathogenesis, epidemiology and control. *Vaccine* 20:3068, 2002.
19. Powers DC, Sears SD, Murphy BR, et al: Systemic and local antibody responses in elderly subjects given live or inactivated influenza A virus vaccines. *J Clin Microbiol* 27:2666, 1989.
20. Kaesberg PR, Ershler WB: The importance of immune senescence in the incidence and malignant properties of cancer in hosts of advanced age. *J Gerontol* 44:63, 1989.
21. Miller RA: The cell biology of aging: Immunological models. *J Gerontol* 44:B4, 1989.
22. Radl J: Age-related monoclonal gammopathies: Clinical lessons from the aging C57BL mouse. *Immunol Today* 11:234, 1990.
23. Martin GM: The genetics of aging. *Hosp Pract (Off Ed)* 32:47, 55, 59 passim, 1997.
24. Yu CE, Oshima J, Fu YH, et al: Positional cloning of the Werner's syndrome gene. *Science* 272:258, 1996.
25. Yu CE, Oshima J, Wijsman EM, et al: Mutations in the consensus helicase domains of the Werner syndrome gene. Werner's Syndrome Collaborative Group. *Am J Hum Genet* 60:330, 1997.
26. Merideth MA, Gordon LB, Clauss S, et al: Phenotype and course of Hutchinson-Gilford progeria syndrome. *N Engl J Med* 358:592, 2008.

27. Kennedy BK, Guarente L: Genetic analysis of aging in *Saccharomyces cerevisiae. Trends Genet* 12:355, 1996.
28. Szilard L: On the nature of the aging process. *Proc Natl Acad Sci U S A* 45:30, 1959.
29. Morley AA: Is ageing the result of dominant and co-dominant mutations? *J Theor Biol* 98:469, 1982.
30. Cummings DJ: Mitochondrial DNA in *Podospora anserina*. A molecular approach to cellular senescence. *Monogr Dev Biol* 17:254, 1984.
31. Fairweather DS, Fox M, Margison GP: The *in vitro* life span of MRC-5 cells is shortened by 5-azacytidine-induced demethylation. *Exp Cell Res* 168:153, 1987.
32. Burnet M: *Intrinsic Mutagenesis: A Genetic Approach for Aging.* Wiley, New York, 1974.
33. Hart RW, Setlow RB: Correlation between deoxyribonucleic acid excision-repair and life-span in a number of mammalian species. *Proc Natl Acad Sci U S A* 71:2169, 1974.
34. Orgel LE: The maintenance of the accuracy of protein synthesis and its relevance to ageing. *Proc Natl Acad Sci U S A* 49:517, 1963.
35. Allsopp RC, Vaziri H, Patterson C, et al: Telomere length predicts replicative capacity of human fibroblasts. *Proc Natl Acad Sci U S A* 89:10114, 1992.
36. Longo DL: Telomere dynamics in aging: Much ado about nothing? [guest editorial]. *J Gerontol A Biol Sci Med Sci*. 64A:963, 2009.
37. Bjorkstein J: Cross linkage and the aging process, in *Theoretical Aspects of Aging*, edited by M Rothstein, p 43. Academic Press, New York, 1974.
38. Kohn RR: *Principles of Mammalian Aging*, 2 ed. Prentice Hall, Englewood Cliffs, NJ, 1978.
39. Kreisle RA, Stebler BA, Ershler WB: Effect of host age on tumor-associated angiogenesis in mice. *J Natl Cancer Inst* 82:44, 1990.
40. Harman D: Aging: A theory based on free radical and radiation chemistry. *J Gerontol* 11:298, 1956.
41. Harman D: The aging process. *Proc Natl Acad Sci U S A* 78:7124, 1981.
42. Sohal RS, Svensson I, Sohal BH, Brunk UT: Superoxide anion radical production in different animal species. *Mech Ageing Dev* 49:129, 1989.
43. Sohal RS, Sohal BH, Brunk UT: Relationship between antioxidant defenses and longevity in different mammalian species. *Mech Ageing Dev* 53:217, 1990.
44. Sohal RS, Weindruch R: Oxidative stress, caloric restriction, and aging. *Science* 273:59, 1996.
45. Perez VI, Van Remmen H, Bokov A, et al: The overexpression of major antioxidant enzymes does not extend the life span of mice. *Aging Cell* 8:73, 2009.
46. Lee CM, Chung SS, Kaczkowski JM, et al: Multiple mitochondrial DNA deletions associated with age in skeletal muscle of rhesus monkeys. *J Gerontol* 48:B201, 1993.
47. Melov S, Shoffner JM, Kaufman A, Wallace DC: Marked increase in the number and variety of mitochondrial DNA rearrangements in aging human skeletal muscle. *Nucleic Acids Res* 23:4122, 1995.
48. Schwarze SR, Lee CM, Chung SS, et al: High levels of mitochondrial DNA deletions in skeletal muscle of old rhesus monkeys. *Mech Ageing Dev* 83:91, 1995.
49. Li Y, Huang TT, Carlson EJ, et al: Dilated cardiomyopathy and neonatal lethality in mutant mice lacking manganese superoxide dismutase. *Nat Genet* 11:376, 1995.
50. Epstein CJ, Avraham KB, Lovett M, et al: Transgenic mice with increased Cu/Zn-superoxide dismutase activity: Animal model of dosage effects in Down syndrome. *Proc Natl Acad Sci U S A* 84:8044, 1987.
51. Harris TB, Kiel D, Roubenoff R, et al: Association of insulin-like growth factor-I with body composition, weight history, and past health behaviors in the very old: The Framingham Heart Study. *J Am Geriatr Soc* 45:133, 1997.
52. Birkenhager-Gillesse EG, Derksen J, Lagaay AM: Dehydroepiandrosterone sulphate (DHEAS) in the oldest old, aged 85 and over. *Ann N Y Acad Sci* 719:543, 1994.
53. Rudman D, Drinka PJ, Wilson CR, et al: Relations of endogenous anabolic hormones and physical activity to bone mineral density and lean body mass in elderly men. *Clin Endocrinol (Oxf)* 40:653, 1994.
54. Hobbs CJ, Plymate SR, Rosen CJ, Adler RA: Testosterone administration increases insulin-like growth factor-I levels in normal men. *J Clin Endocrinol Metab* 77:776, 1993.
55. Rudman D, Feller AG, Nagraj HS, et al: Effects of human growth hormone in men over 60 years old. *N Engl J Med* 323:1, 1990.
56. Walford R: *The Immunological Theory of Aging.* Williams and Wilkins, Baltimore, MD, 1969.
57. Makinodan T, Kay MM: Age influence on the immune system. *Adv Immunol* 29:287, 1980.
58. Smith GS, Walford RL: Influence of the main histocompatibility complex on ageing in mice. *Nature* 270:727, 1977.
59. Hirokawa K: Understanding the mechanism of the age-related decline in immune function. *Nutr Rev* 50:361, 1992.
60. Christensen K, Vaupel JW: Determinants of longevity: Genetic, environmental and medical factors. *J Intern Med* 240:333, 1996.
61. World Health Prospects: *The 2006 Revision*. Population Division, Department of Economic and Social Affairs, United Nations, 2007. Available at www.un.org/esa/population/ordering.htm.
62. Orr WC, Sohal RS: Extension of life-span by overexpression of superoxide dismutase and catalase in Drosophila melanogaster. *Science* 263:1128, 1994.
63. Anderson RM, Shanmuganayagam D, Weindruch R: Caloric restriction and aging: Studies in mice and monkeys. *Toxicol Pathol* 37:47, 2009.
64. Mattson MP: Dietary factors, hormesis and health. *Ageing Res Rev* 7:43, 2008.
65. Ramsey JJ, Colman RJ, Binkley NC, et al: Dietary restriction and aging in rhesus monkeys: The University of Wisconsin study. *Exp Gerontol* 35:1131, 2000.
66. Lane MA, Roth GS, Ingram DK: Caloric restriction mimetics: A novel approach for biogerontology. *Methods Mol Biol* 371:143, 2007.
67. Heilbronn LK, de Jonge L, Frisard MI, et al: Effect of 6-month calorie restriction on biomarkers of longevity, metabolic adaptation, and oxidative stress in overweight individuals: A randomized controlled trial. *JAMA* 295:1539, 2006.
68. Redman LM, Martin CK, Williamson DA, Ravussin E: Effect of caloric restriction in non-obese humans on physiological, psychological and behavioral outcomes. *Physiol Behav* 94:643, 2008.
69. Fowler CG, Chiasson KB, Hart DB, et al: Tympanometry in rhesus monkeys: Effects of aging and caloric restriction. *Int J Audiol* 47:209, 2008.
70. Raman A, Ramsey JJ, Kemnitz JW, et al: Influences of calorie restriction and age on energy expenditure in the rhesus monkey. *Am J Physiol Endocrinol Metab* 292:E101, 2007.
71. Hayflick L: The limited *in vitro* lifetime of human diploid cell strains. *Exp Cell Res* 37:614, 1965.
72. Cristofalo VJ, Lorenzini A, Allen RG, et al: Replicative senescence: A critical review. *Mech Ageing Dev* 125:827, 2004.
73. Rohme D: Evidence for a relationship between longevity of mammalian species and life spans of normal fibroblasts *in vitro* and erythrocytes *in vivo*. *Proc Natl Acad Sci U S A* 78:5009, 1981.
74. Lichtman MA, Rowe JM: The relationship of patient age to the pathobiology of the clonal myeloid diseases. *Semin Oncol* 31:185, 2004.
75. Beghe C, Wilson A, Ershler WB: Prevalence and outcomes of anemia in geriatrics: A systematic review of the literature. *Am J Med* 116 Suppl 7A:3S, 2004.
76. Cesari M, Penninx BW, Lauretani F, et al: Hemoglobin levels and skeletal muscle: Results from the InCHIANTI study. *J Gerontol A Biol Sci Med Sci* 59:249, 2004.
77. Cesari M, Penninx BW, Pahor M, et al: Inflammatory markers and physical performance in older persons: The InCHIANTI study. *J Gerontol A Biol Sci Med Sci* 59:242, 2004.
78. Hakim FT, Gress RE: Immunosenescence: Deficits in adaptive immunity in the elderly. *Tissue Antigens* 70:179, 2007.
79. Linton PJ, Dorshkind K: Age-related changes in lymphocyte development and function. *Nat Immunol* 5:133, 2004.
80. Hartsock RJ, Smith EB, Petty CS: Normal variations with aging of the amount of hematopoietic tissue in bone marrow from the anterior iliac crest. A study made from 177 cases of sudden death examined by necropsy. *Am J Clin Pathol* 43:326, 1965.
81. Ricci C, Cova M, Kang YS, et al: Normal age-related patterns of cellular and fatty bone marrow distribution in the axial skeleton: MR imaging study. *Radiology* 177:83, 1990.
82. Steinmann GG, Klaus B, Muller-Hermelink HK: The involution of the ageing human thymic epithelium is independent of puberty. A morphometric study. *Scand J Immunol* 22:563, 1985.
83. Haynes BF, Sempowski GD, Wells AF, Hale LP: The human thymus during aging. *Immunol Res* 22:253, 2000.
84. Tavian M, Coulombel L, Luton D, et al: Aorta-associated CD34+ hematopoietic cells in the early human embryo. *Blood* 87:67, 1996.
85. Abe J: Immunocytochemical characterization of lymphocyte development in human embryonic and fetal livers. *Clin Immunol Immunopathol* 51:13, 1989.
86. Campagnoli C, Fisk N, Overton T, et al: Circulating hematopoietic progenitor cells in first trimester fetal blood. *Blood* 95:1967, 2000.
87. Kurtzberg J, Denning SM, Nycum LM, et al: Immature human thymocytes can be driven to differentiate into nonlymphoid lineages by cytokines from thymic epithelial cells. *Proc Natl Acad Sci U S A* 86:7575, 1989.
88. Fowlkes BJ, Pardoll DM: Molecular and cellular events of T cell development. *Adv Immunol* 44:207, 1989.
89. Donskoy E, Goldschneider I: Thymocytopoiesis is maintained by blood-borne precursors throughout postnatal life. A study in parabiotic mice. *J Immunol* 148:1604, 1992.
90. Rothenberg EV: The development of functionally responsive T cells. *Adv Immunol* 51:85, 1992.
91. Charbord P, Tavian M, Humeau L, Peault B: Early ontogeny of the human marrow from long bones: An immunohistochemical study of hematopoiesis and its microenvironment. *Blood* 87:4109, 1996.
92. Harrison DE, Astle CM: Loss of stem cell repopulating ability upon transplantation. Effects of donor age, cell number, and transplantation procedure. *J Exp Med* 156:1767, 1982.
93. Harrison DE: Long-term erythropoietic repopulating ability of old, young, and fetal stem cells. *J Exp Med* 157:1496, 1983.
94. de Haan G, Van Zant G: Dynamic changes in mouse hematopoietic stem cell numbers during aging. *Blood* 93:3294, 1999.
95. Harrison DE, Astle CM, Stone M: Numbers and functions of transplantable primitive immunohematopoietic stem cells. Effects of age. *J Immunol* 142:3833, 1989.
96. Liang Y, Van Zant G, Szilvassy SJ: Effects of aging on the homing and engraftment of murine hematopoietic stem and progenitor cells. *Blood* 106:1479, 2005.
97. Sudo K, Ema H, Morita Y, Nakauchi H: Age-associated characteristics of murine hematopoietic stem cells. *J Exp Med* 192:1273, 2000.
98. Leng SX, Hung W, Cappola AR, et al: White blood cell counts, insulinlike growth factor-1 levels, and frailty in community-dwelling older women. *J Gerontol A Biol Sci Med Sci* 64A:499, 2009.

99. Justesen J, Stenderup K, Ebbesen EN, et al: Adipocyte tissue volume in bone marrow is increased with aging and in patients with osteoporosis. *Biogerontology* 2:165, 2001.
100. Verma S, Rajaratnam JH, Denton J, et al: Adipocytic proportion of bone marrow is inversely related to bone formation in osteoporosis. *J Clin Pathol* 55:693, 2002.
101. De Meyer T, De Buyzere ML, Langlois M, et al: Lower red blood cell counts in middle-aged subjects with shorter peripheral blood leukocyte telomere length. *Aging Cell* 7:700, 2008.
102. Greider CW: Telomeres and senescence: The history, the experiment, the future. *Curr Biol* 8:R178, 1998.
103. Frenck RW Jr, Blackburn EH, Shannon KM: The rate of telomere sequence loss in human leukocytes varies with age. *Proc Natl Acad Sci U S A* 95:5607, 1998.
104. Gattermann N: Mitochondrial DNA mutations in the hematopoietic system. *Leukemia* 18:18, 2004.
105. Kadenbach B, Munscher C, Frank V, et al: Human aging is associated with stochastic somatic mutations of mitochondrial DNA: *Mutat Res* 338:161, 1995.
106. Bolognesi C, Abbondandolo A, Barale R, et al: Age-related increase of baseline frequencies of sister chromatid exchanges, chromosome aberrations, and micronuclei in human lymphocytes. *Cancer Epidemiol Biomarkers Prev* 6:249, 1997.
107. Lamberts SW, van den Beld AW, van der Lely AJ: The endocrinology of aging. *Science* 278:419, 1997.
108. French RA, Broussard SR, Meier WA, et al: Age-associated loss of bone marrow hematopoietic cells is reversed by GH and accompanies thymic reconstitution. *Endocrinology* 143:690, 2002.
109. Nissenson AR, Goodnough LT, Dubois RW: Anemia: Not just an innocent bystander? *Arch Intern Med* 163:1400, 2003.
110. Balducci L, Ershler WB, Bennett JM, eds. *Anemia in the Elderly*. Springer, New York, 2007.
111. Blanc B, Finch CA, Hallberg L: Nutritional anaemias. Report of a WHO Scientific Group. *World Health Organ Tech Rep Ser* 405:1, 1968.
112. Ania BJ, Suman VJ, Fairbanks VF, et al: Incidence of anemia in older people: An epidemiologic study in a well defined population. *J Am Geriatr Soc* 45:825, 1997.
113. Chaves PH, Ashar B, Guralnik JM, Fried LP: Looking at the relationship between hemoglobin concentration and prevalent mobility difficulty in older women. Should the criteria currently used to define anemia in older people be reevaluated? *J Am Geriatr Soc* 50:1257, 2002.
114. Culleton BF, Manns BJ, Zhang J, et al: Impact of anemia on hospitalization and mortality in older adults. *Blood* 107:3841, 2006.
115. Izaks GJ, Westendorp RG, Knook DL: The definition of anemia in older persons. *JAMA* 281:1714, 1999.
116. Zakai NA, Katz R, Hirsch C, et al: A prospective study of anemia status, hemoglobin concentration, and mortality in an elderly cohort: The Cardiovascular Health Study. *Arch Intern Med* 165:2214, 2005.
117. Penninx BW, Pahor M, Woodman RC, Guralnik JM: Anemia in old age is associated with increased mortality and hospitalization. *J Gerontol A Biol Sci Med Sci* 61:474, 2006.
118. Beutler E, West C: Hematologic differences between African-Americans and whites: The roles of iron deficiency and alpha-thalassemia on hemoglobin levels and mean corpuscular volume. *Blood* 106:740, 2005.
119. Patel KV, Harris TB, Faulhaber M, et al: Racial variation in the relationship of anemia with mortality and mobility disability among older adults. *Blood* 109:4663, 2007.
120. Chaves PH, Xue QL, Guralnik JM, et al: What constitutes normal hemoglobin concentration in community-dwelling disabled older women? *J Am Geriatr Soc* 52:1811, 2004.
121. Guralnik JM, Eisenstaedt RS, Ferrucci L, et al: Prevalence of anemia in persons 65 years and older in the United States: Evidence for a high rate of unexplained anemia. *Blood* 104:2263, 2004.
122. Artz AS, Fergusson D, Drinka PJ, et al: Prevalence of anemia in skilled-nursing home residents. *Arch Gerontol Geriatr* 39:201, 2004.
123. Gaskell H, Derry S, Andrew Moore R, McQuay HJ: Prevalence of anaemia in older persons: Systematic review. *BMC Geriatr* 8:1, 2008.
124. Pandya N, Bookhart B, Mody SH, et al: Study of anemia in long-term care (SALT): Prevalence of anemia and its relationship with the risk of falls in nursing home residents. *Curr Med Res Opin* 24:2139, 2008.
125. Robinson B, Artz AS, Culleton B, et al: Prevalence of anemia in the nursing home: Contribution of chronic kidney disease. *J Am Geriatr Soc* 55:1566, 2007.
126. Ferrucci L, Maggio M, Bandinelli S, et al: Low testosterone levels and the risk of anemia in older men and women. *Arch Intern Med* 166:1380, 2006.
127. Ferrucci L, Guralnik JM, Woodman RC, et al: Proinflammatory state and circulating erythropoietin in persons with and without anemia. *Am J Med* 118:1288, 2005.
128. Artz AS, Fergusson D, Drinka PJ, et al: Mechanisms of unexplained anemia in the nursing home. *J Am Geriatr Soc* 52:423, 2004.
129. Strom SS, Velez-Bravo V, Estey EH: Epidemiology of myelodysplastic syndromes. *Semin Hematol* 45:8, 2008.
130. Mori M, Murai Y, Hirai M, et al: Serum erythropoietin titers in the aged. *Mech Ageing Dev* 46:105, 1988.
131. Kario K, Matsuo T, Nakao K: Serum erythropoietin levels in the elderly. *Gerontology* 37:345, 1991.
132. Kario K, Matsuo T, Kodama K, et al: Reduced erythropoietin secretion in senile anemia. *Am J Hematol* 41:252, 1992.
133. Ershler WB, Sheng S, McKelvey J, et al: Serum erythropoietin and aging: A longitudinal analysis. *J Am Geriatr Soc* 53:1360, 2005.
134. Lipschitz DA, Udupa KB, Milton KY, Thompson CO: Effect of age on hematopoiesis in man. *Blood* 63:502, 1984.
135. Nagel JE, Pyle RS, Chrest FJ, Adler WH: Oxidative metabolism and bactericidal capacity of polymorphonuclear leukocytes from normal young and aged adults. *J Gerontol* 37:529, 1982.
136. Leng SX, Xue QL, Tian J, et al: Inflammation and frailty in older women. *J Am Geriatr Soc* 55:864, 2007.
137. MacGregor RR, Shalit M: Neutrophil function in healthy elderly subjects. *J Gerontol* 45:M55, 1990.
138. Rao KM, Currie MS, Padmanabhan J, Cohen HJ: Age-related alterations in actin cytoskeleton and receptor expression in human leukocytes. *J Gerontol* 47:B37, 1992.
139. MacKinney AA Jr: Effect of aging on the peripheral blood lymphocyte count. *J Gerontol* 33:213, 1978.
140. Pawelec G, Akbar A, Caruso C, et al: Human immunosenescence: Is it infectious? *Immunol Rev* 205:257, 2005.
141. Lugada ES, Mermin J, Kaharuza F, et al: Population-based hematologic and immunologic reference values for a healthy Ugandan population. *Clin Diagn Lab Immunol* 11:29, 2004.
142. Nilsson-Ehle H, Jagenburg R, Landahl S, et al: Haematological abnormalities and reference intervals in the elderly. A cross-sectional comparative study of three urban Swedish population samples aged 70, 75 and 81 years. *Acta Med Scand* 224:595, 1988.
143. Lee SJ, Lindquist K, Segal MR, Covinsky KE: Development and validation of a prognostic index for 4-year mortality in older adults. *JAMA* 295:801, 2006.
144. Takubo T, Tatsumi N: [Reference values for hematologic laboratory tests and hematologic disorders in the aged]. *Rinsho Byori* 48:207, 2000.
145. Haverkate F, Thompson SG, Duckert F: Haemostasis factors in angina pectoris; relation to gender, age and acute-phase reaction. Results of the ECAT Angina Pectoris Study Group. *Thromb Haemost* 73:561, 1995.
146. Kario K, Matsuo T, Kobayashi H: Close relationship between hemostatic factors and acute-phase reaction as normal aging process. *J Am Geriatr Soc* 44:614, 1996.
147. Mari D, Mannucci PM, Coppola R, et al: Hypercoagulability in centenarians: The paradox of successful aging. *Blood* 85:3144, 1995.
148. Scarabin PY, Van Dreden P, Bonithon-Kop C, et al: Age-related changes in factor VII activation in healthy women. *Clin Sci (Lond)* 75:341, 1988.
149. Balleisen L, Bailey J, Epping PH, et al: Epidemiological study on factor VII, factor VIII and fibrinogen in an industrial population: I: Baseline data on the relation to age, gender, body-weight, smoking, alcohol, pill-using, and menopause. *Thromb Haemost* 54:475, 1985.
150. Conlan MG, Folsom AR, Finch A, et al: Associations of factor VIII and von Willebrand factor with age, race, sex, and risk factors for atherosclerosis. The Atherosclerosis Risk in Communities (ARIC) Study. *Thromb Haemost* 70:380, 1993.
151. Ernst E, Resch KL: Fibrinogen as a cardiovascular risk factor: A meta-analysis and review of the literature. *Ann Intern Med* 118:956, 1993.
152. Cadroy Y, Daviaud P, Saivin S, et al: Distribution of 16 hemostatic laboratory variables assayed in 100 blood donors. *Nouv Rev Fr Hematol* 32:259, 1990.
153. Gudnason T, Hrafnkelsdottir T, Wall U, et al: Fibrinolytic capacity increases with age in healthy humans, while endothelium-dependent vasodilation is unaffected. *Thromb Haemost* 89:374, 2003.
154. Sundell IB, Nilsson TK, Ranby M, et al: Fibrinolytic variables are related to age, sex, blood pressure, and body build measurements: A cross-sectional study in Norsjo, Sweden. *J Clin Epidemiol* 42:719, 1989.
155. Dolan G, Neal K, Cooper P, et al: Protein C, antithrombin III and plasminogen: Effect of age, sex and blood group. *Br J Haematol* 86:798, 1994.
156. Pieper CF, Rao KM, Currie MS, et al: Age, functional status, and racial differences in plasma D-dimer levels in community-dwelling elderly persons. *J Gerontol A Biol Sci Med Sci* 55:M649, 2000.
157. Juhan-Vague I, Renucci JF, Grimaux M, et al: Thrombin-activatable fibrinolysis inhibitor antigen levels and cardiovascular risk factors. *Arterioscler Thromb Vasc Biol* 20:2156, 2000.
158. Schatteman KA, Goossens FJ, Scharpe SS, et al: Assay of procarboxypeptidase U, a novel determinant of the fibrinolytic cascade, in human plasma. *Clin Chem* 45:807, 1999.
159. Mehta J, Mehta P, Lawson D, Saldeen T: Plasma tissue plasminogen activator inhibitor levels in coronary artery disease: Correlation with age and serum triglyceride concentrations. *J Am Coll Cardiol* 9:263, 1987.
160. Eliasson M, Evrin PE, Lundblad D: Fibrinogen and fibrinolytic variables in relation to anthropometry, lipids and blood pressure. The Northern Sweden Monica study. *J Clin Epidemiol* 47:513, 1994.
161. Cawkwell RD: Patient's age and the activated partial thromboplastin time test. *Thromb Haemost* 39:780, 1978.
162. Bauer KA, Weiss LM, Sparrow D, et al: Aging-associated changes in indices of thrombin generation and protein C activation in humans. Normative Aging Study. *J Clin Invest* 80:1527, 1987.
163. Kario K, Matsuo T, Kobayashi H: Which factors affect high D-dimer levels in the elderly? *Thromb Res* 62:501, 1991.
164. Gurwitz JH, Avorn J, Ross-Degnan D, et al: Aging and the anticoagulant response to warfarin therapy. *Ann Intern Med* 116:901, 1992.
165. Deguchi K, Deguchi A, Wada H, Murashima S: Study of cardiovascular risk factors and hemostatic molecular markers in elderly persons. *Semin Thromb Hemost* 26:23, 2000.

166. Scarabin PY, Aillaud MF, Amouyel P, et al: Associations of fibrinogen, factor VII and PAI-1 with baseline findings among 10,500 male participants in a prospective study of myocardial infarction—The PRIME Study. Prospective Epidemiological Study of Myocardial Infarction. *Thromb Haemost* 80:749, 1998.
167. Hager K, Platt D: Fibrin degeneration product concentrations (D-dimers) in the course of ageing. *Gerontology* 41:159, 1995.
168. Tracy RP, Bovill EG, Fried LP, et al: The distribution of coagulation factors VII and VIII and fibrinogen in adults over 65 years. Results from the Cardiovascular Health Study. *Ann Epidemiol* 2:509, 1992.
169. Laharrague PF, Cambus JP, Fillola G, Corberand JX: Plasma fibrinogen and physiological aging. *Aging (Milano)* 5:445, 1993.
170. Hager K, Felicetti M, Seefried G, Platt D: Fibrinogen and aging. *Aging (Milano)* 6:133, 1994.
171. Takeshita K, Yamamoto K, Ito M, et al: Increased expression of plasminogen activator inhibitor-1 with fibrin deposition in a murine model of aging, "Klotho" mouse. *Semin Thromb Hemost* 28:545, 2002.
172. Tofler GH, Massaro J, Levy D, et al: Relation of the prothrombotic state to increasing age (from the Framingham Offspring Study). *Am J Cardiol* 96:1280, 2005.
173. Cushman M, Yanez D, Psaty BM, et al: Association of fibrinogen and coagulation factors VII and VIII with cardiovascular risk factors in the elderly: The Cardiovascular Health Study. Cardiovascular Health Study Investigators. *Am J Epidemiol* 143:665, 1996.
174. Tracy RP, Arnold AM, Ettinger W, et al: The relationship of fibrinogen and factors VII and VIII to incident cardiovascular disease and death in the elderly: Results from the cardiovascular health study. *Arterioscler Thromb Vasc Biol* 19:1776, 1999.
175. Cohen HJ, Harris T, Pieper CF: Coagulation and activation of inflammatory pathways in the development of functional decline and mortality in the elderly. *Am J Med* 114:180, 2003.
176. McDermott MM, Greenland P, Green D, et al: D-dimer, inflammatory markers, and lower extremity functioning in patients with and without peripheral arterial disease. *Circulation* 107:3191, 2003.
177. Wilson CJ, Cohen HJ, Pieper CF: Cross-linked fibrin degradation products (D-dimer), plasma cytokines, and cognitive decline in community-dwelling elderly persons. *J Am Geriatr Soc* 51:1374, 2003.
178. Rafnsson SB, Deary IJ, Smith FB, et al: Cognitive decline and markers of inflammation and hemostasis: The Edinburgh Artery Study. *J Am Geriatr Soc* 55:700, 2007.
179. McDermott MM, Ferrucci L, Liu K, et al: D-dimer and inflammatory markers as predictors of functional decline in men and women with and without peripheral arterial disease. *J Am Geriatr Soc* 53:1688, 2005.
180. Yamamoto K, Shimokawa T, Yi H, et al: Aging and obesity augment the stress-induced expression of tissue factor gene in the mouse. *Blood* 100:4011, 2002.
181. Kop WJ, Gottdiener JS, Tangen CM, et al: Inflammation and coagulation factors in persons >65 years of age with symptoms of depression but without evidence of myocardial ischemia. *Am J Cardiol* 89:419, 2002.
182. Panagiotakos DB, Pitsavos C, Chrysohoou C, et al: Inflammation, coagulation, and depressive symptomatology in cardiovascular disease-free people; the ATTICA study. *Eur Heart J* 25:492, 2004.
183. von Kanel R, Dimsdale JE, Mills PJ, et al: Effect of Alzheimer caregiving stress and age on frailty markers interleukin-6, C-reactive protein, and D-dimer. *J Gerontol A Biol Sci Med Sci* 61:963, 2006.
184. von Kanel R, Mills PJ, Fainman C, Dimsdale JE: Effects of psychological stress and psychiatric disorders on blood coagulation and fibrinolysis: A biobehavioral pathway to coronary artery disease? *Psychosom Med* 63:531, 2001.
185. Walston J, McBurnie MA, Newman A, et al: Frailty and activation of the inflammation and coagulation systems with and without clinical comorbidities: Results from the Cardiovascular Health Study. *Arch Intern Med* 162:2333, 2002.
186. Folsom AR, Boland LL, Cushman M, et al: Frailty and risk of venous thromboembolism in older adults. *J Gerontol A Biol Sci Med Sci* 62:79, 2007.
187. Aspinall R: Longevity and the immune response. *Biogerontology* 1:273, 2000.
188. Tyan ML: Age-related decrease in mouse T cell progenitors. *J Immunol* 118:846, 1977.
189. Aspinall R: Age-associated thymic atrophy in the mouse is due to a deficiency affecting rearrangement of the TCR during intrathymic T cell development. *J Immunol* 158:3037, 1997.
190. Lacorazza HD, Guevara Patino JA, Weksler ME, et al: Failure of rearranged TCR transgenes to prevent age-associated thymic involution. *J Immunol* 163:4262, 1999.
191. Hartwig M, Steinmann G: On a causal mechanism of chronic thymic involution in man. *Mech Ageing Dev* 75:151, 1994.
192. Plum J, De Smedt M, Leclercq G, et al: Interleukin-7 is a critical growth factor in early human T-cell development. *Blood* 88:4239, 1996.
193. Le PT, Kurtzberg J, Brandt SJ, et al: Human thymic epithelial cells produce granulocyte and macrophage colony-stimulating factors. *J Immunol* 141:1211, 1988.
194. Le PT, Lazorick S, Whichard LP, et al: Human thymic epithelial cells produce IL-6, granulocyte-monocyte-CSF, and leukemia inhibitory factor. *J Immunol* 145:3310, 1990.
195. Le PT, Tuck DT, Dinarello CA, et al: Human thymic epithelial cells produce interleukin 1. *J Immunol* 138:2520, 1987.
196. Gruver AL, Hudson LL, Sempowski GD: Immunosenescence of ageing. *J Pathol* 211:144, 2007.
197. Cakman I, Rohwer J, Schutz RM, et al: Dysregulation between TH1 and TH2 T cell subpopulations in the elderly. *Mech Ageing Dev* 87:197, 1996.
198. Hodes RJ: Aging and the immune system. *Immunol Rev* 160:5, 1997.
199. Perussia B, Kobayashi M, Rossi ME, et al: Immune interferon enhances functional properties of human granulocytes: Role of Fc receptors and effect of lymphotoxin, tumor necrosis factor, and granulocyte-macrophage colony-stimulating factor. *J Immunol* 138:765, 1987.
200. Sokolov VV, Kaplunova OA, Ovseenko TE: [Age factors in architectonics of the splenic arterial vessels]. *Morfologiia* 124:57, 2003.
201. Luscieti P, Hubschmid T, Cottier H, et al: Human lymph node morphology as a function of age and site. *J Clin Pathol* 33:454, 1980.
202. Effros RB, Cai Z, Linton PJ: CD8 T cells and aging. *Crit Rev Immunol* 23:45, 2003.
203. Globerson A, Effros RB: Ageing of lymphocytes and lymphocytes in the aged. *Immunol Today* 21:515, 2000.
204. Grubeck-Loebenstein B, Wick G: The aging of the immune system. *Adv Immunol* 80:243, 2002.
205. Vallejo AN: Age-dependent alterations of the T cell repertoire and functional diversity of T cells of the aged. *Immunol Res* 36:221, 2006.
206. Mascarucci P, Taub D, Saccani S, et al: Age-related changes in cytokine production by leukocytes in rhesus monkeys. *Aging (Milano)* 13:85, 2001.
207. Mascarucci P, Taub D, Saccani S, et al: Cytokine responses in young and old rhesus monkeys: Effect of caloric restriction. *J Interferon Cytokine Res* 22:565, 2002.
208. Daynes RA, Araneo BA, Ershler WB, et al: Altered regulation of IL-6 production with normal aging. Possible linkage to the age-associated decline in dehydroepiandrosterone and its sulfated derivative. *J Immunol* 150:5219, 1993.
209. Fagiolo U, Cossarizza A, Scala E, et al: Increased cytokine production in mononuclear cells of healthy elderly people. *Eur J Immunol* 23:2375, 1993.
210. Kania DM, Binkley N, Checovich M, et al: Elevated plasma levels of interleukin-6 in postmenopausal women do not correlate with bone density. *J Am Geriatr Soc* 43:236, 1995.
211. Straub RH, Konecna L, Hrach S, et al: Serum dehydroepiandrosterone (DHEA) and DHEA sulfate are negatively correlated with serum interleukin-6 (IL-6), and DHEA inhibits IL-6 secretion from mononuclear cells in man in vitro: Possible link between endocrinosenescence and immunosenescence. *J Clin Endocrinol Metab* 83:2012, 1998.
212. Young DG, Skibinski G, Mason JI, James K: The influence of age and gender on serum dehydroepiandrosterone sulphate (DHEA-S), IL-6, IL-6 soluble receptor (IL-6sR) and transforming growth factor beta 1 (TGF-beta1) levels in normal healthy blood donors. *Clin Exp Immunol* 117:476, 1999.
213. Chorinchath BB, Kong LY, Mao L, McCallum RE: Age-associated differences in TNF-alpha and nitric oxide production in endotoxic mice. *J Immunol* 156:1525, 1996.
214. O'Mahony L, Holland J, Jackson J, et al: Quantitative intracellular cytokine measurement: Age-related changes in proinflammatory cytokine production. *Clin Exp Immunol* 113:213, 1998.
215. Roubenoff R, Harris TB, Abad LW, et al: Monocyte cytokine production in an elderly population: Effect of age and inflammation. *J Gerontol A Biol Sci Med Sci* 53:M20, 1998.
216. Wu WC, Schifftner TL, Henderson WG, et al: Preoperative hematocrit levels and postoperative outcomes in older patients undergoing noncardiac surgery. *JAMA* 297:2481, 2007.
217. Kollman C, Howe CW, Anasetti C, et al: Donor characteristics as risk factors in recipients after transplantation of bone marrow from unrelated donors: The effect of donor age. *Blood* 98:2043, 2001.
218. Makipour S, Kanapuru B, Ershler WB: Unexplained anemia in the elderly. *Semin Hematol* 45:250, 2008.
219. Penninx BW, Guralnik JM, Onder G, et al: Anemia and decline in physical performance among older persons. *Am J Med* 115:104, 2003.
220. Penninx BW, Kritchevsky SB, Newman AB, et al: Inflammatory markers and incident mobility limitation in the elderly. *J Am Geriatr Soc* 52:1105, 2004.
221. Penninx BW, Pahor M, Cesari M, et al: Anemia is associated with disability and decreased physical performance and muscle strength in the elderly. *J Am Geriatr Soc* 52:719, 2004.
222. Penninx BW, Pluijm SM, Lips P, et al: Late-life anemia is associated with increased risk of recurrent falls. *J Am Geriatr Soc* 53:2106, 2005.
223. Ezekowitz JA, McAlister FA, Armstrong PW: Anemia is common in heart failure and is associated with poor outcomes: Insights from a cohort of 12,065 patients with new-onset heart failure. *Circulation* 107:223, 2003.
224. Bernstein E, Kaye D, Abrutyn E, et al: Immune response to influenza vaccination in a large healthy elderly population. *Vaccine* 17:82, 1999.
225. Gross PA, Quinnan GV Jr, Weksler ME, et al: Relation of chronic disease and immune response to influenza vaccine in the elderly. *Vaccine* 7:303, 1989.
226. McElhaney JE, Meneilly GS, Lechelt KE, et al: Antibody response to whole-virus and split-virus influenza vaccines in successful ageing. *Vaccine* 11:1055, 1993.
227. Murasko DM, Bernstein ED, Gardner EM, et al: Role of humoral and cell-mediated immunity in protection from influenza disease after immunization of healthy elderly. *Exp Gerontol* 37:427, 2002.
228. Muszkat M, Friedman G, Dannenberg HD, et al: Response to influenza vaccination in community and in nursing home residing elderly: Relation to clinical factors. *Exp Gerontol* 38:1199, 2003.
229. Yamamoto K, Takeshita K, Shimokawa T, et al: Plasminogen activator inhibitor-1 is a major stress-regulated gene: Implications for stress-induced thrombosis in aged individuals. *Proc Natl Acad Sci U S A* 99:890, 2002.

230. Tracy RP, Bovill EG, Yanez D, et al: Fibrinogen and factor VIII, but not factor VII, are associated with measures of subclinical cardiovascular disease in the elderly. Results from The Cardiovascular Health Study. *Arterioscler Thromb Vasc Biol* 15:1269, 1995.
231. Harris TB, Ferrucci L, Tracy RP, et al: Associations of elevated interleukin-6 and C-reactive protein levels with mortality in the elderly. *Am J Med* 106:506, 1999.
232. Taaffe DR, Harris TB, Ferrucci L, et al: Cross-sectional and prospective relationships of interleukin-6 and C-reactive protein with physical performance in elderly persons: MacArthur studies of successful aging. *J Gerontol A Biol Sci Med Sci* 55:M709, 2000.
233. Yaffe K, Lindquist K, Penninx BW, et al: Inflammatory markers and cognition in well-functioning African-American and white elders. *Neurology* 61:76, 2003.
234. Abbatecola AM, Ferrucci L, Grella R, et al: Diverse effect of inflammatory markers on insulin resistance and insulin-resistance syndrome in the elderly. *J Am Geriatr Soc* 52:399, 2004.
235. Cesari M, Leeuwenburgh C, Lauretani F, et al: Frailty syndrome and skeletal muscle: Results from the Invecchiare in Chianti study. *Am J Clin Nutr* 83:1142, 2006.
236. Pai JK, Pischon T, Ma J, et al: Inflammatory markers and the risk of coronary heart disease in men and women. *N Engl J Med* 351:2599, 2004.
237. Shlipak MG, Fried LF, Crump C, et al: Elevations of inflammatory and procoagulant biomarkers in elderly persons with renal insufficiency. *Circulation* 107:87, 2003.
238. Ding C, Parameswaran V, Udayan R, et al: Circulating levels of inflammatory markers predict change in bone mineral density and resorption in older adults: A longitudinal study. *J Clin Endocrinol Metab* 93:1952, 2008.
239. Spranger J, Kroke A, Mohlig M, et al: Inflammatory cytokines and the risk to develop type 2 diabetes: Results of the prospective population-based European Prospective Investigation into Cancer and Nutrition (EPIC)-Potsdam Study. *Diabetes* 52:812, 2003.
240. Finch CE, Landfield PW: Neuroendocrine and autonomic functions in aging mammals, in *Handbook of the Biology of Aging*, edited by CE Finch, EL Schenider, p 567. Van Nostrand Reinhold, New York, 1985.
241. Ferrucci L, Guralnik JM, Bandinelli S, et al: Unexplained anaemia in older persons is characterised by low erythropoietin and low levels of pro-inflammatory markers. *Br J Haematol* 136:849, 2007.
242. Denny SD, Kuchibhatla MN, Cohen HJ: Impact of anemia on mortality, cognition, and function in community-dwelling elderly. *Am J Med* 119:327, 2006.
243. Joosten E, Pelemans W, Hiele M, et al: Prevalence and causes of anaemia in a geriatric hospitalized population. *Gerontology* 38:111, 1992.

PART IV

Molecular and Cellular Hematology

CHAPTER 9
GENETIC PRINCIPLES AND MOLECULAR BIOLOGY

Ernest Beutler

SUMMARY

The understanding of hematology is more than ever dependent upon an appreciation of genetic principles and the tools that can be used to study genetic variation. All of the genetic information that makes up an organism is encoded in the DNA. This information is transcribed into messenger ribonucleic acid (mRNA) and then the triplet code of those mRNAs that encode proteins is translated into protein. Changes that affect the DNA or RNA sequence or its expression, either in the germ line or acquired after birth, can cause many hematologic disorders. These may be mutations that change the DNA sequence, including single base changes, deletions, insertion, and duplications, or they may be epigenetic changes that affect gene expression without any change in the DNA sequence.

The detection of defined mutations that cause a variety of diseases is now possible and has become a routine method for the diagnosis of some disorders. The development of methods to disrupt or to prevent expression of specific genes has made it possible to produce mouse models of human hematologic diseases, and such models have the potential to serve as means to better understand pathophysiology and to study treatment strategies.

Inheritance patterns depend upon the biologic effect and chromosomal location of the mutation. Common autosomal recessive hematologic diseases include sickle cell disease, the thalassemias, and Gaucher disease. Hereditary spherocytosis, thrombophilia caused by factor V Leiden, most forms of von Willebrand disease, and acute intermittent porphyria are characterized by autosomal dominant inheritance. Mutations that cause glucose-6-phosphate dehydrogenase deficiency, hemophilia A and B, and the most common form of chronic granulomatous disease, are all carried on the X chromosome and therefore manifest X-linked inheritance, with transmission of the disease state from a heterozygous mother to her son. Understanding the genetics of a disorder is necessary for accurate genetic counseling.

Acronyms and abbreviations that appear in this chapter include: ARMS, amplification refractory mutation system; ASOH, allele-specific oligonucleotide hybridization; BACs, bacterial artificial chromosomes; bp, base pairs; cDNA, complementary DNA; CRM, cross-reacting material; CpG, cytosine phosphate guanine; ENU, *N*-ethyl-*N*-nitrosourea; G-6-PD, glucose-6-phosphate dehydrogenase; GTP, guanosine triphosphate; IAP, intra-cisternal A particle; HUMARA, human androgen receptor X-chromosome inactivation assay; mRNA, messenger ribonucleic acid; miRNA, microribonucleic acid; mtDNA, mitochondrial DNA; NADH, nicotinamide adenine dinucleotide (reduced form); PACs, P1-derived artificial chromosomes; PCR, polymerase chain reaction; PNH, paroxysmal nocturnal hemoglobinuria; RF, release factor; RFLP, restriction fragment length polymorphism; RISC, RNA-induced silencing complex; RNAi, RNA interference; rRNA, ribosomal ribonucleic acid; RT-PCR, reverse transcriptase polymerase chain reaction; siRNA, small interfering ribonucleic acid; SNP, single nucleotide polymorphism; SSCP, single stranded conformation polymorphism; TpG, thymine phosphate guanine; tRNA, transfer ribonucleic acid; UDP, uridine diphosphate; YAC, yeast artificial chromosome.

Many of the hematologic diseases described in this text have a genetic basis. Often the disease is caused by a mutation in a single gene. Some of these disorders, such as sickle cell disease (Chap. 48), thalassemia (Chap. 47), glucose-6-phosphate dehydrogenase deficiency (Chap. 46), and factor V Leiden (Chap. 125), are extremely common whereas others, such as congenital dyserythropoietic anemia type I (Chap. 39), chronic granulomatous disease (Chap. 66), and afibrinogenemia (Chap. 126), are rare, but all are caused by mutations in a gene that result in the formation of a defective protein or an insufficient amount of a normal protein. The principal focus of this chapter is such genetic disorders. However, a number of acquired hematologic diseases, including lymphomas, leukemias, and paroxysmal nocturnal hemoglobinuria, are the consequence of acquired damage to the genetic apparatus. Understanding these diseases requires an appreciation of how the genetic apparatus functions.

All of the information required for the development of a complete adult organism is encoded in the DNA of a single cell—the zygote. This information, designated the *genome*, includes the data needed for the synthesis of all enzymes; all the plasma proteins, including the clotting factors, complement components, and the transport proteins; all the membrane proteins, including receptors; and all of the cytoskeletal proteins. The units of information into which the genome is organized are the *genes*. Genetic diseases are the result of changes, or *mutations* in these genes.

THE PATTERN OF INHERITANCE

The inheritance of each genetic disease follows a distinctive pattern. The concept of dominant and recessive inheritance is one of the most deeply ingrained in our genetic thinking. It has long played a primary role in the introduction of every high school student of biology to genetics and is used extensively in the classification of genetic disease. A dominant disease is one that is expressed when the patient has only a single copy of the mutant gene, that is, in the heterozygous state. A recessive disease, on the other hand, is expressed only when both copies of the gene are abnormal. If the mutations on both alleles are the same, then the patient is *homozygous*. If two different abnormal alleles have been inherited, then the patient is a *compound heterozygote*. It is often implied that genes are dominant or recessive. This is incorrect. It is disease states or phenotypes that are dominant or recessive. The gene for sickle cell hemoglobin is expressed in the heterozygous state, so that the carrier of this gene has sickle cell trait. Sickle cell trait is therefore dominant, but sickle cell disease, which occurs in the homozygote, is recessive. By definition, the phenotype of an individual heterozygous for a mutation causing recessive disease does not differ from the phenotype of an individual homozygous for the normal gene.

The principles of dominant and recessive disease can be readily applied to mutations occurring on the *autosomes* (chromosomes other than the X chromosome), but the situation is somewhat different when dealing with genes on the X chromosome. Although the X chromosome is involved in the sex-determination process, most of the genes on the X chromosome have nothing whatsoever to do with sex determination. Some of the hematologically more important of these "X-linked" genes include those which code for glucose-6-phosphate dehydrogenase (G-6-PD), phosphoglycerate kinase, factor VIII, factor IX, Bruton-type agammaglobulinemia, one form of chronic granulomatous disease, and one of the enzymes required for the synthesis of the phosphatidylinositol anchor that is involved in the etiology of paroxysmal nocturnal hemoglobinuria (PNH).

THE FAMILY HISTORY

The family history can give a physician considerable insight into the nature of a hematologic disorder. One should ascertain whether another member of the family has had a similar disease. In the case of patients with anemia, this is often difficult, because so many women have a history of anemia, usually as a result of iron deficiency. To estimate the severity of anemia it is particularly germane to inquire whether transfusion was required. A history of gallstones, particularly at an early age, may indicate that a hemolytic disorder was present. Similarly, episodes of jaundice in family members may be the only clue to the existence of familial hemolytic anemia.

Presence of the disease in one of the parents strongly suggests a dominant mode of transmission. If neither parent is affected, but one or more siblings have the disease, an autosomal recessive transmission is more likely. Consanguinity of the patient's parents makes it highly probable that a disease is an autosomal recessive disorder. Occurrence primarily in male siblings and maternal uncles, with mild or absent manifestations of the disease in the mother, suggests an X-linked mode of inheritance. Father-to-son transmission rules out X linkage.

Lack of any family history does not rule out the genetic basis of a disease. In some instances, the disease may be so mild in other family members that it is not recognized. Whenever possible, the family members should be examined, rather than relying solely on history. Occasionally the gene mutation causing the disorder may have arisen in the generation in which the disease presents (*denovo* mutation).

Once the mode of genetic transmission is clear, the diagnostic alternatives have been narrowed considerably. For example, methemoglobinemia transmitted as an autosomal dominant disorder is a result of hemoglobin M, whereas methemoglobinemia transmitted as an autosomal recessive disorder is a result of cytochrome b5 reductase (the reduced form of nicotinamide adenine dinucleotide [NADH] diaphorase) deficiency (Chap. 49). Hemolytic anemia with autosomal dominant transmission is likely to be a result of hereditary spherocytosis, but sex-linked transmission of the hemolytic state suggests a deficiency of G-6-PD or, more rarely, phosphoglycerate kinase. A bleeding disorder that is transmitted in an X-linked fashion may be caused by a deficiency of factor VIII or factor IX, but autosomal recessive inheritance should suggest to the physician a deficiency of other clotting factors, such as factor X, XI, or V. Careful analysis of the family history not only will make possible more appropriate genetic counseling to the patient and family, but also will shorten the road to a correct diagnosis.

LINKAGE

In human somatic cells, chromosomes are present in pairs: 1 pair of sex chromosomes (2 X chromosomes in females and an X and Y in males) and 22 pairs of autosomes. One chromosome of each pair is distributed into the gametes, so that eggs and sperm of humans each contains 23 chromosomes.

If two genes are located on different chromosomes or are far apart on the same chromosome, they are said to be unlinked. This means the chance of inheriting each of the genes is independent of the other. For example, if a parent is a carrier of pyruvate kinase deficiency and sickle cell trait, caused by genes on different autosomes, the chance of an offspring inheriting pyruvate kinase deficiency is 1 in 2 and the chance of an offspring inheriting sickle cell trait is 1 in 2. Consequently, one-fourth of the offspring will inherit both pyruvate kinase deficiency and sickle cell trait, one-fourth will inherit neither, one-fourth will inherit only sickle cell trait, and one-fourth will inherit only pyruvate kinase deficiency.

If the two genes in question are close together on the same chromosome, however, the situation may be quite different. For example, the genes encoding glucocerebrosidase (Gaucher disease) and pyruvate kinase are both on the long arm of chromosome 1. If a parent carries mutations in both these genes on the same chromosome, the probability of the parent's child inheriting either both of the abnormal genes or neither of the abnormal genes is much greater than the probability of the child's inheriting one or the other. Yet the inheritance of only one of these two genes is not an impossibility because of the phenomenon of crossing-over during meiosis. In the course of the formation of germ cells, homologous pairs of chromosomes come into side-by-side apposition and regularly exchange chromosomal material. Thus two genes that were originally on the same chromosome may find themselves on separate chromosomes after germ cell formation. The probability of their being separated during meiosis is a function of their distance from one another on the chromosome, and this distance is expressed in terms of map units or Morgans. One-hundredth of a Morgan, a centimorgan (cM), represents the genetic distance that gives a 1 percent probability per generation of a crossover between the two genes. A rule of thumb is that this corresponds to a physical distance of 1 megabase (1,000,000 base pairs), but the actual physical distance represented by a centimorgan varies a great deal from one location in the genome to another. In fact, the correlation between physical distance and recombination distance varies a great deal even at the same location between the sexes.[1] It is not unusual for genes on the same chromosome to be so far apart that the probability of their finding themselves in separate germ cells is just as great as though they had been on separate chromosomes. The genes encoding red cell pyruvate kinase and glucocerebrosidase are very tightly linked[2] and, not surprisingly, the physical distance between their 5′ ends is only 71,000 base pairs.[3]

X LINKAGE AND X INACTIVATION

The chromosomal complement of males differs from that of females in that males have one X chromosome and one Y chromosome, whereas females have two X chromosomes. However, early in embryonic development, most of the genes on one of the two X chromosomes of somatic cells of female mammals becomes randomly transcriptionally inactive, thus in some cells the paternally derived chromosome is inactivated, in others, the maternally derived chromosome is inactivated.[4,5] Inactivation remains fixed, so that all the progeny of the cell in which the maternally derived X chromosome is inactive show only the gene products from the paternal X. Female heterozygotes for X-linked genes such as G-6-PD deficiency, phosphoglycerate kinase deficiency, factor VIII, or factor IX deficiency are, therefore, a mosaic of cells, some of which manifest the full-blown deficiency, as it is found in affected males, and some of which are normal. Inactivation is a process controlled by the *XIST* gene[6,7]; the final proportion of cells with one or the other X chromosome active depends upon random factors, and on selection between cell populations which may occur following the inactivation process.[8,9] The process of X inactivation is not only useful in understanding the expression of X-linked diseases in women, but has been valuable in studying the possible clonal origin of a variety of disorders. As shown in Figure 9–1, the progeny of a single cell of a female heterozygous for an X-linked gene will manifest only the phenotype of the original cell. Examination of electrophoretically distinguishable variants of G-6-PD and/or of polymorphic mRNA transcripts has made it possible to demonstrate that the red cells are a clone in chronic myelogenous leukemia,[10] essential thrombocythemia,[11] paroxysmal nocturnal hemoglobinuria,[12] polycythemia vera,[11] and probably in acute myelogenous leukemia.[13,14] This implies that each of these disorders arises through transformation of a single cell and that, in the case of the

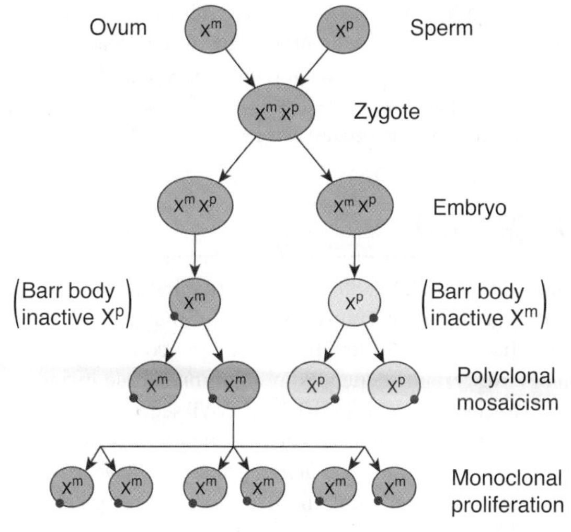

FIGURE 9–1. At fertilization, the female zygote inherits one maternal chromosome (Xm) and one paternal X chromosome (XP). At some time early in embryogenesis, one X in each cell is inactivated at random and condenses to form the Barr body. The active X remains active not only for the lifetime of that cell but for the lifetime of all of its progeny. A tumor with a clonal origin will consist entirely of cells in all of which either X^m or X^P is active. A tumor with a multicentric origin may contain both X^m and X^P cells.

myelogenous leukemias, both erythroid cells and leukocytes are part of the malignant clone.

With the development of DNA-based technology it has been possible to use X-linked genes as a clonal marker even when there is not a different protein product from the two alleles. A different pattern of methylation of cytidines distinguishes the active from the inactive X chromosome.[15] This fact, together with the existence of restriction endonucleases that distinguish methylated from unmethylated cytidine, has made it possible to utilize restriction fragment length polymorphisms (RFLPs) to determine the clonal origin of neoplasms,[16] even when no polymorphism involving an X-linked enzyme is available. The existence of polymorphisms involving the coding region of genes also makes possible the detection of clones by reverse transcription and amplification of mRNA,[17,18] and this approach more accurately reflects the pattern of inactivation than commonly used differential methylation of human androgen receptor X-chromosome inactivation assay (HUMARA) gene locus.[19]

The pattern of genetic transmission of X-linked genes is characteristic: A father cannot transmit an X-linked gene to his son; the offspring is a boy by virtue of the fact that he inherited the father's Y chromosome, not his X chromosome. Conversely, it is a truism that males always inherit X-linked genes from their mother and that the mother therefore must be either heterozygous or homozygous for the gene. Because X inactivation is random, however, the degree of expression of mutant alleles of X-linked genes in females is highly variable. This is why, even with the most sophisticated phenotypic assessment, it is not always possible to detect the heterozygous state in the mother of an affected individual. It also explains why even twin carriers of diseases such as factor VIII deficiency can have very different levels of the factor VIII.

MITOCHONDRIAL INHERITANCE

The vast majority of the genetic material in cells is encoded in the chromosomal nuclear DNA. However, mitochondria have their own replicating DNA. Apparently having arisen from symbiotic bacteria over a billion years ago, the DNA of mitochondrial DNA (mtDNA) exists as a closed circular molecule of 16,569 nucleotides. This DNA encodes 13 polypeptides, all of which are subunits of the mitochondrial energy-producing pathway, a small and a large ribosomal RNA, and 22 transfer RNAs.[20] Some proteins found in mitochondria are, however, encoded in nuclear DNA. Because mitochondria are transmitted through the egg, inheritance is entirely maternal.[21] Cells contain several hundred mitochondria, each with several copies of mtDNA. To become clinically significant, mitochondrial mutations must confer some selective advantage upon the mitochondrion with the mutation; mutations that affect only a few of the hundreds of mitochondria in each cell are unlikely to produce a phenotype. Mitochondrial mutations, often consisting of deletions, are responsible for a number of neurologic diseases.[21] Some of the childhood marrow-failure syndromes,[22,23] particularly Pearson marrow-pancreas syndrome,[24] are hematologic manifestations of mitochondrial mutations.

EPIGENETICS

(For more details regarding epigenetics, see Chap. 10.)

Even genetically identical individuals may differ in their phenotype. For example, genetically identical mice homozygous for the agouti gene may differ markedly in their coat color, and this has been attributed to random inactivation of an upstream retrotransposon.[25] The inactivation of the X chromosome by [6,7] is another example. The factors that produce epigenetic changes are incompletely understood, but most attention has been paid to methylation of cytosine phosphate guanine (CpG) dinucleotides and the acetylation of histones.[26]

One of the targets of epigenetic regulation is the CpG-rich islands of the promoter regions of housekeeping genes. Methylation of the cytidines in these islands may result in inactivation or activation of the downstream gene. Other important targets are transposable elements, and imprinted genes. An outstanding example of the effect of transposable elements is the variable phenotype of genetically identical agouti mice (Fig. 9–2).[25]

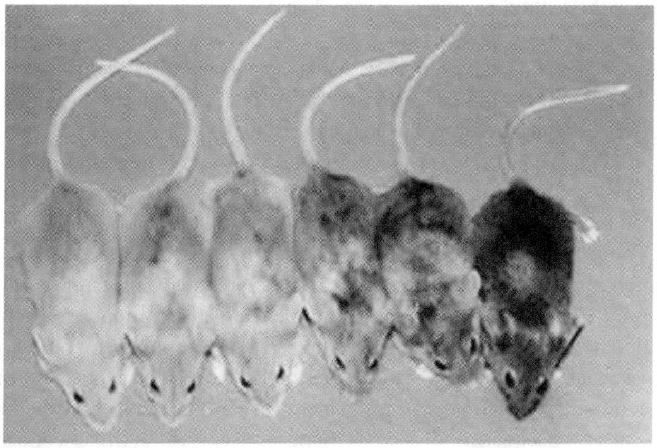

FIGURE 9–2. Yellow agouti (Avy) mice display a range of coat color phenotypes although they are genetically identical. C57BL/6 *Avy/a* littermates, the strain had been maintained by brother–sister mating for more than 30 generations. In *Avy*, an intracisternal A particle (IAP) retrotransposon has inserted 100 kb upstream from the agouti hair cycle-specific promoters. When the IAP is silent, the agouti protein is expressed specifically in the hair follicle during a particular stage of the hair cycle, and the fur is agouti (*right*). When the IAP is active, *A* is transcribed from a cryptic promoter in the long terminal repeat of the IAP, the normal program of *A* expression is abrogated and the agouti protein is expressed pancellularly. Mice in which the IAP is completely silent are phenotypically indistinguishable from agouti mice. *(Reprinted by permission from Macmillan Publishers Ltd.,* Nature Genetics *2001.*[25]*)*

It was proposed 45 years ago that, like those on the X-chromosome, only one of the two autosomal genes might be expressed at some loci.[27] Using modern genomic methods, that has proven to be the case for a considerable number of alleles.[28] Some of these alleles are *imprinted*, that is, they are regularly active or inactive depending on the state of the allele in a specific parent—the mother in the case of some alleles; the father in others (see Chap. 10).

DNA AND THE GENETIC CODE

Understanding how the massive amount of information required to allow a complex organism to grow and survive is coded has been one of the major advances of modern biology. The information is contained in the polynucleotide, DNA, and, to some extent, in the epigenetic changes induced by DNA methylation, modification of histones, and possibly other as yet unknown factors. DNA contains only four different bases: adenine (A), guanine (G), thymine (T), and cytosine (C). DNA exists as a double helix in which A is always paired with T, and G is always paired with C.

The two ends of a strand of DNA are not the same. The nucleosides that make up each strand are linked to each other through a molecule of phosphoric acid, attached to the 3′ carbon of the deoxyribose of one nucleoside and to the 5′ carbon of the next one. A linear strand of DNA thus has one end in which the hydroxyl group attached to the 5′ carbon is free; at the other end the hydroxyl group attached to the 3′ carbon is not involved in a link. These ends are designated the 5′ and 3′ ends, respectively. By convention, the 5′ end is depicted at the left and is called the "upstream" end, and the 3′ end is designated as "downstream." In the pairing of two complementary strands of DNA the polarity of the two strands is opposite (antiparallel), that is, the 5′ end of each strand is paired with the 3′ end of the other. By convention, the strand shown at the top is the coding, or "sense," strand, but the strand at the bottom is the one that actually serves as a template for RNA synthesis. Thus the sequence of the mRNA corresponds to that of the top strand, and the triplet code may be read from this strand.

It is the faithful pairing of A with T and C with G in double-stranded DNA that makes possible the accurate replication of the genetic code. When cells divide, the two DNA strands separate. As this occurs, the bases of the separate strands pair with the complementary purine or pyrimidine nucleotide which becomes linked to each other, forming a complementary strand of nucleotides. In this way the cell forms two double strands that are identical with the original double strand. Extensive proofreading and repair mechanisms serve to maintain the fidelity of the code.

The sequence of base pairs in the DNA strand specifies the sequence of amino acids in proteins. Each base cannot represent a single amino acid, as only 4 bases are found in DNA and there are 20 commonly occurring amino acids in proteins. Thus a triplet code is the minimum number of bases that is required to code for 20 amino acids and the genetic code has been found, in fact, to consist of triplets: each amino acid is specified by one or more sequences of 3 bases. Long stretches of the triplet code are colinear with the amino acid sequence of the protein whose synthesis of the gene specifies, but these stretches are separated by *intervening sequences* or *introns* that do not encode the amino acid sequence of the protein. Moreover, DNA does not directly assemble amino acids into protein. This is achieved through a mechanism that involves another polynucleotide, RNA. There are two differences between the nucleotide composition DNA and RNA. First, the nucleotide units contain ribose instead of deoxyribose. Second, in RNA uridine (U) is used instead of the thymidine (T) component of DNA. Moreover, single-stranded RNA is very flexible and has a tendency to form a complex loop-stem structure that can actually assume enzymatic activity, so-called *ribozymes*. mRNA is synthesized with a base sequence determined by the DNA, which serves as a template in a copying process that is designated as *transcription*. The mRNA is then *translated* into protein. Non-coding RNAs, small interfering ribonucleic acids (siRNAs), and microribonucleic acids (miRNAs) play important regulatory roles (see "Interfering RNA" below).

TRANSCRIPTION

The transcription of DNA into mRNA is the first step in gene expression. For a gene to be transcribed, a promoter must be located "upstream" (i.e., in the 5′ direction) from the coding region. Typical promoters have certain sequences in common. These include a "CAT box," the cytosine- and guanine-rich CCAAT sequence, and a TAATA box, an adenine- and thymine-rich sequence. Mutations in these regions impair transcription of a gene; such lesions have been identified as causes of the thalassemias, and are discussed in greater detail in Chap. 47. The effectiveness of a promoter may be increased by more distant DNA sequences, known as enhancers, which may be either upstream or downstream of the gene. The identification of sequences that enhance expression of the globin genes has been of particular importance in designing vectors for gene transfer to remedy the hemoglobinopathies (see Chaps. 27, 47, and 48).[29,30]

RNA PROCESSING

The mRNA that is formed on the DNA template by RNA polymerase is not ready to be translated to a polypeptide. First it must be processed, adding a cap to the 5′ end and a poly-A tail to the 3′ end and by removing introns. Capping consists of formation of an atypical 5′ to 5′ triphosphate bond between the 5′ terminus of the mRNA and a molecule of 7-methylguanosine. The addition of a poly-A tail serves to stabilize the mRNA. Recognition of a sequence (AAUAAA) serves as a signal that a poly-A tail should be added at a point that is approximately 15 bases downstream from the signal when another consensus sequence, YGTGTTYY (where Y stands for a pyrimidine, i.e., thymine or cytidine), is present farther downstream. Sometimes more than one adenylation signal is present, and then additional species of mRNA with 3′ portions differing in length may be formed.

Excision of introns is particularly important, since they interrupt the coding sequence. The first (5′) bases of the intron are always GpU and the last (3′) bases are always ApG (the p represents the phosphate bond between the nucleosides). But there are many such couplets in the RNA and additional information is required for an actual splice site to exist. The nature of this information has not been clearly defined, but a "consensus" sequence that most splice sites resemble closely has been defined. Removal of the intron is a complex enzymatic process.[31] Splicing of a given normal mRNA does not always occur in the same manner. Sometimes "alternative splicing" occurs, so that after processing, some of the mRNA molecules contain an exon that is missing from other messenger molecules. This is a powerful mechanism that allows a single gene to direct the synthesis of more than one polypeptide. Potentially the type of polypeptide made can be modulated according to need, and different tissues and different developmental stages may use different splice sites to make tissue-specific polypeptides. Alternative splicing has been important, for example, in producing different forms of erythrocyte membrane band 4.1[32] and different forms of pyruvate kinase for the liver and for the erythrocyte.[33] It is a powerful mechanism that allows that body to produce more than 100,000 proteins from some 30,000 genes. On the other hand, mutations may cause missplicing. Usually this results in decreased protein production, as in hemoglobin E disease, no protein production as in some Gaucher disease mutations and thalassemia (see Chap. 47), and, in rare cases, increased protein production, as in dominant thrombocythemia.[34]

TRANSLATION

Processed mRNA contains the code for the synthesis of proteins, and an elaborate mechanism has evolved for the *translation* of the triplet code in the mRNA into protein. A ribosomal complex, consisting of ribosomal RNA (rRNA) subunits and protein components attaches to the 5′ end of the mRNA. The transport of the needed amino acids to the ribosomal complex is achieved by clover-shaped RNA molecules designated transfer RNA (tRNA). tRNA molecules contain a recognition site that binds to a triplet on mRNA and a site that carries the amino acid appropriate for that triplet to the mRNA, where the ribosomal complex creates the peptide bond between it and the amino acid that is immediately 5′ to it. The initiation of protein synthesis is almost always at an AUG codon,[35] usually one quite near the 5′ end of the messenger RNA. A consensus sequence[35] around this codon marks it for the starting point of protein synthesis. The ribosome moves down the mRNA, adding amino acids to the nascent protein chain as it goes, until it reaches a termination codon, which serves as the signal to stop protein synthesis. The ribosome is then released and can begin the synthesis of another protein molecule. This complex process requires the presence of initiation factors (elongation factors, as well as a release factor [RF]), ATP, and guanosine triphosphate (GTP).[36]

Because the initiation codon AUG codes for methionine, the amino terminus of the primary translated protein is always a methionine, but this is usually cleaved from the protein during *processing*. Modification of the protein occurs in the endoplasmic reticulum and in the Golgi apparatus and may include changes such as the removal of a presequence and/or a leader sequence that directs the protein to the proper intra- or extracellular location, the addition of sugars to glycoproteins, the addition of fatty acids, and the formation of internal sulfhydryl bonds.

REGULATION

Many genes are highly specialized in their function. Hemoglobin is made only by erythrocyte precursors, crystallin only by the lens, and immunoglobulins only by lymphoid cells. Such genes must be silenced in other types of cells. On the other hand, so-called *housekeeping genes* produce their products in all cells. The latter include the enzymes of the basic metabolic processes that provide energy to all cells, such as hexokinase, phosphoglycerate kinase, and G-6-PD, or genes that encode basic structural proteins.

Clearly, an elaborate system for the regulation of protein production exists in all organisms, and this system is only beginning to be understood. Regulation of transcription determines to a large extent whether a protein will be synthesized.[37] Promoters and enhancers are activated by transcription factors that are produced by the cell. Such factors, in turn, may be activated or inactivated by phosphorylation and by other processes. Regulation also occurs at the translational level. The mRNA of ferritin contains an iron responsive element that binds to a 87-kDa regulatory protein in the absence of iron, effectively shutting off translation.[38] The same type of binding site in the 3′ untranslated region of the transferrin receptor mRNA serves to stabilize the message by allowing the protein to bind in the absence of iron.[39] Similarly, a UA-rich portion in the 3′ untranslated portion of the tumor necrosis factor gene serves to inhibit translation of that mRNA.[40] It is also likely that the stability of the mRNA itself is regulated by nucleases.[41–44]

THE METHODS OF MOLECULAR BIOLOGY

CLONING DNA

The sequencing of DNA and the preparation of probes requires that a fragment of DNA is amplified manyfold to provide a relatively pure sample for study. The classical method by which this is achieved, *cloning*, is a central technique of molecular biology. It is generally accomplished by inserting the DNA into a vector, a bacteriophage or plasmid, that normally replicates within a bacterial cell. When such a phage or plasmid contains a foreign DNA fragment, the fragment also undergoes replication and can then be purified in greatly amplified form.

If the DNA is not available in pure form to begin with, it must be purified from a collection of DNA fragments that is designated a *library*. An adequate genomic library consists of millions of fragments of the genetic material of a cell that have been ligated into a suitable vector. Another valuable type of library is made by transcribing mRNA from a tissue into complementary DNA (cDNA) using the enzyme reverse transcriptase. Such a cDNA library is particularly useful for the isolation of genes because in it are represented only the intron-free portions of genes that are being actively transcribed in a tissue. In contrast, a genomic library represents all of the genetic material, coding and noncoding, transcribed and nontranscribed.

Many different vectors have been designed and they possess the capacity to replicate fragments of DNA of widely differing sizes. The largest of these are yeast artificial chromosomes (YACs), which may incorporate a million or more base pairs of DNA into a vector that is grown in a yeast host.[45] Such vectors are very useful in mapping genes because of their very large size, but there is a tendency for the DNA in YACs to be rearranged, which can lead to errors. Other vectors that also incorporate large fragments of DNA, ranging to about 100,000 base pairs (bp) in length, are bacterial artificial chromosomes (BACs), P1-derived artificial chromosomes (PACs), and cosmids (20,000 to 30,000 bp). Much smaller inserts, ranging in size from approximately 3000 to 12,000 bp can be cloned into bacteriophages. Bacteria transfected with a library are plated on a semisolid culture medium and the desired DNA fragment is identified with a labeled probe consisting of synthetic complementary sequence. The precise base sequence cannot be deduced from the amino acid sequence, because there is more than one codon for most amino acids. However, if an appropriate portion of amino acid sequence is selected, several different complementary sequences encompassing all of the possibilities may be used as probes.

Antibodies against the gene product may also serve as probes by using an "expression vector" in which a promotor is present upstream from the cloned DNA. When the fragment is in the correct orientation and when it is "in frame" so that the triplets are read correctly, sufficient gene product may be formed to allow detection by the use of antibodies or reaction with a ligand. Colonies (or, in the case of phage vectors, plaques) that react with the probe are selected and subcultured at lower density until a single reactive colony or plaque is isolated.

The Polymerase Chain Reaction

Amplification of the desired part of the genome may be achieved, when some of the sequence is already known, by using the polymerase chain reaction (PCR), a technique that is much simpler than cloning. For example, one may wish to determine the sequence of a portion of a gene for diagnostic purposes, but cloning the gene(s) of interest is too time-consuming and labor intensive to be practical. Two primers matching opposite strands of DNA on either side of the region of interest are used to amplify the intervening segment of DNA by more than a million fold. Successive cycles of DNA synthesis from the primers and chain separation by heating between the cycles are the basis of this powerful technique.[46,47] PCR is so sensitive that under optimal conditions the DNA from a single cell may be amplified. Moreover, the stability of DNA is such that very old preserved material may be used. Thus, it is possible to amplify the DNA from blood films,[48] mummies, and other ancient biologic material.[49] Amplifying by PCR cDNA produced by reverse-transcribing mRNA in tissue extracts (reverse transcriptase polymerase chain reaction [RT-PCR]) provides a very sensitive means for measuring the expression of genes in tissues.

In the early cycles of PCR, the rate of amplification is a function of the amount of template; thus it allows for quantification of mRNA or DNA. For this purpose, a housekeeping mRNA is also measured and the ratio of this reference mRNA to tested mRNA is used. Thus, the slope of the curve can be used to measure the amount of mRNA or DNA in a specimen. This process, which has been designated *real-time PCR*, has been automated by using fluorescent probes that are destroyed during the amplification process or a dye that binds only to double-stranded DNA.[50]

Cutting DNA with Restriction Endonucleases

The discovery that many bacteria elaborate enzymes that cleave double-stranded DNA at the sites of very specific sequences greatly facilitated the study of DNA. Such enzymes generally recognize palindromes, that is, DNA sequences that read the same in one direction on the upper strand and in the opposite direction in the lower strand. Figure 9–3 illustrates how one such palindrome is cleaved by the commonly used restriction endonuclease, EcoRI. Several hundred restriction endonucleases are now commercially available.

Restriction endonucleases are useful both for cloning DNA and for analyzing its structure. Many of the restriction endonucleases produce fragments with overlapping ends (see, e.g., EcoRI in Fig. 9–3). Such "sticky ends" may be used for the ligation (i.e., splicing) of DNA fragments into a vector by using a vector with complementary sticky ends. The seal is made permanent with the enzyme DNA ligase.

The size of restriction fragments produced after digesting whole genomic DNA with restriction endonucleases may be appreciated using the technique of Southern blotting, a useful procedure named after the investigator who developed it.[51] The DNA is digested with one or more restriction endonucleases and then subjected to electrophoresis in a gel that separates fragments by size. It is then transferred to a membrane that binds DNA, and the appropriate DNA fragments are detected using labeled probes. Alternatively, the segment of DNA that is of interest may be amplified using the PCR technique and digested by a restriction endonuclease to determine whether or not target sites are present.

One of the most powerful uses of restriction endonucleases is in the detection of genetic variability. Changes in nucleotides may create or abolish restriction sites. Thus, they change the size of fragments that are formed when the DNA is digested. Such areas of variability represent RFLPs. In some cases, the changes in nucleotide sequence may be the ones that cause the disease itself. For example, the sickle cell mutation causes disappearance of a restriction site recognized by the enzyme *Mst* II,[52] and the G-6-PD A- mutation causes the formation of a restriction

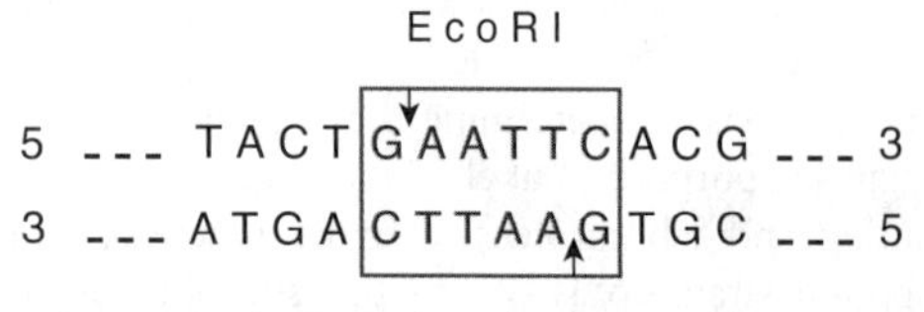

FIGURE 9–3. A representation EcoRI cleavaging its recognition sequence (outlined by the rectangle). Whenever this restriction endonuclease encounters the palindromic sequence GAATTC, DNA is cleaved at the position shown by the *arrows*.

site recognized by *Nla* III; such changes have proved valuable in diagnosis (see Chaps. 46–49), although they are gradually being replaced by automatic sequencing, as it has become generally available.

Deletions of chromosomal material, as occur in α-thalassemia, also produce changes in fragment sizes. Larger fragments may appear if the deleted fragment contains a restriction site, or smaller fragments if it does not. If the area covered by the probe is deleted in its entirety, as occurs in hydrops fetalis (see Chap. 47), no band will be seen at all. Even when the lesion that causes the disease does not directly affect a restriction site, RFLPs may be valuable in disease detection by virtue of close linkage to a disease-causing gene. Multiple restriction sites near the gene of interest produce haplotypes that may unequivocally identify a chromosome. Such haplotypes are particularly useful in the prenatal diagnosis of the thalassemias (see Chap. 47). Because haplotypes are stable over many generations, they can be used to deduce whether a mutation occurred only once and then expanded ("founder effect"), or whether it arose independently several times. Sickle cell disease represents a situation in which the mutation occurs in the context of several different haplotypes, so that there were several founders (see Chap. 48), factor IX, in which instance each of the common mutations had its own founder (Chap. 125). The extent to which rearrangements have taken place within a haplotype by crossing over permits estimates to be made of when the founder mutation occurred.

Sequencing

The chain termination technique[53] is commonly used to determine the sequence of DNA. It depends upon synthesizing a labeled strand of DNA, with the DNA to be sequenced serving as the template. The mixture of nucleotides used contains a nucleotide analogue that results in chain termination when incorporated. Gel electrophoresis of the labeled products produces "ladders" of polynucleotides. The size of each fragment depends on the point at which there exists a nucleotide corresponding to the chain terminating analogue in the mixture. In modern centers, sequencing can be done rapidly and accurately by automated methods in which the elongation of the strand is terminated by a fluorescent nucleotide.[54]

Although DNA sequencing formerly required cloning of the fragment to be studied, amplification by PCR serves as a simpler alternative.

Detecting Mutations in Individual Patients or in Population Studies

Increasingly the method of choice in detecting mutations in individual patients is PCR amplification of genomic DNA. The use of the other PCR- or restriction enzyme-based methods is usually more practical in performing surveys of patient or other populations. The use of restriction sites in detecting mutations in individual patients was discussed above (see "Cutting DNA with Restriction Endonucleases"), but because many substitutions neither abolish nor create restriction sites, the use of restriction endonucleases is not feasible in every case. However, a mismatch in one of the primers used in amplifying DNA by PCR, selected so as to create a restriction site where none existed before, is a technique that has been used successfully to detect mutations.[55] Using amplifying primers that fit one genotype but not the other has been used in "color PCR"[56] and in the "amplification refractory mutation system (ARMS)."[57] The failure of fragments of DNA to ligate when aligned on a template in which there is a misfit of the terminal nucleotide also has been used to detect mutations.[58] The hybridization of labeled oligonucleotide probes with a defined sequence to an amplified DNA target, a method designated allele-specific oligonucleotide hybridization (ASOH), is also very useful.[59] Probes containing approximately 17 nucleotides fitting either the normal or the mutant sequence are hybridized to PCR-amplified DNA. A single mismatch in an oligonucleotide of this size produces a sufficient change in melting temperature (i.e., the temperature at which the strands of DNA separate) that the two sequences can be distinguished from one another.

When the mutation is not known, other techniques may prove useful in narrowing the region that needs to be sequenced. Single-stranded conformation polymorphism (SSCP) analysis takes advantage of the fact that a single base substitution will usually change the conformation of single-stranded DNA and change its migration in a gel when subjected to electrophoresis. Denaturing high-pressure liquid chromatography is a more automated embodiment of this technique that appears to be highly efficient in detecting mutations.[60]

Interference with Gene Expression

Antisense RNA and DNA It is possible to interdict the expression of a gene at several different levels. The translation of mRNA can be inhibited and the mRNA degraded by *antisense* RNA or DNA, molecules that have a sequence complementary to the mRNA that is to be inactivated. When such oligonucleotides are present, they inhibit gene expression through a variety of mechanisms. For example, they form a double strand with the RNA, just as two complementary strands of DNA will hybridize to form the normal double-stranded form of DNA. Because the double-stranded form cannot be translated and is probably degraded rapidly, the production of its protein product is inhibited specifically. In experimental systems, antisense DNA or stable DNA analogues, such as the methylphosphonates,[61] can be transfected directly into cells or the RNA can be made off of a plasmid with the appropriate DNA template and a promoter. Originally this approach was used, for example, to suppress lymphoma growth with DNA oligonucleotides antisense to introns of the oncogene c-myc,[62] to suppress marrow cells from patients with chronic myelogenous leukemia by antisense DNA directed at the BCR-ABL junction,[63] or to suppress BCL-2–positive lymphoma cells in culture by BCL-2 antisense.[64] Because antisense RNA can be produced in vivo by transcribing the sense strand of a gene, it may represent a natural regulatory mechanism.[65,66]

Interfering RNA It has become apparent, however, that RNA plays a much broader role in the physiologic regulation of genes than merely the formation of antisense mRNAs. siRNAs and the closely related miRNAs represent a more recently discovered mechanism for silencing of genes, through a process known as RNA interference (RNAi; see references 67 and 68 for reviews). In the case of siRNA, double-stranded RNA is cleaved by the "dicer" enzyme into approximately 22 base pair segments that trigger the destruction through the RNA-induced silencing complex (RISC) of the homologous targeted mRNA. Although siRNAs tend to operate through RISC and slice the targeted mRNA, the miRNAs that represent endogenous duplexes can decrease the amount of target mRNA(s) or can also posttranscriptionally regulate gene expression by complexing with the same RISC and interfering with the targeted mRNAs translation. miRNAs may play an important role in hematopoietic differentiation[69] and seem to be widely used as a gene regulatory and antiviral measure. The use of siRNA has become very useful to molecular biologists as a powerful method for the downregulation of genes in experimental systems.

Ribozymes Cleaving RNA at defined sequences, much as restriction endonucleases cleave DNA, is one of the known enzymatic functions of RNA, and this function provides a means by which the expression of a gene can be interdicted in experimental systems. This *ribozyme* approach has been used, for example, in preventing replication of the HIV-1 virus[70,71] and by cleaving BCR-ABL with a view to developing a treatment for chronic myelogenous leukemia.[72] DNA may assume a similar enzymatic function.[73]

Transgenic and Knockout Animal Models The insertion of DNA fragments into the nucleus of a fertilized ovum provides a means for altering the genetic constitution of animals. Animals that have been engineered in this manner are referred to as *transgenic*. The use of promoters that are inducible or tissue specific permits studies of the effect of a gene product that might be lethal if expressed in all tissues or at all times during embryogenesis. Transgenic mice that carry the human sickle β-globin gene have been produced and when superimposed on a murine thalassemic genotype produce high enough levels of human hemoglobin S to have some potential as an animal model of sickle disease (Chaps. 47 and 48).[74]

Another valuable technique for the study of gene function is targeted disruption ("knocking out") of genes. In this technique, a DNA construct that contains regions homologous to the gene being targeted and selectable markers is transfected into an embryonic mouse stem cell. Once a cell in which recombination has occurred within a gene is found, it can be implanted into a blastocyst, with the hope that some of the progeny of the implanted cell will become germ cells. If this does occur, the knockout can be propagated and homozygous animals bred. The value of the technique is often limited by the fact that the knockout may be lethal (e.g., G-6-PD[75] deficiency and Gaucher disease[76]) or may not have any abnormal phenotype. But in some diseases, such as hemochromatosis,[77–80] knockout models of various forms of the disease are valuable resources. In situations in which a knockout proves to be lethal, or where it would be useful to limit the deficiency to a single organ system, the Cre/LoxP site-specific recombination system has proven to be very useful.[81] The LoxP sequence, a 13-base pair inverted repeat, is inserted so that it flanks the gene that is to be removed. Site-specific recombination is catalyzed by the P-1 bacteriophage Cre-recombinase, excising the intervening DNA targeted by the LoxP sequence and ligating the remaining 5′ and 3′ DNA. Tissue-specific excision can be achieved by inserting the Cre-recombinase downstream from a tissue-specific promoter. Random mutagenesis with agents such as *N*-ethyl-*N*-nitrosourea (ENU) can identify functions of genes whose role in a metabolic pathway was unsuspected. For example, a mutation in a membrane serine protease of unknown function revealed that it was a negative regulator of hepcidin.[82] Subsequent investigations revealed that mutations of this gene caused hereditary iron deficiency in humans.[83]

MUTATIONS

Types of Mutations

Mutations can occur in structural genes (the part of the DNA that specifies the amino acid sequence of protein), in the poorly understood regulatory apparatus that determines whether or not a gene will be available for transcription, in introns, or in portions of the DNA between genes that have no known function. As shown in Table 9–1, hematologic diseases provide examples of every known mechanism for causing mutations.

A change of one nucleotide to another without a change in the number of nucleotides in the sequence is called a *point mutation* or a *single nucleotide polymorphism* (SNP). Point mutations may change a codon so it specifies a different amino acid than does a normal codon; such mutations are designated as *missense* mutations. If the point mutation changes a codon that specified an amino acid to a stop codon, it is designated as a *nonsense* mutation. But some codon changes, particularly those in the third position, do not alter the amino acid that is specified by the triplet. Such mutations are called *synonymous* or *silent* mutations, and are often ignored as being of no importance. However, such point mutations can be of functional importance: (1) they can introduce splicing sites, and result in missplicing; (2) they can change the confirmation of the mRNA and thereby stability[84]; (3) they can

TABLE 9–1. Examples of Genetic Mechanisms in Hematologic Disease

Diseases caused by inherited mitochondrial mutations		
Sideroblastic anemias	del	Chap. 58
Diseases caused by inherited X-linked mutations		
G-6-PD deficiency	del, spl, pm	Chap. 46
Chronic granulomatous disease	pm, del, spl, ins	Chap. 66
Bruton agammaglobulinemia	pm, del, spl, ins	Chap. 82
Hemophilia	pm, del, spl, ins, tr	Chap. 124
Inherited autosomal dominant diseases		
Hereditary spherocytosis	pm, del, spl, ins	Chap. 45
Unstable hemoglobinopathies	pm, del	Chap. 48
Acute intermittent porphyria	pm, del, spl, ins	Chap. 57
von Willebrand disease	pm, del, ins	Chap. 127
Factor V Leiden	pm	Chap. 131
Inherited autosomal recessive diseases		
Pyruvate kinase deficiency	pm, del, spl, ins	Chap. 46
Thalassemia major	pm, del, spl, ins	Chap. 47
Sickle cell disease	pm	Chap. 48
Gaucher disease	pm, del, spl, ins, tr	Chap. 73
Diseases caused by acquired X-linked mutations		
PNH	pm, del, spl, ins	Chap. 40
Diseases caused by acquired autosomal dominant mutations		
Chronic myelogenous leukemia	tr	Chap. 90
Mantel cell lymphoma	tr	Chap. 102

del = deletion; ins = insertion; pm = point mutation; spl = splicing mutation; tr = translocation.

decrease the efficiency of protein synthesis, because the abundance of different tRNAs differs vastly; and (4) possibly because of changes in the rate of protein synthesis, abnormalities in folding may occur.[85]

Other types of mutations are deletions, inversions and insertions (e.g., duplication of stretches of DNA in a gene). Such changes account for the majority of the known mutations in hemophilia A (Chap. 124). *Microsatellites* are a special form of deletion or insertion. These are repeating units of one to six nucleotides, for example, ATATATATAT. Such sequences are unstable in evolution of a species and tend to be very polymorphic. Instead of only two possible genotypes, as in the case of most SNPs, there may be 5, 10, or more different numbers of repeats at a given locus in different individuals. As a result, microsatellites are very useful in genetic mapping. Single nucleotide mutations do not occur at random. Changes in the dinucleotide CpG to TpG are particularly common because invertebrate DNA cytidines followed by guanine are often methylated and the methylcytosine formed is susceptible to oxidation to thymine. Thus, an unusually high proportion of point mutations are found in CpG dinucleotides in hemophilia A[86] and G-6-PD deficiency.[87] Deletions or duplications of portions of genes tend to occur in areas in which the same sequence is repeated more than once. Thus, there are "hot spots" in the genome in which, for one reason or another, mutations are particularly likely to occur.

Another mechanism by which mutation appears to occur is that of *gene conversion*. This poorly understood phenomenon results in the sequence of one gene being transferred *en bloc* to another. This phenomenon is thought to account for the maintenance of identical sequence between duplicated genes.[88]

Many mutations affect the amount of processed mRNA that is formed. For example, mutations that cause abnormal splicing may produce a messenger that cannot be translated. Regulatory mutations that impair the rate at which a gene is transcribed into mRNA can be the consequence of mutations in promoter or enhancer elements. Mutations that cause thalassemia by impairing transcription of the hemoglobin locus are the best characterized of these (Chap. 47). A premature stop codon introduced by a nonsense mutation will often result in a decrease in the amount of mRNA through a complex process that has been called *nonsense-mediated decay*. However, most mutations causing hematologic disease seem to be structural mutations, those in which the sequence of the coding region of the gene is altered.

Errors in the coding sequence of a gene may result in failure to form any of the protein, in the formation of a very unstable protein that may never appear in the fully assembled form, or in the formation of an abnormal protein. The latter circumstance appears to be the most common. The abnormal protein may maintain all, some, or none of the functional properties of the normal protein. Even when it has lost the functional properties of the original protein, it may retain its antigenic properties, and it is then designated *cross-reacting material* (CRM). Occasionally the mutation may create a gene product that interferes with the function of the normal protein or that serves as a "poison" subunit that prevents functioning of the protein. Such mutations are known as dominant negative, and they are inherited in a dominant fashion. Mutations that result in the formation of normal amounts of stable proteins with normal functional properties are not clinically significant, but they may be very valuable from the point of view of population and family studies, or as genetic markers for various types of biologic investigations. Some "deficiencies" of enzymes are also clinically harmless. For example, genetic absence of the glycosyl transferases that convert the H antigen to the A or B antigen (see Chap. 137) results in the appearance of blood group O, surely a clinical state that cannot be considered a disease. Genetic variants that reach a frequency of more than 1 percent in a population are known as *polymorphisms*. Sometimes genetic variants, such as the sickle cell gene or the G-6-PD deficiency gene, reach polymorphic levels because the deleterious effects that they may have are counterbalanced by beneficial effects on survival, such as increased resistance to malaria. They are known as *balanced polymorphisms*.

All cells receive the same complement of genes. Nonetheless, some proteins are tissue-specific. Several circumstances can account for this. Some enzymes that appear to perform the same function are encoded by different genes in different tissues. For example, the pyruvate kinase of leukocytes and that of erythrocytes are under separate genetic control (see Chap. 46). In other cases, alternative splicing of the primary mRNA can produce different polypeptides, a phenomenon that is particularly prominent with some of the red cell membrane proteins.[89] Differences in posttranslational processing, including proteolysis and glycosylation of the same polypeptide by different enzymes in different tissues, can lead to different final products. However, in most instances a mutation that affects an enzyme in one type of blood cell will also affect the same enzyme in other blood cells, in liver, in brain, and in other tissues.

The types of enzyme deficiencies encountered clinically are limited by the ability of the affected individual to survive. Thus complete absence of a key glycolytic enzyme from all tissues is incompatible with the basic process of energy metabolism and would almost surely be lethal long before birth. In contrast, the inheritance of enzyme deficiencies that are manifested only in erythrocytes are apparently quite compatible with survival and thus, many of the enzyme defects that are observed in humans are ones that only affect the red blood cell.

Mutation Nomenclature

Historically, mutations were first detected by sequencing the protein, usually hemoglobin. Indeed, the mutation in sickle cell disease was described before the genetic code had been deciphered. Thus, mutations were designated by indicating the amino acid change. Amino acid–based nomenclature does not unambiguously define the mutation, as the same amino acid substitution can be caused by different nucleotide substitutions. Further ambiguity is introduced by the fact that three different starting points for the numbering of amino acids in protein are commonly employed: (1) The methionine start codon; (2) the amino acid after the methionine start codon; and (3) the amino terminal amino acid of the processed protein. Finally, there are many mutations, such as those that change splice sites or promoters that cannot be designated by an amino acid substitution. Nonetheless, amino acid–based mutation has been so widely used that they serve as useful "nicknames" for mutations; the nucleotide-based designation would simply not be recognized by workers in the field. Moreover, knowing the amino acid change sometimes provides valuable information regarding the effect of the mutation at the protein level. Therefore, while the more robust nucleotide-based mutation is preferred in this text, the amino acid–based notation is used when it is the one that is generally recognized. Standards have been established for the different notations that are in use.[90–93]

Gene Duplication

Crossing-over during meiosis usually occurs with great precision. Homologous genes pair with each other, and although genes which were together on the chromosome before meiosis may now be on opposite chromosomes of the pair, each chromosome still contains a complete set of genes (see Fig. 9–1). Occasionally, however, an error occurs and pairing during meiosis is imperfect. Under these circumstances—unequal crossing-over (see Fig. 47–8)—one of the daughter chromosomes contains a duplicated gene, while the other one exists with a gene deleted.

Once a duplication has occurred, further duplications occur more readily, because pairing of the first of the duplicate genes on one chromosome with the second gene of the duplicate on the other produces one chromosome with a triplicated gene and one with a single gene (Chap. 47). Duplication has probably played a very important role in the course of evolution,[94] because the presence of two genes with the same function allows experiments of nature: Mutations can accumulate on one of the genes while the original function is still provided by the duplicate. Examples of the results of gene duplication abound in hematology, particularly with respect to the hemoglobin loci. The α-chain loci are duplicated, and there are also two nearly identical copies of the γ-chain locus (see Chap. 47). Furthermore, the close similarity of their amino acid sequence and the fact that they are tightly linked indicate that the β, γ, and δ loci represent the result of duplication of a single ancestral gene. The process of unequal crossing-over takes place not only between genes, but also within genes. When this occurs, one would anticipate that a portion of the amino acid sequence of a protein is represented twice on one chromosome and is missing on the other. The Lepore hemoglobins, leading to a thalassemic clinical state, are an example of this type of unequal crossing-over (see Fig. 47–8). These abnormal hemoglobins have the amino acid sequence of the δ chain at the amino end, and the sequence of the β chain at the carboxyl end. The complement to this kind of abnormality, the "anti-Lepore" hemoglobin, also has also been found (see Chaps. 47 and 48). Similarly, a mutation of the glucocerebrosidase gene causing Gaucher disease has been found to be the result of a crossover between the active gene and the pseudogene.[95] The two types of haptoglobin represent an ancestral gene and one in which a major part of that gene has been duplicated.[96]

Pseudogenes Pseudogenes are DNA sequences that resemble the corresponding functional genes, but do not form a gene product. Pseudogenes exist, for example, for the β globin chain, von Willebrand factor, ferritin, and glucocerebrosidase. These pseudogenes apparently arose by gene duplication and simulate the true gene, even in having introns. They have apparently lost their ability to function, either through mutations in the coding region or in their promoters. Some pseudogenes are devoid of introns. They may well have arisen in evolution as a result of the reverse transcription of a processed mRNA by retroviral reverse transcriptase. Unlike genes that arose by tandem duplication as a result of unequal crossover, such pseudogenes can be found anywhere in the genome. For example, a functional glutathione-S-transferase gene is on chromosome 11 and a pseudogene is located on chromosome 12.[97]

Genotype–Phenotype Correlations Even before detection of mutations at the DNA level was feasible, clinicians could deduce that the same genotype did not always produce the same clinical disease picture (phenotype). Sibs inheriting autosomal recessive disorders from their parents often have been observed to have discordant clinical presentations—one severely affected, one mildly so—even though the same pair of disease-producing genes were inherited. With the development of the ability to define genotypes directly, the great degree of genotype–phenotype dissociation has become even more evident. Thus, persons inheriting the same sickle, G-6-PD, factor VIII, or glucocerebrosidase mutations may have mild or severe sickle disease, hemolytic anemia, hemophilia A, or Gaucher disease, respectively. The factors that modify disease expression are usually not understood.[98] In the case of G-6-PD deficiency, a second mutation, one in the uridine diphosphate (UDP) glucuronyltransferase-1 gene has been shown to determine whether severe jaundice will be present.[99,100] Thrombophilia is much more likely to occur in patients with factor V Leiden if a second mutation of a gene encoding another coagulation factor such as protein C is coinherited.[101,102] Environmental factors may play a role; clinically significant hemochromatosis is probably more common in alcoholics and thrombophilia in women receiving oral contraceptives. Epigenetic factors have been shown to be important in the case of imprinted genes, such as the *KCNQ10T1* gene of Beckwith-Wiedemann syndrome (see Chap. 10).[103]

GENOMICS AND PROTEOMICS

Genomics and proteomics are catchphrases to describe the large-scale analysis of gene sequence and protein production, respectively. Much, but not all, of the human genome sequence is known. There are many areas with extensive duplications in which the sequence is incorrect and there are still gaps in the sequence. Nonetheless, much of the sequence is accurate and it is now possible to use powerful computer programs to search for new members of gene families that have been found to be important, or DNA or amino acid-sequence motifs that are known or believed to serve specific functions. Another application of genomics is the hybridization of the mRNA from a tissue with microarrays of fragments of thousands of DNA sequences. This technology, known as *expression profiling,* has been used to characterize gene expression in tissues or cells under different conditions. These data may sometimes be useful in understanding a disease state, and this approach has been used, for example, in an attempt to provide predictive data about lymphomas.[104]

Gene sequences only predict the unprocessed sequence of a protein, and give only indirect information about the important posttranslational changes that create the final functional protein. *Proteomics* provides techniques for the separation of proteins and for their rapid identification by means such as the characterization of tryptic fragments by mass spectrometry and their comparison with a large computerized library of data.[100]

REFERENCES

1. Fain PR, Goldgar DE, Wallace MR, et al: Refined physical and genetic mapping of the NF1 region on chromosome 17. *Am J Hum Genet* 45:721, 1989.
2. Glenn D, Gelbart T, Beutler E: Tight linkage of pyruvate kinase (*PKLR*) and glucocerebrosidase (*GBA*) genes. *Hum Genet* 93:635, 1994.
3. Demina A, Boas E, Beutler E: Structure and linkage relationships of the region containing the human L-type pyruvate kinase (*PKLR*) and glucocerebrosidase (*GBA*) genes. *Hematopathol Mol Hematol* 11:63, 1998.
4. Beutler E, Yeh M, Fairbanks VF: The normal human female as a mosaic of X-chromosome activity: Studies using the gene for G-6-PD deficiency as a marker. *Proc Natl Acad Sci U S A* 48:9, 1962.
5. Lyon MF: Sex chromatin and gene action in the mammalian X-chromosome. *Am J Hum Genet* 14:135, 1962.
6. Wutz A, Gribnau J: X inactivation Xplained. *Curr Opin Genet Dev* 17:387, 2007.
7. Willard HF: X chromosome inactivation, XIST, and pursuit of the X-inactivation center. *Cell* 86:5, 1996.
8. Gartler SM, Linder D: Developmental and evolutionary implications of the mosaic nature of the G-6-PD system. *Cold Spring Harb Symp Quant Biol* 29:253, 1964.
9. Beutler E: The distribution of gene products among populations of cells in heterozygous humans. *Cold Spring Harb Symp Quant Biol* 29:261, 1964.
10. Fialkow PJ, Gartler SM, Yoshida A: Clonal origin of chronic myelocytic leukemia in man. *Proc Natl Acad Sci U S A* 58:1468, 1967.
11. Liu E, Jelinek J, Pastore YD, et al: Discrimination of polycythemias and thrombocytoses by novel, simple, accurate clonality assays and comparison with PRV-1 expression and BFU-E response to erythropoietin. *Blood* 101:3294, 2003.
12. Oni SB, Osunkoya BO, Luzzatto L: Paroxysmal nocturnal hemoglobinuria: Evidence for monoclonal origin of abnormal red cells. *Blood* 36:145, 1970.
13. Beutler E, West C, Johnson C: Involvement of the erythroid series in acute myeloid leukemia. *Blood* 53:1203, 1979.
14. Fialkow PJ, Singer JW, Raskind WH, et al: Clonal development, stem-cell differentiation, and clinical remissions in acute nonlymphocytic leukemia. *N Engl J Med* 317:468, 1987.
15. Lindsay S, Monk M, Holliday R, et al: Differences in methylation on the active and inactive human X chromosomes. *Ann Hum Genet* 49:115, 1985.
16. Gilliland DG, Blanchard KL, Bunn HF: Clonality in acquired hematologic disorders. *Annu Rev Med* 42:491, 1991.
17. Curnutte JT, Hopkins PJ, Kuhl W, Beutler E: Studying X-inactivation. *Lancet* 339:749, 1992.
18. Prchal JT, Guan YL, Prchal JF, Barany F: Transcriptional analysis of the active X-chromosome in normal and clonal hematopoiesis. *Blood* 81:269, 1993.
19. Swierczek SI, Agarwal N, Nussenzveig RH, et al: Hematopoiesis is not clonal in health elderly women. *Blood* 112:3001, 2008.
20. Wallace DC: Mitochondrial DNA sequence variation in human evolution and disease. *Proc Natl Acad Sci U S A* 91:8739, 1994.
21. Wallace DC: Mitochondrial diseases in man and mouse. *Science* 283:1482, 1999.
22. Bader-Meunier B, Rotig A, Mielot F, et al: Refractory anaemia and mitochondrial cytopathy in childhood. *Br J Haematol* 87:381, 1994.
23. Superti-Furga A, Schoenle E, Tuchschmid P, et al: Pearson bone marrow-pancreas syndrome with insulin-dependent diabetes, progressive renal tubulopathy, organic aciduria and elevated fetal haemoglobin caused by deletion and duplication of mitochondrial DNA. *Eur J Pediatr* 152:44, 1993.
24. Cormier V, Rötig A, Quartino AR, et al: Widespread multi-tissue deletions of the mitochondrial genome in the Pearson marrow-pancreas syndrome. *J Pediatr* 117:599, 1990.
25. Whitelaw E, Martin DI: Retrotransposons as epigenetic mediators of phenotypic variation in mammals. *Nat Genet* 27:361, 2001.
26. Ordway JM, Curran T: Methylation matters: Modeling a manageable genome. *Cell Growth Differ* 13:149, 2002.
27. Beutler E: Autosomal inactivation. *Lancet* 1:1242, 1963.
28. Gimelbrant A, Hutchinson JN, Thompson BR, Chess A: Widespread monoallelic expression on human autosomes. *Science* 318:1136, 2007.
29. Jarman AP, Wood WG, Sharpe JA, et al: Characterization of the major regulatory element upstream of the human alpha-globin gene cluster. *Mol Cell Biol* 11:4679, 1991.
30. Orkin SH: Globin gene regulation and switching: circa 1990. *Cell* 63:665, 1990.
31. Faustino NA, Cooper TA: Pre-mRNA splicing and human disease. *Genes Dev* 17:419, 2003.
32. Conboy JG, Chan J, Mohandas N, Kan YW: Multiple protein 4.1 isoforms produced by alternative splicing in human erythroid cells. *Proc Natl Acad Sci U S A* 85:9062, 1988.
33. Noguchi T, Yamada K, Inoue H, et al: The L- and R-type isozymes of rat pyruvate kinase are produced from a single gene by use of different promoters. *J Biol Chem* 262:14366, 1987.
34. Wiestner A, Schlemper RJ, van der Maas AP, Skoda RC: An activating splice donor mutation in the thrombopoietin gene causes hereditary thrombocythaemia. *Nat Genet* 18:49, 1998.
35. Kozak M: Compilation and analysis of sequences upstream from the translational start site in eukaryotic mRNAs. *Nucleic Acids Res* 12:857, 1984.
36. Steitz TA: A structural understanding of the dynamic ribosome machine. *Nat Rev Mol Cell Biol* 9:242, 2008.
37. Maniatis T, Goodbourn S, Fischer JA: Regulation of inducible and tissue-specific gene expression. *Science* 236:1237, 1987.
38. Cazzola M, Skoda RC: Translational pathophysiology: A novel molecular mechanism of human disease. *Blood* 95:3280, 2000.
39. Meyron-Holtz EG, Ghosh MC, Rouault TA: Mammalian tissue oxygen levels modulate iron regulatory protein activities in vivo. *Science* 306:2087, 2004.
40. Han J, Brown T, Beutler B: Endotoxin-responsive sequences control cachectin/tumor necrosis factor biosynthesis at the translational level. *J Exp Med* 171:465, 1990.
41. Han J, Beutler B, Huez G: Complex regulation of tumor necrosis factor mRNA turnover in lipopolysaccharide-activated macrophages. *Biochim Biophys Acta* 1090:22, 1991.
42. Liebhaber SA: mRNA stability and the control of gene expression. *Nucleic Acids Symp Ser* 29, 1997.
43. Caput D, Beutler B, Hartog K, et al: Identification of a common nucleotide sequence in the 3′-untranslated region of mRNA molecules specifying inflammatory mediators. *Proc Natl Acad Sci U S A* 83:1670, 1986.
44. Shaw G, Kamen R: A conserved AU sequence from the 3′ untranslated region of GM-CSF mRNA mediates selective mRNA degradation. *Cell* 46:659, 1986.
45. Heaney JD, Bronson SK: Artificial chromosome-based transgenes in the study of genome function. *Mamm Genome* 17:791, 2006.
46. Amplification of nucleic acid sequences: The choices multiply. *J NIH Res* 3:81, 1991.
47. *PCR Protocols: A Guide to Methods and Applications*. Academic Press, San Diego, 1990.
48. de Melo MB, Sales TS, Lorand-Metze I, Costa FF: Rapid method for isolation of DNA from glass slide smears for PCR. *Acta Haematol* 87:214, 1992.
49. Paabo S, Poinar H, Serre D, et al: Genetic analyses from ancient DNA. *Annu Rev Genet* 38:645, 2004.
50. Vanguilder H, Vrana K, Freeman W: Twenty-five years of quantitative PCR for gene expression analysis. *Biotechniques* 44:619, 2008.
51. Southern E: Gel electrophoresis of restriction fragments. *Methods Enzymol* 68:152, 1979.
52. Chang JC, Kan YW: Antenatal diagnosis of sickle cell anaemia by direct analysis of the sickle mutation. *Lancet* 2:1127, 1981.
53. Sanger F, Nicklen S, Coulson AR: DNA sequencing with chain-terminating inhibitors. *Proc Natl Acad Sci U S A* 74:5463, 1977.
54. Sterky F, Lundeberg J: Sequence analysis of genes and genomes. *J Biotechnol* 76:1, 2000.
55. Kumar R, Dunn LL: Designed diagnostic restriction fragment length polymorphisms for the detection of point mutations in ras oncogenes. *Oncogene Res* 4:235, 1989.
56. Chehab FF, Kan YW: Detection of specific DNA sequences by fluorescence amplification: A color complementation assay. *Proc Natl Acad Sci U S A* 86:9178, 1989.
57. Mistry PK, Smith SJ, Ali M, et al: Genetic diagnosis of Gaucher's disease. *Lancet* 339:889, 1992.
58. Barany F: Genetic disease detection and DNA amplification using cloned thermostable ligase. *Proc Natl Acad Sci U S A* 88:189, 1991.
59. Beutler E, Gelbart T: Large-scale screening for HFE mutations: Methodology and cost. *Genet Test* 4:131, 2000.
60. Fruchon S, Bensaid M, Borot N, et al: Use of denaturing HPLC and a heteroduplex generator to detect the HFE C282Y mutation associated with genetic hemochromatosis. *Clin Chem* 49:822, 2003.
61. Smith CC, Aurelian L, Reddy MP, et al: Antiviral effect of an oligo (nucleoside methylphosphonate) complementary to the splice junction of herpes simplex virus type 1 immediate early pre-mRNAs 4 and 5. *Proc Natl Acad Sci U S A* 83:2787, 1986.
62. McManaway ME, Neckers LM, Loke SL, Al-Nasser AA, Redner RL, Shiramizu BT, Goldschmidts WL, Huber BE, Bhatia K, Magrath IT: Tumour-specific inhibition of lymphoma growth by an antisense oligodeoxynucleotide. *Lancet* 335:808, 1990.
63. Szczylik C, Skorski T, Nicolaides NC, et al: Selective inhibition of leukemia cell proliferation by BCR-ABL antisense oligodeoxynucleotides. *Science* 253:562, 1991.
64. Cotter FE, Johnson P, Hall P, et al: Antisense oligonucleotides suppress B-cell lymphoma growth in a SCID-hu mouse model. *Oncogene* 9:3049, 1994.
65. Weintraub HM: Antisense RNA and DNA. *Sci Am* 262:40, 1990.
66. Simons RW: Naturally occurring antisense RNA control—A brief review. *Gene* 72:35, 1988.
67. Fabbri M, Garzon R, Andreeff M, et al: MicroRNAs and noncoding RNAs in hematological malignancies: molecular, clinical and therapeutic implications. *Leukemia* 22:1095, 2008.

68. Kim D, Rossi J: RNAi mechanisms and applications. *Biotechniques* 44:613, 2008.
69. Chen CZ, Li L, Lodish HF, Bartel DP: MicroRNAs modulate hematopoietic lineage differentiation. *Science* 303:83, 2004.
70. Chen CJ, Banerjea AC, Harmison GG, et al: Multitarget-ribozyme directed to cleave at up to nine highly conserved HIV-1 env RNA regions inhibits HIV-1 replication—Potential effectiveness against most presently sequenced HIV-1 isolates. *Nucleic Acids Res* 20:4581, 1992.
71. Heidenreich O, Eckstein F: Hammerhead ribozyme-mediated cleavage of the long terminal repeat RNA of human immunodeficiency virus type 1. *J Biol Chem* 267:1904, 1992.
72. Soda Y, Tani K, Bai Y, et al: A novel maxizyme vector targeting a BCR-ABL fusion gene induced specific cell death in Philadelphia chromosome-positive acute lymphoblastic leukemia. *Blood* 104:356, 2004.
73. Abdelgany A, Wood M, Beeson D: Hairpin DNAzymes: A new tool for efficient cellular gene silencing. *J Gene Med* 9:727, 2007.
74. Beuzard Y: Mouse models of sickle cell disease. *Transfus Clin Biol* 15:7, 2008.
75. Longo L, Vanegas OC, Patel M, et al: Maternally transmitted severe glucose 6-phosphate dehydrogenase deficiency is an embryonic lethal. *EMBO J* 21:4229, 2002.
76. Tybulewicz VLJ, Tremblay ML, LaMarca ME, et al: Animal model of Gaucher's disease from targeted disruption of the mouse glucocerebrosidase gene. *Nature* 357:407, 1992.
77. Zhou XY, Tomatsu S, Fleming RE, et al: HFE gene knockout produces mouse model of hereditary hemochromatosis. *Proc Natl Acad Sci U S A* 95:2492, 1998.
78. Nicolas G, Bennoun M, Devaux I, et al: Lack of hepcidin gene expression and severe tissue iron overload in upstream stimulatory factor 2 (USF2) knockout mice. *Proc Natl Acad Sci U S A* 98:8780, 2001.
79. Niederkofler V, Salie R, Arber S: Hemojuvelin is essential for dietary iron sensing, and its mutation leads to severe iron overload. *J Clin Invest* 115:2180, 2005.
80. Huang FW, Pinkus JL, Pinkus GS, Fleming MD, Andrews NC: A mouse model of juvenile hemochromatosis. *J Clin Invest* 115:2187, 2005.
81. Yu Y, Bradley A: Engineering chromosomal rearrangements in mice. *Nat Rev Genet* 2:780, 2001.
82. Du X, She E, Gelbart T, et al: The serine protease TMPRSS6 is required to sense iron deficiency. *Science* 320:1088, 2008.
83. Melis MA, Cau M, Congiu R, et al: A mutation in the TMPRSS6 gene, encoding a transmembrane serine protease that suppresses hepcidin production, in familial iron deficiency anemia refractory to oral iron. *Haematologica* 93:1473, 2008.
84. Capon F, Allen MH, Ameen M, et al: A synonymous SNP of the corneodesmosin gene leads to increased mRNA stability and demonstrates association with psoriasis across diverse ethnic groups. *Hum Mol Genet* 13:2361, 2004.
85. Kimchi-Sarfaty C, Oh JM, Kim IW, et al: A "silent" polymorphism in the MDR1 gene changes substrate specificity. *Science* 315:525, 2007.
86. Youssoufian H, Kazazian HH Jr, Phillips DG, et al: Recurrent mutations in haemophilia A give evidence for CpG mutation hotspots. *Nature* 324:380, 1986.
87. Vulliamy TJ, D'Urso M, Battistuzzi G, et al: Diverse point mutations in the human glucose 6-phosphate dehydrogenase gene cause enzyme deficiency and mild or severe hemolytic anemia. *Proc Natl Acad Sci U S A* 85:5171, 1988.
88. Hess JF, Schmid CW, Shen CK: A gradient of sequence divergence in the human adult alpha-globin duplication units. *Science* 226:67, 1984.
89. Benz EJ Jr, Huang SC: Role of tissue specific alternative pre-mRNA splicing in the differentiation of the erythrocyte membrane. *Trans Am Clin Climatol Assoc* 108:78, 1997.
90. Ad Hoc Committee on Mutation Nomenclature: Update on nomenclature for human gene mutations. *Hum Mutat* 8:197, 1996.
91. Antonarakis SE: Recommendations for a nomenclature system for human gene mutations. Nomenclature Working Group. *Hum Mutat* 11:1, 1998.
92. Beutler E, McKusick VA, Motulsky AG, et al: Mutation nomenclature: Nicknames, systematic names, and unique identifiers. *Hum Mutat* 8:203, 1996.
93. den Dunnen JT, Paalman MH: Standardizing mutation nomenclature: Why bother? *Hum Mutat* 22:181, 2003.
94. Ohno S: *Evolution by Gene Duplication*. Springer Verlag, Berlin, 1970.
95. Zimran A, Sorge J, Gross E, et al: A glucocerebrosidase fusion gene in Gaucher disease. Implications for the molecular anatomy, pathogenesis and diagnosis of this disorder. *J Clin Invest* 85:219, 1990.
96. Manoharan A: Congenital haptoglobin deficiency. *Blood* 90:1709, 1997.
97. Board PG, Coggan M, Woodcock DM: The human Pi class glutathione transferase sequence at 12q13-q14 is a reverse-transcribed pseudogene. *Genomics* 14:470, 1992.
98. Beutler E: Discrepancies between genotype and phenotype in hematology: An important frontier. *Blood* 98:2597, 2001.
99. Kaplan M, Renbaum P, Levy-Lahad E, et al: Gilbert syndrome and glucose-6-phosphate dehydrogenase deficiency: A dose-dependent genetic interaction crucial to neonatal hyperbilirubinemia. *Proc Natl Acad Sci U S A* 94:12128, 1997.
100. Sampietro M, Lupica L, Perrero L, et al: The expression of uridine diphosphate glucuronosyltransferase gene is a major determinant of bilirubin level in heterozygous beta-thalassaemia and in glucose-6-phosphate dehydrogenase deficiency. *Br J Haematol* 99:437, 1997.
101. Lane DA, Grant PJ: Role of hemostatic gene polymorphisms in venous and arterial thrombotic disease. *Blood* 95:1517, 2000.
102. Rosendaal FR: Venous thrombosis: A multicausal disease. *Lancet* 353:1167, 1999.
103. Weksberg R, Shuman C, Caluseriu O, et al: Discordant KCNQ1OT1 imprinting in sets of monozygotic twins discordant for Beckwith-Wiedemann syndrome. *Hum Mol Genet* 11:1317, 2002.
104. Lossos IS, Levy R: Diffuse large B-cell lymphoma: insights gained from gene expression profiling. *Int J Hematol* 77:321, 2003.

CHAPTER 10
GENOMICS AND EPIGENETICS

Lynn B. Jorde

SUMMARY

The ability to analyze data obtained from the entire human genome (genomics) is having a significant impact on hematology and on medicine in general. This chapter provides a basic description of microarray technology and how this technology can be used to study disease-associated genetic variation, copy number variation, gene expression, and patterns of epigenetic modification. In addition, the principles of epigenetics, in which the expression of genes is altered by chemical modifications such as methylation, are reviewed. Several disease examples are given in which epigenetic modifications have significant clinical effects.

Acronyms and abbreviations that occur in this chapter include: DMR, differentially methylated region; IGF2, insulin-like growth factor 2; mRNA, messenger ribonucleic acid; SNP, single nucleotide polymorphism.

GENOMICS AND EPIGENETICS

Increasingly, genetic variation is being assessed at the level of the entire genome. Studies of genome-wide variation are part of the now well-known science of *genomics*.[1] During the past decade, several important tools have emerged that allow investigators to collect and analyze genomic data.

The most widely used of these tools is the *microarray* (Fig. 10–1).[2,3] To make a DNA microarray, single-stranded DNA sequences consisting of about 20 bases (oligonucleotides, from "a few" nucleotides) are robotically placed on a small glass slide. A single slide (1 cm^2) can contain millions of different oligonucleotides. These oligonucleotides correspond to different alleles (DNA sequences at a specific chromosome location) in populations. Typically these alleles are *single-nucleotide polymorphisms* (SNPs). Some of the oligonucleotides may contain known disease-causing mutations. Fluorescently labeled single-stranded DNA from a subject is hybridized with the oligonucleotides on the slide to determine, for a specific region in the genome, which DNA sequence undergoes complementary base pairing with that of the subject. The pattern of hybridization signals is analyzed by a computer, providing a detailed profile of genetic variation specific to an individual's DNA. With current technology, enough probes can be placed on a single microarray to analyze variation in one million SNPs in an individual.

SNP microarrays are now used routinely to perform *genome-wide association studies*, in which the frequencies of each SNP are compared in disease cases and unaffected controls.[4] SNPs that show significant frequency differences in cases and controls may lie within or near a gene that contributes to disease susceptibility. The design of these studies has been made considerably more efficient as a result of the International Haplotype Map Project (HapMap).[5] This large-scale international effort was designed to help identify a set of SNPs that provide maximum information about potential disease associations, with minimal correlation among different SNPs. This helps to ensure that each SNP provides as much independent information as possible.

Microarrays are also used to examine *copy number variants*, *methylation patterns* in an individual's genome, and *genetic variation* among species and in various pathogenic infectious organisms. An important diagnostic tool for many hematologic cancers is *array comparative genomic hybridization*, in which DNA from a tumor sample is compared with normal DNA (see Chap. 11) by hybridization to a microarray, to determine which regions of the genome are amplified or deleted in the tumor sample.[6,7]

Another application of DNA microarrays is to determine which genes are being expressed (i.e., transcribed) in a given tissue sample (e.g., from a tumor).[8] Messenger RNA (mRNA) from the tissue is extracted and used as a template to form a complementary DNA sequence, which is then hybridized on the slide with oligonucleotides representing many different genes. The pattern of positive hybridization signals indicates which genes are expressed in the tissue sample. These "expression arrays" can be used, for example, to test which genes are actively expressed in lymphoma or leukemia cells, and expression profiles can help to predict the aggressiveness of an individual's cancer.[9] Abnormal expression of microRNAs (small noncoding RNA sequences that can regulate gene expression [see Chap. 9]) can lead to leukemias and other malignancies, and microarrays are also used to assess microRNA expression.[10]

Importantly, microarrays typically test for known SNPs that are incorporated in oligonucleotide probes. A rare, previously unidentified mutation will not be detected by conventional microarrays. There is now growing interest in *high-throughput DNA sequencing* technologies that permit direct sequencing of all exons in the genome (the *exome*), or even the entire DNA sequence of an individual.[11–15] With complete DNA sequencing, all variants, both common and rare, should be detected. This is the goal, for example, of the ongoing, publicly funded 1000 Genomes Project, in which the genomes of more than 1000 humans will be resequenced and analyzed.[16] The cost of resequencing an entire genome is declining rapidly, and whole-genome sequences will be available for clinical application in the near future.

Considering the large volume of data that is produced by a single microarray, or the even larger amount produced by the sequencing of an individual's entire 3-billion-base genome, it is not surprising that sophisticated *bioinformatic* tools have been developed to deal with such data. These algorithms deal with issues such as DNA base calling and genotype inference (missing genotypes), sequence alignment, and gene annotation.[12,17,18]

EPIGENETICS AND DISEASE

Traditionally, geneticists have focused on the ways in which mutations of DNA sequences can lead to disease (Chap. 9), and this has been a major goal of the genomic approaches just discussed. However, the same DNA sequence can sometimes produce dramatically different phenotypes, as a consequence of chemical modifications that alter the expression of genes (the nature and effects of these modifications are collectively termed *epigenetics*). An important example of such a modification is DNA *methylation*, the attachment of methyl groups to cytosine bases followed by guanine bases (CG) in the DNA sequence (Fig. 10–2).[19] When the DNA sequence near a gene becomes heavily methylated, the DNA is less likely to be transcribed into mRNA. Methylation, along with histone hypoacetylation and condensation of chromatin, inhibits the binding of proteins that promote transcription. In other words, the gene becomes transcriptionally inactive. This process is similar in many ways to X chromosome inactivation, which is discussed in Chap. 9.

Epigenetic alteration of gene activity can have important disease consequences. For example, a major cause of one form of inherited colon cancer (hereditary nonpolyposis colorectal cancer) is the methylation of

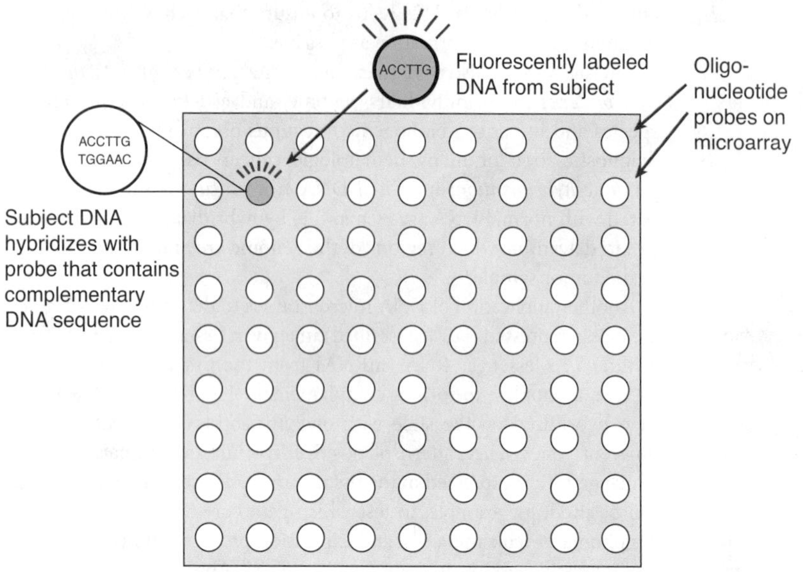

FIGURE 10–1. Schematic of a microarray, in which oligonucleotides are placed or synthesized on a glass slide and then hybridized with labeled single-stranded DNA from a subject. Complementary base pairing will occur between the subject DNA fragment and the oligonucleotide on the slide only if the sequences are complementary to one another. A fluorescent label on the subject's DNA marks the location on the microarray at which the subject's DNA undergoes hybridization, thus indicating the DNA sequence of the subject at a specific location in the genome. *(From Jorde LB, Carey JC, Bamshad MJ:* Medical Genetics, *4th ed. Mosby/Elsevier, Philadelphia, 2010. With permission.)*

the promoter region of a gene, *MLH1*, whose protein product repairs damaged DNA. When *MLH1* becomes inactive, damaged DNA accumulates, resulting eventually in colon tumors.[20] Methylation, and therefore silencing, of tumor-suppressor genes is an important mechanism that can increase cancer risk (e.g., *RB1*, associated with retinoblastoma; *BRCA1*, associated with breast cancer; and *VHL*, associated with von Hippel-Lindau disease).[21]

A recent study showed that identical (monozygotic) twins accumulate different methylation patterns in the DNA sequences of their somatic cells as they age, causing increasing numbers of phenotypic differences.[22] Intriguingly, twins with significant lifestyle differences (e.g., smoking vs. nonsmoking) accumulated larger numbers of differences in their methylation patterns. The twins, despite having identical DNA sequences, become more and more different as a result of epigenetic changes, which in turn affect the expression of genes.

GENOMIC IMPRINTING

Gregor Mendel's experiments with garden peas demonstrated that the phenotype is the same whether a given allele is inherited from the mother or the father. This principle, which has long been part of the central dogma of genetics, does not always hold. For some human genes, the gene is transcriptionally active on only one copy of a chromosome (e.g., the copy inherited from the father). On the other copy of the chromosome (the one inherited from the mother) the gene is transcriptionally inactive. This process of gene silencing, in which genes are silenced depending on which parent transmits them, is known as *imprinting*, and the transcriptionally silenced genes are said to be "imprinted."[23,24] At least several dozen human genes, and perhaps as many as 200 or so, are thought to be imprinted. When genes are imprinted, they are usually heavily methylated (in contrast to the nonimprinted copy of the allele, which is typically not methylated), so this is another example of an epigenetic modification of the DNA sequence. Microarray techniques, discussed above, are used increasingly to study methylation patterns at the level of the entire genome. Several important human diseases can be caused by abnormal imprinting patterns.

Prader-Willi and Angelman Syndromes

A well-known disease example of imprinting is associated with a deletion of about 4 million base pairs (Mb) of the long arm of chromosome 15. When this deletion is inherited from the father, the child manifests Prader-Willi syndrome, whose features include short stature, hypotonia, small hands and feet, obesity, mild to moderate mental retardation, and hypogonadism (Fig. 10–3A).[25] The same 4-Mb deletion, when inherited from the mother, causes Angelman syndrome, which is characterized by severe mental retardation, seizures, and an ataxic gait (Fig. 10–3B).[26] These diseases are each seen in approximately 1 of every 15,000 livebirths, and chromosome deletions are responsible for approximately 70 percent of cases of both diseases. The deletions that cause Prader-Willi and Angelman syndromes are indistinguishable at the DNA sequence level and affect the same group of genes.

For several decades, it was unclear how the same deletion could produce such disparate results in different patients. Further analysis showed that the 4-Mb deletion (the *critical region*) contains several genes that normally are transcribed only on the copy of chromosome 15 that is inherited from the father.[27] These genes are transcriptionally inactive (imprinted) on the copy of chromosome 15 inherited from the mother. Similarly, other genes in the critical region are transcriptionally active only on the chromosome copy inherited from the mother and are inactive on the chromosome inherited from the father. Thus, several genes in this region are normally active on only one chromosome copy (Fig. 10–4). If the single active copy of one of these genes is lost because of a chromosome deletion, then no gene product is produced at all, resulting in disease.

Molecular analysis has revealed much about genes in this critical region of chromosome 15.[28,29] The gene responsible for Angelman syndrome encodes a ligase involved in ubiquitin-mediated protein

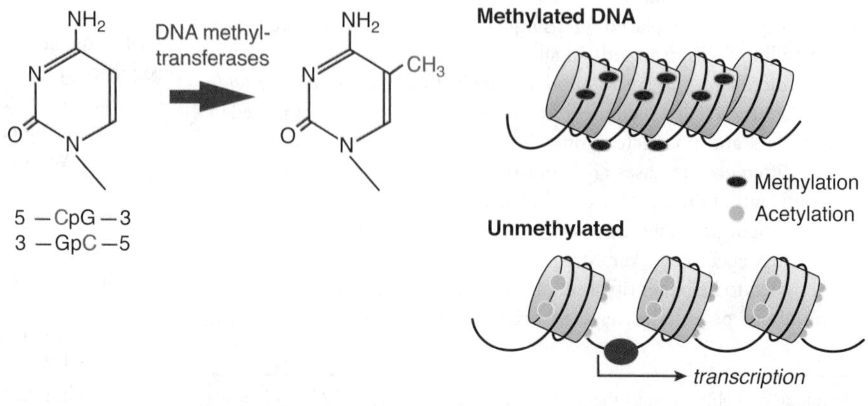

FIGURE 10–2. DNA methylation. Methyl groups attach to the cytosine base (C) when it is followed by a guanine base (G), helping to inactivate an associated gene. *(From Taylor SM: p53 and deregulation of DNA methylation in cancer.* Cell Sci Rev *2:82, 2006. With permission.)*

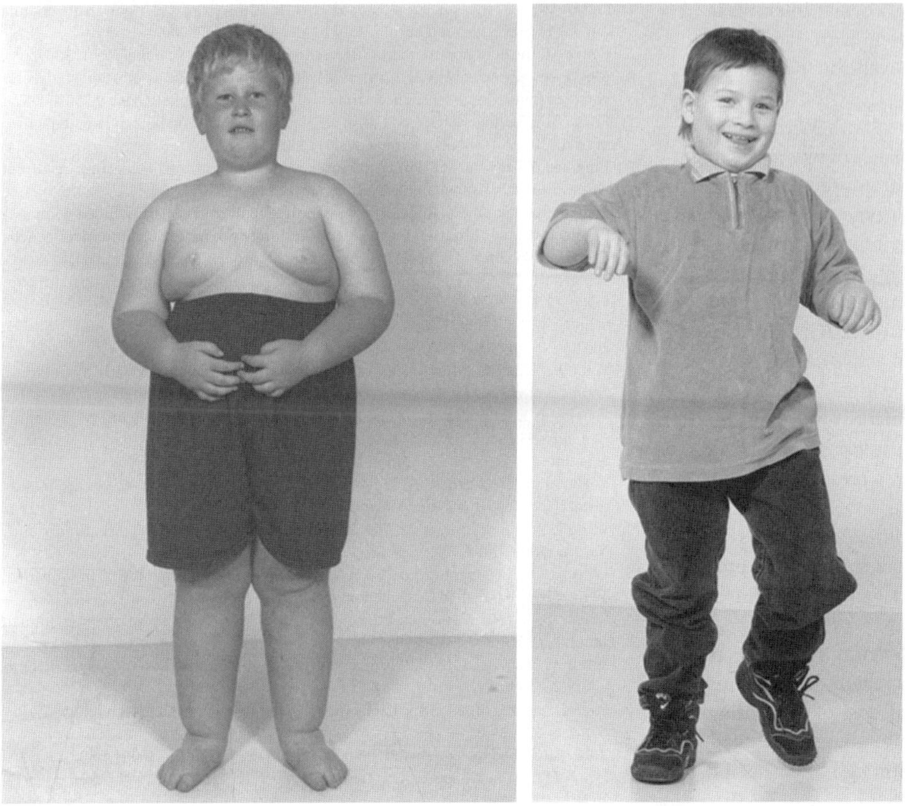

A B

FIGURE 10–3. **A.** A child with Prader-Willi syndrome (truncal obesity, small hands and feet, inverted V-shaped upper lip). **B.** A child with Angelman syndrome (characteristic posture, ataxic gait, bouts of uncontrolled laughter). *(From Jorde LB, Carey JC, Bamshad MJ:* Medical Genetics*, 4th ed. Mosby/Elsevier, Philadelphia, 2010. With permission.)*

degradation during brain development (consistent with the mental retardation and ataxia observed in this disorder). In brain tissue, this gene is active only on the chromosome copy inherited from the mother. Consequently, a maternally transmitted deletion removes the single active copy of this gene. Several genes in the critical region are associated with Prader-Willi syndrome, and they are transcribed only on the chromosome transmitted by the father. A paternally transmitted deletion removes the only active copies of these genes, producing the features of Prader-Willi syndrome.

Several mechanisms in addition to chromosome deletions can cause Prader-Willi and Angelman syndromes.[29] One mechanism is *uniparental disomy*, a condition in which the individual inherits two copies of a chromosome from one parent and no copy from the other. When two copies of the maternal chromosome 15 are inherited, Prader-Willi syndrome results because no active paternally transmitted genes are present. Conversely, disomy of the paternal chromosome 15 produces Angelman syndrome. When it occurs during mitotic division, *acquired uniparental disomy* can lead to cancer because of a reduction in tumor-suppressor gene expression or an increase in oncogene expression.[30,31] Uniparental disomy can also cause homozygous *JAK2* V617F in polycythemia vera (see Chap. 86[31]). DNA sequence mutations in the identified Angelman syndrome gene can also produce disease. Finally, approximately 1 percent of cases of Prader-Willi syndrome result from a small deletion of the region that contains an imprinting control center on chromosome 15, which is the DNA sequence that helps to set and reset the imprint itself.

Beckwith-Wiedemann Syndrome

Another well-known example of imprinting is Beckwith-Wiedemann syndrome, an overgrowth condition that is accompanied by an increased predisposition to cancer. Beckwith-Wiedemann syndrome is usually identifiable at birth because of large size for gestational age, neonatal hypoglycemia, a large tongue, creases on the ear lobe, and omphalocele.[32] Children with Beckwith-Wiedemann syndrome have an increased risk of developing Wilms tumor or hepatoblastoma. Both of these tumors can be treated

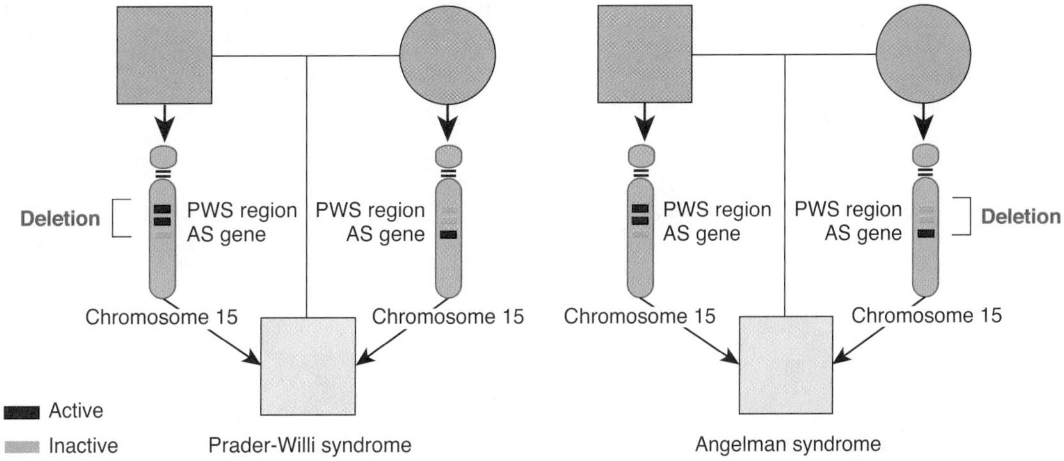

FIGURE 10–4. These pedigrees illustrate the inheritance patterns of Prader-Willi syndrome, which can be caused by a 4-Mb deletion of chromosome 15q when inherited from the father. In contrast, Angelman syndrome can be caused by the same deletion, but only when it is inherited from the mother. The reason for this difference is that different genes in this region are normally imprinted (inactivated) in the copies of 15q transmitted by the mother and the father. *(From Jorde LB, Carey JC, Bamshad MJ:* Medical Genetics*, 4th ed. Mosby/Elsevier, Philadelphia, 2010. With permission.)*

effectively if they are detected early, so screening at regular intervals is an important part of management. Some children with Beckwith-Wiedemann syndrome also develop asymmetrical overgrowth of a limb or one side of the face or trunk (hemihyperplasia).

As with Angelman syndrome, a minority of Beckwith-Wiedemann syndrome cases (~20–30%) are caused by the inheritance of two copies of a chromosome from the father and no copy of the chromosome from the mother (uniparental disomy, in this case affecting chromosome 11). Several genes on the short arm of chromosome 11 are imprinted on either the paternally or maternally transmitted chromosome. These genes are found in two separate, differentially methylated regions (DMRs). In DMR1, the gene that encodes insulin-like growth factor 2 (IGF2) is inactive on the maternally transmitted chromosome but active on the paternally transmitted chromosome. Thus, a normal individual has only one active copy of *IGF2*. When two copies of the paternal chromosome are inherited (i.e., paternal uniparental disomy) or there is loss of imprinting on the maternal copy of *IGF2*, an active *IGF2* gene is present in double dose. This produces increased levels of IGF2 during fetal development, contributing to the overgrowth features of Beckwith-Wiedemann syndrome. (Unlike Prader-Willi and Angelman syndromes, which are produced by a missing gene product, Beckwith-Wiedemann syndrome is caused, in part, by overexpression of a gene product.)

In 50 to 60 percent of cases, Beckwith-Wiedemann syndrome is caused by a loss of the paternal imprint of DMR2, a region that contains several genes including *KCNQ1* and *CDKN1C*. This loss of imprinting is thought to result in silencing of growth inhibitors and thus overgrowth and increased cancer predisposition, although the specific mechanisms remain unknown.

Russell-Silver Syndrome

Russell-Silver syndrome is characterized by growth retardation, proportionate short stature, leg length discrepancy, and a small, triangular-shaped face. About one-third of Russell-Silver syndrome cases are caused by imprinting abnormalities of chromosome 11p15.5 that lead to down-regulation of IGF2 and therefore diminished growth. Another 10 percent of cases of Russell-Silver syndrome are caused by maternal uniparental disomy. Thus, while upregulation, or extra copies, of active IGF2 causes overgrowth in Beckwith-Wiedemann syndrome, downregulation of IGF2 causes the diminished growth seen in Russell-Silver syndrome.

REFERENCES

1. Jorde LB, Little PFR, Dunn MJ, Subramaniam S, eds: *Encyclopedia of Genetics, Genomics, Proteomics and Bioinformatics.* John Wiley, Chichester, UK, 2005.
2. Trevino V, Falciani F, Barrera-Saldana HA: DNA microarrays: A powerful genomic tool for biomedical and clinical research. *Mol Med* 13:527, 2007.
3. Dufva M: Introduction to microarray technology. *Methods Mol Biol* 529:1, 2009.
4. McCarthy MI, Abecasis GR, Cardon LR, et al: Genome-wide association studies for complex traits: Consensus, uncertainty and challenges. *Nat Rev Genet* 9:356, 2008.
5. Frazer KA, Ballinger DG, Cox DR, et al: A second generation human haplotype map of over 3.1 million SNPs. *Nature* 449:851, 2007.
6. Emanuel BS, Saitta SC: From microscopes to microarrays: Dissecting recurrent chromosomal rearrangements. *Nat Rev Genet* 8:869, 2007.
7. Higgins RA, Gunn SR, Robetorye RS: Clinical application of array-based comparative genomic hybridization for the identification of prognostically important genetic alterations in chronic lymphocytic leukemia. *Mol Diagn Ther* 12:271, 2008.
8. Wiltgen M, Tilz GP: DNA microarray analysis: Principles and clinical impact. *Hematology* 12:271, 2007.
9. Staudt LM: Molecular Diagnosis of the Hematologic Cancers. *N Engl J Med* 348:1777, 2003.
10. Yin JQ, Zhao RC, Morris KV: Profiling microRNA expression with microarrays. *Trends Biotechnol* 26:70, 2008.
11. Pettersson E, Lundeberg J, Ahmadian A: Generations of sequencing technologies. *Genomics* 93:105, 2009.
12. Shendure J, Ji H: Next-generation DNA sequencing. *Nat Biotechnol* 26:1135, 2008.
13. Voelkerding KV, Dames SA, Durtschi JD: Next-generation sequencing: From basic research to diagnostics. *Clin Chem* 55:641, 2009.
14. Wang J, Wang W, Li R, et al: The diploid genome sequence of an Asian individual. *Nature* 456:60, 2008.
15. Wheeler DA, Srinivasan M, Egholm M, et al: The complete genome of an individual by massively parallel DNA sequencing. *Nature* 452:872, 2008.
16. Kuehn BM: 1000 Genomes Project promises closer look at variation in human genome. *JAMA* 300:2715, 2008.
17. Simon R: Microarray-based expression profiling and informatics. *Curr Opin Biotechnol* 19:26, 2008.
18. Pop M, Salzberg SL: Bioinformatics challenges of new sequencing technology. *Trends Genet* 24:142, 2008.
19. Robertson KD: DNA methylation and human disease. *Nat Rev Genet* 6:597, 2005.
20. Lynch HT, de la Chapelle A: Hereditary colorectal cancer. *N Engl J Med* 348:919, 2003.
21. Esteller M: Epigenetics in cancer. *N Engl J Med* 358:1148, 2008.
22. Fraga MF, Ballestar E, Paz MF, et al: Epigenetic differences arise during the lifetime of monozygotic twins. *Proc Natl Acad Sci U S A* 102:10604, 2005.
23. Jaenisch R, Bird A: Epigenetic regulation of gene expression: How the genome integrates intrinsic and environmental signals. *Nat Genet* 33:245, 2003.
24. da Rocha ST, Ferguson-Smith AC: Genomic imprinting. *Curr Biol* 14:R646, 2004.
25. Wattendorf DJ, Muenke M: Prader-Willi syndrome. *Am Fam Physician* 72:827, 2005.
26. Williams CA, Beaudet AL, Clayton-Smith J, et al: Angelman syndrome 2005: Updated consensus for diagnostic criteria. *Am J Med Genet A* 140:413, 2006.
27. Horsthemke B, Buiting K: Imprinting defects on human chromosome 15. *Cytogenet Genome Res* 113:292, 2006.
28. Jiang Y-H, Bressler J, Beaudet AL: Epigenetics and human disease. *Annu Rev Genomics Hum Genet* 5:479, 2004.
29. Horsthemke B, Wagstaff J: Mechanisms of imprinting of the Prader-Willi/Angelman region. *Am J Med Genet A* 146A:2041, 2008.
30. Tuna M, Knuutila S, Mills GB: Uniparental disomy in cancer. *Trends Mol Med* 15:120, 2009.
31. Kralovics R, Guan Y, Prchal JT: Acquired uniparental disomy of chromosome 9p is a frequent stem cell defect in polycythemia vera. *Exp Hematol* 30:229, 2002.
32. Weksberg R, Shuman C, Smith AC: Beckwith-Wiedemann syndrome. *Am J Med Genet C Semin Med Genet* 137:12, 2005.

CHAPTER 11
CYTOGENETICS AND MOLECULAR ABNORMALITIES

Lucy A. Godley and Michelle M. Le Beau

SUMMARY

Cytogenetic analysis provides pathologists and clinicians with a powerful tool for the diagnosis and classification of hematologic malignant diseases. The detection of an acquired, somatic mutation establishes the diagnosis of a neoplastic disorder and rules out hyperplasia, dysplasia, or morphologic changes caused by toxic injury or vitamin deficiency. Specific cytogenetic abnormalities have been identified that are very closely, and sometimes uniquely, associated with morphologically distinct subsets of leukemia or lymphoma, enabling clinicians to predict their clinical course and likelihood of responding to particular treatments. The detection of one of these recurring abnormalities is helpful in establishing the diagnosis and adds information of prognostic importance. In many cases, the prognostic information derived from cytogenetic analysis is independent of that provided by other clinical features. Patients with favorable prognostic features benefit from standard therapies with well-known spectra of toxicities, whereas those with less favorable clinical and cytogenetic characteristics may be better treated with more intensive or investigational therapies. Pretreatment cytogenetic analysis also can be useful in choosing between postremission therapies that differ widely in cost, acute and chronic morbidity, and effectiveness. The appearance of new abnormalities in the karyotype of a patient under observation often signals clonal evolution and more aggressive behavior. The disappearance of a chromosomal abnormality present at diagnosis is an important indicator of complete remission following treatment, and its reappearance may herald disease recurrence.

GENETIC CONSEQUENCES OF GENOMIC REARRANGEMENTS

Over the past two decades, the genes that are located at the breakpoints of a number of the recurring chromosomal translocations have been identified. Alterations in the expression of the genes or in the properties of the encoded proteins resulting from the rearrangement play an integral role in the process of malignant transformation.[1,2] The altered genes fall into several functional classes, including tyrosine or serine protein kinases, cell surface receptors, growth factors, and the largest class, transcription factors. These latter proteins are involved in the induction or repression of gene transcription, often functioning in a tissue-specific fashion to regulate growth and differentiation.

There are two general mechanisms by which chromosomal translocations result in altered gene function. The first is deregulation of gene expression. This mechanism is characteristic of the translocations in lymphoid neoplasms that involve the immunoglobulin genes in B-lineage tumors and the T-cell receptor genes in T-lineage tumors. These rearrangements result in the inappropriate or constitutive expression of an oncogene. The second mechanism is the expression of a novel fusion protein, resulting from the juxtaposition of coding sequences from two genes that are normally located on different chromosomes. Such chimeric proteins are "tumor-specific" in that the fusion gene typically does not exist in nonmalignant cells. Thus, the detection of such a fusion gene or protein product can be important in diagnosis and in the detection of residual disease or early relapse. Moreover, they may also be appropriate targets for tumor-specific therapies. An example is the chimeric BCR-ABL1 protein resulting from the t(9;22) in chronic myeloid leukemia (CML) (see "Methods of Cell Preparation" below). All of the translocations cloned to date in the myeloid leukemias result in a fusion protein.

Chromosomal translocations result in the activation of genes in a dominant fashion. A number of human tumors are believed to result from homozygous, recessive mutations. These mutations lead to the absence of a functional protein product, suggesting that these genes function as "suppressor" genes whose normal role(s) is to limit cellular proliferation. The hallmark of tumor-suppressor genes is the loss of genetic material in malignant cells, resulting from chromosomal loss or deletion, as well as from other genetic mechanisms.[1]

Extensive experimental evidence indicates that, with the possible exception of CML, more than one mutation is required for the pathogenesis of hematologic malignancies. That is, expression of translocation-specific fusion genes or deregulated expression of oncogenes is required, but insufficient to induce leukemia. Thus, an important aspect of leukemia biology is the elucidation of the spectrum of chromosomal and molecular mutations that cooperate in the pathways leading to leukemogenesis. Where known, we describe the cooperating mutations associated with specific cytogenetic subsets of leukemia or lymphoma.

Acronyms and abbreviations that appear in this chapter include: ALCL, anaplastic large cell lymphoma; ALL, acute lymphocytic or lymphoblastic leukemia; AML, acute myelogenous leukemia; BL, Burkitt lymphoma; CDS, commonly deleted segment; CLL, chronic lymphocytic leukemia; CML, chronic myelogenous leukemia; DAPI, 4,6-diamidino-2-phenylindole-dihydrochloride; del, deletion; DLBCL, diffuse large B-cell lymphoma; EBV, Epstein-Barr virus; EFS, event-free survival; FAB, French-American-British; FISH, fluorescence *in situ* hybridization; IGH, immunoglobulin heavy chain; inv, inversion; ITD, internal tandem duplication; LOH, loss of heterozygosity; MDS, myelodysplastic syndrome; NHL, non-Hodgkin lymphoma; qRT-PCR, quantitative reverse transcriptase polymerase chain reaction; RA, refractory anemia; RAEB, refractory anemia with excess blasts; RARS, refractory anemia with ringed sideroblasts; RCMD, refractory cytopenia with multilineage dysplasia; SKY, spectral karyotyping; t, translocation; t-, therapy-related; WHO, World Health Organization.

METHODS OF CELL PREPARATION

Cytogenetic analysis of malignant diseases should be based upon the study of the tumor cells themselves. In leukemia, the specimen is usually obtained by marrow aspiration and is either processed immediately (direct preparation) or cultured for 24 to 72 hours. When a marrow aspirate cannot be obtained, a marrow biopsy (bone core specimen) or a blood sample for patients who have circulating immature myeloid or lymphoid cells can often be processed successfully. An involved lymph node or tumor mass specimen may be processed for the analysis of lymphoma cells.

For specimen collection, 1 to 5 mL of marrow are aspirated aseptically into a syringe coated with preservative-free sodium heparin and transferred to a sterile 15-mL centrifuge tube containing 5 mL of culture medium (RPMI 1640, 100 units sodium heparin). The use of Vacutainer tubes should be avoided, as the heparin in Vacutainers contains preservatives that suppress cell growth. Approximately 75 percent of marrow biopsies will yield adequate numbers of metaphase cells for complete analysis. For blood specimens, 10 mL are drawn aseptically by venipuncture into a syringe coated with preservative-free heparin. To avoid loss of cell viability, it is critical that the specimen be transported at room temperature to the cytogenetics laboratory without delay. Overnight shipment of specimens frequently results in loss of cell viability, and most laboratories experience a high proportion (25–50%) of inadequate analyses using such specimens. For optimally handled specimens, approximately 95 percent of all cases should be adequate for cytogenetic analysis. Those cases that are inadequate generally represent samples from patients with hypocellular marrows.

METHODS THAT COMPLEMENT KARYOTYPE ANALYSIS

FLUORESCENCE IN SITU HYBRIDIZATION

Cytogenetic analysis of human tumors is often technically difficult because of the presence of multiple abnormalities and requires highly skilled personnel. These factors have led investigators to seek alternative methods for identifying chromosomal abnormalities, such as fluorescence *in situ* hybridization (FISH).[3] The FISH technique is based on the same principle as Southern blot analysis, namely, the ability of single-stranded DNA to anneal to complementary DNA.[3] FISH can be performed on marrow or blood films, or fixed and sectioned tissue, as it does not require dividing cells. The target DNA is the nuclear DNA of interphase cells, or the DNA of metaphase chromosomes that are affixed to a glass microscope slide. Commercially available probes are now directly labeled with fluorochrome, which simplifies the technique by eliminating the probe preparation and detection steps. With the development of dual- and triple-pass filters, most laboratories now have the capacity to hybridize and detect two to three probes simultaneously. Table 11–1 summarizes the commercially available FISH probes. Several types of probes can be used to detect chromosomal abnormalities by FISH. Hybridization of centromere-specific probes has been used to detect monosomy, trisomy, and other aneuploidies in both leukemias and solid tumors, as well as the sex chromosome complement in the transplant setting (Fig. 11–1).

Chromosome-specific libraries, which paint the chromosomes, are particularly useful in identifying marker chromosomes (rearranged chromosomes of unidentified origin), or structural rearrangements, such as translocations. Translocations and deletions can also be identified in interphase or metaphase cells by using genomic probes that are derived from the breakpoints of recurring translocations or within the deleted segment (see Fig. 11–1). In some cases, FISH analysis provides more sensitivity, in that cytogenetic abnormalities have been identified by FISH in samples that appeared to be normal by conventional cytogenetic analyses. Advantages of FISH include (1) the rapid nature of the method and the ability to analyze large numbers of cells; (2) its high sensitivity and specificity; and (3) the ability to obtain cytogenetic data from samples with a low mitotic index or terminally differentiated cells. The major disadvantage is the inability to interrogate more than a few abnormalities. FISH is most powerful when the analysis is targeted toward those abnormalities that are known to be associated with a particular tumor or disease. In a clinical setting, cytogenetic analysis could be performed at the time of diagnosis to identify the chromosomal abnormalities in an individual patient's malignant cells. Thereafter, FISH with the appropriate probes could be used to detect residual disease or early relapse, and to assess the efficacy of therapeutic regimens. For example, the use of FISH to detect the t(9;22) in CML patients following therapy with an oral tyrosine kinase inhibitor, or sex chromosome determination after a sex-mismatched transplant, is widespread. Material from patients newly presenting are often analyzed most efficiently by conventional cytogenetic analysis, combined with quantitative reverse transcriptase polymerase chain reaction (qRT-PCR) analysis if a specific chromosome rearrangement is suspected, for example, a *BCR-ABL1* fusion. Molecular qRT-PCR monitoring of the blood and marrow of CML patients is now part of the recommended testing for patient followup.[4]

Spectral Karyotype Analysis

In spectral karyotyping (SKY), also known as multiplex FISH, 24 differentially labeled painting probes representing each chromosome are cohybridized, and Fourier spectroscopy is used to distinguish each spectrally overlapping probe, allowing the identification of numerical and structural abnormalities (see Fig. 11–1).[1] SKY has remained largely a research tool because of the labor-intensive nature and the requirement for specialized equipment.

MICROARRAY ANALYSIS

Emerging technologies that are likely to play a major role in the future diagnosis and management of hematologic disorders include microarray-based gene expression profiling and proteomic analysis.[5] Virtually all of the hematopoietic malignancies have been studied by microarray technology, revealing complex, but unique, expression profiles for each disease subtype. Microarray technology has enabled high-resolution genomewide genotyping using single-nucleotide polymorphisms (SNPs). This technology facilitates genomewide association studies for the identification of disease susceptibility loci, as well as the identification of acquired abnormalities, such as genetic imbalances (e.g., cryptic deletions and duplications), and loss of heterozygosity (LOH) that occurs without concurrent changes in the gene copy number, which can be attributed to somatic mitotic recombination (referred to as copy-neutral LOH). Several studies have validated the diagnostic utility of this technology, suggesting that future diagnostic tests and management decisions will be based on the initial genomic and/or proteomic profiling of individual patients.[6]

CHROMOSOME NOMENCLATURE

Chromosomal abnormalities are described according to the International System for Human Cytogenetic Nomenclature (Table 11–2).[7] To describe the chromosomal complement, the total chromosome number is listed first, followed by the sex chromosomes, and numerical and structural abnormalities in ascending order. The observation of at least two cells with the same structural rearrangement, for example, translocations, deletions, or inversions, or gain of the same chromosome, or three cells each showing loss of the same chromosome, is considered evidence for the presence of an abnormal clone. However, one cell with a normal karyotype is considered evidence for the presence of a normal cell line. Patients whose cells show no alteration or nonclonal (single cell) abnormalities are considered to be normal. An exception to this is a single cell characterized by a recurring structural abnormality. In such instances, it is likely that this represents the karyotype of the malignant cells in that particular patient.

SPECIFIC CLONAL DISORDERS

CHRONIC MYELOID LEUKEMIA (CML)

The first consistent chromosomal abnormality in any malignant disease was identified in CML (see Chap. 90). The Philadelphia (Ph) chromosome results from a translocation involving chromosomes 9 and 22

TABLE 11–1. Selected FISH Probes to Detect Recurring Chromosomal Abnormalities

Disease*	Abnormality	Probe†	Format‡
AML-M2	t(8;21)	RUNX1/ETO	Two-color dual fusion
AML-M4Eo	inv(16)/t(16;16)	CBFB	Two-color break-apart
AML-M3	t(15;17)	PML/RARA	Two-color dual fusion
AML	t(11q23)	MLL	Two-color break-apart
	inv(3)/t(3;3)	EVI1/HTERC	Two-color break-apart
AML/MDS	−5/del(5q)	EGR1/5p	Two-color deletion
	−7/del(7q)	D7S522/CEP7	Two-color deletion
	7q22.1/7q31		Two-color deletion
	del(20q)	D20S108	Single color
	20q12/20q13.12		Two-color deletion
	+8	CEP8	Single color
CML	t(9;22)	BCR/ABL	Two-color dual fusion
	del(9q)	LSI9q34	Single color
	+8	CEP8	Single color
	i(17q)	HER2/CEP17	Two color (17q/centromere)
ALL	t(12;21)	TEL/AML1	Two-color extra signal
			Two-color dual fusion
	t(11q23)	MLL	Two-color break-apart
	t(8;14)	IGH/MYC/CEP8	Tri-color dual fusion
	t(9;22)	BCR/ABL	Two-color dual fusion
	del(9p)/t(9p)	CDKN2A(p16)/D9Z3	Two-color
	t(1;19)	TCF3/PBX1	Two-color dual fusion
		TCF3 (E2A)	Two-color break-apart

Disease*	Abnormality	Probe†	Format‡
CLL, Myeloma	+12	CEP12/D12Z1	Single color
	del(13q)	D13S319/13q34	Single color
		13q14.3/D13S1825	Two-color deletion
	del(11q)	ATM	Single color
		D11Z1/ATM	Two-color deletion
	−17/del(17p)	TP53	Single color
		D17Z1/TP53	Two-color deletion
	del(6q)	MYB/D6Z1	Two-color deletion
	t(14q32)	IGH	Two-color break-apart
Myeloma	t(4;14)	IGH/FGFR3	Two-color dual fusion
	t(14;16)	IGH/MAF	Two-color dual fusion
NHL	t(11;18)	API2(BIRC3)/MALT1	Two-color dual fusion
	t(14;18)	IGH/BCL2	Two-color dual fusion
		BCL2	Two-color break-apart
	t(8;14)	IGH/MYC/CEP8	Tri-color dual fusion
		MYC	Two-color break-apart
	t(3;14)	BCL6	Two-color break-apart
	t(14q32)	IGH	Two-color break-apart
	t(14q11.2)	TCRA/D	Two-color break-apart
MCL, Myeloma	t(11;14)	CCND1/IGH	Two-color dual fusion
ALCL	t(2;5)	ALK	Two-color break-apart
Miscellaneous			
Stem cell transplants		CEPX/CEPY	Single color or two color
		DXZ1/DYZ1	

*ALCL, anaplastic large cell lymphoma; ALL, acute lymphoblastic leukemia; AML, acute myeloid leukemia; CLL, chronic lymphocytic leukemia; CML, chronic myeloid leukemia; MCL, mantle cell lymphoma; MDS, myelodysplastic syndrome; NHL, non-Hodgkin lymphoma.

†FISH probes are marketed by several companies, including Abbott Molecular Diagnostics (www.abbottmolecular.com), Cytocell (www.cytocell.co.uk), and Stretton Scientific (www.strettonscientific.co.uk). Vysis probes are now marketed by Abbott Molecular Diagnostics.

‡In two-color break-apart probes, DNA sequences from the 5′ and 3′ regions of a single gene/region are labeled and detected with red and green fluorochromes. In the germ line configuration, a yellow fusion signal is observed, whereas individual red and green signals are observed when the sequences are separated as a result of a translocation. With two-color fusion probes, DNA sequences flanking the breakpoints of the involved genes are brought together to form either one (single-fusion probes) or two (dual-fusion probes) yellow fusion signal(s). With the two-color extra-signal probes, DNA sequences flanking the breakpoint on the partner chromosomes are brought together to form a fusion yellow signal; however, part of the DNA sequences recognized by one of the probes may remain at the original site, giving rise to an extra signal in a single color.

(t(9;22)(q34;q11.2); Fig. 11–2A), and arises in a pluripotential stem cell that gives rise to both lymphoid and myeloid lineage cells. The standard t(9;22) is identified in approximately 92 percent of CML patients, whereas 6 to 8 percent have variant translocations that involve a third chromosome in addition to chromosomes 9 and 22. The genetic consequence of the t(9;22) or the complex translocations is to move a segment of the Abelson (*ABL1*) oncogene on chromosome 9 next to a segment of the *BCR* gene on 22. Analyses of leukemia cells from rare patients with typical CML who lack the t(9;22) have revealed a rearrangement involving *ABL1* and *BCR* that is detectable only at the molecular level (1–2% of cases).[8]

The t(9;22) and resultant *BCR-ABL1* fusion is the *sine qua non* of CML.[8] The BCR-ABL1 fusion protein is located on the cytoplasmic surface of the cell membrane and acquires a novel function in transmitting growth-regulatory signals to the nucleus via the RAS/MAPK, PI3K/AKT, and JAK/STAT signal transduction pathways. The tyrosine kinase activity of the BCR-ABL1 fusion protein can be specifically inhibited by several commercially available oral tyrosine kinase inhibitors: imatinib mesylate (Gleevec/STI571, Novartis Pharmaceuticals, East Hanover, NJ), dasatinib (Sprycel, BMS-354825, Bristol-Myers Squibb, Princeton, NJ), and nilotinib (Tasigna, AMN107, Novartis Pharmaceuticals, East Hanover, NJ). Additional oral agents are also being tested in clinical trials.[9] Imatinib has shown remarkable activity in all phases of CML and is the preferred therapy for most patients with newly diagnosed CML (see Chap. 90).[10] The *BCR-ABL1* translocation can be detected by cytogenetic and FISH analysis, qRT-PCR, and Southern blot analysis to diagnose the disease and detect residual disease. Studies of patients treated with imatinib show a strong correlation

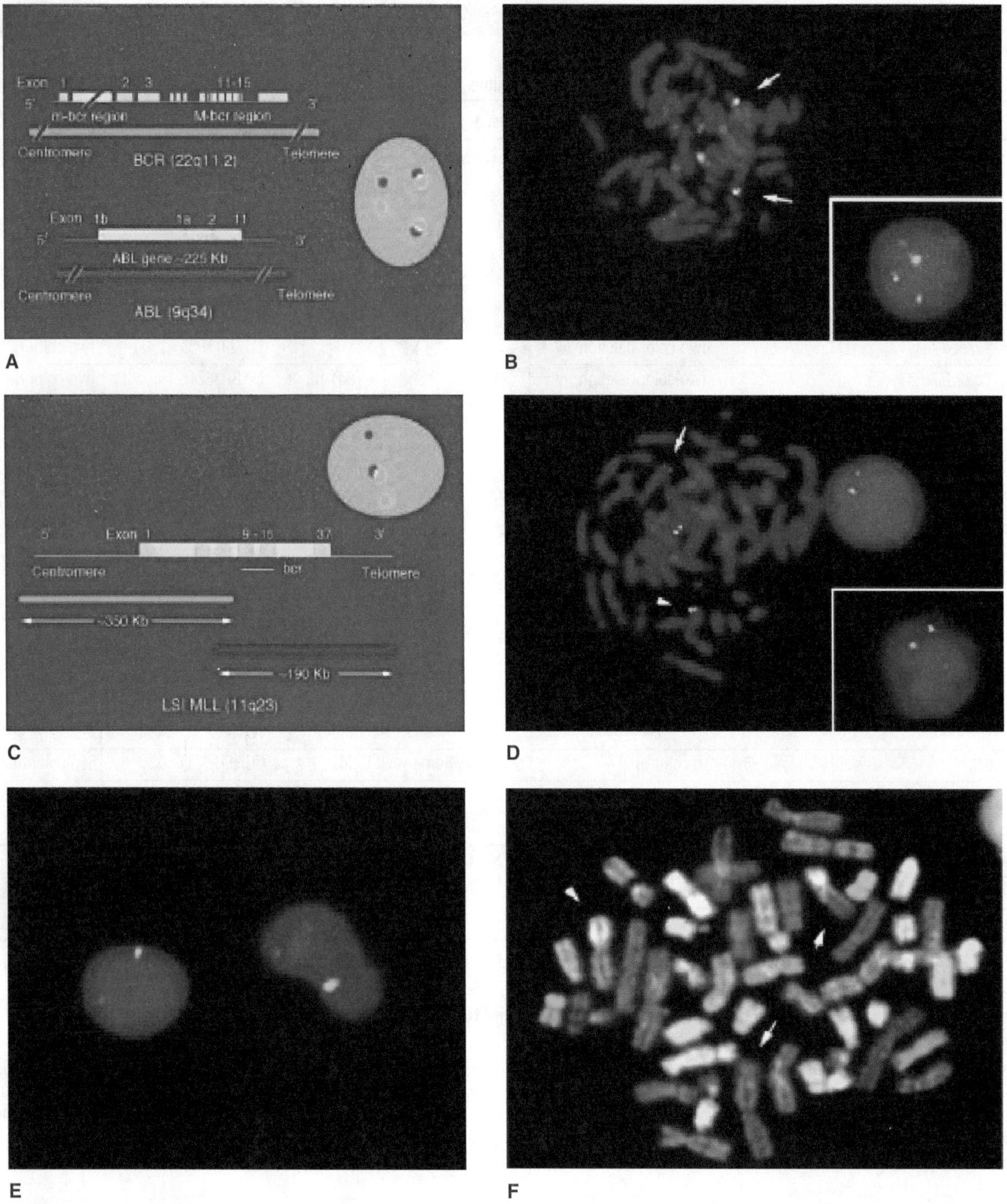

FIGURE 11–1. Fluorescence *in situ* hybridization and spectral karyotyping analysis. Panels *B, D*, and *E* illustrate images of metaphase and interphase cells following FISH; the cells are counterstained with 4,6-diamidino-2-phenylindole-dihydrochloride (DAPI). **A.** Schematic of the *BCR* and *ABL1* loci, location of the *BCR* and *ABL1* dual fusion probe (Vysis, Inc.), and configuration of signals in interphase cells. **B.** Hybridization of the *BCR-ABL1* dual fusion probe to metaphase and interphase cells with the t(9;22). In cells with the t(9;22), only one green and one red signal is observed on the normal 9 and 22 homologues, and two yellow fusion signals (*arrows*) are observed on the der(9) and the der(22) (Ph) chromosomes as a result of the juxtaposition of the *ABL1* and *BCR* sequences. **C.** Schematic of the *MLL* gene, location of the *MLL* break-apart probe (Vysis, Inc.), and configuration of signals in interphase cells. **D.** Hybridization of the *MLL* break-apart probe to metaphase and interphase cells with a t(11q23). In cells with a *MLL* translocation, a yellow fusion signal is observed for the germ line configuration on the normal chromosome 11 homologue, a green signal is observed on the der(11) chromosome, and a red signal is observed on the partner chromosome. **E.** Hybridization of a directly labeled centromere-specific probe for the X (CEPX™ Spectrum Green, Vysis, Inc.) and Y (CEPX™ Spectrum Orange, Vysis, Inc.) chromosomes (*arrows*) to metaphase and interphase cells from a marrow aspirate of a female patient with acute myelogenous leukemia (AML) who received a marrow transplant from a male donor. Centromere-specific probes hybridize to the repetitive DNA sequences that are present at the centromeres of human chromosomes. **F.** Spectral karyotyping analysis of a metaphase cell from an AML-M7. Twenty-four differentially labeled probes representing each human chromosome are cohybridized, and imaging analysis software assigns a unique color to each. A complex karyotype was identified by conventional cytogenetic analysis, including a derivative chromosome 1 with additional material of unknown origin on 1p, a deletion of 8p, a derivative chromosome 11 resulting from an unbalanced translocation involving 1 and 11, and a derivative chromosome 12, consisting of 11q and 12q. The results of spectral karyotyping confirmed the identity of the rearranged chromosome 12 (*arrowhead*), but clarified the other abnormalities. The additional material on 1p was derived from chromosome 8 (long arrow, blue signal), and the der(11) actually consisted of material from chromosomes 1, 11, and 12 (*short arrow*, 11p white signal; chromosome 12 brown signal; 1p blue-pink signal).

TABLE 11–2. Glossary of Cytogenetic Terminology

Aneuploidy—An abnormal chromosome number caused by either gain or loss of chromosomes.

Banded chromosomes—Chromosomes with alternating dark and light segments because of special stains or pretreatment with enzymes before staining. Each chromosome pair has a unique pattern of bands.

Breakpoint—A specific site on a chromosome containing a DNA break that is involved in a structural rearrangement, such as a translocation or deletion.

Centromere—The chromosome constriction that is the site of the spindle fiber attachment. The position of the centromere determines whether chromosomes are *metacentric* (X-shaped, e.g., chromosomes 1–3, 6–12, X, 16, 19, 20) or *acrocentric* (inverted V-shaped, e.g., chromosomes 13–15, 21, 22, Y). During mitosis, the two exact copies of the DNA in each chromosome are separated by shortening of the spindle fibers attached to opposite sides of the dividing cell.

Clone—In the cytogenetic sense, this is defined as two cells with the same additional or structurally rearranged chromosome, or three cells with loss of the same chromosome.

Deletion—A segment of a chromosome is missing as the result of two breaks and loss of the intervening piece (interstitial deletion). Molecular studies of many recurring deletions have shown that, in each case, the deletions were interstitial, rather than terminal (single break with loss of the terminal segment).

Diploid—Normal chromosome number and composition of chromosomes.

Haploid—Only one-half the normal complement, i.e., 23 chromosomes.

Hyperdiploid—Additional chromosomes; therefore, the modal number is 47 or greater.

Hypodiploid—Loss of chromosomes with a modal number of 45 or less.

Inversion—Two breaks occur in the same chromosome with rotation of the intervening segment. If both breaks were on the same side of the centromere, it is called a paracentric inversion. If they were on opposite sides, it is called a pericentric inversion.

Isochromosome—A chromosome that consists of identical copies of one chromosome arm with loss of the other arm. Thus, an isochromosome for the long arm of no. 17 [i(17)(q10)] contains two copies of the long arm (separated by the centromere) with loss of the short arm of the chromosome.

Karyotype—Arrangement of chromosomes from a particular cell according to an internationally established system such that the largest chromosomes are first and the smallest ones are last. A normal female karyotype is described as 46,XX and a normal male karyotype is 46,XY. An *idiogram* is an idealized representation (diagram) of the chromosomes.

Pseudodiploid—A diploid number of chromosomes accompanied by structural abnormalities.

Recurring abnormality—A numerical or structural abnormality noted in multiple patients who have a similar neoplasm. Such abnormalities are characteristic or diagnostic of distinct subtypes of leukemia and lymphoma that have unique morphologic and/or immunophenotypic features. Recurring abnormalities represent genetic mutations that are involved in the pathogenesis of the corresponding diseases; many recurring abnormalities have prognostic significance.

Translocation—A break in at least two chromosomes with exchange of material. In a reciprocal translocation, there is no obvious loss of chromosomal material. Translocations are indicated by t; the chromosomes involved are noted in the first set of brackets and the breakpoints in the second set of brackets. The Ph translocation is t(9;22)(q34;q11.2).

Nomenclature symbols:

- p—Short arm
- q—Long arm
- +—If before the chromosome, indicates a gain of a whole chromosome (e.g., +8).
- −—If before the chromosome, indicates a loss of a whole chromosome (e.g., −7) and if after the chromosome indicates loss of part of the chromosome (e.g., 5q−, loss of part of the long arm of chromosome 5)
- ?—Indicates uncertainty about the identity of the chromosome or band listed just after the ?.
- t—translocation
- del—deletion
- inv—inversion
- i—isochromosome
- mar—marker chromosome
- r—ring chromosome

SOURCE: Modified with permission from Rowley JD: Chromosome abnormalities in human cancer, in *Practice and Principles of Oncology*, 3rd ed, edited by VT De Vita, S Hellman, S Rosenberg, pp. 81–97. JP Lippincott, Philadelphia, 1989.

between *BCR-ABL1* levels as measured in the blood by qRT-PCR and the percentage of Ph^+ cells in the marrow.[10]

Several types of genetic changes are associated with imatinib resistance, including point mutations leading to amino acid substitutions in the BCR-ABL1 kinase domain that interfere with imatinib binding, as well as the acquisition of additional copies of the Ph chromosome or *BCR-ABL1* gene amplification, both of which can be detected by FISH.[10] Although some patients who achieve a complete cytogenetic response on imatinib develop clonal karyotypic abnormalities, most commonly +8, −7, or del(20q), the majority of them do not go on to develop the clinical features of a myelodysplastic syndrome.[11] The significance of these early findings will be elucidated by the analysis of a large number of patients who have had complete cytogenetic responses to imatinib and are being followed prospectively.

As they enter the more aggressive stages of accelerated and blast phase disease, most CML patients (80%) show karyotypic evolution with the appearance of new chromosomal abnormalities in very distinct patterns in addition to the Ph chromosome. A change in the karyotype is considered to be a grave prognostic sign.[12] With the exception of an isochromosome of the long arm of chromosome 17 [i(17)(q10)], which is usually associated with myeloid blast transformation, there is no association of a particular karyotype with lymphoid or myeloid blast transformation. The most common changes, a gain of chromosomes 8 or 19, or a second Ph (by gain of the first), or an i(17q), frequently occur in combination to produce modal chromosome numbers of 47 to 50. Other genetic changes identified in CML in blast crisis include mutations in the *TP53, RB1, MYC, CDKN2A* (*p16*), *KRAS/NRAS*, or *RUNX1/AML1* genes.

Rarely, marrow biopsies from patients will appear similar to those patients with CML, but will lack a Ph chromosome or the *BCR-ABL1* fusion. Most often these patients have a myelodysplastic syndrome (MDS) or myeloproliferative neoplasm (MPN), most commonly chronic myelomonocytic leukemia, refractory anemia with excess blasts, or the

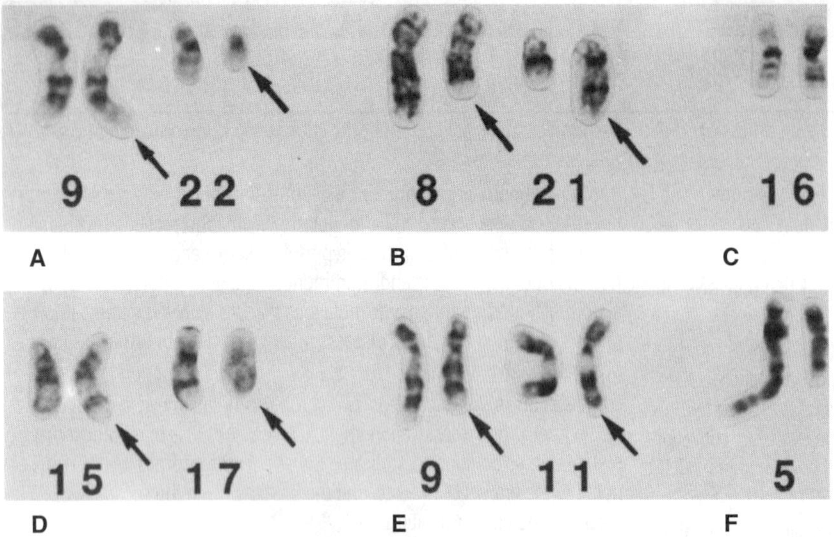

FIGURE 11–2. Partial karyotypes from trypsin-Giemsa-banded metaphase cells depicting recurring chromosomal rearrangements observed in myeloid leukemias. The rearranged chromosomes are identified with *arrows*. **A.** t(9;22)(q34;q11.2), CML. **B.** t(8;21)(q22;q22), AML-M2. **C.** inv(16)(p13.1q22), AMMoL-M4Eo. **D.** t(15;17)(q22;q12–21.1), APL. **E.** t(9;11)(p22;q23), AMoL-M5. **F.** del(5)(q13q33), t-AML.

poorly understood disorder of "atypical CML." Cytogenetic analysis of marrow biopsies from these patients commonly have a normal karyotype, +8, +13, del(20q), or i(17q). These patients have a substantially shorter survival than do those whose cells have the t(9;22). Because each of the oral tyrosine kinase inhibitors blocks kinase activities in addition to BCR-ABL1, they have proven to be effective in other disorders, including chronic myeloproliferative diseases with platelet-derived growth factor receptor (PDGFR)-β rearrangements, a myeloproliferative variant of hypereosinophilic syndrome that expresses the FIP1L1-PDGFRA fusion protein, and in rare patients with mast cell malignancies that have a *KIT* mutation (see Chap. 90).[13]

■ OTHER MYELOPROLIFERATIVE NEOPLASMS

A cytogenetically abnormal clone is present in 15 percent of untreated polycythemia vera patients compared with 40 percent of treated patients.[14] When the disease transforms to acute myeloid leukemia (AML), almost 100 percent have an abnormal clone. The presence of a chromosome abnormality at diagnosis does not necessarily predict a short survival or the development of leukemia. However, a change in the karyotype may be an ominous sign. Marrow cells frequently contain additional chromosomes (+8 or +9). Trisomy 8 and 9 may occur together which is otherwise rare.[14] Structural rearrangements most often involve a del(13q) or del(20q), noted in 30 percent of patients. Loss of chromosome 7 (20% of patients) and del(5q) (40% of patients) are often observed in the leukemic phase, and may be related to the prior treatment received by these patients (see Chap. 86).

Cytogenetic analysis of cells from patients with primary myelofibrosis has revealed clonal abnormalities in 60 percent of patients (see Chap. 91).[14] These abnormalities are similar to those noted in other myeloid disorders. The most common anomalies are +8, −7, or a del(7q), del(11q), del(13q), and del(20q).[14] A change in the karyotype may signal evolution to AML. Fewer than 10 percent of patients with essential thrombocythemia have an abnormal clone (see Chap. 87). Recurring abnormalities include +8 and del(13q). Although del(5q) and inv(3)/t(3;3) are associated with thrombocytosis, they are characteristic of MDS or AML, rather than essential thrombocythemia.

Mutant JAK2 (JAK2^{V617F}) is a constitutively active tyrosine kinase that activates the STAT, PI3K, and MAPK signalling pathways downstream of the erythropoietin receptor, thrombopoietin receptor, or the granulocyte colony-stimulating factor (G-CSF) receptor, to promote proliferation and transformation of hematopoietic progenitor cells. *JAK2* mutations occur in approximately 95% of patients with polycythemia vera, essential thrombocythemia (50–70% of cases), and myelofibrosis (40–50% of cases) (see Chaps. 86, 87, and 91).[15] In refractory anemia with ringed sideroblasts with thrombocytosis (RARS-T), a myelodysplastic/myeloproliferative syndrome, classified by the World Health Organization (WHO), 60 percent of patients have the *JAK2*^{V617F} mutation.[16] RARS-T patients with *JAK2*^{V617F} mutations present with higher white blood cell and platelet counts (see Chap. 88).

■ PRIMARY MYELODYSPLASTIC SYNDROMES

The MDSs are a heterogeneous group of diseases, including refractory cytopenia with unilineage dysplasia, refractory anemia with ring sideroblasts (RARS), refractory cytopenia with multilineage dysplasia (RCMD), refractory anemia with excess blasts (RAEB–1,2), myelodysplastic syndrome with isolated del(5q), myelodysplastic syndrome unclassifiable, and childhood myelodysplastic syndrome, including refractory cytopenia of childhood (see Chap. 88).[17] Clonal chromosome abnormalities can be detected in marrow cells of 40 to 100 percent of patients with primary MDS at diagnosis (refractory anemia [RA], 25%; RARS, 10%; RCMD, 50%; RAEB–1,2, 50–70%; MDS with isolated del(5q), 100%).[18,19] The proportion varies with the risk that a subtype will transform to AML, which is highest for RCMD and RAEB. The common chromosome changes, +8, −5/del(5q), −7/del(7q), and del(20q), are similar to those seen in AML *de novo*. The recurring translocations that are closely associated with the distinct morphologic subsets of AML *de novo* are almost never seen in MDS. With the exception of MDS with isolated del(5q), the chromosome changes show no close association with the specific subtypes of MDS. MDS with isolated del(5q) occurs in a subset of older patients, frequently women, with RA, generally low blast counts, and normal or elevated platelet counts.[20] These patients have an interstitial deletion of 5q, typically as the sole abnormality. These patients can have a relatively benign course that extends over several years (see Chap. 88).[20]

Cytogenetic abnormalities in MDS are predictive of survival and progression to AML.[19] Patients with a "good outcome" have normal karyotypes, −Y alone, del(5q) alone, or del(20q) alone, those with an "intermediate outcome" have other abnormalities, and those with a "poor outcome" have complex karyotypes (≥3 abnormalities, typically with abnormalities of chromosome 5 and/or 7), or chromosome 7 abnormalities.[19] With larger datasets, more rare recurring cytogenetic abnormalities may be examined allowing a refining of the cytogenetic risk groups, and providing the clinician with more information to predict the expected outcome for their patient.[21]

■ ACUTE MYELOID LEUKEMIA *DE NOVO*

Clonal chromosomal abnormalities are detected in 80 to 90 percent of patients with acute myelogenous leukemia (AML). The most frequent abnormalities are +8 and −7, which are seen in most subtypes of AML.[1] Specific rearrangements are closely associated with particular subtypes

TABLE 11–3. Recurring Chromosome Abnormalities in Malignant Myeloid Diseases.

Disease*	Chromosome Abnormality	Frequency†	Involved Genes‡		Consequence§
CML	t(9;22)(q34;q11.2)	~98% (100%)¶	*ABL1*	*BCR*	Fusion protein–altered cytokine signaling pathways
CML blast phase	t(9;22) with +8, +Ph, +19, or i(17q)	~70%			
AML-M2	t(8;21)(q22;q22)	18% (30%)	*RUNX1T1/ETO*	*RUNX1/AML1*	Fusion protein–altered transcriptional regulation
AML-M3, M3V	t(15;17)(q22;q12–21.1)	14% (98%)	*PML*	*RARA*	Fusion protein–altered transcriptional regulation
AMMoL-M4Eo	inv(16)(p13.1q22) or t(16;16)(p13.1;q22)	8% (~100%)	*MYH11*	*CBFB*	Fusion protein–altered transcriptional regulation
AMMoL-M4, AMoL-M5	t(9;11)(p22;q23)	11% (30%) for all t(11q23)	*MLLT3/AF9*	*MLL*	MLL fusion proteins–altered transcriptional regulation
	t(10;11)(p11-p15;q23)		*MLLT10/AF10*	*MLL*	
	t(11;17)(q23;q25)		*MLL*	*MLLT6/AF17*	
	t(11;19)(q23;p13.3)		*MLL*	*MLLT1/ENL*	
	t(11;19)(q23;p13.1)		*MLL*	*ELL*	
	t(6;11)(q27;q23)		*MLLT4/AF6*	*MLL*	
	Other t(11q23)		*MLL*		
	del(11q23)				
AML	+8	10%			
	+11	1–2%	*MLL*		Internal tandem duplication
	−7 or del(7q)	10%			
	−5 or del(5q)	10%			
	t(6;9)(p23;q34)	1%	*DEK*	*NUP214/CAN*	
	inv(3)(q21q26.2) or t(3;3)	2%	*EVI1*		
	del(20q)	5%			
	t(12p) or del(12p)	2%			
Therapy-related AML	−7 or del(7q) and/or −5 or del(5q)	75%			
	der(1;7)(q10;p10)	2%			
	t(9;11)(p22;q23)/t(11q23)	3%	*MLL*		MLL fusion protein–altered transcriptional regulation
	t(21q22)	2%	*RUNX1/AML1*		Fusion protein–altered transcriptional regulation
CMMoL	t(5;12)(q32;p13)	2–5%	*PDGFRB*	*ETV6/TEL*	Fusion protein–altered signaling pathways

*AML-M2, acute myeloblastic leukemia with maturation; AMMoL, acute myelomonocytic leukemia; AMMoL-M4Eo, acute myelomonocytic leukemia with abnormal eosinophils; AMoL, acute monoblastic leukemia; AML, acute myeloid leukemia; APL-M3, M3V, hypergranular (M3) and micrgranular (M3V) acute promyelocytic leukemia; CML, chronic myeloid leukemia; CMMoL, chronic myelomonocytic leukemia.

†The percentage refers to the frequency within the disease overall. The numbers in the parentheses refer to the frequency within the morphologic or immunologic subtype of the disease.

‡Genes are listed in order of citation in the karyotype, e.g., for CML, *ABL1* is at 9q34 and *BCR* at 22q11.2.

§Consequence refers to the expected consequence of the chromosomal abnormality at the molecular and cellular level.

¶Some patients with CML have an insertion of *ABL1* adjacent to *BCR* in a normal-appearing chromosome 22.

of AML as recognized by the WHO and French-American-British (FAB) classification schemes (Table 11–3; see Chap. 89).[22]

Translocation 8;21

The 8;21 translocation [t(8;21)(q22;q22)], described in 1973, was the first translocation identified in AML (see Fig. 11–2B). The t(8;21) is common and is observed in 5 to 10 percent of all AML cases with an abnormal karyotype and in 10 percent of M2 patients. This translocation is the most frequent abnormality in children with AML and occurs in 15 to 20 percent of karyotypically abnormal cases. Loss of a sex chromosome (−Y in males, −X in females), or a del(9q) with loss of 9q22 accompanies the t(8;21) in 75 percent of cases. The presence of the t(8;21) identifies a morphologically and clinically distinct subset of AML, and most cases with the t(8;21) are classified as AML with maturation (M2). AML with the t(8;21) has a favorable prognosis in adults (overall 5-year survival of 70%), but the outcome in children is poor.[23] At the molecular level, the t(8;21) involves the *RUNX1/AML1* gene, which encodes a transcription factor, also known as core-binding factor, that is essential for hematopoiesis. The *RUNX1* gene on chromosome 21 is fused to the *RUNX1T1/ETO* gene on chromosome 8 and results in a RUNX1-RUNX1T1 chimeric protein. Transformation by RUNX1-RUNX1T1 likely results from transcriptional repression of normal RUNX1 target genes via aberrant recruitment of nuclear transcriptional corepressor complexes.[23]

Inversion 16 and Translocation 16;16

Another clinical–cytogenetic association involves acute myelomonocytic leukemia with abnormal eosinophils, including large and irregular basophilic granules, and positive reactions with periodic acid-Schiff and chloroacetate esterase. Most patients have an inversion of chromosome 16, inv(16)(p13.1q22) (see Fig. 11–2C), but some have a t(16;16)(p13.1;q22), and the WHO classification system now recognizes these as a distinct form of AML (see Chap. 89). These aberrations are relatively common, occurring in 5 percent of AML and 25 percent of AMMoL (acute myelomonocytic leukemia) patients.[1] These patients have a good response to intensive chemotherapy with a complete remission rate of approximately 90 percent and an overall 5-year survival of 60 percent.[23] The breakpoint at 16q22 occurs within the *CBFB* gene, which encodes one subunit of the RUNX1/CBFB transcription factor. Thus, like the t(8;21), the inv(16) disrupts the RUNX1/AML1 pathway regulating hematopoiesis. Secondary cooperating mutations of *KIT, KRAS,* and *NRAS* are common in core-binding factor-associated leukemias, although only *KIT* mutations confer a poor prognosis.[23]

Translocation 15;17

The t(15;17)(q22;q12–21.1) (see Fig. 11–2D) is highly specific for acute promyelocytic leukemia (APL) and has not been found in any other disease.[24] Rare variant translocations, which occur in less than 2 percent of cases, include the t(11;17)(q23;q12–21.1) and t(5;17)(q34;q12–21.1), which result in the ZBTB16 (PLZF)-RARA and NPM1-RARA fusion proteins, respectively. Establishing the diagnosis of APL with the typical t(15;17) is important, because this disease is sensitive to therapy with all-*trans* retinoic acid, whereas other cases of AML and some of the APL-like disorders associated with the variant translocations do not respond to this treatment (see Chap. 89). The t(15;17) results in a fusion retinoic acid receptor-α protein (PML-RARA). The oncogenic potential of the APL fusion proteins appears to result from the aberrant repression of RARA-mediated gene transcription through histone deacetylase (HDAC)-dependent chromatin remodeling. Genetic mutations that cooperate with PML-RARA include *FLT3* internal tandem duplications (ITDs), observed in 35 percent of patients.

Translocations Involving 11q

Recurring translocations involving 11q23 are seen in approximately 35 percent of M5 patients and are of great interest in acute leukemia for at least three reasons.[1,25] First, there are more than 50 different recurring rearrangements that involve 11q23 and, thus, along with 14q32, 11q23 is one of the bands most frequently involved in rearrangements in human tumor cells.[25,26] The breakpoints in the translocation partners include 1p32, 4q21, and 19p13.3 in acute lymphoblastic leukemia (ALL; see Chap. 93), and 1q21, 2q21, 6q27, 9p22, 10p11, 17q25, 19p13.3, and 19p13.1 in AML (see Chap. 89). Second, these translocations occur in both lymphoid and myeloid leukemias. One common translocation in infants, t(4;11)(q21;q23), has a lymphoblastic phenotype, whereas other translocations, such as the t(9;11)(p22;q23) (see Fig. 11–2E) and t(11;19)(q23;p13.1), are common in monoblastic leukemias. Finally, translocations involving 11q23 have a very unusual age distribution, comprising about three-quarters of the chromosome abnormalities in leukemia cells of children younger than 1 year of age.[25] With the exception of the t(9;11), which may have an intermediate outcome, translocations of 11q23 are associated with a poor outcome.[22] Translocations of 11q23 involve *MLL,* a very large gene (>100 kb) with multiple transcripts of 12 to 15 kb. The MLL protein is a histone methyltransferase that assembles in protein complexes that regulate gene transcription via chromatin remodeling.[26] All of the *MLL* translocations identified to date result in fusion proteins.

Trisomy 11

Trisomy 11 is a rare abnormality, noted as a sole aberration in 1 to 2 percent of MDS or AML, and confers an unfavorable outcome.[27] It is notable that an ITD of the *MLL* gene is detected in 90 percent of AMLs with +11 as the sole abnormality and in 10 percent of AML cases with a normal karyotype. The rearrangement is the result of a duplication of *MLL* exons 2 to 6 or 2 to 8 mediated by recombination between *Alu* repetitive elements and may produce a partially duplicated protein.

Inversion 3 and t(3;3)

Each of the other recurring rearrangements in AML occurs in fewer than 3 percent of patients. A unique feature of abnormalities involving the long arm of chromosome 3 [inv(3)(q2lq26.2) or t(3;3)(q2l;q26.2)] is the presence of platelet counts above 100,000/μL, sometimes over $10^6/\mu$L, and an increase in marrow megakaryocytes, especially micromegakaryocytes.[1] It is noteworthy that most of the recurring translocations described above occur in younger patients with a median age in the thirties, whereas other abnormalities, such as –5/del(5q), or –7/del(7q), occur in patients with a median age older than 50 years. Moreover, many of the latter patients have occupational exposure to mutagenic agents, such as solvents, petroleum, and pesticides.

Mutations

The prognosis of patients with AML is also determined by mutations, most commonly of the *FLT3, NPM1, CEBPA,* or *KIT* genes (Table 11–4).[28]

TABLE 11–4. Frequency of Gene Mutations in MDS and AML

	Disease		
Mutated Gene	MDS (% of patients)	AML (% of patients)	t-MDS/t-AML (% of patients)
FLT3 (ITD)	2.4	15–35	0
FLT3 (TKD)	1	5–8	<1
NRAS	10–15	10	10
KIT^{D816}	~1	2	NA
MLL (ITD)	3	7	2–3
RUNX1	10–15	12	15–30
TP53	5–10	5–10	25–30
PTPN11	~1	~1	3
NPM1	Rare	35	4–5
CEBPA	1–8	6–18	Rare
JAK2^{V617F}	2–5	2–5	2–5

Mutations of FMS-like tyrosine kinase 3 (FLT3), including both ITDs and point mutations within the tyrosine kinase domain, are among the most common genetic changes seen in AML, occurring in 15 to 35 percent of cases. *FLT3*-ITD mutations may occur in any subtype of AML, but are most common in APL and AML with a normal karyotype, and are associated with a poor prognosis, particularly in those cases with loss of the remaining wild type *FLT3* allele.[29] Mutations of the FLT3 tyrosine kinase domain (codons 835 or 836 of the second tyrosine kinase domain) are noted in 5 to 8 percent of AML.[29] Mutations of *NPM1* also occur frequently in AML (35% of adult cases, and 80–90% of acute monocytic leukemia), but are less frequent in patients with recurring cytogenetic abnormalities. In the absence of *FLT3* mutations, *NPM1* mutations are associated with a favorable prognosis.[30] *NPM1* mutations, most commonly involve exon 12, resulting in alterations at the C-terminus, that is, replacement of tryptophan(s) at position 288 and 290, and aberrant localization of the protein to the cytoplasm. *CEBPA* mutations (6–15% of all AMLs), are often biallelic, and are usually associated with intermediate risk cytogenetics but are generally associated with a favorable prognosis.[28] Mutations of *KIT* are noted in 2 percent of AMLs, 22 to 38 percent of patients with inv(16)/t(16;16), and in 12 to 47 percent of patients with t(8;21), where they are associated with a poor prognosis.[23] With respect to epigenetic changes, transcriptional silencing via DNA methylation of the *CDKN2B* (*p15*^{INK4B}) gene is observed in a high percentage of patients with AML or therapy-related (t-)MDS/t-AML, and is associated with −7/del(7q), and a poor prognosis.[31]

THERAPY-RELATED MYELOID NEOPLASMS (T-MDS AND T-AML)

Therapy-related myeloid neoplasms, or t-MDS/t-AML, have been recognized as a late complication of cytotoxic therapy used in the treatment of both malignant and nonmalignant diseases.[32] In patients who received alkylating agents, the characteristic recurring chromosome abnormalities observed are loss of part or all of chromosomes 5 and/or 7 [−5/del(5q) or −7/del(7q)] (see Fig. 11–2F). Clinically, these patients have a long latency period (5 years), present with MDS, which often progresses rapidly to AML with multilineage dysplasia, and a poor prognosis. In our experience, 92 percent of t-MDS/t-AML patients had an abnormal karyotype and 70 percent had an abnormality of one or both chromosome 5 and 7[33]; these observations have been confirmed in other series.[34] In contrast, only approximately 16 percent of patients with AML *de novo* have a similar abnormality of chromosomes 5 or 7 or both.[1]

By cytogenetic and molecular analysis, investigators have defined a 970-kb commonly deleted segment (CDS) containing 21 genes on the long arm of chromosome 5 (5q31) predicted to contain a myeloid tumor-suppressor gene.[35] A second, nonoverlapping, CDS in 5q32 is implicated in the 5q− syndrome.[36] Parallel studies have revealed a 2.5-Mb CDS within 7q22 containing 16 genes. Molecular analysis of the genes within these regions did not reveal inactivating mutations in the remaining alleles, nor was there evidence of transcriptional silencing.[35] These observations are compatible with a haploinsufficiency model (gene dosage effect resulting from the loss of one allele), and several candidate haploinsufficient genes (*EGR1, CTNNA1, RPS14*) have been identified on 5q. The EGR1 transcription factor is downstream of cytokine signaling pathways. In a mouse model, loss of a single allele of *Egr1* cooperates with mutations induced by an alkylating agent in the development of myeloid diseases.[37] The gene encoding α-catenin (*CTNNA1*) is expressed at lower levels in AML or MDS with a del(5q) than in other AMLs or normal hematopoietic stem cells (HSCs).[38] *RPS14* encodes an essential component of the 40S subunit of ribosomes, and haploinsufficiency of this gene appears to be responsible for the defect in erythropoiesis in the 5q− syndrome.[39] These studies raise the possibility that haploinsufficiency for one or more of these genes in HSCs may contribute to the pathogenesis of MDS or AML with a del(5q).

A second subtype of t-AML has been identified that is distinctly different from the more common leukemia that follows alkylating agents or irradiation. This type of t-AML is seen in patients receiving drugs known to inhibit topoisomerase II, such as etoposide, teniposide, and doxorubicin. Clinically, these patients have a shorter latency period (1–2 years), present with overt leukemia, often with monocytic features, without a preceding myelodysplastic phase, and have a more favorable response to intensive induction therapy. Balanced translocations involving the *MLL* gene at 11q23, or the *RUNX1/AML1* gene at 21q22 are common in this subgroup.[32] Figure 11–3 shows the relative frequency of recurring cytogenetic abnormalities in *de novo* AML and therapy-related MDS and AML.

ACUTE LYMPHOBLASTIC LEUKEMIA (ALL)

ALL is the most frequent leukemia in children (see Chap. 93). In both childhood and adult ALL, the identification of prognostic subgroups based on recurring cytogenetic abnormalities (Table 11–5) and molecular markers has resulted in the application of risk-adapted therapies.[40] The most useful prognostic indicators are karyotype (including ploidy), age, white blood cell count, and response to initial therapy (day 14 marrow response and end-induction minimal residual disease). Based on these parameters, the Children's Oncology Group has defined four risk groups: lower risk (5-year event-free survival [EFS], at least

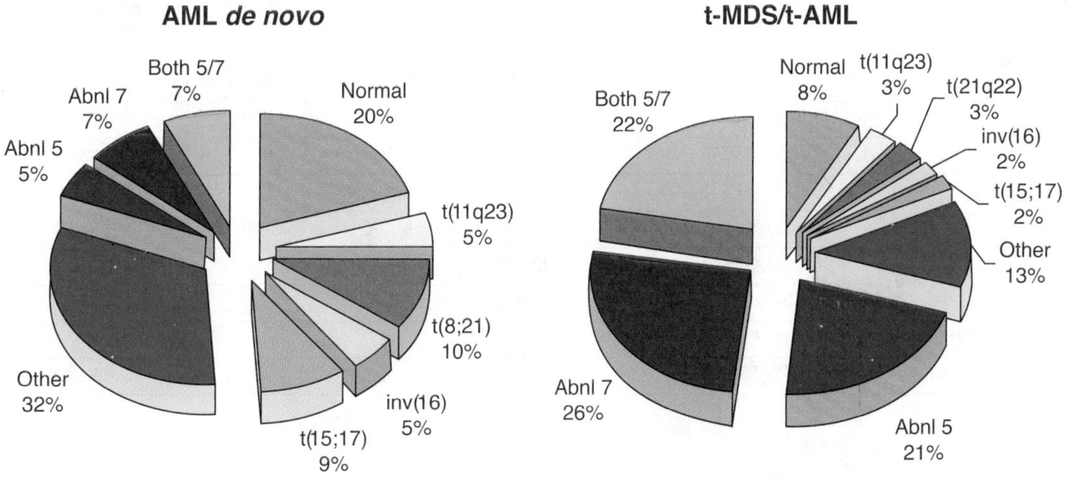

FIGURE 11–3. Frequency of recurring chromosome abnormalities in *de novo* AML and in therapy-related AML and MDS. Abnl, abnormal.

TABLE 11–5. Cytogenetic-Immunophenotypic Correlations in Malignant Lymphoid Diseases

Disease*	Chromosome Abnormality	Frequency†	Involved Genes‡		Consequence§
Acute lymphoblastic leukemia:					
Precursor B	t(12;21)(p13;q22)	25%	*ETV6/TEL*	*RUNX1/AML1*	Fusion protein–TF
	t(9;22)(q34;q11.2)	10%¶	*ABL1*	*BCR*	Fusion protein–altered cytokine signaling pathways
	t(4;11)(q21;q23)	5%	*AFF14*	*MLL*	Fusion protein–TF
	t(17;19)(q21–22;p13.3)	1%	*HLF*	*TCF3 (E2A)*	Fusion protein–TF
	t(11;19)(q23;p13.3)	1%	*MLL*	*MLLT1/ENL*	Fusion protein–TF
Pre-B	t(1;19)(q23;p13.3)	6% (30%)	*PBX1*	*TCF3 (E2A)*	Fusion protein–TF
B(SIg+)	t(8;14)(q24.1;q32)	5% (95%)	*MYC*	*IGH@*	Deregulated expression–TF
	t(2;8)(p12;q24.1)	<1% (1%)	*IGK@*	*MYC*	Deregulated expression–TF
	t(8;22)(q24.1;q11.2)	<1% (4%)	*MYC*	*IGL@*	Deregulated expression–TF
Other	Hyperdiploidy$^{50-60}$	10%			
	del(12p),t(12p)	10%			
T	t(11;14)(p15;q11.2)	1%	*LMO1*	*TRA@*	Deregulated expression–TF
	t(11;14)(p13;q11.2)	3%	*LMO2*	*TRA@*	Deregulated expression–TF
	t(8;14)(q24.1;q11.2)	<1%	*MYC*	*TRA@*	Deregulated expression–TF
	inv(14)(q11.2q32)	<1%	*TRA@*	*TCL1A*	Deregulated expression–TF
	t(10;14)(q24;q11.2)	3%	*TLX1*	*TRD@*	Deregulated expression–TF
	t(1;14)(p32;q11.2)	1%	*TALI*	*TRD@*	Deregulated expression–TF
	t(7;9)(q34;q34)	2%	*TRB@*	*NOTCH1*	Deregulated expression–TF
	t(7;19)(q34;p13.3)	<1%			
	del(9p),t(9p)	<1% (10%)	*CDKN2A/ CDKN2B*		Tumor suppressor gene–cell-cycle regulation
Non-Hodgkin lymphoma:					
B-cell NHL					
Burkitt	t(8;14)(q24.1;q32)	95%	*MYC*	*IGH@*	Deregulated expression–TF
	t(2;8)(p12;q24.1)	1%	*IGK@*	*MYC*	Deregulated expression–TF
	t(8;22)(q24.1;q11.2)	4%	*MYC*	*IGL@*	Deregulated expression–TF
Follicular SNCL	t(14;18)(q32;q21.3)	80%	*IGH@*	*BCL2*	Deregulated expression–antiapoptosis protein
DLBCL	t(14;18)(q32;q21.3)	20%	*IGH@*	*BCL2*	Deregulated expression–antiapoptosis protein
DLBCL	t(3;22)(q27;q11.2)	45% for all t(3q27)	*BCL6*	*IGL@*	Deregulated expression–TF
	t(3;14)(q27;q32)		*BCL6*	*IGH@*	Deregulated expression–TF
	t(3q27)				
MCL	t(11;14)(q13;q32)	~100%	*CCND1*	*IGH@*	Deregulated expression–cell-cycle regulation
LPL	t(9;14)(p13;q32)		*PAX5*	*IGH@*	Deregulated expression–TF
SLL	t(14;19)(q32;q13.3)		*IGH@*	*BCL3*	Deregulated expression–TF
MALT	t(11;18)(q21;q21)	40–50%	*BIRC3/API2*	*MALT1*	Fusion protein–increased NF-κB activation
	t(1;14)(p22;q32)	10%	*BCL10*	*IGH@*	Deregulated expression–increased NF-κB activation
	t(14;18)(q32;q21)	10–20%	*IGH@*	*MALT1*	
	t(3;14)(p14.1;q32)	10%	*FOXP1*	*IGH@*	
T-cell NHL					
(Ki-l+) ALCL	t(2;5)(p23;q35)	75%	*ALK*	*NPM1*	Deregulated expression–tyrosine kinase

(continued)

TABLE 11–5. Cytogenetic-Immunophenotypic Correlations in Malignant Lymphoid Diseases (Continued)

Disease*	Chromosome Abnormality	Frequency†	Involved Genes‡		Consequence§
Chronic lymphocytic leukemia:					
B	t(11;14)(q13;q32)	10%	*CCND1*	*IGH@*	Deregulated expression–cell-cycle regulation
	t(14;19)(q32;q13.2)	10%	*IGH@*	*BCL3*	Deregulated expression–increased NF-κB activation
	t(2;14)(p13;q32)	5%		*IGH@*	
	t(14q32)	20%			
	del(13q)	30%			
	+12	30%			
T	t(8;14)(q24.1;q11.2)	5%	*MYC*	*TRA@*	Deregulated expression–TF
	inv14(q11.2q32)	5%	*TRA@/TRD@*	*IGH@*	Deregulated expression
	inv14(q11.2q32)	5%	*TRA@/TRD@*	*TCL1A*	Deregulated expression–TF
Multiple myeloma:					
B	−13/del(13q)	40%			
	t(4;14)(p16;q32)	15%	*FGFR3*	*IGH@*	Deregulated expression–Growth factor receptor
	t(14;16)(q32;q23)	5%	*IGH@*	*MAF*	Deregulated expression–TF
	t(6;14)(p21;q32)	4%	*CCND3*	*IGH@*	Deregulated expression–cell-cycle regulation
	t(11;14)(q13;q32)	15%	*CCND1*	*IGH@*	Deregulated expression–cell-cycle regulation
	t(14q32)	50%	*IGH@*		
	hyperdiploidy, +3,+5,+7,+9,+11	20%			
Adult T-cell leukemia/lymphoma:					
	t(14;14)(q11.2;q32)		*TRA@*	*IGH@*	Deregulated expression
	inv(14)(q11.2q32)		*TRA@/TRD@*	*IGH@*	Deregulated expression
	+3				

*ALCL, anaplastic large cell lymphoma; CTCL, cutaneous T-cell lymphoma; DLBCL, diffuse large B-cell lymphoma; Ki-1, anti-CD30 antibody; LPL, lymphoplasmacytoid lymphoma; MALT, mucosa-associated lymphoid tumor; MCL, mantle cell lymphoma; SIg, surface immunoglobulin; SLL, small lymphocytic lymphoma.

†The percentage refers to the frequency within the disease overall. The number in the parentheses refers to the frequency within the morphologic or immunologic subtype of the disease.

‡Genes are listed in order of citation in karyotype; for example, for precursor B ALL, *ETV6/TEL* is at 12p13 and *RUNX1/AML1* is at 21q22.

§Consequence refers to the expected consequence of the chromosomal abnormality at the molecular and cellular level.

¶By cytogenetic analysis, the frequency in children is approximately 5%, and in adults approximately 25%; using molecular probes, this frequency is 30% in adults overall, and 50% in adults older than 60 years of age.

85%) with either the *ETV6/RUNX1* fusion or simultaneous trisomies of chromosomes 4, 10, and 17; standard and high risk (those remaining in the respective National Cancer Institute risk groups); and very high risk (5-year EFS, 45% or below) with extreme hypodiploidy (fewer than 44 chromosomes), or the *BCR/ABL1* fusion, and induction failure.[41]

TRANSLOCATION 9;22

The incidence of the t(9;22) in ALL is 30 percent in adults (the incidence may approach 50% in adults older than 60 years of age) and 5 percent in children. Thus, the Ph chromosome is the most frequent rearrangement in adult ALL. Approximately 70 percent of the patients show additional abnormalities, a frequency that is substantially higher than that observed in CML with +der(22)t(9;22),+21, abnormalities of 9p, +8, −7, and +X (noted in descending frequency). Monosomy 7 is associated with a poorer outcome.[42] A chromosomally normal cell line is frequently noted in the marrow of Ph+ ALL patients (70%), but is rare in untreated CML. Most cases have a B-lineage phenotype (CD10+, CD19+, and TdT+), but there is frequent expression of myeloid-associated antigens (CD13 and CD33). The disease in both adults and children is characterized by high white blood cell counts, a high percentage of circulating blasts, and a poor prognosis. As in CML, the t(9;22) in ALL results in a *BCR-ABL1* fusion gene. However, in over half of the patients, the break in *BCR* is more proximal, resulting in a smaller fusion protein with even greater tyrosine kinase activity ($BCR\text{-}ABL1^{p190}$).

TRANSLOCATIONS INVOLVING 11q

Translocations involving the *MLL* gene at 11q23 are observed in 5 percent of ALL patients.[43] Of these, the most common is the t(4;11)(q21;q23) (Fig. 11–4A). The t(11;19)(q23;p13.3) is second in frequency. However, this rearrangement is not limited to ALL in that approximately 50 percent of these cases have AML, usually monoblastic. Of note is the high frequency of translocations involving 11q23 in infant ALL (60–80%). Patients with the t(4;11) have a pro-B

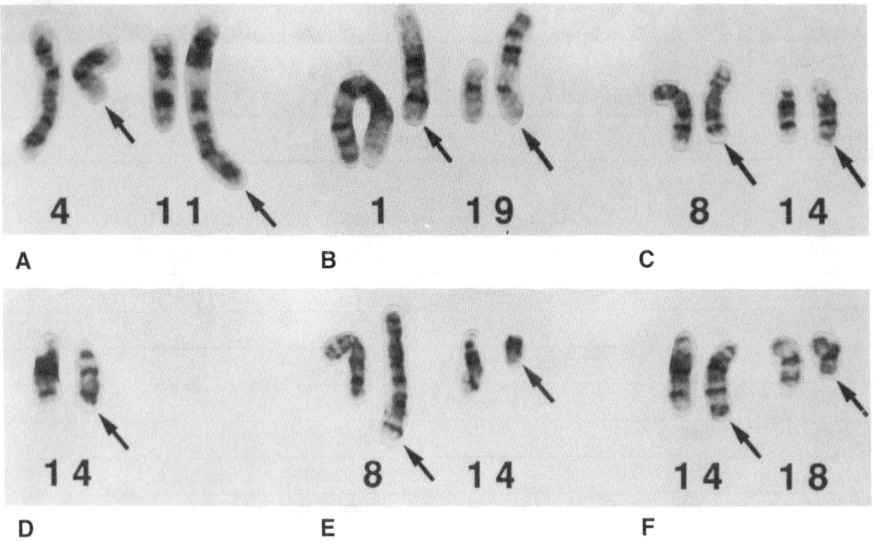

FIGURE 11–4. Partial karyotypes of trypsin-Giemsa-banded metaphase cells depicting recurring chromosomal rearrangements observed in lymphoid malignant diseases. The rearranged chromosomes are identified with *arrows*. **A.** t(4;11)(q21;q23) in ALL. **B.** t(1;19)(q21;p13.3) in pre-B cell ALL. **C.** t(8;14)(q24.1;q32) in B-cell ALL and Burkitt lymphoma. **D.** inv(14)(q11.2q32) in T-cell leukemia/lymphoma. **E.** t(8;14)(q24.1;q11.2) in T-cell leukemia/lymphoma. **F.** t(14;18)(q32;q21.3) in B-cell NHL.

phenotype (CD10–, CD19+), with coexpression of monocytic (CD15+) or, less commonly, T-cell markers. Clinically, both children and adults have aggressive features with hyperleukocytosis, extramedullary disease, and a poor response to conventional chemotherapy.[43] Adults with the t(4;11) have a remission rate of 75 percent, but a median EFS of only 7 months. Rearrangements affecting *MLL* represent a major class of mutations in acute leukemia and identify patients with a poor outcome.

TRANSLOCATION 12;21

The t(12;21)(p13;q22) has been identified in a high proportion (~25%) of childhood precursor B leukemia, but is uncommon in adults (~4% of ALL cases).[44] The translocation is not easily detected by cytogenetic analysis because of the similarity in size and banding pattern of 12p and 21q. However, the rearrangement can be detected reliably using reverse-transcriptase polymerase chain reaction (RT-PCR) or FISH analysis. The t(12;21) defines a distinct subgroup of patients characterized by an age between 1 and 10 years, B-lineage immunophenotype (CD10+, CD19+, HLA-DR+), and a favorable outcome, particularly when other favorable risk factors are present. In a recent series, patients with the t(12;21) had a 5-year EFS of 91 percent as compared to 65 percent for patients without this rearrangement. However, the t(12;21) may be associated with late disease recurrences. The t(12;21) results in a fusion protein containing the N-terminus of ETV6/TEL, a transcriptional repressor of the ETS family, and most of the RUNX1/AML1 transcription factor.

HYPERDIPLOIDY

The leukemia cells of some patients with ALL are characterized by a gain of many chromosomes. Two distinct subgroups are recognized: a group with 1 to 4 extra chromosomes,[47–50] and the more common group with >50 chromosomes. Chromosome numbers usually range from 51 to 60, and a few patients may have up to 65 chromosomes. Hyperdiploidy (>50 and usually <66 chromosomes) is common in children (~30%), but is rarely observed in adults (<5%). Certain additional chromosomes are common (X chromosome, and chromosomes 4, 6, 10, 14, 17, 18, and 21). Chromosome 21 is gained most frequently (100% of cases). Patients who have hyperdiploidy with >50 chromosomes have all of the previously recognized clinical factors that indicate a good prognosis, including age between 1 and 9 years, low white blood cell count (median: 6700/μL), and favorable immunophenotype (early pre-B or pre-B).[45] The favorable prognosis associated with high hyperdiploidy has been associated with gains of chromosomes 4, 10, and 17, whereas a gain of chromosome 5 and i(17q) are associated with a poor outcome.[45]

TRANSLOCATION 1;19

The t(1;19)(q23;pl3.3) has been identified in approximately 6 percent of children with a B-lineage leukemia. The leukemia cells have cytoplasmic immunoglobulin and are CD10+, CD19+, CD34–, and CD9+ (see Fig. 11–4B). A reciprocal translocation involving the long arms of chromosomes 8 and 14 [t(8;14)(q24.1;q32)] is observed in mature B-cell ALL (see Fig. 11–4C).[46] These patients have a high incidence of central nervous system involvement and/or abdominal nodal involvement at diagnosis. Although the outcome for both children and adults with a t(8;14) has been poor, the use of high-intensity chemotherapy has markedly improved the outcome (EFS of 80% in children).[46]

PROFILING SINGLE NUCLEOTIDE POLYMORPHISMS

Genomewide profiling studies using SNP arrays has revealed DNA copy-number abnormalities in pediatric ALL that disrupt pathways controlling B-cell development and differentiation, including deletions of *PAX5* (in 32% of cases), *IKZF1* (*IKAROS*, in 29%), and *EBF1* (in 8%). Genetic alteration of *IKZF1* was associated with a very poor outcome in B-cell progenitor ALL. The gene expression profile of this group had increased expression of HSC genes, and was similar to the signature of *BCR-ABL1*-positive ALL, another high-risk subtype of ALL with a high frequency of *IKZF1* deletions. [6]

T-CELL ACUTE LYMPHOBLASTIC LEUKEMIA

T-lymphoblastic leukemia/lymphoma has a distinct pattern of recurring karyotypic abnormalities.[47] Rearrangements involving 14q11.2 (see Fig. 11–4D) and two regions of chromosome 7 (7q34) and 7p14) are particularly frequent in T-cell malignancies (see Table 11–5). The most common are the t(10;11)(q24;q11.2) (7% of child and 30% of adult patients, *TLX1* gene); the cryptic t(5;14)(q35;q32) (*TLX3*, 20% of child and 10–15% of adult cases), t(11;14) (p13;q11.2) (~3%, *LMO2* gene), and t(7;9)(q34;q34) (~2%, *NOTCH1* gene). Approximately 30 percent of patients have activating mutations of the *NOTCH1* gene. Patients with T-cell ALL are most often young males and often have a mediastinal tumor mass, high white blood cell count, and leukemia cells in the cerebrospinal fluid. These same clinical characteristics are associated with lymphoblastic lymphoma, another T-cell malignancy. Figure 11–5 shows the relative frequency of cytogenetic abnormalities in ALL.

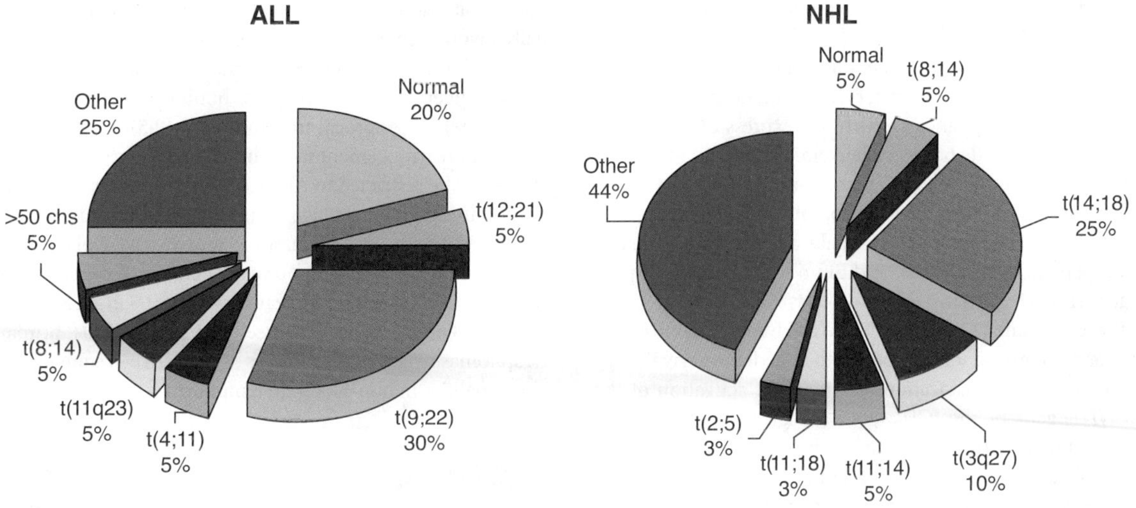

FIGURE 11–5. Frequency of recurring chromosome abnormalities in ALL and non-Hodgkin lymphoma. chs, chromosomes.

CHRONIC LYMPHOCYTIC LEUKEMIA

The chromosomal abnormalities associated with chronic lymphocytic leukemia (CLL) have been delineated through the use of FISH.[48] When conventional cytogenetic techniques are used, only 50 percent of CLL patients have detectable chromosomal abnormalities. The most common abnormality is trisomy 12 (present in 20–60% of cases), followed by structural abnormalities of 13q and 14q. However, when FISH analysis is used to study specific abnormalities, chromosomal abnormalities can be detected in greater than 80 percent of patients. The most frequent chromosomal changes seen by FISH are loss or deletion of 13q (present in 55% of cases); deletion of 11q, the location of the *ATM* gene (18%); trisomy of 12q (16%); deletion of 17p, the location of the *TP53* gene (7%); and deletion of 6q (6%). Patient survival correlates with cytogenetic subtype, with a shorter median survival observed in patients with 17p (32 months) or 11q (79 months) deletions, than in those with no detectable abnormality (111 months), trisomy of 12q (114 months), or −13/del(13q) (133 months). Two microRNA genes (miR-16–1 and miR-15a) are possible target genes in the 13q14.3 region. FISH probes capable of detecting the deletions of 11q, 13q, and 17p, trisomy 12, and *IGH* translocations are commercially available, and facilitate the application of risk-adapted treatment strategies.

The prognosis of patients with CLL is also determined by two other molecular abnormalities: the status of the immunoglobulin heavy-chain variable region (*IGHv*) and the expression level of CD38. Patients whose CLL cells express *IGHv* genes containing somatic mutations have a 24-year median survival compared to only 6 to 8 years in those patients who do not have somatic *IGHv* gene mutations.[49] This simple grouping of patients based on the mutation status of the *IGHv* gene may reflect the fact that CLL cells that have few or no *IGHv* mutations also often contain chromosomal aberrations that confer a poor prognosis, for example, deletions of 11q or 17p, or trisomy 12, whereas CLL cells with *IGHv* mutations often contain deletions of 13q, which confer a more favorable clinical course. Unfortunately, testing for somatic mutations in the *IGHv* gene is not widely used. ZAP-70, an enzyme normally expressed in T lymphocytes and critical for T-cell activation, is upregulated in CLL cells that contain unmutated *IGHv* genes, conferring a poor prognosis.[50] Patients whose CLL cells have mutated IGHv and lack expression of ZAP-70 and CD38, a membrane protein with signaling activity, have the longest treatment-free period after initial diagnosis.[51]

T-cell CLL and large granular lymphocytic leukemia are uncommon disorders in which the malignant lymphocytes have a T-cell immunophenotype. Rearrangements involving band 14q11.2 with or without an accompanying break in 14q32 have been reported in T-CLL as well as in T-cell lymphomas (see Table 11–5).[47] The most common is inv(14)(q11.2q32).

NON-HODGKIN LYMPHOMA

Cytogenetic analyses of non-Hodgkin lymphoma (NHL) have demonstrated that greater than 90 percent of cases are characterized by clonal chromosomal abnormalities and, more importantly, many of the recurring abnormalities correlate with histology and immunophenotype (see Table 11–5).[52] For example, the t(14;18) is observed in a high proportion of follicular small, cleaved cell lymphomas (70–90%); most patients with a t(3;22)(q27;q11.2) or t(3;14)(q27;q32) have diffuse large B-cell lymphomas (DLBCL); and patients with a t(8;14)(q24.1;q32) have either small, noncleaved cell lymphoma or DLBCL. Band 14q32, the location of *IGHv*, is frequently involved in translocations in B-cell neoplasms (~70% of patients). In contrast, a large proportion of T-cell neoplasms are characterized by rearrangements that involve 14q11.2, 7q34, or 7p14, the locations of the T-cell receptor genes. Gene expression profiling has proven useful in distinguishing unique genetic subtypes of lymphoma.[53]

The t(8;14) is characteristic of both endemic and nonendemic Burkitt lymphoma (BL), as well as Epstein-Barr virus (EBV)-negative and EBV-positive tumors (see Fig. 11–4E). Moreover, the t(8;14) has also been observed in other lymphomas, particularly small, noncleaved cell (non-Burkitt) and large cell immunoblastic lymphomas, AIDS-associated BL (100% of patients) and AIDS-related DLBCL (30%).[54] Two other variant translocations also occur in BL: t(2;8)(p12;q24.1) and t(8;22)(q24.1;q11.2). All three translocations involve chromosome band 8q24.1. As discussed earlier, these same translocations have been seen in some patients with B-cell ALL. The t(8;14) involves a break within the *IGH* locus on chromosome 14, and a break either 5′ or within *MYC* on chromosome 8, and relocates the *MYC* coding exons to chromosome 14. MYC is a transcription factor that plays a critical role in a number of cellular processes including DNA replication, proliferation, and apoptosis; its oncogenic properties are due to its constitutive expression.

Between 70 and 90 percent of follicular lymphomas and 20 percent of DLBCL have the t(14;18) (see Fig. 11–4F), in which the *BCL2* gene at 18q21.3 is juxtaposed to the *IGH* J segment, leading to the deregulated expression of *BCL2*.[55] Common secondary abnormalities include −7, +18, and del(6q). Other malignancies which overexpress *BCL2*, but do not harbor the t(14;18), include hairy cell leukemia and CLL. The *BCL2* gene encodes a 26-kDa mitochondrial membrane protein that functions to increase cell survival through antiapoptotic mechanisms.

The t(11;14) (q13;q32) is observed in virtually all cases of mantle cell lymphoma, in 3 percent of myelomas, and in up to 20 percent of prolymphocytic leukemias.[56,57] Many cases also have deletions or point mutations of the *ATM* gene (11q22.3). Mantle cell lymphomas are currently regarded as a poor prognostic group with a median survival from diagnosis of 3 years. This translocation results in the activation of the cyclin D1 (*CCND1*) gene by the *IGH@* gene (J region).[56] The *CCND1* gene is located 100 to 130 kb away from the breakpoint on 11q13. A variety of growth factors promote cell proliferation by activating the D-type cyclins, causing cells to go through the restriction start point of the cell cycle at G_1 and committing them to divide via phosphorylation and inactivation of RB1.

The *BCL6* gene was cloned from the recurring breakpoint at 3q27 in cells characterized by a t(3;22)(q27;q11.2), t(3;14)(q27;q32), or, rarely, t(2;3)(p12;q27).[52] *BCL6* rearrangements occur in 40 percent of DLBCLs and, in some series, up to 10 percent of follicular lymphomas. The translocations lead to the truncation of the *BCL6* gene within the first exon or the first intron, substitution of its promoter sequences with an *Ig* promoter, and deregulated expression. The *BCL6* gene product is a 96-kDa POZ/Zn finger, nuclear protein that acts as a potent transcriptional repressor. It is predominantly expressed in the B-cell lineage, particularly in mature B cells, and may suppress genes involved in lymphocyte activation, differentiation, cell cycle arrest, and apoptosis. Somatic mutations have been identified in the 5′ regulatory regions of *BCL6* in approximately 20 percent of DLBCLs without translocations leading to deregulation of *BCL6*, suggesting that overexpression of *BCL6* is more broadly involved than initially recognized.[58]

Extranodal marginal zone B-cell lymphomas of mucosa-associated lymphoid tissue (MALT lymphoma) are comprised of several genetic subgroups, one characterized by trisomy 3 plus other abnormalities (60% of patients), and another by the t(11;18)(q21;q21) (25–50%) and its variants.[59] Of note is that the t(11;18) is not observed in primary large B-cell gastric lymphoma. The t(11;18) results in the fusion of the apoptosis-inhibitor gene *BIRC3 (API2)*, to a novel gene at 18q21, *MALT1*, whose product activates the NF-κB (nuclear factor-κB) pathway.

A number of recurring chromosomal abnormalities have been recognized in T-cell leukemias and lymphomas (see Table 11–5). Similar to B-cell neoplasms, in which rearrangements frequently involve the chromosomal bands containing the immunoglobulin gene loci, T-cell neoplasms often have rearrangements involving band 14q11.2, the site of the T-cell receptor α-chain and δ-chain genes (*TXPα, TCRδ*) or, less often, one of two regions of chromosome 7 (7q34 and 7p14) to which the T-cell receptor β-chain (*TCR*) and γ-chain (*TCR*) genes have been localized, respectively.[52] These translocations result from aberrant V-D-J recombination events. With few exceptions, the involved gene on the partner chromosome encodes a transcription factor, whose expression is deregulated or activated as a result of the rearrangement (see Table 11–5). As a consequence of a chromosomal rearrangement that brings an oncogene under the controlling influence of promoters or enhancers that are active for immunoglobulin synthesis in B cells or in T-cell receptor synthesis, T cells may gain a proliferative advantage, resulting in malignant clonal expansion.

Anaplastic large cell lymphoma (ALCL), a distinctive subtype of NHL, is characterized by a young age at presentation and skin and/or lymph node infiltration by large, often bizarre lymphoma cells, which preferentially involve the paracortical areas and lymph node sinuses. The majority of such tumors express one or more T-cell antigens, a minority express B-cell antigens, and some express both T- and B-cell antigens (the null phenotype). A reciprocal translocation, t(2;5)(p23;q35), t(1;2)(q25;p23), or variant rearrangement involving the *ALK* tyrosine kinase gene at 2p23 appears to be restricted to ALCL of either T-cell or null phenotype, and is present in a high percentage of these cases.[60] The tumor cells are positive for CD30 on the cell membrane and in the Golgi region, and ALK expression is detectable in 60 to 85 percent of cases, where it confers a more favorable outcome (5-year survival: 80% in ALK+ vs. 40% in ALK− tumors). The t(2;5) has also been found in CD30+ primary cutaneous lymphomas. Figure 11–5 shows the relative frequency of cytogenetic abnormalities in non-Hodgkin lymphoma.

MYELOMA

As in CLL, the application of molecular cytogenetic tools, such as FISH, has led to the discovery of numerous chromosomal abnormalities in essential monoclonal gammopathy, myeloma, and plasma cell leukemia.[57,61] Essential monoclonal gammopathy is characterized by chromosomal aneuploidy, *IgH* translocations (45% of patients), and deletions of 13q (15–50% of patients; see Chap. 108). Plasma cell myeloma is a malignancy of postfollicular B cells and is characterized by the acquisition of complex chromosomal rearrangements. As in monoclonal gammopathy, the earliest changes involve deletions of 13q14, and translocations of the *IGH* gene, which deregulate the expression of oncogenes located near the translocation breakpoints. Loss of chromosome 13 or a del(13q) are the most frequently observed chromosomal losses in myeloma and confer a poor prognosis.[57] With the use of FISH, deletions of 13q are detected in 40 to 50 percent of patients with multiple myeloma and may be associated with specific 14q translocations.

Among the most frequent chromosomal rearrangements noted in plasma cell malignancies are translocations involving the *IGH* locus on 14q32. *IgH* translocations are detectable by interphase FISH analysis in approximately 50 percent of patients with monoclonal gammopathy, 60 to 75 percent of patients with myeloma, and more than 80 percent of patients with plasma cell leukemia.[57] The t(11;14)(q13;q32) is found in 15 percent of cases, and results in cyclin D1 overexpression and may deregulate expression of *MYEOV* (myeloma overexpressed gene). The t(4;14)(p16;q32) is noted in approximately 15 percent of patients and deregulates the expression of the fibroblast growth factor receptor 3 gene *(FGFR3)* translocated to the der(14), and the *MMSET* domain remaining on the der(4) chromosomes. The t(14;16)(q32;q23), noted in 5 percent of cases, results in the overexpression of the *MAF* transcription factor gene. Cyclin D3 overexpression occurs in the context of the t(6;14)(p21;q32), and is observed in 4 percent of patients. The translocation partners for the remaining 40 percent of multiple myeloma cases are currently unknown. The t(4;14) and t(14;16) are both associated with a poor clinical outcome, whereas the t(11;14) confers a favorable prognosis. Translocations involving unknown partners confer an intermediate prognosis.

Additional events occur with disease progression, including mutations of *NRAS* and *KRAS*, *MYC* deregulation, and epigenetic alterations. Activating mutations of *NRAS* or *KRAS* have been identified in MGUS (~5%), and at a higher frequency in myeloma (30–40%); but the frequency may be higher in patients who relapse (80%).[62] Several genes are silenced through aberrant promoter hypermethylation in both monoclonal gammopathy and myeloma, including *DAPK1* (67% of patients), *SOCS1*, *CDKN2B (p15)*, and *CDKN2A (p16)*.[57]

REFERENCES

1. Carlson KM and Le Beau MM. Cytogenetics/fluorescent *in situ* hybridization, in *Clinical Hematology*, edited by NS Young, SL Gerson, KA High, p 1336. Elsevier, Mosby, 2005.
2. Gilliland DG: Molecular genetics of human leukemias: New insights into therapy. *Semin Hematol* 39:6, 2002.
3. Gozzetti A, Le Beau MM: Fluorescence *in situ* hybridization: Uses and limitations. *Semin Hematol* 37:320, 2000.
4. Radich JP, Oehler V: Monitoring chronic myelogenous leukemia in the age of tyrosine kinase inhibitors. *J Natl Compr Canc Netw* 5:497, 2007.
5. Braziel RM, Shipp MA, Feldman AL, et al: Molecular diagnostics. *Hematology (Am Soc Hematol Educ Program)* 279, 2003.
6. Mullighan CG, Su X, Zhang J, et al: Deletion of IKZF1 and prognosis in acute lymphoblastic leukemia. *N Engl J Med* 360:470, 2009.
7. Shaffer LG, Tommerup N: *ISCN: 2005: An International System for Human Cytogenetic Nomenclature*. S. Karger, Basel, Switzerland, 2005.
8. Melo JV, Barnes DJ: Chronic myeloid leukaemia as a model of disease evolution in human cancer. *Nat Rev Cancer* 7:441, 2007.
9. O'Hare T, Eide CA, Deininger MW: New BCR-ABL inhibitors in chronic myeloid leukemia: Keeping resistance in check. *Expert Opin Investig Drugs* 17:865, 2008.
10. Deininger MW: Milestones and monitoring in patients with CML treated with imatinib. *Hematology Am Soc Hematol Educ Program* 419, 2008.
11. Deininger MW, Cortes J, Paquette R, et al: The prognosis for patients with chronic myeloid leukemia who have clonal cytogenetic abnormalities in Philadelphia chromosome-negative cells. *Cancer* 110:1509, 2007.
12. Barnes DJ, Melo JV: Cytogenetic and molecular genetic aspects of chronic myeloid leukaemia. *Acta Haematol* 108:180, 2002.
13. Tefferi A: Molecular drug targets in myeloproliferative neoplasms: Mutant ABL1, JAK2, MPL, KIT, PDGFRA, PDGFRB and FGFR1. *J Cell Mol Med* 13:215, 2009.
14. Adeyinka A, Dewald GW: Cytogenetics of chronic myeloproliferative disorders and related myelodysplastic syndromes. *Hematol Oncol Clin North Am* 17:1129, 2003.
15. Levine RL, Pardanani A, Tefferi A, et al: Role of JAK2 in the pathogenesis and therapy of myeloproliferative disorders. *Nat Rev Cancer* 7:673, 2007.
16. Zipperer E, Wulfert M, Germing U, et al: MPL 515 and JAK2 mutation analysis in MDS presenting with a platelet count of more than 500 × 10(9)/L. *Ann Hematol* 87:413, 2008.
17. Vardiman JW, Thiele J, Arber DA, et al: The 2008 revision of the WHO classification of myeloid neoplasms and acute leukemia: Rationale and important changes. *Blood* 114:937, 2009.
18. Olney HJ, Le Beau MM: Evaluation of recurring cytogenetic abnormalities in the treatment of myelodysplastic syndromes. *Leuk Res* 31:427, 2007.
19. Greenberg P, Cox C, LeBeau MM, et al: International scoring system for evaluating prognosis in myelodysplastic syndromes. *Blood* 89:2079, 1997.
20. Nimer SD: Clinical management of myelodysplastic syndromes with interstitial deletion of chromosome 5q. *J Clin Oncol* 24:2576, 2006.
21. Haase D, Germing U, Schanz J, et al: New insights into the prognostic impact of the karyotype in MDS and correlation with subtypes: Evidence from a core dataset of 2124 patients. *Blood* 110:4385, 2007.
22. Mrozek K, Bloomfield CD: Clinical significance of the most common chromosome translocations in adult acute myeloid leukemia. *J Natl Cancer Inst Monogr* 39:52, 2008.
23. Mrozek K, Marcucci G, Paschka P, et al: Advances in molecular genetics and treatment of core-binding factor acute myeloid leukemia. *Curr Opin Oncol* 20:711, 2008.
24. Mistry AR, Pedersen EW, Solomon E, et al: The molecular pathogenesis of acute promyelocytic leukaemia: Implications for the clinical management of the disease. *Blood Rev* 17:71, 2003.
25. Olney HJ, Mitelman F, Johansson B, et al: Unique balanced chromosome abnormali ties in treatment-related myelodysplastic syndromes and acute myeloid leukemia: Report from an international workshop. *Genes Chromosomes Cancer* 33:413, 2002.
26. Krivtsov AV, Armstrong SA: MLL translocations, histone modifications and leukaemia stem-cell development. *Nat Rev Cancer* 7:823, 2007.
27. Farag SS, Archer KJ, Mrozek K, et al: Isolated trisomy of chromosomes 8, 11, 13 and 21 is an adverse prognostic factor in adults with de novo acute myeloid leukemia: Results from Cancer and Leukemia Group B 8461. *Int J Oncol* 21:1041, 2002.
28. Dohner K, Dohner H: Molecular characterization of acute myeloid leukemia. *Haematologica* 93:976, 2008.
29. Bacher U, Haferlach T, Kern W, et al: A comparative study of molecular mutations in 381 patients with myelodysplastic syndrome and in 4130 patients with acute myeloid leukemia. *Haematologica* 92:744, 2007.
30. Falini B, Mecucci C, Tiacci E, et al: Cytoplasmic nucleophosmin in acute myelogenous leukemia with a normal karyotype. *N Engl J Med* 352:254, 2005.
31. Christiansen DH, Andersen MK, Pedersen-Bjergaard J: Methylation of p15INK4B is common, is associated with deletion of genes on chromosome arm 7q and predicts a poor prognosis in therapy-related myelodysplasia and acute myeloid leukemia. *Leukemia* 17:1813, 2003.
32. Godley LA, Larson RA: Therapy-related myeloid leukemia. *Semin Oncol* 35:418, 2008.
33. Smith SM, Le Beau MM, Huo D, et al: Clinical-cytogenetic associations in 306 patients with therapy-related myelodysplasia and myeloid leukemia: The University of Chicago series. *Blood* 102:43, 2003.
34. Pedersen-Bjergaard J, Andersen MK, Christiansen DH: Therapy-related acute myeloid leukemia and myelodysplasia after high-dose chemotherapy and autologous stem cell transplantation. *Blood* 95:3273, 2000.
35. Lai F, Godley LA, Joslin J, et al: Transcript map and comparative analysis of the 1.5-Mb commonly deleted segment of human 5q31 in malignant myeloid diseases with a del(5q). *Genomics* 71:235, 2001.
36. Boultwood J, Fidler C, Strickson AJ, et al: Narrowing and genomic annotation of the commonly deleted region of the 5q− syndrome. *Blood* 99:4638, 2002.
37. Joslin JM, Fernald AA, Tennant TR, et al: Haploinsufficiency of EGR1, a candidate gene in the del(5q), leads to the development of myeloid disorders. *Blood* 110:719, 2007.
38. Liu TX, Becker MW, Jelinek J, et al: Chromosome 5q deletion and epigenetic suppression of the gene encoding alpha-catenin (CTNNA1) in myeloid cell transformation. *Nat Med* 13:78, 2007.
39. Ebert BL, Pretz J, Bosco J, et al: Identification of RPS14 as a 5q− syndrome gene by RNA interference screen. *Nature* 451:335, 2008.
40. Harrison CJ: Cytogenetics of paediatric and adolescent acute lymphoblastic leukaemia. *Br J Haematol* 144:147, 2009.
41. Schultz KR, Pullen DJ, Sather HN, et al: Risk- and response-based classification of childhood B-precursor acute lymphoblastic leukemia: A combined analysis of prognostic markers from the Pediatric Oncology Group (POG) and Children's Cancer Group (CCG). *Blood* 109:926, 2007.
42. Wetzler M, Dodge RK, Mrozek K, et al: Additional cytogenetic abnormalities in adults with Philadelphia chromosome-positive acute lymphoblastic leukaemia: A study of the Cancer and Leukaemia Group B. *Br J Haematol* 124:275, 2004.
43. Pui CH, Chessells JM, Camitta B, et al: Clinical heterogeneity in childhood acute lymphoblastic leukemia with 11q23 rearrangements. *Leukemia* 17:700, 2003.
44. Rubnitz JE, Downing JR, Pui CH, et al: TEL gene rearrangement in acute lymphoblastic leukemia: A new genetic marker with prognostic significance. *J Clin Oncol* 15:1150, 1997.
45. Sutcliffe MJ, Shuster JJ, Sather HN, et al: High concordance from independent studies by the Children's Cancer Group (CCG) and Pediatric Oncology Group (POG) associating favorable prognosis with combined trisomies 4, 10, and 17 in children with NCI Standard-Risk B-precursor Acute Lymphoblastic Leukemia: A Children's Oncology Group (COG) initiative. *Leukemia* 19:734, 2005.
46. Faderl S, Jeha S, Kantarjian HM: The biology and therapy of adult acute lymphoblastic leukemia. *Cancer* 98:1337, 2003.
47. Graux C, Cools J, Michaux L, et al: Cytogenetics and molecular genetics of T-cell acute lymphoblastic leukemia: From thymocyte to lymphoblast. *Leukemia* 20:1496, 2006.
48. Caporaso N, Goldin L, Plass C, et al: Chronic lymphocytic leukaemia genetics overview. *Br J Haematol* 139:630, 2007.
49. Zenz T, Mertens D, Dohner H, et al: Molecular diagnostics in chronic lymphocytic leukemia—Pathogenetic and clinical implications. *Leuk Lymphoma* 49:864, 2008.
50. Crespo M, Bosch F, Villamor N, et al: ZAP-70 expression as a surrogate for immunoglobulin-variable-region mutations in chronic lymphocytic leukemia. *N Engl J Med* 348:1764, 2003.
51. Morilla A, Gonzalez de Castro D, Del Giudice I, et al: Combinations of ZAP-70, CD38 and IGHV mutational status as predictors of time to first treatment in CLL. *Leuk Lymphoma* 49:2108, 2008.
52. Campbell LJ: Cytogenetics of lymphomas. *Pathology* 37:493, 2005.
53. Lenz G, Wright GW, Emre NC, et al: Molecular subtypes of diffuse large B-cell lymphoma arise by distinct genetic pathways. *Proc Natl Acad Sci U S A* 105:13520, 2008.
54. Haralambieva E, Boerma EJ, van Imhoff GW, et al: Clinical, immunophenotypic, and genetic analysis of adult lymphomas with morphologic features of Burkitt lymphoma. *Am J Surg Pathol* 29:1086, 2005.
55. Viardot A, Barth TF, Moller P, et al: Cytogenetic evolution of follicular lymphoma. *Semin Cancer Biol* 13:183, 2003.
56. Bertoni F, Zucca E, Cotter FE: Molecular basis of mantle cell lymphoma. *Br J Haematol* 124:130, 2004.
57. Chng WJ, Glebov O, Bergsagel PL, et al: Genetic events in the pathogenesis of multiple myeloma. *Best Pract Res Clin Haematol* 20:571, 2007.
58. Pasqualucci L, Migliazza A, Basso K, et al: Mutations of the BCL6 proto-oncogene disrupt its negative autoregulation in diffuse large B-cell lymphoma. *Blood* 101:2914, 2003.
59. Starostik P, Patzner J, Greiner A, et al: Gastric marginal zone B-cell lymphomas of MALT type develop along 2 distinct pathogenetic pathways. *Blood* 99:3, 2002.
60. Chiarle R, Voena C, Ambrogio C, et al: The anaplastic lymphoma kinase in the pathogenesis of cancer. *Nat Rev Cancer* 8:11, 2008.
61. Shaughnessy JD Jr, Zhan F, Burington BE, et al: A validated gene expression model of high-risk multiple myeloma is defined by deregulated expression of genes mapping to chromosome 1. *Blood* 109:2276, 2007.
62. Rasmussen T, Kuehl M, Lodahl M, et al: Possible roles for activating RAS mutations in the MGUS to MM transition and in the intramedullary to extramedullary transition in some plasma cell tumors. *Blood* 105:317, 2005.

CHAPTER 12
APOPTOSIS

Roberta A. Gottlieb

SUMMARY

Apoptosis is a term originally coined by Wyllie, Kerr, and Currie to describe a form of cell death characterized by cell shrinkage and nuclear condensation, and is derived from the Greek term for the shedding of leaves or petals. This physiologic, tightly regulated process is initiated by eukaryotic cells in response to internal or external cues. Apoptosis occurs in all multicellular organisms as the means to balance cell proliferation in continuously renewing tissues in order to maintain a constant organ size, and to eliminate cells that are unneeded, or defective. In the hematopoietic system, cell production is delicately balanced against cell death and removal through the monocyte–macrophage system. A panoply of cytokines and growth factors regulate cell survival, proliferation, and apoptosis. Stem cell factor, Flt ligand, erythropoietin, thrombopoietin, granulocyte colony-stimulating factor (G-CSF), granulocyte-macrophage colony-stimulating factor (GM-CSF), interleukin (IL)-3, IL-5, IL-6, IL-7, and IL-11, amongst others, variably suppress apoptosis and stimulate cell cycling. Tumor necrosis factor-α, Fas ligand, tumor necrosis factor-related apoptosis-inducing ligand, and interferon-γ promote apoptosis of cells expressing the appropriate receptors. Failure of apoptosis leads to tumorigenesis, and many oncogenes and tumor suppressors regulate apoptosis, including p53 and c-myc.

Apoptosis, a term coined by Wyllie, Kerr, and Currie,[1] occurs at defined times and locations during development, thus earning it the name *programmed cell death*.[2] It is a critical process during embryogenesis, where tissue remodeling requires highly regulated cell death. For example, programmed cell death takes place during the elimination of interdigital webs in mammalian development, and in the regression of the tadpole's tail as it develops into a frog. Three of the most important genes that control apoptosis were first identified through detailed studies of development in the nematode *Caenorhabditis elegans*. Two of them, designated *C. elegans* death *(ced)-3* and *ced-4*, are essential for programmed cell death to occur, and one gene, *ced-9*, is essential for opposing cell death.[3,4] These genes were subsequently found to be conserved throughout evolution and are represented by large families of mammalian homologues. Ced-3 is a cysteine protease with the unusual characteristic of cleaving peptides after aspartic acid residues. The first mammalian homologue of Ced-3 to be identified was interleukin-1β–converting enzyme (ICE). Subsequently, a family of more than 10 related cysteine proteases ("death proteases") was identified; they are designated caspases, for cysteine aspartases.[5] The nematode death gene, *ced-4*, encodes a protein that controls the activation of the caspase, ced-3.

Abbreviations and acronyms that appear in this chapter include: AML: acute myelogenous leukemia; Apaf-1, apoptotic peptidase-activating factor 1; Bak, Bcl-2 homologous antagonist killer; Bax, Bcl-2–associated X protein; B-CLL, B-cell chronic lymphocytic leukemia; Bcl, B-cell lymphoma; BH, Bcl-2 homology; Bid, BH3 interacting domain death agonist; ced, *Caenorhabditis elegans* death; CML, chronic myelogenous leukemia; CrmA, cowpox response-modifier protein A; FADD, Fas-associated death domain; IAP, inhibitor of apoptosis protein; ICE, interleukin-1β-converting enzyme; IL, interleukin; TNF, tumor necrosis factor.

Ced-4 is, in turn, regulated through interaction with ced-9.[6] Apoptotic peptidase activating factor 1 (Apaf-1) is the mammalian homologue of ced-4. B-cell lymphoma (Bcl)-2 is the mammalian homologue of the antiapoptosis gene, *ced-9*, and was first identified as an oncogene created by a chromosomal 8;14 translocation in B-cell lymphoma.[7] Studies of the mammalian homologues of the *C. elegans* death genes have led to an understanding of the critical elements of the "death machinery" of apoptosis.

FEATURES OF PROGRAMMED CELL DEATH

Mitochondrial alterations, caspase activation, and chromatin fragmentation are among the key events that characterize apoptosis. Upon initiation of the death program, cells undergo dramatic volume loss, membrane blebbing, cytoplasmic acidification, rearrangement of the cytoskeleton, and loss of contact with adjacent cells and extracellular matrix. Cells exhibit disordered ion homeostasis characterized by diminished proton elimination (and/or increased proton production), and volume loss accomplished largely through potassium and chloride efflux, which is accompanied by water loss. Calcium homeostasis is also disturbed, because mitochondrial sequestration of calcium is impaired. Membrane blebbing and phosphatidylserine externalization are attributed to proteolytic cleavage of the membrane cytoskeletal protein fodrin (a spectrin homologue) and to activation of the phospholipid scramblase, which is activated by low pH and elevated calcium levels. Cytoskeletal alterations are partly caused by proteolytic cleavage of actin, as well as by changes in the activity of kinases and G proteins that regulate the state of assembly of cytoskeletal components. A variety of signaling pathways that participate in survival signaling are proteolytically inactivated.[8]

The cell is marked for ingestion by neighboring cells or professional phagocytes through the upregulation of certain adhesion markers and through scramblase-mediated externalization of phosphatidylserine. In the intact organism, apoptotic cells are removed before membrane integrity is lost, thereby preventing spillage of cellular contents. The magnitude and efficiency of this clearance process is exemplified by the clearance of inflammatory cells during the resolution of pneumonia.[9]

■ MITOCHONDRIAL ALTERATIONS

In addition to their role in ATP production, the mitochondria play a key role in the regulation of apoptosis. The mitochondria are complex organelles consisting of an outer membrane, an inner membrane, an intermembrane space, and the matrix, which is enclosed by the inner membrane. The outer membrane is highly permeable to small molecules, which can transit through voltage-dependent anion channel, the highly abundant porin. The antiapoptotic Bcl-2 family members may limit ATP hydrolysis in mitochondria by regulating outer membrane permeability to adenine nucleotides through voltage-dependent anion channel.[10,11] Sequestered in the space between the inner and outer mitochondrial membranes are Smac/DIABLO (second mitochondrial activator of caspases/direct inhibitor of apoptosis protein binding protein with a low isoelectric point), a factor that relieves the inhibition of caspases by inhibitor of apoptosis protein (IAP); Omi/HtrA2, a serine protease that may also interact with IAPs; and apoptosis-inducing factor and endonuclease G, both of which promote DNA fragmentation and chromatin condensation; and cytochrome *c*, which is a cofactor for caspase activation.[12]

The release of these proapoptotic factors from the mitochondria is regulated by members of the Bcl-2 family, some of which oppose apoptosis while others promote it. In general, their function is to regulate

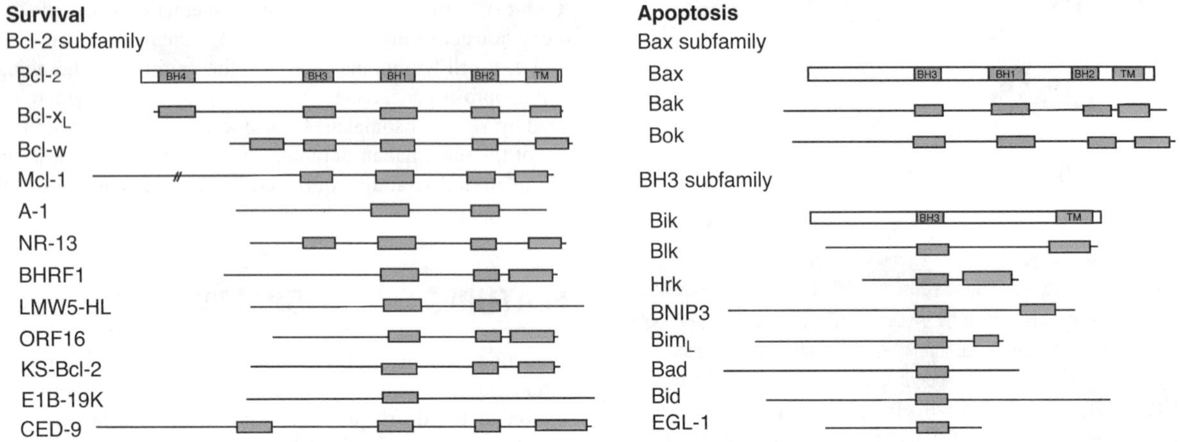

FIGURE 12–1. Bcl-2 family members and their role in apoptosis regulation. Bcl-2 homology (BH) domains represent conserved sequences among family members. *TM* designates the transmembrane domain. The Bcl-2 subfamily promotes cell survival. Proapoptotic members are grouped into the Bax subfamily and the BH3 subfamily, which has high sequence divergence outside the BH3 domain. *(Adapted from Adams JM, Cory S,[58] with permission.)*

mitochondrial outer membrane permeability. The Bcl-2 family members have in common up to four regions of homology, termed Bcl-2 homology (BH) domains. In general, antiapoptotic Bcl-2 family members possess all four BH domains, whereas proapoptotic Bcl-2–associated X protein (Bax) and Bcl-2 homologous antagonist killer (Bak) lack BH domain 4 (BH4). Another subset of proapoptotic members share homology only in the BH3 domain, including BH3 interacting domain death agonist (Bid), Bcl-2-associated death promoter (Bad), and Bim. Apoptosis is regulated by interactions between Bcl-2 (or other antiapoptotic family members) and Bax or Bak. The BH3-only proteins signal apoptosis by interacting with Bcl-2 (thereby liberating Bax/Bak to promote apoptosis), or by directly activating Bax/Bak. Bcl-2, which opposes apoptosis, is able to prevent the release of cytochrome *c* from mitochondria, while the proapoptotic Bax promotes cytochrome *c* release.[13,14] Proteolytic processing of Bid or dephosphorylation of Bad results in its translocation to the mitochondria, where it causes cytochrome *c* release. Bax also translocates from cytosol to mitochondria during apoptosis. Because these molecules bear structural similarity to the pore-forming colicins, much attention has been directed toward their potential role as pore formers in the outer mitochondrial membrane. Bcl-2 family members and their function (pro- or antiapoptotic) are shown in Figure 12–1 and reviewed in reference 15.

CASPASE ACTIVATION

The caspases can be grouped into three functional categories. The first group includes ICE (also designated caspase-1) and two related caspases: caspase-4 and caspase-5. Although ICE primarily participates in cytokine processing, the roles of the other members of this group are not clear. The second group consists of the effector caspases, such as caspase-3, which possess a short prodomain (<3 kDa). The effector caspases are responsible for cleaving many of the important intracellular protein substrates that are degraded during apoptosis.[16] The third, and perhaps most interesting, group includes the signaling caspases, which possess a large prodomain. Most cells express multiple caspases, probably related to the observed redundancy in pathways that initiate cell death; it also appears that the caspases may work in a cascade fashion, perhaps analogous to the amplification seen in the coagulation system. Figure 12–2 diagrams the caspase family.

Caspases are synthesized as proenzymes with an amino-terminal prodomain that is removed by proteolytic processing. The enzyme is further processed into large (~20 kDa) and small (~10 kDa) fragments that form a heterodimer. Two heterodimers assemble to form the active tetrameric protease (Fig. 12–3). Caspases are capable of autoprocessing under certain circumstances. Although effector caspases are dependent on proteolytic activation, the signaling caspases are dependent on interaction with a cofactor, as exemplified by the interaction of caspase-9 with Apaf-1.[17]

Activation of caspases may be accomplished through multiple pathways, two of which have been worked out in detail (Fig. 12–4). The receptor-mediated pathway involves a cell surface receptor, such as Fas or the receptor for tumor necrosis factor (TNF)-α. Occupancy of the receptor with its ligand causes recruitment of a cytosolic adapter molecule containing a protein-protein interaction region termed the death domain. The adapter molecule (e.g., Fas-associated death domain [FADD] or tumor necrosis factor receptor-associated death domain) then recruits a signaling procaspase such as caspase-8 or caspase-10 that docks with the adapter molecule and undergoes proximity-induced processing. Caspase-8 or caspase-10 may directly activate caspase-3 and related effector caspases. It may be possible to target these so-called death receptors for anticancer therapy.[18]

An alternative pathway exists involving activation of caspase-9 through interaction of Apaf-1, which must bind cytochrome *c* and deoxyadenosine

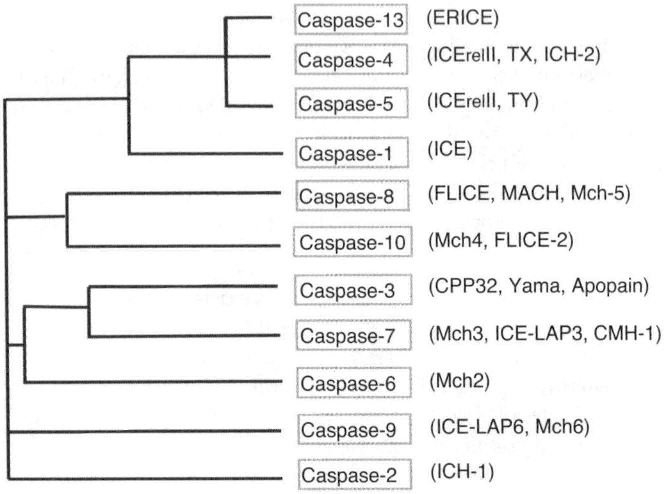

FIGURE 12–2. Phylogenetic tree for the caspase family. Caspase designations and their aliases are shown. *(Adapted from Wang Y, Gu X,[59] with permission.)*

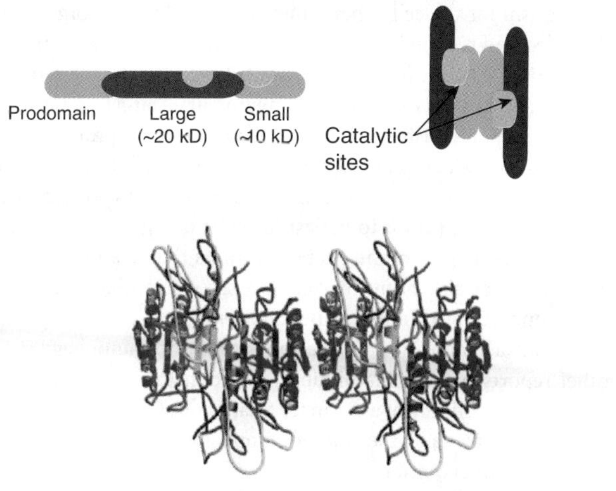

FIGURE 12–3. Diagram of caspase processing and assembly. Members of the cysteine aspartate protease (caspase) family are characterized by an amino-terminal prodomain (*hatched area*) and a catalytic domain (*dotted area*), which is processed by cleavage after Asp residues to release large (~20 kDa) and small (~10 kDa) subunits. The two fragments assemble into a heterodimer. Two heterodimers form a tetramer in the active form of the caspase. A stereo pair image of the crystal structure of a typical caspase is shown. *(Reprinted with permission from Riedl SJ, Fuentes-Prior P, Renatus M, et al.[60])*

triphosphate or ATP (Fig. 12–5).[19] Apaf-1, which has homology to ced-4, is present in the cytosol and inactive until cytochrome *c* is available for interaction. It possesses a caspase activation and recruitment domain that is essential for its function. This pathway is termed the intrinsic or mitochondrial pathway because it depends upon the release of cytochrome *c* from the mitochondria. Bcl-2 family members regulate mitochondrial outer membrane permeability and release of cytochrome *c*. However, there is crosstalk with the death receptor pathway, as caspase-8 can proteolytically activate Bid, leading to cytochrome *c* release.[20]

Cytotoxic T lymphocytes inject granzyme B into cells to trigger apoptosis. Granzyme B is a serine protease that cleaves caspases after Asp residues to generate active caspases. The introduction of granzyme B into the cytosol of target cells results in the rapid activation of caspase-3 and subsequent cell death. Granzyme B also cleaves Bid to an active fragment, thereby triggering the mitochondrial pathway. Cytotoxic T lymphocytes are protected from their own granzyme B by expression of a serpin (serine protease inhibitor protein), and adenovirus type 5 also encodes an inhibitor of granzyme B, thereby allowing escape from this mechanism of immune surveillance.[21]

It is generally believed that activation of proteases constitutes an irreversible event and that the caspases are the ultimate effectors of apoptotic cell destruction. However, inhibition of caspases may not always prevent cell death. There are also conditions in which caspase activation functions in a physiologic (nonapoptotic) role. For example, caspase-3 is activated in a subset of T cells and participates in processing of interleukin (IL)-16 without leading to apoptosis, and caspase-1 processes IL-1β.[22]

NUCLEAR ALTERATIONS

The classic histologic manifestations of apoptosis are the condensation of nuclear chromatin and fragmentation of the nucleus. DNA condensation and classic apoptotic body formation depend on proteolysis of lamin by one or more caspases.[23] DNA digestion is accomplished by several distinct endonucleases, eventually resulting in fragments representing multiples of the approximately 200-bp nucleosome (the so-called nucleosomal ladder). The search for the responsible endonucleases has yielded several candidates, including DNase I and DNase II. DNA fragmentation factor consists of a 40-kDa caspase-activated DNase bound to its 45-kDa inhibitor. Cleavage of caspase-activated DNase releases it from caspase-activated DNase inhibitor, thereby enabling it to function as an endonuclease.[24] Apoptosis-inducing factor and endonuclease G can also mediate DNA fragmentation. Although DNA fragmentation is commonly observed in apoptosis, it is not an essential feature.

In addition to the characteristic morphologic changes in the nucleus, it is possible to detect DNA fragmentation using a histologic method known as ***terminal deoxynucleotidyl transferase deoxyuridine triphosphate nick-end labeling***, in which labeled deoxynucleotides are incorporated into nuclear DNA at sites of nicking. The incorporated nucleotides are then detected using conventional histochemical staining or fluorescence detection. This method is widely used to detect DNA fragmentation in tissue sections and in cell suspensions evaluated by flow cytometry. DNA fragmentation is also reflected by a subdiploid DNA content.

ENDOGENOUS PREVENTION OF APOPTOSIS

Cells have evolved a variety of safeguards to prevent inappropriate apoptosis. Viruses have also exploited these safeguards to prevent the cell from undergoing apoptosis in response to the presence of the virus. Bcl-2, which opposes apoptosis, has corresponding viral homologues, including E1B-19K. The cell also has IAPs, which bind to caspases and inhibit their activity. The cowpox response-modifier protein A (CrmA) is a viral gene product that performs the same function. Transcriptional

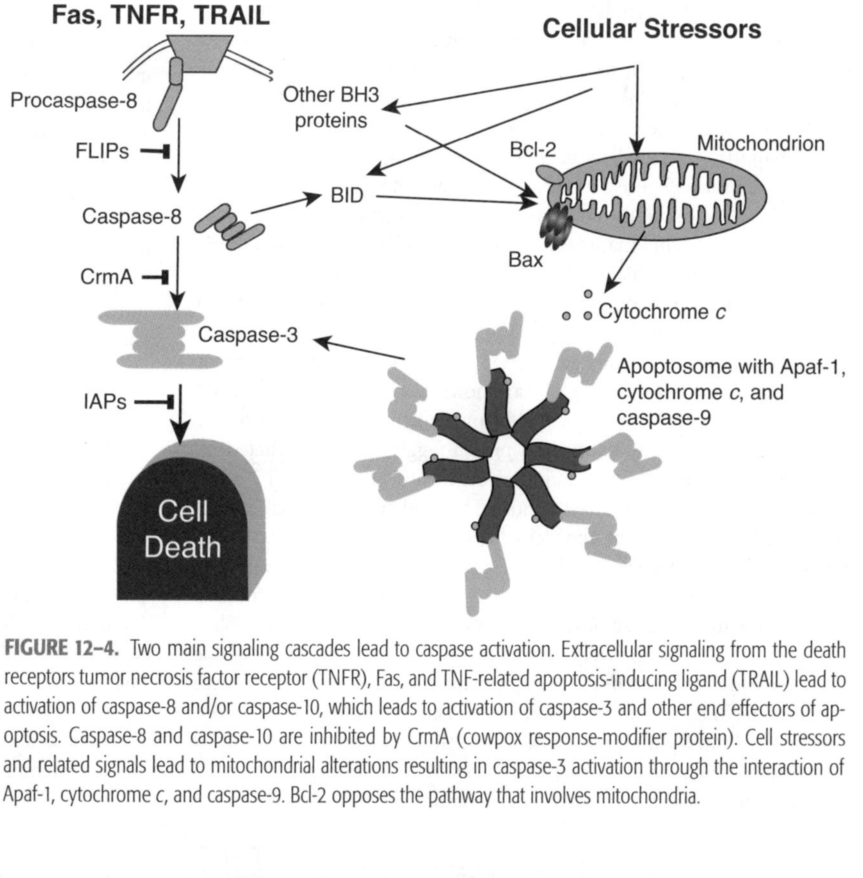

FIGURE 12–4. Two main signaling cascades lead to caspase activation. Extracellular signaling from the death receptors tumor necrosis factor receptor (TNFR), Fas, and TNF-related apoptosis-inducing ligand (TRAIL) lead to activation of caspase-8 and/or caspase-10, which leads to activation of caspase-3 and other end effectors of apoptosis. Caspase-8 and caspase-10 are inhibited by CrmA (cowpox response-modifier protein). Cell stressors and related signals lead to mitochondrial alterations resulting in caspase-3 activation through the interaction of Apaf-1, cytochrome *c*, and caspase-9. Bcl-2 opposes the pathway that involves mitochondria.

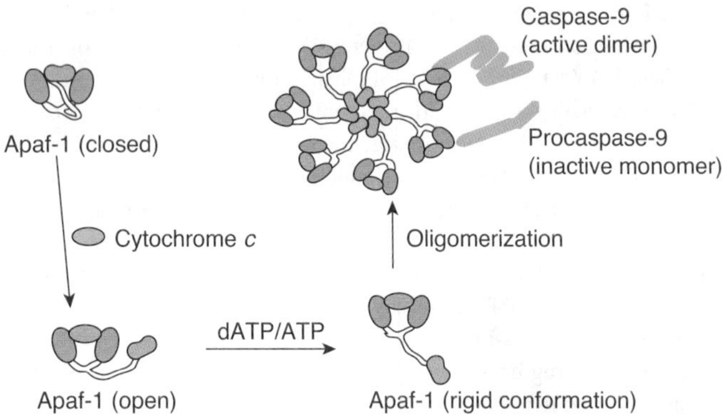

FIGURE 12–5. Model for caspase-9 activation by Apaf-1. In healthy cells, Apaf-1 exists in an autoinhibited conformation (*top left*). In response to an apoptotic signal, cytochrome *c* is released from mitochondria. Cytochrome *c* converts Apaf-1 from a "closed" monomer to an open conformer. The subsequent binding of deoxyadenosine triphosphate (dATP)/ATP results in oligomerization to a heptamer that recruits procaspase-9. An inactive procaspase-9 monomer on one spoke of the apoptosome is presumed to recruit another monomer to create the asymmetric dimer having a single active site. *(Adapted from Acehan D, Jiang X, Morgan DG, et al,[61] with permission.)*

regulation of antiapoptotic genes is mediated in part through nuclear factor-κB, which is mimicked by the viral transcription factor v-Rel.

AUTOPHAGY

MOLECULAR FEATURES

Autophagy is an important factor in determining life span, and is important in handling protein aggregates. It is also critically important in mitochondrial quality control, as it is the mechanism by which damaged mitochondria are eliminated.[25] Autophagy is an intracellular housekeeping process for bulk degradation of proteins and organelles that involves the *de novo* formation of a double-membrane structure that engulfs its target and then routes it to the lysosome, where the contents are proteolytically degraded. The process involves a complex system of proteins involved in membrane trafficking, as well as two enzyme systems resembling ubiquitin ligases. Many of these genes are tightly conserved from yeast to mammals. Figure 12–6 is an abbreviated description of the process, and is reviewed in the context of cancer.[26] Initiation of autophagy is mediated by a protein kinase (Atg1) and the class III phosphatidyl inositol-3 kinase complex which includes Beclin 1. Mutation or inactivation of one allele of *beclin 1* is commonly seen in breast and ovarian cancers, and may occur in other malignancies.[27] Initiation of the double-membrane structure requires autophagy genes Atg5, -7, -12, and -16, while further maturation is mediated by Atg8 (also known as microtubule-associated light chain 3 or LC3) and the oxidation-reduction-sensitive protease Atg4. Recognition of ubiquitinated protein aggregates is mediated by p62, whereas recognition of damaged organelles is mediated by additional factors still under investigation. These adaptor proteins interact with Atg8/LC3 to recruit the cup-shaped phagophore membrane to engulf the target. Once the double-membrane structure encircles its target, the autophagosome is shuttled to the lysosome via microtubules. Thus agents that paralyze or disrupt the microtubule network (vinblastine, nocodazole) will interfere with autophagy. Fusion with the lysosome requires acidification of both compartments and can be prevented with chloroquine or the specific inhibitor of the vacuolar proton pump, Bafilomycin A1. Proteolytic degradation within the lysosome is mediated by cathepsins, which have a pH optimum below 4. Autophagy is induced rapidly under conditions of nutrient limitation and represents a survival mechanism for the cell, where unwanted proteins and organelles can be degraded and recycled for new protein synthesis or as substrates for ATP production. Its close linkage to the nutritional state of the cell is reflected by the fact that it is inhibited by mammalian target of rapamycin and activated by adenosine monophosphate-activated protein kinase. The ability to induce autophagy appears to be beneficial in solid tumors experiencing metabolic stress, as it allows cells at the hypoxic and nutrient-limited core of a tumor to persist for extended periods of time. In contrast (and perhaps more in keeping with its role as a tumor suppressor), autophagy has also been invoked as a second mechanism of cell death, and a number of chemotherapeutic agents have been shown to induce cell death accompanied by the upregulation of autophagy.[28] However, other reports indicate that inhibiting autophagy (e.g., with chloroquine) increases the efficacy of anticancer treatments. Clearly more work is necessary to understand the role of autophagy and the proper context for therapeutic intervention.

Our knowledge of the role of autophagy in the hematopoietic system is at an early stage. However, given its fundamental importance to cellular homeostasis, its role in a myriad of diseases and physiologic processes is likely to be better appreciated in the coming years, particularly as new methods to measure and manipulate the process are introduced.

APOPTOSIS IN THE HEMATOPOIETIC SYSTEM

NEUTROPHILS

Neutrophils are produced and destroyed at extremely high rates, and their elimination is accomplished through apoptosis. Growth factors such as granulocyte-macrophage colony-stimulating factor drive increased neutrophil production but also suppress apoptosis. In the case of mature neutrophils, apoptosis is a default program requiring no new protein synthesis. Excessive neutrophil apoptosis occurs in myelokathexis, a congenital disorder characterized by severe chronic leukopenia and neutropenia. Defective expression of Bcl-x_L has been implicated in this disorder. Excessive apoptosis of myeloid progenitor cells has been described in cyclic neutropenia and severe congenital neutropenia (Kostmann syndrome), as well as in myelokathexis.[29] Increased numbers of autophagosomes are noted during certain phases of the neutropenic cycle.

Delayed neutrophil apoptosis is observed in chronic neutrophilic leukemia and chronic myelogenous leukemia (CML; Chap. 90). Inefficient clearance of apoptotic neutrophils contributes to inflammation in rheumatoid arthritis and systemic lupus erythematosus, and may predispose to formation of autoantibodies against neutrophil granule proteins (antineutrophil cytoplasmic autoantibodies). Certain autoantibodies also induce autophagic cell death. Defective clearance of neutrophils from airways may exacerbate inflammation in cystic fibrosis and bronchiectasis and may permit survival of ingested pathogens.

PLATELETS

Maximal platelet production coincides with the onset of apoptosis in mature megakaryocytes (Chap. 113). However, detailed studies have been hampered by the difficulty of studying megakaryocytes *in vitro*. However, the proapoptotic stimuli nitric oxide and TNF-α trigger platelet production, whereas caspase inhibition or overexpression of antiapoptotic Bcl-x_L block proplatelet formation. The process of platelet formation may require additional coordination, because staurosporine, a kinase inhibitor that triggers apoptosis in a wide range of cell types, causes megakaryocyte apoptosis without proplatelet formation.[30] Platelets, once shed from megakaryocytes, possess mitochondria with normal membrane potential, exhibit normal transbilayer orientation of phosphatidylserine, and lack caspase-9. When deprived of survival fac-

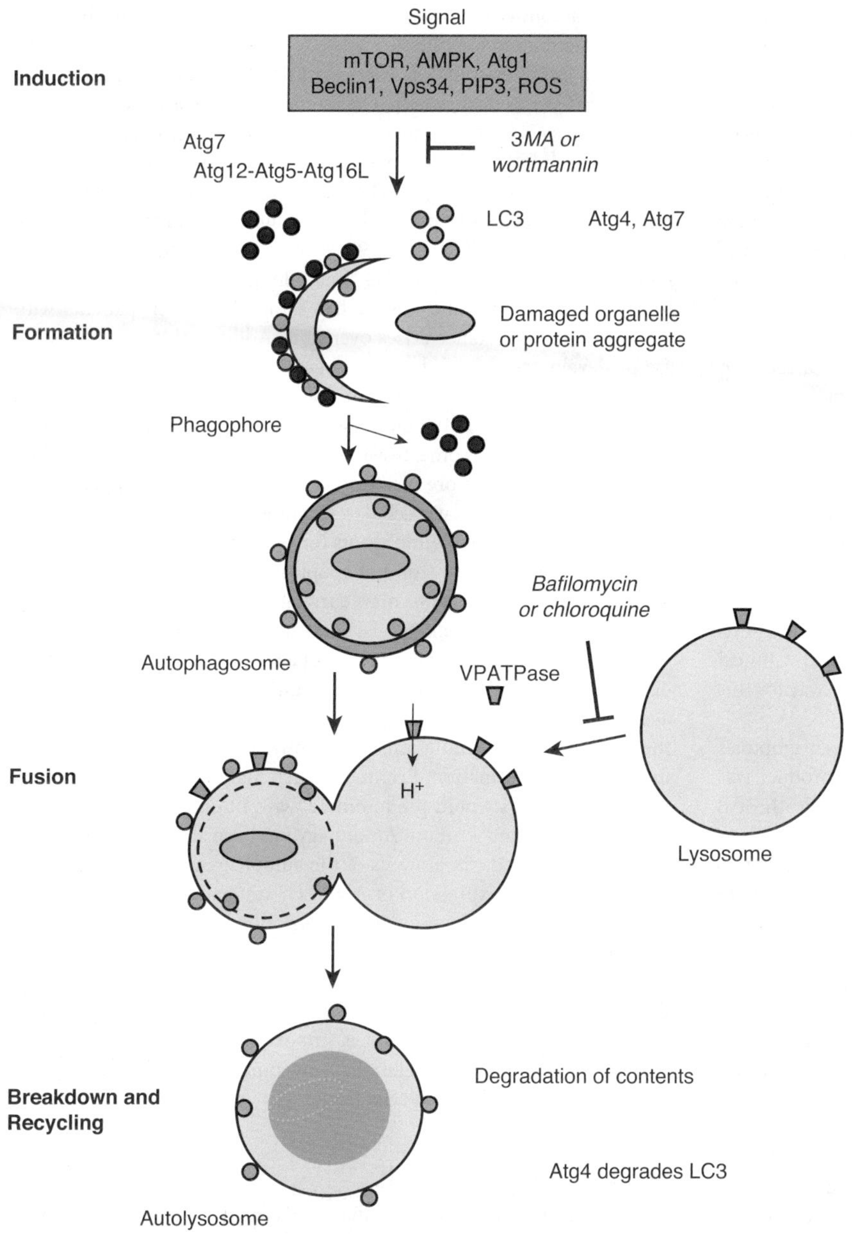

FIGURE 12–6. Key elements of autophagy. Signaling through Beclin1/Vps34, Atg1, energy deprivation, inhibition of mTOR (mammalian target of rapamycin), or reactive oxygen can initiate autophagy. Atg7 conjugates Atg12 onto a lysine residue of Atg5, which complexes with Atg16L. Atg4 activates LC3, which is then conjugated to phosphatidylethanolamine by Atg7. The growing ends of the phagophore engulf a target, then join together to form the autophagosome, which has a double membrane. Acidification is required for fusion with a lysosome, after which acidic hydrolases degrade the contents. The degradation products are then exported out of the autolysosome. AMPK, adenosine monophosphate-activated protein kinase.

tors in plasma, these anucleate cells undergo a form of cell death that is independent of caspases. It has been suggested that megakaryocytes regulate cell death in a localized, organelle-specific fashion.[31]

ERYTHROCYTES

The process of erythrocyte production involves chromatin condensation and removal of the nucleus. This parallel with apoptosis has prompted speculation that erythrocyte maturation and senescence represent "apoptosis in slow motion." In support of that notion, it has been shown that Raf-1 suppresses caspase activation in erythroid progenitors, and that Raf-1 downregulation and caspase activation are required for red cell production.[32] Removal of senescent red cells by the spleen depends on phosphatidylserine externalization (Chap. 32).[33] Erythropoietin, which stimulates erythropoiesis (Chap. 31), prolongs red cell survival by inducing the expression of Bcl-x_L and by inhibiting a volume-sensitive cation channel that activates phosphatidylserine externalization. Elimination of mitochondria from erythroid precursors requires the participation of the BH3-only protein Nix, which triggers mitochondrial depolarization and removal by autophagy.[34]

APOPTOSIS IN HUMAN DISEASE

The occurrence of apoptosis in pathophysiologic settings, or its absence in physiologic settings, results in human disease. More simply, many diseases can be grouped according to whether there is too much apoptosis or too little.

INSUFFICIENT APOPTOSIS

Because apoptosis must occur at defined times during development, a failure of apoptosis to occur in the appropriate settings would be expected to give rise to developmental defects. However, genetically defined abnormalities in known elements of the process of apoptosis have not been identified in human developmental disorders. Some insights have been derived from gene knockout studies in mice. Deletion of the gene encoding caspase-3, arguably the most important death protease, results in mice that die in utero or soon after birth with an excess of brain tissue, owing to a failure of normal programmed cell death during neural development.

In the immune system, deletion of self-reactive T cells is essential to prevent autoimmune disorders.[35] Signaling for lymphocyte deletion is accomplished through engagement of one or more cell surface receptors, including a molecule known as Fas/APO-1/CD95. Engagement of Fas by its ligand results in aggregation of proteins (FADD and caspase-8) through self-association regions known as death domains, culminating in caspase activation and death of the cell. Fas expression on lymphocytes provides a means by which unwanted T cells can be eliminated. Mutation of Fas or its ligand in mice results in a disease that strongly resembles systemic lupus erythematosus. In humans, mutations of Fas occur in the heritable autoimmune lymphoproliferative syndrome, in which CD3+/CD4−/CD8− T cells fail to undergo apoptosis and contribute to autoimmune disease.[36] Many of the cellular proteins that are autoantigens are selectively cleaved by granzyme B to generate unique fragments.[37] Cleavage by granzyme B contributes to the autoantigenic properties of distinct cellular targets in a range of autoimmune disorders including myasthenia gravis, systemic sclerosis, Jo-1 autoantibody-associated myositis, and Sjögren syndrome.

In areas of immune sanctuary, such as the testis, Sertoli cells express high levels of Fas ligand to prevent invading T cells from surviving long enough to mount an immune response against sperm cells (which the body recognizes as foreign). A similar mechanism of protection is involved in limiting inflammatory responses in viral infections in sensitive organs such as the eye. Immune-mediated rejection of transplanted organs rests in part on the induction of apoptosis in the foreign cells. This mechanism has been exploited by genetic manipulation to express Fas ligand on pancreatic islet cells to prevent induction of apoptosis in the transplanted cells, with resulting prolonged survival of the allograft.

A number of viral proteins block apoptosis signaling or effector pathways. Baculovirus p35 and cowpox viral protein CrmA directly inhibit caspases, adenovirus E1B inhibits caspase-3 activation, and herpesvirus-poxvirus caspase-8 inhibitor proteins block downstream death domain signaling. The function of these proteins may be critical to viral virulence by blocking host defense against viral replication; infected cells engage the apoptotic machinery and mark themselves for phagocytic ingestion, thus limiting the extent of viral infection. Numerous Bcl-2 homologues have been identified in γ-herpesviruses, thus explaining their persistence and propensity for malignant transformation.[38]

Polycythemia vera is characterized by an abnormal clone of hematopoietic cells that are hypersensitive to growth factors such as erythropoietin (Chap. 86). These clonal cells overexpress Bcl-x_L, which prevents apoptosis and may contribute to the survival of erythroid progenitors in the absence of erythropoietin. Most patients with polycythemia vera have a somatic gain-of-function mutation of Janus kinase 2, which initiates anti-apoptotic signaling, including upregulation of Bcl-x_L. Clinical trials with Janus kinase 2 (JAK2) kinase inhibitors are under way for this and other myeloproliferative disorders.[39]

Tumor growth rate is determined by the imbalance between apoptosis and mitosis. For example, the function of the Bcl-2 gene product was discovered because its overexpression prevents the normal death of B cells, leading to a lymphoma associated with a normal rate of proliferation but reduced apoptosis.[40] Epstein-Barr virus encodes at least two Bcl-2 homologues and is associated with Burkitt lymphoma, Hodgkin lymphoma, AIDS-related lymphoma, and nasopharyngeal carcinoma. Human herpesvirus 8 expresses a Bcl-2 homologue and is associated with AIDS-related Kaposi sarcoma. A malignant cell may arise when a cell fails to undergo apoptosis when it should have. Loss of a necessary growth factor or removal from the normal extracellular matrix should trigger a cell to commit suicide. If, however, the cell fails to die, it may survive and proliferate sufficiently for its progeny to acquire other mutations, including loss of p53 and activation of other oncogenes. Thus, the first step in oncogenesis may be a failure of apoptosis. The tumor-suppressor p53 gene product is a transcription factor activated by DNA damage to induce a family of p53-dependent genes that regulate the cell cycle and induce apoptosis through a mitochondrial-dependent pathway.[41] However, it has been recognized that mitochondria may regulate the activity of p53.[42] Although mutations of p53 have been found in many malignant tumors and in some families with hereditary cancer syndromes, it is mutated in less than 20 percent of hematologic malignancies, most commonly in acute myelogenous leukemia (AML; Chap. 89), myelodysplastic syndrome (Chap. 88), and CML (Chap. 90) in blast crisis.[43] This suggests that p53 is a relatively weak apoptosis regulator in myeloid cells, or that other signaling pathways in hematopoietic cells can override p53-mediated death signals. However, given the central importance of p53 inactivation in many cancers, considerable work is focused on strategies to restore p53 function.[44,45]

In B-cell chronic lymphocytic leukemia (B-CLL), small mature B cells accumulate as a result of diminished apoptosis. In part this is mediated through an autocrine loop involving survival factors of the tumor necrosis factor family, such as B-cell activation factor. These autocrine factors are secreted by B cells and bind to their receptors to suppress apoptosis, drive proliferation, and increase resistance to chemotherapeutic drugs.[46] Disruption of this autocrine loop may represent an effective therapeutic approach in B-CLL, certain B-cell lymphomas, and some autoimmune disorders including systemic lupus erythematosus and rheumatoid arthritis.[47]

Modulation of apoptosis is widely considered a key target for cancer therapy. Efforts to decrease their resistance to apoptosis are directed at targets such as Bcl-2 family members, mitochondria, or the death receptors.[18,48,49] Inhibition of survival signaling through phosphatidyl inositol 3-kinases is at an early stage.[50] These avenues have been accelerated as a result of the success of tyrosine kinase inhibitors, which were initially developed to target CML (Chap. 90).[51] In CML the activity of the BCR-ABL oncogene prevents apoptosis. Imatinib mesylate, a potent inhibitor of the BCR-ABL tyrosine kinase, has shown benefit in patients with CML; however, resistance arises over time. Additional kinase inhibitors are in development, and the range of indications is expanding. Resistance to imatinib arises as the result of a variety of cellular alterations, including the induction of autophagy, and inhibition of autophagy with chloroquine can overcome resistance.[52] Although malignant cells are generally considered more resistant to the induction of apoptosis, they still possess the necessary cellular machinery and, when exposed to appropriate chemotherapeutic agents (or radiation), usually die by apoptosis, not necrosis.[53] Evaluation of apoptosis and autophagy in response to chemotherapeutic agents may correlate with prognosis and might eventually direct the selection of agents on an individualized basis.

One hypothesis about mechanisms of aging is that too little apoptosis occurs, permitting the survival of cells that have sustained DNA damage. Such damaged cells would function inefficiently at best, owing to the accumulation of mutations in essential genes, and could undergo malignant transformation. Eventually, such marginally functioning and precancerous cells would predominate, with more generalized cellular dysfunction as time went on. Autophagy has been strongly linked to life span. Rate-limiting components of the autophagy machinery diminish with age, and overexpression of Atg8/LC3 can extend life span considerably in lower life forms.[54] Caloric restriction and agents that activate sirtuins (such as resveratrol) may extend life span through the upregulation of autophagy.[55] Impaired autophagy is accompanied by the development of aggregopathies, DNA damage, heart failure, and shortened life span. In this regard, it is important to note that the caloric excess that accompanies metabolic syndrome will suppress autophagy in most tissues and could accelerate aging.

EXCESSIVE APOPTOSIS

Excessive cell death is of particular concern in organs that are populated by terminally differentiated, nondividing cells. Any cells lost, whether by apoptosis or necrosis, are irreplaceable. In settings where cell death is inevitable, inhibiting the enzymatic processes of apoptosis may not salvage the cell but may merely convert its demise to a necrotic form. However, if a cell is damaged beyond repair, a tidy, noninflammatory apoptotic death may still be preferable, avoiding collateral damage from inflammation.

Excessive apoptosis is now being recognized in a variety of hematopoietic disorders. Megaloblastic anemia as a result of deficiency of folate or vitamin B_{12} is characterized by ineffective erythropoiesis with increased early erythrocyte progenitors and failure to mature into reticulocytes (Chap. 41). Animal studies reveal that folate deficiency results in insufficient purines for DNA synthesis, and mismatch repair is affected early, leading to apoptosis.[56]

In some cases, excessive apoptosis may be a result of unavailability of a necessary growth factor, an inability to respond to the growth factor, or alterations in the balance of proapoptotic and antiapoptotic Bcl-2 family members. The myelodysplastic syndromes (Chap. 88), which are characterized by peripheral cytopenias and (at least in the early stages) marrow hypercellularity, are associated with defects in DNA repair or cell-cycle regulation. They are also associated with excessive apoptosis throughout myeloid differentiation, resulting in ineffective myelopoiesis. Stromal cells also show increased apoptosis. In the natural course of the disease, apoptosis-resistant clones eventually emerge, with concomitant progression to AML. Therapeutic approaches include promoting differentiation, modulating the immune system, increasing cell survival in the early phase, and promoting apoptosis in the late phase.[57] Fanconi anemia is accompanied by increased susceptibility to apoptosis mediated by Fas and TNF-α (Chap. 34). It seems likely that additional myeloid disorders will be recognized to possess abnormalities in apoptosis.

REFERENCES

1. Wyllie AH, Kerr JFR, Currie AR: Cell death: The significance of apoptosis. *Int Rev Cytol* 68:251, 1980.
2. Wickremasinghe RG, Hoffbrand AV: Biochemical and genetic control of apoptosis: Relevance to normal hematopoiesis and hematological malignancies. *Blood* 93:3587, 1999.
3. Ellis HM, Horvitz HR: Genetic control of programmed cell death in the nematode *C. elegans*. *Cell* 44:817, 1986.
4. Metzstein MM, Stanfield GM, Horvitz HR: Genetics of programmed cell death in *C. elegans*: Past, present and future. *Trends Genet* 14:410, 1998.
5. Alnemri ES, Livingston DJ, Nicholson DW, et al: Human ICE/CED-3 protease nomenclature [letter to the editor]. *Cell* 87:171, 1996.
6. Putcha GV, Johnson EM Jr: Men are but worms: Neuronal cell death in *C. elegans* and vertebrates. *Cell Death Differ* 11:38, 2004.
7. Korsmeyer SJ: Chromosomal translocations in lymphoid malignancies reveal novel protooncogenes. *Annu Rev Immunol* 10:785, 1992.
8. Wolf BB, Green DR: Suicidal tendencies: Apoptotic cell death by caspase family proteinases. *J Biol Chem* 274:20049, 1999.
9. Savill J, Haslett C: Granulocyte clearance by apoptosis in the resolution of inflammation. *Semin Cell Biol* 6:385, 1995.
10. McClintock DS, Santore MT, Lee VY, et al: Bcl-2 family members and functional electron transport chain regulate oxygen deprivation-induced cell death. *Mol Cell Biol* 22:94, 2002.
11. Steenbergen C, Das S, Su J, et al: Cardioprotection and altered mitochondrial adenine nucleotide transport. *Basic Res Cardiol* 104:149, 2009.
12. Festjens N, van Gurp M, van Loo G, et al: Bcl-2 family members as sentinels of cellular integrity and role of mitochondrial intermembrane space proteins in apoptotic cell death. *Acta Haematol* 111:7, 2004.
13. Kluck RM, Bossy-Wetzel E, Green DR, Newmeyer DD: The release of cytochrome c from mitochondria: A primary site for Bcl-2 regulation of apoptosis. *Science* 275:1132, 1997.
14. Yang J, Liu X, Bhalla K, et al: Prevention of apoptosis by Bcl-2: Release of cytochrome c from mitochondria blocked. *Science* 275:1129, 1997.
15. Susnow N, Zeng L, Margineantu D, Hockenbery DM: Bcl-2 family proteins as regulators of oxidative stress. *Semin Cancer Biol* 19:42, 2009.
16. Tewari M, Quan LT, O'Rourke K, et al: Yama/CPP32 beta, a mammalian homolog of CED-3, is a CrmA-inhibitable protease that cleaves the death substrate poly(ADP-ribose) polymerase. *Cell* 81:801, 1995.
17. Salvesen GS, Riedl SJ: Caspase mechanisms. *Adv Exp Med Biol* 615:13, 2008.
18. Papenfuss K, Cordier SM, Walczak H: Death receptors as targets for anti-cancer therapy. *J Cell Mol Med* 12:2566, 2008.
19. Li P, Nijhawan D, Budihardjo I, et al: Cytochrome c and dATP-dependent formation of Apaf-1/Caspase-9 complex initiates an apoptotic protease cascade. *Cell* 91:479, 1997.
20. Yin XM: Bid, a BH3-only multi-functional molecule, is at the cross road of life and death. *Gene* 369:7, 2006.
21. Chavez-Galan L, Arenas-Del Angel MC, Zenteno E, et al: Cell death mechanisms induced by cytotoxic lymphocytes. *Cell Mol Immunol* 6:15, 2009.
22. Franchi L, Eigenbrod T, Munoz-Planillo R, Nunez G: The inflammasome: A caspase-1-activation platform that regulates immune responses and disease pathogenesis. *Nat Immunol* 10:241, 2009.
23. Lazebnik YA, Takahashi A, Moir RD, et al: Studies of the lamin proteinase reveal multiple parallel biochemical pathways during apoptotic execution. *Proc Natl Acad Sci U S A* 92:9042, 1995.
24. Sakahira H, Enari M, Nagata S: Cleavage of CAD inhibitor in CAD activation and DNA degradation during apoptosis [see comments]. *Nature* 391:96, 1998.
25. Twig G, Elorza A, Molina AJ, et al: Fission and selective fusion govern mitochondrial segregation and elimination by autophagy. *EMBO J* 27:433, 2008.
26. Kondo Y, Kondo S: Autophagy and cancer therapy. *Autophagy* 2:85, 2006.
27. Shi YH, Ding ZB, Zhou J, Qiu SJ, Fan J: Prognostic significance of beclin 1-dependent apoptotic activity in hepatocellular carcinoma. *Autophagy* 5:380, 2009.
28. Chen N, Karantza-Wadsworth V: Role and regulation of autophagy in cancer. *Biochim Biophys Acta* 1793:1516, 2009.
29. Carlsson G, Aprikyan AA, Tehranchi R, et al: Kostmann syndrome: Severe congenital neutropenia associated with defective expression of Bcl-2, constitutive mitochondrial release of cytochrome c, and excessive apoptosis of myeloid progenitor cells. *Blood* 103:3355, 2004.
30. de Botton S, Sabri S, Daugas E, et al: Platelet formation is the consequence of caspase activation within megakaryocytes. *Blood* 100:1310, 2002.
31. Kaluzhny Y, Ravid K: Role of apoptotic processes in platelet biogenesis. *Acta Haematol* 111:67, 2004.
32. Kolbus A, Pilat S, Husak Z, et al: Raf-1 antagonizes erythroid differentiation by restraining caspase activation. *J Exp Med* 196:1347, 2002.
33. Boas FE, Forman L, Beutler E: Phosphatidylserine exposure and red cell viability in red cell aging and in hemolytic anemia. *Proc Natl Acad Sci U S A* 95:3077, 1998.
34. Chen M, Sandoval H, Wang J: Selective mitochondrial autophagy during erythroid maturation. *Autophagy* 4:926, 2008.
35. Los M, Wesselborg S, Schulze-Osthoff K: The role of caspases in development, immunity, and apoptotic signal transduction: Lessons from knockout mice. *Immunity* 10:629, 1999.
36. Fleisher TA: The autoimmune lymphoproliferative syndrome: An experiment of nature involving lymphocyte apoptosis. *Immunol Res* 40:87, 2008.
37. Casciola-Rosen L, Miagkov A, Nagaraju K, et al: Granzyme B: Evidence for a role in the origin of myasthenia gravis. *J Neuroimmunol* 201–202:33, 2008.
38. Ivanovska I, Galonek HL, Hildeman DA, Hardwick JM: Regulation of cell death in the lymphoid system by Bcl-2 family proteins. *Acta Haematol* 111:42, 2004.
39. Pardanani A: JAK2 inhibitor therapy in myeloproliferative disorders: Rationale, preclinical studies and ongoing clinical trials. *Leukemia* 22:23, 2008.
40. Hockenbery D, Nunez G, Milliman C, et al: Bcl-2 is an inner mitochondrial membrane protein that blocks programmed cell death. *Nature* 348:334, 1990.
41. el-Deiry WS: Regulation of p53 downstream genes. *Semin Cancer Biol* 8:345, 1998.
42. Holley AK, St Clair DK: Watching the watcher: Regulation of p53 by mitochondria. *Future Oncol* 5:117, 2009.
43. Boyapati A, Kanbe E, Zhang DE: p53 alterations in myeloid leukemia. *Acta Haematol* 111:100, 2004.
44. Lu C, El-Deiry WS: Targeting p53 for enhanced radio- and chemo-sensitivity. *Apoptosis* 14:597, 2009.
45. Bell HS, Ryan KM: Targeting the p53 family for cancer therapy: "Big brother" joins the fight. *Cell Cycle* 6:1995, 2007.
46. Kern C, Cornuel JF, Billard C, et al: Involvement of BAFF and APRIL in the resistance to apoptosis of B-CLL through an autocrine pathway. *Blood* 103:679, 2004.
47. Sun J, Lin Z, Feng J, et al: BAFF-targeting therapy, a promising strategy for treating autoimmune diseases. *Eur J Pharmacol* 597:1, 2008.
48. Gogvadze V, Orrenius S, Zhivotovsky B: Mitochondria as targets for chemotherapy. *Apoptosis* 14:624, 2009.
49. Kang MH, Reynolds CP: Bcl-2 inhibitors: Targeting mitochondrial apoptotic pathways in cancer therapy. *Clin Cancer Res* 15:1126, 2009.
50. Maira SM, Stauffer F, Schnell C, Garcia-Echeverria C: PI3K inhibitors for cancer treatment: where do we stand? *Biochem Soc Trans* 37:265, 2009.
51. Zhang J, Yang PL, Gray NS: Targeting cancer with small molecule kinase inhibitors. *Nat Rev Cancer* 9:28, 2009.
52. Mishima Y, Terui Y, Taniyama A, et al: Autophagy and autophagic cell death are next targets for elimination of the resistance to tyrosine kinase inhibitors. *Cancer Sci* 99:2200, 2008.
53. Brown JM, Wouters BG: Apoptosis, p53, and tumor cell sensitivity to anticancer agents. *Cancer Res* 59:1391, 1999.
54. Vellai T: Autophagy genes and ageing. *Cell Death Differ* 16:94, 2009.
55. Salminen A, Kaarniranta K: SIRT1: Regulation of longevity via autophagy. *Cell Signal* 21:1356, 2009.
56. Li GM, Presnell SR, Gu L: Folate deficiency, mismatch repair-dependent apoptosis, and human disease. *J Nutr Biochem* 14:568, 2003.
57. Melchert M, List A: Targeted therapies in myelodysplastic syndrome. *Semin Hematol* 45:31, 2008.
58. Adams JM, Cory S: The Bcl-2 protein family: Arbiters of cell survival. *Science* 281:1322, 1998.
59. Wang Y, Gu X: Functional divergence in the caspase gene family and altered functional constraints: Statistical analysis and prediction. *Genetics* 158:1311, 2001.
60. Riedl SJ, Fuentes-Prior P, Renatus M, et al: Structural basis for the activation of human procaspase-7. *Proc Natl Acad Sci U S A* 98:14790, 2001.
61. Acehan D, Jiang X, Morgan DG, et al: Three-dimensional structure of the apoptosome: Implications for assembly, procaspase-9 binding, and activation. *Mol Cell* 9:423, 2002.
62. Adams JM, Cory S: Apoptosomes: Engines for caspase activation. *Curr Opin Cell Biol* 14:715, 2002.

CHAPTER 13

CELL-CYCLE REGULATION AND HEMATOLOGIC DISORDERS

Mathias Schmid and Dennis A. Carson

SUMMARY

Complex feedback pathways regulate the passage of cells through the G_1, S, G_2, and M phases of the growth cycle. Two key checkpoints control the commitment of cells to replicate DNA synthesis and to mitosis. Many oncogenes and tumor-suppressor genes promote malignant change by stimulating cell-cycle entry, or disrupting the checkpoint response to DNA damage. Advances in the understanding of epigenetic gene expression regulation provide the basis for novel therapeutic approaches. This chapter presents the pathways as well as the genetic and epigenetic alterations that regulate cell replication and tabulates the various oncogenes and tumor-suppressor genes that are involved in hematologic malignancies.

Cellular mitosis is the final step of a defined program—the cell cycle—that can be separated into four phases: the G_1, S, G_2, and M phases (Fig. 13–1). A number of surveillance systems (checkpoints) control the cell cycle and interrupt its progression when DNA damage occurs or when the cells have failed to complete a necessary event.[1] These checkpoints have been given an empirical definition: When the occurrence of an event B is dependent on the completion of prior event A, the dependence is a result of a checkpoint if a loss-of-function mutation can be found that relieves the dependence.[1] Three major cell-cycle checkpoints have been discovered: the DNA damage checkpoint, the spindle checkpoint, and the spindle-pole body duplication checkpoint.[2–4] The functional consequence of failure to "satisfy" the requirements of a cell-cycle checkpoint is usually death by apoptosis. However, small numbers of genetically altered cells may survive. Cells with defective checkpoints have an advantage when selection favors multiple genetic changes. Cancer cells are often missing one or more checkpoints, which facilitates a greater rate of genomic evolution.[5]

A disturbance of cell-cycle regulation is an important pathway in the development of many hematologic malignancies as a result of mutations in tumor-suppressor genes or oncogenes. Until the end of the 20th century, it was believed that the only mechanism by which the "gatekeepers" of the cell cycle could be inactivated was deletion or mutation (gain-of-function or loss-of-function mutations). Progress in the understanding of the regulation of gene expression put emphasis on another mechanism of gene inactivation, called *epigenetic regulation* (see Chap. 10). This term summarizes several molecular modifications, including histone deacetylation, CpG-island hypermethylation, ubiquitination, and phosphorylation.

Acronyms and abbreviations that appear in this chapter include: AML, acute myelogenous leukemia; APL, acute promyelocytic leukemia; cdk, cyclin-dependent kinase; CML, chronic myelogenous leukemia; HAT, histone acetylases; HDAC, histone deacetylase; HDACi, histone deacetylase inhibitor; INK4, inhibitor of kinase 4; MTAP, methylthioadenosine phosphorylase; PLZF, promyelocytic leukemia Kruppel-like zinc finger; RARα, retinoic acid receptor-α; rPTK, receptor protein-tyrosine kinase; TGF-β, transforming growth factor-β.

CYCLINS AND CYCLIN-DEPENDENT KINASES (Table 13–1)

Early experiments on the control of mitosis in human cells provided evidence for the existence of factors called *M-phase* and *S-phase promoting factors*.[6] The key element of S-phase promoting factor was thought to be cdc2. Experiments performed in *Xenopus* eggs showed that cdc2 is an M-phase–specific histone H1 kinase,[7] but is just one subunit of a regulatory complex. A second component is cyclin B, which is synthesized in interphase and degraded in mid-mitosis. More than 10 members of the mammalian cyclin family have been cloned. Most of these cyclins interact with a group of cdc2-related kinases called *cyclin-dependent kinases* (cdks),[8,9] while others are involved in alternate splicing processes.[10] Phosphorylation of tyrosine 15 is the key event in regulating human cdc2 activity. Threonine 14 also is phosphorylated in G_2 phase. Both phosphorylation sites are required for mitotic initiation. Cdc2 interacts with cyclin B in mitosis, whereas the cdc2/cyclin A complex is formed before mitosis and probably is required for progression through late G_2 phase.[11] Thus, cyclins A and B are also called the *mitotic* cyclins, because they are upregulated in late G_2 or G_2/M phase and undergo proteolysis in M phase. The exit from mitosis is characterized by the abrupt ubiquitination and subsequent degradation of cyclin B. Cells with a defective cyclin B degradation mechanism or without mitotic cyclin B easily become aneuploid. The exact role of the other mitotic cyclin, cyclin A, is still unclear. There is evidence that it both acts at the G_2/M transition and binds cdk2 in S phase. Cyclin A is mandatory for the downregulation of APC (anaphase-promoting complex).[12] Overexpression of cyclin A in G_1 phase leads to an accelerated entry into S phase.[13] Because cdc2 is able to interact with mitotic and G_1 cyclins, it is likely that one protein kinase potentially can fulfill several different functions in the cell cycle at various checkpoints. There are several cdc2-related protein kinases in humans that interact with the corresponding cyclins. Originally, three cdc2-related proteins were isolated, which were able to replace deficient cdc28 function in budding yeast: cdk1, cdk2, and cdk3.[14–16] Another group of cdks that bind to cyclin D (a G_1 cyclin) are named cdk4,[17] cdk5,[18] and cdk6.[19] Cdk4 has been in the focus of tumor-suppressor gene research for the past several years, because it complexes with cyclin D1. This complex is an important element in the $p16^{INK4A}$-retinoblastoma (RB) gene pathway, which is commonly disrupted in cancer. Three other cyclin-dependent kinases have been partially characterized: cdk7 ($p40^{MO15}$) interacts with cyclin H and is responsible for phosphorylating cdc2 on threonine 161.[20] Cdk8 interacts with cyclin C, Med12, and Med13, and forms a complex called "CDK8" subcomplex. Several substrates for cdk8, when complexed with the above-mentioned proteins, have been detected, including RNA polymerase II and histone H3.[21] Cdk8 directly antagonizes the repression of β-catenin transcription by the transcription factor E2F1 in colorectal cancer.[22] The suppression of β-catenin by E2F1 contributes to apoptosis. Therefore, overexpression of cdk8 (and also RB) accounts for a reduced rate of apoptosis and increased cell growth.[22] Cdk9 binds cyclin T1 and displays a tissue-specific expression pattern.[23] That cdk9/cyclin T1 specifically interacts with the tat element of HIV-1 links this cyclin-dependent kinase directly to the replication pathway of HIV, and circumstantially to HIV-1–related malignancies (e.g., Kaposi sarcoma).[24] Cdk10[25] and cdk11[26] define a novel class of cyclin-dependent kinases, Both cdks interact with apoptosis-related factors[26] or transcription factors such as ets.[27] Cdk10 has two isoforms

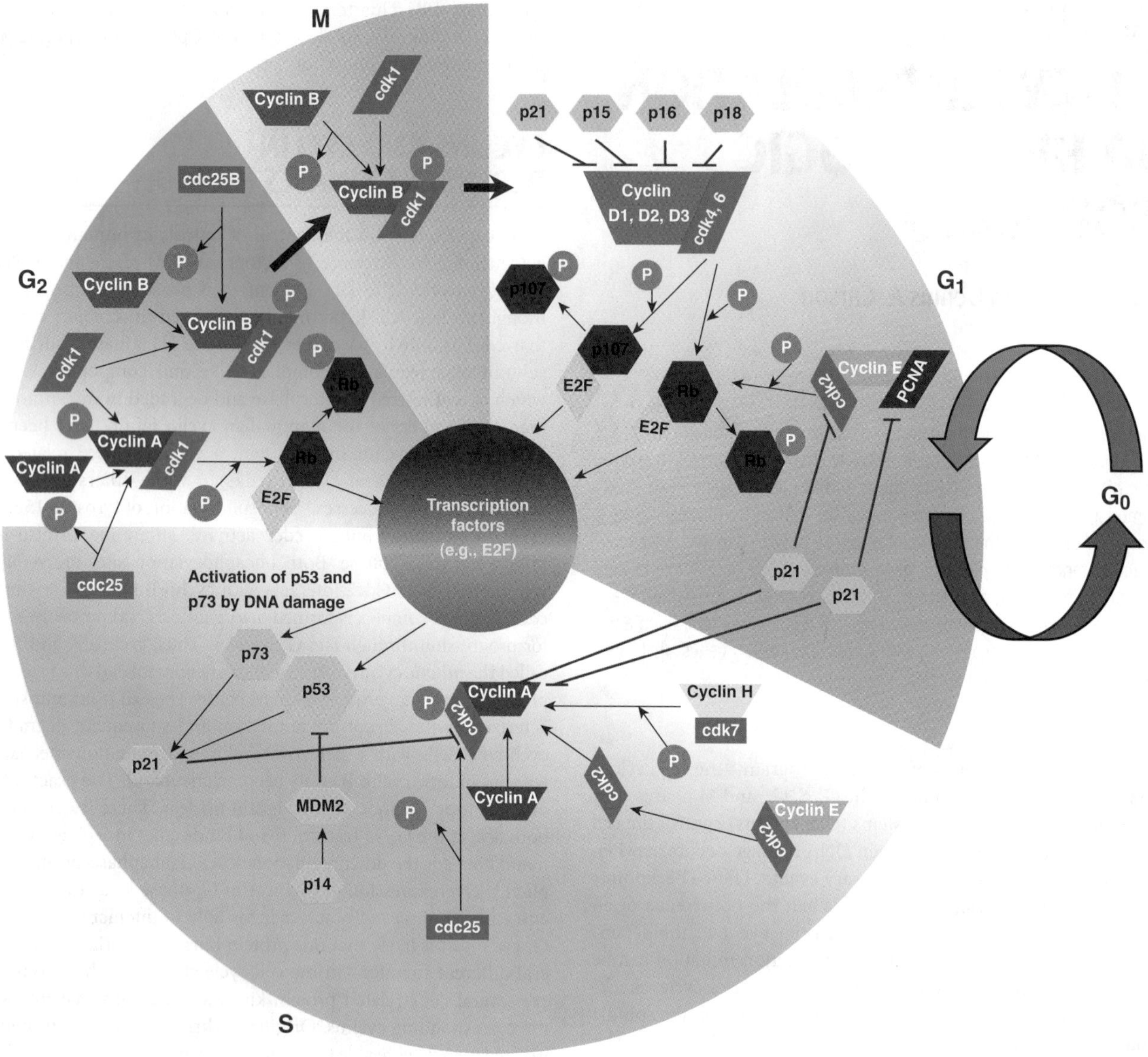

FIGURE 13–1. Cell-cycle regulation in mammalian cells.

with different functions. A role at the G_2/M transition has been suggested for the first isoform of cdk10, whereas the alternative splicing form interacts with the N-terminus of the Ets2 transcription factor. It has been shown in a mouse model, that this interaction affects the G_2/M transition.[28] Two known cyclin-dependent kinases, cdk12 and cdk13, interact with both forms of cyclin L (cyclin L1 and L2). This complex seems to be involved in alterative RNA-splicing,[10,29] and thus is involved in the premessenger RNA processing machinery. All cyclins share an approximately 150-amino-acid region, called the *cyclin box*, which interacts with the cdks.[30] The G_1 cyclins (C, D, and E) and the mitotic cyclins (A and B)[31] form distinct categories, although cyclin H, cyclins L_1 and L_2, and the type T cyclins (T_1, T_2a, and T_2b) fall outside these two major groups.

Cyclin A binds and activates cdk2 mainly in S phase. However, microinjection of anticyclin A antibodies into cells causes cell cycle arrest just before S phase.[11] This observation, together with the finding that overexpression of cyclin A leads to accelerated S-phase entry, suggests that cyclin A is involved in transformation.[13] Cyclin A is able to compensate cyclin E function. Cyclin E is important for the duplication of centrosomes. In cyclin E-defective cells, cyclin A can take over the function of cyclin E in S-phase, whereas cyclin A is important for centrosome amplification in G_2-arrested cells, irrespective of cyclin E.[32] The importance of cyclin A in cell division is underlined by recent reports.[33] In addition to its role at the G_1/S boundary, cyclin A acts in late G_2 phase, where it complexes with cdk1. Cyclin E, the other cyclin that interacts with cdk2, may control the progression from G_1 to S phase, but the exact time point when cdk2 "switches" from cyclin E to cyclin A binding is unknown. Cells overexpressing cyclin E progress much faster through G_1 into S phase, but the time required for DNA synthesis remains normal.[34] Cyclin E levels also are regulated by environmental factors, including transforming growth factor-β (TGF-β) and irradiation. These effects are, in part, mediated by small proteins, the cyclin-dependent kinase inhibitors. Cyclin E accumulates at the G_1/S boundary of the cell cycle, where it stimulates functions associated with entry into and progression through S phase.[35] In normal cells, cyclin E levels are highly regulated so that peak cyclin E–cdk2 kinase activity occurs only for a short interval near the G_1/S boundary.[35] Cyclin E–cdk2 complexes become active during S phase and are then rapidly ubiquitinated after phosphorylation.[36] The fatal overexpression of cyclin E has been observed in variety of human malignancies,[37] leading

TABLE 13–1. CDKs, Associated Cyclins, and the Stage of the Cell Cycle Where They Act

Cdk	Associated Cyclin	Cell-Cycle Stage
Cdk1	Cyclin A, B	G_2/M
Cdk2	Cyclin A, D, E; cyclin H	G_1/S; S; G_2/M
Cdk3	Ik3-1, Ik3-2	G_1
Cdk4	Cyclin D	G_1/S; S
Cdk5	Cyclin D	G_1/S
Cdk6	Cyclin D	G_1/S; S
Cdk7	Cyclin H	G_1/S; transcriptional regulation
Cdk8	Cyclin C	G_1/S; G_2/M, transcriptional regulation
Cdk9	Cyclin T1, T2	Acts on differentiation, interaction with tat, the transcriptional regulator of the HIV virus
Cdk10	Interacts with ets-2[25]	G_2/M[27]
Cdk11	RanBPM, RNPS1[26] casein kinase[58], cyclin L	Promotes apoptosis
Cdk12	Cyclin L1 and L2	Regulates alternative splicing[29]
Cdk13	Cyclin L	Regulates alternative splicing[10]

to a high cyclin E level throughout the cell cycle. The direct linkage between cyclin E overexpression and tumorigenesis is poorly understood. It has been suggested that the cyclin E–cdk2 complex phosphorylates and inactivates the retinoblastoma protein[38] or leads to genomic instability via the generation of aneuploid cells.[39] Cyclin E overexpression delays progression through early phases of mitosis and causes mitosis to be executed aberrantly, regulating mitotic progression.[40]

The B-type cyclins associate with cdk1 and cdk2 to form the classical mitotic cyclin–cdk complexes.[41] Cyclin B is synthesized in S phase and accumulates together with cdk2, and is ubiquitinated, followed by degradation, allowing the cell to exit from mitosis. The cyclin B/cdk2 checkpoint is very often defective in malignant cells, leading to uncontrolled M-phase entry and aneuploidy. The cellular localization of the cdk1–cyclin B complexes is strictly cell-cycle–dependent. Although the complexes accumulate in the cytoplasm during G_2 and S phase, they move to the nucleus in mitosis and bind to the mitotic spindle.[42,43] The cyclin B family has different family members with distinct functions. At mitotic entry, cyclin B1–cdk1 promotes chromosome condensation, nuclear membrane dissolution, mitotic aster assembly, and Golgi breakdown, whereas cyclin B2–cdk1 can only induce Golgi disassembly.[44] At prophase, cyclin B1 accumulates in the nucleus[45] and then localizes to condensed chromatin, spindle microtubules, centrosomes, and chromatin during prometaphase.[46] Distinct sequence elements are responsible for the localization of cyclin B1 to the chromatin, centrosomes, and kinetochores during mitosis.[47]

The three cyclin D molecules—D_1, D_2, and D_3—function mainly in late G_1 phase, where they bind cdk4 and cdk6. These complexes phosphorylate RB, restraining its inhibitory effects on E2F and related transcription factors. Cyclin D_1 is the major D cyclin in most cell types. All three cyclin D molecules act in late G phase, just before entry into S phase. Many tumors have high cyclin D_1 levels without amplification or mutation of the cyclin D_1 structural gene. Instead, cyclin D levels may be regulated by a feedback loop dependent on RB. Alterations of the RB gene in cancer may secondarily cause upregulation of cyclin D transcription. As a result of its central role in cell-cycle control, the cyclin D–cdk4 complex is an important target for anticancer drugs. Mice lacking cyclin D1 are completely resistant to ErbB-2–driven breast cancer.[48] ErbB-2–induced mammary tumor development is also prohibited by the inactivation of the cyclin D1 partner cdk4, underlining the role of this complex in human malignancies.[49] Another member of the cdk family, cdk9, partners with cyclin T, an 87-kDa cyclin C-type protein with three subunits.[50] The so-called cdk9-related pathway comprises two cdk9 isoforms (cdk9–42 and cdk9–55), cyclin T1, cyclin T2a, cyclin T2b and cyclin K.[23] Cdk9 and its binding partner cyclin T1 comprise the positive transcription elongation factor β.[51] Positive transcription elongation factor β can hyperphosphorylate the C-terminal domain of RNA polymerase II. In addition, positive transcription elongation factor β forms a complex with the HIV tat protein that binds the transactivation response element. The modification of RNA polymerase II by cdk9/cyclin T facilitates the efficient multiplication of the viral genome.[52] Other binding partners of cdk9 include tumor necrosis factor signal-transducer molecule and tumor necrosis factor receptor-associated factor 2,[53] as well as MAQ1 and 7SK RNA.[54] In addition, cdk9 is expressed throughout the cell cycle[55] and is also involved in viral (HIV, herpes) replication.[23]

The cdk10 gene encodes two different cdk-like putative kinases; it is postulated that they exert their function at the G_2/M transition.[25] These two isoforms predominate in human tissues, except in brain and muscle, and the relative isoform levels do not vary during the cell cycle.[25] Cdk10 interacts with the N-terminus of the Ets2 transcription factor, which contains the highly conserved pointed transactivation domain. The pointed domain is implicated in protein-protein interactions and Ets2 requires an intact pointed domain to bind Cdk10, which inhibits Ets2 transactivation in mammalian cells.[27] This could be an important factor for the development of follicular lymphoma, because it could be shown that cdk10 is overexpressed in this entity.[56] In addition, CDK10 silencing increases ETS2-driven transcription of c-RAF, resulting in mitogen-activated protein kinase (MAPK) pathway activation and loss of tumor cell reliance upon estrogen signaling.[57] Cdk10 promotors are frequently hypermethylated in malignant tumors, resulting in low expression levels of cdk10 and impaired cell-cycle regulation.[57]

Cdk11 is associated with cyclin L.[58] It is part of the large family of p34(cdc2)-related kinases whose functions appear to be linked with cell-cycle progression, tumorigenesis, and apoptotic signaling. Cdk11 interacts with the p47 subunit of eukaryotic initiation factor 3 during apoptosis and is therefore directly involved in cell death mechanisms.[59] Casein kinase 2 phosphorylates the cdk11 amino-terminal domain, suggesting that cdk11 participates in signaling pathways that include casein kinase 2 and that its function may help to coordinate the regulation of RNA transcription and processing events.[58] So far two isoforms of cdk11 have been identified, a larger p110 and a smaller p46 isoform. During Fas- or tumor necrosis factor-α-induced apoptosis, the caspase-processed p46 isoform is generated from the larger p110 isoform and it promotes apoptosis when it is ectopically expressed in human cells. Cdk11 also stabilizes the microtubule assembly of cells[60]; cdk11 is therefore mandatory for the maintenance of sister chromatid cohesion[61] and its disruption can contribute to the development of cancer.[62]

SUBSTRATES AND INHIBITORS OF CYCLIN-DEPENDENT KINASES

Many cyclin-cdk substrates have been identified by immunoprecipitation or two-hybrid assays, but only a few of them are thought to exert a direct function in cell-cycle control. The regulation of the cell cycle has been studied extensively during the last decade and a consensus paradigm of cell-cycle regulation has been suggested.[45,63] According to this consensus paradigm, the important switch of the cell cycle is the RB

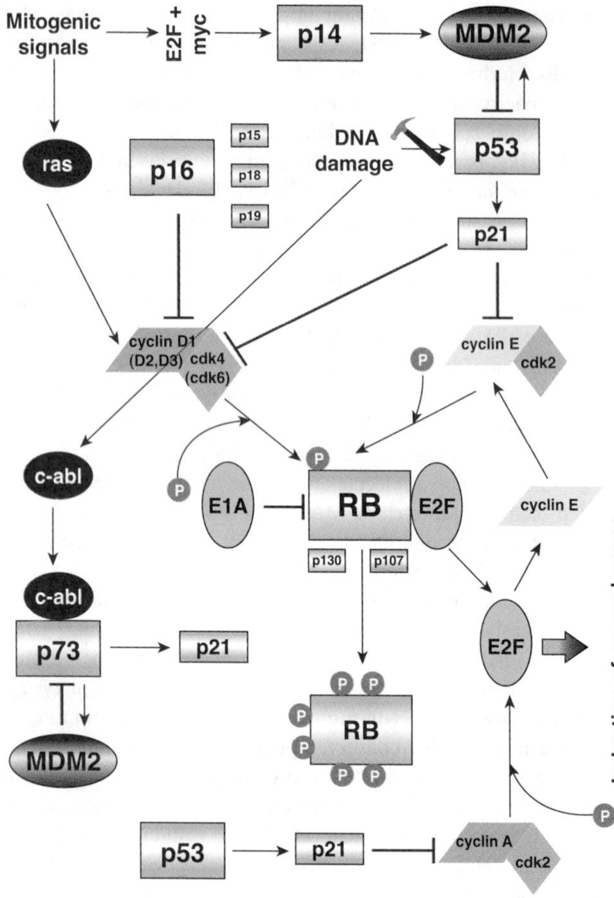

FIGURE 13–2. Interactions between cyclin-dependent kinase inhibitors (p16, p14, p21), p53, and the retinoblastoma protein (RB).

family of proteins (Fig. 13–2). In its hypophosphorylated state, RB binds to and inhibits a class of transcription factors, of which the best characterized is the E2F transcription factor. Hyperphosphorylation causes RB to detach from its binding site, permitting transcriptional activation of genes necessary for DNA synthesis and cell division. This phosphorylation of RB is regulated in a cell-cycle–dependent manner.[64] A widely accepted model suggests that RB is phosphorylated by different regulators such as cyclin E/cdks and p27 at the so-called "R" point, a time point during G_1 when mitosis becomes independent of exogenous stimuli.[65] Interference with RB function impairs G_1 checkpoint regulation, fosters unrestrained cell growth, a nearly universal characteristic of malignancy. RB controls the activity of several other cell-cycle regulatory elements such as Skp2.[66] The Skp2 regulation follows an autocrine loop where Skp2 triggers p27 degradation, followed by cyclin E/cdk2 activation, consecutive cdk2-induced RB-phosphorylation, and further E2F-dependent Skp2 expression.[67] Causes of reduced RB activity include changes in the structural gene, the sequestration and inactivation of the protein by viral oncogene products, and hyperphosphorylation of RB as a result of increased cdk4 and cyclin D activity or deletion of the gene for the $p16^{INK4A}$ inhibitor of cdk4. Deletions, mutations, and translocations of RB are common in various malignancies, while homozygous deletions of the $p16^{INK4A}$ gene are even more frequent. Many different transforming viruses (papillomavirus, simian virus 40) produce proteins that interact with RB. Both cyclin D_1–cdk4 and cyclin $D_1(D_2, D_3)$–cdk6 complexes are able to phosphorylate RB.[68,69] The time point of RB phosphorylation correlates strongly with the appearance of the cyclin D_1–cdk4 complex.[70] The link between RB and cyclin D is supported by the observation that loss of RB function leads to a decrease in the cellular cyclin D level.[71] However, cyclin D is not the only cyclin that is involved in the RB regulatory pathway.[66,69] Ectopic expression of both cyclin A and cyclin E restores RB hyperphosphorylation and causes cell-cycle arrest in cancer cell lines. Perhaps the cdk2–cyclin A complex contributes to additional phosphorylation of RB, whereas the cdk2–cyclin E complex prolongs the phosphorylation time.[72] The key regulatory element for the G_1 to S transition is the RB:E2F complex. After RB is phosphorylated by cdk4 and/or cdk6 complexes during G_1 phase and cdk2 at G_1/S interphase, E2F proteins are released and promote the transcription of genes essential for the transition to S phase.[66,73] As mentioned above the $p16^{INK4A}$/cyclin D_1/cdk4/RB/E2F cascade is probably one of the most important cascades in cell-cycle control, and is frequently affected in human cancer. For example, this pathway is defective in nearly 100 percent of acute myelogenous leukemia (AML) cell lines and most of the primary AML samples, although the exact mechanism of inactivation is not always clear. Two RB-related proteins, p107 and p130, form complexes with the transcription factor E2F,[74] bind to the region of the adenovirus E1A protein required for transformation, and are able to induce G_1 arrest when they are overexpressed in human malignant cell lines.[75,76] Unlike RB, the p107 and p130 proteins contain a so-called spacer region that interacts with cdk2/cyclin A and cdk2/cyclin E,[77] although it seems to be unlikely that these two complexes regulate the activity of p107 and p130.[72] Instead, p107 may bind and inactivate the cyclin A and cyclin E complexes. Thus, p107 may regulate the cell cycle by several different mechanisms. Because both p107 and p130 are regulated through phosphorylation, efficient cell-cycle entry is accompanied by phosphorylation of all the RB-related proteins.[78]

In addition to its cell-cycle regulatory properties, RB also influences hematopoietic differentiation.[79] RB interacts with the transcription factor PU.1, which blocks erythroid differentiation in the proerythroblast stage when ectopically overexpressed in marrow cells,[80,81] and represses GATA-1 activity.[82] An important interaction in this differentiation process is the interaction between hematopoietic stem cells and the microenvironment of the marrow. In addition, hypophosphorylated RB promotes monocytic over neutrophilic differentiation in bipotent progenitor cells, an event that is switched to neutrophilic differentiation if RB expression is inhibited. This finding points to an important property of RB independent of cell-cycle control.[83]

Besides regulation by phosphorylation, specific protein inhibitors of cdk enzymatic activity have been identified.[84] The cyclin-dependent kinase inhibitors cause cells to arrest in G_1 phase, followed by differentiation and/or senescence. The first cyclin-dependent kinase inhibitor identified was $p21^{cip1}$.[85] It binds to several cyclin/cdk complexes, including cyclin A/cdk2, cyclin D/cdk4, and cyclin E/cdk2 (see Fig. 13–2).[64,86] Several different cell-cycle regulatory pathways are affected by $p21^{cip1}$. The molecule has a p53 binding site in its promoter, and an increase in p53 levels results in transcriptional activation of $p21^{cip1}$, slowing cell-cycle progression. In addition to this p53-dependent pathway, $p21^{cip1}$ is also regulated in a p53-independent manner. Several binding partners of $p21^{cip1}$, including pim-1, have been identified. Pim-1 associates with and phosphorylates $p21^{cip1}$ *in vivo*, which influences the subcellular localization of $p21^{cip1}$.[87] $p21^{cip1}$ is phosphorylated by pim-1 at two distinct sites, Thr^{145} and Ser^{146}; phosphorylation on Thr^{145} results in a nuclear localization of $p21^{cip1}$ and a disruption of the cell cycle, while phosphorylation on Ser^{146} leads to a cytoplasmic localization of $p21^{cip1}$,[88] suggesting that overexpression of pim-1 in certain tumors plays a key role in tumorigenesis.[89] Like RB, expression and function of $p21^{cip1}$ is also affected by several different mechanisms, including mutation and histone deacetylation (see "The Role of Histone Deacetylases in Cell-Cycle Regulation" below). Other members of the

$p21^{cip1}$ family of cyclin-dependent kinase inhibitors include $p27^{kip1}$ and $p57^{kip1}$.[68,90] As a CDK inhibitor, $p27^{kip1}$ has tumor-suppressor activity. Besides cdks, $p27^{kip1}$ regulates additional cellular processes, including cell motility, some of which seem to mediate the oncogenic activities of $p27^{kip1}$. These activities of $p27^{kip1}$ are regulated through multiple phosphorylation sites. The multiple functions of $p27^{kip1}$ are dependent on a number of different conditions, and dictate whether the protein displays anti- or protumorigenic properties.[91] High-level expression of $p27^{kip1}$ leads to a cell-cycle block in G_1 phase after treatment of cells with TGF-β. One major difference between $p21^{cip1}$ and $p27^{kip1}$ is that the former binds predominantly to cdk2 whereas the latter binds cdk4.

The cellular levels of a number of cell-cycle regulators, including $p21^{cip1}$ and $p27^{kip1}$ are regulated by ubiquitination and subsequent proteolysis. Polyubiquitinated proteins are degraded by the 26S proteasome complex. There are two major ubiquitination systems in the cell, designated *SCF* and *APC*.[75,77] SCF is named for three of its core components, Skp1, Cdc53, and an F-box-containing protein. Important examples of SCF substrates are Cln1, Sic1, Wee1, Cdc6/Cdc18, E2F, cyclin D_1, cyclin E, $p21^{cip1}$, $p27^{kip1}$, and $p57^{kip2}$.[92]

A second group of cyclin-dependent kinase inhibitors belong to the inhibitor of the kinase 4 (INK4) family and include $p15^{INK4B}$, $p16^{INK4A}$, $p18^{INK4C}$, and $p19^{INK4D}$.[71,74,93,94] They all bind and inhibit the cyclin D_1–cdk4 and/or cyclin D_1–cdk6 complex, which regulates cell-cycle progression via RB.[71,93] TGF-β also is a potent inducer of $p15^{INK4B}$,[71] one of the mechanisms by which the cytokine regulates the proliferation of hematopoietic cells (see Chap. 16). $p16^{INK4A}$ is probably the most important cyclin-dependent kinase inhibitor, because the gene is inactivated by several mechanisms (deletion, mutation, hypermethylation) in many different human cancers.[95] Surprisingly, $p16^{INK4A}$ and $p14^{ARF}$ are overexpressed in some cases of human hematologic malignancies.[96] This overexpression is probably a result of defects downstream of $p16^{INK4A}$, particularly caused by mutations in the RB gene.[97] In hematologic malignancies, the highest frequencies of $p14^{ARF}$, $p15^{INK4B}$, or $p16^{INK4A}$ inactivations are found in T-cell acute lymphoblastic leukemia,[98] secondary high-grade lymphomas, and mantle cell lymphomas.[99,100] The potency of $p14^{ARF}$ and $p16^{INK4A}$ in terms of tumorigenicity becomes obvious because the reexpression of both genes by either retroviral transfection or demethylation of the promoter regions results in a complete reversion of the malignant phenotype.[101,102] $p14^{ARF}$ has multiple tumor-suppressor functions, some of which are mediated by signaling to p53. On the other hand, it has been shown that $p14^{ARF}$ is able to drive tumor progression in a p53-independent fashion, especially in myc-driven lymphomas.[103]

ONCOGENES (Table 13–2)

The complicated cell-cycle network has its parallel in the several different oncogenes and tumor-suppressor genes that influence carcinogenesis and tumor progression. The products of oncogenes, the oncoproteins, lead to or facilitate the transformation of a normal into a malignant cell. Oncogenes can be carried into the cell by viruses or they can arise from mutations in normal cellular genes. In addition, they can also arise from leukemia- or lymphoma-associated translocations where two usually separated genes are fused together and form a novel fusion protein. The familiar concept of this kind of protooncogene activation can be blurred by the fusion proteins because they possess unique capabilities not shared by either of the individual fusion partners. Oncoproteins can interact directly with cell-cycle regulatory proteins or control their activity by phosphorylation and dephosphorylation. Not all mutations in oncogenes lead to an altered function of the resulting product. The nomenclature in the oncogene tumor-suppressor gene field is not always clear. As a general guideline, if a mutation causes a functional loss of the gene product (loss of function), and the recessive loss of function leads directly to uncontrolled cell division, the underlying gene can be named a *tumor-suppressor gene*. On the other hand, if the mutation leads to an altered gene product (gain of function) that interacts abnormally with other proteins to influence the cell cycle, this gene is an *oncogene*, acting in a dominant fashion. Translocations are typical of oncogenes, whereas homozygous deletions and hypermethylation of CpG-nucleotide repeats are characteristic features of tumor suppressor genes.

Probably more than 200 oncogenes/oncogene candidates have been described in the literature, and most of them are involved in the pathogenesis and development of all kinds of tumors, especially the hematologic malignancies. Among the chromosomal translocations, the most well-studied are found in AML. They include t(8;21)(q22;q22), del[4](q12;q12), t(5;12)(q31-q32;p13), t(15;17)(q22;12), inv16(p13;q22), t(9;11)(p22;q23), t(9;22)(q34;q11), t(3;3)(q21;q26), t(8;16)(p11;p13), t(6;9)(p23;q34), t(7;11)(p15;p15), t(6;11)(q27;q23), t(11;19)(q23;p13.1), t(11;19)(q23;p13.3), t(16;16)(p13;q22), t(16;21)(p11;q22), and t(1;22)(p13;q13).[104,105] In contrast, in secondary myeloid leukemias recurrent numerical and unbalanced cytogenetic abnormalities predominate such as del(5q), del(7q), −7, and del(20q), and are often associated with a poor prognosis.[105,106] Table 13–2 lists some of the fusion partners. Next to the chromosomal translocations in AML as described above, there also aberrant fusion proteins in acute lymphoblastic leukemia (ALL), such as t(9;21), which is also found in chronic myelogenous leukemia (CML), t(4;11) in prolymphoblastic leukemia, and t(12;22) in childhood ALL. Some lymphomas are characterized by t(8;14) (Burkitt lymphoma), t(11;14) (mantle cell lymphoma), or t(14;18) (follicular lymphoma; for a review see reference 89).[107] An excellent overview of chromosomal rearrangements in cancer and the affected genes is given by Fröhling and Döhner.[105]

The exact mechanism by which the fusion proteins lead to tumorigenesis is not always well understood. Nevertheless, in patients with AML abnormal expression of the transcription factor RUNX1 (AML1) is able to promote cell-cycle progression by shortening G_1 phase and by repressing $p21^{cip1}$ promoter activity. RUNX1 is absolutely required for the establishment of adult-type hematopoiesis[108]; it regulates genes specific to the lymphoid, myeloid, and megakaryocyte lineages,[109] and mice lacking RUNX1 do not develop definitive hematopoiesis, indicating a role in adult hematopoietic stem cell formation.[110] In contrast, the fusion product AML1/ETO, derived from the t(8;21), slows down cell-cycle progression, suggesting that one gene in different "fusion situations" can cause different effects on the cell cycle.[111] Activation of the RUNX1-repression domain or fusing the gene to ETO results in downregulation of cdk4 and myc, directly linking this fusion protein to cell-cycle checkpoints.[111] Additional evidence for the direct involvement of RUNX1 in cell-cycle control comes from the observation that the transcription factor binds to the $p19^{INK4D}$ promoter and downregulates $p19^{INK4D}$ expression in megakaryocytes.[112] Inhibiting the oligomerization domain of ETO interferes with RUNX1/ETO oncogenic activity and these cells lose their progenitor cell characteristics, arrest cell-cycle progression, and undergo cell death.[113] Another interesting chromosomal translocation fusion product that affects cell-cycle control is found in patients with acute promyelocytic leukemia (APL) or its variant form (vAPL). The promyelocytic leukemia-retinoic acid receptor-α (PML-RARα), which results from t(15;17)(q22;12), upregulates cyclin A_1 expression, whereas PML itself seems to be a negative regulator of cell growth because its overexpression leads to growth suppression and G_1 arrest in a variety of different cell types.[114] PML is crucial for the growth-inhibiting activity of retinoic acid and its absence abrogates the retinoic acid-dependent transactivation of $p21^{cip1}$.[115] Another mechanism by which PML elicits irreversible growth arrest is believed to

TABLE 13–2. Oncogenes Involved in Human Hematologic Malignancies and Their Chromosomal Localization

Oncogene	Description	Locus	Function	Associated Malignancies
ab11; ab12	Abelson murine leukemia virus	9q34.1; 1q24-q25	tyr protein kinase	Lymphoid and myeloid neoplasms
akt1; akt2	Murine thymoma virus	14q32.3; 19q13.1	ser/thr kinase	Breast cancer, thymoma
Alk	Receptor tyrosine kinase	2p23	tyr kinase	Lymphomas
am11	AML-associated protein	21q22.3	Transcription factor	Acute myeloid leukemia
Axl	Receptor tyrosine kinase	19q13.1-q13.2	tyr kinase	Acute leukemias
bc12, bc13	B-cell leukemia-associated oncogenes	18q21;19q13.1-q13.2	Apoptosis regulation	B-cell leukemias, lymphomas
EGFR	Epidermal growth factor receptor	7p12	Growth factor receptor	Several human neoplasms
erb	Avian erythroblastic leukemia viral oncogene	17q21.1	EGF receptor	Brain tumors, breast cancer, several others
erg	v-ets avian erythroblastosis virus	21q22.3	Transcription factor	Acute myeloid leukemia
eto	Involved in the t(8;21) in acute myeloid leukemia	8q22	Transcription factor?	Acute myeloid leukemia
fes	Feline sarcoma virus	15q26.1	tyr kinase	Sarcoma?
fgr	Gardner-Rasheed feline sarcoma virus	1p36.2-p36.1	tyr kinase	Myeloid leukemias
fos	Murine osteosarcoma virus	14q24.3	Transcription factor	Several human neoplasms
fyn	Oncogene related to src, fgr yes	6q21	tyr kinase	Several human neoplasms
Jak-2	Tyrosine protein kinase	9p24	tyr kinase	Myeloproliferative disorders
jun	Avian sarcoma virus 17	1p32-p31	Transcription factor	Ovarian, breast, colon, lung, leukemia, several others
kit	Hardy-Zuckerman 4 feline sarcoma virus	4p11-p12	Receptor tyr kinase	Acute myeloid leukemia
lyn	Yamaguchi sarcoma virus related	8q13	tyr kinase	Lymphoid and myeloid neoplasms
myb	Avian myeloblastosis virus	6q22-q23	Transcription factor	Hematologic disorders, several human neoplasms
myc	MC29 myelocytoma virus	8q24.12-q24.13	Transcription factor	Myeloid, lymphatic neoplasms, renal cancer
npm1	Nucleophosmin (nuclear phosphoprotein)	5q35	tyr kinase	Childhood acute myeloid leukemia
pim-1	Murine leukemia virus	6p21.2	ser/thr kinase	T-cell lymphoma
pml	Involved in t(15;17) in promyelocytic leukemia	15q22	Transcription factor	Promyelocytic leukemia
raf	Murine leukemia virus	3p25	ser/thr kinase	Several human neoplasms
rar	Retinoic acid receptor	17q12	Transcription factor	(Pro-)myelocytic leukemia
ras	Harvey sarcoma viral oncogene	Several	G-protein	Myeloid neoplasms, several human neoplasms
ret	Receptor tyrosine kinase	10q11.2	tyr kinase	Multiple endocrine neoplasia type A/B; Hirschsprung disease
spi	Spleen focus forming virus	11p12-p11.22	Transcription factor	Myeloid leukemias, lymphomas?
src	Rous sarcoma virus	20q11.2-q12	tyr kinase	Lymphomas
tax1	Human T-cell leukemia virus-binding protein	7q13	Binding protein	Acute T-cell leukemia
tel	t(5;12) involved oncogene	12p13	Transcription factor	Myeloid leukemia
tm11	TCL1/MTCP1-like protein	14q32.1	?	T-cell leukemia, lymphoma

involve activation of the tumor-suppressor pathway $p16^{INK4A}$/RB.[116] Recent data point toward a linkage between PML and the nucleoporins, especially Nup98 and Nup214. In some AML specimens, these nucleoporins were expressed as oncogenic fusion proteins and become directed—complexed with PML—to common cytoplasmic compartments during the M-to-G_1 transition of the cell cycle. In promyelocytic leukemia cells, the loss of function of normal PML causes an increase in cytoplasmic-bound versus nuclear-membrane-bound nucleoporins.[117] Consequently, PML by itself is a tumor-suppressor gene that positively regulates cell-cycle progression. Further evidence for a tumor-suppressor gene function of PML comes from transgenic mice models where $PML^{-/-}$ mouse embryonic fibroblasts are enriched in S phase and the G_0/G_1 phase is minimized.[118] In APL, this regulatory role is disrupted by the fusion to RARα. One mechanism by which this fusion protein (and also the promyelocytic leukemia Kruppel-like zinc finger [PLZF]-RARα fusion derived from the rare t(11;17)) affects cell-cycle control is its strong interaction with SMRT or N-CoR, two corepressor elements that are important for the recruitment of histone deacetylases, as described below in "The Role of Histone Deacetylases in Cell-Cycle Regulation."[114] In accordance with this is the finding that retrovirally transduced PML-RARα induces a maturation arrest in the corresponding cells, implying that these cells are unable to express certain transcription factors as a consequence of the conformational changes caused by the recruitment of the histone deacetylases (HDACs).[119] A variant of this chromosomal translocation results in a fusion protein between RARα and the PLZF protein, which is observed in a subset of patients with APL.[119,120]

The translocation t(9:22), which fuses the *BCR* gene to the c-*ABL* gene, is a characteristic feature of CML (see Chap. 88). The chromosome 9 breakpoints, where the c-abl gene is located, involves a large region of about 200 kb, but fusion genes invariably include the abl exon 2. The corresponding breakpoints on chromosome 22 are located in a much smaller region, including the bcr-gene.[121] The bcr-abl fusion protein localizes to the cytoskeleton and displays enhanced tyrosine kinase activity.[122] It is also found in some cases of ALL and in occasional cases of AML.[123,124] Bcr-abl not only regulates cell proliferation, apoptosis, differentiation, and adhesion, but also induces resistance to cytostatic drugs by modulation of DNA repair mechanisms, cell-cycle checkpoints, and Bcl-2 protein family members. Upon DNA damage bcr-abl enhances repair of DNA lesions and prolongs activation of cell-cycle checkpoints (e.g., G_2/M), providing more time for repair of otherwise lethal lesions, so that these cells have a significant survival advantage.[123] The bcr-abl fusion product is so far the only oncogenic product that is sufficient to induce malignant growth *in vivo* without the presence of other abnormal molecular changes. Several reports have shown that bcr-abl–positive cells display pronounced G_2/M delay in response to various chemotherapeutics and irradiation. The exact mechanism of G_2/M delay in bcr-abl–positive cells has not been characterized in detail but it seems that the cdc2-cyclin B_1 regulation is affected. The bcr-abl signaling transduction involves adapter molecules such as GRB2 and GAB2 as well as signaling pathways (phosphatidylinositol 3′-kinase [PI3K], Janus-type kinase [JAK]-signal transducer and activator of transcription [STAT]).[122] In addition, although there is no direct evidence that the abnormal bcr-abl product affects the M checkpoint itself, some data suggest that bcr-abl–positive CML cells contain elevated MAD2 and BUB1-levels, genes that inhibit the APC and therefore cause mitotic spindle arrest.[125] Amplification of the fusion sequence is frequently used to detect minimal residual disease in patients under therapy with interferon-α, the tyrosine kinase inhibitor STI571,[126] and after blood stem cell transplantation.[127] The etv6 gene is the only known non-bcr fusion partner of abl, sometimes observed as etv6-abl in ALL or myeloproliferative syndromes (t(9;12)(q34;p13)).[128] The affected cells show only a minor response to imatinib.

Mutant-activated receptor protein-tyrosine kinases (rPTK) comprise a family of very well characterized oncogenes. The constitutive activation of rPTK usually is achieved by mutations that lead to the dimerization and activation of their cytoplasmic catalytic domains.[129] Another possible cause of rPTK dimerization is chromosomal translocations that create chimeric proteins. In the t(2;5) translocation, found in several anaplastic large-cell lymphomas, N-terminal nucleophosmin sequences on the long arm of chromosome 5 are fused to the cytoplasmic domain of the Alk protein on chromosome 2.[130,131] The characteristic translocation of chronic myelomonocytic leukemia, t(5;12), fuses sequences from the transcription factor Tel to the cytoplasmic domain of the platelet-derived growth factor-β receptor (*TEL-PDGFβR*), resulting in the formation of a TEL-PDGFβR fusion protein and the constitutive activation of the RTK,[132] and targeting Id1 (inhibitor of DNA-binding 1).[133] Patients with the t(5;12) translocation respond to imatinib, as the drug also inhibits the platelet-derived growth factor receptor. The chromosomal area surrounding the *TEL* gene is a fragile site, because the Tel gene is involved in several other translocations in human acute leukemias (e.g., t(12;9)). One of the TGF-β receptors also is involved in oncogenesis, because mutations are frequently found in colon cancer. TGF-β receptor signaling acts through the Smad family of transcription factors.

Two important oncogene families encode the Ras and Rho family proteins. Ras itself is a G protein, and activating mutations in H-Ras, K-Ras, and N-Ras have been found in nearly all kinds of human cancers. Several different Ras mutations are able to transform normal cells in tissue culture.[134,135] Mutations in many different Ras family members have been identified in cancer (e.g., Raf1, p110 PI3K, Rin1, Mekk1), but the exact downstream signaling effects of each mutation are still unclear. The Ras and the Rho families of oncoproteins are linked by a small G protein called *Rac*, which is required for transformation by Ras.[136,137] The normal formation of actin filaments is required for G_1/S-phase entry. Recent data have shown the Rho-guanosine triphosphatases play a key role in the Wnt-signaling pathway, where they are involved in cellular polarization processes.[138] Thus, alterations in the Rho pathway may lead to premature entry into S phase by interference with cytoskeletal organization. The Ras/Raf/Mek/Erk cascade couples signals from the surface to the intracellular space and triggers cell proliferation signals that influence the cell cycle. Abnormal activation of this cascade occurs in several leukemias because of activating mutations in the Ras protooncogene.[139] Ectopic overexpression of Raf proteins is associated with cell proliferation whereas overexpression of activated Raf is associated with cell-cycle arrest in G_1 phase.[140,141] Different *Raf* genes have different functions in cells, although A-Raf and B-Raf share three conserved domains termed CR1, CR2, and CR3.[142] A-Raf is able to upregulate the expression of cyclin D_1, cdk2, cyclin E, and cdk4, whereas B-Raf and Raf-1 induce $p21^{cip1}$, leading to a G_1 arrest.[139,142] The mode of action of these Raf molecules is not fully understood but one explanation why they act differently may be because they activate different downstream pathways, namely the MAPK (MEK [MAP/ERK (extracellular response kinase)]). The three different MAPK cascades are the ERK–, JNK/SAPK–, and the p38 pathways. The MAP kinase pathways consist of three types of kinases in a series, MAPKKK, MAPKK, and MAPK (ERK), each sequentially activating the next kinase. The MAPK cascades all transmit responses from several different surface receptors to the nucleus.[143] One explanation for the oncogenic effects of the MAPK pathway is that ERK activates c-myc via phosphorylation on serine 62.[144] In addition, repression of c-myc is required for terminal differentiation of many cell types, including hematopoietic cells. Thus, deregulated expression of c-myc in both M_1 AML cells and in normal myeloid cells derived from murine marrow blocks terminal differentiation and its associated growth arrest, and also induces apoptosis, which is dependent on the Fas/CD95 pathway. New data suggest a linkage between c-myc downregulation, the $p16^{INK4A}$/cyclinD1/RB–, and the SMAC/Diabolo apoptotic pathway.[145] Several different transcription factors have been implicated in the downregulation of c-myc expression during differentiation, including C/EBPα, CTCF, BLIMP-1, and RFX1. Alterations in the expression and/or function of these transcription factors, or of the c-myc and Max interacting proteins, such as MM-1 and Mxi1, can influence the neoplastic process.[146,147]

Experiments on oncoproteins have focused on apoptosis, the lethal response of a cell to either DNA damage or to signaling through cell surface "death" receptors. Key regulators of apoptosis induced by DNA damage are the multiple members of the bcl family of proteins, which include Bcl, Bcl-x_L, Bax, and Bad. Bcl-2 is involved in the t(14;18) chromosomal translocation, which is found in many leukemias and lymphomas of B-cell origin.[148] The disruption of these loci increases expression of Bcl, and results in the uncontrolled accumulation of malignant B cells, because of an impaired balance between growth and apoptosis.[149,150] It has also been shown that Bcl-x_L, Bax, and Bad are

TABLE 13–3. Characterization of Human Tumor Suppressor Genes

Tumor-Suppressor Gene	Chromosome Locus	Diseases	Major Mechanism(s) of Inactivation
Cadherin 1 (E-cadherin)	16q22.1	Malignomas of the gastrointestinal tract	Hypermethylation of CpG islands, mutation
CDKN1A (p21, Cip1)	6p21.2	Several human malignant and nonmalignant diseases	Homozygous deletion?
CDKN1C (p57, Kip2)	11p15.5	Breast cancer?, Wilms tumor	Hypermethylation of CpG islands, mutations?
CDKN2A (p16)	9p21	Several human cancers	Homozygous deletion, hypermethylation of CpG islands, mutations
CDKN2B (p15)	9p21	Several human cancers	Homozygous deletion, hypermethylation of CpG islands
$p14^{ARF}$	9p21	Several human cancers	Homozygous deletion, hypermethylation of CpG islands, mutations
p53	17p13.1	Several human cancers	Mutations
WT1	11p13	Wilms tumor, nephroblastoma	Homozygous deletion, mutation
DMBT1	10q25.3–26.1	Malignant brain tumors	Homozygous deletion
PTEN	10q23	Glioblastoma, breast cancer	Mutation
p73	1p36	Leukemia, lymphoma	Hypermethylation of CpG islands, mutation?
VHL	3p	von Hippel-Lindau disease	Hypermethylation of CpG islands
H19	11p15.5	Hepatoblastoma, Wilms tumor	Hypermethylation of CpG islands
HIC1	17p13	AML, HCC, breast cancer	Hypermethylation of CpG islands
RB	13q14.2	Several human cancers	Mutation
nm23	17q21.3–22	Neuroblastoma, breast, prostate cancer, melanoma	Mutation, hypermethylation of CpG islands?
H-cadherin	16q24	Lung cancer	Hypermethylation of CpG islands
N33	8p22	Glioblastoma multiforme	Hypermethylation of CpG-islands, mutation
S100A2	1q21	Breast cancer	Hypermethylation of CpG-islands, mutation
APC	5q21-q22	Adenomatosis polyposis coli	Homozygous deletion, mutation hypermethylation of CpG islands,
NF-1, NF-2	17q11.2,22q12.2	Neurofibromatosis, bilateral acoustic neuroma	Mutation

involved in the regulation of AML cells. For example, the ratio between Bax and Bcl-2 is a prognostic factor in this myeloid neoplasm.[151] The nuclear histone deacetylase complex, which regulates the structural conformation of DNA and therefore the activation of several genes, is targeted by ETO, the fusion partner of the RUNX1 gene in patients with AML. The t(8;21) translocation that occurs in such patients allows the formation of a stable complex between the histone deacetylase complex and ETO, contributing to leukemogenesis.[152,153] PLZF, PLZF-RARα, and BCL-6 are other oncogenes that target the histone deacetylase complex.[154,155]

TUMOR-SUPPRESSOR GENES (Table 13–3)

Almost every cancer harbors one or more abnormalities of tumor-suppressor genes. These include mutations, translocations, deletions or epigenetic modifications. In addition, at least two epigenetic mechanisms—the hypermethylation of CpG islands in the promoter and the aberrant acetylation of histones (especially histone H_4)—can silence tumor-suppressor genes in a variety of human cancer cell lines and primary tumors.

The products of the three most important tumor suppressor genes (*RB*, *P53*, and *p16*^{INK4A}) are interconnected biochemically. The *RB* gene maps to chromosome 13q14 and has several downstream effectors, among which the transcription factor E2F is the best characterized.[156] The *RB* gene family consists of three closely related proteins, RB, p107, and p130. All three proteins are able to interact with several E2F family members.

Transcriptional activation and repression are mediated via complexes consisting of RB family members, E2F family members, and so-called DP proteins.[157] Besides its role in cell-cycle control, RB can modulate RNA polymerase activity, thus linking cell-cycle progression to transcriptional regulation. More than 30 separate cellular proteins have been identified that bind to RB. These proteins can be divided into different groups, including transcription factors, growth factors, protein kinases, protein phosphatases, and nuclear matrix proteins. Mutations of RB are frequent in leukemias; soft-tissue sarcomas; and breast, esophagus, prostate, and renal carcinomas.[158] Several viral or oncoproteins can bind to and inactivate RB.[159,160]

The p53 gene has therefore been called a "guardian" of the genome because it transmits signals arising from these various forms of DNA damage, leading to cell-cycle arrest or apoptosis. p53 protein is also the target of leukemogenic mutations. Damaging factors, such as hypoxic stress, chemicals, or irradiation either alter the p53 protein itself or can stabilize its cellular inhibitor, MDM2 (mouse double-minute 2; in humans, HDM2).[161] The MDM2 protein inhibits p53 transcription and stimulates p53 degradation.[162,163] Moreover, MDM2 is able to affect chromosomal stability independently of p53.[164] The MDM2 binding region includes several phosphorylation sites, although the exact mechanism by which MDM2 regulates p53 degradation is still not clear.[165] The *p14*^{ARF} tumor-suppressor gene, which is encoded within the *p16*^{INK4A} locus by alternate splicing, controls MDM2 activity.[166] The *p14*^{ARF} gene shares exons 2 and 3 with *p16*^{INK4A} but has a distinct exon 1. The discovery that two important tumor-suppressor genes are encoded by the same chromosomal locus and share several exons was unexpected and is unique in human biology. The *p16*^{INK4A} gene function depends on p53, because overexpression of *p16*^{INK4A} causes cell-cycle arrest in p53 wild-type cells but not in p53-dependent cells.[167] The transcription of *p16*^{INK4A} is regulated by E2F, which is under the control of RB.[168] This indicates the existence of yet another feedback loop, which links the RB pathway to p53.[169] The Ras protein is another identified *p16*^{INK4A} factor involved in MDM2-p53-p21-RB regulation.[170,171] Different signaling routes that connect DNA damage with p53 include a cascade of Ser/Thr kinases, for example, ATM, ATR, Chk1 and Chk2, which phosphorylate p53.[172] Abnormalities of p53 are found in slightly more than 50 percent of all human tumors and, surprisingly, even in some normal cells. It is unclear if these "normal" cells represent a pool of premalignant cells in an otherwise healthy individual or, more likely, p53 changes are just one step in multistage tumorigenesis. Two different p53 homologues, p63 and p73, have been described, which show DNA binding, transactivation, and oligomerization domains similar to p53.[173] This similarity in the DNA binding domain allows p63 and p73 to regulate p53 target genes, induce cell-cycle arrest and apoptosis, and therefore act as tumor suppressors.[174] The p73 gene has been localized to chromosome 1p36, a common region of cytogenetic changes in cancer. p73 protein also can bind p53, inhibiting its transcriptional regulatory activity.[175] Although p53 mutations are found frequently in all cancers, p63 and p73 mutations are much more rare.[174,176] However, the p73 gene is inactivated by hypermethylation of CpG islands in its promoter region in both leukemias and lymphomas.[177]

Homozygous deletions of the *p16*^{INK4A}/*p14*^{ARF} gene locus on human chromosome 9p21 have been detected in gliomas,[74,178] primary cancers of the lung,[74,179] bladder,[180] head and neck,[181] as well as in acute T-cell leukemias[182,183] and mesotheliomas.[184] Because inherited mutations of *p16*^{INK4A} exon 2 may interfere with its expression and/or function, without causing an amino acid change in *p14*^{ARF}, it is clear that *p16*^{INK4A} inactivation alone is an important step in the evolution of malignant disease. However, in established tumor cell lines, nearly all chromosome 9p21 deletions disable the entire *p16*^{INK4A}/*p14*^{ARF} locus. Both proteins act as suppressors of the G_1-S transition, even though they function in two different pathways: *p16*^{INK4A} acts as an inhibitor of cyclin D_1/cdk4[6] complexes whereas *p14*^{ARF} stabilizes p53 by inhibition of MDM2. Several models provide insight into the different modes of action of *p16*^{INK4A} and *p14*^{ARF} on cell-cycle regulation. Interestingly, if the entire p19^{ARF}/p16^{INK4A} locus is disrupted in mice (the mouse homologue of p14^{ARF} is p19^{ARF}), the mice develop lymphomas, lymphoid leukemias, and sarcomas, suggesting that these tumor-suppressor genes do not act in a lineage-specific manner on cell-cycle regulation but in a more general one. Retroviral expression of p16^{INK4A} restores the normal phenotype in some cell types underlining the strong tumor-suppressor potency of p16^{INK4A}. The *p15*^{INK4B} gene, also located on chromosome 9p21, approximately 20 kb centromeric of *p16*^{INK4A}, is deleted somewhat less frequently. Analyses of primary tumors, however, show that not all 9p21 deletions encompass these three tumor suppressor genes. One mechanism for disruption of the *p15*^{INK4B}/*p14*^{ARF}/*p16*^{INKA} region in T-cell leukemias may be the action of an illegitimate V(D)J recombinase.[185] Several new binding partners of p16^{INK4A} have been identified.[186] The RB gene interacts with one of these factors, BRG1, to remodel chromatin structures. BRG1 also acts upstream of RB with p16^{INK4A} and functions as a tumor suppressor.[186]

The p15^{INK4B}/p16^{INK4A}/p14^{ARF} locus on chromosome 9p21 is a real hotspot in the development of human cancer and approximately 50 percent of all human malignancies show abnormalities in at least one of these tumor-suppressor genes. Another gene lies about 100 kb telomeric of p16^{INK4A}, and this gene, methylthioadenosine phosphorylase (MTAP), encodes an important enzyme in the purine metabolism. Some early gliomas show MTAP deletions without deletions of other genes on 9p21, suggesting that MTAP by itself has tumor-suppressor properties. The reexpression of MTAP in breast cancer cells severely inhibits their ability to form colonies in soft agar or collagen, supporting this hypothesis.[187] In addition, MTAP-expressing cells are suppressed for tumor formation when implanted into severe combined immune deficiency mice. Recent findings suggest that the enzyme ornithine decarboxylase (ODC) is overexpressed in MTAP-deleted tumors, providing evidence for a new pathway in tumorigenesis. Overexpression of ODC has been observed in many tumors and is linked to the ras pathway.[188] Reexpression of MTAP in ODC overexpressing cells decreases ODC levels and inhibits tumor cell growth.[189] In addition, Stevens and colleagues showed that high levels of 5′-deoxy-5′-(methylthio)adenosine (MTA) induce matrix metalloproteinase and growth factor gene expression in melanoma cells leading to enhanced invasion and vasculogenic mimicry. In addition, MTA induced the secretion of *β*-fibroblast growth factor and the upregulation of activator protein-1, demonstrating a tumor-supporting role of MTA, which is increased in MTAP-deficient cells.[190]

The mechanisms by which the above-mentioned genes are inactivated are rather different. Especially in permanent cell lines, *p15*^{INK4B}/*p14*^{ARF}/*p16*^{INKA} and MTAP are homozygously deleted. One allele of MTAP is also deleted in AML lines, but not in primary AML samples. Mutations in *p15*^{INK4B}/*p14*^{ARF}/*p16*^{INKA} genes are rare, and if present, occur in exon 2. Hypermethylation of CpG islands in the promoter areas of both *p15*^{INK4B}/*p14*^{ARF}/*p16*^{INKA} are frequently found in hematologic malignancies.[191–193] The availability of demethylating agents such as 5-aza-2′-deoxycytidine (decitabine) makes this phenomenon an interesting target for chemotherapy.[194,195] Decitabine has been used to treat patients suffering from different hematologic malignancies and was reported to have activity in advanced myelodysplastic syndrome, accompanied by demethylation of the *p16*^{INK4A} promoter.[195] However, p16^{INK4A} and p15^{INK4B} are not the only targets of these demethylating agents in hematologic malignancies.[196] Transcriptional regulation by methylation is mediated by a multiprotein complex consisting of a MeCP2, a methylcytosine-binding protein with a transcriptional repressor domain that binds the corepressor mSin3A, which is itself one element of a multiprotein complex that includes HDAC1 and HDAC2.[197,198] Therefore, reexpression of silenced genes can be achieved by demethylating DNA or by destabilizing HDACs, and it could be demonstrated that both mechanisms are tightly linked. Histone deacetylase inhibitors (HDACi) and demethylating agents act synergistically to induce genes silenced in cancer by hypermethylation.[102] Another new mechanism of gene regulation and inactivation *in vivo* is degradation by microRNAs. This has also been shown for several members of the p16^{INK4A}-CDK4/cyclin D_1/RB pathway.[199]

THE ROLE OF HISTONE DEACETYLASES IN CELL-CYCLE REGULATION

HDACs catalyze the deacetylation of lysine residues in the histone N-terminal tails and are found in large multiprotein complexes with transcriptional corepressors. Human HDACs are grouped into three classes based on their similarity to known yeast factors: class I HDACs are similar to the yeast transcriptional repressor yRPD3; class II HDACs are

TABLE 13–4. Different Types and Classes of Histone Deacetylases

Enzyme	Mechanism of Deacetylase Activity	Tissue Expression	Interacting Protein
Class I			
HDAC1	Zn^{2+} dependent	Ubiquitous	RB, p53, MYOD, NF-κB, DNMT1, DNMT3A, MBD2, SP1, BRCA1, MeCP2, ATM
HDAC2	Zn^{2+} dependent	Ubiquitous	RB, NF-κB, BRCA1, DNMT1
HDAC3	Zn^{2+} dependent	Ubiquitous	RB, NF-κB
HDAC8	Zn^{2+} dependent	Ubiquitous	EST1B, Hsp70
HDAC11	Zn^{2+} dependent?	Tissue specific	Interleukin 10
Class II			
HDAC4	Zn^{2+} dependent	Tissue specific	MEF2
HDAC5	Zn^{2+} dependent	Tissue specific	MEF2
HDAC6	Zn^{2+} dependent	Tissue specific	Hsp90?
HDAC7	Zn^{2+} dependent	Tissue specific	MEF2
HDAC9	Zn^{2+} dependent?	Tissue specific	MEF2
HDAC10	Zn^{2+} dependent?	Ubiquitous	RB
Class III			
Sirt1–7	NAD^+ dependent	?	p53

HDAC, histone deacetylase; NAD, nicotinamide adenine dinucleotide; NF-κB, nuclear factor kappa B; RB, retinoblastoma.

similar to the yeast transcriptional repressor yHDA1; and class III HDACs are similar to the yeast transcriptional repressor ySIR2 (Table 13–4, Fig. 13–3).[200,201] Eleven different HDACs have been identified so far. The physiologic counterparts of the HDACs are histone acetylases (HATs). In the nucleosome, positively charged hypoacetylated histones bind tightly to the phosphate backbone of the DNA and maintain the chromatin in an inactive, silent state. Both HAT and HDAC activities are recruited to target genes in complexes with sequence-specific transcription factors and their cofactors. Examples of these cofactors include NCoR or SMRT (Fig. 13–4). Several different transcription factors are assembled with these complexes, including bcl-6, Mad-1, PML, and ETO.[200] HDACs are involved in different cellular mechanisms, including proliferation and differentiation. Irregular activation of HDACs leads to the loss of cell-cycle control.[202] Gene silencing by HDAC complexes is an important mechanism in the development of AML, most notably acute promyelocytic leukemia. The PML-RARα fusion protein is an oncoprotein which represses retinoic acid-dependent transcription by recruitment of HDAC to RAR-regulated genes (Fig. 13–4B), halting myeloid maturation because of cell-cycle arrest. In the PML-RARα fusion protein, the RARα is not responsive to physiologic concentrations of retinoic acid and supraphysiologic doses of all-*trans*-retinoic acid are necessary to overcome the tight HDAC-recruitment and the consequent cell-cycle block.[200] The rare translocation t(11;17) fuses the RARα gene to the PLZF gene, which directly interacts with the NCoR–mSin3a–HDAC complex to suppress gene transcription. This block can only be overcome by the addition of a HDACi. Another well-known example of transcriptional silencing by the recruitment of an HDAC repressor is the AML1-ETO fusion protein which results from the t(8;21) translocation. As already described, the addition of an HDACi can relieve ETO-mediated transcriptional repression.[203] Although 11 HDACs have been described so far, only limited information is available about their redundant biologic and physiologic functions. As shown in Figure 13–4B, inhibitors of HDAC activity lead to the reexpression of silenced genes and to the induction of differentiation. Most of these inhibitors, like depsipeptide or SAHA,[204] do not exhibit isoenzyme selectivity and are therefore of limited therapeutic value. However, the HDACi valproic acid is the first drug within this group that selectively inhibits one HDAC, namely HDAC2.[205] Valproic acid induces proteasomal degradation of HDAC2. Basal and valproic acid-induced HDAC2 turnover strongly depend on the E2 ubiquitin conjugase Ubc8 and the E3 ubiquitin ligase RLIM. Thus, polyubiquitination and proteasomal degradation provide an isoenzyme-selective mechanism for downregulation of HDAC2.[205] This also underlines the importance of another cell-cycle element and leads to the last part of this chapter, to the proteasome.

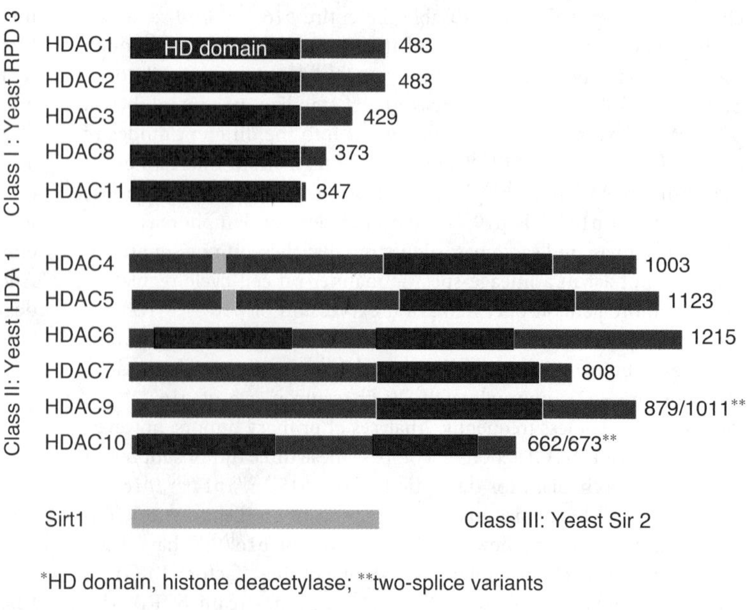

FIGURE 13–3. Classes of human histone deacetylases.

THE PROTEASOME: THE RECYCLING MACHINERY

The proteasome is a 2.4 mDa, multicentric protease complex with an important role in cellular protein regulation. Its structure consists of a cylindrical core, the so-called 20S particle, composed of four stacked rings with a total of seven proteins in each ring. The second part of the proteasome, two copies of the so-called 19S particle are bound to the 20S core. Only proteins that have been ubiquitinated can be degraded in the proteasome. The ubiquitination of different substrate proteins involves the sequential action of three enzymes: E1 (an adenosine triphosphate [ATP]-dependent ubiquitin-activating enzyme), E2 (a ubiquitin-conjugating enzyme), and E3 (ubiquitin-protein ligase). The ubiquitin-proteasome pathway plays a critical role in the degradation of

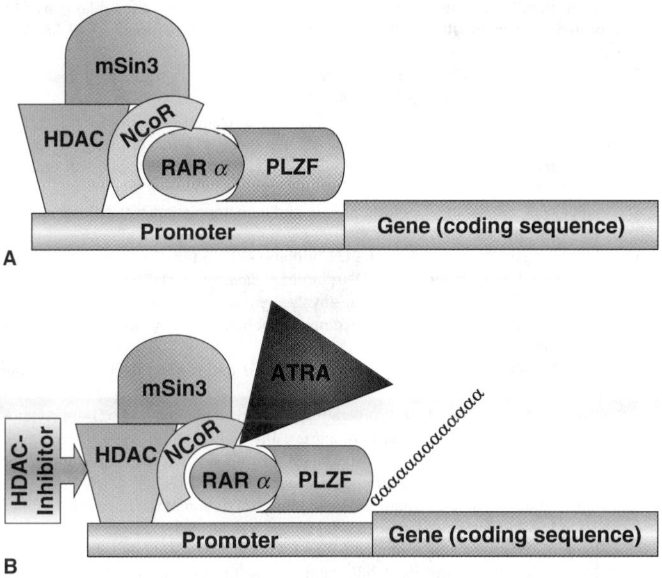

FIGURE 13–4. A. Transcriptional silencing by the recruitment of histone deacetylases (HDACs) in AML with t(11;17). See text for further description. **B.** Transcriptional reactivation and induction of differentiation by histone deacetylase inhibitors and all-*trans*-retinoic acid (ATRA) in AML with t(11;17). See text for further description.

intracellular proteins involved in cell-cycle control, transcription factor activation, apoptosis, and tumor growth through an ATP-dependent mechanism (the proteasome-ubiquitin pathway).[206] Proteins such as HDAC2 are tagged with several ubiquitin molecules and then degraded in the machinery.[205] Several tumors depend on rapid cell cycling, which requires expression and degradation of numerous regulatory proteins. Some of the proteins that undergo proteasome-mediated degradation include cyclins (cyclins A, B, D, E), cdk inhibitors ($p27^{kip1}$, $p21^{cip1}$), p53, RB, cdc25 phosphatase, and others.[207] The rapid turnover of these proteins triggers the rapid growth rate of certain human malignancies, thus the proteasome is an excellent new target for the development of new drugs, as attested by the success of the proteasome inhibitor bortezomib in patients with multiple myeloma. These substances inhibit the proteolytic activity of the proteasome and so cells accumulate in the G_2-M phase of the cell cycle with a decrease of cells in G_1.[207,208] For example, $p27^{kip1}$, $p21^{cip1}$are upregulated in multiple myeloma cells after the treatment with bortezomib, leading to cell-cycle arrest and apoptosis.[209]

The proteasome is also required for activation of the nuclear transcription factor nuclear factor-κB, which plays a role in maintaining cell viability through the transcription of inhibitors of apoptosis in response to environmental stress or cytotoxic agents. Based on these observations, targeting the proteasome has become a novel new approach to cancer therapy and with a better understanding of the human cell-cycle machinery it will be possible in the future to identify new targets for antineoplastic therapies.

REFERENCES

1. Hartwell LH, Weinert TA: Checkpoints: Controls that ensure the order of cell cycle events. *Science* 246:629, 1989.
2. Elledge SJ: Cell cycle checkpoints: Preventing an identity crisis. *Science* 274:1664, 1996.
3. Russell P: Checkpoints on the road to mitosis. *Trends Biochem Sci* 23:399, 1998.
4. Murray AW: The genetics of cell cycle checkpoints. *Curr Opin Genet Dev* 5:5, 1995.
5. Hartwell LH, Kastan MB: Cell cycle control and cancer. *Science* 266:1821, 1994.
6. Rao PN, Johnson RT: Mammalian cell fusion: Studies on the regulation of DNA synthesis and mitosis. *Nature* 225:159, 1970.
7. Lohka MJ, Hayes MK, Maller JL: Purification of maturation-promoting factor, an intracellular regulator of early mitotic events. *Proc Natl Acad Sci U S A* 85:3009, 1988.
8. Sherr CJ: Mammalian G1 cyclins. *Cell* 73:1059, 1993.
9. Pines J: Cyclins and cyclin-dependent kinases: Take your partners. *Trends Biochem Sci* 18:195, 1993.
10. Chen HH, Wong YH, Geneviere AM, et al: CDK13/CDC2L5 interacts with L-type cyclins and regulates alternative splicing. *Biochem Biophys Res Commun* 354:735, 2007.
11. Pagano M, Pepperkok R, Verde F, et al: Cyclin A is required at two points in the human cell cycle. *EMBO J* 11:961, 1992.
12. Rape M, Kirschner MW: Autonomous regulation of the anaphase-promoting complex couples mitosis to S-phase entry. *Nature* 432:588, 2004.
13. Resnitzky D, Hengst L, Reed SI: Cyclin A-associated kinase activity is rate limiting for entrance into S phase and is negatively regulated in G1 by p27Kip1. *Mol Cell Biol* 15:4347, 1995.
14. Meyerson M, Enders GH, Wu CL, et al: A family of human cdc2-related protein kinases. *EMBO J* 11:2909, 1992.
15. Solomon MJ: Activation of the various cyclin/cdc2 protein kinases. *Curr Opin Cell Biol* 5:180, 1993.
16. Lew J, Wang JH: Neuronal cdc2-like kinase. *Trends Biochem Sci* 20:33, 1995.
17. Matsushime H, Ewen ME, Strom DK, et al: Identification and properties of an atypical catalytic subunit (p34PSK-J3/cdk4) for mammalian D type G1 cyclins. *Cell* 71:323, 1992.
18. Xiong Y, Zhang H, Beach D: D type cyclins associate with multiple protein kinases and the DNA replication and repair factor PCNA. *Cell* 71:505, 1992.
19. Meyerson M, Harlow E: Identification of G1 kinase activity for cdk6, a novel cyclin D partner. *Mol Cell Biol* 14:2077, 1994.
20. Fesquet D, Labbe JC, Derancourt J, et al: The MO15 gene encodes the catalytic subunit of a protein kinase that activates cdc2 and other cyclin-dependent kinases (cdks) through phosphorylation of Thr161 and its homologues. *EMBO J* 12:3111, 1993.
21. Knuesel MT, Meyer KD, Donner AJ, et al: The human CDK8 subcomplex is a histone kinase that requires Med12 for activity and can function independently of mediator. *Mol Cell Biol* 29:650, 2009.
22. Morris EJ, Ji JY, Yang F, et al: E2F1 represses beta-catenin transcription and is antagonized by both pRB and CDK8. *Nature* 455:552, 2008.
23. Romano G, Giordano A: Role of the cyclin-dependent kinase 9-related pathway in mammalian gene expression and human diseases. *Cell Cycle* 7:3664, 2008.
24. Chen D, Fong Y, Zhou Q: Specific interaction of Tat with the human but not rodent P-TEFb complex mediates the species-specific Tat activation of HIV-1 transcription. *Proc Natl Acad Sci U S A* 96:2728, 1999.
25. Sergere JC, Thuret JY, Le Roux G, et al: Human CDK10 gene isoforms. *Biochem Biophys Res Commun* 276:271, 2000.
26. Hu D, Mayeda A, Trembley JH, et al: CDK11 complexes promote pre-mRNA splicing. *J Biol Chem* 278:8623, 2003.
27. Kasten M, Giordano A: Cdk10, a Cdc2-related kinase, associates with the Ets2 transcription factor and modulates its transactivation activity. *Oncogene* 20:1832, 2001.
28. Bagella L, Giacinti C, Simone C, et al: Identification of murine cdk10: Association with Ets2 transcription factor and effects on the cell cycle. *J Cell Biochem* 99:978, 2006.
29. Chen HH, Wang YC, Fann MJ: Identification and characterization of the CDK12/cyclin L1 complex involved in alternative splicing regulation. *Mol Cell Biol* 26:2736, 2006.
30. Hunt T: Cyclins and their partners: From a simple idea to complicated reality. *Semin Cell Biol* 2:213, 1991.
31. Lees EM, Harlow E: Sequences within the conserved cyclin box of human cyclin A are sufficient for binding to and activation of cdc2 kinase. *Mol Cell Biol* 13:1194, 1993.
32. Hanashiro K, Kanai M, Geng Y, et al: Roles of cyclins A and E in induction of centrosome amplification in p53-compromised cells. *Oncogene* 27:5288, 2008.
33. Krug U, Yasmeen A, Beger C, et al: Cyclin A1 regulates WT1 expression in acute myeloid leukemia cells. *Int J Oncol* 34:129, 2009.
34. Ohtsubo M, Roberts JM: Cyclin-dependent regulation of G1 in mammalian fibroblasts. *Science* 259:1908, 1993.
35. Ekholm SV, Reed SI: Regulation of G(1) cyclin-dependent kinases in the mammalian cell cycle. *Curr Opin Cell Biol* 12:676, 2000.
36. Strohmaier H, Spruck CH, Kaiser P, et al: Human F-box protein hCdc4 targets cyclin E for proteolysis and is mutated in a breast cancer cell line. *Nature* 413:316, 2001.
37. Ekholm-Reed S, Mendez J, Tedesco D, et al: Deregulation of cyclin E in human cells interferes with prereplication complex assembly. *J Cell Biol* 165:789, 2004.
38. Zhang HS, Postigo AA, Dean DC: Active transcriptional repression by the Rb-E2F complex mediates G1 arrest triggered by p16INK4a, TGFbeta, and contact inhibition. *Cell* 97:53, 1999.
39. Rajagopalan H, Jallepalli PV, Rago C, et al: Inactivation of hCDC4 can cause chromosomal instability. *Nature* 428:77, 2004.
40. Keck JM, Summers MK, Tedesco D, et al: Cyclin E overexpression impairs progression through mitosis by inhibiting APC(Cdh1). *J Cell Biol* 178:371, 2007.
41. McGowan CH, Russell P, Reed SI: Periodic biosynthesis of the human M-phase promoting factor catalytic subunit p34 during the cell cycle. *Mol Cell Biol* 10:3847, 1990.
42. Buendia B, Draetta G, Karsenti E: Regulation of the microtubule nucleating activity of centrosomes in Xenopus egg extracts: Role of cyclin A-associated protein kinase. *J Cell Biol* 116:1431, 1992.

43. Gallant P, Nigg EA: Cyclin B2 undergoes cell cycle-dependent nuclear translocation and, when expressed as a non-destructible mutant, causes mitotic arrest in HeLa cells. *J Cell Biol* 117:213, 1992.
44. Draviam VM, Orrechia S, Lowe M, et al: The localization of human cyclins B1 and B2 determines CDK1 substrate specificity and neither enzyme requires MEK to disassemble the Golgi apparatus. *J Cell Biol* 152:945, 2001.
45. Pines J: The cell cycle kinases. *Semin Cancer Biol* 5:305, 1994.
46. Arnaoutov A, Dasso M: The Ran GTPase regulates kinetochore function. *Dev Cell* 5:99, 2003.
47. Bentley AM, Normand G, Hoyt J, et al: Distinct sequence elements of cyclin B1 promote localization to chromatin, centrosomes, and kinetochores during mitosis. *Mol Biol Cell* 18:4847, 2007.
48. Yu Q, Sicinska E, Geng Y, et al: Requirement for CDK4 kinase function in breast cancer. *Cancer Cell* 9:23, 2006.
49. Landis MW, Pawlyk BS, Li T, et al: Cyclin D1-dependent kinase activity in murine development and mammary tumorigenesis. *Cancer Cell* 9:13, 2006.
50. Wei P, Garber ME, Fang SM, et al: A novel CDK9-associated C-type cyclin interacts directly with HIV-1 Tat and mediates its high-affinity, loop-specific binding to TAR RNA. *Cell* 92:451, 1998.
51. Peng J, Zhu Y, Milton JT, et al: Identification of multiple cyclin subunits of human P-TEFb. *Genes Dev* 12:755, 1998.
52. Fujinaga K, Cujec TP, Peng J, et al: The ability of positive transcription elongation factor B to transactivate human immunodeficiency virus transcription depends on a functional kinase domain, cyclin T1, and Tat. *J Virol* 72:7154, 1998.
53. MacLachlan TK, Sang N, De Luca A, et al: Binding of CDK9 to TRAF2. *J Cell Biochem* 71:467, 1998.
54. Michels AA, Nguyen VT, Fraldi A, et al: MAQ1 and 7SK RNA interact with CDK9/cyclin T complexes in a transcription-dependent manner. *Mol Cell Biol* 23:4859, 2003.
55. Garriga J, Bhattacharya S, Calbo J, et al: CDK9 is constitutively expressed throughout the cell cycle, and its steady-state expression is independent of SKP2. *Mol Cell Biol* 23:5165, 2003.
56. Husson H, Carideo EG, Neuberg D, et al: Gene expression profiling of follicular lymphoma and normal germinal center B cells using cDNA arrays. *Blood* 99:282, 2002.
57. Iorns E, Turner NC, Elliott R, et al: Identification of CDK10 as an important determinant of resistance to endocrine therapy for breast cancer. *Cancer Cell* 13:91, 2008.
58. Trembley JH, Hu D, Slaughter CA, et al: Casein kinase 2 interacts with cyclin-dependent kinase 11 (CDK11) *in vivo* and phosphorylates both the RNA polymerase II carboxyl-terminal domain and CDK11 *in vitro*. *J Biol Chem* 278:2265, 2003.
59. Shi J, Feng Y, Goulet AC, et al: The p34cdc2-related cyclin-dependent kinase 11 interacts with the p47 subunit of eukaryotic initiation factor 3 during apoptosis. *J Biol Chem* 278:5062, 2003.
60. Yokoyama H, Gruss OJ, Rybina S, et al: Cdk11 is a RanGTP-dependent microtubule stabilization factor that regulates spindle assembly rate. *J Cell Biol* 180:867, 2008.
61. Hu D, Valentine M, Kidd VJ, et al: CDK11(p58) is required for the maintenance of sister chromatid cohesion. *J Cell Sci* 120:2424, 2007.
62. Chandramouli A, Shi J, Feng Y, et al: Haploinsufficiency of the cdc2l gene contributes to skin cancer development in mice. *Carcinogenesis* 28:2028, 2007.
63. Sherr CJ: Cancer cell cycles. *Science* 274:1672, 1996.
64. Gu Y, Turck CW, Morgan DO: Inhibition of CDK2 activity in vivo by an associated 20K regulatory subunit. *Nature* 366:707, 1993.
65. Blagosklonny MV, Pardee AB: The restriction point of the cell cycle. *Cell Cycle* 1:103, 2002.
66. Assoian RK, Yung Y: A reciprocal relationship between Rb and Skp2: Implications for restriction point control, signal transduction to the cell cycle and cancer. *Cell Cycle* 7:24, 2008.
67. Yung Y, Walker JL, Roberts JM, et al: A Skp2 autoinduction loop and restriction point control. *J Cell Biol* 178:741, 2007.
68. Nourse J, Firpo E, Flanagan WM, et al: Interleukin-2-mediated elimination of the p27Kip1 cyclin-dependent kinase inhibitor prevented by rapamycin. *Nature* 372:570, 1994.
69. Santamaria D, Ortega S: Cyclins and CDKS in development and cancer: Lessons from genetically modified mice. *Front Biosci* 11:1164, 2006.
70. Genovese C, Trani D, Caputi M, et al: Cell cycle control and beyond: Emerging roles for the retinoblastoma gene family. *Oncogene* 25:5201, 2006.
71. Serrano M, Hannon GJ, Beach D: A new regulatory motif in cell-cycle control causing specific inhibition of cyclin D/CDK4 [see comments]. *Nature* 366:704, 1993.
72. Chan FK, Zhang J, Cheng L, et al: Identification of human and mouse p19, a novel CDK4 and CDK6 inhibitor with homology to p16ink4. *Mol Cell Biol* 15:2682, 1995.
73. DeGregori J, Leone G, Ohtani K, et al: E2F-1 accumulation bypasses a G1 arrest resulting from the inhibition of G1 cyclin-dependent kinase activity. *Genes Dev* 9:2873, 1995.
74. Nobori T, Miura K, Wu DJ, et al: Deletions of the cyclin-dependent kinase-4 inhibitor gene in multiple human cancers. *Nature* 368:753, 1994.
75. Bai C, Sen P, Hofmann K, et al: SKP1 connects cell cycle regulators to the ubiquitin proteolysis machinery through a novel motif, the F-box. *Cell* 86:263, 1996.
76. Feldman RM, Correll CC, Kaplan KB, et al: A complex of Cdc4p, Skp1p, and Cdc53p/cullin catalyzes ubiquitination of the phosphorylated CDK inhibitor Sic1p [see comments]. *Cell* 91:221, 1997.
77. Skowyra D, Koepp DM, Kamura T, et al: Reconstitution of G1 cyclin ubiquitination with complexes containing SCFGrr1 and Rbx1 [see comments]. *Science* 284:662, 1999.
78. Sun A, Bagella L, Tutton S, et al: From G0 to S phase: A view of the roles played by the retinoblastoma (Rb) family members in the Rb-E2F pathway. *J Cell Biochem* 102:1400, 2007.
79. Krug U, Ganser A, Koeffler HP: Tumor suppressor genes in normal and malignant hematopoiesis. *Oncogene* 21:3475, 2002.
80. Hagemeier C, Bannister AJ, Cook A, et al: The activation domain of transcription factor PU.1 binds the retinoblastoma (RB) protein and the transcription factor TFIID *in vitro*: RB shows sequence similarity to TFIID and TFIIB. *Proc Natl Acad Sci U S A* 90:1580, 1993.
81. Walkley CR, Sankaran VG, Orkin SH: Rb and hematopoiesis: Stem cells to anemia. *Cell Div* 3:13, 2008.
82. Zhang P, Zhang X, Iwama A, et al: PU.1 inhibits GATA-1 function and erythroid differentiation by blocking GATA-1 DNA binding. *Blood* 96:2641, 2000.
83. Bergh G, Ehinger M, Olsson I, et al: Involvement of the retinoblastoma protein in monocytic and neutrophilic lineage commitment of human bone marrow progenitor cells. *Blood* 94:1971, 1999.
84. Sherr CJ, Roberts JM: Inhibitors of mammalian G1 cyclin-dependent kinases. *Genes Dev* 9:1149, 1995.
85. Zhang H, Xiong Y, Beach D: Proliferating cell nuclear antigen and p21 are components of multiple cell cycle kinase complexes. *Mol Biol Cell* 4:897, 1993.
86. Li Y, Jenkins CW, Nichols MA, et al: Cell cycle expression and p53 regulation of the cyclin-dependent kinase inhibitor p21. *Oncogene* 9:2261, 1994.
87. Wang Z, Bhattacharya N, Mixter PF, et al: Phosphorylation of the cell cycle inhibitor p21Cip1/WAF1 by Pim-1 kinase. *Biochim Biophys Acta* 1593:45, 2002.
88. Zhang Y, Wang Z, Magnuson NS: Pim-1 kinase-dependent phosphorylation of p21Cip1/WAF1 regulates its stability and cellular localization in H1299 cells. *Mol Cancer Res* 5:909, 2007.
89. Ellwood-Yen K, Graeber TG, Wongvipat J, et al: Myc-driven murine prostate cancer shares molecular features with human prostate tumors. *Cancer Cell* 4:223, 2003.
90. Kato JY, Matsuoka M, Polyak K, et al: Cyclic AMP-induced G1 phase arrest mediated by an inhibitor (p27Kip1) of cyclin-dependent kinase 4 activation. *Cell* 79:487, 1994.
91. Vervoorts J, Luscher B: Post-translational regulation of the tumor suppressor p27(KIP1). *Cell Mol Life Sci* 65:3255, 2008.
92. Koepp DM, Harper JW, Elledge SJ: How the cyclin became a cyclin: Regulated proteolysis in the cell cycle. *Cell* 97:431, 1999.
93. Hirai H, Roussel MF, Kato JY, et al: Novel INK4 proteins, p19 and p18, are specific inhibitors of the cyclin D-dependent kinases CDK4 and CDK6. *Mol Cell Biol* 15:2672, 1995.
94. Hannon GJ, Beach D: P15ink4b is a potential effector of TGF-beta-induced cell cycle arrest [see comments]. *Nature* 371:257, 1994.
95. Adams L, Roth MJ, Abnet CC, et al: Promoter methylation in cytology specimens as an early detection marker for esophageal squamous dysplasia and early esophageal squamous cell carcinoma. *Cancer Prev Res (Phila Pa)* 1:357, 2008.
96. Lee YK, Park JY, Kang HJ, et al: Overexpression of p16INK4A and p14ARF in haematological malignancies. *Clin Lab Haematol* 25:233, 2003.
97. Drexler HG: Review of alterations of the cyclin-dependent kinase inhibitor INK4 family genes p15, p16, p18 and p19 in human leukemia-lymphoma cells. *Leukemia* 12:845, 1998.
98. Sulong S, Moorman AV, Irving JA, et al: A comprehensive analysis of the CDKN2A gene in childhood acute lymphoblastic leukemia reveals genomic deletion, copy number neutral loss of heterozygosity, and association with specific cytogenetic subgroups. *Blood* 113:100, 2009.
99. Diccianni MB, Batova A, Yu J, et al: Shortened survival after relapse in T-cell acute lymphoblastic leukemia patients with p16/p15 deletions. *Leuk Res* 21:549, 1997.
100. Belaud-Rotureau MA, Marietta V, Vergier B, et al: Inactivation of p16INK4a/CDKN2A gene may be a diagnostic feature of large B cell lymphoma leg type among cutaneous B cell lymphomas. *Virchows Arch* 452:607, 2008.
101. Bender CM, Pao MM, Jones PA: Inhibition of DNA methylation by 5-aza-2′-deoxycytidine suppresses the growth of human tumor cell lines. *Cancer Res* 58:95, 1998.
102. Cameron EE, Bachman KE, Myohanen S, et al: Synergy of demethylation and histone deacetylase inhibition in the re-expression of genes silenced in cancer. *Nat Genet* 21:103, 1999.
103. Humbey O, Pimkina J, Zilfou JT, et al: The ARF tumor suppressor can promote the progression of some tumors. *Cancer Res* 68:9608, 2008.
104. Mrozek K, Heinonen K, Bloomfield CD: Clinical importance of cytogenetics in acute myeloid leukaemia. *Best Pract Res Clin Haematol* 14:19, 2001.
105. Frohling S, Dohner H: Chromosomal abnormalities in cancer. *N Engl J Med* 359:722, 2008.
106. Dann EJ, Rowe JM: Biology and therapy of secondary leukaemias. *Baillieres Best Pract Res Clin Haematol* 14:119, 2001.
107. Vega F, Medeiros LJ: Chromosomal translocations involved in non-Hodgkin lymphomas. *Arch Pathol Lab Med* 127:1148, 2003.
108. Ichikawa M, Asai T, Chiba S, et al: Runx1/AML-1 ranks as a master regulator of adult hematopoiesis. *Cell Cycle* 3:722, 2004.
109. Elagib KE, Racke FK, Mogass M, et al: RUNX1 and GATA-1 coexpression and cooperation in megakaryocytic differentiation. *Blood* 101:4333, 2003.
110. Okuda T, van Deursen J, Hiebert SW, et al: AML1, the target of multiple chromosomal translocations in human leukemia, is essential for normal fetal liver hematopoiesis. *Cell* 84:321, 1996.
111. Scandura JM, Boccuni P, Cammenga J, et al: Transcription factor fusions in acute leukemia: Variations on a theme. *Oncogene* 21:3422, 2002.

112. Gilles L, Guieze R, Bluteau D, et al: P19INK4D links endomitotic arrest and megakaryocyte maturation and is regulated by AML-1. *Blood* 111:4081, 2008.
113. Wichmann C, Chen L, Heinrich M, et al: Targeting the oligomerization domain of ETO interferes with RUNX1/ETO oncogenic activity in t(8;21)-positive leukemic cells. *Cancer Res* 67:2280, 2007.
114. Lin RJ, Sternsdorf T, Tini M, et al: Transcriptional regulation in acute promyelocytic leukemia. *Oncogene* 20:7204, 2001.
115. Le XF, Vallian S, Mu ZM, et al: Recombinant PML adenovirus suppresses growth and tumorigenicity of human breast cancer cells by inducing G1 cell cycle arrest and apoptosis. *Oncogene* 16:1839, 1998.
116. Bischof O, Nacerddine K, Dejean A: Human papillomavirus oncoprotein E7 targets the promyelocytic leukemia protein and circumvents cellular senescence via the Rb and p53 tumor suppressor pathways. *Mol Cell Biol* 25:1013, 2005.
117. Jul-Larsen A, Grudic A, Bjerkvig R, et al: Cell-cycle regulation and dynamics of cytoplasmic compartments containing the promyelocytic leukemia protein and nucleoporins. *J Cell Sci* 122:1201, 2009.
118. Salomoni P, Pandolfi PP: The role of PML in tumor suppression. *Cell* 108:165, 2002.
119. Hayakawa F, Abe A, Kitabayashi I, et al: Acetylation of PML is involved in histone deacetylase inhibitor-mediated apoptosis. *J Biol Chem* 283:24420, 2008.
120. Chen Z, Brand NJ, Chen A, et al: Fusion between a novel Kruppel-like zinc finger gene and the retinoic acid receptor-alpha locus due to a variant t(11;17) translocation associated with acute promyelocytic leukaemia. *EMBO J* 12:1161, 1993.
121. Tefferi A, Gilliland DG: Oncogenes in myeloproliferative disorders. *Cell Cycle* 6:550, 2007.
122. Ren R: Mechanisms of BCR-ABL in the pathogenesis of chronic myelogenous leukaemia. *Nat Rev Cancer* 5:172, 2005.
123. Skorski T: BCR/ABL regulates response to DNA damage: The role in resistance to genotoxic treatment and in genomic instability. *Oncogene* 21:8591, 2002.
124. Gleissner B, Thiel E: Molecular genetic events in adult acute lymphoblastic leukemia. *Expert Rev Mol Diagn* 3:339, 2003.
125. Chi YH, Ward JM, Cheng LI, et al: Spindle assembly checkpoint and p53 deficiencies cooperate for tumorigenesis in mice. *Int J Cancer* 124:1483, 2009.
126. Fabbro D, Ruetz S, Buchdunger E, et al: Protein kinases as targets for anticancer agents: From inhibitors to useful drugs. *Pharmacol Ther* 93:79, 2002.
127. Spinelli O, Peruta B, Tosi M, et al: Clearance of minimal residual disease after allogeneic stem cell transplantation and the prediction of the clinical outcome of adult patients with high-risk acute lymphoblastic leukemia. *Haematologica* 92:612, 2007.
128. Tirado CA, Sebastian S, Moore JO, et al: Molecular and cytogenetic characterization of a novel rearrangement involving chromosomes 9, 12, and 17 resulting in ETV6 (TEL) and ABL fusion. *Cancer Genet Cytogenet* 157:74, 2005.
129. Rodrigues GA, Park M: Dimerization mediated through a leucine zipper activates the oncogenic potential of the met receptor tyrosine kinase. *Mol Cell Biol* 13:6711, 1993.
130. Fujimoto J, Shiota M, Iwahara T, et al: Characterization of the transforming activity of p80, a hyperphosphorylated protein in a Ki-1 lymphoma cell line with chromosomal translocation t(2;5). *Proc Natl Acad Sci U S A* 93:4181, 1996.
131. Amin HM, Lai R: Pathobiology of ALK+ anaplastic large-cell lymphoma. *Blood* 110:2259, 2007.
132. Golub TR, Barker GF, Lovett M, et al: Fusion of PDGF receptor beta to a novel ets-like gene, tel, in chronic myelomonocytic leukemia with t(5;12) chromosomal translocation. *Cell* 77:307, 1994.
133. Tam WF, Gu TL, Chen J, et al: Id1 is a common downstream target of oncogenic tyrosine kinases in leukemic cells. *Blood* 112:1981, 2008.
134. Graham SM, Cox AD, Drivas G, et al: Aberrant function of the Ras-related protein TC21/R-Ras2 triggers malignant transformation. *Mol Cell Biol* 14:4108, 1994.
135. Saxena N, Lahiri SS, Hambarde S, et al: RAS: Target for cancer therapy. *Cancer Invest* 26:948, 2008.
136. Khosravi-Far R, Solski PA, Clark GJ, et al: Activation of Rac1, RhoA, and mitogen-activated protein kinases is required for Ras transformation. *Mol Cell Biol* 15:6443, 1995.
137. Yip SC, El-Sibai M, Coniglio SJ, et al: The distinct roles of Ras and Rac in PI 3-kinase-dependent protrusion during EGF-stimulated cell migration. *J Cell Sci* 120:3138, 2007.
138. Schlessinger K, Hall A, Tolwinski N: Wnt signaling pathways meet Rho GTPases. *Genes Dev* 23:265, 2009.
139. Chang F, Steelman LS, Lee JT, et al: Signal transduction mediated by the Ras/Raf/MEK/ERK pathway from cytokine receptors to transcription factors: Potential targeting for therapeutic intervention. *Leukemia* 17:1263, 2003.
140. Crump M: Inhibition of raf kinase in the treatment of acute myeloid leukemia. *Curr Pharm Des* 8:2243, 2002.
141. Davis RK, Chellappan S: Disrupting the Rb-Raf-1 interaction: A potential therapeutic target for cancer. *Drug News Perspect* 21:331, 2008.
142. Thiel G, Ekici M, Rossler OG: Regulation of cellular proliferation, differentiation and cell death by activated Raf. *Cell Commun Signal* 7:8, 2009.
143. Johnson NL, Gardner AM, Diener KM, et al: Signal transduction pathways regulated by mitogen-activated/extracellular response kinase kinase induce cell death. *J Biol Chem* 271:3229, 1996.
144. Seth A, Gonzalez FA, Gupta S, et al: Signal transduction within the nucleus by mitogen-activated protein kinase. *J Biol Chem* 267:24796, 1992.
145. Amendola D, De Salvo M, Marchese R, et al: Myc down-regulation affects cyclin D1/cdk4 activity and induces apoptosis via Smac/Diablo pathway in an astrocytoma cell line. *Cell Prolif* 42:94, 2009.
146. Hoffmann I, Clarke PR, Marcote MJ, et al: Phosphorylation and activation of human cdc25-C by cdc2—Cyclin B and its involvement in the self-amplification of MPF at mitosis. *EMBO J* 12:53, 1993.
147. Zhang H, Gao P, Fukuda R, et al: HIF-1 inhibits mitochondrial biogenesis and cellular respiration in VHL-deficient renal cell carcinoma by repression of C-MYC activity. *Cancer Cell* 11:407, 2007.
148. Kramer MH, Hermans J, Wijburg E, et al: Clinical relevance of BCL2, BCL6, and MYC rearrangements in diffuse large B-cell lymphoma. *Blood* 92:3152, 1998.
149. Bonnotte B, Favre N, Moutet M, et al: Bcl-2-mediated inhibition of apoptosis prevents immunogenicity and restores tumorigenicity of spontaneously regressive tumors. *J Immunol* 161:1433, 1998.
150. Yin DX, Schimke RT: Inhibition of apoptosis by overexpressing Bcl-2 enhances gene amplification by a mechanism independent of aphidicolin pretreatment. *Proc Natl Acad Sci U S A* 93:3394, 1996.
151. Del Principe MI, Del Poeta G, Venditti A, et al: Apoptosis and immaturity in acute myeloid leukemia. *Hematology* 10:25, 2005.
152. Gelmetti V, Zhang J, Fanelli M, et al: Aberrant recruitment of the nuclear receptor corepressor-histone deacetylase complex by the acute myeloid leukemia fusion partner ETO. *Mol Cell Biol* 18:7185, 1998.
153. Wang J, Hoshino T, Redner RL, et al: ETO, fusion partner in t(8;21) acute myeloid leukemia, represses transcription by interaction with the human N-CoR/mSin3/HDAC1 complex. *Proc Natl Acad Sci U S A* 95:10860, 1998.
154. Wong CW, Privalsky ML: Components of the SMRT corepressor complex exhibit distinctive interactions with the POZ domain oncoproteins PLZF, PLZF-RARalpha, and BCL-6. *J Biol Chem* 273:27695, 1998.
155. David G, Alland L, Hong SH, et al: Histone deacetylase associated with mSin3A mediates repression by the acute promyelocytic leukemia-associated PLZF protein. *Oncogene* 16:2549, 1998.
156. Yunis JJ, Ramsay N: Retinoblastoma and subband deletion of chromosome 13. *Am J Dis Child* 132:161, 1978.
157. Grana X, Garriga J, Mayol X: Role of the retinoblastoma protein family, pRB, p107 and p130 in the negative control of cell growth. *Oncogene* 17:3365, 1998.
158. Bookstein R, Lee WH: Molecular genetics of the retinoblastoma suppressor gene. *Crit Rev Oncog* 2:211, 1991.
159. Chellappan S, Kraus VB, Kroger B, et al: Adenovirus E1A, simian virus 40 tumor antigen, and human papillomavirus E7 protein share the capacity to disrupt the interaction between transcription factor E2F and the retinoblastoma gene product. *Proc Natl Acad Sci U S A* 89:4549, 1992.
160. Krug U, Ganser A, Koeffler HP: Tumor suppressor genes in normal and malignant hematopoiesis. *Oncogene* 21:3475, 2002.
161. Stommel JM, Wahl GM: Accelerated MDM2 auto-degradation induced by DNA-damage kinases is required for p53 activation. *EMBO J* 23:1547, 2004.
162. Kubbutat MH, Jones SN, Vousden KH: Regulation of p53 stability by Mdm2. *Nature* 387:299, 1997.
163. Eischen CM, Lozano G: P53 and MDM2: Antagonists or partners in crime? *Cancer Cell* 15:161, 2009.
164. Bouska A, Eischen CM: Mdm2 affects genome stability independent of p53. *Cancer Res* 69:1697, 2009.
165. Roth J, Dobbelstein M, Freedman DA, et al: Nucleo-cytoplasmic shuttling of the hdm2 oncoprotein regulates the levels of the p53 protein via a pathway used by the human immunodeficiency virus rev protein. *EMBO J* 17:554, 1998.
166. Quelle DE, Zindy F, Ashmun RA, et al: Alternative reading frames of the INK4a tumor suppressor gene encode two unrelated proteins capable of inducing cell cycle arrest. *Cell* 83:993, 1995.
167. Kamijo T, Zindy F, Roussel MF, et al: Tumor suppression at the mouse INK4a locus mediated by the alternative reading frame product p19ARF. *Cell* 91:649, 1997.
168. Bates S, Phillips AC, Clark PA, et al: P14arf links the tumour suppressors Rb and p53 [letter]. *Nature* 395:124, 1998.
169. Palmero I, Pantoja C, Serrano M: P19arf links the tumour suppressor p53 to Ras [letter]. *Nature* 395:125, 1998.
170. Prives C: Signaling to p53: Breaking the MDM2-p53 circuit. *Cell* 95:5, 1998.
171. Sherr CJ: Tumor surveillance via the ARF-p53 pathway. *Genes Dev* 12:2984, 1998.
172. Kurz EU, S.P. Lees-Miller, DNA damage-induced activation of ATM and ATM-dependent signaling pathways. *DNA Repair (Amst)* 3:889, 2004.
173. Senoo M, Manis JP, Alt FW, et al: P63 and p73 are not required for the development and p53-dependent apoptosis of T cells. *Cancer Cell* 6:85, 2004.
174. Deyoung MP, Ellisen LW: P63 and p73 in human cancer: Defining the network. *Oncogene* 26:5169, 2007.
175. Di Como CJ, Gaiddon C, Prives C: P73 function is inhibited by tumor-derived p53 mutants in mammalian cells. *Mol Cell Biol* 19:1438, 1999.
176. Melino G, Lu X, Gasco M, et al: Functional regulation of p73 and p63: Development and cancer. *Trends Biochem Sci* 28:663, 2003.
177. Kawano S, Miller CW, Gombart AF, et al: Loss of p73 gene expression in leukemias/lymphomas due to hypermethylation. *Blood* 94:1113, 1999.
178. Olopade OI, Jenkins RB, Ransom DT, et al: Molecular analysis of deletions of the short arm of chromosome 9 in human gliomas. *Cancer Res* 52:2523, 1992.
179. Schmid M, Malicki D, Nobori T, et al: Homozygous deletions of methylthioadenosine phosphorylase (MTAP) are more frequent than p16INK4A (CDKN2) homozygous deletions in primary non- small cell lung cancers (NSCLC). *Oncogene* 17:2669, 1998.

180. Stadler WM, Olopade OI: The 9p21 region in bladder cancer cell lines: Large homozygous deletion inactivate the CDKN2, CDKN2B and MTAP genes. *Urol Res* 24:239, 1996.
181. Gonzalez MV, Pello MF, Lopez-Larrea C, et al: Deletion and methylation of the tumour suppressor gene p16/CDKN2 in primary head and neck squamous cell carcinoma. *J Clin Pathol* 50:509, 1997.
182. Yamada Y, Hatta Y, Murata K, et al: Deletions of p15 and/or p16 genes as a poor-prognosis factor in adult T- cell leukemia. *J Clin Oncol* 15:1778, 1997.
183. Hori Y, Hori H, Yamada Y, et al: The methylthioadenosine phosphorylase gene is frequently co-deleted with the p16INK4a gene in acute type adult T-cell leukemia. *Int J Cancer* 75:51, 1998.
184. Kratzke RA, Otterson GA, Lincoln CE, et al: Immunohistochemical analysis of the p16INK4 cyclin-dependent kinase inhibitor in malignant mesothelioma. *J Natl Cancer Inst* 87:1870, 1995.
185. Cayuela JM, Gardie B, Sigaux F: Disruption of the multiple tumor suppressor gene MTS1/p16(INK4a)/CDKN2 by illegitimate V(D)J recombinase activity in T-cell acute lymphoblastic leukemias. *Blood* 90:3720, 1997.
186. Becker TM, Haferkamp S, Dijkstra MK, et al: The chromatin remodelling factor BRG1 is a novel binding partner of the tumor suppressor p16INK4a. *Mol Cancer* 8:4, 2009.
187. Christopher SA, Diegelman P, Porter CW, et al: Methylthioadenosine phosphorylase, a gene frequently codeleted with p16(cdkN2a/ARF), acts as a tumor suppressor in a breast cancer cell line. *Cancer Res* 62:6639, 2002.
188. Lan L, Trempus C, Gilmour SK: Inhibition of ornithine decarboxylase (ODC) decreases tumor vascularization and reverses spontaneous tumors in ODC/Ras transgenic mice. *Cancer Res* 60:5696, 2000.
189. Subhi AL, Diegelman P, Porter CW, et al: Methylthioadenosine phosphorylase regulates ornithine decarboxylase by production of downstream metabolites. *J Biol Chem* 23:23, 2003.
190. Stevens AP, Spangler B, Wallner S, et al: Direct and tumor microenvironment mediated influences of 5′-deoxy-5′-(methylthio)adenosine on tumor progression of malignant melanoma. *J Cell Biochem* 106:210, 2009.
191. Jaffrain-Rea ML, Ferretti E, Toniato E, et al: P16 (Ink4a, Mts-1) gene polymorphism and methylation status in human pituitary tumours. *Clin Endocrinol (Oxf)* 51:317, 1999.
192. Baylin SB, Herman JG, Graff JR, et al: Alterations in DNA methylation: A fundamental aspect of neoplasia. *Adv Cancer Res* 72:141, 1998.
193. Boultwood J, Wainscoat JS: Gene silencing by DNA methylation in haematological malignancies. *Br J Haematol* 138:3, 2007.
194. Timmermann S, Hinds PW, Munger K: Re-expression of endogenous p16ink4a in oral squamous cell carcinoma lines by 5-aza-2′-deoxycytidine treatment induces a senescence-like state. *Oncogene* 17:3445, 1998.
195. Hennessy BT, Garcia-Manero G, Kantarjian HM, et al: DNA methylation in haematological malignancies: The role of decitabine. *Expert Opin Investig Drugs* 12:1985, 2003.
196. Xiong J, Epstein RJ: Growth inhibition of human cancer cells by 5-aza-2′-deoxycytidine does not correlate with its effects on INK4a/ARF expression or initial promoter methylation status. *Mol Cancer Ther* 8:779, 2009.
197. Razin A: CpG methylation, chromatin structure and gene silencing-a three-way connection. *EMBO J* 17:4905, 1998.
198. Jones PL, Veenstra GJ, Wade PA, et al: Methylated DNA and MeCP2 recruit histone deacetylase to repress transcription. *Nat Genet* 19:187, 1998.
199. Bueno MJ, de Castro IP, Malumbres M: Control of cell proliferation pathways by microRNAs. *Cell Cycle* 7:3143, 2008.
200. Vigushin DM, Coombes RC: Histone deacetylase inhibitors in cancer treatment. *Anticancer Drugs* 13:1, 2002.
201. Thiagalingam S, Cheng KH, Lee HJ, et al: Histone deacetylases: Unique players in shaping the epigenetic histone code. *Ann N Y Acad Sci* 983:84, 2003.
202. Haberland M, Montgomery RL, Olson EN: The many roles of histone deacetylases in development and physiology: Implications for disease and therapy. *Nat Rev Genet* 10:32, 2009.
203. Wang J, Saunthararajah Y, Redner RL, et al: Inhibitors of histone deacetylase relieve ETO-mediated repression and induce differentiation of AML1-ETO leukemia cells. *Cancer Res* 59:2766, 1999.
204. Zhou W, Zhu WG: The changing face of HDAC inhibitor depsipeptide. *Curr Cancer Drug Targets* 9:91, 2009.
205. Kramer OH, Zhu P, Ostendorff HP, et al: The histone deacetylase inhibitor valproic acid selectively induces proteasomal degradation of HDAC2. *EMBO J* 22:3411, 2003.
206. McBride WH, Iwamoto KS, Syljuasen R, et al: The role of the ubiquitin/proteasome system in cellular responses to radiation. *Oncogene* 22:5755, 2003.
207. Richardson PG, Mitsiades C, Hideshima T, et al: Proteasome inhibition in the treatment of cancer. *Cell Cycle* 4:290, 2005.
208. Elliott PJ, Ross JS: The proteasome: A new target for novel drug therapies. *Am J Clin Pathol* 116:637, 2001.
209. Pei XY, Dai Y, Grant S: Synergistic induction of oxidative injury and apoptosis in human multiple myeloma cells by the proteasome inhibitor bortezomib and histone deacetylase inhibitors. *Clin Cancer Res* 10:3839, 2004.

CHAPTER 14
SIGNAL TRANSDUCTION PATHWAYS

Kenneth Kaushansky

SUMMARY

Essentially all external influences upon cells of any organ are mediated by biochemical and molecular mechanisms that are triggered by interactions with membrane, cytoplasmic, or nuclear receptors. Our understanding of the receptors and the intermediate molecules that couple them with cellular pathways that influence the proliferation, activation, differentiation, or survival of hematopoietic cells has expanded significantly. Proteins on the surface of blood cells that transmit vital information from the extracellular environment include single-pass, homodimeric, heterodimeric, and heterotrimeric transmembrane proteins that do, or do not, contain intrinsic kinase activity, but either way signal by inducing the tyrosine phosphorylation of a multitude of cytoplasmic proteins, seven transmembrane domain proteins that signal though G proteins, heterodimeric integrins that recruit large focal adhesions, and large families of heterodimeric proteins that induce serine and threonine phosphorylation. This chapter describes the receptors that influence blood cell production and function, the secondary mediators and the biochemical modifications they undergo to alert the cell to an external influence, the molecular mechanisms that allow for the coordination of multiple signals impacting a cell simultaneously, and the processes upon which they impact.

AN OVERVIEW OF CELL SIGNALING

Blood cells and their marrow-based progenitors are exquisitely responsive to their environment. A wide variety of cues are detected by mature blood cells that impact significantly on their function. For example, leukocytes respond to noxious stimuli by chemokine-induced migration toward inflammatory stimuli, cross endothelial cell barriers and the extracellular matrix by engaging integrins, and then respond to chemotactic gradients to enter inflammatory foci to contact and engulf microorganisms on encountering bacterial products. Likewise, platelets adhere to reactive endothelial surfaces or denuded subendothelial cell matrix by engagement of extracellular adhesive proteins. Adherent platelets can also recruit additional platelets and aggregate with them through interactions with platelet integrins, secrete growth factors that will recruit cells that mediate repair of vascular injury and then contract to strengthen the platelet plug by engagement of numerous granule substances. Even the anucleate erythrocyte responds to mechanical deformation and hypoxemia with adenosine triphosphate (ATP) release. Adrenergic receptors also play important roles in the normal erythrocyte response to parasitic infection or in the pathologic red cell's interactions with endothelial cell surfaces (e.g., patients with hemoglobinopathies). Each of these events induces an intracellular signal that leads to further cellular reactivity toward the initiating stimulus, or that prepares the cell for subsequent functional events. Like the functional activation of mature blood cells, the generation of blood cells is under tight regulation, mediated by soluble hematopoietic growth factors, cytokines, and components of the marrow microenvironment. Here again, the erythropoietin (EPO) response to anemia is sensed by hematopoietic progenitor cell surface receptors; their coordinated reaction involves a myriad of signals that impact on the survival, growth, and differentiation of both undifferentiated and lineage-committed cells. Although anemia induces red cell production and inflammation leads to the production and functional activation of leukocytes, many of the intracellular signals that mediate these two responses overlap substantially. This chapter illustrates a number of principles that mediate the growth and functional responses of blood cells and their progenitors in health and disease. A better understanding of how blood cells respond to their environment can lead to improved strategies to intervene in pathologic processes in which too many or too few blood cells are produced, or in which the functional activation of blood cells is insufficient or overly exuberant and leads to disease. Moreover, a thorough knowledge of how the signaling pathways that mediate growth and cell survival are disrupted in the hematologic malignancies has begun to allow the rational intervention in such diseases.

Acronyms and abbreviations that appear in this chapter include: BCR, B-cell antigen receptor; BMP, bone morphogenic protein; CT-1, cardiotrophin-1; CNTF, ciliary neurotrophic factor; DD, death domain; DR, death receptor; EPO, erythropoietin; EPOR, erythropoietin receptor; ERK, extracellular response kinase; FADD, Fas-associated death domain; FAK, focal adhesion kinase; G-CSF, granulocyte colony-stimulating factor; Gab, Grb binding; GH, growth hormone; GM-CSF, granulocyte-macrophage colony-stimulating factor; GPCR, G-protein-coupled receptor; HCR, hematopoietic cytokine receptor; IAP, inhibitors of apoptosis; IKK, I-κB kinase; IL, interleukin; IRS, Insulin receptor substrate; ITAM, immunoreceptor tyrosine-based activation motif; ITIM, immunoreceptor tyrosine-based inhibitory motif; JAK, Janus family kinase; JNK, c-Jun N-terminal kinase; LIF, leukemia inhibitory factor; M-CSF, macrophage colony-stimulating factor; MAPK, mitogen-activated protein kinase; NR, nuclear receptor; OSM, oncostatin M; PI3K phosphoinositol 3 kinase; PIAS, protein inhibitor of activated STATs; PIP, phosphoinositol phosphate; PKC, protein kinase C; PTP, protein tyrosine phosphatases; RACK, receptor for activated C kinase; RTK, receptor tyrosine kinase; SCID, severe combined immunodeficiency; SH2, Src homology 2; SOCS, suppressors of cytokine signaling; STATs, signal transducers and activators of transcription; SUMO, small ubiquitin-like modifier; TNF, tumor necrosis factor; TGF, transforming growth factor; TM, transmembrane; TPO, thrombopoietin; TRADD, TNF receptor death domain; TRAF, TNF receptor-associated factor; TRAIL, tumor necrosis factor-related apoptosis-inducing ligand.

TYPES OF RECEPTORS AND THEIR MECHANISMS OF ACTIVATION

THE TYPE I HEMATOPOIETIC CYTOKINE RECEPTORS

The Erythropoietin Receptor

The erythropoietin receptor (EPOR) was cloned in 1989,[1] settling several controversies and setting many important paradigms in receptor biology. Like other hematopoietic cytokines of this class (granulocyte colony-stimulating factor [G-CSF], thrombopoietin [TPO], and growth hormone [GH]), EPO binds to a homodimeric receptor[2,3] with picomolar affinity.[4] Numerous studies in these and multiple other cell-signaling systems demonstrate the importance of phosphorylation of vital cytoplasmic mediators in signal transduction,[5–7] yet one initial conundrum was that the cloned EPOR bears no kinase domain.[1] Rather, subsequent studies revealed that the EPOR employs a cytoplasmic kinase of the Janus family (JAK) to initiate signaling.[8] Although cytokine binding to the receptor was initially thought to recruit JAKs to the cytoplasmic domain motifs termed *Box1* and *Box2* domains, it is almost certain that inactive kinase molecules are tethered to the receptor prior to ligand engagement. This information, along with the availability of the tertiary structure of

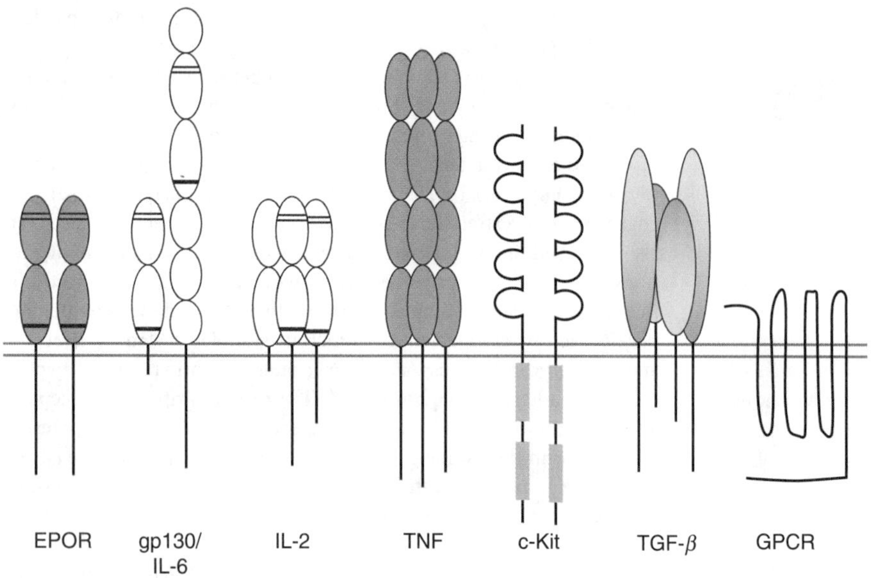

FIGURE 14–1. An illustration of cell surface receptors. Each member of the cell surface receptors is depicted as an extracellular region of one or multiple domains, with conserved disulfide bonds indicated by *thin cross lines*, and the conserved WS box indicated by a *thick cross line*. The founding member of each receptor class is indicated. EPOR, erythropoietin receptor; GPCR, G-protein couple receptor; gp130, glycoprotein 130; IL, interleukin; TGF, transforming growth factor; TNF, tumor necrosis factor.

EPOR and of EPO bound to EPOR,[9,10] has provided a key insight into the initiation of signal transduction. EPOR exists as a preformed cell surface dimer (see Fig. 14–1), in a conformation that separates the two cytoplasmic domains of the subunits (and hence the two tethered JAK molecules) by 73 Å (angstroms). EPO binds sequentially to the two subunits of the preformed EPOR dimer at two distinct faces of the molecule, first to one subunit with the high-affinity face of the ligand (also termed *site I*), and then to the second subunit of EPOR with a lower-affinity face (termed *site II*), but an interaction that reduces the off-rate of the ligand. Upon engagement of the two EPOR subunits, a stunning conformational change ensues, shifting the distance between the two cytoplasmic domains of the receptor subunits from 73 Å to 39 Å, a shift that appears to bring the two inactive JAK molecules into sufficiently close juxtaposition to allow cross-phosphorylation and kinase activation. Once the two tethered JAK molecules are active, multiple additional tyrosine residues become phosphorylated, residues of the receptor itself and those on a number of tethered signaling molecules, events that trigger the totality of cellular EPO responses. Although direct proof for this model of signal initiation is not available for other cytokines of this class, it is widely assumed that a variety of growth factors, interleukins, and hormones activate cellular events in the same manner.

The understanding that a single molecule of EPO can bind simultaneously to two EPOR molecules, and the realization that multiple other cytokines employ a similar stoichiometry of activation has allowed for therapeutic engineering of cytokines into antagonists. Following EPO binding to a first molecule of EPOR through site I, the receptor conformational change becomes dependent on binding of EPO site II to a second EPOR subunit. By altering the residues at site II, it is possible to block this engagement. If site I is altered to increase its affinity for binding to a first receptor subunit so that the affinity of the mutant protein rivals that of the intact molecule, a potent rationally designed antagonist is generated. This strategy has been successfully employed to create pegvisomant, a GH antagonist useful for the treatment of acromegaly and a forerunner of the interleukin (IL)-5 antagonists for eosinophil-mediated disorders currently under development.

The engagement of two receptor subunits by a cognate ligand is one mechanism of inducing the receptor conformational change necessary for JAK activation, but several other mechanisms exist that have been exploited by man and nature. Small molecules and dimeric antibodies can induce signaling through the EPOR and at least for the former, can serve as EPO mimetics for therapeutic use.[11] Moreover, the 55-kDa glycoprotein (gp55) of the Friend erythroleukemia virus hijacks the EPOR for virus-induced proliferation[12] by directly binding to EPOR and (presumably) by inducing the same receptor conformational changes as induced by the authentic hormone. Thus, there are many ways to activate EPOR, and many subtleties dependent on the actual tertiary structural changes induced.[13]

The Interleukin-6 Receptor Family The IL-6 family of cytokine receptors displays several properties distinct from those of EPOR and its related receptors.[14,15] Unlike the receptors discussed thus far, the IL-6R is composed of a heterodimer. One subunit is termed IL-6Rα, which binds IL-6 with modest affinity, but despite a short cytoplasmic domain IL-6Rα plays no role in signaling. Instead, the second receptor subunit, termed gp130 based on its apparent molecular weight (Mr), a molecule that alone has no affinity for IL-6 but together with IL-6Rσ enhances the binding affinity of the heterodimeric receptor, is responsible for initiating signal transduction in the presence of ligand. In addition, soluble forms of the IL-6R, if loaded with IL-6, can bind to cells bearing only gp130 and activate the latter.[16] Like EPOR and other members of that subfamily, gp130 engages JAKs to initiate signal transduction.[17] Moreover, it is almost certain that the mature IL-6R complex is composed of at least two molecules of IL-6R and two of gp130,[18] the latter required to bring the requisite two JAK molecules to the signaling complex. An additional feature of the IL-6 family is that gp130 serves as the signaling receptor subunit for several cytokines, including IL-11, oncostatin M (OSM), leukemia inhibitory factor (LIF), ciliary neurotrophic factor (CNTF), and cardiotrophin-1 (CT-1). Similar to its role in the IL-6R, gp130 binds to each of these ligands only in the additional presence of a cytokine-specific receptor subunit (e.g., IL-11R, LIF-R) to form the holoreceptor. As a consequence of this shared coreceptor physiology, when two or more of the cytokine-specific receptors are present on a cell, the two corresponding ligands can compete for a limiting amount of gp130, and hence for cytokine-specific signaling. This physiology also allows therapeutically engineered cytokine-receptor complexes to stimulate signaling in all cells that express gp130.[19] Furthermore, the same principles that allow the rationale design of an EPO or GH antagonist can be used to engineer IL-6 antagonists for treatment of pathologic states dependent on interactions with receptors that require gp130 for receptor signaling.[20,21]

The Interleukin-2 Receptor Family The IL-2 family of receptors is also quite complex, in most cases sharing one and even two subunits with receptors for other cytokines of the same class (see Fig. 14–1). IL-2Rβ is shared with the IL-15R, and IL-2Rγ (also termed γ_C [for common]) is shared with the IL-4, IL-7, IL-9, IL-15, and IL-21 receptors.[22] Another feature of the IL-2R not yet discussed for the EPOR or IL-6R families is that of a devoted JAK. While JAK2 is employed by all the EPOR subfamily members along with some of the IL-6R subfamily members, and JAK1 and TYK2 are also shared amongst these latter receptors, the fourth and final JAK family member, JAK3, is engaged only by γ_C. In addition to providing a more fundamental understanding of the principles of signal transduction, careful investigation of the IL-2 family of receptors also has afforded detailed insights into a number of clinically important immunodeficiency states.[23] The complexity of this family of receptors was illustrated by the progressive investigation into the origins of severe combined immunodeficiency (SCID).[24] As is discussed in Chap. 82, SCID is a severe loss of natural killer (NK) and T lymphocytes and has been traced to deficiencies of either γ_C or JAK3, a phenotype recapitulated quite well (but not perfectly) by genetic elimination of the same molecules in mice. However, genetic elimination of IL-2 leads to a phenotype quite different than SCID of humans or engineered mice. Instead, of the multiple cytokines for which γ_C and JAK3 support signaling, only elimination of IL-7 or the IL-7R recapitulates the phenotype,[25,26] a finding now consistent with the finding that IL-7 affects common lymphoid progenitors (Chap. 16), while other cytokines in the family affect more differentiated lymphoid cells.

THE TUMOR NECROSIS FACTOR RECEPTOR SUPERFAMILY

At present the tumor necrosis factor (TNF) superfamily of receptors and ligands comprises at least 30 receptors and 20 ligands,[27,28] and illustrates several novel points in signal transduction pathways: trimeric binding (see Fig. 14–1), receptor promiscuity, and decoy receptors. Although many TNF ligand family members (TNF-α, TNF-β, CD40L [CD154], receptor activator of nuclear factor-κB ligand [RANKL; osteoprotegerin ligand (OPGL)], OX40L, etc.) can bind to several receptors, the ligands are, for the most part, subfamily specific. For example, TNF-α only binds to the six TNF-α receptors and tumor necrosis factor-related apoptosis-inducing ligand (TRAIL) binds to the five TRAIL receptors,[29] although it can also bind to the receptor termed *osteoprotegerin* (OPG).[30] Ligands in this family bind as trimers to homotrimeric receptors, leading to recruitment of secondary signaling molecules to the cytoplasmic domain of the receptors. In general, there are two classes of cytoplasmic domains in these receptors, based on whether they contain the death domain (DD), a region capable of binding signaling mediators that initiate apoptosis (see Chap. 12). As such, receptors that do not contain a DD or other signaling domain can function as "decoy receptors," diverting ligand from initiating programmed cell death in the target cell. For example, among the TNF-α receptors, TNFRI (DR2) contains a DD, and among the five TRAIL receptors, DR4 and DR5 contain DDs, whereas TNFR2 and DcR1 and DcR2 and OPG act as decoy receptors for TNF and TRAIL, respectively. The biologic consequences of ligand binding to individual TNFR family members depend on the relative affinity of their cytoplasmic domains for multiple adaptor proteins; tumor necrosis factor receptor death domain (TRADD) and Fas-associated death domain (FADD) engagement trigger apoptosis pathways, whereas recruitment of one of the six TNF receptor-associated factor (TRAF) family members leads to activation of transcription factors such as nuclear factor-κB (NF-κB) and kinases such as c-Jun N-terminal kinase (JNK) that lead to cell survival, proliferation, and activation of inflammation.

THE RECEPTOR TYROSINE KINASES

The receptor tyrosine kinases (RTKs) comprise another class of receptors that contains members vital for hematopoiesis and mature blood cell function (see Fig. 14–1). The first hematopoietic member of this family to be identified was the eukaryotic version of the *v-fms* oncogene, designated *c-fms*. Further study revealed that the protooncogene is the sole receptor for macrophage colony-stimulating factor (M-CSF),[31] and although somewhat distinct in possessing a split kinase domain, was immediately grouped with other RTKs, such as the receptors for insulin, vascular endothelial cell growth factor and epidermal growth factor, among several others. Subsequently, two additional hematopoietic receptor family members have been identified, c-Kit and Flt-3. These receptors were each cloned based on their homology to the viral oncogene *v-kit* or *c-fms*, respectively.[32,33] Like all other members of the family, upon engagement of their cognate ligand the kinase domains of homodimeric RTKs become activated, leading to the phosphorylation of receptor cytoplasmic domain tyrosine residues and other tethered substrates. In an apparent example of convergent evolution, like members of the hematopoietic cytokine receptor (HCR) family, RTKs were also found to employ JAKs in their signaling pathways[34]; as a result, many of the same secondary signaling pathways are activated by both classes of receptors. But perhaps serving as an even more striking example of convergent evolution, the tertiary structure of the index ligand for a hematopoietic RTK, M-CSF, bears substantial homology to essentially all the ligands of the hematopoietic cytokine receptor family, such as granulocyte-macrophage colony-stimulating factor (GM-CSF).[35]

TRANSFORMING GROWTH FACTOR β RECEPTORS

The transforming growth factor (TGF) receptor family consists of seven type I and five type II receptors that heterodimerize to form receptors for multiple TGF-β family members, including the TGF-β/activin/nodal and bone morphogenic protein (BMP) subfamilies. The precise stoichiometry of binding involves a ligand dimer, stabilized by disulfide and/or hydrophobic bonds, and two type I and two type II subunits (see Fig. 14–1); the tertiary structure of the complex has been carefully investigated.[36] Both type I and type II receptors contain an N-terminal ligand binding, transmembrane, and cytoplasmic ser/thr kinase domains; the type I receptors additionally contain a Gly/Ser (GS)-rich domain.[36] For TGF-β subfamily members, the type II subunit bears a high-affinity ligand binding site, which on TGF-β or activin engagement recruits type I receptors, bringing the two cytoplasmic domains into close juxtaposition, enabling the type II kinase to phosphorylate Ser residues on the type I receptor GS domain, thereby activating the type I kinase. Cell-surface-bound coreceptors also exist and aid in generating the signaling complex for TGF-β, but not activin or BMP ligands. For BMP family members, the type I receptor bears the high-affinity ligand binding site, such that BMP initially binds to type I receptor, with the type II subunit subsequently recruited to form the signaling complex. Once the two receptor kinases are activated, they recruit and phosphorylate the SMAD (Sma- and Mad-related protein) adaptor proteins, allowing their nuclear translocation and transcriptional activation. However, SMAD-independent TGF-β signaling pathways also exist.[37]

G-PROTEIN-COUPLED RECEPTORS

Several molecules that play essential roles in blood cell development or function signal by engaging G-protein-coupled receptors (GPCRs), clearly the largest family of cell surface receptors in organisms as diverse as yeast and humans, estimated to comprise approximately 1000 distinct gene products, or approximately 3 percent of the human genome. Also termed *serpentine* or *heptahelical receptors* (for their seven transmembrane domains that form four extracellular and three intracellular loops; see Fig. 14–1), GPCRs are so named because they use three small "G" proteins (G, G, and G) for signal transduction. In the unstimulated state, all three G proteins bind to the intracellular loops of the receptor. Individual ligands engage GPCR in one of many different ways. For example, small lipophilic molecules (e.g., epinephrine) bind to transmembrane (TM) domains of the receptor, disrupting the interactions between TM3 and TM6, leading to conformational changes that alter G protein binding.[38] Other GPCRs use additional extracellular domains (e.g., the "Venus flytrap" domain)[39] to bind and dimerize receptors. Still others, which are engaged by proteases, are activated by protease cleavage of the receptor amino terminus, leading to the "unmasking" of a hexapeptide at the new amino terminus, which then interacts with one of the receptor extracellular or transmembrane domains.[40] By each of these and other mechanisms a conformational change occurs in the GPCR, allowing monomeric G and dimeric G to dissociate from the intracellular loops and each to engage secondary signaling pathways.[41] Examples of critical molecules that employ GPCRs and display hematologic activity are thrombin, adrenergic hormones, and chemokines. The outcomes of such engagement include cellular growth and survival, functional activation, and migration.

INTEGRINS AND OTHER ADHESION MOLECULES

Although adhesion molecules play a vital structural role in tissue cohesion, physically bridging cells in the marrow with each other and with extracellular matrix macromolecules, and at sites at which mature blood cells interact with the endothelium, engagement of blood and progenitor cell integrins and other adhesion molecules also generates vital signals within the cell that affect its survival, proliferation, and functional activation.[42–44] In fibroblasts, cell adhesion is most clearly manifest at contact sites termed focal adhesions, and the signaling complexes that form on cytoplasmic domains of the integrins that support them are termed focal adhesion complexes.[45] Within such complexes are components of the actin cytoskeleton, kinases both specific for focal adhesions and several others found in other cytoplasmic sites,[46–48] and a number of scaffolding molecules upon which adhesion strengthening and signaling take place. Moreover, growth factor receptors functionally interact with integrins, adding to signaling complexity. Thus, adhesion molecules must also be considered as signaling receptors.

NUCLEAR RECEPTORS

Nuclear receptors (NRs) are nascent transcription factors that play a wide variety of roles in cellular physiology by binding small lipophilic hormones. Some NRs, such as glucocorticoid hormone receptors, remain sequestered in the cytoplasm in the absence of their cognate ligand, and upon ligand engagement translocate to the nucleus and bind and activate palindromic, direct repeat, or inverted palindromic sequences that comprise nucleotide hormone response elements.[49] Other NRs, such as receptors for vitamin A metabolites (retinoids), remain bound to nuclear DNA and repress transcription, until engaged by ligand upon which nuclear coactivators are recruited leading to enhancement of gene transcription.[50–52] Although sex, glucocorticoid, and thyroid hormones may play subtle roles in blood cell biology, retinoid receptors, which most commonly bind as heterodimers with the RXR receptor to retinoid response elements of the form PuGTTCA(N)2,5PuGTTCA, play vital developmental roles in a myriad of cell systems, and play similar roles in hematopoiesis. Amongst the hematopoietic targets of retinoid receptors are c-myc, C/EBPε, and p21.[53] However, because this class of receptors represents a nearly direct pathway from stimulus to response, without intervening signaling, they are not discussed further in this chapter.

THE DIVERSITY OF DOWNSTREAM SIGNALS

PROTEIN PHOSPHORYLATION

Protein phosphorylation is the critical first and vital response to engagement of signaling molecules of nearly all classes of cell surface receptors, including those that affect blood cell production and function. Numerous studies reveal that protein tyrosine phosphorylation is detectible within a minute of the addition of a wide variety of hematopoietic cytokines to blood cells and their progenitors. Evidence from nearly all studies employing chemical inhibitors of kinase function or various knockout and knockin strategies shows that JAK activation is critical for hematopoietic cell survival, growth, and differentiation, and mature cell response to a wide range of stimuli (Fig. 14–2).[54,55] Several studies have elucidated an important mechanism of regulation of JAK kinases, one which is altered in the myeloproliferative diseases polycythemia vera, essential thrombocytosis and idiopathic myelofibrosis (see Chaps. 86, 87, and 91).

Based on homologies to a number of other proteins JAK kinases display 7 domains. These include (1) the domains that tether the kinase to the cytoplasmic domain of the cytokine receptor (JH3-JH7), (2) the kinase domain (JH1), and (3) a pseudokinase domain (JH2), so termed because of its homology to other tyrosine kinases but lack of kinase activity. Nevertheless, despite its lack of kinase activity, the pseudokinase domain inhibits the kinase activity of the kinase domain, as shown by single and double domain expression studies.[56] Based on the known structure of the kinase domain of a fibroblast growth factor receptor tyrosine kinase, the kinase and pseudokinase domains of JAK2 have been modeled.[57] The structure indicates several potential sites of interaction between the activation loop of the kinase domain and the pseudokinase domain. Of great interest, one such interaction exists between Val_{617} in the pseudokinase domain, a residue somatically mutated to Phe in the hematopoietic cells of virtually all patients with polycythemia vera and approximately half with essential thrombocythemia and idiopathic myelofibrosis (see Chaps. 86, 87, and 91).[58-62]

Among the phosphorylation targets of JAKs and other immediately responsive kinases in both normal and neoplastic hematopoiesis are the signaling receptor itself, perhaps the rate-limiting step in signaling,[63] adaptor molecules (Shc, Grb2, IRS, Gab) that once modified recruit additional signaling substrates, regulatory subunits of secondary kinases (p85 phosphoinositol 3 kinase [PI3K]), latent transcription factors (signal transducers and activators of transcription [STATs]), and several phosphatases (SHP2, SHIP). By catalyzing the phosphorylation of Tyr residues present in certain receptor motifs, RTKs and JAK2 modify many signaling proteins to acquire the capacity to bind Src homology (SH)-2 domain-containing proteins. Perhaps equally important are ser/thr phosphorylation sites induced by activated TGF-β receptors. However, most of the downstream signaling components of all of the receptors that use JAK2 and other kinases to transduce growth and differentiation cues have been derived from candidate gene approaches; the availability of antibodies to specific signaling mediators has dictated the molecules that have been studied. An unbiased approach to identifying the entire "signaling space" used by all of the receptors noted above is required if we are to fully understand the influence of the extracellular milieu on hematopoiesis.

MEMBRANE LIPID MODIFICATION

Upon recruitment to a doubly phosphorylated receptor cytoplasmic domain or adapter protein the regulatory subunit of PI3K undergoes conformational changes enabling the binding of its 110-kDa kinase subunit, resulting in activation of the kinase (see Fig. 14–2).[64] The major target of PI3K is membrane inositols, perhaps most importantly $PI_{4,5}$ phosphate (PIP2), converting the latter into $PI_{3,4,5}P$ (PIP3). Once present in adequate amounts, PIP3 recruits proteins with pleckstrin homology domains to the inner cytoplasmic membrane, which become phosphorylated by their juxtaposition to another PH domain containing kinase, PDK.[65] Among the best known of the recruited proteins are protein kinase B (also termed Akt), a kinase that phosphorylates a broad range of

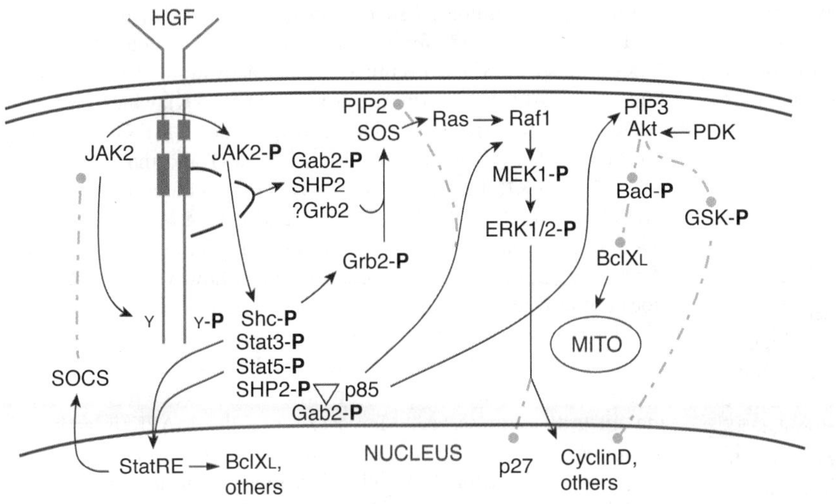

FIGURE 14–2. An illustration of signal transduction pathways. Signal transduction ensues when a hematopoietic growth factor (HGF) binds to its cognate receptor, resulting in a change in receptor conformation bringing two tethered JAK molecules into close proximity (attachment site to receptor is indicated by two *green boxes*, representing the box1 and box2 motifs). Molecules that become phosphorylated upon activation are indicated by **P**. A multiprotein complex that forms on a scaffolding molecule, such as Gab2, is indicated by the *triangle*. Stimulatory pathways (vis-à-vis cell proliferation) are indicated by *solid lines with arrow heads*. Inhibitory pathways are indicated by *broken lines with ball heads*. The nucleus and the mitochondria (MITO) are indicated.

substrates in a wide variety of cells, all with the ultimate effect of enhancing cell survival and/or cell cycling.[66] For example, Akt phosphorylates Bad, a proapoptotic protein that once so modified is targeted for degradation.[67] Akt indirectly activates NF-κB,[67] a transcription factor that influences several cell cycle and survival proteins,[68] including the antiapoptotic Bcl and IAP (inhibitors of apoptosis) proteins and the cell cycle activators c-Myc and cyclin D. In addition, forkhead family members, which when present enhance transcription of cell cycle inhibitors such as p27 and the proapoptotic protein Fas ligand, are phosphorylated and inactivated by Akt.[69] Akt is activated by the bcr-abl oncogene in blood cells of patients with chronic myelogenous leukemia (CML), and blockade of PI3K reduces their proliferation substantially.[70]

NUCLEAR TRANSLOCATION

In addition to the posttranslational modification of signaling molecules illustrated in the preceding examples, relocalization of signaling molecules is also a vital process that conveys information within the cell. This cellular strategy is well illustrated by the activation of NF-κB,[68] a family of transcription factors activated by growth factor, nuclear, TGF/BMP family, and integrin receptors that affect genes vital for cell survival and growth. In the unstimulated cell, NF-κB subunits reside in the cytoplasm, sequestered from their nuclear targets by virtue of its binding to I-κB. Upon cellular activation of Akt, I-κB kinase is activated by phosphorylation, which then phosphorylates I-κB, thereby releasing NF-κB and targeting I-κB for proteasomal destruction, allowing NK-κB to translocate to the nucleus and bind and activate target genes.

A second example of cytoplasmic sequestration blocking nuclear function involves the SMAD proteins that mediate TGF-β receptor signaling.[36] Once recruited to the phosphorylated type I TGF-β receptor, SMAD2 is phosphorylated, reducing its affinity for SARA, a molecule that helps tether SMAD2 to the receptor. Once free of SARA, a SMAD2/SMAD4 complex forms, which is competent to translocate to the nucleus, either by the generation of a nuclear localization signal or because of the elimination of the SARA blockade of the SMAD2 nuclear pore complex interaction site. In addition to ingress, the formation of a SMAD2/SMAD4 complex also blocks a nuclear export signal present on the latter.[71]

ENGAGEMENT OF ADAPTOR PROTEINS

Another general theme to emerge from numerous studies on signal transduction is that multimolecular complexes of signaling intermediaries often assemble on scaffolding or adaptor proteins, which develop the capacity to assemble signaling complexes upon phosphorylation.[72] Insulin receptor substrates (IRSs) were the first such adaptors identified, and are phosphorylated by the activated insulin receptor.[73] IRS proteins are also modified by several other receptor-activated kinases, including JAKs.[54] Grb-binding (Gab) proteins are a family of at least three adapters, so named because of their ability to bind to the adaptor Grb2, a signaling intermediate necessary for Ras activation.[74] Both IRS and Gab proteins present multiple sites for phosphorylation, and once so modified present numerous SH2-binding and other protein–protein interacting motifs (see Fig. 14–2), which allow assembly of signaling complexes. Additional molecules serve this function in other signaling receptors, such as paxillin binding on the cytoplasmic tails of α-integrin.[48] Paxillin presents four different types of protein–protein interaction domains (SH3, SH2, LD [Leu-Asp], and LIM [lin-11/Isl-1/Mec-3]) enabling it to bind downstream kinases (focal adhesion kinase [FAK], the related Pyk2 kinase, Src kinase, and paxillin-associated kinase [PAK]), other adaptor molecules (Crk, PIX, PKL), and phosphatases (PTP-PEST). As many cellular kinases can phosphorylate adaptor proteins (e.g., in addition to integrin engagement, GH binding leads to paxillin phosphorylation), such complexes can function as a nexus to coordinate multiple cellular stimuli into a concerted response.

Another example of the capacity of adaptor proteins to translate extracellular signals into intracellular physiologic change is found in the response to TNF ligands. The capacity of receptors that bear DDs to induce apoptosis is dependent on the binding of the adaptor protein FADD to the cytoplasmic domain of TNF receptor (TNFR), which then recruits and activates the initiating caspases 8 and 10, leading to activation of the executioner caspases 3, 6, and 7 (see Chap. 12).[28,29,75] This extracellular signal-mediated apoptotic pathway stands in contrast to a second, cell-intrinsic apoptosis pathway, in which DNA damage, cell-cycle checkpoint defects, or loss of survival factors leads to enhanced expression of proapoptotic bcl family members (bax, bad, bclXs, bid). Once proapoptotic proteins overcome the level of antiapoptotic family members (bc12, BclXL), mitochondrial transmembrane potential declines, leading to leakage of cytochrome c and SMAC, the former engaging the apoptotic protease-activating factor (APAF) adaptor, thereby activating caspase 9 and, subsequently, the executioner family of caspases, the latter inhibiting members of the IAP family that otherwise attenuate caspase action. It should also be noted that although these two apoptosis pathways can be discussed as distinct entities, merging at the level of caspase 3, they interact. For example, activation of caspase 8 by TNF family members can also cleave bid to cause mitochondrial leakage of cytochrome c, thereby engaging the cell intrinsic pathway, serving to amplify the extracellular signal pathway to programmed cell death.

Binding of TNF family members to their receptors does not always result in apoptosis. Although there are likely many mechanisms for this finding, one is mediated by the binding of adaptors. Different TNF family receptors employ one of six TRAFs to engage and activate I-κB kinase (IKK), which leads to the release of NF-κB, a transcription factor that induces expression of several prosurvival and proliferation-associated genes.[68]

SIGNALING SPECIFICITY WITHIN EACH RECEPTOR FAMILY

Once a large number of receptor/cytokine systems were identified and tools to study some of their downstream signaling events developed, it became clear that most cytokine receptors stimulate a very similar cadre of signaling events as other members of the same family. For example, EPO, TPO, GH, GM-CSF, IL-6, and leptin all stimulate the phosphorylation of JAK2, yet lead to quite different cellular effects. One theory of hematopoiesis posits that growth factors merely serve to prevent apoptosis; the stochastic induction of one or another set of transcription factors is responsible for the distinct lineage differentiation events of hematopoiesis.[76] If this is true, then overlapping signaling events supported by a diverse range of cytokines might not be surprising as they would subserve the same end point, inhibition of programmed cell death. However, it is also clear that some cytokines and extracellular stimuli induce changes in critical transcription factors, and that the fate of multipotent progenitor cells can be influenced by the cytokines to which they are exposed; if so, each cytokine would need to induce distinct signals. Careful studies of signaling events have supported this hypothesis. For example, JAK3 is engaged only by cytokine receptors that use γ_C,[77] and although EPO activates the same JAK as TPO (JAK2), the former leads to activation of STAT5,[78] whereas the latter leads to STAT5 and STAT3 activation,[79] which targets a different set of genes. Moreover, engagement of integrin $\alpha_5\beta_1$ stimulates EPO-induced erythroid development, while stimulation of integrin $\alpha_4\beta_1$ mediates signals that inhibit erythropoiesis and enhances TPO-induced megakaryocyte growth.[80,81] Additional examples of relative signaling specificity that separates sets of cytokines are the predominance of STAT5 activation by IL-2, compared with STAT1 and STAT3 by the closely related IL-21,[82] and the almost exclusive engagement of STAT4 by IL-12 and STAT6 by IL-4 and IL-13.[83,84] Consequently, because our understanding of the entirety of downstream signals is far from complete, the cytoplasmic domains of cytokine receptors bear almost no homology other than that required to engage JAKs, and there already exists a modest degree of signaling specificity, it is likely that although several cytokines engage overlapping sets of signaling intermediaries, each will result in a unique set of signaling events. It is almost certain that the use of unbiased screens of the entirety of signaling molecules will be required to decipher all the interactions induced by ligand engagement of the multiple receptor families described in this chapter. Such efforts have been described for the epidermal growth factor receptor family,[85] and should be highly informative in studies of hematopoietic signaling.

SIGNALING INSULATION

Many of the kinases and other intermediaries that play important roles in signal transduction are not absolutely substrate specific; nevertheless, they do participate in specific pathways free from interference from other pathways. Perhaps the best example of this is found in the mitogen-activated protein kinase (MAPK) pathway.[86] At least three major MAPK pathways operate in most cells, the p42/p44 ERK (extracellular response kinase), p38, and JNK, each of which is triggered by distinct stimuli (mitogens such as cytokines for ERK, inflammatory mediators and hypoxia for p38, and stress and noxious stimuli for JNK), but all of which eventuate in the activation of a cascade of kinases, a MAPK kinase kinase (also termed MEKK), which phosphorylates and activates a MAPK kinase (also termed a MEK), and finally the MAPK. The MAPKKK for ERK1/2 is Raf-1 and the MAPKK for ERK1/2 is MEK1, the MAPKKK for p38 is MEKK1 and the MAPKK is MKK3, and for JNK they are MEKK1 and MKK4 or MKK7, respectively. Because each of these kinases display only limited substrate specificity *in vitro*, it would be difficult to explain how MEKK1 activation does not lead to ERK activation without some mechanism to insulate the signals. Several scaffolding proteins have now been identified that assemble specific MAPKKK, MAPKK, and MAPKs.[87] By forming complexes of the cascade on pathway-specific scaffolding molecules, signaling integrity is preserved. Moreover, once the MAPK is activated, additional scaffolding molecules can link the specific MAPK to its target transcription factors.[88] Additional examples of "insulating" signaling scaffolds include those for NF-κB and the TNF receptor,[89] the B-cell antigen receptor (termed BLNK),[90] and protein kinase C and integrins (termed RACKs).[91]

EXTINGUISHING SIGNALS

In addition to initiating signaling by extracellular ligands, the cell must also be able to extinguish the stimulus to prepare for additional events and to guard against continuous cell growth. Several mechanisms have been identified that extinguish the signals initiated by extracellular stimuli.

RECEPTOR DOWN-MODULATION

Shortly after binding to ligand, hematopoietic cytokine receptors and receptor tyrosine kinases are rapidly internalized,[92] serving to down-modulate further signaling.[93] Receptor internalization is dependent on membrane clathrin,[93] which represents a major mechanism of endocytosis of cell-surface proteins, and on at least one element of ligand-induced signaling.[94] The sites on hematopoietic receptors responsible for internalization are mapped,[95] potentially allowing intervention in this process. For example, activation of c-Mpl by TPO leads to engagement of the adaptor protein 2 (AP2) complex, which results in clathrin binding and receptor internalization. The kinetics of this process is delayed, taking approximately 30 minutes for near complete internalization, allowing the TPO signal to persist only a short time.[96]

PHOSPHATASES

As discussed earlier in "The Diversity of Downstream Signals," phosphorylation of numerous proteins and membrane lipids plays a vital role in signal transduction within the cell. Thus, elimination of these modifications through the action of phosphatases would be expected to terminate such signals. Moreover, because some of the same signals are activated in malignant transformation, protein tyrosine phosphatases (PTPs) might also be expected to play an important antioncogenic role. Several cellular phosphatases have been identified that play roles in signal termination and as tumor suppressors.

Hematopoietic cell phosphatase (also termed SHP1) bears two SH2 domains that interact with cytokine and inhibitory immune coreceptors at ITIM (immunoreceptor tyrosine-based inhibitory motif) sites that have been modified by Tyr phosphorylation. Once so engaged, SHP1 becomes activated and dephosphorylates associated phosphotyrosine activation sites on receptors, adaptor molecules, and their associated kinases.[97] One of the earliest clues that SHP1 plays an important role in hematopoietic signaling came from the discovery that the moth-eaten mouse phenotype is a result of a genetic loss of function of SHP1.[98] These mice demonstrate a massive expansion and tissue accumulation of monocytes and myeloid cells, resulting in chronic inflammation, massive immune defects, and premature death. Careful analysis of the mice revealed they manifest defective controls over the cellular activation and proliferation response to exogenous stimuli, such as that induced by engagement of the B-cell antigen receptor (BCR) complex. At steady state SHP1 is thought to engage the BCR (through presently unclear mechanisms) and maintains the antigen-binding subunits (immunoglobulin [Ig]α and Igβ) in a dephosphorylated, quiescent state. The phosphatase is displaced from the complex upon antigen engagement, but is later re-recruited to the complex once ITIM containing inhibitory coreceptors such as CD22, PIR-B, CD72, and FcγRIIb are phosphorylated and recruited to the activated complex.[99] Once recruited to the BCR complex, SHP1 removes the activating Tyr phosphate sites on the ITAM (immunoreceptor tyrosine-based activation motif) sites of Igα/β, the coreceptor CD19, the adaptor BLNK and Lyn kinase, and the BCR returns to its quiescent state. Similar roles for SHP1 have been identified in T cells,[100] NK cells,[101] monocytes and macrophages,[102] and erythroid cells.[103] The latter is of particular interest, as mutation of the site on EPOR to which SHP1 binds causes familial erythrocytosis, as a result of reduction of EPO signaling. Of interest, this mutation was identified in a family containing a two-time Olympic gold medalist.[104]

SOCS Proteins

Another mechanism of growth factor signal termination is mediated by the suppressors of cytokine signaling (SOCS) proteins. The cloning of a STAT-inducible gene, CIS,[105] and several additional genes that bear substantial sequence homology,[106,107] has yielded a family of proteins that can directly suppress growth factor receptor-induced signals. The engagement of either hematopoietic cytokine receptors or receptor tyrosine kinases leads to STAT activation, as discussed earlier in "The Diversity of Downstream Signals." One of the transcriptional targets of STATs are the SOCS and PIAS (protein inhibitor of activated STATs) genes (see Fig. 14–2), which upon transcription and translation bind to phosphotyrosine residues and inhibit either JAK kinases, STATs, or the phosphorylated receptors themselves, blocking recruitment of signaling adaptor molecules.[108] Ubiquitin and SUMO (small ubiquitin-like modifier) also have been shown to play a vital role in SOCS- and PIAS-mediated repression of cytokine signaling.[108,109]

INHIBITORY SIGNALS

Finally, some signals impact adversely on signals derived from alternate receptors. One example is the interaction of growth factors and TGF-β-derived signals. One of the major hematopoietic effects of TGF-β on hematopoietic stem cells is to reduce cell cycling. In contrast, many growth factors, such as SCF, Flt3 ligand, and TPO enhance stem cell cycling and induce their proliferation. As TGF-β is constitutively expressed in the marrow stroma, one mechanism by which growth factors can overcome cell cycle suppression is mediated by growth factor-induced ERK1/2 activation. The cell cycling effects of TGF-β are mediated by nuclear SMAD2–SMAD4, and nuclear localization of the complex is determined, at least in part, by the blockade of a nuclear export signal on the complex. As growth factor-induced MAPK leads to the phosphorylation of several sites on the linker region of SMAD2, the balance of nuclear and cytoplasmic SMAD is tipped toward the latter, leading to reduced suppressive effects of TGF-β on the cell cycle.[110] Another form of this type of cross-talk between cytokines is illustrated by TPO and interferon alpha (IFN-α), the latter suppressing megakaryopoiesis driven by the former. By induction of SOCS-1, not usually induced by TPO, IFN-α inhibits TPO mediated signaling.[111]

SIGNAL COORDINATION AND CROSS-TALK

In the foregoing discussion several examples of the convergence of signaling pathways and receptor crosstalk were summarized. Over the past decade, two types of cell membrane-based supramolecular organizations have been identified, lipid rafts and tetraspanin webs. In their seminal fluid–mosaic model of the cell membrane, Singer and Nicolson posited that integral membrane proteins float in a random array of membrane lipids.[112] This model was modified to account for local heterogeneity of the lipid bilayer. Lipid rafts, local concentrations of specific membrane lipids and proteins, are defined by the methods to isolate them—the insoluble components of a cold detergent extraction in which raft components "float" to the top of a density gradient.[113] Upon discovery that many of the proteins present in such rafts were involved in signal transduction, it became apparent that these membrane subdomains could represent a structural basis for communication between seemingly disparate components of the signal transduction apparatus. This hypothesis was best validated in hematopoietic cells.[37,114,115]

A second level of membrane-based structural organization of signaling molecules has been elucidated—the tetraspanin-enriched microdomain or "web." The tetraspanin family of membrane proteins is characterized by four transmembrane domains punctuating two extracellular regions, a CCG motif, and several other conserved cysteine residues in the extracellular domain. The tetraspanins now include more than 30 members,[116] most or all of which interact with other cell surface molecules, and have been functionally linked to cell adhesion, migration, differentiation, and signal transduction. Members of this family are thought to act as molecular facilitators of protein–protein interaction by associating with "partners," the bimolecular complexes then interact with others in a slightly less avid manner, and the complexes loosely associate in microdomains. CD9, CD63, and CD81 are the tetraspanins most closely linked to hematopoietic cell function, are usually found in association with β_1 and β_3 integrins,[117] affect many hematopoietic cell types,[118–120] and act in concert with multiple signaling receptors, kinases, and phosphatases.[121,122]

REFERENCES

1. D'Andrea AD, Lodish HF, Wong GG: Expression cloning of the murine erythropoietin receptor. *Cell* 57:277, 1989.
2. Watowich SS, Hilton DJ, Lodish HF: Activation and inhibition of erythropoietin receptor function: Role of receptor dimerization. *Mol Cell Biol* 14:3535, 1994.
3. Livnah O, Stura EA, Middleton SA, et al: Crystallographic evidence for preformed dimers of erythropoietin receptor before ligand activation. *Science* 283:987, 1999.
4. Broudy VC, Lin N, Egrie J, et al: Identification of the receptor for erythropoietin on human and murine erythroleukemia cells and modulation by phorbol ester and dimethyl sulfoxide. *Proc Natl Acad Sci U S A* 85:6513, 1988.
5. Kanakura Y, Druker B, Cannistra SA, et al: Signal transduction of the human granulocyte-macrophage colony-stimulating factor and interleukin-3 receptors involves tyrosine phosphorylation of a common set of cytoplasmic proteins. *Blood* 76:706, 1990.
6. Spivak JL, Fisher J, Isaacs MA, et al: Protein kinases and phosphatases are involved in erythropoietin-mediated signal transduction. *Exp Hematol* 20:500, 1992.
7. Otani H, Erdos M, Leonard WJ: Tyrosine kinase(s) regulate apoptosis and bcl-2 expression in a growth factor-dependent cell line. *J Biol Chem* 268:22733, 1993.
8. Witthuhn BA, Quelle FW, Silvennoinen O, et al: JAK2 associates with the erythropoietin receptor and is tyrosine phosphorylated and activated following stimulation with erythropoietin. *Cell* 74:227, 1993.
9. Syed RS, Reid SW, Li C, et al: Efficiency of signalling through cytokine receptors depends critically on receptor orientation. *Nature* 395:511, 1998.
10. Cheetham JC, Smith DM, Aoki KH, et al: NMR structure of human erythropoietin and a comparison with its receptor bound conformation. *Nat Struct Biol* 5:861, 1998.

11. Wrighton NC, Farrell FX, Chang R, et al: Small peptides as potent mimetics of the protein hormone erythropoietin. *Science* 273:458, 1996.
12. Li JP, D'Andrea AD, Lodish HF, et al: Activation of cell growth by binding of Friend spleen focus-forming virus gp55 glycoprotein to the erythropoietin receptor. *Nature* 343:762, 1990.
13. Livnah O, Johnson DL, Stura EA, et al: An antagonist peptide-EPO receptor complex suggests that receptor dimerization is not sufficient for activation. *Nat Struct Biol* 5:993, 1998.
14. Taga T, Kishimoto T: Gp130 and the interleukin-6 family of cytokines. *Annu Rev Immunol* 15:797, 1997.
15. Hirano T: Interleukin 6 and its receptor: Ten years later. *Int Rev Immunol* 16:249, 1998.
16. Jones SA, Rose-John S: The role of soluble receptors in cytokine biology: The agonistic properties of the sIL-6R/IL-6 complex. *Biochim Biophys Acta* 1592:251, 2002.
17. Stahl N, Boulton TG, Farruggella T, et al: Association and activation of Jak-Tyk kinases by CNTF-LIF-OSM-IL-6 beta receptor components. *Science* 263:92, 1994.
18. Pflanz S, Kurth I, Grotzinger J, et al: Two different epitopes of the signal transducer gp130 sequentially cooperate on IL-6-induced receptor activation. *J Immunol* 165:7042, 2000.
19. Baiocchi M, Marcucci I, Rose-John S, et al: An IL-6/IL-6 soluble receptor (IL-6R) hybrid protein (H-IL-6) induces EPO-independent erythroid differentiation in human CD34(+) cells. *Cytokine* 12:1395, 2000.
20. Adachi Y, Yoshio-Hoshino N, Nishimoto N. The blockade of IL-6 signaling in rational drug design. *Curr Pharm Des* 14:1217, 2008.
21. Tassone P, Galea E, Forciniti S, et al: The IL-6 receptor super-antagonist Sant7 enhances antiproliferative and apoptotic effects induced by dexamethasone and zoledronic acid on multiple myeloma cells. *Int J Oncol* 21:867, 2002.
22. Waldmann TA: T-cell receptors for cytokines: Targets for immunotherapy of leukemia/lymphoma. *Ann Oncol* 11(Suppl 1):101, 2000.
23. Leonard WJ: The molecular basis of X-linked severe combined immunodeficiency: Defective cytokine receptor signaling. *Annu Rev Med* 47:229, 1996.
24. Uribe L, Weinberg KI: X-linked SCID and other defects of cytokine pathways. *Semin Hematol* 35:299, 1998.
25. von Freeden-Jeffry U, Vieira P, Lucian LA, et al: Lymphopenia in interleukin (IL)-7 gene-deleted mice identifies IL-7 as a nonredundant cytokine. *J Exp Med* 181:1519, 1995.
26. Appasamy PM: Biological and clinical implications of interleukin-7 and lymphopoiesis. *Cytokines Cell Mol Ther* 5:25, 1999.
27. Ashkenazi A: Targeting death and decoy receptors of the tumour-necrosis factor superfamily. *Nat Rev Cancer* 2:420, 2002.
28. Aggarwal BB: Signalling pathways of the TNF superfamily: A double-edged sword. *Nat Rev Immunol* 3:745, 2003.
29. Wang S, El-Deiry WS: TRAIL and apoptosis induction by TNF-family death receptors. *Oncogene* 22:8628, 2003.
30. Emery JG, McDonnell P, Burke MB, et al: Osteoprotegerin is a receptor for the cytotoxic ligand TRAIL. *J Biol Chem* 273:14363, 1998.
31. Sherr CJ: The role of the CSF-1 receptor gene (C-*fms*) in cell transformation. *Leukemia* 2:132S, 1988.
32. Lyman SD, Jacobsen SE: c-Kit ligand and Flt3 ligand: Stem/progenitor cell factors with overlapping yet distinct activities. *Blood* 91:1101, 1998.
33. Broudy VC: Stem cell factor and hematopoiesis. *Blood* 90:1345, 1997.
34. Linnekin D: Early signaling pathways activated by c-Kit in hematopoietic cells. *Int J Biochem Cell Biol* 31:1053, 1999.
35. Pandit J, Bohm A, Jancarik J, et al: Three-dimensional structure of dimeric human recombinant macrophage colony-stimulating factor. *Science* 258:1358, 1992.
36. Shi Y, Massague J: Mechanisms of TGF-beta signaling from cell membrane to the nucleus. *Cell* 113:685, 2003.
37. Feng XH, Derynck R. Specificity and versatility in tgf-beta signaling through Smads. *Annu Rev Cell Dev Biol* 21:659, 2005.
38. Chen S, Lin F, Xu M, et al: Phe(303) in TMVI of the alpha(1B)-adrenergic receptor is a key residue coupling TM helical movements to G-protein activation. *Biochemistry* 41:588, 2002.
39. Bessis AS, Rondard P, Gaven F, et al: Closure of the Venus flytrap module of mGlu8 receptor and the activation process: Insights from mutations converting antagonists into agonists. *Proc Natl Acad Sci U S A* 99:11097, 2002.
40. Coughlin S. Protease-activated receptors in hemostasis, thrombosis and vascular biology. *J Thromb Haemost* 3:1800, 2005.
41. Slupsky JR, Quitterer U, Weber CK, et al: Binding of Gbetagamma subunits to cRaf1 downregulates G-protein-coupled receptor signalling. *Curr Biol* 9:971, 1999.
42. Levesque JP, Simmons PJ: Cytoskeleton and integrin-mediated adhesion signaling in human CD34+ hemopoietic progenitor cells. *Exp Hematol* 27:579, 1999.
43. Martin KH, Slack JK, Boerner SA, et al: Integrin connections map: To infinity and beyond. *Science* 296:1652, 2002.
44. Rose DM, Alon R, Ginsberg MH. Integrin modulation and signaling in leukocyte adhesion and migration. *Immunol Rev* 218:126, 2007.
45. Mitra SK, Schlaepfer DD. Integrin-regulated FAK-Src signaling in normal and cancer cells. *Curr Opin Cell Biol* 18:516, 2006.
46. Sastry SK, Burridge K: Focal adhesions: A nexus for intracellular signaling and cytoskeletal dynamics. *Exp Cell Res* 261:25, 2000.
47. Schwartz MA, Ginsberg MH: Networks and crosstalk: Integrin signalling spreads. *Nat Cell Biol* 4:E65, 2002.
48. Schaller MD: Paxillin: A focal adhesion-associated adaptor protein. *Oncogene* 20:6459, 2001.
49. Aranda A, Pascual A: Nuclear hormone receptors and gene expression. *Physiol Rev* 81:1269, 2001.
50. Mehta K: Retinoids as regulators of gene transcription. *J Biol Regul Homeost Agents* 17:1, 2003.
51. Ahuja HS, Szanto A, Nagy L, et al: The retinoid X receptor and its ligands: Versatile regulators of metabolic function, cell differentiation and cell death. *J Biol Regul Homeost Agents* 17:29, 2003.
52. Carlberg C: Current understanding of the function of the nuclear vitamin D receptor in response to its natural and synthetic ligands. *Recent Results Cancer Res* 164:29, 2003.
53. Collins SJ: Retinoic acid receptors, hematopoiesis and leukemogenesis. *Curr Opin Hematol* 15:346, 2008.
54. Ihle JN, Kerr IM: Jaks and Stats in signaling by the cytokine receptor superfamily. *Trends Genet* 11:69, 1995.
55. Parganas E, Wang D, Stravopodis D, et al: Jak2 is essential for signaling through a variety of cytokine receptors. *Cell* 93:385, 1998.
56. Saharinen P, Vihinen M, Silvennoinen O: Autoinhibition of Jak2 tyrosine kinase is dependent on specific regions in its pseudokinase domain. *Mol Biol Cell* 14:1448, 2003.
57. Lindauer K, Loerting T, Liedl KR, Kroemer RT. Prediction of the structure of human Janus kinase 2 (JAK2) comprising the two carboxy-terminal domains reveals a mechanism for autoregulation. *Protein Eng* 14:27, 2001.
58. James C, Ugo V, LeCouedic JP, et al: A unique clonal JAK2 mutation leading to constitutive signaling causes polycythaemia vera. *Nature* 434:1144, 2005.
59. Baxter EJ, Scott LM, Campbell PJ, et al.: Acquired mutation of the tyrosine kinase JAK2 in human myeloproliferative disorders. *Lancet* 365:1054, 2005.
60. Kralovics R, Passamonti F, Buser AS, et al.: A gain-of-function mutation of JAK2 in myeloproliferative disorders. *N Engl J Med* 352:1779, 2005.
61. Levine RL, Wadleigh M, Cools J, et al: Activating mutation in the tyrosine kinase JAK2 in polycythemia vera, essential thrombocythemia, and myeloid metaplasia with myelofibrosis. *Cancer Cell* 7:387, 2005.
62. Kaushansky K: On the molecular origins of the chronic myeloproliferative disorders: It all makes sense. *Blood* 105:4187, 2005.
63. Rane SG, Reddy EP: Janus kinases: Components of multiple signaling pathways. *Oncogene* 19:5662, 2000.
64. Rameh LE, Cantley LC: The role of phosphoinositide 3-kinase lipid products in cell function. *J Biol Chem* 274:8347, 1999.
65. Vanhaesebroeck B, Alessi DR: The PI3K-PDK1 connection: More than just a road to PKB. *Biochem J* 346 Pt 3:561, 2000.
66. Chang F, Lee JT, Navolanic PM, et al: Involvement of PI3K/Akt pathway in cell cycle progression, apoptosis, and neoplastic transformation: A target for cancer chemotherapy. *Leukemia* 17:590, 2003.
67. Datta SR, Brunet A, Greenberg ME: Cellular survival: A play in three Akts. *Genes Dev* 13:2905, 1999.
68. Karin M, Lin A: NF-kappaB at the crossroads of life and death. *Nat Immunol* 3:221, 2002.
69. Tothova Z, Gilliland DG: FoxO transcription factors and stem cell homeostasis: insights from the hematopoietic system. *Cell Stem Cell* 1:140, 2007. .
70. Kawauchi K, Ogasawara T, Yasuyama M, et al: Involvement of Akt kinase in the action of STI571 on chronic myelogenous leukemia cells. *Blood Cells Mol Dis* 31:11, 2003.
71. Inman GJ, Nicolas FJ, Hill CS: Nucleocytoplasmic shuttling of Smads 2, 3, and 4 permits sensing of TGF-beta receptor activity. *Mol Cell* 10:283, 2002.
72. Pawson T, Scott JD: Signaling through scaffold, anchoring, and adaptor proteins. *Science* 278:2075, 1997.
73. White MF: The IRS-1 signaling system. *Curr Opin Genet Dev* 4:47, 1994.
74. Gu H, Neel BG: The "Gab" in signal transduction. *Trends Cell Biol* 13:122, 2003.
75. Micheau O, Tschopp J: Induction of TNF receptor I-mediated apoptosis via two sequential signaling complexes. *Cell* 114:181, 2003.
76. Cantor AB, Orkin SH: Hematopoietic development: A balancing act. *Curr Opin Genet Dev* 11:513, 2001.
77. Liu KD, Gaffen SL, Goldsmith MA, et al: Janus kinases in interleukin-2-mediated signaling: JAK1 and JAK3 are differentially regulated by tyrosine phosphorylation. *Curr Biol* 7:817, 1997.
78. Wakao H, Harada N, Kitamura T, et al: Interleukin 2 and erythropoietin activate STAT5/MGF via distinct pathways. *EMBO J* 14:2527, 1995.
79. Drachman JG, Sabath DF, Fox NE, et al: Thrombopoietin signal transduction in purified murine megakaryocytes. *Blood* 89:483, 1997.
80. Kapur R, Cooper R, Zhang L, et al: Cross-talk between alpha(4)beta(1)/alpha(5)beta(1) and c-Kit results in opposing effect on growth and survival of hematopoietic cells via the activation of focal adhesion kinase, mitogen-activated protein kinase, and Akt signaling pathways. *Blood* 97:1975, 2001.
81. Fox N, Kaushansky K: Engagement of integrin alpha 4 beta 1 but not alpha 5 beta 1 enhances thrombopoietin (TPO)-induced megakaryocyte (MK) growth. *Blood* 98:292a, 2001.
82. Habib T, Nelson A, Kaushansky K: IL-21: A novel IL-2-family lymphokine that modulates B, T, and natural killer cell responses. *J Allergy Clin Immunol* 112:1033, 2003.
83. Bacon CM, Petricoin EF 3rd, Ortaldo JR, et al: Interleukin 12 induces tyrosine phosphorylation and activation of STAT4 in human lymphocytes. *Proc Natl Acad Sci USA* 92:7307, 1995.

84. Quelle FW, Shimoda K, Thierfelder W, et al: Cloning of murine Stat6 and human Stat6, Stat proteins that are tyrosine phosphorylated in responses to IL-4 and IL-3 but are not required for mitogenesis. *Mol Cell Biol* 15:3336, 1995.
85. Jones RB, et al: A quantitative protein interaction network for the ErbB receptors using protein microarrays. *Nature* 439:168, 2006.
86. Cobb MH, Goldsmith EJ: How MAP kinases are regulated. *J Biol Chem* 270:14843, 1995.
87. Whitmarsh AJ, Davis RJ: Structural organization of MAP-kinase signaling modules by scaffold proteins in yeast and mammals. *Trends Biochem Sci* 23:481, 1998.
88. Lee CM, Onesime D, Reddy CD, et al: JLP: A scaffolding protein that tethers JNK/p38MAPK signaling modules and transcription factors. *Proc Natl Acad Sci U S A* 99:14189, 2002.
89. Soond SM, Terry JL, Colbert JD, et al: TRUSS, a novel tumor necrosis factor receptor 1 scaffolding protein that mediates activation of the transcription factor NF-kappaB. *Mol Cell Biol* 23:8334, 2003.
90. Chiu CW, Dalton M, Ishiai M, et al: BLNK: Molecular scaffolding through "cis"-mediated organization of signaling proteins. *EMBO J* 21:6461, 2002.
91. Besson A, Wilson TL, Yong VW: The anchoring protein RACK1 links protein kinase Cepsilon to integrin beta chains. Requirements for adhesion and motility. *J Biol Chem* 277:22073, 2002.
92. Yee NS, Langen H, Besmer P: Mechanism of kit ligand, phorbol ester, and calcium-induced down-regulation of c-kit receptors in mast cells. *J Biol Chem* 268:14189, 1993.
93. Vieira AV, Lamaze C, Schmid SL: Control of EGF receptor signaling by clathrin-mediated endocytosis. *Science* 274:2086, 1996.
94. Broudy VC, Lin NL, Liles WC, et al: Signaling via Src family kinases is required for normal internalization of the receptor c-Kit. *Blood* 94:1979, 1999.
95. Dahlen DD, Broudy VC, Drachman JG: Internalization of the thrombopoietin receptor is regulated by 2 cytoplasmic motifs. *Blood* 102:102, 2003.
96. Hitchcock I, Chen M, Fox NE, Kaushansky K: YRRL motifs in the cytoplasmic domain of the thrombopoietin receptor regulate receptor internalization and degradation. *Blood* 112:2222, 2008
97. Zhang J, Somani AK, Siminovitch KA: Roles of the SHP-1 tyrosine phosphatase in the negative regulation of cell signalling. *Semin Immunol* 12:361, 2000.
98. Tsui HW, Siminovitch KA, De Souza L, et al: Motheaten and viable motheaten mice have mutations in the haematopoietic cell phosphatase gene. *Nat Genet* 4:124, 1993.
99. Otipoby KL, Draves KE, Clark EA: CD22 regulates B cell receptor-mediated signals via two domains that independently recruit Grb2 and SHP-1. *J Biol Chem* 276:44315, 2001.
100. Pani G, Fischer KD, Mlinaric-Rascan I, et al: Signaling capacity of the T cell antigen receptor is negatively regulated by the PTP1C tyrosine phosphatase. *J Exp Med* 184:839, 1996.
101. Binstadt BA, Brumbaugh KM, Dick CJ, et al: Sequential involvement of Lck and SHP-1 with MHC-recognizing receptors on NK cells inhibits FcR-initiated tyrosine kinase activation. *Immunity* 5:629, 1996.
102. Kim CH, Qu CK, Hangoc G, et al: Abnormal chemokine-induced responses of immature and mature hematopoietic cells from motheaten mice implicate the protein tyrosine phosphatase SHP-1 in chemokine responses. *J Exp Med* 190:681, 1999.
103. Sharlow ER, Pacifici R, Crouse J, et al: Hematopoietic cell phosphatase negatively regulates erythropoietin-induced hemoglobinization in erythroleukemic SKT6 cells. *Blood* 90:2175, 1997.
104. Longmore GD: Erythropoietin receptor mutations and Olympic glory. *Nat Genet* 4:108, 1993.
105. Yoshimura A, Ohkubo T, Kiguchi T, et al: A novel cytokine-inducible gene CIS encodes an SH2-containing protein that binds to tyrosine phosphorylated interleukin 3 and erythropoietin receptors. *EMBO J* 14:2816, 1995.
106. Naka T, Narazaki M, Hirata M, et al: Structure and function of a new STAT-induced STAT inhibitor. *Nature* 387:924, 1997.
107. Starr R, Willson TA, Viney EM, et al: A family of cytokine-inducible inhibitors of signalling. *Nature* 387:917, 1997.
108. Wormald S, Hilton DJ: Inhibitors of cytokine signal transduction. *J Biol Chem* 279:821, 2004.
109. Schmidt D, Muller S: PIAS/SUMO: New partners in transcriptional regulation. *Cell Mol Life Sci* 60:2561, 2003.
110. Grimm OH, Gurdon JB: Nuclear exclusion of Smad2 is a mechanism leading to loss of competence. *Nat Cell Biol* 4:519, 2002.
111. Wang Q, Miyakawa Y, Fox N, et al: Interferon-alpha directly represses megakaryopoiesis by inhibiting thrombopoietin-induced signaling through induction of SOCS-1. *Blood* 96:2093, 2000.
112. Singer SJ, Nicolson GL: The fluid mosaic model of the structure of cell membranes. *Science* 175:720, 1972.
113. Brown DA, Rose JK: Sorting of GPI-anchored proteins to glycolipid-enriched membrane subdomains during transport to the apical cell surface. *Cell* 68:533, 1992.
114. Viola A, Schroeder S, Sakakibara Y, et al: T lymphocyte costimulation mediated by reorganization of membrane microdomains. *Science* 283:680, 1999.
115. Bodin S, Viala C, Ragab A, et al: A critical role of lipid rafts in the organization of a key FcgammaRIIa-mediated signaling pathway in human platelets. *Thromb Haemost* 89:318, 2003.
116. Hemler ME: Tetraspanin proteins mediate cellular penetration, invasion, and fusion events and define a novel type of membrane microdomain. *Annu Rev Cell Dev Biol* 19:397, 2003.
117. Cook GA, Longhurst CM, Grgurevich S, et al: Identification of CD9 extracellular domains important in regulation of CHO cell adhesion to fibronectin and fibronectin pericellular matrix assembly. *Blood* 100:4502, 2002.
118. Miyazaki T, Muller U, Campbell KS: Normal development but differentially altered proliferative responses of lymphocytes in mice lacking CD81. *EMBO J* 16:4217, 1997.
119. Clay D, Rubinstein E, Mishal Z, et al: CD9 and megakaryocyte differentiation. *Blood* 97:1982, 2001.
120. Anzai N, Lee Y, Youn BS, et al: C-kit associated with the transmembrane 4 superfamily proteins constitutes a functionally distinct subunit in human hematopoietic progenitors. *Blood* 99:4413, 2002.
121. Skubitz KM, Campbell KD, Iida J, et al: CD63 associates with tyrosine kinase activity and CD11/CD18, and transmits an activation signal in neutrophils. *J Immunol* 157:3617, 1996.
122. Kurita-Taniguchi M, Hazeki K, Murabayashi N, et al: Molecular assembly of CD46 with CD9, alpha3-beta1 integrin and protein tyrosine phosphatase SHP-1 in human macrophages through differentiation by GMCSF. *Mol Immunol* 38:689, 2002.

CHAPTER 15
THE CLUSTER OF DIFFERENTIATION ANTIGENS

Thomas J. Kipps

SUMMARY

The cluster of differentiation (CD) antigens are cellular molecules that are each recognized by monoclonal antibodies (mAbs) that allow for the identification of each molecule's biochemical properties and cellular distribution. The CD number for each molecule is defined at international workshops that exchange such mAbs and compare their ability to react with human cells and/or human cell molecules. This chapter provides an overview of the approximately 350 CD antigens defined as of the eighth international workshop, listing the other names for these CD antigens along with their biochemistry, membrane-orientation, genetics, cellular distribution, and physiology.

Acronyms and abbreviations that appear in this chapter include: act., activated; ADAM, a disintegrin and metalloprotease; AF, accessory factor; Ag, antigen; ALK, anaplastic lymphoma kinase; ALL, acute lymphocytic leukemia; APC, antigen-presenting cell; APO-1, apoptosis antigen ligand-1; APRIL, a proliferation-inducing ligand; ART1, ADP-ribosyltransferase 1; BAFF, B-cell activating factor of the tumor necrosis factor family; BCMA, B-cell maturation antigen; BMP, bone morphogenetic protein; BMPR, bone morphogenetic protein receptor; C-type lectin, Ca2+-dependent lectin; CA, carcinoma; Ca2+, ionized calcium; CALLA, common acute leukemia antigen; CCR, chemokine C-C motif receptor; CD, cluster of differentiation; CEA, carcinoembryonic antigen; CMRF, epitope recognized by the CMRF-35 mAB; CMV, cytomegalovirus; CNS, central nervous system; CRTH2, chemoattractant receptor-homologous molecule; CTL, cytotoxic T lymphocytes; CTLA-4, cytotoxic T-lymphocyte–associated protein-4; CXCR, chemokine CXC motif receptor; DAF, decay accelerating factor; DC, dendritic cell; DNAM, DNAX accessory molecule; ELAM, endothelial leukocyte adhesion molecule; eos, eosinophil; EBV, Epstein-Barr virus; ECM, extracellular matrix; esp., especially; FDC, follicular dendritic cells; FGF, fibroblast growth factor; FGFR, fibroblast growth factor receptor; GC, germinal center; G-CSF, granulocyte colony-stimulating factor; GI, gastrointestinal; GM-CSF, granulocyte-macrophage colony-stimulating factor; gp, glycoprotein; GPI, glycosylphosphatidylinositol; HA, hyaluronan; HCL, hairy cell leukemia; hsp, heat shock protein; Hep., heptaspan; HEV, high endothelial venules; HGM-CSFR, human granulocyte-macrophage colony-stimulating factor; HIgR, herpesvirus immunoglobulin-like receptor; HIV, human immunodeficiency virus; HLA, human leukocyte antigen; HML, human mucosal lymphocyte; HSC, hematopoietic stem cells; HSV, herpes simplex virus; IAP, integrin associated protein; ICAM, intercellular adhesion molecule; IEL, intraepithelial lymphocytes; IFN, interferon; IGF, insulin-like growth factor; IgSF, immunoglobulin superfamily; IL, interleukin; ILT, immunoglobulin-like transcript; IRF3, interferon regulatory factor 3; IRTA, immunoglobulin superfamily receptor translocation associated; ITAM, immune tyrosine-based activating motifs; ITGAE, integrin alpha E; ITIM, immune tyrosine-based inhibitory motifs; ITSM, immune tyrosine-based switch motifs; JAM, junctional adhesion molecule-1; KIR, killer cell inhibitory receptor; LAMP, lysosomal membrane-associated glycoprotein; LARC, liver and activation-regulated chemokine; LDL, low-density lipoprotein; LECAM, leukocyte endothelial cell adhesion molecule; LFA, leukocyte function antigen; LGL, large granular lymphocyte; LIF, leukemia inhibitory factor; LIR, leukocyte immunoglobulin-like receptor; LPS, lipopolysaccharide; mAb, monoclonal antibody; MCP, monocyte chemoattractant protein; MDR, multidrug resistance; MHC, major histocompatibility complex; MICA, major histocompatibility complex class I chain A; MICB, major histocompatibility complex class I chain B; MIP-1, macrophage inflammatory protein; MMP, matrix metalloproteinase; MRP, mobility-related protein; MSP, macrophage-stimulating protein; MSP-R, macrophage-stimulating protein receptor; MUC-1, mucin-1; MØ, macrophages; NCAM, neural cell adhesion molecule; NF-κB, nuclear factor-kappa B; NK, natural killer; O, orientation/anchorage of the antigen in the plasma membrane; PAMP, pathogen-associated molecular pattern; PDC, plasmacytoid dendritic cell; PDGF, platelet-derived growth factor; PECAM, platelet endothelial cell adhesion molecule; PHN, paroxysmal nocturnal hemoglobinuria; PI-PLC, phosphatidylinositol phospholipase C; plts, platelets; PMN, polymorphonuclear leukocytes; PRR1, poliovirus receptor-related 1 protein; PRR2, poliovirus receptor-related 2 protein; PVRL, poliovirus receptor-like; RAET1E, retinoic acid early transcript 1E; RAIDD, receptor-interacting protein-associated ICH-1/CED-3-homologous protein with a death domain; RANTES, regulated on activation, normal T-cell expressed, and secreted protein; RasGAP, Ras guanosine triphosphatase-activating protein; RBC (rbc), red blood cell; Rc, receptor; RGD, amino acid sequence, arginine-glycine-aspartic acid; RIP, receptor-interacting protein; RON, Récepteur d'Origine Nantaise; SCR, steel factor receptor; SDF-1α, stromal-derived factor-1α; Sema, semaphorin; Siglec, sialic acid-binding immunoglobulin-like lectin; SLAM, signaling lymphocytes activation molecule; SLC, secondary lymphoid tissue chemokine; sIg, surface immunoglobulin; TACI, transmembrane activator and calcium modulator and cyclophilin-ligand interactor; TACTILE, T-cell activation increased late expression; TALLA-1, T-cell–acute lymphoblastic leukemia antigen-1; TAPA, target of antiproliferative antibody; TCR, T-cell receptor; Tet., tetraspan; TFPI, tissue factor pathway inhibitor; TGF, transforming growth factor; THANK, tumor necrosis factor homologue that activates apoptosis, nuclear factor-kappa B, and c-Jun NH2-terminal kinase; TLR, toll-like receptor; TLX, trophoblast leukocyte-common antigen; TNF, tumor necrosis factor; TNFR, tumor necrosis factor receptor; TNFRSF, tumor necrosis factor receptor superfamily; TNFSF, tumor necrosis factor superfamily; TRADD, tumor necrosis factor receptor superfamily 1A-associated via death domain; TRANCE, tumor necrosis factor-related activation-induced cytokine; T_{reg}, regulatory T cells; TRIF, toll/interleukin-1 receptor domain-containing adapter inducing interferon-β; ULBP, cytomegalovirus UL-16 binding protein; uPA, urokinase plasminogen activator; VCAM, vascular cell adhesion molecule; VEGF, vascular endothelial growth factor; VLA, very-late antigen; VWF, von Willebrand factor; WBC, white blood cell.

DEFINITION AND HISTORY

The advent of monoclonal antibody (mAb) technology revolutionized the classification of cell surface antigens. The availability of virtually unlimited quantities of monospecific typing reagents permitted the identification and study of previously unrecognized lymphoid and myeloid-specific surface proteins. However, as the number of mAbs detecting cell-surface differentiation antigens grew, the need for an international standardization became apparent.

Accordingly, eight international workshops have been held to exchange mAbs to compare their ability to react with human cells and/or human cell protein tissues or cell types.[1] An antigen that is recognized by a cluster of antibodies can be assigned a "cluster of differentiation" (CD) number. If only one mAb defines a cluster or if all mAbs defining a cluster originate from the same laboratory, a suffix "w" is added to the CD designation. The last conference, held in Adelaide, Australia, in December 2004, compiled the data obtained from testing hundreds of different mAbs.[1] The conference culminated in the classification of scores of new CD antigens.

Table 15–1 presents all CD antigens defined at this and previous workshops and any common names used before a CD number was assigned (column marked "Other Names"). Table 15–1 summarizes what is known about each CD antigen's molecular size(s) ("Size"), orientation or attachment to the plasma membrane ("O"), tissue distribution ("Distribution"), and known or suspected physiology ("Physiology"). Table 15–1 also indicates the chromosomal location of the gene(s) encoding each CD antigen. Below the chromosomal location is the official name of the human gene encoding the CD, provided in italics. Below the gene name is the "Entrez Gene" number. This number allows for retrieval of updated information about the gene and its genetics in the "Gene" database of the National Center for Biotechnology Information, which is available at: www.ncbi.nlm.nih.gov/sites/entrez. Other useful websites for analyzing protein or genomic structure are SWISSPROT protein structure database (available at http://us.expasy.org), or the central repository for genomic mapping data from the Human Genome Project Information (available at www.ornl.gov/sci/techresources/Human_Genome/home.shtml).

GENERAL STRUCTURE OF MEMBRANE ANTIGENS

Membrane antigens are classified into different groups, depending on how they orient or anchor themselves to the plasma membrane (Fig. 15–1).[1,2]

TYPE I TRANSMEMBRANE PROTEINS

Type I transmembrane molecules have their COOH-termini in the cytoplasm and their NH_2-termini outside the cell. Each of these molecules generally has a signal sequence at the NH_2-terminus that is cleaved off after the molecule passes into the endoplasmic reticulum. Afterward, it may be glycosylated in the Golgi apparatus (if it contains glycosylation sites) and then expressed on the cell surface. These proteins commonly serve as cell surface receptors and/or ligands. Many belong to the immunoglobulin superfamily (see Chaps. 77 and 78).

Each type I protein generally has a transmembrane domain of approximately 25 hydrophobic amino acid residues followed by a cluster of basic amino acids that bind the protein to phospholipid head groups inside the surface membrane bilayer. The transmembrane domain does not contain any charged amino acid residues, such as Arg, Asn, Asp, Glu, Gln, His, or Lys, except when it associates with the transmembrane domain of another cell surface protein(s) to form a multimeric complex. An example of this formation is the multimeric complex formed by the CD3 proteins, CD247, and the two chains of the T-cell receptor for antigen (see Chap. 78).

TYPE II TRANSMEMBRANE PROTEINS

Type II transmembrane proteins have an orientation opposite to that of type I transmembrane proteins. The NH_2-terminus is located inside the cell and the COOH-terminus is located extracellularly. These proteins often have uncleaved signal sequences for transmembrane domains, allowing for their cleavage and release from the cell surface. As such, these proteins may double as cell surface antigens and plasma proteins, each often having a physiologic effect(s) on cells bearing the respective ligand(s).

TYPE III TRANSMEMBRANE PROTEINS

Type III transmembrane proteins cross the plasma membrane more than once. Some pass through the bilayer as many as 12 times, such as the multidrug-resistant transporter protein MDR-1, now designated as CD243. Because these proteins cross the membrane multiple times, the molecules can form channels that often are used to transport ions or small molecules through the lipid bilayer.

Important subgroups of type III transmembrane proteins that commonly are found on leukocytes are the tetraspan family and the seven transmembrane domain proteins. The tetraspan proteins each pass through the surface bilayer four times and have both COOH-termini and NH_2-termini inside the cell. Many of the type III transmembrane proteins listed in Table 15–1 belong to this family, which are identified in the table in the membrane organization column as "Tet." An example is CD20, a molecule postulated to form a calcium channel that is required for B-cell activation. The transmembrane domain proteins pass through the plasma membrane seven times and typically have their COOH-termini in the cytoplasm and their NH_2-termini outside the cell. These proteins are identified in Table 15–1 in the membrane organization column as "III Hep." Such proteins generally are G-protein–coupled receptors for external ligands. When such receptors bind to their specific ligand they undergo a conformational change, resulting in activation of the G protein, which binds guanosine triphosphate (GTP).

TYPE IV TRANSMEMBRANE PROTEINS

Type IV proteins can be distinguished from type III proteins by the presence of a water-filled transmembrane channel. None of the current CD antigens have such a membrane organization.

TYPE V GLYCOSYLPHOSPHATIDYLINOSITOL-ANCHORED PROTEINS

Type V proteins use lipid to attach themselves to the plasma membrane. The most common attachment for extracellular proteins in this category is the glycosylphosphatidylinositol (GPI) anchor. The GPI anchor can be cleaved by the bacterial enzyme phosphatidylinositol phospholipase C (PI-PLC). Release of an antigen from the cell surface by treatment with PI-PLC often is used to verify that the surface protein has a GPI anchor. However, this criterion is not absolute, as some GPI-anchored proteins are resistant to PI-PLC.

Newly synthesized proteins destined to receive a GPI anchor each contains a secretion signal sequence at the NH_2-terminus and another signal sequence at the COOH-terminus. The latter directs cleavage and subsequent appendage of a GPI anchor soon after the molecule's biosynthesis and extrusion into the endoplasmic reticulum. This biosynthetic pathway is defective in paroxysmal nocturnal hemoglobinuria (PNH; see Chap. 40).

The site of attachment for GPI generally precedes a hydrophobic domain of 7 to 20 amino acids that sometimes doubles as an actual transmembrane domain. In this case, the molecule may exist as either of two isoforms, one attached to the membrane via a GPI anchor and another as a type I transmembrane protein. Because GPI-anchored proteins associate specifically with sphingomyelin lipids, follow a different path of transport to the cell surface than type I transmembrane proteins, are excluded from coated pits, and are not able to associate directly with intracellular proteins, a GPI isoform of a given surface protein usually has a physiology that is distinct from that of its respective type I transmembrane isoform.

TISSUE DISTRIBUTION OF MEMBRANE ANTIGENS

The tissue distributions for each CD antigen listed in Table 15–1 summarize the work of many laboratories. However, comprehensive analysis of the full gamut of different tissues has not been performed for several CD antigens. As such, the cell types listed in the distribution column for a particular CD antigen should not necessarily be considered as the only cell types that can express that CD antigen, particularly in pathologic settings when there can be aberrant protein expression.

TABLE 15–1. Cluster of Differentiation Antigens Defined as of the Eighth International Workshop on Leukocyte Typing

Antigen	Other Names	Size	O	Genetics	Distribution	Physiology
CD1a→e	CD1a: T6/leu-6; R4; HTA1; CD1b: R1; CD1c: M241; R7; CD1d: R3; CD1e: R2	1a:49 1b:45 1c:43 1d:38 1e:36	I	1q22-q23 *CD1A-E* A: 909 B: 910 C: 911 D: 912 E: 913	Cortical thymocytes, DC, Langerhans cells (CD1a), brain astrocytes, dermal epithelial cells (CD1d), some B cells (CD1c, d)	CD1 can associate with β_2-microglobulin (β_2-M) to present "nonclassical" antigens, e.g., lipids and glycolipids, to T cells. There are six isoforms encoded by separate exons. CD1a, CD1b, and CD1c are in group 1, which is expressed primarily on Ag-presenting cells. CD1d is in group 2, which does not always associate with β_2-M.
CD2	Sheep red blood cell-Rc; Leukocyte Function Ag-2 (LFA-2); Leu-5; T11; Tp50	45–58	I	1p13.1 *CD2* 914	Thymocytes, T cells, NK cells, some B cells	Serves as a ligand for CD48 and CD58 (LFA-3) that enhances adhesion between T cells and Ag-presenting cells (APC) and also plays a role in signal transduction
CD3	CD3δ CD3ε CD3γ	20 20 25–28	I I I	11q23 *CD3D-G* D: 915 E: 916 G: 917	Pan–T-cell	CD3 defines a family of proteins that, together with CD247, form the signal transduction complex of the T-cell Rc for Ag (see Chap. 78).
CD4	T4; Leu-3; L3T4	55	I	12pter-p12 *CD4* 920	Thymocytes, helper/inducer T cells, monocytes, MØ, DC, and some PMN	CD4 serves as an Rc for HLA class II that facilitates recognition of peptide antigens. It also is a co-Rc for HIV gp120 and an Rc for IL-16 (see Chap. 78).
CD5	Tp67; Leu-1; T1	67	I	11q13 *CD5* 921	T cells and some B cells	Scavenger Rc previously thought to serve as ligand for CD72 that modulates signals transduced by the Rc for Ag.
CD6	T12; Tp120	105, 130	I	11q13 *CD6* 923	T cells, some B cells, medullary thymocytes, some cortical thymocytes, brain	Scavenger Rc that serves as ligand for CD166 that plays role in T-cell development.
CD7	gp40; Tp41	40	I	17q25.2-q25.3 *CD7* 924	Some hemopoietic stem cells (denotes commitment to B or NK cells), some T cells, monocytes, NK cells	Associates with PI3 kinase via YXXM motif upon crosslinking, implying that it may be involved in cell activation and serves as an Rc for K12 protein and galectin-1.
CD8α	T8; Leu-2α chain	68 (32–34)	I	2p12 *CD8A* 925	Cytotoxic/suppressor T cells, some γ/δ T cells, some NK cells, most thymocytes	Forms a homodimer on γ/δ T cells or a heterodimer with CD8β to serve as co-Rc for HLA class I that facilitates recognition of peptide antigens presented in the context of HLA class I. The cytoplasmic domain can bind lck (see Chap. 78).
CD8β	β chain of CD8 heterodimer	68 (32–34)	I	2p12 *CD8B1* 926	Cytotoxic/suppressor T cells, some NK cells, most thymocytes	Forms a heterodimer with CD8α to act as Rc for HLA class I (see above). Unlike CD8α, CD8β cannot form homodimers.
CD9	p24; DRAP-27; MRP-1	24	III Tet.	12p13.3 *CD9* 928	plts, pre-B, act. T cells, eos., basophils, endothelia and epithelial cells, brain, peripheral nerves, vascular smooth muscle, cardiac muscle, ovocytes	Plays role in signal transduction leading to cell activation, adhesion, and/or aggregation. Associates with other tetraspan proteins (CD63, CD81, CD82) or with CD41/CD61 in plts to trigger activation. Required on ova for fusion with sperm.
CD10	Membrane metalloendopeptidase (MME); neutral endopeptidase; encephalinase; CALLA	95–100	II	3q25.1-q25.2 *MME* 4311	Pre-B and pre-T cells, GC B cells, marrow stroma, some PMN, epithelial cells	A neutral endopeptidase that cleaves biologically act. peptides on the amino side of hydrophobic amino acids, thereby reducing the local concentration of peptide hormones.

(*continued*)

TABLE 15–1. Cluster of Differentiation Antigens Defined as of the Eighth International Workshop on Leukocyte Typing (Continued)

Antigen	Other Names	Size	O	Genetics	Distribution	Physiology
CD11a	Integrin αL (ITGAL); leukocyte function Ag-1 (LFA-1)	180	I	16p11.2 *ITGAL* 3683	Lymphocytes, monocytes, MØ, PMN (weak)	Complexes with CD18 to form Rc for CD50, CD54, or CD102, thereby facilitating homotypic or heterotypic adhesion and cell activation.
CD11b	Integrin, αM (ITGAM); complement Rc 3 (CR3); C3biR; Mac-1; Mo-1; αM chain of β_2 integrins	165–170	I	16p11.2 *ITGAM* 3684	Monocytes, MØ, PMN, DC, some B and T cells, and NK cells	Complexes with CD18 to form a Rc for C3bi, clotting factor X, fibrinogen, CD54, or CD102, thereby facilitating homotypic or heterotypic adhesion, cell activation, phagocytosis, and/or chemotaxis.
CD11c	Integrin α–X (ITGAX); Leu M5; CR4; Axb2; SLEB6	145–150	I	16p11.2 *ITGAX* 3687	Expression strong on monocytes MØ, and NK cells, moderate on PMN, and weak on some B and T cells	Complexes with CD18 to form an adhesion Rc for fibrinogen and Rc for C3bi. Also can bind LPS, CD54, CD23, and fibrinogen. Binding induces cellular adhesion and chemotaxis, and helps trigger neutrophil respiratory burst.
CD11d	Integrin α–D (ITGAD); ADB2; FLJ39841	150	I	16p11.2 *ITGAD* 3681	Myelomonocytic cells, red pulp MØ (strong), blood WBC (moderate)	Forms a heterodimer with CD18 to make an Rc for CD50 (ICAM-3), but not CD54 or CD106.
CDw12	p90–120	150–160 (120)		– *CDW12* 23444	Monocytes, PMN, NK cells (weak)	A phosphoprotein of unknown function.
CD13	Alanyl (membrane) aminopeptidase (ANPEP); APN; gp150 (EC 3.4.11.2)	150–170	II	15q25–26 *ANPEP* 290	Myeloid cells, endothelial and epithelial cells, osteoclasts, marrow stroma, LGL, fibroblasts, brain	A zinc-binding metalloprotease that trims peptides bound to HLA class II and removal of N-terminal amino acids from biologically active peptides, thereby reducing their local concentration. Is also Rc for coronaviruses and cytomegalovirus.
CD14	gp55; GPI-liked gp; LPS Rc	53–55	GPI	5q22-q32 *CD14* 929	Monocytes (strong), DC, osteoclast progenitors, PMN (moderate), B cells (weak)	Associates with TLR4 to form Rc for lipopolysaccharide (LPS) that can transduce signal(s), leading to oxidative burst and/or synthesis of tumor necrosis factor alpha.
CD15	Lewis x (Le^X); 3-fucosyl-*N*-acetyl-lactosamine (3-FAL)	185–260	–	11q21 *FUT4* 2526	PMN, eos, monocytes	A carbohydrate determinant that is found on several gps (e.g., CD11/CD18, CD66) and is dependent on the activity of $\alpha_{1,3}$-fucosyltransferase (*FUT4*).
CD15s	sialyl Lewis X (sLe^X)	185–260	–	9q34.3 *FUT7* 2529	PMN, basophils, eosinophils, monocytes, myeloid cells, some T cells (weak)	The sialylated form of CD15, is a ligand for CD62E (ELAM-1), and is dependent upon fucosyl transferase 7 (*FUT7*).
CD15su	6′ sulphosialyl Lewis X	185–260	–		Similar to CD15s	Structurally the same as CD15 except that it possesses a sulfate group on GlcNAc.
CD15u	3′ sulpho-Lewis X	185–260	–		Similar to CD15s	Structurally the same as CD15 except that it possesses a sulfate group on the terminal galactose.
CD16a	Fc of IgG, low-affinity IIIA, Rc (FCGR3A); transmembrane form of FcγRIIIA (low-affinity FcRc)	50–65	I	1q23 *FCGR3A* 2214	NK cells, MØ, activated monocytes, mast cells, and γ/δ T cells	Complexes with the FcεRIγ on phagocytes and mast cells and CD3ζ, on NK cells to form low-affinity Rc for Fc of IgG_1 or IgG_3 in mediating antibody-dependent cytotoxicity (ADCC).
CD16b	Fc of IgG, low-affinity IIIB, Rc (FCGR3B); GPI-anchored form of FcγRIII (low-affinity FcRc); FcγRIIIB	48–60	GPI	1q23 *FCGR3B* 2215	PMN	This is the GPI isoform of CD16 that is deficient in patients with PNH. Has no intrinsic signaling function, but is capable of inducing ADCC of rbc.

(*continued*)

TABLE 15–1. Cluster of Differentiation Antigens Defined as of the Eighth International Workshop on Leukocyte Typing (Continued)

Antigen	Other Names	Size	O	Genetics	Distribution	Physiology
CD17	Lactosylceramide (LacCer)	150–160 (120)	–	–	PMN (strong), basophils, plts, monocytes, some B cells, tonsillar DC	Can mediate homotypic adhesion, serve as Rc for GM3 gangliosides, and facilitate phagocytosis of bacteria.
CD18	Integrin, β_2 (ITGB2); β chain of the β_2 integrins	90–95	I	21q22.3 *ITGB2* 3689	Same as CD11a-d combined	Complexes with one of several α chains (CD11a→d) and is essential for correct leukocyte adhesion and signaling.
CD19	B4; Bgp95	120 (95)	I	16p11.2 *CD19* 930	All B cells and B cell precursors, some FDC	Forms part of the B-cell Rc (BCR) complex with CD21, CD81, and Leu13 to facilitate BCR signal transduction. The cytoplasmic domain can associate with PI-3K, Vav, and Src family kinases Lyn and Fyn.
CD20	Membrane-spanning 4-domains, subfamily A, member 1 (MS4A1); B1; Bp35; Leu-16	33, 35, 37	III Tet.	11q12 *MS4A1* 931	B cells but not plasma cells	May act as a Ca^{2+} channel involved in regulating cell-cycle progression that can be targeted by mAb for therapy of B cell lymphomas.
CD21	Complement Rc 2 (CR2); EBV-Rc; C3d-Rc; gp140	145	I	1q32 *CR2* 1380	B cells, FDC (strong), pharyngeal and cervical epithelial cells (weak), some T cells, fetal astrocytes	Rc for C3d, C3dg, C3bi, and Epstein-Barr virus. Binding of C3d to CD21 enhances BCR signal transduction. Can associate with CD23 to regulate production of IgE.
CD22	Bgp135; B lymphocyte cell adhesion molecule (BL-CAM); Leu-14; Lyb-8; LPAP	110–130	I	19p13.1 *CD22* 933	Mature B cells but not plasma cells	A siglec that binds sialoglyco-conjugates (NeuAcα2→6Galβ_1→4GlcNAc) on some CD45 isoforms and gps to provide inhibitory signaling via its cytoplasmic ITIMs.
CD23	Fc of IgE, low affinity Rc II (FCER2); FcεRII; BLAST-2; (alternatively spliced forms are called FcεRIIa and FcεRIIb); Leu-20; B6	45–50	II	19p13.3 *FCER2* 2208	sIgM$^+$/sIgD$^+$ B cells, monocytes, some T cells, FDC, eos., NK cells, plts	A Ca^{2+}-dependent (C-type) lectin with low affinity for IgE, CD21, CD11a, and CD11b, that plays a role in the regulation of IgE synthesis and in cell-cell adhesion. Secreted form of CD23 may act as B-cell growth factor.
CD24	Heat-stable Ag (HSA); BA-1	35–45	GPI	6q21 *CD24* 934	B cells, pre-B cells, PMN, epithelium, ≤ 2% of thymocytes	Regulates the binding of CD49d/CD29 (VLA-4), binds CD62P, and can facilitate cellular activation, adhesion, and memory B cell formation.
CD25	IL-2 Rcα (IL2RA); TAC-Ag; α-chain of the IL-2 Rc	55	I	10p15-p14 *IL2RA* 3559	Regulatory CD4/CD25+ T cells, act. T and act. B cells, some thymocytes, early myeloid cells, and MØ	A low-affinity Rc for IL-2 that can associate with CD122 and CD132 to form a heterotrimeric Rc with high-affinity for IL-2.
CD26	Dipeptylpeptidase IV (DPPA); (EC 3.4.14.5); adenosine deaminase-binding protein	110, 120	II	2q24.3 *DPPA* 1803	Intestinal epithelial cells, renal proximal tubule, bile duct, prostate, memory or act. T cells, medullary thymocytes, some B cells, NK cells	A serine-type exopeptidase that cleaves dipeptides from the amino-termini of proteins with a penultimate proline or alanine residue. With an intracellular domain that associates with adenosine deaminase, it also can function as a T-cell costimulatory molecule. Also binds collagen, fibroblast activation protein (FAP), and HIV Tat.
CD27	S152; T14; Tp55; TNFRSF7	110 (55)	I	12p13 *CD27* 939	Naïve T cells, memory-type B cells, NK cells, medullary thymocytes, hemopoietic stem cells and early progenitor cells	A ligand for CD70 that can serve as a costimulatory molecule leading to activation of NF-κB and stress-activated protein kinase (SAPK)/c-Jun N-terminal kinase (JNK).
CD28	Tp44 Ag; T44	90 (44)	I	2q33 *CD28* 940	95% of CD4 T cells, 50% of CD8 T cells, most plasma cells	A ligand for CD80 and CD86 involved in T cell costimulation and stabilization of IL-2 mRNA.

(continued)

TABLE 15–1. Cluster of Differentiation Antigens Defined as of the Eighth International Workshop on Leukocyte Typing (Continued)

Antigen	Other Names	Size	O	Genetics	Distribution	Physiology
CD29	Integrin, β_1 (ITGB1); very-late Ag (VLA) β chain (VLAB); platelet GPIIa; integrin β_1 subunit	110–130	I	10p11.2 *ITGB1* 3688	plts and all leukocytes with higher levels on memory T cells	Assembles into a heterodimer with one of several α chains (CD49a→f or CD51) to form Rc involved in cell–cell or cell–matrix adhesion. Plays critical role in embryogenesis, development, and HSC differentiation.
CD30	TNF Rc superfamily, member 8 (TNFRSF8); Ki-1 Ag; Ber-H2	120 (105)	I	1p36 *TNFRSF8* 943	act. T, B, and NK cells, monocytes, Reed-Sternberg cells, embryonal CA	Upon binding its ligand, CD153, CD30 can activate NF-κB, Jun N-terminal kinase (JNK), and p38. Can play a role in TCR-mediated apoptosis.
CD31	Platelet endothelial cell adhesion molecule-1 (PECAM-1); GPIIa; endocam	130–140	I	17q23 *PECAM1* 5175	Monocytes, myeloid cells, plts, cell–cell junctions of vascular endothelium, some T cells, PMN	Interacts with itself and with integrin $\alpha V/\beta 3$ and glycosaminoglycans. Facilitates cell-to-cell adhesion involved in leukocyte transendothelial migration to sites of inflammation.
CD32	FcγRIIa (FCGR2A) FcγRIIb (FCGR2B) FcγRIIc (FCGR2C)	40	I	1q23 *FCGR2A* 2212 *FCGR2B* 2213 *FCGR2C* *9103*	FCGR2A: myeloid cells, plts, epithelia, FCGR2B: B cells, MØ, monocytes DC, some T cells FCGR2C: NK cells	Low-affinity Rc for IgG that can bind aggregated IgG. FCGR2B and FCGR2C have cytoplasmic ITIMs, which can provide an inhibitory signal, whereas the FCGR2A has cytoplasmic ITAMs, which can provide a costimulatory signal. Some individuals lack expression of *FCGR2C* because of allelic polymorphism.
CD33	gp67; My9; p67; Siglec3	150 (67)	I	19q13.3 *CD33* 945	Cells of myelomonocytic lineage but not stem cells	Binds to sialoglyco conjugates NeuAcα_2→3Galβ_1→3(4)GlcNAc and NeuAcα_2→3Galβ_1→3GalNAc and may mediate cell-cell adhesion. Has intracellular ITIMs that can exert an inhibitory effect on signal transduction.
CD34	My10; Spg90	110	I	1q32 *CD34* 947	1–4% of marrow cells including HSC, endothelium	Possibly facilitates cytoadhesion through its ability to bind CD62L and CD62E. Is used as a marker for stem-cell enrichment.
CD35	Complement Rc 1 (CR1); C3b/C4b Rc; Immune adherence Rc; C3BR; KN	160–285	I	1q32 *CR1* 1378	Monocytes, PMN, DC, rbc, B cells, some T cells, some astrocytes, glomerular podocytes	Facilitates phagocytosis and/or binding to immune complexes or cells coated with C3b, CD3bi, CD3g or C4b. CD35 is one of the few CD antigens with allotypic polymorphism resulting in varied molecular sizes.
CD36	Platelet GPIV; GPIIIb; OKM-5; PASIV	88–113 (85)	I	7q11.2 *CD36* 948	plts, monocytes, MØ, adipocytes, some epithelial, endothelial cells, some DC, pancreatic β cells	Signal-transducing scavenger Rc for thrombospondin, collagen, oxidized low-density lipoprotein, fatty acids, anionic phospholipids, *Plasmodium falciparum* infected rbc, and bacterial diacylglycerides
CD37	gp52–40; T-span -26	40–64	III Tet.	19p13.3 *CD37* 951	Mature B cells, some T cells/ monocytes (weak)	Complexes with HLA class II, CD53, CD81, and CD82 in B-cell membrane, suggesting role in signal transduction and/or Ag transport.
CD38	T10; ADP-ribosyl cyclase; gp45	39–45	II	4p15 *CD38* 952	Plasma cells, early or act. B and T cells, thymocytes, monocytes, NK cells, brain, myeloid progenitors	Can synthesize cyclic ADP-ribose (ADPR) from nicotinamide adenine dinucleotide and hydrolyze cADPR to ADP-ribose and bind CD31 and hyaluronic acid. May play a role cell activation, proliferation, or apoptosis, depending on cellular environment. Anti-CD38 found in some diabetics.

(continued)

TABLE 15–1. Cluster of Differentiation Antigens Defined as of the Eighth International Workshop on Leukocyte Typing (Continued)

Antigen	Other Names	Size	O	Genetics	Distribution	Physiology
CD39	Ectonucleotide triphosphate diphosphohydrolase 1 (ENTPD1); vascular ATP diphosphohydrolase; ATPDase apyrase; gp80; EC 3.6.1.5	78	III	10q24 *ENTPD1* 953	Endothelial cells, MØ, DC, act. cells of the NK, mantle zone B cells, act. T cells, neurons, plts	Ectoapyrase that hydrolyzes extracellular ATP and ADP, thereby inhibiting ADP-induced inflammation, thrombosis, and/or plt aggregation. Thrombin inactivates CD39 on endothelial cells.
CD40	Bp50; TNF Rc Superfamily, member 5 (TNFRSF5)	85 (48)	I	20q12–13.2 *CD40* 958	Mature B cells, monocytes, MØ, DC, some epithelial cells, CD34 stem cells	Rc for CD154, which can induce cell activation, isotype switching (B cells), and expression of immune costimulatory molecules on antigen-presenting cells.
CD41	Integrin, α_{2b} (ITGA2B); αIIβ integrin; GPIIb of the GPIIb/GPIIIa complex	135 (120, 23)	I	17q21.32 *ITGA2B* 3674	plts and megakaryocytes	Associates with CD61 to form Rc for fibrinogen, fibronectin, vitronectin, VWF, and thrombospondin to facilitate platelet adhesion and aggregation.
CD42a	Glycoprotein IX (GPIX); gp9	22 (17–22)	I	3q21.3 *GP9* 2815	plts and megakaryocytes	CD42a complexes with CD42b, CD42c, and CD42d with a 2:2:2:1 stoichiometry to form the GP1b complex that binds to subendothelial VWF and thrombin, allowing for plt adhesion to damaged blood vessels. Mutations in CD42 can result in Bernard-Soulier syndrome (see Chap. 121).
CD42b	Glycoprotein Ib, α chain (GP1BA); CD42bα; GPIbα; glycocalicin	160 (145)	I	17pter-p12 *GP1BA* 2811	plts and megakaryocytes	A mucin that serves as binding site of the GP1b complex for VWF and thrombin by forming disulfide-linked heterodimer with CD42c that noncovalently associates with CD42a and CD42d.
CD42c	Glycoprotein Ib, β chain (GP1BB); CD42bβ; GPIbβ	160 (24)	I	22q11–21-q11.23 *GP1BB* 2812	plts and megakaryocytes	Forms disulfide-linked heterodimer with CD42b that associates with CD42a and CD42d to form an Rc for VWF and thrombin.
CD42d	Glycoprotein V (GPV)	82	I	3q29 *GP5* 2814	plts and megakaryocytes	Complexes with CD42a, CD42b, and CD42c to form Rc for VWF and thrombin.
CD43	Sialophorin (SPN); leukosialin; leukocyte sialoglycoprotein; gp95; gpL115	95–135	I	16p11.2 *SPN* 6693	Thymocytes, T cells, PMN, MØ, monocytes, NK cells, plts, brain, act. B cells (weak), plasma cells, hemopoietic stem cells	Sialoglycoprotein that can interact with CD54, HLA class I, CD62P, or hyaluronic acid, serve to inhibit excessive cell–cell adhesion, help regulate T-cell activation, and act as a counter-Rc for CD169.
CD44	Phagocytic gp-1 (Pgp-1); Hermes Ag; extracellular matrix Rc type III (ECMRIII); HUTCH-1; gp80–95	90	I	11p13 *CD44* 960	most cell types except plts, hepatocytes, cardiac muscle, renal tubular epithelium, testis	An Rc for hyaluronate that facilitates lymphocyte binding to high endothelial venules (HEV). Variants of CD44 have attached chondroitin sulfate and are able to bind fibronectin, laminin, and collagen. Also is Rc for chemotactic cytokine osteopontin.
CD44R	CD44R1; Restricted (exon 9 of CD44); CD44v1–10	85–200	I	11p13 *CD44* 960	Epithelial cells, rbc, monocytes, act. leukocytes	Serves as the protein backbone of rbc Lutheran Ag and, like CD44, may be involved in leukocyte attachment and rolling on endothelium for homing to lymphoid tissue and sites of inflammation.
CD45	Protein tyrosine phosphatase, Rc type, C (PTPRC); T200; leukocyte common Ag (LCA); EC 3.1.34	180–220	I	1q31–32 *PTPRC* 5788	All hematopoietic cells except rbc	A surface tyrosine phosphatase that can associate with CD2, CD3, and CD4 and can modulate signal transduction by surface Ag Rc.

(*continued*)

TABLE 15–1. Cluster of Differentiation Antigens Defined as of the Eighth International Workshop on Leukocyte Typing (Continued)

Antigen	Other Names	Size	O	Genetics	Distribution	Physiology
CD45RA	B220	220	I	See CD45	B cells, subset of naïve CD4 T cells, monocytes	A surface tyrosine phosphatase formed by joining the 8-amino-acid NH_2-terminal sequence to that encoded by exons A, B, and C. This is the largest of the CD45 isoforms.
CD45RB	T200	205, 220	I	See CD45	Memory T-cell subset, monocytes, PMN (weak)	A surface tyrosine phosphatase formed by joining the 8-amino-acid NH_2-terminal sequence to that encoded by exon band C.
CD45RC		190, 205, 220	I	See CD45	Some T cells	A surface tyrosine phosphatase formed by joining the 8-amino-acid NH_2-terminal sequence to that encoded by exon C.
CD45RO	Restricted T200	180	I	See CD45	Thymocytes act., some memory T-cells	A surface tyrosine phosphatase formed by joining the 8-amino-acid NH_2-terminal sequence to the CD45 backbone without A, B, or C. This is the smallest of the CD45 isoforms.
CD46	Membrane cofactor protein (MCP); HuLy-m5; trophoblast leukocyte-common Ag (TLX)	46–63 (51–68)	I	1q32 *CD46* 4179	All nucleated cells except unfertilized oocytes	Acts as cofactor for factor I mediated proteolytic cleavage of C3b, and C4b, thereby protecting against complement-mediated damage. Serves as Rc for several pathogens, including measles virus, Herpes virus, *Streptococcus pyogenes*, and *Neisseria* sp.
CD47	Integrin-associated protein (IAP); MEM-133; ovarian CA Ag (OA3); Rh-associated protein; CDw149	45–60 (50–55)	III Tet.	3q13.1-q13.2 *CD47* 961	All human cells except Rh_{null} rbc	Associates with CD61-integrins to form Rc for thrombospondin or leukocyte-inhibitory-Rc signal-regulatory protein (SIRPα), leading to either activation or apoptosis via heterotrimeric Gi-protein-signaling. Forms part of the Rh complex.
CD48	HuLym3; OX45; BLAST-1BCM1; MEM-102	45	GPI	1q21.3-q22 *CD48* 962	All hematopoietic cells except PMN, plts, or rbc.	Low-affinity Rc for CD2 and ligand for CD244 that can inhibit NK effector functions. In T cells may promote signal transduction via cytoplasmic interaction with *lck* and *fyn* tyrosine kinases.
CD49a	Integrin α_1 subunit (ITGA1); very-late Ag (VLA)-1 α subunit	200 (210)	I	5q11.2 *ITGA1* 3672	Monocytes, endothelium, smooth muscle, act. T and B cells	Assembles into a heterodimer with CD29 to form a Rc for type IV collagen and laminin involved in leukocyte extravasation.
CD49b	Integrin $\alpha 2$ (ITGA2); GPIa; Ia subunit of platelet gp Ia-IIa; very-late Ag (VLA)-2 α subunit; ECMRI	160	I	5q23-q31 *ITGA2* 3673	plts, megakaryocytes, monocytes, act. T and B cell, NK cells, thymocytes, fibroblasts, endothelium, osteoclasts, epithelium	Assembles with CD29 to form an Rc for type I collagen, VLA-3, and E-cadherin. Also acts as Rc for echovirus.
CD49c	Integrin α_3 (ITGA3); very-late Ag (VLA)-3 α subunit	150 (30/125)	I	17q21.33 *ITGA3* 3675	Monocytes, T and B cells, kidney glomerulus, thyroid, some basement membranes	Assembles with CD29 to form an Rc for laminin-5 and epilgrin (kalinin) that also binds weakly to collagen and fibronectin. May play role in cell–cell adhesion and/or signal transduction.
CD49d	Integrin α_4 (ITGA4); very-late Ag (VLA)-4 α subunit	150 (145)	I	2q31.3 *ITGA4* 3676	T, B, and NK cells, eos., monocytes, erythroblasts, thymocytes, mast cells, DC, basophils, myeloblasts	Assembles with CD29 or $\beta 7$ integrin to form VLA-4 or $\alpha 4\beta 7$, which respectively bind VCAM-1 (CD106), connecting segment-1 (CS-1, an isoform of fibronectin), invasin, and thrombospondin, or mucosal addressin MAdCAM-1 and CS-1. These integrins help regulate the inflammatory response and play a role in T-cell activation.

(*continued*)

TABLE 15–1. Cluster of Differentiation Antigens Defined as of the Eighth International Workshop on Leukocyte Typing (Continued)

Antigen	Other Names	Size	O	Genetics	Distribution	Physiology
CD49e	Integrin α_5 (ITGA5); very-late Ag (VLA)-5 α subunit; Ic subunit of GPIc-IIa	155 (135/25)	I	12q11-q13 *ITGA5* 3678	Thymocytes, T cells, monocytes, plts, act. or very early B cells, DC, but not plts	Assembles with CD29 to form a Rc for fibronectin and neural adhesion molecule L1 via binding to RGD. Upon binding, it activates the Na^+/H^+ antiporter and can provide costimulatory signal to T cells.
CD49f	Integrin α_6 (ITGA6); very-late Ag (VLA)-6 α subunit; subunit of laminin Rc; platelet GPIc	140 (120/30)	I	2p31.1 *ITGA6* 3655	plts, megakaryocytes, MØ, monocytes, thymocytes, T cells, adherent epithelia	Assembles with CD29 or the β_4 integrin chain (CD104) to form an Rc for invasin, merosin, and laminin on basement membranes. Plays role in embryogenesis, cell adhesion, migration, and cell signaling.
CD50	Intercellular adhesion molecule-3 (ICAM-3)	120–160	I	19p13.3–2 *ICAM3* 3385	Thymocytes, T and B cells, monocytes, PMN, endothelial cells, Langerhans cells	CD50 is a ligand for activated LFA-1 (CD11a/CD18) and that, when engaged, can provide a costimulatory signal for cell activation and/or HIV replication.
CD51	Integrin α_v (ITGAV); vitronectin Rc	150 (125/24)	I	2q31-q32 *ITGAV* 3685	Endothelial cells, monocytes, MØ, plts (weak), some B cells (weak)	Can assemble with CD29 (β1), CD61(β_3), β_5, β_6, or β_8 integrins. The CD51/CD61 complex binds RGD motifs in ECM proteins, vitronectin, fibrinogen, VWF factor, laminin, bone sialoprotein (Bsp1), thrombospondin, or neural adhesion molecule L1. CD51/CD29 or CD51/β_6 bind vitronectin and fibronectin. These Rc facilitate plt aggregation and/or leukocyte adhesion and migration through the subendothelium. Involved in bone resorption by facilitating osteoclast adhesion to osteopontin.
CD52	Campath-1, HE-5	25–29	GPI	1p36 *CDW52* 1043	Lymphocytes, monocytes, PMN (weak), eos (strong), seminal vesicles, epididymis, spermatozoa	Some anti-CD52 mAbs are strongly mitogenic, suggesting that CD52 plays a role in signal transduction.
CD53	OX-44, tetraspanin-25, Tspan-25	32–42	III Tet.	1p13 *CD53* 963	Leukocytes (highest on B cells)	Can transduce signals in B cells, monocytes, and PMN, causing Ca^{++} mobilization leading to cell activation.
CD54	Intercellular adhesion molecule-1 (ICAM-1); BB2' P3.58	80–114	I	19p13.3-p13.2 *ICAM1* 3383	Leukocytes, endothelial and epithelial cells, expression increased with activation	Functions as a ligand for LFA-1 (CD11a/CD18), Mac-1 (CD11b/CD18), and CD11c/CD18 (p150,95). CD54 also is an Rc for rhinovirus, can bind CD43, and can bind to *Plasmodium falciparum*-infected rbc.
CD55	Decay accelerating factor (DAF); CR; CROM; TC	55–70	GPI	1q32 *DAF* 1604	All cells in contact with serum, CNS, epithelial cells	Neutralizes complement activation on autologous tissue by preventing the assembly of C3 convertase or accelerating disassembly of preformed convertase. CD55 can bind C3b/C3Bb convertase, C4b/C4b/2a convertase, CD97, coxsackie viruses (G1, B3, B5), echoviruses (type 7) enterovirus 70, and *Escherichia coli* Dr-adhesins.
CD56	Neural cell adhesion molecule-1 (NCAM); Leu19; NKH1; MSK39	140 or 180; 120 (GPI)	I or GPI	11q23.1 *NCAM1* 4684	NK cells, embryonic cells, muscle, neural cells, epithelium, some act. T cells	Facilitates homotypic and heterotypic adhesion and may play a role in contact-dependent growth inhibition, neuronal development, and NK cell cytotoxicity. CD56 can bind NCAM-1, heparin sulphate, and chondroitin sulfated proteoglycans.

(*continued*)

TABLE 15–1. Cluster of Differentiation Antigens Defined as of the Eighth International Workshop on Leukocyte Typing (Continued)

Antigen	Other Names	Size	O	Genetics	Distribution	Physiology
CD57	Human natural killer-1 (HNK-1); Leu 7; NK-1; GLCATP; GlcUAT-P	110	–	11q25 *B3GAT1* 27087	NK cells, some T, few B, some Schwann cells	A carbohydrate structure, 2-*O*-sulfoglucuronic acid β_1-3Gal β_1-4GlcNAc, which requires $\beta_{1,3}$-glucuronyltransferase 1, encoded by *B3GAT1*. CD57 may be attached to several gps (e.g., CD56, myelin gp), where it can bind laminin, CD62P, or CD62L.
CD58	Leukocyte function associated-3 (LFA-3); FLJ43722	45–70	I or GPI	1p13 *CD58* 965	Most hemopoietic cells, fibroblasts, endothelial and epithelial cells	Binds CD2 and enhances T-cell Ag recognition. The CD58 homolog on sheep rbc allows these cells to form rosettes with human T cells.
CD59	Complement protectin; IF-5Ag; EJ16; MIRL; MIN1; EL32; MACIF; HRF20; MIC11; MSK21	19–25	GPI	11p13 *CD59* 966	leukocytes, rbc, endothelial and epithelial cells, placenta, spermatozoa, body fluids	Inhibits complement membrane attack by binding to activated C8 and C9. It also is a minor ligand for CD2 and may be involved in T-cell signal transduction.
CD60a	GD3; SIAT8; SIAT8A	–	–	12p12.1-p11.2 *ST8SIA1* 6489	Melanocytes, glial cells, neurons, pancreatic islet cells, plts, adrenal medulla, thymocytes, some T cells, B cells (weak)	Oligosaccharide sequence of the ganglioside GD3: NeuAcα_2–8NeuAc-α_2–3Gal-β_1–4Glcβ_1-Cer, which requires the enzyme α-*N*-acetyl-neurminade $\alpha_{2,8}$-sialytransferase1, encoded by *ST8SIA1*. It may help regulate of apoptosis and mitochondrial permeability.
CD60b	9-*O*-acetyl GD3	–	–	–	Some T cells, act B cells, neuroectodermal cells in thymus epithelium and skin	Epitope formed by 9-*O*-acetyl GD3 and related disialosyl structures linked to lactosylceramide or its analogues.
CD60c	7-*O*-acetyl GD3		–	–	T cells	Epitope formed by 7-*O*-acetyl-GD3 and related disialosyl structures linked either to lactosylceramide or its analogues.
CD61	Integrin, β_3 (ITGB3); GPIIIa; β_3 integrin; vitronectin Rc β chain; 9-*O*-acetyl-GD3	90 (110)	I	17q21.32 *ITGB3* 3690	Complexed with CD41 on plts and megakaryocytes, complexed with CD51 on monocytes, MØ, endothelial cells, plts, some B cells, osteoclasts, some mast cells, fibroblasts	Associates with CD41 to form the GPIIb-IIIa heterodimer on plts that facilitates aggregation. Absent or dysfunctional CD41/CD61 leads to Glanzmann thrombasthenia (see Chap. 121). Also complexes with CD51 to form a Rc for RGD motifs in ECM proteins (e.g., vitronectin, fibronectin, and VWF).
CD62E	Selectin E (SELE); endothelial leukocyte adhesion molecule-1 (ELAM-1); LECAM-2; ESEL	107–115 (97)	I	1q22-q25 *SELE* 6401	act. endothelial cells, skin, placenta, marrow endothelium	Facilitates adhesion and leukocyte extravasation of PMN, monocytes, and some T cells to vascular endothelium by binding carbohydrate ligands (e.g., CD15s) on various molecules, including GlyCAM1, CD34, CD107a, and CD162.
CD62L	Selectin L (SELL); Mel-14; TQ1; leukocyte adhesion molecule-1 (LAM-1); LNHR; LECAM-1; Leu-8	65 (74–95)	I	1q23-q25 *SELL* 6402	B cells, T cells, PMN, thymocytes monocytes, eos., basophils, erythroid and myeloid progenitor cells, some NK cells	Recognizes carbohydrate ligands (e.g., CD15s) found on various gps (e.g., MAdCAM-1, GlyCAM-1, CD34) to facilitate "rolling" of leukocytes on act. endothelium at inflammatory sites or at high endothelial venules (HEV) of peripheral lymph nodes.
CD62P	Selectin P (SELP); GMP-140; LECAM-3; PADGEM; CD62; GRMP; PSEL; FLJ45155	120 (140)	I	1q21–24 *SELP* 6403	act. plts, act. endothelium, megakaryocytes	Binds CD15s or other carbohydrate ligands of CD24 or CD162, which permits the tethering and rolling of leukocytes that precedes their extravasation. Binding to CD24 also may play role in tumor metastases. CD62P also binds unrelated polyanions.

(*continued*)

TABLE 15–1. Cluster of Differentiation Antigens Defined as of the Eighth International Workshop on Leukocyte Typing (Continued)

Antigen	Other Names	Size	O	Genetics	Distribution	Physiology
CD63	Lysosomal membrane-associated gp 3 (LAMP 3); LIMP; gp55; granulophysin; OMA81H; MLA1; ME491	40–60	III Tet.	12q12-q13 *CD63* 967	act. plts, monocytes, MØ, secretory granules (Weibel-Palade bodies) of vascular endothelial cells, platelet dense granules, fibroblasts, osteoclasts, smooth muscle, brain, synovium	Lysosomal protein that translocates to the cell surface upon cellular activation to associate with VLA-3, -4, or -6, or with CD11/CD18, CD9, or CD81 to facilitate adhesion with various ligands in the ECM.
CD64	Fc of IgG, high affinity Rc 1A (FCGR1A); FcγRI; FcRI	72	I	1q21.2-q21.3 *FCGR1A* 2209	Monocytes, MØ, act. PMN, FDC	High-affinity Rc for the Fc of IgG that mediates antibody-dependent cellular cytotoxicity, phagocytosis of immune complexes, and release of cytokines (e.g., IL-1, IL-6, or TNF-α), and/or reactive oxygen intermediates.
CD65 CD65s	Ceramide-dodecasaccharide 4c; (sialylated-CD65 is CD65s; VIM-2)	–	–	–	Myeloid cells, some monocytic cells	CD65s is a carbohydrate determinant with a minimal epitope consisting of NeuAc$\alpha_2\rightarrow$3Gal$\beta_1\rightarrow$4GlcNAc$\beta_1\rightarrow$3Gal$\beta_1\rightarrow$4GlcNAc(Fuc$\alpha_1\rightarrow$3)$\beta_1\rightarrow$3Galβ. CD65 lacks the terminal sialic acid. The gp(s) that have these determinants may be involved in signal transduction leading to formation of the respiratory burst.
CD66a	CEA-related cell adhesion molecule 1 (CEACAM1); phosphorylated gp; biliary glycoprotein-1 (BGP-1); nonspecific cross-reacting Ag-160 (NCA-160)	140–180 (113,96, 74)	I	19q13.2 *CEACAM1* 634	PMN, histiocytes, some myeloid progenitor cells, brush border of colonic epithelial cells	A biliary gp member of the carcinoembryonic Ag family of adhesion molecules that can bind CD62E, mannose-sensitive adhesin of gut microbes, CD66a, CD66c, or CD66e to facilitate Ca^{2+}-independent homotypic or heterotypic adhesion and/or neutrophil activation. Also, is a Rc for *Neisseria meningitis* and *Neisseria gonorrhoeae*.
CD66b	Formerly CD67; CEA-related cell adhesion molecule 8 (CEACAM8); CGM6; p100; nonspecific cross-reacting Ag-95 (NCA-95)	95–100	GPI	19q13.2 *CEACAM8* 1088	Granulocytes	CD66b is a GPI isoform of CD66 that can facilitate heterotypic adhesion by binding the core protein of CD66c, CD62E, and/or galectins.
CD66c	CEA-related cell adhesion molecule 6 (CEACAM6); nonspecific cross-reacting Ag-90 (NCA-90)	90	GPI	19q13.2 *CEACAM6* 4680	Myeloid and epithelial cells	CD66c is a GPI isoform of CD66 that can facilitate homotypic adhesion through binding the core protein of CD66c, or heterotypic adhesion through binding to CD66a-e, CD62E, and/or galectins. Also, is a Rc for *Neisseria meningitis* and *Neisseria gonorrhoeae*, pathogenic *Neisseria* sp., or *Escherichia coli*.
CD66d	CEA-related cell adhesion molecule 3 (CEACAM3); CGM1; CEA; W264; MGC119875	35	I	19q13.2 *CEACAM* 1084	Granulocytes	Member of carcinoembryonic Ag family of adhesion molecules that facilitates homotypic adhesion and neutrophil activation. Also binds the opacity-associated (Opa) proteins of pathogenic *Neisseria* sp.
CD66e	CEA-related cell adhesion molecule 5 (CEACAM5); carcinoembryonic Ag (CEA); meconium Ag100	180–200	GPI	19q13.1-q13.2 *CEACAM5* 1048	Embryonic tissues, adult colon epithelial cells (very weak)	Can facilitate Ca^{2+}-independent homotypic and heterotypic adhesion during embryogenesis. CD66e can bind CD66a, CD66c, CD66e, or the opacity-associated (Opa) proteins of pathogenic *Neisseria* sp.

(continued)

TABLE 15–1. Cluster of Differentiation Antigens Defined as of the Eighth International Workshop on Leukocyte Typing (Continued)

Antigen	Other Names	Size	O	Genetics	Distribution	Physiology
CD66f	Pregnancy-specific glycoprotein 1 (PSG1); SP-1; PSBG1; PSGGA; DHFRP2; PSGIIA; FLJ90598	54–72	GPI	19q13.2 *PSG1* 5669	Placental syncytiotrophoblasts, tissues derived from all three germ layers during embryogenesis, adult colon epithelial cells (very weak)	Member of carcinoembryonic Ag family of adhesion molecules that may protect the fetus from maternal immune recognition and is essential for successful pregnancy.
CD67	See CD66b.	95–100	GPI	19q13.2 *CEACAM8* 1088	Granulocytes	Same as CD66b.
CD68	gp110; macrosialin (mouse)	110	I	17p13 *CD68* 968	Mostly confined to cytoplasmic granules of monocytes/MØ, DC, granulocytes, osteoclasts, mast cells, act. lymphocytes, myeloid progenitor cells, nurse-like cells	A sialomucin belonging to a family of highly glycosylated, acidic lysosomal gps that include LAMP-1 (CD107a) and LAMP-2 (CD107b). It may protect the lysosomal membranes from attack by hydrolases, bind oxidative low-density lipoprotein, and contribute to foam cell formation in atherosclerosis.
CD69	Activation inducer molecule (AIM); early activation Ag (EA1); MLR3; gp34/28; Leu-23; VEA; CLEC2C	60 (28, 33)	II	12p13-p12 *CD69* 969	plts, act. lymphocytes, act. granulocytes, CD4+ or CD8+ thymocytes	Member of the Ca^{2+}-dependent (C-type) lectin superfamily of type II transmembrane proteins. Forms a homodimer that may function as signal transducer that can enhance $Ca+^{2}+$ flux, cell activation, and/or platelet aggregation.
CD70	Ki-24 Ag; CD27-ligand; TNFSF7	50	II	19p13.3 *CD70* 970	act. B and some act. T cells, act. NK cells	Member of the TNFSF that binds CD27 and may provide a costimulatory signal for T-cell activation and generation of T-cell memory.
CD71	Transferrin Rc (TFRC); TFR; TFR1; TRFR; T9	190 (95)	II	3q29 *TFRC* 7037	act. or proliferating cells, reticulocytes, brain, capillary endothelium	Binds serum iron-transport protein ferrotransferrin at neutral pH and iron-free apotransferrin at acidic intracellular pH to facilitate cellular iron uptake.
CD72	LYB2; CD72b	45	II	9p13.3 *CD72* 971	All B cells (except plasma cells), MØ (weak), DC (weak)	A member of the $Ca+^{2}+$-dependent (C-type) lectin superfamily that can bind CD100. CD72 may attenuate B-cell Rc (BCR) signaling via its phosphorylated cytoplasmic ITIM domains, which recruit SHP-1. Binding to CD100 can lead to dephosphorylation of ITIM and enhance BCR signaling. CD72 also putatively binds CD5.
CD73	5′-Nucleotidase, ecto (NT5E); ecto-5′-nucleotidase	69–72	GPI	6q14-q21 *NT5E* 4907	Most B cells, some T cells, thymocytes (weak), some epithelial and endothelial cells, FDC	Catalyses 5′ dephosphorylation of pyrimidine and purine ribo- and deoxyribonucleoside monophosphates to nucleosides. May contribute to lymphocyte adhesion and/or activation.
CD74	MHC class II-associated invariant chain; class II-specific chaperone; invariant chain (Ii)	33, 35, 41 (43)	II	5q32 *CD74* 972	B cells, monocytes (weak), DC, act. T cells	Associates with the α and β chains of HLA class II proteins in the endoplasmic reticulum to prevent binding of endogenous peptides. It is released from the HLA protein in the acidic lysosomal compartment.
CD75	Lactosamine; NeuAc $\alpha_{2,6}$-Gal$\beta_{1,4}$ GlcNAc core epitope; CD75s (indicates sialylated lactosamine); CDw76	67 and 85	–	–	CD75—germinal-center B cells, subsets of endothelial and epithelial cells, few T cells, rbc, most mature B cells (weak), but not plasma cells	CD75 defines lactosamine structures and CD75s defines sialylated lactosamines (e.g. NeuAcα_2–6Galβ_1–4GlcNAcβ_1–3Galβ_1–4Glc-β_1–1′Cer) that each are found on various glycosphingolipids and gps. CD75s requires β-galactoside $\alpha_{2,6}$-sialyltransferase (SiaT-1) activity in the Golgi to produce the $\alpha_{2,6}$-sialylated form of CD75.

(continued)

TABLE 15–1. Cluster of Differentiation Antigens Defined as of the Eighth International Workshop on Leukocyte Typing (Continued)

Antigen	Other Names	Size	O	Genetics	Distribution	Physiology
CD75s	–	–	–	–	CD75s most mature B cells, but not germinal-center B cells or plasma cells	–
CDw76	HD66, CRIS-4	–	–	–	See CD75 (CD75s)	CD75s, but formerly considered distinct because of its reactivity with different antibodies.
CD77	Globotriaosylceramide ($G\beta_3$); Pk blood group; Burkitt lymphoma-associated Ag (BLA); ceramide trihexoside (CTH)	1	–	–	Germinal-center B cells (esp. centroblasts), FDC, endothelium, some epithelial cells	A globotriaosylceramide, which possibly binds CD19, that is formed by action of $\alpha_{1,4}$-galactosyltransferase, which transfers a galactose to the $\alpha_{1,4}$ position of lactosylceramide. Rc for verotoxin of *Escherichia coli* and the Shiga toxin of *Shigella dysenteriae.* May help eliminate germinal-center B cells that fail to make antibodies that fail to bind Ag.
CDw78	Ba	–	–	–	B cells (increased after activation), monocytes, MØ, DC	Provisional designation dropped since mAbs assigned to this specificity were found to bind epitopes on HLA class II molecules.
CD79a	mb-1; IGA; Ig-α	32–33	I	19q13.2 *CD79A* 973	B cells	An accessory molecule of the B-cell Rc (BCR) complex required for sIg expression and signal transduction (see Chap. 77).
CD79b	B29; IGB; Ig-β	37–39	I	17q23 *CD79B* 974	B cells	An accessory molecule that mediates sIg expression and signal transduction (see Chap. 77).
CD80	B7; B7–1; BB1; LAB7; CD28LG1	60	I	3q13.3-q21 *CD80* 941	act. B cells, monocytes, blood-derived DC, FDC, MØ, act. T cells (weak)	Interacts with CD28 or CD152 (CTLA-4) for costimulation or inhibition of T-cell activation, respectively (see Chap. 78).
CD81	Target of antiproliferative antibody-1 (TAPA-1); M38	26	III Tet.	11p15.5 *CD81* 975	All leukocytes, esp. lymphocytes (strong), endothelia	Member of the CD19/CD21/Leu-13 signal transduction complex that is involved in B-cell signaling. CD81 also can serve as the Rc for hepatitis C virus.
CD82	R2; IA4; 4F9; C33; KAI1; TSPAN27; ST6	50–53	III Tet.	11p11.2 *CD82* 3732	Epithelia, endothelia, monocytes, PMN, plts, act. lymphocytes, fibroblasts	Complexes with CD37, CD53, CD81, integrins, and/or HLA to play a role in signal transduction.
CD83	HB15; BL11	43	I	6p23 *CD83* 9308	DC (not FDC) (strong), Langerhans cells, B cells (weak), interdigitating reticular cells	May play a role in Ag presentation or lymphocyte activation. Good marker for mature DC.
CD84	SLAM family; member 5 (SLAMF5); p75; GR6; Hly9-β	64–82	I	1q24 *CD84* 8832	Monocytes, MØ, GC B cells (strong), mantle zone B cells (weak), plts	Has structural similarities to adhesion molecules such as CD2 and CD48, suggesting role in intercellular interactions/signaling.
CD85	See CD85j.	110	I	19q13.4	See CD85j.	See CD85j (see Chap. 79).
CD85a	Leukocyte-Ig-like Rc, subfamily B, member 3 (LILRB3); Ig-like transcript-5 (ILT5); HL9	110	I	19q13.4 *LILRB3* 11025	NK cells, monocytes, MØ, DC, granulocytes, and some T cells	Polymorphic Rc for HLA class I molecules with cytoplasmic ITIMs that inhibits Rc-signaling and/or cytotoxicity upon binding.
CD85b	Leukocyte-Ig-like Rc, subfamily A, member 6 (LILRA6); LIR6; ILT8; ILT5	110	I	19q13.4 *LILRA6* 79168	NK cells	Ig-like molecule that lacks cytoplasmic ITIMs.
CD85c	Leukocyte-Ig-like Rc, subfamily B, member 5 (LILRB5); LIR5; ILT8	110	I	19q13.4 *LILRB5* 10990	NK cells	Polymorphic Rc for HLA class I molecules with cytoplasmic ITIMs that inhibits Rc-signaling and/or cytotoxicity upon binding.

(continued)

TABLE 15–1. Cluster of Differentiation Antigens Defined as of the Eighth International Workshop on Leukocyte Typing (Continued)

Antigen	Other Names	Size	O	Genetics	Distribution	Physiology
CD85d	Leukocyte-Ig-like Rc, subfamily B, member 2 (LILRB2); LIR2; ILT4; MIR10; LILRA6; MIR-10	110	I	19q13.4 *LILRB2* 10288	NK cells, monocytes, MØ, some DC, myeloid cells, PMN (weak)	Polymorphic Rc for HLA class I molecules with cytoplasmic ITIMs that inhibits Rc-signaling and/or cytotoxicity upon binding. Also binds trophoblast-restricted HLA-G1 to inhibit potential maternal–fetal immune reactions.
CD85e	Leukocyte-Ig-like Rc, subfamily A, member 3 (LILRA3); LIR4; ILT6; HM31	110	I	19q13.4 *LILRA3* 11026	–	Soluble Ig-like protein without transmembrane or cytoplasmic domains.
CD85f	Leukocyte-Ig-like Rc, subfamily A, member 5 (LILRA5); LIR5; ILT11	110	I	19q13.4 *LILRA5* 353514	NK cells	Ig-like molecule without cytoplasmic ITIMs.
CD85g	Leukocyte-Ig-like Rc, subfamily A, member 4 (LILRA4); ILT7	110	I	19q13.4 *LILRA4* 23547	plasmacytoid DC, monocytes, act. B	Ig-like protein without cytoplasmic ITIMs that associates with FcεRIγ chain to form an Rc.
CD85h	Leukocyte-Ig-like Rc, subfamily A, member 2 (LILRA2); LIR7; ILT1	110	I	19q13.4 *LILRA2* 11027	Myeloid cells, monocytes	Ig-like protein without cytoplasmic ITIMs.
CD85i	Leukocyte-Ig-like Rc, subfamily A, member 1 (LILRA1); LIR6	110	I	19q13.4 *LILRA1* 11024	B cells, monocytes	Ig-like protein without cytoplasmic ITIMs that associates with FcεRIγ chain to form an Rc.
CD85j	Leukocyte-Ig-like Rc, subfamily B, member 1 (LILRB1); LIR1; ILT2; MIR7; CD85	110	I	19q13.4 *LILRB1* 10859	NK cells, DC, monocytes, most T cells, plasma cells, B cells (weak)	Polymorphic Rc for HLA class I molecules with cytoplasmic ITIMs that can inhibit Rc-signaling and/or cytotoxicity upon binding. Binds trophoblast-restricted HLA-G1 to inhibit potential maternal-fetal immune reactions. Also binds the class-I-like protein UL18 of CMV.
CD85k	Leukocyte-Ig-like Rc, subfamily B, member 4 (LILRB4); LIR5; ILT3; HM18	60	I	19q13.4 *LILRB4* 11006	Monocytes, mast cells, MØ, DC cells, PMN, B cells, NK cells, endothelial cells	Is a putative inhibitory Rc with unknown ligand that has cytoplasmic ITIMs.
CD86	B7–2; B70; LAB72; CD28LG2; MGC34413	80	I	3q21 *CD86* 942	Interdigitating DC cells, act. B cells, act. monocytes, act. blood-derived DC cells	Interacts with CD28 to provide a costimulatory signal or with CD152 (CTLA-4) to provide an inhibitory signal for T-cell activation.
CD87	Plasminogen activator, urokinase Rc (PLAUR); urokinase plasminogen activator Rc (uPAR); Mo3	35–68 (32–66)	GPI	19q13 *PLAUR* 5329	Leading-edge of migrating leukocytes (monocytes, PMN, DC cells, act. T cells, LGL), fibroblasts, endothelia, smooth muscle, keratinocyte, placental trophoblasts, hepatocytes	Rc for uPA that can retain and concentrate uPA at the plasma membrane, allowing for local conversion of plasminogen to plasmin, which binds and hydrolyses ECM. Binds vitronectin, β_1 and β_2 integrins, and kininogen, and facilitates cell adhesion.
CD88	Complement component 5a Rc 1 (C5R1); Rc for C5a; C5a-Rc	40	III Hep.	19q13.3–13.4 *C5R1* 728	Granulocytes, monocytes, MØ, DC cells, astrocytes, microglia	A G-protein–coupled Rc that triggers chemotaxis, activation, respiratory burst, and degranulation, upon binding to C5a. Also binds anaphylatoxin.
CD89	FcRc for IgA; FcαRc (FCAR)	45–100	I	19q13.2- q13.4 *FCAR* 2204	Granulocytes, monocytes, MØ, DC cells	Associates with CD11b/CD18 to form a low-affinity Rc for IgA_1 or IgA_2 that can trigger granulocyte respiratory burst, phagocytosis, and release of inflammatory cytokines upon binding Fc of IgA in immune complexes.

(continued)

TABLE 15–1. Cluster of Differentiation Antigens Defined as of the Eighth International Workshop on Leukocyte Typing (Continued)

Antigen	Other Names	Size	O	Genetics	Distribution	Physiology
CD90	Thy-1; theta Ag	25–35 (25–29)	GPI	11q22.3-q23 *THY1* 7070	HSC, brain, some fetal thymocytes, act. endothelial cells esp. high endothelial venules	May play role in development of neuron memory, help regulate growth and/or differentiation of HSC, and facilitate transendothelial leukocyte migration during inflammation.
CD91	Low-density lipoprotein (LDL)-related protein 1 (LEP1); α_2-macroglobulin Rc (α_2M-R)	600 (515/85)	I	12q13-q14 *LEP1* 4035	Monocytes, MØ, hepatocytes, neurons, astrocytes, fibroblasts, epithelia, syncytiotrophoblasts, Alzheimer plaques, atherosclerotic plaques	Member of the LDL Rc family that can bind to α_2 macroglobulin-proteinase complexes, inhibitor-complexed urokinase and tissue-plasminogen activators, LPL, chylomicron remnants, *Pseudomonas* exotoxin A, and various hsps (e.g., gp96, hsp90, calreticulin). Mediates uptake and metabolism of its ligands.
CD92	Solute carrier family 44, member 1 (SLC44A1); choline transporter-like protein 1 (CHTL1); p70	70	III	9q31.2 *SLC44A1* 23446	Monocytes, blood-derived DC, PMN, lymphocytes (weak), endothelium (weak)	Transports choline for synthesis of membrane phospholipids. Has one cytoplasmic ITIM that potentially may provide inhibitory signaling.
CD93	C1q Rc precursor (C1qRP); GR11	110 (126)		20p11.21 *CD93* 22918	NK cells, monocytes, granulocytes, plts, endothelial cells	Rc for C1q that potentially may assist phagocytosis of cells coated with complement.
CD94	Killer cell lectin-like Rc subfamily D, member 1 (KLRD1); Kp43	30	II	12p13 *KLRD1* 3824	NK (increased upon activation), a few T cells	C-type lectin that complexes with CD159a or CD159c to form Rc for HLA class I molecules and/or peptides derived from HLA class I molecules. Functions as an inhibitory Rc for NK cells (see Chap. 79).
CD95	Apo-1; FAS; TNFRSF6; APT1; apoptosis Ag 1	45,90 (45)	I	10q24.1 *FAS* 355	act. lymphocytes, fibroblasts, monocytes, PMN, liver	Rc for CD178, which can induce apoptosis of cells bearing CD95.
CD96	T-cell activation increased late expression (TACTILE)	240, 180, 160 (160)	I	3q13.13-q13.2 *CD96* 10225	T and NK cells (increased upon activation)	Expressed primarily upon activation, suggesting it plays a role in cell adhesion during late phases of intercellular cognate interactions.
CD97	BL-KDD/F12	74–89 (75–86)	III Hep.	19p13 *CD97* 976	act. lymphocytes, PMN, monocytes, DC, MØ, smooth muscle cells	Rc for CD55 and chondroitin sulfate that may be involved in cell adhesion and/or signaling after leukocyte activation. May play role in PMN migration.
CD98	Solute carrier family 3, member 2 (SLCA2); 4F2; FRP-1; RL-388	125 (45/ 80)	II	11q13 *SLC3A2* 6520	Strong on monocytes, myocardial cells, act. T cells, and proliferating cells, but weak on T, B, and NK cells	Two-chain, disulfide-linked molecule that can serve as a chaperone for actin-associated amino acid transporters. Binds and complexes with β_1 integrins to help regulate their adhesive functions.
CD99	MIC2; E2; 12E7; HuLy-m6; FMC29; CD99R	32	I	Xp22.33 and Yp11.3 *CD99* 4267	Most hematopoietic cells, esp. thymocytes; CD99 is found on surface of Xg(a+) rbc and in cytoplasm of Xg(a–) rbc. CD99R on myeloid cells, NK cells, and CD4/CD8+ thymocytes	Adhesion molecule that facilitates positive selection of thymocytes and transendothelial migration of leukocytes at sites of inflammation Also, involved in rosette formation with sheep rbc. CD99 signaling also may induce apoptosis.

(continued)

TABLE 15–1. Cluster of Differentiation Antigens Defined as of the Eighth International Workshop on Leukocyte Typing (Continued)

Antigen	Other Names	Size	O	Genetics	Distribution	Physiology
CD100	Semaphorin 4D (SEMA4D); collapsin 4; Coll4	300 (150)	I	9q22.2 *SEMA4D* 10507	Myeloid cells, T cells, act. DC, act. B cells, brain, kidney, heart	A semaphorin Rc for CD72 and plexin-B1 that can modify the signaling activity of other receptors (e.g., in B cells it can modify CD40-CD154 interactions, downmodulate CD23, and mitigate the inhibitory effect of CD72). Soluble CD100 promotes B-cell activation. Binding to plexin-B1/Met plays a role in invasive epithelial cell growth.
CD101	Ig superfamily, member 2 (IGSF2); V7; p126	240 (126)	I	1p13 *IGSF2* 9398	Granulocytes, monocytes, DC, some mucosal T cells, act. T	Ligation of CD101 can promote cellular activation.
CD102	Intercellular adhesion molecule-2 (ICAM-2)	54–68	I	17q23-q25 *ICAM2* 3384	Endothelial cells (strong), plts (strong), subset of lymphocytes, monocytes, DC, splenic sinusoids	Ligand for LFA-1 (CD11a/CD18) and CR3 (CD11b/CD18) that plays role in the homing of cells to sites of inflammation. Interaction with integrins also can play an immune co-stimulatory role.
CD103	Integrin α_E-subunit (ITGAE); human mucosal lymphocyte-1 integrin (HML-1); integrin α_E chain	175 (150,25)	I	17p13 *ITGAE* 3682	Intraepithelial lymphocytes, 1–2% of blood lymphocytes, testis, prostate ovary, pancreas, HCL	Associates with the β_7 integrin to form a Rc that binds CD324 to facilitate adhesion to epithelia. Useful in diagnosis of HCL.
CD104	Integrin *β4* ($ITGB_4$); TSP-1180	210 (220)	I	17q25 *ITGB4* 3691	Basal epithelia of skin and gastrointestinal tract, endothelia during angiogenesis, thymocytes, Schwann cells, few neurons	Associates with α_6 (CD49f) to form a Rc for keratins and laminins (and possibly epiligrin), facilitating adhesion of cells to the ECM.
CD105	Endoglin (ENG); Rc for transforming growth factor-beta (TGF-β) types I and III	180 (90)	II	9q33-q34.1 *ENG* 2022	Vascular endothelium (particularly during angiogenesis), MØ, act. monocytes, FDC, syncytiotrophoblasts, proerythroblast, fibroblasts, cardiac mesenchymal cells	Complexes with TGF-β Rc I or Rc II to form Rc for TGF-β_1 and/or TGF-β_3. Plays role is the regulation of cell differentiation, migration, and possibly angiogenesis.
CD106	Vascular cell adhesion molecule-1 (VCAM-1); INCAM-110	100–110	I	1p31-p32 *VCAM1* 7412	act. endothelial cells, some MØ, FDC, marrow stroma, cardiac and skeletal myoblasts, some MØ, kidney, placenta, brain	Serves as a ligand for VLA-4 ($\alpha_4\beta_1$ integrin or CD49d/CD29) and $\alpha_4\beta_7$, which are involved in leukocyte adhesion, transmigration, and immune costimulation. Plays a role in the interactions of marrow stromal cells and HSCs.
CD107a	Lysosome-associated membrane protein-1 (LAMP-1)	120	I	13q34 *LAMP1* 3916	Lysosomal membrane gps of metabolically act. cells, act. plts, PMN, T cells, MØ, DC, endothelial cells, tonsillar epithelium	Ligand for galectin-3 that might play a role in bringing molecules into lysosomes for degradation. The carbohydrates attached to CD107 include sialylated Lewis^X, which can be recognized by lectins and selectins (e.g., CD62L, E, or P).
CD107b	Lysosome-associated membrane protein-2 (LAMP-2)	120	I	Xq24 *LAMP2* 3920	See CD107a	See CD107a above. Deficiency causes Danon disease.
CD108	Semaphorin 7A (SEMA7A); John-Milton-Hagen rbc blood group Ag; Selm L; GPI-gp80;	76 (80)	GPI	15q22.3-q23 *SEMA7A* 8482	RBC, act. lymphocytes, blood lymphocytes (weak)	A membrane-bound semaphorin that might play a role in induction of proinflammatory cytokines (e.g., IL-6, IL-8, TNF-α).

(continued)

TABLE 15–1. Cluster of Differentiation Antigens Defined as of the Eighth International Workshop on Leukocyte Typing (Continued)

Antigen	Other Names	Size	O	Genetics	Distribution	Physiology
CD109	Gov[a/b] alloantigen; 8A3; E123; 7D1	170	GPI	6q13 *CD109* 135228	Endothelium; plts; act. T cell; hematopoietic and mesenchymal stem cells	Member of the α_2-macroglobulin/C3; C4; C5 family of thioester-containing proteins.
CD110	Myeloproliferative leukemia virus oncogene (MPL); thrombopoietin Rc; TPO-R	85–92	I	1p34 *MPL* 4352	HSCs; megakaryocytes; plts	Rc for thrombopoietin that signals for megakaryocyte proliferation and differentiation or stem cell survival.
CD111	Poliovirus Rc-related 1 protein (PRR1); nectin-1; Hve C1; HIgR	75	I	11q23.3 *PVRL1* 5818	Myelomonocytic cells; megakaryocytes; plts; epithelial and neuronal cells	Binds itself and/or related nectin-2, -3, or -4, or the poliovirus Rc CD155 to facilitate homotypic and heterotypic adhesion. Also serves as an Rc for herpes simplex virus 1 and 2 and pseudorabies virus.
CD112	Poliovirus Rc-related 2 protein (PRR2); nectin-2; Hve B; PRR2	72; 64	I	19q13.2 *PVRL2* 5819	Hematopoietic; endothelial; epithelial; and neuronal cells	Binds itself and/or related nectin-1 and -3, or the poliovirus Rc CD155 to facilitate homotypic and heterotypic adhesion. Also serves as an Rc for herpes simplex virus 1 and pseudorabies virus.
CD113	Poliovirus Rc-like 3 (PVRL3); nectin-3	61	I	3q13 *PVRL3* 25945	Epithelial cells, placenta, testis, thyroid, brain (weak)	Binds itself and/or related nectin-1 and -2, or the poliovirus Rc CD155 to facilitate homotypic and heterotypic adhesion.
CD114	Granulocyte-colony stimulating factor Rc (CSF3R)	130–150	I	1p35-p34.3 *CSF3R* 1441	Monocytes; MØ; PMN and their precursors	Rc for G-CSF involved in regulating myeloid differentiation and proliferation.
CD115	Colony-stimulating factor-1 Rc (CSF1R); macrophage colony-stimulating factor Rc (M-CSFR); c-fms	150	I	5q33-q35 *CSF1R* 1436	Placenta; MØ; monocytes and their precursors; DC, osteoclasts, neurons, microglia, astrocytes.	Rc for M-CSF, which induces tyrosine phosphorylation of CD115, leading to the proliferation and differentiation of monocytes and their progenitors.
CD116	Colony-stimulating factor-2 Rc, α subunit (CSF2RA); granulocyte-macrophage colony-stimulating factor Rc α subunit	80	I	Xp22.32; Yp11.3; pseudo-autosomal *CSF2RA* 1438	Myeloid precursors; monocytes; PMN; endothelial cells; DC; fibroblasts	Low-affinity Rc for GM-CSF that forms high-affinity Rc for GM-CSF when complexed with CD131.
CD117	Rc for stem cell factor (SCFR); c-kit; steel factor Rc (SCR)	145	I	4q11-q12 *KIT* 3815	Hemopoietic progenitors; mast cells; melanocytes; spermatogonia; oocytes; some NK cells	Rc for stem-cell factor (SCF) that is required for normal hematopoiesis, reproduction, pigmentation, or gastrointestinal function.
CD118	Leukemia inhibitory factor Rc (LIFR)	190 (membrane form)	I	5p13-p12 *LIFR* 3977	Broad tissue expression except lymphocytes	Low-affinity Rc for leukemia inhibitory factor (LIF) that can form a high-affinity Rc for LIF when complexed with CD130.
CD119	IFN-gamma Rc (IFNγR, IFNGR1)	90–100	I	6q23.3 *IFNGR1* 3459	MØ; monocytes; T; B; and NK cells; PMN; epithelial cells; endothelium; fibroblasts	High-affinity Rc for IFN-γ, but cannot transduce a signal in transfected cell lines without IFN-γ accessory factor-1 (AF-1).
CD120a	Tumor necrosis factor Rc superfamily, member 1A (TNFRSF1A); TNF-α Rc of 55 kDa (TNFRp55); TNFRI	55	I	12p13.2 *TNFRSF1A* 7132	Many cell types—highest levels on epithelial cells; GC dendritic reticulum cells	High-affinity Rc for tumor necrosis factor-alpha (TNF-α) and tumor necrosis factor-beta (TNF-β), which can trigger recruitment of TRADD and RAIDD to induce caspase-dependent apoptosis. Defects in CD120a causes autosomal dominant familial *Hibernian fever*, which also is called TNF-Rc-associated periodic syndrome (TRAPS).

(*continued*)

TABLE 15–1. Cluster of Differentiation Antigens Defined as of the Eighth International Workshop on Leukocyte Typing (Continued)

Antigen	Other Names	Size	O	Genetics	Distribution	Physiology
CD120b	Tumor necrosis factor Rc superfamily, member 1B (TNFRSF1B); TNF-α Rc of 75 kDa (TNFRp75); TNFRII	75	I	1p36.3-p36.2 *TNFRSF1B* 7133	Highest on myeloid cells, but also on many other cell types	High-affinity Rc for tumor necrosis factor-alpha (TNF-α) and tumor necrosis factor-beta (TNF-β) or lymphotoxin α, which can induce activation of NF-κB.
CDw121a	IL-1 Rc type 1 (ILIR1); IL-1R	80	I	2q12 *IL1R1* 3554	T cells, thymocytes, chondrocytes, synovial cells, endothelial cells, fibroblasts, hepatocytes keratinocytes	Rc for interleukin-1 alpha (IL-1α) and interleukin-1 beta (IL-1β) that induces cellular activation and/or proliferation upon binding IL-1.
CDw121b	IL-1 Rc type 2 (ILIR2); IL-1R (type II)	60–68	I	2q12-q22 *IL1R2* 7850	B cells, monocytes, PMN, skin epithelial basal cells, ureter, female reproductive tract	Decoy Rc for IL-1α and IL-1β that may inhibit IL-1 effects by competing with CD120a for IL-1 binding. Soluble form acts as an antagonist.
CD122	IL-2 Rc β (IL2RB); p75; IL-2Rβ	70–75	I	22q13.1 *IL2RB* 3560	NK cells; act. T cells; B cells; monocytes	Complexes with CD132 to form intermediate-affinity Rc for IL-2 and IL-15 or with CD25 and CD132 to form high-affinity Rc for these cytokines.
CD123	IL-3 Rc α chain (IL3RA)	70	I	Xp22.3; Yp13.3 *IL3RA* 3563	Pluripotent stem cells and committed hemopoietic progenitor cells, mast cells, MØ, some B cells (weak)	Low-affinity Rc for IL-3 that can complex with CD131 to form a high-affinity Rc for IL-3 that, upon binding this cytokine, can stimulate cell proliferation and/or differentiation.
CD124	IL-4 Rc (IL4R)	140	I	16p12.1-p11.2 *IL4R* 3566	Mature B cells, T cells, epithelium, endothelium, hemopoietic precursors, fibroblasts	Complexes with CD132 to form a high-affinity Rc for IL-4, which can induce cellular differentiation and/or activation. Can complex with the IL-13 Rc α_1 chain to form a Rc for IL-4 and IL-13.
CD125	IL-5 Rc α chain (IL5RA)	60	I	3p26-p24 *IL5RA* 3568	eos., basophils, act. B cells, B1 B cells	Low-affinity Rc for IL-5 that can associate with CD131 to form a high-affinity IL-5 Rc that can stimulates proliferation and/or differentiation upon binding IL-5.
CD126	IL-6 Rc (IL6R)	80	I	1q21 *ILR6* 3570	Plasma cells (high), act. B (high), WBC (weak), epithelial cells fibroblasts, neural cells, hepatocytes	Associates with CD130 to form Rc for IL-6 that can stimulate cell growth and/or differentiation upon binding IL-6. Soluble CD126, generated by selected proteinases, can serve as antagonist to IL-6.
CD127	IL-7 Rc (IL7R); p90; IL-7Rα	80	I	5p13 *IL7R* *3575*	B-cell precursors; thymocytes; mature T cells; monocytes	Associates with CD132 to form high-affinity Rc for IL-7, which plays critical role in lymphoid development.
CD128A					See CD181.	
CD128B					See CD182.	
CD129	IL-9 Rc (IL9R)	64	I	Xq28; Yq12 *IL9R* 3581	act. T cells, B cells, eos., myeloid- and erythroid-progenitors, MØ, mast cells, epithelial cells, neurons	Associates with CD132 to form a Rc for IL-9 that stimulates cell growth and/or differentiation.
CD130	Interleukin-6 signal transducer (IL6ST); gp130; oncostatin-M Rc	130–140	I	5q11 *IL6ST* 3572	Most WBC, epithelial cells, fibroblasts, hepatocytes, neural cells	Common and signaling chain of heterodimeric Rc for oncostatin-M, IL-6, leukemia inhibitory factor, IL-11, ciliary neurotrophic factor, and cardiotrophin I.

(continued)

TABLE 15–1. Cluster of Differentiation Antigens Defined as of the Eighth International Workshop on Leukocyte Typing (Continued)

Antigen	Other Names	Size	O	Genetics	Distribution	Physiology
CD131	Colony-stimulating factor 2 Rc β (CSF2RB); common β-chain of Rc for IL-3, IL-5, or GM-CSF	120–140	I	22q13.1 *CSF2RB* 1439	Myeloid cells, pre-B cells, hematopoietic progenitor cells	Common chain of heterodimeric Rc for IL-3, IL-5, GM-CSF Rc.
CD132	Interleukin 2 Rc γ (IL2RG); Common γ chain of Rc for IL-2, IL-4, IL-7, IL-9, or IL-15	64–70	I	Xq13.1 *IL2RG* 3561	Thymocytes, most WBC, increased with activation	Common γ chain for three-chain Rc for IL-2, IL-4, IL-7, IL-9, or IL-15. Mutations in CD132 can cause X-linked severe combined immune deficiency (XSCID).
CD133	Prominin mouse-like I (PROML1); AC133	120	III	4p15.32 *PROM1* 8842	Hematopoietic tissues (esp. stem cells), epithelial cells, neural stem cells	Pentaspan membrane protein that can be used for positive selection of HSC.
CD134	Tumor necrosis factor Rc superfamily, member 4 (TNFRS4); OX40; Rc for OX40-ligand	48	I	1p36 *TNFRS4* 7293	Medullary thymocytes, act. T cells, fibroblasts hematopoietic progenitors	Member of TNF-Rc family that is the Rc for CD252. Ligation of CD134 inhibits apoptosis and can enhance cell activation.
CD135	Fms-related tyrosine kinase 3 (FLT3); flk-2; STK-1	130 (160)	I	13q12 *FLT3* 2322	HSC	CD135 is a type I tyrosine kinase that serves as Rc for FLT3-ligand.
CD136	MØ-stimulating 1 Rc (MST1R); Récepteur d'Origine Nantaise (RON)	180 (150/40)	I	3p21.3 *MST1R* 4486	Monocytes, granulocytes, epithelial cells, MØ	Heterodimeric two-chain Rc for macrophage-stimulating protein (MSP).
CD137	Tumor necrosis factor Rc superfamily, member 9 (TNFRS9); ILA (induced by lymphocyte act.); 4–1BB	83 (39)	I	1p36 *TNFRSF9* 3604	act. T cells, thymocytes, monocytes, FDC	Member of TNF-Rc family that is the Rc for 4–1BBL that can provide costimulatory signal for T-cell growth.
CD138	Syndecan-1 (SDC1); heparan sulfate proteoglycan; B-B4	100–250	I	2p24.1 *SDC1* 6382	Immature B cells, plasma cells, endothelial cells, mesenchymal cells, act. keratinocytes	CD138-heparan sulphate can serve as Rc for ECM proteins (e.g., fibronectin, collagen, thrombospondin, collagens, basic fibroblast growth factor) and play a role in cell adhesion.
CD139		209 (228)		*CD139* 23448	B cells, monocytes, FDC, PMN, endothelial cells	Unknown
CD140a	Platelet-derived growth factor Rc α chain (PDGFRA)	180	I	4q11–12 *PDGFRA* 5156	Erythroid and myeloid precursors, monocytes, megakaryocytes, plts, osteoblasts, glial cells	Forms a homodimeric Rc for PDGF-AA, PDGF-AB, PDGF-BB, and PDGF-CC, or a heterodimeric Rc with CD140b for PDGF-AB, PDGF-BB, and PDGF-CC.
CD140b	Platelet-derived growth factor Rc β chain (PDGFRB)	180	I	5q31-q32 *PDGFRB* 5159	Mesenchymal cells, monocytes, PMN, various cancers	Same as CD140a except that CD140b has preferential binding to RasGAP and less binding than CD140a to Crk.
CD141	Thrombomodulin (THBD); fetomodulin	105 (75)	I	20p11.2 *THBD* 7056	Endothelial cells, PMN, keratinocytes, smooth muscle, myeloid cells, plts, synovial lining, syncytiotrophoblasts	CD141 binds thrombin, inhibiting its fibrinolytic activity and allowing it to activate protein C, which degrades factors Va and VIIIa and reduces the amount of thrombin generated.
CD142	Coagulation factor III (F3); tissue factor; thromboplastin	42–47	I	1p22-p21 *F3* 2152	Keratinocytes, epithelia, adventitia, mesenchymal stromal cells, Schwann cells, act. monocytes, blood-vessel adventitia, astrocytes, myocardium	High-affinity Rc for factor VII (FVII), which when bound to CD142 is converted to FVIIa by serine proteases. Factor Xa/TFPI can bind and inhibit the activity of the CD142/FVIIa complex.

(continued)

TABLE 15–1. Cluster of Differentiation Antigens Defined as of the Eighth International Workshop on Leukocyte Typing (Continued)

Antigen	Other Names	Size	O	Genetics	Distribution	Physiology
CD143	Angiotensin-converting enzyme (ACE); peptidyl dipeptidase A	170	I	17q23.3 *ACE* 1636	Endothelial cells, proximal renal tubules, neuronal cells, mesenchymal tissues, some T cells, germinal cells, epididymis, act. MØ	Metallopeptidase that can metabolize angiotensin or bradykinin and cleave the C-terminal dipeptide from substance P, LH-RH, and other dipeptides. Plays role in sperm binding and penetration of ovocytes.
CD144	Cadherin 5 (CDH5); VE-cadherin	135 (130)	I	16q22.1 *CDH5* 1003	Endothelium	Ca^{+2}+-dependent homotypic cell adhesion molecule that plays a role in contact inhibition.
CDw145		110; 90; 25		*None assigned*	Endothelium, stromal cells	Unknown.
CD146	Melanoma cell adhesion molecule (MCAM); Muc 18; S-ENDO; Mel-CAM; A32	118 (130)	I	11q23.3 *MCAM* 4162	Endothelium, sm. muscle, some act. T cells, FDC, myofibroblasts, ganglion cells, cerebellar cortex, some epithelial cells, extravillous trophoblast	Potential cell-adhesion molecule, esp. of neural crest cells during development.
CD147	BSG basigin (BSG); M6; Extracellular matrix metalloproteinase inducer (EMMPRIN)	54 (65)	I	19p13.3 *BSG* 682	Many types of nonhematopoietic cells, act. lymphocytes, monocytes, resting WBC (weak)	Binds to integrins and may facilitate cell adhesion and activation. Plays a role in odor perception, immune function, and memory development.
CD148	Protein tyrosine phosphates, Rc type, J (PTPRJ); HTPT-η; p260; Density-enhanced phosphotyrosine phosphatase-1 (DEP-1)	200–250	I	11p11.2 *PTPRJ* 5795	Monocytes, PMN, DC, plts, nerve cells, Kupffer cells, fibroblasts, act. lymphocytes	Phosphotyrosine phosphatase activated on contact between cells that may play role in contact inhibition, lymphocyte signal transduction, or T-cell activation.
CDw149	CD47R; MEM-133			see CD47	Blood lymphocytes, weakly on plts, PMN, monocytes	mAbs that defined this specificity actually recognize CD47 with low affinity on a subset of CD47-positive cells (see CD47).
CD150	Signaling lymphocyte act. molecule family member 1 (SLAMF1); SLAM	65–80 (70–95)	I	1q22-q23 *SLAMF1* 6504	Thymocytes, resting CD45RO+ T cells, some B, act. lymphocytes, DC	Binds itself to play role in homotypic cell adhesion and activation. Also, can serve as an Rc for measles virus.
CD151	Platelet-endothelial tetraspan Ag-3 (PETA-3); Tspan-24; SFA-1	28–32	III Tet.	11p15.5 *CD151* 977	plts, megakaryocytes, monocytes, epithelial and endothelial cells, muscle	Associates with β_1 (CD29) integrins and may play a role in homotypic adhesion.
CD152	Cytotoxic T lymphocyte Ag-4 (CTLA-4)	50 (33)	I	2q33 *CTLA4* 1493	act. T cells, CD4+CD25+ T_{reg} cells	High-affinity ligand for CD80 and CD86 that negatively regulates T-cell activation.
CD153	CD30-ligand; TNFSF8	40	II	9q33 *TNFSF8* 944	act. T cells, act. MØ, granulocytes, B cells, some myeloid progenitors (weak)	High-affinity ligand for CD30, which can enhance Ag-induced proliferation and cytokine production.
CD154	CD40-ligand (CD40LG); gp39; TNF-related activation protein (TRAP); TNFSF5	39	II	Xq26 *CD40LG* 959	act. $CD4^+$ T cells, few act. $CD8^+$ T cells, act. plts	Ligand for CD40 that induces activation, proliferation, and/or differentiation of CD40-expressing cells and plays important role in immune activation.
CD155	Poliovirus Rc (PVR), nectin-like 5	80–90	I	19q13.2 *PVR* 5817	Monocytes, endothelial cells, epithelial cells, neuronal cells	Can complex with CD113 to bind $\alpha_v\beta_3$ integrin or bind vitronectin, CD56 and/or CD226 to nectin-1 and/or -2 to play role in homotypic adhesion. Also can bind CMV and serve as Rc for poliovirus.

(continued)

TABLE 15–1. Cluster of Differentiation Antigens Defined as of the Eighth International Workshop on Leukocyte Typing (Continued)

Antigen	Other Names	Size	O	Genetics	Distribution	Physiology
CD156a	A disintegrin and metalloprotease 8 (ADAM8); MS2	69	I	10q26.3 *ADAM8* 101	Monocytes, PMN	A disintegrin and metalloprotease (ADAM) that may be involved in leukocyte extravasation and neurodegeneration.
CD156b	A disintegrin and metalloprotease 17 (ADAM17); TNF-α converting enzyme (TACE)	100	I	2p25 *ADAM17* 6868	Monocytes, MØ, PMN, T cells, myocytes, endothelial cells	A disintegrin and metalloprotease (ADAM) that can cleave membrane-bound TNF-α and TGF-α into a soluble cytokine.
CD156c	A disintegrin and metalloprotease 10 (ADAM10)	65 (70)	I	15q22 *ADAM10* 102	Broad range of expression with high levels in thymus, liver, and muscle	An endopeptidase that can cleave and thereby release membrane proteins (e.g., TNF-α or Ephrin A_2).
CD157	Bone marrow stromal cell Ag 1 (BST-1); BP-3/IF7; cADPr hydrolase 2; Mo5	42–45	GPI	4p15 *BST1* 683	Monocytes, PMN, MØ, marrow stroma, FDC, synovial cells, endothelial cells	ADP-ribosyl cyclase and cADP-ribose hydrolase, which use NAD and cyclic ADP-ribose as substrates.
CD158a-z	Killer-inhibitory Rc (KIR) family. Individual proteins are designated: CD158a, CD158b, CD158c, CD158d, CD158E1, CD158f, CD158g, CD158h, CD158i, CD158j, CD158k, or CD158z	50–70	I	19q13.4 a: *KIR2DL1* b: *KIR2DL2/L3* c: *KIR2DS6* d: *KIR2DL4* e: *KIR3DL1* f: *KIR2DL5A* g: *KIR2DS5* h: *KIR2DS1* i: *KIR2DS4* j: *KIR2DS2* k: *KIR3DL2* z: *KIR3DL7*	NK cells, some T cells (see Chap. 79)	The KIR family of polymorphic proteins is comprised of at least 15 members. Each is named based on the number of extracellular Ig-like domains (KIR2D or KIR3D) and for whether the protein has a long (L) or short (S) cytoplasmic domain or is secreted (P). Many KIR bind polymorphic epitopes on HLA class I molecules. When bound, L-type KIR have cytoplasmic ITIMs and are inhibitory, whereas S-type KIR may facilitate cell activation.
CD159a	Killer-cell Ig-like Rc, 2 domains, long cytoplasmic tail 1 (KIR2DL1, KLRC1); NKAT; NKG2A	43	I	19q13.4 *KIR2DL1* 3802	NK cells, some T cells	Covalently associates with CD94 to form Rc for HLA class I molecules that has cytoplasmic ITIMs and can inhibit NK-cell mediated cytotoxicity.
CD159c	Killer cell lectin-like Rc subfamily C, member 2 (KLRC2); NKG2C	36	II	12p13 *KLRC2* 3822	NK cells, few T cells	Covalently associates with CD94 to for Rc for HLA class I molecules that can inhibit NK cell-mediated cytotoxicity.
CD160	BY55; NK1; NK28	27 (80)	GPI	1q21.1 *CD160* 11126	γ/δ T cells, CD8 T cells, $CD56^{dim}$CD16+ NK cells, intestinal intraepithelial lymphocytes	Ligand for classical and nonclassical HLA class I molecules that serves as costimulatory molecules for cytotoxic effector cells.
CD161	Killer cell lectin-like Rc subfamily B1 (KLRB1); NKR-P1A	40–44	II	12p13 *KLRB1* 3820	NK cells, some T cells (weak)	Ligand for polymorphic determinants on HLA class I.
CD162	Selectin P ligand (SELPLG); P-selectin glycoprotein ligand 1 (PSGL-1)	250 (120)	I	12q24 *SELPLG* 6404	PMN, monocytes, most T cells, some B cells	Binds to CD62P, CD62E, and CD62L, and helps facilitate leukocyte rolling and extravasation.
CD162R	CD162 with PEN5 epitope	250 (120)	I	12q24 *SELPLG* 6404	$CD56^{dim}$CD16+NK cells, oligodendrocyte precursors	Posttranslational modification of CD162 that adds the PEN5 epitope, allowing it to better bind CD62L.

(continued)

TABLE 15–1. Cluster of Differentiation Antigens Defined as of the Eighth International Workshop on Leukocyte Typing (Continued)

Antigen	Other Names	Size	O	Genetics	Distribution	Physiology
CD163	M130 Ag; GHI/61; Ki-M8; SM4; D11; Ber-Mac3; RM3/1	110 (130)	I	12p13.3 *CD163* 9332	Monocytes, most MØ	Scavenger Rc group B family member that may play a role in the regulation of the immune response in inflammatory processes.
CD164	Multiglycosylated core protein 24 (MGC-24); sialomucin	160 (80)	I	6q21 *CD164* 8763	Epithelial cells, monocytes, marrow stroma, many embryonic tissues, HSC	Mucin-like molecule that may mediate adhesion between marrow stroma and hemopoietic progenitors and may also be involved in negatively regulating growth of CD34+ hematopoietic progenitors.
CD165	AD2; gp37; SN2	37 (42)	N/A	– *CD165* 23449	plts, thymocytes, T (weak), NK cells (weak), some monocytes,	May play a role in intercellular adhesion between thymocytes and thymic epithelial cells.
CD166	Activated leukocyte cell adhesion molecule (ALCAM)	100–105	I	3q13.1 *ALCAM* 214	Thymic epithelial cells, act. T cells, CD34+ marrow cells, endothelial cells	Can bind itself or CD6 to play role in homotypic or heterotypic cell adhesion.
CD167a	Discoidin domain Rc tyrosine kinase 1 (DDR1); Tyrosine kinase Rc E (TRKE); cell adhesion kinase (CAK)	125	I	6p21.3 *DDR1* 780	Epithelial cells, B cells (weak)	Binds all types of collagen (types I–VI and VIII) to help determine cell morphology and tissue infiltration.
CD167b	Discoidin domain Rc tyrosine kinase 2 (DDR2)	130	I	1q23.3 *DDR2* 4921	Widely expressed, but highest in skin, kidney, cardiac or skeletal muscle	Binds fibrillar collagens (types I–III and V) and plays role in induction of MMP-1 and -2.
CD168	Hyaluronan-mediated motility Rc (HMMR); IHABP; RHAMM	88, 84, 88	I	5q33.2-qter *HMMR* 3161	Subset of thymocytes, act. T and B cells, monocytes, G-CSF mobilized blood cells	Rc for hyaluronan (HA) involved in HA-directed cell motility. Also interacts with the mitotic spindle to play role in the cell cycle.
CD169	Sialic acid-binding Ig-like lectin 1 (SIGLEC1); sialoadhesin (Sn)	180 (200)	I	20p13 *SIGLEC1* 6614	Stromal MØ, particularly those in spleen, lymph nodes, and marrow	A sialoadhesin that binds sialylated ligands (e.g., MUC-1), esp. sialic acid in the $\alpha_{2,3}$-glycosidic linkage on *N*- and *O*-glycans, thereby enhancing cell–cell adhesion.
CD170	Sialic acid-binding Ig-like lectin 5 (SIGLEC5); OBBP2; CD33L2	140 (70)	I	19q13.3 *SIGLEC5* 8778	PMN, act. MØ	Binds $\alpha_{2,3}$- and $\alpha_{2,6}$-like sialic acid and glycophorin A on rbc to downregulate cell activation.
CD171	L1 cell adhesion molecule (L1CAM); neuronal adhesion molecule	200–230	I	Xq28 *L1CAM* 3897	Neurons, Schwann cells, CD4 T cells (weak), some B cells, monocytes, FDC, epithelia	Binds itself or neurocan, chondroitin-sulfate-containing proteoglycans, laminin, or integrins $\alpha_V\beta_3$, $\alpha_{II}b\beta_3$, $\alpha_5\beta_1$, or $\alpha_9\beta_1$, to facilitate homotypic or heterotypic adhesion. Also can serve as a T-cell costimulatory molecule.
CD172a	Signal regulatory protein α (SIRPα); SHPS-1	85–90	I	20p13 *SIRPA* 140885	Monocytes, MØ, HSC, neuronal tissue	Can bind CD47 and lung surfactant proteins SP-A and SP-D. With cytoplasmic ITIMs it can serve as inhibitory Rc to suppress various cell functions (e.g., anchorage-independent cell growth).
CD172b	Signal regulatory protein β_1 (SIRPβ_1)	110–120	I	20p13 *SIRB1* 10326	Myeloid cells	Can associate with DAP-12 homodimers to play a role in cell activation.
CD172g	Signal regulatory protein γ (SIRPγ); SIRPβ_2	55	I	20p13 *SIRPG* 55423	Most T cells, some B cells	Can bind CD47 with lower affinity than CD172a and may play a role in intercellular T-cell signaling.

(*continued*)

TABLE 15–1. Cluster of Differentiation Antigens Defined as of the Eighth International Workshop on Leukocyte Typing (Continued)

Antigen	Other Names	Size	O	Genetics	Distribution	Physiology
CD173	Blood group H type 2; Galβ_1→ 4GlcNAc β-R			Carbohydrate Ag	Hematopoietic progenitors, endothelial cells, rbc, some basal epithelial cells	Carbohydrate specificity that is generated by the activity of β-D-galactoside2-L-fucosyl transferase (FUT1) that may play role in cell adhesion.
CD174	Fucosyltransferase 3 (FUT3); Lewis^Y; Le^Y			19p13.3 *FUT3* 2525	Epithelial cells and HSC	A difucosylated tetrasaccharide found on type 2 blood group oligosaccharides on glycolipids or glycoproteins formed by $\alpha_{1,2}$- and $\alpha_{1,3}$-fucosyltransferase (FUT3)
CD175	Tn Ag (T-Ag novelle)			Carbohydrate Ag	Hematopoietic cells and a variety of carcinoma cell lines	Carbohydrate specificity consisting of a monosaccharide attached in an *O*-linked fashion that serves as the precursor for ABO Ag and CD176.
CD175s	Sialyl-Tn			Carbohydrate Ag	Hematopoietic cells esp. in CFU-E to erythroblasts	Carbohydrate specificity that is dependent upon sialyltransferase ST6GalNAcI implicated in tumor-cell invasiveness.
CD176	Thomsen-Friedenreich (TF) Ag; pan-CA Ag; Galβ_1→3Gal NAc α_1-R			Carbohydrate Ag	Epithelium, hematopoietic cells, variety of carcinoma and leukemia cell lines	A disaccharide, Galβ_1-$_3$GalNAcα_1, attached to various protein carriers via *O*-glycosyl linkage that binds to asialoglycoprotein Rc on hepatocytes and is implicated in tumor-cell invasiveness.
CD177	Polycythemia vera rubra 1 (PRV1); NB1; HNA-2a	49–55 (56–64)	GPI	19q13.2 *PRV1* 57126	Most PMN and some myeloid precursors, overexpressed in polycythemia vera	Unknown function, but can be the target of alloantibodies in patients who are CD177-negative, resulting in severe acute lung injury after transfusion from CD177+ donor.
CD178	Fas ligand (FASLG); APO-1; TNFSF6	40	II	1q23 *FASLG* 356	act. T cells, act. NK, PMN, eye parenchyma, astrocytes, placenta	Ligand for CD95 that can induce caspase-dependent apoptosis of cells bearing CD95.
CD179a	VpreB; prelymphocyte gene 1 (VPREB1); Ig iota (ι) chain (IGVPB)	16–18	–	22q11.22 *VPREB1* 7441	Pro-B and pre-B cells	Associates noncovalently with CD179b to form an Ig light-chain–like structure on developing pro-B and pre-B cells to play a critical role in B-cell development.
CD179b	Ig lambda (λ)-like polypeptide 1 (IGLL1); Ig lambda5; Ig omega chain	22	–	22q11.23 *IGLL1* 3543	Pro-B and early pre-B cells	Associates noncovalently with CD179a to form an Ig light-chain–like structure on developing pro-B and pre-B cells to play a critical role in B-cell development.
CD180	RP105; LY64; Bgp95	95–105	I	5q12 *CD180* 4064	Mantle zone and marginal zone B cells, monocytes, DC	A toll-like Rc that, upon ligation with LPS, induces activation that leads to upregulation of CD80 and CD86 and increase in cell size.
CD181	IL-8 Rc α (IL-8RA) ; formerly CD128a; CXCR1	58–67	III Hep.	2q35 *IL8RA* 3577	PMN, basophils, monocytes (weak), keratinocytes, some T cells, NK cells (weak)	A G-protein-coupled CXC-chemokine Rc for IL-8 that induces chemotaxis and/or cell activation upon binding IL-8.
CD182	IL-8 Rc β (IL-8RB); CXCR2; formerly CDw128B	58–67	III Hep.	2q35 *IL8RB* 3579	PMN, basophils, monocytes (weak), NK cells (weak), various epithelia, some neurons	A G-protein-coupled CXC-chemokine Rc for IL-8, GRO α, β, γ, and NAP-2 that induces chemotaxis and/or cell activation.
CD183	Chemokine (C-X-C-motif) Rc 3 (CXCR3); G-protein-coupled Rc 9 (GPR9); CXC-L2; IP10-R; Mig-R	41	III Hep.	Xq13 *CXCR3* 2833	act. T cells, act. NK cells, transformed B cells, plasmacytoid DC	G-protein-coupled CXC-chemokine Rc for IP10 (INF-γ-inducible 10-kDa protein), Mig (monokine induced by IFN- γ), and I-TAC (IFN-inducible T-cell α-chemoattractant).
CD184	Chemokine (C-X-C-motif) Rc 4 (CXCR4); fusin; LESTR; NPY3R; HM89; FB22; LCR1; HUMSTR	40	III Hep.	2q21 *CXCR4* 7852	B and T cells, monocytes, MØ, DC, PMN, endothelial and epithelial cells, astrocytes	G-protein-coupled CXC-chemokine Rc for CXCL12 (stromal-derived factor-1α [SDF-1α]) and co-Rc for HIV (see Chap. 83).

(continued)

TABLE 15–1. Cluster of Differentiation Antigens Defined as of the Eighth International Workshop on Leukocyte Typing (Continued)

Antigen	Other Names	Size	O	Genetics	Distribution	Physiology
CD185	Chemokine (C-X-C-motif) Rc 5 (CXCR5); Burkitt lymphoma Rc 1 (BLR1)	52	III Hep.	11q23.3 *CXCR5* 643	B cells, monocytes, Burkitt lymphoma cells (strong)	G-protein-coupled CXC-chemokine Rc for CXCL13.
CD186	Chemokine (C-X-C-motif) Rc 6 (CXCR6); BONZO; STRL33; TYM-STR	39	III Hep.	3p21 *CXCR6* 10663	Activated T cells	G-protein-coupled CXC-chemokine Rc for CXCL16 and co-Rc for HIV-1, HIV-2, and SIV (see Chap. 83).
CD191	Chemokine (C-C motif) Rc 1 (CCR1); CC-CKR-1	41	III Hep.	3p21 *CCR1* 1230	Low levels in most tissues, T cells	G-protein-coupled CC-chemokine Rc for MIP-1α, RANTES, MCP-3, and MPIF-1.
CD192	Chemokine (C-C motif) Rc 2 (CCR2); MCP-1-R; CKR2	42	III Hep.	3p21.31 *CCR2* 729230	Monocytes, act. T and B cells	G-protein-coupled CC-chemokine Rc for MCP-1 and co-Rc for HIV (see Chap. 83).
CD193	Chemokine (C-C motif) Rc 3 (CCR3); CKR3; eosinophil eotaxin Rc	41	III Hep.	3p21.31 *CCR3* 1232	eos., basophils, epithelial cells, some T (Th2) cells	G-protein-coupled CC-chemokine Rc for CCL11, MCP-4, RANTES, and MCP-3.
CD194	Chemokine (C-C motif) Rc 4 (CCR4); CKR4; K5-5	41	III Hep.	3p24 *CCR4* 1233	CD4+CD25+ T_{reg} and CLA+ T cells, IL-2-act. NK cells, MØ, basophils	G-protein-coupled CC-chemokine Rc for MIP-1, RANTES, TARC and MCP-1.
CD195	Chemokine (C-C motif) Rc 5 (CCR5); CKR5	37	III Hep.	3q21.31 *CXCR5* 1234	T cells, MØ, monocytes, endothelial/epithelial cells, some neurons, astrocytes	G-protein-coupled CC-chemokine Rc for MCP-2, MIP-1α, MIP-1β, and RANTES, that also may play a role in cell proliferation/differentiation and co-Rc for HIV (see Chap. 83).
CD196	Chemokine (C-C motif) Rc 6 (CCR6); CKR6; LARC Rc	42	III Hep.	6q27 *CCR6* 1235	Memory T cells, immature DC, some B cells	G-protein-coupled CC-chemokine Rc for CCL20 or LARC.
CD197	Chemokine (C-C motif) Rc 7 (CCR7); BLR2; EBI1	40	III Hep.	17q12-q21.2 *CCR7* 1236	Lymphocytes, thymus, blood-derived DC, MØ, monocytes,	G-protein-coupled CC-chemokine Rc for CCL19 (ECL), MIP-3β, or CCL21 (SLC) that is upregulated by infection with Epstein-Barr virus
CDw198	Chemokine (C-C motif) Rc 8 (CCR8); CKRL1	41	III Hep.	3p22 *CCR8* 1237	Thymus, NK cells, monocytes, monocyte-derived DC	G-protein-coupled CC-chemokine Rc for SCYA1/I-309 and minor co-Rc for HIV (see Chap. 83).
CDw199	Chemokine (C-C motif) Rc 9 (CCR9)	42	III Hep.	3p21.3 *CCR9* 10803	Thymus, weak in marrow or spleen	G-protein-coupled CC-chemokine Rc for SCYA25 (TECK) and minor co-Rc for HIV (see Chap. 83).
CD200	OX2; MRC	33	I	3q12-q13 *CD200* 4345	Thymocytes, B cells, act. T cells, FDC, neurons, endothelium, kidney glomeruli, smooth muscle	Binds the OX2 Rc found on MØ, PMN, monocytes, DC, and microglia, causing downregulation of cell activation.
CD201	Protein C Rc (PROCR); endothelial protein C Rc (EPCR)	50	I	20q11,2 *PROCR* 10544	Endothelium of large vessels; trophoblast cells at fetal–maternal boundary	Binds to protein C to enhance its thrombin-thrombomodulin-mediated activation on endothelial surfaces. Soluble CD201 in plasma can inhibit anticoagulant activity of protein C. Also complexes with proteinase 3 and phospholipids(s) to form Rc for Mac-1 on act. PMN that reduces endothelial adhesion.

(continued)

TABLE 15–1. Cluster of Differentiation Antigens Defined as of the Eighth International Workshop on Leukocyte Typing (Continued)

Antigen	Other Names	Size	O	Genetics	Distribution	Physiology
CD202b	Tunica internal endothelia cell kinase (TEK); tyrosine kinase with Ig and EGF homology domains (TIE2)	145	I	9p21 *TEK* 7010	Endothelial cells, angioblasts, subset of HSC	Rc for angiopoietins 1, 2, and 4 that are involved in angiogenesis. Also may play a role in maintaining viability of HSC.
CD203c	Ectonucleotide pyrophosphatase/phosphodiesterase 3 (ENPP3); B10; PDNP3	270 (130, 150)	II	6q22 *ENPP3* 5169	Basophils, mast cells, uterus, pancreas, intestine, liver, immature glial cells, hematopoietic progenitor cells	An ectoenzyme that catalyzes the hydrolysis of extracellular nucleotides (e.g., nucleoside phosphates, NAD, and oligonucleotides).
CD204	MØ scavenger Rc 1 (MSR1), SR-A	220	I	8q22 *MSR1* 4481	Tissue MØ	Rc for acetylated and oxidized low-density lipoprotein and glycated collagen type IV, and may function in the recognition of pathogenic microorganisms.
CD205	Lymphocyte Ag 75 (LY75); DEC-205; gp200-MR6	205	I	2q24 *LY75* 4065	Tingible body MØ, interdigitating and blood-derived DC, thymic epithelium	Recycled endocytic Rc that helps direct extracellular Ag into endosomes for presentation by HLA class I proteins.
CD206	Mannose Rc, C type 1 (MRC1); mannose Rc, C-type lectin	162–175	I	10p12.33 *MRC1* 4360	Some mononuclear phagocytes, endothelial cells, immature DC, retinal epithelium, mesangial cells	Rc involved in phagocytosis and endocytosis of particles containing lysosomal hydrolases, glycans, sulphated sugars, etc. (e.g., microbial pathogens).
CD207	Langerin; CLEC4K	40	II	2p13 *CD207* 50489	Langerhans DC (particularly immature DC)	Binds mannose-bearing gps and glycolipids found on microbial pathogens, including gp120 of HIV.
CD208	Lysosomal-associated protein 3 (LAMP3)	70–79	I	3q26.3-q27 *LAMP3* 27074	DC and CD40-activated B cells, testis (weak)	May play a role in processing exogenous Ag for presentation by HLA class II molecules.
CD209	DC-Specific ICAM-3 grabbing nonintegrin (DC-SIGN)	44	II	19p13 *CD209* 30835	Immature monocyte-derived DC, placental MØ	High-affinity Rc for CD50 (ICAM-1) and CD102 (ICAM-2) that may facilitate DC-induced T-cell activation and DC-transendothelial migration. It also can act as a Rc for many different pathogens.
CDw210a	IL-10 Rc α (IL10RA); IL-10R1	90–110	I	11q23 *IL10RA* 3587	Hematopoietic cells, lymphocytes, monocytes, MØ	High-affinity Rc for IL-10 that forms signaling complex with CDw210b
CDw210b	IL-10 Rc β (IL10RB); IL-10R2	90–110	I	21q22 *IL10RB* 3588	hematopoietic cells, lymphocytes, monocytes, MØ	Does not bind IL-10 by itself, but forms complex with CDw210a to allow for IL-10–induced tyrosine phosphorylation of JAK1 and TYK2 kinases. Also has a high-affinity Rc for IL-22 and possibly IL-26, IL-28A and B, and IL-29.
CD212	IL-12 Rc β_1 (IL12RB1)	85	I	19p13.1 *IL12RB1* 3594	act. T cells, NK cells, and some monocytes	Rc for IL-12 that forms high-affinity IL-12 Rc when complexed with the IL-12 Rc β_2 chain.
CD213α1	IL-13 Rc α_1 (IL13RA1)	65	I	Xq24 *IL13RA1* 3597	Most hematopoietic cells, heart, liver, ovary, CNS	Low-affinity Rc for IL-13 that forms high-affinity IL-13 when complexed with CD124 to mediate signaling via JAK1, STAT3, and STAT6.
CD213α2	IL-13 Rc α_2 (IL13RA2)	50	I	Xq13.1-q28 *IL13RA2* 3598	Cord-blood lymphocytes, immature DC, some blood lymphocytes	High-affinity Rc for IL-13 that lacks a cytoplasmic domain, but with CD213α_1 can play a role in binding and internalization of IL-13.

(continued)

TABLE 15–1. Cluster of Differentiation Antigens Defined as of the Eighth International Workshop on Leukocyte Typing (Continued)

Antigen	Other Names	Size	O	Genetics	Distribution	Physiology
CD217	IL-17 Rc A (IL17RA)	128–158	I	22q11.1 *IL17RA* 23765	Thymocytes, leukocytes, fibroblast-like synoviocytes	Low-affinity Rc for IL-17.
CD218a	IL-18 Rc 1 (IL18R1); IL-1RRP	68	I	2q12 *IL18R1* 8809	Throughout the immune system, lung, heart, liver gut	Together with CD218b forms a Rc for IL-18 that can activate NF-κB.
CD218b	IL-18 Rc accessory protein (IL18RAP)	68	I	2q12 *IL18RAP* 8807	Act. T cells (more selective distribution than CD218a), lung, heart, liver gut	Together with CD218a forms a Rc for IL-18 that can activate NF-κB.
CD220	Insulin Rc (INSR)	400 (135/ 95)	I	1q21-q23 *INSR* 3645	Widely expressed on many tissues	Rc for insulin and insulin-like growth factor-2 (IGF-2), which induces glucose uptake.
CD221	Insulin-like growth factor 1 Rc (IGF1R)	135/ 90	I	15q26.3 *IGF1R* 3480	Widely expressed on many tissues and overexpressed in many cancers	Rc for insulin and insulin-like growth factors 1 and 2 (IGF-1 and IGF-2), which can induce mitogenic signaling.
CD222	Insulin-like growth factor type-2 Rc (IGF2R); manose-6-phosphate Rc (MPR1)	250 (300)	I	6q26 *IGF2R* 3482	Ubiquitous	Can bind and internalize a variety of different ligands into lysosomes and complex with CD87 and plasminogen to regulate the activity of TGF-β, serve as Rc for IGF-2, or bind *Chlamydia pneumoniae* to facilitate infection.
CD223	Lymphocyte-activation Protein (LAG-3)	70	I	12p13.32 *LAG3* 3902	NK, act. T cells	Can bind HLA class II proteins and serve as a costimulatory/adhesion molecule in Ag presentation.
CD224	γ-Glutamyl transferase 1 (GGT); EC2.3.2.2	100 (55–60 / 21–30)	II	22q11.23 *GGT1* 2678	Renal tubular cells, pancreas, epididymis, vascular endothelium, alveolar epithelial cells, some B cells, MØ	A two-chain ectoenzyme involved in the degradation and neosynthesis of glutathione and conversion of leukotriene C_4 to leukotriene D_4. It also can convert nitric oxide donor, GSNO, to s-nitrocysteinylglycine, providing nitric oxide to the cell.
CD225	IFN-induced transmembrane protein 1 (IFIM1)	17	I	11p15.5 *IFITM1* 8519	B and T cells, NK cells, vascular endothelial cells	Complexes with CD21, CD19, and CD81 on B cells to regulate cell activation, but complexes with CD81 on other cell types.
CD226	Platelet and T cell activation Ag 1 (PTA1); TLiSA1; DNAM-1	65	I	18q22.3 *CD226* 10666	act. NK cells, plts, monocytes, and some T cells and thymocytes	Associates with LFA-1 and actin-binding protein 4.1G to form Rc for CD112 and CD155, facilitating cell activation and/or adhesion.
CD227	Mucin 1 (MUC1); episialin; peanut-reactive urinary protein (PUN); DF3; H23; polymorphic epithelial mucin (PEM)	220–700 (25)	I	1q21 *MUC1* 4582	Apical surface of all glandular epithelial cells, act. T cells, monocytes, some B cells, FDC, some hematopoietic cells	A transmembrane epithelial mucin that can bind various other proteins (e.g., CD54, selectins, CD169, Grb2, β-catenin, GSK-3β) that can hinder intercellular interactions and help lubricate the cell-surface membrane.
CD228	Melanotransferrin, p97	80–90	GPI	3q28-q29 *MF12* 4241	Melanomas, myoepithelial cells, liver parenchyma, brain capillary endothelium	Structurally related to transferrin, CD228 may help sequester iron at the cell surface membrane.
CD229	Lymphocyte Ag 9 (LY9)	120	I	1q21.3-q22 *LY9* 4063	Mature T and B cells	Interacts with itself to facilitate homotypic intercellular adhesion.

(*continued*)

TABLE 15–1. Cluster of Differentiation Antigens Defined as of the Eighth International Workshop on Leukocyte Typing (Continued)

Antigen	Other Names	Size	O	Genetics	Distribution	Physiology
CD230	Prion protein (PRNP); PrPc	30–40	GPI	20p13 *PRNP* 5621	widely expressed on most cell types, esp. on neurons	Sialoglycoprotein that facilitates homotypic adhesion and that can undergo a conformational change to form a protease-resistant aggregate in prion disease.
CD231	Tetraspan 7 (TSPAN7); TALLA-1; SN1; SN1a; TM4SF2	150 (32–45)	III Tet.	Xq11.4 *TSPAN7* 7102	Neurons, neuroblastoma, and T-cell ALL	Tetraspan protein used as marker for T-cell ALL.
CD232	Plexin C1 (PLXNC1); Virus-encoded semaphorin protein Rc (VESP R)	200	I	12q23.3 *PLXNC1* 10154	Monocytes, some DC, some B cells, neuronal cells	Rc semaphoring 7A that also can bind a virus encoded semaphorin, A39R, which can inhibit integrin-mediated adhesion and migration.
CD233	Solute carrier family 4, anion exchanger, member 1 (SLC4A1); band 3; Diego blood group; EPB3; anion exchanger 1 (AE1)	95–110	III	17q21-q22 *SLC4A1* 6521	RBC, a truncated form is expressed in the renal distal tubules	CD233 functions as a bicarbonate transporter/anion exchanger and as an attachment site for the rbc cytoskeleton. Mutations in CD233 can result in hereditary spherocytosis, renal tubular acidosis, or novel rbc Ags (e.g., Diego blood group).
CD234	Fu-glycoprotein; Duffy blood group chemokine Rc (DARC)	36	III Hep.	1q21-q22 *DARC* 2532	RBC, postcapillary venules, high-endothelial venules, endothelium of spleen and marrow, Purkinje cells, renal collecting ducts, lung alveoli, thyroid	Rc for CC chemokines (RANTES, MCP-1) and CXC chemokines (IL-8, MSGA) to modulate the level(s) of these proinflammatory molecules. Also can serve as Rc for *Plasmodium vivax* and *Plasmodium knowlesi* to facilitate infection.
CD235a	Glycophorin A (GYPA); PAS-2; sialoglycoprotein A, MN sialoglycoprotein	66 (28–31)	I	4q28.2-q31.1 *GYPA* 2993	RBC, all erythroid cells, HSC	A major sialoglycoprotein that bears the antigenic determinants of the MN blood group. It can bind CD170, influenza, and *Plasmodium falciparum*.
CD235b	Glycophorin B (GYPB); PAS-3, sialoglycoprotein δ, ss-active sialoglycoprotein	20	I	4q28.2-q31 *GYPB* 2994	rbc	A major sialoglycoprotein that bears the antigenic determinants of the S/s blood group.
CD236	Glycophorin C/D (GYPC/D); Gerbich blood group Ag; Webb and Duch Ag	30	I	2q14-q21 *GYPC* 2995	rbc	The Gerbich and Yus phenotypes are a result of deletion of exon 3 and 2 of *GYPC*, respectively. The Webb and Duch antigens, also known as glycophorin D, result from single point mutations of the glycophorin C gene, *GYPC* (see CD236R).
CD236R	Glycophorin C (GYPC)	40	I	2q14-q21 *GYPC* 2995	rbc	CD236 and CD236R complex with p55 and the rbc-cytoskeletal-protein band 4.1 to help maintain rbc mechanical stability and deformability. It also can bind *Plasmodium falciparum* erythrocyte-binding protein 2 (PfEBP-2).
CD238	Kell blood group, metalloendopeptidase (KEL)	115–200 (93)	II	7q33 *KEL* 3792	RBC, testis, weak on various other tissues (e.g., brain, heart, skeletal muscle)	Polymorphic zinc endopeptidase that cleaves precursor of endothelin-3 to its bioactive form as a potent vasoconstrictor.
CD239	B-cell adhesion molecule (BCAM); Lutheran blood group Ag	85, 78	I	19q13.2 *BCAM* 4059	RBC, basal epithelium, vascular endothelium, pancreas, many other cell types (weak)	Binds the α_5-chain of laminin 10/11 to facilitate adhesion and/or intracellular signaling.
CD240CE	Rh blood group, CcEe Ag (RHCE); Rh; RhC	30	III	1p36.11 *RHCE* 6006	RBC, erythroid progenitors at the CFU-E stage	Closely associates with CD241, CD242, CD47, and CD235b to form the Rh complex that may help maintain rbc mechanical stability in association with ankyrin-R.

(*continued*)

TABLE 15–1. Cluster of Differentiation Antigens Defined as of the Eighth International Workshop on Leukocyte Typing (Continued)

Antigen	Other Names	Size	O	Genetics	Distribution	Physiology
CD240D	Rh blood group, D Ag (RHD); Rh30D; Rhesus blood group Ag	30	III	1p36.11 *RHD* 6007	RBC; erythroid progenitors at the CFU-E stage	(See CD240CE.) Loss of the CD240D results in the Rh-negative rbc phenotype.
CD240DCE	Rh30D/CE	30	III	1p36.11	RBC; erythroid progenitors at the CFU-E stage	(See CD240CE.) CD240CDE is encoded by a hybrid gene *RHD-RHCE* created when a portion of the *RHD* gene is replaced by an equivalent portion of *RHCE*.
CD241	Rh-associated gp (RHAG); Rh2; Rh50	50	III	6p21.1-p11 *RHAG* 6005	Erythroid progenitors at the BFU-E stage to mature rbc	Essential for expression of Rh blood group Ag, it forms complex of two CD241 subunits and two Rh subunits that is noncovalently associated with CD47, CD235b, and CD242 and that may help maintain rbc mechanical stability in association with ankyrin-R.
CD242	Intercellular adhesion molecule 4 (ICAM-4); Landsteiner-Wiener (LW) blood group	42	I	19p13.2-cen *ICAM4* 3386	Erythroid progenitors at the BFU-E stage to mature rbc	Forms part of the Rh complex (see CD241) and carries the LW blood group Ag. It also is an adhesion molecule that may promote sickle cell adhesion to the endothelium.
CD243	ATP-binding cassette, subfamily B, member 1 (ABCB1) multidrug resistance protein 1 (MDR-1); P-gp, pgp 170	170	III	7q21.1 *ABCB1* 5243	Widely expressed on epithelia and endothelia	Member of the ATP-binding cassette (ABC) transporters involved in the cellular efflux of various molecules that are potentially toxic to the cell.
CD244	2B4; NK activation-inducing ligand (NAIL); p38	70	I	1q23.3 *CD244* 51744	NK cell, $\gamma\delta$ T cells, some thymocytes, some CD8+ T cells, basophils, monocytes	It binds CD48 with high affinity and possesses 4 cytoplasmic ITSMs that can inhibit NK-cell effector functions to allow for non–HLA-restricted NK-cell cytotoxicity.
CD245	P220/240; DY12; DY35	220–250		Not assigned	Mononuclear leukocytes, PMN (weak), plts (weak), T cells (weak)	It may be involved in signal transduction and costimulation of T and NK cells.
CD246	Anaplastic lymphoma Rc tyrosine kinase (ALK); Ki-1	200	I	2p23 *ALK* 238	Scattered cells in the adult brain; otherwise absent from normal adult tissues	It is a putative Rc for growth factors pleiotrophin (PTN) and midkine (MK) that can activate the mitogen-activated protein kinase (MAPK) pathway.
CD247	Zeta (ζ) chain; CD3ζ	16	I	1q22-q23 *CD3Z* 919	T cells, CD3$^-$CD56+CD16+ NK cells	It forms a dimeric signaling molecule that associates with the TCR-CD3 complex to play an essential role in T-cell activation.
CD248	Tumor endothelial marker-1 (TEM-1); endosialin; CD164 sialomucin-like-1 (CD164L1)	175	I	11q13 *CD248* 57124	Endothelial cells, α-smooth muscle cells in some vessels	It may play a role in cell–cell interactions, during angiogenesis and tumor metastasis.
CD249	Glutamyl aminopeptidase A; APA; gp160	160	II	4q25 *ENPEP* 2028	Endothelial cells, epithelial cells, renal proximal tubule cells, renal glomeruli	It is an ectoenzyme that catalyses release from peptides of the N-terminal glutamate, plays catabolic role in the renin–angiotensin pathway, is involved in formation of brain angiotensin III, and plays regulatory role in angiogenesis.
CD252	TNFSF4; OX-40 ligand (OX40L); gp34; CD134 ligand (CD134L)	34	II	1q25 *TNFSF4* 7292	B cells, DC, endothelial cells	It binds OX40 on T cells to provide immune costimulatory signal that apparently favors Th2-type responses.

(continued)

TABLE 15–1. Cluster of Differentiation Antigens Defined as of the Eighth International Workshop on Leukocyte Typing (Continued)

Antigen	Other Names	Size	O	Genetics	Distribution	Physiology
CD253	TNFSF10; TNF-related apoptosis-inducing ligand (TRAIL); Apo-2L; TNF-like-2 (TL2)	48, 19	II	3q26 *TNFSF10* 8743	act. T cells, act. NK cells, monocytes, DC, and weakly on other cell types	It can bind CD261 and CD262 to induce caspase-dependent apoptosis. It also can bind to decoy-Rc CD263 and CD264, and to osteoprotegerin (OPG).
CD254	TNFSF11; TRANCE; Rc activator for nuclear factor κB ligand (RANKL); CD265-ligand	35	II	13q14 *TNFSF11* 8600	act. T cells, marrow (weak), brain (weak)	It can bind either osteoprotegerin (TNFRSF11B), to stimulate osteoclast differentiation and activation, or CD265, to provide survival stimulus to DC and help in T-dependent immune responses.
CD255	TNFSF12; TNF-related weak inducer of apoptosis (TWEAK); APO3-ligand	18	II	17p13 *TNFSF12* 8742	Endothelial cells, CNS, muscle, pancreas, fibroblasts, IFNγ-stimulated lymphocytes, monocytes	It can bind to CD266 to promote proliferation and endothelial migration or to APO3 (TNFRSF12) to induce apoptosis.
CD256	TNFSF13; a proliferation-inducing ligand (APRIL); TALL-2	28	II	17p13.1 *TNFSF13* 8741	Secreted by monocytes, MØ, and nurse-like cells (NLC)	It can bind CD269 or CD267 to activate the canonical NF-κB pathway, inducing cell activation and resistance to apoptosis.
CD257	TNFS13B; B-cell activating factor of the TNF-family (BAFF); TALL-1; B-lymphocyte stimulator (BLyS)	31	II	13q32–34 *TNFSF13B* 10673	Monocytes, nurse-like cells (NLC), MØ, act. B cells (weak), placenta (weak), lung (weak), heart (weak)	It can bind CD269, CD267, or CD268 to induce canonical and noncanonical NF-κB, inducing cell activation and resistance to apoptosis.
CD258	TNFSF14; LIGHT; herpesvirus entry mediator ligand (HVEM-L)	29	II	19p13.3 *TNFSF14* 8740	act. leukocytes (strong), resting leukocytes (weak)	It can bind CD270 or lymphotoxin-β Rc (LTbR) to costimulate T-cell and DC activation. It also may play a role in intestinal inflammation and IgA nephropathy.
CD261	TNFRSF10A; TRAIL-R1; death Rc 4 (DR4)	50	I	8p21 *TNFRSF10A* 8797	Widely expressed on lymphoid and gut tissue	Rc for CD253, which can induce caspase-dependent apoptosis.
CD262	TNFRSF10B; TRAIL-R2; death Rc 5 (DR5)	48	I	8p22–21 *TNFRSF10B* 8794	Lymphocytes, MØ, monocytes, granulocytes	Rc for CD253, which can induce caspase-dependent apoptosis.
CD263	TNFRSF10C; TRAIL-R3; DcR1; LIT; TRID	65	I	8p22-p21 *TNFRS10C* 8794	Lymphocytes, MØ, PMN, monocytes, hepatocytes, neurons, Leydig cells, muscle, lung, heart	Decoy Rc for CD253 that does not activate caspase-dependent apoptosis.
CD264	TNFRSF10D; TRAIL-R4; DcR2	35	I	8p21 *TNFRS10D* 8793	Lymphocytes, MØ, PMN, monocytes, testis, ovary, placenta, prostate, intestine, pancreas, lung, heart, kidney	Decoy Rc for CD253 that does not activate caspase-dependent apoptosis.
CD265	TNFRSF11A; RANK; TRANCE-R; ODFR; OFE; FEO; EOF; PDB2	97	I	18q22.1 *TNFRSF11A* 8792	Broad tissue distribution, except not on stem cells or rbc	Rc for CD254 that can induce osteoclast differentiation and activation (enhancing bone resorption), enhance antiapoptotic signaling, and play role in lymph node development.
CD266	TNFRSF12A; TWEAK-R; FN14; Fn14; TWEAKR	14	I	16p13.3 *TNFRSF12A* 51330	Broad tissue distribution, including cells that can express TWEAK	Rc for TWEAK (CD255) that can induce proliferation, endothelial cell migration, and cellular activation.
CD267	TNFRSF13B; TACI; CVID	32	I	17p11.2 *TNFRSF13B* 23495	B cells	Rc for CD256 and CD257, which can activate the canonical NF-κB pathway, enhancing cell survivals.

(*continued*)

TABLE 15–1. Cluster of Differentiation Antigens Defined as of the Eighth International Workshop on Leukocyte Typing (Continued)

Antigen	Other Names	Size	O	Genetics	Distribution	Physiology
CD268	TNFRSF13C; BAFF Rc; BR3		I	22q13.1–13.31 *TNFRSF13C* 115650	B cells, some CD4 T cells	Rc for only CD257, which can activate both canonical and noncanonical NF-κB pathways, enhancing cell survival/activation.
CD269	TNFRSF17; BCMA; BCM	27	I	16p13.1 *TNFRSF17* 608	B cells, plasma cells, GC-B cells (strong)	Rc for CD256 and CD257, which can activate the canonical NF-κB pathway, enhancing cell survival.
CD270	TNFRSF14; LIGHT-R; herpes virus entry mediator (HVEM)	30	I	1p36.3–36.2 *TNFRSF14* 8764	T cells, immature DC, monocytes	As Rc for CD258, CD272, lymphotoxin-α_3, and gp D (gD) of HSV-1 and HSV-2, it can provide costimulatory signal or facilitate HSV entry into the cell.
CD271	Nerve growth factor Rc (NGFR); TNFRSF16; p75; LNGFR	75	I	17q21–22 *NGFR* 4804	Neurons, stromal cells, FDC	As Rc to all neurotrophins, pro-NGF, brain-derived neurotrophic factor (BDNR), pro-BDNF, NT3 and NT4/5, β-amyloid, and aggregated CD230 (prion protein), it has pleiotropic functions.
CD272	B- and T-lymphocyte attenuator (BTLA)	33	I	3q13.2 *BTLA* 151888	Lymphocytes, splenic MØ, blood-derived DC	Rc for CD270, which induces recruitment of phosphatases to its cytoplasmic ITIMs, thereby providing an inhibitory signal.
CD273	Programmed cell death 1 ligand 2 (PDCD1LG2); B7-DC; PD-L2	25	I	9p24.2 *PDCD1LG2* 80380	DC, act. monocytes and T cells, heart, lung, liver	Rc for CD279, which can provide coinhibitory signal, and for an unidentified ligand, which can provide a costimulatory signal.
CD274	B7-H1; PD-L1; PDCD1LG1	40	I	9p24 *CD274* 29126	DC, act. T cells, act. monocytes, muscle, placenta, lung	Rc for CD279, which can provide coinhibitory signal, and for an unidentified ligand, which can provide a costimulatory signal.
CD275	ICOS ligand (ICOSLG); splice variants hGL50 and B7-homologue 2 (B7-H2); B7-related protein-1 (B7RP-1); ligand for ICOS (LICOS)		I	21q22.3 *ICOSLG* 23308	B cells, monocytes, MØ, endothelial cells, DC	It can bind CD278 to costimulate CD278-bearing T cells, enhancing cytokine production and T-cell helper function.
CD276	B7-H3 (long); 4Ig-B7-H3	110	I	15q23-q24 *CD276* 80381	NK cells, DC, T cells, B cells, act. monocytes	Rc of the B7 family that provides coinhibitory signaling.
CD277	BT3.1; BTF5	56	I	6p22.1 *BTN3A1* 11119	Lymphocytes, DC, monocytes, some stem cells	Rc of the B7 family that may help regulate T-cell activation.
CD278	Inducible costimulator (ICOS)	55–60	I	2q33 *ICOS* 29851	act. T cells, thymic medulla	Upon binding its ligand CD275, it provides for T-cell costimulation, leading to production of cytokines such as IL-4, IL-5, IL-6, INFγ, TNF-α, GM-CSF, but not IL-2.
CD279	Programmed cell death 1 (PDC1 or PD-1)	55	I	2q37.3 *PDCD1* 5133	CD4–/CD8–double-negative γ/δ thymocytes, act. T cells, act. B cells, NK-T cells (weak)	It binds CD273 and CD274 to provide an inhibitory signal via its intracellular ITIM and ITSM domains, which might help mitigate autoimmunity.
CD280	Mannose Rc, C type 2 (MRC2) endo180; TWM22; MRC2; UPARAP; KIAA0709	180	I	17q23.2 *MRC2* 9902	Myeloid progenitors, fibroblasts, some endothelial cells, some MØ, mesenchymal cells	It binds gelatin and collagen (types I, II, IV, and V) in the ECM to facilitate uptake and lysosomal degradation. It forms complex with urokinase plasminogen activator and its Rc CD87 to play role in CD87-dependent cell migration.

(continued)

TABLE 15–1. Cluster of Differentiation Antigens Defined as of the Eighth International Workshop on Leukocyte Typing (Continued)

Antigen	Other Names	Size	O	Genetics	Distribution	Physiology
CD281	Toll-like Rc 1 (TLR1); TIL	90	I	4p14 *TLR1* 7096	Monocytes, PMN, breast milk	Toll-like Rc for pathogen-associated molecular patterns (PAMP) (e.g., mycobacterial 19-kDa lipoprotein, triacylated lipopeptides, *Borrelia burgdorferi* outer surface protein A lipoprotein), which can help trigger the innate immune response.
CD282	Toll-like Rc 2 (TLR2); TIL4	85	I	4q32 *TLR2* 7097	Monocytes (strong), WBC, lung, fetal liver, breast milk	Toll-like Rc for pathogen-associated molecular patterns (PAMP) (e.g., protozoan, fungal, bacterial lipoproteins), which can help trigger the innate immune response. Can cooperate with CD286 to form Rc for microbial diacyl-lipopeptides.
CD283	Toll-like Rc 3 (TLR3)	100	I	4q35 *TLR3* 7098	Fibroblasts, blood-derived DC, microglia, astrocytes, pancreas and placenta cells, breast milk	Mostly intracellular toll-like Rc for double-stranded RNA of viruses, which recruits TRIF to induce activation of NF-κB and IRF3, leading to production of type I interferons.
CD284	Toll-like Rc 4 (TLR4)	85	I	9q32-q33 *TLR4* 7099	Monocytes, MØ, granulocytes, DC, act. CD4+ T cells, breast milk	Toll-like Rc for lipopolysaccharide (found in bacterial pathogens) to trigger production of inflammatory cytokines.
CD285	Toll-like Rc 5 (TLR5); TIL3	120	I	1q41-q42 *TLR5* 7100	Mucosal epithelium, WBC, monocytes, ovary, prostate, tests, breast milk	Toll-like Rc for flagellin of bacterial pathogens (e.g., *Legionella pneumophila*, *Pseudomonas aeruginosa*), which triggers release of inflammatory cytokines and is implicated in progression of inflammatory bowel disease.
CD286	Toll-like Rc 6 (TLR6)	85	I	4p14 *TLR6* 10333	Monocytes, immature myeloid DC, breast milk	Associates with CD282 to form Toll-like Rc for microbial diacyl-lipopeptides (see CD282).
CD287	Toll-like Rc 7 (TLR7)	120	I	Xp22.3 *TLR7* 51284	Endosomes of plasmacytoid DC, B cells, myeloid DC	Toll-like Rc for GU-rich ssRNA found in many viruses, which helps trigger innate immune response to virus infection and is implicated in autoimmune response to RNA-associated auto-Ag (e.g., Sm and ribonucleoprotein).
CD288	Toll-like Rc 8 (TLR8)	83	I	Xp22 *TLR8* 51311	Endosomal and lysosomal compartments of MØ, some DC	Toll-like Rc for GU-rich ssRNA found in many viruses, which helps trigger innate immune response to virus infection and is implicated in autoimmune response to RNA-associated auto-Ag (e.g., Sm and ribonucleoprotein).
CD289	Toll-like Rc 9 (TLR9)	115–120	I	3p21.3 *TLR9* 54106	plasmacytoid DC (strong), other WBC (moderate to weak)	Toll-like Rc for unmethylated CpG DNA motifs found in pathogens, which helps trigger the innate immune response to infection.
CD290	Toll-like Rc 10 (TLR10)	91–100	I	4p14 *TLR10* 81793	B cells, plasmacytoid DC, lymphoid tissues	Toll-like Rc for pathogen-associated molecular patterns (PAMP).
CD291	Toll-like Rc 11 (TLR11)	97	I	– *TLR11* 442887	Expressed in mouse, but not in humans	*TLR11* is not found expressed in humans because of a stop codon.
CD292	Bone morphogenetic protein Rc, type 1A (BMPR1A); ALK-3	50–58	I	10q22.3 *BMPR1A* 657	Chondrocytes, bone progenitors, epithelial cells of the epidermis, skeletal muscle, hair follicles, intestine	Complexes with bone morphogenetic protein (BMP) Rc II (BMPRII) to form heterodimeric Rc for BMP-2 and BMP-4 to help regulate bone development and chondrogenesis.

(*continued*)

TABLE 15–1. Cluster of Differentiation Antigens Defined as of the Eighth International Workshop on Leukocyte Typing (Continued)

Antigen	Other Names	Size	O	Genetics	Distribution	Physiology
CDw293	Bone morphogenetic protein Rc, type 1B (BMPR1B); ALK-6	50–58	I	4q22-q24 *BMPR1B* 658	Bone progenitor cells, chondrocytes, embryonic tissue cells	Complexes with bone morphogenetic protein (BMP) Rc II (BMPRII) to form heterodimeric Rc for BMP-2 and BMP-4 to help regulate bone development and chondrogenesis.
CD294	G-protein-coupled Rc 44 (GPR44); CRTH2	43	III Hep.	11q12-q13.3 *GPR44* 11251	Th2 type T cells, eosinophils, basophils, many other tissues outside immune system	G-protein-coupled Rc for prostaglandin D2 that can play a role in cell activation.
CD295	Leptin Rc (LEPR); OBR; B219	130–150	I	1p31 *LEPR* 3953	Most cell types	Rc for leptin that helps regulate food intake and lipid metabolism.
CD296	ADP-ribosyl-transferase 1 (ART1)	37	GPI	11p15 *ART1* 417	Epithelial cells, some T cells, heart, skeletal muscle	An ectoenzyme that catalyzes the transfer of a single ADP-ribose group from NAD onto an arginine of a target protein (e.g., α_7-integrin, defensin-1, CD11a, CD18, ADP-ribosylate guanidine-containing substrates).
CD297	ADP-ribosyl-transferase 4 (ART4); DOK1; DO; Dombrock blood group	38	I	12p13-p12 *ART4* 420	RBC, erythroblasts, act. monocytes	An ectoenzyme that catalyzes the transfer of a single ADP-ribose group from NAD onto an arginine, thereby reversibly modifying the protein's function.
CD298	ATPase, Na+/K+ transporting, β_3 (ATP1B3)	32	II	3q23 *ATP1B3* 483	All leukocytes	β_3 subunit of the Na-K-ATPase involved in Na+/K+ transport and increased upon activation.
CD299	C-type lectin domain family 4, member M (CLEC4M); DC-SIGN2; L-SIGN; CD209L	40	II	19p13 *CLEC4M* 10332	Liver sinusoidal endothelial cells (LSECs), lymph nodes, the placenta, type II alveolar cells, and lung	Member of the C-type lectin family. Binds to CD50, several complex pathogens such as HIV-type I. May be a pathogen recognition Rc. Can mediate in trans-delivery of pathogens to other cellular targets.
CD300a, c, e	**a**: CMRF-35H; CMRF35H9; IRC1; IRC2; IRp60 **c**: LIR; CMRF35; IGSF16; CMRF35A; CMRF-35[a]; CMRF35A1 **e**: CMRL35L1	20–60	I	17q25.1 *CD300A,C,E* a: 11314 c: 10871 e: 342510	CD300a: monocytes, neutrophils, some T and B cells CD300c: LGL, some T and B cells, monocytes, MØ, granulocytes, DC CD300e: monocytes, MØ, DC	300a: Ig-like Rc of the CMRF family with cytoplasmic ITIMs that can provide a signal that inhibits activation or cytolytic activity. 300c: Ig-like Rc of the CMRF family that may help regulate release of inflammatory cytokines (e.g., type I IFN, TNF-α). 300e: Ig-like Rc of the CMRF family that mediates activating signals by interacting with DAP12.
CD300LB CD300LD CD300LG	**LB**: CLM7; IREM3; TREM5; CD300LB **LD**: LIR; CMRF35; IGSF16; CMRF35A; CMRF-35[a]; CMRF35A1 **LG**: CLM9; TREM4; NEPMUCIN; CD300LG	20–60	I	17q21-q25 *CD300LB, LD, LG* LB: 124599 LD: 100131439 LG: 146894	CD300LB: monocytes, neutrophils, some T and B cells CD300LD: not characterized CD300LG: most hematopoietic cells, capillary endothelium	300LB: Ig-like Rc of the CMRF-like family that can provide costimulatory signal for cell activation. 300LD: Ig-like Rc of the CMRF-like family of unknown function. 300LG: Ig-like Rc of the CMRF-like family that might play a role in molecular traffic across the capillary endothelium.
CD301	C-type lectin domain family 10, member A (CLEC10A); HML2; HML	38	II	17p13.1 *CLEC10A* 10462	Immature DC, MØ	C-type lectin that binds to carbohydrates with terminal galactose and *N*-acetylgalactosamine residues and plays role in Rc-mediated endocytosis of glycosylated proteins.
CD302	DCL1	30	I	2q24.2 *CD302* 9936	Granulocytes, MØ, monocytes, DC	Binds glycosylated antigens and plays a role in Rc-mediated endocytosis of glycosylated proteins.

(continued)

TABLE 15–1. Cluster of Differentiation Antigens Defined as of the Eighth International Workshop on Leukocyte Typing (Continued)

Antigen	Other Names	Size	O	Genetics	Distribution	Physiology
CD303	C-type lectin domain family 4, member C (CLEC4C); DLEC; BDCS-2; CLECSF11	38	II	12p13.2-p12.3 *CLEC4C* 170482	Plasmacytoid dendritic cells (PDCs)	C-type lectin that captures and targets Ag for processing and presentation to T cells.
CD304	Neuropilin-1 (NRP1); BDCA-4; VEGF165R	140	I	10p12 *NRP1* 8829	Endothelial cells, neurons, plasmacytoid dendritic cells (PDCs), many carcinomas	Rc for VEGF-A and semaphoring-3A (sema-3a) that plays a role in angiogenesis or axonal growth (neurons).
CD305	Leukocyte-associated Ig-like Rc 1 (LAIR1)	31	I	19q13.4 *LAIR1* 3903	Most lymphocytes (except GC B cells), monocytes, DC	Rc with cytoplasmic ITIMs that provides signal upon binding unknown ligand that can inhibit cell activation.
CD306	Leukocyte-associated Ig-like Rc 2 (LAIR2)	16	I	19q13.4 *LAIR2* 3904	Monocytes	Ig-like Rc with cytoplasmic ITIMs that provides signal upon binding unknown ligand that can inhibit cell activation.
CD307	Fc Rc-like 5 (FCRL5); Ig-superfamily Rc translocation-associated (IRTA)-2; FcRH5; BXMAS1	100	I	1q21 *FCRL5* 83416	B cells	Member of IRTA gene family that binds aggregated IgG (esp. IgG_1) in immune complexes. It has cytoplasmic ITIMs for signaling that may inhibit cell activation.
CD308	Fms-related tyrosine kinase 1 (FLT1); vascular endothelial growth factor Rc 1 (VEGFR1)	152	I	13q12 *FLT1* 2321	Vascular endothelium, monocytes, osteoblasts, trophoblasts	Rc for VEGF, VEGF-A/B, and placental growth factor (PlGF) involved in angiogenesis, regulation of stem-cell mobilization, and/or osteoblast proliferation.
CD309	Kinase insert domain Rc (KDR); vascular endothelial growth factor Rc 2 (VEGFR2)	230	I	4q11-q12 *KDR* 3791	Embryonic tissues, adult endothelium associated with pathologic lymphangiogenesis (e.g., CA, diabetic retinopathy)	Rc for endothelial growth factors (e.g., VEGF and its isoforms) that is involved in regulation of lymphangiogenesis.
CD310	Fms-related tyrosine kinase 4 (FLT4); vascular endothelial growth factor Rc 3 (VEGFR3); PCL	146	I	5q35.3 *FLT4* 2324	Lymphatic endothelium of normal and malignant tissues; spindle cells of Kaposi sarcoma	Critical for angiogenesis in embryos and plays a role in angiogenesis and lymphangiogenesis in adults.
CD311	Epidermal growth factor module-containing mucin-like Rc 1 (EMR1)	98	III Hep.	19p13.3 *EMR1* 2015	Monocytes, MØ	Seven transmembrane domains resembling G-protein-coupled Rc of unknown function.
CD312	Epidermal growth factor module-containing mucin-like Rc 2 (EMR2)	90	III Hep.	19p13.1 *EMR2* 30817	Myeloid cells, act. lymphocytes	Seven transmembrane domains resembling G-protein-coupled Rc for glycosaminoglycans (GAG) chondroitin sulphate, and dermatan sulphate.
CD313	Epidermal growth factor module-containing mucin-like Rc 3 (EMR3)	80–90	III Hep.	19p13.1 *EMR3* 84658	PMN (high), monocytes MØ, spleen, lung, RBC, placenta, marrow	Seven transmembrane domains resembling G-protein-coupled Rc that may play role in inflammation.
CD314	Killer cell lectin-like Rc subfamily K, member 1 (KLR1); NKG2D	26	II	12p13.2-p12.3 *KLRK1* 22914	NK cells, CD8+ T cells, few CD4+ T cells, γ/δ T cells	C-type lectin Rc for HLA class I-related proteins expressed on virus-infected cells (e.g., MICA, MICB, ULBP-1, -2, -3, and -4, and the RAET1E-1) that can facilitate cell-mediated killing.
CD315	Prostaglandin F2 Rc-negative regulator (PTGFRN); FPRP; CD9P1; SMAP6; KIAA1436	135	I	1p13.1 *PTGFRN* 5738	B cells, act. monocytes, CA cell-lines	It can associate with tetraspanin molecules CD9 and CD81 and may be involved in regulation of cell motility and polarity.

(continued)

TABLE 15–1. Cluster of Differentiation Antigens Defined as of the Eighth International Workshop on Leukocyte Typing (Continued)

Antigen	Other Names	Size	O	Genetics	Distribution	Physiology
CD316	Ig superfamily, member 8 (IgSF8); PGRL; EWI-2; CD81P3	63	I	1q23.1 *IGSF8* 93185	Lymphocytes, many nonhematologic tissues	It forms complex with tetraspanin molecules CD9 and CD81 that may function in oocyte fertilization, nervous system development, cell proliferation, and myogenesis.
CD317	Bone marrow stromal cell Ag 2 (BST2); HM1.24	29–33	II	19p13.2 *BST2* 684	Lymphocytes, marrow stroma, monocytes, DC	It may be involved in pre–B-cell growth and lymphoid–stroma interactions.
CD318	CUB domain containing protein 1 (CDCP-1); SIMA135	140	I	3p21.31 *CDCP1* 64866	CD34+ CD133+ marrow cells, keratinocytes, colorectal CA lines	It may play role in early hematopoiesis and wound healing.
CD319	SLAM family member 7 (SLAMF7); 19A; 19A24; CRACC; CS1	66	I	1q23.1-q24.1 *SLAMF7* 57823	CTL, act. B cells, NK cells, mature DC	It can help trigger cell-mediated cytotoxicity and/or play role homotypic cell adhesion.
CD320	8D6	29	I	19p13.3-p13.2 *CD320* 51293	FDC	It may play a role in FDC-mediated plasma cell proliferation.
CD321	F11Rc (F11R); junctional adhesion molecule-1 (JAM-1)	32–35	I	1q21.2-q21.3 *F11R* 50848	PMN, monocytes, lymphocytes, many nonhematologic cell types	It can serve as ligand for LFA-1 and play role in the formation of tight junctions between cells.
CD322	Junctional adhesion molecule-2 (JAM-2)	45	I	21q21.2 *JAM2* 58494	Endothelial cells, B cells, some T cells, muscle	It can associate with CD321 and CD323, play role in the formation of tight junctions between cells, and promote lymphocyte extravasation.
CD323	Junctional adhesion molecule-3 (JAM-3); JAM-C; FLJ14529	43	I	11q25 *JAM3* 83700	plts, T cells, NK cells, endothelial cells, many nonhematologic tissues	It can associate with CD321 and CD322, play role in the formation of tight junctions between cells, and promote leukocyte extravasation.
CD324	Cadherin-1, type 1 (CDH1), E-cadherin (ECAD); CDHE; CDH1; uvomorulin (UVO); Arc-1	120	I	16q22.1 *CDH1* 999	Nonneural epithelial cells, stem cells, erythroblasts	Cadherin with cytoplasmic domain that binds β-catenin that is involved in Ca^{2+}-dependent homotypic adhesion, cell differentiation, and polarity. It also can bind integrins $\alpha e\beta 7$ and $\alpha 2\beta 1$.
CD325	Cadherin 2, type 1 (CDH2); N-cadherin (NCAD); CDHM; CDH2	140	I	18q11.2 *CDH2* 1000	Neurons, endothelial cells, osteoblasts, stem cells, cells that lack expression of C234 and P-cadherin	Cadherin with cytoplasmic domain that binds β-catenin that is involved in synapse formation and homotypic adhesion. It is necessary during gastrulation for left-right asymmetry in the CNS.
CD326	Epithelial cell adhesion molecule (EPCAM); EGP; ESA; KSA; M4S1; MK-1; EGP-2; EGP40	40	I	2p21 *EPCAM* 4072	Most types of epithelium except adult squamous, GI CA	"CA-associated Ag" involved in homotypic adhesion that may help maintain position of cells during proliferation.
CD327	Sialic acid binding Ig-like lectin 6 (siglec-6); OB-BP1; CD33L; CD33L1	49	I	19q13.3 *SIGLEC6* 946	Splenic and intestinal B cells, PMN (weak), placental trophoblast	A siglec that can bind sialyl-Tn motifs (e.g., Neu5Ac-α2-6GalNAc-α) and leptin, and play a role in cell–cell recognition and inhibit signaling via its cytoplasmic ITIM.
CD328	Sialic acid binding Ig-like lectin 7 (siglec-7); AIRM1; p75; QA79; D-siglec	75	I	19q13.3 *SIGLEC7* 27036	NK cells, placenta, liver, ling and spleen, low levels in monocytes, granulocytes	A siglec that can bind α2,3- and α2,6-linked sialic acids and disialogangliosides and play an inhibitory signaling role via its cytoplasmic ITIM.

(continued)

TABLE 15–1. Cluster of Differentiation Antigens Defined as of the Eighth International Workshop on Leukocyte Typing (Continued)

Antigen	Other Names	Size	O	Genetics	Distribution	Physiology
CD329	Sialic acid binding Ig-like lectin 9 (siglec-9); OBBP-Like	50.1	I	19q13.41 *SIGLEC9* 27180	PMN, monocytes, some B cells (weak), most T cells (weak), NK cells (weak)	A siglec that can bind α2,3- and α2,6-linked sialic acids and provide an inhibitory signal via its cytoplasmic ITIM.
CD330	Sialic acid-binding Ig-like lectin 10 (siglec 10); siglec-like protein 2 (SLG2); PRO940; MGC126774	90–120	I	19q13.3 *SIGLEC10* 89790	Eosinophils, PMN, monocytes, spleen, T and B cells (Sv3 isoform), NK cells (Sv4 isoform)	A siglec that can bind α2,3- and α2,6-sialylated glycoconjugates and play an inhibitory role in cell signaling via its cytoplasmic ITIMs. Alternative RNA splicing can make 6 different isoforms (long, Sv1–4, 6) that are differentially expressed by various cell types.
CD331	Fibroblast growth factor Rc 1 (FGFR1); FLT2; FLG; OGD; KAL2; BFGFR; HBGFR; N-SAM; FLJ99988	130	I	8p11.2-p11.1 *FRFR1* 2260	Fibroblasts, epithelial and endothelial cells	Tyrosine-kinase Rc with 2 main cell-type specific isoforms generated via differential RNA splicing: FGFR1b or FGFR1c, which bind FGF-1, -2, -3, and -10, or FGF-1, -2, -4, -5, and -6, respectively, to mediate pleiotropic effects (e.g., embryonic morphogenesis, adult tissue repair, wound healing, tumor angiogenesis). Point mutations in CD331 can cause Pfeiffer syndrome causing craniosynostosis and broad digits.
CD332	Fibroblast growth factor Rc 2 (FGFR2); KGFR; TK14; BEK; KSAM-1; JWS; CEK3; CFD1; ECT1; KGFR; TK14; TK25; BFR-1; K-SAM; FLJ98662	115–135	I	10q26 *FGFR2* 2263	Epithelial cells (FGFR2b isoform), mesenchymal cells (FGFR2c isoform)	Tyrosine-kinase Rc with 2 main cell-type specific isoforms generated via differential RNA splicing: FGFR2b or FGFR2c, which bind FGF-1, -3, -7, -10, and -22, or FGF-1, -2, -4, -6, -9, -17, and -18, respectively, to mediate pleiotropic effects (e.g., embryonic morphogenesis, adult tissue repair, wound healing, tumor angiogenesis). Point mutations in CD332 can cause various syndromes (e.g., Crouzon, Jackson-Weiss, Apert, Beare-Stevenson cutis gyrata, Pfeiffer).
CD333	Fibroblast growth factor Rc 3 (FGFR3); ACH; CEK2; JTK4; HSFGFR3EX	115–135	I	4p16.3 *FGFR3* 2261	Fibroblasts, epithelial cells (FGFR3b isoform)	Tyrosine-kinase Rc with 2 main cell-type specific isoforms generated via differential RNA splicing: FGFR3b or FGFR3c, which bind FGF-9, or FGF-1, -2, -4, -6, -8, -9, -16, -17, 18, and -19, respectively, to mediate pleiotropic effects (e.g., embryonic morphogenesis, adult tissue repair, wound healing, tumor angiogenesis).
CD334	Fibroblast growth factor Rc 4 (FGFR4); TKF; JTK2; MGC20292	110	I	5q35.1-qter *FGFR4* 2264	Epithelial cells, fibroblasts, skeletal muscles	Tyrosine-kinase Rc with high-affinity for acidic FGFs (e.g., FGF-1, -2, -4, -6, -8, -9 -16, -17, -18, and -19) that mediates pleiotropic effects and plays a role in muscle differentiation.
CD335	Natural cytotoxicity triggering Rc 1 (NCR1); NKp46; Ly94; FLJ99094	46	I	19q13.42 *NCR1* 9437	NK cells	Major lysis Rc of NK cells that can bind influenza hemagglutinin (HA) or HA-neuraminidase and mediate direct lysis of tumor or virus-infected cells.
CD336	Natural cytotoxicity triggering Rc 2 (NCR2); NKp44; Ly95; DJ149M18.1	44	I	6p21.1 *NCR2* 9436	IL-2 act. NK cells, some γ/δ T cells	NK cell Rc that can bind influenza hemagglutinin (HA) or HA-neuraminidase and help mediate direct lysis of tumor or virus-infected cells.
CD337	Natural cytotoxicity triggering Rc 3 (NCR3); NKp30; Ly117; 1C7; MALS	30	I	6p21.3 *NCR3* 259197	NK cells	NK cell Rc that may bind membrane-associated heparan sulphate proteoglycans and help mediate direct lysis of tumor or virus-infected cells.

(continued)

TABLE 15–1. Cluster of Differentiation Antigens Defined as of the Eighth International Workshop on Leukocyte Typing (Continued)

Antigen	Other Names	Size	O	Genetics	Distribution	Physiology
CD338	ATP-binding cassette, subfamily G, member 2 (ABCG2); MRX; MXR; ABCP; BCRP; ABC15; BCRP1; EST157481	72	III	4q22 *ABCG2* 9429	Subset of HSC, tissue stem cells, placental trophoblast, small intestinal epithelium, endothelium of CNS vasculature	ATP-dependent efflux transporter protein that can transport organic anions (e.g., various drugs, toxic chemicals) across the cell membrane against a concentration gradient and account for resistance to some types of CA chemotherapy.
CD339	Jagged 1 (JAG1); JAGL1; hJ1; MGC104644; AWS; AHD; AGS	150	I	20p12.1-p11.23 *JAG1* 182	Stromal cells, epithelium	Rc for Notch1, Notch2, and Notch3 that can mediate Notch signaling. Mutations in CD339 can cause tetralogy of Fallot (pulmonary stenosis, ventricular septal defects, dextroposition of the aorta, right ventricular hypertrophy) or Alagille syndrome, which affects multiple tissues (e.g., heart, liver, skeleton, kidney, eyes).
CD340	v-Erb-B2 erythroblastic leukemia viral oncogene homolog 2 (ERBB2); HER-2; HER-2/neu; NGL; p185^{HER2}	185	I	17q11.2-q12; 17q21.1 *ERBB2* 2064	Epithelial cells, marrow mesenchymal stem cells, overexpressed in a subset of many different CAs (e.g., breast, lung, ovary, colon, cervix)	Forms heterodimers with other members of the Erb-B family or plexin-B1, which can effect signaling leading to activation of MAP kinases and phosphoinositide-3-kinase (PI-3K). Can form homodimers when overexpressed as in some CA.
CD344	Frizzled-4 (FZD4); Fz-4; hFz-4; FzE4; EVR1; FEVR; GPCR; FZD4S; MGC34390	45	III Hep.	11q14.2 *FZD4* 8322	Kidney, liver, lung, CNS, neuronal stem cells	G-protein-coupled Rc for various Wnt proteins and norrin (Norrie disease pseudoglioma homolog) that can activate the Wnt/β-catenin pathway and help regulate cell polarity, proliferation, and/or development. Mutations in CD344 can cause familial exudative vitreoretinopathy.
CD349	Frizzled-9 (FZD9); Fz-9; FZD3	45	III Hep.	7q11.23 *FZD9* 8326	Brain, testis, eye, skeletal muscle, kidney	G-protein-coupled Rc for Wnt-2 and Wnt-7a that can activate the Wnt/β-catenin pathway and help regulate cell polarity, proliferation, and CNS development.
CD350	Frizzled-10 (FZD10); Fz10; hFz10; FzE7	45	III Hep.	12q24.3 *FZD10* 11211	Placental syncytiotrophoblast, colon and cervical CA	G-protein-coupled Rc for various Wnt proteins that can activate the Wnt/β-catenin pathway and help regulate cell polarity, proliferation, and embryonic development.

The CD designation is listed in the far left column labeled "Antigen." Common names of an antigen before it was given CD status are listed in the column labeled "Other Names." The molecular size(s) of the nonreduced CD antigen is listed in the column labeled "Size." If the molecular size(s) of the reduced CD antigen is different, then the size is provided in parentheses. The orientation or anchorage to the plasma membrane of each protein is listed in the column labeled "O." For type III proteins, the term "Tet." is used to distinguish proteins of the tetraspan family and "Hep." (Heptaspan) is used to mark proteins with seven transmembrane domains. In the column labeled "Genetics" is listed first the chromosomal location of the gene(s) encoding the CD antigen, followed by the official name of the human gene (provided in italics) and then the Entrez Gene identification number, which allows for retrieval of updated information about the genetics of the CD antigen in the "Gene" database of the National Center for Biotechnology Information available at: http://www.ncbi.nlm.nih.gov/sites/entrez. Tissue and cell types that are known to express a particular CD are listed in the column marked "Distribution." The proposed or known physiology of a CD antigen is listed in the column labeled "Physiology." For an explanation of the abbreviations used in this table, see the list of acronyms and abbreviations at the beginning of the chapter.

A review of the tissues recognized by the mAbs used to define the CD antigen is provided in the summary books published after each workshop.[1,3–5] References to these books are implied, but not necessarily cited, for each CD antigen listed.

Some surface antigens are useful for delineating the cell lineage of leukocytes. Unique assignment of a surface antigen to a particular lineage is best when the antigen is related to a unique functional property of a given cell type. The CD3 surface antigens form part of the T-cell receptor complex for antigen (see Chap. 78). As such, CD3 is expressed exclusively by mature lymphocytes of the T-cell lineage. In a similar vein, surface immunoglobulin (sIg) is a B-cell lineage-specific marker. The presence of sIg on a given cell may be misleading, however, because of expression on diffuse cell types of Fc receptors for soluble and/or aggregated Ig. Instead, expression of CD79α and CD79β, two chains that associate with sIg to form part of the B-cell surface antigen receptor, may be more precise in defining B-lineage cells (see Chap. 77).

Many CD antigens are expressed at varying levels by many different cell types. Rather than the exclusive expression of a single CD antigen

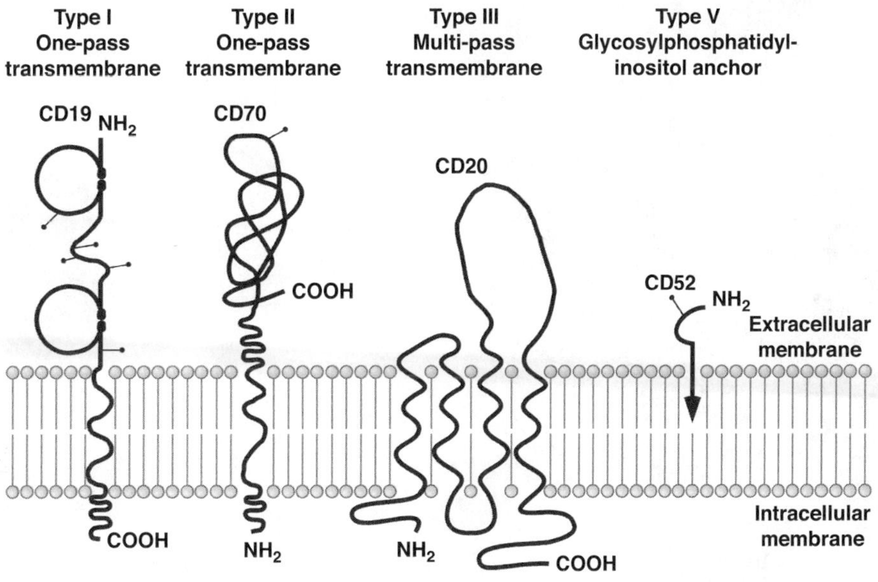

FIGURE 15–1. Major different types of surface proteins with respect to how they integrate into the membrane bilayer. The types of membrane protein are indicated at the *top*. The *straight lines* attached to the *open circles* represent the lipid bilayer. The *colored lines* represent the polypeptide backbones. The *thin pegs* extending from the polypeptide backbone represent carbohydrates. CD19 (*far left*) is a type I transmembrane protein that passes through the membrane once. It has its C-terminus (COOH) in the cytoplasm and N-terminus (NH_2) outside the cell. CD70 (*second from left*) is a type II single-pass transmembrane protein with the N-terminus inside the cell. CD20 (*second from right*) is a type III multispan protein that also is a tetraspan molecule in that it traverses the lipid bilayer four times. The tetraspan proteins have both the N-terminus and C-terminus in the cytoplasm. CD52 (*far right*) is a glycosylphosphatidylinositol (GPI)-anchored protein. *Labels at the far right* indicate the extracellular and intracellular membranes.

with a particular cell type, the peculiar constellation of surface antigens expressed by a given cell helps assign the cell to a particular lineage or sublineage of cells. Increasingly, the resolution of many important cell subpopulations requires use of mAb combinations that can define expression of more than one CD antigen in multiparameter flow cytometric analyses.

REFERENCES

1. Zola H, Swart B, Nicholson I, et al: *Leukocyte and Stromal Cell Molecules*. John Wiley and Sons, Hoboken, NJ, 2007.
2. Barclay A, Brown M, Law S, et al: *The Leukocyte Antigen Facts Book*, 2nd ed. Academic Press, San Diego, CA, 1997.
3. Scholossman S, Boumsell L, Gilks W, et al: *Leukocyte Typing V, White Cell Differentiation Antigens*. Oxford University Press, Oxford, 1995.
4. Kishimoto T, Kikutani H, von der Borne A, et al: *Leukocyte Typing VI, White Cell Differentiation Antigens*. Garland Science, New York, 1998.
5. Mason D, Simmons D, Buckley C, et al: *Leukocyte Typing VII, White Cell Differentiation Antigens*. Oxford University Press, Oxford, 2002.

CHAPTER 16

HEMATOPOIETIC STEM CELLS, PROGENITORS, AND CYTOKINES

Kenneth Kaushansky

SUMMARY

Blood cell production is an enormously complex process in which a small number of hematopoietic stem cells expand and differentiate into an excess of 10^{11} cells each day. Based on a number of strategies available to the experimental hematologist a hierarchy of hematopoietic stem, progenitor, and mature blood cells is emerging in which each successive developmental stage loses the potential to differentiate into a specific type or class of cells. The characteristics of the stem and progenitor cells that give rise to the formed elements of the blood are the subject of this chapter, including the roles played by transcription factors and external signals in lineage fate determination, the cytokines and cell adhesion molecules that support cell survival, self-renewal, expansion, and differentiation, and the cell surface properties that allow for their purification, and biochemical and genetic characterization. A thorough understanding of hematopoietic stem and progenitor cells and their supportive microenvironment can provide critical insights into developmental biology of multiple cell systems, favorably impact blood cell development for therapeutic benefit, impact genetic therapy for a number of blood and other disorders of man, and potentially even provide the tools necessary to allow the regeneration of multiple organs.

Acronyms and abbreviations that appear in this chapter include: AGM, aorta-gonad-mesonephros; BFU-E, burst forming unit–erythroid; BFU-Meg, burst forming unit–megakaryocyte; CAFC, cobblestone area forming cell; CAR, CXCL12-abundant reticular; CLP, common lymphoid progenitor; CFC, colony-forming cell; CFU-E, colony forming unit–erythroid; CFU-GM, colony forming unit–granulocyte-macrophage; CFU-Meg, colony-forming unit–megakaryocyte; CLP, common lymphoid progenitor; CMP, common myeloid progenitor; EBF, early B-cell factor; EGF, endothelial growth factor; ECM, extracellular matrix; EPO, erythropoietin; EPOR, erythropoietin receptor; FAK, focal adhesion kinase; FL, FLT-3 ligand; G-CSF, granulocyte colony-stimulating factor; G-CSF-R, granulocyte colony-stimulating factor receptor; GM-CSF, granulocyte-macrophage colony-stimulating factor; GM-CSF-R, granulocyte-monocyte colony-stimulating factor receptor; GMP, granulocyte-macrophage progenitor; HSC, hematopoietic stem cell; Ig, immunoglobulin; IRF4, interferon regulatory factor 4; IL, interleukin; LEF, lymphoid-enhancer binding factor; LR, laminin receptor; LTC, long-term culture; LTC-IC, long-term culture initiating cell; M-CSF, macrophage colony-stimulating factor; Meg, megakaryocyte; MEP, megakaryocyte-erythroid progenitor; R, receptor; RAG, recombination activating gene; SCF, stem cell factor; SCL, stem cell leukemia; SDF-1, stromal-derived factor-1; SLAM, signaling lymphocyte activation molecule; TCF, T-cell factor; TGF, transforming growth factor; TPO, thrombopoietin; VCAM, vascular cell adhesion molecule; VLA, very-late antigen.

AN OVERVIEW OF HEMATOPOIESIS

Blood cell production is an enormous and complex process. Based on the adult blood volume (5 L), the number of each of the blood cell types per microliter of blood, and their circulatory half-life, it can be calculated that each day an adult human produces 2×10^{11} erythrocytes, 1×10^{11} leukocytes, and 1×10^{11} platelets. Over the past 4 decades experimental hematologists have developed a model of blood cell production in which a hierarchical developmental progression of primitive, multipotential hematopoietic stem cells (HSCs) gradually lose one or more developmental potentials and ultimately become committed to a single cell lineage, which matures into the corresponding blood cell type.[1] Perhaps one of the most compelling arguments supporting this model of hematopoiesis is derived from extensive purification schemes using cell surface markers that yield cells at each predicted developmental stage[2] (Fig. 16–1). Although hematopoietic development is considered by most investigators as an irreversible stepwise and progressive loss of developmental potentials, studies now suggest that cells undergoing apparent differentiation steps might oscillate between different stages depending on their position in the cell cycle.[3] But regardless of the precise relationships between different stages of hematopoietic development, the availability of this model and the data leading to its construction have provided important insights into the biology and clinical uses of hematopoietic stem and progenitor cells. This chapter focuses on our understanding of the molecular basis for blood cell development, beginning with the HSC and its offspring, the lineage-committed progenitor cells.

DEVELOPMENTAL BIOLOGY OF HEMATOPOIESIS

Blood cell production begins in the yolk sac,[4] where extraembryonic mesoderm develops into angioblasts and primitive erythroid precursors at day 7 postcoitum of the mouse; cells of the outer layer of the undifferentiated mesoderm at this time flatten and become endothelial cells, and the inner cells round up to become clusters of erythroid precursors,[5] termed *blood islands*. Like in the embryo proper, there is much evidence to suggest that these two cells are derived from a common precursor (the hemangioblast).[6] Once adjacent blood islands begin to coalesce on day 8, the endothelial cells form vascular channels, which by day 8.5 connect with the embryonic vasculature, allowing yolk sac blood cells to exit the blood islands, complete their maturation, and enucleate in the embryonic bloodstream.[7] In both mouse and man there is a stage of embryonic development where both primitive erythrocytes (as characterized by ζ globin phenotype) and definitive red cells are produced in the yolk sac, although the former appears only very transiently. Although not as well characterized, yolk sac myelopoiesis and thrombopoiesis also occur, perhaps as part of the development of multipotent progenitors that appear by day 8.5 postcoitum. Cells capable of differentiating into multiple cell lineages become recognizable early during yolk sac hematopoiesis.[8] However, such cells reproducibly engraft only in the marrow of myeloablated embryonic animals and not in adults,[9] making it unlikely that such cells are true HSCs, although this topic remains controversial. By day 11 postcoitum repopulating HSCs are clearly present in the yolk sac, but the relationship of these cells and the HSCs that are clearly demonstrable a day earlier in the aorta-gonad-mesonephros (AGM) region is not certain. By day 12.5, postcoitum hematopoiesis in the murine yolk sac is eliminated.

Although it was long believed that the developmental origin of the adult mammalian hematopoietic system was the yolk sac, subsequent research has shown that the first adult-type HSCs are derived from

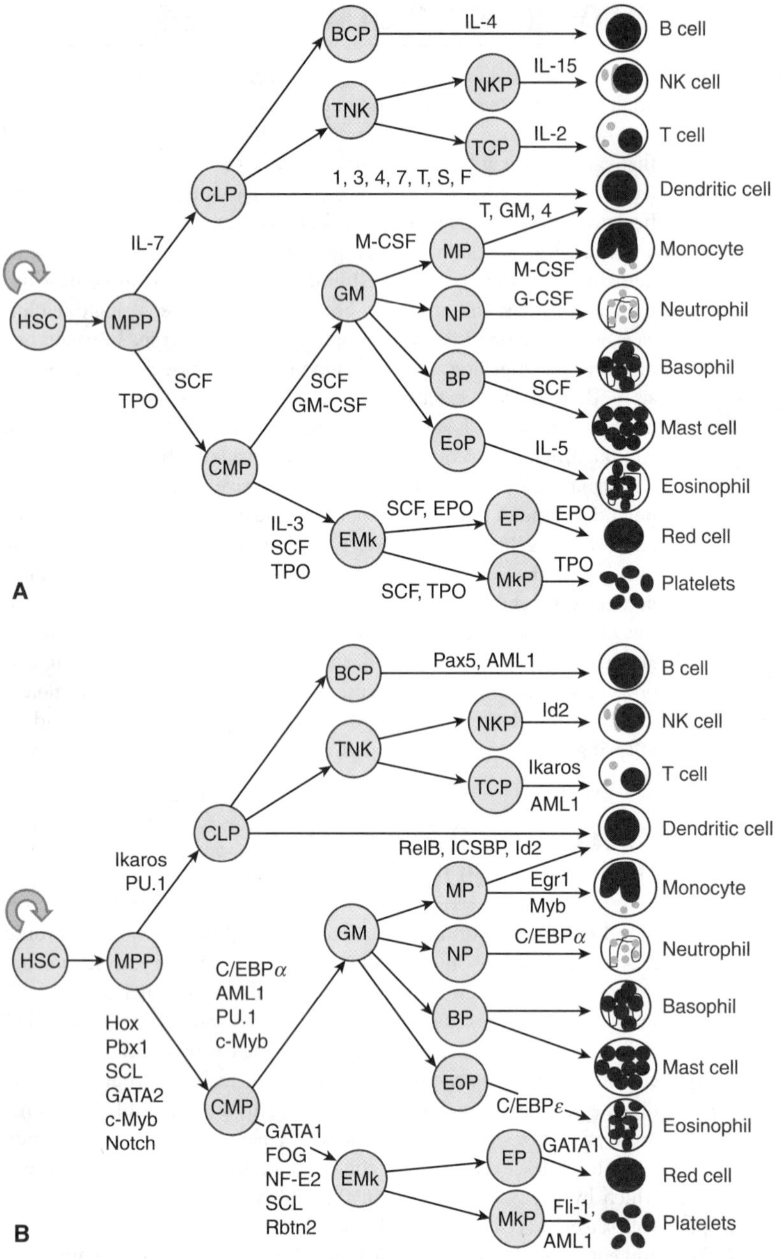

FIGURE 16–1. The figure displays the hematopoietic progenitors that have been defined by in vitro assays or by more complex tissue-based assays. In **(A)** the growth factors responsible for cell survival and proliferation at each corresponding stage of hematopoietic development are shown, and in **(B)** the corresponding transcription factors are illustrated. See text for definitions, except that T,GM,4 represents tumor necrosis factor alpha (TNF-α), GM-CSF and IL-4, and 1,3,4,7,T,S,F represents IL-1, IL-3, IL-4, IL-7, TNF-α, SCF, and Flt3 Ligand. Although a single type of macrophage is illustrated, the blood monocyte can differentiate into a plethora of tissue specific macrophage types, including the hepatic Kupffer cell, the brain microglia, and the bone osteoclast (see Chaps. 67 and 69 for details). Similarly, a single dendritic cell is shown, but of two distinct origins, lymphoid or myeloid (see Chap. 18).

mesodermal cells within a region of the embryonic paraaortic splanchnopleure known as the AGM, particularly from the ventral wall of the dorsal aorta.[10–12] The AGM remains a source of hematopoiesis between days 9.5 and 11.5 postcoitum in the mouse and days 30 and 37 in the human.[13,14] Of interest, the development of hematopoietic cells in this region (as well as in the yolk sac) occurs in a "reverse" direction, that is, single lineage-committed progenitors appear prior to multilineage progenitors, which appear prior to stem cells. This region also has cells that express a number of molecules in common with endothelial cells, including CD34, the transcription factors SCL and GATA-2, and the receptors c-kit and FLK-1.[15] Moreover, cell culture experiments have established that such cells display combined endothelial and hematopoietic potential, establishing them as "hemangioblasts," the postulated combined endothelial cell–hematopoietic precursor.[16]

Approximately 2 days following the appearance of HSCs in the AGM region, hematopoiesis begins in the fetal liver. Careful dissection experiments of the 1970s indicate that fetal liver hematopoiesis is dependent on an exogenous source of hematopoietic cells,[17] which populate the fetal liver in two waves, consisting of erythroid and multilineage progenitors around day 9 of murine gestation and committed progenitors and true HSCs at day 11.[18] Although there is no direct proof, the temporal appearance of these cell types in the AGM approximately 1 to 2 days prior to their appearance in the fetal liver strongly suggests that the former is the source for populating the latter. In humans the fetal liver becomes the major source of blood cells around 5 weeks gestation, and the marrow begins to populate with hematopoietic cells at 8 weeks gestation. Unlike the random pattern of cells seen in the yolk sac, hematopoiesis in the fetal liver is well organized; erythroid cells are usually found in clusters surrounding a central macrophage and CD15+ myelopoietic cells localize mainly around portal triad vessels, although lymphoid precursors fail to demonstrate a specific localization pattern and are randomly found amongst heaptocytes.[19] Up to 50 percent of the fetal liver is composed of hematopoietic cells at days 12 to 14 of murine embryonic life, a proportion that begins to decrease as hepatocytes replace hematopoietic cells and the latter shift to the marrow, prior to birth.

The final shift in the site of hematopoiesis occurs before birth; although the marrow begins to populate with liver derived hematopoietic cells at day 16 in the mouse and at 8 weeks gestation in the human, it is mostly myeloid in nature and contributes little to the circulating blood until just before birth.[20] Hematopoietic stem and progenitor cells circulate in large numbers during fetal life, as clinically witnessed by the use of umbilical cord blood as a rich source of HSCs for transplantation. However, shortly after birth neonatal blood has very few primitive hematopoietic cells, as they begin to home to and lodge in the marrow. Genetic studies reveal that marrow localization of HSCs is dependent on stromal cell-derived factor (SDF)-1[21] as elimination of the chemokine or its receptor (CXCR4) leads to marrow hypoplasia.[22] The shifts in localization of hematopoiesis during mammalian development are likely the result of changes both in the cell surface adhesion molecules on hematopoietic stem and progenitors that occur during ontogeny, and the characteristics of stromal cells of the yolk sac, AGM, fetal liver, and adult marrow that provide the microenvironmental support of HSC survival, homing and lodgment, self-renewal, proliferative expansion, and differentiation.

THE HEMATOPOIETIC STEM CELL

FUNCTIONAL DEFINITION

Although the concept of a common "mother cell" of all blood elements in the adult dates to Maximov in 1909, and its potential for participation in disease as proposed by Danchakoff in 1916,[23] the basic concepts of a hierarchical organization of stem and progenitor cells leading to mature blood cell production were congealed by Till and McCulloch using a spleen colony-forming assay, experimentally establishing the existence of multipotential hematopoietic cells.[24] The capacity to transplant marrow cells and reconstitute all aspects of hematopoiesis in myeloablated recipients provided an *in vivo* assay for the HSC, but it was not until the development of clonal *in vitro* assays of lineage committed progenitors that a coherent model of blood cell production began to emerge. The pioneering work of Pluznik and Sachs[25] and of Bradley and Metcalf[26] provided methods to enumerate and characterize marrow cells committed to the hematopoietic lineage. These investigators independently developed culture conditions that allowed colonies of leukocytes to develop from single progenitors. However, as a result of the more fastidious conditions required for erythropoiesis and megakaryopoiesis *in vitro*, the description of methods to culture these progenitors did not occur for another decade or more.[27–31] Work using density fractionation, cell sorting, and fluorescent dye exclusion methods has yielded purified populations of stem cells,[32–36] common myeloid[37] and lymphoid[38] progenitors, and lineage-restricted hematopoietic progenitors[39,40]—methods that have greatly advanced our understanding of the cell and molecular biology of blood cell development. Figure 16–1 depicts a working model of this process.

STEM CELL KINETICS

Based on transplantation data indicating that there are a remarkably similar total-body number of HSCs in mice and cats, it has been estimated that all mammals, including humans, possess 2×10^4 stem cells,[41] and because only a small fraction of these are cycling (and therefore contributing to blood cell production) at any given time, it is also clear that daily blood cell development from the few cycling stem cells to produce the approximately 4×10^{11} mature blood cells represents a massive amplification process. However, the capacity of HSCs to contribute to hematopoiesis changes with age. The number of HSCs increases with age in some but not all strains of mice.[42,43] Also, HSC differentiation in aged animals is skewed towards the myeloid rather than lymphoid lineage.[44] The molecular basis for these changes are undergoing intense study.[45–48]

Another measure of stem cell kinetics is the time it takes for transplanted marrow cells to repopulate a lethally irradiated animal. Studies using retroviral markers suggest that HSCs can be divided into short-term and long-term repopulating cells, based on the timing of their appearance in the blood following intravenous transplantation (fewer than or more than 3 months following transplantation in mice).[49] However, a rapidly repopulating stem cell has been identified using a direct marrow injection strategy, a cell capable of generating large numbers of erythroid and myeloid cells within 2 weeks of injection.[50] Moreover, by transplanting luciferase-labeled single stem cells, a strategy that allows the serial tracking of the cells during life, initially detected foci were found to expand locally, seed other sites in the marrow or spleen, and then recede with different kinetics.[51] From these experimental approaches it is clear that HSCs are heterogeneous.

STEM CELL ASSAYS

Transplantation Assays

Assays of Murine Stem Cells Experimental transplantation in animals affords the clearest estimation of HSC properties as the capacity to durably regenerate all of hematopoiesis in an otherwise lethally irradiated animal remains the gold standard for the field; moreover, the technique can be made quantitative. Typically, either 2×10^5 genetically marked, whole murine marrow cells, or reduced numbers of variably purified cells are infused intravenously into recipient animals who had previously received 90 to 110 cGy of whole-body irradiation. Blood cells and marrow are monitored for hematopoietic recovery in the following weeks and months, and the success of the transplant is measured by survival, and long-range contribution to hematopoiesis in the recipient. The contribution of donor cells to recovery is established by analysis of the posttransplant blood or marrow cells; the most common method of distinguishing donor from residual recipient blood and marrow cells is the use of flow cytometry against isoforms of the cell membrane-bound phosphatase CD45, present on virtually all hematopoietic cells. In a more quantitative embodiment of the strategy, limiting numbers of the genetically distinct cells (e.g., CD45.1+) are mixed with a "just adequate" (for full recovery) number of alternately marked cells (e.g., CD45.2+) and the proportion of CD45.1 to total CD45.1+ plus CD45.2+ cells is assessed following transplantation, yielding a calculation of the number of stem cells in the initial inoculum, an approach termed *competitive repopulation*.[52] Because there exist both "short-term" and "long-term" repopulating cells, the degree of donor cell chimerism is tested 3 or more months following transplantation, to be certain that only the latter are evaluated. For example, transplantation of megakaryocyte-erythroid progenitor (MEP) cells allows for survival in a lethally irradiated mouse, as these cells allow sufficient time for endogenous recovery of the small number of relatively radio-resistant HSCs in the recipient mouse.[53] Consequently, survival alone following cell transplantation is not a sufficient measure of the presence of stem cells in a given population. Thus, with the appropriate caveats, this approach allows an assessment of the numbers or "quality" of HSCs in the test population (i.e., some genetically altered stem cell populations repopulate less robustly than wild-type cells as a consequence of defects in cytokine receptors or other genes that affect the self-renewal, survival, or proliferation of stem cells). Based on the use of these experimental tools, we know most about murine HSCs. Obviously, this approach is not available to assess human HSCs. Instead, a number of alternate experimental approaches have been developed.

Assays of Human HSCs Severely immunocompromised mice can be engrafted by human HSCs, provided their survival can be supported in a strictly controlled animal care environment and that the experiments take place prior to the development of other untoward effects in such animals (e.g., tumor formation). The first assay employing this strategy relies on the combined immunodeficiency created by the severe combined immunodeficiency (SCID) and nonobese diabetic (NOD) genetic mutations.[54] Subsequently, these mice were found to bear some ability to reject or alter the developmental characteristics of human cell repopulation, leading other investigators to add genetic defects to the NOD-SCID background that improve the engraftment of normal and pathologic human marrow cells, such as β_2-microglobulin null,[55] γC null,[56] or crossing with mice that also express human hematopoietic cytokines.[57] Such animal models have allowed the assessment of (a) stem cell numbers in human CD34+ cells from mobilized blood or umbilical cord blood,[58] (b) assessment of the effects of gene therapy vectors,[59,60] cell cycle inhibitors,[61] or cytokine cocktails designed to expand stem cell numbers[58–64] on the retention of repopulating capacity, or (c) allows the study of fundamental biological properties of human HSCs *in vivo*, such as the cell-cycle restriction of repopulating cells.[65]

Surrogate In Vitro Stem Cell Assays

Although *in vivo* assays remain the gold standard, NOD-SCID and more severely immunocompromised mice are difficult to maintain and remain expensive and quite cumbersome methods to assess human HSC quality and quantity. As a result, a number of culture-based methods have been developed to more quickly and quantitatively evaluate human HSC function. Generally, each relies on long-term cell growth in culture and other special features to establish their validity as a model of the human HSC.

The ability to grow marrow cells in culture for extended periods of time provided an important tool to explore HSC biology.[66] In long-term cultures human or murine marrow is incubated in serum-containing medium under defined conditions, and after several weeks the stromal layer that has developed is recharged with fresh marrow cells, which then produce mature blood cells and their progenitors for many months. Cell fractionation studies show that the HSC resides adherent to the stromal cell layer in such cultures,[67] and that enzymatic disruption of the stromal layer will allow one to reseed a secondary stromal cell layer with the capacity to produce hematopoietic cells for a period of weeks to months, thereby defining an *in vitro* assayable cell termed the *long-term culture-initiating cell* (LTC-IC).[68] A second assay that has been developed based on similar principles is the cobblestone area-forming cell (CAFC), which, when evaluated by phase-contrast microscopy, gives rise to complex colonies of multiple hematopoietic cell types under the stromal cell layer of long-term cultures.[69] Unfortunately, when careful comparisons are made between these assays and transplantation studies the true HSCs comprise only a fraction of the repopulating cells found in marrow. Thus, conclusions about stem cell behavior from such *in vitro* assays cannot be considered rigorous.

■ CELL SURFACE PHENOTYPE

Numerous investigators have used monoclonal antibodies to an increasing number of hematopoietic cell surface proteins to negatively and/or positively enrich for stem and primitive hematopoietic progenitor cells. Although the function of only a few of these stem cell markers is known, it has not impeded their use for research and/or therapeutic benefit. Others have taken advantage of the capacity of primitive hematopoietic cells to extrude fluorescent organic chemicals or on their buoyant density to obtain purified populations of these scarce marrow cells; most successful stem cell purification strategies employ several such techniques.

The antigenic proteins and glycoproteins that exclusively or predominantly present on HSCs include (1) CD34, a 90- to 110-kDa type I glycoprotein that is postulated to mediate cell adhesion and/or cell cycle arrest[70–72]; (2) CD90 (Thy1),[73] a heavily glycosylated glycophosphoinositol-linked protein that participates in T cell adhesion to stromal cells[74]; (3) CD117 (the c-Kit receptor),[75] which supports primitive hematopoietic cell survival and proliferation[76,77]; (4) AA4,[34] a murine molecule homologous to the human phagocyte C1q complement receptor[78]; (5) Sca1,[79] a murine surface molecule shown by knockout studies to be necessary for normal stem cell development[80]; (6) CD133,[81] a 115-kDa pentaspan cell surface glycoprotein expressed on the apical surface of neuroepithelial and HSCs that has been proposed to function in establishing or maintaining plasma membrane protrusions[82]; (7) CD164,[83] a cell surface sialomucin that is present in several alternately spliced isoforms and that enhances blood cell homing and inhibits CD34+/CD38– cell proliferation[84]; CD150, a member of the signaling lymphocyte activation molecule (SLAM) family of lymphocyte proliferation receptors[85]; and (8) CD110 (the thrombopoietin [TPO] receptor c-Mpl)[86] present on virtually all repopulating HSCs,[87] and established to be vital for human HSC physiology as genetic elimination of the receptor leads to congenital amegakaryocytic thrombocytopenia at birth and aplastic anemia shortly thereafter.[88]

Many or most of the surface membrane proteins found on HSCs are also present on cells that have begun to differentiate towards specific lineages, precluding the exclusive use of positive selection alone for stem cell purification. Thus, a number of stem cell purification strategies include negative selection, based on cell surface markers absent on HSCs but present on mature blood cells and their corresponding unilineage-committed progenitors. Typically, cocktails of negatively selecting antibodies include CD38, HLA-DR, CD3, CD4, CD5, or CD8 for T lymphocytes; CD11b, CD14, or Gr-1 to exclude macrophages and granulocytes; CD10, CD19, CD20, or B220 to eliminate B lymphocytes; and glycophorin A or Ter119 to remove erythroid cells. The products that result from the use of such combinations of negative-selecting antibodies are termed *Lin*$^-$ cells.

A particularly difficult problem is presented by separating true HSCs from their progeny committed to the lymphoid or myeloid lineage, but not differentiated beyond that stage. Recent studies clarify the cell surface profile of the common lymphoid progenitor (CLP) as Lin$^-$/interleukin (IL)-7R(receptor)α^+/Thy1$^-$/Sca-110^{w}/c-kit^{low}[37] and the common myeloid progenitor (CMP) as Lin$^-$/IL-7Rα^-/c-Kit $^+$/Sca-1$^-$.[36] The cell surface phenotype of human HSCs includes CD34+/CD38–/KDR(VEGFR2)$^+$/Thy1$^+$/CD133+/Lin^{-2}, although most of these markers require careful clinical assessment before their widespread use in patients can be considered.

■ STEM CELL INTEGRINS

Integrins are a family of heterodimeric single-pass transmembrane proteins (18 α and 8 β subunits form more than 20 different cell surface adhesion receptors in humans) characterized by multiple immunoglobin (Ig)-like extracellular domains that allow two-way communication between a cell and its environment.[89] A large number of cell types require contact for survival; *in vitro*, this is usually manifest as integrin-dependent cell adhesion, either to extracellular matrix protein(s) or to other cells. In such cultures, disruption of adherence causes programmed cell death; for example, endothelial cells undergo apoptosis upon forced detachment *in vitro*, as a result of disruption of multiple integrins.[90] Integrins also influence the proliferation of cells by affecting the G_1 to S phase transition of the cell cycle.[91] These effects also operate *in vivo*; α_1 integrin (a component of the $\alpha_1\beta_1$ collagen receptor) null mice have a hypoplastic dermis, and the growth of α_1 –/– fibroblasts on collagen is substantially reduced.[92]

Hematopoietic stem and progenitor cells express multiple integrins, including $\alpha_4\beta_1$ (also termed *very-late antigen* [VLA] 4), which binds to either vascular cell adhesion molecule (VCAM) 1 or fibronectin, and $\alpha_5\beta_1$ (VLA5), which binds to a region of fibronectin distinct from the $\beta_1\beta_1$ binding domain. Moreover, primitive hematopoietic cells are thought to express integrin αIIbβ_3, the platelet fibrinogen receptor, based on the death of multiple hematopoietic lineages in mice expressing a suicide transgene under control of the integrin αIIb promoter.[93] However, the physiologic significance of this finding is uncertain at present.

The avidity of progenitor cell-integrin interactions can be altered by external effectors; numerous cytokines and chemokines, including cytokines critical for stem cell function (stem cell factor [SCF], TPO and SDF-1), enhance integrin-mediated binding.[94–96] Counterreceptors for both integrins, such as VCAM1 and fibronectin (FN), are highly expressed in the marrow matrix and on marrow stromal cells (see "Matrix Proteins" in "The Hematopoietic Microenvironment" below). Integrin-based interactions with the stroma are responsible for homing and retention of stem and primitive progenitor cells in the marrow, as antibodies that interfere with the interaction can mobilize stem and progenitor cells into the blood.[97] However, it is uncertain whether integrins can influence the survival or growth of HSCs, or affect their ultimate developmental fate.

■ METABOLISM-BASED CHARACTERISTICS

One of the hallmarks of HSCs is their resistance to chemotherapy-induced cytotoxicity. A primary reason for this property is high-level expression of drug efflux pumps of the multidrug resistance class of proteins.[98,99] The presence of these verapamil-sensitive efflux pumps has enabled the separation of HSCs based on their low-level retention of various fluorescent markers such as rhodamine 123 and Hoechst 33342, the "Rh^{lo}/Ho^{lo}" population of murine cells[100] and the side population (SP) of cells in human marrow.[101] However, before such maneuvers can be used for clinical stem cell enrichment procedures, the lack of toxicity of the fluorescent dyes must be confirmed. Nevertheless, such experimental strategies continue to shed important insights into HSC biology.

CELL CYCLE CHARACTERISTICS

Adult hematopoietic cells display altered engraftment capacity dependent on their phase in the cell cycle. Using primitive hematopoietic cell populations several investigators have demonstrated that only quiescent G_0/G_1 phase cells engraft into lethally irradiated recipient animals; cells in the S and early G_2 phase display minimal engraftment capacity,[102,103] a situation that can be experimentally manipulated; elimination of p21, a key cell-cycle progression gene, enhances stem cell expansion.[104] This finding correlates well with findings that the profile of expressed genes in a highly selected population of primitive hematopoietic cells shifts when they are induced from $G_{0/1}$ phase into the cell cycle.[105] However, although this cell-cycle dependence of engraftment of stem cells is true for adult cells, the corresponding cell populations derived from umbilical cord blood or fetal liver is not cell-cycle dependent.[106] A better understanding of these findings is very likely to shed important new insights into the genes that regulate engraftment.

GENE EXPRESSION PROFILE

It can be argued that the most critical feature of the HSC is its ability to quantitatively balance its three fates, apoptosis, self-renewal and differentiation into the mature elements of the blood. Moreover, the undifferentiated cell must express (at the least) the initiating genes responsible for all possible developmental lineages. A useful conceptual framework for this process can be constructed by considering the gene expression profiles of stem and committed hematopoietic progenitors that develop into the multiple hematopoietic differentiation pathways. At each developmental step genes associated with the adopted pathway should remain expressed or be up regulated, while the genes that specify the alternate lineage(s) are likely silenced. A thorough understanding of these gene expression profiles should help to explain the circuitry of specific aspects of hematopoiesis, and of developmental biology in general.

Initial studies using immortalized multipotent hematopoietic cell lines reinforced this conceptual framework; pluripotency is characterized by the expression of multiple genes associated with multiple cell fates.[107] Studies of purified HSCs and lineage-committed progenitors have also strengthened this hypothesis, revealing coexpression of several different lineage-affiliated gene sets in single primitive hematopoietic cells.[108] In contrast, the downstream progenitors of HSCs were found to express only lineage-appropriate transcripts, such as for the granulocyte colony-stimulating factor receptor (G-CSF-R) in granulocyte-macrophage progenitors (GMPs), or β-globin and the erythropoietin receptor (EPOR) in committed erythroid progenitors.[36] Similar findings were reported for lymphoid committed cells, although some promiscuity was detected in B-cell progenitors.[109]

With these principles established, more ambitious efforts to catalog all the genes expressed by each stage of hematopoietic development have been made possible by advances in microarray approaches to gene expression.[110] On an even broader scale, and as might be expected, comparisons of different types of stem cells reveals an overlap in the expressed genes, supporting the hypothesis that the mechanisms responsible for critical stem cell properties, such as self-renewal, are shared among the cells derived from multiple organs.[111] This observation also provides a powerful tool to identify such proteins. Such studies have also begun to identify novel genes expressed in HSCs, potentially allowing our better understanding of their role in hematopoiesis.

TRANSCRIPTION FACTOR PROFILE

An important goal of modern cell biology is to provide a molecular explanation for the gene or sets of genes required to orchestrate specific developmental events. Fundamental to this process is an understanding of the proteins present in cells that regulate gene transcription in a lineage-, ontogenic stage-, and developmental level-specific manner. Unlike what is claimed for many organ-specific programs, no single lineage-unique family of master regulators exerts executive control over hematopoiesis. Rather, an assemblage of specific and nonunique factors and signals converge to determine lineage and differentiation patterns. Several transcription factors have been identified in stem cell populations or have been shown to affect stem cell differentiation into the lymphoid and myeloid lineages. In addition to transcription factors that regulate HSC expansion, a number of epigenetic changes have been identified that affect gene expression in these cells. The polychrome group gene BMI1 encodes a protein that forms part of a polychrome group repressor complex, which represses a number of important target genes including the cell-cycle regulator p16/INK4a, a pathway that regulates HSC function in normal and malignant hematopoiesis.[112] In addition, methylation can affect HSC gene expression, as the DNA methyltransferases DNMT3A and DNMT3B affect HSC self-renewal.[113]

HSC Self-Renewal and Expansion

Members of the Hox family of transcription factors are important regulators of hematopoietic cell decisions, at least at the level of self-renewal/expansion, based on (1) a similar role in multiple organ systems[114]; (2) their lineage- and differentiation-stage-specific expression pattern in hematopoietic cells[115]; (3) disruption of their usual level or pattern of expression that leads to hematologic expansion or malignancies[116,117]; and (4) their elimination,[118] or elimination of the gene(s) that regulate them,[119] which leads to significant defects in hematopoiesis. In addition, members of the extradenticle family of homeodomain-containing proteins serve as cofactors for Hox proteins, altering their cellular localization, DNA-binding affinities, and specificities. Like Hox genes, genetic elimination of some of these cofactor proteins can lead to HSC defects. For example, Pbx1 null mice display greatly reduced numbers of CMPs,[120] and overexpression or altered expression of MEIS1 is associated with hematologic malignancy.[121]

HSC to CLP Commitment

The Ikaros gene encodes a family of lymphoid-restricted zinc-finger transcription factors related to the Drosophila hunchback gene.[122] All isoforms of Ikaros contain a highly conserved carboxyl-terminal activation domain and two zinc-finger domains that mediate their dimerization. However, only isoforms 1 to 3 of the six known alternately spliced forms contain more than three of the four N-terminal zinc fingers required for DNA binding to the consensus DNA core motif GGGA.[123] The PU.1 gene is 1 of approximately 30 members of the Ets family of transcription factors that bind to the purine-rich sequence 5′-GGAA-3′.[122] Genetic elimination of the Ikaros and PU.1 genes have established their critical role in commitment of HSCs to the lymphoid lineage; fetal stem cells in Ikaros −/− mice fail to generate any definitive T or B lymphocyte precursors,[124] and although thymocyte precursors can be identified postnatally, they undergo aberrant differentiation or fail to develop into the CD4, dendritic and some $\gamma\delta$T-cell subsets in adult mice. Consequently, Ikaros is essential for all of lymphopoiesis early during ontogeny, and for several subsets of lymphocytes later in life. In a similar fashion, PU.1-deficient mice also lack any definitive T- and B-cell precursors in their lymphoid organs at birth (and myeloid cells; see "HSC to CMP Commitment" below),[125] and if knockout mice are maintained on antibiotics and survive the first 48 hours of life, they begin to develop normal-appearing T cells 3 to 5 days later. In contrast, mature B cells and macrophages remain undetectable in the older mice, indicating absolute tissue dependence for this lineage.

HSC to CMP Commitment

The SCL (stem cell leukemia) gene encodes one of the transcription factors responsible for the initial stages of myeloid development, a gene first identified at the site of chromosomal rearrangement in a patient with stem cell leukemia.[126] SCL belongs to the helix-loop-helix family of transcription factors, which form dimers and bind DNA at consensus E-box motifs (CANNTG).[127] Although initially identified as a gene rearranged in T-cell acute lymphocytic leukemia, an essential role for SCL in hematopoietic development was established by gene ablation studies, which revealed a complete absence of primitive blood cells and lethality in scl–/– embryos at day 9.5 postcoitum.[128] Consistent with this pan-hematopoietic phenotype, previous studies showed that SCL is downregulated in differentiating granulocytic and monocytic progenitor cells and that forced expression of the gene in hematopoietic cell lines inhibits cytokine-induced granulocytic and monocytic differentiation.[129,130] Consistent with their respective roles in promoting stem cell and mature cell survival and proliferation, SCF sustains SCL expression in primary CD34+ cells, maintaining them in an undifferentiated state, whereas granulocyte-monocyte colony-stimulating factor (GM-CSF) downregulates SCL levels and favors granulocyte and monocyte differentiation.[130,131] Together, these results suggest that SCL expression is required for HSC and CMP maintenance, and that down-modulation of the transcription factor is essential for myeloid differentiation.

The GATA transcription factor family contains six members possessing a highly related DNA-binding domain composed of two conserved zinc-finger motifs.[132] GATA1 and GATA2 are present in hematopoietic cells, GATA2 is found in the same cells as SCL, with GATA1 expression restricted to latter stages of erythroid/megakaryocytic (MEP) differentiation. Because genetic elimination of GATA2 is lethal as a result of numerous nonhematopoietic defects, and because individual hematopoietic lineage-specific knockouts have not yet been engineered, the role of GATA2 in early hematopoiesis is uncertain. However, like SCL, elimination of GATA2 expression is required for hematopoietic cell maturation.[133]

As noted above, numerous lines of evidence indicate that HSCs express the TPO receptor, c-Mpl, as best exemplified by its expression on all AA4$^+$/Sca$^+$ cells that are capable of long-term hematopoietic repopulation.[87] Several investigators have shown that the 5′ flanking region of the c-mpl gene contains a functionally important GATA site and that GATA1 transactivates the gene in hematopoietic cell lines.[134,135] Because GATA1 does not appear in hematopoietic cells until they have lost their repopulating capacity, it is possible that GATA2 fulfills this role in HSCs, although there is no evidence yet available establishing that this protein can transactivate the c-mpl GATA site.[136]

THE HEMATOPOIETIC MICROENVIRONMENT

It has been estimated that the concentration of cells within the marrow is 10^9/mL; as a result, multiple cell–cell and cell–matrix interactions occur.[137] A major advance in experimental hematology has been the capacity to grow hematopoietic cells in long-term culture.[138] When high concentrations of marrow cells are placed in serum-containing cultures, a stromal cell layer and extracellular proteinaceous matrix form, and when subsequently recharged with fresh marrow cells, these long-term cultures (LTCs) are capable of supporting hematopoiesis for months with simple demi-depletion and replacement of culture medium. It is assumed that the cell–cell and cell–matrix interactions that develop in such cultures more closely resemble those found *in vivo*, helping to explain the longevity of such cultures and their capacity to maintain hematopoietic stem and primitive progenitor cells far longer *ex vivo* than do nonstromal cell-containing cultures. The molecular basis for the improved hematopoietic environment of LTCs is thought to rely on stromal cell surface molecules that promote cell–cell contact, prevent programmed cell death, and regulate growth.

The microenvironmental effects on stem cells have far reaching clinical implications as well; our ability to mobilize marrow stem cells for transplantation has greatly changed the way we treat hematologic and other malignancies, and ultimate success in the efforts of experimental hematologists to expand HSCs *ex vivo* with cocktails of cytokines and stromal cells for applications in gene therapy and regenerative medicine will undoubtedly derive only from a thorough understanding of the molecular bases for the interaction of HSCs with their microenvironment.

Marrow stromal cells influence hematopoiesis in a number of ways, by producing several cytokines that positively or negatively affect hematopoietic cell growth,[139–142] including some, like SCF, that are expressed on their cell surfaces, resulting in enhanced biologic activity.[143] Stromal cells are the origin of a number of extracellular matrix proteins that either directly affect hematopoietic cells, or do so indirectly by binding growth factors and presenting them in a functional context.[144] They also bear the Jagged/Delta family ligands that stimulate Notch proteins to undergo cleavage and translocation into the nucleus, events that are critical mediators of cell fate decision making,[145,146] including for hematopoietic cells.[147] Cell–cell interactions mediated by integrins present on hematopoietic cells and counter-receptors on stromal cells are also very important for hematopoiesis.[65,72] In addition to bringing hematopoietic cells into close proximity to cells producing soluble or cell-bound cytokines, and hence raising the local concentration of these growth promoting proteins, integrin engagement leads to intracellular signaling, usually promoting entry into the cell cycle and preventing programmed cell death.[148] Reflecting the vital and sometimes lineage specific roles of the hematopoietic microenvironment, the extracellular matrix and stromal cells reside in a highly organized structure.

ANATOMY

Hematopoiesis is highly compartmentalized within areas of red marrow, with erythropoiesis occurring in clusters surrounding a central macrophage,[149] granulocyte development associated with stromal cells,[150] and megakaryopoiesis occurring adjacent to the endothelial sinusoidal cells.[151] In the adult marrow, the specialized niche in which HSCs develop into differentiated progeny has been termed the *hematon* by Peault, a structure that includes Str01$^+$ mesenchymal cells, desmin-positive perivascular lipocytes, Flk1$^+$ endothelial cells, macrophages, and hematopoietic progenitors.[152] From these structures can be derived all lineages of committed colony-forming cells (e.g., colony-forming unit-granulocyte-macrophage [CFU-GM] and burst-forming unit-erythroid [BFU-E]) and primitive cells that score positive in CAFC assays, LTC-IC, and high proliferative potential colony-forming cell assays (see Chap. 4).

STROMAL CELLS

Fibroblasts are perhaps the best-studied of the marrow stromal cells, and can bind to primitive hematopoietic cells[153] by engaging cell surface integrins.[154] Marrow endothelial cells also support primitive hematopoietic cells, including LTC-IC.[155] The CXCL12-abundant reticular (CAR) cells, which surround the sinusoidal endothelial cells *in vivo*, are also likely to play the critical niche function of the vascular wall.[156] However, based on their ability to increase the number of HSCs when experimentally increased, osteoblasts, which line trabecular bone and reside adjacent to primitive hematopoietic cells,[157] are thought to provide a critical role in serving as the HSC supportive niche.[158] The origin of all of these cell types is thought to reside in the mesenchymal stem cell, a functionally defined entity that under specific conditions can be induced to form fibroblasts, endothelial cells, CAR cells, and osteoblasts, amongst others,[159] and hold promise to therapeutically manipulate hematopoiesis.[160] Mesenchymal stem cells are discussed more extensively in Chap. 28.

Marrow stromal cells affect HSCs in multiple ways. Each of these cells is known to produce a number of cytokines critical for primitive and mature hematopoietic cell development. For example, although a number of organs produce TPO constitutively,[161] marrow stromal cells are induced to produce the hormone in states of thrombocytopenia.[162,163] Stromal cells produce SCF constitutively in both soluble and membrane bound forms,[76] and FLT-3 ligand (FL) is produced both constitutively by stromal cells and lymphocytes and can be induced to high levels in the presence of pancytopenia.[164]

Besides growth factor production, stromal cells are also known to display counterreceptors for the integrins present on hematopoietic cells, including VCAM1,[165] interactions that promote cell survival and proliferation in several ways.[166] Osteoblast-derived annexin II serves as an adhesion molecule for HSCs.[167] Stromal cells also elaborate extracellular matrix components, including collagen, laminin, fibronectin, heparins, hyaluronan, and tenascin, which display important effects on HSCs (see "Matrix Proteins" below). These substances, in turn, engage a number of HSC integrins and other cell surface molecules, and form a solid matrix on which hematopoietic cells firmly attach. Of considerable clinical interest, it appears that interference with cell–matrix interactions,[168] or digestion of the extracellular matrix itself,[169,170] is involved in mobilizing HSCs by some agents such as granulocyte colony-stimulating factor (G-CSF) and IL-8.

Cytokines

The regulation of stem cell survival, proliferation, and differentiation has been difficult to address because of the rarity of stem cells and the requirement that they be assessed using cumbersome transplantation assays. Several cytokines are able to exert effects on HSCs. The pursuit of the cytokines that affect HSCs is of more than pure physiologic interest, as the availability of the right combination of such proteins could allow expansion of the cells for therapeutic use without sacrificing their pluripotent and self-renewal capacities. Three proteins—SCF, FL, and TPO—and their corresponding receptors (c-Kit, Flt3, and c-Mpl, respectively) exert important effects on the number and/or growth of HSCs both *in vitro* and *in vivo* (Table 16–1).

Stem Cell Factor The molecule termed SCF, steel factor, mast cell growth factor, or c-Kit ligand was cloned by several groups based on its binding to a cell surface receptor encoded by the protooncogene c-Kit,[76] previously identified as responsible for the severe defects in hematopoiesis, pigmentation, and gametogenesis in W mice. As the phenotype of mice bearing alleles of W was quite similar to those of steel (Sl), but in transplantation studies one strain displayed a stem cell autonomous defect (W) while the other was not (Sl), it had been hypothesized that the two genes represented the receptor for a growth factor and the cytokine itself, respectively,[171] a tenet proven true with the cloning of SCF.

SCF is synthesized by marrow fibroblasts and other cell types. Soluble SCF is a highly glycosylated 36-kDa protein released from its initial site on the cell membrane by proteolytic processing. An alternatively spliced form of SCF messenger RNA (mRNA), that does not encode the cleavage site, remains on the cell membrane, and is a more potent stimulus of c-Kit-receptor-bearing cells.[140] The ratio of soluble to membrane encoding SCF mRNA varies widely in different tissues, ranging from 10:1 in the brain, to 4:1 in the marrow, to 0.4:1 in the testis.[172]

The importance of SCF to hematopoiesis is easily demonstrated; although nullizygous mice (Sl/Sl) are embryonic lethal because of a number of developmental defects, the presence of a partially functional allele (Sl^d) allows compound heterozygotes (Sl/Sl^d) to survive into adulthood, albeit with severe anemia[171] because of diminished numbers/quality of HSCs.[173] In addition to its critical role in the development of embryonic and fetal hematopoiesis, treatment of adult mice with an antibody that neutralizes the SCF receptor, c-Kit, also results in severe pancytopenia,[174] indicating an important hematopoietic role for the receptor/ligand pair throughout life.

When present in culture SCF alone can maintain the long-term repopulating ability of murine $Sca\text{-}1^+/Rh^{lo}/Lin^-$ hematopoietic cells,

TABLE 16–1. Cytokines and Hormones Active on Stem Cells and Progenitors

Cytokine	Principal Activities
IL-1	Induces production of other cytokines from many cells, works in synergy with other cytokines on primitive hematopoietic cells
IL-2	T-cell growth factor
IL-3	Stimulates the growth of multiple myeloid cell types, involved in delayed type hypersensitivity
IL-4	Stimulates B cell growth and modulates the immune response by affecting immunoglobulin class switching
IL-5*	Eosinophil growth factor and affects mature cell function
IL-6	Stimulates B lymphocyte growth; works in synergy with other cytokines on megakaryocytic progenitors
IL-7*	Principal regulator of early lymphocyte growth
IL-9	Produced by Th2 lymphocytes; costimulates the growth of multiple myeloid cell types
IL-11	Shares activities with IL-11; also affects the gut mucosa
IL-15*	Modulates T lymphocyte activity and stimulates natural killer cell proliferation
IL-21	Affects growth and maturation of B, T, and natural killer cells
SCF*	Affects primitive hematopoietic cells of all lineages and the growth of basophils and mast cells
EPO*	Stimulates the proliferation of erythroid progenitors
M-CSF*	Promotes the proliferation of monocytic progenitors
G-CSF*	Stimulates growth of neutrophilic progenitors, acts in synergy with IL-3 on primitive myeloid cells and activates mature neutrophils
GM-CSF	Affects granulocyte and macrophage progenitors and activates macrophages
TPO*	Affects hematopoietic stem cells and megakaryocytic progenitors

*Primary regulator of the corresponding cell lineage.

suggesting that the cytokine can promote the survival of hematopoietic stem cells *in vitro*.[175] However, alone, SCF is only a weak stimulator of cell proliferation, primarily inducing the development of mast cells both *in vitro* and *in vivo*. Nevertheless, in the additional presence of IL-3, IL-6, IL-11, G-CSF, or TPO, SCF exerts profound effects on the generation of hematopoietic progenitor cells of all lineages,[176–178] pointing to primitive hematopoietic cells as critical targets. The molecular mechanisms of such synergy are beginning to emerge.[179] A physical association of c-Kit and EPOR has been detected following SCF stimulation of cells bearing both receptors, an event that is essential for their functional synergy.[180]

Flt3 Ligand FL was cloned as the binding partner for a then newly identified novel orphan receptor,[181] a protein most closely related to the receptors for macrophage colony-stimulating factor (M-CSF) (hence the term flt = fms like tyrosine kinase), and c-Kit. FL is expressed by T lymphocytes and marrow stromal cells.[164,181] The Flt3 receptor is a 160-kDa cell surface molecule expressed primarily on primitive hematopoietic cells.[182] Of considerable clinical interest, from 11 percent to 25 percent of the abnormal cells from patients with myelodysplastic syndromes or acute myelogenous leukemia express an aberrant form of Flt3 receptor that bears an internal tandem duplication,[183–185] resulting in the constitutive activation of the receptor and a reduced likelihood of patient survival. This observation has lead to an attempt to control the growth of such mutant-receptor-bearing cells with specific Flt3 kinase inhibitors.[186]

FL was initially cloned using a soluble form of the receptor to identify ligand-bearing cells.[187] As their receptors bear a number of common structural features, it was not surprising to find that FL shares significant structural homology, as well as biologic properties with both M-CSF and SCF. Like the other two cytokines, FL displays a 4α-helix bundle tertiary structure and exists in both membrane-bound and soluble states, the result of alternate splicing of the primary transcript that does or does not include a cleavage site for its release from the cell membrane.[188]

Unlike SCF levels which remain relatively static regardless of blood cell counts,[76] blood concentrations of FL can rise more than 25-fold in response to pancytopenia.[189] Interestingly, only pancytopenia, and not individual lineage deficiencies cause an increase in blood FL concentrations, suggesting that the cytokine is a bone fide regulator of stem or primitive hematopoietic cells. Consistent with this conclusion, transplantation data indicate that HSCs from Flt3-deficient mice do not effectively reconstitute the hematopoietic system,[190] being three- to eightfold less efficient in repopulation as wild-type cells, a conclusion reinforced by its genetic combination with c-Kit mutant mice.[190]

Like SCF, FL appears to act on HSCs only in synergy with other hematopoietic cytokines,[191,192] a finding particularly true for its combination with TPO.[193,194] In addition, FL is a potent stimulus of B lymphopoiesis and granulocyte-macrophage proliferation and development, particularly of the latter towards the dendritic cell lineage.[195,196]

Thrombopoietin TPO is a 45- to 70-kDa hormone that was cloned by both traditional biochemical purification and expression cloning strategies based on the use of a then orphan class I cytokine receptor, first identified as the cellular homologue of the murine-transforming oncogene v-mp1.[197] Thrombopoietin bears extensive sequence homology to erythropoietin (EPO), sharing 20 percent identity and an additional 25 percent similarity. The hormone is produced in several organs, including the liver, kidney, skeletal muscle, and the marrow stroma. Based on murine liver transplantation studies about half of steady-state TPO production occurs in that organ,[198] but in states of thrombocytopenia the marrow stroma increases production substantially.[160,163] The hormone acts on megakaryocyte (Meg) progenitors to enhance their survival and proliferation and on immature megakaryocytes to promote their differentiation, but surprisingly not on mature cells during platelet formation.[199] Multiple lines of evidence also indicate that TPO can exert profound effects on the HSC. The hormone also supports the survival of candidate HSC populations, and acts in synergy with IL-3 and SCF to induce these cells into the cell cycle and increase their output of both primitive and committed hematopoietic progenitor cells of all lineages.[200,201] These properties are also seen *in vivo*. For example, administration of the hormone to myelosuppressed animals leads to more rapid recovery of all hematopoietic lineages, including primitive cells,[202–205] and genetic elimination of TPO or its receptor severely reduces the number of marrow stem and progenitor cells of all lineages to 15 to 25 percent of normal values.[87,206,207] In addition, as noted in "Flt3 Ligand" above, TPO acts in synergy with FL to expand primitive hematopoietic cells in suspension culture, and when used to supplement LTC, the hormone maintained HSC numbers for up to 2 months,[207] compared to standard LTCs in which repopulating HSCs are no longer detectable at this time.

Stromal Cell Derived Factor 1 SDF1 is produced by a number of the cells that occupy the hematopoietic microenvironment, and has profound effects on HSC localization to the stem cell niche.[22] However, SDF1 is also thought to display direct effects on the survival and proliferation of hematopoietic stem and progenitor cells, both alone and in synergy with other hematopoietic cytokines.[208,209]

Notch Ligands The human homologue of Drosophila Notch was identified as an altered gene product in T-cell leukemia.[210] The discovery that the hematopoietic microenvironment displays Notch ligands, and that Notch isoforms appear on primitive hematopoietic cells[211,212] opened the possibility that Notch affects HSCs. This assertion has been directly proven: The Notch ligands Delta1 and Delta4 expand primitive hematopoietic cells.[213,214] It is possible that the favorable effect of marrow osteoblasts on HSCs is a result of their expression of Notch ligands, as inhibition of Notch processing blocks the expansion in LTC-IC seen in mice in which osteoblasts have been experimentally expanded.[158]

Wnt Proteins A role for Wnt proteins in hematopoiesis was suggested by their localization at sites of fetal blood cell production and their ability to expand hematopoietic progenitor cells.[215] Wnt 3a has been shown to expand long-term repopulating HSCs.[216,217] As Wnt proteins are expressed on primitive hematopoietic cells,[218] it is also possible that in addition to classical paracrine signaling, Wnts could act in an autocrine fashion in HSC biology.

Transforming Growth Factor β The transforming growth factor (TGF) family of ligands (TGF-β, activins, bone morphogenetic proteins [BMP]) bind to members of the TGF-β receptor family and trigger activation of the SMAD (Sma- and Mad-related protein) group of intracellular mediators.[219] Unlike the cytokines discussed above, TGF-β members inhibit HSC cycling,[220,221] and so blunt cell expansion, at least *in vitro*. Nevertheless, the situation *in vivo* is complex; genetic elimination of TGF-β does not alter HSC self-renewal or regeneration *in vivo*,[222] likely because of redundancy in the TGF-β system of ligands.[223] In contrast, genetic elimination of several of the SMAD proteins disrupts normal HSC homeostasis.[224,225] Recent data suggests that BMP4 might be the critical member of the TGF family that affects HSC biology.[226]

The mechanisms by which these cytokines exert their effects on HSCs are only now beginning to be understood at the molecular level, but it is already clear that effects on the transcription factors that govern HSC survival, self-renewal, and expansion likely play critical roles. It has long been understood that Wnt proteins act to stimulate an increase in intracellular levels of β-catenin, a nascent transcription factor. Upon being liberated from proteasomal degradation in the presence of Wnt, β-catenin translocates to the nucleus and alters transcription of genes displaying the T-cell factor (TCF)/lymphoid-enhancer binding factor (LEF) consensus sequence.[227] Moreover, TGF-β-induced alterations in SMAD protein phosphorylation affects their ability to activate transcription directly.[228] However, most of the cytokine receptors that affect HSCs do not directly affect transcription factors; rather, several cytokines affect signaling pathways that alter the expression, activity, or subcellular localization of HSC transcription factors.

As discussed in "HSC to CMP Commitment" above, SCL is a helix-loop-helix transcription factor critical for hematopoiesis. SCF enhances the survival of primitive hematopoietic cells in culture by maintaining their expression of SCL,[131] which enhances expression of the SCF receptor c-Kit.[229] Two additional transcription factors that play vital roles in HSC expansion, HOXB4 and HOXA9, are both affected by cytokines. Exogenous expression of HOXB4 to levels only twice normal are associated with a marked and rapid expansion of transduced HSCs on their transplantation into lethally irradiated recipients.[116] In both model cell lines and primitive hematopoietic cells TPO doubles the expression of HOXB4, in a p38 mitogen-activated protein kinase (MAPK) fashion.[230] Of probably greater significance is the effect of TPO on HOXA9, a gene that also induces rapid expansion of HSCs on its introduction into these cells, and whose genetic elimination leads to a profound deficit in numbers of HSC *in vivo*.[118] Although the hormone fails to affect total cellular levels of HOXA9 in either model cells or primary primitive murine HSC populations, TPO greatly enhances HOXA9 nuclear translocation by inducing expression of its translocation partner, MEIS1, and leading to ERK1/2 MAPK-induced MEIS1 phosphorylation.[231]

A third mechanism by which cytokines affect HSC expansion is through global inhibitors of signaling. In addition to its direct effects on HSC survival and self-renewal pathways, TPO has been shown to interact with the adaptor protein LNK,[232] which inhibits signaling pathways derived from a broad range of hematopoietic cytokines,[233,234] including TPO.[235] From these data is appears that TPO and LNK alternately regulate HSC expansion and each other.[236]

MATRIX PROTEINS

Fibronectin

Fibronectin is a 450-kDa fibril-forming glycoprotein composed of two subunits that is a major component of the hematopoietic microenvironment. Fibronectin is produced by both marrow stromal (endothelial cells and fibroblasts) and blood cells,[237] and is implicated in marrow homing of hematopoietic cells.[238] Distinct domains of fibronectin have been identified that interact with different integrins, for example, those for integrin $\alpha_4\beta_1$ and for integrin $\alpha_5\beta_1$.[148] HSCs display multiple integrins and their engagement contributes to cell survival and/or expansion. For example, *ex vivo* culture of human CD34+ cells on fibronectin maintains the repopulating capacity of HSCs, whereas growing the cells in suspension obliterates their ability to repopulate hematopoiesis.[239] Fibronectin binding to $\alpha_4\beta_1$ integrins also enhances the generation of large numbers of committed hematopoietic progenitors[240] and LTC-IC[241] from primitive precursors. Multiple molecular mechanisms for the effects of fibronectin on integrin bearing cells have been identified, and serve as a paradigm for the supportive effects of this entire class of microenvironmental signals.

Integrin engagement by fibronectin triggers a number of intracellular signaling events that affect the cellular cytoskeleton and transcriptional events. Complexes composed of kinases, adaptors, and cytoskeletal components are recruited to sites of integrin engagement, initiated by interactions with integrin cytoplasmic domains.[89] A critical molecule for integrin-based signaling is paxillin, a 68-kDa protein that contains a number of protein–protein binding domains, and which binds to the cytoplasmic domain of the integrin.[242] Additional binding partners also help trigger intracellular signaling, including focal adhesion kinase (FAK) and the closely related Pyk2 kinase. Upon recruitment, FAK and Pyk2 are activated and initiate Tyr phosphorylation of paxillin and other associated molecules, creating additional protein binding sites and activating tethered secondary messenger molecules. One vital signaling pathway downstream of FAK and Pyk2 is phosphoinositol 3 kinase (PI3K), which is mediated by the association of its regulatory p85 subunit with the adhesion kinases (see Chap. 14).[243] FAK also directly activates a pathway that results in upregulation of the cyclin D promoter,[244] affecting cell proliferation. Integrin engagement also leads to Src activation, engagement of Grb2, and activation of Ras,[245] pathways also activated by SCF and TPO, and potentially providing a mechanism by which diverse extrinsic stimuli of HSCs may converge.

Hyaluronan

Another stromal cell matrix glycoprotein is hyaluronan, which binds to two hematopoietic cell surface receptors, RHAMM and CD44. Although most CD34+ marrow cells express CD44, only a fraction of them adhere to hyaluronan,[246] a process that can be mediated by cytokines, as a result of either increased surface expression of CD44 or an alteration in its conformation. Consistent with the latter notion, certain epitopes on CD44 have been shown to be inducible,[247] and antibodies to CD44 can alter the adherence of CD34+ cells to marrow stroma.[248] Nevertheless, other data suggests that RHAMM is the primary receptor for hyaluronan.[249] It is also of considerable interest that primitive hematopoietic cells also express hyaluronan, and that it plays an important role in their lodgment in the marrow and subsequent proliferation.[250]

Heparan Sulfate

Long-term cultures that support hematopoiesis develop a heparan sulfate proteoglycan layer. Immunochemical analysis has shown that marrow stromal cell lines synthesize and secrete numerous members of the syndecan family of heparan sulfate, including glypican, betaglycan, and perlecan.[18] Evidence is accumulating that heparan sulfate-containing proteoglycans may be vital components of the stem cell niche. For example, the structure of the heparan sulfate secreted from stromal cell lines that support long-term hematopoiesis are significantly larger and more highly sulfated than heparan sulfate from nonsupportive stromal cell lines, and when used alone in long-term cultures, the former can support LTC-IC whereas desulfated heparan sulfate cannot.[251]

Tenascin

Tenascins are large, extracellular matrix (ECM) glycoproteins found in several tissues, synthesis of which is upregulated in response to tissue regeneration. Tenascins are multimeric proteins composed of numerous modules. For example, tenascin-C is composed of six subunits linked like spokes in a wheel by their C-terminal fibrinogen-like domains, each subunit being composed of multiple epidermal growth factor (EGF)-like and fibronectin type III modules. Two forms of tenascin of Mr 280 and 220 kDa are also expressed at high levels by marrow stromal cells.[252] Marrow cells can adhere to tenascin-C within the fibrinogen-like and to two sets of the fibronectin type III-like repeats, and when so engaged, they undergo a proliferative response.[253] Genetic elimination of tenascin leads to modest deficiencies in marrow hematopoietic progenitor cells,[254] although as the levels of fibronectin in such mice are also reduced, it is unclear if direct tenascin engagement of hematopoietic cells is responsible, or the defect is a result of the secondary reduction of fibronectin engagement of β_1 integrins.

Laminins

Laminins are heterotrimeric ($\alpha\beta\gamma$) extracellular proteins that regulate cellular function by adhesion to integrin and nonintegrin receptors. At present, 5 α chains, 3 β chains, and 2 γ chains have been characterized, which combine to form at least 12 distinct laminin isoforms.[255] Laminins containing γ_2 and either β_1 and α_5 chains are expressed in marrow, but only the latter (laminin-10/11) binds to $\alpha_6\beta_1$ integrin on primitive hematopoietic cell lines[256] and to primary human CD34+/CD38− stem and progenitor cells.[257] A second, nonintegrin laminin receptor (LR) also binds laminins, as well as other components of the extracellular matrix, such as fibronectin, collagen, and elastin, and is composed of an acylated dimer of 32-kDa subunits.[258] Although not an integrin, the LR associates with integrins (e.g., integrin $\alpha_6\beta_4$) to modulate laminin binding.[259] Functionally, laminin-10/11 facilitates SDF-1α-stimulated transmigration of CD34+ cells,[260] and displays mitogenic activity toward human hematopoietic progenitor cells.[255] The nonintegrin LR associates with the GM-CSF receptor (GM-CSF-R) to modulate its signaling properties, down-modulating receptor signaling in the absence of laminin, and releasing the inhibition when bound by its ligand.[261] This arrangement could provide a novel molecular explanation for how laminins affect cell proliferation; whether this physiology extends to other cytokines that affect HSCs is under investigation.

Collagen Types I, III, V, and VI

Collagen types I, III, IV, and VI have been identified in LTC or in situ from marrow sections by a number of methods.[35,262] Most of the marrow-derived collagen types are assembled into long fibrils, which form the fine, background reticulin staining seen on marrow biopsies, although type IV collagen is assembled into a meshwork seen most commonly as part of basement membranes. Collagens also interact with laminins in the marrow. Collagen types I and VI are strong adhesive substrates for various hematopoietic cell lines and marrow mononuclear cells, including committed myeloid and erythroid progenitors.[262,263] Classic collagen receptors on blood cells are of two types, the β_1 integrins ($\alpha_1\beta_1$ and $\alpha_2\beta_1$) and the nonintegrin glycoprotein VI, present predominantly on platelets.

CONTROVERSIES IN HEMATOPOIESIS

LINEAGE FATE DETERMINATION

One of the most contentious issues in hematopoiesis is the origin of stem cell commitment to specific blood cell lineages. Two schools of thought exist: extrinsic and intrinsic control. The former, championed by Metcalf and others,[264] argues that cytokines, extracellular matrix, or other stimuli instruct the hematopoietic stem or progenitor cell to differentiate into specific cell types. In contrast, Dexter and others[265] argue that a hierarchy of transcription factors direct a cell toward a specific lineage, mechanistically explained by a stochastic rise in one or more of a mutually antagonistic set of transcription factors, that drive developmental pathways by enhancing expression of the genes that characterize that pathway, and by interfering with the levels or function of the transcription factors that drive the alternate lineage fate choice.

The Case for Transcription Factors

A strong case has been made for intrinsic control of stem cell lineage determination.[265] As Enver and colleagues state: "Simply put, the question is this: Is unilineage commitment the result of a cell-autonomous, internally driven program, or rather is it the consequence of a cell responding to an external, environmentally imposed agenda?" These and several other investigators argue that the stochastic rise in one or another lineage determining transcription factor in the multilineage progenitor leads to its ultimate lineage commitment.

It is abundantly clear that transcription factors can direct lineage commitment in hematopoietic cells. A partial list of transcription factors restricted to specific hematopoietic lineages includes Pax5 (B cells),[266] Ikaros (B/T cells),[267] PU.1 and C/EBPα (myeloid and B cells),[268,269] GATA1 (erythrocytes and megakaryocytes),[132,270] Fli1 (megakaryocytes),[271] and C/EBPε (granulocytes).[272] A number of loss-of-function studies have revealed the nonredundant role of these proteins in development of the corresponding cell lineage. For example, genetic elimination of Pax5 eliminates B cells[273,274]; elimination of Ikaros leaves a mouse devoid of fetal T cells, fetal and adult B cells, and their progenitors[124]; and loss of C/EBPα leads to absolute neutropenia.[275] Moreover, the exogenous expression of several transcription factors in lineage committed progenitor cells can redirect cell fate. For example, C/EBPα is expressed in myeloid progenitor cells, and introduction of a regulatable C/EBPα gene into purified erythroid progenitors causes their switch to the myeloid lineage.[276] In further support of this hypothesis, several lines of evidence have been gathered, including the finding that forced expression of the antiapoptotic gene bcl_2 in a growth factor-dependent multipotential hematopoietic cell line resulted in growth factor independence and spontaneous differentiation into all of the possible cell lineages that develop when the corresponding growth factor(s) are added to the wild-type cells.[277]

In addition to providing these and other arguments in favor of a transcription factor-based intrinsic regulatory mechanism of stem cell fate, proponents of the intrinsic hypothesis point to feed-forward switch-like molecular mechanisms in which a stochastic increase in one of a binary set of such transcription factors reduces the level or activity of those transcription factors responsible for alternate cell fates. An example of this physiology is illustrated by the mutually antagonistic effects of the erythroid transcription factor GATA1 and the myeloid transcription factor PU.1; GATA1 acts to inhibit the myeloid activation potential of PU.1,[278] and PU.1 blocks the binding of GATA1 to its genetic target sites.[279] Thus, when the level of GATA1 stochastically rises above that of PU.1 in a CMP, the granulocyte-macrophage potential would be extinguished and the MEP potential of the cell would march forward, unfettered. Alternately, CMPs in which PU.1 levels rise above that of GATA1 would develop along the myeloid lineages, both through the direct stimulation of myeloid gene expression by PU.1, and indirectly by the blockade of GATA1-mediated erythroid and megakaryocytic gene expression programs.

The Case for Humoral Mediators

Although much evidence has been garnered in favor of an intrinsic mechanism of stem and progenitor cell fate determination, proponents of an extrinsic instructive hypothesis have also generated a large amount of compelling evidence in favor of the importance of extrinsic signals. One illustrative example of the capacity of certain extrinsic signals to impact specific patterns of differentiation is that the exogenous expression of an IL-2Rβ transgene in CLPs induces their differentiation into myeloid cells.[280] Subsequent studies revealed that the presence of the exogenous receptor leads to upregulation of the GM-CSF-R in the CLP, and that exogenous expression of GM-CSF-R could also lead a CLP toward monocyte/macrophage development.[2] In separate studies, other cytokines were shown to direct myeloid lineage fate determination; compared to the differentiation profile seen when marrow cells were cultured with SCF alone, an antiapoptotic stimulus, the addition of IL-5 greatly enhanced the number of marrow progenitor cells that gave rise to eosinophilic colonies, whereas the addition of TPO induced a predominance of megakaryocytic colonies, without significant changes in the number of apoptotic cells in any of the three culture conditions. These results were interpreted to indicate that while the SCF could keep nearly all progenitor cells alive under the cell culture conditions employed, the second cytokine directed the multilineage progenitors into specific cell fates.[281]

A number of external signaling events have been found to directly impact the transcriptional apparatus of the cell. For example, as previously noted, two transcription factors that lead to the self-renewal and expansion of HSCs, HOXB4, and HOXA9 are induced to higher levels of expression or to translocate into the nucleus of stem cells in response to TPO.[235,236] Moreover, SCL, a transcription factor that when expressed in maturing hematopoietic cells inhibits cytokine-induced granulocytic and monocytic differentiation, maintaining them in an undifferentiated state, is enhanced by SCF and down-modulated by GM-CSF.[131] Thus, strong evidence supporting both extrinsic and intrinsic control of lineage determination has been presented, and like the case for most conflicts in biology, it is most likely that elements of both mechanisms operate in hematopoiesis.

STEM CELL EXPANSION, SELF-RENEWAL, OR DIFFERENTIATION

The ability to divide symmetrically to generate identical daughters is a feature of most cells, including HSCs. However, the multipotent stem cell possesses an added ability to undergo asymmetric cell divisions, yielding one committed progenitor daughter and one stem cell daughter, or two differentiating progeny; regulating the balance between symmetric and asymmetric stem cell divisions becomes critical in maintaining proper HSC numbers and in meeting the demand for differentiated cells. A question related to the previous discussion of whether intrinsic or extrinsic factors determine HSC lineage fate, is whether intrinsic or extrinsic factors determine the possible outcomes for a dividing HSC (two HSC progeny [stem cell expansion], one HSC and one differentiating cell [a self-renewal division], or two differentiating progeny). It is clear that feedback mechanisms exist that govern the size of the stem cell pool, as following myeloablation and transplantation of a limited number of HSCs the pool expands toward that seen in a normal individual but not beyond, even when subjected to forced overexpression of genes that enhance HSC expansion.[282] HSCs do not appear to have a limit on their capacity for expansion; experiments using serial transplantation of marrow cells revealed that even after four such maneuvers the transplantation of a limiting number of HSCs was associated with a tenfold expansion in the recipient,[283] a level of expansion remarkably consistent from one serial transplant to the next. Thus, there does not appear to be an intrinsic limit on HSC expansion that sets the size of the stem cell pool. Rather, evidence from quantitative transplants suggests that there exist both intrinsic and extrinsic controls on the size of the stem cell pool.

Using a competitive repopulation strategy Pawliuk and colleagues showed that following transplantation the degree to which a limiting number of transplanted HSCs expand depends on the source of the cells; fetal liver cells expand to a far greater degree than a similar number of adult marrow-derived HSCs,[284] suggesting to these investigators that an intrinsic mechanism governs stem cell expansion divisions. However, evidence for an extrinsic mechanism that regulates stem cell expansion also exists, as the transplantation of a smaller number of either fetal liver or adult marrow HSCs resulted in slower marrow recovery but ultimately greater levels of HSC expansion than did infusion of larger numbers of cells. These results were interpreted to suggest that the more rapid recovery of marrow function associated with the administration of a larger marrow inoculum, with its increased numbers of stem cells, prematurely shut down HSC expansion, calling attention to an extrinsic regulatory mechanism. Moreover, the differences in expansion capacity amongst fetal and adult stem cells might also reflect the influence of extrinsic factors When adult human marrow cells are transplanted, they retain their stem cell capacity only if quiescent at the time of transfer.[285] In contrast, fetal liver and cord blood stem cells contribute to long-term hematopoiesis regardless of the phase of the cell cycle in which they reside at the time of harvest.[286] It is postulated that this latter property of fetal stem cells depends on the fetal hematopoietic microenvironment, making it likely that extrinsic factors play the key role in the decision to self-renew or differentiate. Strong experimental evidence has been generated indicating that stem cell numbers in an individual are governed by the number of hematopoietic niches.[287] This data strongly suggests that, at the very least, the availability of stem cell niches places an upper limit upon HSC expansion.

Clues from the developmental biology of lower organisms may also shed important insights into the mechanisms that regulate the decision between symmetric and asymmetric HSC divisions.[288] Within the niche of developing Drosophila gonadal tissue exist hierarchies of cells. When female gonadal stem cells divide, the cell directly contacting the niche supportive cells remains a stem cell, the daughter that loses contact differentiates and initiates oogenesis. A similar niche architecture also sets the stage for gonadal stem cell retention in the fly testis and in many tissues of many organisms. The developing principle is that a stem cell in contact with the stem cell determining niche stromal cell, or residing in a region of the niche possessing the highest concentration of a stem cell determining soluble factor, will remain a stem cell, and those removed from contact or soluble factor will differentiate. In such a niche, the axis of stem cell division then determines cell fate; if the axis of cell division is parallel to the front of stem cell determining contact or soluble mediator gradient, the proximal cell will remain a stem cell while the distal cell differentiates; if the axis of cell division is perpendicular, both cells will remain under the influence of the "stemness" factor(s), and remain stem cells. Consequently, spindle-polarizing signals could be responsible for the fate of the daughters of stem cell division, a focus of much research, but at present, few established mechanisms.

STEM CELL PLASTICITY

A remarkable observation has been repeatedly made in patients who underwent sex-mismatched (male into female) marrow transplantation, subsequent organ damage, and careful study at the time of their eventual death. In such settings, Y chromosome-bearing cells were identified at the site of repair of previous myocardial infarctions, strokes, and other organ damage. These observations suggest that hematopoietic cells can contribute to the replacement of damaged cells of multiple organs. More direct experimentation has lent additional support to this idea; several investigators have found that marrow cells are capable of giving rise to cells of multiple organs, including nerve,[289,290] liver,[291,292] skeletal muscle,[293] and cardiac muscle,[294] in a process termed *transdifferentiation*. However, direct evidence establishing this conclusion is lacking, as most such studies have assayed only partially purified cell populations that might also contain alternate types of stem cells,[295] and almost none have been performed using single cells, a requirement for robust proof of their multipotency. An alternate explanation for the presence of marked hematopoietic cells at nonhematopoietic sites of organ damage has been termed *cell fusion*. It has long been appreciated that marrow cells (especially macrophages) can fuse with other cells, and spontaneous *in vitro* fusion of embryonic stem cells with marrow-derived cells yields hybrids that display stem cell function[296,297]; further experimentation is required to prove or disprove the concept of HSC plasticity,[300] a proof that will have far reaching implications for regenerative medicine.

HEMATOPOIETIC PROGENITORS

The loss of one or more developmental potentials of the HSC results in a progenitor committed to any number of specific hematopoietic cell lineages. Besides the loss of pluripotency, committed hematopoietic progenitors display a number of characteristics that differ from their parents, including the lack of capacity for self-renewal, a higher fraction of cells traversing the cell cycle, reduced ability to efflux foreign substances, and a change in their surface protein profile. On the genetic level, the transition of HSCs to committed progenitors is marked by the downregulation of a large number of HSC-associated genes and progressive upregulation of a limited number of lineage-specific genes. This section highlights some of the features of specific lineage-committed progenitors that allow for their purification, characterization, and, potentially, their manipulation for therapeutic benefit. Details of the morphologic, biochemical, and genetic aspects of the differentiation of each of these progenitors is found in the chapters corresponding to their mature blood cell types.

PROGENITOR CELL ASSAYS

Assays for most hematopoietic progenitor cells consist of marrow or (occasionally) blood cells, either unfractionated or purified to varying degrees, a semisolid support (either methylcellulose or agar, which prevents cellular migration), and a source of hematopoietic growth factors. The cultures are incubated in a humidified environment at 37°C (98.6°F) for 2 to 7 days for murine cells, or 5 to 14 days for human cells, during which time the vast majority of the cells that began culture as mature blood cells die, allowing the few hematopoietic progenitors present to proliferate and differentiate into mature blood cells. As the cells in such culture systems are immobilized by the semisolid supporting matrix, all of the progeny in the resultant colonies are derived from a single progenitor, allowing one to retrospectively determine the developmental capacity of that cell, termed a *colony-forming cell* (CFC) or *unit* (CFU). The requirement for a source of hematopoietic growth factors was initially fulfilled by using cellular underlayers containing fibroblasts, lymphocytes, or monocytes, or tissue culture medium conditioned by a variety of normal and neoplastic cellular sources, but essentially all the requisite growth factors are now available in purified recombinant form. Despite substantial progress in our understanding of the developmental requirements of committed hematopoietic progenitors, we still do not have an adequate *in vitro* colony-forming assay for some well-characterized hematopoietic progenitor cells (e.g., those committed to the T lymphocytic or natural killer [NK] cell lineages) that still require more complex assays (e.g., fetal thymus explant assay).

CHARACTERISTICS OF SPECIFIC PROGENITOR CELL TYPES

Lymphoid Progenitors

Common Lymphoid Progenitors (CLP) The existence of a population of cells committed to all lymphoid lineages but devoid of myeloid capacity was theorized to exist based on a number of analyses. For example, patients with adenosine deaminase deficiency, or mice with genetic elimination of the γ_C receptor, the signaling kinase JAK3, or the transcription factor Ikaros lack T and B lymphocytes and have few, if any, myeloid defects, arguing that the defects in these disorders might affect a CLP; however, this does not prove the existence of a cell common for all. Work using cell sorting for CD10+/CD34+/Thy$^-$/c-Kit$^-$/Lin$^-$ human marrow cells revealed the capacity to develop into T, B, NK, and lymphoid dendritic cell progenitors,[298] but the report did not demonstrate a common progenitor capable of giving rise to each lineage on a clonal level.

More recent work, based upon the importance of IL-7 for all single-lineage lymphoid progenitor cells, and on the severe lymphopenia seen when the gene was eliminated in mice,[299] has indicated that the IL-7R marks a CLP that can be used in flow cytometry to isolate a population of IL7R$^+$/Lin$^-$/Thy$^-$/Sca^{lo}/Kit^{lo} cells that engrafts all of lymphopoiesis but no myelopoiesis in congenic mice.[37] For example, the injection of 2000 such CD45.1+ cells plus 1×10^5 whole-marrow CD45.2+ cells into lethally irradiated CD45.2 recipients lead to 3 to 20 percent CD45.1+ B and T lymphocytes, which disappear after approximately 6 months. In contrast, this strategy never results in the appearance of CD45.1+ myeloid cells. When limiting dilution studies were performed, about 1 in 20 such cells could give rise to short-term B-lymphopoiesis when injected intravenously, and an equal number could give rise to T-lymphopoiesis when injected into the thymus. In colony-forming assays using IL-7, SCF, and FL, approximately 20 percent of such cells gave rise to pre-B and pro-B cell colonies *in vitro*. Thus, given the low likelihood of proper homing when injected into mice, it is almost certain that the CLP exists and is IL7R$^+$/Lin$^-$/Thy$^-$/Sca^{lo}/Kit^{lo}. When a genetic expression analysis was performed comparing HSC to CLP, the latter demonstrated a down-modulation of many molecules associated with HSCs, such as the cell surface receptors c-Mpl, β_1-integrin, and Tie2 and the transcription factors HOXA9 and EGR1, and upregulation of the IL-7R and the recombination activating protein RAG2.[300]

T Lymphocyte/NK Cell, T Lymphocyte, and NK Cell Progenitors Simple colony-forming assays for mixed T/NK cell progenitors have not been developed, but the existence of the bipotent progenitor can be inferred from studies in which CD44+CD25–FcγRII/III$^-$ fetal thymic cells are cultured with genetically marked, deoxyguanosine treated fetal thymic lobes under 70 percent oxygen at 37°C (98.6°F). Without cytokine supplementation, such cultures yield primarily CD3+/Thy1$^+$ T cells, but if IL-2 plus IL-15 are added, the NK cell potential (CD3–/NK1.1$^+$) of these cells is realized, and if IL-7 is also added, the number of single cells that yield cells of both lineages increases significantly.[301] As this type of readout is possible from single day 12 fetal thymus cells, such studies establish that bipotent T/NK cell progenitors exist.

E box binding proteins consisting of HEB, E2–2, and the E2A gene products E12 and E47 form a distinct subgroup within the large family of basic helix-loop-helix transcription factors.[302] Heterodimers or homodimers form between family members through their HLH region, and through their basic regions bind to canonical E-box DNA sequences and thereby affect gene expression, including T cell targets such as CD4[303] and the pre-Tα,[304] and assist in recombination of the $\gamma\delta$ T-cell receptors.[305] It is now clear that E2A is required for the transition from the bipotent T/NK progenitor to committed T-cell progenitors as its genetic elimination leads to preservation of the former but elimination of the latter.[301]

Another important subgroup of HLH proteins is the Id family, which contain an HLH region but lack a DNA binding domain, thereby acting as a sink for functional HLH proteins and thus negatively regulating the function of E proteins.[306] Id proteins appear to be essential for NK cell development, as genetic elimination of Id2 leads to a profound loss of NK cell progenitors[307] and forced overexpression of Id3 leads to a shift of T/NK cells preferentially into the NK cell lineage.[308]

It is also clear that Notch activation plays a vital role in T-cell lineage commitment from the CLP. Overexpression of active Notch1 directs marrow stem cells into immature CD4+/CD8+ T cells and inhibits B-lymphocyte development.[309] Overexpression of Notch1 in RAG-deficient precursors also results in differentiation to the T-cell lineage, although only to the immature CD4–/CD8– stage, indicating that Notch cannot substitute for pre-T-cell receptor signaling.[310]

B-Lymphocyte Progenitors B-cell progenitors include the proB cell, the earliest cell irreversibly committed to the lineage, which are CD34+/CD10+/CD38+/CD19+/CD20+, the pre-B cell, which displays the initial stages of Ig rearrangement, expresses immunoglobulin heavy chains in their cytoplasm and are CD34–/CD10+/CD19+/CD20+/CD38–, and immature B cells which begin immunoglobulin light chain production, express cell surface IgM, and are CD10+/CD19+/CD20+. Pro-B cells can be detected in a simple colony-forming assay.[311] Normally, B-cell precursor development occurs in contact with the hematopoietic microenvironment, mediated by precursor cell integrin $\beta_1\beta_1$ and stromal cell VCAM or matrix fibronectin. A number of cytokines affect B-cell progenitor proliferation,[312] including IL-7,[313] insulin-like growth factor (IGF)-1,[314] SDF1,[315] and SCF,[316] although based on genetic knockout studies, B cells are absolutely dependent only on IL-7[299] and SDF1.[22]

A number of cytokines also inhibit B-cell precursor development, including interferon alpha/beta (IFN-α/β),[317] IFN-γ,[318] IL-4,[319] and TGF-β.[320] The role of these and other inhibitory cytokines in B lymphopoiesis is complex, as in some situations a cytokine can inhibit one stage and stimulate another stage of development, and some might act indirectly.

A number of transcription factors are required for mature B cell function, including PU.1, nuclear factor-κB (NF-κB), early B-cell factor (EBF), interferon regulatory factor 4 (IRF4), and Oct2, many of which bind to the promoters and enhancers involved in immunoglobulin gene expression. In contrast to these relatively later stage effects, E2A is required for commitment to the lineage.[321] The marrow of E2A-deficient mice is devoid of CD19 B cells, as well as most B lineage-specific genes, including Rag1/2, Pax5, EBF, and VpreB. Moreover, no immunoglobulin rearrangement is detectable, and there are no IL-7 responsive cells. Reintroduction of E2A into the marrow cells of null mice reconstitutes pre-B-cell development.[322]

E2A sits upon a hierarchy of B-cell lineage-specific genes and transcription factors[323]; E2A directly regulates the expression of Rag1, λ5, D-J_H, V-Jκ and the transcription factor EBF, the latter, in turn, regulating VpreB, mb-1, D-J_H, V-Jκ, and the transcription factor Pax5, which, in turn, regulates CD19 and LEF1 and shuts down genes associated with alternate lineages, such as M-CSF-R (monocytic), myeloperoxidase (neutrophilic), GATA1 (MEP), and pTα (T lymphocytic). As noted in "Notch Ligands" above, a critical condition for B-cell commitment is the absence of Notch signaling.

Myeloid Progenitors

Common Myeloid Progenitors Flow cytometry has also been extensively used to purify myeloid progenitors; an IL-7R$^-$/Lin$^-$/c-Kit$^+$/Sca-1$^-$ population of murine marrow cells, which by virtue of being Sca1$^-$ excludes HSCs, develop into all myeloid lineages.[36] Based on expression of CD34 and the FcγRII/III, three distinct subpopulations can be identified by further flow cytometry, IL-7Rα^-/Lin$^-$/c-Kit$^+$/Sca-1$^-$/CD34+/FcRγ^{lo}, IL-7Rα^-/Lin$^-$/c-Kit$^+$/Sca-1$^-$/CD34–/FcRγ^{lo}, and IL-7Rα^-/Lin$^-$/c-Kit$^+$/Sca-1$^-$/CD34+/FcRγ^{hi}. When tested in colony-forming assays in the presence of SCF, FL, IL-11, IL-3, GM-CSF, EPO, and TPO, each cell population yielded distinct mature cell types.[36] IL-7Rα^-/Lin$^-$/c-Kit$^+$/Sca-1$^-$/CD34+/FcRγ^{lo} cells give rise to all myeloid colony types, including CFU-Mix, BFU-E, CFU-megakaryocyte (CFU-Meg), MEP, CFU-GM, CFU-granulocyte (CFU-G), and CFU-macrophage (CFU-M), consistent with that expected for the CMP. In contrast, IL-7Rα^-/Lin$^-$/c-Kit$^+$/Sca-1$^-$/CD34+/FcRγ^{hi} cells form only CFU-M-, CFU-G-, and CFU-GM-derived colonies in response to any of the growth factors, alone or in combination, and thus represent granulocyte/macrophage lineage-restricted progenitors (GMP). Finally, IL-7Rα^-/Lin$^-$/c-Kit$^+$/Sca-1$^-$/CD34–/FcRγ^{lo} cells form only BFU-E-, CFU-Meg-, and mixed megakaryocyte-erythroid colonies, leading to their designation as MEP. To demonstrate their capacity to differentiate *in vivo*, limiting numbers of each cell population were transplanted into congenic mice; in such studies, cell fate outcomes correspond strictly with those of the *in vitro* colony assays. For example, 6 days after injection of 5000 CMPs, both donor-derived Gr-1$^+$/Mac-1$^+$ myelomonocytic cells and TER119$^+$ erythroid cells were detectable in recipients. In contrast, when 5000 GMPs were transplanted, only Gr-1$^+$/Mac-1$^+$ cells were recovered, and only for a transient period of time. Likewise, megakaryocytic-erythroid progenitors (MEPs) reconstituted only TER119$^+$ cells in similar experiments, and the genetically marked progeny from each of these progenitor populations disappear within 4 weeks of transplantation, indicating their limited self-renewal capacity.

Erythroid/Megakaryopoietic, Erythroid, and Megakaryopoietic Progenitors Culture conditions necessary for *in vitro* erythropoiesis have been known for nearly 35 years,[324,325] with colony morphologies ranging from small compact clusters of 20 to 50 erythrocytes developing with 2 to 5 days in murine and human marrow plasma clot cultures (colony forming unit–erythroid [CFU-E]), to large highly complex colonies containing up to thousands of cells taking from 7 to 14 days to develop in methylcellulose or agar (BFU-E). The cytokine requirement for the former is simple—EPO; whereas a cytokine that stimulates earlier cells, such as IL-3 or SCF, is required for the latter progenitor cell type.

Culture conditions that support the proliferation of Meg progenitors have been established for both mouse and man.[29,31] Using either methylcellulose, agar, or a plasma clot, two colony morphologies that contain exclusively megakaryocytes have been described. The CFU-Meg is a cell that develops into a simple colony containing from 3 to 50 mature Megs, larger, more complex colonies that include satellite collections of Megs and contain up to several hundred cells are derived from the burst-forming unit–megakaryocyte (BFU-Meg). Because of the difference in their proliferative potential and by analogy to erythroid progenitors, BFU-Meg and CFU-Meg are thought to represent primitive and mature progenitors restricted to the Meg lineage. And like their erythroid counterparts, the cytokine requirements for CFU-Meg are simple: TPO stimulates the growth of 75 percent of all CFU-Meg, with IL-3 being required along with TPO for the remainder,[77] whereas IL-3 or SCF is required alone with TPO for more complex, larger Meg colony formation from their more primitive progenitors.

Progenitors for erythrocytes and Megs display many common features: they share a number of transcription factors (SCL, GATA1, GATA2, NF-E2), cell surface molecules (TER119), and cytokine receptors (for IL-3, SCF, EPO, and TPO), and most erythroid and Meg leukemia cell lines display, or can be induced to display features of the alternate lineage.[326] Moreover, the cytokines most responsible for development of these two lineages—EPO and TPO—are the two most closely related proteins in the hematopoietic cytokine family[148] and display synergy in stimulating the growth of progenitors of both lineages.[77] For these and other reasons it has been postulated that erythropoiesis and megakaryopoiesis share a common progenitor cell,[327] a hypothesis now established[36] with the identification of IL-7Rα^-/Lin$^-$/c-Kit$^+$/Sca-1$^-$/CD34–/FcRγ^{lo} cells.

Like other primitive hematopoietic cells, bipotent MEP progenitors resemble small lymphocytes but can be distinguished by a specific pattern of cell surface protein display. As noted above, MEPs are IL-7Rα^-/Lin$^-$/c-Kit$^+$/Sca-1$^-$/CD34–/FcRγ^{lo}. Cells committed to the Meg lineage then begin to express CD41 and CD61 (integrin αIIbβ_3), CD42 (glycoprotein Ib), and glycoprotein V. Those that are committed to the erythroid lineage begin to express CD41 and the transferrin receptor (CD71), and as they mature lose CD41 expression but express the thrombospondin receptor (CD36), glycophorin, and, ultimately, globin.[328] These and other cell surface markers provide experimental hematologists several strategies to purify committed Meg[39,329] and erythroid[330] progenitors. Another useful method to identify megakaryoblasts is histochemical staining for von Willebrand factor, and in rodents, acetylcholinesterase.[331]

The transcription factors expressed by erythroid and Meg progenitors that allow for their commitment to the lineage are becoming increasingly well understood. GATA1 is an X-linked gene encoding a 50-kDa polypeptide that contains two zinc fingers required for DNA binding.[270] Genetic elimination of the transcription factor established the critical role of this transcription factor in hematopoiesis; GATA1 –/– mice are embryonic lethal as a consequence of failure of erythropoiesis,[332] and Meg-specific elimination of GATA1 leads to severe thrombocytopenia as a consequence of dysmegakaryopoiesis.[333] GATA1 acts in concert with another protein that affects transcription without binding to DNA, Friend of GATA (FOG).[334] The importance of this interaction to megakaryopoiesis is clear: several different mutations of the site on GATA1 responsible for FOG binding lead to congenital thrombocytopenia.[335]

The ets family of transcription factors includes about 30 members that bind to a purine box sequence, proteins that interact in both positive and antagonistic ways. For example, PU.1, initially termed Spi-1 based on its association with spleen focus-forming virus-induced erythroleukemias, blocks erythroid differentiation, although it appears important for megakaryocyte development.[336] Moreover, the ets factor Fli-1 is essential for megakaryopoiesis[337] and mutations in the transcription factor are also associated with congenital thrombocytopenia in man.[271]

Granulocyte/Monocytic, Granulocyte, and Monocytic Progenitors As noted above, GMPs (CFU-GM) are IL-7Rα^-/Lin$^-$/c-Kit$^+$/Sca-1$^-$/CD34+/FcRγ^{hi}, reflecting their beginning differentiation towards phagocytic cells (i.e., FcRγ positive). In the human, GMP are CD34+/CD33+/CD13+ markers, which are of clinical significance. For example, CD33 is also termed Siglec-2, a member of a family of sialic-acid-binding surface membrane proteins of the immunoglobulin superfamily that are involved in cell–cell interactions and signaling. Although the role of CD33 is not yet known with certainty, it has become a therapeutic target because of its high-level expression on the blasts of several forms of acute myelogenous leukemia[338]; the use of gemtuzumab ozogamicin, in which a humanized anti-CD33 monoclonal antibody has been fused to *N*-acetyl-gamma calicheamicin 1,2-dimethyl hydrazine dichloride, a potent antitumor antibiotic, has resulted in a complete remission rate of 15 to 20 percent as a single agent in patients with relapsed disease.[339] These initial successes have prompted its testing in earlier stage disease along with other active agents.[340] When marrow grafts are purged of CD33-bearing cells durable engraftment occurs, but is often quite delayed, indicating that CD33 is not present on the HSC, but that the presence of GMPs in a transplantation product is vital for rapid engraftment.

CD13 is also termed aminopeptidase N, an ectopeptidase present in many organs other than the marrow, a member of a family of proteases that play an important role in cell growth by virtue of their cleavage of biologically important peptides, in some cases inactivating, and in some cases activating them, and by serving a cell adhesive function as well. CD13 is present on early hematopoietic cells, including myeloid and lymphoid lineage progenitors, but disappears from the latter class of cells and its expression rises as monocytes mature. Although it functions to scavenge peptides in the intestinal brush border and degrade endorphins and enkephalins in the synaptic cleft, its role in hematopoiesis is less clear, although IL-8 is a substrate of its proteolytic activity.

Once bipotent GMPs differentiate, they further restrict their developmental potential. Monocytic progenitors are characterized by a predominance of PU.1, whereas granulocytic cells by members of the C/EBP family—C/EBPα and C/EBPε—are vital for the expression of neutrophil and eosinophil granule proteins.[272,341] A recent study suggests that the developmental decision of a bipotent GMP into each of the two lineages might be mediated by alterations in the relative levels of PU.1 and C/EBP expression[342]; haploinsufficiency of PU.1 (PU.1$^{+/-}$) results in a reduction in CFU-M frequency in the marrow and an increase in CFU-G levels, even ameliorating the neutropenia seen in G-CSF null mice. Moreover, by increasing expression of C/EBPα, a transcription factor that drives granulocytic differentiation, G-CSF further influences the choice between the granulocytic and monocytic lineages. However, it is also clear that PU.1 plays an important role in both lineages, and it is likely that additional investigation will yield new insights into the molecular mechanisms that establish the ordered process we term *myelopoiesis*.

REFERENCES

1. Ogawa M: Differentiation and proliferation of hematopoietic stem cells. *Blood* 81:2844, 1993.
2. Kondo M, Wagers AJ, Manz MG, et al: Biology of hematopoietic stem cells and progenitors: Implications for clinical application. *Annu Rev Immunol* 21:759, 2003.
3. Colvin GA, Lambert JF, Moore BE, et al: Intrinsic hematopoietic stem cell/progenitor plasticity: Inversions. *J Cell Physiol* 199:20, 2004.
4. Moore MA, Metcalf D: Ontogeny of the haemopoietic system: Yolk sac origin of *in vivo* and *in vitro* colony forming cells in the developing mouse embryo. *Br J Haematol* 18:279, 1970.
5. Flamme I, Frolich T, Risau W: Molecular mechanisms of vasculogenesis and embryonic angiogenesis. *J Cell Physiol* 173:206, 1997.
6. Jaffredo T, Gautier R, Eichmann A, et al: Intraaortic hemopoietic cells are derived from endothelial cells during ontogeny. *Development* 125:4575, 1998.
7. Palis J, Yoder MC: Yolk-sac hematopoiesis: The first blood cells of mouse and man. *Exp Hematol* 29:927, 2001.
8. Huang H, Zettergren LD, Auerbach R: *In vitro* differentiation of B cells and myeloid cells from the early mouse embryo and its extraembryonic yolk sac. *Exp Hematol* 22:19, 1994.
9. Cumano A, Dieterlen-Lievre F, Godin I: Lymphoid potential, probed before circulation in mouse, is restricted to caudal intraembryonic splanchnopleura. *Cell* 86:907, 1996.
10. Peault B, Oberlin E, Tavian M: Emergence of hematopoietic stem cells in the human embryo. *C R Biol* 325:1021, 2002.
11. Robin C, Ottersbach K, de Bruijn M, et al: Developmental origins of hematopoietic stem cells. *Oncol Res* 13:315, 2003.
12. Galloway JL, Zon LI: Ontogeny of hematopoiesis: Examining the emergence of hematopoietic cells in the vertebrate embryo. *Curr Top Dev Biol* 53:139, 2003.
13. Wood HB, May G, Healy L, et al: CD34 expression patterns during early mouse development are related to modes of blood vessel formation and reveal additional sites of hematopoiesis. *Blood* 90:2300, 1997.
14. Tavian M, Coulombel L, Luton D, et al: Aorta-associated CD34+ hematopoietic cells in the early human embryo. *Blood* 87:67, 1996.
15. Marshall CJ, Moore RL, Thorogood P, et al: Detailed characterization of the human aorta-gonad-mesonephros region reveals morphological polarity resembling a hematopoietic stromal layer. *Dev Dyn* 215:139, 1999.
16. Marshall CJ, Kinnon C, Thrasher AJ: Polarized expression of bone morphogenetic protein-4 in the human aorta-gonad-mesonephros region. *Blood* 96:1591, 2000.
17. Johnson GR, Moore MA: Role of stem cell migration in initiation of mouse foetal liver haemopoiesis. *Nature* 258:726, 1975.
18. Dzierzak E, Medvinsky A: Mouse embryonic hematopoiesis. *Trends Genet* 11(9):359, 1995.
19. Timens W, Kamps WA: Hemopoiesis in human fetal and embryonic liver. *Microsc Res Tech* 39:387, 1997.
20. Clapp DW, Freie B, Lee WH, et al: Molecular evidence that in situ-transduced fetal liver hematopoietic stem/progenitor cells give rise to medullary hematopoiesis in adult rats. *Blood* 86:2113, 1995.
21. Ara T, Tokoyoda K, Sugiyama T, et al: Long-term hematopoietic stem cells require stromal cell-derived factor-1 for colonizing bone marrow during ontogeny. *Immunity* 19:257, 2003.
22. Nagasawa T, Hirota S, Tachibana K, et al: Defects of B-cell lymphopoiesis and bone-marrow myelopoiesis in mice lacking the CXC chemokine PBSF/SDF-1. *Nature* 382:635, 1996.
23. Danchakoff V: Origin of the blood cells. Development of the haematopoietic organs and regeneration of the blood cells from the standpoint of the monophyletic school. *Anat Rec* 10:397, 1916.
24. Till JE, McCulloch CE: A direct measurement of the radiation sensitivity of normal mouse bone marrow cells. *Radiat Res* 14:213, 1961.
25. Pluznik DH, Sachs L: The cloning of normal "mast" cells in tissue culture. *J Cell Physiol* 66:319, 1965.
26. Bradley TR, Metcalf D: The growth of mouse bone marrow cells *in vitro*. *Aust J Exp Biol Med Sci* 44:287, 1966.
27. Silver RK, Erslev AJ: The action of erythropoietin on erythroid cells *in vitro*. *Scand J Haematol* 13:338, 1974.
28. Hara H, Ogawa M: Erthropoietic precursors in mice with phenylhydrazine-induced anemia. *Am J Hematol* 1:453, 1976.
29. Metcalf D, MacDonald HR, Odartchenko N, et al: Growth of mouse megakaryocyte colonies *in vitro*. *Proc Natl Acad Sci USA* 72:1744, 1975.
30. McLeod DL, Shreve MM, Axelrad AA. Induction of megakaryocyte colonies with platelet formation *in vitro*. *Nature* 261:492, 1976.

31. Vainchenker W, Bouguet J, Guichard J, et al: Megakaryocyte colony formation from human bone marrow precursors. *Blood* 54:940, 1979.
32. Spangrude GJ, Heimfeld S, Weissman IL: Purification and characterization of mouse hematopoietic stem cells. *Science* 241:58, 1988.
33. Civin CI, Strauss LC, Fackler MJ, et al: Positive stem cell selection—Basic science. *Prog Clin Biol Res* 333:387; discussion 402, 1990.
34. Matthews W, Jordan CT, Wiegand GW, et al: A receptor tyrosine kinase specific to hematopoietic stem and progenitor cell-enriched populations. *Cell* 65:1143, 1991.
35. Penn PE, Jiang DZ, Fei RG, et al: Dissecting the hematopoietic microenvironment. IX. Further characterization of murine bone marrow stromal cells. *Blood* 81:1205, 1993.
36. Kiel MJ, Yilmaz OH, Iwashita T, et al: SLAM family receptors distinguish hematopoietic stem and progenitor cells and reveal endothelial niches for stem cells. *Cell* 121:1109, 2005.
37. Akashi K, Traver D, Miyamoto T, et al: A clonogenic common myeloid progenitor that gives rise to all myeloid lineages. *Nature* 404:193, 2000.
38. Kondo M, Weissman IL, Akashi K: Identification of clonogenic common lymphoid progenitors in mouse bone marrow. *Cell* 91:661, 1997.
39. Muta K, Krantz SB, Bondurant MC, et al: Distinct roles of erythropoietin, insulin-like growth factor I, and stem cell factor in the development of erythroid progenitor cells. *J Clin Invest* 94:34, 1994.
40. Nakorn TN, Miyamoto T, Weissman IL: Characterization of mouse clonogenic megakaryocyte progenitors. *Proc Natl Acad Sci USA* 100:205, 2003.
41. Abkowitz JL, Catlin SN, McCallie MT, et al: Evidence that the number of hematopoietic stem cells per animal is conserved in mammals. *Blood* 100:2665, 2002.
42. Yilmaz OH, Kiel MJ, Morrison SJ: SLAM family markers are conserved among hematopoietic stem cells from old and reconstituted mice and markedly increase their purity, *Blood* 107:924, 2006.
43. Chen J, Astle CM, Harrison DE: Genetic regulation of primitive hematopoietic stem cell senescence. *Exp Hematol* 28:442, 2000.
44. Roobrouck VD, Ulloa-Montoya F, Verfaillie CM: Self-renewal and differentiation capacity of young and aged stem cells. *Exp Cell Res* 314:1937, 2008.
45. Dykstra B, de Haan G: Hematopoietic stem cell aging and self-renewal. *Cell Tissue Res* 331:91, 2008.
46. Chambers SM, Shaw CA, Gatza C, et al: Aging hematopoietic stem cells decline in function and exhibit epigenetic dysregulation. *PLoS Biol* 5:e201, 2007
47. Rossi DJ, Bryder D, Seita J, et al: Deficiencies in DNA damage repair limit the function of haematopoietic stem cells with age. *Nature* 447:725, 2007.
48. Nijnik A, Woodbine L, Marchetti C, et al: DNA repair is limiting for haematopoietic stem cells during ageing. *Nature* 447:686, 2007.
49. Mazurier F, Gan OI, McKenzie JL, et al: Lentivector-mediated clonal tracking reveals intrinsic heterogeneity in the human hematopoietic stem cell compartment and culture-induced stem cell impairment. *Blood* 103:545, 2004.
50. Mazurier F, Doedens M, Gan OI, et al: Rapid myeloerythroid repopulation after intrafemoral transplantation of NOD-SCID mice reveals a new class of human stem cells. *Nat Med* 9:959, 2003.
51. Cao YA, Wagers AJ, Beilhack A, et al: Shifting foci of hematopoiesis during reconstitution from single stem cells. *Proc Natl Acad Sci USA* 101:221, 2004.
52. Harrison DE: Competitive repopulation: A new assay for long-term stem cell functional capacity. *Blood* 55:77, 1980.
53. Nakorn TN, Traver D, Weissman IL, Akashi K: Myeloerythroid restricted progenitors are sufficient to confer radioprotection and provide the majority of day 8 CFU-S. J Clin Invest 109:1579, 2002.
54. Larochelle A, Vormoor J, Hanenberg H, et al: Identification of primitive human hematopoietic cells capable of repopulating NOD/SCID mouse bone marrow: Implications for gene therapy. *Nat Med* 2:1329, 1996.
55. Thanopoulou E, Cashman J, Kakagianne T, et al: Engraftment of NOD/SCID-$_2$ microglobulin null mice with multi-lineage neoplastic cells from patients with myelodysplastic syndrome. *Blood* 103:4285, 2004.
56. Ito M, Hiramatsu H, Kobayashi K, et al: NOD/SCID/gamma©(null) mouse: An excellent recipient mouse model for engraftment of human cells. *Blood* 100:3175, 2002.
57. Feuring-Buske M, Gerhard B, Cashman J, et al: Improved engraftment of human acute myeloid leukemia progenitor cells in beta 2-microglobulin-deficient NOD/SCID mice and in NOD/SCID mice transgenic for human growth factors. *Leukemia* 17:760, 2003.
58. Tanavde VM, Malehorn MT, Lumkul R, et al: Human stem-progenitor cells from neonatal cord blood have greater hematopoietic expansion capacity than those from mobilized adult blood. *Exp Hematol* 30:816, 2002.
59. Miyoshi H, Smith KA, Mosier DE, et al: Transduction of human CD34+ cells that mediate long-term engraftment of NOD/SCID mice by HIV vectors. *Science* 283:682, 1999.
60. Scherr M, Battmer K, Blomer U, et al: Lentiviral gene transfer into peripheral blood-derived CD34+ NOD/SCID-repopulating cells. *Blood* 99:709, 2002.
61. Cashman J, Dykstra B, Clark-Lewis I, et al: Changes in the proliferative activity of human hematopoietic stem cells in NOD/SCID mice and enhancement of their transplantability after *in vivo* treatment with cell cycle inhibitors. *J Exp Med* 196:1141, 2002.
62. Guenechea G, Segovia JC, Albella B, et al: Delayed engraftment of nonobese diabetic/severe combined immunodeficient mice transplanted with *ex vivo*-expanded human CD34(+) cord blood cells. *Blood* 93:1097, 1999.
63. Ueda T, Tsuji K, Yoshino H, et al: Expansion of human NOD/SCID-repopulating cells by stem cell factor, Flk2/Flt3 ligand, thrombopoietin, IL-6, and soluble IL-6 receptor. *J Clin Invest* 105:1013, 2000.
64. Zielske SP, Gerson SL: Cytokines, including stem cell factor alone, enhance lentiviral transduction in nondividing human LTCIC and NOD/SCID repopulating cells. *Mol Ther* 7:325, 2003.
65. Glimm H, Oh IH, Eaves CJ: Human hematopoietic stem cells stimulated to proliferate *in vitro* lose engraftment potential during their S/G(2)/M transit and do not reenter G(0). *Blood* 96:4185, 2000.
66. Dexter TM, Allen TD, Lajtha LG: Conditions controlling the proliferation of haemopoietic stem cells *in vitro*. *J Cell Physiol* 91:335, 1977.
67. Coulombel L, Eaves AC, Eaves CJ: Enzymatic treatment of long-term human marrow cultures reveals the preferential location of primitive hemopoietic progenitors in the adherent layer. *Blood* 62:291, 1983.
68. Sutherland HJ, Lansdorp PM, Henkelman DH, et al: Functional characterization of individual human hematopoietic stem cells cultured at limiting dilution on supportive marrow stromal layers. *Proc Natl Acad Sci USA* 87:3584, 1990.
69. Ploemacher RE, van der Sluijs JP, Voerman JS, et al: An *in vitro* limiting-dilution assay of long-term repopulating hematopoietic stem cells in the mouse. *Blood* 74:2755, 1989.
70. Fackler MJ, Krause DS, Smith OM, et al: Full-length but not truncated CD34 inhibits hematopoietic cell differentiation of M1 cells. *Blood* 85:3040, 1995.
71. Krause DS, Fackler MJ, Civin CI, et al: CD34: Structure, biology, and clinical utility. *Blood* 87:1, 1996.
72. Verfaillie CM: Adhesion receptors as regulators of the hematopoietic process. *Blood* 92:2609, 1998.
73. Baum CM, Weissman IL, Tsukamoto AS, et al: Isolation of a candidate human hematopoietic stem-cell population. *Proc Natl Acad Sci USA* 89:2804, 1992.
74. Barda-Saad M, Rozenszajn LA, Ashush H, et al: Adhesion molecules involved in the interactions between early T cells and mesenchymal bone marrow stromal cells. *Exp Hematol* 27:834, 1999.
75. Sanchez MJ, Holmes A, Miles C, et al: Characterization of the first definitive hematopoietic stem cells in the AGM and liver of the mouse embryo. *Immunity* 5:513, 1996.
76. Broudy VC: Stem cell factor and hematopoiesis. *Blood* 90:1345, 1997.
77. Broudy VC, Lin NL, Kaushansky K: Thrombopoietin (c-mpl ligand) acts synergistically with erythropoietin, stem cell factor, and interleukin-11 to enhance murine megakaryocyte colony growth and increases megakaryocyte ploidy *in vitro*. *Blood* 85:1719, 1995.
78. Dean YD, McGreal EP, Akatsu H, et al: Molecular and cellular properties of the rat AA4 antigen, a C-type lectin-like receptor with structural homology to thrombomodulin. *J Biol Chem* 275:34382, 2000.
79. Uchida N, Weissman IL: Searching for hematopoietic stem cells: Evidence that Thy-1.110 Lin− Sca-1+ cells are the only stem cells in C57BL/Ka-Thy-1.1 bone marrow. *J Exp Med* 175:175, 1992.
80. Ito CY, Li CY, Bernstein A, et al: Hematopoietic stem cell and progenitor defects in Sca-1/Ly-6A-null mice. *Blood* 101:517, 2003.
81. Miraglia S, Godfrey W, Yin AH, et al: A novel five-transmembrane hematopoietic stem cell antigen: Isolation, characterization, and molecular cloning. *Blood* 90:5013, 1997.
82. Fargeas CA, Florek M, Huttner WB, et al: Characterization of prominin-2, a new member of the prominin family of pentaspan membrane glycoproteins. *J Biol Chem* 278:8586, 2003.
83. Watt SM, Buhring HJ, Rappold I, et al: CD164, a novel sialomucin on CD34(+) and erythroid subsets, is located on human chromosome 6q21. *Blood* 92:849, 1998.
84. Zannettino AC, Buhring HJ, Niutta S, et al: The sialomucin CD164 (MGC-24v) is an adhesive glycoprotein expressed by human hematopoietic progenitors and bone marrow stromal cells that serves as a potent negative regulator of hematopoiesis. *Blood* 92:2613, 1998.
85. Kiel MJ, Yilmaz OH, Iwashita T, et al: SLAM family receptors distinguish hematopoietic stem and progenitor cells and reveal endothelial niches for stem cells. *Cell* 121:1109, 2005.
86. Zeigler FC, de Sauvage F, Widmer HR, et al: *In vitro* megakaryocytopoietic and thrombopoietic activity of c-mpl ligand (TPO) on purified murine hematopoietic stem cells. *Blood* 84:4045, 1994.
87. Solar GP, Kerr WG, Zeigler FC, et al: Role of c-mpl in early hematopoiesis. *Blood* 92:4, 1998.
88. Ballmaier M, Germeshausen M, Schulze H, et al: C-mpl mutations are the cause of congenital amegakaryocytic thrombocytopenia. *Blood* 97:139, 2001.
89. Hynes RO: Integrins: Versatility, modulation, and signaling in cell adhesion. *Cell* 69:11, 1992.
90. Fukai F, Mashimo M, Akiyama K, et al: Modulation of apoptotic cell death by extracellular matrix proteins and a fibronectin-derived antiadhesive peptide. *Exp Cell Res* 242:92, 1998.
91. Fang F, Orend G, Watanabe N, et al: Dependence of cyclin E-CDK2 kinase activity on cell anchorage. *Science* 271:499, 1996.
92. Pozzi A, Wary KK, Giancotti FG, et al: Integrin alpha$_1$beta$_1$ mediates a unique collagen-dependent proliferation pathway *in vivo*. *J Cell Biol* 142:587, 1998.
93. Tropel P, Roullot V, Vernet M, et al: A 2.7-kb portion of the 5′ flanking region of the murine glycoprotein alphaIIb gene is transcriptionally active in primitive hematopoietic progenitor cells. *Blood* 90:2995, 1997.

94. Kovach NL, Lin N, Yednock T, et al: Stem cell factor modulates avidity of alpha 4 beta 1 and alpha 5 beta 1 integrins expressed on hematopoietic cell lines. *Blood* 85:159, 1995.
95. Zauli G, Bassini A, Vitale M, et al: Thrombopoietin enhances the alpha IIb beta 3-dependent adhesion of megakaryocytic cells to fibrinogen or fibronectin through PI 3 kinase. *Blood* 89:883, 1997.
96. Peled A, Kollet O, Ponomaryov T, et al: The chemokine SDF-1 activates the integrins LFA-1, VLA-4, and VLA-5 on immature human CD34(+) cells: Role in transendothelial/stromal migration and engraftment of NOD/SCID mice. *Blood* 95:3289, 2000.
97. Papayannopoulou T: Mechanisms of stem-/progenitor-cell mobilization: The anti-VLA-4 paradigm. *Semin Hematol* 37:11, 2000.
98. Chaudhary PM, Roninson IB: Expression and activity of P-glycoprotein, a multidrug efflux pump, in human hematopoietic stem cells. *Cell* 66:85, 1991.
99. Scharenberg CW, Harkey MA, Torok-Storb B: The ABCG2 transporter is an efficient Hoechst 33342 efflux pump and is preferentially expressed by immature human hematopoietic progenitors. *Blood* 99:507, 2002.
100. Wolf NS, Kone A, Priestley GV, et al: *In vivo* and *in vitro* characterization of long-term repopulating primitive hematopoietic cells isolated by sequential Hoechst 33342-rhodamine 123 FACS selection. *Exp Hematol* 21:614, 1993.
101. Uchida N, Fujisaki T, Eaves AC, et al: Transplantable hematopoietic stem cells in human fetal liver have a CD34(+) side population (SP)phenotype. *J Clin Invest* 108:1071, 2001.
102. Habibian HK, Peters SO, Hsieh CC, et al: The fluctuating phenotype of the lympho-hematopoietic stem cell with cell cycle transit. *J Exp Med* 188:393, 1998.
103. Orschell-Traycoff CM, Hiatt K, Dagher RN, et al: Homing and engraftment potential of Sca-1(+)lin() cells fractionated on the basis of adhesion molecule expression and position in cell cycle. *Blood* 96:1380, 2000.
104. Stier S, Cheng T, Forkert R, et al: *Ex vivo* targeting of p21Cip1/Waf1 permits relative expansion of human hematopoietic stem cells. *Blood* 102:1260, 2003.
105. Lambert JF, Liu M, Colvin GA, et al: Marrow stem cells shift gene expression and engraftment phenotype with cell cycle transit. *J Exp Med* 197:1563, 2003.
106. Wilpshaar J, Falkenburg JH, Tong X, et al: Similar repopulating capacity of mitotically active and resting umbilical cord blood CD34(+) cells in NOD/SCID mice. *Blood* 96:2100, 2000.
107. Hu M, Krause D, Greaves M, et al: Multilineage gene expression precedes commitment in the hemopoietic system. *Genes Dev* 11:774, 1997.
108. Miyamoto T, Iwasaki H, Reizis B, et al: Myeloid or lymphoid promiscuity as a critical step in hematopoietic lineage commitment. *Dev Cell* 3:137, 2002.
109. Nutt SL, Heavey B, Rolink AG, et al: Commitment to the B-lymphoid lineage depends on the transcription factor Pax5. *Nature* 401:556, 1999.
110. Phillips RL, Ernst RE, Brunk B, et al: The genetic program of hematopoietic stem cells. *Science* 288:1635, 2000.
111. Terskikh AV, Easterday MC, Li L, et al: From hematopoiesis to neuropoiesis: Evidence of overlapping genetic programs. *Proc Natl Acad Sci USA* 98:7934, 2001.
112. Lessard, J, Sauvageau, G. Bmi-1 determines the proliferative capacity of normal and leukaemic stem cells. *Nature* 423:255, 2003.
113. Tadokoro Y, Ema H, Okano M, Li E, Nakauchi H: *De novo* DNA methyltransferase is essential for self-renewal, but not for differentiation, in hematopoietic stem cells. *J Exp Med* 204:715, 2007.
114. Cillo C, Cantile M, Faiella A, et al: Homeobox genes in normal and malignant cells. *J Cell Physiol* 188:161, 2001.
115. Magli MC, Largman C, Lawrence HJ: Effects of HOX homeobox genes in blood cell differentiation. *J Cell Physiol* 173:168, 1997.
116. Sauvageau G, Thorsteinsdottir U, Eaves CJ, et al: Overexpression of HOXB4 in hematopoietic cells causes the selective expansion of more primitive populations *in vitro* and *in vivo*. *Genes Dev* 9:1753, 1995.
117. Buske C, Humphries RK: Homeobox genes in leukemogenesis. *Int J Hematol* 71:301, 2000.
118. Lawrence HJ, Helgason CD, Sauvageau G, et al: Mice bearing a targeted interruption of the homeobox gene HOXA9 have defects in myeloid, erythroid, and lymphoid hematopoiesis. *Blood* 89:1922, 1997.
119. Yagi H, Deguchi K, Aono A, et al: Growth disturbance in fetal liver hematopoiesis of Mll-mutant mice. *Blood* 92:108, 1998.
120. DiMartino JF, Selleri L, Traver D, et al: The Hox cofactor and proto-oncogene Pbx1 is required for maintenance of definitive hematopoiesis in the fetal liver. *Blood* 98:618, 2001.
121. Calvo KR, Knoepfler PS, Sykes DB, et al: Meis1a suppresses differentiation by G-CSF and promotes proliferation by SCF: Potential mechanisms of cooperativity with Hoxa9 in myeloid leukemia. *Proc Natl Acad Sci USA* 98:13120, 2001.
122. Georgopoulos K: Transcription factors required for lymphoid lineage commitment. *Curr Opin Immunol* 9:222, 1997.
123. Molnar A, Georgopoulos K: The Ikaros gene encodes a family of functionally diverse zinc finger DNA-binding proteins. *Mol Cell Biol* 14:8292, 1994.
124. Wang JH, Nichogiannopoulou A, Wu L, et al: Selective defects in the development of the fetal and adult lymphoid system in mice with an Ikaros null mutation. *Immunity* 5:537, 1996.
125. McKercher SR, Torbett BE, Anderson KL, et al: Targeted disruption of the PU.1 gene results in multiple hematopoietic abnormalities. *EMBO J* 15:5647, 1996.
126. Begley CG, Aplan PD, Denning SM, et al: The gene SCL is expressed during early hematopoiesis and encodes a differentiation-related DNA-binding motif. *Proc Natl Acad Sci USA* 86:10128, 1989.
127. Lecuyer E, Hoang T: SCL: From the origin of hematopoiesis to stem cells and leukemia. *Exp Hematol* 32:11, 2004.
128. Shivdasani RA, Mayer EL, Orkin SH: Absence of blood formation in mice lacking the T-cell leukaemia oncoprotein tal-1/SCL. *Nature* 373:432, 1995.
129. Brady G, Billia F, Knox J, et al: Analysis of gene expression in a complex differentiation hierarchy by global amplification of cDNA from single cells. *Curr Biol* 5:909, 1995.
130. Hoang T, Paradis E, Brady G, et al: Opposing effects of the basic helix-loop-helix transcription factor SCL on erythroid and monocytic differentiation. *Blood* 87:102, 1996.
131. Caceres-Cortes JR, Krosl G, Tessier N, et al: Steel factor sustains SCL expression and the survival of purified CD34+ bone marrow cells in the absence of detectable cell differentiation. *Stem Cells* 19:59, 2001.
132. Martin DI, Tsai SF, Orkin SH: Increased gamma-globin expression in a nondeletion HPFH mediated by an erythroid-specific DNA-binding factor. *Nature* 338:435, 1989.
133. Persons DA, Allay JA, Allay ER, et al: Enforced expression of the GATA-2 transcription factor blocks normal hematopoiesis. *Blood* 93:488, 1999.
134. Deveaux S, Filipe A, Lemarchandel V, et al: Analysis of the thrombopoietin receptor (MPL) promoter implicates GATA and Ets proteins in the coregulation of megakaryocyte-specific genes. *Blood* 87:4678, 1996.
135. Yamaguchi Y, Zon LI, Ackerman SJ, et al: Forced GATA-1 expression in the murine myeloid cell line M1: Induction of c-Mpl expression and megakaryocytic/erythroid differentiation. *Blood* 91:450, 1998.
136. Yamaguchi Y, Ackerman SJ, Minegishi N, et al: Mechanisms of transcription in eosinophils: GATA-1, but not GATA-2, transactivates the promoter of the eosinophil granule major basic protein gene. *Blood* 91:3447, 1998.
137. Long MW: Blood cell cytoadhesion molecules. *Exp Hematol* 20:288, 1992.
138. Dexter TM: Haemopoiesis in long-term bone marrow cultures. A review. *Acta Haematol* 62:299, 1979.
139. Kaushansky K, Lin N, Adamson JW: Interleukin 1 stimulates fibroblasts to synthesize granulocyte-macrophage and granulocyte colony-stimulating factors. Mechanism for the hematopoietic response to inflammation. *J Clin Invest* 81:92, 1988.
140. Toksoz D, Zsebo KM, Smith KA, et al: Support of human hematopoiesis in long-term bone marrow cultures by murine stromal cells selectively expressing the membrane-bound and secreted forms of the human homolog of the steel gene product, stem cell factor. *Proc Natl Acad Sci USA* 89:7350, 1992.
141. Selleri C, Maciejewski JP, Sato T, et al: Interferon-gamma constitutively expressed in the stromal microenvironment of human marrow cultures mediates potent hematopoietic inhibition. *Blood* 87:4149, 1996.
142. Guerriero A, Worford L, Holland HK, et al: Thrombopoietin is synthesized by bone marrow stromal cells. *Blood* 90:3444, 1997.
143. Miyazawa K, Williams DA, Gotoh A, et al: Membrane-bound Steel factor induces more persistent tyrosine kinase activation and longer life span of c-kit gene-encoded protein than its soluble form. *Blood* 85:641, 1995.
144. Gordon MY, Riley GP, Watt SM, et al: Compartmentalization of a haematopoietic growth factor (GM-CSF) by glycosaminoglycans in the bone marrow microenvironment. *Nature* 326:403, 1987.
145. Artavanis-Tsakonas S, Matsuno K, Fortini ME: Notch signaling. *Science* 268:225, 1995.
146. Nye JS, Kopan R: Developmental signaling. Vertebrate ligands for Notch. *Curr Biol* 5:966, 1995.
147. Karanu FN, Murdoch B, Miyabayashi T, et al: Human homologues of Delta-1 and Delta-4 function as mitogenic regulators of primitive human hematopoietic cells. *Blood* 97:1960, 2001.
148. Kapur R, Cooper R, Zhang L, et al: Cross-talk between alpha(4)beta(1)/alpha(5)beta(1) and c-Kit results in opposing effect on growth and survival of hematopoietic cells via the activation of focal adhesion kinase, mitogen-activated protein kinase, and Akt signaling pathways. *Blood* 97:1975, 2001.
149. Shaklai M, Tavassoli M: Cellular relationship in the rat bone marrow studied by freeze fracture and lanthanum impregnation thin-sectioning electron microscopy. *J Ultrastruct Res* 69:343, 1979.
150. Westen H, Bainton DF: Association of alkaline-phosphatase-positive reticulum cells in bone marrow with granulocytic precursors. *J Exp Med* 150:919, 1979.
151. Tavassoli M, Aoki M: Localization of megakaryocytes in the bone marrow. *Blood Cells* 15:3, 1989.
152. Blazsek I, Chagraoui J, Peault B: Ontogenic emergence of the hematon, a morphogenetic stromal unit that supports multipotential hematopoietic progenitors in mouse bone marrow. *Blood* 96:3763, 2000.
153. Verfaillie C, Blakolmer K, McGlave P: Purified primitive human hematopoietic progenitor cells with long-term *in vitro* repopulating capacity adhere selectively to irradiated bone marrow stroma. *J Exp Med* 172:509, 1990.
154. Simmons PJ, Masinovsky B, Longenecker BM, et al: Vascular cell adhesion molecule-1 expressed by bone marrow stromal cells mediates the binding of hematopoietic progenitor cells. *Blood* 80:388, 1992.
155. Rafii S, Shapiro F, Pettengell R, et al: Human bone marrow microvascular endothelial cells support long-term proliferation and differentiation of myeloid and megakaryocytic progenitors. *Blood* 86:3353, 1995.
156. Sugiyama T, Kohara H, Noda M, Nagasawa T: Maintenance of the hematopoietic stem cell pool by CXCL12-CXCR4 chemokine signaling in bone marrow stromal cell niches. *Immunity* 25:977, 2006.

157. Islam A, Glomski C, Henderson ES: Bone lining (endosteal) cells and hematopoiesis: A light microscopic study of normal and pathologic human bone marrow in plastic-embedded sections. *Anat Rec* 227:300, 1990.
158. Calvi LM, Adams GB, Weibrecht KW, et al: Osteoblastic cells regulate the haematopoietic stem cell niche. *Nature* 425:841, 2003.
159. Keating A: Mesenchymal stromal cells. *Curr Opin Hematol* 13:419, 2006.
160. Dazzi F, Horwood NJ: Potential of mesenchymal stem cell therapy. *Curr Opin Oncol* 19:650, 2007.
161. Lok S, Kaushansky K, Holly RD, et al: Cloning and expression of murine thrombopoietin cDNA and stimulation of platelet production *in vivo*. *Nature* 369:565, 1994.
162. McCarty JM, Sprugel KH, Fox NE, et al: Murine thrombopoietin mRNA levels are modulated by platelet count. *Blood* 86:3668, 1995.
163. Sungaran R, Markovic B, Chong BH: Localization and regulation of thrombopoietin mRNa expression in human kidney, liver, bone marrow, and spleen using in situ hybridization. *Blood* 89:101, 1997.
164. Solanilla A, Dechanet J, El Andaloussi A, et al: CD40-ligand stimulates myelopoiesis by regulating flt3-ligand and thrombopoietin production in bone marrow stromal cells. *Blood* 95:3758, 2000.
165. Quirici N, Soligo D, Caneva L, et al: Differentiation and expansion of endothelial cells from human bone marrow CD133(+) cells. *Br J Haematol* 115:186, 2001.
166. Yanai N, Sekine C, Yagita H, et al: Roles for integrin very late activation antigen-4 in stroma-dependent erythropoiesis. *Blood* 83:2844, 1994.
167. Jung Y, Wang J, Song J, et al: Annexin II expressed by osteoblasts and endothelial cells regulates stem cell adhesion, homing, and engraftment following transplantation. *Blood* 110:82, 2007.
168. Scott LM PG, Koni P, Papayannopoulou T: Adult mice with conditional VCAM-1 ablation show altered hemopoietic progenitor biodistribution, homing and regeneration patterns. *Blood* 102, 2003.
169. Carstanjen D, Ulbricht N, Iacone A, et al: Matrix metalloproteinase-9 (gelatinase B) is elevated during mobilization of peripheral blood progenitor cells by G-CSF. *Transfusion* 42:588, 2002.
170. Fibbe WE, Pruijt JF, van Kooyk Y, et al: The role of metalloproteinases and adhesion molecules in interleukin-8-induced stem-cell mobilization. *Semin Hematol* 37:19, 2000.
171. Russell ES: Hereditary anemias of the mouse: A review for geneticists. *Adv Genet* 20:357, 1979.
172. Huang EJ, Nocka KH, Buck J, et al: Differential expression and processing of two cell associated forms of the kit-ligand: KL-1 and KL-2. *Mol Biol Cell* 3:349, 1992.
173. Miller CL, Rebel VI, Helgason CD, et al: Impaired steel factor responsiveness differentially affects the detection and long-term maintenance of fetal liver hematopoietic stem cells *in vivo*. *Blood* 89:1214, 1997.
174. Ogawa M, Matsuzaki Y, Nishikawa S, et al: Expression and function of c-kit in hemopoietic progenitor cells. *J Exp Med* 174:63, 1991.
175. Li CL, Johnson GR: Stem-cell factor enhances the survival but not the self-renewal of murine hematopoietic long-term repopulating cells. *Blood* 84:408, 1994.
176. Bernstein ID, Andrews RG, Zsebo KM: Recombinant human stem-cell factor enhances the formation of colonies by CD34+ and CD34+Lin cells, and the generation of colony-forming cell progeny from CD34+Lin cells cultured with interleukin-3, granulocyte colony-stimulating factor, or granulocyte-macrophage colony-stimulating factor. *Blood* 77:2316, 1991.
177. Brandt J, Briddell RA, Srour EF, et al: Role of c-Kit ligand in the expansion of human hematopoietic progenitor cells. *Blood* 79:634, 1992.
178. Ariyama Y, Misawa S, Sonoda Y: Synergistic effects of stem-cell factor and interleukin-6 or interleukin-11 on the expansion of murine hematopoietic progenitors in liquid suspension-culture. *Stem Cells* 13:404, 1995.
179. Kent D, Copley M, Benz C, et al: Regulation of hematopoietic stem cells by the steel factor/KIT signaling pathway. *Clin Cancer Res* 14:1926, 2008.
180. Wu H, Klingmuller U, Acurio A, et al: Functional interaction of erythropoietin and stem cell factor receptors is essential for erythroid colony formation. *Proc Natl Acad Sci USA* 94:1806, 1997.
181. Lyman SD, James L, Johnson L, et al: Cloning of the human homolog of the murine Flt3 ligand—A growth factor for early hematopoietic progenitor cells. *Blood* 83:2795, 1994.
182. Rosnet O, Schiff C, Pebusque MJ, et al: Human Flt3/Flk2 gene—CDNA cloning and expression in hematopoietic cells. *Blood* 82:1110, 1993.
183. Yokota S, Kiyoi H, Nakao M, et al: Internal tandem duplication of the FLT3 gene is preferentially seen in acute myeloid leukemia and myelodysplastic syndrome among various hematological malignancies. A study on a large series of patients and cell lines. *Leukemia* 11:1605, 1997.
184. Thiede C, Steudel C, Mohr B, et al: Analysis of FLT3-activating mutations in 979 patients with acute myelogenous leukemia: Association with FAB subtypes and identification of subgroups with poor prognosis. *Blood* 99:4326, 2002.
185. Zwaan CM, Meshinchi S, Radich JP, et al: FLT3 internal tandem duplication in 234 children with acute myeloid leukemia: Prognostic significance and relation to cellular drug resistance. *Blood* 102:2387, 2003.
186. O'Farrell AM, Foran JM, Fiedler W, et al: An innovative phase I clinical study demonstrates inhibition of FLT3 phosphorylation by SU11248 in acute myeloid leukemia patients. *Clin Cancer Res* 9:5465, 2003.
187. Lyman SD, James L, Vanden Bos T, et al: Molecular cloning of a ligand for the flt3/flk-2 tyrosine kinase receptor: A proliferative factor for primitive hematopoietic cells. *Cell* 75:1157, 1993.
188. Lyman SD, James L, Escobar S, et al: Identification of soluble and membrane-bound isoforms of the murine flt3 ligand generated by alternative splicing of mRNAs. *Oncogene* 10:149, 1995.
189. Lyman SD, Seaberg M, Hanna R, et al: Plasma/serum levels of flt3 ligand are low in normal individuals and highly elevated in patients with Fanconi anemia and acquired aplastic anemia. *Blood* 86:4091, 1995.
190. Mackarehtschian K, Hardin JD, Moore KA, et al: Targeted disruption of the flk2/flt3 gene leads to deficiencies in primitive hematopoietic progenitors. *Immunity* 3:147, 1995.
191. Rasko JE, Metcalf D, Rossner MT, et al: The flt3/flk-2 ligand: Receptor distribution and action on murine haemopoietic cell survival and proliferation. *Leukemia* 9:2058, 1995.
192. Robinson S, Mosley RL, Parajuli P, et al: Comparison of the hematopoietic activity of flt-3 ligand and granulocyte-macrophage colony-stimulating factor acting alone or in combination. *J Hematother Stem Cell Res* 9:711, 2000.
193. Kobayashi M, Laver JH, Kato T, et al: Thrombopoietin supports proliferation of human primitive hematopoietic cells in synergy with steel factor and/or interleukin-3. *Blood* 88:429, 1996.
194. Piacibello W, Sanavio F, Garetto L, et al: Extensive amplification and self-renewal of human primitive hematopoietic stem cells from cord blood. *Blood* 89:2644, 1997.
195. Namikawa R, Muench MO, de Vries JE, et al: The FLK2/FLT3 ligand synergizes with interleukin-7 in promoting stromal-cell-independent expansion and differentiation of human fetal pro-B cells *in vitro*. *Blood* 87:1881, 1996.
196. Strobl H, Bello-Fernandez C, Riedl E, et al: Flt3 ligand in cooperation with transforming growth factor-beta1 potentiates *in vitro* development of Langerhans-type dendritic cells and allows single-cell dendritic cell cluster formation under serum-free conditions. *Blood* 90:1425, 1997.
197. Kaushansky K: Thrombopoietin: The primary regulator of platelet production. *Blood* 86:419, 1995.
198. Qian S, Fu F, Li W, et al: Primary role of the liver in thrombopoietin production shown by tissue-specific knockout. *Blood* 92:2189, 1998.
199. Kaushansky K: Thrombopoietin. *N Engl J Med* 339:746, 1998.
200. Sitnicka E, Lin N, Priestley GV, et al: The effect of thrombopoietin on the proliferation and differentiation of murine hematopoietic stem cells. *Blood* 87:4998, 1996.
201. Kobayashi M, Laver JH, Kato T, et al: Recombinant human thrombopoietin (Mpl ligand) enhances proliferation of erythroid progenitors. *Blood* 86:2494, 1995.
202. Kaushansky K, Broudy VC, Grossmann A, et al: Thrombopoietin expands erythroid progenitors, increases red cell production, and enhances erythroid recovery after myelosuppressive therapy. *J Clin Invest* 96:1683, 1995.
203. Akahori H, Shibuya K, Obuchi M, et al: Effect of recombinant human thrombopoietin in nonhuman primates with chemotherapy-induced thrombocytopenia. *Br J Haematol* 94:722, 1996.
204. Neelis KJ, Hartong SC, Egeland T, et al: The efficacy of single-dose administration of thrombopoietin with coadministration of either granulocyte/macrophage or granulocyte colony-stimulating factor in myelosuppressed rhesus monkeys. *Blood* 90:2565, 1997.
205. Farese AM, Hunt P, Grab LB, et al: Combined administration of recombinant human megakaryocyte growth and development factor and granulocyte colony-stimulating factor enhances multilineage hematopoietic reconstitution in nonhuman primates after radiation-induced marrow aplasia. *J Clin Invest* 97:2145, 1996.
206. Alexander WS, Roberts AW, Nicola NA, et al: Deficiencies in progenitor cells of multiple hematopoietic lineages and defective megakaryocytopoiesis in mice lacking the thrombopoietic receptor c-Mpl. *Blood* 87:2162, 1996.
207. Yagi M, Ritchie KA, Sitnicka E, et al: Sustained *ex vivo* expansion of hematopoietic stem cells mediated by thrombopoietin. *Proc Natl Acad Sci USA* 96:8126, 1999.
208. Broxmeyer HE, Kohli L, Kim CH, et al: Stromal cell-derived factor-1/CXCL12 directly enhances survival/antiapoptosis of myeloid progenitor cells through CXCR4 and G(alpha)i proteins and enhances engraftment of competitive, repopulating stem cells. *J Leukoc Biol* 73:630, 2003.
209. Lee Y, Gotoh A, Kwon H-J, et al. Enhancement of intracellular signaling associated with hematopoietic progenitor cell survival in response to SDF-1/CXCL12 in synergy with other cytokines. *Blood* 99:4307, 2002.
210. Ellisen LW, Bird J, West DC, et al: TAN-1, the human homolog of the Drosophila notch gene, is broken by chromosomal translocations in T lymphoblastic neoplasms. *Cell* 66(4):649, 1991.
211. Milner LA, Kopan R, Martin DI, Bernstein ID: A human homologue of the Drosophila developmental gene, Notch, is expressed in CD34 hematopoietic precursors. *Blood* 83:2057, 1994.
212. Karanu FN, Murdoch B, Gallacher L, et al: The notch ligand jagged-1 represents a novel growth factor of human hematopoietic stem cells. *J Exp Med* 192:1365, 2000.
213. Karanu FN, Murdoch B, Miyabayashi T, et al: Human homologues of Delta-1 and Delta-4 function as mitogenic regulators of primitive human hematopoietic cells. *Blood* 97:1960, 2001.
214. Varnum-Finney B, Brashem-Stein C, Bernstein ID: Combined effects of Notch signaling and cytokines induce a multiple log increase in precursors with lymphoid and myeloid reconstituting ability. *Blood* 101:1784, 2003.
215. Austin TW, Solar GP, Ziegler FC, et al: A role for the Wnt gene family in hematopoiesis: Expansion of multilineage progenitor cells. *Blood* 89:3624, 1997.
216. Willert K, Brown JD, Danenberg E, et al: Wnt proteins are lipid-modified and can act as stem cell growth factors. *Nature* 423:448, 2003.

217. Reya T, Duncan AW, Ailles L, et al: A role for Wnt signaling in self-renewal of hematopoietic stem cells. *Nature* 423:409, 2003.
218. Van Den Berg DJ, Sharma AK, Bruno E, Hoffman R: Role of members of the Wnt gene family in human hematopoiesis. *Blood* 92:3189, 1998.
219. Shi Y, Massague J: Mechanisms of TGF-beta signaling from cell membrane to the nucleus. *Cell* 113:685, 2003.
220. Sitnicka E, Ruscetti FW, Priestley GV, et al: Transforming growth factor beta 1 directly and reversibly inhibits the initial cell divisions of long-term repopulating hematopoietic stem cells. *Blood* 88:82, 1996.
221. Batard P, Monier MN, Fortunel N, et al: TGF-(beta)1 maintains hematopoietic immaturity by a reversible negative control of cell cycle and induces CD34 antigen up-modulation. *J Cell Sci* 113(Pt 3):383, 2000.
222. Larsson J, Blank U, Helgadottir H, et al: TGF-beta signaling-deficient hematopoietic stem cells have normal self-renewal and regenerative ability *in vivo* despite increased proliferative capacity *in vitro*. *Blood* 102:3129, 2003.
223. Larsson J, Karlsson S: The role of Smad signaling in hematopoiesis. *Oncogene* 29:5676, 2005.
224. Blank U, Karlsson G, Moody JL, et al: Smad7 promotes self-renewal of hematopoietic stem cells *in vivo*. *Blood* 108:4246, 2006.
225. Karlsson G, Blank U, Moody JL, et al: Smad4 is critical for self-renewal of hematopoietic stem cells. *J Exp Med* 204:467, 2007.
226. Lengerke C, Schmitt S, Bowman TV, et al: BMP and Wnt specify hematopoietic fate by activation of the Cdx-Hox pathway. *Cell Stem Cell* 2:72, 2008.
227. Timm A, Grosschedl R: Wnt signaling in lymphopoiesis. *Curr Top Microbiol Immunol* 290:225, 2005.
228. Ross S, Hill CS: How the Smads regulate transcription. *Int J Biochem Cell Biol* 40:383, 2008.
229. Krosl G, He G, Lefrancois M, et al: Transcription factor SCL is required for c-kit expression and c-Kit function in hemopoietic cells. *J Exp Med* 188:439, 1998.
230. Kirito K, Fox N, Kaushansky K: Thrombopoietin stimulates Hoxb4 expression: An explanation for the favorable effects of TPO on hematopoietic stem cells. *Blood* 102:3172, 2003.
231. Kirito K, Fox N, Kaushansky K: Thrombopoietin (TPO) induces the nuclear translocation of HoxA9 in hematopoietic stem cells (HSC): A potential explanation for the favorable effects of TPO on HSCs. *Mol Cell Biol* 24:6751, 2004.
232. Tong W, Lodish HF: Lnk inhibits Tpo-mpl signaling and Tpo-mediated megakaryocytopoiesis. *J Exp Med* 200(5):569, 2004.
233. Tong W, Zhang J, Lodish HF. Lnk inhibits erythropoiesis and EPO-dependent JAK2 activation and downstream signaling pathways. *Blood* 105:4604, 2005.
234. Takaki S, Sauer K, Iritani BM, et al: Control of B cell production by the adaptor protein lnk: Definition of a conserved family of signal-modulating proteins. *Immunity* 13:599, 2000.
235. Seita J, Ema H, Ooehara J, et al: Lnk negatively regulates self-renewal of hematopoietic stem cells by modifying thrombopoietin-mediated signal transduction. *Proc Natl Acad Sci USA* 104:2349, 2007.
236. Buza-Vidas N, Antonchuk J, Qian H, et al: Cytokines regulate postnatal hematopoietic stem cell expansion: opposing roles of thrombopoietin and LNK. *Genes Dev* 20:2018, 2006.
237. Schick PK, Wojenski CM, Bennett VD, et al: The synthesis and localization of alternatively spliced fibronectin EIIIB in resting and thrombin-treated megakaryocytes. *Blood* 87:1817, 1996.
238. Prosper F, Stroncek D, McCarthy JB, et al: Mobilization and homing of peripheral blood progenitors is related to reversible downregulation of alpha4 beta1 integrin expression and function. *J Clin Invest* 101:2456, 1998.
239. Dao MA, Hashino K, Kato I, et al: Adhesion to fibronectin maintains regenerative capacity during *ex vivo* culture and transduction of human hematopoietic stem and progenitor cells. *Blood* 92:4612, 1998.
240. Yokota T, Oritani K, Mitsui H, et al: Growth-supporting activities of fibronectin on hematopoietic stem/progenitor cells *in vitro* and *in vivo*: Structural requirement for fibronectin activities of CS1 and cell-binding domains. *Blood* 91:3263, 1998.
241. Bhatia R, Williams AD, Munthe HA: Contact with fibronectin enhances preservation of normal but not chronic myelogenous leukemia primitive hematopoietic progenitors. *Exp Hematol* 30:324, 2002.
242. Liu S, Kiosses WB, Rose DM, et al: A fragment of paxillin binds the alpha 4 integrin cytoplasmic domain (tail) and selectively inhibits alpha 4-mediated cell migration. *J Biol Chem* 277:20887, 2002.
243. Sarkar S, Svoboda M, de Beaumont R, et al: The role of Aktand RAFTK in beta1 integrin mediated survival of precursor B-acute lymphoblastic leukemia cells. *Leuk Lymphoma* 43:1663, 2002.
244. Zhao J, Bian ZC, Yee K, et al: Identification of transcription factor KLF8 as a downstream target of focal adhesion kinase in its regulation of cyclin D1 and cell cycle progression. *Mol Cell* 11:1503, 2003.
245. Schlaepfer DD, Hunter T: Focal adhesion kinase overexpression enhances ras-dependent integrin signaling to ERK2/mitogen-activated protein kinase through interactions with and activation of c-Src. *J Biol Chem* 272:13189, 1997.
246. Legras S, Levesque JP, Charrad R, et al: CD44-mediated adhesiveness of human hematopoietic progenitors to hyaluronan is modulated by cytokines. *Blood* 89:1905, 1997.
247. Bendall LJ, James A, Zannettino A, et al: A novel CD44 antibody identifies an epitope that is aberrantly expressed on acute lymphoblastic leukaemia cells. *Immunol Cell Biol* 81:311, 2003.
248. Bendall LJ, Kirkness J, Hutchinson A, et al: Antibodies to CD44 enhance adhesion of normal CD34+ cells and acute myeloblastic but not lymphoblastic leukaemia cells to bone marrow stroma. *Br J Haematol* 98:828, 1997.
249. Pilarski LM, Pruski E, Wizniak J, et al: Potential role for hyaluronan and the hyaluronan receptor RHAMM in mobilization and trafficking of hematopoietic progenitor cells. *Blood* 93:2918, 1999.
250. Nilsson SK, Haylock DN, Johnston HM, et al: Hyaluronan is synthesized by primitive hemopoietic cells, participates in their lodgment at the endosteum following transplantation, and is involved in the regulation of their proliferation and differentiation *in vitro*. *Blood* 101:856, 2003.
251. Gupta P, Oegema TR Jr, Brazil JJ, et al: Structurally specific heparan sulfates support primitive human hematopoiesis by formation of a multimolecular stem cell niche. *Blood* 92:4641, 1998.
252. Klein G, Beck S, Muller CA: Tenascin is a cytoadhesive extracellular matrix component of the human hematopoietic microenvironment. *J Cell Biol* 123:1027, 1993.
253. Seiffert M, Beck SC, Schermutzki F, et al: Mitogenic and adhesive effects of tenascin-C on human hematopoietic cells are mediated by various functional domains. *Matrix Biol* 17:47, 1998.
254. Ohta M, Sakai T, Saga Y, et al: Suppression of hematopoietic activity in tenascin-C-deficient mice. *Blood* 91:4074, 1998.
255. Siler U, Seiffert M, Puch S, et al: Characterization and functional analysis of laminin isoforms in human bone marrow. *Blood* 96:4194, 2000.
256. Gu Y, Sorokin L, Durbeej M, et al: Characterization of bone marrow laminins and identification of alpha5-containing laminins as adhesive proteins for multipotent hematopoietic FDCP-Mix cells. *Blood* 93:2533, 1999.
257. Siler U, Rousselle P, Muller CA, et al: Laminin gamma2 chain as a stromal cell marker of the human bone marrow microenvironment. *Br J Haematol* 119:212, 2002.
258. Landowski TH, Dratz EA, Starkey JR: Studies of the structure of the metastasis-associated 67 kDa laminin binding protein: Fatty acid acylation and evidence supporting dimerization of the 32 kDa gene product to form the mature protein. *Biochemistry* 34:11276, 1995.
259. Ardini E, Tagliabue E, Magnifico A, et al: Co-regulation and physical association of the 67-kDa monomeric laminin receptor and the alpha6beta4 integrin. *J Biol Chem* 272:2342, 1997.
260. Gu YC, Kortesmaa J, Tryggvason K, et al: Laminin isoform-specific promotion of adhesion and migration of human bone marrow progenitor cells. *Blood* 101:877, 2003.
261. Chen J, Carcamo JM, Borquez-Ojeda O, et al: The laminin receptor modulates granulocyte-macrophage colony-stimulating factor receptor complex formation and modulates its signaling. *Proc Natl Acad Sci USA* 100:14000, 2003.
262. Klein G, Muller CA, Tillet E, et al: Collagen type VI in the human bone marrow microenvironment: A strong cytoadhesive component. *Blood* 86:1740, 1995.
263. Koenigsmann M, Griffin JD, DiCarlo J, et al: Myeloid and erythroid progenitor cells from normal bone marrow adhere to collagen type I. *Blood* 79:657, 1992.
264. Metcalf D: Lineage commitment and maturation in hematopoietic cells: The case for extrinsic regulation. *Blood* 92:345; discussion 352, 1998.
265. Enver T, Heyworth CM, Dexter TM: Do stem cells play dice? *Blood* 92:348; discussion 352, 1998.
266. Souabni A, Cobaleda C, Schebesta M, et al: Pax5 promotes B lymphopoiesis and blocks T cell development by repressing Notch1. *Immunity* 17:781, 2002.
267. Georgopoulos K, Moore DD, Derfler B: Ikaros, an early lymphoid-specific transcription factor and a putative mediator for T cell commitment. *Science* 258:808, 1992.
268. Hromas R, Orazi A, Neiman RS, et al: Hematopoietic lineage- and stage-restricted expression of the ETS oncogene family member PU.1. *Blood* 82:2998, 1993.
269. Hohaus S, Petrovick MS, Voso MT, et al: PU.1 (Spi-1) and C/EBP alpha regulate expression of the granulocyte-macrophage colony-stimulating factor receptor alpha gene. *Mol Cell Biol* 15:5830, 1995.
270. Martin DI, Zon LI, Mutter G, et al: Expression of an erythroid transcription factor in megakaryocytic and mast cell lineages. *Nature* 344:444, 1990.
271. Hart A, Melet F, Grossfeld P, et al: Fli-1 is required for murine vascular and megakaryocytic development and is hemizygously deleted in patients with thrombocytopenia. *Immunity* 13:167, 2000.
272. Gombart AF, Kwok SH, Anderson KL, et al: Regulation of neutrophil and eosinophil secondary granule gene expression by transcription factors C/EBP epsilon and PU.1. *Blood* 101:3265, 2003.
273. Thevenin C, Nutt SL, Busslinger M: Early function of Pax5 (BSAP) before the pre-B cell receptor stage of B lymphopoiesis. *J Exp Med* 188:735, 1998.
274. Enver T: B-cell commitment: Pax5 is the deciding factor. *Curr Biol* 9:R933, 1999.
275. Zhang DE, Zhang P, Wang ND, et al: Absence of granulocyte colony-stimulating factor signaling and neutrophil development in CCAAT enhancer binding protein alpha-deficient mice. *Proc Natl Acad Sci USA* 94:569, 1997.
276. Cammenga J, Mulloy JC, Berguido FJ, et al: Induction of C/EBPalpha activity alters gene expression and differentiation of human CD34+ cells. *Blood* 101:2206, 2003.
277. Fairbairn LJ, Cowling GJ, Reipert BM, et al: Suppression of apoptosis allows differentiation and development of a multipotent hemopoietic cell line in the absence of added growth factors. *Cell* 74:823, 1993.
278. Nerlov C, Querfurth E, Kulessa H, et al: GATA-1 interacts with the myeloid PU.1 transcription factor and represses PU.1-dependent transcription. *Blood* 95:2543, 2000.
279. Zhang P, Zhang X, Iwama A, et al: PU.1 inhibits GATA-1 function and erythroid differentiation by blocking GATA-1 DNA binding. *Blood* 96:2641, 2000.

280. Kondo M, Scherer DC, Miyamoto T, et al: Cell-fate conversion of lymphoid-committed progenitors by instructive actions of cytokines. *Nature* 407:383, 2000.
281. Metcalf D: Lineage commitment in the progeny of murine hematopoietic preprogenitor cells: Influence of thrombopoietin and interleukin 5. *Proc Natl Acad Sci USA* 95:6408, 1998.
282. Thorsteinsdottir U, Sauvageau G, Humphries RK. Enhanced *in vivo* regenerative potential of HOXB4-transduced hematopoietic stem cells with regulation of their pool size. *Blood* 94:2605, 1999.
283. Iscove NN, Nawa K. Hematopoietic stem cells expand during serial transplantation *in vivo* without apparent exhaustion. *Curr Biol* 7:805, 1997.
284. Pawliuk R, Eaves C, Humphries RK: Evidence of both ontogeny and transplant dose-regulated expansion of hematopoietic stem cells *in vivo*. *Blood* 88:2852, 1996.
285. Gothot A, van der Loo JC, Clapp DW, et al: Cell cycle-related changes in repopulating capacity of human mobilized peripheral blood CD34(+) cells in non-obese diabetic/severe combined immune-deficient mice. *Blood* 92:2641, 1998.
286. Wilpshaar J, Bhatia M, Kanhai HH, et al: Engraftment potential of human fetal hematopoietic cells in NOD/SCID mice is not restricted to mitotically quiescent cells. *Blood* 100:120, 2002.
287. Czechowicz A, Kraft D, Weissman IL, Bhattacharya D: Efficient transplantation via antibody-based clearance of hematopoietic stem cell niches. *Science* 318:1296, 2007.
288. Fuchs E, Tumbar T, Guasch G: Socializing with the neighbors: Stem cells and their niche. *Cell* 116:769, 2004.
289. Mezey E, Chandross KJ, Harta G, et al: Turning blood into brain: Cells bearing neuronal antigens generated *in vivo* from bone marrow. *Science* 290:1779, 2000.
290. Brazelton TR, Rossi FM, Keshet GI, et al: From marrow to brain: Expression of neuronal phenotypes in adult mice. *Science* 290:1775, 2000.
291. Lagasse E, Connors H, Al-Dhalimy M, et al: Purified hematopoietic stem cells can differentiate into hepatocytes *in vivo*. *Nat Med* 6:1229, 2000.
292. Alison MR, Poulsom R, Jeffery R, et al: Hepatocytes from non-hepatic adult stem cells. *Nature* 406:257, 2000.
293. Ferrari G, Cusella-De Angelis G, Coletta M, et al: Muscle regeneration by bone marrow-derived myogenic progenitors. *Science* 279:1528, 1998.
294. Orlic D, Kajstura J, Chimenti S, et al: Bone marrow cells regenerate infarcted myocardium. *Nature* 410:701, 2001.
295. Jiang Y, Jahagirdar BN, Reinhardt RL, et al: Pluripotency of mesenchymal stem cells derived from adult marrow. *Nature* 418:41, 2002.
296. Ying QL, Nichols J, Evans EP, et al: Changing potency by spontaneous fusion. *Nature* 416:545, 2002.
297. Terada N, Hamazaki T, Oka M, et al: Bone marrow cells adopt the phenotype of other cells by spontaneous cell fusion. *Nature* 416:542, 2002.
298. Galy A, Travis M, Cen D, et al: Human T, B, natural killer, and dendritic cells arise from a common bone marrow progenitor cell subset. *Immunity* 3:459, 1995.
299. von Freeden-Jeffry U, Vieira P, Lucian LA, et al: Lymphopenia in interleukin (IL)-7 gene-deleted mice identifies IL-7 as a nonredundant cytokine. *J Exp Med* 181:1519, 1995.
300. Terskikh AV, Miyamoto T, Chang C, et al: Gene expression analysis of purified hematopoietic stem cells and committed progenitors. *Blood* 102:94, 2003.
301. Ikawa T, Kawamoto H, Fujimoto S, et al: Commitment of common T/Natural killer (NK) progenitors to unipotent T and NK progenitors in the murine fetal thymus revealed by a single progenitor assay. *J Exp Med* 190:1617, 1999.
302. Massari ME, Murre C: Helix-loop-helix proteins: Regulators of transcription in eucaryotic organisms. *Mol Cell Biol* 20:429, 2000.
303. Sawada S, Littman DR: A heterodimer of HEB and an E12-related protein interacts with the CD4 enhancer and regulates its activity in T-cell lines. *Mol Cell Biol* 13:5620, 1993.
304. Takeuchi A, Yamasaki S, Takase K, et al: E2A and HEB activate the pre-TCR alpha promoter during immature T cell development. *J Immunol* 167:2157, 2001.
305. Bain G, Romanow WJ, Albers K, et al: Positive and negative regulation of V(D)J recombination by the E2A proteins. *J Exp Med* 189:289, 1999.
306. Norton JD: ID helix-loop-helix proteins in cell growth, differentiation and tumorigenesis. *J Cell Sci* 113 Pt 22:3897, 2000.
307. Yokota Y, Mansouri A, Mori S, et al: Development of peripheral lymphoid organs and natural killer cells depends on the helix-loop-helix inhibitor Id2. *Nature* 397:702, 1999.
308. Heemskerk MH, Blom B, Nolan G, et al: Inhibition of T cell and promotion of natural killer cell development by the dominant negative helix loop helix factor Id3. *J Exp Med* 186:1597, 1997.
309. Pui JC, Allman D, Xu L, et al: Notch1 expression in early lymphopoiesis influences B versus T lineage determination. *Immunity* 11:299, 1999.
310. Allman D, Karnell FG, Punt JA, et al: Separation of Notch1 promoted lineage commitment and expansion/transformation in developing T cells. *J Exp Med* 194:99, 2001.
311. Denis KA, Witte ON: *In vitro* development of B lymphocytes from long-term cultured precursor cells. *Proc Natl Acad Sci USA* 83:441, 1986.
312. Takatsu K: Cytokines involved in B-cell differentiation and their sites of action. *Proc Soc Exp Biol Med* 215:121, 1997.
313. Namen AE, Lupton S, Hjerrild K, et al: Stimulation of B-cell progenitors by cloned murine interleukin-7. *Nature* 333:571, 1988.
314. Gibson LF, Piktel D, Landreth KS: Insulin-like growth factor-1 potentiates expansion of interleukin-7-dependent pro-B cells. *Blood* 82:3005, 1993.
315. Nagasawa T, Kikutani H, Kishimoto T: Molecular cloning and structure of a pre-B-cell growth-stimulating factor. *Proc Natl Acad Sci USA* 91:2305, 1994.
316. McNiece IK, Langley KE, Zsebo KM: The role of recombinant stem cell factor in early B cell development. Synergistic interaction with IL-7. *J Immunol* 146:3785, 1991.
317. Gongora R, Stephan RP, Zhang Z, et al: An essential role for Daxx in the inhibition of B lymphopoiesis by type I interferons. *Immunity* 14:727, 2001.
318. Yoshikawa H, Nakajima Y, Tasaka K: IFN-gamma induces the apoptosis of WEHI 279 and normal pre-B cell lines by expressing direct inhibitor of apoptosis protein binding protein with low pI. *J Immunol* 167:2487, 2001.
319. Mitchell PL, Clutterbuck RD, Powles RL, et al: Interleukin-4 enhances the survival of severe combined immunodeficient mice engrafted with human B-cell precursor leukemia. *Blood* 87:4797, 1996.
320. Lee G, Namen AE, Gillis S, et al: Normal B cell precursors responsive to recombinant murine IL-7 and inhibition of IL-7 activity by transforming growth factor-beta. *J Immunol* 142:3875, 1989.
321. Bain G, Maandag EC, Izon DJ, et al: E2A proteins are required for proper B cell development and initiation of immunoglobulin gene rearrangements. *Cell* 79:885, 1994.
322. Bain G, Robanus Maandag EC, te Riele HP, et al: Both E12 and E47 allow commitment to the B cell lineage. *Immunity* 6:145, 1997.
323. Kee BL, Quong MW, Murre C: E2A proteins: Essential regulators at multiple stages of B-cell development. *Immunol Rev* 175:138, 2000.
324. Iscove NN, Sieber F: Erythroid progenitors in mouse bone marrow detected by macroscopic colony formation in culture. *Exp Hematol* 3:32, 1975.
325. Clarke BJ, Housman D: Characterization of an erythroid precursor cell of high proliferative capacity in normal human peripheral blood. *Proc Natl Acad Sci USA* 74:1105, 1977.
326. Long MW, Heffner CH, Williams JL, et al: Regulation of megakaryocyte phenotype in human erythroleukemia cells. *J Clin Invest* 85:1072, 1990.
327. McDonald TP, Sullivan PS: Megakaryocytic and erythrocytic cell lines share a common precursor cell. *Exp Hematol* 21:1316, 1993.
328. Nakahata T, Okumura N: Cell surface antigen expression in human erythroid progenitors: Erythroid and megakaryocytic markers. *Leuk Lymphoma* 13:401, 1994.
329. Hodohara K, Fujii N, Yamamoto N, et al: Stromal cell-derived factor-1 (SDF-1) acts together with thrombopoietin to enhance the development of megakaryocytic progenitor cells (CFU-MK). *Blood* 95:769, 2000.
330. Sawada K, Krantz SB, Dai CH, et al: Purification of human blood burst-forming units-erythroid and demonstration of the evolution of erythropoietin receptors. *J Cell Physiol* 142:219, 1990.
331. Sporn LA, Chavin SI, Marder VJ, et al: Biosynthesis of von Willebrand protein by human megakaryocytes. *J Clin Invest* 76:1102, 1985.
332. Pevny L, Simon MC, Robertson E, et al: Erythroid differentiation in chimaeric mice blocked by a targeted mutation in the gene for transcription factor GATA-1. *Nature* 349:257, 1991.
333. Shivdasani RA, Fujiwara Y, McDevitt MA, et al: A lineage-selective knockout establishes the critical role of transcription factor GATA-1 in megakaryocyte growth and platelet development. *EMBO J* 16:3965, 1997.
334. Tsang AP, Visvader JE, Turner CA, et al: FOG, a multitype zinc finger protein, acts as a cofactor for transcription factor GATA-1 in erythroid and megakaryocytic differentiation. *Cell* 90:109, 1997.
335. Nichols KE, Crispino JD, Poncz M, et al: Familial dyserythropoietic anaemia and thrombocytopenia due to an inherited mutation in GATA1. *Nat Genet* 24:266, 2000.
336. Doubeikovski A, Uzan G, Doubeikovski Z, et al: Thrombopoietin-induced expression of the glycoprotein IIb gene involves the transcription factor PU.1/Spi-1 in UT7-Mpl cells. *J Biol Chem* 272:24300, 1997.
337. Athanasiou M, Clausen PA, Mavrothalassitis GJ, et al: Increased expression of the ETS-related transcription factor FLI-1/ERGB correlates with and can induce the megakaryocytic phenotype. *Cell Growth Differ* 7:1525, 1996.
338. Giles F, Estey E, O'Brien S: Gemtuzumab ozogamicin in the treatment of acute myeloid leukemia. *Cancer* 98:2095, 2003.
339. Pagano L, Fianchi L, Caira M, Rutella S, Leone G: The role of gemtuzumab ozogamicin in the treatment of acute myeloid leukemia patients. *Oncogene* 26:3679, 2007.
340. Stasi R. Gemtuzumab ozogamicin: an anti-CD33 immunoconjugate for the treatment of acute myeloid leukaemia. *Expert Opin Biol Ther* 8:527, 2008.
341. Khanna-Gupta A, Zibello T, Sun H, et al: C/EBP epsilon mediates myeloid differentiation and is regulated by the CCAAT displacement protein (CDP/cut). *Proc Natl Acad Sci USA* 98:8000, 2001.
342. Dahl R, Walsh JC, Lancki D, et al: Regulation of macrophage and neutrophil cell fates by the PU.1:C/EBPalpha ratio and granulocyte colony-stimulating factor. *Nat Immunol* 4:1029, 2003.

CHAPTER 17
THE INFLAMMATORY RESPONSE

Jeffrey S. Warren and Peter A. Ward

SUMMARY

The inflammatory response is characterized by a rapid but relatively short-lived increase in local blood flow, an increase in microvascular permeability, and the sequential recruitment of different types of leukocytes. Superimposed is a series of reparative processes (e.g., angiogenesis, production of extracellular matrix, parenchymal regeneration, and scar formation). The early hemodynamic changes at a site of inflammation establish low shear conditions that enable marginated leukocytes to engage in low-affinity selectin-mediated rolling interactions with endothelial cells. In response to locally produced soluble and cell surface mediators, endothelial cells and rolling leukocytes become activated and sequentially express sets of complementary adhesion molecules that include β_2 integrins, selectins, and members of the immunoglobulin superfamily. Leukocyte and endothelial cell adhesion molecules mediate the high-affinity adhesive interactions necessary for leukocyte emigration from the vascular space and along chemotactic gradients. Analogous, temporally regulated, soluble mediators and cellular adhesion molecules also orchestrate succeeding monocyte- and lymphocyte-rich chronic inflammatory responses. This basic paradigm is modulated by numerous surface-active and soluble inflammatory mediators. Recruited leukocytes and cells indigenous to the anatomic site of inflammation both play critical roles in host defense and tissue repair.

HISTORY

The sentinel clinical features of acute inflammation—rubor, calor, tumor, and dolor—have been recognized for 5000 years.[1] Dr. John Hunter, the renowned late-18th-century Scottish surgeon, observed that the inflammatory response is not a disease *per se* but rather a nonspecific and salutary response to a variety of insults. Through his microscopic examinations of transparent vital membrane preparations, Julius Cohnheim concluded that the inflammatory response is fundamentally a vascular phenomenon. Phagocytosis was described in the late 19th century by Eli Metchnikoff and his colleagues. Morphologic studies, using both live animals and fixed histologic preparations, transformed our understanding of inflammation and led to the currently held concepts of inflammation-associated hemodynamic alterations, "acute" inflammation, and "chronic" inflammation.[1,2] During the past 5 decades, the modern techniques of biochemistry, tissue culture, monoclonal antibody production, recombinant DNA technology, and the genetic manipulation of isolated cells and whole animals have enabled a more detailed understanding of the cellular and molecular mechanisms that characterize the inflammatory response. These studies, in concert with "experiments of nature" such as chronic granulomatous disease (see Chap. 66) and the leukocyte adhesion deficiency disorders (see Chap. 66), have permitted the formulation of complex, yet elegant, models of acute and chronic inflammation and led to the promise of incisive therapeutic approaches. A vast array of human diseases is marked by either defects in the development of the inflammatory response or the deleterious effects of the inflammatory response itself.

Acronyms and abbreviations that appear in this chapter include: BPI, bactericidal/permeability-increasing protein; CAP37, cationic antimicrobial protein; CD, cluster of differentiation; eNOS, endothelial nitric oxide synthase; HEV, high endothelial venules; HPETE, hydroperoxyeicosatetraenoic acid; ICAM, intercellular adhesion molecule; Ig, immunoglobulin; IL, interleukin; iNOS, inducible nitric oxide synthase; LT, leukotriene; LTB_4 / C_4 / D_4 / E_4, leukotriene B_4 / C_4 / D_4 / E_4; MASP, mannan-binding lectin-associated serine protease; MBL, mannan-binding lectin; NADPH, nicotinamide adenine dinucleotide phosphate (reduced); nNOS, neuronal nitric oxide synthase; NO, nitric oxide; NOS, nitric oxide synthase; PAF, platelet-activating factor; PSGL-1, P-selectin glycoprotein ligand-1; RGD, arginine-glycine-aspartic acid peptide sequence; TNF, tumor necrosis factor; VCAM, vascular cell adhesion molecule; VLA, very-late antigen.

GENERAL CHARACTERISTICS OF INFLAMMATION

Although necessarily contrived, it is useful to consider inflammation as an acute or chronic process. "Acute" inflammation lasts from minutes to a few days and is characterized by pronounced local hemodynamic and microvascular changes and leukocyte accumulation.[2] The acute inflammatory response is consistently marked by microvascular leakage and the accumulation of neutrophils. The four cardinal signs of inflammation, alluded to above, can be accounted for within the physiologic terms of acute inflammation. The systemic effects of inflammation, particularly acute inflammation, account for the familiar clinical findings of fever, the acute phase response, and altered sensorium.

The chronic inflammatory response, which lasts much longer and is more varied in its effects, is marked by the growth of new capillaries and the proliferation of resident fibroblasts.[2] Cellular infiltrates include primarily lymphocytes and monocytes, but there are many variations in the cellular composition, anatomic distribution, and tempo of development of chronic inflammatory lesions. Chronic inflammatory processes are classified according to these variations. For example, granulomatous inflammation is a chronic process marked by nodular aggregates of mononuclear phagocytes that have become "transformed" into so-called epithelioid histiocytes because of their similar appearance to epithelial cells. Granulomas may be distributed along blood vessels (e.g., angiocentric), along airways (e.g., bronchocentric), or randomly throughout the interstitium or parenchyma of an organ. Other chronic inflammatory processes are marked by a preponderance of plasma cells or eosinophils. In contrast to the more stereotyped appearance of an acute inflammatory lesion, the particular appearance of a chronic inflammatory lesion can sometimes provide insight into its cause (e.g., caseating granulomas in tuberculosis, eosinophil-rich infiltrates in a parasitic infection, and plasma cell-rich infiltrates in viral hepatitis).

Superimposed upon the acute and chronic inflammatory response is repair.[2] Repair may entail the regeneration of parenchymal cells damaged as the direct result of an insult *per se* or as "bystanders" to the inflammatory response. Repair is characterized by the growth of new capillaries (angiogenesis) and the activation of fibroblasts which produce extracellular matrix (e.g., scar tissue). In some circumstances an inflammatory response is self-limited (e.g., sunburn), whereas in other situations the response can persist for years (e.g., tuberculous granulomas). The persistence or elimination of an insult has a major influence on outcome—whether complete regeneration, persistence of inflammation, or scar formation.

This chapter first addresses acute inflammation, which encompasses localized changes in blood flow, alterations in microvascular permeability, and neutrophil exudation. There has been great progress in understanding the processes of endothelial cell activation, low avidity leukocyte–endothelial adhesion, high-affinity or stationary leukocyte–endothelial adhesive interactions, leukocyte emigration, leukocyte activation, and the subsequent dampening of an inflammatory response. The second section of this chapter introduces the vast array of soluble and surface-active mediators that regulate both acute and chronic inflammatory responses. These mediators include substances that range from short-lived reactive oxygen and nitrogen intermediates to entire regulatory systems (e.g., complement system and coagulation cascade). Many regulatory mediators of inflammation have become targets for rational therapeutic strategies. Finally, a brief overview of chronic inflammation and tissue repair is provided. This chapter provides a framework for understanding the basic processes of inflammation while promoting an appreciation for the highly complex and integrated nature of the regulated inflammatory response.

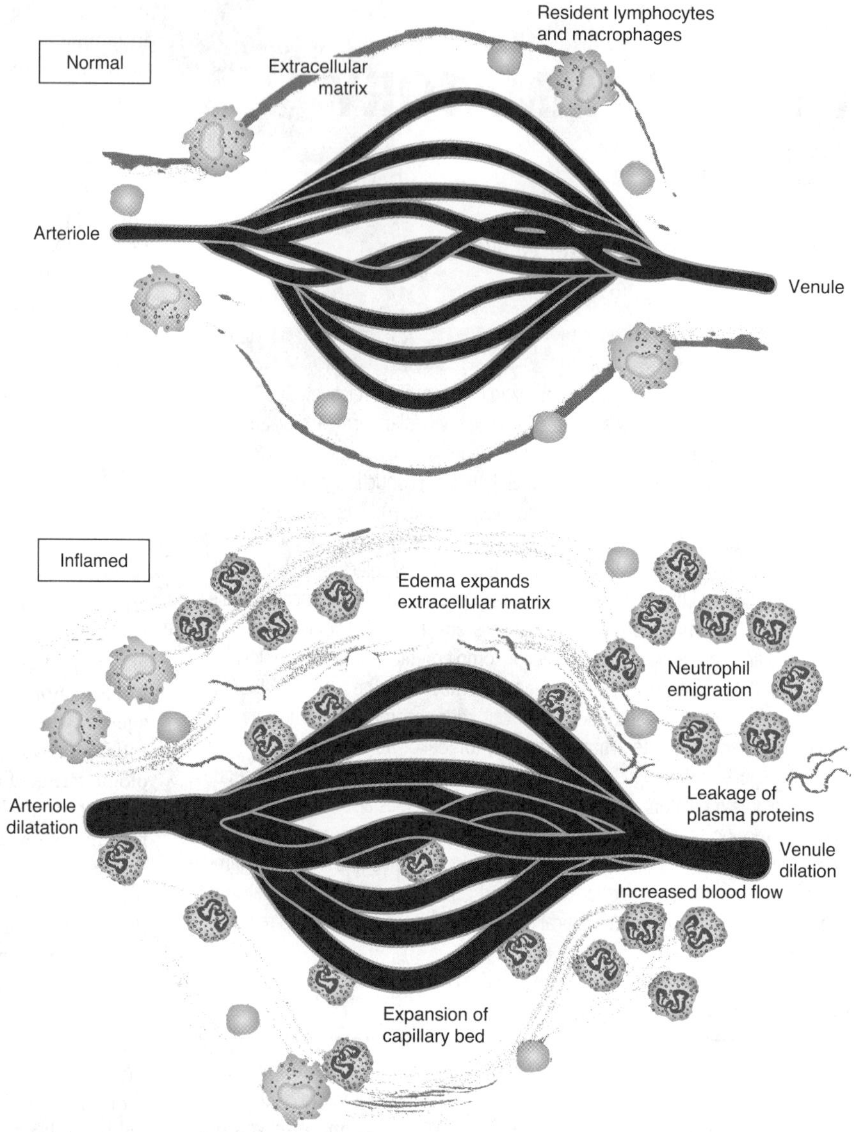

FIGURE 17–1. Early hemodynamic events in acute inflammation. Vascular dilatation, increased microvascular permeability, fluid transudation, and leukocyte recruitment and emigration occur after a transient period of arteriolar vasoconstriction. *(Modified and redrawn with permission from Cotran RS, Kumar V, Collins T, Robbins SL (eds):* Robbins Pathologic Basis of Disease, *6th ed. WB Saunders, Philadelphia, 1999.[39])*

ACUTE INFLAMMATION

HEMODYNAMIC CHANGES

The hemodynamic changes that occur early in the acute phase of inflammation include arteriolar vasodilation and a localized increase in microvascular permeability (Fig. 17–1). In many circumstances, arteriolar vasodilation follows a rapid and transient period of vasoconstriction.[2] Arteriolar vasodilation results in increased blood flow, thus explaining the familiar redness and warmth which characterize a site of acute inflammation. The increase in blood flow, coupled with increases in microvascular permeability, results in hemoconcentration and a localized increase in blood viscosity. These localized hemodynamic changes are critical to subsequent leukocyte emigration because selectin-mediated, low-affinity, rolling leukocyte–endothelial adhesive interactions can efficiently occur only under conditions of reduced shear force. Experimental studies using *in vitro* flow chambers and semitransparent vital membrane preparations in live animals indicate that selectin-mediated leukocyte–endothelial rolling adhesive interactions cannot occur in the face of the shear forces exerted by normal blood flow. Increased microvascular permeability leads to protein-rich plasma exudation, which is characteristic of acute inflammation. Microvascular leakage occurs through a variety of temporally regulated mechanisms, including rapid and short-lived venular endothelial cell contraction, which is accompanied by widening of intercellular junctions; so-called endothelial cell retraction, which is less-well understood but involves long-lived cytokine-mediated cytoskeletal changes; leukocyte-mediated endothelial cell injury; direct endothelial cell injury by physical trauma; and leakage via new capillaries that do not yet possess fully "closed" intercellular junctions.[2,3] An increase in the rate of transcytosis in which plasma constituents cross endothelial cells in vesicles or vacuoles (vesiculovacuolar organelles) has a role in neoplastic blood vessels and may play a role in inflammation.[4] Alterations in local blood flow occur at the level of arterioles, which are regulated largely by the autonomic nervous system, NO, vasoactive peptides, and eicosanoids. A variety of soluble mediators can induce increases in microvascular permeability through several of the above-mentioned mechanisms.

LEUKOCYTE RECRUITMENT

The orchestrated recruitment of leukocytes into a site of inflammation is a fundamental characteristic of the inflammatory response.[5] The importance of white blood cells in host defense is highlighted in patients with leukocyte deficiencies or defects in white cell function. Leukocytes are critical because of their central role in the phagocytosis and containment or killing of microbes and in the digestion of necrotic tissue debris. Leukocyte-derived products such as proteolytic enzymes and reactive oxygen intermediates contribute to tissue injury.

Leukocyte Adhesion and Transmigration

When vascular stasis occurs as the result of the hemodynamic changes of early acute inflammation, leukocytes are displaced from the central

TABLE 17–1. Adhesion Molecules in Inflammation

Family	Structure	Members	Tissue Distribution	Counterreceptor
Selectin	N-terminal lectin domain, epidermal growth factor domain, multiple complement regulatory repeats, transmembrane, and short cytoplasmic tail	P-selectin	Endothelium, platelets	PSGL-1, SLe^x glycoprotein
		E-selectin	Endothelium	PSGL-1, SLe^x glycoprotein
		L-selectin	Leukocytes	GlyCam-1, MAdCAM-1, CD34
Immunoglobulin superfamily	Multiple immunoglobulin domains, transmembrane region and cytoplasmic tail	ICAM-1	Endothelium	CD11a/CD18
		ICAM-2		CD11b/CD18
		ICAM-3		
		VCAM-1	Endothelium	VLA-4
		CD31 (PECAM)	Endothelium	CD31
Integrin (β_2; leukocyte)	Heterodimers: distinct α subunits with common β subunits	CD11a/CD18 (LFA-1)	Neutrophils, monocytes, macrophages, and lymphocytes	ICAM-1
				ICAM-2
				ICAM-3
		CD11b/CD18 (Mac-1)	Neutrophils, monocytes, and macrophages	ICAM-1, iC3b, LPS, and fibronectin
		VLA-4	Monocytes and lymphocytes	VCAM-1 and fibronectin

CD, cluster of differentiation; ICAM, intercellular adhesion molecule; LFA-1, leukocyte function-associated antigen-1; LPS, lipopolysaccharide; PECAM, platelet endothelial cell adhesion molecule; PSGL-1, P-selectin glycoprotein ligand-1; sLe^x, sialyl Lewis X; VCAM, vascular cell adhesion molecule; VLA, very-late antigen.

axial column of blood cells to positions along the endothelial surface. This process, called margination, is enhanced under conditions of slow blood flow.[2] Individual leukocytes adhere transiently and weakly to the endothelial surface. Studies using vital membrane preparations and flow chamber studies using endothelial cell monolayers and suspensions of purified leukocytes reveal that cells literally tumble and roll along the endothelial surface.[6] Rolling neutrophil–endothelial adhesive interactions occur within minutes of the initiation of an acute inflammatory response and can, depending on the time within the evolution of an inflammatory response, involve neutrophils, lymphocytes, monocytes, basophils, or eosinophils. The leukocyte–endothelial cell-rolling adhesive interaction is a specific and necessary step that precedes high-affinity, or so-called stationary, adhesion and emigration.[5,6] Early rolling adhesive interactions are mediated largely by selectins and their carbohydrate-rich counterreceptors.[6] In turn, the cell surface expression of selectins (and other intercellular adhesion molecules; see below) is regulated by a number of locally produced proinflammatory mediators.[6,7]

Selectins contain an extracellular N-terminal carbohydrate-binding region that is homologous to mammalian lectins, an epidermal growth factor-like domain, a series of complement regulatory domains, and a lipophilic transmembrane domain (Table 17–1).[6] P-selectin is expressed by endothelial cells and platelets, E-selectin by endothelial cells, and L-selectin by most white blood cells. P-selectin is stored in endothelial intracytoplasmic granules called Weibel-Palade bodies.[5] When endothelial cells are exposed to histamine, thrombin, or platelet-activating factor (PAF), preformed P-selectin is rapidly (within minutes) translocated to the endothelial surface where it engages marginated leukocytes via carbohydrate moieties that contain sialic acid residues (e.g., P-selectin glycoprotein ligand-1 [PSGL-1]).[6] This transient, low-affinity, binding interaction, which can withstand only the low-flow shear force conditions found in stasis, accounts in part for the early rolling interactions (Fig. 17–2). The development of single knockout mice (i.e., lack individual selectins [P/; E/; or L/], double knockout mice (e.g., E/P/), and even triple knockout mice, has confirmed that rolling can be almost completely accounted for by selectins.[8,9] Exposure of endothelial cells to tumor necrosis factor (TNF)-α or interleukin (IL)-1β results in protein synthesis-dependent expression of E-selectin, a response that occurs within 1 to 2 hours and peaks at 4 to 6 hours.[5] As in the case of P-selectin–mediated leukocyte adhesion, E-selectin–mediated adhesion occurs via a series of sialylated

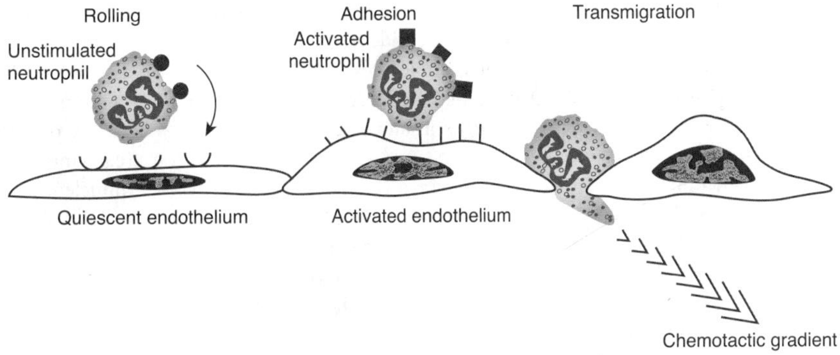

FIGURE 17–2. Leukocyte–endothelial adhesive interactions. Early in the acute inflammatory response, marginated leukocytes engage in transient, low-affinity, selectin-mediated adhesive interactions with endothelial cells. As the response evolves, activated leukocytes and endothelial cells engage in high-affinity β_2-integrin and immunoglobulin superfamily mediated adhesive interactions. A variety of chemotactic factors can provide the motive force for leukocyte emigration.

and fucosylated carbohydrate moieties related to the sialyl Lewis X and sialyl Lewis A blood group antigens but found on leukocytes (Table 17–1).[6] The selectin counterreceptors consist of mucin-like glycoproteins coated with various sialyl moieties.[6,10] L-selectin is constitutively expressed by leukocytes, participates in white blood cell–endothelial homing (e.g., lymphocyte homing to lymph nodes via high endothelial venules [HEV]) and leukocyte–leukocyte adhesive interactions via mucin-like glycoproteins, and is shed by means of "sheddase" enzymes such as ADAM-17(TACE) when the leukocyte is activated (Table 17–1).[10] Key mucin-like glycoproteins include MadCAM-1, GlyCAM-1, and CD34. L-selectin shedding facilitates leukocyte emigration by allowing the white blood cell to detach from the endothelium. Low-affinity rolling adhesive interactions set the stage for β-integrin and immunoglobulin superfamily mediated, high-affinity adhesive interactions and leukocyte transmigration.[5,7,11]

Relatively weak selectin-mediated and high-affinity stationary adhesive interactions are not temporally or mechanistically discrete. For example, TNF-α and IL-β induce E-selectin, which is not expressed by quiescent cells, and increase endothelial expression of intercellular adhesion molecule (ICAM)-1 and vascular cell adhesion molecule (VCAM)-1, which are constitutively expressed in low concentrations and, in the case of ICAM-1, are involved in the recruitment of all types of leukocytes, and in the case of VCAM-1, are involved in the recruitment of all types of chronic inflammatory leukocytes (lymphocytes, monocytes, eosinophils, and basophils).[5] ICAM-1 binds to β_2 (leukocyte) integrins, which are heterodimeric structures that contain varied α chains (CD11a, CD11b, CD11c, CD11d) and a common β chain (CD18).[11] VCAM-1 binds to β_1 integrins (e.g., VLA-4/$\alpha_4\beta_1$) (see Table 17–1).[12] Activated endothelial cells secrete PAF and IL-8, which activate overlying leukocytes.[12] Leukocyte CD11b/CD18 (Mac-1) is upregulated in terms of number and undergoes a transient conformational change that increases its binding affinity for endothelial ICAM-1. CD11a/CD18 also exhibits an increase in binding avidity, but there is no increase in number of surface molecules. CD11c/CD18 binds to iC3b (see below) and initiates phagocytosis, but plays a lesser role in neutrophils than do CD11a/CD18 and CD11b/CD18.

Intercellular adhesion molecules are found on a variety of cell types aside from endothelial cells. CD11a/CD18 interacts with both ICAM-1 and ICAM-2, whereas CD11b/CD18 binds to ICAM-1 and the complement activation product iC3b (see below). The roles of CD11c/CD18, CD11d/CD18, and ICAM-3 in leukocyte–endothelial adhesion are less-well established. β_1 Integrins, notably very-late antigen (VLA)-4, are found on chronic inflammatory leukocytes (e.g., lymphocytes, monocytes, basophils, and eosinophils) and mediate leukocyte binding via VCAM-1.[11,12] β_1-Integrin–mediated adhesive interactions occur via arginine-glycine-aspartic acid peptide sequences (RGDs) within VCAM-1, as well as within matrix molecules (e.g., fibronectin). β_2-Integrin-ICAM– and β_1-VCAM-1–mediated adhesive interactions occur later (hours to days) in the inflammatory response than do selectin-mediated interactions.

Additional adhesive interactions are also involved in leukocyte transmigration.[5] The functional importance of the various complementary leukocyte–endothelial adhesive interactions has been clarified by *in vitro* leukocyte–endothelial binding studies and *in vivo* studies that employed neutralizing antibodies directed against adhesion molecules, pharmacologic antagonists of adhesion molecules, and knockout mice.[5] The functional importance of leukocyte integrins (CD11a/ CD18, CD11b/CD18, CD11c/CD18) has also been highlighted by clinical and experimental observations in patients with leukocyte adhesion deficiencies (see Chap. 66).

Leukocyte diapedesis through interendothelial spaces is at least partially dependant on CD31 (platelet endothelial cell adhesion molecule [PECAM]-1).[13] In turn, extravascular leukocytes bind to extracellular matrix molecules via β_1 integrins and CD44.[2] The life span of neutrophils, normally 4 to 10 hours, can be greatly extended (up to 48 hours) following emigration into an inflammatory site. Various soluble cytokines (see "Leukocyte Chemotaxis and Activation" below) can alter the basal rate of neutrophil apoptosis, thus providing a means for localized increases or decreases in duration of survival.

Leukocyte Chemotaxis and Activation

Leukocytes tightly bound to endothelium emigrate from the vascular space into the interstitium by extending pseudopods between intercellular junctions (see Fig. 17–2).[14] Secreted neutral proteases, such as elastase, cathepsin G, and proteinase 3, play a role in the passage or "invasion" of leukocytes through the subendothelial extracellular matrix. Collagenases are particularly important in leukocyte transmigration through basement membranes. As is detailed later, a variety of matrix metalloproteinases also play a role in tissue remodeling. This group of enzymes includes mediators produced by a variety of cell types. Leukocyte emigration and subsequent movement through the interstitium follow chemical concentration gradients; processes facilitated by binding interactions between leukocyte integrins and complementary sites on extracellular matrix molecules (e.g., fibronectin).[7] A wide variety of soluble mediators can provide trigger for this process.[15] Chemotactic factors for neutrophils include peptides from bacteria (e.g., *N*-formyl peptides), complement-derived peptides (e.g., C5a), cell membrane-derived chemotactic lipids (e.g., PAF), and cytokines and chemokines produced by a variety of cell types (e.g., IL-8 from endothelial cells).[15] Chemotactic factors vary with respect to their specificity for different types of leukocytes. For example, *N*-formyl peptides and C5a both induce neutrophil and monocyte chemotaxis, IL-8 induces neutrophil chemotaxis, and monocyte chemoattractant protein-1 (MCP-1) induces chemotactic responses in monocytes and a specific subset of memory T lymphocytes. Each of these chemotactic factors activates "target" cells by engaging specific cell surface receptors, which, in turn, are linked to the contractile cell motility apparatus.[15]

In addition to chemotaxis, soluble and cell surface mediators induce leukocyte activation, which is manifested by a wide array of changes in cellular function (e.g., leukocyte integrin upregulation and increased binding avidity [e.g., CD11a/CD18], selectin shedding [e.g., L-selectin], lysosome degranulation, and initiation of the respiratory burst). Great advances in understanding of the biochemical pathways involved in chemotaxis, cell activation, and degranulation have occurred. Although there are many nuances in the signal transduction pathways involved in these processes, several themes have emerged. Cell surface receptors are activated by specific ligands (e.g., C5a, leukotriene B_4 [LTB_4], IL-8) and receptor activation is transduced via specific G proteins and membrane-associated phospholipases, which lead to mobilization of intracellular calcium, influx of extracellular calcium, and protein phosphorylation. A variety of rare diseases linked to genetic receptor and effector defects (e.g., interferon [IFN]-γ receptor deflects and nicotinamide adenine dinucleotide [reduced form] [NADPH] oxidase defects) have provided insight into leukocyte function and the importance of such specific activities in host defense.

The principal result of neutrophil and monocyte recruitment is to provide (1) high concentrations of activated leukocytes that can release lytic substances and reactive oxygen and nitrogen intermediates needed to destroy foreign invaders, and (2) a vehicle to contain foreign particulates through phagocytosis. The products and functions of activated inflammatory cells are at once salutary because they contain and destroy invaders and deleterious because they cause tissue damage.

Leukocyte activation, especially that of neutrophils and mononuclear phagocytes, results in the secretion of many microbicidal peptides (e.g., defensins, bactericidal/permeability-increasing protein [BPI], cationic antimicrobial protein [CAP37]) and lytic enzymes (e.g., myeloperoxidase, elastase, cathepsin G).[16] The release of such granular constituents is accompanied by the generation of reactive oxygen and nitrogen intermediates (e.g., O_2^-, H_2O_2, NO), the generation of arachidonate metabolites (e.g., leukotrienes and prostaglandins), and the production of other mediators (see below).[16,17] In some circumstances these materials are released into phagolysosomes, where they contribute to the destruction of engulfed microbes, while in other circumstances they are secreted into the extracellular milieu, where they amplify the inflammatory response and cause tissue damage. The different types of neutrophil granules (primary azurophilic, secondary specific, tertiary gelatinase-containing, and secretory vesicles) are released in a coordinated differential fashion.[16]

Phagocytosis involves three distinct steps: recognition and attachment, engulfment, and degradation (killing) of the ingested material.[18] Phagocytosis is enhanced greatly when particles (e.g., bacteria) are coated with opsonins, which, in turn, function as ligands for leukocyte surface receptors. The major opsonins include the Fc domain of immunoglobulin (Ig) G and IgM and the complement-derived fragments C3b and iC3b, which are generated via activation of the complement cascades and covalently bond to the surfaces of particles and large molecules. There are a variety of Fc receptors (FcγRI, FcγRII, FcγRIIIB, etc.) and complement receptors (e.g., CR1, CR3, CR4) that specifically engage their respective opsonins when the latter coat foreign particulates.[19,20] In addition to facilitating receptor-mediated phagocytosis of opsonized particles, Fc receptors trigger cell activation with the attendant release of granular constituents and the generation of reactive oxygen intermediates.[19,20] Other important recognition molecules expressed by leukocytes include integrins, the C1q receptor, mannose receptors, and scavenger receptors.[2] Mannose receptors bind to mannose and fucose moieties which are present on some microbes but not mammalian cells while scavenger receptors bind to a variety of microbes as well as oxidized and acetylated low-density lipoproteins.[2] Some enhanced phagocytic reactions occur independently of opsonins. The engulfment, degranulation, and oxidative burst triggered as the result of engagement of FcR is enhanced by the concurrent engagement of complement receptors. In some circumstances, engulfment is enhanced by the simultaneous binding of the leukocyte to specific extracellular matrix molecules (e.g., fibronectin) or soluble cytokines. Engulfment results in the formation of phagosomes, which fuse with lysosomes to form phagolysosomes in which the foreign particle is oxidized and degraded. Numerous mechanisms for killing and/or degradation of microbes have been elucidated (Table 17–2). Although these mechanisms are classified as either oxygen-dependent or oxygen-independent, both types of processes may be involved in the destruction of a given microorganism, and a given microorganism may vary greatly in its susceptibility to various mechanisms of destruction.[16–20] Extracellular release of reactive oxygen and nitrogen intermediates, lysosomal enzymes, lipid mediators, and cationic proteins can all contribute to inflammation-related tissue injury.

TABLE 17–2. Killing and Degradation of Microorganisms in Phagocytes

Oxygen-Dependent		Oxygen-Independent
Superoxide anion	(O_2^-)	Arachidonate metabolites (prostaglandins, leukotrienes)
Hydrogen peroxide	(H_2O_2)	Platelet-activating factor
Hydroxyl radical	(HO•)	Lysosomal proteases
Singlet oxygen	($^1O_2$)	Lactoferrin
N-chloramines	(R-NHC1, R-NCl_2)	Lysozyme
Hypohalous acids	(HO-X)	Cationic proteins (e.g., bactericidal permeability increasing protein, major basic protein, defensins)
Nitric oxide	(NO)	
Peroxynitrite	($ONOO^-$)	

REGULATION OF THE INFLAMMATORY RESPONSE

The foregoing sections provide a conceptual framework for the inflammatory response, specifically, the hemodynamic alterations, mechanisms of specific leukocyte–endothelial adhesive interactions, chemotaxis, leukocyte activation, phagocytosis, and intracellular microbial killing mechanisms. The many steps that constitute this paradigm are regulated by a variety of soluble mediators that are produced by endothelial cells and leukocytes at a site of inflammation, by other resident cells (e.g., tissue macrophages, fibroblasts, mast cells), and as byproducts of bloodborne proteins (e.g., complement system, coagulation cascade; Table 17–3).

Reactive Oxygen Intermediates

Since the early 1970s it has been recognized that activated phagocytes exhibit a transient but marked increase in oxygen consumption and in the generation of reduced oxygen metabolites.[17] Although small quantities of reactive oxygen intermediates are produced as byproducts of a variety of biochemical pathways, the chief source is the leukocyte membrane-associated NADPH oxidase, an enzyme complex that is defective in patients with chronic granulomatous disease (see Chap. 66). Reactive oxygen intermediates include superoxide anion (O_2^-), hydrogen peroxide (H_2O_2), hydroxyl radical (HO•), and singlet oxygen ($^1O_2$).[17] These reduced oxygen products play a major role in intraphagolysosomal killing of microorganisms, and when released extracellularly, are directly or indirectly responsible for a variety of inflammatory processes, including endothelial cell lysis, extracellular matrix degradation, activation of latent proteolytic enzymes (collagenase, gelatinase), inactivation of antiproteases, interaction with toxic metabolites of L-arginine, and generation of chemotactic factors from arachidonic acid and the complement component C5.[21] In addition to their role in endothelial cytotoxicity, reactive oxygen intermediates are cytotoxic for fibroblasts, erythrocytes, tumor cells, and various parenchymal cells.[21] The biochemical mechanisms implicated include lipid peroxidation, formation of carbonyl moieties and nitrosylation products, intracellular enzyme inactivation, protein oxidation, and oxidant-mediated DNA damage. Reactive oxygen intermediates (e.g., O_2^-) can also undergo reactions with reactive nitrogen intermediates (e.g., nitric oxide [NO]; see "Reactive Nitrogen Intermediates" below) to generate toxic NO derivatives.[22] Within limits, host cells are protected by antioxidant defense systems (e.g., superoxide dismutase, catalase, reduced glutathione).[21]

Reactive Nitrogen Intermediates

Described in 1980 as endothelium-derived relaxing factor (EDRF), NO is the soluble, gaseous, short-acting biosynthetic product of L-arginine, O_2, NADPH, and nitric oxide synthase (NOS). As suggested by its original name, NO mediates vascular smooth muscle relaxation. NO binds to the heme moiety of guanylyl cyclase to trigger the generation of intracytoplasmic cyclic guanosine monophosphate (cGMP) and, through the activation of a series of kinases, induces smooth-muscle

TABLE 17–3. Inflammatory Mediator Systems

Mediator System	Source	Major Actions
Reactive oxygen intermediates (O_2^-, H_2O_2, HOX, HO)	Leukocytes, endothelial cells	Tissue damage through cytolysis, matrix degradation, activation of complement, and generation of chemotactic lipids
Reactive nitrogen intermediates (NO, $ONOO^-$, NO_2^-, NO_3^-)	Monocytes, macrophages, lymphocytes, endothelial cells	Cytostasis of cells, inhibition of DNA synthesis, inhibition of mitochondrial respiration, and formation of OH
Lysosomal granule constituents (proteases, lysozyme, lactoferrin, cationic proteins)	Neutrophils, monocytes	Tissue damage through proteolysis, matrix degradation, and catalysis of oxidant-generating reactions
Cytokines and chemokines (TNF, IL-1, IL-8, MCP-1, etc.)	Monocytes, macrophages, and endothelial cells	Cell activation, induction of adhesion, chemotaxis, fever, and acute-phase response
Platelet-activating factor	Leukocytes, endothelial cells	Vascular permeability and cell activation
Arachidonic acid metabolites (prostaglandins, 5-HPETE, leukotrienes)	Cell membranes (endothelial cells, platelets, leukocytes)	Coagulation, vasodilation, vascular permeability, cell activation, and chemotaxis
Kinins (bradykinin, kallikrein)	Plasma	Pain, vascular permeability, and vasodilation
Vasoactive amines (serotonin, histamine)	Platelets, mast cells, and basophils	Vascular permeability, induction of adhesion
Complement	Plasma, macrophages	Chemotaxis, vascular permeability, and cell activation
Coagulation	Plasma	Chemotaxis, vascular permeability, and complement activation

5-HPETE, 5 hydroperoxyeicosatetraenoic acid; MCP-1, monocyte chemoattractant protein-1.

relaxation and vasodilation.[24] Three different forms of NOS have been characterized:[24] endothelial (eNOS), neuronal (nNOS), and inducible (iNOS). Nitric oxide can be produced either constitutively (eNOS, nNOS) or induced (iNOS) in a wide variety of cell types (e.g., endothelial cells, neurons, macrophages, respectively). Nitric oxide produced by eNOS plays a particularly important role in the localized regulation of vascular tone, whereas NO derived from nNOS is important in neuronal signal transduction.[24] NO also plays important roles in the inhibition of smooth-muscle proliferation and in inflammation.[22] The roles of NO in inflammation include inhibition of most cell-mediated inflammation, reduction in platelet aggregation and adhesion, and as a regulator of leukocyte recruitment.[22] Specifically, NO produced by cytokine-iNOS reduces leukocyte recruitment into sites of inflammation.[22,24] NO can react with reactive oxygen intermediates to form both reactive oxygen and nitrogen species (e.g., $NO + O_2^- \; NO_2^- + HO\bullet$), it can inhibit DNA synthesis, it can directly kill microbes and tumor cells, and it can inactivate cytosolic glutathione and a number of sulfhydryl enzymes.[22,24] NO and its generating enzymes, eNOS, nNOS, and iNOS, represent a regulatory system that has varied effects on the inflammatory response depending upon location and setting.

Lysosomal Granule Constituents

The activation of neutrophils, monocytes, and macrophages results in the release, either through exocytosis or as the result of cell death, of a wide variety of proinflammatory mediators that have important roles in the inflammatory response. Neutrophils contain three major types of granules and also secretory vesicles (see Chaps. 59 and 60).[16] Large, primary (azurophilic) granules contain myeloperoxidase, lysozyme, a variety of cationic proteins, defensins, phospholipase, acid hydrolases, and neutral proteases (e.g., proteinase 3, collagenases, elastase). Smaller, secondary (specific) granules contain lactoferrin, lysozyme, type IV collagenase, subunits of NADPH oxidase, and the β_2-integrin CD11b/CD18. Tertiary granules contain gelatinase, subunits of NADPH oxidase, and CD11b/CD18. Acid proteases function most efficiently within phagolysosomes where the pH is low, whereas neutral proteases can function efficiently within extracellular inflammatory exudates. Lysosomal granule constituents contribute to the inflammatory response and tissue injury through a wide array of mechanisms (e.g., degradation of extracellular matrix, proteolytic generation of chemotactic peptides, and catalysis of reactive oxygen metabolite generation).

Cytokines and Chemokines

Cytokines are relatively small (5–20-kDa) proteins that are produced by many cell types and modulate the function of other cell types. Individual cells may produce many different cytokines, and an individual cytokine may exert a wide variety of effects; they are pleiotropic.[25] In addition to their important roles in regulating various aspects of the immune response (e.g., lymphocyte activation and differentiation), many cytokines participate in natural immunity (e.g., TNF-α, IL-1α, type I interferons), activate inflammatory cells (e.g., γ-interferon), and participate in hematopoiesis (e.g., IL-3, granulocyte-monocyte colony-stimulating factor, granulocyte colony-stimulating factor, macrophage colony-stimulating factor).[25] Among the most thoroughly characterized cytokines are IL-1 and TNF-α. IL-1 and TNF-α are structurally dissimilar but share many biologic activities and can function as autocrine, paracrine, and endocrine mediators of inflammation (Table 17–4).[25] IL-1 and TNF-α are produced by various cell types and are pleiotropic. Their most important functions in inflammation include endothelial, leukocyte, and fibroblast activation.[25]

IL-1 and TNF-α are key proximal mediators of the "acute-phase response." Stimuli such as bacterial endotoxin (lipopolysaccharide), toxins, immune complexes, and physical factors (e.g., heat or trauma) can induce macrophages (and other cell types) to secrete IL-1 and TNF-α. In turn, IL-1 and TNF-α mediate fever, somnolence, increased production of proteins such as α_1-antiprotease and α_2-macroglobulin, and decreased production of proteins such as albumin and transferrin.[25] The acute phase response is a stereotyped host metabolic response to a wide variety of insults. In clinical medicine, the above changes in specific protein synthesis yield a characteristic set of changes visible by serum protein electrophoresis. In addition to the

TABLE 17–4. Interleukin-1 and Tumor Necrosis Factor in Inflammation

Acute-phase response
Fever
Shock
Neutrophilia
Somnolence
Anorexia
Acute-phase proteins
Endothelial activation
Induction of IL-1, IL-6, IL-8
Procoagulant phenotype
Leukocyte adherence
Fibroblast activation
Proliferation
Collagen synthesis
Collagenase and protease induction

systemic acute-phase response, IL-1 and TNF-α induce endothelial activation marked by increases in leukocyte adherence and a procoagulant state, leukocyte activation marked by cytokine secretion, and fibroblast activation marked by proliferation, collagen synthesis, and collagenase production.[25] These actions are critical components of inflammation and wound healing, and they exemplify the linkage between the inflammatory response and the coagulation system.

IL-1, which exhibits a wide variety of biologic activities, was initially termed endogenous pyrogen because of its ability to induce temperature elevation and the acute-phase response.[25] IL-1 is now known to be relevant to acute inflammation because of its ability to induce cytokine production in monocytes, macrophages, fibroblasts, and endothelial cells (TNF-α, IL-1, and IL-6). IL-1 can also induce NOS. As noted previously, IL-1 can activate endothelial cells, resulting in the expression of adhesion molecules and a procoagulant phenotype.[25]

TNF-α, originally identified as "cachectin," can induce cytokine production in a variety of cells. TNF-α can induce neutrophil activation and the expression of adhesion molecules on endothelial cells.[25] In contrast to IL-1, TNF-α also possesses potent cytotoxic activities for certain types of cells. Both IL-1 and TNF-α are produced in response to endotoxemia and both can mediate a systemic shock-like response.

Chemokines, or "intercrines," are small proteins, which, in addition to the more general properties of cytokines, exhibit prominent chemotactic activities.[26] Chemokines are grouped into four classes based on the arrangements of conserved cysteine (C) residues in mature peptides.[27] The two most studied subfamilies include the alpha, or "C-X-C" chemokines, and the beta, or "C-C" chemokines. "C-X-C" chemokines are so designated because the first two N-terminal cystine residues are separated by a single amino acid. Alpha chemokines, of which IL-8 is the prototype, consistently exhibit neutrophil chemotactic activity, whereas the beta, or "C-C" chemokines, of which MCP-1 is the prototype, exhibit monocyte chemotactic activity (Table 17–5).[26] Both *in vitro* and *in vivo* studies have provided insight into the roles of chemokines in inflammation. For example, MCP-1 knockout mice (MCP-1 –/–) exhibit reductions in monocyte influx into sites of experimentally induced peritonitis and delayed-type hypersensitivity.[28] Complementary studies using knockout mice devoid of the MCP-1 receptor CCR2 (C-C chemokine receptor 2), do not form typical granulomas.[29] These types of studies, as well as many studies that have employed specific chemokine-neutralizing antibodies or soluble chemokine receptor antagonists, have provided valuable insight into the pathophysiology of inflammation. Seemingly contradictory experimental results suggest that leukocyte recruitment mechanisms are multiple, overlapping, or redundant, and certainly not completely understood. Chemokines activate leukocytes through a family of membrane receptors (serpentines) that contain seven transmembrane domains and are linked to heterotrimeric G proteins.[26]

Inflammatory Lipids

Lipid mediators of inflammation, derived from cell membranes, can act either intracellularly or extracellularly, the latter in a localized, short-lived manner.[30] Arachidonic acid, a 20-carbon polyunsaturated fatty acid (5,8,11,14-eicosatetraenoic acid) derived either from dietary sources or by conversion from linoleic acid, is maintained in cell membranes as an esterified phospholipid.[30] Three families of inflammatory mediators derived from arachidonic acid are generated via the cyclooxygenase and lipoxygenase pathways.[30] Arachidonic acid is released from membrane phospholipids via cellular phospholipases such as phospholipase A_2. Phospholipase activation is triggered by mechanical/physical or chemical stimuli. Arachidonic acid can be metabolized via the cyclooxygenase pathway to prostaglandins (e.g., PGG_2, PGH_2,

TABLE 17–5. Chemokines

Family	Members	Abbreviation(s)	Primary Target Cell(s)
α-Chemokines (C-X-C)	Interleukin-8	IL-8	Neutrophils
	Platelet factor 4	PF4	Neutrophils
	Melanocyte growth-stimulatory activity	MGSA or GROα	Neutrophils
	Neutrophil-activating peptide-2	NAP-2	Neutrophils
	γ-Interferon-inducible protein	γ-IP-10	Neutrophils
β-Chemokines (C-C)	Monocyte chemoattractant protein-1	MCP-1/MCAF or JE	Monocytes, basophils
	Regulated on activation, normal T-cell expressed and presumably secreted	RANTES	Monocytes, eosinophils, basophils
	Macrophage inflammatory protein-1α	MIP-1α	Monocytes, eosinophils
	Macrophage inflammatory protein-1β	MIP-1β	Monocytes

PGD_2, PGE_2, PGF_2), prostacyclin (PGI_2), or thromboxane (TXA_2).[30] Prostacyclins mediate vasodilation and the inhibition of platelet aggregation, thromboxanes have the opposite effects, and PGD_2, PGE_2, and PGF_2 mediate vasodilation and edema. Activation of the lipoxygenase pathway results in the synthesis of 5-hydroperoxyeicosatetraenoic acid (5-HPETE), which is a potent chemoattractant of neutrophils and can be modified to yield a series of other leukotrienes. LTB_4 induces neutrophil chemotaxis, aggregation, degranulation, and adherence, while LTC_4, LTD_4, and LTE_4 trigger smooth-muscle constriction, increases in vascular permeability and bronchoconstriction.[30] Members of both of these families of lipid-derived mediators have been detected in inflammatory exudates. Lipoxins (A_4 [LXA_4] and B_4 [LXB_4]) are generated via the 12-lipooxygenase branch of the lipoxygenase pathway and a unique transcellular biosynthetic pathway.[31] Neutrophils generate LTA_4 via the 5-lipooxygenase pathway; in turn, lipoxins (LXA_4 and LXB_4) are generated through the action of platelet 12-lipooxygense on neutrophil LTA_4. Prevention of neutrophil-platelet binding interrupts this pathway. Lipoxins inhibit neutrophil chemotaxis and adhesion to endothelium.[31]

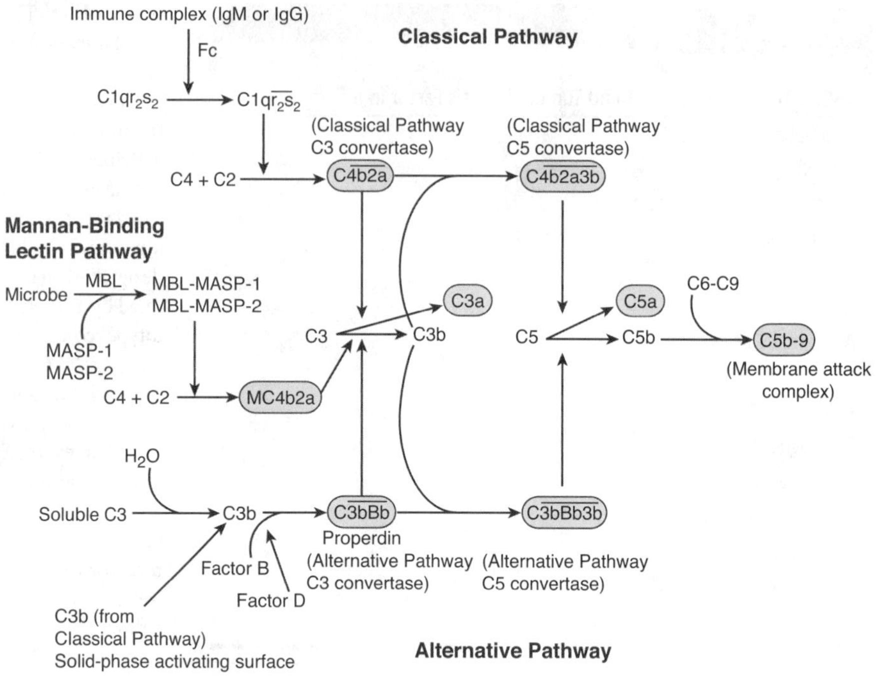

FIGURE 17–3. The complement system. The complement system consists of a series of soluble and surface-associated mediators that are functionally organized into the classical, alternative, and mannan-binding lectin (MBL) pathways. The three pathways of complement converge and lead to the production of the pore-forming membrane attack complex. The classical pathway is most often activated by IgG- and IgM-containing immune complexes, the alternative pathway can be activated by a variety of particulates, and the MBL pathway by various carbohydrate surfaces. In all three cases, complex multicomponent enzyme complexes, called C3 and C5 convertases, are formed. A variety of proinflammatory peptide fragments (e.g., C3a, C5a) are generated as a result of complement activation.

PAF is a potent proinflammatory lipid produced by a variety of cell types, including neutrophils, monocytes, endothelial cells, and IgE-sensitized basophils.[32] Derived from the cell membrane constituent choline phosphoglyceride, PAF is an acetyl glycerol ether phosphocholine that is synthesized following the activation of phospholipase A_2. PAF triggers platelet aggregation and degranulation, increases vascular permeability, and promotes leukocyte accumulation and activation. *In vivo* studies using specific PAF antagonists have suggested a role for PAF in a variety of acute inflammatory lesions.[32]

Kinins

The kinin system is activated by contact activation of clotting factor XII (Hageman factor) (see Chaps. 115 and 116).[33] Activation of the kinin system results in the generation of bradykinin, the nine amino-acid vasoactive peptide. Bradykinin possesses several activities, including the capacity to increase vascular permeability, to induce smooth-muscle contraction, to trigger vasodilation, and to cause pain.[33] Activated Hageman factor (factor XIIa), also known as the prekallikrein activator, converts plasma prekallikrein to kallikrein. In turn, kallikrein cleaves high-molecular-weight kininogen to produce bradykinin. Models of septic shock reveal decreases in plasma kininogen that parallel decreases in peripheral arterial resistance.[33]

Vasoactive Amines

Histamine and serotonin (5-hydroxytryptamine) are low-molecular-weight vasoactive amines. Histamine is contained in mast cell and basophil granules, whereas platelets are the chief source of serotonin.[34] Localized release of histamine results in wheal formation as a consequence of increases in vascular permeability. Histamine induces the formation of reversible openings in endothelial tight junctions, triggers the formation of prostacyclin by endothelial cells, and induces NO release from the endothelium. In addition, histamine, like thrombin, can induce the rapid upregulation of endothelial P-selectin.[34] Serotonin, which acts through receptors on vascular smooth-muscle cells, is responsible for vasoconstriction, whereas interaction with endothelial receptors results in vasodilation (via release of NO) and increased permeability.[2] Release of histamine and serotonin from mast cells and platelets can be triggered by IgE-mediated type I hypersensitivity reactions, directly by C3a or C5a, and directly by neutrophil-granule-derived cationic proteins.

Complement

The complement system, including its soluble and cell membrane-associated regulators, consists of nearly two dozen plasma proteins that give rise to mediators of chemotaxis, increased vascular permeability, opsonic activity, phagocytic activation, and cytolysis.[35] In a manner analogous to coagulation, the complement system is activated through a cascade of proteolytic cleavage reactions. There are three convergent pathways (Fig. 17–3). The first of these, the "classical pathway," is initiated primarily by complement-fixing immune complexes (IgG and IgM), whereas the second, the "alternative pathway," is triggered by a variety of substances that include IgA aggregates, endotoxin, cobra venom factor, and the polysaccharide components of some bacterial and fungal cell walls. The third pathway, the "mannan-binding" lectin (MBL) pathway, is activated when MBL binds to a carbohydrate-coated microorganism. Upon binding, MBL activates MBL-associated serine proteases (e.g., MASP-1, MASP-2), which function in a manner analogous to C1r and C1s of the classical pathway. MBL recognizes carbohydrate moieties infrequently present in mammalian hosts, thus constituting a system for recognizing foreign particulates. The classical pathway is initiated by the fixation of C1 ($C1qr_2s_2$) by the Fc portion of surface-bound IgG or IgM immunoglobulins. Activated C1 ($C1qr_2s_2$) cleaves C2 and C4, which leads to the formation of the "classical pathway" C3 convertase C4b2a. Activation of the alternative pathway results in the formation of an "alternative pathway" C3 convertase following direct cleavage of C3 and subsequent interactions of C3b with factors B and D in the presence of Mg^{2+}. The resulting complex, C3bBb, is stabilized by properdin, leading to the stable C3 convertase C3bBbP. C3 convertases generated via any of the three pathways can cleave C3 to form C3a and C3b. C3b can bind to either the classical or alternative pathway C3 convertase to form a C5 convertase, which cleaves C5 into C5a and C5b. C5a is released into the fluid phase, like C3a, whereas C5b combines first with C6 and then C7 to form C5b-7, which, in turn, binds with C8 and multiple C9 molecules to form C5b-9, the membrane attack complex. In addition to the cell-activating and cytolytic activities of C5b-9, individual complement cleavage products and complexes perform a variety of specific and potent proinflammatory activities.[35] These various functions, combined with the rapid amplification in numbers of complement-derived mediators, emphasize the vital role of complement in acute inflammation. The most important activation products of complement appear to be C5a, the major chemotactic factor, and the anaphylatoxins (C3a, C4a, C5a), of which C3a is the most abundant. C5b-9 appears to be a major cytotoxic product, provided that this complex is assembled on the surface of a susceptible cell (e.g., bacterium). A series of soluble and cell membrane-associated complement proteins play important roles in the regulation of the complement cascade.[35]

Coagulation System

The coagulation system is reviewed in detail in Chaps. 115, 116, and 117. The interrelationships among the coagulation system and inflammatory mediator systems are important in the context of host defense and the pathophysiology of septic shock. Activation of the clotting cascade results in the generation of fibrinopeptides, which increase vascular permeability and are chemotactic for leukocytes. Thrombin induces endothelial expression of P-selectin, resulting in increased neutrophil adhesion.[10] In addition, plasmin is responsible for the activation of Hageman factor, which then can activate the kinin system, and can cleave C3 into its active components.[33] It can also generate fibrin-split products. The induction of procoagulant activity in endothelial cells exposed to TNF-α and IL-1 further links the coagulation system to the inflammatory response.[25]

CHRONIC INFLAMMATION AND REPAIR

The chronic inflammatory response and repair processes are, like the acute inflammatory response, highly regulated. By definition, "chronic" inflammation connotes a process that lasts for weeks to months, and sometimes for years. Chronic inflammation is characterized by the recruitment of mononuclear cells including lymphocytes, monocytes, and plasma cells, as well as by the proliferation of new capillaries (angiogenesis) and increases in the deposition of extracellular matrix. Replacement of damaged tissue by new small blood vessels and extracellular matrix constitutes a fundamental aspect of chronic inflammation and, simultaneously, is an integral part of wound healing and repair. The recruitment of this wide variety of cell types is achieved by complex interactions among cytokines, chemokines, and indigenous cells. Great advances in understanding of angiogenesis and extracellular matrix molecule metabolism have been made in recent years.

Chronic inflammation can be caused by persistent infections with a wide variety of microorganisms (e.g., *Treponema pallidum, Mycobacterium tuberculosis*). In contrast to highly virulent organisms that trigger acute pyogenic infections (e.g., *Streptococcus pneumoniae, Haemophilus influenzae*), organisms that induce chronic inflammation typically exhibit relatively low intrinsic toxicity, are poorly cleared, and provoke a delayed-type hypersensitivity reaction. Chronic inflammation is also triggered by long-term exposure to insoluble exogenous particles (e.g., carbon dust, silica).[2] The initiation of other chronic inflammatory processes such as atherosclerosis and autoimmune diseases (e.g., rheumatoid arthritis, systemic lupus erythematosus) is less-well understood, but it is clear that a variety of environmental factors (e.g., diet in atherosclerosis) and genetic factors (e.g., human leukocyte antigen [HLA]-linked susceptibility is rheumatoid arthritis) are important. The characteristics of individual chronic inflammatory responses are dependent on the location of the injury and the type of injurious agent. As noted throughout this chapter, the recruitment of mononuclear cells into an inflammatory lesion is governed by the same types of mechanisms that orchestrate the recruitment of neutrophils into sites of acute inflammation. Unlike most acute conditions, chronic inflammatory processes are often marked by a relatively specific morphology (e.g., granuloma formation in tuberculosis, eosinophil infiltration in parasitic infections) and by the coexistence of tissue repair (i.e., angiogenesis and extracellular matrix production).

A key cell type in chronic inflammatory processes is the macrophage.[36] Tissue macrophages are derived from circulating blood monocytes and can adopt relatively specific functions based on their differentiation in selected body sites (e.g., hepatic Kupffer cells, alveolar macrophages, central nervous system microglia). In the setting of chronic inflammation, tissue macrophages can be activated by immunologic means (γ-interferon secreted by antigen-activated T lymphocytes) and by nonimmunologic means (microbial endotoxin, extracellular matrix proteins, and foreign particulates; see Chap. 68). In turn, activated macrophages enlarge, become more metabolically active, exhibit enhanced phagocytosis, and secrete a large array of mediators.[36] Mediators secreted by activated macrophages include proteases, reactive oxygen and nitrogen intermediates, coagulation factors, arachidonic acid-derived lipids, and cytokines. These mediators, as detailed in preceding sections, participate in inflammation. Activated macrophages also secrete collagenases that participate in tissue remodeling, angiogenic factors (e.g., fibroblast growth factor), and profibrogenic growth factors (fibroblast growth factor, transforming growth factor-β, platelet-derived growth factor).[36] Consequently, activated tissue macrophages participate in inflammation *per se*, tissue remodeling, angiogenesis, and fibrosis.

Although macrophages play a central role in all facets of chronic inflammation, other cell types are also important. Lymphocytes, both B and T cells, are recruited into chronic inflammatory lesions via leukocyte–endothelial adhesive interactions and via chemotactic mechanisms analogous to those involved in neutrophil recruitment. Antigen-activated T lymphocytes produce γ-interferon, which, as discussed above, is an important soluble activator of tissue macrophages.[37] Activated lymphocytes produce a variety of proinflammatory mediators that are involved in lymphocyte proliferation (e.g., IL-2) and in immune regulation (e.g., IL-5 in IgE production).[37]

Eosinophils and mast cells also play important roles in some types of chronic inflammation. Mast cells, which tend to be distributed along small blood vessels, possess high-affinity FcεRI receptors for IgE.[38] Engagement of mast cell-bound IgE triggers degranulation that leads to histamine and arachidonic acid-derived lipid release (see Chap. 63). Eosinophils are characteristically formed in IgE-mediated allergic reactions and in parasitic infections (see Chap. 62). Eotaxin, a C-C chemokine, binds to and activates eosinophils via CCR3.[38] Recruited eosinophils secrete various granule proteins that help kill parasites, but which can also cause tissue damage. As inferred above, the histopathologic appearance of many chronic inflammatory lesions can provide insight into their pathogenesis and cause. A variety of poorly degraded, intrinsically low toxicity agents can induce granulomatous inflammation (e.g., *M. tuberculosis*). Many parasites induce an eosinophilic response (e.g., *Toxocara canis*). Finally, the induction of tissue remodeling, angiogenesis, and fibrosis can contribute to both tissue damage and repair, and can also suggest underlying etiology (e.g., lung fibrosis associated with asbestos). The tremendous advances in understanding of the inflammatory response hold great promise for the future of both diagnostics and therapeutics.

REFERENCES

1. Weissman G: Inflammation: Historical perspectives, in *Inflammation: Basic Principles and Clinical Correlates*, 2d ed, edited by JJ Gallin, IM Goldstein, R Snyderman, p 5. Raven Press, New York, 1992.
2. Acute and chronic inflammation, in *Robbins and Cotran Pathologic Basis of Disease*, 7th ed, edited by V Kumar, AK Abbas, N Fausto, p 47. Saunders Elsevier, Philadelphia, 2005.
3. Lentsch AB, Ward PA: Regulation of inflammatory vascular damage. *J Pathol* 190:343, 2000.
4. Dvorak AM, Feng D: The vesiculo-vacuolar organelle (vvo). A new endothelial cell permeability organelle. *J Histochem Cytochem* 49:419, 2001.
5. Muller WA: Leukocyte-endothelial cell interactions in the inflammatory response. *Lab Invest* 82:521, 2002.
6. Chen S, Springer TA: Selectin receptor-ligand bonds: Formation limited by shear rate and dissociation governed by the Bell model. *Proc Natl Acad Sci U S A* 98:950, 2001.
7. Hynes RO: Integrins: Bidirectional, allosteric signaling machines. *Cell* 110:673, 2002.
8. Jung U, Key K: Mice lacking two or all three selectins demonstrate overlapping and distinct functions for each selectin. *J Immunol* 162:6755, 1999.
9. Jung U, Ramos CL, Bullard DC, Ley K: Gene-targeted mice reveal importance of L-selectin-dependent rolling for neutrophil adhesion. *Am J Physiol Heart Circ Physiol* 274:H1785, 1998.
10. McEver RP: Selectins: Lectins that initiate cell adhesion under flow. *Curr Opin Cell Biol* 14:581, 2002.
11. Takagi J, Springer TA: Integrin activation and structural rearrangement. *Immunol Rev* 186:141, 2002.
12. Shimaoka M, Takagi J, Springer TA: Conformational regulation of integrin structure and function. *Annu Rev Biophys Biomol Struct* 31:485, 2002.
13. Muller WA: Migration of leukocytes across endothelial junctions: some concepts and controversies. *Microcirculation* 8:118, 2001.
14. Luscinskas FW, Ma S, Nusrat A,et al: Leukocyte transendothelial migration: A junctional affair. *Semin Immunol* 14:105, 2002.
15. Ciacchetti G, Allen PG, Glogauer M: Chemotactic signaling pathways in neutrophils: from receptor to actin assembly. *Crit Rev Oral Biol Med* 13:220, 2002.
16. Faurschou M, Borregaard N: Neutrophil granules and secretory vesicles in inflammation. *Microbes Infect* 5:1317, 2003.
17. Babior BM, Lambeth JD, Nauseef W: The neutrophil NADPH oxidase. *Arch Biochem Biophys* 397:342, 2002.
18. Underhill DM, Ozinsky A: Phagocytosis of microbes: Complexity in action. *Annu Rev Immunol* 20:825, 2002.
19. Digstelbluem HM, Kallenberg CGM, Van de Winkel JGJ: Inflammation in autoimmunity: Receptors for IgG. *Trends Immunol* 22:510, 2001.
20. Baumann U, Schmidt RE: The role of Fc receptors and complement in autoimmunity. *Adv Exp Med Biol* 495:219, 2001.
21. Babior BM: Phagocytes and oxidative stress. *Am J Med* 109:33, 2003.
22. Beckman JS, Koppenol WH: Nitric oxide, superoxide, and peroxynitrite: The good, the bad, and the ugly. *Am J Physiol* 271: C1424, 1996.
23. Furchgott RF, Zawadzki JV: The obligatory role of endothelial cells in the relaxation of arterial smooth muscle by acetylcholine. *Nature* 288:373, 1980.
24. Laroux FS, Pavlick KP, Hines IN, et al: Role of nitric oxide in inflammation. *Acta Physiol Scand* 173:113, 2001.
25. Abbas AK, Lichtman AH: *Cellular and Molecular Immunology*, 3rd ed, p 249. WB Saunders, Philadelphia, 1999.
26. Rossi D, Zlotnik A: The biology of chemokines and their receptors. *Annu Rev Immunol* 18:217, 2000.
27. Zlotnik A, Yoshie O: Chemokines: A new classification system and their role in immunity. *Immunity* 12:121, 2000.
28. Lu B, Rutledge BJ, Gu L, et al: Abnormalities in monocyte recruitment and cytokine expression in monocyte chemoattractant protein 1-deficient mice. *J Exp Med* 187:601, 1998.
29. Kuziel WA, Morgan SJ, Dawson TC, et al: Severe reduction in leukocyte adhesion and monocyte extravasation in mice deficient in CC chemokine receptor 2. *Proc Natl Acad Sci U S A* 94:12053, 1997.
30. Zurier RB: Prostaglandins, leukotrienes, and related compounds, in *Kelley's Textbook of Rheumatology*, 6th ed, edited by ED Harris Jr, RC Budd, GS Firestein, MC Genovese, JS Sargent, S Ruddy, p 356. Saunders Elsevier, Philadelphia, 2005.
31. Levy BD, Serhan CN: Polyisoprenyl phosphates: Natural antiinflammatory lipid signals. *Cell Mol Life Sci* 59:729, 2002.
32. Prescott SM, Zimmerman GA, Stafforini DM, McIntyre TM: Platelet-activating factor and related lipid mediators. *Annu Rev Biochem* 69:419, 2000.
33. Couture R, Harrisson M, Vianna RM, Cloutier F: Kinin receptors in pain and inflammation. *Eur J Pharmacol* 429:161, 2001.
34. Repka-Ramirez MS, Baraniuk JN: Histamine in health and disease. *Clin Allergy Immunol* 17:1, 2002.
35. Holers MV: Complement, in *Clinical Immunology: Principles and Practice*, 2nd ed, edited by RR Rich, TT Fleisher, WT Shearer, BL Kotizn, HW Schroeder Jr, p 21.1. Mosby, London, 2001.
36. Thomas R, Arend WP: Antigen-presenting cells, in *Kelley's Textbook of Rheumatology*, 6th ed, edited by ED Harris Jr, RC Budd, GS Firestein, MC Genovese, JS Sargent, S Ruddy, p 101. Elsevier Saunders, Philadelphia, 2005.
37. Kumar V, Abbaas AK, Fausto N: Diseases of immunity, in *Robbins and Cotran Pathologic Basis of Disease*, 7th ed, p 193. Saunders Elsevier, Philadelphia, 2005.
38. Gould HJ, Sutton BJ, Beavil AJ, et al: The biology of IgE and the basis of allergic disease. *Annu Rev Immunol* 21:579, 2003.
39. Cellular pathology II: Adaptations, intracellular accumulations, and cell aging, in *Robbins Pathologic Basis of Disease*, 6th ed, edited by Cotran RS, Kumar V, Collins T, Robbins SL, p 31. WB Saunders, Philadelphia, 1999.

CHAPTER 18
INNATE IMMUNITY

Bruce Beutler

SUMMARY

The innate immune system provides immediate protection against infection and serves an essential antigen-presenting role that allows the adaptive immune response to occur during the days and weeks that follow. The sensory apparatus that allows detection of infectious microbes has been deciphered in large part, and it is now known that toll-like receptors (TLRs), NOD-like receptors (NLRs), and RIG-I–like helicases (RLHs) permit recognition of specific molecules of microbial origin. Much has also been learned of the biochemical events that follow activation of these sensors. Susceptibility to infection in humans is strongly heritable, and among the many loci that influence it, those that encode proteins vital to the innate immune response are of central importance. Moreover, autoinflammatory and autoimmune diseases are dependent upon the activation of innate immune signaling pathways.

INNATE IMMUNITY VERSUS ADAPTIVE IMMUNITY

In humans, as in all mammals, resistance to microbial infection is based partly upon lymphocytes, which yield highly specific responses to microbial antigens: either the production of antibodies or the expansion of T-cell cell clones that are directly cytotoxic to infected cells (see Chaps. 77 and 78). This, the *adaptive* immune response, is a recent fixture in evolution, witnessed only in vertebrates and traceable to the development of a mechanism for recombination of genomic DNA that arose approximately 450 million years ago. A more fundamental type of immunity, known as *innate* immunity, is represented in one form or another in all multicellular organisms. For this reason, much progress in the innate immunity field has come from the study of model animals, such as *Drosophila melanogaster*, and model plants, such as *Arabidopsis thaliana*. Despite the vast evolutionary divergence between these organisms from *Homo sapiens*, both species utilize defensive proteins and signaling pathways that are ancestrally related to those in humans.

Abbreviations and acronyms that appear in this chapter include: AD, acidic activation domain; BIR, baculovirus inhibitor of apoptosis repeat; CARD, caspase activation and recruitment domain; CD, cluster of differentiation; CMV, cytomegalovirus; CTLA, cytotoxic T lymphocyte antigen; DAI, DNA-dependent activator of IRFs; ERK, extracellular signal-regulated kinase; FADD, Fas-associated death domain; FIIND, F-interacting domain; IFN, interferon; IFN-β promoter stimulator 1; I-κB, inhibitor of κB; IKK, I-κB kinase; IL, interleukin; IPAF, ice-protease activating factor; IPS-1, IRAK, interleukin-1 receptor-associated kinase; IRF, interferon response factor; JAK, Janus-associated kinase; JNK, c-Jun N-terminal kinase; LPS, lipopolysaccharide; LRR, leucine-rich repeat; MAL, MyD88 adaptor-like; MCMV, mouse cytomegalovirus; MDA5, melanoma differentiation-associated gene 5; MDP, muramyl dipeptide; MyD88, myeloid differentiation 88; NACHT, a nucleotide-binding domain present in NAIP, CIITA, HET-E, and TP-1; NAD, NACHT-associated domain; NADPH, nicotinamide adenine dinucleotide phosphate; NBS, nucleotide binding sequence; NEMO, NF-κB essential modulator; NF-κB, nuclear factor-κB; NK, natural killer; NLR, NOD-like receptor; NOD, nucleotide-binding oligomerization domain; PAR-2, proteinase-activated G-protein-coupled receptor; PRAT4A, protein associated with TLR4; PYD, pyrin domain; RIG-I, retinoic acid inducible gene I; RIP, receptor-interacting protein; RLH, RIG-I like helicase; SARM, sterile-alpha and armadillo motif; SOCS-1, suppressor of cytokine synthesis 1; STAT, signal transducer and activator of transcription; STING, stimulator of interferon genes; TAK-1, transforming growth factor B activating kinase 1; TBK1, TANK-binding kinase 1; TIR, toll/interleukin-1 receptor/resistance; TLR, toll-like receptor; TNF, tumor necrosis factor; Tpl2, tumor progression locus 2; TRAF, tumor necrosis factor receptor-associated factor; TRAM, TRIF-related adaptor molecule; TRIF, toll-interleukin 1 receptor (TIR) domain-containing adaptor inducing IFN-β; UCM, upregulation of costimulatory molecules.

Like the adaptive immune system, the innate immune system is endowed with a means of detecting microbes, destroying microbes, and at the same time, exercising self-tolerance. These mechanisms are far older than the analogous adaptive immune mechanisms, and as a consequence, are more refined. Although it is sometimes called the "primitive" immune system, the innate immune system is both sophisticated and highly effective. Moreover, adaptive immunity is largely dependent upon innate immunity in the sense that antigen presentation and adaptive immune activation depend upon innate immune cells.

Innate immunity, which acts immediately to protect the host in the event of microbial inoculation, fills a temporal gap that would otherwise exist in the global immune response. Days or weeks are required for an effective adaptive immune response to develop when the naïve host encounters a new pathogen. During this time, innate immunity alone protects the host. Indeed, innate immunity is objectively more important than adaptive immunity. In a nonsterile environment, survival would be impossible without it (Table 18–1).

TYPES OF INNATE IMMUNITY

Innate immunity embraces a large number of host resistance mechanisms. It is possible to divide the innate immune system into cellular and noncellular components, and also into afferent and effector components. Noncellular components of innate immunity include antimicrobial peptides, which selectively disrupt microbial cell membranes, complement, components of which also disrupt cell membranes, and such proteins as hemopexin and haptoglobin, which deny iron to invasive microbes. Cellular components include cells of myeloid origin (*granulocytes*, *monocyte/macrophages*, *mast cells*, and *dendritic cells*) and lymphoid cells (*natural killer [NK] cells* and *NKT cells*). As such, it can be seen that despite their recent evolutionary origin, some lymphoid cells have been coopted to serve in the innate immune system rather than the adaptive immune system. Many other cells are also endowed with some degree of innate (often "cell-autonomous") immune function. For example, fibroblasts can sense viral infection and respond with interferon production.

It is difficult to cleanly divide innate immune responses into "afferent" and "effector" functions, as a response, once initiated, runs its course in a preprogrammed fashion, proceeding from microbe sensing all the way through to microbial killing. However, the proteins responsible for microbial recognition, signaling, and the development of a transcriptional response within innate immune cells are generally considered "afferent" components; the cytokines that mediate the response and the cellular weaponry that is used to destroy viruses and bacteria may be considered "effector" components.

This chapter focuses largely on the afferent arm of cellular innate immunity, as the effector mechanisms (neutrophil-mediated killing, complement, and antimicrobial peptides) are covered in other chapters (see Chaps. 16, 60, 66, and 68).

TABLE 18–1. Comparisons between Innate and Adaptive Immunity

	Innate Immunity	Adaptive Immunity
Sensing mechanism	TLRs, NK receptors, NLRs, RLHs, fMLP receptor	Immunoglobulins, T-cell receptors
Cellular components	Macrophages, dendritic cells, granulocytes, mast cells, NK cells	T cells, B cells
Efferent mechanisms	Cytokine production, inflammatory response, phagocytosis, pathogen killing	Antibody production, cytokine production, cell killing
Purpose	Alert other innate and adaptive immune cells to pathogen presence; directly kill pathogen; encourage the development of an adaptive immune response	Assist in efficacy of innate immune response, produce highly specific ligands for pathogens
Time scale of response	Quick (maximal in minutes to hours)	Slow (maximal in days to weeks)
Specific memory	No	Yes
Phylogeny	Ancient (all multicellular organisms)	Recent (vertebrates only)

fMLP, *N*-formyl-methionyl-leucyl-phenylalanine; NK, natural killer; NLR, NOD (nondefinitive)-like receptor; RLH, RIG (retinoic acid-inducible gene)-I–like helicases; TLR, toll-like receptors.

MICROBE RECOGNITION BY THE TOLL-LIKE RECEPTORS

Discovery of the Mammalian Toll-Like Receptors as the Primary Sensors of the Innate Immune System

The toll-like receptors (TLRs) collectively mediate the recognition of most microbes. The substances recognized by each of these TLRs have been defined in part for 9 of the 10 TLRs identified in the human genome. Although some publications suggest that the TLRs (notably TLRs 2 and 4) detect dozens of molecules, the evidence favoring most of these interactions is slender, and a conservative viewpoint is preferred; hence, Table 18–2 presents only those interactions that appear validated.

The microbe-sensing function of the mammalian TLRs was discovered as a result of inquiry into the mechanism of endotoxin sensing. Endotoxin (later identified as lipopolysaccharide [LPS]) was first described by Pfeiffer as a toxic component of *Vibrio cholerae* more than 100 years ago.[1] Its chemical structure was established many years later (reviewed in reference 2), and a toxic "lipid A" moiety of LPS was synthesized artificially in 1985 and found to have full biologic activity.[3] The identity of the LPS receptor was established in 1998, through the positional cloning of *Lps*, a locus required for all cellular responses to endotoxin, and for the effective clearance of Gram-negative bacterial infections[4] in laboratory mice. Mice that were unresponsive to LPS were found to have inactivating mutations in the *Tlr4* locus.[5] It had previously been recognized that toll, a *Drosophila* protein also known for its developmental effects,[6] was required for the innate immune response to fungal infection in flies.[7] Hence, the discovery of an LPS sensing function for TLR4, a homologue of toll, made good evolutionary sense.

Other molecules of microbial origin (for example, di- and tri-acylated lipopeptides and lipoproteins, lipoteichoic acid, unmethylated DNA bearing cytosine phosphate guanine [CpG] dinucleotides in a particular context, flagellin, and double-stranded RNA [dsRNA]) can elicit responses qualitatively similar to those elicited by LPS. Reverse genetic methods established that each of these molecules was recognized by a particular TLR or heteromeric combination of TLRs.[8–12] Moreover, genetic complementation analyses demonstrated that at least some microbial ligands directly engage the TLRs in order to elicit a signal.[13,14] On the other hand, other molecules enhance the signal, and also participate in ligand recognition. Dectin-1 is a type II membrane C-type lectin that recognizes glucans present in the cell walls of fungi and enhances TLR2/6 signaling.[15] Similarly, proteinase-activated G-protein-coupled receptor (PAR-2) signaling enhances TLR4 responses to LPS.[16] Other examples include the binding of CD14 to LPS[17] and the augmentation of LPS responses,[18] as well as the enhancement of responses to bacterial diacylglycerides by CD36.[19] It is likely that these accessory molecules form complexes with the TLRs, which are responsible for transducing the signal across the cell membrane. TLR4, alone among the TLRs, is known to exist as a tight complex with MD-2, a small secreted protein that is required for TLR4 to reach the cell surface and for LPS sensing.[20]

Structure of the TLRs

The TLRs are single-spanning transmembrane proteins with leucine-rich repeat (LRR) motifs in their extracellular domains and a characteristic TIR (toll/interleukin-1 receptor/resistance) motif in their cytoplasmic domains. The TIR domain is based on an ancient protein fold[21] evident

TABLE 18–2. Toll-Like Receptors, Microbial Specificities, and Transducers

TLR	Known Macromolecular Associations	Ligand(s)	Adapter Use	Reference
1	TLR2	Tri-acyl lipopeptides	MyD88, MAL	10, 117–119
2	TLRs 1 or 6, or homodimer	Lipopeptides, lipoteichoic acid, zymosan, protozoal GPI	MyD88, MAL	8
3	–	dsRNA	TRIF	12, 36, 100
4	CD14, MD-2	LPS	MyD88, MAL, TRIF, TRAM	5, 17, 35, 36, 100, 120
5	–	Flagellin	MyD88	11
6	TLR2	Di-acyl lipopeptides, glucans, lipoteichoic acid	MyD88, MAL	121
7	–	ssRNA, imidazoquinolines	MyD88	122
8	–	ssRNA, imidazoquinolines	MyD88	123
9	–	Unmethylated CpG motifs	MyD88	9
10	–	Unknown	Unknown	124

CpG, cytosine phosphate guanine; dsRNA, double-stranded ribonucleic acid; GPI, glycosylphosphatidylinositol; LPS, lipopolysaccharide; MAL, MyD88 adaptor-like; MyD88, myeloid differentiation factor 88; ssRNA, single-stranded ribonucleic acid; TRAM, TRIF-related adaptor molecule; TRIF, toll/interleukin-1 receptor domain-containing adaptor inducing interferon-*β*.

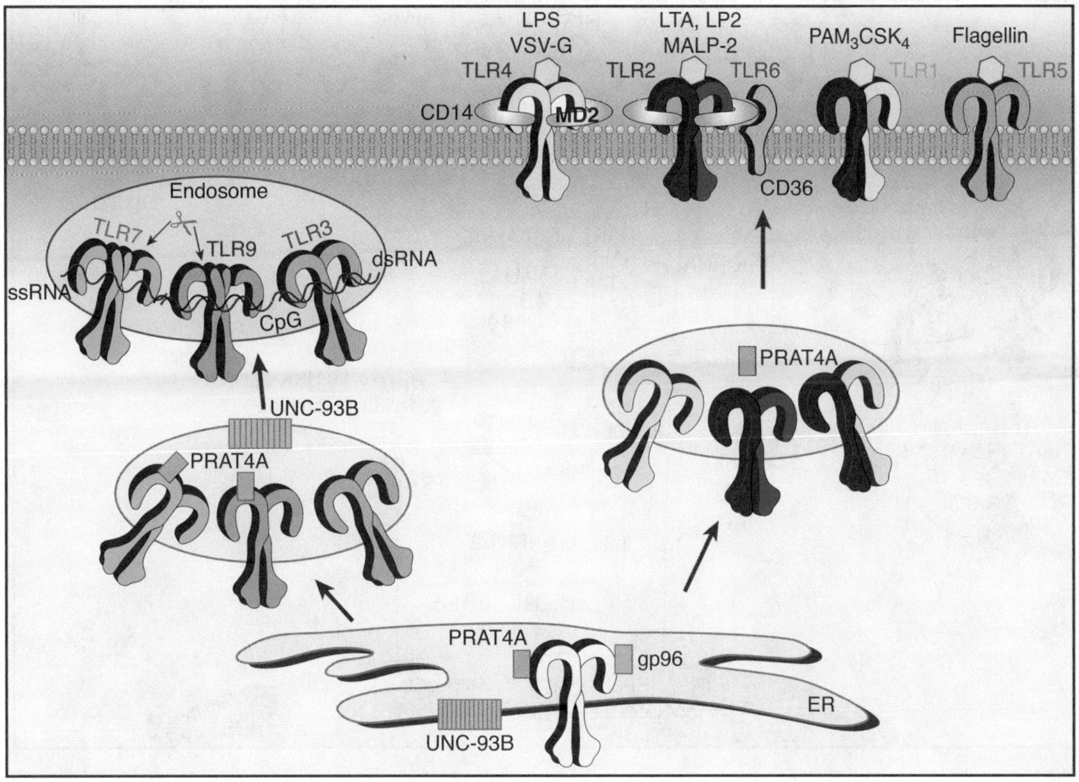

FIGURE 18–1. The toll-like receptors (TLRs). The TLRs exist in homo- or heterodimeric form and are capable of sensing diverse molecules derived from pathogenic organisms. TLRs 1, 2, 4, 5, and 6 are located at the cell surface, whereas TLRs 3, 7, and 9 are located in the endosome. All TLR maturation is dependent on the chaperone protein gp96 in the endoplasmic reticulum (ER). Two other ER proteins, PRAT4A and UNC-93B, play important roles in TLR trafficking. PRAT4A is necessary for TLRs 1, 2, 4, 7, and 9 responses, whereas UNC-93B is required for TLRs 3, 7, and 9 trafficking. At the cell surface, a TLR4 complex composed of TLR4, MD2, and CD14 specifically binds to lipopolysaccharide (LPS) and vesicular stomatitis virus glycoprotein G (VSV-G). The TLR2/6 heterodimer, along with CD36 and CD14, recognizes diacylated lipopeptides and lipoteichoic acid (LTA). The TLR1/2 heterodimer senses triacylated lipopeptides (PAM_3CSK_4), and TLR5 recognizes flagellin. TLR7 is able to bind to single-stranded RNA, TLR9 to CpG DNA, and TLR3 to double-stranded RNA. Proteolysis of both TLR7 and TLR9 occurs in the endolysosome, and at least in the case of TLR9, is required for function. Abbreviations are as used in the text.

in cytosolic plant disease resistance proteins (where it often is represented together with a nucleotide binding sequence [NBS] and/or LRR motifs). The TIR domain is found in proteins of the interleukin (IL)-1 and IL-18 receptor family, the adapter proteins that carry signals from TLRs, and the TLRs themselves.

The structure of the TLR2/1, 2/6, 3, and 4 ectodomains has been determined by X-ray crystallography. Each molecule is horseshoe-shaped, and each is a homodimer or heterodimer. The nature of the ligand receptor interaction appears to be very different in each case. To activate TLR4, LPS interacts with MD-2, which has a hydrophobic pocket that accommodates the lipid A moiety of LPS.[22,23] TLR2/1 heterodimers are "crosslinked" by the engagement of two acyl chains by TLR1 and a single acyl chain by TLR2.[24] TLR3 molecules bind a linear, negatively charged dsRNA oligonucleotide, which triggers activation.[25]

Little (TLR3) or no (TLRs 7 and 9) surface expression of TLRs 3, 7, 8, and 9 can be detected, and tagged versions of the molecules are found to reside within the interior of transfected cells.[26] The ectodomains of these TLRs project into endocytic vesicles and detect foreign molecules there rather than within the extracellular space. TLRs 3, 7, 8, and 9 depend upon UNC-93B, a 12-spanning endoplasmic reticulum (ER) membrane protein, to gain access to the endosomal compartment.[27] Proteolysis of TLR7 and 9 occurs in the endolysosome, and at least for TLR9, this cleavage is necessary for activating downstream signaling pathways.[28,29] UNC-93B can serve a chaperone function, escorting these molecules and perhaps others to their destination in the cell.[30] The protein associated with TLR4, PRAT4A (encoded by *TNRC5*), serves to play a critical role in chaperoning multiple TLRs to their destination,[31] while the ER chaperone protein, gp96 (also called GRP94 or HSP90B1), is critical for all TLR maturation (Fig. 18–1).[32]

TIR Adapter Signaling

The signaling events initiated by the TLRs are increasingly complex (reviewed in references 33 and 34). Figure 18–2 illustrates TLR signaling pathways as they are presently understood. It must be recognized that not all TLRs operate within the same cells, nor are all cells equivalent in their responses to TLR ligation. Notably macrophages and conventional (myeloid) dendritic cells respond to different stimuli than either lymphoid cells or plasmacytoid dendritic cells (which are specialized for type I interferon production). Moreover, some cells not usually regarded as "professional" components of the innate immune system are capable of responding to TLR ligands in one way or another.

A total of five TIR adapter proteins are encoded in the human genome. These adapters are myeloid differentiation factor 88 (MyD88); MyD88 adaptor-like (MAL), also known as toll/interleukin-1 receptor domain containing adaptor protein (TIRAP); TIR domain-containing adaptor inducing interferon-β (TRIF), also known as TICAM-1 and first identified by a mutant allele known as *Lps2*; TRIF-related adaptor molecule (TRAM), also known as TICAM-2; and sterile-alpha and armadillo motif (SARM). The function of SARM remains unknown. However, the four remaining adapters have well-defined roles in signal transduction. All four of these adapters are required for normal signaling

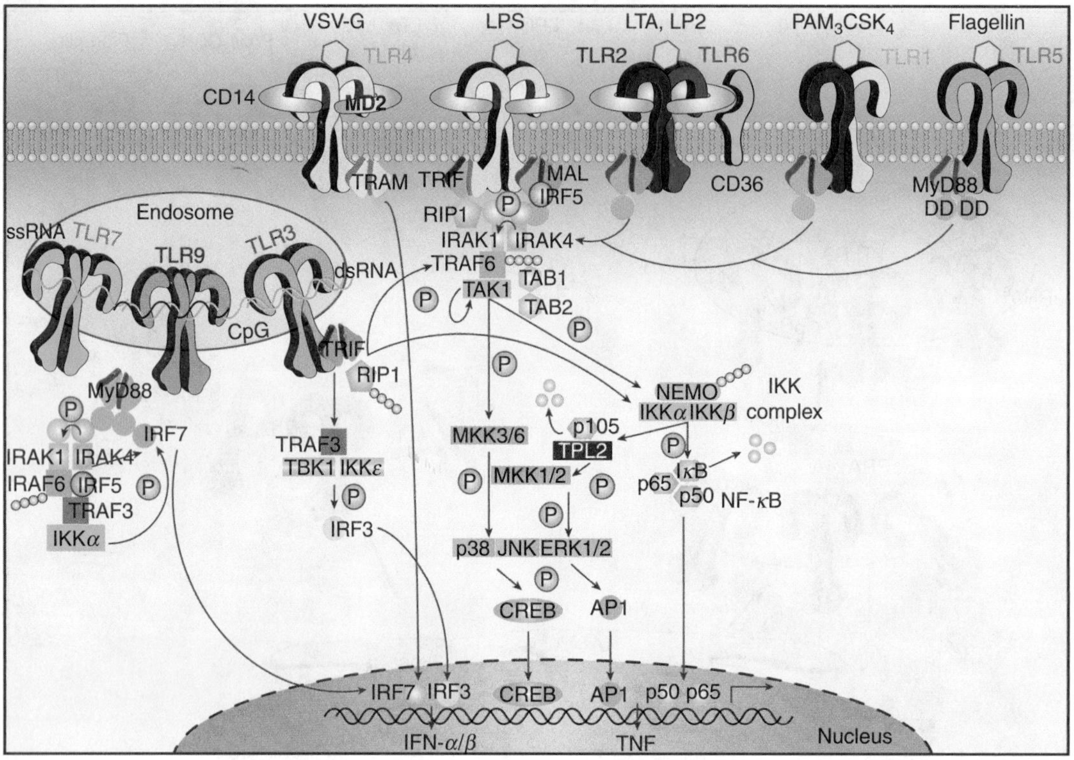

FIGURE 18–2. Overview of TLR signaling pathways. Shown are the activating events downstream of TLR activation that ultimately lead to the induction of thousands of genes including TNF and type I IFN, which are critical in activating innate and adaptive immune responses. Once TLR complexes recognize a specific molecule, they recruit combinations of adaptor proteins (MyD88, TRIF, TRAM, MAL) and initiate activation of downstream signaling molecules. Please see text for details of MyD88-dependent signaling. Activation of NF-κB by TRIF requires polyubiquitinated RIP1, which interacts with the TRAF6/TAK1 complex. RIP1 is not required for TRIF-dependent activation of IRF3, which requires TRAF3, and the IKK-related kinases, TBK1 and IKK-i/ε. When bound to vesicular stomatitis virus glycoprotein G (VSV-G), TLR4 can signal through TRAM to induce IRF7 activation, a process that is partially dependent on TRIF. K63 ubiquitination is represented by *chained circles*. *Small circles* represent protein degradation. LTA, lipoteichoic acid; LP2, lipopeptide 2. PAM_3CSK_4 is a triacyl lipopeptide. Phosphorylation events are represented by *P*-labeled circles. Abbreviations are as used in the text.

from the LPS receptor, TLR4. MyD88 and MAL act in concert with one another, and TRIF and TRAM act together, so that two primary "branches" of the LPS signaling pathway diverge at the level of the receptor.[35,36] TRIF alone serves TLR3 signaling; MyD88 and MAL (but neither TRIF nor TRAM) serve TLR2; and MyD88 alone serves TLRs 7, 8, and 9 (see Fig. 18–2). Mutational inactivation of MyD88 creates a severe immunodeficiency state in mice and humans,[37,38] and compound homozygosity for mutations at both MyD88 and TRIF loci causes immunodeficiency that is still more severe, in which animals are essentially unable to sense the presence of most microbes.[36]

It is probable that the adapter proteins exist as dimers in a total of five homomeric and heteromeric complexes with one another. While this has not been established by rigorous methods, the existence of dimers would best explain the diversity of signals that are observed to emanate from the TLRs. MAL and TRAM may function as "bridges" joining MyD88 and TRIF, respectively, to the TLR4 receptor. However, MyD88 can directly engage other receptors (TLRs 7, 8, and 9, for example), and TRIF can directly engage TLR3.[39] MAL/MyD88 signaling is very different from TRAM/TRIF signaling in several respects.

MyD88, when activated, recruits interleukin-1 receptor-associated kinase (IRAK) 4, a serine kinase, through an interaction involving death domains on each molecule.[33,34] This, in turn, leads to the phosphorylation of IRAK (IRAK1), and to the recruitment of tumor necrosis factor receptor-associated factor (TRAF) 6, a cellular scaffold protein that coordinates the recruitment of several other protein kinases. TRAF6 is endowed with E3 ubiquitin ligase activity, and in conjunction with the E2 ligases Ubc13/Uev1A, Ubc4, and Ubc5, adds chains of K63-linked polyubiquitin to itself, as well as inhibitor of κB (I-κB) kinase γ (IKKγ; also called NEMO [NF-κB essential modulator]), to TRAF2, and to RIP (receptor-interacting protein; reviewed in reference 40). Transforming growth factor-β activating kinase 1 (TAK-1) is also recruited to the TRAF6 complex, and phosphorylates IKKγ, which in complex with IKKα and IKKβ phosphorylates I-κB (an inhibitor of the p65 form of nuclear factor-κB [NF-κB]), leading to its K48-ubiquitin–mediated degradation.[40] Nuclear translocation of homo- or heterodimers composed of p65 and/or p50 NF-κB ensues. NF-κB drives the transcription of hundreds of genes encoding proteins that form the inflammatory response.

At the same time, the IKK complex phosphorylates the p105 form of NF-κB, which is complexed with MAP3K8 (also known as Tpl2). This leads to the degradation of p105 NF-κB, and to the activation of MAP3K8.[41,42] MAP3K8 activates MEK1 and MEK2, while independently MEK3 and MEK6 are activated by TAK1.[34] The MEKs activate mitogen-activated protein kinase (MAPK) family members, including extracellular signal-regulated kinase (ERK) 1 and ERK2, c-Jun N-terminal kinase (JNK), and p38 kinases. These kinases trigger the activation of other transcription factors. Among these is c-Jun, which together with c-Fos forms the transcription factor AP1. Also members of the cyclic adenosine monophosphate response element binding protein (CREB) family are activated.

Still other transcription factors are also activated following TLR stimulation. Interferon response factor (IRF) 1, IRF3, and IRF7 are among these, and are activated in different ways, depending on which TLR initiates the signal. TLRs 3 and 4 activate primarily IRF3, which is phosphorylated by TANK-binding kinase 1 (TBK1) and IKK (both distantly homologous to the IKKs),[43,44] while IRFs 1 and 7 are activated

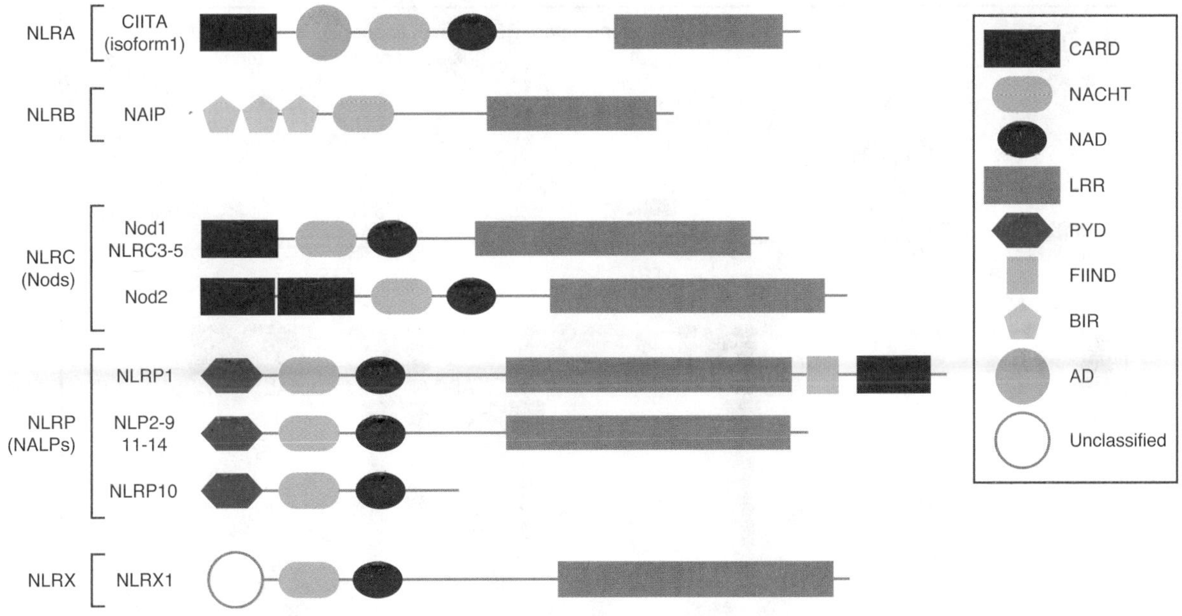

FIGURE 18–3. Domain structure of NOD-like receptors (NLRs). The various members of the NOD-like receptor family are grouped into subfamilies based on domain structure and homology by the Human Genome Gene Nomenclature Committee (HGNC), although sometimes domain classifications and homologies remain unclear. The LRR domain contains variable numbers of LRR repeats. Isoform 1 of CIITA contains an N-terminal CARD domain. Abbreviations are used in the text.

by TLRs 7 and 9, through the action of kinases that have not been fully characterized.[45,46] Activation of IRFs 1 and 3 can initiate expression of the interferon (IFN)-β gene.[45,47] IFN-β mediates antiviral effects, and is also required for the upregulation of costimulatory proteins (e.g., CD40, CD80, and CD86) that enhance the activation of an adaptive immune response. Hence, the adjuvant effects of LPS and dsRNA are dependent upon the type I IFN receptor.[48] IRF7 induces the expression of the IFN-α genes.[46,47] Both α and β IFNs bind to the type I interferon receptor, rendering similar if not identical biologic responses. For reasons that remain unclear, the heteromeric MyD88/MAL complex is incapable of driving type I IFN gene expression.

Countervailing Influences in TIR Adapter Signaling IRAK-M, a homologue of IRAKs 1, 2, and 4, is an inhibitor of TIR domain signaling and may participate in feedback inhibition of signaling known as *endotoxin tolerance*.[49] In addition, suppressor of cytokine synthesis 1 (SOCS-1) inhibits signal transduction from the Janus-associated kinase/signal transducer and activator of transcription (JAK/STAT) pathway, activated by type I IFN, one of the key cytokines elicited in the course of an innate immune response.[50] A20 and CYLD, both deubiquitination enzymes, remove the K63 ubiquitin tails from TRAF6, NEMO, and RIP, inhibiting the activation cascade.[40] Still more distally, inhibition of signaling via antiinflammatory cytokines (such as IL-10 or transforming growth factor-β) act to limit responses initiated by the TLRs.

SENSORS OF THE NUCLEOTIDE-BINDING OLIGOMERIZATION DOMAIN-LIKE RECEPTOR FAMILY

An extensive family of proteins defined by their motif structure caspase activation and recruitment domain (CARD), Pyrin, or baculovirus inhibitor of apoptosis repeat (BIR) domains followed by nucleotide binding "NACHT" domains, and LRR domains arranged in tandem participate in innate immune responses to intracellular microbes, as well as noninfectious inflammatory stimuli, including, for example, uric acid crystals and aluminum hydroxide particles. Collectively called the nucleotide-binding oligomerization domain (NOD)-like receptors (NLRs), the proteins have been assigned to several subfamilies (Fig. 18–3).[51] Mutations within different representatives of the family produce dominant or semidominant inflammatory diseases. In some cases there is limited penetrance and strong dependence upon the presence of mutations in other genes. For example, *NOD2* mutations have been clearly shown to enhance the likelihood of Crohn disease[52] and to cause Blau syndrome,[53] whereas distinct *NLPR3* mutations are the proximal cause of cold-induced autoinflammatory syndrome (CIAS) 1, chronic infantile neurologic, cutaneous, and articular (CINCA) syndrome, and neonatal-onset multisystem inflammatory disease (NOMID).[54–56] Mutations in the structurally related *MEFV* (pyrin-encoding) gene are responsible for familial Mediterranean fever.[57] Pyrin has been shown to interact with the adaptor protein PSTPIP1 (proline-serine-threonine phosphatase-interacting protein 1). Mutations in the gene encoding this protein also cause an inflammatory disorder, pyogenic sterile arthritis, pyoderma gangrenosum, and acne (PAPA) syndrome.[58]

The inflammatory potential of the NLR superfamily is exerted through two signaling pathways: the "inflammasome" pathway and the "NOD1/2" pathway. Each is less-fully elucidated at present than the TLR signaling pathways. Moreover, each likely interacts with the TLR signaling pathways, and in the case of the inflammasome, is dependent on the TLR signaling for full expression of activity.

The Inflammasome Pathway

The "inflammasome" pathway (Fig. 18–4) is induced by at least three proteins, but possibly others as well. Ice-protease activating factor (IPAF/NLRC4; encoded by *CARD12*), NACHT (a nucleotide-binding domain present in NAIP, CIITA, HET-E, and TP-1) domain-, leucine-rich repeat-, and pyrin domain-containing protein 1 (NLRP1, also known as CARD7), and NLRP3 (also known as *cyropyrin*) each trigger the inflammasome response. Diverse cellular perturbations probably lead to activation of IPAF, NLRP1, and NLRP3. However, cytosolic flagellin introduced via type III or type IV bacterial secretion systems activates IPAF.[59] Anthrax lethal factor and muramyldipeptide (MDP), introduced via pore-forming toxins, activate NLRP1.[60,61] Peptidoglycan

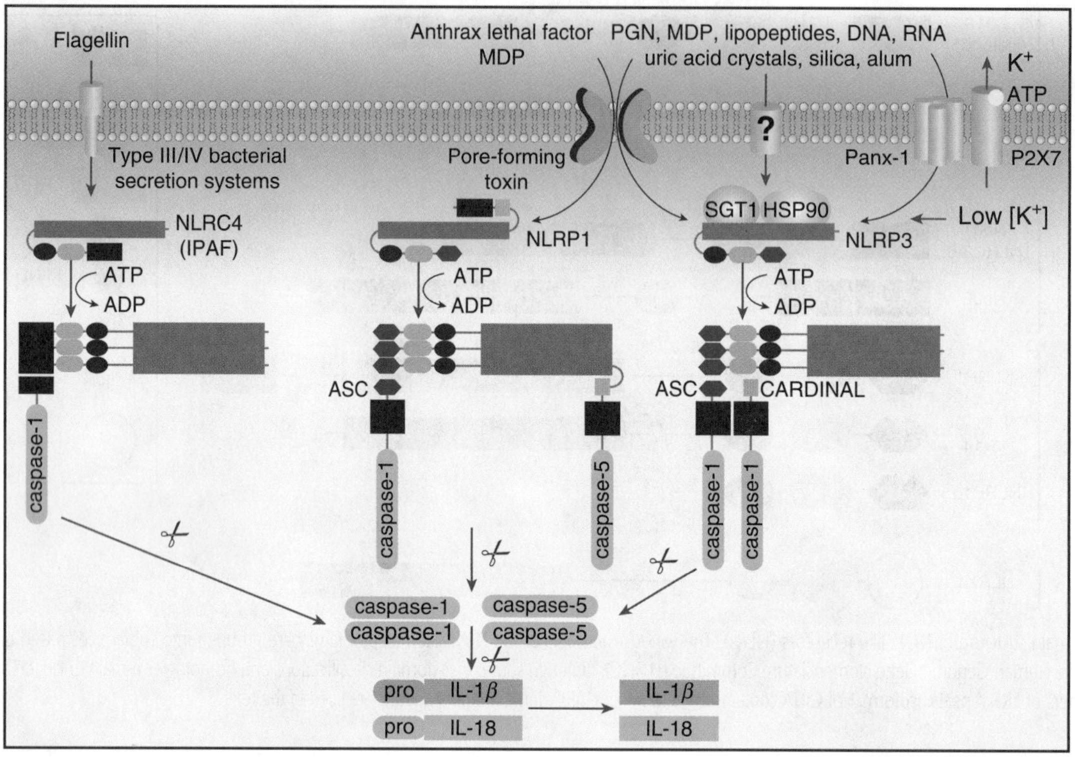

FIGURE 18–4. Inflammasome complexes formed by NLRP1 (NALP1), NLRP3 (NALP3), and NLRC4 (IPAF). In the absence of activating signals, NLRs are present in the cytosol in inactive conformations. The SGT1/HSP90 chaperone complex associates with and keeps NLRP3 in an activation-ready state. Upon activation, binding and hydrolysis of ATP result in oligomerization and inflammasome formation. NLRP1 and NLRP3 engage procaspase-1 through adaptor proteins (ASC or ASC/CARDINAL for NLRP3), whereas NLRC4 is able to bind procaspase-1 directly. NLRP1 is also able to engage procaspase-5. Cleavage by the inflammasome releases activated caspases, which are then able to process and activate inflammatory cytokines. Protein domains for the NLR proteins are the same as in Figure 18–3. The long tan rectangles indicate LRR domains, dark blue ovals indicate NAD domains, light tan ovals indicate NACHT domains, the red rectangles indicate CARD domains, light green squares indicate FIIND domains, and the green hexagons indicate the PYD domains. Abbreviations are used in the text.

(PGN), MDP, lipopeptides, nucleic acids, uric acid crystals, alum, and other foreign substances activate NLRP3.[62–66] Full activation of NLRP3 depends upon a drop in cytosolic potassium concentration, mediated in part by the potassium-exporting channel P2X7. Activation of P2X7 recruits the gap junction channel Pannexin-1 (Panx-1), allowing entry of bacterial products and other molecules into the cell.[67] Although it is not clear whether or not the inducers have direct contact with the NLRPs or IPAF, the latter undergo oligomerization (mediated by the NACHT domain). They then signal either directly (in the case of IPAF) or via adapter proteins (ASC in the case of NLRP1, and both ASC and CARDINAL in the case of NLRP3) to activate the cytosolic cysteine proteases caspase-1 and/or caspase-5. Activation occurs through CARD interactions. Homodimeric caspase-1 and caspase-5 act to convert the inflammatory cytokine pro–IL-1β into its active form. Importantly, inflammasome signaling does not initially activate expression of the IL-1β encoding gene. However, TLR signaling, which activates NF-κB, or signaling by IL-1β itself, can do so.[51]

IL-1β signals via its receptor to activate a signaling pathway similar to those used by the TLRs, dependent upon MyD88 and its downstream signaling cascade components. As such, IL-1β may be viewed as an endogenous ligand that elicits a response similar to those elicited by microbial ligands. This signal initially may initially be induced by a focal infection operating in conjunction with a noninfectious inflammatory stimulus.

The NOD Pathway

NOD1 (CARD4) and NOD2 (CARD15) proteins have been mentioned as sensors of γ-D-glutamyl diaminopimelic acid (DAP) and MDP, respectively, both components of microbial cell walls. They apparently detect intracellular bacteria or bacterial fragments.[68–70] NOD2 has been strongly implicated in the pathogenesis of Crohn disease through linkage disequilibrium mapping and sequence analysis,[52] but mutations of NOD2 cause disease with low penetrance, suggesting the importance of other genetic and environmental factors. No clear disease association has been defined for NOD1. The NOD proteins do not form the core of inflammasomes, although recent data suggest that NOD2 is able to associate with NLRP1 and caspase-1 upon stimulation with MDP.[71] In response to microbial stimuli, the NOD proteins oligomerize and signal via TRAF2 and TRAF5 (for NOD1) or via TRAF6 (for NOD2) to cause K63 ubiquitination of RICK2 (also known as RIP2, or CARDIAK), a protein with a domain structure similar to receptor interacting protein (RIP), known for its involvement in tumor necrosis factor (TNF) signal transduction. RICK2 activates TAK1, and by way of TAK1, elicits the activation of both NF-κB and the MAPK cascade, leading activation of the transcription factor AP1 (Fig. 18–5).

SENSORS OF THE RLH PATHWAYS

Although TLRs are capable of detecting nucleic acids within the endosomal compartment and do make an essential contribution to the detection of some viruses (notably herpesviruses), other viruses are detected chiefly or entirely by cytosolic receptors. Among these are the RIG-I–like helicases (RLHs), including retinoic acid-inducible gene I (RIG-I), melanoma differentiation-associated gene 5 (MDA5), and LGP2, which are the best-known sensors and are believed to undergo direct interaction with nucleic acids to initiate a response. These proteins have RNA helicase domains (involved in binding nucleic acids), as

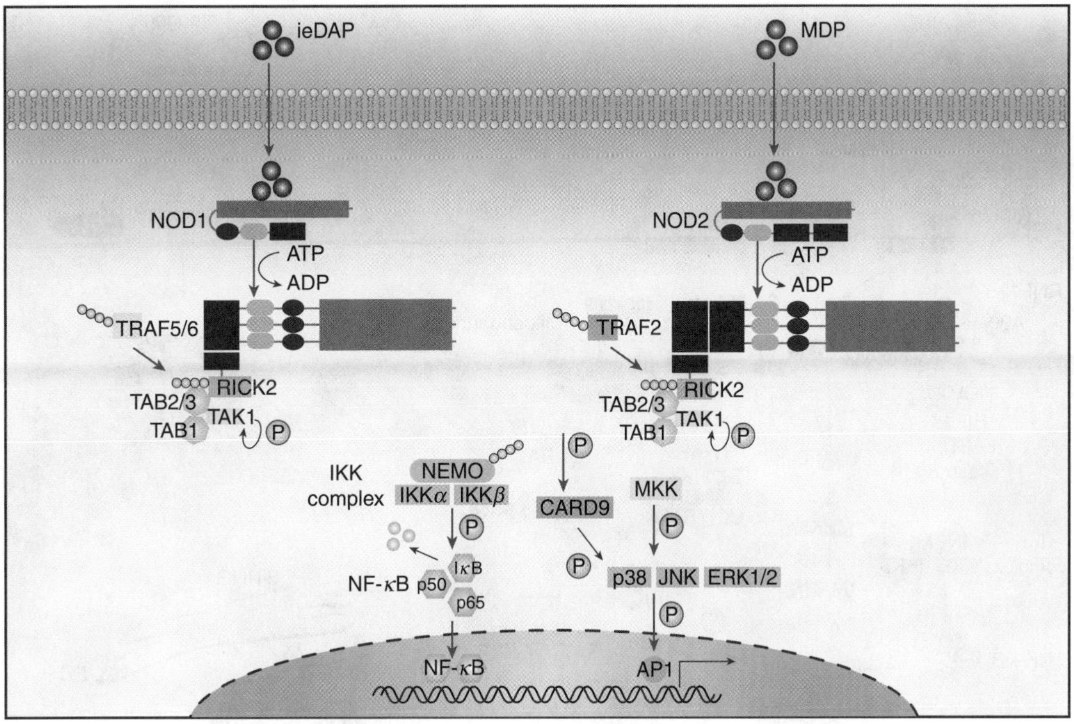

FIGURE 18–5. The NOD1/2 signaling pathways. Upon sensing PGN-derived motifs in the cytosol (DAP and MDP), NOD1 and NOD2 oligomerize and form complexes with the CARD domain-conaining serine threonine kinase RICK2. Signaling through TRAFs (E3 ubiquitin ligases) results in K63 ubiquitination (*chained circles*) of RICK2, and TAK1 recruitment. Activation of the TAK1 complex leads to IKK and MKK activation, resulting in signaling cascades similar to those activated in response to TLR ligands. CARD9 is important for p38 activation downstream of NOD2. NLR protein domains shown are the same as in Figure 18–3. The long tan rectangles indicate LRR domains, dark blue ovals indicate NAD domains, light tan ovals indicate NACHT domains, and the red rectangles indicate CARD domains. Phosphorylation events are represented by *P*-labeled circles. Abbreviations are as used in the text.

well as a regulatory domain (RD) that has been implicated in inhibiting downstream signaling,[72] but is also necessary for RNA sensing.[73,74] Both RIG-I and MDA5 have more proximal CARD domains involved in signaling, whereas LGP2 does not. On this basis it was initially believed that LGP2 might have an inhibitory function.[75] However, it appears to contribute to sensing in a positive manner, and may augment MDA5 signaling.[74,76]

Although TLR3 can detect dsRNA and its synthetic analogue poly I:C, the dominant sensor of poly I:C *in vivo* is MDA5.[77] While long poly I:C polymers are detected by MDA5, shorter polymers are better detected by RIG-I. RIG-I is able to form stable complexes with dsRNA molecules containing blunt ends or 5′ overhangs, whereas dsRNA with 3′ overhangs are unwound by its helicase activity.[73] RIG-I additionally recognizes single-stranded RNA (ssRNA) molecules, distinguishing them from host RNA by detecting 5′-triphosphate structures present on the former, such as is found in ssRNA from the influenza virus.[78,79] RIG-I must be activated by T-cell receptor-interacting molecule 25 (TRIM25), a host resistance factor that K63 ubiquitinates the former protein.

The RLHs signal by CARD domain-mediated interaction with IFN-β promoter stimulator (IPS)-1 (also known as MAVS, VISA, and CARDIF).[80–83] IPS-1 is an integral protein of the mitochondrial outer membrane with a CARD domain that projects into the cytoplasm. It is capable of activating three different pathways when stimulated by the RLHs. One pathway mimics the TNF signaling pathway, and includes the adaptor protein tumor necrosis factor receptor death domain (TRADD), Fas-associated death domain protein (FADD), RIP1, caspase-8, and caspase-10, and leads to IKK complex and NF-κB activation. A second pathway recruits TRAF6 and mitogen-activated kinase kinase (MEKK)1, leading to activation of the MAPKs and AP1. These two pathways are responsible for inflammatory cytokine production. The third pathway entails activation of TBK1 and IKK, and leads to the activation of IRF3 and IRF7, with ensuing type I IFN production (Fig. 18–6).

A pathway for responses to cytoplasmic double-stranded DNA (dsDNA) also exists in mammalian cells. STING is a penta-spanning ER membrane protein that appears to have nonredundant function in detection of dsDNA, although it may not represent the sensor itself, and has no obvious motifs that would recognize DNA.[84] A putative cytosolic DNA sensor DAI (for DNA-dependent activator of IRFs) has also been described. DAI contains DNA binding domains, and enhances DNA-mediated induction of type I IFNs *in vitro*.[85] However, the role of DAI as a sensor of cytoplasmic DNA appears to be redundant.[86] Whatever the pathway involved, dsDNA responses entail only IFN production (and not inflammatory cytokine production) and are entirely dependent upon TBK1 (see Fig. 18–6).

KEY EFFECTOR CYTOKINES IN THE INNATE IMMUNE RESPONSE

Cells of the innate immune system exhibit a measure of autonomy (e.g., neutrophils directly engulf and destroy pathogens), but also initiate the adaptive immune response to microbes and summon "reinforcements" to the site of infection. These functions depend upon the production of cytokines, too numerous to describe in this chapter. However, a few of the key mediators are listed here.

Tumor Necrosis Factor-α

A homotrimeric cytokine that is made by many cells, TNF is synthesized in greatest amounts by mononuclear phagocytes that have been

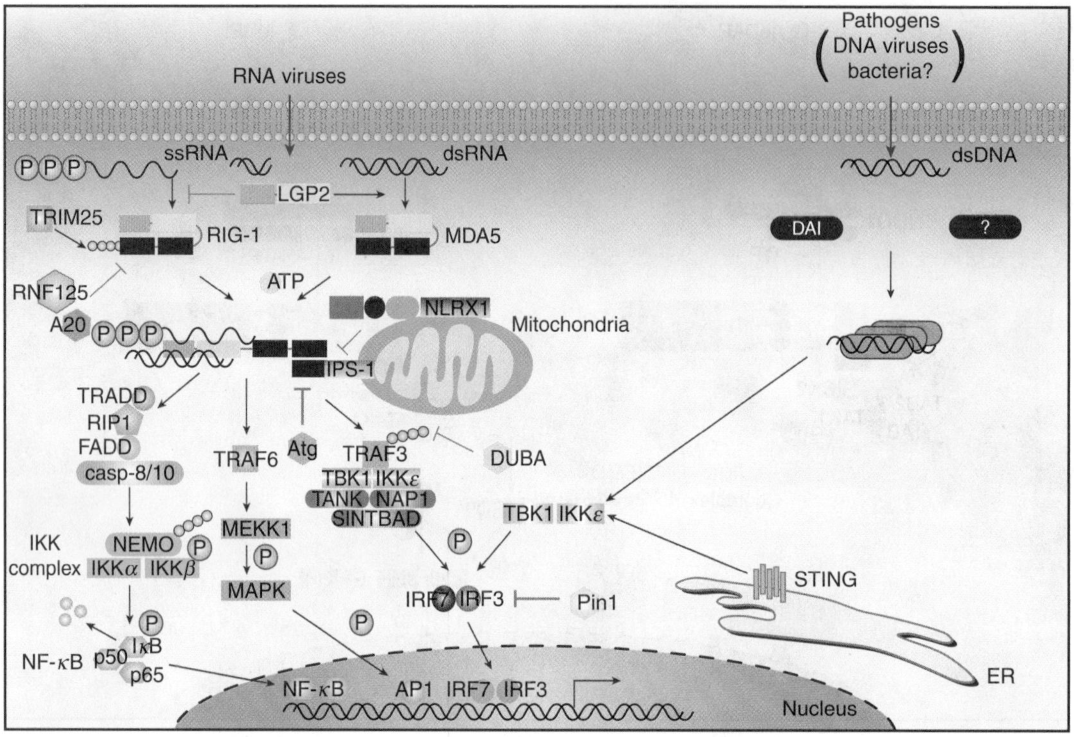

FIGURE 18–6. Cytosolic sensors and signaling pathways. RIG-I and MDA5 respond to different viral infections, recognizing ssRNA and dsRNA, respectively. RIG-I also detects short dsRNA sequences. LGP2 is also able to bind to dsRNA, and appears to modulate RIG-I and MDA5 signaling. Full RIG-I activity requires K63 ubiquitination (*chained circles*) by TRIM25. RIG-I and MDA5 activate IPS-1, which interacts with a complex containing RIP1, FADD, and TRADD, as well as TRAF6, and TRAF3. Association of FADD with procaspase-8 or procaspase-10 results in cleavage to the mature, active caspase-8 or caspase-10, which go on to activate NF-κB. Recruitment of TRAF6 leads to activation of the MAPK pathway and AP1, whereas K63 ubiquitinated TRAF3 activates IRF3 and IRF7 through the kinases IKKi/ε and TBK. The latter also associate with TRAF family member-associated NF-κB activator (TANK), NAK-associated protein 1 (NAP1), and similar to NAP1 TBK1 adaptor (SINTBAD). IPS-1 is negatively regulated by the autophagy conjugate Atg12–Atg5, and potentially by NLRX1, whereas RIG-I is negatively regulated by the IFN-inducible ubiquitin ligases RNF125 and A20. The TRAF3-dependent pathway is negatively controlled by the deubiquitinase DUBA. The peptidyl-prolyl-isomerase Pin1 triggers phosphorylated IRF3 ubiquitination and degradation. Double-stranded DNA can also be sensed via cytosolic sensors such as DAI. The ER membrane protein STING is necessary for cytosolic DNA sensing, although the mechanism is unknown. STING also associates with RIG-I (not shown). CARD domains are indicated by the red rectangles, helicase domains by the light blue rectangles, RD domains by the light green rectangles. NLRX1 domains are the same as in Figure 18–3 except for the unclassified domain, which is shown inserted into the mitochondrial membrane and appears in green. The tan rectangle indicates the LRR domain, the dark blue circle indicates the NAD domain, and the light tan oval indicates the NACHT domain. Phosphorylation events are represented by *P*-labeled circles. Abbreviations are as used in the text.

exposed to LPS or other TLR-activating stimuli. It was recognized as a key endogenous mediator of endotoxicity,[87] and later, as a mediator of other forms of inflammation (including sterile inflammation, as observed in rheumatoid arthritis, Crohn disease, ankylosing spondylitis, and psoriasis). The TNF signaling pathway depends upon two receptors, involves NF-κB activation, and is ancestrally related to the *Drosophila Imd* (immunodeficiency) pathway for recognition of Gram-negative bacteria.[88] The ancient phylogenetic origins of TNF signaling, its large representation in distant species, the remarkable therapeutic efficacy of TNF neutralization in the diseases just mentioned, and the immunocompromising effects of TNF and TNF receptor mutations in animals all suggest that TNF is one of the most important of the cytokines utilized by the innate immune system for effective containment of infection.

Interleukin-1α and β

Once known as pleiotropic inflammatory cytokines, IL-1α and IL-1β, two distantly related ligands that share the same set of receptors, are produced in response to innate immune stimuli and evoke fever, swelling, and neutrophil adhesion in the region of an infectious nidus. The type I IL-1 receptor, responsible for most or all of the agonist activity of the IL-1 proteins, has two chains, each of which is endowed with a cytoplasmic TIR domain. The receptor complex signals via MyD88 and no other adapters are known to be required. IL-1 signaling may act as an amplification mechanism that augments the primary infectious signal, and transmits awareness of infection to cells that lack the innate immune sensors required for detection of microbes.

Interleukin-6

Signaling via a receptor that utilizes the JAK/STAT pathway, IL-6 activates many elements of the "acute phase response"; that is, hepatic production of fibrinogen, serum amyloid A protein, and C-reactive protein. It also has thrombopoietic activity, which may assist in the generation of platelets, which are often consumed in the course of a serious infection (see Chap. 113).

Interleukin-12

A cytokine made in abundance in response to TLR stimulation, IL-12 activates the production of interferon-γ by lymphoid cells, which, in turn, increases the microbicidal activity of mononuclear phagocytes. Unlike most cytokines, IL-12 is a heterodimeric protein, and the IL-12 p40 subunit is subject to induction, whereas the p35 subunit is synthesized even under nonstimulated conditions. Mutations of the genes encoding IL-12 or its receptor, or the interferon-γ or its receptor, are known to cause relatively severe susceptibility to infection by mycobacteria and other intracellular infections. Hence the IL-12–interferon-γ feedback loop is considered one of the most important innate/adaptive immune interactions.

Chemokines

A family of small proteins, highly redundant in receptor specificity and organized into CC and CXC subfamilies as based on the spacing of two highly conserved cysteine residues, the chemokines are induced by primary microbial stimuli and by TNF and IL-1. Binding to G-protein-coupled receptors, some chemokines exhibit neutrophil chemotactic activity, and are believed to contribute to the egress of neutrophils from blood into infected tissue.

Granulocyte Colony-Stimulating Factor and Granulocyte-Macrophage Colony-Stimulating Factor

The central hematopoietic response is attuned to events in the peripheral tissues, and granulocyte colony-stimulating factor and granulocyte-macrophage colony-stimulating factor encourage the production, release, and activation of granulocytes and monocytes to cope with an infectious challenge. These cytokines are produced in direct response to TLR signaling, and also in response to secondary cytokines such as TNF. They signal via JAK/STAT-coupled receptors.

Interferons

Type I interferons (IFN-α and IFN-β) are expressed immediately in response to LPS, dsRNA, or unmethylated DNA, and have broad activity in the containment of viral infections. LPS-induced type I IFN production depends upon TLR4 and the adapters TRIF and TRAM. dsRNA-induced type I IFN depends upon TLR3 and TRIF (but not TRAM). Unmethylated CpG motifs in DNA stimulate type I IFN production depends upon MyD88. Although many cells are induced to an antiviral state as the result of interferon stimulation, NK cells, which are specialized for the elimination of virus-infected targets, are particularly dependent upon type I IFN signaling,[89] and require it for the elimination of specific pathogens such as cytomegalovirus.[90] The type I IFNs are also involved in protection against bacterial infection,[91] and type I IFN signaling has been shown to be important to the development of endotoxic shock.[92] Plasmacytoid dendritic cells are a particularly important source of type I IFN.[93]

Type II interferon (IFN-γ) has less antiviral activity than type I interferon, is produced by T cells in response to IL-12 receptor stimulation, and is crucial for the elimination of intracellular pathogens, such as mycobacteria, which reside within macrophages of the infected host.

THE ACTIVATION OF ADAPTIVE IMMUNITY

The adjuvant effect of microbes has been known since the classic studies of Lewis and Loomis[94] who coined the term "allergic irritability" to describe the augmented production of antibodies against a protein antigen in guinea pigs infected with *Mycobacterium tuberculosis.* Freund and McDermott[95] demonstrated that heat-killed mycobacteria were capable of eliciting an exaggerated antibody response as well when coadministered with a protein antigen, a fact that indicated that molecular components of microbes (rather than infection *per se*) were responsible for adjuvanticity. LPS was shown to be endowed with adjuvant activity by Condie and associates in 1955,[96] and by 1975 the *Lps* locus was shown to be required for this effect of LPS (as it was required for all other cellular effects of LPS).[97] By deduction, the positional cloning of *Lps* thus revealed the essential role of TLR4 in LPS adjuvanticity.[5]

Activation of an adaptive immune response to a specific antigen has long been known to depend upon two signals that occur in the course of antigen presentation. First, the T-cell receptor must be activated. In addition, costimulatory molecules upregulated on the antigen-presenting cell (e.g., CD40, CD69, CD80, and CD86) are known to interact with receptors (or in some cases ligands) on the T cell (see Chap. 78). An exchange of signals occurs over a period of approximately 12 hours,[98] ultimately leading to autonomous expansion of the T cell clone, and, in turn, activation of specific B cells. Some of these signals are well characterized. For example, CD80 and CD86 both engage CD28 and cytotoxic T-lymphocyte antigen on the T-cell surface, and abrogation of signaling via these costimulatory receptors is known to substantially attenuate the adaptive immune response.[99]

Upregulation of costimulatory molecules (UCM) is therefore essential, although not by itself sufficient, for activation of the adaptive immune response. LPS depends upon TRIF (and specifically, upon TRIF-mediated type I interferon gene expression) to elicit UCM,[36,48,100] and absent TRIF, LPS cannot exert an adjuvant effect. TRAM is also required for UCM.[35] While MyD88 does not elicit UCM, it does contribute to LPS-induced adjuvanticity in an experimental setting.[48] It is likely that IL-12, a cytokine that is largely MyD88-dependent, also contributes to the adjuvant effect, along with other proteins yet to be identified.

Although several studies suggested that TLR signaling is required for adaptive immune responses to occur, it was observed later that mice lacking all TLR signaling are quite capable of mounting adaptive immune responses, including antibody responses and recall responses to defined antigens administered with diverse adjuvants.[101] It is now evident that there is much redundancy in adaptive immune responses, and several innate immune pathways can independently trigger such responses.

DISEASES CAUSED BY INNATE IMMUNE DEFECTS

Premature death from infection is strongly heritable in humans.[102] Defects of the innate immune sensing apparatus are expected to cause hypersusceptibility to infection in humans as they clearly do in mice, and specific examples of such mutations have come to light, including the previously discussed NLR disorders. Missense mutations of TLR4 that are very rare among the normal white population are quite common in patients with systemic meningococcal disease, and have been assigned a role in susceptibility on this basis.[103] A nonsense mutation of TLR5 was found to be overrepresented in patients who developed Legionnaire disease as compared to a comparably exposed population that remained disease free.[104] Mutations of IRAK4 and MyD88 have been shown to create susceptibility to suppurative Gram-positive infections.[38,105] In humans, both TLR3[106] and UNC93B1[107] mutations cause susceptibility to recurrent herpes simplex virus encephalitis, and presumably to other diseases as well.

On the effector side, examples of immunocompromise from innate immune defects are far better known, and include diseases caused by mutations affecting IFN-γ,[108] IL-12[109] and its receptor,[110,111] defects of granule formation,[112] and defects of the reduced form of nicotinamide adenine dinucleotide phosphate oxidase (see Chap. 66).[113]

THE GENERAL STRATEGY OF INNATE IMMUNE RESPONSES AND THE CONCEPT OF FORWARD FEEDBACK LOOPS IN AUTOIMMUNITY

Although the term *autoimmunity* is reserved for inappropriate adaptive immune responses that damage tissues of the host, the innate immune system may also cause injury or death, and typically does so when systemic activation occurs in the course of a serious infection. Innate immune responses, which entail cytokine-mediated inflammation and coagulation, evolved to contain small inoculates of microorganisms by encouraging the influx of granulocytes to engulf and destroy these pathogens, and by stimulating the development of an adaptive immune response. The mechanisms that are employed to these ends can be lethal if they are generalized rather than focal. In several examples, the importance of microbes as drivers of inflammation has been cited, and forward–feedback loops may perpetuate inflammation or autoimmunity. It has been reported, for example, that endogenous DNA, signaling via TLR9, is responsible for the generation and perpetuation of antinucleoprotein antibodies in a mouse model of systemic lupus erythematosus.[114] The involvement of TLRs 3 and 7 may also be important. In hemophagocytic lymphohistiocytosis, an amplification loop involving a microbial driver, cytotoxic T lymphoctye expansion, and interferon-γ-driven myeloid expansion has been well described in mice.[115] In SHP1 deficiency in mice, autoimmunity and inflammation also depend upon a microbial driver and activation of TIR domain signaling pathways.[116] Beyond this, the innate immune system may indeed contribute to sterile inflammation (autoinflammatory disease), as witnessed in many human diseases that have so far eluded etiologic decipherment.

REFERENCES

1. Pfeiffer R: Untersuchungen Uber das Choleragift. *Z Hygiene* 11:393, 1892.
2. Raetz CR, Whitfield C: Lipopolysaccharide endotoxins. *Annu Rev Biochem* 71:635, 2002.
3. Galanos C, Luderitz O, Rietschel ET, et al: Synthetic and natural *Escherichia coli* free lipid A express identical endotoxic activities. *Eur J Biochem* 148:1, 1985.
4. Rosenstreich DL, Weinblatt AC, O'Brien AD: Genetic control of resistance to infection in mice. *Crit Rev Immunol* 3:263, 1982.
5. Poltorak A, He X, Smirnova I, et al: Defective LPS signaling in C3H/HeJ and C57BL/10ScCr mice: Mutations in *Tlr4* gene. *Science* 282:2085, 1998.
6. Anderson KV, Bokla L, Nusslein-Volhard C: Establishment of dorsal-ventral polarity in the Drosophila embryo: The induction of polarity by the Toll gene product. *Cell* 42:791, 1985.
7. Lemaitre B, Nicolas E, Michaut L, et al: The dorsoventral regulatory gene cassette spatzle/Toll/cactus controls the potent antifungal response in *Drosophila* adults. *Cell* 86:973, 1996.
8. Takeuchi O, Kaufmann A, Grote K, et al: Preferentially the R-stereoisomer of the mycoplasmal lipopeptide macrophage-activating lipopeptide-2 activates immune cells through a Toll-like receptor 2- and MyD88-dependent signaling pathway. *J Immunol* 164:554, 2000.
9. Hemmi H, Takeuchi O, Kawai T, et al: A Toll-like receptor recognizes bacterial DNA. *Nature* 408:740, 2000.
10. Takeuchi O, Sato S, Horiuchi T, et al: Cutting edge: Role of Toll-like receptor 1 in mediating immune response to microbial lipoproteins. *J Immunol* 169:10, 2002.
11. Hayashi F, Smith KD, Ozinsky A, et al: The innate immune response to bacterial flagellin is mediated by Toll-like receptor 5. *Nature* 410:1099, 2001.
12. Alexopoulou L, Holt AC, Medzhitov R, Flavell RA: Recognition of double-stranded RNA and activation of NF-kappaB by Toll-like receptor 3. *Nature* 413:732, 2001.
13. Poltorak A, Ricciardi-Castagnoli P, Citterio A, Beutler B: Physical contact between LPS and Tlr4 revealed by genetic complementation. *Proc Natl Acad Sci U S A* 97:2163, 2000.
14. Bauer S, Kirschning CJ, Hacker H, et al: Human TLR9 confers responsiveness to bacterial DNA via species-specific CpG motif recognition. *Proc Natl Acad Sci U S A* 98:9237, 2001.
15. Gantner BN, Simmons RM, Canavera SJ, et al: Collaborative induction of inflammatory responses by dectin-1 and Toll-like receptor 2. *J Exp Med* 197:1107, 2003.
16. Rallabhandi P, Nhu QM, Toshchakov VY, et al: Analysis of proteinase-activated receptor 2 and TLR4 signal transduction: A novel paradigm for receptor cooperativity. *J Biol Chem* 283:24314, 2008.
17. Wright SD, Ramos RA, Tobias PS, et al: CD14, a receptor for complexes of lipopolysaccharide (LPS) and LPS binding protein. *Science* 249:1431, 1990.
18. Haziot A, Ferrero E, Kontgen F, et al: Resistance to endotoxin shock and reduced dissemination of Gram-negative bacteria in CD14-deficient mice. *Immunity* 4:407, 1996.
19. Hoebe K, Georgel P, Rutschmann S, et al: CD36 is a sensor of diacylglycerides. *Nature* 433:523, 2005.
20. Nagai Y, Akashi S, Nagafuku M, et al: Essential role of MD-2 in LPS responsiveness and TLR4 distribution. *Nat Immunol* 3:667, 2002.
21. Xu Y, Tao X, Shen B, et al: Structural basis for signal transduction by the Toll/interleukin-1 receptor domains. *Nature* 408:111, 2000.
22. Kim HM, Park BS, Kim JI, et al: Crystal structure of the TLR4-MD-2 complex with bound endotoxin antagonist Eritoran. *Cell* 130:906, 2007.
23. Ohto U, Fukase K, Miyake K, Satow Y: Crystal structures of human MD-2 and its complex with antiendotoxic lipid IVa. *Science* 316:1632, 2007.
24. Jin MS, Kim SE, Heo JY, et al: Crystal structure of the TLR1-TLR2 heterodimer induced by binding of a tri-acylated lipopeptide. *Cell* 130:1071, 2007.
25. Liu L, Botos I, Wang Y, et al: Structural basis of toll-like receptor 3 signaling with double-stranded RNA. *Science* 320:379, 2008.
26. Ahmad-Nejad P, Hacker H, Rutz M, et al: Bacterial CpG-DNA and lipopolysaccharides activate Toll-like receptors at distinct cellular compartments. *Eur J Immunol* 32:1958, 2002.
27. Tabeta K, Hoebe K, Janssen EM, et al: The Unc93b1 mutation 3d disrupts exogenous antigen presentation and signaling via Toll-like receptors 3, 7 and 9. *Nat Immunol* 7:156, 2006.
28. Ewald SE, Lee BL, Lau L, et al: The ectodomain of Toll-like receptor 9 is cleaved to generate a functional receptor. *Nature* 456:658, 2008.
29. Park B, Brinkmann MM, Spooner E, et al: Proteolytic cleavage in an endolysosomal compartment is required for activation of Toll-like receptor 9. *Nat Immunol* 9:1407, 2008.
30. Kim YM, Brinkmann MM, Paquet ME, Ploegh HL: UNC93B1 delivers nucleotide-sensing toll-like receptors to endolysosomes. *Nature* 452:234, 2008.
31. Takahashi K, Shibata T, Akashi-Takamura S, et al: A protein associated with Toll-like receptor (TLR) 4 (PRAT4A) is required for TLR-dependent immune responses. *J Exp Med* 204:2963, 2007.
32. Yang Y, Liu B, Dai J, et al: Heat shock protein gp96 is a master chaperone for toll-like receptors and is important in the innate function of macrophages. *Immunity* 26:215, 2007.
33. Beutler B, Jiang Z, Georgel P, et al: Genetic analysis of host resistance: Toll-like receptor signaling and immunity at large. *Annu Rev Immunol* 24:353, 2006.
34. Kawai T, Akira S: TLR signaling. *Semin Immunol* 19:24, 2007.
35. Yamamoto M, Sato S, Hemmi H, et al: TRAM is specifically involved in the Toll-like receptor 4-mediated MyD88-independent signaling pathway. *Nat Immunol* 4:1144, 2003.
36. Hoebe K, Du X, Georgel P, et al: Identification of Lps2 as a key transducer of MyD88-independent TIR signaling. *Nature* 424:743, 2003.
37. Takeuchi O, Hoshino K, Akira S: Cutting edge: TLR2-deficient and MyD88-deficient mice are highly susceptible to *Staphylococcus aureus* infection. *J Immunol* 165:5392, 2000.
38. von Bernuth H, Picard C, Jin Z, et al: Pyogenic bacterial infections in humans with MyD88 deficiency. *Science* 321:691, 2008.
39. Oshiumi H, Matsumoto M, Funami K, et al: TICAM-1, an adaptor molecule that participates in Toll-like receptor 3-mediated interferon-beta induction. *Nat Immunol* 4:161, 2003.
40. Chen ZJ: Ubiquitin signalling in the NF-kappaB pathway. *Nat Cell Biol* 7:758, 2005.
41. Waterfield M, Jin W, Reiley W, et al: IkappaB kinase is an essential component of the Tpl2 signaling pathway. *Mol Cell Biol* 24:6040, 2004.
42. Beinke S, Deka J, Lang V, et al: NF-kappaB1 p105 negatively regulates TPL-2 MEK kinase activity. *Mol Cell Biol* 23:4739, 2003.
43. Fitzgerald KA, McWhirter SM, Faia KL, et al: IKKepsilon and TBK1 are essential components of the IRF3 signaling pathway. *Nat Immunol* 4:491, 2003.
44. Sato S, Sugiyama M, Yamamoto M, et al: Toll/IL-1 receptor domain-containing adaptor inducing IFN-beta (TRIF) associates with TNF receptor-associated factor 6 and TANK-binding kinase 1, and activates two distinct transcription factors, NF-kappa B and IFN-regulatory factor-3, in the Toll-like receptor signaling. *J Immunol* 171:4304, 2003.
45. Negishi H, Fujita Y, Yanai H, et al: Evidence for licensing of IFN-gamma-induced IFN regulatory factor 1 transcription factor by MyD88 in Toll-like receptor-dependent gene induction program. *Proc Natl Acad Sci U S A* 103:15136, 2006.
46. Kaisho T: Type I interferon production by nucleic acid-stimulated dendritic cells. *Front Biosci* 13:6034, 2008.
47. Honda K, Ohba Y, Yanai H, et al: Spatiotemporal regulation of MyD88-IRF-7 signalling for robust type-I interferon induction. *Nature* 434:1035, 2005.
48. Hoebe K, Jannsen EM, Kim SO, et al: Upregulation of costimulatory molecules induced by lipopolysaccharide and double-stranded RNA occurs by Trif-dependent and Trif-independent pathways. *Nat Immunol* 4:1223, 2003.
49. Kobayashi K, Hernandez LD, Galan JE, et al: IRAK-M is a negative regulator of Toll-like receptor signaling. *Cell* 110:191, 2002.
50. Kinjyo I, Hanada T, Inagaki-Ohara K, et al: SOCS1/JAB is a negative regulator of LPS-induced macrophage activation. *Immunity* 17:583, 2002.
51. Ye Z, Ting JP: NLR, the nucleotide-binding domain leucine-rich repeat containing gene family. *Curr Opin Immunol* 20:3, 2008.
52. Hugot JP, Chamaillard M, Zouali H, et al: Association of NOD2 leucine-rich repeat variants with susceptibility to Crohn's disease. *Nature* 411:599, 2001.
53. Miceli-Richard C, Lesage S, Rybojad M, et al: CARD15 mutations in Blau syndrome. *Nat Genet* 29:19, 2001.
54. Hoffman HM, Mueller JL, Broide DH, et al: Mutation of a new gene encoding a putative pyrin-like protein causes familial cold autoinflammatory syndrome and Muckle-Wells syndrome. *Nat Genet* 29:301, 2001.
55. Feldmann J, Prieur AM, Quartier P, et al: Chronic infantile neurological cutaneous and articular syndrome is caused by mutations in CIAS1, a gene highly expressed in polymorphonuclear cells and chondrocytes. *Am J Hum Genet* 71:198, 2002.

56. Neven B, Callebaut I, Prieur AM, et al: Molecular basis of the spectral expression of CIAS1 mutations associated with phagocytic cell-mediated autoinflammatory disorders CINCA/NOMID, MWS, and FCU. *Blood* 103:2809, 2004.
57. The International FMF Consortium: Ancient missense mutations in a new member of the RoRet gene family are likely to cause familial Mediterranean fever. *Cell* 90:797, 1997.
58. Wise CA, Gillum JD, Seidman CE, et al: Mutations in CD2BP1 disrupt binding to PTP PEST and are responsible for PAPA syndrome, an autoinflammatory disorder. *Hum Mol Genet* 11:961, 2002.
59. Miao EA, Andersen-Nissen E, Warren SE, Aderem A: TLR5 and Ipaf: Dual sensors of bacterial flagellin in the innate immune system. *Semin Immunopathol* 29:275, 2007.
60. Boyden ED, Dietrich WF: Nalp1b controls mouse macrophage susceptibility to anthrax lethal toxin. *Nat Genet* 38:240, 2006.
61. Bruey JM, Bruey-Sedano N, Luciano F, et al: Bcl-2 and Bcl-XL regulate proinflammatory caspase-1 activation by interaction with NALP1. *Cell* 129:45, 2007.
62. Martinon F, Agostini L, Meylan E, Tschopp J: Identification of bacterial muramyl dipeptide as activator of the NALP3/cryopyrin inflammasome. *Curr Biol* 14:1929, 2004.
63. Mariathasan S, Newton K, Monack DM, et al: Differential activation of the inflammasome by caspase-1 adaptors ASC and Ipaf. *Nature* 430:213, 2004.
64. Cassel SL, Eisenbarth SC, Iyer SS, et al: The Nalp3 inflammasome is essential for the development of silicosis. *Proc Natl Acad Sci U S A* 105:9035, 2008.
65. Eisenbarth SC, Colegio OR, O'Connor W, et al: Crucial role for the Nalp3 inflammasome in the immunostimulatory properties of aluminium adjuvants. *Nature* 453:1122, 2008.
66. Dostert C, Petrilli V, Van Bruggen R, et al: Innate immune activation through Nalp3 inflammasome sensing of asbestos and silica. *Science* 320:674, 2008.
67. Pelegrin P, Barroso-Gutierrez C, Surprenant A: P2X7 receptor differentially couples to distinct release pathways for IL-1beta in mouse macrophage. *J Immunol* 180:7147, 2008.
68. Girardin SE, Boneca IG, Carneiro LA, et al: Nod1 detects a unique muropeptide from gram-negative bacterial peptidoglycan. *Science* 300:1584, 2003.
69. Girardin SE, Boneca IG, Viala J, et al: Nod2 is a general sensor of peptidoglycan through muramyl dipeptide (MDP) detection. *J Biol Chem* 278:8869, 2003.
70. Girardin SE, Travassos LH, Herve M, et al: Peptidoglycan molecular requirements allowing detection by Nod1 and Nod2. *J Biol Chem* 278:41702, 2003.
71. Hsu LC, Ali SR, McGillivray S, et al: A NOD2-NALP1 complex mediates caspase-1-dependent IL-1beta secretion in response to *Bacillus anthracis* infection and muramyl dipeptide. *Proc Natl Acad Sci U S A* 105:7803, 2008.
72. Saito T, Hirai R, Loo YM, et al: Regulation of innate antiviral defenses through a shared repressor domain in RIG-I and LGP2. *Proc Natl Acad Sci U S A* 104:582, 2007.
73. Takahasi K, Yoneyama M, Nishihori T, et al: Nonself RNA-sensing mechanism of RIG-I helicase and activation of antiviral immune responses. *Mol Cell* 29:428, 2008.
74. Pippig DA, Hellmuth JC, Cui S, et al: The regulatory domain of the RIG-I family ATPase LGP2 senses double-stranded RNA. *Nucleic Acids Res* 37:2014, 2009.
75. Rothenfusser S, Goutagny N, Diperna G, et al: The RNA helicase Lgp2 inhibits TLR-independent sensing of viral replication by retinoic acid-inducible gene-I. *J Immunol* 175:5260, 2005.
76. Venkataraman T, Valdes M, Elsby R, et al: Loss of DExD/H box RNA helicase LGP2 manifests disparate antiviral responses. *J Immunol* 178:6444, 2007.
77. Gitlin L, Barchet W, Gilfillan S, et al: Essential role of mda-5 in type I IFN responses to polyriboinosinic:polyribocytidylic acid and encephalomyocarditis picornavirus. *Proc Natl Acad Sci U S A* 103:8459, 2006.
78. Hornung V, Ellegast J, Kim S, et al: 5′-Triphosphate RNA is the ligand for RIG-I. *Science* 314:994, 2006.
79. Pichlmair A, Schulz O, Tan CP, et al: RIG-I-mediated antiviral responses to single-stranded RNA bearing 5′-phosphates. *Science* 314:997, 2006.
80. Kawai T, Takahashi K, Sato S, et al: IPS-1, an adaptor triggering RIG-I- and Mda5-mediated type I interferon induction. *Nat Immunol* 6:981, 2005.
81. Seth RB, Sun L, Ea CK, Chen ZJ: Identification and characterization of MAVS, a mitochondrial antiviral signaling protein that activates NF-kappaB and IRF 3. *Cell* 122:669, 2005.
82. Xu LG, Wang YY, Han KJ, et al: VISA is an adapter protein required for virus-triggered IFN-beta signaling. *Mol Cell* 19:727, 2005.
83. Meylan E, Curran J, Hofmann K, et al: Cardif is an adaptor protein in the RIG-I antiviral pathway and is targeted by hepatitis C virus. *Nature* 437:1167, 2005.
84. Ishikawa H, Barber GN: STING is an endoplasmic reticulum adaptor that facilitates innate immune signalling. *Nature* 455:674, 2008.
85. Takaoka A, Wang Z, Choi MK, et al: DAI (DLM-1/ZBP1) is a cytosolic DNA sensor and an activator of innate immune response. *Nature* 448:501, 2007.
86. Wang Z, Choi MK, Ban T, et al: Regulation of innate immune responses by DAI (DLM-1/ZBP1) and other DNA-sensing molecules. *Proc Natl Acad Sci U S A* 105:5477, 2008.
87. Beutler B, Milsark IW, Cerami A: Passive immunization against cachectin/tumor necrosis factor (TNF) protects mice from the lethal effect of endotoxin. *Science* 229:869, 1985.
88. Georgel P, Naitza S, Kappler C, et al: Drosophila immune deficiency (IMD) is a death domain protein that activates antibacterial defense and can promote apoptosis. *Dev Cell* 1:503, 2001.
89. Orange JS, Biron CA: Characterization of early IL-12, IFN-alphabeta, and TNF effects on antiviral state and NK cell responses during murine cytomegalovirus infection. *J Immunol* 156:4746, 1996.
90. Andrews DM, Scalzo AA, Yokoyama WM, et al: Functional interactions between dendritic cells and NK cells during viral infection. *Nat Immunol* 4:175, 2003.
91. Mancuso G, Midiri A, Biondo C, et al: Type I IFN signaling is crucial for host resistance against different species of pathogenic bacteria. *J Immunol* 178:3126, 2007.
92. Karaghiosoff M, Steinborn R, Kovarik P, et al: Central role for type I interferons and Tyk2 in lipopolysaccharide-induced endotoxin shock. *Nat Immunol* 4:471, 2003.
93. Cella M, Jarrossay D, Facchetti F, et al: Plasmacytoid monocytes migrate to inflamed lymph nodes and produce large amounts of type I interferon. *Nat Med* 5:919, 1999.
94. Lewis PA, Loomis D: The formation of anti-sheep hemolytic amboceptor in the normal and tuberculous guinea pig. *J Exp Med* 40:503, 1924.
95. Freund J, Gottschalk R: Standardization of tuberculin with the aid of guinea pigs sensitized by killed tuberculosis bacilli in liquid petroleum. *Arch Pathol* 34:73, 1942.
96. Condie RM, Zak SJ, Good RA: Effect of Meningococcal Endotoxin on the Immune Response. *Proc Soc Exp Biol Med* 90:355, 1955.
97. Skidmore BJ, Chiller JM, Morrison DC, Weigle WO: Immunologic properties of bacterial lipopolysaccharide (LPS): Correlation between the mitogenic, adjuvant, and immunogenic activities. *J Immunol* 114:770, 1975.
98. Germain RN, Jenkins MK: *In vivo* antigen presentation. *Curr Opin Immunol* 16:120, 2004.
99. Borriello F, Sethna MP, Boyd SD, et al: B7-1 and B7-2 have overlapping, critical roles in immunoglobulin class switching and germinal center formation. *Immunity* 6:303, 1997.
100. Yamamoto M, Sato S, Hemmi H, et al: Role of adaptor TRIF in the MyD88-independent toll-like receptor signaling pathway. *Science* 301:640, 2003.
101. Gavin AL, Hoebe K, Duong B, et al: Adjuvant-enhanced antibody responses in the absence of toll-like receptor signaling. *Science* 314:1936, 2006.
102. Sorensen TI, Nielsen GG, Andersen PK, Teasdale TW: Genetic and environmental influences on premature death in adult adoptees. *N Engl J Med* 318:727, 1988.
103. Smirnova I, Mann N, Dols A, et al: Assay of locus-specific genetic load implicates rare Toll-like receptor 4 mutations in meningococcal susceptibility. *Proc Natl Acad Sci U S A* 100:6075, 2003.
104. Hawn TR, Verbon A, Lettinga KD, et al: A common dominant TLR5 stop codon polymorphism abolishes flagellin signaling and is associated with susceptibility to Legionnaires' disease. *J Exp Med* 198:1563, 2003.
105. Picard C, Puel A, Bonnet M, et al: Pyogenic bacterial infections in humans with IRAK-4 deficiency. *Science* 299:2076, 2003.
106. Zhang SY, Jouanguy E, Ugolini S, et al: TLR3 deficiency in patients with herpes simplex encephalitis. *Science* 317:1522, 2007.
107. Casrouge A, Zhang SY, Eidenschenk C, et al: Herpes simplex virus encephalitis in human UNC-93B deficiency. *Science* 314:308, 2006.
108. Jouanguy E, Altare F, Lamhamedi S, et al: Interferon-gamma-receptor deficiency in an infant with fatal bacille Calmette-Guerin infection. *N Engl J Med* 335:1956, 1996.
109. Picard C, Fieschi C, Altare F, et al: Inherited interleukin-12 deficiency: IL12B genotype and clinical phenotype of 13 patients from six kindreds. *Am J Hum Genet* 70:336, 2002.
110. Altare F, Durandy A, Lammas D, et al: Impairment of mycobacterial immunity in human interleukin-12 receptor deficiency. *Science* 280:1432, 1998.
111. De Jong R, Altare F, Haagen IA, et al: Severe mycobacterial and Salmonella infections in interleukin-12 receptor-deficient patients. *Science* 280:1435, 1998.
112. Barbosa MD, Nguyen QA, Tchernev VT, et al: Identification of the homologous beige and Chédiak-Higashi syndrome genes. *Nature* 382:262, 1996.
113. Royer-Pokora B, Kunkel LM, Monaco AP, et al: Cloning the gene for an inherited human disorder—chronic granulomatous disease—on the basis of its chromosomal location. *Nature* 322:32, 1986.
114. Leadbetter EA, Rifkin IR, Hohlbaum AM, et al: Chromatin-IgG complexes activate B cells by dual engagement of IgM and Toll-like receptors. *Nature* 416:603, 2002.
115. Crozat K, Hoebe K, Ugolini S, et al: *Jinx*, an MCMV susceptibility phenotype caused by disruption of *Unc13d*: A mouse model of type 3 familial hemophagocytic lymphohistiocytosis. *J Exp Med* 204:853, 2007.
116. Croker BA, Lawson BR, Berger M, et al: Inflammation and autoimmunity caused by a SHP1 mutation depend on IL-1, MyD88, and a microbial trigger. *Proc Natl Acad Sci U S A* 105:15028, 2008.
117. Fitzgerald KA, Palsson-McDermott EM, Bowie AG, et al: Mal (MyD88-adapter-like) is required for Toll-like receptor-4 signal transduction. *Nature* 413:78, 2001.
118. Horng T, Barton GM, Medzhitov R: TIRAP: An adapter molecule in the Toll signaling pathway. *Nat Immunol* 2:835, 2001.
119. Yamamoto M, Sato S, Hemmi H, et al: Essential role for TIRAP in activation of the signalling cascade shared by TLR2 and TLR4. *Nature* 420:324, 2002.
120. Poltorak A, Smirnova I, He XL, et al: Genetic and physical mapping of the *Lps* locus—Identification of the toll-4 receptor as a candidate gene in the critical region. *Blood Cells Mol Dis* 24:340, 1998.
121. Takeuchi O, Kawai T, Muhlradt PF, et al: Discrimination of bacterial lipoproteins by Toll-like receptor 6. *Int Immunol* 13:933, 2001.
122. Hemmi H, Kaisho T, Takeuchi O, et al: Small anti-viral compounds activate immune cells via the TLR7 MyD88-dependent signaling pathway. *Nat Immunol* 3:196, 2002.
123. Jurk M, Heil F, Vollmer J, et al: Human TLR7 or TLR8 independently confer responsiveness to the antiviral compound R-848. *Nat Immunol* 3:499, 2002.
124. Chuang T, Ulevitch RJ: Identification of hTLR10: A novel human Toll-like receptor preferentially expressed in immune cells. *Biochim Biophys Acta* 1518:157, 2001.

CHAPTER 19

DENDRITIC CELLS AND THE CONTROL OF INNATE AND ADAPTIVE IMMUNITY

Madhav Dhodapkar and Ralph M. Steinman

SUMMARY

The term *dendritic cell* defines a multifunctional group of cells that serve as sentinels, adjuvants, and controllers of many immune functions. The cells play important roles in both innate and adaptive immune response to invading pathogens and other clinically important situations, such as malignancy. Dendritic cells have receptors for substances found in the environment, providing the cells with the capacity to respond rapidly to pathogens and certain endogenous stimuli, such as antigen-antibody complexes. In this capacity, they can play an important role in activation of innate immune effector mechanisms involved as the first-line defense against infection. In addition, these cells can serve as highly effective antigen-presenting cells that can induce T-cell proliferation (activation) or lack of activation (tolerance) in response to recognition of peptides presented by the dendritic cells' major histocompatibility complex antigens. As such, the cells help regulate the responses to antigen by the adaptive immune system involving T and B lymphocytes. This chapter describes the varied types and functions of this important class of cells.

FUNCTIONS OF DENDRITIC CELLS

Host defense against pathogens, both infectious and neoplastic, is mediated by innate and adaptive responses, often in concert. Innate immune mechanisms act quickly to resist pathogens but do not develop improved function or memory following an initial exposure. Adaptive responses by B and T lymphocytes are acquired over days to months and are capable of memory, that is, improved responses upon pathogen reexposure (see Chaps. 77 and 78). Dendritic cells (DCs) are important mediators of both innate and adaptive immunity and often are responsible for linking together these two forms of resistance.[1–3]

DENDRITIC CELLS AND INNATE IMMUNITY

Among the many mechanisms of innate resistance (Table 19–1), DCs participate by producing large amounts of protective cytokines, including interleukin (IL)-12 and type I interferons, and by activating innate lymphocytes such as natural killer (NK) cells, NK T cells, and $\gamma\delta$ T cells. The innate response of DCs, particularly cytokine and chemokine production, frequently is mediated by distinct "pattern-recognition receptors" (see Chap. 18). These respond to evolutionarily conserved molecular signatures of microbes, parasites and viruses[4–11] and include toll-like receptors (TLRs), nucleotide-binding oligomerization domain-like receptors, retinoic acid-inducible gene 1-like receptors, as well as numerous C-type lectins. Innate pattern recognition receptors do not have the exquisite specificity provided by the antigen receptors for adaptive immunity on B and T cells, but they do recognize specific classes of ligands such as single- or double-stranded RNA, lipopolysaccharides, and other microbial constituents. DCs express these receptors, as do many cell types. Distinctively, DCs respond to agonists for pattern recognition receptors by becoming potent immunostimulatory cells, including the presentation of captured antigens. DCs also respond to noninfectious stimuli, which include certain particulates such as uric acid crystals, heat shock and chromatin proteins, and different types of lymphocytes involved in innate responses. These noninfectious stimuli may be important for activating DCs to initiate host responses following transplantation or in disease states such as cancer or allergy.

Acronyms and abbreviations that appear in this chapter include: CD, cluster of differentiation; CMV, cytomegalovirus; DC, dendritic cell; GM-CSF, granulocyte-monocyte colony-stimulating factor; Ig, immunoglobulin; IL, interleukin; MHC, major histocompatibility complex; NK, natural killer; TLR, toll-like receptor; TNF, tumor necrosis factor.

DENDRITIC CELLS AND THE CONTROL OF ADAPTIVE IMMUNITY

Adaptive immunity comprises several major activities of B and T lymphocytes (Table 19–2). DCs control many features of adaptive immunity. Adaptive lymphocytes have exquisite diversity and specificity by virtue of antibody and immunoglobulin-like receptors for antigen on B cells and T cells, respectively. The receptor genes undergo rearrangements and other somatic diversification mechanisms to create an immense array of antigen receptors. This array might be thought of as the largest combinatorial library of specificities in the world!

An essential counterpart to adaptive immunity is adaptive tolerance, which is the silencing of cells with receptors that are reactive to self or harmless environmental antigens. DCs play a role here, especially with regard to T cells. T cells develop tolerance centrally in the thymus and peripherally in lymphoid organs.[12–15]

During immunization, DCs initiate the clonal expansion of T cells and can directly and indirectly influence the growth of B cells. In addition, DCs can control the subsequent differentiation of lymphocytes, such that the properties of the lymphocytes are appropriate to the invading pathogen.[16] For example, under the influence of DCs, T cells can be polarized to produce either interferon-γ (T-helper [Th] type 1 cells) to activate macrophages to resist infection by intracellular microbes; or IL-4, IL-5, and IL-13 (Th2 cells) to mobilize white cells to resist helminths; or IL-7 (Th17 cells) to mobilize phagocytes at body surfaces to resist extracellular bacteria (see Chap. 78). DCs can also drive T cells to suppress immunity by expressing IL-10 (Tr1 cells) or FOXP3.

Adaptive immunity imparts memory to the host. The memory can be induced by antigen-bearing DCs, but the mechanisms are obscure. Nevertheless, memory provides a population of lymphocytes that allow the host to respond more rapidly and effectively to rechallenge with antigen. As a result of memory, the frequency and function of antigen-specific lymphocytes are improved, leading to more rapid production of protective antibodies, cytokines, or killer molecules.

DENDRITIC CELL FUNCTIONS

DCs function as sentinels of the immune system, conductors of the immune orchestra, and nature's adjuvants (Table 19–3).[1,3,17,18] As sentinels, DCs sense a variety of environmental stimuli, producing cytokines, such as IL-12 and type I interferons that help stimulate immune responses.[19] DCs express most types of TLRs although there are subsets of DCs that differentially express TLRs, e.g., plasmacytoid DCs are major sites for TLR-7 and TLR-9 expression.[20] DCs also can respond to a number of endogenous stimuli, ranging from inflammatory cytokines, including tumor necrosis factor-alpha (TNF-α), IL-1, or interferons, to

TABLE 19–1. Some Innate Mechanisms of Host Resistance

Phagocytic cells: granulocytes and macrophages
Innate lymphocytes: natural killer (NK) cells, NK T cells, $\gamma\delta$ T cells
Mast cells
Complement
Microbial-binding lectins and pentraxins
Cytokines, including interferons
Chemokines and antimicrobial peptides

endogenous stimuli mentioned above. DCs capture microbes and tumor cells, processing their component antigens for presentation to the adaptive immune system. In addition to antigen processing and presentation, sentinel DCs produce chemokines and cytokines. They migrate to lymphoid tissues, recruiting naïve antigen-specific lymphocytes and instructing their subsequent development.

On the other hand, DCs can silence self-reactive T cells, either deleting or anergizing (paralyzing) the lymphocytes.[21,22] Moreover, DCs can recruit antigen-specific regulatory lymphocytes that suppress immune responses by other so-called effector cells.[23]

DCs can activate innate lymphocytes, such as NK and NK T cells (see Chap. 79). Such activation contributes to an expansion in cell numbers as well as enhanced NK and NK T-cell killing activity and cytokine production. Reciprocally, these innate cells act back on DCs, enhancing DC maturation and the initiation of adaptive immune responses. Interaction of DCs with such lymphocytes is an example of cross-talk between cell types and involves multiple cell-surface molecules and cytokines.[24–27]

DCs are a critical bridge between innate and adaptive immunity including memory. As part of the innate response, DCs differentiate or mature to become potent initiators of adaptive immunity. The type of mature DC varies according to the challenge, for example, some parasite products cause DCs to induce a Th2 type of T-cell response, whereas some viruses and bacteria cause DCs to induce Th1 type of immunity. In short, the presence of antigen and lymphocytes often is insufficient to induce many innate and adaptive responses. A third party, the DC system of antigen-presenting cells, typically is pivotal.

LIFE HISTORY AND HETEROGENEITY OF DENDRITIC CELLS

TISSUE DISTRIBUTION

Homeostasis of DCs requires replacement by DC progenitors, and pathways for this are just being identified. For some populations, such

TABLE 19–2. Some Features of Adaptive Immunity by B and T Lymphocytes

Diversity and specificity: somatically rearranged immunoglobulin receptors
Tolerance: specific silencing to self and harmless environmental antigens
Clonal expansion and its regulation: increased, then decreased, numbers of antigen-specific lymphocytes during an immune response
Appropriateness: pathogen-relevant, differentiation of lymphocytes
Memory: long-lived capacity for improved function upon reexposure to antigen

TABLE 19–3. Some Key Consequences of Dendritic Cell Function

Sensors: rapid and appropriate differentiation in response to pathogen-associated molecular patterns and other signals
Sentinels: positioned in peripheral tissues to optimize antigen capture and migrate to lymphoid tissues
Tolerance: deletion and anergy of self-reactive lymphocytes and induction of regulatory T cells
Innate resistance: activation of innate lymphocytes, including NK and NK T cells, secretion of protective cytokines
Adaptive immunity: differentiation of quiescent, naïve T cells to form effectors, establishment of memory lymphocytes, antibody responses

as epidermal Langerhans cells, self-renewal contributes to steady-state homeostasis.[28] In the steady state, DCs in lymphoid tissues originate from marrow progenitors[29–31] that are distinct from monocytes and circulate in the blood.[29,32] However, monocytes also contribute to DC formation at certain mucosal surfaces[33,34] and during some infections.[35,36] The production and proliferation of several DC subsets in lymphoid tissues during the steady-state is controlled by FLT3 ligand, whereas during inflammation, another cytokine, granulocyte-macrophage colony-stimulating factor (GM-CSF) seems to play a role in mobilizing DCs.[37,38]

Most of the DCs in tissues during steady state are considered "immature" because they are not yet able to act as potent initiators of immunity. Nevertheless, immature DCs are specialized cells. They express numerous receptors for environmental stimuli, such as TLRs and cytokine receptors, and endocytic receptors that can facilitate antigen uptake and processing. Immature DCs line body surfaces, such as the airway and intestine. They also are found in the interstitial spaces of most organs, including the heart and kidney. Some DCs continually traffic through tissues in the steady state, typically moving via the afferent lymphatics to lymph nodes. The traffic can increase upon appropriate stimulation, as initially revealed by research on contact allergens. In the steady state, the migration of DCs, such as through the intestinal and airway epithelium, allows DCs to carry samples of self and environmental antigens to regional lymph nodes,[39–41] with the potential of tolerizing the T-cell repertoire. The DCs extend their processes between mucosal epithelial cells, without disrupting the barrier function of the epithelium while allowing the DCs to sample the environment.[42–44] In contrast, under certain conditions inducing their maturation, such as infection with influenza in the lung,[41] the migrating DCs are the critical link for initiating immunity in the draining lymphoid tissues.

This general scheme of the life history of DCs must be placed in the context of DC heterogeneity, because there are many types of DCs (Table 19–4), including monocyte-derived DCs and plasmacytoid DCs. Subtypes of so-called conventional or classical DCs also exist, with the cluster of differentiation (CD)8+ and CD8– subsets in mouse spleen being the most intensively studied, and the CD103+ and CD103– subsets in tissues such as lung and intestine and skin. Nevertheless, much of the research on subsets of DCs takes place in mice, and translation into humans, e.g., for CD8+ and CD8– classical DCs, remains limited.

DENDRITIC CELL PRECURSORS IN MARROW AND BLOOD

Progenitors for DCs express FLT3, a receptor tyrosine kinase that is activated upon binding to FLT3 ligand.[30,38,45,46] Activation of FLT3 greatly expands the numbers of DCs.[47] At the precursor level in the

TABLE 19–4. Dendritic Cell Heterogeneity: Origin, Subsets, and Nomenclature

Marrow: committed progenitors, e.g., monocyte and dendritic cell progenitor, common dendritic cell progenitor, predendritic cell
Blood: plasmacytoid and "classical" subsets
Peripheral tissues: epidermal (epithelial) and dermal (interstitial) subsets
Lymphoid tissues: plasmacytoid and other subsets
Other: interdigitating cells, monocyte-derived dendritic cells

blood, distinct subsets of DCs, as described above, can be distinguished by their differential expression of several marker proteins and distinctive functions. Most classical DCs in human blood express the CD11c integrin and BDCA-1, whereas the plasmacytoid subset of human DCs lacks CD11c and expresses the lectin BDCA-2.[48] An important feature of plasmacytoid DCs is their ability to produce very high levels of type I interferons upon contact with enveloped viruses, including ultraviolet-inactivated viruses.[49,50] The DCs are signaled following ligation of TLR-7 and TLR-9 by viral RNA[51,52] and DNA, respectively.[53,54] Many investigators are now identifying the transcriptional controls for the generation of these different types of DCs, and this will undoubtedly illuminate the programs for DC subset development and function.[55–57]

■ DENDRITIC CELLS IN PERIPHERAL TISSUES

As illustrated by the skin, distinct subsets of DCs are associated with epithelia (e.g., epidermal Langerhans cells) and interstitial spaces (dermal DCs).[58–60] These subsets have different markers, including molecules with a potential role in antigen presentation. Langerhans cells express a C-type lectin called *langerin/CD207*, which can be internalized into special compartments called *Birbeck granules*.[61] These cells also express the CD1a member of the CD1 family of glycolipid-presenting molecules. Dermal DCs in contrast express abundant mannose receptor/CD206 and the CD1b and CD1c forms of glycolipid-presenting molecules.[58] Langerin expression is not restricted to Langerhans cell, as subsets of DCs in lymphoid and nonlymphoid tissues that express langerin have also been identified. The origins, identification and functions of different subsets of skin DCs, and DCs in other peripheral tissues, are areas of active research.

■ DENDRITIC CELLS IN LYMPHOID TISSUES, ESPECIALLY PERIPHERAL LYMPHOID ORGANS

Representatives of the Langerhans cells and plasmacytoid DCs, along with additional subsets of so-called classical DCs, are present in the lymphoid tissues. For example, in mouse spleen,[62] one subset of DCs lacks the integrin CD11b but selectively expresses endocytic receptors, termed DEC-205/CD205[63] and CLEC9A,[64–66] as well as treml4.[67] This subset is specialized to take up dying cells, including targets killed by NK lymphocytes.[68] Another subset of mouse DCs expresses CD11b and is capable of some phagocytic and pinocytic activity, but it lacks DEC-205 and appears not to ingest many types of dying cells.

In mice, DC subsets have different capacities for antigen presentation. For example, CD8+DEC205+ DCs are more effective at processing antigens for presentation on major histocompatibility complex (MHC) class I to CD8+ T cells, whereas DCs expressing another C-type lectin receptor, DCIR2, are more efficient at processing antigens for presentation on MHC class II to CD4+ T cells.[69] The subset of DCs expressing CD8a is selectively depleted in mice lacking a transcription factor Batf3, suggesting distinct requirements for their development.[70] Human counterparts of these DC subsets are also being distinguished in blood and in skin as BDCA-1+ and BDCA-3+,[48,59] but functional studies remain to be reported.

By electron microscopy, DCs in lymphoid tissues often are termed "interdigitating cells." These cells appear as large stellate cells with a lucent "empty"-appearing cytoplasm. The DEC205/CD205 lectin receptor is currently the best marker for these DCs in human lymph nodes.[71]

DCs involved in induction of immune tolerance can be called "tolerogenic DCs." Tolerogenic DCs may represent a distinct subset, but more likely many types of DCs are capable of inducing tolerance. The type of tolerance depends on the state of DC maturation and the environments in which the DCs are located.

The biology (homeostasis and function) of DCs and their subsets is likely influenced by specific location (e.g., mucosal, liver) and context (e.g., inflammation, steady state). The marrow is an example of a tissue relevant to hematology where the biology of dendritic cells is distinct. In that location, a subset of perivascular DCs, expressing migration inhibitor factor, may serve as a specialized extrafollicular niche for B cells.[72]

■ MEANING OF DENDRITIC CELL HETEROGENEITY

The significance of the heterogeneity of DCs is an active area of research. In one view, DC subsets are precommitted to carry out select innate responses and, in turn, perhaps, distinct types of adaptive immunity. Plasmacytoid DCs are a major source of type I interferons, particularly with inactivated viruses[49,73] yet other DCs can be a rich source of interferon after certain live viral infections and signaling through protein kinase R.[74] Some evidence indicates different subsets of DCs polarize helper T cells to either the Th1- or Th2-type pathway of differentiation.[75–77] In contrast, other data indicate these same subsets are plastic, influenced by the pathogen to bring about different types of innate and adaptive immunity.[78] The field of DC subsets is limited by the relative lack of direct analyses of DCs *in vivo*, as opposed to data on DCs studied *ex vivo* or following reinfusion, especially in humans.

ELEMENTS OF DENDRITIC CELL FUNCTION FOR INITIATION OF IMMUNITY

DCs are "antigen-presenting cells." An antigen-presenting cell is *any* cell that uses its MHC products (or other antigen-presenting molecules, such as the CD1 molecules that present glycolipids and lipoglycans) to bind and display (i.e., "present") fragments of antigen to lymphocytes. DCs are much more specialized or professional than other antigen-presenting cells. This means that DCs have efficient and regulated pathways for antigen uptake and processing, and the DCs express dozens of other features that allow them to initiate and control immunity. For example, when DCs mature in response to infection, hundreds and even thousands of gene transcripts can be upregulated or downregulated.[79,80] Most of the early attention on the function of DCs was on their ability to stimulate T-cell immunity, but the significant roles of DCs in the induction of tolerance and in the regulation of other types of lymphocytes, such as NK, NK T cells, $\gamma\delta$ T cells, and B cells, are increasingly evident (Table 19–5).

■ ANTIGEN CAPTURE

Many different endocytic receptors are expressed by DCs, where they enhance the efficiency of antigen capture, processing, and presentation.[81] One example, which has been pursued *in vivo* in mice, involves

TABLE 19–5. Some Important Components of Dendritic Cell Function

Cell processes or dendrites and motility: numerous and continually probing
Antigen handling: specialized antigen uptake receptors and processing pathways for classic (MHC) and nonclassic (CD1 and others) presenting molecules, including cross-presentation onto MHC class I and CD1
MHC class II products: high and regulated expression
Migration in lymphatics to lymphoid organs and localization to T-cell areas
Environmental sensing: multiple receptors for microbial and nonmicrobial products and exaggerated responses to the products
Cytokine receptors, including hematopoietins (flt3L and GM-CSF, but not monocyte colony-stimulating factor, granulocyte colony-stimulating factor)
Chemokine receptors, especially for homing to tissues (CCR6) and lymph nodes (CCR7, CCR2)
Induction of peripheral tolerance via intrinsic and extrinsic pathways
Activation of innate lymphocytes (e.g., NK cells)

the engineering of antigens into antibodies that bind to the endocytic receptor DEC205/CD205. The modified antibody then targets the antigen selectively to DCs in lymphoid tissues.[21,75,82] Antibody-mediated targeting to DCs in lymphoid tissues enhances presentation of the associated antigen more than 100-fold to CD8+ and CD4+ T cells. In other words, although DCs are positioned to pick up antigens and process them for presentation in lymphoid organs, receptor-based pathways exist through which antigen capture (and in some cases, antigen processing) can be improved to a major extent.

Many potential antigen uptake receptors are predicted to be C-type lectins,[64,65,83] but in many cases their natural ligands have not been identified. DCs also express Fcγ and Fcε receptors for immune complexes and several scavenger receptors. Recognition of pathogens by DC receptors can have two outcomes. One outcome is antigen presentation. In the second outcome, the pathogen may use the receptor to exploit and evade the host. An example studied in tissue culture is the lectin DC-SIGN/CD209, which is expressed by monocyte-derived DCs. DC-SIGN is commandeered by different agents, such as HIV-1 and cytomegalovirus (CMV), to be transmitted to T cells and endothelial cells, respectively[84,85]; by Dengue virus to replicate within DCs[86]; and by *Mycobacterium tuberculosis* to trigger production of the suppressive cytokine IL-10.[87,88]

ANTIGEN PROCESSING

Following uptake, efficient processing of antigen yields peptides that bind to MHC class II and class I products. The terminology can be confusing, but by definition, "exogenous" antigens are processed directly following uptake, whereas "endogenous" antigens are processed following biosynthesis in the antigen-presenting cell. The more classic or earliest defined routes involved processing of "exogenous" antigens for presentation of MHC II–peptide complexes to CD4+ T lymphocytes and "endogenous" antigens for presentation of MHC class I–peptide complexes to CD8+ T cells.

However, a more recently appreciated route leads to the presentation of exogenous antigens on MHC I products. This pathway is termed "cross-presentation" and can be particularly well developed in DCs, especially those cells in lymphoid tissues *in vivo* where cross-presentation leads efficiently to either tolerance or immunity in CD8+ T lymphocytes, depending upon the DC maturation stimulus.[82,89] The exogenous pathway is illustrated by the uptake of dying cells,[89,90] which models the capture of cell-associated antigens from transplants, tumors, foci of infection, and self tissues. The pathway is called "cross-presentation" because antigens located in a dying cell "crossover" to the processing and presentation machinery of the DC. Nevertheless, cross-presentation of antigens onto MHC class I can involve the proteasome and transporters for antigenic peptides, which are used in the presentation of endogenous antigens.

DCs are a major cell type involved in cross-presentation of both proteins[70,91] and probably lipids.[92,93] Cross-presentation has been observed with nonreplicating microbes, dying cells, ligands for the DEC205 receptor, and immune complexes including antibody-coated tumor cells. These examples allow DCs to induce tolerance or immunity to antigens that are not synthesized *de novo* in these cells. Fcγreceptors, in addition to mediating presentation, can influence DC maturation, either enhancing maturation through activating forms of the receptor or preventing maturation through inhibitory forms.[94] Such consequences of antibody binding to DC Fc receptors, with regard to DC maturation and cross-presentation, must be considered when trying to understand the use of antibodies as therapeutic agents in patients.

DCs are a major site for expression of the CD1 family of antigen-presenting molecules, although individual CD1 molecules can be restricted to subsets of DCs. For example, CD1a typically is found on epidermal Langerhans cells in skin, whereas CD1b and CD1c are expressed on dermal DCs. CD1 molecules present glycolipids, whereas microbial glycolipids are the best studied to date with regard to CD1a, CD1b, and CD1c.[95] In addition, CD1d molecules on DCs efficiently present the synthetic glycolipid α-galactosylceramide. This process leads to activation of distinct lymphocytes with a restricted T-cell repertoire, the NK T cells.[96] NK T cells have significant potential as effector cells because they can produce large amounts of interferon-$\gamma$and lyse tumor targets.

A newer "nonclassical" pathway for antigen presentation involves the presentation of "endogenous" proteins on MHC class II.[97] This pathway involves autophagy and also is well developed in DCs.[98] It allows nuclear, mitochondrial and cytoplasmic proteins to be presented from digestive compartments, including as a first example, the EBNA1 nuclear antigen from the Epstein-Barr virus.[99]

REGULATION AND MATURATION OF DENDRITIC CELLS

Maturation refers to the stimulus-dependent differentiation of DCs that allows differentiation of lymphocytes for immunity and memory. Immature DCs efficiently take up antigen but do not induce immunity, that is, the production of immune effectors and the establishment of memory. For immune induction to occur, DCs require additional stimuli that lead to an intricate differentiation process called "maturation." Maturation comprises changes in the endocytic and antigen processing machineries, the production of chemokines and cytokines, and the expression of many cell surface molecules, including those of the B7, TNF, and Notch ligand families. Therefore, DCs can separate in time two of the vital components for initiating immunity: antigen uptake by immature DCs and expression of costimulatory functions for lymphocytes by mature cells.[100,101]

In the case of DCs derived from marrow and monocyte precursors, DC maturation is accompanied by exquisite changes in the endocytic system with attendant consequences for antigen processing and presentation. Lysosomal processing is activated by assembly of an active proton pump.[102] This adenosine triphosphatase acidifies the lysosome so that processing of antigens and the MHC class II associated invariant chain can proceed. The MHC–peptide complexes form within the endocytic system of the maturing DCs[103] which then traffic in distinct nonlysosomal compartments to the cell surface.[104] Also, internalization and degradation of MHC II occurs via ubiquitination in immature but not mature DCs.[105] DC maturation also increases presentation on MHC I. One change is the formation of an "immunoproteasome," a combinatorial form of proteasome that increases the spectrum of peptides destined to be presented on MHC I.[106] Another regulated process involves the uptake or endocytosis step itself. During maturation, uptake is dampened as a result of inactivation of a rho-guanosine triphosphatase termed cdc42.[107] Therefore, DCs have an endocytic system that is tightly regulated and devoted to presentation of captured antigens, rather than clearance and scavenging.

A hallmark of DC maturation in response to several stimuli is upregulation of costimulatory molecules such as CD80 and CD86.[108] The upregulation seems to result from production of inflammatory cytokines, particularly TNF-α.[96] Nonetheless, CD86 upregulation should not be equated directly with immunogenicity, which requires other DC functions, such as those triggered by CD40 ligation, cytokines such as IL12 or type I interferons, or engagement of other receptors such as CD70.[96]

ACTIVATION OF INNATE LYMPHOCYTES

Increasing attention is now being paid to crosstalk between DCs and other innate effectors such as NK cells.[109] DCs can prime resting NK cells, which, after activation, might induce further maturation of DCs. NK-mediated killing of virus-infected cells or tumor cells may provide a source of antigens for generation of T-cell responses via DCs, further linking innate and adaptive immunity. NK cells also negatively regulate DC function by killing immature DCs.[110] A significant proportion of NK cells reside in the T-cell regions of lymphoid tissues, thereby providing an opportunity for direct interaction between DC and NK cells *in vivo*.[111]

GENERATION OF ANTIBODY-FORMING B CELLS

DCs enhance antibody formation by several mechanisms, the classical pathway involving induction of antigen-specific CD4+ helper T cells which then help B-cell growth and antibody secretion.[112] In addition, DCs can have direct effects on B cells that greatly enhance immunoglobulin (Ig) secretion and isotype switching, including production of the IgA class of antibodies, which contribute to mucosal immunity.[113,114] DCs can induce a B-cell class switch in a CD40-independent manner, through production of ligands such as B-lymphocyte stimulator (B-cell activating factor belonging to the tumor necrosis factor family [BAFF]) and a proliferation-induced ligand (APRIL), including T cell-independent induction of IgA antibodies to commensal organisms.[115] Plasmacytoid DCs stimulate antibody responses to influenza virus in culture.[116] Production of antibodies by any of these mechanisms may lead to interaction with DC FcγR and thereby an adaptive response by T cells.

POSITIONING AND MIGRATION OF DENDRITIC CELLS

DCs are strategically positioned as immature cells along body surfaces (skin, airway, gut) and in the interstitial spaces of many organs, such as the heart and kidneys. As mentioned, DCs are able to extend their processes through the tight junctions in epithelia, without altering the epithelial barrier, which allows them to sample antigens from harmless environmental antigens and commensal microorganisms. In the steady state, DCs appear to migrate continuously from tissues into afferent lymphatics and probably blood. Steady-state traffic of DCs may allow the DCs to sample self and environmental antigens for purposes of tolerance. One possibility is that the "tolerogenic" DC may not be the migratory cell itself. Instead, the migrating DC may die in the lymph node and be processed by resident DCs in that organ[90] or additional mechanisms may transfer antigen and MHC peptide complexes to more "resident" DCs.[117] Most DCs in a lymph node often are assumed to represent immigrants from the tissues, but it now appears that most DCs in the T-cell areas are derived from blood progenitors.[29,118]

TOLEROGENIC PROPERTIES OF DENDRITIC CELLS

Much of the early focus on DCs was on their immunogenic properties, but increasing evidence indicates DCs *in situ* can mediate antigen-specific unresponsiveness or tolerance in the central lymphoid organs and in the periphery. In the thymus, DCs generate tolerance by deleting self-reactive T cells.[119] Other cells, particularly the specialized epithelium of the thymic medulla,[120] are important in deletional tolerance or negative selection.

DCs also induce tolerance in peripheral lymphoid organs. For example, DCs may induce tolerance to antigens present in dying self tissues. Uptake, especially when receptor mediated, leads to presentation of antigens on MHC class I and II products.[21,82,89] In mice, the targeting of antigens to receptors on resting DCs can lead to deletion of the corresponding T cells and unresponsiveness to antigenic challenge. However, if a stimulus for DC maturation is coadministered, the mice develop immunity. DCs also can contribute to the expansion and differentiation of T cells that can suppress or regulate other immune cells.[121,122] One possibility is that distinct developmental stages and subsets of DCs account for the different pathways, leading to peripheral tolerance, such as deletion or suppression of self-reactive T cells. The tolerogenic capacities of DCs may be linked to their metabolic properties. For example, DCs convert vitamin A and D to retinoic acid and 1,25-dihydroxyvitamin D_3, which may be important for their ability to induce suppressor T cells.[123,124]

DENDRITIC CELLS IN IMMUNOTHERAPY

At this time, the principal hematologic field addressed from the perspective of DC biology is the host response to malignancy and associated strategies for immunotherapy of cancer. The features of DCs outlined in Table 19–5 explain their relevance to these fields. Two major underpinnings for immunotherapy are, first, malignant cells express a large number of alterations that are viewed as antigens by the immune system, and, second, there are many immune mechanisms—antibodies, T cells, and NK cells—that can act against tumors. Moreover, immune resistance is specific, nonnoxious and durable, and it can be coupled with other strategies that reduce the immune evasive features of tumors. Although immune antibodies now represent a major advance in the treatment of cancer, cell-mediated immune mechanisms are currently underexplored and undersupported, a major imbalance in the cancer field.

DCs can efficiently process antigens from a variety of different sources, such as tumor cells, and initiate responses by the different kinds of innate and adaptive lymphocytes, especially NK and T cells. Therefore, harnessing DCs to manipulate the host response to tumors and to other hematologic antigens seems logical. It is a distinct and promising approach to cancer prevention and therapy because it allows multiple immune processes to be mobilized against the tumor, and multiple targets within the tumor making evasion by tumor mutation more difficult.

An example is myeloma, in which both T cells and tumor cells from the marrow can be studied. In the premalignant state, termed *essential monoclonal gammopathy*, myeloma-reactive T cells are detected in the marrow.[125] Using DCs to present myeloma cells as antigens, the presence of both CD4+ helper T cells and CD8+ killer T cells in the marrow can be detected. In contrast, myeloma-reactive T cells cannot be detected in patients with advanced myeloma. Nonetheless, myeloma-reactive CD4+ and CD8+ T cells can be generated when the T cells are cultured for 1 to 2 weeks in the presence of DCs that have captured myeloma cells.[126] The presentation of myeloma cells is greatly enhanced when they are coated with antisyndecan antibodies.[126,127]

DCs have important potential roles in immunotherapy.[3,128,129] Several approaches are being used to generate DCs under clinical-grade conditions, load them with tumor antigens *ex vivo*, and reinfuse the cells to actively immunize patients against cancer antigens or, more broadly, to study several aspects of the human immune response to cancer.

One approach to DC-based immunotherapy utilizes blood DCs that are differentiated and charged with tumor antigens. A second approach generates DCs *ex vivo* from proliferating progenitors within CD34+ populations. This process provides a composite of cells with properties of epidermal and dermal DCs. A third approach differentiates DCs from blood monocytes (see Chap. 25).

Ex vivo-derived and antigen-loaded DCs have been used to expand antigen-specific T-cell responses in healthy volunteers[130,131] and in cancer patients.[132–135] These early studies have yielded some evidence of clinical activity, with tumor regressions in patients with either solid tumors or hematologic malignancies. An important advantage of the *ex vivo* approach to immunotherapy is that several key parameters of DC function can be controlled and researched, such as the loading of DCs with multiple antigens (from whole tumor cells or with RNA from whole tumor cells) and the control of the DC maturation state. Injection of immature DCs may lead to inhibition of T-cell responses and induction of regulatory T cells.[136] Furthermore, DCs can boost innate lymphocytes such as NK cells[111] and glycolipid-reactive NK T cells.[27]

Another approach, still in the preclinical setting, targets antigens to DCs directly *in situ*. This objective can be achieved by incorporating the antigens into monoclonal antibodies specific for receptors expressed selectively or at much higher levels on DCs or DC subsets. Targeting via the DEC-205 receptor is an early example and stresses the need to simultaneously consider the maturation state of the antigen-capturing DCs. In the steady state, tolerance can ensue.[21,137] For immunity, a complex process of maturation must be induced, for example, by the actions of agonistic anti-CD40 antibodies,[82] TLR ligands,[138] or innate lymphocytes.[96]

A setting where the biology of DCs plays a central role in hematology is allogeneic stem cell transplantation. The immunologic activity of donor T cells in allogeneic stem cell transplantation is a critical factor for eradicating residual malignancy, a process termed *graft-versus-leukemia*, but can also lead to detrimental graft-versus-host disease. There is considerable evidence that both graft-versus-host and graft-versus-leukemia are dependent on remaining host antigen-presenting cells of which DCs are the most potent.[139]

REFERENCES

1. Steinman RM, Banchereau J: Taking dendritic cells into medicine. *Nature* 449:419, 2007.
2. Belkaid Y, Oldenhove G: Tuning microenvironments: Induction of regulatory T cells by dendritic cells. *Immunity* 29:362, 2008.
3. Melief CJ: Cancer immunotherapy by dendritic cells. *Immunity* 29:372, 2008.
4. Lemaitre B, Hoffmann J: The host defense of *Drosophila melanogaster*. *Annu Rev Immunol* 25:697, 2007.
5. Akira S, Uematsu S, Takeuchi O: Pathogen recognition and innate immunity. *Cell* 124:783, 2006.
6. Beutler BA: TLRs and innate immunity. *Blood* 113:1399, 2009.
7. Rakoff-Nahoum S, Medzhitov R: Toll-like receptors and cancer. *Nat Rev Cancer* 9:57, 2009.
8. Ting JP, Kastner DL, Hoffman HM: CATERPILLERs, pyrin and hereditary immunological disorders. *Nat Rev Immunol* 6:183, 2006.
9. Meylan E, Tschopp J, Karin M: Intracellular pattern recognition receptors in the host response. *Nature* 442:39, 2006.
10. Kanneganti TD, Lamkanfi M, Nunez G: Intracellular NOD-like receptors in host defense and disease. *Immunity* 27:549, 2007.
11. Kawai T, Akira S: The roles of TLRs, RLRs and NLRs in pathogen recognition. *Int Immunol* 21:317, 2009.
12. Dhodapkar MV, Steinman RM, Krasovsky J, et al: Antigen-specific inhibition of effector T cell function in humans after injection of immature dendritic cells. *J Exp Med* 193:233, 2001.
13. Steinman RM, Hawiger D, Nussenzweig MC: Tolerogenic dendritic cells. *Annu Rev Immunol* 21:685, 2003.
14. Lambrecht BN: Dendritic cells and the regulation of the allergic immune response. *Allergy* 60:271, 2005.
15. Morelli AE, Thomson AW: Tolerogenic dendritic cells and the quest for transplant tolerance. *Nat Rev Immunol* 7:610, 2007.
16. Zhu J, Paul WE: CD4, T cells: Fates, functions, and faults. *Blood* 112:1557, 2008.
17. Pulendran B: Modulating vaccine responses with dendritic cells and toll-like receptors. *Immunol Rev* 199:227, 2004.
18. Banchereau J, Palucka AK: Dendritic cells as therapeutic vaccines against cancer. *Nat Rev Immunol* 5:296, 2005.
19. Reis e Sousa C, Hieny S, Scharton-Kersten T, et al: *In vivo* microbial stimulation induces rapid CD40L-independent production of IL-12, by dendritic cells and their re-distribution to T cell areas. *J Exp Med* 186:1819, 1997.
20. Gilliet M, Cao W, Liu YJ: Plasmacytoid dendritic cells: sensing nucleic acids in viral infection and autoimmune diseases. *Nat Rev Immunol* 8:594, 2008.
21. Hawiger D, Inaba K, Dorsett Y, et al: Dendritic cells induce peripheral T cell unresponsiveness under steady state conditions *in vivo*. *J Exp Med* 194:769, 2001.
22. Probst HC, McCoy K, Okazaki T, et al: Resting dendritic cells induce peripheral CD8+ T cell tolerance through PD-1, and CTLA-4. *Nat Immunol* 6:280, 2005.
23. Yamazaki S, Dudziak D, Heidkamp GF, et al: CD8+ CD205+ splenic dendritic cells are specialized to induce Foxp3+ regulatory T cells. *J Immunol* 181:6923, 2008.
24. Walzer T, Dalod M, Robbins SH, et al: Natural-killer cells and dendritic cells: "L'union fait la force." *Blood* 106:2252, 2005.
25. Terme M, Ullrich E, Delahaye NF, et al: Natural killer cell-directed therapies: moving from unexpected results to successful strategies. *Nat Immunol* 9:486, 2008.
26. Münz C, Steinman RM, Fujii S: Dendritic cell maturation by innate lymphocytes: Coordinated stimulation of innate and adaptive immunity. *J Exp Med* 202:203, 2005.
27. Fujii S, Shimizu K, Hemmi H, Steinman RM: Innate Valpha14(+) natural killer T cells mature dendritic cells, leading to strong adaptive immunity. *Immunol Rev* 220:183, 2007.
28. Merad M, Manz MG, Karsunky H, et al: Langerhans cells renew in the skin throughout life under steady-state conditions. *Nat Immunol* 3:1135, 2002.
29. Liu K, Victora GD, Schwickert TA, et al: *In vivo* analysis of dendritic cell development and homeostasis. *Science* 324:392, 2009.
30. Onai N, Obata-Onai A, Schmid MA, et al: Identification of clonogenic common $Flt3^+M\text{-}CSFR^+$ plasmacytoid and conventional dendritic cell progenitors in mouse bone marrow. *J Exp Med* 193:233, 2007.
31. Naik SH, Sathe P, Park HY, et al: Development of plasmacytoid and conventional dendritic cell subtypes from single precursor cells derived *in vitro* and *in vivo*. *Nat Immunol* 8:1217, 2007.
32. Liu K, Waskow C, Liu X, et al: Origin of dendritic cells in peripheral lymphoid organs of mice. *Nat Immunol* 8:578, 2007.
33. Varol C, Landsman L, Fogg DK, et al: Monocytes give rise to mucosal, but not splenic, conventional dendritic cells. *J Exp Med* 204:171, 2007.
34. Jakubzick C, Tacke F, Ginhoux F, et al: Blood monocyte subsets differentially give rise to $CD103^+$ and $CD103^-$ pulmonary dendritic cell populations. *J Immunol* 180:3019, 2008.
35. Leon B, Lopez-Bravo M, Ardavin C: Monocyte-derived dendritic cells formed at the infection site control the induction of protective T helper 1, responses against *Leishmania*. *Immunity* 26:519, 2007.
36. Serbina NV, Salazar-Mather TP, Biron CA, et al: TNF/iNOS-producing dendritic cells mediate innate immune defense against bacterial infection. *Immunity* 19:59, 2003.
37. Merad M, Manz MG: Dendritic cell homeostasis. *Blood* 113:3418, 2009.
38. Shortman K, Naik SH: Steady-state and inflammatory dendritic-cell development. *Nat Rev Immunol* 7:19, 2007.
39. Huang F-P, Platt N, Wykes M, et al: A discrete subpopulation of dendritic cells transports apoptotic intestinal epithelial cells to T cell areas of mesenteric lymph nodes. *J Exp Med* 191:435, 2000.
40. Vermaelen KY, Carro-Muino I, Lambrecht BN, Pauwels RA: Specific migratory dendritic cells rapidly transport antigen from the airways to the thoracic lymph nodes. *J Exp Med* 193:51, 2001.
41. Brimnes MK, Bonifaz L, Steinman RM, Moran TM: Influenza virus-induced dendritic cell maturation is associated with the induction of strong T cell immunity to a coadministered, normally nonimmunogenic protein. *J Exp Med* 198:133, 2003.
42. Rescigno M, Urbano M, Valzasina B, et al: Dendritic cells express tight junction proteins and penetrate gut epithelial monolayers to sample bacteria. *Nat Immunol* 2:361, 2001.
43. Niess JH, Brand S, Gu X, et al: CX3CR1-mediated dendritic cell access to the intestinal lumen and bacterial clearance. *Science* 307:254, 2005.
44. Chieppa M, Rescigno M, Huang AYC, Germain RN: Dynamic imaging of dendritic cell extension into the small bowel lumen in response to epithelial cell TLR engagement. *J Exp Med* 203:2841, 2006.

45. D'Amico A, Wu L: The early progenitors of mouse dendritic cells and plasmacytoid predendritic cells are within the bone marrow hemopoietic precursors expressing Flt3. *J Exp Med* 198:293, 2003.
46. Onai N, Obata-Onai A, Tussiwand R, et al: Activation of the Flt3, signal transduction cascade rescues and enhances type I interferon-producing and dendritic cell development. *J Exp Med* 203:227, 2006.
47. Pulendran B, Banchereau J, Burkeholder S, et al: Flt3-ligand and granulocyte colony-stimulating factor mobilize distinct human dendritic cell subsets *in vivo*. *J Immunol* 165:566, 2000.
48. Dzionek A, Fuchs A, Schmidt P, et al: BDCA-2, BDCA-3, and BDCA-4: Three markers for distinct subsets of dendritic cells in human peripheral blood. *J Immunol* 165:6037, 2000.
49. Siegal FP, Kadowaki N, Shodell M, et al: The nature of the principal type 1, interferon-producing cells in human blood. *Science* 284:1835, 1999.
50. Asselin-Paturel C, Boonstra A, Dalod M, et al: Mouse type I IFN-producing cells are immature APCs with plasmacytoid morphology. *Nat Immunol* 2:1144, 2001.
51. Diebold SS, Kaisho T, Hemmi H, et al: Innate antiviral responses by means of TLR7-mediated recognition of single-stranded RNA. *Science* 303:1529, 2004.
52. Heil F, Hemmi H, Hochrein H, et al: Species-specific recognition of single-stranded RNA via toll-like receptor 7, and 8. *Science* 303:1526, 2004.
53. Lund J, Sato A, Akira S, et al: Toll-like receptor 9-mediated recognition of herpes simplex virus-2, by plasmacytoid dendritic cells. *J Exp Med* 198:513, 2003.
54. Tabeta K, Georgel P, Janssen E, et al: Toll-like receptors 9, and 3, as essential components of innate immune defense against mouse cytomegalovirus infection. *Proc Natl Acad Sci U S A* 101:3516, 2004.
55. Tamura T, Tailor P, Yamaoka K, et al: IFN regulatory factor-4, and -8, govern dendritic cell subset development and their functional diversity. *J Immunol* 174:2573, 2005.
56. Aliberti J, Schulz O, Pennington DJ, et al: Essential role for ICSBP in the *in vivo* development of murine CD8alpha + dendritic cells. *Blood* 101:305, 2003.
57. Cisse B, Caton ML, Lehner M, et al: Transcription factor E2–2, is an essential and specific regulator of plasmacytoid dendritic cell development. *Cell* 135:37, 2008.
58. Ebner S, Ehammer Z, Holzmann S, et al: Expression of C-type lectin receptors by subsets of dendritic cells in human skin. *Int Immunol* 16:877, 2004.
59. Zaba LC, Fuentes-Duculan J, Steinman RM, et al: Normal human dermis contains distinct populations of $CD11c^{+}BDCA\text{-}1^{+}$ dendritic cells and $CD163^{+}FXIIIA^{+}$ macrophages. *J Clin Invest* 117:2517, 2007.
60. Kissenpfennig A, Henri S, Dubois B, et al: Dynamics and function of Langerhans cells in vivo: dermal dendritic cells colonize lymph node areas distinct from slower migrating Langerhans cells. *Immunity* 22:643, 2005.
61. Valladeau J, Ravel O, Dezutter-Dambuyant C, et al: Langerin, a novel C-type lectin specific to Langerhans cells, is an endocytic receptor that induces the formation of Birbeck granules. *Immunity* 12:71, 2000.
62. Vremec D, Shortman K: Dendritic cells subtypes in mouse lymphoid organs. Cross-correlation of surface markers, changes with incubation, and differences among thymus, spleen, and lymph nodes. *J Immunol* 159:565, 1997.
63. Jiang W, Swiggard WJ, Heufler C, et al: The receptor DEC-205, expressed by dendritic cells and thymic epithelial cells is involved in antigen processing. *Nature* 375:151, 1995.
64. Caminschi I, Proietto AI, Ahmet F, et al: The dendritic cell subtype-restricted C-type lectin Clec9A is a target for vaccine enhancement. *Blood* 112:3264, 2008.
65. Sancho D, Joffre OP, Keller AM, et al: Identification of a dendritic cell receptor that couples sensing of necrosis to immunity. *Nature* 458:899, 2009.
66. Huysamen C, Willment JA, Dennehy KM, Brown GD: CLEC9A is a novel activation C-type lectin-like receptor expressed on BDCA3+ dendritic cells and a subset of monocytes. *J Biol Chem* 283:16693, 2008.
67. Hemmi H, Idoyaga J, Suda K, et al: A new triggering receptor expressed on myeloid cells (Trem) family member, Trem-like 4, binds to dead cells and is a DNAX activation protein 12-linked marker for subsets of mouse macrophages and dendritic cells. *J Immunol* 182:1278, 2009.
68. Iyoda T, Shimoyama S, Liu K, et al: The $CD8^{+}$ dendritic cell subset selectively endocytoses dying cells in culture and *in vivo*. *J Exp Med* 195:1289, 2002.
69. Dudziak D, Kamphorst AO, Heidkamp GF, et al: Differential antigen processing by dendritic cell subsets *in vivo*. *Science* 315:107, 2007.
70. Hildner K, Edelson BT, Purtha WE, et al: Batf3 deficiency reveals a critical role for CD8+ dendritic cells in cytotoxic T cell immunity. *Science* 322:1097, 2008.
71. Granelli-Piperno A, Pritsker A, Pack M, et al: Dendritic cell-specific intercellular adhesion molecule 3-grabbing nonintegrin/CD209, is abundant on macrophages in the normal human lymph node and is not required for dendritic cell stimulation of the mixed leukocyte reaction. *J Immunol* 175:4265, 2005.
72. Sapoznikov A, Pewzner-Jung Y, Kalchenko V, et al: Perivascular clusters of dendritic cells provide critical survival signals to B cells in bone marrow niches. *Nat Immunol* 9:388, 2008.
73. Cella M, Jarrossay D, Facchetti F, et al: Plasmacytoid monocytes migrate to inflamed lymph nodes and produce large amounts of type I interferon. *Nat Med* 5:919, 1999.
74. Diebold SS, Montoya M, Unger H, et al: Viral infection switches non-plasmacytoid dendritic cells into high interferon producers. *Nature* 424:324, 2003.
75. Soares H, Waechter H, Glaichenhaus N, et al: A subset of dendritic cells induces $CD4^{+}$ T cells to produce IFN-γ by an IL-12-independent but CD70-dependent mechanism *in vivo*. *J Exp Med* 204:1095, 2007.
76. Moser M, Murphy KM: Dendritic cell regulation of T_H1-T_H2, development. *Nat Immunol* 1:199, 2000.
77. Pulendran B, Smith JL, Caspary G, et al: Distinct dendritic cell subsets differentially regulate the class of immune responses *in vivo*. *Proc Natl Acad Sci U S A* 96:1036, 1999.
78. Boonstra A, Asselin-Paturel C, Gilliet M, et al: Flexibility of mouse classical and plasmacytoid-derived dendritic cells in directing T helper type 1, and 2, cell development: dependency on antigen dose and differential toll-like receptor ligation. *J Exp Med* 197:101, 2003.
79. Granucci F, Vizzardelli C, Pavelka N, et al: Inducible IL-2, production by dendritic cells revealed by global gene expression analysis. *Nat Immunol* 2:882, 2001.
80. Huang Q, Liu do N, Majewski P, et al: The plasticity of dendritic cell responses to pathogens and their components. *Science* 294:870, 2001.
81. Mellman I, Steinman RM: Dendritic cells: Specialized and regulated antigen processing machines. *Cell* 106:255, 2001.
82. Bonifaz LC, Bonnyay DP, Charalambous A, et al: *In vivo* targeting of antigens to maturing dendritic cells via the DEC-205, receptor improves T cell vaccination. *J Exp Med* 199:815, 2004.
83. Figdor CG, van Kooyk Y, Adema GJ: C-type lectin receptors on dendritic cells and Langerhans cells. *Nat Rev Immunol* 2:77, 2002.
84. Geijtenbeek TBH, Kwon DS, Torensma R, et al: DC-SIGN, a dendritic cell specific HIV-1, binding protein that enhances *trans*-infection of T cells. *Cell* 100:587, 2000.
85. Halary F, Amara A, Lortat-Jacob H, et al: Human cytomegalovirus binding to DC-SIGN is required for dendritic cell infection and target cell trans-infection. *Immunity* 17:653, 2002.
86. Tassaneetrithep B, Burgess TH, Granelli-Piperno A, et al: DC-SIGN (CD209) mediates dengue virus infection of human dendritic cells. *J Exp Med* 197:823, 2003.
87. van Kooyk Y, Geijtenbeek TB: DC-SIGN: Escape mechanism for pathogens. *Nat Rev Immunol* 3:697, 2003.
88. Tailleux L, Schwartz O, Herrmann J-L, et al: DC-SIGN is the major *Mycobacterium tuberculosis* receptor on human dendritic cells. *J Exp Med* 197:121, 2003.
89. Liu K, Iyoda T, Saternus M, et al: Immune tolerance after delivery of dying cells to dendritic cells *in situ*. *J Exp Med* 196:1091, 2002.
90. Inaba K, Turley S, Yamaide F, et al: Efficient presentation of phagocytosed cellular fragments on the MHC class II products of dendritic cells. *J Exp Med* 188:2163, 1998.
91. Jung S, Unutmaz D, Wong P, et al: *In vivo* depletion of $CD11c^{+}$ dendritic cells abrogation priming of $CD8^{+}$ T cells by exogenous cell-associated antigens. *Immunity* 17:211, 2002.
92. Wu DY, Segal NH, Sidobre S, et al: Cross-presentation of disialoganglioside GD3 to natural killer T cells. *J Exp Med* 198:173, 2003.
93. Shimizu K, Kurosawa Y, Taniguchi M, et al: Cross presentation of tumor cells loaded with -galactosylceramide leads to potent and long lived T cell mediated immunity via dendritic cells. *J Exp Med* 204:2641, 2007.
94. Kalergis AM, Ravetch JV: Inducing tumor immunity through the selective engagement of activating Fcγreceptors on dendritic cells. *J Exp Med* 195:1653, 2002.
95. Vincent MS, Gumperz JE, Brenner MB: Understanding the function of CD1-restricted T cells. *Nat Immunol* 4:517, 2003.
96. Fujii S, Liu K, Smith C, et al: The linkage of innate to adaptive immunity via maturing dendritic cells in vivo requires CD40, ligation in addition to antigen presentation and CD80/86, costimulation. *J Exp Med* 199:1607, 2004.
97. Schmid D, Munz C: Innate and adaptive immunity through autophagy. *Immunity* 27:11, 2007.
98. Schmid D, Pypaert M, Münz C: Antigen-loading compartments for major histocompatibility complex class II molecules continuously receive input from autophagosomes. *Immunity* 26:79, 2007.
99. Paludan C, Schmid D, Landthaler M, et al: Endogenous MHC class II processing of a viral nuclear antigen after autophagy. *Science* 307:593, 2005.
100. Schuler G, Steinman RM: Murine epidermal Langerhans cells mature into potent immunostimulatory dendritic cells in vitro. *J Exp Med* 161:526, 1985.
101. Romani N, Koide S, Crowley M, et al: Presentation of exogenous protein antigens by dendritic cells to T cell clones: intact protein is presented best by immature, epidermal Langerhans cells. *J Exp Med* 169:1169, 1989.
102. Trombetta ES, Ebersold M, Garrett W, et al: Activation of lysosomal function during dendritic cell maturation. *Science* 299:1400, 2003.
103. Inaba K, Turley S, Iyoda T, et al: The formation of immunogenic major histocompatibility complex class II-peptide ligands in lysosomal compartments of dendritic cells is regulated by inflammatory stimuli. *J Exp Med* 191:927, 2000.
104. Chow A, Toomre D, Garrett W, Mellman I: Dendritic cell maturation triggers retrograde transport of MHC class II transport from lysosomes to the plasma membrane. *Nature* 418:988, 2002.
105. Shin JS, Ebersold M, Pypaert M, et al: Surface expression of MHC class II in dendritic cells is controlled by regulated ubiquitination. *Nature* 444:115, 2006.
106. Morel S, Levy F, Burlet-Schiltz O, et al: Processing of some antigens by the standard proteasome but not by the immunoproteasome results in poor presentation by dendritic cells. *Immunity* 12:107, 2000.
107. Garrett WS, Chen LM, Kroschewski R, et al: Developmental control of endocytosis in dendritic cells by Cdc42. *Cell* 102:325, 2000.
108. Inaba K, Witmer-Pack M, Inaba M, et al: The tissue distribution of the B7–2, costimulator in mice: abundant expression on dendritic cells in situ and during maturation *in vitro*. *J Exp Med* 180:1849, 1994.
109. Zitvogel L: Dendritic and natural killer cells cooperate in the control/switch of innate immunity. *J Exp Med* 195:F9-F14, 2002.

110. Ferlazzo G, Tsang ML, Moretta L, et al: Human dendritic cells activate resting NK cells and are recognized via the NKp30, receptor by activated NK cells. *J Exp Med* 195:343, 2002.
111. Ferlazzo G, Münz C: NK cell compartments and their activation by dendritic cells. *J Immunol* 172:1333, 2004.
112. Inaba K, Steinman RM: Protein-specific helper T lymphocyte formation initiated by dendritic cells. *Science* 229:475, 1985.
113. Tezuka H, Abe Y, Iwata M, et al: Regulation of IgA production by naturally occurring TNF/iNOS-producing dendritic cells. *Nature* 448:929, 2007.
114. Fayette J, Dubois B, Vandenabelle S, et al: Human dendritic cells skew isotype switching of CD40-activated naive B cells towards IgA1, and IgA2. *J Exp Med* 185:1909, 1997.
115. Macpherson AJ, Uhr T: Induction of protective IgA by intestinal dendritic cells carrying commensal bacteria. *Science* 303:1662, 2004.
116. Jego G, Palucka AK, Blanck JP, et al: Plasmacytoid dendritic cells induce plasma cell differentiation through type I interferon and interleukin 6. *Immunity* 19:225, 2003.
117. Qu C, Nguyen VA, Merad M, Randolph GJ: MHC class I/peptide transfer between dendritic cells overcomes poor cross-presentation by monocyte-derived APCs that engulf dying cells. *J Immunol* 182:3650, 2009.
118. Jakubzick C, Bogunovic M, Bonito AJ, et al: Lymph-migrating, tissue-derived dendritic cells are minor constituents within steady-state lymph nodes. *J Exp Med* 205:2839, 2008.
119. Zal T, Volkmann A, Stockinger B: Mechanisms of tolerance induction in major histocompatibility complex class II-restricted T cells specific for a blood-borne self-antigen. *J Exp Med* 180:2089, 1994.
120. Kyewski B, Derbinski J, Gotter J, Klein L: Promiscuous gene expression and central T-cell tolerance: more than meets the eye. *Trends Immunol* 23:364, 2002.
121. Yamazaki S, Iyoda T, Tarbell K, et al: Direct expansion of functional $CD25^+$ $CD4^+$ regulatory T cells by antigen processing dendritic cells. *J Exp Med* 198:235, 2003.
122. Tarbell KV, Yamazaki S, Olson K, et al: $CD25^+$ $CD4^+$ T cells, expanded with dendritic cells presenting a single autoantigenic peptide, suppress autoimmune diabetes. *J Exp Med* 199:1467, 2004.
123. Coombes JL, Siddiqui KR, Arancibia-Carcamo CV, et al: A functionally specialized population of mucosal $CD103^+$ DCs induces $Foxp3^+$ regulatory T cells via a TGF-β- and retinoic acid-dependent mechanism. *J Exp Med* 204:1757, 2007.
124. Sun CM, Hall JA, Blank RB, et al: Small intestine lamina propria dendritic cells promote *de novo* generation of Foxp3, T reg cells via retinoic acid. *J Exp Med* 204:1775, 2007.
125. Dhodapkar MV, Krasovsky J, Osman K, Geller MD: Vigorous premalignancy-specific effector T cell response in the bone marrow of patients with monoclonal gammopathy. *J Exp Med* 198:1753, 2003.
126. Dhodapkar MV, Krasovsky J, Olson K: T cells from the tumor microenvironment of patients with progressive myeloma can generate strong, tumor-specific cytolytic responses to autologous, tumor-loaded dendritic cells. *Proc Natl Acad Sci U S A* 99:13009, 2002.
127. Dhodapkar KM, Krasovsky J, Williamson B, Dhodapkar MV: Anti-tumor monoclonal antibodies enhance cross-presentation of cellular antigens and the generation of myeloma-specific killer T cells by dendritic cells. *J Exp Med* 195:125, 2002.
128. Figdor CG, De Vries IJ, Lesterhuis WJ, Melief CJ: Dendritic cell immunotherapy: Mapping the way. *Nat Med* 10:475, 2004.
129. Melief CJ, van der Burg SH: Immunotherapy of established (pre)malignant disease by synthetic long peptide vaccines. *Nat Rev Cancer* 8:351, 2008.
130. Dhodapkar MV, Bhardwaj N: Active immunization of humans with dendritic cells. *J Clin Immunol* 20:167, 2000.
131. Dhodapkar MV, Krasovsky J, Steinman RM, Bhardwaj N: Mature dendritic cells boost functionally superior $CD8^+$ T-cell in humans without foreign helper epitopes. *J Clin Invest* 105:R9, 2000.
132. Hsu FJ, Benike C, Fagnoni F, et al: Vaccination of patients with B-cell lymphoma using autologous antigen-pulsed dendritic cells. *Nat Med* 2:52, 1996.
133. Nestle FO, Alijagic S, Gilliet M, et al: Vaccination of melanoma patients with peptide- or tumor lysate-pulsed dendritic cells. *Nat Med* 4:328, 1998.
134. Thurner B, Haendle I, Roder C, et al: Vaccination with mage-3A1, peptide-pulsed mature, monocyte-derived dendritic cells expands specific cytotoxic T cells and induces regression of some metastases in advanced stage IV melanoma. *J Exp Med* 190:1669, 1999.
135. Banchereau J, Palucka AK, Dhodapkar M, et al: Immune and clinical responses in patients with metastatic melanoma to $CD34^+$ progenitor-derived dendritic cell vaccine. *Cancer Res* 61:6451, 2001.
136. Dhodapkar MV, Steinman RM: Antigen-bearing, immature dendritic cells induce peptide-specific, $CD8^+$ regulatory T cells *in vivo* in humans. *Blood* 100:174, 2002.
137. Hawiger D, Masilamani RF, Bettelli E, et al: Immunological unresponsiveness characterized by increased expression of CD5, on peripheral T cells induced by dendritic cells *in vivo*. *Immunity* 20:695, 2004.
138. Trumpfheller C, Caskey M, Nchinda G, et al: The microbial mimic polyIC induces durable and protective $CD4^+$ T cell immunity together with a dendritic cell targeted vaccine. *Proc Natl Acad Sci U S A* 105:2574, 2008.
139. Merad M, Hoffmann P, Ranheim E, et al: Depletion of host Langerhans cells before transplantation of donor alloreactive T cells prevents skin graft-versus-host disease. *Nat Med* 10:510, 2004.

PART V

Therapeutic Principles

CHAPTER 20

PHARMACOLOGY AND TOXICITY OF ANTINEOPLASTIC DRUGS

Bruce A. Chabner, Jeffrey Barnes, James Cleary, Andrew Lane, Constantine Mitsiades, and Paul Richardson

SUMMARY

The safe and effective use of anticancer drugs in the treatment of hematologic malignancies requires an in-depth knowledge of the pharmacology of these agents. In this field of medicine, the margin of safety is narrow and the potential for serious toxicity is real. At the same time, anticancer drugs cure many hematologic malignancies and provide palliation for others. The discovery and development of treatments for leukemia and lymphoma have provided a paradigm for approaches to the improved treatment of the more common solid tumors.

The intelligent use of these drugs begins with an understanding of their mechanism of action. Most anticancer drugs inhibit the synthesis of DNA or directly attack its integrity through the formation of DNA adducts or enzyme-mediated breaks. These DNA-directed actions are recognized by repair processes and by the checkpoints that monitor DNA integrity, including most prominently p53. If DNA damage cannot be repaired, and if the DNA damage reaches thresholds for activating programmed cell death, then DNA damage is translated into tumor regression. Attention has turned to the possibility of identifying molecular targets unique to tumor cells, or dramatically overexpressed in those cells, including molecules involved in cell signaling and cell cycle control, but the principles of drug action and resistance to these compounds remain the same. Resistance to drug action can arise from alterations in any one of the critical steps required for drug activity; these steps include drug uptake and distribution through the bloodstream or across the blood–brain barrier; transport across the cell membrane; transformation of the parent drug to its active form within the tumor cell or in the liver; interaction of the drug with its target protein or nucleic acid; enzymatic or chemical inactivation of the agent; drug transport out of the cell; and elimination of the agent from the body through the kidneys or through metabolic transformation. The underlying mutability of tumors leads to the spontaneous generation of cells with alterations in drug uptake, transformation, inactivation, and target binding. In the presence of the selective pressure of a cytotoxic drug, drug-resistant tumors grow out as the dominant tumor population. Combination chemotherapy evades resistance that carries specificity for single agents, but the expression of multidrug resistance genes, as well as loss of the apoptotic response, can result in resistance even to combination drug therapy.

In addition to the molecular determinants of drug action, pharmacokinetics (the disposition of drugs in humans) plays a critical role in determining drug effectiveness and toxicity. Drug regimens are designed to achieve a maximally effective concentration in plasma and tumor cells for an effective duration of exposure. Because of the potential of these agents for toxicity, it is critical for oncologists to understand the pathways of drug clearance and to adjust dose in the presence of compromised organ function. Drugs such as methotrexate, hydroxyurea, and the newer purine antagonists (fludarabine and cladribine) are eliminated primarily by renal excretion and should not be used in full doses in patients with renal dysfunction. Similarly, hepatic dysfunction with elevated serum bilirubin concentrations should alert clinicians to decrease doses of the taxanes, vinca alkaloids, and (with less certainty) the anthracyclines. In addition, clinicians must be alert to the potential for drug interactions, particularly the ability of drugs that induce or inhibit cytochrome P450 3A4 and 2B6 to alter the metabolism of taxanes.

A growing body of knowledge indicates inherited genetic variations in drug-metabolizing enzymes may lead to differences in drug toxicity and response. The most important of these familial syndromes affecting treatment of leukemia is the deficiency of thiopurine methyltransferase, which slows the elimination of 6-mercaptopurine and leads to unanticipated toxicity during maintenance chemotherapy for acute lymphocytic leukemia. Pharmacokinetic monitoring has a standard role in the use of certain therapies, particularly high-dose methotrexate, and in the evaluation of new drugs or new drug combinations. Major cancer centers must have the capability of performing pharmacokinetic studies in conjunction with their clinical research programs.

To assure appropriate dose reduction, regimen choice, and management of toxicity, there is no substitute for therapy based on standard protocols and peer-reviewed clinical trials. Adherence to protocols ensures that the pharmacologic and pharmacogenetic variables affecting cancer chemotherapy can be recognized early in the course of treatment and that serious untoward events can be avoided while maintaining effective therapy.

Acronyms and abbreviations that appear in this chapter include: ABVD, Adriamycin (doxorubicin), bleomycin, vinblastine, and dacarbazine; ADCC, antibody-dependent cellular cytotoxicity; ALL, acute lymphocytic leukemia; AML, acute myelogenous leukemia; APL, acute promyelocytic leukemia; ara-C, cytarabine; ara-CTP, cytarabine triphosphate; ara-G, arabinosylguanine; ara-U, arabinosyluracil; ATRA, all-*trans*-retinoic acid; BCNU, bischloroethylnitrosourea; CLL, chronic lymphocytic leukemia; CML, chronic myelogenous leukemia; CYP, cytochrome P450; dCK, deoxycytidine kinase; DHFR, dihydrofolate reductase; HDAC, histone deacetylase; IC_{50}, inhibiting growth by concentration 50 percent; IL, interleukin; MDR, multidrug resistance; MP, mercaptopurine; MRP, multidrug resistance-associated protein; MTD, maximum tolerated dose; RARα, retinoic acid receptor-α; 6-TG, 6-thioguanine.

The leukemias and lymphomas have been the proving ground for cancer chemotherapy. Perhaps because of their rapid rates of proliferation, the lack of surgical treatment options, the ready access to malignant cells, and the availability of mouse models of leukemia, the hematologic malignancies drew the attention of early investigators interested in treating cancer with drugs. There was no surgical option for treating these patients, and most were not curable with radiation therapy. The first evidence for activity of a chemical antitumor agent came in 1942, from the experimental work and subsequent clinical trials conducted by Goodman, Gilman, and colleagues at Yale, and their observation that nitrogen mustard caused tumor regression in a patient with Hodgkin lymphoma.[1] Six years later, Sidney Farber, a pathologist at Children's Hospital in Boston, made the even more startling discovery of remission induction by aminopterin and then methotrexate in acute lymphocytic leukemia. His work ushered in the modern era of chemotherapy.[2] Over the next 20 years, clinical trials in these diseases established the basic principles of cyclic combination therapy and dose intensification,[3] developed effective strategies for management of infectious and hemorrhagic complications, and led to the cure of these diseases with chemotherapy. High-dose chemotherapy with marrow reconstitution has further extended the cure rate in leukemias and lymphomas. As our understanding of the biologic and molecular basis for malignancy has advanced, the concept of molecularly targeted therapy achieved its first striking success with the development of imatinib mesylate for chronic myelogenous leukemia.[4] Studies of relapsing patients on imatinib provided the first clear evidence for target mutation as a mechanism of clinical drug resistance.[5] The first effective use of a monoclonal antibody, Rituxan, has extended the cure rate for large cell lymphomas, and the first clear demonstration of drug-induced differentiation by all-*trans*-retinoic acid has led to a remarkable improvement in the cure rate of acute promyelocytic leukemia.[6] Other noncytotoxic drugs, such as arsenic trioxide, thalidomide, and bortezomib, with unusual mechanisms of action, have become valuable components of regimens for specific kinds of hematologic malignancies. It is likely that molecular studies of the abnormalities in pathways that control proliferation, survival, and migration of lymphomas and leukemias will reveal distinct subsets of disease, and will identify new targets for future therapies.

BASIC PRINCIPLES OF CANCER CHEMOTHERAPY

The safe and effective use of chemotherapy in clinical practice requires a thorough understanding of the basic aspects of drug action as well as knowledge of the important clinical toxicities, pharmacokinetics, and drug interactions of the various agents. Antineoplastic chemotherapy is a complex undertaking, with the potential for serious or fatal side effects. Patients are best served if their treatment is based on evidence from clinical trials which define optimal doses, schedules, and drug combinations. The specific protocol chosen for treatment should be appropriate not only for the stage and histology of the tumor but should consider individual patient comorbidities, age, and susceptibility to specific potential toxicities. Thus, bleomycin is usually not an appropriate choice for a patient with serious underlying renal or lung disease, nor is doxorubicin an appropriate drug for use in a patient with a history of congestive heart failure, and even in patients with normal cardiac or pulmonary function, total dose limits should be respected for these agents. While clinical trials define the benefit and risks of a cohort of patients of a defined age range and physiology, these results may not be easily extrapolated to patients at the extreme ends of the spectrum. Depending on the major route of drug clearance, doses should be modified for renal or hepatic dysfunction (Table 20–1). In patients with extreme obesity (body mass index >30), drug clearance does not increase in proportion to the increase in body mass, and doses are usually capped at no more than 75 percent of a dose based on body surface area.

Changes in the dose and schedule of a drug offer potentially greater antitumor effects, but often lead to unique toxicities. With marrow or blood stem cell storage and reinfusion, potentially lethal doses of chemotherapy can be administered in an attempt to cure malignancies refractory to standard chemotherapy. In general, these regimens may produce organ toxicities not seen at conventional doses—including pneumonitis, cardiac failure, vascular endothelial damage, and hepatic and renal insufficiency—and are ordinarily reserved for patients of younger age and with normal baseline organ function (see Chap. 21).

The success of chemotherapy in curing hematologic malignancy is incompletely understood. Although targeted therapies exploit clear differences in biology conferred by mutations or amplification of key genes, an explanation for the differential effects of cytotoxic drugs on tumor versus normal tissues is less obvious. The greater susceptibility of malignant cells to drug toxicity, as reflected in the phenomenon of leukemia remission induction, with restoration of normal marrow function, may result from the relative resistance of normal marrow stem cells to drug injury. These stem cells exist in a nonreplicating phase of the cell cycle, where they are less susceptible to damage by DNA-directed agents, and they express genes that protect against chemical and hypoxic damage. In addition, there is growing evidence that cancer cells lack cell-cycle checkpoints that recognize DNA damage and activate repair of DNA strand breaks, base deletions, or other lesions induced by chemotherapy. This differential in repair capability may allow normal cells to repair damage and recovery from chemotherapy-induced injury.

TABLE 20–1. Dose Modification in Patients with Renal or Hepatic Dysfunction

Renal dysfunction (creatinine clearance <60 mL/min)

Reduce dose in proportion to reduction in creatinine clearance.

Drugs

1. Methotrexate
2. Cisplatin
3. Carboplatin
4. Bleomycin
5. Etoposide
6. Hydroxyurea
7. Deoxycoformycin
8. Fludarabine phosphate
9. Cladribine
10. Topotecan
11. Gleevec
12. Dasatinib (likely, but no guidelines available)
13. Lenalidomide

Hepatic dysfunction

For bilirubin >1.5 mg/dL reduce initial dose by 50%.

For bilirubin >3.0 mg/dL reduce initial dose by 75%.

Drugs

1. Amsacrine
2. Doxorubicin
3. Daunorubicin
4. Vincristine
5. Vinblastine
6. Paclitaxel and docetaxel
7. Mitoxantrone
8. Gleevec
9. Dasatinib

COMBINATION CHEMOTHERAPY

Most leukemias and lymphomas are highly drug sensitive, but, with the exception of the curability of Burkitt lymphoma (treated with cyclophosphamide) and hairy cell leukemia (treated with cladribine), are rarely, if ever, cured with single-agent chemotherapy. Combination chemotherapy forestalls the emergence of drug-resistant cells and thus is curative in settings where individual agents are ineffective. Empirical principles have resulted from the clinical experience of the past four decades of combination therapy. In general, drugs selected for combination therapy should have demonstrable antineoplastic activity, or at least biologic effects, against the tumor in question. The lone exception may be targeted drugs that inhibit signal transduction or angiogenesis; these drugs may exhibit limited antitumor activity on their own, but may significantly augment the action of cytotoxic agents.[7] Individual agents in a combination should have different mechanisms of action and should not share a common mechanism of resistance such as multidrug resistance (MDR). The dose-limiting toxicities of the agents chosen should not overlap; otherwise, they could not be used together at or near full doses. The clinical use of specific combinations should be based on preclinical evidence of synergistic interaction. Favorable molecular or biochemical drug interactions may be dependent on specific sequences and schedules of administration. Pharmacokinetic interactions should be defined in initial trials of drug combinations so as to avoid under- or overdosing of individual agents.

Another important consideration in designing clinical protocols is dose intensity, the dose administered per unit time, which should be maintained throughout a treatment regimen. Achieving this objective may require the use of hematopoietic growth factors to hasten marrow recovery, prevent repeated episodes of febrile neutropenia, and allow on-time administration of the next treatment cycle.

Interdigitation of chemotherapy with surgery and irradiation makes it possible to take advantage of favorable cytokinetic or radiosensitizing effects of chemotherapy, while avoiding enhancement of toxicity. Thus, 5-fluorouracil and cisplatin are potent radiosensitizers used with radiation therapy to enhance local tumor control in malignancies of the head and neck,[8] esophagus,[9] rectum,[10] and anus.[11] Surgical reduction of tumor bulk increases the response rate of ovarian tumors to chemotherapy, perhaps by eliminating poorly perfused tumor masses.[12] In the treatment of lymphomas, the toxicity of radiation therapy to sensitive organs such as skin, lung, heart, and brain may be significantly increased by concurrent administration of anthracyclines, a consideration that has prompted the use of radiation therapy either before or after anthracycline antibiotics, but not concurrently. Likewise, bleomycin sensitizes the lungs to damage by high inspired O_2 during surgery. Antiangiogenic therapies are associated with an increased risk of bowel perforation in patients who have recently undergone intraabdominal surgery.

■ CELL KINETICS AND CANCER CHEMOTHERAPY

The cell-killing characteristics of cancer chemotherapeutic agents vary according to their mechanism of action. Many of the most effective agents in antileukemic therapy belong to the antimetabolite class, including cytosine arabinoside and methotrexate. These drugs kill cells most effectively during the DNA-synthetic phase (S phase) of the cell cycle. For these agents, a prolonged period of tumor exposure to drug is essential so as to maximize the number of cells exposed during the vulnerable period of the cell cycle. As would be predicted, the antimetabolite drugs are primarily active against rapidly dividing tumors such as acute leukemias and intermediate and high-grade lymphomas. Other anticancer drugs, such as the topoisomerase inhibitors and alkylating agents, do not require cells to be exposed during a specific phase of the cell cycle, although like the antimetabolites, these drugs are generally more effective against actively proliferating cells as compared to resting cells. Still others, most notably the nitrosoureas and busulfan, are equally toxic to dividing and nondividing cells, and at the same time, deplete marrow stem cells. In general, the toxicity of alkylating agents is determined by the total dose of drug, whereas for the cell-cycle-specific drugs (such as methotrexate and cytosine arabinoside), both drug concentration and duration of exposure determine cytocidal effect. However, for drugs that act through alternate mechanisms, such as the taxanes, myelosuppression correlates best with the duration of exposure above a threshold plasma concentration, which is approximately 50 to 100 nM for paclitaxel and 200 nM for docetaxel.[13]

High-dose regimens achieve a number of worthwhile objectives for these agents, including an enhancement of cross-membrane transport, saturation of anabolic pathways inside the cell, and prolongation of the period of effective drug concentration. However, achieving these objectives is realized at the cost of increased toxicity to normal proliferating marrow precursor cells and may produce significant and unexpected damage to normal organs, such as hepatic venoocclusive disease (alkylating agents), cerebellar toxicity (cytosine arabinoside), or pulmonary toxicity (nitrosoureas and alkylating agents). Because hematopoietic stem cells can be harvested, stored, and reinfused, dose-limiting toxicities of high-dose chemotherapy are generally those affecting nonhematologic organs.

The choice of an appropriate dose and schedule of drug administration depends on a number of factors: (1) the drug's cell-cycle dependence; (2) the often empirically derived relationship between antitumor effects, drug dose, and schedule; (3) pharmacokinetic behavior and the need to maintain a specific drug concentration for a given period of time; (4) potential interactions with other components of the treatment regimen; and (5) patient tolerance. Clinical trials, often empirical in their design, provide the necessary information.

■ DRUG RESISTANCE

Inadequate treatment of a sensitive tumor tends to select for the outgrowth of drug-resistant clones of the original tumor. The reasons for emergence of drug resistance are manifold. Cancer cells often harbor basic defects in DNA repair as one of their hallmark mutations and spontaneously generate drug resistant mutants, even in the absence of drug exposure. Thus it has been demonstrated in the specific example of imatinib treatment of chronic myelogenous leukemia (CML) that drug-resistant cells, carrying specific mutations in the *BCR-ABL* gene, can be identified in marrow prior to treatment and are subsequently selected by exposure to drug.[5] A similar finding of pretreatment mutations explains drug resistance to inhibitors to the epidermal growth factor receptor in non–small-cell lung cancer.[14] In addition, many cancer drugs, especially alkylating agents, and irradiation are mutagenic and increase the rate of generation of drug-resistant mutants. To discourage the outgrowth of resistant cells, multiple agents with differing mechanisms of resistance should be used simultaneously, because the likelihood of there being a doubly or triply resistant cell is the product of the probabilities of the independent drug-resistant mutations occurring at the same time in a single cell. The probability of a cell division resulting in mutation at any given genetic locus is approximately 10^{-6} for somatic cells; thus the probability of multiple independent mutations arising in the same cell is 10^{-12} or lower. Mutation rates may be distinctly higher in tumor cells and may be further increased by exposure to alkylating agents and irradiation. Some mutations, such as those affecting apoptosis, may confer resistance to diverse agents. Thus, the probability of encountering MDR cells is much higher in reality.

In choosing drugs for combination therapy, one must bear in mind potential mechanisms of resistance. Classical MDR occurs as a consequence, of increased expression of drug efflux pumps such as the P-glycoprotein or the multidrug resistance-associated proteins (MRPs)[15,16] and confers resistance to a broad spectrum of agents derived from natural products, including taxanes, anthracyclines, vinca alkaloids, and epipodophyllotoxins. Other mechanisms of resistance that induce amplification of a target gene, such as dihydrofolate reductase[17] or *BCR-ABL* kinase,[18] may be highly specific for a single drug. Table 20–2 lists the common mechanisms of resistance. Although none of these biochemical changes are routinely measured either prior to or following therapy, these mechanisms should be considered in developing new protocols and in choosing new therapy for patients who relapse from primary treatment.

In addition to drug-specific mechanisms of resistance, mutations that abolish recognition of DNA damage, such as the loss of components of the mismatch repair gene complex,[19] seem to block initiation of apoptosis by cisplatin, thiopurines, or alkylating agents. Other mutations that block the induction of apoptosis, such as loss of p53[20] or overexpression

TABLE 20–2. Mechanisms of Resistance to Anticancer Drugs

Mechanisms	Drugs Affected	Clinical Role
1. Decreased drug uptake		
Reduced folate transporter	Methotrexate	ALL
Nucleoside transporter	Cytosine arabinoside	AML
2. Increased drug efflux		
MDR transporter (P-glycoprotein)	Anthracyclines, vinca alkaloids, taxanes, etoposide	Myeloma, AML, non-Hodgkin lymphoma
MRP transporters, breast cancer-resistant protein	Anthracyclines, vinca alkaloids, taxanes, etoposide	Breast cancer
3. Decreased drug activation in tumor		
Deoxycytidine kinase deletion	Cytarabine, fludarabine, cladribine, clofarabine	AML, CLL, hairy cell leukemia
Hypoxanthine phosphoribosyltransferase deletion	6-Mercaptopurine	Uncertain
Folylpolyglutamation	Methotrexate	Acute leukemias
4. Increased drug inactivation		
Thiopurine methyltransferase	6-Mercaptopurine	ALL
Bleomycin hydrolase	Bleomycin	Uncertain
Glutathione transferase	Alkylating agents	Uncertain
5. Decreased target enzyme		
Topoisomerase I	Camptothecins	Uncertain
Topoisomerase II	Anthracyclines, etoposide	Uncertain
6. Increased target enzyme		
Dihydrofolate reductase	Methotrexate	Acute leukemia, small-cell lung cancer
Thymidylate synthase	5-Fluorouracil	Solid tumors
Adenosine deaminase	Deoxycoformycin	Uncertain
7. Mutated intracellular target		
BCR-ABL kinase	Imatinib mesylate, dasatinib	CML
Tubulin	Vinca alkaloids, taxanes	Uncertain
Topoisomerase I	Camptothecins	Uncertain
Topoisomerase II	Anthracyclines, etoposide	Uncertain
8. Increase DNA repair		
Guanine-0-6-methyltransferase	Procarbazine, nitrosoureas temozolomide	Brain tumors
Nucleotide excision repair	Platinating drugs	Ovarian cancer
9. Decreased DNA damage recognition		
p53 mutation	Many cancer drugs, radiation	Leukemias, lymphomas
Mismatch DNA repair mutations	Platinating agents, methylating drugs, thiopurines	Colon cancer, glioblastoma, leukemias

ALL, acute lymphocytic leukemia; AML, acute myelogenous leukemia; CML, chronic myelogenous leukemia. See text for references and explanation.

of the antiapoptotic factors such as BCL-2,[21] may render tumor cells insensitive to a broad array of drugs and modalities, including ionizing irradiation, alkylating agents, antimetabolites, and anthracyclines. Although the specific contribution of p53 mutation and altered apoptosis to clinical resistance is still uncertain, emerging evidence suggests that these factors are commonly associated with clinical resistance and aggressive tumor growth and may be more relevant causes of drug resistance in the clinic than are the classical drug-specific mechanisms found in experimental tumors.

The contribution of tumor stem cells to treatment resistance and disease recurrence is an intriguing, but as yet undefined, possibility. It is clear that many tissues, including marrow, contain stem cells capable of repopulating organs, even from single cells.[22] Likewise, many tumors contain stem cells, which, on careful evaluation, preserve many of the surface antigens of their normal counterpart, and display resistance to DNA damage, irradiation, and natural products.[23] It is possible, but still to be established, that these drug-resistant stem cells represent the ultimate barrier to successful cancer treatment.

CELL-CYCLE-SPECIFIC AGENTS

■ METHOTREXATE

Farber and associates showed that the folate antagonist aminopterin induced a complete remission in children with acute lymphoblastic leukemia (ALL), thereby launching the modern era of chemotherapy. Unfortunately, these remissions were short-lived, and the leukemia invariably became resistant within months to further treatment. Subsequently, methotrexate, a 4-amino, N-10 methyl analogue of folic acid, supplanted aminopterin because it had a better therapeutic index. Methotrexate continues to be a key drug in the induction and maintenance therapy of ALL, in the intrathecal prophylaxis and treatment of central nervous system (CNS) leukemia, in the primary treatment of CNS lymphomas, and in combination therapy of intermediate- and high-grade lymphomas.

Mechanisms of Action

Methotrexate enters cells through an active uptake process mediated in most tumor cells by the reduced folate transporter[24] and is actively effluxed from cells by the MRP class of exporters.[25] A second uptake transporter, the membrane folate-binding protein, has lower affinity for methotrexate, but may contribute to uptake of other antifolates. A third, low pH transporter may also participate in methotrexate influx, but its role is uncertain.[26] By virtue of its 4-amino substitution, methotrexate potently inhibits the enzyme dihydrofolate reductase (DHFR), which recycles oxidized dihydrofolate to its active tetrahydrofolate state. Inhibition of DHFR leads to rapid depletion of the intracellular tetrahydrofolate coenzymes required for thymidylate and purine biosynthesis (see Chap. 41). As a result, DNA synthesis is blocked and cell replication stops. Methotrexate is retained in tumor cells for many hours as a

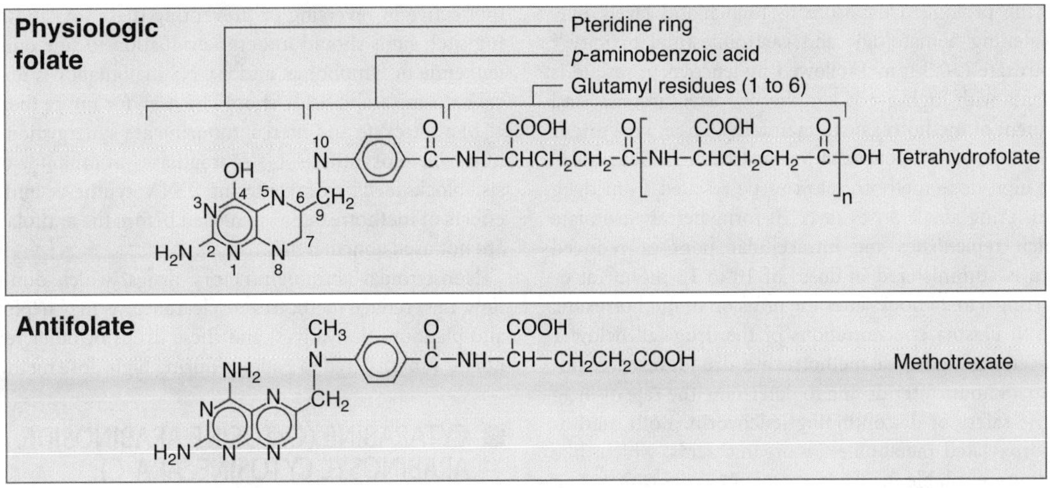

FIGURE 20–1. Structures of folate, tetrahydrofolate, and its analogue methotrexate. The vitamin is absorbed as a monoglutamate and converted intracellularly to a polyglutamate, in which form it is both physiologically active and is stored in cells. Methotrexate, the 2,4-diamino analogue of folic acid, is shown in the bottom panel and is also converted to a polyglutamate intracellularly. *(Reproduced from Brunton L, Lazo J, Parker K:* Goodman & Gilman's The Pharmacological Basis of Therapeutics, *11th ed, chap 51. McGraw-Hill, New York, 2006. With permission from the publisher.)*

consequence of an enzymatic process that adds up to six glutamate moieties in an unusual peptide linkage to the γ-carboxyl group of the drug (Fig. 20–1). Polyglutamation is an important determinant of methotrexate selectivity. Methotrexate polyglutamates, in addition to their long persistence in cells and their potent inhibition of DHFR, have greatly increased inhibitory effects on other folate-dependent enzymes, including thymidylate synthase and enzymes that synthesize purines (Fig. 20–2). Cells that convert the drug to polyglutamates efficiently, such as leukemic myeloblasts and lymphoblasts, are more susceptible to the drug than are normal myeloid precursors, which have limited capability for polyglutamation.[27] Accumulation of polyglutamates correlates with increased cytotoxicity and treatment response in childhood lymphoblastic leukemia.[28] Hyperdiploid ALLs are particularly efficient in transporting methotrexate and in producing polyglutamated species, factors that may contribute to their favorable prognosis.[29] Polyglutamates are slowly degraded to their readily effluxed monoglutamate form by γ-glutamyl hydrolase, and a polymorphism (T127I) that deceases γ-glutamyl hydrolase activity is associated with enhanced polyglutamate accumulation in leukemic cells.[30] Acquired resistance to methotrexate in patients with leukemia is associated with increased levels of dihydrofolate reductase as a consequence of gene amplification,[17] defective polyglutamation,[31] and impaired drug uptake,[32] or increased efflux by the MRP class of transporters.[33]

Clinical Pharmacology

Methotrexate is well absorbed when administered orally at low doses (5–10 mg/m^2), but when doses exceed 30 mg/m^2, absorption is variable. Consequently, doses greater than 25 mg/m^2 should be administered parenterally.

The concentration of methotrexate in plasma declines in a polyexponential manner. A very rapid initial disposition phase persists for only a few minutes after intravenous administration. The intermediate disposition phase has a 2- to 3-hour half-life and persists for 12 to 24 hours after dosing. The terminal phase of drug decay is considerably slower, with an 8- to 10-hour half-life, and this phase becomes important in determining drug toxicity and the effectiveness of leucovorin rescue in patients treated with high-dose methotrexate. Methotrexate is primarily excreted unchanged by the kidney, although a minor fraction of the drug (7–30%) is inactivated by hepatic hydroxylation at the 7 position. Thus, patients with renal impairment should not be treated with meth-

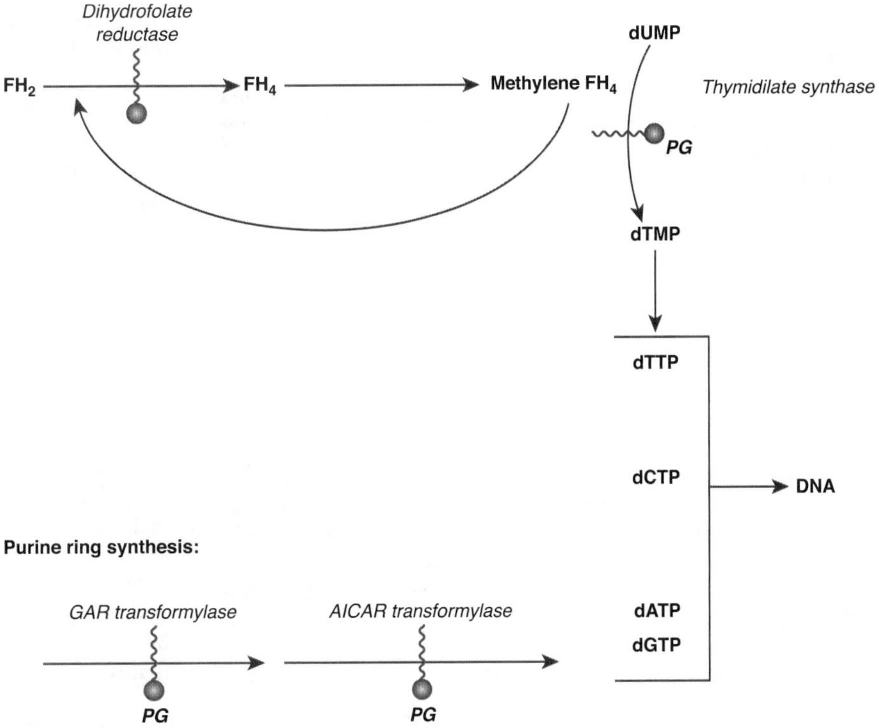

FIGURE 20–2. Mechanism of methotrexate action. Sites of enzyme inhibition by methotrexate (~~●) and its polyglutamates (*PG* ●~~). AICAR, aminoimidazole-carboxamide ribonucleotide; dUMP, deoxyuridine monophosphate; FH_2, dihydrofolate; FH_4, tetrahydrofolate; GAR, glycine amide ribonucleotide.

otrexate, because the prolonged exposure to high blood levels may result in life-threatening hematologic and gastrointestinal toxicity.[34] High-dose methotrexate (>0.5 g/m^2) followed by leucovorin rescue is used to treat patients with high-grade lymphoma, osteosarcoma, and ALL. Dose adjustment of methotrexate to maintain a target area under the concentration × time (C × T) curve improves treatment outcome.[35] Patients receiving high-dose methotrexate can be rescued from drug toxicity by administering small doses of *N*-10-formyltetrahydrofolate (leucovorin), which replenishes the intracellular pool of reduced folates. Leucovorin is administered in doses of 10 to 15 mg/m^2 at 6-hour intervals, starting 6 to 24 hours after the infusion of methotrexate, and continuing until plasma concentrations of the drug fall below 1 μM. In patients receiving high-dose methotrexate, drug levels are routinely assayed 24 to 48 hours after dosing to determine the rate of drug elimination and the safety of discontinuing leucovorin. Both methotrexate and its hydroxylated metabolite are organic acids, which, like uric acid, are much more soluble in alkaline urine. In patients receiving such therapy, renal toxicity may result from intrarenal precipitation of the parent drug or its 7-OH metabolite, and is generally the cause of decreased drug clearance. Renal dysfunction can be prevented by alkalinizing the urine to pH 7 with intravenous sodium bicarbonate prior to and during therapy, and patients should be given intensive hydration, as well. If drug concentrations in plasma exceed 1 μM at 48 hours after high-dose therapy, leucovorin should be continued at higher doses of 50 to 100 mg/m^2 every 6 hours until methotrexate concentrations fall below 0.1 μM. The higher doses of leucovorin are necessary to compete with methotrexate for transport and polyglutamation. In cases of extreme renal failure, with stable drug levels in the 10 μM range, leucovorin will not be effective. In this setting, continuous flow hemodialysis may provide a sustained reduction in drug levels.[36] An alternative effective measure in this circumstance is the administration of carboxypeptidase G, a bacterial enzyme that degrades antifolates.[37] (The enzyme can be obtained from the Cancer Therapy Evaluation Program of the National Cancer Institute [301–496–6138] and may be lifesaving.)

Adverse Effects

The dose-limiting toxicities of methotrexate are myelosuppression and gastrointestinal toxicity. Toxic doses of methotrexate can induce thrombocytopenia and/or leukopenia, although leukopenia is more common. An early indication of methotrexate toxicity to the gastrointestinal tract is oral mucositis, whereas more severe toxicity may be manifested as diarrhea and gastrointestinal bleeding. Less common toxic effects of methotrexate are skin rash (10%), pneumonitis, and chemical hepatitis. Transaminase elevations are frequently seen after high-dose methotrexate but rapidly return to normal in most patients, and without sequelae, but low-dose chronic administration, as routinely employed to treat psoriasis or rheumatoid arthritis, may lead to portal fibrosis and cirrhosis in a small percentage of patients.

Methotrexate, given intrathecally in doses of 12 mg every 4 days for children older than age 3 years and for adults, is used to prevent or treat meningeal leukemia and lymphoma. Dose adjustment is required for children younger than age 3 years, and should be made according to established protocols. Because the drug distributes poorly into the ventricular system after spinal injection, patients with active meningeal leukemia are frequently treated through an indwelling ventricular reservoir. Toxicities caused by intrathecal administration of methotrexate include acute arachnoiditis with nuchal rigidity and headache, as well as more chronic CNS toxicities, such as dementia, motor deficits, seizures, and coma.[38] Rarely, these neurotoxicities develop hours after intrathecal drug administration, but more commonly they occur in the days or weeks after initiation of intrathecal treatment, and are most often seen in patients with active meningeal leukemia. Leucovorin is ineffective in reversing or preventing these toxicities. Patients exhibiting such signs should undergo evaluation to rule out progressive CNS leukemia or lymphoma, and if CNS malignancy is not found, intrathecal cytosine arabinoside should be used for future therapy.

Methotrexate and mercaptopurine are synergistic in their inhibition of purine biosynthesis. L-Asparaginase, an inhibitor of protein synthesis, blocks cells from entering DNA synthesis and antagonizes the effects of methotrexate, when used before the antifolate. The two drugs are not used concurrently.

Nonsteroidal antiinflammatory drugs, which diminish renal blood flow, may reduce methotrexate clearance, as may nephrotoxic antibiotics and platinum derivatives, and these drugs or other renal toxins should not be administered to patients during high-dose methotrexate therapy.

■ CYTARABINE (CYTOSINE ARABINOSIDE, ARABINOSYL CYTOSINE, ARA-C)

Cytarabine is an antimetabolite analogue of cytidine, differing in the configuration at the substituent on C_2' position of the sugar, in which the C_2'-hydroxyl group is *cis*-oriented relative to the C_1'-*N*-glycosyl bond, in contrast to the *trans* configuration of the ribose nucleoside. Cytarabine is a mainstay in the induction of remission in patients with acute myelogenous leukemia (AML).

High doses (1–3 g/m^2) of cytarabine given at 12-hour intervals for 6 to 12 doses are more effective alone or in a combination with anthracyclines than conventional doses (100–150 mg/m^2 q12h) in consolidation therapy of AML, and they confer particular benefit in patients with cytogenetic abnormalities [t(8:21), inv[16], t(9:16), and del(16)] related to the core binding factor that regulates hematopoiesis.[39] Other subsets of leukemia may have increased sensitivity to ara-C. ALL patients with MLL gene translocations have upregulation of the hENT nucleoside transporter and have a greater sensitivity to ara-C.[40] AML patients with RAS mutations seem to derive greater benefit from high dose ara-C than do patients with wild-type RAS in their tumors.[41] Cytarabine has also been used to treat ALL, lymphoma, and both the chronic and the blast phases of CML, but its exact role in the treatment of these malignancies is less well defined.

Mechanism of Action

Cytarabine is converted to the nucleoside triphosphate (ara-CTP) intracellularly. The first step is catalyzed by deoxycytidine kinase; polymorphisms of the CdK gene may affect the rate of activation, and ultimately response.[42] Ara-CTP is an inhibitor of DNA polymerase and is also incorporated into DNA, where it terminates strand elongation.[43] If repair is unsuccessful, apoptosis is initiated. Cytarabine and its mononucleotide are deaminated and inactivated by two intracellular enzymes, cytidine deaminase and deoxycytidylate deaminase, respectively. The arabinosyluracil (ara-U) formed as a consequence of cytarabine deamination clears more slowly from plasma than does cytarabine and may inhibit subsequent inactivation of cytarabine in high-dose regimens.

Acquired cytarabine resistance in experimental leukemias consistently results from the loss of deoxycytidine kinase.[44] Other changes implicated in experimental tumors include decreased drug uptake because of decreased expression of the equilibrative nucleoside transporter, increased deamination, increased pool size of competitive deoxycytidine triphosphate, and inhibition of the apoptotic pathway. Some of these changes have been reported in studies of human leukemia, but these results have not been confirmed in definitive trials.[45]

Clinical Pharmacology

Cytarabine is administered intravenously either as a bolus injection or a continuous infusion. It is not orally bioavailable because of its degradation by cytidine deaminase, which is present in the gastrointestinal epithelium and liver. Two standard schedules of ara-C administration are used: (1) rapid infusion of 100 mg/m^2 every 12 hours for 7 days; or (2) continuous infusion of 100 to 200 mg/m^2 per day for 5 to 7 days. Cytarabine distributes rapidly throughout total-body water and is eliminated from plasma with a biologic half-life of 7 to 20 minutes. Most of the dose is excreted as ara-U, an inactive metabolite, which is formed in plasma, the liver, granulocytes, and other tissues. Inhibition of cytarabine deamination by ara-U may be responsible for the prolongation of the biologic half-life of the drug as larger doses are administered.[46] Single-bolus injections and short infusions (30 minutes to 1 hour duration) at doses as high as 5 g/m^2 produce little myelotoxicity because of the drug's rapid clearance, whereas continuous intravenous infusion of only 1 g/m^2 over 48 hours produces severe marrow toxicity. Unlike most drugs, a relatively high concentration of cytarabine is achieved in the cerebrospinal fluid after intravenous administration, and may approach 50 percent of the corresponding concentration in plasma.

Cytarabine is also used intrathecally to treat meningeal leukemia. Doses of 50 to 70 mg in adults are usually employed and afford cerebrospinal fluid levels of the drug near 1 mM, which decline with a half-life of 2 hours. Cytarabine (50 mg given every 2 weeks) has been impregnated into a gel matrix, in a formulation called DepoCyt, for sustained release into the cerebrospinal fluid, thus avoiding the need for repeated spinal taps. Initial clinical results in spinal lymphomatous meningitis indicate that it has efficacy equal to that of methotrexate.[47]

Adverse Effects

The dose-limiting toxicity for conventional dosing regimens of cytarabine, 100 to 150 mg/m^2 per day for 5 to 10 days, is myelosuppression. Nausea and vomiting also occur at these doses, the severity of which increases markedly when higher doses are employed, although repeated administration of the drug results in some tolerance. The nadir of the white count and platelet count occurs at about days 7 to 10 after the last dose of drug. Neurologic, gastrointestinal, and liver toxicity have also been observed when high-dose regimens are used. Hepatotoxicity ranges from abnormalities in serum transaminase levels to frank jaundice. The severity of these effects increases as the duration of therapy is prolonged; however, toxic effects rapidly subside upon discontinuation of treatment. Pulmonary infiltrates as a result of noncardiogenic pulmonary edema, and occasionally associated with severe pulmonary dysfunction, occur in leukemic patients receiving cytarabine, as do gastrointestinal ulcerations with bleeding and infrequently perforation. Cytarabine treatment is also reported to predispose to *Streptococcus viridans* pneumonia.[48]

In patients older than 60 years of age, high-dose cytarabine (3 g/m^2 every 12 hours for six doses) causes cerebellar toxicity, manifested as ataxia and slurred speech.[49] Confusion and dementia may supervene, leading to a fatal outcome. Cerebellar toxicity is more frequent in patients with abnormal renal function because of slowed elimination of ara-U, with consequent inhibition of cytarabine deamination. Intrathecal cytarabine is usually well tolerated, but neurologic side effects have been reported (seizures, alterations in mental status).

GEMCITABINE

Although primarily used for solid tumors, gemcitabine, a 2′-2′-difluoro analogue of deoxycytidine, has significant activity against Hodgkin lymphoma. Its mechanism of action is similar to cytarabine, in that, as a nucleotide, it competes with deoxycytidine triphosphate for incorporation into the elongating DNA strand, where it terminates DNA synthesis. It is also self-potentiating in that at a second site of action, it reduces competitive pools of deoxycytidine triphosphate through inhibition of ribonucleotide reductase. It achieves higher nucleotide levels in tumor cells than does ara-CTP, and has a longer intracellular half-life. Its clinical pharmacokinetics are determined primarily by its rapid deamination by cytidine deaminase, yielding a short plasma half-life ($t_{1/2}$) of 15 minutes. Standard schedules use 1000 mg/m^2 infused over 30 minutes, and produced peak drug concentrations of 20–60 μM in plasma. Longer infusion times may produce higher intracellular triphosphate concentrations, but the benefit is uncertain.[50]

Resistance in solid tumors arises from low expression of the influx transporter hENT, increased expression of ribonucleotide reductase, and low levels of the initial activating enzyme, deoxycytidine kinase. Gemcitabine is an extremely potent radiosensitizer and should not be used concurrently with radiation therapy except in clinical trials.

Toxicities are mainly acute myelosuppression, mild hepatic enzyme elevations, uncommonly a reversible pneumonitis, and with prolonged usage, a progressive hemolytic uremic syndrome with capillary leak, leading to pleural effusions, ascites, and renal failure.[51]

5-AZACYTIDINE AND 5-AZA-2′-DEOXYCYTIDINE

Both 5-azacytidine and decitabine (5-aza-2′-deoxycytidine), its closely related deoxy analogue, exhibit cytotoxic activity and also induce differentiation of malignant cells at low doses. The latter action results from their incorporation into DNA and their covalent inactivation of DNA methyltransferase. The resulting inhibition of methylation of cytosine bases in DNA leads to enhanced transcription of otherwise silent genes.[52] The differentiating effects of 5-azacytidine are the basis for the induction of fetal hemoglobin synthesis in patients with sickle cell anemia and thalassemia[53] and its approved use in low-dose therapy of myelodysplastic syndromes. The usual doses of 5-azacytidine are 75 mg/m^2 per day for 7 days, repeated every 28 days, whereas decitabine is used in doses of 20 mg intravenously every day for 5 days every 4 weeks. Responses become apparent in myelodysplasia after two to five courses.

5-Azacytidine and decitabine are rapidly deaminated and converted to a chemically unstable metabolite that immediately degrades into inactive products. Pharmacologic activity results from phosphorylation of the parent compound by cytidine kinase (for 5-azacytidine) or deoxycytidine kinase (for decitabine), with subsequent conversion to a triphosphate nucleotide that becomes incorporated into RNA and DNA. The primary clinical toxicities of both 5-azacytidine and decitabine[54] include reversible myelosuppression, nausea and vomiting with higher doses, hepatic dysfunction, myalgia, and fever and rash. Resistance likely results from defects in drug activation or alternative mechanisms for gene silencing, such as histone methylation or acetylation.

PURINE ANALOGUES

Purine analogues (Fig. 20–3) have won an important role in remission induction and maintenance for ALL, and in the past decade new analogues have shown remarkable activity in chronic leukemias and small cell lymphomas. With methotrexate, 6-mercaptopurine (6-MP) is a critical component in the maintenance phase of curative therapy of childhood ALL. Other clinically useful purine analogues include azathioprine, a 6-MP precursor and potent immunosuppressive agent; allopurinol, an inhibitor of xanthine oxidase, useful in the prevention of uric acid nephropathy; 2-chlorodeoxyadenosine, effective in the treatment of hairy cell leukemia and other lymphoid malignancies; 6-thioguanine (6-TG), an antileukemic agent; and fludarabine phosphate (2-fluoroara-adenosine monophosphate), an effective agent for chronic lymphocytic leukemia and follicular lymphomas, and for suppression of graft-versus-host disease in transplantation. A new purine analogue, nelarabine, is an ara-guanine prodrug, with strong activity against T-cell diseases, includ-

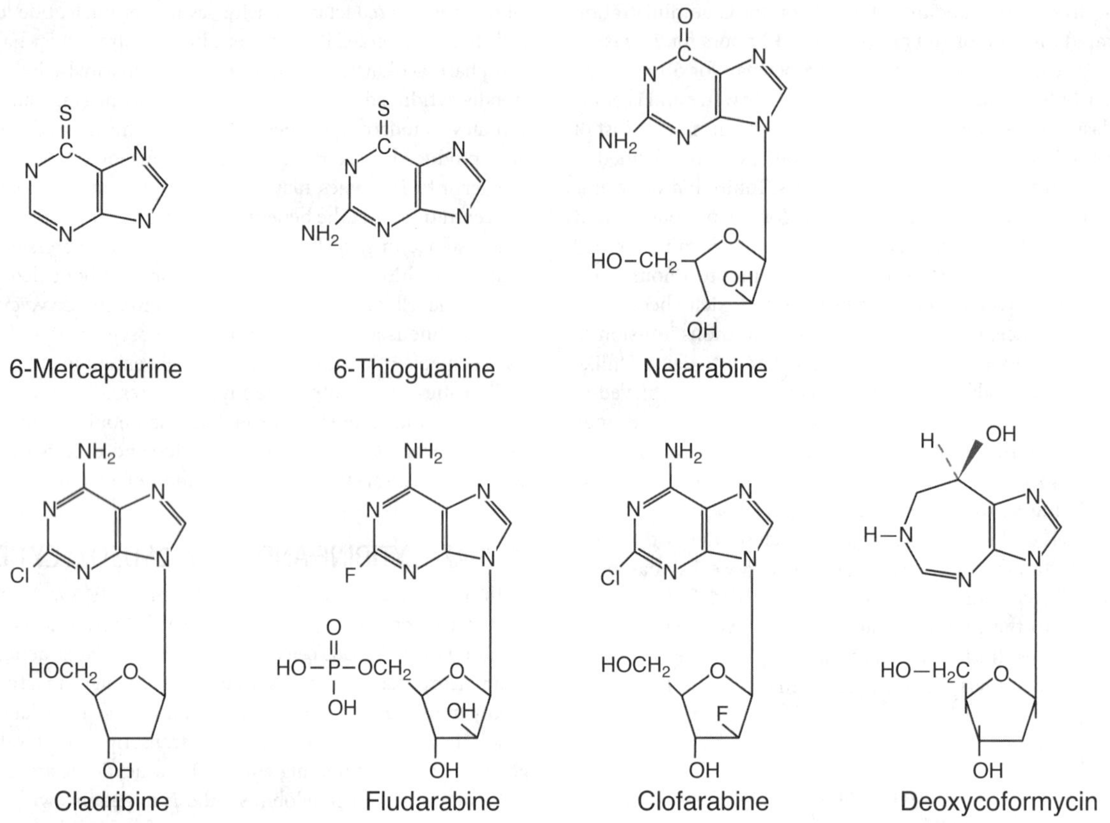

FIGURE 20–3. Purine analogues.

ing lymphoblastic leukemias and lymphomas.[55] The basis for this T-cell sensitivity appears to be the resistance of arabinosylguanine (ara-G) to degradation by the catabolic enzyme, purine nucleoside phosphorylase. High levels of arabinosylguanine triphosphate (ara-GTP) accumulate in T-cell neoplasms, leading to Fas ligand-mediated apoptosis. The most recent addition, clofarabine, also an adenosine analogue, has notable activity against childhood ALL and adult AML. Deoxycoformycin, a potent inhibitor of adenosine deaminase, is also effective in the treatment of T-cell malignancies and hairy cell leukemia.

Mechanism of Action of 6-Thiopurines

Both 6-MP and 6-TG have a thiol group substituted for the 6-oxo or 6-hydroxy group of hypoxanthine or guanine, respectively, and are converted to nucleotides by hypoxanthine guanine phosphoribosyltransferase. They block synthesis of purines. The nucleotides of both 6-MP and 6-TG are incorporated into DNA, where they become methylated and are recognized by the mismatch repair system. Cells proceed through at least two further cycles of proliferation before undergoing apoptosis.[56] Cell death correlates with the extent of their incorporation into DNA.

In experimental tumor cells, resistance is most commonly caused by decreased activity of hypoxanthine guanine phosphoribosyltransferase, by increased efflux by the transporter MRP-4, and by the absence of an effective mismatch repair process. Resistance in human leukemia is poorly understood. Patients differ in their rates of metabolic clearance of 6-MP and in their ability to efflux 6-thiopurines from cells. Rapid systemic clearance of the drug, as mediated by methylation of the thiol group by 5-thiopurine-methyltransferase (TMPT),[57] is associated with a high leukemia recurrence rate in ALL maintenance therapy. Low levels of red blood cell thiopurine nucleotides correlate with a high level of activity of TMPT and a high risk of clinical relapse in patients with ALL,[58] whereas decreased activity of TMPT, because of an inherited polymorphism, is associated with increased drug toxicity. A commercial test for enzyme polymorphism is available. A second polymorphism of significance involves the cellular efflux protein, MRP-4; an inactive variant is associated with high 6-TG nucleotide concentrations in cells, and may be responsible for great sensitivity of Japanese patients to 6-thiopurines, as the variant occurs in 18 percent of the Japanese population.[59] A polymorphism affecting the inosine triphosphate pyrophosphorylase enzyme (rs41320251) responsible for degrading a thiopurine nucleotide intermediate is associated with increased methyl-mercaptopurine nucleotides and a high incidence of febrile neutropenia in children with ALL.[60]

Methotrexate and 6-MP are highly synergistic, possibly because methotrexate blocks the *de novo* synthesis of purines and enhances the use of preformed purines and purine analogues such as 6-MP. 6-Thiopurines inhibit the anticoagulant effect of warfarin in some patients, leading to a requirement for higher doses of warfarin in patients receiving chronic 6-thiopurine therapy.

Clinical Pharmacology of 6-Thiopurines

Both 6-TG and 6-MP are given orally at doses of 50 to 100 mg/m^2 per day. Oral absorption of 6-MP is erratic, as only 16 to 50 percent of an oral dose is systemically available.[61] Food and antibiotics may decrease absorption. Both 6-MP and 6-TG are inactivated by metabolism, and have half-lives of approximately 1 hour in plasma. During 6-TG treatment, 6-thioguanine nucleotides accumulate to much higher levels in leukemic cells, as compared to 6-MP treatment, but 6-thiomethyl nucleotides are almost 30-fold higher after 6-MP, and do have reduced, but significant, inhibitory activity.[62] 6-MP is inactivated by metabolism to 6-thiouric acid, a reaction catalyzed by xanthine oxidase. Allopurinol inhibits the metabolic inactivation of 6-MP, but not of 6-TG. Therefore, it is generally recommended that dosages of orally administered 6-MP must be reduced by 75 percent in patients receiving allopurinol. 6-TG is inactivated primarily by S-methylation, followed by oxidation and desulfuration. Dose reduction is not necessary when 6-TG and allopurinol are administered together.

Adverse Effects of 6-Thiopurines

Both 6-TG and 6-MP are myelotoxic, producing nadirs of white blood cells and platelets at 7 to 10 days after treatment.[63] Moderate nausea and vomiting may also be observed. Patients may experience mild but rapidly reversible hepatotoxicity after treatment with either compound. Cirrhosis has occurred in some children with leukemia who are receiving long-term therapy with 6-MP. TMPT, which inactivates 6-thiopurines, occurs in several polymorphic forms that fail to metabolize the analogues. Approximately 1 person in 10 of the white population is heterozygous for ineffective polymorphic forms of the enzyme and will have significantly greater myelosuppression, whereas 1 patient in 300 is homozygous for the inactive forms, accumulates high concentrations of thioguanine nucleotides in both tumor and normal cells, and is at risk for overwhelming toxicity, even with greatly reduced doses of 6-MP.[64]

Other toxicities may occur, including hypersensitivity reactions (fever, rash); interstitial pneumonitis; pancreatitis; opportunistic infection, and an increased incidence of AML in patients receiving chronic immunosuppressive treatment with 6-MP.

FLUDARABINE PHOSPHATE

Originally synthesized as a deamination-resistant analogue of adenosine, fludarabine phosphate contains two important substitutions: a fluorine attached to the purine ring, which renders the drug stable to deamination, and an arabinose sugar in place of deoxyribose, which leads to its pharmacologic activity as an inhibitor of DNA synthesis and ribonucleotide reductase. It has outstanding activity in chronic lymphocytic leukemia (CLL).[65] It is strongly immunosuppressive, like the other purine analogues, and is frequently used for this purpose in nonmyeloablative allogeneic marrow transplantation[66] and in the treatment of collagen vascular diseases.

The pharmacology of fludarabine phosphate requires removal of the phosphate group in plasma to allow cellular uptake by nucleoside transporters, and then intracellular rephosphorylation. Fludarabine is activated to the monophosphate level by deoxycytidine kinase. The triphosphate inhibits DNA polymerase and becomes incorporated into both DNA and RNA.[67] Its mechanism of cytotoxicity results from DNA chain termination and induction of apoptosis, although it also inhibits ribonucleotide reductase (RNR), a self-potentiating activity that increases its incorporation into DNA.[68] Its triphosphate has a long intracellular half-life of 15 hours in CLL cells. Resistance has been ascribed to decreased active uptake, a deficiency of activating deoxycytidine kinase (dCK), increased efflux, or increased RNR activity.

The drug is available in the United States as an intravenous preparation, and for oral use. It has 60 to 80 percent bioavailability. Because it is resistant to adenosine deaminase, fludarabine is eliminated primarily by renal excretion (60%), with a terminal $t_{1/2}$ of 10 hours. For patients treated with fludarabine, the standard intravenous dose is 25 mg/m^2 daily for 5 days, **whereas the approved oral dose is 40 mg/m^2 daily for 5 days.** In patients with renal impairment, a 20 percent dose reduction for a creatinine clearance of 17 to 40 mL/min/m^2, and a 40 percent dose reduction for a creatinine clearance less than 17 mL/min/m^2 yields an area under the curve (AUC) approximately equal to that seen in patients with normal renal function receiving full doses of fludarabine.[69,70]

The recommended oral dose is 40 mg/m^2 per day. In CLL, the recommended doses are 25 mg/m^2 per day for 5 days given as 2-hour infusions and repeated every 4 weeks. When administered at these doses, fludarabine causes only moderate myelosuppression. In CLL patients, its antileukemic effect will lead to a progressive improvement in marrow function over a period of two to three cycles of treatment, with a median time to disease progression of 31 months. However, the drug also exerts cytotoxic effects against both B and T lymphocytes, lowering CD4 T cell counts to 150 to 200 cells/μL and predisposing patients to opportunistic infection. In patients with a large tumor burden, rapid tumor lysis may rarely lead to hyperuricemia, renal failure, and hypocalcemia (tumor lysis syndrome).[71] Thus, patients should be well hydrated and their urine alkalinized prior to beginning therapy. The primary toxicity is acute and reversible myelosuppression. Peripheral sensory and motor neuropathy may occur during standard-dose therapy; autoimmune phenomena, including prolonged neutropenia and hemolytic anemia with both warm and cold antibodies, have been reported.[72] Approximately 10 percent of CLL patients receiving fludarabine may develop a hypersensitivity syndrome of pulmonary infiltrates, hypoxemia, and fever, responsive to glucocorticoids.[73] At higher doses (125 mg/m^2 per day for 5 days) altered mental status, seizures, coma, and optic neuritis have been reported. Myelodysplasia and acute leukemias have been reported as late complications.[74]

CLADRIBINE (2-CHLORODEOXYADENOSINE, 2-CDA)

The extreme sensitivity of normal and malignant lymphocytes to deamination-resistant purine analogues is further exemplified by the potent activity of cladribine in hairy cell leukemia, CLL, and low-grade lymphomas.[75] A single course of cladribine, typically 0.09 mg/kg per day for 7 days by continuous intravenous infusion, induces complete response in 80 percent of patients with hairy cell leukemia, and partial responses in the remainder. Administration by subcutaneous injection or by 2-hour intravenous infusions for 5 days to the same total dose achieves similar results. The drug has much the same intracellular fate as fludarabine, undergoing phosphorylation by dCK and further conversion to a triphosphate that becomes incorporated into DNA. The triphosphate of cladribine has a very long intracellular half-life of 9.7 hours in CLL cells isolated from patients treated with the drug.[76] The triphosphate also accumulates in mitochondria, disrupting oxidative phosphorylation, and inhibits RNR and depletes nicotinamide adenine dinucleotide levels in tumor cells. All of these actions might help explain the drug's toxicity to slowly dividing lymphoid malignancies such as hairy cell leukemia and CLL. The actual mechanisms by which cladribine induces DNA strand breaks are not completely understood. However, similar to fludarabine, it inhibits DNA chain extension and daughter strand synthesis.[77] Furthermore, the drug's inhibition of RNR lowers levels of the competitive nucleotide deoxyadenosine triphosphate. The cumulative effects of cladribine induce apoptosis (programmed cell death).

Cladribine is eliminated primarily (>50%) by renal excretion, with a terminal plasma half-life of 7 hours. In a patient with renal failure, continuous flow hemodialysis effectively cleared the drug and prevented serious myelosuppression.[78] Cladribine retains effectiveness in at least a fraction of hairy cell leukemia patients resistant to deoxycoformycin or fludarabine, although clinical experience with sequential use of these drugs is limited. Toxicities of cladribine include transient myelosuppression, fever, tumor lysis syndrome, and occasional opportunistic infections possibly related to immunosuppression. The development of cumulative thrombocytopenia during treatment with repeated courses of the drug may limit its use. Resistance develops in experimental tumors through decreased uptake, loss of the activating enzyme dCK, increased RNR activity, increased efflux,[79] or by induction of 5′-nucleotidase activity.

CLOFARABINE (2-CHLORO-2′FLUORO-ARABINOSYLADENINE)

This analogue has halogen substitutions on both the purine ring and arabinose sugar, resulting in a ready uptake and activation, to a highly stable intracellular triphosphate (half-life of 24 hours), which terminates DNA synthesis, inhibits RNR, and induces apoptosis. The usual adult dose of 52 mg/m^2 given as a 2-hour infusion daily for 5 days has a plasma half-life of 6.5 hours. The primary route of clearance is through renal excretion, and dose adjustment according to creatinine clearance is recommended for patients with abnormal renal function.

Toxicities are myelosuppression; uncommonly, fever, hypotension, and pulmonary edema, suggestive of capillary leak caused by cytokine release; hepatic transaminitis; hypokalemia; and hypophosphatemia. As a single agent, the drug is well tolerated by elderly AML patients in whom it produces remission rates of 30 percent.[80]

NELARABINE (6-METHOXY-ARABINOSYLGUANINE)

The only guanine nucleoside analogue, nelarabine has relatively specific activity as a secondary agent for T-cell lymphoblastic lymphoma and acute T-cell leukemias. Its mode of action is similar to the other purine analogues, in that it becomes incorporated into DNA and terminates DNA synthesis. Its selective action for T cells may relate to the ability of T cells to activate purine nucleosides and the lack of susceptibility of this drug to purine nucleoside phosphorylase, a degradative reaction.

Usual doses are an intravenous 2-hour infusion of 1500 mg/m^2 for adults on days 1, 3, and 5, and a lower dose of 650 mg/m^2 per day for 5 days for children. The drug is rapidly activated by demethylation after administration, yielding the arabinosyl guanine, which has a longer plasma half-life of 3 hours. It is then converted intracellularly to its triphosphate[81] which becomes incorporated into DNA. It is eliminated primarily by degradation to the guanine base, and to a lesser extent by renal excretion. Doses should be reduced proportionately for patients with renal impairment and creatinine clearance less than 50 mL/min.

The primary toxicities are myelosuppression and abnormal liver function tests, but the drug may cause a spectrum of neurologic abnormalities, including seizures, delirium, somnolence, and the Guillain-Barré syndrome of ascending paralysis.

PENTOSTATIN (2′-DEOXYCOFORMYCIN)

Pentostatin contains a unique seven-carbon primary ring system that closely resembles the transition-state intermediate of the adenosine deaminase reaction. As such, pentostatin is a potent inhibitor of the enzyme, leading to accumulation of intracellular adenosine and deoxyadenosine nucleotides. In addition, the triphosphate of pentostatin is incorporated into DNA. The imbalance in purine nucleotide pools produced by pentostatin probably accounts for its cytotoxicity.

Although initial trials of pentostatin demonstrated striking renal and neurologic toxicities at doses of 10 mg/m^2 per day or greater, lower doses (4 mg/m^2 biweekly) are extremely effective in inducing pathologically confirmed complete responses in hairy cell leukemia. At this lower dose, severe depletion of normal T cells occurs and may predispose to opportunistic infection.[82] The optimal dose may be lower than 4 mg/m^2 biweekly. The drug is eliminated entirely by renal excretion, necessitating proportional dose reduction in patients with reduced creatinine clearance.

RIBONUCLEOTIDE REDUCTASE INHIBITOR: HYDROXYUREA

Hydroxyurea inhibits RNR, the enzyme that converts ribonucleotide diphosphates to deoxyribonucleotides. It chelates iron, an essential cofactor in the RNR reaction. In malignant disease, hydroxyurea is most commonly used for treating polycythemia vera, essential thrombocythemia, and the chronic phase of CML and to lower the leukocyte count rapidly during blast crisis of CML. It has also become the standard agent for preventing painful crisis and reducing hospitalization in patients with sickle cell disease and in thalassemia patients with hemoglobin (Hgb) C/SS. Its antisickling activity results from induction of Hgb F through its activation of a specific promoter for the γ-globin gene. It may also exert antisickling activity and decrease occlusion of small vessels through its generation of nitric oxide, a vasodilator, and through decreased expression of adhesion molecules such as L-selectin, on neutrophils.[83] Resistance to hydroxyurea occurs in experimental tumors as a consequence of an increase in the catalytic subunit of RNR or through mutations that produce an enzyme that binds the drug with decreased affinity.

Clinical Pharmacology

Hydroxyurea is usually administered orally. It is well absorbed, even when large doses such as 50 to 75 mg/kg are given for rapid lowering of the white blood cell count in patients with chronic myelogenous leukemia. In chronic therapy of myeloproliferative disease, starting doses of 15 mg/kg orally are adjusted upward or downward based on neutrophil counts. In managing patients with sickle cell disease, neutrophils should be maintained above 2000 per milliliter.[84] Hydroxyurea may also be given intravenously to rapidly lower the white blood cell count in patients with extreme leukemic leukocytosis or thrombocytosis. Peak plasma levels following oral administration are achieved at about 1 hour and decline with a $t_{1/2}$ of 3 to 4 hours thereafter. Renal excretion is the major route of drug elimination, and doses should be modified for patients with decreased renal function in proportion to the deficit in creatinine clearance.

Adverse Effects

The major toxicities of hydroxyurea are leukopenia and the induction of megaloblastic changes. Nausea, drug fever, pneumonitis, maculopapular skin rash, and painful leg ulcers have been observed with this drug, although it is generally very well tolerated. Hydroxyurea, like cytosine arabinoside, is an S-phase–specific agent. Accordingly, single large doses effect little toxicity other than myelosuppression. The nadir of the leukocyte count occurs 6 to 7 days after a single dose of drug, and the leukocyte count recovers rapidly. It is a potent teratogen and should not be used in women of childbearing age. Its potential to cause leukemic transformation is not established, but small cases series suggest this may occur.[85]

ANTITUBULINS

VINCA ALKALOIDS

Among the many vinca alkaloids that have been extensively evaluated during the past four decades, vinblastine and vincristine are the only ones commonly used in the treatment of hematologic neoplasms: vinblastine because of its excellent activity in the treatment of Hodgkin lymphoma and vincristine in lymphomas and childhood leukemia. Both drugs have broader spectra of activity in solid-tumor therapy, particularly in treating childhood sarcomas (vincristine), and testicular cancer (vinblastine).

Mechanism of Action

The vinca alkaloids exert their cytotoxic action by their binding to tubulin, a structural protein found in the cytoplasm of cells. Microtubules, assembled through polymerization of tubulin dimers, form the spindle along which the chromosomes migrate during mitosis and become an important structural component of neuronal axons. Binding of the vinca alkaloids to tubulin leads to inhibition of formation of the mitotic spindle,[86] arresting cells in metaphase and inducing apoptosis. Resistance to the vinca alkaloids may be acquired through the expression of multidrug resistance, which causes increased efflux of the drugs from the resistant cells. Alternatively, resistant cells may contain mutant tubulin with decreased avidity of vinca binding.[87] The clinical importance of these resistance mechanisms, however, is still uncertain.

Clinical Pharmacology

Vincristine and vinblastine are both administered by the intravenous route. The average single dose of vincristine is 1.4 mg/m^2 and that of vinblastine 8 to 9 mg/m^2. Sequential doses of the drugs are usually given at weekly or every 2 weeks during a cycle of therapy. These doses provide peak plasma drug concentrations of approximately 1 μM. The plasma pharmacokinetics of both vinca analogues are characterized by a very rapid initial disposition phase followed by a slow terminal phase of decay, with half-lives of 20 to 85 hours. Almost 70 percent of a dose of vincristine is metabolized by the liver and excreted in the feces. Cytochrome P450 (CYP)-mediated metabolism is also the major route of inactivation of vinblastine, producing a variety of inactive metabolic products that are excreted in the bile. Inducers of CYP 3A4, such as Dilantin or carbamazepine, enhance clearance, while inhibitors delay clearance and increase toxicity. Accordingly, the dose of vincristine or vinblastine should be reduced in patients with hepatic impairment. Although specific guidelines for dose reduction have not been developed, a 50 percent decrease in dose is recommended for patients presenting with a bilirubin level of 1.5 to 3 mg/dL and a 75 percent reduction for levels greater than 3 mg/dL. Dose reduction is not necessary for patients with impaired renal function, as very little intact drug is excreted in urine.

Adverse Effects

The dose-limiting side effect of vincristine is neurotoxicity, which usually occurs when the total dose received exceeds 6 mg/m^2. The initial signs of neurotoxicity are paresthesia of the fingers and lower extremities and loss of deep tendon reflexes. Continued administration may lead to profound loss of motor strength, such as weakness of dorsiflexion of the foot and extension of the wrists. Elderly patients are particularly susceptible to such toxicities. Occasionally, cranial nerve palsies may lead to vocal chord paralysis or diplopia, and severe jaw pain may result from vincristine administration. At high doses of vincristine (>3 mg total single dose), autonomic neuropathy may cause obstipation and paralytic ileus. Sensory changes and reflex abnormalities slowly improve when the drug is discontinued; motor impairment improves less rapidly and may be irreversible. Inappropriate antidiuretic hormone release resulting in symptomatic dilutional hyponatremia has been ascribed to vincristine.

While marrow suppression is not common with vincristine administration, myelosuppression may be noted in patients with impaired marrow function as a consequence of prior treatment with other drugs. Platelet counts are relatively unaffected.

The primary toxicity of vinblastine is leukopenia. The white count reaches a nadir at day 7 and reverses rapidly thereafter. Mucositis may result from higher doses (>8 mg/m^2) of vinblastine or when it is used in combination with other cytotoxic drugs. Neurotoxicity is rare, but ileus can occur at high doses.

Both drugs cause severe pain and local toxicity if extravasated. Neither drug should ever be given intrathecally. Vincristine administered inadvertently into the cerebrospinal fluid causes acute neurologic dysfunction, coma, and death. Attempts at replacement of the cerebral spinal fluid with an electrolyte solution, Ringer lactate, supplemented with 15 mL/L of fresh-frozen plasma, have been reported to avert a fatal outcome, but do not prevent severe neurologic sequelae.[88]

■ TAXANES

The taxanes, paclitaxel (Taxol) and docetaxel (Taxotere), are a second class of antimitotic compounds that differ in mechanism and toxicity profile from the vinca alkaloids. Paclitaxel was purified from an extract of the bark of *Taxus brevifolia,* whereas docetaxel is a closely related semisynthetic derivative. Neither drug has won an important role in the treatment of hematologic malignancies. They bind to the β-tubulin subunit of microtubules and promote the polymerization of microtubules, leading to disordered mitotic spindle formation and a block in the progression through mitosis.[89] Both drugs induce apoptosis in tumor cells irrespective of the p53 status of the cells and kill cells at 10-nM concentrations in cell culture in a time-dependent manner.[90] In experimental settings, resistance is related to increased drug efflux, mutations in β-tubulin, or increased expression of antiapoptotic proteins such as survivin,[91] or of the mitosis-related aurora kinase.[92]

The taxanes are subject to multidrug resistance mediated by the *mdr* and *mrp* genes, as well as to β-tubulin mutations. Because they are highly insoluble in aqueous solution, both drugs are formulated in lipid-based solvents that cause occasional hypersensitivity reactions. Thus, paclitaxel is given after pretreatment with antihistamines (cimetidine, Benadryl), and dexamethasone. Both drugs are cleared primarily by hepatic CYP metabolism, although by different isoenzymes (paclitaxel predominantly by CYP 2B6 and docetaxel by CYP 3A4) with terminal plasma half-lives of 10 to 13 hours. Their metabolism is stimulated by phenytoin (Dilantin) and other CYP-inducing drugs and inhibited by ketoconazole. Their major toxicities, aside from hypersensitivity, are a sharp but brief leukopenia, milder thrombocytopenia, and mucositis. High-dose or repeated cycles of the taxanes cause a sensory and motor peripheral neuropathy that is reversible with drug discontinuation. Occasional patients have experienced atrial conduction block or atrial or ventricular arrhythmias after paclitaxel administration, and the combination of paclitaxel with doxorubicin may produce a greater incidence of congestive heart failure than seen with doxorubicin alone.[93] A syndrome of progressive fluid retention and peripheral edema occurs in patients receiving multiple cycles of docetaxel and can be at least partially prevented by pretreatment with glucocorticoids.[94]

Although the taxanes have not found a valuable role in the treatment of hematologic malignancy, a number of analogues and new formulations are under development. Abraxane, consisting of Taxol bound to albumen microparticles, does not require a lipid solvent, is virtually free of hypersensitivity as a side effect, and enters cells by a separate albumen mediated transporter. It is approved for treatment of relapsed breast cancer. An entirely new class of natural products, the epothilones, have a similar mechanism of action, are less susceptible to MDR, and have activity against solid tumors, particularly breast and prostate cancer.[95]

TOPOISOMERASE I INHIBITORS

■ CAMPTOTHECINS

This group of compounds includes synthetic derivatives of 20 (*S*)-camptothecin, a naturally occurring compound initially isolated from the *Camptotheca acuminata* bush. The campothecins interact with a unique target, topoisomerase I, stabilizing the enzyme's complex with DNA and preventing the resealing of DNA single-strand breaks induced by the enzyme. Resistance arises through mutation, deletion, or decreased expression of the topoisomerase I gene. The primary agents in clinical use are irinotecan, which is approved for treatment of colon cancer, and topotecan, approved for use against ovarian cancer and small-cell lung cancer. Irinotecan, most commonly administered intravenously at a dose of 125 mg/m^2 once each week for 4 weeks every 42 days, has shown promise against lymphomas in phase II trials performed in Japan.[96] Response rates of 42 percent in previously treated patients with non-Hodgkin lymphoma, and of 38 percent in patients with refractory or relapsed adult T-cell leukemia-lymphoma, were reported. These encouraging results remain to be confirmed. Topotecan has remission-inducing activity in patients with myelodysplasia and chronic myelomonocytic leukemia, both as a single agent (1.5 mg/m^2 per day for 5 days) and in combination with cytarabine.[97,98] Objective responses have also been observed in phase I clinical trials in patients with acute myelogenous leukemia.[99] The two drugs differ substantially in their profile of toxicities and pharmacokinetic behavior. Irinotecan is a water-soluble prodrug that converts to the active species, SN-38, by carboxyl esterase-mediated cleavage of the parent drug. SN-38 and its parent drug are eliminated by biliary excretion, either directly after glucuronidation of the parent or its active metabolite SN-38. Therefore, irinotecan must be used with caution and at lower doses in patients with Gilbert disease or hepatic dysfunction.[100] In contrast to the hepatic extraction and excretion of irinotecan, approximately two-thirds of the dose of topotecan is eliminated by renal excretion, with the remainder being cleared by biliary excretion. Dose adjustment proportional to creatinine clearance is indicated in patients with renal failure.[101] Topotecan toxicity consists mainly of myelosuppression and, to a lesser degree, mucositis, whereas irinotecan causes a profound diarrhea, which is responsive to loperamide, and a more modest myelosuppression. The maximum tolerated dose of topotecan for the daily 30-minute IV infusion × 5 schedule in patients hematologic malignancies is 4.5 mg/m^2 per day.[102] This is considerably greater than the approved dose for solid tumors, and gastrointestinal side effects, such as mucositis and diarrhea, become dose-limiting at these higher doses.

TOPOISOMERASE II INHIBITORS

■ ANTHRACYCLINE ANTIBIOTICS

The anthracyclines are a unique class of natural products that inhibit topoisomerase II (Topo II), an enzyme important in DNA strand passage, the untangling of DNA prior to replication or repair. Doxorubicin, daunorubicin, idarubicin, and epirubicin are closely related in structure, each possessing a rigid planar core to which is linked a Daunosamine sugar. The molecules differ in side chain substitutions attached to the anthracycline ring system, and exhibit different spectra of antitumor activity and toxicity. Mitoxantrone, a closely related, nonglycosidic anthracenedione, has very similar pharmacologic properties to those of the anthracyclines. The anthracyclines are produced by a *Streptomyces* species, whereas mitoxantrone is a synthetic compound. Doxorubicin (Adriamycin) has broad activity against solid and hematologic malignancies. It is an important component of the standard multidrug regimens used to treat Hodgkin lymphoma (ABVD [doxorubicin, bleomycin, vinblastine and dacarbazine]) and aggressive non-Hodgkin lymphoma (CHOP [cyclophosphamide, doxorubicin, vincristine, and prednisone]). Daunorubicin and idarubicin are used almost exclusively in combination with cytarabine for the treatment of AML, whereas epirubicin is primarily effective against solid tumors. Mitoxantrone is employed for the treatment of AML and breast cancer, and as an immunosuppressive for patients with multiple sclerosis.

Mechanism of Action

Anthracyclines target the replication and structural integrity of DNA. Their primary mechanism of toxicity stems from their interaction with Topo II, an enzyme that creates DNA strand breaks and promotes strand passage through those breaks. Strand passage is essential in untangling DNA in preparation for replication and repair. Once the strand passage and unwinding is complete, Topo II reseals the broken DNA strands. The anthracyclines inhibit the resealing step by forming a complex with Topo II and the broken DNA strand to which the enzyme is linked. Accumulation of strand breaks activates apoptosis. The planar molecular structure of these drugs promotes their intercalation between opposing strands of the DNA helix and may contribute to the specificity of sites of DNA breakage. In addition to their inhibition of Topo II, the anthracyclines generate free radicals by virtue of the oxidation-reduction cycling of their quinone groups, an action catalyzed by the binding of Fe^{2+}. Free radical generation is thought to be responsible for their cardiac toxicity.

The importance of the presence of Topo II in determining response to anthracyclines is best illustrated by the greater benefit of anthracycline-based breast cancer treatment in patients with amplification of the target enzyme.[103] The gene coding for Topo II is located within the frequently amplified region on chromosome 17 that includes the Her-2 gene. Thus anthracycline-containing regimens are particularly effective in Her-2–amplified breast cancers.[104]

The anthracyclines enter cells through a passive transport process. The lipophilic structure of anthracyclines allows them to achieve high intracellular concentrations. Anthracyclines are pumped out of the cell by a series of ATP-dependent transporters, including the P-glycoprotein or MDR transporter and related efflux pumps.[16] Other mechanisms for anthracycline resistance include decreased Topo II activity or Topo II mutations in the enzyme that inhibit drug binding.

Clinical Pharmacology

Doxorubicin and daunorubicin are converted to active hydroxyl metabolites, and thereafter to a spectrum of inactive products in the liver. Their major metabolic products are aglycones, side-chain-modified products, glucuronides, sulphates, and oxidative metabolites. The only active metabolic product is the alcohol resulting from oxidation of a side-chain carbonyl by aldoketoreductase. Only a minor fraction of the dose of either drug is excreted in the urine as the parent drug or active metabolite. The pharmacokinetics of the clinically useful anthracyclines are predominantly influenced by their terminal disposition phase, which exceed 24 hours. Although prolongation of the half-life of doxorubicin has been reported in studies of patients with compromised liver function, no clear correlations with toxicity have been established. However, it is wise to begin therapy of patients with elevated serum bilirubin levels at 50 percent doses of doxorubicin or daunorubicin, and adjust according to tolerance. Idarubicin, the only anthracycline that appears amenable to oral administration, has an oral bioavailability of 20 percent for the parent drug and 40 percent for parent plus idarubicinol, the primary active metabolite. Idarubicinol has a very prolonged biologic half-life, ranging from 50 to 60 hours, and is likely responsible for the antitumor activity of this drug. In contrast to the metabolites of doxorubicin and daunorubicin, idarubicinol is eliminated primarily by renal excretion.

Mitoxantrone has a long terminal half-life of 23 to 42 hours. Only a minor fraction of unchanged drug is excreted in the urine (<10%) or stool (<20%). The majority of the drug is metabolized or bound to tissues. Patients with impaired hepatic function may have a more prolonged elimination of mitoxantrone.

The usual dose of doxorubicin when administered as a single agent by bolus intravenous injection is 60 to 75 mg/m^2 every 3 to 4 weeks. Less cardiac toxicity may result from schedules that avoid high peak plasma concentrations, such as weekly doses (15–25 mg/m^2) or continuous intravenous infusion over 48 to 96 hours, as in the EPOCH (etoposide, prednisone, vincristine, cyclophosphamide, and doxorubicin) regimen.[105] When given in combination with other myelotoxic agents such as cyclophosphamide, the dose of doxorubicin is usually decreased because of overlapping marrow toxicity. Daunorubicin has been used as the anthracycline of choice in the treatment of AML. To minimize the cardiotoxic effects of daunorubicin, in standard "3+7" therapy in AML the daunorubicin dosage (30 mg/m^2 per day) is given over 3 days to avoid high peak concentrations.

Adverse Effects

Myelosuppression is the primary acute toxicity of this class of drugs, with a nadir occurring 7 to 10 days after single-dose administration and recovery by 2 weeks. Mitoxantrone produces less nausea and vomiting than does either daunorubicin or doxorubicin. Doxorubicin may cause mucositis, especially when used in maximally tolerated divided doses given over 2 to 3 days or when used in combination with other drugs that cause mucositis. Anthracyclines can also cause radiation recall in previously irradiated tissues, especially when the drug is administered just prior to or in the weeks following irradiation. Alopecia often occurs. Extravasation of these drugs can result in tissue necrosis so they should be administered with through an indwelling central venous catheter. Patients taking doxorubicin should also be warned that their urine may turn red.

Cardiotoxicity is the major late toxic effect of anthracyclines.[106] Cardiotoxicity results from free radical formation catalyzed by the anthracycline's quinone moiety. Clinically, anthracycline-induced cardiotoxicity presents as either acute or subacute/chronic damage to cardiac myocytes. The acute effects are manifest as arrhythmias, conduction abnormalities, or a "pericarditis-myocarditis syndrome." On the other hand, the more common long-term consequence is congestive heart failure (CHF), which can develop during treatment or months after treatment. Studies in breast cancer have demonstrated a 0.5 to 1 percent risk of cardiomyopathy in patients treated with anthracyclines.[107] The risk is higher in patients receiving trastuzumab (Herceptin) or paclitaxel in combination with doxorubicin.

The risk of anthracycline-induced cardiotoxicity increases with total dose, but is difficult to estimate for any individual patient. In patients with normal cardiac function prior to treatment, the subsequent rate of doxorubicin-induced CHF reaches 0.14 percent at total doses of 400 mg/m^2, but climbs thereafter to 7 to 20 percent at total doses of 550 mg/m^2.[108] The threshold for cardiotoxicity varies among the different anthracyclines. For example, the threshold for daunorubicin (600–700 mg/m^2) is significantly higher than for doxorubicin (400 mg/m^2). However, it should be remembered that these thresholds are based on population studies, and for any individual patient the risk is difficult to predict. The clinician must pay close attention to symptoms of CHF, such as dyspnea, cough, orthopnea, and the presence of weight gain or ankle edema, throughout a course of treatment and irrespective of total dose.

Besides the cumulative dose of anthracycline, other risk factors for anthracycline-induced cardiomyopathy include mediastinal (mantle) radiation, preexisting heart disease, and patient age, the risk being highest in children younger than the age of 4 years. Children who receive greater than 300 mg/m^2 have a significant risk of having decreased myocardial contractility, decreased ventricular dimension, and an increased incidence of cardiac events (such as myocardial infarction and CHF) in their adult years. For this reason, it is recommended that the total anthracycline dose be limited to 300 mg/m^2 in children. In addition, children treated with anthracyclines should have long-term cardiology followup.[109]

Ejection fraction measurements have been helpful as a noninvasive technique for demonstrating a decline in myocardial function, a sign of impending myocardial failure. Ejection fraction measurements, usually by multigated acquisition scan (MUGA radionuclide angiography), should be performed to verify normal cardiac function prior to starting anthracycline-based chemotherapy, and should be repeated at the earliest sign of cardiac dysfunction and before every two cycles of treatment when the total dose exceeds 300 mg/m^2. Anthracyclines should be discontinued if the ejection fraction falls below 40 percent, or if the ejection fraction drops a total of 20 percent from pretreatment levels.

As cardiotoxicity of anthracyclines results from the generation of free radicals by an anthracycline-iron complex, dexrazoxane, an iron chelator, decreases free radical formation *in vitro* and decreases the risk of cardiotoxicity in children receiving treatment for ALL and in adult patients with metastatic breast cancer.[109] Fortunately, dexrazoxane does not cause any apparent diminution of antitumor activity. The addition of dexrazoxane to an anthracycline-based regimen represents an alternative to discontinuing anthracyclines in patients who are approaching higher total-dose thresholds of drug, but who still require treatment.

Treatment with Topo II inhibitors, including anthracyclines, mitoxantrone, and the epipodophyllotoxins (discussed below), increases the risk of AML. AML typically develops 6 months to 5 years after exposure to the Topo II inhibitor.[107] This heightened risk derives from the increased DNA double-strand breaks generated by the Topo II inhibitor. These double-stranded DNA breaks can give rise to balanced chromosomal translocations.[111] Anthracyclines and mitoxantrone have affinity for specific DNA sequences and cause translocations at specific hot spots in the genome, including a 6-base pair breakpoint region in the PML gene causing the 15;17 translocation, the 11q23 translocation involving the MLL gene, and the 11;20 translocation involving the NUP98 gene.[110,111]

■ EPIPODOPHYLOTOXINS

Two semisynthetic derivatives of podophyllotoxin, VP-16 (etoposide) and VM-26 (teniposide), inhibit Topo II and have significant clinical activity in hematologic malignancies. Etoposide has been incorporated into combination therapy regimens for Hodgkin lymphoma, large cell lymphomas, leukemias, and various solid tumors, and is a frequent component of high-dose chemotherapy regimens. Teniposide has limited value in clinical oncology. Its use is generally restricted to childhood acute leukemia, where it appears to be synergistic with cytarabine. These compounds induce double-stranded breaks in DNA through their sequence-specific binding to DNA in complex with Topo II.[112] One mechanism of resistance is increased expression of the MDR phenotype.[16] A second mechanism results from decreased Topo II activity or mutation of the enzyme, resulting in decreased drug binding.[113,114]

Clinical Pharmacology

Etoposide is administered in doses of 100 to 120 mg/m^2 per day for 3 days, either consecutively or every other day. Approximately 30 to 40 percent of an intravenous dose of etoposide is excreted intact in the urine; thus, doses of etoposide require modification for patients with compromised renal function but not hepatic dysfunction.[115] The half-life of etoposide is 15 hours. The clinical activity of etoposide is highly schedule dependent. Single conventional doses are essentially without antitumor effect as compared to consecutive daily doses for 3 to 5 days. The oral administration of 50 mg/day for 2 to 3 weeks is a commonly used regimen that takes advantage of that schedule dependency.

The pharmacokinetics of teniposide are very similar to those of etoposide, with a terminal plasma half-life of 20 to 48 hours. However, little parent drug appears intact in the urine, and dose modification for patients with renal dysfunction is unnecessary.

Adverse Effects

When administered intravenously, both etoposide and teniposide should be infused over a 30-minute period to avoid hypotensive episodes. The major toxicity of both drugs is leukopenia, which is rapidly reversible. Thrombocytopenia is less common. Nausea and vomiting often follow etoposide administration. Alopecia may occur with both drugs. Other toxicities, such as fever, mild elevation of liver function tests, and peripheral neuropathy, are relatively uncommon. Because the major toxicity of etoposide is limited to the marrow, this drug is a valuable component of high-dose regimens used with marrow transplantation. In high-dose etoposide protocols (3–4 g/m^2 given over 3–5 days) oropharyngeal mucositis becomes a prominent toxicity. Less frequent high-dose toxicities include hepatocellular damage and, rarely, anaphylactic-like symptoms, probably related to the chromophore-based vehicle. Secondary AML associated with translocation at 11q23 may follow etoposide treatment in children with ALL[116] and in adults with solid tumors.[117]

AGENTS ACTIVE THROUGHOUT THE CELL CYCLE

THE ALKYLATING DRUGS

These drugs are important in the treatment of hematopoietic malignancies either as single agents or as components of standard- or high-dose regimens. Their role as treatment for both acute and chronic hematologic malignancies results from their unique mechanism of cell killing and their lack of cell cycle specificity. They may eradicate noncycling cells that escape cycle-active components of the treatment.

Although these agents share the common property of forming covalent bonds with electron-rich sites on DNA (oxygen and nitrogen substituents), they exhibit important differences in their intrinsic reactivity, route of cellular uptake, favored sites of alkylation on DNA bases, and the specific mechanism of DNA repair that determines cell survival. These differences are borne out in experimental settings, where cross-resistance to alkylating agents is incomplete. Thus, protocols employing multiple alkylators, particularly in high-dose regimens, have a rational basis.[118] Alkylating agents differ as well in their patterns of toxicity. The majority of these drugs cause myelosuppression and mucositis as their primary acute toxicities, as well as delayed pulmonary fibrosis and late secondary leukemias. These leukemias often arise after a period of myelodysplasia, are usually highly drug resistant AML, and carry defects in chromosomes 5 or 7. Busulfan, bischloroethylnitrosourea (BCNU), and cyclophosphamide are most likely to cause vascular endothelial damage (hepatic venoocclusive disease) when used in high doses. However, these same drugs are often used in high-dose regimens, as they cause less mucositis than other alkylating agents. 4-Hydroperoxycyclophosphamide, an activated analogue of cyclophosphamide, appears to spare marrow stem cells relative to tumor cells and has been used for *in vitro* purging of marrow in autologous transplantation.[119]

Although platinum analogues are not true alkylating agents in that they form metal adducts rather than carbon adducts with DNA, RNA, and protein, their range of toxicities and mechanisms of resistance have much in common with the classical alkylators. They have limited use in hematologic malignancy, carboplatin having a role in high-dose chemotherapy for lymphomas. Their DNA adducts are subject to repair by nucleotide excision repair and double-strand break repair, processes dependent on functional p53 activity.[120] Polymorphisms of the repair pathways, especially the mismatch repair process, may be associated with drug resistance,[121] whereas errors in double-strand break repair, such as found in BRCA1- and BRCA2-related breast cancers and ovarian cancer, may lead to greater sensitivity to platinating drugs.

Mechanism of Action

All alkylating agents (Fig. 20–4) have in common the generation of highly reactive carbonium intermediates that attack electron-rich sites on DNA, such as the *N*-7, *O*-2, and *O*-6 positions of guanine and the *N*-1, *N*-3, and *N*-7 positions of adenine. For many of these agents, the alkylating group must undergo a preliminary activation reaction mediated either by chemical rearrangement of the molecule, as in the case of nitrogen mustard and the nitrosoureas, or by metabolic activation followed by chemical rearrangement, as for cyclophosphamide, ifosfamide, and procarbazine. In most alkylating agents the molecule is bifunctional, usually containing two chloroethyl groups, and these drugs form intrastrand and, less frequently, interstrand crosslinks.

A second class of alkylating drugs, exemplified by busulfan, dimethyltriazenoimidazole carboxamide (DTIC) and the closely related temozolomide, and procarbazine, produce only single-strand alkylation but may be highly carcinogenic, as, for example, procarbazine. In general, all the commonly used alkylating drugs, including cyclophosphamide, ifosfamide, melphalan, chlorambucil, and the methylating drugs, produce the same spectrum of myelosuppressive, carcinogenic, and

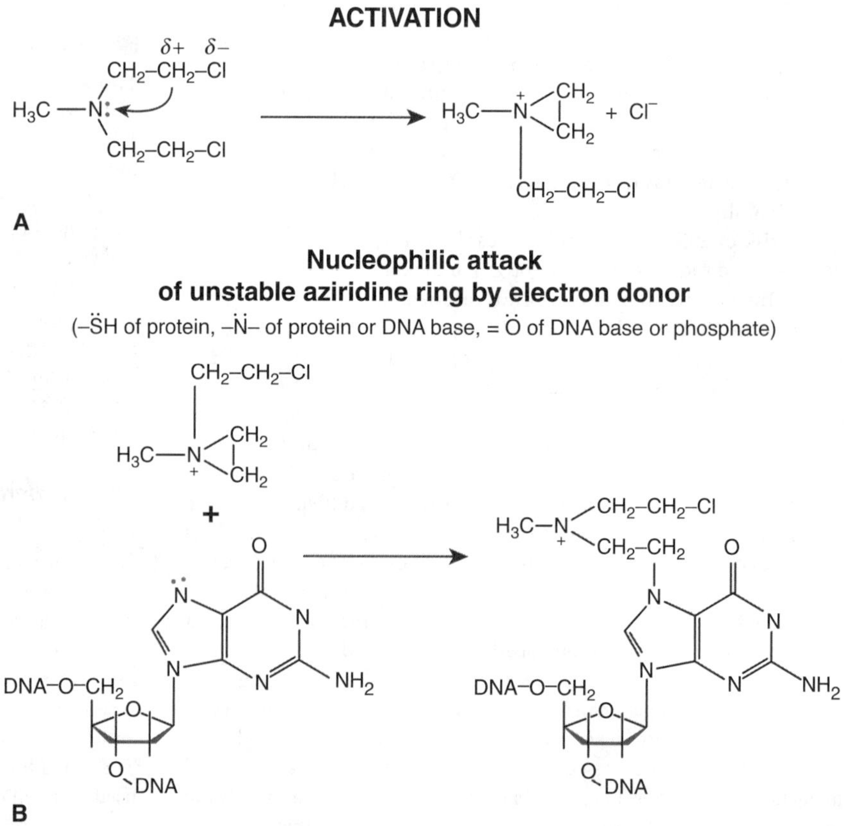

FIGURE 20–4. Mechanism of action of alkylating agents. *(Reproduced from Brunton L, Lazo J, Parker K:* Goodman & Gilman's The Pharmacological Basis of Therapeutics, *11th ed, chap 51. McGraw-Hill, New York, 2006. With permission from the publisher.)*

genotoxic actions, and depend on an intact mismatch repair system to recognize their adducts and initiate apoptosis.

Experimental systems have elucidated the mechanisms of resistance to alkylating agents.[122] Some mechanisms are specific for certain alkylating agents (e.g., impaired uptake of nitrogen mustard as a consequence of an alteration in the membrane carrier for choline, or deletion of the amino acid carrier used by melphalan), whereas others appear to be less specific (e.g., drug inactivation associated with an increase in intracellular sulfhydryl compounds, and enhanced nucleotide-excision repair of DNA adducts). The primary resistance mechanisms for various alkylating drugs, as documented in experimental tumors, include increased degradation by aldehyde dehydrogenase (specifically for cyclophosphamide)[123]; increased conjugation of the reactive intermediates with glutathione or glutathione transferase (all chloroethylating agents and platinum analogues); increased repair of the *O*-6 guanine alkyl lesions by a specific alkyl transferase (nitrosoureas, procarbazine, temozolomide, and dacarbazine)[124]; increased nucleotide excision repair (all platinum derivatives and chloroethylating agents, except possibly nitrosoureas); decreased uptake (melphalan, nitrogen mustard); decreased ability to recognize DNA damage because of defective mismatch repair, especially the loss of the MLH6 component[125] (most alkylating agents and platinum derivatives); and defective initiation of apoptosis (p53 loss of function mutants), which affects all alkylators. The basis of alkylating agent resistance in the clinic is still incompletely understood.

Clinical Pharmacology

In general, the alkylating agents and their reactive intermediates have short residence times in the systemic circulation and within cells. They are eliminated predominantly by hydrolysis, by chemical or biochemical conjugation to the sulfhydryl groups of glutathione or proteins, or by oxidative metabolism in the case of ifosfamide and cyclophosphamide. Therefore, dose reduction is not required in patients with diminished renal function, or with hepatic dysfunction.

A few of the drugs require enzymatic activation. Cyclophosphamide and ifosfamide are closely related molecules that undergo hepatic CYP-mediated activation. Their active metabolites include a highly labile phosphoramide mustard and a second toxic metabolite, acrolein, which is excreted in the urine.[126] To counteract toxicity to kidneys and bladder, mercaptoethane sulfonate (MESNA) is administered simultaneously in equivalent doses to patients receiving ifosfamide or high-dose cyclophosphamide. Procarbazine and DTIC require metabolic activation by hepatic CYP isoenzymes, whereas temozolomide, a structural congener of DTIC, spontaneously activates to a methylating intermediate, and has become the preferred drug for treating glioblastomas.

Nitrogen mustard is a highly reactive compound in its parent form, and thus can be administered topically for treatment of skin cancers and cutaneous lymphoma. It is a potent vesicant, and care must be taken in the mixing and administering the drug. Extravasation may lead to severe tissue injury. The second-generation alkylating agents, which include cyclophosphamide, melphalan, busulfan, and chlorambucil, are more chemically stable and absorbed reasonably well when given orally.

The newest alkylating drug, bendamustine, is now approved for both chronic lymphocytic leukemia and relapsed lymphomas, and consists of a purine base with a *bis*-chloroethyl side chain. In experimental systems it is only partially cross-resistant with other alkylators, and produces a bulky DNA adduct that is slowly repaired by base excision repair. It strongly induces p53 phosphorylation and apoptosis, as well as cell necrosis, a distinct cell death response.[127] Bendamustine metabolism produces two minor toxic metabolites through hydroxylation of its 4 position and *N*-demethylation. The bulk of drug is eliminated through its reactivity with sulfhydryls and adduct formation. The drug displays much the same pattern of toxicity of other alkylating drugs, with perhaps less myelosuppression.

Carboplatin, often used in high-dose therapy of lymphomas, is primarily excreted by the kidneys. Its dose should be based on renal function, aiming at a specific AUC of 5 to 7, according to the formula:

$$\text{Dose (mg/m}^2\text{)} = \text{AUC} \times (\text{glomerular filtration rate} + 25)$$

Adverse Effects

Marrow toxicity, which is cumulative and a function of total dose, is the most important toxic effect of these compounds. Other toxicities include denudation of the gastrointestinal epithelium, as well as lung, cardiac, and endothelial damage. Because alkylating agents all react with DNA, mutations and secondary leukemias are major long-term effects of these agents. This hazard appears to be related to the total dose administered. The monofunctional methylating agents (e.g., procarbazine) are especially potent in this regard and may have a major role in the increased incidence of secondary malignancies noted in patients who have been treated with chemotherapy. The dose-limiting toxicity of one of these drugs, dacarbazine, is nausea and vomiting rather than marrow suppression.

Nitrosoureas produce a characteristic delayed myelosuppression that reaches a nadir 4 to 6 weeks after administration. Busulfan, like the nitrosoureas, depletes stem cells and can cause profound marrow hypoplasia or permanent aplasia when administered over prolonged periods of time and must be used with caution. All alkylating agents, but particularly busulfan and the nitrosoureas, may produce pulmonary fibrosis. An increased expression of platelet-derived growth factor-β and insulin-like growth factor-1 on hyperplastic alveolar macrophages and hyperplastic type II pneumocytes may play an important role in the fibrogenesis induced by nitrosoureas. The nitrosoureas also cause nephrotoxicity, particularly after total doses of 1200 mg/m^2 BCNU, whereas cyclophosphamide and ifosfamide cause chronic bladder toxicity, hemorrhage, and, in rare cases, bladder carcinomas.

Carboplatin causes an acute thrombocytopenia, as well as a more chronic sensory neuropathy.

High-Dose Alkylating Agent Therapy

The development of marrow stem cell rescue techniques has made it possible to administer doses of chemotherapy that would otherwise produce life-threatening aplasia. To be of benefit, however, high-dose therapy must employ agents that have a relatively steep dose–response relationship and must not have lethal extramedullary toxicity at high doses. Among the classes of cytotoxics, alkylators have a particularly favorable linear relationship between dose and cytotoxicity in experimental systems. Their hematopoietic toxicity is generally limiting within standard-dose ranges, and high-dose regimens with cyclophosphamide appear to spare marrow stem cells. Other organ toxicities are infrequent until doses are increased manyfold, making them ideal candidates for high-dose regimens. When agents are administered with stem cell rescue, marrow toxicity ceases to be dose limiting and extramedullary toxic effects become dose limiting. Depending on the agent and the toxicity profile, doses may only be escalated by as little as twofold, as seen with cisplatin because of renal toxicity, or to as high as 18-fold in the case of thiotepa (Table 20–3).[128–134] However, when agents are combined into a high-dose regimen, overlapping extramedullary toxicities of the agents must be considered so as to avoid serious new additive and/or synergistic toxicities (Table 20–4).[135–139] Overlapping extramedullary toxicities (particularly the risk of pulmonary or hepatic dysfunction or secondary leukemia) cannot be completely avoided, but rational drug selection can minimize the dose reductions of the individual agents, compared to their single-agent maximum tolerated dose (MTD), while at the same time ensuring safety of the combination

TABLE 20–3. Dose-Limiting Extramedullary Toxicities of Single-Agent Chemotherapy

Drug	Maximum Tolerated Dose, mg/m²*	Increase Over Standard Dose†	Major Toxicities‡
Cyclophosphamide	7000	7.0	Cardiac
Ifosfamide	16,000	2.7	Renal, CNS
Thiotepa§	1005	18.0	GI, CNS
Melphalan§	180	5.6	GI
Busulfan§	640	9.0	GI, hepatic
BCNU§	1050	5.3	Lung, hepatic
Cisplatin	200	2.0	Renal, neuropathy
Carboplatin§	2000	5.0	Hepatic, renal
Etoposide	3000	6.0	GI
Cytarabine	3000	10–30	Neurologic, mucositis

BCNU, bischloroethyl nitrosourea; CNS, central nervous system; GI, gastrointestinal.

*Independent of hematopoietic toxicity. Dose may be given over multiple days.

†Fold increase. This is an approximation because standard doses may vary.

‡All drugs listed in this table cause vascular endothelial damage and venoocclusive disease, as well as late secondary leukemias.

§With stem cell support.

regimen. This is illustrated in Table 20–4, which shows the fraction of the single-agent MTD that can be administered in combination with other drugs. As might be expected, this fraction is quite variable depending on the drug combinations, with the average fractional MTD used in combination ranging from 0.5 to 1. Depending on the regimen, significant gastrointestinal, pulmonary, hepatic, and/or renal toxicities are encountered and become dose limiting. For these reasons, high-dose regimens are safest in patients who are younger (<70 years) and who have had minimal prior chemotherapy and radiation therapy.

AGENTS OF DIVERSE MECHANISMS

■ BLEOMYCIN

Bleomycin is a mixture of cytotoxic peptides produced by the fungus *Streptomyces verticillis*.[140] Because it has antitumor effects with little or no marrow toxicity, it is commonly used as part of combination regimens (such as ABVD) to treat Hodgkin lymphoma, the aggressive lymphomas, and with cisplatin and vinblastine to treat germ cell tumors. Bleomycin acts by causing both single- and double-strand breaks in DNA. These breaks form as a consequence of a bleomycin:Fe (II) complex that undergoes oxidation-reduction cycling with molecular oxygen. The drug avidly binds to DNA and its reactive center abstracts a proton from deoxyribose, leading to cleavage of the sugar at the 3′-carbon.[141] In experimental tumors, resistance to bleomycin has been attributed to increased tumor cell concentrations of an aminohydrolase that cleaves and inactivates the drug.[142] Some resistant cell lines exhibit enhanced capacity to repair strand breaks, and in others, resistance results from decreased drug accumulation. Additional factors, such as increased free radical detoxification, may also influence toxicity. The tumor specificity of bleomycin, its severe cutaneous and pulmonary toxicity, and its lack of toxicity to marrow and the gastrointestinal tract may be a result of widely differing levels of a bleomycin hydrolase enzyme in these tissues. A polymorphism in the hydrolase gene, identified by SNP A1450G, is believed to confer resistance to the drug through its enhancement of hydrolase activity.[143] Cell killing occurs throughout the cell cycle.

Clinical Pharmacology

Bleomycin may be administered intravenously or intramuscularly in doses of 10 to 20 units/m² per week to cumulative doses of 250 units for systemic therapy, as well as intrapleurally or intraperitoneally for control of malignant effusions. The half-life of drug elimination from plasma is estimated to be 2 to 3 hours. After a single intravenous injection, more than half the dose is excreted, unchanged, in the urine within 24 hours.[144] Bleomycin elimination may be markedly impaired in patients with poor renal function; such patients are at risk of overwhelming skin and lung toxicity. Dose reduction proportional to creatinine clearance should be considered in patients with a creatinine clearance lower than 60 mL/min.

Adverse Effects

Bleomycin has few or no effects on normal marrow; however, in patients given other myelosuppressive drugs or who are recovering from marrow toxicity from these agents, additional mild myelosuppression may be observed. The primary toxicities that result from bleomycin are pulmonary fibrosis and skin changes. In experimental settings, the drug

TABLE 20–4. Toxicities and Doses of High-Dose Regimens Administered with Stem Cell Support

Regimen	Dose (mg/m²)	Fraction of MTD*	Major Toxicities	Tumor Targets	Reference
Cyclophosphamide	6000	0.86	GI, cardiac	Breast	135
Thiotepa	500	0.5			
Carboplatin	800	0.4			
Cyclophosphamide	6000	0.86	Lung, GI	Lymphomas	136
BCNU	300	0.29			
Etoposide	750	0.25			
Busulfan	640	1.0	Lung, GI, hepatic	Lymphoma	137
Cyclophosphamide	8000	1.0			
Ifosfamide	16,000	1.0	Renal, hepatic, GI	Lymphomas	138
Carboplatin	1800	0.9			
Etoposide	1500	0.5			
Cyclophosphamide	5625	0.8	Cardiac, hepatic, renal	Breast	139
BCNU	600	0.57			
Cisplatin	164	0.82			

BCNU, bischloroethylnitrosourea; GI, gastrointestinal; MTD, maximum tolerated dose.

*This is the fraction of the single-agent MTD (see Table 20–3, Col. 2).

induces the secretion of numerous cytokines, including interleukin (IL)-6, tumor necrosis factor-α and transforming growth factor-β, by alveolar macrophages and inflammatory cells, leading to collagen deposition.[145] The risk of pulmonary toxicity is related to the cumulative dose administered, increasing to 10 percent in patients given more than 450 mg. Risk is also greater in patients older than age 70 years, in patients with underlying lung disease, in patients receiving bleomycin who are given high oxygen concentrations, and in patients who have had previous radiotherapy to the lungs. Single doses of 25 mg/m^2 or more predispose to this toxic effect. Symptoms of pulmonary toxicity include cough and dyspnea. Chest radiographs show nonspecific infiltrates, especially in the lower lobes. Chest computed tomography changes may show more extensive infiltrates, fibrosis in later stages of evolution, atelectasis, or cavitation. Positron emission tomography scans are strongly positive. Open-lung biopsy may be required to distinguish bleomycin pulmonary toxicity from infection or malignant disease. Findings of bleomycin toxicity include an inflammatory alveolar infiltrate with edema, pulmonary hyaline formation, and squamous metaplasia of the alveolar lining cells. These changes progress to intraalveolar and interstitial fibrosis over a period of months. Patients with bleomycin lung toxicity have a measurable decrease in carbon monoxide diffusing capacity, a test of possible value in predicting potential pulmonary toxicity.[146] Because there is no specific therapy for patients with bleomycin lung toxicity, close attention should be paid to early pulmonary symptoms and radiographic changes. In patients with bleomycin pulmonary toxicity, some improvement may be seen on discontinuation of the drug, but the pulmonary fibrosis is usually not reversible. Glucocorticoids may decrease inflammation, but are of no proven benefit once fibrosis has occurred. O_2 supplementation must be avoided, as it promotes the oxidation-reduction injury to pulmonary tissue.

The dermatologic toxicity of bleomycin is also dose related. Erythema, hyperpigmentation, hyperkeratosis, and even ulceration may occur when the drug is given in conventional daily doses for longer than 2 to 3 weeks. Areas of skin pressure, especially of the hands, fingers, and joints, are initially affected, and Raynaud phenomenon may become apparent in the distal digits. Nail changes and alopecia may also occur with continued use of the drug. In combination regimens (e.g., ABVD) where bleomycin is used intermittently, skin toxicity is rarely a problem.

Fever and malaise are common symptoms and may be alleviated with the use of acetaminophen. Hypersensitivity reactions have also been observed. Idiosyncratic cardiovascular collapse has been rarely noted. A 1- or 2-mg test dose administered to such susceptible patients may result in hypotension, tachycardia, pulmonary insufficiency, or anaphylactoid reactions within 30 to 60 minutes. Their occurrence precludes further treatment with bleomycin.

L-ASPARAGINASE

The enzyme L-asparaginase is used clinically in the treatment of lymphoid malignancies, particularly in poor-risk B-cell ALL, T-cell ALL, and in high grade lymphomas.

Mechanism of Action

The cells causing these lymphoid malignancies require exogenous L-asparagine for growth; they obtain this amino acid from the systemic pool of amino acids generated by the liver. The enzyme L-asparaginase, which catalyzes the hydrolysis of asparagine to aspartic acid and ammonia, rapidly depletes L-asparagine from plasma and induces an asparagine deficiency in lymphoid malignant cells. Resistant tumors are able to respond by induction of asparagine synthetase,[147] thereby restoring intracellular pools of asparagine. For reasons not well understood, hyperdiploid ALL cells are particularly sensitive to L-asparaginase, whereas cells containing the BCR-ABL translocation are more resistant.[148] *In vitro* incubation of leukemic cells with drug appears to predict sensitivity,[149] but is unproven as a useful tool for choosing therapy.

Three L-asparaginase preparations are available in the United States.[150] The product purified from *Escherichia coli* is employed as a first-line agent, while a second preparation (pegaspargase), derived by attachment of polyethylene glycol to the *E. coli* enzyme, is used for first-time therapy and for patients hypersensitive to the unmodified enzyme. A third preparation, purified from *Erwinia chrysanthemi*, can be obtained from the National Cancer Institute of the United States for patients hypersensitive to the *E. coli* enzyme, but is rarely used. The various preparations differ in their pharmacokinetics, immunogenicity, and recommended doses. The *E. coli* enzyme is usually given in doses of 6000 to 10,000 IU every third day for 3 to 4 weeks, although much higher doses (25,000 IU once weekly) may be more effective in ALL treatment. Levels are maintained continuously above 0.2 IU/mL plasma, leading to total abolition of asparagine in the systemic circulation. The *E. coli* enzyme has an elimination half-life of 14 to 24 hours. Monomethoxypolyethylene glycol (PEG) conjugated to the enzyme reduces its immunogenicity and extends its half-life to 6 days. PEG-asparaginase is used in patients hypersensitive to the unmodified enzyme, in doses of 2500 IU/m^2 intramuscularly every 2 weeks. Single doses deplete L-asparagine from plasma for 2 to 3 weeks. Some patients remain hypersensitive to both preparations of *E. coli* enzyme; enzyme from *Erwinia* has a low incidence of hypersensitivity and approximately equal catalytic activity to the *E. coli* preparation, but a more rapid clearance. Consequently, the *Erwinia* enzyme must be used in higher doses.

Adverse Effects

Reactions to the first dose are uncommon, but after two or more doses of the drug, hypersensitivity may develop in up to 20 percent of patients, varying from urticarial reactions to hypotension, laryngospasm, and cardiac arrest. Skin testing to predict allergic reactions is helpful in some, but not all, cases, and should be performed to confirm a clinical suspicion of hypersensitivity. Hypersensitive patients may have antibodies to L-asparaginase in their plasma. More than half the patients with such circulating antibodies will not display an overt allergic reaction to the drug, but these patients may have more rapid disappearance of drug from plasma and an inadequate clearance of asparagine from plasma and cells, leading to therapeutic failure. Patients who are treated with L-asparaginase should be observed carefully for several hours after dosing, and epinephrine should be available in case anaphylactic reactions occur. Anaphylaxis is less likely when L-asparaginase is given intramuscularly than when it is administered intravenously. PEG-asparaginase has much reduced immunogenicity and hypersensitivity reactions are uncommon.

The other major toxic effects of L-asparaginase are a consequence of the ability of this drug to inhibit protein synthesis in normal tissues. Inhibition of protein synthesis in the liver will result in hypoalbuminemia, a decrease in clotting factors, a decrease in serum lipoproteins, and a marked increase in plasma triglycerides. Inhibition of insulin production may lead to hyperglycemia. The clotting abnormalities that are regularly observed as a consequence of L-asparaginase treatment include initial decreases in the anticoagulant factors antithrombin III, protein C, and protein S, leading to either arterial or venous thrombosis in occasional patients, and a predilection to thrombosis of cortical sinus vessels.[151] With more prolonged therapy, bleeding sequelae may result from inhibition of the synthesis of procoagulant proteins such as fibrinogen and factors II, VII, IX, and X. Consequently, monitoring of coagulation factors is recommended. High doses of L-asparaginase may cause cerebral dysfunction that manifests as confusion, stupor, seizures, or coma, and cortical sinus thrombosis has been documented by magnetic resonance imaging scan in such patients.[152] Clinical thromboembolic episodes may occur in up to 35 percent of children with ALL.[153] These events are mostly asymptomatic thrombi associated with central venous catheters; less frequently, cortical sinus and atrial thrombi may occur. Preexisting clotting abnormalities, such as antiphospholipid antibodies or factor V Leiden, may predispose to thromboembolic complications.[154]

Acute nonhemorrhagic pancreatitis occurs as a complication of L-asparaginase treatment, especially in patients who have extreme elevations of plasma triglycerides (>2 g/dL).[155]

Because L-asparaginase manifests little toxicity in marrow or gastrointestinal mucosa, it has been used in combination with other drugs that do have such toxicities.

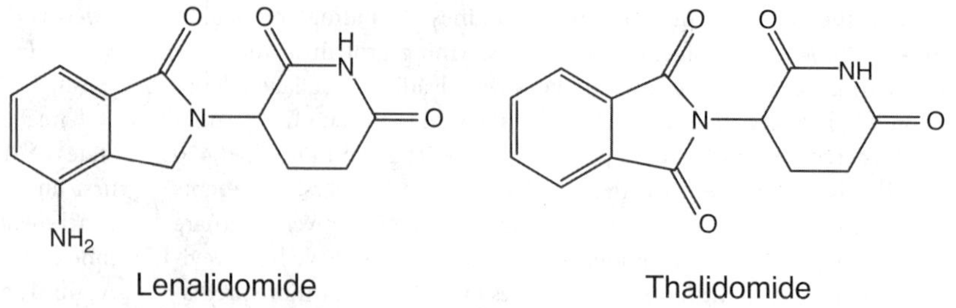

FIGURE 20–5. Thalidomide and lenalidomide. *(Reproduced from Brunton L, Lazo J, Parker K: Goodman & Gilman's The Pharmacological Basis of Therapeutics, 11th ed, chap 51. McGraw-Hill, New York, 2006. With permission from the publisher.)*

THALIDOMIDE AND LENALIDOMIDE

Thalidomide (α-phthalimidoglutarimide; Fig. 20–5), approved in 1953 as a sedative, was withdrawn shortly thereafter because of its teratogenicity. It causes dysmelia (i.e., stunted limb growth) when used during early pregnancy. However, it has since resurfaced as an antibacterial and antitumor agent, with clear effectiveness against leprosy and myeloma,[156] and its close analogue, lenalidomide has proven to be less toxic, and potentially more effective. Lenalidomide is approved for treating relapsed patients with myeloma, as well as for myelodysplasia in patients with the 5q− variant of this syndrome.

The mechanism of action of thalidomide and the newer analogue, lenalidomide, is poorly understood, and indeed may differ in various clinical settings, but there is considerable preclinical evidence for a number of different actions, including a prominent antiangiogenic effect against tumors,[157] immune modulation, and inhibition of cytokine secretion. It inhibits neovascularization in the mouse cornea, blocks proliferation of endothelial cells in culture,[158] and inhibits secretions of vascular endothelial growth factor and other angiogenic cytokines[159]; antiangiogenic effects have also been ascribed to lenalidomide. Thalidomide potently stimulates phosphorylation and activation of the CD28 costimulatory molecule.[160] This effect can lead to enhancement of T-cell function and activation of signaling pathways. Thalidomide has inhibitory effects on cytokine secretion, lowering levels of tumor necrosis factor-α and γ-interferon in leprosy patients. In addition it enhances natural killer cell numbers and function, suppresses T-regulatory cells, and stimulates cytolytic T-cell function. Although lenalidomide has not been studied as extensively as thalidomide, it likely has the same spectrum of action.

Clinical Pharmacology of Thalidomide and Its Congeners

Thalidomide consists of two enantiomers that rapidly interconvert in solution and biological fluid. Its two imide bonds are unstable and undergo hydrolysis in solution. The poorly soluble drug undergoes slow and somewhat variable oral absorption with peak levels achieved in 2.9 to 4.3 hours[161,162] after doses ranging from 50 to 400 mg. There is no evidence for induction of metabolism on a daily dosing regimen. Drug concentrations in plasma decay with a half-life of 5 to 7 hours, the major pathways for elimination including spontaneous hydrolysis of the imide esters, and further CYP-mediated metabolism by the liver. At high doses of 1200 mg, the rate of clearance of drug from plasma decreases. Less than 1 percent of the drug is excreted unchanged in the urine. No dose adjustment is required for renal dysfunction, although its neuropathy may aggravate an underlying neuropathy secondary to renal failure or amyloidosis.

Lenalidomide is well absorbed orally in doses up to 400 mg, and exhibits a plasma half-life of 3 hours. Approximately 70 percent of administered drug is excreted unchanged by the renal route. Dose adjustments are recommended for patients in moderate (10 mg/day for creatinine clearance of 30–50 mL/min) or severe (10 mg every other day for creatinine clearance <30 mL/min) renal failure.

Clinical Use

Thalidomide has been evaluated against a number of human malignancies, with occasional responses in brain tumors, renal cell cancer, hepatoma, and Kaposi sarcoma. It has established value in treating multiple myeloma refractory to first-line chemotherapy.[163,164] In responding patients, all aspects of the disease, including marrow infiltration with tumor cells, anemia, and performance status, improved with therapy. Thalidomide has synergistic myeloma-inhibiting activity with glucocorticoids, interferon-α, bortezomib, and cytotoxic agents. However, lenalidomide, which has less prominent side effects and probably equal efficacy, will likely replace thalidomide in first-line regimens for myeloma.

Thalidomide is generally well tolerated in doses of 50 to 1200 mg daily. In treating myeloma, a 1-month trial is usually sufficient to observe a decline in paraprotein and an improvement in symptoms. Doses can usually be escalated 200 mg every 2 weeks until dose-limiting toxicity is reached at 600 to 800 mg/day. Patients older than age 65 years are less tolerant of side effects, particularly sedation, constipation, fatigue, and peripheral sensory neuropathy, and receive a median dose of 400 mg/day,[165] whereas younger patients may tolerate up to a median of 800 mg/day. At doses below 400 mg/day, the peripheral neuropathy, primarily sensory in nature and related to cumulative dose, may become bothersome with extended treatment, but usually improves with dose reduction or drug discontinuation. To avoid undue sedation, the drug is given either in divided doses, morning and evening, or as a single evening dose. Other side effects include rash, dizziness and orthostatic hypotension, neutropenia, mood changes or depression, and nausea. Hypersensitivity and bradycardia also have been reported. Rarely patients may develop an interstitial pneumonitis or fulminant hepatic failure.

Trials of thalidomide in combination with cytotoxic drugs or biologics have disclosed unexpected toxicities.[166] Thalidomide in combination with doxorubicin or with prednisone is associated with an increased incidence of thromboembolism, a complication that can be prevented by concurrent treatment with low-molecular-weight heparin or aspirin.[167] Because of its teratogenicity, patients of childbearing age should take precautions to prevent pregnancy while on therapy. In trials of thalidomide and interferon against renal cell carcinoma, in which high doses of interferon (9 million IU subcutaneously three times per week) were used, 4 of 13 patients developed complex partial seizures and visual disturbances.[168] Two of 19 patients on low-dose interferon (1.5 to 3 million IU three times weekly) developed complex partial seizures in a trial against melanoma.

In the United States, thalidomide is approved for use under a special restricted distribution program, the System for Thalidomide Education and Prescribing Safety (STEPS).

The analogue, lenalidomide, with significant activity against myeloma, causes much less sedation, constipation, and neurotoxicity, but prominent myelosuppression in 20 percent of patients. It is proving to be highly effective in remission induction with bortezomib and prednisone or with prednisone alone. Used in doses of 25 mg/day for 21 of 28 days, it is dramatically effective in normalizing hematologic parameters in the subset of patients with myelodysplasia who have a 5q− deletion on cytogenetics. A gene expression profile characteristic of lenalidomide responders has been reported.[169] Lenalidomide produces dramatic tumor swelling (tumor flare reaction) and tumor lysis in patients with CLL, a potentially fatal complication, even in patients with disease refractory to conventional agents. In CLL, it is equally effective in patients with poor prognostic cytogenetics (chromosomes 11 and 17 deletions). To avoid acute tumor responses, it must be used in low doses (beginning at 2.5 to 5 mg/day and escalating thereafter) to avoid tumor flare reaction and renal failure.[170] It has rarely been associated with severe hepatic and renal toxicity.

Like thalidomide, lenalidomide in combination with anthracyclines or glucocorticoids causes a 15 percent incidence of thrombotic events, and in these combinations should be administered with low-molecular-weight heparin, although prospective trials of anticoagulation are lacking.[171]

DIFFERENTIATING AGENTS

Certain chemical agents have the ability to cause terminal differentiation (maturation) of malignant cells.[172,173] The most prominent among these are members of the vitamin A family (carotenes and retinoids), vitamin D and its analogues, phenylacetic acid, various cytotoxic agents used in low concentrations (such as hydroxyurea), inhibitors of DNA methylation such as 5-azacytidine and 5-aza-2′deoxycytidine or decitabine, and inhibitors of histone deacetylase, exemplified by vorinostat, depsipeptide, and various benzamides.[174] In addition, biologic agents such as the interferons and interleukins induce terminal differentiation of both malignant and normal cells, but the role of terminal differentiation in the anticancer action of these drugs in humans is uncertain, as they have multiple biologic effects.

■ RETINOIDS

As the first effective terminal differentiating agent in cancer therapy, all-*trans*-retinoic acid (ATRA) induces complete responses in a high percentage of patients with acute promyelocytic leukemia (APL), and has become a standard member of the combination regimen for treatment and cure of this disease.[175] ATRA acts through binding to a nuclear receptor formed by the heterodimerization of the retinoic acid receptor-α (RARα) and its partner, the retinoid X receptor. In APL, an abnormal fusion protein, composed of portions of the RARα and a unique transcription factor (the *PML* gene product) results from the characteristic 15;17 chromosomal translocation found in this disease.[176] The fusion protein has a lower affinity for retinoids than does the wild-type molecule. High concentrations of retinoids are required to displace a corepressor bound to the protein, and activate key differentiation factors such as C/EBP and PU.1.[177] The fusion protein forms a variety of homo- and heterodimers that regulate genes and increase leukemic stem cell renewal, suppress apoptosis and DNA repair, further contributing to progression of leukemia. In experimental settings, resistance to ATRA differentiating activity results from mutation or loss of retinoid binding in the *PML-RARα* fusion gene, indicating that the fusion gene product plays a role in retinoid responsiveness, and sensitivity can be restored by transfection of a functional *RARα* gene.[178]

ATRA is administered to APL patients in doses of 25 to 45 mg/m^2 per day until complete remission is achieved and reaches peak serum levels of 300 ng/mL 1 to 2 hours after administration.[179] It is also used in remission maintenance, with 6-MP, methotrexate, or ara-C. The parent drug disappears from serum with a half-life of less than 1 hour during the initial course of treatment, but its rate of clearance greatly accelerates with continued treatment, a factor that may contribute to resistance to ATRA therapy. Induction of CYP 26A1-mediated metabolism is suspected to underlie this accelerated clearance, and may account for the high rate of disease recurrence if ATRA is used as a single agent.[180] The primary toxicities of ATRA resemble those of other retinoids and vitamin A, specifically dry skin, cheilitis, mild and reversible hepatic dysfunction, bone tenderness and hyperostosis on radiography, hypercalcemia, hyperlipidemia, and occasional cases of pseudotumor cerebri. Imidazole antifungals block the degradation of ATRA and may lead to hypercalcemia and renal failure. In addition, approximately 15 percent of patients with APL, particularly those with an initial leukemic cell count greater than 5000/μL, develop a syndrome of hyperleukocytosis, fever, altered mental status, pleural and pericardial effusions, and respiratory failure (the "retinoic acid syndrome").[181] Hyperleukocytosis results from a rapid increase in the number of mature leukemic cells in the blood and from the increased expression of integrins on the leukemic cell surface and secretion of cytokines in response to ATRA. In patients with white blood cell counts above 20 × 10^3 cells/μL, pleural and pericardial effusions and peripheral edema develop rapidly, and respiratory distress, cardiac failure, and renal insufficiency may lead to death. Anecdotal reports indicate that high-dose glucocorticoids reverse this syndrome, which is mediated by leukocyte adhesion and clogging of small vessels and/or by cytokine release.[182] The early introduction of cytotoxic chemotherapy during remission induction, and the use of dexamethasone sodium phosphate (10 mg twice daily for 3 or more days in patients with initial leukemic counts of greater than 5000 cells/μL), drastically lower the incidence of the syndrome and improve the safety of ATRA therapy.

■ ARSENIC TRIOXIDE

In the 1930s, arsenic was used to treat CML and other malignancies with little effect. Based on further clinical trials of arsenic trioxide (As_2O_3) in Harbin, China, in 1992, it resurfaced as an impressively effective treatment for relapsed APL, and appears to also be active against multiple myeloma and myelodysplasia.[183,184] Its mechanism of action probably stems from its ability to promote free radical production.[185] It inhibits the detoxification of free radicals and inactivates glutathione, an important radical scavenger.[186] It promotes degradation of the PML-RARα fusion protein,[187] and upregulates p53 and proapoptotic proteins. The cumulative effect is to induce maturation and promote apoptosis in APL cells. In addition, it has antiangiogenic effects. The sum of these actions is potent antitumor activity in some but not all tumor cells. In APL patients refractory to ATRA and conventional chemotherapy (see Chap. 89), it produces strikingly durable complete responses, and is therefore under study as a part of primary treatment regimens for this disease.[186]

Patients are treated with a 2-hour IV infusion of 10 mg/day for 60 days, or until marrow remission is achieved, with further consolidation therapy beginning 3 weeks after remission. Remissions appear in 2 to 3 months after beginning doses of 0.15 mg/kg per day for 25 days every 3 to 6 weeks, with evidence of leukemic cell differentiation and a progressive blood leukocytosis after 2 weeks of therapy.[188] Side effects of arsenic trioxide in APL may include hyperglycemia, elevated liver enzymes, and hypokalemia, none of which require discontinuation of therapy. Occasional patients complain of fatigue, dysesthesias, and lightheadedness.

A pulmonary distress syndrome, similar to that encountered with APL cell maturation after ATRA therapy, occurs in approximately 10 percent of patients, and is managed with glucocorticoids, oxygen, and temporary withholding of arsenic trioxide. Arsenic trioxide prolongs the cardiac QT interval, and uncommonly produces atrial or ventricular arrhythmias; it is important to maintain serum K^+ at normal concentrations during arsenic trioxide therapy, and to avoid use of other drugs that prolong the QT interval, such as macrolide antibiotics, methadone, or quinidine.

Torsade de pointes occurs infrequently during arsenic trioxide treatment, but requires immediate treatment with intravenous magnesium sulfate, K^+ repletion, and defibrillation if the arrhythmia and hemodynamic instability persist.[189]

A maximum plasma concentration of 5.5 to 7.3 μM was achieved in the initial studies from China, and small amounts of drug and the methylated metabolite are eliminated in the urine, the rest remaining in tissues.[190]

INHIBITORS OF HISTONE DEACETYLASE

The most recent addition to the list of differentiating agents approved for clinical use against hematologic malignancies is vorinostat, or SAHA (suberoylanilide hydroxamic acid).[191] Vorinostat was derived from a series of planar-polar compounds that chelate Zn^{2+} and thereby inhibit the Zn^{2+}-dependent enzymatic activity of histone deacetylases (HDACs). This family of enzymes removes acetyl groups from amino groups of the lysines found in chromatin, thus promoting the compacting of chromatin and DNA and preventing gene expression; inhibitors of HDACs, such as vorinostat, decompact DNA from chromatin, promote the transcription of DNA, and cause terminal differentiation and apoptosis of tumor cells, with minimal effects on normal tissue. Vorinostat also inhibits the removal of acetyl groups from nonhistone proteins, but this activity has uncertain significance.

FDA approval of Vorinostat was based upon its ability to cause partial or complete responses in 30 percent of patients with cutaneous T-cell lymphoma (CTCL) after their tumor had progressed on at least two prior regimens.[192] Responses required a median of 55 days of treatment on a schedule of a single oral 400 mg per day, and lasted a median of 5.5 months. The drug undergoes inactivation by glucuronidation, followed by oxidation of its aliphatic side chain. The parent compound has a terminal half-life of 2 hours, although histones remain hyperacetylated for as long as 10 hours after an oral dose.

The drug causes minimal toxicity: mild to moderate fatigue, diarrhea, anemia, and minor decreases in the platelet count. Clinically significant thrombocytopenia occurs in 6 percent. Hydroxamic acids as a class cause lengthening of the QT interval, but no cardiac arrhythmias have not been attributed to vorinostat in its initial evaluation.

Other HDAC inhibitors, including depsipeptide, a complex natural product, have produced consistent responses in CTCL and peripheral T-cell lymphoma, and have entered advanced stages of clinical evaluation. Depsipeptide (Romidepsin, Istodax) has won approval for cutaneous T-cell lymphoma based on a 30 to 40 percent response rate in previously treated patients. Its toxicities include T-wave changes on EKG, QTc prolongation, mild myelosuppression, and fatigue.

SMALL MOLECULES WITH SPECIAL MOLECULAR TARGETS

■ BCR-ABL TYROSINE KINASE INHIBITORS

The first molecularly targeted drug to make a major impact on cancer treatment was imatinib mesylate (Gleevec), an inhibitor of ABL tyrosine kinase activity and notably the mutant ABL characteristic of the BCR-ABL fusion protein in chronic myelogenous leukemia. The uniform effectiveness of this agent has been ascribed to the unique role of the 9:22 translocation and the resultant BCR-ABL fusion protein in CML. This single molecular event produces growth factor independence and by itself is sufficient to cause and maintain malignant transformation in experimental settings.[193] The drug was selected for clinical study by scientists at Ciba-Geigy (later Novartis) based on a high throughput screen for kinase inhibition. Imatinib was the first drug of this class approved in 2001 for the treatment of CML based on the large phase III IRIS trial (International Randomized Study of Interferon and STI571), which showed induction of durable remissions in a large proportion of patients.[194,195] Since then two additional agents dasatinib (Sprycel) and nilotinib (Tasigna) have been approved for imatinib-refractory or intolerant patients (Table 20–5).

Mechanism of Action

Imatinib, nilotinib, and dasatinib (Fig. 20–6) are all inhibitors of the BCR-ABL kinase, as well as the c-KIT kinase[196] and the platelet-derived growth factor receptor kinase. The c-KIT kinase is the target for imatinib in the treatment of gastrointestinal stromal tumors,[197] while activating mutations of platelet-derived growth factor receptor are targeted by imatinib in the treatment of hypereosinophilia syndrome,[198] chronic myelomonocytic leukemia,[199] and dermatofibrosarcoma protuberans.[200] Dasatinib also inhibits the Src family kinases, an important secondary target in CML.[201] Dasatinib (IC_{50} [inhibiting growth by concentration 50%] = <1 nM)[201] and nilotinib (IC_{50} = <20 nM)[202] are both more potent inhibitors of BCR-ABL compared to imatinib (IC_{50} = 100 nM). Crystallographic and mutagenesis studies indicate that imatinib and nilotinib bind to a segment of the BCR-ABL tyrosine kinase domain that fixes the enzyme in a closed or inactive state, in which the protein is unable to bind its substrate, ATP.[202–204] The contact points between imatinib and the enzyme become sites of mutations in drug-resistant leukemic cells, preventing tight binding of the drug and locking the enzyme in its active configuration, in which it has access to substrate. Nilotinib has been modified to overcome 32 of the 33 point mutations to imatinib.[200–202] Dasatinib is unique in that it is able to bind BCR-ABL in both the active and inactive configuration, which may be one of the mechanisms that allows it to overcome resistance.[201]

Clinical Pharmacology

The BCR-ABL kinase inhibitors are all well absorbed by the oral route and subject to clearance by hepatic CYP 3A4 metabolism. Dasatinib's absorption is pH dependent and may be affected by the use of H_2 blockers or proton pump inhibitors. The bioavailability of nilotinib is increased if taken with meals and should therefore be taken on an empty stomach. Clearance is delayed in patients with renal dysfunction, apparently as a result of decreased P450 activity in the presence of renal failure. Limited data indicate that imatinib penetrates poorly into the cerebrospinal fluid, achieving concentrations of 1 percent of simultaneous drug levels in the systemic circulation.[205] There are no data about the penetration of nilotinib or dasatinib in the cerebral spinal fluid.

All three drugs are more than 96 percent protein bound, largely by α_1-acid glycoprotein, a binding protein present in higher concentrations in humans than in mice.[206] Thus therapeutic studies in mice may overpredict drug activity. α_1-Acid glycoprotein concentrations vary over a fourfold range in human subjects, and total drug concentrations in plasma appear to be a function of α_1-acid glycoprotein levels. Clindamycin displaces imatinib mesylate from binding to α_1-acid glycoprotein and, in mice, increases the concentration of drug found in cells.

Resistance to the tyrosine kinase inhibitors arises from point mutations in three separate segments of the kinase domain.[207] The most relevant of these mutations are those that hold the enzyme in its active conformation and maintain kinetic activity. The most common mutations associated

TABLE 20–5. Tyrosine Kinase Inhibitors in Treatment of CML

	Targets	Unique Pharmacokinetics	Mechanism of Clearance	Half-Life	Dosing	Drug Interactions	Toxicity
Imatinib	BCR-ABL, c-Kit, platelet-derived growth factor receptor (PDGFR)	98% bioavailability Transport via OCT-1	Hepatic Dose adjustments for severe hepatic and renal impairment	18 hours	Once daily 400–800 mg	CYP3A4 inducers (dexamethasone, phenytoin, carbamazepine, etc.) CYP3A4 inhibitors (aprepitant, clarithromycin, itraconazole etc.)	Dose-related fluid retention, heart failure, hepatotoxicity, nausea and vomiting, diarrhea, abdominal pain, skin reactions, myelosuppression
Dasatinib	BCR-ABL, c-Kit, PDGFR, Src family kinases	pH-dependent absorption	Hepatic	3–5 hours	Once daily at 100 mg or twice daily at 70 mg	CYP3A4 inducers (dexamethasone, phenytoin, carbamazepine, etc.) CYP3A4 inhibitors (aprepitant, clarithromycin, itraconazole etc.) Antacids, H_2 blockers, proton pump inhibitors	Fluid retention (>20%) including pleural and pericardial effusions, heart failure, hepatotoxicity, nausea and vomiting, diarrhea, abdominal pain, skin reactions, myelosuppression, QT prolongation (*in vitro*), hypocalcemia, hypophosphatemia
Nilotinib	BCR-ABL, c-Kit, PDGFR	Increased bioavailability if taken with food	Hepatic	17 hours	Twice daily at 400 mg	CYP3A4 inducers (dexamethasone, phenytoin, carbamazepine, etc.) CYP3A4 inhibitors (aprepitant, clarithromycin, itraconazole etc.) Drugs that prolong the QT interval	Fluid retention, heart failure, hepatotoxicity, nausea and vomiting, diarrhea, abdominal pain, skin reactions, myelosuppression, QT prolongation, hypocalcemia, hypophosphatemia, elevated serum lipase and amylase

with clinical resistance affect amino acids 255 and 315, both of which serve as contact points; these mutations confer high-level resistance to imatinib and nilotinib. Dasatinib can bind to both the active and inactive conformation and can overcome resistance to substitution at 255 but not 315.[204] Other mutations affect the phosphate-binding region and the "activation loop" of the domain with varying degrees of associated resistance. Some mutations, such as at amino acids 351 and 355, confer low levels of resistance to imatinib, with these tumor cells remaining sensitive to higher drug doses and also sensitive to both nilotinib and dasatinib.[204,208] This may explain the clinical response of some resistant patients to dose escalation of imatinib. Experimental studies of enzyme mutagenesis indicate that mutations in regions outside the kinase domain, and affecting interactions with proteins that dock with the kinase, can also confer resistance, but these have uncertain relevance to clinical resistance.[209]

Kinase mutations known to cause drug resistance may be detected in some patients prior to initiation of therapy, particularly in patients with Philadelphia chromosome-positive ALL[210,211] or CML progressing to blastic crisis. This finding strongly supports the hypothesis that drug-resistant cells arise through spontaneous mutation, and are further selected by drug exposure. Among CML patients, mutations are detectable in some patients receiving imatinib mesylate, including one-third of those undergoing treatment in the accelerated phase and in late (longer than 4 years from diagnosis) chronic phase CML.[212] Most patients with mutations demonstrate clinical resistance at the time a mutation is detected, or shortly thereafter. Mutations involving the phosphate binding loop are associated with rapid disease progression and death within a median of 4.5 months.

In addition to kinase mutation, amplification of the wild-type kinase gene, leading to overexpression of the enzyme, has been identified in tumor samples from a few patients with resistance to treatment.[213] The *MDR* gene, which codes for a drug efflux protein, confers resistance to imatinib experimentally[214]; thus far this mechanism has not been implicated in clinical resistance. In addition to efflux mechanisms, influx mechanisms may also play an important role. Recent studies indicate that imatinib but not nilotinib or dasatinib is taken into cells via the organic cation transporter-1 (OCT1) and that downregulation of this pathway may confer resistance.[215]

Not all resistance is explained by kinase amplification or mutation, or by pharmacokinetic factors. There is a growing awareness of the appearance of mutant Philadelphia chromosome-negative clones carrying the karyotype of myelodysplastic cells in patients receiving imatinib for CML, and a few cases of progression to myelodysplastic syndrome and AML have been reported.[216,217] Ongoing research into novel agents for resistant CML includes evaluation of histone deacetylase inhibitors, heat shock protein inhibitors, and third-generation kinase inhibitors.

Adverse Effects

Imatinib, dasatinib, and nilotinib have modest toxicity. All cause low levels of gastrointestinal distress including diarrhea, nausea, and vomiting. All can promote fluid retention including edema and pleural effusions, with dasatinib causing significantly more edema than the other drugs of this class.[218,219] Nilotinib causes a prolongation of the QT interval that is not seen in patients receiving imatinib.[219] All three drugs can induce neutropenia and anemia that can require transfusion support, dose reduction, or discontinuation. In addition, all three drugs in this class can be associated with hepatotoxicity. Most nonhematologic adverse reactions are self-limited and respond to dose adjustments. After the adverse events have resolved, many times the drug may be retitrated back to initial dosing.

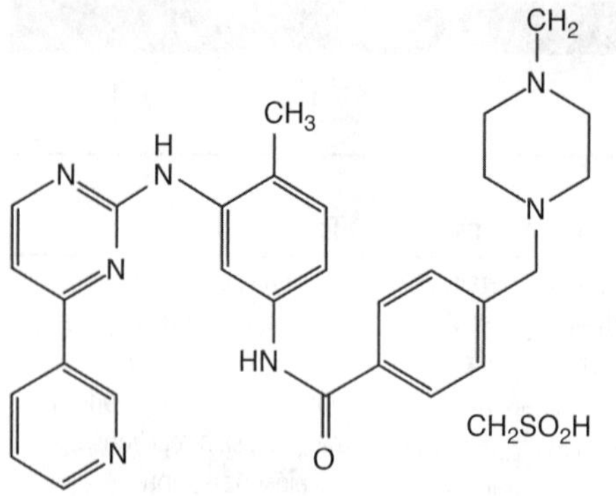

Imatinib

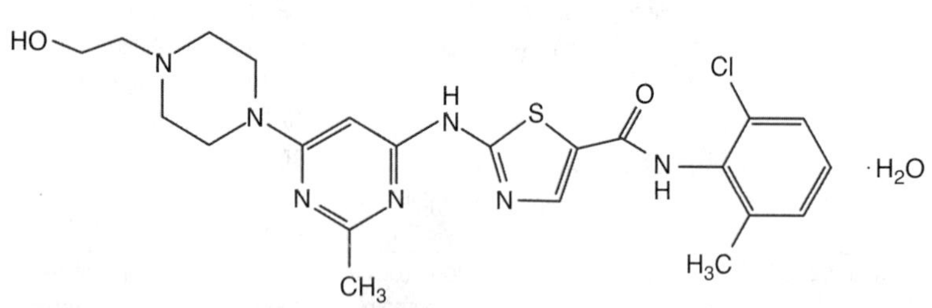

Dasatinib

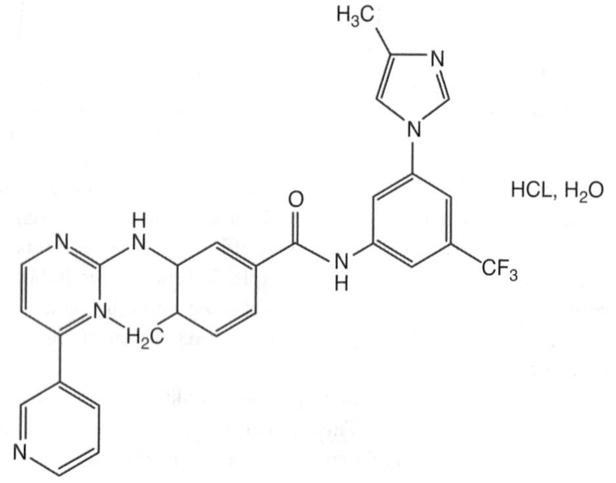

Nilotinib

FIGURE 20–6. BCR-ABL tyrosine kinase inhibitors.

■ BORTEZOMIB

As an unusual chemical entity with a unique mechanism of action, bortezomib (formerly referred to as PS-341) has attracted great interest in the field of cancer chemotherapy and now plays a central role in the therapy of myeloma. It is indicated for treatment of myeloma patients with relapsed or refractory disease,[220] for second therapy in myeloma,[221] and for previously untreated patients with myeloma, as well as for relapsed or refractory mantle cell lymphoma.[222] Bortezomib inhibits the chymotryptic-like activity of the 20S subunit of the proteasome, thereby altering the balance of intracellular expression of regulators of proliferation and survival in a manner conducive to rapid and irreversible commitment of myeloma cells to their death. As the first-in-class proteasome inhibitor, bortezomib validates the pathways for intracellular regulation of protein homeostasis as a therapeutic target for myeloma and mantle cell lymphoma, and potentially other cancers.

Mechanism of Action

Bortezomib is a dipeptide in which boron is covalently bound to a pyrazinyl-carbonyl side chain, which, in turn is attached to a phenyl group (Fig. 20–7). It inhibits the proteasome, a central regulator of the process of degradation of intracellular proteins. The proteosome consists of a multimeric 20S core particle that exhibits 3 distinct proteolytic activities (chymotryptic, tryptic and post-glutamyl peptide hydrolytic-like activities). Bortezomib potently (Ki = 0.6 nM) and reversibly inhibits chymotryptic-like activity through its binding to the β_5 subunit of the 20S core. This inhibition leads to accumulation of undegraded ubiquitinated proteins and interrupts the orderly recycling of their amino acid constituents. Accumulation of ubiquitinated protein triggers a state of cellular stress to which myeloma cells are typically quite sensitive because of their excessive production of myeloma protein. The bortezomib-induced accumulation of IκB, a proteasomal substrate, and the ensuing IκB inhibition of nuclear factor-κB may play a role in its antimyeloma activity, given the importance of nuclear factor-κB in myeloma pathophysiology, but this action cannot account for the full spectrum of effects triggered by proteasome inhibition. Thus, bortezomib induces accumulation of negative regulators of tumor cell proliferation, survival and drug resistance, such as IκB, p21, p27; it causes a perturbation in adhesive interactions of tumor cells with their neighboring stromal cells and downregulates cytokine production and inhibits angiogenesis.[223,224] The composite outcome of these actions is an irreversible commitment of MM cells to apoptosis.[223,224] Bortezomib sensitizes tumor cells to a broad array of other therapies including alkylators,[225] anthracyclines,[226] thalidomide and its derivatives,[227] and histone deacetylase inhibitors. Bortezomib is only a weak substrate for the MDR drug efflux system.

Clinical Pharmacology

The standard schedule of bortezomib administration is an intravenous injection at a maximum tolerated dose of 1.3 mg/m^2 on days 1, 4, 8, and 11 (twice weekly for 2 weeks, with a 10-day rest period). This dose inhibits the proteasome function of blood mononuclear cells by approximately 60 to 80 percent, and is associated with an acceptable safety profile and antitumor activity in both preclinical studies and clinical settings.[220,221] Indeed, at doses that demonstrate clinical activity, side effects are manageable and include thrombocytopenia (typically with nadir of platelet count toward the end of the

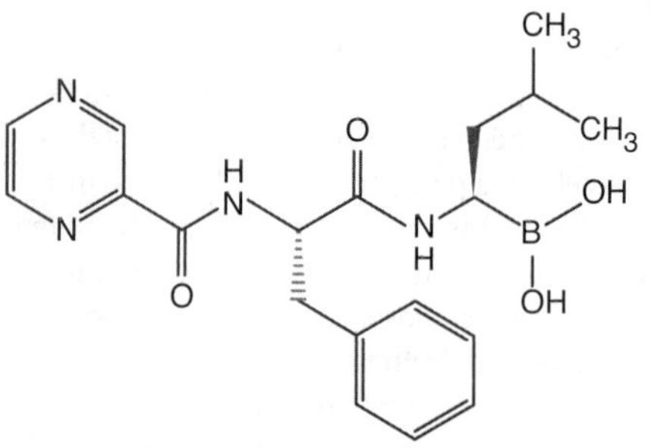

FIGURE 20–7. Bortezomib.

second week of each cycle and recovery by the end of the cycle), diarrhea, and fatigue.[220,221] Approximately 15 percent of bortezomib-treated patients may develop a painful sensory peripheral neuropathy, for which vigilant monitoring for detection of early patient symptoms and ensuing dose reductions are warranted. After each bortezomib use, proteasome function in healthy tissues returns to its baseline within 2 to 3 days. This observation is the basis for the administration of successive bortezomib doses at least 72 hours apart.

Bortezomib has a terminal $t_{1/2}$ of 5.45 hours and undergoes *in vivo* deboronation (which neutralizes its inhibitory effect on the proteasome) and then is hydroxylated by CYP 3A4 and 2D6. Because the parent compound is not excreted by the kidneys, bortezomib does not have to be dose-reduced in myeloma patients with renal dysfunction. Bortezomib has now become a key component of many regimens in which it is combined with other agents, such as prednisone, melphalan, lenalidomide, or thalidomide.[225–227] These combinations regimens have manageable side effects and produce impressive rates, depth, and durability of clinical response, even in patients with relapsed/refractory myeloma resistant to individual agent(s) of the respective regimens.

THERAPEUTIC MONOCLONAL ANTIBODIES

Monoclonal antibodies are an important class of agents for the treatment of hematologic malignancies. As a group, lymphoid cells express a variety of antigens that are attractive targets for monoclonal-based therapy, as shown in Table 20–5. Development of monoclonal antibodies against specific targets has been largely accomplished by the empiric method of immunizing mice against human tumor cells and screening the hybridomas for antibodies of interest. Because murine antibodies have a short half-life and induce a human antimouse antibody immune response, they are partially or fully humanized when used as therapeutic reagents. Presently, several monoclonal antibodies have received FDA approval for non-Hodgkin lymphoma and CLL, including rituximab and alemtuzumab. Although several mechanism(s) of action have been described for monoclonal antibodies, including direct induction of apoptosis, antibody-dependent cellular cytotoxicity (ADCC), and complement-dependent cytotoxicity, the clinically important mechanisms for most antibodies remain uncertain.[228]

Monoclonal antibodies may also be engineered to combine the antibody with a toxin (immunotoxin), or a radioactive isotope (radioimmunoconjugates), or to contain a second specificity (bispecific antibodies; Table 20–6).[229–231] For example, it is possible to conjugate an antibody with specificity to B-cell lymphomas with an antibody against CD3, which binds to and activates normal T cells, so as to enhance T-cell–mediated lysis of the lymphoma cell. One such example of a bispecific antibody contains anti-CD3 and anti-CD19 specificity. Monoclonal antibodies raised against the immunoglobulin idiotype on a B-cell lymphoma represent another therapeutic strategy, which was first reported in 1982 by Miller and associates.[232]

NAKED MONOCLONAL ANTIBODIES

Rituximab

Rituximab, the first monoclonal to receive FDA approval, is a chimeric antibody containing the human immunoglobulin G_1 and κ constant regions with murine variable regions. Rituximab targets the B-cell antigen CD20 expressed on the surface of normal B cells and on more than 90 percent of B-cell neoplasms, and is present from the pre–B-cell stage through terminal differentiation to plasma cells.[233] To date, the biologic functions of CD20 remain uncertain, although incubation of B cells with anti-CD20 antibody has variable effects on cell-cycle progression, depending on the monoclonal antibody type.[234,235] Monoclonal antibody binding to CD20 generates transmembrane signals that produce a number of events including autophosphorylation and activation of serine/tyrosine protein kinases, and induction of c-myc oncogene expression and major histocompatibility complex class II molecules.[236] CD20 promotes transmembrane Ca^{2+} conductance through its possible function as a Ca^{2+} channel.[237] These studies demonstrate the importance of CD20 in B-cell regulation, but do not in themselves indicate how ligation of the receptor produces cell death independent of ADCC or complement-mediated pathways.

Rituximab was initially approved as a single agent for relapsed indolent lymphomas, but has activity in other clinical settings: (1) in combination with chemotherapy for the initial treatment of follicular and diffuse large B-cell lymphoma; (2) in combination with chemotherapy for other indolent B-cell non-Hodgkin lymphomas (NHLs), including chronic lymphocytic leukemia, mantle cell lymphoma, Waldenström macroglobulinemia, and marginal lymphomas[238]; (3) and in combination with salvage chemotherapy for many indolent and aggressive B-cell NHLs.[240] Maintenance rituximab has gained increased acceptance based on its demonstrated ability to delay time to progression and more to improve overall survival.[240,241]

Rituximab is infused IV both as a single agent and in combination with chemotherapy at a dose of 375 mg/m^2. As a single agent it is given weekly for 4 weeks with maintenance doses every 3 to 6 months. It has a half-life of approximately 22 days.[242] Pretreatment with antihistamines, acetaminophen, and glucocorticoids have become a standard measure to modulate infusion reactions. During the first administration, the rate must be increased slowly to prevent infusional reactions. Infusions

TABLE 20–6. Monoclonal Antibody-Based Drugs

Target Antigen and Primary Cell Type	Function	Unlabeled	Radioisotope Based	Toxin Based
CD20: B cells	Proliferation/differentiation	Rituximab (chimeric)	^{131}I-tositumomab ^{90}Y-ibritumomab tiuxetan	None
CD22: B cells	Activation	Epratuzumab (humanized)	LL2 ^{131}Iodine, LL2 ^{90}Yttrium	BL-22 (*Pseudomonas* toxin)
CD52: B and T cells	Unknown	Alemtuzumab (humanized)	None	None
High-affinity IL-2R (CD25 α subunit): B and T cells	Activation	Daclizumab (humanized)	None	Denileukin diftitox (diphtheria toxin)

begin at 50 mg/h and in the absence of reactions, the rate increases in 50 mg/h increments every 30 minutes to a maximum rate of 400 mg/h. On subsequent cycles in the absence of reactions, infusions may start at 100 mg/h and increase in 100 mg/h increments every 30 minutes to a maximum rate of 400 mg/h. Patients with a large number of circulating tumor cells are at increased risk for tumor lysis syndrome and should receive a reduced dose of 50 mg/m^2 on day 1 of treatment in addition to standard tumor lysis prophylaxis. The remainder of the dose can then be given on day 3.

Resistance to rituximab may occur by down regulation of CD20, impaired ADCC, decreased complement activation, limited effects on signaling and induction of apoptosis, or inadequate blood levels.[228,243] Studies in relapsed indolent B-cell NHL suggest a correlation between higher mean serum rituximab levels and clinical responses,[244] implying that dose escalation may overcome rituximab resistance in some patients. Also polymorphisms in two of the receptors for the antibody Fc region responsible for complement activation, FcγRIIIa and FcγRIIa, predict the clinical response to rituximab monotherapy in patients with follicular lymphoma but not in patients with CLL.[245,246]

Toxicities Rituximab infusion causes reactions as a result of the murine component, which can be life-threatening in the absence of pretreatment with antihistamines. With pretreatment, symptoms are usually mild and include fever, chills, throat itching, urticaria, and mild hypotension, all of which can respond to decreased infusion rates and antihistamines. Rarely, rituximab infusion leads to severe mucocutaneous skin reactions (Stevens-Johnson syndrome). Rituximab, as a result of immune suppression, may reactivate hepatitis B infection, prompting the recommendation to screen patients for hepatitis B infection prior to initiation of therapy. It may lead, also, to progressive and fatal multifocal leukoencephalopathy caused by Jacob-Creutzfeldt virus.[248] Hypogammaglobulinemia and delayed neutropenia may appear 1 to 5 months after administration.[249,250]

Alemtuzumab

Alemtuzumab (Campath) is a humanized monoclonal antibody targeted against the CD52 antigen present on the surface of normal neutrophils and lymphocytes as well as most B- and T-cell lymphomas.[251] CD52 is expressed at reasonable levels and does not modulate with antibody binding, making it a good target for unconjugated monoclonal antibodies. Alemtuzumab can induce tumor cell death through ADCC and complement-dependent cytotoxicity.[25] The antibody is most useful in treating low-grade lymphomas and CLL, particularly in patients with disease refractory to fludarabine.[252,253] In refractory CLL, overall response rates are approximately 38 percent with complete responses of 6 percent in multiple series. In untreated CLL, overall response rates reach 83 percent, including complete responses of 24 percent.[253] The most concerning side effects are acute infusion reactions and depletion of normal neutrophils and T cells (Table 20–7). Opportunistic infections present a serious threat, particularly in patients previously teated with fludarabine.[254,255] Patients should receive prophylactic antibiotic against *Pneumocystis carinii* and herpes virus during treatment, and should be monitored for cytomegalovirus infection. Significant infectious complications have limited studies of alemtuzumab in combination with chemotherapy in T-cell lymphomas.[255]

IMMUNOTOXINS

Immunotoxins combine immune proteins such as antibodies, antibody Fab fragments, or interleukins and toxins (see Tables 20–6 and 20–7) such as ricin A chain or *Pseudomonas* exotoxin. These molecules have the advantage of the high specificity of the protein for its receptor or antigen, and its ability to internalize once bound to its receptor, together with the potency of the toxin molecule. As an example, one particularly potent molecule consists of bioengineered immunotoxin incorporating a single-chain variable-domain fragment fused to a 38-kDa truncated form of *Pseudomonas* exotoxin A (PE38). This molecule has particular efficacy against refractory hairy cell leukemia,[256] although it is not yet FDA approved.

Denileukin Diftitox

Denileukin diftitox (Ontak, DAB389 IL-2) combines IL-2 and the catalytically active fragment of diphtheria toxin.[257] The toxin fragment crosses into the target cell, carried in with its fusion partner which binds with high affinity to the human IL-2 receptor. Malignant T- and B-cell tumors express the high affinity form of the IL-2R, which is not expressed on normal resting T cells but is upregulated by antigen activation. The limited tissue expression of the high-affinity IL-2R makes this a selective target for cancer treatments. Denileukin diftitox causes hypersensitivity reactions, a vascular leak syndrome, and constitutional toxicities including fever, chills, and fatigue; glucocorticoid premedication significantly decreases toxicity. It may produce loss of color vision and diminished visual acuity. Antibody reactions to denileukin diftitox can be detected in virtually all patients after treatment, but do not preclude clinical benefit with continued treatment. Denileukin diftitox clearance accelerates in later cycles of treatment by two- to threefold as a result of development of antibodies, but its serum levels are greater than those required to produce cell death in IL-2R–expressing cells lines (1 to 10 ng/mL

TABLE 20–7. Dose and Toxicity of FDA-Approved Monoclonal Antibody-Based Drugs

Drug	Mechanism	Dose and Schedule	Major Toxicity
Rituximab	Antibody-dependent cytotoxicity, complement activation, induction of apoptosis	375 mg/m^2 IV infusion weekly × 4	Infusion related; late-onset neutropenia
Alemtuzumab	Complement activation, antibody-dependent cytotoxicity, possible induction of apoptosis	Escalation 3, 10, 30 mg/m^2 IV TIW followed by 30 mg/m^2 TIW for 4 to 12 weeks	Infusion-related toxicity with fever, rash, and dyspnea; T-cell depletion with increased infections
^{90}Y-ibritumomab tiuxetan	Targeted radiotherapy	0.4 mCi/kg IV	Hematologic toxicity, myelodysplasia
^{131}I-tositumomab	Targeted radiotherapy	Patient-specific dosimetry	Hematologic toxicity, myelodysplasia
Denileukin diftitox	Targeted diphtheria toxin with inhibition of protein synthesis	9–18 mcg/kg per day IV × 5 every 21 days	Fever, arthralgia, asthenia, hypotension

for longer than 90 minutes). Patients with a history of hypersensitivity reactions to diphtheria toxin or IL-2 should not be treated.

Clinically, denileukin diftitox produced an overall response rate of 49.1 percent at a dose of 18 mcg/kg per day in a double-blind, placebo-controlled phase III trial in 144 heavily pretreated patients with CTCL.[258] Denileukin diftitox received FDA approval for use in patients with recurrent CTCL in 2008. Its role in other T-cell lymphomas and in graft-versus-host disease is currently under investigation.

The vitamin A analogue, bexarotene, increases the level of high affinity IL-2 receptor expression on malignant T cells, a finding that has prompted studies of combinations of these agents.[259]

Gemtuzumab Ozogamicin

An alternative to unarmed antibody, or radiolabeled antibody, a potent chemical agent, which would otherwise become lethal to the host, may be linked to an antibody, and thereby directed to the specific tissue displaying the antigen. The success of this approach depends on stability of the antibody-toxin conjugate, the specificity of binding to tumor, and the ability of the bound antigen to internalize the antibody and release the chemical inside the cell. Gemtuzumab ozogamicin (Mylotarg), a humanized mouse antibody covalently linked to a potent chemical toxin, calicheamicin, exemplifies this approach. The antibody recognizes CD33, an antigen expressed by more than 90 percent of AML cells but not expressed on normal marrow hematopoietic stem cells (although it is expressed on myeloid progenitor cells). Calicheamicin dissociates from the antibody inside the cell and binds to the minor groove of DNA, producing strand breaks and caspase-9-dependent apoptosis.[260] Activation of calicheamicin depends on reduction of an internal disulfide, producing a di-radical that links to deoxyribose sugars on opposing DNA strands.[261]

The antibody conjugate produced a 30 percent complete response rate in relapsed AML, when administered at a dose of 9 mg/m^2 for up to three doses at 2-week intervals.[262] Most patients require two to three doses to achieve remission. It is currently approved in patients older than age 60 years with AML in first relapse who are not candidates for other therapies. Its primary toxicities include myelosuppression in all patients treated, and hepatocellular damage in 30 to 40 percent of patients, manifested by hyperbilirubinemia and enzyme elevations. Patients may manifest a syndrome that resembles hepatic venoocclusive disease when they subsequently undergo myeloablative therapy, or when gemtuzumab ozogamicin follows high-dose chemotherapy.[263,264] The cause of hepatic damage appears to be direct injury to sinusoids rather than venules. Defibrotide may prevent severe or fatal hepatic injury in patients receiving a stem cell transplantation following gemtuzumab ozogamicin.[265] Prolonged myelosuppression, particularly that affecting platelet recovery, has followed remission induction with gemtuzumab ozogamicin.[266] Trials are investigating gemtuzumab ozogamicin in combination with standard AML induction chemotherapy in the upfront setting in both older and younger adults.[266–269]

The pharmacokinetics of gemtuzumab ozogamicin are incompletely understood. Some free toxin is released in the bloodstream and undergoes hepatic degradation, perhaps accounting for the hepatic toxicity. Resistance to Mylotarg may result from export of the calicheamicin by the MDR transporter in tumor cells, modulation of CD33 expression,[270] or failure to saturate a high density of CD33 antigen on tumor cells.[271]

RADIOIMMUNOCONJUGATES

Radioimmunoconjugates allow monoclonal antibodies to deliver radioactive particles to specifically targeted tumor cells (see Tables 20–6 and 20–7).[229,230] ^{131}Iodine (^{131}I) is commonly used because it is readily available, inexpensive, and easily conjugated to a monoclonal antibody. The gamma particles emitted by ^{131}I are useful for imaging and therapy, but have the drawbacks of releasing free ^{131}I and ^{131}I-tyrosine into the blood and present a potential health hazard to caregivers. The beta-emitter ^{90}yttrium (^{90}Y) has emerged as an attractive alternative to ^{131}I, based on its higher energy and longer path length, and effectiveness in larger tumors. It also has a short half-life and remains tightly conjugated to antibody, even after endocytosis, providing a safer profile for outpatient use. Murine antibodies with either ^{131}I (tositumomab or Bexxar) or ^{90}Y (ibritumomab tiuxetan or Zevalin) have impressive responses rates of 65 to 80 percent in relapsed lymphomas.[229,230,272] Both drugs require significant collaboration between medical oncologists and nuclear medicine departments for administration. The administration of either Zevalin or Bexxar requires two steps: first a test dose to determine biodistribution and allow dose calculation, and a second step of actual therapeutic dosing. In each step, unlabeled antibody is first administered to saturate nontumor binding sites. When using Zevalin, an initial dose of Rituximab precedes an imaging dose of Zevalin conjugated to indium-111. Images are then collect by a gamma camera over a several day period. Once the conjugate's biodistribution is determined, a second dose of unconjugated rituximab saturates the low-affinity binding sites and the appropriate dose of Zevalin ^{90}Y is administered and distributes to high-affinity sites on the tumor. Bexxar administration follows a similar pattern of a dosimetric study, followed by a therapeutic step. These radioimmunoconjugates produce few side effects aside from marrow suppression related to the radionuclide. However, worrisome reports of secondary leukemias have dampened enthusiasm for their use. The anti-CD20 radioimmunoconjugates are being investigated as a consolidation therapy after chemotherapy, and for high-dose tumor ablation prior to stem cell transplantation.

REFERENCES

1. Goodman LS, Wintrobe MM, Dameshek W, et al: Nitrogen mustard therapy: Use of methyl bis (B-chlorethyl) amino hydrochloride for Hodgkin's disease, lymphosarcoma, leukemia and certain allied and miscellaneous disorders. *JAMA* 132:126, 1946.
2. Farber S, Diamond LK, Mercer RD, et al: Temporary remissions in acute leukemia in children produced by folic acid antagonist, 4-aminopteroylglutamic acid (aminopterin). *N Engl J Med* 238:787, 1948.
3. Devita V, Serpick A, Carbone P: Combination chemotherapy in the treatment of advanced Hodgkin's disease. *Ann Intern Med* 73:881, 1970.
4. Druker BJ, Tamura S, Buchdunger E, et al: Effects of a selective inhibitor of the ABL tyrosine kinase on the growth of BCR-ABL positive cells. *Nat Med* 2:561, 1996.
5. Shah NP, Skaggs BJ, Branford S, et al: Sequential ABL kinase inhibitor therapy selects for compound drug-resistant BCR-ABL mutations with altered oncogenic potency. *J Clin Invest* 117:2562, 2007.
6. Tallman MS: Treatment of relapsed or refractory acute promyelocytic leukemia. *Best Pract Res Clin Haematol* 20:57, 2007.
7. Slamon DJ, Leyland-Jones B, Shak S, et al: Use of chemotherapy plus a monoclonal antibody against HER2 for metastatic breast cancer that overexpresses HER2. *N Engl J Med* 344:783, 2001.
8. Vokes EE, Schilsky RL, Weichselbaum RR, et al: Induction chemotherapy with cisplatin, fluorouracil, and high-dose leucovorin for locally advanced head and neck cancer: A clinical and pharmacologic analysis. *J Clin Oncol* 8:241, 1990.
9. Seitz JF, Giovanni M, Padaut-Cesana J, Fuentes C: Inoperable nonmetastatic squamous cell carcinoma of the esophagus managed by concomitant chemotherapy (5-fluorouracil and cisplatin) and radiation therapy. *Cancer* 66:214, 1990.
10. Sauer R, Becker H, Hohenberger W, et al: Preoperative versus postoperative chemoradiotherapy for rectal cancer. *N Engl J Med* 351:1731, 2004.
11. Leichman L, Nigro N, Vaitkevicius VK, et al: Cancer of the anal canal: Model for preoperative adjuvant combined modality therapy. *Am J Med* 78:211, 1985.
12. Omura GA, Bundy BN, Berek JS, et al: Randomized trial of cyclophosphamide plus cisplatin with or without doxorubicin in ovarian carcinoma: A Gynecologic Oncology Group study. *J Clin Oncol* 7:457, 1989.
13. Bruno R, Hille D, Riva A, et al: Population pharmacokinetics/pharmacodynamics of docetaxel in phase II studies in patients with cancer. *J Clin Oncol* 16:187, 1998.
14. Maheswaran S, Sequist LV, Nagrath S, et al: Detection of mutations in EGFR in circulating lung-cancer cells. *N Engl J Med* 359:366, 2008.
15. Kruh GD, Zeng H, Rea PA, et al: MRP subfamily transporters and resistance to anticancer agents. *J Bioenerg Biomembr* 33:493, 2001.
16. Boorst P, Oude Elferink R: Mammalian ABC transporters in health and disease. *Annu Rev Biochem* 71:537, 2002.

17. Goker E, Waltham M, Kheradpour A, et al: Amplification of the dihydrofolate reductase gene is a mechanism of acquired resistance to methotrexate in patients with acute lymphoblastic leukemia and is correlated with p53 gene mutations. *Blood* 86:677, 1995.
18. Nimmanapalli R, Bhalla K: Mechanisms of resistance to imatinib mesylate in Bcr-Abl-positive leukemias. *Curr Opin Oncol* 14:616, 2002.
19. Fink D, Aebi S, Howell S: The role of DNA mismatch repair in drug resistance. *Clin Cancer Res* 4:1, 1998.
20. Kirsch D, Kastan M: Tumor-suppressor p53: Implications for tumor development and prognosis. *J Clin Oncol* 16:3158, 1998.
21. Holleman A, den Boer ML, de Menezes RX, et al: The expression of 70 apoptosis genes in relation to lineage, genetic subtype, cellular drug resistance, and outcome in childhood acute lymphoblastic leukemia. *Blood* 07:769, 2006.
22. Leong KG, Wang B-E, Johnson L, Geo W-Q: Generation of a prostate from a single adult stem cell. *Nature* 456:804, 2008.
23. Diehn M, Cho RW, Lobo NA, et al: Association of reactive oxygen species levels and radioresistance in cancer stem cells. *Nature* 458:780, 2009.
24. Moscow JA, Connolly T, Myers TG, et al: Reduced folate carrier gene (RFC1) expression and anti-folate resistance in transfected and non-selected cell lines. *Int J Cancer* 72:184, 1997.
25. Barrado JC, Synold TW, Laver J, et al: Co-administration of probenecid, an inhibitor of a cMOAT/MRP-like plasma membrane ATPase, greatly enhanced the efficacy of a new 10-deazaaminopterin against human solid tumors *in vivo*. *Clin Cancer Res* 6:3705, 2000.
26. Zhao R, Qiu A, Tsai E, et al: The proton-coupled folate transporter: Impact on pemetrexed transport and on antifolates activities compared with the reduced folate carrier. *Mol Pharmacol* 74:854, 2008.
27. Galpin A, Schuetz J, Mason E, et al: Differences in folylpolyglutamate synthetase and dihydrofolate reductase expression in human B-lineage versus T-lineage leukemic lymphoblasts: Mechanisms for lineage differences in methotrexate polyglutamylation and cytotoxicity. *Mol Pharmacol* 52:155, 1997.
28. Masson E, Relling MV, Synold TW, et al: Accumulation of methotrexate polyglutamates in lymphoblasts is a determinant of antileukemic effects *in vivo*. A rationale for high-dose methotrexate. *J Clin Invest* 97:73, 1996.
29. Synold TW, Relling MV, Boyett JM, et al: Blast cell methotrexate polyglutamate accumulation *in vivo* differs by lineage, ploidy, and methotrexate dose in acute lymphoblastic leukemia. *J Clin Invest* 94:1996, 1994.
30. Cheng Q, Wu B, Kager L, et al: A substrate specific functional polymorphism of human gamma-glutamyl hydrolase alters catalytic activity and methotrexate polyglutamate accumulation in acute lymphoblastic leukaemia cells. *Pharmacogenetics* 14:557, 2004.
31. Longo GS, Gorlick R, Tong WP, et al: Gamma-glutamyl hydrolase and folylpolyglutamate synthetase activities predict polyglutamylation of methotrexate in acute leukemia. *Oncol Res* 9:259, 1997.
32. Ge Y, Haska CL, LaFiura K, et al: Prognostic role of the reduced folate carrier, the major membrane transporter for methotrexate, in childhood acute lymphoblastic leukemia: A report from the Children's Oncology Group. *Clin Cancer Res* 13:451, 2007.
33. Assaraf YG, Rothem L, Hooijberg JH, et al: Loss of multidrug resistance protein 1 expression and folate efflux activity results in a highly concentrative folate transport in human leukemia cells. *J Biol Chem* 278:6680, 2003.
34. Stoller RG, Hande KR, Jacobs SA, et al: Use of plasma pharmacokinetics to predict and prevent methotrexate toxicity. *N Engl J Med* 297:630, 1977.
35. Evans W, Crom W, Abromowitch M, et al: Clinical pharmacodynamics of high-dose methotrexate in acute lymphocytic leukemia: Identification of a relation between concentration and effect. *N Engl J Med* 314:471, 1986.
36. Wall SM, Johansen MJ, Maloney DA, et al: Effective clearance of methotrexate using high-flux hemodialysis membranes. *Am J Kidney Dis* 28:846, 1996.
37. Schwartz S, Borner K, Müller K, et al: Glucarpidase (carboxypeptidase g2) intervention in adult and elderly cancer patients with renal dysfunction and delayed methotrexate elimination after high-dose methotrexate therapy. *Oncologist* 12:1299, 2007.
38. Shapiro WR, Allen JC, Horten BC: Chronic methotrexate toxicity to the central nervous system. *Clin Bull* 10:49, 1980.
39. Bloomfield CD, Lawrence D, Byrd JC, et al: Frequency of prolonged remission duration after high-dose cytarabine intensification in acute myeloid leukemia varies by cytogenetic subtype. *Cancer Res* 58:4173, 1998.
40. Stam RW, Den Boer ML, Meijerink JPP, et al: Differential mRNA expression of Ara-C sensitivity in MLL gene-rearranged infant acute lymphoblastic leukemia. *Blood* 101:1270, 2003.
41. Neubauer A, Maharry K, Mrózek K, et al: Patients with acute myeloid leukemia and RAS mutations benefit most from postremission high-dose cytarabine: A Cancer and Leukemia Group B study. *J Clin Oncol* 26:4603, 2008.
42. Lamba JK, Crews K, Pounds S, et al: Pharmacogenetics of deoxycytidine kinase: Identification and characterization of novel genetic variants. *J Pharmacol Exp Ther* 323:935, 2007.
43. Kufe DW, Munroe D, Herrick D, et al: Effects of 1-β-D-arabinofuranosylcytosine incorporation on eukaryotic DNA template function. *Mol Pharmacol* 26:128, 1984.
44. Owens JK, Shewach DS, Ullman B, Mitchell RS: Resistance to 1-β-D-arabinofuranosylcytosine in human T-lymphoblasts mediated by mutations within the deoxycytidine kinase gene. *Cancer Res* 52:2389, 1992.
45. Flasshove M, Strumberg D, Ayscue L, et al: Structural analysis of the deoxycytidine kinase gene in patients with the acute myeloid leukemia and resistance to cytosine arabinoside. *Leukemia* 8:780, 1993.
46. Capizzi RL, Powell BL: Sequential high-dose ara-C and asparaginase versus high-dose ara-C alone in the treatment of patients with relapsed and refractory acute leukemias. *Semin Oncol* 14(Suppl 1):40, 1987.
47. Cole BF, Glantz MJ, Jaeckle KA, et al: Quality-of-life-adjusted survival comparison of sustained-release cytosine arabinoside versus intrathecal methotrexate for treatment of solid tumor neoplastic meningitis. *Cancer* 97:3053, 2003.
48. Kern W, Kurrle E, Schmeiser T: Streptococcal bacteremia in adult patients with leukemia undergoing aggressive chemotherapy. A review of 55 cases. *Infection* 18:138, 1990.
49. Herzig RH, Hines JD, Herzig GP, et al: Cerebellar toxicity with high-dose cytosine arabinoside. *J Clin Oncol* 5:927, 1987.
50. Gandhi V: Questions about gemcitabine dose rate: Answered or unanswered? *J Clin Oncol* 25:5691, 2007.
51. Walter RB, Joerger M, Pestalozzi BC: Gemcitabine-associated hemolytic-uremic syndrome. *Am J Kidney Dis* 40(4):E16, 2002.
52. Claus R, Lubbert M: Epigenetic targets in hematopoietic malignancies. *Oncogene* 22:6489, 2003.
53. Ley TJ, DeSimone J, Anagnon NP, et al: 5-Azacytidine selectively increases gamma chain synthesis in a patient with β-thalassemia. *N Engl J Med* 307:1469, 1982.
54. Kantarjian HM, O'Brien S, Cortes J, et al: Results of decitabine (5-aza-2′-deoxycytidine) therapy in 130 patients with chronic myelogenous leukemia. *Cancer* 98:522, 2003.
55. Rodriguez CO Jr, Stellrecht CM, Gandhi V: Mechanisms for T-cell selective cytotoxicity of arabinosylguanine. *Blood* 102:1842, 2003.
56. Karran P, Attard N: Thiopurines in current medical practice: Molecular mechanisms and contributions to therapy-related cancer. *Nat Rev Cancer* 8:24, 2008.
57. Lennard L, Lillyman JS: Are children with lymphoblastic leukaemia given enough 6-mercaptopurine? *Lancet* 2:785, 1987.
58. Lennard L, Lilleyman JS, Van Loon J, Weinshilboum RM: Genetic variation in response to 6-mercaptopurine for childhood acute lymphoblastic leukaemia. *Lancet* 336:225, 1990.
59. Krishnamurthy P, Schwab M, Takenaka K, et al: Transporter-mediated protection against thiopurine-induced hematopoietic toxicity. *Cancer Res* 68:4983, 2008.
60. Stocco G, Cheok MH, Crews KR, et al: Genetic polymorphism of inosine triphosphate pyrophosphatase is a determinant of mercaptopurine metabolism and toxicity during treatment for acute lymphoblastic leukemia. *Clin Pharmacol Ther* 85:164, 2009.
61. Zimm S, Collins JM, Riccardi R, et al: Variable bioavailability of oral 6-mercaptopurine: Is maintenance chemotherapy in acute lymphoblastic leukemia being optimally delivered? *N Engl J Med* 308:1005, 1983.
62. Erb N, Janka-Schaub G: Pharmacokinetics and metabolism of thiopurines in children with acute lymphoblastic leukemia receiving 6-thioguanine versus 6-mercaptopurine. *Cancer Chemother Pharmacol* 42:266, 1998.
63. Harms DO, Gobel U, Spaar HJ, et al: Thioguanine offers no advantage over mercaptopurine in maintenance treatment of childhood ALL: Results of the randomized trial COALL-92. *Blood* 102:2736, 2003.
64. Jones TS, Yang W, Evans WE, Relling MV: Using HapMap tools in pharmacogenomic discovery: The thiopurine methyltransferase polymorphism. *Clin Pharmacol Ther* 81:729, 2007.
65. Keating MJ, O'Brien S, Lerner S, et al: Long-term follow-up of patients with chronic lymphocytic leukemia (CLL) receiving fludarabine regimens as initial therapy. *Blood* 92:1165, 1998.
66. Slavin S, Nagler A, Naparstek E, et al: Nonmyeloablative stem cell transplantation and cell therapy as an alternative to conventional bone marrow transplantation with lethal cytoreduction for the treatment of malignant and nonmalignant hematologic diseases. *Blood* 91:756, 1998.
67. Brockman RW, Cheng Y-C, Schabel FM Jr, et al: Metabolism and chemotherapeutic activity of 9-β-D-arabinofuranosyl-2-fluoroadenine against murine leukemia L1210 and evidence for its phosphorylation by deoxycytidine kinase. *Cancer Res* 40:3610, 1980.
68. Gandhi V, Plunkett W: Cellular and clinical pharmacology of fludarabine. *Clin Pharmacokinet* 41:93, 2002.
69. Martell RE, Peterson BL, Cohen HJ, et al: Analysis of age, estimated creatinine clearance and pretreatment hematologic parameters as predictors of fludarabine toxicity in patients treated for chronic lymphocytic leukemia: A CALGB (9011) coordinated intergroup study. *Cancer Chemother Pharmacol* 50:37, 2002.
70. Lichtman SM, Etcubanas E, Budman DR, et al: The pharmacokinetics and pharmacodynamics of fludarabine phosphate in patients with renal impairment: A prospective dose adjustment study. *Cancer Invest* 20:904, 2002.
71. Cheson B, Frame J, Vena D, et al: Tumor lysis syndrome: An uncommon complication of fludarabine therapy of chronic lymphocytic leukemia. *J Clin Oncol* 16:2313, 1998.
72. Cheson BD: Immunologic and immunosuppressive complications of purine analogue therapy. *J Clin Oncol* 13:2431, 1995.
73. Helman DL Jr, Byrd JC, Ales NC, et al: Fludarabine-related pulmonary toxicity: A distinct clinical entity in chronic lymphoproliferative syndromes. *Chest* 122:785, 2002.

74. Tam CS, O'Brien S, Wierda W, et al: Long-term results of the fludarabine, cyclophosphamide, and rituximab regimen as initial therapy of chronic lymphocytic leukemia. *Blood* 112:975, 2008.
75. Estey EH, Kurzrock R, Kantarjin HM, et al: Treatment of hairy cell leukemia with 2-chlorodeoxyadenosine (2-CdA). *Blood* 79:882, 1992.
76. Albertoni F, Lindemalm S, Reichelova V, et al: Pharmacokinetics of cladribine in plasma and its 5-monophosphate and 5-triphosphate in leukemic cells of patients with chronic lymphocytic leukemia 1. *Clin Cancer Res* 4:653, 1998.
77. Beutler E: Cladribine (2-chlorodeoxyadenosine). *Lancet* 340:952, 1992.
78. Crews KR, Wimmer PS, Hudson JQ, et al: Pharmacokinetics of 2-chlorodeoxyadenosine in a child undergoing hemofiltration and hemodialysis for acute renal failure. *J Pediatr Hematol Oncol* 24:677, 2002.
79. de Wolf C, Jansen R, Yamaguchi H, et al: Contribution of the drug transporter ABCG2 (breast cancer resistance protein) to resistance against anticancer nucleosides. *Mol Cancer Ther* 7:3092, 2008.
80. Bonate PL, Arthaud L, Cantrell WR Jr, et al: Discovery and development of clofarabine: A nucleoside analogue for treating cancer. *Nat Rev Drug Discov* 5:855, 2006.
81. Sanford M, Lyseng-Williamson KA: Nelarabine. *Drugs* 68:439; 2008.
82. Steis R, Urba WJ, Kopp WC, et al: Kinetics of recovery of CD4+ cells in peripheral blood of deoxycoformycin-treated patients. *J Natl Cancer Inst* 83:1678, 1992.
83. Halsey C, Roberts IA: The role of hydroxyurea in sickle cell disease. *Br J Haematol* 120:177, 2003.
84. Platt OS: Hydroxyurea for the treatment of sickle cell anemia. *N Engl J Med* 358:1362, 2008.
85. Sterkers Y, Preudhomme C, Lai J-L, et al: Acute myeloid leukemia and myelodysplastic syndromes following essential thrombocythemia treated with hydroxyurea: High proportion of cases with 17p deletion. *Blood* 91:616, 1998.
86. Madoc-Jones H, Mauro F: Interphase action of vinblastine and vincristine: Differences in their lethal action through the mitotic cycle of cultured mammalian cells. *J Cell Physiol* 72:185, 1968.
87. Cabral FR, Brady RC, Schiber MJ: A mechanism of cellular resistance to drugs that interfere with microtubule assembly. *Ann N Y Acad Sci* 46:748, 1986.
88. Dyke RW: Treatment of inadvertent intrathecal administration of vincristine. *N Engl J Med* 321:1270, 1989.
89. Rowinsky EK, Donehower RC: Paclitaxel (Taxol). *N Engl J Med* 332:1004, 1995.
90. Lopes NM, Adams EG, Pitts TW, et al: Cell kill kinetics and cell cycle effects of Taxol on human hamster ovarian cell lines. *Cancer Chemother Pharmacol* 32:235, 1993.
91. Zaffaroni N, Pennati M, Colella G, et al: Expression of the anti-apoptotic gene survivin correlates with Taxol resistance in human ovarian cancer. *Cell Mol Life Sci* 59:1406, 2002.
92. Anand S, Penrhyn-Lowe S, Venkitaraman AR: AURORA-A amplification overrides the mitotic spindle assembly checkpoint, inducing resistance to Taxol. *Cancer Cell* 3:51, 2003.
93. Gianni L, Vigano L, Locatelli A, et al: Human pharmacokinetic characterization and in vitro study of the interaction between doxorubicin and paclitaxel in patients with breast cancer. *J Clin Oncol* 15:1906, 1997.
94. Semb K, Aamdal S, Oian P: Capillary protein leak syndrome appears to explain fluid retention in cancer patients who receive docetaxel treatment. *J Clin Oncol* 16:3426, 1998.
95. Rivera E, Lee J, Davies A: Clinical development of ixabepilone and other epothilones in patients with advanced solid tumors. *Oncologist* 13:1207, 2008.
96. Ohno R, Okada K, Masaoka T, et al: An early phase II study of CPT-11: A new derivative of camptothecin, for the treatment of leukemia and lymphoma. *J Clin Oncol* 8:1907, 1990.
97. Beran M, Kantarjian H, Obrien S, et al: Topotecan, a topoisomerase I inhibitor, is active in the treatment of myelodysplastic syndrome and chronic myelomonocytic leukemia. *Blood* 88:2473, 1996.
98. Beran M, Estey E, O'Brien S, et al: Topotecan and cytarabine is an active combination regimen in myelodysplastic syndromes and chronic myelomonocytic leukemia. *J Clin Oncol* 17:2819, 1999.
99. Kantarjian HM, Beran M, Ellis A, et al: Phase I study of topotecan, a new topoisomerase I inhibitor, in patients with refractory or relapsed acute leukemia. *Blood* 81:1146, 1993.
100. Iyer L, King C, Whitington P, et al: Genetic predisposition to the metabolism of irinotecan (CPT-11). Role of uridine glucuronosyltransferase isoform 1A1 in the glucuronidation of its active metabolite (SN-38) in human liver microsomes. *J Clin Invest* 101:847, 1998.
101. Grochow LB, Rowinski EK, Johnson R, et al: Pharmacokinetics and pharmacodynamics of topotecan in patients with advanced cancer. *Drug Metab Dispos* 20:706, 1992.
102. Rowinsky EK, Kaufmann SH, Baker, SD, et al: A phase I and pharmacological study of topotecan infused over 30 minutes for five days in patients with refractory acute leukemia. *Clin Cancer Res* 2:1921, 1996.
103. O'Malley FP, Chia S, Tu D, et al: Topoisomerase II alpha and responsiveness of breast cancer to adjuvant chemotherapy. *J Natl Cancer Inst* 101:644, 2009.
104. Slamon DJ, Press MF: Alterations in the TOP2A and HER2 genes: Association with adjuvant anthracycline sensitivity in human breast cancers. *J Natl Cancer Inst* 101:615, 2009.
105. Gutierrez M, Chabner BA, Pearson D, et al: Role of a doxorubicin-containing regimen in relapsed and resistant lymphomas: An 8-year follow-up study of EPOCH. *J Clin Oncol* 18:3633, 2000.
106. Moreb JS, Oblon DJ: Outcome of clinical congestive heart failure induced by anthracycline chemotherapy. *Cancer* 70:2637, 1992.
107. Burstein HJ, Winer EP: Primary care for survivors of breast cancer. *N Engl J Med* 343:1086, 2000.
108. Shan K, Lincoff AM, Young JB: Anthracycline-induced cardiotoxicity. *Ann Intern Med* 125:47, 1996.
109. Lipshultz SE, Alvarez JA, Scully RE: Anthracycline associated cardiotoxicity in survivors of childhood cancer. *Heart* 94:525, 2008.
110. Mistry AR, Felix CA, Whitmarsh RJ, et al: DNA topoisomerase ii in therapy-related acute promyelocytic leukemia. *N Engl J Med* 352:1529, 2005.
111. Pedersen-Bjergaard J: Insights into leukemogenesis from therapy-related leukemia. *N Engl J Med* 352:1591, 2005.
112. Capranico G, Zunino F: Antitumor inhibitors of DNA topoisomerases. *Curr Pharm Des* 1:1, 1995.
113. Zwelling LA, Hinds M, Chan D, et al: Characterization of an amsacrine-resistant line of human leukemia cells. Evidence for a drug resistant form of topoisomerase II. *J Biol Chem* 264:16411, 1989.
114. Buggs BY, Danks MK, Beck WT, Suttle DP: Expression of a mutant topoisomerase II in CCRF-CEM human leukemia cells selected for resistance to teniposide. *Proc Natl Acad Sci U S A* 88:7654, 1991.
115. Stewart CF, Arbuck SG, Fleming RA, et al: Changes in the clearance of total and unbound etoposide in patients with liver dysfunction. *J Clin Oncol* 8:1874, 1990.
116. Winick N, McKenna R, Shuster JJ, et al: Secondary acute myeloid leukemia in children with B-lineage acute lymphoblastic leukemia treated with an epipodophyllotoxin. *J Clin Oncol* 11:209, 1993.
117. Ratain MJ, Kaminer LS, Bitran JD, et al: Acute nonlymphocytic leukemia following etoposide and cisplatin combination chemotherapy for advanced non-small-cell carcinoma of the lung. *Blood* 70:1412, 1987.
118. Peters WP, Shpall EJ, Jones RB, et al: High-dose combination alkylating agents with bone marrow support as initial treatment for metastatic breast cancer. *J Clin Oncol* 6:1368, 1988.
119. Yeager AM, Kaizer H, Santos GW, et al: Autologous bone marrow transplantation in patients with acute nonlymphocytic leukemia using *ex vivo* marrow treatment with 4-hydroperoxycyclophosphamide. *N Engl J Med* 315:141, 1986.
120. Reed E: Platinum-DNA adduct, nucleotide excision repair and platinum based anticancer chemotherapy. *Cancer Treat Rev* 24:331, 1998.
121. Gurubhagavatula S, Liu G, Park S, et al: XPD and XRCC1 genetic polymorphisms are prognostic factors in advanced non-small cell lung cancer patients treated with platinum chemotherapy. *J Clin Oncol* 22:2594, 2004.
122. Tew KD, Colvin M, Jones RB: Alkylating agents, in *Cancer Chemotherapy and Biotherapy: Principles and Practice*, 4th ed, edited by BA Chabner, DL Longo, p 297. Lippincott, Philadelphia, 2006.
123. Hilton J: Role of aldehyde dehydrogenase in cyclophosphamide-resistant L1210 leukemia. *Cancer Res* 44:5156, 1984.
124. Erickson L: The role of *O*-6 methylguanine DNA methyltransferase (MGMT) in drug resistance and strategies for its inhibition. *Semin Cancer Biol* 2:257, 1991.
125. Hunter C, Smith R, Cahill DP, et al: A hypermutation phenotype and somatic MSH6 mutations in recurrent human malignant gliomas after alkylator chemotherapy. *Cancer Res* 66:3987, 2006.
126. Droller MJ, Saral R, Santos G: Prevention of cyclophosphamide-induced hemorrhagic cystitis. *Urology* 20:256, 1982.
127. Leoni LM, Bailey B, Reifert J, et al: Bendamustine (Treanda) displays a distinct pattern of cytotoxicity and unique mechanistic features compared with other alkylating agents. *Clin Cancer Res* 14:309, 2008.
128. Gianni AM, Bregni M, Siena S, et al: Recombinant human granulocyte-macrophage colony stimulating factor reduces hematologic toxicity and widens clinical applicability of high-dose cyclophosphamide treatment in breast cancer and non-Hodgkin's lymphoma. *J Clin Oncol* 8:768, 1990.
129. Elias AD, Eder JP, Shea T, et al: High-dose ifosfamide with mesna uroprotection: A phase I study. *J Clin Oncol* 8:170, 1990.
130. Lazarus HM, Reed MD, Spitzer TR, et al: High-dose IV thiotepa and cryopreserved autologous bone marrow transplantation for therapy of refractory cancer. *Cancer Treat Rep* 71:689, 1987.
131. Peters WP, Henner WD, Grochow LB, et al: Clinical and pharmacologic effects of high dose single agent busulfan with autologous bone marrow support in the treatment of solid tumors. *Cancer Res* 47:6402, 1987.
132. Phillips GL, Wolff SN, Fay JW, et al: Intensive 1,3-bis(2-chloroethyl)-1-nitrosourea (BCNU) monochemotherapy and autologous marrow transplantation for malignant glioma. *J Clin Oncol* 4:639, 1986.
133. Ozols RF, Corden BJ, Jacob J, et al: High dose cisplatin in hypertonic saline. *Ann Intern Med* 100:19, 1984.
134. Shea TC, Flaherty M, Elias A, et al: A phase I clinical and pharmaco-kinetic study of carboplatin and autologous bone marrow support. *J Clin Oncol* 7:651, 1989.
135. Eder JP, Elias A, Shea TC, et al: A phase I-II study of cyclophosphamide, thiotepa, and carboplatin with autologous bone marrow transplantation in solid tumor patients. *J Clin Oncol* 8:1239, 1990.
136. Kessinger A, Armitage JO, Smith DM, et al: High-dose therapy and autologous peripheral blood stem cell transplantation for patients with lymphoma. *Blood* 74:1260, 1989.
137. Jones RJ, Piantadosi S, Mann RB, et al: High-dose cytotoxic therapy and bone marrow transplantation for relapsed Hodgkin's disease. *J Clin Oncol* 8:527, 1990.

138. Wilson WH, Jain V, Bryant G, et al: Phase I and II study of high-dose ifosfamide, carboplatin, and etoposide with autologous bone marrow rescue in lymphomas and solid tumors. *J Clin Oncol* 10:1712, 1992.
139. Dunphy FR, Spitzer G, Buzdar AU, et al: Treatment of estrogen receptor-negative or hormonally refractory breast cancer with double high-dose chemotherapy intensification and bone marrow support. *J Clin Oncol* 8:1207, 1990.
140. Umezawa H, Maeda K, Takeuchi T, et al: New antibiotics, bleomycin A and B. *J Antibiot (Tokyo)* 19:200, 1966.
141. Burger R: Cleavage of nucleic acids by bleomycin. *Chem Rev* 98:1153, 1998.
142. Sebti SM, Jani JP, Mistry JS, et al: Metabolic inactivation: A mechanism of human tumor resistance to bleomycin. *Cancer Res* 51:227, 1991.
143. de Haas EC, Zwart N, Meijer C, et al: Variation in bleomycin hydrolase gene is associated with reduced survival after chemotherapy for testicular germ cell cancer. *J Clin Oncol* 26:1817, 2008.
144. Alberts DS, Chen HSG, Liu R, et al: Bleomycin pharmacokinetics in man: I. Intravenous administration. *Cancer Chemother Pharmacol* 1:177, 1978.
145. Karmiol S, Remick DG, Kunkel SL, Phan SL: Regulation of rat pulmonary endothelial cell interleukin-6 production by bleomycin: Effects of cellular fatty acid composition. *Am J Respir Cell Mol Biol* 9:628, 1993.
146. Comis RL: Detecting bleomycin pulmonary toxicity: A continued conundrum. *J Clin Oncol* 8:765, 1990.
147. Hutson RG, Kitoh T, Moraga Amador DA: Amino acid control of asparagine synthetase: Relation to asparaginase resistance in human leukemia cells. *Am J Physiol* 272:1691, 1997.
148. Kaspers GJ, Veerman AJ, Pieters R, et al: *In vitro* cellular drug resistance and prognosis in newly diagnosed childhood acute lymphoblastic leukemia. *Blood* 90:2723, 1997.
149. Den Boer ML, Harms DO, Pieters R, et al: Patient stratification based on prednisolone-vincristine-asparaginase resistance profiles in children with acute lymphoblastic leukemia. *J Clin Oncol* 21:3262, 2003.
150. Holle LM: Pegaspargase: An alternative? *Ann Pharmacother* 31:616, 1997.
151. Semeraro N, Montemurro P, Giordano P, et al: Unbalanced coagulation fibrinolysis potential during L-asparaginase therapy in children with acute lymphoblastic leukaemia. *Thromb Haemost* 64:38, 1990.
152. Bushara KO, Rust RS: Reversible MRI lesions due to pegaspargase treatment of non-Hodgkin's lymphoma. *Pediatr Neurol* 17:185, 1997.
153. Michell LG, PARKAA Group: A prospective cohort study determining the prevalence of thrombotic events in children with acute lymphoblastic leukemia and a central venous line who are treated with L-asparaginase. *Cancer* 97:508, 2003.
154. Nowak-Gottl U, Wermes C, Junker R, et al: Prospective evaluation of the thrombotic risk in children with acute lymphoblastic leukemia carrying the MTHFR TT 677 genotype, the prothrombin G20210A variant, and further prothrombotic risk factors. *Blood* 93:1595, 1999.
155. Parsons SK, Skapek SX, Neufeld EJ, et al: Asparaginase-associated lipid abnormalities in children with acute lymphoblastic leukemia. *Blood* 89:1886, 1997.
156. Strobeck M. Multiple myeloma therapies. *Nat Rev Drug Discov* 6:181, 2007.
157. D'Amato RJ, Loughnan MS, Flynn E, et al: Thalidomide is an inhibitor of angiogenesis. *Proc Natl Acad Sci U S A* 91:4082, 1994.
158. Moreira AL, Friedlander DR, Shif B, et al: Thalidomide and a thalidomide analogue inhibit endothelial cell proliferation *in vitro*. *J Neurooncol* 43:109, 1999.
159. Mueller G, Chen R, Huang SY. et al: Amino-substituted thalidomide analogs: Potent inhibitors of TNF-alpha production. *Bioorg Med Chem Lett* 9:1625, 1999.
160. LeBlanc R, Hideshia T, Catley L, et al: Immunomodulatory drug co-stimulates T-cells via B7-CD28 pathway. *Blood* 103:1787, 2004.
161. Richardson PG, Schlossman RL, Weller E, et al: Immunomodulatory drug CC-5013 Overcomes drug resistance and is well tolerated in patients with relapsed multiple myeloma. *Blood* 100:3063, 2002.
162. Teo SK, Scheffler MR, Kook KA, et al: Thalidomide dose proportionality assessment following single doses to healthy subjects. *J Clin Pharmacol* 41:662, 2001.
163. Piscitelli SC, Figg WD, Hahn B, et al: Single-dose pharmacokinetics of thalidomide in human immunodeficiency virus-infected patients. *Antimicrob Agents Chemother* 41:2797, 1997.
164. Singhal S, Mehta J, Desikan R, et al: Antitumor activity of thalidomide in refractory multiple myeloma. *N Engl J Med* 341:1565, 1999.
165. Mileshikin L, Biagi J, Underhil C, et al: Multicenter phase 2 trial of thalidomide in relapsed/refractory multiple myeloma: Adverse prognostic impact of advanced age. *Blood* 102:69, 2003.
166. Rajkumar SV, Hayman S, Gertz M, et al: Combination therapy with thalidomide plus dexamethasone for newly diagnosed myeloma. *J Clin Oncol* 20:4319, 2002.
167. Musallam KM, Dahdaleh FS, Shamseddine AI, Taher AT: Incidence and prophylaxis of venous thromboembolic events in multiple myeloma patients receiving immunomodulatory therapy. *Thromb Res* 123:679, 2008.
168. Nathan PD, Gore ME, Eisen TG: Unexpected toxicity of combination thalidomide and interferon-alpha-2a treatment in metastatic renal cell carcinoma. *J Clin Oncol* 20:1429, 2002.
169. Ebert BL, Galili N, Tamayo P, et al: An erythroid differentiation signature predicts response to lenalidomide in myelodysplastic syndrome. *PLoS Med* 5:e35, 2008.
170. Andritsos LA, Johnson AJ, Lozanski G, et al: Higher doses of lenalidomide are associated with unacceptable toxicity including life-threatening tumor flare in patients with chronic lymphocytic leukemia. *J Clin Oncol* 26:2519, 2008.
171. Weber DM, Chen C, Niesvizky R, et al: Lenalidomide plus dexamethasone for relapsed multiple myeloma in North America. *N Engl J Med* 357:2133, 2007.
172. Kizaki M, Nakazato T, Ito K, et al: A novel therapeutic approach for hematological malignancies based on cellular differentiation and apoptosis. *Int J Hematol* 1(Suppl 1):250, 2002.
173. Parkinson DR, Smith MA: Retinoid therapy for acute promyelocytic leukemia: A coming of age for the differentiation therapy of malignancy [editorial]. *Ann Intern Med* 117:338, 1992.
174. Sandor V, Bakke S, Robey RW, et al: Phase I trial of the histone deacetylase inhibitor, depsipeptide (FR901228, NSC 630176), in patients with refractory neoplasms. *Clin Cancer Res* 8:718, 2002.
175. Warrell RP Jr, Frankel SR, Miller WH Jr, et al: Differentiation therapy of acute promyelocytic leukemia with tretinoin (all-*trans*-retinoic acid). *N Engl J Med* 324:1385, 1991.
176. Kazizuka A, Miller WH Jr, Umesono K, et al: Chromosomal translocation t(15;17) in human acute promyelocytic leukemia fuses RARα with a novel putative transcription factor, PML. *Cell* 66:663, 1991.
177. Collins SJ: Retinoic acid receptors, hematopoiesis and leukemogenesis. *Curr Opin Hematol* 15:346, 2008.
178. Robertson KA, Emami B, Collins SJ: Retinoic acid-resistant HL-60R cells harbor a point mutation in the retinoic acid receptor ligand binding domain that confers dominant negative activity. *Blood* 80:1885, 1992.
179. Muindi JRF, Frankel SR, Huselton C, et al: Clinical pharmacology of oral all-*trans*-retinoic acid in patients with acute promyelocytic leukemia. *Cancer Res* 52:2138, 1992.
180. Muindi J, Frankel SR, Miller WH Jr, et al: Continuous treatment with all-*trans*-retinoic acid causes a progressive reduction in plasma drug concentrations: Implications for relapse and retinoid "resistance" in patients with acute promyelocytic leukemia. *Blood* 79:299, 1992.
181. Frankel SR, Eardley A, Lauwers G, et al: The "retinoic acid syndrome" in acute promyelocytic leukemia. *Ann Intern Med* 117:292, 1992.
182. De Botton S, Dombret H, Sanz M, et al: Incidence, clinical features, and outcome of all-*trans*-retinoic acid syndrome in 413 cases of newly diagnosed acute promyelocytic leukemia. *Blood* 92:2712, 1998.
183. Soignet SL, Maslak P, Wang Z-G, et al: Complete remission after treatment of acute promyelocytic leukemia with arsenic trioxide. *N Engl J Med* 339:1341, 1998.
184. List AF, Schiller GJ, Mason J, et al: Trisenox (arsenic trioxide) in patients with myelodysplastic syndromes (MDS): Preliminary findings in a phase 2 clinical study [abstract]. *Blood* 102:423a, 2003.
185. Miller WH Jr, Schipper HM, Lee JS, et al: Mechanisms of action of arsenic trioxide. *Cancer Res* 62:3893, 2002.
186. Wang ZY, Chen Z: Acute promyelocytic leukemia: From highly fatal to highly curable. *Blood* 111:2505, 2008.
187. Lallemand-Breitenbach V, Jeanne M, Benhenda S, et al: Arsenic degrades PML or PML-RARalpha through a SUMO-triggered RNF4/ubiquitin-mediated pathway. *Nat Cell Biol* 10:547, 2008.
188. Chen G-Q, Shi X-G, Tang W, et al: Use of arsenic trioxide (As_2O_3) in the treatment of acute promyelocytic leukemia (APL): I. As_2O_3 exerts dose-dependent dual effects on APL cells. *Blood* 89:3345, 1997.
189. Gupta A, Lawrence AT, Krishnan K, et al: Current concepts in the mechanisms and management of drug-induced QT prolongation and torsade de pointes. *Am Heart J* 153:891, 2007.
190. Shen Z-X, Chen G-Q, Ni J-H, et al: Use of arsenic trioxide (As_2O_3) in the treatment of acute promyelocytic leukemia (APL): II. Clinical efficacy and pharmacokinetics in relapsed patients. *Blood* 89:3354, 1997.
191. Minucci S, Pelicci: PG Histone Deacetylase Inhibitors and the Promise of Epigenetic (and more) Treatments for Cancer. *Nat Rev Cancer* 6:38, 2006.
192. Mann BS, Johnson JR, Cohen, MH, et. al: FDA approval summary: Vorinostat for treatment of advanced primary cutaneous T-cell lymphoma. *Oncologist* 12:1247, 2007.
193. Druker BJ: Perspectives on the development of a molecularly targeted agent. *Cancer Cell* 1:31, 2002.
194. O'Brien SG, Guilhot F, Larson RA, et al: Imatinib compared with interferon and low-dose cytarabine for newly diagnosed chronic-phase chronic myeloid leukemia. *N Engl J Med* 348:994, 2003.
195. Druker BJ, Guilhot F, O'Brien SG, et al: Five-year follow-up of patients receiving imatinib for chronic myeloid leukemia. *N Engl J Med* 355:2408, 2006.
196. Heinrich MC, Griffith DJ, Druker BJ, et al: Inhibition of c-kit receptor tyrosine kinase activity by STI 571, a selective tyrosine kinase inhibitor. *Blood* 96:925, 2000.
197. Demetri GD, von Mehren M, Blanke CD, et al: Efficacy and safety of imatinib mesylate in advanced gastrointestinal stromal tumors. *N Engl J Med* 347:472, 2002.
198. Cools J, DeAngelo DJ, Gotlib J, et al: A tyrosine kinase created by fusion of the PDGFRA and FIP1L1 genes as a therapeutic target of imatinib in idiopathic hypereosinophilic syndrome. *N Engl J Med* 348:1201, 2003.
199. Magnusson MK, Meade KE, Nakamura R, et al: Activity of STI571 in chronic myelomonocytic leukemia with a platelet-derived growth factor beta receptor fusion oncogene. *Blood* 100:1088, 2002.
200. Sirvent N, Maire G, Pedeutour F: Genetics of dermatofibrosarcoma protuberans family of tumors: From ring chromosomes to tyrosine kinase inhibitor treatment. *Genes Chromosomes Cancer* 37:1, 2003.
201. Shah NP, Tran C, Lee FY, et al: Overriding imatinib resistance with a novel ABL kinase inhibitor. *Science* 305:399, 2004.
202. Weisberg E, Manley PW, Breitenstein W, et al: Characterization of AMN107, a selective inhibitor of native and mutant bcr-abl. *Cancer Cell* 7:129, 2005.
203. Wisniewski D, Lambek CL, Liu C, et al: Characterization of potent inhibitors of the bcr-abl and the c-kit receptor tyrosine kinases. *Cancer Res* 62:4244, 2002.

204. O'Hare T, Walters DK, Stoffregen EP, et al: *In vitro* activity of bcr-abl inhibitors AMN107 and BMS-354825 against clinically relevant imatinib-resistant abl kinase domain mutants. *Cancer Res* 65:4500, 2005.
205. Takayama N, Sato N, O'Brien SG, et al: Imatinib mesylate has limited activity against the central nervous system involvement of Philadelphia chromosome-positive acute lymphoblastic leukaemia due to poor penetration into cerebrospinal fluid. *Br J Haematol* 119:106, 2002.
206. Gambacorti-Passerini C, Zucchetti M, Russo D, et al: Alpha1 acid glycoprotein binds to imatinib (STI571) and substantially alters its pharmacokinetics in chronic myeloid leukemia patients. *Clin Cancer Res* 9:625, 2003.
207. Shah NP, Nicoll JM, Nagar B, et al: Multiple BCR-ABL kinase domain mutations confer polyclonal resistance to the tyrosine kinase inhibitor imatinib (STI571) in chronic phase and blast crisis chronic myeloid leukemia. *Cancer Cell* 2:117, 2002.
208. Corbin AS, La Rosee P, Stoffregen EP, et al: Several bcr-abl kinase domain mutants associated with imatinib mesylate resistance remain sensitive to imatinib. *Blood* 101:4611, 2003.
209. Azam M, Latek RR, Daley GQ: Mechanisms of autoinhibition and STI-571/imatinib resistance revealed by mutagenesis of BCR-ABL. *Cell* 112:831, 2003.
210. Roche-Lestienne C, Lai JL, Darre S, et al: A mutation conferring resistance to imatinib at the time of diagnosis of chronic myelogenous leukemia. *N Engl J Med* 348:2265, 2003.
211. Hofmann WK, Komor M, Wassmann B, et al: Presence of the BCR-ABL mutation Glu255Lys prior to STI571 (imatinib) treatment in patients with Ph+ acute lymphoblastic leukemia. *Blood* 102:659, 2003.
212. Branford S, Rudzki Z, Walsh S, et al: Detection of BCR-ABL mutations in patients with CML treated with imatinib is virtually always accompanied by clinical resistance, and mutations in the ATP phosphate-binding loop (P-loop) are associated with a poor prognosis. *Blood* 102:276, 2003.
213. Morel F, Bris MJ, Herry A, et al: Double minutes containing amplified bcr-abl fusion gene in a case of chronic myeloid leukemia treated by imatinib. *Eur J Haematol* 70:235, 2003.
214. Mahon FX, Belloc F, Lagarde V, et al: MDR1 gene overexpression confers resistance to imatinib mesylate in leukemia cell line models. *Blood* 101:2368, 2003.
215. White DL, Saunders VA, Dang P, et al: OCT-1-mediated influx is a key determinant of the intracellular uptake of imatinib but not nilotinib (AMN107): Reduced OCT-1 activity is the cause of low in vitro sensitivity to imatinib. *Blood* 108:697, 2006.
216. Bumm T, Muller C, Al-Ali HK, et al: Emergence of clonal cytogenetic abnormalities in Ph– cells in some CML patients in cytogenetic remission to imatinib but restoration of polyclonal hematopoiesis in the majority. *Blood* 101:1941, 2003.
217. Andersen MK, Pedersen-Bjergaard J, Kjeldsen L, et al: Clonal Ph-negative hematopoiesis in CML after therapy with imatinib mesylate is frequently characterized by trisomy 8. *Leukemia* 16:1390, 2002.
218. Talpaz M, Shah NP, Kantarjian H, et al: Dasatinib in imatinib-resistant Philadelphia chromosome-positive leukemias. *N Engl J Med* 354:2531, 2006.
219. Kantarjian HM, Giles F, Gattermann N, et al: Nilotinib (formerly AMN107), a highly selective BCR-ABL tyrosine kinase inhibitor, is effective in patients with Philadelphia chromosome-positive chronic myelogenous leukemia in chronic phase following imatinib resistance and intolerance. *Blood* 110:3540, 2007.
220. Richardson PG, Barlogie B, Berenson J, et al: A phase 2 study of bortezomib in relapsed, refractory myeloma. *N Engl J Med* 348:2609, 2003.
221. Richardson PG, Sonneveld P, Schuster MW, et al: Bortezomib or high-dose dexamethasone for relapsed multiple myeloma. *N Engl J Med* 352:2487, 2005.
222. O'Connor OA, Wright J, Moskowitz C, et al: Phase II clinical experience with the novel proteasome inhibitor bortezomib in patients with indolent non-Hodgkin's lymphoma and mantle cell lymphoma. *J Clin Oncol* 23:676, 2005.
223. Mitsiades N, Mitsiades CS, Poulaki V, et al: Molecular sequelae of proteasome inhibition in human multiple myeloma cells. *Proc Natl Acad Sci U S A* 99:14374, 2002.
224. Hideshima T, Richardson P, Chauhan D, et al: The proteasome inhibitor PS-341 inhibits growth, induces apoptosis, and overcomes drug resistance in human multiple myeloma cells. *Cancer Res* 61:3071, 2001.
225. San Miguel JF, Schlag R, Khuageva NK, et al: Bortezomib plus melphalan and prednisone for initial treatment of multiple myeloma. *N Engl J Med* 359:906, 2008.
226. Orlowski RZ, Nagler A, Sonneveld P, et al: Randomized phase III study of pegylated liposomal doxorubicin plus bortezomib compared with bortezomib alone in relapsed or refractory multiple myeloma: Combination therapy improves time to progression. *J Clin Oncol* 25:3892, 2007.
227. Richardson P, Jagannath S, Raje N, et al: Lenalidomide, bortezomib, and dexamethasone (Rev/Vel/Dex) in patients with relapsed or relapsed/refractory multiple myeloma (MM): Preliminary results of a phase II study. *Blood* 110:797A, 2007.
228. Maloney DG, Smith B, Rose A: Rituximab: Mechanism of action and resistance. *Semin Oncol* 29(1 Suppl 2):2, 2002.
229. Horning SJ, Younes A, Jain V, et al. Efficacy and safety of tositumomab and iodine-131 tositumomab (Bexxar) in B-cell lymphoma, progressive after rituximab. *J Clin Oncol* 23:712, 2005.
230. Witzig TE, Gordon LI, Cabanillas F, et al: Randomized controlled trial of yttrium-90-labeled ibritumomab tiuxetan radioimmunotherapy versus rituximab immunotherapy for patients with relapsed or refractory low-grade, follicular, or transformed B-cell non-Hodgkin's lymphoma. *J Clin Oncol* 20:2453, 2002.
231. Dang NH, Pro B, Hagemeister FB, et al: Phase II trial of denileukin diftitox for relapsed/refractory T-cell non-Hodgkin lymphoma. *Br J Haematol* 136:439, 2007.
232. Miller RA, Maloney DG, Warnke R, Levy R: Treatment of B-cell lymphoma with monoclonal anti-idiotype antibody. *N Engl J Med* 306:517, 1982.
233. Stashenko P, Nadler LM, Hardy R, Schlossman SF: Characterization of a human B lymphocyte-specific antigen. *J Immunol* 125:1678, 1980.
234. Tedder TF, Forsgren A, Boyd AW, et al: Antibodies reactive with the B1 molecule inhibit cell cycle progression but not activation of human B lymphocytes. *Eur J Immunol* 16:881, 1986.
235. Smeland E, Godal T, Ruud E, et al: The specific induction of myc protooncogene expression in normal human B cells is not a sufficient event for acquisition of competence to proliferate. *Proc Natl Acad Sci U S A* 82:6255, 1985.
236. Deans JP, Schieven GL, Shu GL, et al: Association of tyrosine and serine kinases with the B cell surface antigen CD20. induction via CD20 of tyrosine phosphorylation and activation of phospholipase C-gamma 1 and PLC phospholipase C-gamma 2. *J Immunol* 151:4494, 1993.
237. Marcus R, Imrie K, Belch A, et al: CVP chemotherapy plus rituximab compared with CVP as first-line treatment for advanced follicular lymphoma. *Blood* 105:1417, 2005.
238. Habermann TM, Weller EA, Morrison VA, et al: Rituximab-CHOP versus CHOP alone or with maintenance rituximab in older patients with diffuse large B-cell lymphoma. *J Clin Oncol* 24:3121, 2006.
239. Davis TA, Grillo-Lopez AJ, White CA, et al: Rituximab anti-CD20 monoclonal antibody therapy in non-Hodgkin's lymphoma: Safety and efficacy of re-treatment. *J Clin Oncol* 18:3135, 2000.
240. van Oers MHJ, Klasa R, Marcus RE, et al: Rituximab maintenance improves clinical outcome of relapsed/resistant follicular non-Hodgkin lymphoma in patients both with and without rituximab during induction: Results of a prospective randomized phase 3 intergroup trial. *Blood* 108:3295, 2006.
241. Hainsworth JD, Litchy S, Burris HA 3rd, et al: Rituximab as first-line and maintenance therapy for patients with indolent non-Hodgkin's lymphoma. *J Clin Oncol* 20:4261, 2002.
242. Maloney D, Grillo-Lopez A, Bodkin D, et al: IDEC-C2B8: Results of a phase I multiple-dose trial in patients with relapsed non-Hodgkin's lymphoma. *J Clin Oncol* 15:3266, 1997.
243. Cartron G, Watier H, Golay J, Solal-Celigny P: From the bench to the bedside: Ways to improve rituximab efficacy. *Blood* 104:2635, 2004.
244. Berinstein NL, Grillo-Lopez AJ, White CA, et al: Association of serum rituximab (IDEC-C2B8) concentration and anti-tumor response in the treatment of recurrent low-grade or follicular non-Hodgkin's lymphoma. *Ann Oncol* 9:995, 1998.
245. Cartron G, Dacheux L, Salles G, et al: Therapeutic activity of humanized anti-CD20 monoclonal antibody and polymorphism in IgG fc receptor fcgamma RIIIa gene. *Blood* 99:754, 2002.
246. Farag SS, Flinn IW, Modali R, et al: Fc{gamma}RIIIa and fc{gamma}RIIa polymorphisms do not predict response to rituximab in B-cell chronic lymphocytic leukemia. *Blood* 103:1472, 2004.
247. Lowndes S, Darby A, Mead G, Lister A: Stevens-Johnson syndrome after treatment with rituximab. *Ann Oncol* 13:1948, 2002.
248. Carson KR, Evens AM, Richey EA, et al: Progressive multifocal leukoencephalopathy after rituximab therapy in HIV-negative patients: A report of 57 cases from the Research on Adverse Drug Events and Reports project. *Blood* 113:4834, 2009
249. Cattaneo C, Spedini P, Casari S, et al: Delayed-onset peripheral blood cytopenia after rituximab: Frequency and risk factor assessment in a consecutive series of 77 treatments. *Leuk Lymphoma* 47:1013, 2006.
250. Cabanillas F, Liboy I, Pavia O, Rivera E: High incidence of non-neutropenic infections induced by rituximab plus fludarabine and associated with hypogammaglobulinemia: A frequently unrecognized and easily treatable complication. *Ann Oncol* 17:1424, 2006.
251. Kumar S, Kimlinger TK, Lust JA, et al: Expression of CD52 on plasma cells in plasma cell proliferative disorders. *Blood* 102:1075, 2003.
252. Villamor N, Montserrat E, Colomer D: Mechanism of action and resistance to monoclonal antibody therapy. *Semin Oncol* 30:424, 2003.
253. Hillmen P, Skotnicki AB, Robak T, et al: Alemtuzumab compared with chlorambucil as first-line therapy for chronic lymphocytic leukemia. *J Clin Oncol* 25:5616, 2007.
254. Keating MJ, Flinn I, Jain V, et al: Therapeutic role of alemtuzumab (campath-1H) in patients who have failed fludarabine: Results of a large international study. *Blood* 99:3554, 2002.
255. Gallamini A, Zaja F, Patti C, et al: Alemtuzumab (campath-1H) and CHOP chemotherapy as first-line treatment of peripheral T-cell lymphoma: Results of a GITIL (Gruppo Italiano Terapie Innovative nei Linfomi) prospective multicenter trial. *Blood* 110:2316, 2007.
256. Kreitman RJ, Wilson WH, Bergeron K, et al: Efficacy of the anti-CD22 recombinant immunotoxin BL22 in chemotherapy-resistant hairy-cell leukemia. *N Engl J Med* 345:241, 2001.
257. Foss FM: Interleukin-2 fusion toxin: Targeted therapy for cutaneous T cell lymphoma. *Ann N Y Acad Sci* 941:166, 2001.
258. Negro-Vilar A, Dziewanowska Z, Groves ES, et al: Efficacy and safety of denileukin diftitox (dd) in a phase III, double-blind, placebo-controlled study of CD25+ patients with cutaneous T-cell lymphoma (CTCL) [abstract]. *J Clin Oncol* 25(18 Suppl):8026, 2007.
259. Gorgun G, Foss F: Immunomodulatory effects of RXR rexinoids: Modulation of high-affinity IL-2R expression enhances susceptibility to denileukin diftitox. *Blood* 100:1399, 2002.
260. Prokop A, Wrasidlo W, Lode H, et al: Induction of apoptosis by enediyne antibiotic calicheamicin thetaII proceeds through a caspase-mediated mitochondrial amplification loop in an entirely bax-dependent manner. *Oncogene* 22:9107, 2003.

261. Zein N, Sinha AM, McGahren WJ, Ellestad GA: Calicheamicin gamma 1I: An antitumor antibiotic that cleaves double-stranded DNA site specifically. *Science* 240:1198, 2008.
262. Sievers EL, Larson RA, Stadtmauer EA, et al: Efficacy and safety of gemtuzumab ozogamicin in patients with CD33-positive acute myeloid leukemia in first relapse. *J Clin Oncol* 19:3244, 2001.
263. McKoy JM, Angelotta C, Bennett CL, et al: Gemtuzumab ozogamicin-associated sinusoidal obstructive syndrome (SOS): An overview from the research on adverse drug events and reports (RADAR) project. *Leuk Res* 31:599, 2007.
264. Wadleigh M, Richardson PG, Zahrieh D, et al: Prior gemtuzumab ozogamicin exposure significantly increases the risk of veno-occlusive disease in patients who undergo myeloablative allogeneic stem cell transplantation. *Blood* 102:1578, 2003
265. Versluys B, Bhattacharaya R, Steward C, et al: Prophylaxis with defibrotide prevents veno-occlusive disease in stem cell transplantation after gemtuzumab ozogamicin exposure. *Blood* 103:1968, 2004.
266. Larson RA, Sievers EL, Stadtmauer EA, et al: Final report of the efficacy and safety of gemtuzumab ozogamicin (Mylotarg) in patients with CD33-positive acute myeloid leukemia in first recurrence. *Cancer* 104:1442, 2005.
267. Kell WJ, Burnett AK, Chopra R, et al: A feasibility study of simultaneous administration of gemtuzumab ozogamicin with intensive chemotherapy in induction and consolidation in younger patients with acute myeloid leukemia. *Blood* 102:4277, 2003.
268. Burnett AK, Kell WJ, Goldstone AH, et al: The addition of gemtuzumab ozogamicin to induction chemotherapy for AML improves disease free survival without extra toxicity: Preliminary analysis of 1115 patients in the MRC AML15 trial. *Blood* 108:11, 2006.
269. Stadtmauer EA: Trials with gemtuzumab ozogamicin (Mylotarg) combined with chemotherapy regimens in acute myeloid leukemia. *Clin Lymphoma* 2:S24, 2002.
270. Naito K, Takeshita A, Shigeno K, et al: Calicheamicin-conjugated humanized anti-CD33 monoclonal antibody (gemtuzumab zogamicin, CMA-676) shows cytocidal effect on CD33-positive leukemia cell lines, but is inactive on P-glycoprotein-expressing sublines. *Leukemia* 14:1436, 2000.
271. van der Velden VH, Boeckx N, Jedema I, et al: High CD33-antigen loads in peripheral blood limit the efficacy of gemtuzumab ozogamicin (Mylotarg) treatment in acute myeloid leukemia patients. *Leukemia* 18:983, 2004.
272. Horning SJ, Weller E, Kim K, et al: Chemotherapy with or without radiotherapy in limited-stage diffuse aggressive non-Hodgkin's lymphoma: Eastern cooperative oncology group study 1484. *J Clin Oncol* 22:3032, 2004.

CHAPTER 21
PRINCIPLES OF HEMATOPOIETIC CELL TRANSPLANTATION

Robert Lowsky and Robert S. Negrin

SUMMARY

Over the past 60 years the field of hematopoietic cell transplantation (HCT) has evolved from experimental animal models of marrow transplantation to curative therapy for tens of thousands of people yearly who are affected by a wide variety of marrow failure states, myeloid and lymphoid malignant diseases, immune deficiencies, and inborn errors of metabolism. Advances in transplantation immune biology combined with improvements in supportive care have made this evolution possible and have ushered in the modern era of HCT. This chapter discusses the biologic principles and clinical applications of HCT along with its future applications. Selected results demonstrating important principles are highlighted.

HISTORY

The successful clinical application of hematopoietic cell transplantation (HCT) to the therapeutic armamentarium of the hematologist required a century of key developmental discoveries (Table 21–1).

Between the years of 1868 and 1906 European and American investigators established that marrow cells were the source of blood cell production. In 1939, the first documented human marrow transplant was performed in a patient with gold-induced marrow aplasia.[1] The patient was infused intravenously with marrow from a brother with an identical blood group. The transplantation was not successful and the patient died 5 days after the marrow infusion.

In 1922, a Danish investigator carried out studies on modifying radiation injury in guinea pigs by shielding their femora against radiation and prevented the typical depression of platelet count and hemorrhage.[2] This work went essentially unnoticed for more than two decades. The period of 1949 to 1954 was marked by a political climate concerned with the threat of continued atomic warfare and this concern stimulated support for experiments studying the effects of irradiation and led to the development of the field of organ and marrow transplantation. Jacobson and colleagues found that mice could survive an otherwise lethal irradiation exposure if the spleen (a hematopoietic organ in the mouse) was protected by lead foil.[3] Soon afterwards, Lorenz and colleagues showed that lethally irradiated mice and guinea pigs were protected by the administration of syngeneic marrow after irradiation, thereby demonstrating therapeutic efficacy of allogeneic and xenogeneic marrow suspensions.[4] These investigators and others considered that chemicals and/or components from the shielded spleen or infused marrow stimulated endogenous hematopoietic cell recovery after total body irradiation.[5–7] In 1954, Barnes and Loutit showed that if mice were immunized to marrow cells from mice of another strain and then lethally irradiated, no protection was observed by the injection of marrow cells from the strain to which they were immunized.[8] However, if nonimmunized mice were lethally irradiated and injected with the same marrow cells, normal protection was seen and all mice survived more than 60 days. This experiment supported the cellular hypothesis of hematopoiesis and was the first to consider that hematopoietic recovery resulted from cell transplantation repopulation and not humoral factors.[9]

In 1956, Barnes and associates described the treatment of murine leukemia by supralethal irradiation and marrow grafting.[10] Researchers pointed out that the irradiation alone would not kill all leukemia cells, but that residual leukemia cells might be eliminated by colonizing cells through immunologic mechanisms, and the term *adoptive immune therapy* was coined. Their publication stimulated tremendous interest and the period from 1956 to 1959 was characterized by a general realization of the potential application of marrow grafting to treat individuals exposed to lethal irradiation, and to treat human leukemia. In Cooperstown, NY, Thomas and colleagues began studies in terminal leukemia patients, and reported in 1957 six patients treated with irradiation and intravenous infusion of marrow from healthy donors.[11] Only two patients developed transient detectable donor hematopoietic cells and none of the six survived beyond 100 days from the cell infusion. In 1959, Thomas and associates reported a twin with terminal leukemia who received total-body irradiation (TBI) and an intravenous infusion of marrow from the healthy twin.[12] The patient showed prompt hematopoietic recovery and disappearance of the leukemia for 4 months, confirming for the first time that lethal irradiation followed by compatible marrow could have an antileukemic effect and restore normal marrow function. In the same year Mathé and associates reported the infusion of marrow into six patients exposed to potentially lethal irradiation in a reactor accident in Belgrade, Serbia.[13] Five patients survived, yet there was no clear evidence to support engraftment of donor marrow, and thus there was no firm agreement over the contribution made by marrow transfusions to patient recovery.

The first attempts at autologous marrow transplantation appeared during this time. In 1958, Kurnick and colleagues described two patients with metastatic cancer whose marrow was collected and stored by freezing.[14] Following intensive radiation therapy, the marrow was thawed and infused intravenously. One patient died from transplantation complications yet the other showed hematopoietic recovery after a moderately long period of pancytopenia. In Philadelphia, an autologous marrow transplantation was carried out after high-dose nitrogen mustard conditioning in a patient with malignant lymphoma who lived for more than 30 years after transplantation, and the majority of this time was in a state of complete remission.[15]

Despite the many successful preclinical models of marrow transplantation and the predictive value of *in vitro* histocompatibility testing, the

Acronyms and abbreviations that appear in this chapter include: ALL, acute lymphoblastic leukemia; AML, acute myelogenous leukemia; BCNU, carmustine; BuCy, busulfan and cyclophosphamide; c-GVHD, chronic graft-versus-host disease; CIBMTR, Center for International Blood and Marrow Transplantation Research; CML, chronic myelogenous leukemia; CMV, cytomegalovirus; CR1, first complete remission; CXCR4, chemokine-related receptor; DLI, donor leukocyte infusion; FK506, tacrolimus; G-CSF, granulocyte colony-stimulating factor; GVHD, graft-versus-host disease; GVT, graft-versus-tumor; HCT, hematopoietic cell transplantation; HL, Hodgkin lymphoma; HLA, human leukocyte antigen; HSC, hematopoietic stem cell; HSV, herpes simplex virus; ^{131}I, radioactive iodine; Ig, immunoglobulin; IL, interleukin; MMF, mycophenolate mofetil; MSC, mesenchymal stromal cell; NHL, non-Hodgkin lymphoma; NK, natural killer; NRM, nonrelapse mortality; PBMC, blood mononuclear cells; PCR, polymerase chain reaction; RIC, reduced-intensity conditioning; SOS, sinusoidal obstructive syndrome; TBI, total-body irradiation; Th, T-cell helper; TREC, T-cell–receptor excision circle; T_{reg}, T-regulatory cell; UCB, umbilical cord blood; VCAM-1, vascular cell adhesion molecule; VP-16, etoposide; VZV, varicella-zoster virus.

TABLE 21–1. Key Historical Periods in Hematopoietic Cell Transplantation

Years	Event
1868–1906	Discovery that marrow was the source of the various blood cell types
1896–1900	Discovery of ABO system making blood transfusions possible
1939	First documented clinical marrow transplant
1949–1954	Development of preclinical models of marrow and organ transplantation
1956–1959	Early efforts of marrow grafting to treat human diseases
1960–1965	Development of the hierarchical stem/progenitor cell model of hematopoiesis
1960s	Period of pessimism for the clinical application of marrow grafting for the treatment of human diseases
1968–1969	First successful allogeneic HCT in patients with SCID
1975	First successful series of allogeneic HCT for leukemia
1978	First successful series of autologous HCT for leukemia
1988	Isolation of the murine HSC
1990	Nobel Prize in Physiology or Medicine awarded to Dr. E.D. Thomas
2008	More than 700,000 patients worldwide transplanted, more than 125,000 have survived 5 years or beyond after transplantation

HCT, hematopoietic cell transplantation; HSC, hematopoietic stem cell; SCID, severe combined immunodeficiency.

period of 1960 to 1967 was marked by increasing pessimism about allogeneic marrow grafting in human patients. In a published compendium of 203 human allogeneic marrow grafts carried out throughout the 1950s and 1960s, none were considered successful.[16]

The first positive results came from studies of children with an immunologic deficiency. In 1968, Gatti and colleagues performed the first successful allogeneic marrow HCT in a patient with severe combined immunodeficiency.[17] The graft of lymphoid elements from the donor corrected the immunodeficiency, and two similar cases were reported shortly thereafter.[18,19] These patients remained alive and well and were reported in followup 25 years later.[20]

These successes stimulated a resurgence of enthusiasm for marrow transplantation and by 1975 strikingly improved results were published from the Seattle team.[21] These investigators reported the outcomes of 37 patients with aplastic anemia and 73 patients with leukemia who had reached an advanced stage of their disease before transplantation. This study stressed the importance of histocompatibility and proper preparation of the patient before transplantation, detailed the technique of marrow transplantation, emphasized posttransplantation immune suppression and supportive care, and raised the possibility of using unrelated donors. This report ushered in the modern era of HCT. In 1977 and 1980, the first successful HCT procedures from unrelated marrow donors were reported.[22,23] At the end of 1978, the first series of successful autologous HCT for lymphoma were reported.[24,25] Based on the body of his collected work in the field of marrow transplantation, the Nobel Prize in Physiology or Medicine was award to Dr. E.D. Thomas in 1990. By 2008, more than 700,000 patients worldwide had undergone transplantation during the previous three decades and more than 125,000 patients survived 5 years or longer after transplantation.[26]

STEM CELL MODEL OF HEMATOPOIESIS

At the single-cell level, stem cells self-renew into more stem cells and give rise to progeny that differentiate into functional cells carrying out specific functions (Chap. 16).[27] Progenitor cells can be multipotent, oligopotent, or unipotent yet lack self-renewal capabilities. Hematopoietic stem cells (HSCs) are cells that give rise to more HSCs and form all elements of the blood. HSCs are entirely responsible for the development, maintenance, and regeneration of blood-forming tissues for life, and are the most important, if not the only cells required for successful engraftment in hematopoietic transplants.[27] In the adult mouse marrow, all HSC activity is contained in a population marked by the composite phenotype of c-kit^{+}, Thy-1.1^{lo}, lineage marker$^{-/lo}$, and Sca-1^{+} (designated KTLS).[28,29] When transplanted at the single-cell level into irradiated mice, KTLS HSC gave rise to lifelong hematopoiesis, including a steady state of thousands of HSC with more than 10^9 blood cells produced daily.[28–30] In humans the combination of positive selection for CD34, Thy-1, and negative selection for lineage markers, identified a homologous HSC population.[31] Following the success in rodent models, purified populations of human HSC were tested in three separate clinical trials of patients with myeloma, non-Hodgkin lymphoma (NHL), and metastatic breast cancer.[32–34] The goal was to purify HSC and thereby reduce the risk of occult malignant cells as a significant percentage of marrow or blood mononuclear cells are contaminated with malignant cells in all three diseases. These trials presented technical challenges primarily because of the rarity of HSC in marrow and granulocyte colony-stimulating factor (G-CSF) mobilized blood; however, adequate numbers of HSCs could be isolated which were tumor free, from the majority of patients. The time to neutrophil and platelet recovery following purified HSC infusion was comparable to engraftment times using unmanipulated marrow as a graft source, yet there was a significant delay in T-cell recovery, especially of CD4+ T cells, of up to 6 months in almost all patients. A number of patients developed unusual infections (i.e., severe cases of influenza, respiratory syncytial virus, cytomegalovirus and *Pneumocystis* pneumonia), thus, raising caution of using a "pure" HSC product as the sole source of hematopoietic reconstitution in clinical transplantation. Although too few patients were transplanted to evaluate whether the infusion of a product free of contaminating tumor cells impacted outcomes on event-free and overall survival, results appeared favorable.

TRAFFICKING AND HOMING OF HEMATOPOIETIC STEM CELLS

The ability of HSCs to circulate and migrate from marrow to blood and back is an aspect of the hematopoietic system that has been conserved through evolution. Although the biologic role and physiologic significance of this constitutive HSC circulation remains unclear, it is this capacity to traffic that leads to hematopoietic cell reconstitution and forms the essential requirement for success of HCT in the treatment of hematologic and nonhematologic diseases.

The restoration of adequate blood cell production after transplantation requires a series of balanced interactions between the infused HSC and its complex supporting marrow microenvironment (Chap. 4). The initial step requires infused HSC to adhere to the marrow endothelium with sufficient strength to overcome the shear forces of blood flow.[35] The dominant HSC cell surface molecules that mediate adhesion and arrest are the selectin ligands P-selectin glycoprotein ligand-1, and the hematopoietic cell L- and E-selectin ligands that interact principally with endothelial E-selectin.[36–38] Other HSC surface adhesion molecules that mediate adherence to the marrow endothelium are a subset of the integrin superfamily, principally very late antigen-4, $\alpha_4\beta_7$, and lymphocyte function antigen-1, that interact with endothelial immunoglobulin (Ig) superfamily receptors (e.g., vascular cell adhesion molecule [VCAM]-1), and the hyaluronate receptor CD44.[39,40] HSCs that are null for the β integrins cannot migrate to their marrow niche even though they proliferate and differentiate in the fetal liver.[41] Following firm adherence, the transendothelial movement and intraparenchymal homing to hematopoietic niches located within the inner endosteal surface of the bone are predominantly regulated by a gradient of extracellular matrix bound stromal cell-derived factor-1 (also known as CXCL12) binding to the chemokine-related receptor (CXCR4) on HSCs.[42] The requirement for CXCR4 expression on HSCs for homing and engraftment is well documented[43] and forms the basis for new agents that help mobilize marrow stem cells for clinical use. Mice deficient in CXCR4 develop fetal liver hematopoiesis but die prenatally as a consequence of the lack of marrow hematopoiesis.[42] Following successful homing, the initial adhesion of the HSC within the hematopoietic niche appears regulated at least in part by annexin II as inhibitors reduce binding to the marrow microenvironment.[44] The marrow niche is a complex biologic unit composed of different cell types that include potentially self-renewing mesenchymal stromal cells (MSCs), as well as cells with the defined phenotype of parathyroid hormone receptor-bearing osteoblasts.[45,46] MSCs promote engraftment when cotransplanted with HSCs.[47] Osteoblasts, possibly in conjunction with sinusoidal endothelial cells, appear to also play a pivotal role in the regulation of HSC engraftment by producing a number of molecules, such as annexin II, VCAM-1, intercellular adhesion molecule-1, CD44, CD164, and osteopontin, which promote engraftment.[44,48–50] Stimulation of osteoblasts with parathyroid hormone following transplantation results in a cyclic adenosine monophosphate-mediated expansion of the HSC pool that enhances engraftment and improves survival of lethally irradiated animals.[45,51] In addition to the regulators of HSC adhesion and homing, the function of HSC is further regulated by intrinsic genetic programs for quiescence, self-renewal, proliferation, differentiation, and apoptosis that are dependent on communication with a network of interacting cells localized in the marrow microenvironment, including various T-cell subpopulations, adipocytes, and fibroblasts. Given the complexity of HSC trafficking and control, it is surprising that clinical HCT in general has a relatively low rate of graft failure.

SOURCES OF HEMATOPOIETIC STEM CELLS

For human transplantation protocols, HSCs can be collected from a variety of sources including the marrow, blood, and umbilical cord blood obtained at the time of delivery.

■ MARROW

Marrow is the traditional source of HSCs for allogeneic and autologous transplantation.[52] The marrow is typically aspirated by repeated placement of large bore needles into the posterior iliac crest, generally 50 to 100 aspirations simultaneously on both sides, while under regional or general anesthesia. The lowest cell dose to ensure stable long-term engraftment has not been defined with certainty, and a typical collection standard contains more than 2×10^8 nucleated marrow cells/kg recipient body weight. Current guidelines indicate that a volume of up to 20 mL/kg donor body weight is considered safe.

Marrow harvesting is considered a very safe procedure and serious side effects are rare. A review of almost 10,000 unrelated healthy adult donors reported to the National Marrow Donor Program (NMDP) revealed that 70 percent of donors fully recovered by 2 weeks and the risk of serious complications were 1.2 percent; most of which were mechanical with nerve, bone, or tissue injury and resolved within 6 weeks.[53] Death has been reported in the days following healthy donor harvesting at an estimated incidence of 1 per 10,000 donations, yet it is difficult to attribute this, with certainty, as a consequence of the marrow harvest.[54] The use of G-CSF to mobilize stem cells in patients with sickle cell anemia is contraindicated. Evaluation of pediatric marrow donor safety is limited to small single-institution studies.[55–57] As with adults, serious complications in donors younger than age 20 years were rare. The majority of marrow donors younger than age 2 years required allogeneic blood products after donation because of the large volume of marrow required for older, larger recipients. A survey of pediatric transplantation hematologists confirmed that 90 percent of centers were willing to perform a marrow harvest on children, even on those younger than 6 months old.[55]

■ BLOOD

Hematopoietic stem cells are present in the blood at very low levels; however a number of different stimuli including chemotherapy, various hematopoietic growth factors and inhibitors of certain chemokine receptors, result in the mobilization of HSCs from marrow to blood. Once in the blood, the HSCs can be collected by apheresis, and this product has been termed *peripheral blood progenitor cells* (PBPCs) to differentiate from the term *blood stem cells*, which should be reserved for instances where the HSC population itself has been isolated. Agents used for mobilization include G-CSF, granulocyte-monocyte colony-stimulating factor (GM-CSF), interleukin (IL)-3, thrombopoietin, and the CXCR4 antagonist AMD3100.[58–61]

The most common method to harvest autologous and allogeneic PBPCs is by using G-CSF with or without chemotherapy. Like marrow harvesting, this procedure is very safe and in a review of 5930 normal donors, serious side effects were rare (<1%).[62] Splenic rupture has been reported with an estimated incidence of 1 in 10,000 donors, yet with increased awareness this risk will likely decrease.[63,64] Splenic rupture has not been reported in children.

Theoretical concerns exist about the use of short-term growth factor therapy increasing the risk of leukemia in normal donors. Studies in normal adult donors have shown no late effects of short-term G-CSF therapy with 9 years of followup.[65] A detailed white cell subset analysis by fluorescent-activated cell sorting of healthy donors performed 1 year after donation showed no changes in B-, T-, and natural killer (NK) cells or monocytes and neutrophils compared with analysis before G-CSF administration.[66]

The measurement of the absolute number of CD34+ cells/kg recipient body weight collected is a reliable and practical method for determining the adequacy of the PBPC product. Most laboratories measure CD34+ cell content by fluorescent-activated cell sorting. The infusion of $>2 \times 10^6$ CD34+ cells/kg was suggested as the minimum target dose for acceptable engraftment kinetics following autologous HCT yet a more rapid platelet reconstitution is consistently observed by the infusion of higher CD34+ cell doses.[67–69] Platelet recovery appears most affected by grafts with low CD34+ cell numbers. Although inadequate mobilization of healthy donors is rare, patients with malignancies undergoing mobilization for autologous HCT often have difficulty collecting adequate numbers of CD34+ cells. Approximately 10 to 20 percent of patients do not mobilize sufficient numbers of CD34+ cells using G-CSF alone or in combination with chemotherapy. Unfortunately, it has been relatively difficult to prospectively identify these individuals, although most such individuals have been moderately or heavily pretreated with cytotoxic therapies. For patients with NHL, Hodgkin lymphoma (HL), and myeloma who failed mobilization with G-CSF alone, the majority proceeded to collect a transplantable dose

($>2 \times 10^6$ cells/kg) of CD34+ cells when remobilized with AMD3100 plus G-CSF.[70] Studies of allogeneic HCT using AMD3100 mobilized grafts have also confirmed prompt and stable donor cell engraftment.[71]

There is increasing evidence that circadian activity in the hypothalamus regulates the cyclic release of HSC by altering the expression of extracellular matrix bound CXCL12 in the marrow microenvironment.[72–74] Circadian adrenergic signals arising in the suprachiasmatic nuclei are delivered by nerves located in the marrow to stromal cells and result in the rapid downregulation of CXCL12 that is antiphase with the rhythmic release of HSCs; the peak time for HSC release in humans is the evening. A recent study enumerating the CD34+ and CD34+CD38− cell subsets confirmed more abundant ($p < 0.001$) collections from healthy human donors following short course G-CSF administration when harvested at 8 PM compared to 8 AM.[72] Data from 82 healthy donors that underwent G-CSF mobilization for allogeneic HCT confirmed that the average CD34+ cell yield was significantly higher when apheresis was performed in the late afternoon compared to the yield from morning procedures.[72] It remains to be determined whether a simple adjustment in the time of harvesting and cell infusion will have a significant clinical impact.

Mobilized PBPCs versus Marrow

The use of mobilized PBPCs has had a major impact on autologous transplantation. In this clinical setting, there is little debate that mobilized PBPCs are a superior product compared to marrow. A number of phase II clinical trials have documented accelerated engraftment with PBPC products that contain $>2 \times 10^6$ CD34+ cells/kg.[75,76] Randomized clinical trials have confirmed these results.[77–79] In these studies, recovery of absolute neutrophil and platelet count, and red blood cell transfusion requirements have all improved with the use of mobilized PBPC. In a randomized trial of patients with advanced HL or high-grade NHL who received either PBPCs or marrow, the time to absolute neutrophil count of $>5 \times 10^9$/L was reduced from 14 days with marrow to 11 days with PBPCs ($p = 0.005$).[77] The time to platelet recovery of $>20 \times 10^9$/L was 23 days for patients who received marrow compared to 16 days in the PBPC group ($p = 0.02$). Patients who received PBPC also required fewer red blood cell and platelet transfusions and spent less time in the hospital. Overall survival was similar in the two groups. On the basis of these and other results, most transplantation centers use mobilized PBPCs and have adopted a CD34 cell minimum of $>1 \times 10^6$ CD34+ cells/kg with a preferred content of $>2 \times 10^6$ CD34+ cells/kg. An absolute minimum CD34+ cell dose below which autologous HCT would not be recommended has not been defined, and it is the opinion of the authors that marrow harvesting to supplement the PBPC graft be considered for patients with a CD34+ cell dose below 1×10^6 cells/kg.

In the allogeneic setting, the situation is considerably more complex. The approximately 10-fold greater number of T cells contained in PBPC grafts led to the concern that higher number of T cells may result in increased incidence and severity of graft-versus-host disease (GVHD). In the initial phase II studies the incidence and severity of GVHD were similar among patients who received G-CSF mobilized PBPCs compared to historical cohorts of patients who received marrow.[80,81] In a series of prospective studies, most reported no clear difference in the incidence of acute GVHD (grades II to IV).[79–82] The observation that the infusion of 10-fold greater number of T cells did not increase the risk of acute GVHD may in part be related to findings that G-CSF can induce functional immune tolerance *in vivo* in healthy individuals. Purified T cells from G-CSF–mobilized PBPC donors were analyzed by gene-expression profiling and immunophenotyping that showed a predominantly immune-tolerant profile with upregulation of genes related to T-cell helper type 2 (Th2) and T-regulatory (T_{reg}) cells, and downregulation of genes associated with Th1 cells, cytotoxicity, antigen presentation, and GVHD.[86]

Similar to the autologous setting, hematopoietic reconstitution was significantly more rapid in patients who received allogeneic mobilized PBPCs compared to allogeneic marrow.[79–82] These studies were largely performed with patients who had histocompatibility locus antigen (HLA)-compatible siblings, and there are relatively few data yet in the unrelated donor setting, although a large randomized clinical trial through the Marrow Transplantation Clinical Trials Network is ongoing.

The risk of chronic GVHD (limited and extensive) is more controversial. Some studies have not shown a significant difference, including a randomized collaborative study from the Fred Hutchinson Cancer Research Center, the City of Hope National Medical Center, and Stanford University.[87] In this study, the incidence of chronic GVHD for patients who received mobilized blood was 46 percent compared to 35 percent in the patients receiving marrow ($p = 0.54$). In other studies, the risk of chronic GVHD was significantly increased in patients who received G-CSF–mobilized PBPCs.[85] Additional followup of these patients is important to help resolve this issue.

There may be specific reasons to use mobilized PBPCs. For example, in patients with high-risk disease, more rapid hematopoietic reconstitution following PBPC transplantation could result in improved outcomes. Bensinger and colleagues published that patients with high-risk disease (acute myelogenous leukemia [AML] beyond first complete remission [CR1] or after first chronic phase of chronic myelogenous leukemia [CML]) had improved overall survival if they received PBPCs compared to patients with advanced disease characteristics who received marrow.[83] Patients with standard risk (AML in CR1 or first chronic phase of CML) disease had similar outcomes with PBPC and marrow. Consequently, some centers have used an approach where patients with high-risk disease receive mobilized PBPC, whereas those with standard-risk disease continue to receive marrow. In the unrelated donor setting, several randomized clinical trials are ongoing in an effort to address this important question.

■ UMBILICAL CORD BLOOD

Umbilical cord blood (UCB) collected from the umbilical vessels in the placenta at the time of delivery is a rich source of HSCs. Because these cells are immunologically relatively naïve, recipients may have satisfactory outcomes, even when crossing major histocompatibility barriers, thus extending the donor pool to individuals for whom finding allele-matched adult donors can be difficult if not impossible.[89] Registries have been established that can be searched for histocompatible cord blood units. A significant advantage of UCB is that the cells are fully typed before cryopreservation and, therefore, are available, avoiding long search times. A major limitation has been the relatively small number of cells available in the cord blood unit, which has made transplantation feasible mainly for pediatric patients.[90–93] A limited number of studies have been performed in adults and most confirmed prolonged engraftment times.[92,94,95] An analysis of approximately 100 UCB transplants showed that recipients who received $<1.7 \times 10^7$ cells/kg body weight had a high rate of graft failure that led to high nonrelapse mortality (NRM).[91] Thus, it is prudent to anticipate the need for a backup graft given that UCB transplantation is associated with an increased risk of graft failure even when using well-matched, suitably sized, cord blood units. The majority of patients who had graft failure were rescued by this type of a planned approach initiated before day +50 after transplantation. Double-unit UCB transplantation with two closely and suitably matched cord bloods may provide better engraftment by providing a higher CD34+ and CD3+ cell dose.[96] Efforts have also been made to expand HSC from cord blood or potentially use multiple cord blood samples for transplantation to accelerate hematopoietic immune reconstitution.[97]

HAPLOIDENTICAL DONORS

The almost always present yet overlooked donor is the haplotype matched sibling, parent, or offspring. Haploidentical related donor HCT has been evaluated for more than two decades as an alternative option for the approximately 70 percent of patients who do not have an HLA-identical sibling donor. The advantages are that nearly all patients have an immediately available donor and that a strong graft-versus-tumor effect may be realized with HLA disparity. Early attempts at allogeneic HCT from haplotype matched donors were associated with significant GVHD in non–T-cell-depleted transplants and with graft rejection in T-cell-depleted products.[98–100] Extensive *ex vivo* immune cell depletion with anti-CD3+ coated and anti-CD19+ coated microbeads, coupled with mega-dose CD34+ cells can successfully overcome the barriers to engraftment.[100,101] In these protocols, the extensive T-cell depletion that largely prevented GVHD would also be expected to result in weak or no graft-versus-tumor reactions. Yet despite the lack of T-cell–mediated alloreactivity and the unfavorable prognostic features at the time of transplantation, relapse rates in the Perugia protocol remained at less than 18 percent and 30 percent, respectively, in AML and acute lymphoblastic leukemia (ALL) patients transplanted in complete remission.[102] The low rate of relapse was attributed to a strong antitumor effect mediated by donor-versus-recipient NK cell alloreactivity. Transplantation from NK cell alloreactive donors was associated with a significantly lower leukemia relapse rate and improved overall survival; therefore, some authorities recommended selecting NK cell alloreactive donors for haploidentical transplantation.[103] However, the widespread acceptance of haploidentical HCT remains hampered by the prolonged immune reconstitution and a high risk of serious infection.[104] Future directions will focus on efficacy in diseases other than leukemia, developing improved conditioning regimens, and promoting effective and timely posttransplantation immune reconstitution.

MESENCHYMAL STROMAL CELLS

The founding principles of HCT are that infused HSCs home and engraft in the marrow microenvironment and expand and proliferate to reconstitute all of the blood lineages. Yet it may be that another cellular component of the marrow microenvironment, namely the MSC, has the potential to synergize with current HCT regimens and positively impact the field of HCT. Clinical trials with MSCs are ongoing. Chap. 28 discusses this topic more extensively.

Owen was the first to propose that nonhematopoietic MSCs with fibroblastic, osteogenic, and adipocytic potential reside in the marrow microenvironment.[105] At present, MSCs are considered a heterogeneous population of cells because no specific marker or combination of markers is accepted to uniquely define these cells, although surface expression of the three antigens, CD105, CD73, and CD90 (Thy1), appear important.[106] Similarly, there is no single functional assay to distinguish MSCs, analogous to the repopulation assay for HSCs. The lack of a consensus on features to characterize these cells makes it difficult to compare and contrast study outcomes, and this slows the progress of the field. Nonetheless, MSCs are recognized to have diverse biologic properties, suggesting remarkable potential as cellular therapy. In particular, the cytokine-generating and immunomodulatory properties of MSCs hold promise for clinical applications in HCT.[107–109]

MSCs are most commonly isolated from marrow but can be obtained from placenta, UCB, adipose tissue, and fetal lung and blood.[110–115] The current opinion is that MSCs do not circulate in cytokine-mobilized blood. For isolation from the marrow, mononuclear cells are placed in tissue culture and the MSCs adhere to the plastic surface of the tissue culture vessels while the nonadherent cells are easily removed by changing the culture media. Once isolated, MSCs are expanded *in vitro* prior to preparation for a clinical trial; this extensive cell replication raises theoretical concern about malignant transformation.[116,117] However, malignant transformation of MSCs after infusion into human subjects in a clinical trial has not been reported.

The first clinical application of MSCs was to determine if these cells could foster autologous and allogeneic engraftment of HSCs because the cytotoxic effects of chemotherapy and irradiation contained in transplantation preparative regimens damage the marrow microenvironment, including the HSC niche.[45,118] Therefore, infusions of *ex vivo* expanded MSCs may, in principle, help repair the microenvironment and enhance HSC engraftment and immune reconstitution. The infusion of cancer patients undergoing autologous HCT with *ex vivo* expanded autologous MSCs 4 hours prior to the hematopoietic graft resulted in rapid platelet and neutrophil recovery.[119] *Ex vivo* expanded MSCs obtained from HLA-matched siblings could facilitate rapid myeloid and platelet engraftment after cotransplantation with marrow or G-CSF–mobilized PBPCs in patients with leukemia.[120] The time to neutrophil and platelet recovery appeared faster in these single-arm studies, yet it is difficult to draw firm clinical conclusions because these studies lacked control cohorts. Nonetheless, both studies demonstrated that the coadministration of millions of *ex vivo* expanded MSC did not impede engraftment.

Studies in children undergoing haploidentical HCT confirmed that the coadministration of *ex vivo* expanded MSCs 4 hours prior to infusion of the donor hematopoietic cell graft resulted in rapid neutrophil and platelet engraftment and appeared to decrease the likelihood of graft failure.[121] Studies with the use of parental haploidentical MSCs cotransplanted with unrelated UCB grafts to determine if MSCs have the capacity to enhance engraftment and immune reconstitution confirm similar findings.[122]

CONCEPTS OF CURATIVE THERAPY

AUTOLOGOUS HCT

The relationship between the dose of chemotherapy and/or radiation and the number of tumor cells killed has been extensively studied *in vitro* and in preclinical animal models, and forms the basis for the decision to pursue autologous HCT.[123–126] For chemosensitive tumors such as NHL, HL, and leukemia, a relatively steeply rising dose–response curve is observed, meaning that as the dose of the cytoxic agent is increased the number of tumor cells killed is also increased. The possibility for cure following autologous HCT, therefore, is derived from the beneficial effects of the high doses of chemotherapy and/or radiation therapy administered during transplant conditioning that enhance tumor cell kill and overcomes drug resistance. Dose escalation of therapy in autologous HCT is possible because the dose-limiting toxicities on hematopoiesis are circumvented by the infusion of the hematopoietic cell graft.

Autologous HCT is associated with relatively low NRM. The use of mobilized PBPCs has decreased the duration of neutropenia and when combined with improved supportive care the NRM of approximately 8 to 10 percent with marrow in earlier studies has been reduced to 1 to 3 percent with mobilized PBPCs in most centers. In addition, the reduced risks and faster engraftment times have allowed many centers to pursue outpatient transplantation, further easing the difficulty of patients undergoing this procedure, as well as possibly reducing costs.

Tumor Contamination in the Autograft

A consistent concern in autologous transplantation is the possibility that residual clonogenic tumor cells may contaminate the HSC product and contribute to tumor relapse. The relative contributions of tumor cell contamination from the cell product and residual disease in the patient are difficult, if not impossible, to discern. One approach to determine if residual malignant cells do indeed contribute to relapse is to mark the HSC product at the time of harvest and then assay if the marker gene is present in malignant cells at the time of a subsequent relapse. Studies using this approach have been performed in patients with leukemia, lymphoma, and myeloma. In these studies, marrow (or blood-derived) HSCs were marked with either the LNL6 or the closely related GlNa retroviral vector, which encode the neomycin resistance gene.[127–130] This marker gene can subsequently be detected in transduced cells either phenotypically, because it confers resistance to the neomycin analogue G418, or genotypically by polymerase chain reaction (PCR). Data from these studies indicated that marrow harvested from patients whose disease was in "apparent" complete remission likely contained residual tumorigenic cells, because these cells contributed to disease recurrence at medullary and extramedullary sites. The implication is that effective purging may be one requirement for improving the outcome of autologous HCT.

Purging Strategies for an Autologous Product A number of pharmacologic purging techniques have been used for the *in vitro* elimination of tumor cells from the HSC product. The most widely used agents have been the *in vitro* active analogues of the oxazophosphorines ifosfamide and cyclophosphamide. The initial concept was based on the demonstrated relative sparing of HSCs *in vitro* by cyclophosphamide and by activated derivatives of cyclophosphamide as a result of high levels of expression of aldehyde dehydrogenase in stem cells and the ability of this enzyme to inactivate the active metabolites of cyclophosphamide.[131] For patients with AML in first and second remission, phase II studies reported greater than 50 percent long-term leukemia-free survival using purged autografts, a percentage that appeared considerably better than autotransplantation studies that used unpurged marrow.[132,133] There are no randomized trials comparing purged to unpurged products. The widespread adoption of *in vitro* chemical purging, however, was hampered by its negative effects on hematopoietic cell recovery after transplantation and thus it has largely been abandoned.

Other strategies to remove potential malignant cells from the autograft involve immunologic methods. Generally a cocktail of monoclonal antibodies directed against determinants on the tumor cells is used, such as anti–B-cell monoclonal antibodies for patients with B-cell NHL. Sensitive PCR-based methods have been used to evaluate the efficacy of tumor cell removal.[134,135] In one retrospective analysis, patients who had been successfully depleted of PCR positive products were compared with patients who remained PCR positive.[136] This study demonstrated significantly improved outcomes with lower relapse rates for the patients who received a PCR-negative product.

An alternative approach to tumor removal has been to select for HSCs from the autograft to be infused. Positive HSC selection has resulted in a significant reduction in tumor cell contamination through the use of sensitive immunohistochemical and molecular analyses. The most widely used strategy has been to select for CD34+ cells with immunomagnetic techniques in diseases where the tumor does not express the CD34 antigen. Clinical application of CD34-selected cells resulted in rapid multilineage engraftment.[137,138] However, clinical trials failed to document improved clinical outcome for patients who received CD34+-selected autografts as compared to those patients who received unmanipulated autografts in a randomized prospective study of 190 patients with myeloma.[139] CD34 selection is not without potential complications as some studies suggest that CD34-selected grafts in the setting of autologous HCT may result in an increased risk of infection.[140,141] Without prospective randomized clinical trials favoring graft manipulation, many centers find it difficult to justify these procedures and the additional costs associated with them. However, given that disease relapse is the greatest risk of failure following autologous HCT, removal of tumor cells in the graft continues to be an important goal for future development.

Another strategy to decrease tumor contamination of the graft has been *in vivo* purging followed by collecting cells at a time when there is relatively low tumor burden. Two such strategies have been employed. The first uses combination chemotherapy for mobilization, largely in patients with acute leukemia, where cells are collected at a time of early recovery following the mobilization chemotherapy. Several studies have documented that these collections appear to be relatively free of contaminating tumor cells.[142,143] For patients with B-cell lymphoid malignant diseases, an alternative approach has been to use rituximab, the anti–B-cell monoclonal antibody that can be combined with mobilizing agents such as cyclophosphamide. In several studies, tumor cell contamination based on sensitive PCR-based methods revealed significant tumor reduction following rituximab-based mobilization strategies.[144,145] In a randomized study for patients with B-cell NHL *in vivo* purging with rituximab provided equivalent elimination of B cells from the infusate, as did CD34 cell selection.[146] *In vivo* purging with rituximab was associated with a more rapid time to neutrophil and platelet recovery compared to CD34 selection, but immunoglobulin recovery was significantly delayed.

■ ALLOGENEIC HCT

Allogeneic HCT is a considerably more complicated procedure than autologous HCT; it involves more pretransplantation preparation, poses a greater risk for complications to the patient, is associated with a significantly higher NRM rate, and the period of intensive posttransplantation followup is considerably longer. The decision to pursue allogeneic HCT is based on the type, prognosis, and remission status of the underlying disease, the performance status of the patient, and the availability of an appropriate donor. HLA-matched siblings, and matched unrelated donors obtained through national and international registries are frequently used for allogeneic HCT. To establish donor-derived hematopoiesis, there must be a source of HSC and most commonly this is accomplished using unmanipulated marrow or G-CSF–mobilized PBPCs.

A major obstacle that must be overcome in allogeneic HCT is the immune competence of the recipient. This potential to reject infused donor cells is mediated predominantly through regimen-resistant host T and NK cells.[147,148] Strategies to reduce host immunity and promote donor hematopoietic cell engraftment include the choice of chemotherapy and radiation used in the transplantation preparative regimen, and posttransplantation immune suppression medications. Donor T cells in the allograft promote hematopoietic engraftment as depletion of T lymphocytes from the donor graft before transplantation is associated with a substantial increase in the occurrence of graft rejection.[149–151] Other strategies that enhance donor cell engraftment under investigation are the use of monoclonal antibodies directed against T-cell determinants, antibodies conjugated with radioactive isotopes, and infusions of subsets of donor immune cells that facilitate engraftment without promoting GVHD.

Graft-versus-Tumor Effect

An important mechanism of cancer eradication following allogeneic HCT is from the immunologic-based recognition of residual host tumor cells by donor-derived immune cells contained in the donor graft. This phenomenon, termed the graft-versus-tumor (GVT) effect, has been demonstrated beyond dispute and represents one of the most significant biologic findings with implications well beyond the transplant setting. Table 21–2 highlights the lines of evidence supporting this concept.

Another commonly used RIC approach to transplantation from HLA-matched sibling donors consists of fludarabine (between 90 and 150 mg/m^2) and cyclophosphamide (between 900 and 2000 mg/m^2).[197] This type of regimen when combined with rituximab provided excellent long-term event-free survival in patients with indolent lymphoma and potentially with mantle cell lymphoma.[198] Fludarabine combined with busulfan at 4 to 8 mg/kg, with/or without anti–T-lymphocyte globulin, is yet a third RIC regimen that may be more efficacious in patients with myelodysplastic and myeloproliferative syndromes compared to other RIC regimens.[199]

Yet despite RIC, clinical outcomes remain limited by the risks of GVHD and NRM, albeit most patients transplanted using RIC protocols are considered ineligible for full-dose transplantation. Following RIC, the incidence of clinically significant acute GVHD ranged from 20 to 65 percent, accounting for approximately half of NRM.[200–203]

Investigators at Stanford University developed a rodent model of marrow transplantation that used conditioning with fractionated low-dose total-lymphoid irradiation combined with depletive T-cell antibodies (antithymocyte serum and showed that recipients were protected from GVHD induction by donor-derived T cells.[204,205] In the rodent model, as many as 1000 times the number of donor-derived T cells was infused and recipients failed to develop acute lethal GVHD. In this model, total-lymphoid irradiation and antithymocyte serum altered residual host T-cell subsets to favor regulatory NK T cells that suppress GVHD by polarizing the infused donor conventional T cells toward secretion of noninflammatory cytokines such as IL-4, and by promoting expansion of donor CD4+CD25+FoxP3+ regulatory T cells.[206] This skewing of host T-cell subsets was a result of NK T-cell resistance to radiation-induced apoptosis caused by increased expression of antiapoptotic genes.[207] This murine model was successfully translated to clinical transplantation where cancer patients who received total-lymphoid irradiation and antithymocyte globulin conditioning were infused with grafts from HLA-matched related and unrelated donors.[208,209] The majority of patients in these trials developed sustained donor-derived hematopoiesis and had a very low incidence of acute GVHD and NRM.

Mixed Chimerism Following Transplantation with RIC

A common feature to all RIC protocols is the incomplete eradication, at least initially, of host hematopoietic elements. As a consequence a significant percentage of patients have multilineage mixed chimerism for months after transplantation before converting, if ever, to complete donor type. It is difficult to assess the impact of sustained mixed chimerism on the risk of disease recurrence yet most reports indicated that irrespective of the transplant regimen and type of cancer, persistent mixed chimerism was a significant risk factor for disease relapse.[209,210] Interventions such as posttransplantation immunosuppressive drug withdrawal, CD34+-selected donor cell boost, or DLI have been used to convert mixed chimerism to complete donor type. These interventions are not without risk and can result in the development of GVHD. A significant percentage of patients who received Campath-containing RIC required DLI to promote conversion to complete donor type and protect against immune-mediated graft rejection, yet the risk of developing post-DLI GVHD was significant.[211] Mixed chimerism is not unique to RIC as prior to the addition of antithymocyte globulin; almost 60 percent of patients who received a marrow allograft following high-dose conditioning for severe aplastic anemia had mixed chimerism, of which two-thirds eventually converted to complete donor-type hematopoiesis while the remainder experienced late graft failure.[212]

Persistent mixed chimerism may have a role in allogeneic transplantation for noncancer patients. In organ transplantation, tolerance, defined as immune suppression drug withdrawal without graft rejection, was achieved in kidney transplant recipients who received the same donor marrow when sustained mixed chimerism was established, and not in recipients who experienced donor hematopoietic graft loss.[213] The relative merits of RIC compared with alternative therapies such as autologous or full-dose allogeneic HCT are currently under evaluation.

EVALUATION AND SELECTION OF CANDIDATES FOR TRANSPLANTATION

Most transplant candidates are referred by hematologists or oncologists to the tertiary center where the transplantation procedure will be performed. Patients considered for transplantation require in-depth counseling by experienced transplantation physicians, nurses, and social workers who are knowledgeable in the field. Information regarding the prior course, including initial diagnostic studies, previous drug and radiation treatments, and responses to these interventions, as well as a psychosocial assessment of the patient and their caregivers, are of the utmost importance. Table 21–3 highlights the issues and topics that should be addressed during the counseling meetings with transplantation candidates and their families or friends.[214]

Important factors have been identified that consistently impact results following HCT and include, but are not limited to, disease status

TABLE 21–3. Topics Addressed during Counseling Meetings with Transplant Candidate and Care Provider

I.	Rationale for why transplantation is a therapeutic option
II.	How the transplantation is performed
	Autologous
	Allogeneic—choice for full-dose versus RIC
III.	Source of cells
	Marrow versus blood versus other source
IV.	Risks of procedure
V.	Graft failure and graft rejection
VI.	Risk of GVHD
	Acute and chronic forms, compatibility of graft
	Likelihood for long-term immune suppression medication
VII.	Nonrelapse mortality at 100 days and 1 year
VIII.	Risks of relapse
IX.	Timing of transplant
X.	Projected result
XI.	Requirement for dedicated care provider
XII.	Other
	Financial implications
	Durable power of attorney
	Banking of sperm, *in vitro* fertilized eggs
	Duration of stay near the transplantation center
	Return to home and work
	Sexual activity
	Quality-of-life issues
	Habits such as smoking, alcohol, and drug addiction

GVHD, graft-versus-host disease; RIC, reduced-intensity conditioning.

at transplantation, type and compatibility of donor, recipient's age, and comorbid medical conditions.

DISEASE STATUS AT THE TIME OF TRANSPLANTATION

Disease status at the time of transplantation is perhaps the most powerful predictor of long-term disease-free survival following allogeneic and autologous HCT. Early transplantation studies of allogeneic HCT were performed using predominantly patients whose disease failed to respond to a variety of other treatment strategies.[172] Although a small percentage of these patients were salvaged, transplantation was unsuccessful in the majority of patients. Results following treatment of patients earlier in the course of disease are superior. Figure 21–1, for example, is based on HLA identical sibling transplant data from a Center for International Blood and Marrow Transplantation Research (CIBMTR) report covering the period 1998–2004; following with full-dose conditioning for acute myelogenous leukemia, patient survival was related to disease status in patients older than 20 years.[215] Disease status, as determined by positron emission tomography (PET), was an important predictor of progression-free survival for patients with diffuse large B-cell lymphoma and HL undergoing autologous HCT (Fig. 21–2).[216] Evidence of residual disease by PET prior to transplantation was associated with a significantly increased risk for relapse after autologous HCT. These two scenarios highlight a general truism: that patients who have advanced stages or poorly controlled disease at the start of transplant conditioning have significantly inferior outcomes compared to patients transplanted earlier in the course of their disease and to those who have achieved good, albeit temporary, control of their disease. Attempts at salvaging patients with advanced disease who have failed multiple therapies are rarely successful and if transplantation is to be considered as a treatment strategy, it is best to consider this modality early in the course of therapy. These discussions are complex as earlier transplantation, especially allogeneic HCT, carries significant risks to the patient. A number of other disease-specific considerations are important in determining the appropriate timing for transplantation, including the presence and/or persistence of cytogenetic and molecular abnormalities, the immune phenotype, and evidence of extramedullary or extranodal disease. Advanced genetic characterization of leukemia and lymphoma may provide improved insight into cohorts of patients likely to fare well versus poorly with standard therapies for which HCT should be performed earlier in the course of disease.

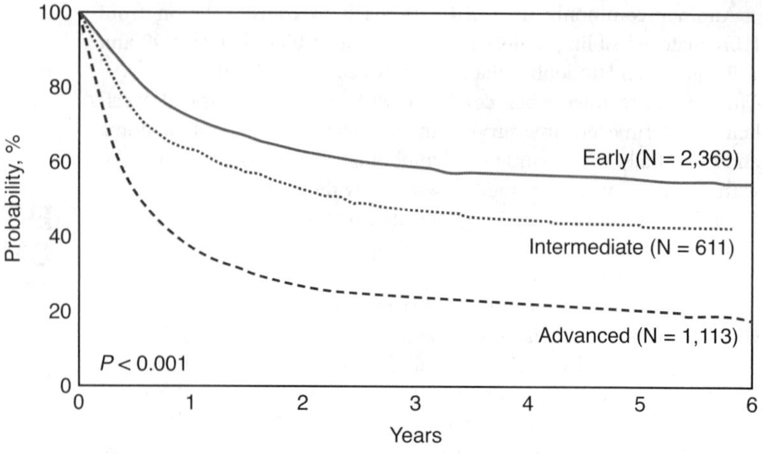

FIGURE 21–1. Probability of survival by disease status following human leukocyte antigen-identical sibling transplants with full-dose conditioning for acute myelogenous leukemia in patients age >20 years during the period 1998–2004.

HISTOCOMPATIBLE DONORS

Over the years the increased precision in HLA typing has resulted in clinically notable improvements in outcome as accurate matching at the MHC is considered essential to minimize GVHD and graft failure.[217] Comparing studies that evaluated the impact of HLA compatibility with the risk of GVHD and other transplantation outcomes is challenging. The main reason relates to the difficulty in assessing the true degree of incompatibility in the earlier studies; when newer molecular-based typing methods were applied to archived specimens, allele disparities were uncovered among phenotypically identical individuals, and these allele disparities were reportedly functionally relevant.[218,219]

Siblings are the preferred donor source. However, patients who do not have siblings, or who do not have a match following HLA analysis, should be considered for an unrelated donor search. Because finding a suitably matched unrelated donor may require 3 to 6 months, early searching is critical in avoiding unnecessary delays in pursuing an allogeneic transplant. An alternative approach in selected patients has been to perform transplantation using cells from a half-matched or haploidentical donor. Cord blood transplantation is another option, especially for children who do not have HLA-matched sibling donors (see section on Umbilical Cord Blood above).

AGE

Among adult and pediatric patients, older age at the time of transplantation is an important determinant that adversely affects NRM following autologous and full-dose allogeneic transplant conditioning.[220–226] In a

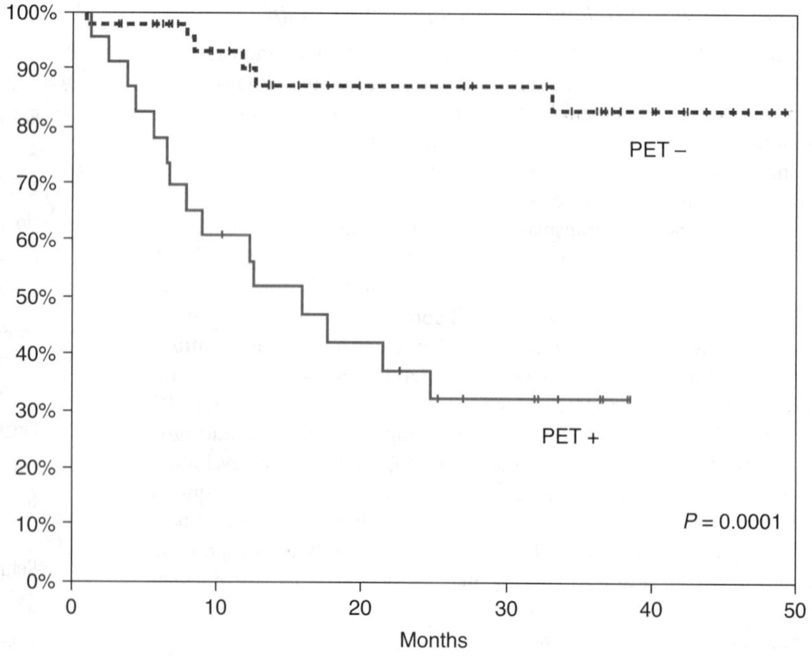

FIGURE 21–2. Progression-free survival curve of 48 patients who had negative positron emission tomography (PET–) scans compared with 24 patients who had positive pretransplantation PET scans (PET+).

study of 52 highly selected patients between 60 and 68 years of age, the 1-year NRM following full-dose allogeneic HCT approached 40 percent,[220] a number considerably higher than the NRM reported in younger transplant recipients. In a single-institution evaluation of 500 autologous transplant recipients, age 50 years or older was associated was a fourfold increase in the 100-day NRM compared to younger patients.[224]

Yet older age does not appear to negatively impact NRM following allogeneic HCT using RIC.[227] For these reasons, full-dose allogeneic HCT is generally offered to patients younger than 50 to 55 years of age, whereas older allotransplantation patients are considered for RIC, which is better tolerated and has been successfully performed in patients into their seventh decade of life. Careful screening for comorbid medical conditions, such as heart, lung, kidney, and liver disease, remains important for all patients being considered for HCT.

COMORBID MEDICAL CONDITIONS

Comorbid medical conditions can have a significant impact on transplantation outcomes. Routine screening of heart and lung function to detect occult abnormalities is of critical importance, especially in older patients. Evaluation of liver and kidney function, as well as exposures to potential pathogens such as cytomegalovirus, hepatitis B and hepatitis C, herpes viruses, and HIV are routine and should be performed in all patients. A new pre-HCT evaluation system, the Charlson Comorbidity Index, was reported and clinically tested to evaluate the influence of comorbidities on HCT outcomes.[228] Although not yet widely used, this tool will likely become valuable in the risk assessment of transplant candidates.

Another major factor impacting outcome following transplantation is the nutritional status of the patient, as extremes such as cachexia or obesity require special considerations. Malnourished patients may require pretransplantation enteral or parenteral nutrition to improve their general condition and patients with excessive obesity (body mass index >35) may be advised to reduce their body weight under the guidance of a dietician. A large clinical study of 2238 patients at the Fred Hutchison Cancer Research Center demonstrated that pretransplantation body weight significantly impacted NRM following allogeneic HCT.[229] Patients, whose actual body weight ranged between 95 and 145 percent of ideal, experienced comparable NRM, whereas patients who weighed less than 95 percent or greater than 145 percent had decreased survival. A similar study of 473 patients undergoing autologous HCT reported that patients who were malnourished and those who were excessively obese fared the worst.[230]

Every effort should be made to encourage potential patients to maintain good health practices, including discontinuation of alcohol and smoking, and avoiding illicit drug use permanently. Attention to the medical evaluation and management of pretransplantation conditions and complications will help improve outcomes after HCT.

DISEASES TREATED WITH TRANSPLANTATION

Table 21–4 presents an extensive list of the diseases treated with HCT. The results obtained with transplantation are reviewed in detail in the disease-specific chapters in this book.

The choice of performing autologous versus allogeneic HCT in patients with hematolymphoid malignancies depends, in part, on the disease being treated, its response to conventional-dose chemotherapy, and the availability of a histocompatible donor. In general terms, autologous transplantation is recommended for patients whose malignancy exhibits chemosensitivity to conventional dose therapy and does not extensively involve the marrow; included are many of the histologic subtypes of lymphoma including HL, germ cell tumors, and other selected pediatric tumors. In these instances tumor eradication is a result of dose escalation of cytotoxic therapy in the transplant regimen, and the autograft serves as hematopoietic cell rescue. In contrast, allogeneic transplantation is generally pursued for hematologic malignancies and disorders that primarily originate in the marrow, such as acute and chronic leukemia, aplastic anemia, and the myelodysplastic and myeloproliferative syndromes. For some diseases with extensive marrow tumor involvement, such as the low-grade lymphomas and myeloma, the decision to pursue autologous or allogeneic HCT is more complex. In general terms, in these settings allogeneic transplantation has been more successful in controlling disease recurrence and has been associated with a significant reduction in disease relapse risk. However, the risks associated with allogeneic transplantation, which include GVHD, increased infections, and regimen toxicities are significant and negatively impact the overall survival of patients. Thus, the decision to pursue

TABLE 21–4. List of Diseases Treated by Hematopoietic Cell Transplantation

Disease/Condition	Allogeneic HCT	Autologous HCT
Malignant disease		
Acute myelogenous leukemia	+	+
Acute lymphoblastic leukemia	+	−
Chronic myelogenous leukemia	+	+
Chronic lymphocytic leukemia	+	+
Myelodysplastic syndromes	+	−
Myeloproliferative syndromes	+	−
Non-Hodgkin lymphoma	+	+
Hodgkin lymphoma	+	+
Myeloma	+	+
Amyloidosis	−	+
Waldenström macroglobulinemia	+	+
Hairy cell leukemia	+	−
Selected solid tumors (testicular cancer, pediatric tumors)	−	+
Neuroblastoma	−	+
Nonmalignant diseases		
Acquired aplastic anemia	+	−
Congenital pure red cell aplasia	+	−
Fanconi anemia	+	−
Thalassemia	+	−
Sickle cell anemia	+	−
Paroxysmal nocturnal hemoglobinuria	+	−
Severe combined immunodeficiency	+	−
Wiskott-Aldrich	+	−
Congenital leukocyte dysfunction	+	−
Osteopetrosis	+	−
Familial erythrophagocytic lymphohistiocytosis	+	−
Glanzmann disease	+	−
Hereditary storage diseases	+	−
Selected autoimmune diseases	+	+

an allogeneic or autologous HCT for patients with these diseases depends on the combination of patient characteristics such as comorbidities and age, availability of a suitable donor, disease-specific characteristics, and often patient preference. Also, for diseases where there the GVT effects are considered more powerful, allogeneic transplantation is favored. Examples include patients with CML, AML, and ALL, and multiply recurrent low-grade lymphoma.[231] For some hematologic conditions, such as the myelodysplastic and myeloproliferative disorders, only allogeneic transplants can be considered.

In addition, patients with selected solid tumors, such as testicular cancer, neuroblastomas, and other pediatric tumors, have had successful outcomes with autologous HCT.[232–234] Studies in women with breast and ovarian carcinoma, and limited studies in patients with renal cell carcinoma and small-cell lung cancer failed to demonstrate a role for HCT.[235–237]

A variety of acquired nonmalignant and congenital disorders can be successfully treated with HCT. Most notable is allogeneic HCT for patients with severe aplastic anemia where outstanding results have been achieved for those individuals who have an HLA-matched sibling donor; upwards of 80 to 90 percent of these patients enjoy long-term disease-free control and complete hematologic remissions.[238,239] Hematopoietic cell transplantation for patients with clinically significant hemoglobin disorders, such as thalassemia major, has been very successful, especially in patients without significant liver disease.[240,241] Likewise, allogeneic HCT is considered a treatment option for young patients with severe forms of sickle cell disease.[242] In patients with hemoglobin disorders, transplantation serves as a form of gene therapy that uses allogeneic hematopoietic cells as vectors for genes essential for normal hematopoiesis. Eventually the vector may well be autologous stem cells transformed by the insertion of normal genes, yet there is no indication that this will occur in the near future.[243]

For patients with severe combined immunodeficiency syndrome and other congenital lymphoid immunodeficiencies, allogeneic HCT remains the treatment of choice.[244,245] The role of allogeneic HCT for patients with storage diseases, a diverse group of disorders that typically involve a single gene defect in a lysosomal hydrolytic enzyme or peroxisomal function, is evolving and it appears that subsets of selected mucopolysaccharidoses derive the most benefit.[246,247] Autologous and allogeneic HCT is currently being evaluated in clinical trials for some autoimmune diseases in which patients have had life-threatening events or critical organ damage.

SELECTED RESULTS OF HEMATOPOIETIC CELL TRANSPLANTATION

A comprehensive discussion of transplantation outcomes is beyond the scope of this chapter. Please refer to other disease-focused chapters of this text for more complete information. A brief overview of transplantation-related outcomes in a number of diseases is presented.

ACUTE MYELOGENOUS LEUKEMIA

Hematopoietic cell transplantation has a significant role in the treatment of AML patients. Many studies have consistently demonstrated that relapse rates are markedly impacted by allogenic HCT. With improved prognosis afforded by cytogenetic and genetic analysis of the leukemic cells, patients with higher risk of disease recurrence can be better selected for transplantation-based therapies.

Induction Failure/Refractory Relapse

The likelihood for long-term survival is very low in AML patients whose disease fails to achieve remission following induction therapy (primary induction failure), or whose disease initially responds yet subsequently relapses and remains refractory to reinduction therapy (refractory relapse). Studies in younger (i.e., <60 years of age) patients with induction failure AML or refractory relapse consistently confirm an event-free survival of 15 to 30 percent following allogeneic HCT from a matched sibling or unrelated donor.[248–250] The timing for transplantation is often determined by logistical issues, such as donor availability. Most authorities in the field suggest that little is gained by persisting with standard chemotherapy if a complete response is not achieved after two cycles of conventional dose induction.[251]

SECOND OR SUBSEQUENT REMISSION

Selected young patients with AML in second remission may have long-term event-free survival, yet this is generally limited to patients with favorable cytogenetics and those who had a long first remission. Data reported from the CIBMTR in 2007 highlighted a 5-year 50 percent (2% SD) overall survival for adult patients with AML in second or subsequent remission transplanted from an HLA-matched sibling donor.[215] There have been no comparable improvements in non–transplantation-based strategies for recurrent AML, indicating that the advantage of allogeneic HCT in second remission or beyond persists. Patients with AML beyond CR1 who lack a matched sibling donor are candidates for either matched unrelated donor or autologous HCT, yet no studies that compared autologous to unrelated donor transplantation for AML patients in second or subsequent remission are available.

First Remission

A question of significant practical importance is how best to treat a younger AML patient who achieved a first remission following induction chemotherapy. Numerous large prospective trials were conducted with the general design that all newly diagnosed AML patients received induction therapy and once in first remission patients with an HLA-matched sibling were allocated to allogeneic HCT, while those without donors were randomized to either autologous HCT or best-of-care chemotherapy. A meta-analysis focused on the comparative outcomes of allogeneic HCT versus chemotherapy and included all such studies conducted between 1995 and 2003, provided the trials were reported in English, followed the intent-to-treat principle, and presented survival data.[252] Five studies were identified that comprised 3100 patients of whom 1151 received an allogeneic HCT and 1949 received best-of-care chemotherapy.[253–257] A survival benefit in favor of the transplantation arm was reported for patients with unfavorable-risk cytogenetics (hazard ratio: 1.24). For patients with favorable-risk cytogenetics, chemotherapy without transplantation was the preferred initial treatment choice. There was a nonsignificant trend (hazard ratio: 1.09) in favor of allogeneic HCT for patients with intermediate-risk cytogenetics. Randomized prospective clinical trials that compared autologous HCT to best-of-care chemotherapy for AML patients in first remission provided little compelling data to support the widespread use of autologous HCT.[253,258–261]

Treatment algorithms for adults younger than 60 years of age with newly diagnosed AML currently consider the cytogenetic risk assignment and whether mutations in any of the commonly evaluated transcription factors (NPM1, CEBPA, MLL-PTD) or tyrosine kinases (FLT3-ITD, FLT3-TKD, NRAS, c-KIT) are identified (see Chaps. 11 and 89). Allogeneic HCT following RIC versus best-of-care nontransplantation therapy is currently being evaluated in randomized prospective trials in the United States and Europe for older AML patients in first remission.

ACUTE LYMPHOBLASTIC LEUKEMIA

Allogeneic HCT has been widely pursued in adult patients with ALL, especially those patients with high-risk features typically defined as elevated white blood cell count at diagnosis, non–T-cell disease, adverse cytogenetics, extramedullary disease, and failure to achieve remission within 30 days of treatment (Chap. 93). Many studies have generally demonstrated an important role for allogeneic HCT in this clinical setting with consistent reduction in relapse rates and often improvement in expected overall survival.[181,262,263] A large prospective trial has also demonstrated an improvement in overall survival for adult ALL patients with standard-risk features.[264] The study included patients between 15 and 55 years of age although the age threshold, if there is one, at which "adult" ALL begins and "childhood" ALL ceases is a matter of current controversy. Indeed, there may be evidence that patients up to the age of 25 years might achieve better outcomes on pediatric protocols.[265,266] In the authors' opinion allogeneic HCT from an HLA-matched sibling donor should be considered for the majority of adult patients with ALL in CR1.

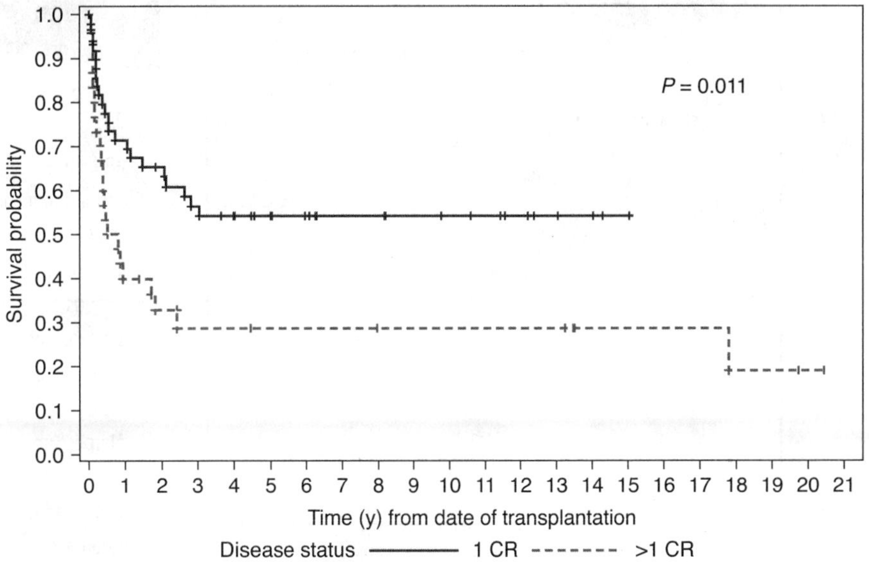

FIGURE 21–3. Overall survival by remission status at transplantation. 1CR, first complete remission; y, years.

Philadelphia Chromosome-Positive Acute Lymphoblastic Leukemia

Historically, the poor outcome with chemotherapy led to trials evaluating the role of allogeneic HCT for the treatment of adult Philadelphia chromosome-positive (Ph+) ALL. A study conducted from City of Hope and Stanford University of 23 Ph+ ALL patients transplanted while in first complete remission, using a graft from HLA-matched siblings reported a 3-year probability of event-free survival and relapse of 65 percent and 12 percent, respectively.[267] Additional followup of 67 patients has continued to show that these patients fare well with allogeneic HCT despite their dismal prognosis with chemotherapy alone (Fig. 21–3).[268] Several studies report that imatinib combined with multiagent chemotherapy in newly diagnosed Ph+ ALL with subsequent allogeneic HCT improved survival and decreased relapse rates even further[269]; these observations suggest that eradication of pretransplantation minimal residual disease is desirable. Currently, trials are being developed to compare combination chemotherapy and a tyrosine kinase inhibitor to allogeneic HCT. Beyond first remission, allogeneic HCT is curative in a smaller percentage of patients but also remains the treatment of choice.

■ MULTIPLE MYELOMA

Autologous HCT within the first year of initiating treatment has been the standard of care for patients younger than 70 years of age with newly diagnosed myeloma. Although neither chemotherapy nor autologous HCT produces a cure, event-free and overall survival were prolonged following autologous HCT when compared to treatment with conventional chemotherapy alone.[270,271] Yet with the incorporation of the new chemotherapeutic agents (e.g., bortezomib, thalidomide, lenalidomide) as initial therapy, the response rate for patients with advanced stage myeloma has improved and survival with chemotherapy alone is improving. Whether the use of these newer agents, alone or in combination, will delay or possibly even eliminate the need for HCT in patients with myeloma is not known at this time. In addition, survival with HCT is improving for certain populations with the incorporation of double (tandem) autologous HCT.[272,273] Consequently, the use of tandem transplantion is currently being compared to autologous transplantation followed by reduced-intensity conditioning allogeneic transplantation in patients with myeloma through the U.S. Clinical Trials Network.

■ NON-HODGKIN LYMPHOMA AND HODGKIN LYMPHOMA

Patients with chemosensitive moderate- and high-grade lymphoma beyond first complete remission have an improved overall survival with high-dose therapy followed by autologous HCT compared to best-of-care salvage chemotherapy.[274,275] Improvement in survival for patients with B-cell NHL may further be achieved with inclusion of rituximab as an *in vivo* purging strategy and perhaps in the posttransplantation setting.[276] Autologous transplantation has also been pursued with encouraging results in patients in first remission with high-risk malignancies that fare relatively poorly with standard chemotherapy, such as diffuse large B-cell lymphoma patients with high-risk features, mantle cell lymphoma, and some T-cell lymphomas.[277–279] Additional studies that address the question of whether performing autologous HCT in first complete remission improves outcomes for lymphoma patients with disease that is slow to respond and remains PET-positive are ongoing. The use of PET scanning following salvage chemotherapy for relapsed NHL and HL patients may help to identify patients who are at high risk of relapse despite autologous transplantation where other options may be pursued such as combined auto/reduced-intensity transplantation or posttransplant immunotherapy.

Relapse of lymphoma after autologous HCT is the major reason for treatment failure. Several phase II studies reported that patients who suffer a relapse of lymphoma after autologous transplantation could still be salvaged and experienced long-term survival of greater than 45 percent using RIC and allogeneic transplantation from matched related and unrelated donors (Fig. 21–4).[209,280] Larger studies are required to better define the strength of the GVT effect among the different lymphoma subtypes.

COMPLICATIONS OF HEMATOPOIETIC CELL TRANSPLANTATION

Table 21–5 lists the complications associated with HCT; the more common issues are discussed below. The first 100 days following the cell infusion is typically the time of greatest risk for recipients of autologous and allogeneic HCT. Care by physicians skilled in the management of patients undergoing these procedures is of critical importance. Progress

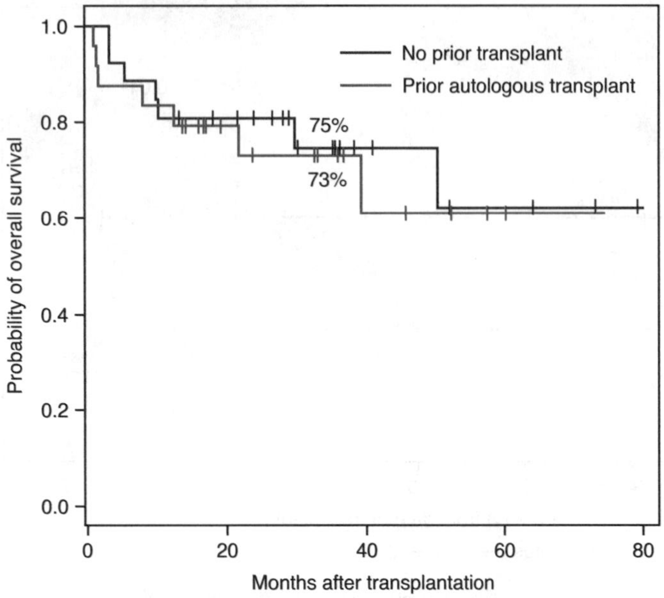

FIGURE 21–4. Probability of survival following RIC conditioning and allogeneic HCT from matched related and unrelated donors in 32 patients with lymphoid malignant diseases that had relapsed from a prior autologous transplant. Results are compared to 32 lymphoma patients who underwent RIC without having had a prior autologous transplant.

in the supportive care of patients is critically important in improving overall outcomes.

GRAFT FAILURE

Graft failure is defined as the lack of hematopoietic cell engraftment following autologous and allogeneic HCT. Criteria are predominantly operational and graft failure is divided into primary (early) and secondary (late) phases. The consequences of graft failure are significant and include a high risk of mortality, often as a consequence of infection and hemorrhage related to cytopenias.

Primary (Early) and Secondary (Late) Graft Failure

Myeloid engraftment is commonly defined as the first of three consecutive days on which the absolute neutrophil count exceeds 5×10^8/L.[191] Myeloid engraftment typically occurs within 21 days of the graft infusion, irrespective of whether the product represents autologous marrow or blood, or is from an allogeneic matched related or unrelated donor. Platelet recovery is more loosely defined and is the first day of a platelet count of at least 20, 50, or 100×10^9/L, sustained without transfusion for 7 days.[281,282] Platelet recovery may be substantially delayed compared with myeloid recovery or sometimes not achieved at all especially if the higher platelet value (100×10^9/L) is used as the threshold. A hemoglobin level of at least 8 g/dL without transfusion support is an accepted threshold for red cell engraftment.[282]

Primary graft failure is defined as a failure to achieve these threshold counts beyond day +28 posttransplantation. An isolated cytopenia does not necessarily invoke graft failure as this may be a transitory phenomenon related to infection, a medication, a lineage-specific immune-mediated cytopenia, or GVHD.

Patients who meet criteria for initial engraftment but subsequently developed loss of a previously functioning graft defined by at least two cytopenic lines were considered to have late or secondary graft failure.[210] Late graft failure is more often associated with allogeneic HCT than with autologous transplantation. Some possible causes for late graft failure include graft rejection related to residual host immunity, persistent or progressive disease, low donor cell yield, medication side effect, infection, or GVHD.

TABLE 21–5. Complications of Hematopoietic Cell Transplantation

Vascular access complications
Graft failure
Blood group incompatibilities and hemolytic complications
Acute GVHD
Chronic GVHD
Infectious complications
Bacterial infections
Fungal infections
Cytomegalovirus infection
Herpes simplex virus infections
Varicella-zoster virus infections
Epstein-Barr virus infections
Adenovirus, respiratory viruses, HHV-6, -7, -8, and other viruses
Gastrointestinal complications
Mucosal ulceration/bleeding
Nutritional support
Hepatic complications
Sinusoidal obstructive syndrome
Hepatitis: infectious versus noninfectious
Lung injury
Interstitial pneumonitis: infectious versus noninfectious
Diffuse alveolar hemorrhage
Engraftment syndrome
Bronchiolitis obliterans
Kidney and bladder complications
Endocrine complications
Drug–drug interactions
Growth and development
Late onset nonmalignant complications
Osteoporosis/osteopenia, avascular necrosis, dental problems, cataracts, chronic fatigue, psychosocial effects, and rehabilitation
Secondary malignancies
Neurologic complications
Infectious, transplant conditioning and immune suppression medication toxicities

GVHD, graft-versus-host disease; HHV, human herpes virus subtypes.

Graft Rejection and Poor Graft Function

Graft rejection is a term that is unique to allogeneic HCT. It is the immune-mediated rejection of the donor cells by residual host effector cells that occurs because of the genetic disparity between the recipient and the donor.[148,283,284] Graft rejection is a possible cause of primary or secondary graft failure following allogeneic HCT. The determination of graft rejection requires analysis of blood or marrow for chimerism as graft rejection is defined as the inability to detect a meaningful percentage of donor hematopoietic elements. In contrast to graft rejection, poor graft function describes the failure to achieve adequate blood counts following allogeneic HCT in the presence of complete donor hematopoietic cell chimerism.

Graft Failure Following Reduced-Intensity Conditioning

Allogeneic HCT following RIC is associated with incomplete eradication of host hematopoietic elements. As a consequence a significant percentage of patients have multilineage mixed chimerism for several months after transplantation before converting to complete donor type.[210] Primary engraftment following allogeneic HCT using RIC is defined by neutrophil, platelet, and hemoglobin count recovery as outlined above, in addition to achievement of ∏5 percent donor T cells (CD3+) by day +28 after transplantation. A failure to surpass the 5 percent threshold at any time after transplantation is considered primary graft failure, whereas secondary graft failure is reserved for cases that initially surpass the 5 percent threshold but the T-cell chimerism subsequently falls below this level. Mixed chimerism describes patients enumerating 5 to 95 percent donor T cells, and full or complete chimerism is considered the achievement of greater than 95 percent donor T-cell origin. There remains a lack of consensus regarding the use of these terms.

Incidence of Graft Failure

The incidence of graft failure varies widely in published reports as often the consequences associated with graft failure (i.e., morbidity and mortality caused by infection, hemorrhage, and disease progression) are reported and not the graft failure itself. To estimate the incidence of graft failure following autologous HCT it is reasonable to consider that in most centers the 100-day NRM is 10 percent or less, of which only a small subset can be attributed to graft failure. Another surrogate marker for estimating the incidence of graft failure following autologous HCT is the requirement for hematopoietic cell rescue using a backup product. A study of 300 patients who underwent autologous HCT revealed that 4.7 percent required their backup product.[285] Unmanipulated marrow, AML, and CD34+ selection of G-CSF–mobilized blood mononuclear cells collected by apheresis were risk factors for graft failure in this study. Thus, it is reasonable to estimate that the incidence of graft failure following autologous HCT is between 1 and 5 percent.

Graft failure following allogeneic HCT is more complex than graft failure after autologous HCT because of the presence of confounding factors such as histocompatibility and ABO matching, graft-versus-host and host-versus-graft reactions, and the use of posttransplantation immune suppression.[284,286,287] These factors increase the risk of immune-mediated graft rejection such that the risk of graft failure following allogeneic HCT is reported to occur in 5 to 20 percent of patients.

Table 21–6 highlights strategies for the treatment for early and late graft failure following autologous and allogeneic HCT.

TABLE 21–6. Treatment Strategies for Graft Failure

Graft failure following autologous HCT
Autologous backup should be available for manipulated products
Hematopoietic growth factor support
Consideration for allogeneic HCT
Graft failure following allogeneic HCT
Autologous backup
Hematopoietic growth factor support
Alterations in immune suppression medication to convert mixed to full donor chimerism
Donor lymphocyte infusion to convert to full donor type
CD34+ cell boost for poor graft function
Regrafting using same or alternate donor

■ REGIMEN-RELATED ORGAN TOXICITIES

The severity of organ toxicities associated with HCT is in part related to the intensity of the specific agents administered, the amount of prior therapy received, patient comorbidities before transplantation, and the presence of posttransplantation factors, including the use of posttransplantation medications such as immune suppression drugs and antimicrobial agents.

Mucositis

Mucositis occurs in more than 90 percent of patients receiving high-dose regimens and is often regarded as the most difficult issue from the patient's perspective.[288,289] Current management is unsatisfactory and includes frequent rinsing with antimicrobial and antifungal medications, antiviral treatment for patients with history of herpes simplex virus (HSV) seropositivity, and pain control often with continuous intravenous infusions of narcotic drugs. Improvement typically occurs around the time of hematopoietic reconstitution. Fully ablative regimens, TBI-based conditioning, and the administration of posttransplantation methotrexate for GVHD prevention are associated with more severe mucositis.[289] Severe mucositis may result in significant tissue edema leading to upper airway obstruction and/or aspiration pneumonitis, although, fortunately, these complications of mucositis are rare. Gastroenteritis induced by the regimen results in nausea, vomiting, and diarrhea, which may persist for weeks after the transplant.[290,291] Breaches in the mucosal lining predispose to bacterial translocation from the gastrointestinal tract with increased risk of bacteremia and sepsis. Central lines are placed before HCT for administration of fluids, drugs, and hyperalimentation because most often during the period of therapy-induced mucositis and gastroenteritis patients are unable to maintain adequate caloric and fluid intake. Novel strategies, including the use of growth factors such as keratinocyte growth factor has been effective in the autologous transplantation setting using aggressive TBI-based conditioning.[292] In addition to impacting mucositis, this agent has also prevented GVHD in murine models.[293]

Sinusoidal Obstructive Syndrome/Venoocclusive Disease

Sinusoidal obstructive syndrome (SOS) is a clinical syndrome of tender hepatomegaly, fluid retention, weight gain, and elevated serum bilirubin that follows autologous or allogeneic HCT.[294] This syndrome is also called venoocclusive disease of the liver, but this term inaccurately describes the underlying pathobiology, as the liver injury is initiated in the hepatic sinusoids, and obstruction of hepatic venules is not essential to the development of the clinical signs and symptoms.[295]

The incidence of SOS varies significantly with the intensity of the regimen; from less than 10 percent with RIC to as high as 50 percent following regimens that use cyclophosphamide combined with TBI of greater than 14 Gy.[296] An important contributor to the variability in the incidence of SOS is the large variations in the metabolism of cyclophosphamide from patient to patient.[297] Severe forms of SOS generally represent a fraction of all cases: Among patients with myeloid malignancies the incidence of severe SOS was 7 percent following cyclophosphamide 120 mg/kg plus TBI 12 to 13.2 Gy and was 2 percent following targeted busulfan and cyclophosphamide 120 mg/kg.[298] Gemtuzumab ozogamicin may cause sinusoidal liver injury when used to treat patients with AML.[299] Pretransplantation liver injury is a risk factor for SOS; and the risk of SOS was almost 40 percent when higher-dose gemtuzumab ozogamicin was given in close proximity to a cyclophosphamide-containing transplant regimen.[300] Lowering the dose of gemtuzumab ozogamicin appeared to eliminate this risk.

The severity of SOS is somewhat arbitrary and generally is classified as mild (clinically apparent yet resolves without treatment), moderate (requiring diuretics and pain medication for abdominal discomfort yet completely resolves), or severe (requires specific therapies but does not resolve before day 100 or death).[296]

An important component of therapy for SOS is the management of sodium and water balance with diuretics, preservation of renal blood flow, and paracenteses for ascites that is associated with significant discomfort or pulmonary compromise. Patients with a poor prognosis can be recognized quickly after SOS onset by the steep rises in serum bilirubin, body weight and other liver enzymes, hepatic venous pressure measurement of over 20 torr, development of portal vein thrombosis, and multiorgan failure requiring mechanical ventilation or renal dialysis.[301] There is a lack of satisfactory therapies for severe SOS; the best results are thought to be with the use of intravenous defibrotide, a mixture of single-stranded porcine oligodeoxyribonucleotides that induces antithrombotic and profibrinolytic effects in preclinical models.[302,303] Its mechanism of action in the treatment of SOS remains unknown. An experience of 88 patients with moderate and severe SOS treated with defibrotide resulted in complete resolution in 36 percent of patients with relatively low toxicity.[302] Other approaches involve the administration of thrombolytic therapy with tissue plasminogen activator, *N*-acetylcysteine, activated protein C, prednisone, topical nitrates, and glutamine, yet none of these therapies have shown convincing evidence of efficacy.

Prevention of sinusoidal injury is likely to be the more effective strategy. Efforts to develop protocols that reduce the incidence and severity of SOS by possibly protecting against sinusoidal injury have been made. Heparin has been explored by low-dose continuous infusion in a prospective randomized clinical trial of 161 patients who underwent allogeneic or autologous HCT. Patients were randomized to low-dose heparin (100 U/kg total dose per day) by continuous intravenous infusion or placebo. The heparin was initiated prior to the start of the preparative regimen and continued until 30 days after HCT, or until neutrophil engraftment was achieved, whichever was less. A significantly lower incidence of venoocclusive disease was noted in the heparin-treated group of 2.5 percent versus 13.7 percent in the control group.[304] There was no increased risk of bleeding or other toxicities in the patients treated with heparin. Yet the beneficial effect of heparin has not been observed in other prospective studies.[305] Another approach has been to use ursodeoxycholic acid throughout the peritransplant period to reduce the incidence of SOS. In a prospective randomized clinical trial in patients undergoing full-dose allogeneic transplant conditioning, prophylaxis with ursodeoxycholic acid did not affect the risk of venoocclusive disease; unexpectedly, however, prophylaxis did result in reduced NRM from acute GVHD and improved overall survival.[306]

Pulmonary Complications

Noncardiogenic diffuse lung injury, also referred to as idiopathic pulmonary syndrome, remains a significant problem following autologous or allogeneic HCT. Historically, approximately 50 percent of lung injury after HCT was from infection, yet with the judicious use of broad-spectrum antimicrobial agents noninfectious causes are more prevalent.[307]

Idiopathic pulmonary syndrome occurs in 10 to 15 percent of transplant recipients.[308] Risk factors for idiopathic pulmonary syndrome include high-dose conditioning compared to RIC, the administration of TBI, the development of GVHD, older recipient age, prior history of cigarette smoking, prior thoracic/mediastinal irradiation, and a pretransplantation diffusion lung capacity of carbon monoxide that is reduced from below the normal range.[309,310] Treatment for idiopathic pulmonary syndrome is generally supportive and also includes glucocorticoids combined with broad spectrum antimicrobial agents.[308] Antibodies against tumor necrosis factor (TNF)-α have also been explored in animal models and initial studies in patients are promising.[311]

Idiopathic pulmonary syndrome comprises a spectrum of clinical presentations. In a small subset of patients, diffuse pulmonary hemorrhage develops, more often in the immediate posttransplantation period, and is characterized by progressive shortness of breath, cough, and hypoxemia.[312] Classically, diffuse alveolar hemorrhage is defined by the demonstration of progressively bloodier aliquots in bronchoalveolar lavage fluid.[313] Mortality from this complication is high (often >75 percent) despite the use of high-dose steroids. Alveolar hemorrhage can be from infectious and noninfectious causes.[314] Another subset of patients with idiopathic pulmonary syndrome develop periengraftment respiratory distress, clinically characterized by symptoms that are identical to alveolar hemorrhage, yet bronchoscopy fails to identify blood.[315] Periengraftment respiratory distress, by definition, occurs within 1 week of neutrophil engraftment. In the autologous setting, the symptoms respond promptly to steroids, whereas in the allogeneic setting, patients respond less well, indicating that perhaps some cases may be complicated by GVHD.[315,316]

Lung inflammation following the administration of 1,3-*bis*(2-choloroethyl)-1-nitrosurea (BCNU) and transfusion-associated lung injury are two other forms of noninfectious lung injury that technically do not fit idiopathic pulmonary syndrome as they have distinct etiologies.[317,318] BCNU-induced pneumonitis is often characterized by a nonproductive cough with increasing dyspnea and bilateral pulmonary infiltrates on chest radiography with or without fevers, and often occurs 30 to 60 days after transplantation.[317] Pulmonary function tests reveal a restrictive pattern of lung injury and a decrease in the diffusion lung capacity of carbon monoxide compared to the pretransplantation value. Treatment with glucocorticoids early in the clinical course promptly reduces mortality and morbidity and is the key for a successful outcome. If untreated or recognized late significant pulmonary fibrosis may develop. Plasma-containing blood products are commonly administered to transplant recipients and transfusion-associated lung injury is estimated to occur in 1 in 1000 to 1 in 5000 transfusions.[318] Symptoms present acutely, with the onset of dyspnea and respiratory distress within 8 hours following transfusion. Glucocorticoid administration, forced diuresis, and respiratory support result in complete recovery in most patients within 2 to 4 days.

INFECTIONS

Susceptibility to infection is a significant challenge in the clinical management of transplant recipients. The essential principles are prevention, judicious monitoring, and expeditiously treating all bacterial, fungal, and viral infections. These basic principles are widely accepted, yet the day-to-day strategy for achieving these principles varies widely from center to center and physician to physician.

Two important measures for reducing infections in immune-compromised transplant recipients are an effective hand-washing policy, and a strategy for preventing transmission of respiratory infections, including metapneumovirus, respiratory syncytial virus, parainfluenza, and influenza.[319,320] Screening the blood supply has reduced the incidence of transfusion-related infections, especially hepatitis C and cytomegalovirus (CMV) for seronegative recipients.[320]

The duration of neutropenia and severity of oral and gastrointestinal mucosal damage from the conditioning regimen are risk factors for infection before neutrophil recovery has occurred.[319] Following neutrophil recovery, the persistent B- and T-cell–mediated immune deficiency increases susceptibility to opportunistic infections. Immune recovery following autologous HCT is relatively rapid compared to after allogeneic transplantation. Most autologous transplant recipients recover T-cell immunity specific for herpes viruses, including CMV by 3 months after the transplant.[321] The degree and duration of immune deficiency following allogeneic HCT are influenced, in part, by the type of immune-suppressive therapy and severity of GVHD. Chronic GVHD imparts chronic B- and T-cell immune deficiencies that may persist for years, and Ig production and reticuloendothelial function may also be impaired.[322–326]

Bacterial Infections

Bacterial infections are common during the period of immediate neutropenia that follows the preparative transplant regimen, and are mostly caused by Gram-positive organisms, although Gram-negative infections also occur.[327] The increased risk is caused not only by the neutropenia, but also by the presence of indwelling catheters and tissue injury from the preparative regimen. Patient and staff hygiene is important at reducing infection risk.[320] Some centers also institute other measures such as gowning and masking, although there is little evidence that these actions reduce infection risk. Removal of venous catheters is sometimes required for patients who do not respond promptly to treatment. Chap. 22 reviews specific strategies and regimens for treating bacterial infections in neutropenic patients.

Patients who require ongoing immune-suppressive therapy for the control of chronic GVHD are at risk for recurrent bacteremia with encapsulated bacteria and sinopulmonary infections.[328,329] Strategies for prevention of bacterial infections beyond 90 days after allogeneic HCT include the daily use of penicillin or trimethoprim-sulfamethoxazole until immune-suppressive drug withdrawal.[320] Infrequent bacterial infections that should also be considered, especially in the presence of a pulmonary infiltrate or nodule, are *Legionella*, *Nocardia*, *Mycobacterium tuberculosis*, and atypical mycobacteria.

Fungal Infections

Fungal infections can be serious complications following HCT and are more commonly observed in recipients of allografts as a result of the requirement for posttransplantation immune-suppression medication. The incidence of fungal infection varies considerably among transplantation centers because of a variety of factors, including geographic location, nearby construction, and the prophylactic regimen employed. *Candida* and *Aspergillus* represent the most common fungal pathogens; however, other organisms can also cause life-threatening infections.[330] Chap. 22 discusses the treatment and prophylaxis of fungal infections.

Fluconazole prophylaxis decreases the incidence of invasive and superficial *Candida albicans* infections and may decrease the 100-day mortality in allogeneic HCT recipients.[331] Fluconazole has limited activity against *Candida krusei*, *Torulopsis glabrata*, and *Aspergillus* species. Also, some centers reported an increased incidence of resistant *Candida* infections in patients receiving prophylactic fluconazole.[332] Hepatosplenic candidiasis is not a contraindication to transplantation if antifungal therapy is given during the period of neutropenia and continued thereafter.

Invasive aspergillosis is emerging as a frequent cause of mortality from infection.[333] Risk factors for the development of aspergillosis are older age, acute and chronic GVHD, treatment with prednisone, and prolonged neutropenia.[334,335] The respiratory tract is the most common portal of entry, and clinical manifestations are typically pneumonia and sinusitis.[336] *Aspergillus* is the most common cause of brain abscesses in patients after HCT.[337] High-efficiency particulate air filtration systems can reduce the risk of nosocomial *Aspergillus* infections.

Viral Infections

Infection from the herpesvirus family members can cause significant morbidity and mortality and is a common phenomenon following HCT. Most of the infections are a result of reactivation and the temporal pattern of reactivation follows a relatively predictable course; HSV causes clinically apparent disease at about 2 to 3 weeks, CMV disease usually occurs during the second to third months after transplantation, and varicella-zoster virus (VZV) recurrences present at a median of 5 months after HCT.[338,339]

CMV is an important viral pathogen after HCT. Infection occurs from reactivation of latent virus or is newly acquired from the donor graft or blood transfusions.[340,341] Before effective prevention strategies were introduced, 70 percent of CMV-seropositive transplant recipients and 32 percent of CMV-seronegative recipients developed CMV infections.[342]

During the first 100 days after transplantation, patients with viremia are at high risk for developing CMV pneumonitis or gastroenteritis.[339] First-line therapy for patients with CMV pneumonia or gastroenteritis is ganciclovir combined with IV Ig.[343] Cidofovir and foscarnet can be considered as second-line therapy for CMV disease. Because treatment of established CMV disease with antiviral agents has not been satisfactory, strategies for prophylaxis have been emphasized.[344] Sensitive screening tests using CMV-specific antigenemia or PCR assays are readily available and in routine use. The strategy of preemptively treating patients who develop positive results with these tests is established therapy.

The incidence of late CMV disease after transplantation has increased perhaps because the early use of ganciclovir blunts the recovery of CMV-specific immunity.[345] Among seropositive patients who survived 3 months, approximately 18 percent developed late CMV disease. For patients who received treatment for GVHD with prednisone, the incidence exceeded 30 percent.[346] In view of this, patients with chronic active GVHD require monitoring for reactivation for 1 year or longer after transplantation.

Major questions remain with respect to the duration of therapy, and the relative merits of oral preparations of ganciclovir. Other approaches for prevention of CMV that have been pursued include the early restoration or the adoptive transfer of CMV-specific T cells.[347]

Two other members of the herpesvirus family that cause significant morbidity in the posttransplantation setting are HSV and VZV. The pathogenesis of these viruses is explained by their shared characteristics of latency, reactivation, and neurotropism.

Virtually all HSV disease occurring after HCT is a result of reactivation, and the serologic status of the recipient determines risk for disease and the requirement for prophylaxis.[348] Without acyclovir prophylaxis, HSV infections occur in 80 percent of seropositive patients.[349] Oral mucositis, cutaneous infections, esophagitis, genital herpes, and pneumonia are the most common clinical manifestations. Acyclovir is very effective for the prevention and treatment of HSV and the recommended dosing from the American Society for Blood and Marrow Transplantation is 200 mg orally three times a day or 250 mg/m^2 intravenously every 12 hours.[350] It is also recommended that acyclovir be started at the beginning of conditioning therapy and continue until engraftment or mucositis resolves. Acyclovir is well tolerated immediately after transplantation with no effect on the recovery of neutrophil counts. The duration of HSV prophylaxis remains controversial as "rebound" reactivation after cessation of prophylaxis is relatively common.[350] Valacyclovir 500 mg orally twice daily is a recommended alternative to acyclovir. If a patient is receiving maribavir, foscarnet, valganciclovir, or cidofovir for treatment of another virus, acyclovir is not necessary.

The reported incidence of VZV infection after HCT ranges from 16 to 63 percent.[351–354] The risk of developing recurrent VZV disease after transplantation appears the same for recipients of autologous and allogeneic HCT provided GVHD is not present. Important risk factors for VZV reactivation include the presence of continued immune-suppression medication for the treatment of chronic GVHD, and recipients of cord blood transplants.[355] The initial manifestations of recurrence are localized in approximately half of patients. Treatment with acyclovir within 24 to 48 hours of the onset of herpes zoster prevents dissemination and shortens the course of cutaneous disease.[354,356] The failure of VZV infections to resolve quickly or their recurrence shortly after acyclovir therapy is discontinued is usually a function of the limited host immune response and should not be attributed to acyclovir resistance in most cases. When resistance occurs it is usually mediated by thymidine kinase mutations; as a result, valacyclovir and famciclovir are not effective for treating VZV infections caused by acyclovir-resistance strains.[357] Foscarnet has activity against isolates that are not inhibited by acyclovir, yet its clinical use is complicated by potential nephrotoxicity.[358]

Varicella-zoster immune globulin is an antibody preparation containing IgG antibodies obtained from high-titer immune human serum. Treatment with this immune globulin results in the passive transfer of antibody which is important for prophylaxis following exposure of seronegative immune-compromised HCT recipients who have not had previous VZV infection. This product, however, is no longer commercially available in the United States because production was discontinued by its only licensed manufacturer. There is no evidence to support that passive antibody prophylaxis will reduce the risk of VZV reactivation after HCT in patients who have serologic evidence of prior VZV infection.[359]

The efficacy of acyclovir prophylaxis for preventing recurrent VZV infection in HCT recipients has been evaluated in multiple randomized placebo-controlled and nonrandomized studies where the dose of acyclovir ranged from 400 to 3200 mg/day and the duration varied from 6 to 12 months.[360–362] All studies confirmed that during the period of treatment, VZV infection was reduced, yet there was a rapid recurrence of herpes zoster when the drugs were discontinued. None of the placebo recipients had fatal dissemination likely because the prompt initiation of acyclovir for the treatment of recurrent VZV infection was very effective. As a result clinical practice remains varied with some institutions electing to use acyclovir for suppression of VZV infection after HCT and other centers opting not to use routine prophylaxis.

The live-attenuated varicella vaccine approved for administration to healthy children in the United States cannot be given to immune-compromised HCT patients. However, the vaccine can be heat inactivated without loss of immunogenicity.[363] Immunization with this product may help boost VZV-specific T-cell responses after HCT and decrease the risk of herpes zoster in this population by acting as a substitute for the "natural" resensitization caused by VZV reactivation. When the inactivated vaccine was given to autologous HCT patients pretransplantation as well as at 30, 60, and 90 days posttransplantation, the risk of herpes zoster was reduced and protection correlated with reconstitution of VZV CD4 T-cell immunity.[363]

IMMUNE RECONSTITUTION

The reconstitution of a competent immune system after HCT is essential for a clinical successful outcome. Without appropriate immune reconstitution transplant recipients are at increased risk of infection with opportunistic viruses, bacteria, and fungi, and at increased risk for tumor relapse.[364,365] Recipients of autologous and allogeneic HCT have their preexisting lymphoid immunity eliminated by the immune-suppressive medications, irradiation, and chemotherapeutic agents used in transplant preparative regimens. Lymphoid immune reconstitution comes from two sources: there is the passive transfer of the mature T and B lymphocytes present in the graft, and a recapitulation of normal lymphoid immunity derived from the newly engrafted HSC.[364]

The assessment of immune reconstitution following HCT can be done by the detailed immunophenotypic analyses of the T and B lymphocytes with characterization of their state of differentiation.[366] Functional immune capacity that predicts against infection is determined by the presence of antigen-specific T lymphocytes, which are detected by using antigen-specific blastogenesis or cytokine capture assays to tetanus toxoid, *Candida*, and the herpes viruses (CMV, HSV, and VZV). The presence of a positive blastogenic response confirms antigen-specific T lymphocytes and that adequate amounts of IL-2 are secreted to support cell proliferation.[367] Restoration of cytotoxic T-lymphocyte function to CMV and VZV often requires more than 6 months, even in the absence of GVHD, yet HSV-specific immunity can be seen as early as 3 months after transplantation.

The thymus contributes to late immune reconstitution; it exports newly generated T cells to the periphery. Quantification of a DNA excision circle, generated during T-cell receptor rearrangement (TREC), can be used as a measure of thymic function.[368] As TRECs are lost with each cell division, cells in which they are present can be identified as recent thymic emigrants, and thymic output can thereby be quantitated. High TREC levels consistent with increased thymic output were associated with an increased number of naïve T cells and a broader T-cell repertoire. Young patients have a more rapid recovery and higher TREC levels after HCT than older patients.[323] Low TREC levels correlate with the presence of chronic GVHD and severe opportunistic infections. The extent of the thymic rebound correlates with the patient's capacity to respond to vaccinations.[369] Measures to enhance thymic output after transplantation, especially in older patients, may enhance immune reconstitution and decrease the risk of infections.

Specific antibody production after HCT can be determined by evaluating responses to immunization with a neoantigen (ΦX174), reimmunization with protein antigens (tetanus toxoid), or natural stimulation with bacterial polysaccharide antigens (pneumococcal and meningococcal polyribophosphates).[370] Defects in Ig production persist beyond 6 months even in recipients whose posttransplantation course has not been complicated. In these patients, serum IgG and IgM achieve normal levels by 1 year after transplantation, yet serum IgA may remain low for a period of 2 years. The use of immune-suppressive medication for chronic GVHD control contributes further to a delay in Ig recovery.[370,371]

Improving Immune Reconstitution

Animal experiments have shown that thymic function can be protected from the harmful effects of irradiation and busulfan by the administration of keratinocyte growth factor.[372] Clinical trials are now underway to demonstrate whether the peritransplant administration of this cytokine will result in more rapid immune reconstitution.

IL-7 is a cytokine essential for T-cell development in mice and humans, as well as for T-cell homeostasis. IL-7 levels rise in serum and tissues after T-cell depletion and fall upon recovery. In preclinical studies, posttransplantation administration of IL-7 had marked effects on T-cell immune reconstitution and improved reconstitution in mice and primates, yet did not aggravate GVHD.[373] Clinical trials are now underway to determine if peritransplant IL-7 administration will result in improved immune reconstitution after HCT.

Immunizations

Immune responses to influenza, pneumococcal polysaccharide, inactivated polio virus, diphtheria, pertussis, tetanus toxoid, *Haemophilus influenzae*–type B conjugate vaccines, and hepatitis B are likely to be meaningful 1 year after autologous HCT and in recipients of an allograft who do not have chronic GVHD.[350] Only a minority of patients receiving immune-suppressive medication for the treatment of chronic GVHD may have an adequate response after vaccination. Immunization with a live-attenuated measles, mumps, and rubella vaccine can be given safely when administered 2 years after autologous HCT and is not recommended for recipients of an allograft who are maintained on immune-suppressive medication.[350]

ACUTE GRAFT-VERSUS-HOST DISEASE

Acute GVHD remains one of the most serious and challenging complications following allogeneic HCT. The requirements for acute GVHD have been known for more than 40 years and include that the graft must contain immunologically competent cells, the recipient must express tissue antigens not found in the donor, and the recipient must be immunologically suppressed enough that an effective response against transplanted cells cannot be made.[374]

An important aspect of the graft-versus-host reaction involves the recognition of the host's disparate major and minor histocompatibility antigens by T cells in the donor graft.[374–376] There are two primary classes of MHC antigens: HLA class I antigens that have a broad distribution and are expressed on all cells, and HLA class II antigens that are expressed on antigen-presenting cells, including macrophages, dendritic cells, B cells, and activated T cells.[219] Minor histocompatibility antigens are genetic polymorphisms of endogenous cellular proteins presented as small peptides bound in the grooves of the major histocompatibility antigens to donor T cells.[377] Some minor histocompatibility antigens associated with acute GVHD include CD31, HA-1, and the male-specific DBY gene with a female donor.[378,379]

The most important risk factor for the development of acute GVHD is the degree of HLA disparity between donor and recipient.[376] The increased incidence of acute GVHD in patients transplanted from fully HLA-matched unrelated donors compared to related donors is likely related to an increased disparity in minor histocompatibility antigens or unrecognized disparities of the phenotypically matched major histocompatibility loci.[380] Other risk factors for acute GVHD development include older patient age, gender disparity (in some studies, males receiving cells from female donors increased the risk), and the type of immune prophylaxis used.[381,382] The graft source with respect to marrow versus PBPC does not seem to impact the risk of acute GVHD development. Yet within the PBPC group of transplant recipients, some centers reported that a higher CD34+ cell dose is an independent risk factor for acute GVHD.[383,384]

To facilitate the study and prognostication of acute GVHD, a clinical staging and grading system was developed.[385] According to this classic definition, acute GVHD occurred prior to day 100 and primarily affected skin, gastrointestinal tract, and liver. The severity score was clinically based and ranged between grades 0 and IV, as defined by involvement of each organ system. Biopsies of affected organs are helpful to establish a definitive diagnosis. The staging and grading system of acute GVHD has been updated.[386,387] The most notable amendments include the following: acute GVHD can be diagnosed beyond day +100 after transplantation, and patients who have anorexia, nausea, and vomiting as their only manifestation combined with a positive upper gastrointestinal tract biopsy for acute GVHD are included under overall grade II acute GVHD. Consistently, grade I or very limited acute GVHD has a favorable prognosis and does not require treatment with systemic therapy.[388] Acute GVHD, overall grades II to IV, is considered clinically significant because it is moderately severe, and usually consists of multiorgan disease. Grade II acute GVHD is not typically associated with a poor outcome; however, severe (grades III and IV) acute GVHD is associated with a high risk of mortality and decreased patient survival.[388]

Pathophysiology

The current model for acute GVHD development requires three steps.[376,389] In step 1, the transplant conditioning regimen (chemotherapy and/or irradiation) damages and activates host tissues leading to increased secretion of the inflammatory cytokines TNF-α and IL-1. These cytokines enhance donor T-cell recognition of the host by upregulating the expression of major and minor host tissue histocompatibility antigens and also affect other molecules on host antigen-presenting cells. An important aspect of tissue injury from the transplant regimen occurs in the gastrointestinal tract and results in leakage of endotoxins such as lipopolysaccharides into the systemic circulation that serve as inflammatory stimuli.[376] Full-dose preparative regimens, especially those that include TBI are important in this process because of the associated endothelial and epithelial damage in the gastrointestinal tract.

In step 2 of acute GVHD, resting donor T-cells become activated in secondary lymphoid organs by host-activated protein C (endogenous direct antigen presentation) or donor-activated protein C (exogenous indirect antigen presentation) that present alloantigens to the T-cell receptors in context of peptides in the MHC groove.[376] Costimulatory signals are required for full T-cell activation. Donor T-cell activation is characterized by a cellular proliferation and predominance of Th1 cells and the secretion of IL-2 and IFN-γ. Several laboratories have identified that naïve (CD62L+) T cells induce experimental acute GVHD, whereas memory (CD62L–) T cells do not.[390,391] Murine models of marrow transplantation show that simultaneous infusions of T_{regs} limited the proliferation and clonal expansion of activated donor T cells and protected against acute GVHD development in murine models.[392] These insights are currently being translated to human transplantation.

In step 3, the cellular effectors mediate tissue injury and destruction in the target organs of acute GVHD resulting in its clinical manifestations.[376] This step involves the continued release of inflammatory cytokines that direct specific antihost donor-derived T cells to migrate to the target tissues—skin, liver, and gut—of acute GVHD. Other effector cell populations that contribute to local tissue injury by amplifying the proinflammatory response include neutrophils and mononuclear phagocytes.

Acute Graft-versus-Host Disease Prevention

The mainstay of acute GVHD prevention is prophylaxis with immunosuppressive drugs and all patients undergoing allogeneic HCT with a T-cell–replete graft require prophylaxis. Primary prophylaxis with cyclosporine-methotrexate or FK506 (tacrolimus)-methotrexate is the commonly used standard to prevent acute GVHD.[393–395] A randomized clinical trial using HLA-matched related and unrelated donors confirmed a modest reduction in the incidence of acute GVHD with FK506-methotrexate compared to cyclosporine-methotrexate yet this did not result in improved survival.[396] A randomized trial comparing cyclosporine and methotrexate to the combination of cyclosporine, prednisone, and methotrexate did not show any significant difference in acute GVHD incidence, relapse risk, and overall survival.[397] Currently, FK506-methotrexate is being compared to sirolimus and FK506 in a randomized prospective trial through the Marrow Transplantation Clinical Trials Network.

An alternative approach for the prevention of acute GVHD has been to deplete donor T cells from the graft prior to infusion.[398] A variety of techniques have been employed, including physical separation, density gradient centrifugation, monoclonal antibody-based depletion methods, and CD34-cell-positive selection. Although extensive removal of donor-derived T cells was effective in eradicating acute GVHD, it was associated with a higher risk of graft rejection, opportunistic infection, and relapse, such that overall survival was not improved.[399,400]

The concept of partial marrow T-cell depletion as accomplished by counterflow elutriation and T10B9 antibody plus complement was evaluated in a multicenter randomized trial of 405 transplant recipients of HLA-matched unrelated donor grafts.[401] Patients in the partial T-cell depletion arm received a prescribed CD3+ cell dose of 5×10^5 cells/kg which represented a mean of a 1– log depletion compared to patients in the unmanipulated marrow arm. The cumulative incidence of acute GVHD grades II to IV was significantly lower in the partial T-cell depletion arm, 39 percent compared to 63 percent for those who received unmanipulated marrow. Yet partial marrow T-cell depletion did not improve event-free and overall survival. The risk of chronic GVHD was similar in both arms.

Another approach to establish partial T-cell depletion of the donor graft used Campath 1H antibody, an IgM antibody that binds to CD52, a molecule expressed on a variety of cells, including T cells.[211] Although acute GVHD risk was low, patients who received *in vitro* or *in vivo* partial T-cell depletion with Campath were at increased risk for opportunistic infections, graft loss, and relapse.

Treatment of Established Acute Graft-versus-Host Disease

The most common agent used to treat acute GVHD is a glucocorticoid administered as methylprednisolone or prednisone at a dose of 1 to 2 mg/kg per day with subsequent tapering once disease activity resolves.[388] Higher doses of methylprednisolone (10 mg/kg per day) do not prevent evolution to grade III or IV acute GVHD or improve survival.[388] A complete remission of acute GVHD is reported in less than 50 percent of cases after primary treatment with glucocorticoids and the likelihood for long-term survival is low among individuals who developed glucocorticoid-refractory acute GVHD. A variety of other approaches have been explored in the treatment of acute GVHD, including the use of other immunosuppressive agents, antibody-based therapies either to T-cells or cytokines, and photopheresis, all administered in combination with prednisone. When a CD5-specific immunotoxin was added to prednisone at the start of treatment to help eradicate activated donor T-cells, acute GVHD manifestations were more effectively controlled during the first 5 weeks only compared to prednisone alone.[388] Similarly, no long-term benefit was observed when anti–T-lymphocyte globulin was added to prednisone as primary therapy.[388,402] Other immune-suppressive agents have been studied in patients with glucocorticoid-dependent acute GVHD and include daclizumab, rapamycin, MMF, ABX-CBL (CD147-specific monoclonal antibody), and visilizumab. Yet the survival outcomes reported at 6 and 12 months for glucocorticoid-dependent GVHD were poor and associated with a high NRM rate.[402] A recent phase II study from the clinical trials network compared the efficacy of MMF, pentostatin, anti-TNF, and anti-IL2 receptor antibodies in combination with glucocorticoids for patients with new onset grades II to IV acute GVHD.[403] It was reported that the addition of MMF to steroids induced the best responses and plans to compare the addition of steroids with and without MMF for the treatment of newly diagnosed acute GVHD are underway.

The immunomodulatory properties of MSCs suggest that these cells may have a role in preventing or treating acute GVHD. The index case, without a prior preclinical model, was a 9-year-old patient with severe glucocorticoid refractory gut and liver acute GVHD after a matched unrelated donor transplant was treated with *ex vivo* expanded MSCs from his haploidentical mother.[404] While continuing with broad-spectrum immune-suppression medication, the infusion of MSCs was followed by prompt resolution acute GVHD. The acute GVHD flared with immune-suppression drug withdrawal and was controlled again with a second infusion of MSCs. Since this report, several phase I/II studies have confirmed the capacity of MSCs obtained from HLA-identical siblings, unrelated donors, or haploidentical family members to successfully treat GVHD.[120,121,405] The results of several ongoing large controlled clinical studies are anticipated.

Chronic Graft-versus-Host Disease

Chronic GVHD is another significant complication following allogeneic HCT.[406] By convention many transplantation groups use day 100 after cell infusion as a convenient divider between acute and chronic GVHD. However, it is recognized that manifestations of chronic GVHD may occur before day 100.

The clinical manifestations of chronic GVHD are broad and share overlapping features with a variety of autoimmune disorders, such as scleroderma, lichen planus, and dermatomyositis.[406] Indeed, autoantibody production is commonly observed after allogeneic HCT. Clinical features of chronic GVHD include skin lesions that may initially resemble lichen planus and that may progress to generalized scleroderma, keratoconjunctivitis, buccal mucositis, esophageal and vaginal strictures, intestinal abnormalities, chronic liver disease, pulmonary insufficiency secondary to bronchiolitis obliterans, and a wasting syndrome. If generalized scleroderma occurs, it may lead to joint contractures and debility. Elevations in alkaline phosphatase and serum bilirubin are often the first indication of hepatic involvement with chronic GVHD. Damage to the bile ducts has a similar histopathology to that seen in primary biliary cirrhosis. Liver biopsies are often helpful in establishing a diagnosis.

A staging system for chronic GVHD that classified patients into none, limited, and extensive categories was developed.[407] The utilization of this classification system was difficult because many patients were not classifiable by strict organ criteria and followup studies reported a poor correlation with predicting late NRM.[408] Poor prognostic factors for survival are extensive skin involvement, thrombocytopenia, and progressive-type onset following acute GVHD.[408,409] Patients with extensive chronic GVHD have an increased mortality rate, especially patients with platelet counts less than 100×10^9/L on day 100 and those patients with low serum albumin. Revisions to staging chronic GVHD were proposed and are being adopted.[410]

The lack of animal models that reproduce critical aspects of chronic GVHD has limited the ability to understand the pathophysiology of this complication. T cells from animals with a syndrome resembling chronic GVHD produce an unusual pattern of cytokines, such as IL-4 and IFN-γ but not IL-2, which is consistent with the notion that cells with a Th2 phenotype are important mediators of this problem.[322] One proposed mechanism to induce autoimmunity might be the failure to develop normal regulatory controls after allogeneic HCT in the setting of thymic damage and/or immune-suppression medication.[322,411]

To prevent the development of chronic GVHD, patients without GVHD at day 80 after transplantation were randomized to a 24-month course of cyclosporine and compared to a group receiving cyclosporine for 6 months.[412] At the end of therapy no significant differences between the groups in the incidence of chronic GVHD, transplantation-related survival, or overall survival was reported. It was therefore concluded that patients without GVHD at day 80 would have a standard taper of cyclosporine to discontinuation at 6 months.

The mainstay of treatment for established chronic GVHD continues to be prednisone. Because of the chronic nature of this disease, long-term treatment is often required. Alternate-day dosing has been found to help reduce some of the toxicity associated with prolonged glucocorticoid use.[413] Treatment of chronic GVHD is an art and remains a balance between the slow taper of immune-suppressive medications against the risk of GVHD flare and infection. A variety of newer agents are being explored for the treatment of chronic GVHD. Psoralen plus ultraviolet A was used to treat chronic GVHD with some success, especially in some patients with sclerodermatous-like skin changes.[414] Rapamycin has efficacy in some patients with chronic GVHD.[415] Recent data showed that antibodies to the platelet-derived growth factor receptor induced constitutive activation of this tyrosine kinase that was associated with to collagen deposition in patients with scleroderma.[416] In similar fashion, patients with scleroderma-like GVHD showed excellent responses when treated with the tyrosine kinase inhibitor imatinib.[417] Studies evaluating the role of these agents are ongoing. The presence of antibodies to minor histocompatibility antigens in patients with chronic GVHD suggested a role that donor B cells have productive interactions with donor T cells in this disease.[418] B cells can act directly as antigen-presenting cells in their ability to process and present limiting amounts of antigen to T cells. Rituximab is the subject of ongoing clinical trials to prevent and treat chronic GVHD.

■ RELAPSE OF DISEASE AFTER HCT

Relapse following autologous and allogeneic HCT is an ominous clinical event. Every effort should be made to carefully and completely document relapse as it is common for patients to have residual radiographic abnormalities following transplantation, especially patients with lymphoma. Patients with myeloma have a gradual reduction in the paraprotein level which may take several months after autologous transplant to reach maximal response. Following RIC, the allogeneic GVT effects may take weeks to months to result in tumor eradication, and it may be difficult to distinguish persistent yet slowly regressing disease from slowly progressive disease. Molecular evidence of CML at less than 3 months after allogeneic HCT was not associated with an increased risk of relapse, and moreover minimal residual disease by quantitative PCR can be detected in up to 50 percent of patients beyond 3 years of transplant transplantation without impacting on their risk of relapse.[419–421] Therefore, because patients are highly sensitized to the possibility of disease relapse, clear and unequivocal documentation is required prior to declaring a patient has in fact relapsed.

Relapse after Autologous HCT

The most important cause of treatment failure following autologous HCT remains disease relapse. Relapse often occurs at sites of previous disease, suggesting that residual cells within the patient are responsible for the recurrence.[422] Patients who have disease relapse after autologous HCT can be considered candidates to receive additional salvage therapy with chemotherapy, irradiation, immunomodulators, and monoclonal antibodies. In patients who continue to show chemosensitivity, relatively reasonable survival may be achieved. A second HCT is a feasible option, with allogeneic RIC being increasingly offered in this setting and multiple reports documenting 2- to 3-year event-free survival of more than 50 percent (see Fig. 21–4).[209]

Strategies to reduce disease recurrence have been explored. The use of early posttransplantation radiation therapy to sites of prior bulk or persistent disease might reduce the likelihood of disease recurrence.[422,423] Immunologic interventions have been used in an effort to generate an "autologous GVT response" and thereby decrease the risk of recurrence following autologous HCT.[424] Yet results from a randomized clinical trial in patients with poor-risk NHL and HL failed to demonstrate a difference in event-free and overall survival for patients in the IL-2 induction arm compared to patients in the noninduction arm. Vaccination strategies, such as using idiotype-pulsed dendritic cells and other vaccination approaches, have been explored in early phase clinical trials and have shown relative safety and immunologic responses in some patients.[425] Ongoing studies are being conducted that will determine whether patients who develop an immunologic response will predict or influence overall disease outcome.

Other adoptive cellular therapeutic approaches including the use of allogeneic NK cells, cytokine-induced killer cells, and anti–Epstein-Barr virus-reactive T cells in patients with HL who have evidence of Epstein-Barr virus expression are under clinical investigation.

The use of monoclonal antibody-based therapies directed at the tumor cells appears a promising strategy to reduce the risk of disease recurrence. This strategy is most feasible in patients with B-cell NHL where rituximab is an effective therapy. The administration of post-transplantation rituximab beginning 6 weeks following autologous HCT and continuing for 6 months in patients with refractory B-cell NHL resulted in excellent disease-free and overall survival.[276]

The antibody-drug conjugate cAC10-vcMMAE (SGN-35) consists of a tubulin inhibitor monomethylauristatin E (MMAE) conjugated to the chimeric anti-CD30 monoclonal antibody cAC10 and has shown objective responses in more than 45 percent of patients when administered as a single agent to patients with Hodgkin lymphoma who had disease progression after autologous HCT.[426] Using a similar approach to what is being done with rituximab, SGN-35 will be tested in a randomized study to determine if posttransplantation administration to patients at high risk for disease relapse will demonstrate improved event-free survival compared to patients receiving no additional post-transplantation chemotherapy.

Relapse after Allogeneic HCT

The treatment of disease relapse following allogeneic HCT has generally been unsuccessful. The use of chemotherapy can result in disease responses; however, this is unlikely to be durable. Performing a second myeloablative transplantation procedure has largely been unsuccessful because of excessive toxicity and the nonrelapse transplantation-related mortality can be greater than 50 percent.[427,428] One exception may be children or adolescents who had disease relapse beyond 2 years from a prior autologous transplant.[429]

Most published reports regarding the successful application of DLI involved patients with relapsed CML, which is the malignancy known to be most sensitive to the GVT effects. Disease status at the time of DLI was a key predictor of response and patients with relapsed chronic phase CML had sustained rates of response of more than 75 percent in most reports.[430] For patients with more advanced stages of relapse of CML, DLI alone is unlikely to be associated with a durable remission.[161] Imatinib administered concomitantly with DLI was shown to more rapidly induce a complete molecular response and should be considered as a synergistic approach in all patients with posttransplantation relapse of CML irrespective of disease status.[431]

The use of DLI is not without toxicity and the concern of inducing serious GVHD remains a risk.[160] The onset of GVHD development following DLI is typically 1 month after the cell infusion. Marrow aplasia is another risk associated with DLI and is reported in 20 to 50 percent of patients who received this therapy.[160] Marrow aplasia is thought to occur when donor lymphocytes ablate the recipient tumor and hematopoietic cells, but there are too few donor hematopoietic cells to support adequate hematopoiesis. Therefore, the use of DLI is cautioned in patients who have disease relapse and chimerism reveals mostly recipient-type multi-lineage blood or marrow cells.

A retrospective analysis of 307 consecutive patients who had recurrent or persistent high-risk leukemia (chronic phase CML excluded) or myelodysplastic syndrome after allogeneic HCT and who received at least one relapse-directed intervention that included withdrawal of immunosuppression, chemotherapy, or DLI, was reported.[432] Transplants were performed at a single institution and outcomes were analyzed according to time intervals from transplantation to detection of malignancy: "early," less than 100 days (n = 111); intermediate," 100 to 200 days (n = 73); and "late," greater than 200 days (n = 123). The overall remission rate was 30 percent and the 2-year overall survival estimates for patients with early, intermediate, and late recurrence were 3 percent,

9 percent, and 19 percent, respectively. Individual types or combinations of these nonrandomly assigned relapse-directed interventions were not associated with higher or lower probabilities of remission or survival. Therefore, more effective strategies are needed for the treatment of recurrent hematologic malignancies after HCT. In the absence of innovative clinical trials, patients with early recurrence should be counseled to consider foregoing further interventions in favor of palliative care.

The potency of DLI for the treatment of some forms of recurrent malignancy after allogeneic HCT and its frequent serious toxicities, GVHD and marrow hypoplasia, have generated intense interest in the development of selective adoptive transfer of donor-derived cell therapies that may have greater antitumor efficacy yet minimal toxicity.

The use of "activated DLI" has been explored; donor T cells underwent *ex vivo* costimulation and expansion by exposure to magnetic beads coated with anti-CD3 and anti-CD28 monoclonal antibodies and were infused in allogeneic transplantation recipients who had disease relapse other than CML.[433] Approximately 35 percent of patients achieved a response and none developed life-threatening GVHD. Ongoing studies using these cells will include dose escalation and repetitive dosing to minimize late recurrence.

Cytokine-induced killer cells are cytotoxic effector cells expressing the T-cell marker CD3+ and the NK cell marker CD56+ and have shown potent activity against a variety of human tumor cell lines with a markedly reduced capacity to induce GVHD in murine models.[434] Cytokine-induced killer cells are generated *in vitro* by culture of blood lymphocytes with IFN-, IL-2, and anti-CD3. In culture, T-cell expansion and activation occur, resulting in cells with cytolytic function related to NKG2D-mediated recognition, a T-cell-receptor-independent mechanism.[435] Because cytokine-induced killer cells generated from patients with AML have demonstrated cytotoxic function against autologous leukemic blasts, these cells may also have a role in decreasing relapse following autologous HCT.[436] A variety of additional strategies are under investigation, including the generation of antigen-specific T cells, memory CD4+ T cells, and NK cells. The use of cytokines such as IL-2 with or without IFN-γ, monoclonal antibodies, and vaccination strategies are all areas of active research.

FUTURE DIRECTIONS

Understanding the mechanisms and targets of GVT reactions continues to be an area of intense interest. In addition, understanding the complexities of immunologic reactions has revealed that not only are T-cell populations responsible for the effector phase, but also other T-cell populations regulate these responses. The concept of using T_{regs} to control adverse effects such as GVHD has been successful in murine models and holds significant promise in its application to the treatment of patients.

Other defined cellular populations, cytokines, and vaccination strategies show promise in reducing the risk of disease relapse following autologous and allogeneic HCT. In addition, improved strategies to reduce the risk of acute and chronic GVHD could enable extension of allogeneic HCT beyond the treatment of patients with hematologic malignancies. For example, animal models of autoimmune diseases demonstrated that these disorders can be effectively treated with HCT and preliminary evidence in patients is supportive. In addition, animal studies demonstrate that combined same-donor organ and marrow transplantation results in tolerance to the transplanted organ in recipients who had persistent mixed chimerism. Early reports of this work in humans suggest that extension of allogeneic HCT to these and other disease settings could provide new therapeutic concepts to improve outcomes for patients with diverse clinical problems.

The near future holds that rather than transplanting all of the cells that are mobilized or aspirated from the marrow, clinicians and researchers in the field will isolate the cell type(s) needed for optimal results, and this will differ depending on the disease and the outcome being sought.

REFERENCES

1. Osgood EE, Riddle MC, Mathew TJ: Aplastic anemia treated with daily transfusions and intravenous marrow; case report. *Ann Intern Med* 13:357, 1939.
2. Fabricius-Moller J: *Experimental Studies of the Hemorrhagic Diathesis from X-Ray Sickness*. Levin and Munksgaard Forlag, Copenhagen, 1922.
3. Jacobson LO, Marks EK, Robson MJ, et al: The effect of spleen protection on mortality following X-irradiation. *J Lab Clin Med* 34:1538, 1949.
4. Lorenz E, Uphoff D, Reid TR, et al: Modification of irradiation injury in mice and guinea pigs by marrow injections. *J Natl Cancer Inst* 12:197, 1951.
5. Cole LJ, Fishler MC, Bond VP: Subcellular fractionation of mouse spleen radiation protection activity. *Proc Natl Acad Sci U S A* 39:759, 1953.
6. Hilfinger MF Jr, Ferguson JH, Riemenschneider PA: The effect of homologous marrow emulsion on rabbits after total body irradiation. *J Lab Clin Med* 42:581, 1953.
7. Lorenz E, Congdon CC: Modification of lethal irradiation injury in mice by injection of homologous or heterologous bone. *J Natl Cancer Inst* 14:955, 1954.
8. Barnes DWH, Loutit JF: What is the recovery factor of the spleen? *Nucleon* 12:68, 1954.
9. Barnes DWH, Loutit JF: *Spleen Protection: The Cellular Hypothesis. Radiobiology Symposium*, p 134. Butterworth, London, 1955.
10. Barnes DW, Corp MJ, Loutit JF, et al: Treatment of murine leukaemia with X rays and homologous marrow; preliminary communication. *Br Med J* 2:626, 1956.
11. Thomas ED, Lochte HL Jr, Lu WC, et al: Intravenous infusion of marrow in patients receiving radiation and chemotherapy. *N Engl J Med* 257:491, 1957.
12. Thomas ED, Lochte HL Jr, Cannon JH, et al: Supralethal whole body irradiation and isologous marrow transplantation in man. *J Clin Invest* 38:1709, 1959.
13. Mathe G, Jammet H, Pendic B, et al: [Transfusions and grafts of homologous marrow in humans after accidental high dosage irradiation]. *Rev Fr Etud Clin Biol* 4:226, 1959.
14. Kurnick NB, Montano A, Gerdes JC, et al: Preliminary observations on the treatment of postirradiation hematopoietic depression in man by the infusion of stored autogenous marrow. *Ann Intern Med* 49:973, 1958.
15. Haurani FI: Thirty-one-year survival following chemotherapy and autologous marrow in malignant lymphoma. *Am J Hematol* 55:35, 1997.
16. Bortin MM: A compendium of reported human marrow transplants. *Transplantation* 9:571, 1970.
17. Gatti RA, Meuwissen HJ, Allen HD, et al: Immunological reconstitution of sex-linked lymphopenic immunological deficiency. *Lancet* 2:1366, 1968.
18. De Koning J, Van Bekkum DW, Dicke KA, et al: Transplantation of bone-marrow cells and fetal thymus in an infant with lymphopenic immunological deficiency. *Lancet* 1:1223, 1969.
19. Bach FH, Albertini RJ, Joo P, et al: Bone-marrow transplantation in a patient with the Wiskott-Aldrich syndrome. *Lancet* 2:1364, 1968.
20. Bortin MM, Bach FH, van Bekkum DW, et al: 25th Anniversary of the first successful allogeneic marrow transplants. *Bone Marrow Transplant* 14:211, 1994.
21. Thomas ED, Storb R, Clift RA, et al: Bone-marrow transplantation (parts I and II). *N Engl J Med* 292:832, 1975.
22. Hansen JA, Clift RA, Thomas ED, et al: Transplantation of marrow from an unrelated donor to a patient with acute leukemia. *N Engl J Med* 303:565, 1980.
23. O'Reilly RJ, Dupont B, Pahwa S, et al: Reconstitution in severe combined immunodeficiency by transplantation of marrow from an unrelated donor. *N Engl J Med* 297:1311, 1977.
24. Appelbaum FR, Herzig GP, Ziegler JL, et al: Successful engraftment of cryopreserved autologous marrow in patients with malignant lymphoma. *Blood* 52:85, 1978.
25. Appelbaum FR, Deisseroth AB, Graw RG Jr, et al: Prolonged complete remission following high dose chemotherapy of Burkitt's lymphoma in relapse. *Cancer* 41:1059, 1978.
26. Research CFIBaMT (CIBMTR). *Annual Progress Report 2008*. Available at: www.cibmtr.org.
27. Weissman IL: Stem cells: Units of development, units of regeneration, and units in evolution. *Cell* 100:157, 2000.
28. Spangrude GJ, Heimfeld S, Weissman IL: Purification and characterization of mouse hematopoietic stem cells. *Science* 241:58, 1988.
29. Ikuta K, Weissman IL: Evidence that hematopoietic stem cells express mouse c-kit but do not depend on steel factor for their generation. *Proc Natl Acad Sci U S A* 89:1502, 1992.
30. Osawa M, Hanada K, Hamada H, et al: Long-term lymphohematopoietic reconstitution by a single CD34-low/negative hematopoietic stem cell. *Science* 273:242, 1996.
31. Baum CM, Weissman IL, Tsukamoto AS, et al: Isolation of a candidate human hematopoietic stem-cell population. *Proc Natl Acad Sci U S A* 89:2804, 1992.
32. Negrin RS, Atkinson K, Leemhuis T, et al: Transplantation of highly purified CD34+Thy-1+ hematopoietic stem cells in patients with metastatic breast cancer. *Biol Blood Marrow Transplant* 6:262, 2000.

33. Vose JM, Bierman PJ, Lynch JC, et al: Transplantation of highly purified CD34+Thy-1+ hematopoietic stem cells in patients with recurrent indolent non-Hodgkin's lymphoma. *Biol Blood Marrow Transplant* 7:680, 2001.
34. Michallet M, Philip T, Philip I, et al: Transplantation with selected autologous peripheral blood CD34+Thy1+ hematopoietic stem cells (HSCs) in myeloma: Impact of HSC dose on engraftment, safety, and immune reconstitution. *Exp Hematol* 28:858, 2000.
35. Hidalgo A, Robledo MM, Teixido J: CD44-mediated hematopoietic progenitor cell adhesion and its complex role in myelopoiesis. *J Hematother Stem Cell Res* 11:539, 2002.
36. Katayama Y, Hidalgo A, Furie BC, et al: PSGL-1 participates in E-selectin-mediated progenitor homing to marrow: Evidence for cooperation between E-selectin ligands and alpha4 integrin. *Blood* 102:2060, 2003.
37. Sackstein R: The marrow is akin to skin: HCELL and the biology of hematopoietic stem cell homing. *J Investig Dermatol Symp Proc* 9:215, 2004.
38. Frenette PS, Subbarao S, Mazo IB, et al: Endothelial selectins and vascular cell adhesion molecule-1 promote hematopoietic progenitor homing to marrow. *Proc Natl Acad Sci U S A* 95:14423, 1998.
39. Papayannopoulou T, Craddock C, Nakamoto B, et al: The VLA4/VCAM-1 adhesion pathway defines contrasting mechanisms of lodgement of transplanted murine hemopoietic progenitors between marrow and spleen. *Proc Natl Acad Sci U S A* 92:9647, 1995.
40. Vermeulen M, Le Pesteur F, Gagnerault MC, et al: Role of adhesion molecules in the homing and mobilization of murine hematopoietic stem and progenitor cells. *Blood* 92:894, 1998.
41. Hirsch E, Iglesias A, Potocnik AJ, et al: Impaired migration but not differentiation of haematopoietic stem cells in the absence of beta1 integrins. *Nature* 380:171, 1996.
42. Nagasawa T, Hirota S, Tachibana K, et al: Defects of B-cell lymphopoiesis and bone-marrow myelopoiesis in mice lacking the CXC chemokine PBSF/SDF-1. *Nature* 382:635, 1996.
43. Lapidot T: Mechanism of human stem cell migration and repopulation of NOD/SCID and B2mnull NOD/SCID mice. The role of SDF-1/CXCR4 interactions. *Ann N Y Acad Sci* 938:83, 2001.
44. Jung Y, Wang J, Song J, et al: Annexin II expressed by osteoblasts and endothelial cells regulates stem cell adhesion, homing, and engraftment following transplantation. *Blood* 110:82, 2007.
45. Calvi LM, Adams GB, Weibrecht KW, et al: Osteoblastic cells regulate the haematopoietic stem cell niche. *Nature* 425:841, 2003.
46. Mendes SC, Robin C, Dzierzak E: Mesenchymal progenitor cells localize within hematopoietic sites throughout ontogeny. *Development* 132:1127, 2005.
47. Zhang Y, Adachi Y, Suzuki Y, et al: Simultaneous injection of marrow cells and stromal cells into marrow accelerates hematopoiesis *in vivo*. *Stem Cells* 22:1256, 2004.
48. Jung Y, Wang J, Havens A, et al: Cell-to-cell contact is critical for the survival of hematopoietic progenitor cells on osteoblasts. *Cytokine* 32:155, 2005.
49. Nilsson SK, Johnston HM, Whitty GA, et al: Osteopontin, a key component of the hematopoietic stem cell niche and regulator of primitive hematopoietic progenitor cells. *Blood* 106:1232, 2005.
50. Zannettino AC, Buhring HJ, Niutta S, et al: The sialomucin CD164 (MGC-24v) is an adhesive glycoprotein expressed by human hematopoietic progenitors and marrow stromal cells that serves as a potent negative regulator of hematopoiesis. *Blood* 92:2613, 1998.
51. El-Badri NS, Wang BY, Cherry, et al: Osteoblasts promote engraftment of allogeneic hematopoietic stem cells. *Exp Hematol* 26:110, 1998.
52. Thomas ED, Storb R: Technique for human marrow grafting. *Blood* 36:507, 1970.
53. Horowitz MM, Confer DL: Evaluation of hematopoietic stem cell donors. *Hematology Am Soc Hematol Educ Program* 469, 2005.
54. Anderlini P, Rizzo JD, Nugent ML, et al: Peripheral blood stem cell donation: An analysis from the International Marrow Transplant Registry (IBMTR) and European Group for Blood and Marrow Transplant (EBMT) databases. *Bone Marrow Transplant* 27:689, 2001.
55. Chan KW, Gajewski JL, Supkis D Jr, et al: Use of minors as marrow donors: Current attitude and management. A survey of 56 pediatric transplantation centers. *J Pediatr* 128:644, 1996.
56. Sanders J, Buckner CD, Bensinger WI, et al: Experience with marrow harvesting from donors less than two years of age. *Bone Marrow Transplant* 2:45, 1987.
57. Pulsipher MA, Levine JE, Hayashi RJ, et al: Safety and efficacy of allogeneic PBSC collection in normal pediatric donors: The pediatric blood and marrow transplant consortium experience (PBMTC) 1996–2003. *Bone Marrow Transplant* 35:361, 2005.
58. Siena S, Bregni M, Brando B, et al: Circulation of CD34+ hematopoietic stem cells in the peripheral blood of high-dose cyclophosphamide-treated patients: Enhancement by intravenous recombinant human granulocyte-macrophage colony-stimulating factor. *Blood* 74:1905, 1989.
59. Chao NJ, Schriber JR, Grimes K, et al: Granulocyte colony-stimulating factor "mobilized" peripheral blood progenitor cells accelerate granulocyte and platelet recovery after high-dose chemotherapy. *Blood* 81:2031, 1993.
60. Glaspy JA, Shpall EJ, LeMaistre CF, et al: Peripheral blood progenitor cell mobilization using stem cell factor in combination with filgrastim in breast cancer patients. *Blood* 90:2939, 1997.
61. Liles WC, Broxmeyer HE, Rodger E, et al: Mobilization of hematopoietic progenitor cells in healthy volunteers by AMD3100, a CXCR4 antagonist. *Blood* 102:2728, 2003.
62. Pulsipher MA, Nagler A, Iannone R, et al: Weighing the risks of G-CSF administration, leukopheresis, and standard marrow harvest: Ethical and safety considerations for normal pediatric hematopoietic cell donors. *Pediatr Blood Cancer* 46:422, 2006.
63. Becker PS, Wagle M, Matous S, et al: Spontaneous splenic rupture following administration of granulocyte colony-stimulating factor (G-CSF): Occurrence in an allogeneic donor of peripheral blood stem cells. *Biol Blood Marrow Transplant* 3:45, 1997.
64. Falzetti F, Aversa F, Minelli O, et al: Spontaneous rupture of spleen during peripheral blood stem-cell mobilisation in a healthy donor. *Lancet* 353:555, 1999.
65. Confer DL, Miller JP: Long-term safety of filgrastim (rhG-CSF) administration. *Br J Haematol* 137:77, 2007.
66. Storek J, Dawson MA, Maloney DG: Normal T, B, and NK cell counts in healthy donors at 1 year after blood stem cell harvesting. *Blood* 95:2993, 2000.
67. Shpall EJ, Champlin R, Glaspy JA: Effect of CD34+ peripheral blood progenitor cell dose on hematopoietic recovery. *Biol Blood Marrow Transplant* 4:84, 1998.
68. Weaver CH, Hazelton B, Birch R, et al: An analysis of engraftment kinetics as a function of the CD34 content of peripheral blood progenitor cell collections in 692 patients after the administration of myeloablative chemotherapy. *Blood* 86:3961, 1995.
69. Weaver CH, Potz J, Redmond J, et al: Engraftment and outcomes of patients receiving myeloablative therapy followed by autologous peripheral blood stem cells with a low CD34+ cell content. *Bone Marrow Transplant* 19:1103, 1997.
70. Calandra G, McCarty J, McGuirk J, et al: AMD3100 plus G-CSF can successfully mobilize CD34+ cells from non-Hodgkin's lymphoma, Hodgkin's disease and myeloma patients previously failing mobilization with chemotherapy and/or cytokine treatment: Compassionate use data. *Bone Marrow Transplant* 41:331, 2008.
71. Devine SM, Vij R, Rettig M, et al: Rapid mobilization of functional donor hematopoietic cells without G-CSF using AMD3100, an antagonist of the CXCR4/SDF-1 interaction. *Blood* 112:990, 2008.
72. Lucas D, Battista M, Shi PA, et al: Mobilized hematopoietic stem cell yield depends on species-specific circadian timing. *Cell Stem Cell* 3:364, 2008.
73. Mendez-Ferrer S, Lucas D, Battista M, et al: Haematopoietic stem cell release is regulated by circadian oscillations. *Nature* 452:442, 2008.
74. Quesenberry PJ, Dooner GJ, Dooner MS: Problems in the promised land: Status of adult marrow stem cell biology. *Exp Hematol* 37:775, 2009.
75. Taylor KM, Jagannath S, Spitzer G, et al: Recombinant human granulocyte colony-stimulating factor hastens granulocyte recovery after high-dose chemotherapy and autologous marrow transplantation in Hodgkin's disease. *J Clin Oncol* 7:1791, 1989.
76. Watts MJ, Sullivan AM, Jamieson E, et al: Progenitor-cell mobilization after low-dose cyclophosphamide and granulocyte colony-stimulating factor: An analysis of progenitor-cell quantity and quality and factors predicting for these parameters in 101 pretreated patients with malignant lymphoma. *J Clin Oncol* 15:535, 1997.
77. Schmitz N, Linch DC, Dreger P, et al: Randomised trial of filgrastim-mobilised peripheral blood progenitor cell transplantation versus autologous bone-marrow transplantation in lymphoma patients. *Lancet* 347:353, 1996.
78. Kanteti R, Miller K, McCann J, et al: Randomized trial of peripheral blood progenitor cell vs marrow as hematopoietic support for high-dose chemotherapy in patients with non-Hodgkin's lymphoma and Hodgkin's disease: A clinical and molecular analysis. *Bone Marrow Transplant* 24:473, 1999.
79. Smith TJ, Hillner BE, Schmitz N, et al: Economic analysis of a randomized clinical trial to compare filgrastim-mobilized peripheral-blood progenitor-cell transplantation and autologous marrow transplantation in patients with Hodgkin's and non-Hodgkin's lymphoma. *J Clin Oncol* 15:5, 1997.
80. Schmitz N, Bacigalupo A, Labopin M, et al: Transplantation of allogeneic peripheral blood progenitor cells—The EBMT experience. *Bone Marrow Transplant* 17(Suppl 2):S40, 1996.
81. Barge AJ: A review of the efficacy and tolerability of recombinant haematopoietic growth factors in marrow transplantation. *Bone Marrow Transplant* 11(Suppl 2):1, 1993.
82. Couban S, Simpson DR, Barnett MJ, et al: A randomized multicenter comparison of marrow and peripheral blood in recipients of matched sibling allogeneic transplants for myeloid malignancies. *Blood* 100:1525, 2002.
83. Bensinger WI, Martin PJ, Storer B, et al: Transplantation of marrow as compared with peripheral-blood cells from HLA-identical relatives in patients with hematologic cancers. *N Engl J Med* 344:175, 2001.
84. Powles R, Mehta J, Kulkarni S, et al: Allogeneic blood and bone-marrow stem-cell transplantation in haematological malignant diseases: A randomised trial. *Lancet* 355:1231, 2000.
85. Blaise D, Kuentz M, Fortanier C, et al: Randomized trial of marrow versus lenograstim-primed blood cell allogeneic transplantation in patients with early-stage leukemia: A report from the Societe Francaise de Greffe de Moelle. *J Clin Oncol* 18:537, 2000.
86. Toh HC, Sun L, Soe Y, et al: G-CSF induces a potentially tolerant gene and immunophenotype profile in T cells *in vivo*. *Clin Immunol* 132:83, 2009.
87. Flowers ME, Parker PM, Johnston LJ, et al: Comparison of chronic graft-versus-host disease after transplantation of peripheral blood stem cells versus marrow in allogeneic recipients: Long-term follow-up of a randomized trial. *Blood* 100:415, 2002.
88. Schmitz N, Beksac M, Hasenclever D, et al: Transplantation of mobilized peripheral blood cells to HLA-identical siblings with standard-risk leukemia. *Blood* 100:761, 2002.
89. Gluckman E, Rocha V, Boyer-Chammard A, et al: Outcome of cord-blood transplantation from related and unrelated donors. Eurocord Transplant Group and the European Blood and Marrow Transplantation Group. *N Engl J Med* 337:373, 1997.

90. Barker JN, Davies SM, DeFor T, et al: Survival after transplantation of unrelated donor umbilical cord blood is comparable to that of human leukocyte antigen-matched unrelated donor marrow: Results of a matched-pair analysis. *Blood* 97:2957, 2001.
91. Wagner JE, Barker JN, DeFor TE, et al: Transplantation of unrelated donor umbilical cord blood in 102 patients with malignant and nonmalignant diseases: Influence of CD34 cell dose and HLA disparity on treatment-related mortality and survival. *Blood* 100:1611, 2002.
92. Long GD, Laughlin M, Madan B, et al: Unrelated umbilical cord blood transplantation in adult patients. *Biol Blood Marrow Transplant* 9:772, 2003.
93. Rodrigues CA, Sanz G, Brunstein CG, et al: Analysis of risk factors for outcomes after unrelated cord blood transplantation in adults with lymphoid malignancies: A study by the Eurocord-Netcord and lymphoma working party of the European group for blood and marrow transplantation. *J Clin Oncol* 27:256, 2009.
94. Takahashi S, Iseki T, Ooi J, et al: Single-institute comparative analysis of unrelated marrow transplantation and cord blood transplantation for adult patients with hematologic malignancies. *Blood* 104:3813, 2004.
95. Laughlin MJ, Barker J, Bambach B, et al: Hematopoietic engraftment and survival in adult recipients of umbilical-cord blood from unrelated donors. *N Engl J Med* 344:1815, 2001.
96. Barker JN: Umbilical cord blood (UCB) transplantation: An alternative to the use of unrelated volunteer donors? *Hematology Am Soc Hematol Educ Program* 55, 2007.
97. Haylock DN, Nilsson SK: Expansion of umbilical cord blood for clinical transplantation. *Curr Stem Cell Res Ther* 2:324, 2007.
98. Ash RC, Horowitz MM, Gale RP, et al: Marrow transplantation from related donors other than HLA-identical siblings: Effect of T cell depletion. *Bone Marrow Transplant* 7:443, 1991.
99. Gale RP, Reisner Y: Graft rejection and graft-versus-host disease: Mirror images. *Lancet* 1:1468, 1986.
100. Aversa F, Velardi A, Tabilio A, et al: Haploidentical stem cell transplantation in leukemia. *Blood Rev* 15:111, 2001.
101. Aversa F, Tabilio A, Velardi A, et al: Treatment of high-risk acute leukemia with T-cell-depleted stem cells from related donors with one fully mismatched HLA haplotype. *N Engl J Med* 339:1186, 1998.
102. Aversa F: Haploidentical haematopoietic stem cell transplantation for acute leukaemia in adults: Experience in Europe and the United States. *Bone Marrow Transplant* 41:473, 2008.
103. Ruggeri L, Capanni M, Urbani E, et al: Effectiveness of donor natural killer cell alloreactivity in mismatched hematopoietic transplants. *Science* 295:2097, 2002.
104. Aversa F, Reisner Y, Martelli MF: The haploidentical option for high-risk haematological malignancies. *Blood Cells Mol Dis* 40:8, 2008.
105. Owen M: Histogenesis of bone cells. *Calcif Tissue Res* 25:205, 1978.
106. Dominici M, Le Blanc K, Mueller I, et al: Minimal criteria for defining multipotent mesenchymal stromal cells. The International Society for Cellular Therapy position statement. *Cytotherapy* 8:315, 2006.
107. Nauta AJ, Fibbe WE: Immunomodulatory properties of mesenchymal stromal cells. *Blood* 110:3499, 2007.
108. Le Blanc K, Ringden O: Immunobiology of human mesenchymal stem cells and future use in hematopoietic stem cell transplantation. *Biol Blood Marrow Transplant* 11:321, 2005.
109. Nolta JA, Hanley MB, Kohn DB: Sustained human hematopoiesis in immunodeficient mice by cotransplantation of marrow stroma expressing human interleukin-3: Analysis of gene transduction of long-lived progenitors. *Blood* 83:3041, 1994.
110. Pittenger MF, Mackay AM, Beck SC, et al: Multilineage potential of adult human mesenchymal stem cells. *Science* 284:143, 1999.
111. Zuk PA, Zhu M, Mizuno H, et al: Multilineage cells from human adipose tissue: Implications for cell-based therapies. *Tissue Eng* 7:211, 2001.
112. Izadpanah R, Trygg C, Patel B, et al: Biologic properties of mesenchymal stem cells derived from marrow and adipose tissue. *J Cell Biochem* 99:1285, 2006.
113. Zhang Y, Li C, Jiang X, et al: Human placenta-derived mesenchymal progenitor cells support culture expansion of long-term culture-initiating cells from cord blood CD34+ cells. *Exp Hematol* 32:657, 2004.
114. Ghodsizad A, Klein HM, Borowski A, et al: Intraoperative isolation and processing of BM-derived stem cells. *Cytotherapy* 6:523, 2004.
115. Bieback K, Kern S, Kluter H, et al: Critical parameters for the isolation of mesenchymal stem cells from umbilical cord blood. *Stem Cells* 22:625, 2004.
116. Aguilar S, Nye E, Chan J, et al: Murine but not human mesenchymal stem cells generate osteosarcoma-like lesions in the lung. *Stem Cells* 25:1586, 2007.
117. Miura M, Miura Y, Padilla-Nash HM, et al: Accumulated chromosomal instability in murine marrow mesenchymal stem cells leads to malignant transformation. *Stem Cells* 24:1095, 2006.
118. Kumagai M, Manabe A, Coustan-Smith E, et al: Use of stroma-supported cultures of leukemic cells to assess antileukemic drugs. II: Potent cytotoxicity of 2-chlorodeoxyadenosine in acute lymphoblastic leukemia. *Leukemia* 8:1116, 1994.
119. Koc ON, Gerson SL, Cooper BW, et al: Rapid hematopoietic recovery after coinfusion of autologous-blood stem cells and culture-expanded marrow mesenchymal stem cells in advanced breast cancer patients receiving high-dose chemotherapy. *J Clin Oncol* 18:307, 2000.
120. Lazarus HM, Koc ON, Devine SM, et al: Cotransplantation of HLA-identical sibling culture-expanded mesenchymal stem cells and hematopoietic stem cells in hematologic malignancy patients. *Biol Blood Marrow Transplant* 11:389, 2005.
121. Ball LM, Bernardo ME, Roelofs H, et al: Cotransplantation of ex vivo expanded mesenchymal stem cells accelerates lymphocyte recovery and may reduce the risk of graft failure in haploidentical hematopoietic stem-cell transplantation. *Blood* 110:2764, 2007.
122. Macmillan ML, Blazar BR, DeFor TE, et al: Transplantation of ex-vivo culture-expanded parental haploidentical mesenchymal stem cells to promote engraftment in pediatric recipients of unrelated donor umbilical cord blood: Results of a phase I-II clinical trial. *Bone Marrow Transplant* 43:447, 2009.
123. Durkin WJ, Ghanta VK, Balch CM, et al: A methodological approach to the prediction of anticancer drug effect in humans. *Cancer Res* 39:402, 1979.
124. Frei E 3rd, Canellos GP: Dose: A critical factor in cancer chemotherapy. *Am J Med* 69:585, 1980.
125. Santos GW, Owens AH Jr: Allogeneic marrow transplants in cyclophosphamide treated mice. *Transplant Proc* 1:44, 1969.
126. Frei EI: Pharmacologic strategies for high-dose chemotherapy, in: *High-dose Cancer Therapy: Pharmacology, Hematopoietins, Stem Cells*, edited by JO Armitage, KH Antman, p 3. Williams & Wilkins, Baltimore, MD, 1995.
127. Rill DR, Moen RC, Buschle M, et al: An approach for the analysis of relapse and marrow reconstitution after autologous marrow transplantation using retrovirus-mediated gene transfer. *Blood* 79:2694, 1992.
128. Brenner MK, Rill DR, Moen RC, et al: Gene-marking to trace origin of relapse after autologous bone-marrow transplantation. *Lancet* 341:85, 1993.
129. Alici E, Bjorkstrand B, Treschow A, et al: Long-term follow-up of gene-marked CD34+ cells after autologous stem cell transplantation for myeloma. *Cancer Gene Ther* 14:227, 2007.
130. Bachier CR, Giles RE, Ellerson D, et al: Hematopoietic retroviral gene marking in patients with follicular non-Hodgkin's lymphoma. *Leuk Lymphoma* 32:279, 1999.
131. Nissen-Meyer R, Host H: A comparison between the hematological side effects of cyclophosphamide and nitrogen mustard. *Cancer Chemother Rep* 9:51, 1960.
132. Gorin NC, Aegerter P, Auvert B, et al: Autologous marrow transplantation for acute myelocytic leukemia in first remission: A European survey of the role of marrow purging. *Blood* 75:1606, 1990.
133. Gorin NC, Aegerter P, Auvert B: Autologous marrow transplantation for acute leukemia in remission: An analysis of 1322 cases. *Haematol Blood Transfus* 33:660, 1990.
134. Negrin RS, Blume KG: The use of the polymerase chain reaction for the detection of minimal residual malignant disease. *Blood* 78:255, 1991.
135. Negrin RS, Pesando J: Detection of tumor cells in purged marrow and peripheral-blood mononuclear cells by polymerase chain reaction amplification of bcl-2 translocations. *J Clin Oncol* 12:1021, 1994.
136. Gribben JG, Freedman AS, Neuberg D, et al: Immunologic purging of marrow assessed by PCR before autologous marrow transplantation for B-cell lymphoma. *N Engl J Med* 325:1525, 1991.
137. Anderson KC, Andersen J, Soiffer R, et al: Monoclonal antibody-purged marrow transplantation therapy for myeloma. *Blood* 82:2568, 1993.
138. Vescio R, Schiller G, Stewart AK, et al: Multicenter phase III trial to evaluate CD34(+) selected versus unselected autologous peripheral blood progenitor cell transplantation in myeloma. *Blood* 93:1858, 1999.
139. Stewart AK, Vescio R, Schiller G, et al: Purging of autologous peripheral-blood stem cells using CD34 selection does not improve overall or progression-free survival after high-dose chemotherapy for myeloma: Results of a multicenter randomized controlled trial. *J Clin Oncol* 19:3771, 2001.
140. Holmberg LA, Boeckh M, Hooper H, et al: Increased incidence of cytomegalovirus disease after autologous CD34-selected peripheral blood stem cell transplantation. *Blood* 94:4029, 1999.
141. Crippa F, Holmberg L, Carter RA, et al: Infectious complications after autologous CD34-selected peripheral blood stem cell transplantation. *Biol Blood Marrow Transplant* 8:281, 2002.
142. Carella AM, Congiu AM, Gaozza E, et al: High-dose chemotherapy with autologous marrow transplantation in 50 advanced resistant Hodgkin's disease patients: An Italian study group report. *J Clin Oncol* 6:1411, 1988.
143. Carella AM, Dejana A, Lerma E, et al: In vivo mobilization of karyotypically normal peripheral blood progenitor cells in high-risk MDS, secondary or therapy-related acute myelogenous leukaemia. *Br J Haematol* 95:127, 1996.
144. Flinn IW, O'Donnell PV, Goodrich A, et al: Immunotherapy with rituximab during peripheral blood stem cell transplantation for non-Hodgkin's lymphoma. *Biol Blood Marrow Transplant* 6:628, 2000.
145. Lazzarino M, Arcaini L, Bernasconi P, et al: A sequence of immuno-chemotherapy with Rituximab, mobilization of *in vivo* purged stem cells, high-dose chemotherapy and autotransplant is an effective and non-toxic treatment for advanced follicular and mantle cell lymphoma. *Br J Haematol* 116:229, 2002.
146. van Heeckeren WJ, Vollweiler J, Fu P, et al: Randomised comparison of two B-cell purging protocols for patients with B-cell non-Hodgkin lymphoma: *In vivo* purging with rituximab versus *ex vivo* purging with CliniMACS CD34 cell enrichment device. *Br J Haematol* 132:42, 2006.
147. Bordignon C, Kernan NA, Keever CA, et al: The role of residual host immunity in graft failures following T-cell-depleted marrow transplants for leukemia. *Ann N Y Acad Sci* 511:442, 1987.
148. Murphy WJ, Kumar V, Bennett M: Acute rejection of murine marrow allografts by natural killer cells and T cells. Differences in kinetics and target antigens recognized. *J Exp Med* 166:1499, 1987.

149. Kernan NA, Bordignon C, Heller G, et al: Graft failure after T-cell-depleted human leukocyte antigen identical marrow transplants for leukemia: I: Analysis of risk factors and results of secondary transplants. *Blood* 74:2227, 1989.
150. Kernan NA, Flomenberg N, Dupont B, et al: Graft rejection in recipients of T-cell-depleted HLA-nonidentical marrow transplants for leukemia. Identification of host-derived antidonor allocytotoxic T lymphocytes. *Transplantation* 43:842, 1987.
151. Patterson J, Prentice HG, Brenner MK, et al: Graft rejection following HLA matched T-lymphocyte depleted marrow transplantation. *Br J Haematol* 63:221, 1986.
152. Fefer A, Sullivan K, Weiden P, et al: Graft versus leukemia effect in man. The relapse rate of acute leukemia is lower after allogeneic than after syngeneic marrow transplantation, in *Cellular Immunotherapy of Cancer*, edited by R Truit, RP Gale, M Bortin, p 401. Alan R Liss, New York, 1987.
153. Fefer A, Einstein AB, Thomas ED, et al: Bone-marrow transplantation for hematologic neoplasia in 16 patients with identical twins. *N Engl J Med* 290:1389, 1974.
154. Gale RP, Horowitz MM, Ash RC, et al: Identical-twin marrow transplants for leukemia. *Ann Intern Med* 120:646, 1994.
155. Martin PJ, Hansen JA, Buckner CD, et al: Effects of *in vitro* depletion of T cells in HLA-identical allogeneic marrow grafts. *Blood* 66:664, 1985.
156. Weiden PL, Flournoy N, Thomas ED, et al: Antileukemic effect of graft-versus-host disease in human recipients of allogeneic-marrow grafts. *N Engl J Med* 300:1068, 1979.
157. Goldman JM, Gale RP, Horowitz MM, et al: Marrow transplantation for chronic myelogenous leukemia in chronic phase. Increased risk for relapse associated with T-cell depletion. *Ann Intern Med* 108:806, 1988.
158. Martin PJ, Clift RA, Fisher LD, et al: HLA-identical marrow transplantation during accelerated-phase chronic myelogenous leukemia: Analysis of survival and remission duration. *Blood* 72:1978, 1988.
159. Kolb HJ, Mittermuller J, Clemm C, et al: Donor leukocyte transfusions for treatment of recurrent chronic myelogenous leukemia in marrow transplant patients. *Blood* 76:2462, 1990.
160. Kolb HJ, Schattenberg A, Goldman JM, et al: Graft-versus-leukemia effect of donor lymphocyte transfusions in marrow grafted patients. *Blood* 86:2041, 1995.
161. Dazzi F, Szydlo RM, Cross NC, et al: Durability of responses following donor lymphocyte infusions for patients who relapse after allogeneic stem cell transplantation for chronic myeloid leukemia. *Blood* 96:2712, 2000.
162. Hauch M, Gazzola MV, Small T, et al: Anti-leukemia potential of interleukin-2 activated natural killer cells after marrow transplantation for chronic myelogenous leukemia. *Blood* 75:2250, 1990.
163. Bellucci R, Wu CJ, Chiaretti S, et al: Complete response to donor lymphocyte infusion in myeloma is associated with antibody responses to highly expressed antigens. *Blood* 103:656, 2004.
164. Halverson DC, Schwartz GN, Carter C, et al: In vitro generation of allospecific human CD8+ T cells of Tc1 and Tc2 phenotype. *Blood* 90:2089, 1997.
165. Faber LM, van der Hoeven J, Goulmy E, et al: Recognition of clonogenic leukemic cells, remission marrow and HLA-identical donor marrow by CD8+ or CD4+ minor histocompatibility antigen-specific cytotoxic T lymphocytes. *J Clin Invest* 96:877, 1995.
166. Warren EH, Greenberg PD, Riddell SR: Cytotoxic T-lymphocyte-defined human minor histocompatibility antigens with a restricted tissue distribution. *Blood* 91:2197, 1998.
167. Scheibenbogen C, Letsch A, Thiel E, et al: CD8 T-cell responses to Wilms tumor gene product WT1 and proteinase 3 in patients with acute myelogenous leukemia. *Blood* 100:2132, 2002.
168. Delmon L, Ythier A, Moingeon P, et al: Characterization of antileukemia cells' cytotoxic effector function. Implications for monitoring natural killer responses following allogeneic marrow transplantation. *Transplantation* 42:252, 1986.
169. Hercend T, Takvorian T, Nowill A, et al: Characterization of natural killer cells with antileukemia activity following allogeneic marrow transplantation. *Blood* 67:722, 1986.
170. Higuchi CM, Thompson JA, Cox T, et al: Lymphokine-activated killer function following autologous marrow transplantation for refractory hematological malignancies. *Cancer Res* 49:5509, 1989.
171. Thomas ED, Bryant JI, Buckner CD, et al: Allogeneic marrow grafting using HL-A matched donor-recipient sibling pairs. *Trans Assoc Am Physicians* 84:248, 1971.
172. Thomas ED, Buckner CD, Banaji M, et al: One hundred patients with acute leukemia treated by chemotherapy, total body irradiation, and allogeneic marrow transplantation. *Blood* 49:511, 1977.
173. Vriesendorp HM: Radiobiological speculations on therapeutic total body irradiation. *Crit Rev Oncol Hematol* 10:211, 1990.
174. Thomas ED, Clift RA, Hersman J, et al: Marrow transplantation for acute nonlymphoblastic leukemic in first remission using fractionated or single-dose irradiation. *Int J Radiat Oncol Biol Phys* 8:817, 1982.
175. Clift RA, Buckner CD, Appelbaum FR, et al: Long-term follow-up of a randomized trial of two irradiation regimens for patients receiving allogeneic marrow transplants during first remission of acute myelogenous leukemia. *Blood* 92:1455, 1998.
176. Duell T, van Lint MT, Ljungman P, et al: Health and functional status of long-term survivors of marrow transplantation. EBMT Working Party on Late Effects and EULEP Study Group on Late Effects. European Group for Blood and Marrow Transplantation. *Ann Intern Med* 126:184, 1997.
177. Appelbaum FR, Badger CC, Bernstein ID, et al: Is there a better way to deliver total body irradiation? *Bone Marrow Transplant* 10(Suppl 1):77, 1992.
178. Shank B, O'Reilly RJ, Cunningham I, et al: Total body irradiation for marrow transplantation: The Memorial Sloan-Kettering Cancer Center experience. *Radiother Oncol* 18 Suppl 1:68, 1990.
179. Shank B, Chu FC, Dinsmore R, et al: Hyperfractionated total body irradiation for marrow transplantation. Results in seventy leukemia patients with allogeneic transplants. *Int J Radiat Oncol Biol Phys* 9:1607, 1983.
180. Blume KG, Forman SJ: High-dose etoposide (VP-16)-containing preparatory regimens in allogeneic and autologous marrow transplantation for hematologic malignancies. *Semin Oncol* 19:63, 1992.
181. Jamieson CH, Amylon MD, Wong RM, et al: Allogeneic hematopoietic cell transplantation for patients with high-risk acute lymphoblastic leukemia in first or second complete remission using fractionated total-body irradiation and high-dose etoposide: A 15-year experience. *Exp Hematol* 31:981, 2003.
182. Storb R: Preparative regimens for patients with leukemias and severe aplastic anemia (overview): Biological basis, experimental animal studies and clinical trials at the Fred Hutchinson Cancer Research Center. *Bone Marrow Transplant* 14(Suppl 4):S1, 1994.
183. Brochstein JA, Kernan NA, Groshen S, et al: Allogeneic marrow transplantation after hyperfractionated total-body irradiation and cyclophosphamide in children with acute leukemia. *N Engl J Med* 317:1618, 1987.
184. Press OW, Eary JF, Appelbaum FR, et al: Radiolabeled-antibody therapy of B-cell lymphoma with autologous marrow support. *N Engl J Med* 329:1219, 1993.
185. Pecego R, Hill R, Appelbaum FR, et al: Interstitial pneumonitis following autologous marrow transplantation. *Transplantation* 42:515, 1986.
186. Horning SJ, Chao NJ, Negrin RS, et al: The Stanford experience with high-dose etoposide cytoreductive regimens and autologous marrow transplantation in Hodgkin's disease and non-Hodgkin's lymphoma: Preliminary data. *Ann Oncol* 2(Suppl 1):47, 1991.
187. Gulati SC, Shank B, Black P, et al: Autologous marrow transplantation for patients with poor-prognosis lymphoma. *J Clin Oncol* 6:1303, 1988.
188. Jagannath S, Dicke KA, Armitage JO, et al: High-dose cyclophosphamide, carmustine, and etoposide and autologous marrow transplantation for relapsed Hodgkin's disease. *Ann Intern Med* 104:163, 1986.
189. Santos GW, Tutschka PJ, Brookmeyer R, et al: Marrow transplantation for acute nonlymphocytic leukemia after treatment with busulfan and cyclophosphamide. *N Engl J Med* 309:1347, 1983.
190. Tutschka PJ, Copelan EA, Klein JP: Marrow transplantation for leukemia following a new busulfan and cyclophosphamide regimen. *Blood* 70:1382, 1987.
191. Clift RA, Buckner CD, Thomas ED, et al: Marrow transplantation for chronic myeloid leukemia: A randomized study comparing cyclophosphamide and total body irradiation with busulfan and cyclophosphamide. *Blood* 84:2036, 1994.
192. Kashyap A, Wingard J, Cagnoni P, et al: Intravenous versus oral busulfan as part of a busulfan/cyclophosphamide preparative regimen for allogeneic hematopoietic stem cell transplantation: Decreased incidence of hepatic venoocclusive disease (HVOD), HVOD-related mortality, and overall 100-day mortality. *Biol Blood Marrow Transplant* 8:493, 2002.
193. Slattery JT, Clift RA, Buckner CD, et al: Marrow transplantation for chronic myeloid leukemia: The influence of plasma busulfan levels on the outcome of transplantation. *Blood* 89:3055, 1997.
194. Storb R, Yu C, Wagner JL, et al: Stable mixed hematopoietic chimerism in DLA-identical littermate dogs given sublethal total body irradiation before and pharmacological immunosuppression after marrow transplantation. *Blood* 89:3048, 1997.
195. Sandmaier B, Maloney DG, Hegenbart U, et al: Allografting with non-myeloablative conditioning for HLA-matched related allografts for hematologic malignancies. *Blood* 96:479a, 2000.
196. Maloney DG, Molina AJ, Sahebi F, et al: Allografting with nonmyeloablative conditioning following cytoreductive autografts for the treatment of patients with myeloma. *Blood* 102:3447, 2003.
197. Khouri IF, Keating M, Korbling M, et al: Transplant-lite: Induction of graft-versus-malignancy using fludarabine-based nonablative chemotherapy and allogeneic blood progenitor-cell transplantation as treatment for lymphoid malignancies. *J Clin Oncol* 16:2817, 1998.
198. Khouri IF, McLaughlin P, Saliba RM, et al: Eight-year experience with allogeneic stem cell transplantation for relapsed follicular lymphoma after nonmyeloablative conditioning with fludarabine, cyclophosphamide, and rituximab. *Blood* 111:5530, 2008.
199. Schetelig J, Bornhauser M, Kiehl M, et al: Reduced-intensity conditioning with busulfan and fludarabine with or without antithymocyte globulin in HLA-identical sibling transplantation—A retrospective analysis. *Bone Marrow Transplant* 33:483, 2004.
200. McSweeney PA, Niederwieser D, Shizuru JA, et al: Hematopoietic cell transplantation in older patients with hematologic malignancies: Replacing high-dose cytotoxic therapy with graft-versus-tumor effects. *Blood* 97:3390, 2001.
201. Hegenbart U, Niederwieser D, Sandmaier BM, et al: Treatment for acute myelogenous leukemia by low-dose, total-body, irradiation-based conditioning and hematopoietic cell transplantation from related and unrelated donors. *J Clin Oncol* 24:444, 2006.
202. Maris MB, Sandmaier BM, Storer BE, et al: Allogeneic hematopoietic cell transplantation after fludarabine and 2 Gy total body irradiation for relapsed and refractory mantle cell lymphoma. *Blood* 104:3535, 2004.
203. Mielcarek M, Martin PJ, Leisenring W, et al: Graft-versus-host disease after nonmyeloablative versus conventional hematopoietic stem cell transplantation. *Blood* 102:756, 2003.
204. Lan F, Zeng D, Higuchi M, et al: Predominance of NK1.1+TCR alpha beta+ or DX5+TCR alpha beta+ T cells in mice conditioned with fractionated lymphoid irradiation protects against graft-versus-host disease: "Natural suppressor" cells. *J Immunol* 167:2087, 2001.

205. Lan F, Zeng D, Higuchi M, et al: Host conditioning with total lymphoid irradiation and antithymocyte globulin prevents graft-versus-host disease: The role of CD1-reactive natural killer T cells. *Biol Blood Marrow Transplant* 9:355, 2003.
206. Pillai AB, George TI, Dutt S, et al: Host NKT cells can prevent graft-versus-host disease and permit graft antitumor activity after marrow transplantation. *J Immunol* 178:6242, 2007.
207. Yao Z, Liu Y, Jones J, et al: Differences in Bcl-2 expression by T-cell subsets alter their balance after in vivo irradiation to favor CD4+Bcl-2hi NKT cells. *Eur J Immunol* 39:763, 2009.
208. Lowsky R, Takahashi T, Liu YP, et al: Protective conditioning for acute graft-versus-host disease. *N Engl J Med* 353:1321, 2005.
209. Kohrt HE, Turnbull BB, Heydari K, et al: TLI and ATG conditioning with low risk of graft-versus-host disease retains anti-tumor reactions after allogeneic hematopoietic cell transplantation from related and unrelated donors. *Blood* 114:1099, 2009.
210. Baron F, Little MT, Storb R: Kinetics of engraftment following allogeneic hematopoietic cell transplantation with reduced-intensity or nonmyeloablative conditioning. *Blood Rev* 19:153, 2005.
211. Morris E, Thomson K, Craddock C, et al: Outcomes after alemtuzumab-containing reduced-intensity allogeneic transplantation regimen for relapsed and refractory non-Hodgkin lymphoma. *Blood* 104:3865, 2004.
212. Hill RS, Petersen FB, Storb R, et al: Mixed hematologic chimerism after allogeneic marrow transplantation for severe aplastic anemia is associated with a higher risk of graft rejection and a lessened incidence of acute graft-versus-host disease. *Blood* 67:811, 1986.
213. Scandling JD, Busque S, Dejbakhsh-Jones S, et al: Tolerance and chimerism after renal and hematopoietic-cell transplantation. *N Engl J Med* 358:362, 2008.
214. Blume K, Krance R: The evaluation and counseling of candidates for hematopoietic cell transplantation, in *Thomas' Hematopoietic Cell Transplantation*, 4th ed, edited by FR Appelbaum, SJ Forman, RS Negrin, KG Blume, p 445. Wiley-Blackwell, Hoboken, NJ, 2009.
215. Center for International Blood and Marrow Transplant Research, 2007. Available at: www.cibmtr.org.
216. Derenzini E, Musuraca G, Fanti S, et al: Pretransplantation positron emission tomography scan is the main predictor of autologous stem cell transplantation outcome in aggressive B-cell non-Hodgkin lymphoma. *Cancer* 113:2496, 2008.
217. Petersdorf EW, Mickelson EM, Anasetti C, et al: Effect of HLA mismatches on the outcome of hematopoietic transplants. *Curr Opin Immunol* 11:521, 1999.
218. Petersdorf EW, Hansen JA, Martin PJ, et al: Major-histocompatibility-complex class I alleles and antigens in hematopoietic-cell transplantation. *N Engl J Med* 345:1794, 2001.
219. Petersdorf EW: HLA matching in allogeneic stem cell transplantation. *Curr Opin Hematol* 11:386, 2004.
220. Wallen H, Gooley TA, Deeg HJ, et al: Ablative allogeneic hematopoietic cell transplantation in adults 60 years of age and older. *J Clin Oncol* 23:3439, 2005.
221. Du W, Dansey R, Abella EM, et al: Successful allogeneic marrow transplantation in selected patients over 50 years of age—A single institution's experience. *Bone Marrow Transplant* 21:1043, 1998.
222. Gandemer V, Auclerc MF, Perel Y, et al: Impact of age, leukocyte count and day 21-marrow response to chemotherapy on the long-term outcome of children with Philadelphia chromosome-positive acute lymphoblastic leukemia in the pre-imatinib era: Results of the FRALLE 93 study. *BMC Cancer* 9:14, 2009.
223. de la Camara R, Alonso A, Steegmann JL, et al: Allogeneic hematopoietic stem cell transplantation in patients 50 years of age and older. *Haematologica* 87:965, 2002.
224. Kusnierz-Glaz CR, Schlegel PG, Wong RM, et al: Influence of age on the outcome of 500 autologous marrow transplant procedures for hematologic malignancies. *J Clin Oncol* 15:18, 1997.
225. Miller CB, Piantadosi S, Vogelsang GB, et al: Impact of age on outcome of patients with cancer undergoing autologous marrow transplant. *J Clin Oncol* 14:1327, 1996.
226. Blume KG, Forman SJ, Nademanee AP, et al: Marrow transplantation for hematologic malignancies in patients aged 30 years or older. *J Clin Oncol* 4:1489, 1986.
227. Corradini P, Zallio F, Mariotti J, et al: Effect of age and previous autologous transplantation on nonrelapse mortality and survival in patients treated with reduced-intensity conditioning and allografting for advanced hematologic malignancies. *J Clin Oncol* 23:6690, 2005.
228. Sorror ML, Maris MB, Storer B, et al: Comparing morbidity and mortality of HLA-matched unrelated donor hematopoietic cell transplantation after nonmyeloablative and myeloablative conditioning: Influence of pretransplantation comorbidities. *Blood* 104:961, 2004.
229. Deeg HJ, Seidel K, Bruemmer B, et al: Impact of patient weight on non-relapse mortality after marrow transplantation. *Bone Marrow Transplant* 15:461, 1995.
230. Dickson TM, Kusnierz-Glaz CR, Blume KG, et al: Impact of admission body weight and chemotherapy dose adjustment on the outcome of autologous marrow transplantation. *Biol Blood Marrow Transplant* 5:299, 1999.
231. Sandmaier BM, Mackinnon S, Childs RW: Reduced intensity conditioning for allogeneic hematopoietic cell transplantation: Current perspectives. *Biol Blood Marrow Transplant* 13:87, 2007.
232. Matthay KK, Reynolds CP, Seeger RC, et al: Long-term results for children with high-risk neuroblastoma treated on a randomized trial of myeloablative therapy followed by 13-*cis*-retinoic acid: A children's oncology group study. *J Clin Oncol* 27:1007, 2009.
233. Ladenstein R, Potschger U, Hartman O, et al: 28 Years of high-dose therapy and SCT for neuroblastoma in Europe: Lessons from more than 4000 procedures. *Bone Marrow Transplant* 41 Suppl 2:S118, 2008.
234. Lazarus HM, Stiff PJ, Carreras J, et al: Utility of single versus tandem autotransplants for advanced testes/germ cell cancer: A center for international blood and marrow transplant research (CIBMTR) analysis. *Biol Blood Marrow Transplant* 13:778, 2007.
235. Banna GL, Simonelli M, Santoro A: High-dose chemotherapy followed by autologous hematopoietic stem-cell transplantation for the treatment of solid tumors in adults: A critical review. *Curr Stem Cell Res Ther* 2:65, 2007.
236. Crump M, Gluck S, Tu D, et al: Randomized trial of high-dose chemotherapy with autologous peripheral-blood stem-cell support compared with standard-dose chemotherapy in women with metastatic breast cancer: NCIC MA:16. *J Clin Oncol* 26:37, 2008.
237. Demirer T, Barkholt L, Blaise D, et al: Transplantation of allogeneic hematopoietic stem cells: An emerging treatment modality for solid tumors. *Nat Clin Pract Oncol* 5:256, 2008.
238. Storb RF, Lucarelli G, McSweeney PA, et al: Hematopoietic cell transplantation for benign hematological disorders and solid tumors. *Hematology Am Soc Hematol Educ Program* 372, 2003.
239. Deeg HJ, Leisenring W, Storb R, et al: Long-term outcome after marrow transplantation for severe aplastic anemia. *Blood* 91:3637, 1998.
240. Lucarelli G, Clift RA, Galimberti M, et al: Marrow transplantation in adult thalassemic patients. *Blood* 93:1164, 1999.
241. Gaziev J, Sodani P, Lucarelli G: Hematopoietic stem cell transplantation in thalassemia. *Bone Marrow Transplant* 42(Suppl 1):S41, 2008.
242. Bhatia M, Walters MC: Hematopoietic cell transplantation for thalassemia and sickle cell disease: Past, present and future. *Bone Marrow Transplant* 41:109, 2008.
243. Sadelain M, Boulad F, Lisowki L, et al: Stem cell engineering for the treatment of severe hemoglobinopathies. *Curr Mol Med* 8:690, 2008.
244. Buckley RH, Schiff SE, Schiff RI, et al: Hematopoietic stem-cell transplantation for the treatment of severe combined immunodeficiency. *N Engl J Med* 340:508, 1999.
245. Antoine C, Muller S, Cant A, et al: Long-term survival and transplantation of haemopoietic stem cells for immunodeficiencies: Report of the European experience 1968–99. *Lancet* 361:553, 2003.
246. Souillet G, Guffon N, Maire I, et al: Outcome of 27 patients with Hurler's syndrome transplanted from either related or unrelated haematopoietic stem cell sources. *Bone Marrow Transplant* 31:1105, 2003.
247. Peters C, Shapiro EG, Anderson J, et al: Hurler syndrome: II: Outcome of HLA-genotypically identical sibling and HLA-haploidentical related donor marrow transplantation in fifty-four children. The Storage Disease Collaborative Study Group. *Blood* 91:2601, 1998.
248. Biggs JC, Horowitz MM, Gale RP, et al: Marrow transplants may cure patients with acute leukemia never achieving remission with chemotherapy. *Blood* 80:1090, 1992.
249. Fung HC, Stein A, Slovak M, et al: A long-term follow-up report on allogeneic stem cell transplantation for patients with primary refractory acute myelogenous leukemia: Impact of cytogenetic characteristics on transplantation outcome. *Biol Blood Marrow Transplant* 9:766, 2003.
250. Appelbaum FR, Clift RA, Buckner CD, et al: Allogeneic marrow transplantation for acute nonlymphoblastic leukemia after first relapse. *Blood* 61:949, 1983.
251. Milligan DW, Grimwade D, Cullis JO, et al: Guidelines on the management of acute myelogenous leukaemia in adults. *Br J Haematol* 135:450, 2006.
252. Yanada M, Matsuo K, Emi N, et al: Efficacy of allogeneic hematopoietic stem cell transplantation depends on cytogenetic risk for acute myelogenous leukemia in first disease remission: A metaanalysis. *Cancer* 103:1652, 2005.
253. Reiffers J, Stoppa AM, Attal M, et al: Allogeneic vs autologous stem cell transplantation vs chemotherapy in patients with acute myelogenous leukemia in first remission: The BGMT 87 study. *Leukemia* 10:1874, 1996.
254. Keating S, de Witte T, Suciu S, et al: The influence of HLA-matched sibling donor availability on treatment outcome for patients with AML: An analysis of the AML 8A study of the EORTC Leukaemia Cooperative Group and GIMEMA. European Organization for Research and Treatment of Cancer. Gruppo Italiano Malattie Ematologiche Maligne dell'Adulto. *Br J Haematol* 102:1344, 1998.
255. Slovak ML, Kopecky KJ, Cassileth PA, et al: Karyotypic analysis predicts outcome of preremission and postremission therapy in adult acute myelogenous leukemia: A Southwest Oncology Group/Eastern Cooperative Oncology Group Study. *Blood* 96:4075, 2000.
256. Burnett AK, Wheatley K, Goldstone AH, et al: The value of allogeneic marrow transplant in patients with acute myelogenous leukaemia at differing risk of relapse: Results of the UK MRC AML 10 trial. *Br J Haematol* 118:385, 2002.
257. Suciu S, Mandelli F, de Witte T, et al: Allogeneic compared with autologous stem cell transplantation in the treatment of patients younger than 46 years with acute myelogenous leukemia (AML) in first complete remission (CR1): An intention-to-treat analysis of the EORTC/GIMEMAAML-10 trial. *Blood* 102:1232, 2003.
258. Burnett AK, Goldstone AH, Stevens RM, et al: Randomised comparison of addition of autologous bone-marrow transplantation to intensive chemotherapy for acute myelogenous leukaemia in first remission: Results of MRC AML 10 trial. UK Medical Research Council Adult and Children's Leukaemia Working Parties. *Lancet* 351:700, 1998.
259. Levi I, Grotto I, Yerushalmi R, et al: Meta-analysis of autologous marrow transplantation versus chemotherapy in adult patients with acute myelogenous leukemia in first remission. *Leuk Res* 28:605, 2004.
260. Zittoun RA, Mandelli F, Willemze R, et al: Autologous or allogeneic marrow transplantation compared with intensive chemotherapy in acute myelogenous leukemia.

European Organization for Research and Treatment of Cancer (EORTC) and the Gruppo Italiano Malattie Ematologiche Maligne dell'Adulto (GIMEMA) Leukemia Cooperative Groups. *N Engl J Med* 332:217, 1995.

261. Cassileth PA, Harrington DP, Appelbaum FR, et al: Chemotherapy compared with autologous or allogeneic marrow transplantation in the management of acute myelogenous leukemia in first remission. *N Engl J Med* 339:1649, 1998.
262. Attal M, Blaise D, Marit G, et al: Consolidation treatment of adult acute lymphoblastic leukemia: A prospective, randomized trial comparing allogeneic versus autologous marrow transplantation and testing the impact of recombinant interleukin-2 after autologous marrow transplantation. BGMT Group. *Blood* 86:1619, 1995.
263. Doney K, Fisher LD, Appelbaum FR, et al: Treatment of adult acute lymphoblastic leukemia with allogeneic marrow transplantation. Multivariate analysis of factors affecting acute graft-versus-host disease, relapse, and relapse-free survival. *Bone Marrow Transplant* 7:453, 1991.
264. Goldstone AH, Richards SM, Lazarus HM, et al: In adults with standard-risk acute lymphoblastic leukemia, the greatest benefit is achieved from a matched sibling allogeneic transplantation in first complete remission, and an autologous transplantation is less effective than conventional consolidation/maintenance chemotherapy in all patients: Final results of the International ALL Trial (MRC UKALL XII/ECOG E2993). *Blood* 111:1827, 2008.
265. Barry E, DeAngelo DJ, Neuberg D, et al: Favorable outcome for adolescents with acute lymphoblastic leukemia treated on Dana-Farber Cancer Institute Acute Lymphoblastic Leukemia Consortium Protocols. *J Clin Oncol* 25:813, 2007.
266. Schiffer CA: Differences in outcome in adolescents with acute lymphoblastic leukemia: A consequence of better regimens? Better doctors? Both? *J Clin Oncol* 21:760, 2003.
267. Snyder DS, Nademanee AP, O'Donnell MR, et al: Long-term follow-up of 23 patients with Philadelphia chromosome-positive acute lymphoblastic leukemia treated with allogeneic marrow transplant in first complete remission. *Leukemia* 13:2053, 1999.
268. Laport GG, Alvarnas JC, Palmer JM, et al: Long-term remission of Philadelphia chromosome-positive acute lymphoblastic leukemia after allogeneic hematopoietic cell transplantation from matched sibling donors: A 20-year experience with the fractionated total body irradiation-etoposide regimen. *Blood* 112:903, 2008.
269. Lee S, Kim YJ, Min CK, et al: The effect of first-line imatinib interim therapy on the outcome of allogeneic stem cell transplantation in adults with newly diagnosed Philadelphia chromosome-positive acute lymphoblastic leukemia. *Blood* 105:3449, 2005.
270. Attal M, Harousseau JL, Stoppa AM, et al: A prospective, randomized trial of autologous marrow transplantation and chemotherapy in myeloma. Intergroupe Francais du Myelome. *N Engl J Med* 335:91, 1996.
271. Child JA, Morgan GJ, Davies FE, et al: High-dose chemotherapy with hematopoietic stem-cell rescue for myeloma. *N Engl J Med* 348:1875, 2003.
272. Cavo M, Tosi P, Zamagni E, et al: Prospective, randomized study of single compared with double autologous stem-cell transplantation for myeloma: Bologna 96 clinical study. *J Clin Oncol* 25:2434, 2007.
273. Attal M, Harousseau JL, Facon T, et al: Single versus double autologous stem-cell transplantation for myeloma. *N Engl J Med* 349:2495, 2003.
274. Philip T, Armitage JO, Spitzer G, et al: High-dose therapy and autologous marrow transplantation after failure of conventional chemotherapy in adults with intermediate-grade or high-grade non-Hodgkin's lymphoma. *N Engl J Med* 316:1493, 1987.
275. Yuen AR, Rosenberg SA, Hoppe RT, et al: Comparison between conventional salvage therapy and high-dose therapy with autografting for recurrent or refractory Hodgkin's disease. *Blood* 89:814, 1997.
276. Horwitz SM, Negrin RS, Blume KG, et al: Rituximab as adjuvant to high-dose therapy and autologous hematopoietic cell transplantation for aggressive non-Hodgkin lymphoma. *Blood* 103:777, 2004.
277. Chen AI, McMillan A, Negrin RS, et al: Long-term results of autologous hematopoietic cell transplantation for peripheral T cell lymphoma: The Stanford experience. *Biol Blood Marrow Transplant* 14:741, 2008.
278. Khouri IF, Saliba RM, Okoroji GJ, et al: Long-term follow-up of autologous stem cell transplantation in patients with diffuse mantle cell lymphoma in first disease remission: The prognostic value of beta2-microglobulin and the tumor score. *Cancer* 98:2630, 2003.
279. Verdonck LF, van Putten WL, Hagenbeek A, et al: Comparison of CHOP chemotherapy with autologous marrow transplantation for slowly responding patients with aggressive non-Hodgkin's lymphoma. *N Engl J Med* 332:1045, 1995.
280. Devetten MP, Hari PN, Carreras J, et al: Unrelated donor reduced-intensity allogeneic hematopoietic stem cell transplantation for relapsed and refractory Hodgkin lymphoma. *Biol Blood Marrow Transplant* 15:109, 2009.
281. Davies SM, Kollman C, Anasetti C, et al: Engraftment and survival after unrelated-donor marrow transplantation: A report from the national marrow donor program. *Blood* 96:4096, 2000.
282. Wulff JC, Santner TJ, Storb R, et al: Transfusion requirements after HLA-identical marrow transplantation in 82 patients with aplastic anemia. *Vox Sang* 44:366, 1983.
283. Nakamura H, Gress RE: Graft rejection by cytolytic T cells. Specificity of the effector mechanism in the rejection of allogeneic marrow. *Transplantation* 49:453, 1990.
284. Anasetti C, Amos D, Beatty PG, et al: Effect of HLA compatibility on engraftment of marrow transplants in patients with leukemia or lymphoma. *N Engl J Med* 320:197, 1989.
285. Pottinger B, Walker M, Campbell M, et al: The storage and re-infusion of autologous blood and BM as back-up following failed primary hematopoietic stem-cell transplantation: A survey of European practice. *Cytotherapy* 4:127, 2002.
286. McCann SR, Bacigalupo A, Gluckman E, et al: Graft rejection and second marrow transplants for acquired aplastic anaemia: A report from the Aplastic Anaemia Working Party of the European Marrow Transplant Group. *Bone Marrow Transplant* 13:233, 1994.
287. Storb R, Longton G, Anasetti C, et al: Changing trends in marrow transplantation for aplastic anemia. *Bone Marrow Transplant* 10 Suppl 1:45, 1992.
288. McGuire DB, Johnson J, Migliorati C: Promulgation of guidelines for mucositis management: Educating health care professionals and patients. *Support Care Cancer* 14:548, 2006.
289. Vera-Llonch M, Oster G, Ford CM, et al: Oral mucositis and outcomes of allogeneic hematopoietic stem-cell transplantation in patients with hematologic malignancies. *Support Care Cancer* 15:491, 2007.
290. DiBaise JK, Lyden E, Tarantolo SR, et al: A prospective study of gastric emptying and its relationship to the development of nausea, vomiting, and anorexia after autologous stem cell transplantation. *Am J Gastroenterol* 100:1571, 2005.
291. Wu D, Hockenberry DM, Brentnall TA, et al: Persistent nausea and anorexia after marrow transplantation: A prospective study of 78 patients. *Transplantation* 66:1319, 1998.
292. Spielberger R, Stiff P, Bensinger W, et al: Palifermin for oral mucositis after intensive therapy for hematologic cancers. *N Engl J Med* 351:2590, 2004.
293. Rossi S, Blazar BR, Farrell CL, et al: Keratinocyte growth factor preserves normal thymopoiesis and thymic microenvironment during experimental graft-versus-host disease. *Blood* 100:682, 2002.
294. DeLeve LD, Shulman HM, McDonald GB: Toxic injury to hepatic sinusoids: Sinusoidal obstruction syndrome (veno-occlusive disease). *Semin Liver Dis* 22:27, 2002.
295. Shulman HM, Fisher LB, Schoch HG, et al: Veno-occlusive disease of the liver after marrow transplantation: Histological correlates of clinical signs and symptoms. *Hepatology* 19:1171, 1994.
296. McDonald GB, Hinds MS, Fisher LD, et al: Veno-occlusive disease of the liver and multiorgan failure after marrow transplantation: A cohort study of 355 patients. *Ann Intern Med* 118:255, 1993.
297. McDonald GB, McCune JS, Batchelder A, et al: Metabolism-based cyclophosphamide dosing for hematopoietic cell transplant. *Clin Pharmacol Ther* 78:298, 2005.
298. McCune JS, Batchelder A, Deeg HJ, et al: Cyclophosphamide following targeted oral busulfan as conditioning for hematopoietic cell transplantation: Pharmacokinetics, liver toxicity, and mortality. *Biol Blood Marrow Transplant* 13:853, 2007.
299. McKoy JM, Angelotta C, Bennett CL, et al: Gemtuzumab ozogamicin-associated sinusoidal obstructive syndrome (SOS): An overview from the research on adverse drug events and reports (RADAR) project. *Leuk Res* 31:599, 2007.
300. Wadleigh M, Richardson PG, Zahrieh D, et al: Prior gemtuzumab ozogamicin exposure significantly increases the risk of veno-occlusive disease in patients who undergo myeloablative allogeneic stem cell transplantation. *Blood* 102:1578, 2003.
301. Bearman SI, Anderson GL, Mori M, et al: Venoocclusive disease of the liver: Development of a model for predicting fatal outcome after marrow transplantation. *J Clin Oncol* 11:1729, 1993.
302. Richardson PG, Murakami C, Jin Z, et al: Multi-institutional use of defibrotide in 88 patients after stem cell transplantation with severe veno-occlusive disease and multisystem organ failure: Response without significant toxicity in a high-risk population and factors predictive of outcome. *Blood* 100:4337, 2002.
303. Kornblum N, Ayyanar K, Benimetskaya L, et al: Defibrotide, a polydisperse mixture of single-stranded phosphodiester oligonucleotides with lifesaving activity in severe hepatic veno-occlusive disease: Clinical outcomes and potential mechanisms of action. *Oligonucleotides* 16:105, 2006.
304. Attal M, Huguet F, Rubie H, et al: Prevention of hepatic veno-occlusive disease after marrow transplantation by continuous infusion of low-dose heparin: A prospective, randomized trial. *Blood* 79:2834, 1992.
305. Carreras E, Bertz H, Arcese W, et al: Incidence and outcome of hepatic veno-occlusive disease after blood or marrow transplantation: A prospective cohort study of the European Group for Blood and Marrow Transplantation. European Group for Blood and Marrow Transplantation Chronic Leukemia Working Party. *Blood* 92:3599, 1998.
306. Ruutu T, Eriksson B, Remes K, et al: Ursodeoxycholic acid for the prevention of hepatic complications in allogeneic stem cell transplantation. *Blood* 100:1977, 2002.
307. Afessa B, Litzow MR, Tefferi A: Bronchiolitis obliterans and other late onset noninfectious pulmonary complications in hematopoietic stem cell transplantation. *Bone Marrow Transplant* 28:425, 2001.
308. Kantrow SP, Hackman RC, Boeckh M, et al: Idiopathic pneumonia syndrome: Changing spectrum of lung injury after marrow transplantation. *Transplantation* 63:1079, 1997.
309. Crawford SW, Longton G, Storb R: Acute graft-versus-host disease and the risks for idiopathic pneumonia after marrow transplantation for severe aplastic anemia. *Bone Marrow Transplant* 12:225, 1993.
310. Weiner RS, Horowitz MM, Gale RP, et al: Risk factors for interstitial pneumonia following marrow transplantation for severe aplastic anaemia. *Br J Haematol* 71:535, 1989.
311. Yanik G, Hellerstedt B, Custer J, et al: Etanercept (Enbrel) administration for idiopathic pneumonia syndrome after allogeneic hematopoietic stem cell transplantation. *Biol Blood Marrow Transplant* 8:395, 2002.
312. Lewis ID, DeFor T, Weisdorf DJ: Increasing incidence of diffuse alveolar hemorrhage following allogeneic marrow transplantation: Cryptic etiology and uncertain therapy. *Bone Marrow Transplant* 26:539, 2000.

313. Robbins RA, Linder J, Stahl MG, et al: Diffuse alveolar hemorrhage in autologous marrow transplant recipients. *Am J Med* 87:511, 1989.
314. Majhail NS, Parks K, Defor TE, et al: Diffuse alveolar hemorrhage and infection-associated alveolar hemorrhage following hematopoietic stem cell transplantation: Related and high-risk clinical syndromes. *Biol Blood Marrow Transplant* 12:1038, 2006.
315. Capizzi SA, Kumar S, Huneke NE, et al: Peri-engraftment respiratory distress syndrome during autologous hematopoietic stem cell transplantation. *Bone Marrow Transplant* 27:1299, 2001.
316. Cahill RA, Spitzer TR, Mazumder A: Marrow engraftment and clinical manifestations of capillary leak syndrome. *Bone Marrow Transplant* 18:177, 1996.
317. Alessandrino EP, Bernasconi P, Colombo A, et al: Pulmonary toxicity following carmustine-based preparative regimens and autologous peripheral blood progenitor cell transplantation in hematological malignancies. *Bone Marrow Transplant* 25:309, 2000.
318. Silliman CC, Boshkov LK, Mehdizadehkashi Z, et al: Transfusion-related acute lung injury: Epidemiology and a prospective analysis of etiologic factors. *Blood* 101:454, 2003.
319. Baden L, Rubin R: Infection in the hematopoietic stem cell transplant recipient, in *Stem Cell Transplantation for Hematologic Malignancies*, edited by RJ Soiffer, p 237. Humana Press, Totowa, NJ, 2004.
320. Dykewicz CA: Guidelines for preventing opportunistic infections among hematopoietic stem cell transplant recipients: Focus on community respiratory virus infections. *Biol Blood Marrow Transplant* 7(Suppl)9S, 2001.
321. Reusser P, Attenhofer R, Hebart H, et al: Cytomegalovirus-specific T-cell immunity in recipients of autologous peripheral blood stem cell or marrow transplants. *Blood* 89:3873, 1997.
322. Zhang C, Todorov I, Zhang Z, et al: Donor CD4+ T and B cells in transplants induce chronic graft-versus-host disease with autoimmune manifestations. *Blood* 107:2993, 2006.
323. Douek DC, Vescio RA, Betts MR, et al: Assessment of thymic output in adults after haematopoietic stem-cell transplantation and prediction of T-cell reconstitution. *Lancet* 355:1875, 2000.
324. Kapoor N, Chan R, Weinberg KI, et al: Defective anticarbohydrate antibody responses to naturally occurring bacteria following marrow transplantation. *Biol Blood Marrow Transplant* 5:46, 1999.
325. Dulude G, Roy DC, Perreault C: The effect of graft-versus-host disease on T cell production and homeostasis. *J Exp Med* 189:1329, 1999.
326. Lum LG, Seigneuret MC, Storb R: The transfer of antigen-specific humoral immunity from marrow donors to marrow recipients. *J Clin Immunol* 6:389, 1986.
327. Collin BA, Leather HL, Wingard JR, et al: Evolution, incidence, and susceptibility of bacterial bloodstream isolates from 519 marrow transplant patients. *Clin Infect Dis* 33:947, 2001.
328. Ochs L, Shu XO, Miller J, et al: Late infections after allogeneic marrow transplantations: Comparison of incidence in related and unrelated donor transplant recipients. *Blood* 86:3979, 1995.
329. Kulkarni S, Powles R, Treleaven J, et al: Chronic graft versus host disease is associated with long-term risk for pneumococcal infections in recipients of marrow transplants. *Blood* 95:3683, 2000.
330. Ascioglu S, Rex JH, de Pauw B, et al: Defining opportunistic invasive fungal infections in immunocompromised patients with cancer and hematopoietic stem cell transplants: An international consensus. *Clin Infect Dis* 34:7, 2002.
331. Marr KA, Seidel K, Slavin MA, et al: Prolonged fluconazole prophylaxis is associated with persistent protection against candidiasis-related death in allogeneic marrow transplant recipients: Long-term follow-up of a randomized, placebo-controlled trial. *Blood* 96:2055, 2000.
332. van Burik JH, Leisenring W, Myerson D, et al: The effect of prophylactic fluconazole on the clinical spectrum of fungal diseases in marrow transplant recipients with special attention to hepatic candidiasis. An autopsy study of 355 patients. *Medicine (Baltimore)* 77:246, 1998.
333. Post MJ, Lass-Floerl C, Gastl G, et al: Invasive fungal infections in allogeneic and autologous stem cell transplant recipients: A single-center study of 166 transplanted patients. *Transpl Infect Dis* 9:189, 2007.
334. Ng TT, Robson GD, Denning DW: Hydrocortisone-enhanced growth of *Aspergillus* spp.: Implications for pathogenesis. *Microbiology* 140(Pt 9):2475, 1994.
335. Martino R, Parody R, Fukuda T, et al: Impact of the intensity of the pretransplantation conditioning regimen in patients with prior invasive aspergillosis undergoing allogeneic hematopoietic stem cell transplantation: A retrospective survey of the Infectious Diseases Working Party of the European Group for Blood and Marrow Transplantation. *Blood* 108:2928, 2006.
336. Machida U, Kami M, Kanda Y, et al: Aspergillus tracheobronchitis after allogeneic marrow transplantation. *Bone Marrow Transplant* 24:1145, 1999.
337. Hagensee ME, Bauwens JE, Kjos B, et al: Brain abscess following marrow transplantation: Experience at the Fred Hutchinson Cancer Research Center, 1984–1992. *Clin Infect Dis* 19:402, 1994.
338. Rizzo JD, Wingard JR, Tichelli A, et al: Recommended screening and preventive practices for long-term survivors after hematopoietic cell transplantation: Joint recommendations of the European Group for Blood and Marrow Transplantation, the Center for International Blood and Marrow Transplant Research, and the American Society of Blood and Marrow Transplantation. *Biol Blood Marrow Transplant* 12:138, 2006.
339. Ljungman P, Perez-Bercoff L, Jonsson J, et al: Risk factors for the development of cytomegalovirus disease after allogeneic stem cell transplantation. *Haematologica* 91:78, 2006.
340. Bowden RA, Slichter SJ, Sayers MH, et al: Use of leukocyte-depleted platelets and cytomegalovirus-seronegative red blood cells for prevention of primary cytomegalovirus infection after marrow transplant. *Blood* 78:246, 1991.
341. Meyers JD: Prevention of cytomegalovirus infection after marrow transplantation. *Rev Infect Dis* 11 Suppl 7:S1691, 1989.
342. Neiman PE, Reeves W, Ray G, et al: A prospective analysis interstitial pneumonia and opportunistic viral infection among recipients of allogeneic marrow grafts. *J Infect Dis* 136:754, 1977.
343. Fraser GA, Walker, II: Cytomegalovirus prophylaxis and treatment after hematopoietic stem cell transplantation in Canada: A description of current practices and comparison with Centers for Disease Control/Infectious Diseases Society of America/American Society for Blood and Marrow Transplantation guideline recommendations. *Biol Blood Marrow Transplant* 10:287, 2004.
344. Zaia J, Molinder K: Advances in CMV diagnostic testing and their implications for the management of CMV infection in transplant recipients, in *Infectious Complications in Transplant Patients*, edited by N Singh, JM Aguado, p 75. Kluwer Academic Publishers, Boston, 2000.
345. Boeckh M, Leisenring W, Riddell SR, et al: Late cytomegalovirus disease and mortality in recipients of allogeneic hematopoietic stem cell transplants: Importance of viral load and T-cell immunity. *Blood* 101:407, 2003.
346. Nichols WG, Corey L, Gooley T, et al: High risk of death due to bacterial and fungal infection among cytomegalovirus (CMV)-seronegative recipients of stem cell transplants from seropositive donors: Evidence for indirect effects of primary CMV infection. *J Infect Dis* 185:273, 2002.
347. Micklethwaite K, Hansen A, Foster A, et al: *Ex vivo* expansion and prophylactic infusion of CMV-pp65 peptide-specific cytotoxic T-lymphocytes following allogeneic hematopoietic stem cell transplantation. *Biol Blood Marrow Transplant* 13:707, 2007.
348. Meyers JD, Flournoy N, Thomas ED: Infection with herpes simplex virus and cell-mediated immunity after marrow transplant. *J Infect Dis* 142:338, 1980.
349. Saral R, Burns WH, Laskin OL, et al: Acyclovir prophylaxis of herpes-simplex-virus infections. *N Engl J Med* 305:63, 1981.
350. Guidelines for preventing opportunistic infections among hematopoietic stem cell transplant recipients. *MMWR Recomm Rep* 49:1, 2000.
351. Locksley RM, Flournoy N, Sullivan KM, et al: Infection with varicella-zoster virus after marrow transplantation. *J Infect Dis* 152:1172, 1985.
352. Ljungman P, Lonnqvist B, Gahrton G, et al: Clinical and subclinical reactivations of varicella-zoster virus in immunocompromised patients. *J Infect Dis* 153:840, 1986.
353. Schuchter LM, Wingard JR, Piantadosi S, et al: Herpes zoster infection after autologous marrow transplantation. *Blood* 74:1424, 1989.
354. Arvin AM: Varicella-zoster virus. *Clin Microbiol Rev* 9:361, 1996.
355. Tomonari A, Iseki T, Takahashi S, et al: Varicella-zoster virus infection in adult patients after unrelated cord blood transplantation: A single institute experience in Japan. *Br J Haematol* 122:802, 2003.
356. Balfour HH Jr, Bean B, Laskin OL, et al: Acyclovir halts progression of herpes zoster in immunocompromised patients. *N Engl J Med* 308:1448, 1983.
357. Balfour HH Jr, Benson C, Braun J, et al: Management of acyclovir-resistant herpes simplex and varicella-zoster virus infections. *J Acquir Immune Defic Syndr* 7:254, 1994.
358. Lietman PS: Clinical pharmacology: Foscarnet. *Am J Med* 92:8S, 1992.
359. Weinstock DM, Boeckh M, Sepkowitz KA: Postexposure prophylaxis against varicella zoster virus infection among hematopoietic stem cell transplant recipients. *Biol Blood Marrow Transplant* 12:1096, 2006.
360. Boeckh M, Kim HW, Flowers ME, et al: Long-term acyclovir for prevention of varicella zoster virus disease after allogeneic hematopoietic cell transplantation—A randomized double-blind placebo-controlled study. *Blood* 107:1800, 2006.
361. Kanda Y, Mineishi S, Saito T, et al: Long-term low-dose acyclovir against varicella-zoster virus reactivation after allogeneic hematopoietic stem cell transplantation. *Bone Marrow Transplant* 28:689, 2001.
362. Thomson KJ, Hart DP, Banerjee L, et al: The effect of low-dose acyclovir on reactivation of varicella zoster virus after allogeneic haemopoietic stem cell transplantation. *Bone Marrow Transplant* 35:1065, 2005.
363. Hata A, Asanuma H, Rinki M, et al: Use of an inactivated varicella vaccine in recipients of hematopoietic-cell transplants. *N Engl J Med* 347:26, 2002.
364. Parkman R: Antigen-specific immunity following hematopoietic stem cell transplantation. *Blood Cells Mol Dis* 40:91, 2008.
365. Parkman R, Cohen G, Carter SL, et al: Successful immune reconstitution decreases leukemic relapse and improves survival in recipients of unrelated cord blood transplantation. *Biol Blood Marrow Transplant* 12:919, 2006.
366. Crooks GM, Weinberg K, Mackall C: Immune reconstitution: From stem cells to lymphocytes. *Biol Blood Marrow Transplant* 12:42, 2006.
367. O'Reilly RJ, Keever CA, Small TN, et al: The use of HLA-non-identical T-cell-depleted marrow transplants for correction of severe combined immunodeficiency disease. *Immunodefic Rev* 1:273, 1989.
368. Douek DC, McFarland RD, Keiser PH, et al: Changes in thymic function with age and during the treatment of HIV infection. *Nature* 396:690, 1998.
369. Hazenberg MD, Otto SA, de Pauw ES, et al: T-cell receptor excision circle and T-cell dynamics after allogeneic stem cell transplantation are related to clinical events. *Blood* 99:3449, 2002.
370. Witherspoon RP, Storb R, Ochs HD, et al: Recovery of antibody production in human allogeneic marrow graft recipients: Influence of time posttransplantation, the

presence or absence of chronic graft-versus-host disease, and antithymocyte globulin treatment. *Blood* 58:360, 1981.
371. Abrahamsen IW, Somme S, Heldal D, et al: Immune reconstitution after allogeneic stem cell transplantation: The impact of stem cell source and graft-versus-host disease. *Haematologica* 90:86, 2005.
372. Min D, Taylor PA, Panoskaltsis-Mortari A, et al: Protection from thymic epithelial cell injury by keratinocyte growth factor: A new approach to improve thymic and peripheral T-cell reconstitution after marrow transplantation. *Blood* 99:4592, 2002.
373. Alpdogan O, Schmaltz C, Muriglan SJ, et al: Administration of interleukin-7 after allogeneic marrow transplantation improves immune reconstitution without aggravating graft-versus-host disease. *Blood* 98:2256, 2001.
374. Billingham R: The biology of graft-versus-host disease. *Harvey Lect* 62:21, 1966–1967.
375. Grebe SC, Streilein JW: Graft-versus-host reactions: A review. *Adv Immunol* 22:119, 1976.
376. Ferrara JL, Levine JE, Reddy P, et al: Graft-versus-host disease. *Lancet* 373:1550, 2009.
377. den Haan JM, Sherman NE, Blokland E, et al: Identification of a graft versus host disease-associated human minor histocompatibility antigen. *Science* 268:1476, 1995.
378. Miklos DB, Kim HT, Zorn E, et al: Antibody response to DBY minor histocompatibility antigen is induced after allogeneic stem cell transplantation and in healthy female donors. *Blood* 103:353, 2004.
379. Behar E, Chao NJ, Hiraki DD, et al: Polymorphism of adhesion molecule CD31 and its role in acute graft-versus-host disease. *N Engl J Med* 334:286, 1996.
380. Kernan NA, Bartsch G, Ash RC, et al: Analysis of 462 transplantations from unrelated donors facilitated by the National Marrow Donor Program. *N Engl J Med* 328:593, 1993.
381. Nash RA, Pepe MS, Storb R, et al: Acute graft-versus-host disease: Analysis of risk factors after allogeneic marrow transplantation and prophylaxis with cyclosporine and methotrexate. *Blood* 80:1838, 1992.
382. Weisdorf D, Hakke R, Blazar B, et al: Risk factors for acute graft-versus-host disease in histocompatible donor marrow transplantation. *Transplantation* 51:1197, 1991.
383. Przepiorka D, Smith TL, Folloder J, et al: Risk factors for acute graft-versus-host disease after allogeneic blood stem cell transplantation. *Blood* 94:1465, 1999.
384. Baron F, Maris MB, Storer BE, et al: High doses of transplanted CD34+ cells are associated with rapid T-cell engraftment and lessened risk of graft rejection, but not more graft-versus-host disease after nonmyeloablative conditioning and unrelated hematopoietic cell transplantation. *Leukemia* 19:822, 2005.
385. Przepiorka D, Weisdorf D, Martin P, et al: 1994 Consensus conference on acute GVHD grading. *Bone Marrow Transplant* 15:825, 1995.
386. Cahn JY, Klein JP, Lee SJ, et al: Prospective evaluation of 2 acute graft-versus-host (GVHD) grading systems: A joint Societe Francaise de Greffe de Moelle et Therapie Cellulaire (SFGM-TC), Dana Farber Cancer Institute (DFCI), and International Marrow Transplant Registry (IBMTR) prospective study. *Blood* 106:1495, 2005.
387. Rowlings PA, Przepiorka D, Klein JP, et al: IBMTR Severity Index for grading acute graft-versus-host disease: Retrospective comparison with Glucksberg grade. *Br J Haematol* 97:855, 1997.
388. Bacigalupo A: Management of acute graft-versus-host disease. *Br J Haematol* 137:87, 2007.
389. Reddy P, Ferrara JL: Immunobiology of acute graft-versus-host disease. *Blood Rev* 17:187, 2003.
390. Anderson BE, McNiff J, Yan J, et al: Memory CD4+ T cells do not induce graft-versus-host disease. *J Clin Invest* 112:101, 2003.
391. Chen BJ, Cui X, Sempowski GD, et al: Transfer of allogeneic CD62L$^-$ memory T cells without graft-versus-host disease. *Blood* 103:1534, 2004.
392. Edinger M, Hoffmann P, Ermann J, et al: CD4+CD25+ regulatory T cells preserve graft-versus-tumor activity while inhibiting graft-versus-host disease after marrow transplantation. *Nat Med* 9:1144, 2003.
393. Storb R, Deeg HJ, Farewell V, et al: Marrow transplantation for severe aplastic anemia: Methotrexate alone compared with a combination of methotrexate and cyclosporine for prevention of acute graft-versus-host disease. *Blood* 68:119, 1986.
394. Storb R, Deeg HJ, Whitehead J, et al: Methotrexate and cyclosporine compared with cyclosporine alone for prophylaxis of acute graft versus host disease after marrow transplantation for leukemia. *N Engl J Med* 314:729, 1986.
395. Nash RA, Pineiro LA, Storb R, et al: FK506 in combination with methotrexate for the prevention of graft-versus-host disease after marrow transplantation from matched unrelated donors. *Blood* 88:3634, 1996.
396. Ratanatharathorn V, Nash RA, Przepiorka D, et al: Phase III study comparing methotrexate and tacrolimus (Prograf, FK506) with methotrexate and cyclosporine for graft-versus-host disease prophylaxis after HLA-identical sibling marrow transplantation. *Blood* 92:2303, 1998.
397. Chao NJ, Schmidt GM, Niland JC, et al: Cyclosporine, methotrexate, and prednisone compared with cyclosporine and prednisone for prophylaxis of acute graft-versus-host disease. *N Engl J Med* 329:1225, 1993.
398. Filipovich AH, Vallera DA, Youle RJ, et al: *Ex-vivo* treatment of donor marrow with anti-T-cell immunotoxins for prevention of graft-versus-host disease. *Lancet* 1:469, 1984.
399. Papadopoulos EB, Carabasi MH, Castro-Malaspina H, et al: T-cell-depleted allogeneic marrow transplantation as postremission therapy for acute myelogenous leukemia: Freedom from relapse in the absence of graft-versus-host disease. *Blood* 91:1083, 1998.
400. Jakubowski AA, Small TN, Young JW, et al: T cell depleted stem-cell transplantation for adults with hematologic malignancies: Sustained engraftment of HLA-matched related donor grafts without the use of antithymocyte globulin. *Blood* 110:4552, 2007.
401. Wagner JE, Thompson JS, Carter SL, et al: Effect of graft-versus-host disease prophylaxis on 3-year disease-free survival in recipients of unrelated donor marrow (T-cell Depletion Trial): A multi-centre, randomised phase II-III trial. *Lancet* 366:733, 2005.
402. Deeg HJ: How I treat refractory acute GVHD. *Blood* 109:4119, 2007.
403. Alousi A, Weisdorf D, Logan B, et al: A Phase II randomized trial evaluating etanercept, mycophenolate mofetil, denileukin diftitox, and pentostatin in combination with corticosteroids in 180 patients with newly diagnosed acute GVHD. *Blood* 112:55a, 2008.
404. Le Blanc K, Rasmusson I, Sundberg B, et al: Treatment of severe acute graft-versus-host disease with third party haploidentical mesenchymal stem cells. *Lancet* 363:1439, 2004.
405. Ringden O, Uzunel M, Rasmusson I, et al: Mesenchymal stem cells for treatment of therapy-resistant graft-versus-host disease. *Transplantation* 81:1390, 2006.
406. Lee SJ, Vogelsang G, Flowers ME: Chronic graft-versus-host disease. *Biol Blood Marrow Transplant* 9:215, 2003.
407. Shulman HM, Sullivan KM, Weiden PL, et al: Chronic graft-versus-host syndrome in man. A long-term clinicopathologic study of 20 Seattle patients. *Am J Med* 69:204, 1980.
408. Lee SJ, Klein JP, Barrett AJ, et al: Severity of chronic graft-versus-host disease: Association with treatment-related mortality and relapse. *Blood* 100:406, 2002.
409. Akpek G, Lee SJ, Flowers ME, et al: Performance of a new clinical grading system for chronic graft-versus-host disease: A multicenter study. *Blood* 102:802, 2003.
410. Filipovich AH, Weisdorf D, Pavletic S, et al: National Institutes of Health consensus development project on criteria for clinical trials in chronic graft-versus-host disease: I: Diagnosis and staging working group report. *Biol Blood Marrow Transplant* 11:945, 2005.
411. Sakaguchi S, Sakaguchi N: Thymus and autoimmunity. Transplantation of the thymus from cyclosporin A-treated mice causes organ-specific autoimmune disease in athymic nude mice. *J Exp Med* 167:1479, 1988.
412. Kansu E, Gooley T, Flowers ME, et al: Administration of cyclosporine for 24 months compared with 6 months for prevention of chronic graft-versus-host disease: A prospective randomized clinical trial. *Blood* 98:3868, 2001.
413. Sullivan KM, Witherspoon RP, Storb R, et al: Alternating-day cyclosporine and prednisone for treatment of high-risk chronic graft-v-host disease. *Blood* 72:555, 1988.
414. Furlong T, Leisenring W, Storb R, et al: Psoralen and ultraviolet A irradiation (PUVA) as therapy for steroid-resistant cutaneous acute graft-versus-host disease. *Biol Blood Marrow Transplant* 8:206, 2002.
415. Couriel DR, Saliba R, Escalon MP, et al: Sirolimus in combination with tacrolimus and corticosteroids for the treatment of resistant chronic graft-versus-host disease. *Br J Haematol* 130:409, 2005.
416. Baroni SS, Santillo M, Bevilacqua F, et al: Stimulatory autoantibodies to the PDGF receptor in systemic sclerosis. *N Engl J Med* 354:2667, 2006.
417. Olivieri A, Locatelli F, Zecca M, et al: Imatinib for refractory chronic graft-versus-host-disease with fibrotic features. *Blood* 114:709, 2009.
418. Miklos DB, Kim HT, Miller KH, et al: Antibody responses to H-Y minor histocompatibility antigens correlate with chronic graft-versus-host disease and disease remission. *Blood* 105:2973, 2005.
419. Pichert G, Roy DC, Gonin R, et al: Distinct patterns of minimal residual disease associated with graft-versus-host disease after allogeneic marrow transplantation for chronic myelogenous leukemia. *J Clin Oncol* 13:1704, 1995.
420. Radich JP, Gehly G, Gooley T, et al: Polymerase chain reaction detection of the BCR-ABL fusion transcript after allogeneic marrow transplantation for chronic myeloid leukemia: Results and implications in 346 patients. *Blood* 85:2632, 1995.
421. Radich JP, Gooley T, Bryant E, et al: The significance of bcr-abl molecular detection in chronic myeloid leukemia patients "late," 18 months or more after transplantation. *Blood* 98:1701, 2001.
422. Mundt AJ, Sibley G, Williams S, et al: Patterns of failure following high-dose chemotherapy and autologous marrow transplantation with involved field radiotherapy for relapsed/refractory Hodgkin's disease. *Int J Radiat Oncol Biol Phys* 33:261, 1995.
423. Pezner RD, Nademanee A, Forman SJ: High-dose therapy and autologous marrow transplantation for Hodgkin's disease patients with relapses potentially treatable by radical radiation therapy. *Int J Radiat Oncol Biol Phys* 33:189, 1995.
424. Bolanos-Meade J, Garrett-Mayer E, Luznik L, et al: Induction of autologous graft-versus-host disease: Results of a randomized prospective clinical trial in patients with poor risk lymphoma. *Biol Blood Marrow Transplant* 13:1185, 2007.
425. Davis TA, Hsu FJ, Caspar CB, et al: Idiotype vaccination following ABMT can stimulate specific anti-idiotype immune responses in patients with B-cell lymphoma. *Biol Blood Marrow Transplant* 7:517, 2001.
426. Bartlett N, Forero-torres A, Rosenblatt J, et al: Complete remissions with weekly dosing of SGN-35, a novel antibody-drug conjugate (ADC) targeting CD30, in a phase I dose-escalation study in patients with relapsed or refractory Hodgkin lymphoma or systemic anaplastic large cell lymphoma. *J Clin Oncol* 27:8500a, 2009.
427. Tsai T, Goodman S, Saez R, et al: Allogeneic marrow transplantation in patients who relapse after autologous transplantation. *Bone Marrow Transplant* 20:859, 1997.
428. Radich JP, Gooley T, Sanders JE, et al: Second allogeneic transplantation after failure of first autologous transplantation. *Biol Blood Marrow Transplant* 6:272, 2000.
429. Hale GA, Tong X, Benaim E, et al: Allogeneic marrow transplantation in children failing prior autologous marrow transplantation. *Bone Marrow Transplant* 27:155, 2001.
430. Porter DL, Collins RH Jr, Shpilberg O, et al: Long-term follow-up of patients who achieved complete remission after donor leukocyte infusions. *Biol Blood Marrow Transplant* 5:253, 1999.

431. Savani BN, Montero A, Kurlander R, et al: Imatinib synergizes with donor lymphocyte infusions to achieve rapid molecular remission of CML relapsing after allogeneic stem cell transplantation. *Bone Marrow Transplant* 36:1009, 2005.
432. Mielcarek M, Storer BE, Flowers ME, et al: Outcomes among patients with recurrent high-risk hematologic malignancies after allogeneic hematopoietic cell transplantation. *Biol Blood Marrow Transplant* 13:1160, 2007.
433. Porter DL, Levine BL, Bunin N, et al: A phase 1 trial of donor lymphocyte infusions expanded and activated *ex vivo* via CD3/CD28 costimulation. *Blood* 107:1325, 2006.
434. Schmidt-Wolf IG, Negrin RS, Kiem HP, et al: Use of a SCID mouse/human lymphoma model to evaluate cytokine-induced killer cells with potent antitumor cell activity. *J Exp Med* 174:139, 1991.
435. Groh V, Rhinehart R, Randolph-Habecker J, et al: Costimulation of CD8alphabeta T cells by NKG2D via engagement by MIC induced on virus-infected cells. *Nat Immunol* 2:255, 2001.
436. Linn YC, Lau LC, Hui KM: Generation of cytokine-induced killer cells from leukaemic samples with *in vitro* cytotoxicity against autologous and allogeneic leukaemic blasts. *Br J Haematol* 116:78, 2002.

CHAPTER 22
TREATMENT OF INFECTIONS IN THE IMMUNOCOMPROMISED HOST

Steven Beutler and Lisa Beutler

SUMMARY

Infection is a major cause of morbidity and mortality in patients with severe inherited or acquired neutropenia or aplastic anemia, qualitative disorders of neutrophils, and, notably, those persons receiving chemotherapy for treatment of hematologic neoplasms. Severe neutropenia and monocytopenia often result from the combined effects of replacement of marrow with malignant cells and superimposed intense chemotherapy. The severity and duration of the neutropenia determine the risk of infection. Bacterial infections may result in rapid clinical deterioration and, if not treated appropriately, death. Fungal, viral, and parasitic infections also may result in potentially lethal complications during or after chemotherapy. Methods of diagnosis of bacterial, fungal, viral, and protozoal infection are considered and treatment regimens described. The use of home antibiotic may be appropriate for certain patients. Because prevention of infection during periods of neutropenia should reduce morbidity and improve outcome, attention is focused on prophylaxis therapy against bacterial, parasitic, viral, and/or fungal infections.

The risk of infection exists in many persons with hematologic diseases, including patients with severe inherited or acquired neutropenia or aplastic anemia, qualitative disorders of neutrophils, and those persons receiving intensive, marrow-suppressive chemotherapy. The profound pancytopenia that results from cytoreductive chemotherapy is a common manifestation of hematopoietic suppression. During the periods of neutropenia that follow such chemotherapy, infection develops in most patients. Patients with neoplasms of the lymphoid system commonly manifest altered humoral and cellular immunity, resulting in an increased incidence of nonbacterial infection.

RISK FACTORS AND INFECTING ORGANISMS

SEVERITY OF NEUTROPENIA

Bacterial, fungal, viral, and parasitic organisms may cause infection in neutropenic patients. Bacterial infections are the most frequent and usually the most serious. The risk for bacterial infection increases when the neutrophil count falls to less than 500/μL (0.5×10^9/L) and becomes especially pronounced at neutrophil counts less than 100/μL (0.1×10^9/L).[1] The rate of decline and duration of neutropenia are important in determining the risk of bacterial infection. Disruption of mucosal barriers, especially in the oral cavity, esophagus, and bowel, further favors the development of infection by providing portals of entry.

> Acronyms and abbreviations that appear in this chapter include: CMV, cytomegalovirus; MRSA, methicillin-resistant *Staphylococcus aureus*; RSV, respiratory syncytial virus.

BACTERIAL PATHOGENS

Historically, Gram-negative bacilli have been the most commonly isolated pathogens. These organisms include *Klebsiella, Escherichia coli, Pseudomonas,* and *Proteus*. These bacteria are responsible for a variety of infections, including pneumonia, soft-tissue infections, perirectal infections, and primary bacteremia. Urinary tract infections are less frequent unless a urinary catheter is present or urinary tract obstruction has developed. Meningitis is uncommon.

At present, roughly half of all documented infections in neutropenic patients are caused by Gram-positive pathogens. Staphylococcal species and enterococcus are now the pathogens most frequently isolated from neutropenic patients.[2] This finding may result, in part, from the popularity of semipermanent venous catheters and from the use of prophylactic regimens that are active against Gram-negative rods. Several reports document the increasing frequency of *Streptococcus viridans* as a major pathogen in neutropenic patients,[3] especially in those receiving a marrow transplant, perhaps because these patients have a higher incidence of mucositis. Septic shock may occur in these patients.[4] Anaerobic infections are less common unless periodontal or gastrointestinal pathology coexists.

Patients with Hodgkin lymphoma, other lymphomas, or chronic lymphocytic leukemia primarily suffer from impaired cell-mediated immunity and diminished antibody production.[5] Consequently, the spectrum of infections in these patients differs from that found in neutropenic patients. Bacterial infections, when they occur, tend to result from encapsulated organisms such as *Pneumococcus* or *Haemophilus*. *Listeria* and *Nocardia* infections also are seen more frequently in this group of patients.

FUNGAL PATHOGENS

Fungal infections are common during periods of prolonged neutropenia and in patients with lymphomas or chronic lymphocytic leukemia. *Candida* species are most frequently isolated. Historically, *Candida albicans* has been the most common isolate; however, in recent years the number of non-*albicans Candida* infections has increased, partly as a consequence of widespread prophylaxis activity against *C. albicans*.[6] The gastrointestinal tract serves as a reservoir for *Candida*, and erosive esophagitis may develop. *Candida* may enter the bloodstream via indwelling catheters.

Aspergillus and *Phycomycetes* also may cause invasive disease. These organisms tend to colonize and infect the sinuses and bronchopulmonary tree.

Because cell-mediated immunity is required for defense against fungal infections, infections with *Cryptococcus, Aspergillus, Coccidioides, Histoplasma*, and *Candida* are more common in patients with leukemia or lymphoma who require chronic glucocorticoid treatment.

VIRAL PATHOGENS

Viral infections are especially frequent in patients with impaired cell-mediated immunity. Among viruses that cause infections in immunocompromised hosts, herpes simplex, varicella zoster, cytomegalovirus (CMV), and adenoviruses are the most important. Cutaneous lesions and mucositis often are caused by herpes simplex. Herpes zoster infections may be especially severe and have a propensity for dissemination. Left untreated, primary varicella infections are associated with a high mortality rate. CMV may cause febrile illnesses associated with pneumonia, hepatitis, and/or gastrointestinal tract ulcerations. Respiratory infections resulting from respiratory syncytial virus (RSV) have been documented in approximately 18 percent of marrow transplant recipients with pulmonary symptoms during the winter months.[7] Influenza virus, picornavirus, and other viruses have been isolated from such patients.

PROTOZOAL PATHOGENS

Pneumocystis jiroveci, formerly called *Pneumocystis carinii*, is a ubiquitous, endogenous parasite that may cause pneumonia in neutropenic patients and in those with defective cell-mediated immunity. It often becomes clinically evident after glucocorticoids have been tapered or discontinued. *Toxoplasma gondii*, another protozoan parasite, may be responsible for brain abscesses in patients with lymphoma or chronic lymphocytic leukemia, especially in those treated with glucocorticoids. Glucocorticoid-treated patients from endemic areas also are at risk for *Strongyloides* hyperinfection.

MYCOBACTERIAL INFECTIONS

The association between lymphoid malignancies and tuberculosis, particularly among patients born outside the United States, has been recognized for more than a century. It threatens to become a more frequent, serious problem with the resurgence of tuberculosis and the increased prevalence of drug-resistant strains.[8,9] Atypical mycobacterial infections are very common in HIV-positive patients but are rare in patients receiving chemotherapy.

RECOGNITION AND DIAGNOSIS OF INFECTION

The development of an infection in a neutropenic patient may be accompanied by dramatic clinical manifestations or by none at all. Any fever that develops is very suggestive of infection. However, hypothermia, declining mental status, myalgia, or lethargy also may indicate infection in these patients. The usual local signs of infection, such as pus formation, may be absent or delayed because they are mediated by neutrophils.[10]

A careful physical examination should be performed when such a change in condition is observed. Special attention should be paid to the mouth and teeth for evidence of thrush or periodontal disease. The skin should be examined in detail. Innocuous-appearing skin lesions may be septic emboli. Ordinarily trivial injuries inflicted by venipuncture or intravenous catheters may become infected and result in septicemia. An increased incidence of perianal and perirectal infection is observed in neutropenic patients.[11] Examination of the rectum may provide a clue to the source of fever in patients without other clinical findings. Although such examinations should not be performed unnecessarily on an immunocompromised patient, rectal or pelvic examination should not be deferred when searching for a cause of fever.

Chest radiographic films should be obtained initially and may need to be repeated, although this practice has been questioned in patients without respiratory complaints.[12] Chest computed tomography may reveal lesions not detected on routine radiograms.[13] Sinus radiographic films may be helpful if relevant symptoms are present.

Blood cultures should be collected prior to institution of antibiotic therapy, and periodically thereafter if fever persists. If an indwelling venous catheter is present, some of the cultures should be obtained from the catheter. The common practice of separating blood cultures by 10 to 15 minutes does not seem to have any physiologic or experimental basis. However, obtaining two to three cultures improves the likelihood of recovering fastidious organisms. To improve the likelihood of isolating fungal pathogens, the specimens should be retained by the laboratory for at least 10 days. Urine and sputum cultures may be helpful. Results of the latter, however, must be interpreted with caution, because the results may reflect the flora colonizing the oropharynx rather than the pathogens infecting the lung. Skin lesions of a suspicious nature should be biopsied and cultured. Stools should be examined for *Clostridium difficile* toxin in patients with diarrhea. Potentially infected intravenous lines should be cultured upon removal. Nasal cultures may be useful in predicting pulmonary aspergillosis.[14] Fungal and viral infections, which may be difficult to document using conventional culture techniques, may be diagnosed by polymerase chain reaction and antigen detection.[15,16]

Open-lung biopsies once were advocated for further evaluation of neutropenic patients with pulmonary infiltrates.[17] However, this procedure should not be routinely performed in immunocompromised patients with pneumonia because the result rarely establishes a treatable diagnosis. The procedure may be useful under certain limited circumstances, for example, when further empiric therapy would be unacceptably toxic in a patient whose clinical condition is deteriorating.

Transbronchial lung biopsies are generally considered unsafe in patients with thrombocytopenia because of the high risk of uncontrolled bleeding. Obtaining material via bronchial brushing or lavage carries a lower risk and may yield useful information.[18]

TREATMENT AND PREVENTION

INITIAL TREATMENT

Bacterial Infections

Many different regimens have been evaluated and found to be acceptable for empiric therapy in patients with febrile neutropenia. Generally, combination therapy has been favored for initial empiric therapy, but single-drug therapy also may be efficacious in patients with less profound neutropenia, those who are not overtly septic, and those who may have problems tolerating aminoglycosides. Use of single-drug therapy cannot be recommended for all patients with stem cell failure and severe neutropenia and monocytopenia who appear to be infected.

Imipenem,[19] meropenem,[20] cefepime,[21,22] and ceftazidime[23] have each been studied as a single agent. These drugs are active against most of the virulent pathogens infecting neutropenic patients. Two newer carbapenems, doripenem and ertapenem, remain to be studied as single agents for empiric therapy in neutropenic patients.[24] Differences in institutional sensitivity patterns should guide initial antibiotic selection, and subsequent modification of therapy can optimize treatment.

Development of resistant organisms during single-drug therapy is of concern. Aminoglycosides may provide synergy against Gram-negative bacilli and further broaden the spectrum of antimicrobial activity, but they increase the risk of nephrotoxicity. No good evidence supports the simultaneous use of two β-lactam drugs. Quinolones, usually in conjunction with another antibiotic, are effective in patients who have not received quinolone prophylaxis.[25]

Not all patients require empiric therapy for Gram-positive pathogens. Patients with catheters, patients presenting with sepsis, and other high-risk patients should be treated empirically for Gram-positive infections. Among patients without these risk factors, Gram-positive coverage should be added if fever persists for more than 3 to 5 days after Gram-negative treatment is initiated.[2]

The emergence of multidrug-resistant organisms will, over the next several years, influence the approach to empiric therapy. Approximately 60 percent of the hospital-acquired strains of *Staphylococcus aureus* now are methicillin-resistant *S. aureus* (MRSA), as are a growing number of community-acquired strains.[26] Vancomycin, Synercid (quinupristin/dalfopristin),[27] linezolid,[28] daptomycin,[29] and tigecycline[30] are active against MRSA. Ceftobiprole is a soon-to-be-approved, broad-spectrum cephalosporin that is also active against MRSA.[31] In addition, there are a number of drugs currently in clinical trials that have activity against MRSA. Among the most promising are iclaprim,[32] a dihydrofolate reductase inhibitor, and dalbavancin,[33] a second-generation glycopeptide that can be administered once per week. The emergence of vancomycin-resistant *S. aureus* strains may limit the use of vancomycin in the treatment of *S. aureus* infections in the future.[34] Linezolid causes thrombocytopenia and therefore must be used with caution in patients who are receiving chemotherapy. Treatment with linezolid has also been tied to peripheral neuropathy and serotonin syndrome.[35]

Vancomycin-resistant enterococcus is being isolated with increasing frequency and presents a major challenge, particularly among neutropenic patients.[36] Cefepime and ceftazidime lack activity against enterococcus. Synercid (quinupristin/dalfopristin),[27] linezolid,[37] daptomycin,[38] and tigecycline[39] are the only agents currently available for treatment of this pathogen. The latter two have not received FDA approval for this indication.

Drug resistance among Gram-negative pathogens is also of great clinical concern in neutropenic patients. Enteric pathogens, particularly *Klebsiella*, which produce extended-spectrum β lactamases, increasingly have become a clinical problem.[40] These organisms are resistant to all cephalosporins and exhibit varying and unpredictable degrees of sensitivity to aminoglycosides and quinolones. The carbapenems (imipenem, meropenem, doripenem, ertapenem) are active against these pathogens. Carbapenemase-producing organisms, currently relatively rare, may become an important clinical problem in the future. Treatment options for infections caused by these organisms may be limited to aminoglycosides, colistin, and possibly tigecycline.[41]

Studies on empiric antibiotic treatment published before 2005 may have limited validity in today's environment. Furthermore, there are limited data regarding the efficacy and spectrum of adverse effects of many newer agents in the neutropenic patient population.

Fungal Infections

Systemic fungal infections are relatively common in neutropenic patients, and empiric antifungal therapy should be considered in febrile patients if empiric antibiotic therapy is not effective within 3 to 5 days.[42] Amphotericin B deoxycholate has been the drug of choice for the majority of fungal infections that develop in neutropenic hosts, although its position has been challenged by the introduction of newer azole drugs and echinocandins. The dose of amphotericin should be advanced rapidly so that the full therapeutic dose is given by the first or second day. Serum creatinine, potassium, and magnesium levels should be monitored.[43] Fever and chills associated with administration of this drug may be treated or prevented with meperidine or diphenhydramine hydrochloride and acetaminophen. This will not be necessary in all patients, and systemic reactions tend to decrease after several doses. Twenty-five to 50 mg of hydrocortisone added to the infusion may attenuate the reactions.[44] Infusions have traditionally been given over 4 to 6 hours; however, some data show that prolonged infusion over 24 hours reduces both infusion complications and nephrotoxicity associated with the drug without affecting the efficacy of the drug.[45,46]

There are three lipid-associated formulations of amphotericin currently available in the United States. AmBisome (liposomal amphotericin B); Abelcet (amphotericin B lipid complex); and Amphotec/Amphocil (amphotericin B colloidal dispersion). These three agents are not interchangeable. These formulations, particularly AmBisome, are less nephrotoxic, and appear to be at least as efficacious as nonlipid formulations. Infusion-related symptoms are not consistently less common with these preparations, but are generally manageable.[47,48] These data come from studies in which the nonlipid formulation was administered over 4 hours. It will be important to determine whether nephrotoxicity of the newer preparations is lower than that of nonlipid preparations infused over 24 hours.[49] Lipid preparations of amphotericin B are significantly more expensive than amphotericin B deoxycholate. However, the cost of managing renal complications is also significant, so AmBisome, Abelcet, or Amphotec may actually be cost-effective in many cases.[50]

Fluconazole, an azole drug that can be administered orally or intravenously, is approved for treatment of *C. albicans, Candida neoformans*, and *Coccidioides immitis*. It is less active against non-*albicans Candida* species and is completely inactive against *Candida krusei*. It also lacks activity against *Aspergillus*.[51] It can be used to treat patients with sensitive strains of fungus who cannot tolerate or do not respond to amphotericin B.

Voriconazole is a newer azole drug, which is also available in intravenous and oral formulations. A large study concluded that voriconazole is as effective as liposomal amphotericin B as empiric therapy for febrile neutropenia, but these results are controversial.[52,53] Oral voriconazole may be a good alternative to the intravenous formulation in neutropenic patients with uncomplicated persistent fever.[54] It is one of the drugs used as first-line therapy against *Aspergillus*.[38] The intravenous preparation may result in the acute development of visual loss, which is generally temporary and reversible. This may be related to high blood levels of the drug.[55]

Posaconazole is the newest approved azole. It can only be administered orally and is predominantly used prophylactically; however, it has shown promise as salvage therapy for invasive aspergillosis.[56]

The echinocandins, which include caspofungin, micafungin, and anidulafungin, are a class of drugs that has activity against a wide variety of *Candida* species as well as *Aspergillus*. They are generally well tolerated, and may become especially important as the prevalence of non-*albicans Candida* infections rises.[57] Currently, only caspofungin is approved for first-line empirical use in febrile neutropenia.[58] Caspofungin is also the only echinocandin approved as salvage therapy for aspergillosis; however, mounting evidences suggests that micafungin is also effective in the treatment of invasive *Aspergillus* infections.[59] The echinocandins may have synergy with other antifungal agents against *Aspergillus* species, but randomized, prospective clinical trials evaluating echinocandins as a part of combination therapy in *Aspergillus* treatment have yet to be performed.[60] Anidulafungin, the newest approved echinocandin, has shown excellent efficacy in the treatment of candidiasis[61]; its clinical efficacy in the treatment of aspergillosis remains to be tested.

Although currently not as large a problem as drug-resistant bacteria, the development of drug-resistant fungal organisms is a potential clinical threat. Prophylactic use of antifungals likely contributes breakthrough infection with uncommon antifungal-resistant species.[62] Cross-resistance within and between classes of antifungals is also another potentially important problem, which is deserving of clinical study.[63]

Viral Infections

A limited number of options are available for treatment of viral infections. Acyclovir is active against herpes simplex and, at higher doses, against varicella zoster. It is not useful against CMV or Epstein-Barr virus. Other agents, such as famciclovir and valacyclovir, are as effective in treating herpes simplex infections, and may be administered less frequently, but are not available for intravenous administration.[64]

Ganciclovir, valganciclovir, and foscarnet have efficacy in treatment of CMV disease and are also active against herpes simplex.[65] They are most effective when they are used early in the course of the infection. Hence, frequent screening for antigenemia and early treatment in high-risk patients, such as transplant recipients, may allow for improved outcomes.[66] Both agents have been used successfully in conjunction with CMV immunoglobulin for treatment of CMV pneumonia in marrow transplant patients.[67] Ganciclovir results in neutropenia in a significant percentage of patients who receive it. Foscarnet therapy may be complicated by azotemia and electrolyte abnormalities.

Ribavirin can be used to treat RSV. Oseltamivir and zanamivir can be used if influenza A is suspected. However, the use of these agents in neutropenic patients with hematologic malignancies has not been evaluated.

Protozoal Infections

P. jiroveci may be treated with trimethoprim-sulfamethoxazole. Pentamidine should be used in patients who are allergic to or otherwise intolerant of trimethoprim-sulfamethoxazole.[68] Other regimens, including dapsone-trimethoprim, primaquine-clindamycin, and atovaquone, have proved efficacious in patients with AIDS but are largely untested in patients with chemotherapy-related immunosuppression.

Mycobacterial Infections

Rates of *Mycobacterium tuberculosis* infection are high among patients with hematologic malignancy worldwide, and should be ruled out in neutropenic patients with lung infiltrates who have entered the United States from underdeveloped countries. First-line therapy for tuberculosis includes rifampin, isoniazid, pyrazinamide, and ethambutol. Combination therapy is recommended.[69]

Infections with multidrug-resistant tuberculosis are difficult to treat and are associated with poor prognoses. The prevalence of multidrug-resistant tuberculosis varies tremendously by country, ranging from nearly 0 percent to more than 25 percent.[70] Drugs used to treat multidrug-resistant tuberculosis include fluoroquinolones, amikacin, capreomycin, and kanamycin. Extensively drug-resistant *M. tuberculosis*, which is defined as being resistant to fluoroquinolones and at least one injectable second-line agent, is a potentially huge clinical problem.[71]

Table 22–1 lists the drugs used as empiric therapy in neutropenic patients.

■ ADJUSTING THERAPY

Adjustment or modification of the initial antimicrobial regimen may be necessary for several reasons. Results of cultures may suggest another regimen would be more active or less toxic. All cultures may remain negative while the patient fails to respond to the regimen. Fever may recur following an initial response to therapy, raising the possibility of a superinfection.

Adjusting therapy based on a culture report usually is straightforward, but the other two situations may pose dilemmas. In these circumstances, resistant organisms or noninfectious causes of fever must be considered. Repeat cultures and careful clinical reappraisal may prove helpful. Empiric modification of the antibiotic regimen to enhance the effect on Gram-positive or fungal pathogens may be successful. Vancomycin is active against Gram-positive organisms. Antifungal therapy should be strongly considered if a combination of antibacterial agents proves ineffective after 5 to 7 days of treatment.[2] A brief therapeutic trial of a nonsteroidal antiinflammatory agent may eliminate fever caused by tumor or tumor lysis. Adrenal insufficiency should also be ruled out.

■ DURATION OF THERAPY

Antibiotics usually should be discontinued when the neutropenia resolves or clinical evidence of infection is no longer present. Often, however, the fever resolves, while neutropenia is expected to continue for a prolonged period. Antibiotic therapy is commonly continued until the granulocyte count reaches 500/μL (0.5×10^9/L). Although this therapy reduces the number of relapsing infections, it likely increases the risk of superinfection and antibiotic toxicity. Marrow recovery may be delayed by cephalosporins and sulfa drugs. Therefore, discontinuing antibiotics after an appropriate course in patients who have responded promptly and completely to therapy is reasonable.[72,73] If antibiotics are discontinued, close observation is required, and therapy should be reinstituted at any suggestion of recurrent infection.

The duration of antifungal therapy varies considerably. Infection with *Pneumocystis* requires 2 to 3 weeks of therapy. Herpetic infections generally are treated for 7 days.

■ FEVER FOLLOWING RECOVERY FROM CHEMOTHERAPY

Fevers occasionally persist after the granulocyte count has returned to normal levels. Drug fever is a consideration in this setting, but more commonly a deep-seated infection is present.[74] Hepatosplenic candidiasis[75] and indwelling catheter infections must be considered in these patients. Elevated serum alkaline phosphatase levels and a characteristic image on computed tomography are common with hepatic involvement.[76] Hepatic ultrasonography[77] and magnetic resonance imaging[78] are diagnostically useful, but biopsy may be required to establish the diagnosis. Hepatosplenic candidiasis requires prolonged therapy. Several regimens have been proposed, including fluconazole,[79] caspofungin,[80] and liposomal amphotericin B.[81] Cure is difficult to achieve regardless of the regimen used. In one study, roughly 20 percent of patients diagnosed with hepatosplenic candidiasis died as a result of the infection by 10 months postdiagnosis.[82]

Indwelling catheter infection should be considered when fevers continue after marrow recovery. Diagnosing catheter infections remains a major challenge, and the use of catheter-sparing diagnostic techniques should be considered, as the need to remove catheters is patient and organism dependent. Coagulase-negative *Staphylococcus* spp. are most commonly isolated. Minor exit site infections generally respond promptly to antibiotic therapy. Infection of indwelling catheters with *Staphylococcus epidermidis* and other pathogens often can be cured with 5 to 7 days of vancomycin. If the catheter is to be retained, a 10- to 14-day course of antibiotics is recommended.[83]

If a tunnel infection is present, successful therapy is less likely. Gram-negative infections[84] or fungal infections[85] of the catheter usually necessitate its removal. This may be followed, if necessary, by insertion of a new catheter at a different site. Catheters impregnated with antibiotics may resist infection but have not been widely studied in neutropenic patients.[86] Chlorhexidine and silver-impregnated central venous catheters do not appear to prevent bloodstream infections in neutropenic patients.[87] Chlorhexidine-gluconate impregnated sponges have not been studied in neutropenic patients specifically, but may be effective at preventing minor cutaneous infections.[88] Use of antibiotic-coated catheters may lead to false-negative culture results. Catheter infections and their management are reviewed elsewhere.[89]

■ OUTPATIENT THERAPY

Ten years ago, treatment of the febrile neutropenic patient outside of the hospital would have been unthinkable. Economic pressures, coupled with the widespread availability of home infusion services and more potent oral antibiotics, have made outpatient therapy an option for some of these patients.[90] The future availability of long acting antibiotics such as dalbavancin (see "Initital Treatment" above) will provide additional alternatives for outpatient treatment of certain infections.[91]

Outcomes among patients with neutropenic fever treated as outpatients seem to be comparable to those observed in hospitalized patients, provided the patients are selected properly and appropriate monitoring can be ensured. Suitable candidates for home therapy include patients who are expected to have a short-duration of neutropenia and who have few comorbidities.[92] Individuals who remain febrile, who require multiple antibiotics, or who are unreliable are not candidates for home

TABLE 22–1. Maximum Recommended Doses of Antibiotics

Drug Category	Drug	Brand Name	Dose	Adjustment for Renal Insufficiency	Activity	Toxicity
Antipseudomonal penicillins	Piperacillin-tazobactam	Zosyn	4.5 g q6h	+	Methicillin-sensitive *Staphylococcus, Streptococcus,* anaerobes, *Pseudomonas aeruginosa*	Hypokalemia, antiplatelet effect
Antipseudomonal cephalosporins	Ceftazidime	Fortaz	2 g q8h	+++	*Pseudomonas aeruginosa,* enteric Gram-negative rods, methicillin-sensitive *staphylococcus*	
	Cefepime	Maxipime	2 g q8–12h			
Aminoglycosides	Amikacin	Amikin	15 mg/kg per day*	+++	Enteric Gram-negative rods, *Pseudomonas aeruginosa*	Nephrotoxicity, ototoxicity
	Tobramycin	Nebcin	4–5 mg/kg per day*			
	Gentamicin	Garamycin	4–5 mg/kg per day*			
Glycopeptide	Vancomycin	Vancocin	30 mg/kg per day in 2 doses*	+++	*Staphylococcus* (including MRSA), *Streptococcus, Corynebacterium*	Ototoxicity, red-man syndrome with rapid infusion
	Dalbavancin	Zeven	1 g × 1, then 500 mg weekly	+(?)		
Carbapenem	Imipenem	Primaxin	0.5–1 g q6h	++ to +++	Gram-negative rods, *Pseudomonas aeruginosa (except for ertapenem)*, methicillin sensitive, *Staphylococcus,* enterococcus, anaerobes	Nausea, seizures (Primaxin)
	Meropenem	Merrem	1 g q8h	++		
	Ertapenem	Invanz	1 g q24h	++		
	Doripenem	Doribax	0.5 g q8h	++		
Monobactam	Aztreonam	Azactam	2 g q6h	+	Gram-negative rods, *Pseudomonas aeruginosa*	
Sulfonamides	Trimethoprim-sulfamethoxazole	Bactrim; Septra	10–20 mg/kg per day (based on trimethoprim) in 2–4 doses/day	++	*Pneumocystis carinii,* Gram-negative rods, *Haemophilus, Staphylococcus*	Sulfa allergy, increased creatinine, nausea, rash
Fluoroquinolones	Ciprofloxacin	Cipro	500–750 mg q12h PO or 200–400 mg IV q12h	+	Gram-negative rods, *Pseudomonas aeruginosa*	Nausea; not for use in children
	Levofloxacin	Levaquin	750 mg PO or IV q24h	+++	Gram-negative rods	Nausea; not for use in children
Nucleosides	Acyclovir	Zovirax	15 mg/kg per day IV (30 mg/kg per day IV for encephalitis or for herpes zoster) in 3 divided doses; comparable oral dose approximately twice as high	+ to ++	Herpes simplex and zoster	Crystalluria
	Valacyclovir	Valtrex	1000 mg BID (TID in herpes zoster) PO	++	Herpes simplex and zoster	
	Famciclovir	Famvir	250–500 mg TID PO	+++	CMV, herpes simplex	
	Ganciclovir	Cytovene	10 mg/kg per day in 2 divided doses IV or 1000 mg PO TID	++		Neutropenia
Phosphonoformate	Foscarnet	Foscavir	180 mg/kg per day in 3 doses	++	CMV	Renal failure, electrolyte abnormalities
Polyene antifungals	Amphotericin B	Fungizone	0.7–1.0 mg/kg per day in a single daily dose over 2–6 h	0	*Candida, Aspergillus, Torulopsis,* other fungus	Nausea, vomiting, chills, fever, renal failure hypokalemia, hypomagnesemia
	Ampho B lipid complex	Abelcet	5 mg/kg per day		*Candida, Aspergillus, Torulopsis,* other fungus	Fever, chills, nausea, vomiting, increased creatinine

(*continued*)

TABLE 22–1. Maximum Recommended Doses of Antibiotics (Continued)

Drug Category	Drug	Brand Name	Dose	Adjustment for Renal Insufficiency	Activity	Toxicity
Polyene antifungals (continued)	Ampho B cholesteryl sulfate complex	Amphocil/ Amphotec	4–6 mg/kg per day		*Candida, Aspergillus, Torulopsis,* other fungus	Fever, chills, nausea, vomiting, increased creatinine
	Ampho B liposomal ampho	AmBisome	5 mg/kg per day		*Candida, Aspergillus, Torulopsis,* other fungus	Fever, chills, nausea, vomiting, increased creatinine
Azole	Fluconazole	Diflucan	400 mg/day PO/IV	++	*Candida albicans, Cryptococcus, Coccidioides immitis,* histoplasmosis	LFT abnormality
	Voriconazole	Vfend	300 mg bid IV or PO			Loss of vision with IV prep
	Posaconazole	Noxafil	200 mg PO TID or 400 mg PO BID	0		Nausea, diarrhea, LFT abnormality
Echinocandin	Caspofungin	Cancidas	70 mg × 1, then 50 mg qd	0	Aspergillus, candida	
	Micafungin	Mycamine	100–150 mg IV qd	0		
	Anidulafungin	Eraxis	200 mg IV × 1, then 100 mg q24h	0		
Diamidine	Pentamidine	Pentam	4 mg/kg q24h IV	++(*)	*Pneumocystis carinii*	Renal failure, hypotension, hypoglycemia
Oxazolidinone	Linezolid	Zyvox	600 mg q12h PO or IV	0	MRSA, VRE	Thrombocytopenia, anemia
Lipopeptide	Daptomycin	Cubicin	4–6 mg/kg q24h IV	++	MRSA	

BID, twice per day; CMV, cytomegalovirus; ESBL, extended-spectrum β-lactamase; IV, intravenous; LFT, liver function tests; MRSA, methicillin-resistant *Staphylococcus aureus*; TID, three times per day; VRE, vancomycin-resistant *enterococcus*; (?), insufficient information; (*), should consider discontinuing if kidney function deteriorates.

*Adjust dose based on levels.

NOTE: 0, no adjust ment required; +, small adjustment for creatinine clearance <20; ++, moderate adjustment required; +++, nearly complete renal excretion; dose to be reduced proportionately to renal function.

therapy. Nurses should be experienced in the evaluation of chemotherapy patients and familiar with catheter care and maintenance. Rigorous family education is crucial for a successful outcome.

PREVENTION OF INFECTIONS

Bacterial Infections

In view of the high mortality rate associated with infections in neutropenic patients, preventive measures remain a priority. Careful attention to sterile technique and personal hygiene is of the utmost importance in the prevention of bacterial infection during neutropenia. Instrumentation should be avoided whenever possible. Intravenous access sites should be carefully maintained. In addition, systemic antibiotics are currently widely used as prophylaxis against Gram-negative infections in neutropenic patients. This practice reduces the incidence of bacterial infections, and may be associated with a decrease in all-cause mortality.[93]

The use of prophylactic antibiotics reduces the number of Gram-negative infections in high-risk patients who are expected to have prolonged, severe neutropenia. By contrast, the use of antibiotic prophylaxis in lower-risk patients is of much less certain benefit, and may not be necessary in most cases.[94] Several studies have shown a reduction in mortality in high-risk patients given prophylactic antibiotics, but the contribution of this practice to the emergence of drug-resistant pathogens must be taken into account when deciding whether to employ it.[93,95] Furthermore, although the agents employed for this purpose are generally safe, the risk of drug toxicity must also be taken into consideration. Adverse events associated with antibiotic prophylaxis include drug fever, rash, cytopenias, and infection with *C. difficile*.[96] The latter deserves strong consideration, as drug-resistant, hypervirulent strains of this organism have become more prevalent over the last several years.[97] The incidence of *C. difficile* is extraordinarily high in cancer patients on a broad variety of antibiotics, including fluoroquinolones and cephalosporins.[98]

Trimethoprim-sulfamethoxazole has been well studied and is beneficial for some patients. The therapy has the additional advantage of preventing *Pneumocystis*, which is significant in institutions with a high prevalence of this organism.[99] Trimethoprim-sulfamethoxazole also has activity against Gram-positive organisms,[100] but does not have activity against *Pseudomonas aeruginosa*. It causes a rash in 5 to 10 percent of individuals, its use may be associated with infections with resistant organisms, and it may result in delayed marrow recovery.[101]

The fluorinated quinolones, particularly ciprofloxacin and levofloxacin, have received considerable attention for their ability to prevent Gram-negative infections in neutropenic patients.[100] Ciprofloxacin has more activity against *Pseudomonas*, whereas levofloxacin is more active against Gram-positive organisms. Unfortunately, indiscriminate use of these agents in the community, as well as prophylactic use, has led to a greatly increased prevalence of quinolone-resistant Gram-negative organisms. Up to 80 percent of *E. coli* isolates from patients with febrile neutropenia are resistant to quinolones,[102] and quinolone prophylaxis has resulted in an increased incidence of bacteremia with quinolone-resistant *S. viridans*.[103] Prophylactic use also eliminates these agents from therapeutic use in the same patient.[104] For these reasons, some centers abandoned the use of prophylactic quinolones in some patients.[105,106] In at least one case, however, institutional cessation of quinolone prophylaxis resulted in an increased incidence of bacteremia caused by Gram-negative organisms, which was reversed by reinstitution of fluoroquinolone prophylaxis.[107] In summary, there is, at present, a clear role for quinolone prophylaxis in some patients. However, because of increasing resistance to these drugs, it is important to continuously monitor their efficacy and discourage their indiscriminate use.

Isoniazid hydrazide therapy is recommended for all tuberculin-positive patients who require chemotherapy unless they have been treated previously.

The ability of granulocyte-macrophage colony-stimulating factor and granulocyte colony-stimulating factor to raise the granulocyte count in neutropenic patients may reduce the risk bacterial infections in this group of patients. However, there is no evidence that prophylaxis with these agents reduces infection-related mortality.[108] Although a subset of patients may benefit from this therapy,[109] definitive methods for selecting such patients are lacking.

Low bacteria diets are often recommended to patients expected to experience neutropenia, but their effectiveness at preventing infection has not been shown.[110] Similarly the efficacy of reverse isolation, though often employed as a prophylactic measure, has not been demonstrated.[111]

Parasitic Infections

P. jiroveci pneumonia can be prevented with trimethoprim-sulfamethoxazole.[112] Pentamidine administered intravenously or monthly in aerosolized form may be effective in patients who cannot tolerate trimethoprim-sulfamethoxazole.[113,114] Dapsone and atovaquone have each been used as a second-line prophylactic agent in hematopoietic stem cell transplant recipients.[115,116] Although *P. jiroveci* is a ubiquitous organism, institutional variability in the incidence of infection is observed; therefore, the need for prophylaxis varies.

Viral Infections

Acyclovir and its prodrug valacyclovir are effective at preventing recurrent herpes simplex infections in patients receiving chemotherapy.[117] Such prophylaxis probably is unnecessary in patients who lack antibodies to herpes simplex virus. Long-term treatment with acyclovir also prevents reactivation of varicella zoster virus in hematopoietic stem cell transplant recipients,[118] as well as in patients undergoing chemotherapy for multiple myeloma.[119] Varicella zoster immunoglobulin given to previously seronegative individuals may in some cases reduce the incidence of varicella following exposure.[120]

Hematopoietic stem cell transplant recipients have a high risk of CMV infection. Patients at particular risk include those who are seropositive before transplantation, seronegative patients who receive transplants from seropositive donors, and those who receive highly immunosuppressive conditioning regimens prior to transplantation.[121,122] The use of CMV seronegative blood components can markedly decrease the transmission of CMV by transfusion; white blood cell reduction also seems to be of value.[123] Treatment with ganciclovir[124] and its prodrug valganciclovir[125] has been used to prevent CMV infection in transplant recipients. Oral valacyclovir is an equally effective alternative.[126] These drugs can cause myelosuppression, which may be of concern in neutropenic patients.[127] In addition, the emergence of ganciclovir- and valganciclovir-resistant CMV has been reported in association with preventive treatment.[128] Foscarnet may be equally effective at preventing CMV infection in transplantation patients and has less hematotoxicity.[129] Similar results have been reported among solid-organ transplant recipients.[130] CMV prophylaxis among patients receiving conventional chemotherapy has not been as widely studied, but currently there is no evidence supporting its use in this population.[131] Prophylactic immunotherapy has potential benefit but is not currently in widespread use.[132]

Active immunizations with killed vaccines such as influenza are of some benefit. Attenuated vaccines, such as measles and zoster,[133] should be avoided.

Fungal Infections

The high mortality rate of invasive fungal infections in neutropenic patients makes their prevention extremely important. Antifungal prophylaxis in these patients has been studied for more than two decades, yet there is still a great deal of controversy surrounding its efficacy.[134] Studies on prevention of fungal infections in neutropenic patients are difficult to evaluate. Results of the various studies have been conflicting, partly because different definitions and outcomes were applied, different doses of antifungal agents were administered, and the numbers of study patients have often been small.

As with antibacterial prophylaxis, the clearest benefit of antifungal prophylaxis is seen in patients expected to have severe, prolonged neutropenia, particularly allogeneic transplant recipients. Antifungal prophylaxis is not indicated in patients who are undergoing chemotherapy with low levels of myelotoxicity.[135] When deciding whether to treat prophylactically, drug toxicity must be taken into account. In addition, prophylactic use of antifungal agents may select for more resistant strains of fungus and lead to breakthrough infection with organisms inherently resistant to the agent used for prophylaxis. For example, certain prophylactic regimens active against *Candida* may actually increase the incidence of *Aspergillus* infections.[136] Antifungal prophylaxis does appear to diminish the incidence of mucositis; however, close observation and early treatment of mucositis also provide a reasonable approach to this problem.[135] The ability of antifungal agents to prevent systemic infection in high-risk patients has been shown in several studies, but their ability to reduce all-cause mortality has not been established.[137]

Several azole drugs have been studied as prophylactic agents. A number of studies document a statistically significant reduction in superficial and invasive fungal infections when fluconazole is used prophylactically.[138,139] However, breakthrough infection with *Aspergillus*, *Torulopsis glabrata*, and *C. krusei* have occurred with fluconazole prophylaxis.[140] Itraconazole[141] and voriconazole[142] have a broader spectrum of activity, are more effective at preventing *Aspergillus* infection, and are generally well tolerated. Prophylaxis with posaconazole is associated with a lower risk of *Aspergillus* infection, and a trend toward lower mortality; however, incidence of serious side effects with this drug may be higher than with the other azoles.[143]

Echinocandins have become popular antifungal prophylactic agents. Caspofungin has been shown to be as effective as itraconazole in preventing *Aspergillus* and *Candida* infections, and is similarly well tolerated.[144] Micafungin was shown to be superior to fluconazole at preventing systemic fungal infections in hematopoietic stem cell transplant recipients, although the two agents were equally effective at preventing *Candida* infections.[145] Anidulafungin, the newest echinocandin, remains to be studied as a prophylactic agent.

Low-dose amphotericin B is as effective as fluconazole at preventing invasive candidiasis, but its use is limited because it is not as well tolerated as the other antifungals.[146] Aerosolized amphotericin B shows promise as an agent to prevent invasive pulmonary aspergillosis among neutropenic patients.[147]

Although prophylaxis with a variety of agents appears to reduce the incidence of invasive fungal infections, close monitoring with aggressive treatment at the earliest signs of fungal infection may be as effective. Microbiologic, molecular, and radiologic monitoring for early signs of fungal infection are being evaluated as alternatives to routine prophylactic treatment with antifungal agents.[148] Measurement of the fungal cell wall components 1,3-β-D-glucan[149] and galactomannan[150] in the blood has shown promise as an fungal infection surveillance technique. Real-time polymerase chain reaction of fungal gene products is another technique that appears to have high sensitivity and specificity for detecting candidemia, though it will require standardization before widespread use is possible.[151]

INFECTIONS IN HEMATOPOIETIC STEM CELL TRANSPLANTATION RECIPIENTS

Patients receiving hematopoietic stem cell transplants are at risk for the same infections occurring in patients rendered neutropenic by chemotherapy. Graft-versus-host disease and the immunosuppressive agents used to treat it result in a particularly high incidence of infection in this group of patients. Viral infections, especially CMV and varicella zoster virus, are especially troublesome. Infection in such patients has been reviewed[152,153] and is discussed in Chap. 21.

REFERENCES

1. Bodey GP, Buckley M, Sathe YS, Freireich EJ: Quantitative relationships between circulating leukocytes and infection in patients with acute leukemia. *Ann Intern Med* 64:328, 1966.
2. Bal AM, Gould IM: Empirical antimicrobial treatment for chemotherapy-induced febrile neutropenia. *Int J Antimicrob Agents* 29:501, 2007.
3. Reilly AF, Lange BJ: Infections with viridans group streptococci in children with cancer. *Pediatr Blood Cancer* 49:774, 2007.
4. Martino R, Manteiga R, Sanchez I, et al: Viridans streptococcal shock syndrome during bone marrow transplantation. *Acta Haematol* 94:69, 1995.
5. Wadhwa PD, Morrison VA: Infectious complications of chronic lymphocytic leukemia. *Semin Oncol* 33:240, 2006.
6. Hachem R, Hanna H, Kontoyiannis D, et al: The changing epidemiology of invasive candidiasis: *Candida glabrata* and *Candida krusei* as the leading causes of candidemia in hematologic malignancy. *Cancer* 112:2493, 2008.
7. Whimbey E, Champlin RE, Couch RB, et al: Community respiratory virus infections among hospitalized adult bone marrow transplant recipients. *Clin Infect Dis* 22:778, 1996.
8. Kamboj M, Sepkowitz KA: The risk of tuberculosis in patients with cancer. *Clin Infect Dis* 42:1592, 2006.
9. De La Rosa GR, Jacobson KL, Rolston KV, et al: Mycobacterium tuberculosis at a comprehensive cancer centre: Active disease in patients with underlying malignancy during 1990–2000.*Clin Microbiol Infect* 10:749, 2004.
10. Sickles EA, Greene WH, Wiernik PH: Clinical presentation of infection in granulocytopenic patients. *Arch Intern Med* 135:715, 1975.
11. Cohen JS, Paz IB, O'Donnell MR, Ellenhorn JD: Treatment of perianal infection following bone marrow transplantation. *Dis Colon Rectum* 39:981, 1996.
12. Korones DN, Hussong MR, Gullace MA: Routine chest radiography of children with cancer hospitalized for fever and neutropenia: Is it really necessary? *Cancer* 80:1160, 1997.
13. Heussel CP, Kauczor HU, Heussel G, et al: Early detection of pneumonia in febrile neutropenic patients: Use of thin-section CT. *AJR Am J Roentgenol* 169:1347, 1997.
14. Aisner J, Murillo J, Schimpff SC, Steere AC: Invasive aspergillosis in acute leukemia: Correlation with nose cultures and antibiotic use. *Ann Intern Med* 90:4, 1979.
15. Maschmeyer G, Beinert T, Buchheidt D, et al: Diagnosis and antimicrobial therapy of lung infiltrates in febrile neutropenic patients: Guidelines of the infectious diseases working party of the German Society of Haematology and Oncology. *Eur J Cancer* 45:2462, 2009.
16. Cuenca-Estrella M, Meije Y, Diaz-Pedroche C, et al: Value of serial quantification of fungal DNA by a real-time PCR-based technique for early diagnosis of invasive Aspergillosis in patients with febrile neutropenia. *J Clin Microbiol* 47:379, 2009.
17. Toledo-Pereyra LH, DeMeester TR, Kinealey A, et al: The benefits of open lung biopsy in patients with previous non-diagnostic transbronchial lung biopsy. A guide to appropriate therapy. *Chest* 77:647, 1980.
18. Pagano L, Pagliari G, Basso A, et al: The role of bronchoalveolar lavage in the microbiological diagnosis of pneumonia in patients with haematological malignancies. *Ann Med* 29:535, 1997.
19. Klastersky JA: Use of imipenem as empirical treatment of febrile neutropenia. *Int J Antimicrob Agents* 21:393, 2003.
20. Feld R, DePauw B, Berman S, et al: Meropenem versus ceftazidime in the treatment of cancer patients with febrile neutropenia: A randomized, double-blind trial. *J Clin Oncol* 18:3690, 2000.
21. Raad II, Escalante C, Hachem RY, et al: Treatment of febrile neutropenic patients with cancer who require hospitalization: A prospective randomized study comparing imipenem and cefepime. *Cancer* 98:1039, 2003.
22. Yamamura D, Gucalp R, Carlisle P, et al: Open randomized study of cefepime versus piperacillin-gentamicin for treatment of febrile neutropenic cancer patients. *Antimicrob Agents Chemother* 41:1704, 1997.
23. Egerer G, Goldschmidt H, Salwender H, et al: Efficacy of continuous infusion of ceftazidime for patients with neutropenic fever after high-dose chemotherapy and peripheral blood stem cell transplantation. *Int J Antimicrob Agents* 15:119, 2000.
24. Zhanel GG, Wiebe R, Dilay L, et al: Comparative review of the carbapenems. *Drugs* 67:1027, 2007.
25. Bliziotis IA, Michalopoulos A, Kasiakou SK, et al: Ciprofloxacin vs an aminoglycoside in combination with a beta-lactam for the treatment of febrile neutropenia: A meta-analysis of randomized controlled trials. *Mayo Clin Proc* 80:1146, 2005.
26. Klein E, Smith DL, Laxminarayan R: Hospitalizations and deaths caused by methicillin-resistant *Staphylococcus aureus*, United States, 1999–2005. *Emerg Infect Dis* 13:1840, 2007.
27. Klastersky J: Role of quinupristin/dalfopristin in the treatment of Gram-positive nosocomial infections in haematological or oncological patients. *Cancer Treat Rev* 29:431, 2003.
28. Falagas ME, Siempos II, Vardakas KZ: Linezolid versus glycopeptide or beta-lactam for treatment of Gram-positive bacterial infections: Meta-analysis of randomised controlled trials. *Lancet Infect Dis* 8:53, 2008.
29. Bamberger DM: Bacteremia and endocarditis due to methicillin-resistant Staphylococcus aureus: The potential role of daptomycin. *Ther Clin Risk Manag* 3:675, 2007.
30. Florescu I, Beuran M, Dimov R, et al: Efficacy and safety of tigecycline compared with vancomycin or linezolid for treatment of serious infections with methicillin-resistant *Staphylococcus aureus* or vancomycin-resistant enterococci: A Phase 3, multicentre, double-blind, randomized study. *J Antimicrob Chemother* 62 Suppl 1:i17, 2008.
31. Stein RA, Goetz RM, Ganea GM: Ceftobiprole: A new beta-lactam antibiotic. *Int J Clin Pract* 63:930, 2009.
32. Sader HS, Fritsche TR, Jones RN: Potency and bactericidal activity of iclaprim against recent clinical Gram-positive isolates. *Antimicrob Agents Chemother* 53:2171, 2009.
33. Pope SD, Roecker AM: Dalbavancin: A novel lipoglycopeptide antibacterial. *Pharmacotherapy* 26:908, 2006.
34. Appelbaum PC: Reduced glycopeptide susceptibility in methicillin-resistant *Staphylococcus aureus* (MRSA). *Int J Antimicrob Agents* 30:398, 2007.
35. Beekmann SE, Gilbert DN, Polgreen PM, IDSA Emerging Infections Network: Toxicity of extended courses of linezolid: Results of an Infectious Diseases Society of America Emerging Infections Network survey. *Diagn Microbiol Infect Dis* 62:407, 2008.
36. DiazGranados CA, Jernigan JA: Impact of vancomycin resistance on mortality among patients with neutropenia and enterococcal bloodstream infection. *J Infect Dis* 191:588, 2005.
37. Smith PF, Birmingham MC, Noskin GA, et al: Safety, efficacy and pharmacokinetics of linezolid for treatment of resistant Gram-positive infections in cancer patients with neutropenia. *Ann Oncol* 14:795, 2003.
38. Rolston KV: Review: Daptomycin for the treatment of gram-positive infections in neutropenic cancer patients. *Clin Adv Hematol Oncol* 6:815, 2008.
39. Garrison MW, Nuemiller JJ: *In vitro* activity of tigecycline against quinolone-resistant *Streptococcus pneumoniae*, methicillin-resistant *Staphylococcus aureus* and vancomycin-resistant enterococci. *Int J Antimicrob Agents* 29:191, 2007.
40. Nicasio AM, Kuti JL, Nicolau DP: The current state of multidrug-resistant Gram-negative bacilli in North America. *Pharmacotherapy* 28:235, 2008.
41. Nordmann P, Cuzon G, Naas T: The real threat of *Klebsiella pneumoniae* carbapenemase-producing bacteria. *Lancet Infect Dis* 9:228, 2009.
42. Schiel X, Link H, Maschmeyer G, et al: A prospective, randomized multicenter trial of the empirical addition of antifungal therapy for febrile neutropenic cancer patients: Results of the Paul Ehrlich Society for Chemotherapy (PEG) Multicenter Trial II. *Infection* 34:118, 2006.
43. Rapp RP: Changing strategies for the management of invasive fungal infections. *Pharmacotherapy* 24:4S, 2004.
44. Oto OA, Paydas S, Disel U, et al: Amphotericin B deoxycholate (d-AMB) use in cases with febrile neutropenia and fungal infections: Lower toxicity with suitable premedication. *Mycoses* 50:135, 2007.
45. Peleg AY, Woods ML: Continuous and 4 h infusion of amphotericin B: A comparative study involving high-risk haematology patients. *J Antimicrob Chemother* 54:803, 2004.
46. Slavin MA, Szer J, Grigg AP, et al: Guidelines for the use of antifungal agents in the treatment of invasive *Candida* and mould infections. *Intern Med J* 34:192, 2004.
47. Subira M, Martino R, Gomez L, et al: Low-dose amphotericin B lipid complex vs. conventional amphotericin B for empirical antifungal therapy of neutropenic fever in patients with hematologic malignancies—A randomized, controlled trial. *Eur J Haematol* 72:342, 2004.

48. Ostrosky-Zeichner L, Marr KA, Rex JH, Cohen SH: Amphotericin B: Time for a new "gold standard." *Clin Infect Dis* 37:415, 2003.
49. Schneemann M, Bachli EB: Continuous infusion of amphotericin B deoxycholate: A cost-effective gold standard for therapy of invasive fungal infections? *Clin Infect Dis* 38:303, 2004.
50. Kleinberg M: What is the current and future status of conventional amphotericin B? *Int J Antimicrob Agents* 27 Suppl 1:12, 2006.
51. Cuenca-Estrella M, Arendrup MC, Chryssanthou E, et al: Multicentre determination of quality control strains and quality control ranges for antifungal susceptibility testing of yeasts and filamentous fungi using the methods of the Antifungal Susceptibility Testing Subcommittee of the European Committee on Antimicrobial Susceptibility Testing (AFST-EUCAST). *Clin Microbiol Infect* 13:1018, 2007.
52. Walsh TJ, Pappas P, Winston DJ, et al: Voriconazole compared with liposomal amphotericin B for empirical antifungal therapy in patients with neutropenia and persistent fever. *N Engl J Med* 346:225, 2002.
53. Marr KA: Empirical antifungal therapy—New options, new tradeoffs. *N Engl J Med* 346:278, 2002.
54. Przepiorka D, Buadi FK, McClune B: Oral voriconazole for empiric antifungal treatment in patients with uncomplicated febrile neutropenia. *Pharmacotherapy* 28:58, 2008.
55. Pascual A, Calandra T, Bolay S, et al: Voriconazole therapeutic drug monitoring in patients with invasive mycoses improves efficacy and safety outcomes. *Clin Infect Dis* 46:201, 2008.
56. Raad II, Hanna HA, Boktour M, et al: Novel antifungal agents as salvage therapy for invasive aspergillosis in patients with hematologic malignancies: Posaconazole compared with high-dose lipid formulations of amphotericin B alone or in combination with caspofungin. *Leukemia* 22:496, 2008.
57. Cappelletty D, Eiselstein-McKitrick K: The echinocandins. *Pharmacotherapy* 27:369, 2007.
58. Eschenauer G, Depestel DD, Carver PL: Comparison of echinocandin antifungals. *Ther Clin Risk Manag* 3:71, 2007.
59. Chandrasekar PH, Sobel JD: Micafungin: A new echinocandin. *Clin Infect Dis* 42:1171, 2006.
60. Dennis CG, Greco WR, Brun Y, et al: Effect of amphotericin B and micafungin combination on survival, histopathology, and fungal burden in experimental aspergillosis in the p47phox–/– mouse model of chronic granulomatous disease. *Antimicrob Agents Chemother* 50:422, 2006.
61. Reboli AC, Rotstein C, Pappas PG, et al: Anidulafungin versus fluconazole for invasive candidiasis. *N Engl J Med* 356:2472, 2007.
62. Lionakis MS, Lewis RE, Torres HA, et al: Increased frequency of non-fumigatus Aspergillus species in amphotericin B- or triazole-pre-exposed cancer patients with positive cultures for aspergilli. *Diagn Microbiol Infect Dis* 52:15, 2005.
63. Rodriguez-Tudela JL, Alcazar-Fuoli L, Mellado E, et al: Epidemiological cutoffs and cross-resistance to azole drugs in *Aspergillus fumigatus*. *Antimicrob Agents Chemother* 52:2468, 2008.
64. Glenny AM, Fernandez Mauleffinch LM, Pavitt S, Walsh T: Interventions for the prevention and treatment of herpes simplex virus in patients being treated for cancer. *Cochrane Database Syst Rev* 1:CD006706, 2009.
65. Biron KK: Antiviral drugs for cytomegalovirus diseases. *Antiviral Res* 71:154, 2006.
66. Almyroudis NG, Jakubowski A, Jaffe D, et al: Predictors for persistent cytomegalovirus reactivation after T-cell-depleted allogeneic hematopoietic stem cell transplantation. *Transpl Infect Dis* 9:286, 2007.
67. Ljungman P: Cytomegalovirus pneumonia: Presentation, diagnosis, and treatment. *Semin Respir Infect* 10:209, 1995.
68. Shankar SM, Nania JJ: Management of Pneumocystis jiroveci pneumonia in children receiving chemotherapy. *Paediatr Drugs* 9:301, 2007.
69. Al-Anazi KA, Al-Jasser AM, Evans DA: Infections caused by mycobacterium tuberculosis in patients with hematological disorders and in recipients of hematopoietic stem cell transplant, a twelve year retrospective study. *Ann Clin Microbiol Antimicrob* 6:16, 2007.
70. Wright A, Zignol M, Van Deun A, et al: Epidemiology of antituberculosis drug resistance 2002–07: An updated analysis of the Global Project on Anti-Tuberculosis Drug Resistance Surveillance. *Lancet* 373:1861, 2009.
71. Jassal M, Bishai WR: Extensively drug-resistant tuberculosis. *Lancet Infect Dis* 9:19, 2009.
72. DiNubile MJ: Stopping antibiotic therapy in neutropenic patients. *Ann Intern Med* 108:289, 1988.
73. Cornelissen JJ, Rozenberg-Arska M, Dekker AW: Discontinuation of intravenous antibiotic therapy during persistent neutropenia in patients receiving prophylaxis with oral ciprofloxacin. *Clin Infect Dis* 21:1300, 1995.
74. Barton TD, Schuster MG: The cause of fever following resolution of neutropenia in patients with acute leukemia. *Clin Infect Dis* 22:1064, 1996.
75. Sallah S: Hepatosplenic candidiasis in patients with acute leukemia: Increasingly encountered complication. *Anticancer Res* 19:757, 1999.
76. Thaler M, Pastakia B, Shawker TH, et al: Hepatic candidiasis in cancer patients: The evolving picture of the syndrome. *Ann Intern Med* 108:88, 1988.
77. Karthaus M, Huebner G, Elser C, et al: Early detection of chronic disseminated Candida infection in leukemia patients with febrile neutropenia: Value of computer-assisted serial ultrasound documentation. *Ann Hematol* 77:41, 1998.
78. Sallah S, Semelka R, Kelekis N, et al: Diagnosis and monitoring response to treatment of hepatosplenic candidiasis in patients with acute leukemia using magnetic resonance imaging. *Acta Haematol* 100:77, 1998.
79. Torres-Valdivieso MJ, Lopez J, Melero C, et al: Hepatosplenic candidosis in an immunosuppressed patient responding to fluconazole. *Mycoses* 37:443, 1994.
80. Arda B, Soyer N, Sipahi OR, et al: Possible hepatosplenic candidiasis treated with liposomal amphotericin B and caspofungin combination. *J Infect* 52:387, 2006.
81. Walsh TJ, Whitcomb P, Piscitelli S, et al: Safety, tolerance, and pharmacokinetics of amphotericin B lipid complex in children with hepatosplenic candidiasis. *Antimicrob Agents Chemother* 41:1944, 1997.
82. Chen CY, Chen YC, Tang JL, et al: Hepatosplenic fungal infection in patients with acute leukemia in Taiwan: Incidence, treatment, and prognosis. *Ann Hematol* 82:93, 2003.
83. Raad I, Hanna H, Maki D: Intravascular catheter-related infections: Advances in diagnosis, prevention, and management. *Lancet Infect Dis* 7:645, 2007.
84. Hanna H, Afif C, Alakech B, et al: Central venous catheter-related bacteremia due to gram-negative bacilli: Significance of catheter removal in preventing relapse. *Infect Control Hosp Epidemiol* 25:646, 2004.
85. Raad I, Hanna H, Boktour M, et al: Management of central venous catheters in patients with cancer and candidemia. *Clin Infect Dis* 38:1119, 2004.
86. Chatzinikolaou I, Hanna H, Graviss L, et al: Clinical experience with minocycline and rifampin-impregnated central venous catheters in bone marrow transplantation recipients: Efficacy and low risk of developing staphylococcal resistance. *Infect Control Hosp Epidemiol* 24:961, 2003.
87. Logghe C, Van Ossel C, D'Hoore W, et al: Evaluation of chlorhexidine and silver-sulfadiazine impregnated central venous catheters for the prevention of bloodstream infection in leukaemic patients: A randomized controlled trial. *J Hosp Infect* 37:145, 1997.
88. Garland JS, Alex CP, Mueller CD, et al: A randomized trial comparing povidone-iodine to a chlorhexidine gluconate-impregnated dressing for prevention of central venous catheter infections in neonates. *Pediatrics* 107:1431, 2001.
89. Mermel LA, Allon M, Bouza E, et al: Clinical practice guidelines for the diagnosis and management of intravascular catheter-related infection: 2009 Update by the Infectious Diseases Society of America. *Clin Infect Dis* 49:1, 2009.
90. Elting LS, Lu C, Escalante CP, et al: Outcomes and cost of outpatient or inpatient management of 712 patients with febrile neutropenia. *J Clin Oncol* 26:606, 2008.
91. Billeter M, Zervos MJ, Chen AY, et al: Dalbavancin: A novel once-weekly lipoglycopeptide antibiotic. *Clin Infect Dis* 46:577, 2008.
92. Moores KG: Safe and effective outpatient treatment of adults with chemotherapy-induced neutropenic fever. *Am J Health Syst Pharm* 64:717, 2007.
93. Pascoe J, Steven N: Antibiotics for the prevention of febrile neutropenia. *Curr Opin Hematol* 16:48, 2009.
94. Freifeld A, Sepkowitz K: The conundrum of fluoroquinolone prophylaxis. *Nat Clin Pract Oncol* 3:524, 2006.
95. Hammond SP, Baden LR: Antibiotic prophylaxis for patients with acute leukemia. *Leuk Lymphoma* 49:183, 2008.
96. van Vliet MJ, Tissing WJ, Dun CA, et al: Chemotherapy treatment in pediatric patients with acute myeloid leukemia receiving antimicrobial prophylaxis leads to a relative increase of colonization with potentially pathogenic bacteria in the gut. *Clin Infect Dis* 49:262, 2009.
97. Cookson B: Hypervirulent strains of *Clostridium difficile*. *Postgrad Med J* 83:291, 2007.
98. Gerding DN: Clindamycin, cephalosporins, fluoroquinolones, and *Clostridium difficile*-associated diarrhea: This is an antimicrobial resistance problem. *Clin Infect Dis* 38:646, 2004.
99. Green H, Paul M, Vidal L, Leibovici L: Prophylaxis for Pneumocystis pneumonia (PCP) in non-HIV immunocompromised patients. *Cochrane Database Syst Rev* 3:CD005590, 2007.
100. van de Wetering MD, de Witte MA, Kremer LC, et al: Efficacy of oral prophylactic antibiotics in neutropenic afebrile oncology patients: A systematic review of randomised controlled trials. *Eur J Cancer* 41:1372, 2005.
101. Kovatch AL, Wald ER, Albo VC, et al: Oral trimethoprim/sulfamethoxazole for prevention of bacterial infection during the induction phase of cancer chemotherapy in children. *Pediatrics* 76:754, 1985.
102. Cattaneo C, Quaresmini G, Casari S, et al: Recent changes in bacterial epidemiology and the emergence of fluoroquinolone-resistant *Escherichia coli* among patients with haematological malignancies: Results of a prospective study on 823 patients at a single institution. *J Antimicrob Chemother* 61:721, 2008.
103. Prabhu RM, Piper KE, Litzow MR, et al: Emergence of quinolone resistance among viridans group streptococci isolated from the oropharynx of neutropenic peripheral blood stem cell transplant patients receiving quinolone antimicrobial prophylaxis. *Eur J Clin Microbiol Infect Dis* 24:832, 2005.
104. Baden LR: Prophylactic antimicrobial agents and the importance of fitness. *N Engl J Med* 353:1052, 2005.
105. Gomez L, Garau J, Estrada C, et al: Ciprofloxacin prophylaxis in patients with acute leukemia and granulocytopenia in an area with a high prevalence of ciprofloxacin-resistant *Escherichia coli*. *Cancer* 97:419, 2003.
106. Baum HV, Franz U, Geiss HK: Prevalence of ciprofloxacin-resistant *Escherichia coli* in hematologic-oncologic patients. *Infection* 28:278, 2000.
107. Kern WV, Klose K, Jellen-Ritter AS, et al: Fluoroquinolone resistance of Escherichia coli at a cancer center: Epidemiologic evolution and effects of discontinuing prophylactic fluoroquinolone use in neutropenic patients with leukemia. *Eur J Clin Microbiol Infect Dis* 24:111, 2005.
108. Sung L, Nathan PC, Alibhai SM, et al: Meta-analysis: Effect of prophylactic hematopoietic colony-stimulating factors on mortality and outcomes of infection. *Ann Intern Med* 147:400, 2007.

109. Repetto L, Biganzoli L, Koehne CH, et al: EORTC Cancer in the Elderly Task Force guidelines for the use of colony-stimulating factors in elderly patients with cancer. *Eur J Cancer* 39:2264, 2003.
110. Gardner A, Mattiuzzi G, Faderl S, et al: Randomized comparison of cooked and noncooked diets in patients undergoing remission induction therapy for acute myeloid leukemia. *J Clin Oncol* 26:5684, 2008.
111. Russell JA, Poon MC, Jones AR, et al: Allogeneic bone-marrow transplantation without protective isolation in adults with malignant disease. *Lancet* 339:38, 1992.
112. Green H, Paul M, Vidal L, Leibovici L: Prophylaxis of Pneumocystis pneumonia in immunocompromised non-HIV-infected patients: Systematic review and meta-analysis of randomized controlled trials. *Mayo Clin Proc* 82:1052, 2007.
113. Kim SY, Dabb AA, Glenn DJ, et al: Intravenous pentamidine is effective as second line Pneumocystis pneumonia prophylaxis in pediatric oncology patients. *Pediatr Blood Cancer* 50:779, 2008.
114. Marras TK, Sanders K, Lipton JH, et al: Aerosolized pentamidine prophylaxis for Pneumocystis carinii pneumonia after allogeneic marrow transplantation. *Transpl Infect Dis* 4:66, 2002.
115. Sangiolo D, Storer B, Nash R, et al: Toxicity and efficacy of daily dapsone as Pneumocystis jiroveci prophylaxis after hematopoietic stem cell transplantation: A case-control study. *Biol Blood Marrow Transplant* 11:521, 2005.
116. Colby C, McAfee S, Sackstein R, et al: A prospective randomized trial comparing the toxicity and safety of atovaquone with trimethoprim/sulfamethoxazole as Pneumocystis carinii pneumonia prophylaxis following autologous peripheral blood stem cell transplantation. *Bone Marrow Transplant* 24:897, 1999.
117. Warkentin DI, Epstein JB, Campbell LM, et al: Valacyclovir versus acyclovir for HSV prophylaxis in neutropenic patients. *Ann Pharmacother* 36:1525, 2002.
118. Boeckh M, Kim HW, Flowers ME, et al: Long-term acyclovir for prevention of varicella zoster virus disease after allogeneic hematopoietic cell transplantation—A randomized double-blind placebo-controlled study. *Blood* 107:1800, 2006.
119. Vickrey E, Allen S, Mehta J, Singhal S: Acyclovir to prevent reactivation of varicella zoster virus (herpes zoster) in multiple myeloma patients receiving bortezomib therapy. *Cancer* 115:229, 2009.
120. Weinstock DM, Boeckh M, Boulad F, et al: Postexposure prophylaxis against varicella-zoster virus infection among recipients of hematopoietic stem cell transplant: Unresolved issues. *Infect Control Hosp Epidemiol* 25:603, 2004.
121. Boeckh M, Nichols WG: The impact of cytomegalovirus serostatus of donor and recipient before hematopoietic stem cell transplantation in the era of antiviral prophylaxis and preemptive therapy. *Blood* 103:2003, 2004.
122. Boeckh M, Nichols WG, Papanicolaou G, et al: Cytomegalovirus in hematopoietic stem cell transplant recipients: Current status, known challenges, and future strategies. *Biol Blood Marrow Transplant* 9:543, 2003.
123. Vamvakas EC: Is white blood cell reduction equivalent to antibody screening in preventing transmission of cytomegalovirus by transfusion? A review of the literature and meta-analysis. *Transfus Med Rev* 19:181, 2005.
124. van der Heiden PL, Kalpoe JS, Barge RM, et al: Oral valganciclovir as pre-emptive therapy has similar efficacy on cytomegalovirus DNA load reduction as intravenous ganciclovir in allogeneic stem cell transplantation recipients. *Bone Marrow Transplant* 37:693, 2006.
125. Ayala E, Greene J, Sandin R, et al: Valganciclovir is safe and effective as pre-emptive therapy for CMV infection in allogeneic hematopoietic stem cell transplantation. *Bone Marrow Transplant* 37:851, 2006.
126. Winston DJ, Yeager AM, Chandrasekar PH, et al: Randomized comparison of oral valacyclovir and intravenous ganciclovir for prevention of cytomegalovirus disease after allogeneic bone marrow transplantation. *Clin Infect Dis* 36:749, 2003.
127. Ar MC, Ozbalak M, Tuzuner N, et al: Severe bone marrow failure due to valganciclovir overdose after renal transplantation from cadaveric donors: Four consecutive cases. *Transplant Proc* 41:1648, 2009.
128. Allice T, Busca A, Locatelli F, et al: Valganciclovir as pre-emptive therapy for cytomegalovirus infection post-allogenic stem cell transplantation: Implications for the emergence of drug-resistant cytomegalovirus. *J Antimicrob Chemother* 63:600, 2009.
129. Reusser P, Einsele H, Lee J, et al: Randomized multicenter trial of foscarnet versus ganciclovir for preemptive therapy of cytomegalovirus infection after allogeneic stem cell transplantation. *Blood* 99:1159, 2002.
130. Hodson EM, Craig JC, Strippoli GF, Webster AC: Antiviral medications for preventing cytomegalovirus disease in solid organ transplant recipients. *Cochrane Database Syst Rev* 2:CD003774, 2008.
131. Sandherr M, Einsele H, Hebart H, et al: Antiviral prophylaxis in patients with haematological malignancies and solid tumours: Guidelines of the Infectious Diseases Working Party (AGIHO) of the German Society for Hematology and Oncology (DGHO). *Ann Oncol* 17:1051, 2006.
132. Micklethwaite KP, Clancy L, Sandher U, et al: Prophylactic infusion of cytomegalovirus-specific cytotoxic T lymphocytes stimulated with Ad5f35pp65 gene-modified dendritic cells after allogeneic hemopoietic stem cell transplantation. *Blood* 112:3974, 2008.
133. Curtis KK, Connolly MK, Northfelt DW: Live, attenuated varicella zoster vaccination of an immunocompromised patient. *J Gen Intern Med* 23:648, 2008.
134. Glasmacher A, Prentice AG: Evidence-based review of antifungal prophylaxis in neutropenic patients with haematological malignancies. *J Antimicrob Chemother* 56 Suppl 1:i23, 2005.
135. Cornely OA, Ullmann AJ, Karthaus M: Evidence-based assessment of primary antifungal prophylaxis in patients with hematologic malignancies. *Blood* 101:3365, 2003.
136. Maschmeyer G: The changing face of febrile neutropenia-from monotherapy to moulds to mucositis. Prevention of mould infections. *J Antimicrob Chemother* 63 Suppl 1:i27, 2009.
137. Michallet M, Ito JI: Approaches to the management of invasive fungal infections in hematologic malignancy and hematopoietic cell transplantation. *J Clin Oncol* 27:3398, 2009.
138. Goodman JL, Winston DJ, Greenfield RA, et al: A controlled trial of fluconazole to prevent fungal infections in patients undergoing bone marrow transplantation. *N Engl J Med* 326:845, 1992.
139. Rotstein C, Bow EJ, Laverdiere M, et al: Randomized placebo-controlled trial of fluconazole prophylaxis for neutropenic cancer patients: Benefit based on purpose and intensity of cytotoxic therapy. The Canadian Fluconazole Prophylaxis Study Group. *Clin Infect Dis* 28:331, 1999.
140. Wingard JR, Merz WG, Rinaldi MG, et al: Increase in *Candida krusei* infection among patients with bone marrow transplantation and neutropenia treated prophylactically with fluconazole. *N Engl J Med* 325:1274, 1991.
141. Potter M: Strategies for managing systemic fungal infection and the place of itraconazole. *J Antimicrob Chemother* 56 Suppl 1:i49, 2005.
142. Vehreschild JJ, Bohme A, Buchheidt D, et al: A double-blind trial on prophylactic voriconazole (VRC) or placebo during induction chemotherapy for acute myelogenous leukaemia (AML). *J Infect* 55:445, 2007.
143. Cornely OA, Maertens J, Winston DJ, et al: Posaconazole vs. fluconazole or itraconazole prophylaxis in patients with neutropenia. *N Engl J Med* 356:348, 2007.
144. Mattiuzzi GN, Alvarado G, Giles FJ, et al: Open-label, randomized comparison of itraconazole versus caspofungin for prophylaxis in patients with hematologic malignancies. *Antimicrob Agents Chemother* 50:143, 2006.
145. van Burik JA, Ratanatharathorn V, Stepan DE, et al: Micafungin versus fluconazole for prophylaxis against invasive fungal infections during neutropenia in patients undergoing hematopoietic stem cell transplantation. *Clin Infect Dis* 39:1407, 2004.
146. Wolff SN, Fay J, Stevens D, et al: Fluconazole vs. low-dose amphotericin B for the prevention of fungal infections in patients undergoing bone marrow transplantation: A study of the North American Marrow Transplant Group. *Bone Marrow Transplant* 25:853, 2000.
147. Rijnders BJ, Cornelissen JJ, Slobbe L, et al: Aerosolized liposomal amphotericin B for the prevention of invasive pulmonary aspergillosis during prolonged neutropenia: A randomized, placebo-controlled trial. *Clin Infect Dis* 46:1401, 2008.
148. Almyroudis NG, Segal BH: Prevention and treatment of invasive fungal diseases in neutropenic patients. *Curr Opin Infect Dis* 22:385, 2009.
149. Senn L, Robinson JO, Schmidt S, et al: 1,3-Beta-D-glucan antigenemia for early diagnosis of invasive fungal infections in neutropenic patients with acute leukemia. *Clin Infect Dis* 46:878, 2008.
150. Pfeiffer CD, Fine JP, Safdar N: Diagnosis of invasive aspergillosis using a galactomannan assay: A meta-analysis. *Clin Infect Dis* 42:1417, 2006.
151. McMullan R, Metwally L, Coyle PV, et al: A prospective clinical trial of a real-time polymerase chain reaction assay for the diagnosis of candidemia in nonneutropenic, critically ill adults. *Clin Infect Dis* 46:890, 2008.
152. Aschan J: Allogeneic haematopoietic stem cell transplantation: Current status and future outlook. *Br Med Bull* 77–78:23, 2006.
153. Appelbaum FR, Forman SJ, Negrin RS, Blume KG: *Thomas' Hematopoietic Cell Transplantation*. Wiley-Blackwell, Malden, MA, 2009.

CHAPTER 23
PRINCIPLES OF ANTITHROMBOTIC THERAPY

Charles W. Francis and Mark Crowther

SUMMARY

Antithrombotic drugs are among the most commonly used in medicine and are generally separated into anticoagulants, fibrinolytic agents, and platelet inhibitors based on their primary mechanism of action. At the time of writing, warfarin is the only oral anticoagulant available in the United States, although other agents are available in Europe and Canada. Warfarin acts by inhibiting vitamin K action, has a prolonged effect, requires monitoring, and is widely used for prevention and treatment. Rivaroxaban and apixaban are novel oral inhibitors of factor Xa, whereas dabigatran is an orally available inhibitor of thrombin. Unfractionated heparin and the low-molecular-weight heparins are the most commonly used rapidly acting parenteral anticoagulants; they inhibit activated serine proteases through antithrombin. One synthetic agent in this class, fondaparinux, is specific for inhibition of factor Xa, and is effective for prevention and treatment of venous thromboembolism. Several parenteral direct thrombin inhibitors have excellent anticoagulant action and offer an alternative to heparins. Several fibrinolytic agents are available, all of which convert plasminogen to plasmin to accelerate clot lysis. Differences among them include their degree of fibrin specificity, half-life, and antigenicity. Antiplatelet agents play an important role in prevention and treatment of arterial thrombosis. Aspirin is a cyclooxgenase-1 inhibitor that is effective and widely used in the prevention of stroke and myocardial infarction. Drugs that modulate cyclic adenosine monophosphate (cAMP) levels include dipyridamole, pentoxifylline, and cilostazol, and are primarily used in treatment of peripheral vascular disease. Adenosine diphosphate (ADP) receptor blockers such as ticlopidine, clopidogrel, and prasugrel are effective in treatment of coronary and peripheral arterial disease. Examples of inhibitors of fibrinogen interaction with $\alpha_{IIb}\beta_3$ are abciximab, tirofiban, and eptifibatide. These drugs are highly effective in treatment of patients with acute coronary syndromes.

OVERVIEW

Antithrombotic agents are highly effective and are among the most commonly used drugs in medicine because thrombotic diseases are the leading cause of mortality and morbidity in Western countries. Antithrombotic agents are characterized separately as anticoagulants, antiplatelet agents, or fibrinolytic drugs, depending on their primary mechanism, although there is overlap in their activities (Table 23–1). Their greatest use is in prevention of thrombosis in patients at high risk, but they also have important applications for treating acute thrombosis. For many agents, the risk-to-benefit ratio is narrow, with the result that bleeding complications occur. Bleeding is the most common adverse effect of anticoagulation. Consequently, the clinician should carefully weigh the risks and benefits for each patient when selecting treatment. Generally, these drugs do not cause bleeding by themselves, but rather they exacerbate preexisting bleeding or predispose to bleeding from pathologic lesions that may be found in the gastrointestinal or genitourinary tracts or central nervous system. A careful review of comorbid conditions that may increase bleeding risk is important when deciding on therapy.

Acronyms and abbreviations that appear in this chapter include: ACT, activated clotting time; ADP, adenosine diphosphate; aPTT, activated partial thromboplastin time; cAMP, cyclic adenosine monophosphate; COX, cyclooxygenase; CYP, cytochrome P450; DVT, deep vein thrombosis; HIT, heparin-induced thrombocytopenia; INR, international normalized ratio; ISI, international sensitivity index; LMWH, low-molecular-weight heparin; MI, myocardial infarction; NSAID, nonsteroidal antiinflammatory drug; PE, pulmonary embolism; PG, prostaglandin; PGI_2, prostacyclin; PRP, platelet-rich plasma; PT, prothrombin time; SQ, subcutaneous; TNK, tenecteplase; t-PA, tissue-type plasminogen activator.

Anticoagulant therapy acts to decrease fibrin formation by inhibiting the formation and action of thrombin, and its most common use is in preventing systemic embolization in patients with atrial fibrillation and for secondary prevention of venous thromboembolism. Anticoagulant therapy is often monitored using coagulation testing because of marked biologic variation in effect. Antiplatelet agents act to inhibit platelet function, and their primary uses are in preventing thrombotic complications of cerebrovascular and coronary artery disease. They also have a role in treatment of acute myocardial infarction and some effect in preventing venous thrombosis. Fibrinolytic agents accelerate lysis of thrombi by increasing conversion of plasminogen to plasmin, and are primarily used in the acute management of myocardial infarction, in clearing occluded catheters and also in selected patients with stroke or venous thromboembolism. Fibrinolytic therapy is associated with a higher risk of bleeding complications than treatment with either anticoagulants or antiplatelet agents. Treatment of acute thrombosis often involves combinations of agents with multiple actions for maximum effect.

Antithrombotic therapy is an area of intense research in new drug development with many promising agents in clinical trials. These efforts are based on scientific developments in recent years that have elucidated details of the biochemistry and cell and molecular biology of the hemostatic system. Newer agents are typically targeted toward specific enzymes, whereas older drugs affect multiple sites.

VITAMIN K ANTAGONISTS

The development of vitamin K antagonists as oral anticoagulants began in the 1920s with investigation of a hemorrhagic disease in cattle, the cause of which was eventually traced to ingestion of moldy hay leading to hypoprothrombinemia.[1] A coumarin that inhibited vitamin K was purified and eventually introduced into clinical practice in the 1940s. Several coumarin derivatives with differing pharmacologic properties are now available as anticoagulants worldwide, and are collectively referred to as vitamin K antagonists, but warfarin is nearly universally used in North America. These agents are widely used to prevent or treat common thrombotic diseases and represent the most commonly used oral anticoagulant currently available.[2,3]

PHARMACOLOGY

The coumarins are competitive inhibitors of vitamin K. They inhibit γ-carboxylation reactions required for synthesis of several coagulation proteins, including factors II, VII, IX, and X, as well as proteins C and S, which are involved in inhibitory regulation of hemostasis. The synthesis of these proteins requires a posttranslational modification of several glutamic acid residues, converting them to γ-carboxylated glutamic acid, which is required for proper membrane interaction and biologic

TABLE 23–1. Types and Function of Antithrombotic Agents

Anticoagulants–decrease fibrin formation by inhibiting thrombin or thrombin formation
- Agents
  - Oral–warfarin and other vitamin K antagonists; dabigatran (direct thrombin inhibitor) and rivaroxaban (direct X_a inhibitor)
  - Parenteral–heparin, low-molecular-weight heparins, fondaparinux, direct thrombin inhibitors (argatroban, desirudin, bivalirudin)

Antiplatelet agents–inhibit platelet function
- Agents
  - Aspirin, clopidogrel, prasugrel, dipyridamole, abciximab, eptifibatide, tirofiban
  - Primary use is preventing and treating arterial thrombosis

Fibrinolytic agents–plasminogen activators that convert plasminogen to plasmin and accelerate clot lysis
- Agents
  - Streptokinase, urokinase, alteplase, reteplase, tenecteplase
  - Primary use is in treatment of acute myocardial infarction; also used in selected patients with stroke, pulmonary embolism, and deep vein thrombosis

activity (see Chap. 115).[4–7] The carboxylation reaction requires reduced vitamin K, which is converted to vitamin K epoxide in the reaction. Vitamin K epoxide subsequently undergoes reduction by an enzyme that is inhibited by warfarin.[8–10] Therefore, treatment with warfarin causes reduced γ-carboxylation, leading to synthesis of molecules with impaired activity.[11–13]

Warfarin preparations consist of a racemic mixture of S and R enantiomers in approximately equal proportion in an oral formulation with high bioavailability. Warfarin is water soluble and rapidly absorbed after oral administration, reaching a peak concentration after 60 to 90 minutes. An intravenous preparation is also available for patients who cannot take oral medications or who have malabsorption. It is tightly bound to plasma proteins with a half-life of 35 to 45 hours, with only the free, nonbound form having biologic activity.[2] Warfarin is metabolized through the cytochrome P450 system, the activity of which is influenced by environmental factors and also by genetic polymorphisms that alter the structure of common enzymes. Other vitamin K antagonists have similar activities but exhibit differences in absorption and elimination.

Because warfarin is a vitamin K antagonist, its action is influenced by the vitamin K content of the diet. Naturally occurring vitamin K is found in a variety of vegetables, and changes in diet can affect the vitamin K availability and warfarin effect.[14] This may be seen particularly in patients receiving warfarin who are on strict weight reduction diets or in those with little oral intake because of illness. Also, diarrhea can affect vitamin K availability as can administration of broad-spectrum antibiotics leading to marked warfarin sensitivity in hospitalized patients. Ingestion of vitamin K in dietary supplements or vitamins also affects sensitivity to warfarin. Liver disease can increase sensitivity to warfarin because of impaired synthesis of coagulation factors, and hyper- or hypometabolic states may also alter sensitivity. Hereditary resistance to warfarin has been described and related to specific mutations in vitamin K epoxide reductase.[15–17] Many drug interactions can influence the pharmacodynamics of warfarin by altering synthesis or clearance of vitamin K-dependent coagulation factors or interfering with warfarin metabolism, and patients should be advised to consult their physician or pharmacist about effects on anticoagulation when changing drug therapy or starting new medication (Table 23–2).[14] Other commonly used drugs affecting hemostasis such as aspirin, nonsteroidal antiinflammatory agents, heparins, and other anticoagulants can potentiate the antihemostatic effects of warfarin and can lead to bleeding.

■ ADMINISTRATION AND MONITORING

The anticoagulant effect of warfarin is the result of decreased levels of vitamin K-dependent coagulation factors, and their concentration represents a balance of synthesis and metabolism. Warfarin administration impairs synthesis, and levels of vitamin K-dependent factors fall in relation to their metabolism. This is short for factor VII, with a half-life of approximately 5 hours, but longer for factors X and IX ($t_{1/2}$ = 24 hours) and longest for factor II (prothrombin) with a half-life of approximately 72 hours. The desired anticoagulant effect results from a balanced reduction of all factors and requires several days to achieve. Imbalances in reduction of coagulation factors may occur during initiation

TABLE 23–2. Effect of Drugs on Warfarin Response

Potentiate Effect	
α-Methyldopa	Indomethacin
Acetaminophen	Isoniazid
Acetohexamide	Mefenamic acid
Allopurinol	Methimazole
Androgenic and anabolic steroids	Methotrexate
Antibiotics that disrupt intestinal flora (tetracyclines, streptomycin, erythromycin, kanamycin, nalidixic acid, neomycin)	Methylphenidate
	Nalidixic acid
	Nortriptyline
	Oxyphenbutazone
Cephaloridine	*p*-Aminosalicylic acid
Chloral hydrate	Paromomycin
Chloramphenicol	Phenylbutazone
Chlorpromazine	Phenyramidol
Chlorpropamide	Phenytoin
Cimetidine	Propylthiouracil
Clofibrate	Quinidine
Diazoxide	Salicylate
Disulfiram	Sulfinpyrazone
Ethacrynic acid	Sulfonamides
Glucagon	Thyroid hormone
Guanethidine	Tolbutamide
Depress Effect	
Antipyrine	Glutethimide
Azathioprine	Griseofulvin
Barbiturates	Haloperidol
Carbamazepine	Phenobarbital
Digitalis	Prednisone
Ethanol	Rifampin
Ethchlorvynol	Vitamin K

of therapy as factor VII level falls rapidly, whereas others, especially factor II, decline more slowly. The initial rapid fall in factor VII level may lead to an early elevation in the prothrombin time (PT) expressed as international normalized ratio (INR) without reflecting the desired anticoagulant effect. Because protein C is a natural inhibitor of coagulation with a short half-life (approximately 8 hours), its level may fall rapidly, theoretically inducing a procoagulant state during initiation of therapy.

As a result of the delayed anticoagulant effect of warfarin, therapy must be initiated with a rapidly acting agent such as heparin or low-molecular-weight heparin (LMWH) if immediate anticoagulation is needed. For example, patients with venous thromboembolism are typically given heparin or a LMWH for rapid effect, and warfarin is also administered within the first 24 hours. After a period of 5 or more days, the necessary anticoagulant effect of warfarin is achieved, and the parenteral anticoagulant can be stopped. Anticoagulation is initiated with a dose close to the expected daily maintenance requirement, which is usually between 5 and 10 mg.[18–21] There is, however, great variability in the doses required, and smaller amounts should be used for frail, elderly, or poorly nourished patients or those with an increased bleeding risk. Large "loading doses" of warfarin were recommended in the past, but these are inappropriate and may cause hemorrhage without shortening the time to achieve adequate anticoagulation. In patients with a low level of protein C or protein S as a result of an inherited deficiency, initiation of warfarin therapy without concomitant heparin or other immediately acting anticoagulant can lead to very low levels of these natural anticoagulants with ensuing thrombosis such as skin necrosis.

The anticoagulant effect of the vitamin K antagonists is monitored using the PT, which is sensitive to decreases in vitamin K–dependent factors and is progressively lengthened as the vitamin K–dependent factors reach lower levels. A critical component of the PT is the thromboplastin reagent that is used. Variability in thromboplastin composition leads to variation in results. The widespread introduction of the INR has improved standardization of results.[22–24] Manufacturers determine the potency of thromboplastins by measuring the international sensitivity index (ISI), and this is used as a correction factor for the responsiveness of the thromboplastin in the PT. The INR represents the ratio of the patient PT to control PT corrected by the ISI. By this method, INR values obtained in different laboratories can be reliably compared for therapeutic monitoring.

During initiation of therapy, the INR is checked every 2 to 3 days for 1 to 2 weeks until a stable therapeutic effect is achieved. The target INR for most indications is 2.5 with a desirable therapeutic range from 2 to 3 (Table 23–3). A higher INR is recommended for patients with mechanical heart valve replacement and for those who failed anticoagulant therapy despite well-documented INR values in the 2 to 3 range. During chronic therapy, the INR should be monitored regularly, depending on stability of the response, and minor dose adjustments are frequently needed. Monitoring can also be performed using portable instruments that are suitable for home use, enabling selected patients to learn to modify their warfarin doses in response to their INR value.[25–28] Specialized clinics devoted to monitoring warfarin typically achieve better results in maintaining patients within the therapeutic range, resulting in fewer bleeding complications.[29–32] Problems with keeping patients within the therapeutic range often result from failure of compliance, changes in diet, medication or alcohol intake, or intercurrent illnesses.

Warfarin sensitivity is affected by polymorphisms in cytochrome P450 (CYP) and vitamin K epoxide reductase complex (VKORC), and pharmacogenomics may become important in dosing. The clearance of warfarin is the result of hepatic metabolism and CYP2C9 is the most important enzyme mediating its clearance.[33,34] A number of polymorphisms have been identified, but the most important are CYP2C9*2 and CYP2C9*3, which are found in approximately 11 percent and 7 percent of patients and result in reductions of enzymatic activity of approximately 30 percent and 80 percent, respectively.[35–39] This reduced metabolic clearance leads to increased drug levels and an increased anticoagulant effect. VKORC1 converts oxidized Vitamin K to the active reduced form as required for posttranslational carboxylation. VKORC1 is the target of warfarin, which functions as a competitive inhibitor. Numerous coding polymorphisms have been identified that can affect the response to warfarin.[40,41] Common haplotypes can be separated into low (A)- and high (B)-dose groups with different sensitivities to warfarin.

TABLE 23–3. Recommended INR Values during Oral Anticoagulant Therapy

Condition	Target INR (Range)
Deep vein thrombosis treatment	2.5 (2.0–3.0)
Pulmonary embolism treatment	2.5 (2.0–3.0)
Deep venous thrombosis prophylaxis	2.5 (2.0–3.0)
Atrial fibrillation	2.5 (2.0–3.0)
Cardiac valve replacement	
Tissue valves	2.5 (2.0–3.0)
Mechanical valves	3.0 (2.5–3.5)
Acute myocardial infarction	2.5 (2.0–3.0)

Evidence is clear that polymorphisms in either CYP2C9 or VKORC1 affect warfarin sensitivity. Typical studies have performed genotyping in patients on stable anticoagulation and related genotype to warfarin dose and outcomes.[42–45] These have shown that patients with at least one variant allele have an increased risk of INRs over the desired range and the variant groups also require more time to achieve stable dosing compared to patient with wild type allele. Although these retrospective studies indicate that CYP2C9 and VKORC1 genotype clearly effect warfarin sensitivity, any clinical value would derive from the potential to use genotyping as a guide in warfarin dosing. Prospective studies have incorporated genotyping for CYP2C9 and VKORC1 into algorithms that typically include clinical variables such as age, gender, and drug interactions. Incorporation of CYP2C9 and VKORC1 polymorphisms significantly improves the ability to predict warfarin doses but has not been shown to impact important patient outcomes when compared with warfarin dosing algorithms that do not incorporate genotypic information.[46–50]

Complications

The most serious and common complication of oral anticoagulation is bleeding, and its risk is related primarily to patient characteristics, the intensity of the anticoagulation, and the length of therapy. Risk factors for bleeding include older age, recent surgery or trauma, a history of recent gastrointestinal bleeding, renal insufficiency, hypertension, cerebrovascular disease, and use of drugs with potentiating activity (see Table 23–2). The intensity of anticoagulation as reflected by the INR is the most important predictor of bleeding risk, which is low in the therapeutic range but increases as the INR prolongs further. The cumulative risk of bleeding increases with a longer duration of treatment, whereas the absolute risk is greatest early, possibly caused by pathologic lesions present at the time therapy is started. Overall, the total risk of major bleeding with a 6-month course of anticoagulation for venous thromboembolism is less than 3 percent in recent trials.[51] A rare complication of warfarin therapy is skin necrosis that usually occurs early in the course of anticoagulation.[52,53] Typical initial complaints are burning and tingling at the affected site, which usually involves a region with a large amount of subcutaneous tissue, such as the breast, buttock, or thigh. Painful hemorrhagic full-thickness skin infarction develops and frequently requires skin grafting. Thrombosis in dermal and subdermal venules is the underlying cause, and this may be caused by disproportionately rapid reduction in proteins C and S. Other complications from warfarin are rare. Occasional patients report alopecia; hypersensitivity reactions are rare and are almost uniformly caused by the dye used in the pill rather than by the warfarin itself.

Warfarin use in patients with heparin-induced thrombocytopenia (HIT) may be complicated by limb gangrene caused by occlusive venous thrombosis; this effect is likely a result of a combination of inadequate parenteral anticoagulant effect and reduced levels of protein C, in concert with relatively preserved levels of factors II and X that are seen early in warfarin treatment.[54] This complication highlights the need for parenteral anticoagulants to be continued in patients with HIT until the coagulopathy has largely resolved as indicated by a return of the platelet count to normal or near normal levels,

Oral anticoagulation should be avoided in pregnancy because warfarin crosses the placenta, and exposure during organogenesis in the first trimester can lead to fetal embryopathy with significant cranial bone malformations.[55,56] The impact of the novel anticoagulants, which are small molecules that could cross the placenta during pregnancy, is unknown. Anticoagulation during pregnancy increases bleeding complications, especially later in pregnancy. Warfarin may be considered during the second trimester, but heparin or a LMWH is a preferable alternative in most situations. Vitamin K antagonists are safe during lactation; the safety of novel agents during lactation is unknown.[57]

Reversal of Anticoagulation

Anticoagulation must be reversed for episodes of bleeding, surgery, trauma, or overdosage. Appropriate interventions for patients with excessively prolonged INRs without bleeding include holding warfarin doses, administering low doses of vitamin K (0.5–1.0 mg), and increasing the frequency of monitoring (Table 23–4).[58] Serious bleeding and major warfarin overdosage requires factor replacement and larger vitamin K doses that may need to be given intravenously. Anticoagulated patients who need invasive procedures represent management problems, and decisions about periprocedural anticoagulation should be based on balancing the risk of thromboembolism with that of bleeding from the procedure. The goal is to reduce the intensity of anticoagulation during and immediately after surgery, while avoiding thromboembolism caused by the underlying disease. Generally, the risk of recurrence is greatest in the period shortly after an episode of acute thrombosis and declines progressively over time. If possible, elective surgery and other invasive procedures associated with a high bleeding risk should be postponed during the first several months following acute thrombosis. Generally, the bleeding risk is highest during surgery and decreases rapidly to baseline after approximately 7 to 10 days. Most surgery can be done with a minimal bleeding risk in patients receiving warfarin and an INR of 1.5 or less. Patients at moderate or high risk of thrombotic recurrence should receive heparin or LMWH "bridging therapy" when their INR becomes subtherapeutic. Postprocedural bridging therapy should be undertaken only in patients in whom the risks of this therapy (principally bleeding) are less than the perceived benefits (a reduced risk of thromboembolism). Full anticoagulation can be resumed after the invasive procedure when the bleeding risk declines. Evidence-based guidelines for bridging therapy are available.[59–62]

TABLE 23–4. Reversing Warfarin Therapy

Indication	Action
INR <6	Lower the dose, consider withholding one or more doses
	Recheck in 3 to 7 days
INR 6–10	Lower the dose and withhold 1 to 3 doses
	Consider administering vitamin K, 1–2 mg orally
	Recheck INR in 24–48 hours
INR >10	Withhold doses until INR in desired range and cause of elevation ascertained
	Give vitamin K, 2–4 mg orally
	Recheck INR in 24 hours
Serious bleeding and major overdose	Consider fresh-frozen plasma or prothrombin complex concentrate, and give 5–10 mg vitamin K intravenously

HEPARIN AND LOW-MOLECULAR-WEIGHT HEPARINS

PHARMACOLOGY

Heparin and the related LMWHs are the most widely used, rapidly acting, parenteral anticoagulants. Heparin derives its name from its original description as an aqueous extract of liver (hepar) that exhibited anticoagulant activity *in vitro*.[63] It is a mixture of sulfated glycosaminoglycans composed of chains of alternating residues of D-glycosamine and iduronic acid. Heparin is very heterogeneous in composition and includes molecules varying in chain lengths (average chain length: 50 saccharide units) with molecular weights between 5000 and 30,000 daltons (average Mr: approximately 15,000 daltons). It is extracted from lungs and intestinal tissue of cows and swine and assayed biologically by its ability to prolong blood clotting *in vitro*.[64] Heparin has no direct anticoagulant effect, but it acts through antithrombin (AT), a serine protease inhibitor. Only about one-third of heparin molecules contain the necessary unique pentasaccharide sequence required to interact with AT and have anticoagulant activity.[65,66]

AT inhibits thrombin, factor Xa, and other coagulation serine proteases in a reaction that is slow by itself, but is accelerated approximately 1000-fold in the presence of heparin.[67,68] To inhibit thrombin, heparin binds to both the enzyme and AT, forming a ternary complex. The inhibition of factor Xa, however, occurs through binding to heparin–AT complex without the requirement for heparin binding directly also to factor Xa. The requirement for a ternary heparin–AT–thrombin complex requires heparin molecules with 19 or more saccharide units, whereas smaller heparin molecules are effective in promoting factor Xa inactivation. Heparin also stimulates release of tissue factor pathway inhibitor from endothelial cells, which might contribute to anticoagulant activity.[69,70] Thrombin and factor Xa are relatively protected from inhibition by the heparin–AT complex when they are surface immobilized within thrombi or on cells.[71–73] Heparin also interacts with heparin cofactor II; high concentrations of heparin accelerate thrombin inhibition by heparin cofactor II.[74]

Heparin is not absorbed after oral ingestion, so it must be given either subcutaneously or intravenously. Following parenteral administration, heparin exerts an immediate anticoagulant effect. It interacts with proteins and cells in the blood, resulting in complex pharmacokinetics characterized by rapid equilibration and slower clearance.[75–77] The initial binding to cells is saturable within concentrations used clinically, resulting in a dose-dependent half-life that increases from approximately 1 hour at a dose of 100 U/kg to 2.5 hours at 400 U/kg. Pharmacodynamics varies among individuals and also depends on the method of administration. After subcutaneous injection, bioavailability may be less than 50 percent in low doses, but increases at higher, therapeutic doses.

ADMINISTRATION AND MONITORING

To achieve a full anticoagulant effect rapidly, heparin is usually administered intravenously. A common protocol uses an initial intravenous bolus of 5000 units or 75 U/kg, followed by a maintenance infusion of 1250 to 1660 U/h or 18 U/kg per hour. Clinical studies demonstrate a lower occurrence of bleeding complications with continuous intravenous rather than intermittent bolus therapy. The anticoagulant effect is immediate, but laboratory monitoring is needed because of the variability in response among patients. Monitoring is most convenient with the activated partial thromboplastin time (aPTT), which is sensitive to plasma heparin concentrations of 0.1 U/mL or higher. Because different reagents and measuring systems have differing sensitivities to heparin, it is recommended that the therapeutic range be established for each laboratory by calibrating the aPTT to a plasma heparin concentration of 0.2 to 0.4 units by protamine sulfate titration, or 0.3 to 0.7 U/mL using an antifactor Xa assay.[64] The usual aPTT range for heparin therapy is between 1.5 and 2.5 times the mean of the normal range. Clinically useful nomograms are available for adjusting the heparin dose using either fixed- or weight-based dosing.[78,79] Alternatively, monitoring can be performed using anti-Xa levels, which is a useful approach when the aPTT is unreliable, as in patients with baseline prolongation of the aPTT as a consequence of lupus anticoagulant. Rapid achievement of a therapeutic level as reflected by the aPTT or anti-Xa is important in ensuring an adequate anticoagulant effect.

Some patients appear to respond poorly to heparin, with inadequate prolongation of the aPTT despite apparently adequate or even high heparin dosage. This phenomenon is termed *heparin resistance* and is usually caused by an acute-phase response that results in high levels of procoagulant proteins, including factor VIII. The antithrombotic effect of heparin correlates best with plasma heparin levels, which may be adequate in these circumstances despite a subtherapeutic aPTT.[80] For patients who require heparin doses of greater than 35,000 U/day to increase the aPTT into the therapeutic range, consideration should be given to using heparin levels determined by an anti-Xa assay. Substitution of LMWH for unfractionated heparin is another consideration. Although AT deficiency may cause heparin resistance, most AT-deficient patients can be adequately anticoagulated with heparin in usual doses. No monitoring is recommended when low doses of heparin are used for prophylaxis of venous thromboembolic disease, although minimal prolongation of the aPTT may occur. Care is required in very lightweight patients, particularly the frail elderly who may be anticoagulated with usual "prophylactic" doses of unfractionated heparin; aPTT monitoring might be considered in such patients.

A large study demonstrated that patients with acute venous thromboembolism can be safely treated with fixed, weight-adjusted heparin doses without aPTT monitoring.[81] In this study, 708 patients were allocated randomly to receive either unfractionated heparin with a subcutaneous bolus dose of 333 U/kg followed by a twice-daily dose of 250 U/kg, or LMWH over 3 months of followup. Recurrent venous thromboembolism occurred in 13 patients who were allocated to unfractionated heparin and in 12 who were allocated to LMWH. Major bleeding occurred in 4 and 5 patients, respectively. This study calls into question the need for routine aPTT monitoring of therapeutic dose, weight-adjusted unfractionated heparin and warrants validation.

Reversal

Heparin has a short half-life, and its anticoagulant effect disappears several hours after discontinuation of an intravenous infusion. Therefore, stopping the infusion and local measures are usually adequate to control bleeding. However, in major or life-threatening bleeding, the anticoagulant effect can be neutralized with protamine sulfate, which is a basic polypeptide that binds tightly to the acidic heparin molecule. The usual dose of protamine required is 1 mg to neutralize 100 units of heparin. The dose to be administered is based on the amount of heparin remaining in the circulation. Protamine is routinely used to neutralize heparin after cardiopulmonary bypass using standard formulas and activated clotting time monitoring.

Adverse Effects

The most frequent complication of heparin administration is bleeding, which is related to the dose and intensity of treatment, as well as to patient characteristics.[51] HIT is an immune-mediated platelet consumption caused by an antibody directed against a complex of heparin and platelet factor 4 (see Chap. 133). Despite thrombocytopenia, HIT is more commonly associated with thrombotic complications than bleeding, and it occurs in approximately 3 percent of patients when defined as a 50 percent reduction in baseline platelet count or development of a platelet count of less than 150,000/μL during therapy.[82,83] Platelet counts should be monitored during treatment and heparin discontinued if thrombocytopenia occurs. An alternative anticoagulant that does not interact with the heparin-platelet factor 4 complexes should be administered. Vitamin K antagonists should be given only after the platelet count has risen over 150,000/μL. Long-term heparin therapy can also cause osteoporosis, and radiographic evidence of bone loss occurs in approximately 15 percent of women who receive prolonged treatment during pregnancy, with symptomatic vertebrae fractures in approximately 2 percent. The bone loss may resolve after heparin is discontinued.

LOW-MOLECULAR-WEIGHT HEPARIN

Limitations of unfractionated heparin led to studies correlating structural and functional relationships of heparin, and this eventually resulted in the development of LMWHs, several of which are now available. LMWH preparations are produced by treating heparin chemically or enzymatically to decrease the size of the polysaccharide chains, yielding products with restricted molecular weight distributions with a mean of approximately 4000 to 5000 daltons.[84] Like heparin, LMWHs exert antithrombotic effects through interaction with AT. In the presence of LMWH, AT inactivates factor Xa in the same way as unfractionated heparin, but it is less able to inactivate thrombin because the shorter polysaccharide length does not allow formation of the necessary ternary complex. Consequently, LMWHs have a greater proportion of antifactor Xa than antithrombin activity.

LMWHs also have different pharmacokinetic properties than unfractionated heparin.[64] Following subcutaneous administration, LMWHs are nearly completely absorbed, a clear benefit over unfractionated heparin, which exhibits variable and dose-dependent absorption. LMWHs also exhibit less binding to plasma proteins and cells than unfractionated heparin, resulting in more predictable blood levels and anticoagulant effects.[64,84] LMWHs have a longer plasma half-life than unfractionated heparins, allowing once or twice daily subcutaneous administration for many applications.

LMWHs have significant renal clearance, and high levels can accumulate in patients with renal insufficiency. Care must be taken in dosing LMWHs in patients with reduced renal function as bleeding risks are increased,[85] and monitoring with antifactor Xa levels may be needed. Similarly, monitoring may be necessary to achieve appropriate levels in very obese patients, although weight-based dosing probably achieves better anticoagulation.[64] Protamine sulfate does not completely reverse the anticoagulant effect of LMWH but is partially effective and can be useful in patients with serious hemorrhage.[86] Several LMWH preparations are available and approved for both prophylaxis and treatment of venous and arterial thrombotic diseases. Each preparation differs slightly and is pharmacologically unique, although the agents are likely similarly effective for the treatment and prevention of venous thrombosis. Table 23–5 lists the doses used for common indications.

Similar to unfractionated heparin, the most common adverse effect is bleeding, which occurs at approximately the same frequency and severity when used in similar patient groups for the same indication. HIT is much less common than with unfractionated heparin,[82,83] occurring only in 0.3 to 0.45 percent of patients. However, cross-reactivity of the antibody occurs, and LMWH is not an acceptable choice for continued anticoagulation in patients with HIT. Animal studies suggest that osteoporosis may be less common with LMWH, and this is reported by several small clinical trials.[87]

TABLE 23–5. Low-Molecular-Weight Heparin Regimens[†,*]

	Drug[†]	Regimen
Prophylaxis of VTE		
General surgery		
Low risk	Dalteparin	2500 U, 1 or 2 h preoperation and daily
	Enoxaparin	40 mg, 2 h preoperation and daily
	Fondaparinux	2.5 mg daily (start 6–8 h postoperation)
High risk	Dalteparin	5000 U, 10–14 preoperation and daily
		2500 U, 1–2 h preoperation and after 12 h; then 5000 U daily (with malignancy)
	Enoxaparin	40 mg, 2 h preoperation and daily
	Fondaparinux	2.5 mg daily (start 6–8 h postoperation)
Orthopedic surgery	Dalteparin	2500 U, 4–8 h postoperation and 5000 U daily; or 2500 U , 2 h preoperation and 2500 U 4–8 h postoperation and 5000 U daily; or 5000 U, 10–14 preoperation and 5000 U daily
	Enoxaparin	30 mg BID starting 12–24 h postoperation; 40 mg 9–15 h preoperation and once daily
	Fondaparinux	2.5 mg daily (start 6–8 h postoperation)
Medical patients	Enoxaparin	40 mg once daily
Treatment of VTE	Fondaparinux	weight <50 kg: 5 mg daily; 50–100 kg: 7.5 daily; >75 kg: 10 mg daily
	Dalteparin (VTE with cancer)	200 U/kg daily × 1 month; then, 150 U/kg daily for up to 6 months
	Enoxaparin	1 mg/kg q12h; 1.5 mg/kg daily
	Tinzaparin	175 U/kg daily
Acute coronary syndrome unstable angina and non-STEMI	Dalteparin	120 U/kg (max 10,000 U) q12h
	Enoxaparin	
	STEMI	30 mg IV bolus plus 1mg/kg SQ q12h (older than age 75 y: initial 0.75 mg/kg with no IV bolus)
	Unstable angina and non-STEMI	1 mg/kg 12 h

STEMI, ST-segment elevation myocardial infarction; VTE, venous thromboembolism.

*Consult package insert for more detailed dosing information. Only FDA approved-indications are included.

[†]Drug brand names: dalteparin, Fragmin; enoxaparin, Lovenox; fondaparinux, Arixtra; tinzaparin, Innohep.

CHOICE OF HEPARIN OR LOW-MOLECULAR-WEIGHT HEPARIN

The factors governing the choice of heparin or LMWH concern effectiveness, safety, convenience, and cost. LMWH is more effective than heparin in patients placed in high-risk settings, such as those with major trauma and those undergoing major orthopedic surgery. For treatment of venous thromboembolic disease, the safety and efficacy of heparin and LMWH are comparable, but LMWH offers better convenience because subcutaneous administration permits outpatient treatment, which is preferable for most patients. LMWHs may be difficult to use in patients with renal insufficiency because of decreased clearance, and intravenous heparin may offer advantages in such patients. LMWHs are incompletely reversed by protamine sulfate, making them more difficult to use for cardiac bypass surgery. Unfractionated heparin may be preferable in patients who require an invasive procedure on an urgent basis because of its shorter half-life. LMWHs may offer some advantages for patients with acute coronary syndromes.

Danaparoid

Danaparoid is a mixture of glycosaminoglycans and is composed of approximately 84 percent heparan sulfate, 12 percent dermatan sulfate, and 4 percent chondroitin sulfate. It is an AT-dependent anticoagulant with predominant antifactor Xa activity. The plasma half-life is approximately 24 hours with predominant renal clearance. Danaparoid is not reversed by protamine sulfate. Danaparoid differs structurally from heparin and it has been used successfully to treat patients with HIT. Although there is *in vitro* cross-reactivity of 10 to 20 percent of heparin antibodies with danaparoid, this is of uncertain clinical relevance. Danaparoid is administered subcutaneously, and levels may be monitored with anti-factor Xa assays performed using a danaparoid standard curve. At the time of writing danaparoid has not been approved in the United States, and availability elsewhere was limited.

Fondaparinux

Fondaparinux is a unique heparin-like anticoagulant with highly selective AT dependent anti-factor Xa activity.[64] It is a completely synthetic pentasaccharide whose structure is based on the heparin sequence that interacts with AT. It binds reversibly and with high affinity to AT, resulting in a conformational change that renders it effective in inhibiting factor Xa but not thrombin. Whereas unfractionated heparin and all LMWHs are derived from animal sources, fondaparinux is synthesized in a structurally homogenous form containing no animal products. Consequently, fondaparinux does not induce allergic responses. Because it inhibits factor Xa but has no direct action on thrombin, its mechanism of action depends on reducing thrombin generation.

Pharmacologic studies show that maximum plasma levels are reached approximately 2 hours after subcutaneous administration with an elimination half-life of approximately 17 hours independent of the dose.[88,89] Bioavailability is nearly complete after subcutaneous or intravenous administration. There is a low intra- and intersubject variability with little accumulation after multiple daily doses. Because elimination is primarily renal and the agent is excreted unchanged in the urine, fondaparinux is contraindicated in patients with severe renal impairment. Fondaparinux plasma levels can be measured with the anti-factor Xa assay, but there is no effect on other coagulation assays including the activated clotting time (ACT), aPTT, or thrombin clotting time.

Clinical studies have evaluated the use of fondaparinux in several conditions, and it is approved by the FDA for prevention of venous thromboembolism in patients undergoing major orthopedic surgery or with hip fracture, prophylaxis after abdominal surgery, and treatment of deep venous thrombosis (DVT) or pulmonary embolism (PE). For prophylaxis it is administered subcutaneously in a dose of 2.5 mg once daily, whereas a weight-adjusted dose is used for treatment of venous thromboembolism. Although not approved at the time of writing for use in patients with unstable coronary syndromes, fondaparinux at a dose of 2.5 mg per day is equivalently effective to, but safer than, enoxaparin.[90]

The principal adverse effect is bleeding, and its frequency and severity have been comparable to those observed with LMWH. Elevated levels may occur in patients with renal insufficiency, and caution should be exercised in using fondaparinux in patients with renal compromise. Cross-reactivity with antibodies causing HIT does not occur,[91,92] and fondaparinux may be a good choice for an anticoagulant in patients with HIT, particularly those needing subcutaneous administration, although it is not approved by the FDA for this purpose.[93]

DIRECT THROMBIN INHIBITORS

LEPIRUDIN

Lepirudin is closely related to hirudin, a natural anticoagulant found in the salivary glands of the leech. Lepirudin is composed of 65 amino acids and is identical to natural hirudin except for substitution of leucine for isoleucine at the N-terminus of the molecule and the absence of a sulfate group on tyrosine 63. Lepirudin has bioavailability of approximately 88 percent after subcutaneous administration with peak plasma levels after a single dose in 1.3 to 2.5 hours. The half-life is 1 to 3 hours in normal volunteers with predominantly renal catabolism, but it may be as long as 2 days in dialysis-dependent patients.[64,94–96] Lepirudin prolongs the aPTT in a concentration-dependent manner,[97] but the ecarin clotting time may be better as a measure of blood levels.[98]

Lepirudin is approved for use in treatment of HIT (Table 23–6) and has also been used successfully in clinical trials for other nonapproved indications, including prevention and treatment of DVT and in patients with acute coronary syndromes. It has no structural homology with heparin and exhibits no cross-reactivity with HIT antibodies. The recommended dosing depends on renal function. For patients with normal function, treatment is initiated with a bolus of 0.4 mg/kg followed by an infusion to maintain the aPTT at 1.5 to 2.5 times normal. With renal insufficiency, both the bolus and infusion rate should be decreased.

The primary adverse effect is bleeding. Antihirudin antibodies occur in approximately 40 percent of HIT patients treated with lepirudin, which may decrease drug clearance and thus increase the anticoagulant effect, possibly because of delayed renal elimination of lepirudin-antibody complexes, which retain anticoagulant properties.[99–102] There is no available agent to reverse the effects of lepirudin. The infusion should be discontinued in case of bleeding complications or overdosage and aPTT and other coagulation parameters monitored as appropriate. Hemofiltration or hemodialysis may be useful with very high levels or renal compromise. Also, factor VIIa decreases bleeding in patients receiving lepirudin.

TABLE 23–6. Clinical Indications and Use of Direct Thrombin Inhibitors

Agent	Clinical Indication	Regimen	Monitoring
Lepirudin	HIT	0.4 mg/kg bolus 0.15 mg/kg/h	aPTT
Bivalirudin	Angioplasty, PCI with HIT	0.75 mg/kg/bolus; then 1.75 mg/kg/h	ACT
Argatroban	HIT	2 mcg/kg/min	aPTT
	HIT with PCI	350 mcg/kg/min bolus, then 15 to 400 mcg/kg/min	ACT

ACT, activated clotting time; aPTT, activated partial thromboplastin time; HIT, heparin-induced thrombocytopenia; PCI, percutaneous coronary intervention.

BIVALIRUDIN

Bivalirudin, a recombinant protein based on the structure of hirudin, is composed of a dodecapeptide analogue of the carboxy-terminal region of hirudin linked by a four-glycine residue to a structure directed to the active site of thrombin.[103] The glycine bridge permits easy cleavage of the molecule, providing a more reversible interaction with the catalytic site of thrombin than hirudin,[103] which may result in fewer bleeding complications. Pharmacokinetic studies show that plasma clearance is rapid (4.6 mL/min/kg) in patients with normal renal function with a volume of distribution of 0.2 L/kg and elimination of half-life of approximately 30 minutes.[64,104] There is dose-dependent prolongation of the ACT and aPTT that correlates with plasma concentrations. There are both renal and hepatic clearance, and consequently, dose modification is recommended for patients with moderate-to-severe functional impairment or patients who are dialyzed.

Bivalirudin is effective when used with aspirin in patients with unstable angina or postinfarction angina undergoing angioplasty, and it is approved for this use.[105] It is also approved for patients with HIT undergoing percutaneous coronary intervention (see Table 23–6). In some clinical trials, bivalirudin also shows efficacy in preventing restenosis after coronary angioplasty, as an adjunct to streptokinase in acute myocardial infarction, and in preventing venous thrombosis after orthopedic surgery and in patients with HIT. However, these are nonapproved indications. The most common adverse effect is bleeding, and no specific antidote is available. The infusion should be discontinued in patients with bleeding complications and blood levels monitored with the aPTT or other coagulation parameters. Antibivalirudin antibodies have not been detected following therapy.

ARGATROBAN

Argatroban is a small-molecule arginine derivative that reversibly inhibits thrombin by binding directly to the active catalytic site with a K_i of 3.9×10^{-8} mol/L.[64,106] Because of its small size, argatroban is an effective inhibitor of thrombin, both bound to surfaces and in solution.[107] The anticoagulant effect can be assessed with either the aPTT or ACT, and both correlate with plasma concentrations of the drug.[108] Argatroban is approximately 50 percent protein bound and has a volume of distribution of 0.2 L/kg and an elimination half-life of 39 to 51 minutes.[109,110] Metabolism is primarily hepatic, and the clearance and half-life are prolonged in patients with hepatic functional abnormalities requiring dose reduction. Renal function has less effect on argatroban pharmacokinetics.

Argatroban is approved for treatment and prophylaxis of HIT and for percutaneous interventions in patients with HIT (see Table 23–6). It also shows some benefit in patients with thrombotic stroke in clinical trials. For treatment of HIT, argatroban is administered at 2 mcg/kg per hour and adjusted to maintain the aPTT at 1.5 to 3 times baseline. For patients with HIT who are undergoing percutaneous coronary interventions, the drug is administered as a bolus of 350 mcg/kg followed by a continuous infusion of 15 to 400 mcg/kg per minute for a target ACT of 300 to 450 seconds. As with other direct thrombin inhibitors, the main side effect is bleeding, and no specific agent is available to reverse its action. The anticoagulant effect may be prolonged in patients with hepatic impairment. If overdosage or excess bleeding occurs, the infusion should be discontinued and the aPTT and other coagulation parameters monitored.

The transition from argatroban to warfarin in patients requiring long-term anticoagulation is complicated because argatroban has a significant effect on both the PT and the aPTT.[111] In patients transitioning to warfarin an INR should be measured; if it is greater than 4.0, the argatroban should be stopped for several hours and the INR remeasured. If the INR is still greater than 2.0, the argatroban can be discontinued; if it is less than 2.0, the argatroban should be reinstituted and the same procedure followed on the next day.

DABIGATRAN ETEXILATE

Dabigatran etexilate is a double prodrug with a bioavailability of approximately 6 percent after oral administration. The absorbed drug is rapidly converted by esterases to dabigatran. Peak levels occur 1 to 2 hours after an oral dose; the half-life is approximately 12 hours. Dabigatran does not require a cofactor and reversibly inhibits the active site of thrombin.[112] Dabigatran does not interfere with drugs that are metabolized by the cytochrome P450 enzyme system and it produces a predictable anticoagulant response,[113] which allows therapy without the need for monitoring. Dabigatran prolongs the ecarin clotting time, aPTT, and PT.[114,115]

The major side effect of dabigatran is hemorrhage. No specific antidote is available. Consequently, bleeding complications are managed symptomatically. Although not well studied, dialysis or hemoperfusion likely removes this compound from the circulation, and the administration of activated coagulation factor complexes such as FEIBA (factor VIII inhibitor bypassing activity), Autoplex, or recombinant activated factor VII (factor VIIa) may overcome its anticoagulant effect.[116]

Dabigatran etexilate (220 mg or 150 mg once daily) is as effective as enoxaparin (40 mg once daily) for the prevention of venous thromboembolism after total hip replacement, and has a similar safety profile.[117] In a second study, dabigatran was found to be as effective as enoxaparin for the prevention of venous thromboembolism in patients who underwent total knee replacement.[118] Dabigatran was inferior to enoxaparin when enoxaparin was used at a dose of 30 mg subcutaneously twice daily.[119] Dabigatran is in late phase III evaluation for the prevention of stroke in patients with atrial fibrillation and for long-term secondary prevention of recurrent venous thrombosis at the time of this writing.

DIRECT FACTOR Xa INHIBITORS

RIVAROXABAN

Rivaroxaban is an available orally administered direct factor Xa inhibitor that produces its anticoagulant effect through reversible binding with the factor Xa molecule. Rivaroxaban can inhibit both free and thrombus-associated factor Xa. Like dabigatran, it is dependent on renal excretion, and bioaccumulation may occur in patients with renal insufficiency.

Rivaroxaban produces its peak anticoagulant effect within 4 hours of oral administration and has a terminal elimination half-life of 5.7 to 9.2 hours. Rivaroxaban prolongs the PT and the aPTT to an extent roughly proportionate to the amount of drug present, as measured by inhibition of factor Xa.[120]

The principal side effect of rivaroxaban therapy is bleeding; in a randomized clinical trial comparing rivaroxaban 10 mg once daily with enoxaparin 40 mg once daily, begun preoperatively, major bleeding occurred in less than 1 percent of rivaroxaban- and placebo-treated patients.[121] Similarly, in a randomized phase II study comparing rivaroxaban (10 to 40 mg orally twice daily or 40 mg orally once daily) with enoxaparin (1 mg/kg subcutaneously twice daily), both followed by warfarin, major bleeding occurred in 1.7 to 3.3 percent of rivaroxaban-treated patients and in no patients receiving enoxaparin.[122] There is no antidote for the anticoagulant effect of rivaroxaban.

In four phase III clinical trials, rivaroxaban significantly reduced venographically detected deep vein thrombosis when compared with enoxaparin administered at doses of 40 mg once daily or 30 mg twice daily.[121–125] Based on these results rivaroxaban has been approved for venous thromboembolism prophylaxis in patients who are undergoing orthopedic surgery in Canada and Europe.

FIBRINOLYTIC THERAPY

Fibrinolytic therapy is administered by infusing high doses of a plasminogen activator to accelerate the conversion of plasminogen to the active fibrinolytic enzyme plasmin, which proteolytically degrades fibrin (see Chap. 136). The specific biochemical and pharmacologic properties of different agents are important determinants of the administration regimen, the efficacy of clot lysis, and the nature of adverse effects. For example, some fibrinolytic drugs are bacterial products that are antigenic and can cause allergic responses, whereas others are recombinant human proteins. Some agents activate plasminogen prominently, both in blood and at the clot surface, and induce a systemic fibrinolytic state in addition to accelerating clot lysis. In contrast, the activity of other agents is more specifically limited to the clot surface with fewer systemic effects. Fibrinolytic therapy is used for treatment of both venous and arterial thrombosis and represents standard treatment for many patients presenting with acute myocardial infarction because it accelerates reperfusion, decreases mortality, and reduces morbidity (Chap. 135). Thrombolytic therapy has also become standard for many patients presenting with thrombosis of peripheral arteries, bypass grafts, and catheters.[126] It is used for treatment of selected patients with thrombotic stroke. Fibrinolytic therapy improves outcome in selected hemodynamically unstable patients with large pulmonary emboli associated (Chap. 136).

The evolution of fibrinolytic therapy, including a historical perspective on its clinical evolution, has been reviewed.[127]

STREPTOKINASE

Streptokinase was the first plasminogen activator used clinically. It is derived from β-hemolytic streptococci and has a unique indirect mechanism of action. By itself, streptokinase has no enzymatic activity, but it combines with plasminogen to form an equimolar streptokinase–plasminogen complex that can then convert other plasminogen molecules to plasmin. Additionally, the streptokinase–plasminogen complex can undergo proteolytic cleavage itself, resulting in activation. When administered in therapeutic doses, streptokinase is an effective thrombolytic agent. The streptokinase–plasmin(ogen) complex can bind to fibrin through the "kringle" domains of plasmin and activate clot-bound plasminogen to accelerate clot lysis (see Chap. 136), but can also act on plasminogen in the blood to produce plasmin, giving rise to systemic proteolysis termed the *lytic state*. This results in consumption of plasminogen and α_2-antiplasmin, degradation of fibrinogen, factor V, and VIII, proteolysis of platelet membrane proteins by plasmin, and platelet activation. Streptokinase has a rapid plasma clearance with a half-life of approximately 20 minutes, but the duration of the proteolytic effect is more prolonged.[127]

Streptokinase can be used to treat either venous or arterial thrombosis. Higher doses given over a shorter time are typically used for arterial disease. For either venous or arterial thrombosis, a sufficient dose must be administered to overcome circulating neutralizing antibodies, which are common because of the frequency of streptococcal infections in the population. Occasionally, individuals have a high titer of antibodies that neutralize this amount of streptokinase, resulting in resistance. Streptokinase is antigenic, and high-titer antibodies develop 1 to 2 weeks after use, precluding retreatment until the titer declines. High titers can also cause febrile or hypotensive reactions. The first large study to demonstrate the utility of coronary reperfusion employed streptokinase.[128] Although not widely used in North America, streptokinase is still extensively used given its low cost, widespread availability, and familiarity.

TISSUE-TYPE PLASMINOGEN ACTIVATOR AND RECOMBINANT TISSUE PLASMINOGEN ACTIVATOR (ALTEPLASE)

Tissue-type plasminogen activator (t-PA) is a naturally occurring plasminogen activator that is structurally and immunologically distinct from urokinase. t-PA is synthesized by endothelial cells as a single-chain polypeptide and was originally produced from cell culture for pharmacologic use, but is now synthesized by recombinant techniques (alteplase). t-PA directly converts plasminogen to plasmin in a reaction that is accelerated several hundred fold in the presence of fibrin. In the absence of fibrin, t-PA has much less activity, and this property accounts for the relative "fibrin specificity" of t-PA observed physiologically. However, when administered pharmacologically in a high dose, significant proteolysis of plasma fibrinogen often occurs, but this is typically less prominent than observed with treatment using either streptokinase or urokinase. The half-life of t-PA following intravenous administration is about 5 minutes, which requires a constant infusion to maintain therapeutic plasma levels. t-PA is not antigenic because it is a physiologic enzyme.[127]

t-PA has been evaluated in treatment of DVT, PE, myocardial infarction, stroke, catheter thrombosis, and peripheral arterial occlusion. In patients with PE, a regimen of 100 mg intravenously over 2 hours results in a high rate of clot lysis and hemodynamic improvement. t-PA has been evaluated in many large studies for acute myocardial infarction and administration results in improved mortality and morbidity. t-PA has also been evaluated in treatment of stroke and results in significant benefit in highly selected patients who are treated within hours of symptom onset (see Chap. 136).

RETEPLASE

Recombinant technology has been used to engineer many t-PA mutants in an attempt to improve pharmacologic properties. The structural modifications in reteplase include removal of the finger, kringle 1, and EGF (epidermal growth factor) receptor domains. These changes result in enhanced firbrin specificity and a significantly longer half-life of 15 minutes compared to 4 minutes with t-PA, so it can be administered as an intravenous bolus rather than a continuous infusion. Its mode of administration (two 10-U IV boluses given over 2 minutes, 30 minutes apart) make it particularly useful for prehospital administration in remote areas, or areas with limited access to primary percutaneous coronary interventions.[129]

TENECTEPLASE

Tenecteplase (TNK-tissue plasminogen activator) is another bioengineered variant of t-PA with a longer half-life, increased resistance to inactivation by plasminogen activator inhibitor-1, and improved fibrin specificity. Advantages include a longer half-life, greater fibrin specificity, ease and rapidity of administration, and similar clinical efficacy as t-PA for treatment of acute myocardial infarction. It has a half-life of more than 30 minutes and can be administered as a single IV bolus. Large studies have shown it to be equivalently effective as other t-PA derivatives.[127]

OTHER PLASMINOGEN ACTIVATORS

Many other plasminogen activators have been characterized, prepared for clinical use, and tested in limited trials. These include a variety of genetically engineered mutants of t-PA and urokinase-plasminogen activator, as well as chimeric forms of t-PA and urokinase-plasminogen activator and bifunctional agents that include antiplatelet agents. A particularly interesting plasminogen activator is staphylokinase, a 15.5-kDa protein produced by *Staphylococcus aureus* and known for many years to have fibrinolytic properties. Similar to streptokinase, it is an indirect activator and forms a 1:1 stoichiometric complex with plasminogen, which then forms plasmin. It is much more fibrin-specific than streptokinase, producing high rates of clot lysis without significant effects on the levels of fibrinogen, plasminogen, or α_2-antiplasmin. It is, however, antigenic, and neutralizing antibodies develop following therapy. Another novel but naturally occurring plasminogen activator is derived from the vampire bat, which secretes plasminogen activators in its saliva. One form was developed for possible clinical use and shows high potency and fibrin specificity with very few systemic effects. Lanoteplase, another bioengineered variant of t-PA, is active and showed promise in clinical trials, but has not been approved and marketed.

ANTIPLATELET DRUGS

Platelets play an important role in hemostasis and thrombosis and inhibitors of platelet function are important therapeutic agents (see Chaps. 114, 122, and 135). Platelets adhere to exposed subendothelium, become activated, release contents of their dense and α granules, and form aggregates. Additional platelets from the circulating blood are then recruited by adenosine diphosphate (ADP), which is released from dense granules, and also by thromboxane A_2 synthesized by activated platelets in the aggregate. Simultaneous with the initial platelet adhesion and aggregation, thrombin generation is initiated. The activated platelet phospholipid membrane is an effective surface for binding of coagulation factors to enhance the rate of thrombin generation. As thrombin is formed it activates additional platelets and also cleaves fibrinopeptides from fibrinogen to form fibrin in and around the platelet plug, consolidating it. The role of platelets in initiating thrombosis is greater in the arterial circulation than in the venous circulation because higher shear forces present in arteries activate platelets. Therefore, antiplatelet drugs are more effective in arterial than in venous thrombosis. Tables 23–7 and 23–8 summarize the types of drug, their use in clinical settings, their mechanism of action, and their dosages.

TABLE 23–7. Antiplatelet Agents by Mechanism of Action and Clinical Use

Cyclooxygenase inhibitors	
Aspirin	Coronary and cerebrovascular disease
Agents that increase cAMP	
Dipyridamole	Coronary, cerebrovascular, peripheral arterial disease
Pentoxifylline	Peripheral arterial disease
Cilostazol	Peripheral arterial disease
ADP receptor blockers	
Ticlopidine	Cerebrovascular disease
Clopidogrel	Coronary, cerebrovascular disease, PCI
Prasugrel	Not approved in United States at time of this writing
ADP mimetic	
Cangrelor	Not approved in United States at time of this writing
$\alpha_{IIb}\beta_3$ inhibitors	
Abciximab	ACS, PCI
Eptifibatide	ACS, PCI
Tirofiban	ACS, PCI

ACS, acute coronary syndrome; cAMP, cyclic adenosine monophosphate; PCI, percutaneous coronary intervention.

TABLE 23–8. Antiplatelet Agents, Approved Dosing

Agent	Usual Dose	Duration of Effect
Aspirin	75–650 mg daily	7–10 days (life of the platelet)
Dipyridamole	75–100 mg QID	$t_{1/2}$ 40 min
Pentoxifylline	400 mg BID	$t_{1/2}$ l–1.6 h
Cilostazol	100 mg BID	$t_{1/2}$ 11–13 h
Ticlopidine	250 mg BID	7–10 days (life of the platelet)
Clopidogrel	75 mg daily, loading dose 300 mg*	7–10 days (life of the platelet)
Abciximab	0.25 mg/kg, then 10 mcg/kg/min	<0 min and 30 min
Eptifibatide	ACS 180 mcg/kg, then 2 mcg/kg/min PCI 180 mcg/kg, then 2 mcg/kg/min with 180 mcg/kg at 10 min†	$t_{1/2}$ 2.5 h
Tirofiban	0.4 mcg/kg/min × 30 min, then 0.1 mcg/kg/min*	$t_{1/2}$ 2 h

ACS, acute coronary syndrome; PCI, percutaneous coronary intervention; $t_{1/2}$, half-life.

*Larger loading and maintenance dosing is being studied.

†Decrease infusion rate by 50% for renal dysfunction.

CYCLOOXYGENASE-1 INHIBITORS

Cyclooxygenase-1 (COX-1) is an enzyme that is present in most cells. It converts arachidonic acid released from phospholipids by phospholipase A_2 or phospholipase C and diacylglycerol to prostaglandin G_2 (see Chap. 114). A peroxidase converts prostaglandin G_2 to prostaglandin H_2, which is then converted by thromboxane synthase in platelets to thromboxane A_2. Thromboxane A_2 is a potent activator of platelets. In endothelial cells, prostaglandin H_2 is converted to prostacyclin, a potent inhibitor of platelet function, through an increase in intraplatelet cyclic adenosine monophosphate (cAMP).

Aspirin (acetylsalicylic acid) was recognized as an inhibitor of platelet function in the 1960s, although the mechanism of its action was unknown at that time. It prolonged the bleeding time in normal subjects slightly, although usually not out of the normal range, and its effect lasted for several days. It was demonstrated that acetylation of cyclooxygenase is important in platelet inhibition by aspirin. Because platelets cannot synthesize new COX, irreversible enzyme inhibition by aspirin means that inhibition persists for the life span of the platelet. Most cells have two forms of COX, known as COX-1 and COX-2. COX-1 is synthesized constitutively, whereas COX-2 is only synthesized under stress conditions. Both COX-1 and COX-2 are inhibited by aspirin and most nonsteroidal antiinflammatory drugs (NSAIDs), with aspirin acetylating both forms. The nonaspirin COX inhibitors are reversible inhibitors, so they are active only while in the circulation. It was thought initially that only COX-1 is found in platelets, but COX-2 has been detected in platelets and its effect is particularly apparent when there was a rapid platelet turnover. Because COX-1 is the major COX in platelets, COX-2–specific inhibitors have minimal effect on platelet function.

Aspirin and several of the commonly used NSAIDs (e.g., indomethacin, ibuprofen, and naproxen) have similar *in vitro* effects on platelet function. Platelet aggregometry demonstrates that the second wave of aggregation induced by ADP or epinephrine in citrated platelet-rich plasma (PRP) is abolished after aspirin ingestion and that aggregation induced by low concentrations of collagen is markedly decreased. Arachidonic acid-induced aggregation is abolished after aspirin ingestion. Additionally, secretion of dense granule components (ADP, ATP, and serotonin) and of α-granule proteins by ADP, epinephrine, collagen, and arachidonic acid is inhibited in citrated PRP after aspirin ingestion or with addition of indomethacin to citrated PRP. Because of these *in vitro* effects of aspirin, the drug has been used extensively as an inhibitor of platelet function *in vivo*, with beneficial effects in primary and secondary prevention and in treatment of myocardial infarction (see Chap. 135). Aspirin is also beneficial in stroke prevention with carotid artery disease and embolic stroke, although anticoagulation with warfarin or its analogues is generally more effective than aspirin in embolic stroke in most patients with a cardiac embolic source.[130] Aspirin is rarely used to prevent venous thrombosis although it does have some efficacy in this domain. Other drugs that inhibit COX-1 are not used to prevent either arterial or venous thrombosis.

Aspirin was traditionally administered at a very high dose (doses as high as 650 mg four times per day have been described). However, a series of clinical trials, supported by laboratory evidence have failed to find support for larger aspirin doses.[131] At present, and for most indications, a daily dose of 81 mg to 325 mg is recommended as lower-dose aspirin appears as effective and may be associated with a lower risk of gastrointestinal bleeding than higher doses.[132,133] Broadly, aspirin is currently recommended for primary and secondary prevention of a wide variety of atherosclerotic outcomes including stroke, myocardial infarction, and peripheral vascular disease. As this field changes rapidly, interested readers are invited to review current management guidelines in locations such as the National Guidelines Clearinghouse (www.guideline.gov).

DRUGS THAT MODULATE CYCLIC ADENOSINE MONOPHOSPHATE LEVELS

cAMP in platelets is formed from ATP by the action of adenylate cyclase and degraded by cAMP phosphodiesterase, and basal levels of cAMP in platelets are low. Elevated levels of intraplatelet cAMP are induced by inhibition of cAMP phosphodiesterase, or by stimulation of adenylate cyclase activity, resulting in inhibition of platelet activation through several pathways: (1) modulation of phosphorylation of specific proteins; (2) inhibition of several steps in metabolism of phosphoinositol phosphates; and (3) lowering of intracellular Ca^{2+}, and accumulation of Ca^{2+} by platelet microsomes. Agents that inhibit the cAMP phosphodiesterase include theophylline, papaverine, and dipyridamole, as well as pentoxifylline and cilostazol. Several prostaglandins stimulate adenylate cyclase, including prostaglandin E_1 (PGE_1), PGD_2, and PGI_2 (prostacyclin). Drugs that elevate cAMP levels are dipyridamole, pentoxifylline, and cilostazol. Dipyridamole can be used alone or in combination with aspirin. A very large study of dipyridamole in combination with low-dose aspirin (25 mg) found the combination equivalently effective to clopidogrel for the secondary prevention of noncardioembolic stroke.[134] Recent systematic reviews have also suggested that the combination of dipyridamole and aspirin is superior to aspirin alone for the prevention of cerebrovascular events.[135]

The other two phosphodiesterase inhibitors (pentoxifylline and cilostazol) are used primarily in patients with peripheral vascular disease. In addition to their inhibitory effect on platelets they may exert a beneficial effect on blood rheology and the microcirculation by increasing red cell deformability, thereby reducing blood viscosity. Cilostazol increases vascular endothelial growth factor levels, which may lead to an increase in collateral circulation. Pentoxifylline inhibits vascular smooth-muscle cell proliferation and collagen synthesis, which may enhance vasodilation.

Cilostazol probably increases walking distance in patients with peripheral vascular disease; its effect on cardiovascular outcomes is unknown.[136] Pentoxifylline probably is an effective treatment for ulcers associated with peripheral vascular disease; however, it is only modestly (if at all) effective for treatment of peripheral vascular disease.[137,138]

ADENOSINE DIPHOSPHATE RECEPTOR BLOCKERS

The third class of platelet inhibitors is the ADP receptor blockers, which include ticlopidine, clopidogrel, and prasugrel. These agents are thienopyridines and they selectively inhibit platelet activation induced by ADP. Hepatic metabolism is necessary for clopidogrel activity and the CYP01A pathway is involved; drugs that affect this pathway may enhance clopidogrel clearance and reduce its activity.[139] There are three ADP receptors on platelet membranes (see Chap. 114), with the thienopyridines inhibiting one of them, the P2Y12 receptor. The inhibition of binding of ADP to the P2Y12 receptor results in inhibition of adenylate cyclase.

In addition to ticlopidine, clopidogrel, and prasugrel, several other direct inhibitors of ADP mediated inactivation of platelets are being studied. These include AZD6140, a reversible ADP receptor blocker and cangrelor, which is a rapidly acting ADP receptor blocker that is administered intravenously.

Ticlopidine was available for clinical use before clopidogrel. The Canadian American Ticlopidine Study was a randomized, placebo-controlled, double-blind study of the efficacy and safety of ticlopidine in patients with recent stroke. The primary outcome efficacy variable was recurrent stroke, myocardial infarction, or vascular death. There was a risk reduction of 30.2 percent with ticlopidine. In terms of safety, there was a 1 percent incidence of severe neutropenia with ticlopidine and 2 percent incidence of skin rash and of diarrhea. A review of four trials of ticlopidine plus aspirin versus oral anticoagulants for coronary stenting showed benefit to the combination in terms of reduced risk of nonfatal myocardial infarction and revascularization at 30 days, combined negative events (mortality, myocardial infarction, revascularization at 30 days), and major bleeding, but increased the risk of thrombocytopenia and neutropenia. Ticlopidine plus aspirin also reduced the risk of stent thrombosis. Strict monitoring of blood cell counts was recommended. Drug reactions included thrombotic thrombocytopenia purpura, thrombocytopenia, marrow aplasia, anemia, pancytopenia, agranulocytosis, and neutropenia. In clinical practice fear of toxicity has largely led ticlopidine to be abandoned in favor of clopidogrel. Recommendations for ticlopidine use have been revised and published.[140,141]

The first clinical trial of clopidogrel was the Clopidogrel Versus Aspirin in Patients at Risk of Ischemic Events (CAPRIE) trial, a large randomized, blinded trial of clopidogrel versus aspirin in 19,000 patients at risk of ischemic events. Patients were enrolled after recent myocardial infarction or stroke or if they had symptomatic peripheral arterial disease. The primary outcome was the occurrence of ischemic stroke, myocardial infarction, or vascular death. With a mean followup of 1.91 years, there was a relative risk reduction of 8.7 percent in the clopidogrel group ($p = 0.043$). No major differences were noted in terms of safety. Neutropenia occurs rarely with clopidogrel.[142]

Clopidogrel is also used in acute coronary syndromes, based on the Clopidogrel in Unstable Angina to Prevent Recurrent Events (CURE) study.[143] The CREDO study also examined aspirin with and without clopidogrel in acute coronary syndromes and showed a consistent benefit of extended treatment with clopidogrel for each component of the composite endpoint of cardiovascular death, myocardial infarction, or stroke. Clopidogrel use is increasing in patients after a first ischemic stroke. Clopidogrel in combination with aspirin is also indicated after coronary stenting, in particular with drug eluting stents. Interested readers are referred to recent guidelines for evidence and recommendations in this rapidly changing therapeutic area. A comprehensive clearinghouse can be found at www.guideline.gov.[132,133,140,141] Patients' degree of platelet inhibition after clopidogrel therapy varies. Larger loading doses of clopidogrel appear to reduce variability in response; the safety and efficacy of such doses are being compared in ongoing studies.[144]

Prasugrel is a "third-generation" P2Y12 blocking agent that is approved in Europe but not in North America. Unlike clopidogrel it can be converted to its active metabolite via esterases present in either the liver or the gut. Like clopidogrel it irreversibly blocks the P2Y12 receptor.[144] Evidence for the use of prasugrel comes predominately from one large study of prasugrel compared with clopidogrel. This study randomized 13,608 patients with moderate-to-high-risk acute coronary syndromes and who were scheduled to undergo percutaneous coronary intervention to receive prasugrel (a 60-mg loading dose and a 10-mg daily maintenance dose) or clopidogrel (a 300-mg loading dose and a 75-mg daily maintenance dose) for up to 15 months.[145] Although prasugrel significantly reduced death from cardiovascular causes, nonfatal myocardial infarction and nonfatal stroke, it significantly increased all forms of bleeding, including major and fatal hemorrhage.

AZD6140 and cangrelor are two additional inhibitors of ADP-mediated platelet activation. Cangrelor is the first parenteral ADP blocker to enter large scale clinical evaluation. It is an ATP analogue that has a very short half-life (less than 10 minutes). After its administration is stopped platelet function returns to normal within 20 minutes. Cangrelor appears to have limited interindividual differences in treatment response and, if proven safe and effective, it would provide the ability to rapidly inhibit and recover platelet function in patients with dynamic thrombotic states. AZD6140 is another investigational antiplatelet agent. It is unique amongst P2Y12 receptor antagonists insofar as it provides reversible inhibition after oral administration without the need for metabolic activation.[144] Both AZD6140 and cangrelor are being evaluated in large phase III clinical trials after promising results in phase II evaluations.

$\alpha_{IIB}\beta_3$ BLOCKERS

Fibrinogen binds specifically and saturably to the surface of activated platelets, and the $\alpha_{IIb}\beta_3$ complex is the fibrinogen receptor. This complex mediates platelet aggregation induced by all physiologic agonists. The critical amino acids on fibrinogen for binding to the $_{IIb}\beta_3$ complex are located in the C-terminal dodecapeptide of the γ chain and an arginine-glycine-aspartic acid (RGD) sequence of the α chain. Of the monoclonal antibodies that have been developed against $\alpha_{IIb}\beta_3$ complex, some react with the complex on resting or activated platelets, whereas others react better after platelets have been activated, for example, by ADP. Fibrinogen binds only to the activated conformation of the receptor $\alpha_{IIb}\beta_3$.

Because monoclonal antibodies against the $\alpha_{IIb}\beta_3$ receptor block platelet aggregation by preventing ligand binding to the receptor, they were introduced as antiplatelet agents. The first two antibodies developed were 10E5 and 7E3, but the latter had better pharmacologic properties. The clinical version of 7E3, called *abciximab*, is the Fab'$_2$ fragment of a chimeric mouse-human antibody. Initial human pharmacodynamic studies were performed in patients with unstable angina and in patients undergoing high-risk coronary angioplasty, and dose-related inhibition of platelet function was found. No spontaneous bleeding was observed, despite prolongation of the template bleeding time. Because of the mouse component of abciximab, it may induce antimouse antibodies, preventing repeated use in patients.

The first large clinical trial of abciximab was the Evaluation of c7E3 for the Prevention of Ischemic Complications (EPIC) trial, published in 1994, in which the drug was used in patients with high-risk coronary angioplasty. Abciximab reduced ischemic events after angioplasty when given together with heparin and aspirin, but it also increased the risk of bleeding. A subsequent study of patients undergoing percutaneous coronary intervention, the Evaluation in PTCA to Improve Long-term Outcome with Abciximab GP IIb/IIIa ($\alpha_{IIb}\beta_3$) Blockade (EPILOG) study, demonstrated efficacy in both low-risk and high-risk patients without any increase in major bleeding.[146,147]

Other types of inhibitors of fibrinogen binding to platelets have also been developed. Those in clinical use are eptifibatide, a cyclic heptapeptide based on a rattlesnake venom peptide, and tirofiban, a non-peptide derivative of tyrosine. Animal studies of eptifibatide were performed in a canine model of coronary thrombosis, showing suppression of platelet-dependent flow reduction. Pharmacokinetic and pharmacodynamic studies in animals and humans showed a rapid onset of action, short plasma half-life, and rapid reversibility of action The pharmacodynamics of eptifibatide are substantially altered by anticoagulants that chelate calcium, and pharmacokinetic modeling suggests that optimal dosing is obtained by giving a second bolus 10 minutes after the first bolus. Eptifibatide is not immunogenic.

The first major clinical trial of eptifibatide was the Integrilin to Minimize Platelet Aggregation and Coronary Thrombosis (IMPACT) II trial in patients undergoing any kind of coronary intervention.[148] There was a highly significant reduction in the composite endpoint of death, myocardial infarction, coronary artery bypass grafting, repeat urgent or emergent coronary intervention, or stent placement for abrupt closure at 24 hours with both eptifibatide dosing arms. There was no increase in major bleeding. The effect was no longer significant at 30 days on intention-to-treat analysis.

Animal studies with tirofiban were performed in dogs. Dose-dependent inhibition of *ex vivo* platelet aggregation was achieved, with rapid reversibility at the end of the infusion. Electrically induced coronary artery thrombosis was markedly reduced by tirofiban infusion, without significant extension of the bleeding time. Pharmacokinetic and pharmacodynamic studies in humans showed that tirofiban provided a well-tolerated reversible means of inhibiting platelet function. Bleeding time was prolonged, and ADP-induced aggregation was blocked by at least 80 percent in normal volunteers. The plasma half-life was 1.6 hours. ADP- and collagen-induced platelet aggregation in normal volunteers returned to 55 percent and 89 percent of baseline, respectively, by 3 hours after the end of infusion. Similar results were found in a dose-ranging study in patients undergoing coronary angioplasty. Based on these results tirofiban has been extensively studied as an adjunct to therapies for patients with, or at risk of, acute coronary syndromes. Clinical results for patients treated with tirofiban have been reviewed.[149]

THROMBIN RECEPTOR BLOCKERS

Platelet activation occurs through a variety of cell surface receptors. The thrombin receptor is a particularly potent platelet activator. SCH 530348 is the first of the thrombin receptor inhibitors to be evaluated in large-scale clinical trials in humans. This drug has shown promise in early phase investigations and is now the subject of two large-scale phase III studies. If successful, this drug will represent a new therapeutic option for the treatment and prevention of atherosclerotic vascular diseases. [144]

COMBINED ANTIPLATELET THERAPY

Potent platelet inhibition is more effectively achieved with combination therapy than with any one agent. As a result, use of multiple antiplatelet agents has become routine in patients with acute coronary syndromes, and in those with coronary stents. In general, these studies found that combination therapy is more effective than monotherapy at a cost of increased bleeding. Agents used in combination therapy include aspirin, dipyridamole, clopidogrel, $\alpha_{IIb}\beta_3$ inhibitors, warfarin, rivaroxaban, and novel agents such as SCH 530348.[150] Combination therapy with aspirin and clopidogrel reduces stent restenosis after percutaneous coronary interventions, and is the standard of practice in this area. Combination therapy with aspirin (162–325 mg daily) and clopidogrel is recommended essentially for all patients with acute coronary syndromes, although the duration of clopidogrel therapy varies and is related to the nature of the patient and the type of intervention.[133] Dual or multiple antiplatelet therapy does not offer advantages over single agents in some settings; thus in selected patients who are at high risk of cerebrovascular disease, combination therapy with aspirin and clopidogrel increases bleeding without a reduction of stroke.[151,152] Triple therapy with warfarin, aspirin, and clopidogrel is also used in some patients, particularly in those patients with atrial fibrillation and coronary artery disease. This therapy has not been tested in large studies but is associated with a significant risk of bleeding. With the advent of novel agents, other combinations of therapy, such as the addition of rivaroxaban to aspirin (with or without clopidogrel), are likely to become more common. Although such combinations may offer increased efficacy, this increase is likely to come at the expense of increased complications including bleeding.

REFERENCES

1. Link KP: The discovery of dicumarol and its sequels. *Circulation* 19:97, 1959.
2. Ansell J, Hirsh J, Hylek E, et al: Pharmacology and management of the vitamin K antagonists: American College of Chest Physicians Evidence-Based Clinical Practice Guidelines (8th edition). *Chest* 133(6 Suppl):160S, 2008.
3. Hirsh J, Fuster V, Ansell J, et al: American Heart Association/American College of Cardiology Foundation guide to warfarin therapy. *Circulation* 107:1692, 2003.
4. Nelsestuen GL, Zytkovicz TH, Howard JB: The mode of action of vitamin K: Identification of gamma-carboxyglutamic acid as a component of prothrombin. *J Biol Chem* 249:6347, 1974.
5. Stenflo I, Fernlund P, Egan W, et al: Vitamin K dependent modifications of glutamic acid residues in prothrombin. *Proc Natl Acad Sci U S A* 71:2730, 1974.
6. Freedman SJ, Blostein MD, Baleja JD, et al: Identification of the phospholipid binding site in the vitamin K-dependent blood coagulation protein factor IX. *J Biol Chem* 271:16227, 1996.

7. Magnusson S, Sottrup-Jensen L, Petersen TE, et al: Primary structure of the vitamin K-dependent part of prothrombin. *FEBS Lett* 44:189, 1974.
8. Whitlon DS, Sadowski JA, Suttie JW: Mechanism of coumarin action: Significance of vitamin K epoxide reductase inhibition. *Biochemistry* 17:1371,1978.
9. Fasco MJ, Hildebrandt EF, Suttie JW: Evidence that warfarin anticoagulant action involves two distinct reductase activities. *J Biol Chem* 257:11210, 1982.
10. Morris DP, Soute BA, Vermeer C, et al: Characterization of the purified vitamin K-dependent gamma-glutamyl carboxylase. *J Biol Chem* 268:8735, 1993.
11. Paul B, Oxley A, Brigham K, et al: Factor II, VII, IX and X concentrations in patients receiving long-term warfarin. *J Clin Pathol* 40:94, 1987.
12. Malhotra OP: Dicoumarol-induced prothrombins containing 6, 7, and 8 gamma-carboxyglutamic acid residues: Isolation and characterization. *Biochem Cell Biol* 67:411, 1989.
13. Ratcliffe JV, Furie B, Furie BC: The importance of specific gamma-carboxyglutamic acid residues in prothrombin. Evaluation by site-specific mutagenesis. *J Biol Chem* 268:24339, 1993.
14. Holbrook AM, Pereira JA, Labiris R, et al: Systematic overview of warfarin and its drug and food interactions. *Arch Intern Med* 165:1095, 2005.
15. Loebstein R, Dvoskin I, Halkin H, et al: A coding VKORC1 Asp36Tyr polymorphism predisposes to warfarin resistance. *Blood* 109:2477, 2007.
16. Harrington DJ, Underwood S, Morse C, et al: Pharmacodynamic resistance to warfarin associated with a Val66Met substitution in vitamin K epoxide reductase complex subunit 2. *Thromb Haemost* 93:23, 2005.
17. Rost S, Fregin A, Ivaskevicious V, et al: Mutations in VKORC1 cause warfarin resistance and multiple coagulation factor deficiency type 2. *Nature* 427:537, 2004.
18. Harrison L, Johnston M, Massicotte MP, et al: Comparison of 5-mg and 10-mg loading doses in initiation of warfarin therapy. *Ann Intern Med* 126:133, 1997.
19. Crowther MA, Ginsberg J, Kearon C, et al: A randomized trial comparing 5 mg and 10 mg warfarin loading doses. *Arch Intern Med* 159:46, 1999.
20. Kovacs MJ, Rodger M, Anderson DR, et al: Comparison of 10-mg and 5-mg warfarin initiation nomograms together with low-molecular-weight heparin for outpatient treatment of acute venous thromboembolism. A randomized, double-blind, controlled trial. *Ann Intern Med* 138:714, 2003.
21. Ageno W, Turpie AGG, Steidl L: Comparison of a daily fixed 2.5 mg warfarin dose with a 5 mg, international normalized ratio adjusted, warfarin dose initially following heart valve replacement. *Am J Cardiol* 88:40, 2001.
22. Loeliger EA, van den Besselaar AM, Lewis SM: Reliability and clinical impact of the normalization of the prothrombin times in oral anticoagulant control. *Thromb Haemost* 53:148, 1985.
23. Kovacs MJ, Wong A, MacKinnon K, et al: Assessment of the validity of the INR system for patients with liver impairment. *Thromb Haemost* 71:727, 1994.
24. Johnston M, Harrison L, Moffat K, et al: Reliability of the international normalized ratio for monitoring the induction phase of warfarin: Comparison with the prothrombin time ratio. *J Lab Clin Med* 128:214, 1996.
25. Siebenhofer A, Berghold A, Sawicki PT: A systematic review of studies of self-management of oral anticoagulation. *Thromb Haemost* 91:225, 2004.
26. Heneghan C, Alonso-Coello P, Garcia-Alamino JM, et al: Self-monitoring of oral anticoagulation: A systematic review and meta-analysis. *Lancet* 367:404, 2006.
27. White RH, McCurdy A, Marensdorff H, et al: Home prothrombin time monitoring after the initiation of warfarin therapy: A randomized, prospective study. *Ann Intern Med* 111:730, 1989.
28. Ansell J, Hasenkam JM, Voller H: Guidelines for implementation of patient self-testing and patient self-management of oral anticoagulation. *Int J Cardiol* 99:37, 2004.
29. Matchar DB, Samsa GP, Cohen SJ, et al: Improving the quality of anticoagulation of patients with atrial fibrillation in managed care organizations: Results of the managing anticoagulation services trial. *Am J Med* 113:42, 2002.
30. Wilson SJ, Wells PS, Kovacs MJ, et al: Comparing the quality of oral anticoagulant management by anticoagulation clinics and by family physicians: A randomized controlled trial. *CMAJ* 169:293, 2003.
31. Gadisseur AP, Breukink-Engbers WG, van der Meer FJ, et al: Comparison of the quality of oral anticoagulant therapy through patient self-management and management by specialized anticoagulation clinics in the Netherlands: A randomized clinical trial. *Arch Intern Med* 163:2639, 2003.
32. Cromheecke ME, Levi M, Colly LP, et al: Oral anticoagulation self-management and management by a specialist anticoagulation clinic: A randomised cross-over comparison. *Lancet* 356:97, 2000.
33. Kaminsky LS, Zhang ZY: Human P450 metabolism of warfarin. *Pharmacol Ther* 73:67, 1997.
34. Yamazaki H, Shimada T: Human liver cytochrome P450 enzymes involved in the 7-hydroxylation of R- and S- warfarin enantiomers. *Biochem Pharmacol* 54:1195, 1997.
35. Veenstra DL, Blough DK, Higashi MK, et al: CYP2C9 haplotype structure in European American warfarin patients and association with clinical outcomes. *Clin Pharmacol Ther* 77:353, 2005.
36. Moridani M, Fy L, Selby R, et al: Frequency of CYP2C9 polymorphisms affecting warfarin metabolism in a large anticoagulant clinic cohort. *Clin Biochem* 39:606, 2006.
37. Crespi CL, Miller VP: The R144C change in the CYP2C9*2 allele alters interaction of the cytochrome P450 with NADPH:cytochrome P450 oxidoreductase. *Pharmacogenetics* 7:203, 1997.
38. Takanashi K, Tainaka H, Kobayashi K, et al: CYP2C9 lie359 and Leu359 variants: Enzyme kinetic study with seven substrates. *Pharmacogenetics* 10:95, 2000.
39. Yasar U, Eliasson E, Dahl ML, et al: Validation of methods for CYP2C9 genotyping: Frequencies of mutant alleles in a Swedish population. *Biochem Biophys Res Commun* 254:628, 1999.
40. D'Andrea G, D'Ambrosio RL, Di Perna P, et al: A polymorphism in the VKORC1 gene is associated with an interindividual variability in the dose-anticoagulant effect of warfarin. *Blood* 105:645, 2005.
41. Rieder MJ, Reiner AP, Gage BG, et al: Effect of VKORC1 haplotypes on transcriptional regulation and warfarin dose. *N Engl J Med* 352:2285, 2005.
42. Higashi MK, Veenstra DL, Kondo LM, et al: Association between CYP2C9 genetic variants and anticoagulation-related outcomes during warfarin therapy. *JAMA* 287:1690, 2002.
43. Sconce EA, Khan TI, Wynne HA, et al: The impact of CYP2C9 and VKORC1 genetic polymorphism and patient characteristics upon warfarin dose requirements: Proposal for a new dosing regimen. *Blood* 106:2329, 2005.
44. Carlquist JF, Horne BD, Muhlestein JB, et al: Genotypes of the cytochrome p450 isoform, CYP2C9, and the vitamin K epoxide reductase complex subunit 1 conjointly determine stable warfarin dose: A prospective study. *J Thromb Thrombolysis* 22:191, 2006.
45. Gage BF, Eby C, Milligan PE: Use of pharmacogenetics and clinical factors to predict the maintenance dose of warfarin. *Thromb Haemost* 91:87, 2004.
46. Anderson JL, Horne BD, Stevens SM, et al: Randomized trial of genotype-guided versus standard warfarin dosing in patients initiating oral anticoagulation. *Circulation* 116:2563, 2007.
47. Schwarz UI, Ritchie MD, Bradford Y, et al: Genetic determinants of response to warfarin during initial anticoagulation. *N Engl J Med* 358:999, 2008.
48. Caldwell MD, Awad T, Johnson JA, et al: CYP4F2 genetic variant alters required warfarin dose. *Blood* 111:4106, 2008.
49. Wadelius M, Chen LY, Lindh JD, et al: The largest prospective warfarin-treated cohort supports genetic forecasting. *Blood* 113:784, 2009.
50. Klein TE, Altman RB, Eriksson N, et al: Estimation of the warfarin dose with clinical and pharmacogenetic data. *N Engl J Med* 360:753, 2009.
51. Schulman S, Beyth RJ, Kearon C, et al: Hemorrhagic complications of anticoagulant and thrombolytic treatment: American College of Chest Physicians Evidence-Based Clinical Practice Guidelines (8th edition). *Chest* 133(6 Suppl):257S, 2008.
52. Sallah S, Thomas DP, Roberts HR: Warfarin and heparin-induced skin necrosis and the purple toe syndrome: Infrequent complications of anticoagulant treatment. *Thromb Haemost* 78:785, 1997.
53. Egred M, Rodrigues E: Purple digit syndrome and warfarin-induced skin necrosis. *Eur J Intern Med* 16:294, 2005.
54. Warkentin TE, Sikov WM, Lillicrap DP: Multicentric warfarin-induced skin necrosis complicating heparin-induced thrombocytopenia [review; 36 refs]. *Am J Hematol* 62:44, 1999.
55. Bates SM, Greer IA, Pabinger I: Venous thromboembolism, thrombophilia, antithrombotic therapy, and pregnancy. *Chest* 133(6 Suppl):845S, 2008.
56. Marik PE, Plane LA: Venous thromboembolic disease and pregnancy. *N Engl J Med* 359:2025, 2008.
57. Ito S: Drug therapy for breast-feeding women. *N Engl J Med* 343:118, 2000.
58. Douketis JD, Berger PB, Dunn AS, et al: The perioperative management of antithrombotic therapy: American College of Chest Physicians Evidence-Based Clinical Practice Guidelines (8th edition). *Chest* 133(6 Suppl):299S, 2008.
59. Dunn AS, Spuropoulos A, Turpie AG: Bridging therapy in patients on long-term oral anticoagulants who require surgery: The Prospective Peri-operative Enoxaparin Cohort Trial (PROSPECT). *J Thromb Haemost* 5:22, 2007.
60. Woods K, Douketis JD, Kathirgamanathan K, et al: Low-dose oral vitamin K to normalize the international normalized ratio prior to surgery in patients who require temporary interruption of warfarin. *J Thromb Thrombolysis* 24:93, 2007.
61. Jaffer AK, Ahmed M, Brotman DJ, et al: Low-molecular-weight-heparins as periprocedural anticoagulation for patients on long-term warfarin therapy: A standardized bridging therapy protocol. *J Thromb Thrombolysis* 20:11, 2005.
62. Spandorfer JM, Lynch S, Weitz HH, et al: Use of enoxaparin for the chronically anticoagulated patient before and after procedures. *Am J Cardiol* 84:478, 1999.
63. Howell WH: Heparin as an anticoagulant. *Am J Physiol* 63:434, 1923.
64. Hirsh J, Bauer KA, Donati MB, et al: Parenteral anticoagulants: American College of Chest Physicians Evidence-Based Clinical Practice Guidelines (8th edition). *Chest* 133(6 Suppl):141S, 2008.
65. Casu B, Oreste P, Torri G, et al: The structure of heparin oligosaccharide fragments with high anti-(factor Xa) activity containing the minimal antithrombin III-binding sequence. Chemical and ^{13}C nuclear-magnetic-resonance studies. *Biochem J* 197:599, 1981.
66. Choay J, Lormeau JC, Petitou M, et al: Structural studies on a biologically active hexasaccharide obtained from heparin. *Ann N Y Acad Sci* 370:644, 1981.
67. Abildgaard U: Highly purified antithrombin 3 with heparin cofactor activity prepared by disc electrophoresis. *Scand J Clin Lab Invest* 21:89, 1968.
68. Rosenberg RD, Damus PS: The purification and mechanism of action of human antithrombin-heparin cofactor. *J Biol Chem* 248:6490, 1973.
69. Lupu C, Poulsen E, Roquefeuil S, et al: Cellular effects of heparin on the production and release of tissue factor pathway inhibitor in human endothelial cells in culture. *Arterioscler Thromb Vasc Biol* 19:2251, 1999.
70. Gori AM, Pepe G, Attanasio M, et al: Tissue factor reduction and tissue factor pathway inhibitor release after heparin administration. *Thromb Haemost* 81:589, 1999.

71. Teitel JM, Rosenberg RD: Protection of factor Xa from neutralization by the heparin-antithrombin complex. *J Clin Invest* 71:1383, 1983.
72. Hogg PJ, Jackson CM: Fibrin monomer protects thrombin from inactivation by heparin- antithrombin III: Implications for heparin efficacy. *Proc Natl Acad Sci U S A* 86:3619, 1989.
73. Weitz JI, Hudoba M, Massel D, et al: Clot-bound thrombin is protected from inhibition by heparin- antithrombin III but is susceptible to inactivation by antithrombin III-independent inhibitors. *J Clin Invest* 86:385, 1990.
74. Tollefsen DM, Majerus DW, Blank MK: Heparin cofactor II: Purification and properties of a heparin-dependent inhibitor of thrombin in human plasma. *J Biol Chem* 257:2162, 1982.
75. Lane DA, Denton J, Flynn AM, et al: Anticoagulant activities of heparin oligosaccharides and their neutralization by platelet factor 4. *Biochem J* 218:725, 1984.
76. Young E, Prins M, Levine MN, et al: Heparin binding to plasma proteins, an important mechanism for heparin resistance. *Thromb Haemost* 67:639, 1992.
77. de Swart CAM, Nijmeyer B, Roelofs JMM, et al: Kinetics of intravenously administered heparin in normal humans. *Blood* 60:1251, 1982.
78. Cruickshank MK, Levine MN, Hirsh J, et al: A standard heparin nomogram for the management of heparin therapy. *Arch Intern Med* 151:333, 1991.
79. Raschke RA, Reilly BM, Guidry JR, et al: The weight-based heparin dosing nomogram compared with a "standard-care" nomogram: A randomized controlled trial. *Ann Intern Med* 119:874, 1993.
80. Levine MN, Hirsh J, Gent M, et al: A randomized trial comparing activated thromboplastin time with heparin assay in patients with acute venous thromboembolism requiring large daily doses of heparin. *Arch Intern Med* 154:49, 1994.
81. Kearon C, Ginsberg JS, Julian JA, et al: Comparison of fixed-dose weight-adjusted unfractionated heparin and low-molecular-weight heparin for acute treatment of venous thromboembolism. *JAMA* 296:935, 2006.
82. Warkentin TE, Greinacher A: *Heparin-induced thrombocytopenia, Third edition.* Marcel Dekker, New York, 2004.
83. Warkentin TE, Greinacher A, Koster A, et al: Treatment and prevention of heparin-induced thrombocytopenia: American College of Chest Physicians Evidence-Based Clinical Practice Guidelines (8th edition). *Chest* 133(6 Suppl):340S, 2008.
84. Weitz JI: Low-molecular-weight heparins. *N Engl J Med* 337:688, 1997.
85. Lim W, Dentali F, Eikelboom JW, et al: Meta-analysis: Low-molecular-weight heparin and bleeding in patients with severe renal insufficiency. *Ann Intern Med* 144:673, 2006.
86. Van Ryn-McKenna J, Cai L, Ofosu FA, et al: Neutralization of enoxaparin-induced bleeding by protamine sulfate. *Thromb Haemost* 63:271, 1990.
87. Rajgopal R, Bear M, Butcher MK, et al: The effects of heparin and low molecular weight heparins on bone. *Thromb Res* 122:293, 2008.
88. Boneu B, Necciari J, Cariou R, et al: Pharmacokinetics and tolerance of the natural pentasaccharide (SR90107/Org31540) with high affinity to antithrombin III in man. *Thromb Haemost* 74:1468, 1995.
89. Donat F, Duret JP, Santoni A, et al: The pharmacokinetics of fondaparinux sodium in healthy volunteers. *Clin Pharmacokinet* 41 Suppl 2:1, 2002.
90. Mehta SR, Granger CB, Eikelboom JW, et al: Efficacy and safety of fondaparinux versus enoxaparin in patients with acute coronary syndromes undergoing percutaneous coronary intervention: Results from the OASIS-5 trial. *J Am Coll Cardiol* 50:1742, 2007.
91. Amiral J, Lormeau JC, Marfaing-Koka A, et al: Absence of cross-reactivity of SR90107A/ORG31540 pentasaccharide with antibodies to heparin-PF4 complexes developed in heparin-induced thrombocytopenia. *Blood Coagul Fibrinolysis* 8:114, 1997.
92. Elalamy I, Lecrubier C, Potevin F, et al: Absence of *in vitro* cross-reaction of pentasaccharide with the plasma heparin-dependent factor of twenty-five patients with heparin-associated thrombocytopenia. *Thromb Haemost* 74:1384, 1995.
93. Parody R, Oliver A, Souto JC, et al: Fondaparinux (ARIXTRA) as an alternative anti-thrombotic prophylaxis when there is hypersensitivity to slow molecular weight and unfractionated heparins. *Haematologica* 88:ECR32, 2003.
94. Cardot JM, Lefevre GY, Godbillon JA: Pharmacokinetics of rec-hirudin in healthy volunteers after intravenous administration. *J Pharmacokinet Biopharm* 22:147, 1994.
95. Zoldhelyi P, Webster MW, Fuster V, et al: Recombinant hirudin in patients with chronic, stable coronary artery disease. Safety, half-life, and effect on coagulation parameters. *Circulation* 88:2015, 1993.
96. Verstraete M, Nurmohamed M, Kienast J, et al: Biologic effects of recombinant hirudin (CGP 39393) in human volunteers. European Hirudin in Thrombosis Group. *J Am Coll Cardiol* 22:1080, 1993.
97. Tripodi A, Chantarangkul V, Arbini AA, et al: Effects of hirudin on activated partial thromboplastin time determined with ten different re-agents. *Thromb Haemost* 70:286, 1993.
98. Potzsch B, Hund S, Madlener K, et al: Monitoring of recombinant hirudin: Assessment of a plasma-based ecarin clotting time assay. *Thromb Res* 86:373, 1997.
99. Huhle G, Hoffmann U, Song X, et al: Immunologic response to recombinant hirudin in HIT type II patients during long-term treatment. *Br J Haematol* 106:195, 1999.
100. Huhle G, Liebe V, Hudek R, et al: Anti-r-hirudin antibodies reveal clinical relevance through direct functional inactivation of r-hirudin or prolongation of r-hirudin's plasma half-life. *Thromb Haemost* 86:936, 2001.
101. Song X, Huhle G, Wang L, et al: Generation of anti-hirudin antibodies in heparin-induced thrombocytopenic patients treated with r-hirudin. *Circulation* 100:1528, 1999.
102. Eichler P, Friesen HJ, Lubenow N, et al: Antihirudin antibodies in patients with heparin-induced thrombocytopenia treated with lepirudin: Incidence, effects on aPTT, and clinical relevance. *Blood* 96:2373, 2000.
103. Maraganore JM, Bourdon P, Jablonski J, et al: Design and characterization of hirulogs: A novel class of bivalent peptide inhibitors of thrombin. *J Clin Invest* 29:7095, 1990.
104. Fox I, Dawson A, Loynds P, et al: Anticoagulant activity of Hirulog, a direct thrombin inhibitor, in humans. *Thromb Haemost* 69:157, 1993.
105. Warkentin TE, Grenacher A, Koster A: Bivalirudin. *Thromb Haemost* 99:830, 2008.
106. Kikumoto R, Tamao Y, Tezuka T, et al: Selective inhibition of thrombin by (2R, 4R)-4-methyl-1-[N2-[(3-methyl-1,2,3,4-tetrahydro-8-quinolinyl+++)sulfony1]-1-arginyl)]-2-piperidinecarboxylic acid. *Biochemistry* 23:85, 1984.
107. Berry CN, Girardot C, Lecoffre C, et al: Effects of the synthetic thrombin inhibitor argatroban on fibrin- or clot-incorporated thrombin: Comparison with heparin and recombinant Hirudin. *Thromb Haemost* 72:381, 1994.
108. Hursting MJ, Alford KL, Becker JC, et al: Novastan (brand of argatroban): A small-molecule, direct thrombin inhibitor. *Semin Thromb Hemost* 23:503, 1997.
109. McKeage K, Plosker GL: Argatroban [review; 36 refs]. *Drugs* 61:515, 2001.
110. Swan SK, Hursting MJ: The pharmacokinetics and pharmacodynamics of argatroban: Effects of age, gender, and hepatic or renal dysfunction. *Pharmacotherapy* 20:318, 2000.
111. Gosselin RC, Dager WE, King JH, et al: Effect of direct thrombin inhibitors, bivalirudin, lepirudin, and argatroban, on prothrombin time and INR values. *Am J Clin Pathol* 121:593, 2004.
112. Gross PL, Weitz JI: New anticoagulants for treatment of venous thromboembolism. *Arterioscler Thromb Vasc Biol* 28:380, 2008.
113. Blech S, Ebner T, Ludwig-Schwellinger E, et al: The metabolism and disposition of the oral direct thrombin inhibitor, dabigatran, in humans. *Drug Metab Dispos* 36:386, 2008.
114. Stangier J, Stahle H, Rathgen K, et al: Pharmacokinetics and pharmacodynamics of the direct oral thrombin inhibitor dabigatran in healthy elderly subjects. *Clin Pharmacokinet* 47:47, 2008.
115. Wienen W, Stassen JM, Priepke H, et al: *In-vitro* profile and *ex-vivo* anticoagulant activity of the direct thrombin inhibitor dabigatran and its orally active prodrug, dabigatran etexilate. *Thromb Haemost* 98:155, 2007.
116. Wienen W, Stassen JM, Priepke H, et al: Effects of the direct thrombin inhibitor dabigatran and its orally active prodrug, dabigatran etexilate, on thrombus formation and bleeding time in rats. *Thromb Haemost* 98:333, 2007.
117. Eriksson BI, Dahl OE, Rosencher N, et al: Dabigatran etexilate versus enoxaparin for prevention of venous thromboembolism after total hip replacement: A randomised, double-blind, non-inferiority trial. *Lancet* 370:949, 2007.
118. Eriksson BI, Dahl OE, Rosencher N, et al: Oral dabigatran etexilate vs. subcutaneous enoxaparin for the prevention of venous thromboembolism after total knee replacement: The RE-MODEL randomized trial. *J Thromb Haemost* 5:2178, 2007.
119. Ginsberg JS, Davidson BL, Comp PC, et al: Oral thrombin inhibitor dabigatran etexilate vs North American enoxaparin regimen for prevention of venous thromboembolism after knee arthroplasty surgery. *J Arthroplasty* 24:1, 2009.
120. Kubitza D, Becka M, Wensing G, et al: Safety, pharmacodynamics, and pharmacokinetics of BAY 59–7939—an oral, direct Factor Xa inhibitor—after multiple dosing in healthy male subjects. *Eur J Clin Pharmacol* 61:873, 2005.
121. Lassen MR, Ageno W, Borris LC, et al: Rivaroxaban versus enoxaparin for thromboprophylaxis after total knee arthroplasty. *N Engl J Med* 358:2776, 2008.
122. Agnelli G, Gallus A, Goldhaber SZ, et al: Treatment of proximal deep-vein thrombosis with the oral direct factor Xa inhibitor rivaroxaban (BAY 59–7939): The ODIXa-DVT (Oral Direct Factor Xa Inhibitor BAY 59–7939 in Patients With Acute Symptomatic Deep-Vein Thrombosis) study. *Circulation* 116:180, 2007.
123. Eriksson BI, Borris LC, Friedman RJ, et al: Rivaroxaban versus enoxaparin for thromboprophylaxis after hip arthroplasty. *N Engl J Med* 358:2765, 2008.
124. Kakkar AK, Brenner B, Dahl OE, et al: Extended duration rivaroxaban versus short-term enoxaparin for the prevention of venous thromboembolism after total hip arthroplasty: A double-blind, randomized controlled trial. *Lancet*, 372:31, 2008.
125. Buller HR, Lensing AW, Prins MH, et al: A dose-ranging study evaluating once-daily oral administration of the factor Xa inhibitor rivaroxaban in the treatment of patients with acute symptomatic deep vein thrombosis: the Einstein-DVT Dose-Ranging Study. *Blood* 112:2242, 2008.
126. Hilleman DE, Dunlay RW, Packard KA: Reteplase for dysfunctional hemodialysis catheter clearance. *Pharmacotherapy* 23:137, 2003.
127. Van de Werf FJ, Topol EJ, Sobel BE: The impact of fibrinolytic therapy for ST-segment-elevation acute myocardial infarction. *J Thromb Haemost* 7:14, 2009.
128. Effectiveness of intravenous thrombolytic treatment in acute myocardial infarction. Gruppo Italiano per lo Studio della Streptochinasi nell'Infarto Miocardico (GISSI). *Lancet* 1:397, 1986.
129. Simpson D, Siddiqui MA, Scott LJ, et al: Spotlight on reteplase in thrombotic occlusive disorders. *BioDrugs* 21:65, 2007.
130. Singer DE, Albers GW, Dalen JE, et al: Antithrombotic therapy in atrial fibrillation: American College of Chest Physicians Evidence-Based Clinical Practice Guidelines (8th edition). *Chest* 133(6 Suppl):546S, 2008.
131. Gurbel PA, Bliden KP, DiChiara J, et al: Evaluation of dose-related effects of aspirin on platelet function: Results from the Aspirin-Induced Platelet Effect (ASPECT) Study. *Circulation* 115:3156, 2007.
132. Sacco RL, Adams R, Albers G, et al: Guidelines for prevention of stroke in patients with ischemic stroke or transient ischemic attack: A statement for healthcare professionals from the American Heart Association/American Stroke Association Council on Stroke: Co-sponsored by the Council on Cardiovascular Radiology and Interven-

tion: The American Academy of Neurology affirms the value of this guideline. *Stroke* 37:577, 2006.
133. Antman EM, Hand M, Armstrong PW, et al: 2007 Focused update of the ACC/AHA 2004 guidelines for the management of patients with st-elevation myocardial infarction: A report of the American College of Cardiology/American Heart Association Task Force on Practice Guidelines: Developed in collaboration with the Canadian Cardiovascular Society endorsed by the American Academy of Family Physicians: 2007 Writing Group to Review New Evidence and Update the ACC/AHA 2004 guidelines for the management of patients with st-elevation myocardial infarction, writing on behalf of the 2004 Writing Committee. *Circulation* 117:296, 2008.
134. Sacco RL, Diener HC, Yusuf S, et al: Aspirin and extended-release dipyridamole versus clopidogrel for recurrent stroke. *N Engl J Med* 359:1238, 2008.
135. Verro P, Gorelick PB, Nguyen D: Aspirin plus dipyridamole versus aspirin for prevention of vascular events after stroke or TIA: A meta-analysis. *Stroke* 39:1358, 2008.
136. Robless P, Mikhailidis DP, Stansby GP: Cilostazol for peripheral arterial disease. *Cochrane Database Syst Rev* CD003748, 2008.
137. Jull A, Arroll B, Parag V, et al: Pentoxifylline for treating venous leg ulcers. *Cochrane Database Syst Rev* CD001733, 2007.
138. Moher D, Pham B, Ausejo M, et al: Pharmacological management of intermittent claudication: A meta-analysis of randomised trials. *Drugs* 59:1057, 2000.
139. Juurlink DN, Gomes T, Ko DT, et al: A population-based study of the drug interaction between proton pump inhibitors and clopidogrel. *CMAJ* 180:713, 2009.
140. Becker RC, Meade TW, Berger PB, et al: The primary and secondary prevention of coronary artery disease: American College of Chest Physicians Evidence-Based Clinical Practice Guidelines (8th edition). *Chest* 133(6 Suppl):776S, 2008.
141. Albers GW, Amarenco P, Easton JD, et al: Antithrombotic and thrombolytic therapy for ischemic stroke: American College of Chest Physicians Evidence-Based Clinical Practice Guidelines (8th edition). *Chest* 133(6 Suppl):630S, 2008.
142. The CAPRIE steering committee: A randomised, blinded, trial of clopidogrel versus aspirin in patients at high risk of ischaemic events (CAPRIE). *Lancet* 348:1329, 1996.
143. Fox KA, Mehta SR, Peters R, et al: Benefits and risks of the combination of clopidogrel and aspirin in patients undergoing surgical revascularization for non-ST-elevation acute coronary syndrome: The Clopidogrel in Unstable Angina to Prevent Recurrent Ischemic Events (CURE) Trial. *Circulation* 110:1202, 2004.
144. Sabatine MS: Novel antiplatelet strategies in acute coronary syndromes. *Cleve Clin J Med* 76:S8, 2009.
145. Wiviott SD, Braunwald E, McCabe CH, et al: Prasugrel versus clopidogrel in patients with acute coronary syndromes. *N Engl J Med* 357:2001, 2007.
146. Anonymous: Use of a monoclonal antibody directed against the platelet glycoprotein IIb/IIIa receptor in high-risk coronary angioplasty. The EPIC Investigation [see comments]. *N Engl J Med* 330:956, 1994.
147. The EPILOG investigators: Platelet glycoprotein IIb/IIIa receptor Blockade and Low-dose heparin during percutaneous coronary revascularization. *N Engl J Med* 336:1689, 1997.
148. Anonymous: Randomised placebo-controlled trial of effect of eptifibatide on complications of percutaneous coronary intervention: IMPACT-II: Integrilin to Minimise Platelet Aggregation and Coronary Thrombosis-II: *Lancet* 349:1422, 1997.
149. van 't Hof AW, Valgimigli M: Defining the role of platelet glycoprotein receptor inhibitors in STEMI: Focus on tirofiban. *Drugs* 69:85, 2009.
150. Witkowski A, Maciejewski P, Wasek W, et al: Influence of different antiplatelet treatment regimens for primary percutaneous coronary intervention on all-cause mortality. *Eur Heart J* 30:1687,2009.
151. Hart RG: What's new in stroke? The top 10 studies of 2006–2008. Part II. *Pol Arch Med Wewn* 118:747, 2008.
152. Hart RG: What's new in stroke? The top 10 studies of 2006–2008. Part I. *Pol Arch Med Wewn* 118:650, 2008.

CHAPTER 24

PRINCIPLES OF IMMUNE CELL THERAPY

Carolina Berger and Stanley R. Riddell

SUMMARY

Antigen-specific T cells, which recognize processed fragments of proteins presented in association with major histocompatibility complex molecules, represent an important component of the host response to pathogens and tumors. Adoptive T-cell therapy, in which T cells are administered to augment or establish an immune response, shows efficacy for the treatment of infectious and malignant diseases. The clinical application of T-cell transfer has been facilitated by identification of target antigens expressed by viruses and tumors, improved strategies for the isolation and genetic engineering of antigen-specific T cells with intrinsic qualities that enable their persistence *in vivo*, and the recognition that transferring T cells into a lymphopenic environment improves the efficiency of cell transfer and treatment efficacy. The development of cell based vaccines that can elicit a tumor-reactive T-cell response *in vivo* to treat cancer remains an area of investigation. Dendritic cells (DCs) are specialized antigen-presenting cells that elicit and regulate specific T-cell responses. Strategies that employ DCs that have taken up tumor antigens *in vitro* as vaccines or that target antigen to DCs *in vivo* to elicit a response are being investigated. Insight into the obstacles to routinely achieving an effective antitumor response either by T-cell therapy or vaccination have been derived from careful analysis of clinical trials, and it is likely that further development of immune cell therapy will be combined with interventions that target specific regulatory or inhibitory pathways.

ADOPTIVE CELLULAR THERAPY OF VIRAL DISEASES

Two broad subsets of antigen-specific T cells cooperate to terminate acute viral infections and control reactivation of latent viruses. CD8+ cytotoxic T lymphocytes (CTLs) recognize viral peptides presented by major histocompatibility complex (MHC) class I molecules and lyse infected cells, and produce inflammatory cytokines. CD4+ T-helper (Th) cells recognize viral peptides presented by class II MHC molecules and produce cytokines that amplify T-cell responses or promote B-cell proliferation and antibody production. A deficiency of CD8+ and CD4+ T cells occurs after allogeneic hematopoietic stem cell transplantation (HSCT) as a consequence of the administration of intensive chemoradiotherapy, anti–T-cell monoclonal antibodies (mAbs), and/or immunosuppressive drugs, and these patients are at risk for life-threatening viral infection.[1] T-cell therapy for human viruses requires knowledge of the antigens presented by infected cells, strategies for isolating and propagating T cells of the appropriate phenotype and specificity, and methods for monitoring the *in vivo* activity of transferred cells (Fig. 24–1). Clinical trials have now established that adoptive T-cell therapy has antiviral activity against cytomegalovirus (CMV), Epstein-Barr virus (EBV), and adenovirus infection in immunocompromised allogeneic HSCT recipients.

Acronyms and abbreviations that appear in this chapter include: APC, antigen-presenting cell; cDNA, complementary DNA; CML, chronic myelogenous leukemia; CMV, cytomegalovirus; CTL, cytotoxic T lymphocyte; DC, dendritic cell; EBV, Epstein-Barr virus; GVHD, graft-versus-host disease; GVL, graft-versus-leukemia; HSCT, hematopoietic stem cell transplantation; LPD, lymphoproliferative disease; mAbs, monoclonal antibodies; mHAgs, minor histocompatibility antigens; MHC, major histocompatability complex; PBMC, peripheral blood mononuclear cells; SNP, single nucleotide polymorphism; TCR, T-cell receptor; Th, T helper; TIL, tumor-infiltrating lymphocyte.

T-CELL THERAPY OF CYTOMEGALOVIRUS INFECTION

CMV is a DNA virus that infects many cell types *in vivo*, including hematopoietic progenitors, monocytes, and endothelium. To evade complete elimination by host immunity, CMV encodes proteins that interfere with antigen presentation in cells that are replicating virus, and establishes latency in a subset of infected cells.[2] Normal CMV+ individuals maintain high levels of CD8+ and CD4+ T cells that are specific for CMV antigens, and these responses are essential to control infection.[3–5] CMV frequently reactivates in individuals with a T-cell immunodeficiency, such as after allogeneic HSCT and solid-organ transplantation, and contributes to morbidity and mortality. Lymphocytopenia and a deficiency of functional CMV-specific T cells persist for several months in many HSCT recipients, and CMV reactivation is frequent.[6] The administration of ganciclovir or foscarnet to treat viral reactivation reduces CMV disease early after HSCT, but disease may occur later when antiviral drugs are discontinued.[6–8] Thus, suppression of CMV replication with antiviral drugs provides only temporary control of reactivation, and restoration of immune function is essential to contain CMV infection.

Target Antigens for Cytomegalovirus-Specific T Cells

Studies of the specificity of CMV-specific T cells isolated from immunocompetent CMV seropositive individuals have identified antigens to target in T-cell therapy. The majority of CD8+ CTLs elicited by *in vitro* stimulation with autologous CMV-infected cells are specific for virion proteins, including the pp65 and pp150 matrix proteins that are introduced into the cytoplasm of cells immediately following viral entry and are rapidly processed and presented for T-cell recognition. CTLs specific for pp65 and pp150 can lyse infected cells before class I MHC is down-regulated by viral immune evasion genes.[9] Although virion proteins are important targets for CD8+ T cells, stimulation of blood mononuclear cells (PBMC) from normal CMV+ donors with panels of CMV peptides or with cells infected with a CMV strain that is deleted of the immune evasion genes identified a significant CD8+ T-cell response to intermediate-early (IE) or early (E) viral proteins.[3,4] IE and E are not efficiently presented to T cells *in vitro* by cells replicating wild-type CMV, but evidence from a murine model suggests that IE-specific T cells recognize cells that are reactivating CMV from latency.[10] Thus, reconstitution of responses both to virion and IE or E antigens may be necessary to restore control of both the latent and replicating pools of virus in immunodeficient hosts.

CD4+ Th cells are required for optimal CD8+ CTL cell responses and may eliminate CMV-infected cells that express class II MHC *in vivo*. The specificity of the CD4+ Th cell response to CMV is not as well characterized as for CD8+ T cells. Studies using recombinant CMV proteins or peptide panels have identified CD4+ T cell responses to pp65, IE-1, glycoprotein B, and the major capsid protein (UL86) in normal CMV+ individuals.[3,11,12]

Techniques for Isolation and Adoptive Transfer of CMV-Specific T Cells

The application of T-cell therapy for CMV in allogeneic HSCT recipients required the development of approaches to reliably isolate CMV-specific

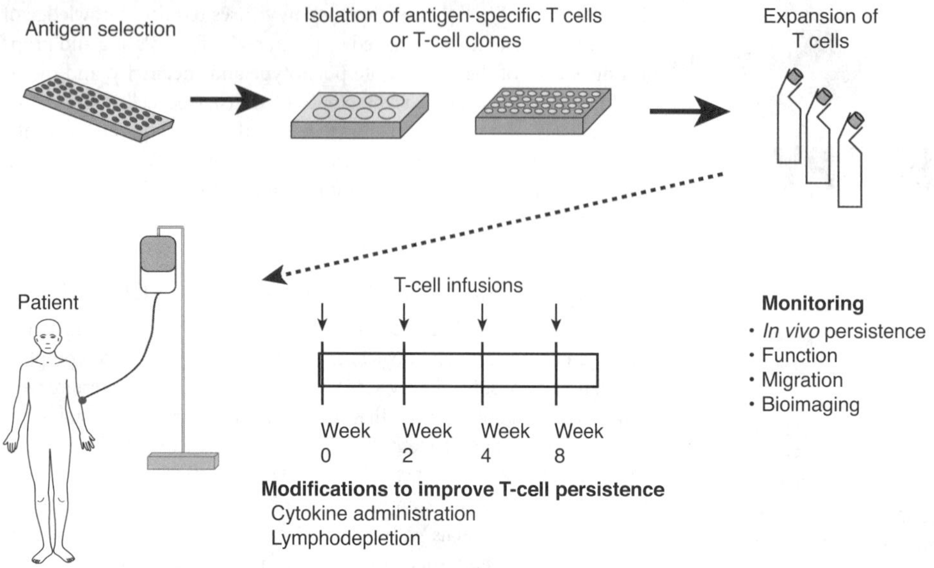

FIGURE 24–1. Scheme for adoptive T-cell therapy with antigen-specific T cells. T cells are selected based on antigen specificity, phenotype, and function, and expanded by *in vitro* culture. Patients receiving T cells are monitored after each cell infusion for toxicity, persistence, and migration of transferred cells and for efficacy.

T cells from the stem cell donor, and to remove potentially alloreactive T cells that could cause graft-versus-host disease (GVHD). The first clinical trial of T-cell therapy employed CD8+ CMV-specific T-cell clones that were isolated and expanded by *in vitro* culture of donor lymphocytes with autologous CMV-infected fibroblasts.[13] The T-cell clones were screened to exclude reactivity with noninfected recipient cells prior to adoptive transfer, making it unlikely that therapy would cause GVHD. In a phase I study, 14 allogeneic HSCT recipients received four escalating weekly doses ($3.3 \times 10^7 - 1 \times 10^9/m^2$) of CD8+ CMV-specific CTL clones as prophylaxis for CMV disease. The treatment did not cause toxicity or exacerbate GVHD. In 11 patients who were deficient in CTL responses immediately prior to infusion, CMV-specific cytolytic activity was increased after therapy to levels equivalent to those in the donor.[14] Transferred CTLs were detected for more than 12 weeks after infusion, but the magnitude of the response declined in the subset of patients who did not recover endogenous CD4+ CMV-specific Th-cell responses, suggesting that CD4+ Th cells may be required for CD8+ T-cell persistence.[14] None of the 14 patients developed CMV viremia or disease, which in the absence of antiviral drug therapy was expected to occur approximately 50 percent or 40 percent of these patients, respectively.[14]

The results of the initial trial of adoptive T-cell therapy for CMV suggested this approach can provide an alternative to antiviral drugs for controlling CMV infection in HSCT recipients. More efficient culture methods have now been developed for isolating T cells for therapy that circumvents the use of live virus and dermal fibroblasts as antigen-presenting cells (APCs), improvements that have enabled broader application of this approach.[15,16] Clinical trials of T-cell therapy with polyclonal CD4+ or CD8+ T cells, or both CD4+ and CD8+ T cells, have been performed at several centers, and the results confirm the efficacy of adoptive therapy for CMV (Table 24–1).[15,17–20] Moreover, very low doses (10^5/kg) of polyclonal CMV-specific CD4+ and CD8+ T cells infused early after HSCT result in a dramatic *in vivo* expansion of CMV-specific T cells and prevention of subsequent CMV reactivation.[15,20] These patients were severely lymphopenic at the time the CMV-specific T cells were infused because an anti-T cell MAb was given prior to transplantation as part of the conditioning regimen. Thus, the *in vivo* proliferation of CMV-specific T cells may have been promoted in part by homeostatic mechanisms that operate in lymphopenia to restore T-cell numbers.

T-CELL THERAPY OF EPSTEIN-BARR VIRUS INFECTION

EBV infection occurs in more than 90 percent of individuals in the United States and can cause an infectious mononucleosis syndrome (see Chap. 84), but is commonly not clinically apparent, as the virus is rapidly contained by the normal host immune response. However, EBV is never completely

TABLE 24–1. Adoptive T-Cell Therapy for Viral Infection after Allogeneic Stem Cell Transplant

Virus	No. of Patients	Trial Design	Cell Phenotype and Dose	Antiviral Activity	Ref.
CMV	14	Prophylaxis	$CD8^+$ T cell clones (3.3×10^7–$1\times109/m^2$)	No CMV disease	14
CMV	16	Post viral reactivation	$CD8^+$ and $CD4^+$ polyclonal ($.2\times10^5$–1×10^5/kg)	2/16 patients had subsequent reactivation	15
CMV	9	Post viral reactivation	$CD8^+$ tetramer selected (1.7×10^3–3.3×10^4/kg)	Reduction in viremia, no CMV disease	20
CMV	8	Persistent viremia	$CD4^+$ and $CD8^+$ polyclonal ($10^7/m^2$)	Decreased viral load in 6/8 patients	19
CMV	12	Prophylaxis	$CD4^+$ and $CD8^+$ polyclonal ($2\times10^7/m^2$)	Low titer reactivation in 4/12 patients, no CMV disease	17
EBV	10	Prophylaxis or treatment	$CD4^+$ and $CD8^+$ polyclonal (10^7–$10^8/m^2$)	Resolution of viremia and LPD (1 patient)	31
EBV	39	Prophylaxis	$CD4^+$ and $CD8^+$ polyclonal (10^7–$10^8/m^2$)	No EBV LPD (expected incidence 11%)	33
EBV, CMV, Adenovirus	11	Prophylaxis or treatment	Multispecific $CD4^+$ and $CD8^+$ (5×10^6–$10^8/m^2$)	Antiviral activity against all three viruses	18
Adenovirus	9	Treatment	$CD4^+$ and $CD8^+$ (1.2–5×10^3/kg)	Clearance of virus in 5/6 patients	39

cleared and persists in a latent form in B lymphocytes. Some latently infected B cells express only the EBNA-1 protein, which has glycine-alanine repeats that inhibit its translation and processing for presentation to CD8+ T cells.[21] Infected B cells may activate the latency III program of viral genes that includes EBNA-1, EBNA-2, EBNA-3A, EBNA-3B, EBNA-3C, LMP-1, LMP-2A, and LMP-2B, and which induce cell proliferation.[22] EBV-specific CD8+ and CD4+ T cells are essential to prevent the growth of EBV+ B cells in immunocompetent hosts.[23] Thus, tumors comprised of proliferating EBV+ B cells can arise in individuals with a T-cell deficiency.

Retrospective analysis showed that allogeneic HSCT recipients who received a transplant from a partially human leukocyte antigen (HLA)-matched relative or an unrelated donor were at high risk of EBV-lymphoproliferative disease (LPD) because of the severe immunodeficiency caused by T-cell depletion to prevent GVHD, or intensive immunosuppression administered to treat GVHD.[24] Solid-organ graft recipients are also at risk for EBV-LPD, particularly those who require anti–T-cell mAbs to treat graft rejection. Historically, patients with EBV-LPD have had a grave prognosis, responding poorly to both antiviral drug therapy and chemotherapy. Treatment with mAb specific for B-cell molecules, such as CD20, can be effective, particularly if accompanied by a reduction in immunosuppressive drugs.[25] However, restoration of EBV-specific T cells is critical for long-term control of the virus infection.

Target Antigens for Epstein-Barr Virus-Specific T Cells

The CD8+ CTL response to EBV infection in normal hosts is mainly directed against lytic viral proteins and the EBNA-3A, -3B, and -3C latency proteins.[26] The CD4+ Th-cell response to EBV is similarly directed against both lytic and latent EBV antigens, and may contribute to eliminating class II MHC+ EBV-infected cells *in vivo*.[27] A quantitative deficiency of EBV-specific CTLs frequently exists in the first 6 months after allogeneic HSCT, and is especially severe if T-cell depletion is used as part of the conditioning regimen.[28] This deficiency of EBV-specific T cells allows the unimpeded lytic infection of memory B cells that can spread to additional B cells, some of which may activate the latency III program and undergo proliferation characteristic of LPD.[29]

Techniques for Isolation and Adoptive Transfer of EBV-Specific T Cells

The efficacy of T-cell therapy for EBV-LPD was first demonstrated in a study in which unselected donor lymphocytes were administered to five patients with EBV-LPD after T-cell–depleted allogeneic HSCT. A dose of approximately 1×10^6 CD3+ T cells/kg was infused because of the concern that higher T-cell doses would cause severe GVHD. This treatment resulted in complete resolution of EBV-LPD in all patients.[30] Unfortunately, therapy was complicated by fatal respiratory failure in two patients with EBV-LPD involving the lungs, and all the patients developed GVHD, which suggested that future studies should focus on selection of EBV-specific T cells for therapy to avoid transferring alloreactive T cells.[30]

In vitro culture techniques have been developed to generate EBV-specific T-cell lines from allogeneic HSCT donors using autologous EBV-lymphoblastoid cell lines (LCLs) for stimulation. The T-cell lines become oligoclonal and highly EBV-specific after repeated stimulations *in vitro* and are depleted of alloreactive T cells that cause GVHD. The adoptive transfer of such EBV-specific T-cell lines was effective in 2 of 3 HSCT recipients with established EBV-LPD without causing GVHD.[31] One patient had progressive LPD despite T-cell infusions; analysis of this patient's tumor revealed a mutation in the EBNA-3B gene that eliminated the region encoding the epitopes targeted by the major CTL response in the T-cell line.[32] This finding illustrates the problem of targeting only a few antigenic epitopes, particularly when treating a large tumor burden that may contain escape variants.

Prophylactic infusion of EBV-specific T cells should diminish the probability that escape variants would emerge. A subsequent study administered donor EBV-specific T-cell lines to patients at risk for EBV-LPD after T-cell–depleted allogeneic HSCT.[33] No GVHD was observed, and this strategy was highly effective in preventing EBV-LPD. Based on historical controls, LPD was expected to occur in 14 percent of the patients, but there were no cases of LPD in the treated cohort.[33] A subset of patients exhibited rising plasma EBV DNA before the T cells were administered, and the viral load promptly declined after T-cell therapy. A second study administered EBV-specific CTLs to recipients of T-cell–depleted HSCT only after high EBV-DNA levels had developed. A reduction of EBV DNA was observed in 4 of 5 recipients, whereas 1 patient, who received a T-cell line that lacked an EBV-specific component, progressed to EBV-LPD.[34] Thus, transfer of EBV-specific T cells safely and rapidly reconstituted immunity, mediated antiviral activity, and protected the majority of patients from EBV-LPD (see Table 24–1).

T-CELL THERAPY OF ADENOVIRUS INFECTION

Adenovirus infection is a serious complication of allogeneic HSCT, particularly in pediatric recipients who receive a T-cell depleted stem cell graft, and is not adequately controlled with available antiviral drugs.[35] There is inferential evidence that T-cell immunity is critical for protection against adenovirus infection,[36] which has encouraged several groups to pursue the development of specific adoptive T-cell therapy. There are a large number of adenovirus serotypes, and a key issue is to identify broadly conserved T-cell epitopes. Target antigens encoded by adenovirus are now being defined, with most attention focused on the abundant hexon virion protein.[37,38] Preliminary reports of adoptive T-cell therapy for adenovirus infection are encouraging. Feuchtinger and colleagues used γ-interferon capture techniques to isolate adenovirus-specific CD8+ and CD4+ T cells from the transplant donor, and demonstrated that infusion of such T cells correlated with a decrease in viral load.[39] Leen and associates used a culture method in which a recombinant adenovirus that encodes the CMV pp65 protein is used to infect EBV-LCL for use in stimulating T cells from HSCT donors.[18] This culture method results in the simultaneous expansion of T cells specific for adenovirus, CMV, and EBV, and the infusion of such T cells into HSCT recipients augmented T-cell responses to all three viruses and promoted virus clearance.

MONITORING PERSISTENCE, FUNCTION, AND MIGRATION OF VIRUS-SPECIFIC T CELLS AFTER ADOPTIVE THERAPY

Transferred T cells must persist as functional memory T cells and migrate to sites of virus replication to be effective. Methods based on functional or structural properties of T cells have been developed for tracking transferred T cells in the blood. In the study of adoptive therapy with CD8+ CMV-specific T-cell clones, assays of cytolytic activity provided a semiquantitative analysis of T-cell function.[14] New approaches that use flow cytometry after staining of blood samples with HLA tetramers folded with viral peptides or intracellular staining to detect cytokines produced after antigen stimulation can now be employed to enumerate and analyze the function of cells on a single-cell level.[4] Endogenous or introduced genetic markers can also be useful for tracking transferred T cells *in vivo*. The unique DNA sequences of the rearranged T-cell receptor (TCR) $V\alpha$ or $V\beta$ genes were used to evaluate survival of transferred T cells in the first trial of CMV-specific T-cell therapy.[14] Real-time polymerase chain reaction with TCR-specific primers that flank the unique CDR3 sequence can provide precise quantitation of transferred T cells in blood samples.

Monitoring the trafficking of virus-specific T cells to tissue sites is a more formidable problem. A retrovirus encoding the neomycin phosphotransferase gene (*neo*) was introduced into a subset of the infused EBV-specific T cells to provide a genetic marker. This enables investigators to monitor for persistence and migration of the transferred cells. *Neo*+ T cells were detected 80 months after infusion, confirming that at least some of the transferred T cells were capable of persisting for more than a year after transfer.[40] In patients treated for established EBV-LPD with *Neo*+ T cells, biopsy of the tumor after therapy revealed infiltration of T cells containing the marker gene. Gene marking is effective in very immunodeficient hosts, but expression of a foreign marker gene can be complicated by an immune response to the transferred cells leading to their elimination.[41,42] Dynamic and sensitive imaging modalities to examine *in vivo* migration of adoptively transferred cells would be useful in a variety of settings. However, the available imaging modalities are useful only in small animals.[43] Positron emission tomography imaging has permitted repeated *in vivo* assessment of the migration of adoptively transferred T cells in murine studies.[44]

FUTURE DIRECTIONS IN VIRUS-SPECIFIC T-CELL THERAPY

T-cell therapy is established as an important modality to prevent or treat viral infections in allogeneic HSCT recipients. The use of T-cell therapy for EBV-LPD in solid-organ transplantation recipients is difficult to implement because of the lack of a donor from whom to generate T cells for therapy, and the need for continuing immunosuppression to prevent organ rejection. Use of EBV-specific T cells from unrelated donors is being pursued,[45] and the use of TCR gene transfer to engineer EBV specificity in autologous T cells might be beneficial.[46]

A subset of malignancies that occur in immunocompetent hosts, including Hodgkin lymphoma and nasopharyngeal carcinoma, are associated with EBV.[22] These tumors express a limited number of EBV proteins that are recognized by a low frequency of T cells in normal hosts. Preliminary studies demonstrate the feasibility of isolating, expanding, and infusing these T cells.[47,48] However, effective therapy of sporadic EBV+ tumors may require strategies that can overcome immune evasion mechanisms employed by these tumors.

A key issue for T-cell therapy of opportunistic viruses is to improve the feasibility and broaden the application of this approach. In this regard, techniques have been developed for rapidly isolating antigen-specific T cells directly from the blood of the donor using HLA/peptide tetramers that bind T cells based on TCR specificity, or using mAbs to capture T cells that produce interferon-γ or that have upregulated activation markers in response to antigen stimulation.[49–51]

ADOPTIVE CELLULAR THERAPY OF MALIGNANCY

There is evidence from murine models that the host immune system has a dynamic relationship with a developing tumor and can recognize, control, and even eliminate cancer.[52] Studies in animal models have also demonstrated that the adoptive transfer of T cells, particularly CD8+ CTLs specific for antigens expressed on tumor cells, can eradicate disseminated tumors. Immunogenic proteins in human tumors have now been identified by screening of tumor complementary DNA (cDNA) libraries with tumor-specific T cells isolated from the blood or tumor environment,[53] or by screening of patient sera for antibody responses to tumor-associated proteins.[54] Distinct categories of tumor antigens have been uncovered, and several are being investigated as targets for T-cell therapy or vaccination (Table 24–2). However, the clinical translation of adoptive T-cell therapy and other immunotherapeutic modalities for human cancers has proven to be more challenging than for opportunistic viral infections. This reflects many issues including the difficulty isolating highly avid tumor-specific T cells from cancer patients, and evasion mechanisms that tumors employ to avoid immune elimination including the local recruitment of regulatory T cells (T_{REG}) or other

TABLE 24–2. Categories of Tumor Antigens

Antigen	Tumor	Expression in Normal Tissues
Antigens arising from mutations or gene rearrangements		
p21Ras	Acute leukemia, others	–
p53	~50% of tumors	–
BCR/ABL	CML	
PML/RARα	APL	
CDK-4, MUM-1	Melanoma	–
β-Catenin	Melanoma, lung, others	–
Tissue-specific differentiation antigens		
Tyrosinase	Melanoma	Melanocytes
MART-1/Melan-A	Melanoma	Melanocytes
GP100	Melanoma	Melanocytes
MUC1	Colon, breast, others	Many epithelial tissues
Cancer-testis antigens		
MAGE-1, MAGE-2, MAGE-3	Melanoma	Testis, placenta
GAGE and others	Melanoma	Testis, placenta
NY-ESO-1	Melanoma, breast cancer	Testis, placenta
Nonmutated overexpressed proteins		
HER-2/neu	Breast cancer, ovarian cancer	Breast tissue, ovary
Telomerase catalytic protein	Colon cancer, others	Liver, others
Prostatic acid phosphatase	Prostate	Prostate
CD20, idiotype proteins	Immunoglobulin molecule of B cells	B lymphocytes
Oncofetal proteins		
CEA	Colon cancer, others	Liver, others
AFP	Liver cancer	–
Viral proteins		
HPV E6 and E7	Cervical cancer	–
EBV LMP-1 and EBNA-1 proteins	Hodgkin lymphoma, nasopharyngeal lymphoma	–

suppressor cells, loss of antigen or HLA expression, and expression or secretion of inhibitory molecules or cytokines.[55] Additionally, a problem distinct from the results of T-cell therapy for viruses, is that tumor-reactive T cells persisted only transiently *in vivo* after adoptive transfer in the majority of clinical trials, even if high-dose interleukin (IL)-2 was given to support their survival.[56–60]

The development of immune cell therapy for malignancy has focused on melanoma because target antigens have been identified and this tumor has responded to nonspecific immune therapy with IL-2,[61] and on amplifying the graft-versus-leukemia (GVL) effect after allogeneic HSCT because of the evidence that donor T cells mediate tumor eradication in this setting.[62] The ability to engineer T cells to have tumor specificity by introducing TCR genes that recognize tumor-associated antigens, or chimeric antigen receptor genes that encodes a single chain monoclonal antibody domain linked to the CD3 zeta chain of the TCR, and confers recognition of a tumor-associated, cell-surface molecule, is facilitating the broader application of T-cell therapy for human cancers.[63,64]

CELLULAR THERAPY OF MELANOMA

Early studies demonstrated that the adoptive transfer of autologous polyclonal tumor-infiltrating lymphocytes (TILs), isolated and expanded from resected melanoma specimens, combined with the administration of high-dose IL-2 resulted in a 31 percent response rate in patients with advanced melanoma.[65] Most of the responses were transient, but these results validated the potential to eradicate a human solid tumor with immunotherapy. These results also encouraged efforts to define the antigens recognized by TILs in responding patients, and to refine the approaches to augmenting T-cell responses to tumor antigens.

Target Antigens for Melanoma-Specific T Cells

Melanoma has served as a model for the discovery of human tumor antigens because T cells specific for melanoma cells can often be detected in the blood or the tumor microenvironment. A landmark in cancer immunotherapy was the identification by cDNA expression cloning of MAGE-1, a tumor-specific gene product recognized by T cells derived from a melanoma patient.[53] Several additional melanoma antigens recognized by CD8+ and/or CD4+ T cells have been discovered, including proteins that function in normal melanocyte physiology such as tyrosinase, gp100, and MART-1; cancer testis antigens such as MAGE-1, NY-ESO-1, and others; and mutated proteins that arise as a consequence of the genetic instability of tumors.[53,66,67] Studies in other tumors have associated T-cell infiltration with favorable prognosis. Also, antigens in breast, ovarian, and prostate cancer have been identified.[68,69]

Techniques for Isolation and Adoptive Transfer of Melanoma-Specific T Cells

The adoptive transfer of tumor-specific T-cell clones or oligoclonal populations of T cells expanded *ex vivo* can, in principle, allow control over the magnitude and function of the tumor-reactive T-cell response in the patient. Methods have been developed for isolating melanoma-specific T cells *in vitro*. If the tumor is easily accessible, T cells can be isolated directly from the tumor biopsies by culture in high-dose IL-2.[70] Alternatively, autologous dendritic cells (DCs) pulsed with synthetic peptides corresponding to defined melanoma antigens can be used as stimulators to expand reactive T cells from the blood.[71] A problem with the latter approach is that T cells with low avidity for the antigen are often isolated. T cells with higher avidity can be preferentially expanded using lower concentrations of peptide, by varying the cytokines used for T-cell expansion, or by using APCs transfected with the genes encoding the antigen or pulsed with lysates of the tumor.[72,73]

Early clinical trials of T-cell therapy for melanoma have evaluated the adoptive transfer of CD8+ T-cell clones specific for MART-1 or gp100; or polyclonal melanoma-reactive T cells derived and expanded from TIL. In a study of 10 patients, four infusions of autologous CD8+ T-cell clones at a dose of $3.3 \times 10^9/m^2$ were administered at 14- to 21-day intervals.[74] A peak frequency of 2.2 percent of all CD8+ T cells was achieved in the blood after the T-cell infusions, but the transferred cells did not persist long-term. Low-dose IL-2 was administered for 14 days following some infusions and improved the persistence of transferred CTLs without causing toxicity. The T cells localized to tumor sites and mediated transient antitumor activity in some patients with advanced disease.[74] The response rate was higher in patients treated with polyclonal TIL and high-dose IL-2, and included some complete responses.[75] These studies identified several issues that may have limited efficacy of T-cell therapy. Most notable was that transferred T cells persisted poorly in most treated patients despite the infusion of large numbers (up to 10^{11}) of T cells.[56,74,75] The inability of T cells to persist *in vivo* could reflect an inadequate antigen-specific CD4+ Th response, terminal differentiation of T cells during expansion, activation-induced T-cell death at the tumor site, or cell death as a consequence of IL-2 withdrawal.[56,76]

A major advance in the field was the demonstration that the persistence of transferred T cells and therapeutic efficacy could be improved by the administration of cyclophosphamide and fludarabine to deplete endogenous lymphocytes prior to infusing melanoma-reactive T cells that were expanded from TIL. In these studies, high-dose IL-2 was administered daily after T-cell transfer until toxicity required it be discontinued, and a subset of the patients achieved prolonged high-level engraftment of one or a few tumor-reactive CD8+ T cell clonotypes present in the infused polyclonal T-cell product.[77–80] Several mechanisms make the lymphopenic environment favorable for T-cell transfer, including less competition for cytokines such as IL-15 and IL-7 that promote lymphocyte survival,[81,82] and the elimination of CD4+ CD25+ or other regulatory T cells.[83] Studies in murine models have confirmed that lymphodepletion can be exploited to improve the antitumor efficacy of transferred T cells.[84]

Melanoma patients who received 2 Gy or 12 Gy of total-body irradiation in addition to cyclophosphamide and fludarabine before transfer of TIL had a response rate of 52 percent and 72 percent, respectively.[85] The antitumor activity correlated with the persistence of high levels of transferred tumor-reactive CD8+ T cells. These remarkable results in a metastatic tumor that is unresponsive to conventional therapy were achieved with modest toxicity, which was primarily related to autoimmunity induced against apparently normal melanocytes.[85] Most of the efforts in melanoma have focused on the CD8+ T-cell response to tumor antigens. CD4+ T cells can mediate antitumor effects in animal models and a recent study reported a durable regression of melanoma after the infusion of a CD4+ T-cell clone specific for the NY-ESO-1 antigen.[86]

CELLULAR THERAPY OF LEUKEMIA

Allogeneic donor T cells contained in or derived from the stem cell graft can mount a GVL effect that can contribute to the eradication of malignancy.[87] This underscores studies an the antitumor effects of infusions of unselected donor lymphocytes given to patients who relapse after allogeneic HSCT. Such donor lymphocytic infusions can have potent antitumor effects in patients with relapsed chronic myeloid leukemia (CML), but less effective in acute leukemias, and are often complicated by the development or exacerbation of acute and chronic GVHD.[88] Research is ongoing to identify leukemia-associated target antigens that can be used to direct adoptive T-cell therapy to promote a GVL without causing GVHD.

Target Antigens for Leukemia-Specific T Cells

GVHD and GVL effects usually coexist, but a GVL effect can be observed after HSCT in the absence of GVHD.[87] Thus, it is presumed there are antigens that are expressed by leukemia cells that can be targeted by allogenic T cells. Several categories of such antigens have been identified. These include (1) minor histocompatibility antigens (mHAgs) that are selectively expressed in hematopoietic cells including leukemic cells, (2) tumor-specific proteins resulting from chromosome translocations or mutations, and (3) normal proteins that are overexpressed in leukemic cells. Proteins in the latter two classes could be targets both in the transplantation and nontransplantation setting, whereas mHAgs are only relevant after allogeneic HSCT.

Minor Histocompatibility Antigens

The increased potency of the GVL effect after allogeneic HSCT compared with syngeneic HSCT emphasizes the importance of disparity in major HLA and mHAgs for immune-mediated eradication of malignancy.[87] Class I and class II molecules on recipient T cells display mHAgs, which are peptides derived from proteins that differ between the donor and recipient as a result of genetic polymorphism.[62] In murine models, the adoptive transfer of T cells specific for a single mHAg eradicated leukemia without causing GVHD.[89] In humans, donor T cells reactive with recipient mHAgs can be isolated after transplantation from most allogeneic HSCT recipients.[90] Analysis of the specificity of such T-cell clones shows that many mHAgs are expressed preferentially in hematopoietic cells, including leukemic blasts, and might permit the separation of GVL from GVHD (Fig. 24–2).[90] mHAg-specific CD8+ CTLs prevent engraftment of human leukemia in nonobese diabetic/severe combined immune deficiency mice, providing evidence that the leukemic stem cell can be recognized by allogeneic T cells.[91]

Most mHAgs result from nonsynonymous single nucleotide polymorphisms (SNPs) in the coding sequence of donor and recipient genes that alter the HLA binding or TCR contact of HLA-bound peptides. There are several million SNPs with an allele frequency of >5 percent in the human genome, including approximately 50,000 SNPs that lead to amino acid changes in proteins.[92] Identification of the polymorphic genes that encode mHAgs is facilitated by the data on genetic variation from the human HapMap project, which has enabled the use of whole genome association analysis for mHAg discovery in addition to conventional techniques for antigen discovery.[62,93] Identifying the subset of mHAgs that will be the most useful to target to augment the GVL effect requires consideration of several factors, including the allele frequency of the mHAg encoding gene, the HLA restricting allele that presents the mHAg, and the expression and presentation of the mHAg in leukemia cells and nonhematopoietic tissues.[94] Most mHAg discovery thus far has focused on CD8+ T cells, but CD4+ T cells are likely to play a key role either as direct effector cells in the GVL response, or to support the function and persistence of CD8+ T cells, and efforts to define class II MHC-restricted mHAgs remain an important area of investigation.

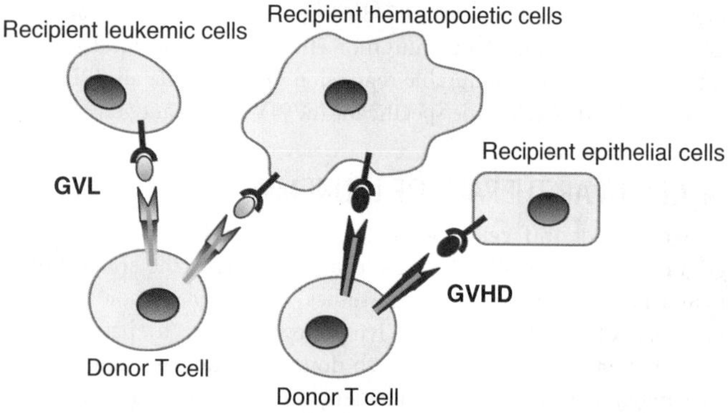

FIGURE 24–2. Tissue-specific expression of minor histocompatibility antigens may permit separation of GVHD from GVL effects. The genes that encode mHAgs may be ubiquitously expressed on recipient tissues and be targets for both GVHD and GVL effects or be selectively expressed on hematopoietic cells and be targets for a GVL effect without GVHD.

Autosome-encoded mHAgs that could be targets for therapy of leukemia after allogeneic HSCT include HA-1 and HA-2, which are encoded by *KIAA0023* and *MY01G*, respectively, and presented by HLA-A2; peptides encoded by *BCL2A1*, which encodes two mHAgs presented by HLA A24 and HLA B44, respectively; LRH-1, encoded by the *P2X5* gene and presented by HLA B7; SP110, which is derived by a novel peptide-splicing mechanism and presented by HLA A3; and PANE-1, which is presented by HLA A3 and selectively expressed on B-lymphoid malignancies.[62,94,95] Direct evidence for a role of these mHAgs in the GVL effect is provided by studies using HLA-A/peptide tetramers to detect expansion of mHAg-reactive T cells in patients who responded to treatment with donor lymphocyte infusions for treatment of relapse following transplantation.[96,97]

There is also evidence for a role of Y-chromosome–encoded mHAgs in the GVL effect. Male recipients of allogeneic HSCT from female donors have a higher risk of GVHD but exhibit a lower risk of leukemia relapse than do other donor/recipient gender combinations, even after controlling for GVHD.[98] Several H-Y antigens are ubiquitously expressed in tissues, providing an explanation for the increased GVHD. However, a mHAg encoded by the Y-chromosome gene *UTY* and presented by HLA-B8 is preferentially expressed in hematopoietic cells including acute myeloid leukemia, and has not been associated with GVHD.[91,99] *UTY* is likely to encode peptides that bind to other HLA alleles, suggesting that it may be a broadly applicable target for a GVL response in male recipients of HSCT from female donors.

Leukemia-Associated Proteins

Leukemia-associated proteins that could be targets for cellular therapy have been identified.[100] These include mutated proteins such as p21/Ras or the products of chromosome translocations such as BCR/ABL and the promyelocytic leukemia-retinoic acid receptor α protein (PML-RARα), which can provide unique peptides that represent potential tumor-specific targets.[101,102] Nonpolymorphic proteins, such as proteinase 3 (PR-3) and Wilms tumor antigen-1 (WT-1), which are overexpressed in some leukemias, also represent potential targets for T-cell therapy.[103,104] CD8+ T cells reactive with an epitope of PR-3 presented by HLA-A2 have been isolated from normal donors by stimulation of PBMCs with a synthetic peptide termed PR-1.[103] PR-1–specific CTLs were sufficiently avid to lyse CML cells and inhibit leukemic colony formation *in vitro*, but did not affect normal hematopoietic progenitors.[105] Expansion of functional PR-1–specific T cells was observed in patients with CML who responded to interferon-α or allogeneic HSCT, suggesting that these T cells may have contributed to the response.[106] T cells specific for WT-1, which is expressed at high levels in myeloid leukemias but at low levels in normal hematopoietic cells, have also been isolated from normal donors by *in vitro* stimulation of PBMCs with synthetic peptides.[107] WT-1–specific CTL selectively lysed leukemic blasts and prevented engraftment of leukemia in immunodeficient mice, suggesting that these T cells may mediate an antileukemic effect without affecting normal hematopoiesis *in vivo*.[104,108] Recent work has identified WT-1–specific T cells after HLA-identical sibling HSCT and correlated these cells with a GVL effect.[109] Thus, nonpolymorphic epitopes derived from both PR-3 and WT-1 could serve as targets for T-cell therapy, and several groups are conducting trials of adoptive T-cell therapy targeting these antigens.

FUTURE DIRECTIONS IN T-CELL THERAPY OF CANCER

Patient Conditioning and Cytokines

Significant progress has been made in cellular therapy for melanoma, but additional studies are necessary to define the optimal and safest regimens for adoptive therapy with tumor-reactive T cells. Advances in our understanding of the role of individual cytokines in T-cell survival *in vitro* and *in vivo*, and of the regulation of T-cell activation and homeostasis will surely provide new opportunities for improving the persistence of *in vitro*-expanded T cells after transfer, perhaps obviating use of toxic chemoradiotherapy to deplete lymphocytes before T-cell infusions. IL-15 is an attractive cytokine for promoting T-cell survival and may soon be available for clinical investigation.[110] Combining T-cell therapy with targeted depletion of regulatory T cells, checkpoint inhibitors, and vaccines is also under investigation, and may help overcome mechanisms by which tumors evade elimination by limiting the quantity and quality of the host response.

Genetic Retargeting of T Cells with T-Cell Receptor Genes

Extending cellular therapy to patients from whom tumor-reactive T cells cannot be isolated and to other malignancies can be accomplished using gene transfer approaches to retarget patient T cells to recognize tumor antigens. A direct approach involves the use of retroviral or lentiviral vectors to transfer of TCR α and β chain genes isolated from tumor-reactive T cells into T cells obtained from the patient. The transfer of TCR genes into T cells to impart specificity to viral antigens, tumor-associated antigens, or mHAgs has been demonstrated.[46,111–113] It is often difficult to achieve the same surface level of TCR expression in transduced T cells as observed in the parental T-cell clone from which the TCR genes were isolated. This problem was apparent in the first clinical trial in which this approach was used to generate T cells to treat melanoma and likely contributed in part to the limited antitumor activity of the transferred gene-modified T cells.[114] Many of the reasons for poor expression of introduced TCRs have been identified and approaches have been developed to improve expression.[115] Another potential problem is that the transfer of TCR genes endows T cells with additional rearranged TCR chains, leading to T cells that could potentially express four different TCR molecules on the cell surface: the natural endogenous TCR, the exogenously introduced TCR, and two mixed heterodimers consisting of endogenous and exogenous TCR chains. Such mismatched TCRs could result in potentially deleterious self-reactive specificities. This problem can be mitigated by the introduction of cysteine residues into the extracellular constant region of the α and β TCR chains to provide for disulfide bond formation and promote preferential pairing of the introduced chains[116,117]; or by using murine constant domains in place of the human constant regions.[118] These modifications of the introduced TCR chains provide for more stable pairing during assembly and export, and better competition for limiting components of the TCR complex, such as CD3ζ or the human tripartite motif protein (TRIM).[119]

Chimeric antigen receptors fashioned by fusing single-chain antibody domains to the TCR ζ chain alone or in combination with costimulatory signaling domains, can also be introduced into T cells to target surface molecules expressed on tumors.[120–122] This approach is now being investigated for treatment of B-lineage malignancies that express CD20, which has already been validated as a target for mAb therapy, or CD19 that is B-lineage specific and expressed on acute lymphocytic leukemia, chronic lymphocytic leukemia, and B-cell lymphomas.[63]

Intrinsic Programming of T Cells in Adoptive Therapy

The quality of the T cells that are selected for adoptive transfer or genetic modification is a critical factor that determines the persistence of transferred effector cells. The T-lymphocyte pool from which T cells for adoptive immunotherapy potentially could be isolated contains CD45RA+ CD62L+ naïve (T_N), CD45RO+ CD62L+ central memory (T_{CM}), and CD62L– effector memory (T_{EM}) subsets that differ in phenotype, function, and homing.[123] Studies in animal models have demonstrated that the origin of CD8+ T_E cells has a profound influence on their ability to persist *in vivo* after adoptive transfer. T-cell clones derived from T_{CM} were uniquely capable of persisting in the blood long-term after adoptive transfer, and of migrating to memory T-cell niches in the lymph nodes and marrow. Moreover, these cells reacquired phenotypic properties of memory cells, and responded to antigen challenge.[124] These results have implications for the types of T cells that should be selected for adoptive transfer, and for strategies to derive tumor-reactive T cells for immunotherapy by genetic retargeting. The demonstration of the superior engraftment properties of T_E derived from T_{CM} would suggest that selection or enrichment of T_{CM} prior to gene insertion will provide a superior T-cell product for adoptive therapy, and may overcome the inconsistent T-cell persistence observed in initial studies.[63,114]

Suicide Genes for Conditional Ablation

Adoptive T-cell therapy is not without risk, which includes the potential for inducing GVHD in trials of therapy targeting mHAgs and damage to normal tissues when self-proteins are targeted. An approach that may improve the safety of T-cell therapy is to introduce a suicide gene into the T cells that could be activated if toxicity occurred. Introduction of the herpes simplex virus-thymidine kinase (*HSV-TK*) gene has been effective in reversing GVHD after donor-lymphocyte infusion.[125] However, the viral thymidine kinase is immunogenic and can result in premature elimination of transferred T cells that do not cause toxicity.[41,42] Suicide genes based on inducing cell death through activation of CD95 (Fas) or caspases using a chemical dimerizer to activate an engineered chimeric human CD95 or caspase transgene product have been developed and may circumvent the problem of immunogenicity.[126–128]

CELLULAR VACCINES

An alternative or complementary approach to the adoptive transfer of tumor-reactive T cells is to elicit antitumor responses *in vivo* by vaccination (see Chap. 25). Although vaccines may be broadly applicable and have been effective in animal models, human trials have revealed significant limitations of current approaches including the difficulty eliciting an immune response that is qualitatively and quantitatively adequate for eradicating established tumors.[80] The response rates to vaccines comprised of tumor associated peptides admixed with adjuvants has been relatively poor in solid-tumor patients, although vaccination with PR-1 or WT-1 peptides of patients who had relapsed with leukemia has shown promise.[129]

It is conceivable that autologous DCs loaded *ex vivo* with tumor antigens or tumor cells modified to express molecules that recruit DCs may have advantages over peptide vaccines.[61,80,130] DCs have been identified as potent APCs, and when appropriately activated and matured, display a unique ability to initiate immune responses of both CD8+ and CD4+ T cells.[131] In murine models, DCs have been pulsed with tumor lysates or peptides, transfected with RNA- or DNA-encoding tumor antigens, or fused to tumor cells for use in vaccination, and have induced protective tumor-specific immunity.[131] Similarly, vaccination with allogeneic tumor cells genetically modified to express cytokines that enhance immunogenicity by recruiting DC or promoting T cell activation have shown promise in animal models and in humans.[132,133]

DC-based vaccine strategies are being actively pursued for therapy of melanoma and a variety of other tumors.[134] Immunization with *ex vivo*-generated DCs has proven feasible and safe and has resulted in the augmentation of tumor-specific T-cell responses and the regression of disease in a subset of melanoma patients.[135] Multiple strategies can be used for introducing antigens into DCs, and it is unclear which strategy will be most effective. Among the variables being evaluated for improving immunogenicity and clinical efficacy are the subsets of DCs used for vaccination, activation and maturation signals that are delivered, vaccine schedule, and strategies to direct migration of DCs to secondary lymphoid organs *in vivo* or to overexpress costimulatory molecules. Alternatively, vaccine strategies that obviate *ex vivo* culture of DCs by directing antigen to these cells *in situ* have been proposed.[135,136] Studies in animal models demonstrate that vaccination can enhance the efficacy of adoptive T-cell therapy,[137] and it is likely that this approach will be evaluated in clinical trials.

REFERENCES

1. Einsele H, Hebart H: Cellular immunity to viral and fungal antigens after stem cell transplantation. *Curr Opin Hematol* 9:485, 2002.
2. Powers C, DeFilippis V, Malouli D, et al: Cytomegalovirus immune evasion. *Curr Top Microbiol Immunol* 325:333, 2008.
3. Sylwester AW, Mitchell BL, Edgar JB, et al: Broadly targeted human cytomegalovirus-specific CD4+ and CD8+ T cells dominate the memory compartments of exposed subjects. *J Exp Med* 202:673, 2005.
4. Manley TJ, Luy L, Jones T, et al: Immune evasion proteins of human cytomegalovirus do not prevent a diverse CD8+ cytotoxic T cell response in natural infection. *Blood* 104:1075, 2004.
5. Li CR, Greenberg PD, Gilbert MJ, et al: Recovery of HLA-restricted cytomegalovirus (CMV)-specific T cell responses after allogeneic bone marrow transplant: Correlation with CMV disease and effect of ganciclovir prophylaxis. *Blood* 83:1971, 1994.
6. Boeckh M, Leisenring W, Riddell SR, et al: Late cytomegalovirus disease and mortality in recipients of allogeneic hematopoietic stem cell transplants: Importance of viral load and T cell immunity. *Blood* 101:407, 2003.
7. Boeckh M, Nichols WG, Papanicolaou G, et al: Cytomegalovirus in hematopoietic stem cell transplant recipients: Current status, known challenges, and future strategies. *Biol Blood Marrow Transplant* 9:543, 2003.
8. Griffiths P, Whitley R, Snydman DR, et al: Contemporary management of cytomegalovirus infection in transplant recipients: Guidelines from an IHMF workshop, 2007. *Herpes* 15:4, 2008.
9. Riddell SR, Greenberg PD: T-cell therapy of cytomegalovirus and human immunodeficiency virus infection. *J Antimicrob Chemother* 45 Suppl T3:35, 2000.
10. Simon CO, Holtappels R, Tervo HM, et al: CD8 T cells control cytomegalovirus latency by epitope-specific sensing of transcriptional reactivation. *J Virol* 80:10436, 2006.
11. Fuhrmann S, Streitz M, Reinke P, et al: T cell response to the cytomegalovirus major capsid protein (UL86) is dominated by helper cells with a large polyfunctional component and diverse epitope recognition. *J Infect Dis* 197:1455, 2008.
12. Crompton L, Khan N, Khanna R, et al: CD4+ T cells specific for glycoprotein B from cytomegalovirus exhibit extreme conservation of T cell receptor usage between different individuals. *Blood* 111:2053, 2008.
13. Riddell SR, Watanabe KS, Goodrich JM, et al: Restoration of viral immunity in immunodeficient humans by the adoptive transfer of T cell clones. *Science* 257:238, 1992.
14. Walter EA, Greenberg PD, Gilbert MJ, et al: Reconstitution of cellular immunity against cytomegalovirus in recipients of allogeneic bone marrow by transfer of T cell clones from the donor. *N Engl J Med* 333:1038, 1995.
15. Peggs KS, Verfuerth S, Pizzey A, et al: Adoptive cellular therapy for early cytomegalovirus infection after allogeneic stem-cell transplantation with virus-specific T cell lines. *Lancet* 362:1375, 2003.
16. Kleihauer A, Grigoleit U, Hebart H, et al: Ex vivo generation of human cytomegalovirus-specific cytotoxic T cells by peptide-pulsed dendritic cells. *Br J Haematol* 113:231, 2001.
17. Micklethwaite KP, Clancy L, Sandher U, et al: Prophylactic infusion of cytomegalovirus-specific cytotoxic T lymphocytes stimulated with Ad5f35pp65 gene-modified dendritic cells after allogeneic hemopoietic stem cell transplantation. *Blood* 112:3974, 2008.
18. Leen AM, Myers GD, Sili U, et al: Monoculture-derived T lymphocytes specific for multiple viruses expand and produce clinically relevant effects in immunocompromised individuals. *Nat Med* 12:1160, 2006.
19. Einsele H, Roosnek E, Rufer N, et al: Infusion of cytomegalovirus (CMV)-specific T cells for the treatment of CMV infection not responding to antiviral chemotherapy. *Blood* 99:3916, 2002.
20. Cobbold M, Khan N, Pourgheysari B, et al: Adoptive transfer of cytomegalovirus-specific CTL to stem cell transplant patients after selection by HLA-peptide tetramers. *J Exp Med* 202:379, 2005.
21. Yin Y, Manoury B, Fahraeus R: Self-inhibition of synthesis and antigen presentation by Epstein-Barr virus-encoded EBNA1. *Science* 301:1371, 2003.
22. Thorley-Lawson DA, Gross A: Persistence of the Epstein-Barr virus and the origins of associated lymphomas. *N Engl J Med* 350:1328, 2004.
23. Tan LC, Gudgeon N, Annels NE, et al: A re-evaluation of the frequency of CD8+ T cells specific for EBV in healthy virus carriers. *J Immunol* 162:1827, 1999.
24. Curtis RE, Travis LB, Rowlings PA, et al: Risk of lymphoproliferative disorders after bone marrow transplantation: A multi-institutional study. *Blood* 94:2208, 1999.
25. Kuehnle I, Huls MH, Liu Z, et al: CD20 monoclonal antibody (rituximab) for therapy of Epstein-Barr virus lymphoma after hemopoietic stem-cell transplantation. *Blood* 95:1502, 2000.
26. Annels NE, Callan MF, Tan L, et al: Changing patterns of dominant TCR usage with maturation of an EBV-specific cytotoxic T cell response. *J Immunol* 165:4831, 2000.
27. Amyes E, Hatton C, Montamat-Sicotte D, et al: Characterization of the CD4+ T cell response to Epstein-Barr virus during primary and persistent infection. *J Exp Med* 198:903, 2003.
28. Meij P, van Esser JW, Niesters HG, et al: Impaired recovery of Epstein-Barr virus (EBV)-specific CD8+ T lymphocytes after partially T-depleted allogeneic stem cell transplantation may identify patients at very high risk for progressive EBV reactivation and lymphoproliferative disease. *Blood* 101:4290, 2003.
29. Timms JM, Bell A, Flavell JR, et al: Target cells of Epstein-Barr-virus (EBV)-positive post-transplant lymphoproliferative disease: Similarities to EBV-positive Hodgkin's lymphoma. *Lancet* 361:217, 2003.
30. Papadopoulos EB, Ladanyi M, Emanuel D, et al: Infusions of donor leukocytes to treat Epstein-Barr virus-associated lymphoproliferative disorders after allogeneic bone marrow transplantation. *N Engl J Med* 330:1185, 1994.
31. Rooney CM, Smith CA, Ng CY, et al: Use of gene-modified virus-specific T lymphocytes to control Epstein-Barr-virus-related lymphoproliferation. *Lancet* 345:9, 1995.
32. Gottschalk S, Edwards OL, Sili U, et al: Generating CTLs against the subdominant Epstein-Barr virus LMP1 antigen for the adoptive immunotherapy of EBV-associated malignancies. *Blood* 101:1905, 2003.
33. Rooney CM, Smith CA, Ng CY, et al: Infusion of cytotoxic T cells for the prevention and treatment of Epstein-Barr virus-induced lymphoma in allogeneic transplant recipients. *Blood* 92:1549, 1998.
34. Gustafsson A, Levitsky V, Zou JZ, et al: Epstein-Barr virus (EBV) load in bone marrow transplant recipients at risk to develop posttransplant lymphoproliferative disease: Prophylactic infusion of EBV-specific cytotoxic T cells. *Blood* 95:807, 2000.
35. Leen AM, Bollard CM, Myers GD, et al: Adenoviral infections in hematopoietic stem cell transplantation. *Biol Blood Marrow Transplant* 12:243, 2006.
36. Chakrabarti S, Mautner V, Osman H, et al: Adenovirus infections following allogeneic stem cell transplantation: Incidence and outcome in relation to graft manipulation, immunosuppression, and immune recovery. *Blood* 100:1619, 2002.
37. Leen AM, Christin A, Khalil M, et al: Identification of hexon-specific CD4 and CD8 T cell epitopes for vaccine and immunotherapy. *J Virol* 82:546, 2008.
38. Feuchtinger T, Richard C, Joachim S, et al: Clinical grade generation of hexon-specific T cells for adoptive T cell transfer as a treatment of adenovirus infection after allogeneic stem cell transplantation. *J Immunother* 31:199, 2008.
39. Feuchtinger T, Matthes-Martin S, Richard C, et al: Safe adoptive transfer of virus-specific T cell immunity for the treatment of systemic adenovirus infection after allogeneic stem cell transplantation. *Br J Haematol* 134:64, 2006.
40. Heslop HE, Ng CY, Li C, et al: Long-term restoration of immunity against Epstein-Barr virus infection by adoptive transfer of gene-modified virus-specific T lymphocytes. *Nat Med* 2:551, 1996.
41. Riddell SR, Elliott M, Lewinsohn DA, et al: T cell mediated rejection of gene-modified HIV-specific cytotoxic T lymphocytes in HIV-infected patients. *Nat Med* 2:216, 1996.
42. Berger C, Flowers ME, Warren EH, et al: Analysis of transgene-specific immune responses that limit the in vivo persistence of adoptively transferred HSV-TK-modified donor T cells after allogeneic hematopoietic cell transplantation. *Blood* 107:2294, 2006.
43. Shu CJ, Guo S, Kim YJ, et al: Visualization of a primary anti-tumor immune response by positron emission tomography. *Proc Natl Acad Sci U S A* 102:17412, 2005.
44. Brentjens RJ, Latouche JB, Santos E, et al: Eradication of systemic B-cell tumors by genetically targeted human T lymphocytes co-stimulated by CD80 and interleukin-15. *Nat Med* 9:279, 2003.
45. Haque T, Wilkie GM, Jones MM, et al: Allogeneic cytotoxic T-cell therapy for EBV-positive posttransplantation lymphoproliferative disease: Results of a phase 2 multicenter clinical trial. *Blood* 110:1123, 2007.
46. Schumacher TN: T cell-receptor gene therapy. *Nat Rev Immunol* 2:512, 2002.
47. Gottschalk S, Heslop HE, Rooney CM: Adoptive immunotherapy for EBV-associated malignancies. *Leuk Lymphoma* 46:1, 2005.
48. Bollard CM, Gottschalk S, Leen AM, et al: Complete responses of relapsed lymphoma following genetic modification of tumor-antigen presenting cells and T-lymphocyte transfer. *Blood* 110:2838, 2007.
49. Wolfl M, Kuball J, Ho WY, et al: Activation-induced expression of CD137 permits detection, isolation, and expansion of the full repertoire of CD8+ T cells responding to antigen without requiring knowledge of epitope specificities. *Blood* 110:201, 2007.
50. Keenan RD, Ainsworth J, Khan N, et al: Purification of cytomegalovirus-specific CD8 T cells from peripheral blood using HLA-peptide tetramers. *Br J Haematol* 115:428, 2001.
51. Becker C, Pohla H, Frankenberger B, et al: Adoptive tumor therapy with T lymphocytes enriched through an IFN-gamma capture assay. *Nat Med* 7:1159, 2001.
52. Koebel CM, Vermi W, Swann JB, et al: Adaptive immunity maintains occult cancer in an equilibrium state. *Nature* 450:903, 2007.

53. van der Bruggen P, Traversari C, Chomez P, et al: A gene encoding an antigen recognized by cytolytic T lymphocytes on a human melanoma. *Science* 254:1643, 1991.
54. Chen YT, Scanlan MJ, Sahin U, et al: A testicular antigen aberrantly expressed in human cancers detected by autologous antibody screening. *Proc Natl Acad Sci U S A* 94:1914, 1997.
55. Drake CG, Jaffee E, Pardoll DM: Mechanisms of immune evasion by tumors. *Adv Immunol* 90:51, 2006.
56. Dudley ME, Wunderlich J, Nishimura MI, et al: Adoptive transfer of cloned melanoma-reactive T lymphocytes for the treatment of patients with metastatic melanoma. *J Immunother* 24:363, 2001.
57. Park JR, Digiusto DL, Slovak M, et al: Adoptive transfer of chimeric antigen receptor re-directed cytolytic T lymphocyte clones in patients with neuroblastoma. *Mol Ther* 15:825, 2007.
58. Yee C, Thompson JA, Roche P, et al: Melanocyte destruction after antigen-specific immunotherapy of melanoma: Direct evidence of T cell-mediated vitiligo. *J Exp Med* 192:1637, 2000.
59. Kershaw MH, Westwood JA, Parker LL, et al: A phase I study on adoptive immunotherapy using gene-modified T cells for ovarian cancer. *Clin Cancer Res* 12:6106, 2006.
60. Robbins PF, Dudley ME, Wunderlich J, et al: Cutting edge: Persistence of transferred lymphocyte clonotypes correlates with cancer regression in patients receiving cell transfer therapy. *J Immunol* 173:7125, 2004.
61. Rosenberg SA: Progress in human tumour immunology and immunotherapy. *Nature* 411:380, 2001.
62. Bleakley M, Riddell SR: Molecules and mechanisms of the graft-versus-leukaemia effect. *Nat Rev Cancer* 4:371, 2004.
63. Till BG, Jensen MC, Wang J, et al: Adoptive immunotherapy for indolent non-Hodgkin lymphoma and mantle cell lymphoma using genetically modified autologous CD20-specific T cells. *Blood* 112:2261, 2008.
64. Pule MA, Savoldo B, Myers GD, et al: Virus-specific T cells engineered to coexpress tumor-specific receptors: Persistence and antitumor activity in individuals with neuroblastoma. *Nat Med* 14:1264, 2008.
65. Rosenberg SA, Aebersold P, Cornetta K, et al: Gene transfer into humans—Immunotherapy of patients with advanced melanoma, using tumor-infiltrating lymphocytes modified by retroviral gene transduction. *N Engl J Med* 323:570, 1990.
66. Rosenberg SA: A new era for cancer immunotherapy based on the genes that encode cancer antigens. *Immunity* 10:281, 1999.
67. Engelhard VH, Bullock TN, Colella TA, et al: Antigens derived from melanocyte differentiation proteins: Self-tolerance, autoimmunity\1\4 use for cancer immunotherapy. *Immunol Rev* 188:136, 2002.
68. Wang W, Epler J, Salazar LG, et al: Recognition of breast cancer cells by CD8+ cytotoxic T cell clones specific for NY-BR-1. *Cancer Res* 66:6826, 2006.
69. Kao H, Marto JA, Hoffmann TK, et al: Identification of cyclin B1 as a shared human epithelial tumor-associated antigen recognized by T cells. *J Exp Med* 194:1313, 2001.
70. Dudley ME, Wunderlich JR, Shelton TE, et al: Generation of tumor-infiltrating lymphocyte cultures for use in adoptive transfer therapy for melanoma patients. *J Immunother* 26:332, 2003.
71. Yee C, Savage PA, Lee PP, et al: Isolation of high avidity melanoma-reactive CTL from heterogeneous populations using peptide-MHC tetramers. *J Immunol* 162:2227, 1999.
72. Parkhurst MR, DePan C, Riley JP, et al: Hybrids of dendritic cells and tumor cells generated by electrofusion simultaneously present immunodominant epitopes from multiple human tumor-associated antigens in the context of MHC class I and class II molecules. *J Immunol* 170:5317, 2003.
73. Meyer zum Buschenfelde C, Nicklisch N, Rose-John S, et al: Generation of tumor-reactive CTL against the tumor-associated antigen HER2 using retrovirally transduced dendritic cells derived from CD34+ hemopoietic progenitor cells. *J Immunol* 165:4133, 2000.
74. Yee C, Thompson JA, Byrd D, et al: Adoptive T-cell therapy using antigen-specific CD8+ T cell clones for the treatment of patients with metastatic melanoma: In vivo persistence, migration, and antitumor effect of transferred T cells. *Proc Natl Acad Sci U S A* 99:16168, 2002.
75. Rosenberg SA, Packard BS, Aebersold PM, et al: Use of tumor-infiltrating lymphocytes and interleukin-2 in the immunotherapy of patients with metastatic melanoma. A preliminary report. *N Engl J Med* 319:1676, 1988.
76. Gattinoni L, Klebanoff CA, Palmer DC, et al: Acquisition of full effector function *in vitro* paradoxically impairs the *in vivo* antitumor efficacy of adoptively transferred CD8+ T cells. *J Clin Invest* 115:1616, 2005.
77. Dudley ME, Wunderlich JR, Robbins PF, et al: Cancer regression and autoimmunity in patients after clonal repopulation with antitumor lymphocytes. *Science* 298:850, 2002.
78. Dudley ME, Wunderlich JR, Yang JC, et al: Adoptive cell transfer therapy following non-myeloablative but lymphodepleting chemotherapy for the treatment of patients with refractory metastatic melanoma. *J Clin Oncol* 23:2346, 2005.
79. Huang J, Khong HT, Dudley ME, et al: Survival, persistence, and progressive differentiation of adoptively transferred tumor-reactive T cells associated with tumor regression. *J Immunother* 28:258, 2005.
80. Rosenberg SA, Yang JC, Restifo NP: Cancer immunotherapy: Moving beyond current vaccines. *Nat Med* 10:909, 2004.
81. Tan JT, Dudl E, LeRoy E, et al: IL-7 is critical for homeostatic proliferation and survival of naive T cells. *Proc Natl Acad Sci U S A* 98:8732, 2001.
82. Tan JT, Ernst B, Kieper WC, et al: Interleukin (IL)-15 and IL-7 jointly regulate homeostatic proliferation of memory phenotype CD8+ cells but are not required for memory phenotype CD4+ cells. *J Exp Med* 195:1523, 2002.
83. Colombo MP, Piconese S: Regulatory-T cell inhibition versus depletion: The right choice in cancer immunotherapy. *Nat Rev Cancer* 7:880, 2007.
84. Wrzesinski C, Paulos CM, Gattinoni L, et al: Hematopoietic stem cells promote the expansion and function of adoptively transferred antitumor CD8 T cells. *J Clin Invest* 117:492, 2007.
85. Dudley ME, Yang JC, Sherry R, et al: Adoptive cell therapy for patients with metastatic melanoma: Evaluation of intensive myeloablative chemoradiation preparative regimens. *J Clin Oncol* 26:5233, 2008.
86. Hunder NN, Wallen H, Cao J, et al: Treatment of metastatic melanoma with autologous CD4+ T cells against NY-ESO-1. *N Engl J Med* 358:2698, 2008.
87. Horowitz MM, Gale RP, Sondel PM, et al: Graft-versus-leukemia reactions after bone marrow transplantation. *Blood* 75:555, 1990.
88. Kolb HJ, Schmid C, Barrett AJ, et al: Graft-versus-leukemia reactions in allogeneic chimeras. *Blood* 103:767, 2004.
89. Fontaine P, Roy-Proulx G, Knafo L, et al: Adoptive transfer of minor histocompatibility antigen-specific T lymphocytes eradicates leukemia cells without causing graft-versus-host disease. *Nat Med* 7:789, 2001.
90. Warren EH, Greenberg PD, Riddell SR: Cytotoxic T-lymphocyte-defined human minor histocompatibility antigens with a restricted tissue distribution. *Blood* 91:2197, 1998.
91. Bonnet D, Warren EH, Greenberg PD, et al: CD8(+) minor histocompatibility antigen-specific cytotoxic T lymphocyte clones eliminate human acute myeloid leukemia stem cells. *Proc Natl Acad Sci U S A* 96:8639, 1999.
92. Carlson CS, Eberle MA, Rieder MJ, et al: Additional SNPs and linkage-disequilibrium analyses are necessary for whole-genome association studies in humans. *Nat Genet* 33:518, 2003.
93. Kamei M, Nannya Y, Torikai H, et al: HapMap scanning of novel human minor histocompatibility antigens [comment]. *Blood* 21:113, 2009.
94. Spierings E, Hendriks M, Absi L, et al: Phenotype frequencies of autosomal minor histocompatibility antigens display significant differences among populations. *PLoS Genet* 3:e103, 2007.
95. Warren EH, Vigneron NJ, Gavin MA, et al: An antigen produced by splicing of noncontiguous peptides in the reverse order. *Science* 313:1444, 2006.
96. Marijt WA, Heemskerk MH, Kloosterboer FM, et al: Hematopoiesis-restricted minor histocompatibility antigens HA-1- or HA-2-specific T cells can induce complete remissions of relapsed leukemia. *Proc Natl Acad Sci U S A* 100:2742, 2003.
97. de Rijke B, van Horssen-Zoetbrood A, Beekman JM, et al: A frameshift polymorphism in P2X5 elicits an allogeneic cytotoxic T lymphocyte response associated with remission of chronic myeloid leukemia. *J Clin Invest* 115:3506, 2005.
98. Randolph SS, Gooley TA, Warren EH, et al: Female donors contribute to a selective graft-versus-leukemia effect in male recipients of HLA-matched, related hematopoietic stem cell transplants. *Blood* 103:347, 2004.
99. Warren EH, Gavin MA, Simpson E, et al: The human UTY gene encodes a novel HLA-B8-restricted H-Y antigen. *J Immunol* 164:2807, 2000.
100. Barrett AJ: Understanding and harnessing the graft-versus-leukaemia effect. *Br J Haematol* 142:877, 2008.
101. Van Elsas A, Nijman HW, Van der Minne CE, et al: Induction and characterization of cytotoxic T-lymphocytes recognizing a mutated p21ras peptide presented by HLA-A*0201. *Int J Cancer* 61:389, 1995.
102. Bocchia M, Korontsvit T, Xu Q, et al: Specific human cellular immunity to bcr-abl oncogene-derived peptides. *Blood* 87:3587, 1996.
103. Molldrem J, Dermime S, Parker K, et al: Targeted T-cell therapy for human leukemia: Cytotoxic T lymphocytes specific for a peptide derived from proteinase 3 preferentially lyse human myeloid leukemia cells. *Blood* 88:2450, 1996.
104. Bellantuono I, Gao L, Parry S, et al: Two distinct HLA-A0201-presented epitopes of the Wilms tumor antigen 1 can function as targets for leukemia-reactive CTL. *Blood* 100:3835, 2002.
105. Molldrem JJ, Clave E, Jiang YZ, et al: Cytotoxic T lymphocytes specific for a nonpolymorphic proteinase 3 peptide preferentially inhibit chronic myeloid leukemia colony-forming units. *Blood* 90:2529, 1997.
106. Molldrem JJ, Lee PP, Wang C, et al: Evidence that specific T lymphocytes may participate in the elimination of chronic myelogenous leukemia. *Nat Med* 6:1018, 2000.
107. Menssen HD, Renkl HJ, Entezami M, et al: Wilms' tumor gene expression in human CD34+ hematopoietic progenitors during fetal development and early clonogenic growth. *Blood* 89:3486, 1997.
108. Gao L, Bellantuono I, Elsasser A, et al: Selective elimination of leukemic CD34(+) progenitor cells by cytotoxic T lymphocytes specific for WT1. *Blood* 95:2198, 2000.
109. Rezvani K, Yong AS, Savani BN, et al: Graft-versus-leukemia effects associated with detectable Wilms tumor-1 specific T lymphocytes after allogeneic stem-cell transplantation for acute lymphoblastic leukemia. *Blood* 110:1924, 2007.
110. Waldmann TA: The biology of interleukin-2 and interleukin-15: Implications for cancer therapy and vaccine design. *Nat Rev Immunol* 6:595, 2006.
111. Cooper LJ, Kalos M, Lewinsohn DA, et al: Transfer of specificity for human immunodeficiency virus type 1 into primary human T lymphocytes by introduction of T cell receptor genes. *J Virol* 74:8207, 2000.
112. Engels B, Uckert W: Redirecting T lymphocyte specificity by T cell receptor gene transfer—A new era for immunotherapy. *Mol Aspects Med* 28:115, 2007.
113. Stanislawski T, Voss RH, Lotz C, et al: Circumventing tolerance to a human MDM2-derived tumor antigen by TCR gene transfer. *Nat Immunol* 2:962, 2001.
114. Morgan RA, Dudley ME, Wunderlich JR, et al: Cancer regression in patients after transfer of genetically engineered lymphocytes. *Science* 314:126, 2006.

115. Leisegang M, Engels B, Meyerhuber P, et al: Enhanced functionality of T cell receptor-redirected T cells is defined by the transgene cassette. *J Mol Med* 86:573, 2008.
116. Cohen CJ, Li YF, El-Gamil M, et al: Enhanced antitumor activity of T cells engineered to express T cell receptors with a second disulfide bond. *Cancer Res* 67:3898, 2007.
117. Kuball J, Dossett ML, Wolfl M, et al: Facilitating matched pairing and expression of TCR chains introduced into human T cells. *Blood* 109:2331, 2007.
118. Cohen CJ, Zhao Y, Zheng Z, et al: Enhanced antitumor activity of murine-human hybrid T cell receptor (TCR) in human lymphocytes is associated with improved pairing and TCR/CD3 stability. *Cancer Res* 66:8878, 2006.
119. Kirchgessner H, Dietrich J, Scherer J, et al: The transmembrane adaptor protein TRIM regulates T cell receptor (TCR) expression and TCR-mediated signaling via an association with the TCR zeta chain. *J Exp Med* 193:1269, 2001.
120. Sadelain M, Riviere I, Brentjens R: Targeting tumours with genetically enhanced T lymphocytes. *Nat Rev Cancer* 3:35, 2003.
121. Kershaw MH, Teng MW, Smyth MJ, et al: Supernatural T cells: Genetic modification of T cells for cancer therapy. *Nat Rev Immunol* 5:928, 2005.
122. Brentjens RJ, Santos E, Nikhamin Y, et al: Genetically targeted T cells eradicate systemic acute lymphoblastic leukemia xenografts. *Clin Cancer Res* 13:5426, 2007.
123. Sallusto F, Geginat J, Lanzavecchia A: Central memory and effector memory T cell subsets: Function, generation, and maintenance. *Annu Rev Immunol* 22:745, 2004.
124. Berger C, Jensen MC, Lansdorp PM, et al: Adoptive transfer of effector CD8+ T cells derived from central memory cells establishes persistent T cell memory in primates. *J Clin Invest* 118:294, 2008.
125. Bonini C, Ferrari G, Verzeletti S, et al: HSV-TK gene transfer into donor lymphocytes for control of allogeneic graft-versus-leukemia. *Science* 276:1719, 1997.
126. Straathof KC, Pule MA, Yotnda P, et al: An inducible caspase 9 safety switch for T-cell therapy. *Blood* 105:4247, 2005.
127. de Witte MA, Jorritsma A, Swart E, et al: An inducible caspase 9 safety switch can halt cell therapy-induced autoimmune disease. *J Immunol* 180:6365, 2008.
128. Berger C, Blau CA, Huang ML, et al: Pharmacologically regulated Fas-mediated death of adoptively transferred T cells in a nonhuman primate model. *Blood* 103:1261, 2004.
129. Mailander V, Scheibenbogen C, Thiel E, et al: Complete remission in a patient with recurrent acute myeloid leukemia induced by vaccination with WT1 peptide in the absence of hematological or renal toxicity. *Leukemia* 18:165, 2004.
130. Rosenberg SA, Yang JC, Schwartzentruber DJ, et al: Immunologic and therapeutic evaluation of a synthetic peptide vaccine for the treatment of patients with metastatic melanoma. *Nat Med* 4:321, 1998.
131. Banchereau J, Briere F, Caux C, et al: Immunobiology of dendritic cells. *Annu Rev Immunol* 18:767, 2000.
132. Jaffee EM, Hruban RH, Biedrzycki B, et al: Novel allogeneic granulocyte-macrophage colony-stimulating factor-secreting tumor vaccine for pancreatic cancer: A phase I trial of safety and immune activation. *J Clin Oncol* 19:145, 2001.
133. Fukuda T, Chen L, Endo T, et al: Antisera induced by infusions of autologous Ad-CD154-leukemia B cells identify ROR1 as an oncofetal antigen and receptor for Wnt5a. *Proc Natl Acad Sci U S A* 105:3047, 2008.
134. Engell-Noerregaard L, Hansen TH, Andersen MH, et al: Review of clinical studies on dendritic cell-based vaccination of patients with malignant melanoma: Assessment of correlation between clinical response and vaccine parameters. *Cancer Immunol Immunother* 58:1, 2009.
135. Cerundolo V, Hermans IF, Salio M: Dendritic cells: A journey from laboratory to clinic. *Nat Immunol* 5:7, 2004.
136. Merad M, Sugie T, Engleman EG, et al: *In vivo* manipulation of dendritic cells to induce therapeutic immunity. *Blood* 99:1676, 2002.
137. Overwijk WW, Theoret MR, Finkelstein SE, et al: Tumor regression and autoimmunity after reversal of a functionally tolerant state of self-reactive CD8+ T cells. *J Exp Med* 198:569, 2003.

CHAPTER 25
PRINCIPLES OF VACCINE THERAPY

Sattva S. Neelapu and Larry W. Kwak

SUMMARY

Vaccines are biologic substances that are designed to stimulate the host immune system to elicit a neutralizing response against clinically relevant targets. Active immunotherapy with vaccines has been extremely effective as prevention against self-limiting infectious pathogens. However, effective vaccine therapy of chronic infectious diseases or cancer, in the therapeutic setting, remains a promising but largely unrealized goal. Hematologic malignancies are an excellent model system for vaccine therapies, in part because of accessibility and susceptibility to immune effector mechanisms and availability of tumor cells for studies of mechanism.

ADVANTAGES OF CANCER VACCINE THERAPY

Immunity elicited by therapeutic cancer vaccines offers several advantages over passive immunotherapy using monoclonal antibodies. In active immune therapy, all components of the effector immune response are host derived (without murine or xenogeneic components that could cause indirect toxicity). The lack of foreign components also allows the host response to be sustained. Also, if the vaccine contains more than a single determinant of the target antigen, the immune response could be broad in scope, recognizing more than a single epitope in the antigen (polyclonal). This feature might be of particular importance for cancer immunotherapy, as mutation of individual peptide epitopes is a possible mechanism of immune evasion by tumors. In addition to inducing antibodies, which can recognize intact proteins on the surface of tumor cells, vaccines activate T cells that can recognize peptide fragments derived from proteins, which may be endogenously processed and presented on the surface of tumor cells. Such T cells have various effector mechanisms capable of neutralizing tumor cells, including lysis of the tumor cell by cell-to-cell contact and the local production of cytokines that might directly neutralize tumor cells (e.g., interferon-γ).

COMPONENTS OF THERAPEUTIC CANCER VACCINES

Most therapeutic cancer vaccines that are being tested in clinical trials have at least three components: antigenic material derived from the tumor, a carrier, and an adjuvant. The antigenic material is usually a protein or peptide derived from the tumor that is either uniquely expressed or is overexpressed in the tumor, compared with normal tissues. A unique tumor antigen or the overexpression of the antigen to prevent the tumor is necessary to prevent the induction of an unwanted autoimmune response against normal tissues following vaccination. The carrier is necessary for delivery of the tumor antigen to antigen-presenting cells, such as dendritic cells, in order to induce the immune response against the tumor antigen. The third component of a cancer vaccine, the adjuvant, is usually a cytokine or other nonspecific immune stimulant to facilitate an enhanced immune response against the tumor antigen.

Acronyms and abbreviations that appear in this chapter include: cDNA, complementary DNA; GM-CSF, granulocyte-monocyte colony-stimulating factor; HLA, human leukocyte antigen; IL, interleukin; KLH, keyhole limpet hemocyanin; PD-L, programmed death ligand.

ANTIGEN DISCOVERY

Both conventional and novel technologies used to define cancer-associated antigens, such as serologic analysis by recombinant expression cloning (SEREX), serial analysis of gene expression (SAGE), screening tumor complementary DNA (cDNA) libraries with tumor-reactive T cells, and characterization of peptides eluted from tumor-derived human leukocyte antigen (HLA) molecules, have resulted in a rapidly growing list of candidate tumor antigens for various hematologic malignancies (Table 25–1). The majority of these candidate antigens have been identified since 1998. Furthermore, the application of genomic and proteomic techniques, combined with the feasibility of isolating sufficient quantities of clonogenic tumor cells from individual patients, should identify additional targets that are differentially expressed in tumors as compared with normal tissues (see Chap. 15).

Desirable characteristics for candidate target antigens for immune therapy include antigens that are selectively expressed by the tumor or that are required to maintain the malignant cell phenotype or cell survival. Host T-cell recognition of such antigens requires that they are naturally processed and presented by tumor cells into peptides that bind host HLA molecules. Optimally, the candidate antigen should contain both CD4+ and CD8+ T-cell epitopes. Antigens recognized by humoral immune responses must be expressed on the tumor cell surface, and the relevant epitopes must be accessible to antibody molecules. Candidate tumor antigens should be immunogenic (capable of being recognized by the host immune system).

Vaccine therapy does not necessarily require a completely defined tumor antigen. Vaccines can consist of whole tumor cells or subcellular components containing putative antigens. For example, autologous tumor cells engineered to overexpress cytokines such as granulocyte-macrophage colony-stimulating factor (GM-CSF),[15,16] or activated *ex vivo* by CD40 receptor engagement,[17] can be effective at inducing tumor-specific T cells with as yet undefined antigen specificity. Similarly, transfer of the gene encoding CD40– ligand into chronic lymphocytic leukemia cells induced CD4+ and CD8+ T-cell responses in human patients.[18] Vaccination with membrane proteins extracted from tumor cells and incorporated into liposomes along with interleukin (IL)-2 is another strategy that is currently in clinical testing.[19]

VACCINE DELIVERY

Effective delivery of the target antigen to the immune system is critical for the successful induction of immunity. For most tumor antigens, this is a daunting challenge, as most antigens (with the exception of viral antigens associated with cancers) are weakly immunogenic, self, or tissue differentiation antigens.

Many vaccine-delivery strategies use dendritic cells. These key antigen-presenting cells are principally responsible for initiating a host immune response.[20] The cells, represented in minute quantities, have the powerful capacity to take up antigens, and once activated, to present processed peptides to T cells. Accordingly, optimizing the delivery of tumor antigens to specialized antigen-presenting cells is critical. Such

TABLE 25–1. Examples of Candidate Human Tumor Antigens for Hematologic Cancers

Antigen	Reference
Minor histocompatibility antigens (HA-1, HA-2)	1
Proteinase-3	2
Wilms tumor antigen-1	3
B-cell receptor (immunoglobulin idiotype)	4
Anaplastic lymphoma kinase	5
Sperm protein 17	6
Sperm protein associated with the nucleus on X chromosome (SPAN-X)	7
CML-66	8
Survivin	9
HM1.24	10
Immature laminin receptor protein	11
BCR-ABL fusion protein	12
Aurora kinase	13
Fibromodulin	14

efforts have included isolation of dendritic cells from blood, followed by physical loading with protein or peptide antigens, or introducing the genes for candidate antigens by transfection with cDNA or messenger RNA, or by fusion with whole tumor cells. Loaded dendritic cells have been administered to patients as vaccines.[21]

An alternative strategy is to target the delivery of antigens to dendritic cells *in vivo*. Traditional approaches focused on attempts to make the antigen look foreign to the host immune system; for example, by chemical linkage to larger, highly immunogenic proteins (carriers) or incorporation into liposomes. Rational approaches to increase the efficiency of antigen delivery to dendritic cells have included genetic fusion of the gene encoding the antigen to one encoding biologically active molecules that has the ability to target cell surface receptors on antigen-presenting cells. Such targeting molecules have included cytokines, chemokines, antibody Fc or Fab fragments, transferrin, CD40, and mannose, which serve as ligands for specific receptors on antigen-presenting cells.[22] Such molecular vaccines can be administered as naked DNA or as fusion proteins. Other promising approaches to target dendritic cells *in vivo* are represented by recombinant viral or bacterial vectors or virus-like particles.[23,24]

■ IMMUNOSTIMULANTS TO ENHANCE VACCINE EFFICACY

Traditionally, immunologic adjuvants, described by the late Charles Janeway as "immunology's dirty little secret," such as alum and oil-in-water emulsions (e.g., incomplete Freund adjuvant), provide a physical depot for slow release of antigen. Adjuvants also serve as general immune stimulants by providing a danger signal to activate antigen-presenting cells. This feature describes classical adjuvant components, such as bacterial cell wall extracts, as well as unmethylated CpG DNA sequences, which deliver maturation signals to dendritic cells through toll-like receptors (see Chap. 18).[25] The incorporation of either recombinant cytokines or their genes into vaccine formulations may increase vaccine potency by broadly enhancing the function of either antigen-presenting cells or T cells. Consequently, cytokines, such as interferon-γ, IL-2, and IL-15, may be useful as components of vaccines.[26] Such cytokines also can help direct the type of immune response elicited. For example, IL-12 elicits primarily T-helper (Th) type 1 cell responses, whereas the inclusion of IL-4 or IL-10 generally induces predominantly Th2 cell responses (see Chap. 78). Some cytokines, such as GM-CSF, which can induce dendritic cell differentiation, can also function as an adjuvant by recruiting antigen-presenting cells to local vaccination sites.[27]

CLINICAL TRIAL DESIGN

Cancer vaccine trials might not fit into the paradigm developed for chemotherapeutic agents, which have direct effects on tumor and normal host cells. For example, studies in heavily pretreated patients with terminal disease might be inappropriate for vaccines, which generally require an intact host immune system. For this reason, even safety cannot be evaluated completely in patients who cannot make an immune response, because any toxicity will likely be indirect, resulting from the immune response elicited. In addition, animal models show that the immune system may be more effective at clearing minimal residual disease than at clearing advanced tumor cell burdens. Accordingly, several late-stage clinical trials of cancer vaccines are testing this approach in the setting of clinical remission, after primary surgery or chemotherapy.

Although conventional clinical trials generally test one experimental agent at a time, vaccine formulations may contain several components. The simultaneous optimization of multiple variables (e.g., vaccine and adjuvant dose and schedule, and routes of administration) in a single clinical study often requires the application of novel, more flexible clinical trial design.[28]

ASSAYS OF VACCINE EFFICACY

The development of surrogate measures of vaccine efficacy has potential value for answering the scientific question of whether it is even possible to vaccinate human patients against a candidate antigen. Traditional assays of immune response, including simple lymphoproliferation and cytotoxicity assays, requiring prolonged periods of prior stimulation, are being replaced by quantitative assays that can measure effector function of T cells directly sampled from blood (e.g., enzyme-linked immunospot assay [ELISPOT]) and by sensitive tetramer binding assays (Table 25–2).[29] In some cases, tetramer-binding assays have been combined with intracellular cytokine production to provide both quantitative and functional analyses of antigen-specific T cells.[30] An important aim of clinical trials is to determine which, if any, of these measures of immune response are valid surrogates for vaccine efficacy.

B-CELL ANTIGEN-RECEPTOR VACCINES AS SCIENTIFIC PROOF OF PRINCIPLE

B cells are clonally restricted to express surface immunoglobulin receptors that have unique epitopes present in the antibody variable region termed idiotypes (see Chap. 77). Idiotypes expressed by B-cell malignancies are clonally distributed and thus can serve as tumor-specific target antigen for specific immunotherapy. Idiotypes were initially validated as tumor-rejection antigens in mouse models of myeloma and lymphoma,[31,32] and the first clinical trial testing this approach in human patients with lymphoma was reported in 1992.[33,34] Customized idiotype proteins were isolated by heterohybridoma fusion, conjugated chemically to keyhole limpet hemocyanin (KLH), which functioned as

TABLE 25–2. Monitoring of Human Immune Responses

Type of Response	Representative Assay
CD4+ T cells	Cytokine induction
	Cytokine ELISPOT (IFN-γ)
	Intracellular cytokine
	Proliferation
CD8+ T cells	Cytotoxicity
	Limiting dilution analysis
	Tetramer
	Cytokine ELISPOT (IFN-γ)
	Intracellular cytokine
Antibody	ELISA
	Flow cytometry
	ELISPOT
Multiple	Microarray
	Cytokine mRNA by RT-PCR
	T-cell spectratyping

ELISA, enzyme-linked immunoabsorbent assay; ELISPOT, enzyme-linked immunospot assay; IFN, interferon; mRNA, messenger RNA; RT-PCR, reverse transcriptase polymerase chain reaction.

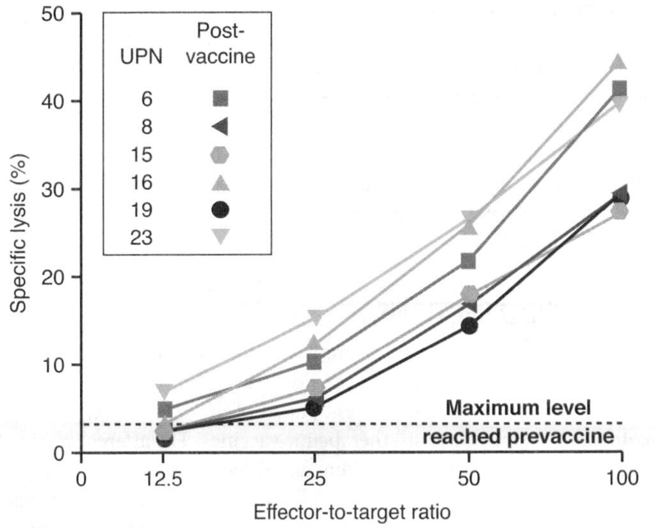

FIGURE 25–2. T-cell–mediated lysis of human autologous lymphoma cells after vaccination with idiotype KLH protein plus GM-CSF. Representative results are shown from six individual patients, designated by unique patient number (*UPN*). *(Adapted from Bendandi M, Gocke CD, Kobrin CB, et al,[4] with permission.)*

a carrier, and emulsified in a simple oil-in-water emulsion. These vaccines elicited predominantly antibody responses.

Subsequently, guided by additional data from murine lymphoma models (Fig. 25–1), recombinant GM-CSF protein was substituted as the immunologic adjuvant. Soluble GM-CSF, initially mixed with the vaccine and then administered for three additional daily doses subcutaneously as close as possible to the original site of immunization, significantly enhanced vaccine potency, consistent with previous gene therapy studies.[35] The cellular mechanism of this effect required CD8+ and CD4+ T cells.[36]

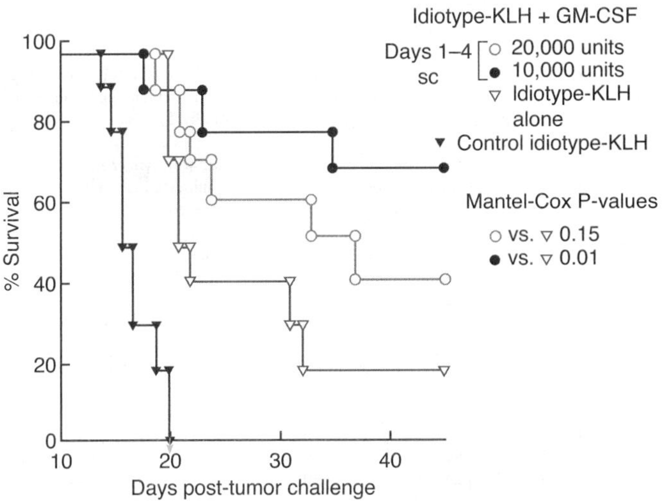

FIGURE 25–1. GM-CSF enhances lymphoma vaccine potency. Mice were vaccinated subcutaneously with idiotype KLH protein, together with or without various doses of GM-CSF and challenged with a lethal dose of syngeneic lymphoma cells. The use of 10,000 units of GM-CSF plus idiotype KLH conjugate on days 1 to 4 (*closed dots*) resulted in a significantly longer survival after tumor challenge than did idiotype KLH conjugate vaccination alone.

A phase II study was designed to test these vaccines in the setting of minimal residual disease, defined as first remission after chemotherapy in follicular lymphoma patients.[4] Previously untreated patients first received treatment with uniform chemotherapy to achieve complete remission. After a 6-month break to allow for immune reconstitution, idiotype proteins conjugated with KLH plus GM-CSF vaccines were administered in five monthly doses. Surrogate assays for vaccine efficacy were developed that used autologous lymphoma cells as targets for both B- and T-cell responses. In 19 patients (86%), vaccination elicited CD8+ cytotoxic T-lymphocyte cells reactive with the lymphoma cell (Fig. 25–2). More than half of the patients remain in continuous first complete remission, even after a median followup of more than 7 years. A randomized, controlled phase III trial testing this vaccine formulation in follicular lymphoma patients in first remission was reported to improve disease-free survival as compared with controls suggesting that therapeutic cancer vaccines could induce meaningful clinical benefit in cancer patients.[37]

IMPEDIMENTS TO VACCINE THERAPY

Despite the success of the idiotype vaccine phase III trial in follicular lymphoma, most other phase III trials of cancer vaccines have been disappointing and objective clinical response rates have been low. Potential reasons for the failure despite the high immunogenicity of vaccines[38] may be categorized into factors affecting the afferent or priming phase of the immune response and factors influencing the efferent or effector phase of the immune response. For instance, during the afferent phase of the immune response, it is possible that the magnitude of the T-cell response or the avidity of the induced T-cells was not high enough following vaccination. During the effector phase of the immune response, it is possible that the antitumor T cells may not have trafficked to the tumor site or, if they trafficked, they may not have been able to overcome newly recognized immunosuppressive mechanisms present in the tumor microenvironment. Several immunosuppressive mechanisms were shown to impair the function of tumor-specific effector T cells in the tumor microenvironment in various animal models and in some human cancers.[39] Important negative regulatory pathways that inhibit T-cell function include extrinsic suppression by regulatory T cells (T_{regs}); direct inhibition through inhibitory ligands such as cytotoxic T-lymphocyte antigen (CTLA)-4, programmed death-ligand 1 (PD-L1), PD-L2, and B7-H4; soluble factors such as transforming growth factor β and IL-10; and metabolic dysregulation of essential amino acids such as tryptophan.[39]

FUTURE DIRECTIONS

Advances in understanding of immune tolerance and tumor-induced immunosuppression have now provided several novel agents to augment both the afferent and efferent phases of the immune responses in combination strategies with therapeutic vaccines. The afferent phase of the immune response could be enhanced by using more potent vaccines with novel adjuvants such as toll-like receptor ligands, or by vaccinating donors of transplant recipients who have a healthy immune system as opposed to patients who may be immunocompromised either from the cancer or from therapy.[40] Alternatively, vaccines could be used in combination with agents that inhibit the immunosuppressive mechanisms, such as coinhibitory receptors/ligands[41] and/or deplete regulatory T cells,[42] to augment the afferent and/or effector phase of the immune response. The use of these agents in combination with therapeutic cancer vaccines may lead to enhanced antitumor immunity and improved clinical outcome.

REFERENCES

1. Marijt WA, Heemskerk MH, Kloosterboer FM, et al: Hematopoiesis-restricted minor histocompatibility antigens HA-1- or HA-2-specific T cells can induce complete remissions of relapsed leukemia. *Proc Natl Acad Sci U S A* 100:2742, 2003.
2. Molldrem JJ, Komanduri K, Wieder E: Overexpressed differentiation antigens as targets of graft-versus-leukemia reactions. *Curr Opin Hematol* 9:503, 2002.
3. Bellantuono I, Gao L, Parry S, et al: Two distinct HLA-A0201-presented epitopes of the Wilms tumor antigen 1 can function as targets for leukemia-reactive CTL. *Blood* 100:3835, 2002.
4. Bendandi M, Gocke CD, Kobrin CB, et al: Complete molecular remissions induced by patient-specific vaccination plus granulocyte-monocyte colony-stimulating factor against lymphoma. *Nat Med* 5:1171, 1999.
5. Passoni L, Scardino A, Bertazzoli C, et al: ALK as a novel lymphoma-associated tumor antigen: Identification of 2 HLA-A2.1-restricted CD8+ T-cell epitopes. *Blood* 99:2100, 2002.
6. Lim SH, Wang Z, Chiriva-Internati M, et al: Sperm protein 17 is a novel cancer-testis antigen in multiple myeloma. *Blood* 97:1508, 2001.
7. Wang Z, Zhang Y, Liu H, et al: Gene expression and immunologic consequence of SPAN-Xb in myeloma and other hematologic malignancies. *Blood* 101:955, 2003.
8. Yang XF, Wu CJ, Mclaughlin S, et al: CML66, a broadly immunogenic tumor antigen, elicits a humoral immune response associated with remission of chronic myelogenous leukemia. *Proc Natl Acad Sci U S A* 98:7492, 2001.
9. Zeis M, Siegel S, Wagner A, et al: Generation of cytotoxic responses in mice and human individuals against hematological malignancies using survivin-RNA-transfected dendritic cells. *J Immunol* 170:5391, 2003.
10. Chiriva-Internati M, Liu Y, Weidanz JA, et al: Testing recombinant adeno-associated virus-gene loading of dendritic cells for generating potent cytotoxic T lymphocytes against a prototype self-antigen, multiple myeloma HM1.24. *Blood* 102:3100, 2003.
11. Siegel S, Wagner A, Kabelitz D, et al: Induction of cytotoxic T-cell responses against the oncofetal antigen-immature laminin receptor for the treatment of hematologic malignancies. *Blood* 102:4416, 2003.
12. Pinilla-Ibarz J, Cathcart K, Korontsvit T, et al: Vaccination of patients with chronic myelogenous leukemia with bcr-abl oncogene breakpoint fusion peptides generates specific immune responses. *Blood* 95:1781, 2000.
13. Ochi T, Fujiwara H, Suemori K, et al: Aurora-A kinase: A novel target of cellular immunotherapy for leukemia. *Blood* 113:66, 2009.
14. Mayr C, Bund D, Schlee M, et al: Fibromodulin as a novel tumor-associated antigen (TAA) in chronic lymphocytic leukemia (CLL), which allows expansion of specific CD8+ autologous T lymphocytes. *Blood* 105:1566, 2005.
15. Levitsky HI, Montgomery J, Ahmadzadeh M, et al: Immunization with granulocyte-macrophage colony-stimulating factor-transduced, but not B7-1-transduced, lymphoma cells primes idiotype-specific T cells and generates potent systemic antitumor immunity. *J Immunol* 156:3858, 1996.
16. Dranoff G: Cytokines in cancer pathogenesis and cancer therapy. *Nat Rev Cancer* 4:11, 2004.
17. von Bergwelt-Baildon MS, Vonderheide RH, Maecker B, et al: Human primary and memory cytotoxic T lymphocyte responses are efficiently induced by means of CD40-activated B cells as antigen-presenting cells: Potential for clinical application. *Blood* 99:3319, 2002.
18. Wierda WG, Cantwell MJ, Woods SJ: CD40-ligand (CD154) gene therapy for chronic lymphocytic leukemia. *Blood* 96:2917, 2000.
19. Neelapu SS, Gause BL, Harvey L, et al. A novel proteoliposomal vaccine induces antitumor immunity against follicular lymphoma. *Blood* 109:5160, 2007.
20. Liu YJ: Dendritic cell subsets and lineages, and their functions in innate and adaptive immunity. *Cell* 106:259, 2001.
21. Cerundolo V, Hermans IF, Salio M: Dendritic cells: A journey from laboratory to clinic. *Nat Immunol* 5:7, 2004.
22. Biragyn A, Kwak LW: Designer cancer vaccines are still in fashion. *Nat Med* 6:966, 2000.
23. Tartour E, Benchetrit F, Haicheur N, et al: Synthetic and natural non-live vectors: Rationale for their clinical development in cancer vaccine protocols. *Vaccine* 20(Suppl 4):A32, 2002.
24. Zhang L, Tang Y, Akbulut H, et al: An adenoviral vector cancer vaccine that delivers a tumor-associated antigen/CD40-ligand fusion protein to dendritic cells. *Proc Natl Acad Sci U S A* 100:15101, 2003.
25. Kreig AM: CpG motifs in bacterial DNA and their immune effects. *Annu Rev Immunol* 20:709, 2002.
26. Waldmann TA, Dubois S, Tagaya Y: Contrasting roles of IL-2 and IL-15 in the life and death of lymphocytes: Implications for immunotherapy. *Immunity* 14:105, 2001.
27. Pardoll DM: Spinning molecular immunology into successful immunotherapy. *Nat Rev Immunol* 2:227, 2002.
28. Simon RM, Steinberg SM, Hamilton M, et al: Clinical trial designs for the early clinical development of therapeutic cancer vaccines. *J Clin Oncol* 19:1848, 2001.
29. Lyerly HK: Quantitating cellular immune responses to cancer vaccines. *Semin Oncol* 30(3 Suppl 8):9, 2003.
30. Lee PP, Yee C, Savage PA, et al: Characterization of circulating T cells specific for tumor-associated antigens in melanoma patients. *Nat Med* 5:677, 1999.
31. Lynch RG, Graff RJ, Sirisinha S, et al: Myeloma proteins as tumor-specific transplantation antigens. *Proc Natl Acad Sci U S A* 69:1540, 1972.
32. Stevenson GT, Elliott EV, Stevenson FK: Idiotypic determinants on the surface of immunoglobulin of neoplastic lymphocytes: A therapeutic target. *Fed Proc* 36:2268, 1977.
33. Kwak LW, Campbell MJ, Czerwinski DK, et al: Induction of immune responses in patients with B-cell lymphoma against the surface-immunoglobulin idiotype expressed by their tumors. *N Engl J Med* 327:1209, 1992.
34. Hsu FJ, Caspar CB, Czerwinski D, et al: Tumor-specific idiotype vaccines in the treatment of patients with B-cell lymphoma—Long-term results of a clinical trial. *Blood* 89:3129, 1997.
35. Dranoff G, Jaffee E, Lazenby A, et al: Vaccination with irradiated tumor cells engineered to secrete murine granulocyte-macrophage colony-stimulating factor stimulates potent, specific, and long-lasting anti-tumor immunity. *Proc Natl Acad Sci U S A* 90:3539, 1993.
36. Kwak LW, Young HA, Pennington RW, et al: Vaccination with syngeneic lymphoma-derive immunoglobulin idiotype combined with granulocyte/macrophage colony-stimulating factor primes mice for a protective T-cell response. *Proc Natl Acad Sci U S A* 93:10972, 1996.
37. Schuster SJ, Neelapu SS, Gause BL, et al. Idiotype vaccine therapy (BiovaxID) in follicular lymphoma in first complete remission: Phase III clinical trial results. *J Clin Oncol* 27(Suppl):18s, 2009.
38. Neelapu SS, Kwak LW, Kobrin CB, et al. Vaccine-induced tumor-specific immunity despite severe B-cell depletion in mantle cell lymphoma. *Nat Med* 11:986, 2005.
39. Zou W. Immunosuppressive networks in the tumour environment and their therapeutic relevance. *Nat Rev Cancer* 5:263, 2005.
40. Neelapu SS, Munshi NC, Jagannath S, et al. Tumor antigen immunization of sibling stem cell donors in multiple myeloma. *Bone Marrow Transplant* 36:315, 2005.
41. Phan GQ, Yang JC, Sherry RM, et al: Cancer regression and autoimmunity induced by cytotoxic T lymphocyte-associated antigen 4 blockade in patients with metastatic melanoma. *Proc Natl Acad Sci U S A* 100:8372, 2003.
42. Dannull J, Su Z, Rizzieri D, et al. Enhancement of vaccine-mediated antitumor immunity in cancer patients after depletion of regulatory T cells. *J Clin Invest* 115:3623, 2005.

CHAPTER 26

PRINCIPLES OF THERAPEUTIC APHERESIS: INDICATIONS, EFFICACY, AND COMPLICATIONS

Bruce C. McLeod

SUMMARY

Therapeutic apheresis provides a means to rapidly alter the composition of blood components. It can be a valuable and safe initial treatment of a number of illnesses associated with quantitative and/or qualitative abnormalities of blood cells or plasma. Cell depletions are useful in symptomatic thrombocythemia and hyperleukocytosis, or to provide autologous or allogeneic stem and progenitor cells for hematopoietic reconstitution or immunocytes for immunomodulation. Plasma exchange is useful in certain paraproteinemias, antibody-mediated disorders, and toxin-mediated diseases. It also can be used to replace a deficient plasma constituent. Red cell exchange is used primarily for severe manifestations of sickle cell disease. Selective extraction techniques are available for immunoglobulin G and low-density lipoprotein, and modulation of certain immune responses is possible with photopheresis. Adverse effects with current techniques are infrequent and usually mild.

Therapeutic apheresis comprises a set of related techniques in which the amount or composition of a blood component is manipulated for a therapeutic purpose, usually with a continuous-flow centrifugal blood separation instrument. Available techniques are divided into three main categories: blood cell depletion, blood component exchange, and blood component modification (Table 26–1). Cell-depletion procedures usually target excess platelets or leukocytes. These procedures currently are undertaken almost exclusively for hematologic diseases. Similar techniques adapted for autologous or allogeneic leukocyte donation provide cells for transplantation and/or immunotherapy. Blood component exchanges target plasma or red cells. Plasma exchange is beneficial in a number of antibody-mediated conditions, many of which are not usually considered hematologic diseases. Specialized techniques have been developed for online selective extraction of certain individual constituents, such as immunoglobulin (Ig) G and low-density lipoproteins (LDLs), from plasma separated by an apheresis instrument, and for photochemical modification of separated lymphocytes (photopheresis).

Acronyms and abbreviations that appear in this chapter include: ADAMTS13, von Willebrand cleaving metalloproteinase; ALL, acute lymphocytic leukemia; AML, acute myelogenous leukemia; ANCAs, antineutrophil cytoplasmic antibodies; BPC, blood progenitor cell; CML, chronic myelogenous leukemia; CTCL, cutaneous T-cell lymphoma; HLA, human leukocyte antigen; HPA, human platelet alloantigen; Ig, immunoglobulin; LDL, low-density lipoprotein; MNC, mononuclear cell; SPS, stiff person syndrome; TTP, thrombotic thrombocytopenic purpura.

The goal of therapeutic apheresis is usually therapeutic depletion. Candidate entities for therapeutic depletion should be pathogenic and susceptible to meaningful depletion by apheresis. The latter provision implies that a substantial portion of the total body burden is intravascular and that the half-life is relatively long. In practice, this limits utility to blood cells and large, slowly catabolized plasma proteins, such as immunoglobulins and LDLs.[1] In some instances, infusion of normal blood constituents in quantity may be important. Apheresis therapy depletes rapidly but does not decrease production of an abnormal blood constituent. In most illnesses, therefore, apheresis therapy is best used acutely to control symptoms until more definitive therapy takes effect. Chronic apheresis therapy is seldom appropriate unless more convenient treatments are ineffective or contraindicated.

Adverse effects of therapeutic apheresis with modern instruments occur infrequently and are generally mild. Symptomatic hypotension occurs in 1 to 2 percent of patients. Hypocalcemia as a result of citrate infusion can occur. Urticaria may be seen when donor plasma is infused in plasma exchange. Deaths are extremely rare. Most deaths are attributable to central venous catheter placement or to the progression of the disease rather than to apheresis therapy per se.[2–5] Table 26–2 lists the overall nonaccess-related adverse effect rates for common procedures observed in one large multicenter study.[3]

CELL DEPLETION

PLATELETPHERESIS

Thrombocythemia can usually be managed pharmacologically with hydroxyurea or anagrelide. However, therapeutic plateletpheresis can be valuable in patients with symptomatic thrombocythemia who require rapid reduction of platelet count or who cannot tolerate drug therapy.[6] Platelet count usually can be lowered by approximately 50 percent with each procedure, although the decrement may be less if platelets are mobilized from an enlarged spleen during apheresis. Plateletpheresis can reverse clinical manifestations of myocardial or cerebral ischemia, pulmonary embolism, and gastrointestinal bleeding. Multiple procedures at intervals of a few days are usually needed until chemotherapy takes effect. Whether or not prophylactic plateletpheresis lowers the incidence of thrombosis or hemorrhage is not known; however, prophylactic plateletpheresis may prevent placental infarction and fetal death in pregnant patients with thrombocythemia.[7] Long-term plateletpheresis is logistically and financially burdensome and is seldom indicated as the sole therapy for thrombocythemia (see Chap. 87).

LEUKAPHERESIS

The most common therapeutic application of leukapheresis is removal of malignant leukocytes. Leukapheresis has been performed in acute and chronic leukemias and in the leukemic phase of lymphoma. The usual goal of leukapheresis is relieving or forestalling acute symptoms of hyperleukocytosis, but leukapheresis occasionally has been used as a primary method of disease control.[6] Immunomodulation by removal of nonmalignant lymphocytes also has been attempted,[8,9] but has not become an accepted treatment of any illness. A putative antiinflammatory effect, to be derived from adsorption/depletion of modest numbers of granulocytes and monocytes from anticoagulated whole blood by a filter-type device, has not proven beneficial in controlled trials in ulcerative colitis.[10]

The threshold white cell count for pulmonary and/or cerebral dysfunction (leukostasis) in patients with leukemia is not known. The count may depend on rheologic variables that differ among different leukemias and even among patients with the same type of leukemia.

TABLE 26-1. Therapeutic Apheresis Techniques

- I. Cell Depletion
  - A. Plateletpheresis
  - B. Leukapheresis
    1. Therapeutic white blood cell removal
    2. Blood progenitor cell collection
    3. Immunocyte collection
- II. Blood Component Exchange
  - A. Plasma exchange (plasmapheresis)
  - B. Red cell exchange
- III. Blood Component Modification
  - A. Selective extraction of a plasma constituent
  - B. Photopheresis

Clinical manifestations of hyperleukocytosis may occur in acute myelogenous leukemia (AML) when the white cell count is 75×10^9/L[11,12] but more likely occur when the white cell count exceeds 200×10^9/L.[13] Although controlled trials documenting benefit are lacking, therapeutic leukapheresis often is performed urgently in patients with AML if the white cell count is greater than 100×10^9/L because this is a risk factor for early death.[14] Patients with acute lymphocytic leukemia (ALL) often are treated similarly, even though symptoms occur less frequently in this condition. In one study of ALL patients, leukapheresis led to a lower incidence of electrolyte abnormalities.[15] However, several observational studies of prophylactic leukapheresis in AML have failed to show either prevention of coagulopathy or tumor lysis syndrome, or improvement in overall survival.[16–18]

White cell removal in chronic myelogenous leukemia (CML) was one of the earliest applications of apheresis instruments in patients.[19] Repeated leukapheresis as therapy for CML also provided leukocytes for transfusion to infected neutropenic patients with acute leukemia.[20] Some CML patients experienced reduced organomegaly and amelioration of constitutional symptoms, but chronic leukapheresis did not prolong life or delay onset of blast transformation.[21] Logistical and financial issues make this approach impractical except in unusual circumstances, such as pregnancy,[22] in which delayed chemotherapy is desirable. Leukapheresis therapy for CML is usually reserved for patients who have white cell counts of 300 to 500×10^9/L and signs of leukostasis. Even higher white cell counts are tolerated in chronic lymphocytic leukemia.[23]

TABLE 26-2. Nonaccess-Related Adverse Effect Rates for Common Therapeutic Apheresis Procedures

Procedure	Adverse Effect Rate, %
Plasma exchange	
Without plasma infusion	3.4
With plasma infusion	7.8
Leukapheresis	5.7
Plateletpheresis	0.0
Red cell exchange	10.0
Blood progenitor cell collection	1.7

Adapted from McLeod et al.[3]

In Sézary syndrome, a leukemic phase of cutaneous T-cell lymphoma (CTCL), repeated leukapheresis reduces the number of circulating malignant (Sézary) cells and improves or resolves skin lesions.[24,25] Photopheresis (extracorporeal photochemotherapy) has been used to treat CTCL, especially in the erythrodermic phase.[26] In photopheresis, leukocytes removed by apheresis are exposed to ultraviolet A light in the presence of 8-methoxypsoralen and then returned to the patient. Photochemical damage to DNA is believed to render the malignant cells immunomodulatory, thereby stimulating host antitumor immunity.[27] Photopheresis has resulted in sustained remissions in CTCL[28] and has become an accepted therapy for this illness.[29]

The extent to which the white cell count should be lowered is not known with certainty for any application of therapeutic leukapheresis. Processing at least two patient blood volumes has been recommended, with white cell count reductions of 15 to 86 percent reported in acute leukemias.[6] Predicting the outcome of a procedure is difficult because of mobilization of cells into the bloodstream, underestimation of patient blood volume by standard formulas, and patient-specific differences in the behavior of leukemic cells in a centrifugal instrument. In practice, it is worthwhile to monitor the white cell count during a procedure and to continue the procedure until a 30 to 50 percent decline is achieved.

MONONUCLEAR CELL COLLECTION

Leukapheresis techniques optimized for mononuclear cell (MNC) depletion have been adapted for collection of stem and progenitor cells and various immunocytes from circulating blood. These techniques are described here, although the therapeutic effect derives from subsequent infusion (transplantation) of cells rather than from depletion, even in the autologous setting.

Blood Progenitor Cell Collection

Stem and progenitor cells in quantities adequate to support hematopoietic reconstitution after myeloablative therapy can be obtained from most individuals by MNC collection. Prospective donors are pretreated with conventional chemotherapy (autologous only) and/or hematopoietic growth factors (autologous or allogeneic) to "mobilize" the desired cells from the marrow into the circulating blood. Unlike marrow harvest, blood progenitor cell (BPC) collection does not require general anesthesia. Also, BPC collection yields cells that engraft more rapidly after transplantation than marrow-derived cells. The latter two properties are significant advantages. As a result, BPC collection has largely supplanted marrow harvest for allogeneic and autologous stem cell transplantation. BPC transplants contain more T cells and may cause more frequent and/or more severe graft-versus-host disease in the allogeneic setting; however, this potential disadvantage does not offset the perceived advantages for donor and recipient (see Chap. 21).[30] BPCs are a convenient substrate for some instances of gene insertion therapy (see Chap. 27).[31] Although complications of BPC collection occur infrequently (see Table 26–2),[3] mobilization with granulocyte colony-stimulating factor has led to splenic rupture[32] and to fatal sickle cell crisis in an allogeneic donor with mild hemoglobin SC disease.[33]

Immunocyte Collection

MNC collection from individuals who have not been "mobilized" still can serve as a source of T cells, natural killer cells, dendritic cells, and other cells having a role in the immune response to tumors or infectious agents (see Chap. 24). Deliberate infusion of T cells from a matched allogeneic stem cell donor (donor lymphocyte infusion) can enhance the graft-versus-tumor effect in preventing or combatting relapse (see Chap. 21).[34] Methods whereby autologous MNCs are manipulated *ex vivo* to boost a specific immune response to tumor or microbial antigens and then reinfused[35] are being explored (see Chap. 25).

BLOOD COMPONENT EXCHANGES

■ PHYSIOLOGY

Therapeutic blood component exchange reduces the concentration of a harmful blood constituent by removing patient material and simultaneously replacing it with a substitute lacking the unwanted constituent. In a plasma exchange, the extent of depletion of an unwanted macromolecule X can be estimated at any point by the formula[36]:

$$X_n = X_o e^{-n}$$

where X_o = starting concentration of X; n = volume exchanged, expressed in patient plasma volumes; X_n = concentration of X after exchange of n plasma volumes; and e = base natural log.

This formula describes an asymptotic function that predicts (assuming equilibration with extravascular substance is slow) exchange of one plasma volume lowers the intravascular concentration of a substance by approximately 65 percent, whereas exchange of a second plasma volume lowers the intravascular concentration only approximately 23 percent more. Removal is more efficient in the early portion of an exchange, so many exchanges are limited to a single plasma volume. For IgG antibodies, the existence of a substantial extravascular reservoir provides a further rationale for a series of single plasma volume exchanges separated by intervals adequate to allow reequilibration between intravascular and extravascular spaces. Applied in a reciprocal manner, the formula works equally well for predicting the outcome of a red cell exchange, although the final concentration of normal red cells can be increased efficiently beyond the predicted level by removing some red cells while infusing a plasma substitute at the beginning of a procedure and infusing red cells while removing plasma at the end of a procedure.[37]

A protein-containing replacement fluid must be given during plasma exchange. Usually either normal plasma or 5 percent albumin is chosen. For most applications, 5 percent albumin is preferred because it does not transmit viral infections or cause urticarial reactions, and it can be administered without regard to blood type. As expected, IgG levels fall by approximately 65 percent after a single plasma volume exchange for albumin and then take several weeks to recover. Coagulation factor levels also fall, with transient prolongation of the prothrombin time and partial thromboplastin time. However, clinical bleeding usually is not encountered, and all coagulant proteins except fibrinogen return to the normal range within 6 to 24 hours after an exchange.[31] Because most other plasma protein levels also recover quickly between exchanges, a series of thrice-weekly exchanges of patient plasma for 5 percent albumin produces selective depression in immunoglobulin levels.[38] Plasma replacement may be necessary in certain illnesses, such as thrombotic thrombocytopenic purpura (TTP), to achieve the desired therapeutic effect. Plasma may be given in the final portion of an exchange to replete coagulation factors when a patient has a preexisting bleeding diathesis.

■ PLASMA EXCHANGE

Therapeutic plasma exchange has been used to treat several types of plasma constituent abnormalities (Table 26–3). In most instances, the goal is to remove a pathogenic immunoglobulin from the patient's blood. Cases can be subdivided based on whether the antigenic specificity of the immunoglobulin or an abnormal physical property imparted to the blood by its presence (e.g., hyperviscosity) mediates the disease process. In a few instances, plasma exchange can help by removing substances other than immunoglobulin (e.g., LDL). Lastly, plasma exchange can replete a deficient factor to a higher level than plasma infusion alone.

TABLE 26–3. Indication Categories for Plasma Exchange

Goal	Example
Immunoglobulin removal	
Abnormal physical properties	Hyperviscosity syndrome
Specific antibody	Goodpasture syndrome
Nonimmunoglobulin constituent removal	Familial hypercholesterolemia
Factor replacement	Thrombotic thrombocytopenic purpura

Immunoglobulins with Pathogenic Physical Properties

Almost all of the conditions in this category are caused by monoclonal proteins. The hyperviscosity syndrome, which can be a feature of macroglobulinemia and rarely results from the effects of species of IgG or IgA, probably is the oldest indication for therapeutic apheresis.[39,40] It is particularly amenable to plasma exchange because IgM is distributed largely in the plasma and not in the extravascular fluid. Because the relationship between paraprotein concentration and viscosity is nonlinear, reduced viscosity sufficient to relieve both hemorrhagic and ischemic symptoms can be achieved with an exchange of only 500 to 1000 mL of plasma by manual bag techniques. Larger automated exchanges are even more effective. Plasma exchange can reverse clinical manifestations of cryoglobulinemia, such as vasculitis, glomerulonephritis, and Raynaud phenomenon.[41,42] In both instances, plasma exchange is best used as a temporizing strategy until more definitive therapy directed at the protein-producing cells takes effect. However, long-term treatment can be effective in unusual circumstances.

Plasma exchange has been used in renal failure associated with myeloma in hopes of depleting nephrotoxic free light chains.[43,44] In one prospective, randomized study of oliguric patients requiring dialysis, only patients treated with plasma exchange and chemotherapy recovered renal function.[44] However, a subsequent randomized trial in 104 myeloma patients presenting with renal failure showed no advantage for those assigned to receive 5 to 7 plasma-exchange treatments.[45] The effectiveness of plasma exchange in depleting light chains has been questioned.[46]

Immunoglobulins with Pathogenic Specificity

A number of diseases are mediated by circulating antibody specific for a host tissue antigen. Although autoreactive, some of these antibodies probably are stimulated by exposure to alloantigens (e.g., anti-human platelet antigen [HPA]-1a in posttransfusion purpura). Plasma exchange therapy is useful in many such illnesses, including the examples listed in Table 26–4.

Hematologic Diseases In posttransfusion purpura, thrombocytopenia develops abruptly about 1 week after a blood transfusion, in association with an alloantibody response to a platelet-specific antigen. The thrombocytopenia may occur even more rapidly in previously pregnant patients or in those who have had the reaction previously. The mechanism by which

TABLE 26–4. Examples of Specific Antibodies in Diseases Treated with Plasma Exchange

Antibody Specificity	Disease
Autoantibodies	
Motor endplate acetylcholine receptor	Myasthenia gravis
Nerve-ending calcium-channel active zone	Lambert-Eaton myasthenic syndrome
Peripheral nerve myelin	Guillain-Barré syndrome, chronic inflammatory demyelinating polyneuropathy
Red cell I/i	Cold agglutinin disease
Factor VIII	Acquired hemophilia
α_3 Chain of type IV collagen	Goodpasture syndrome
Alloantibodies	
HPA-1a or other platelet antigen	Posttransfusion purpura
Anti-A, anti-B	ABO-incompatible transplant
Anti-D	Hydrops fetalis
Factor VIII	Hemophilia A inhibitor

the patient's antigen-negative platelets are destroyed is not clear.[47] Plasma exchange hastens recovery from this self-limited syndrome, as does IV γ-globulin infusion.[48]

Plasma exchange reportedly was beneficial in some trials of acute idiopathic thrombocytopenic purpura,[49,50] but has since been superseded by IV γ-globulin.[51]

Plasma exchange is not routinely recommended for warm autoimmune hemolytic anemia but has been reported to be helpful in refractory cases when used in combination with IV γ-globulin or pulse cyclophosphamide. In cold agglutinin disease, significant but transient reductions in antibody titer and hemolysis severity have been reported. In such cases, warming the extracorporeal circuit and replacement fluids is very important. A case control study suggests that plasma exchange does not improve responsiveness to transfusion in either illness.[52,53]

Coagulation factor inhibitors (autoantibodies and alloantibodies) can be removed by plasma exchange. Removal alone will not control bleeding caused by a high-titer inhibitor but may reduce the titer enough to allow replacement factor to circulate temporarily. The replacement fluid for such exchanges should be fresh-frozen plasma.[54,55] Repeated IgG antibody removal by online immunoadsorption with a protein A/Sepharose affinity column, in combination with factor replacement and immunosuppression, have induced tolerance in alloimmunized hemophiliacs[56–58]; however, other methods of immune tolerance induction are now preferred (see Chap. 124).[59]

Plasma exchange has been attempted in patients with disorders of blood cell production that can be linked to circulating antibody, including aplastic anemia and pure red cell aplasia.[58]

Removal of alloantibodies to red blood cells can be accomplished by therapeutic apheresis. Plasma exchange and isoagglutinin-specific immunoadsorption have been used to prepare patients for ABO-incompatible marrow transplants[60–62] and to treat pure red cell aplasia occurring after such transplants.[63] Apheresis instruments can also be used to remove red cells from the graft; this has become the preferred alternative because it involves a single manipulation that does not inconvenience the patient.[64] In sensitized Rh-negative women, removal of maternal IgG by plasma exchange during pregnancy to ameliorate destruction of fetal red cells has largely been supplanted by intrauterine transfusion of compatible cells.[65] Plasma exchange may still be attempted if therapy is needed prior to 18 to 20 weeks gestation, when intrauterine transfusion is not technically feasible.[66,67]

Neurologic Diseases Neurologic diseases account for many plasma exchange treatments. The effectiveness of plasma exchange complements other evidence supporting an autoimmune etiology for several neuropathic and neuromuscular disorders.

In Guillain-Barré syndrome, early treatment with plasma exchange clearly hastens recovery from an illness in which antibodies to myelin are frequently found, possibly in response to infection with *Campylobacter jejuni*.[68] Antimyelin antibodies may be found in chronic inflammatory demyelinating polyneuropathy[69]; a controlled trial showed patients treated with plasma exchange improved significantly. Chronic neuropathy in the context of a monoclonal gammopathy may also respond to plasma exchange.[68]

Myasthenia gravis and Lambert-Eaton syndrome are mediated by autoantibodies to structures in the neuromuscular junction. In the former, the target is the acetylcholine receptor on the muscle cell, whereas in the latter antibodies are directed against structures in the nerve ending. Both illnesses respond to plasma exchange, which has been most useful in severe myasthenia gravis.[68]

Autoantibodies that may block central nervous system neurotransmission are implicated in other neurologic diseases. Many patients with stiff person syndrome (SPS) make an antibody to glutamic acid decarboxylase that may inhibit synthesis of the neurotransmitter γ-aminobutyric acid. Paraneoplastic SPS may be caused by antibody to one of two synaptic proteins, amphiphysin or gephyrin. In Rasmussen encephalitis, antibodies to the Glu R3 receptor for the neurotransmitter glutamate are present. Plasma exchange reportedly benefits individual patients with these antibodies.[70]

Several other paraneoplastic syndromes with neurologic manifestations are associated with autoantibodies to neural antigens, such as encephalomyelitis with anti-Hu, cerebellar degeneration with anti-Yo, opsoclonus-myoclonus with anti-Ri, and retinal degeneration with anti-CAR. Results from plasma exchange have been disappointing.[71,72]

Renal and Rheumatic Diseases Goodpasture syndrome of glomerulonephritis and lung hemorrhage is caused by linear deposition of autoantibody to a collagen found in pulmonary and renal basement membranes. Prompt intervention with plasma exchange and cyclophosphamide is the treatment of choice.[73] By contrast, controlled trials of nephritis associated with systemic lupus erythematosus have shown that oral cyclophosphamide and plasma exchange are no better than oral cyclophosphamide alone.[74,75] One study of pauci-immune rapidly progressive glomerulonephritis suggested benefit from plasma exchange in patients with dialysis-dependent renal failure.[76] These patients had rapidly progressive glomerulonephritis without an apparent cause but had associated systemic signs of vascular inflammation (systemic vasculitis); some cases were characterized only by renal disease. A distinct feature of these cases was the virtual absence of antibody deposition after immunofluorescence staining of the biopsy specimens, which led to the label "pauci-immune" rapidly progressive glomerulonephritis. More than 80 percent of patients with pauci-immune progressive glomerulonephritis have circulating antineutrophil cytoplasmic antibodies (ANCAs), and, thus, this form of progressive glomerulonephritis is now termed *ANCA-associated vasculitis*. A more recent trial in patients with severe renal dysfunction in ANCA-associated vasculitis showed better outcomes with plasma exchange than with pulse methylprednisolone.[77] Plasma exchange has been attempted in patients with several other categories of severe vasculitis,[78–80] but studies of severe nonrenal lupus erythematosus reported excess deaths from infection when plasma exchange was added to pulse intravenous cyclophosphamide therapy.[81,82] Multiple controlled trials have shown that plasma exchange is ineffective in reversing unselected episodes of renal transplant rejection.[83] However, favorable outcomes in uncontrolled series of patients with circulating donor-specific antibody have rekindled interest in this topic.[84–86] Pretransplant plasma exchange may allow successful transplantation despite human leukocyte antigen (HLA) or ABO incompatibility.[87]

Nonimmunoglobulin Constituents

Removal of LDLs by plasma exchange can lower cholesterol levels and promote resorption of xanthomas and atheromas in patients with familial hypercholesterolemia.[88,89] Online selective extraction of lipoproteins from patient plasma can be accomplished by chemical or immunologic means.[90] Two methods—dextran sulfate absorption[91] and heparin-induced LDL precipitation[92]—are approved by the FDA for patients with severe hypercholesterolemia resistant to dietary and drug therapy. Removal of phytanic acid by plasma exchange[93] or selective LDL extraction[94] can prevent or reverse neurologic manifestations in Refsum disease. Plasma exchange can remove excessive levels of low-molecular-weight drugs, toxins, and hormones bound to plasma proteins.[83]

Normal Factor Replacement

Conceptually, plasma exchange (normal plasma for the patient's deficient plasma) can be employed to correct a deficiency of any plasma factor that is not available in a concentrated form. Plasma exchange can achieve higher levels (theoretically 65 percent of normal with a single plasma volume exchange) than simple plasma infusion, without inducing volume overload. Repletion of coagulation factors is part of the rationale for using plasma exchange to support patients with acute liver failure until recovery or liver transplantation.[95]

TTP was found empirically to respond to daily plasma exchange with normal plasma replacement.[96–98] Results of treatment are better with plasma exchange but some patients respond to simple plasma infusion,[99] suggesting that replacement of a deficient plasma factor is an important element of the therapeutic effect. The success of plasma exchange in TTP led to its application in patients with thrombocytopenia and microangiopathy whose clinical features suggest hemolytic uremic syndrome or are difficult to classify.

Many patients with TTP have severe deficiency (<5% of normal activity) of the von Willebrand cleaving metalloproteinase ADAMTS13, which limits the size of circulating von Willebrand factor multimers.[100,101] In adult patients with "acquired" TTP, the deficiency is caused by an IgG autoantibody inhibitor,[100,101] which provides a basis for a variety of immunosuppressive therapies. Simultaneous depletion of inhibitor and infusion of enzyme provide an especially strong and satisfying rationale for plasma exchange (see Chap. 133). In other patients with thrombotic microangiopathy, ADAMTS13 levels are not severely depressed[100–102]; the rationale for plasma exchange in such patients remains uncertain. Nondeficient patients with the clinical picture of idiopathic TTP have higher platelet counts and serum creatinines than do ADAMTS13-deficient patients.[103–104] Patients in both categories are likely to be treated with plasma exchange as well as immunosuppressive and/or antiplatelet agents. Surprisingly the nondeficient patients improve sooner and relapse less often; indeed, the rarity of relapse has been taken to argue against an autoimmune process. Thus these clinical differences suggest a different etiology for non–ADAMTS13-deficient TTP that might not provide a rationale for plasma exchange.[105] For those with hemolytic uremic syndrome, the efficacy of plasma exchange is doubtful.[106]

A rapid assay for ADAMTS13 might be useful to guide plasma exchange and other immunosuppressive measures in patients with thrombotic microangiopathy. In one retrospective report on a heterogenous group of 142 patients, ADAMTS13 levels did not seem predictive of response to plasma exchange; however, only 13 percent of the patients were severely deficient, and most did not receive initial glucocorticoid therapy.[107] In another report from the same center, 27 percent of patients treated for thrombotic microangiopathy had serious therapy-related complications (2% fatal); 84 percent of the complications were attributed to central venous catheters placed for plasma exchange.[108] This degree of risk emphasizes the need for prospective studies addressing the efficacy of plasma exchange and other immunosuppressive treatments, especially in patients without severe ADAMTS13 deficiency, to refine future management practices.

RED CELL EXCHANGE

Most red cell exchanges are performed in patients with complications of sickle cell disease (see Chap. 48). The goal of exchanging patient cells for cells containing hemoglobin A is creating a red cell mixture that has far fewer hemoglobin SS cells. This change may interrupt the vicious cycle of sickling, stasis, vasoocclusion, and progressive ischemia.[109] The ratio of hemoglobin AA cells to hemoglobin SS cells needed to accomplish a salutary effect is not known, but red cell exchanges should aim for a posttreatment blood hemoglobin A level greater than 70 percent so that a level greater than 50 percent persists for several weeks. Exchange may be indicated in severe crises such as stroke,[110] chest syndrome,[111] cholestasis,[112,113] and priapism.[114,115] Exchange in priapism sometimes is associated with neurologic events occurring up to 11 days later.[116] Exchange is not indicated for simple pain crisis,[117] but prophylactic exchanges may prevent future events in patients with frequent or overlapping crises. Prophylactic red cell exchange has been recommended for pregnant patients and prior to general anesthesia, but these two indications are controversial.[118] Long-term maintenance of a hemoglobin A level greater than 70 percent is recommended for pediatric patients who have sustained a stroke or have imaging evidence of brain ischemia.[118,119] Prophylactic red cell exchange can achieve this level with a far lower risk of iron overload than frequent transfusion but requires exposure to more red cell units.[120]

In other applications, red cell exchange can lower parasite load in severe falciparum malaria and babesiosis.[109] Exchange of red cells for a plasma substitute can lower hematocrit rapidly, without hypovolemia, in polycythemic states,[121] and deplete iron more rapidly than simple phlebotomy in hemochromatosis.[122] Exchange of plasma for red cells can rapidly raise hematocrit without producing hypervolemia.[123] Exchange of red cells can treat high-risk acute methemoglobinemia refractory to methylene blue therapy.[124]

REFERENCES

1. McLeod BC: An approach to evidenced-based therapeutic apheresis. *J Clin Apher* 17:124, 2002.
2. Strauss RG, McLeod BC: Complications of therapeutic apheresis, in *Transfusion Reactions*, 3rd ed, edited by MA Popovsky, p 405. AABB Press, Bethesda, MD, 2007.
3. McLeod BC, Price TH, Owen H, et al: Frequency of immediate adverse effects associated with therapeutic apheresis. *Transfusion* 39:282, 1999.
4. Bolan CD, Greer SE, Cecco SA, et al: Comprehensive analysis of citrate effects during plateletpheresis in normal donors. *Transfusion* 41:1165, 2001.
5. Bolan CD, Cecco SA, Wesley RA, et al: Controlled study of citrate effects and response to i.v. calcium administration during allogeneic peripheral blood progenitor cell donation. *Transfusion* 42:935, 2002.
6. Hester J: Therapeutic cell depletion, in *Apheresis: Principles and Practice*, 2nd ed, edited by BC McLeod, TH Price, R Weinstein, p 283. AABB Press, Bethesda, MD, 2003.
7. Mercer B, Drouin J, Jolly E, D'Anjou G: Primary thrombocythemia in pregnancy: A report of two cases. *Am J Obstet Gynecol* 159:127, 1988.
8. Klippel JH: Apheresis: Biotechnology and the rheumatic diseases. *Arthritis Rheum* 27:1081, 1984.

9. McFarland HF, Rose JW: Lymphocytapheresis in the treatment of multiple sclerosis. *Plasma Ther Transfus Technol* 3:411, 1982.
10. Sands BE, Sandborn WJ, Feagon B, et al: A randomized, double-blind, sham-controlled study of granulocyte/monocyte apheresis for active ulcerative colitis. *Gastroenterology* 135:400, 2008.
11. Fritz RD, Forkner GE, Freireich EJ, et al: The association of fatal intracranial hemorrhage and blastic "crisis" in patients with acute leukemia. *N Engl J Med* 261:59, 1959.
12. Freireich E, Thomas L, Rei E, et al: A distinctive type of intracerebral hemorrhage associated with "blastic crisis" in patients with leukemia. *Cancer* 13:146, 1960.
13. McKee LC, Collins RD: Intravascular leukocyte thrombi and aggregates as a cause of morbidity and mortality in leukemia. *Medicine (Baltimore)* 53:463, 1974.
14. Ventura GJ, Hester JP, Smith TL, Keating MJ: Acute myeloblastic leukemia with hyperleukocytosis: Risk factors for early mortality in induction. *Am J Hematol* 27:34, 1988.
15. Maurer HS, Steinharz PG, Gaynon PS, et al: The effect of initial management of hyperleukocytosis on early complications and outcome of children with acute lymphoblastic leukemia. *J Clin Oncol* 6:1425, 1988.
16. Porcu P, Farag S, Marcucci G, et al: Leukocytoreduction for acute leukemia. *Ther Apher* 6:15, 2002.
17. Chang M-C, Chen T-Y, Tang J-L, et al: Leukapheresis and cranial irradiation in patients with hyperleukocytic acute myeloid leukemia: No impact on early mortality and intracranial hemorrhage. *Am J Hematol* 82:976, 2007.
18. Bug G, Anaggrou K, Tonn T, et al: Impact of leukapheresis on early death rate in adult acute myeloid leukemia presenting with hyperleukocytosis. *Transfusion* 47:1843, 2007.
19. Morse EE, Carbone PP, Freireich EJ, et al: Repeated leukapheresis of patients with chronic myelocytic leukemia. *Transfusion* 6:175, 1966.
20. Morse EE, Freireich EJ, Carbone PP, et al: The transfusion of leukocytes from donors with chronic myelocytic leukemia to patients with leukopenia. *Transfusion* 6:183, 1966.
21. Hester JP, McCredie KB, Freireich EJ: Response to chronic leukapheresis procedures and survival of chronic myelogenous leukemia patients. *Transfusion* 22:305, 1982.
22. Caplan SM, Coco FV, Berkman EM: Management of chronic myelocytic leukemia in pregnancy by cell pheresis. *Transfusion* 18:120, 1978.
23. Lichtman MA, Rowe JM: Hyperleukocytic leukemias: Rheological, clinical, and therapeutic considerations. *Blood* 60:279, 1982.
24. Edelson R, Factor M, Andrews A, et al: Successful management of the Sézary syndrome. *N Engl J Med* 291:293, 1974.
25. Belter SV, Knop J, Bruske K, Sorg C: Leukapheresis in the treatment of cutaneous T-cell lymphomas. *Br J Dermatol* 115:159, 1986.
26. Edelson RL, Berger C, Gasparro F, et al: Treatment of cutaneous T-cell lymphoma by extracorporeal photochemotherapy. *N Engl J Med* 316:297, 1987.
27. Marks DI, Rockman SP, Oziemski MA, Fox RM: Mechanisms of lymphocytotoxicity induced by extracorporeal photochemistry for cutaneous T cell lymphoma. *J Clin Invest* 86:2080, 1990.
28. Lim HW, Edelson RL: Photopheresis for the treatment of cutaneous T-cell lymphoma. *Hematol Oncol Clin North Am* 9:1117, 1995.
29. Scarisbrick JJ, Taylor P, Holtick U, et al: UK consensus statement on the use of extracorporeal photopheresis for treatment of cutaneous T-cell lymphoma and chronic graft-versus-host disease. *Br J Dermatol* 158:659, 2008.
30. Mechanic SA, Krause D, Proytcheva MA, Snyder EL: Mobilization and collection of peripheral blood progenitor cells, in *Apheresis: Principles and Practice*, 2nd ed, edited by BC McLeod, TH Price, R Weinstein, p 503. AABB Press, Bethesda, MD, 2003.
31. Klein HG: Cellular gene therapy, in *Apheresis: Principles and Practice*, 2nd ed, edited by BC McLeod, TH Price, R Weinstein, p 643. AABB Press, Bethesda, MD, 2003.
32. Verappan R, Morrison M, Williams S, Variakojis D: Splenic rupture in a patient with plasma cell myeloma following G-CSF/GM-CSF administration for stem cell transplantation and review of the literature. *Bone Marrow Transplant* 40:361, 2007.
33. Adler BK, Salzman DE, Carabasi H, et al: Fatal sickle cell crisis after granulocyte colony-stimulating factor administration. *Blood* 97:3313, 2001.
34. Porter DL, Antin JH. Donor leukocyte infusions in myeloid malignancies: New strategies. *Baillieres Best Pract Res Clin Haematol* 19:737, 2006.
35. Ribas A, Butterfield LH, Glaspy JA, Economou JS: Current developments in cancer vaccines and cellular immunotherapy. *J Clin Oncol* 21:2415, 2003.
36. Weinstein R: Basic principles of therapeutic blood exchange, in *Apheresis: Principles and Practice*, 2nd ed, edited by BC McLeod, TH Price, R Weinstein, p 295. AABB Press, Bethesda, MD, 2003.
37. Rawal A, Anderson C, Rodgers ZR, et al: Isovolemic hemodilution followed by red cell exchange in patients with sickle cell disease [abstract]. *J Clin Apher* 17:153, 2002.
38. McLeod BC, Sassetti RJ, Stefoski D, Davis FA: Partial plasma protein replacement in therapeutic plasma exchange. *J Clin Apher* 1:115, 1983.
39. Schwab PJ, Fahey JL: Treatment of Waldenström's macroglobulinemia by plasmapheresis. *N Engl J Med* 263:574, 1960.
40. Solomon A, Fahey JL: Plasmapheresis therapy in macroglobulinemia. *Ann Intern Med* 58:789, 1963.
41. Berkman EM, Orlin JB: Use of plasmapheresis and partial plasma exchange in the management of patients with cryoglobulinemia. *Transfusion* 20:171, 1980.
42. McLeod BC, Sassetti RJ: Plasmapheresis with return of cryoglobulin-depleted autologous plasma (cryoglobulinpheresis) in cryoglobulinemia. *Blood* 55:866, 1980.
43. Wahlin A, Lofvenberg E, Holm J: Improved survival in multiple myeloma with renal failure. *Acta Med Scand* 221:205, 1987.
44. Johnson WJ, Kyle RA, Pineda AA, et al: Treatment of renal failure associated with multiple myeloma. *Arch Intern Med* 150:863, 1990.
45. Clark WF, Stewart AK, Rock GA, et al: Plasma exchange when myeloma presents as renal failure: A randomized, controlled trial. *Ann Intern Med* 143:777, 2005.
46. Cserti C, Haspel R, Stowell C, Dzik W: Light chain removal by plasmapheresis in myeloma-associated renal failure. *Transfusion* 47:511, 2007.
47. McCrae KR, Herman JH: Posttransfusion purpura: Two unusual cases and a literature review. *Am J Hematol* 52:205, 1996.
48. Mueller-Eckhardt C, Kiefel V: High dose IgG for post-transfusion purpura revisited. *Blut* 57:163, 1988.
49. Marder VJ, Nusbacher J, Anderson FW: One-year follow-up of plasma exchange therapy in 14 patients with idiopathic thrombocytopenic purpura. *Transfusion* 21:291, 1981.
50. Blanchette VS, Hogan VA, McCombie NE, et al: Intensive plasma exchange therapy in ten patients with idiopathic thrombocytopenic purpura. *Transfusion* 24:388, 1984.
51. Bussel JB: Autoimmune thrombocytopenic purpura. *Hematol Oncol Clin North Am* 4:179, 1990.
52. Koo AP: Therapeutic apheresis in autoimmune and rheumatic disorders. *J Clin Apher* 15:18, 2000.
53. McLeod BC: Evidence based therapeutic apheresis in autoimmune and other hemolytic anemias. *Curr Opin Hematol* 14:647, 2007.
54. Nilsson IM, Berntorp E, Freiburghaus C: Treatment of patients with factor VIII and IX inhibitors. *Thromb Haemost* 70:56, 1993.
55. Cohen AJ, Kessler CM: Acquired inhibitors. *Baillieres Clin Haematol* 9:331, 1996.
56. Nilsson IM, Berntorp E, Zettervoll O: Induction of immune tolerance in patients with hemophilia and antibodies to factor VIII by combined treatment with intravenous IgG, cyclophosphamide, and factor VIII. *N Engl J Med* 318:947, 1988.
57. Uehlinger J, Button GR, McCarthy JM, et al: Immunoadsorption for coagulation factor inhibitors. *Transfusion* 31:269, 1991.
58. Grima KM: Therapeutic apheresis in hematological and oncological diseases. *J Clin Apher* 15:28, 2000.
59. Hay CRM, Brown S, Collins, PW, et al: The diagnosis and management of factor VIII and IX inhibitors: A guideline from the United Kingdom haemophilia centre doctors organisation. *Br J Haematol* 133:591, 2006.
60. Berkman EM, Caplan W, Kim GS: ABO-incompatible bone marrow transplantation: Preparation by plasma exchange and in vivo antibody absorption. *Transfusion* 18:504, 1978.
61. Bensinger WL, Baker DA, Buckner CD, et al: Immunoadsorption for removal of A and B blood group antibodies. *N Engl J Med* 304:160, 1981.
62. Bensinger WL, Baker DA, Buckner CD, et al: In vitro and in vivo removal of anti-A erythrocyte antibody by adsorption to a synthetic immunoadsorbent. *Transfusion* 21:335, 1981.
63. Helbig G, Stella-Holowiecka B, Wojnar J, et al: Pure red cell aplasia following major and bidirectional ABO-incompatible allogeneic stem cell transplantation: recovery of donor-derived erythropoiesis after long-term treatment using different strategies. *Ann Hematol* 86:677, 2007.
64. Braine HG, Sensenbrenner LL, Wright SK, et al: Bone marrow transplantation with major ABO incompatibility using erythrocyte depletion of marrow prior to infusion. *Blood* 60:420, 1982.
65. Rock G, Lafreniere I, Chan L, McCombie N: Plasma exchange in the treatment of hemolytic disease of the newborn. *Transfusion* 21:546, 1981.
66. Watson WJ, Katz VL, Bowes WA: Plasmapheresis during pregnancy. *Obstet Gynecol* 76:451, 1990.
67. Ruma MS, Moise KJ, Kim E, et al: Combined plasmapheresis and intravenous immunoglobulin for the treatment of several maternal red cell alloimmunization. *Am J Obstet Gynecol* 196:138.el, 2007.
68. Lehmann HC, Hartung H-P, Hetzel GR, et al: Plasma exchange in neuroimmunological disorders. Part 2: Treatment of neuromuscular disorders. *Arch Neurol* 63:1066, 2006.
69. Allen D, Giannopoulos K, Gray I, et al: Antibodies to peripheral nerve myelin proteins in chronic inflammatory demyelinating polyradiculopathy. *J Peripher Nerv Syst* 10:174, 2005.
70. Lehmann HC, Hartung H-P, Hetzel GR, et al: Plasma exchange in neurological disorders. Part 1: Rationale and treatment of inflammatory central nervous system disorders. *Arch Neurol* 63:930, 2006.
71. Moll JWB, Vecht CJ: Immune diagnosis of paraneoplastic neurological disease. *Clin Neurol Neurosurg* 97:71, 1995.
72. Das A, Hochberg FH, McNelis S: A review of the therapy of paraneoplastic neurologic syndromes. *J Neurooncol* 41:181, 1999.
73. Pusey CD. Anti-glomerular basement membrane disease. *Kidney Int* 64:1535, 2003.
74. Lewis EJ, Hunsicker LG, Lan S-P, et al: A controlled trial of plasmapheresis therapy in severe lupus nephritis. *N Engl J Med* 326:1373, 1992.
75. Doria A, Piccoli A, Vesco P, et al: Therapy of lupus nephritis. *Ann Med Interne (Paris)* 145:307, 1994.
76. Pusey CD, Rees AJ, Evans DJ, et al: Plasma exchange in focal necrotizing glomerulonephritis without anti-GBM antibodies. *Kidney Int* 40:757, 1991.
77. Jayne DR, Gaskin G, Rasmussen N, et al: Randomized trial of plasma exchange of high-dosage methylprednisolone as adjunctive therapy for severe renal vasculitis. *J Am Soc Nephrol* 18:2180, 2007.
78. Gerraty RP, McKelvie PA, Byrne E: Aseptic meningoencephalitis in primary Sjögren's syndrome. *Acta Neurol Scand* 88:309, 1993.

79. Jenkins HR, Jewkes F, Vujanic GM: Systemic vasculitis complicating infantile autoimmune enteropathy. *Arch Dis Child* 71:534, 1994.
80. Fauci AS, Leavitt RY: Systemic vasculitis, in *Current Therapy in Allergy, Immunology and Rheumatology*, edited by LM Liechtenstein, AS Fauci, p 149. Decker, Toronto, 1988.
81. Aringer M, Smolen J, Graninger W: Severe infections in plasmapheresis-treated systemic lupus erythematosus. *Arthritis Rheum* 41:414, 1998.
82. Schroeder JO, Schwab U, Zennet R, et al: Plasmapheresis and subsequent pulse cyclophosphamide in severe systemic lupus erythematosus. Preliminary results of the LPSG-Trial. *Arthritis Rheum* 40:S325, 1997.
83. Winters JL, Pineda A, McLeod BC, Grima K: Therapeutic apheresis in renal and metabolic diseases. *J Clin Apher* 15:53, 2000.
84. Crespo M, Pascual M, Tolkoff-Rubin N, et al: Acute humoral rejection in renal allograft recipients: I. Incidence, serology and clinical characteristics. *Transplantation* 71:652, 2001.
85. Montgomery RA, Zachary AA, Racusen LC, et al: Plasmapheresis and intravenous immune globulin provides effective rescue therapy for refractory humoral rejection and allows kidneys to be successfully transplanted into crossmatch-positive recipients. *Transplantation* 70:887, 2000.
86. White NB, Greenstein SM, Contafio AW, et al: Successful rescue therapy with plasmapheresis and intravenous immunoglobulin for acute humoral renal transplant rejection. *Transplantation* 78:772, 2004.
87. Rahman T, Harper L: Plasmapheresis in nephrology. *Curr Opin Nephrol Hypertens* 15:603, 2006.
88. Ginsberg HN: Update on the treatment of hypercholesterolemia, with a focus on HMG-CoA reductase inhibitors and combination regimens. *Clin Cardiol* 18:307, 1995.
89. Mabuchi H, Koizumi J, Michishita I, et al: Effects on coronary atherosclerosis of long-term treatment of familial hypercholesterolemia by LDL-apheresis. *Beitr Infusionther* 23:87, 1988.
90. Thompson GR, HEART-UK LDL Apheresis working group. Recommendations for the use of LDL apheresis. *Atherosclerosis* 198:247, 2008.
91. Gordon BR, Kelsey SF, Dan P, et al: Long-term effects of low-density lipoprotein apheresis using an automated dextran sulfate cellulose adsorption system. *Am J Cardiol* 81:407, 1998.
92. Lane DM, McConathy WJ, Laughlin LO, et al: Weekly treatment of diet/drug-resistant hypercholesterolemia with the heparin-induced extra-corporeal low-density lipoprotein precipitation (HELP) system by selective plasma low-density lipoprotein removal. *Am J Cardiol* 71:816, 1993.
93. Gibberd FB: Plasma exchange for Refsum's disease. *Transfus Sci* 14:23, 1993.
94. Gutsche H-U, Siegmund JB, Hoppmann I: Lipapheresis: An immunoglobulin-sparing treatment for Refsum's disease. *Acta Neurol Scand* 94:190, 1996.
95. Kondrup J, Almdal T, Vilstrup H, et al: High volume plasma exchange in fulminant hepatic failure. *Int J Artif Organs* 15:669, 1992.
96. Byrnes JJ, Moake JL, Periman P: Effectiveness of the cryosupernatant fraction of plasma in the treatment of refractory thrombotic thrombocytopenic purpura. *Am J Hematol* 34:169, 1990.
97. Welborn JL, Emrick P, Acevedo M: Rapid improvement of thrombotic thrombocytopenic purpura with vincristine and plasmapheresis. *Am J Hematol* 35:18, 1990.
98. Rock G, Shumak K, Kelton J, et al: Thrombotic thrombocytopenic purpura: Outcome in 24 patients with renal impairment treated with plasma exchange. *Transfusion* 32:710, 1992.
99. Rock GA, Shumak KH, Buskard NA, et al: Comparison of plasma exchange with plasma infusion in the treatment of thrombotic thrombocytopenic purpura. *N Engl J Med* 325:393, 1991.
100. Furlan M, Robles R, Galbusera M, et al: Von Willebrand factor-cleaving protease in thrombotic thrombocytopenic purpura and the hemolytic-uremic syndrome. *N Engl J Med* 339:1578, 1998.
101. Tsai H-M, Lian EC-Y: Antibodies to von Willebrand factor-cleaving protease in acute thrombotic thrombocytopenic purpura. *N Engl J Med* 339:1585, 1998.
102. Veyradier A, Obert B, Houllier A, et al: Specific von Willebrand factor-cleaving protease in thrombotic microangiopathies: A study of 111 cases. *Blood* 98:1765, 2001.
103. Raife T, Atkinson B, Montgomery R, et al: Severe deficiency of vWF-cleaving protease (ADAMTS13) activity defines a distinct population of thrombotic microangiopathy patients. *Transfusion* 44:142, 2004.
104. Zakarija A, Bandarenko N, Kwaan H, et al: Risk factors for thrombotic thrombocytopenic purpura: results of surveillance, epidemiology and risk factors for TTP (SERF-TTP) group [abstract]. *J Clin Apher* 22:51, 2007.
105. Sadler JE: Von Willebrand factor, ADAMTS13 and thrombotic thrombocytopenic purpura. *Blood* 112:11, 2008.
106. McLeod BC: Thrombotic microangiopathies in bone marrow and organ transplant patients. *J Clin Apher* 17:118, 2002.
107. Vesely SK, George JN, Lämmele B, et al: ADAMTS13 activity in thrombotic thrombocytopenic purpura-hemolytic uremic syndrome: Relation to presenting features and clinical outcomes in a prospective cohort. *Blood* 102:60, 2003.
108. McMinn JR Jr, Thomas IA, Terrell DR, et al: Complication of plasma exchange in thrombotic thrombocytopenic purpura-hemolytic uremic syndrome. A study of 78 additional patients. *Transfusion* 43:415, 2003.
109. Pepkowitz S: Red cell exchange and other therapeutic alterations of red cell mass, in *Apheresis: Principles and Practice*, 2nd ed, edited by BC McLeod, TH Price, R Weinstein, p 411. AABB Press, Bethesda, MD, 2003.
110. Adams RJ: Stroke prevention and treatment in sickle cell disease. *Arch Neurol* 58:565, 2001.
111. Gladwin MT, Vichinsky E: Pulmonary complications of sickle cell disease. *N Engl J Med* 359:2254, 2008.
112. Rossof AH, McLeod BC, Holmes AW, Fried W: Intrahepatic sickling crisis in hemoglobin SC disease: Management by partial exchange transfusion. *Plasma Ther* 2:7, 1981.
113. Sheehy TW, Law DE, Wade BH: Exchange transfusion for sickle cell intrahepatic cholestasis. *Arch Intern Med* 140:1364, 1980.
114. Hamre MR, Harmon EP, Kirkpatrick DV, et al: Priapism as a complication of sickle cell disease. *J Urol* 145:1, 1991.
115. Chakrabarty A, Upadhyay J, Dhabuwala CB, et al: Priapism associated with sickle cell hemoglobinopathy in children: Long-term effects on potency. *J Urol* 155:1419, 1996.
116. Rackoff WR, Ohene-Frempong K, Month S, et al: Neurologic events after partial exchange transfusion for priapism in sickle cell disease. *J Pediatr* 120:882, 1992.
117. Kleinman SH, Hurvitz CG, Goldfinger D: Use of erythrocytapheresis in the treatment of patients with sickle cell disease. *J Clin Apher* 2:170, 1984.
118. Telen MJ: Principles and problems of transfusion in sickle cell disease. *Semin Hematol* 38:315, 2001.
119. Cohen AR, Martin MB, Silber JH, et al: A modified transfusion program for prevention of stroke in sickle cell disease. *Blood* 79:1657, 1992.
120. Vichinsky E: Consensus document for transfusion-related iron overload. *Semin Hematol* 38:2, 2001.
121. Kaboth U, Rumph KW, Liersch T, et al: Advantages of isovolemic large-volume erythrocytapheresis as a rapidly effective and long-lasting treatment modality for red blood cell depletion in patients with polycythemia vera. *Ther Apher* 1:131, 1997.
122. Cesana M, Mandelli C, Tiribelli C, et al: Concomitant primary hemochromatosis and β-thalassemia trait: Iron depletion by erythrocytapheresis and desferrioxamine. *Am J Gastroenterol* 84:150, 1989.
123. McLeod BC, Reed SR, Viernes AV, Valentino L: Rapid red cell transfusion by apheresis. *J Clin Apher* 9:142, 1994.
124. Golden PJ, Weinstein R: Treatment of high-risk, refractory acquired methemoglobinemia with automated red blood cell exchange. *J Clin Apher* 13:28, 1998.

CHAPTER 27
PRINCIPLES OF GENE TRANSFER FOR THERAPY

Januario E. Castro and Thomas J. Kipps

SUMMARY

The term *gene therapy* describes treatment resulting from insertion of a gene(s) into somatic cells. High-level expression of a transferred gene (or transgene) can be achieved in almost any type of mammalian cell. Once inside the cell, the transgene can direct synthesis of an intracellular cell surface or secreted protein that can complement a genetic deficiency or confer upon the cell a desired phenotype or function. Alternatively, the transferred genetic material can repress expression of genes encoding unwanted or mutated proteins through "gene interference" or gene complementation. Conceivably, transfer and expression of appropriate genes could correct genetic deficiencies or generate somatic cells with a desired characteristic(s) that can result in therapeutic benefit. Many clinical trials have involved gene therapy for patients with various hematologic diseases, such as leukemia, lymphoma, Gaucher disease, aplastic anemia, hemoglobinopathies, or coagulation factor deficiencies. Results from some clinical trials suggest gene therapy may be useful for treatment of a variety of genetic or acquired diseases, including hematologic disorders. This chapter reviews the basic principles of gene transfer and the results of selected preclinical and clinical studies.

MECHANISM OF GENE TRANSFER

■ VIRUS VECTORS

Vectors can be derived from viruses such as retroviruses or adenoviruses. Such vectors can transfer their genetic material into somatic cells with high efficiency. Virus entry can be accomplished by binding to cell surface receptors or through nonspecific attachment. Typically, such viruses bind and enter host cells via receptor-mediated endocytosis, allowing for efficient entry of the virus genetic material into the cell. Table 27–1 lists the cell receptors for specific virus vectors.

Virus vectors generally use viruses that are modified such that they are unable to generate progeny virus except in specific cell lines. The cell lines that can propagate such virus vectors generally have been genetically modified to complement the replication defect of the virus vector. These so-called packaging cell lines express a gene(s) that is deleted or mutated in the virus vector that is essential for generating progeny virus capable of infecting other cells. Ordinary somatic cells that lack this gene(s) cannot complement the genetic defect of such virus vectors and therefore cannot produce infectious progeny virus. One exception to this is the oncolytic vectors, which selectively replicate in and lyse human tumor cells, providing a promising means for targeted tumor destruction. This idea has rapidly evolved from the discovery of an E1B-deleted adenovirus (ONYX-015) capable of replicating in p53-deficient cells to a larger list of candidate vectors that are currently in clinical development.[1]

Virus vectors also can be produced by packaging cells that are genetically modified to synthesize and replace the virus vector's envelope proteins with those of another virus, such as vesicular stomatitis virus-G.[2] These modified, virus particles are called *pseudotyped* viruses because they have the envelope protein(s) of virus that is distinct from that of the genetic material confined within the particle. Generally, the envelope protein(s) selected for generating pseudotyped viruses is derived from viruses that have a broader or more-desired tissue tropism and/or more resilient physical characteristics. Table 27–1 lists some examples of pseudotyped virus and their receptors.

Upon binding and entry into the target cell, the virus vector inserts its genetic material into the infected cell. The RNA of retroviruses must first be modified prior to its transport to the nucleus. For this purpose, retroviruses carry a reverse transcriptase that converts the virus single-stranded RNA into copy or complementary DNA (cDNA). DNA viruses, such as adenovirus or adeno-associated virus (AAV), on the other hand, do not require such modification. In any case, during productive infection, the virus genome or its cDNA is transported to the nucleus, where it usurps host cellular machinery to direct the synthesis of virus-specific proteins and assembly of new virus particles (Fig. 27–1).

Retrovirus Vectors

Retrovirus vectors are lipid-enveloped particles containing a positive-sense, single-stranded RNA that typically is 7 to 11 kilobases (kb) in length. These vectors produce stable, high-level transgene expression in the infected cell and its progeny.

The *Retroviridae* family includes several members that are used as vectors in gene therapy. The viruses initially evaluated were the mammalian and avian C-type retroviruses (oncoretroviruses). In addition, spumavirus and lentivirus, which includes HIV, have been modified for use in gene transfer.

The preintegration nuclear protein complex of oncoretroviruses, such as murine leukemia virus, is relatively unstable and cannot be used for effecting transgene expression in nondividing cells. In contrast, the preintegration complex of lentiviruses is more stable and can transit through the intact nuclear membrane.[3] Therefore, lentivirus-derived vectors have an advantage over previously used retrovirus vectors in that their cDNA can enter into the nucleus of nondividing cells,[4] where it can integrate into the host cell's genome, a requirement for retrovirus transgene expression.

Both oncoretrovirus and lentivirus vectors integrate into the host cell genome, a requirement for expression of virus-encoded transgenes. Insertions in or near host cell genes can result in "insertional mutagenesis." Such insertional mutagenesis has been implicated in the development of leukemia in pediatric patients with X-linked severe combined immune deficiency who were treated with lentivirus-vectors encoding the interleukin (IL)-2 receptor gene *IL-2RG*.[5,6] Two independent studies showed that the leukemic blast in those patients contained vector insertions in at least one protooncogene site (LMO2, BMI, CCND2). However, additional genetic abnormalities also were present, suggesting deregulation of the network that controls growth of T-cell progenitors. Most patients with post-gene therapy leukemia achieved complete and sustained remissions following treatment with chemotherapy. Such remissions were associated with restoration of polyclonal transduced T-cell populations.[5,6]

Acronyms and abbreviations that appear in this chapter include: AAV, adeno-associated virus; ADA, adenosine deaminase; AML, acute myelogenous leukemia; ASCT, autologous stem cell transplant; CAR, coxsackie adenovirus receptor; cDNA, copy or complementary DNA; CLL, chronic lymphocytic leukemia; dsDNA, double-stranded DNA; dsRNA, double-stranded RNA; GM-CSF, granulocyte-monocyte colony-stimulating factor; HSV, herpes simplex virus; IFN, interferon; IL, interleukin; IL-2RG, interleukin-2 receptor gene; NPM-ALK, nucleophosmin-anaplastic lymphoma kinase; OS, overall survival; RFS, relapse-free survival; RNAi, RNA interference; siRNA, small interfering RNA; TNF, tumor necrosis factor.

TABLE 27–1. Vectors Used in Gene Therapy and Their Receptors

Vector	Cellular Receptors
Retroviruses	
Amphotropic retrovirus	Sodium-phosphate symporters (e.g., Ram-1)
Ecotropic retrovirus	Cationic amino acid transport proteins (e.g., CAT 1 or Rec-1)
Lentivirus (HIV-1)	CD4 and CCR5 or CXCR4
Viruses Used to Make *Pseudotyped* Vectors	
Vesicular stomatitis virus (VSV)	Phosphatidylserine
Gibbon ape leukemia virus (GAL V)	Sodium-phosphate symporters (e.g., Glvr-1)
Adenovirus serotype 27 (Ad37)	(see Ad37 below)
Adeno-associated virus serotype 6 (AAV-6)	(see AAV-6 below)
Adenovirus	
Ad2, Ad4, Ad5, Ad17 serotypes	Coxsackievirus/adenovirus receptor (CAR) (1° receptor) and integrins $\alpha_\gamma\beta_3$ or $\alpha_\gamma\beta_5$ (2° receptors for internalization)
Ad11, Ad16, Ad21, Ad35 serotypes	Complement regulatory protein CD46 and/or receptors other than CAR
Ad37 serotype	Sialic acid residues or a 50-kDa membrane receptor protein that appears more broadly expressed than CAR
Adeno-Associated Virus (AAV)	
AAV-2, AAV-3	Heparan sulfate (1° receptor) or fibroblast growth factor receptor-1 (alternative receptor for AAV-2) and integrin $\alpha_\gamma\beta_5$ (2° receptor for internalization)
AAV-6	Receptor other than that used by AAV-2 that is expressed at high level on skeletal muscle
Herpes Simplex Virus (HSV)	
HSV-1	Herpesvirus entry mediator-A (Hve-A), nectin-1 (Hve-C/CD111), and/or 3-*O*- sulfated glucosamine residues
HSV-2	Nectin-2

Retrovirus vectors can be used for delivery of small interfering RNA (siRNA) and/or microRNAs (miRNAs), which mediate sequence-specific RNA cleavage and represents a potential approach to treat human diseases in general. Using designed miRNAs that target different regions in the HIV-1 genome inhibited HIV-1 replication *in vitro*.[7] This promising strategy is currently under clinical investigation.

Adenovirus Vectors

Adenovirus vectors also are used for gene therapy. More than 50 different human adenovirus serotypes exist, but current vectors primarily are derived from serotypes 2 and 5.[8] In some cases, these vectors have deletions in important replication genes, making the virus unable to replicate in most cells and creating space for insertion of a desired transgene(s).[9] In contrast to retrovirus vectors, adenovirus vectors do not pose a risk for insertional mutagenesis because they do not integrate into the host cell's genome.[8]

Several qualities make adenoviruses good candidates for gene therapy. Adenoviruses can be produced and purified with high titers.[10] They can generate high levels of transgene expression in nonproliferating cells, and their double-stranded DNA (dsDNA) genome remains as an episome, mitigating the problem of insertional mutagenesis.[11]

However, adenovirus vectors have some disadvantages, including low-level expression of the transgene without a suitable promoter/enhancer to direct gene expression, the inability to transfer the transgene to successive generations of progeny daughter cells, and the capacity to induce T-cell–directed immune responses against virus-infected cells that often lead to clearance of transgene-expressing cells.[12,13] Furthermore, antibodies that develop against adenovirus proteins following the initial infection can neutralize the capacity of adenovirus vectors to infect cells *in vivo*.[14] On the other hand, the so-called immunogenicity of adenovirus-infected cells can be considered an advantage because immunogenicity may enhance development of antitumor immunity in response to adenovirus-infected tumor cells.[14,15]

Efficient infection by adenovirus type 5 requires the coxsackie-adenovirus receptor (CAR) protein.[16–18] Because many human cells express little or no CAR protein, different serotypes of adenovirus vectors that do not use CAR are being studied, along with engineered type 5 adenovirus vectors that have modified fiber proteins or that are encapsulated in liposomal nanoparticles, allowing such vectors to infect cells in a CAR-independent manner. These vectors have shown some success *in vitro* as well as *in vivo*.[19–21]

Adeno-Associated Virus

AAV is a human parvovirus that initially was discovered as a contaminant in adenovirus preparations. AAV requires a helper virus, such as adenovirus, to mediate a productive infection.[22] Of the 11 known human virus serotypes, AAV-2 is the best studied.[23]

AAV vectors have a number of qualities that make them highly suitable for gene therapy. The viral dsDNA may remain as an episome or integrate into the host cell's genome. AAV-2, and presumably other serotypes, has been reported to integrate at a specific site in the q arm of chromosome 19 (AAVS1). However, current AAV vectors do not have this ability (they lack the sequences required both in *trans* and in *cis*), and integration, which has been observed to occur at a low frequency, is random.[23] AAV genome integration has the risk of inducing mutagenesis but also offers the advantage of persistent gene expression in nondividing cells and long-term transgene expression in successive generations of daughter cells after.[24–27] Another major advantage of using AAV is that the parent virus is not known to cause human disease.[27]

AAV, however, have a major limitation, and this is their small capacity for transgene insertion (<5 kb). New vector engineering had made possible to insert very large transgenes into AAV vectors. It is feasible to have split vectors in which one construct has slight sequence overlap with a second construct so that recombination after vector nuclear entry leads to the intact transgene product being expressed.[28]

AAV has become increasingly popular for use as a vector in human clinical trials. As of 2008, the Recombinant DNA Advisory Committee and the Food and Drug Administration (FDA) had approved 38 clinical protocols involving use of AAV. AAV vectors are being examined for gene therapy of Parkinson disease, α_1-antitrypsin deficiency, heart failure, prostate cancer, hemophilia, and epilepsy.[23,29,30] The increased popularity of AAV vectors reflects the appreciation of the long-term transgene expression observed in animal models and the relative lack of adverse effects noted in preclinical animal models.

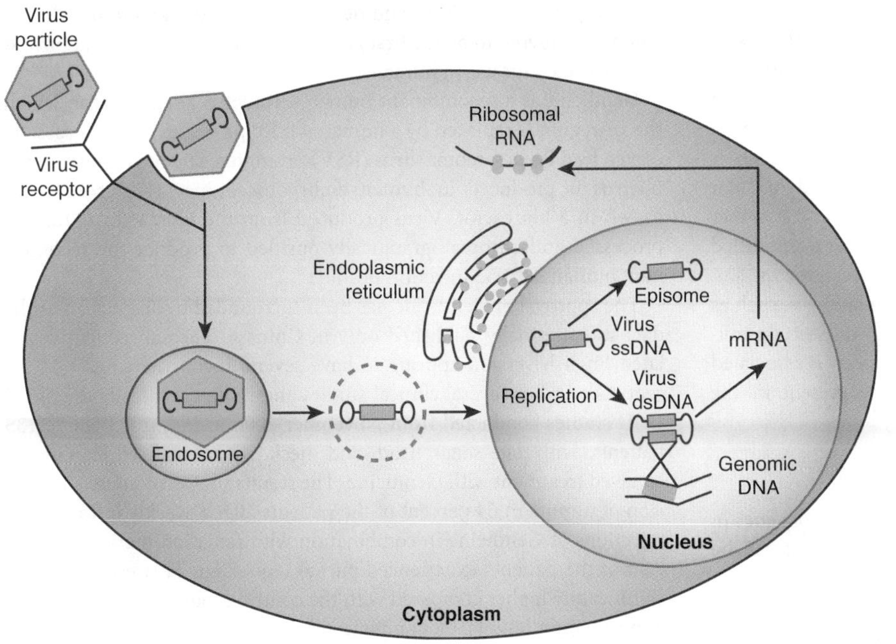

FIGURE 27–1. Interaction of vector with target cells. Virus vector binding to the target cell, its passage through the cell membrane, and subsequent release of the vector genome from the endosome are shown. Following trafficking of the vector genome to the nucleus, the genes within the episomal or integrated vector genome can be transcribed, allowing for production of transgene RNA, which then can be translated into protein. dsDNA, double-stranded DNA; ssDNA, single-stranded DNA.

Herpes Simplex Virus

Herpes viruses are DNA viruses that can be modified for use as vehicles for gene transfer into somatic cells. Among this family of virus, herpes simplex virus type 1 (HSV-1) is the most extensively studied for potential use in human gene therapy. Its genome consists of 152 kb of linear dsDNA containing at least 84 contiguous genes, of which only 50 percent is essential for virus replication. For this reason, HSV-1 vectors can carry very large transgene inserts (approximately 30 kb), potentially allowing HSV-1 vectors to contain multiple transgenes that can be individually or coordinately expressed.[31]

After deletion of the immediate early gene region, HSV vectors can be grown only in specially engineered packaging cell lines. Such HSV vectors can infect a broad range of somatic cells that, in turn, cannot produce infectious virus particles.[32] Another attractive feature of HSV vectors is that they can effect high-level expression of a transgene in many different cell types.[33]

Three different classes of vectors can be derived from HSV-1: replication-competent attenuated vectors, replication-incompetent recombinant vectors, and defective helper-dependent vectors known as *amplicons*. Amplicons consist of the transgene sequence cloned directly into a eukaryotic expression plasmid that contains one HSV origin of replication and a packaging signal. This process enables the amplicon to replicate and undergo packaging with the HSV gene products encoded by a cotransfected helper HSV vector.[34]

HSV offers advantages in cellular systems where other vectors are less effective. For example, chronic lymphocytic leukemia (CLL) cells, which are relatively resistant to infection with retroviruses or adenovirus, are highly sensitive to infection with HSV-1 vectors.[35] The sensitivity of CLL cells and some other lymphoid cells to infection by HSV-1 is in part a result of their high-level expression of the herpes virus entry mediator-A (Hve-A) protein, one of the known receptors for HSV-1.

Several clinical studies are under way using a genetically engineered oncolytic HSV-1 vector in glioblastoma and other cancers.[34,36,37] Such vectors have been injected directly into the tumor or tumor vasculature, but the clinical benefit of this approach remains to be established.

NONVIRUS-MEDIATED GENE TRANSFER AND INTERFERENCE

Nonvirus vectors use different combinations of DNA or RNA. In general, these systems are easier to produce than are virus vectors.[38] Such nonvirus vectors generally lack the efficiency of virus vector-mediated gene delivery systems. However, multiple strategies are being developed to improve gene delivery by nonvirus vectors, including those using cationic lipids,[39] *in vivo* electroporation,[40,41] hydrodynamic injection of isotonic saline,[42] cell-penetrating peptides,[40] liposome encapsulation,[43] neoglycoproteins, glycosylated plasmids,[44] or bacterial vectors.[45] Conceivably, any one or a combination of these techniques someday may improve the efficacy of nonvirus vector systems to levels approaching those of virus-based vector delivery systems.

Plasmid DNA Expression Vectors

DNA plasmid expression vectors can be used for gene transfer.[46] Generally, the transgene is placed downstream of a strong promoter, such as the heterologous cytomegalovirus promoter/enhancer region and upstream of a polyadenylation signal sequence to allow for appropriate RNA processing and transport from the nucleus.

The efficiency of gene expression following intravascular or intramuscular delivery of naked DNA generally is highest in muscle and liver. High-level transgene expression can be achieved in larger animals, including primates. Improved DNA expression vectors may allow for sustained transgene expression over prolonged periods.[47] Finally, DNA fusion vaccines containing immune-stimulatory sequences can augment the immune response to vector-encoded transgene antigens.[48–50]

DNA minicircles are novel supercoiled minimal expression cassettes, derived from conventional plasmids for the use in nonvirus gene therapy and vaccination. Minicircle DNA lacks some of the bacterial backbone sequence (antibiotic resistance gene, an origin of replication, and inflammatory sequences intrinsic to bacterial DNA). DNA minicircles appear safe and may provide for enhanced efficiency of gene transfer and expression.[51,52]

Oligonucleotides

Oligonucleotides are short pieces of synthetic, generally single-stranded DNA. Oligonucleotides can be generated with a phosphorothioate backbone that resists degradation by nucleases that otherwise rapidly metabolize standard, single-stranded pieces of DNA and enhances the oligonucleotide half-life.

Oligonucleotides can produce "gene interference" or inhibition of expression of aberrant or undesired genes.[53] Gene interference involves oligonucleotide binding to complementary sequences in a target RNA sequence, thereby inhibiting its processing or expression. The FDA approved the first *antisense oligonucleotide* product in 1998 for treatment of patients with cytomegalovirus retinitis.[54,55] Several other oligonucleotides with antisense sequences are being evaluated in clinical trials applied to solid tumors and hematologic malignancies.[56,57]

Aptamers, also called decoys or "chemical antibodies," represent an emerging class of short DNA or RNA oligonucleotides or peptides with potential therapeutical applications. They can assume a specific and stable three-dimensional shape *in vivo*, thereby providing specific tight binding to protein targets. The first aptamer approved for use in clinical trials was a RNA-based molecule (Macugen, pegaptanib), which is administered into the vitreous of patients with age-related macular degeneration to target vascular endothelial growth factor.[58] Another aptamer with apparent clinical activity is AS1411, a 26-mer unmodified guanosine-rich oligonucleotide that can inhibit cancer cell growth.[59]

Certain oligonucleotides/aptamers can directly stimulate cells, such as macrophages, dendritic cells, or B cells, by interacting with certain toll-like receptors, such as TLR-9 (see Chap. 18).[60] This property is associated with nonmethylated CpG dinucleotides that may be present in the sequence of the oligonucleotide.[61,62]

RNA Interference

Double-stranded RNA (dsRNA) can cause selective silencing of genes in multiple cell types.[63] The interference of gene expression that can be affected by dsRNA is termed *RNA interference* (RNAi).[64]

Several mechanisms have been proposed to account for the mechanism(s) underlying RNAi:[65] dsRNA-directed destruction of target RNA[66,67]; dsRNA suppression of gene transcription by affecting the chromatin structure of the targeted genes[68,69]; dsRNA-directed methylation and silencing of genomic regions that contain the target genes[65,68,70]; dsRNA-directed inhibition of translation of target genes[71]; and dsRNA-mediated chromosomal rearrangements.[72]

RNAi may have application in gene therapy. RNAi can suppress replication of HIV or other RNA viruses in human cells.[73,74] In addition, RNAi may be used to silence unwanted genes more efficiently than antisense oligonucleotide.[75,76]

dsRNA is an unstable molecule with a relatively short half-life. Several systems are being developed to overcome the problem of dsRNA's instability. For example, one system generates siRNA by virus vectors that produce small stem-loop RNA,[77,78] which can be transcribed using either polymerase II or III promoters. The vector-encoded RNA can be processed inside the cells by the Dicer enzyme into siRNA, which, in turn, can regulate the expression of selected target genes.[78,79]

A widely held assumption is that inhibition of oncogenes or genes encoding angiogenesis factors or inhibitors of tumor-cell apoptosis should block the uncontrolled proliferation of tumor cells. RNAi directed at such genes apparently can slow tumor cell growth *in vitro* and in experimental animals.[80] Also, RNAi directed at the multidrug resistance (*MDR*) gene expressed in many tumors apparently can sensitize resistant tumor cells to chemotherapy agents or radiation. The first clinical using RNAi involved patients with glioblastoma multiforme using a dsRNA to target tenascin-C, an extracellular matrix glycoprotein that contributes to tumor-cell adhesion, invasion, migration, and proliferation. The RNAi treatment apparently delayed tumor growth and/or reduced symptoms of recurrent disease and was associated with an improvement in overall survival (OS) and quality of life.[81,82] Other clinical studies using this strategy are currently under way.[80]

GENE THERAPY APPLICATIONS

APPROVAL OF THE FIRST GENE THERAPY PRODUCT

The number of clinical trials in gene therapy conducted in the United States, Europe, and Asia has grown exponentially during the last decade (1999–2009). As a result of this, in October 2003, China's State Food and Drug Administration approved Gendicine (Ad-p53) for the treatment of patients with head and neck squamous cell carcinoma. Gendicine is considered to be the first gene therapy compound ever approved and marketed for use in humans.

Gendicine is a recombinant human serotype 5 adenovirus in which the E1 region is replaced by a human wild-type p53 expression cassette driven by a Rous sarcoma virus (RSV) promoter. The recombinant adenovirus is produced in human embryonic kidney (HEK) 293 cells grown in a bioreactor. Virus produced from the bioreactor is further processed and chromatographically purified to produce the recombinant human Ad-p53 injection product.

The approval of Gendicine has been surrounded by skepticism as the data was originally published only in Chinese. The subsequent translated English version appears to have several inconsistencies.[83,84] This report describes several clinical studies and more specifically the phase II/III studies conducted from November 2000 to May 2003 where 135 patients with late-stage head and neck squamous cell carcinoma received treatment with Gendicine. The results showed complete regression of tumors in 64 percent of the patients after 8 weekly intratumoral injections of Gendicine in combination with radiation therapy; 29 percent of the patients experienced partial regression. This numbers were significantly higher compared with the control group that received radiation therapy only (19% complete response and 60% partial response rates in treated patients). Approximately 75 percent of the patients enrolled in this study had advanced nasopharyngeal carcinoma, which is a subclassification of head and neck cancer.

Another related product, Oncorine (H101) was also approved in 2005 by the SFDA in China for the treatment of patients with head and neck small-cell cancer. Oncorine is a E1B-55k, E3 gene-deleted adenovirus very similar to Onyx-015. This oncolytic vector is capable of replicating and inducing lysis of cells that have inactivating mutations in *p53*. Oncorine (H101) injected into the tumor as an adjunct to chemotherapy enhanced the clinical response to chemotherapy.[1]

HEMATOPOIETIC STEM CELLS

Hematopoietic stem cells can be modified with gene therapy protocols to treat a variety of diseases, including primary immune deficiency disease (see Chap. 82), hemoglobinopathies (see Chaps. 47 and 48), metabolic diseases, and various genetic disorders.[85–87] The main advantage of modifying hematopoietic stem cells is that these cells can undergo self-renewal and/or differentiate into mature cells of different lineages.[88–90]

Gene Marking of Hematopoietic Stem Cells

The initial clinical trials on the application of hematopoietic stem cells used gene marking to investigate the origin of relapse of leukemia patients subjected to autologous hematopoietic cell transplantation. These studies demonstrated that clinical relapse in patients with acute myelogenous leukemia (AML) and chronic myelogenous leukemia resulted from the presence of contaminating residual leukemia cells in the transplanted stem cell collection.[91–93] The data from patients treated in these early studies have provided information on the long-term safety of various approaches that could be used for therapeutic gene transfer.

INHERITED DISORDERS

Adenosine Deaminase Deficiency

Adenosine deaminase (ADA) deficiency is a fatal disorder of purine metabolism and immunodeficiency that causes severe combined immunodeficiency (SCID) in newborns (see Chap. 82). Currently, ADA-deficient patients who lack an appropriate hematopoietic stem cell donor are treated with pegylated ADA. This expensive treatment is required throughout life and cannot restore the capacity of all treated patients to generate protective immunity.

The genetic treatment of ADA-deficient patients was the first attempt to cure an inherited disease by a gene therapy approach. Retrovirus transduction of the normal ADA gene into blood T lymphocytes of affected patients corrected the deficiency *in vitro* and suggested the feasibility of a gene transfer approach *in vivo*.[94] Subsequently, clinical studies showed encouraging results after transfer of the ADA gene into blood lymphocytes of ADA-deficient patients[95] or when patients were treated with autologous ADA-transduced umbilical cord stem cells.[96]

A later protocol showed the relevance of nonmyeloablative conditioning as a procedure to facilitate engraftment of ADA-transduced CD34+ stem cells with a retrovirus vector containing the ADA gene.[97,98] In this trial, investigators observed in treated patients a sustained engraftment of transduced hematopoietic stem cells, increased leukocyte counts, and improved immune function. All 10 patients were alive and healthy after a median followup of 4.0 years (range: 1.8–8.0). Furthermore, all patients could develop antigen-specific antibody in response to vaccines and most have not required continued enzyme-replacement therapy or intravenous immune globulin infusions.[98]

X-Linked Severe Combined Immune Deficiency

X-linked SCID is caused by mutations in the *IL-2RG* X-linked gene that encodes the common γ-chain (γc) of the lymphocyte receptors for IL-2 and other cytokines (see Chap. 82).[99] The only therapy available for this form of SCID is allogeneic hematopoietic cell transplantation,[100] which is predicated upon finding a suitable donor (see Chap. 21).

The initial work in humans used retrovirus-transduced CD34+ autologous hematopoietic stem cells. In treated patients, transgene expression was detectable for prolonged periods and was associated with normalization of immune repertoire of T cells, B cells, and natural killer cells.[101] These encouraging findings were confirmed in a followup study of six more patients treated under the same protocol. Nine of 11 treated children experienced sustained improvements in immune function.[102]

Some of the patients, however, experienced a late serious adverse effect of therapy. In 2002, two patients who had received gene therapy and achieved immune reconstitution developed T-cell acute lymphoblastic leukemia almost 3 years later.[103,104] Both of these patients had leukemia T cells with insertions of the vector genetic material near *LMO2*, resulting in dysregulated *LMO2* gene expression.[102,103,105] In both cases, the leukemia T cells expressed abnormal amounts of the LMO2 protein, which previously had been linked to murine and human lymphocytic leukemias.[106] In January 2005, a third treated patient developed acute lymphoblastic leukemia with a very similar clinical presentation. The leukemia cells also had insertion of the genetic vector near the *LMO2* gene. However, the pathogenic significance of this insertion was less certain as the leukemia cells also had insertions of the vector near three other protooncogenes.[107] Nevertheless, these cases suggest that mutagenesis caused by insertion of the vector into the genome can contribute to leukemia development.

Hemoglobinopathies

High-level regulated globin gene expression is required for therapy of severely affected patients with sickle cell disease (see Chap. 48) or β-thalassemia (see Chap. 47).[108]

Two research groups have achieved transfer and expression of curative levels of β-globin in the red cell progeny of murine stem cells in animal models of β-thalassemia and sickle cell disease.[109,110]

Another study evaluated the use of lentivirus vectors encoding a β-globin transgene to transduced, human progenitor stem cells from patients lacking normal β-globin genes. After transfer to immunodeficient mice, the β-globin–transduced human stem cells were able to produce erythroid cells with stable levels of β-globin expression. These animals produced erythroid cells that expressed human β-globin at levels that should be therapeutic in patients with sickle cell anemia or β-thalassemia.[111]

Gaucher Disease

Gaucher disease is a lysosomal storage disorder resulting from a deficiency of glucocerebrosidase (see Chap. 79). Transduction of murine hematopoietic stem cells has been achieved, with long-term expression of the glucocerebrosidase gene in macrophages of transplanted mice.[112,113] Two clinical trials using Maloney-based retrovirus vectors targeted to human CD34+ cells yielded similar results with low transduction of blood cells.[114,115]

Using AAV- and HIV-1–derived lentivirus vectors, stable expression of human glucocerebrosidase protein has been achieved in the blood and liver of experimental animals and in fibroblast derived from patients with Gaucher disease.[116,117]

Fanconi Anemia

Fanconi anemia is an inherited chromosomal recessive syndrome characterized by marrow failure and cellular hypersensitivity to DNA crosslinking agents, which results in aplastic anemia and an increased incidence of malignancy. Fanconi anemia is caused by mutations in a DNA repair pathway, including at least 13 Fanconi anemia-complementing genes (see Chap. 34). The A and C genes (*FANCA* and *FANCC*) have been genetically engineered into retrovirus and AAV vectors.[118] Recombinant lentivirus vectors have been tested in FANCA–/– and FANCC–/– mice.[119] For these particular experiments, long-term repopulating hematopoietic progenitors were transduced with lentivirus vectors encoding the normal gene. Following lentivirus transduction, resistance to DNA-damaging agents was restored, allowing for *in vivo* selection of the corrected cells with nonmyeloablative doses of cyclophosphamide. This approach requires validation using human cells.

Hemophilia

Sustained therapeutic levels of clotting factors VIII and IX could significantly affect the clinical course of patients with hemophilia (see Chap. 124).

Initial efforts concentrated on the replacement of factor IX, because the coding region and regulatory sequences could readily be encapsidated in the AAV vector. A factor IX AAV vector could "cure" mice with hemophilia B[120] and performed well in a canine model of hemophilia.[121] Patients with hemophilia B have received intramuscular injections of a recombinant AAV encoding factor IX. No evidence of local or systemic toxicity has been observed up to 40 months after the initial injection. Preexisting high-titer antibodies to AAV did not prevent gene transfer or expression. Despite evidence for gene transfer and expression, circulating levels of factor IX were less than 2 percent in all cases.[122,123] Another study evaluated the use of AAV encoding factor IX injected directly into the hepatic artery. One of the treated patients experienced a transient, but significant, improvement of the serum levels of factor IX, suggesting the route of administration may be a factor in the efficiency of this approach.[124] The treated patients also experienced transient transaminitis, most likely as a result of cell-mediated immunity against hepatocytes that had taken up the vector and expressed virus proteins.[125]

Twelve patients with hemophilia A received intravenous infusion of retrovirus encoding factor VIII.[126] Plasma factor VIII levels increased in six of the treated patients and were associated with a reduced tendency for bleeding. An *ex vivo* approach using nonvirus plasmid transfection of autologous fibroblasts in culture also has been reported.[127] Four of 12 patients with hemophilia A had transient improvement in factor VIII plasma levels.

In general, the outcomes of human trials have been inferior to results observed in animals. Further development in gene delivery and expression systems is required to achieve serum levels of clotting factors that are clinically relevant.

■ ACQUIRED DISORDERS

Acquired Immunodeficiency Syndrome

HIV/AIDS currently is best treated with pharmaceutical inhibitors of reverse transcriptase and virus proteases (see Chap. 83). Nevertheless, concerns exist over the long-term efficacy of such treatment, the need for chronic drug administration, the lack of compliance of some patients, and long-term toxicity of the medications. Alternative genetic therapies that could overcome such problems are the subject of much interest.

The potential for generation of a cytotoxic response to HIV-specific elements in HIV patients has provided the bases for vaccination protocols. One study evaluated the activity of autologous fibroblasts modified to express envelope proteins of HIV IIIB as artificial antigen-presenting cells.[128] The study demonstrated that HIV-specific cytotoxic T-lymphocyte responses could be generated by this protocol. No local or systemic side effects related to treatment were observed.[129]

Other investigators have studied the use of T lymphocytes transduced with vectors expressing the chimeric protein CD4/CD3ζ, which is assembled using the extracellular domain of CD4 and the intracellular domain of the ζ-chain of the T-cell receptor. In theory, this chimeric molecule could bind to HIV and, after engagement of the receptor, generate signaling events similar to those elicited by specific antigen binding. In a phase II clinical trial, HIV patients infused with CD4/CD3ζ-transduced T lymphocytes experienced decreased virus load in reservoir sites, such as the rectal mucosa.[130,131]

In another trial using CD34+ hematopoietic stem cells derived from patients with HIV-associated lymphomas, the investigators transduced hematopoietic stem cells with a *trans*-dominant Rev protein.[132] These approaches generated relatively few transduced hematopoietic stem cells, which also provided for only short-term engraftment.

Retrovirus vectors encoding miRNAs that target genes in different regions of the HIV-1 genome could inhibit HIV-1 replication *in vitro* and potentially *in vivo.*[133] Retrovirus vectors encoding a HIV entry-inhibitory peptide (maC46) also have been used to transduce the T lymphocytes of patients with advance stage AIDS *ex vivo*. Intravenous infusions of these vector-modified, autologous T cells were well tolerated and did not produce severe adverse effects. However, such infusions resulted in a significant increase of CD4 counts that persisted for up to one year after therapy.[134]

Results of early phase I trials of retroviral vectors encoding a *tat*/viral protein R-targeting ribozyme showed the gene transfer procedure to be safe and technically feasible, and suggested that the vectors were maintained in mature hematopoietic cells for up to 4 years.[135] The clinical benefit of this strategy was not evaluated.

Another potential strategy for treatment of patients with HIV/AIDS is to use RNA decoys that mimic RNA structures that are necessary for the virus life cycle. Studies demonstrate that it is feasible to transduce cells with retroviral vectors that encode such RNA decoys.[136]

■ LEUKEMIA AND LYMPHOMA

Gene Interference

Strategies using antisense oligonucleotides currently are under evaluation in clinical trials. For example, antisense oligonucleotides targeting the open reading frame of the *BCL-2* messenger RNA can downregulate its expression, resulting in increased susceptibility to apoptosis.[137] Phase I to III clinical trials have been conducted with Oblimersen, an 18-base phosphorothioate *BCL-2* antisense oligonucleotide, in patients with adult leukemias. A randomized clinical study involving patients with CLL demonstrated that the addition of oblimersen to fludarabine monophosphate and cyclophosphamide increased the rates of complete responses and nodular partial responses of patients with relapsed or refractory disease.[138] On the other hand, patients with acute or chronic myelogenous leukemia have experienced only marginal clinical benefit from the use of this agent (see Chaps. 9 and 10).[139,140]

Other antisense oligonucleotides targeting *BCR-ABL*, protein kinase C-α, human telomerase reverse transcriptase, and ribonucleotide reductase have been evaluated in preclinical studies and in phase I and II clinical trials.[141–144] The results of these studies show the feasibility and safety of this approach, and in some cases, partial responses to the treatment modality.

Studies also have evaluated the activity of siRNA in leukemia and lymphoma cells. In one study, three different chemically synthesized siRNAs were used to target the nucleophosmin-anaplastic lymphoma kinase (NPM-ALK) fusion gene that is expressed in anaplastic large cell lymphomas. The siRNAs decreased expression of NPM-ALK protein and increased susceptibility to apoptosis.[145] Similar results were observed in a different study that evaluated siRNA targeting the multidrug resistance mediated by P-glycoprotein.[146]

Similarly, there is growing interest to regulate the expression of miRNAs. These small RNAs regulate multiple critical biologic functions in normal and cancer cells. Several studies demonstrated that miRNA expression profiles can be used to distinguish normal cells from cancer cells.[147] Particularly in CLL, a unique microRNA expression signature composed of 13 genes (of 190 analyzed) was associated with prognostic factors and disease progression.[148] Similar miRNA expression profiles have been described in other types of leukemia, lymphomas, and other cancers.[149] Preclinical and early clinical studies targeting miRNA in cancer are currently in progress.[150,151]

Gene Transfer for Development of Tumor Vaccines

Studies have evaluated the use of lymphoma or leukemia cells transduced with immune-stimulatory genes to generate enhanced antitumor responses. Some examples include the use of vectors encoding IL-2, IL-12, interferon (IFN)-γ, and granulocyte-macrophage colony-stimulating factor, and genes for immune accessory molecules, including tumor necrosis factor (TNF)-α, CD80, and the ligand for CD40 (CD154).

Immune Costimulatory Surface Molecules Transduction of CLL B cells with an adenovirus encoding CD154 (Ad-CD154) can induce leukemia cells to express immune costimulatory molecules, thereby enhancing their capacity to present antigens to cytotoxic T lymphocytes.[152] Eleven patients received a single infusion of autologous CLL cells transduced *ex vivo* with Ad-CD154.[153] Nearly all treated patients exhibited increased serum levels of IL-12 and IFN-γ, enhanced expression of immune costimulatory molecules on bystander leukemia cells, increased absolute numbers of blood T cells, and reduced blood leukemia cell counts and lymph node size. After additional infusions of Ad-CD154–transduced cells, patients showed disease stabilization, with delayed disease progression and the need for further treatment. Two of the treated patients did not require additional therapy 4 years after treatment.[154]

Using a membrane-stable chimeric homolog of CD154 (ISF35) Wierda and colleagues conducted a clinical study in subjects with CLL using a dose escalation administration of autologous leukemia cells transduced with Ad-ISF35. Similarly to what was observed in patients receiving Ad-CD154, the infusions were well tolerated and clinical benefit was observed in the majority of patients including subjects with high-risk CLL that have 17p–. The administration of Ad-ISF35 via direct intranodal administration also has been investigated. In a phase I clinical study, 15 patients with CLL received intranodal injection of Ad-ISF35 with a single ultrasonography-guided intranodal injection of 1 to 30 × 10^{10} Ad-ISF35 viral particles in four different dose cohorts. Injections were well-tolerated, with some patients developing local swelling, erythema, and "flu-like" symptoms. Some patients in the highest-dose cohorts had transient and asymptomatic hypophosphatemia and neutropenia. Ad-ISF35 intranodal injection resulted in significant reductions in blood leukemia cell counts, lymphadenopathy, and splenomegaly in the majority of patients. Although there was no evidence for dissemination of Ad-ISF35 beyond the injected lymph node, direct intranodal injection of Ad-ISF35 induced blood CLL cells to express death receptors, proapoptotic proteins, and immune costimulatory molecules, suggesting the presence of a "bystander" and systemic effect.[155]

A study evaluated the safety and efficacy of an IL-2– and CD154 (CD40-ligand)-expressing recipient-derived tumor vaccine consisting of leukemic blasts admixed with skin fibroblasts transduced with adenoviral vectors encoding human IL-2 (hIL-2) and hCD154. Ten patients (including 7 children) with high-risk acute myeloid (n = 4) or lymphoblastic (n = 6) leukemia in remission (after allogeneic stem cell transplantation [n = 9] or chemotherapy alone [n = 1]) received up to six subcutaneous injections of the IL-2/CD40L vaccine. No severe adverse reactions were noted. Immunization produced a 10- to 890-fold increase in T cells reactive against recipient-derived blasts and in some patients an increase in immunoglobulin G antibodies that bound to the patients' blasts. Eight patients remained disease free for 27 to 62 months after treatment (5-year OS: 90%).[156]

Immune Stimulatory Cytokines Human leukemia cells typically express negligible levels of CD80 and low levels of CD86, causing the cells to be ineffective at stimulating T cells in response to presented antigens.[157] Primary human leukemic cells from patients with AML can be transduced with retrovirus vectors to express CD80. *In vitro*, such transduced leukemia cells could stimulate proliferation of allogeneic T cells in mixed lymphocyte culture.[158] CLL B cells transduced with HSV-based amplicon vectors encoding CD80 can stimulate allogeneic T cells in mixed lymphocyte reactions and stimulate T cells to produce IL-2 and IFN-γ.[159] Studies performed in animal models using transduced leukemia cells with CD80 or CD86 show modest antitumor immunity.[160–162] To date, results of clinical trials using this approach have not been reported.

Murine B lymphoma cells transduced to express IL-2 and the lymphotactic chemokine lymphotactin are better able to induce antitumor immunity than nontransduced lymphoma cells or lymphoma cells transduced to express IL-2 alone.[163] Two clinical trials using transduction of IL-2 in prostate cancer have been reported.[164,165]

Preclinical studies have shown that mouse lymphoma B cells (A20) transduced with a retrovirus encoding IL-12 could induce immunity against A20 cells in syngeneic mice more efficiently than A20 cells transduced with control vectors.[166] Additionally, dendritic cells transfected with a plasmid encoding IL-12 are an effective alternative for generating enhanced antigen presentation and antitumor immune responses in a murine model of lymphoma.[167]

Transduction of cells with TNF-α inhibits the development or progression of leukemia in experimental animals.[168,169] However, systemic administration of TNF-α induces serious toxicities that limit its clinical application.[170,171] Membrane-bound TNF molecules may lack the undesirable side effects of soluble TNF-α. Coincubation of CLL cells expressing a membrane-stabilized form of TNF-α induced bystander CLL cells to express immune accessory molecules, such as CD80 and CD54. Conceivably, such modified forms of active TNF-α that resist cleavage from the plasma membrane may be used in gene therapy of various hematologic cancers.

Preclinical models have demonstrated the efficacy of granulocyte-monocyte colony-stimulating factor (GM-CSF)-secreting cancer immunotherapies (GVAX platform) accompanied by immunotherapy-primed lymphocytes following autologous stem cell transplant (ASCT) in hematologic malignancies. A phase II study evaluated the use of autologous leukemia cells admixed with GM-CSF-secreting K562 cells (K562/GM) followed by ASCT. Fifty-four subjects were enrolled, 46 (85%) achieved a complete remission and 28 (52%) received the pretransplantation immunotherapy. For all patients who achieved a complete response, the 3-year relapse-free survival (RFS) was 47.4 percent and OS was 57.4 percent. For the 28 immunotherapy treated patients, the RFS and OS were 61.8 and 73.4 percent, respectively. Posttreatment induction of delayed-type hypersensitivity reactions to autologous leukemia cells was associated with longer 3-year RFS (100% vs. 48%). Minimal residual disease was monitored by quantitative analysis of WT1, a leukemia-associated gene. A decrease in WT1 transcripts in blood was noted in 69 percent of patients following the first immunotherapy dose and was also associated with longer 3-year RFS (61% vs. 0%). Collectively, this study shows that modified K562/GM cells have potential therapeutic potential in patients with AML when used in combination with primed lymphocytes and ASCT.[172]

REFERENCES

1. Crompton AM, Kirn DH: From ONYX-015 to armed vaccinia viruses: The education and evolution of oncolytic virus development. *Curr Cancer Drug Targets* 7:133, 2007.
2. Abe A, Emi N, Kanie T, et al: Expression cloning of oligomerization-activated genes with cell-proliferating potency by pseudotype retrovirus vector. *Biochem Biophys Res Commun* 320:920, 2004.
3. Naldini L, Blomer U, Gage FH, et al: Efficient transfer, integration, and sustained long-term expression of the transgene in adult rat brains injected with a lentiviral vector. *Proc Natl Acad Sci U S A* 93:11382, 1996.
4. Naldini L, Blomer U, Gallay P, et al: In vivo gene delivery and stable transduction of nondividing cells by a lentiviral vector [see comments]. *Science* 272:263, 1996.
5. Hacein-Bey-Abina S, Garrigue A, Wang GP, et al: Insertional oncogenesis in 4 patients after retrovirus-mediated gene therapy of SCID-Xl. *J Clin Invest* 118:3132, 2008.
6. Howe SJ, Mansour MR, Schwarzwaelder K, et al: Insertional mutagenesis combined with acquired somatic mutations causes leukemogenesis following gene therapy of SCID-Xl patients. *J Clin Invest* 118:3143, 2008.
7. Lo HL, Chang T, Yam P, et al: Inhibition of HIV-1 replication with designed miRNAs expressed from RNA polymerase II promoters. *Gene Ther* 14:1503, 2007.
8. Douglas JT: Adenovirus-mediated gene delivery: An overview. *Methods Mol Biol* 246:3, 2004.
9. Curiel DT: Strategies to adapt adenoviral vectors for targeted delivery. *Ann N Y Acad Sci* 886:158, 1999.
10. Kamen A, Henry O: Development and optimization of an adenovirus production process. *J Gene Med* 6 Suppl 1:S184, 2004.
11. Nasz I, Adam E: Recombinant adenovirus vectors for gene therapy and clinical trials. *Acta Microbiol Immunol Hung* 48:323, 2001.
12. Yang Y, Ertl HC, Wilson JM: MHC class I-restricted cytotoxic T lymphocytes to viral antigens destroy hepatocytes in mice infected with E1-deleted recombinant adenoviruses. *Immunity* 1:433, 1994.
13. Yang Y, Wilson JM: Clearance of adenovirus-infected hepatocytes by MHC class I-restricted CD4+ CTLs *in vivo*. *J Immunol* 155:2564, 1995.
14. Sumida SM, Truitt DM, Kishko MG, et al: Neutralizing antibodies and CD8+ T lymphocytes both contribute to immunity to adenovirus serotype 5 vaccine vectors. *J Virol* 78:2666, 2004.
15. Borgland SL, Bowen GP, Wong NC, et al: Adenovirus vector-induced expression of the C-X-C chemokine IP-10 is mediated through capsid-dependent activation of NF-kappaB. *J Virol* 74:3941, 2000.
16. Hidaka C, Milano E, Leopold PL, et al: CAR-dependent and CAR-independent pathways of adenovirus vector-mediated gene transfer and expression in human fibroblasts. *J Clin Invest* 103:579, 1999.
17. McDonald D, Stockwin L, Matzow T, et al: Coxsackie and adenovirus receptor (CAR)-dependent and major histocompatibility complex (MHC) class I-independent uptake of recombinant adenoviruses into human tumour cells. *Gene Ther* 6:1512, 1999.
18. Santis G, Legrand V, Hong SS, et al: Molecular determinants of adenovirus serotype 5 fibre binding to its cellular receptor CAR. *J Gen Virol* 80:1519, 1999.
19. Yang L, Wang L, Su XQ, et al: Suppression of ovarian cancer growth via systemic administration with liposome-encapsulated adenovirus-encoding endostatin. *Cancer Gene Ther* 17(1):49–57, 2010.

20. Stoff-Khalili MA, Stoff A, Rivera AA, et al: Gene transfer to carcinoma of the breast with fiber-modified adenoviral vectors in a tissue slice model system. *Cancer Biol Ther* 4:1203, 2005.
21. Meier O, Greber UF: Adenovirus endocytosis. *J Gene Med* 6 Suppl 1:S152, 2004.
22. Muzyczka N: Use of adeno-associated virus as a general transduction vector for mammalian cells. *Curr Top Microbiol ImmunolMicrobiol Immunol* 158:97, 1992.
23. Daya S, Berns KI: Gene therapy using adeno-associated virus vectors. *Clin Microbiol Rev* 21:583, 2008.
24. Duan D, Sharma P, Yang J, et al: Circular intermediates of recombinant adeno-associated virus have defined structural characteristics responsible for long-term episomal persistence in muscle tissue. *J Virol* 72:8568, 1998.
25. Flotte TR: Gene therapy progress and prospects: Recombinant adeno-associated virus (rAAV) vectors. *Gene Ther* 11:805, 2004.
26. Nakai H, Iwaki Y, Kay MA, Couto LB: Isolation of recombinant adeno-associated virus vector-cellular DNA junctions from mouse liver. *J Virol* 73:5438, 1999.
27. Mueller C, Flotte TR: Clinical gene therapy using recombinant adeno-associated virus vectors. *Gene Ther* 15:858, 2008.
28. Yan Z, Zhang Y, Duan D, Engelhardt JF: Trans-splicing vectors expand the utility of adeno-associated virus for gene therapy. *Proc Natl Acad Sci U S A* 97:6716, 2000.
29. Sarkar R, Mucci M, Addya S, et al: Long-term efficacy of adeno-associated virus serotypes 8 and 9 in hemophilia a dogs and mice. *Hum Gene Ther* 17:427, 2006.
30. High KA: Adeno-associated virus-mediated gene transfer for hemophilia B. *Int J Hematol* 76:310, 2002.
31. Krisky DM, Marconi PC, Oligino TJ, et al: Development of herpes simplex virus replication-defective multigene vectors for combination gene therapy applications. *Gene Ther* 5:1517, 1998.
32. Wolfe D, Goins WF, Kaplan TJ, et al: Herpesvirus-mediated systemic delivery of nerve growth factor. *Mol Ther* 3:61, 2001.
33. Burton EA, Huang S, Goins WF, Glorioso JC: Use of the herpes simplex viral genome to construct gene therapy vectors. *Methods Mol Med* 76:1, 2003.
34. Marconi P, Argnani R, Berto E, et al: HSV as a vector in vaccine development and gene therapy. *Hum Vaccin* 4:91, 2008.
35. Eling DJ, Johnson PA, Sharma S, et al: Chronic lymphocytic leukemia B cells are highly sensitive to infection by herpes simplex virus-1 via herpesvirus-entry-mediator A. *Gene Ther* 7:1210, 2000.
36. Mace AT, Ganly I, Soutar DS, Brown SM: Potential for efficacy of the oncolytic herpes simplex virus 1716 in patients with oral squamous cell carcinoma. *Head Neck* 30:1045, 2008.
37. Harrow S, Papanastassiou V, Harland J, et al: HSV1716 injection into the brain adjacent to tumour following surgical resection of high-grade glioma: Safety data and long-term survival. *Gene Ther* 11:1648, 2004.
38. Seow Y, Wood MJ: Biological gene delivery vehicles: Beyond viral vectors. *Mol Ther* 17:767, 2009.
39. Tranchant I, Thompson B, Nicolazzi C, et al: Physicochemical optimisation of plasmid delivery by cationic lipids. *J Gene Med* 6 Suppl 1:S24, 2004.
40. Jarver P, Langel U: The use of cell-penetrating peptides as a tool for gene regulation. *Drug Discov Today* 9:395, 2004.
41. Bloquel C, Fabre E, Bureau MF, Scherman D: Plasmid DNA electrotransfer for intracellular and secreted proteins expression: New methodological developments and applications. *J Gene Med* 6 Suppl 1:S11, 2004.
42. Andrianaivo F, Lecocq M, Wattiaux-De Coninck S, et al: Hydrodynamics-based transfection of the liver: Entrance into hepatocytes of DNA that causes expression takes place very early after injection. *J Gene Med* 6:877, 2004.
43. Zou W, Luo C, Zhang Z, et al: A novel oncolytic adenovirus targeting to telomerase activity in tumor cells with potent. *Oncogene* 23:457, 2004.
44. Monsigny M, Mayer R, and Roche AC: Sugar-lectin interactions: Sugar clusters, lectin multivalency and avidity. *Carbohydr Lett* 4:35, 2000.
45. Jia LJ, Hua ZC: Development of bacterial vectors for tumor-targeted gene therapy. *Methods Mol Biol* 542:131, 2009.
46. Herweijer H, Wolff JA: Progress and prospects: Naked DNA gene transfer and therapy. *Gene Ther* 10:453, 2003.
47. Miao CH, Thompson AR, Loeb K, Ye X: Long-term and therapeutic-level hepatic gene expression of human factor IX after naked plasmid transfer *in vivo*. *Mol Ther* 3:947, 2001.
48. Rice J, Elliott T, Buchan S, Stevenson FK: DNA fusion vaccine designed to induce cytotoxic T cell responses against defined peptide motifs: Implications for cancer vaccines. *J Immunol* 167:1558, 2001.
49. Stevenson FK, Rosenberg W: DNA vaccination: A potential weapon against infection and cancer. *Vox Sang* 80:12, 2001.
50. Zhu D, Rice J, Savelyeva N, and Stevenson FK: DNA fusion vaccines against B-cell tumors. *Trends Mol Med* 7:566, 2001.
51. Stenler S, Andersson A, Simonson OE, et al: Gene transfer to mouse heart and skeletal muscles using a minicircle expressing human vascular endothelial growth factor. *J Cardiovasc Pharmacol* 53(1):18–23, 2009.
52. Mayrhofer P, Schleef M, Jechlinger W: Use of minicircle plasmids for gene therapy. *Methods Mol Biol* 542:87, 2009.
53. Yuen AR, Sikic BI: Clinical studies of antisense therapy in cancer. *Front Biosci* 5:D588, 2000.
54. Henry SP, Miner RC, Drew WL, et al: Antiviral activity and ocular kinetics of antisense oligonucleotides designed to inhibit CMV replication. *Invest Ophthalmol Vis Sci* 42:2646, 2001.
55. Roehr B: Fomivirsen approved for CMV retinitis. *J Int Assoc Physicians AIDS Care* 4:14, 1998.
56. Plummer R, Vidal L, Griffin M, et al: Phase I study of MG98, an oligonucleotide antisense inhibitor of human DNA methyltransferase 1, given as a 7-day infusion in patients with advanced solid tumors. *Clin Cancer Res* 15:3177, 2009.
57. Dean E, Jodrell D, Connolly K, et al: Phase I trial of AEG35156 administered as a 7-day and 3-day continuous intravenous infusion in patients with advanced refractory cancer. *J Clin Oncol* 27:1660, 2009.
58. Das M, Mohanty C, and Sahoo SK: Ligand-based targeted therapy for cancer tissue. *Expert Opin Drug Deliv* 6:285, 2009.
59. Bates PJ, Laber DA, Miller DM, et al: Discovery and development of the G-rich oligonucleotide AS1411 as a novel treatment for cancer. *Exp Mol Pathol* 86:151, 2009.
60. Hemmi H, Takeuchi O, Kawai T, et al: A Toll-like receptor recognizes bacterial DNA. *Nature* 408:740, 2000.
61. Krieg AM: CpG motifs: The active ingredient in bacterial extracts? *Nat Med* 9:831, 2003.
62. Wu CC, Castro JE, Motta M, et al: Selection of oligonucleotide aptamers with enhanced uptake and activation of human leukemia B cells. *Hum Gene Ther* 14:849, 2003.
63. Mello CC, Conte D Jr: Revealing the world of RNA interference. *Nature* 431:338, 2004.
64. Rocheleau CE, Downs WD, Lin R, et al: Wnt signaling and an APC-related gene specify endoderm in early C. elegans embryos. *Cell* 90:707, 1997.
65. Haddad E, Landais, P, Friedrich W, et al: Long-term immune reconstitution and outcome after HLA-nonidentical T-cell-depleted bone marrow transplantation for severe combined immunodeficiency: A European retrospective study of 116 patients. Blood 91:3646, 1998.
66. Parrish S, Fleenor J, Xu S, et al: Functional anatomy of a dsRNA trigger: Differential requirement for the two trigger strands in RNA interference. *Mol Cell* 6:1077, 2000.
67. Zamore PD, Tuschl T, Sharp PA, Bartel DP: RNAi: Double-stranded RNA directs the ATP-dependent cleavage of mRNA at 21 to 23 nucleotide intervals. *Cell* 101:25, 2000.
68. Tabara H, Sarkissian M, Kelly WG, et al: The rde-1 gene, RNA interference, and transposon silencing in *C. elegans*. *Cell* 99:123, 1999.
69. Pal-Bhadra M, Bhadra U, Birchler JA: Cosuppression in *Drosophila*: Gene silencing of Alcohol dehydrogenase by white-Adh transgenes is polycomb dependent. *Cell* 90:479, 1997.
70. Mette MF, Aufsatz W, van der Winden J, et al: Transcriptional silencing and promoter methylation triggered by double-stranded RNA. *EMBO J* 19:5194, 2000.
71. Olsen PH, Ambros V: The lin-4 regulatory RNA controls developmental timing in Caenorhabditis elegans by blocking LIN-14 protein synthesis after the initiation of translation. *Dev Biol* 216:671, 1999.
72. Mochizuki K, Fine NA, Fujisawa T, Gorovsky MA: Analysis of a piwi-related gene implicates small RNAs in genome rearrangement in tetrahymena. *Cell* 110:689, 2002.
73. Gitlin L, Karelsky S, Andino R: Short interfering RNA confers intracellular antiviral immunity in human cells. *Nature* 418:430, 2002.
74. Novina CD, Murray MF, Dykxhoorn DM, et al: SiRNA-directed inhibition of HIV-1 infection. *Nat Med* 8:681, 2002.
75. Wright P: Antisense and siRNA Technologies—SMi's Second Annual Conference. 16–17 February 2003, London, UK. *IDrugs* 7:233, 2004.
76. Stephens AC, Rivers RP: Antisense oligonucleotide therapy in cancer. *Curr Opin Mol Ther* 5:118, 2003.
77. Brummelkamp TR, Bernards R, Agami R: A system for stable expression of short interfering RNAs in mammalian cells. *Science* 296:550, 2002.
78. Paddison PJ, Caudy AA, Bernstein E, et al: Short hairpin RNAs (shRNAs) induce sequence-specific silencing in mammalian cells. *Genes Dev* 16:948, 2002.
79. Devroe E, Silver PA: Retrovirus-delivered siRNA. *BMC Biotechnol* 2:15, 2002.
80. Kim DH, Rossi JJ: Strategies for silencing human disease using RNA interference. *Nat Rev Genet* 8:173, 2007.
81. Wyszko E, Rolle K, Nowak S, et al: A multivariate analysis of patients with brain tumors treated with ATN-RNA. *Acta Pol Pharm* 65:677, 2008.
82. Zukiel R, Nowak S, Wyszko E, et al: Suppression of human brain tumor with interference RNA specific for tenascin-C. *Cancer Biol Ther* 5:1002, 2006.
83. Peng Z: Current status of Gendicine in China: Recombinant human Ad-p53 agent for treatment of cancers. *Hum Gene Ther* 16:1016, 2005.
84. Wilson JM: Gendicine: The first commercial gene therapy product. *Hum Gene Ther* 16:1014, 2005.
85. Bueren JA, Guenechea G, Casado JA, et al: Genetic modification of hematopoietic stem cells: Recent advances in the gene therapy of inherited diseases. *Arch Med Res* 34:589, 2003.
86. Ott MG, Seger R, Stein S, et al: Advances in the treatment of Chronic Granulomatous Disease by gene therapy. *Curr Gene Ther* 7:155, 2007.
87. Papapetrou EP, Zoumbos NC, and Athanassiadou A: Genetic modification of hematopoietic stem cells with nonviral systems: Past progress and future prospects. *Gene Ther* 12 Suppl 1:S118, 2005.
88. Mollah ZU, Aiba S, Manome H, et al: Cord blood CD34+ cells differentiate into dermal dendritic cells in co-culture with cutaneous fibroblasts or stromal cells. *J Invest Dermatol* 118:450, 2002.
89. Krivit W, Sung JH, Shapiro EG, Lockman LA: Microglia: The effector cell for reconstitution of the central nervous system following bone marrow transplantation for lysosomal and peroxisomal storage diseases. *Cell Transplant* 4:385, 1995.
90. Matayoshi A, Brown C, DiPersio JF, et al: Human blood-mobilized hematopoietic precursors differentiate into osteoclasts in the absence of stromal cells. *Proc Natl Acad Sci U S A* 93:10785, 1996.

91. Deisseroth AB, Zu Z, Claxton D, et al: Genetic marking shows that Ph+ cells present in autologous transplants of chronic myelogenous leukemia (CML) contribute to relapse after autologous bone marrow in CML. *Blood* 83:3068, 1994.
92. Brenner MK, Rill DR, Moen RC, et al: Gene-marking to trace origin of relapse after autologous bone-marrow transplantation. *Lancet* 341:85, 1993.
93. Tey SK, Brenner MK: The continuing contribution of gene marking to cell and gene therapy. *Mol Ther* 15:666, 2007.
94. Kantoff PW, Kohn DB, Mitsuya H, et al: Correction of adenosine deaminase deficiency in cultured human T and B cells by retrovirus-mediated gene transfer. *Proc Natl Acad Sci U S A* 83:6563, 1986.
95. Blaese RM: Development of gene therapy for immunodeficiency: Adenosine deaminase deficiency. *Pediatr Res* 33:S49; discussion S53, 1993.
96. Kohn DB, Hershfield MS, Carbonaro D, et al: T lymphocytes with a normal ADA gene accumulate after transplantation of transduced autologous umbilical cord blood CD34+ cells in ADA-deficient SCID neonates. *Nat Med* 4:775, 1998.
97. Aiuti A, Slavin S, Aker M, et al: Correction of ADA-SCID by stem cell gene therapy combined with nonmyeloablative conditioning. *Science* 296:2410, 2002.
98. Aiuti A, Cattaneo F, Galimberti S, et al: Gene therapy for immunodeficiency due to adenosine deaminase deficiency. *N Engl J Med* 360:447, 2009.
99. Noguchi M, Yi H, Rosenblatt HM, et al: Interleukin-2 receptor gamma chain mutation results in X-linked severe combined immunodeficiency in humans. *Cell* 73:147, 1993.
100. Haddad E, Landais P, Friedrich W, et al: Long-term immune reconstitution and outcome after HLA-nonidentical T-cell-depleted bone marrow transplantation for severe combined immunodeficiency: A European retrospective study of 116 patients. *Blood* 91:3646, 1998.
101. Cavazzana-Calvo M, Hacein-Bey S, de Saint Basile G, et al: Gene therapy of human severe combined immunodeficiency (SCID)-X1 disease. *Science* 288:669, 2000.
102. Hacein-Bey-Abina S, Le Deist F, Carlier F, et al: Sustained correction of X-linked severe combined immunodeficiency by *ex vivo* gene therapy. *N Engl J Med* 346:1185, 2002.
103. Hacein-Bey-Abina S, von Kalle C, Schmidt M, et al: A serious adverse event after successful gene therapy for X-linked severe combined immunodeficiency. *N Engl J Med* 348:255, 2003.
104. Hacein-Bey-Abina S, Von Kalle C, Schmidt M, et al: LMO2-associated clonal T cell proliferation in two patients after gene therapy for SCID-X1. *Science* 302:415, 2003.
105. McCormack MP, Forster A, Drynan L, et al: The LMO2 T-cell oncogene is activated via chromosomal translocations or retroviral insertion during gene therapy but has no mandatory role in normal T-cell development. *Mol Cell Biol* 23:9003, 2003.
106. Rabbitts TH, Bucher K, Chung G, et al: The effect of chromosomal translocations in acute leukemias: The LMO2 paradigm in transcription and development. *Cancer Res* 59:1794s, 1999.
107. Hacein-Bey-Abina S, Schmidt M, Le Deist F, et al: Gene therapy for severe combined immunodeficiency X1. *Blood* 106:60a, 2005.
108. von Kalle C, Baum C, Williams DA: Lenti in red: Progress in gene therapy for human hemoglobinopathies. *J Clin Invest* 114:889, 2004.
109. May C, Rivella S, Callegari J, et al: Therapeutic haemoglobin synthesis in beta-thalassaemic mice expressing lentivirus-encoded human beta-globin. *Nature* 406:82, 2000.
110. Pawliuk R, Westerman KA, Fabry ME, et al: Correction of sickle cell disease in transgenic mouse models by gene therapy. *Science* 294:2368, 2001.
111. Imren S, Fabry ME, Westerman KA, et al: High-level beta-globin expression and preferred intragenic integration after lentiviral transduction of human cord blood stem cells. *J Clin Invest* 114:953, 2004.
112. Nolta JA, Sender LS, Barranger JA, Kohn DB: Expression of human glucocerebrosidase in murine long-term bone marrow cultures after retroviral vector-mediated transfer. *Blood* 75:787, 1990.
113. Enquist IB, Nilsson E, Ooka A, et al: Effective cell and gene therapy in a murine model of Gaucher disease. *Proc Natl Acad Sci U S A* 103:13819, 2006.
114. Barranger JA, Rice EO, Swaney WP: Gene transfer approaches to the lysosomal storage disorders. *Neurochem Res* 24:601, 1999.
115. Dunbar CE, Kohn DB, Schiffmann R, et al: Retroviral transfer of the glucocerebrosidase gene into CD34+ cells from patients with Gaucher disease: *In vivo* detection of transduced cells without myeloablation. *Hum Gene Ther* 9:2629, 1998.
116. Hong YB, Kim EY, Yoo HW, Jung SC: Feasibility of gene therapy in Gaucher disease using an adeno-associated virus vector. *J Hum Genet* 49:536, 2004.
117. Kim EY, Hong YB, Lai Z, et al: Expression and secretion of human glucocerebrosidase mediated by recombinant lentivirus vectors *in vitro* and *in vivo*: Implications for gene therapy of Gaucher disease. *Biochem Biophys Res Commun* 318:381, 2004.
118. Croop JM: Gene therapy for Fanconi anemia. *Curr Hematol Rep* 2:335, 2003.
119. Galimi F, Noll M, Kanazawa Y, et al: Gene therapy of Fanconi anemia: Preclinical efficacy using lentiviral vectors. *Blood* 100:2732, 2002.
120. Herzog RW, Hagstrom JN, Kung SH, et al: Stable gene transfer and expression of human blood coagulation factor IX after intramuscular injection of recombinant adeno-associated virus. *Proc Natl Acad Sci U S A* 94:5804, 1997.
121. Herzog RW, Yang EY, Couto LB, et al: Long-term correction of canine hemophilia B by gene transfer of blood coagulation factor IX mediated by adeno-associated viral vector. *Nat Med* 5:56, 1999.
122. Kay MA, Manno CS, Ragni MV, et al: Evidence for gene transfer and expression of factor IX in haemophilia B patients treated with an AAV vector. *Nat Genet* 24:257, 2000.
123. Manno CS, Chew AJ, Hutchison S, et al: AAV-mediated factor IX gene transfer to skeletal muscle in patients with severe hemophilia B. *Blood* 101:2963, 2003.
124. Kay MA, High K, Glader B, et al: A phase I/II clinical trial for liver directed AAV-mediated gene transfer for hemophilia B. *Blood* 100:115a, 2002.
125. Manno CS, Pierce GF, Arruda VR, et al: Successful transduction of liver in hemophilia by AAV-Factor IX and limitations imposed by the host immune response. *Nat Med* 12:342, 2006.
126. Powell JS, Ragni MV, White GC 2nd, et al: Phase 1 trial of FVIII gene transfer for severe hemophilia A using a retroviral construct administered by peripheral intravenous infusion. *Blood* 102:2038, 2003.
127. Roth DA, Tawa NE Jr, O'Brien JM, et al: Nonviral transfer of the gene encoding coagulation factor VIII in patients with severe hemophilia A. *N Engl J Med* 344:1735, 2001.
128. Galpin JE, Casciato DA, Richards SB: A phase I clinical trial to evaluate the safety and biological activity of HIV-IT (TAF) (HIV-1IIIB env-transduced, autologous fibroblasts) in asymptomatic HIV-1 infected subjects. *Hum Gene Ther* 5:997, 1994.
129. Ziegner UH, Peters G, Jolly DJ, et al: Cytotoxic T-lymphocyte induction in asymptomatic HIV-1-infected patients immunized with retro vector-transduced autologous fibroblasts expressing HIV-1IIIB Env/Rev proteins. *AIDS* 9:43, 1995.
130. Deeks SG, Wagner B, Anton PA, et al: A phase II randomized study of HIV-specific T-cell gene therapy in subjects with undetectable plasma viremia on combination antiretroviral therapy. *Mol Ther* 5:788, 2002.
131. Walker RE, Bechtel CM, Natarajan V, et al: Long-term in vivo survival of receptor-modified syngeneic T cells in patients with human immunodeficiency virus infection. *Blood* 96:467, 2000.
132. Kang EM, de Witte M, Malech H, et al: Nonmyeloablative conditioning followed by transplantation of genetically modified HLA-matched peripheral blood progenitor cells for hematologic malignancies in patients with acquired immunodeficiency syndrome. *Blood* 99:698, 2002.
133. Lo HL, Chang T, Yam P, Marcovecchio PM, et al: Inhibition of HIV-1 replication with designed miRNAs expressed from RNA polymerase II promoters. *Gene Ther* 14(21): 1503-12, 2007.
134. van Lunzen J, Glaunsinger T, Stahmer I, et al: Transfer of autologous gene-modified T cells in HIV-infected patients with advanced immunodeficiency and drug-resistant virus. *Mol Ther* 15:1024, 2007.
135. Macpherson JL, Boyd MP, Arndt AJ, et al: Long-term survival and concomitant gene expression of ribozyme-transduced CD4+ T-lymphocytes in HIV-infected patients. *J Gene Med* 7:552, 2005.
136. Eberhardy SR, Goncalves J, Coelho S, et al: Inhibition of human immunodeficiency virus type 1 replication with artificial transcription factors targeting the highly conserved primer-binding site. *J Virol* 80:2873, 2006.
137. Cotter FE, Johnson P, Hall P, et al: Antisense oligonucleotides suppress B-cell lymphoma growth in a SCID-hu mouse model. *Oncogene* 9:3049, 1994.
138. Wierda WG, O'Brien S, Wang X, et al: Prognostic nomogram and index for overall survival in previously untreated patients with chronic lymphocytic leukemia. *Blood* 109:4679, 2007.
139. Wetzler M, Donohue KA, Odenike OM, et al: Feasibility of administering oblimersen (G3139; Genasense) with imatinib mesylate in patients with imatinib resistant chronic myeloid leukemia—Cancer and leukemia group B study 10107. *Leuk Lymphoma* 49:1274, 2008.
140. Moore J, Seiter K, Kolitz J, et al: A Phase II study of Bcl-2 antisense (oblimersen sodium) combined with gemtuzumab ozogamicin in older patients with acute myeloid leukemia in first relapse. *Leuk Res* 30:777, 2006.
141. Rao S, Watkins D, Cunningham D, et al: Phase II study of ISIS 3521, an antisense oligodeoxynucleotide to protein kinase C alpha, in patients with previously treated low-grade non-Hodgkin's lymphoma. *Ann Oncol* 15:1413, 2004.
142. Skorski T, Nieborowska-Skorska M, Nicolaides NC, et al: Suppression of Philadelphia1 leukemia cell growth in mice by BCR-ABL antisense oligodeoxynucleotide. *Proc Natl Acad Sci U S A* 91:4504, 1994.
143. Yuan Z, and Mei HD: Inhibition of telomerase activity with hTERT antisense increases the effect of CDDP-induced apoptosis in myeloid leukemia. *Hematol J* 3:201, 2002.
144. Klisovic RB, Blum W, Wei X, et al: Phase I study of GTI-2040, an antisense to ribonucleotide reductase, in combination with high-dose cytarabine in patients with acute myeloid leukemia. *Clin Cancer Res* 14:3889, 2008.
145. Ritter U, Damm-Welk C, Fuchs U, et al: Design and evaluation of chemically synthesized siRNA targeting the NPM-ALK fusion site in anaplastic large cell lymphoma (ALCL). *Oligonucleotides* 13:365, 2003.
146. Peng Z, Xiao Z, Wang Y, et al: Reversal of P-glycoprotein-mediated multidrug resistance with small interference RNA (siRNA) in leukemia cells. *Cancer Gene Ther*. 2004.
147. Calin GA, Croce CM: MicroRNA signatures in human cancers. *Nat Rev Cancer* 6:857, 2006.
148. Calin GA, Ferracin M, Cimmino A, et al: A MicroRNA signature associated with prognosis and progression in chronic lymphocytic leukemia. *N Engl J Med* 353:1793, 2005.
149. Lu J, Getz G, Miska EA, et al: MicroRNA expression profiles classify human cancers. *Nature* 435:834, 2005.
150. Visone R, Croce CM: MiRNAs and cancer. *Am J Pathol* 174:1131, 2009.
151. Gondi CS, Rao JS: Concepts in *in vivo* siRNA delivery for cancer therapy. *J Cell Physiol* 220:285, 2009.
152. Kato K, Cantwell MJ, Sharma S, Kipps TJ: Gene transfer of CD40-ligand induces autologous immune recognition of chronic lymphocytic leukemia B cells. *J Clin Invest* 101:1133, 1998.
153. Wierda WG, Cantwell MJ, Woods SJ, et al: CD40-ligand (CD154) gene therapy for chronic lymphocytic leukemia. *Blood* 96:2917, 2000.

154. Castro JE, Cantwell MJ, Prussak CE, et al: Long-term follow up of chronic lymphocytic leukemia patients treated with CD40-ligand (CD154) gene therapy [abstract]. *Blood* 102:1790, 2003.
155. Castro JE, Sandoval-Sus JD, Melo-Cardenas J, et al: Phase I study of intranodal direct injection of adenovirus encoding recombinant CD40-ligand (Ad-ISF35) in patients with chronic lymphocytic leukemia [abstract]. *J Clin Oncol* 27(Suppl):3003, 2009.
156. Rousseau RF, Biagi E, Dutour A, et al: Immunotherapy of high-risk acute leukemia with a recipient (autologous) vaccine expressing transgenic human CD40L and IL-2 after chemotherapy and allogeneic stem cell transplantation. *Blood* 107:1332, 2006.
157. Hirano N, Takahashi T, Ohtake S, et al: Expression of costimulatory molecules in human leukemias. *Leukemia* 10:1168, 1996.
158. Hirst WJ, Buggins A, Darling D, et al: Enhanced immune costimulatory activity of primary acute myeloid leukaemia blasts after retrovirus-mediated gene transfer of B7.1. *Gene Ther* 4:691, 1997.
159. Tolba KA, Bowers WJ, Hilchey SP, et al: Development of herpes simplex virus-1 amplicon-based immunotherapy for chronic lymphocytic leukemia. *Blood* 98:287, 2001.
160. Dunussi-Joannopoulos K, Weinstein HJ, Arceci RJ, Croop JM: Gene therapy with B7.1 and GM-CSF vaccines in a murine AML model. *J Pediatr Hematol Oncol* 19:536, 1997.
161. Hirano N, Takahashi T, Azuma M, et al: Protective and therapeutic immunity against leukemia induced by irradiated B7–1 (CD80)-transduced leukemic cells. *Hum Gene Ther* 8:1375, 1997.
162. Stripecke R, Cardoso AA, Pepper KA, et al: Lentiviral vectors for efficient delivery of CD80 and granulocyte- macrophage- colony-stimulating factor in human acute lymphoblastic leukemia and acute myeloid leukemia cells to induce antileukemic immune responses. *Blood* 96:1317, 2000.
163. Dilloo D, Bacon K, Holden W, et al: Combined chemokine and cytokine gene transfer enhances antitumor immunity. *Nat Med* 2:1090, 1996.
164. Pantuck AJ, van Ophoven A, Gitlitz BJ, et al: Phase I trial of antigen-specific gene therapy using a recombinant vaccinia virus encoding MUC-1 and IL-2 in MUC-1-positive patients with advanced prostate cancer. *J Immunother* 27:240, 2004.
165. Pantuck AJ, Belldegrun AS: Phase I clinical trial of interleukin 2 (IL-2) gene therapy for prostate cancer. *Curr Urol Rep* 2:33, 2001.
166. Nishimura T, Watanabe K, Yahata T, et al: The application of IL-12 to cytokine therapy and gene therapy for tumors. *Ann N Y Acad Sci* 795:375, 1996.
167. Chen HW, Lee YP, Chung YF, et al: Inducing long-term survival with lasting antitumor immunity in treating B cell lymphoma by a combined dendritic cell-based and hydrodynamic plasmid-encoding IL-12 gene therapy. *Int Immunol* 15:427, 2003.
168. Gautam SC, Xu YX, Pindolia KR, et al: TNF-alpha gene therapy with myeloid progenitor cells lacks the toxicities of systemic TNF-alpha therapy. *J Hematother* 8:237, 1999.
169. Gautam SC, Pindolia KR, Xu YX, et al: Antileukemic activity of TNF-alpha gene therapy with myeloid progenitor cells against minimal leukemia. *J Hematother* 7:115, 1998.
170. Villani F, Galimberti M, Mazzola G, et al: Pulmonary toxicity of alpha tumor necrosis factor in patients treated by isolation perfusion. *J Chemother* 7:452, 1995.
171. Krigel RL, Padavic-Shaller KA, Rudolph AA, et al: Hemorrhagic gastritis as a new dose-limiting toxicity of recombinant tumor necrosis factor. *J Natl Cancer Inst* 83:129, 1991.
172. Borrello IM, Levitsky HI, Stock W, et al: GM-CSF secreting cellular immunotherapy in combination with autologous stem cell transplant (ASCT) as post-remission therapy for acute myeloid leukemia (AML). *Blood* 114:1736, 2009.

CHAPTER 28

REGENERATIVE MEDICINE: PRINCIPLES OF MULTIPOTENTIAL CELL THERAPY FOR TISSUE REPLACEMENT

Armand Keating

SUMMARY

The discipline of regenerative medicine is developing rapidly, is based on evolving principles of stem cell biology, and is characterized by rapid clinical investigation with rationales that lag behind the numerous laboratory studies that have emerged. This chapter reviews the areas of cell biology that have contributed to regenerative medicine and briefly discusses clinical applications. Despite the advances, the field is associated with numerous conflicting studies and a somewhat undisciplined approach to the use of the term *stem cells*. Nevertheless, laboratory studies have stimulated clinical trials, including prospective randomized trials to treat various types of tissue damage. The potential for this novel therapy is great, but much work is required to reduce the technology to routine clinical practice. The design of more appropriate preclinical models will better inform clinical trials design and move this field forward even more rapidly, in a manner analogous to the development of marrow transplantation 50 years ago.

DEFINITION AND HISTORY

Regenerative medicine arose from the convergence of several disciplines over the last 20 years, including stem cell biology; tissue engineering; materials science; cell, tissue, and organ transplantation; and developmental and molecular biology.[1,2] It has been defined as "an interdisciplinary field of research and clinical applications focused on the repair, replacement or regeneration of cell, tissues or organs to restore impaired function resulting from any cause, including congenital defects, disease, trauma or ageing."[2] Four important developments have influenced the field: (1) demonstration of putative differentiation of hematopoietic stem/progenitor cells along lineages leading to nonhematopoietic tissues; (2) differentiation of mesenchymal stromal cells found in the marrow and other sites to tissues of mesodermal and even nonmesodermal origin; (3) manipulation of embryonic stem cell differentiation; and (4) the ability to reprogram adult somatic cells-induced pluripotent stem (iPS) cells to embryonic-like cells, which in turn, can differentiate along specific lineages. The features of an ideal stem cell for clinical tissue regeneration have been identified[3] as: (1) abundant (available in up to the billions); (2) can be harvested in a minimally invasive manner; (3) able to differentiate along multiple lineage pathways reproducibly; (4) able to be transplanted safely and effectively from allogeneic and autologous sources; and (5) able to be manufactured in a Good Manufacturing Practice–compliant manner.

Acronyms and abbreviations that appear in this chapter include: G-CSF, granulocyte colony-stimulating factor; HSCs, hematopoietic stem cells; iPS, induced pluripotent stem cells; MSCs, mesenchymal stromal cells.

HEMATOPOIETIC CELLS

In the first decade of the 21st century a number of studies suggested that hematopoietic cells, specifically hematopoietic stem cells (HSCs), could undergo "transdifferentiation" into cells of other lineages. The notion of a one-way HSC lineage differentiation pathway in which cells followed an orderly progression from less to more differentiated states came to be questioned (see Fig. 28–1).

One of the earliest studies suggestive of transdifferentiation showed that purified HSCs appeared to differentiate into hepatocytes *in vivo*.[4] In a murine tyrosinemia model in which mice develop liver failure as a consequence of a lack of fumarylacetoacetate hydrolase, transplantation with HSCs defined by the immunophenotype, c-Kit+Sca1+Lin–, is curative. Moreover, numerous donor-derived hematopoietic cells were incorporated into the hepatic parenchyma. A subsequent study from the same group, however, showed that the marrow-derived donor repopulating hepatocytes in this model arose by cell fusion and not by differentiation of HSCs.[5]

Other contemporaneous studies indicated that CD34+Sca-1+ self-renewing HSCs could differentiate into epithelial cells of the liver, lung, gastrointestinal tract, and skin.[6] In another study,[7] marrow-derived c-Kit+ Lin– cells when injected into mouse myocardium after an experimentally induced acute myocardial infarction showed coexpression of the donor cell marker (green fluorescence protein) and cardiomyocyte determinants, inferring transdifferentiation of HSC to cardiac muscle cells. Evidence of regenerating myocardium in this model suggested the possible role of the HSCs in tissue repair. Work from other laboratories suggested that the data could be explained, as in the case of the donor hepatocytes, by cell fusion.[8,9] This phenomenon, however, may not provide the entire explanation, because of the low frequency of cell fusion, which has ranged from 1 per 100,000 to 1 per 10 in published studies. Nevertheless, several groups have shown rigorously that transdifferentiation does not occur in the injured mouse myocardium model, especially when using methodologies that preclude potentially false-positive results from the autofluorescence of donor cells.[10,11] In another negative study, no benefit was shown by the stem/progenitor cell mobilization from granulocyte colony-stimulating factor (G-CSF) administration after experimental acute myocardial infarction in a nonhuman primate model.[12] This area nonetheless remains controversial as reports of marrow cells adopting cardiomyocyte characteristics *in vivo* continue to be documented.[13]

Despite the conflicting data, numerous studies have been initiated with marrow-derived cells, especially for the regeneration of injured myocardium. Few laboratory studies, however, have attempted to identify the specific cell types within the marrow most responsible for tissue regeneration. An exception was a study suggesting that the marrow cells responsible were CD34–cKit+Sca-1+ cells, consistent with mesenchymal stromal cell (MSC) population.[14]

MESENCHYMAL STROMAL CELLS

Historical Context

Burgeoning research in mesenchymal stromal cells has its origins in the work of Alexander Freidenstein. Freidenstein identified an osteogenic precursor in the marrow[15] and developed a clonal assay for marrow stromal cells—the colony-forming unit–fibroblast[16]—which Maureen

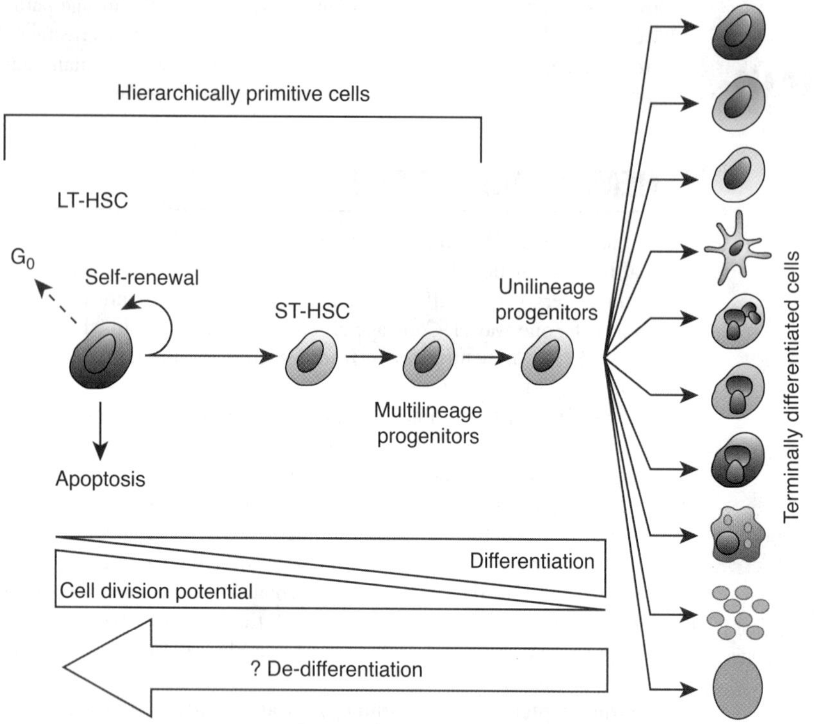

FIGURE 28–1. The conventional unidirectional stem cell lineage differentiation pathway was questioned as a result of data showing "transdifferentiation" of hematopoietic cells into committed cells of other lineages. LT-HSC, long-term hematopoietic stem cell; ST-HSC, short-term hematopoietic stem cell. *(From Pina C, Enver T: Differential contributions of haematopoietic stem cells to foetal and adult haematopoiesis: Insights from functional analysis of transcriptional regulators.* Oncogene *26:6750, 2007. Adapted by permission from Macmillan Publishers Ltd.,* Oncogene, *copyright 2007.)*

Owen suggested represents a stromal stem cell.[17] A similar assay was developed for human marrow-derived cells.[18] Subsequent studies demonstrated the ability of this cultured plastic-adherent population derived from marrow mononuclear cells to undergo differentiation to adipocytes and chondrocytes, in addition to osteogenic cells.[19] Studies by Caplan redirected much of the work on MSCs in the late 1990s toward tissue regeneration based on the notion that they consisted of stem cells capable of differentiating along all the mesodermal lineages.[20]

Definition of Mesenchymal Stromal Cells

Confusion regarding the nature of the cells Caplan described as "mesenchymal stem cells" led to the adoption of new terminology and a formal definition.[21,22] The cells, termed *mesenchymal stromal cells* (still MSCs), are a heterogeneous population (i.e., not all are stem cells) of plastic-adherent cells that exhibit multipotential (adipogenic, osteogenic, and chondrogenic) differentiation *in vitro* and have the immunophenotype (CD105 [endoglin; SH2]$^+$; CD73 [ecto-5′-nucleotidase]; SH3$^+$; and CD90 [Thy1]$^+$) and are negative for cell surface markers (CD45; CD14 or CD11b; CD79 or CD19; HLA-DR).

There are, however, no known specific markers for MSCs, although low-affinity nerve growth factor receptor (CD271),[23] GD2,[24] gp130[25], and the embryonic stem cell marker, SSEA-4,[26] are present unexpectedly. The STRO-1 antibody identifies MSC precursors but cross-reacts with some hematopoietic cells,[27] and after two decades of study, the antigen is still unknown. Primary cultured MSCs appear equivalent to those freshly isolated from the marrow.[28] They have the immunophenotype CD45^{lo}, CD271+, CD73+, CD105+, and CD10+, and may be regarded as adventitial reticular cells or vascular pericytes.[28]

Cells with an immunophenotype similar to marrow-derived MSC can also be isolated from many other tissues including fat,[29] placenta,[30] skin,[31] umbilical cord blood,[32] and the human umbilical cord itself, either from the perivascular region[33] or within Wharton's jelly,[34] as well as from the synovium[35] and dental pulp.[36]

Differentiation Potential of Mesenchymal Stromal Cells

Numerous *in vitro* studies provide evidence showing the ability of MSCs to differentiate into many cell types, including myocytes,[37] neurons,[38] hepatocytes,[39] cardiomyocytes,[40] lung epithelial cells,[41] and endothelial cells,[42] among others, in addition to the well-documented osteogenic, adipogenic, and chondrogenic lineages. The differentiative capacity of MSCs may be explained in part by their derivation from the mesoderm, although studies suggest a neural crest origin in part.[43] The data infer a potential and partly hypothetical, stem cell-lineage hierarchy for MSCs, according to Figure 28–2.[44]

The isolation of true stem cells from the MSC population has been challenging, especially MSCs from human sources. Nonetheless, the clonal derivation of human MSCs from human umbilical cord perivascular cells has been accomplished *in vitro*, and confirmed *in vivo* in an immune-deficient mouse model.[45] The studies reveal a deterministic stem progenitor cell hierarchy with a varying ability of precursors to give rise to fat, muscle, cartilage, bone, and fibrous tissue. Figure 28–3 shows a hierarchical scheme of stem-progenitor cell differentiation for the human umbilical cord perivascular MSCs.[31]

Bioactive Molecules from Mesenchymal Stromal Cells

Until recently, MSCs were thought to mediate tissue regeneration by differentiating into the specific cells damaged, and then functionally integrating into the affected organ. An alternative explanation is that MSCs act to promote tissue repair through engraftment and subsequent secretion of soluble mediators, which stimulate the recovery of endogenous cells and/or their progenitors. This latter mechanism is gaining experimental support. For example, multiple studies demonstrate that MSCs produce many biologically active substances, including hormones, chemokines, and components of the extracellular matrix. MSCs secrete a variety of cytokines including interleukin (IL)-6, IL-7, IL-8, IL-11, IL-12, IL-14, IL-15, stem cell factor, FLT-3 ligand, IL-1α, leukemia inhibitory factor, granulocyte-macrophage colony-stimulating factor, and G-CSF.[46] They also secrete chemokines and chemokine ligands as well as stromal-derived factor-1, involved in HSC homing to the stem cell niche.[46] Several angiogenic factors are also expressed by both murine and human MSCs.[47] Extracellular matrix molecules such as proteoglycans, glycosaminoglycans, and basal lamina and interstitial collagen types are actively produced by MSCs.[48,49] These, and other factors yet to be discovered, may be important mediators of tissue regeneration released by the donor MSCs.

Immunomodulatory Properties of Mesenchymal Stromal Cells

The immunomodulatory properties of MSCs have received considerable attention, as the cells affect a wide spectrum of immune cells, of both the innate and adaptive immune systems.[44] Interactions between MSCs and immune cells have been extensively reviewed[44,50] and are

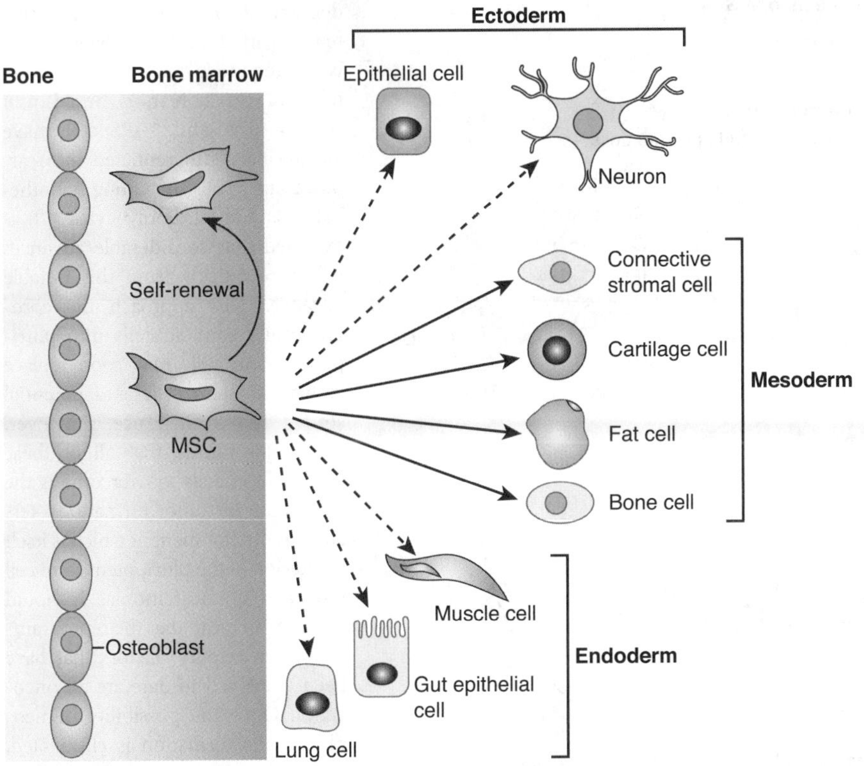

FIGURE 28–2. A schematic representation of the differentiation potential of mesenchymal stromal cells (MSCs). The range of potential cell types includes those normally derived from all three primordial germ layers, ectoderm, mesoderm, and endoderm. *(From Uccelli A, Moretta L, Pistoia V.[44] Reprinted by permission from Macmillan Publishers Ltd.,* Nature Reviews Immunology, *copyright 2008.)*

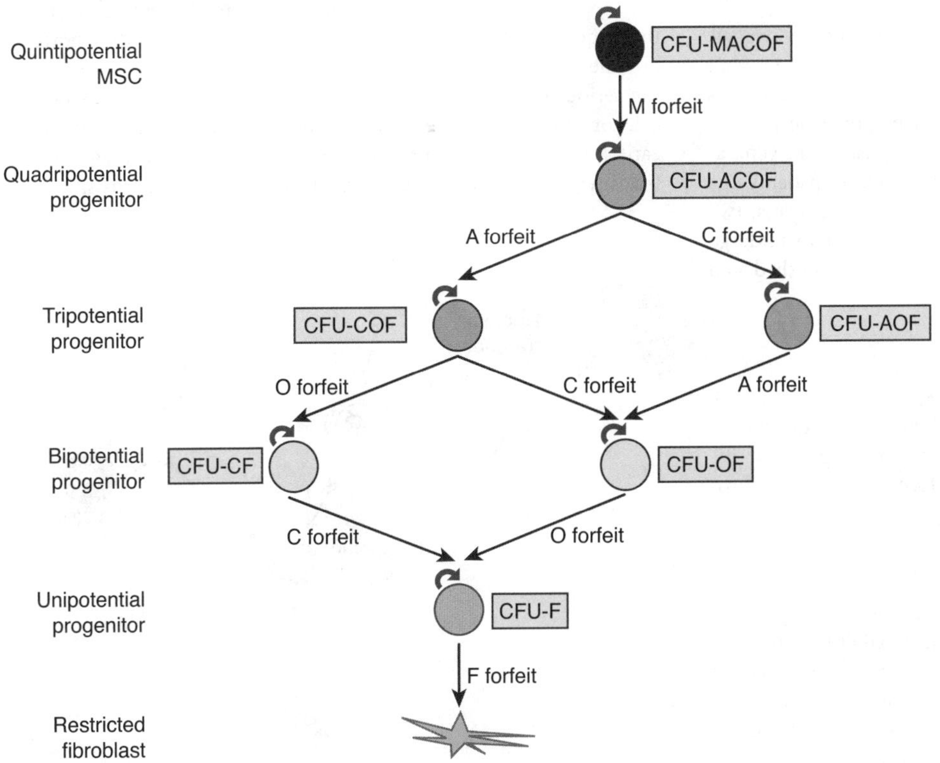

FIGURE 28–3. Hierarchy of mesenchymal stromal cell (MSC) differentiation involving five lineages: M, myogenic; A, adipogenic; C, chondrogenic; O, osteogenic; F, fibrogenic. The multipotent MSC progressively loses differentiation potential. CFU , colony-forming unit. *(Reproduced with permission from Sarugaser R, Hanoun L, Keating A, et al.[45])*

represented in Figure 28–4.[36] The immunomodulatory properties of MSCs may be important in facilitating tissue regeneration, in part by suppressing inflammatory responses, such as in the early period (3–5 days) after acute myocardial infarction.[51,52]

Preclinical Models of Tissue Regeneration with Mesenchymal Stromal Cells

An extensive literature exists of experimental models investigating the role of MSCs in the regeneration of myocardium,[53] neuronal tissue,[54] bone,[55] and liver,[56] among other tissues. Organ regeneration with MSCs has been most extensively studied for the myocardium and serves to highlight the issues and challenges common to this field.

Early studies suggested that MSCs differentiate into cardiomyocytes under appropriate conditions *in vitro*, especially after coincubation with the demethylating agent 5-azacytidine.[57] Subsequent studies indicate that stromal characteristics may be retained despite the acquisition of cardiac myocyte markers.[58] Moreover, the electrophysiology of the differentiated MSCs may not be characteristic of cardiomyocytes but rather of the original stromal cell.[58] Despite these limitations, numerous studies show hemodynamic improvement in rat[59] and pig[60] models of ischemic injury. In numerous examples the presence of donor MSCs in the ischemic area is short-lived, and improvement in ventricular function can be achieved with the infusion of cell extract alone,[61] supporting the notion of a paracrine effect. Further improvement in cardiac function was demonstrated when MSCs were engineered to overexpress the prosurvival gene Akt, but this enhancement could also be accounted for by soluble mediators.[62]

■ GENERATION OF PLURIPOTENCY IN SOMATIC CELLS BY NUCLEAR REPROGRAMMING

There are several approaches to the generation of pluripotent stem cells from somatic cells, and recent technical advances argue that the field is no longer restricted to producing embryonic stem cells. Figure 28–5 summarizes the approaches.[68]

Nuclear Transfer

Embryonic stem cell lines were first isolated from the inner cell mass of blastocyst stage embryos.[49,50] They can be propagated *in vitro* indefinitely and have the theoretical capacity to become any cell in the body.[51] Human embryonic stem cells were first generated in 1998;[52] can now be cultured successfully without xenogeneic feeder layers; and are able to differentiate into neural, hematopoietic, and pancreatic progenitor cells.[51] A limitation of the clinical use of

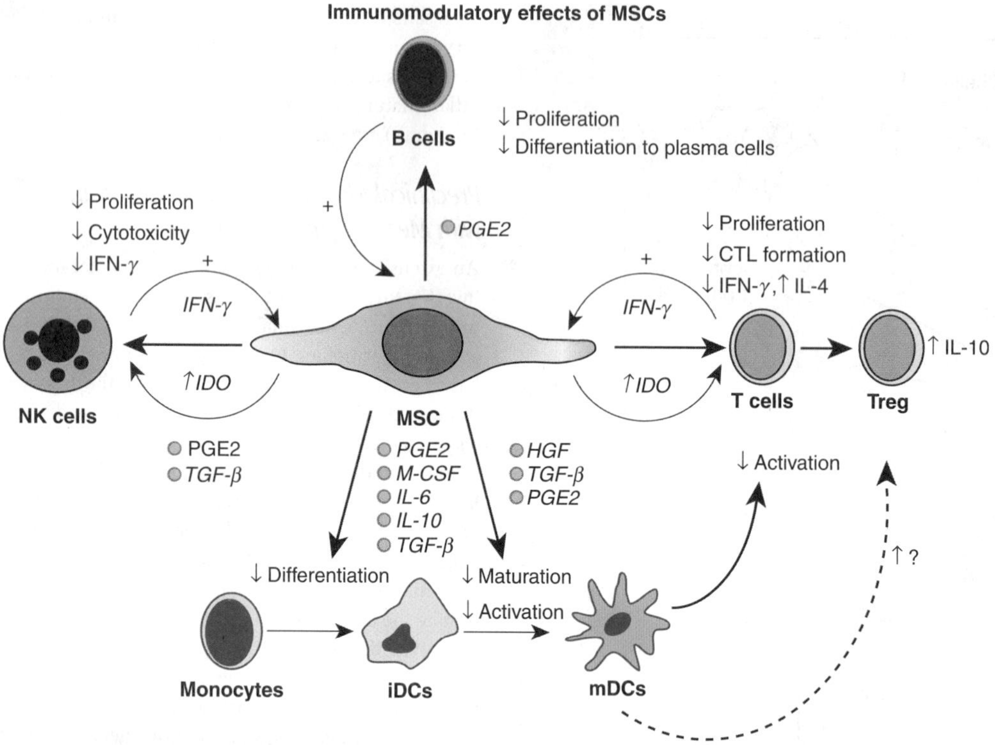

FIGURE 28–4. The immunomodulatory effects of mesenchymal stromal cells (MSCs). The MSC has the capacity to elaborate a wide range of soluble mediators of cellular differentiation, which affect B and T lymphocytes, natural killer (NK) cells, dendritic cells, and monocytes and macrophages. CTL, cytotoxic T lymphocyte; iDCs, immature dendritic cells; IDO, indoleamine 2,9-dioxygenase; HGF, hepatocyte growth factor; IFN, interferon; M-CSF, macrophage colony-stimulating factor; mDCs, mature dendritic cells; PGE2, prostaglandin E_2; TGF, transforming growth factor; Treg, T-regulatory cell. *(This research was originally published in* Blood. *From Nauta A, Fibbe WE[50] with permission of the American Society of Hematology.)*

established embryonic stem cell lines however, as with most allogeneic tissue, is rejection. This can be overcome by the transfer of an adult somatic cell nucleus to generate an embryonic stem cell line that is genetically identical to the patient's cells, but such approaches remain challenging. Although initially thought to be accomplished, the generation of cloned embryonic stem cells from the skin cells of patients in a Korean experiment was shown to be fraudulent.[53] Nevertheless, two other ways to manipulate adult somatic cells or nuclei to undergo reprogramming and induce a pluripotent state are now established, and are shown schematically in Figure 28–5.[68]

Embryonic Stem Cell–Somatic Cell Fusion

Several studies show the feasibility of reprogramming somatic cell nuclei from mammalian cells.[68] It is unclear whether the factors inducing pluripotency reside in the embryonic stem cell cytoplasm or the somatic cell nucleus. It is noteworthy that the fused cell contains chromosomes from both cell types.

Induced Pluriopotent Stem Cells from Factors

Yamanaka and colleagues revolutionized the approach to nuclear reprogramming by inducing pluripotent stem cells from adult somatic cells. They showed that four genes, *c-Myc, Oct4, Sox2,* and *Klf4,* were sufficient to reprogram murine fibroblasts into embryonic stem cell-like cells.[69] The adoption of this strategy has been extraordinarily rapid and innovative (see Chap. 27), leading a number of investigators to replace retroviral gene transfer with potentially more efficient and safer systems involving lentiviral,[70] adenoviral,[71] or plasmid[72] vectors, a transposon approach that eliminates transgenes through transposase expression[73] and direct delivery of the reprogramming proteins themselves.[74] Moreover, c-Myc is not required,[75] and a combination of Oct4, Sox2, Nanog, and Lin28 is also successful.[76] iPS cells have already been differentiated into cardiovascular cells, including endothelial cells and cardiomyocytes.[77] It is expected that considerable advances will arise quickly from this notable advance. This approach of reprogramming somatic cells into pluripotent stem cells may soon replace embryonic stem cells as a potential source for clinical use. However, the major hurdle that all of these approaches needs to overcome is the prevention of tumor formation—teratomas, development of which is itself a criterion of the pluripotent stem cell state, and teratocarcinomas. It should be borne in mind that the reprogramming transcription factors that have been employed to date are all oncogenes. Once the possibility of neoplastic transformation is eliminated, there will be rapid translation of these exciting observations to patients.

■ CLINICAL APPLICATIONS

Most clinical trials in tissue regeneration are small single-arm studies that require confirmation in prospective trials. Some studies, however, provide convincing proof-of-principle, such as the use of MSCs in healing serious skin wounds.[78] Most of the trials involve marrow-derived cells or MSCs for a wide variety of indications, including acute myocardial infarction, chronic congestive heart failure, cartilage defects, fractures, delayed surgical wound healing, osteoporosis, aseptic

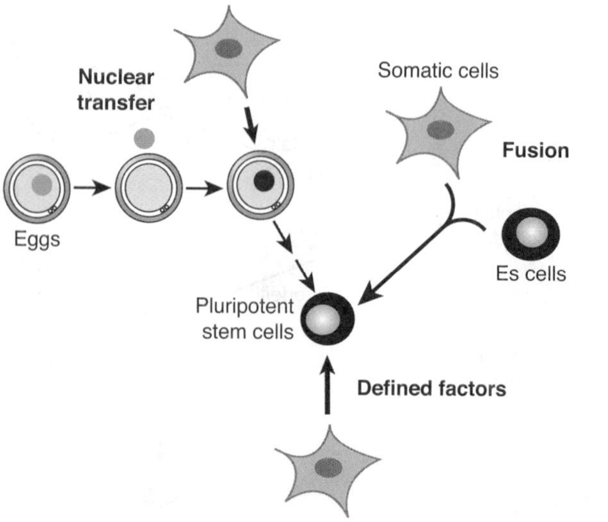

FIGURE 28–5. Methods for inducing pluripotency in somatic cells. The figure illustrates the two most common routes to obtain pluripotent cells for therapeutic application. *(From Yamanaka S[68] with permission of The Royal Society.)*

TABLE 28–1. Clinical Trials of Mesenchymal Stem Cells in Cardiac Disease

LVESV	Reduced by 4.74 mL	$p = 0.003$
MI lesion area	Reduced by 3.51%	$p = 0.004$
LVEF	Improved by 2.99%	$p = 0.0007$
LVEDV	Reduced by 2.47%	$p = 0.13$

LVEDV, left ventricular end-diastolic volume; LVEF, left ventricular ejection fraction; LVESV, left ventricular end-systolic volume; MI, myocardial infarction.

The table shows changes in hemodynamic endpoints identified in the 13 randomized clinical trials of MSCs in patients with ischemic cardiac disease.

SOURCE: Based on Martin-Rendon E, Brunskill SJ, Hyde CJ, et al.[82]

necrosis of the femoral head, stroke, and severe peripheral vascular disease, among others.

Of all clinical studies, the treatment of ischemic heart injury has been the most extensive and the most mature, and include prospective randomized placebo-controlled trials. The majority of the randomized controlled trials for cardiac regeneration employed marrow-derived cells. Both prospective randomized controlled trials of G-CSF mobilization after acute myocardial infarction, such as the Regenerate Vital Myocardium by Vigorous Activation of Bone Marrow Stem Cells (REVIVAL-2)[79] and the Stem Cells in Myocardial Infarction (STEMMI) trials,[80] showed no difference in ventricular function, infarct size, frequency of coronary artery restenosis, or target-vessel revascularization. Two systematic reviews have analyzed the use of marrow-derived cells for cardiac regeneration. In one, 12 randomized controlled trials and 6 cohort studies of a total of 999 patients were analyzed.[81] An improvement in left ventricular ejection fraction of 3.7 percent and a reduction of 4.8 mL in left ventricular end-systolic volume were noted. In addition, infarct scar size was reduced by 5.5 percent. The Cochrane Collaboration conducted a systematic review of 13 randomized controlled trials involving 811 patients treated with autologous marrow-derived cells.[82] Table 28–1 summarizes the changes in hemodynamic end-points.

From these systematic analyses it can be concluded that improvements in physiologic and anatomical endpoints in the experimental versus conventional treatment arms were modest. The procedure appeared to be safe, at least in the short-term. It remains to be determined whether or not it is clinically significant. Given the relatively small changes however, further preclinical investigation is required to identify approaches and cell types that will yield more clinically meaningful outcomes.

REFERENCES

1. Nose Y, Okubo H: Artificial organs versus regenerative medicine: Is it true? *Artif Organs* 27:765, 2003.
2. Daar AS, Greenwood HL: A proposed definition of regenerative medicine. *J Tissue Eng Regen Med* 1:179, 2007.
3. Gimble JM: Adipose tissue-derived therapeutics. *Expert Opin Biol Ther* 3:705, 2003.
4. Lagasse E, Connors H, Al-Dhalimy, et al: Purified hematopoietic stem cells can differentiate into hepatocytes in vivo. *Nat Med* 6:1229, 2000.
5. Wang X, Willenbring H, Akkari Y, et al: Cell fusion is the principal source of bone-marrow-derived hepatocytes. *Nature* 422:897, 2003.
6. Krause DS, Theise ND, Collector MI, et al: Multi-organ, multi-lineage engraftment by a single bone marrow-derived stem cell. *Cell* 105:369, 2001.
7. Orlic D, Kajstsure J, Chimenti S, et al: Bone marrow cells regenerate infracted myocardium. *Nature* 410:701, 2001.
8. Terada N, Hamazaki T, Oka M, et al: Bone marrow cells adopt the phenotype of other cells by spontaneous cell fusion. *Nature* 416:542, 2002.
9. Alvarez-dolado M, Pardal R, Garcia-Verdugo JM, et al: Fusion of bone-marrow-derived cells with Purkinje neurons, cardiomyocytes and hepatocytes. *Nature* 425:968, 2003.
10. Murry CE, Soonpaa MH, Reinecke H, et al: Haematopoietic stem cells do not transdifferentiate into cardiac myocytes in myocardial infarcts. *Nature* 428:664, 2004.
11. Balsam LB, Wagers AJ, Christensen JL, et al: Haematopoietic stem cells adopt mature haematopoietic fates in ischaemic myocardium. *Nature* 428:668, 2004.
12. Norol F, Merlet P, Isnard R, et al: Influence of mobilized stem cells on myocardial infarct repair in a nonhuman primate model. *Blood* 102:4361, 2003.
13. Rota M, Kajsture J, Hosoda T, et al: Bone marrow cells adopt the cardiomyogenic fate in vivo. *Proc Natl Acad Sci U S A* 104:17783, 2007.
14. Kawada H, Fujita J, Kinjo K, et al: Nonhematopoietic mesenchymal stem cells can be mobilized and differentiate into cardiomyocytes after myocardial infarction. *Blood* 104:3581, 2004.
15. Friedenstein AJ, Petrakova KV, Kurolesova AI, et al: Heterotopic of bone marrow. Analysis of precursor cells for osteogenic and hematopoietic tissues. *Transplantation* 6:230, 1968.
16. Friedenstein AJ, Deriglasova UF, Kulagina NN, et al: Cursors for fibroblasts in different populations of hematopoietic cells as detected by the *in vitro* colony assay method. *Exp Hematol* 2:83, 1974.
17. Owen M: Marrow stromal stem cells. *J Cell Sci* 10(Suppl):63, 1988.
18. Castro-Malaspina H, Gay RE, Resnick E, et al: Characterization of human bone marrow fibroblast colony-forming cells (CFU-F) and their progeny. *Blood* 56:289, 1980.
19. Pittenger MF, MacKay AM, Beck SC, et al: Multilineage potential of adult human mesenchymal stem cells. *Science* 284:143, 1999.
20. Caplan AI: Mesenchymal stem cells. *J Orthop Res* 9:641, 1991.
21. Horwitz E, Le BK, Dominici M, et al: Clarification of the nomenclature for MSC: The International Society for Cellular Therapy position statement. *Cytotherapy* 7:393, 2005.
22. Dominici M, Le BK, Mueller I, et al: Minimal criteria for defining multipotent mesenchymal stromal cells. The International Society for Cellular Therapy position statement. *Cytotherapy* 8:315, 2006.
23. Jones EA, Kinsey SE, English A, et al: Isolation and characterization of bone marrow multipotential mesenchymal progenitor cells. *Arthritis Rheum* 46:3349, 2002.
24. Martinez G, Hoffman T, Marino R, et al: Human bone marrow mesenchymal stem cells express neuronal ganglioside GD2: A novel surface marker for the identification of MSCs. *Blood* 109:4245, 2007.
25. Erices A, Conget P, Rojas C, et al: Gp130 Activation by soluble interlukin-6 receptor/interleukin-6 enhances osteoblastic differentiation of human bone marrow-derived mesenchymal stem cells. *Exp Cell Res* 280:24, 2002.
26. Battula VL, Bareiss PM, Treml S, et al: Human placenta and bone marrow derived MSC cultures in serum-free, b-FGF-containing medium express cell surface frizzled-9 and SSEA-4 and give rise to multilineage differentiation. *Differentiation* 75:279, 2007.
27. Simmons PJ, Torok-Storb B: Identification of stromal cell precursors in human bone marrow by a novel monoclonal antibody, STRO-1. *Blood* 78:55, 1991.
28. Jones E, McGonagle D: Human bone marrow mesenchymal stem *in vivo*. *Rheumatology* 47:126, 2008.
29. Zuk PA, Zhu M, Ashjian P, et al: Human adipose tissue is a source of multipotent stem cells. *Mol Biol Cell* 13:4279, 2002.
30. In't Anker PS, Scherjon SA, Klejburg-van der Keur C, et al: Isolation of mesenchymal stem cells of fetal or maternal origin from human placenta. *Stem Cells* 22:1338, 2004.
31. Shih DT, Lee DC, Chen SC, et al: Isolation and characterization of neurogenic mesenchymal stem cells in human scalp tissue. *Stem Cells* 7:1012, 2005.
32. Erices A, Conget P, Minguell JJ: Mesenchymal progenitor cells in human umbilical cord blood. *Br J Haematol* 109:235, 2000.
33. Sarugaser R, Lickorish D, Baksh D, et al: Human umbilical cord perivascular (HUCPV) cells: A source of mesenchymal progenitors. *Stem Cells* 23:220, 2005.
34. Wang HS, Hung SC, Peng ST, et al: Mesenchymal stem cells in the Wharton's jelly of the human umbilical cord. *Stem Cells* 22:1330, 2004.
35. De Bari C, Dell'Accio F, Tylzanowski P, et al: Multipotent mesenchymal stem cells from adult human synovial membrane. *Arthritis Rheum* 44:1928, 2001.
36. Gronthos S, Mankani M, Brahim J, et al: Postnatal human dental pulp stem cells (DPSCs) *in vitro* and *in vivo*. *Proc Natl Acad Sci U S A* 97:13625, 2000.
37. Wakitani S, Saito T, Caplan AI: Myogenic cells derived from rat bone marrow mesenchymal stem cells exposed to 5-azacytidine. *Muscle Nerve* 18:1417, 1995.
38. Woodbury D, Schwartz EJ, Prockop DJ, et al: Adult rat and human bone marrow stromal cells differentiate into neurons. *J Neurosci Res* 61:364, 2000.
39. Weng YS, Lin HY, Hsiang Weng YS, et al: The effects of different growth factors on human bone marrow stromal cells differentiating into hepatocyte-like cells. *Adv Exp Med Biol* 534:119, 2003.
40. Toma C, Pittenger MF, Cahill KS, et al: Human mesenchymal stem cells differentiate to a cardiomyocyte phenotype in the adult murine heart. *Circulation* 105:93, 2002.
41. Sueblinvong V, Loi R, Eisenhauer PL, et al: Derivation of lung epithelium from human cord blood-derived mesenchymal stem cells. *Am J Respir Crit Care Med* 177:701, 2008.
42. Oswald J, Broxberger S, Jorgensen B, et al: Mesenchymal stem cells can be differentiated into endothelial cells *in vitro*. *Stem Cells* 22:377, 2004.
43. Morikawa S, Mabuchi Y, Kunimichi N, et al: Development of mesenchymal stem cells partially originate from the neural crest. *Biochem Biophys Res Commun* 379:1114, 2009.
44. Uccelli A, Moretta L, Pistoia V: Mesenchymal stem cells in health and disease. *Nat Rev Immunol* 8:726, 2008.
45. Sarugaser R, Hanoun L, Keating A, et al: Human mesenchymal stem cells self-renew and differentiate according to a deterministic hierarchy. *PLoS ONE* 4:e6498, 2009.

46. Horwitz EM, Dominici M: How do mesenchymal stromal cells exert their therapeutic benefit? *Cytotherapy* 10:771, 2008.
47. Phinney DG: Biochemical heterogeneity of mesenchymal stem cell populations. *Cell Cycle* 6:2884, 2007.
48. Keating A, Singer JW, Killen PD, et al: Donor origin of the *in vivo* hematopoietic microenvironment after marrow transplantation in man. *Nature* 298:280, 1982.
49. Clark BR, Keating A: Biology of bone marrow stroma. *Ann N Y Acad Sci* 770:70, 1995.
50. Nauta A, Fibbe WE: Immunomodulatory properties of mesenchymal stromal cells. *Blood* 110:3499, 2007.
51. Tolar J, Wang X, Braunlin E: The host immune response is essential for the beneficial effect of adult stem cells after myocardial ischemia. *Exp Hematol* 35:1153, 2007.
52. Mishra PK: Bone marrow-derived mesenchymal stem cells for treatment of heart failure: Is it all paracrine actions and immunomodulation? *J Cardiovasc Med* 9:122, 2008.
53. Atsma DE, Fibbe WE, Rabelink TJ: Opportunities and challenges for mesenchymal stem cell-mediated heart repair. *Curr Opin Lipidol* 18:645, 2007.
54. Parr AM, Tator CH, Keating A: Bone marrow-derived mesenchymal stromal cells for the repair of central nervous system injury. *Bone Marrow Transplant* 40:609, 2007.
55. Jones KB, Seshadri T, Krantz R, et al: Cell based therapies for osteonecrosis of the femoral head. *Biol Blood Marrow Transplant* 14:1081, 2008.
56. Sgodda M, Aurich H, Kleist S, et al: Hepatocyte differentiation of mesenchymal stem cells from rat peritoneal adipose tissue *in vitro* and *in vivo*. *Exp Cell Res* 313:2875, 2007.
57. Makino S, Fukuda K, Miyoshi S, et al: Cardiomyocytes can be generated from marrow stromal cells in vitro. *J Clin Invest* 103:697, 1999.
58. Rose RA, Jiang H, Wang XH, et al: Bone marrow-derived mesenchymal stromal cells express cardiac-specific markers, retain the stromal phenotype and do not become functional cardiomyocytes. *Stem Cells* 26:2884, 2008.
59. Ma J, Ge J, Zhang S, et al: Time course of myocardial stromal cell-derived factor 1 expression and beneficial effects of intravenously administered bone marrow stem cells in rats with experimental myocardial infarction. *Basic Res Cardiol* 100:217, 2005.
60. Shake JG, Gruber PJ, Baumgartner WA, et al: Mesenchymal stem cell implantation in a swine myocardial infarct model: Engraftment and functional effects. *Ann Thorac Surg* 73:1919, 2002; discussion 73:1926, 2002.
61. Yeghiazarians Y, Zhang Y, Prasad M, et al: Injection of bone marrow cell extract into infracted hearts results in functional improvement comparable to intact cell therapy. *Mol Ther* 17:1250, 2009.
62. Gnecchi M, He H, Liang OD, et al: Paracrine action accounts for marked protection of ischemic heart by Akt-modified mesenchymal stem cells. *Nat Med* 11:367, 2005.
63. Evans MJ, Kaufman MH: Establishment in culture of pluripotential cells from mouse embryos. *Nature* 292:154, 1981.
64. Martin GR: Isolation of a pluripotent cell line from early mouse embryos cultured in medium conditioned by teratocarcinoma stem cells. *Proc Natl Acad Sci U S A* 78:7634, 1981.
65. Hochedlinger K, Jaenisch R: Nuclear transplantation, embryonic stem cells, and the potential for cell therapy. *N Engl J Med* 349:275, 2003.
66. Thomson JA, Itskovitz-Eldor J, Shapiro SS: Embryonic stem cell lines derived from human blastocysts. *Science* 282:1145, 1998.
67. Hwang WS, et al: Evidence of a pluripotent human embryonic stem cell line derived from a cloned blastocyst. *Science* 303:1669, 2004.
68. Yamanaka S: Pluripotency and nuclear reprogramming. *Philos Trans R Soc Lond B Biol Sci* 363:2079, 2008.
69. Takahashi K, Yamanaka S: Induction of pluripotent stem cells from mouse embryonic and adult fibroblast cultures by defined factors. *Cell* 126:663, 2006.
70. Hotta A, Cheung AYL, Farra N, et al: Isolation of human iPS cells using EOS lentiviral vectors to select for pluripotency. *Nat Methods* 6:370, 2009.
71. Stadtfeld M, Nagaya M, Utikal M, et al: Induced pluripotent stem cells generated without viral integration. *Science* 322:945, 2008.
72. Okita K, Nakagawa M, Hyenjong H, et al: Generation of mouse induced pluripotent stem cells without viral vectors. *Science* 322:949, 2008.
73. Woltjen K, Michael IP, Mohseni P, et al: *PiggyBac* transposition reprograms fibroblasts to induce pluripotent stem cells. *Nature* 458:766, 2009.
74. Zhou H, Wu S, Joo JY, et al: Generation of induced pluripotent stem cells using recombinant proteins. *Cell Stem Cell* 4:381, 2009.
75. Nakagawa M, Koyanagi M, Tanabe K, et al: Generation of induced pluripotent stem cells without Myc from mouse and human fibroblasts. *Nat Biotechnol* 26:101, 2008.
76. Yu J, Vodyanik MA, Smuga-Otto K, et al: Induced pluripotent stem cell lines derived from human somatic cells. *Science* 318:1917, 2007.
77. Narazaki G, Uosaki H, Teranishi M, et al: Directed and systematic differentiation of cardiovascular cells from mouse induced pluripotent stem cells. *Circulation* 118:498, 2008.
78. Yoshikawa T, Mitsuno H, Nonaka I, et al: Wound therapy by marrow mesenchymal cell transplantation. *Plast Reconstr Surg* 121:860, 2008.
79. Zohlnhöfer D, Ott I, Mehilli J, et al: Stem cell mobilization by granulocyte colony-stimulating factor in patients with acute myocardial infarction. *JAMA* 295:1003, 2006.
80. Ripa RS, Jørgensen E, Wang Y, et al: Stem cell mobilization induced by subcutaneous granulocyte-colony stimulating factor to improve cardiac regeneration after acute ST-elevation myocardial infarction: Result of the double-blind, randomized, placebo-controlled stem cells in myocardial infarction (STEMMI) trial. *Circulation* 113:1983, 2006.
81. Abdel-Latif A, Bolli R, Tleyjeh I, et al: Adult bone marrow-derived cells for cardiac repair. *Arch Intern Med* 167:989, 2007.
82. Martin-Rendon W, Brunskill SJ, Hyde CJ, et al: Autologous bone marrow stem cells to treat acute myocardial infarction: A systemic review. *Eur Heart J* 29:1807, 2008.

PART VI

The Erythrocyte

CHAPTER 29

MORPHOLOGY OF THE ERYTHRON

Brian S. Bull and Paul C. Herrmann

SUMMARY

Collectively, the progenitor and adult red cells are termed the *erythron* to reinforce the idea that they function as an organ. The widely dispersed cells comprising this organ arise from undifferentiated, pluripotential stem cells. Following commitment, erythroid progenitors progress through several replicative stages, each having a characteristic ultrastructural morphology. As the cells mature, hemoglobin is synthesized with increasing intensity. The nucleus becomes more pyknotic and eventually is extruded. The mature erythrocyte adopts a variety of forms within two sequences—from discocyte to echinocyte and from discocyte to stomatocyte. These series are stages through which a single erythrocyte can pass reversibly as a result of changes in pH, plasma protein levels, and presence of amphipathic drugs. Other shapes, once acquired, are irreversible and frequently represent a particular pathophysiologic process. Names derived from Greek terms have been attached to these erythrocyte shapes because there is significant benefit to standardized terminology.

ERYTHRON

The mass of circulating erythrocytes constitutes an organ responsible for the transport of oxygen. Because the oxygen concentration per unit volume of blood is indistinguishable from the volume percent of oxygen in air, each cell of the multicellular organism that is the human body has gas (O_2, CO_2) exchange equivalent to that which would be available to a unicellular organism. Collectively, the progenitor and adult red cells making up this organ are termed the *erythron,* which arises from undifferentiated, pluripotential stem cells. Following commitment, erythroid progenitors progress through several replicative stages, becoming more functionally specialized with maturation. In the process, they acquire many of the human blood group antigens.[1] Eventually the reticulocyte and finally the mature circulating erythrocyte are produced.

In the adult stage of development, the total number of circulating erythrocytes is in steady state unless perturbed by pathologic or environmental insult. This is not so during growth *in utero*, particularly in the early stages of embryonic development. Consequently, erythrocyte production in the adult differs markedly from that in the embryo/fetus.

THE EARLIEST ERYTHRON

In the very early stages of human growth and development, there are two forms of red cell maturation: primitive and definitive (see Chap. 6).[2–6] The primitive stage originates from mesothelial cells that migrate through the primitive streak in the yolk sac. The primitive erythron supplies the embryo with oxygen during the phase of rapid growth before the definitive form of maturation has had a chance to develop and seed an appropriate niche. The hallmark of this primitive erythron is a semisynchronous release of nucleated erythroid precursors containing primitive hemoglobin. Although primitive in the sense that the cells contain nuclei when released into the circulation, this form of maturation differs from avian and reptilian erythropoiesis in that the nucleus is eventually expelled from the mammalian cells as they circulate. The presence of a nucleus in the cells of the primitive erythron decreases the efficiency of gas exchange in the lungs and microvasculature because the nucleus prevents the red cell from behaving as a fluid droplet.[7] Hence, these cells are less-efficient oxygen carriers than the anucleate cells of the definitive erythron that follows.

The definitive stage of maturation makes its appearance around week 5 of embryogenesis when multipotential stem cells develop in the endoderm and lining of the embryonic blood vessels. These seed the liver with the burst-forming unit–erythroid (BFU-E), which maintains the erythron for most of fetal life. In later fetal life, skeletal development provides marrow niches for the erythron to which it relocates forming erythroblastic islands.[8] The definitive stage of erythroid maturation predominates during the remainder of fetal development and is the only type of maturation present through childhood and adult life.

Acronyms and abbreviations that appear in this chapter include: BFU-E, burst-forming unit–erythroid; CFU-E, colony-forming unit–erythroid; DIC, disseminated intravascular coagulation; DMT1, divalent metal transporter 1; ICAM-4, intercellular adhesion molecule-4; ISC, irreversibly sickled cell; MCHC, mean corpuscular hemoglobin concentration; MCV, mean corpuscular volume; TTP, thrombotic thrombocytopenic purpura.

ERYTHROID PROGENITORS AND STIMULATING FACTORS

BURST-FORMING UNIT–ERYTHROID

The earliest characterized progenitor committed to the erythroid lineage is the BFU-E. BFU-E is defined *in vitro* by its ability to create a "burst" on semisolid media—that is, a colony consisting of several hundred to thousands of cells in 10 to 14 days (see Chap. 31, Fig. 31–1). This progenitor requires a number of factors for proliferation, prevention of apoptosis, and differentiation (see Chap. 31). In addition, it supplies a number of factors necessary for the specialized macrophages that appear to nurse the erythropoietic development in the erythroblastic island described below.[9] The BFU-E requires interleukin-3, granulocyte-macrophage colony-stimulating factor, erythropoietin, and other factors for proliferation, prevention of apoptosis, and differentiation to morphologically recognizable erythroid precursors (see Chap. 16).

COLONY-FORMING UNIT–ERYTHROID

As maturation progresses, a late progenitor, colony forming unit–erythroid (CFU-E), can be defined *in vitro* (see Chap. 31, Fig. 31–1). CFU-E is very sensitive to erythropoietin (see Chaps. 16 and 31) and can undergo only a few divisions. Thus, CFU-E forms a small colony of morphologically recognizable erythroid precursors in 2 to 5 days. Adhesion between erythroid cells and macrophages occurs at the CFU-E stage of maturation.[10]

ERYTHROBLASTIC ISLAND

The anatomical unit of erythropoiesis in the normal adult is the *erythroblastic island.*[11] The erythroblastic island consists of one or two centrally located macrophages surrounded by maturing erythroid cells (Fig. 29–1). A number of binding proteins are implicated in the cell–cell adhesions important to this process.[12] The ligand LW gp, a member of the intercellular adhesion molecule family that is virtually restricted in its expression to erythroid cells, appears at this stage and may help stabilize the erythroblastic island.[13] Intercellular adhesion molecule-4

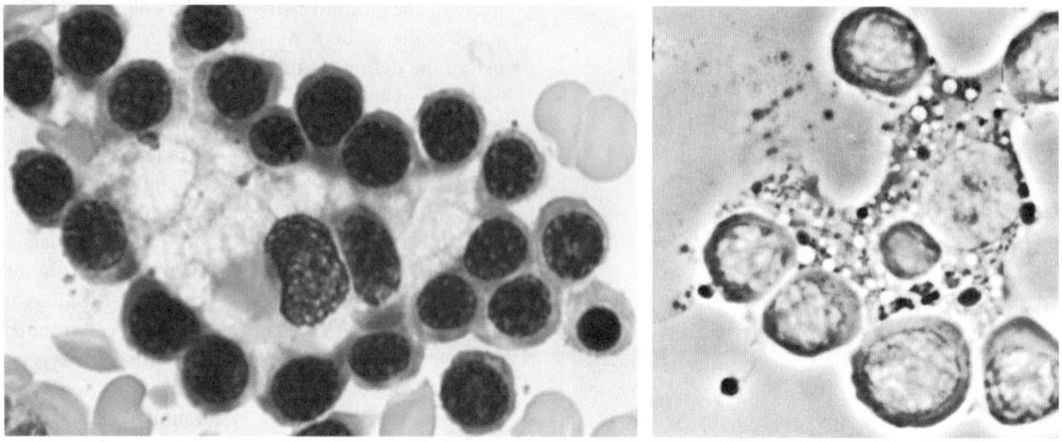

FIGURE 29–1. Erythroblastic island. **A.** Erythroblastic island as seen in Wright-Giemsa-stained marrow. Note central macrophage surrounded by a cohort of attached erythroblasts. **B.** Erythroblastic island in the living state examined by phase-contrast microscopy. The macrophage shows dynamic movement in relation to its surrounding erythroblasts.

(ICAM-4) is critical for island formation.[14] Phase-contrast microcinematography reveals that the macrophage is far from passive or immobile. Intriguing evidence suggests that either erythroblastic islands migrate or that erythroid precursors move from island to island, as islands near sinusoids are composed of more acidophilic, mature erythroblasts while islands more distant from the sinusoids are composed of proerythroblasts.[15] The macrophage's pseudopodium-like cytoplasmic extensions move rapidly over cell surfaces of the surrounding wreath of erythroblasts. On scanning electron micrographs, the central macrophage of the erythroblastic island appears sponge-like, with surface invaginations in which the erythroblasts lie. As the erythroblast matures, it moves along a cytoplasmic extension of the macrophage away from the main body. When the erythroblast is sufficiently mature for nuclear expulsion, the erythroblast makes contact with an endothelial cell, passes through a pore in the cytoplasm of the endothelial cell via an unclear mechanism, and enters the circulation as a reticulocyte (see Chap. 4). The nucleus is ejected prior to egress from the marrow, phagocytized, and degraded by the marrow macrophages in a process very like eryptosis (the physiologic death of erythrocytes; see "Eryptosis—Red Cell Suicide" below).[16,17]

In addition to the unique cytological features described above, the macrophage of the erythroblastic island is also molecularly distinct as demonstrated by a unique immunophenotypic signature, pronounced adhesive properties, ability for avid endocytosis, and lack of a respiratory burst.[18] In addition, the macrophage of the erythroblastic island appears to play a stimulatory role in erythropoiesis independent of erythropoietin. The anemias of chronic inflammation and myelodysplasia appear to result, at least in part, from inadequate stimulation of erythropoiesis by the macrophages.[19]

In addition to fibronectin,[20,21] a cell-to-cell recognition system is almost certainly critical to the formation and maintenance of the erythroblastic island. Maturing erythroid cells express adhesion molecules including integrins, selectins, sialomucins, cadherins, and molecules belonging to the immunoglobulin superfamily.[13] Marrow macrophages express hemagglutinin ligands, sialoadhesins, and erythroblast receptors.[22] The cell recognition system also is operative *in vitro*. Erythroblastic islands form in long-term marrow cultures with an adherent stromal cell layer. Likewise, erythroblasts grown from BFU-E in methylcellulose or in plasma clots form erythroid islands if the clots are lysed, permitting erythroblast–macrophage association.[23,24] Despite the central role of erythroid islands in erythropoiesis, morphologically normal development of erythroid cells occurs *in vitro* without these structures as long as developing cells are provided with appropriate cytokines and growth factors.[25] Such growth, however, occurs at a much slower rate than that observed *in vivo*, when erythroblasts form erythroblastic islands.[12]

The erythroblastic island is a fragile structure. It is usually disrupted in the process of obtaining a marrow specimen by needle aspiration and is commonly seen in marrow films only in clinical situations with accelerated erythroblastic activity, such as acute hemolytic anemia and erythroleukemia.

MARROW IRON METABOLISM

Chap. 42 discusses the details of iron metabolism. In normal humans, the marrow macrophage plays a major role in iron conservation. Aged and damaged erythrocytes, identified and trapped within the marrow microcirculation, are phagocytosed by the macrophage. Lysosomes release their lytic enzymes into the primary phagosome of the macrophage. Digestion of the engulfed red cell is virtually complete within 60 minutes. The membrane is reduced to multiple myelin laminae, and erythrocyte iron is transformed into aggregates of ferritin (Fig. 29–2).

Ferritin is a 440-kDa protein consisting of 24 subunits arranged to form a hollow sphere. The central cavity can store 4500 iron atoms[26] in the form of electron-dense particles of approximately 6 nm (60 Å) (see Fig. 29–2). Microdiffraction techniques have shown that the iron cores display a hexagonal structure.[27] Under the light microscope, hemosiderin is the intracellular, yellowish, iron-containing pigment in iron-loaded tissues. Under the electron microscope, hemosiderin is largely composed of dense clusters of ferritin, most of which are membrane enclosed.[28] Ferritin in lysosomes is converted into hemosiderin upon partial degradation of its protein shell by lysosomal enzymes.[29] By contrast, ferritin that is degraded within the cytosol results in complete release of the iron.[30]

The outer membrane of erythroblasts possesses transferrin receptors on clathrin-coated pits. Adherence of transferrin to these portions of the cell membrane initiates a local membrane invagination, and intracytoplasmic vesicles are formed. The vesicles rapidly shed their clathrin coats and fuse with lysosomes, forming endosomes.[26,31] The acid pH in the endosome permits release of iron from transferrin.[26] DMT1 protein is present in the endosomal membrane where it transports iron

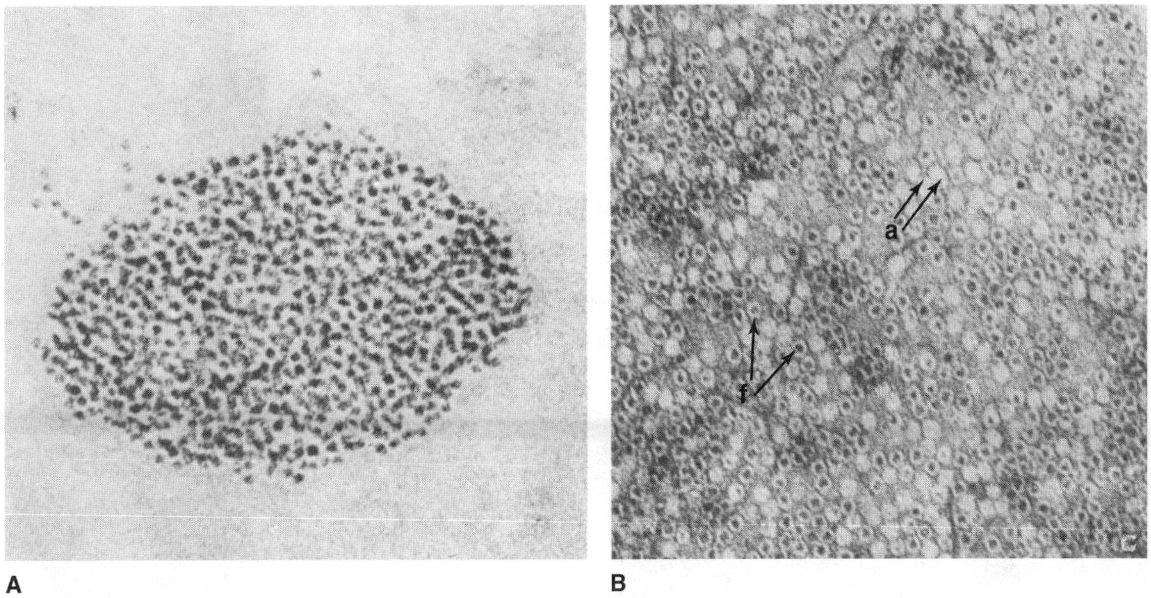

FIGURE 29–2. Ultrastructural aspects of ferritin. **A.** Electron micrograph of a membrane-bound erythroblast siderosome showing that the siderosome is composed of individual ferritin molecules. **B.** Electron micrograph of negatively stained ferritin and apoferritin mixture showing the ferritin molecule (*f*) with its protein coat and central dense iron core. Apoferritin molecules (*a*) lack the central iron cores. *(From Bessis MC, Breton-Gorius J,[166] with permission.)*

released from the transferrin complex into the cytoplasm for heme synthesis (see Chap. 42). Direct mitochondria–endosome interaction is involved[32] and may also involve the protein mobilferrin.[33] Apotransferrin and transferrin receptor molecules are cycled back to the cell membrane, where apotransferrin is released into the extracellular medium. Immunocytochemical labeling of transferrin receptors has shown that the same pit can contain the transferrin receptors and ferritin molecules.[34] Calculations suggest that the coated vesicle transfers 1000 times more iron via ferritin than via transferrin.[31]

Despite the efficiency of this transfer mechanism, it is not clear whether ferritin iron can support the biosynthesis of heme in mitochondria.[35,36] Possibly the cytosolic ferritin in early red cell precursors is used for hemoglobin synthesis, while the ferritin clusters in mature erythroblasts represent storage of excess iron. The H ferritin (see Chap. 42) messenger RNA accumulates specifically during early erythroid differentiation.[37]

In the presence of oxygen, uncomplexed iron catalyzes superoxide formation and forms a lethal mixture containing reactive hydroxyl radicals.[38,39] Hydroxyl radicals cause lipid peroxidation and DNA strand breakage, establishing a self-amplifying and autocatalytic redox reaction capable of destroying the developing erythroid cell.[40] A similar catalysis by hemin creating reactive oxygen species is responsible for the devastating cutaneous manifestation of acute porphyria attacks and illustrates the potential harm of a loose oxygen-activating catalyst. Such disastrous outcomes are normally thwarted because iron is kept in the safe, bound, ferric form (extracellular transferrin, intracellular ferritin, membrane-encapsulated hemosiderin)[41] and the bound iron is transferred directly from endosomes to mitochondria.[40,41]

ERYTHROBLASTIC SERIES

■ EARLY PROGENITORS

Numerically, BFU-E and CFU-E represent only a minute proportion of human marrow cells. In mice, CFU-E can be generated in large numbers and then enriched by centrifugal elutriation and Percoll density gradient centrifugation. Under the electron microscope, these cells show large nucleoli, abundant polyribosomes, and large mitochondria (Fig. 29–3).[42] Isolation of CD34+ cells from cord blood and marrow has replaced the laborious elutriation/density gradient centrifugation process. *In vitro* cultures using CD34+ cells as the starting material have identified the critical cytokines required for differentiation and maturation[25,43,44] and enabled identification and tracing of pure cohorts of erythroid precursors (see Chaps. 16 and 31) through all the morphologic stages. The erythroid precursor cells in marrow are shown with light microscopy in Figure 29–4. The ultrastructure of each precursor is described in the sections that immediately follow.[45]

Proerythroblasts

On stained films, the proerythroblast (Fig. 29–5) appears as a large cell, 20 to 25 μm in diameter, irregularly rounded or slightly oval. The nucleus occupies approximately 80 percent of the cell area and contains fine chromatin delicately distributed in small clumps. One or several well-defined nucleoli are present.

Polyribosomes arranged in groups of two to six are numerous in the cytoplasm and are typical of this stage. The high concentration of polyribosomes gives the cytoplasm of these cells its characteristic intense basophilia. At high magnification, ferritin molecules are seen dispersed singly throughout the cytoplasm and lining the clathrin-coated pits on the cell membrane (Fig. 29–5).

Three to 12 granules present in the Golgi zone contain ferritin molecules.[46] The granules stain for acid phosphatase, indicating their lysosomal nature, and differ from another class of small granules, the catalase-containing granules. Diffuse cytoplasmic density on sections stained for peroxidase indicates hemoglobin is already present. Dispersed glycogen particles are present in the cytoplasm.[47]

Basophilic Erythroblasts

Basophilic erythroblasts are smaller than proerythroblasts, measuring 16 to 18 μm (Figs. 29–4 and 29–6). The nucleus occupies three-fourths

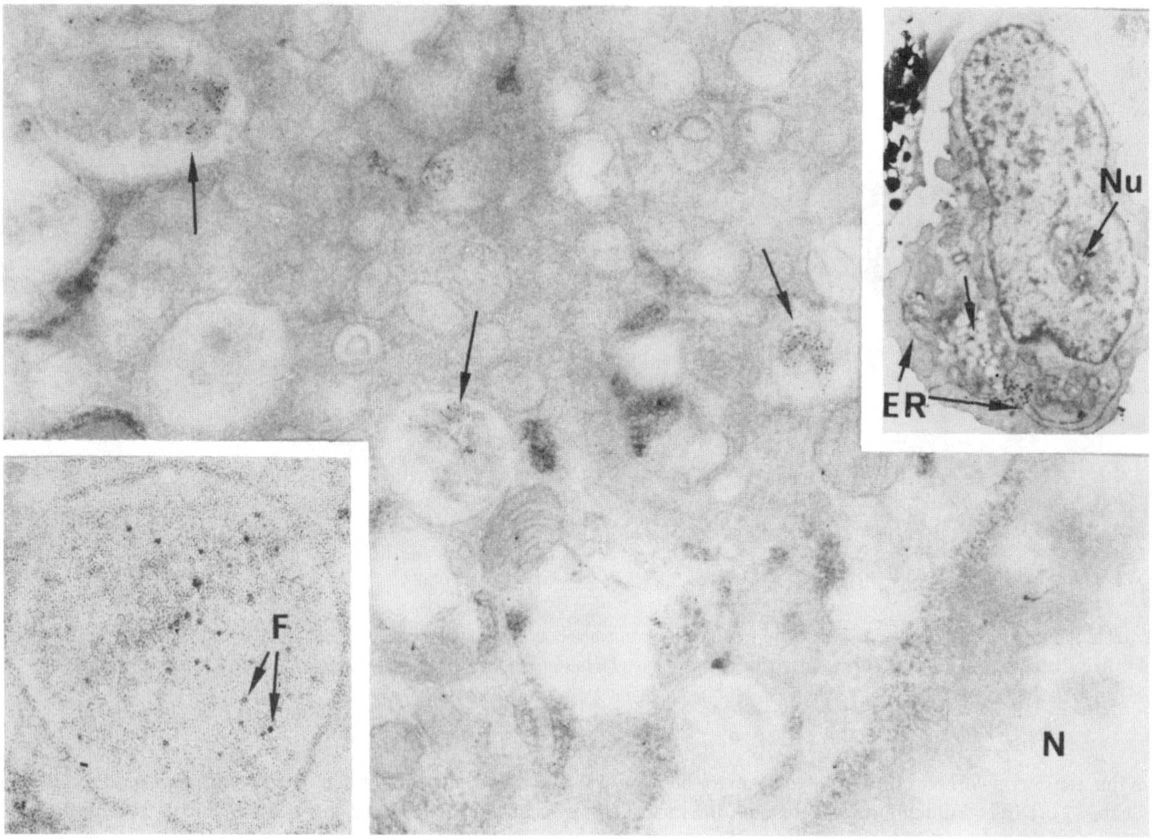

FIGURE 29–3. *Right inset*: Unstained section of a normal presumptive CFU-E that was enriched by panning from marrow, using the monoclonal antibody FA-152.[167] This blast has a large nucleolus (*Nu*). Incubation in diaminobenzidine medium reveals weak peroxidase activity in the endoplasmic reticulum (*ER*). In the Golgi zone, several granules appear as vacuoles (*arrow*). *Main figure*: On enlargement of the Golgi zone, a portion of the nucleus (*N*) is seen surrounded by a perinuclear cistern containing weak peroxidase activity. Several granules with a pale matrix contain ferritin molecules (*arrows*). *Left inset*: High magnification of a granule showing ferritin molecules (*F*) of characteristic structure and density. *(Adapted from Breton-Gorius J, Villeval JL, Mitjavila MT, et al,[168] with permission.)*

of the cell area and is composed of characteristic dark violet heterochromatin interspersed with pink-staining clumps of euchromatin linked by irregular strands. The whole arrangement often resembles wheel spokes or a clock face. The cytoplasm stains deep blue, leaving a perinuclear halo that expands into a juxtanuclear clear zone around the Golgi apparatus.

Cytoplasmic basophilia at this stage results from the continued presence of polyribosomes. Microtubules are often seen connecting two erythroblasts in mitosis.

Polychromatophilic Erythroblasts

Following the second mitotic division of the erythropoietic series, the cytoplasm changes from blue to pink as hemoglobin dilutes the polyribosome content (Figs. 29–4 and 29–7). Cells at this stage are smaller than basophilic erythroblasts, measuring approximately 12 to 15 μm in diameter. The nucleus occupies less than half of the cell area. The heterochromatin is located in well-defined clumps spaced regularly about the nucleus, producing a checkerboard pattern. The nucleolus is lost, but the perinuclear halo persists.

Electron microscopy of the polychromatophilic erythroblast reveals increased aggregation of nuclear heterochromatin. Active ferritin transport across the cell membrane is always evident, and siderosomes along with dispersed ferritin molecules can be identified within the cytoplasm.[11] This normal distribution of ferritin iron in the erythroblast characterizes the *normal sideroblast*. Mitochondrial iron usually is not apparent, even though the iron is incorporated into protoporphyrin in the mitochondria. The Golgi apparatus becomes quite small and may contain lysosomes.

Orthochromic Erythroblasts

After the final mitotic division of the erythropoietic series, the concentration of hemoglobin increases within the erythroblast. More than any of its predecessors, the orthochromic erythroblast stains like a mature erythrocyte (Figs. 29–4 and 29–8); however, it is always somewhat polychromatophilic because of residual polyribosomes.

Under the light microscope, the nucleus appears almost completely dense and featureless. It is measurably decreased in size. This cell is the smallest of the erythroblastic series, varying from 10 to 15 μm in diameter. The nucleus occupies approximately one-fourth of the cell area and is eccentric.

A surprising motility can be appreciated under the phase-contrast microscope. Round projections appear suddenly in different parts of the cell periphery and are just as quickly retracted. The movements probably are made in preparation for ejection of the nucleus.[11]

The cell ultrastructure is characterized by irregular borders, reflecting its motile state. The heterochromatin forms large masses. The cytoplasmic ribosomes are further dispersed with an increase in the relative proportion of diribosomes and monoribosomes. Mitochondria are reduced in number and size. Hemoglobin is present within the nucleus itself.[47,48]

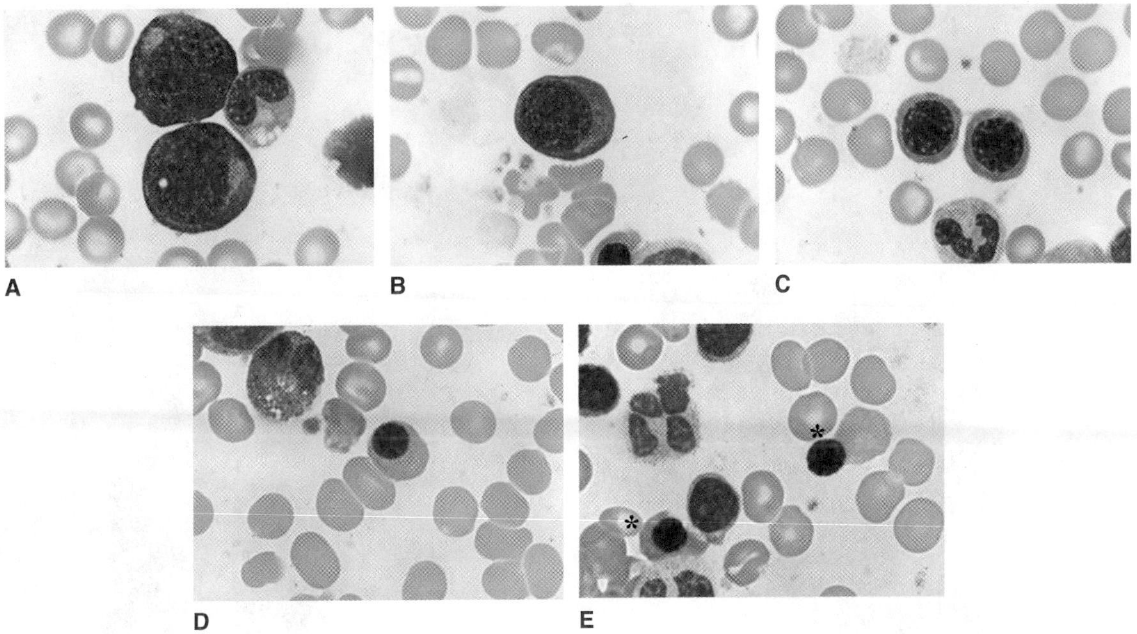

FIGURE 29–4. Human erythrocyte precursors. Light microscopic appearance. Marrow films stained with Wright stain. There are five stages of erythroblast development recognizable by light microscopy. **A.** Proerythroblasts. Two are present in this field. They are the largest red cell precursor, with a fine nuclear chromatin pattern, nucleoli, basophilic cytoplasm, and often a clear area at the site of the Golgi apparatus. **B.** Basophilic erythroblast. The cell is smaller than the proerythroblast, the nuclear chromatin is slightly more condensed and cytoplasm is basophilic. **C.** Polychromatophilic erythroblasts. The cell is smaller on average than its precursors. The nuclear chromatin is more condensed with a checkerboard pattern developing. Nucleoli are not apparent, usually. The cytoplasm is gray, reflecting the staining modulation induced by hemoglobin synthesis, which adds cytoplasmic content that takes an eosinophilic stain, admixed with the residual basophilia of the fading protein synthetic apparatus. **D.** Orthochromic normoblast. Smaller on average than its precursor, increased condensation of nuclear chromatin, with homogeneous cytoplasmic coloration approaching that of a red cell. **E.** Late orthochromatic erythroblasts (asterisks). The orthochromatic erythroblast to the right is undergoing apparent enucleation. The other three mononuclear cells are lymphocytes. A degenerating four-lobed neutrophil is also present. *(Used with permission from* Lichtman's Atlas of Hematology, *www.accessmedicine.com.)*

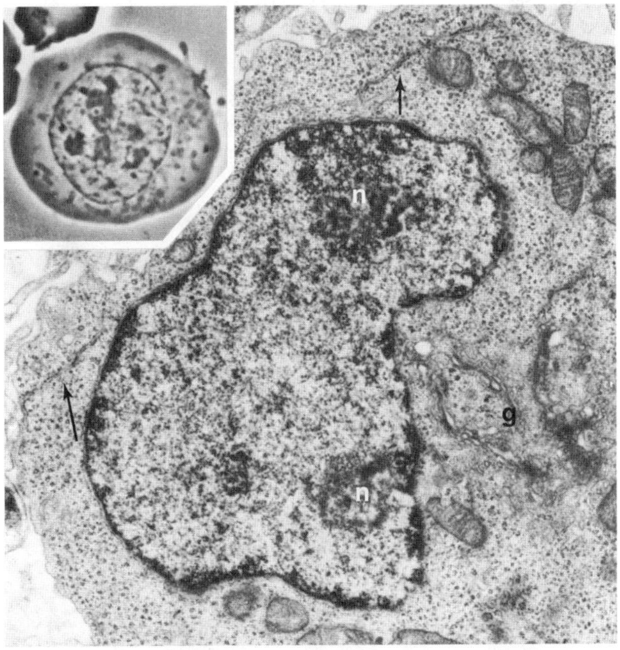

FIGURE 29–5. Proerythroblast. Phase-contrast micrograph (*inset*) of a proerythroblast showing the immature nucleus with nucleoli and finely dispersed nuclear chromatin. The centrosome (juxtanuclear clear zone) is apparent with its dense accumulation of mitochondria. Electron microscopic section of the proerythroblast shows nucleoli (*n*) in contact with the nuclear membrane. Chromatin is finely dispersed and forms small aggregates in the fixed nuclear membrane. The perinuclear canal is narrow but well defined. Polyribosome groups, many in helical configuration, are dispersed throughout the cytoplasm. The Golgi apparatus (*g*) is well developed, and regions of endoplasmic reticulum (*arrows*) are seen.

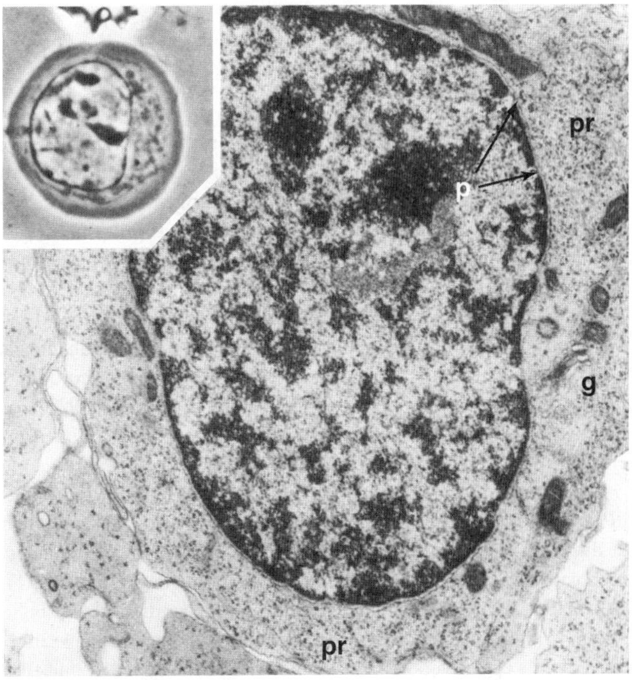

FIGURE 29–6. Basophilic erythroblast. Phase-contrast photomicrograph (*inset*) shows increased clumping of the nuclear chromatin and further rounding of the cell, with aggregation of the mitochondria and centrosome into the regions of nuclear indentation. Electron microscopic section shows clumping of the nuclear chromatin, nuclear pores (*p*), organization of the nucleoli, increased density of polyribosomes (*pr*), well-developed Golgi apparatus (*g*), and a decrease in smooth endoplasmic reticulum.

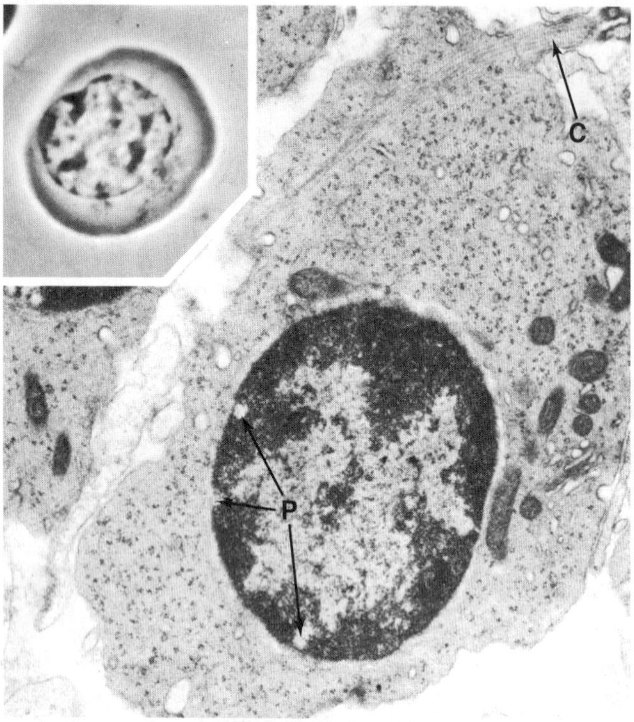

FIGURE 29–7. Polychromatophilic erythroblast. Phase-contrast micrograph (*inset*) demonstrates diminished size of this cell compared with its precursor. Further clumping of nuclear chromatin gives the nucleus a checkerboard appearance. The centrosome is condensed, and a perinuclear halo has developed. Electron microscopic section demonstrates relative reduction of the density of polyribosomes and dilution by the moderately osmiophilic hemoglobin in the cytoplasm. Nuclear chromatin shows a marked increase in clumping, and nuclear pores (*P*) are enlarged.

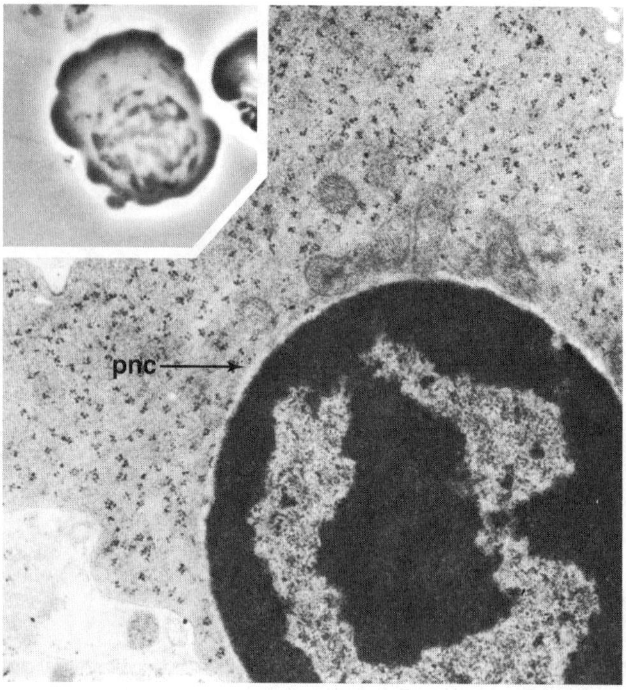

FIGURE 29–8. Orthochromic erythroblast. Phase-contrast appearance of this cell in the living state (*inset*) shows the irregular borders indicative of its characteristic motility, the eccentric nucleus making contact with the plasmalemma, further pyknosis of the nuclear chromatin, and condensation of the centrosome. Electron microscopic section shows further dilution of polyribosomes, some of which appear to be disintegrating into monoribosomes, by the increasing hemoglobin. The number of mitochondria is decreased, and some mitochondria are degenerating. Nuclear chromatin is clumped into large masses, and a perinuclear canal (*pnc*) is seen.

RETICULOCYTE

Birth

Prior to enucleation, intermediate filaments and the marginal band of microtubules disappear. Tubulin and actin become concentrated at the point where the nucleus will exit.[49] These changes, accompanied by microtubular rearrangements, play a role in nuclear expulsion.[50,51]

Expulsion of the nucleus *in vitro* is not an instantaneous phenomenon; it requires a period of minutes.[11] The process begins with several vigorous contractions around the midportion of the cell, followed by a division of the cell into unequal portions. The smaller portion consists of the expelled nucleus accompanied by a thin rim or "corona" of hemoglobinized cytoplasm. Loss of the "corona" of hemoglobin from the expelled nucleus leads, in part, to an increase in the "early peak" of stercobilin when the rate of erythropoiesis is increased.[52]

In vivo, expulsion of the nucleus may occur while the erythroblast is still part of an erythroblastic island (Fig. 29–9), or the nucleus may be lost during passage through the wall of a marrow sinus. The nucleus, which cannot traverse the small opening, remains in the marrow. The outer leaflet of the bilaminar membrane surrounding the expelled nucleus is high in phosphatidylserine, a signal for macrophage ingestion. There is controversy as to whether or not the expelled nucleus is ingested by the macrophage of the erythroblastic island or by other macrophages resident in marrow.[16]

Two proposals have been advanced to explain how the reticulocyte exits the marrow. The precise mechanism is unknown. The reticulocyte may actively traverse the sinus epithelium.[53] More likely, however, the reticulocyte may be driven across by a pressure differential because it appears incapable of directed amoeboid motion.[54,55] The electron microscope pictures of red cells traversing endothelial pores or slits typically show the intraluminal (intrasinusoidal) portion to be tense and roughly spherical and the interstitial (marrow) portion to be flac-

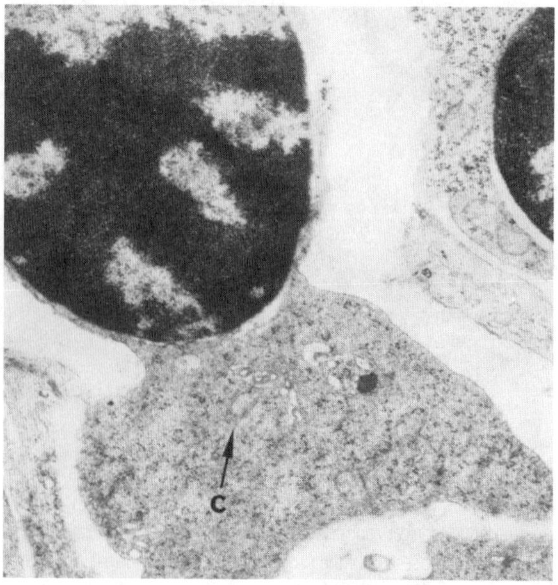

FIGURE 29–9. Orthochromic erythroblast ejecting its nucleus. A thin rim of cytoplasm surrounds the nucleus. In the cytoplasm, a single centriole (*c*) is partially encircled by some Golgi saccules.

cid, suggesting that hydraulic pressure on the viscous hemoglobin solution within the cell is driving the process.[56,57]

Maturation

The reticulocyte, as it enters the circulation, retains mitochondria, small numbers of ribosomes, the centriole, and remnants of the Golgi apparatus. It contains no endoplasmic reticulum. Supravital staining with brilliant cresyl blue or new methylene blue produces aggregates of ribosomes, mitochondria, and other cytoplasmic organelles. These artifactual aggregates stain deep blue and, arranged in reticular strands, give the reticulocyte its name. *In vitro* maturation is similar to *in vivo* maturation. However, in a plasma clot culture, the naked nuclei remain undamaged (Fig. 29–10). If the clot is lysed, the macrophages in the culture immediately recognize and phagocytose the expelled nuclei. Maturation of the circulating reticulocyte requires 24 to 48 hours. During this period, approximately 20 percent of the ultimate hemoglobin content

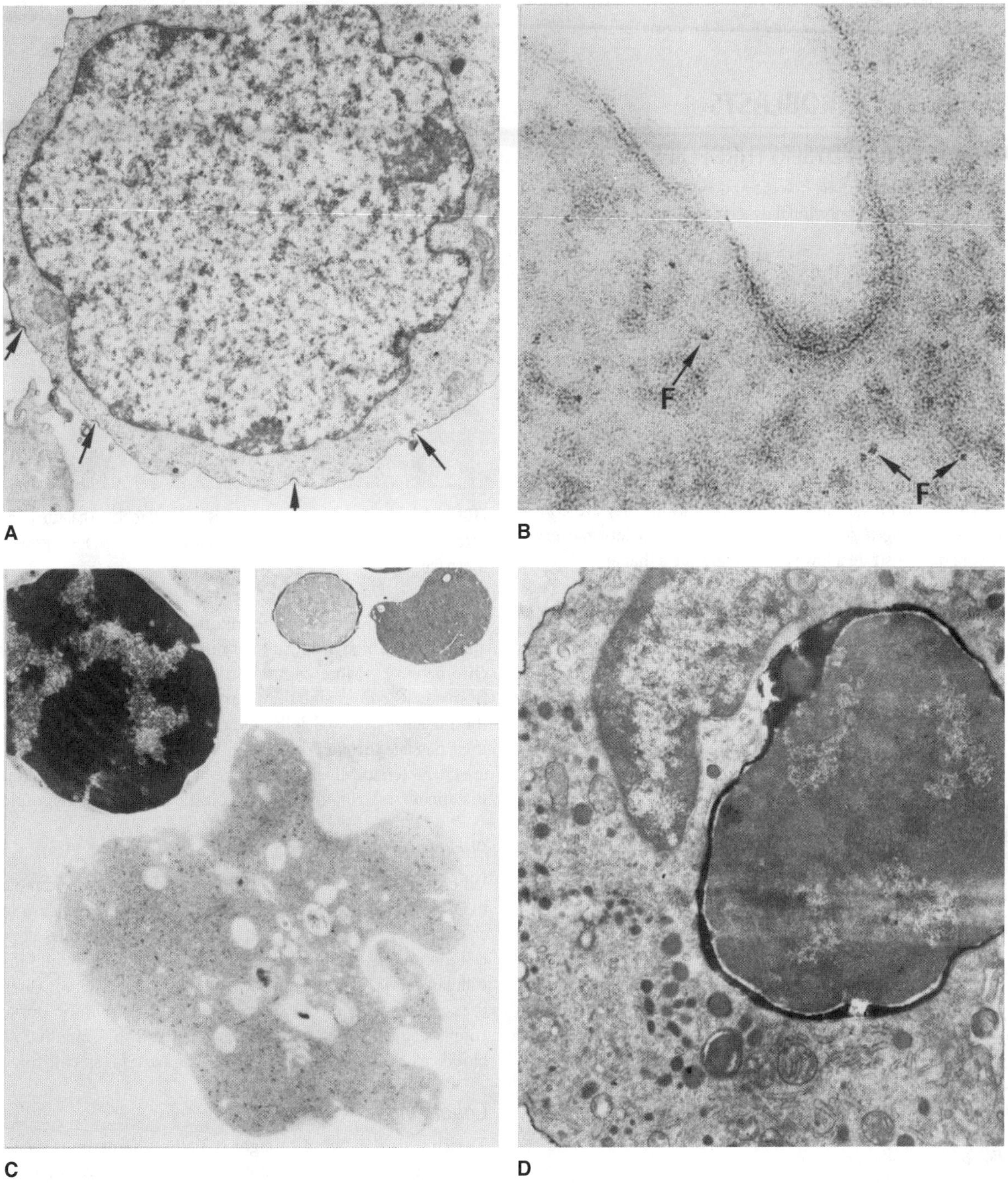

FIGURE 29–10. Erythroblast maturation in an *in vitro* plasma clot from BFU-E. **A.** At day 9 of culture, a cell resembling the *in vivo* proerythroblast exhibits numerous ferritin-coated membrane invaginations (*arrows*). **B.** One invagination seen at high magnification. Note the numerous ferritin molecules (*F*) dispersed in the cytoplasm. **C.** At day 12 of culture, an extruded nucleus is seen close to a reticulocyte. *Inset*: When the hemoglobin is emphasized by cytochemical staining, the thin rim of cytoplasm surrounding the nucleus is clearly visible. **D.** In the cell suspension produced by clot lysis, a macrophage phagocytoses a hemoglobin-rimmed erythroblast nucleus that was recently extruded. *(Panels C and D adapted from Breton-Gorius J, Guichard J, Vainchenker W,[23] with permission.)*

is synthesized and the final assembly of the submembrane skeleton completed.[11] Living reticulocytes observed by phase-contrast microscopy are slightly motile, irregularly shaped cells with a characteristically puckered exterior. Examined by electron microscopy, reticulocytes are irregularly shaped and contain many remnant organelles. The organelles, small smooth vesicles, and an occasional centriole are grouped in the hilar region. In "young" reticulocytes, the vast majority of ribosomes dispersed throughout the cytoplasm are in the form of polyribosomes. As protein synthesis diminishes during maturation, the polyribosomes gradually transform into monoribosomes. Simultaneously, loss of transferrin receptors occurs,[58,59] and eventually the capacity for endocytosis disappears.[60]

PATHOLOGIC ERYTHROBLASTS

MEGALOBLASTS AND DYSERYTHROPOIESIS

Chaps. 39 and 41 describe the morphologic abnormalities characterizing megaloblastic maturation and polyclonal dyserythropoietic anemias.

PATHOLOGIC SIDEROBLASTS

A heterogeneous group of erythrocyte maturation disorders is accompanied by ineffective erythropoiesis and hyperferremia. Erythrocyte maturation disorders include acquired idiopathic sideroblastic anemia, pyridoxine-responsive anemia, alcohol-induced sideroblastic anemia, lead intoxication, dyserythropoietic anemia, and certain hemoglobinopathies (see Chaps. 39, 48, 51, and 58). These conditions are characterized by the presence of pathologic sideroblasts. When stained for iron, these cells show small iron-containing granules that might be arranged in a ring around the nucleus. For this reason, they are commonly referred to as *ringed sideroblasts*.[61] Iron stains of normal erythroid precursors demonstrate a few very fine granules that are difficult to see without carefully focusing up and down through the cell.

Electron microscopic studies show that granules in ringed sideroblasts are iron-loaded mitochondria containing a unique form of ferritin—mitochondrial ferritin (see Chaps. 42 and 58). Because mitochondrial iron is distinct from ferritin antigenically, ultrastructurally, and by electron probe analysis, mitochondrial iron is termed *ferruginous micelles*.[11] In hereditary sideroblastic anemia, mitochondrial iron deposits occur primarily in late polychromatophilic erythroblasts. In acquired sideroblastic anemia, iron overload affects the early proerythroblast.[62] In cells with iron-loaded mitochondria, many ferritin molecules are deposited between adjacent erythroblast membranes (Fig. 29–11).[63]

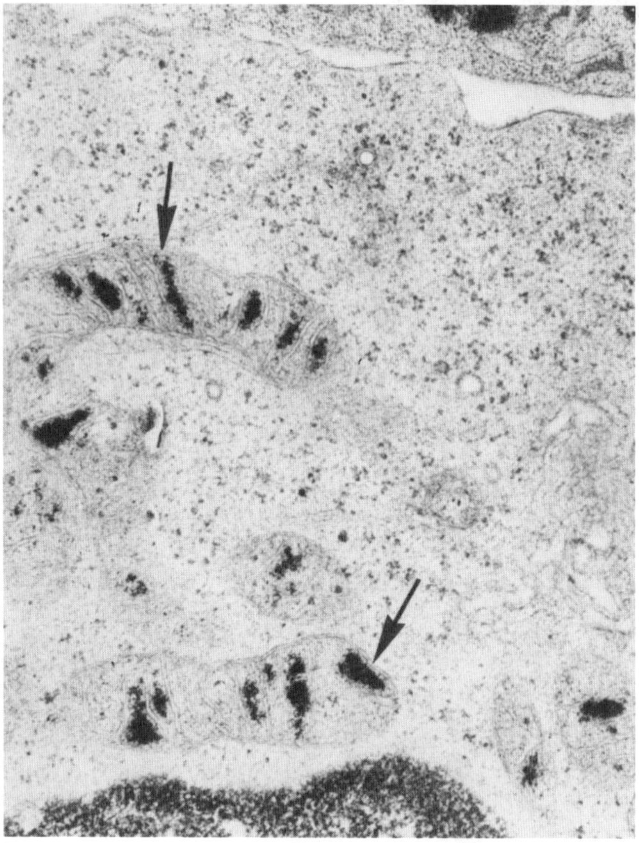

FIGURE 29–11. Pathologic sideroblast is an erythroblast characterized by the presence of mitochondrial deposits of iron-containing ferruginous micelles (*arrows*) between the cristae.

PATHOLOGY OF THE RETICULOCYTE AND ERYTHROCYTE

The reticulocyte may show pathologic alterations in size or staining properties. The reticulocyte may contain inclusions visible by light microscopy or identifiable only on ultrastructural analysis. Most pathologic inclusions usually attributed to erythrocytes are actually found within reticulocytes (Table 29–1) and are nuclear or cytoplasmic remnants derived from late-stage normoblasts. In splenectomized patients, they may also be found in mature erythrocytes.

Howell-Jolly Bodies

Howell-Jolly bodies[64] are small nuclear remnants that have the color of a pyknotic nucleus on Wright-stained films (Fig. 29–12A) and give a positive Feulgen reaction for DNA.[65] They are spherically shaped, randomly distributed in the red cell,[66] and usually no larger than 0.5 μm in diameter. Howell-Jolly bodies may be numerous, although generally only one is present. In pathologic situations, they appear to represent chromosomes that have separated from the mitotic spindle during abnormal mitosis, and contain a high proportion of centromeric material along with heterochromatin.[66,67] More commonly, during normal maturation they arise from nuclear fragmentation (karyorrhexis) or incomplete expulsion of the nucleus.[68] Howell-Jolly bodies are pitted from the reticulocytes in their passage through the interendothelial slits of the splenic sinus. They are characteristically present in the blood of splenectomized persons and in patients suffering from megaloblastic anemia, and hyposplenic states.

Pocked (or Pitted) Red Cells

When viewed by interference-phase microscopy, pocked red cells appear to have surface membrane "pits" or craters.[69] The vesicles or indentations characterizing these cells represent autophagic vacuoles adjacent to the cell membrane.[70] The vacuoles appear to be instrumental in disposal of cellular debris as the erythrocyte passes through the microcirculation of the spleen.[71] Within 1 week following splenectomy, pocked red cell counts begin to rise, reaching a plateau at 2 to 3 months.[72] Pocked red blood cell counts sometimes are used as a test for splenic function.

Cabot Rings

The ring-like or figure-of-eight structures sometimes seen in megaloblastic anemia within reticulocytes and in an occasional, heavily stippled, late intermediate megaloblast[73] are designated *Cabot rings* (Fig. 29–12D). Their exact composition is questionable. Some investigators have suggested that Cabot rings originate from spindle material that was mishandled during abnormal mitosis.[74] Others have found no indication of DNA or spindle filaments but have shown the rings are associated with adherent granular material containing arginine-rich

TABLE 29–1. Erythrocyte and Reticulocyte Inclusions

Inclusions	Composition	Cell Type	Appearance on Wright-Stained Film	Comments	Reference
"Reticulofilamentous substance"	Artifactual aggregation of ribosomes	Reticulocytes	Invisible	Visible after supravital staining	11
Howell-Jolly bodies	Nuclear fragment containing aberrant chromosomes	Reticulocytes; rarely erythrocytes	Dense blue spherical granule(s)	Visible in unstained cells	64–68
Cabot rings	Spindle remnant or histone-rich and iron-rich "cytoplasmic currents"	Reticulocytes; heavily stippled late intermediate megaloblasts	Ring or figure-of-eight strand stained purple	Visible in some hemolytic states	11, 73–75
Basophilic stippling	Pathologic precipitation of ribosomes	Reticulocytes	Dispersed blue granulations		76
Heinz bodies	Denatured hemoglobin	Erythrocytes; occasionally reticulocytes	Rarely visible	Refractile inclusions after staining with methylene or Nile blue dyes	77, 78
Hemoglobin H inclusions	Denatured hemoglobin (induced *in vitro* by exposure to brilliant cresyl blue, methylene blue, new methylene blue)	Erythrocytes; reticulocytes	Invisible	Gives "golf-ball" appearance to erythrocytes after incubation with appropriate supravital stains	79–83

histone and nonhemoglobin iron.[75] Because histone biosynthesis and iron metabolism/mobilization are abnormal in pernicious anemia, Cabot rings may simply be markers of aberrant "cytoplasmic currents" within the cell.[11]

Basophilic Stippling

Basophilic stippling consists of granulations of variable size and number that stain deep blue with Wright stain (Fig. 29–12B). Electron microscopic studies have shown that *punctate basophilia* represents aggregated ribosomes.[76] Clumps form during the course of drying and postvital staining of the cells, much as "reticulum" in reticulocytes precipitates from ribosomes during supravital staining. The clumped ribosomes may include degenerating mitochondria and siderosomes. In conditions such as lead intoxication and thalassemia, the altered reticulocyte ribosomes have a greater propensity to aggregate. As a result, basophilic granulation appears larger and is referred to as *coarse basophilic stippling*.

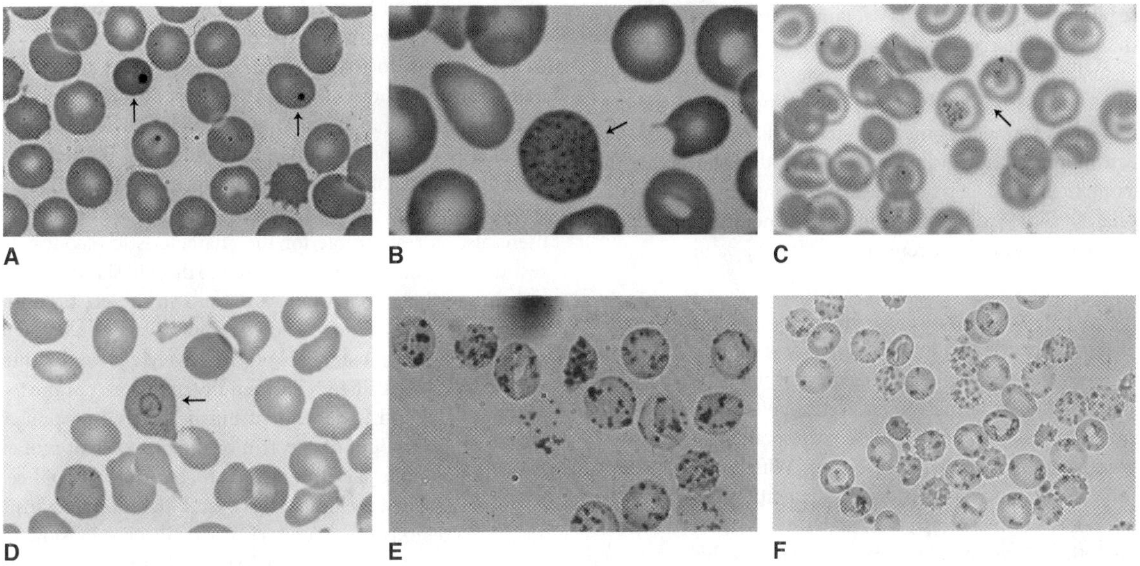

FIGURE 29–12. Red cell inclusions. Blood films. **A.** Red cells with Howell-Jolly bodies (*arrows*) postsplenectomy. The crisp circular border, dark blue color, and peripheral location are characteristic. **B.** Basophilic stippling. These basophilic inclusions may be fine or coarse. In this case, the cell contains coarse stippling seen in lead poisoning (*arrow*). **C.** Siderocyte. These cells contain purple granules when stained with Wright's stain (Pappenheimer bodies). Compared to basophilic stippling, siderotic granules are usually fewer in number and sometimes clustered. These Prussian blue stained cells confirm that the granules contain iron (blue reaction product). Arrow points to two siderocytes. **D.** Cabot ring. Rare red cell inclusion (*arrow*). See text for further description. **E.** Heinz bodies. These cells from a patient with glucose-6-phosphate dehydrogenase deficiency were incubated with a supravital dye, which stains the denatured globin precipitates. **F.** Red cells from a patient with hemoglobin H disease (α-thalassemia). The hemoglobin precipitates are stained with brilliant cresyl blue. *(Used with permission from* Lichtman's Atlas of Hematology, *www.accessmedicine.com.)*

Heinz Bodies

Heinz bodies are composed of denatured proteins, primarily hemoglobin, that form in red cells as a result of chemical insult (see Chap. 51); in hereditary defects of the hexose monophosphate shunt (see Chap. 46); in the thalassemias (see Chap. 47); and in unstable hemoglobin syndromes (see Chap. 48).[77] Heinz bodies are not seen on ordinary Wright- or Giemsa-stained blood films. Heinz bodies are readily visible in red cells stained supravitally with brilliant cresyl blue or crystal violet (Fig. 29–12E). They tend to adhere to the interior of the red cell membrane and protrude into the cytoplasm. On dried and stained blood films, they are characteristically located about one third of the distance in from the edge of the disc, where membrane curvature is at a minimum, presumably because of the membrane stiffening they cause. Membrane stiffening is also likely responsible for their removal as red cells traverse the interepithelial slits of the splenic sinus.[78]

Hemoglobin H Inclusions

Hemoglobin H is composed of β_4 tetramers, indicating that β chains are present in excess as a result of impaired α-chain production. Exposure to redox dyes such as brilliant cresyl blue, methylene blue, or new methylene blue, results in denaturation and precipitation of abnormal hemoglobin.[79] Brilliant cresyl blue causes the formation of a large number of small membrane-bound inclusions, giving the cell a characteristic "golf ball–like" appearance when viewed by light microscopy (Fig. 29–12F). Methylene blue and new methylene blue generate a smaller number of variably sized membrane-bound and floating inclusions.[80] These changes are seen most frequently in α-thalassemia but also can be found in patients with unstable hemoglobin[81] (see Chaps. 47 and 48) and in rare cases of erythroleukemia.[82,83]

Siderosomes and Pappenheimer Bodies

Normal or pathologic cells containing siderosomes ("iron bodies") usually are reticulocytes. The iron granulations are larger and more numerous in the pathologic state. Electron microscopy has shown that many of these bodies are mitochondria containing ferruginous micelles rather than the ferritin aggregates characterizing normal siderocytes.[84] Siderosomes usually are found in the cell periphery, whereas basophilic stippling tends to be distributed homogeneously throughout the cell. Pappenheimer bodies are siderosomes that stain with Wright stain (Fig. 29–12C). Electron microscopy of Pappenheimer bodies shows that the iron often is contained within a lysosome, as confirmed by the presence of acid phosphatase. Siderosomes may contain degenerating mitochondria, ribosomes, and other cellular remnants.

Macroreticulocytes

"Stress" reticulocytes are released into the circulation during an intense erythropoietin response to acute anemia or experimentally in response to large doses of exogenously administered erythropoietin.[85] These cells may be twice the normal volume, with a corresponding increase in hemoglobin content (see Chap. 31, Fig. 31–2). Whether the increase results from one less mitotic division during maturation or from some other process is not clear. In contrast, even under moderate erythropoietic stress, some reticulocytes in the marrow pool shift to the circulating pool. These "shift" reticulocytes contain a higher-than-normal RNA content and now can be quantified. Quantification is commonly performed by applying a fluorescent stain to the aggregated ribosomal material and then dividing reticulocytes into high-, medium-, and low-fluorescence categories using a fluorescence-sensitive flow cytometer. The "stress" reticulocytes of the older literature likely fall in the high- and medium-fluorescence categories.[85]

STRUCTURE AND SHAPE OF ERYTHROCYTES

The normal resting shape of the erythrocyte is a biconcave disc. Variations in the shape and dimensions of the red cell are useful in the differential diagnosis of anemias (see Chaps. 33 and 45). Normal human red cells have a diameter of 7.5 to 8.7 μm, and the diameter decreases slightly with cell age. The size decrease likely results from removal of membrane and hemoglobin throughout the erythrocyte life span by spleen-facilitated vesiculation.[86] The cells have an average volume of 90 fl[87] and a surface area of approximately 136 μm^2.[88] The membrane is present in sufficient excess to allow the cell to swell to a sphere of approximately 150 fl or to enter a capillary with a diameter of 2.8 μm. The normal erythrocyte stains reddish-brown in Wright-stained blood films and pink with Giemsa stain. The central third of the cell appears relatively pale compared with the periphery, reflecting its biconcave shape. Red cells on dried blood films are 0.6 μm thick, having lost about two-thirds of their normal thickness.[11] Many artifacts can be produced in the preparation of the blood film. They may result from contamination of the glass slide or coverslip with traces of fat, detergent, or other impurities.[89] Friction and surface tension involved in the preparation of the blood film produce fragmentation, "doughnut cells" or anulocytes, and crescent-shaped cells.[89] Observed under the phase-contrast or interference microscope, the red cell shows a characteristic internal scintillation known as *red cell flicker*.[90] The scintillation results from thermally excited undulations of the red cell membrane. Frequency analysis of the surface undulations has provided an estimate of the membrane curvature elastic constant and of changes in this constant resulting from alcohol, cholesterol loading, and exposure to cross-linking agents.[91]

■ RED CELL SHAPE AND SURVIVAL IN THE CIRCULATION

The red cell spends most of its circulatory life within the capillary channels of the microcirculation. During its 100- to 120-day life span, the red cell travels approximately 250 km and loses 15 to 20 percent of its hemoglobin.[86,92] The mechanism whereby the hemoglobin is lost without an inordinate quantity of cell membrane going with it remains one of the enigmas of hematology.[92] The long survival of the red cell is at least partially a result of the unique capacity of its membrane to "tank tread"—that is, to rotate around the red cell contents.[7] This arrangement transmits shocks from wall contact through the membrane to the viscous hemoglobin solution in the interior rather than concentrating the energy of contact in the membrane. The physical arrangement of membrane skeletal proteins in a uniform shell[93] of highly folded hexagonal/pentagonal units[94–96] permits this unusual behavior. The arrangement also is responsible for the characteristic biconcave shape of the resting cell.[97] Subtle differences in the discoid shape assumed by resting cells are probably related to variations in the elastic properties of the submembrane skeleton.[88] Red cells must also be able to withstand large shear forces and must be able to massively deform to enter the microcirculation. The resiliency and fluidity of the membrane to deformation requires ATP and is dependant on the skeletal proteins.[98–100] A deficiency in the amount of spectrin or the presence of mutant spectrin in the submembrane skeleton results in abnormal discoid cells in hereditary spherocytosis, elliptocytosis, and pyropoikilocytosis (see Chap. 45).[101] In regions of circulatory standstill or very slow flow, red cells travel in aggregates of two to a dozen cells, forming rouleaux.[102] Within large vessels, aggregation is disrupted by increased shear forces.

■ NOMENCLATURE OF COMMON RED CELL SHAPES

An international terminology using uniform Greek word stems has been introduced to describe cells based on their three-dimensional morphology (Table 29–2).[103]

TABLE 29–2. Nomenclature of Red Cell Shapes and Associated Disease States

Terminology (Greek Meaning)	Old Terms, Synonyms	Description	Micrograph	Associated Disease States
Discocyte (disc)	Biconcave disc	Biconcave disc form of RBC	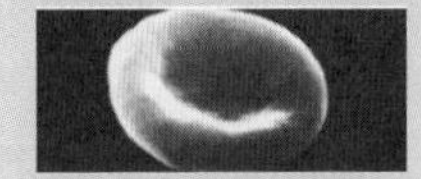	
Echinocyte (I–III) (sea urchin)	"Burr cell," crenated cell, "berry cell"	Spiculated RBC with short, equally spaced projections over entire surface; progressing from the "crenated disc" (echinocyte I) to the crenated sphere (echinocyte IV—not shown) with nearly complete loss of spicules	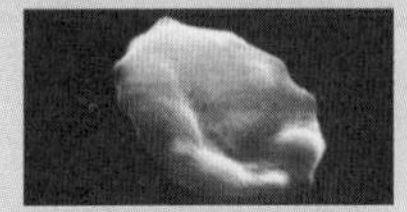 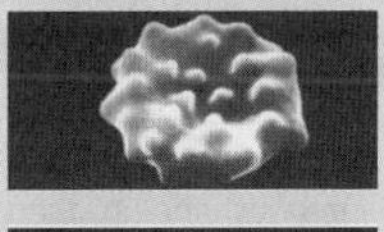 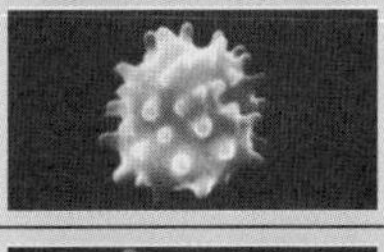	Uremia, liver disease Low-potassium red cells Immediately posttransfusion with aged or metabolically depleted blood Carcinoma of stomach and bleeding peptic ulcers
Acanthocyte (spike)	"Spur cell," acanthoid cell, acanthrocyte	Irregularly spiculated RBC with projections of varying length and position	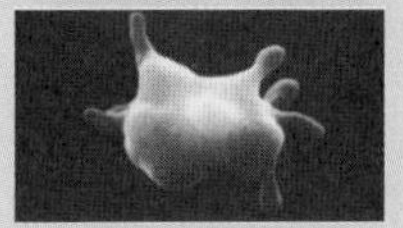	Abetalipoproteinemia Alcoholic liver disease Postsplenectomy state Malabsorptive states
Stomatocyte (I–III) (mouth)	Mouth cell, cup form, mushroom cap, uniconcave disc, microspherocyte	Bowled-shaped RBC with single concavity; progressing from shallow bowl (I) to near sphere with small dimple (seen as mouth-shaped form in peripheral film)	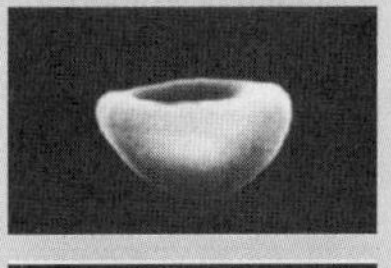 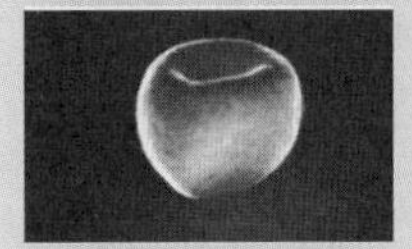	Hereditary spherocytosis Hereditary stomatocytosis Alcoholism, cirrhosis, obstructive liver disease Erythrocyte sodium-pump defect
Spherostomatocyte (sphere)	Spherocyte, prelytic sphere, microspherocyte	Spherical RBC with dense hemoglobin content; scanning electron microscopy shows a persistent minimal dimple	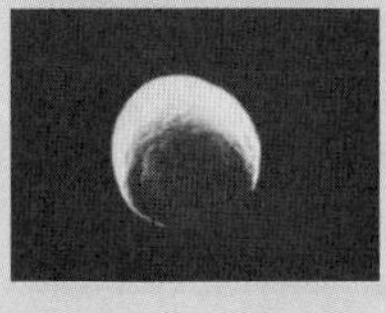	Hereditary spherocytosis (cells actually spherostomatocytes) Immune hemolytic anemia Posttransfusion Heinz body hemolytic anemia Water-dilution hemolysis Fragmentation hemolysis
Schizocyte (cut)	Schistocyte, helmet cell, fragmented cell	Split RBC, often showing half-disc shape with two or three pointed extremities; may be small, irregular fragment	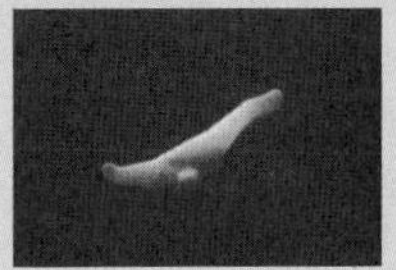	Microangiopathic hemolytic anemia (TTP, DIC, vasculitis, glomerulonephritis, renal graft rejection) Carcinomatosis Heart-valve hemolysis (prosthetic or pathologic valves) Severe burns March hemoglobinuria
Elliptocyte (oval)	Ovalocyte	Oval to elongated ellipsoid RBC (with polarization of hemoglobin)	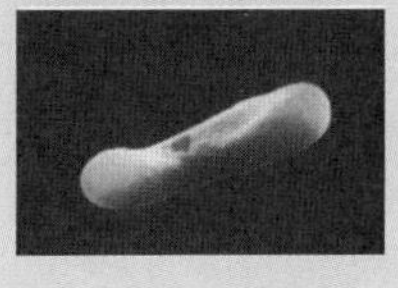	Hereditary elliptocytosis Thalassemia Iron deficiency Myelophthisic anemias Megaloblastic anemias

(*continued*)

TABLE 29–2. Nomenclature of Red Cell Shapes and Associated Disease States (Continued)

Terminology (Greek Meaning)	Old Terms, Synonyms	Description	Micrograph	Associated Disease States
Drepanocyte (sickle)	Sickle cell	RBC containing polymerized hemoglobin S; showing varying shapes from bipolar, spiculated forms to holly-leaf and irregularly spiculated forms	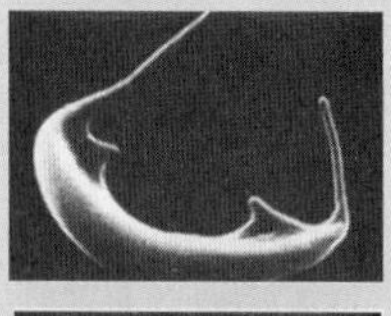 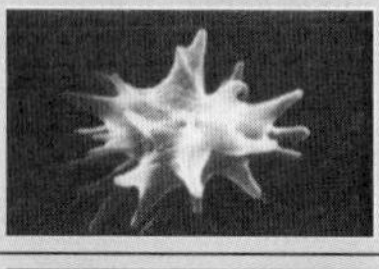	Sickle cell disorders (SS, S trait, SC, SD, S thalassemia, etc.) Hemoglobin C-Harlem Hemoglobin Memphis/S
Codocyte (bell)	Target cell	Bell-shaped RBC that assumes a target shape on dried films of blood	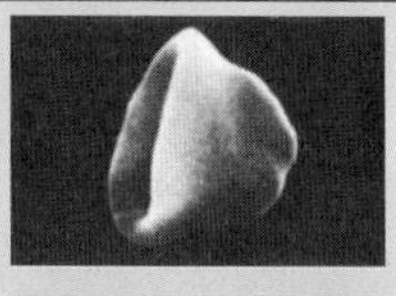 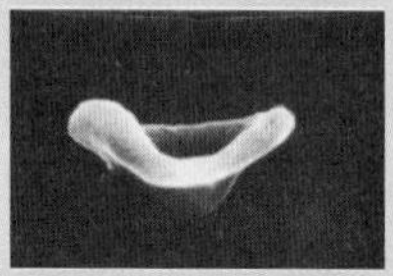	Obstructive liver disease Hemoglobinopathies (S, C) Thalassemia Iron deficiency Postsplenectomy state Lecithin cholesterol acetyltransferase deficiency
Dacryocyte (tear)	Teardrop cell	RBC with a single elongated or pointed extremity	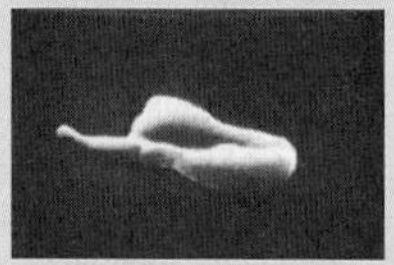	Primary myelofibrosis Myelophthisic anemias Thalassemia
Leptocyte (thin)	Thin cell, wafer cell	Thin, flat RBC with hemoglobin at periphery	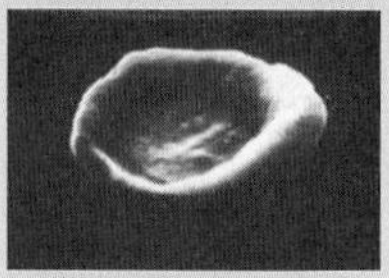	Thalassemia Obstructive liver disease (±iron deficiency)
Keratocyte (horn)	Horn cell	RBC with spicules resulting from ruptured vacuole; cell appears half-moon shaped or spindle shaped	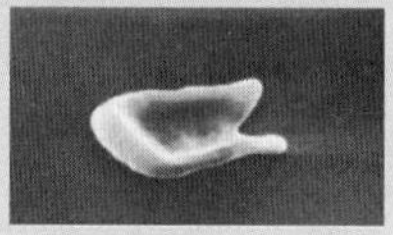	DIC or vascular prosthesis

DIC, disseminated intravascular coagulation; RBC, red blood cell; TTP, thrombotic thrombocytopenic purpura.

The *discocyte* is the form assumed by a red cell when it is not subjected to external deforming stress. It is a smooth, biconcave disc (Fig. 29–13A). A discocyte can be reversibly and rapidly transformed by a variety of environmental agents into two other forms: the *stomatocyte*, a uniconcave cup-shaped cell (Fig. 29–13B), and the *echinocyte*, covered by 10 to 30 short, hemispherical projections evenly spaced over the cell surface (Fig. 29–13C). In general, these changes can be superimposed on other red cell shapes, which suggests they represent membrane energy equilibrium states.[97]

The *acanthocyte* is irregularly shaped, with 2 to 10 hemispherically tipped spicules of variable length and diameter (Fig. 29–13D). The bases of the spicules on the acanthocyte are of varying girth, unlike the spicules on echinocytes, which have remarkably uniform dimensions.

Notwithstanding the time-honored use of the word, the *spherocyte* is not a truly spherical cell (Fig. 29–13E). Its thickness is greatly increased so that the central concavity is significantly reduced and may be overlooked. On scanning electron microscopic examination, the spherocyte frequently bears a small dimple or irregular area suggesting derivation from a stomatocyte.

The *schistocyte* refers to a red cell fragment that characteristically assumes a half-disc shape with two or three pointed extremities (Fig. 29–13F). Because it is produced by the sealing of two opposing membrane surfaces followed by physical cleavage or fragmentation of a red cell, the schistocyte is smaller than the normal discocyte and may display one or more regions of stiffened and distorted membrane where the sealing and cleavage occurred.

The *drepanocyte* (*sickle cell*) describes the sickle cell and a variety of shapes induced by polymerization of sickle hemoglobin. Drepanocytes vary in shape, ranging from bipolar, spiculated forms to cells with long, irregular spicules and holly-leaf configurations (Fig. 29–13G).

The *elliptocyte* (ovalocyte) basically is an oval biconcave disc. It shows varying degrees of elliptical aberration, ranging from a slightly oval to an almost cylindrical, bipolar, elongated shape (Fig. 29–13H).

A relative excess of membrane in the *codocyte* (*target cell*) results in membrane recurvature in the center of the dimple. Hemoglobin accumulates where the upper and lower cell membranes separate when the cell is on a blood film, forming the central density, or "bull's-eye," of the target (Fig. 29–13I).

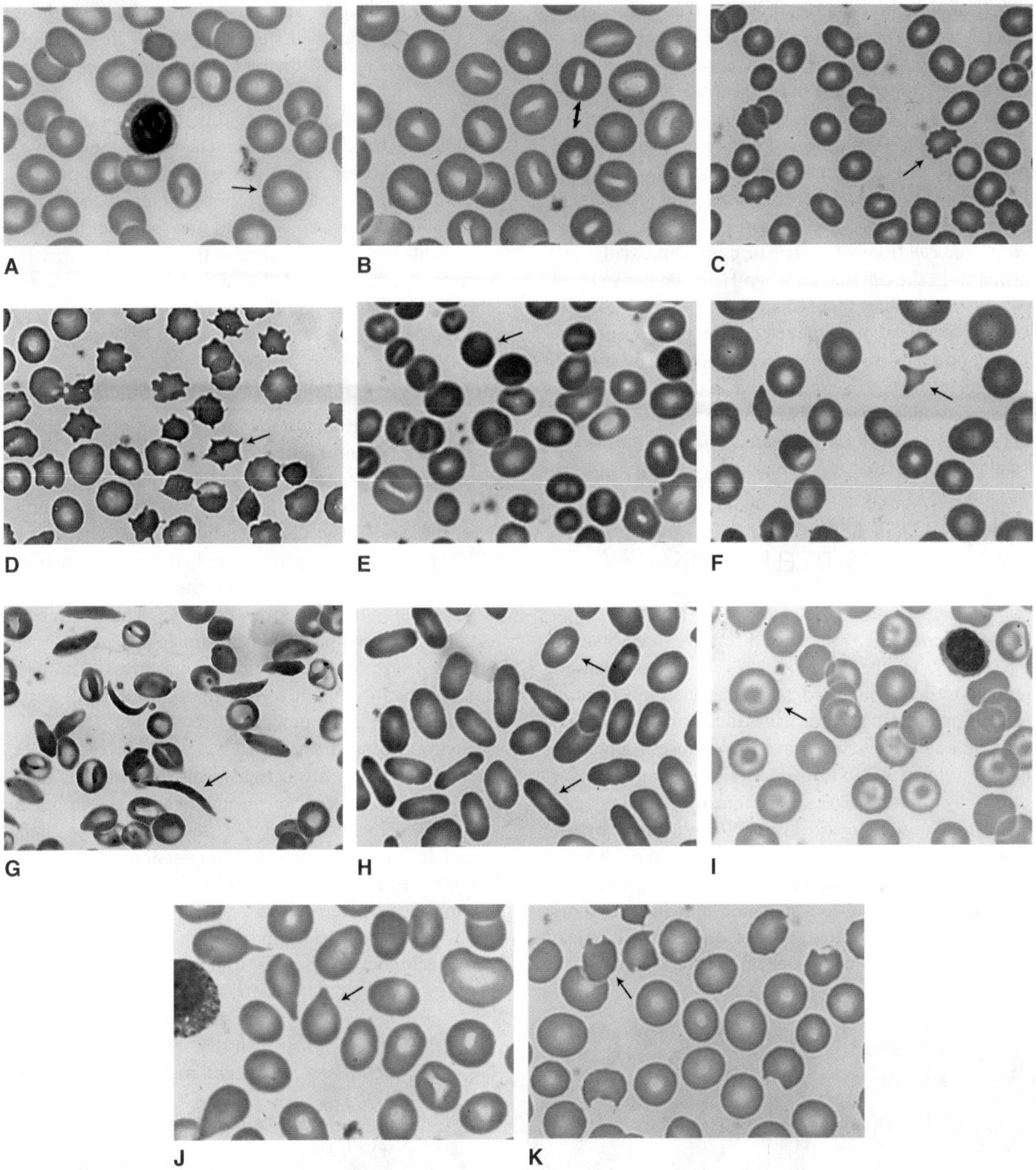

FIGURE 29–13. A. Normal blood. Arrow points to a normochromic-normocytic discocyte. **B.** Stomatocytes. The double arrow points to the two morphologic types of stomatocyte: upper cell with a slit-shaped pale area and lower cell with a small central circular pale area. **C.** Echinocytes. The field has several such cells. The arrow points to one example with evenly distributed, blunt, short, circumferentially-positioned, projections. **D.** Acanthocytes. The arrow points to one example with a few spike-shaped projections, unevenly distributed and of varying lengths. **E.** Spherocytes. Small, circular, densely-staining (hyperchromic) cells which, when fully developed, show no central pallor. **F.** Schizocytes (schistocytes, helmet cells, fragmented red cells). These microcytic cell fragments may assume varied shapes. The arrow points to a triangular shape, but two others of different shape are also present in the field. Despite being damaged and very small, they frequently maintain a biconcave appearance as witnessed by their central pallor. **G.** Drepanocytes (sickle cells). Numerous sickle cells are shown. Two are in the classic shape of the blade on the agricultural sickle (arrow). Many red cells that have undergone the transformation to a "sickle" cell take the slightly less extreme form of elliptical cells with a very narrow diameter with condensed hemoglobin in the center (para-crystallization). About eight such cells are in the field. **H.** Elliptocytes and ovalocytes. The lower arrow points to an elliptocyte (cigar-shaped). The upper arrow points to an ovalocyte (football-shaped). Because both forms may be seen together in a case of inherited disease (same gene mutation resulting in both shapes), as shown here, it has been proposed that all such shapes be called elliptocytes with a Roman numeral to designate the severity of the shape change toward the elliptical, that is, elliptocytes I, II, III. **I.** Codocytes (target cells). The arrow points to one characteristic example among several in the field. The hemoglobin concentration corralled by membrane recurvature in the center of the cell gives it the appearance of an archery target. **J.** Dacryocytes (tear drop cells). Three dacryocytes are in this field. One example is indicated by the arrow. **K.** Keratocyte (horn cell). Several examples are in the field. The arrow points to a typical such cell with two sharp projections. *(Used with permission from* Lichtman's Atlas of Hematology, *www.accessmedicine.com.)*

The *dacryocyte* (tear-drop erythrocyte) refers to a cell characterized by a single elongated or pointed extremity (Fig. 29–13J). This cell shape has been referred to as a *teardrop, racket*, or *tail poikilocyte*.

The *leptocyte* is a wafer-thin cell that has a generally large diameter, displays a thin rim of hemoglobin at the periphery, and has a large area of central pallor. Such a cell reflects an increased surface-to-volume ratio.

The *keratocyte* is a red cell with a relatively normal cell volume that was deformed by removal of a region of apposed and sealed membranes so that the cell presents with two or more points (Fig. 29–13K).

The *"bite" cell* is a red cell from which one or more semicircular portions were removed from the cell margin when Heinz bodies were pitted out by the splenic macrophages (see Chap. 46).[104]

If necessary, any shape variation of the red cell can be described precisely using compound terms such as *spherostomatocyte*. Addition of modifiers such as *micro-* or *macro-* to denote a changed volume may add to descriptive precision, as in *microspherocyte* or *macroleptocyte*.

Variability in the size of red cells is designated *anisocytosis*. Any type of shape abnormality is designated as *poikilocytosis* (see Chap. 2).

NORMAL PHYSIOLOGY AND PATHOPHYSIOLOGY OF RED CELL SHAPES

Biconcave Discs

A healthy red blood cell maintains its normal biconcave shape by minimizing bending energy in the membrane.[105] As the suspending medium becomes more hypotonic, red cells change from biconcave discs to spheres. This mathematically tractable transformation gave rise to the original hypothesis that the biconcave shape arose as a bending energy minimum. Developments in mathematical modeling of the various shapes assumed by a red cell have shown that, by including bending rigidity and stretch and shear elasticity contributed by the membrane skeleton,[106,107] the minimization-of-energy approach can reproduce, with surprising fidelity, all red cell shapes along the "main sequence" of shape transformation from stomatocyte to biconcave disc to echinocytes I, II, and III.[108,109] Additional evidence that the major mechanical forces are now reasonably well understood comes from "non-main sequence" shapes such as *knizocytes* (three-dimpled cell) and triangular-mouthed stomatocytes, which also can be mathematically modeled by considering bending rigidity, stretch, and shear elasticity (see Fig. 29–14).[109]

The source of membrane rigidity remains elusive, however. Does the resistance to bending arise from changes in the relative surface area of the inner and outer leaflets of the bilaminar plasma membranes, as the original "bilayer couple" hypothesis contemplates,[110] perhaps by incorporation of a cytoplasmic protein into the inner bilayer?[111] Or does the remarkable bending resistance of the membrane arise from interaction between the bilayer and the underlying spectrin cytoskeleton,[112–115] with the latter undergoing expansion or contraction as a result of a morphologic change of the anion exchanger band 3?

Stomatocyte-Echinocyte-Discocyte Equilibrium

At physiologic pH and in the presence of normal plasma protein levels (particularly albumin), healthy red cells are always smooth, biconcave discs (Fig. 29–15). As the pH is raised, the albumin concentration lowered, or in the presence of lysolecithin or anionic phenothiazine derivatives, the rim of the disc becomes bumpy. The bumps are low and widely spaced, and they involve only the membrane of the red cell rim. This form is an echinocyte I. Further environmental stress results in transformation to echinocytes II and III. These cells bear 10 to 30 projections of surprisingly uniform dimensions, equally spaced over the entire cell surface. If the environmental stress is sufficiently intense or is of sufficient duration so that the echinocyte III becomes a spheroechinocyte I or II, the process is irreversible.

Environmental stress caused by low pH, excess albumin, or cationic phenothiazine derivatives transforms the discocyte into an intermediate form having deeper biconcavities and then into a cup-shaped cell with only a single concavity—a stomatocyte. The changes are readily reversible, but if the single deep depression on the stomatocyte surface is obliterated by membrane loss, the transformation becomes irreversible and a spherostomatocyte results.

A wide array of agents, in addition to pH and albumin, cause stomatocytic-echinocytic changes in red cell shape. The agents include amphiphilic drugs and detergents, competitive transport inhibitors/affinity labels of band 3, and antibodies directed toward integral membrane constituents.[115]

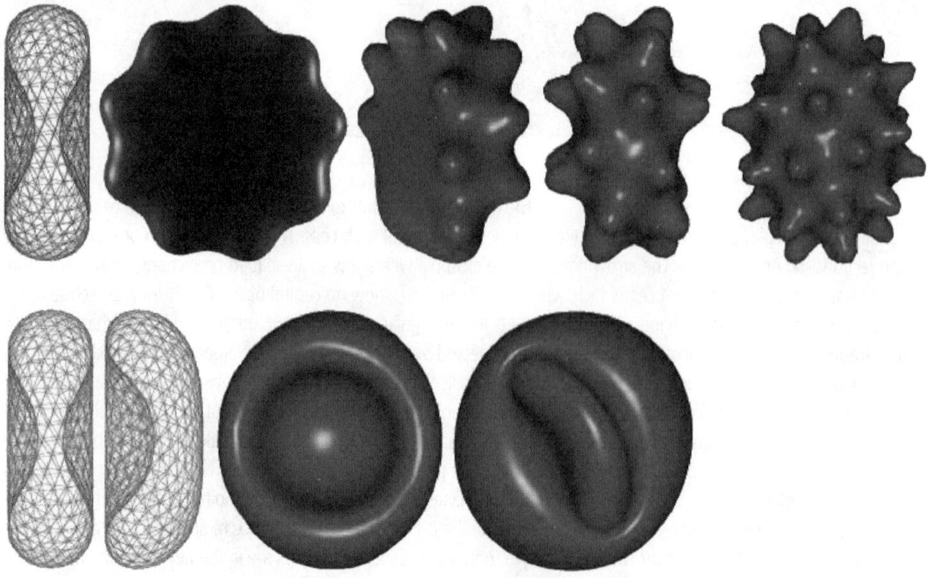

FIGURE 29–14. Discocyte-echinocyte and discocyte-stomatocyte transformation generated mathematically.[108,109] The match between real shapes depicted in Fig. 29–15 and those generated mathematically is exceptionally good, even to the first appearance of the crenation spicules over the rim rather than in the dimple of the biconcave disc. *(Adapted from Lim HWG, Wortis M, Mukhopadhyay R,[109] with permission.)*

Aged Cells

The reticulocyte loses membrane as it matures into a discocyte. Membrane loss by vesiculation continues throughout the erythrocyte life span. The vesiculation process results in loss of up to 20 percent of the cell's hemoglobin with preferential loss of hemoglobin A_{1c} and hemoglobin A_{1e2}.[86] As erythrocytes age, the hemoglobin accumulates in endovesicles, which are removed by the spleen. These vesicles remain in the erythrocyte in asplenia. The notion that erythrocyte aging is synonymous with membrane loss, increasing mean corpuscular hemoglobin concentration (MCHC), and decreasing deformability largely results from studies on density-separated cells and the equating of dense cells with aged cells. Indeed, dense cells are dense because their MCHC is elevated, and an elevated MCHC exerts a profoundly

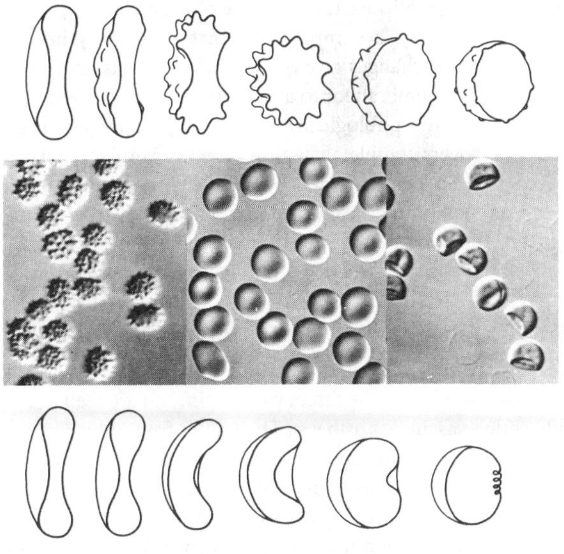

FIGURE 29–15. Discocyte-echinocyte and discocyte-stomatocyte transformation. *Upper panel* schematically depicts the echinocytic transformation as induced by a rise in pH, a lack of albumin in the suspension, or exposure to an anionic phenothiazine derivative. Note that the low protuberances heralding echinocytogenic transformation appear preferentially over the rim of the biconcave disc. *Lower panel* schematically depicts stomatocyte formation as induced by a cationic phenothiazine derivative, a lowering of pH, or an excess of albumin in the suspending medium. Note that the intermediate form between the disc and the early cup is not a bent disc but rather a bowtie form with very steep sides to the dimples.[169] *Center panel* shows the microscopic appearance in wet preparations of stomatocytes (*right*), discocytes (*middle*), and echinocytes (*left*).

depressant effect on red cell deformability. Thus, dense cells are always relatively nondeformable, but whether they are aged is not settled. One thing is clear: unlike the reticulocyte, the aged red cell is not easily distinguished morphologically. Chap. 32 discusses red cell aging and senescence.

Codocytes

Codocytes may be seen in obstructive liver disease, hemoglobinopathies (S and C), thalassemia, iron deficiency, postsplenectomy, and lecithin cholesterol acetyltransferase deficiency.

In the circulation, the codocyte is a bell-shaped cell that assumes a target configuration when it is dried on a slide in the preparation of a blood film.[89] On a flat surface, the codocyte tends to evert its concavity into a central projection into which hemoglobin redistributes. This results in a central density (target) on the blood film. The codocyte is characterized by relative membrane excess because of either increased red cell surface area or decreased intracellular hemoglobin. In patients with obstructive liver disease, lecithin cholesterol acetyltransferase activity is depressed. This increases the cholesterol-to-phospholipid ratio[116] and produces an absolute increase in the surface area of the red cell membrane. In contrast, membrane excess is only relative in patients with iron-deficiency anemia and thalassemia because of the reduced quantity of intracellular hemoglobin.

Acanthocytes

Acanthocytes may be seen in abetalipoproteinemia, alcoholic liver disease, postsplenectomy state, and malabsorptive states.

Acanthocytes are generated from normal red blood cells under conditions that alter their membrane lipid content, possibly by loss of glycerophospholipids resulting in a relative increase of sphingomyelin.[117] Once produced, the shape is irreversible except in the rare McLeod syndrome (see Chaps. 45 and 137), where incubation of the acanthocytic cells with phosphatidylserine or chlorpromazine restores the discoid shape.[118] A markedly increased membrane cholesterol-to-lecithin ratio is common in acanthocytes from patients with hepatocellular disease and abetalipoproteinemia (see Chap. 45).

Discocyte–Drepanocyte Transformation

The sickle cell, or drepanocyte, displays a characteristic variation of form on stained blood films (see Chap. 48). The fusiform cell in the crescent shape with two pointed extremities is encountered most commonly. Examination by phase-contrast microscopy of deoxygenated sickle cell blood reveals varied cell forms characterized by pointed extremities in holly leaf and poikilocytic configurations, many with multiple spicules several micrometers long. The spicules are fragile and easily avulsed from the cell. If sickle cell formation is observed by phase-contrast microscopy, the earliest change with deoxygenation is loss of flicker,[119] followed by slight deformation at the discocyte border with displacement of the hemoglobin to one region of the cell. The cell then elongates and becomes rigid as a result of polymerization of hemoglobin S in rods or filaments.[120] The rods are 15 to 18 nm (150–180 Å) in diameter and composed of monomolecular filaments 6 to 7 nm (60–70 Å) in diameter, intertwined into a six-stranded helix.[121] In partially sickled cells, the polymers display random orientation. As polymerization increases, the polymeric filaments undergo lateral reorientation into rods that are generally aligned with the long axis of the drepanocyte. Upon reoxygenation, the drepanocyte resumes the discocyte form and, in so doing, loses membrane by microspherulation and fragmentation during retraction of long spicules.[122] Evidence suggests that the more typical sickle-shaped cells form under slow deoxygenation. Thus, the cell membrane is maximally stressed, and more of the membrane is lost during the unsickling cycle after slow deoxygenation.[123] The unsickling process also leads to formation of micro Heinz bodies that adhere to the internal surface of the red cell membrane and contribute to increased membrane rigidity and cation leak.[77] With each sickle–unsickle cycle, membrane damage accumulates, as signaled by increasing amounts of an altered membrane protein β-actin. The alteration results from formation of a disulfide bond between ^{284}Cys and ^{373}Cys residues. This altered protein has been designated ISC β-actin to link it to the reduced membrane deformability of irreversibly sickled cells (ISCs).[124] These cells are incapable of reversion to the biconcave disc shape, even when fully oxygenated.[125] They have an increased hemoglobin concentration, increased cation permeability, decreased potassium, and increased sodium. In addition to ISCs, the blood of patients with sickle cell anemia contains small numbers of another rigid, membrane-damaged cell—the *sequestrocyte.* Sequestrocytes are characterized by linear zones of membrane fusion that entrap lakes of hemoglobin. They appear massively vacuolated under the light microscope. Sequestrocytes presumably arise from a combination of physical damage from sickle–unsickle cycles and oxidative membrane damage that causes transcellular cross-bonding of the cell membrane.[126]

Schistocytes

Schistocytes are seen in microangiopathic hemolytic anemias (thrombotic thrombocytopenic purpura [TTP], disseminated intravascular coagulation [DIC], vasculitis, glomerulonephritis, renal graft rejection), carcinomatosis, heart valve hemolysis (prosthetic or pathologic valves), severe burns, and March hemoglobinuria.

Fibrin strands in damaged blood vessels can be arrayed so that they sieve the passing red cells. If a passing red cell folds over or otherwise attaches to the strand, the bloodstream pulls on the arrested cell, stretches it, and eventually fragments it.[127,128] If the two inner surfaces of the red cell membrane become approximated prior to rupture, the torn membrane seals[129] and the schistocyte contains hemoglobin. The more rigid schistocytes and those with a low relative surface area are rapidly removed by the spleen; the remainder may circulate for many days.

Spherocytes and Stomatocytes

Spherocytes are seen in hereditary spherocytosis, immune hemolytic anemia, posttransfusion, Heinz body hemolytic anemia, water-dilution hemolysis, and fragmentation hemolysis. Stomatocytes are seen in hereditary stomatocytosis as well as in hereditary spherocytosis, alcoholism, cirrhosis, obstructive liver disease, and erythrocyte sodium pump defects.

Red cells sensitized with antibodies, complement, or immune complexes lose cholesterol and surface area. As a result, they are less deformable and more osmotically fragile.[130] Heinz body formation leads to membrane depletion by fragmentation, with spherocyte formation.[131] A spherogenic mechanism common to Heinz body hemolytic anemias and immune hemolysis is partial phagocytosis of portions of the cell containing aggregates of denatured hemoglobin[131] and portions of the sensitized membrane,[132] respectively.

Stomatocytosis is a rare form of spherocytosis.[133] The anomaly is caused by abnormal permeability of the red cell membrane to the univalent cations Na^+ and K^+. The group of disorders is heterogenous and includes overhydrated and dehydrated hereditary stomatocytosis, cryohydrocytosis, and familial pseudohyperkalemia.[134] Chap. 45 discusses these disorders in more detail.

A spectrum of abnormal cells varying from normal discocytes to stomatocytes, spherostomatocytes, and dense microspherocytes is seen in hereditary spherocytosis.[135]

Heat-Induced Shape Changes

Heating red cells to temperatures greater than 49°C depolymerizes spectrin. If the heating episode is brief and the inner surfaces of the biconcavities are in contact, the surfaces fuse upon cooling.[136] More vigorous heating causes marked spherulation of the entire cell. Microspherocytes bud from the cell surface, and the entire cell is transformed into small spherical fragments (*pyropoikilocytes*). The fragments can be recovered from the blood after severe burns (see Chap. 51, Fig. 51–1A).

Elliptocytes

Elliptocytes are seen in hereditary elliptocytosis as well as in thalassemia, iron deficiency, myelophthisic anemia, and megaloblastic anemia.

In blood films of normal subjects, elliptical or oval cells usually constitute less than 1 percent of the erythrocytes. In various pathologic situations, with or without anemia (thalassemia trait, folate and iron deficiency), the number of elliptocytes can increase to 10 percent. Exceptionally, as in dyserythropoiesis, the proportion can be as high as 50 percent. In hereditary elliptocytosis (see Chap. 45), the number of elliptical erythrocytes varies greatly, from 0 to 98 percent.[137] Such fluctuations have forced hematologists to substitute a biochemical and functional (rheologic) definition of hereditary elliptocytosis for the original morphologic definition.[137] Qualitative and quantitative anomalies of spectrin, band 3,[101,138–140] and protein 4.1,[141,142] the major proteins of the membrane skeleton, are associated with hereditary elliptocytosis. As a consequence, rheologic membrane properties are impaired.[139,143] Severe hemolytic anemia is seen only in the homozygous form of the disease (hereditary pyropoikilocytosis) where *pyropoikilocytes* typically are present.

Dacryocytes

Dacryocytes are seen in primary myelofibrosis, myelophthisic anemia, and thalassemia.

Dacryocytes typically are found in the bloodstream of patients with marrow fibrosis, often accompanied by extramedullary hemopoiesis. How these marrow changes give rise to dacryocytes is unknown. Aspiration of red cell membrane into a micropipette of appropriate dimensions produces a morphologically similar shape change; however, the cell usually recovers completely within minutes. Similar deformation in a reticulocyte can be permanent because the deformation occurred while the submembrane skeleton was being assembled. A delay during egress from the marrow or from extramedullary sites, such as in primary myelofibrosis (see Chap. 91), provides such an opportunity.

Keratocytes ("Horn Cells," "Burr Cells," or "Helmet Cells")

Keratocytes are erythrocytes from which one or more roughly circular bites were removed from the discocyte margin, and are seen in DIC or in patients with a vascular prosthesis. They differ from schistocytes in that their hemoglobin content is normal or only slightly lower than normal. They are not formed by sectioning of a red cell. Rather, they appear to arise when all the hemoglobin is squeezed out of a portion near the edge of a discocytic red cell and the two opposite membrane surfaces fuse.[144] The process forms a pseudovacuole that soon ruptures, probably because of stiffening of the membrane skeleton in the fused portion. The result is a notch with bordering spicules or horns. Experimentally, membrane fusion with pseudovacuole formation can be produced by temperatures greater than 49°C[136] and by mechanical stress.[129] *In vitro* exposure to diamide and *N*-ethylmaleimide[145] also produces this characteristic form.

"Bite" Cells

"Bite" cells are seen in Heinz body hemolytic anemias, and are formed when the Heinz bodies are pitted from the cells by splenic macrophages.[104] Emphasis on the missing portion rather than on the horns that remain led to the term *bite cell*.[146] *In vivo* exposure to sulfonamide drugs such as dapsone and sulfasalazine and the urinary tract antiseptic phenazopyridine results in "bite" cells in susceptible individuals.[147] Bite cells are a form of keratocyte. Bite cells should be distinguished from other keratocytes because bite cell formation involves removal of denatured hemoglobin (and membrane), whereas keratocytes in general appear to be formed by membrane apposition and subsequent removal of the apposed membranes.

Crystals of Hemoglobin C Disease

In splenectomized patients with homozygous hemoglobin C disease, up to 10 percent of the circulating cells may contain tetrahedral crystals (see Chap. 48, Fig. 48–7).[148] Crystal-containing cells are rare or absent in blood films from nonsplenectomized patients.[149] The efficiency in splenic removal may be a result of spherocyte formation from release of osmotically active particles as hemoglobin C crystals "melt" while undergoing deoxygenation in the spleen. "Melting" of hemoglobin C crystals upon deoxygenation occurs readily *in vitro*, behavior opposite to that of sickle hemoglobin crystals.[150] *In vitro* dehydration of hemoglobin C-containing cells for a 24-hour period between slide and coverslip[151] or hypertonic dehydration of red cells in 3 percent NaCl buffer for 4 to 12 hours readily produces crystals. In homozygous hemoglobin C disease, up to 75 percent of cells may show crystals. Lower percentages of crystals occur in hemoglobin SC and other hemoglobin C variants. Molecular subunits in a tetragonal or hexagonal arrangement may be identified within hemoglobin C crystals.[152] Hemoglobin Setif, like hemoglobin C, may precipitate as intracellular crystals when the tonicity of the suspending medium is raised.[153] The process occurs in oxygenated solutions and at osmolarities achieved in the renal medulla. No clinical symptoms among heterozygous carriers of the Setif gene have been reported.

OSMOTIC BEHAVIOR

The red cell behaves as an osmometer.[154] Red cells placed into a hypertonic solution shrink, and the inner surfaces of the biconcavities touch over a progressively larger central region. When red cells in hypotonic solutions reach their critical hemolytic volume, holes or pores greater than 10 nm (100 Å) in diameter appear[155] and the hemoglobin exits. The probability of pore formation is affected by elastic membrane properties and is delayed in thalassemic cells.[156] Following hemolysis (exit of the hemoglobin), the holes or tears close, and the cell resumes its original biconcave shape.

DEFORMABILITY

An important determinant of red cell survival in the circulation is the cell's deformability. The deformability of the intact cell consists of contributions from the intrinsic deformability of the membrane itself, the internal viscosity (for practical purposes, the MCHC), and the surface-to-volume ratio of the cell. The deformability of the intact cell can be measured by the time needed for a red cell suspension to traverse a filter of known pore size.[157] Alternatively, the cells can be suspended in a viscous medium and exposed to a shear force. The change in shape can be observed microscopically, as in the rheoscope,[158] or by laser diffraction, as in the ektacytometer.[159] Additional information can be obtained from ektacytometric analysis by varying the osmolarity of the suspending medium, which changes the surface-to-volume ratio and the internal viscosity of the cells during the analytical procedure.[160] Alternatively, the red cell can be folded over a spiderweb strand in the presence of rapidly flowing buffer. The deformability of the membrane can be estimated from the relationship between the flow rate of the buffer and the deformation of the red cell.[161]

A 20 percent increase in MCHC results in an approximately 600 percent increase in internal viscosity.[162] An increase of this magnitude still leaves the red cell with sufficient deformability to survive in the circulation, although such nondeformable cells probably experience a prolonged transit time through the spleen. This is not the case for erythrocytes from patients with xerocytosis (desiccytosis). In such patients, the erythrocytes are always perilously close to the upper limits of internal viscosity, consistent with traversing the vasculature.[163]

In the circulation, the primary cause of decreased red cell deformability is likely insufficient membrane (spherocytosis) rather than stiffening of the membrane. The interendothelial slits of the splenic sinus stress cells with a normal surface-to-volume ratio, and splenic phagocytes remove cells with a lower-than-normal ratio. It is self-evident that a perfectly spherical red cell will be rigid no matter how low the MCHC or how flexible the isolated membrane.

ERYTHROCYTOLYSIS

Eryptosis—Red Cell Suicide

Physiologic red cell death has been dubbed *eryptosis*. It is likely similar to the mechanism responsible for nuclear extrusion in erythroid development. The process begins when prostaglandin E_2 forms in the erythrocyte. The prostaglandin E_2 activates a calcium permeable ion channel. Equilibration of calcium concentration across the erythrocyte membrane activates calcium sensitive potassium channels causing hyperpolarization. Calcium equilibration also stimulates a scramblase enzyme that allows phosphatidylserine, usually confined to the inner membrane leaflet, to transfer to the outer leaflet. The presence of increased quantities of phosphatidylserine on the outer leaflet signals macrophages to engulf and destroy the erythrocyte. The activity of scramblase is further enhanced by ceramide. Because ceramide is formed by sphingomyelinase, the process becomes linked to several stressors including osmotic shock and platelet-activating factor, which affect sphingomyelinase activity.[164,165]

REFERENCES

1. Southcott MJG, Tanner MJA, Anstee DJ: The expression of human blood group antigens during erythropoiesis in a cell culture system. *Blood* 93:4425, 1999.
2. McGrath K, Palis J: Ontogeny of erythropoiesis in the mammalian embryo. *Curr Top Dev Biol* 82:1, 2008.
3. McGrath KE, Palis J: Hematopoiesis in the yolk sac: More than meets the eye. *Exp Hematol* 33:1021, 2005.
4. Palis J: Ontogeny of erythropoiesis. *Curr Opin Hematol* 15:155, 2008.
5. Tavian M, Peault B: Embryonic development of the human hematopoietic system. *Int J Dev Biol* 49:243, 2005.
6. Zambidis ET, Peault B, Park TS, et al: Hematopoietic differentiation of human embryonic stem cells progresses through sequential hematoendothelial, primitive, and definitive stages resembling human yolk sac development. *Blood* 106:860, 2005.
7. Schmid-Schonbein H, Wells R: Fluid drop-like transition of erythrocytes under shear. *Science* 165:288, 1969.
8. Pereda J, Niimi G: Embryonic erythropoiesis in human yolk sac: Two different compartments for two different processes. *Microsc Res Tech* 71:856, 2008.
9. Sadahira Y, Mori M: Role of the macrophage in erythropoiesis. *Pathol Int* 49:841, 1999.
10. Breton-Gorius J, Vuillet-Gaugler MH, Coulombel L, et al: Association between leukemic erythroid progenitors and bone-marrow macrophages. *Blood Cells* 17:127, 1991.
11. Bessis M: *Living Blood Cells and Their Ultrastructure.* Springer-Verlag, Berlin, 1973.
12. Chasis JA, Mohandas N: Erythroblastic islands: Niches for erythropoiesis. *Blood* 112, 2008.
13. Spring FA, Parsons SF: Erythroid cell adhesion molecules. *Transfus Med Rev* 14:351, 2000.
14. Lee G, Lo A, Short SA, et al: Targeted gene deletion demonstrates that the cell adhesion molecule ICAM-4 is critical for erythroblastic island formation. *Blood* 108:2064, 2006.
15. Yokoyama T, Etoh T, Kitagawa H, et al: Migration of erythroblastic islands toward the sinusoid as erythroid maturation proceeds in rat bone marrow. *J Vet Med Sci* 65:449, 2003.
16. Hristoskova S, Holzgreve W, Hahn S, Rusterholz C: Human mature erythroblasts are resistant to apoptosis. *Exp Cell Res* 313:1024, 2007.
17. Yoshida H, Kawane K, Koike M et al: Phosphatidylserine-dependent engulfment by macrophages of nuclei from erythroid precursor cells. *Nature* 437:754, 2005.
18. Manwani D, Bieker JJ: The erythroblastic island. *Curr Top Dev Biol* 82:23, 2008.
19. Rhodes MM, Kopsombut P, Bondurant MC, et al: Adherence to macrophages in erythroblastic islands enhances erythroblast proliferation and increases erythrocyte production by a different mechanism than erythropoietin. *Blood* 111:1700, 2008.
20. Wright SD, Meyer BC: Fibronectin receptor of human macrophages recognizes the sequence Arg-Gly-Asp-Ser. *J Exp Med* 162:762, 1985.
21. Patel VP, Lodish HF: The fibronectin receptor on mammalian erythroid precursor cells—Characterization and developmental regulation. *J Cell Biol* 102:449, 1986.
22. Fraser IP, Gordon S: Murine erythroleukemia (Mel) cells bear ligands for the sialoadhesin and erythroblast receptor macrophage hemagglutinins. *Eur J Cell Biol* 64:217, 1994.
23. Breton-Gorius J, Guichard J, Vainchenker W: Absence of erythroblastic islands in plasma clot culture and their possible reconstitution after clot lysis. *Blood Cells* 5:461, 1979.
24. Parmley RT, Ogawa M, Spicer SS, et al: Human marrow erythropoiesis in culture. 3. Ultrastructural and cytochemical studies of cellular interactions. *Exp Hematol* 6:78, 1978.
25. Panzenbock B, Bartunek P, Mapara MY, Zenke M: Growth and differentiation of human stem cell factor/erythropoietin-dependent erythroid progenitor cells *in vitro*. *Blood* 92:3658, 1998.
26. Klausner RD, Harford JB, Rao K: Molecular aspects of the regulation of cellular iron metabolism, in *Proteins of Iron Storage and Transport* edited by G Spik, J Montreuil, RR Crichton, J Mazurier, p 111. Elsevier Science, Amsterdam, 1985.
27. Quintana C, Bonnet N, Jeantet AY, Chemelle P: Crystallographic study of the ferritin molecule—New results obtained from natural crystals *in situ* (mollusk oocyte) and from isolated molecules (horse spleen). *Biol Cell* 59:247, 1987.
28. Iancu TC: Iron and neoplasia—Ferritin and hemosiderin in tumor cells. *Ultrastruct Pathol* 13:573, 1989.
29. Richter GW: Studies of iron overload—Rat-liver siderosome ferritin. *Lab Invest* 50:26, 1984.
30. Koorts AM, Viljoen M: Ferritin and ferritin isoforms I: Structure–function relationships, synthesis, degradation and secretion. *Arch Physiol Biochem* 113:30, 2007.
31. Pearse BM: Coated vesicles from human placenta carry ferritin, transferrin, and immunoglobulin G. *Proc Natl Acad Sci U S A* 79:451, 1982.
32. Ponka P, Sheftel AD, Zhang AS: Iron targeting to mitochondria in erythroid cells. *Biochem Soc Trans* 30:735, 2002.
33. Conrad ME, Umbreit JN, Moore EG, Heiman D: Mobilferrin is an intermediate in iron transport between transferrin and hemoglobin in K562 cells. *J Clin Invest* 98:1449, 1996.

34. Parmley RT, Hajdu I, Denys FR: Ultrastructural localization of the transferrin receptor and transferrin on marrow cell surfaces. *Br J Haematol* 54:633, 1983.
35. Grasso JA, Hillis TJ, Mooneyfrank JA: Ferritin is not a required intermediate for iron utilization in heme synthesis. *Biochim Biophys Acta* 797:247, 1984.
36. Speyer BE, Fielding J: Ferritin as a cytosol iron transport intermediate in human reticulocytes. *Br J Haematol* 42:255, 1979.
37. Drysdale J, Jain SK, Boyd D: Human ferritins: Genes and proteins, in *Proteins of Iron Storage and Transport* edited by G Spik, J Montreuil, RR Crichton, J Mazurier, p 343. Elsevier Science, Amsterdam, 1985.
38. Fenton HJH: Oxidation of tartaric acid in presence of iron. *J Chem Soc Trans* 65:899, 1894.
39. Haber F, Weiss J: Uber die Katalyse des Hydroperoxydes. *Naturwissenschaften* 20:948, 1932.
40. Scott MD, Eaton JW: Thalassemic erythrocytes—Cellular suicide arising from iron and glutathione-dependent oxidation reactions. *Br J Haematol* 91:811, 1995.
41. Harrison PM, Arosio P: Ferritins: Molecular properties, iron storage function and cellular regulation. *Biochim Biophys Acta* 1275:161, 1996.
42. Nijhof W, Wierenga PK: Isolation and characterization of the erythroid progenitor cell: CFU-E. *J Cell Biol* 96:386, 1983.
43. Malik P, Fisher TC, Barsky LL, et al: An *in vitro* model of human red blood cell production from hematopoietic progenitor cells. *Blood* 91:2664, 1998.
44. Sato T, Maekawa T, Watanabe S, et al: Erythroid progenitors differentiate and mature in response to endogenous erythropoietin. *J Clin Invest* 106:263, 2000.
45. Kie JH, Jung YJ, Woo SY, et al: Ultrastructural and phenotypic analysis of *in vitro* erythropoiesis from human cord blood CD34+ cells. *Ann Hematol* 82:278, 2003.
46. Bessis M, Breton-Gorius J: Ultra-structure du pro-erythroblaste. *Nouv Rev Fr Hematol* 1:529, 1961.
47. Breton-Gorius J, Reyes F: Ultrastructure of human bone marrow cell maturation. *Int Rev Cytol* 46:251, 1976.
48. Dvorak AM, Dvorak HF, Karnovsky MJ: Cytochemical localization of peroxidase activity in the developing erythrocyte. *Am J Pathol* 67:303, 1972.
49. Xue SP, Zhang SF, Du Q, et al: The role of cytoskeletal elements in the two-phase denucleation process of mammalian erythroblasts *in vitro* observed by laser confocal scanning microscope. *Cell Mol Biol (Noisy-le-grand)* 43:851, 1997.
50. Chasis JA, Prenant M, Leung A, Mohandas N: Membrane assembly and remodeling during reticulocyte maturation. *Blood* 74:1112, 1989.
51. Lazarides E: From genes to structural morphogenesis—The genesis and epigenesis of a red blood cell. *Cell* 51:345, 1987.
52. Bessis M, Breton-Gorius J, Thiery JP: Role possible de l'hemoglobine accompagnant le noyau des erythroblastes dans l'origine de la stercobiline élimnée précocement. *C R Acad Sci III* 252:2300, 1961.
53. Wilson JG, Tavassoli M: Microenvironmental factors involved in the establishment of erythropoiesis in bone marrow. *Ann N Y Acad Sci* 718:271, 1994.
54. Lichtman MA, Santillo P: Red cell egress from the marrow—Vis-à-tergo. *Blood Cells* 12:11, 1986.
55. Waugh RE, Hsu LL, Clark P, Clark A: Analysis of cell egress in bone marrow, in *White Cell Mechanics: Basic Science and Clinical Aspects* edited by HJ Meiselman, MA Lichtman, PL LaCelle, p 221. Alan R. Liss, New York, 1984.
56. Chamberlain JK, Lichtman MA: Marrow cell egress: Specificity of the site of penetration into the sinus. *Blood* 52:959, 1978.
57. Waugh RE: Reticulocyte rigidity and passage through endothelial-like pores. *Blood* 78:3037, 1991.
58. Nunez MT, Glass J, Fischer S, et al: Transferrin receptors in developing murine erythroid cells. *Br J Haematol* 36:519, 1977.
59. Pan BT, Johnstone RM: Fate of the transferrin receptor during maturation of sheep reticulocytes *in vitro*: Selective externalization of the receptor. *Cell* 33:967, 1983.
60. Zweig S, Singer SJ: Concanavalin A-induced endocytosis in rabbit reticulocytes, and its decrease with reticulocyte maturation. *J Cell Biol* 80:487, 1979.
61. Bowman WD Jr: Abnormal ("ringed") sideroblasts in various hematologic and non-hematologic disorders. *Blood* 18:662, 1961.
62. Hines JD, Grasso JA: The sideroblastic anemias. *Semin Hematol* 7:86, 1970.
63. Flandrin G, Daniel MT, Breton-Gorius J, et al: Ilôt érythroblastique anormal dû au développement de jonctions intercellulaires (synartèse érythroblastique). Un nouveau mécanisme d'anémie. Problèmes posés par le diagnostic. *Nouv Rev Fr Hematol* 14:161, 1974.
64. Jolly JMJ: Recherches sur la formation des globules rouges des mammiféres. *Arch Anat Microsc* 9:133, 1907.
65. Discombe G: L'origine des corps de Howell-Jolly et des anneaux de cabot. *Sang.* 19:262, 1948.
66. Felka T, Lemke J, Lemke C, et al: DNA degradation during maturation of erythrocytes—Molecular cytogenetic characterization of Howell-Jolly bodies. *Cytogenet Genome Res* 119:2, 2007.
67. Rondanelli EG, Trenta A, Magliulo E, et al: Morphogénèse des micronoyaux supplémentaires (pseudo-corps de Jolly) dans les cellules érythropoïétiques irradiées. Recherches cinémicrographiques en contraste de phase. *Acta Haematol* 35:232, 1966.
68. Koyama S: Studies on Howell-Jolly body. *Acta Haemat Jpn* 23:20, 1960.
69. Koyama S, Kihira H, Aoki S, Ohnishi H: Postsplenectomy vacuole: A new erythrocytic inclusion body. *Mie Med J* 11:425, 1962.
70. Holroyde CP, Gardner FH: Acquisition of autophagic vacuoles by human erythrocytes. Physiological role of the spleen. *Blood* 36:566, 1970.
71. O'Grady JG, Harding B, Egan EL, et al: "Pitted" erythrocytes: Impaired formation in splenectomized subjects with congenital spherocytosis. *Br J Haematol* 57:441, 1984.
72. Buchanan GR, Holtkamp CA, Horton JA: Formation and disappearance of pocked erythrocytes: Studies in human subjects and laboratory animals. *Am J Hematol* 25:243, 1987.
73. Kass L: Origin and composition of Cabot rings in pernicious anemia. *Am J Clin Pathol* 64:53, 1975.
74. Van Oye E: L'Origine des anneaux de Cabot. *Rev Hematol* 9:173, 1954.
75. Kass L, Gray RH: Ultrastructural visualization of Cabot rings in pernicious anemia. *Experientia* 32:507, 1976.
76. Jensen WN, Moreno GD, Bessis MC: An electron microscopic description of basophilic stippling in red cells. *Blood* 25:933, 1965.
77. Lessin LS, Wallas CH: Biochemical basis for membrane alterations in irreversibly sickled cells (ISC). *Blood* 42:978, 1973.
78. Heinz R: Uber Blutdegeneration und Regeneration. *Beitr Pathol* 29:299, 1901.
79. Chinprasertsuk S, Piankijagum A, Wasi P: *In vivo* induction of intraerythrocytic inclusion bodies in hemoglobin H disease: An electron microscopic study. *Birth Defects Orig Artic Ser* 23:317, 1987.
80. Wickramasinghe SN, Hughes M, Fucharoen S, Wasi P: The morphology of redox-dye-treated HbH-containing red cells: Differences between cells treated with brilliant cresyl blue, methylene blue and new methylene blue. *Clin Lab Haematol* 7:353, 1985.
81. Sansone G, Sciarratta GV, Ivaldi G, Chiappara G: Hb H-like inclusions in red cells of patients with unstable haemoglobin. *Haematologica* 72:481, 1987.
82. Beaven GH, Coleman PN, White JC: Occurrence of haemoglobin H in leukaemia: A further case of erythroleukaemia. *Acta Haematol* 59:37, 1978.
83. Wickramasinghe SN, Hughes M, Higgs DR, Weatherall DJ: Ultrastructure of red cells containing haemoglobin H inclusions induced by redox dyes. *Clin Lab Haematol* 3:51, 1981.
84. Bessis MC, Breton-Gorius J: Iron particles in normal erythroblasts and normal and pathological erythrocytes. *J Biophys Biochem Cytol* 3:503, 1957.
85. Brecher G, Haley JE, Prenant M, Bessis M: Macronormoblasts, Macroreticulocytes and Macrocytes. *Blood Cells* 1:547, 1975.
86. Willekens FLA, Roerdinkholder-Stoelwinder B, Groenen-Dopp YAM, et al: Hemoglobin loss from erythrocytes *in vivo* results from spleen-facilitated vesiculation. *Blood* 101:747, 2003.
87. Bull BS, Hay KL: Are red blood cell indexes international. *Arch Pathol Lab Med* 109:604, 1985.
88. Korpman RA, Dorrough DC, Brailsford JD, Bull BS: Red cell shape as an indicator of membrane structure—Ponders rule reexamined. *Blood Cells* 3:315, 1977.
89. Bessis M: *Blood Smears Reinterpreted*. Springer, New York, 1977.
90. Burton AL, Anderson WL, Andrews RV: Quantitative studies on flicker phenomenon in erythrocytes. *Blood* 32:819, 1968.
91. Fricke K, Wirthensohn K, Laxhuber R, Sackmann E: Flicker spectroscopy of erythrocytes—A sensitive method to study subtle changes of membrane bending stiffness. *Eur Biophys J* 14:67, 1986.
92. Willekens FL, Werre JM, Groenen-Dopp YA, et al: Erythrocyte vesiculation: A self-protective mechanism? *Br J Haematol* 141:549, 2008.
93. Brailsford JD, Korpman RA, Bull BS: Red cell shape from discocyte to hypotonic spherocyte—Mathematical delineation based on a uniform shell hypothesis. *J Theor Biol* 60:131, 1976.
94. Byers TJ, Branton D: Visualization of the protein associations in the erythrocyte membrane skeleton. *Proc Natl Acad Sci U S A* 82:6153, 1985.
95. Liu SC, Derick LH, Palek J: Visualization of the hexagonal lattice in the erythrocyte membrane skeleton. *J Cell Biol* 104:527, 1987.
96. Shen BW, Josephs R, Steck TL: Ultrastructure of the intact skeleton of the human erythrocyte membrane. *J Cell Biol* 102:997, 1986.
97. Bull BS, Brailsford JD: Red blood cell shape, in *Red Blood Cell Membranes: Structure, Function, Clinical Implications* edited by P Agre, JC Parker, p 401. Marcel Dekker, New York, 1989.
98. Borghi N, Brochard-Wyart F: Tether extrusion from red blood cells: Integral proteins unbinding from cytoskeleton. *Biophys J* 93:1369, 2007.
99. Hsu YJ, Goodman SR: Spectrin and ubiquitination: A review. *Cell Mol Biol (Noisy-le-grand).* Suppl 51:OL801, 2005.
100. Li J, Lykotrafitis G, Dao M, Suresh S: Cytoskeletal dynamics of human erythrocyte. *Proc Natl Acad Sci U S A* 104:4937, 2007.
101. Liu SC, Derick LH, Agre P, Palek J: Alteration of the erythrocyte membrane skeletal ultrastructure in hereditary spherocytosis, hereditary elliptocytosis, and pyropoikilocytosis. *Blood* 76:198, 1990.
102. Branemark PI, Bagge U: Intravascular rheology of erythrocytes in man. *Blood Cells* 3:11, 1977.
103. Bessis M: Red cell shapes: An illustrated classification and its rationale, in *Red Cell Shape: Physiology, Pathology, Ultrastructure* edited by M Bessis, R Weed, P LeBlond, p 1. Springer-Verlag, New York, 1973.
104. Prasad AS: Acquired hemolytic anemias, in *Hematology: Clinical and Laboratory Practice* edited by RL Bick, p 391. Mosby Year Book, St. Louis, 1993.
105. Canham PB: The minimum energy of bending as a possible explanation of the biconcave shape of the human red blood cell. *J Theor Biol* 26:61, 1970.
106. Iglic A: A possible mechanism determining the stability of spiculated red blood cells. *J Biomech* 30:35, 1997.
107. Iglic A, Kralj-Iglic V, Hagerstrand H: Amphiphile induced echinocyte-spheroechinocyte transformation of red blood cell shape. *Eur Biophys J* 27:335, 1998.

108. Lim GHW: *A numerical study of morphologies and morphological transformations of human erythrocyte based on membrane mechanics* [PhD Thesis]. Simon Fraser University, British Columbia, 2003.
109. Lim HWG, Wortis M, Mukhopadhyay R: Stomatocyte-discocyte-echinocyte sequence of the human red blood cell: Evidence for the bilayer-couple hypothesis from membrane mechanics. *Proc Natl Acad Sci U S A* 99:16766, 2002.
110. Sheetz MP, Painter RG, Singer SJ: Biological-membranes as bilayer couples. 3. Compensatory shape changes induced in membranes. *J Cell Biol* 70:193, 1976.
111. Gedde MM, Yang EY, Huestis WH: Resolution of the paradox of red cell shape changes in low and high pH. *Biochim Biophys Acta* 1417:246, 1999.
112. Gimsa J, Ried C: Do band-3 protein conformational changes mediate shape changes of human erythrocytes. *Mol Membr Biol* 12:247, 1995.
113. Gimsa J: A possible molecular mechanism governing human erythrocyte shape. *Biophys J* 75:568, 1998.
114. Wong P: Mechanism of control of erythrocyte shape—A possible relationship to band-3. *J Theor Biol* 171:197, 1994.
115. Wong P: A basis of echinocytosis and stomatocytosis in the disc-sphere transformations of the erythrocyte. *J Theor Biol* 196:343, 1999.
116. Cooper RA, Jandl JH: Bile salts and cholesterol in the pathogenesis of target cells in obstructive jaundice. *J Clin Invest* 47:809, 1968.
117. Clark MR, Aminoff MJ, Chiu DTY, et al: Red cell deformability and lipid composition in 2 forms of acanthocytosis—Enrichment of acanthocytic populations by density gradient centrifugation. *J Lab Clin Med* 113:469, 1989.
118. Redman CM, Huima T, Robbins E, et al: Effect of phosphatidylserine on the shape of Mcleod red cell acanthocytes. *Blood* 74:1826, 1989.
119. Padilla F, Bromberg PA, Jensen WN: Sickle-unsickle cycle—Cause of cell fragmentation leading to permanently deformed cells. *Blood* 41:653, 1973.
120. Bessis M, Nomarski G, Thiery JP, Breton-Gorius J: Etude sur la falciformation des globules rouges au microscope polarisant et au microscope électronique. II. L'intérieur du globule; comparaison avec les cristaux intra-globulaires. *Rev Hematol* 13:249, 1958.
121. White JG: The fine structure of sickled hemoglobin *in situ*. *Blood* 31:561, 1968.
122. Jensen WN, Lessin LS: Membrane alterations associated with hemoglobinopathies. *Semin Hematol* 7:409, 1970.
123. Horiuchi K, Ballas SK, Asakura T: The effect of deoxygenation rate on the formation of irreversibly sickled cells. *Blood* 71:46, 1988.
124. Abraham A, Bencsath FA, Shartava A, et al: Preparation of irreversibly sickled cell beta-actin from normal red blood cell beta-actin. *Biochemistry* 41:292, 2002.
125. Bertles JF, Milner PF: Irreversibly sickled erythrocytes: A consequence of the heterogeneous distribution of hemoglobin types in sickle-cell anemia. *J Clin Invest* 47:1731, 1968.
126. Weinstein RS, Warth JA, Near K, Marikovsky Y: Sequestrocytes—A manifestation of trans cellular cross-bonding of the red cell membrane in sickle cell anemia. *J Cell Sci* 94:593, 1989.
127. Bull BS, Kuhn IN: Production of schistocytes by fibrin strands (a scanning electron microscope study). *Blood* 35:104, 1970.
128. Young TW, Keeney GL, Bull BS: Red cell fragmentation in human disease (a light and scanning electron microscope study). *Blood Cells* 10:493, 1984.
129. Bull BS, Weinstein RS, Korpman RA: On the thickness of the red cell membrane skeleton—Quantitative electron microscopy of maximally narrowed isthmus regions of intact cells. *Blood Cells* 12:25, 1986.
130. Cooper RA: Loss of membrane components in pathogenesis of antibody-induced spherocytosis. *J Clin Invest* 51:16, 1972.
131. Rifkind RA, Danon D: Heinz body anemia—An ultrastructural study. I. Heinz body formation. *Blood* 25:885, 1965.
132. Rabinovitch M: Phagocytosis: The engulfment stage. *Semin Hematol* 5:134, 1968.
133. Lock SP, Smith RS, Hardisty RM: Stomatocytosis: A hereditary red cell anomally associated with haemolytic anaemia. *Br J Haematol* 7:303, 1961.
134. Delaunay J, Stewart G, Iolascon A: Hereditary dehydrated and overhydrated stomatocytosis: Recent advances. *Curr Opin Hematol* 6:110, 1999.
135. Leblond PF, de Boisfleury A, Bessis M: La forme des erythrocytes dans la sphèrocytose héréditaire. *Nouv Rev Fr Hematol* 13:873, 1973.
136. Bull B: Holey red cells: A brief note—A commentary. *Blood Cells* 9:173, 1983.
137. Dhermy D, Feo C, Garbarz M, et al: Prenatal diagnosis of hereditary elliptocytosis with molecular defect of spectrin. *Prenat Diagn* 7:471, 1987.
138. Coetzer T, Palek J, Lawler J, et al: Structural and functional heterogeneity of alpha-spectrin mutations involving the spectrin heterodimer self-association site—Relationships to hematologic expression of homozygous hereditary elliptocytosis and hereditary pyropoikilocytosis. *Blood* 75:2235, 1990.
139. Dhermy D, Garbarz M, Lecomte MC, et al: Hereditary elliptocytosis—Clinical, morphological and biochemical studies of 38 cases. *Nouv Rev Fr Hematol* 28:129, 1986.
140. Marchesi SL, Knowles WJ, Morrow JS, et al: Abnormal spectrin in hereditary elliptocytosis. *Blood* 67:141, 1986.
141. Agre PC, Zinkham WH, Casella JF, Bennett V: Spectrin deficiency is common to all forms of hereditary spherocytosis (HS): The degree of deficiency correlates with osmotic fragility [abstract]. *Blood* 62(Suppl 1):42a, 1983.
142. Marchesi SL, Conboy J, Agre P, et al: Molecular analysis of insertion/deletion mutations in protein 4.1 in elliptocytosis. I. Biochemical identification of rearrangements in the spectrin/actin binding domain and functional characterizations. *J Clin Invest* 86:516, 1990.
143. Bull B, Feo C, Bessis M: Behavior of elliptocytes under shear stress in the rheoscope and ektacytometer. *Cytometry* 3:300, 1983.
144. Santillo PA, Lichtman MA: Holey red cells: A brief note. *Blood Cells* 9:169, 1983.
145. Fischer TM: Role of spectrin in cross bonding of the red cell membrane. *Blood Cells* 13:377, 1988.
146. Greenberg MS: Heinz body hemolytic anemia—Bite cells—Clue to diagnosis. *Arch Intern Med* 136:153, 1976.
147. Yoo D, Lessin LS: Drug-associated bite cell hemolytic anemia. *Am J Med* 92:243, 1992.
148. Diggs LW, Kraus AP, Morrison DB, Rudnicki RPT: Intraerythrocytic crystals in a white patient with hemoglobin C in the absence of other types of hemoglobin. *Blood* 9:1172, 1954.
149. Fabry ME, Kaul DK, Raventos C, et al: Some aspects of the patho-physiology of homozygous Hb-CC erythrocytes. *J Clin Invest* 67:1284, 1981.
150. Hirsch RE, Raventos-Suarez C, Olson JA, Nagel RL: Ligand state of intraerythrocytic circulating HbC crystals in homozygote CC patients. *Blood* 66:775, 1985.
151. Charache S, Conley CL, Waugh DF, et al: Pathogenesis of hemolytic anemia in homozygous hemoglobin C disease. *J Clin Invest* 46:1795, 1967.
152. Lessin LS, Jensen WN, Ponder E: Molecular mechanism of hemolytic anemia in homozygous hemoglobin C disease—Electron microscopic study by freeze-etching technique. *J Exp Med* 130:443, 1969.
153. Charache S, Raik E, Holtzclaw D, et al: Pseudosickling of hemoglobin Setif. *Blood* 70:237, 1987.
154. Ponder E: *Hemolysis and Related Phenomena*. Grune & Stratton, New York, 1948.
155. Seeman P: Transient holes in erythrocyte membrane during hypotonic hemolysis and stable holes in membrane after lysis by saponin and lysolecithin. *J Cell Biol* 32:55, 1967.
156. Pribush A, Hatskelzon L, Kapelushnik J, Meyerstein N: Osmotic swelling and hole formation in membranes of thalassemic and spherocytic erythrocytes. *Blood Cells Mol Dis* 31:43, 2003.
157. Stuart J, Bull BS, Juhan-Vague I: Microrheological techniques for the measurement of erythrocyte deformability, in *Investigative Microtechniques in Medicine and Biology* edited by J Chayen, L Bitensky, p 297. Marcel Dekker, New York, 1984.
158. Schmid-Schonbein H, von Gosen J, Heinich L, et al: A counter-rotating "rheoscope chamber" for the study of the microrheology of blood cell aggregation by microscopic observation and microphotometry. *Microvasc Res* 6:366, 1973.
159. Bessis M, Mohandas N, Feo C: Automated ektacytometry: A new method of measuring red cell deformability and red cell indices. *Blood Cells* 6:315, 1980.
160. Mohandas N, Clark MR, Jacobs MS, Shohet SB: Analysis of factors regulating erythrocyte deformability. *J Clin Invest* 66:563, 1980.
161. Bull BS, Brailsford JD: A new method of measuring deformability of red cell membrane. *Blood* 45:581, 1975.
162. Williams AR, Morris DR: The internal viscosity of the human erythrocyte may determine its life span *in vivo*. *Scand J Haematol* 24:57, 1980.
163. Clark MR, Mohandas N, Caggiano V, Shohet SB: Effects of abnormal cation transport on deformability of desiccytes. *J Supramol Struct* 8:521, 1978.
164. Foller M, Huber SM, Lang F: Erythrocyte programmed cell death. *IUBMB Life* 60:661, 2008.
165. Lang KS, Lang PA, Bauer C, et al: Mechanisms of suicidal erythrocyte death. *Cell Physiol Biochem* 15:195, 2005.
166. Bessis MC, Breton-Gorius J: Iron metabolism in bone marrow as seen by electron microscopy—A critical review. *Blood* 19:635, 1962.
167. Edelman P, Vinci G, Villeval JL, et al: A monoclonal antibody against an erythrocyte ontogenic antigen identifies fetal and adult erythroid progenitors. *Blood* 67:56, 1986.
168. Breton-Gorius J, Villeval JL, Mitjavila MT, et al: Ultrastructural and cytochemical characterization of blasts from early erythroblastic leukemias. *Leukemia* 1:173, 1987.
169. Jay AWL: Geometry of human erythrocyte. 1. Effect of albumin on cell geometry. *Biophys J* 15:205, 1975.

CHAPTER 30

COMPOSITION OF THE ERYTHROCYTE

Ernest Beutler

SUMMARY

Quantitative data have been published about many of the components of the red cell, including minerals, carbohydrates, enzymes and other proteins, vitamins, and lipids. Some of these are marred by the failure to rigorously remove white cells from the red cell pellet, but this chapter provides access to some of the large amount of data that is available.

The erythrocyte is a complex cell. The membrane is composed of lipids and proteins, and the interior of the cell contains metabolic machinery designed to sustain the cell through its 120-day life span and maintain the integrity of hemoglobin function. Each component of red blood cells may be expressed as a function of red cell volume, grams of hemoglobin, or square centimeters of cell surface. These expressions are usually interchangeable, but under certain circumstances each may have specific advantages. However, because disease may produce changes in the average red cell size, hemoglobin content, or surface area, the use of any of these measurements individually may, at times, be misleading.

For convenience and uniformity, data in the accompanying tables (Tables 30–1 through 30–9) are expressed in terms of cell constituent per milliliter of red cell and per gram of hemoglobin. In many instances, this process required recalculation of published data. These recalculations assume a hematocrit value of 45 percent and 33 g of hemoglobin per deciliter of red cells. To obtain concentration per gram of hemoglobin, the concentration per milliliter red blood cell (RBC) can be multiplied by 3.03. The tables list only some of the most commonly referred to constituents of the erythrocyte. The reference on which each value is based is the first number presented in the last column of each table. Where applicable, additional confirmatory references are given. Additional data and references may be found elsewhere.[1,2] In some instances, only the percentage of the total of the type of constituent present is given. Chap. 46 presents data regarding activities of red cell enzymes.

TABLE 30–1. Human Erythrocyte Protein and Water Content

Component	mg/mL RBC	Reference
Water	721 ± 17.3	3, 4
Total protein	371	4, 5
Nonhemoglobin protein	9.2	4, 6
Insoluble stroma protein	6.3	6
Enzyme proteins	2.9	6
Extensive study by proteomic methods		7, 8

Acronyms and abbreviations that appear in this chapter include: RBC, red blood cell.

TABLE 30–2. Human Erythrocyte Lipids

Fatty Acids as Percent of Total Fatty Acid		Reference
Lauric (n-C_{12})	0.3	9
Myristic (n-C_{14})	0.8	9
Pentoenoic (n-C_{15})	0.3	9
Palmitoleic (16:1)	1.1	9
Palmitic (n-C_{16})	41.0	9
(C_{17}) branched	0.3	9
(n-C_{17})	0.3	9
Linoleic	15.3	9
Oleic	18.9	9
Oleic isomer	Trace	9
Stearic (n-C_{18})	7.9	9
Arachidonic (20:4)	7.9	9
C_{22} unsaturated (a)	2.5	9
C_{22} unsaturated (b)	2.0	9
Long-Chain Aldehydes as Percent of Total Aldehydes		**Reference**
n-C_{14}	Trace	9
Branched C_{15}	0.8	9
n-C_{15}	0.6	9
Highly branched C_{16}	Trace	9
C_{16} monoene	0.4	9
n-C_{16}	24.2	9
Highly branched C_{17}	1.7	9
Branched C_{17}	7.5	9
n-C_{17}	1.3	9
C_{18} monoene	6.0	9
Isomeric C_{18} monoene	2.8	9
n-C_{18}	42.5	9
Unknown C_{19}	2.9	9
Unknown C_{20}	3.1	9
Unknown C_{21}	5.6	9
Fatty Acids as Percent of Total Neutral Lipids Fatty Acids		**Reference**
n-C_{10}	0.0–0.6	10
n-C_{12}	1.1–2.2	10
n-C_{14}	5.9–17.3	10
16:1	3.2–6.0	10
n-C_{16}	15.2–22.6	10
18.2 and 3	11.4–21.1	10
18:1	28.8–29.1	10
n-C_{18}	5.7–10.7	10
Unsaturated C_{19}A	Trace	10
Arachidonic	7.4–8.3	10
Polyunsaturated C_{20}	Trace	10

TABLE 30–3. Human Erythrocyte Phospholipids

Lipid	Amount	Reference
Total phospholipids	2.98 ± 0.20 mg/mL RBC	11
Cephalin	1.17 (0.38–1.91) mg/mL RBC	11
Ethanolamine phosphoglyceride	29% of total phospholipid	11
Mean plasmalogen content	67% of ethanolamine phosphoglyceride	11
Serine phosphoglyceride	10% of total phospholipid	11
Mean plasmalogen content	8% of serine phosphoglyceride	11
Lecithin	0.32 (0.03–0.95) mg/mL	12
Sphingomyelin	0.12–1.13 mg/mL	12
Lysolecithin	1.82% of total phospholipids	13

NOTE: Some results are given as mean ± standard deviation.

TABLE 30–5. Nucleotides

Compound	μmol/mL RBC	Reference
Adenosine monophosphate	0.021 ± 0.003	14–20
Adenosine diphosphate	0.216 ± 0.036	14–19
Adenosine triphosphate	1.35 ± 0.035	16–18, 20–23
Cyclic adenosine monophosphate	0.015 ± 0.0024	24
Cyclic guanosine monophosphate	0.013 ± 0.0042	24
Guanosine diphosphate	0.018 ± 0.005	16
Guanosine triphosphate	0.052 ± 0.012	15, 16
Inosine monophosphate	0.031 ± 0.005	16–20
Nicotinamide adenine dinucleotide		25, 26
Reduced	0.0018 ± 0.001	25, 26
Oxidized	0.049 ± 0.006	25, 26
Nicotinamide adenine dinucleotide phosphate		25, 26
Reduced	0.032 ± 0.002	
Oxidized	0.0014 ± 0.0011	
S-adenosylmethionine	0.005	27
Total nucleotide	1.534 ± 0.033	28
Uridine diphosphoglucose	0.031 ± 0.005	16, 29
Uridine diphosphate *N*-acetyl glucosamine	0.018	29

NOTE: Some results are given as mean ± standard deviation.

TABLE 30–4. Fatty Acid Compositions of Erythrocyte Phospholipids[6,7] (mol %)

Shorthand Designation*	Mixed Phospholipids Methanol Fraction	Ethanolamine	Serine	Choline
12:0	0.1	. . .	. . .	0.1
14:0	0.5	0.2	Trace	0.5
14:0	0.3	0.2	Trace	0.3
16:0	28.8	18.9	7.1	33.0
cis $16{:}1^{9}$	0.7	0.6	0.4	0.1
17:0	0.4	Trace	0.3	0.5
18:0	15.1	8.0	41.6	11.7
cis $18{:}1^{9}$	18.3	21.6	7.9	17.9
trans $18{:}1^{9}$	2.9	3.6	5.1	2.7
cis,cis $18{:}2^{9,12}$	10.6	7.0	2.8	18.2
cis,cis,cis $18{:}3^{9,12,15}$	. . .	Trace	. . .	. . .
19:0 iso or ante-iso	Trace	0.2	. . .	. . .
20:0	0.1	. . .	Trace	0.2
$20{:}1^{11}$	0.2	0.3	Trace	0.2
$20{:}2^{8,11}$	. . .	Trace	. . .	. . .
$20{:}2^{11,14}$	0.1	0.1	. . .	0.2
$20{:}3^{5,8,11}$	1.6	1.0	2.1	1.6
$20{:}4^{5,8,11,14}$	10.8	21.9	19.7	5.0
$20{:}5^{5,8,11,14,17}$	0.8	1.4	0.3	0.5
(22:unsat.?)	1.7	4.7	2.2	0.3
22:5	0.7	0.8	0.9	1.7
22:5	2.3	2.3	2.0	2.7
$22{:}5^{7,10,13,16,19}$	1.0	. . .	. . .	1.0
$22.6^{4,7,10,13,16,19}$	2.1	3.9	4.2	1.1
14:0	Trace	. . .	. . .	0.8
Branched 15:0	2.8	2.6	5.5	. . .
15:0 iso or ante-iso	0.1	. . .	0.4	. . .
15:0	0.2	0.3	. . .	. . .
Unknown	0.1	. . .	1.6	1.0
cis $16{:}1^{9}$	Trace	. . .	. . .	0.2
16:0	18.2	15.9	17.1	49.8
Branched 17:0 unsat.?	0.9	1.5	. . .	. . .
Branched 17:unsat.?	2.4	3.0	. . .	. . .
Branched 17:0	5.8	5.5	11.3	6.9
17:0 iso or ante-iso	1.1	0.8	0.7	2.9
cis,cis $18{:}2^{9,12}$	Trace	. . .	1.4	. . .
cis $18{:}1^{9}$	6.8	7.0	5.4	5.3
18:1 isomer	13.2	18.8	10.5	7.7
18:0	37.1	40.4	32.3	19.2
Unknown	1.3	2.1	. . .	. . .

TABLE 30–6. Amino Acids and Other Nitrogen-containing Compounds

Compound	μmol/mL RBC	Reference
Alanine	0.275 ± 0.060	29–33
α-Amino butyrate	0.016 ± 0.009	30–32
Arginine	0.040 ± 0.013	30–32, 34, 35
Asparagine	0.121 ± 0.041	30, 31
Aspartate*	0.306 ± 0.081	30
Carnitine	0.23	36, 37
Citrulline	0.036 ± 0.005*	30
Glutamate	0.265 ± 0.089	30, 32, 38
Glutamine	0.624 ± 0.136	32, 39, 40
Glycine	0.347 ± 0.070	30, 31
Histidine	0.086 ± 0.013	30, 32, 35, 41
Isoleucine	0.058 ± 0.013	30, 31
Leucine	0.110 ± 0.009	30, 31
Lysine	0.139 ± 0.032	30, 32, 35
Methionine	0.015 ± 0.006	30, 32, 35
Ornithine	0.120 ± 0.028	30,32
Phenylalanine	0.049 ± 0.006	30–32, 35
Proline	0.137 ± 0.035	30–32
Serine	0.149 ± 0.032	30,31
Taurine	0.349 ± 0.057	30
Threonine	0.116 ± 0.022	30–32
Tyrosine	0.059 ± 0.009	30–32, 35
Valine	0.171 ± 0.028	30–32, 35
Creatine	0.33 ± 0.11	42
Creatinine	0.159	43
Cystine	0.016 ± 0.002	35
Ergothioneine	0.355 ± 0.112	32
Ethanolamine	0.007	32
Glutathione oxidized	0.0036 ± 0.0014	44, 45
Glutathione reduced	2.234 ± 0.354	14
Tryptophan	0.024 ± 0.004	32, 34, 35, 46
Uric acid	0.113	32, 43
Urea	4.121 ± 0.420	32

*Measured in samples treated with sodium sulfite before analysis.

NOTE: Some results are given as mean ± standard deviation.

TABLE 30–7. Human Erythrocyte Coenzyme and Vitamins

Compound	μmol/mL RBC	Reference
Ascorbic acid	0.02892 ± 0.00431	47
Choline free	Trace	48
Cocarboxylase	0.00021	49
Coenzyme A	0.0027	50
Nicotinic acid	0.105	51
Pantothenic acid	0.001 ± 0.00028	52
Pyridoxal phosphate	$20\times10^{-6} \pm 2\times10^{-6}$	53
Pyridoxal	$11\times10^{-6} \pm 3\times10^{-6}$	53
Total vitamin B_6 aldehydes	$30\times10^{-6} \pm 8\times10^{-6}$	53
Pyridoxamine phosphate	$8\times10^{-6} \pm 8\times10^{-6}$	53
4-Pyridoxic acid	$4\times10^{-6} \pm 4\times10^{-6}$	53
Riboflavin	0.00059 ± 0.00021	54
Flavin adenine dinucleotide	0.000398 ± 0.000042	55
Thiamine	0.00027	56

NOTE: Some results are given as mean ± standard deviation.

Tables 30–8 and 30–9 appear on page 432.

REFERENCES

1. Friedemann H, Rapoport SM: Enzymes of the red cell: A critical catalogue, in *Cellular and Molecular Biology of Erythrocytes*, edited by H Yoshikawa, SM Rapoport, p 181. University Park Press, Baltimore, MD, 1974.
2. Pennell RB: Comparison of normal human red cells, in *The Red Blood Cell*, edited by DM Surgenor, p 98. Academic Press, New York, 1974.
3. Nichols G, Nichols N: Electrolyte equilibrium in erythrocytes during diabetic acidosis. *J Clin Invest* 32:113, 1953.
4. Ponder E: *Hemolysis and Related Phenomena*. Grune & Stratton, New York, 1948.
5. Silverman L, Glick D: Measurement of protein concentration by quantitative electron microscopy. *J Cell Biol* 40:773, 1969.
6. Behrendt H: *Chemistry of Erythrocytes*. Charles C Thomas, Springfield, IL, 1957.
7. Tyan YC, Jong SB, Liao JD, et al: Proteomic profiling of erythrocyte proteins by proteolytic digestion chip and identification using two-dimensional electrospray ionization tandem mass spectrometry. *J Proteome Res* 4:748, 2005.
8. Prabakaran S, Wengenroth M, Lockstone HE, et al: 2-D DIGE analysis of liver and red blood cells provides further evidence for oxidative stress in schizophrenia. *J Proteome Res* 6:141, 2007.
9. Kates M, Allison AC, James AT: Phosphatides of human blood cells and their role in spherocytosis. *Biochim Biophys Acta* 48:571, 1961.
10. James AT, Lovelock JE, Webb JPW: The lipids of whole blood. I. Lipid biosynthesis in human blood in vitro. *Biochem J* 73:106, 1959.
11. Farquhar JW: Human erythrocytes phosphoglycerides. I. Quantification of plasmalogens, fatty acids and fatty aldehydes. *Biochim Biophys Acta* 60:80, 1962.
12. Kirk E: The concentration of lecithin, cephalin, ether-insoluble phosphatide, and cerebrosides in plasma and red blood cells of normal adults. *J Biol Chem* 123:637, 1938.
13. Phillips GB, Roome NS: Quantitative chromatographic analysis of the phospholipids of abnormal human red blood cells. *Proc Soc Exp Biol Med* 109:360, 1962.
14. Beutler E: *Red Cell Metabolism: A Manual of Biochemical Methods*. Grune & Stratton, New York, 1984.
15. Bishop C, Rankine D, Talbott JH: The nucleotides in normal human blood. *J Biol Chem* 234:1233, 1959.
16. Mandel P, Chambon P, Karon H, et al: Nucleotides libres des globules rouges et des reticulocytes. *Folia Haematol Int Mag Klin Morphol Blutforsch* 78:525, 1962.
17. Bartlett GR: Human red cell glycolytic intermediates. *J Biol Chem* 234:449, 1959.
18. Gerlach E, Fleckenstein A, Gross E: Der Intermediaere Phosphat-Stoffwechsel des Menschen-Erythrocyten. *Pflugers Arch* 266:528, 1958.
19. Löhr GW, Waller HD: The biochemistry of erythrocyte aging. *Folia Haematol Int Mag Klin Morphol Blutforsch* 78:384, 1961.
20. Yoshikawa H, Nakano M, Miyamoto K, Tatibana M: Phosphorus metabolism in human erythrocyte. II. Separation of acid-soluble phosphorus compounds incorporating p32, by column chromatography with ion exchange resin. *J Biochem* (Tokyo). 47:635, 1960.
21. Beutler E, Mathai CK: A comparison of normal red cell ATP levels as measured by the firefly system and the hexokinase system. *Blood* 30:311, 1967.
22. Minakami S, Suzuki C, Saito T, Yoshikawa H: Studies on erythrocyte glycolysis I, determination of the glycolytic intermediates in human erythrocytes. *J Biochem* 58:543, 1965.
23. Ramos JLA, Nonoyama K, Quintal VS, Barretto OCDO: Red cell enzymes and intermediates in AGA term newborns, AGA preterm newborns and SGA term newborns. *Acta Paediatr Scand* 79:32, 1990.
24. Patterson WD, Hardman JG, Sutherland EW: A comparison of cyclic nucleotide levels in plasma and cells of rat and human blood. *Endocrinology* 95:325, 1974.
25. Canepa L, Ferraris AM, Miglino M, Gaetani GF: Bound and unbound pyridine dinucleotides in normal and glucose-6-phosphate dehydrogenase-deficient erythrocytes. *Biochim Biophys Acta* 1074:101, 1991.
26. Micheli V, Simmonds HA, Bari M, Pompucci G: HPLC determination of oxidized and reduced pyridine coenzymes in human erythrocytes. *Clin Chim Acta* 220:1, 1993.

TABLE 30–8. Human Erythrocyte Carbohydrates, Organic Acids, and Metabolites

Compound	μmol/mL RBC	Reference
Deoxyribonucleic acid	Trace	57
Dihydroxyacetone phosphate	0.0094 ± 0.0028	14
2,3-Diphosphoglycerate	4.171 ± 0.636	14, 18, 22, 23
Fructose	0.000354 ± 0.0000191	58
Fructose 6-phosphate	0.0093 ± 0.002	14, 17, 22, 59
Fructose 3-phosphate	0.013 ± 0.001	60, 61
Fructose 2,6-diphosphate*	48 ± 13	62
Fructose 1,6-diphosphate	0.0019 ± 0.0006	14, 17, 18, 22, 59
Glucuronic acid	Trace	63
Glucose	In equilibrium with plasma	64, 65
Glucose 6-phosphate	0.0278 ± 0.0075	14, 17, 22, 59
Glucose 1,6-diphosphate	0.18–0.30	17, 66
Glyceraldehyde 3-phosphate	Not detectable	14
Lactic acid	0.932 ± 0.211	6, 14, 67
Mannose 1,6-diphosphate	0.150	66
Octulose 1,8-diphosphate	Trace	68
Pyruvate	0.0533 ± 0.0215	14
3-Phosphoglycerate	0.0449 ± 0.0051	14, 22
2-Phosphoglycerate	0.0073 ± 0.0025	14, 22
Phosphoenol pyruvate	0.0122 ± 0.0022	14
Ribonucleic acid	1.355 mg	69
Ribose 1,5-diphosphate	<0.02	70, 71
Ribulose 5-phosphate	Trace	72
Sedoheptulose 7-phosphate	Trace	72
Sedoheptulose diphosphate	Trace	73
Sialic acid	0.825 ± 0.028	70
Sorbitol	31.1 ± 5.3	58, 60, 74
Sorbitol 3-phosphate	0.013 ± 0.001	61

*Values are given in picomoles.

NOTE: Some results are given as mean ± standard deviation.

TABLE 30–9. Human Erythrocyte Electrolytes

Electrolyte	μmol/mL RBC	Reference
Aluminum	0.0026	75
Bromide	0.1225	76, 77
Calcium	0.0089 ± 0.0030	77–79
Chloride	78	77, 80
Chromium	0.0004	81
Cobalt	0.0002	77, 82
Copper	0.018	81, 83, 84
Fluoride	0.0131	85
Iodine, protein-bound	0.0013	86
Lead	0.0082	75, 77, 83, 87
Magnesium	3.06	81, 88–90
Manganese	0.0034	75, 91
Nickel	0.0009	81
Phosphorus (acid soluble):		
Total P	13.2	92
Inorganic P	0.466	92
Lipid P	3.840	93
Unidentified P	0.955	92
Potassium	102.4 ± 3.9	88, 94–98
Rubidium	0.054	77
Silicon	0.036–0.060*	99
Silver	Trace	75
Sodium	6.2 ± 0.8	94–96
Sulfur	0.0044	100
Tin	0.0022	75
Zinc	0.153	81, 101, 102

*Obtained by subtracting plasma concentration from whole-blood concentration.

NOTE: Some results are given as mean ± standard deviation.

27. Lagendijk J, Ubbink JB, Vermaak WJH: Quantification of erythrocyte *S*-adenosyl-L-methionine levels and its application in enzyme studies. *J Chromatogr B Biomed Appl* 576:95, 1992.
28. Overgard-Hansen K, Jorgensen S: Determination and concentration of adenine nucleotides in human blood. *Scand J Clin Lab Invest* 12:10, 1960.
29. Mills GC: Uridine diphosphate glucose and uridine diphosphate *N*-acetylglucosamine in erythrocytes. *Tex Rep Biol Med* 18:446, 1960.
30. Hagenfeldt L, Arvidsson A: A distribution of amino acids between plasma and erythrocytes. *Clin Chim Acta* 100:133, 1980.
31. Leighton WP, Rosenblatt S, Chanley JD: Determination of erythrocyte amino acids by gas chromatography. *J Chromatogr* 164:427, 1979.
32. McMenamy RH, Lund CC, Neville GJ, Wallach DFH: Studies of unbound amino acid distributions in plasma, erythrocytes, leukocytes and urine of normal human subjects. *J Clin Invest* 39:1675, 1960.
33. Wiss O, Kruger R: Der Einfluss Enteral und Parenteral Verabreichter Glucose auf den Alaningehalt des Blutes. *Helv Chim Acta* 31:1774, 1948.
34. Hier SW, Bergeim O: The microbiological determination of certain free amino acids in human and dog plasma. *J Biol Chem* 163:129, 1946.
35. Johnson CA, Bergeim O: The distribution of free amino acids between erythrocytes and plasma in man. *J Biol Chem* 188:833, 1951.
36. Borum PR, York CM, Bennett SG: Carnitine concentration of red blood cells. *Am J Clin Nutr* 41:653, 1985.
37. Reichmann H, V.Lindeneiner N: Carnitine analysis in normal human red blood cells, plasma, and muscle tissue. *Eur Neurol* 34:40, 1994.
38. Divino Filho JC, Hazel SJ, Furst P, et al: Glutamate concentration in plasma, erythrocyte and muscle in relation to plasma levels of insulin-like growth factor (IGF)-I, IGF binding protein-1, and insulin in patients on haemodialysis. *J Endocrinol* 156:519, 1998.
39. Preisler H, Browman G, Henderson E, et al: Treatment of acute myelocytic leukemia: Effects of early intensive consolidation. *ASCO Abstracts* 443, 1980.
40. Iyer GYN: Distribution of glutamine, glutamic acids, and aspartic acid between erythrocytes and plasma. *Indian J Med Res* 44:201, 1956.
41. von Euler H, Heller L: Free histidine in the blood serum of normal and Jensen sarcoma-bearing rats. *Arch Miner Geol* 24A:23, 1947.
42. Griffiths WJ, Fitzpatrick M: The effect of age on the creatine in red cells. *Br J Haematol* 13:175, 1967.
43. Jellinek EM, Looney JM: Statistics of some biochemical variables on healthy men in the age range of twenty to forty-five years. *J Biol Chem* 128:621, 1939.
44. Srivastava SK, Beutler E: Oxidized glutathione levels in erythrocytes of glucose-6-phosphate dehydrogenase-deficient subjects. *Lancet* 2:23, 1968.
45. Rossi R, Milzani A, Dalle-Donne I, et al: Blood glutathione disulfide: In vivo factor or in vitro artifact? *Clin Chem* 48:742, 2002.
46. Steele BF, Reynolds MS, Baumann CA: Amino acids in the blood and urine of human subjects ingesting different amounts of the same proteins. *J Nutr* 40:145, 1950.
47. Westerman MP, Zhang Y, McConnell JP, et al: Ascorbate levels in red blood cells and urine in patients with sickle cell anemia. *Am J Hematol* 65:174, 2000.

48. Luecke R, Pearson PB: The microbiological determination of free choline in plasma and urine. *J Biol Chem* 153:259, 1944.
49. Beerstecher E, Spangler S, Granick S, et al: Blood vitamins, hormones, enzymes. Blood coenzymes: Vertebrates, in *Blood and Other Body Fluids*, edited by PL Altman, DS Dittmer, p 108. Federation of American Societies for Experimental Biology, Washington, DC, 1961.
50. Kaplan NO, Lipmann F: The assay of distribution of coenzyme A. *J Biol Chem* 174:37, 1948.
51. Klein JR, Perlzweig WA, Handler P: Determination of nicotinic acid in blood cells and plasma. *J Biol Chem* 145:27, 1942.
52. Pearson PB: The pantothenic acid content of the blood of mammalia. *J Biol Chem* 140:423, 1941.
53. Masse PG, Mahuren JD, Tranchant C, Dosy J: B-6, vitamers and 4-pyridoxic acid in the plasma, erythrocytes, and urine of postmenopausal women. *Am J Clin Nutr* 80:946, 2004.
54. Burch HB, Bessey OA, Lowry OH: Fluorometric measurements of riboflavin and its natural derivatives in small quantities of blood serum and cells. *J Biol Chem* 175:457, 1948.
55. Beutler E: Glutathione reductase: Stimulation in normal subjects by riboflavin supplementation. *Science* 165:613, 1969.
56. Burch HB, Bessey OA, Love RH, Lowry OH: The determination of thiamine and thiamine phosphates in small quantities of blood and blood cells. *J Biol Chem* 198:477, 1952.
57. Metais P, Mandel P: Teneur en acide desoxypentosenucleique des leucocytes chez l'homme normal et a l'etat pathologique. *C R Seances Soc Biol Fil* 144:277, 1950.
58. Liang HR, Takagaki T, Foltz RL, Bennett P: Quantitative determination of endogenous sorbitol and fructose in human erythrocytes by atmospheric-pressure chemical ionization LC tandem mass spectrometry. *J Chromatogr B Analyt Technol Biomed Life Sci* 824:36, 2005.
59. Lionetti FJ, McLellan WL, Fortier NL, Foster JM: Phosphate esters produced from inosine in human erythrocyte ghosts. *Arch Biochem* 94:7, 1961.
60. Kawaguchi M, Fujii T, Kamiya Y, et al: Effects of fructose ingestion on sorbitol and fructose 3-phosphate contents of erythrocytes from healthy men. *Acta Diabetol* 33:100, 1996.
61. Petersen A, Szwergold BS, Kappler F, et al: Identification of sorbitol 3-phosphate and fructose 3-phosphate in normal and diabetic human erythrocytes. *J Biol Chem* 265:17424, 1990.
62. Colomer D, Pujades A, Carballo E, Vives Corrons JL: Erythrocyte fructose 2, 6-bisphosphate content in congenital hemolytic anemias. *Hemoglobin* 15:517, 1991.
63. Deichmann WB, Dierker M: The spectrophotometric estimation of hexuronates (expressed as glucuronic acid) in plasma or serum. *J Biol Chem* 163:753, 1946.
64. Jung CY: Carrier-mediated glucose transport across human red cell membranes, in *The Red Blood Cell*, edited by DM Surgenor, p 705. Academic Press, New York, 1975.
65. Lacko L, Wittke B, Geck P: The temperature dependence of the exchange transport of glucose in human erythrocytes. *J Cell Physiol* 82:213, 1973.
66. Bartlett GR: Glucose and mannose diphosphates in the red blood cell. *Biochim Biophys Acta* 156:231, 1968.
67. Johnson RE, Edward HT, Dill DB, Wilson JW: Blood as a physicochemical system. XIII. The distribution of lactate. *J Biol Chem* 157:461, 1945.
68. Bartlett GR, Bucolo G: Octulose phosphates from the human red blood cell. *Biochem Biophys Res Commun* 3:474, 1960.
69. Mandel P, Métals P: Les acides nucléiques du plasma sanguin chez l'homme. *C R Seances Soc Biol Fil* 142:241, 1948.
70. Aminoff D, Anderson J, Dabich L, Gathmann WD: Sialic acid content of erythrocytes in normal individuals and patients with certain hematologic disorders. *Am J Hematol* 9:381, 1980.
71. Vanderheiden BS: Ribosediphosphate in the human erythrocyte. *Biochem Biophys Res Commun* 6:117, 1961.
72. Bruns FH, Noltmann E, Vahlhaus E: Über den Stoffwechsel von Ribose-5-phosphat in Hämolysaten. I. Aktivitäts-messung und Eigenschaften der Phosphoribose-isomerase. II. Der Pentosephosphate-Cyclus in roten Blutzellen. *Biochem Z* 330:483, 1958.
73. Bucolo G, Bartlett GR: Sedoheptulose diphosphate formation by the human red blood cell. *Biochem Biophys Res Commun* 3:620, 1960.
74. Inoue S, Lin SL, Chang T et al: Identification of free deaminated sialic acid (2-keto-3-deoxy-D-glycero-D-galacto-nononic acid) in human red blood cells and its elevated expression in fetal cord red blood cells and ovarian cancer cells. *J Biol Chem* 273:27199, 1998.
75. Kehoe RA, Cholak J, Story RV: A spectrochemical study of the normal ranges of concentration of certain trace metals in biological materials. *J Nutr* 19:579, 1940.
76. Hunter G: Micro-determination of bromide in body fluids. *Biochem J* 60:261, 1955.
77. Ojo JO, Oluwole AF, Durosinmi MA, et al: Baseline levels of elemental concentrations in whole blood, plasma, and erythrocytes of Nigerian subjects. *Biol Trace Elem Res* 43–44:461, 1994.
78. Bernard J-F, Bournier O, Boivin P: Human erythrocytic calcium concentration in hemolytic anemia. *Biomedicine* 23:431, 1975.
79. Shoji S, Komiyama A, Nakamura M, Nomoto S: Calcium content of healthy human erythrocytes. *Clin Chem* 35:1264, 1989.
80. Bernstein RE: Potassium and sodium balance in mammalian red cells. *Science* 120:459, 1954.
81. Herring WB, Leavell BS, Paizao LM, Yoe JH: Trace metals in human plasma and red blood cells: A study of magnesium, chromium, nickel, copper and zinc. I. Observations of normal subjects. *Am J Clin Nutr* 8:846, 1960.
82. Heyrovsky A: The biochemistry of cobalt. III. Amounts of cobalt in plasma, erythrocytes, urine, and feces of normal subjects. *Cas Lek Cesk* 91:680, 1952.
83. Mahalingam TR, Vijayalakshmi S, Prabhu RK et al: Studies on some trace and minor elements in blood—A survey of the Kalpakkam (India) population. 2. Reference values for plasma and red cells, and correlation with coronary risk index. *Biol Trace Elem Res* 57:207, 1997.
84. Lahey ME, Gubler CJ, Cartwright GE, Wintrobe MM: Studies on copper metabolism. VI. Blood copper in normal human subjects. *J Clin Invest* 32:322, 1953.
85. Largent EJ, Cholak J: Blood electrolytes. Man, in *Blood and Other Body Fluids*, edited by PL Altman, DS Dittmer, p 21. Federation of American Societies for Experimental Biology, Washington, DC, 1961.
86. McClendon JF, Foster WC: Protein-bound iodine in erythrocytes and plasma and elsewhere. *Am J Med Sci* 207:549, 1944.
87. Jensovsky L, Roth Z: Der normale Bleigehalt im menschlichen Blute. *Naturwissenschaften* 48:382, 1961.
88. McCance RA, Widdowson EM: The effect of development, anaemia, and undernutrition on the composition of the erythrocyte. *Clin Sci* 15:409, 1956.
89. Huijgen HJ, Sanders R, van Olden RW, et al: Intracellular and extracellular blood magnesium fractions in hemodialysis patients: Is the ionized fraction a measure of magnesium excess? *Clin Chem* 44:639, 1998.
90. Martin BJ, Lyon TD, Fell GS, McKay P: Erythrocyte magnesium in elderly patients: Not a reliable guide to magnesium status. *J Trace Elem Med Biol* 11:44, 1997.
91. Miller DO, Yoe JH: Spectrophotometric determination of manganese in human plasma and red cells with benzohydroxamic acid. *Anal Chim Acta* 26:224, 1962.
92. Bartlett GR, Savage E, Hughes L, Marlow AA: Carbohydrate intermediates and related cofactors with benzohydroxamic acid. *J Appl Physiol* 6:51, 1953.
93. Ferranti F, Giannetti O: The microdetermination of phosphorus (inorganic, acid-soluble, lipoid and total) in the blood and excretions. *Diagn Tec Lab Napoli Riv Mens* 4:664, 1933.
94. Overman RR, Davis AK: The application of flame photometry to sodium and potassium determinations in biological fluids. *J Biol Chem* 168:641, 1947.
95. Mayer KDF, Starkey BJ: Simpler flame photometric determination of erythrocyte sodium and potassium: The reference range for apparently healthy adults. *Clin Chem* 23:275, 1977.
96. Bernard JF, Bournier O, Renoux M, et al: Unclassified haemolytic anaemia with splenomegaly and erythrocyte cation abnormalities—A disease of the spleen? *Scand J Haematol* 17:231, 1976.
97. Hald PM: Notes on the determination and distribution of sodium and potassium in cells and serum of normal human blood. *J Biol Chem* 163:429, 1946.
98. Streef GM: Sodium and calcium content of erythrocytes. *J Biol Chem* 129:661, 1939.
99. Tamada T: An indirect spectrophotometric method for the determination of silicon in serum, whole blood and erythrocytes. *Anal Sci* 19:1291, 2003.
100. Reed L, Denis W: On the distribution of the non-protein sulfur of the blood between serum and corpuscles. *J Biol Chem* 73:623, 1927.
101. Vallee BL, Gibson JG: The zinc content of normal human whole blood, plasma, leucocytes, and erythrocytes. *J Biol Chem* 176:445, 1948.
102. Zak B, Nalbandian RM, Williams LA, Cohen J: Determination of human erythrocyte zinc: Hemoglobin ratios. *Clin Chim Acta* 7:634, 1962.

CHAPTER 31
PRODUCTION OF ERYTHROCYTES

Josef T. Prchal

SUMMARY

Production of red cells or *erythropoiesis*, is a tightly regulated process by which hematopoietic stem cells differentiate into erythroid progenitors and then mature into red cells. Erythropoiesis generates ~2 × 10^{11} new erythrocytes to replace the 2 × 10^{11} red cells (~1% of the total red cell mass) removed from the circulation each day. Red cell production increases severalfold after blood loss or hemolysis.

When one of the progeny of the multipotential hematopoietic stem becomes committed to the erythroid lineage, this early erythroid progenitor undergoes a series of divisions that eventually result in morphologically recognizable erythroblasts. After expulsion of the nucleus, a polychromatophilic macrocyte (a reticulocyte if stained with new methylene blue) leaves the marrow. During the first 24 hours in the circulation, polychromatophilic macrocytes lose their residual organelles (mitochondria and ribosomes) through the action of degradative enzymes and become indistinguishable from other red cells of any age by light microscopy. Erythropoiesis is controlled by transcription factors and cytokines, the principal ones being GATA 1 and erythropoietin (EPO), which influence the rate of lineage commitment, proliferation, apoptosis, differentiation, and number of divisions from the earliest progenitor to late erythroblasts. The number of red cells produced varies in response to tissue oxygenation that determines the level of the transcription factors, hypoxia-inducible factors (HIF), HIF-1 and HIF-2, the principal regulators of the response to hypoxia. HIFs modulate erythropoiesis by regulation of EPO production and iron metabolism.

HISTORY

Erythrocytes evolved largely for the purpose of transporting oxygen to tissues. Thus, the size of the red cell mass and the rate of red cell production must be closely related to supply and demand for oxygen in the tissues. Toward the end of the 19th century, French mountaineers and physiologists established that a low tissue tension of oxygen stimulates red cell production.[1] In 1906, Paul Carnot, a professor at the Sorbonne, and Mademoiselle DeFlandre, his associate, suggested that hypoxia generates a humoral factor capable of stimulating red cell production.[2] Based on questionable experimental data, influential biochemist Friederich Miescher[3] erroneously proposed that marrow hypoxia directly stimulates red cell production. Finally, in 1950, in an ingenious study on parabiotic rats, Kurt Reissmann[4] provided evidence for the existence of an indirect humoral mechanism. This work and work of Erslev and colleagues,[5,6] who demonstrated that the plasma from anemic rabbits and primates contains an erythrocyte-stimulating factor, provided a strong basis for an existence of the factor appropriately named erythropoietin (EPO). In 1957, Jacobson and coworkers[7] reported that EPO was produced by the kidney, a finding that raised the possibility that EPO isolated in adequate amounts might be of therapeutic benefit to uremic patients. After *EPO* cloning and production of recombinant EPO in therapeutic quantities, EPO has proved to not only have indications for therapy of anemia, but also has extraerythroid side effects that are yet to be fully elucidated, such as its purported effect on cancer growth. Widespread use of EPO for the treatment of anemia has surpassed original expectations.

Acronyms and abbreviations that appear in this chapter include: ACEI, angiotensin-converting enzyme inhibitors; AngII, angiotensin II; Bcl-x_L, an antiapoptotic factor; BFU–E, burst-forming unit–erythroid; CFU–E, colony-forming unit–erythroid; CIS, a signal transduction protein that downregulates activity of erythropoietin receptor; CPM, counts per minute; EPO, erythropoietin; EPOR, EPO receptor; FOG, "friend of GATA," a GATA-1 interacting protein; GATA-1 transcription factor; HCP, hematopoietic cell phosphatase; Hct, hematocrit; HIF, hypoxia-inducible transcription factor; ICSH, International Committee on Standardization in Hematology; JAK2, a tyrosine kinase that interacts with erythropoietin receptor; miRNAs, microRNAs are small molecular noncoding RNA molecules; OS-9, osteosarcoma protein 9; PU.1, transcription factor; RACK1, receptor of activated protein kinase C; RAS, the renin–angiotensin system; RCM, red cell mass; RSUME, RWD-containing sumoylation enhancer; SOCS3, a signal transduction protein (also known as CIS3) that downregulates activity of erythropoietin receptor; SSAT, spermidine/spermine-*N*-acetyltransferase; VHL, von Hippel-Lindau protein.

PHYLOGENY OF RED CELL PRODUCTION

HEMOGLOBIN AND RED CELLS

Hemoglobin is present in the most primitive animal forms, such as *Paramecium* and *Tetrahymena*. Some crustaceans, such as *Daphnia*, are capable of developing an oxygen transport system without circulating red cells.[8] One interesting exception is an Antarctic ice fish (*Chaenocephalus aceratus*) lacking hemoglobin.[9] These ice fish compensate for the absence of hemoglobin by their unusual nitric oxide metabolism.[10–12] They have very large hearts and unusually large diameter capillaries. This permits a large volume of blood to circulate at high flow rate and at low vascular pressure because of decreased peripheral resistance. This permits their survival in the very high oxygen content of Antarctic waters.[10]

An erythroid cell that can synthesize, carry, and protect hemoglobin from oxidation was found only with the development of a circulatory system. Circulating nucleated erythrocytes first appear in the worms of the phylum Nemertina and in the sessile marine creatures of the phylum Phoronida. Erythropoiesis in these primitive invertebrates takes place near or on the peritoneal surface, derived from endothelial cells.[13] Nonnucleated red cells are observed for the first time in the more advanced phylum Annelida. However, the evolutionary advantage derived from enucleation appears to be slight. Nucleated red cells are observed in more advanced animals, such as reptiles and birds.[14] All mammalian erythrocytes are nonnucleated and in most species are disc shaped, but are oval in some species.[15] The emergence of red cells appears to be related to the protective and regulatory effect of intracellular compounds on hemoglobin and its oxygen affinity.

In premammalian species, the spleen is the fundamental erythropoietic organ. However, in some fish, the kidneys also are involved in red cell production.[16,17] In vertebrates, an evolutionary shift occurred from the spleen to the liver and from the liver to the hollow bones.[18] The homeostatic regulation of blood or hemoglobin production has been studied in *Daphnia*,[8] where a balance exists between oxygen need and hemoglobin production. In higher animals, this relationship is maintained by adjusting red cell production. Studies of birds,[19] fish,[20] and mammals[21] indicate red cell production is controlled by EPO, which is capable of adjusting red cell production to the demands for oxygen in the tissues. EPO of mammals has considerable biologic similarity and genetic homology.[22]

ONTOGENY OF RED CELL PRODUCTION

EMBRYONIC AND FETAL ERYTHROPOIESIS

The environment within the bone apparently is optimal for cellular proliferation and maturation. However, bone cavities do not develop until the fifth fetal month. Other, presumably less favorable, sites are responsible for red cell production during early embryonic life (see Chap. 6). In the human, large nucleated blood cells are first formed in the yolk sac[23] and some enucleate.[24] During the second gestational month, erythropoiesis moves to fetal liver, wherein smaller, but still macrocytic, nonnucleated cells are produced.[25,26] At birth, the hepatic phase of blood cell production ceases, and erythropoiesis moves to the marrow. Refer to Chaps. 6 and 48 for details of developmental switching of embryonic, fetal, and adult globin expression.

During the neonatal period, the volume of available marrow space is almost the same as the total volume of hematopoietic cells and marrow vasculature.[27] This process continues for a few years until the growth of bones and bone cavities exceeds the growth of hematopoietic mass. However, whenever the demand on erythropoiesis increases (blood loss, hypoxia, thalassemia, or hemolysis), the lack of reserve space in neonates and small children reactivates extramedullary erythropoiesis in the liver and spleen.[28] In adults, expansion of marrow space continues, and the amount of fatty tissue gradually increases in all bone cavities. Because of the abundant marrow space, compensatory reactivation of extramedullary sites rarely occurs in later life. Extramedullary hematopoiesis during adult years indicates pathologic rather than compensatory blood formation, such as seen in primary myelofibrosis (Chap. 91) wherein the stem cells have abnormal interaction with the extracellular matrix.[29] During fetal life, EPO production is primarily hepatic.[30] At birth, a gradual switch to renal production of EPO occurs. In the adult, the kidney is responsible for approximately 85 percent of total production (see Chap. 36).[31,32]

CELLULAR COMPONENTS OF ERYTHROPOIESIS

PROGENITOR CELLS

Our ability to evaluate early erythropoiesis rests on functional assays of hematopoietic progenitors. The developmentally earliest defined erythroid progenitor is the burst-forming unit–erythroid (BFU–E). It was initially termed a burst because it contains cells still capable of migration. These cells form smaller clusters around a larger central colony, giving the appearance of a sunburst with satellite colonies (Fig. 31–1). However, all the cells in the colony and its satellites are derived from a single BFU–E and, thus, are clonal. BFU–E takes longer than more mature erythroid progenitors to form a colony of erythroblasts (~10–14 days) and form a relatively large BFU–E colony (~2000 cells). BFU–E expresses EPO receptors (EPORs). BFU–E then mature into colony-forming unit–erythroids (CFU–E), the more mature erythroid progenitor. CFU–E is the later, more differentiated erythroid progenitor that is identified *in vitro* by smaller colonies (50–200 cells) that mature in 3 to 5 days. However, EPOR density and EPO dependency increase gradually as progenitor cells mature, culminating at the level of the CFU–E.[33] BFU–E and CFU–E cannot be identified by microscopy (see Chap. 29), but they can be studied *in vitro* by their ability to generate microscopically recognizable hemoglobinized precursors (i.e., erythroblasts) by so-called clonogenic assays on semisolid media.

PRECURSOR CELLS

In contrast, cells that constitute the latter stages of erythropoiesis can be identified by light microscopy (see Chap. 29). The number of erythroid precursor cells determines to a great extent the number of red cells produced. The proerythroblasts also contain EPORs that, in the presence of higher than normal levels of EPO, may accelerate their entry into their first mitotic division. This process may lead to a shortened marrow transit time of erythroblasts[34] and result in release of still immature erythrocytes (polychromatophilic macrocytes), so-called stress reticulocytes (Fig. 31–2).[35] Creation of a normal red cell is the end result of an orderly transformation of a proerythroblast with a large nucleus and a volume of approximately 900 fl to a hemoglobinized anucleate disc-shaped cell with a volume of approximately 90 fl. Although cytoplasmic maturation is continuous, the interposed mitotic divisions cause a stepwise reduction in cytoplasmic and nuclear volumes, enabling recognition of proerythroblasts, erythroblasts, and polychromatophilic macrocytes (reticulocytes) with light microscopy (see Chap. 29). Direct measurements of the number of marrow erythroblasts and reticulocytes have shown approximately 50 erythroblasts and approximately 124 reticulocytes for each proerythroblast (Table 31–1).[36,37] This distribution conforms to the number of cells in a theoretic erythroid pyramid (Table 31–1, Fig. 31–3). In the pyramid, each erythroblast undergoes five mitotic divisions over 5 days before the orthochromatic erythroblast loses its nucleus and enters a 2- to 3-day period of maturation before its release from the marrow. The size and shape of these erythroid pyramids undoubtedly vary, but such variations play a role in the physiologic control of red cell production. When production is suppressed, as in anemia of chronic renal disease (caused by lack of EPO), the distribution of erythroblasts appears normal, with no morphologic or ferrokinetic evidence

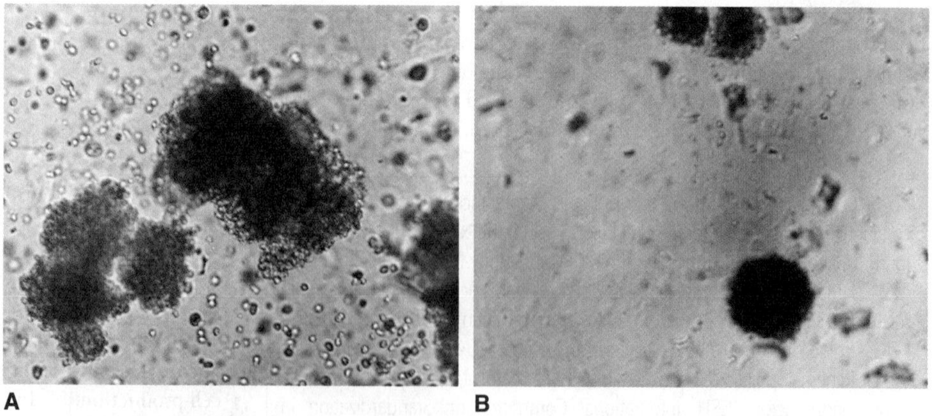

FIGURE 31–1. BFU–E and CFU–E. Erythroid colony growth in methylcellulose medium in presence of erythropoietin. Normal human marrow. The colonies are stained for hemoglobin. **A.** Burst-forming unit–erythroid (BFU–E). This colony grows from a single marrow erythroid progenitor cell (BFU–E). It was photographed at 14 days in culture. The BFU–E is a differentiated cell, committed to the erythroid lineage. The BFU–E is a more primitive progenitor in the erythroid maturation pathway than the colony-forming unit–erythroid (CFU–E). The colony it forms is large, compared to the CFU–E, has spreading margins, and often satellite colonies. **B.** CFU–E. This colony was photographed at day 7 in culture. The CFU–E originates from a more mature single progenitor cell than the BFU–E. The CFU–E is smaller and grows typically in a tight, dense colony, compared to the BFU–E. The sequence established in the erythroid lineage is BFU–E, CFU–E, erythrocyte precursors (proerythroblast, etc.). *(Used with permission from* Lichtman's Atlas of Hematology, *www.accessmedicine.com.)*

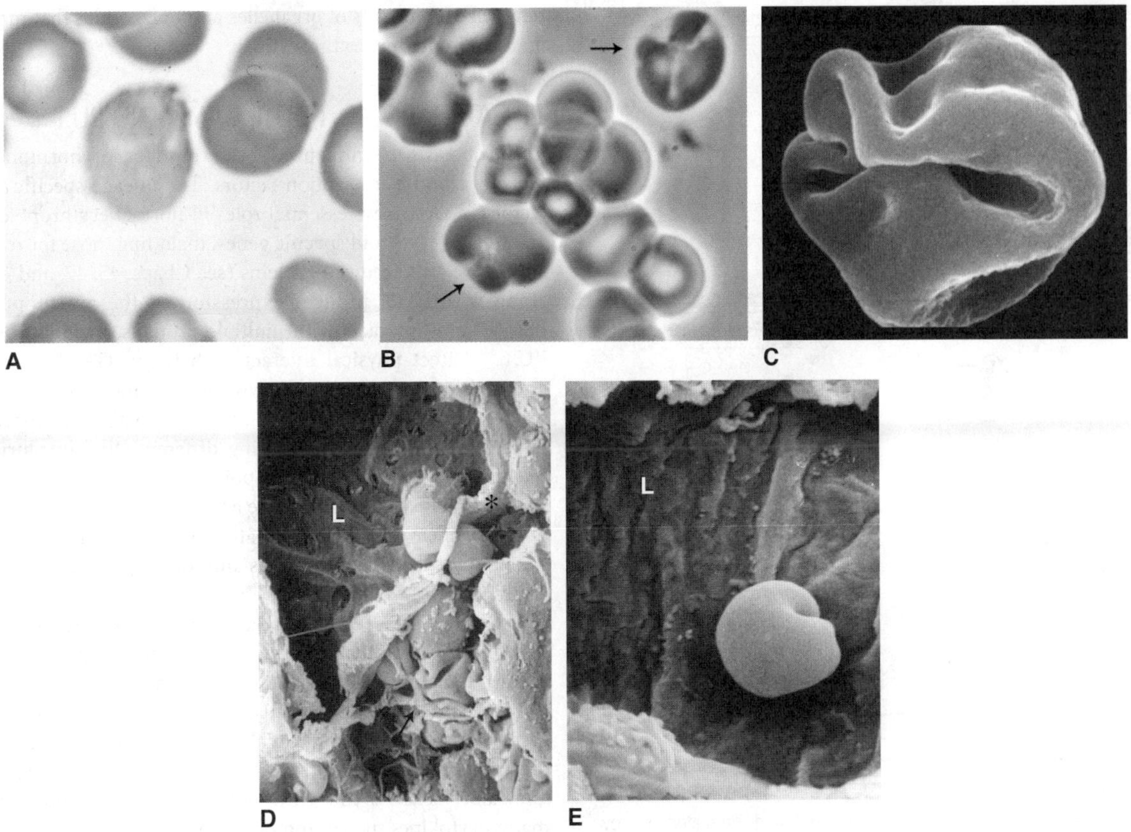

FIGURE 31–2. Stress reticulocytes. **A.** Blood film. Hemolytic anemia. The polychromatophilic macrocyte with puckering evident by the cloverleaf-shaped clear areas (folds) is a characteristic stress erythrocyte, so named because they are prematurely released from the marrow by high levels of erythropoietin, usually as a result of a hemolytic anemia. They are large, intensely polychromatophilic, and often have evidence of excess surface area as evident by folds. **B.** Phase contrast microscopy of the blood cells in suspension from a case of hemolytic anemia. The *arrows* point to two macrocytes with puckered (folded) surfaces, characteristic of stress reticulocytes. **C.** A scanning electron micrograph of a stress reticulocyte. Note the markedly increased surface area to volume relationship for a red cell. **D.** Scanning electron micrograph of a marrow sinus of a mouse. *L* denotes the sinus lumen. The *asterisk* is the edge of the endothelial lining of the sinus, torn in preparation for microscopy. The *arrow* points to two anucleate red cells folded amidst the reticular cell extensions that make up the stroma of marrow. Note the severe folding of reticulocytes *in situ*. Note similarity between folds of the cell to the scanning image in **(C)**. Just below the *asterisk* is an enucleated red cell (reticulocyte) half in the hematopoietic space and half in the lumen, presumptively in egress. Note the surface folding required when traversing the narrow pore in endothelium. **E.** A marrow sinus with an anucleate red cell emerging into the lumen. Note the folding required to negotiate the narrow pore through which the cell is exiting. (See Chap. 4 for details of erythrocyte egress.) *(Used with permission from* Lichtman's Atlas of Hematology, *www.accessmedicine.com.)*

of ineffective erythropoiesis or abnormal erythroblast apoptosis.[34] When production is increased, as in severe hemolytic anemia, the erythroblastic pyramids also appear normal, with no evidence of additional mitotic divisions. Consequently, the rate of red cell production largely depends on the number of erythroid progenitors formed.

TABLE 31–1. Erythroid Pools

	Cell Number × 10[8] per kg/Body Weight	
Cell Type	Observed*	Theoretic Model (Fig. 31–3)
Proerythroblasts	1	1
Erythroblasts	49	58
Marrow reticulocytes	82	64
Blood reticulocytes	31	32
Mature red cells	3300	3800

Adapted from Donohue et al[31] and Finch et al.[32]

As the erythroblast matures, its synthetic activities increase rapidly, producing all proteins characteristic of mature red blood cells, particularly globin. Eventually 95 percent of all protein in the red cell is hemoglobin, almost all hemoglobin A ($\alpha_2\beta_2$) in adults, with only small amounts of hemoglobin F ($\alpha_2\gamma_2$) and hemoglobin A_2 ($\alpha_2\delta_2$). Hemoglobin F is unequally distributed and is present only in some erythrocytes, designated as F cells (see Chaps. 47 and 48).

EPOR density declines sharply on early erythroblasts, and EPORs are absent from the more mature erythroblast forms while the number of receptors for transferrin increases, reflecting the increased demands for iron for heme synthesis. The microenvironment may be important for proliferation and maturation of erythroblasts. However, *in situ* secreted or circulating growth factors and cytokines appear to be less important for precursor cells than for progenitor cells. Intercellular adhesion molecules secure the structural integrity of the marrow, and fibronectin is of special importance for erythroblasts.[38] Loss of fibronectin receptors heralds the migration of polychromatophilic macrocytes (reticulocytes) into blood, but some newly emerging erythrocytes remain sticky even after release and are temporarily sequestered by the spleen (see Chap. 5). Because erythroid colonies developed *in vitro* consist mainly of nucleated red cells, enucleation may primarily be induced by marrow stromal cells (see Chaps. 4 and 29).

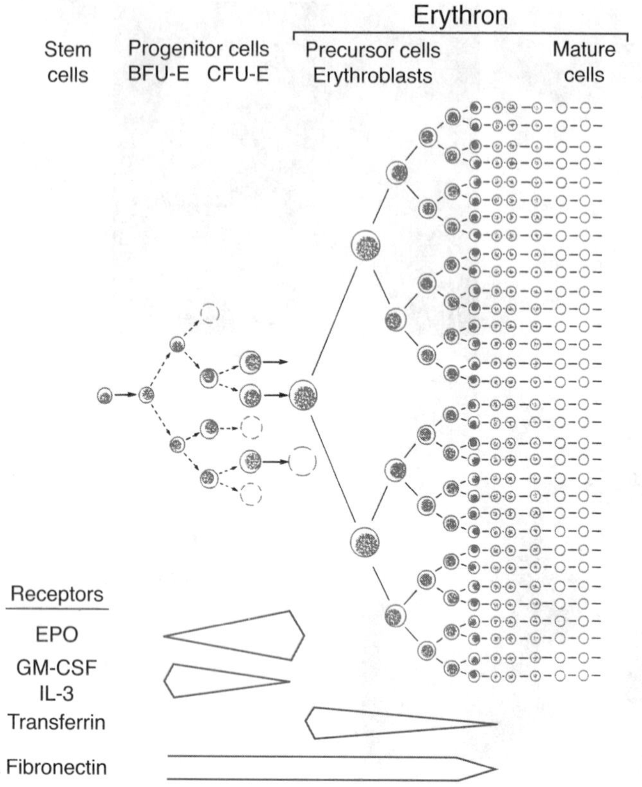

FIGURE 31–3. Theoretical model of proliferation of erythroid-committed marrow cells, including their most important receptors. GM-CSF, granulocyte-macrophage colony-stimulating factor; IL, interleukin.

Microscopic determination of marrow cellularity and proportion of erythroblasts permits semiquantitative evaluation of erythropoiesis. However, in disease states the presence of ineffective erythropoiesis, as seen in iron deficiency, anemia of chronic disease, megaloblastic anemias, and thalassemias, makes the morphologic approach misleading (see Chaps. 37, 41, 42, and 47). Red cell production can be accurately estimated by ferrokinetic studies using ^{59}Fe. Similarly, the amount of the final product of erythropoiesis, the red cell mass, can also be accurately measured. Unfortunately, the ever-increasing regulation of even minute amounts of radioisotopes used *in vivo* makes these methods available in only a few specialized centers.

Chaps. 6, 47, and 48 discuss developmental control of erythropoiesis, differential use of globin genes, and the crucial differences between embryonic yolk sac and fetal/adult definite erythropoiesis. This chapter focuses mainly on adult erythropoiesis.

REGULATION OF ERYTHROPOIESIS

Erythropoiesis is a tightly regulated system, but the details are still not fully elucidated. Much remains to be learned from uncovering the molecular basis of many congenital and acquired mutations that disrupt the control of erythropoiesis.

Erythropoiesis can be viewed as composed of three stages. In the initial stage, commitment of pluripotential hematopoietic progenitors to committed erythroid precursors takes place. The second stage is characterized by expansion of erythroid progenitors that is largely regulated by EPO and is made effective by the appearance of EPOR on surface of these progenitors. The expression of EPOR peaks in early erythroblasts and then declines. The terminal stage consists of enucleation and removal of remnants of organelles and nucleotides that may be toxic to mature circulating erythrocytes.

GATA-1, BCL-X_L, FOG-1, GAS6, AND PU.1

Erythropoiesis is influenced by a number of hormones/cytokines, receptors, and transcription factors. The lineage-specific transcription factor GATA-1 plays essential roles in normal erythropoiesis and activates many erythroid specific genes, including those for α and β globin and cytoskeletal red cell proteins (see Chaps. 45, 47, and 48). GATA-1, along with EPO, induces expression of the antiapoptotic protein Bcl-x_L[39] and interacts with multiple proteins, including FOG-1[40] and PU.1.[41] Direct physical interaction between GATA-1 and FOG-1 is essential for normal human erythroid and megakaryocyte maturation *in vivo*.[42] In contrast, GATA-1 interaction with PU.1 appears to counteract erythropoiesis by inducing differentiation of pluripotent stem cell to myeloid and B lymphopoiesis and inhibition of erythropoiesis.[41,43,44] Whereas PU.1 absence appears to be required for completion of terminal erythroid differentiation, low levels of PU.1 expression are essential for fetal erythropoiesis and for proper augmentation of adult erythropoiesis at times of stress.[45]

Growth arrest-specific 6 (Gas6) protein is a secreted vitamin K-dependent protein that interacts with cell membranes and leads to intracellular signaling (via its receptor tyrosine kinases). Gas6 receptors are expressed in hematopoietic tissue, megakaryocytes, myelomonocytic precursors, and marrow stromal cells. Gas6 has been shown to amplify the erythropoietic response to EPO using a mouse model of Gas6 knockout.[46] Gas6 is known to downregulate the expression of inflammatory cytokines such as tumor necrosis factor-α by macrophages.[47]

Multipotent progenitors (see Chap. 16) and primitive erythroid progenitors, the BFU–E, require stem cell factor, interleukin-3, granulocyte-macrophage colony-stimulating factor, and thrombopoietin for growth and survival (Fig. 31–4).

ERYTHROPOIETIN, OXYGEN SENSING, AND HYPOXIA-INDUCIBLE FACTOR

Erythropoietin

The principal hormone regulating erythropoiesis is EPO, which is produced principally in the kidney.[7] Erythroid progenitors express their own EPO.[48] Different levels of kidney-produced EPO are optimal for various stages of erythroid maturation.[49] Purification of EPO provided a partial protein sequence that led to cloning of the gene and permitted mass production of the recombinant protein.[50] EPO and its recombinant form are heavily glycosylated α-globulins with a molecular mass of 34,000 daltons and a specific activity of approximately 200,000 IU/mg.[51,52] Sixty percent of the molecular weight of the recombinant protein is contributed by amino acids; the remaining 40 percent is composed of carbohydrate. Using molecular probes for *EPO*, messenger RNA (mRNA) enabled the localization of the synthesis of EPO to renal cortical interstitial cells[53,54] of endothelial or fibroblastic lineage. The cells appear to function in an all-or-none fashion, with the overall production of mRNA dependent on the number of cells activated.[55]

Certain 5′ sequences located 6000 to 12,000 bp upstream also affect EPO gene transcription.[56] These sequences are not hypoxia sensitive but appear necessary for tissue and cellular specificity.[56] Hepatic production is contributed primarily by hepatocytes but is a less important source than is the kidney.[57] During fetal life, however, hepatic EPO production is of major importance for red cell production (see Chap. 6).[58,59] EPO production is regulated almost exclusively by hypoxia at the transcription level. EPO is not stored but secreted immediately.[53–55] Circulating recombinant EPO and presumably native EPO have a

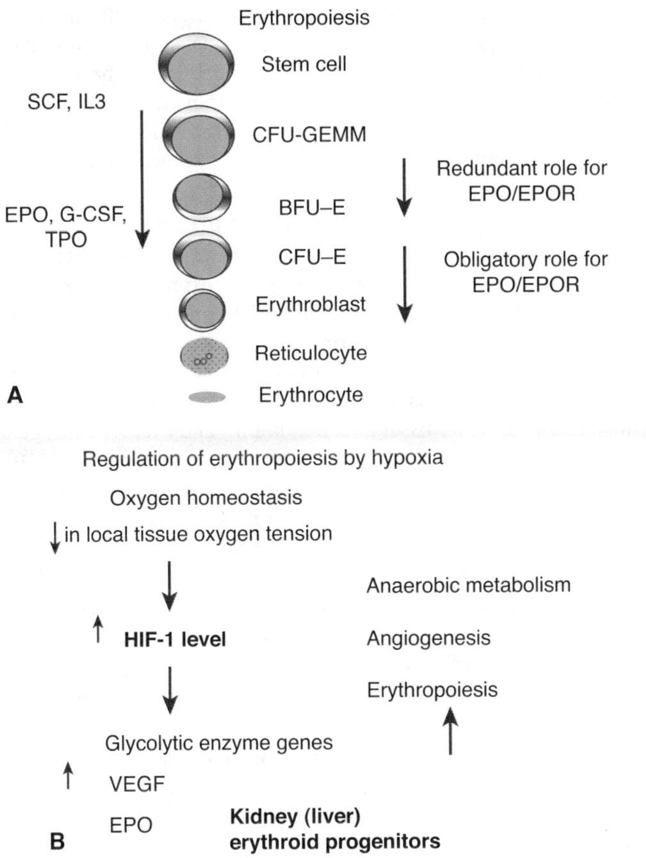

FIGURE 31–4. A. Cytokine influence on hematopoiesis. CFU-GEMM, colony-forming unit–growing granulocyte, erythrocyte, megakaryocyte, and macrophage precursors; G-CSF, granulocyte colony-stimulating factor; IL3, interleukin-3; SCF, stem cell factor; TPO, thrombopoietin. **B.** Regulation of erythropoiesis by hypoxia. HIF-1, hypoxia inducible factor-1; VEGF, vascular endothelial growth factor I.

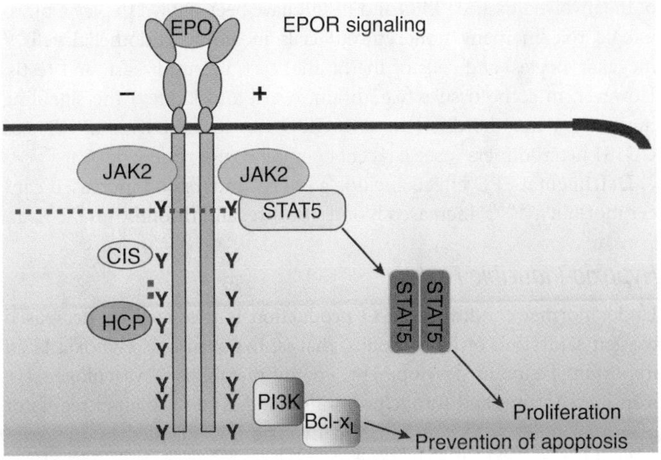

FIGURE 31–5. Outline of erythropoietin–erythropoietin receptor (EPO–EPOR) signaling. Activation of JAK2 and STAT5 represents erythropoiesis-promoting signals. Interaction of CIS and HCP inhibit erythropoiesis. PI3 kinase (PI3K) activation of Bcl-x_L inhibits apoptosis of erythroid progenitors. HCP, hematopoietic cell phosphatase.

half-life ($T_{1/2}$) of 4 to 12 hours, with a volume of distribution slightly larger than that of the plasma volume.[60] EPO is degraded after it binds to EPOR (see "Erythropoietin Receptor" below).[61]

Erythropoietin Receptor

Interaction of EPO with its receptor EPOR results in (1) stimulation of erythroid cell division, (2) erythroid differentiation by induction of erythroid-specific protein expression, and (3) prevention of erythroid progenitor apoptosis (reviewed in reference 72). [62] Earlier models of this interaction were based on the ligand (EPO)-induced homodimerization of EPOR. In reality, EPOR is a preformed homodimer that undergoes a major conformational change upon binding,[63] which initiates the EPO-specific erythroid signal transduction cascade (Fig. 31–5). The cytoplasmic portion of EPOR contains a positive regulatory domain that interacts with Janus kinase 2 (JAK2).[64] Immediately after EPO binding, JAK2 cross-phosphorylates the EPOR itself, and other proteins such as STAT5, thus initiating a cascade of erythroid-specific signaling.[65] JAK2/STAT5 signaling plays an essential role in EPO–EPOR-mediated regulation of erythropoiesis (Fig. 31–5).[66] Deficiency of EPO–EPOR is lethal by abrogating fetal liver erythropoiesis (but not the "primitive" yolk sac erythropoiesis). However, in these *EPO* or *EPOR* knockout mice, differentiation of pluripotential stem cells to BFU–E occurs, but not the subsequent erythroid differentiation. This occurrence demonstrates the crucial role of EPO in terminal erythroid maturation and differentiation.[67–69] The C-terminal cytoplasmic portion of EPOR also possesses a domain essential for prevention of apoptosis (Fig. 31–5) by inducing expression of Bcl-x_L via phosphoinositide 3 kinase.[39] However, the cytoplasmic portion of EPOR also contains a negative regulatory domain[70] that interacts with hematopoietic cell phosphatase (HCP, also known as SHP1) and down-modulates signal transduction.[71] Once recruited by EPOR tyrosine (Y)429, HCP attaches to the cytoplasmic EPOR domain and dephosphorylates JAK2. Inactivation of the HCP binding site leads to prolonged phosphorylation of JAK2/STAT5.[71,72] CIS3 (also known as SOCS3), another negative regulator of erythropoiesis, binds to the cytoplasmic portion of the EPOR Y401 and suppresses EPO-dependent JAK2/STAT5 signaling.[73,74] Thus, deletion of the distal C-terminal cytoplasmic portion of EPOR results in a truncated EPOR, abolishes negative regulatory elements, and results in increased proliferation of erythroid progenitor cells. Gain-of-function mutations resulting from deletion of the negative regulatory domain of the *EPOR* gene (see Chap. 56) have been demonstrated in a proportion of patients with primary familial and congenital polycythemia, but are rarely found in erythroleukemia.[75]

Because the activation signal after EPO binding to its receptor is downregulated and EPO rapidly disappears after binding to EPOR, EPO–EPOR internalization is one mechanism of downregulation of EPO signaling.[61] After EPO binds to the receptor, EPO–EPOR complexes are ubiquinated, internalized, and targeted for degradation. This process involves two proteolytic systems, the proteosomes that remove part of the intracellular domain of EPOR at the cell surface and the lysosomes that degrade the EPO–EPOR complex in the cytoplasm.[76]

Another incompletely understood mechanism of erythropoiesis regulation is the presence of several EPOR isoforms, some of which may have an inhibitory function on erythropoiesis.[77–79]

Nonerythroid Effect of Erythropoietin Signaling

Soon after the erythroid effects of recombinant EPO were described, nonerythroid effects were identified.[80] Some of these effects are beneficial, including roles in neural, cardiovascular, and retinal tissues and in immune function and in tissue repair. It has been claimed that the hormone also exerts beneficial effects on athletic performance and improved neurocognition, but these are not convincingly substantiated. The effects of EPO in nonerythroid tissues are the result of EPO binding to EPOR, and, as in erythroid cells, the EPO–EPOR interaction initiates a signal transduction process that regulates the survival, growth, and differentiation of the involved tissue.[81] EPO and EPOR have been shown to play a physiologic role in many nonerythroid cells including endothelial cells,[82] megakaryocytes, and cells of the brain, heart, uterus, breast, and testis. However, in some tissues (e.g., brain, heart, and kidney) the signaling mechanism may be different since EPO can interact with EPOR and CD131 heterodimers[83]; see a recent comprehensive review.[84]

Detrimental EPO effects include a poorly understood increased cancer mortality,[64,85,86] increased blood pressure, and thromboses.[84]

Hypoxia-Inducible Factors

Under normal conditions, EPO production is mediated by decreased oxygen saturation of hemoglobin, that is, hypoxemia.[49] Hypoxia is an important factor in development, energy metabolism, vasculogenesis, iron metabolism, and tumor promotion and is the principal regulator of erythropoiesis. The response to hypoxia is controlled by hypoxia-inducible factors (HIF) transcriptional factors.[87,88] Adaptive physiologic responses to hypoxia serve to (1) increase O_2 delivery to cells, (2) allow cells to survive under reduced O_2 by activating glycolysis, and (3) reduce the formation of reactive oxygen species.[89] The transcription factor HIF-1 is induced in hypoxic cells and binds to the *cis*-acting nucleotide sequence referred to as *hypoxia-responsive element* (HRE), first identified in the 3′-flanking region of the human *EPO* gene.[90] Many hypoxia-inducible genes are directly regulated by HIF-1. Approximately 3 percent of all genes expressed in endothelial tissue are HIF-1 regulated.[91] HIF-1 is a heterodimeric transcription factor composed of a highly-regulated HIF-1α subunit and a constitutively expressed HIF-1β subunit (Fig. 31–6). The HIF-1β subunit belongs to the basic helix-loop-helix containing the PER-ARNT-SIM (PAS)-domain family of transcription factors. Only the α subunits of HIF-1 and HIF-2 are hypoxia regulated and exist only in HIF heterodimers; consequently, they are the key subunits in determining the hypoxia-modulated quantity and activity of HIF-1 and HIF-2 heterodimers. They regulate the resultant transcription of hypoxia-inducible genes. The half-life of HIF-1α in the cell is minutes under normoxic conditions. HIF-1 and HIF-2 α subunits are rapidly degraded by the von Hippel-Lindau (VHL) protein-ubiquitin-proteasome pathway.[92] The targeting and subsequent polyubiquitination of HIF α subunits requires VHL, iron, O_2, and proline hydroxylase activity, and, as depicted in Figure 31–6, this complex constitutes the oxygen sensor.[93,94]

This degradation of HIF-1α is initiated by a posttranslational hydroxylation event at residue proline 564 (P564) that is mediated by one of several iron-containing proline hydroxylases (PHDs). The hydroxylation of HIF-1α facilitates binding to the VHL protein and subsequent ubiquitination and proteasomal degradation. Osteosarcoma protein 9 (OS-9) binds to both HIF-1α and PHD2 and is required for efficient prolyl hydroxylation.[95] Under hypoxic conditions, HIF-1 and HIF-2 α proteins are not degraded and are translocated to the cell nucleus where they dimerize with HIF-β to form the HIF heterodimer that activates transcription through binding to specific HREs on target genes. Another regulatory step involves O_2-dependent asparaginyl-hydroxylation of asparagine (N) 803 in HIF-1α that requires the enzyme FIH-1 (factor inhibiting HIF-1, also known as HIF-3). Hydroxylation of N803 during normoxia blocks the binding of transcription factors p300 and CBP to HIF-1, resulting in inhibition of HIF-1–mediated gene transcription. Under hypoxic conditions, HIF-α is not hydroxylated. The unmodified protein escapes VHL-binding, ubiquitination, and degradation (see Fig. 31–6). When N803 of HIF-1α is not asparaginyl-hydroxylated, p300 and CBP can bind to the HIF-1 heterodimer, allowing transcriptional activation of HIF-1 target genes.

HIF-2 Transcription Factor HIF-1α and HIF-2α exhibit a high degree sequence homology but have differing mRNA expression patterns: HIF-1α is expressed ubiquitously, whereas HIF-2α expression is restricted to certain tissues.[87,96] Both HIF-1α and HIF-2α are regulated by identical mechanisms by hypoxia and form a heterodimer with the same HIF-β subunit. The kidney is the main site of EPO production (i.e., renal interstitial cells), and HIF-1 is the principal regulator of *EPO* transcription in the kidney.[87] In other tissues, such as brain[97] and liver[59] (which generates ~15% of circulating EPO), *EPO* gene transcription is HIF-2-dependent.[96] The discovery of an iron-responsive element in the 5′ untranslated region of *HIF-2α* reveals a novel regulatory link between iron availability and *HIF-2α* expression[98] that may also influence control of erythropoiesis. Therefore, when the iron supply is limited, HIF-2α decreases, and when iron is abundant, liver HIF-2α increases, thereby increasing liver-synthesized EPO production and further promoting erythropoiesis. The importance of HIF-2α in regulation of *EPO* gene was demonstrated by a gain-of-function *HIF-2α* mutation causing erythrocytosis (see Chap. 56).[99]

Hypoxia-Independent Regulation of HIF While O_2-dependent regulation of the HIF-1α-subunit is mediated by prolyl hydroxylases, VHL protein, and the proteasomal complex, hypoxia-independent regulation of HIF-1α has been uncovered. This novel mechanism involves the receptor of activated protein kinase C (RACK1) as a HIF-1α–interacting protein that promotes prolyl hydroxylase/VHL-independent proteasomal degradation of HIF-1α. RACK1 competes with heat shock protein 90 (HSP90) for binding to the PAS-A domain of HIF-1α. HIF-1α degradation is abolished by loss-of-function RACK1. RACK1 binds to the proteasomal

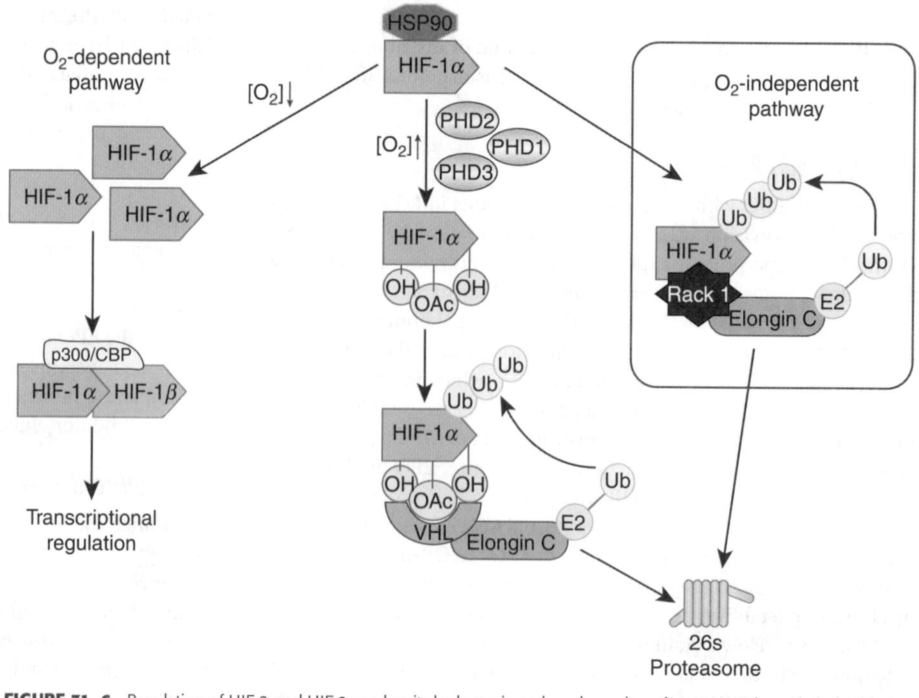

FIGURE 31–6. Regulation of HIF-2 and HIF-2α subunits by hypoxic and nonhypoxic pathways. HIF, hypoxia-inducible factor; HSP90, heat shock protein 90; PHDs, proline hydroxylases; p300 and CBP, cofactors of hypoxia response transcription with HIF-1; RACK1, receptor of activated protein kinase C; ub, ubiquitin residues; VHL, von Hippel-Lindau protein.

subunit, elongin-C, and promotes ubiquitination of HIF-1α (see Fig. 31–6). Therefore, RACK1 and HSP90 are the essential components of an O_2/PHD/VHL-independent mechanism for regulating HIF-1α.[100]

Hypoxia-Dependent and -Independent HIF-1α Regulation Treatment of cells with HSP90 inhibitors induces degradation of HIF-1α even under hypoxic conditions. HSP90 competes with RACK1 for binding to spermidine/spermine-*N*-acetyltransferase-2 (SSAT2) that binds to HIF-1α and promotes its ubiquitination/degradation by stabilizing the interaction of VHL and elongin C. SSAT1, which shares a 46 percent amino acid identity with SSAT2, also binds to HIF-1α and promotes its ubiquitination/degradation. However, in contrast to SSAT2, SSAT1 acts by stabilizing the interaction of HIF-1α with RACK1. Thus, SSAT1 and SSAT2 play complementary roles in promoting O_2-independent and O_2-dependent degradation of HIF-1α. Similarly, elongin-C can be recruited by both oxygen-dependent and -independent binding to HIF-1α (see Fig. 31–6).

Another novel mechanism of HIF-1α regulation has also been described: (1) RSUME (RWD-containing sumoylation enhancer) is induced by hypoxia and enhances the sumoylation of HIF-1α, promoting its stabilization and transcriptional activity during hypoxia[101]; and (2) calcineurin which, along with calcium and calmodulin-dependent serine/threonine phosphatase, inhibits the ubiquitination and proteasomal degradation of HIF-1α.[102]

A third pathway has been proposed to account *for the degradation of HIF-1α* in cells treated with immunophilins and histone deacetylase inhibitors, based on studies suggesting that these agents induce HIF-1α degradation by an O_2-independent mechanism that is also ubiquitin independent.[103]

The rapid degradation of HIF is complex and tightly regulated, and mutations affecting the genes that encode the regulatory factors may underlie some of the unexplained congenital polycythemias.

This complex (see Chaps. 33 and 56 and Fig. 33–6) constitutes the oxygen sensor.[104–106]

INSULIN-LIKE GROWTH FACTOR-1, RENIN–ANGIOTENSIN SYSTEM, AND HEMATOPOIESIS

Although *in vitro* studies of erythropoiesis have provided crucial information about the regulation of erythropoiesis, many experiments were performed in the presence of serum and serum-component proteins capable of stimulating and inhibiting erythropoiesis.[107,108] Using serum-free conditions, insulin-like growth factor-1 (IGF-1) can partially substitute for EPO in BFU–E cultures. Furthermore, anephric nonanemic patients with no detectable EPO have elevated levels of IGF-1.[109]

The renin–angiotensin system (RAS) regulates fluid and electrolyte homeostasis and blood pressure.[110] The primary function of angiotensin during development is modulation of tissue growth and differentiation.[111] Angiotensin II (AngII) is a ligand for two distinct receptors, type 1 (AT1) and type 2. AT1 appears to have a major role in modulating cell proliferation.[112] The role of the RAS in regulating erythropoiesis has been long suspected, although the controlling mechanisms are complex and not fully elucidated. The RAS was first postulated to regulate erythropoiesis in the 1980s after the discovery that use of angiotensin-converting enzyme inhibitors (ACEIs) for treatment of hypertension could cause anemia.[113] This hypothesis is based on the presumption that reduced oxygen pressure in the kidneys triggers HIF-1α to induce EPO release.[114] However, AngII significantly modulates erythropoiesis directly. Whereas AngII directly stimulated proliferation of hematopoietic progenitors *in vitro*,[115] inhibition of its effects using ACEIs induced apoptosis of erythroid progenitors in renal transplant patients.[116] In an *in vivo* laboratory model, mice with angiotensin-converting enzyme gene knockout developed normocytic anemia that was fully reversed with AngII infusion.[117]

ROLE OF APOPTOSIS IN ERYTHROPOIESIS

Prevention of apoptosis is a well-recognized mechanism assuring productive early erythropoiesis and preventing anemia; however, the importance of proapoptotic processes for *productive terminal erythropoiesis* has been demonstrated. Bnip3L is a proapoptotic Bcl-2 family member. The knockout of this gene in *Bnip3L*$^{-/-}$ mice, resulted in expansion of erythroid precursors[118]; however, unexpectedly, the mice had anemia. This was caused by a decreased red cell survival and to the Bnip3L failure to target the mitochondria into autophagosomes for degradation during erythroid maturation.

MICRORNAS IN ERYTHROPOIESIS

MicroRNAs (miRNAs) are small, noncoding, 18 to 22 nt RNAs that regulate gene expression by inhibiting protein translation or by destabilizing target mRNAs; they are important regulators of hematopoiesis. The role of miRNAs in regulation of erythropoiesis is currently being defined. Some miRNAs are mainly expressed in early stages of erythropoiesis, others in late stages, and some have biphasic expression during erythroid differentiation. Some appear to have erythroid-specific expression.[119] miRNAs exact role in erythropoiesis and their molecular targets are currently being defined at many laboratories.[120] One miRNA, miR-223, declines during erythroid differentiation and reduces expression of LIM domain-only protein 2 (LMO2). LMO2 protein was discovered from its involvement by chromosomal translocation in T-cell acute lymphoblastic leukemia. This suggests that LMO2 and its down-modulation of miR-223 is required for erythroid differentiation.[121]

MEASUREMENTS OF RED CELL MASS

The red cell mass is maintained and regulated by the kidney and marrow, which under steady-state conditions precisely replaces cells lost by senescence. Red cell mass defines anemia and polycythemia. The kinetics of red cell production and destruction helps establish their pathogenesis. A number of tests have been developed to measure the three main components of red cell kinetics: red cell mass, rate of red cell production, and rate of red cell destruction. Some of these tests are simple but indirect and only semiquantitative, such as hematocrit, reticulocyte count, haptoglobin, lactic dehydrogenase, and unconjugated bilirubin concentration. Examination of the marrow allows assessment of total cellularity and relative erythroid contribution but is limited in that the kinetics of cell production cannot be inferred from a single static image, obtained from a very small fraction of the whole marrow. These tests are very useful in the aggregate but can be supplemented by more complex but direct quantitation; however, most require use of radioisotopes.

HEMATOCRIT

Packed red cell volume is commonly referred as the *hematocrit*. It can be measured as volume of blood composed of erythrocytes in 1 mL of blood. Total body hematocrit is the volume of red cells in the body divided by the total blood volume. Blood hematocrit is the simplest and most widely used test for estimating the size of red cell mass. In most anemic patients, blood hematocrit gives an excellent approximation of total red cell mass and a functional estimation of the oxygen-carrying capacity and whole blood viscosity. Its main drawback is that it is an indirect measure that is influenced by changes in plasma volume and may not reflect the size of the red cell mass in dehydrated patients. Dehydration usually is clinically apparent and in most cases can be taken into account when evaluating the significance of a specific hematocrit determination. Only direct measurement of red cell mass can differentiate between relative and absolute polycythemia. However, when the hematocrit is greater than 60 percent, almost all patients have an increase in total red cell mass.[122] The extent of the increase cannot be estimated accurately from a hematocrit measurement alone.

RED CELL MASS AND PLASMA VOLUME

A more direct and accurate estimate of the size of the red cell mass is obtained from labeling a known volume of red cells and determining the dilution of this label in blood. Radioactive iron is an excellent label of red cells because it is biosynthetically incorporated into hemoglobin *in vivo*. In experimental animals, radioactive iron can be given to a donor animal and the donor's cells transfused into the animal whose red cell volume is being assessed. However, the radiation exposure to the donor and the hazards of transfusing allogeneic cells preclude its use in humans. Thus, almost all current clinical methods use labeling of autologous red cells *in vitro* by any one of a number of isotopes. If studies must be performed in radiation-sensitive individuals, such as pregnant women, red cell labeling can be performed by nonradioactive chromium-123 or by biotin, which is detected with streptavidin coupled to a fluorochrome.[124] Among the isotopes available, chromium-51 (^{51}Cr) is the most widely used label, although technetium-99m (^{99m}Tc) is convenient and accurate.[125] Chromium in the form of the chromate ion (CrO_2^-) readily enters the red cell and binds to globin chains. Excess isotope in the incubation mixture can be removed by washing or by using ascorbic acid to reduce the chromate ion to a nonpermeant chromic ion. Approximately 15 minutes after injection of a known amount of labeled cells, a sample of blood is obtained; its volume, hematocrit, and radioactivity are determined; and the total red cell volume is calculated from the equation:

$$\text{Red cell mass (mL)} = \frac{\text{CPM of isotype injected}}{\text{CPM of red cells in sample}}$$

where CPM = counts per minute. Sampling time is generally 15 minutes. Chromium also labels white cells; thus, one should centrifuge and remove the buffy coat before labeling if the white cell count is elevated ($>25 \times 10^9$/L).

No theoretical objection exists to measuring the red cell mass using labeled cells. It is independent of the hematocrit of the blood utilized to measure radioactivity, and replicate determination can be made with a coefficient of variation of approximately 1.5 percent.[126] The principal problem lies in reporting the measured red cell mass. The total red cell mass can be expressed as a volume related to body surface (mL/m^2) or as a volume related to body weight (mL/kg). A committee of the International Committee on Standardization in Hematology (ICSH) has extensively examined existing data and concluded that the most reproducible expressions of red cell mass are related to body surface area estimated from height and weight:[127]

$$RCM_{Males} = (1486 \times S) - 285$$

$$RCM_{Females} = (822 \times S) + (1.06 \times Age)$$

where RCM = red cell mass, S = body surface area in square meters, and Age = age in years. The calculated values ± 25 percent included 98 percent of the measured male values and 99 percent of the measured female values.[13]

Despite the ICSH recommendation, the most common method is to report red cell mass values in terms of milliliters per kilogram. However, this method of expression gives erroneously low values in obese individuals because fat is hypovascular. A better method might be to express the red cell mass in terms of lean weight. In general, lean weight is 20 percent less than actual weight in normal males and 25 percent less in normal females.[125] However, estimation of lean weight in obese individuals is inaccurate. From a practical point of view, RCM probably is best reported in terms of actual weight, with mental adjustments made based on body configuration. In general, the RCM of normal females ranges from 23 to 29 mL/kg body weight and of normal males ranges from 26 to 32 mL/kg.[127]

PLASMA LABELS

Red cell mass also can be estimated from plasma volume. Radioactive iodine (^{125}I) is used to label albumin and measure its distribution volume.[128] Other radioactive isotopes of iodine other than ^{99m}Tc have been used, but ^{125}I has virtually supplanted all other plasma labels. Albumin labeled with radioactive iodine is commercially available, and a known amount is injected intravenously. Several blood samples are obtained within the first 15 minutes and centrifuged. CPM per milliliter of plasma is measured, plotted on semilogarithmic paper, and extrapolated to zero time. This procedure is necessary because, in contradistinction to labeled red cells, labeled albumin is removed gradually, beginning immediately after injection. Plasma volume is calculated according to the equation:

$$\text{Plasma volume (mL)} = \frac{\text{CPM of labeled albumin injected}}{\text{CPM/mL plasma at 0 hour}}$$

The continuous exchange of intravascular with extravascular albumin is the major problem encountered when plasma volume is measured with labeled albumin. Even with extrapolation to 0 hour, plasma volume is somewhat larger than that measured with a strictly intravascular protein such as fibrinogen.[129] Consequently, if measurement of the plasma volume is used to calculate the size of the total red cell mass, it is a less-reliable measure than determining red cell mass directly with tagged red cells. This inaccuracy is further aggravated by the fact that the venous hematocrit used to calculate red cell mass from measured plasma volume does not reflect accurately the distribution of plasma and red cells in the body. However, from a practical point of view, the results of estimating RCM from plasma volume are surprisingly accurate and have been advocated based on simplicity and low cost.[128]

TOTAL-BODY HEMATOCRIT

When total RCM is measured with labeled red cells, the value is approximately 10 percent lower than that calculated from plasma volume and the hematocrit of blood. In fact, the mean hematocrit of blood in all of the vessels (total-body hematocrit) clearly is somewhat lower than the hematocrit measured from blood obtained from large vessels; these differences are a result of varying proportions of plasma in different size vessels.

Generally, the ratio of total-body hematocrit as estimated by direct measurements of red cell volume and plasma volume to the large-vessel hematocrit ranges from 0.89 to 0.92.[130] Consequently, when using the determined plasma volume to calculate RCM and total blood volume, a correction factor is necessary, and a value of 0.90 is generally used:

$$\text{Corrected red cell mass} = \frac{\text{Hct} \times \text{plasma volume} \times 0.90}{100 - \text{Hct}}$$

where Hct = hematocrit.

Recommended procedures for determination and evaluation of blood volume are outlined by the ICSH.[131]

MEASUREMENTS OF RED CELL PRODUCTION

Under normal circumstances, most human red cells produced in the marrow live, or have the potential to live, a normal life span. Under certain conditions, however, a fraction of red cell production is ineffective, with destruction of nonviable red cells either within the marrow or shortly after the cells reach the blood.[34]

EFFECTIVE RED CELL PRODUCTION

Effective erythropoiesis is most simply estimated by determining the reticulocyte count. This count usually is expressed as the percentage of red cells that are reticulocytes, but it also can be expressed as the total number of circulating reticulocytes per unit of blood (absolute reticulocyte count and corrected reticulocyte counts; equations 1 and 2 below).

Equation 1

$$\text{Absolute reticulocyte count} = \frac{\%\ \text{reticulocytes} \times \text{red cell count}}{100}$$

Equation 2

$$\text{Corrected reticulocyte \%} = \text{reticulocyte \%} \times \frac{\text{actual hematocrit}}{\text{normal hematocrit}}$$

A simple clinical method to estimate effective erythropoiesis uses the reticulocyte count to calculate the reticulocyte index (see equation 3 below).[132] This measurement depends on several assumptions: (1) the human red cell life span is approximately 100 days (actually approximately 115); (2) the life span is finite and, thus, the oldest 1 of 100 or 1 percent of red cells is removed (and replaced) each day; (3) the reticulocyte is identifiable as such in the blood for 1 day using supravital stain; and (4) the reticulocyte count of 1 percent in a person with a normal hematocrit represents normal red cell production and thus "1" is the basal reticulocyte index.

In anemic patients, two calculations are needed to measure the reticulocyte index and compare it to the normal of 1 in the basal state. To correct the reticulocyte percentage for the lower red cell count in anemic subjects, the reticulocyte percent is multiplied by the ratio of the patient's hematocrit over the normal mean hematocrit, providing a corrected reticulocyte percent.

Conversion of the corrected reticulocyte count (see equation 2 above) the reticulocyte index (equation 3 below) is achieved by taking into account the estimated life span of reticulocytes. The life span of reticulocytes in blood in a normal individual is approximately 1 day. However, when red cell production is increased under conditions of erythropoietic stress, for example, in severe anemia, reticulocytes are released prematurely and circulate as reticulocytes for 2 to 4 days, except in situations with low EPO levels, as in renal insufficiency.

Equation 3

$$\text{Reticulocyte index} = \frac{\text{corrected reticulocyte \%}}{\text{correction factor (usually 2)}}$$

Accordingly, the elevated reticulocyte count may give an erroneous impression of the actual rate of daily red cell production. To take this situation into account when estimating the rate of red cell production in anemic patients with high reticulocyte counts, dividing the absolute reticulocyte count by a factor may provide a more accurate estimate of red cell production.[132] For simplicity, an average factor of 2 often is used; however, the factor depends on the degree of anemia: 1.5 in mild cases, 2.5 in moderate cases, and 3.0 in severe cases.

An example follows: A patient with autoimmune hemolytic anemia has a hematocrit of 10 and reticulocyte count of 70 percent. The marrow cannot increase production by 70-fold. To measure the approximate true increase, we calculate the reticulocyte index as follows: corrected reticulocyte count = 70 × 10/45 = 15, and reticulocyte index = 15/3= 5 × basal. Thus, marrow erythroid production in response to this severe anemia has increased fivefold, a plausible response to this severity of hemolytic anemia.

INEFFECTIVE RED CELL PRODUCTION

Ineffective erythropoiesis is suspected when the reticulocyte count is normal or only slightly increased despite erythroid hyperplasia of the marrow. Ineffective erythropoiesis was first recognized as an entity from the study of isotope incorporation into fecal urobilin following administration of labeled glycine, a precursor of heme.[133] Two peaks were observed: an early peak at 3 to 5 days and a late peak at 100 to 120 days. One of the sources of the early labeled peak was suggested to be the hemoglobin of red cells that had never completed their development, having been destroyed either in the marrow or shortly after reaching the blood. Subsequent studies revealed that in certain disorders, such as pernicious anemia, thalassemia, and sideroblastic anemia, ineffective erythropoiesis is a major component of total erythropoiesis. This component can be quantitated by measuring ^{15}N-labeled glycine incorporation into the early bilirubin peaks[133,134] or ferrokinetics.[34] Calculated from bilirubin peaks and turnover, ineffective erythropoiesis under normal conditions amounts to approximately 4 to 12 percent of total erythropoiesis. Using ferrokinetic methods, ineffective erythropoiesis is calculated as the difference between total plasma iron turnover and erythrocyte iron turnover plus storage iron turnover (see "Ferrokinetics" below and Fig. 31–7). The values estimated from such studies in normal subjects are higher, ranging from 14 to 34 percent.[34] However, the results, both high and low, probably are misleading because none of the methods actually measures cell death, only the turnover of heme and iron. It is possible that little premature death of cells occurs in normal subjects, but much of the early release of bilirubin and iron is derived from the rim of hemoglobin extruded during enucleation of erythroblasts (see Chap. 29).

TOTAL ERYTHROPOIESIS

Total erythropoiesis, which is the sum of effective and ineffective red cell production, can be estimated from a marrow examination. Films or sections from marrow aspirates and biopsies are first examined for relative content of fat and hematopoietic tissue. This examination gives an estimate of overall hematopoietic activity within the marrow space. A differential count then is performed, determining the ratio between granulocytic and erythroid precursors (M:E ratio). In a normal adult, the ratio is approximately 3:1 to 5:1. The ratio can be used to estimate whether erythropoiesis is normal, increased, or decreased (see Chap. 3).

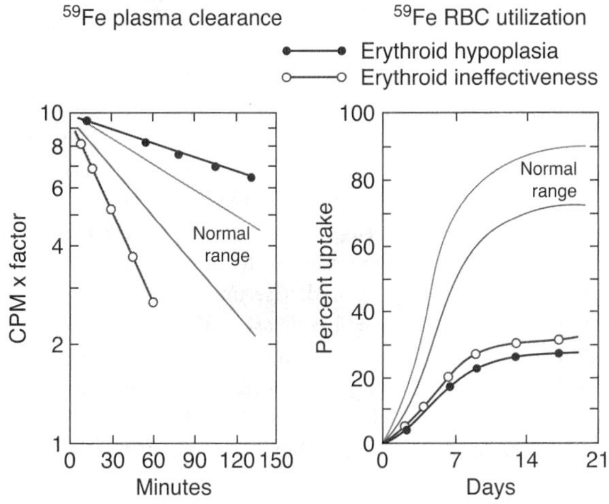

FIGURE 31-7. Iron clearance and iron utilization in normal subjects, patients with decreased effective red cell production (erythroid hypoplasia), and patients with ineffective red cell production. CPM, counts per minute; RBC, red blood cell.

The ratio is only an approximation of total erythroid activity because the ratio can be altered by changing the myeloid and erythroid components, and an aspirate or biopsy of a small segment of the marrow may not always reflect total marrow activity. These assumptions are valid as long as the marrow reflects the steady state, if the marrow is recovering from aplasia, or is developing aplasia, it will not accurately reflect output of mature red cells. However, when used in conjunction with determination of red blood cell count and reticulocyte count, under most circumstances the ratio provides qualitative information about the rate and effectiveness of red blood cell production. A more accurate quantitation of total erythropoiesis can be made by measuring the rate of production of red cells (ferrokinetics; see Fig. 31–7) or, in steady-state conditions, the rate of destruction of red cells (red cell life span, bilirubin production, carbon monoxide excretion).

FERROKINETICS

In 1950, Huff and associates[135] described a method for measuring the rate of red cell production utilizing a simple model of iron metabolism (Fig. 31–8; see Chap. 42). In this method, radioactive iron is complexed to transferrin *in vitro* and injected intravenously. Alternatively, ^{59}Fe can be injected directly intravenously as the gluconate without preincubation with the patient's own plasma, providing enough unbound transferrin is available, because binding is almost instantaneous. The rate of clearance of the transferrin-bound iron from the plasma (^{59}Fe plasma $T_{1/2}$) and the subsequent uptake in the red cells are measured. From these two values and from determinations of plasma iron concentration and plasma volume, the rate of formation of red cells can be calculated.[34]

The initial clearance of iron is exponential, and sampling during this period can be used to calculate $T_{1/2}$. In normal individuals, initial clearance averages approximately 90 minutes. Initial clearance is shorter in patients with hyperplasia of the erythropoietic tissue and longer in patients with marrow hypoplasia (see Fig. 31–7). However, the clearance rate is not a direct measurement of erythropoietic activity because it depends on the size of the pool of unlabeled, circulating iron. Consequently, calculation of the plasma iron turnover rate must include the plasma iron concentration. Clearance is expressed in milligrams of iron. The point of reference can be hemoglobin mass, blood volume, or weight, but a commonly used expression is micrograms of iron per deciliters of whole blood per day:

$$\text{Plasma iron turnover rate (mg iron/dL blood/24 h)} = \frac{\text{plasma iron (mg/dL)} \times (100 - \text{Hct})}{T_{1/2}(\text{min}) \times 100}$$

Under normal conditions, radioactive iron is incorporated into newly formed red cells after a few days and reaches a maximum approximately 10 to 14 days after injection (see Fig. 31–7). Normal utilization is 70 to 90 percent on day 10 to 14, a value that is so high that further increases have little significance. However, decreased utilization is an important finding and suggests immature red cells are destroyed in the marrow before they are released to the circulation (ineffective erythropoiesis; see Fig. 31–7) or that serum iron is diverted to nonerythropoietic tissues (marrow hypoplasia). The shape of the red cell utilization curve also is important. An early and steep rise (rapid marrow transit time) suggests a high EPO level. Finally, an early rise in utilization with a subsequent falloff suggests hemolysis.

When calculating utilization, the blood volume must be known:

$$\text{Red cell iron utilization (\%)} = \frac{\text{CPM of 1 mL blood} \times \text{blood volume} \times 100}{\text{CPM of } ^{59}\text{Fe injected}}$$

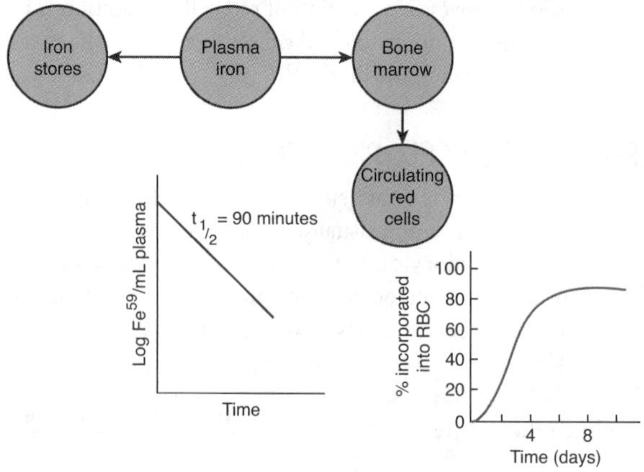

FIGURE 31–8. Single dynamic pool model of iron metabolism. Radioactive iron injected into the plasma iron pool is cleared from the plasma as a single exponential, and approximately 80 percent is incorporated into circulating blood cells.

Using the plasma iron clearance and utilization of iron, the red cell turnover in milligrams per deciliter blood for 24 hours is calculated as follows:

$$\text{Red cell iron turnover (mg iron/dL blood/24 h)} = \text{plasma iron turnover} \times \text{maximal red cell iron utilization}$$

The normal value of red cell iron turnover is 0.30 to 0.70 mg/dL blood per 24 hours.[34] This range fits very well with a crude estimation of the iron used for maintaining the red cell mass in 1 dL of blood or 45 mL of packed red cells. The daily red cell production must equal the daily red cell destruction (45 mL/120 = 0.38 mL), assuming a red cell life span of 120 days. Because 1 mL of packed red cells contains approximately 1 mg of iron, a daily plasma iron turnover of 0.38 mg is needed by 1 dL of blood to maintain homeostasis.

Calculating red cell iron turnover has provided useful information about the total volume and effectiveness of erythroid tissue (Table 31–2). However, an elevated serum iron concentration gives erroneous impressions of the state of erythropoiesis. Moreover, more prolonged sampling of plasma following an intravenous injection of ^{59}Fe has shown that clearance is not a single exponential but must be represented by several exponential components.[136] This finding has led to the introduction of more complex models of iron kinetics with a single pool of plasma iron exchanging with a number of extravascular erythroid and nonerythroid pools. Careful analysis of such models has

TABLE 31–2. Plasma Radioactive Iron Clearance and Red Blood Cell Uptake

Condition	Plasma ^{59}FE $T_{1/2}$	Red Blood Cell Uptake (%)
Normal	90 min	80–90
Increased erythropoiesis	Rapid (10–40 min)	80–90
Hemolytic anemia	Rapid	20–90*
Ineffective erythropoiesis	Normal to rapid	10–30
Iron-deficiency anemia	Normal to rapid	100
Decreased erythropoiesis	Slow (≥180 min)	0–20

*Variability a result of variability in intensity of hemolysis and size of iron stores.

generated computer-supported methods calculating the degree and effectiveness of erythroid activity.[137] Although possibly more accurate than the conventional method of calculating iron turnover, the models appear to be too cumbersome for clinical use. Moreover, even these sophisticated methods may not give an accurate account of the state of erythropoiesis. Despite a constant rate of red cell production, the plasma iron turnover was found to increase with increasing plasma iron and transferrin saturation. This finding was first thought to result from increased nonerythroid iron uptake and led to the introduction of various correction factors in the calculation of red cell iron turnover.[136] However, the iron in plasma is present in two pools, a diferric and a monoferric transferrin pool (see Chap. 42), and the erythroid and nonerythroid receptors have a four times greater avidity for diferric transferrin than for monoferric transferrin. Consequently, total plasma iron turnover depends on the degree of saturation and does not necessarily reflect the number of transferrin receptors, presumably a critical measure of erythropoietic capacity.[138] To measure the number of transferrin receptors, adjusting the plasma iron turnover equations for both nonerythroid uptake and degree of transferrin saturation and expressing the plasma turnover in terms of transferrin rather than iron have been proposed.[139] Normal erythroid uptake of transferrin is 60 ± 12 μmol per liter of blood per day, a value that has appropriately decreased and increased in patients with hypoplastic and hyperplastic marrow.

REFERENCES

1. Erslev AJ: Blood and mountains, in *Blood, Pure and Eloquent,* edited by MM Wintrobe, p 257. McGraw-Hill, New York, 1980.
2. Carnot P, Deflandre C: Sur l'activité hématopoiétique des serum au cours de la régénération du sang. *Acad Sci Med* 3, 1906.
3. Miescher F: Über die Beziehungen Zwischen Meereshohe und Beschaffenheit des Blutes. *Koresp Bltt Schweitz Aerzte* 24, 1893.
4. Reissmann KR: Studies on the mechanism of erythropoietic stimulation in parabiotic rats during hypoxia. *Blood* 5:372, 1950.
5. Erslev A: Humoral regulation of red cell production. *Blood* 8:349, 1953.
6. Erslev A, Lavietes PH, Van Wagenen G: Erythropoietic stimulation induced by anemic serum. *Proc Soc Exp Biol Med* 83:548, 1953.
7. Jacobson LO, Goldwasser E, Fried W, et al: Role of the kidney in erythropoiesis. *Nature* 179:633, 1957.
8. Fox H: The hemoglobin of *Daphnia. Proc R Soc Lond (Biol)* 135:195, 1948.
9. Hemmingsen EA, Douglas EL: Respiratory characteristics of the hemoglobin-free fish *Chaenocephalus aceratus. Comp Biochem Physiol* 33:733, 1970.
10. Sidell BD, O'Brien KM: When bad things happen to good fish: The loss of hemoglobin and myoglobin expression in Antarctic icefishes. *J Exp Biol* 209:1791, 2006.
11. Garofalo F, Amelio D, Cerra MC, et al: Morphological and physiological study of the cardiac NOS/NO system in the Antarctic (Hb-/Mb-) icefish *Chaenocephalus aceratus* and in the red-blooded *Trematomus bernacchii. Nitric Oxide* 20:69, 2009.
12. Garofalo F, Pellegrino D, Amelio D, et al: The Antarctic hemoglobinless icefish, fifty five years later: A unique cardiocirculatory interplay of disaptation and phenotypic plasticity. *Comp Biochem Physiol A Mol Integr Physiol.* 154:10, 2009.
13. Scott RB: Comparative hematology: The phylogeny of the erythrocyte. *Blut* 12:340, 1966.
14. Andrew W: *Comparative Hematology.* Grune & Stratton, New York, 1965.
15. Bolliger A: Observations on the blood of a monotreme *Tachyglossus aculeatus. Aust J Sci* 22:1959.
16. Iorio RJ: Some morphologic and kinetic studies of the developing erythroid cells of the common gold fish *Carassius auratus. Cell Tissue Kinet* 2:319, 1969.
17. Jordan HE: Comparative hematology, in *Handbook of Hematology,* edited by H Downey, p 703. Hoeber-Harper, New York, 1938.
18. Robb-Smith AHT: *The Growth of Knowledge of the Functions of the Blood,* edited by RG Macfarlane, AHT Robb-Smith. Academic Press, New York, 1961.
19. Rosse WF, Waldmann TA: Factors controlling erythropoiesis in birds. *Blood* 27:654, 1966.
20. Zanjani ED, Yu ML, Perlmutter A, et al: Humoral factors influencing erythropoiesis in the fish (blue gourami, *Trichogaster trichopterus*). *Blood* 33:573, 1969.
21. Erslev AJ: Control of red cell production. *Annu Rev Med* 11:1959.
22. Shoemaker CB, Mitsock LD: Murine erythropoietin gene: Cloning, expression, and human gene homology. *Mol Cell Biol* 6:849, 1986.
23. Le Douarin NM: Cell migrations in embryos. *Cell* 38:353, 1984.
24. Kingsley PD, Malik J, Emerson RL, et al: "Maturational" globin switching in primary primitive erythroid cells. *Blood* 107:1665, 2006.
25. Hoyes AD, Riches DJ, Martin BG: The fine structure of haemopoiesis in the human fetal liver. I. The haemopoietic precursor cells. *J Anat* 115:99, 1973.
26. Palis J, Robertson S, Kennedy M, et al: Development of erythroid and myeloid progenitors in the yolk sac and embryo proper of the mouse. *Development* 126:5073, 1999.
27. Hudson G: Bone-marrow volume in the human foetus and newborn. *Br J Haematol* 11:446, 1965.
28. Brannon D: Extramedullary hematopoiesis in anemia. *Bull Johns Hopkins Hosp* 41:1927.
29. Erslev AJ: Medullary and extramedullary blood formation. *Clin Orthop Relat Res* 52:25, 1967.
30. Zanjani ED, Poster J, Burlington H, et al: Liver as the primary site of erythropoietin formation in the fetus. *J Lab Clin Med* 89:640, 1977.
31. Flake AW, Harrison MR, Adzick NS, et al: Erythropoietin production by the fetal liver in an adult environment. *Blood* 70:542, 1987.
32. Zanjani ED, Ascensao JL, McGlave PB, et al: Studies on the liver to kidney switch of erythropoietin production. *J Clin Invest* 67:1183, 1981.
33. Sawyer ST, Penta K: Erythropoietin cell biology. *Hematol Oncol Clin North Am* 8:895, 1994.
34. Finch CA, Deubelbeiss K, Cook JD, et al: Ferrokinetics in man. *Medicine (Baltimore)* 49:17, 1970.
35. Noble NA, Xu QP, Hoge LL: Reticulocytes II: Reexamination of the *in vivo* survival of stress reticulocytes. *Blood* 75:1877, 1990.
36. Donohue DM, Reiff RH, Hanson ML, et al: Quantitative measurement of the erythrocytic and granulocytic cells of the marrow and blood. *J Clin Invest* 37:1571, 1958.
37. Finch CA, Harker LA, Cook JD: Kinetics of the formed elements of human blood. *Blood* 50:699, 1977.
38. Goltry KL, Patel VP: Specific domains of fibronectin mediate adhesion and migration of early murine erythroid progenitors. *Blood* 90:138, 1997.
39. Gregory T, Yu C, Ma A, et al: GATA-1 and erythropoietin cooperate to promote erythroid cell survival by regulating bcl-xL expression. *Blood* 94:87, 1999.
40. Tsang AP, Visvader JE, Turner CA, et al: FOG, a multitype zinc finger protein, acts as a cofactor for transcription factor GATA-1 in erythroid and megakaryocytic differentiation. *Cell* 90:109, 1997.
41. Nerlov C, Querfurth E, Kulessa H, et al: GATA-1 interacts with the myeloid PU.1 transcription factor and represses PU.1-dependent transcription. *Blood* 95:2543, 2000.
42. Ohneda K, Yamamoto M: Roles of hematopoietic transcription factors GATA-1 and GATA-2 in the development of red blood cell lineage. *Acta Haematol* 108:237, 2002.
43. Cantor AB, Orkin SH: Transcriptional regulation of erythropoiesis: An affair involving multiple partners. *Oncogene* 21:3368, 2002.
44. Xie H, Ye M, Feng R, et al: Stepwise reprogramming of B cells into macrophages. *Cell* 117:663, 2004.
45. Back J, Dierich A, Bronn C, et al: PU.1 determines the self-renewal capacity of erythroid progenitor cells. *Blood* 103:3615, 2004.
46. Angelillo-Scherrer A, Burnier L, Lambrechts D, et al: Role of Gas6 in erythropoiesis and anemia in mice. *J Clin Invest* 118:583, 2008.
47. Lemke G, Lu Q: Macrophage regulation by Tyro 3 family receptors. *Curr Opin Immunol* 15:31, 2003.
48. Stopka T, Zivny JH, Stopkova P, et al: Human hematopoietic progenitors express erythropoietin. *Blood* 91:3766, 1998.
49. Krantz SB: Erythropoietin. *Blood* 77:419, 1991.
50. Lappin TR, Rich IN: Erythropoietin—The first 90 years. *Clin Lab Haematol* 18:137, 1996.
51. Jelkmann W: Erythropoietin: Structure, control of production, and function. *Physiol Rev* 72:449, 1992.
52. Jelkmann W, Metzen E: Erythropoietin in the control of red cell production. *Ann Anat* 178:391, 1996.
53. Koury ST, Bondurant MC, Koury MJ: Localization of erythropoietin synthesizing cells in murine kidneys by *in situ* hybridization. *Blood* 71:524, 1988.
54. Lacombe C, Da Silva JL, Bruneval P, et al: Peritubular cells are the site of erythropoietin synthesis in the murine hypoxic kidney. *J Clin Invest* 81:620, 1988.
55. Koury ST, Koury MJ, Bondurant MC, et al: Quantitation of erythropoietin-producing cells in kidneys of mice by *in situ* hybridization: Correlation with hematocrit, renal erythropoietin mRNA, and serum erythropoietin concentration. *Blood* 74:645, 1989.
56. Semenza GL, Dureza RC, Traystman MD, et al: Human erythropoietin gene expression in transgenic mice: Multiple transcription initiation sites and *cis*-acting regulatory elements. *Mol Cell Biol* 10:930, 1990.
57. Schuster SJ, Koury ST, Bohrer M, et al: Cellular sites of extrarenal and renal erythropoietin production in anaemic rats. *Br J Haematol* 81:153, 1992.
58. Mole DR, Radcliffe PJ: Regulation of endogenous erythropoietin production, in *Erythropoietins and Erythropoiesis,* 2nd ed, edited by G Molineux, MA Foote, SG Elliot, p 19. Birkhäuser-Verlag AG, Basel, 2009.
59. Rankin EB, Biju MP, Liu Q, et al: Hypoxia-inducible factor-2 (HIF-2) regulates hepatic erythropoietin *in vivo. J Clin Invest* 117:1068, 2007.
60. Flaharty KK, Caro J, Erslev A, et al: Pharmacokinetics and erythropoietic response to human recombinant erythropoietin in healthy men. *Clin Pharmacol Ther* 47:557, 1990.
61. Sawyer ST, Krantz SB, Goldwasser E: Binding and receptor-mediated endocytosis of erythropoietin in Friend virus-infected erythroid cells. *J Biol Chem* 262:5554, 1987.
62. Ebert BL, Bunn HF: Regulation of the erythropoietin gene. *Blood* 94:1864, 1999.

63. Constantinescu SN, Keren T, Socolovsky M, et al: Ligand-independent oligomerization of cell-surface erythropoietin receptor is mediated by the transmembrane domain. *Proc Natl Acad Sci U S A* 98:4379, 2001.
64. Witthuhn BA, Quelle FW, Silvennoinen O, et al: JAK2 associates with the erythropoietin receptor and is tyrosine phosphorylated and activated following stimulation with erythropoietin. *Cell* 74:227, 1993.
65. Damen JE, Wakao H, Miyajima A, et al: Tyrosine 343 in the erythropoietin receptor positively regulates erythropoietin-induced cell proliferation and Stat5 activation. *EMBO J* 14:5557, 1995.
66. Parganas E, Wang D, Stravopodis D, et al: Jak2 is essential for signaling through a variety of cytokine receptors. *Cell* 93:385, 1998.
67. Divoky V, Prchal JT: Mouse surviving solely on human erythropoietin receptor (EpoR): Model of human EpoR-linked disease. *Blood* 99:3873, 2002.
68. Lin CS, Lim SK, D'Agati V, et al: Differential effects of an erythropoietin receptor gene disruption on primitive and definitive erythropoiesis. *Genes Dev* 10:154, 1996.
69. Wu H, Liu X, Jaenisch R, et al: Generation of committed erythroid BFU-E and CFU-E progenitors does not require erythropoietin or the erythropoietin receptor. *Cell* 83:59, 1995.
70. D'Andrea AD, Yoshimura A, Youssoufian H, et al: The cytoplasmic region of the erythropoietin receptor contains nonoverlapping positive and negative growth-regulatory domains. *Mol Cell Biol* 11:1980, 1991.
71. Klingmuller U, Lorenz U, Cantley LC, et al: Specific recruitment of SH-PTP1 to the erythropoietin receptor causes inactivation of JAK2 and termination of proliferative signals. *Cell* 80:729, 1995.
72. Arcasoy MO, Harris KW, Forget BG: A human erythropoietin receptor gene mutant causing familial erythrocytosis is associated with deregulation of the rates of Jak2 and Stat5 inactivation. *Exp Hematol* 27:63, 1999.
73. Marine JC, McKay C, Wang D, et al: SOCS3 is essential in the regulation of fetal liver erythropoiesis. *Cell* 98:617, 1999.
74. Sasaki A, Yasukawa H, Shouda T, et al: CIS3/SOCS-3 suppresses erythropoietin (EPO) signaling by binding the EPO receptor and JAK2. *J Biol Chem* 275:29338, 2000.
75. Prchal JT, Gregg XT: Erythropoiesis. Genetic Abnormalities, in *Erythropoietins and Erythropoiesis*, 2nd ed, edited by G Molineux, MA Foote, SG Elliot, p 61. Birkhäuser-Verlag AG, Basel, 2009.
76. Walrafen P, Verdier F, Kadri Z, et al: Both proteosomes and lysosomes degrade the activated erythropoietin receptor. *Blood* 105:600, 2005.
77. Arcasoy MO, Jiang X, Haroon ZA: Expression of erythropoietin receptor splice variants in human cancer. *Biochem Biophys Res Commun* 307:999, 2003.
78. Barron C, Migliaccio AR, Migliaccio G, et al: Alternatively spliced mRNAs encoding soluble isoforms of the erythropoietin receptor in murine cell lines and bone marrow. *Gene* 147:263, 1994.
79. Nakamura Y, Nakauchi H: A truncated erythropoietin receptor and cell death: A reanalysis. *Science* 264:588, 1994.
80. Prchal JT, Semenza GL, Prchal J, et al: Familial polycythemia. *Science* 268:1831, 1995.
81. Noguchi CT, Wang L, Rogers HM, et al: Survival and proliferative roles of erythropoietin beyond the erythroid lineage. *Expert Rev Mol Med* 10:e36, 2008.
82. Anagnostou A, Lee ES, Kessimian N, et al: Erythropoietin has a mitogenic and positive chemotactic effect on endothelial cells. *Proc Natl Acad Sci U S A* 87:5978, 1990.
83. Brines M, Cerami A: Discovering erythropoietin's extra-hematopoietic functions: Biology and clinical promise. *Kidney Int* 70:246, 2006.
84. Arcasoy MO: The non-haematopoietic biological effects of erythropoietin. *Br J Haematol* 141:14, 2008.
85. Agarwal N, Gordeuk VR, Prchal JT: Are erythropoietin receptors expressed in tumors? Facts and fiction—More careful studies are needed. *J Clin Oncol* 25:1813, 2007.
86. Hardee ME, Cao Y, Fu P, et al: Erythropoietin blockade inhibits the induction of tumor angiogenesis and progression. *PLoS ONE* 2:e549, 2007.
87. Hirota K, Semenza GL: Regulation of angiogenesis by hypoxia-inducible factor 1. *Crit Rev Oncol Hematol* 59:15, 2006.
88. Yoon D, Pastore YD, Divoky V, et al: Hypoxia-inducible factor-1 deficiency results in dysregulated erythropoiesis signaling and iron homeostasis in mouse development. *J Biol Chem* 281:25703, 2006.
89. Fukuda R, Zhang H, Kim JW, et al: HIF-1 regulates cytochrome oxidase subunits to optimize efficiency of respiration in hypoxic cells. *Cell* 129:111, 2007.
90. Beck I, Ramirez S, Weinmann R, et al: Enhancer element at the 3′-flanking region controls transcriptional response to hypoxia in the human erythropoietin gene. *J Biol Chem* 266:15563, 1991.
91. Manalo DJ, Rowan A, Lavoie T, et al: Transcriptional regulation of vascular endothelial cell responses to hypoxia by HIF-1. *Blood* 105:659, 2005.
92. Maxwell P, Wiesener MS, Chang GW, et al: The tumour suppressor protein VHL targets hypoxia-inducible factors for oxygen-dependent proteolysis. *Nature* 399:271, 1999.
93. Jaakkola P, Mole DR, Tian YM, et al: Targeting of HIF-alpha to the von Hippel-Lindau ubiquitylation complex by O_2-regulated prolyl hydroxylation. *Science* 292:468, 2001.
94. Ivan M, Kondo, K, Yang, H, et al: HIF alpha targeted for VHL-mediated destruction by proline hydroxylation: Implications for O_2 sensing. *Science* 292:464, 2001.
95. Baek JH, Liu YV, McDonald KR, et al: Spermidine/spermine N(1)-acetyltransferase-1 binds to hypoxia-inducible factor-1alpha (HIF-1alpha) and RACK1 and promotes ubiquitination and degradation of HIF-1alpha. *J Biol Chem* 282:33358, 2007.
96. Gruber M, Hu CJ, Johnson RS, et al: Acute postnatal ablation of Hif-2alpha results in anemia. *Proc Natl Acad Sci U S A* 104:2301, 2007.
97. Chavez JC, Baranova O, Lin J, et al: The transcriptional activator hypoxia inducible factor 2 (HIF-2/EPAS-1) regulates the oxygen-dependent expression of erythropoietin in cortical astrocytes. *J Neurosci* 26:9471, 2006.
98. Sanchez M, Galy B, Muckenthaler MU, et al: Iron-regulatory proteins limit hypoxia-inducible factor-2alpha expression in iron deficiency. *Nat Struct Mol Biol* 14:420, 2007.
99. Percy MJ, Furlow PW, Lucas GS, et al: A gain-of-function mutation in the HIF2A gene in familial erythrocytosis. *N Engl J Med* 358:162, 2008.
100. Liu YV, Baek JH, Zhang H, et al: RACK1 competes with HSP90 for binding to HIF-1alpha and is required for O(2)-independent and HSP90 inhibitor-induced degradation of HIF-1alpha. *Mol Cell* 25:207, 2007.
101. Carbia-Nagashima A, Gerez J, Perez-Castro C, et al: RSUME, a small RWD-containing protein, enhances SUMO conjugation and stabilizes HIF-1alpha during hypoxia. *Cell* 131:309, 2007.
102. Liu YV, Hubbi ME, Pan F, et al: Calcineurin promotes hypoxia-inducible factor 1alpha expression by dephosphorylating RACK1 and blocking RACK1 dimerization. *J Biol Chem* 282:37064, 2007.
103. Kong X, Alvarez-Castelao B, Lin Z, et al: Constitutive/hypoxic degradation of HIF-alpha proteins by the proteasome is independent of von Hippel Lindau protein ubiquitylation and the transactivation activity of the protein. *J Biol Chem* 282:15498, 2007.
104. Epstein AC, Gleadle JM, McNeill LA, et al: *C. elegans* EGL-9 and mammalian homologs define a family of dioxygenases that regulate HIF by prolyl hydroxylation. *Cell* 107:43, 2001.
105. Ivan M, Kondo K, Yang H, et al: HIFalpha targeted for VHL-mediated destruction by proline hydroxylation: Implications for O_2 sensing. *Science* 292:464, 2001.
106. Jaakkola P, Mole DR, Tian YM, et al: Targeting of HIF-alpha to the von Hippel-Lindau ubiquitylation complex by O_2-regulated prolyl hydroxylation. *Science* 292:468, 2001.
107. Correa PN, Eskinazi D, Axelrad AA: Circulating erythroid progenitors in polycythemia vera are hypersensitive to insulin-like growth factor-1 *in vitro*: Studies in an improved serum-free medium. *Blood* 83:99, 1994.
108. Mirza AM, Ezzat S, Axelrad AA: Insulin-like growth factor binding protein-1 is elevated in patients with polycythemia vera and stimulates erythroid burst formation in vitro. *Blood* 89:1862, 1997.
109. Brox AG, Congote LF, Fafard J, et al: Identification and characterization of an 8-kd peptide stimulating late erythropoiesis. *Exp Hematol* 17:769, 1989.
110. Gomez RA, Norwood VF: Developmental consequences of the renin-angiotensin system. *Am J Kidney Dis* 26:409, 1995.
111. Ray PE, Aguilera G, Kopp JB, et al: Angiotensin II receptor-mediated proliferation of cultured human fetal mesangial cells. *Kidney Int* 40:764, 1991.
112. Tufro-McReddie A, Gomez RA: Ontogeny of the renin-angiotensin system. *Semin Nephrol* 13:519, 1993.
113. Verhaaren HA, Vande Walle J, Devloo-Blancquaert A: Captopril in severe childhood hypertension—Reversible anaemia with high dosage. *Eur J Pediatr* 144:554, 1986.
114. Wang AY, Yu AW, Lam CW, et al: Effects of losartan or enalapril on hemoglobin, circulating erythropoietin, and insulin-like growth factor-1 in patients with and without posttransplant erythrocytosis. *Am J Kidney Dis* 39:600, 2002.
115. Mrug M, Stopka T, Julian BA, et al: Angiotensin II stimulates proliferation of normal early erythroid progenitors. *J Clin Invest* 100:2310, 1997.
116. Glezerman I, Patel H, Glicklich D, et al: Angiotensin-converting enzyme inhibition induces death receptor apoptotic pathways in erythroid precursors following renal transplantation. *Am J Nephrol* 23:195, 2003.
117. Cole J, Ertoy D, Lin H, et al: Lack of angiotensin II-facilitated erythropoiesis causes anemia in angiotensin-converting enzyme-deficient mice. *J Clin Invest* 106:1391, 2000.
118. Sandoval H, Thiagarajan P, Dasgupta SK, et al: Essential role for Nix in autophagic maturation of erythroid cells. *Nature* 454:232, 2008.
119. Bruchova H, Yoon D, Agarwal AM, et al: Regulated expression of microRNAs in normal and polycythemia vera erythropoiesis. *Exp Hematol* 35:1657, 2007.
120. Bruchova H, Merkerova M, Prchal JT: Aberrant expression of microRNA in polycythemia vera. *Haematologica* 93:1009, 2008.
121. Felli N, Pedini F, Romania P, et al: MicroRNA 223-dependent expression of LMO2 regulates normal erythropoiesis. *Haematologica* 94:479, 2009.
122. Pearson TC, Botterill CA, Glass UH, et al: Interpretation of measured red cell mass and plasma volume in males with elevated venous PCV values. *Scand J Haematol* 33:68, 1984.
123. Sioufi HA, Button LN, Jacobson MS, et al: Nonradioactive chromium technique for red cell labeling. *Vox Sang* 58:204, 1990.
124. Cavill I, Trevett D, Fisher J, et al: The measurement of the total volume of red cells in man: A non-radioactive approach using biotin. *Br J Haematol* 70:491, 1988.
125. Jones J, Mollison PL: A simple and efficient method of labelling red cells with 99mTc for determination of red cell volume. *Br J Haematol* 38:141, 1978.
126. Chaplin H Jr: Precision of red cell volume measurement using ^{32}P-labelled cells. *J Physiol* 123:22, 1954.
127. Pearson TC, Guthrie DL, Simpson J, et al: Interpretation of measured red cell mass and plasma volume in adults: Expert Panel on Radionuclides of the International Council for Standardization in Haematology. *Br J Haematol* 89:748, 1995.
128. Fairbanks VF, Klee GG, Wiseman GA, et al: Measurement of blood volume and red cell mass: Re-examination of ^{51}Cr and ^{125}I methods. *Blood Cells Mol Dis* 22:169, 1996.
129. Larsen OA: Studies of the body hematocrit phenomenon: Dynamic hematocrit of large vessel and initial distribution space of albumin and fibrinogen in the whole body. *Scand J Clin Lab Invest* 22:189, 1968.

130. Button LN, Gibson JG 2nd, Walter CW: Simultaneous determination of the volume of red cells and plasma for survival studies of stored blood. *Transfusion* 5:143, 1965.
131. Recommended methods for measurement of red-cell and plasma volume: International Committee for Standardization in Haematology. *J Nucl Med* 21:793, 1980.
132. Hillman RS, Finch CA: Erythropoiesis: Normal and abnormal. *Semin Hematol* 4:327, 1967.
133. Samson D, Halliday D, Nicholson DC, et al: Quantitation of ineffective erythropoiesis from the incorporation of [15N] delta-aminolaevulinic acid and [15N] glycine into early labelled bilirubin. I. Normal subjects. *Br J Haematol* 34:33, 1976.
134. Samson D, Halliday D, Nicholson DC, et al: Quantitation of ineffective erythropoiesis from the incorporation of [15N] delta-aminolaevulinic acid and [15N] glycine into early labelled bilirubin. II. Anaemic patients. *Br J Haematol* 34:45, 1976.
135. Huff RL, Hennessy TG, Austin RE, et al: Plasma and red cell iron turnover in normal subjects and in patients having various hematopoietic disorders. *J Clin Invest* 29:1041, 1950.
136. Cook JD, Marsaglia G, Eschbach JW, et al: Ferrokinetics: A biologic model for plasma iron exchange in man. *J Clin Invest* 49:197, 1970.
137. Ricketts C, Cavill I, Napier JA, et al: Ferrokinetics and erythropoiesis in man: An evaluation of ferrokinetic measurements. *Br J Haematol* 35:41, 1977.
138. Bauer W, Stray S, Huebers H, et al: The relationship between plasma iron and plasma iron turnover in the rat. *Blood* 57:239, 1981.
139. Beguin Y: The soluble transferrin receptor: Biological aspects and clinical usefulness as quantitative measure of erythropoiesis. *Haematologica* 77:1, 1992.

CHAPTER 32
DESTRUCTION OF ERYTHROCYTES

Ernest Beutler

SUMMARY

The survival of red cells in the circulation can be measured in a variety of ways: (1) by labeling with isotopes, particularly ^{51}Cr, and assessing the disappearance of the tag from the circulation over time; (2) by labeling the erythrocytes with biotin or fluorescent dye and measuring this marker over time; (3) by determining the disappearance of transfused allogeneic erythrocytes using immunologic markers; and (4) by measuring the excretion of carbon monoxide (CO), a product of heme catabolism.

Such studies show that normal human red cells have a finite life span averaging 120 days, with very little random destruction. During maturation of the reticulocyte, cell density increases, but after a few days of intravascular life span there is little further increase in density or other changes in the physical property of the red cells. Thus cell density is not a good marker for aged red cells. This has made the senescent changes in the red cell that mark it for destruction difficult to study. Candidates for such changes include changes in membrane band 3 and exposure of phosphatidylserine on the membrane, which may be of major importance.

RED CELL DESTRUCTION

MEASUREMENT OF RED CELL DESTRUCTION

Red Cell Life Span

The original method for the measurement of the red cell life span consisted in the transfusion of cells that were compatible but identifiable immunologically—the Ashby technique; type O red cells were infused into individuals with type A or B cells and the recipients' own cells were removed using anti-A or anti-B serum.[1] During World War II and shortly after, this method was used extensively, but in recent years, because of the hazards associated with the administration of allogeneic erythrocytes, it has been completely replaced by techniques based on labeling of autologous blood.

In 1946, Shemin and Rittenberg demonstrated that the incorporation of nitrogen (^{15}N)-labeled glycine into heme could be used to measure the life span of the red cells.[2] Since then a number of other isotopic methods have been developed. These can be divided into three groups: (1) those that label a cohort of cells, (2) those that label cells randomly, and (3) those that use indirect measurements such as the rate of production of red cells or the rate of heme breakdown. The first two classes yield information about the nature of the shortening of the red cell life span, age-dependent or random. The last group yields only mean life span.

Acronyms and abbreviations that appear in this chapter include: ADP, adenosine diphosphate; AMP, adenosine monophosphate; C_3, third component of complement; ^{14}C, radioactive carbon; CO, carbon monoxide; ^{51}Cr, chromium-51; ^{50}Cr, chromium-50; DFP, diisopropylfluorophosphate; ^{55}Fe or ^{59}Fe, radioactive iron; G-6-PD, glucose-6-phosphate dehydrogenase; Ig, immunoglobulin; ^{111}In, indium-111; ^{15}N, nitrogen; PK, pyruvate kinase; ^{99m}Tc, technetium-99m.

Cohort Methods

Cohort methods depend on the biosynthetic incorporation of the label into the developing red cells. In these methods a group of cells of approximately the same age is labeled. The labels used are glycine-containing labeled ^{15}N,[2] radioactive carbon (^{14}C),[3] or radioactive iron (either ^{55}Fe or ^{59}Fe).[4–6] The main disadvantage of cohort labeling is the need for prolonged periods of sampling, especially if the life span is only moderately reduced (Fig. 32–1). In addition, radioiron from destroyed red cells may be reutilized making it difficult to interpret results.

Random-Label Methods

The random-label methods are the Ashby differential agglutination technique,[1] which uses an immunologic marker, and or the use of various red cell labels such as chromium (^{50}Cr, ^{51}Cr, or ^{53}Cr),[7–9] diisopropylfluorophosphate (DFP) labeled with ^{32}P, ^{103}H,[11] or ^{14}C,[12] ^{14}C cyanate,[13] a lipophilic dye,[14,15] or biotin.[16,17]

By far the most commonly used radioactive isotope for the measurement of the red cell life span is ^{51}Cr. As the chromate ion penetrates the red cell membrane it binds to the β and γ chains of globin. Unfortunately, these bonds are not covalent and there is a continuous elution of the isotope, varying from 0.5 to 2.9 percent per day.[18] DFP, on the other hand, is irreversibly bound to red cell cholinesterase. There is some elution of unbound DFP during the first 2 to 3 days of study, but after that, DFP disappearance closely matches red cell destruction.[19,20] Nevertheless, because sample preparation is somewhat complicated, this label is not commonly used.

To accurately calculate red cell life span using a random label method requires steady-state conditions or that correction can be made for concurrent blood loss or blood transfusion. Fortunately, it is usually possible to gain an accurate estimate of red cell half-life by sampling three times a week for 1 to 2 weeks.

In the normal human the red cell life span is finite with an average of about 120 days, with very little random destruction, that is, loss irrespective of cell age (0.06 to 0.4 percent per day). In some mammalian species the amount of random destruction is much greater.[21] The survival curve of randomly labeled human red cells should consequently be nearly linear from day 0 to day 120, with a half-life of 60 days. When ^{51}Cr is used as the label, approximately 1 percent of label elutes per day and the survival curve becomes exponential with a half-life of approximately 30 days (see Fig. 32–1). For clinical use, the red cell life span is usually expressed as chromium $T_{1/2}$ and compared to the normal of 30 days.

Because merely expressing the red cell life span measured by chromium as chromium $T_{1/2}$ will not give information as to the character of destruction, senescence versus random, it has been recommended that in addition a correction factor for chromium elution be used and the data recorded using linear coordinates.[22] If the data lie on a straight line, the destruction is by senescence and the life span can be calculated as twice the half-life. If the data indicate exponential disappearance and it is necessary to use a semilogarithmic paper in order to depict the data on a straight line, the destruction is random and the life span is 1.44 times the half-life. One objection to this method is that the degree of chromium elution is not a constant but varies from day to day and from disease to disease.[18] Furthermore, the best fit of data is rarely linear or exponential, but somewhere between. Although computer-assisted methods can resolve ambiguities, the inherent biologic and technical variations in measuring red cell life span are such that it is better to rely on chromium $T_{1/2}$ with intuitive adjustments based on clinical findings.

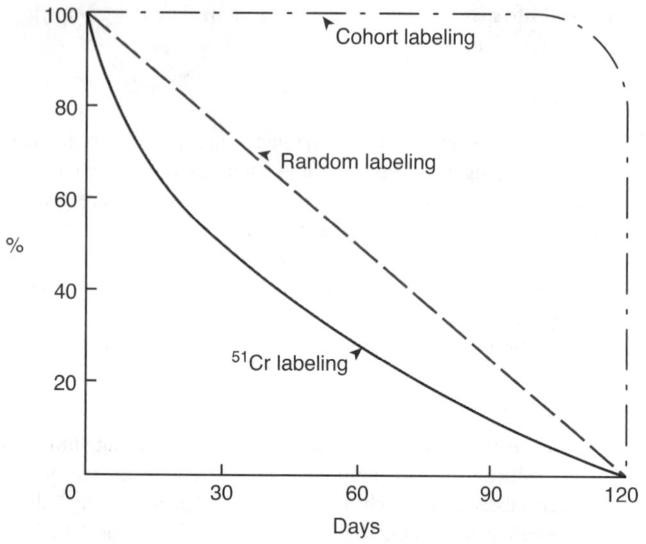

FIGURE 32–1. Red cell life span measured by cohort labeling or random labeling. When red cells are labeled randomly with chromium-51 (^{51}Cr) there is a daily 1 percent elution which needs to be corrected for in the calculation of total red cell life span.

Indirect Methods

There are two approaches to the calculation of the red cell life span by indirect methods: from a measurement of the rate of production of red cells utilizing radioactive iron and from a measurement of the rate of breakdown of heme to bilirubin[23], that is, the release of carbon monoxide from catabolized heme.[24] Both of these compounds are derived almost exclusively from catabolized hemoglobin and measurements of their rate of production have provided useful information about the red cell life span. There are too many variables that affect the serum bilirubin level to make it a reliable, quantitative measurement of red cell destruction. The measurement of CO production was formerly very tedious, requiring elaborate rebreathing apparatus. With the development of newer technologies[25,26] measuring CO levels has become more practical. An advantage of the measurement of blood CO as an indication of the rate of red cell destruction is that it gives the rate of destruction at a single point in time.

In Situ Localization of Red Cell Production and Destruction

As part of routine erythrokinetic studies both radioactive iron and radioactive chromium may be used to localize red cell production and red cell destruction. This is accomplished by positioning probes for external counting over the sacrum, liver, spleen, and heart and measuring the distribution of radioactivity in the body.[27]

In a normal subject, ^{59}Fe injected intravenously is cleared rapidly from the plasma, and within 24 hours approximately 85 percent of the radioactivity can be accounted for in the marrow. The liver and the spleen divide the remaining 15 percent. Over the next 10 days the marrow radioactivity decreases gradually as a result of the release into circulating blood of red cells labeled with radioactive hemoglobin. Patterns showing different uptake and distribution of the radioactive iron have been found for various hematologic disorders.[28] In hypersplenism, the trapping and destruction of iron-labeled cells in the spleen increases splenic radioactivity rapidly, and in patients with erythroid hypoplasia the distribution of radioactive iron between liver and marrow is reversed (Fig. 32–2).

More effective methods demonstrating in situ erythropoiesis involve imaging marrow, liver, and spleen with a technetium-99m (^{99m}Tc) sulfur colloid or indium-111 (^{111}In).[29] Although these isotopes label primarily the monocyte-macrophage system, their uptake is similar to that of ^{59}Fe and they can be used as surrogate markers to estimate the distribution of erythroid tissue.

Surface counting for chromium-51 (^{51}Cr)-labeled red cells provides a characteristic organ distribution of radioactivity and has been used to demonstrate the degree of red cell sequestration and destruction in an enlarged spleen (Fig. 32–2).[30] This approach has been used to predict the results of elective splenectomy, but the utility of this method has been challenged.[31] The in situ localization of red cell sequestration or destruction can also be determined by following the tissue distribution of ^{59}Fe-labeled red cells, especially if the red cell life span is very short.

SENESCENCE OF NORMAL ERYTHROCYTES

Methodologic Considerations

Labeling a cohort of human erythrocytes with ^{59}Fe and centrifuging the cells in a density gradient demonstrates that reticulocytes and young red cells are less dense than mature red cells.[32,33] However, at the end of the life span of the labeled cohort, radioactivity is fairly evenly distributed throughout red cells of all densities, with only a slight tendency of the radioactivity to be concentrated in the more dense cells. Unfortunately, many studies of the properties of senescent cells in the past have been based upon the characteristics of the most dense fraction of erythrocytes, using various fractionating techniques. In fact, the most dense fraction of red cells is only slightly enriched with old erythrocytes.[34,35] A combination of density separation and elutriation seemed to provide results superior to density separation alone using hemoglobin A_{1C} content as a marker, but the degree of enrichment with older cells has not

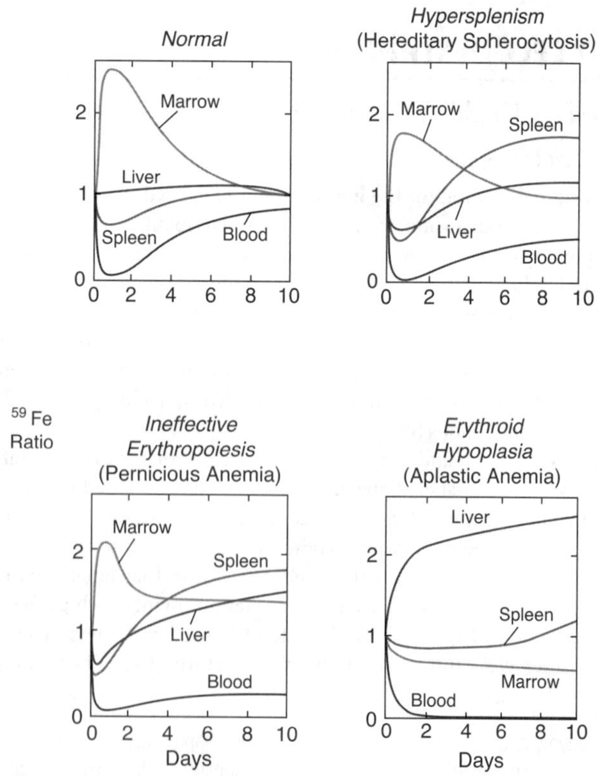

FIGURE 32–2. Tissue distribution of ^{59}Fe in normal subjects, hypersplenic patients, and anemic patients with ineffective and effective erythropoiesis. The radioactivity is expressed on the ordinate as a ratio relative to the radioactivity measured in the same organ 15 minutes after the intravenous administration of the isotope. *(Redrawn from RS Hillman and CA Finch,[28] with permission.)*

been documented using actual old red cells as separated by biotinylation or by the mouse hypertransfusion technique.[36]

There are two animal models and one human disease model that provide cells that are truly aged. In mice, in vivo aged cells have been produced by serially transfusing mice, maintaining polycythemia to suppress virtually all erythropoiesis.[37] In other species, particularly the rabbit, red cells have been labeled with traces of biotin, which allows them to be recovered from the circulation.[38] The human model is transient erythroblastopenia of childhood (Chaps. 35 and 54), a disorder in which there is cessation of all erythropoiesis for several months; however, the density and deformability of the aged cells in erythroblastopenia of childhood is normal.[34] The use of the latter model has been criticized because this disorder is not fully understood and the red cells in the circulation may not be entirely normal.[39] However, the results that have been obtained are consistent with those obtained in animal models and are probably reliable (see "Properties of Aged Cells" below).

Properties of Aged Cells Although the activities of a large number of enzymes, including hexokinase, glucose-6-phosphate dehydrogenase (G-6-PD), and pyruvate kinase (PK), are higher in reticulocytes than in mature erythrocytes, the activities of these enzymes do not normally continue to decline during the aging of the erythrocyte.[38,40] Pyrimidine-5′-nucleotidase[41,42] and adenosine monophosphate (AMP)-deaminase[43–45] appear to be exceptions to this rule in that there is continuing decline of enzyme activity throughout the life span of the red cell. This stability of many of the red cell enzymes during the aging of normal erythrocytes contrasts to the circumstances that are brought about by mutations in enzymes such as G-6-PD and PK, where instability of the abnormal enzyme leads to accelerated decay in the amount of enzyme protein, a factor that surely plays an important role in the ultimate demise of the cell (Chap. 46). Fluorescent sorting of blood type NN erythrocytes transfused into humans shows that the most dense fractions are only minimally enriched with old cells,[46] and biotinylated aged cells of rabbits have been found to have only a modestly decreased surface area, volume, cell water, and density and therefore slightly decreased deformability.[35,47]

A small number of red cell vesicles, approximately 190 per microliter blood, have been harvested from the circulation, and it was proposed that the loss of such a membrane in hemoglobin vesicles may play a role in the aging process.[48]

Mechanism of Destruction of Normal, Aged Cells

Several different mechanisms of destruction of red cells when they reach the end of their normal, physiologic life span have been proposed. Determining the actual mechanism(s) is especially difficult because the cells that are marked for removal are bound to be present at very low concentrations or not at all in the circulating blood—they have been removed. Many of the earlier data are predicated upon the isolation of dense cells and the consideration that they are "old"; we now recognize that they are not (see "Methodologic Considerations" above). Moreover, it is likely that there is more than one mechanism that serves to remove effete red cells from the circulation; there is no known mutation that lengthens red cell life span.

Band 3 Clustering Models

It has been proposed that an altered membrane band 3 serves as a receptor for antibodies directed against a neoantigen, designated senescent-cell antigen, and that possibly after-binding complement marks the senescent cell for destruction. But much, if not all, of the evidence for these models depends upon the assumption that dense cells are old, and the uptake of cells by monocytes as a surrogate for their being marked for destruction.[49] However, immunoglobulin levels on aged, biotinylated rabbit cells are not increased,[50] and the fact that red cell life span has never been demonstrated to be prolonged in agammaglobulinemic patients casts serious doubt upon the concept that immunoglobulins mediate removal of senescent red cells.

Phosphatidylserine Exposure Models The exposure of phosphatidylserine on the outer leaflet of the cell membrane is one of the signals that allows macrophages to recognize apoptotic cells. It is likely that this is, indeed, at least one of the signals by which macrophages recognize senescent erythrocytes,[51–53] a process that has been designated as *erythroptosis*.[54] Data from a biotinylated rabbit erythrocyte model suggests that the average time during which phosphatidylserine is exposed is only 0.3 to 0.5 days, so that few cells with increased exposure of the phospholipid are in the circulation at any time.[52] An increase of phosphatidylserine exposure has also been documented in humans descending from high altitudes,[55] a circumstance in which there is accelerated destruction of young erythrocytes, a circumstance that has been referred to as *neocytolysis*,[56] originally observed during space travel at zero gravity and subsequently in descent from high altitudes. A proposed model for the destruction of newly formed cells was that endothelial cells might respond to changes in circulating erythropoietin by influencing the interaction of phagocytes with young red cells, targeting the cells by surface adhesion molecules.[56] A study in mice, using somewhat different methods, suggested that phosphatidylserine exposure is greatest in young erythrocytes, and does not increase with aging.[57] It is not yet clear whether phosphatidylserine exposure is the only or even the primary signal that indicates that a cell has reached the end of its life span, but it is the only major difference between senescent and nonsenescent erythrocytes that has been documented clearly.[53]

Another model that has been proposed is based upon a slight increase in green autofluorescence, believed to represent the result of oxidative damage, which has been observed in aging murine erythrocytes.[58] Interaction of erythrocyte ACD 44 with a hyaluronic acid may play a role in the clearance of aged erythrocytes from the circulation, but such clearance seems limited to primates, and a patient with CD 44 deficiency manifested congenital dyserythropoietic anemia.[59]

■ MECHANISMS OF DESTRUCTION

The previous section ("Senescence of Normal Erythrocytes") enumerated some mechanisms that may be involved in normally terminating the life of the effete erythrocyte. It has sometimes been assumed that the mechanisms by which red cells are destroyed prematurely in disease states reflect these normal mechanisms. Although there may well be some overlap, the mechanisms of red cell destruction in disease states are likely different. The assumption that the mechanisms that bring around hemolytic anemia represent premature aging of the erythrocyte is no more logical than to suggest that an animal's death through pneumonia, renal failure, or cancer represents premature aging.

Intravascular Destruction

If the red cell membrane is breached in the circulation the red cell is destroyed. This mode of demise of the erythrocyte occurs at a low frequency normally, but may be the predominant mode of destruction in some hemolytic disorders, for example, ABO-incompatible transfusions (Chaps. 53 and 137) and paroxysmal nocturnal hemoglobinuria (Chap. 40) where the complement complex creates holes in the red cell membrane, and in cardiac valve hemolysis (Chap. 50) and microangiopathic hemolytic anemia (Chaps. 50 and 130) where the shear stress may be so strong as to break open the membrane.

Extravascular Destruction

Most commonly the life of the red cell comes to an end when it is ingested by a macrophage. Clearly, signals that allow the macrophage to distinguish the younger normal red cell from a damaged or senescent cell must exist. Such signals may consist of decreased deformability and/or altered surface properties.

Decreased Deformability The red cell does not circulate as the biconcave disc customarily observed under the microscope. Instead, it is normally greatly distorted by the shear stresses in the circulation and such distortion is an absolute requirement for the red cell to be able to negotiate the narrow slits that separate the splenic pulp from the sinuses (Chaps. 5 and 55). The deformability of the erythrocyte can be measured clinically using the ektacytometer, an instrument that displays the diffraction pattern of a red cell suspension under shear stress.[60,61] The red cell membrane, a lipid bilayer, bends readily but has very little capacity to stretch. Thus, deformability is largely a function of the excess red cell membrane intrinsic to the biconcave disc shape of the cell, membrane composition, and to some extent, of the viscosity of the hemoglobin solution within the cell. As the red cell loses membrane it assumes a spherical shape and loses its ability to deform. Hereditary spherocytosis and hereditary elliptocytosis are prototypic of hemolytic anemias in which decreased deformability as a result of a decreased surface-to-volume ratio plays a key role in red cell destruction (Chap. 45). However, loss of membrane plays a role in many types of pathologic hemolysis, including autoimmune hemolytic anemia (Chap. 53). In sickle cell disease and hemoglobin C disease (Chap. 48) the internal viscosity of the cell is increased. Loss of water from the red cell, as may occur when the membrane is damaged and leaks potassium as in hereditary xerocytosis (Chap. 45), also markedly impairs the deformability of the cell.

Altered Surface Properties

The surface of the red cell membrane can be altered by binding of antibodies to surface antigens, by binding of complement components, and by chemical alterations, particularly oxidation of membrane components. Immunoglobulin (Ig) G-coated red cells[62] and red cells coated by the third component of complement (C_3)[63,64] are bound by Fc receptors on macrophages and undergo partial phagocytosis. This results in the formation of a spherocyte.

In vitro oxidation of red cells with phenylhydrazine or adenosine diphosphate (ADP) plus iron causes clustering of band 3 protein in the membrane. Although the physiologic significance of this is far from clear, it has been suggested that the clustered protein serves as a recognition site for the binding of IgG.[65,66] Oxidative damage to the membrane may play a role in the removal of sickle cells (Chap. 48) and thalassemic cells from the circulation (Chap. 47).

■ FATE OF DESTROYED RED CELLS

Intravascular Destruction

Hemoglobin When red cells are destroyed in the vascular compartment the hemoglobin escaping into the plasma is bound to haptoglobin. A dimeric glycoprotein, each molecule of haptoglobin can bind two hemoglobin dimers. The haptoglobin–hemoglobin complex is cleared from the plasma with a $T_{1/2}$ of 10 to 30 minutes. After the complex is carried to the liver parenchyma, the heme of the hemoglobin is converted to iron and biliverdin by heme oxygenase and the biliverdin is further catabolized to bilirubin. CO is released in the course of cleavage of heme by heme oxygenase.[67]

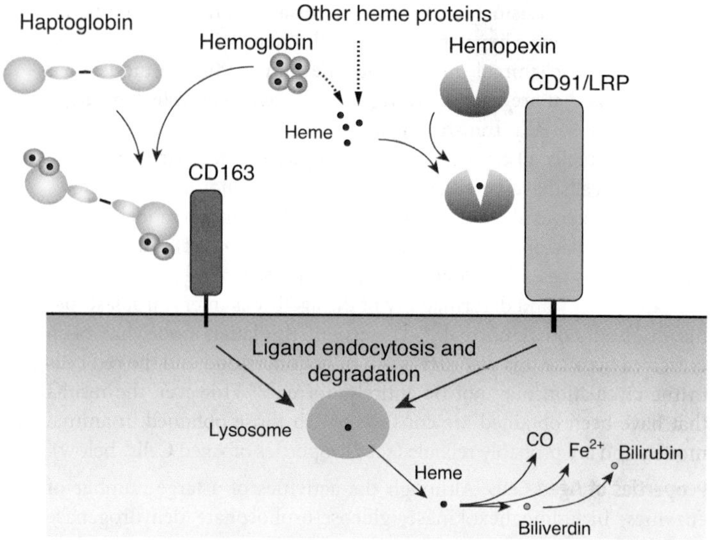

FIGURE 32–3. Overview of the receptor pathways for endocytosis of extracellular heme and hemoglobin in complex with hemopexin and haptoglobin, respectively. LRP/CD91 and CD163 represent two pathways for uptake of extracellular heme incorporated in hemopexin-heme and haptoglobin-hemoglobin. Both receptors are highly expressed in phagocytic macrophages, which are known to metabolize heme into bilirubin, Fe, and CO. In addition to the expression in macrophages, LRP/CD91 is highly expressed in several other cell types including hepatocytes, neurons, and syncytiotrophoblasts. *(From V Hvidberg, MB Maniecki, C Jacobsen, et al,[71] with permission.)*

Free haptoglobin, in contrast to the hemoglobin–haptoglobin complex, has a $T_{1/2}$ of 5 days, and when large amounts of the rapidly turned over haptoglobin–hemoglobin complex are formed, the haptoglobin content of the plasma is depleted. The haptoglobin content of the plasma is diminished not only in the plasma of patients undergoing frank intravascular hemolysis, but also from the plasma of patients who, like those with sickle cell disease, have accelerated red cell destruction occurring primarily within macrophages. Presumably there is either enough intravascular hemolysis in such hemolytic disorders to lower the plasma haptoglobin level or sufficient leakage from the phagocytic cells into the plasma to bind to haptoglobin. Thus the measurement of plasma haptoglobin levels has some usefulness in diagnosing the presence of hemolysis.

Heme Free heme that is released into the circulation is bound in a 1:1 ratio to the plasma glycoprotein hemopexin,[68] which is cleared from the plasma with a $T_{1/2}$ of 7 to 8 hours.[69,70] The heme–hemopexin complex is taken up by a low-density lipoprotein-related receptor, CD91.[71] Figure 32–3 illustrates the parallel functions of hemopexin and haptoglobin. When the capacity of hemopexin to bind heme is saturated, excess heme may bind to albumin to form methemalbumin.[72]

Extravascular Destruction

Red cells that are engulfed by phagocytic cells are degraded within lysosomes into lipids, protein, and heme. The proteins and lipids are reprocessed in their respective catabolic pathways and the heme is cleaved by a microsomal heme oxygenase[73] into iron and biliverdin. The latter is catabolized to bilirubin.

Bilirubin Excretion

Regardless of the site of destruction of hemoglobin one of the final products is bilirubin, and this is excreted through the bile into the gastrointestinal tract where it is converted to urobilinogens by bacterial reduction.[74] A small fraction of urobilinogen is reabsorbed and excreted into the urine. Thus, the fecal and urinary urobilinogen excretion have been used as an indicator of the rate of hemolysis, but are only uncommonly used for this purpose in modern practice because the collections are cumbersome and because alternative degradative pathways detract severely from the accuracy of the estimates of the rate of heme catabolism.

REFERENCES

1. Ashby W: The determination of the length of life of transfused blood corpuscles in man. *J Exp Med* 29:267, 1919.
2. Shemin D, Rittenberg D: Life span of human red blood cell. *J Biol Chem* 166:627, 1946.
3. Berlin NI, Meyer LM, Lazarus M: Life span of the rat red blood cell as determined by glycine-2-C^{14}. *Am J Physiol* 165:565, 1951.
4. Beutler E, Dern RJ, Alving AS: The hemolytic effect of primaquine. IV. The relationship of cell age to hemolysis. *J Lab Clin Med* 44:439, 1954.
5. Birgens HS, Hansen OP, Henriksen JH, Wantzin P: Quantitation of erythropoiesis in myelomatosis. *Scand J Haematol* 22:357, 1979.
6. Weinstein IM, Beutler E: The use of Cr-51 and Fe-59 in a combined procedure to study erythrocyte production and destruction in normal human subjects and in patients with hemolytic or aplastic anemia. *J Lab Clin Med* 45:616, 1955.
7. Silver HM, Seebeck MA, Cowett RM, et al: Red cell volume determination using a stable isotope of chromium. *J Soc Gynecol Investig* 4:254, 1997.
8. Lindsell CJ, Franco RS, Smith EP, Joiner CH, Cohen RM: A method for the continuous calculation of the age of labeled red blood cells. *Am J Hematol* 83:454, 2008.
9. Beutler E, West C: Measurement of the viability of stored red cells by the single-isotope technique using 51-Cr: Analysis of validity. *Transfusion* 24:100, 1984.
10. Cohen JA, Warringa MGPJ: The fate of P^{32} labeled diisopropyl fluorophosphonate in the human body and its use as a labeling agent in study of turnover of blood plasma and red cells. *J Clin Invest* 33:459, 1954.
11. Cline MJ, Berlin NI: Measurement of red cell survival with tritiated diisopropyl fluorophosphate. *J Lab Clin Med* 60:826, 1962.
12. Milner PF, Charache S: Life span of carbamylated red cells in sickle cell anemia. *J Clin Invest* 52:3161, 1973.
13. Eschbach JW, Korn D, Finch CA: ^{14}C cyanate as a tag for red cell survival in normal and uremic man. *J Lab Clin Med* 89:823, 1977.
14. Horan PK, Slezak SE: Stable cell membrane labelling. *Nature* 340:167, 1989.
15. Slezak SE, Horan PK: Fluorescent in vivo tracking of hematopoietic cells. Part I. Technical considerations. *Blood* 74:2172, 1989.
16. Suzuki T, Dale GL: Biotinylated erythrocytes: In vivo survival and in vitro recovery. *Blood* 70:791, 1987.
17. Strauss RG, Mock DM, Widness JA, et al: Posttransfusion 24-hour recovery and subsequent survival of allogeneic red blood cells in the bloodstream of newborn infants. *Transfusion* 44:871, 2004.
18. Bentley SA, Glass HI, Lewis SM, Szur L: Elution correction in ^{51}Cr red cell survival studies. *Br J Haematol* 26:179, 1974.
19. Cline MJ, Berlin NI: Simultaneous measurement of the survival of two populations of erythrocytes with the use of labelled diisopropyl fluorophosphate. *J Lab Clin Med* 61:249, 1963.
20. McCurdy PR, Sherman AS: Irreversibly sickled cells and red cell survival in sickle cell anemia: A study with both DF32P and 51CR. *Am J Med* 64:253, 1978.
21. Eadie GS, Brown IW Jr: Red blood cell survival studies. *Blood* 8:1110, 1953.
22. International Committee for Standardization in Haematology: Recommended method for radioisotope red-cell survival studies. *Br J Haematol* 45:659, 1980.
23. Berlin NI, Berk PD: Quantitative aspects of bilirubin metabolism for hematologists. *Blood* 57:983, 1981.
24. Doyle J, Vreman HJ, Stevenson DK, et al: Does vitamin C cause hemolysis in premature newborn infants? Results of a multicenter double-blind, randomized, controlled trial. *J Pediatr* 130:103, 1997.
25. Furne JK, Springfield JR, Ho SB, Levitt MD: Simplification of the end-alveolar carbon monoxide technique to assess erythrocyte survival. *J Lab Clin Med* 142:52, 2003.
26. Vreman HJ, Stevenson DK: Carboxyhemoglobin determined in neonatal blood with a CO-oximeter unaffected by fetal oxyhemoglobin. *Clin Chem* 40:1522, 1994.
27. ICSH Panel on Diagnostic Applications of Radioisotopes in Hematology: Recommended methods for surface counting to determine sites of red cell destruction. *Br J Haematol* 30:249, 1975.
28. Hillman RS, Finch CA: Erythropoiesis: Normal and abnormal. *Semin Hematol* 4:327, 1967.
29. Datz FL, Taylor AJ: The clinical use of radionuclide bone marrow imaging. *Semin Nucl Med* 15:239, 1985.
30. Jandl JH, Greenberg MS, Yonemoto RH, Castle WB: Clinical determination of the sites of red cell sequestration in hemolytic anemias. *J Clin Invest* 35:842, 1956.
31. Ferrant A, Cauwe F, Michaux JL, et al: Assessment of the sites of red cell destruction using quantitative measurements of splenic and hepatic red cell destruction. *Br J Haematol* 50:591, 1982.
32. Borun ER, Figueroa WG, Perry SM: The distribution of Fe^{59} tagged human erythrocytes in centrifuged specimens as a function of cell age. *J Clin Invest* 36:676, 1957.
33. Luthra MG, Friedman JM, Sears DA: Studies of density fractions of normal human erythrocytes labeled with iron-59 in vivo. *J Lab Clin Med* 94:879, 1979.
34. Linderkamp O, Friederichs E, Boehler T, Ludwig A: Age dependency of red blood cell deformability and density: Studies in transient erythroblastopenia of childhood. *Br J Haematol* 83:125, 1993.
35. Dale GL, Norenberg SL: Density fractionation of erythrocytes by Percoll/hypaque results in only a slight enrichment for aged cells. *Biochim Biophys Acta* 1036:183, 1990.
36. Bosch FH, Werre JM, Roerdinkholder-Stoelwinder B, et al: Characteristics of red blood cell populations fractionated with a combination of counterflow centrifugation and Percoll separation. *Blood* 79:254, 1992.
37. Ganzoni AM, Oakes R, Hillman RS: Red cell aging in vivo. *J Clin Invest* 50:1373, 1971.
38. Suzuki T, Dale GL: Senescent erythrocytes: Isolation of in vivo aged cells and their biochemical characteristics. *Proc Natl Acad Sci U S A* 85:1647, 1988.
39. Haram S, Carriero D, Seaman C, Piomelli S: The mechanism of decline of age-dependent enzymes in the red blood cell. *Enzyme* 45:47, 1991.
40. Zimran A, Forman L, Suzuki T, Dale GL, Beutler E: In vivo aging of red cell enzymes: Study of biotinylated red blood cells in rabbits. *Am J Hematol* 33:249, 1990.
41. Beutler E, Hartman G: Age-related red cell enzymes in children with transient erythroblastopenia of childhood and hemolytic anemia. *Pediatr Res* 19:44, 1985.
42. Beutler E: The relationship of red cell enzymes to red cell life-span. *Blood Cells* 14:69, 1988.
43. Dale GL, Norenberg SL: Time-dependent loss of adenosine 5′-monophosphate deaminase activity may explain elevated adenosine 5′-triphosphate levels in senescent erythrocytes. *Blood* 74:2157, 1989.
44. Paglia DE, Valentine WN, Nakatani M, Brockway RA: AMP deaminase as a cell-age marker in transient erythroblastopenia of childhood and its role in the adenylate economy of erythrocytes. *Blood* 74:2161, 1989.
45. Dale GL, Norenberg SL, Suzuki T, Forman L: Altered adenine nucleotide metabolism in senescent erythrocytes from the rabbit. *Prog Clin Biol Res* 319:259, 1989.
46. Clark MR, Corash L, Jensen RH: Density distribution of aging, transfused human red cells. *Blood* 74(Suppl 1):217a, 1989.
47. Waugh RE, Narla M, Jackson CW, et al: Rheologic properties of senescent erythrocytes: Loss of surface area and volume with red blood cell age. *Blood* 79:1351, 1992.
48. Willekens FL, Werre JM, Groenen-Dopp YA, et al: Erythrocyte vesiculation: a self-protective mechanism? *Br J Haematol* 141:549, 2008.
49. Arese P, Turrini F, Schwarzer E: Band 3/complement-mediated recognition and removal of normally senescent and pathological human erythrocytes. *Cell Physiol Biochem* 16:133, 2005.
50. Dale GL: Does surface bound immunoglobulin mediate erythrocyte death? Commentary. *Blood Cells* 14:36, 1988.
51. Connor J, Pak CC, Schroit AJ: Exposure of phosphatidylserine in the outer leaflet of human red blood cells. Relationship to cell density, cell age, and clearance by mononuclear cells. *J Biol Chem* 269:2399, 1994.
52. Boas FE, Forman L, Beutler E: Phosphatidyl serine exposure and red cell viability in red cell aging and in hemolytic anemia. *Proc Natl Acad Sci U S A* 95:3077, 1998.
53. Kuypers FA, De Jong K: The role of phosphatidylserine in recognition and removal of erythrocytes. *Cell Mol Biol* 50:147, 2004.
54. Daugas E, Cande C, Kroemer G: Erythrocytes: Death of a mummy. *Cell Death Differ* 8:1131, 2001.
55. Risso A, Turello M, Biffoni F, Antonutto G: Red blood cell senescence and neocytolysis in humans after high altitude acclimatization. *Blood Cells Mol Dis* 38:83, 2007.
56. Rice L, Alfrey CP: The negative regulation of red cell mass by neocytolysis: Physiologic and pathophysiologic manifestations. *Cell Physiol Biochem* 15:245, 2005.
57. Khandelwal S, Saxena RK: A role of phosphatidylserine externalization in clearance of erythrocytes exposed to stress but not in eliminating aging populations of erythrocyte in mice. *Exp Gerontol* 43:764, 2008.
58. Khandelwal S, Saxena RK: Age-dependent increase in green autofluorescence of blood erythrocytes. *J Biosci* 32:1139, 2007.
59. Kerfoot SM, McRae K, Lam F, et al: A novel mechanism of erythrocyte capture from circulation in humans. *Exp Hematol* 36:111, 2008.
60. Rigal CS: The place of instruments in the scientific work of Marcel Bessis (1917–1994): The electron microscope and the ektacytometer. *Hematol Cell Ther* 42:250, 2000.
61. Shin S, Hou JX, Suh JS, Singh M: Validation and application of a microfluidic ektacytometer (RheoScan-D) in measuring erythrocyte deformability. *Clin Hemorheol Microcirc* 37:319, 2007.
62. Lo Buglio AF, Cotran RS, Jandl JH: Red cells coated with immunoglobulin G: Binding and sphering by mononuclear cells in man. *Science* 158:1582, 1967.
63. Jandl JH, Tomlinson AS: The destruction of red cells by antibodies in man. II. Pyrogenic, leukocytic and dermal responses to immune hemolysis. *J Clin Invest* 37:1202, 1958.
64. Lutz HU, Stammler P, Kock D, Taylor RP: Opsonic potential of C3b-anti-band 3 complexes when generated on senescent and oxidatively stressed red cells or in fluid phase, in *Red Blood Cell Aging*, edited by M Magnani, A DeFlora, p 367. Plenum Press, New York, 1991.
65. Low PS, Waugh SM, Zinke K, Drenckhahn D: The role of hemoglobin denaturation and band 3 clustering in red blood cell aging. *Science* 227:531, 1985.

66. Beppu M, Mizukami A, Nagoya M, Kikugawa K: Binding of anti-band 3 autoantibody to oxidatively damaged erythrocytes. Formation of senescent antigen on erythrocyte surface by an oxidative mechanism. *J Biol Chem* 265:3226, 1990.
67. Carter K, Worwood M: Haptoglobin: A review of the major allele frequencies worldwide and their association with diseases. *Int J Lab Hematol* 29:92, 2007.
68. Piccard H, Van den Steen PE, Opdenakker G: Hemopexin domains as multifunctional liganding modules in matrix metalloproteinases and other proteins. *J Leukoc Biol* 81:870, 2007.
69. Sears DA: Disposal of plasma heme in normal man and patients with intravascular hemolysis. *J Clin Invest* 49:5, 1970.
70. Wochner RD, Spilberg I, Iio A, et al: Hemopexin metabolism in sickle-cell disease, porphyrias and control subjects—Effects of heme injection. *N Engl J Med* 290:822, 1974.
71. Hvidberg V, Maniecki MB, Jacobsen C, et al: Identification of the receptor scavenging hemopexin-heme complexes. *Blood* 106:2572, 2005.
72. Rosen H, Sears DA: Spectral properties of hemopexin-heme: The Schumm test. *J Lab Clin Med* 74:941, 1969.
73. Maines MD: The heme oxygenase system: A regulator of second messenger gases. *Annu Rev Pharmacol Toxicol* 37:517, 1997.
74. Elder G, Gray CH, Nicholson DG: Bile pigment fate in gastrointestinal tract. *Semin Hematol* 9:71, 1972.

CHAPTER 33

CLINICAL MANIFESTATIONS AND CLASSIFICATION OF ERYTHROCYTE DISORDERS

Josef T. Prchal

SUMMARY

Anemias are characterized by a decrease and polycythemias by an increase of the red cell mass. Because the anemias have their principal effect by decreasing the oxygen-carrying capacity of blood, they are best expressed in terms of hemoglobin concentration. Anemia may cause symptoms because of tissue hypoxia (e.g., fatigue, dyspnea on exertion). These manifestations are also caused by compensatory attempts to ameliorate hypoxia (e.g., hyperventilation, tachycardia, and increased cardiac output). Tissue hypoxia sensing is ubiquitous and it is signaled by an increased level of transcription factors, hypoxia-inducible transcription factors HIF-1 and HIF-2. HIFs upregulate transcription of many genes that are involved in angiogenesis, energy metabolism, and iron balance, as well as erythropoiesis, including the principal erythropoietic factor, erythropoietin. The classification of anemia is evolving, as it should take into account new kinetic and molecular findings.

The polycythemias (erythrocytoses) are best expressed in terms of the packed red cell volume (hematocrit), as their clinical manifestations are primarily related to the expanded red cell mass and resulting increased viscosity of blood, and specific features related to the pathophysiology stemming from the molecular causative defect (e.g., thrombosis in polycythemia vera, cyanosis in congenital methemoglobinemia). The polycythemias are either caused by an aberrant function of hematopoietic progenitors—primary polycythemias (e.g., a monoclonal expansion of a multipotential hematopoietic cell [polycythemia vera] or gain-of-function mutations of erythroid progenitors)—or are caused by increased levels of circulating erythropoiesis-stimulating factors, usually erythropoietin—secondary polycythemias (e.g., chronic pulmonary disease, cobalt poisoning or high oxygen affinity hemoglobin mutants). Some polycythemias have hypersensitive erythroid progenitors as well as increased levels of erythropoietin, and thus share features of both primary and secondary polycythemia; that is, Chuvash polycythemia. Persons with relative (spurious) polycythemia have a contracted plasma volume and normal red cell mass.

ANEMIA

■ PATHOPHYSIOLOGY AND MANIFESTATIONS

Effect on Oxygen Transport

The clinical manifestations of anemia are a function of the degree of tissue hypoxia and the etiology and pathogenesis of the specific anemia (e.g., splenomegaly characteristic of hereditary spherocytosis, neurologic degeneration, or gastric atrophy of pernicious anemia). Decreased oxygen-carrying capacity mobilizes compensatory mechanisms designed to prevent or ameliorate tissue anoxia. The red cells also carry carbon dioxide from the tissues to the lungs and help distribute nitric oxide throughout the body (see Chap. 49), but transport of these gases does not appear to be dependent on the number of red cells available and remains normal in anemic patients. Tissue hypoxia occurs when the pressure of oxygen in the capillaries is too low to provide cells with enough oxygen for the cells' metabolic needs. In an average person, the red cell mass must provide the total body tissues with approximately 250 mL/min of oxygen to support life. Because the oxygen-carrying capacity of normal blood is 1.34 mL per gram of hemoglobin (approximately 200 mL per liter of normal blood) and cardiac output is approximately 5000 mL/min, 1000 mL/min of oxygen is available at the tissue level. Extraction of one-fourth of this amount reduces the oxygen tension of 100 torr in the arterial end of the capillary to 40 torr in the venous end. This partial extraction ensures the presence of sufficient diffusion pressure throughout the capillaries to provide all cells with enough oxygen for the cells' metabolic needs (Fig. 33–1). In anemia, extraction of the same amount of oxygen leads to greater hemoglobin desaturation and lower oxygen tension at the venous end of the capillary. The resulting anoxia in the immediate vicinity initiates a number of compensatory, and frequently symptomatic, adjustments in the supply of blood and oxygen.

Acronyms and abbreviations used in this chapter include: HIF, hypoxia-inducible factor.

Hypoxia-Inducible Transcription Factor 1 Hypoxia-inducible transcription factor 1 (HIF-1) and its homologue with tissue-restricted expression HIF-2 play a central role in the body's response to hypoxia (see Chaps. 31 and 56). HIF-1 was first identified as a factor regulating the transcriptional activity of the erythropoietin gene (see Chap. 31).[1] The essential role of this transcriptional factor in global regulation of protection against hypoxia soon became clear. Its actions include respiratory control, transcriptional regulation of glycolytic enzyme genes, angiogenesis, and energy metabolism.[2–4] The prediction that hypoxia-regulated subunit of HIF-1 (HIF-1α) degradation is controlled by an enzyme sensitive to the presence or absence of oxygen[5] proved to be prescient. Chap. 31 describes the current knowledge of hypoxia sensing in greater detail. Tissue-specific and known and unknown factors are responsible for tissue-specific mobilization of the compensatory mechanisms listed below that permit survival under hypoxic conditions. Figure 33–2 outlines the regulation of some physiologic processes by hypoxia.

Decreased Oxygen Consumption

Energy metabolism at the optimal oxygen supply is sustained by efficient oxidative phosphorylation. In hypoxia, energy is produced by less-efficient glycolysis accomplished by upregulation of transcription of glycolytic enzyme genes[4] and increased glucose transport, a process known as the *Pasteur effect*. The Pasteur effect and its cancer exception, that is, the Warburg effect, are explained at the molecular level by changes in HIF-1 levels.[4,6–8]

Decreased Oxygen Affinity

Efficient increase of tissue oxygen delivery is accomplished by decreasing the affinity of hemoglobin for oxygen (right-shifted hemoglobin oxygen dissociation curve). This action permits increased oxygen extraction from the same amount of hemoglobin (see Chap. 48).[9] Acutely, a very small shift in pH produces a large effect on the dissociation curve because of the Bohr effect. In chronic anemia, increased oxygen tissue delivery is accomplished by increased amounts of 2,3-bisphosphoglycerate (see Chap. 46).[9] The increased synthesis of 2,3-bisphosphoglycerate in anemia is accomplished by increasing the intracellular pH of red cells (see Chap. 46) by respiratory alkalosis resulting from increased respiration. This effect is clearly demonstrated in individuals with high-altitude hypoxemia.[10]

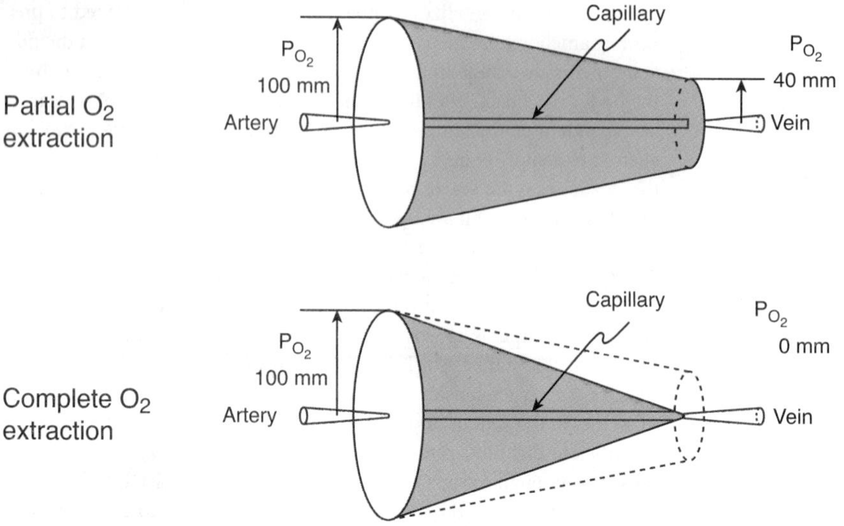

FIGURE 33–1. Theoretical tissue segment provided with oxygen from one capillary. With an arterial diffusion pressure of oxygen of 100 torr and partial oxygen extraction resulting in a venous oxygen pressure of 40 torr, one capillary can provide oxygen to cells within a truncated cone segment. With complete oxygen extraction, however, oxygen cannot be supplied to cells within a rim of tissue around the apex of the cone.

Increased Tissue Perfusion

The effect of decreased oxygen-carrying capacity on the tissue tension of oxygen can be compensated by increasing tissue perfusion by changing vasomotor activity and angiogenesis.[2] Because in chronic anemia the blood volume is not changed (Fig. 33–3),[11] increased tissue perfusion is organ selective, accomplished by shunting the blood from nonvital donor areas to oxygen-sensitive essential recipient organs. In acute anemia, the major donor areas for redistribution of blood are the mesenteric and iliac beds.[12] In chronic anemia in humans, the donor areas are the cutaneous tissue[13] and the kidneys.[14] Vasoconstriction and oxygen deprivation in the skin causes characteristic pallor of anemia. In the kidneys, the oxygen supply under normal conditions exceeds oxygen demands. The arteriovenous oxygen difference in the kidney is as low as 1.4 mL/dL (compared with the myocardium, where the difference can be as high as 20 mL/dL), indicating that even a severe reduction in kidney perfusion can be tolerated. Nevertheless, enough renal hypoxia must be present to activate HIF-1 and stimulate increased erythropoietin production and erythropoiesis (see Chaps. 31 and 36). The effect on renal excretory mechanisms is slight because the reduction in renal blood flow is offset by high plasmacrit. Even in severe anemia in which renal blood flow is reduced by almost 50 percent, the total renal plasma flow is only moderately reduced. Thus, organs with the most pressing need for oxygen, such as myocardium, brain, and muscles, are largely unimpeded by a moderate reduction in oxygen-carrying capacity. Severe anemia can cause retinal hemorrhages.[15]

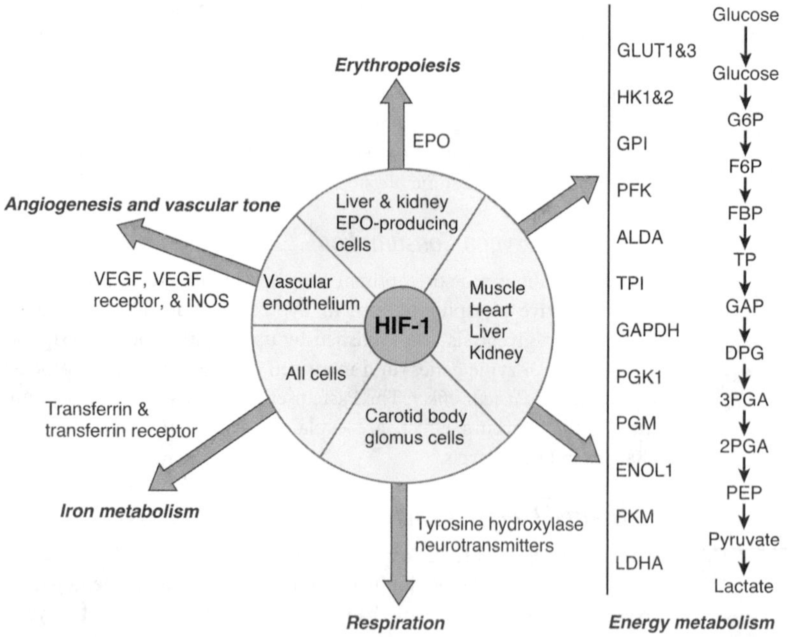

FIGURE 33–2. Regulation of erythropoiesis, angiogenesis, iron metabolism, respiration, and energy metabolism by HIF-1 are examples of physiologic processes regulated by hypoxia. iNOS, inducible nitrous oxide synthase; VEGF, vascular endothelial growth factor. *Right panel, left column*: GLUT1&3, glucose transporters 1 and 3; glycolytic enzymes: HK1&2, hexokinase 1 and 2; GPI, glucose phosphate isomerase; PFK, phosphofructokinase; ALDA, aldolase A; TPI, triosephosphate isomerase; GAPDH, glycerol phosphate dehydrogenase; PGK1, phosphoglycerate kinase; PGM, phosphoglycerate mutase; ENOL1, enolase 1; PKM, pyruvate kinase M isoform; LDHA, lactic dehydrogenase A isoform. *Right column*: Metabolic intermediates generated by the depicted enzymes.

Increased Cardiac Output

Increased cardiac output is an excellent but metabolically expensive compensatory device.[16] It decreases the fraction of oxygen that must be extracted during each circulation, thereby maintaining higher oxygen pressure. Because the viscosity of blood in anemia is decreased and selective vascular dilatation decreases peripheral resistance, high cardiac output can be maintained without any increase in blood pressure.[17] In an otherwise healthy person, a measurable increase in resting cardiac output does not occur until hemoglobin concentration is less than 7 g/dL, and clinical signs of cardiac hyperactivity usually are not present until hemoglobin concentration reaches even lower levels.[18]

Signs of cardiac hyperactivity include tachycardia, increased arterial and capillary pulsation, and hemodynamic "flow" murmurs.[19] The murmurs usually are heard during systole at the apex, over the pulmonary valve area, or at the pulmonary valve area. Murmurs and bruits have been described in many regions, such as over the jugular vein, the closed eye, and the parietal region of the skull, and may be sensed by the patient as roaring in the ears (tinnitus), especially at night. They disappear promptly after the hemoglobin concentration is restored to normal.[19] The myocardium tolerates a prolonged period of sustained hyperactivity. However, angina pectoris and high-output failure may supervene if anemia is so extreme that it exceeds myocardial oxygen demands or if the patient has coronary artery disease. Cardiomegaly, pulmonary congestion, ascites, and edema have been observed, and they require prompt treatment with oxygen, transfusion of packed red cells, and other appropriate measures.

Increased Pulmonary Function

Significant anemia leads to compensatory increase in respiratory rate that decreases the oxygen gradient from

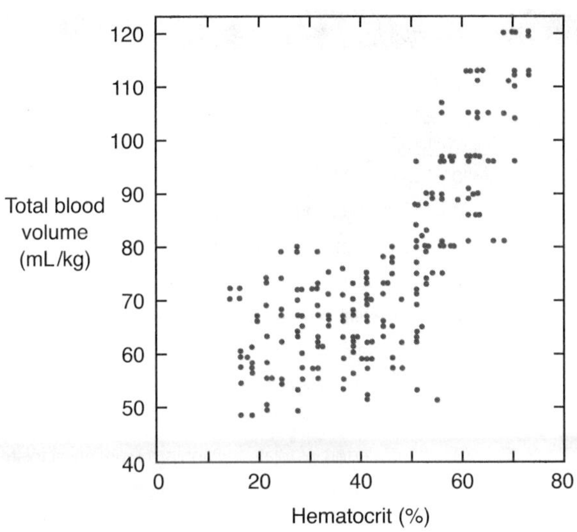

FIGURE 33–3. Relationship between hematocrit and total blood volume in normal individuals and in patients with anemia and polycythemia. *(Reproduced from Huber H, Lewis SM, and Szur Ls.[11])*

ambient air to alveolar air and increases the amount of oxygen available to oxygenate a greater than normal cardiac output. Consequently, exertional dyspnea and orthopnea are characteristic clinical manifestations of moderate to severe anemia.[18–21]

Increased Red Cell Production

The most appropriate response to anemia is a compensatory increase of red cell production, which may increase about twofold to threefold acutely and fourfold to sixfold chronically, and occasionally as much as 10-fold in the latter case. The increase is mediated by increased production of erythropoietin. The rate of erythropoietin synthesis is inversely and logarithmically related to hemoglobin concentration (see Chap. 31). Erythropoietin concentration can increase from approximately 10 mU/mL at normal hemoglobin concentrations to 10,000 mU/mL in severe anemia (Fig. 33–4).[22,23] The change in erythropoietin levels ensures that red cell production balances red cell destruction (compensated hemolysis) or chronic moderate blood loss. Augmented erythroid activity expands marrow space, which, if intense, can cause sternal tenderness and diffuse bone pains. The proportion and number of reticulocytes increase. Because erythroid transit time through the marrow is shortened, "stress reticulocytes" having increased cell volume and surface area appear. They develop characteristic surface folds as a result of the increased surface-area-to-volume ratio that can be identified in the blood film. Nucleated red cells may be observed in the blood in severe anemia.[24]

Administration of human recombinant erythropoietin augments or replaces endogenous synthesis. In pharmacologic amounts, the effect on hemoglobin concentration is most noticeable if endogenous production is subnormal as a result of renal failure or systemic illnesses (see Chaps. 36 and 37). In severe anemia where endogenous erythropoietin production (providing production is not impaired) has already increased red cell production maximally, administration of erythropoietin generally does not help, and the patients require transfusion.[23]

Uncorrected Tissue Hypoxia

A certain residual degree of tissue hypoxia remains despite mobilization of compensatory mechanisms. Hypoxia is essential for initiation of adequate cardiovascular and erythropoietic compensation mechanisms, but severe tissue hypoxia can cause the following symptoms: dyspnea on exertion or even at rest; angina; intermittent claudication; muscle cramps, typically at night; headache; light-headedness; and fatigue. A number of diffuse gastrointestinal and genitourinary symptoms are associated with anemia (e.g., abdominal cramps, nausea), but whether the symptoms should be attributed to tissue hypoxia, compensatory redistribution of blood, or the underlying cause of anemia is uncertain.

■ CLASSIFICATION

Based on determination of the red cell mass, anemia can be classified as (1) *relative* or (2) *absolute*. Relative anemia is characterized by a normal total red cell mass. The conditions usually are not thought of as hematologic disorders but rather as disturbances in plasma volume regulation. However, dilution anemia is of clinical and differential diagnostic importance for the hematologist.

Classification of the *absolute anemias* with decreased red cell mass is difficult because the classification has to consider kinetic, morphologic, and pathophysiologic interacting criteria. Initially, all anemias should be divided into anemias caused by decreased production and anemias caused by increased destruction of red cells. The differentiation is based largely on the reticulocyte count. Subsequent diagnostic breakdown can be based on either morphologic or pathophysiologic criteria.

Morphologic classification subdivides anemia into (1) macrocytic anemia, (2) normocytic anemia, and (3) microcytic hypochromic anemia. The main advantages of this classification are that the classification is simple, is based on readily available red cell indices (mean corpuscular volume [MCV] and mean corpuscular hemoglobin concentration [MCHC]), and forces the physician to consider the most important types of curable anemia: vitamin B_{12}, folic acid, and iron-deficiency anemias. Such practical considerations have led to wide acceptance of this classification. *Pathophysiologic classification* (Table 33–1) is best suited for relating disease processes to potential treatment. In addition, anemia resulting from vitamin or iron-deficiency states occurs in a significant proportion of patients with normal indices.

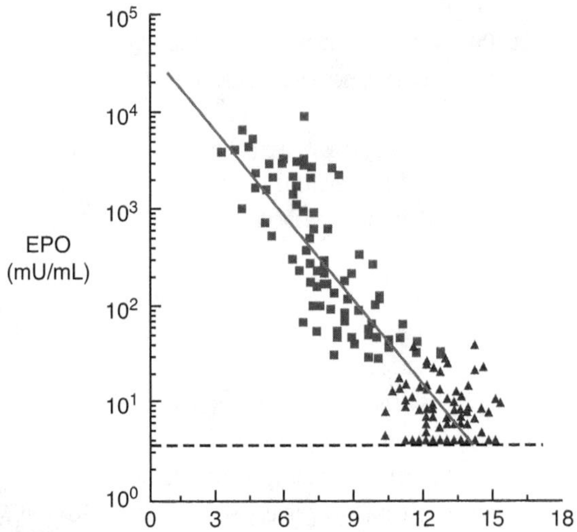

FIGURE 33–4. Erythropoietin levels in plasma of normal individuals and patients with anemia uncomplicated by renal or inflammatory disease. The lower limit of accuracy of the erythropoietin assay is 3 mU/mL and is indicated by the broken line. ■, anemias; ▲, normals.

TABLE 33–1. Classification of Anemia

I. Absolute Anemia (decreased red cell volume)

A. Decreased red cell production

1. Acquired

a. Pluripotential stem cell failure

(1) Aplastic anemia (see Chap. 34)

(a) Radiation induced

(b) Drugs and chemicals (chloramphenicol, benzene, etc.)

(c) Viruses (hepatitis, Epstein-Barr virus, etc.)

(d) Idiopathic

(2) Anemia of leukemia and of myelodysplastic syndromes (see Chaps. 88, 89, and 93)

(3) Anemia associated with marrow infiltration (see Chap. 44)

(4) Postchemotherapy (see Chap. 20)

b. Erythroid progenitor cell failure

(1) Pure red cell aplasia (parvovirus B19 infection, drugs, associated with thymoma, autoantibodies, etc. [see Chap. 35])

(2) Endocrine disorders (see Chap. 38)

(3) Acquired sideroblastic anemia (drugs, copper deficiency, etc. [see Chaps. 58 and 88])

c. Functional impairment of erythroid and other progenitors due to nutritional and other causes

(1) Megaloblastic anemias (see Chap. 41)

(a) B_{12} deficiency

(b) Folate deficiency

(c) Acute megaloblastic anemia because of nitrous oxide (N_2O)

(d) Drug-induced megaloblastic anemia (pemetrexed, methotrexate, phenytoin toxicity, etc.)

(2) Iron-deficiency anemia (see Chap. 42)

(3) Anemia resulting from other nutritional deficiencies (see Chap. 43)

(4) Anemia of chronic disease and inflammation (see Chap. 37)

(5) Anemia of renal failure (see Chap. 36)

(6) Anemia caused by chemical agents (lead toxicity [see Chap. 51])

(7) Acquired thalassemias (seen in some clonal hematopoietic disorders [see Chaps. 47 and 88])

(8) Erythropoietin antibodies (see Chap. 35)

2. Hereditary

a. Pluripotential stem-cell failure (see Chap. 34)

(1) Fanconi anemia

(2) Shwachman syndrome

(3) Dyskeratosis congenita

b. Erythroid progenitor cell failure

(1) Diamond-Blackfan syndrome (see Chap. 34)

(2) Congenital dyserythropoietic syndromes (see Chap. 39)

c. Functional impairment of erythroid and other progenitors from nutritional and other causes

(1) Megaloblastic anemias (see Chap. 41)

(a) Selective malabsorption of vitamin B_{12} (Imerslund-Gräsbeck disease)

(b) Congenital intrinsic factor deficiency

(c) Transcobalamin II deficiency

(d) Inborn errors of cobalamin metabolism (methylmalonic aciduria, homocystinuria, etc.)

(e) Inborn errors of folate metabolism (congenital folate malabsorption, dihydrofolate deficiency, methyltransferase deficiency, etc.)

(2) Inborn purine and pyrimidine metabolism defects (Lesch-Nyhan syndrome, hereditary orotic aciduria, etc.)

(3) Disorders of iron metabolism (see Chap. 42)

(a) Hereditary atransferrinemia

(b) Hypochromic anemia caused by divalent metal transporter (DMT)-1 mutation

(4) Hereditary sideroblastic anemia (see Chap. 58)

(5) Thalassemias (see Chap. 47)

B. Increased red cell destruction

1. Acquired

a. Mechanical

(1) Macroangiopathic (march hemoglobinuria, artificial heart valves [see Chap. 50])

(2) Microangiopathic (disseminated intravascular coagulation [DIC]; thrombotic thrombocytopenic purpura [TTP]; vasculitis [see Chaps. 50, 123, and 130])

(3) Parasites and microorganisms (malaria, bartonellosis, babesiosis, *Clostridium perfringens*, etc. [see Chap. 52])

b. Antibody mediated

(1) Warm-type autoimmune hemolytic anemia (see Chap. 53)

(2) Cryopathic syndromes (cold agglutinin disease, paroxysmal cold hemoglobinuria, cryoglobulinemia [see Chaps. 53 and 137])

(3) Transfusion reactions (immediate and delayed [see Chaps. 53 and 137])

c. Hypersplenism (see Chap. 55)

d. Red cell membrane disorders (see Chap. 45)

(1) Spur cell hemolysis

(2) Acquired acanthocytosis and acquired stomatocytosis, etc.

e. Chemical injury and complex chemicals (arsenic, copper, chlorate, spider, scorpion, and snake venoms, etc. [see Chap. 51])

f. Physical injury (heat, oxygen, radiation [see Chap. 51])

2. Hereditary

a. Hemoglobinopathies (see Chap. 48)

(1) Sickle cell disease

(2) Unstable hemoglobins

(continued)

TABLE 33–1. Classification of Anemia (Continued)

b. Red cell membrane disorders (see Chap. 45)
   (1) Cytoskeletal membrane disorders (hereditary spherocytosis, elliptocytosis, pyropoikilocytosis)
   (2) Lipid membrane disorders (hereditary abetalipoproteinemia, hereditary stomatocytosis, etc.)
   (3) Membrane disorders associated with abnormalities of erythrocyte antigens (McLeod syndrome, Rh deficiency syndromes, etc.)
   (4) Membrane disorders associated with abnormal transport (hereditary xerocytosis)
c. Red cell enzyme defects (pyruvate kinase, 5′ nucleotidase, glucose-6-phosphate dehydrogenase deficiencies, other red cell enzyme disorders [see Chap. 46])
d. Porphyrias (congenital erythropoietic and hepatoerythropoietic porphyrias, rarely congenital erythropoietic protoporphyria [see Chap. 57])
1. Acute blood loss
2. Splenic sequestration crisis (see Chap. 55)

II. Relative (increased plasma volume)
   A. Macroglobulinemia (see Chap. 111)
   B. Pregnancy (see Chap. 7)
   C. Athletes (see Chap. 32)
   D. Postflight astronauts (see Chap. 32)

This chapter presents a classification based on our present concepts of normal red cell production and red cell destruction. Figure 33–5 outlines the cascade of proliferation, differentiation, and maturation underlying the transformation of a multipotential stem cell, first to erythroid progenitor cells, then to erythroid precursor cells, and finally to mature red cells. Each of these steps can become impaired and cause anemia. Therapeutic intervention depends on identifying the defective step and instituting the specific therapy. The limitation of such a classification is that, in most anemias, the pathogenesis involves several steps. For example, a decreased rate of production most often results in production of defective red cells with a shortened life span. Thus, the outline provided is a conceptual guide to our present understanding of the processes underlying the production and destruction of red cells.

POLYCYTHEMIA (ERYTHROCYTOSIS)

■ PATHOPHYSIOLOGY

The production and presence of an increased number of red cells are associated with general and specific effects generated by changes in blood viscosity and blood volume.

At hematocrit readings greater than 50 percent, the viscosity of blood increases logarithmically (Fig. 33–6). The resulting decrease in blood flow reduces the transport of oxygen, with optimal values at hematocrit readings between 40 and 45 percent.[25,26] In a study of red cells from a number of animal species, the optimal value of oxygen transport corresponded closely to their normal hematocrits,[27] which may explain the evolutionary choice of certain hematocrit levels as optimal.[28] However, before concluding that polycythemia always is a suboptimal condition, realize that it may be premature to correlate viscosity readings, derived from blood tested in a rigid glass viscosimeter (Ostwald) or even in a cone-plate viscosimeter, with those in flowing blood through tiny distensible vessels *in vivo*.[29] First, the flow through these narrow channels is rapid (high shear rate), which in a non-Newtonian fluid such as blood causes a marked decrease in viscosity. Second, blood flowing through narrow channels *in vivo* is axial, with a central core of packed red cells sliding over a peripheral layer of lubricating low-viscosity plasma. Finally, and most important, absolute polycythemia is not normovolemic but is accompanied by increased

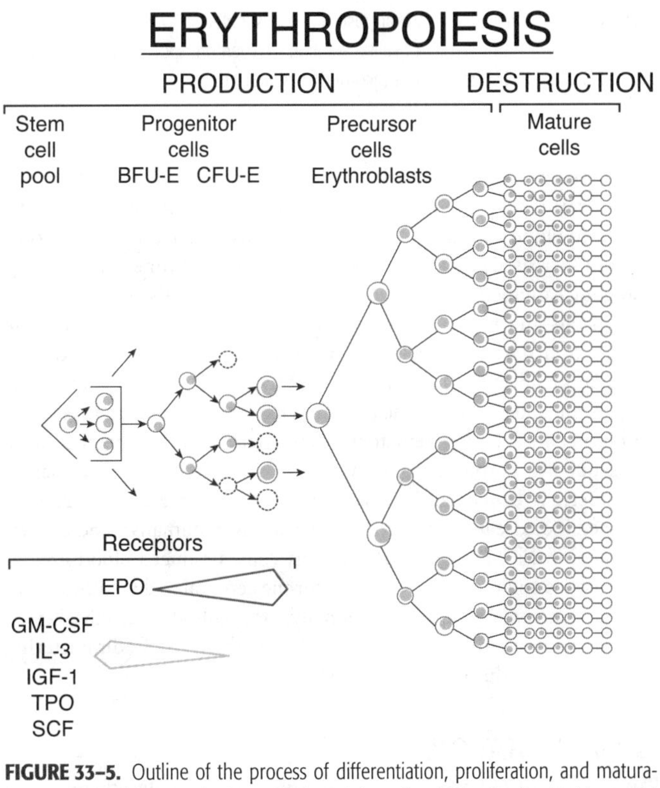

FIGURE 33–5. Outline of the process of differentiation, proliferation, and maturation underlying the production and destruction of red blood cells. Multipotential stem cells responding to a number of growth factors, including granulocyte-monocyte colony-stimulating factors (GM-CSF), interleukin 3 (IL-3), insulin growth factor 1 (IGF-1), thrombopoietin (TPO), and stem cell factor (SCF), differentiate to progenitor cells committed to erythroid development. Progenitor cells, burst-forming unit–erythroid (BFU-E), and colony-forming unit–erythroid (CFU-E) proliferate under the control of erythropoietin (EPO) and finally differentiate to precursor cells (erythroblasts). In the presence of adequate amounts of nutrients, such as vitamin B_{12}, folic acid, and iron, precursor cells proliferate and mature into nucleated red cells, reticulocytes, and mature red blood cells. After a 120-day life span, these cells age and are destroyed.

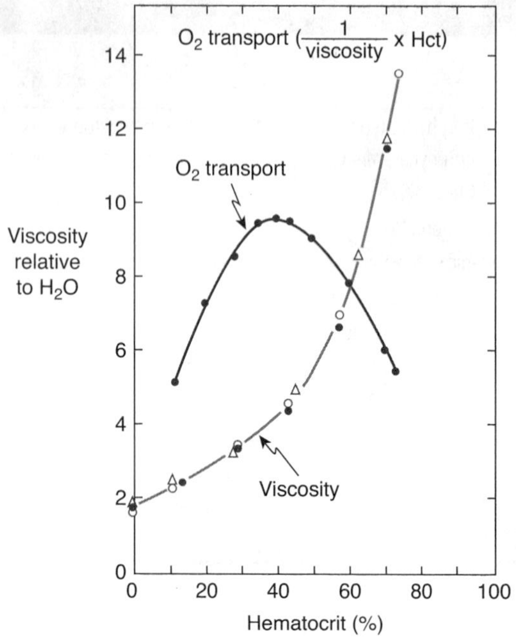

FIGURE 33–6. Viscosity of heparinized normal human blood related to hematocrit (Hct). Viscosity is measured with an Ostwald viscosimeter at 37°C (98.6°F) and expressed in relation to viscosity of saline solution. Oxygen transport is computed from hct and O_2 flow (1/viscosity) and is recorded in arbitrary units.

blood volume, which, in turn, enlarges the vascular bed and decreases peripheral resistance. Because blood pressure remains stable, the increased blood volume must be associated with increased cardiac output and increased oxygen transport (cardiac output times hematocrit). Using measurements of cardiac output in dogs[30] and tissue oxygen tension in rats and mice,[29] construction of curves (Fig. 33–7) that relate oxygen transport to hematocrit in normovolemic and hypervolemic states is possible. The curves show that hypervolemia *per se* increases oxygen transport and that the optimum oxygen transport in these conditions occurs at higher hematocrit values than in normovolemic states. Consequently, despite the increased viscosity, a moderate increase in hematocrit is beneficial. The same may not be true of a more pronounced increase in hematocrit. Observations in humans[31] and experimental animals[30] indicate high viscosity causes reduced blood flow to most tissues and may be responsible for the cerebral and cardiovascular impairment experienced occasionally by high-altitude dwellers,[32] patients with severe polycythemia,[33,34] and athletes self-administering overdoses of erythropoietin (see Chap. 56).

MANIFESTATIONS

The rate of red cell production is increased in true polycythemias, but changes in marrow morphology can be unimpressive, although marrow is hypercellular in a typical patient with polycythemia vera. Under normal conditions, the rate of red cell production is adjusted to maintain the red cell mass at about 30 mL per kilogram of body weight. Because the life span of red cells in polycythemia is normal, a mere doubling of the daily rate of red cell production is adequate to maintain a polycythemic red cell mass of 60 mL/kg. Consequently, the morphology and volume of the marrow are only moderately altered in polycythemia compared with the changes observed in some types of hemolytic anemia, in which the rate of red cell production can be four to six times normal. In erythrocytosis, the number of red cells destroyed daily merely causes a slight increase in bilirubin levels. The presence of secondary gout and splenomegaly usually are signs of a myeloproliferative disorder rather than of erythrocytosis alone. Although considerable homology exists between erythropoietin and thrombopoietin,[35] erythropoietin-driven erythrocytosis is not associated with increased platelet production.

The increased viscosity and vascular space are responsible for many of the signs and symptoms of polycythemia. The characteristic *rubor* in patients with polycythemia vera is caused by excessive deoxygenation of blood flowing sluggishly through dilated cutaneous vessels. Nonspecific symptoms such as headaches, dizziness, tinnitus, and a feeling of fullness of the face and head probably are caused by a combination of increased viscosity and vascular dilatation. In extreme polycythemia and some specific types of polycythemia (e.g., methemoglobinemia; see Chap. 49), *cyanosis* can result from greater than 4 g/dL of deoxygenated hemoglobin (accomplished more easily at higher hemoglobin concentrations [see "blue bloaters" and "pink puffers" in Chap. 56]) or greater than 1.5 g/dL of methemoglobin (see Chap. 49).

Hemorrhages from the nose or stomach in patients with normal platelets and coagulation proteins can be attributed to capillary distention. However, circulatory stagnation causing ischemia and necrosis may contribute. Thromboses are common in polycythemia vera but are not seen at similar frequencies in other types of polycythemias (see Chaps. 56 and 86). Coronary blood flow is decreased in polycythemia,[33] so the risk of coronary thrombosis in patients with a high hematocrit is assumed to be increased; however, statistical analyses have yielded equivocal results.[34,36,37] Polycythemia reportedly does not pose

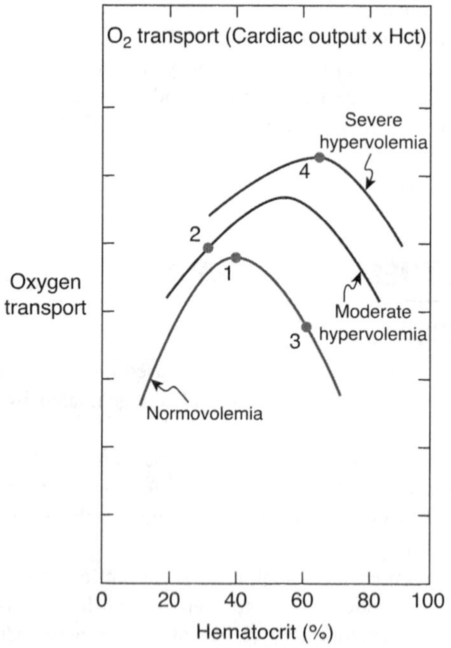

FIGURE 33–7. Oxygen transport at various hematocrit (Hct) levels in normovolemia, mild hypervolemia, and severe hypervolemia. Oxygen transport is estimated by multiplying hematocrit by cardiac output. (1) Optimal oxygen transport for normovolemic subjects is at a hematocrit of approximately 45 percent, with a progressive increase in optimal hematocrit as blood volume increases. (2) Suboptimal hematocrit in a hypervolemic person (anemia of pregnancy) may be associated with higher oxygen transport than in a normovolemic person with normal hematocrit. (3) High hematocrit without an increase in blood volume may be associated with an absolute reduction in oxygen transport and tissue hypoxia. (4) Only high hematocrit coupled with high blood volume enhances oxygen transport to the tissues. *(Adapted from Murray JF, Gold P, and Johnson BL Jr.,[28] and Thorling and Erslev.[29])*

TABLE 33–2. Classification of Polycythemia

I. Absolute (true) Polycythemia (increased red cell volume) (see Chap. 56)	
A. Primary polycythemia	
1. Acquired	
a. Polycythemia vera (see Chap. 86)	
2. Hereditary (see Chap. 56)	
a. Primary familial and congenital polycythemia	
(1) Erythropoietin receptor mutations	
(2) Unknown gene mutations	
B. Secondary polycythemia	
1. Acquired (see Chap. 56)	
a. Hypoxemia	
(1) Chronic lung disease	
(2) Sleep apnea	
(3) Right-to-left cardiac shunts	
(4) High altitude	
(5) Smoking	
b. Carboxyhemoglobinemia (see Chap. 49)	
(1) Smoking	
(2) Carbon monoxide poisoning	
c. Autonomous erythropoietin production (see Chap. 56)	
(1) Hepatocellular carcinoma	
(2) Renal cell carcinoma	
(3) Cerebellar hemangioblastoma	
(4) Pheochromocytoma	
(5) Parathyroid carcinoma	
(6) Meningioma	
(7) Uterine leiomyoma	
(8) Polycystic kidney disease	
d. Exogenous erythropoietin administration ("EPO doping") (see Chap. 56)	
e. Complex or uncertain etiology	
(1) Postrenal transplant (probable abnormal angiotensin II signaling) (see Chap. 56)	
(2) Androgen/anabolic steroids (see Chaps. 28 and 56)	
2. Hereditary	
a. High-oxygen affinity hemoglobins (see Chap. 48)	
b. 2,3-Bisphosphoglycerate deficiency (see Chap. 46)	
c. Congenital methemoglobinemias (recessive, i.e., cytochrome b5 reductase deficiency, dominant globin mutations [see Chap. 49])	
d. Recessive high erythropoietin polycythemias not due to von Hippel-Lindau gene mutations (see Chap. 56)	
e. Autosomal dominant high erythropoietin polycythemias not due to von Hippel-Lindau gene mutations (see Chap. 56)	
C. Mixed primary and secondary polycythemia (see Chap. 56)	
1. Proven or suspected congenital disorders of hypoxia sensing	
a. Chuvash polycythemia	
b. High erythropoietin polycythemias due to mutations of von Hippel-Lindau gene other than Chuvash mutation	
II. Relative (spurious) Polycythemia (normal red cell volume) (see Chap. 56)	
A. Dehydration	
B. Diuretics	
C. Smoking	
D. Gaisböck syndrome	

a risk in surgical patients.[38] Although cerebral blood flow is materially reduced in patients with moderately elevated hematocrit,[31,39] such reductions may have little practical significance.

CLASSIFICATION

Polycythemia, or *erythrocytosis*, is a condition in which the hematocrit percentage is above the upper limit of normal: greater than 51 percent in men and greater than 48 percent in women. Polycythemia can be classified as relative, in which the red cell mass is normal but the plasma volume is decreased, or absolute, in which the red cell mass is increased above normal (see Chap. 56). Table 33–2 outlines the polycythemic states.

Differentiation of absolute from relative polycythemia can be difficult at hematocrits of less than 60 percent. Designation of a measured red cell mass as normal is imprecise because the red cell mass depends on the patient's age, sex, weight, height, and body frame, and because only increases above the mean of greater than 25 percent are considered abnormal.

Primary Polycythemias

Primary or secondary polycythemias are caused by either acquired (polycythemia vera) or congenital mutations (such as gain-of-function erythropoietin receptor causing primary familial and congenital polycythemia) expressed within hematopoietic progenitors that proliferate independently or excessively in response to extrinsic regulators leading to increased production of red cells.

Secondary Polycythemias

Secondary polycythemias are caused by augmentation of erythropoiesis by circulating stimulatory factors such as erythropoietin (polycythemia of high altitude), cobalt, or insulin-like growth factor 1 (see Chap. 56).

Chuvash Polycythemia

Chuvash polycythemia has features of primary and secondary polycythemia (see Chap. 56).

REFERENCES

1. Semenza GL, Nejfelt MK, Chi SM, Antonarakis SE: Hypoxia-inducible nuclear factors bind to an enhancer element located 3′ to the human erythropoietin gene. *Proc Natl Acad Sci U S A* 88:5680, 1991.
2. Guillemin K, Krasnow MA: The hypoxic response: Huffing and HIFing. *Cell* 89:9, 1997.
3. Hochachka PW, Buck LT, Doll CJ, Land SC: Unifying theory of hypoxia tolerance: Molecular/metabolic defense and rescue mechanisms for surviving oxygen lack. *Proc Natl Acad Sci U S A* 93:9493, 1996.

4. Semenza GL: O2-regulated gene expression: Transcriptional control of cardiorespiratory physiology by HIF-1. *J Appl Physiol* 96:1173, 2004.
5. Srinivas V, Zhu X, Salceda S, et al: Hypoxia-inducible factor 1α (HIF-1α) is a non-heme iron protein. *J Biol Chem* 273:18019, 1998.
6. Ivan M, Kondo K, Yang H, et al: HIF-alpha targeted for VHL-mediated destruction by proline hydroxylation: Implications for O_2 sensing. *Science* 292:464, 2001.
7. Jaakkola P, Mole DR, Tian Y, et al: Targeting of HIF-alpha to the von Hippel-Lindau ubiquitylation complex by O_2-regulated prolyl hydroxylation. *Science* 292:468, 2001.
8. Epstein AC, Gleadle JM, McNeill LA, et al: *C. elegans* EGL-9 and mammalian homologs define a family of dioxygenases that regulate HIF by propyl hydroxylation. *Cell* 107:43, 2001.
9. Edwards MJ, Novy MJ, Walters CL, Metcalfe J: Improved oxygen release: An adaptation of mature red cells to hypoxia. *J Clin Invest* 47:1851, 1968.
10. Moore LG, Brewer GJ: Beneficial effect of rightward hemoglobin-oxygen dissociation curve shift for short-term high-altitude adaptation. *J Lab Clin Med* 98:145, 1981.
11. Huber H, Lewis SM, Szur L: The influence of anaemia, polycythaemia and splenomegaly on the relationship between venous haematocrit and red-cell volume. *Br J Haematol* 10:567, 1964.
12. Vatner SF: Effects of hemorrhage on regional blood flow distribution in dogs and primates. *J Clin Invest* 54:225, 1974.
13. Abramson DJ, Fierst SM, Flachs K: Resting peripheral blood flow in the anemic state. *Am Heart J* 25:609, 1954.
14. Bradley SE, Bradley GP: Renal function during chronic anemia in man. *Blood* 2:192, 1947.
15. Merin S, Freund M: Retinopathy in severe anemia. *Am J Ophthalmol* 66:1102, 1968.
16. Duke M, Abelman WH: The hemodynamic response to chronic anemia. *Circulation* 39:503, 1969.
17. Sharpey-Schafer EP: Cardiac output in severe anemia. *Clin Sci* 5:125, 1944.
18. Wintrobe MM: The cardiovascular system in anemia. *Blood* 1:121, 1946.
19. Wales RT, Martin EA: Arterial bruits in anemia. *Br Med J* 2:1444, 1963.
20. Blumgart HL, Altschule MD: Clinical significance of cardiac and respiratory adjustments in chronic anemia. *Blood* 3:329, 1948.
21. Fatemian M, Gamboa A, Leon-Velarde F, et al: Selected contribution: Ventilatory response to CO2 in high-altitude natives and patients with chronic mountain sickness. *J Appl Physiol* 94:1279, 2003.
22. Adamson JW: The erythropoietin/hematocrit relationship in normal and polycythemic man: Implications of marrow regulation. *Blood* 32:597, 1968.
23. Erslev AJ: Erythropoietin. *N Engl J Med* 324:1339, 1991.
24. Ward HP, Halman J: The association of nucleated red cells in the peripheral smear with hypoxemia. *Ann Intern Med* 67:1190, 1967.
25. Dintenfass I: A preliminary outline of the blood high viscosity syndromes. *Arch Intern Med* 118:427, 1966.
26. Stone HO, Thompson HK Jr, Schmidt-Nielson K: Influence of erythrocytes on blood viscosity. *Am J Physiol* 221:913, 1968.
27. Erslev AJ, Caro J, Schuster SJ: Is there an optimal hemoglobin level? *Transfus Med Rev* 3:237, 1989.
28. Murray JF, Gold P, Johnson BL Jr: The circulatory effects of hematocrit variations in normovolemic and hypervolemic dogs. *J Clin Invest* 42: 1150, 1963.
29. Thorling EB, Erslev AJ: The "tissue" tension of oxygen and its relation to hematocrit and erythropoiesis. *Blood* 31:332, 1968.
30. Fan FC, Chen RYZ, Schuessler GB, Chien S: Effects of hematocrit variations on regional hemodynamics and oxygen transport in the dog. *Am J Physiol* 238:H545, 1980.
31. Pearson TC, Humphrey PRD, Thomas DJ, et al: Hematocrit, blood viscosity, cerebral blood flow, and vascular occlusion, in *Clinical Aspects of Blood Viscosity and Cell Deformability*, edited by GDO Lowe, p 97. Springer-Verlag, New York, 1981.
32. Monge CM, Monge CC: *High Altitude Diseases: Mechanism and Management*, p 34. Thomas, Springfield, IL, 1966.
33. Kershenovich S, Modiano M, Ewy GA: Markedly decreased coronary blood flow in secondary polycythemia. *Am Heart J* 123:521, 1992.
34. Conley CL, Russell RP, Thomas CB, Tumulty PA: Hematocrit values in coronary artery disease. *Arch Intern Med* 113:170, 1969.
35. Kaushansky K: Thrombopoietin. *N Engl J Med* 339:749, 1998.
36. Mayer GA: Hematocrit and coronary heart disease. *CMAJ* 93:1151, 1965.
37. Hershberg PJ, Wells RE, McGandy RB: Hematocrit and prognosis in patients with acute myocardial infarction. *JAMA* 219:855, 1972.
38. Lubarsky DA, Gallagher CJ, Berend JL: Secondary polycythemia does not increase the risk of perioperative hemorrhagic or thrombotic complications. *J Clin Anesth* 3:99, 1991.
39. Thomas DJ, Marshall J, Russell RWR, et al: Cerebral blood flow in polycythemia. *Lancet* 2:161, 1977.

CHAPTER 34
APLASTIC ANEMIA: ACQUIRED AND INHERITED

George B. Segel and Marshall A. Lichtman

SUMMARY

Acquired aplastic anemia is a clinical syndrome in which there is a deficiency of red cells, neutrophils, monocytes, and platelets in the blood, and fatty replacement of the marrow with a near absence of hematopoietic precursor cells. Reticulocytopenia, neutropenia, monocytopenia, and thrombocytopenia, when severe, are life-threatening because of the risk of infection and bleeding, complicated by severe anemia. Most cases occur without an evident precipitating cause and are the result of the expression of autoreactive cytotoxic T lymphocytes that suppress or destroy primitive CD34+ multipotential hematopoietic cells. The disorder also can occur after (1) prolonged high-dose exposure to certain toxic chemicals (e.g., benzene), (2) after specific viral infections (e.g., Epstein-Barr virus), (3) as an idiosyncratic response to certain pharmaceuticals (e.g., ticlopidine, chloramphenicol), (4) as a feature of a connective tissue or autoimmune disorder (e.g., lupus erythematosus), or, (5) rarely, in association with pregnancy. The final common pathway may be through cytotoxic T-cell autoreactivity, whether idiopathic or associated with an inciting agent since they all respond in a similar fashion to immunosuppressive therapy. The differential diagnosis of acquired aplastic anemia includes the hypoplastic marrow that can accompany paroxysmal nocturnal hemoglobinuria or hypoplastic oligoblastic (myelodysplastic syndrome) or polyblastic myelogenous leukemia. Allogeneic hematopoietic stem cell transplantation is curative in approximately 80 percent of younger patients with high-resolution human leukocyte antigen (HLA)-matched sibling donors although the posttransplant period may be severely complicated by graft-versus-host disease. The disease may be significantly ameliorated or occasionally cured by immunotherapy, especially a regimen coupling antithymocyte globulin with cyclosporine. However, after successful treatment with immunosuppressive agents, the disease may relapse or evolve into a clonal myeloid disorder, such as paroxysmal nocturnal hemoglobinuria, a clonal cytopenia, or oligoblastic or polyblastic myelogenous leukemia. Several uncommon inherited disorders, including Fanconi anemia, Shwachman-Diamond syndrome, dyskeratosis congenita and others have as a primary manifestation aplastic hematopoiesis.

Acronyms and abbreviations that appear in this chapter include: A, adenine; ALG, antilymphocyte globulin; ALL, acute lymphocytic leukemia; AML, acute myelogenous leukemia; ATG, antithymocyte globulin; ATR, ataxia-telangiectasia mutated and rad3-related kinase; BFU–E, erythroid burst-forming units; CD, cluster of differentiation; CFU-GM, colony-forming unit–granulocyte-macrophage; CMV, cytomegalovirus; EBV, Epstein-Barr virus; G, guanine; G-CSF, granulocyte colony-stimulating factor; HHV, human herpes virus; HIV, human immunodeficiency virus; HLA, human leukocyte antigen; IL, interleukin; LDH, lactic dehydrogenase; NMRI, nuclear magnetic resonance imaging; PCP, pentachlorophenol; PNH, paroxysmal nocturnal hemoglobinuria; SCF, stem cell factor; T, thymine; TNF, tumor necrosis factor; TNT, trinitrotoluene; TPO, thrombopoietin.

ACQUIRED APLASTIC ANEMIA

DEFINITION AND HISTORY

Aplastic anemia is a clinical syndrome that results from a marked diminution of marrow blood cell production. The latter results in reticulocytopenia, anemia, granulocytopenia, monocytopenia, and thrombocytopenia. The diagnosis usually requires the presence of pancytopenia with a neutrophil count fewer than 1500/μL (1.5×10^9/L), a platelet count fewer than 50,000/μL (50×10^9/L), a hemoglobin concentration less than 10 g/dL (100 g/L), and an absolute reticulocyte count fewer than 40,000/μL (40×10^9/L), accompanied by a hypocellular marrow without abnormal or malignant cells or fibrosis.[1] For the purpose of therapeutic decision making, comparative clinical trials, and international sharing of data, the disease has been stratified into moderately severe, severe, and very severe acquired aplastic anemia based on the blood counts (especially the neutrophil count) and the degree of marrow hypocellularity (Table 34–1). Most cases of aplastic anemia are acquired; fewer cases are the result of an inherited disorder, such as Fanconi anemia, Shwachman-Diamond syndrome, and others (see "Hereditary Aplastic Anemia" below).

Aplastic anemia was first recognized by Ehrlich in 1888.[2] He described a young, pregnant woman who died of severe anemia and neutropenia. Autopsy examination revealed a fatty marrow with essentially no hematopoiesis. The name *aplastic anemia* was subsequently applied to this disease by Chauffard, a French hematologist, in 1904,[3] and although an anachronistic term because the morbidity is the result of pancytopenia, especially neutropenia and thrombocytopenia, the designation is entrenched in medical usage. For the next 40 years, many conditions that caused pancytopenia were confused with aplastic anemia based on incomplete or inadequate histologic study of the patient's marrow.[4] The development of improved instruments for percutaneous marrow biopsy in the last half of the 20th century improved diagnostic precision. In 1972, Thomas and his colleagues established that marrow transplantation from a histocompatible sibling could cure the disease.[5] The disease initially was thought to result from an atrophy or chemical injury of primitive marrow hematopoietic cells. The unexpected recovery of marrow recipients who were given immunosuppressive conditioning therapy but who did not engraft with donor stem cells raised the possibility that the disease may not be intrinsic to primitive hematopoietic cells but the result of a suppression of hematopoietic cells by immune cells, notably T lymphocytes.[6] The requirement to treat the recipient of a marrow transplant from an identical twin with immunosuppressive conditioning therapy for optimal results of transplant, buttressed this suspicion.[7] This supposition was confirmed by a clinical trial that established antilymphocyte globulin (ALG) capable of ameliorating the disease in the majority of patients.[8] Since that time, compelling evidence for a cellular autoimmune mechanism has accumulated (see the main section "Etiology and Pathogenesis" below).

EPIDEMIOLOGY

The International Aplastic Anemia and Agranulocytosis Study and a French study found the incidence rate of acquired aplastic anemia to be about 2 per 1,000,000 persons per year.[1,9] This approximate annual incidence rate has been confirmed in studies in Spain (Barcelona),[10] Brazil (State of Parana),[11] and Canada (British Columbia).[12] The highest frequency of aplastic anemia occurs in persons between the ages of 15 and 25 years; a second peak occurs between the ages of 65 and 69.[1] Aplastic anemia is more prevalent in the Far East where the incidence is approximately 7 per 1,000,000 in parts of China,[13] approximately 4 per 1,000,000 in sections of Thailand,[14] approximately 5 per 1,000,000 in areas of Malaysia,[15] and approximately 7 per 1,000,000 among children of Asian descent living in a province of Canada.[12] The explanation for a

TABLE 34–1. Degree of Severity of Acquired Aplastic Anemia

Diagnostic Categories	Hemoglobin	Reticulocyte Concentration	Neutrophil Count	Platelet Count	Marrow Biopsy	Comments
Moderately severe	<100 g/L	$<40 \times 10^9$/L	$<1.5 \times 10^9$/L	$<50 \times 10^9$/L	Marked decrease of hematopoietic cells.	At the time of diagnosis at least 2 of 3 blood counts should meet these criteria.
Severe	<90 g/L	$<30.0 \times 10^9$/L	$<0.5 \times 10^9$/L	$<30.0 \times 10^9$/L	Marked decrease or absence of hematopoietic cells.	Search for a histocompatible sibling should be made if age permits.
Very Severe	<80 g/L	$<20.0 \times 10^9$/L	$<0.2 \times 10^9$/L	$<20.0 \times 10^9$/L	Marked decrease or absence of hematopoietic cells.	Search for a histocompatible sibling should be made if age permits.

NOTE: These values are approximations and must be considered in the context of an individual patient's situation. (In some clinical trials, the blood count thresholds for moderately severe aplastic anemia are higher, e.g., platelet count $<100 \times 10^9$/L and absolute reticulocyte count $<60{,}000 \times 10^9$/L.) The marrow biopsy may contain the usual number of lymphocytes and plasma cells; "hot spots," focal areas of erythroid cells, may be seen. No fibrosis, abnormal cells, or malignant cells should be evident in the marrow. Dysmorphic features of blood or marrow cells are not features of acquired aplastic anemia. Ethnic differences in the lower limit of the absolute neutrophil count should be considered. (See Chap. 65.)

twofold or greater incidence in the Orient compared to the Occident may be multifactorial,[16] but a predisposition gene or genes is a likely component.[12,17] Studies have not established the use of chloramphenicol in Asia as a cause. Poorly regulated exposure of workers to benzene is a factor,[18] but the attributable risk from benzene and other toxic exposures does not explain the magnitude of the difference in the incidence in Asia compared to that in Europe and South America.[16,17] A relationship to impure water use in Thailand has led to speculation of an infectious etiology, although no agent, including seronegative hepatitis, a known association with the onset of acquired aplastic anemia,[16] has been identified. Seronegative viral hepatitis is a forerunner of approximately 7 percent of cases of acquired aplastic anemia.[17] The male-to-female incidence ratio of aplastic anemia in most studies is approximately one.[17]

ETIOLOGY AND PATHOGENESIS

Table 34–2 lists the potential causes for aplastic anemia.

The final common pathway to the clinical disease is a decrease in blood cell formation in the marrow. The number of marrow CD34+ cells (multipotential hematopoietic progenitors) and their derivative colony-forming unit–granulocyte-macrophage (CFU-GM) and burst-forming unit–erythroid (BFU-E) are reduced markedly in patients with aplastic anemia.[19–22] Long-term culture-initiating cells, an *in vitro* surrogate assay for hematopoietic stem cells, also are reduced to approximately 1 percent of normal values.[22] Potential mechanisms responsible for acquired marrow cell failure include (1) direct toxicity to hematopoietic multipotential cells, (2) a defect in the stromal microenvironment of the marrow required for hematopoietic cell development, (3) impaired production or release of essential multilineage hematopoietic growth factors, (4) cellular or humoral immune suppression of the marrow multipotential cells, and (5) progressive erosion of chromosome telomeres. There is little experimental evidence for a stromal microenvironmental defect or a deficit of critical hematopoietic growth factors, and the role of telomerase mutations with consequent telomere shortening is unclear, although present in as much as 40 percent of patients.[23] Deficiencies in telomere repair could predispose to aplastic anemia by affecting the size of the multipotential hematopoietic cell compartment and by decreasing the multipotential cell's response to a marrow injury, and could play a role in the evolution of aplastic anemia to a clonal myeloid disease by contributing to genome instability.[23] Thus, reduced hematopoiesis in most cases of aplastic anemia results from cytotoxic T-cell-mediated immune suppression of very early CD34+ hematopoietic multipotential progenitor or stem cells.[24] A small fraction of cases is initiated by a toxic exposure, drug exposure, or viral infection, but in these cases the pathogenesis also

TABLE 34–2. Etiologic Classification of Aplastic Anemia

- Acquired
- Autoimmune
- Drugs
  - See Table 34–3
- Toxins
  - Benzene
  - Chlorinated hydrocarbons
  - Organophosphates
- Viruses
  - Epstein-Barr virus
  - Non-A, -B, -C, -D, -E, or -G hepatitis virus
  - Human immunodeficiency virus (HIV)
- Paroxysmal nocturnal hemoglobinuria
- Autoimmune/connective tissue disorders
  - Eosinophilic fasciitis
  - Immune thyroid disease (Graves disease, Hashimoto thyroiditis)
  - Rheumatoid arthritis
  - Systemic lupus erythematosus
- Thymoma
- Pregnancy
- Iatrogenic
  - Radiation
  - Cytotoxic drug therapy
- Hereditary
  - Fanconi anemia
  - Dyskeratosis congenita
  - Shwachman-Diamond syndrome
  - Other rare syndromes (see Table 34–8)

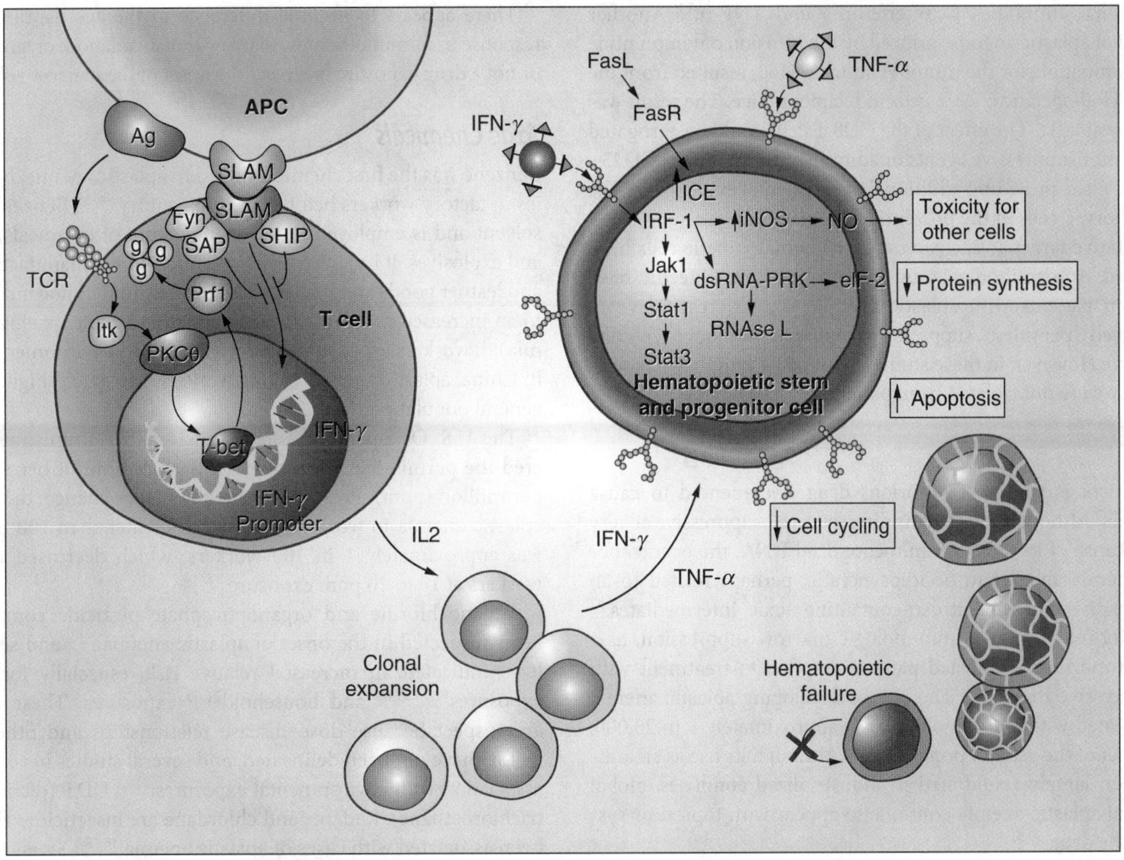

FIGURE 34–1. Immune pathogenesis of apoptosis of CD34 multipotential hematopoietic cells in acquired aplastic anemia. Antigens are presented to T lymphocytes by antigen-presenting cells (APCs). This triggers T cells to activate and proliferate. T-bet, a transcription factor, binds to the interferon-γ (IFN-γ) promoter region and induces gene expression. SLAM-associated protein (SAP) binds to Fyn and modulates the signaling lymphocyte activation molecule (SLAM) activity on IFN-γ expression, diminishing gene transcription. Patients with aplastic anemia show constitutive T-bet expression and low SAP levels. IFN-γ and tumor necrosis factor-α (TNF-α) upregulate both the T cell's cellular receptors and the Fas receptor. Increased production of interleukin-2 leads to polyclonal expansion of T cells. Activation of the Fas receptor by the Fas ligand leads to apoptosis of target cells. Some effects of IFN-γ are mediated through interferon regulatory factor 1 (IRF-1), which inhibits the transcription of cellular genes and entry into the cell cycle. IFN-γ is a potent inducer of many cellular genes, including inducible nitric oxide synthase (NOS), and production of nitric oxide (NO) may diffuse its cytotoxic effects. These events ultimately lead to reduced cell cycling and cell death by apoptosis. *(Reproduced from Young NS, Calado RT, Scheinberg P: Current concepts in the pathophysiology and treatment of aplastic anemia.* Blood *108:2509, 2006, with permission of The American Society of Hematology.)*

may relate to autoimmunity as there is evidence of immune dysfunction in seronegative hepatitis, after benzene exposure, and many such patients respond to anti–T-cell therapy.[24]

Autoreactive Cytotoxic T Lymphocytes

In vitro and clinical observations have resulted in the identification of a cytotoxic T-cell-mediated attack on multipotential hematopoietic cells in the CD34+ cellular compartment as the basis for acquired aplastic anemia.[25] Cellular immune injury to the marrow after drug-, viral-, or toxin-initiated marrow aplasia could result from the induction of neoantigens that provoke a secondary T-cell-mediated attack on hematopoietic cells. This mechanism could explain the response to immunosuppressive treatment in cases that follow exposure to an exogenous agent. Spontaneous or mitogen-induced increases in mononuclear cell production of interferon-γ,[26,27] interleukin (IL)-2,[27] and tumor necrosis factor-α (TNF-α)[28,29] occur. Elevated serum levels of interferon-γ are present in 30 percent of patients with aplastic anemia, and interferon-γ expression has been detected in the marrow of most patients with acquired aplastic anemia.[30] Addition of antibodies to interferon-γ enhances *in vitro* colony growth of marrow cells from affected patients.[31] Long-term marrow cultures manipulated to elaborate exaggerated amounts of interferon-γ, markedly reduced the frequency of long-term culture-initiating cells.[24] These observations indicate that acquired aplastic anemia is the result of cellular immune-induced apoptosis of primitive CD34+ multipotential hematopoietic progenitors, mediated by cytotoxic T lymphocytes, in part, through the expression of T-helper type 1 (Th1) inhibitory cytokines, interferon-γ, and TNF-α (Fig. 34–1).[32] The secretion of interferon-γ is a result of the upregulation of transcription regulatory factor T-bet,[33] and apoptosis of CD34+ cells is, in part, mediated through a FAS-dependent pathway.[24] Because HLA-DR2 is more prevalent in patients with aplastic anemia, antigen recognition may be a factor in those patients. A variety of other potential factors have been found in some patients, including nucleotide polymorphisms in cytokine genes, overexpression of perforin in marrow cells, and decreased expression of SAP, a modulator protein that inhibits interferon-γ secretion.[24]

A decrease in regulatory T cells contributes to the expansion of an autoreactive CD8+CD28– T-cell population, which induces apoptosis of autologous hematopoietic multipotential hematopoietic cells.[34] One mouse model of immune-related marrow failure, induced by infusion of parental lymph node cells into F1 hybrid recipients, caused a fatal aplastic anemia. The aplasia could be prevented by immunotherapy or with monoclonal antibodies to interferon-γ and TNF-α.[24] Another mouse model of aplastic anemia induced by the infusion of lymph node cells histoincompatible for the minor H antigen, H60, resulted from the expansion of H60-specific CD8 T cells in recipient mice. The result was severe marrow aplasia. The effect of the CD8 T cells could be abrogated by either immunosuppressive agents or administration of CD4+CD25+ regulatory T cells,[35] providing additional experimental evidence for the role of regulatory T cells in the prevention of aplastic anemia.

Several putative target antigens on affected hematopoietic cells have been identified. Autoantibodies to one putative antigen, kinectin, have been found in patients with aplastic anemia. T cells, responsive to kinectin-derived peptides, suppress granulocyte-monocyte colony growth *in vitro*. However, in these studies cytotoxic T lymphocytes with that specificity were not isolated from patients.[36]

Drugs

Chloramphenicol is the most notorious drug documented to cause aplastic anemia. Although this drug is directly myelosuppressive at very high dose because of its effect on mitochondrial DNA, the occurrence of aplastic anemia appears to be idiosyncratic, perhaps related to an inherited sensitivity to the nitroso-containing toxic intermediates.[37] This sensitivity may produce immunologic marrow suppression, as a substantial proportion of affected patients respond to treatment with immunosuppressive therapy.[38] The risk of developing aplastic anemia in patients treated with chloramphenicol is approximately 1 in 20,000, or 25 times that of the general population.[39] Although its use as an antibiotic has been largely abandoned in industrialized countries, global reports of fatal aplastic anemia continue to appear with topical or systemic use of the drug.[50,51]

Epidemiologic evidence established that quinacrine (Atabrine) increased the risk of aplastic anemia.[40] This drug was administered to all U.S. troops in the South Pacific and Asiatic theaters of operations as prophylaxis for malaria during 1943 and 1944. The incidence of aplastic anemia was 7 to 28 cases per 1,000,000 personnel per year in the prophylaxis zones, whereas untreated soldiers had 1 to 2 cases per 1,000,000 personnel per year. The aplasia occurred during administration of the offending agent and was preceded by a characteristic rash in nearly half the cases. Many other drugs have been reported to increase the risk of aplastic anemia, but owing to incomplete reporting of information and the infrequency of the association, the spectrum of drug-induced aplastic anemia may not be fully appreciated. Table 34–3 is a partial list of drugs that have been implicated.[41–51]

Many of these drugs are known to also induce selective cytopenias, such as agranulocytosis, which usually are reversible after discontinuation of the offending agent. These reversible reactions are not correlated with the risk of aplastic anemia, casting doubt on the effectiveness of routine monitoring of blood counts as a strategy to avoid aplastic anemia.

Because aplastic anemia is a rare event with drug use, it may occur because of an underlying metabolic or immunologic predisposition (gene polymorphism) in susceptible individuals. In the case of phenylbutazone-associated marrow aplasia, there is delayed oxidation and clearance of a related compound, acetanilide, as compared to either normal controls or those with aplastic anemia from other causes. This finding suggests excess accumulation of the drug as a potential mechanism for the aplasia. In some cases, drug interactions or synergy may be required to induce marrow aplasia. Cimetidine, a histamine H_2-receptor antagonist, is occasionally implicated in the onset of cytopenias and aplastic anemia, perhaps owing to a direct effect on early hematopoietic progenitor cells.[52] This drug accentuates the marrow-suppressive effects of the chemotherapy drug carmustine.[53] In several instances, it has been reported as a possible cause of marrow aplasia when given with chloramphenicol.

There appears to be little difference in the age distribution, gender, response to immunotherapy, marrow transplantation, or survival whether or not a drug exposure preceded the onset of the marrow aplasia.

Toxic Chemicals

Benzene was the first chemical linked to aplastic anemia, based on studies in factory workers before the 20th century.[54–59] Benzene is used as a solvent and is employed in the manufacture of chemicals, drugs, dyes, and explosives. It has been a vital chemical in the manufacture of rubber and leather goods and has been used widely in the shoe industry, leading to an increased risk for aplastic anemia (and acute myelogenous leukemia) in workers exposed to a poorly regulated environment.[56] In studies in China, aplastic anemia among workers was sixfold higher than in the general population.[18]

The U.S. Occupational Safety and Health Administration has lowered the permissible atmospheric exposure limit of benzene to 1 part per million (ppm). Previous to that regulatory change, the frequency of aplastic anemia in workers exposed to greater than 100 ppm benzene was approximately 1 in 100 workers, which decreased to 1 in 1000 workers at 10 to 20 ppm exposure.[55]

Organochlorine and organophosphate pesticide compounds have been suspected in the onset of aplastic anemia[57,58] and several studies have indicated an increased relative risk, especially for agricultural exposures[11,16,59,60] and household[11,60] exposures. These relationships are suspect because dose–disease relationships and other important factors have not been delineated, and several studies have not found an association with environmental exposures.[12,61] DDT (dichlorodiphenyltrichloroethane), lindane, and chlordane are insecticides that have also been associated with cases of aplastic anemia.[16,58] Occasional cases still occur following heavy exposure at industrial plants or after its use as a pesticide.[62] Lindane is metabolized in part to pentachlorophenol (PCP), another potentially toxic chlorinated hydrocarbon that is manufactured for use as a wood preservative. Many cases of aplastic anemia and related blood disorders have been attributed to PCP over the past 25 years.[58,63] Prolonged exposures to petroleum distillates in the form of Stoddard solvent[64] and acute exposure to toluene through the practice of glue sniffing[65,66] also have been reported to cause marrow aplasia. Trinitrotoluene (TNT), an explosive used extensively during World Wars I and II, is absorbed readily by inhalation and through the skin.[67] Fatal cases of aplastic anemia were observed in munitions workers exposed to TNT in Great Britain[68] from 1940 to 1946. In most cases, these conclusions have not been derived from specific studies but from accumulation of case reports or from patient histories, making conclusions provisional, although the argument for minimizing exposures to potential toxins is logical in any case.

Viruses

Non-A, -B, -C, -D, -E, -G Hepatitis Virus A relationship between hepatitis and the subsequent development of aplastic anemia has been the subject of a number of case reports, and this association was emphasized by two major reviews in the 1970s.[69,70] In the aggregate, these reports summarized findings in more than 200 cases. In many instances, the hepatitis was improving or had resolved when the aplastic anemia was noted 4 to 12 weeks later. Approximately 10 percent of cases occurred more than 1 year after the initial diagnosis of hepatitis. Most patients were young (ages 18 to 20 years); two-thirds were male, and their survival was short (10 weeks). Although hepatitis A and B have been implicated in aplastic anemia in a small number of cases, most cases are related to non-A, non-B, non-C hepatitis.[71–73] Severe aplastic anemia developed in 9 of 31 patients who underwent liver transplantation for non-A, non-B, non-C hepatitis,

TABLE 34–3. Drugs Associated with Aplastic Anemia

Category	High Risk	Intermediate Risk	Low Risk
Analgesic			Phenacetin, aspirin, salicylamide
Antiarrhythmic			Quinidine, tocainide
Antiarthritic		Gold salts	Colchicine
Anticonvulsant		Carbamazepine, hydantoins, felbamate	Ethosuximide, phenacemide, primidone, trimethadione, sodium valproate
Antihistamine			Chlorpheniramine, pyrilamine, tripelennamine
Antihypertensive			Captopril, methyldopa
Antiinflammatory		Penicillamine, phenylbutazone, oxyphenbutazone	Diclofenac, ibuprofen, indomethacin, naproxen, sulindac
Antimicrobial			
Antibacterial		Chloramphenicol	Dapsone, methicillin, penicillin, streptomycin, β-lactam antibiotics
Antifungal			Amphotericin, flucytosine
Antiprotozoal		Quinacrine	Chloroquine, mepacrine, pyrimethamine
Antineoplastic drugs			
Alkylating agent	Busulfan, cyclophosphamide, melphalan, nitrogen mustard		
Antimetabolite	Fluorouracil, mercaptopurine, methotrexate		
Cytotoxic antibiotic	Daunorubicin, doxorubicin, mitoxantrone		
Antiplatelet			Ticlopidine
Antithyroid			Carbimazole, methimazole, methylthiouracil, potassium perchlorate, propylthiouracil, sodium thiocyanate
Sedative and tranquilizer			Chlordiazepoxide, chlorpromazine (and other phenothiazines), lithium, meprobamate, methyprylon
Sulfa derivative		Sulfonamides	
Antibacterial			Numerous sulfonamides
Diuretic		Acetazolamide	Chlorothiazide, furosemide
Hypoglycemic			Chlorpropamide, tolbutamide
Miscellaneous			Allopurinol, interferon, pentoxifylline, penicillamine

NOTE: Drugs that invariably cause marrow aplasia with high doses are termed *high risk;* drugs with 30 or more reported cases are listed as moderate risk; others are less often associated with aplastic anemia (low risk).

SOURCE: This list was compiled from the AMA Registry,[41] publications of the International Agranulocytosis and Aplastic Anemia Study,[42–46] other reviews and studies,[24,47–50] previous compilations of offending agents,[51] and selected reports. An additional comprehensive source for potentially offending drugs can be found in *The Drug Etiology of Agranulocytosis and Aplastic Anemia,* Oxford, UK: Oxford University Press, 1991.

but in none of 1463 patients transplanted for other indications.[75] Several lines of evidence indicate there is no causal association with hepatitis C virus, suggesting that an unknown viral agent is involved.[16,75,76] Hepatitis virus B or C can be a secondary infection, if carefully screened blood products are not used for transfusion. In 15 patients with posthepatitic aplastic anemia, no evidence was found for hepatitis A, B, C, D, E, or G, transfusion-transmitted virus, or parvovirus B19.[76] Several reports suggest a relationship of parvovirus B19 to aplastic anemia,[77,78] whereas others have not.[79] This relationship has not been established (see Chap. 35). The effect of seronegative hepatitis may be mediated through an autoimmune T-cell effect because of evidence of T-cell activation and cytokine elaboration.[24] These patients also have a similar response to combined immunotherapy as does idiopathic aplastic anemia (see "TREATMENT, Combination Immunotherapy").

Epstein-Barr Virus Epstein-Barr virus (EBV) has been implicated in the pathogenesis of aplastic anemia.[80,81] The onset usually occurs within 4 to 6 weeks of infection. In some cases, infectious mononucleosis is subclinical, with a finding of reactive lymphocytes in the blood film and serological results consistent with a recent infection (see Chap. 84). EBV has been detected in marrow cells,[81] but it is uncertain whether marrow aplasia results from a direct effect or an immunologic response by the host. Patients have recovered following therapy with antithymocyte globulin.[81]

Other Viruses Human immunodeficiency virus (HIV) infection frequently is associated with varying degrees of cytopenia. The marrow is often cellular, but occasional cases of aplastic anemia have been noted.[82–84] In these patients, marrow hypoplasia may result from viral suppression and from the drugs used to control viral replication in this disorder. Human herpes virus (HHV)-6 has caused severe marrow aplasia subsequent to marrow transplantation for other disorders.[85]

Autoimmune Diseases

The incidence of severe aplastic anemia was sevenfold greater than expected in patients with rheumatoid arthritis.[47] It is uncertain whether the aplastic anemia is related directly to rheumatoid arthritis or to the various drugs used to treat the condition (gold salts, D-penicillamine, and nonsteroidal antiinflammatory agents). Occasional cases of aplastic anemia are seen in conjunction with systemic lupus erythematosus.[86] *In vitro* studies found either the presence of an antibody[87] or suppressor cell[88,89] directed against hematopoietic progenitor cells. Patients have recovered after plasmapheresis,[87] glucocorticoids,[89] or cyclophosphamide therapy,[88,90] which is compatible with an immune etiology.

Eosinophilic fasciitis, an uncommon connective tissue disorder with painful swelling and induration of the skin and subcutaneous tissue, has been associated with aplastic anemia.[91,92] Although it may be antibody-mediated in some cases, it has been largely unresponsive to therapy.[91] Nevertheless, (1) stem cell transplantation, (2) immunosuppressive therapy using cyclosporine,[91] (3) immunosuppressive therapy using antithymocyte globulin (ATG), or (4) immunosuppressive therapy with ATG and cyclosporine cures or significantly ameliorates the disease in a few patients.[92]

Severe aplastic anemia also has been reported coincident with immune thyroid disease (Graves disease)[93–97] and the aplasia has been reversed with treatment of the hyperthyroidism. Aplastic anemia has occurred in association with thymoma.[98–103] Autoimmune renal disease and aplastic anemia have occurred concurrently. The underlying relationship may be the role of cytotoxic T lymphocytes in the pathogenesis of several autoimmune diseases and in aplastic anemia.[104]

Pregnancy

There are a number of reports of pregnancy-associated aplastic anemia, but the relationship between the two conditions is not always clear.[105–110] In some patients, preexisting aplastic anemia is exacerbated with pregnancy, only to improve following termination of the pregnancy.[105,106] In other cases, the aplasia develops during pregnancy with recurrences during subsequent pregnancies.[106,107] Termination of pregnancy or delivery may improve the marrow function, but the disease may progress to a fatal outcome even after delivery.[105–107] Therapy may include elective termination of early pregnancy, supportive care, immunosuppressive therapy, or marrow transplantation after delivery. Pregnancy in women previously treated with immunosuppression for aplastic anemia can result in the birth of a normal newborn.[110] In this latter study of 36 pregnancies, 22 were uncomplicated, 7 were complicated by a relapse of the marrow aplasia, and 5 without marrow aplasia required red cell transfusion during delivery.[110] One death occurred from cerebral thrombosis in a patient with paroxysmal nocturnal hemoglobinuria (PNH) and marrow aplasia.

Iatrogenic Causes

Although marrow toxicity from cytotoxic chemotherapy or radiation produces direct damage to stem cells and more mature cells, resulting in marrow aplasia, most patients with acquired aplastic anemia cannot relate an exposure that would be responsible for marrow damage.

Chronic exposure to low doses of radiation or use of spinal radiation for ankylosing spondylitis is associated with an increased, but delayed, risk of developing aplastic anemia and acute leukemia.[111,112] Patients who were given thorium dioxide (Thorotrast) as an intravenous contrast medium suffered numerous late complications, including malignant liver tumors, acute leukemia, and aplastic anemia.[113] Chronic radium poisoning with osteitis of the jaw, osteogenic sarcoma, and aplastic anemia was seen in workers who painted watch dials with luminous paint when they moistened the brushes orally.[114]

Acute exposures to large doses of radiation are associated with the development of marrow aplasia and a gastrointestinal syndrome.[115,116] Total body exposure to between 1 and 2.5 Gy leads to gastrointestinal symptoms and depression of leukocyte counts, but most patients recover. A dose of 4.5 Gy leads to death in half the individuals (LD_{50}) owing to marrow failure. Higher doses in the range of 10 Gy are universally fatal unless the patient receives extensive supportive care followed by marrow transplantation. Aplastic anemia associated with nuclear accidents was seen after the disaster that occurred at the Chernobyl nuclear power station in the Ukraine in 1986.[117]

Antineoplastic drugs such as alkylating agents, antimetabolites, and certain cytotoxic antibiotics have the potential for producing marrow aplasia. In general, this is transient, is an extension of their pharmacologic action, and resolves within several weeks of completing chemotherapy. Although unusual, severe marrow aplasia can follow use of the alkylating agent, busulfan, and may persist indefinitely. Patients may develop marrow aplasia 2 to 5 years after discontinuation of alkylating agent therapy. These cases often evolve into hypoplastic myelodysplastic syndromes.

Stromal Microenvironment and Growth Factors

Short-term clonal assays for marrow stromal cells have shown variable defects in stromal cell function. Serum levels of stem cell factor (SCF) have been either moderately low or normal in several studies of aplastic anemia.[118,119] Although SCF augments the growth of hematopoietic colonies from aplastic anemia patient's marrows, its use in patients has not led to clinical remissions. Another early acting growth factor, FLT-3 ligand, is 30- to 100-fold elevated in the serum of patients with aplastic anemia.[120] Fibroblasts grown from patients with severe aplastic anemia have subnormal cytokine production. However, serum levels of granulocyte colony-stimulating factor,[121] erythropoietin,[122] and thrombopoietin (TPO)[123] are usually high. Synthesis of IL-1, an early stimulator of hematopoiesis, is decreased in mononuclear cells from patients with aplastic anemia.[124] Studies of the microenvironment have shown relatively normal stromal cell proliferation and growth factor production.[125] These findings, coupled with the limited response of patients with aplastic anemia to growth factors, suggest that cytokine deficiency is not the etiologic problem in most cases. The most compelling argument is that most patients transplanted for aplastic anemia are cured with allogeneic donor stem cells and autologous stroma.[126]

A rare exception is the homozygous or mixed heterozygous mutation of the TPO receptor gene, *MPL*, which can cause amegakaryocytic thrombocytopenia that evolves, later, into aplastic anemia (see Chap. 119).

■ CLINICAL FEATURES

The onset of symptoms of aplastic anemia may be gradual with pallor, weakness, dyspnea, and fatigue as a result of the anemia. Dependent petechiae, bruising, epistaxis, vaginal bleeding, and unexpected bleeding at other sites secondary to thrombocytopenia are frequent presenting signs of the underlying marrow disorder. Rarely, it may be more dramatic with fever, chills, and pharyngitis or other sites of infection resulting from neutropenia and monocytopenia. Physical examination generally is unrevealing except for evidence of anemia (e.g., conjunctival and cutaneous pallor, resting tachycardia) or cutaneous bleeding (e.g., ecchymoses and petechiae), gingival bleeding and intraoral purpura. Lymphadenopathy and

TABLE 34–4. Approach to Diagnosis

History and Physical Examination
• Complete blood counts, reticulocyte count, and examination of the blood film
• Marrow aspiration and biopsy
• Marrow cell cytogenetics to evaluate clonal myeloid disease
• Fetal hemoglobin level and DNA stability test as markers of Fanconi anemia
• Immunophenotyping of red and white cells, especially for CD55, CD59 to exclude PNH
• Direct and indirect Coombs test to rule out immune cytopenia
• Serum lactate dehydrogenase (LDH) and uric acid that if increased may reflect neoplastic cell turnover
• Liver function tests to assess evidence of any recent hepatitis virus exposure
• Screening tests for hepatitis viruses A, B, and C
• Screening tests for EBV, cytomegalovirus (CMV), and HIV
• Serum B12 and red cell folic acid levels to rule out megaloblastic pancytopenia
• Serum iron, iron-binding capacity, and ferritin as a baseline prior to chronic transfusion therapy

splenomegaly are not features of aplastic anemia; such findings suggest an alternative diagnosis such as a clonal myeloid or lymphoid disease.

LABORATORY FEATURES

Blood Findings

Patients with aplastic anemia have varying degrees of pancytopenia. Anemia is associated with a low reticulocyte index. The relative reticulocyte count is usually less than 1 percent and may be zero despite the high levels of erythropoietin. Absolute reticulocyte counts are usually fewer than 40,000/μL (40 × 10^9/L). Macrocytes may be present. The absolute neutrophil and monocyte count are low. An absolute neutrophil count fewer than 500/μL (0.5 × 10^9/L) along with a platelet count fewer than 30,000/μL (30 × 10^9/L) is indicative of severe disease and a neutrophil count below 200/μL (0.2 × 10^9/L) denotes very severe disease (see Table 34–1). Lymphocyte production is thought to be normal, but patients may have mild lymphopenia. Platelets function normally. Significant qualitative changes of red cell, leukocyte, or platelet morphology are not features of classical acquired aplastic anemia. On occasion, only one cell line is depressed initially, which may lead to an early diagnosis of red cell aplasia or amegakaryocytic thrombocytopenia. In such patients, other cell lines will fail shortly thereafter (days to weeks) and permit a definitive diagnosis. Table 34–4 is a plan for initial laboratory investigation.

Plasma Findings

The plasma contains high levels of hematopoietic growth factors, including erythropoietin, thrombopoietin, and myeloid colony-stimulating factors. Plasma iron values are usually high, and ^{59}Fe clearance is prolonged, with decreased incorporation into red cells.

Marrow Findings

Morphology The marrow aspirate typically contains numerous spicules with empty, fat-filled spaces, and relatively few hematopoietic cells. Lymphocytes, plasma cells, macrophages, and mast cells may be present. On occasion, some spicules are cellular or even hypercellular ("hot spots"), but megakaryocytes usually are reduced. These focal areas of residual hematopoiesis do not appear to be of prognostic significance. Residual granulocytic cells generally appear normal, but it is not unusual to see mild macronormoblastic erythropoiesis, presumably as a result of the high levels of erythropoietin. Marrow biopsy is essential to confirm the overall hypocellularity (Fig. 34–2), as a poor yield of spicules and cells occurs in marrow aspirates in other disorders, especially if fibrosis is present.

In severe aplastic anemia, as defined by the International Aplastic Anemia Study Group, less than 25 percent cellularity or less than 50 percent cellularity with less than 30 percent hematopoietic cells is seen in the marrow.

Progenitor Cell Growth *In vitro* CFU-GM and BFU-E colony assays reveal a marked reduction in progenitor cells.[19–22]

Cytogenetic Studies Cytogenetic analysis may be difficult to perform owing to low cellularity; thus, multiple aspirates may be required to

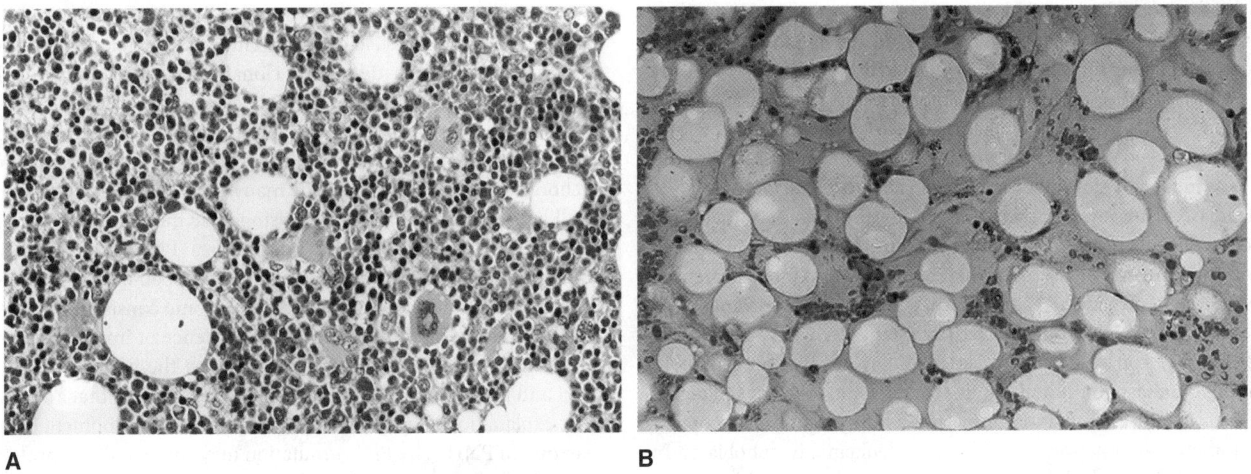

FIGURE 34–2. Marrow biopsy in aplastic anemia. **A.** A normal marrow biopsy section of a young adult. **B.** The marrow biopsy section of a young adult with very severe aplastic anemia. The specimen is devoid of hematopoietic cells and contains only scattered lymphocytes and stromal cells. The hematopoietic space is replaced by reticular cells (pre-adipocytic fibroblasts) converted to adipocytes.

provide sufficient cells for study. The results are normal in aplastic anemia. Clonal cytogenetic abnormalities in otherwise apparent aplastic anemia is indicative of an underlying hypoaccumulative clonal myeloid disease.[127]

Imaging Studies Magnetic resonance imaging can be used to distinguish between marrow fat and hematopoietic cells.[128] This may be a more useful overall estimate of marrow hematopoietic cell density than morphologic techniques and may help differentiate hypoplastic myelogenous leukemia from aplastic anemia.[128]

DIFFERENTIAL DIAGNOSIS

Any disease that can present with pancytopenia may mimic aplastic anemia if only the blood counts are considered. Measurement of the reticulocyte count and an examination of the blood film and marrow biopsy are essential early steps to arrive at a diagnosis. A reticulocyte percentage of 0.5 percent to zero is strongly indicative of aplastic erythropoiesis, and when coupled with leukopenia and thrombocytopenia, points to aplastic anemia. Absence of qualitative abnormalities of cells on the blood film and a markedly hypocellular marrow are characteristic of acquired aplastic anemia. The disorders most commonly confused with severe aplastic anemia include the approximately 5 to 10 percent of patients with myelodysplastic syndromes who present with a hypoplastic rather than a hypercellular marrow. Myelodysplasia should be considered if there is abnormal blood film morphology consistent with myelodysplasia (e.g., poikilocytosis, basophilic stippling, neutrophils with the pseudo-Pelger-Hüet anomaly). Marrow erythroid precursors in myelodysplasia may have dysmorphic features. Pathologic sideroblasts are inconsistent with aplastic anemia and a frequent feature of myelodysplasia. Granulocyte precursors may have reduced or abnormal granulation. Megakaryocytes may have abnormal nuclear lobulation (e.g., unilobular micromegakaryocytes; see Chap. 88). If clonal cytogenetic abnormalities are found, a clonal myeloid disorder, especially myelodysplastic syndrome or hypocellular myelogenous leukemia is likely. Magnetic resonance imaging (MRI) studies of bone may be useful in differentiating severe aplastic anemia from clonal myeloid syndromes. The former gives a fatty signal and the latter a diffuse cellular pattern.

A hypocellular marrow frequently is associated with PNH. PNH is characterized by an acquired mutation in the *PIG-A* gene that encodes an enzyme that is required to synthesize mannolipids. The latter deficiency prevents the synthesis of the glycosyl-phosphatidylinositol anchor precursor. This moiety anchors several proteins, including inhibitors of the complement pathway to blood cell membranes, and its absence accounts for the complement-mediated hemolysis in PNH. As many as 50 percent of patients with otherwise typical aplastic anemia have evidence of glycosyl-phosphatidylinositol molecule defects and diminished phosphatidylinositol-anchored protein on leukocytes and red cells as judged by flow cytometry, analogous to that seen in PNH.[129] The decrease or absence of these membrane proteins may make the PNH clone of cells resistant to the acquired immune attack on normal marrow components, or the phosphatidylinositol-anchored protein(s) on normal cells provides an epitope that initiates an aberrant T-cell attack, leaving the PNH clone relatively resistant (see Chap. 40).[24]

Occasionally, apparent aplastic anemia may be the prodrome to childhood[130] or, less commonly, adult[131] acute lymphoblastic leukemia. Sometimes, careful examination of marrow cells by light microscopy or flow cytometry will uncover a population of leukemic lymphoblasts. In other cases, the acute leukemia may appear later. Hairy-cell leukemia, Hodgkin disease, or another lymphoma subtype, rarely, may be preceded by a period of marrow hypoplasia. Immunophenotyping of marrow and blood cells by flow cytometry for CD25 may uncover the presence of hairy cells. Other clinical features may be distinctive (see Chap. 95). Organomegaly such as lymphadenopathy, hepatomegaly, or splenomegaly are inconsistent with the atrophic (hypoproliferative) features of aplastic anemia. Large granular lymphocytic leukemia has also been associated with aplastic anemia. Rare cases of typical acquired aplastic anemia have been followed by t(9;22)-positive acute lymphocytic leukemia (ALL), or chronic myelogenous leukemia (CML).[131]

RELATIONSHIP AMONG APLASTIC ANEMIA, PNH, AND CLONAL MYELOID DISEASES

In addition to the diagnostic difficulties occasionally presented by patients with hypoplastic myelodysplastic syndromes, hypoplastic acute myelogenous leukemia (AML), or PNH with hypocellular marrows, there may be a more fundamental relationship among these three diseases and aplastic anemia. The development of clonal cytogenetic abnormalities such as monosomy 7 or trisomy 8 in a patient with aplastic anemia portends the evolution of a myelodysplastic syndrome or acute leukemia. Occasionally, these cytogenetic markers have been transient, and in cases with disappearance of monosomy 7, hematologic improvement has occurred as well.[132] Persistent monosomy 7 carries a poor prognosis as compared to trisomy 8.[133,134]

As many as 15 to 20 percent of patients with aplastic anemia have a 5-year probability of developing myelodysplasia.[132] If one excludes any transformation to a clonal myeloid disorder that occurs up to 6 months after treatment to avoid misdiagnosis among the hypoplastic clonal myeloid diseases, the frequency of a clonal disorder was nearly 15 times greater in patients treated with immunosuppression as compared to those treated with marrow transplantation after 39 months of observation.[135] This finding suggests either that immune suppression by anti–T-cell therapy enhances the evolution of a neoplastic clone or that it does not suppress the intrinsic tendency of aplastic anemia to evolve to a clonal disease, but provides the increased longevity of the patient required to express that potential. The latter interpretation is more likely as patients successfully treated solely with androgens develop clonal disease as frequently as those treated with immunosuppression.[136] Transplantation may reduce the potential to clonal evolution in patients with aplastic anemia by reestablishing robust lymphohematopoiesis.

Telomere shortening also may play a pathogenetic role in the evolution of aplastic anemia into myelodysplasia. Patients with aplastic anemia have shorter telomere lengths than matched controls, and patients with aplastic anemia with persistent cytopenias had greater telomere shortening over time than matched controls. Three of five patients with telomere lengths less than 5 kb developed clonal cytogenetic changes, whereas patients with longer telomeres did not develop such diseases.[23,137]

The relationship of PNH to aplastic anemia remains enigmatic. Because hematopoietic stem cells lacking the phosphatidylinositol-anchored proteins are present in many or all normal persons in very small numbers,[138] it is not surprising that more than 50 percent of patients with aplastic anemia may have a PNH cell population as detected by immunophenotyping.[129] The probability of patients with aplastic anemia developing a clinical syndrome consistent with PNH is 10 to 20 percent, and this is not a consequence of immunosuppressive treatment.[132] Patients also may present with the hemolytic anemia of PNH and later develop progressive marrow failure so that any pathogenetic explanation should consider both types of development of aplastic marrows in PNH. The *PIG-A* mutation may confer either a proliferative or survival advantage to PNH cells.[139] A survival advantage could result if the anchor protein or one of its ligands served as an epitope for the T-lymphocyte cytotoxicity inducing the marrow aplasia. In this case, the presenting event could either reflect cytopenias or the sensitivity of red

TABLE 34–5. Initial Management of Aplastic Anemia

- Discontinue any potential offending drug and use an alternative class of agents if essential.
- Anemia: transfusion of leukocyte-depleted, irradiated red cells as required for very severe anemia.
- Very severe thrombocytopenia or thrombocytopenic bleeding: consider ε-aminocaproic acid; transfusion of platelets as required.
- Severe neutropenia; use infection precautions.
- Fever (suspected infection): microbial cultures; broad-spectrum antibiotics if specific organism not identified, granulocyte colony-stimulating factor (G-CSF) in dire cases. If child or small adult with profound infection (e.g., gram-negative bacteria, fungus, persistent positive blood cultures) can consider neutrophil transfusion from a G-CSF pretreated donor.
- Immediate assessment for allogeneic stem cell transplantation: Histocompatibility testing of patient, parents, and siblings. Search databases for unrelated donor, if appropriate.

cells to complement lysis and hemolysis, depending on the intrinsic proliferative potential of the PNH clone.

Within our current state of knowledge, aplastic anemia is an autoimmune process, and any residual hematopoiesis is presumably polyclonal. This is a critical distinction from hypoplastic leukemia and PNH, which are clonal (neoplastic) diseases. The environment of the aplastic marrow, however, may favor the eventual evolution of a mutant (malignant) clone, especially if immunotherapy is used, whereas hematopoietic stem cell transplantation may either ablate threatening minor clones or establish more robust hematopoiesis, an environment less conducive to clonal evolution.

TREATMENT

Approach to Therapy

Severe anemia, bleeding from thrombocytopenia, and, rarely at the time of diagnosis, infection secondary to granulocytopenia and monocytopenia require prompt attention to remove potential life-threatening conditions and improve patient comfort (Table 34–5). More specific treatment of the marrow aplasia involves two principal options: (1) syngeneic or allogeneic hematopoietic stem cell transplantation or (2) combination immunosuppressive therapy with ATG and cyclosporine. The selection of the specific mode of treatment depends on several factors, including the patient's age and condition and the availability of a suitable allele-level HLA-matched hematopoietic stem cell donor. In general, transplantation is the preferred treatment for children and most otherwise healthy younger adults. Early histocompatibility testing of siblings is of particular importance because it establishes whether there is an optimal donor available to the patient for transplantation. The preferred stem cell source is a histocompatible sibling matched at the HLA-A, B, C, and DR loci.

Supportive Care

The Use of Blood Products Although it was recommended that red cell and platelet transfusions be used sparingly in potential transplant recipients to minimize sensitization to histocompatibility antigens, this has become less important since ATG and cyclophosphamide have been used as the preparative regimen for transplantation in aplastic anemia, as their use has markedly reduced the problem of graft rejection.[140]

Cytomegalovirus (CMV)-reduced risk red cells and platelets should be given to a potential transplant recipient to minimize problems with CMV infections after transplantation. Once a patient is shown to be CMV-positive, this restriction is no longer necessary. Leukocyte-depletion filters or CMV serotesting are equivalent methods of decreasing the risk of transmitting CMV.

Red Cell Transfusion Packed red cells to alleviate symptoms of anemia usually are indicated at hemoglobin values below 8 g/dL (80 g/L), unless comorbid medical conditions require a higher hemoglobin concentration. These products should be leukocyte-depleted to lessen leukocyte and platelet sensitization and to reduce subsequent transfusion reactions and radiated to reduce the potential for a graft-versus-host reaction. It is important not to transfuse patients with red cells (or platelets) from family members if transplantation within the family is remotely possible, as this approach may sensitize patients to minor histocompatibility antigens, increasing the risk of graft rejection after marrow transplantation. Following a marrow transplant, or in those individuals in whom transplantation is not a consideration, family members may be ideal donors for platelet products. Because each unit of red cells adds approximately 200 to 250 mg of iron to the total body iron, over the long-term transfusion-induced iron overload may occur. This is not a major problem in patients who respond to transplantation or immunosuppressive therapy, but it is an issue in nonresponders who require continued transfusion support. In the latter case, consideration should be given to iron chelation therapy. Newer oral agents will make this procedure easier to effect (see Chap. 47).[141]

Platelet Transfusion It is important to assess the risk of bleeding in each patient. Most patients tolerate platelet counts of 10,000/μL (10×10^9/L) without undue bruising or bleeding, unless a systemic infection is present.[142,143] A traumatic injury or surgery requires transfusion to >50,000/μL or >100,000/μL, respectively. Administration of ε-aminocaproic acid, 100 mg/kg per dose every 4 hours (maximum dose 5 g) orally or intravenously, may reduce the bleeding tendency.[144] Pooled random-donor platelets may be used until sensitization ensues, although it is preferable to use single-donor platelets from the onset to minimize sensitization to HLA or platelet antigens. Subsequently, single-donor apheresis products or HLA-matched platelets may be required.

Platelet refractoriness is a major problem with long-term transfusion support.[145] This may occur transiently, with fever or infection, or as a chronic problem secondary to HLA sensitization. In the past, this occurred in approximately 50 percent of patients after 8 to 10 weeks of transfusion support. Filtration of blood and platelet concentrates to remove leukocytes reduces this problem to approximately 15 percent of patients receiving chronic transfusions.[145,146] Patient's should also get ABO-identical platelets because this enhances platelet survival and further decreases refractoriness to platelet transfusion. Single-donor HLA-matched apheresis-harvested platelets may be necessary in previously pregnant or transfused patients who are already allosensitized or who become so after treatment with leukoreduced platelets. The frequency of either of these events is less than 10 percent. Approaches to chronic platelet transfusion are discussed in Chap. 141. The utility of TPO receptor agonists in the thrombocytopenia of aplastic anemia is yet to be determined.

Management of Neutropenia Neutropenic precautions should be applied to hospitalized patients with a severe depression of the neutrophil count. The level of neutrophils requiring precautions is fewer than 500/μL (0.5×10^9/L). One approach is to use private rooms, with requirements for face masks and handwashing with antiseptic soap. Unwashed fresh fruits and vegetables should be avoided as they are sources of bacterial contamination. It is uncommon for patients with aplastic anemia to present with a significant infection. When patients with aplastic anemia become febrile, cultures should be obtained from the throat, sputum (if any), blood, urine, stool, and any suspicious lesions. Broad-spectrum bacteriocidal antibiotics should be initiated promptly, without awaiting culture results. The choice of antibiotics depends on the prevalence of organisms and their antibiotic sensitivity in the local setting. Organisms of concern usually include *Staphylococcus aureus* (notably methicillin- and oxacillin-resistant strains), *Staphylococcus epidermidis* (in patients with venous access devices), and gram-negative organisms. Patients with persistent culture-negative fevers should be considered for antifungal treatment (see Chap. 22).

In the past, leukocyte transfusions were used on a daily basis to reduce the short-term mortality from infections. It was unusual to detect more than 100 to 200 neutrophils per microliter for more than a few hours after transfusion. The yield of neutrophils can be increased by administering granulocyte colony-stimulating factor (G-CSF) to the donor,[147] but most physicians avoid using white cell products because present-day antibiotics are usually sufficient to treat a patient for an episode of sepsis. Notable exceptions include documented invasive aspergillosis unresponsive to amphotericin (particularly in the posttransplant setting), infections with organisms resistant to all known antibiotics, and if blood cultures remain positive in spite of antibiotic treatment. Leukocyte transfusion is more effective in children and adults with smaller body size, as transfused leukocytes have a smaller distribution space, which results in higher blood and tissue concentrations.

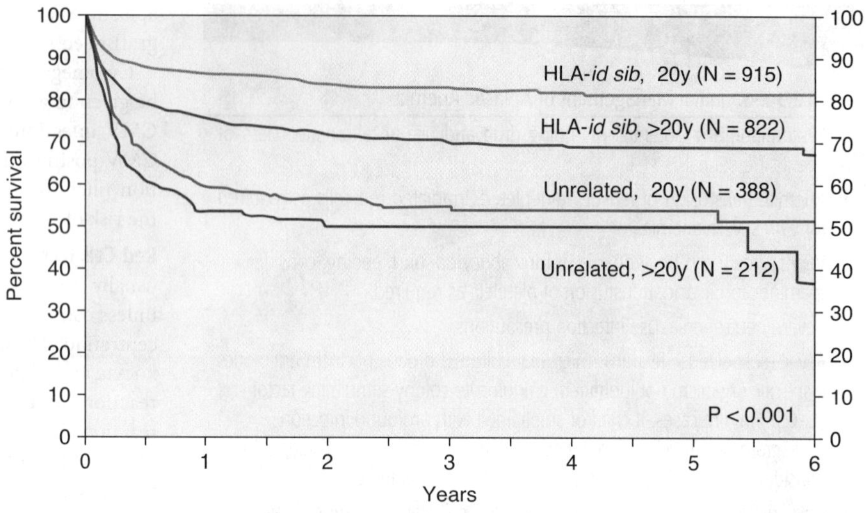

FIGURE 34–3. Probability of survival after hematopoietic stem cell transplantation for severe aplastic anemia by donor type and age, 1998–2004. Patients receiving marrow from a matched sibling had better outcomes if they were equal to or less than 20 years of age, compared to those older than 20 years of age. Patients receiving marrow from a matched sibling fared better than those who received marrow from a matched unrelated donor, at any age. Patients younger than 20 or older than 20 years of age did not have a significant difference in outcome if they received marrow from an unrelated matched donor. *Id*, identical; *sib*, sibling. *(Figure reproduced from the Center for International Transplant Research data on the National Marrow Donor Program website. http://www.marrow.org/PATIENT/Undrstnd_Disease_Treat/Lrn_about_Disease/Aplastic_Anemia/AA_Tx_Outcomes/index.html. Last accessed February 2009.)*

Hematopoietic Stem Cell Transplantation Prompt therapy usually is indicated for patients with severe aplastic anemia. The major curative approach is hematopoietic stem cell transplantation from a histocompatible sibling.[148–150] This treatment modality is described in Chap. 21. Only 20 to 30 percent of patients in the United States have compatible sibling donors (related to average family size). In the unusual case of an identical twin donor, conditioning is required to obliterate the immune disease in the recipient, but it can be limited to cyclophosphamide. In this setting, an 80 to 90 percent survival is expected. Marrow stem cells seem to perform better than blood stem cells when used as a source for patients with aplastic anemia, although this is under continued study. The results of transplantation are best in patients younger than age 20 years (80 to 90 percent long-term survival) but decrease every decade of age thereafter. Posttransplant mortality is increased and survival decreased with increasing age (Fig. 34–3). In patients older than age 40 years, survival in matched sibling transplant is reduced to approximately 50 percent.[151] There are still uncertainties about the optimal conditioning program in younger and older patients. ATG, cyclophosphamide, total-body radiation, and fludarabine are among the agents being studied.[148,150,151] The longer the delay between diagnosis and transplant, the less salutary the outcome, probably as a result of a greater number of transfusions and a higher likelihood of pretransplant infection. Acute and chronic graft-versus-host disease are serious complications, and therapy to prevent or ameliorate them is a standard part of posttransplant treatment.[148,151] Transplants have been performed using stem cells from partially matched siblings or unrelated, histocompatible donors recruited through the National Marrow Donor Program or similar organizations in other countries.[152] Umbilical cord blood is an alternative source of stem cells from unrelated donors (or, rarely, siblings) for transplantation in children. The use of high-resolution, HLA typing of a matched, unrelated donor markedly improves the prognosis for transplantation.[153] High-resolution DNA matching at HLA-A, -B, -C, and -DRB1 (8 of 8 allele) is considered the lowest level of matching consistent with the highest level of survival. If there is an HLA mismatch at one or more loci, especially HLA-A or -DRB1, the outcome is compromised,[153] and immunosuppression with combined therapy may be preferred initially, depending on patient age, cytomegalovirus status, and disease severity. The use of hematopoietic stem cell transplantation can be considered for patients who do not respond or who no longer respond to immunotherapy.[151] If the patient in question is a candidate for stem cell transplantation based on all relevant factors, transplantation could be considered at any age for a patient with a syngeneic donor; transplantation could be considered as a first-choice therapy up to age 50 years for a patient with an HLA allele-level matched sibling donor; and transplantation could be considered a first-choice therapy if an allele-level HLA-matched unrelated donor is available for patients younger than age 20 years.[151]

Components of Anti–T-Lymphocyte (Immunosuppressive) Therapy

Antilymphocyte Serum and Antithymocyte Globulin ATG and ALG act principally by reducing cytotoxic T cells. This involves ATG-induced apoptosis through both FAS and TNF pathways.[154] Cathepsin B also plays a role in T-cell cytotoxicity at clinical concentrations of ATG, but may involve an independent apoptosis pathway.[155] ATG and ALG also release hematopoietic growth factors from T cells.[156,157] Horse and rabbit ATG are licensed in the United States. Skin tests against horse serum should be performed prior to administration.[158] If positive, the patient may be desensitized. ATG therapy is given daily for 4 to 10 days with doses of 15 to 40 mg/kg. Fever and chills are common during the first day of treatment. Concomitant treatment with glucocorticoids, such as methylprednisolone or dexamethasone lessens the reaction to ATG. Studies are under way to compare equine to rabbit ATG in the immunotherapy of aplastic anemia.

ATG treatment may accelerate platelet destruction, reduce the absolute neutrophil count, and cause a positive direct antiglobulin test. This effect may lead to an increase in transfusion requirements during the 4- to 10-day treatment interval. Serum sickness, characterized by spiking fevers, skin rashes, and arthralgias, occurs commonly 7 to 10 days from the first dose. The clinical manifestations of serum sickness can be diminished by increasing the glucocorticoid dose from day 10 to day 17 after treatment. Approximately one-third of patients no longer require transfusion support after treatment with ATG alone.[159–161]

Of 358 patients responding to immunosuppressive therapy, principally ATG alone, 74 (21%) relapsed after a mean of 2.1 years. The actuarial incidence of relapse was 35 percent at 10 years.[162] Similar results were observed when 227 patients were treated with immunosuppression, primarily ATG alone.[163] The actuarial survival at 15 years was 38 percent following immunosuppression.[162] However, a combination of immunosuppressive agents provides more effective therapy than ATG alone (see "Combination Immunotherapy" below).

Twenty-eight (22%) of 129 patients treated with ALG developed myelodysplasia, leukemia, paroxysmal nocturnal hemoglobinuria, or combined disorders.[164] This tendency to relapse and to develop clonal hematologic disorders was reviewed by the European Cooperative Group for Bone Marrow Transplantation in 468 patients, most of whom received ATG.[165] The risk of a hematologic complication increased continuously and reached 57 percent at 8 years after immunosuppressive therapy. A further survey found 42 (5%) malignancies in 860 patients treated with immunosuppression, whereas only 9 (1%) malignancies were seen in 748 patients who received marrow transplants.[166]

Cyclosporine Administration of cyclosporine, a cyclic polypeptide that inhibits IL-2 production by T lymphocytes and prevents expansion of cytotoxic T cells in response to IL-2, is another approach to immunotherapy. After the initial report of its ability to induce remission in 1984,[167] several groups have used cyclosporine as either (1) primary treatment,[168–171] (2) in patients refractory to ATG or glucocorticoids,[169–174] (3) in combination with granulocyte colony-stimulating factors,[175,176] or (4) in varying combinations with other modes of therapy.[177] Cyclosporine is administered orally at 10 to 12 mg/kg per day for at least 4 to 6 months. Dosage adjustments may be required to maintain trough blood levels of 200 to 400 ng/mL. Renal impairment is common and may require increased hydration or dose adjustments to keep creatinine values below 2 mg/dL. Cyclosporine also may cause moderate hypertension, a variety of neurological manifestations, and other side effects. Several drug classes interact with cyclosporine to either increase (e.g., some antibiotics and antifungals) or decrease (e.g., some anticonvulsants) blood levels. Responses usually are seen by 3 months and may range from achieving transfusion independence to complete remission. Approximately 25 percent of patients respond to this agent when used alone, but the response rate has ranged from 0 to 80 percent in various reports.[177]

Although immunosuppression with ALG or ATG has been used the longest and has a seemingly better response rate, there are certain advantages to cyclosporine. This drug does not require hospitalization or use of central venous catheters. Fewer platelet transfusions are required during the first few weeks of therapy compared to treatment with ALG or ATG. A French cooperative trial showed equal effectiveness of ATG plus prednisone compared to cyclosporine.[178] In this crossover study of newly diagnosed patients, survival of approximately 65 percent was observed 12 months after diagnosis.

Combination Immunotherapy Combination treatment of severe aplastic anemia usually includes, for example, ATG, 40 mg/kg per day, for 4 days; cyclosporine, 10 to 12 mg/kg per day, for 6 months and methylprednisolone, 1 mg/kg per day, for 2 weeks.[179] The dose of cyclosporine is adjusted to maintain a trough level of 200–400 ng/mL. Prophylaxis for *Pneumocystis carinii* with daily trimethoprim-sulfamethoxazole or with monthly pentamidine inhalations should be considered for these patients as they receive immunosuppressive therapy.

The addition of cyclosporine to the combination of ALG and glucocorticoids improves response rates to approximately 70 percent of patients (Table 34–6).[180,181] G-CSF added to the combined immunosuppressive therapy does not increase response rate or survival.[183] Response is usually defined as a significant improvement in red cells, white cells, and platelets to eliminate risk of infection and bleeding and the requirement for red cell transfusions.

TABLE 34–6. Response to Immunotherapy in Patients with Severe Aplastic Anemia

Year of Publication	Principal Drugs Used	No. Pts (Age-range, yrs)	Significant Response No. (%)	Survival at 5/10 Years (%)	Relapse at 5 Years (Cum%)	Comments	Reference
2008	ATG + CYA	77 (<18)	57 (74)	83/80	25	8.5% evolved to clonal myeloid disease	180
2007	ATG + CYA	44 (NR)	31 (70)	NR/88	NR	All cases were associated with hepatitis	181
2007	ATG + CYA	47 (19–75)	31 (66)	80/NR	45	No late clonal diseases at 5 years	182
2007	ATG + CYA + G-CSF	48 (19–74)	37 (77)	90/NR	15	No late clonal diseases at 5 years	182
2006	ATG + CYA	47 (8–71)	37 (79)	80/75	NR	No late clonal diseases at 10 years	183
2006	ATG + CYA + G-CSF + rhuEPO	30 (5–68)	22 (73)	80/75	NR	One patient developed clonal myeloid disease	183

ATG, antithymocyte globulin; Cum%, cumulative percent; CYA, cyclosporine A, G-CSF, granulocyte colony-stimulating factor; No. Pts, number of patients; NR, not reported; rhuEPO, recombinant human erythropoietin.

NOTE: In some cases response, survival, and relapse percentages are very close approximations, read off the published graphs. Significant response combines complete and partial remissions, which usually means the platelet and red cell count are high enough to avoid transfusions and neutrophil count over a critical level. Some protocols used short periods of glucocorticoid treatment to ameliorate reactions to ATG. There is a significant frequency of relapses or progression to clonal myeloid disease after 5 to 10 years postimmunotherapy.

The 5-year survival after completion of combination immunosuppressive therapy may approximate that after stem cell transplantation.[184] Forty-eight children treated between 1983 and 1992 had a 10-year survival of approximately 75 percent for marrow transplantation and approximately 75 percent for combined immunosuppressive therapy, although there were only half the number of severely affected patients in the immunosuppressive therapy group.[185] Thus, immunosuppression may be preferable for patients who are older than 30 years of age and in those who may experience a delay in finding a suitable donor. Marrow transplants are, however, curative for aplastic anemia, whereas more frequent sequelae have been found after immunosuppressive therapy,[186–188] notably a substantial rate of evolution to a myelodysplastic syndrome or acute myelogenous leukemia.

A recent National Institutes of Health protocol was designed to increase immune tolerance by specific deletion of activated T lymphocytes that target primitive hematopoietic progenitor cells.[24] Concurrent administration of cyclosporine with ATG may diminish the ATG effect so that in this program cyclosporine is introduced at a later time. The addition of new immunosuppressive agents, such as mycophenolate mofetil, rapamycin, or monoclonal antibodies, to the IL-2 receptor may be more effective in decreasing cytotoxic T cells, sparing the targeted hematopoietic stem cells.[24]

For the 30 to 40 percent of patients who relapse after immunotherapy, retreatment with ATG and cyclosporine is effective in 50 to 60 percent of them.[189,190]

High-Dose Glucocorticoid Treatment Marrow recovery can occur after very high doses of glucocorticoids.[191,192] Methylprednisolone in the range of 500 to 1000 mg daily for 3 to 14 days has been successful, but the side effects, which include marked hyperglycemia and glycosuria, electrolyte disturbances, gastric irritation, psychosis, increased infections, and aseptic necrosis of the hips, can be severe. Glucocorticoids at lower doses commonly are used only as a component of combination therapy for aplastic anemia to ameliorate the toxic effects of ATG and in providing additional lymphocyte suppression.

High-Dose Cyclophosphamide Therapy High-dose cyclophosphamide has been used as a form of immunosuppression.[193] Although it would seem inappropriate to administer high doses of chemotherapy to patients with severe marrow aplasia, this approach was based on observations of autologous recovery after preparative therapy for allogeneic transplants.[6] Ten patients received cyclophosphamide at 45 mg/kg per day intravenously for 4 days with or without cyclosporine for an additional 100 days. Gradual neutrophil and platelet recovery ensued over 3 months. Seven patients responded completely and remained in remission 11 years after treatment. High-dose cyclophosphamide treatment may spare hematopoietic stem cells, which have high levels of aldehyde dehydrogenase and are relatively resistant to cyclophosphamide.[194,195] Thus, cyclophosphamide in this situation may be more immunosuppressive than myelotoxic. The most extensive trial of high-dose cyclophosphamide resulted in 65 percent of patients responding completely at 50 months.[196] However, the role of this regimen as initial therapy is not clear because of early toxicity that may exceed that of the ATG-cyclosporine combination.[197] The probability of a durable remission may be superior, but there are insufficient data (comparative clinical trials) to conclude whether high-dose cyclophosphamide provides better long-term results than ATG and cyclosporine. The latter approach is favored at this time.

Rituximab A case report of the successful use of the anti-CD20 humanized mouse antibody rituximab has provided preliminary evidence for its potential effectiveness in treating aplastic anemia.[198] Clinical trials should examine its efficacy compared to standard immunotherapy (ATG and cyclosporine), in patients refractory to standard therapy, or as a third drug in an immunotherapy regimen. The role of B lymphocytes in the pathogenesis of aplastic anemia has not been defined.

Androgens Randomized trials have not shown efficacy when androgens were used as primary therapy for severe or moderately severe aplastic anemia.[199,200]

Androgens stimulate the production of erythropoietin, and their metabolites stimulate erythropoiesis when added to marrow cultures *in vitro*. High doses of androgens were beneficial in some patients with moderately severe aplasia.[199] Series of patients were reported in which survival seemed improved as compared with historical controls, but this could have resulted from improved supportive care.[136] Masculinization and other androgen side effects can be severe. Long-term survivors after androgen therapy have essentially the same progression to clonal hematologic disorders as patients treated with immunosuppressive agents.[136] These agents have been replaced by immunosuppression or allogeneic hematopoietic stem cell transplantation.

Cytokines Despite their effectiveness in accelerating recovery from chemotherapy, these agents have been far less effective in achieving long-term benefits in patients with severe aplastic anemia. Daily treatment with G-CSF[201,202] has improved marrow cellularity and increased neutrophil counts approximately 1.5- to 10-fold. Unfortunately, in nearly all patients, the blood counts return to baseline within several days of cessation of therapy. Although occasional patients show evidence of trilineage marrow recovery with long-term therapy, the vast majority do not respond. Therapy with myeloid growth factors is probably best reserved for episodes of severe infection or as a preventive measure prior to dental work or other procedures that would compromise mucosal barriers in patients who have not responded to stem cell transplant or immunotherapy. Prophylactic use of growth factors is not warranted. G-CSF in a dose of 5 μg/kg by subcutaneous injection is easiest to administer and seems to be associated with the fewest side effects. The drug can be given daily or fewer times per week depending on the response. Newer pegylated preparations have greater longevity and usually are administered at less frequent, every-other-week intervals.

IL-1, a potent stimulator of marrow stromal cell production of other cytokines, and IL-3 have been ineffective in small numbers of patients with severe aplastic anemia.[204,205] These disappointing results with cytokines are not unexpected, as previous work has found high serum levels of growth factors in patients with aplastic anemia. Moreover, the majority of patients have suppression of very primitive progenitors, which may be unresponsive to individual factors that act on more mature progenitor cells.

Splenectomy Removal of the spleen does not increase hematopoiesis but may increase neutrophil and platelet counts two- to threefold and improve survival of transfused red cells or platelets in highly sensitized individuals.[206] The surgical morbidity and mortality in patients with few platelets and white cells makes this a questionable therapeutic procedure. Because there are more successful methods of therapy that attack the fundamental problem, this approach would not be used today.

Other Therapy High doses of intravenous gamma globulin have been given to small numbers of patients with severe aplastic anemia[207,208] because of its success in treating certain cases of antibody-mediated pure red cell aplasia. Some improvement was noted in 4 of 6 patients treated. Another treatment that is occasionally successful is lymphocytapheresis to deplete T cells.[209,210]

Course and Prognosis

At diagnosis, the prognosis is largely related to the absolute neutrophil and platelet count. The absolute neutrophil count is the most important prognostic feature, with a count of fewer than 500/μL (0.5×10^9/L) considered severe aplastic anemia and a count of fewer than 200/μL ($0.2 \times$

10^9/L) very severe aplastic anemia, the latter associated with a poor response to immunotherapy and usually a dire prognosis if early successful allogeneic transplant is not available. In the past, the prognosis appeared worse when the disease followed hepatitis.[69,70] But more comprehensive results with immunosuppression[191] or hematopoietic stem cell transplantation[211] show an equivalent response to that seen with idiopathic or drug-induced cases.

Before marrow transplantation and immunosuppressive therapy, more than 25 percent of the patients with severe aplastic anemia died within 4 months of diagnosis; half succumbed within 1 year.[212,213] Marrow transplantation is curative for approximately 80 to 90 percent of patients younger than 20 years of age, approximately 70 percent if between the ages of 20 and 40 years, and approximately 50 percent if older than age 40 years.[151,214] Unfortunately, as many as 40 percent of transplant survivors suffer the deleterious consequences of chronic graft-versus-host disease,[151] and the risk of subsequent cancer can be as high as 10 percent in older patients or after immunotherapy prior to hematopoietic stem cell transplantation.[215] The best outcomes occur in those patients who have an allele-based HLA-matched sibling, have not been exposed to immunosuppressive therapy prior to transplantation, have not been exposed and sensitized to blood cell products, have had marrow rather than a blood stem cell donor product, and have not been subjected to high-dose radiation in the conditioning regimen for transplantation.[151,215–217]

Combination immunosuppressive therapy with ATG and cyclosporine leads to a marked improvement in approximately 70 percent of the patients. Although some patients have normal blood counts, many continue with moderate anemia or thrombocytopenia. In as many as 40 percent of patients initially responding to immunosuppressive therapy, their disease may relapse or progress over 10 years to paroxysmal nocturnal hemoglobinuria, a myelodysplastic syndrome, or acute myelogenous leukemia.[162–169,195–197] Moreover, the beneficial effects of immunotherapy are often lost 10 years after treatment. In 168 transplanted patients the actuarial survival at 15 years was 69 percent, and in 227 patients receiving immunosuppressive therapy it was 38 percent.[162]

Treatment with high-dose cyclophosphamide produces early results similar to that seen with the combination of ATG and cyclosporine.[218] However, cyclophosphamide has greater early toxicity and slower hematologic recovery, but may generate more durable remissions. Its use has been too limited to reach a firm conclusion on its relative merits and it is rarely used as first choice immunotherapy.

HEREDITARY APLASTIC ANEMIA

■ FANCONI ANEMIA

Definition and History

Fanconi anemia is the most common form of constitutional aplastic anemia and was initially described in three brothers by Fanconi in 1927.[219] It is inherited as an autosomal recessive condition that results from defects in genes that modulate the stability of DNA.

Epidemiology

Fanconi Anemia is an uncommon disorder and is estimated to be present in 1 in 1 million individuals. It is far more frequent in Afrikaners of European descent.[220] This unusually high frequency has been attributed to a founder effect.

Etiology and Pathogenesis

Thirteen complementation groups, defined by somatic cell hybridization, are associated with the development of Fanconi anemia.[221] A complementation group is a genetic subgroup. Identifying a complementation group requires adding a gene to the genome of a cell to correct (complement) the genetic defect. This procedure can be done by cell fusion studies. After fusing two cells together, thereby joining their genetic material, one can test the cells for the genetic defect. In the case of Fanconi anemia, this would be with the diepoxybutane test. Hybrids in which the hypersensitivity to diepoxybutane is corrected (complemented) can be assumed to result from the fusion of cells from different genetic subgroups (complementation groups), whereas hybrids that still show the sensitivity are the result of fusion of cells from the same subgroup. Because one can determine the complementation group without knowing the gene involved, this approach is the first step in understanding the genetic basis of a disease. Once the genes are known, one does not need to use cell fusion studies; rather, retroviral vectors can be used to insert corrected genes into the cells.

The complementation groups have been designated *FANCA, B, C, D1, D2, E, F, G, I, J, L, M,* and *N.* Table 34–7 lists the gene mutations corresponding to these complementation groups. The great majority of patients have mutations of *FANCA, FANCC,* or *FANCG.*[222] It has been proposed that the A and C gene products, which are cytoplasmic proteins, form an "FA core complex" with the products of genes B, E, F, G, L, and M, which are adaptors or phosphorylators.[222,223] The complex translocates to the nucleus, where it is required for the ubiquitylation of FANCD2 and protects the cell from DNA cross-linking and participates in DNA repair (Fig. 34–4). DNA damage initiates activation of the FA/BRCA pathway and ubiquitylation of FANCD2, which is targeted to the altered DNA and facilitates repair by interacting with DNA repair proteins, BRCA1, FANCD1/BRCA2, FANCN/PALB2, and RAD51. In the presence of a mutant gene product, normal function is disturbed leading to damaging effects in sensitive tissues, including hematopoietic cells. In addition to the genetic defects leading to DNA instability and an inability to repair DNA, TNF-α and -γ are overexpressed in the marrow of Fanconi anemia patients.[224] The excess TNF-α may play a role in the suppression of erythropoiesis in these patients.

Clinical Features

Growth retardation results in short stature, and skeletal anomalies are common. Absent, misshapen, or supernumerary thumbs and dysplastic radii occur in half the patients. Hip and vertebral abnormalities also may occur. Septal heart defects, eye abnormalities, and absent, misshapen, or fused kidneys may be present. Learning disability is frequent, and microcephaly and mental retardation may be a feature. Hypogonadism also may be evident. The skin may be generally hyperpigmented or may have areas of abnormal skin pigmentation referred to as *café-au-lait* spots, which are flat, light brown, and from 1 to 12 centimeters in diameter. Hepatosplenomegaly is not a feature of the disease. Some patients have no or minor phenotypic abnormalities and may be diagnosed as a result of the onset of marrow failure or a cancer involving any of many sites as late as the fifth decade of life.

The onset of marrow failure is gradual and usually is evident during the last half of the first decade of life. The manifestations of anemia, including weakness, fatigue, and dyspnea on exertion, and of thrombocytopenia with epistaxis, purpura, or other unexpected bleeding, are the principal findings. Hematologic and visceral manifestations are combined eventually in more than a third of patients, but some may have cytopenias and inconspicuous somatic changes, whereas others may have somatic anomalies with no or a nominal disorder of blood cell formation for months or years. Some who carry the gene may be virtually unaffected.[225–227] In a review of the more than 1300 patients in the literature, 100 patients or fewer than 7 percent without anomalies were identified by chromosome breakage studies (see "Laboratory Features" below) because of affected siblings.[227] In the past, children in

TABLE 34–7. Gene Mutations Found in Fanconi Anemia

Gene	Chromosome Location	% of Patients	Inheritance	Protein Function
FANCA	16q24.3	~65*	AR	FA Core Complex
FANCB	Xp22.31	rare	XLR	FA Core Complex
FANCC	9q22.3	~10	AR	FA Core Complex
FANCDI (BRCA2)	13q12.3	rare	AR	RAD51 Recruitment
FANCD2	3p25.3	rare	AR	Monoubiquitinated protein
FANCE	6p21.3	~10	AR	FA Core Complex
FANCF	11p15	rare	AR	FA Core Complex
FANCG (XRCC9)	9p13	~10	AR	FA Core Complex
FANCI (KIAA1794)	15q25–26	rare	AR	Monoubiquitination of FANCD2
FANCJ (BACH1/BRIP1)	17q22.3	rare	AR	5′ to 3′ DNA helicase/ATPase
FANCL (PHF9/POG)	2q16.1	rare	AR	FA Core Complex, E3 Ubiquitin ligase
FANCM (Hef)	14q21.3	rare	AR	FA Core Complex, ATPase/translocase, DNA helicase motifs
FANCN (PALB2)	16q12.1	rare	AR	Regulation of BRCA2 localization
To be identified		~5		

AR, autosomal recessive; ATPase, adenosine triphosphatase; XLR, X-linked recessive.

*There are more than 100 mutant FANCA alleles, approximately 40% of which are large intragenic deletions. This table was made using material from references 221–223.

Fanconi families with an onset of aplastic anemia without congenital somatic abnormalities were thought to have a different disorder termed *Estren-Dameshek syndrome.*[228] However, these children, whose lymphocytes show sensitivity to diepoxybutane, are considered to have Fanconi anemia without skeletal abnormalities.

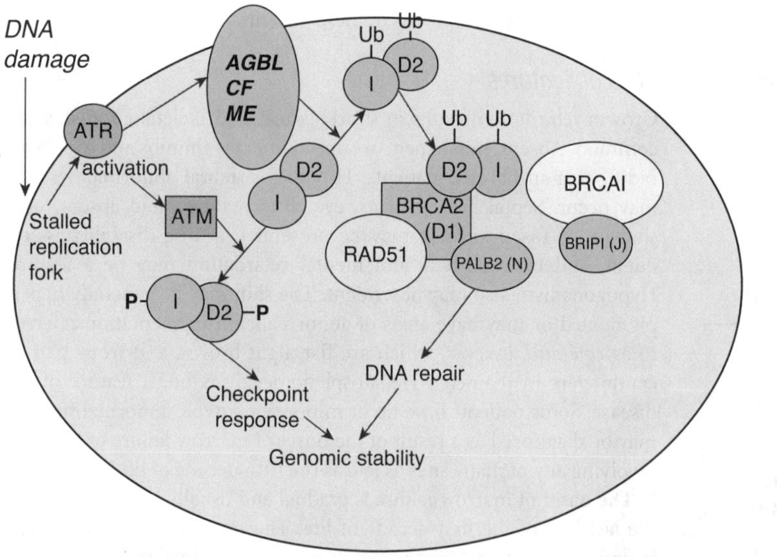

FIGURE 34–4. Representation of the "FA/BRCA pathway." Following DNA damage when a replication fork encounters a DNA cross-link, ATR (ataxia telangiectasia and rad3-related protein) is activated. This leads to the activation of the FA pathway as well as cell-cycle checkpoint activation via the ATM (Ataxia Telangiectasia Mutated) protein. Activation of the FA pathway leads to the formation of the "FA core complex" (consisting of the FA proteins A, B, C, E, F, G, L, and M). This activated FA core complex leads to the monoubiquitination of FANCD2 (FANCD2-Ub) and FANCI (I-Ub). The I-Ub/FANCD2-Ub complex is then targeted to the chromatin containing the cross link where it interacts with BRCA2 and possibly other DNA repair proteins (e.g., RAD51, J, N) leading to the repair of the DNA damage. Proteins mutated in the different FA subtypes are shown in yellow. *(Reproduced from reference 221 with permission of Elsevier.)*

Laboratory Features

Blood counts and marrow cellularity are often normal until 5 to 10 years of age, when pancytopenia develops over an extended interval. Macrocytosis with anisocytosis and poikilocytosis may be present before any cytopenia occurs. Thrombocytopenia may precede the development of granulocytopenia and anemia. The marrow becomes hypocellular, and *in vitro* colony assays reveal a decrease in CFU-GM and BFU-E.[227]

Random chromatid breaks are present in myeloid cells, lymphocytes, and chorionic villus biopsy samples. This chromosome damage is intensified after exposure to DNA cross-linking agents such as mitomycin C or diepoxybutane. The hypersensitivity of the chromosomes of marrow cells or lymphocytes to the latter agent is used as a diagnostic test for this condition. Cell-cycle progression is prolonged at the G2 to M transition, and the cells are more susceptible to oxygen toxicity when cultured *in vitro.* It is important to test the lymphocytes from pediatric patients with aplastic anemia for sensitivity to diepoxybutane, because therapy for Fanconi anemia differs from that used for acquired aplastic anemia.

In the near future, clinical laboratories will be able to genotype suspected patients. Determining the specific gene mutation responsible in a patient (see Table 34–7) is important because it confirms the diagnosis, identifies the genotype linked to BRCA2 that may predispose to a cancer (e.g. breast, ovary), and permits carrier detection.[229]

Differential Diagnosis

The differential diagnosis of Fanconi anemia includes other causes of aplastic anemia, particularly those familial syndromes

TABLE 34–8. Other Rare Syndromes Associated with Aplastic Anemia

Disorder	Findings	Inheritance	Mutated Gene	References
Ataxia-pancytopenia (myelocerebellar disorder)	Cerebellar atrophy and ataxia; aplastic pancytopenia; ± monosomy 7; increased risk of AML	AD	Unknown	256–258
Congenital amegakaryocytic thrombocytopenia	Thrombocytopenia; absent or markedly decreased marrow megakaryocytes; hemorrhagic propensity; elevated thrombopoietin; propensity to progress to aplastic pancytopenia; propensity to evolve to clonal myeloid disease	AR (compound heterozygotes)	*MPL*	259, 260
DNA ligase IV deficiency	Pre- and postnatal growth delay; dysmorphic facies; aplastic pancytopenia	AR (compound heterozygotes)	*LIG4*	261–263
Dubowitz syndrome	Intrauterine and post-partum growth failure; short stature; microcephaly; mental retardation; distinct dysmorphic facies; aplastic pancytopenia; increased risk of AML and ALL	AR	Unknown	264, 265
Nijmegen breakage syndrome	Microcephaly; dystrophic facies; short stature; immunodeficiency; radiation sensitivity; aplastic pancytopenia; predisposition to lymphoid malignancy	AR	*NBS1*	266, 267
Reticular dysgenesis (type of severe immunodeficiency syndrome)	Lymphopenia; anemia and neutropenia; corrected by hematopoietic stem cell transplantation	XLR	Unknown	268, 269
Seckel syndrome	Intrauterine and post- partum growth failure; microcephaly; characteristic dysmorphic facies (bird-headed profile); aplastic pancytopenia; ? increased risk of AML	AR	*ATR* (and *RAD3*-related gene); *PCNT*	270–273
WT syndrome	Radial/ulnar abnormalities; aplastic pancytopenia; increased risk of AML	AD	Unknown	274

AD, autosomal dominant; ALL, acute lymphocytic leukemia; AML, acute myelogenous leukemia; AR, autosomal recessive; XLR, X-linked recessive.

NOTE: The listed clinical findings in each syndrome are not comprehensive. The designated clinical findings may not be present in all cases of the syndrome. Isolated cases of familial aplastic anemia with or without associated anomalies that are not consistent with Fanconi anemia or other defined syndromes have been reported.[227]

associated with skeletal anomalies and other dysmorphic features. Other familial types of aplastic anemia have been reported with or without associated anomalies. In those instances in which no sensitivity to DNA damaging agents is observed, the syndrome does not represent Fanconi anemia. Several uncommon syndromes of this type are described below and are tabulated in Table 34–8.

Therapy and Course

Most patients with Fanconi anemia do not respond to ATG or cyclosporine but do improve with androgen preparations, often for as long as several years. Cytokines may provide some improvement in blood counts, but their effect may wane. Studies in a mouse model also suggest that cytokine effects may not be sustained.[230] The cumulative median survival is about 20 years from progressive marrow failure, conversion to myelodysplastic syndrome, acute myelogenous leukemia (approximately 10 percent of patients), or the development of a variety of other cancers such as genitourinary system, digestive system (especially liver), head and neck.[231] Multiple cancers in an individual patient also occur. Cancers may occur as late as the fifth decade of life and precede the diagnosis of Fanconi anemia in 25 percent of patients.[231] The presence of a clonal cytogenetic abnormality or marrow morphology consistent with myelodysplasia markedly reduces the 5-year survival.[232] Allogeneic hematopoietic stem cell transplantation is curative for the marrow manifestations of Fanconi anemia.[232–235] A marked reduction in dosage of the marrow-conditioning regimen of cyclophosphamide and radiation is necessary owing to the undue sensitivity of the tissues to DNA-damaging exposures. The risk of cancer is so high that, where practical, surveillance should be used, for example, frequent pelvic exams in females, hepatic ultrasonography to detect adenomas, and careful oropharyngeal examinations. Therapy of cancer in patients with Fanconi anemia needs to consider the marked sensitivity of their cells to DNA cross-linking agents and radiotherapy.

Normal cDNA has been transferred into cells from patients with restoration of resistance to DNA damaging agents.[236,237] Difficulties in this approach include the paucity of stem cells in these patients, as well as the potential toxicity of the gene transfer methodology.

■ DYSKERATOSIS CONGENITA

Definition

This inherited disorder is characterized by cutaneous and mucous membrane abnormalities, progressive marrow insufficiency, and a predisposition to malignant transformation. It is much more common in males than in females, and occurs in about 1 per 1 million population.[221,238]

Pathogenesis

Dyskeratosis usually is inherited as a recessive X-chromosome–linked disorder although rare cases can have autosomal dominant or autosomal recessive inheritance (Table 34–9). The disease is a reflection of telomere complex dysfunction,[239,240] and it results from defective telomerase activity resulting from mutations in the telomerase-related genes (Fig. 34–5).[240] The telomerase complex maintains the length of telomeres, which are nucleotide tandem repeat structures residing at the termini of eukaryotic chromosomes (e.g., 5′-TTAGGG-3′). Telomerase restores the G-rich telomere repeats that are lost as a result of end-processing during

TABLE 34–9. Gene Mutations in Dyskeratosis Congenita

Gene	Chromosome Location	% of Patients	Inheritance	Protein Function
DKC1	Xq28	30	XLR	Essential part of snoRNPs and telomerase
TERC	3q26	<5	AD	RNA 3′ end processing and stability
TERT	5p15.33	<6	AD, AR	Reverse transcriptase component of telomerase
NOP10 (NOLA3)	15q14-q15	<1	AR	RNA binding
TINF2	14q11.2	11	AD	? Binds to TRF1 to regulate telomere length
To be identified		~50%		

AD, autosomal dominant; AR, autosomal recessive; XLR, X-linked recessive.

NOTE: Table prepared from data in references 221, 223, and 273. Percent of patients is approximate because of continuing identification of mutations.

normal cell division. Combined with protein, located at the ends of chromosomes, they maintain chromosome integrity by preventing end-to-end chromosome fusion, preventing chromosome degradation, and preventing chromosome instability.

In dyskeratosis congenita, the telomeres are markedly shortened resulting in genomic instability and cell (including marrow cell) apoptosis. Rapidly proliferating cells are at highest risk for dysfunction. Mutations of the *DKC1* gene are responsible for the X-linked recessive form. *DKC1* encodes dyskerin, which is a conserved multifunctional protein component of the telomerase complex. Mutations of the *TERT, TERC,* and *TINF2* genes are the principal abnormalities in the autosomal dominant form. TERC is the RNA component of the telomerase reverse transcriptase that TERT, the reverse transcriptase, uses to synthesize the 6-bp repeats on the 3′ end of telomeric DNA. *TINF2* is a component of the shelterin complex. The latter permits the distinction of telomeres from sites of DNA damage, preventing their otherwise inappropriate processing. Recessive mutations in *NOP10*, which encodes small ribonucleoproteins associated with the telomerase complex, have been described in a consanguineous family.[241] Homozygous recessive mutations in the telomerase reverse transcriptase (*TERT*) produce a severe variant, referred to as the Høyeraal-Hreidarsson syndrome.[275]

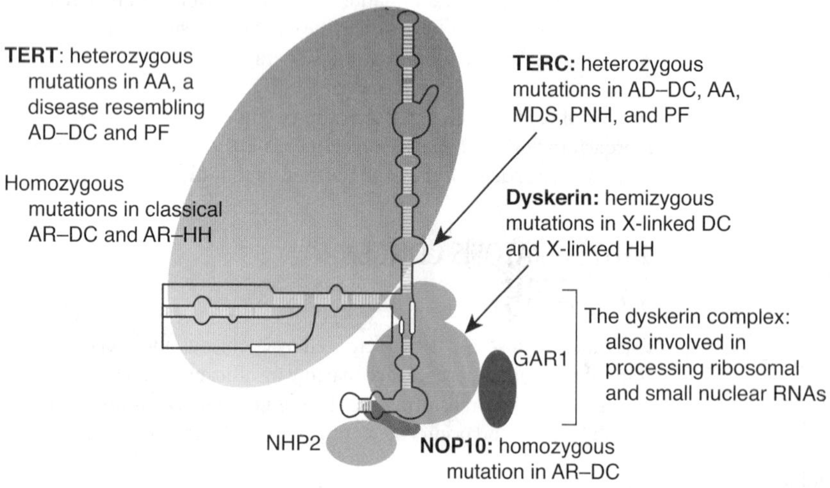

FIGURE 34–5. Representation of the interaction between dyskerin and the other molecules (GAR1, NHP2, NOP10, TERC, and TERT) of the telomerase complex (and their association with different disease categories). Telomerase is an RNA-protein complex because TERC is an RNA molecule that is never translated. The other molecules (dyskerin, GAR1, NHP2, NOP10 and TERT) are proteins. The minimal active telomerase enzyme is composed of two molecules each of TERT, TERC, and dyskerin. Dyskerin, GAR1, NHP2, and NOP10 are important for the stability of the telomerase complex. AA, aplastic anemia; AD–DC, autosomal dominant dyskeratosis congenita; AR–DC, autosomal recessive dyskeratosis congenita; AR–HH, autosomal recessive Høyeraal-Hreidarsson syndrome; MDS, myelodysplasia; PNH, paroxysmal nocturnal hemoglobinuria; PF, pulmonary fibrosis; X-linked DC, X-linked dyskeratosis congenita; X-linked HH, X-linked Høyeraal-Hreidarsson syndrome. *(Reprinted from reference 221 with permission of Elsevier.)*

Clinical Findings

The cutaneous findings usually appear after 5 years of age and include reticulated, tan to gray, hyperpigmented and hypopigmented cutaneous macules; alopecia of scalp, eyelashes, and eyebrows; adermatoglyphia (loss of dermal ridges on fingers and toes); hyperkeratosis of palms and soles; mucosal leukoplakia in 75 percent of patients; and dystrophic nails in more than 85 percent of patients.[221,238,239] Other mucosal sites, such as conjunctiva, lacrimal duct, esophagus, urethra, vagina, and anus, can be involved, sometimes with stenosis and, for example, dysphagia or dysuria. Pulmonary vascular involvement occurs in a significant minority of affected children. Aplastic anemia usually develops in late childhood or early adulthood and is evident in the classical blood and marrow findings described under acquired aplastic anemia, above. Female carriers of X-linked dyskeratosis congenital may have slight abnormalities such as a dystrophic nail, a single area of hypopigmentation, or slight leukoplakia.[238]

Diagnosis

The diagnosis results from the combination of phenotypic findings and blood cell deficiencies. Genetic analysis for telomerase complex gene mutations should be used to confirm the clinical conclusion. Shortened telomere length in leukocytes also can be assessed by flow cytometric fluorescence in situ hybridization studies.[242]

Management

Stem cell hematopoietic transplantation has had inconsistent results because of frequent and severe posttransplantation complications.[243] Nonmyeloablative transplantation might improve results.[244,245] Transplantation might improve the cytopenias but not the abnormalities of other organs or the frequency of secondary nonhematopoietic cancer.

Course and Prognosis

The incidence of squamous cell carcinoma of mucosal sites is increased and they often originate in sites of leukoplakia in the skin, gastrointestinal, or genitourinary tracts. These usually develop between the ages of 20 and 30 years. Mortality from neutropenic infection or thrombocytopenic hemorrhage occurs in about two-thirds of patients with aplastic anemia. Median survival is about 30 years.

SHWACHMAN-DIAMOND SYNDROME

Definition

An uncommon inherited disorder that is estimated to occur once in every 100,000 births, manifesting exocrine pancreatic insufficiency with secondary steatorrhea, blood cell deficiencies, and skeletal abnormalities. It was first described in 1964.[247,249]

Pathogenesis

Shwachman-Diamond syndrome results from mutations in the *SBDS* gene on chromosome 7q11, which induces accelerated cellular apoptosis via the FAS pathway.[249] The resulting hyperproliferation may account for the abnormal telomere shortening that has been documented in the leukocytes in this condition.[250] The pathogenetic mechanism that (1) prevents development of pancreatic acinar cells, (2) results in abnormal bone morphogenesis, and (3) causes marrow impairment of blood cell production is not understood. *SBDS* knockdown in experimental animals affects expression of genes involved in brain, bone, and marrow development, and may be the result of the gene's role in RNA processing.[251,252] The mutations also result in abnormalities in neutrophil motility and chemotaxis, but pus formation *in vivo* seems adequate.

Clinical Findings

Pancreatic insufficiency, steatorrhea, and neutropenia are present in most patients at the time of diagnosis.[247,248] Pallor may reflect anemia and easy bruising; epistaxis or bleeding from other sites reflect thrombocytopenia. Neutropenia occurs in approximately 95 percent, anemia in approximately 50 percent, and thrombocytopenia in approximately 35 percent of patients.[249] Thus, a substantial plurality of patients has bicytopenia or tricytopenia with an hypoplastic marrow. Fetal hemoglobin levels are elevated in approximately 75 percent of the patients, perhaps secondary to erythroid hypoplasia. Cytogenetic abnormalities involving chromosomes 7 and 20 have been described in marrow cells. Nutritional inadequacies related to intestinal malabsorption result in a failure to thrive. Short stature is characteristic. Skeletal abnormalities are present in most patients, notably osteopenia, but also syndactyly, supernumerary metatarsals, coax vera deformity, and dental enamel defects and caries. Delayed puberty is common. The neutropenia and chemotactic abnormality may result in recurrent infections, including sinusitis, otitis, pneumonia, osteomyelitis, and others. Pancreatic cell lipase production improves with age, and as many as half the patients may have improvement in lipid absorption in the small bowel with time.

Management

Supportive care, particularly with supplemental pancreatic enzymes, to provide proper nutrition, and appropriate and prompt treatment of bacterial infections with antibiotics is important. Many agents, including G-CSF, glucocorticoids, pancreatic extract, vitamins, have been tried to improve the neutropenia with erratic results. Some agents have potential risks, such as G-CSF fostering clonal evolution and glucocorticoids fostering immunodeficiency. Severe hematopoietic dysfunction and cytopenias can be corrected with allogeneic hematopoietic stem cell transplantation.[253]

Course and Prognosis

Death from overwhelming sepsis is common. These patients, especially males, have a significant risk of progression to a myelodysplastic syndrome or acute myelogenous leukemia.[248,254,255] Survival is a function of the severity of the cytopenias. If the cytopenias are mild, survival is not uncommon into the fourth or fifth decade of life. If symptomatic pancytopenia, especially neutropenia, is present, median survival is about 20 to 30 years.[248,255]

OTHER INHERITED APLASTIC ANEMIAS

Several other rare syndromes are associated with aplastic pancytopenia, and these are described in Table 34–8. Congenital amegakaryocytic thrombocytopenia results from mutations in the thrombopoietin receptor gene, *MPL*.[259,260] Reticular dysgenesis results from a pluripotential stem cell defect as both lymphoid and myeloid progenitors are affected.[268,269] The Seckel syndrome results from mutations in the *ATR* gene, and marrow cells exhibit heightened sister chromatid exchange.[270–273] The ataxia-telangiectasia mutated and rad3-related (ATR) kinase orchestrates cellular responses to DNA damage and replication stress. The genetic basis of marrow failure in these four syndromes that involve aplastic pancytopenia is not yet known, but may be related to defects in the ATR-dependent DNA damage-repair pathway.[259] Most of these syndromes can be treated by marrow transplantation, but this step, if successful, does not correct somatic abnormalities, only the hematopoietic defect. The restoration of robust hematopoiesis by transplantation may decrease their propensity to undergo clonal evolution to a clonal myeloid or, in some cases, lymphoid disorder.

REFERENCES

1. The International Agranulocytosis and Aplastic Anemia Study. Incidence of aplastic anemia: The relevant diagnostic criteria. *Blood* 70:1718, 1987.
2. Ehrlich P: Über einen Fall von Anamie mit Bemerkungen über regenerative Veranderungen des Knochenmarks. *Charite Ann* 13:300, 1888.
3. Chauffard M: Un cas d'anémie pernicieuse aplastique. *Bull Soc Med Hop Paris* 21:313, 1904.
4. Scott JL, Cartwright GE, Wintrobe MM: Acquired aplastic anemia: an analysis of thirty-nine cases and review of the pertinent literature. *Medicine (Baltimore)* 38:119, 1959.
5. Thomas ED, Storb R, Fefer A, et al: Aplastic anemia treated by bone marrow transplantation. *Lancet* 1: 284, 1972.
6. Thomas ED, Storb R, Giblett B et al: Recovery from aplastic anemia following attempted marrow transplantation. *Exp Hematol* 4:97, 1976.
7. Champlin RE, Feig SA, Sparkes RS, Gale RP: Bone marrow transplantation from identical twins in the treatment of aplastic anaemia: Implication for the pathogenesis of the disease. *Br J Haematol* 56:455, 1984.
8. Speck B, Gluckman E: Treatment of aplastic anemia by antilymphocyte globulin with and without allogeneic bone marrow infusions. *Lancet* II:1145–1148, 1977.
9. Mary JY, Baumelou E, Guiguet M: Epidemiology of aplastic anemia in France: A prospective multicenter study. *Blood* 75:1646, 1990.
10. Montané E, Ibáñez L, Vidal X, et al: Epidemiology of aplastic anemia: A prospective multicenter study. *Haematologica* 93:518, 2008.
11. Maluf EM, Pasquini R, Eluf JN, et al: Aplastic anemia in Brazil: Incidence and risk factors. *Am J Hematol* 71:268, 2002.
12. McCahon E, Tang K, Rogers PC, McBride ML, Schultz KR: The impact of Asian descent on the incidence of acquired severe aplastic anaemia in children. *Br J Haematol* 121:170, 2003.
13. Chongli Y and Ziaobo Z: Incidence survey of aplastic anemia in China. *Chin Med Sci J* 6:203, 1991.
14. Issaragrisil S: Epidemiology of aplastic anemia in Thailand. Thai Aplastic Anemia Study Group. *Int J Hematol* 70:137, 1999.
15. Yong AS, Goh AS, Rahman M, et al: Epidemiology of aplastic anemia in the state of Sabah, Malaysia. *Med J Malaysia* 53:59, 1998.
16. Issaragrisil S, Kaufman DW, Anderson T, et al: The epidemiology of aplastic anemia in Thailand. *Blood* 107:1299, 2006.

17. Young NS, Kaufman DW: The epidemiology of acquired aplastic anemia. *Haematologica* 93:489, 2008.
18. Yin SN, Hayes RB, Linet MS, et al: A cohort study of cancer among benzene-exposed workers in China: overall results. *Am J Ind Med* 29:227, 1996.
19. Kagan WA, Ascensao J, Pahwa R, et al: Aplastic anemia: presence in human bone marrow of cells that suppress myelopoiesis. *Proc Natl Acad Sci U S A* 73:2890, 1976.
20. Maciejewski JP, Anderson S, Katevas P, Young NS: Phenotypic and functional analysis of bone marrow progenitor cell compartment in bone marrow failure. *Br J Haematol* 87:227, 1994.
21. Scopes J, Bagnara M, Gordon-Smith EC, et al: Haemopoietic progenitor cells are reduced in aplastic anaemia. *Br J Haematol* 86:427, 1994.
22. Maciejewski JP, Selleri C, Sato T, et al: A severe and consistent deficit in marrow and circulating primitive hematopoietic cells (long-term culture-initiating cells) in acquired aplastic anemia. *Blood* 88:1983, 1996.
23. Young NS, Scheinberg P, Calado RT: Aplastic anemia. *Curr Opin Hematol* 15:162, 2008.
24. Young NS, Calado RT, Scheinberg P: Current concepts in the pathophysiology and treatment of aplastic anemia. *Blood* 108:2509, 2006.
25. Young NS, Maciejewski J: Mechanisms of disease: The pathophysiology of acquired aplastic anemia. *N Engl J Med* 336:1365, 1997.
26. Laver J, Castro-Malaspina H, Kernan NA, et al: In vitro interferon-gamma production by cultured T-cells in severe aplastic anaemia: Correlation with granulomonopoietic inhibition in patients who respond to anti-thymocyte globulin. *Br J Haematol* 69:545, 1988.
27. Gascon P, Zoumbos NC, Scala G, et al: Lymphokine abnormalities in aplastic anemia: implications for the mechanism of action of antithymocyte globulin. *Blood* 65:407, 1985.
28. Hinterberger W, Adolf G, Bettelheim P, et al: Lymphokine overproduction in severe aplastic anemia is not related to blood transfusions. *Blood* 74:2713, 1989.
29. Shinohara K, Ayame H, Tanaka M, et al: Increased production of tumor necrosis factor alpha by peripheral blood mononuclear cells in the patients with aplastic anemia. *Am J Hematol* 37:75, 1991.
30. Nistico, A, Young, NS: Gamma-interferon gene expression in the bone marrow of patients with aplastic anemia. *Ann Intern Med* 120:463, 1994.
31. Zoumbos N, Gascon P, Djeu J, Young NS: Interferon is a mediator of hematopoietic suppression in aplastic anemia in vitro and possibly in vivo. *Proc Natl Acad Sci U S A* 82:188, 1985.
32. Sloand E, Kim S, Maciejewski JP, et al: Intracellular interferon-gamma in circulating and marrow T cells detected by flow cytometry and the response to immunosuppressive therapy in patients with aplastic anemia. *Blood* 100:1185, 2002.
33. Solomou EE, Keyvanfar K, Young NS: T-bet, a Th1 transcription factor, is up-regulated in T cells from patients with aplastic anemia. *Blood* 107:3983, 2006.
34. Risitano AM, Maciejewski JP, Green S, et al: In vivo dominant immune responses in aplastic anaemia: Molecular tracking of putatively pathogenetic T-cell clones by TCR beta-CDR3 sequencing. *Lancet* 364:355, 2004.
35. Chen J, Ellison FM, Eckhaus MA, et al: Minor antigen h60-mediated aplastic anemia is ameliorated by immunosuppression and the infusion of regulatory T cells. *J Immunol* 178:4159, 2007.
36. Hirano N, Butler MO, Von Bergwelt-Baildon MS, et al: Autoantibodies frequently detected in patients with aplastic anemia. *Blood* 102:4567, 2003.
37. Smick K, Condit PK, Proctor RL, Sutcher V: Fatal aplastic anemia: An epidemiological study of its relationship to the drug chloramphenicol. *J Chronic Dis* 17:899, 1964.
38. Modan B, Segal S, Shani M, Sheba C: Aplastic anemia in Israel: Evaluation of the etiological role of chloramphenicol on a community-wide basis. *Am J Med Sci* 270:441, 1975.
39. Yunis AA Chloramphenicol toxicity: 25 years of research. *Am J Med* 87:44N, 1989.
40. Custer RP: Aplastic anemia in soldiers treated with Atabrine (quinacrine). *Am J Med Sci* 212:211, 1946.
41. Best WR: Drug-associated blood dyscrasias. *JAMA* 185:286, 1963.
42. The International Agranulocytosis and Aplastic Anemia Study: Risks of agranulocytosis and aplastic anemia: A first report of their relation to drug use with special reference to analgesics. *JAMA* 256:1749, 1986.
43. Retsagi G, Kelly JP, Kaufman DW: Risk of agranulocytosis and aplastic anaemia in relation to use of antithyroid drugs: International Agranulocytosis and Aplastic Anaemia Study. *BMJ* 297:262, 1988.
44. International Agranulocytosis and Aplastic Anemia Study: Anti-infective drug use in relation to the risk of agranulocytosis and aplastic anemia. *Arch Intern Med* 149:1036, 1989.
45. Kelly JP, Kaufman DW, Shapiro S: Risks of agranulocytosis and aplastic anemia in relation to the use of cardiovascular drugs: The International Agranulocytosis and Aplastic Anemia Study. *Clin Pharmacol Ther* 49:330, 1991.
46. Kaufmann DW, Kelly JP, Jurgelon JM, et al: Drugs in the aetiology of agranulocytosis and aplastic anaemia. *Eur J Haematol* 57(Suppl):23, 1996.
47. Baumelou E, Guiguet M, Mary JY, et al: Epidemiology of aplastic anemia in France: A case control study. I. Medical history and medication use. *Blood* 81:1471, 1993.
48. Bithell TC, Wintrobe MM: Drug-induced aplastic anemia. *Semin Hematol* 4:194, 1967.
49. Williams DM, Lynch RE, Cartwright GE: Drug-induced aplastic anemia. *Semin Hematol* 10:195, 1973.
50. Heimpel H, Heit W: Drug-induced aplastic anaemia. *Clin Haematol* 9:641, 1980.
51. Williams DM: Pancytopenia, aplastic anemia and pure red cell aplasia, in *Wintrobe's Clinical Hematology*, 10th ed, edited by GR Lee, J Foerster, J Lukens, et al, pp 1452–1459. Williams & Wilkins, Baltimore, 1999.
52. Tonkonow B, Hoffman R: Aplastic anemia and cimetidine. *Arch Intern Med* 140:1123, 1980.
53. Volkin RL, Shadduck RK, Winkelstein A, et al: Potentiation of carmustine-cranial-irradiation-induced myelosuppression by cimetidine. *Arch Intern Med* 142:243, 1982.
54. Khan HA: Benzene toxicity: A consolidated short review of human and animal studies. *Hum Exp Toxicol* 26:677, 2007.
55. Smith MT: Overview of benzene-induced aplastic anemia. *Eur J Haematol* 60:107, 1996.
56. Snyder R: Benzene and leukemia. *Crit Rev Toxicol* 32:155, 2002.
57. Fleming LE, Timmeny MA: Aplastic anemia and pesticides. An etiologic association? *J Occup Med* 35:1106, 1993.
58. Rugman FP, Cosstick R: Aplastic anaemia associated with organochlorine pesticide: Case reports and review of evidence. *J Clin Pathol* 43:98, 1990.
59. Muir KR, Chilvers CE, Harriss C, et al: The role of occupational and environmental exposures in the aetiology of acquired severe aplastic anaemia: A case control investigation. *Br J Haematol* 123:906, 2003.
60. Valdez Salas B, Garcia Duran EI, Wiener MS: Impact of pesticides use on human health in Mexico: A review. *Rev Environ Health* 15:399, 2000.
61. Ahamed M, Anand M, Kumar A, Siddiqui MK: Childhood aplastic anaemia in Lucknow, India: Incidence, organochlorines in the blood and review of case reports following exposure to pesticides. *Clin Biochem* 39:762, 2006.
62. Rauch AE, Kowalsky SF, Lesar TS, et al: Lindane (Kwell)-induced aplastic anemia. *Arch Intern Med* 150:2393, 1990.
63. Roberts HJ: Pentachlorophenol-associated aplastic anemia, red cell aplasia, leukemia and other blood disorders. *J Fla Med Assoc* 77:86, 1990.
64. Prager D, Peters C: Development of aplastic anemia and the exposure to Stoddard solvent. *Blood* 35:286, 1970.
65. Powers D: Aplastic anemia secondary to glue sniffing. *N Engl J Med* 273:700, 1965.
66. Kirtadze I, Zurabashvili D: Study of chemical composition of glue "RAZI" used by solvent abusers in Tbilisi. *Georgian Med News* 133:65, 2006.
67. Sabbioni G, Sepai O, Norppa H, et al: Comparison of biomarkers in workers exposed to 2,4,6-trinitrotoluene. *Biomarkers* 12:21, 2007.
68. Crawford MAD: Aplastic anaemia due to trinitrotoluene intoxication. *Br Med J* 2:430, 1954.
69. Ajlouni K, Doeblin TD: The syndrome of hepatitis and aplastic anaemia. *Br J Haematol* 27:345, 1974.
70. Hagler L, Pastore RA, Bergin JJ: Aplastic anemia following viral hepatitis: Report of 2 fatal cases and literature review. *Medicine (Baltimore)* 54:139, 1975.
71. Pol S, Driss F, Devergie A, et al: Is hepatitis C virus involved in hepatitis-associated aplastic anemia? *Ann Intern Med* 113:435, 1990.
72. Hibbs JR, Frickhofen N, Rosenfeld SJ, et al: Aplastic anemia and viral hepatitis: Non-A, non-B, non-C? *JAMA* 267:2051, 1992.
73. Honkaniemi E, Gustafsson B, Fischler B, et al: Acquired aplastic anaemia in seven children with severe hepatitis with or without liver failure. *Acta Paediatr* 96:1660, 2007.
74. Tzakis AG, Arditi M, Whitington PF, et al: Aplastic anemia complicating orthotopic liver transplantation for non-A, non-B hepatitis. *N Engl J Med* 319:393, 1988.
75. Brown KE, Tisdale J, Barrett AJ, Dunbar CE, Young NS: Hepatitis-associated aplastic anemia. *N Engl J Med* 336:1059, 1997.
76. Safadi R, Or R, Ilan Y et al: Lack of known hepatitis virus in hepatitis-associated aplastic anemia and outcome after bone marrow transplantation. *Bone Marrow Transplant* 27:183, 2001.
77. Mishra B, Malhotra P, Ratho RK, et al: Human parvovirus B19 in patients with aplastic anemia. *Am J Hematol* 79:166, 2005.
78. Yetgin S, Cetin M, Ozyürek E, et al: Parvovirus B19 infection associated with severe aplastic anemia in an immunocompetent patient. *Pediatr Hematol Oncol* 21:223, 2004.
79. Wong S, Young NS, Brown KE: Prevalence of parvovirus B19 in liver tissue: No association with fulminant hepatitis or hepatitis-associated aplastic anemia. *J Infect Dis* 187:1581, 2003.
80. Lazarus KH, Baehner RL: Aplastic anemia complicating infectious mononucleosis: A case report and review of the literature. *Pediatrics* 67:907, 1981.
81. Baranski B, Armstrong G, Truman JT, et al: Epstein-Barr virus in the bone marrow of patients with aplastic anemia. *Ann Intern Med* 109:695, 1988.
82. Vinters HV, Mah V, Mohrmann R, Wiley CA: Evidence for human immunodeficiency virus (HIV) infection of the brain in a patient with aplastic anemia. *Acta Neuropathol* 76:311, 1988.
83. Samuel D, Castaing D, Adam R, et al: Fatal acute HIV infection with aplastic anaemia, transmitted by liver graft. *Lancet* 1:1221, 1988.
84. Morales CE, Sriram I, Baumann MA: Myelodysplastic syndrome occurring as possible first manifestation of human immunodeficiency virus infection with subsequent progression to aplastic anaemia. *Int J STD AIDS* 1:55, 1990.
85. Rosenfeld CS, Rybka WB, Weinbaum D, et al: Late graft failure due to dual bone marrow infection with variants A and B of human Herpesvirus-6. *Exp Hematol* 23:626, 1995.
86. Pavithran K, Raji NL, Thomas M: Aplastic anemia complicating lupus erythematosis—Report of a case and review of the literature. *Rheumatol Int* 22:253, 2002.

87. Bailey FA, Lilly M, Bertoli LF, Ball GV: An antibody that inhibits in vitro bone marrow proliferation in a patient with systemic lupus erythematosus and aplastic anemia. *Arthritis Rheum* 31:901, 1989.
88. Roffe C, Cahill MR, Samanta A, et al: Aplastic anaemia in systemic lupus erythematosus: A cellular immune mechanism? *Br J Rheumatol* 30:301, 1991.
89. Sumimoto S, Kawai M, Kasajima Y, Hamamoto T: Aplastic anemia associated with systemic lupus erythematosus. *Am J Hematol* 38:329, 1991.
90. Winkler A, Jackson RW, Kay DS, et al: High-dose intravenous cyclophosphamide treatment of systemic lupus erythematosus-associated aplastic anemia [letter]. *Arthritis Rheum* 31:693, 1988.
91. Kim SW, Rice L, Champlin R, Udden MM. Aplastic Anemia in eosinophilic fasciitis: Responses to immunosuppression and marrow transplantation. *Haematologica* 28:131, 1997.
92. Debusscher L, Bitar N, DeMaubeuge J, et al: Eosinophilic fasciitis and severe aplastic anemia: Favorable response to either antithymocyte globulin or cyclosporin A in blood and skin disorders. *Transplant Proc* 20:310, 1988.
93. Kumar M and Goldman J: Severe aplastic anemia and Grave's disease in a paediatric patient. *Br J Haematol* 118:327, 2002.
94. Tomonari A, Tojo A, Iseki T, et al: Severe aplastic anemia with autoimmune thyroiditis showing no hematological response to intensive immunosuppressive therapy. *Acta Haematol* 109:90, 2003.
95. Aydin Y, Berker D, Ustün I, et al: A very rare cause of aplastic anemia: Graves disease. *South Med J* 101:666, 2008.
96. Lima CS, Zantut Wittmann DE, Castro V, et al: Pancytopenia in untreated patients with Graves' disease. *Thyroid* 16:403, 2006.
97. Das PK, Wherrett D, Dror Y: Remission of aplastic anemia induced by treatment for Graves disease in a pediatric patient. *Pediatr Blood Cancer* 49:210, 2007.
98. Dincol G, Saka B, Aktan M, et al: Very severe aplastic anemia following resection of lymphocytic thymoma: effectiveness of antilymphocyte globulin, cyclosporine A and granulocyte-colony stimulating factor. *Am J Hematol* 64:78, 2000.
99. Ritchie DS, Underhill C, Grigg AP. Aplastic anemia as a late complication of thymoma in remission. *Eur J Haematol* 68:389, 2002.
100. Gaglia A, Bobota A, Pectasides E, et al: Successful treatment with cyclosporine of thymoma-related aplastic anemia. *Anticancer Res* 27:3025, 2007.
101. Trisal V, Nademanee A, Lau SK, Grannis FW Jr: Thymoma-associated severe aplastic anemia treated with surgical resection followed by allogeneic stem-cell transplantation. *J Clin Oncol* 25:3374, 2007.
102. Arcasoy MO, Gockerman JP: Aplastic anaemia as an autoimmune complication of thymoma. *Br J Haematol* 137:272, 2007.
103. Park CY, Kim HJ, Kim YJ, et al: Very severe aplastic anemia appearing after thymectomy. *Korean J Intern Med* 18:61, 2003.
104. Abrams EM, Gibson IW, Blydt-Hansen TD: The concurrent presentation of minimal change nephrotic syndrome and aplastic anemia. *Pediatr Nephrol* 24:407, 2009.
105. Aitchison RGM, Marsh JCW, Hows JM, et al: Pregnancy associated aplastic anaemia: A report of 5 cases and review of current management. *Br J Haematol* 73:541, 1989.
106. Pajor A, Kelemen E, Szak'acs Z, Lehoczky D: Pregnancy in idiopathic aplastic anemia (report of 10 patients). *Eur J Obstet Gynecol Reprod Biol* 45:19, 1992.
107. Bourantas K, Makrydimas G, Georgiou I, et al: Aplastic anemia: Report of a case with recurrent episodes in consecutive pregnancies. *J Reprod Med* 42:672, 1997.
108. Kwon JY, Lee Y, Shin JC, et al: Supportive management of pregnancy-associated aplastic anemia. *Int J Gynaecol Obstet* 95:115, 2006.
109. Thakral B, Saluja K, Sharma RR, et al: Successful management of pregnancy-associated severe aplastic anemia. *Eur J Obstet Gynecol Reprod Biol* 131:244, 2007.
110. Tichelli A, Socie G, Marsh J et al: Outcome of pregnancy and disease course among women with aplastic anemia treated with immunosuppression. *Ann Intern Med* 137:164, 2002.
111. Court-Brown WM, Doll R: Leukaemia and aplastic anaemia in patients irradiated for ankylosing spondylitis. 1957. *J Radiol Prot* 27:B15-B154, 2007.
112. Darby SC, Doll R, Gill SK, Smith PG: Long term mortality after a single treatment course with x-rays in patients treated with ankylosing spondylitis. *Br J Cancer* 55:179, 1987.
113. Johnson SAN, Bateman CJT, Beard MEJ, et al: Long-term haematological complications of Thorotrast. *Q J Med* 182:259, 1977.
114. Martland HS: The occurrence of malignancy in radioactive persons: A general review of data gathered in the study of the radium dial painters, with special reference to the occurrence of osteogeneic sarcoma and the inter-relationship of certain blood diseases. *Am J Cancer* 15:2435, 1931.
115. Cronkite EP, Haley TJ: Clinical aspects of acute radiation injury, in *Manual on Radiation Haematology*, pp 169–173. International Atomic Energy Agency, Vienna, 1971.
116. Mettler FA Jr, Moseley RD Jr: *Medical Effects of Ionizing Irradiation*, pp 1–185. Grune and Stratton, New York, 1985.
117. Gale RP: USSR: Follow-up after Chernobyl. *Lancet* 1:401, 1990.
118. Nimer SD, Leung DHY, Wolin MJ, Golde DW: Serum stem cell factor levels in patients with aplastic anemia. *Int J Hematol* 60:185, 1994.
119. Kojima S, Matsuyama T, Kodera Y: Plasma levels and production of soluble stem cell factor by marrow stromal cells in patients with aplastic anaemia. *Br J Haematol* 99:440, 1997.
120. Lyman SD, Seaberg M, Hanna R, et al: Plasma/serum levels of flt3 ligand are low in normal individuals and highly elevated in patients with Fanconi anemia and acquired aplastic anemia. *Blood* 86:4091, 1995.
121. Kojima S, Matsuyama T, Kodera Y, et al: Measurement of endogenous plasma granulocyte colony-stimulating factor in patients with acquired aplastic anemia by a sensitive chemiluminescent immunoassay. *Blood* 87:1303, 1996.
122. Kojima S, Matsuyama T, Kodera Y: Circulating erythropoietin in patients with acquired aplastic anaemia. *Acta Haematol* 94:117, 1995.
123. Emmons RVD, Reid DM, Cohen RL, et al: Human thrombopoietin levels are high when thrombocytopenia is due to megakaryocyte deficiency and low when due to increased platelet destruction. *Blood* 87:4068, 1996.
124. Nakao S, Matsushima K, Young N: Deficient interleukin I production by aplastic anaemia monocytes. *Br J Haematol* 71:431, 1989.
125. Holmberg LA, Seidel K, Leisenring W, Torok-Storb B: Aplastic anemia: Analysis of stromal cell function in long-term marrow cultures. *Blood* 84:3685, 1994.
126. Stute N, Fehse B, Schroder J et al: Human mesenchymal stem cells are not of donor origin in patients with severe aplastic anemia who underwent sex-mismatched allogeneic bone marrow transplant. *J Hematother Stem Cell Res* 11:977, 2002.
127. Applebaum FR, Barrall J, Storb R, et al: Clonal cytogenetic abnormalities in patients with otherwise typical aplastic anemia. *Exp Hematol* 15:1134, 1987.
128. Negendank W, Weissman D, Bey TM, et al: Evidence for clonal disease by magnetic resonance imaging in patients with hypoplastic marrow disorders. *Blood* 78:2872, 1991.
129. Schrezenmeier H, Hertenstein B, Wagner B, et al: A pathogenetic link between aplastic anemia and paroxysmal nocturnal hemoglobinuria is suggested by a high frequency of aplastic anemia patients with a deficiency of phosphatidylinositol glycan anchored proteins. *Exp Hematol* 23:81, 1995.
130. Horsley SW, Colman S, McKinley M, et al: Genetic lesions in a preleukemic aplasia phase in a child with acute lymphoblastic leukemia. *Genes Chromosomes Cancer* 47:333, 2008.
131. Suzan F, Terré C, Garcia I, et al: Three cases of typical aplastic anaemia associated with a Philadelphia chromosome. *Br J Haematol* 112:385, 2001.
132. Socie G, Rosenfeld S, Frickhofen N, et al: Late clonal diseases of aplastic anemia. *Semin Hematol* 37:91–101 2000.
133. Gordon-Smith EC, Marsh JC, Gibson FM: Views on the pathophysiology of aplastic anemia. *Int J Hematol* 76(Suppl 2):163, 2002.
134. Maciejewski JP, Risitano A, Sloand EM, et al: Distinct clinical outcomes for cytogenetic abnormalities evolving from aplastic anemia. *Blood* 99:3129, 2002.
135. Socie G, Henryamar M, Bacigalupo A, et al: Malignant tumors occurring after treatment of aplastic anemia. *N Engl J Med* 329:1152, 1993.
136. Najean Y, Haguenauer O: Long-term (5–20 years) evolution of non-grafted aplastic anemias. *Blood* 76:2222, 1990.
137. Ball SE, Gibson FM, Rizzo S: Progressive telomere shortening in aplastic anemia. *Blood* 91:3582, 1998.
138. Rosse WF: New insights into paroxysmal nocturnal hemoglobinuria. *Curr Opin Hematol* 8:61, 2001.
139. Nakakuma H, Kawaguchi T: Pathogenesis of selective expansion of PNH clones. *Int J Hematol* 77:121, 2003.
140. Storb R, Blume KG, O'Donnell MR, et al: Cyclophosphamide and antithymocyte globulin to condition patients with aplastic anemia for allogeneic marrow transplantation: the experience in four centers. *Biol Blood Marrow Transplant* 7:39, 2001.
141. Metzgeroth G, Dinter D, Schultheis B, et al: Deferasirox in MDS patients with transfusion-caused iron overload-a phase-II study. *Ann Hematol* 88:301, 2009.
142. Sagmeister M, Oec L, Gmur J: A restrictive platelet transfusion policy allowing long-term support of outpatients with severe aplastic anemia. *Blood* 93:3124, 1999.
143. Lawrence JB, Yomtovian RA, Hammons T, et al: Lowering the prophylactic platelet transfusion threshold: a prospective analysis. *Leuk Lymphoma* 41:67, 2001.
144. Zeigler ZR: Effects of epsilon aminocaproic acid on primary haemostasis. *Haemostasis* 21:313, 1991.
145. Hod E, Schwartz J: Platelet transfusion refractoriness. *Br J Haematol* 142:348, 2008.
146. Slichter SJ, Davis K, Enright H, et al: Factors affecting posttransfusion platelet increments, platelet refractoriness, and platelet transfusion intervals in thrombocytopenic patients. *Blood* 105:4106, 2005.
147. Drewniak A, Boelens JJ, Vrielink H, et al: Granulocyte concentrates: prolonged functional capacity during storage in the presence of phenotypic changes. *Haematologica* 93:1058, 2008.
148. Armand P, Antin JH: Allogeneic stem cell transplantation for aplastic anemia. *Biol Blood Marrow Transplant* 13:505, 2007.
149. Georges GE, Storb R. Stem cell transplantation for aplastic anemia. *Int J Hematol* 75:141, 2002.
150. Champlin RE, Perez WS, Passweg JR, et al: Bone marrow transplantation for severe aplastic anemia: A randomized controlled study of conditioning regimens. *Blood* 109:4582, 2007.
151. Locasciulli A, Oneto R, Bacigalupo A, et al: Outcome of patients with acquired aplastic anemia given first line bone marrow transplantation or immunosuppressive treatment in the last decade: A report from the European Group for Blood and Marrow Transplantation (EBMT). *Haematologica* 92:11, 2007.
152. Viollier R, Socié G, Tichelli A, et al: Recent improvement in outcome of unrelated donor transplantation for aplastic anemia. *Bone Marrow Transplant* 41:45, 2008.
153. Lee SJ, Klein J, Haagenson M, Baxter-Lowe LA, et al: High-resolution donor-recipient HLA matching contributes to the success of unrelated donor marrow transplantation. *Blood* 110:4576, 2007.
154. Dubey S and Nityanand S: Involvement of Fas and TNF pathways in the induction of apoptosis of T cells by antithymocyte globulin. *Ann Hematol* 82:496, 2003.

155. Michallet M-C, Saltel F, Preville X, et al: Cathepsin-B-dependent apoptosis triggered by antithymocyte globulins: A novel mechanism of T-cell depletion. *Blood* 102:3719, 2003.
156. Mangan KF, D'Alessandro L, Mullaney MT: Action of antithymocyte globulin on normal human erythroid progenitor cell proliferation in vitro: Erythropoietic growth-enhancing factors are released from marrow accessory cells. *J Lab Clin Med* 107:353, 1986.
157. Kawano Y, Nissen C, Gratwohl A, Speck B: Immunostimulatory effects of different antilymphocyte globulin preparations: A possible clue to their clinical effect. *Br J Haematol* 68:115, 1988.
158. Bielory L, Wright R, Nienhuis AW, et al: Antithymocyte globulin hypersensitivity in bone marrow failure patients. *JAMA* 260:3164, 1988.
159. Camitta B, O'Reilly RJ, Sensenbrenner L: Antithoracic duct lymphocyte globulin therapy of severe aplastic anemia. *Blood* 62:883, 1983.
160. Champlin R, Ho W, Gale RP: Antithymocyte globulin treatment in patients with aplastic anemia: a prospective randomized trial. *N Engl J Med* 308:113, 1983.
161. Young N, Griffin P, Brittain E, et al: A multicenter trial of antithymocyte globulin in aplastic anemia and related diseases. *Blood* 72:1861, 1988.
162. Schrezenmeier H, Marin P, Raghavachar A, et al: Relapse of aplastic anaemia after immunosuppressive treatment: A report from the European Bone Marrow Transplantation Group SAA Working Party. *Br J Haematol* 85:371, 1993.
163. Doney K, Leisenring W, Storb R, Appelbaum FR: Primary treatment of acquired aplastic anemia: Outcomes with bone marrow transplantation and immunosuppressive therapy. *Ann Intern Med* 126:107, 1997.
164. Tichelli A, Gratwohl A, Nissen C, Speck B: Late clonal complications in severe aplastic anemia. *Leuk Lymphoma* 12:167, 1994.
165. De Planque MM, Bacigalupo A, Würsch A, et al: Long-term follow-up of severe aplastic anaemia patients treated with antithymocyte globulin. *Br J Haematol* 73:121, 1989.
166. Socié G, Henry-Amar M, Bacigalupo A, et al: Malignant tumors occurring after treatment of aplastic anemia. *N Engl J Med* 319:1152, 1993.
167. Stryckmans PA, Dumont JP, Velu T, Debusscher L: Cyclosporine in refractory severe aplastic anemia [letter]. *N Engl J Med* 310:655, 1984.
168. Lazzarino M, Morra E, Canevari A, et al: Cyclosporine in the treatment of aplastic anaemia and pure red-cell aplasia. *Bone Marrow Transplant* 4(Suppl 4):165, 1989.
169. Hinterberger-Fischer M, Höcker P, Lechner K, et al: Oral cyclosporin-A is effective treatment for untreated and also for previously immunosuppressed patients with severe bone marrow failure. *Eur J Haematol* 43:136, 1989.
170. Tötterman TH, Höglund M, Bengtsson M, et al: Treatment of pure red-cell aplasia and aplastic anaemia with cyclosporin: Long-term clinical effects. *Eur J Haematol* 42:126, 1989.
171. Leeksma OC, Thomas LLM, van der Lelie J, et al: Effectiveness of low dose cyclosporine in acquired aplastic anaemia with severe neutropenia. *Neth J Med* 41:143, 1992.
172. Leonard EM, Raefsky E, Griffith P, et al: Cyclosporine therapy of aplastic anaemia, congenital and acquired red-cell aplasia. *Br J Haematol* 72:278, 1989.
173. Tong J, Bacigalupo A, Piaggio G, et al: Severe aplastic anemia (SAA): Response to cyclosporin A (CyA) in vivo and in vitro. *Eur J Haematol* 46:212, 1991.
174. Nakao S, Yamaguchi M, Shiobara S, et al: Interferon-g gene expression in unstimulated bone marrow mononuclear cells predicts a good response to cyclosporine therapy in aplastic anemia. *Blood* 79:2531, 1992.
175. Kojima S, Fukada M, Miyajima Y, Matsuyama T: Cyclosporine and recombinant granulocyte colony-stimulating factor in severe aplastic anemia [letter]. *N Engl J Med* 313:920, 1990.
176. Bertrand Y, Amri F, Capdeville R, et al: The successful treatment of two cases of severe aplastic anaemia with granulocyte colony-stimulating factor and cyclosporine A [case report]. *Br J Haematol* 79:648, 1991.
177. Schrezenmeier H, Schlander M, Raghavachar A: Cyclosporin A in aplastic anemia—Report of a workshop. *Ann Hematol* 65:33, 1992.
178. Gluckman E, Esperou-Bourdeau H, Baruchel A, et al: Multicenter randomized study comparing cyclosporine-A alone and antithymocyte globulin with prednisone for treatment of severe aplastic anemia. *Blood* 79:2540, 1992.
179. Rosenfeld S, Follmann D, Nunez O, et al: Antithymocyte globulin and cyclosporine for severe aplastic anemia: Association between hematologic response and long-term outcome. *JAMA* 289:1130, 2003.
180. Scheinberg P, Wu CO, Nunez O, et al: Long-term outcome of pediatric patients with severe aplastic anemia treated with antithymocyte globulin and cyclosporine. *J Pediatr* 153:814, 2008.
181. Osugi Y, Yagasaki H, Sako M, et al: Antithymocyte globulin and cyclosporine for treatment of 44 children with hepatitis associated aplastic anemia. *Haematologica* 92:1687, 2007.
182. Teramura M, Kimura A, Iwase S, et al: Treatment of severe aplastic anemia with antithymocyte globulin and cyclosporin A with or without G-CSF in adults: A multicenter randomized study in Japan. *Blood* 110:1756, 2007.
183. Zheng Y, Liu Y, Chu Y: Immunosuppressive therapy for acquired severe aplastic anemia (SAA): A prospective comparison of four different regimens. *Exp Hematol* 34:826, 2006.
184. Bacigalupo A, Brand R, Oneto R, et al: Treatment of acquired severe aplastic anemia: Bone marrow transplantation compared with immunosuppressive therapy—The European Group for Blood and Marrow Transplantation experience. *Semin Hematol* 37:69, 2000.
185. Gillio AP, Boulad F, Small TN, et al: Comparison of long-term outcome of children with severe aplastic anemia treated with immunosuppression versus bone marrow transplantation. *Biol Blood Marrow Transplant* 3:18, 1997.
186. De Planque MM, Kluin-Nelemans HC, Van Krieken HJM, et al: Evolution of acquired severe aplastic anaemia to myelodysplasia and subsequent leukaemia in adults. *Br J Haematol* 70:55, 1988.
187. Tichelli A, Gratwohl A, Würsch A, et al: Late haematological complications in severe aplastic anaemia. *Br J Haematol* 69:413, 1988.
188. Moore MAS, Castro-Malaspina H: Immunosuppression in aplastic anemia—Postponing the inevitable? *N Engl J Med* 314:1358, 1991.
189. Tichelli A, Passweg J, Nissen C, et al: Repeated treatment with horse antilymphocyte globulin for severe aplastic anaemia. *Br J Haematol* 100:393, 1998.
190. Scheinberg P, Nunez O, Young NS: Retreatment with rabbit anti-thymocyte globulin and ciclosporin for patients with relapsed or refractory severe aplastic anaemia. *Br J Haematol* 133:622, 2006.
191. Bacigalupo A, Van Lint MT, Cerri R, et al: Treatment of severe aplastic anemia with bolus 6-methylprednisolone and antilymphocyte globulin. *Blut* 41:168, 1980.
192. Issaragrisil S, Tangnai-Trisorana Y, Siriseriwan T, et al: Methylprednisolone therapy in aplastic anaemia: Correlation of in vitro tests and lymphocyte subsets with clinical response. *Eur J Haematol* 40:343, 1988.
193. Brodsky RA, Sensenbrenner LL, Jones RJ: Complete remission in severe aplastic anemia after high-dose cyclophosphamide without bone marrow transplantation. *Blood* 87:491, 1996.
194. Jones RJ, Barber JP, Vala MS et al: Assessment of aldehyde dehydrogenase in viable cells. *Blood* 85:2742, 1995.
195. Kastan MB, Schlaffer I, Russo JE, et al: Direct demonstration of aldehyde dehydrogenase in human hematopoietic progenitor cells *Blood* 75:1947, 1990.
196. Brodsky RA, Sensenbrenner LL, Smith BD, et al: Durable treatment-free remission following high-dose cyclophosphamide for previously untreated severe aplastic anemia. *Ann Intern Med* 135:477, 2001.
197. Brodsky RA: High-dose cyclophosphamide for aplastic anemia and autoimmunity. *Curr Opin Oncol* 14:143, 2002.
198. Hansen PB, Lauritzen AM: Aplastic anemia successfully treated with rituximab. *Am J Hematol* 80:292, 2005.
199. French Cooperative Group for the Study of Aplastic and Refractory Anemias: Androgen therapy in aplastic anemia: A comparative study of high and low doses of 4 different androgens. *Scand J Haematol* 36:346, 1986.
200. Champlin RE, Ho WG, Feig SA, et al: Do androgens enhance the response to antithymocyte globulin in patients with aplastic anemia? A prospective randomized trial. *Blood* 66:184, 1985.
201. Sonoda Y, Ohno Y, Fujii H, et al: Multilineage response in aplastic anemia patients following long-term administration of filgrastim (recombinant human granulocyte colony stimulating factor). *Stem Cells* 11:543, 1993.
202. Bessho M, Jinnai I, Hirashima K, et al: Trilineage recovery by combination therapy with recombinant human granulocyte colony-stimulating factor and erythropoietin in patients with aplastic anemia and refractory anemia. *Stem Cells* 12:604, 1994.
203. Socie G, Mary JY, Schrezenmeier H, et al: Granulocyte-stimulating factor and severe aplastic anemia: A survey by the European Group for Blood and Marrow Transplantation (EBMT). *Blood* 109:2794, 2007.
204. Ganser A, Lindemann A, Siepelt G, et al: Effects of recombinant human interleukin-3 in aplastic anemia. *Blood* 76:1287, 1990.
205. Walsh CE, Liu JM, Anderson SM, et al: A trial of recombinant human interleukin-1 in patients with severe refractory aplastic anaemia. *Br J Haematol* 80:106, 1992.
206. Speck B, Tichelli A, Widmer E, et al: Splenectomy as an adjuvant measure in the treatment of severe aplastic anaemia. *Br J Haematol* 92:818, 1996.
207. Sadowitz PD, Dubowy RL: Intravenous immunoglobulin in the treatment of aplastic anemia. *Am J Pediatr Hematol Oncol* 12:198, 1990.
208. Bodenstein H: Successful treatment of aplastic anemia with high-dose immunoglobulin [letter]. *N Engl J Med* 314:1368, 1991.
209. Ito T, Haraiwa M, Ishikawa Y, et al: Lymphocytapheresis in a patient with severe aplastic anaemia. *Acta Haematol* 80:167, 1988.
210. Morales-Polanco MR, Sanchez-Valle E, Guerrero-Rivera S, et al: Treatment results of 23 cases of severe aplastic anemia with lymphocytapheresis. *Arch Med Res* 28:85, 1997.
211. Kiem HP, McDonald GB, Myerson D, et al: Marrow transplantation for hepatitis-associated aplastic anemia: A follow-up of long-term survivors. *Biol Blood Marrow Transplant* 2:93, 1996.
212. Lewis SM: Course and prognosis in aplastic anemia. *Br Med J* 1:1027, 1965.
213. Lynch RE, Williams DM, Reading JC, Cartwright GE: The prognosis in aplastic anemia. *Blood* 45:517, 1975.
214. Horowitz MM: Current status of allogeneic bone marrow transplantation in acquired aplastic anemia. *Semin Hematol* 37:30, 2000.
215. Ades L, Mary J-Y, Robin M, et al: Long-term outcome after bone marrow transplantation for severe aplastic anemia. *Blood* 103:2490, 2004.
216. Schrezenmeier H, Passweg JR, Marsh JC, et al: Worse outcome and more chronic GVHD with peripheral blood progenitor cells than bone marrow in HLA-matched sibling donor transplants for young patients with severe acquired aplastic anemia. *Blood* 110:1397, 2007.
217. Locasciulli A: Acquired aplastic anemia in children: incidence, prognosis and treatment options. *Paediatr Drugs* 4:761, 2002.

218. Tisdale JF, Dunn DE, Maciejewski J: Cyclophosphamide and other new agents for the treatment of severe aplastic anemia. *Semin Hematol* 37:102–109 2000.
219. Fanconi G: Familiäre infantile perniziosaartige anämie (perniziöses blutbild und konstitution). *Jahrbuch Kinderheil* 117:257, 1927.
220. Rosendorff J, Bernstein R, Macdougall L, Jenkins T: Fanconi anemia: another disease of unusually high prevalence in the Afrikaans population of South Africa. *Am J Med Genet* 27:793, 1987.
221. Dokal I, Vulliamy T: Inherited aplastic anaemias/bone marrow failure syndromes. *Blood Rev* 22:141, 2008.
222. Jacquemont C, Taniguchi T: The Fanconi anemia pathway and ubiquitin. *BMC Biochem* 22(8 Suppl 1):S10, 2007.
223. Alter BP, Giri N, Savage SA, et al: Update on inherited bone marrow failure syndromes (IBMFS). *IBMFS Newsletter of the Clinical Genetics Branch*, National Cancer Institute. P.1, Summer 2008.
224. Dufour C, Corcione A, Svahn J, et al: TNF-α and TNF-γ are overexpressed in the bone marrow of Fanconi anemia patients and TNF-α suppresses erythropoiesis in vitro. *Blood* 102:2053, 2003.
225. D'Apolito M, Zelante L, Savoia A: Molecular basis of Fanconi anemia. *Haematologica* 83:533, 1998.
226. Garcia-Higuera I, Kuang Y, D'Andrea AD: The molecular and cellular biology of Fanconi anemia. *Curr Opin Hematol* 6:83, 1999.
227. Young NA, Alter BP: *Aplastic Anemia: Acquired and Inherited*. W.B. Saunders, Philadelphia, 1994.
228. Estren S, Damshek W: Familial hypoplastic anemia of childhood: Report of 8 cases in 2 families with beneficial effects of splenectomy in 1 case. *Am J Dis Child* 73:671, 1947.
229. Swhimamura A, D'Andrea AD: Subtyping of Fanconi anemia patients: Implications for clinical management. *Blood* 102:3459, 2003.
230. Carreau M, Liu L, Gan OI, et al: Short-term granulocyte colony-stimulating factor and erythropoietin treatment enhances hematopoiesis and survival in the mitomycin C-conditioned Fancc(-/-) mouse model, while long-term treatment is ineffective. *Blood* 100:1499, 2002.
231. Alter BP: Cancer in Fanconi anemia. *Cancer* 97:425, 2003.
232. Alter BP, Caruso JP, Drachtman RA, et al: Fanconi anemia: Myelodysplasia as a predictor of outcome. *Cancer Genet Cytogenet* 117:125, 2000.
233. Gluckman E, Wagner JE: Hematopoietic stem cell transplantation in childhood inherited bone marrow failure syndrome. *Bone Marrow Transplant* 41:127, 2008.
234. Huck K, Hanenberg H, Nürnberger W, et al: Favourable long-term outcome after matched sibling transplantation for Fanconi-anemia (FA) and in vivo T-cell depletion. *Klin Padiatr* 220:147, 2008.
235. Ayas M, Al-Jefri A, Al-Seraihi A, et al: Second stem cell transplantation in patients with Fanconi anemia using antithymocyte globulin alone for conditioning. *Biol Blood Marrow Transplant* 14:445, 2008.
236. Kelly PF, Radtke S, von Kalle C, et al: Stem cell collection and gene transfer in Fanconi anemia. *Mol Ther* 15:211, 2007.
237. Dufour C, Svahn J: Fanconi anaemia: New strategies. *Bone Marrow Transplant* 41(Suppl 2):S90, 2008.
238. Dokal I: Dyskeratosis congenita in all its forms. *Br J Haematol* 110:768, 2000.
239. Vulliamy TJ, Dokal I: Dyskeratosis congenita: the diverse clinical presentation of mutations in the telomerase complex. *Biochimie* 90:122, 2008.
240. Savage SA, Alter BP: The role of telomere biology in bone marrow failure and other disorders. *Mech Ageing Dev* 129(1–2):35, 2008.
241. Walne AJ, Vulliamy T, Marrone A, et al: Genetic heterogeneity in autosomal recessive dyskeratosis congenita with one subtype due to mutations in the telomerase-associated protein NOP10. *Hum Mol Genet* 16:1619, 2007.
242. Alter BP, Baerlocher GM, Savage SA, et al: Very short telomere length by flow fluorescence in situ hybridization identifies patients with dyskeratosis congenita. *Blood* 110:1439, 2007.
243. Ghavamzadeh A, Alimoghadam K, Nasseri P, et al: Correction of bone marrow failure in dyskeratosis congenita by bone marrow transplantation. *Bone Marrow Transplant* 23:299, 1999.
244. Cesaro S, Oneto R, Messina C, et al: Haematopoietic stem cell transplantation for Shwachman-Diamond disease: A study from the European Group for Blood and Marrow Transplantation. *Br J Haematol* 131:231, 2005.
245. Güngör T, Corbacioglu S, Storb R, Seger RA: Nonmyeloablative allogeneic hematopoietic stem cell transplantation for treatment of dyskeratosis congenita. *Bone Marrow Transplant* 31:407, 2003.
246. Dror Y, Freedman MH, Leaker M, et al: Low-intensity hematopoietic stem-cell transplantation across human leucocyte antigen barriers in dyskeratosis congenita. *Bone Marrow Transplant* 31:847, 2003.
247. Ginzberg H, Shin J, Ellis L, et al: Shwachman syndrome: Phenotypic manifestations of sibling sets and isolated cases in a large patient cohort are similar. *J Pediatr* 135:81, 1999.
248. Shimamura A: Shwachman-Diamond syndrome. *Semin Hematol* 43:178, 2006.
249. Rujkijyanont P, Watanabe K, Ambekar C, et al: SBDS-Deficient cells undergo accelerated apoptosis through the FAS pathway. *Haematologica* 93:363, 2008.
250. Thornley I, Dror Y, Sung L, et al: Abnormal telomere shortening in leucocytes of children with Shwachman-Diamond syndrome. *Br J Haematol* 117:189, 2002.
251. Ganapathi KA, Shimamura A: Ribosomal dysfunction and inherited marrow failure. *Br J Haematol* 141(3):376, 2008.
252. Ganapathi KA, Austin KM, Lee CS, et al: The human Shwachman-Diamond syndrome protein, SBDS, associates with ribosomal RNA. *Blood* 110:1458, 2007.
253. Bhatla D, Davies SM, Shenoy S, et al: Reduced-intensity conditioning is effective and safe for transplantation of patients with Shwachman-Diamond syndrome. *Bone Marrow Transplant* 42:159, 2008.
254. Dokal I, Rule S, Chen F, et al: Adult onset of acute myeloid leukaemia (M6) in patients with Shwachman-Diamond syndrome. *Br J Haematol* 99:171, 1997.
255. Dror Y, Squire J, Durie P, Freedman MH: Malignant myeloid transformation with isochromosome 7q in Shwachman-Diamond syndrome. *Leukemia* 12:1591, 1998.
256. Li FP, Hecht F, Kaiser-McCaw B et al: Ataxia-pancytopenia: syndrome of cerebellar ataxia, hypoplastic anemia, monosomy 7 and acute myelogenous leukemia. *Cancer Genet Cytogenet* 4:189, 1981.
257. Mahmood F, King MD, Smyth OO, et al: Familial cerebellar hypoplasia and pancytopenia without chromosomal breakages. *Neuropediatrie* 29:302, 1998.
258. González-del AA, Cervera M, Gomez L, et al: Ataxia-pancytopenia syndrome. *Am J Med Genet* 90:252, 2000.
259. Geddis AE: Inherited thrombocytopenia: Congenital amegakaryocytic thrombocytopenia and thrombocytopenia with absent radii. *Semin Hematol* 43:196, 2006.
260. Germeshausen M, Ballmaier M, Welte K: MPL mutations in 23 patients suffering from congenital amegakaryocytic thrombocytopenia: The type of mutation predicts the course of the disease. *Hum Mutat* 27:296, 2006.
261. Pierce AJ, Jasin M: NHEJ deficiency and disease. *Mol Cell* 8:1160, 2001.
262. O'Driscoll M, Gennery AR, Seidel J, et al: An overview of three new disorders associated with genetic instability: LIG4 syndrome, RS-SCID and ATR-Seckel syndrome. *DNA Repair (Amst)* 3:1227, 2004.
263. O'Driscoll M, Jeggo PA: CSA can induce DNA double-strand breaks: Implications for BMT regimens particularly for individuals with defective DNA repair. *Bone Marrow Transplant* 41:983, 2008.
264. Walters TR, Desposito F: Aplastic anemia in Dubowitz syndrome. *J Pediatr* 106:622, 1985.
265. Berthold F, Fuhrmann W, Lampert F: Fatal aplastic anemia in a patient with Dubowitz syndrome. *Eur J Pediatr* 146:605, 1987.
266. Gennery AR, Slatter MA, Bhattacharya A, et al: The clinical and biological overlap between Nijmegen Breakage Syndrome and Fanconi anemia. *Clin Immunol* 113:214, 2004.
267. Gadkowska-Dura M, Dzieranowska-Fangrat K, Dura W, et al: Unique morphological spectrum of lymphomas in Nijmegen breakage syndrome (NBS) patients with high frequency of consecutive lymphoma formation. *J Pathol* 216:337, 2008.
268. Stephan JL, Vlekova V, Le Deist F, et al: Severe combined immunodeficiency: A retrospective single-center study of clinical presentation and outcome in 117 patients. *J Pediatr* 123:564, 1993.
269. Bertrand Y, Muller SM, Casanova JL, et al: Reticular dysgenesis: HLA non-identical bone marrow transplants in a series of 10 patients. *Bone Marrow Transplant* 29:759, 2002.
270. Esperou-Bourdeau H, Leblanc T, Schaison G, et al: Aplastic anemia associated with "bird-headed" dwarfism (Seckel syndrome). *Nouv Rev Fr Hematol* 35:99, 1993.
271. O'Driscoll M, Ruiz-Perez VL, Woods CG, et al: A splicing mutation affecting expression of ataxia-telangiectasia and RAD3-related protein (ATR) results in Seckel syndrome. *Nat Genet* 33:497, 2003.
272. Griffith E, Walker S, Martin CA, et al: Mutations in pericentrin cause Seckel syndrome with defective ATR-dependent DNA damage signaling. *Nat Genet* 40:232, 2008.
273. Hayani A, Suarez CR, Molnar Z, et al: Acute myeloid leukemia in a patient with Seckel syndrome. *J Med Genet* 31:148, 1994.
274. Gonzalez CH, Durkin-Stamm MV, Geimer NF, et al: The WT syndrome—A "new" autosomal dominant pleiotropic trait of radial/ulnar hypoplasia with high risk of bone marrow failure and/or leukemia. *Birth Defects Orig Artic Ser* 13:31, 1977.
275. Walne AJ, Vulliamy TJ, Beswick R, et al: TINF2 mutations result in very short telomeres: Analysis of a large cohort of patients with dyskeratosis congenita and related bone marrow failure syndromes. *Blood* 112:3594, 2008.

CHAPTER 35
PURE RED CELL APLASIA

Neal S. Young

SUMMARY

Pure red cell aplasia is the diagnosis applied to isolated anemia secondary to failure of erythropoiesis. Cardinal findings are a low hemoglobin level, reticulocytopenia, and absent or extremely infrequent erythroid precursor cells in the marrow. Historical names for pure red cell aplasia include *erythroblast hypoplasia, erythroblastopenia, red cell agenesis, hypoplastic anemia,* and *aregenerative anemia. Aplastic anemia* confers the same meaning, of course, but is applied to pancytopenia and an empty marrow (see Chap. 34). Pure red cell aplasia was first separated from aplastic anemia by Kaznelson in 1922. The association of red cell aplasia and thymoma interested physicians in the 1930s and ultimately led to laboratory studies linking pure red cell aplasia to immune mechanisms, including the early identification of antierythroid precursor cell antibodies by Krantz, and later characterization of T cells that inhibited erythropoiesis. Red cell aplasia was recognized in the 1940s as an acute and life-threatening complication of sickle cell disease and other hemolytic anemias, presaging the role of a specific virus in the etiology of both acute and chronic erythropoietic failure. Despite its infrequency, pure red cell aplasia has been a subject of much laboratory research because of its link to an immune mechanism of erythropoietic failure and as a manifestation of parvovirus B19 infection and destruction of marrow red cell progenitors. However, because of its infrequency, pure red cell aplasia has not been the subject of large or controlled clinical trials; as a result, therapeutic recommendations are based on single cases or small series.

INHERITED PURE RED CELL APLASIA (DIAMOND-BLACKFAN ANEMIA)

DEFINITION AND HISTORY

Anemia in infancy and early childhood associated with absent reticulocytes in the blood and erythroid precursor cells in the marrow was described by Joseph[1] in 1936 as a "failure of erythropoiesis" and by Diamond and Blackfan[2] in 1938 as "congenital hypoplastic anemia." Gasser[3] first reported a response of a patient to glucocorticoids in 1951, and Diamond and associates[4] presented a series of treated patients. Genetic linkage studies have identified a causative mutated gene in a subset of patients with inherited red cell aplasia.[5] Hundreds of cases have been reported, and many excellent reviews have been published.[6–15] Although Joseph was the first to describe the disorder, the anemia invariably is referred to as either *Blackfan-Diamond* or *Diamond-Blackfan anemia.*

ETIOLOGY AND PATHOGENESIS

An annual incidence of 5 cases per 1 million livebirths has been estimated from registry data.[16] Well-characterized pedigrees are consistent with an autosomal dominant or, less often, recessive inheritance pattern. Sporadic cases are seen most frequently. Retrospective studies may reveal subtle hematologic or biochemical lesions, or an abnormal gene, in an affected parent or another relative without clinical anemia.[17]

Genetic studies have led to the characterization of Diamond-Blackfan anemia as a disease of ribosomal biogenesis.[18–20] Linkage analyses of several dozen European families mapped to a site on chromosome 19q13[21] and the finding of a translocation in one individual allowed cloning of the *RPS19* gene, which encodes a protein involved in ribosome assembly.[5] Most mutations are whole-gene deletions, translocations, or truncations; this pattern suggests a mechanism of haploinsufficiency, and *RPS19* behaves as a dominant gene.[22] Disruption of both copies of the gene in the mouse prevents implantation.[23] *RPS19* mutations occur in approximately 25 percent of patients with inherited red cell aplasia,[22,24] but mutations subsequently have been identified in other ribosomal biogenesis genes in Diamond-Blackfan anemia (*RPS24, RPS7, RPS17, RPL35A, RPL11, RPL5*) in fewer cases.[22,25] RNA-interference experiments have implicated *RPS14* in one of the myelodysplastic syndromes characterized by loss of 5q.[26]

Precisely how defects in ribosomal protein genes cause constitutional red cell aplasia is uncertain. Historically, Diamond-Blackfan anemia has been characterized by diminished erythroid progenitor cell numbers (colony-forming unit–erythroid [CFU-E] and burst-forming unit–erythroid [BFU-E]).[27,28] In cell-culture analyses, early, relatively erythropoietin-independent erythropoiesis is normal; the major defect is in the late stage of erythropoietin-dependent erythroid cell expansion and maturation.[29] A defect in late erythroid differentiation is compatible with the classic findings of macrocytosis and increased hemoglobin F expression. Granulopoiesis in the granulocyte-macrophage colony-forming unit assay and the earlier hematopoietic progenitors as measured *in vitro* by long-term culture-initiating cell assay (an assay for an early multipotential hematopoietic progenitor) frequently are abnormal but to a lesser degree than CFU-E and BFU-E formation.[30] *RPS19* is expressed ubiquitously, and the apparently specific role of *RSP19* in red cell development has not been elucidated.[20] In tissue-culture experiments, silencing of *RPS19* profoundly affects erythropoietic differentiation and, to lesser degrees, myelopoiesis.[31,32] In a zebrafish model, deficiency of rps19 in early embryogenesis caused a decrease in erythrocytes and also physical anomalies.[33]

Despite responsiveness of patients to glucocorticoids, there is little evidence of an immune mechanism, cellular or humoral, underlying inherited red cell aplasia.

CLINICAL FEATURES

Approximately one-third of patients are diagnosed at birth or within a few weeks of delivery, and almost all are identified within the first year of life.[7] Considerable variations are noted with regard to severity of phenotype, ranging from hydrops fetalis[34,35] to presentation in adulthood, when diagnosis is inferred from associated physical anomalies.[36] No sex predominance exists. Increased rates of prematurity in patients and of miscarriages in families have been inferred from collected cases.[9] Symptoms of anemia in early childhood include pallor, apathy, poor appetite, and "failure to thrive." Physical anomalies occur in approximately one-third of cases; most frequent is craniofacial dysmorphism. The classic appearance described by Cathie[37] is "tow-colored hair, snub nose, wide-set eyes, thick upper lips, and an intelligent expression." Malformations of the thumbs and short stature are followed in frequency of occurence by abnormalities of the urogenital system, web neck, and skeletal and cardiac defects.[7,12,16] These physical anomalies are less prevalent than the abnormalities seen in Fanconi anemia.

Acronyms and abbreviations that appear in this chapter include: BFU-E, burst-forming unit–erythroid; CD20, a cluster differentiation expressed on the surface of all mature B cells; CFU-E, colony-forming unit–erythroid; CLL, chronic lymphocytic leukemia; Ig, immunoglobulin; IL-3, interleukin 3; LGL, large granular lymphocytic leukemia; NK, natural killer cells; *RPS14, RPS19,* genes for the ribosomal subunit proteins; T-cell, thymus-derived lymphocyte.

LABORATORY FEATURES

The degree of anemia is highly variable at diagnosis. Erythrocytes may be macrocytic or normocytic. Reticulocytopenia is profound. The marrow, which usually is devoid of erythroid precursors, may show small numbers of megaloblastoid early erythroid cells with apparent "maturation arrest." Platelets are normal or elevated. Leukocytes may be normal or slightly decreased at presentation. Neutrophils often decline with age, and in adult survivors neutropenia occasionally is severe enough to predispose to fatal infection.[38]

Erythrocyte adenosine deaminase level is elevated in approximately 75 percent of patients but also may be increased in other aregenerative anemias of childhood.[39] Serum erythropoietin level, serum iron level, and total iron-binding capacity are high. Ferritin levels increase after multiple transfusions, and patients develop iron overload if they are not treated with iron chelators.

DIFFERENTIAL DIAGNOSIS

The characteristic triad consists of the clinical diagnostic features of anemia, reticulocytopenia, and a paucity or absence of erythroid precursors in the marrow. These findings may by supplemented by increased activity of red cell adenosine deaminase and ribosomal gene mutation analysis. Fanconi anemia can be excluded by cytogenetic analyses under clastogenic stress and determination of Fanconi anemia gene mutations (see Chap. 34). Transient erythroblastopenia of childhood, which unusually occurs in the first year of life, is characterized by spontaneous recovery. When presentation occurs at older ages, the distinction between inherited and acquired aplastic anemia is somewhat arbitrary[11] because the hematologic features are similar. A positive family history, physical anomalies, and characteristic cytogenetic, enzymatic, or genetic findings strongly indicate an inherited disorder.

THERAPY, COURSE, AND PROGNOSIS

Untreated inherited pure red cell aplasia is fatal; death results from severe anemia and congestive heart failure. Transfusions, glucocorticoids, and allogeneic stem cell transplantation are of proven efficacy. Predictors of a response to glucocorticoids include older age at presentation, a family history, and a normal platelet count. Younger age at presentation and premature birth correlate with continued red cell transfusion dependence.[40] Supportive care consists of red cell transfusions. Injury to visceral organs from iron overload has been a major cause of death in the past. To avoid transfusional hemosiderosis, chelation should be initiated early (see Chap. 42). Red cell transfusions should be leukocyte depleted to avoid alloimmunization (see Chap. 140). Erythrocytes are administered with the goal of eliminating symptoms and permitting normal growth and sexual development, usually achieved by maintaining hemoglobin levels between 7 and 9 g/dL (70–90 g/L).

Glucocorticoids are effective in many patients.[41] Although the mechanism of action of glucocorticoids in this disease is not understood, their toxicities are substantial, and a response is not predictable. Once the diagnosis is established, prednisone is administered at 2 mg/kg daily in three or four divided doses.[8,9,42] A reticulocyte response is seen in the majority of patients 1 to 4 weeks later, followed by a rise in hemoglobin level. Once the hemoglobin level reaches 9 to 10 g/dL (90–100 g/L), very slow reduction of the glucocorticoid dose is undertaken by decreasing the number of daily doses. When a single daily dose is achieved, an alternate-day schedule is adopted. In general, severe anemia can be avoided with continued glucocorticoid administration. The maintenance dose may be low (1–2 mg/day). Some patients may tolerate complete withdrawal of prednisone, but relapse is frequent and most responders become glucocorticoid dependent. A variety of patterns of response have been described, ranging from prompt recovery and apparent cure to refractoriness after years of responsiveness.[9] Conversely, a second trial of glucocorticoids years after an apparent therapeutic failure may be successful. In a series of 76 patients followed for the long term, 59 were treated with prednisone; 31 initially responded, and 2 of the 25 who initially failed later responded.[8] Glucocorticoid responsiveness is strongly associated with better survival, and patients who require low doses of prednisone, or those few who spontaneously remit, may have normal life expectancies. Long-term use of high-dose prednisone results in significant toxicity, including some combination of growth retardation, cushingoid facies, buffalo hump, osteoporosis, aseptic necrosis of the hip and fractures, diabetes, hypertension, and cataracts. Red cell transfusions with iron chelation may be preferable to such an outcome.

Allogeneic stem cell marrow transplantation, when successful, is curative (see Chap. 21), but the procedure has not been widely applied to children responding to medical measures. The median life expectancy of patients requiring transfusions and iron chelation is 30 to 40 years. A less favorable outcome is related to poor compliance and resulting cardiac and hepatic disease from iron overload.[8] Because of the morbidity and mortality associated with allogeneic stem cell transplant, most patients have been transplanted late in their disease course, after large numbers of transfusions, accumulation of heavy iron loads, and alloimmunization. Despite the poor predictive factors, 15 of 19 patients of the first published series of cases survived 5 months to many years post transplantation.[12] Comparable survival rates have been reported from European[43] and Japanese registries.[44] Stem cell transplantation from unrelated stem cell donors or use of cord blood stem cells[43,44] has been less successful. Recurrent red cell aplasia despite full engraftment was reported in one child after transplantation.[42,45]

Other therapies have not gained wide acceptance despite promising pilot studies, including interleukin (IL)-3,[46] high-dose methylprednisolone,[47] cyclosporine and other immunosuppressive agents,[48,49] and prolactin induction by metoclopropamide.[50]

With better survival, the risk of late development of leukemia has become apparent.[20] Four of 76 patients followed at Children's Hospital in Boston died of acute myelogenous leukemia, with a calculated relative risk of greater than 200 times expected.[8]

Gene transfer *in vitro* has functionally corrected cells defective in *RSP19* (gene encoding ribosomal protein[51]). In animal models, corrected cells show improved erythropoiesis and a survival advantage *in vivo*,[52] offering the possibility of gene therapy.

TRANSIENT APLASTIC CRISIS AND TRANSIENT ERYTHROBLASTOPENIA OF CHILDHOOD

DEFINITION AND HISTORY

Temporary failure of erythropoiesis is clinically identical to pure red cell aplasia except for spontaneous resolution of symptoms and of the laboratory findings of normocytic and normochromic anemia and marrow erythroid hypoplasia, usually over the course of a few weeks. Erythrocyte production is halted (1) by acute B19 parvovirus infection, typically in the context of underlying hemolytic disease (called transient aplastic crisis); (2) in normal children, usually after an infection by another (unknown) childhood virus (transient erythroblastopenia of childhood); or (3) as a transient reaction to a drug.

An anemic crisis was described in the 1940s first by Lyngar[53] and then by Owren,[54] Gasser,[3] and Dameshek and Bloom[55] in kindreds with hereditary spherocytosis. Several children within a family suffered anemic crises and exhibited low, rather than the usually high, reticulocyte numbers. Transient aplastic crisis also was noted as a complication of sickle cell disease.[56,57] Marrow examination showed decrease or absence of erythroid precursor cells, and often giant erythroblasts.[54,55] An infectious etiology was suspected from the history of a preceding febrile illness in families and its simultaneous occurrence in siblings. After the serendipitous discovery of B19 parvovirus in a normal blood donor, Pattison and colleagues screened large numbers of stored sera for evidence of recent infection. Immunoglobulin (Ig) M antibody or viral antigen was found in the blood of Jamaican children in London, all of whom had transient aplastic crisis of sickle cell disease.[58] B19 parvovirus later was established as the agent also responsible for fifth disease.[59] In the large cohort of sickle cell patients in Jamaica reported by Serjeant and colleagues,[60,61] virtually all episodes of transient aplastic crisis could be linked to B19 parvovirus. In retrospect, red cell aplasias blamed on kwashiorkor, vitamin deficiency, bacterial infections, and chemical exposures likely represent parvovirus infection.

Gasser (cited in reference 50) described erythroblastopenia in normal children who ultimately recovered[54]; the disease was recognized as an entity by Wranne[62] in the 1970s. Transient erythroblastopenia of childhood has an unclear etiology but may represent a postviral immune-mediated syndrome.

ETIOLOGY AND PATHOGENESIS

B19 parvovirus, a small DNA virus, commonly infects humans. Most of the adult population has IgG antibodies specific to B19.[59] The virus is tropic for erythroid progenitor cells,[63] mainly as a result of their P antigen or globoside, the receptor for entry of B19 into the cell.[64,65] Infection lyses the target cell and abrogates erythropoiesis *in vitro* and *in vivo*. Reticulocytopenia probably accompanies B19 parvovirus infection in all infected persons.[66] Anemia only manifests if red cell survival is decreased. Infection ordinarily is terminated by production of neutralizing antibodies to the virus (when such antibodies are absent, persistence of the virus produces chronic pure red cell aplasia). B19 parvovirus causes epidemics of fifth disease in the normal population and also of transient aplastic crisis in hematology clinics such as those specializing in sickle cell disease.[67,68] In fifth disease, IgM antibody is present in the blood, and virus levels are low or not detectable. Symptoms and signs of a typical "slapped cheek" cutaneous eruption and arthralgia or arthritis are secondary to antibody–virus immune complex deposition.

In contrast, in transient aplastic crisis, high concentrations of virus are present in the circulation, and patients do not develop fifth disease. In children with sickle cell disease, the incidence of B19 parvovirus infection was estimated at approximately 11 percent, and 75 percent of patients were infected by age 20 years.[69] In this setting, parvovirus infection was associated with transient aplastic crisis, a higher frequency of fever, pain, acute chest syndrome, and acute splenic sequestration syndrome.[69] As in normal individuals, parvovirus infection can also be asymptomatic in sickle cell disease.[70]

The origins of transient erythroblastopenia of childhood are poorly understood. An apparent viral prodrome is typical,[71] and temporal and seasonal clustering of cases may occur.[72–74] With rare exception,[75] B19 parvovirus is not the etiology,[76,77] and no other virus has been consistently implicated.[71] Erythroid colony numbers (see Chaps. 29 and 31) usually are low.[78] An immune pathophysiology has been inferred from *in vitro* experiments in which IgG from sera of patients inhibited erythropoiesis.[78,79] Cell-mediated mechanisms also may play a causal role. In one report, T-cell depletion led to a dramatic increase in CFU-E formation.[80] A possible relationship between transient erythroblastopenia of childhood and inherited red cell aplasia has been suggested by the clustering of polymorphic alleles in familial transient erythroblastopenia.[81]

The same drugs implicated in chronic pure red cell aplasia apply to transient erythropoietic failure.[82] Laboratory investigations of red cell aplasia secondary to diphenylhydantoin[83] and rifampicin[84] are consistent with a hapten mechanism, in which serum antibody affects erythroid progenitor cells only in the presence of drug.

CLINICAL FEATURES

Transient aplastic crisis typically occurs in younger patients who are chronically anemic as a result of hereditary spherocytosis, sickle cell disease, or another hemolytic anemia. The decrease in erythropoiesis results in more evident pallor, fatigue, lassitude, and dyspnea on exertion. Gastrointestinal complaints or headache are not uncommon.[85] Parvovirus infection can unmask previously undiagnosed underlying hemolytic anemia. Physical examination may reveal signs of anemia, such as pallor, tachycardia, and a flow murmur. No rash or joint swelling is seen. Elevated serum bilirubin or overt icterus may be a clue to underlying hemolysis. In contrast, transient erythroblastopenia of childhood presents as an acute anemia in a previously well child. The syndrome has an estimated incidence rate of 4 to 5 cases per 1 million of livebirths.[86–88] Transient erythroblastopenia is a frequent diagnosis in children with severe anemia,[87,89] and is the most common cause of acquired red cell aplasia in pediatric patients.[6,86] Most patients are 1 to 3 years old,[6,89] but transient erythroblastopenia of childhood can occur in the first year of life and through adolescence. Rare complications include seizures and transient neurologic abnormalities.[90–92]

LABORATORY EVALUATION

In both syndromes, anemia is the hallmark, and hemoglobin levels may be markedly depressed. Reticulocytes usually are absent from the blood, and erythroid precursor cells are not present or markedly decreased in the marrow. Red cell indices are normal. White blood cell and platelet counts are normal or elevated. An occasional patient will have mild to moderate neutropenia or thrombocytopenia, especially if the patient has intact splenic function, as in hereditary spherocytosis or transient erythroblastopenia of childhood. If the episode is brief and diagnosed during marrow recovery, patients may present with reticulocytosis, and nucleated red blood cells may be seen on the blood film.

DIFFERENTIAL DIAGNOSIS

The reticulocyte count readily distinguishes the cause of increasing anemia in a patient with hemolytic disease as transient aplastic crisis. The most important differential diagnosis for transient erythroblastopenia of childhood is inherited pure red cell aplasia. For the former, the age at presentation is older, the patient usually has no family history except transient erythroblastopenia of childhood that can occur simultaneously in siblings.[93] Physical anomalies are absent, and the syndrome resolves spontaneously. In transient erythroblastopenia of childhood (in contrast to inherited red cell aplasia), erythrocyte adenosine deaminase levels are normal, and red cells do not show "stress" patterns of fetal hemoglobin and i antigen (red cell antigen expressed primarily on feral erythrocytes) expression. The patient's medical history, the red cell indices, and appropriate serum assays should allow prompt exclusion of more common causes of anemia in children, such as iron deficiency or other nutritional deficiencies. When transient erythroblastopenia is associated with neutropenia, acute lymphoblastic leukemia and aplastic anemia may be suspected: marrow examination clarifies the diagnosis.[94] A record of current medications, more important in adults, may provide the basis for a tentative diagnosis of drug-induced rather than idiopathic disease.

THERAPY, COURSE, AND PROGNOSIS

Transient aplastic crisis resolves as neutralizing antibodies to B19 parvovirus are made, usually within 1 to 2 weeks of infection. Ensuing reticulocytosis may be brisk, and the hemoglobin may transiently rise to higher than normal values. White cell and platelet numbers may "rebound," and some bone pain from marrow expansion may be present. Severe anemia requires transfusion of red blood cells (see Chap. 140). No established role for administration of immunoglobins exists unless the patient has an immune deficiency state and the viral infection cannot be eliminated.

Transient erythroblastopenia of childhood typically terminates after a few weeks, but anemia may persist occasionally for months.[6] Transfusions may be required during that interval.

For drug-associated transient failure of erythropoiesis, the suspected offending drug is discontinued and the diagnosis inferred from subsequent clinical improvement.

ACQUIRED PURE RED CELL APLASIA

DEFINITION AND HISTORY

Acquired pure red cell aplasia is an uncommon cause of anemia that occurs principally in older adults. The blood counts and marrow appearance are indistinguishable from the picture of Diamond-Blackfan anemia—that is, anemia, severe reticulocytopenia, and absent marrow erythroid precursor cells. The nosologic origins of acquired pure red cell aplasia are obscure. Early descriptions are intermixed with those of aplastic anemia (in retrospect, a poor term for generalized marrow failure). Kaznelson[95] is credited with the first case report in 1922. Early distinction of the two syndromes was stimulated by the relationship of red cell aplasia to thymoma. Although red cell aplasia shares with aplastic anemia an immune pathophysiology and responsiveness to immunosuppressive therapies, the absence of involvement of neutrophils, monocytes, and platelets makes the diagnostic distinction evident. Many of the diverse clinical associations (Table 35–1) are consistent with an immune-mediated pathophysiology. The mechanism of red cell failure is best understood for T-cell–mediated autoimmune destruction and persistent B19 parvovirus infection.

TABLE 35–1. Classification of Pure Red Cell Aplasia

Fetal red cell aplasia (nonimmune hydrops fetalis)
Parvovirus B19 *in utero*
Inherited (Diamond-Blackfan anemia)
RPS19 mutations (~25% of cases)
Acquired
Transient pure red cell aplasia
Acute B19 parvovirus infection in hemolytic disease (transient aplastic crisis; ~100% of cases)
Transient erythroblastopenia of childhood
Chronic pure red cell aplasia
Idiopathic
Large granular lymphocytic leukemia
Chronic lymphocytic leukemia
Clonal myeloid diseases (especially 5q-syndrome)
Persistent B19 parvovirus infection in immunodeficient host (~15% of cases)
Thymoma
Collagen vascular diseases
Post stem cell transplant
Anti-ABO antibodies
Drug induced
Antierythropoietin antibodies
Pregnancy

ETIOLOGY AND PATHOGENESIS

Immune-Mediated Erythropoietic Failure

Clinical and laboratory evidence supports both antibody and cellular mechanisms of inhibition of erythropoiesis. Red cell aplasia is associated with autoimmune diseases, such as rheumatoid arthritis, systemic lupus erythematosus, myasthenia gravis, autoimmune hemolytic anemia, acquired hypoimmunoglobulinemia, autoimmune polyglandular syndrome, and especially thymoma, and with lymphoproliferative processes, such as chronic lymphocytic leukemia (CLL) and Hodgkin lymphoma, in which immune dysregulation is common. Serum inhibitors can be detected in the laboratory. Krantz and colleagues showed that immunoglobulin fractions from the patient's blood inhibited heme synthesis and red cell progenitor assays *in vitro*.[96] Antibodies that inhibit BFU-E and CFU-E colony formation are present frequently in patients with red cell aplasia. A pathophysiologic role can be inferred, first from the response of patients to favorable response to directed at antibodies, such as plasmapheresis and monoclonal antibody to CD20 (an antigen present on B cells), and second from decreased or absent plasma antibody in recovered patients. Antibodies may be involved in the red cell aplasia of pregnancy.[97]

Autoantibodies to erythropoietin rarely have caused this disease.[98,99] More frequently, red cell aplasia secondary to antibodies is elicited by administration of recombinant erythropoietin to patients undergoing renal dialysis (see Chap. 36).[100–104] Anemia can be profound, and some patients remain transfusion dependent despite discontinuation of hormone therapy. Glycosylation of recombinant erythropoietin is different from the native molecule, but antibodies are directed against conformational epitopes of the protein and not to the sugar moieties; erythropoietin immunogenicity is associated with human leukocyte antigen (HLA) specificities.[105] The second example of antibodies of known specificity causing red cell aplasia occurs after hematopoietic stem cell transplantation using donors mismatched at a major ABO locus, which can lead to delayed donor erythroid engraftment or late erythropoietic failure.[106–109] In most cases of red cell aplasia, however, the target antigen(s) are not known.

Red cell aplasia also might be associated with lymphoproliferative disease. In one survey of patients with red cell aplasia, 6 percent were found to have CLL and 7 percent large granular lymphocytic leukemia (LGL).[111,112] In another series of 47 red cell aplasia patients, four had CLL and nine had LGL.[113] There might be many reasons for this association, some of which likely stem from the pathophysiology and/or treatment of the underlying lymphoproliferative disease, such as leukemia- and/or treatment-associated inhibition of erythropoiesis, disruption of the marrow microenvironment, and/or dysregulation of the adaptive immune system leading to pathologic erythroid-directed autoimmunity (see Chaps. 94 and 96).

In some cases, T cells might contribute to erythropoietic failure.[110] Flow cytometric and molecular methods can sometimes detect clonal T-cell expansion in patients with normal numbers of circulating lymphocytes.[114,115] Lymphocytes from patients with idiopathic pure red cell aplasia,[116–119] or red cell aplasia associated with CLL,[120,121] LGL,[122–124] thymoma,[125] other lymphoid malignancies,[126,127] Epstein-Barr virus infection,[128] and human T-cell leukemia virus 1 infection[129] suppressed erythropoiesis in colony assays. Several mechanisms of cell killing have been suggested.[14,112] Moreover, in some cases, T cells can recognize and kill and/or inhibit erythropoietic progenitor cells in a HLA-class I restricted manner as a result of expression of particular $\alpha\beta$ T-cell receptors that recognize erythroid-specific peptide antigens (see Chap. 78).[130] In another case of chronic red cell aplasia associated with LGL, erythropoiesis was inhibited by non–HLA-restricted $\gamma\delta$ T cells that lysed CFU-E. These T cells downregulated class I HLA antigens, making them susceptible to recognition and lysis by the patients' own natural killer (NK) cells (see Chap. 79).[14]

Persistent B19 Parvovirus Infection

B19 parvovirus specifically infects and is toxic to erythroid progenitor cells. Parvovirus infection normally is terminated by the humoral immune response within 1 to 2 weeks of infection. Linear neutralizing epitopes are localized to a relatively small region of the capsid protein.[131] In the absence of an effective antibody response, infection persists and causes pure red cell aplasia.[59,131] Erythropoietic failure may be the only evidence of parvoviral infection. Persistence of B19 parvovirus infection may occur in the setting of immunodeficiency, most commonly caused by chemotherapeutic and immunosuppressive drugs,[132] human immunodeficiency virus 1 infection,[133] and occasionally with Nezelof syndrome's subtle immunologic abnormalities.[134] Parvovirus at one time may have accounted for approximately 15 percent of severe anemia in patients with acquired immunodeficiency syndrome,[135] but highly effective antiretroviral drug regimens have reduced its role.[136,137] Persistent B19 parvovirus infection can occur in the fetus exposed during the midtrimester of pregnancy. The infection can cause hydrops fetalis as a result of viral cytotoxicity for erythroid progenitors in the fetal liver and death of the newborn as a result of severe anemia and congestive heart failure.[59] In rare instances, parvovirus infected or hydropic infants rescued by red cell transfusion show congenital red cell aplasia or dyserythropoietic anemia.[35]

Intrinsic Cellular Defects Leading to Failed Red Blood Cell Production

Red cell aplasia can be the first or the major manifestation of myelodysplasia.[138] Discrete genetic defects can lead to failure of erythropoiesis. Activating point mutations in *N-RAS* (an oncogene in the RAS group) occur in some cases of myelodysplastic syndrome.[139,140] Mutant *N-RAS in vitro* can induce a proliferative defect in erythroid progenitor cells.[141]

Medications

Idiosyncratic drug reactions account for a far smaller proportion of red cell aplasia than of agranulocytosis (see Chap. 65). Case reports have implicated various agents, such as diphenylhydantoin, sulfa and sulfonamide drugs, azathioprine, allopurinol, isoniazid, procainamide, ticlopidine, ribavirin, and penicillamine. Causality is impossible to assign from case reports. As with nonsteroidal antiinflammatory drugs, gold, and colchicine, the underlying rheumatic syndrome may be the etiologic link.

CLINICAL FEATURES

Symptomatic anemia in the older patient may manifest as pallor, fatigue, lassitude, pulsatile tinnitus, and anginal chest pain. Iatrogenic Cushing syndrome and the physical stigmata of secondary hemochromatosis are seen in patients after prolonged glucocorticoid administration and long-term red cell transfusion therapy. Concomitant diseases include CLL and lymphomas, collagen vascular disorders, myasthenia gravis, especially in the setting of thymoma, and some cancers. Red cell aplasia also may complicate pregnancy. Persistent B19 parvovirus infection should be suspected in the anemic cancer patient after stem cell transplantation, in patients treated with immunosuppressive drugs, in patients with AIDS, and in patients with a family or personal history suggestive of inherited immune disorder. Other viral infections have been implicated in pure red cell aplasia, including infectious mononucleosis and, in some patients, hepatitis (an unknown agent in seronegative hepatitis).

LABORATORY FEATURES

Anemia is either normocytic or macrocytic, reticulocytopenia is profound, and white cell and platelet counts are normal. The marrow has absent or very few erythroid precursor cells but normal granulopoiesis and megakaryopoiesis. Iron saturation and ferritin level frequently are elevated and rise further after repeated red cell transfusions. Erythroid colony assays may predict responsiveness to immunosuppressive treatment. The presence of marrow or blood BFU-E and CFU-E correlates with hematologic improvement,[116,142,143] but these tests are not generally available.

A thymoma should be sought by chest imaging, including computed tomographic scan. The association of thymoma and pure red cell aplasia has been emphasized but is uncommon. One experienced investigator found thymoma in only 2 of 37 patients,[144] and other series reported a low incidence.[110,113] The thymomas usually are encapsulated and have a spindle cell histology. In one series, 10 of 56 cases were considered malignant because of their locally infiltrating character[145]; therefore, the tumors should be surgically excised, if feasible.

Patients with lymphocytosis, lymphadenopathy, and/or unusual lymphocyte morphology on the blood film should undergo evaluation for an associated lymphoproliferative diseases, such as CLL (see Chap. 94) or LGL (see Chap. 96).

Persistent parvovirus infection can be difficult to diagnose. Giant pronormoblasts scattered on the marrow film are characteristic of the condition (Fig. 35–1), but such typical cells may not be observed.

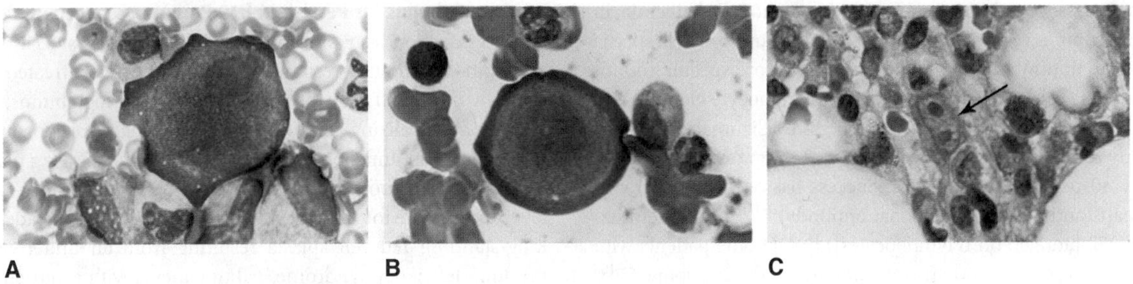

FIGURE 35–1. A and **B.** Giant early erythroblast precursors in the marrow aspirate of a patient with chronic pure red cell aplasia secondary to persistent B19 parvovirus infection. Note the nuclear inclusions (*darker nuclear shading*) representing parvovirus infection. **C.** Marrow biopsy section. The *arrows* point to binucleate erythroid precursor cell with nuclear inclusions representing parvovirus infection. *(Used with permission from* Lichtman's Atlas of Hematology, *www.accessmedicine.com.)*

Marrow morphologies that are dysplastic or suggestive of leukemia also have been described. Serum antibodies specific to the virus are absent or only IgM is positive. Parvovirus DNA should be present in high concentrations in the blood and readily measured by molecular techniques.

DIFFERENTIAL DIAGNOSIS

Distinction between inherited and acquired red cell aplasia may be impossible in the younger patient. Rarely, pure red cell aplasia is difficult to distinguish from more generalized marrow failure if other blood counts are borderline. A dysmorphic marrow smear and abnormal chromosomes point to myelodysplasia as responsible for isolated anemia and reticulocytopenia. B19 parvovirus infection should always be suspected and searched for in any immunosuppressed individual who is anemic because the infection can be treated.

THERAPY, COURSE, AND PROGNOSIS

Treatment

Transfusion Therapy As with inherited red cell aplasia, transfusions and iron chelation are basic to management.[146] In an adult, one unit of packed erythrocytes per week can replace marrow erythropoiesis, which for convenience usually is transfused as two units every 2 weeks. The goal of preventing symptoms of anemia is achievable in most patients if the nadir hemoglobin is greater than 7 g/dL (70 g/L). A goal greater than 9 g/dL (90 g/L) may be preferable in patients with cardiac or pulmonary disease and in older patients. Even refractory pure red cell aplasia is consistent with a prolonged and perhaps even normal life expectancy, and iron chelation therapy can be initiated based on the ferritin level (see Chap. 42).

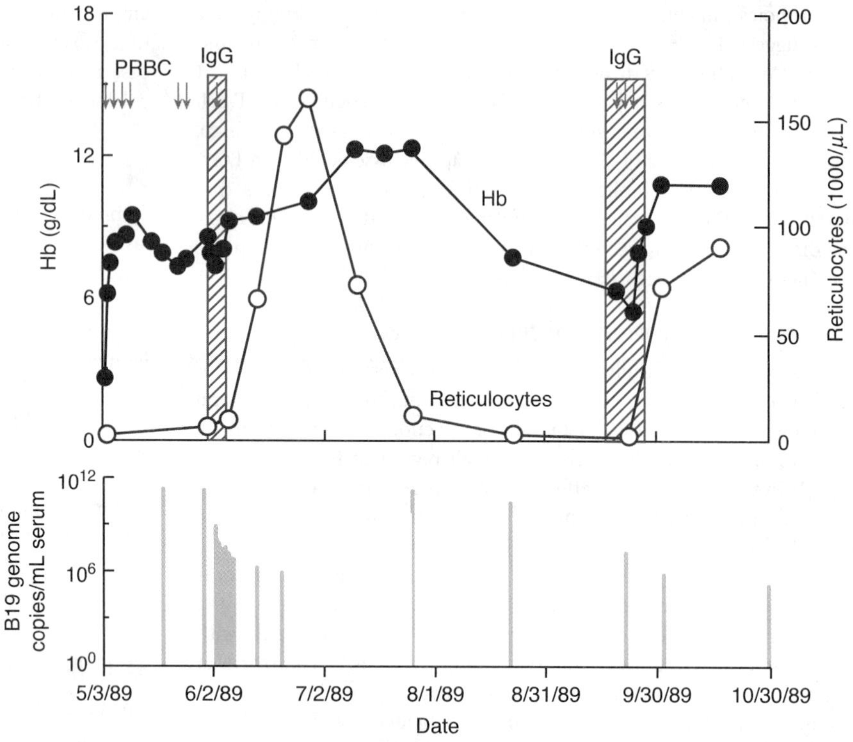

FIGURE 35–2. Diagram of the clinical course of a human immunodeficiency virus-1–infected patient with red cell aplasia caused by B19 persistent parvovirus.[123] Note the increase of the reticulocyte count (*open circles*) to the first infusion of immunoglobulin (*hatched bar*) and the subsequent decline in parvovirus titers. Thereafter, the reticulocyte count and the hemoglobin concentration (*closed circles*) decrease, reflecting the return of the anemia. A second immunoglobulin treatment increases the reticulocyte count and hemoglobin concentration and decreases the parvovirus titers.

Immunosuppression Immunosuppressive agents are used to treat disease with suspected immune origin. Response is likely in the majority of patients, but sequential treatment with a variety of agents often is required. Some patients, however, remain refractory to treatment.[110,146–148] Typically, prednisone 1 to 2 mg/kg per day is given first, and about half of patients improve. A 1- to 2-month trial can be associated with significant toxicity and evidence of Cushing syndrome. Higher response rates have been cited for cyclosporine, and some investigators advocate using this drug first.[48,149–153] Cytotoxic agents, especially azathioprine and cyclophosphamide,[154] can be beneficial but are not the first choice because of their mutagenic and leukemogenic properties. These drugs may be preferred for red cell aplasia associated with large granular lymphocytic leukemia, in which cytoreduction is required.[114,155,156] Acquired pure red cell aplasia often responds to antithymocyte globulin.[116,143,157] More specific monoclonal antibodies have less toxicity than does antilymphocyte globulin and can be administered without hospitalization.[158] Daclizumab, a monoclonal antibody directed against the interleukin-2 receptor, is effective in approximately 40 percent of patients.[159] Success has been reported also using rituximab (anti-CD20 monoclonal antibody)[160–162] and alemtuzumab (anti-CD52 [antigen on B lymphocytes]).[163,164] Some patients with resistant disease also respond to fludarabine and cladribine.[165,166] Plasmapheresis[167,168] has produced long-lasting improvement in a few patients, presumably by removing pathogenic antibodies.[167] The absence of randomized trials and even case series of adequate sample size makes the extrapolation of case reports to quantitative estimates of response problematic for many of these therapies.[146] In cases of red cell aplasia associated with a lymphoproliferative disease, such as CLL or LGL, the therapy should be directed at, or in consideration of, the underlying leukemia/lymphoma (see Chaps. 94, 96, and 97).

A thymoma should be excised to prevent local spread of a malignant tumor, but thymectomy does not necessarily improve marrow function.[145] Red cell aplasia can follow thymectomy. Cyclosporine appears the most effective drug to treat pure red cell aplasia associated with thymoma.[169] Red cell aplasia is rarely an indication for stem cell transplantation because the anemia usually can be managed with less drastic approaches. Unresponsive patients have been cured by infusion of allogeneic stem cells after cyclophosphamide conditioning.[170,171]

Other Therapies Despite early favorable case reports, androgens, erythropoietin, and splenectomy are not routinely used to treat pure red cell aplasia.

Immunoglobulins for Persistent B19 Parvovirus Infection Persistent parvovirus infection results from the inability of the host to mount an effective humoral immune response. It can be effectively treated in almost all cases by administration of commercial immunoglobulins, an excellent source of neutralizing antibodies present in a large proportion of the normal population. Infusion of immunoglobulins at 0.4 g/kg per day for 5 to 10 days should produce brisk reticulocytosis and restore a hemoglobin level appropriate for the patient. A single course may be adequate to cure long-standing red cell aplasia resulting from an underlying inherited immunodeficiency syndrome,[172] but patients with acquired immunodeficiency syndrome may not show complete clearance of parvovirus from the circulation and may relapse, requiring retreatment[133] or maintenance immunoglobulin injections (Fig. 35–2).[133,173] Patients suffering from persistent B19 parvovirus infection do not have typical manifestations of a viral infection, such as fever. In these patients, immunoglobulin infusions can induce fifth disease symptoms of variable severity, including cutaneous eruptions and arthritis. Older case reports of red cell aplasia responsive to immunoglobulin infusions likely represent treatment of patients with previously unrecognized parvovirus infection.

REFERENCES

1. Joseph WH: Anemia of infancy and early childhood. *Medicine (Baltimore)* 15:307, 1936.
2. Diamond LK, Blackfan KD: Hypoplastic anemia. *Am J Dis Child* 464, 1939.
3. Gasser C: Aplasia of erythropoiesis. *Pediatr Clin North Am* 4:445, 1957.
4. Diamond LK, Wang WC, Alter BB: Congenital hypoplastic anemia. *Adv Pediatr* 22:349, 1976.
5. Draptchinskaia N, Gustavsson P, Anderson B, et al: The gene encoding ribosomal protein S19 is mutated in Diamond-Blackfan anaemia. *Nat Genet* 21:169, 1999.
6. Glader BE: Diagnosis and management of red cell aplasia in children. *Hematol Oncol Clin North Am* 1:431, 1987.
7. Halperin SD, Freedman HM: Diamond-Blackfan anemia: Etiology, pathophysiology, and treatment. *Am J Pediatr Hematol Oncol* 11:380, 1989.
8. Janov A, Leong T, Nathan D, et al: Diamond-Blackfan anemia, natural history and sequelae of treatment. *Medicine (Baltimore)* 75:77, 1996.
9. Alter BP: Diamond-Blackfan anemia, in *Aplastic Anemia, Acquired and Inherited*, edited by NS Young, BP Alter, p. 361. WB Saunders, Philadelphia, 1994.
10. Willig TN, Gazda H, Sieff CA: Diamond-Blackfan anemia. *Curr Opin Hematol* 7:85, 2000.
11. Freedman MH: Pure red cell aplasia in childhood and adolescence: Pathogenesis and approaches to diagnosis. (Clinical annotations.) *Br J Haematol* 85:246, 1993.
12. Tisdale J, Dunbar CE: Pure red cell aplasia, in *The Bone Marrow Failure Syndromes*, edited by NS Young, p. 135. WB Saunders, Philadelphia, 2000.
13. Dessypris EN: Aplastic anemia and pure red cell aplasia. *Curr Opin Hematol* 1:157, 1994.
14. Fisch P: Pure red cell aplasia. *Br J Haematol* 111:1010, 2000.
15. Croisille L, Tchernia G, Casadevall N: Autoimmune disorders of erythropoiesis. *Curr Opin Hematol* 8:68, 2001.
16. Ball SE, McGuckin CP, Jenkins G: Diamond-Blackfan anaemia in the U.K.: Analysis of 80 cases from a 20-year birth cohort. *Br J Haematol* 94:645, 1996.
17. Ball S, DBA Study Group: Normal parental results should not be taken as evidence of sporadic de novo DBA: Results of family studies from the *UK DBA Registry. Proceedings of the 5th Annual Diamond Blackfan Anemia International Consensus Conference*, March 2004, New York City.
18. Dianzani I, Loreni F: Diamond-Blackfan anemia: A ribosomal puzzle. *Haematologica* 93:1601, 2008.
19. Ellis SR, Lipton JM: Diamond Blackfan anemia: A disorder of red blood cell development. *Curr Top Dev Biol* 82:217, 2008.
20. Lipton J: Diamond Blackfan anemia: New paradigms for a "not so pure" inherited red cell aplasia. *Semin Hematol* 43:167, 2006.
21. Gustavsson P, Willig TN, Van Haederingen A: Diamond-Blackfan anaemia: Genetic homogeneity for a gene on chromosome 19q13 restricted to 1.8 Mb. *Nat Genet* 16:368, 1997.
22. Campagnoli MF, Ramenghi U, Armiraglio M, et al: RPS19 mutations in patients with Diamond-Blackfan anemia. *Hum Mutat* 29:911, 2008.
23. Matsson H, Davey EJ, Draptchinskaia N, et al: Targeted disruption of the ribosomal protein S19 gene is lethal prior to implantation. *Mol Cell Biol* 24:4032, 2004.
24. Wilig TN, Draptchinskaia N, Dianzani I, et al: Mutations in ribosomal protein S19 gene Diamond-Blackfan anemia: Wide variations in phenotypic expression. *Blood* 94:4294, 1999.
25. Boria I, Quarello P, Avondo F, et al: A new database for ribosomal protein genes which are mutated in Diamond-Blackfan anemia. *Hum Mutat* 29:E263, 2008.
26. Ebert BL, Pretz J, Bosco J, et al: Identification of *RPS1r* as a 5q− syndrome gene by RNA interference screen. *Nature* 451:335, 2008.
27. Perdahl EB, Naprstek BL, Wallace WC, et al: Erythroid failure in Diamond-Blackfan anemia is characterized by apoptosis. *Blood* 83:645, 1994.
28. Casadevall N, Croisille L, Auffray I, et al: Age-related alterations in erythroid and granulopoietic progenitors in Diamond-Blackfan anaemia. *Br J Haematol* 87:369, 1994.
29. Ball S, DBA Study Group: Further definition of the erythroid defect in DBA, and the modulatory effect of steroids and prolactin. *Proceedings of the 5th Annual Diamond Blackfan Anemia International Consensus Conference,* March 2004, New York City.
30. Giri N, Kang E, Tisdale JF, et al: Clinical and laboratory evidence for a trilineage haematopoietic defect in patients with refractory Diamond-Blackfan anaemia. *Br J Haematol* 108:167, 2000.
31. Flygare J, Kiefer T, Miyake K, et al: Diamond-Blackfan anemia phenotype created in healthy CD34+ cells through lentivirus-mediated siRNA silencing of ribosomal protein S19. *Proceedings of the 5th Annual Diamond Blackfan Anemia International Consensus Conference*, March 2004, New York City.
32. Miyake K, Flygare J, Kiefer T, et al: Development of cellular models for ribosomal protein S19 (RPS19)-deficient diamond-blackfan anemia using inducible expression of siRNA against RPS19. *Mol Ther* 11: 627, 2005.
33. Uechi T, Nakajima Y, Chakraborty A, et al: Deficiency of ribosomal protein S19 during early embryogenesis leads to reduction of erythrocytes in a zebrafish model of Diamond-Blackfan anemia. *Hum Mol Genet* 17:3204, 2008.
34. Scimeca PG, Weinblatt ME, Slepowitz G, et al: Diamond-Blackfan syndrome: An unusual cause of hydrops fetalis. *Am J Pediatr Hematol Oncol* 10:241, 1988.
35. Brown KE, Green SW, Antunez-de-Mayolo J, et al: Congenital anemia following transplacental B19 parvovirus infection. *Lancet* 343:895, 1994.
36. Balaban EP, Buchanan GR, et al: Diamond-Blackfan syndrome in adult patients. *Am J Med* 78:533, 1985.
37. Cathie IA: Erythrogenesis imperfecta. *Arch Dis Child* 25:313, 1950.
38. Schofield KP, Evans DIK: Diamond-Blackfan syndrome and neutropenia. *J Clin Pathol* 44:742, 1991.
39. Glader BE, Backer K: Elevated red cell adenosine deaminase activity: A marker of disordered erythropoiesis in Diamond-Blackfan anaemia and other haematologic diseases. *Br J Haematol* 68:165, 1988.
40. Willig TN, Niemeyer CM, Leblanc T, et al: Identification of new prognosis factors from the clinical and epidemiologic analysis of a registry of 229 Diamond-Blackfan anemia patients: DBA group of Sciete d'Hematologic et d'Immunologie Pediatrique (SHIP), Gesellshaft fur Padiatrische Onkologie und Hamatologie (GPOH), and the European Society for Pediatric Hematology and Immunology (ESPHI). *Pediatr Res* 46:553, 1999.
41. Vlachos A, Ball S, Dahl N, et al: Diagnosing and treating Diamond Blackfan anaemia: Results of an international clinical consensus conference. *Br J Haematol* 142:849, 2008.
42. Stern GA, Killingsworth DW: Complications of topical antimicrobial agents. *Int Ophthalmol Clin* 29:137, 1989.
43. Vlachos A, Federman N, Reyes-Haley C, et al: Hematopoietic stem cell transplantation for Diamond Blackfan anemia: A report from the Diamond Blackfan Anemia Registry. *Bone Marrow Transplant* 27:381, 2001.
44. Mugishima H, Ohga S, Ohara A, et al: Hematopoietic stem cell transplantation for Diamond-Blackfan anemia: A report from the Aplastic Anemia Committee of the Japanese Society of Pediatric Hematology. *Pediatr Transplant* 11:601, 2007.
45. Wynn RF, Grainger JD, Carr TF, et al: Failure of allogeneic bone marrow transplantation to correct Diamond-Blackfan anaemia despite haemopoietic stem cell engraftment. *Bone Marrow Transplant* 24:803, 1999.
46. Ball SE, Tchernia G, Wranne L, et al: Is there a role for interleukin-3 Diamond-Blackfan anaemia results of a European multicentre study. *Br J Haematol* 91:313, 1995.
47. Ozsoylu S: High-dose intravenous corticosteroid treatment for patients with Diamond-Blackfan syndrome resistant or refractory to conventional treatment. *Am J Pediatr Hematol Oncol* 10:217, 1988.
48. Leonard EM, Raefsky E, Griffith P, et al: Cyclosporine therapy of aplastic anaemia, congenital and acquired red cell aplasia. *Br J Haematol* 72:278, 1989.
49. Marmont AM: Congenital hypoplastic anaemia refractory to corticosteroids but responding to cyclophosphamide and antilymphocytic globulin. *Acta Haematol* 60:90, 1978.
50. Rutella S, Pierelli L, Bonanno G, et al: Role for granulocyte colony-stimulating factor in the generation of human T regulatory type 1 cells. *Blood* 100:2562, 2002.
51. Hamaguchi I, Ooka A, Brun A, et al: Gene transfer improves erythroid development in ribosomal protein S19-deficient Diamond-Blackfan anemia. *Blood* 100:2724, 2002.
52. Flygare J, Olsson K, Richter J, et al: Gene therapy of Diamond Blackfan anemia CD34+ cells leads to improved erythroid development and engraftment following transplantation. *Exp Hematol* 36:1428, 2008.
53. Lyngar E: Samtidig optreden av anemisk kriser hos 3 barn i en familie med hemolytisk ikterus. *Nord Med* 14:1246, 1942.
54. Owren PA: Congenital hemolytic jaundice: The pathogenesis of the "hemolytic crisis." *Blood* 3:231, 1948.
55. Dameshek W, Bloom ML: The events in the hemolytic crisis of hereditary spherocytosis, with particular reference to the reticulocytopenia, pancytopenia and an abnormal splenic mechanism. *Blood* 3:1381, 1948.
56. Chernoff AI, Josephson AM: Acute erythroblastopenia in sickle-cell anemia and infectious mononucleosis. *Am J Dis Child* 82:310, 1951.
57. Singer K, Motulsky AG, Wile SA: Aplastic crisis in sickle cell anemia. A study of its mechanism and its relationship to other types of hemolytic crises. *J Lab Clin Med* 35:721, 1950.
58. Simmons P, Kaushansky K, Torok-Storb B: Mechanisms of cytomegalovirus-mediated myelosuppression: Perturbation of stromal cell function versus direct infection of myeloid cells. *Proc Natl Acad Sci U S A* 87:1386, 1990.
59. Young NS, Brown KE: Parvovirus B19. *N Engl J Med* 350:586, 2004.
60. Serjeant GR, Topley JM, Mason K, et al: Outbreak of aplastic crises in sickle cell anaemia associated with parvovirus-like agent. *Lancet* 2:595, 1981.
61. Serjeant GR, Serjeant BE, Pattison JR, et al: Sero-epidemiology of human parvovirus infection in homozygous sickle cell disease [abstract]. *Blood* 80:10a, 1992.
62. Wranne L: Transient erythroblastopenia in infancy and childhood. *Scand J Haematol* 7:76, 1970.
63. Young NS, Harrison M, Moore JG, et al: Direct demonstration of the human parvovirus in erythroid progenitor cells infected in vitro. *J Clin Invest* 74:2024, 1984.

64. Brown KE, Anderson SM, Young NS: Erythrocyte P antigen: Cellular receptor for B19 parvovirus. *Science* 262:114, 1993.
65. Brown KE, Hibbs JR, Gallinella G, et al: Resistance to human parvovirus B19 infection due to lack of virus receptor (erythrocyte P antigen). *N Engl J Med* 330:1192, 1993.
66. Anderson MJ, Jones SE, Minson AC: Diagnosis of human parvovirus infection by dot-blot hybridization using cloned viral DNA. *J Med Virol* 15:163, 1985.
67. Young NS, Mortimer PP: Viruses and bone marrow failure. *Blood* 63:729, 1984.
68. Chorba TL, Coccia P, Holman RC, et al: Role of parvovirus B19 in aplastic crisis and erythema infectiosum (fifth disease). *J Infect Dis* 154:383, 1986.
69. Smith-Whitley K, Zhao H, et al: The epidemiology of human parvovirus B19 in children with sickle cell disease. *Blood* 103:422, 2003.
70. Serjeant BE, Hambleton RR, Kerr S, et al: Haematological response to parvovirus B19 infection in homozygous sickle-cell disease. *Lancet* 341:1237, 1993.
71. Skeppner G, Kreuger A, Elinder G: Transient erythroblastopenia of childhood: Prospective study of 10 patients with special reference to viral infections. *J Pediatr Hematol Oncol* 24:294, 2002.
72. Beresford CH, MacFarlane SD: Temporal clustering of transient erythroblastopenia (cytopenia) of childhood. *Aust Paediatr J* 23:351, 1987.
73. Bhambhani K, Inoue S, Sarnaik SA: Seasonal clustering of transient erythroblastopenia of childhood. *Am J Dis Child* 142:175, 1988.
74. Hays T, Lane PA, Shafer F: Transient erythroblastopenia of childhood. A review of 26 cases and reassessment of indications for bone marrow aspirate. *Am J Dis Child* 143:605, 1989.
75. Prassouli A, Papadakis V, Tsakris A, et al: Classic transient erythroblastopenia of childhood with human parvovirus B19 genome detection in the blood and bone marrow. *J Pediatr Hematol Oncol* 27:333, 2005.
76. Young NS, Mortimer PP, Moore GJ, et al: Characterization of a virus that causes transient aplastic crisis. *J Clin Invest* 73:224, 1984.
77. Rogers BB, Rogers ZR, Timmons CF: Polymerase chain reaction amplification of archival material for parvovirus B19 in children with transient erythroblastopenia of childhood. *Pediatr Pathol Lab Med* 16:471, 1996.
78. Gussetis ES, Peristeri J, Kitra V, et al: Clinical value of bone marrow cultures in childhood pure red cell aplasia. *J Pediatr Hematol Oncol* 20:120, 1998.
79. Koenig HM, Lightsey AL, Nelson DP, et al: Immune suppression of erythropoiesis in transient erythroblastopenia of childhood. *Blood* 54:742, 1979.
80. Tamary H, Kaplinsky C, Shvartzmayer S, et al: Transient erythroblastopenia of childhood: Evidence for cell-mediated suppression of erythropoiesis. *Am J Pediatr Hematol Oncol* 15:386, 1993.
81. Gustavsson P, Klar J, Matsson H, et al: Familiar transient erythroblastopenia of childhood is associated with the chromosome 19q13.2 region but not caused by mutations in coding sequences of the ribosomal protein S19 (RPS19) gene. *Br J Haematol* 119:261, 2002.
82. Thompson DF, Gales MA: Drug-induced pure red cell aplasia. *Pharmacotherapy* 16:1002, 1996.
83. Dessypris EN, Redline S, Harris JW, et al: Diphenylhydantoin-induced pure red cell aplasia. *Blood* 65:789, 1985.
84. Mariette Y, Mitjavila MT, Moulinie PR, et al: Rifampicin-induced pure red cell aplasia. *Am J Med* 87:459, 1989.
85. Smith JC, Megason GC, Iyer RV, et al: Clinical characteristics of children with hereditary hemolytic anemias and aplastic crisis: A 7-year review. *South Med J* 87:702, 1994.
86. Kynaston JA, West NC, Reid MM: A regional experience of red cell aplasia. *Eur J Pediatr* 152:306, 1993.
87. Farhi DC, Leubbers E, Rosenthal N: Bone marrow biopsy findings in childhood anemia—Prevalence of transient erythroblastopenia of childhood. *Arch Pathol Lab Med* 122:638, 1998.
88. Skeppner G, Wranne L: Transient erythroblastopenia of childhood in Sweden: Incidence and findings at the time of diagnosis. *Acta Paediatr* 82:574, 1993.
89. Cherrick I, Karayalcin G, Lanzkowsky P: Transient erythroblastopenia of childhood: Prospective study of fifty patients. *Am J Pediatr Hematol Oncol* 16:320, 1994.
90. Michelson Ad, Marshall PC: Transient neurological disorder associated with transient erythroblastopenia of childhood. *Am J Pediatr Hematol Oncol* 9:161, 1987.
91. Young RSK, Rannels E, Hilmi A, et al: Severe anemia in childhood presenting as transient ischemic attacks. *Stroke* 14:622, 1983.
92. Chan GCF, Kanwar VS, Wilimas J: Transient erythroblastopenia of childhood associated with transient neurologic deficit: Report of a case and review of the literature. *J Paediatr Child Health* 34:299, 1998.
93. Skeppner G, Forestier E, Henter JI, et al: Transient red cell aplasia in siblings: A common environmental or a common hereditary factor? *Acta Paediatr* 87:43, 1998.
94. Leuschner S, Bödewaldt-Radzun S, Rister M: Increase of CALLA-positive stimulated lymphoid cells in transient erythroblastopenia of childhood. *Eur J Pediatr* 149:551, 1990.
95. Kaznelson P: Zur Enstehung der Blut Plattchen. *Verh Dtsch Ges Inn Med* 34:557, 1922.
96. Dessypris EN, Krantz SB, Roloff JS, et al: Mode of action of the IgG inhibitor of erythropoiesis in transient erythroblastopenia of childhood. *Blood* 59:114, 1982.
97. Baker RI, Manoharan A, De Luca E, et al: Pure red cell aplasia of pregnancy: A distinct clinical entity. *Br J Haematol* 85:619, 1993.
98. Peschle C, Marmont AM, Marone G, et al: Pure red cell aplasia: Studies on an IgG serum inhibitor neutralizing erythropoietin. *Br J Haematol* 30:411, 1975.
99. Casadevall N, Dupuy E, Molho-Sabatier P, et al: Autoantibodies against erythropoietin in a patient with pure red-cell aplasia. *N Engl J Med* 334:630, 1996.
100. Prabhakar SS, Muhlfelder T: Antibodies to recombinant human erythropoietin causing pure red cell aplasia. *Clin Nephrol* 47:331, 1997.
101. Casadevall N, Nataf J, Viron B, et al: Pure red-cell aplasia and antierythropoietin antibodies in patients treated with recombinant erythropoietin. *N Engl J Med* 346:469, 2002.
102. Locatelli F, del Vecchio L: Pure red cell aplasia secondary to treatment with erythropoietin. *J Nephrol* 16:461, 2003.
103. Pollock C, Johnson DW, Horl WH, et al: Pure red cell aplasia induced by erythropoiesis-stimulating agents. *Clin J Am Soc Nephrol* 3:193, 2008.
104. McKoy JM, Stonecash RE, Cournoyer D, et al: Epoetin-associated pure red cell aplasia: Past, present, and future considerations. *Transfusion* 48:1754, 2008.
105. Fijal B, Ricci D, Vercammen E, et al: Case-control study of the association between select *HLA* genes and anti-erythropoietin antibody-positive pure red-cell aplasia. *Pharmacogenomics* 9:157, 2008.
106. Bolan CD, Leitman SF, Griffith LM, et al: Delayed donor red cell chimerism and pure red cell aplasia following major ABO-incompatible nonmyeloablative hematopoietic stem cell transplantation. *Blood* 98:1687, 2001.
107. Grigg AP, Juneja SK: Pure red cell aplasia with the onset of graft versus host disease. *Bone Marrow Transplant* 32:1099, 2003.
108. Hayden PJ, Gardiner N, Molloy K, et al: Pure red cell aplasia after a major ABO-mismatched bone marrow transplant for chronic myeloid leukaemia: Response to reintroduction of cyclosporin. *Bone Marrow Transplant* 33:459, 2004.
109. Helbig G, Stella-Holowiecka B, Wojnar J, et al: Pure red-cell aplasia following major and bi-directional ABO-incompatible allogeneic stem-cell transplantation: Recovery of donor-derived erythropoiesis after long-term treatment using different therapeutic strategies. *Ann Hematol* 86:677, 2007.
110. Charles RJ, Sabo KM, Kidd PG, et al: The pathophysiology of pure red cell aplasia: Implications for therapy. *Blood* 87:4831, 1996.
111. Chikkappa G, Zarrabi MH, Tsan MF: Pure red-cell aplasia in patients with chronic lymphocytic leukemia. *Medicine* (Baltimore) 65:339, 1986.
112. Go RS, Lust JA, Phyliky RL: Aplastic anemia and pure red cell aplasia associated with large granular lymphocyte leukemia. *Semin Hematol* 40:196, 2003.
113. Lacy MQ, Kurtin PJ, Tefferi A: Pure red cell aplasia: Association with large granular lymphocyte leukemia and the prognostic value of cytogenetic abnormalities. *Blood* 87:3000, 1996.
114. Yamada O: Clonal T cell proliferation in patients with pure red cell aplasia. *Leuk Lymphoma* 35:69, 1999.
115. Fujishima N, Hirokawa M, Fujishima M, et al: Oligoclonal T cell expansion in blood but not in the thymus from a patient with thymoma-associated pure red cell aplasia. *Haematologica* 91(Suppl): ECR47, 2006.
116. Abkowitz JL, Powell JS, Nakamura JM, et al: Pure red cell aplasia: Response to therapy with anti-thymocyte globulin. *Am J Hematol* 23:363, 1986.
117. Abkowitz JL, Kadin ME, Powell JS, et al: Pure red cell aplasia: Lymphocyte inhibition of erythropoiesis. *Br J Haematol* 63:59, 1986.
118. Hanada T, Abe T, Nakamura H, et al: Pure red cell aplasia: Relationship between inhibitory activity of T cells to CFU-E and erythropoiesis. *Br J Haematol* 58:107, 1984.
119. Linch DC, Cawley JC, MacDonald SM, et al: Acquired pure red-cell aplasia associated with an increase of T cells bearing receptors for the Fc of IgG. *Acta Haematol* 65:270, 1981.
120. Mangan KF, D'Alessandro L: Hypoplastic anemia in B cell chronic lymphocytic leukemia: Evolution of T cell-mediated suppression of erythropoiesis in early-stage and late-stage disease. *Blood* 66:533, 1985.
121. Mangan KF, Chikkappa G, Farley PC: T gamma cells suppress growth of erythroid colony-forming units *in vitro* in the pure red cell aplasia of B-cell chronic lymphocytic leukemia. *J Clin Invest* 70:1148, 1982.
122. Hoffman R, Kopel S, Hsu SD, et al: T cell chronic lymphocytic leukemia: Presence in bone marrow and peripheral blood of cells that suppress erythropoiesis in vitro. *Blood* 52:255, 1978.
123. Nagasawa T, Abe T, Nakagawa T: Pure red cell aplasia and hypogammaglobulinemia associated with Tr-cell chronic lymphocytic leukemia. *Blood* 57:1025, 1981.
124. Handgretinger R, Geiselhart A, Moris A: Pure red cell aplasia associated with clonal expansion of granular lymphocytes expressing killer-cell inhibitory receptors. *N Engl J Med* 340:278, 1999.
125. Mangan KF, Volkin R, Winkelstein A: Autoreactive erythroid progenitor-T suppressor cells in the pure red cell aplasia associated with thymoma and panhypogammaglobulinemia. *Am J Hematol* 23:167, 1986.
126. Akard LP, Brandt J, Lu Li, et al: Chronic T cell lymphoproliferative disorder and pure red cell aplasia. *Am J Med* 83:1069, 1987.
127. Reid TJI, Mullancy M, Burrell LM, et al: Pure red cell aplasia after chemotherapy for Hodgkin's lymphoma: *In vitro* evidence for T cell mediated suppression of erythropoiesis and response to sequential cyclosporine and erythropoietin. *Am J Hematol* 46:48, 1994.
128. Socinksi MA, Ershler WB, Tosato G, et al: Pure red blood cell aplasia associated with chronic Epstein-Barr virus infection: Evidence for T-cell–mediated suppression of erythroid colony-forming units. *J Lab Clin Med* 104:995, 1984.
129. Levitt LJ, Reyes GR, Moonka DK, et al: Human T-cell leukemia virus-I–associated T-suppressor cell inhibition of erythropoiesis in a patient with pure red cell aplasia and chronic T-gamma-lymphoproliferative disease. *J Clin Invest* 81:538, 1988.

130. Poll EHA, Arwert F, Kortbeek HT, et al: Fanconi anaemia cells are not uniformly deficient in unhooking of DNA interstrand crosslinks induced by mitomycin C or 8-methoxypsoralen plus UV-A. *Hum Genet* 68:228, 1984.
131. Kurtzman G, Cohen R, Field AM, et al: The immune response to B19 parvovirus infection and an antibody defect in persistent viral infection. *J Clin Invest* 84:1114, 1989.
132. Geetha D, Zachary JB, Baldado HM, et al: Pure red cell aplasia caused by Parvovirus B19 infection in solid organ transplant recipients: A case report and review of literature. *Clin Transplant* 14:586, 2000.
133. Frickhofen N, Abkowitz JL, Safford M, et al: Persistent parvovirus infection in patients infected with human immunodeficiency virus type 1 (HIV-1): A treatable cause of anemia in AIDS. *Ann Intern Med* 113:926, 1990.
134. Caroli J, Bernard J, Bessis M, et al: Hemochromatose avec anemic hypochrome et absence d' hemoglobine anormale. *Presse Med* 65:1991, 1957.
135. Abkowitz JL, Brown KE, Wood RW, et al: Clinical relevance of parvovirus B19 as a cause of anemia in patients with human immunodeficiency virus infection. *J Infect Dis* 176:269, 1997.
136. Mylonakis E, Dickinson BP, Mileno MD, et al: Persistent parvovirus B19 related anemia of seven year's duration in an HIV-infected patient: Complete remission associated with highly active antiretroviral therapy. *Am J Hematol* 60:164, 1999.
137. Morelli P, Bestetti G, Longhi E, et al: Persistent parvovirus B19-induced anemia in an HIV-infected patient under HAART. Case report and review of literature. *Eur J Clin Microbiol Infect Dis* 26:833, 2007.
138. Garcia-Suárez J, Pascual T, Muñoz MA, et al: Myelodysplastic syndrome with erythroid hypoplasia/aplasia: A case report and review of the literature. *Am J Hematol* 58:319, 1998.
139. Hirai H: Molecular pathogenesis of MDS. *Int J Hematol* 76:213, 2002.
140. Pellagatti A, Esoof N, Watkins F: Gene expression profiling in the myelodysplastic syndromes using cDNA microarray technology. *Br J Haematol* 125:576, 2004.
141. Darley RL, Hoy TG, Baines P, et al: Mutant N-RAS induces erythroid lineage dysplasia in human CD34+ cells. *J Exp Med* 185:1337, 1997.
142. Lacombe C, Casadevall N, Muller O, et al: Erythroid progenitors in adult chronic pure red cell aplasia: Relationship of *in vitro* erythroid colonies to therapeutic response. *Blood* 64:71, 1984.
143. Mangan KF, Shadduck RK: Successful treatment of chronic refractory pure red cell aplasia with antithymocyte globulin: Correlation with *in vitro* erythroid culture studies. *Am J Hematol* 17:417, 1984.
144. Clark DA, Dessypris EN, Krantz SB: Studies on pure red cell aplasia. XI. Results of immunosuppressive treatment of 37 patients. *Blood* 63:277, 1984.
145. Hirst E, Robertson TI: The syndrome of thymoma and erythroblastopenic anemia. *Medicine (Baltimore)* 46:225, 1967.
146. Sawada K, Fujishima N, Hirokawa M: Acquired pure red cell aplasia: Updated review of treatment. *Br J Haematol* 142:505, 2008.
147. Firkin FC, Maher D: Cytotoxic immunosuppressive drug treatment strategy in pure red cell aplasia. *Eur J Haematol* 41:212, 1988.
148. Kwong YL, Wong KF, Liang RHS, et al: Pure red cell aplasia: Clinical features and treatment results in 16 cases. *Ann Hematol* 72:137, 1996.
149. Mamiya S, Itoh T, Miura AB: Acquired pure red cell aplasia in Japan. *Eur J Haematol* 59:199, 1997.
150. Yamada O, Motoji T, Mizoguchi H: Selective effect of cyclosporine monotherapy for pure red cell aplasia not associated with granular lymphocyte-proliferative disorders. *Br J Haematol* 106:371, 1999.
151. Raghavachar A: Pure red cell aplasia: Review of treatment and proposal for a treatment strategy. *Blut* 61:47, 1990.
152. Tötterman TH, Höglund M, Bengtsson M, et al: Treatment of pure red-cell aplasia and aplastic anaemia with ciclosporin: Long-term clinical effects. *Eur J Haematol* 42:126, 1989.
153. Sawada K-I, Hirokawa M, Fujishima N, et al: Long-term outcome of patients with acquired primary idiopathic pure red cell aplasia receiving cyclosporine A. A nationwide cohort study in Japan for the PRCA Collaborative Study Group. *Hematol J* 92:1021, 2007.
154. Yamada O, Mizoguchi H, Oshimi K: Cyclophosphamide therapy for pure red cell aplasia associated with granular lymphocyte-proliferative disorders. *Br J Haematol* 97:392, 1997.
155. Go RS, Li C-Y, Tefferi A, et al: Acquired pure red cell aplasia associated with lymphoproliferative disease of granular T lymphocytes. *Blood* 98:483, 2001.
156. Fujishima N, Sawada K-I, Hirokawa M, et al: Long-term responses and outcomes following immunosuppressive therapy in large granular lymphocyte leukemia-associated pure red cell aplasia: A nationwide cohort study in Japan for the PRCA Collaborative Study Group. *Haematologica* 93:1555, 2008.
157. Harris SI, Weinberg JB: Treatment of red cell aplasia with antithymocyte globulin: Repeated inductions of complete remissions in two patients. *Am J Hematol* 20:183, 1985.
158. Robak T: Monoclonal antibodies in the treatment of autoimmune cytopenias. *Eur J Haematol* 72:79, 2004.
159. Sloand EM, Scheinberg P, Maciejewski JP, et al: Brief communication: Successful treatment of pure red-cell aplasia with an anti-interleukin-2 receptor antibody (Daclizumab). *Ann Intern Med* 144:181, 2006.
160. Ghazal H: Successful treatment of pure red cell aplasia with rituximab in patients with chronic lymphocytic leukemia. *Blood* 99:1092, 2002.
161. Auner HW, Wolfler A, Beham-Schmid C, et al: Restoration of erythropoiesis by rituximab in an adult patient with primary acquired pure red cell aplasia refractory to conventional treatment. *Br J Haematol* 116:725, 2002.
162. Scaramucci L, Niscola P, Ales M, et al: Pure red cell aplasia associated with hemolytic anemia refractory to standard measures and resolved by rituximab in an elderly patient. *Int J Hematol* 88:343, 2008.
163. Willis F, Marsh JC, Bevan DH, et al: The effect of treatment with Campath-1H in patients with autoimmune cytopenias. *Br J Haematol* 114:891, 2001.
164. Ru X, Liebman HA: Successful treatment of refractory pure red cell aplasia associated with lymphoproliferative disorders with the anti-CD52 monoclonal antibody alemtuzumab (Campath-1H). *Br J Haematol* 123:278, 2004.
165. Ahn JH, Lee KH, Lee JH, et al: A case of refractory idiopathic pure red cell aplasia responsive to fludarabine treatment. *Br J Haematol* 112:527, 2001.
166. Robak T, Kaszn, Ki M, et al: Pure red cell aplasia in patients with chronic lymphocytic leukaemia treated with cladribine. *Br J Haematol* 112:1083, 2001.
167. Messner HA, Fauser AA, Curtis JE, et al: Control of antibody-mediated pure red-cell aplasia by plasmapheresis. *N Engl J Med* 304:1334, 1981.
168. Freund LG, Hippe E, Strandgaard S, et al: Complete remission in pure red cell aplasia after plasmapheresis. *Scand J Haematol* 35:315, 1985.
169. Hirokawa M, Sawada J-I, Fujishima N, et al: Long-term response and outcome following immuno-suppressive therapy in thymoma-associated pure red cell aplasia: A nationwide cohort study in Japan by the PRCA Collaborative Study Group. *Haematologica* 93:27, 2008.
170. Müller BU, Tichelli A, Passweg JR, et al: Successful treatment of refractory acquired pure red cell aplasia (PRCA) by allogeneic bone marrow transplantation. *Bone Marrow Transplant* 23:1205, 1999.
171. Tseng SB, Lin SF, Chang CS, et al: Successful treatment of acquired pure red cell aplasia (PRCA) by allogeneic peripheral blood stem cell transplantation. *Am J Hematol* 74:273, 2003.
172. Kurtzman GJ, Ozawa K, Cohen B, et al: Chronic bone marrow failure due to persistent B19 parvovirus infection. *N Engl J Med* 317:287, 1987.
173. Ramratnam B, Schiffman FJ, Rintels P, et al: Management of persistent B19 parvovirus infection in AIDS. *Br J Haematol* 91:90, 1995.

CHAPTER 36
ANEMIA OF CHRONIC RENAL DISEASE

Jaime Caro and Ubaldo Martinez Outschoorn

SUMMARY

Anemia is an almost constant result of chronic renal failure. Erythropoietin deficiency is the primary cause. Accumulation of toxic metabolic end products plays a secondary role in the pathogenesis of the anemia; however, the effects of these end products largely can be overcome by exogenous erythropoiesis-stimulating agents (ESAs). Inflammatory cytokines lead to increased hepcidin levels in plasma, which block iron absorption in the gut and iron release from macrophage stores. If adequate iron sources are available, hemoglobin levels of 11 to 12 g/dL can be maintained by subcutaneous or intravenous ESA injections. Hemoglobin levels greater than 12 g/dL should be avoided, as clinical trials have shown increased mortality if that target hemoglobin is used. Approximately 95 percent of patients respond to erythropoietin without significant side effects.

HISTORY AND DEFINITION

Anemia is one of the most common manifestations of chronic renal failure. Untreated anemia can, depending on its severity, be associated with a number of abnormalities, including decreased oxygen delivery to the tissues; increased cardiac output and cardiomegaly; decreased cognition and mental acuity; and overall decrease in patient welfare (see Chap. 33). The degree of anemia appears to be roughly proportional to the severity of renal failure, but there is not a strict linear relationship between hematocrit and creatinine clearance. At creatinine clearances of less than 20 mL/min, the hematocrit (Hct) is frequently less than 30 mL/dL, although there is great variability (Fig. 36–1). In polycystic kidney disease the anemia is usually less severe for the degree of renal failure, and patients who have undergone nephrectomy are frequently more anemic than are patients being treated with hemodialysis. Infectious, neoplastic, immunologic, and metabolic disorders that can accompany renal disease can affect the degree of anemia and its response to treatment.[1]

ETIOLOGY AND PATHOGENESIS

Experimental and clinical observations on the effect of intensive dialysis, bilateral-nephrectomy, and treatment with erythropoietin (EPO) have clarified some of the pathophysiologic mechanisms responsible for the anemia of chronic renal disease. The primary cause of the anemia is decreased production of EPO by the diseased kidneys.[2,3] A diminished capacity to excrete potentially toxic metabolic end products may contribute to the anemia by shortening the red cell life span, by marrow suppression, and by increasing the risk of blood loss.[4,5] Concomitant inflammatory conditions and/or malnutrition may aggravate the anemia and impair its response to therapy.[1] Inflammatory conditions lead to increased hepcidin production and hepcidin inhibits enterocyte iron absorption in the gut and macrophage iron release through ferroportin (see Chap. 42). Decreased serum iron concentration may contribute to the anemia and limit the response to exogenous EPO administration.

Acronyms and abbreviations that appear in this chapter include: ADAMTS-13, a disintegrin and metalloproteinase with thrombospondin domain 13; EPO, erythropoietin; ESA, erythropoiesis-stimulating agent; HIF, hypoxia-inducible factor; HUS, hemolytic uremic syndrome; Na^+-K^+, sodium-potassium; PRCA, pure red cell aplasia; TTP, thrombotic thrombocytopenic purpura; VHL, von Hippel-Lindau.

■ RENAL EXCRETORY FAILURE

The life span of red cells in patients with chronic renal disease is usually shorter than normal. Because the red cells survive normally when they are injected into healthy recipients and normal red cells may have a shortened life span in uremic recipients,[4,5] the metabolic or vascular environment in uremic patients is unfavorable for normal survival of red cells. Because erythropoiesis is compromised in patients with chronic renal disease, the modest shortening of red cell life span contributes to the anemia in some cases.

Metabolic Red Cell Dysfunction

The inverse relationship between blood urea nitrogen and red cell life span and the occasional normalization of the red cell life span after intensive dialysis[6] suggest the presence of an erythrocyte metabolic defect. However, red cell enzymes are normal or increased in patients with uremia and the intracellular level of adenosine triphosphate is high, possibly as a result of a high serum phosphate concentration.[7] The intracellular concentration of 2,3-bisphosphoglycerate is increased in response to anemia and hyperphosphatemia,[8] with a moderate decrease in the affinity of hemoglobin for oxygen.[9] In the presence of uremic acidosis, the decrease in oxygen is augmented by a rightward shift of the oxygen dissociation curve (Bohr effect; see Chaps. 48 and 49). However, acidosis also tends to decrease the concentration of intracellular organic phosphates and 2,3-bisphosphoglycerate, establishing a condition of opposing effects on the oxygen affinity of hemoglobin.[10] Intensive dialysis may initially reduce the concentration of intracellular organic phosphate compounds, possibly because of hypophosphatemia.[11] The result is increased oxygen affinity of hemoglobin and temporary aggravation of tissue hypoxia, which may play a role in the so-called dialysis disequilibrium syndrome.[12] The activity of transketolase, a hexose monophosphate shunt enzyme[13] (see Chap. 46), is decreased in uremia. The decreased response of the hexose monophosphate shunt renders the hemoglobin and red cell membrane excessively sensitive to oxidant drugs or chemicals.[14,15] For example, tap water used for hemodialysis and purified with chloramine can cause the formation of Heinz bodies and hemolytic anemia.[16] Exogenous toxins introduced by dialysis fluids, such as copper, nitrates, and formaldehyde, can contribute to hemolysis and occasionally produce severe, even fatal, hemolytic episodes.[17] Parathyroid hormone levels, often increased in renal failure, may be associated with anemia (see Chap. 38); the etiology of anemia of hyperparathyroidism, however, is multifactorial.[18,19]

■ MECHANICAL RED CELL DESTRUCTION

Despite a metabolic basis for hemolysis, a clear-cut correlation between erythrocyte life span and degree of renal failure has not been identified.[2] Red cell injury and premature destruction may be caused by mechanical trauma rather than metabolic alterations.[20] Normal red cells exposed to strong shearing stress, especially at a fibrin interphase, become deformed

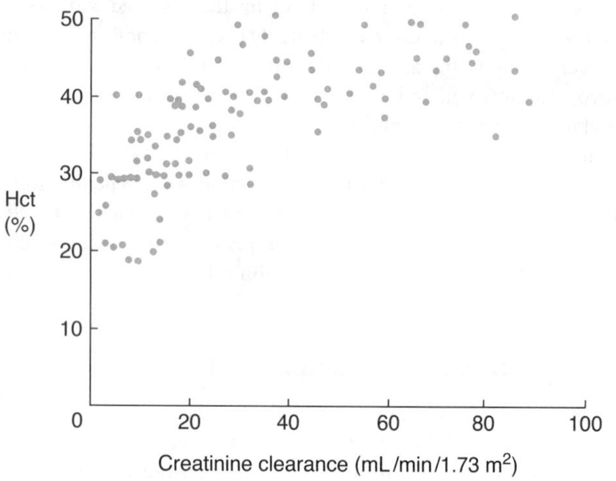

FIGURE 36–1. Relationship between hematocrit and creatinine clearance in patients with chronic renal disease. Anemia is inversely related to the degree of renal impairment in most patients with chronic renal disease. *(Redrawn with permission from Radtke HW, Claussner A, Erbes PM, et al.[2])*

and vulnerable to monocyte-macrophage sequestration. In some cases of malignant hypertension, extensive red cell fragmentation occurs with severe hemolytic anemia,[22] but in most cases of chronic renal disease, the hemolysis and morphologic changes are only moderate. Current understanding relates premature destruction of red cells in uremia with mechanical disruption of metabolically impaired cells.

HEMOLYTIC UREMIC SYNDROME

The hemolysis is not secondary to the uremia, and its manifestations are similar to those found in disseminated intravascular coagulation (see Chap. 130) or other acute microangiopathic disorders (see Chap. 50). The syndrome was first described in 1955 by Gasser and coworkers[22] who found hemolysis and uremia in infants and young children subsequent to episodes of gastrointestinal or upper respiratory infections. Since that time, the syndrome has been recognized in patients of all ages and associated with a variety of exogenous agents, most commonly verotoxin producing *Escherichia coli*.[23,24] The syndrome is initiated by damage to the endothelium of glomerular capillaries and renal arterioles. The damage leads to local platelet deposition, intravascular coagulation, and ischemic renal cortical necrosis.[25] Clinical manifestations are pallor, purpura, jaundice, and oliguria. Laboratory tests reveal anemia. Blood films display many deformed and fragmented red cells (Fig. 36–2), increased numbers of reticulocytes, and occasional nucleated red cells.[24,26] EPO levels usually are increased despite an elevated serum creatinine concentration.[27] Thrombocytopenia and a compensatory increase in marrow megakaryocytes are usually present. Distinguishing hemolytic uremic syndrome (HUS) from the syndrome of thrombotic thrombocytopenic purpura (TTP) can be difficult in many cases (see Chaps. 50 and 133). Normal cleaving of von Willebrand multimers is impaired in TTP because of either a congenital absence of a multimer-cleaving protease (ADAMTS-13 [a disintegrin and metalloprotease with thrombospondin domain 13]) or immunologic inactivation of the protease.[28,29] Most cases of HUS clear spontaneously, but severe cases may cause life-threatening renal failure and are often associated with the use of chemotherapeutic or immunosuppressive agents (see Chaps. 50 and 133), and its prevalence may be increasing.[30]

BLOOD LOSS

Purpura and gastrointestinal and gynecologic bleeding occur in one-third to one-half of all patients with chronic renal failure.[31] In addition, blood is lost during laboratory testing and in discarded dialysis tubing. Iron deficiency frequently contributes to the development of anemia and its response to therapy. The pathogenesis of the bleeding tendency is poorly understood. Thrombocytopenia, when present, is rarely of sufficient magnitude to explain spontaneous blood loss. However, platelet or vascular function as judged from bleeding time, platelet adhesiveness and aggregation, clot retraction, thromboxane formation, or prostacyclin production by vessel walls, is abnormal in the majority of cases and may, alone or in combination, account for the bleeding tendency (see Chaps. 114 and 119).[32] Dialysis corrects or ameliorates both the laboratory and clinical manifestations of abnormal platelet function, but the dialyzable agent responsible has not been identified. Urea or creatinine probably is not involved, but certain guanidine compounds are suspected.[32]

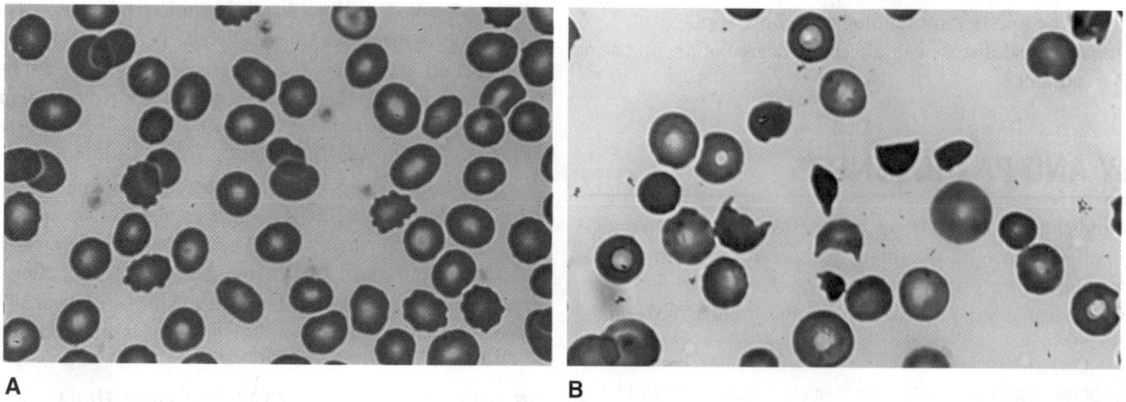

FIGURE 36–2. Blood films. **A.** Chronic renal disease. There is no characteristic red cell change in patients with chronic renal disease. Occasional abnormal cell shapes, such as fragmented cells, target cells, or echinocytes may be seen. The field in this example has several echinocytes, a target cell, several ovalocytes, and a few spherocytes. If iron deficiency or folic acid deficiency complicates the renal disease, blood cell changes compatible with those deficiencies may be superimposed. **B.** Hemolytic-uremic syndrome. Note the high prevalence of schistocytes, the characteristic finding. Several spherocytes are noted. Marked anisocytosis. The large cell is probably a reticulocyte. *(Used with permission from* Lichtman's Atlas of Hematology, *www.accessmedicine.com.)*

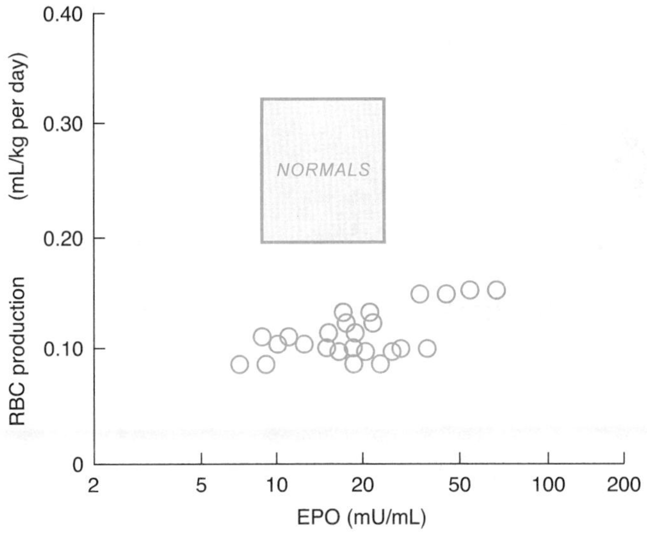

FIGURE 36–3. Relationship between red cell production (RBC) and EPO levels in uremic patients. With stable hematocrits, the rate of red cell production must equal the rate of red cell destruction, which is calculated by dividing red cell mass by red cell life span. The *squares* denote the rate of red cell production in normal individuals at normal EPO levels. Results indicate that uremic patients have decreased red cell production for equivalent serum EPO concentrations compared to normal individuals[40] (see Chap. 31).

MARROW SUPPRESSION

Although EPO deficiency could explain the development of anemia, uremic toxins also may impair erythroid activity and be partly responsible for the development of anemia.[33] Earlier studies have suggested that such uremic toxins exist, but all attempts to identify and isolate the toxins have been unsuccessful.[34] Spermine,[35] an attractive candidate, suppresses all cellular elements, not only the erythroid tissue, when administered in toxic doses. Parathyroid hormone,[36] another contender, causes general marrow suppression and may induce marrow fibrosis.[37] Exogenous EPO is equally effective when administered to patients before and after kidney transplantation.[38] These observations indicate that uremia per se does not affect normal erythroid metabolism *in vivo*. Nevertheless, the response to EPO in stable, well-dialyzed patients is about half the response in normal individuals[39] (Fig. 36–3). Whether the decreased erythroid responsiveness is the result of uremic toxins, associated inflammatory conditions, or relative iron deficiency is not clear. Iron deficiency because of excessive blood loss occurs in most patients with renal failure[40]; therefore, iron supplementation in uremic patients receiving EPO is almost always necessary for their response to therapy.

Aluminum in dialysis water can interfere with iron incorporation in erythroid cells and cause microcytic anemia and occasionally osteomalacia and encephalopathy.[41] In the rare case of nephrotic syndrome, urinary loss of transferrin reportedly causes low iron-binding capacity, with impairment in metabolic cycling of iron,[42] and resulting iron deficiency (see Chap. 42). Folic acid (see Chap. 41) should be repleted in patients who are undergoing intensive dialysis because folic acid is dialyzable and may be lost in the dialysis bath.[43]

FAILURE OF RENAL ENDOCRINE FUNCTION

Erythropoietin

EPO is a 34-kDa glycoprotein hematopoietic growth factor that can control the rate of red cell production by acting on erythroid precursors in the marrow[44] (see Chap. 31).[44] In 1957, Jacobson and coworkers[45] reported that nephrectomized and uremic rats failed to respond to blood loss by releasing EPO, whereas ureter-ligated and equally uremic rats responded in an almost normal manner. This important observation led to the hypothesis that the kidney produces EPO. In the 1970s, studies on isolated perfused kidneys supported the kidney's direct role in EPO production.[46] However, the kidney was not established as an EPO-producing organ until EPO messenger ribonucleic acid (mRNA) was demonstrated in renal tissue.[47–49]

In situ hybridization studies have localized the EPO-producing cells to the cortical interstitium of mouse and rat kidneys.[50,51] Immunoelectron-microscopic techniques show that EPO-expressing cells also express the surface enzyme ecto-5-nucleotidase,[52,53] a marker restricted to fibroblastic cells. An increased number of EPO-producing cells are recruited to express the gene in an all-or-none fashion, with recruitment spreading outward from the corticomedullary boundary as anemia intensifies.[51]

Hypoxia is followed by a measurable accumulation of EPO mRNA in the kidneys, and shortly afterward by an increase in circulating EPO.[54] The molecular mechanisms by which hypoxia-anemia controls production of EPO and other hypoxia-responsive genes are an area of active research (see Chap. 31). A hypoxia-responsive enhancer-sequence element that controls the hypoxia response was identified in the 3-flanking sequence of the human *EPO* gene.[55] This sequence acts as the DNA-binding site for a hypoxia-inducible transcription factor-1 complex (HIF-1), which activates transcription of the *EPO* gene. The HIF-1 complex is formed by two subunits: HIF-α (HIF-1α and HIF-2α), which is expressed only under hypoxic conditions, and HIF-1β, which is constitutively expressed (see Chap. 31).[56] The HIF-α subunits are normally ubiquinated and degraded by the proteasomal system in a process that requires the von Hippel-Lindau (VHL) protein, which acts as an ubiquitin ligase.[57–59] During normoxic conditions, HIF-α proteins are hydroxylated in specific prolyl residues by prolyl-hydroxylase enzymes in an oxygen-dependent reaction.[60–62] Hydroxylation of HIF-α facilitates their interaction with the VHL protein and degradation by the proteasome system. Thus, under hypoxic or anemic conditions, HIF-α's are not degraded and interact with HIF-1β to activate transcription of the *EPO* gene (Fig. 36–4). Patients with VHL mutations

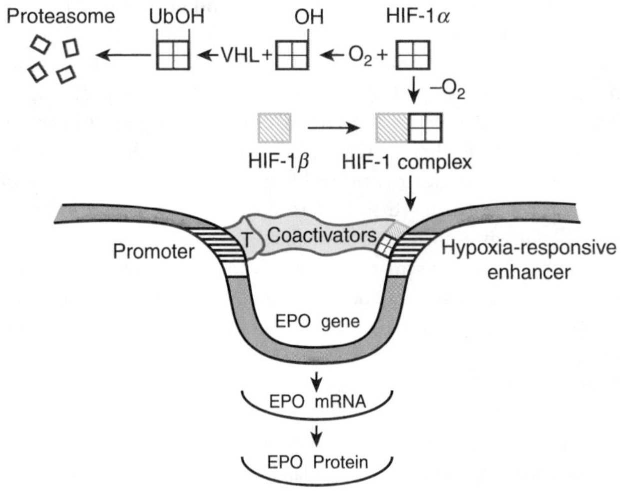

FIGURE 36–4. Molecular control of the *EPO* gene. Schematic of the transcriptional control of the *EPO* gene by the hypoxia-inducible factor 1 (HIF-1) complex. Under normoxic conditions, HIF-1α is hydroxylated (OH) by oxygen- and iron-dependent prolyl-hydroxylase enzymes. Hydroxylated HIF is ubiquinated (Ub) by the von Hippel-Lindau protein (VHL) and degraded by the proteasomal system. During hypoxic or anemic conditions, HIF-1α is not degraded and interacts with HIF-1β to form an active HIF-1 complex that stimulates transcription of the *EPO* gene (EPO mRNA).

overexpress HIF-α proteins and may develop erythrocytosis secondary to increased EPO production.[63] Renal cell carcinomas are usually associated with inactivation of the VHL gene and overexpression of HIF-α proteins.

Extrarenal sites of EPO production exist and account for approximately 15 to 20 percent of total EPO secretion in adult rodents.[64] In humans, very low but still detectable levels of EPO are found in severely anemic anephric individuals (Fig. 36–5),[3] consistent with the presence of extrarenal sites of EPO synthesis. During fetal life, extrarenal production of EPO by the liver predominates, with a gradual change to renal production at birth. In the liver, two types of cells express the *EPO* gene—hepatocytes and the nonparenchymal Ito cells[65–67]—which are morphologically and functionally similar to the interstitial fibroblasts in the kidneys. The genomic determinants of *EPO* gene expression in the kidney are still unclear, but it is known that the kidney requires a 14-kb upstream fragment that is not needed by the liver.[68] Inappropriate production of EPO by renal and extrarenal tumors appears to be accomplished by cells different from those responsible for normal, regulated EPO synthesis. In patients with renal disease, the reduction in EPO production is roughly proportional to the degree of excretory impairment. However, even nonfunctioning kidneys produce some EPO and can maintain hemoglobin levels higher than those found in anephric patients (see Fig. 36–4).[3] The remaining capacity of remnant kidneys to produce EPO is at least partly responsible for the polycythemia (see Chap. 56; postrenal transplant erythrocytosis) that occurs in 10 to 15 percent of patients following kidney transplantation.[69] It also is responsible for the brief but significant increase in EPO levels seen in end-stage uremic patients following episodes of acute hypoxia or blood loss.[70,71]

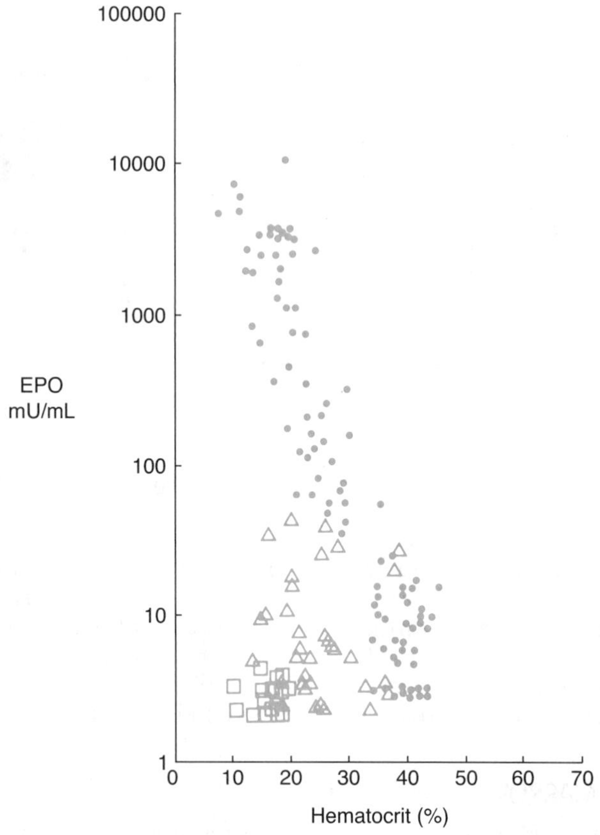

FIGURE 36–5. Circulating EPO levels are decreased in uremic patients. EPO levels in nephric and anephric uremic patients are compared to levels in individuals with intact kidneys. ●, normal subjects and patients with simple anemia; □, anephric patients; △, and uremic-nephric patients. All determinations were made by bioassay of plasma concentrates in hypertransfused mice.[3]

CLINICAL AND LABORATORY FEATURES

The symptoms and physical manifestations of renal failure depend primarily on the underlying disorder. However, anemia almost invariably is present and is of major clinical concern.

■ BLOOD

The anemia is characteristically normocytic and normochromic and is associated with a normal or slightly decreased absolute reticulocyte count for the level of hemoglobin. The blood film usually contains a modest proportion of poikilocytes. Some cells have multiple spicules; others may be microcytic. The former cells, echinocytes or burr cells, were thought to be characteristic of chronic renal failure.[72] However, even normal cells undergo a reversible transformation to burr cell-like echinocytes when exposed to a glass surface or incubated in uremic plasma.[73] Grossly deformed cells, such as acanthocytes with a few large spicules or fragmented schistocytes, are formed in the microcirculation *in vivo*. They are most frequent in the hemolytic uremic syndrome (see Fig. 36–2), but are seen in small numbers on blood films from most uremic patients, especially in the presence of hypertension.

The total and differential leukocyte count and the platelet count are usually normal, but, as with all other hematologic parameters, the underlying disorder plays a modifying role. Uremia and dialysis may have an effect on leukocytes and platelets. The phagocytic activity of granulocytes may be reduced,[74] and complement activation by the hemodialysis membrane may cause pulmonary leukostasis with temporary granulocytopenia.[75] Cell-mediated immunity is depressed, resulting in an increased incidence of infections but also prolonged graft-survival. Platelet function is abnormal and related to the degree of uremia and dialysis. The resulting bleeding tendency may be another pathophysiologic mechanism contributing to anemia.

■ MARROW

The marrow examination is usually normal. The marrow cellularity and proportion of precursors are within the normal range. In effect, marrow erythropoiesis is below that which would be expected if compensation for the anemia occurred.[76] The marrow may be hypocellular or, rarely, even severely hypoplastic.

■ ERYTHROPOIETIN LEVELS

The level of circulating EPO and the iron turnover are within the "normal range," which is inappropriate for the degree of anemia.[3] Iron utilization is regularly decreased in renal insufficiency. Again, these "normal" levels contrast with the increased levels found at similar degrees of anemia but with normal kidney function (see Fig. 36–5). In many cases, the underlying disease causes specific changes in iron kinetics, transferrin, and serum concentrations of folic acid (see Chaps. 41 and 42). These changes modify and aggravate the relative marrow failure that characterize the anemia of chronic renal disease.[77]

THERAPY, COURSE, AND PROGNOSIS

In the past, anemia was often considered a relatively minor problem for patients suffering from the many metabolic consequences of failing kidneys. The development of efficient hospital and home dialysis provided partial relief for many of the metabolic problems, but left the anemia unchanged until recombinant EPO became available.

DIALYSIS

Dialysis per se typically has little effect with regard to correcting the anemia, although a mild increase in hemoglobin concentration may result from the decrease in bleeding tendency. However, for still unexplained reasons, ambulatory peritoneal dialysis may ameliorate and, on occasion, completely correct the anemia.[78]

IRON AND FOLATE SUPPLEMENTATION

Although overt folic acid or iron deficiency may not be evident, these compounds are given routinely to most patients with renal disease. A serum ferritin level of 100 ng/mL must be maintained because effective treatment requires an adequate iron supply to the erythroid precursor cells.

ANDROGEN USE

Androgens had been widely used to stimulate EPO production and action. Even with the advent of appropriate EPO treatment, androgens occasionally are used in apparently resistant patients. Of the many preparations available, nandrolone decanoate[79] and fluoxymesterone[80] usually are effective. However, side effects may occur, and androgen use is now rarely justified given the availability of EPO.

TRANSFUSION THERAPY

Transfusion of red cells may be necessary if there is acute blood loss. Transfusions occasionally are needed to maintain acceptable hemoglobin concentrations in patients who do not respond adequately to EPO.

RECOMBINANT ERYTHROPOIETIN ADMINISTRATION

Replacement therapy with EPO, the most rational approach to treatment of the anemia of renal disease, became a reality in 1987 with the introduction of recombinant human EPO.[81,82] The recombinant product has the same amino acid composition as natural human EPO[83] and an almost identical glycosylation pattern[84]; consequently, antibodies against the recombinant product are rarely found in EPO-treated patients. EPO administration can ameliorate the anemia in almost all patients treated, irrespective of the underlying cause of the renal disorder (Fig. 36–6). The National Kidney Foundation has published detailed guidelines for EPO administration to patients with the anemia of chronic renal diseases.[85] In short, a target hemoglobin (Hgb) level of 11 to 12 g/dL is recommended. The presence of anemia with a hemoglobin of less than 10 g/dL should initiate a thorough search for conditions unrelated to decreased EPO production or action and include measuring iron, iron-binding capacity, ferritin, folic acid, and vitamin B_{12} levels. Determination of EPO levels is not necessary. Complicating chronic illnesses that can aggravate the anemia should be ruled out (see Chap. 37). Because of the availability of venous access in dialysis patients, EPO has been given primarily by the intravenous route. However, pharmacokinetic studies of normal volunteers and patients with chronic renal disease have shown that subcutaneous administration may be equally or more effective.[88,89] The half-life of intravenous EPO is between 6 and 9 hours, with a volume of distribution slightly larger than that of the plasma volume (Fig. 36–7A).[89,90] When the subcutaneous route is used, no peaks are observed, and plasma levels are lower but more sustained (Fig. 36–7B).[91] However, bioavailability after subcutaneous injections appears to be less predictable because of erratic tissue absorption. Subcutaneous EPO administration can maintain a target hemoglobin with use of approximately 30 percent lower doses of EPO.[91,92]

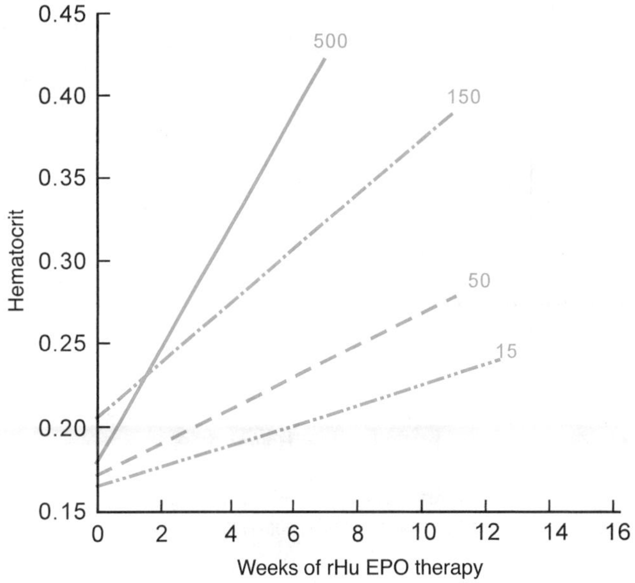

FIGURE 36–6. Erythropoietic response to recombinant human (rHu) EPO therapy in patients with renal disease. The slopes of hematocrit increase in uremic patients after weekly administration of various doses of recombinant EPO. –, 500 units/kg; – · –, 150 units/kg; – – –, 50 units/kg; – ·· –, 15 units/kg. *(Reproduced with permission from Eschbach JW, Egrie JC, Downing MR, et al.[82])*

The FDA recommends that EPO or ESA (erythropoiesis-stimulating agents) be used at the lowest dose to avoid transfusions and not to exceed a hemoglobin of 12g/dL. In addition, the National Kidney Foundation recommends subcutaneous EPO administration as the preferred route, and intravenous, rather than oral, routine iron supplementation to optimize the response. Some physicians have advocated higher-target hemoglobins, close to the normal range, but increased complications and mortality may occur at the near-normal hematocrit range.[93–95] To achieve the target hemoglobin within 3 to 4 months of therapy, the initial EPO dose in adult patients should be 80 to 120 units/kg per week divided into two or three subcutaneous injections or 120 to 180 units/kg per week given as three intravenous injections. The response should be monitored by measuring hematocrit and hemoglobin at least once every 2 weeks. Once the target hemoglobin is reached, most adult patients can be maintained by a total EPO administration of approximately 50 to 100 units/kg per week.[96] Pediatric patients (younger than age 5 years) usually require higher initial and maintenance doses. Newer EPO preparations with a more prolonged plasma half-life have been developed by modifying the sialic content of the EPO molecule (e.g., darbepoetin) or by adding a large methoxy-polyethyleneglycol polymer chain[97] (e.g., continuous erythropoiesis receptor activator [CERA]). Darbepoetin allows for prolongation of the periods between injections, which can now be extended to every 2 weeks. Similar results have been obtained with the pegylated forms where injections at 2- to 4-week intervals are reported to maintain adequate hemoglobin levels.[97]

Other strategies being investigated to stimulate erythropoiesis in renal patients is the use of prolylhydroxylase inhibitors that would stabilize HIF-α proteins and enhance endogenous EPO production.[96] Concern has been raised about the use of these compounds because multiple other genes will also be stimulated. Ultimately, gene therapy using a regulated human *EPO* gene expression system is likely to be

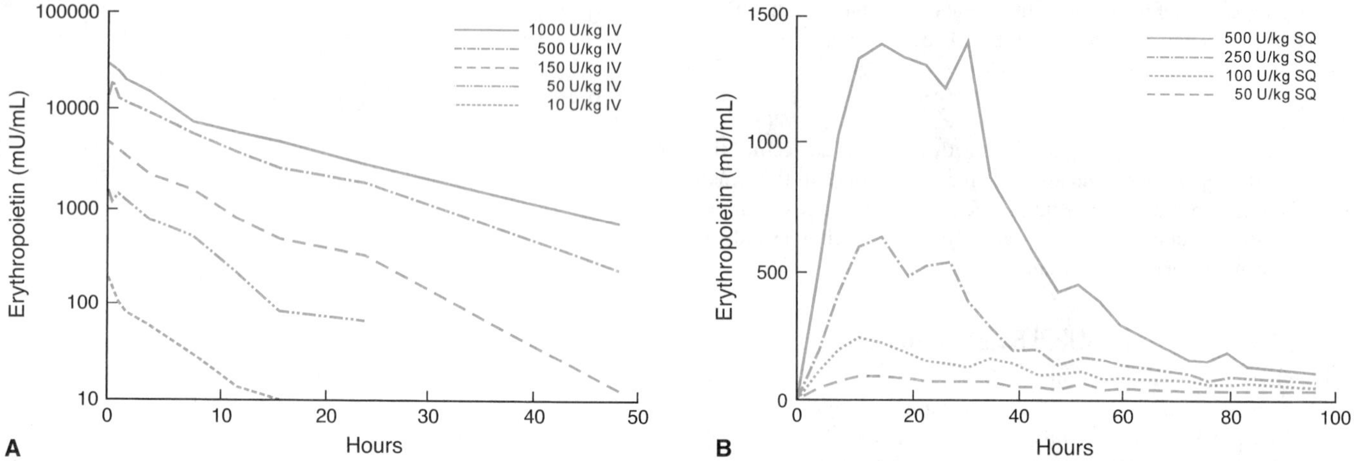

FIGURE 36–7. Pharmacokinetics of plasma EPO in normal volunteers. Plasma concentrations were measured after **(A)** intravenous (IV) administration and **(B)** subcutaneous (SQ) administration. *(Reproduced with permission from Flaherty KK, Caro J, Erslev A, et al.[89])*

used as the ideal treatment for this disease. Anemia in predialysis and dialysis patients can be ameliorated with exogenous EPO and may prevent the development of cardiac hypertrophy without aggravating renal function.[98–100]

Adequate iron supplies must be maintained for sustained erythropoiesis. Intravenous iron is preferred by the National Kidney Foundation because of improved Hgb levels. Many physicians, especially those who administer EPO subcutaneously, prefer an oral iron preparation that provides at least 100 mg of elemental iron per day, although measuring iron is necessary to be sure levels are adequate.[101] The serum iron should be measured at least 24 hours after the previous dose. For patients who are receiving hemodialysis, a diagnosis of absolute or functional iron deficiency should be made before patients are supplemented with intravenous iron. The most widely used criteria include a ferritin level less than 100 mcg/L and/or a transferrin saturation less than 20 percent; however, these recommendations are not based on firm experimental data. A trial showed that patients undergoing hemodialysis who are receiving adequate ESA doses with a Hgb ≤11g/dL, a serum ferritin between 500 and 1200 mcg/mL, a transferrin saturation <25 percent, and who received 1 g sodium ferric gluconate over eight hemodialysis sessions had a better and faster hemoglobin response at 6 weeks of therapy with a mean hemoglobin of 11.9 g/dL compared to 11.3 g/dL.[102] Intravenous iron preparations include iron dextran, iron sucrose, and iron gluconate.[103,104] Ferumoxytol, an iron oxide nanoparticle administered intravenously, has been approved by the FDA for patients with chronic kidney disease.[105] High-molecular-weight iron dextran has a higher rate of anaphylactic reactions (see Chap. 42). Intravenous iron preparations should be administered only by experienced personnel in an appropriate clinical setting.

Hyporesponsiveness to Erythropoietin-Stimulating Agent Treatment

Large multicenter studies show that more than 95 percent of patients respond to EPO therapy. Nevertheless, a small group of patients either do not respond or respond only when larger doses are administered. The most common causes of a poor response are inadequate iron supply, intercurrent infections, inflammatory processes, and splenic red cell sequestration.[106] Aluminum toxicity may be responsible for resistance to treatment and should be suspected in patients with microcytic red cell indices.[107] If the Hgb level is persistently less than 11 g/dL and if ESA doses are greater than EPO 500 IU/kg per week, evaluation for hyporesponsiveness should be carried out.[85] Table 36–1 lists causes of ESA hyporesponsiveness.

Adverse Effects of Erythropoietin

A number of adverse effects were reported during the initial clinical trials, most of which were uncontrolled.[108,109] Some of the adverse effects were not observed in subsequent trials.[110] Hypertension, seizures, thrombosis of arteriovenous fistulas, and high potassium levels in treated patients can occur.[108] Hypertension is the most common complication. It usually represents aggravation of a previously existing condition, but it can occur *de novo*. Blood pressure should be monitored carefully throughout the treatment. Initiation or adjustment of antihypertensive medication and reduction of EPO dosage may be required. Incidence of seizures in patients starting EPO therapy was 3 percent (range: 0–13%); however, the incidence is about the same in EPO-untreated patients.[110] Currently, EPO treatment is not contraindicated in patients with a previous history of seizures. A widespread concern with EPO use is shunt thrombosis in hemodialyzed patients because of higher hematocrits. In a review of 26 studies that enrolled 4100 patients, the average incidence of thrombosis of the access routes in patients receiving EPO was 7.5 percent.[111] This number is well within the accepted values for thrombotic episodes in dialyzed patients who are not receiving EPO. The occurrence of pure red cell aplasia (PRCA)

TABLE 36–1. Common Causes of ESA Hyporesponsiveness
Infection
Cancer, administration of chemotherapy or radiotherapy
Severe secondary hyperparathyroidism
Iron-deficiency anemia
Folate deficiency
Sickle cell anemia
Thalassemia
Hemolytic anemia
Myelodysplastic syndrome

as a result of the development of anti-EPO antibodies initially was very low; only three cases were reported in the first 10 years of EPO use. However, since 1998 the number of reports of patients developing severe anemia as a result of EPO-neutralizing antibodies during the course of EPO treatment have increased.[112,113] Patients with PRCA present with a low absolute reticulocyte count and resistance to EPO treatment. Marrow examinations show a decrease in erythroid precursors. Most of the cases occurred in Europe, and the patients received EPO subcutaneously and most of the patients have responded to immunosuppressive therapy.[113]

The finding of EPO receptors in cells and tissues of nonerythroid origin, including malignant tumors, is potentially important; however, there is no evidence that EPO stimulates tumor growth.[114,115] Several oncology trials show increased mortality with ESA, but the hemoglobin values were at least 13 g/dL and the increased mortality was attributed to cardiovascular complications.[116,117] Despite these caveats, it is clear that amelioration of the anemia has resulted in a variety of beneficial changes[118–120] and has dramatically improved the quality of life of uremic patients.[120–122]

REFERENCES

1. Kalantar-Zadeh K, McAllister CJ, Lehn RS, et al: Effect of malnutrition inflammation complex syndrome on EPO hyporesponsiveness in maintenance hemodialysis patients. *Am J Kidney Dis* 42:761, 2003.
2. Radtke HW, Claussner A, Erbes PM, et al: Serum erythropoietin concentration in chronic renal failure: Relationship to degree of anemia and excretory function. *Blood* 54:877, 1979.
3. Caro J, Brown S, Miller O, et al: Erythropoietin levels in uremic nephric and anephric patients. *J Lab Clin Med* 93:449, 1979.
4. Ragen PA, Hagedorn AB, Owen CA: Radioisotopic study of anemia in chronic renal disease. *Arch Intern Med* 105:518, 1960.
5. Adamson JW, Eschbach J, Finch CA: The kidney and erythropoiesis. *Am J Med* 44:725, 1968.
6. Berry ER, Rambach WA, Alt HL, Del Greco G: Effect of peritoneal dialysis on erythrokinetics and ferrokinetics of azotemic anemia. *Trans Am Soc Artif Intern Organs* 10:415, 1964.
7. Mansell M, Grimes AJ: Red and white cell abnormalities in chronic renal failure. *Br J Haematol* 42:168, 1979.
8. Chillar RK, Desforges JF: Red cell organic phosphates in patients with chronic renal failure on maintenance haemodialysis. *Br J Haematol* 26:549, 1974.
9. Mitchell TR, Pegrum GD: The oxygen affinity of haemoglobin in chronic renal failure. *Br J Haematol* 21:463, 1971.
10. Lichtman MA, Murphy MS, Whitbeck AA, Kearney EA: Oxygen binding to haemoglobin in subjects with hypoproliferative anaemia, with and without chronic renal disease: Role of pH. *Br J Haematol* 27:439, 1974.
11. Lichtman MA, Miller OR, Freeman RB: Erythrocyte adenosine triphosphate depletion during hypophosphatemia in a uremic subject. *N Engl J Med* 280:240, 1969.
12. Torrance JD, Milne FJ, Hurwitz S, et al: Changes in oxygen delivery during hemodialysis. *Clin Nephrol* 3:54, 1975.
13. Lonergan ET, Semar M, Sterzel RB, et al: Erythrocyte transketolase activity in dialyzed patients: A reversible metabolic lesion of uremia. *N Engl J Med* 284:1399, 1971.
14. Yawata Y, Howe R, Jacob HS: Abnormal red cell metabolism causing hemolysis in uremia: A defect potentiated by tap water hemodialysis. *Ann Intern Med* 79:362, 1973.
15. Rosenwund A, Binswanger U, Straub PW: Oxidative injury to erythrocytes, cell rigidity, and splenic hemolysis in hemodialyzed uremic patients. *Ann Intern Med* 82:460, 1975.
16. Eaton JW, Kolpin CF, Swofford HS, et al: Chlorinated urban water: A cause of dialysis-induced hemolytic anemia. *Science* 181:463, 1973.
17. Orringer EP, Mattern WD: Formaldehyde-induced hemolysis in chronic hemodialysis. *N Engl J Med* 294:1416, 1976.
18. Rao DS, Shih M, Mohini R: Effect of serum PTH and bone marrow fibrosis on the response to erythropoietin in uremia. *N Engl J Med* 328:171, 1993.
19. Akmal M, Telfer N, Ansari A, et al: Erythrocyte survival in chronic renal failure: Role of secondary hyperparathyroidism. *J Clin Invest* 76:1695, 1985.
20. Brain MC: The haemolytic-uremic syndrome. *Semin Hematol* 6:162, 1969.
21. Capelli JP, Wesson GL, Erslev AJ: Malignant hypertension and red cell fragmentation syndrome. *Ann Intern Med* 64:128, 1966.
22. Gasser C, Gautier E, Steck A, et al: Hämolytisch-urämische Syndrome: Bilaterale Nierenrindennekrosen bei akuten erworbenen hämolytischen Anämien. *Schweiz Med Wochenschr* 85:905, 1955.
23. Hosler GA, Cusumano AM, Hutchins GM: Thrombotic thrombocytopenic purpura and hemolytic uremic syndrome are distinct pathologic entities. *Arch Pathol Lab Med* 127:834, 2003.
24. Moake JL: Thrombotic microangiopathies. *N Engl J Med* 347:589, 2002.
25. Mitra D, Jaffe EA, Weksler B, et al: Thrombotic thrombocytopenic purpura and sporadic hemolytic-uremic syndrome plasmas induce apoptosis in restricted lineages of human microvascular endothelial cells. *Blood* 89:1224, 1997.
26. Moake JL: Haemolytic-uraemic syndrome. Basic science. *Lancet* 343:393, 1994.
27. Miller RP, Denny WF: Hemolytic anemia during acute renal failure: Observations on plasma erythropoietin levels. *South Med J* 61:29, 1968.
28. Furlan M, Robles R, Galbusera M, et al: Von Willebrand factor–cleaving protease in thrombotic thrombocytopenic purpura and the hemolytic uremic syndrome. *N Engl J Med* 339:1578, 1998.
29. Tsai HM, Lian EC: Antibodies to von Willebrand factor-cleaving protease in acute thrombotic thrombocytopenic purpura. *N Engl J Med* 339:1585, 1998.
30. Lin CC, King KL, Chao YW, et al: Tacrolimus-associated hemolytic uremic syndrome: A case analysis. *J Nephrol* 16:580, 2003.
31. Castaldi PA, Gorman DJ: Disordered platelet function in renal disease, in *Hemostasis and Thrombosis*, edited by RW Colman, J Hirsch, VJ Marder, EW Salzman, p 750. Lippincott, Philadelphia, 1987.
32. Horowitz HI, Stein IM, Cohen BD, White JM: Further studies on the platelet inhibitory effect of guanidinosuccinic acid and its role in uremic bleeding. *Am J Med* 49:336, 1970.
33. Fisher JW: Mechanism of the anemia of chronic renal failure. *Nephron* 25:106, 1980.
34. Bozzini CE, Devoto FCH, Tomio JM: Decreased responsiveness of hematopoietic tissue to erythropoietin in acutely uremic rats. *J Lab Clin Med* 68:411, 1966.
35. Radtke HW, Rege AB, La Marche MB, et al: Identification of spermine as an inhibitor of erythropoiesis in patients with chronic renal failure. *J Clin Invest* 67:1623, 1981.
36. Caro J, Erslev AJ: Uremic inhibitors of erythropoiesis. *Semin Nephrol* 5:128, 1985.
37. Brancaccio D, Cozzolino M, Gallieni M: Hyperparathyroidism and anemia in uremic subjects: A combined therapeutic approach. *J Am Soc Nephrol* 15:S21, 2004.
38. Eschbach JW, Haley NR, Egrie JC, Adamson JW: A comparison of the responses to recombinant human erythropoietin in normal and uremic subjects. *Kidney Int* 42:407, 1992.
39. Erslev AJ, Besarab A: Erythropoietin in the pathogenesis and treatment of the anemia of chronic renal disease. *Kidney Int* 51:622, 1997.
40. Eschbach JW, Cook JD, Schribner BH, Finch CA: Iron balance in hemodialysis patients. *Ann Intern Med* 87:710, 1977.
41. Wills MR, Savory J: Aluminum poisoning: Dialysis encephalopathy, osteomalacia, and anaemia. *Lancet* 2:29, 1983.
42. Rifkind D, Kravetz HM, Knight V, Schade AL: Urinary excretion of iron binding protein in the nephrotic syndrome. *N Engl J Med* 265:115, 1961.
43. Hampers CL, Streiff R, Nathan DG, et al: Megaloblastic hematopoiesis in uremia and in patients on long-term hemodialysis. *N Engl J Med* 276:551, 1967.
44. Erslev AJ: Humoral regulation of red cell production. *Blood* 8:349, 1953.
45. Jacobson LO, Goldwasser E, Fried W, Plazak L: Role of the kidney in erythropoiesis. *Nature* 179:633, 1957.
46. Erslev AJ: *In vitro* production of erythropoietin by kidneys perfused with a serum-free solution. *Blood* 44:77, 1974.
47. Bondurant MC, Koury M: Anemia induces accumulation of erythropoietin mRNA in the kidney and liver. *Mol Cell Biol* 6:2731, 1986.
48. Beru N, McDonald J, Lacombe C, Goldwasser E: Expression of the erythropoietin gene. *Mol Cell Biol* 6:2571, 1986.
49. Schuster SJ, Wilson J, Erslev AJ, Caro J: Physiologic regulation and tissue localization of renal erythropoietin mRNA. *Blood* 70:316, 1987.
50. Lacombe C, DaSilva J-L, Bruneval P, et al: Peritubular cells are the site of erythropoietin synthesis in the murine hypoxic kidney. *J Clin Invest* 81:620, 1988.
51. Koury ST, Bondurant MC, Koury MJ: Localization of erythropoietinsynthesizing cells in murine kidneys by in situ hybridization. *Blood* 71:524, 1988.
52. Maxwell PH, Ferguson DJP, Nicholls LG, et al: Sites of erythropoietin production. *Kidney Int* 51:393, 1997.
53. Maxwell PH, Ratcliffe PJ: The erythropoietin-producing cells. *Exp Nephrol* 4:309, 1996.
54. Schuster SJ, Badiavas E, Costa-Giomi P, et al: Stimulation of erythropoietin gene transcription during hypoxia and cobalt exposure. *Blood* 73:13, 1989.
55. Beck I, Ramirez S, Weinmann R, Caro J: Enhancer element at the 3-flanking region controls transcriptional response to hypoxia in the human erythropoietin gene. *J Biol Chem* 266:15563, 1991.
56. Semenza GL: Hypoxia-inducible factor 1: Master regulator of O_2 homeostasis. *Curr Opin Genet Dev* 8:588, 1998.
57. Salceda S, Caro J: Hypoxia-inducible factor 1alpha (HIF-1alpha) protein is rapidly degraded by the ubiquitin-proteasome system under normoxic conditions. Its stabilization by hypoxia depends on redox-induced changes. *J Biol Chem* 272:22642, 1997.
58. Huang LE, Gu J, Schau M, Bunn HF: Regulation of hypoxia-inducible factor 1alpha is mediated by an O_2-dependent degradation domain via the ubiquitin proteasome pathway. *Proc Natl Acad Sci U S A* 95:7987, 1998.
59. Maxwell PH, Wiesener MS, Chang GW, et al: The tumour suppressor protein VHL targets hypoxia-inducible factors for oxygen-dependent proteolysis. *Nature* 399:271, 1999.

60. Jaakkola P, Mole DR, Tian YM, et al: Targeting of HIF-alpha to the von Hippel-Lindau ubiquitylation complex by O_2-regulated prolyl hydroxylation. *Science* 292:468, 2001.
61. Ivan M, Kondo K, Yang H, et al: HIF-alpha targeted for VHL-mediated destruction by proline hydroxylation: Implications for O_2 sensing. *Science* 292:464, 2001.
62. Epstein AC, Gleadle JM, McNeill LA, et al: *C. elegans* EGL-9 and mammalian homologs define a family of dioxygenases that regulate HIF by prolyl hydroxylation. *Cell* 107:43, 2001.
63. Pastore Y, Jedlickova K, Guan Y, et al: Mutations of von Hippel-Lindau tumor-suppressor gene and congenital polycythemia. *Am J Hum Genet* 73:412, 2003.
64. Erslev AJ, Caro J, Kansu E, Silver R: Renal and extrarenal erythropoietin production in anemic rats. *Br J Haematol* 45:65, 1980.
65. Koury ST, Bondurant MC, Koury MJ, Semenza GL: Localization of cells producing erythropoietin in murine liver by *in situ* hybridization. *Blood* 77:2497, 1991.
66. Schuster SJ, Koury S, Borher M, et al: Cellular sites of extrarenal and renal erythropoietin production in anemic rats. *Br J Haematol* 81:153, 1992.
67. Maxwell PH, Ferguson DJ, Osmond MK, et al: Expression of a homologously recombined erythropoietin-SV40 T antigen fusion gene in mouse liver: Evidence for erythropoietin production by Ito cells. *Blood* 84:1823, 1994.
68. Köchling J, Curtin PT, Madan A: Regulation of human erythropoietin gene induction by upstream flanking sequences in transgenic mice. *Br J Haematol* 103:960, 1998.
69. Dagher FJ, Ramos E, Erslev AJ, et al: Are the native kidneys responsible for erythrocytosis in renal allorecipients? *Transplantation* 28:496, 1979.
70. Walle AJ, Wong GY, Clemons GK, et al: Erythropoietin-hematocrit feedback circuit in the anemia of end-stage renal disease. *Kidney Int* 31:1205, 1987.
71. Eckardt K-U, Druecke T, Leski M, Kurtz A: Unutilized reserves: The production capacity for erythropoietin appears to be conserved in chronic renal disease. *Contrib Nephrol* 88:18, 1991.
72. Schwartz SO, Motto SA: The diagnostic significance of "burr" red blood cells. *Am J Med Sci* 218:563, 1949.
73. Brecher G, Bessis M: Present status of spiculed red cells and their relationship to the discocyte-echinocyte transformation: A critical review. *Blood* 40:333, 1972.
74. Goldblum SE, Reed WP: Host defenses and immunologic alterations associated with chronic hemodialysis. *Ann Intern Med* 93:597, 1980.
75. Craddock PR, Fehr J, Brigham KL, et al: Complement and leukocyte mediated pulmonary dysfunction in hemodialysis. *N Engl J Med* 296:769, 1977.
76. Pasternack A, Wahlberg P: Bone marrow in acute renal failure. *Acta Med Scand* 181:505, 1967.
77. Eschbach JW, Funk D, Adamson JW, et al: Erythropoiesis in patients with renal failure undergoing chronic dialysis. *N Engl J Med* 276:653, 1967.
78. Zappacosta AR, Caro J, Erslev A: The normalization of hematocrit in end-stage renal disease patients on continuous ambulatory peritoneal dialysis: The role of erythropoietin. *Am J Med* 72:53, 1982.
79. Eschbach JW, Adamson JW: Improvement in the anemia of chronic renal failure with fluoxymesterone. *Ann Intern Med* 78:527, 1973.
80. Neff MS, Goldberg J, Slifkin RF, et al: A comparison of androgens for anemia in patients on hemodialysis. *N Engl J Med* 304:871, 1981.
81. Winearls CG, Oliver DO, Pippard MJ, et al: Effect of human erythropoietin derived from recombinant DNA on the anemia of patients maintained by chronic haemodialysis. *Lancet* 2:1175, 1986.
82. Eschbach JW, Egrie JC, Downing MR, et al: Correction of the anemia of end-stage renal disease with recombinant human erythropoietin. *N Engl J Med* 316:73, 1987.
83. Recny MA, Scoble HA, Kim Y: Structural characterization of natural human urinary and recombinant DNA-derived erythropoietin. *J Biol Chem* 262:17156, 1987.
84. Tsuda E, Kawanishi G, Ueda M, et al: The role of carbohydrate in recombinant human erythropoietin. *Eur J Biochem* 188:405, 1990.
85. National Kidney Foundation: KDOQI: Clinical practice guidelines and clinical practice recommendations for anemia in chronic kidney disease. *Am J Kidney Dis* 47(Suppl 3):S11, 2006.
86. National Kidney Foundation: KDOQI: Clinical practice guidelines and clinical practice recommendations for anemia in chronic kidney disease: 2007 Update of hemoglobin target. *Am J Kidney Dis* 50(Suppl 3):471, 2007.
87. Besarab A, Flaharty KK, Erslev A, et al: Clinical pharmacology and economics of recombinant human erythropoietin in end stage renal disease: The case for subcutaneous administration. *J Am Soc Nephrol* 2:1405, 1992.
88. Watson AJ, Gimenez LF, Cotton S, et al: Treatment of anemia of chronic renal failure with subcutaneous recombinant human erythropoietin. *Am J Med* 89:432, 1990.
89. Flaharty KK, Caro J, Erslev A, et al: Pharmacokinetics and erythropoietic response to human recombinant erythropoietin in healthy men. *Clin Pharmacol Ther* 47:557, 1990.
90. Spivak J, Cotes M: Pharmacokinetics of erythropoietin, in *Erythropoietin: Molecular, Cellular, and Clinical Biology*, edited by AJ Erslev, JW Adamson, JW Eschbach, CG Winearls, p 62. Johns Hopkins University Press, Baltimore, MD, 1992.
91. Neumayer HH, Brockmöller J, Fritscka E, et al: Pharmacokinetics of recombinant human erythropoietin after SC administration and in long-term IV treatment in patients on maintenance hemodialysis. *Contrib Nephrol* 76:131, 1989.
92. Kaufman JS, Reda DJ, Fye CL, et al: Subcutaneous compared with intravenous erythropoietin in patients receiving hemodialysis. *N Engl J Med* 339:578, 1998.
93. Besarab A, Bolton WK, Browne JK, et al: The effects of normal as compared with low hematocrit values in patients with cardiac disease who are receiving hemodialysis and epoetin. *N Engl J Med* 339:584, 1998.
94. Singh AK, Szczech L, Tang KL, et al: Correction of anemia with epoetin alfa in chronic kidney disease. *N Engl J Med* 355:2085, 2006.
95. Drueke TB, Locatelli F, Clyne N, et al: Normalization of hemoglobin level in patients with chronic kidney disease and anemia. *N Engl J Med* 355:2071, 2006.
96. Cazzola M: How and when to use erythropoietin. *Curr Opin Hematol* 5:103, 1998.
97. Macdougall IC: Novel erythropoiesis-stimulating agents: A new era in anemia management. *Clin J Am Soc Nephrol* 3:200–207, 2008.
98. Koene R, Frenken LA: Renal function of pre dialysis patients during treatment with human erythropoietin. *Contrib Nephrol* 88:192, 1991.
99. Kuriyama S, Tomonari H, Yoshida H, et al: Reversal of anemia by erythropoietin therapy retards the progression of chronic renal failure, especially in non-diabetic patients. *Nephron* 77:176, 1997.
100. Rossert J, Fouqueray B, Boffa JJ: Anemia management and the delay of chronic renal failure progression. *J Am Soc Nephrol* 14:S173, 2003.
101. Sunder-Plassmann G, Horl WH: Erythropoietin and iron. *Clin Nephrol* 47:141, 1997.
102. Coyne DW Kapoian T, Suki W, et al: Ferric gluconate is highly efficacious in anemic hemodialysis patients with high serum ferritin and low transferrin saturation: Results of the Dialysis Patients' Response to IV Iron with Elevated Ferritin (DRIVE) Study. *J Am Soc Nephrol* 18:975, 2007.
103. Fishbane S: Safety in iron management. *Am J Kidney Dis* 41:18, 2003.
104. Yee J, Besarab A: Iron sucrose: The oldest iron therapy becomes new. *Am J Kidney Dis* 40:1111, 2002.
105. Provenzano R, Schiller B, Rao M, et al: Ferumoxytol as an intravenous iron replacement therapy in hemodialysis patients. *Clin J Am Soc Nephrol* 4:386, 2009.
106. Drueke T: Modulating factors in the hemopoietic response to erythropoietin. *Am J Kidney Dis* 18(Suppl 1):87, 1991.
107. Rosenlof K, Fyhrquist F, Tenhunen R: Erythropoietin, aluminum and anemia in patients on hemodialysis. *Lancet* 335:247, 1990.
108. Casati S, Passerini P, Campise MR, et al: Benefits and risks of protracted treatment with human recombinant erythropoietin in patients having haemodialysis. *Br Med J (Clin Res Ed)* 295:1017, 1987.
109. Eschbach J: The anemia of chronic renal failure: Pathophysiology and the effects of recombinant erythropoietin. *Kidney Int* 35:134, 1989.
110. Buccianti G, Colombi L, Battistel V: Use of recombinant human erythropoietin (rh-EPO) in the treatment of anemia in hemodialysis patients: A multicenter Italian experience. *Haematologica* 78:111, 1993.
111. Laupacis A: Changes in quality of life and functional capacity in hemodialysis patients treated with recombinant human erythropoietin. *Semin Nephrol* 10:11, 1990.
112. Casadevall N, Nataf J, Viron B, et al: Pure red-cell aplasia and antierythropoietin antibodies in patients treated with recombinant erythropoietin. *N Engl J Med* 346:469, 2002.
113. Eckardt K-U, Casadevall N: Pure red-cell aplasia due to anti-erythropoietin antibodies. *Nephrol Dial Transplant* 18:865, 2003.
114. Arcasoy MO, Amin K, Karayal A, et al: Functional significance of erythropoietin receptor expression in breast cancer. *Lab Invest* 82:911, 2002.
115. Brower V: Epoetin for cancer patients: A boon or a danger? *J Natl Cancer Inst* 95:1820, 2003.
116. Leyland-Jones B, Semiglazov V, Pawlicki M, et al. Maintaining normal hemoglobin levels with epoetin alfa in mainly nonanemic patients with metastatic breast cancer receiving first-line chemotherapy: A survival study. *J Clin Oncol* 23:5960, 2005.
117. Henke M, Laszig R, Rube C, et al: Erythropoietin to treat head and neck cancer patients with anaemia undergoing radiotherapy: Randomised, double-blind, placebo-controlled trial. *Lancet* 362:1255, 2003.
118. Moia M, Mannucci PM, Vizotto L, et al: Improvement in the haemostatic defect of uraemia after treatment with recombinant human erythropoietin. *Lancet* 2:1227, 1987.
119. Schaefer R, Kokot F, Heidland A: Impact of recombinant erythropoietin on sexual function in hemodialysis patients. *Contrib Nephrol* 76:273, 1989.
120. Silberberg J, Racine N, Barre P, Sniderman AD: Regression of left ventricular hypertrophy in dialysis patients following correction of anemia with recombinant human erythropoietin. *Can J Cardiol* 6:1, 1990.
121. Evans RW, Rader B, Manninen DL: The quality of life of hemodialysis recipients treated with recombinant human erythropoietin. *JAMA* 263:825, 1990.
122. Adamson JW, Eschbach JW: Erythropoietin for end-stage renal disease [editorial]. *N Engl J Med* 339:625, 1998.

CHAPTER 37
ANEMIA OF CHRONIC DISEASE

Tomas Ganz

SUMMARY

Most patients suffering from chronic infections, chronic inflammations, or some malignancies develop a mild to moderate anemia. This anemia, designated *anemia of chronic disease* or *anemia of inflammation,* is characterized by a low serum iron level, a low to normal transferrin level, and a high to normal ferritin level. The anemia is caused by the inhibitory effects of inflammatory cytokines on erythrocyte production. Among the cytokines, interleukin-6 has a central role, acting by increasing the production of the iron-regulatory hormone hepcidin by hepatocytes. Hepcidin then blocks the release of iron from macrophages and hepatocytes, causing the characteristic hypoferremia associated with this anemia and limiting the availability of iron to the developing erythrocytes. Effective treatment of the underlying disease restores normal erythropoiesis. When this is not possible, and treatment is necessary, therapeutic trials have revealed that the anemia is often responsive to pharmacologic doses of erythropoietin.

DEFINITION AND HISTORY

The terms *anemia of chronic disease* (ACD) or *anemia of chronic disorders* refer to mild to moderately severe anemias (hemoglobin [Hgb] 7–12) associated with chronic infections and inflammatory disorders and some malignancies.[1] The newer name, *anemia of inflammation* (AI), is not only more reflective of the pathophysiology of ACD but also includes *anemia of critical illness,*[2] a condition that presents similarly to *anemia of chronic disease* but develops within days of the onset of illness. An anemia similar to AI is seen in some elderly patients in the absence of a identifiable chronic disease.[3]

AI is characterized by inadequate erythrocyte production in the setting of low serum iron and low iron-binding capacity (i.e., low transferrin) despite preserved or even increased macrophage iron stores in the marrow. The erythrocytes are usually normocytic and normochromic but can be mildly hypochromic and microcytic. Anemia of critical illness[2] can develop acutely (within days) in intensive care settings where the effects of infection or inflammation are exacerbated by disease-related or iatrogenic blood loss or red cell destruction, which by themselves are not sufficiently severe to cause anemia. Anemia of aging[3] is diagnosed in the elderly when a normocytic normochromic anemia with low iron and preserved iron stores develops without an identified underlying disease. Elderly patients in this defined subset typically have an elevated sedimentation rate and/or elevated C-reactive protein (CRP), a high plasma interleukin (IL)-6 concentration, and frailty.

Acronyms and abbreviations that appear in this chapter include: ACD, anemia of chronic disease; AI, anemia of inflammation; CRP, C-reactive protein; EPO, erythropoietin; Hgb, hemoglobin; IDA, iron-deficiency anemia; IL, interleukin; TNF, tumor necrosis factor.

Physicians have known about the pale appearance of patients with chronic infections for hundreds of years. In 19th-century Europe, tuberculosis was the major killer, and the pallor associated with this disease was romanticized in the art literature of the time. The first measurements of red cell mass revealed the association between inflammation and anemia. Discussing "the alterations in the condition of the Blood in Inflammation" in Section 372 of the 1859 edition of the *Principles of Human Physiology*, William B. Carpenter[4] described this connection between inflammation and anemia (author's parentheses): "With this increase in the proportion of fibrin and colorless corpuscles (leukocytes), separately or in combination, there is a diminution of in the proportion of the red corpuscles, albumen and the salts of the blood." In 1961, hundred years later, Maxwell Wintrobe, in the fifth edition of *Clinical Hematology*,[5] used the term "simple chronic anemia" for the normocytic anemia associated with the majority of infections and chronic systemic diseases. He described anemia associated with inflammation as a common subtype. Wintrobe proposed "profound alterations in iron and porphyrin metabolism" as the likely cause, and referred to his own experiments that showed a decrease in erythrocyte survival of only 27 percent, which "could easily be met by increased erythropoiesis if the marrow functional capacity were not impaired." Despite advances in our understanding of the pathophysiology of this very common form of anemia, our knowledge is incomplete.

EPIDEMIOLOGY

The high prevalence of infectious diseases worldwide and the high prevalence of inflammatory and malignant disorders in industrialized countries would suggest that AI is the second or third most common form of anemia after iron-deficiency anemia (IDA) and possibly thalassemia.[6] Although the prevalence of iron deficiency in the industrialized countries is now rapidly decreasing,[6,7] AI is expected to increase as the proportion of the elderly in the population increases. Table 37–1 lists the most common diseases associated with AI.

ETIOLOGY AND PATHOGENESIS

In the chronic setting, AI predominantly results from the body's inability to increase erythrocyte production to compensate for relatively small decrements in erythrocyte survival (reviewed in reference 1). In the steady state, erythrocyte production is sufficiently high so that the resulting anemia is mild to moderate. The anemia associated with acute critical illness has the same pathogenesis as other forms of AI, it develops more rapidly perhaps because of the more extensive erythrocyte destruction and intensive diagnostic phlebotomy common in this setting. The two key questions about the pathogenesis of AI, still only partially answered, are as follows: (1) What accounts for the inability of the AI marrow to increase erythropoiesis? (2) How is this deficit connected to the characteristic hypoferremia and sequestration of iron in macrophages and hepatocytes?

■ RED CELL DESTRUCTION

Human studies indicate that transfused AI erythrocytes have a normal life span in normal recipients but transfused normal erythrocytes have a decreased life span in AI recipients.[1] This finding suggests that increased erythrocyte destruction is caused by the activation of hosts factors such as macrophages that prematurely remove aging erythrocytes from the bloodstream. The explanation is consistent with the predominance of young erythrocytes in AI. Whether extrinsic factors,

TABLE 37–1. Common Conditions Associated with AI

Category	Conditions Associated with AI
Infection	AIDS/HIV, tuberculosis, malaria (contributory), osteomyelitis, chronic abscesses, sepsis
Inflammation	Rheumatoid arthritis, other rheumatologic disorders, inflammatory bowel diseases, systemic inflammatory response syndrome
Malignancy	Carcinomas, myeloma, lymphomas
Cytokine dysregulation	Anemia of aging

such as bacterial toxins and medications, host-derived antibodies, or complement, contribute to this process is unknown.

SUPPRESSIVE EFFECTS OF INFLAMMATION ON ERYTHROPOIETIC PRECURSORS

Some cytokines, chiefly tumor necrosis factor (TNF)-α, IL-1, and the interferons, exert a suppressive effect on erythroid colony formation.[8] The contribution of these mechanisms *in vivo* and the specific pathways that mediate the suppression are not yet known.

INADEQUATE ERYTHROPOIETIN SECRETION AND RESISTANCE TO ERYTHROPOIETIN

The normal response to increased destruction of erythrocytes is transient anemia followed by an increase in erythropoietin (EPO) production and subsequent compensatory increase in erythropoiesis. One proposed explanation for the inadequate marrow response in AI is less EPO production than expected in other types of anemia. Studies of patients with rheumatoid arthritis and AI indicated that EPO levels are increased but less so than in IDA.[9–14] The findings were similar in patients with anemias associated with solid tumors or hematologic malignancies.[15,16] These comparisons did not take into account the potentiating effect of iron deficiency on hypoxia sensing.[17] This effect could increase EPO production in IDA above that in other types of anemia, and make EPO production in AI appear low in comparison. In support of the EPO suppression hypothesis are experiments with EPO-producing cell lines indicate that production of the hormone is inhibited by inflammatory cytokines including TNF-α and IL-1. The inhibition is mediated by the effects of the transcription factor GATA-1 (named after its nucleotide recognition sequence) on the EPO promoter, and the suppression of EPO production can be reversed by a GATA inhibitor.[18] Moreover, both baseline and hypoxia-induced *EPO* gene expression is suppressed in rats treated with bacterial lipopolysaccharide or IL-1β to mimic a septic state.[19] However, suppression of EPO production is not the major mechanism of AI. If it were, administration of relatively small amounts of EPO should be sufficient to reverse the anemia of inflammation. Patients who had renal disease with inflammation, as measured by increased serum CRP greater than 20 mg/L required, on average, 80 percent higher doses of EPO than did patients with simple primary EPO deficiency from renal disease (see Chap. 36 and reference 20). In another study, patients with CRP greater than 50 mg/L reached lower concentrations of hemoglobin than patients with CRP less than 50 mg/L, despite higher doses of EPO.[21] Thus inflammation induces a state of relative resistance to EPO.

ERYTHROPOIESIS RESTRICTION AS A RESULT OF IRON UNAVAILABILITY

Interleukin-6, Hepcidin, and Hypoferremia

Hypoferremia, one of the defining features of AI, develops within hours of the onset of inflammation.[1] Although previous studies of cytokine mediators of hypoferremia of inflammation were inconclusive, subsequent work[22] indicates that the response is dependent on IL-6 which induces the iron-regulatory hormone, hepcidin.[23] Unlike wild-type mice, mice deficient in either hepcidin[24] or IL-6[22] do not become hypoferremic during turpentine-induced inflammation. In human hepatocyte cell cultures, IL-6 is a potent and direct inducer of hepcidin and neither IL-1 nor TNF-α share this activity. The central role of IL-6 is further indicated by the observation that IL-6-deficient mice do not acutely induce hepcidin in response to turpentine inflammation.[22] Infusion of IL-6 into human volunteers induces hepcidin release within hours and causes concomitant hypoferremia.[22] The IL-6–hepcidin axis now appears to be responsible for the induction of hypoferremia during inflammation. However, these studies do not exclude the potential contribution of other cytokines to AI in human diseases or more complex mouse models.

Serum Iron Concentrations Are Dependent on Iron Released from Macrophages and Hepatocytes

In the steady state, almost all of the approximately 20 to 25 mg of iron that daily enters the plasma iron/transferrin pool comes from macrophage recycling of senescent erythrocytes and from hepatocyte iron stores; only about 1 to 2 mg from dietary iron. Only about 2 to 4 mg of iron is bound to transferrin, but the entire daily iron flow transits through this compartment; thus, the iron in this pool turns over every few hours. During inflammation the release of iron from macrophages and probably also from liver stores is markedly inhibited.[25–31] Studies in transgenic mice lacking hepcidin and mice overexpressing hepcidin indicate that the peptide is a negative regulator of iron release from macrophages and of intestinal iron uptake.[32,33] During inflammation, IL-6 induces hepcidin production, which in turn inhibits iron release from macrophages (and probably from hepatocytes), leading to hypoferremia (Fig. 37–1). Hepcidin acts by binding to cell membrane-associated ferroportin molecules that are the only conduits for iron export, and inducing ferroportin internalization and degradation.[34] As hepcidin concentrations increase, less and less ferroportin is available for iron export and the iron release into plasma from macrophages, hepatocytes, and enterocytes decreases.

Erythropoiesis in Anemia of Inflammation Is Limited by Iron

As an intermediate step during the synthesis of heme, iron becomes incorporated into protoporphyrin IX. Zinc is an alternative protoporphyrin ligand. In iron deficiency, the amount of zinc incorporated into protoporphyrin is increased. In AI, zinc protoporphyrin is also increased.[35] In both conditions, insufficient iron reaches the sites of heme synthesis in developing erythrocytes, leading to the substitution of zinc. Moreover, the number of sideroblasts, nucleated erythrocyte precursors that stain for iron with Prussian blue, is decreased in AI.[1] A further indication of the limiting role of iron in patients with AI but no evidence of iron deficiency is that coadministration of parenteral iron can resolve the resistance of AI to EPO.[36,37] Attempts to treat AI with iron alone generally have been unsuccessful, as iron became rapidly trapped in the macrophage compartment.[1,38,39]

Inhibition of Intestinal Absorption of Iron

In long-standing AI, the erythrocytes can become hypochromic and microcytic, partly because progressive depletion of iron stores worsens

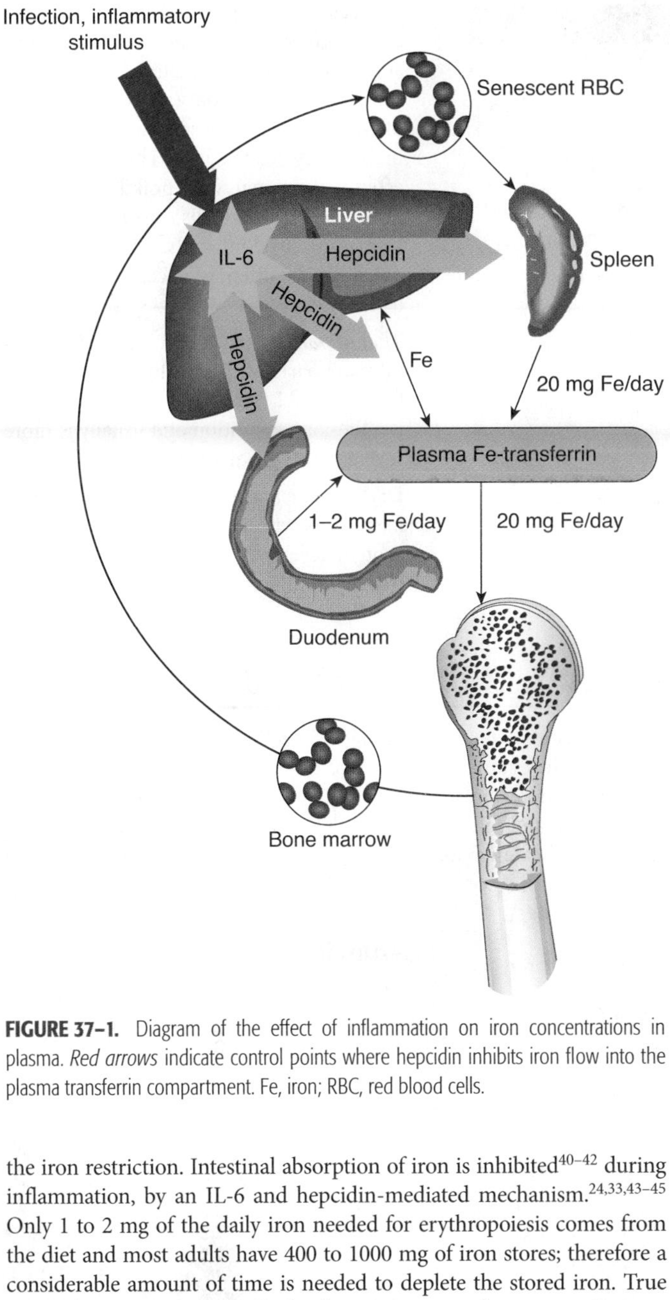

FIGURE 37–1. Diagram of the effect of inflammation on iron concentrations in plasma. *Red arrows* indicate control points where hepcidin inhibits iron flow into the plasma transferrin compartment. Fe, iron; RBC, red blood cells.

the iron restriction. Intestinal absorption of iron is inhibited[40–42] during inflammation, by an IL-6 and hepcidin-mediated mechanism.[24,33,43–45] Only 1 to 2 mg of the daily iron needed for erythropoiesis comes from the diet and most adults have 400 to 1000 mg of iron stores; therefore a considerable amount of time is needed to deplete the stored iron. True iron deficiency can eventually develop in chronic inflammatory diseases, especially in children who have smaller iron stores and additional requirement for iron because of body growth, or in conditions where IL-6 levels are particularly high, such as systemic-onset juvenile chronic arthritis.[46] The anemia in these children was accompanied by an appropriate EPO increase but was unresponsive to oral iron replacement. The anemia was corrected, at least partially, by parenteral iron.

Thus, AI is primarily the result of slightly decreased red cell survival and of macrophage iron sequestration leading to iron-restricted erythropoiesis. In some cases, the condition is compounded by inadequate EPO production, suppressive effect of inflammation on erythropoietic precursors, or depletion of iron stores.

CLINICAL FEATURES

The clinical manifestations of AI usually are obscured by the signs and symptoms of the underlying disease. Moderate anemia (Hgb <10) can exacerbate the symptoms of preexisting ischemic heart disease or respiratory disease, or contribute to fatigue and exertional intolerance. The diagnosis is based on clinical features found in conjunction with typical laboratory abnormalities.

LABORATORY FEATURES

The erythrocytes in AI are usually normocytic and normochromic but, with increasing severity or duration, can become hypochromic and eventually microcytic.[1] The absolute reticulocyte count is normal or slightly elevated.

HYPOFERREMIA AND INCREASED SERUM TRANSFERRIN

Hypoferremia, a decrease in serum iron concentration, is a defining feature of AI. It develops within hours of the onset of infection or severe inflammation. The concentration of the iron-binding protein, transferrin (measured as total iron-binding capacity), is moderately decreased in AI, unlike in IDA, in which transferrin concentration is increased. The decrease in transferrin concentrations develops more slowly than the decrease in serum iron levels because of the longer half-life of transferrin (8–12 days)[47] compared to the half-life of iron (approximately 90 minutes).

INCREASED SERUM FERRITIN

Serum ferritin concentrations, which reflect iron stores and inflammation, are increased in AI but decreased in iron deficiency. Thus, serum ferritin is useful in differential diagnosis in patients with low serum iron concentrations.[48] Depleted iron stores in patients with coexisting inflammation may result in intermediate ferritin levels (Table 37–2 and Fig. 37–2) because ferritin is an acute-phase protein and inflammatory cytokines increase ferritin synthesis. In this situation, iron deficiency should be suspected if ferritin concentrations are less than 60 mcg/L. If the etiology of the anemia remains unclear, the serum transferrin receptor assay[49] may clarify the diagnosis (Table 37–2). Soluble transferrin receptor levels are increased in iron deficiency but, unlike ferritin, are decreased during infection or inflammation.[49]

MARROW IRON STAIN

Marrow aspiration or biopsy is rarely required for the diagnosis of AI. In general, the marrow is normal, unless the underlying disease alters the picture. The most important information obtained from marrow examination is the content and distribution of iron (Chap. 42). Iron in a marrow preparation can be found as storage iron in the cytoplasm of macrophages or as functional iron in nucleated red cells. In normal individuals, a few Prussian blue-staining particles can be found inside or adjacent to many macrophages. Approximately one-third of nucleated red cells contain one to four of these very small blue inclusion bodies and such cells are called *sideroblasts*. Both sideroblasts and macrophage iron are absent in iron deficiency. In contrast, sideroblasts are decreased or absent but macrophage iron is increased in AI. The increase in storage iron in association with a decreased level of circulating iron and a decreased number of sideroblasts is characteristic of AI. Although marrow stain could be considered the gold standard for differential diagnosis of AI and iron deficiency, the discomfort to the patient associated this procedure and the wide availability of the serum ferritin assay have decreased the use of marrow stain in this setting.

TABLE 37–2. Laboratory Studies of Iron Metabolism in Iron Deficiency Anemia and Anemia of Inflammation

	IDA (n = 48)	AI (n = 58)	COMBI (n = 17)
Hemoglobin, g/L	93 ± 16 (96)	102 ± 12 (103)	88 ± 20 (90)
MCV, fl	75 ± 9 (75)	90 ± 7 (91)	78 ± 9 (79)
Iron, μmol/L (10–40)	8 ± 11 (4)	10 ± 6 (9)	6 ± 3 (6)
Transferrin, g/L (2.1–3.4m, 2.0–3.1f)	3.3 ± 0.4 (3.3)	1.9 ± 0.5 (1.8)	2.6 ± 0.6 (2.4)
Transferrin saturation, %	12 ± 17 (5.7)	23 ± 13 (21)	12 ± 7 (8)
Ferritin, mcg/L (15–306m, 5–103f)	21 ± 55 (11)	342 ± 385 (195)	87 ± 167 (23)
TfR, mg/L (0.85–3.05)	6.2 ± 3.5 (5.0)	1.8 ± 0.6 (1.8)	5.1 ± 2.0 (4.7)
TfR/log ferritin	6.8 ± 6.5 (5.4)	0.8 ± 0.3 (0.8)	3.8 ± 1.9 (3.2)

Diagnosis was defined by marrow iron stain and appropriate coexisting disease. Patients with a combination of no stainable marrow iron and either coexisting disease or elevated CRP were classified as "COMBI." Normal ranges for this laboratory for males (m) and females (f) are indicated. Measurements are presented as mean ± SD (median).

SOURCE: Modified from Punnonen K, Irjala K, Rajamaki A,[49] and used by permission.

DIFFERENTIAL DIAGNOSIS

Most patients with chronic infections, inflammatory diseases, or neoplastic disorders are anemic. The diagnosis of AI should only be made if the anemia is mild to moderate, the serum iron and iron-binding capacity are low, and the serum ferritin is elevated. Underlying diseases and their treatments can cause many types of anemia, so other potential causes should be considered.

1. *Drug-induced marrow suppression or drug-induced hemolysis* can complicate infections, inflammatory disorders and cancer. When the marrow is suppressed by cytotoxic drugs or idiopathic toxic reaction, serum iron tends to be high and reticulocyte count low. In hemolysis, reticulocyte counts, haptoglobin, bilirubin, and lactate dehydrogenase often are elevated.

2. *Chronic blood loss* depletes iron stores and decreases serum iron and serum ferritin but increases transferrin (Chap. 42). When AI and chronic blood loss coexist, serum ferritin usually indicates the predominant disorder, although the level can increase as a result of inflammation itself. Testing stool for occult blood and looking for other sources of overlooked blood loss, including phlebotomy and menorrhagia, often identify the source of bleeding. Once this issue is addressed, a successful trial of iron repletion with oral or parenteral iron confirms the diagnosis of combined AI and iron deficiency.

3. *Renal impairment* causes both a deficiency of EPO with resulting decrease of erythropoiesis and a shortened red cell life span (Chap. 36). Although the serum iron level is either normal or high in the anemia of uremia, the diagnosis rests on the finding of increased serum creatinine. AI can coexist with renal failure and should be suspected if there is an underlying inflammatory disorder, there is resistance to EPO therapy, and elevated markers of inflammation such as erythrocyte sedimentation rate or CRP.

4. *Endocrine disorders*, including hypothyroidism and hyperthyroidism, testicular failure and diabetes mellitus, can be associated with a chronic normocytic, normochromic anemia (see Chap. 38). Unless inflammation or associated iron deficiency is present, serum iron should be normal in these disorders.

5. *Anemia resulting from metastatic invasion of the marrow* by tumors can be the presenting symptom of malignancy. The ane-

mia can develop in the setting of a previous diagnosis of carcinoma or lymphoma and by itself is accompanied by normal or increased serum iron (see Chap. 44). It often develops in the setting of preexisting malignancy-related AI. The blood film often is abnormal, with poikilocytes, teardrop-shaped red cells, normoblasts, or immature myeloid cells. Direct marrow examination often is necessary to establish the diagnosis.

6. *Thalassemia* is a common cause of anemia in many parts of the world. It can be confused with AI (see Chap. 47). Microcytosis is a life-long condition and usually is more severe in this group of disorders than in AI.

7. *Dilution anemia* is seen in pregnancy and in patients with severely increased plasma protein levels as a result of myeloma or macroglobulinemia.

THERAPY, COURSE, AND PROGNOSIS

Anemia that presents in the setting of infection, inflammation, or malignancy requires sufficient diagnostic studies to rule out reversible and potentially more threatening causes, such as occult hemorrhage; iron, vitamin B12, and folate deficiency; hemolysis; and drug reaction. If the anemia can be designated as AI after such studies, effective treatment of

Serum ferritin

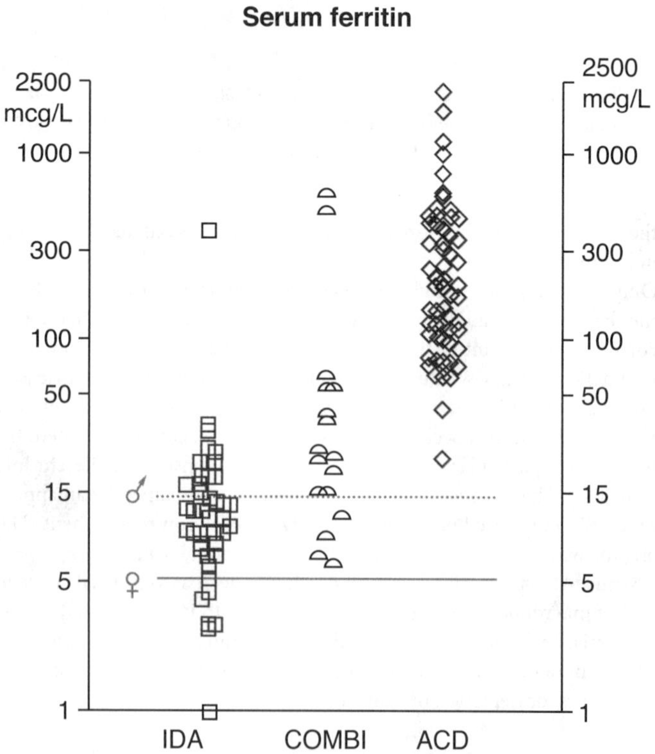

FIGURE 37–2. Distribution of serum ferritin measurements in patients with iron-deficiency anemia (IDA), anemia of chronic disease (ACD = AI), and combined IDA and ACD (COMBI). The horizontal lines indicate lower normal values for healthy men and women. *(Reproduced with permission from Punnonen K, Irjala K, Rajamaki A.[49])*

TABLE 37–3. Treatments of Anemia of Inflammation

Modality	Indications	Typical Setting	Risks and Side Effects	Specific Benefits
Transfusion	Cardiac ischemia Lack of response to other modalities	Hgb <10 g/dL Chest pain and electrocardiogram changes	Infections Volume overload Transfusion reaction	Rapid correction of anemia
Erythropoietin[60]	Fatigue, exertional intolerance	Hgb <10 g/dL Anemia symptoms Balance against side effects in Hgb 10–12 g/dL[61]	Response takes several weeks Rare red cell aplasia with some forms of erythropoietin[67] May worsen outcome in some cancers[68] Increased thromboembolic events[61] Expensive	Usually well tolerated, relatively safe
Iron (oral or parenteral)[37]	Coexisting iron deficiency Resistance to erythropoietin (investigational)	Suspected or documented iron deficiency	Gastrointestinal side effects (oral) Systemic and local reactions (parenteral) May decrease resistance to infections?	Inexpensive, relatively safe

the underlying disease resolves the anemia. If treatment of the underlying disease is not effective and the patient has symptoms or medical complications attributable to anemia, one or more of the available anemia-specific treatment modalities should be considered (Table 37–3).

Acutely, transfusion of erythrocytes is used to correct AI when anemia is moderate to severe and the patient is symptomatic. EPO therapy for the treatment of AI has been tested in the setting of various cancers,[50,51] myeloma and other hematologic malignancies,[16,52,53] rheumatoid arthritis,[54–57] and inflammatory bowel diseases.[58,59] In most reports, more than 50 percent of the patients experienced Hgb increases greater than 2 g/dL. Guidelines for the use of EPO in anemia associated with hematologic and nonhematologic malignancy were published in 2002[60] and updated in 2007,[61] and form a reasonable guide for the EPO treatment of AI. The guidelines (used and quoted here with permission) recommend treating patients with Hgb less than 10 g/dL in whom the treatment of the underlying condition did not alleviate the anemia. For patients with declining Hgb levels but less severe anemia, the decision of whether to use epoetin or darbepoetin immediately or to wait until the Hgb levels fall closer to 10 g/dL should be determined by clinical circumstances (including but not limited to elderly individuals with limited cardiopulmonary reserve, those with underlying coronary artery disease or symptomatic angina, or substantially reduced exercise capacity, energy, or ability to carry out activities of daily living). Because of reports of increased risk of thromboembolism in patients receiving these agents, clinicians should carefully weigh the risks of thromboembolism in patients for whom EPO or darbepoetin are prescribed. The FDA-approved starting dose of epoetin is 150 U/kg three times a week or 40,000 U weekly subcutaneously. The FDA-approved starting dose of darbepoetin is 2.25 mcg/kg weekly or 500 mcg every 3 weeks subcutaneously. Alternative starting doses or dosing schedules have shown no consistent difference in effectiveness on outcomes including transfusion and Hgb response, although they may be considered to improve convenience. Dose escalation should follow FDA-approved labeling; no convincing evidence exists to suggest differences in dose escalation schedules are associated with different effectiveness. Continuing EPO or darbepoetin treatment beyond 6 to 8 weeks in the absence of response (e.g., <1–2 g/dL rise in Hgb), does not appear to be beneficial and EPO therapy should be discontinued. Hgb can be raised to (or near) a concentration of 12 g/dL, at which time the dosage of epoetin or darbepoetin should be titrated to maintain that level. Dose reductions are recommended when Hgb rise exceeds 1 g/dL in any 2-week period or when the Hgb exceeds 11 g/dL. The most specific guidelines for dose reduction are contained in the FDA-approved package insert. Baseline and periodic monitoring of iron, total iron-binding capacity, transferrin saturation, or ferritin levels and instituting iron repletion when indicated may be valuable in limiting the need for EPO, maximizing symptomatic improvement for patients, and determining the reason for failure to respond adequately to EPO.

Coadministration of iron with EPO is a therapeutic strategy based on the idea that iron becomes limiting when marrow production of erythrocytes is stimulated. In some cases, occult iron deficiency coexists with AI.[49,59] In other situations, limited iron stores may become depleted when EPO is initiated.[57] In hemodialysis patients with high ferritin, low transferrin saturation (less than 25%), and above average EPO requirements, iron supplementation of EPO treatment with 1-g loading course (typically 5 treatments of 200 mg) of intravenous ferric gluconate was shown to lead to a small increase in Hgb and decreased dosage of EPO.[62,63] It is not yet certain whether this strategy is applicable to other AI settings.

Existing iron therapies deliver most of the iron to macrophages; only a small percentage of the iron is delivered directly to transferrin.[64] Further studies are needed to determine whether the net effect on the transferrin iron pool is therapeutically important. Pending additional studies, the coadministration of iron with EPO in AI in the absence of demonstrated iron deficiency remains investigational.[37] Concerns exist that iron supplementation in AI increases susceptibility to infections.[65,66]

REFERENCES

1. Cartwright GE: The anemia of chronic disorders. *Semin Hematol* 3:351, 1966.
2. Corwin HL, Krantz SB: Anemia of the critically ill: "Acute" anemia of chronic disease. *Crit Care Med* 28:3098, 2000.
3. Ershler WB: Biological interactions of aging and anemia: A focus on cytokines. *J Am Geriatr Soc* 51:S18, 2003.
4. Carpenter WB: Abnormal forms of the nutritive process-inflammation, in *Principles of Human Physiology,* edited by FG Smith, p 352. Blanchard and Lea, Philadelphia, 1859.
5. Wintrobe MM: *Clinical Hematology,* 5th ed. Lea & Febiger, Philadelphia, 1961.
6. Dallman PR, Yip R, Johnson C: Prevalence and causes of anemia in the United States, 1976 to 1980. *Am J Clin Nutr* 39:437, 1984.
7. Ramakrishnan U, Yip R: Experiences and challenges in industrialized countries: Control of iron deficiency in industrialized countries. *J Nutr* 132:820S, 2002.

8. Means RT Jr, Krantz SB: Inhibition of human erythroid colony-forming units by gamma interferon can be corrected by recombinant human erythropoietin. *Blood* 78:2564, 1991.
9. Baer AN, Dessypris EN, Goldwasser E, et al: Blunted erythropoietin response to anaemia in rheumatoid arthritis. *Br J Haematol* 66:559, 1987.
10. Hochberg MC, Arnold CM, Hogans BB, et al: Serum immunoreactive erythropoietin in rheumatoid arthritis: Impaired response to anemia. *Arthritis Rheum* 31:1318, 1988.
11. Vreugdenhil G, Wognum AW, van Eijk HG, et al: Anaemia in rheumatoid arthritis: The role of iron, vitamin B_{12}, and folic acid deficiency, and erythropoietin responsiveness. *Ann Rheum Dis* 49:93, 1990.
12. Kendall R, Wasti A, Harvey A, et al: The relationship of haemoglobin to serum erythropoietin concentrations in the anaemia of rheumatoid arthritis: The effect of oral prednisolone. *Br J Rheumatol* 32:204, 1993.
13. Noe G, Augustin J, Hausdorf S, et al: Serum erythropoietin and transferrin receptor levels in patients with rheumatoid arthritis. *Clin Exp Rheumatol* 13:445, 1995.
14. Remacha AF, Rodriguez-de la Serna A, Garcia-Die F, et al: Erythroid abnormalities in rheumatoid arthritis: The role of erythropoietin. *J Rheumatol* 19:1687, 1992.
15. Miller CB, Jones RJ, Piantadosi S, et al: Decreased erythropoietin response in patients with the anemia of cancer. *N Engl J Med* 322:1689, 1990.
16. Cazzola M, Messinger D, Battistel V, et al: Recombinant human erythropoietin in the anemia associated with multiple myeloma or non-Hodgkins lymphoma—Dose finding and identification of predictors of response. *Blood* 86:4446, 1995.
17. Safran M, Kaelin WG Jr: HIF hydroxylation and the mammalian oxygen-sensing pathway. *J Clin Invest* 111:779, 2003.
18. Imagawa S, Nakano Y, Obara N, et al: A GATA-specific inhibitor (K-7174) rescues anemia induced by IL-1beta, TNF-alpha, or L-NMMA. *FASEB J* 17:1742, 2003.
19. Frede S, Fandrey J, Pagel H, et al: Erythropoietin gene expression is suppressed after lipopolysaccharide or interleukin-1 beta injections in rats. *Am J Physiol* 273:R1067, 1997.
20. Barany P: Inflammation, serum C-reactive protein, and erythropoietin resistance. *Nephrol Dial Transplant* 16:224, 2001.
21. Macdougall IC, Cooper AC: Erythropoietin resistance: The role of inflammation and pro-inflammatory cytokines. *Nephrol Dial Transplant* 17:39, 2002.
22. Nemeth E, Rivera S, Gabayan V, et al: IL-6 mediates hypoferremia of inflammation by inducing the synthesis of the iron regulatory hormone hepcidin. *J Clin Invest* 113:1271, 2004.
23. Ganz T: Hepcidin, a key regulator of iron metabolism and mediator of anemia of inflammation. *Blood* 102:783, 2003.
24. Nicolas G, Chauvet C, Viatte L, et al: The gene encoding the iron regulatory peptide hepcidin is regulated by anemia, hypoxia, and inflammation. *J Clin Invest* 110:1037, 2002.
25. Freireich EM, Miller A, Emerson CP, et al: The effect of inflammation on the utilization of erythrocyte and transferrin-bound radio-iron for red cell production. *Blood* 12:972, 1957.
26. Haurani FI, Burke W, Martinez EJ: Defective reutilization of iron in the anemia of inflammation. *J Lab Clin Med* 65:560, 1965.
27. O'Shea MJ, Kershenobich D, Tavill AS: Effects of inflammation on iron and transferrin metabolism. *Br J Haematol* 25:707, 1973.
28. Hershko C, Cook JD, Finch CA: Storage iron kinetics. VI. The effect of inflammation on iron exchange in the rat. *Br J Haematol* 28:67, 1974.
29. Zarrabi MH, Lysik R, DiStefano J, et al: The anaemia of chronic disorders: Studies of iron reutilization in the anaemia of experimental malignancy and chronic inflammation. *Br J Haematol* 35:647, 1977.
30. Feldman BF, Kaneko JJ, Farver TB: Anemia of inflammatory disease in the dog: Ferrokinetics of adjuvant-induced anemia. *Am J Vet Res* 42:583, 1981.
31. Fillet G, Beguin Y, Baldelli L: Model of reticuloendothelial iron metabolism in humans: Abnormal behavior in idiopathic hemochromatosis and in inflammation. *Blood* 74:844, 1989.
32. Nicolas G, Bennoun M, Devaux I, et al: Lack of hepcidin gene expression and severe tissue iron overload in upstream stimulatory factor 2 (USF2) knockout mice. *Proc Natl Acad Sci U S A* 98:8780, 2001.
33. Nicolas G, Bennoun M, Porteu A, et al: Severe iron deficiency anemia in transgenic mice expressing liver hepcidin. *Proc Natl Acad Sci U S A* 99:4596, 2002.
34. Nemeth E, Tuttle MS, Powelson J, et al: Hepcidin regulates cellular iron efflux by binding to ferroportin and inducing its internalization. *Science* 306:2090, 2004.
35. Hastka J, Lasserre JJ, Schwarzbeck A, et al: Zinc protoporphyrin in anemia of chronic disorders. *Blood* 81:1200, 1993.
36. Taylor JE, Peat N, Porter C, et al: Regular low-dose intravenous iron therapy improves response to erythropoietin in haemodialysis patients. *Nephrol Dial Transplant* 11:1079, 1996.
37. Goodnough LT, Skikne B, Brugnara C: Erythropoietin, iron, and erythropoiesis. *Blood* 96:823, 2000.
38. Hume R, Currie WJ, Tennant M: Anaemia of rheumatoid arthritis and iron therapy. *Ann Rheum Dis* 24:451, 1965.
39. Beamish MR, Davies AG, Eakins JD, et al: The measurement of reticuloendothelial iron release using iron-dextran. *Br J Haematol* 21:617, 1971.
40. Gubler CJ, Cartwright GE, Wintrobe MM: The anemia of infection. X. The effect of infection on the absorption and storage of iron by the rat. *J Biol Chem* 184:563, 1950.
41. Weber J, Werre JM, Julius HW, et al: Decreased iron absorption in patients with active rheumatoid arthritis, with and without iron deficiency. *Ann Rheum Dis* 47:404, 1988.
42. Weber J, Julius HW, Verhoef CW, et al: Absorption and retention of iron in rheumatoid arthritis. *Ann Rheum Dis* 32:83, 1973.
43. Anderson GJ, Frazer DM, Wilkins SJ, et al: Relationship between intestinal iron-transporter expression, hepatic hepcidin levels and the control of iron absorption. *Biochem Soc Trans* 30:724, 2002.
44. Roe MA, Collings R, Dainty JR, et al: Plasma hepcidin concentrations significantly predict interindividual variation in iron absorption in healthy men. *Am J Clin Nutr* 2009.
45. Young MF, Glahn RP, Riza-Nieto M, et al: Serum hepcidin is significantly associated with iron absorption from food and supplemental sources in healthy young women. *Am J Clin Nutr* 89:533, 2009.
46. Cazzola M, Ponchio L, de Benedetti F, et al: Defective iron supply for erythropoiesis and adequate endogenous erythropoietin production in the anemia associated with systemic-onset juvenile chronic arthritis. *Blood* 87:4824, 1996.
47. Awai M, Brown EB: Studies of the metabolism of I-131–labeled human transferrin. *J Lab Clin Med* 61:363, 1963.
48. Jacobs A, Worwood M: Ferritin in serum. Clinical and biochemical implications. *N Engl J Med* 292:951, 1975.
49. Punnonen K, Irjala K, Rajamaki A: Serum transferrin receptor and its ratio to serum ferritin in the diagnosis of iron deficiency. *Blood* 89:1052, 1997.
50. Ludwig H, Fritz E, Leitgeb C, et al: Prediction of response to erythropoietin treatment in chronic anemia of cancer [see comments]. *Blood* 84:1056, 1994.
51. Smith RE, Tchekmedyian NS, Chan D, et al: A dose- and schedule-finding study of darbepoetin alpha for the treatment of chronic anaemia of cancer. *Br J Cancer* 88:1851, 2003.
52. Dammacco F, Castoldi G, Rodjer S: Efficacy of epoetin alfa in the treatment of anaemia of multiple myeloma. *Br J Haematol* 113:172, 2001.
53. Hedenus M, Adriansson M, San Miguel J, et al: Efficacy and safety of darbepoetin alfa in anaemic patients with lymphoproliferative malignancies: A randomized, double-blind, placebo-controlled study. *Br J Haematol* 122:394, 2003.
54. Peeters HR, Jongen-Lavrencic M, Bakker CH, et al: Recombinant human erythropoietin improves health-related quality of life in patients with rheumatoid arthritis and anaemia of chronic disease; utility measures correlate strongly with disease activity measures. *Rheumatol Int* 18:201, 1999.
55. Peeters HR, Jongen-Lavrencic M, Vreugdenhil G, et al: Effect of recombinant human erythropoietin on anaemia and disease activity in patients with rheumatoid arthritis and anaemia of chronic disease: A randomised placebo controlled double blind 52 weeks clinical trial. *Ann Rheum Dis* 55:739, 1996.
56. Goodnough LT, Marcus RE: The erythropoietic response to erythropoietin in patients with rheumatoid arthritis. *J Lab Clin Med* 130:381, 1997.
57. Kaltwasser JP, Kessler U, Gottschalk R, et al: Effect of recombinant human erythropoietin and intravenous iron on anemia and disease activity in rheumatoid arthritis. *J Rheumatol* 28:2430, 2001.
58. Schreiber S, Howaldt S, Schnoor M, et al: Recombinant erythropoietin for the treatment of anemia in inflammatory bowel disease. *N Engl J Med* 334:619, 1996.
59. Gasche C, Dejaco C, Reinisch W, et al: Sequential treatment of anemia in ulcerative colitis with intravenous iron and erythropoietin. *Digestion* 60:262, 1999.
60. Rizzo JD, Lichtin AE, Woolf SH, et al: Use of epoetin in patients with cancer: Evidence-based clinical practice guidelines of the American Society of Clinical Oncology and the American Society of Hematology. *J Clin Oncol* 20:4083, 2002.
61. Rizzo JD, Somerfield MR, Hagerty KL, et al: Use of epoetin and darbepoetin in patients with cancer: 2007 American Society of Hematology/American Society of Clinical Oncology clinical practice guideline update. *Blood* 111:25, 2008.
62. Kapoian T, O'Mara NB, Singh AK, et al: Ferric gluconate reduces epoetin requirements in hemodialysis patients with elevated ferritin. *J Am Soc Nephrol* 19:372, 2008.
63. Coyne DW, Kapoian T, Suki W, et al: Ferric gluconate is highly efficacious in anemic hemodialysis patients with high serum ferritin and low transferrin saturation: Results of the Dialysis Patients' Response to IV Iron with Elevated Ferritin (DRIVE) study. *J Am Soc Nephrol* 18:975, 2007.
64. Szilagyi G, Erslev AJ: Effect of organic iron compounds on the iron uptake of reticulocytes *in vitro*. *J Lab Clin Med* 75:275, 1970.
65. Jurado RL: Iron, infections, and anemia of inflammation. *Clin Infect Dis* 25:888, 1997.
66. Oppenheimer SJ: Iron and its relation to immunity and infectious disease. *J Nutr* 131:616S, 2001.
67. Rossert J, Casadevall N, Eckardt KU: Anti-erythropoietin antibodies and pure red cell aplasia. *J Am Soc Nephrol* 15:398, 2004.
68. Epoetin: For better or for worse? *Lancet Oncol* 5:1, 2004.

CHAPTER 38

ANEMIA OF ENDOCRINE DISORDERS

Xylina T. Gregg and Josef T. Prchal

SUMMARY

Anemia may be the first manifestation of an endocrine disorder. Anemia caused by endocrine disease is generally mild to moderate; however, a decreased plasma volume in some of these disorders may mask the severity of anemia. It has been proposed that anemia in endocrine-deficiency states may be physiologic because of decreased oxygen requirements, but a direct influence of hormones on erythropoiesis may also contribute to anemia. The pathophysiologic basis of the anemia seen in endocrine disorders may be multifactorial and, thus, not always clear-cut.

THYROID DYSFUNCTION

HYPOTHYROIDISM

Since the 1880s, anemia has been a recognized complication of thyroidectomy[1] and other causes of hypothyroidism.[2] The anemia is usually mild to moderate, with hemoglobin concentrations rarely below 8 to 9 g/dL (80–90 g/L). However, a concomitant decrease in the plasma volume[3] makes the hemoglobin concentration an unreliable indicator of the red cell mass.[4] Dogs subjected to thyroidectomy have a normocytic, normochromic anemia that is associated with reticulocytopenia and marrow erythroid hypoplasia.[5] In humans with hypothyroidism, the associated anemia has been described variably as normocytic, macrocytic, or microcytic;[6] coexisting deficiencies of iron, B_{12}, and folate may explain some of this heterogeneity. Hypothyroidism may contribute to the development of iron deficiency (see Chap. 42) because of an increased predisposition to menorrhagia.[7] Males with hypothyroidism may also be iron deficient, possibly as a result of an associated achlorhydria[8] or because thyroid hormone may augment iron absorption.[9,10] Conversely, iron deficiency impairs thyroid hormone synthesis by reducing the activity of heme-dependent thyroid peroxidase.[11] In patients with coexisting iron-deficiency anemia and subclinical hypothyroidism, the anemia often does not adequately respond to oral iron therapy. In a study in which these patients were randomized to receive 240 mg per day of oral iron alone or 240 mg per day of oral iron plus 75 mcg per day of levothyroxine, the group that received the levothyroxine had statistically significant improvement in the hemoglobin, hematocrit, and ferritin levels.[12]

Although macrocytosis may be seen in uncomplicated anemia of hypothyroidism,[13] significant elevations in the mean corpuscular volume are usually caused by accompanying B_{12} or folate deficiency (see Chap. 41). However, macrocytosis is not a sensitive means of identifying patients with hypothyroidism complicated by B_{12} deficiency.[13] There is an established association of hypothyroidism and pernicious anemia,[14,15] but the underlying mechanism is unknown. In an analysis of 116 hypothyroid patients, 40 percent had low serum vitamin B_{12} levels.[16] Although the mean hemoglobin was slightly lower in the B_{12}-deficient group (11.9 g/L vs. 12.4 g/L), the mean corpuscular volume and prevalence of antithyroid antibodies did not differ between the two groups.

However, when iron deficiency, B_{12} deficiency, and other confounding causes of anemia have been excluded, anemia is also a direct consequence of thyroid hormone deficiency.[17] In hypothyroid humans and thyroidectomized animals, the red cell life span is normal, and results of ferrokinetic studies are compatible with hypoproliferative erythropoiesis.[5,18] Administration of thyroid hormones increases the rate of red cell production in experimental animals,[19] whereas thyroidectomy decreases red cell production.[20] Because thyroid hormones affect the cellular needs for oxygen, these responses are compatible with an appropriate physiologic adjustment. Evidence of a direct effect of thyroid hormones on erythropoiesis exists. *In vitro* studies have shown that triiodothyronine (T_3), and thyroxine (T_4), and noncalorigenic resin triiodothyronine (rT_3) all potentiate the effect of erythropoietin on erythroid colony formation.[21] Thyroid hormones also increase hypoxia-induced production of erythropoietin in the rat kidney and a human hepatoma cell line.[22] Other *in vitro* studies have shown an inhibitory effect of T_3 on erythroid colony formation, particularly in combination with all-*trans* retinoic acid.[23]

The response to thyroid hormone therapy is gradual. Slow improvement in the hemoglobin concentration is seen over a several-month period.[13] White blood cell and platelet counts usually are unaffected in hypothyroidism. However, pancytopenia in association with marrow hypoplasia has been reported in a patient with myxedema coma; the hematologic abnormalities in this patient resolved with thyroid hormone replacement.[24]

HYPERTHYROIDISM

Although thyroid hormone administration increases red cell production in animals,[19] humans with hyperthyroidism generally do not have polycythemia. Anemia is present in 10 to 25 percent of these patients.[25–27] This finding may be the result of increased plasma volume;[3] however, decreased red cell survival[28] and ineffective erythropoiesis[29] also have been described. Patients with Graves disease who were also anemic had higher erythropoietin and lower total iron-binding capacity levels than did the nonanemic patients, but C-reactive protein and ferritin levels did not differ.[27] Antithyroid treatment ameliorates the anemia.[26,27] A patient with autoimmune hemolytic anemia and hyperthyroidism has been described; the hemolysis in this patient abated with treatment of the hyperthyroidism.[30] Pancytopenia rarely occurs but also may respond to treatment of hyperthyroidism.[31,32]

ADRENAL CORTICAL INSUFFICIENCY AND CUSHING SYNDROME

A normocytic normochromic anemia may be seen in primary adrenal insufficiency (Addison disease),[33,34] but the anemia may also be masked by the concomitant reduction in plasma volume that is common in this disease. In a series of patients with Addison disease, untreated patients had normal hemoglobin levels but developed transient anemia after initiation of hormone replacement therapy (presumably secondary to an increased plasma volume).[35]

In experimental animals, adrenalectomy causes a mild anemia that responds to glucocorticoids or erythropoietin.[33,36] The pathophysiologic basis of the anemia and any influence of adrenal cortical hormones on erythropoiesis are not well defined.

Glucocorticoids interact with erythropoietin *in vitro* to enhance erythroid colony proliferation.[37] Glucocorticoid receptors, activated by their cognate ligand, initiate Janus kinase 2 phosphorylation-mediated

Acronyms and abbreviations used in this chapter include: ACTH, adrenocorticotropic hormone; AZT, azidothymidine; T_3, triiodothyronine; T_4, thyroxine.

cytoplasmic signal transduction, which may stimulate erythropoiesis by a mechanism shared with erythropoietin (see Chaps. 31 and 56). Polycythemia has been reported in Cushing syndrome,[38] primary aldosteronism,[39] and Bartter syndrome.[40]

Pheochromocytomas are rarely associated with polycythemia. This finding is believed to be a result of autonomous erythropoietin production by the tumor,[41] often mediated by von Hippel-Lindau mutations that cause or contribute to pheochromocytoma development (see Chap. 56). A syndrome of congenital polycythemia associated with a mutation in the proline hydroxylase type 2 gene and development of pheochromocytoma also has been described.[42]

Pernicious anemia occurs in patients with autoimmune adrenal insufficiency, but is seen primarily in patients with type I polyglandular autoimmune syndrome, whose other manifestations include mucocutaneous candidiasis and hypoparathyroidism.[43] Anemia as a result of primary erythropoietin deficiency was reported in one patient with this syndrome.[44]

ANDROGEN DEFICIENCY

Sexually mature males have higher hemoglobin levels than prepubertal males, older males, and females.[45] The difference is attributed to androgen production. Orchiectomy results in a median decrease in hemoglobin concentration of 1.2 g/dL (12 g/L).[46] "Medical" castration with combined androgen blockade by gonadotropin-releasing agonists and antiandrogens also causes anemia, albeit relatively mild.[47]

The erythropoietic effects of androgens are well documented[48] and have been widely exploited for the treatment of various anemias, especially before the development of recombinant erythropoietin. Androgen therapy reverses anemia and may even cause polycythemia.[48] Testosterone therapy in hypogonadal men increased the mean hematocrit from 38.0 percent to 43.1 percent within 3 months.[49] The mechanism of androgen action appears to be complex, with evidence for stimulation of erythropoietin secretion[50] and a direct effect on the marrow.[51] Androgen receptors have been identified in the marrow cells of human males and females. The cells expressing the receptors included stromal cells, endothelial cells, macrophages, and myeloid precursors, but not erythroid cells.[52]

Estrogens may have a suppressive effect on erythropoiesis. Exogenous administration of large doses of estrogen led to moderately severe anemia.[53,54]

PITUITARY INSUFFICIENCY

The most common cause of pituitary insufficiency is pituitary tumors or consequences of their therapy.[55] Other etiologies include hypothalamic tumors or dysfunction, sarcoidosis or other infiltrative diseases, pituitary hemorrhage or infarct, genetic causes, and idiopathic pituitary failure. Regardless of the cause, hypopituitarism results in a moderately severe normochromic normocytic anemia, with an average hemoglobin of 10 g/dL (100 g/L).[33,56] Anemia and erythroid hypoplasia have also been described in hypophysectomized animals.[57,58]

In rats, removal of the posterior lobe of the pituitary, which secretes vasopressin and oxytocin, does not result in anemia.[59] Thus, the anemia of hypopituitarism presumably results from the absence of the anterior lobe hormones, adrenocorticotropic hormone (ACTH), thyroid-stimulating hormone, follicle-stimulating hormone, luteinizing hormone, growth hormone, and prolactin, although the exact role of each of these hormones in the pathogenesis of anemia is unknown. The resulting deficiencies of thyroid hormones, adrenal hormones, and androgens are likely the major contributors to anemia. Combined adrenalectomy and thyroidectomy in animals results in an anemia that is similar but not identical to that seen after hypophysectomy.[60] A correlation between low testosterone levels and anemia has been observed in human males with hypopituitarism resulting from nonfunctioning pituitary adenomas.[61] The data regarding the role of growth hormone are conflicting. Growth hormone stimulates erythropoietin-induced erythropoiesis *in vitro*.[62,63] Children with isolated growth hormone deficiency become anemic.[64] Growth hormone replacement therapy in patients with growth hormone deficiency increased hemoglobin levels in some studies but not in others.[65,66] Limited information about the influence of prolactin is available.[67] Prolactin administration in mice increased the number of erythroid and myeloid progenitor cells and partially corrected anemia induced by azidothymidine (AZT).[68] Metoclopramide, which stimulates prolactin secretion, improved hemoglobin levels or reduced transfusions in three of nine patients with Diamond-Blackfan anemia.[69] The prolactin receptor can substitute for the erythropoietin receptor in *in vitro* studies of erythroid differentiation.[70,71]

Red cell survival is normal in hypopituitarism, but the marrow is hypoplastic. The results of ferrokinetic studies are consistent with decreased erythropoiesis.[33,72] In addition to anemia, leukopenia and even pancytopenia can occur.[73] Replacement therapy with a combination of thyroid, adrenal, and gonadal hormones usually effectively corrects anemia and other cytopenias.[73,74] Erythropoietin therapy also was effective in one case of postoperative hypopituitarism refractory to hormone replacement therapy.[75]

HYPERPARATHYROIDISM

Anemia not attributable to other causes is present in 3 to 5 percent of patients with primary hyperparathyroidism; these patients usually have severe hyperparathyroidism.[76,77] The anemia is normochromic and normocytic and resolves or improves after parathyroidectomy.[76,77] The cause of the anemia is unknown; marrow fibrosis has been described in a few patients,[76] but is not invariably present.

Although anemia in patients with renal failure is multifactorial, secondary hyperparathyroidism may contribute to refractoriness to erythropoietin therapy. Parathyroidectomy or medical treatment of hyperparathyroidism may improve anemia and decrease requirements for exogenous erythropoietin therapy.[78–80]

REFERENCES

1. Kocher T: Ueber Kropfexstirpation und Ihre Folgen. *Arch Klin Chir* 29:254, 1883.
2. Charcot M: Myxedéme, cachexie pachydermique ou état cretinoide. *Gaz Hop Paris* 54:73, 1881.
3. Muldowney F, Crooks J, Wayne E: The total red cell mass in thyrotoxicosis and myxoedema. *Clin Sci* 16:309, 1957.
4. Das K, Mukherjee M, Sarkar T, et al: Erythropoiesis and erythropoietin in hypo- and hyperthyroidism. *J Clin Endocrinol Metab* 40:211, 1975.
5. Cline M, Berlin N: Erythropoiesis and red cell survival in the hypothyroid dog. *Am J Physiol* 204:415, 1963.
6. Bomford R: Anemia in myxodedem and the role of the thryoid gland in erythropoiesis. *Q J Med* 7:495, 1938.
7. Goldsmith R: The menstrual pattern in thyroid disease. *J Clin Endocrinol Metab* 12:846, 1952.
8. Lerman J, Means J: The gastric secretion in exophthalmic goiter and myxoedema. *J Clin Invest* 11:167, 1932.
9. Pirzio-Biroli G, Bothwell T, Finch C: Iron absorption: II. The absorption of radio iron adminstered with standard meal. *J Lab Clin Med* 51:37, 1958.
10. Donati RM, Fletcher JW, Warnecke MA, et al: Erythropoiesis in hypothyroidism. *Proc Soc Exp Biol Med* 144:78, 1973.
11. Zimmermann M, Kohrle J: The impact of iron and selenium deficiencies on iodine and thyroid metabolism: biochemistry and relevance to public health. *Thyroid* 12:867, 2002.
12. Cinemre H, Bilir C, Gokosmanoglu F, et al: Hematologic effects of levothyroxine in iron-deficient subclinical hypothyroid patients: a randomized, double-blind, controlled study. *J Clin Endocrinol Metab* 94:151, 2009.
13. Horton L, Coburn R, England J, et al: The haematology of hypothyroidism. *Q J Med* 45:101, 1976.

14. Green ST, Ng JP, Chan-Lam D: Insulin-dependent diabetes mellitus, myasthenia gravis, pernicious anaemia, autoimmune thyroiditis and autoimmune adrenalitis in a single patient. *Scott Med J* 33:213, 1988.
15. Carmel R, Spencer CA: Clinical and subclinical thyroid disorders associated with pernicious anemia. Observations on abnormal thyroid-stimulating hormone levels and on a possible association of blood group O with hyperthyroidism. *Arch Intern Med* 142:1465, 1982.
16. Jabbar A, Yawar A, Waseem S, et al: Vitamin B12 deficiency common in primary hypothyroidism. *J Pak Med Assoc* 58:258, 2008.
17. Hines JD, Halsted CH, Griggs RC, et al: Megaloblastic anemia secondary to folate deficiency associated with hypothyroidism. *Ann Intern Med* 68:792, 1968.
18. Kiely JM, Purnell DC, Owen CA Jr: Erythrokinetics in myxedema. *Ann Intern Med* 67:533, 1967.
19. Shalet M, Coe D, Reissmann KR: Mechanism of erythropoietic action of thyroid hormone. *Proc Soc Exp Biol Med* 123:443, 1966.
20. Gordon A, Kadow P, Finkelstein G, et al: The thyroid and blood regeneration in the rat. *Am J Med Sci* 212:385, 1946.
21. Golde D, Bersch N, Chopra I, et al: Thyroid hormones stimulate erythropoiesis in vitro. *Br J Haematol* 37:173, 1977.
22. Fandrey J, Pagel H, Frede S, et al: Thyroid hormones enhance hypoxia-induced erythropoietin production in vitro. *Exp Hematol* 22:272, 1994.
23. Perrin M, Blanchet J, Mouchiroud G: Modulation of human and mouse erythropoiesis by thyroid hormone and retinoic acid: Evidence for specific effects at different steps of the erythroid pathway. *Hematol Cell Ther* 39:19, 1997.
24. Song S, McCallum C, Campbell I: Hypoplastic anaemia complicating myxoedema coma. *Scott Med J* 43:149, 1998.
25. Nightingale S, Vitek PJ, Himsworth RL: The haematology of hyperthyroidism. *Q J Med* 47:35, 1978.
26. Perlman J, Sternthal P: Effect of 131I on the anemia of hyperthyroidism. *J Chronic Dis* 36:405, 1983.
27. Gianoukakis AG, Leigh MJ, Richards P, et al: Characterization of the anaemia associated with Graves' disease. *Clinical Endocrinology* 70:781, 2009.
28. McClellan J, Donegan C, Thorup OA, et al: Survival time of the erythrocyte in myxedema and hyperthyroidism. *J Lab Clin Med* 51:91, 1958.
29. Donati RM, Warnecke MA, Gallagher NI: Ferrokinetics in hyperthyroidism. *Ann Intern Med* 63:945, 1965.
30. Gianoukakis AG, Leigh MJ, Richards P, et al: Characterization of the anemia associated with Graves' disease. *Clin Endocrinol (Oxf)* 2008.
31. Ogihara T, Katoh H, Yoshitake H, et al: Hyperthyroidism associated with autoimmune hemolytic anemia and periodic paralysis: a report of a case in which antihyperthyroid therapy alone was effective against hemolysis. *Jpn J Med* 26:401, 1987.
32. Lima CS, Zantut Wittmann DE, Castro V, et al: Pancytopenia in untreated patients with Graves' disease. *Thyroid* 16:403, 2006.
33. Akoum R, Michel S, Wafic T, et al: Myelodysplastic syndrome and pancytopenia responding to treatment of hyperthyroidism: Peripheral blood and bone marrow analysis before and after antihormonal treatment. *J Cancer Res Ther* 3:43, 2007.
34. Daughaday W, Williams R, Daland G: The effect of endocrinopathies on the blood. *Blood* 3:1342, 1948.
35. Baez-Villasenor J, Rath C, Finch C: The blood picture in Addison's disease. *Blood* 3:769, 1958.
36. Irvine WJ, Stewart AG, Scarth L: A clinical and immunological study of adrenocortical insufficiency (Addison's disease). *Clin Exp Immunol* 2:31, 1967.
37. Van Dyke DC, Contopoulos AN, Williams BS, et al: Hormonal factors influencing erythropoiesis. *Acta Haematol* 11:203, 1954.
38. von Lindern M, Zauner W, Mellitzer G, et al: The glucocorticoid receptor cooperates with the erythropoietin receptor and c-Kit to enhance and sustain proliferation of erythroid progenitors in vitro. *Blood* 94:550, 1999.
39. Plotz CM, Knowlton AI, Ragan C: The natural history of Cushing's syndrome. *Am J Med* 13:597, 1952.
40. Mann DL, Gallagher NI, Donati RM: Erythrocytosis and primary aldosteronism. *Ann Intern Med* 66:335, 1967.
41. Erkelens DW, Statius van Eps LW: Bartter's syndrome and erythrocytosis. *Am J Med* 55:711, 1973.
42. Drenou B, Le Tulzo Y, Caulet-Maugendre S, et al: Pheochromocytoma and secondary erythrocytosis: role of tumour erythropoietin secretion. *Nouv Rev Fr Hematol* 37:197, 1995.
43. Ladroue C, Carcenac R, Leporrier M, et al: PHD2 mutation and congenital erythrocytosis with paraganglioma. *N Engl J Med* 359:2685, 2008.
44. Eisenbarth GS, Gottlieb PA: Autoimmune Polyendocrine Syndromes. *N Engl J Med* 350:2068, 2004.
45. Toonkel R, Levine M, Gardner L: Erythropoietin-deficient anemia associated with autoimmune polyglandular syndrome type I. *Am J Hematol* 75:84, 2004.
46. Hawkins WW, Speck E, Leonard VG: Variation of the hemoglobin level with age and sex. *Blood* 9:999, 1954.
47. Fonseca R, Rajkumar SV, White WL, et al: Anemia after orchiectomy. *Am J Hematol* 59:230, 1998.
48. Bogdanos J, Karamanolakis D, Milathianakis C, et al: Combined androgen blockade-induced anemia in prostate cancer patients without bone involvement. *Anticancer Res* 23:1757, 2003.
49. Shahidi NT: Androgens and erythropoiesis. *N Engl J Med* 289:72, 1973.
50. Snyder P, Peachey H, Berlin J, et al: Effects of testosterone replacement in hypogonadal men. *J Clin Endocrinol Metab* 85:2670, 2000.
51. Alexanian R: Erythropoietin and erythropoiesis in anemic man following androgens. *Blood* 33:564, 1969.
52. Beran M, Spitzer G, Verma D: Testosterone and synthetic and androgens improve the in vitro survival of human marrow progenitor cells in serum-free suspension cultures. *J Lab Clin Med* 99:247, 1982.
53. Mantalaris A, Panoskaltsis N, Sakai Y, et al: Localization of androgen receptor expression in human bone marrow. *J Pathol* 193:361, 2001.
54. Dukes PP, Goldwasser E: Inhibition of erythropoiesis by estrogens. *Endocrinology* 69:21, 1961.
55. Piliero SJ, Medici PT, Haber C: The interrelationships of the endocrine and erythropoietic systems in the rat with special reference to the mechanism of action of estradiol and testosterone. *Ann N Y Acad Sci* 149:336, 1968.
56. Bates A, Van't Hoff W, Jones P, et al: The effect of hypopituitarism on life expectancy. *J Clin Endocrinol Metab* 81:1169, 1996.
57. Grieg H, Metz J, Sunn L: Anemia in hypopituitarism: Treatment with testosterone and cortisone. *S Afr J Lab Clin Med* 2:52, 1956.
58. Crafts RC, Meineke HA: The anemia of hypophysectomized animals. *Ann N Y Acad Sci* 77:501, 1959.
59. Berlin NI, Van Dyke DC, Siri WE, et al: The effect of hypophysectomy on the total circulating red cell volume of the rat. *Endocrinology* 47:429, 1950.
60. Van Dyke DC, Garcia JF, Simpson ME, et al: Maintenance of circulating red cell volume in rats after removal of the posterior and intermediate lobes of the pituitary. *Blood* 7:1005, 1952.
61. Crafts RC: The similarity between anemia induced by hypophysectomy and that induced by a combined thyroidectomy and adrenalectomy in adult female rats. *Endocrinology* 53:465, 1953.
62. Ellegala D, Alden T, Couture D, et al: Anemia, testosterone, and pituitary adenoma in men. *J Neurosurg* 98:974, 2003.
63. Merchav S, Tatarsky I, Hochberg Z: Enhancement of erythropoiesis in vitro by human growth hormone is mediated by insulin-like growth factor I. *Br J Haematol* 70:267, 1988.
64. Golde DW, Bersch N, Li CH: Growth hormone: species-specific stimulation of erythropoiesis in vitro. *Science* 196:1112, 1977.
65. Eugster E, Fisch M, Walvoord E, et al: Low hemoglobin levels in children with in idiopathic growth hormone deficiency. *Endocrine* 18:135, 2002.
66. Ten Have SM, van der Lely AJ, Lamberts SW: Increase in haemoglobin concentrations in growth hormone deficient adults during human recombinant growth hormone replacement therapy. *Clinical Endocrinology* 47:565, 1997.
67. Bergamaschi S, Giavoli C, Ferrante E, et al: Growth hormone replacement therapy in growth hormone deficient children and adults: Effects on hemochrome. *J Endocrinol Invest* 29:399, 2006.
68. Jepson JH, Lowenstein L: Effect of prolactin on erythropoiesis in the mouse. *Blood* 24:726, 1964.
69. Woody M, Welniak L, Sun R, et al: Prolactin exerts hematopoietic growth-promoting effects in vivo and partially counteracts myelosuppression by azidothymidine. *Exp Hematol* 27:811, 1999.
70. Abkowitz JL, Schaison G, Boulad F, et al: Response of Diamond-Blackfan anemia to metoclopramide: Evidence for a role for prolactin in erythropoiesis. *Blood* 100:2687, 2002.
71. Socolovsky M, Fallon A, Lodish H: The prolactin receptor rescues EpoR-/- erythroid progenitors and replaces EpoR in a synergistic interaction with c-kit. *Blood* 92:1491, 1998.
72. Socolovsky M, Dusanter-Fourt I, Lodish H: The prolactin receptor and severely truncated erythropoietin receptors support differentiation of erythroid progenitors. *J Biol Chem* 272:14009, 1997.
73. Degrossi O, Houssay A, Varela J, et al: Erythrokinetic studies in the anemia of thyroid and pituitary insufficiency, in *Advances in Thyroid Research,* edited by R Pitt-Rivers, p 410. Pergamon, New York, 1961.
74. Kim D, Kim J, Park Y, et al: Case of complete recovery of pancytopenia after treatment of hypopituitarism. *Ann Hematol* 83:309, 2004.
75. Ferrari E, Ascari E, Bossolo PA, et al: Sheehan's syndrome with complete bone marrow aplasia: long-term results of substitution therapy with hormones. *Br J Haematol* 33:575, 1976.
76. Nomiyama J, Shinohara K, Inoue H: Improvement of anemia by recombinant erythropoietin in a patient with postoperative hypopituitarism. *Am J Hematol* 47:249, 1994.
77. Boxer M, Ellman L, Geller R, et al: Anemia in primary hyperparathyroidism. *Arch Intern Med* 137:588, 1977.
78. Abarca J, Trigonis C, Hamberger B, et al: Anaemia in primary hyperparathyroidism—Fantasy or reality. *Ann Chir Gynaecol* 74:74, 1985.
79. Barbour GL: Effect of parathyroidectomy on anemia in chronic renal failure. *Arch Intern Med* 139:889, 1979.
80. Argiles A, Mourad G, Lorho R, et al: Medical treatment of severe hyperparathyroidism and its influence on anaemia in end-stage renal failure. *Nephrol Dial Transplant* 9:1809, 1994.
81. Trunzo JA, McHenry CR, Schulak JA, et al: Effect of parathyroidectomy on anemia and erythropoietin dosing in end-stage renal disease patients with hyperparathyroidism. *Surgery* 144:915, 2008.

CHAPTER 39

THE CONGENITAL DYSERYTHROPOIETIC ANEMIAS

Jean Delaunay*

SUMMARY

The congenital dyserythropoietic anemias are a heterogeneous group of uncommon disorders characterized by anemia, the presence of multinuclear erythroid precursors in the marrow, ineffective erythropoiesis, and iron overload. Only the erythroid series shows significant abnormalities, with rare exceptions. Patients have been classified as types I, II, and III, but some patients who appear to fit into the general category of congenital dyserythropoietic anemias do not fit into any of these three groups. Types I and II congenital dyserythropoietic anemias are inherited as autosomal recessive disorders, and type III disease is transmitted as a dominant disorder. Type I disease is caused by mutations of the *CDAN1* gene. Codanin-1, the gene product, is a cell-cycle–regulated protein of currently unknown function. Type II congenital dyserythropoietic anemia is also known as hereditary erythroblastic multinuclearity with a positive acidified serum test, or by its acronym HEMPAS. Abnormal complex carbohydrates are present in patients with the type II disease. *SEC23B* (20p11.23–p12), encoding the SEC23B component of the COPII complex, is the causative gene in most patients. It engenders a vesicle trafficking defect between the endoplasmic reticulum and the *trans*-Golgi and, in turn, a glycosylation abnormality. Although type III disease is clinically milder than the other two forms of congenital dyserythropoietic anemia, it shows a tendency for retinal angioid streaks and myeloma in the long term. There is no specific treatment for these disorders. Management includes red cell transfusion, removal of excess body iron by chelation therapy or judicious phlebotomy, splenectomy, and marrow transplantation. Only in severe forms of type I congenital dyserythropoietic anemia does interferon-α decrease the transfusion needs.

The term *congenital dyserythropoietic anemia*, coined by Heimpel and Wendt,[1] applies to a group of rare hereditary refractory anemias characterized by ineffective erythropoiesis, erythroid multinuclearity, and accumulation of tissue iron. Splenomegaly is common. Anemia is usually first noted in infancy or childhood. The life span of circulating erythrocytes is moderately reduced, and the dominant factor in pathogenesis is a large component of intramedullary cell death. Ineffective erythropoiesis results in an anemia of variable severity associated with a mild macrocytosis, a normal, or at most slightly elevated, absolute reticulocyte count, a moderate increase in unglycosylated (indirect) bilirubin, a low haptoglobin, and a gradual increase in ferritin level. Congenital dyserythropoietic anemias have been classified into three types, named types I, II, and III. In addition, a number of cases that do not fit clearly into any of these three categories have been described.

Acronyms and abbreviations used in this chapter include: *CDAN1* gene, codanin-1; E2F1, transcription factor 1; GDF15, growth differentiation factor 15; HEMPAS, hereditary erythroblastic multinuclearity associated with a positive acidified serum test; *HFE* gene H63D, gene of common hemochromatosis mutation; *SLC4A*, gene encoding band 3; *UGT1A1*, bilirubin UDP-glucuronosyltransferase 1A1 gene.

*Dr. Ernest Beutler wrote this chapter in the previous edition of this textbook. Some of the material from the 7th edition has been retained.

EPIDEMIOLOGY

In 2008, the German, Italian, French, Spanish, Polish, and British registries, covering most European countries, were merged. Eighty-eight cases of type I, 341 cases of type II, and 99 cases of "other types" of congenital dyserythropoietic anemia of either a sporadic or familial type were accumulated into the registry. (In this study, rare type III congenital dyserythropoietic anemia was included in "other types"; Matuschek A, Högel A, Leichtle R, and Heimpel H, personal communication, November 2008.) Type I congenital dyserythropoietic anemia, well documented in whites, has also been described among North Africans, Saudi Arabians, Japanese, Indians, Chinese, and Polynesians. A genetic isolate was discovered among Bedouin tribes living in the Negev region of Israel.[2] Type II congenital dyserythropoietic anemia, reported mostly in whites, also has been observed among Indians, Pakistani, and Polynesians. A genetic isolate may exist in southern Italy.[3] There is a strong recruitment bias by geographical distribution as a result of wide variations in the availability of healthcare services in different regions of the world. One can assume that type I and type II congenital dyserythropoietic anemias, as with most rare genetic disorders, occur in a much wider range of ethnic groups. The geographic distribution of type III congenital dyserythropoietic anemia is more uncertain as it is very rare and phenotypically heterogeneous, making precise diagnosis difficult.

CONGENITAL DYSERYTHROPOIETIC ANEMIA, TYPE I

CLINICAL FINDINGS

Type I congenital dyserythropoietic anemia is inherited as an autosomal recessive disorder (Table 39–1). It can become manifest in infancy, childhood, or adolescence. Anemia is usually moderate (hemoglobin approximately 9.0 g/dL) and is associated with macrocytosis. The spleen size increases with age. Like other hematologic conditions characterized by accelerated intramedullary and peripheral erythrocyte destruction, hepatomegaly and cholelithiasis are common sequelae. Icterus remains mild, but may be aggravated by the A[TA]$_7$TAA polymorphism in the promoter of the *UGT1A1* gene, the cause of Gilbert syndrome.[4]

The disease is often associated with a variety of dysmorphologic features, the most common of which involve the bones of the hand and the foot (syndactyly, hypoplasia of one or several phalanges, presence of a supplementary metatarsal bone, and clubfoot) (Fig. 39–1).[5] A small stature, almond-shaped blue eyes, hypertelorism, micrognathism, and other abnormalities may also be present.

LABORATORY FINDINGS

Blood films usually exhibit a marked poikilocytosis, associated in some cases with a reduction in erythrocyte membrane protein 4.1R.[6] Marrow shows an intense erythroid hyperplasia. Binucleate polychromatic erythroblasts are evident in a frequency of approximately 3 to 7 percent. A highly specific feature is the presence of chromatin bridges linking two nuclei in more or less incompletely separated polychromatic

TABLE 39–1. Main Features of Types I, II, and III Congenital Dyserythropoietic Anemias

CDA Type	Light Microscopy	Electron Microscopy	Serology	Inheritance
I	Most erythroid cells abnormal: double nuclei, internuclear chromatin bridges	Widened nuclear pores, spongy appearance of the heterochromatin, invasion by the cytoplasm containing various organelles	No serologic abnormalities	Autosomal recessive
II	Mature stage erythroblasts with two or more nuclei, lobulated nuclei, karyorrhexis, pseudo-Gaucher cells	Endoplasmic reticulum cisternae lining the inner surface of the red cell plasma membrane	Cells, containing the HEMPAS antigen are lysed by 30% of acidified normal sera; increased agglutinability and lysis with anti-"i" autoantibodies	Autosomal recessive
III	Giant erythroblasts, up to 50 μm in diameter, with up to 12 nuclei, basophilic stippling	Clefts and blebs within nuclear areas, some iron-filled mitochondria, autophagic vacuoles and myelin figures in the cytoplasm	No clearly defined abnormalities	Autosomal dominant (not all cases)

erythroblasts (0.6–2.8 strands per 100 erythroblasts) (Fig. 39–2).[7] Ultrastructural abnormalities consist of a spongy ("Swiss cheese") appearance in up to 60 percent of early and late polychromatic erythroblasts. The nuclei have areas of electrolucency within electron-dense heterochromatin, and contain nuclear membrane-lined cytoplasmic intrusions occasionally with retained cytoplasmic organelles (Fig. 39–3). Higher levels of growth differentiation factor 15 (GDF15) were present in 17 patients so studied. Reduction in serum hepcidin did not reach statistical significance.[8]

GENETICS

One responsible gene, *CDAN1*, has been mapped to 15q15.1-15.3 between markers D15S779 and D15S778[9] and elucidated[10] in the Negev

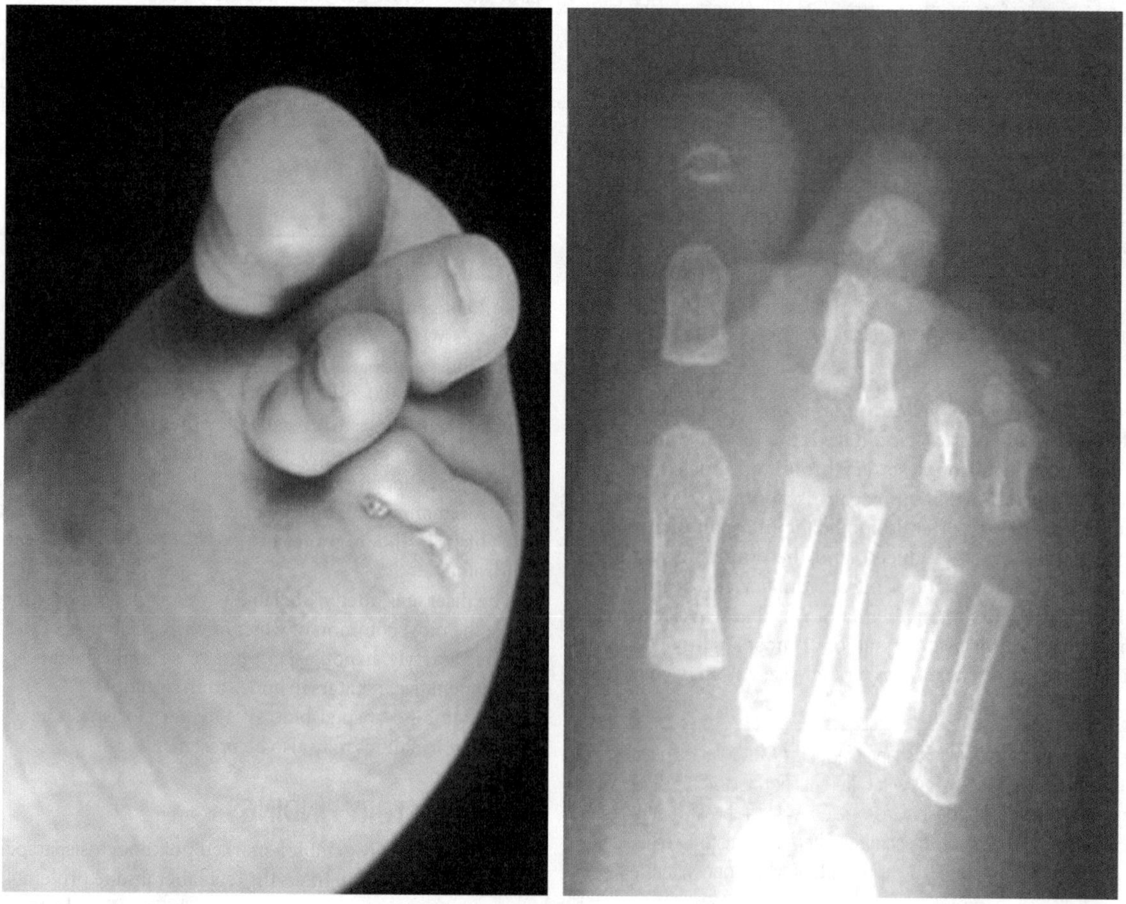

FIGURE 39–1. Foot dysmorphology in CDA I. *Left*. Photograph showing hypoplastic nails, a broad first toe, hypoplastic third finger, and brachysyndactyly of the fourth and the fifth toes. *Right*. Radiograph showing a duplication of the fourth metatarsal bone (both bones being hypoplastic), a duplication of the fourth proximal phalanx, a single middle phalanx for the fourth and fifth toe, and the absence of the fourth distal phalanx. *(From Tamary H, Dgany O, Proust A, et al.[13] By permission of the publisher, Blackwell Publishing, Oxford, UK.)*

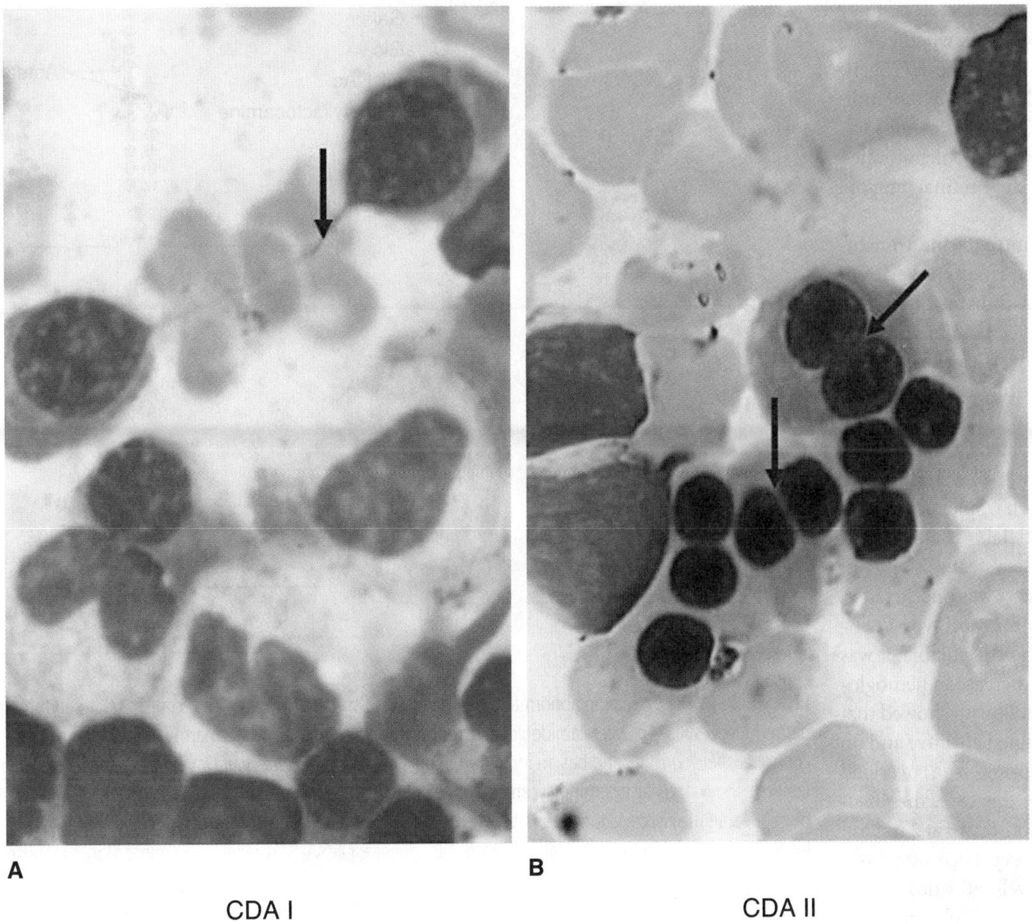

FIGURE 39–2. Light microscopy of marrow. **A.** CDA I. The *arrow* indicates an internuclear chromatin bridge (that is dramatically long in this example). **B.** CDA II. The vertical and oblique *arrows* point to two binucleated erythroblasts. *(Courtesy of Dr. Odile Fenneteau.)*

Bedouin isolate. *CDAN1* spans 15 kbp and has 28 exons. The encoded protein, codanin-1, contains 1227 amino acids. Codanin-1 is a cell-cycle–regulated protein. High levels of codanin-1 are observed in S phase. At mitosis, codanin-1 undergoes phosphorylation and is excluded from condensed chromosomes. The proximal *CDAN1* gene-promoter region appears to be a direct target of E2F1 (transcription factor 1).[11]

Thirty unique mutations have been found in the *CDNA1* gene and affected subjects are either homozygotes or compound heterozygotes for the mutation.[10,12,13] The Bedouin mutation (R1042W) was found once in a white individual born from consanguineous parents[14]; it was located in the hotspot for mutations (the CpG dinucleotide). In all likelihood, it stemmed from a mutational event distinct from that which generated the Bedouin Negev isolate.

In a number of patients, only one *CDAN1* allele is identified with a detectable mutation. In rare subjects, no *CDAN1* mutations were identified. Microsatellite analysis in the 15q15.1-15.3 region, carried out in a group of English patients, suggested that the responsible gene was not linked to *CDAN1* chromosomal region,[15] and the same chromosomal area was also excluded in a Pakistani family.[16] A second gene causative of type I congenital dyserythropoietic anemia is therefore likely.

COURSE AND PROGNOSIS

Severe forms may be present with hydrops fetalis.[17] Pulmonary hypertension has been reported in three Bedouin newborns with CDA I.[18] Iron overload as a result of transfusion, hemosiderosis and/or the enhanced iron absorption characteristic of states of intra- and extramedullary

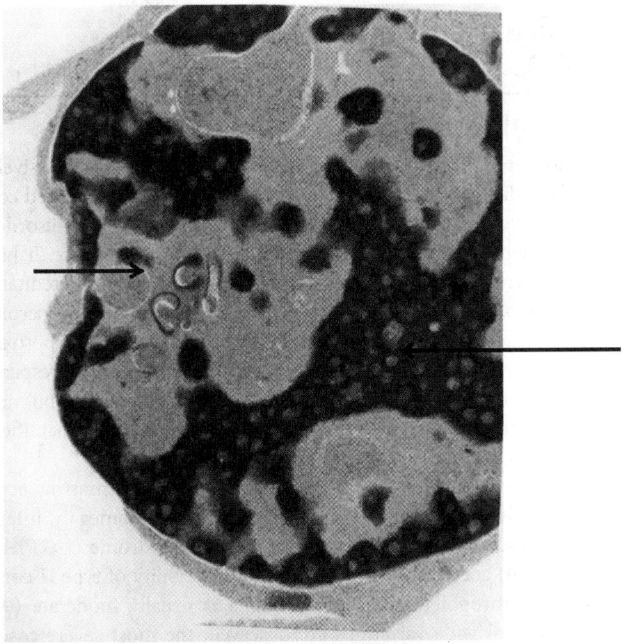

FIGURE 39–3. Ultrastructure of an erythroblast nucleus in CDA I. A typical erythroblast from a patient with CDA I, showing the spongy appearance of the nuclear heterochromatin (*long arrow*) and a cytoplasmic invagination (*short arrow*) inside the nucleus (original magnification ×15,000). *(Courtesy of Prof. Peretz Resnitzky.)*

hemolysis is the main concern as these patients age. It is uncertain whether iron overload is enhanced by the *HFE* gene H63D.[4] Iron chelation may be indicated in those patients who cannot tolerate iron depletion by phlebotomies. Rare patients develop retinal angioid streaks.[14]

In some cases, intrauterine transfusions are warranted by the severity of anemia[17]; however, transfusions are to be avoided whenever possible because of the risk of iron overload. Iron chelation should be instituted when ferritin level exceeds 500 to 1000 μg/L. When anemia is compensated, small-volume regular phlebotomies may be used to decrease body iron. Splenectomy is usually not beneficial.[12] Cholelithiasis requiring cholecystectomy is not unusual. Interferon-α was once used in a child with hepatitis C and type I congenital dyserythropoietic anemia; it was associated with an increase in hemoglobin level. A 9-year followup showed that the treatment remained effective and on repeated liver biopsies, iron overload was normalized. In this case, the effective dose of interferon-α was at 2 million units twice a week. Pegylated interferon could be used as well, at a dose of 30 μg/wk.[19] Allogeneic stem cell transplantation was successful in three transfusion-dependent children who subsequently became transfusion-independent.[20]

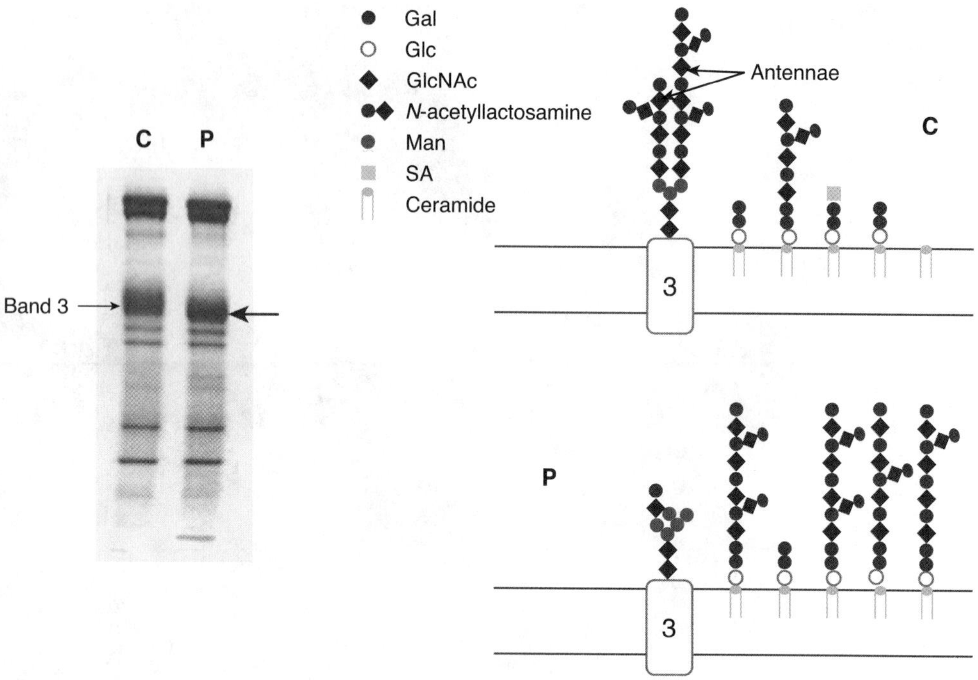

FIGURE 39–4. Glycosylation abnormalities of band 3 and sphingolipids in type II congenital dyserythropoietic anemia. *Left.* Sodium dodecyl sulfate polyacrylamide gel electrophoresis shows that band 3 is narrower in the patient (P, *red arrow*) than in the control (C, *black arrow*), and has an increased anodic migration. *(Courtesy of Dr. Madeleine Fénéant-Thibault.) Right.* In the patient (P), the *N*-acetyllactosaminoglycan antennae are poorly synthesized in band 3 as compared with the control (C). A number of minor side misglycosylations are not shown. As if in counterbalance, the sphingolipids are overglycosylated with *N*-acetyllactosaminoglycans in the patient. Gal, galactose; Glc, glucose; GlcNAc, *N*-acetylglucosamine; Man, mannose; SA, sialic acid.

CONGENITAL DYSERYTHROPOIETIC ANEMIA, TYPE II

CLINICAL FINDINGS

Type II congenital dyserythropoietic anemia is an autosomal recessively inherited condition, although abnormalities in the levels of some red cell membrane glycoconjugates have been found in carriers.[21] The disorder becomes variably manifest in infancy, childhood, or adolescence. It has long been referred to as HEMPAS,[22] a whimsical acronym for *h*ereditary *e*rythroblastic *m*ultinuclearity associated with a *p*ositive *a*cidified *s*erum test. The red cells undergo a positive acidified serum lysis with approximately 30 percent of fresh, compatible, normal sera (which, in this respect, resemble erythrocytes in paroxysmal nocturnal hemoglobinuria), but not with the patient's own serum. The HEMPAS designation and the acidified serum lysis test are obsolete in light of newer diagnostic tools.

The clinical picture includes a hemolytic anemia with marrow erythroid expansion, commonly with splenomegaly, hepatomegaly, intermittent jaundice, and cholelithiasis. The Gilbert syndrome (*UGT1A1* polymorphism) accounts for the phenotypic variability of type II congenital dyserythropoietic anemia.[23] Anemia is usually moderate (9–10g/L), although wide variations are observed, the most severe cases requiring transfusions from birth and thereafter. One case of hydrops fetalis has been reported.[24] Growth differentiation factor GDF15 is increased and the urinary hepcidin is low (Muckenthaler M, Casanovas G, Kiss J, et al, personal communication, November 2008).

LABORATORY FINDINGS

Blood films exhibit a moderate to marked anisocytosis and anisochromia and a number of spherocytes. This, along with the increased percentage of hyperdense cells and a spherocytosis-like ektacytometric curve, may lead to confusion of type II congenital dyserythropoietic anemia with hereditary spherocytosis. In the marrow, from 10 to 30 percent of the erythroblasts, chiefly at the more mature stages, have two or more nuclei or lobulated nuclei (see Fig. 39–2). Karyorrhexis (fragmentation of the nucleus) is common. Gaucher-like cells may develop as a result of phagocytosis of erythroblasts by macrophages. Ringed sideroblasts are present in severe cases. Electronic microscopy shows structures that are often misnamed as a double membrane. These are cisternae of the endoplasmic reticulum that run along the red cell plasma membrane inner surface, and which contain endoplasmic reticulum specific proteins, as shown by immunochemistry labeling.[25] Sodium dodecyl sulfate polyacrylamide gel electrophoresis followed by appropriate immunoblots reveals the presence of calreticulin, glucose-regulated protein 78, and disulfide isomerase, which are specific for the endoplasmic reticulum; these are not detected in normal individuals.

Band 3, the anion exchanger-1, exhibits an increased anodic mobility and a pinched aspect upon sodium dodecyl sulfate polyacrylamide gel electrophoresis (Fig. 39–4). It differs from the band 3 abnormalities seen in some cases of hereditary spherocytosis associated with mutations of the *SLC4A1* gene that result in a uniform reduction of band 3. The band 3 upper edge appears sharp in type II congenital dyserythropoietic anemia because its major glycan moiety has not acquired the normal heterogeneity of length that accounts for its blurred appearance under normal conditions. This finding is the most reliable diagnostic feature of type II congenital dyserythropoietic anemia; however, a marrow aspiration is still needed for diagnosis.

The underglycosylation of band 3 led to an extensive analysis of red cell membrane glycans in general. The polylactosamine antennae, which account for the long, peripheral parts of band 3 glycans, are shortened or missing (see Fig. 39–4). The number of mannosyl residues lying at the base of the antennae is increased. In type II congenital dyserythropoietic anemia, the reduction in band 3 polylactosaminyl moiety, as occurs in the newborn, accounts for the increase in the "i" antigen reactivity, and the reduction in the binding of tomato lectin, of which branched polylactosaminyl are the main target.[26] In addition, the glucose tranporter-1 erythrocyte membrane protein is underglycosylated.[27] Glycosphingolipids are markedly increased.[28,29] They contain, along with a higher amount of long-chain fatty acids, an increase in lactotriosyl- and lactoneotetraosylceramides. Besides, abnormal glycosylation of serum glycoproteins of hepatic origin (transferrin) has also been reported.[30] However, in some congenital disorders of glycosylation (types Ia and Ig), an impaired biosynthesis of *N*-linked oligosaccharide chains in band 3 and glycophorin A was reported without recognizable hematologic defect.[31,32]

Microsomal *N*-acetylglucosaminyltransferase II[33] (GnT II) and Golgi α-mannosidase II[34] (Man II), as well as other enzymes,[35] were found deficient in type II congenital dyserythropoietic anemia. A mouse lacking a functional α-mannosidase II gene developed a dyserythropoietic anemia concurrent with the loss of erythrocyte complex *N*-glycans, resembling the human type II congenital dyserythropoietic anemia.[36]

GENETICS

Mapping of the gene responsible for type II congenital dyserythropoietic anemia to 20q11.21[37] narrowed down the region of the search for enzyme defects. Some genes encoding glycan metabolism enzymes in this chromosomal region (α-mannosidase II, α-mannosidase x, and *N*-acetylglucosaminyl transferase II) and seven genes not all involved in carbohydrate metabolism failed to disclose any mutations.[38,39] The responsible gene, recently relocated to 20p11.23–20p12.1, turned out to be *SEC23B*.[40,40a] It encompasses 54 kbp and has 19 exons. The studied patients were compound heterozygotes or homozygotes for mutations in *SEC23B*. Thirty percent of the mutated alleles carried the E109K substitution. The SEC23B protein (767 amino acids) is a component of the COPII complex. COPII-coated vesicles normally bud out of the endoplasmic reticulum and export proteins to the *trans*-Golgi. Type II congenital dyserythropoietic anemia may be viewed as a disorder of a secretory pathway which, in turn, generates glycosylation abnormalities. The defect in the last abscission of erythroblasts is an additional and important feature yet to be accounted for. Mutations in other COPII components are known but spare the erythroid cell line.

The *retsina* zebra fish that displays a congenital dyserythropoietic anemia with a high number of binucleated erythroblasts, the presence of "double membrane" and an underglycosylation of band 3 has a mutation in the *slc4a1* gene, the zebra fish ortholog of human *SLC4A1*, encoding band 3.[41] Although the zebra fish disease bears some resemblance with human type II congenital dyserythropoietic anemia, its pathogenesis must be different.

COURSE AND PROGNOSIS

The moderate forms of type II congenital dyserythropoietic anemia may have good prognosis with only limited morbidity during pregnancies. Their major complication is iron overload, consistently observed by many investigators, even in the absence of transfusions.[42] In one patient, the combination of the homozygosity for C282Y *HFE* mutation with type II congenital dyserythropoietic anemia resulted in hemochromatosis, simulating a dominantly inherited phenotype.[43] In some cases, a severe phenotype was also the result of additional genetic abnormalities, such as of the coinheritance of glucose-6-phosphate dehydrogenase (G-6-PD) Seattle reported in a Sicilian child.[44]

There are no specific treatments for type II congenital dyserythropoietic anemia. Transfusions may be necessary that may include intrauterine transfusion.[24] The monitoring of iron overload is a key element in the prognosis. Iron chelation should be instituted when ferritin level exceeds 500 to 1000 μg/L. Small volume, periodic phlebotomy may be used in instances in which anemia is moderate and well-compensated.[45] Cholelithiasis may require cholecystectomy. Splenectomy is indicated in the transfusion-dependent cases. However, the criteria for employing splenectomy have not been defined. Marrow transplantation has to be used in some cases.[24,46]

CONGENITAL DYSERYTHROPOIETIC ANEMIA, TYPE III

CLINICAL AND LABORATORY FINDINGS

Type III congenital dyserythropoietic anemia is the least-common congenital dyserythropoietic anemia. One dominantly inherited form was reported as early as in 1951[47] in a woman and her three children, in whom 16 to 22.7 percent of marrow erythroblasts were multinucleated. Giant-size erythrocytes were present in the blood, and giant erythroblasts with coarse basophilic stippling and up to 12 nuclei were present in the marrow. All patients were asymptomatic, with no or minimal anemia. The reticulocyte count was less than 3 percent.

Most of our knowledge about type III congenital dyserythropoietic anemia stems from a large family from the province of Västerbotten in northern Sweden.[48] The diagnosis was made in older children and adults. The condition, also dominantly inherited, was initially coined "hereditary benign erythrocytosis." Patients had a mild to moderate anemia, a mild jaundice, and commonly cholelithiasis. The spleen was not palpable, nor was iron overload recorded. Blood films showed macrocytes and occasional extremely large forms (gigantocytes), and poikilocytes. The marrow had a marked erythroid hyperplasia, with the large multinucleate erythroblasts with big lobulated nuclei, and of giant multinucleate erythroblasts, with up to 12 nuclei. Upon electron microscopy, marrow, in addition to marked multinuclearity, clefts within heterochromatin, autophagic vacuoles, iron-laden mitochondria, and myelin figures in the cytoplasm were noted.[5,7] The size of the Swedish family made it possible to map the responsible gene to 15q22-25.[49] A number of sporadic cases labeled as type III congenital dyserythropoietic anemia have been reported.[50] In the absence of genetic data, it is difficult to assess how these sporadic cases relate to the dominant form.

COURSE AND PROGNOSIS

Stillbirths, including at least one stillborn with hydrops fetalis, were noted in an Indian family,[51] in which the mother, who initially required transfusions, became transfusion independent after splenectomy. In spite of an apparently benign course, type III congenital dyserythropoietic anemia is prone to various long-term complications, including intravascular hemolysis and an increased risk of myeloma and other monoclonal gammapathies,[52] and angioid streaks.[53]

OTHER CONGENITAL DYSERYTHROPOIETIC ANEMIAS

A number of cases of congenital dyserythropoietic anemia that do not have specific features of type I, II, or, to some extent, type III disease

TABLE 39–2. A Classification Frame for Atypical Congenital Dyserythropoietic Anemias

Group	Main Features
IV	Transfusion-dependent anemia
	Pronounced normoblastic erythroid hyperplasia with a slight to moderate increase in the nonspecific dyserythropoietic erythroblasts with irregular or karyorrhectic nuclei
	No precipitated protein within erythroblasts
V	Near-normal hemoglobin with normal or slightly increased mean corpuscular volume
	Predominantly unconjugated hyperbilirubinemia
	Marked normoblastic/slightly megaloblastic hyperplasia
	Little or no erythroid dysplasia
VI	Normal or near-normal hemoglobin with marked macrocytosis
	Erythroid hyperplasia with cobalamin- and folate-independent florid megaloblastic erythropoiesis
VII	Severe transfusion-dependent anemia
	Severe normoblastic erythroid hyperplasia with irregular nuclear shapes in many erythroblasts
	Intraerythroblastic inclusions that resemble precipitated globin but do not contain globin

SOURCE: Based on Wickramasinghe SN, Wood WG,[60] with modifications.

have been reported and reviewed.[54–59] In an attempt to classify all these cases, a method has been proposed based largely on cell morphology (Table 39–2).[60] Progress in classification and in understanding the relationships among individual cases will depend on identification of the mutant genes responsible for the disease.

Biochemical and genetic clues have been found in atypical cases of congenital dyserythropoietic anemia. In a Danish patient[61,62] with persistent embryonic and fetal hemoglobins, and missing CD44, there was a reduction in aquaporin-1–associated Colton antigens (expression reduced by 90%) and increased red cell osmotic fragility. However, no mutations were found in the *AQP1* gene encoding aquaporin-1.[63]

An X-linked dyserythropoietic anemia associated with thrombocytopenia as a result of the V205M mutation in GATA1 on the amino-terminal zinc finger has been described.[64] This mutation occurred at a highly conserved position for the binding of FOG (friend of GATA1). A neighbor mutation in GATA1 (G208S) produced a severe thrombocytopenia but failed to impair erythropoiesis.[65] The mutation, D218G, still on the same zinc-finger domain, was associated with macrothrombocytopenia, macrocytosis, and a mild dyserythropoiesis, but without marked anemia.[66] The R216W mutation led to a congenital erythropoietic porphyria; there was no dyserythropoiesis in a strict sense, but a syndrome akin to β-thalassemia.[67]

DIFFERENTIAL DIAGNOSIS

Congenital dyserythropoietic anemias may be confused with thalassemias and other hemolytic anemias. However, marked anisocytosis, including a macrocytic component, a low or moderate reticulocyte count out of keeping with the degree of anemia and the presence of bizarre morphological abnormalities in the erythroid precursors on marrow examination will point to a correct diagnosis. Because of other diagnostic considerations, hemoglobin and a few red cell enzymes may have been analyzed as a first approach. These studies may show some abnormalities, usually secondary. When *in vitro* globin-chain synthesis was a common test, an imbalance of β-globin-chain synthesis had been found in a number of cases. Type II congenital dyserythropoietic anemia may bear a resemblance to hereditary spherocytosis. Sodium dodecyl sulfate polyacrylamide gel electrophoresis, completed with immunoblots for reticulum endoplasmic proteins, is then the most reliable diagnostic test. In all cases, a marrow aspiration remains indispensable. In some cases, hemochromatosis may be a presenting feature of underlying congenital dyserythropoietic anemia.

REFERENCES

1. Heimpel H, Wendt F: Congenital dyserythropoietic anemia with karyorrhexis and multinuclearity of erythroblasts. *Helv Med Acta* 34:103, 1968.
2. Tamary H, Shalev H, Luria D, et al: Clinical features and studies of erythropoiesis in Israeli Bedouins with congenital dyserythropoietic anemia type I. *Blood* 87:1763, 1996.
3. Iolascon A, Servedio V, Carbone R, et al: Geographic distribution of CDA II: Did a founder effect operate in Southern Italy? *Haematologica* 85:470, 2000.
4. Wickramasinghe SN, Thein SL, Srichairatanakool S, Porter JB: Determinants of iron status and bilirubin levels in congenital dyserythropoietic anaemia type 1. *Br J Haematol* 107:522, 1999.
5. Wickramasinghe SN: Congenital dyserythropoietic anaemias: Clinical features, haematological morphology and new biochemical data. *Blood Rev* 12:178, 1998.
6. Bader-Meunier B, Leverger G, Tchernia G, et al: Clinical and laboratory manifestations of congenital dyserythropoietic anemia type I in a cohort of French children. *J Pediatr Hematol Oncol* 27:416, 2005.
7. Wickramasinghe SN: Congenital dyserythropoietic anemias, in *Blood and Bone Marrow Pathology*, edited by SN Wickramasinghe, J McCullough, p 273. Churchill Livingstone, Elsevier Science, 2003.
8. Tamary H, Shalev H, Perez-Avraham G, et al: Elevated growth differentiation factor 15, expression in patients with congenital dyserythropoietic anemia type I: *Blood* 112:5241, 2008.
9. Tamary H, Shalmon L, Shalev H, et al: Localisation of the gene for congenital dyserythropietic anemia type I to a <1-cM interval on chromosome 15q15.1-15.3. *Am J Hum Genet* 62:1062, 1998.
10. Dgany O, Avidan N, Delaunay J, et al: Congenital dyserythropoietic anemia type I is caused by mutations in codanin-1. *Am J Hum Genet* 71:1467, 2002.
11. Noy-Lotan S, Dgany O, Lahmi R, et al: Codanin-1, the protein encoded by the gene mutated in congenital dyserythropoietic anemia type I (*CDAN1*) is cell cycle modulated. *Haematologica* 94:629, 2009.
12. Heimpel H, Schwarz K, Ebnöther M, et al: Congenital dyserythropoietic anaemia type I (CDA I): Molecular genetics, clinical appearance, and prognosis based on long-term observation. *Blood* 107:334, 2006.
13. Tamary H, Dgany O, Proust A, et al: Clinical and molecular variability in congenital dyserythropoietic anemia type I: *Br J Haematol* 130:625, 2005.
14. Tamary H, Offret H, Dgany O, et al: Congenital dyserythropoietic anaemia, type I, in a Caucasian patient with retinal angioid streaks (homozygous arg1042trp mutation in codanin-1). *Eur J Haematol* 80:271, 2008.
15. Hodges VV, Molloy GY, Wickramasinghe SN: Genetic heterogeneity of congenital dyserythropoietic anemia type I: *Blood* 94:1139, 1999.
16. Ahmed MR, Chehal A, Zahed L, et al: Linkage and mutational analysis of the *CDAN1* gene reveals genetic heterogeneity in congenital dyserythropoietic anemia type I: *Blood* 107:4968, 2006.
17. Parez N, Dommergues M, Zupan V, et al: Severe congenital dyserythropoietic anaemia type 1: Pretenatal management, transfusion support and alpha-interferon therapy. *Br J Haematol* 110:420, 2000.
18. Shalev H, Moser A, Kapelushnik J, et al: Congenital dyserythropoietic anemia type 1, presenting as persistent pulmonary of the newborn. *J Pediatr* 136:553, 2000.
19. Lavabre-Bertrand T, Ramos J, Delfour C, et al: Long-term alpha interferon treatment is effective on anaemia and significantly reduces iron overload in congenital dyserythropoiesis type I. *Eur J Haematol* 73:380, 2004.
20. Ayas M, al-Jefri A, Baothman A, et al: Transfusion-dependent congenital dyserythropoietic anemia type I successfully treated with allogeneic stem cell transplantation. *Bone Marrow Transplant* 29:681, 2002.
21. Zdebska E, Mendek-Czajkowska E, Ploski R, et al: Heterozygosity of CDAN II (HEMPAS) gene may be detected by the analysis of erythrocyte membrane glycoconjugates from healthy carriers. *Haematologica* 87:126, 2002.
22. Crookston JH, Crookston MC, Burnie KL, et al: Hereditary erythroblastic multinuclearity associated with a positive acidified-serum test: A type of congenital dyserythropoietic anaemia. *Br J Haematol* 17:11, 1969.

23. Perrotta S, del Giudice EM, Carbone R, et al: Gilbert's syndrome accounts for the phenotypic variability of congenital dyserythropoietic anemia type II (CDA-II). *J Pediatr* 136:556, 2000.
24. Remacha AF, Badell I, Pujol-Moix N, et al: Hydrops fetalis associated congenital dyserythropoietic anemia treated with intrauterine transfusions and bone marrow transplantation. *Blood* 100:356, 2002.
25. Alloisio N, Texier P, Denoroy L, et al: The cisternae decorating the red cell membrane in congenital dyserythropoietic anemia (Type II) derive from the endoplasmic reticulum. *Blood* 87:4433, 1996.
26. Denecke J, Kranz C, Nimtz M, et al: Characterization of the *N*-glycosylation phenotype of erythrocyte membrane proteins in congenital dyserythropoietic anemia type II (CDA II/HEMPAS). *Glycoconj J* 25:375, 2007.
27. Scartezzini P, Forni GL, Baldi M, et al: Decreased glycosylation of band 3 and band 4.5 glycoproteins of erythrocyte membrane in congenital dyserythropoietic anaemia type II: *Br J Haematol* 51:569, 1982.
28. Bouhours JF, Bouhours D, Delaunay J: Abnormal fatty acid composition of erythrocyte glycosphingolipids in congenital dyserythropoietic anemia type II: *J Lipid Res* 26:435, 1985.
29. Zdebska E, Anselstetter V, Pacuszka T, et al: Glycolipids and glycopeptides of red cell membranes in congenital dyserythropoietic anaemia type II (CDAII). *Br J Haematol* 66:385, 1987.
30. Fukuda MN, Gaetani GF, Izzo P, et al: Incompletely processed N-glycans of serum glycoproteins in congenital dyserythropeitic anaemia type II (HEMPAS). *Br J Haematol* 82:745, 1992.
31. Zdebska E, Musielak M, Jaeken J, Kocielak J: Band 3 glycoprotein and glycophorin A from erythrocytes of children with congenital disorder of glycosylation type-Ia are underglycosylated. *Proteomics* 1:269, 2001.
32. Zdebska E, Bader-Meunier B, Schischmanoff PO, et al: Abnormal glycosylation of red cell membrane band 3 in the congenital disorder of glycosylation type Ig. *Pediatr Res* 54:224, 2003.
33. Fukuda MN, Dell A, Scartezzini P: Primary defect of congenital dyserythropoietic anemia type II: Failure in glycosylation of erythrocyte lactosaminoglycan proteins caused by lowered *N*-acetylglucosaminyltransferase II: *J Biol Chem* 262:7195, 1987.
34. Fukuda MN, Masri KA, Dell A, et al: Incomplete synthesis of N-glycans in congenital dyserythropoietic anemia type II caused by a defect in the gene encoding α-mannosidase II. *Proc Natl Acad Sci U S A* 87:7443, 1990.
35. Fukuda MN: Congenital dyserythropoietic anaemia type II (HEMPAS) and its molecular basis. *Baillieres Clin Haematol* 6:493, 1993.
36. Chui D, Oh-Eda M, Liao YF, et al: Alpha-mannosidase-II deficiency results in dyserythropoiesis and unveils an alternate pathway in oligosaccharide biosynthesis. *Cell* 90:157, 1997.
37. Gasparini P, Miraglia del Giudice E, Delaunay J, et al: Localization of congenital dyserythropoietic anemia II (CDA II) locus to chromosome 20 (20q11.2) by genomewide search. *Am J Hum Genet* 61:1112, 1997.
38. Iolascon A, Miraglia del Giudice E, Perrotta S, et al: Exclusion of three candidate genes as determinants of congenital dyserythropoietic anemia Type II (CDA II). *Blood* 90:4197, 1997.
39. Lanzara C, Ficarella R, Totaro A, et al: Congenital dyserythropoietic anemia type II: Exclusion of seven candidate genes. *Blood Cells Mol Dis* 30:22, 2003.
40. Schwarz K, Iolascon A, Verissimo F, et al: Mutations affecting the secretory COPII coat component SEC23B cause congenital dyserythropoietic anemia type II. *Nat Genet* 41:936, 2009.
40a. Bianchi P, Fermo E, Vercellati C, et al: Congenital dyserythropoietic anemia type II (CDAII) is caused by mutations in the SEC23B gene. *Hum Mutat* 30:1292, 2009.
41. Paw BH, Davidson AJ, Zhou Y, et al: Cell-specific mitotic defect and dyserythropoiesis associated with erythroid band 3, deficiency. *Nat Genet* 34:59, 2003.
42. Heimpel H, Anselstetter V, Chrobak L, et al: Congenital dyserythropoietic anemia type II: Epidemiology, clinical appearance, and prognosis based on long-term observation. *Blood* 102:4576, 2003.
43. Fargion S, Valenti L, Fracanzani AL, et al: Hereditary hemochromatosis in a patient with congenital dyserythropoietic anemia. *Blood* 96:3653, 2000.
44. Gangarossa S, Romano V, Miraglia del Giudice E, et al: Congenital dyserythropoietic anemia type II associated with G6PD Seattle in a Sicilian child. *Acta Haematol* 93:36, 1997.
45. Hofmann WK, Kaltwasser JP, Hoelzer D, et al: Successful treatment of iron overload by phlebotomies in a patient with severe congenital dyserythropoietic anemia type II. *Blood* 89:3068, 1997.
46. Iolascon A, Sabato V, de Mattia D, Locatelli F: Bone marrow transplantation in a case of severe, type II congenital dyserythropoietic anaemia (CDA II). *Bone Marrow Transplant* 27:213, 2001.
47. Wolff JA, von Hofe FH: Familial erythroid multinuclearity. *Blood* 6:1274, 1951.
48. Bergström I, Jacobsson L: Hereditary erythroreticulosis. *Blood* 19:296, 1962.
49. Lind L, Sandström H, Wahlin A, et al: Localization of the gene for congenital dyserythropoietic anemia type III, CDAN3, to chromosome 15q21-q25. *Hum Mol Genet* 4:109, 1995.
50. Accame EA, de Tezanos Pinto M: Congenital dyserythropoiesis with erythroblastic polyploidy. Report of a variety found in Argentinian Mesopotamia [author's transl]. *Sangre (Barc)* 26:545, 1981.
51. Jijina F, Ghosh K, Yavagal D, et al: A patient with congenital dyserythropoietic anaemia type III presenting with stillbirths. *Acta Haematol* 99:31, 1998.
52. Sandström H, Wahlin A, Eriksson M, et al: Intravascular haemolysis and increased prevalence of myeloma and monoclonal gammapathy in congenital dyserythropoietic anemia, type III *Eur J Haematol* 52:42, 1994.
53. Sandström H, Wahlin A, Eriksson M, et al: Angioid streaks are part of a familial syndrome in dyserythropoietic anemia (CDA III). *Br J Haematol* 98:845, 1997.
54. David G, Van Dorpe A: Aberrant congenital dyserythropoietic anaemias, in *Dyserythropoiesis*, edited by SM Lewis, RL Verwilghen, p 93. Academic Press, London, 1977.
55. Bethlenfalvay NC, Hadnagy C, Heimpel H: Unclassified type of congenital dyserythropoietic anaemia (CDA) with prominent peripheral erythroblastosis. *Br J Haematol* 60:541, 1985.
56. Brien WF, Mant MJ, Etches WS: Variant congenital dyserythropoietic anaemia with ringed sideroblasts. *Clin Lab Haematol* 7:231, 1985.
57. Pothier B, Morlé L, Alloisio N, et al: Aberrant pattern of red cell membrane and cytosolic proteins in a case of congenital dyserythropoietic anaemia. *Br J Haematol* 66:393, 1987.
58. Ohisalo JJ, Viitala J, Lintula R, Ruutu T: A new congenital dyserythropoietic anaemia. *Br J Haematol* 68:111, 1988.
59. Woessner S, Trujillo M, Florensa L, et al: Congenital dyserythropoietic anaemia other than type I to III with a peculiar erythroblastic morphology. *Eur J Haematol* 71:211, 2003.
60. Wickramasinghe SN, Wood WG: Advances in the understanding of the congenital dyserythropoietic anaemias. *Br J Haematol* 131:431, 2005.
61. Wickramasinghe SN, Illum N, Wimberley PD: Congenital dyserythropoietic anaemia with novel intra-erythroblastic and intra-erythrocytic inclusions. *Br J Haematol* 79:322, 1991.
62. Parsons SF, Jones J, Anstee DJ, et al: A novel form of congenital dyserythropoietic anemia associated with deficiency of erythroid CD44, and a unique blood group phenotype [In (a-b-), Co (a-b-)]. *Blood* 83:860, 1994.
63. Agre P, Smith BL, Baumgarten R, et al: Human red cell aquaporin CHIP. II: Expression during normal fetal development and in a novel form of congenital dyserythropoietic anemia. *J Clin Invest* 94:1050, 1994.
64. Nichols KE, Crispino JD, Poncz M, et al: Familial dyserythropoietic anaemia and thrombocytopenia due to an inherited mutation in GATA1. *Nat Genet* 24:266, 2000.
65. Mehaffey MG, Newton AL, Gandhi MJ, et al: X-linked thrombocytopenia caused by a novel mutation of GATA-1. *Blood* 98:2681, 2001.
66. Freson K, Devriendt K, Matthijs G, et al: Platelet characteristics in patients with X-linked macrothrombocytopenia because of a novel GATA1, mutation. *Blood* 98:85, 2001.
67. Phillips JD, Steensma DP, Pulsipher MA, et al: Congenital erythropoietic porphyria due to a mutation in GATA1: The first trans-acting mutation causative for a human porphyria. *Blood* 109:2618, 2007.

CHAPTER 40
PAROXYSMAL NOCTURNAL HEMOGLOBINURIA

Charles J. Parker

SUMMARY

In contrast to all other intrinsic abnormalities of the erythrocyte, paroxysmal nocturnal hemoglobinuria (PNH) is an acquired disorder. PNH arises as a consequence of somatic mutation, in one or more hematopoietic stem cells, of *PIGA*, a gene located on the X chromosome that is required for synthesis of the glycosyl phosphatidylinositol (GPI) moiety that anchors some proteins to cell surface. Consequently, all GPI-anchored proteins (GPI-APs) that are normally expressed are deficient on the mutant hematopoietic stem cells and their progeny. The complement-mediated intravascular hemolytic anemia and the resulting hemoglobinuria that are the clinical hallmarks of PNH are a consequence of deficiency of the GPI-anchored complement regulatory proteins, CD55 and CD59. Although PNH is a clonal disease, it is not a malignant disease, and the extent to which the mutant clones expand varies greatly among patients. Thus, the blood of patients with PNH is a mosaic of abnormal and phenotypically normal cells. The size of the mutant clone is an important determinant of the clinical manifestations of the disease that include thrombophilia and marrow failure in addition to hemolysis. The diagnosis of PNH is straightforward using flow cytometry to detect and quantify the percentage of blood erythrocytes and neutrophils that lack GPI-APs. The intravascular hemolysis of PNH can be controlled with eculizumab, a humanized monoclonal antibody that blocks formation of the cytolytic membrane attack complex of complement. Eculizumab, however, has no effect on the underlying disease process. The mutant clone can be eradicated and normal hematopoiesis restored by allogeneic hematopoietic stem cell transplant.

DEFINITION AND EARLY HISTORY

Although commonly regarded as a type of hemolytic anemia, paroxysmal nocturnal hemoglobinuria (PNH) is actually a hematopoietic stem cell disorder. PNH arises as a result of *nonmalignant* clonal expansion of *one or several* hematopoietic stem cells that have acquired a *somatic mutation* of the X-chromosome gene *PIGA* (phosphatidylinositol glycan class A). As a consequence of mutant *PIGA*, progeny of affected stem cells (erythrocytes, granulocytes, monocytes, platelets, and lymphocytes) are deficient in *all* glycosyl phosphatidylinositol-anchored proteins (GPI-APs) that are normally expressed on hematopoietic cells (and all GPI-APs that are normally expressed on hematopoietic cells are deficient on progeny of *PIGA* mutant stem cells). The clinical manifestations of PNH are hemolytic anemia, thrombophilia, and marrow failure, but only the hemolytic anemia is unequivocally a consequence of somatic mutation of *PIGA*.

Acronyms and abbreviations that appear in this chapter include: APC, alternative pathway of complement; DAF, decay accelerating factor; EtN, ethanolamine; GLcN, glucosamine; GPI, glycosyl phosphatidylinositol; GPI-APs, glycosyl phosphatidylinositol-anchored proteins; LDH, lactate dehydrogenase; MAC, membrane attack complex of complement; MDS, myelodysplastic syndrome; MIRL, membrane inhibitor of reactive lysis; *PIGA*, phosphatidylinositol glycan class A; PMN, polymorphonuclear cell; PNH, paroxysmal nocturnal hemoglobinuria; PNH-sc, subclinical PNH; RA, refractory anemia; RAEB, refractory anemia with excess of blasts; RAEB-t, refractory anemia with excess of blasts in transformation; RA-PNH+, RA with a population of PNH cells; RA-PNH−, RA without a population of PNH cells; RARS, refractory anemia with ringed sideroblast; RBCs, red blood cells; RCMD, refractory cytopenias with multilineage dysplasia; RCMD-RS, RCMD with ringed sideroblasts; WHO, World Health Organization.

Comprehensive, scholarly reviews of the history of PNH have been published.[1–4] The first clinical description of PNH is attributed to William Gull in 1866, but he failed to distinguish definitively PNH from paroxysmal cold hemoglobinuria. Paul Strübing, in 1882, clearly recognized PNH as a distinct entity and undertook prescient experiments designed to test his hypothesis that the nocturnal hemoglobinuria was a consequence of acidification of plasma that occurred when carbon dioxide and lactic acid accumulated because of slowing of respiration during sleep. In 1911, A.A. Hijmans van den Berg demonstrated that the hemolysis of PNH is caused by a defect in the red cell rather than by the presence of an abnormal plasma factor (as is the case with paroxysmal cold hemoglobinuria; see Chap. 53). Thomas Hale Ham is credited with discovering, in the late 1930s, that complement mediates the hemolysis of PNH erythrocytes, although it was not until the alternative pathway of complement was identified and characterized in the mid-1950s by Louis Pillemer that the basis of Ham's original observations became apparent. Ham developed the acidified serum lysis test (Ham's test) that along with the sucrose lysis test (sugar water test) of Robert Hartmann and David Jenkins were used as the standard diagnostic tests for PNH until being supplanted in the mid-1990s by flow cytometry. Both Hartmann and William Crosby brought attention to the important role that thrombosis (particularly the Budd-Chiari syndrome) plays in the natural history of PNH, and John Dacie and his pupil and colleague S.M. Lewis first systematically characterized the relationship between PNH and marrow failure.

EPIDEMIOLOGY

The prevalence of PNH is not known with certainty. Prevalence estimates are primarily anecdotal and differ considerably, in large part, because of the heterogeneous nature of the disease. The blood of patients with PNH is a mosaic of normal and abnormal cells, and the extent of the mosaicism varies widely among patients (see "Phenotypic Mosaicism are Characteristic of PNH" below). Patients with small PNH clones have few or no symptoms related to hemolysis. Thus an argument can be made that asymptomatic patients with small clones do not have clinically significant PNH and should be excluded from prevalence estimates. Others, however, may argue that any patient with flow cytometric evidence of a population of GPI-AP deficient cells, regardless of clone size, has PNH and should be included in prevalence estimates. Studies of prevalence that address the issue of disease heterogeneity are needed, but, by any definition, PNH is a rare disease. The prevalence of clinically significant PNH (i.e., classic PNH plus patients with relatively large clones that arise in the setting of another marrow failure syndrome, (see "Clinical Features" below) is likely in the order of <1 case per 200,000 population, easily fulfilling criteria (<1 case per 50,000 population) for classification as an ultraorphan disease.[5] There is a close association between PNH and aplastic anemia, and environmental factors, drugs, and toxins that cause aplastic anemia concordantly increase the risk of developing PNH. Although PNH has been

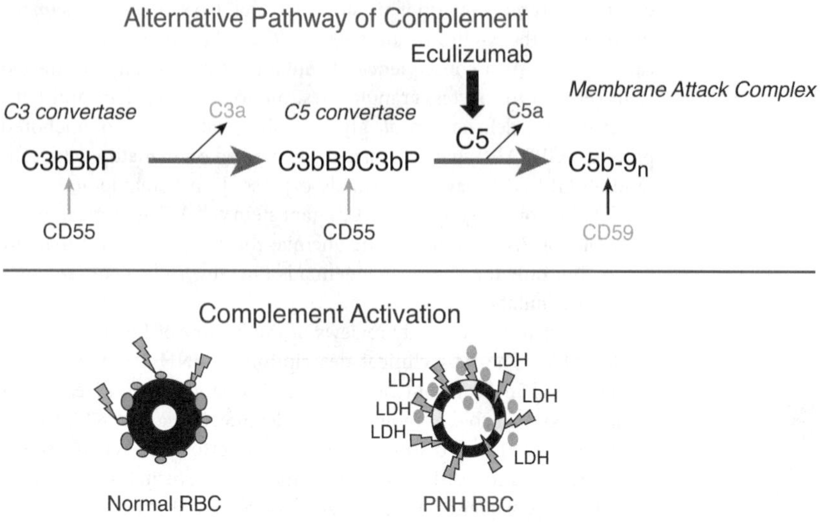

FIGURE 40–1. Complement-mediated lysis of PNH erythrocytes. *Upper panel.* The hemolytic anemia of PNH is Coombs test negative because the process is mediated by the antibody-independent alternative pathway of complement (APC). The C3 convertase of the APC consists of activated C3 (C3b), activated factor B (Bb, the enzymatic subunit of the complex) and factor P (a protein that stabilizes the complex, formally called properdin). The C5 convertase has the same components as the C3 convertase except that two C3b molecules are required to bind and position C5 for cleavage by activated factor B (Bb). C3a and C5a are bioactive peptides that are generated by cleavage of C3 and C5, respectively by their specific activation convertases. The C3 and C5 convertases greatly amplify complement activation by cleaving multiple substrate molecules. The membrane attack complex (MAC) consists of activated C5 (C5b), C6, C7, C8, and multiple molecules of C9 ($C9_n$). The MAC is the cytolytic unit of the complement system. The glycosyl phosphatidylinositol (GPI)-anchored complement regulatory protein CD55 restricts formation and stability of both the C3 and the C5 amplification convertases by destabilizing the interaction between activated factor B (Bb) and C3b (indicated by the *blue arrow*), whereas GPI-anchored CD59 blocks formation of the MAC by inhibiting the binding of C9 to the C5b-8 complex (indicated by the *brown arrow*). Inhibition of MAC formation by the humanized monoclonal anti-C5 antibody eculizumab (indicated by the *red arrow*) ameliorates the intravascular hemolysis of PNH. *Lower panel.* Normal erythrocytes (*left*) are protected against complement-mediated lysis primarily by CD55 (*blue circles*) and CD59 (*green circles*). Deficiency of these GPI-anchored complement regulatory proteins results in APC activation on PNH erythrocytes (*right*). Because of deficiency of CD55 and CD59, the complement cascade activates on the cell surface. Consequently, MACs form pores in the red cell membrane resulting in colloid osmotic lysis and release of hemoglobin (*red circles*) and other contents of the red cell including lactate dehydrogenase (LDH) into the intravascular space. *(Modified with permission from Parker CJ: The pathophysiology of paroxysmal nocturnal hemoglobinuria.* Exp Hematol *35:523, 2007.)*

reported in all age groups, the peak incidence is in the third and fourth decades of life, similar to that of aplastic anemia. PNH is an acquired disorder, and there is no known inherited risk for developing the disease. A number of cases have been reported in which only one of a pair of identical twins was affected.

ETIOLOGY AND PATHOGENESIS

COMPLEMENT AND PNH

The chronic intravascular hemolysis that is the hallmark clinical manifestation of PNH is mediated by the alternative pathway of complement (APC; Fig. 40–1).[6] The APC is a component of innate immunity.[7] This ancient system evolved to protect the host against invasion by pathogenic microorganisms. Unlike the classical pathway of complement that is part of the system of acquired immunity and requires antibody for initiation of activation, the APC is in a state of continuous activation, armed at all times to protect the host (see Chap. 17 for a detailed review of the complement system). The APC cascade can be divided into two functional components: the amplification C3 and C5 convertases and the cytolytic membrane attack complex (MAC). The C3 and C5 convertases (Fig. 40–1, *top panel*) are enzymatic complexes that initiate and amplify the activity of the APC and ultimately generate the MAC (the MAC is the common cytolytic subunit of the classical and lectin pathways of complement as well as the APC [see Chap. 17]).

Because the APC is primed for attack at all times, elaborate mechanisms for self-recognition and for protection of the host against APC-mediated injury have evolved. Both fluid-phase and membrane-bound proteins are involved in these processes. Normal human erythrocytes are protected against APC-mediated cytolysis primarily by decay accelerating factor (DAF, CD55)[8–10] and membrane inhibitor of reactive lysis (MIRL, CD59).[11] These proteins act at different steps in the complement cascade (see Fig. 40–1, *top panel*). CD55 regulates the formation and stability of the C3 and C5 convertases, whereas CD59 blocks the formation of the MAC. Deficiency of CD55 and CD59 on the erythrocytes of PNH is the pathophysiologic basis of the Coombs-negative, intravascular hemolysis that is the clinical hallmark of the disease (Fig. 40–1, *bottom panel*). But why are PNH erythrocytes deficient in the two complement regulatory proteins?

THE MOLECULAR PATHOGENESIS AND GENETIC BASIS OF PNH

PNH is a consequence of clonal expansion of one or more hematopoietic stem cells with mutant *PIGA* (located on Xp22.1).[12] The protein product of *PIGA* is a glycosyl transferase[12–16] that is an obligate constituent of a complex biochemical pathway required for synthesis of the glycosyl phosphatidylinositol (GPI) moiety that anchors individual proteins belonging to diverse functional groups to the cell surface (Fig. 40–2). As a result of mutant *PIGA*, progeny of the affected stem cells are deficient in all GPI-APs. Although more than 20 GPI-APs are expressed by hematopoietic cells, it is deficiency on red blood cells (RBCs) of the two GPI-anchored complement regulatory proteins, CD55 and CD59, that underlies the hemolytic anemia of PNH.[17] RBCs lacking CD55 and CD59 undergo spontaneous intravascular hemolysis as a consequence of unregulated activation of the APC (see Fig. 40–1, *bottom panel*). Thus, the hallmark clinical manifestation of PNH (intravascular hemolysis and the resultant hemoglobinuria) is an epiphenomenon, occurring because the two proteins that regulate complement on erythrocytes happen to be GPI-anchored.

Hypothetically, the PNH phenotype would result from inactivation of any of the more than 25 genes involved in synthesis of the GPI-anchor (see Fig. 40–2), but somatic mutation of no gene involved in GPI-AP synthesis other than *PIGA* has been reported in patients with PNH. This phenomenon is accounted for primarily by the fact that, of the genes involved in the GPI-anchor synthesis pathway, only *PIGA* is located on the X-chromosome. Therefore somatic mutation of only one allele is required for expression of the phenotype as males have one X-chromosome and, as a consequence of X-inactivation during embryogenesis, females have only one functional X-chromosome in somatic tissues. On the other hand, mutation of two alleles would be

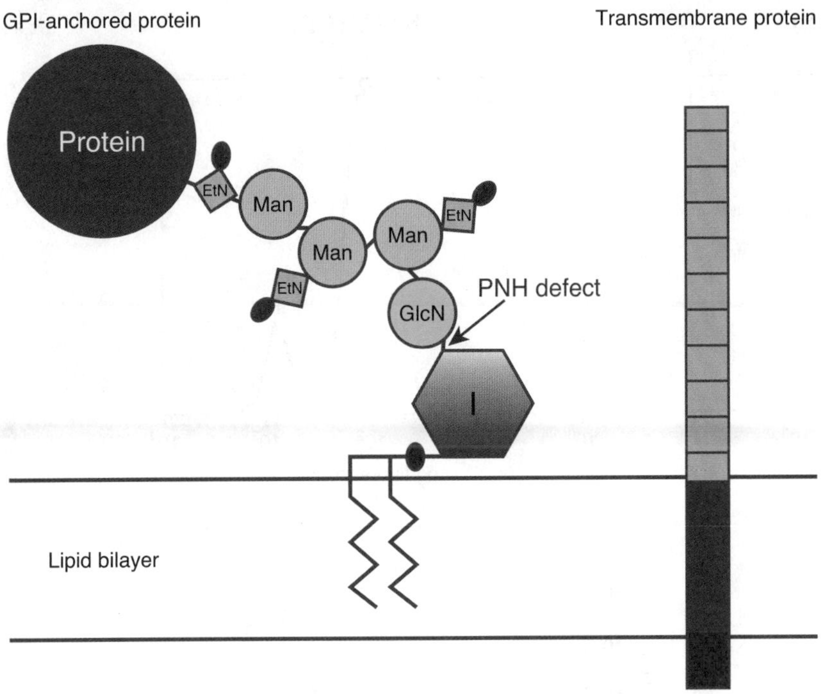

FIGURE 40–2. The molecular and genetic basis of PNH. There are two types of anchoring mechanisms for plasma membrane proteins, transmembrane and GPI. Transmembrane proteins are anchored into the lipid bilayer of the cell by a short series (~25 amino acids) of hydrophobic residues (*blue rectangle*). Transmembrane proteins typically have a short cytoplasmic tail that usually has signaling properties (*red rectangle*). The ectoplasmic portion of the protein is illustrated by the series of *gray-blue squares*. The GPI-APs consists of the following components: phosphatidylinositol (inositol is represented by the *blue hexagon* labeled I and phosphate is represented by the *red oval*); glucosamine (GLcN, *yellow circle*); three mannose (Man, *green circles*); ethanolamine phosphate (EtN, *blue square* with attached phosphate represented by the *red oval*); the protein entity (*blue circle*). The lipid component (indicated by the series of *diagonal lines* within lipid bilayer) is usually 1-alkyl, 2-acylglycerol for mammalian GPI-APs. PNH cells are deficient in all GPI-APs because somatic mutation of the X-chromosome gene *PIGA* disrupts the first step in the biosynthetic pathway (transfer of the nucleotide sugar UDP-GlcNAc to GlcNAc-PI) indicated by the *arrow*.

required for inactivation of any of the autosomal genes involved in the GPI-anchor synthesis pathway.

Cells with *PIGA* mutations do not appear to have a proliferative advantage *in vitro* or in hybrid animal models made with *PIGA* knockouts.[18] They have been found to be relatively resistant to apoptosis in some studies,[19–22] but not in others.[23,24] Thus, the basis of clonal selection and clonal expansion of *PIGA* mutant stem cells in patients with PNH remains largely enigmatic[25] although a number of hypotheses have been proposed (reviewed in reference 17).

■ PHENOTYPIC MOSAICISM IS CHARACTERISTIC OF PNH

The blood of patients with PNH is a mosaic of normal and abnormal cells (Fig. 40–3). Although PNH is a clonal disease, the extent to which the *PIGA*-mutant clone expands varies widely among patients.[17] As an example, in some cases, >90 percent of the blood cells may be derived from the *PIGA*-mutant clone, whereas in others, <10 percent of the blood cells may be GPI-AP deficient. This unique feature (variability in extent of mosaicism) is clinically relevant because patients with relatively small PNH clones have minimal or no symptoms and require no PNH-specific treatment, whereas those with large clones are often debilitated by the consequences of chronic complement-mediated intravascular hemolysis and respond dramatically to complement inhibitory therapy.

Another remarkable feature of PNH is phenotypic mosaicism (see Fig. 40–3A) based on *PIGA* genotype[26] (see Fig. 40–3B) that determines the degree of GPI-AP deficiency.[17] PNH III cells are completely deficient in GPI-APs, PNH II cells are partially (~90%) deficient and PNH I cells express GPI-APs at normal density (putatively, these cells are progeny of residual normal stem cells; see Fig. 40–3A). Phenotype varies among patients (Fig. 40–4). Some patients have only type I and type III cells (the most common phenotype), some have type I, type II, and type III (the second most common phenotype), and some patients have only type I and type II cells (the least common phenotype). Furthermore, the contribution of each phenotype to the composition of the blood varies. Phenotypic mosaicism is clinically relevant because PNH II cells are relatively resistant to spontaneous hemolysis, and patients with a high percentage of type II cells have a relatively benign clinical course (Fig. 40–4).

The anemia of PNH is multifactorial as an element of marrow failure is present in all patients, although the degree of marrow dysfunction is variable.[27] In some patients, PNH arises in the setting of aplastic anemia. In this case, marrow failure is the dominant cause of anemia. In other patients with PNH, evidence of marrow dysfunction may be subtle (e.g., an inappropriately low reticulocyte count) with the degree of anemia being determined primarily by the rate of hemolysis that is, in turn, determined by PNH clone size.

CLINICAL FEATURES

The primary clinical manifestations of PNH are hemolysis, thrombosis, and marrow failure.[27] Constitutional symptoms (fatigue, lethargy, malaise, asthenia) dominate the history, but nocturnal hemoglobinuria is a presenting symptom in only approximately 25 percent of patients.[28] Directed questioning frequently elicits a history of episodic dysphagia and odynophagia, abdominal pain, and male impotence. Venous thrombosis, often occurring at unusual sites (Budd-Chiari syndrome, mesenteric, dermal or cerebral veins), may complicate PNH. Arterial thrombosis is less common.

LABORATORY FEATURES

PNH should be suspected in all patients with nonspherocytic, Coombs negative intravascular hemolysis (Table 40–1).

While the clinical manifestations of PNH depend in large part on the size of the *PIGA* mutant clone, the extent of the associated marrow failure also contributes significantly to disease manifestations. Thus, PNH is not a binary process and based on clinical features, marrow characteristics, and the size of the mutant clone as determined by the percentage of GPI-AP deficient polymorphonuclear cells (PMNs), the International PNH Interest Group recognizes three disease subcategories (Table 40–2).[27]

Reticulocytosis reflects the response to hemolysis, although the reticulocyte count may be lower than expected for the degree of anemia because of underlying marrow failure (see Table 40–1). Serum lactate dehydrogenase (LDH) concentration is always abnormally high in patients with clinically significant hemolysis and serves as an important

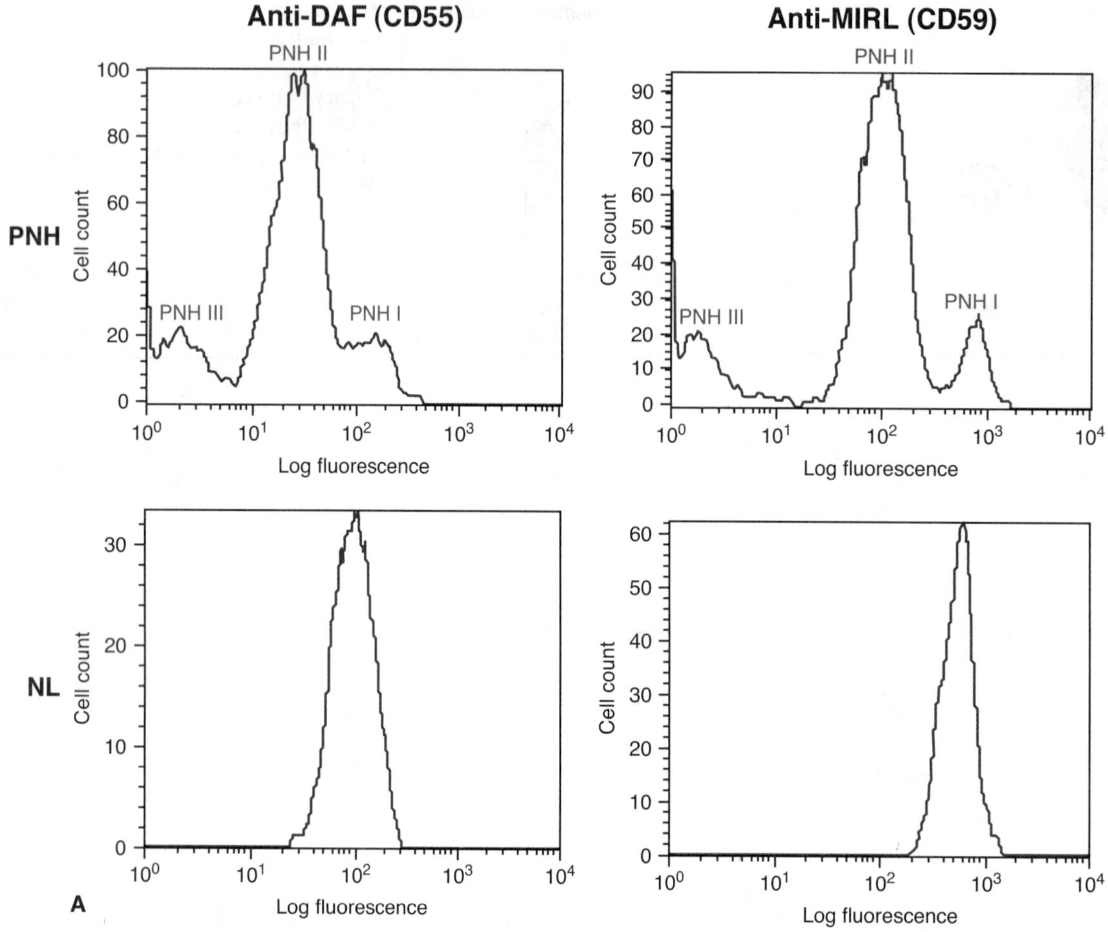

FIGURE 40–3. Phenotypic mosaicism is a characteristic feature of PNH. **A.** The blood of patients with PNH is a mosaic of phenotypically normal and abnormal cells. In some patients, erythrocytes that are partially deficient in GPI-APs (called PNH II) are present in the blood along with cells that are completely deficient (PNH III) and cells that are phenotypically normal (PNH I). In the case illustrated, erythrocytes from a patient with PNH (PNH, *upper panels*) and from a healthy volunteer (NL, *lower panels*) were stained with fluorescently labeled antibodies (anti-CD55, *left panels*; CD59, *right panels*) and analyzed by flow cytometry. (*continued*)

surrogate marker for determining and following the rate of intravascular hemolysis. A close association exists between PNH and aplastic anemia and to a lesser extent between PNH and low-risk myelodysplastic syndromes (see Chaps. 34 and 88 and see "PNH and Marrow Failure" below). By using high-sensitivity flow cytometry, approximately 60 percent of patients with aplastic anemia and 20 percent of patients with low-risk myelodysplastic syndrome (MDS) have been found to have a detectable population of GPI-AP–deficient erythrocytes and granulocytes.[29–31] In approximately 80 percent of these cases, the proportion of GPI-AP deficient cells is <1.0 percent of the total. These patients with very small populations of GPI-AP–deficient erythrocytes have no clinical or biochemical evidence of hemolysis and are designated as subclinical PNH (PNH-sc; see Table 40–2). Varying degrees of leukopenia, thrombocytopenia, and relative reticulocytopenia reflect the extent of marrow insufficiency.

Once suspected, diagnosing PNH is straightforward as deficiency of GPI-APs on blood cells is readily demonstrated by flow cytometry[32] (Fig. 40–5). Although they have much biologic and historic importance, the acidified serum lysis test (Ham test) and the sucrose lysis test (sugar water test) have been largely abandoned as diagnostic assays because they are both less sensitive and less quantitative than flow cytometry. Flow cytometric analysis of both RBCs and PMNs is warranted, as clone size will be underestimated if only RBCs are examined because GPI-AP–deficient red cells are selectively destroyed by complement. Recent transfusion will also affect the estimate of clone size if only RBCs are analyzed, but delineation of PNH phenotypes (i.e., the percentage of types I, II, and III cells) requires flow cytometric analysis of the erythrocyte population.

In addition to flow cytometric analysis, the basic initial evaluation of a patient with PNH should include complete blood count to assess the effects of the disease on production of leukocytes and platelets, as well as on erythrocytes (Table 40–3). In patients with classic PNH, the leukocyte and platelet counts are usually normal or nearly normal, whereas leukopenia, thrombocytopenia, or both invariably accompany PNH/aplastic anemia and PNH/MDS. The reticulocyte count is needed to assess the ongoing capacity of the marrow to respond to the anemia. Although the reticulocyte count is elevated in patients with classic PNH, as noted above, it may be inappropriately low for the degree of anemia, reflecting underlying relative insufficiency of hematopoiesis that is characteristic of the disease. The reticulocyte count is subnormal in patients with PNH with concomitant aplastic anemia or low-risk MDS. Serum LDH is always markedly elevated in classic PNH. The degree of serum LDH elevation is variable in patients with PNH/aplastic anemia and PNH/MDS, depending on the size of the PNH clone (see Table 40–2). By definition, patients with PNH-sc have neither clinical nor biochemical evidence of hemolysis (see Table 40–2). Patients

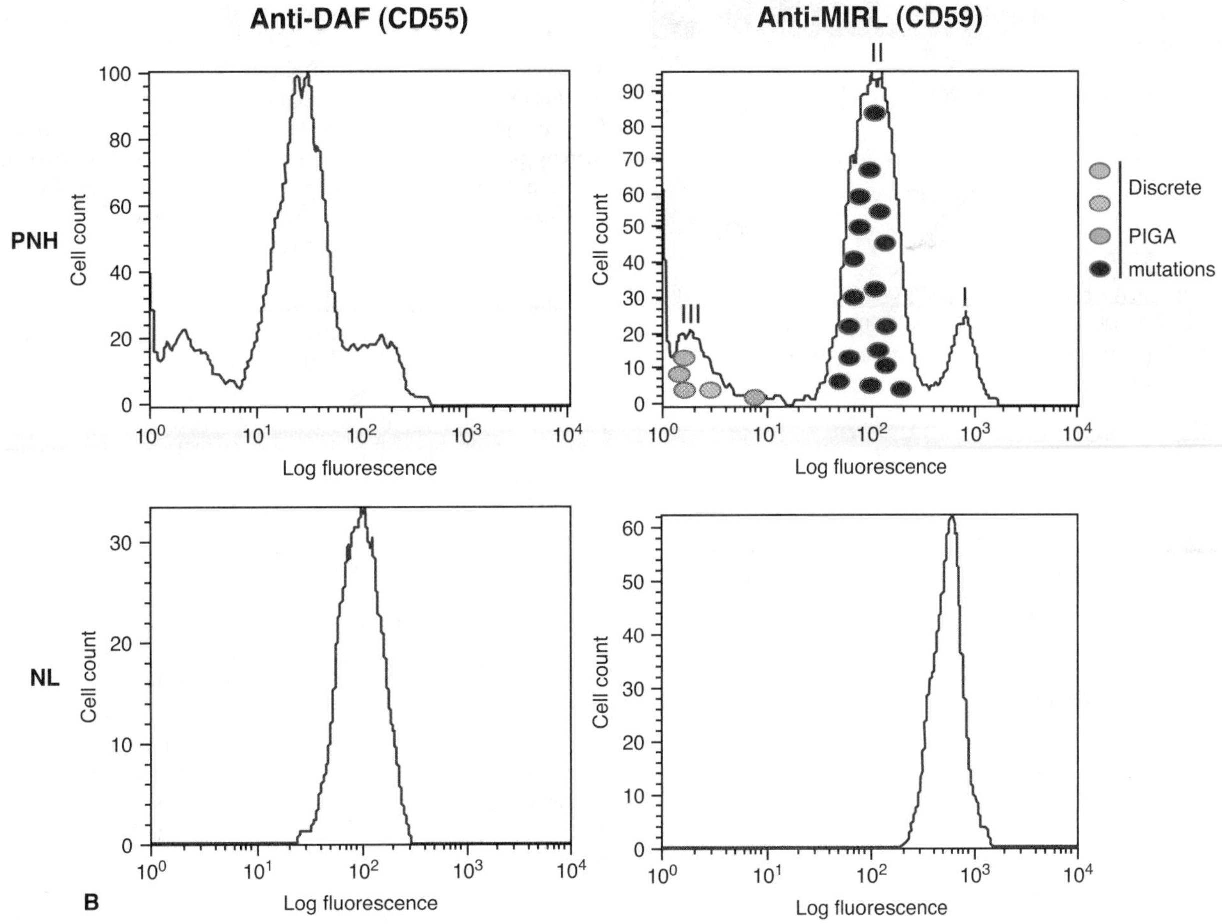

FIGURE 40–3. *(continued)* Phenotypic mosaicism is a characteristic feature of PNH. **B.** *PIGA* genotype determines PNH phenotype. The PNH II phenotype is a consequence of *PIGA* mutation that partially inactivates enzyme function (*red circles*), whereas any *PIGA* mutation that causes complete loss of enzyme function generates the PNH III phenotype (*green, yellow*, and *blue circles*). PNH I cells, have wild-type *PIGA* and are thought to represent the progeny of normal residual hematopoietic stem cells. In a single individual, multiple discrete *PIGA* mutations can be identified, accounting for the phenotypic mosaicism based on GPI-AP expression.

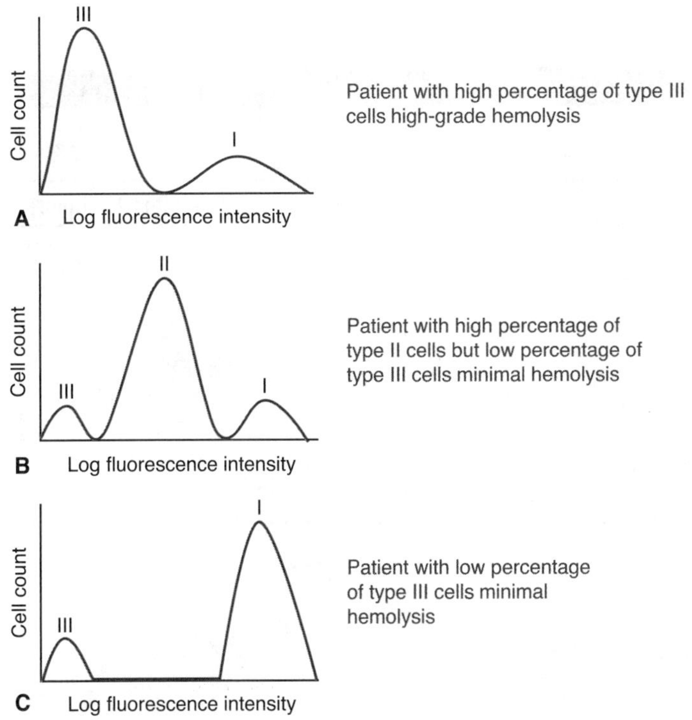

FIGURE 40–4. Clinical manifestations of PNH are determined by clone size and erythrocyte phenotype. Mock flow cytometry histograms of erythrocytes from hypothetical patients with PNH stained with anti-CD59 are illustrated. Both the proportion and type of abnormal erythrocytes vary greatly among patients with PNH, and these characteristics are important determinants of clinical manifestations. **A.** In general, patients with a high percentage of type III erythrocytes have clinically apparent hemolysis. **B.** If the erythrocytes are partially deficient in GPI-AP (PNH II cells), hemolysis may be modest even if the percentage of the affected cells is high. **C.** A patient may have a diagnosis of PNH, but if the proportion of type III cells is low, only biochemical evidence of hemolysis may be observed. (Modified with permission from Parker C, Omine M, Richards S, et al: Diagnosis and management of paroxysmal nocturnal hemoglobinuria. Blood 106:3699, 2005.)

TABLE 40–1. Recommendation for Screening Patients for PNH*

History of episodic hemoglobinuria
Evidence of nonspherocytic, Coombs negative intravascular hemolysis (must have abnormally high serum lactate dehydrogenase)
Patients with aplastic anemia (screen at diagnosis and once yearly even in the absence of intravascular hemolysis)
Patients with refractory anemia (RA) or refractory cytopenias with multilineage dysplasia (RCMD) variants of myelodysplastic syndrome (MDS)†
Patients with venous thrombosis involving unusual sites (usually have evidence of intravascular hemolysis)
• Budd-Chiari syndrome
• Other intraabdominal sites
• Cerebral veins
• Dermal veins

*Screening by flow cytometric analysis of GPI-APs on RBCs and polymorphonuclear cells.

†There is no indication for screening patients with other MDS classifications.

with classic PNH are usually iron deficient as a result of chronic iron loss in the form of hemoglobinuria and hemosiderinuria (see Chap. 42). Marrow aspirate and biopsy are needed to distinguish classic PNH from PNH in the setting of another marrow abnormality. Nonrandom cytogenetic abnormalities are rare in PNH.[25]

DIFFERENTIAL DIAGNOSIS

PNH AND MARROW FAILURE

Although the marrow of patients with classic PNH appears fairly normal morphologically (see Table 40–2), numerous *in vitro* studies have shown that the growth characteristics of marrow-derived stem cells are aberrant.[22,33,34] Moreover, when stem cells are sorted into GPI-AP– and GPI-AP+ populations, compared to the GPI-AP+ population, the growth characteristics of the GPI-AP– population more closely approach those of normal control cells.[22,33] One plausible explanation for this observation is that the GPI-AP– cells are relatively protected from the pathophysiologic process that mediates the marrow injury, thereby providing a basis for natural selection of the *PIGA* mutant clone. In this view of PNH, outgrowth of the *PIGA* mutant clone is seen as an example of Darwinian evolution occurring within the microenvironment of the marrow. Although intellectually appealing, rigorous experimental support for this hypothesis is lacking.

Using high-resolution flow cytometry with the capacity to detect <0.003 percent GPI-AP–deficient erythrocytes and granulocytes, 50 to 60 percent of patients with aplastic anemia can be shown to have a population of PNH cells at diagnosis,[30,35] however, only 10 to 15 percent of patients with aplastic anemia treated with immunosuppressive therapy subsequently develop clinically apparent PNH,[36] and development of clinical disease, when it occurs, typically follows diagnosis of aplastic anemia by several years. In the remainder, GPI-AP– cells persist subclinically or disappear, suggesting that mutant *PIGA* (and the consequent deficiency of GPI-APs) is necessary for clonal selection but is insufficient to account for the clonal expansion required for clinical manifestations of PNH to become apparent. One interpretation of these observations is that factors in addition to mutant *PIGA* determine the clinical phenotype of the disease by affecting the extent to which the *PIGA* mutant stem cells expand. Conceivably, a second genetic event that works additively or synergistically with mutant *PIGA* is required for clonal expansion.[25] That the extent of clonal expansion varies markedly among patients, however, suggests that the second event may have diverse etiologies and could involve somatic mutations, epigenetic phenomenon or stochastic processes.

The basis of the relationship between PNH and aplastic anemia is speculative. Most patients with PNH have some evidence of marrow failure (e.g., thrombocytopenia, leukopenia, or both) during the course of their disease.[37–40] Therefore, marrow injury may play a central role in the development of PNH by providing the conditions that favor the growth/survival of *PIGA*-mutant, GPI-AP–deficient stem cells. Finding a population of GPI-AP–deficient erythrocytes in patients with aplastic anemia is clinically relevant, as these patients have a particularly high probability of

TABLE 40–2. Classification of PNH*

Category	Rate of Intravascular Hemolysis†	Marrow	Flow Cytometry	Benefit from Eculizumab
Classic	Florid (macroscopic hemoglobinuria is frequent or persistent)	Cellular marrow with erythroid hyperplasia and normal or near-normal morphology‡	Large population (>50%) of GPI-AP deficient PMNs¶	Yes
PNH in the setting of another marrow failure syndrome§	Mild to moderate (macroscopic hemoglobinuria is intermittent or absent)	Evidence of a concomitant marrow failure syndrome§	Although variable, the percentage of GPI-AP deficient PMNs¶ is usually relatively small (<30%)	Dependent on the size of the PNH clone
Subclinical	No clinical or biochemical evidence of intravascular hemolysis	Evidence of a concomitant marrow failure syndrome§	Small (<1%) population of GPI-AP deficient PMNs detected by high-resolution flow cytometry	No

*Based on recommendations of the International PNH Interest Group (*Blood* 106:3699, 2005).

†Based on macroscopic hemoglobinuria, serum lactate dehydrogenase concentration, and reticulocyte count.

‡Karyotypic abnormalities are uncommon.

§Aplastic anemia & refractory anemia/MDS are the most commonly associated marrow failure syndromes

¶Analysis of PMNs is more informative than analysis of RBCs because of selective destruction GPI-AP–deficient RBCs.

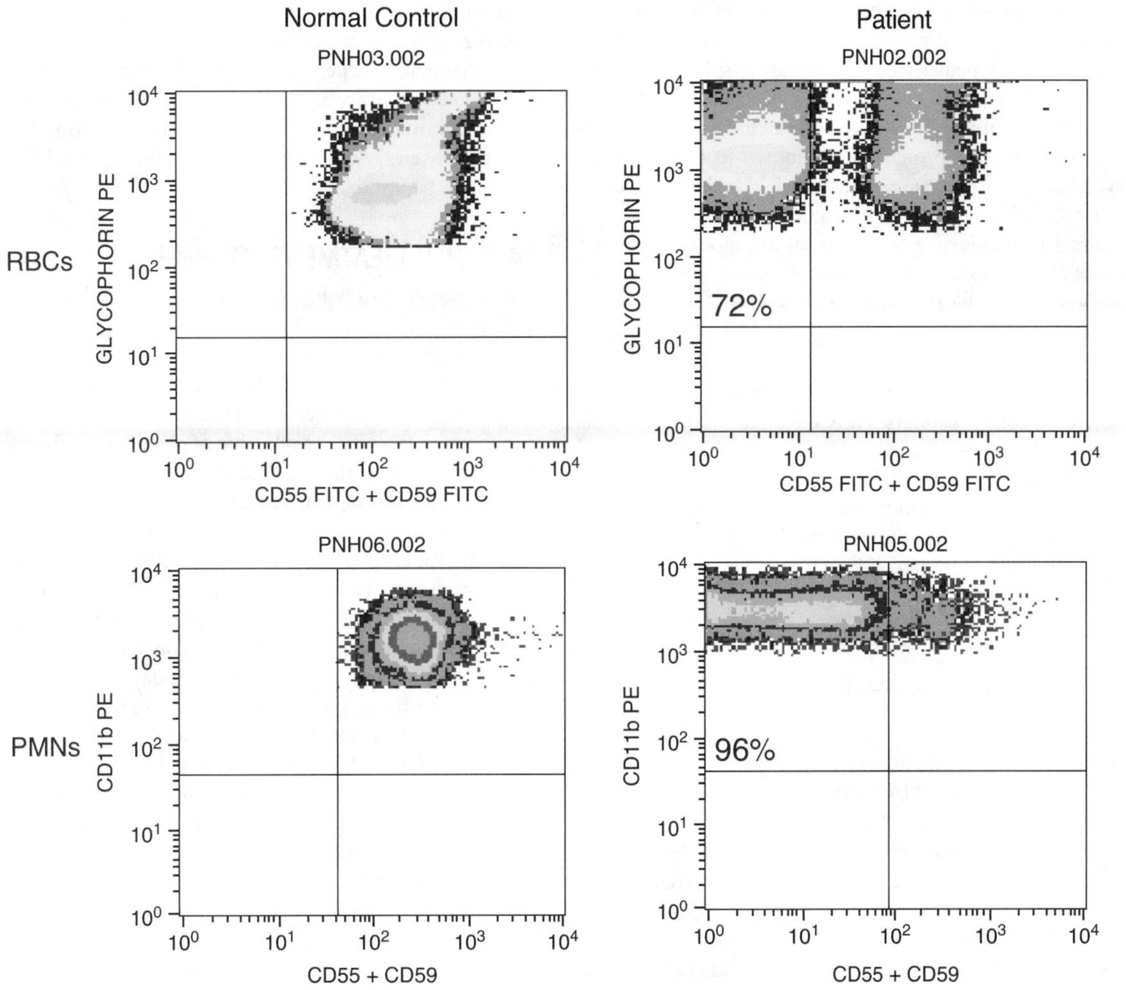

FIGURE 40–5. Diagnosis of PNH by flow cytometry. Erythrocytes (RBCs) and neutrophils (PMNs) from a healthy volunteer and a patient with PNH were analyzed by flow cytometry using antiglycophorin A (*top row, vertical axis*) to identify RBCs and anti-CD11b (*bottom row, vertical axis*) to identify PMNs. GPI-AP expression was detected using a combination of anti-CD55 and anti-CD59 (*top and bottom rows, horizontal axis*). PNH cells are deficient in both CD55 and CD59 (*upper left quadrant of each histogram*). The percentage of GPI-AP–deficient (PNH) cells is shown for each sample.

responding to immunosuppressive therapy and the onset of the response appears to be more rapid compared to patients with aplastic anemia without a population of GPI-AP–deficient erythrocytes.[30,31]

The presence of PNH cells has also been observed in patients with MDS.[29,31,41,42] Of note, the association between PNH and MDS appears to be confined to low-risk categories of MDS, particularly the refractory anemia (RA) variant.[29,31,42] Using high-sensitivity flow cytometry in which ≥0.003 percent GPI-AP–deficient RBCs or PMNs was classified as abnormal, Wang and colleagues reported that 21 of 119 (18%) patients with RA MDS had a population of PNH cells, whereas GPI-AP–deficient cells were not detected in patients with refractory anemia with ringed sideroblast (RARS), refractory anemia with excess of blasts (RAEB), or refractory anemia with excess of blasts in transformation (RAEB-t). Compared to patients with RA without a population of PNH cells (RA-PNH−), patients with RA with a population of PNH cells (RA-PNH+) had a distinct clinical profile characterized by the following features: (1) less-pronounced morphologic abnormalities of blood cells; (2) more severe thrombocytopenia; (3) lower rates of karyotypic abnormalities; (4) higher incidence of HLA-DR15; (5) lower rate of progression to acute leukemia; (6) higher probability of response to cyclosporine therapy.

That a population of PNH cells is associated only with low-risk MDS variants in Japanese patients was confirmed in a North American study of 137 patients[42] classified by World Health Organization (WHO) criteria.[43]

TABLE 40–3. Basic Evaluation for PNH

Flow cytometric evidence of a population of erythrocytes and granulocytes partially or completely deficient in multiple glycosyl phosphatidylinositol-anchored proteins (GPI-APs)*
Complete blood count, reticulocyte count, serum concentration of lactate dehydrogenase (LDH)†, bilirubin (fractionated) and haptoglobin, determination of iron stores
Marrow aspirate, biopsy, and cytogenetics‡

*PNH clone size is determined by the percentage of GPI-AP–deficient PMNs.

†The most important surrogate marker for intravascular hemolysis.

‡Marrow aspirate and biopsy are used to distinguish classic PNH from PNH in the setting of another marrow failure syndrome. Nonrandom karyotypic abnormalities are rare in PNH.

The study found a population of PNH cells in 1 of 5 (20%) patients with 5q− syndrome, in 6 of 17 (35%) patients with RA, and in 2 of 37 (5%) patients with refractory cytopenias with multilineage dysplasia (RCMD), whereas no patient with RARS (0 of 9), RCMD-ringed sideroblasts (0 of 6), RAEB (0 of 26), MDS unspecified (0 of 10), myelodysplastic/myeloproliferative disease (0 of 10), primary myelofibrosis (0 of 5), chronic myelomonocytic leukemia (0 of 5), or acute myeloid leukemia (0 of 6) had a detectable population of GPI-AP–deficient blood cells.

When combined with evidence of polyclonal hematopoiesis (based on the pattern of X-chromosome inactivation in female patients), the presence of a population of PNH cells in patients with MDS predicts a relatively benign clinical course and a high probability of response to immunosuppressive therapy in patients.[29] A relatively good response to immunosuppressive therapy for patients with MDS and aplastic anemia was also predicted by expression of HLA-DR15 in studies of both North American and Japanese patients.[44,45] Together, these observations provide compelling indirect evidence that aplastic anemia and a subgroup of low-risk MDS are immune-mediated diseases and that the immune pathophysiologic process provides the selection pressure that favors the outgrowth of *PIGA* mutant, GPI-AP–deficient stem cells.

THERAPY

ECULIZUMAB

The complement-mediated intravascular hemolysis of PNH can be inhibited by blocking formation of the MAC, the cytolytic component of the complement system (see Fig. 40–1). The MAC consists of complement components C5b, C6, C7, C8, and multiple molecules of C9. Eculizumab (Soliris) is a humanized monoclonal antibody that binds to complement C5, preventing its activation to C5b and thereby inhibiting MAC formation (see Fig. 40–1).[46] In 2007, eculizumab was approved by both the FDA and the European Union Commission for treatment of the hemolysis of PNH. Treatment with eculizumab reduces transfusion requirements, ameliorates the anemia of PNH, and markedly improves quality of life by resolving the debilitating constitutional symptoms (fatigue, lethargy, asthenia) associated with chronic complement-mediated intravascular hemolysis.[47] Following treatment, serum LDH concentration returns to normal, but mild to moderate anemia and reticulocytosis usually persist, likely the result of ongoing extravascular hemolysis mediated by opsonization of PNH erythrocytes by activated complement C3, as eculizumab does not block the activity of the APC C3 convertase (see Fig. 40–1).[48]

Thromboembolic events are the major cause of morbidity and mortality in PNH,[27] and eculizumab appears to ameliorate the thrombophilia of PNH, although the studies that support that conclusion were flawed by suboptimal design.[49]

Eculizumab is given by intravenous infusion on a biweekly schedule following an initial loading period consisting of five weekly treatments. In general, the drug is well tolerated; however, patients with congenital deficiency of complement C5 have an increased risk of infection with *Neisseria* species. For this reasons, patients treated with eculizumab (which blocks the function of C5; see Fig. 40–1) are at risk for meningococcal septicemia. All patients must be inoculated with a meningococcal vaccine 2 weeks before starting therapy, but the vaccine is not 100 percent protective. Whether prophylactic antibiotic therapy aimed at preventing meningococcal infection is justified for a patient receiving eculizumab remains to be determined. Despite the fact that the percentage of GPI-AP–deficient erythrocytes increases during treatment with eculizumab,[50] there have been no reports of catastrophic hemolytic crises in the relatively few PNH patients who have discontinued treatment with eculizumab.[49] This observation supports *in vitro* data showing that complement activation on PNH erythrocytes is attenuated by factor H, the plasma protein that regulates the APC C3 convertase.[51]

Eculizumab is expensive (~$400,000/year in the United States), and it has no effect either on the underlying stem cell abnormality or on the associated marrow failure. Consequently, treatment must continue indefinitely and leukopenia, thrombocytopenia, and reticulocytopenia, if present, persist.

OTHER TREATMENT FOR PNH

Other than eculizumab, there is no specific treatment for PNH, and for patients who are not being treated with eculizumab, management is largely supportive (reviewed in reference 27). Although hemolysis is ameliorated in some patients by treatment with glucocorticoids or androgens, the use of steroids in the management of patients with PNH is controversial.[27] The main value of glucocorticoids may be in attenuating acute hemolytic exacerbations. Under these circumstances, brief pulses of prednisone may reduce the severity and duration of the crisis while avoiding the untoward consequences associated with long-term use. The value of steroids in treating chronic hemolysis is limited by toxicity, and the harm that can accrue from long-term use cannot be overemphasized. An every-other-day schedule may attenuate some of the adverse effects of chronic glucocorticoid use,[52] but patients may note worsening of symptoms on the off day.

Androgen therapy, either alone or in combination with steroids, has been used successfully to treat the anemia of PNH.[52,53] As with glucocorticoids, the mechanism by which androgenic steroids ameliorate the anemia of PNH is not fully understood, although the rapid onset of action is consistent with complement inhibition.[53] Potential complications of androgen therapy include liver toxicity, prostatic hypertrophy, and virilizing effects. The toxicity profile is more favorable for attenuated synthetic androgens such as Danazol, making long-term use of this drug a reasonable management option in responding patients. A starting dose of 400 mg twice a day is recommended, but a lower dose (200–400 mg/day) may be adequate to control chronic hemolysis.[27]

Patients with PNH frequently become iron deficient as a result of both hemoglobinuria and hemosiderinuria.[52,53] Clinically important iron loss from hemosiderinuria can occur (see Chap. 42) even in the absence of gross hemoglobinuria. Replacement is often associated with exacerbation of hemolysis, regardless of the route of administration.[52,53] Compared with parenteral replacement, oral administration of iron may be accompanied by less-severe hemolytic exacerbations, but urinary iron loss may be so great that repletion cannot be achieved through this mechanism.[52] Parenteral repletion is generally safe. Concern for inducing a hemolytic exacerbation should not deter iron repletion, as iron deficiency not only limits erythropoiesis but also exacerbates the hemolysis of PNH.[53] If a hemolytic exacerbation occurs in the setting of iron repletion, the episode can be controlled by treatment with corticosteroids or androgens or by suppression of erythropoiesis by transfusion. There is no concern about iron-replacement therapy inducing a hemolytic exacerbation in patients being treated with eculizumab as hemolysis is inhibited by the drug.

Because the hemolysis is a consequence of a defect intrinsic to patient's erythrocytes, the anemia of PNH responds to red cell transfusion. In addition to increasing the hemoglobin concentration, transfusion may ameliorate hemolysis by suppressing erythropoiesis. Concerns about inducing a hemolytic exacerbation as a consequence of infusion of small amounts of donor plasma that may contaminate red cell preparations appear unwarranted.[54] However, hemofiltration is recommended to prevent transfusion reaction arising from the interaction between donor leukocytes and recipient antibodies. Iatrogenic hemochromatosis from chronic transfusion may be delayed in patients with

PNH as a result of iron loss from hemoglobinuria/hemosiderinuria.[52] In fact, iron overload in patients with classic PNH is rare. But iron overload remains a concern in patients who require chronic transfusion when the anemia is primarily a consequence of marrow failure rather than intravascular hemolysis.

Supplemental folate (5 mg/day) is recommended to compensate for increased utilization (see Chap. 41) associated with heightened erythropoiesis that is a consequence of ongoing hemolysis.[27]

The role of splenectomy in the management of patients with PNH is unclear. Reports of amelioration of hemolysis and improvement in cytopenias following splenectomy are anecdotal. Concerns about lack of proven efficacy and the potential for postoperative complications, particularly thrombosis, have led some to argue that splenectomy has no role in the management of PNH.[27]

HEMATOPOIETIC STEM CELL TRANSPLANTATION

Prior to the availability of eculizumab, the primary indications for transplantation were marrow failure, recurrent, life-threatening thrombosis, and uncontrollable hemolysis (Table 40–4).[27] The latter process can be eliminated by treatment with eculizumab and the thrombophilia of PNH may also respond to inhibition of intravascular hemolysis by eculizumab.[49] Nonetheless, transplant is the only curative therapy for PNH, and the availability of molecularly defined, matched, unrelated donors, less-toxic conditioning regimens, reduction in transplantation-related morbidity and mortality, and improvements in posttransplantation supportive care make this option a viable alternative to medical management. The decision to transplant is complex, however, and requires an understanding of the unique pathobiology of PNH and the input of physicians experienced in transplantation and medical management of PNH.

For patients who are receiving transplantation for marrow failure, the focus of management is on the etiology of the marrow failure (see Table 40–4). For patients with aplastic anemia and a small PNH clone who undergo matched sibling donor allotransplantation, the conditioning regimen of antithymocyte globulin and cyclophosphamide coupled with graft-versus-host effects appear sufficient to eradicate the PNH clone.[27] However, in the unusual situation in which the patient has a syngeneic twin, a more intense conditioning regimen is required, as graft-versus-tumor effect does not contribute to clonal eradication in this circumstance.[55] In the event that a patient with low-risk MDS with a PNH clone requires allotransplantation, the conditioning regimen (marrow ablative or reduced intensity) in combination with graft-versus-tumor effects is sufficient to eradicate the PNH clone.

Transplantation for classic PNH is aimed at eradicating the PNH clone, and both marrow ablative[56–58] and reduced intensity[59,60] conditioning regimens appear to be effective, although experience with the latter is more limited. Successful outcomes have been reported using matched unrelated donors, as well as matched sibling donors.[59,61]

There are no PNH-specific adverse events associated with transplantation; severe, acute graft-versus-host disease (GVHD) occurs in more than one-third of the patients and the incidence of chronic GVHD is roughly 35 percent. Overall survival for unselected PNH patients who undergo transplantation using an human leukocyte antigen (HLA)-matched sibling donor is in the range of 50 to 60 percent.[27]

TABLE 40–4. Hematopoietic Stem Cell Transplantation for PNH

Indications for transplantation
- Marrow failure—approach to management depends primarily on the underlying marrow abnormality (e.g., aplastic anemia) but the treatment regimen must be sufficient to eradicate the PNH clone
- Major complications of PNH
  Refractory, transfusion-dependent hemolytic anemia*
  Recurrent, life-threatening thromboembolic complications†

Conditioning regimens and donors
- Ablative and reduced intensity conditioning regimens have been successful
- For transplantations involving syngeneic twins, an ablative regimen is recommended‡
- Matched unrelated donor transplantations have been successful but experience is limited

Outcomes
- There are no PNH-specific adverse events. Severe, acute graft-versus-host disease occurs in approximately 33% of patients and the incidence of chronic graft-versus-host disease is roughly 35%
- Overall survival for unselected PNH patients who undergo transplantation using an HLA-matched sibling donor is in the range of 50–60%

*Treatment with eculizumab controls the intravascular hemolysis of PNH. Mild to moderate extravascular hemolytic anemia persists in most patients with PNH treated with eculizumab, likely as a consequence of opsonization of erythrocytes by activation and degradation products of complement C3.

†Eculizumab may ameliorate the thrombophilia of PNH.

‡Absence of graft-versus-host effect may render nonablative approaches inadequate.

MANAGEMENT OF THE THROMOPHILIA OF PNH

Thromboembolic complications are the leading cause of morbidity and mortality in PNH.[27] Prophylaxis against thromboembolic events in patients with PNH is an issue of active debate.[27] Current estimates of risk are based on retrospective analysis,[39,49,62–64] but risk appears to correlate with size of the PNH clone (based on flow cytometric determination of the percentage of GPI-AP–deficient PMNs), leading to the recommendation that patients with >50 to 60 percent GPI-AP–deficient PMNs be offered prophylactic anticoagulation.[62,63]

Although arterial thrombosis may be observed,[49] thromboembolic events in patients with PNH usually involve the venous system. Acute thrombotic events require anticoagulation with heparin. Systemic thrombolytic therapy,[65,66] or thrombolytic therapy delivered via canalization directly to the affected site,[67] should be strongly considered in patients with acute onset of Budd-Chiari syndrome.

Thrombocytopenia often complicates PNH, and this issue must be addressed when formulating an anticoagulation management plan. Thrombocytopenia is a relative, but not an absolute, contraindication to anticoagulation, and transfusions should be given to maintain the platelet count in a safe range rather than withholding therapy.[68] Patients with PNH who experience a thromboembolic event should be anticoagulated indefinitely. Recurrent, life-threatening thrombosis merits consideration of marrow transplantation (see Table 40–4).

Eculizumab appears to reduce the risk of thromboembolic complications.[49] For patients being treated with eculizumab who have no prior history of thromboembolic complications, prophylactic anticoagulation may be unnecessary, although it is recommended that anticoagulation continue for those patients who experienced a thromboembolic event prior to initiating therapy with eculizumab.

PREGNANCY AND PNH

Women with PNH can have serious morbidity and increased mortality during pregnancy.[68,69] Because of concerns about fetal/maternal risks from exposure to potentially toxic therapy, transfusion is the mainstay of management. Eculizumab is not approved for use during pregnancy. Moderate to severe thrombocytopenia may complicate the pregnancy, and clinically significant bleeding in this setting necessitates platelet transfusion. The incidence of clinically apparent venous thromboembolism during pregnancy in women with PNH is approximately 10 percent,[68] and these events are associated with a high risk of mortality.[68,69] Similar to nonpregnant patients with PNH, cerebral and hepatic veins are commonly involved sites of thrombosis. Patients who develop thrombosis should be therapeutically anticoagulated, and thrombolytic therapy should be considered for those with Budd-Chiari syndrome. Concurrent thrombocytopenia may necessitate platelet transfusion in patients who require anticoagulation. The role of prophylactic anticoagulation for pregnant women with PNH has not been studied systematically; however, because of the significant morbidity and mortality associated with thromboembolism in this setting, prophylaxis is recommended. Coumadin is contraindicated because of teratogenic potential in the first trimester and hemorrhagic risks later in gestation. Anticoagulation with heparin should begin immediately once the combination of pregnancy and PNH is documented. Low-molecular-weight heparin has a hypothetical advantage over unfractionated heparin because of a lower incidence of drug-induced thrombocytopenia (see Chap. 133). Careful monitoring of the platelet count is required because thrombocytopenia may worsen during the period of anticoagulation. Anticoagulation can be discontinued briefly around the time of delivery. However, it should be restarted as soon as is feasible and continued for at least 6 weeks into the postpartum period, as thrombosis during the puerperium is a major concern.[68,69] Most deliveries can be accomplished vaginally, although premature delivery may be necessary. Despite the many concerns surrounding PNH and pregnancy, successful outcomes appear to be the rule rather than the exception[39,68]; however, management is complicated and should involve the combined efforts of an experienced hematologist and an obstetrician experienced in dealing with high-risk pregnancies.[27]

PEDIATRIC PNH

PNH can occur in the young (approximately 10% of patients are younger than age 21 years at the time of diagnosis).[27] A retrospective analysis of 26 cases underscored the many similarities between childhood and adult PNH.[70] Signs and symptoms of hemolysis, marrow failure, and thrombosis dominate the clinical picture, although gross hemoglobinuria as a presenting symptom may be less common in young patients. A generally good response to immunosuppressive therapy was observed,[70] but based on poor long-term survival, hematopoietic cell transplantation is the recommended treatment for childhood PNH. A more recent study[71] confirmed the common presentation of marrow failure in 11 children with PNH, and reported that 5 patients eventually underwent hematopoietic cell transplant (3 matched unrelated donors and 2 matched family donors), of whom 4 were long-term survivors. Although eculizumab is not approved for PNH patients younger than age 18 years, approval will likely be sought once pharmacodynamic and pharmacokinetic characteristics of the drug are defined for the pediatric/adolescent population. The availability of eculizumab for pediatric PNH may be particularly advantageous as a bridge prior to implementation of more definitive therapy.

COURSE AND PROGNOSIS

The clinical course of PNH is enormously variable. In rare instances, the patient may succumb to this disease within a few months of the first onset of symptoms. Most patients experience a chronic course in which the severity of the disease waxes and wanes as the normal cells and the PNH clone alternately appear to gain ascendancy. Rarely, the abnormal clone disappears altogether, and the patient appears to be cured. Transformation to acute leukemia is uncommon (in the range of 1%). In some instances, but not in others, leukemic blasts are GPI-AP deficient.[72]

As with so many other diseases, initial reports on PNH tended to emphasize the more severely affected patients, so the prognosis was generally deemed to be very grave. As physicians developed a higher index of suspicion concerning this disorder, and as simplified methods for diagnosis became available, milder cases were diagnosed, and these tend to have the better long-term outlook. Nonetheless, even today, the disease must be considered a very serious one, and most patients eventually succumb to its complications. The most commonly lethal of these appear to be thrombotic episodes such as the Budd-Chiari syndrome,[40,64] but the various complications of pancytopenia also may lead to death,[28,38] and in a few patients the terminal episode has been the development of acute leukemia.[72] In a study of 220 patients with PNH followed for up to 46 years, the Kaplan-Meier survival estimate was 65 percent at 10 years and 48 percent at 15 years after diagnosis.[40] In another study of 80 consecutive patients the outlook was similar: the median survival after diagnosis was 10 years, with 28 percent of patients surviving for 25 years.[38] Eight-year cumulative incidence rates of the main complications of pancytopenia, thrombosis, and myelodysplastic syndrome were 15 percent, 28 percent, and 5 percent, respectively. Poor survival was associated with age older than 55 years at the time of diagnosis, the occurrence of thrombosis as a complication, evolution to pancytopenia, a myelodysplastic syndrome or acute leukemia, and thrombocytopenia at diagnosis. The prognosis of patients in whom aplastic anemia antedated PNH was better than in those in whom it did not.[40]

The impact of eculizumab on the natural history and prognosis of PNH has not been determined, although amelioration of thrombotic complications may translate into improved survival.[73]

REFERENCES

1. Crosby WH: Paroxysmal nocturnal hemoglobinuria: A classic description by Paul Strubling in 1882, and a bibliography of the disease. *Blood* 6:270, 1951.
2. Rosse W: A brief history of PNH, in *PNH and the GPI-Linked Proteins*, ed, edited by NS Young, J Moss, p 1. Academic Press, San Diego, 2000.
3. Parker CJ: Paroxysmal nocturnal hemoglobinuria: An historical overview. *Hematology Am Soc Hematol Educ Program* 2008:93, 2008.
4. Parker CJ: Historical aspects of paroxysmal nocturnal haemoglobinuria: "Defining the disease." *Br J Haematol* 117:3, 2002.
5. Hughes DA, Tunnage B, Yeo ST: Drugs for exceptionally rare diseases: Do they deserve special status for funding? *QJM* 98:829, 2005.
6. Parker CJ: Hemolysis in PNH, in *Paroxysmal Nocturnal Hemoglobinuria and the Glycosylphosphatidylinositol-Linked Proteins,* edited by NS Young, J Moss, p 49. Academic Press, San Diego, 2000.
7. Thurman JM, Holers VM: The central role of the alternative complement pathway in human disease. *J Immunol* 176:1305, 2006.
8. Nicholson-Weller A, Burge J, Fearon DT, et al: Isolation of a human erythrocyte membrane glycoprotein with decay-accelerating activity for C3 convertases of the complement system. *J Immunol* 129:184, 1982.
9. Nicholson-Weller A, March JP, Rosenfeld SI, Austen KF: Affected erythrocytes of patients with paroxysmal nocturnal hemoglobinuria are deficient in the complement regulatory protein, decay accelerating factor. *Proc Natl Acad Sci U S A* 80:5066, 1983.
10. Pangburn MK, Schreiber RD, Muller-Eberhard HJ: Deficiency of an erythrocyte membrane protein with complement regulatory activity in paroxysmal nocturnal hemoglobinuria. *Proc Natl Acad Sci U S A* 80:5430, 1983.
11. Holguin MH, Fredrick LR, Bernshaw NJ, et al: Isolation and characterization of a membrane protein from normal human erythrocytes that inhibits reactive lysis of the erythrocytes of paroxysmal nocturnal hemoglobinuria. *J Clin Invest* 84:7, 1989.
12. Kinoshita T, Inoue N, Takeda J: Defective glycosyl phosphatidylinositol anchor synthesis and paroxysmal nocturnal hemoglobinuria. *Adv Immunol* 60:57, 1995.
13. Miyata T, Takeda J, Iida Y, et al: The cloning of PIG-A, a component in the early step of GPI-anchor biosynthesis. *Science* 259:1318, 1993.
14. Miyata T, Yamada N, Iida Y, et al: Abnormalities of PIG-A transcripts in granulocytes from patients with paroxysmal nocturnal hemoglobinuria. *N Engl J Med* 330:249, 1994.

15. Takeda J, Miyata T, Kawagoe K, et al: Deficiency of the GPI anchor caused by a somatic mutation of the PIG-A gene in paroxysmal nocturnal hemoglobinuria. *Cell* 73:703, 1993.
16. Takahashi M, Takeda J, Hirose S, et al: Deficient biosynthesis of *N*-acetylglucosaminyl-phosphatidylinositol, the first intermediate of glycosyl phosphatidylinositol anchor biosynthesis, in cell lines established from patients with paroxysmal nocturnal hemoglobinuria. *J Exp Med* 177:517, 1993.
17. Parker CJ: The pathophysiology of paroxysmal nocturnal hemoglobinuria. *Exp Hematol* 35:523, 2007.
18. Rosti V, Tremml G, Soares V, et al: Murine embryonic stem cells without pig-a gene activity are competent for hematopoiesis with the PNH phenotype but not for clonal expansion. *J Clin Invest* 100:1028, 1997.
19. Brodsky RA, Vala MS, Barber JP, et al: Resistance to apoptosis caused by PIG-A gene mutations in paroxysmal nocturnal hemoglobinuria. *Proc Natl Acad Sci U S A* 94:8756, 1997.
20. Heeney MM, Ormsbee SM, Moody MA, et al: Increased expression of anti-apoptosis genes in peripheral blood cells from patients with paroxysmal nocturnal hemoglobinuria. *Mol Genet Metab* 78:291, 2003.
21. Horikawa K, Nakakuma H, Kawaguchi T, et al: Apoptosis resistance of blood cells from patients with paroxysmal nocturnal hemoglobinuria, aplastic anemia, and myelodysplastic syndrome. *Blood* 90:2716, 1997.
22. Chen R, Nagarajan S, Prince GM, et al: Impaired growth and elevated fas receptor expression in PIGA(+) stem cells in primary paroxysmal nocturnal hemoglobinuria. *J Clin Invest* 106:689, 2000.
23. Ware RE, Nishimura J, Moody MA, et al: The PIG-A mutation and absence of glycosylphosphatidylinositol-linked proteins do not confer resistance to apoptosis in paroxysmal nocturnal hemoglobinuria. *Blood* 92:2541, 1998.
24. Yamamoto T, Shichishima T, Shikama Y, et al: Granulocytes from patients with paroxysmal nocturnal hemoglobinuria and normal individuals have the same sensitivity to spontaneous apoptosis. *Exp Hematol* 30:187, 2002.
25. Inoue N, Izui-Sarumaru T, Murakami Y, et al: Molecular basis of clonal expansion of hematopoiesis in 2 patients with paroxysmal nocturnal hemoglobinuria (PNH). *Blood* 108:4232, 2006.
26. Endo M, Ware RE, Vreeke TM, et al: Molecular basis of the heterogeneity of expression of glycosyl phosphatidylinositol anchored proteins in paroxysmal nocturnal hemoglobinuria. *Blood* 87:2546, 1996.
27. Parker C, Omine M, Richards S, et al: Diagnosis and management of paroxysmal nocturnal hemoglobinuria. *Blood* 106:3699, 2005.
28. Dacie JV, Lewis SM: Paroxysmal nocturnal haemoglobinuria: Clinical manifestations, haematology, and nature of the disease. *Ser Haematol* 5:3, 1972.
29. Ishiyama K, Chuhjo T, Wang H, et al: Polyclonal hematopoiesis maintained in patients with bone marrow failure harboring a minor population of paroxysmal nocturnal hemoglobinuria-type cells. *Blood* 102:1211, 2003.
30. Sugimori C, Chuhjo T, Feng X, et al: Minor population of CD55-CD59- blood cells predicts response to immunosuppressive therapy and prognosis in patients with aplastic anemia. *Blood* 107:1308, 2006.
31. Wang H, Chuhjo T, Yasue S, et al: Clinical significance of a minor population of paroxysmal nocturnal hemoglobinuria-type cells in bone marrow failure syndrome. *Blood* 100:3897, 2002.
32. Richards SJ, Rawstron AC, Hillmen P: Application of flow cytometry to the diagnosis of paroxysmal nocturnal hemoglobinuria. *Cytometry* 42:223, 2000.
33. Chen G, Kirby M, Zeng W, et al: Superior growth of glycophosphatidylinositol-anchored protein-deficient progenitor cells in vitro is due to the higher apoptotic rate of progenitors with normal phenotype *in vivo*. *Exp Hematol* 30:774, 2002.
34. Dunn DE, Liu JM, Young NS: Bone marrow failure in PNH, in *Paroxysmal Nocturnal Hemoglobinuria and the Glycosylphosphatidylinositol-Linked Proteins,* ed, edited by NS Young, J Moss, p 113. Academic Press, San Diego, 2000.
35. Mukhina GL, Buckley JT, Barber JP, et al: Multilineage glycosylphosphatidylinositol anchor-deficient haematopoiesis in untreated aplastic anaemia. *Br J Haematol* 115:476, 2001.
36. Frickhofen N, Heimpel H, Kaltwasser JP, Schrezenmeier H: Antithymocyte globulin with or without cyclosporin A: 11-year follow-up of a randomized trial comparing treatments of aplastic anemia. *Blood* 101:1236, 2003.
37. de Latour RP, Mary JY, Salanoubat C, et al: Paroxysmal nocturnal hemoglobinuria: Natural history of disease subcategories. *Blood* 112:3099, 2008.
38. Hillmen P, Lewis SM, Bessler M, et al: Natural history of paroxysmal nocturnal hemoglobinuria. *N Engl J Med* 333:1253, 1995.
39. Nishimura JI, Kanakura Y, Ware RE, et al: Clinical course and flow cytometric analysis of paroxysmal nocturnal hemoglobinuria in the United States and Japan. *Medicine (Baltimore)* 83:193, 2004.
40. Socie G, Mary JY, de Gramont A, et al: Paroxysmal nocturnal haemoglobinuria: Long-term follow-up and prognostic factors. French Society of Haematology. *Lancet* 348:573, 1996.
41. Dunn DE, Tanawattanacharoen P, Boccuni P, et al: Paroxysmal nocturnal hemoglobinuria cells in patients with bone marrow failure syndromes. *Ann Intern Med* 131:401, 1999.
42. Wang SA, Pozdnyakova O, Jorgensen JL, et al: Detection of paroxysmal nocturnal hemoglobinuria clones in patients with myelodysplastic syndromes and related bone marrow diseases, with emphasis on diagnostic pitfalls and caveats. *Haematologica* 94:29, 2009.
43. Harris NL, Jaffe ES, Diebold J, et al: The World Health Organization classification of neoplastic diseases of the hematopoietic and lymphoid tissues. Report of the Clinical Advisory Committee meeting, Airlie House, Virginia, November, 1997. *Ann Oncol* 10:1419, 1999.
44. Saunthararajah Y, Nakamura R, Nam JM, et al: HLA-DR15 (DR2) is overrepresented in myelodysplastic syndrome and aplastic anemia and predicts a response to immunosuppression in myelodysplastic syndrome. *Blood* 100:1570, 2002.
45. Sugimori C, Yamazaki H, Feng X, et al: Roles of DRB1 *1501 and DRB1 *1502 in the pathogenesis of aplastic anemia. *Exp Hematol* 35:13, 2007.
46. Parker C: Eculizumab for paroxysmal nocturnal haemoglobinuria. *Lancet* 373:759, 2009.
47. Hillmen P, Young NS, Schubert J, et al: The complement inhibitor eculizumab in paroxysmal nocturnal hemoglobinuria. *N Engl J Med* 355:1233, 2006.
48. Risitano AM, Notaro R, Marando L, et al: Complement fraction 3 binding on erythrocytes as additional mechanism of disease in paroxysmal nocturnal hemoglobinuria patients treated by eculizumab. *Blood* 113:4094, 2009.
49. Hillmen P, Muus P, Duhrsen U, et al: Effect of the complement inhibitor eculizumab on thromboembolism in patients with paroxysmal nocturnal hemoglobinuria. *Blood* 110:4123, 2007.
50. Hillmen P, Hall C, Marsh JC, et al: Effect of eculizumab on hemolysis and transfusion requirements in patients with paroxysmal nocturnal hemoglobinuria. *N Engl J Med* 350:552, 2004.
51. Ferreira VP, Pangburn MK: Factor H mediated cell surface protection from complement is critical for the survival of PNH erythrocytes. *Blood* 110:2190, 2007.
52. Rosse WF: Treatment of paroxysmal nocturnal hemoglobinuria. *Blood* 60:20, 1982.
53. Hartmann RC, Jenkins DE Jr, McKee LC, Heyssel RM: Paroxysmal nocturnal hemoglobinuria: Clinical and laboratory studies relating to iron metabolism and therapy with androgen and iron. *Medicine (Baltimore)* 45:331, 1966.
54. Brecher ME, Taswell HF: Paroxysmal nocturnal hemoglobinuria and the transfusion of washed red cells: A myth revisited. *Transfusion* 29:681, 1989.
55. Endo M, Beatty PG, Vreeke TM, et al: Syngeneic bone marrow transplantation without conditioning in a patient with paroxysmal nocturnal hemoglobinuria: *In vivo* evidence that the mutant stem cells have a survival advantage. *Blood* 88:742, 1996.
56. Bemba M, Guardiola P, Garderet L, et al: Bone marrow transplantation for paroxysmal nocturnal haemoglobinuria. *Br J Haematol* 105:366, 1999.
57. Hegenbart U, Niederwieser D, Forman S, et al: Hematopoietic cell transplantation from related and unrelated donors after minimal conditioning as a curative treatment modality for severe paroxysmal nocturnal hemoglobinuria. *Biol Blood Marrow Transplant* 9:689, 2003.
58. Raiola AM, Van Lint MT, Lamparelli T, et al: Bone marrow transplantation for paroxysmal nocturnal hemoglobinuria. *Haematologica* 85:59, 2000.
59. Saso R, Marsh J, Cevreska L, et al: Bone marrow transplants for paroxysmal nocturnal haemoglobinuria. *Br J Haematol* 104:392, 1999.
60. Takahashi Y, McCoy JP Jr, Carvallo C, et al: *In vitro* and *in vivo* evidence of PNH cell sensitivity to immune attack after nonmyeloablative allogeneic hematopoietic cell transplantation. *Blood* 103:1383, 2004.
61. Woodard P, Wang W, Pitts N, et al: Successful unrelated donor bone marrow transplantation for paroxysmal nocturnal hemoglobinuria. *Bone Marrow Transplant* 27:589, 2001.
62. Hall C, Richards S, Hillmen P: Primary prophylaxis with warfarin prevents thrombosis in paroxysmal nocturnal hemoglobinuria (PNH). *Blood* 102:3587, 2003.
63. Moyo VM, Mukina GL, Barrett ES, Brodsky RA: Natural history of paroxysmal nocturnal haemoglobinuria using modern diagnostic assays. *Br J Haematol* 126:133, 2004.
64. Sloand EM, Young NS: Thrombotic complications in PNH, in *Paroxysmal Nocturnal Hemoglobinuria and the Glycosylphosphatidylinositol-Linked Proteins,* edited by NS Young, J Moss, p 101. Academic Press, San Diego, 2000.
65. Griffith JF, Mahmoud AE, Cooper S, et al: Radiological intervention in Budd-Chiari syndrome: Techniques and outcome in 18 patients. *Clin Radiol* 51:775, 1996.
66. McMullin MF, Hillmen P, Jackson J, et al: Tissue plasminogen activator for hepatic vein thrombosis in paroxysmal nocturnal haemoglobinuria. *J Intern Med* 235:85, 1994.
67. Sholar PW, Bell WR: Thrombolytic therapy for inferior vena cava thrombosis in paroxysmal nocturnal hemoglobinuria. *Ann Intern Med* 103:539, 1985.
68. Ray JG, Burows RF, Ginsberg JS, Burrows EA: Paroxysmal nocturnal hemoglobinuria and the risk of venous thrombosis: Review and recommendations for management of the pregnant and nonpregnant patient. *Haemostasis* 30:103, 2000.
69. Tichelli A, Socie G, Marsh J, et al: Outcome of pregnancy and disease course among women with aplastic anemia treated with immunosuppression. *Ann Intern Med* 137:164, 2002.
70. Ware RE, Hall SE, Rosse WF: Paroxysmal nocturnal hemoglobinuria with onset in childhood and adolescence. *N Engl J Med* 325:991, 1991.
71. van den Heuvel-Eibrink MM, Bredius RG, te Winkel ML, et al: Childhood paroxysmal nocturnal haemoglobinuria (PNH), a report of 11 cases in the Netherlands. *Br J Haematol* 128:571, 2005.
72. Harris JW, Koscick R, Lazarus HM, et al: Leukemia arising out of paroxysmal nocturnal hemoglobinuria. *Leuk Lymphoma* 32:401, 1999.
73. Rother RP, Rollins SA, Mojcik CF, et al: Discovery and development of the complement inhibitor eculizumab for the treatment of paroxysmal nocturnal hemoglobinuria. *Nat Biotechnol* 25:1256, 2007.

CHAPTER 41
FOLATE, COBALAMIN, AND MEGALOBLASTIC ANEMIAS

Ralph Green

SUMMARY

Folate in its tetrahydro form is a transporter of one-carbon fragments, which it can carry at any of three oxidation levels: methanol, formaldehyde, and formic acid. The oxidation levels of the folate-bound one-carbon fragments can be altered by oxidation and reduction reactions that require nicotinamide adenine dinucleotide phosphate and nicotinamide adenine dinucleotide phosphate (reduced form, NADPH), respectively. The chief source of the folate-bound one-carbon fragments is serine, which is converted to glycine as it passes its terminal carbon to folate. The one-carbon fragments are used for biosynthesis of purines, thymidine, and methionine. During biosynthesis of purines and methionine, free folate is released in its tetrahydro form. During biosynthesis of thymidine, tetrahydrofolate is oxidized to the dihydro form and must be re-reduced by dihydrofolate reductase in order to continue functioning in one-carbon metabolism. Methotrexate acts as an anticancer agent because it is an exceedingly powerful inhibitor of dihydrofolate reductase.

In the cell, folates are conjugated by the addition of a chain of seven or eight glutamic acid residues. These residues enable the retention of folates in the cell. When folates are absorbed from the intestine, a process that occurs chiefly in the duodenum and proximal jejunum, all but one of the glutamates are removed by the enzyme conjugase. Folates travel in the bloodstream and are taken up by the cells, mainly in the form of unconjugated methyltetrahydrofolate. The newly absorbed folates are rapidly reconjugated in the cell. If reconjugation is prevented, the folates cannot be retained in the cell, resulting in an intracellular folate deficiency.

Cobalamin is required for two reactions: intramitochondrial conversion of methylmalonyl coenzyme A (CoA), a product of catabolism of branched-chain amino acids, and ketogenic amino acids to succinyl CoA, a Krebs cycle intermediate, and cytosolic conversion of homocysteine to methionine, a reaction in which the methyl group of methyltetrahydrofolate is donated to the sulfur atom of homocysteine. In cobalamin deficiency, methyltetrahydrofolate accumulates because, for practical purposes, donation of the methyl group to homocysteine is the only method of generating free tetrahydrofolate from methyltetrahydrofolate. Free tetrahydrofolate is an excellent substrate for the conjugase; methyltetrahydrofolate is a poor substrate. Consequently, much of the methyltetrahydrofolate taken up by a cobalamin-deficient cell leaks out of the cell before it can be conjugated. The megaloblastic anemia of cobalamin deficiency results from an intracellular folate deficiency that arises because of the cell's limited ability to conjugate methyltetrahydrofolate.

Absorption of cobalamin is a highly complex process. Upon arriving in the stomach, cobalamin is taken up by haptocorrin (HC) binder (also called *R binder* or *cobalophilin*), a glycoprotein found in virtually all secretions. When the cobalamin HC complex enters the duodenum, the HC is digested and the cobalamin is released into the intestinal lumen, where it is taken up by intrinsic factor, a glycoprotein secreted by the gastric parietal cells. The cobalamin-intrinsic factor complex is absorbed by cells in the ileum through receptor-mediated endocytosis, involving cubilin and other proteins. The cobalamin is released within lysosomes and transported to the blood stream where it circulates bound to transcobalamin (TC), which delivers its cargo of cobalamin to cells throughout the body. Folic acid (pteroylglutamic acid) and cobalamin (vitamin B_{12}) play key roles in the metabolic machinery of proliferating cells.

Megaloblastic anemia most commonly results from folate or cobalamin (vitamin B_{12}) deficiency. Folate deficiency usually is nutritional in origin. It may be seen in alcoholics and the elderly poor but also is seen in patients on hyperalimentation, with hemolytic anemia, or hemodialysis. In countries in which folic acid fortification of diet has been introduced such as the United States and Canada, the prevalence of folate deficiency has been dramatically reduced. In pregnancy, even a mild folate deficiency may be associated with defects in neural tube closure in the fetus, so pregnant women should always be given folate supplements. The incidence of neural tube defects has fallen considerably in North America since the introduction of folic acid fortification. Diagnosis of folate deficiency is based on measurements of folate in serum, which furnishes information about the current level of folate, and in red cells, which provide data on aggregate folate status over the preceding period during which those red cells were produced. Nutritional folate deficiency is treated with folic acid by mouth.

Folate deficiency as a result of malabsorption occurs in tropical and nontropical sprue. Folate deficiency as a result of tropical sprue is treated with folate supplements and antibiotics. In nontropical sprue, the treatment is folate plus a gluten-free diet.

The most common cause of clinically apparent cobalamin deficiency is pernicious anemia (PA), a condition in which the portion of gastric mucosa that contains the parietal cells is destroyed through an autoimmune mechanism. The parietal cells secrete intrinsic factor, which is essential for cobalamin absorption. Without intrinsic factor, a state of cobalamin deficiency develops over the course of years. Cobalamin deficiency leads not only to megaloblastic anemia but also to a demyelinating disease that manifests itself as peripheral neuropathy, spastic paralysis with ataxia (so-called combined system disease of the spinal cord), dementia, psychosis, or a combination of the foregoing. "Subtle" cobalamin deficiency, often manifested as neurologic symptoms without anemia, appears to be relatively widespread among the elderly. The incidence of gastric cancer is increased by a factor of two to three in patients with PA. Other causes of cobalamin deficiency are gastric resection; stasis of the small intestinal contents as a result of blind loops, strictures, or hypomotility (e.g., as seen in amyloid); and disease or resection of the terminal ileum, the site of vitamin B_{12}-intrinsic factor complex absorption. Patients on a vegan diet become cobalamin deficient. Cobalamin deficiency is diagnosed by measuring the level of either total or TC-bound vitamin in the blood or by measuring serum methylmalonic acid, which accumulates in the bloodstream in patients with cobalamin deficiency. The cause of cobalamin deficiency was determined by the Schilling test, a measure of cobalamin absorption, but the test is obsolete and no replacement is available. In patients with nutritional megaloblastic anemia, folate or cobalamin deficiency as the cause of

Acronyms and abbreviations that appear in this chapter include: AdoCbl, adenosylcobalamin; AICAR, 5-amino-4-imidazole carboxamide ribotide; ATP, adenosine 5′-triphosphate; ATPase, adenosine triphosphatase; AZT, azidothymidine; BFU–E, burst-forming unit–erythroid; CnCbl, cyanocobalamin; CNS, central nervous system; CoA, coenzyme A; CUB, cubilin; CUBAM, the binary ileal cubilin receptor complex consisting of cubilin and amnionless; dTMP, deoxythymidine monophosphate; dU, deoxyuridine; dUMP, deoxyuridine monophosphate; FH_4, tetrahydrofolate; [^{3}H]Thd, [^{3}H]thymidine; HC, haptocorrin; HCl, hydrochloric acid; IM, intramuscular; LDH, lactate dehydrogenase; MCV, mean corpuscular volume; MeCbl, methylcobalamin; MRI, magnetic resonance imaging; MTHFR, methylenetetrahydrofolate reductase; NADP, nicotinamide adenine dinucleotide phosphate; NADPH, nicotinamide adenine dinucleotide phosphate (reduced form); N_2O, nitrous oxide; OHCbl, hydroxocobalamin; PA, pernicious anemia; PteGlu, pteroylglutamic acid (folic acid); SAH, *S*-adenosylhomocysteine; SAM, *S*-adenosylmethionine; TC, transcobalamin; UTP, uridine triphosphate.

the anemia must be determined. If a patient with cobalamin deficiency is treated with folic acid, the anemia may be corrected but the neurologic abnormalities persist or progress. Patients with cobalamin deficiency usually are treated with parenteral cobalamin but large doses of oral cobalamin may be used.

Megaloblastic anemia can develop as an acute disorder with rapid development of leukopenia and/or thrombocytopenia. Nitrous oxide anesthesia is responsible for some cases of acute megaloblastic anemia. The anemia is rarely also seen in patients with a marginal folate status in intensive care units or severe hemolytic anemia through increased folate demand for augmented erythropoiesis. The condition resembles an immune cytopenia but can be ruled out by examining the marrow, which exhibits a floridly megaloblastic picture.

Other causes of megaloblastic anemia include drugs (e.g., hydroxyurea, nucleoside analogues) and certain inborn errors of metabolism. Of the inherited conditions, TC deficiency is singled out because it causes a severe megaloblastic anemia in infants who respond completely to high-dose cobalamin. Irreversible neurologic complications supervene if the deficiency is not detected in time. Megaloblastic-like morphologic features of varying degree are seen in the myelodysplastic syndromes, and in acute leukemia of the erythroleukemia type. Megaloblastic anemia seen in association with refractory anemia with excess sideroblasts sometimes responds to very high doses of pyridoxine.

FOLATE

Folate and cobalamin (vitamin B_{12}) play key roles in the metabolism of all cells, particularly proliferating cells.

CHEMISTRY

The group of compounds consisting of folic acid and its derivatives are referred to as folates. *Folic acid* (pteroylglutamic acid) is composed of a pteridine derivative, a *p*-aminobenzoate residue, and an L-glutamic acid residue (Fig. 41–1A). The first two together are called *pteroic acid*.[1] In nature, folic acid occurs largely as conjugates in which multiple glutamic acids are linked by peptide bonds involving their γ-carboxyl groups (Fig. 41–1B). Additionally, the naturally occurring polyglutamated folates are reduced in the 5, 6, 7, and 8 positions of the pteridine ring (as described below, Fig. 41–1B). Conjugates are named according to the length of the glutamate chain (e.g., pteroylglutamate, pteroyldiglutamate, pteroylhexaglutamate). Therapeutic folic acid (abbreviated PteGlu, or F) has one glutamic acid and the pteridine ring is not reduced.

To form a functional compound, folate must be reduced to tetrahydrofolate (FH_4; see Fig. 41–1B). In this reduction, dihydrofolate (FH_2) is an intermediate. A single enzyme, *dihydrofolate reductase*, catalyzes both $F \rightarrow FH_2$ and $FH_2 \rightarrow FH_4$.

The folate family consists largely of FH_4 derivatives bearing a one-carbon substituent (symbolized as FH_4-C). The varieties of FH_4-C differ with regard to the identity of the one-carbon unit and the site of its attachment to FH_4. Figure 41–2 shows one-carbon substituents of biochemical significance and their major interconversions.

These substituents are attached to FH_4 through N^5, N^{10}, or both (see Fig. 41–2). Specific enzymes interconvert these various FH_4 derivatives through oxidations that require nicotinamide adenine dinucleotide (NADP) and reductions that utilize nicotinamide adenine dinucleotide phosphate (reduced form [NADPH]).

Reduced derivatives of folic acid usually are sensitive to air oxidation. A clinically important exception is N^5-formyl FH_4, also called *citrovorum factor, leucovorin,* or *folinic acid.*

NUTRITION

Sources

Folic acid comes from many sources. The richest vegetable sources are asparagus, broccoli, endive, spinach, lettuce, and lima beans. Each vegetable contains more than 1 mg of folate per 100 g dry weight. The best fruit sources are oranges, lemons, bananas, strawberries, and melons. Folates also are abundant in liver, kidney, yeast, mushrooms, and peanuts. Since the advent of folic acid fortification of the food supply, the median daily intake of folate from an average American diet is estimated to be 350 mcg.[2] Foods are readily depleted of folate by excessive cooking, especially with large amounts of water, discarded before ingestion.

Daily Requirements

In the normal adult, the minimum daily requirement for folic acid is approximately 50 mcg. The average diet contains many times this amount, but some of the folate may be unavailable. Accordingly, the officially recommended dietary allowance of *food* folate for an adult is 0.4 mg.[2] This figure is derived through considerations of the nutrient requirements to satisfy the needs of 97 to 98 percent of healthy individuals and the relative differences in absorption and bioavailability between dietary folate and the more bioavailable synthetic folic acid.

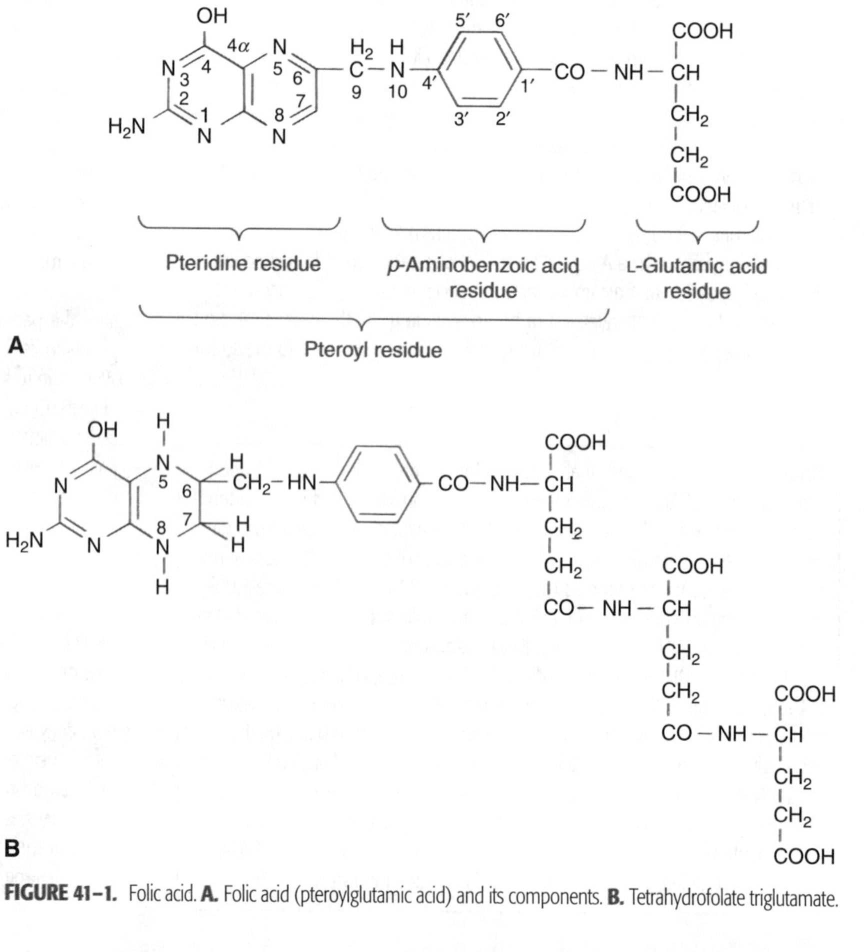

FIGURE 41–1. Folic acid. **A.** Folic acid (pteroylglutamic acid) and its components. **B.** Tetrahydrofolate triglutamate.

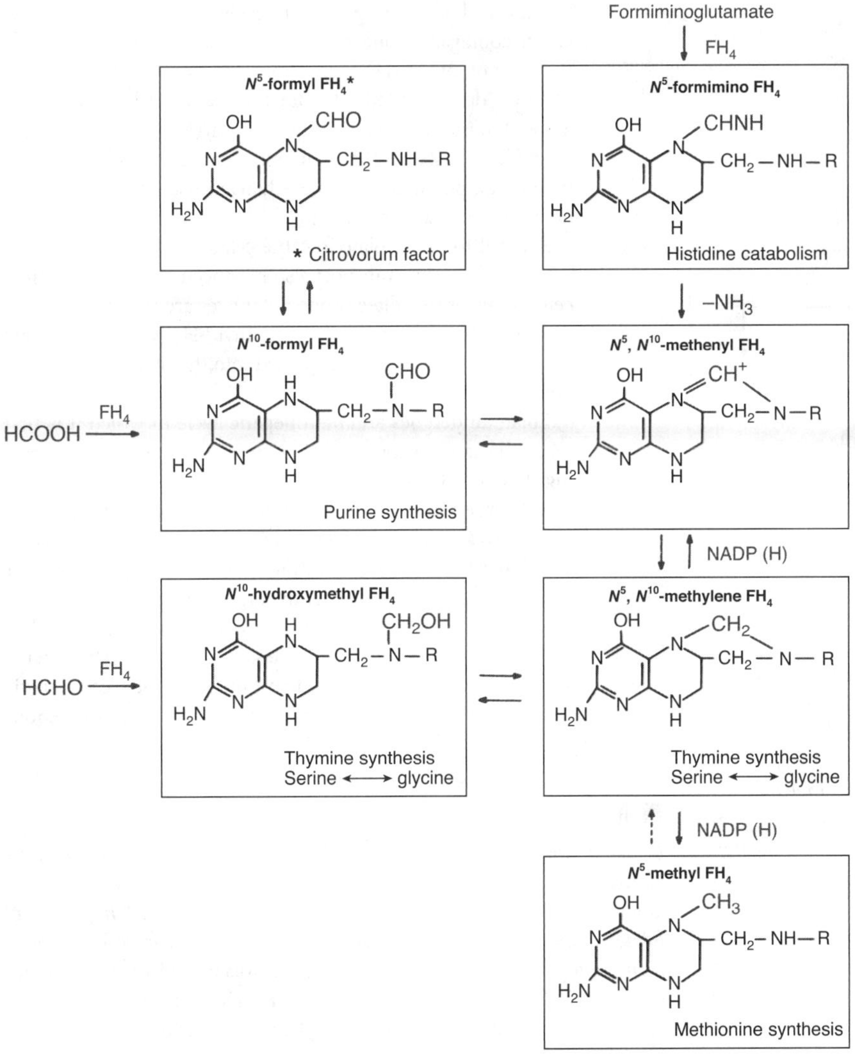

FIGURE 41–2. Derivatives of tetrahydrofolic acid (FH_4), their interconversions, and the metabolic pathways in which they participate. One-carbon substituents are shown in *blue*.

One mcg food folate is the dietary equivalent of 0.6 mcg folic acid added to food. The body is thought to contain approximately 5 mg of folate.[3] When folate intake is reduced to 5 mcg/day, megaloblastic anemia develops in approximately 4 months.[4]

Folic acid requirements increase in hemolytic anemia, leukemia, and other malignant diseases, in alcoholism[5] and during growth; in pregnancy and during lactation requirements increase threefold to sixfold.[6] Adequate folate supplies are particularly important in pregnant and lactating women, in whom the recommended daily allowance is increased to 600 and 500 mcg/day, respectively, to meet requirements.[7]

■ METABOLISM

Folate-Dependent Enzymes

FH_4 is an intermediate in reactions involving the transfer of one-carbon units from a donor to an acceptor. Table 41–1 summarizes the metabolic systems of animal tissues known to require folic acid coenzymes.

One-carbon units enter the folate pool principally via the serine hydroxymethyltransferase reaction[8]

$$\text{Serine} + FH_4 \rightleftharpoons \text{glycine} + N^5, N^{10}\text{-methylene } FH_4 + H_2O$$

which requires pyridoxal phosphate as cofactor.

Among the several one-carbon transfers mediated by folic acid, the transfer that appears to be the most important clinically is the methylation of deoxyuridylate to thymidylate, catalyzed by the enzyme thymidylate synthase.[9] This reaction is an essential step in the synthesis of DNA (Fig. 41–3). In carrying out this reaction, N^5, N^{10}-methylene FH_4 simultaneously transfers and reduces a one-carbon group, itself serving as the hydrogen donor for the reduction.[10] The reaction generates FH_2, which must be reduced again to FH_4 by dihydrofolate reductase and NADPH before it can again be utilized as a coenzyme:

$$\text{dUMP} + N^5, N^{10}\text{-methylene } FH_4 \rightarrow FH_2 + \text{dTMP}$$
$$FH_2 + \text{NADPH} + H^+ \rightarrow FH_4 + \text{NADP}^+$$

where dUMP = deoxyuridine monophosphate; dTMP = deoxythymidine monophosphate; and NADP = nicotinamide adenine dinucleotide phosphate. Limitation of thymidylate synthesis in folic acid deficiency causes incorporation of uracil instead of thymine into DNA.[11]

Folate deficiency diminishes purine biosynthesis by slowing (1) the folate-dependent formylation of glycinamide ribotide to *N*-formylglycinamide ribotide, the reaction that places the C-8 in the purine ring, and (2) the folate-dependent conversion of 5-amino-4-imidazole carboxamide ribotide (AICAR) to 5-formamido-4-imidazole carboxy-amide ribotide, the reaction that places the C-2 in the purine ring.[12] Additional reactions dependent on biopterin, a nonfolate pteridine derivative, that are of potential metabolic importance are hydroxylation of phenylalanine to tyrosine, oxidation of long-chain alkyl ethers of glycerol to fatty acid, hydroxylation of tryptophan to 6-hydroxytryptophan (a precursor of serotonin), 17α-hydroxylation of progesterone,[13] and production of nitric oxide.[14] Tetrahydrofolic acid is weakly active in some of these systems *in vitro*[15]; whether it plays any such role *in vivo* is unknown.

TABLE 41–1. Metabolic Systems Requiring Folic Acid Coenzymes in Animal Cells

System	Related Transformations of Folic Acid Coenzymes
Serine $\rightleftharpoons$ glycine	Serine + $FH_4 \rightleftharpoons N^5, N^{10}$-methylene FH_4 + glycine
Thymidylate synthesis	Deoxyuridylate (dUMP) + N^5, N^{10}-methylene $FH_4 \rightarrow FH_2$ + thymidylate (dTMP)
Histidine catabolism	Formiminoglutamate + $FH_4 \rightarrow N^5$-formimino FH_4 + glutamate
Methionine synthesis	Homocysteine + N^5-methyl $FH_4 \rightarrow FH_4$ + methionine
Purine synthesis	Glycinamide ribotide + N^{10}-formyl $FH_4 \rightarrow FH_4$ + formylglycinamide ribotide
Purine synthesis	5-Amino-4-imidazole carboxamide ribotide + N^{10}-formyl $FH_4 \rightarrow FH_4$ + 5-formamido-4-imidazolecarboxamide ribotide

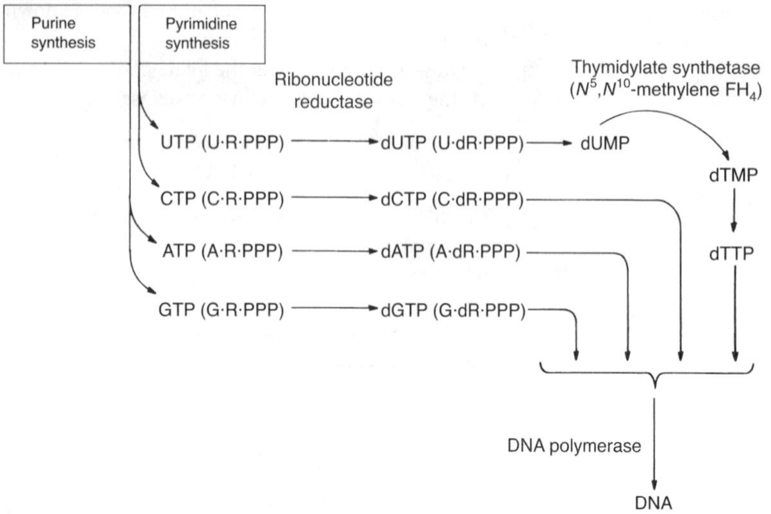

FIGURE 41–3. Pathways of deoxynucleotide and DNA synthesis.

Significance of Folylpolyglutamates

Intracellular folates exist primarily as polyglutamate conjugates.[16] Approximately 75 percent of the folate in human erythrocytes and leukocytes is conjugated.[17] Plasma folate consists largely of the monoglutamate N^5-methyl FH_4 and is transported into the cells in this form.[18] Inside the cells, the polyglutamate chain is added by an ATP-dependent *folylpoly-γ-glutamyl synthase.*[19] The activity of human synthase depends strongly on the form of the folate substrate, declining in the order FH_4 > N^{10}-formyl FH_4 > N^5-methyl FH_4, toward which the enzyme is almost inert.[20] In humans, conjugated folates carry on average seven to eight glutamyl residues.[21] Intracellular folylmonoglutamates leak out of the cells at a fairly rapid rate whereas polyglutamates do not, presumably because of the highly charged polyglutamate tail.[22] Therefore, attachment of the polyglutamylate chain is essential for retaining folates within cells. Folylpolyglutamates are superior to monoglutamates as substrates for folate-dependent enzyme reactions.[17]

■ PHYSIOLOGY

Intestinal Absorption

The proximal jejunum is the principal site of folate absorption. Absorption of a dose of either unconjugated or conjugated folate begins within minutes. Peak levels are reached in 1 to 2 hours. Because only folylmonoglutamate appears in plasma, all folylpolyglutamates are deconjugated during absorption across the intestine.[23] Deconjugating enzymes ("conjugases") play an important but incompletely understood role in the intestinal absorption of folate.[24] Folylpolyglutamate may be hydrolyzed within the lumen of the intestine, and the monoglutamate product may be absorbed subsequently.[25] Alternatively, hydrolysis may occur at the brush border of the intestinal cell (Fig. 41–4). A brush-border conjugase purified from human jejunum catalyzes the Zn^{2+}-dependent deconjugation of folate polyglutamates ranging from $PteGlu_2$ to at least $PteGlu_7$ (K_m = 0.6 μM for both substrates).[26] It is an exopeptidase that successively removes single glutamate residues from the end of the polyglutamate chain, yielding the folylmonoglutamate. A high-affinity folate transporter has been identified that uses a proton-coupled system to facilitate folate absorption.[27] Defects in this proton-coupled folate transporter are the underlying cause of hereditary folate malabsorption.[28]

Conjugases also are found outside the intestine. For example, human plasma contains sufficient conjugase to convert polyglutamates containing more than three glutamyl residues to monoglutamates. Other conjugases appear to be lysosomal carboxypeptidases[29] that are not involved in absorption of folates from the intestine.

Once deconjugated, the folates are actively transported across the intestinal epithelium by a carrier-mediated mechanism (K_m = 1–2 μM) that is independent of Na^+, K^+, and transmembrane potential.[30] The mechanism uses the pH gradient between the jejunal lumen (pH ~6) and the interior of the epithelial cell to drive folate into the cell against a concentration gradient.[31] Passive transport also may occur.[32] In the intestinal cell, the absorbed folate monoglutamates are reduced if necessary, and then converted to N^5-methyl FH_4 (some N^{10}-formyl FH_4 also is made) and transported into the bloodstream without further change.[33]

Folate undergoes an enterohepatic cycle in which it is first secreted against a concentration gradient into the bile, appearing there chiefly as N^5-methyl FH_4 monoglutamate, and then is reabsorbed from the small intestine.[34] Bile contains approximately 2 to 10 times the folate concentration of normal serum, with biliary excretion accounting for up to 0.1 mg of folate per day. This quantity is sufficiently large that interruption of the enterohepatic cycle by biliary diversion causes serum folate levels to fall by more than 50 percent in less than 1 day.[35] The enterohepatic cycle has been proposed to redistribute folate between hepatic stores and peripheral tissues according to the state of the exogenous folate supplies.[36]

■ METABOLISM

Tritiated folylmonoglutamate (^{3}H-F) administered intravenously is almost completely removed from the bloodstream in a few minutes.[37] Uptake involves two classes of folate-binding proteins:[38] *high-affinity folate receptors*[39] that concentrate folate in intracellular vesicles and a *membrane folate transporter* that transports folate from the vesicles into the cytosol. The high-affinity receptors, which are attached to the outer surface of the cell membrane by glycosyl-phosphatidylinositol linkages,[40] bind very tightly (K_d in the nanomolar range) to most physiologic folate monoglutamates,[41] particularly N^5-methyl FH_4, the major circulating folate.[42] Their very high affinity enables the receptors to take up N^5-methyl FH_4 from the plasma, even at its ambient concentration of approximately 10 nM. The membrane folate transporter is a probenecid-inhibitable organic anion carrier that, among other functions, carries reduced folates and methotrexate (but not oxidized folate itself) in and

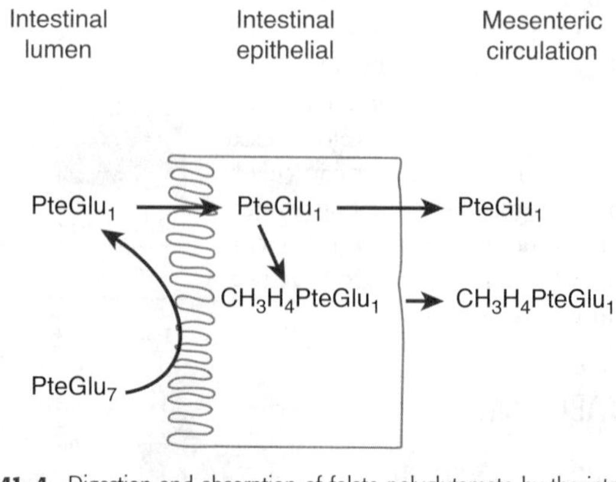

FIGURE 41–4. Digestion and absorption of folate polyglutamate by the intestine. The polyglutamate (in this case, $PteGlu_7$) is hydrolyzed in the intestinal lumen or at the brush border. The resulting pteroylglutamate (PteGlu) is transported into the intestinal cell, where it is reduced and methylated, appearing in the circulation chiefly as N^5-methyl FH_4.

out of the cytoplasm.[38] Its K_m for folate is in the micromolar range. These two classes of receptors cooperate in the following way to transport N^5-methyl FH_4 into the cell:[43] (1) A region of membrane containing a group of folate-loaded high-affinity receptors is internalized as a vesicle (the *caveola*); (2) the caveola is acidified, releasing the folate into the vesicle lumen; (3) the folate is passed from the caveola to the cytoplasm by the membrane folate transporter; and, finally, (4) the caveola recycles to the cell surface, where its high-affinity receptors take on another load of N^5-methyl FH_4. Once internalized, the folates are retained by the cells partly through polyglutamylation[44] but also through tight association with a set of intracellular folate-binding proteins.[45] Three of these proteins are enzymes involved in methyl group metabolism: sarcosine dehydrogenase and dimethylglycine dehydrogenase (mitochondrial)[46] and glycine *N*-methyl transferase (cytosolic).[47] Why these enzymes bind folate so avidly or whether this binding affects overall methyl group metabolism is unknown, although glycine *N*-methyl transferase is speculated to regulate methyl group metabolism by controlling the tissue concentration of *S*-adenosylhomocysteine (SAH), one of its reaction products and a potent inhibitor of most methyltransferases.

Folates have been found in all body tissues that have been analyzed. The principal form of the vitamin in tissues and in blood appears to be the N^5-methyl form.[48] The total folate pool turns over very slowly.[49] Degradation accounts for a portion of this turnover. *p*-Aminobenzoylglutamate has been identified as a breakdown product. The fate of the pteridine moiety is unknown.

FOLATE-BINDING PROTEINS OF SERUM AND MILK

The soluble folate-binding proteins of serum and milk are high-affinity folate receptors that are released from cell membranes by proteolysis.[50] These proteins can be detected in approximately 15 percent of normal individuals[51] and are found at increased levels in some pregnant women, women taking oral contraceptives, folate-deficient alcoholics (but not patients with cobalamin deficiency),[52] and patients with uremia, hepatic cirrhosis, and chronic myelogenous leukemia.[53] In normal subjects, the proteins are approximately two-thirds saturated and have a total folate-binding capacity of approximately 175 pg/mL of serum.[54] The proteins may not be detected in some subjects because of prior saturation of the proteins with unlabeled folate.[55] Serum folate-binding protein has an Mr of 40,000 and prefers oxidized to reduced folates.[53]

Folate-binding proteins have been found in milk and in normal granulocytes.[56] Folate bound to the milk folate binder is absorbed chiefly in the ileum[57] rather than the jejunum, the principal site of absorption of free folate. The milk folate binder, a glycoprotein, also promotes folate transport into the liver via the asialoglycoprotein receptor.[58] The milk folate binder is speculated to protect an infant's folate supply by preventing bacteria from sequestering the vitamin away from the intestinal absorptive surface. The folate-binding protein in granulocytes has been localized to the specific granules, from which it is released when the granulocytes are stimulated.[59]

EXCRETION

Folates are both resorbed and secreted by the kidney. Resorption is accomplished by a membrane-bound high-affinity folate receptor (K_m for N^5-methyl FH_4 = 0.4 nM) located in the brush-borders of the proximal tubules.[60] Filtered folate may thus be returned to the bloodstream. There is resorption of most, but not all, of the filtered folate.

In humans, intact folates and their cleavage products are excreted by the kidney at a rate of 2 to 5 mcg/day.[61] A small percentage of parenterally administered labeled folate is recoverable in the feces and mainly represents overflow from the enterohepatic cycle.[62]

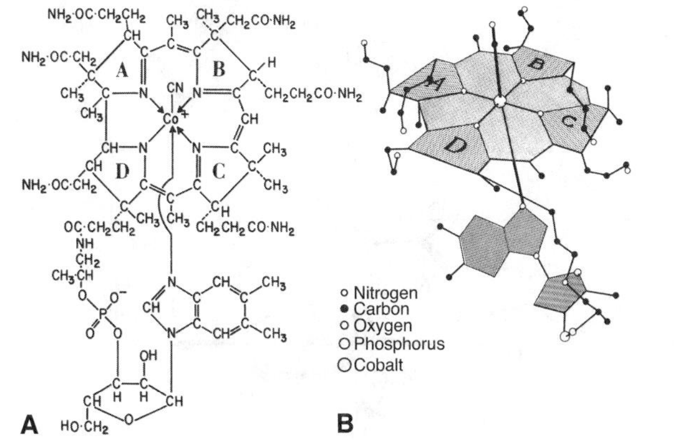

FIGURE 41–5. **A.** Structure of cyanocobalamin (CnCbl; vitamin B_{12}). **B.** Partial structure of CnCbl showing the relationship between the corrin ring and the nucleotide.

ASSAY OF SERUM FOLATE

Folates are measured by chemiluminescent methods using various folate binders. These assays are identical in principle to the radioligand binding assays that they have replaced.

COBALAMIN

CHEMISTRY

Structure and Nomenclature

The cobalamin molecule has two major portions: a porphyrin-like near-planar macrocycle known as corrin, and a nucleotide that lies almost perpendicular to the corrin ring (Fig. 41–5). The corrin moiety contains four reduced pyrrole rings that bind a central cobalt atom whose two remaining coordination positions are occupied by a 5,6-dimethylbenzimidazolyl (5,6-DMB) group, below the ring and various ligands (in this case, —N) above the ring.[63]

Compounds containing the corrin ring are known as *corrinoids*. The cobalamins are corrinoids whose nucleotide contains 5,6-DMB. Two connections exist between the corrin and the nucleotide: (1) a bond between the nucleotide phosphate and a side chain in ring D, and (2) a bond between cobalt and a nitrogen atom of benzimidazole. Figure 41–6 summarizes the numbering and ring designations of the corrin system.

The term *vitamin* B_{12} is sometimes used as a generic term for the cobalamins. The term probably is best reserved, however, as an alternative name for cyanocobalamin, the usual therapeutic cobalamin.

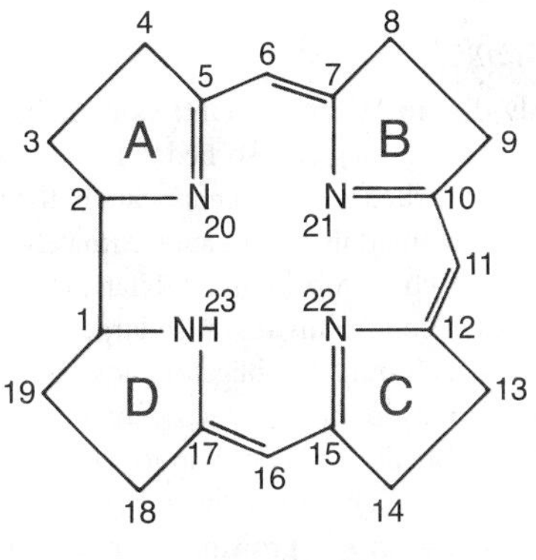

FIGURE 41–6. Corrin ring showing ring designations and standard numbering of the atoms.

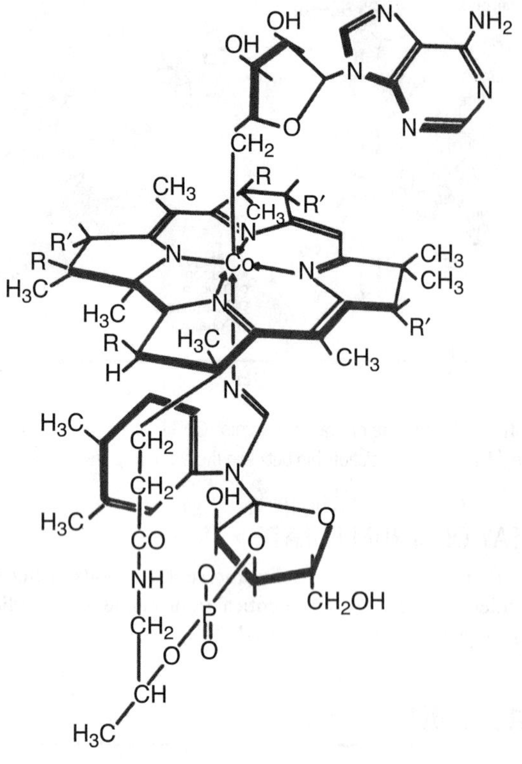

FIGURE 41–7. Adenosylcobalamin (AdoCbl). R = CH_2CONH_2; R′ = $CH_2CH_2CONH_2$.

Four cobalamins are important in animal cell metabolism. Two are *cyanocobalamin* (CnCbl; vitamin B_{12}) and *hydroxocobalamin* (OHCbl) or aquocobalamin (HOH Cbl). The other two cobalamins are alkyl derivatives that are synthesized from OHCbl and serve as coenzymes. In one, *adenosylcobalamin* (AdoCbl), a 5′-deoxyadenosyl replaces OH as the cobalt ligand above the ring (Fig. 41–7).[64] In the second, *methylcobalamin* (MeCbl), the upper ligand is a methyl group. MeCbl is the major form of cobalamin in human blood plasma.[65]

NUTRITION

Sources

Cobalamin is synthesized only by certain microorganisms; animals ultimately depend on microbial synthesis for their cobalamin supply. Foods that contain cobalamin are of animal origin: meat, liver, seafood, and dairy products. Cobalamin has not been found in plants.

Daily Requirements

The average daily diet in Western countries contains 5 to 30 mcg of cobalamin. Of this, 1 to 5 mcg is absorbed.[66] Less than 250 ng appears in the urine; the unabsorbed remainder appears in the feces. Total body content is 2 to 5 mg in an adult,[67] with approximately 1 mg in the liver. The kidneys also are rich in cobalamin.[68] Relative to the daily requirement, body reserves of cobalamin are much larger than those of folate.

Cobalamin has a daily rate of obligatory loss of approximately 0.1 percent of the total-body pool, irrespective of the pool size. For this reason, a deficiency state does not develop for several years after cessation of cobalamin intake. The officially recommended dietary allowance for adults is 2.4 mcg[2]; growth, hypermetabolic states, and pregnancy increase daily requirements. The recommended daily allowance for infants during the first year is 1 to 2 mcg.

ROLE IN METABOLISM

The only two recognized cobalamin-dependent enzymes in human cells are AdoCbl-dependent *methylmalonyl CoA mutase* and MeCbl-dependent *methyltetrahydrofolate-homocysteine methyltransferase.*

Methylmalonyl Coenzyme A Mutase

Methylmalonyl coenzyme A (CoA) mutase is a mitochondrial enzyme that participates in the disposal of the propionate formed during breakdown of valine, isoleucine and odd-carbon fatty acids. The enzyme is a homodimer of a 78-kDa subunit that is encoded by a gene on chromosome 6.[69] In the reaction catalyzed by methylmalonyl CoA mutase, methylmalonyl CoA, which is produced during catabolism of propionate,[70] is converted to succinyl CoA, a Krebs cycle intermediate. In the course of this reaction, a hydrogen on the methyl carbon of the substrate exchanges places with the —COSCoA group (Fig. 41–8).

The coenzyme serves as an intermediate hydrogen carrier, accepting the hydrogen from the substrate in the initial phase of the reaction and returning it to the product after migration of —COSCoA.

N^5-Methyltetrahydrofolate-Homocysteine Methyltransferase

MeCbl participates in cobalamin-dependent synthesis of methionine. *S*-adenosylmethionine (SAM) and methionine synthase reductase are required for methyltransferase activity, probably to reactivate enzyme molecules whose coenzyme is inactivated by oxidation of the cobalt.[71] The reductase converts the oxidized cobalt to the readily alkalizable Co^{1+}, which then accepts a methyl group from SAM, a powerful biologic methylating agent, thereby restoring activity of the methyltransferase. In humans, this pathway also serves as a mechanism critical for converting N^5-methyltetrahydrofolate to tetrahydrofolate required for synthesis of polyglutamates as well as other important one-carbon adducts of folate. The demethylation of N^5-methyl FH_4 is a prerequisite for attachment of the polyglutamate chain to newly acquired folate, which is largely taken up by the cell in the form of N^5-methyl FH_4 monoglutamate.[22] Nitrous oxide (N_2O) impairs methyltransferase by oxidizing cob(I)alamin (a catalytic intermediate in the methyltransferase reaction) to cob(II)alamin. This reaction depletes MeCbl and produces a cobalamin deficiency-like state.

A polymorphic form of methylenetetrahydrofolate reductase (MTHFR), MTHFR 677C→T, is of some clinical importance. The mutation results in a thermolabile form of the enzyme with a higher K_m for its methylene-FH_4 substrate. Retardation of the folate methylation cycle (see Fig. 41–9) affects the levels of homocysteine, an amino acid whose rate of production depends on both folate and cobalamin. These effects are discussed further in "Folate–Cobalamin Relationship" below.

Nonenzymatic Metabolism

Because cobalamin has the capacity to bind cyanide, it may participate in detoxification of cyanide. Tobacco and certain foods (fruits, beans,

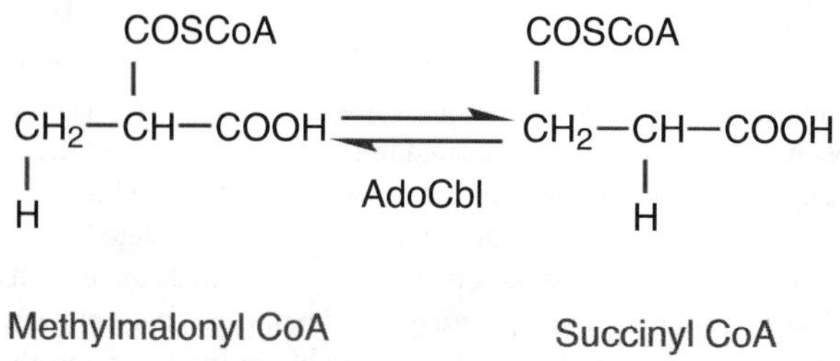

FIGURE 41–8. Methylmalonyl coenzyme A (CoA) mutase reaction.

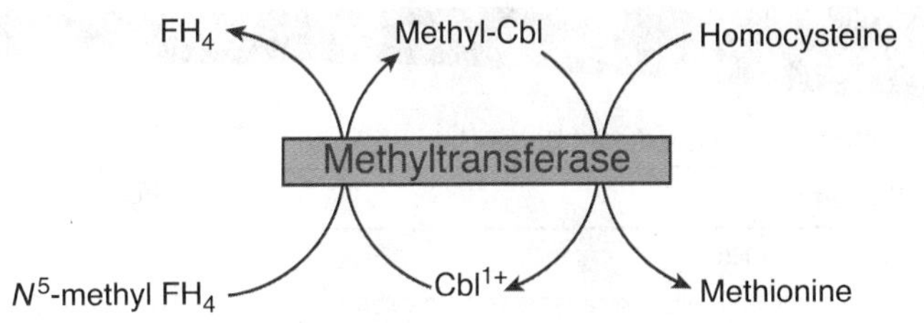

FIGURE 41–9. N^5-methyl FH_4–homocysteine methyltransferase reaction.

tubers, and nuts) contain cyanide in the form of thiocyanate. Although the evidence is inconclusive, cobalamin is believed to play a role in neutralizing cyanide taken in via these substances.[63]

FOLATE–COBALAMIN RELATIONSHIP

In both folate deficiency and cobalamin deficiency, the megaloblastic anemias are fully corrected by treatment with the appropriate vitamin. The megaloblastic anemia of cobalamin deficiency also is variably corrected by folic acid supplementation even if no cobalamin is given, although the remission may be partial and only temporary. Conversely, the anemia of folate deficiency is not helped at all by cobalamin. These clinical observations indicate that the megaloblastic anemia in cobalamin deficiency actually results from an abnormality in folate metabolism.[22] The observation that urinary excretion of formiminoglutamic acid (FIGlu) and AICAR, normally regarded as a sign of folate deficiency, is seen occasionally in pure cobalamin deficiency[72] provides further evidence that folate metabolism is deranged by cobalamin deficiency. Two explanations have been proposed to account for the folate responsiveness of cobalamin-deficient megaloblastic anemia: (1) the *methylfolate trap* hypothesis, which is accepted by the majority of authorities, and (2) the *formate starvation* hypothesis (Fig. 41–10).

METHYLFOLATE TRAP HYPOTHESIS

The methylfolate trap hypothesis[73] is based on the fact that the folate-requiring enzyme N^5-methyl FH_4–homocysteine methyltransferase is also dependent on cobalamin. The hypothesis states that in cobalamin deficiency tissue folates are gradually diverted into the N^5-methyl FH_4 pool because of slowing of the methyltransferase reaction,[74] the only route out of that pool for folate. As N^5-methyl FH_4 levels increase, the levels of other forms of folate decline, with a consequent fall in the rates of reactions in which those forms participate. In particular, because the MTHFR reaction is irreversible, methylene-THF becomes depleted, the synthesis of dTMP is slowed, and megaloblastic anemia ensues.

In its simplest form, the hypothesis predicts that in cobalamin deficiency tissue levels of N^5-methyl FH_4 are abnormally high and those of other forms of folate are abnormally low. Although serum N^5-methyl FH_4 levels are frequently elevated in cobalamin deficiency,[75] tissue folate levels, predominantly polyglutamates, decline.[76] The decreased level appears to be related to the substrate specificity of the folate-conjugating enzyme. This enzyme works very poorly with N^5-methyl FH_4; therefore, it is unable to carry out normal γ-glutamylation of newly internalized N^5-methyl FH_4 monoglutamate in cobalamin-deficient cells because the freshly acquired folate cannot be converted into a suitable substrate (i.e., free FH_4 or formyl FH_4). Thus, although sequestration of tissue folates in an expanded N^5-methyl FH_4 pool may account for some of the effects of the blockade in methyltransferase activity, the major problem seems to be a failure to convert newly acquired folate into a form that can be retained by the cell. The upshot is development of tissue folate deficiency as the unconjugated folate leaks out (Fig. 41–10). The whole process is aggravated by a drop in tissue levels of SAM as the methionine supply is curtailed because of the diminished activity of the methyltransferase.[77] SAM, which is necessary for methyltransferase activity, is also a powerful inhibitor of N^5, N^{10}-methylene FH_4 reductase MTHFR,[78] the enzyme responsible for production of N^5-methyl FH_4. The relief of this inhibition as SAM levels fall accelerates the flow of folates toward N^5-methyl FH_4, further aggravating the metabolic imbalance resulting from impairment in methyltransferase activity.

This problem could be overcome if N^5-methyl FH_4 were converted into a substrate for the conjugating enzyme by another route. In theory, this could be accomplished by reversal of the N^5, N^{10}-methylene FH_4 reductase reaction. For practical purposes, however, the N^5, N^{10}-methylene FH_4 reductase reaction is irreversible *in vivo*[79] and the methylation of biogenic amines by N^5-methyl FH_4 is too slow to provide much relief.

FORMATE STARVATION HYPOTHESIS

This hypothesis holds that formate starvation is the basis for folate responsive megaloblastic anemia of cobalamin deficiency.[80] This theory is based on the diminished capacity of cobalamin-deficient lymphoblasts to incorporate formaldehyde into purine and methionine[77] and on experiments showing that N^5-formyl FH_4 is more effective than

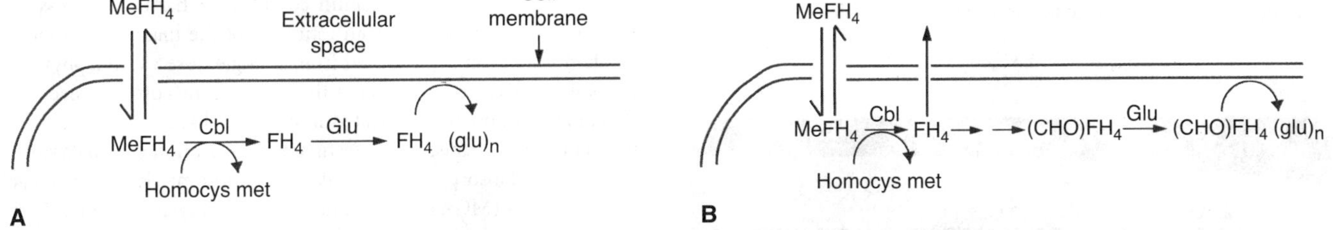

FIGURE 41–10. Methods by which cobalamin deficiency decreases intracellular folate levels. Methyltetrahydrofolate ($MeFH_4$), the principal form of folate in the bloodstream, circulates in the unconjugated form (i.e., it has no polyglutamate side chain). This and other forms of unconjugated FH_4 can be taken into cells but leak out again unless they are conjugated. Methyl FH_4 is not a substrate for the conjugating enzyme, so conjugation cannot occur until the methyl FH_4 is converted to another form of folate. Cobalamin is necessary for this process because it is the cofactor for the reaction that converts methyl FH_4 to FH_4. In cobalamin deficiency, the conversion of methyl FH_4 to FH_4 is defective. Newly transported folate remains in the form of methyl FH_4, which cannot be conjugated and leaks back out of the cell. **A.** According to the *methylfolate trap hypothesis*, all forms of FH_4 other than methyl FH_4 can be conjugated, so methyl FH_4 is the only folate species that leaks out of the cell. **B.** The *formate starvation hypothesis* differs from the methylfolate trap hypothesis solely in assuming that only the formylated folates (N^{10}-formyl FH_4 and/or N^5, N^{10}-methenyl FH_4) can be conjugated, so newly transported methyl FH_4, N^5, N^{10}-methylene FH_4 and free FH_4 leak out of the cell. (CH_2) $FH_4 = N^5$, N^{10}-methylene FH_4; (CHO) $FH_4 = N^{10}$-formyl FH_4 or N^5, N^{10}-methenyl FH_4.

FH_4 at correcting some of the abnormalities in folate metabolism seen in cobalamin deficiency.[81] The hypothesis states that with the decrease in methionine production in cobalamin-deficient conditions, the generation of formate is depressed (because normally the methyl group of excess methionine is rapidly oxidized to formate[82]), leading to a decline in the production of N^5-formyl FH_4.

INTESTINAL ABSORPTION

Intrinsic Factor

Intrinsic factor is one of a number of binding proteins in which cobalamin is ensconced as it makes its way through the body (Table 41–2). Intrinsic factor is needed for the absorption of cobalamins given orally at physiologic dosage levels. Human intrinsic factor is a glycoprotein (Mr approximately 44,000) encoded by a gene on chromosome 11.[83] It has binding sites for cobalamin and a specific ileal receptor, the former situated near the carboxy-terminus and the latter near the amino-terminus of the intrinsic factor molecule.[84] Binding to cobalamin is very tight, and involves the 5,6-DMB lower axial ligand of the molecule. This specificity allows for the exclusion of other non-cobalamin corrinoids during the tightly regulated absorptive process.[63] Table 41–3 summarizes the properties of intrinsic factor. The entrapment of the vitamin alters the conformation of intrinsic factor, producing a more compact form that is resistant to proteolytic digestion.

In humans, intrinsic factor is synthesized and secreted by the parietal cells of the cardiac and fundic mucosa.[85] Secretion of intrinsic factor usually parallels that of hydrochloric acid (HCl). It is enhanced by the presence of food in the stomach, vagal stimulation, and histamine and gastrin. Gastric juice also contains other cobalamin-binding glycoproteins.[86] These proteins were known as the *R proteins* because of their rapid electrophoretic mobility compared with intrinsic factor. Elucidation of the primary protein structure of the R proteins reveals that they belong to the same family of isoproteins as the plasma haptocorrin (HC) binder (previously known as transcobalamins I and III). These HC-like proteins are produced mainly by the salivary glands.

Absorption of Cobalamin: Cubilin

Cobalamins in foods are liberated in the stomach by peptic digestion.[87] They are then bound not to intrinsic factor but to the HC-like protein because cobalamin binds much more tightly to HC than to intrinsic factor at the acid pH of the stomach.[88] Upon entering the duodenum, cobalamin is released from the cobalamin–HC protein complex by digestion with pancreatic proteases, which in normal subjects act by selectively degrading HC and the cobalamin–HC complex while sparing intrinsic factor.[88] At this point, cobalamin finally reaches the intrinsic factor to form the intrinsic factor–cobalamin complex.

TABLE 41–2. Cobalamin-Binding Proteins

Protein	Source	Function
Intrinsic factor	Gastric parietal cells	Promotes absorption uptake of cobalamin by ileum
Transcobalamin	Probably all cells	Promotes uptake of cobalamin by cells
Haptocorrin	Exocrine glands, phagocytes	Helps dispose of cobalamin analogues (?)

TABLE 41–3. Properties of Human Intrinsic Factor

Property	Value
Mr (approximate)	44,000
Cyanocobalamin-binding capacity (mcg/mg)	30.1
Association constant for cyanocobalamin (M^{-1})	1.5×10^{10}
Composition:	
Carbohydrate content (%)	15.0
Hexoses, including fucose (%)	6.9
Hexosamine (residues/mol)	4.1
Sialic acid (residues/mol)	1.7

The intrinsic factor–cobalamin complex, which is very resistant to digestion,[89] traverses the intestine until it reaches the intrinsic factor receptor, *cubilin*,[90] a 460-kDa peripheral membrane glycoprotein located in the microvillus pits of the ileal mucosa brush border that forms part of a multifunctional epithelial receptor complex also found in the yolk sac and renal proximal tubule cells.[91] In the kidney, it appears to serve a role in the overall body economy through tubular reabsorption of cobalamin,[92] but the function of the cubilin receptor complex in the kidney and other polarized epithelial surfaces extends beyond cobalamin. The ileal cubilin receptor complex consists of two proteins, cubilin (CUB) and amnionless (AMN), the product of two distinct genes, *CUB* and *AMN*. Both proteins, which together have been designated the "*CUBAM* complex," colocalize in the endocytic compartment and are required for the process of assimilation of cobalamin,[93] AMN serving as a chaperon for endosomal targeting. Mutations affecting either of the two proteins disrupt the normal process of the intestinal phase of cobalamin absorption. In addition to the tightly embracing components of the CUBAM complex, a distinct large multifunctional protein, megalin, which belongs to the low-density lipoprotein family,[94] also participates in the conformational changes that accompany internalization. The concentration of the CUBAM complex rises progressively to a maximum near the terminal ileum.[95] A specific site on the intrinsic factor molecule avidly attaches to a receptor in a binding reaction that requires a pH of 5.4 or greater and Ca^{2+} (or other divalent cations) but no energy.[96]

The intrinsic factor–cobalamin receptor complex is taken into the ileal mucosal cells over 30 to 60 minutes by endocytosis,[97] where the vitamin is processed and released into the portal blood over many hours. The receptors recycle to the microvillus surface to shuttle another load of intrinsic factor–cobalamin complex.[97] That this process has a limited capacity is evident from estimates of the maximum amount of cobalamin that can be absorbed from a single dose via this physiologic pathway.[63,98] Defects in the genes that regulate the complex mechanism of ileal absorption are implicated in autosomal recessive megaloblastic anemia (MGA1), caused by intestinal malabsorption of cobalamin (see "Selective Malabsorption of Cobalamin, Autosomal Recessive Megaloblastic Anemia (MGA1), Imerslund-Gräsbeck Disease" below).

During its sojourn in the ileal enterocyte, the vitamin first appears in the lysosomes, but by 4 hours most of the vitamin is located in the cytosol.[99] During absorption, the entire intrinsic factor–cobalamin complex appears to be taken into the cell, where the cobalamin is released while the intrinsic factor is degraded.[100]

Cobalamin from a small oral dose (10–20 mcg) starts to appear in the blood after 3 to 4 hours, and the vitamin reaches a peak level in 6 to 12 hours. In the portal blood, the cobalamin is complexed with a cobalamin-transporting protein known as *transcobalamin* (TC) previously known as transcobalamin II.[101] The cobalamin–TC complex is formed in the ileal enterocyte, one of a variety of cells that synthesize TC, or in neighboring vascular endothelial cells in the submucosa.[102] Large oral doses (1 mg) of cobalamin are absorbed by simple diffusion that is not mediated by intrinsic factor.[98] In these instances, vitamin appears in blood within minutes, again as the cobalamin–TC complex.

Like the folates, the cobalamins undergo appreciable enterohepatic recycling.[103] In humans, between 0.5 and 9 mcg/day of cobalamins is secreted into the bile, where the cobalamins bind to protein haptocorrin binder and enter the intestine.[104] In the intestine, the cobalamin–HC complexes of biliary origin are treated exactly like those delivered from the stomach. The cobalamin is released by digestion of the HC by pancreatic proteases, and then is taken up by intrinsic factor and reabsorbed. From 65 to 75 percent of biliary cobalamin is estimated to be reabsorbed by this mechanism.[105] Because of the size of the cobalamin storage pool and the existence of this enterohepatic circulation, a very long time—as long as 20 years—is required for a clinically significant cobalamin deficiency to develop from a diet providing insufficient cobalamin (e.g., a strictly vegetarian diet).[106] Patients who are unable to absorb the vitamin, however, become clinically deficient in only 3 to 6 years because the absorption of both biliary and dietary cobalamin are interdicted.[107]

COBALAMIN IN THE CELL: TRANSCOBALAMIN

Uptake of Cobalamin by Cells

TC is the plasma protein that mediates the transport of cobalamin into the tissues.[108] A β-globulin protein with a calculated molecular weight of 45,538 from the deduced amino acid sequence,[109,110] TC binds cobalamin with exceedingly high affinity ($K_a = 10^{-11}$ *M*).[111] Unlike intrinsic factor, whose binding is relatively specific for cobalamins, TC also can bind certain corrins that are chemically related to the cobalamins but have no function in mammalian systems and are known as cobalamin "analogues."[112] TC is synthesized by many types of cells, including enterocytes, hepatocytes, endothelial cells, mononuclear phagocytes, fibroblasts, and hematopoietic precursors in the marrow.[63] Although circulating TC carries only a minor fraction of the cobalamin in the plasma, it is the protein to which newly acquired cobalamin is first bound. Cobalamin given parenterally associates almost immediately with unsaturated TC,[113] whereas cobalamin absorbed through the intestine probably is carried into the portal blood as the preformed cobalamin–TC complex. These cobalamin–TC complexes are transported into the tissues within minutes of appearing in the bloodstream.[114] The transport process begins with binding of the cobalamin–TC complex to a specific membrane receptor that is present on a wide variety of cells.[115] The protein and gene encoding the TC receptor has been purified from placental membranes and characterized.[116] The receptor belongs to the low-density lipoprotein receptor family and its internalization involves megalin. The receptor-bound complex is internalized by receptor-mediated endocytosis and delivered to a lysosome, where the TC is digested and the cobalamin is freed.[117,118]

Formation of Adenosylcobalamin and Methylcobalamin

To be useful to the cell, CnCbl and OHCbl must be converted to AdoCbl and MeCbl, the coenzymatically active cobalamins. The conversion is accomplished by reduction and alkylation. CnCbl and OHCbl are first reduced to the Co^{2+} form [cob(II)alamin] by NADPH- and nicotinamide adenine dinucleotide (reduced form)-dependent reductases that are present in mitochondria and microsomes.[119] CN^- and OH^- are displaced from the metal during reduction. Some of the cob(II)alamin in the mitochondria is reduced further to the intensely nucleophilic Co^+ form [cob(I)alamin]. This is then alkylated by ATP to form AdoCbl in a reaction in which the 5′-deoxyadenosyl moiety of ATP is transferred to the cobalamin and the three phosphates of ATP are released as inorganic triphosphate (Fig. 41–11). The rest of the cobalamin binds to cytosolic N^5-methyltetrahydrofolate-homocysteine methyltransferase, where it is converted to MeCbl. The several steps involved in the conversion of cobalamin to its coenzymatically active forms are regulated by genes that play a critical role in the processing of the vitamin. There are a number of inherited metabolic errors that correspond to one or more of these specific steps and that result in characteristic syndromes affecting aspects of cobalamin metabolism that are discussed later in this chapter.

PLASMA HAPTOCORRIN (TRANSCOBALAMINS I AND III; "R" PROTEINS)

The haptocorrins (previously known as R proteins) are a group of immunologically related proteins of apparent Mr approximately 60,000 consisting of a single polypeptide species variably substituted with oligosaccharides that terminate with different quantities of sialic acid.[120] They are found in milk, plasma, saliva, gastric juice, and numerous other body fluids. They appear to be synthesized by mucosal cells of the organs that secrete them[121] and by phagocytes.[122] Although the haptocorrins bind cobalamin, they lack intrinsic factor activity, that is, they are unable to promote the intestinal absorption of the vitamin.

Plasma HC carries most (70–90%) of the circulating cobalamin. It contains nine potential glycosylation sites[123] and is encoded by a gene

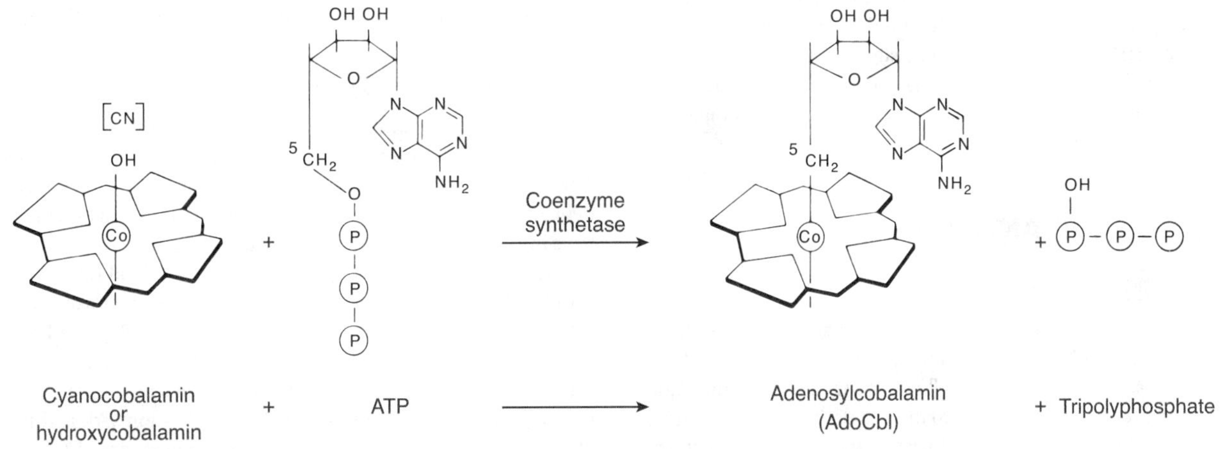

FIGURE 41–11. Biosynthesis of adenosylcobalamin (AdoCbl).

on chromosome 11, the same chromosome that carries the intrinsic factor gene.[124] In contrast to TC, HC clearance from the plasma is very slow (half-life [$T_{1/2}$]: 9–10 days).[125] The asialoglycoprotein receptor carries the cobalamin–HC complexes into the hepatocytes, where they are chiefly eliminated. The complexes are degraded, and their load of cobalamins is excreted in the bile.[103,126] HC binds its ligands more tightly than does either intrinsic factor or TC. Furthermore, HC is less restrictive than either intrinsic factor or TC with respect to ligand specificity; it avidly takes up corrinoids of widely varying structure.[127] The ligand-binding properties of HC and its mode of clearance by the liver suggest that HC helps clear the system of nonphysiologic cobalamin analogues that may have been acquired or may have arisen through degradation of cobalamin.[128,129] As the liver metabolizes analogue–HC complexes, it secretes the analogues into the bile. Because these analogues are bound poorly by intrinsic factor,[127] they are poorly reabsorbed from the intestine and are eliminated in the feces. In reality, the precise role of HC is unknown, although it may play a role in the body economy of cobalamin by facilitating excretion of cobalamin analogues while conserving cobalamin through enterohepatic recycling. Additionally, it has not been shown that HC serves an antimicrobial role.[63] Plasma HC likely consists of half a dozen or more protein species whose isoelectric point (pI) values range from 2.9 to 4.0, and which appear to be derived in large measure from granulocytes.

ASSAY OF SERUM COBALAMIN AND THE TRANSCOBALAMINS

As with folate, cobalamin is usually measured with automated competitive displacement assays using intrinsic factor as a cobalamin-binding protein. The misleading results previously provided by competitive ligand displacement assays were explained by the discovery in serum and tissue of a class of cobalamin analogues that are detected by the radioisotope assay when haptocorrin-type binders were used and not intrinsic factor as the binder.[130] Current assays use intrinsic factor as the binder and give more reliable values for serum cobalamin. The chemical nature and biologic significance of the analogues are unknown,[131] but recent evidence suggests that they may arise in the gastrointestinal tract.[128,129]

TC and HC are present in plasma in trace quantities (approximately 7 and 20 mcg/L, respectively). In fasting plasma, at least 70 percent of the circulating cobalamin is bound to HC.[132] TC binds only 10 to 25 percent of the total plasma cobalamin,[133] but provides the majority (approximately 75 percent) of the total unsaturated cobalamin-binding capacity of plasma.[132] Table 41–4 lists alterations in unsaturated cobalamin-binding capacity and in HC and TC levels in various disease states. In recent years, assays have been developed that measure the fraction of the plasma cobalamin that is bound to TC. This component, known as holotranscobalamin (holoTC), shows improved specificity compared with the standard cobalamin assay for identifying true cobalamin deficiency, although the assays appear to be generally comparable with respect to sensitivity.[134–140]

TABLE 41–4. Levels and Binding Capacity of Cobalamin-Binding Proteins in Disease

Binder	Disease
Increased HC (TCI, R protein)	Myeloproliferative disorders
	Polycythemia vera
	Myelofibrosis
	Benign neutrophilia
	Chronic myelocytic leukemia
	Hepatoma (occasionally)
	Metastatic cancer
Increased TC	Myeloproliferative disorders
	Liver disease
	Inflammatory disorders
	Gaucher disease
	Anti-TC antibodies
Unsaturated cobalamin binders	
Increased	Transient neutropenia
	Elevated HC
Decreased	Liver disease
	Elevated serum cobalamin

Modified from Lawler S, Roberts P, Hoffbrand A,[157] with permission.

MEGALOBLASTIC ANEMIAS

DEFINITION

Megaloblastic anemias are disorders caused by impaired DNA synthesis. The presence of megaloblastic cells is the morphologic hallmark of this group of anemias. Megaloblastic red cell precursors are larger than normal and have more cytoplasm relative to the size of the nucleus. Promegaloblasts show a blue granule-free cytoplasm and a "salt and pepper" granular chromatin that contrasts with the ground-glass texture of its normal counterpart. As the cell differentiates, the chromatin condenses more slowly than normal into darker aggregates that coalesce, but do not fuse homogeneously, giving the nucleus a characteristic fenestrated appearance. The growing maturity of the cytoplasm as it acquires hemoglobin contrasts with the immature-looking nucleus, a feature termed *nuclear-cytoplasmic asynchrony*.

Megaloblastic granulocyte precursors are larger than normal. They show nuclear-cytoplasmic asynchrony, with cytoplasm that looks less mature than the cytoplasm of their normal counterparts. A characteristic cell is the *giant metamyelocyte*, which has a large horseshoe-shaped nucleus, sometimes irregularly shaped, containing ragged open chromatin.

Megaloblastic megakaryocytes may be abnormally large and polylobated, with deficient granulation of the cytoplasm. In severe megaloblastosis, the nucleus may show unattached lobes. Further details are provided in "Laboratory Features" below and in Figures 41–12 and 41–13.

ETIOLOGY AND PATHOGENESIS

Table 41–5 lists the causes of megaloblastic anemia. By far the most common causes worldwide are folate deficiency and cobalamin deficiency. There has, however, been a marked reduction in the prevalence of folate deficiency in North America and a growing number of other regions that have implemented folic acid fortification of the food supply.

Megaloblastic cells have much more cytoplasm and RNA than do their normal counterparts, but they have a relatively normal amount of DNA,[141] suggesting that cytoplasmic constituents (RNA and protein) are synthesized faster than is DNA. Evidence that maturation is retarded in megaloblastic precursors supports this conclusion.[142] DNA synthesis is impaired,[143] and migration of the DNA replication fork and the joining of DNA fragments synthesized from the lagging strand (Okazaki fragments) are delayed,[144] and S phase is prolonged.[143]

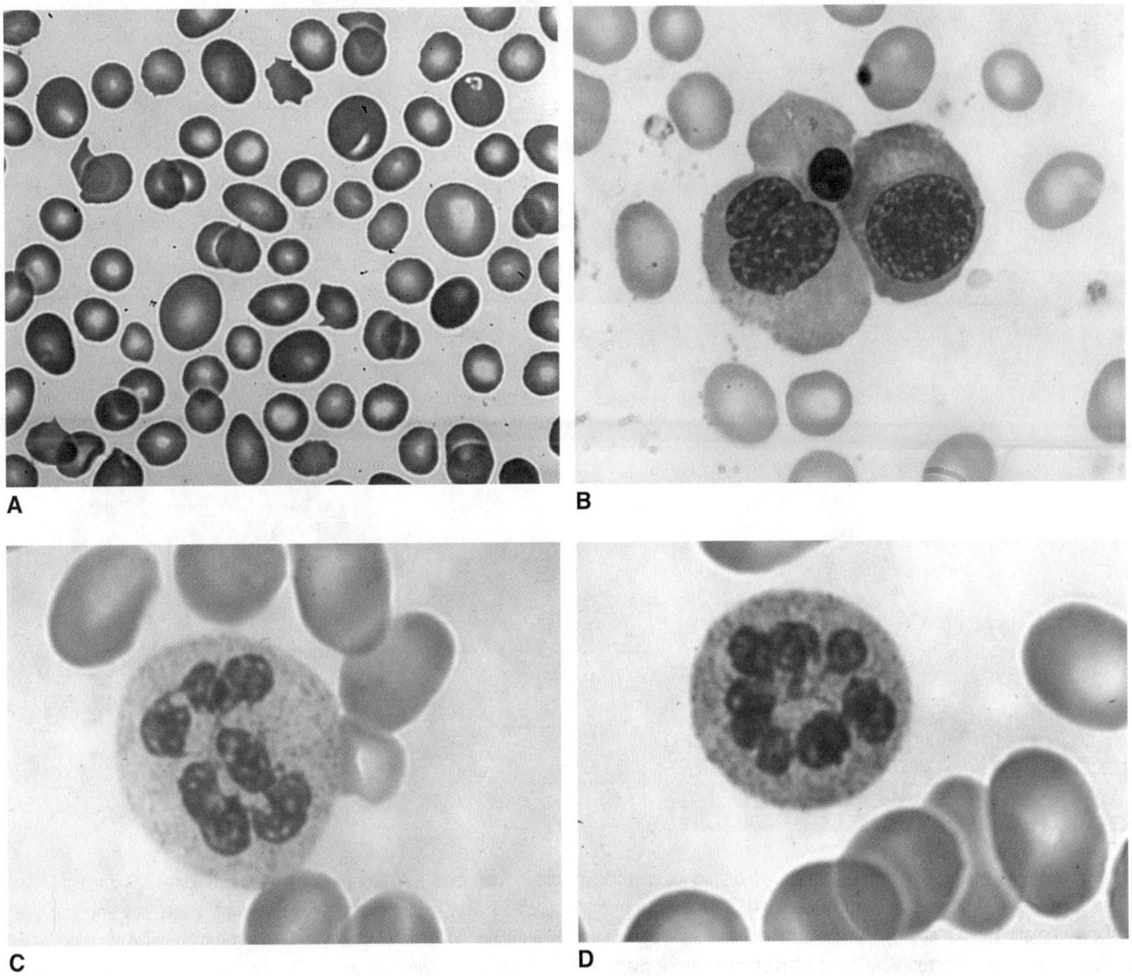

FIGURE 41–12. A. Pernicious anemia. Blood film. Note the striking oval macrocytes, wide variation in red cell size, and poikilocytes. Despite the anisocytosis and microcytes, the mean red cell volume is usually elevated, as in this case (MCV = 121 fl). **B.** Marrow precursors in pernicious anemia. Note very large size of erythroblasts (megaloblasts) and asynchronous maturation. Cell on *right* is a polychromatophilic megaloblast with an immature nucleus for that stage of maturation. Cell on *left* is an orthochromatic megaloblast with a lobulated immature nucleus. An orthochromatic megaloblast with a condensed nucleus is between and above those two cells. **C** and **D.** Two examples of hypersegmented neutrophils characteristic of megaloblastic anemia. The morphology of blood and marrow cells in folate-deficient and vitamin B_{12}-deficient patients is identical. The extent of the morphologic changes in each case is related to the severity of the vitamin deficiency. *(Used with permission from* Lichtman's Atlas of Hematology, *www.accessmedicine.com.)*

Slowing of DNA replication in the megaloblastic anemias of folate and cobalamin deficiency appears to arise from failure of the folate-dependent conversion of dUMP to dTMP. Because of this failure, deoxyuridine triphosphate (dUTP) levels become abundant and because DNA polymerase is promiscuous with respect to its substrate specificity, allows dUTP to become incorporated into the DNA of folate-deficient cells in place of deoxythymidine triphosphate (dTTP).[144] DNA excision-repair mechanisms to repair the DNA by replacing uridine with thymidine fail for the same reason that uridine triphosphate was incorporated into the DNA in the first place. The result is a repetitive iteration of flawed DNA repair that ultimately leads to DNA strand breaks, fragmentation, and apoptotic cell death.[145]

Addition of deoxyuridine (dU) to marrow cells in culture normally decreases the incorporation of tritiated thymidine into DNA, because it is converted via dUMP→dTMP to unlabeled dTTP, which competes with the tritiated thymidine. In megaloblastic cells, this effect of added dU is greatly diminished. This finding is consistent with impairment in the dUMP→dTMP reaction in the megaloblastic cells and is the basis for the *dU suppression test*.[147] The failed excision-repair model following dUTP misincorporation into DNA also explains the chromosome breaks and other abnormalities that occur in megaloblastic cells.[148]

A curious group of findings suggests that the megaloblastic line arises from a more "primitive" precursor than is the case for the normoblastic line. Megaloblasts contain high concentrations of fetal hemoglobin[149] and the fetal isozyme of thymidine kinase.[150] Like megaloblasts, burst-forming unit–erythroid (BFU-E; see Chap. 31) grown with monocyte-conditioned medium are rich in γ-globin chains and appear megaloblastic. BFU–E from the same source but grown with T lymphocytes appear normal and contain the usual proportion of γ-globin chains.[151] The relationship between these observations and the pathogenesis of the nutritional megaloblastic anemias is unclear.

■ CLINICAL FEATURES

All megaloblastic anemias share certain general clinical features. Because the anemia develops slowly, with opportunity for cardiopulmonary and intraerythrocytic compensatory changes,[152] it produces few symptoms until the hematocrit is severely depressed. Symptoms, when they appear, are those of anemia: weakness, palpitation, fatigue,

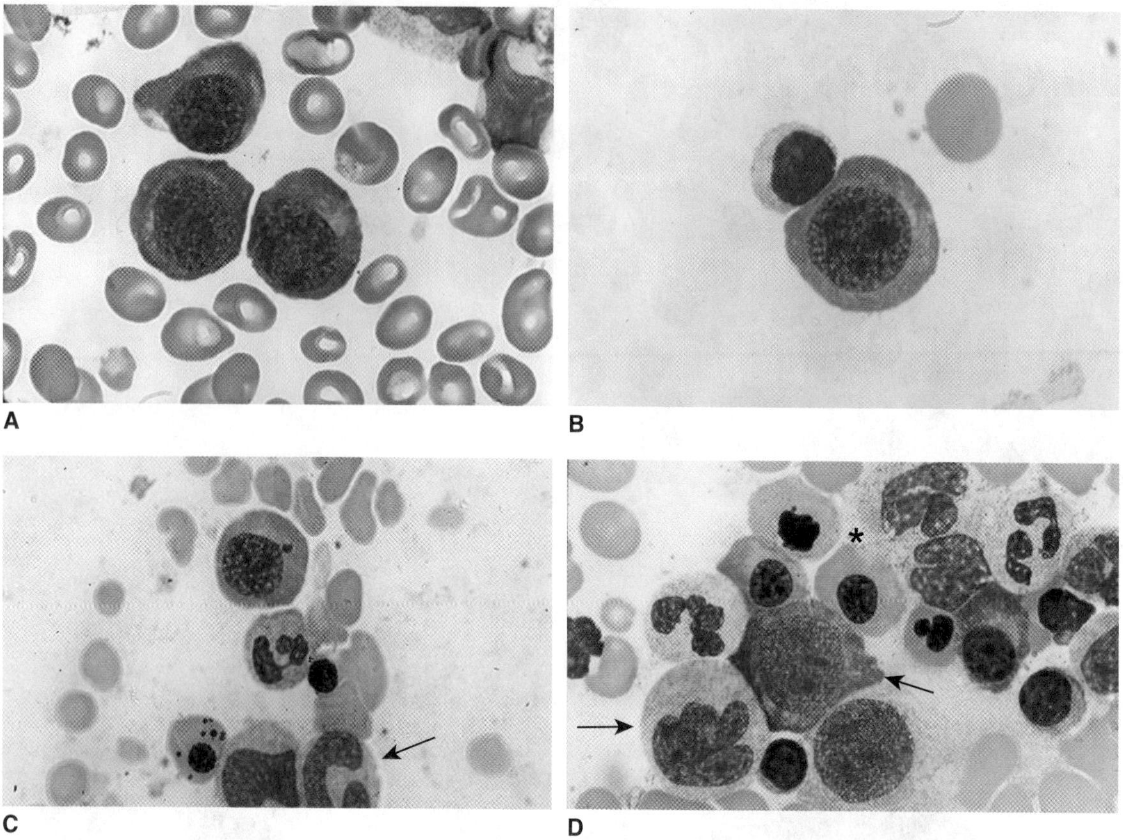

FIGURE 41–13. Marrow films. Megaloblastic anemia. Patient with pernicious anemia (vitamin B_{12} deficiency). **A.** Basophilic megaloblasts. Large cell size, very characteristic nuclear chromatin pattern with exaggerated proportion of euchromatin. **B.** Polychromatophilic megaloblast. Very large cell size for maturational stage. Large nuclear size and abnormally large proportion of euchromatin without appropriate nuclear condensation at this stage of maturation. Adjacent lymphocyte. **C.** Polychromatophilic megaloblast with small nuclear fragment. Arrow indicates giant band neutrophil. At lower left is orthochromatic megaloblast with multiple nuclear fragments. **D.** Oblique arrow indicates promegaloblast. Horizontal arrow indicates giant band neutrophil. To the left of and below the asterisk are four orthochromatic megaloblasts–large cell size for maturational stage. Two with delayed nuclear condensation and two with condensed nuclei with abnormal nuclear margins showing small or large budding nuclei. To the right of the asterisk are two giant band neutrophils. On the right at midfield is a plasma cell below which is a lymphocyte. *(Used with permission from* Lichtman's Atlas of Hematology, *www.accessmedicine.com.)*

light-headedness, and shortness of breath. Severe pallor and slight jaundice caused by a combination of intramedullary and extravascular hemolysis produce a telltale lemon-yellow skin. Leukocyte and platelet counts may be low, but rarely cause clinical problems. Details of the clinical manifestations are given in the sections on the specific forms of megaloblastic anemia later in this chapter.

LABORATORY FEATURES

Blood Cells

All cell lines are affected. Erythrocytes vary markedly in size and shape, often are large and oval, and in severe cases can show basophilic stippling and nuclear remnants (Cabot rings, and Howell-Jolly bodies). Erythroid activity in the marrow is enhanced, although the megaloblastic cells usually die before they are released, accounting for the reduced reticulocyte count. The more severe the anemia, the more pronounced the morphologic changes in the red cells. When the hematocrit is less than 20 percent, erythroblasts with megaloblastic nuclei, including an occasional promegaloblast, may appear in the blood. The anemia is macrocytic (mean corpuscular volume [MCV] = 100–150 fl or more), although coexisting iron deficiency, thalassemia trait,[153] or inflammation can prevent macrocytosis.[154] Slight macrocytosis often is the earliest sign of megaloblastic anemia. Because of the progressive nature of gradual replacement of normocytic red cells with the macrocytic progeny of a megaloblastic marrow, the earliest observable change in red cell indices is an increase in the red cell distribution width (RDW), reflecting an increase in anisocytosis.

Neutrophil nuclei often have more than the usual three to five lobes (Fig. 41–12).[155] Typically, more than 5 percent of the neutrophils have five lobes. Cells may contain six or more lobes, a morphology rarely seen in normal neutrophils but not pathognomonic of megaloblastic hematopoiesis. In nutritional megaloblastic anemias caused by folate deficiency, hypersegmented neutrophils are an early sign of megaloblastosis[4] and persist in the blood for many days after treatment.[155] Neutrophil hypersegmentation was not found to be a sensitive test for mild cobalamin deficiency.[156] Cytogenetic studies show chromosomes that are elongated and broken. Specific therapy corrects these abnormalities, usually within 2 days, although some abnormalities do not disappear for months.[157,158] Platelets are slightly smaller than normal and vary more widely in size (increased platelet distribution width—PDW).[159]

Marrow

Aspirated marrow is cellular and shows striking megaloblastic changes, especially in the erythroid series (Fig. 41–13). Sideroblasts are increased in number and contain increased numbers of iron granules. The ratio

TABLE 41–5. Causes of Megaloblastic Anemias

I. Folate Deficiency	III. Acute Megaloblastic Anemia
A. Decreased intake	A. Nitrous oxide exposure
1. Poor nutrition	B. Severe illness with
2. Old age, poverty, alcoholism	1. Extensive transfusion
3. Hyperalimentation	2. Dialysis
4. Hemodialysis	3. Total parenteral nutrition
5. Premature infants	IV. Drugs
6. Spinal cord injury	A. Dihydrofolate reductase inhibitors
7. Children on synthetic diets	B. Antimetabolites
8. Goat's milk anemia	C. Inhibitors of deoxynucleotide synthesis
B. Impaired absorption	D. Anticonvulsants
1. Nontropical sprue	E. Oral contraceptives
2. Tropical sprue	F. Others, such as long-term exposure to weak folate antagonists (e.g., trimethoprim or low-dose methotrexate)
3. Other disease of the small intestine	
C. Increased requirements	V. Inborn Errors
1. Pregnancy	A. Cobalamin deficiency
2. Increased cell turnover	1. Imerslund-Gräsbeck disease
3. Chronic hemolytic anemia	2. Congenital deficiency of intrinsic factor
4. Exfoliative dermatitis	3. Transcobalamin deficiency
II. Cobalamin Deficiency	B. Errors of cobalamin metabolism
A. Impaired absorption	1. "Cobalamin mutant" syndromes with homocystinuria and/or methylmalonic acidemia
1. Gastric causes	
a. Pernicious anemia	
b. Gastrectomy	C. Errors of folate metabolism
c. Zollinger-Ellison syndrome	1. Congenital folate malabsorption
2. Intestinal causes	2. Dihydrofolate reductase deficiency
a. Ileal resection or disease	3. N^5-methyl FH_4 homocysteine–methyltransferase deficiency
b. Blind loop syndrome	
c. Fish tapeworm	D. Other errors
3. Pancreatic insufficiency	1. Hereditary orotic aciduria
B. Decreased intake	2. Lesch-Nyhan syndrome
1. Vegans	3. Thiamine-responsive megaloblastic anemia
	VI. Unexplained
	A. Congenital dyserythropoietic anemia
	B. Refractory megaloblastic anemia
	C. Erythroleukemia

of myeloid to erythroid precursors falls to 1:1 or lower, and granulocyte reserves may be decreased.[160] In severe cases, promegaloblasts containing an unusually large number of mitotic figures are plentiful. Macrophage iron content often is increased.

Atypical Morphology in Megaloblastic Anemia

Under certain circumstances, megaloblastic anemia may be overlooked because its characteristic morphology is incompletely expressed. For example, a measurable proportion of patients with cobalamin deficiency do not have an MCV above the normal limit.

Coexisting Microcytic Anemia

Many features of megaloblastic anemia may be masked when megaloblastic anemia is combined with a microcytic anemia.[154] The anemia can be normocytic or even microcytic, whereas the blood film may show both microcytes and macroovalocytes (a "dimorphic anemia") or microcytes alone if the microcytic component is sufficiently severe. The marrow may contain "intermediate" megaloblasts[161] that are smaller and look less "megaloblastic" than usual. In this kind of mixed anemia, the microcytic component usually is iron-deficiency anemia,[154] but it may be thalassemia minor[153] or the anemia of chronic disease. Even megaloblastic anemia masked by a severe microcytic anemia usually shows hypersegmented neutrophils in the blood and giant metamyelocytes and bands in the marrow. Neutrophil myeloperoxidase levels are high.[162]

The megaloblastic component of a mixed iron-deficiency anemia can be overlooked, and the patient may be treated only with iron. In this case, the anemia responds only partly to therapy, and megaloblastic features emerge as iron stores fill. The masking of macrocytosis in these situations may be responsible for delay or difficulty in diagnosis of pernicious anemia, particularly in certain geographic areas and ethnic groups where there is a high incidence of thalassemia and microcytic hemoglobinopathies.[153,163,164]

Incomplete Megaloblastic Anemia

If a patient with a full-blown megaloblastic anemia receives cobalamin or folate before marrow aspiration, the anemia persists but the megaloblastic changes may be obscured. Attenuated megaloblastic changes also are seen in patients with early megaloblastic anemia, in patients with coexisting infection,[154] or in patients after transfusion.

Megaloblastic Anemia Misdiagnosed as Acute Leukemia

Occasionally, very severe megaloblastic anemia produces marrow morphology so bizarre as to be mistaken for acute leukemia. The mistaken identification especially occurs if the marrow lacks classic megaloblasts and displays as its principal cell type the bizarre megaloblastic white cell precursors that in a more typical morphologic background, supports the diagnosis of a megaloblastic anemia. In some cases, the erythroid series does not mature, and the megaloblastic pronormoblast dominates the marrow with prominent mitotic figures and dysmorphic forms, raising the possibility of erythroid leukemia.

Megaloblastic Changes in Other Cells

In most forms of megaloblastic anemia, cytologic abnormalities resembling megaloblastosis may appear in other proliferating cells. Epithelial cells from the mouth, stomach, small intestine, and cervix uteri may look megaloblastic, appearing larger than their normal counterparts and containing atypical immature-looking nuclei. Distinguishing these "megaloblastic" changes from the changes of malignancy can be difficult.[165]

Chemical Changes in Body Fluids

Plasma bilirubin, iron, and ferritin levels are increased.[166] Serum lactate dehydrogenase-1 (LDH-1) and LDH-2, both found in red cells, are markedly elevated as a result of rapid intramedullary erythroblast turnover and increase with the severity of the anemia.[167] In megaloblastic anemia LDH-1 is greater than LDH-2, whereas in other anemias LDH-2 is greater than LDH-1.[168] Serum muramidase (lysozyme) levels are high,[169] whereas serum glutamic oxaloacetic transaminase is normal.[170] Erythropoietin levels rise, but less than in other anemias of similar severity.[171] Surprisingly, the elevated erythropoietin levels fall sharply within 1 day of beginning treatment, an interval too short either to have been mediated by the hematocrit or to affect it.

Cytokinetics

Megaloblastic anemia is associated with two pathophysiologic abnormalities: *ineffective erythropoiesis* and *hemolysis.* Ineffective erythropoiesis increases the red cell precursor to reticulocyte ratio, plasma iron turnover,[172] LDH-1 and LDH-2 levels,[168] and "early labeled" bilirubin.[173] Extramedullary hemolysis occurs in megaloblastic anemia, with red cell life span decreased by 30 to 50 percent.[174]

Increased serum muramidase in megaloblastic anemia can be caused by increased granulocyte turnover,[169] possibly induced by disintegration of granulocyte precursors in the marrow (ineffective granulopoiesis). In cobalamin deficiency, platelet production is only 10 percent of that expected from the megakaryocyte mass,[175] perhaps reflecting ineffective thrombopoiesis. Platelets in severe cobalamin deficiency are functionally abnormal.[176]

FOLIC ACID DEFICIENCY

Etiology and Pathogenesis

Folate deficiency is caused by (1) dietary deficiency, (2) impaired absorption, and (3) increased requirements (see Table 41–5).

Decreased Intake Caused by Poor Nutrition Prior to the mid-1990s, inadequate dietary intake was the major cause of folate deficiency. However, in the era of folic acid fortification, the prevalence of folate deficiency has fallen dramatically. In the United States, the prevalence of low plasma folate has dropped from 22 percent to 1.7 percent of the population.[177] Because folate reserves are limited, deficiency develops rapidly in malnourished persons, typically the old, the poor, and the alcoholic. Folate deficiency can occur during hyperalimentation[178] or during hemodialysis, where folate is lost in the dialysis fluid.[179] Subclinical folate deficiency has been reported in subtotal gastrectomy.[180] Folate deficiency can occur in premature infants, especially with infection, diarrhea, or hemolytic anemia[181]; in children on a synthetic diet because of inborn errors[182]; and in infants raised on goat's milk, which is poor in available folate.[183] Destruction of folate through excessive cooking can aggravate folate deficiency.

In alcoholic cirrhosis, megaloblastic anemia usually is caused by folate deficiency.[184] Alcohol may acutely depress serum folate, even if folate stores are replete,[185] and accelerates the development of megaloblastic anemia in persons with early folate deficiency.[186] Alcohol causes acute marrow suppression, decreases in reticulocyte, platelet, and granulocyte levels[187]; reversible vacuolation of erythroid and myeloid precursors; and dysfunction of granulocytes.[188] These changes occur even if large doses of folate are given with the alcohol.[189]

Decreased Intake Caused by Impaired Absorption Nontropical Sprue Nontropical sprue (*celiac disease* in children) is related to ingestion of wheat gluten.[190] Pathologically, nontropical sprue shows atrophy and chronic inflammation of the small intestinal mucosa that is most severe proximally. Findings include weight loss; glossitis (typical of folate deficiency); other signs of a generalized vitamin deficiency; diarrhea; and passage of light-colored, bulky stools with an unusually foul odor caused by steatorrhea. Iron deficiency, hypocalcemia, osteoporosis, and osteomalacia may occur.

Folate malabsorption occurs in most patients with this disorder.[191] Serum folate levels are low,[192] and megaloblastic anemia occurs frequently.

Tropical Sprue Tropical sprue is endemic in the West Indies, southern India, parts of Southern Africa, and Southeast Asia. It can be acquired by travelers to those regions and persists for many years after the travelers return.[193] Tropical sprue is rapidly corrected by folate therapy, even though folate deficiency does not cause the disease. The etiology of tropical sprue is unknown, although the response of the disease to antibiotics suggests infection.[194]

Clinically and pathologically, tropical sprue is like nontropical sprue, except that tropical sprue is more severe in the distal small intestine.[195] Therefore, tropical sprue eventually also leads to cobalamin deficiency[196] and should be strongly considered as a cause of cobalamin deficiency in former residents of the tropics, even though they have been away from the tropics for 20 years or more. Folate malabsorption may occur,[197] possibly because the diseased intestine fails to deconjugate folate polyglutamates.[198] Consequently, megaloblastic anemia is very common in patients with this disease,[199] and may result from both folate and cobalamin deficiency.

Other Intestinal Disorders Malabsorption of folic acid commonly occurs in regional enteritis,[199] after extensive resections of the small intestine,[200] and in conditions such as lymphomatous or leukemic infiltration of the small intestine,[201] Whipple disease,[201] scleroderma and amyloidosis,[202] and diabetes mellitus.[203] Systemic bacterial infections impair folate absorption.[204]

Increased Folate Requirements Pregnancy During pregnancy (see Chap. 7),[205] folate requirements increase five- to tenfold because of transfer of folate to the growing fetus,[206] which draws down maternal folate stores even in the face of severe maternal folate deficiency.[207] Further increases in requirements may result from the presence of multiple fetuses, a poor diet, infection, coexisting hemolytic anemia, or anticonvulsant medication. Lactation aggravates folate deficiency.[208] Consequently, folate deficiency is very common in pregnancy and is the major cause of the megaloblastic anemia of pregnancy,[209] particularly in developing countries.[210]

Folate deficiency is difficult to diagnose in pregnancy because the signs of deficiency are obscured by the normal hematologic changes of pregnancy. During pregnancy, a physiologic "anemia" develops because of increased plasma volume that is only partly offset by an accompanying increase in red cell mass. Hemoglobin levels may fall to 10 g/dL. The anemia is associated with a physiologic macrocytosis; MCV may increase to 120 fl, although the average at term is 104 fl.[211] Serum and red cell folate levels fall steadily during pregnancy, even in well-nourished women who are not taking a folic acid supplement.[212] Conversely, hypersegmented neutrophils, usually a reliable clue to early megaloblastic anemia, are inconspicuous in early megaloblastic anemia of pregnancy.[213]

Increased Cell Turnover Because of increased marrow cell turnover, the folate requirement rises sharply in chronic *hemolytic anemia.*[214] During bouts of acute hemolysis that can occur in these anemias, the marrow may become megaloblastic within days.

Folic acid deficiency may arise in chronic *exfoliative dermatitis,* in which folate losses of 5 to 20 mcg/day may occur.[215] Patients with psoriasis who are treated with methotrexate have an added reason for developing signs of folate deficiency. Pretreating such patients with folate may prevent these signs without impairing the therapeutic effect of methotrexate.[215]

Clinical Features

The clinical picture of folate deficiency includes all the nonspecific manifestations of megaloblastic anemia *plus* the following specific features: (1) a history and laboratory studies indicating folate deficiency, (2) absence of the neurologic signs of cobalamin deficiency (see "Cobalamin Deficiency" below), and (3) a full response to *physiologic* doses of folate.

Laboratory Features

The earliest specific indicator of folate deficiency is a low serum or plasma folate. Raised plasma levels of homocysteine may precede the lowering of plasma folate. However, elevated homocysteine has poor specificity as there are several causes of a raised plasma homocysteine.[216] Plasma folate follows folate intake closely, so a low serum folate (less than approximately 3 ng/mL) may indicate only a drop in folate intake over the preceding few days.[217] Similarly, a low plasma folate, except in malabsorption, rises quickly on refeeding.

A better indicator of the tissue folate status is the red cell folate,[218] which remains relatively unchanged while a red cell is circulating and thus reflects folate status over the preceding 2 to 3 months. Red cell folate usually is quite low in folate-deficient megaloblastic anemia. However, red cell folate also is low in more than 50 percent of patients with cobalamin-deficient megaloblastic anemia[219] owing to the poor retention of methyl THF monoglutamate within the cells[22]; consequently, it cannot be used to distinguish between these two deficiencies. Conversely, red cell folate may be normal in the megaloblastic state that occurs, often with little accompanying anemia, in rapidly developing folate deficiency (see "Acute Megaloblastic Anemia" below).[220]

The dU suppression test has been used in research on pathogenetic mechanisms in megaloblastic states. It adds little to the clinical evaluation of a megaloblastic anemia. The test is further discussed in "Deoxyuridine Suppression" below.

Differential Diagnosis

Macrocytosis occurs in alcoholism without megaloblastic anemia, liver disease, hypothyroidism, aplastic anemia, certain forms of myelodysplasia, pregnancy, and any condition associated with reticulocytosis (e.g., autoimmune hemolytic anemia). However, MCV rarely exceeds 110 fl in these conditions, whereas in folate deficiency, uncomplicated by causes of microcytosis, the MCV is usually over 110 fl.

A full hematologic response to physiologic doses of folate (i.e., 200 mcg daily) distinguishes folate deficiency from cobalamin deficiency, in which a response occurs only at pharmacologic doses of folate (e.g., 5 mg daily). This is not recommended as a diagnostic test because neurologic problems may develop in cobalamin-deficient patients treated with folate alone. Cobalamin may produce a partial response in folate deficiency.[221]

The diagnosis of nontropical sprue rests on (1) the demonstration of malabsorption, (2) a jejunal biopsy showing villus atrophy, and (3) the response to a gluten-free diet. In 80 percent of patients, a gluten-free diet gradually reverses the functional disorder by correcting folate malabsorption.[222]

Nonhematologic Effects of Folate Deficiency

The hematologic problems associated with folate deficiency have been recognized for decades. However, folate deficiency is related to a number of serious disorders not involving the hematopoietic system. Moreover, these disorders occur at folate levels usually regarded as low to normal. They include developmental, neurologic, cardiovascular, and neoplasic diseases.[223]

Abnormalities of Neural Tube Closure

A close association exists between mild folate deficiency and congenital anomalies of the fetus, most notably defects in neural tube closure, but also abnormalities involving the heart, urinary tract, limbs, and other sites.[224] A portion of the neural tube closure defects appear to be associated with antibodies against folate receptors that may be overcome by higher folate intake.[225] Mutations and polymorphisms affecting enzymes of folate metabolism, especially the common 677C→T polymorphism of the *MTHFR* gene (also designated as *MTHFR* 677C→T),[226] also predispose to congenital anomalies. Folic acid fortification programs, which were mandated in the United States and Canada in the mid-1990s, have been highly successful as a public health measure in reducing the incidence of neural tube defect births by between 20 and 50 percent.[227,228]

Cobalamin also plays a significant role as a risk factor for neural tube defects. Levels of TC in normal pregnant women correlate with their likelihood of bearing an infant with a defect in neural tube closure. Patients in the lowest quintile of TC concentration are five times more likely to give birth to a defective infant as patients in the highest quintile.[229] Evidence indicates that in populations exposed to folic acid fortification, there is an approximately threefold increase in the risk of neural tube defects in offspring of mothers in the lowest quartile of TC.[230]

Several poorly defined neuropsychiatric abnormalities that respond to folate therapy have been reported in patients with folate deficiency. The most convincing associations are with depressive illness.[223]

Vascular Disease

A mildly elevated homocysteine level is a major independent risk factor for atherosclerosis and venous thrombosis, possibly because of an effect on the vascular endothelium.[231] Homocysteine levels can decrease with folate, cobalamin, and pyridoxine supplements, possibly reducing the risk of recurrent vascular disease.[232] However, contradictory evidence suggests that supplement use may actually increase the risk of in-stent coronary restenosis[233] or other adverse cardiovascular outcome.[234] An accelerated rate of decrease in stroke mortality has been observed in the United States and Canada that coincided with the introduction of folic acid fortification in these countries.[235] The disparate designs of these studies makes it difficult to draw firm conclusions regarding the question of whether lowering of plasma homocysteine in subjects at risk for cardiovascular disease has any ameliorative or deleterious effect on outcome. Critical factors might relate to several considerations including the preexisting degree of vascular damage and the form and dosage of administered vitamins.

The *MTHFR* polymorphism *MTHFR* 677C→T leads to increased homocysteine levels in subjects with low folate or cobalamin levels,[236] although controversy exists as to whether *MTHFR* 677C→T causes an increased incidence of vascular disease. Like folate, cobalamin seems to be important in decreasing the risk of vascular disease.[237] A 1561C→T polymorphism in the gene for glutamate carboxypeptidase-II increases serum folate and decreases serum homocysteine in the homozygote, possibly protecting against vascular disease.[238]

HELLP Syndrome

Severe folate deficiency reportedly mimics the hemolysis, elevated liver enzymes, low platelets (HELLP) syndrome (preeclampsia with liver swelling and abnormal liver function studies in pregnant women; see Chap. 7).[239] In these patients, the diagnosis of severe folate deficiency can be made based on the presence of anemia and a megaloblastic blood film and marrow. Serum and red cell folate, serum cobalamin, homocysteine, and methylmalonic acid levels all should be assayed before treatment is started. The patient should immediately be given high doses of folate plus cobalamin, the latter in case the megaloblastic anemia actually results from cobalamin deficiency, a possibility rendered more likely in folic acid-fortified populations. A major goal of treatment is preventing preterm delivery of the fetus.

Colon Cancer

A large study of nurses in the United States indicated that supplementation with more than 400 mcg of folic acid per day reduces the incidence of colon cancer by 31 percent.[240] Furthermore, individuals who are homozygous for the 677C→T *MTHFR* mutation also have a decreased incidence for colon cancer compared with 677C→T heterozygotes and normal controls.[241] Other evidence points to possible deleterious effect of folic acid on colon cancer incidence. Although only circumstantial, a recent epidemiologic study reported that after several successive years of a declining incidence of colorectal cancer in the United States and Canada, there was a significant increase in the rate in both countries that coincided with and followed the introduction of folic acid fortification.[242] These apparently contradictory observations may be reconcilable because of the several roles of folate on cellular proliferation and repair as well as on the stage of tumorigenesis.[243] Because folate is critical for *de novo* thymidine synthesis, it plays an important part in DNA repair, thus correcting mutations and DNA strand breaks that could potentially initiate cancer. On the other hand, the growth of established neoplastic clones might be accelerated by additional folate, allowing more rapid tumor progression. The situation is rendered even more complex if the potential role of folate in epigenetic regulation of gene expression is considered. Folate is necessary for synthesis of the universal methyl donor, *S*-adenosyl methionine, which is required for cytosine and histone methylation. In this pathway, too, the role of folate theoretically may be cancer promoting or cancer protective, depending on whether oncogenes or tumor suppressor genes are silenced by methylation of CpG islands in DNA or by conformational changes in chromatin resulting from histone methylation.

Therapy, Course, and Prognosis

Folate 1 to 5 mg/day is given orally, although 1 mg usually is sufficient. At this dose, anemia usually is corrected even in patients with malabsorption. A parenteral preparation containing 5 mg/mL of folate also is available.

Treatment for *tropical sprue* consists of the usual doses of folate, plus cobalamin if indicated. To prevent relapse, treatment should be maintained for at least 2 years. Broad-spectrum antibiotics are helpful adjuncts, although antibiotics alone fail to correct the condition.

Pregnant women must be given at least 400 mcg of folate per day.[244] As to the possibility of overlooking cobalamin deficiency resulting from folate administration, although pernicious anemia (PA) in women of childbearing age is rare in whites, this is not the case among Africans and Hispanics.[245,246] In pregnant women at risk for cobalamin deficiency (e.g., vegans or patients with malabsorption), the deficiency is easily prevented with vitamin B_{12}, 1 mg given parenterally every 3 months during the pregnancy.

Therapeutic doses of folate partially and temporarily correct the hematologic abnormalities in cobalamin deficiency, but the neurologic manifestations can progress, with disastrous results.[247] Therefore, both folate status and cobalamin status must be evaluated early in the workup of a megaloblastic anemia. If treatment is urgent and the nature of the deficiency is unclear, both folate and cobalamin can be given after suitable specimens have been obtained for assay.

Patients who receive low-dose methotrexate therapy as an immunosuppressant may develop side effects, the worst of which is hepatotoxicity. The incidence of side effects, including hepatotoxicity, has been correlated with reduced folate levels.[248] Administration of folic or folinic acid can prevent or greatly diminish the major side effects without reducing the therapeutic effect of low-dose methotrexate.

■ COBALAMIN DEFICIENCY

Etiology and Pathogenesis

Table 41–5 lists disorders that lead to cobalamin deficiency.

Decreased Uptake Caused by Impaired Absorption Cobalamin deficiency most often results from defective absorption, most commonly PA, a condition characterized by failure of gastric intrinsic factor production. Many other causes of defective cobalamin absorption involve mainly the stomach, or small intestine and to lesser extent, the pancreas.

Gastric Disorders Pernicious Anemia PA is a disease of insidious onset that generally begins in middle age or later (usually after age 40 years).[249] In this condition, intrinsic factor secretion fails because of gastric mucosal atrophy. PA is an autoimmune disease. The gastric atrophy of PA probably results from immune destruction of the acid- and pepsin-secreting portion of the gastric mucosa. The term *pernicious anemia* sometimes is used as a synonym for cobalamin deficiency, but it should be reserved for the condition resulting from defective secretion of intrinsic factor by an atrophic gastric mucosa caused by an autoimmune process primarily directed to the parietal cells and their products.

In patients with PA, antibodies occur that recognize the H^+/K^+-adenosine triphosphatase (ATPase), which resides in the secretory membrane of the parietal cell and is responsible for acidifying the stomach contents. These antiparietal cell antibodies occur in approximately 60 percent of patients with simple atrophic gastritis and in 90 percent of patients with PA, but in only 5 percent of a random 30- to 60-year-old population.[250] Antiparietal cell antibodies also occur in a significant percentage of patients with thyroid disease.[251] Conversely, patients with PA have a higher than expected incidence of antibodies against thyroid epithelium, lymphocytes, and renal collecting duct cells.[252]

Antiparietal cell antibodies are not thought to be responsible for the pathogenesis of PA. Rather, studies in mice suggest the gastric atrophy in PA is caused by CD4+ T cells whose receptors recognize the H^+/K^+-ATPase. Thus, thymectomized BALB/c mice develop an autoimmune atrophic gastritis similar to that seen in PA patients. CD4+ T cells from these mice produce atrophic gastritis when injected into nude mice.[253]

Antibodies to intrinsic factor ("type I," or "blocking," antibodies) or the intrinsic factor–cobalamin (Cbl) complex ("type II," or "binding," antibodies) are highly specific to PA patients.[254] Blocking antibodies, which prevent formation of the intrinsic factor–Cbl complex, are found in up to 70 percent of PA sera.[254] Binding antibodies, which prevent the intrinsic factor–Cbl complex from binding to its ileal receptors, are found in about half the sera that contain blocking antibody. Some findings in humans support the idea that T cells are responsible for the gastric atrophy in PA. First, lymphocytes from patients with PA are hyperresponsive to gastric antigens.[255] Second, the correlation between antiparietal cell antibodies and PA is not perfect.[246] Finally, the incidence of PA is higher than expected in patients with agammaglobulinemia, even though their sera contain none of the antibodies typical of PA.[256]

Other Autoimmune Diseases The coexistence of several other autoimmune diseases and PA is further evidence that PA is an autoimmune disease. Antiparietal cell antibodies and PA are unexpectedly frequent in patients with other autoimmune diseases,[257] including autoimmune thyroid disorders (thyrotoxicosis, hypothyroidism, and Hashimoto thyroiditis),[258] type I diabetes mellitus, hypoparathyroidism,[259] Addison disease, postpartum hypophysitis,[260] vitiligo,[261] acquired agammaglobulinemia,[256] infertility in female patients younger than age 40 years,[262] and hypospermia and infertility in males.[263,264] Infertility may, however relate to impairment of DNA synthesis in gonadal cells rather than to an autoimmune mechanism.

Inherited Predisposition to Pernicious Anemia Predisposition to PA can be inherited. The disease is associated with human leukocyte antigen types A2, A3, B7, and B12[265] and with blood group A.[266] PA and antiparietal cell antibodies occur more frequently than expected in the families of PA patients.[267] In one study, gastric atrophy was found in more than 30 percent of the relatives of patients with PA; of these relatives, 65 percent had antiparietal cell antibodies and 22 percent had antiintrinsic factor antibodies.[268] PA occurs relatively frequently in northern Europeans (especially Scandinavians)[269] as well as Africans,[164] but is uncommon in Asians. In Americans of African descent, the disease tends to begin early, occurs with high frequency in women, and often is severe.[164,246]

Stomach and Intestine in Pernicious Anemia Gastric manifestations of PA include achlorhydria, acquired intrinsic factor deficiency previously demonstrable by the Schilling test, and an increased incidence of certain malignancies. There is an approximately twofold increase in the incidence of gastric cancer, similar increases in the incidence of certain hematologic malignancies, and an increase in the incidence of gastric carcinoid.[269] Achlorhydria may precede by many years the loss of intrinsic factor secretion and the development of PA.[270] The absence of achlorhydria excludes the diagnosis of PA. Measurement of gastric acid secretion has been supplanted by serum or plasma, cobalamin, holotranscobalamin, and methylmalonic acid levels.[137,216,271] *Helicobacter pylori*, a microorganism that infects the gastric mucosa, is a major cause of gastritis and peptic ulcers. Evidence is conflicting regarding the role of *H. pylori* in PA. In two studies, cultures of gastric biopsies showed a very low incidence of *H. pylori* infection in PA patients.[272] One study reported that anti-*H. pylori* antibodies were found in only a small fraction of the sera from these patients. The other study reported that these antibodies were present in most of the PA sera, indicating that most of the patients described in the study had been infected previously. Whether *H. pylori* participates in the pathogenesis of PA is an open question. An intriguing hypothesis has been advanced that chronic infection with *H. pylori* may be responsible for triggering an autoimmune reaction directed against the host H+/K+-ATPase protein as a result of molecular mimicry.[273,274]

Fasting plasma gastrin levels are high in most patients with PA, whereas somatostatin levels are low.[275] In biopsies from PA stomachs, however, fundal gastrin and somatostatin levels were high, correlating with increases in argyrophilic cells in the basal crypts; antral gastrin and somatostatin were normal. Gastrin levels are high in simple achlorhydria without PA.[276]

The stomach shows characteristic histologic abnormalities in PA (Fig. 41–14). The mucosa of the cardia and fundus is atrophic, containing few chief (i.e., pepsin-secreting) or parietal cells. The withered mucosa is infiltrated with lymphocytes[277] and plasma cells. In contrast, the antral and pyloric mucosa are normal. Gastric atrophy is partly reversible by glucocorticoid treatment, with some regeneration and return of intrinsic factor secretion, further evidence for the autoimmune nature of PA.[278] Clinical response to administration of glucocorticoids or adrenocorticotropic hormone in patients with neurologic disease may reflect temporary amelioration of underlying and undiagnosed PA.[279]

Megaloblastic changes reversible by cobalamin are seen in the gastrointestinal epithelium. Cells recovered by lavage are large[165] and show atypical nuclei resembling early malignant change.[280] Small intestinal biopsy shows decreased mitoses in crypts, shortening of villi, megaloblastic changes in epithelial cells, and infiltration in the lamina propria.[281] These changes may account for the occasional malabsorption of D-xylose and carotene in PA.[282]

Recognizing pernicious anemia may be difficult. PA combines the general features of megaloblastic anemia and features specific for cobalamin deficiency with unique clinical features related to its (probable) autoimmune etiology and gastric pathology. The disease is easily missed because of its (1) insidious onset, (2) tendency to be masked by the use of multivitamin preparations containing folic acid,[283] and (3) many atypical presentations,[284] including its presentation as a neurologic disease without hematologic findings,[75,285] and its tendency to be overlooked in patients with another autoimmune disease.

Antiparietal cell and antiintrinsic factor antibodies are rarely measured, even though antiintrinsic factor antibodies in particular could be of considerable diagnostic value.[271,286] In the absence of a reliable method to asses vitamin B_{12} absorption, following the demise of the

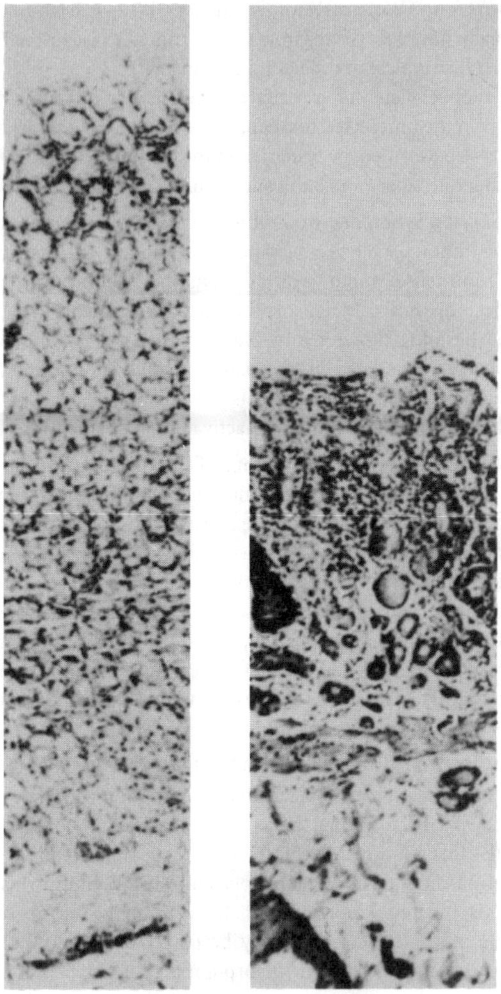

FIGURE 41–14. Gastric histology in pernicious anemia. (*Left*) Normal fundus. The thick mucosa is packed with gastric glands composed mostly of chief cells and parietal cells. The mucus-secreting cells are concentrated in the necks of the glands. (*Right*) Fundus in pernicious anemia. Gastric glands in the atrophic mucosa are sparse and consist mainly of mucus-secreting cells. The mucosa is densely infiltrated by lymphocytes.

Schilling test, measurement of antiintrinsic factor antibodies in serum represents the only available method to confirm a diagnosis of PA Antiintrinsic factor antibody is highly specific for PA (although its sensitivity is only modest), and its presence in a megaloblastic anemia makes the diagnosis of PA almost certain.

Gastrectomy Syndromes Gastric surgery often leads to anemia. Iron-deficiency anemia is most common, but cobalamin deficiency with megaloblastic anemia can occur. After *total gastrectomy*, cobalamin deficiency develops within 5 or 6 years because the operation removes the source of intrinsic factor.[287] The delay between surgery and the onset of cobalamin deficiency reflects the time needed to exhaust cobalamin stores after cobalamin absorption ceases. This may occur more rapidly because of abrogation of the enterohepatic reabsorption of biliary cobalamin.

After *partial gastrectomy*, few patients show frank cobalamin deficiency, but approximately 5 percent have intermediate megaloblastosis, approximately 25 to 50 percent have low serum cobalamin levels, and many have varying degrees of decreased cobalamin absorption.[288] Achlorhydria not present before surgery often develops some years after gastrectomy. Postgastrectomy patients with low serum cobalamin levels usually have low serum iron levels,[289] in contrast to the high iron levels otherwise typical of cobalamin deficiency.

Cobalamin deficiency after partial gastrectomy can be caused by mucosal atrophy in the unresected remnant of the stomach[290] or, if a gastrojejunostomy was performed, by bacterial overgrowth in the afferent loop (see "Competing Intestinal Flora and Fauna: 'Blind Loop Syndrome'" below).

Zollinger-Ellison Syndrome In Zollinger-Ellison syndrome, a gastrin-producing tumor, usually in the pancreas, stimulates the gastric mucosa to secrete immense amounts of HCl. The major clinical problem is a severe ulcer diathesis. Malabsorption of cobalamin occurs when the vast quantities of HCl secreted by the overactive gastric mucosa cannot be completely neutralized by the pancreatic secretions. The resulting acidification of the duodenal contents prevents transfer of Cbl from HC binder to intrinsic factor and also inactivates pancreatic proteases.[291]

Intestinal Diseases Because the terminal ileum is the site for physiologic cobalamin absorption, a number of intestinal disorders can lead to cobalamin deficiency. They include (1) extensive resection of the ileum,[292] (2) inflammatory bowel disease or regional ileitis or other disease affecting the ileum (e.g., lymphoma, radiation damage[293]), (3) cobalamin malabsorption associated with hypothyroidism,[294] or certain drugs,[295] (4) the effects of cobalamin deficiency itself,[296] and (5) sprue, either tropical or, less often, nontropical.[196] In each of these disorders, administration of exogenous intrinsic factor, as was carried out in the Schilling test, would fail to correct subnormal cobalamin absorption.

Competing Intestinal Flora and Fauna: "Blind Loop Syndrome" The *blind loop syndrome* is a state of cobalamin malabsorption with megaloblastic anemia caused by intestinal stasis from anatomic lesions (strictures, diverticula, anastomoses, surgical blind loops) or impaired motility (scleroderma, amyloid).[297] Serum cobalamin is low, but intrinsic factor secretion is normal. Cobalamin malabsorption is not corrected by exogenous intrinsic factor but may be corrected by antibiotic treatment. The defect in cobalamin absorption is caused by colonization of the diseased small intestine by bacteria that take up ingested cobalamin before it can be absorbed from the intestine.[298] Steatorrhea is also seen in the blind loop syndrome.

Another cause of cobalamin deficiency is infestation with the fish tapeworm *Diphyllobothrium latum*. Prevalence is highest near the Baltic Sea, Canada, and Alaska where raw or undercooked fish is consumed. Cobalamin deficiency results from competition between the worm and the host for ingested cobalamin.[299] The clinical picture of *D. latum* infestation ranges from no symptoms to a full-blown megaloblastic anemia with neurologic changes. The infestation is diagnosed by finding tapeworm ova in the feces.

Acquired Immunodeficiency Syndrome A substantial number of patients with AIDS have low serum cobalamin levels with associated evidence of cobalamin malabsorption.[300] In addition, individuals testing seropositive for HIV infection may also have low serum cobalamin and evidence of cobalamin malabsorption.[300] The cause of the malabsorption may be intestinal or gastric or a combination of both.[301,302]

Pancreatic Disease Some degree of cobalamin malabsorption has been demonstrated in 50 to 70 percent of patients with exocrine pancreatic insufficiency.[303] Cobalamin malabsorption in pancreatic insufficiency is caused by a deficiency in pancreatic proteases, resulting in a partial failure to destroy HC–Cbl complexes whose destruction is a prerequisite for the transfer of cobalamin to intrinsic factor. The defect in cobalamin absorption in chronic pancreatitis is corrected by oral trypsin or by presaturating the HC with cobinamide, a cobalamin analogue that is taken up by HC but not by intrinsic factor.[304] Despite the high incidence of abnormal Schilling tests in pancreatic insufficiency, this disorder rarely causes clinically significant cobalamin deficiency.[305]

Dietary Cobalamin Deficiency Dietary cobalamin deficiency is very unusual. It occurs mainly in vegetarians who also do not consume dairy products and eggs (vegans).[306] Low serum cobalamin levels occur in 50 to 60 percent of individuals in this group. The onset of cobalamin deficiency in vegans is slower than in conditions associated with cobalamin malabsorption. Thus it may take 10 to 20 years for an individual consuming a vegan diet to manifest features of cobalamin deficiency.[307] This is because the enterohepatic pathway for biliary cobalamin absorption remains intact, thus conserving body cobalamin stores.[63] Breast-fed infants of vegan mothers also may develop cobalamin deficiency.[308] Cobalamin deficiency in vegans presents with mild megaloblastic anemia, glossitis, and neurologic disturbances.

Cobalamin deficiency may occur in severe general malnutrition. A megaloblastic anemia not related to cobalamin deficiency may accompany kwashiorkor or marasmus.[309]

Neurologic Effects of Cobalamin Deficiency

Formerly, the neurologic abnormalities of cobalamin deficiency were attributed to disordered metabolism of myelin lipids caused by an impaired methylmalonyl CoA mutase reaction.[310] Similar neurologic abnormalities do not, however, occur in patients with inherited methylmalonyl CoA mutase deficiency.[250,311] Authentic combined system disease has occurred in a patient with nutritional folate deficiency[312] and in a patient with N^5, N^{10}-methylene FH_4 reductase deficiency.[313] The latter reports suggest the neurologic lesions of cobalamin deficiency result from deranged methyl group metabolism. Animal studies support this hypothesis. Neurologic disorders closely resembling combined system disease develop in cobalamin-deficient fruit bats,[314] pigs, and monkeys.[315] The development of these disorders is prevented by methionine, which is produced in a cobalamin-dependent reaction and is the precursor of the biologic methylating reagent SAM. A finding that further supports a methylation defect is that brains from cobalamin-deficient pigs contain increased levels of SAH,[316] a powerful methylation inhibitor produced in SAM-dependent methylation reactions:

$$\text{SAM} + \text{RH} \rightarrow \text{SAH} + \text{RCH}_3$$

Against the methylation defect hypothesis is the finding that cobalamin deficiency had no effect on SAM, SAH, or methylation of phospholipids or myelin basic protein[317] in the brains of fruit bats.

CLINICAL FEATURES

The more typical clinical picture of cobalamin deficiency includes the nonspecific manifestations of megaloblastosis, which include anemia, thrombocytopenia, neutropenia, smooth tongue, cardiomyopathy, pale yellow skin and/or weight loss, plus specific features caused by the lack of cobalamin, chiefly neurologic abnormalities. Disturbances in either or both cellular and hormonal immune functions have been reported in cobalamin deficiency.[318,319] Cobalamin deficiency may also contribute to the risk of vascular disease through elevation of homocysteine levels. Other disease associations with cobalamin deficiency have been described. These include a possible increase in breast cancer risk in premenopausal women[320] and in osteoporosis.[321,322] Because cobalamin reserves are large, years may pass between the cessation of cobalamin absorption and the appearance of deficiency symptoms.

Neurologic Abnormalities

Cobalamin deficiency causes a neurologic syndrome that is particularly dangerous because the syndrome can develop in isolation,[323] with no megaloblastic anemia to suggest a lack of cobalamin,[285,324] and because the syndrome cannot be reversed by treatment when it is sufficiently far advanced. The syndrome usually begins with paresthesias in feet and

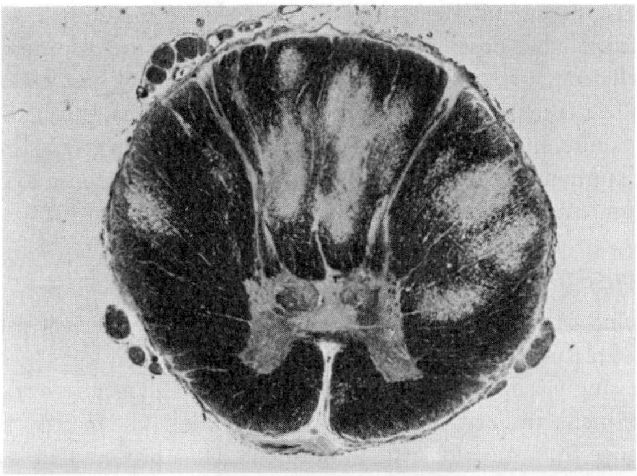

FIGURE 41–15. Degeneration of spinal cord in combined system disease. *(Reproduced with permission from Harris JW, Kellermeyer RW:* The Red Cell: Production, Metabolism, Destruction: Normal and Abnormal, *rev ed. Harvard University Press, Cambridge, 1970.)*

fingers as a result of early peripheral neuropathy and disturbances of vibratory sense and proprioception. The earliest signs, which precede other neurologic findings by months, are loss of position sense in the second toe and loss of vibration sense for a 256-Hz but not a 128-Hz tuning fork.[325] Left untreated, the neurologic disorder progresses to spastic ataxia resulting from demyelination of the dorsal and lateral columns of the spinal cord, so-called *combined system disease* (Fig. 41–15).[326]

The peripheral nerves, the spinal cord, and the brain are affected by cobalamin deficiency. Somnolence and perversion of taste, smell, and vision with occasional optic atrophy are accompanied by slow waves on the electroencephalogram. A dementia mimicking Alzheimer disease can develop.[327] There is recent evidence linking low cobalamin status with brain volume loss and cerebral white matter lesions.[328,329] Psychological derangements, including psychotic depression and paranoid schizophrenia, can occur.[330] Frank psychosis in cobalamin deficiency has been termed *megaloblastic madness*.[331]

The neurologic lesions of cobalamin deficiency can be detected by magnetic resonance imaging (MRI). Demyelination appears as T2-weighted hyperintensity of the white matter.[332] MRI is particularly useful for confirming the diagnosis of a neurologic disorder resulting from cobalamin deficiency. MRI also has been used to follow the progress of neurologic abnormalities during treatment of cobalamin-deficient patients.[332]

Subtle Cobalamin Deficiency

Some observations suggest the existence of a large group of patients who are hematologically normal, with a normal hematocrit and MCV, but who have cobalamin-responsive neuropsychiatric disease.[285] Neuropsychiatric findings include peripheral neuropathy, gait disturbance, memory loss,[329] and psychiatric symptoms, often with abnormal evoked potentials. Serum cobalamin may be normal, borderline, or low, but tissue cobalamin deficiency is suggested by consistently high levels of serum methylmalonic acid and/or homocysteine, very high levels of methylmalonic acid in the cerebrospinal fluid, and an abnormal dU suppression test. Most of the neuropsychiatric abnormalities appear to respond to cobalamin therapy.

LABORATORY FEATURES

Plasma or Serum Cobalamin Levels

Plasma or serum cobalamin is low in most but not all patients with cobalamin deficiency.[216] Cobalamin levels are usually normal in cobalamin deficiency resulting from exposure to nitrous oxide, TC deficiency, and inborn errors of cobalamin metabolism. Levels also may be normal in cobalamin-deficient patients with high HC levels resulting from myeloproliferative diseases. Conversely, plasma cobalamin levels may be low in the presence of normal tissue cobalamins in vegetarians, in subjects taking megadoses of ascorbic acid, in pregnancy (25%), in the presence of HC deficiency,[333,334] and in megaloblastic anemia resulting from folate deficiency (30%).[216] Plasma folate may be high in cobalamin deficiency because of the block in conversion of methyl-THF, which is the predominant form in plasma. Patients deficient in both cobalamin and folate may show normal serum folate levels.

Plasma or Serum Holotranscobalamin

The fraction of the cobalamin in plasma that is bound to transcobalamin constitutes only 10 to 30 percent of the total plasma cobalamin. Even so, it is this fraction that is functionally important and also better reflects the integrity of the cobalamin absorptive status of an individual.[139,335] The major fraction of plasma cobalamin on HC is considered functionally inert and is therefore less relevant for the consideration of cobalamin status. Consequently, and with the development of assays to measure the TC-bound fraction of the plasma cobalamin, an increasing body of evidence has accumulated to validate the usefulness of TC-associated cobalamin (holotranscobalamin).[63,134,137,335,336]

Methylmalonic Acid

Except when caused by an inborn error, methylmalonic aciduria is a reliable indicator of cobalamin deficiency.[337] Normal subjects excrete only traces of methylmalonate (0–3.4 mg/day). In cobalamin deficiency, urine methylmalonate usually is elevated.[338] Cobalamin therapy restores excretion to normal in a few days. Another possible advantage of measurement of urine rather than plasma methylmalonic acid is that in conditions of impaired renal function, when plasma methylmalonic acid may be suspiciously elevated, measurement of the metabolite in urine correlated for creatinine obviates this problem.[339]

Serum or Plasma Methylmalonic Acid and Homocysteine

Elevated plasma or serum methylmalonic acid and homocysteine levels are indicators of *tissue* cobalamin deficiency. Their levels are high in more than 90 percent of cobalamin-deficient patients and rise before plasma cobalamin falls to subnormal levels.[216,340] Elevated plasma methylmalonic acid and/or elevated homocysteine are both indicators of cobalamin deficiency in patients without a congenital disorder in their metabolism. Of the two, methylmalonic acid measurement is both more sensitive and more specific, and elevated methylmalonic acid will persist for several days, even after cobalamin treatment is instituted. Unlike homocysteine levels that rise in folate and pyridoxine deficiencies, as well as in hypothyroidism, methylmalonic acid elevation is seen only in cobalamin deficiency.[216] In renal diseases however, both homocysteine and methylmalonate, acid levels are frequently elevated. Additionally, intestinal bacteria synthesize propionate, a precursor of methylmalonic, and in conditions of bacterial overgrowth, microbial methylmalonic acid may contribute to elevations in plasma methylmalonic acid.[340,341] Although measurement of these metabolites may be used for population screening for evidence of cobalamin deficiency, the finding of an isolated elevation of plasma methylmalonate should not be taken as evidence of clinically attributable cobalamin deficiency.[341,342]

Spinal fluid methylmalonic acid levels are markedly elevated in cobalamin deficiency.[343]

Assays of Cobalamin Absorption and Intrinsic Factor

Despite its numerous shortcomings the previous "gold standard" for assessment of cobalamin absorption was the Schilling test. The Schilling test assessed cobalamin absorption by measuring urinary radioactivity after an oral dose of radioactive cobalamin. The test could be performed even after cobalamin deficiency had been treated. The test consisted of administering a physiologic dose of radiolabeled Co-CnCbl by mouth followed 2 hours later by injection of a large "flushing" dose of unlabeled CnCbl and determination and radioactivity in a 24-hour collection of urine. Subjects with normal absorption excreted 7 percent or more of the radioactivity in the urine. Subjects with subnormal urinary excretion would have the test repeated with addition of an animal-derived intrinsic factor to determine whether the malabsorption could be corrected.[344] The use of the Schilling test has dropped to a point of obsolescence as a consequence of reduced availability of the test components, cost, radioactive waste disposal, and concern about the use of animal-derived tissues for human use, which were required for the intrinsic factor administered in the second part of the test.[63] Replacements for the Schilling test are currently under development. One approach uses measurement of the change in holotranscobalamin following oral administration of non-radiolabeled cobalamin.[335,345] A different approach involves the use of accelerator mass spectrometry and microbially produced C-14 at attomolar concentrations.[346] In this approach, C-14 is measured in blood at the time of peak appearance 6 to 8 hours following the dose. Both methods show promise but are not yet in routine clinical use.

Deoxyuridine Suppression Test

The dU suppression test is based on the finding that unlabeled dU can suppress the uptake of [^{3}H]thymidine ([^{3}H]Thd) into the DNA of cultured lymphocytes or marrow cells through dilution of the label in the thymidine pool.[347] This occurs when the thymidylate synthase reaction is functionally intact, which requires adequate quantities of both folate and cobalamin.

The dU suppression test is chiefly a research tool. It can help diagnose certain special clinical problems,[347] but these problems also can be diagnosed using other laboratory tests, therapeutic trials with vitamins or iron, or watchful waiting. Furthermore, in more than 40 years of use, the test has not moved from the research laboratory into the clinic. The dU suppression test seems unlikely to enjoy more widespread clinical use in the future (Table 41–6).

THERAPY, COURSE, AND PROGNOSIS

Treatment consists of parenteral CnCbl (vitamin B_{12}) or OHCbl to replace daily losses and refill storage pools, which normally contain 2 to 5 mg of cobalamin.[348] Toxicity is highly unusual, and there is no defined upper limit.[2] Doses exceeding 100 mcg saturate the TCs, and the excess is lost in the urine. A typical treatment schedule consists of 1000 mcg cobalamin intramuscular (IM) daily for 2 weeks, then weekly until the hematocrit is normal, and then monthly for life. For neurologic manifestations, 1000 mcg every 2 weeks for 6 months is recommended. Higher doses are given for certain inherited disorders (e.g., TC deficiency). *Transfusion* occasionally is required when the hematocrit is less than 15 percent or the patient is debilitated, infected, or in heart failure. In such instances, packed cells should be given slowly to avoid pulmonary edema. Infections can impair the response to cobalamin and must be treated vigorously.

Response to Treatment and Therapeutic Trial

Following parenteral administration of cobalamin to deficient patients, elevated plasma bilirubin, iron, and LDH levels fall rapidly (Fig. 41–16).[349] Decreasing plasma iron turnover and fecal urobilinogen reflect cessation of ineffective erythropoiesis. Within 12 hours, the marrow begins to change from megaloblastic to normoblastic, a process that is complete in 2 to 3 days. Consequently, morphologic diagnosis may be difficult after treatment is initiated. Reticulocytosis begins on days 3 to 5 and peaks on days 4 to 10.[350] The new red cells come from new normoblasts, not from the old megaloblasts, most of which die before leaving the marrow.[146] Blood hemoglobin concentration becomes normal within 1 to 2 months. If normal values are not achieved by 2 months, another cause of anemia should be sought.

Other changes include the following: (1) prompt and dramatic improvement in the sense of well-being; (2) normalization of leukocyte and platelet counts, although neutrophil hypersegmentation may persist for 10 to 14 days; (3) rise in serum cobalamin and folate. Cobalamin deficiency does not respond to a physiologic dose of folate

TABLE 41–6. Correction of the Deoxyuridine Suppression Test in Nutritional Megaloblastic Anemia

	Corrected By			
Deficiency	CnCbl	Folate	N^5-Formyl FH_4	N^5-Methyl FH_4
Folate	–	+	+	+
Cobalamin	+	+	+	–

CnCbl, cyanocobalamin (vitamin B_{12}); FH_4, tetrahydrofolic acid.

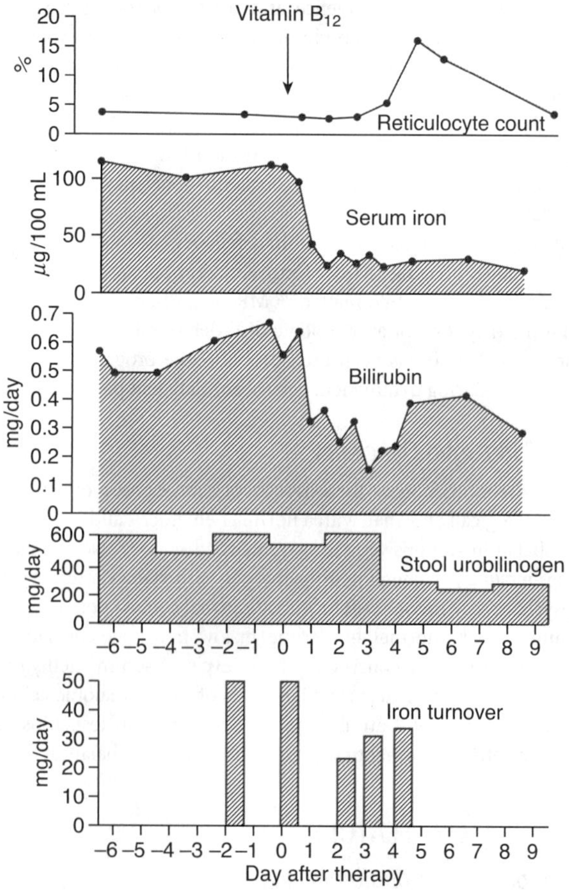

FIGURE 41–16. Effect of cyanocobalamin on reticulocyte count, serum iron, serum bilirubin, stool urobilinogen, and plasma iron turnover. *(Adapted from Coleman D, Donohue D, Finch C, et al. Erythrokinetics in pernicious anemia.* Blood *11:807, 1956.)*

(100–400 mcg/day), although this dose produces a maximal response in folate deficiency. Larger doses of folate (5–15 mg/day) can produce a reticulocytosis and partially or temporarily correct the anemia in cobalamin deficiency.

Special Circumstances

After Gastrectomy Cobalamin should always be given after total gastrectomy. Cobalamin administration is not necessary after partial gastrectomy, but patients need to be watched for megaloblastic anemia, bearing in mind that this anemia can be masked by postgastrectomy iron deficiency.[341,351]

Blind Loop Syndrome The anemia of the blind loop syndrome can be treated by parenteral cobalamin therapy. It also responds after approximately 1 week to oral broad-spectrum antibiotics (cephalexin monohydrate [Keflex] 250 mg QID plus metronidazole 250 mg TID for 10 days),[352] and cobalamin absorption is restored. Successful surgical correction of an anatomic lesion also cures the syndrome.

Fish Tapeworm Treatment consists of a single oral dose of a 50 mg/kg of niclosamide or a dose of 5 to 10 mg/kg of praziquantel.

Rekindled Use of Oral Cobalamin

Much interest has been kindled[353] regarding the possibility of treating cobalamin deficiency with oral cobalamin as had been proposed previously.[354] Oral cobalamin can be used not only for treatment of dietary cobalamin deficiency that occurs in vegans and in patients with very severe general malnutrition, but also for patients with food cobalamin malabsorption[355] and for patients with PA, provided the patients are followed carefully.[356] In patients lacking intrinsic factor, approximately 1 percent of an oral dose of the vitamin is forced across the intestinal epithelium by mass action. Therefore, 1000 to 2000 mcg/day of oral cobalamin supplies most PA patients with their daily cobalamin requirement without the need for injections and their accompanying pain and expense. Cobalamin should be given by mouth to patients with dietary cobalamin deficiency and patients (e.g., hemophiliacs) who cannot take IM injections.

■ ACUTE MEGALOBLASTIC ANEMIA

Megaloblastic anemia usually is a chronic condition that requires weeks or months to develop, but a potentially fatal megaloblastic state resulting from acute tissue folate or cobalamin deficiency can arise over the course of only a few days. Patients with acute megaloblastic anemia present with rapidly developing thrombocytopenia and/or leukopenia and counts that sometimes fall to very low levels, but little change in red cell levels unless another cause of anemia is present. The clinical picture can suggest an immune cytopenia. The diagnosis is made from the marrow aspirate, which is floridly megaloblastic, and confirmed by the rapid response to appropriate replacement therapy.

The most common cause of acute megaloblastic anemia is nitrous oxide (N_2O) anesthesia.[357] N_2O rapidly destroys MeCbl,[358] rapidly leading to a megaloblastic state. AdoCbl eventually is lost, SAM and total folate levels decline, and the proportion of folate in the form of N^5-methyl FH_4 increases.[359] Clinical findings develop quickly. Grossly megaloblastic changes are seen in the marrow after 12 to 24 hours.[360] Hypersegmented neutrophils do not appear until 5 days after exposure but then persist for several days.[361] The effects of N_2O disappear spontaneously after a few days; disappearance can be hastened by folinic acid or cobalamin.[362] Fatalities resulting from N_2O-induced megaloblastosis have occurred in tetanus patients given N_2O for weeks.[357] Long-term recreational use of N_2O has led to a neurologic disorder similar to combined system disease.[363]

Acute megaloblastic anemia occurs in other clinical settings. A rapidly developing megaloblastic state with acute thrombocytopenia has occurred in seriously ill patients, often in intensive care units.[364] Especially at risk are patients who are transfused extensively at surgery,[365] those on dialysis or total parenteral nutrition, and those receiving weak folate antagonists such as trimethoprim. Morphologic clues to the diagnosis (e.g., hypersegmented neutrophils) often are absent from the blood film. Both red cell folate and serum cobalamin levels may be normal, but the marrow is always megaloblastic. A rapid response to therapeutic doses of parenteral folate (5 mg/day) and cobalamin (1 mg) is the rule.

■ MEGALOBLASTIC ANEMIA CAUSED BY DRUGS

Table 41–7 lists the drugs that cause megaloblastic anemia. *Aminopterin* and *methotrexate* are almost structurally identical to folic acid. After they enter cells via the folate carrier[366] and acquire a polyglutamate chain,[367] they act as very powerful inhibitors of dihydrofolate reductase.[368] By blocking the $FH_2 \rightarrow FH_4$ reaction and perhaps inhibiting other enzymes of folate metabolism, they effect the rapid withdrawal of folates from the one-carbon fragment carrier pool, causing a fall in nucleotide (especially thymidine) biosynthesis that leads to a major derangement in DNA replication (see Chaps. 9 and 20).[369]

Toxic effects include necrotic mouth lesions; ulcerations of the esophagus, small intestine, and colon, with abdominal pain, vomiting, and diarrhea; megaloblastic anemia; alopecia; and hyperpigmentation. The drug is excreted by the kidney, so effects and toxicity are prolonged and enhanced if renal function is impaired. Toxicity caused by these folate antagonists is treated with folinic acid (N^5-formyl FH_4). Folate itself is useless because the blocked reductase cannot convert folate to the active tetrahydro form. Folinic acid is already in the tetrahydro form, so folinic acid is effective despite reductase blockade. The usual dose of folinic acid is 3 to 6 mg/day IM. Larger doses are given in chemotherapy protocols that use folinic acid to rescue patients deliberately treated with otherwise fatal doses of methotrexate. Folinic acid was used intrathecally in a patient in whom a large overdose of methotrexate was accidentally delivered into the subarachnoid space.[370]

Zidovudine (azidothymidine [AZT]) is used for HIV infections (AIDS; see Chap. 83).[371] Its principal toxic effect is severe megaloblastic anemia. Anemia or neutropenia produced by zidovudine limits use of this drug.[372]

HIV infection itself suppresses hematopoiesis, leading to pancytopenia with myelodysplastic features (see Chaps. 83 and 88). The blood film shows vacuolated monocytes. Megaloblastosis in HIV infection may result from folate or cobalamin deficiency[373] or AZT or trimethoprim toxicity.

Hydroxyurea is used at high doses to treat chronic myelogenous leukemia, polycythemia vera, and essential thrombocythemia, and at lower doses to treat psoriasis, rheumatoid arthritis, and sickle cell disease (see Chap. 20). It inhibits conversion of ribonucleotides to deoxyribonucleotides.[374] Marked megaloblastic changes are routinely found in the marrow 1 to 2 days after initiating hydroxyurea therapy. These changes are rapidly reversed after the drug is withdrawn. Megaloblastosis as a result of N_2O is discussed in "Acute Megaloblastic Anemia" above.

Long-term use of omeprazole and presumably other H^+/K^+-ATPase inhibitors is associated with reduced serum cobalamin levels, presumably because of the ability of these drugs to inhibit parietal cell function.[375] Reduced serum cobalamin levels are not a problem when these drugs are used for short intervals.[376]

Pemetrexed is an antifolate approved for use in mesothelioma. It also has been used for treatment of non–small cell lung cancer. Like other antifolate agents, pemetrexed can result in a megaloblastic anemia that

TABLE 41–7. Drugs That Cause Megaloblastic Anemia

Agents	Comments	Reference
Antifolates		
Methotrexate	Very potent inhibitor of dihydrofolate reductase	415
Aminopterin	Treat overdose with folinic acid	369
Pyrimethamine	Much weaker than methotrexate and aminopterin	
Trimethoprim	Treat with folinic acid or by withdrawing the drug	416
Sulfasalazine	Can cause acute megaloblastic anemia in susceptible patients, especially those with low folate stores	417
Chlorguanide (Proguanil)		418
Triamterene	Use of folate and cobalamin during pemetrexed treatment reduces toxicity	
Pemetrexed (Alimta)		419
Purine analogues		
6-Mercaptopurine	Megaloblastosis precedes hypoplasia, usually mild	420
6-Thioguanine	Responds to folinic acid but not folate	421
Azathioprine		422
Acyclovir	Megaloblastosis at high doses	423
Pyrimidine analogues		
5-Fluorouracil	Mild megaloblastosis	424
Floxuridine (5-fluorodeoxyuridine)		424
6-Azauridine	Blocks uridine monophosphate production by inhibiting orotidyl decarboxylase; occasional megaloblastosis with orotic acid and orotidine in urine	425
Zidovudine (AZT)	Severe megaloblastic anemia is the major side effect	372
Ribonucleotide reductase inhibitors		
Hydroxyurea	Marked megaloblastosis within 1–2 days of starting therapy; quickly reversed by withdrawing drug	426
Cytarabine (cytosine arabinoside)	Early megaloblastosis is routine	427
Anticonvulsants		
Phenytoin (diphenylhydantoin)	Occasional megaloblastosis, associated with low folate levels; responds to high-dose folate (1–5 mg/day); how anticonvulsants cause low folate is not understood, but may be related to a drug-induced rise in cytochrome P450	428-430
Phenobarbital		428
Primidone		428
Carbamazepine		431
Other drugs that depress folates		
Oral contraceptives	Occasional megaloblastosis; sometimes dysplasia of uterine cervix, corrected with folate	432
Glutethimide		
Cycloserine		
H^+/K^+-ATPase inhibitors		
Omeprazole	Long-term use causes decreased serum cobalamin levels	375
Lansoprazole		
Miscellaneous		
N_2O	See "Acute Megaloblastic Anemia"	357
p-Aminosalicylic acid	Causes cobalamin malabsorption with occasional mild megaloblastic anemia	433
Metformin		434
Phenformin	Causes cobalamin malabsorption but not anemia	
Colchicine		435
Neomycin		436
Arsenic	Causes myelodysplastic hematopoiesis, sometimes with megaloblastic changes	437

is treated with cobalamin and folate. Trimethoprim is a dihydrofolate reductase inhibitor that is designed to act on microbial rather than the mammalian enzyme. Still, in patients with borderline folate status, trimethoprim can precipitate a state of folate deficiency.

MEGALOBLASTIC ANEMIA IN CHILDHOOD

Megaloblastic anemia in childhood is usually the result of genetic disorders affecting either the cobalamin binding proteins or the enzymes concerned with intracellular trafficking of cobalamin or its conversion to coenzymatically active forms. Several recent reviews have dealt comprehensively with this topic.[311,377,378]

Defects Involving Cobalamin-Binding Proteins

Several genetic mutations and polymorphisms exist that affect the key binding proteins for cobalamin. Their effects range from being clinically benign to causing severe cobalamin deficiency with megaloblastic anemia and neurologic complications usually manifesting in infancy or early childhood, occasionally in adolescence or early adulthood. In general, the mutations and deletions affecting the encoded proteins cause serious health consequences whereas the polymorphic variants may be totally inconspicuous or result only in a modified likelihood of disease risk.

Cobalamin malabsorption occurs in four childhood conditions associated with a genetic component: (1) cobalamin malabsorption in the presence of normal intrinsic factor secretion, (2) congenital abnormality of intrinsic factor, (3) TC deficiency, and (4) true PA of childhood. The management of cobalamin deficiency in childhood has been comprehensively reviewed.[378]

Selective Malabsorption of Cobalamin, Autosomal Recessive Megaloblastic Anemia (MGA1), Imerslund-Gräsbeck Disease Imerslund-Gräsbeck disease[379] is an inherited failure of transport of the intrinsic factor–Cbl complex by the ileum, usually accompanied by proteinuria, mostly of albumin.[378] It may be the most common cause of cobalamin deficiency in infancy in some populations.[380] Cobalamin deficiency usually is seen before age 2 years, but may appear earlier or later. Cobalamin malabsorption is not corrected by addition of intrinsic factor. Endogenous intrinsic factor and HCl secretion, TC and HC levels, and gastric and intestinal histology are all normal. Intrinsic factor antibodies are absent. Intrinsic factor–Cbl receptors are present in some but not all patients. The molecular defect responsible for this disease has been elucidated. The ileal phase of cobalamin absorption, two genes code distinct proteins that form part of the cobalamin–IF receptor complex. The first, CUBN, is affected by several mutations described in Finnish patients with MGA1.[93,381] The second, affecting the protein AMN results in a milder MGA1 phenotype and is found in Norwegian patients.[93,382] Again, several mutations in this gene have been described.[93] Patients are treated with IM cobalamin. The anemia is corrected, but proteinuria persists.

Congenital Intrinsic Factor Deficiency Congenital intrinsic factor deficiency is an autosomal recessive disease in which parietal cells fail to produce functionally normal intrinsic factor.[383] Patients present with irritability and megaloblastic anemia when cobalamin stores (<25 mcg at birth) are exhausted. The disease usually presents at age 6 to 24 months. HCl secretion and gastric histology are normal, proteinuria is not present, and antiintrinsic factor antibodies are absent.[384] Abnormal cobalamin absorption is corrected by oral intrinsic factor.[385] Treatment consists of standard doses of IM cobalamin.

Transcobalamin Deficiency Transcobalamin deficiency is an autosomal recessive disorder causing a flagrant megaloblastic anemia that generally presents in early infancy.[386] The disease is dangerously deceptive because it results from a very severe deficiency of tissue cobalamin, usually with normal serum cobalamin levels. Undiagnosed transcobalamin deficiency causes irreversible central nervous system (CNS) damage.[387] Patients are healthy at birth but over the next few weeks develop signs and symptoms of cobalamin deficiency, such as rapidly progressive pancytopenia, mouth ulcers, vomiting, and diarrhea. Recurrent bacterial infections may occur.[386] Neurologic findings are not prominent in the early stages of the disease.[387]

Serum folate and cobalamin are normal (the latter because most cobalamin is carried by HC). Homocysteine and/or methylmalonic acid levels are elevated in the plasma.[388] The marrow is megaloblastic and the cobalamin absorption is usually but not always abnormal and is not corrected by intrinsic factor.[389] The diagnosis is made by measuring plasma TC.[378] Prenatal diagnosis is possible.[390] Serum should be obtained prior to treatment because TC levels in normal individuals drop sharply after cobalamin is given. TC deficiency is treated with cobalamin doses sufficiently large to force enough vitamin into the cells to allow normal function. Initial therapy can consist of oral CnCbl or OHCbl 500 to 1000 mcg twice a week, or IM OHCbl 1000 mcg/week. Blood counts and symptoms should be monitored and doses adjusted upward if necessary.

Several single nucleotide polymorphisms in the TC gene have been described and the allele frequency of the most common form (776 C>G) is high in certain populations.[391,392] Holotranscobalamin levels are lower in individuals homozygous for the G-allele[391] and methylmalonate levels are higher,[392] suggesting that this genotype may be associated with less-favorable cobalamin status.[63]

Haptocorrin Deficiency Congenital deficiency is not associated with clinically manifested cobalamin deficiency, although the plasma or serum cobalamin levels are well below normal,[334] and this is how the condition is recognized. The absence of morbidity in these patients indicates that haptocorrins are not essential for health.

True Juvenile Pernicious Anemia True PA, with gastric atrophy and a defect in intrinsic factor secretion, is exceedingly rare in childhood.[393] Patients usually present in their teens with cobalamin deficiency. Serum antiintrinsic factor antibodies usually are present.[255] The diagnosis and treatment are the same as for PA in adults.

INBORN ERRORS OF COBALAMIN METABOLISM

Cobalamin is converted to AdoCbl and MeCbl by a complex series of transformations involving several steps.[377,388,394] Eight disorders affecting this cobalamin transformation pathway have been described, one for each of the steps. Because the molecular causes of these disorders have not yet been fully characterized, the disorders themselves are not named for a defective protein but instead are designated by sequential capital letters preceded by a *cbl* prefix. The disorders can be grouped into three broad clinical syndromes based on the abnormal metabolites in the patient's urine (Table 41–8). These disorders are usually discovered during investigation of infants with unexplained developmental delay, acidosis, anemia, or unexplained neurologic difficulties. Typically they have normal plasma cobalamin levels.

TABLE 41–8. Cobalamin Mutant Class Syndromes

Syndrome	Methylmalonic Aciduria	Homocystinuria	Megaloblastic Anemia
cblA, cblB, cblH	+	–	–
cblE, cblC	–	+	+
cblC, cblD, cblF	+	+	±

Methylmalonic Aciduria Only (cblA, cblB, and cblH)

In cblA and cblB, AdoCbl production is impaired but MeCbl production is normal. This may result either from an abnormal methylmalonyl CoA mutase (designated mut^{o} or mut^{-}) or from a defect in activation or production of its cofactor, adenosylcobalamin. The cblH variant appears to represent an interallelic variant of cblA.[395] Patients present in infancy with acidosis because they cannot catabolize methylmalonic acid. Symptoms include lethargy and failure to thrive, vomiting, and neurologic problems. Mental retardation is not prominent, and megaloblastic anemia is absent. Most patients respond to 1000 mcg/day of OHCbl or CnCbl, although mut^{o} and mut^{-} patients are unresponsive.

Homocystinuria Only (cblE and cblG)

In these disorders, N^5-methyltetrahydrofolate-homocysteine methyltransferase is defective and lacks the capacity to produce MeCbl.[396] In patients with cblG, methionine synthase is missing or defective.[397] cblE results from failure to reactivate methionine synthase that was inactivated by oxidation of its bound cobalamin.[398] Patients present in infancy with vomiting, mental retardation, and megaloblastic anemia. They have marked homocystinuria and hyperhomocysteinemia without methylmalonic aciduria or methylmalonic acidemia. They respond well to CnCbl 1000 mcg/day or 1000 mcg/week. Infants diagnosed prenatally and treated from birth usually show normal development. On rare occasions, this disorder may first become apparent in adult life.

Methylmalonic Aciduria and Homocystinuria (cblC, cblD, and cblF)

In these disorders, the defect in Cbl transformation affects AdoCbl and MeCbl, probably because reduction of cobalt from Co^{2+} to Co^{1+} is defective. These patients have both hyperhomocysteinemia and methylmalonic acidemia. The age at initial presentation ranges from early infancy to adolescence. In addition to lethargy and failure to thrive, affected infants present with serious neurologic difficulties. Older patients present with psychological problems, progressive dementia, and motor signs and symptoms. cblC disease is the most common of the cobalamin inborn errors. In cblF the defect lies in an inability to release cobalamin from lysosomes.[399] Megaloblastic anemia occurs in about half the cases. Patients respond partially to 1000 mcg/day of OHCbl or CnCbl.

A tentative diagnosis of a cobalamin mutation can be made by demonstrating methylmalonic aciduria and/or homocystinuria in a patient with the clinical findings described above in "Methylmalonic Aciduria Only" or "Homocystinuria Only," respectively. Establishing a diagnosis requires a specialized laboratory equipped to do cultured fibroblast complementation studies.[377] In a patient suspected of having a cobalamin mutation, treatment should be started pending the test results because early high-dose cobalamin treatment is risk-free and may reduce the chance of damage to the CNS. Fetuses with these diseases have been successfully treated *in utero* with very large doses of CnCbl given parenterally to the mother.[400]

INBORN ERRORS OF FOLATE METABOLISM

Megaloblastic anemia in infancy has been described in three inherited disorders of folate metabolism.[28,378,401]

Hereditary Folate Malabsorption

Hereditary folate malabsorption is a rare inherited disorder in which patients cannot absorb folate from the gastrointestinal tract or transport it across the choroid plexus and into the cerebrospinal fluid.[27,28] The molecular basis for this disorder is caused by abnormalities in the proton-coupled folate transporter.[27] Patients present with severe megaloblastic anemia, seizures, mental retardation, and other CNS findings.[402] Folate levels are low in the serum and nil in the cerebrospinal fluid. Folate given parenterally has corrected the anemia and seizures in some patients but has had no effect on other CNS symptoms or on the cerebrospinal fluid folate level. Treatment with daily folinic acid by injection maintains the spinal fluid level and can lead to normal development.[378]

Dihydrofolate Reductase Deficiency

Dihydrofolate reductase deficiency may present isolated megaloblastic anemia within days or weeks after birth. The anemia responds to folinic acid but not to folic acid.[403]

N^5-Methyl FH_4–Homocysteine Methyltransferase Deficiency

Decreased methyltransferase activity was described in a liver biopsy from a child with megaloblastic anemia and mental retardation. The anemia failed to respond to folate, cobalamin, or pyridoxal phosphate.[404] The phenotype of this disorder resembles the inborn errors of cobalamin metabolism affecting the methionine synthesis reaction and has not been well characterized as a distinct entity at the molecular level.

Methylene Tetrahydrofolate Reductase Deficiency

In this rare autosomal recessive disorder there is a severe hyperhomocysteinemia and homocystinuria with low plasma methionine. Patients have neurologic and vascular complications but no megaloblastic anemia or methylmalonic aciduria.[378] The polymorphic variations in MTHFR have been discussed earlier as well as their influence on disease susceptibility.

OTHER INBORN ERRORS

Hereditary Orotic Aciduria

Hereditary orotic aciduria is an autosomal recessive disorder of pyrimidine metabolism[405] characterized by megaloblastic anemia, growth impairment, and excretion of orotic acid in the urine. Cobalamin and folate levels are normal.

Lesch-Nyhan Syndrome

The Lesch-Nyhan syndrome is an X-linked disorder of purine metabolism characterized by hyperuricemia, hyperuricosuria, and a neurologic disease with self-mutilation. It is caused by a hypoxanthine-guanine phosphoribosyltransferase deficiency. One patient described had megaloblastic anemia.[406]

Thiamine-Responsive Megaloblastic Anemia

Seven children with severe megaloblastic anemia, sensorineural deafness, and diabetes mellitus, all beginning in infancy, have been reported. The anemia responded to thiamine (25–100 mg/day). The marrow was reported as myelodysplastic in two patients with the disorder.[407] The gene for this puzzling disorder has been mapped to the long arm of chromosome 1, and the underlying biochemical defect is caused by reduced nucleic acid production through impairment of the thiamine dependent pentose cycle enzyme transketolase that results in cell-cycle arrest and the megaloblastic phenotype.[408] This condition is also discussed in Chap. 43.

OTHER CAUSES OF MEGALOBLASTIC ANEMIA

Congenital Dyserythropoietic Anemia

The congenital dyserythropoietic anemias are lifelong anemias. They often are mild, showing dysplastic changes affecting the red cell line only, most typically multinuclearity of the normoblasts. They appear to result from defects in glycosylation of polylactosaminoglycans linked to membrane proteins and ceramides.[409] Of the three types, two (type I usually[410] and type III occasionally[411]) show megaloblastic red cell precursors (see Chap. 39).

Refractory Megaloblastic Anemia

Refractory megaloblastic anemia is regarded as a manifestation of some sideroblastic anemias (see Chap. 58) and myelodysplastic disorders (see Chap. 88).[412] The megaloblastic changes are atypical. Dysplastic features are confined to the erythroid series. Giant metamyelocytes and bands are absent from the marrow. A few patients with refractory megaloblastic anemia respond to pharmacologic doses of pyridoxine (200 mg/day),[413] perhaps because of an effect on serine transformylase, which requires both pyridoxine and folate.

Acute Erythroid Leukemia

In acute erythroid leukemia, a variety of acute myelogenous leukemia (see Chap 89).[414] Nucleated red cells appear on the blood film, there is usually marked anisocytosis and anisochromia, and macrocytes are usually present. The marrow shows pronounced erythroid hyperplasia involving very bizarre looking megaloblast-like red cell precursors, often containing multiple nuclei or nuclear fragments (see Fig. 89–1). The megaloblastoid erythroid precursors frequently appear vacuolated.

REFERENCES

1. Butterworth CJ, Santini RJ, Frommeyer WJ: The pteroylglutamate components of American diets as determined by chromatographic fractionation. *J Clin Invest* 42:1929, 1963.
2. Institute of Medicine: *Dietary Reference Intakes for Thiamin, Riboflavin, Niacin, Vitamin B6, Folate, Vitamin B12, Pantothenic Acid, Biotin, and Choline*, p 196. The National Academies Press, Washington, DC, 2000.
3. von der Porten A, Gregory Jr, Toth J, et al: *In vivo* folate kinetics during chronic supplementation of human subjects with deuterium-labeled folic acid. *J Nutr* 122:1293, 1992.
4. Herbert V: Minimal daily adult folate requirement. *Arch Intern Med* 110:649, 1962.
5. Halsted C: Folate deficiency in alcoholism. *Am J Clin Nutr* 33:2736, 1980.
6. Alperin J, Hutchinson H, Levin W: Studies of folic acid requirements in megaloblastic anemia of pregnancy. *Arch Intern Med* 117:681, 1966.
7. Schwarz R, Johnston RJ: Folic acid supplementation—When and how. *Obstet Gynecol* 88:886, 1996.
8. Ulevitch R, Kallen R: Purification and characterization of pyridoxal 5'-phosphate dependent serine hydroxymethylase from lamb liver and its action upon beta-phenylserines. *Biochemistry* 16:5342, 1977.
9. Deacon R, Chanarin I, Perry J, Lumb M: Marrow cells from patients with untreated pernicious anaemia cannot use tetrahydrofolate normally. *Br J Haematol* 46:523, 1980.
10. Wahba A, Friedkin M: The enzymatic synthesis of thymidylate. I. Early steps in the purification of thymidylate synthetase of *Escherichia coli*. *J Biol Chem* 237:3794, 1962.
11. Fenech M: The role of folic acid and vitamin B12 in genomic stability of human cells. *Mutat Res* 475:57, 2001.
12. Huennekens F: Folic acid coenzymes in the biosynthesis of purines and pyrimidines. *Vitam Horm* 26:375, 1968.
13. Kaufman S: The phenylalanine hydroxylating system from mammalian liver. *Adv Enzymol Relat Areas Mol Biol* 35:245, 1971.
14. Kwon N, Nathan C, Stuehr D: Reduced biopterin as a cofactor in the generation of nitrogen oxides by murine macrophages. *J Biol Chem* 264:20496, 1989.
15. Banerjee S, Snyder S: Methyltetrahydrofolic acid mediates N- and O-methylation of biogenic amines. *Science* 182:74, 1973.
16. Bird O, McGlohon V, Vaitkus J: Naturally occurring folates in the blood and liver of the rat. *Anal Biochem* 12:18, 1965.
17. Shane B: Folylpolyglutamate synthesis and role in the regulation of one-carbon metabolism. *Vitam Horm* 45:263, 1989.
18. Pratt R, Cooper B: Folates in plasma and bile of man after feeding folic acid—3H and 5-formyltetrahydrofolate (folinic acid). *J Clin Invest* 50:455, 1971.
19. Kisliuk R: Pteroylpolyglutamates. *Mol Cell Biochem* 39:331, 1981.
20. Atkinson I, Garrow T, Brenner A, Shane B: Human cytosolic folylpoly-gamma-glutamate synthase. *Methods Enzymol* 281:134, 1997.
21. Sussman D, Milman G, Shane B: Characterization of human folylpolyglutamate synthetase expressed in Chinese hamster ovary cells. *Somat Cell Mol Genet* 12:531, 1986.
22. Shane B, Stokstad E: Vitamin B12-folate interrelationships. *Annu Rev Nutr* 5:115, 1985.
23. Butterworth CJ, Baugh C, Krumdieck C: A study of folate absorption and metabolism in man utilizing carbon-14–labeled polyglutamates synthesized by the solid phase method. *J Clin Invest* 48:1131, 1969.
24. Rosenberg I, Godwin H: The digestion and absorption of dietary folate. *Gastroenterology* 60:445, 1971.
25. Kesavan V, Noronha J: Folate malabsorption in aged rats related to low levels of pancreatic folyl conjugase. *Am J Clin Nutr* 37:262, 1983.
26. Chandler C, Wang T, Halsted C: Pteroylpolyglutamate hydrolase from human jejunal brush borders. Purification and characterization. *J Biol Chem* 261:928, 1986.
27. Qiu A, Jansen M, Sakaris A, et al: Identification of an intestinal folate transporter and the molecular basis for hereditary folate malabsorption. *Cell* 127:917, 2006.
28. Zhao R, Matherly L, Goldman I: Membrane transporters and folate homeostasis: Intestinal absorption and transport into systemic compartments and tissues. *Expert Rev Mol Med* 11:e4, 2009.
29. Elsenhans B, Ahmad O, Rosenberg I: Isolation and characterization of pteroylpolyglutamate hydrolase from rat intestinal mucosa. *J Biol Chem* 259:6364, 1984.
30. Schron C: pH modulation of the kinetics of rabbit jejunal, brush-border folate transport. *J Membr Biol* 120:192, 1991.
31. Schron C, Washington CJ, Blitzer B: The transmembrane pH gradient drives uphill folate transport in rabbit jejunum. Direct evidence for folate/hydroxyl exchange in brush border membrane vesicles. *J Clin Invest* 76:2030, 1985.
32. Zimmerman J, Selhub J, Rosenberg I: Role of sodium ion in transport of folic acid in the small intestine. *Am J Physiol* 251:G218, 1986.
33. Perry J, Chanarin I: Intestinal absorption of reduced folate compounds in man. *Br J Haematol* 18:329, 1970.
34. Herbert V: Excretion of folic acid in bile. *Lancet* 1:913, 1965.
35. Steinberg S, Campbell C, Hillman R: Kinetics of the normal folate enterohepatic cycle. *J Clin Invest* 64:83, 1979.
36. Steinberg S: Mechanisms of folate homeostasis. *Am J Physiol* 246:G319, 1984.
37. Johns D, Sperti S, Burgen A: The metabolism of tritiated folic acid in man. *J Clin Invest* 40:1684, 1961.
38. Antony A: The biological chemistry of folate receptors. *Blood* 79:2807, 1992.
39. Weitman S, Weinberg A, Coney L, et al: Cellular localization of the folate receptor: Potential role in drug toxicity and folate homeostasis. *Cancer Res* 52:6708, 1992.
40. Luhrs C, Slomiany B: A human membrane-associated folate binding protein is anchored by a glycosyl-phosphatidylinositol tail. *J Biol Chem* 264:21446, 1989.
41. Green T, Ford H: Human placental microvilli contain high-affinity binding sites for folate. *Biochem J* 218:75, 1984.
42. Rothberg K, Ying Y, Kolhouse J, et al: The glycophospholipid-linked folate receptor internalizes folate without entering the clathrin-coated pit endocytic pathway. *J Cell Biol* 110:637, 1990.
43. Matsue H, Rothberg K, Takashima A, et al: Folate receptor allows cells to grow in low concentrations of 5-methyltetrahydrofolate. *Proc Natl Acad Sci U S A* 89:6006, 1992.
44. Hilton J, Cooper B, Rosenblatt D: Folate polyglutamate synthesis and turnover in cultured human fibroblasts. *J Biol Chem* 254:8398, 1979.
45. Zamierowski M, Wagner C: High molecular weight complexes of folic acid in mammalian tissues. *Biochem Biophys Res Commun* 60:81, 1974.
46. Duch D, Bowers S, Nichol C: Analysis of folate cofactor levels in tissues using high-performance liquid chromatography. *Anal Biochem* 130:385, 1983.
47. Cook R, Wagner C: Glycine N-methyltransferase is a folate binding protein of rat liver cytosol. *Proc Natl Acad Sci U S A* 81:3631, 1984.
48. Rosenblatt D, Cooper B, Lue-Shing S, et al: Folate distribution in cultured human cells. Studies on 5,10-CH2-H4PteGlu reductase deficiency. *J Clin Invest* 63:1019, 1979.
49. Stites T, Bailey L, Scott K, et al: Kinetic modeling of folate metabolism through use of chronic administration of deuterium-labeled folic acid in men. *Am J Clin Nutr* 65:53, 1997.
50. Elwood P, Deutsch J, Kolhouse J: The conversion of the human membrane-associated folate binding protein (folate receptor) to the soluble folate binding protein by a membrane-associated metalloprotease. *J Biol Chem* 266:2346, 1991.
51. Colman N, Herbert V: Total folate binding capacity of normal human plasma, and variations in uremia, cirrhosis, and pregnancy. *Blood* 48:911, 1976.
52. Waxman S: Folate binding proteins. *Br J Haematol* 29:23, 1975.
53. Waxman S, Schreiber C: Measurement of serum folate levels and serum folic acid-binding protein by 3H-PGA radioassay. *Blood* 42:281, 1973.
54. Colman N, Herbert V: Folate-binding proteins. *Annu Rev Med* 31:433, 1980.
55. Waxman S, Schreiber C: Characteristics of folic acid-binding protein in folate-deficient serum. *Blood* 42:291, 1973.
56. Rothenberg S: A macromolecular factor in some leukemic cells which binds folic acid. *Proc Soc Exp Biol Med* 133:428, 1970.
57. Mason J, Selhub J: Folate-binding protein and the absorption of folic acid in the small intestine of the suckling rat. *Am J Clin Nutr* 48:620, 1988.
58. Rubinoff M, Abramson R, Schreiber C, Waxman S: Effect of a folate-binding protein on the plasma transport and tissue distribution of folic acid. *Acta Haematol* 65:145, 1981.
59. Colman N, Hebert V: Studies using the calcium ionophore A23187 suggest localization of the human granulocyte folate binder in specific (secondary) granules. *Clin Res* 27:291A, 1979.
60. Selhub J, Nakamura S, Carone F: Renal folate absorption and the kidney folate binding protein. II. Microinfusion studies. *Am J Physiol* 252:F757, 1987.
61. O'Brien J: Urinary excretion of folic and folinic acids in normal adults. *Proc Soc Exp Biol Med* 104:354, 1960.
62. Clifford A, Arjomand A, Dueker S, et al: The dynamics of folic acid metabolism in an adult given a small tracer dose of 14C-folic acid. *Adv Exp Med Biol* 445:239, 1998.
63. Green R, Miller JW: Vitamin B12, in *Handbook of Vitamins*, edited by J Zempleni, RB Rucker, p 413. CRC Press, Boca Raton, FL, 2007.

64. Lenhert P, Hodgkin D: Structure of the 5,6-dimethyl-benzimidazolylcobamide coenzyme. *Nature* 192:937, 1961.
65. Lindstrand K: Isolation of methylcobalamin from natural source material. *Nature* 204:188, 1964.
66. Heyssel R, Bozian R, Darby W, Bell M: Vitamin B12 turnover in man. The assimilation of vitamin B12 from natural foodstuff by man and estimates of minimal daily dietary requirements. *Am J Clin Nutr* 18:176, 1966.
67. Grasbeck R: Calculations on vitamin B12 turnover in man. With a note on the maintenance treatment in pernicious anemia and the radiation dose received by patients ingesting radiovitamin B12. *Scand J Clin Lab Invest* 11:250, 1959.
68. Hsu JM, Kawin B, Minor P, Mitchell JA: Vitamin B12 concentrations in human tissues. *Nature* 210:1264, 1966.
69. Nham S, Wilkemeyer M, Ledley F: Structure of the human methylmalonyl-CoA mutase (MUT) locus. *Genomics* 1990;8:710, 1990.
70. Beck W, Flavin M, Ochoa S: Metabolism of propionic acid in animal tissues. III. Formation of succinate. *J Biol Chem* 229:997, 1957.
71. Taylor R, Weissbach H: Enzymic synthesis of methionine: Formation of a radioactive cobamide enzyme with N5-methyl-14C-tetrahydrofolate. *Arch Biochem Biophys* 119:572, 1967.
72. Knowles J, Prankerd T: Abnormal folic acid metabolism in vitamin B12 deficiency. *Clin Sci* 22:233, 1962.
73. Herbert V, Zalusky R: Interrelations of vitamin B12 and folic acid metabolism: Folic acid clearance studies. *J Clin Invest* 41:1263, 1962.
74. Kano Y, Sakamoto S, Hida K, et al: 5-Methyltetrahydrofolate related enzymes and DNA polymerase alpha activities in bone marrow cells from patients with vitamin B12 deficient megaloblastic anemia. *Blood* 59:832, 1982.
75. Waters A, Mollin D: Observations on the metabolism of folic acid in pernicious anaemia. *Br J Haematol* 9:319,1963.
76. Jeejeebhoy K, Pathare S, Noronha J: Observations on conjugated and unconjugated blood folate levels in megaloblastic anemia and the effects of vitamin B12. *Blood* 26:354, 1965.
77. Boss G: Cobalamin inactivation decreases purine and methionine synthesis in cultured lymphoblasts. *J Clin Invest* 76:213, 1985.
78. Finkelstein JD, Martin JJ: Methionine metabolism is mammals. Adaptation to methionine excess. *J Biol Chem* 261:1582, 1986.
79. Katzen H, Buchanan J: Enzymatic synthesis of the methyl group of methionine. 8. Repression-derepression, purification, and properties of 5,10-methylenetetrahydrofolate reductase from *Escherichia coli*. *J Biol Chem* 240:825, 1965.
80. Chanarin I, Deacon R, Lumb M, Perry J: Vitamin B12 regulates folate metabolism by the supply of formate. *Lancet* 2:505, 1980.
81. Taheri M, Wickremasinghe R, Jackson B, Hoffbrand A: The effect of folate analogues and vitamin B12 on provision of thymine nucleotides for DNA synthesis in megaloblastic anemia. *Blood* 59:634, 1982.
82. Chanarin I, Deacon R, Lumb M, Perry J: Cobalamin and folate: Recent developments. *J Clin Pathol* 45:277, 1992.
83. Hewitt J, Gordon M, Taggart R, et al: Human gastric intrinsic factor: Characterization of cDNA and genomic clones and localization to human chromosome 11. *Genomics* 10:432, 1991.
84. Tang L, Chokshi H, Hu C, et al: The intrinsic factor (IF)-cobalamin receptor binding site is located in the amino-terminal portion of IF. *J Biol Chem* 267:22982, 1992.
85. Levine J, Nakane P, Allen R: Immunocytochemical localization of human intrinsic factor: The nonstimulated stomach. *Gastroenterology* 79:493, 1980.
86. Stenman U: Vitamin B12-binding proteins of R-type, cobalophilin: Characterization and comparison of cobalophilin from different sources *Scand J Haematol* 14:91, 1975.
87. Cooper B, Castle W: Sequential mechanisms in the enhanced absorption of vitamin B12 by intrinsic factor in the rat. *J Clin Invest* 39:199, 1960.
88. Allen R, Seetharam B, Podell E, Alpers D: Effect of proteolytic enzymes on the binding of cobalamin to R protein and intrinsic factor. *In vitro* evidence that a failure to partially degrade R protein is responsible for cobalamin malabsorption in pancreatic insufficiency. *J Clin Invest* 61:47, 1978.
89. Abels J, Schilling R: Protection of intrinsic factor by vitamin B12. *J Lab Clin Med* 64:375, 1964.
90. Moestrup S, Kozyraki R, Kristiansen M, et al: The intrinsic factor-vitamin B12 receptor and target of teratogenic antibodies is a megalin-binding peripheral membrane protein with homology to developmental proteins. *J Biol Chem* 273:5235, 1998.
91. Barth JL, Argraves WS: Cubilin and megalin: Partners in lipoprotein and vitamin metabolism. *Trends Cardiovasc Med* 11:26, 2001.
92. Birn H, Willnow T, Nielsen R, et al: Megalin is essential for renal proximal tubule reabsorption and accumulation of transcobalamin-B(12). *Am J Physiol Renal Physiol* 282:F408, 2002.
93. Fyfe J, Madsen M, Højrup P, et al: The functional cobalamin (vitamin B12)-intrinsic factor receptor is a novel complex of cubilin and amnionless. *Blood* 103:1573, 2004.
94. Christensen E, Birn H: Megalin and cubilin: Multifunctional endocytic receptors. *Nat Rev Mol Cell Biol* 3:256, 2002.
95. Hagedorn C, Alpers D: Distribution of intrinsic factor-vitamin B12 receptors in human intestine. *Gastroenterology* 73:1019, 1977.
96. Kapadia C, Serfilippi D, Voloshin K, Donaldson RJ: Intrinsic factor-mediated absorption of cobalamin by guinea pig ileal cells. *J Clin Invest* 71:440, 1983.
97. Robertson J, Gallagher N: In vivo evidence that cobalamin is absorbed by receptor-mediated endocytosis in the mouse. *Gastroenterology* 88:908, 1985.
98. Chanarin I: *The Megaloblastic Anaemias*, p 140. Blackwell, Oxford, 1969.
99. Horadagoda N, Batt R: Lysosomal localisation of cobalamin during absorption by the ileum of the dog. *Biochim Biophys Acta* 838:206, 1985.
100. Rothenberg S, Weisberg H, Ficarra A: Evidence for the absorption of immunoreactive intrinsic factor into the intestinal epithelial cell during vitamin B12 absorption. *J Lab Clin Med* 79:587, 1972.
101. Hall C: Transcobalamins I and II as natural transport proteins of vitamin B12. *J Clin Invest* 56:1125, 1975.
102. Quadros E, Regec A, Khan K, et al: Transcobalamin II synthesized in the intestinal villi facilitates transfer of cobalamin to the portal blood. *Am J Physiol* 277:G161, 1999.
103. Green R, Jacobsen D, van Tonder S, et al: Enterohepatic circulation of cobalamin in the nonhuman primate. *Gastroenterology* 81:773, 1981.
104. Grasbeck R, Nyberg W, Reizenstein P: Biliary and fecal vit. B12 excretion in man: An isotope study. *Proc Soc Exp Biol Med* 97:780, 1958.
105. Green R, Jacobsen D, Van Tonder S, et al: Absorption of biliary cobalamin in baboons following total gastrectomy. *J Lab Clin Med* 100:771, 1982.
106. Antony A: Vegetarianism and vitamin B-12 (cobalamin) deficiency. *Am J Clin Nutr* 78:3, 2003.
107. Doscherholmen A, Hagen P: A dual mechanism of vitamin B12 plasma absorption. *J Clin Invest* 36:1551, 1957.
108. Seetharam B, Alpers D: Cellular uptake of cobalamin. *Nutr Rev* 43:97, 1985.
109. Quadros EV, Rothenberg SP, Pan YC, Stein S: Purification and molecular characterization of human transcobalamin II. *J Biol Chem* 261:15455, 1986.
110. Platica O, Janeczko R, Quadros E, et al: The cDNA sequence and the deduced amino acid sequence of human transcobalamin II show homology with rat intrinsic factor and human transcobalamin I. *J Biol Chem* 266:7860, 1991.
111. Hippe E, Olesen H: Nature of vitamin B12 binding. 3. Thermodynamics of binding to human intrinsic factor and transcobalamins. *Biochim Biophys Acta* 243:83, 1971.
112. Kolhouse J, Allen R: Absorption, plasma transport, and cellular retention of cobalamin analogues in the rabbit. Evidence for the existence of multiple mechanisms that prevent the absorption and tissue dissemination of naturally occurring cobalamin analogues. *J Clin Invest* 60:1381, 1977.
113. Donaldson RJ, Brand M, Serfilippi D: Changes in circulating transcobalamin II after injection of cyanocobalamin. *N Engl J Med* 296:1427, 1977.
114. Schneider R, Burger R, Mehlman C, Allen R: The role and fate of rabbit and human transcobalamin II in the plasma transport of vitamin B12 in the rabbit. *J Clin Invest* 57:27, 1976.
115. Youngdahl-Turner P, Rosenberg L, Allen R: Binding and uptake of transcobalamin II by human fibroblasts. *J Clin Invest* 61:133, 1978.
116. Quadros E, Nakayama Y, Sequeira J: The protein and the gene encoding the receptor for the cellular uptake of transcobalamin-bound cobalamin. *Blood* 113:186, 2009.
117. Peters TJ, Quinlan A, Hoffbrand AV. Subcellular localization of radioactive vitamin B12 during absorption by guinea-pig ileum. *Clin Sci* 37:568, 1969.
118. Pletsch Q, Coffey J: Properties of the proteins that bind vitamin B12 in subcellular fractions of rat liver. *Arch Biochem Biophys* 151:157, 1972.
119. Watanabe F, Nakano Y: Comparative biochemistry of vitamin B12 (cobalamin) metabolism: Biochemical diversity in the systems for intracellular cobalamin transfer and synthesis of the coenzymes. *Int J Biochem* 23:1353, 1991.
120. Burger R, Allen R: Characterization of vitamin B12-binding proteins isolated from human milk and saliva by affinity chromatography. *J Biol Chem* 249:7220, 1974.
121. Hurlimann J, Zuber C: Vitamin B12-binders in human body fluids. II. Synthesis in vitro. *Clin Exp Immunol* 4:141, 1969.
122. Simons K, Weber T: The vitamin B12-binding protein in human leukocytes. *Biochim Biophys Acta* 117:201, 1966.
123. Johnston J, Bollekens J, Allen R, Berliner N: Structure of the cDNA encoding transcobalamin I, a neutrophil granule protein. *J Biol Chem* 264:15754, 1989.
124. Johnston J, Yang-Feng T, Berliner N: Genomic structure and mapping of the chromosomal gene for transcobalamin I (TCN1): Comparison to human intrinsic factor. *Genomics* 12:459, 1992.
125. Burger R, Schneider R, Mehlman C, Allen R: Human plasma R-type vitamin B12-binding proteins. II. The role of transcobalamin I, transcobalamin III, and the normal granulocyte vitamin B12-binding protein in the plasma transport of vitamin B12. *J Biol Chem* 250:7707, 1975.
126. Guéant J, Monin B, Boissel P, et al: Biliary excretion of cobalamin and cobalamin analogues in man. *Digestion* 30:151, 1984.
127. Gottlieb C, Retief F, Herbert V: Blockade of vitamin B12-binding sites in gastric juice, serum and saliva by analogues and derivatives of vitamin B12 and by antibody to intrinsic factor. *Biochim Biophys Acta* 141:560, 1967.
128. Allen R, Stabler S: Identification and quantitation of cobalamin and cobalamin analogues in human feces. *Am J Clin Nutr* 87:1324, 2008.
129. Green R, Lee K-S, Sutter S, et al: Evidence that physiological doses of vitamin B12 are metabolized or degraded in the gastrointestinal tract: Implications for vitamin B12 bioavailability and fortification. *FASEB J* 335, 2009.
130. Kolhouse J, Kondo H, Allen N, et al: Cobalamin analogues are present in human plasma and can mask cobalamin deficiency because current radioisotope dilution assays are not specific for true cobalamin. *N Engl J Med* 299:785, 1978.
131. Kondo H, Kolhouse J, Allen R: Presence of cobalamin analogues in animal tissues. *Proc Natl Acad Sci U S A* 77:817, 1980.
132. Hom B: Plasma turnover of 57cobalt-vitamin B12 bound to transcobalamin I and II. *Scand J Haematol* 4:321, 1967.

133. Carmel R: The distribution of endogenous cobalamin among cobalamin-binding proteins in the blood in normal and abnormal states. *Am J Clin Nutr* 41:713, 1985.
134. Nexo E, Hvas A, Bleie Ø, et al: Holo-transcobalamin is an early marker of changes in cobalamin homeostasis. A randomized placebo-controlled study. *Clin Chem* 48:1768, 2002.
135. Hvas A, Nexo E: Holotranscobalamin as a predictor of vitamin B12 status. *Clin Chem Lab Med* 41:1489, 2003.
136. Lloyd-Wright Z, Hvas A, Møller J, et al: Holotranscobalamin as an indicator of dietary vitamin B12 deficiency. *Clin Chem* 49:2076, 2003.
137. Obeid R, Herrmann W: Holotranscobalamin in laboratory diagnosis of cobalamin deficiency compared to total cobalamin and methylmalonic acid. *Clin Chem Lab Med* 45:1746, 2007.
138. Herzlich B, Herbert V: Depletion of serum holotranscobalamin II. An early sign of negative vitamin B12 balance. *Lab Invest* 58:332, 1988.
139. Lindgren A, Kilander A, Bagge E, Nexø E: Holotranscobalamin—A sensitive marker of cobalamin malabsorption. *Eur J Clin Invest* 29:321, 1999.
140. Miller JW, Garrod MG, Rockwood AL, et al: Measurement of total vitamin B12 and holotranscobalamin, singly and in combination, in screening for metabolic vitamin B12 deficiency. *Clin Chem* 52:278, 2006.
141. Bertaux O, Mederic C, Valencia R: Amplification of ribosomal DNA in the nucleolus of vitamin B12-deficient Euglena cells. *Exp Cell Res* 195:119, 1991.
142. Rondanelli E, Gorini P, Magliulo E, Fiori G: Differences in proliferative activity between normoblasts and pernicious anemia megaloblasts. *Blood* 24:542, 1964.
143. Steinberg S, Fonda S, Campbell C, Hillman R: Cellular abnormalities of folate deficiency. *Br J Haematol* 54:605, 1983.
144. Wickremasinghe R, Hoffbrand A: Reduced rate of DNA replication fork movement in megaloblastic anemia. *J Clin Invest* 65:26, 1980.
145. Duthie S, McMillan P: Uracil misincorporation in human DNA detected using single cell gel electrophoresis. *Carcinogenesis* 18:1709, 1997.
146. Koury M, Horne D, Brown Z, et al: Apoptosis of late-stage erythroblasts in megaloblastic anemia: Association with DNA damage and macrocyte production. *Blood* 89:4617, 1997.
147. Metz J, Kelly A, Swett V, et al: Deranged DNA synthesis by bone marrow from vitamin B-12-deficient humans. *Br J Haematol* 14:575, 1968.
148. Das K, Mohanty D, Garewal G: Cytogenetics in nutritional megaloblastic anaemia: Prolonged persistence of chromosomal abnormalities in lymphocytes after remission. *Acta Haematol* 76:146, 1986.
149. Forni M, Meyer P, Levy N, et al: An immunohistochemical study of hemoglobin A, hemoglobin F, muramidase, and transferrin in erythroid hyperplasia and neoplasia. *Am J Clin Pathol* 80:145, 1983.
150. Ellims P, Hayman R, Van der Weyden M: Plasma thymidine kinase in megaloblastic anaemia. *Br J Haematol* 44:167, 1980.
151. Reid C, Baptista L, Deacon R, Chanarin I: Megaloblastic change is a feature of colonies derived from an early erythroid progenitor (BFU-E) stimulated by monocytes in culture. *Br J Haematol* 49:551, 1981.
152. Fernandes-Costa F, Green R, Torrance J: Increased erythrocytic diphosphoglycerate in megaloblastic anaemia. A compensatory mechanism? *S Afr Med J* 53:709, 1978.
153. Green R, Kuhl W, Jacobson R, et al: Masking of macrocytosis by alpha-thalassemia in blacks with pernicious anemia. *N Engl J Med* 307:1322, 1982.
154. Spivak J: Masked megaloblastic anemia. *Arch Intern Med* 42:2111, 1982.
155. Lindenbaum J: Megaloblastic anemia and neutrophil hypersegmentation. *Br J Haematol* 44:511, 1980.
156. Carmel R, Green R, Jacobsen DW, Qian GD: Neutrophil nuclear segmentation in mild cobalamin deficiency: Relation to metabolic tests of cobalamin status and observations on ethnic differences in neutrophil segmentation. *Am J Clin Pathol* 106:57, 1996.
157. Lawler S, Roberts P, Hoffbrand A: Chromosome studies in megaloblastic anaemia before and after treatment. *Scand J Haematol* 8:309, 1971.
158. Das K, Mohanty D, Garewal G: Cytogenetics in nutritional megaloblastic anaemia: Prolonged persistence of chromosomal abnormalities in lymphocytes after remission. *Acta Haematol* 76:146, 1986.
159. Bessman J, Williams L, Gilmer PJ: Platelet size in health and hematologic disease. *Am J Clin Pathol* 78:150, 1982.
160. Liu YK Sullivan LW: Marrow granulocyte reserve in pernicious anemia. *Clin Res* 14:321, 1966.
161. Fudenberg H, Estren S: Non-Addisonian megaloblastic anemia; the intermediate megaloblast in the differential diagnosis of pernicious and related anemias. *Am J Med* 25:198, 1958.
162. Gulley M, Bentley S, Ross D: Neutrophil myeloperoxidase measurement uncovers masked megaloblastic anemia. *Blood* 76:1004, 1990.
163. Solanki DL, Jacobson RJ, McKibbon J, Green R: Racial patterns in pernicious anemia. *N Engl J Med* 298:1365, 1978.
164. Solanki D, Jacobson R, Green R, et al: Pernicious anemia in blacks. A study of 64 patients from Washington, D.C., and Johannesburg, South Africa. *Am J Clin Pathol* 75:96, 1981.
165. Boddington M, Spriggs A: The epithelial cells in megaloblastic anaemias. *J Clin Pathol* 12:228, 1959.
166. Hussein S, Laulicht M, Hoffbrand A: Serum ferritin in megaloblastic anaemia. *Scand J Haematol* 20:241, 1978.
167. Emerson P, Wilkinson J: Lactate dehydrogenase in the diagnosis and assessment of response to treatment of megaloblastic anaemia. *Br J Haematol* 12:678, 1996.
168. Winston R, Warburton F, Stott A: Enzymatic diagnosis of megaloblastic anaemia. *Br J Haematol* 19:587, 1970.
169. Hansen N, Karle H: Blood and bone-marrow lysozyme in neutropenia: An attempt towards pathogenetic classification. *Br J Haematol* 21:261, 1971.
170. Heller P, Weinstein H, West M, Zimmerman H: Enzymes in anemia: A study of abnormalities of several enzymes of carbohydrate metabolism in the plasma and erythrocytes in patients with anemia, with preliminary observations of bone marrow enzymes. *Ann Intern Med* 53:898, 1960.
171. de Klerk G, Rosengarten P, Vet R, Goudsmit R: Serum erythropoietin (ESF) titers in polycythemia. *Blood* 58:1171, 1981.
172. Myhre E: Studies on the erythrokinetics in pernicious anemia. *Scand J Clin Lab Invest* 16:391, 1964.
173. Lindahl J: Quantification of ineffective erythropoiesis in megaloblastic anaemia by determination of endogenous production of 14CO after administration of glycine-2–14C. *Scand J Haematol* 24:281, 1980.
174. Hamililton H, Sheets R, Degowin E: Studies with inagglutinable erythrocyte counts. VII. Further investigation of the hemolytic mechanism in untreated pernicious anemia and the demonstration of a hemolytic property in the plasma. *J Lab Clin Med* 51:942, 1958.
175. Harker L, Finch C: Thrombokinetics in man. *J Clin Invest* 48:963, 1969.
176. Obeid R, Geisel J, Schorr H, et al: The impact of vegetarianism on some haematological parameters. *Eur J Haematol* 69:275, 2002.
177. Jacques P, Selhub J, Bostom A, et al: The effect of folic acid fortification on plasma folate and total homocysteine concentrations. *N Engl J Med* 340:1449, 1999.
178. Ballard H, Lindenbaum J: Megaloblastic anemia complicating hyperalimentation therapy. *Am J Med* 56:740, 1974.
179. Whitehead V, Comty C, Posen G, Kaye M: Homeostasis of folic acid in patients undergoing maintenance hemodialysis. *N Engl J Med* 279:970, 1968.
180. Mollin D, Hines J: Late post-gastrectomy syndromes. Observations on the nature and pathogenesis of anaemia following partial gastrectomy. *Proc R Soc Med* 57:575, 1964.
181. Hoffbrand A: Folate deficiency in premature infants. *Arch Dis Child* 45:441, 1970.
182. Royston NJW, Parry, TE: Megaloblastic anaemia complicating dietary treatment of phenylketonuria in infancy. *Arch Dis Child* 37:430,1962. 1962.
183. Ford JD, Scott KJ: The folic acid activity of some milk foods for babies. *J Dairy Res* 35:85, 1968.
184. Savage D, Lindenbaum J: Anemia in alcoholics. *Medicine (Baltimore)* 65:322, 1986.
185. Eichner E, Hillman R: Effect of alcohol on serum folate level. *J Clin Invest* 52:584, 1973.
186. Lieber C: Metabolism and metabolic effects of alcohol. *Semin Hematol* 17:85, 1980.
187. Post R, Desforges J: Thrombocytopenia and alcoholism. *Ann Intern Med* 68:1230, 1968.
188. Liu Y: Effects of alcohol on granulocytes and lymphocytes. *Semin Hematol* 17:130, 1980.
189. Lindenbaum J, Lieber C: Hematologic effects of alcohol in man in the absence of nutritional deficiency. *N Engl J Med* 281:333, 1969.
190. Trier J: Celiac sprue. *N Engl J Med* 325:1709, 1991.
191. Halsted C, Reisenauer A, Romero J, et al: Jejunal perfusion of simple and conjugated folates in celiac sprue. *J Clin Invest* 59:933, 1977.
192. Hjelt K, Krasilnikoff P: The impact of gluten on haematological status, dietary intakes of haemopoietic nutrients and vitamin B12 and folic acid absorption in children with coeliac disease. *Acta Paediatr Scand* 79:911, 1990.
193. Klipstein F: Tropical sprue in New York City. *Gastroenterology* 47:457, 1964.
194. Klipstein F, Schenk E, Samloff I: Folate repletion associated with oral tetracycline therapy in tropical sprue. *Gastroenterology* 51:317, 1966.
195. Klipstein F: Progress in gastroenterology: Tropical sprue. *Gastroenterology* 275, 1968.
196. Sheehy T, Perez-Santiago E, Rubini M: Tropical sprue and vitamin B12. *N Engl J Med* 265:1232, 1961.
197. Klipstein F: Folate in tropical sprue. *Br J Haematol* 23 Suppl:119, 1972.
198. Corcino J, Coll G, Klipstein F: Pteroylglutamic acid malabsorption in tropical sprue. *Blood* 45:577, 1975.
199. Chanarin I, Bennett M: Absorption of folic acid and D-xylose as tests of small-intestinal function. *Br Med J* 1:985, 1962.
200. Booth C: The metabolic effects of intestinal resection in man. *Postgrad Med J* 37:725, 1961.
201. Pitney W, Joske R, Mackinnon N: Folic acid and other absorption tests in lymphosarcoma, chronic lymphocytic leukaemia, and some related conditions. *J Clin Pathol* 13:440, 1960.
202. Hoskins L, Norris H, Gottlieb L, Zamcheck N: Functional and morphologic alterations of the gastrointestinal tract in progressive systemic sclerosis (scleroderma). *Am J Med* 33:459, 1962.
203. Vinnik I, Kern FJ, Struthers JJ: Malabsorption and the diarrhea of diabetes mellitus. *Gastroenterology* 43:507, 1962.
204. Cook G, Morgan J, Hoffbrand A: Impairment of folate absorption by systemic bacterial infections. *Lancet* 2:1416, 1974.
205. Shojania AM: Folic acid and vitamin B12 deficiency in pregnancy and in the neonatal period. *Clin Perinatol* 11:433, 1984.
206. Landon M, Eyre D, Hytten F: Transfer of folate to the fetus. *Br J Obstet Gynaecol* 82:12, 1975.
207. Pritchard J, Scott D, Whalley P, Haling RJ: Infants of mothers with megaloblastic anemia due to folate deficiency. *JAMA* 211:1982, 1970.
208. Shapiro J, Alberts H, Welch P, Metz J: Folate and vitamin B-12 deficiency associated with lactation. *Br J Haematol* 11:498, 1965.

209. Streiff R, Little A: Folic acid deficiency in pregnancy. *N Engl J Med* 276:776, 1967.
210. de Benoist B: Conclusions of a WHO Technical Consultation on folate and vitamin B12 deficiencies. *Food Nutr Bull* 29:S238, 2008.
211. Chanarin I, McFadyen I, Kyle R: The physiological macrocytosis of pregnancy. *Br J Obstet Gynaecol* 84:504, 1977.
212. Avery B, Ledger W: Folic acid metabolism in well-nourished pregnant women. *Obstet Gynecol* 35:616, 1970.
213. Giles C: An account of 335 cases of megaloblastic anaemia of pregnancy and the puerperium. *J Clin Pathol* 19:1, 1966.
214. Lindenbaum J, Klipstein F: Folic acid deficiency in sickle-cell anemia. *N Engl J Med* 269:875, 1963.
215. Hild D: Folate losses from the skin in exfoliative dermatitis. *Arch Intern Med* 123:51, 1969.
216. Green R: Metabolite assays in cobalamin and folate deficiency. *Baillieres Clin Haematol* 8:533, 1995.
217. Herbert V: Experimental nutritional folate deficiency in man. *Trans Assoc Am Physicians* 75:307, 1962.
218. Hoffbrand A, Newcombe F, Mollin D: Method of assay of red cell folate activity and the value of the assay as a test for folate deficiency. *J Clin Pathol* 19:17, 1966.
219. Chanarin I: Folate in blood, cerebrospinal fluid and tissues, in *The Megaloblastic Anaemias*, 3rd ed, p 187. Blackwell Scientific Publications, Oxford, London, 1990.
220. Lindenbaum J: Status of laboratory testing in the diagnosis of megaloblastic anemia. *Blood* 61:624, 1983.
221. Zalusky R, Herbert V, Castle W: Cyanocobalamin therapy effect in folic acid deficiency. *Arch Intern Med* 109:545, 1962.
222. Kinnear D, Macintosh P, Cameron D, et al: Intestinal absorption of tritium-labelled folic acid in idiopathic steatorrhea: Effect of a gluten-free diet. *Can Med Assoc J* 89:975, 1963.
223. Green R, Miller J: Folate deficiency beyond megaloblastic anemia: Hyperhomocysteinemia and other manifestations of dysfunctional folate metabolism. *Semin Hematol* 36:47, 1999.
224. Prevention of neural tube defects: Results of the Medical Research Council Vitamin Study. MRC Vitamin Study Research Group. *Lancet* 338:131, 1991.
225. Rothenberg S, da Costa M, Sequeira J, et al: Autoantibodies against folate receptors in women with a pregnancy complicated by a neural-tube defect. *N Engl J Med* 350:134, 2004.
226. van der Put N, Gabreels F, Stevens E, et al: A second common mutation in the methylenetetrahydrofolate reductase gene: An additional risk factor for neural-tube defects? *Am J Hum Genet* 62:1044, 1998.
227. Honein M, Paulozzi L, Mathews T, et al: Impact of folic acid fortification of the US food supply on the occurrence of neural tube defects. *JAMA* 285:2981, 2001.
228. De Wals P, Tairou F, Van Allen M, et al: Reduction in neural-tube defects after folic acid fortification in Canada. *N Engl J Med* 357:135, 2007.
229. Afman L, van Der Put N, Thomas C, et al: Reduced vitamin B12 binding by transcobalamin II increases the risk of neural tube defects. *QJM* 94:159, 2001.
230. Thompson M, Cole D, Ray J: Vitamin B-12 and neural tube defects: The Canadian experience. *Am J Clin Nutr* 89:697S, 2009.
231. D'Angelo A, Selhub J: Homocysteine and thrombotic disease. *Blood* 90:1, 1997.
232. Schnyder G, Roffi M, Pin R, et al: Decreased rate of coronary restenosis after lowering of plasma homocysteine levels. *N Engl J Med* 345:1593, 2001.
233. Lange H, Suryapranata H, De Luca G, et al: Folate therapy and in-stent restenosis after coronary stenting. *N Engl J Med* 350:2673, 2004.
234. Bønaa K, Njølstad I, Ueland P, et al: Homocysteine lowering and cardiovascular events after acute myocardial infarction. *N Engl J Med* 354:1578, 2006.
235. Yang Q, Botto L, Erickson J, et al: Improvement in stroke mortality in Canada and the United States, 1990 to 2002. *Circulation* 113:1335, 2006.
236. Kluijtmans L, Young I, Boreham C, et al: Genetic and nutritional factors contributing to hyperhomocysteinemia in young adults. *Blood* 101:2483, 2003.
237. Quinlivan E, McPartlin J, McNulty H, et al: Importance of both folic acid and vitamin B12 in reduction of risk of vascular disease. *Lancet* 359:227, 2002.
238. Lievers K, Kluijtmans L, Boers G, et al: Influence of a glutamate carboxypeptidase II (GCPII) polymorphism (1561C$\rightarrow$T) on plasma homocysteine, folate and vitamin B(12) levels and its relationship to cardiovascular disease risk. *Atherosclerosis* 164:269, 2002.
239. Walker S, Wein P, Ihle B: Severe folate deficiency masquerading as the syndrome of hemolysis, elevated liver enzymes, and low platelets. *Obstet Gynecol* 90:655, 1997.
240. Giovannucci E, Stampfer M, Colditz G, et al: Multivitamin use, folate, and colon cancer in women in the Nurses' Health Study. *Ann Intern Med* 129:517, 1998.
241. Ma J, Stampfer M, Giovannucci E, et al: Methylenetetrahydrofolate reductase polymorphism, dietary interactions, and risk of colorectal cancer. *Cancer Res* 57:1098, 1997.
242. Mason J, Dickstein A, Jacques P, et al: A temporal association between folic acid fortification and an increase in colorectal cancer rates may be illuminating important biological principles: A hypothesis. *Cancer Epidemiol Biomarkers Prev* 16:1325, 2007.
243. Kim Y: Will mandatory folic acid fortification prevent or promote cancer? *Am J Clin Nutr* 80:1123, 2004.
244. Rosenberg I: Folic acid and neural-tube defects—Time for action? *N Engl J Med* 327:1875, 1992.
245. Hibbard E, Spencer W: Low serum B12 levels and latent Addisonian anaemia in pregnancy. *J Obstet Gynaecol Br Commonw* 77:52, 1970.
246. Carmel R, Johnson C: Racial patterns in pernicious anemia. Early age at onset and increased frequency of intrinsic-factor antibody in black women. *N Engl J Med* 298:647, 1978.
247. Vilter CF, Vilter RW, Spies TD: The treatment of pernicious and related anemias with synthetic folic acid: I. Observations on the maintenance of a normal hematologic status and on the occurrence of combined system disease at the end of one year. *J Lab Clin Med* 32:262, 1947.
248. Andersen L, Hansen E, Knudsen J, et al: Prospectively measured red cell folate levels in methotrexate treated patients with rheumatoid arthritis: Relation to withdrawal and side effects. *J Rheumatol* 24:830, 1997.
249. Toh B, van Driel I, Gleeson P: Pernicious anemia. *N Engl J Med* 337:1441, 1997.
250. Kano Y, Sakamoto S, MIura Y, Takaaku F: Disorders of cobalamin metabolism. *Crit Rev Oncol Hematol* 3:1, 1985.
251. Irvine W, Davies S, Teitelbaum S, et al: The clinical and pathological significance of gastric parietal cell antibody. *Ann N Y Acad Sci* 124:657, 1965.
252. Gardner P, Heier H: A human autoantibody to renal collecting duct cells associated with thyroid and gastric autoimmunity and possibly renal tubular acidosis. *Clin Exp Immunol* 51:29, 1983.
253. Suri-Payer E, Kehn P, Cheever A, Shevach E: Pathogenesis of post-thymectomy autoimmune gastritis. Identification of anti-H/K adenosine triphosphatase-reactive T cells. *J Immunol* 157:1799, 1996.
254. Kapadia C, Donaldson RJ: Disorders of cobalamin (vitamin B12) absorption and transport. *Annu Rev Med* 36:93, 1985.
255. Chanarin I, James D: Humoral and cell-mediated intrinsic-factor antibody in pernicious anaemia. *Lancet* 1:1078, 1974.
256. Conn H, Binder H, Burns B: Pernicious anemia and immunologic deficiency. *Ann Intern Med* 68:603, 1968.
257. Sharpstone P, James DG: Pernicious anemia and immunologic deficiency. *Ann Intern Med* 68:603, 1968.
258. Ardeman S, Chanarin I, Krafchik B, Singer W: Addisonian pernicious anaemia and intrinsic factor antibodies in thyroid disorders. *Q J Med* 35:421, 1966.
259. Comin D, Hines J, Wieland R: Coexistent pernicious anemia and idiopathic hypoparathyroidism in a women. *JAMA* 207:1147, 1969.
260. Mazzone T, Kelly W, Ensinck J: Lymphocytic hypophysitis. Associated with antiparietal cell antibodies and vitamin B12 deficiency. *Arch Intern Med* 143:1794, 1983.
261. Howitz J, Schwartz M: Vitiligo, achlorhydria, and pernicious anaemia. *Lancet* 1:1331, 1971.
262. Jackson I, Doig W, McDonald G: Pernicious anaemia as a cause of infertility. *Lancet* 2:1159, 1967.
263. Watson A: Seminal vitamin B12 and sterility. *Lancet* 2:644, 1962.
264. Pront R, Margalioth E, Green R, et al: Prevalence of low serum cobalamin in infertile couples. *Andrologia* 41:46, 2009.
265. Ungar B, Mathews J, Tait B, Cowling D: HLA-DR patterns in pernicious anaemia. *Br Med J* 282:768, 1981.
266. Hoskins L, Loux H, Britten A, Zamcheck N: Distribution of ABO blood groups in patients with pernicious anemia, gastric carcinoma and gastric carcinoma associated with pernicious anemia. *N Engl J Med* 273:633, 1965.
267. Wangel A, Callender S, Spray G, Wright R: A family study of pernicious anaemia. I. Autoantibodies, achlorhydria, serum pepsinogen and vitamin B12. *Br J Haematol* 14:161, 1968.
268. Varis K, Ihamäki T, Härkönen M, et al: Gastric morphology, function, and immunology in first-degree relatives of probands with pernicious anemia and controls. *Scand J Gastroenterol* 14:129, 1979.
269. Eriksson S, Clase L, Moquist-Olsson I: Pernicious anemia as a risk factor in gastric cancer. The extent of the problem. *Acta Med Scand* 210:481, 1981.
270. Wilkinson JF: The gastric secretions in pernicious anemia. *Q J Med* 1:361, 1932.
271. Klee G: Cobalamin and folate evaluation: Measurement of methylmalonic acid and homocysteine vs vitamin B(12) and folate. *Clin Chem* 46:1277, 2000.
272. Karnes WJ, Samloff I, Siurala M, et al: Positive serum antibody and negative tissue staining for *Helicobacter pylori* in subjects with atrophic body gastritis. *Gastroenterology* 101:167, 1991.
273. Hershko C, Ronson A, Souroujon M, et al: Variable hematologic presentation of autoimmune gastritis: Age-related progression from iron deficiency to cobalamin depletion. *Blood* 107:1673, 2006.
274. Green R: Protean *H. pylori*: Perhaps "pernicious" too? *Blood* 107:1247, 2006.
275. Slingerland D, Cardarelli J, Burrows B, Miller A: The utility of serum gastrin levels in assessing the significance of low serum B12 levels. *Arch Intern Med* 144:1167, 1984.
276. Ganguli P, Cullen D, Irvine W: Radioimmunoassay of plasmagastrin in pernicious anaemia, achlorhydria without pernicious anaemia, hypochlorhydria, and in controls. *Lancet* 1:155, 1971.
277. Kaye M, Whorwell P, Wright R: Gastric mucosal lymphocyte subpopulations in pernicious anemia and in normal stomach. *Clin Immunol Immunopathol* 28:431, 1983.
278. Rodbro P, Dige-Petersen H, Schwartz M, Dalgaard O: Effect of steroids on gastric mucosal structure and function in pernicious anemia. *Acta Med Scand* 181:445, 1967.
279. Ransohoff R, Jacobsen D, Green R: Vitamin B12 deficiency and multiple sclerosis. *Lancet* 335:1285, 1990.
280. Nieburgs H, Glass G: Gastric-cell maturation disorders in atrophic gastritis, pernicious anemia, and carcinoma. Histologic site of origin and diagnostic significance of abnormal cells. *Am J Dig Dis* 8:135, 1963.

281. Foroozan P, Trier J: Mucosa of the small intestine in pernicious anemia. *N Engl J Med* 277:553, 1967.
282. Bezman A, Kinnear D, Zamcheck N: D-xylose and potassium iodide absorption and serum carotene in pernicious anemia. *J Lab Clin Med* 53:226, 1959.
283. Ellison A: Pernicious anemia masked by multivitamins containing folic acid. *J Am Med Assoc* 173:240, 1960.
284. Carmel R: Subtle and atypical cobalamin deficiency states. *Am J Hematol* 34:108, 1990.
285. Lindenbaum J, Healton E, Savage D, et al: Neuropsychiatric disorders caused by cobalamin deficiency in the absence of anemia or macrocytosis. *N Engl J Med* 318:1720, 1988.
286. Lindenbaum J: Status of laboratory testing in the diagnosis of megaloblastic anemia. *Blood* 61:624, 1983.
287. Maclean L, Sundberg R: Incidence of megaloblastic anemia after total gastrectomy. *N Engl J Med* 254:885, 1956.
288. Gozzard D, Dawson D, Lewis M: Experiences with dual protein bound aqueous vitamin B12 absorption test in subjects with low serum vitamin B12 concentrations. *J Clin Pathol* 40:633, 1987.
289. Van der Weyden M, Rother M, Firkin B: Megaloblastic maturation masked by iron deficiency: A biochemical basis. *Br J Haematol* 22:299, 1972.
290. Lees F, Grandjean L: The gastric and jejunal mucosae in healthy patients with partial gastrectomy. *AMA Arch Intern Med* 101:943, 1958.
291. Shimoda S, Rubin C: The Zollinger-Ellison syndrome with steatorrhea. I. Anticholinergic treatment followed by total gastrectomy and colonic interposition. *Gastroenterology* 55:695, 1968.
292. Kennedy H, Callender S, Truelove S, Warner G: Haematological aspects of life with an ileostomy. *Br J Haematol* 52:445, 1982.
293. Anderson C, Walton K, Chanarin I: Megaloblastic anaemia after pelvic radiotherapy for carcinoma of the cervix. *J Clin Pathol* 34:151, 1981.
294. Tudhope G, Wilson G: Deficiency of vitamin B12 in hypothyroidism. *Lancet* 1:703, 1962.
295. Waxman S, Corcino J, Herbert V: Drugs, toxins and dietary amino acids affecting vitamin B12 or folic acid absorption or utilization. *Am J Med* 48:599, 1970.
296. Lindenbaum J, Pezzimenti JF, Shea N: Small intestinal function in vitamin B12 deficiency. *Ann Intern Med* 80:326, 1974.
297. Cameron D, Watson G, Witts L: The clinical association of macrocytic anemia with intestinal stricture and anastomosis. *Blood* 4:793, 1949.
298. Murphy M, Sourial N, Burman J, et al: Megaloblastic anaemia due to vitamin B12 deficiency caused by small intestinal bacterial overgrowth: Possible role of vitamin B12 analogues. *Br J Haematol* 62:7, 1986.
299. Nyberg W: The influence of Diphyllobothrium latum on the vitamin B12-intrinsic factor complex. I. *In vivo* studies with Schilling test technique. *Acta Med Scand* 167:185, 1960.
300. Harriman G, Smith P, Horne M, et al: Vitamin B12 malabsorption in patients with acquired immunodeficiency syndrome. *Arch Intern Med* 149:2039, 1989.
301. Herzlich B, Schiano T, Moussa Z, et al: Decreased intrinsic factor secretion in AIDS: Relation to parietal cell acid secretory capacity and vitamin B12 malabsorption. *Am J Gastroenterol* 87:1781, 1992.
302. Remacha A, Cadafalch J: Cobalamin deficiency in patients infected with the human immunodeficiency virus. *Semin Hematol* 36:75, 1999.
303. Guéant J, Champigneulle B, Gaucher P, Nicolas J: Malabsorption of vitamin B12 in pancreatic insufficiency of the adult and of the child. *Pancreas* 5:559, 1990.
304. Toskes P, Deren J, Conrad M: Trypsin-like nature of the pancreatic factor that corrects vitamin B12 malabsorption associated with pancreatic dysfunction. *J Clin Invest* 52:1660, 1973.
305. Henderson J, Simpson J, Warwick R, Shearman D: Does malabsorption of vitamin B 12 occur in chronic pancreatitis? *Lancet* 2:241, 1972.
306. Gilois C, Wierzbicki A, Hirani N, et al: The hematological and electrophysiological effects of cobalamin. Deficiency secondary to vegetarian diets. *Ann N Y Acad Sci* 669:345, 1992.
307. Ford M: Megaloblastic anaemia in a vegetarian. *Br J Clin Pract* 34:222, 1980.
308. Michaud J, Lemieux B, Ogier H, Lambert M: Nutritional vitamin B12 deficiency: Two cases detected by routine newborn urinary screening. *Eur J Pediatr* 151:218, 1992.
309. Wickramasinghe S, Akinyanju O, Grange A, Litwinczuk R: Folate levels and deoxyuridine suppression tests in protein-energy malnutrition. *Br J Haematol* 53:135, 1983.
310. Frenkel E: Abnormal fatty acid metabolism in peripheral nerves of patients with pernicious anemia. *J Clin Invest* 52:1237, 1973.
311. Watkins D, Rosenblatt DS: Cobalamin and inborn errors of cobalamin absorption and metabolism. *Endocrinologist* 11:98, 2001.
312. Lever E, Elwes R, Williams A, Reynolds E: Subacute combined degeneration of the cord due to folate deficiency: Response to methyl folate treatment. *J Neurol Neurosurg Psychiatry* 49:1203, 1986.
313. Clayton P, Smith I, Harding B, et al: Subacute combined degeneration of the cord, dementia and parkinsonism due to an inborn error of folate metabolism. *J Neurol Neurosurg Psychiatry* 49:920, 1986.
314. Green R, Van Tonder S, Oettle G, et al: Neurological changes in fruit bats deficient in vitamin B12. *Nature* 254:148, 1975.
315. Weir D, Keating S, Molloy A, et al: Methylation deficiency causes vitamin B12-associated neuropathy in the pig. *J Neurochem* 51:1949, 1988.
316. Molloy A, Orsi B, Kennedy D, et al: The relationship between the activity of methionine synthase and the ratio of S-adenosylmethionine to S-adenosylhomocysteine in the brain and other tissues of the pig. *Biochem Pharmacol* 44:1349, 1992.
317. Deacon R, Purkiss P, Green R, et al: Vitamin B12 neuropathy is not due to failure to methylate myelin basic protein. *J Neurol Sci* 72:113, 1986.
318. Kätkä K: Immune functions in pernicious anaemia before and during treatment with vitamin B12. *Scand J Haematol* 32:76, 1984.
319. Kätkä K, Eskola J, Granfors K, et al: Serum IgA deficiency and anti-IgA antibodies in pernicious anemia. *Clin Immunol Immunopathol* 46:55, 1988.
320. Zhang S, Willett W, Selhub J, et al: Plasma folate, vitamin B6, vitamin B12, homocysteine, and risk of breast cancer. *J Natl Cancer Inst* 95:373, 2003.
321. Dhonukshe-Rutten R, Lips M, de Jong N, et al: Vitamin B-12 status is associated with bone mineral content and bone mineral density in frail elderly women but not in men. *J Nutr* 133:801, 2003.
322. Stone K, Bauer D, Sellmeyer D, Cummings S: Low serum vitamin B-12 levels are associated with increased hip bone loss in older women: A prospective study. *J Clin Endocrinol Metab* 89:1217, 2004.
323. Beck W: Neuropsychiatric consequences of cobalamin deficiency. *Adv Intern Med* 36:33, 1991.
324. Victor M, Lear A: Subacute combined degeneration of the spinal cord; current concepts of the disease process; value of serum vitamin B12; determinations in clarifying some of the common clinical problems. *Am J Med* 20:896, 1956.
325. Herbert V: Biology of disease: Megaloblastic anemias. *Lab Invest* 52:3, 1985.
326. Di Lazzaro V, Restuccia D, Fogli D, et al: Central sensory and motor conduction in vitamin B12 deficiency. *Electroencephalogr Clin Neurophysiol* 84:433, 1992.
327. Fraser T: Cerebral manifestations of Addisonian pernicious anaemia. *Lancet* 2:458, 1960.
328. Vogiatzoglou A, Refsum H, Johnston C, et al: Vitamin B12 status and rate of brain volume loss in community-dwelling elderly. *Neurology* 71:826, 2008.
329. de Lau L, Smith A, Refsum H, et al: Plasma vitamin B12 status and cerebral white-matter lesions. *J Neurol Neurosurg Psychiatry* 80:149, 2009.
330. Shulman R: Psychiatric aspects of pernicious anaemia: A prospective controlled investigation. *Br Med J* 3:266, 1967.
331. Smith ADM: Megaloblastic madness. *Br Med J* 2:1840, 1960.
332. Stojsavljevi N, Levi Z, Drulovi J, Dragutinovi G: A 44-month clinical-brain MRI follow-up in a patient with B12 deficiency. *Neurology* 49:878, 1997.
333. Carmel R: R-binder deficiency. A clinically benign cause of cobalamin pseudodeficiency. *JAMA* 250:1886, 1983.
334. Carmel R: Mild transcobalamin I (haptocorrin) deficiency and low serum cobalamin concentrations. *Clin Chem* 49:1367, 2003.
335. Bor M, Nexo E, Hvas A: Holo-transcobalamin concentration and transcobalamin saturation reflect recent vitamin B12 absorption better than does serum vitamin B12. *Clin Chem* 50:1043, 2004.
336. von Castel-Roberts K, Morkbak A, Nexo E, et al: Holo-transcobalamin is an indicator of vitamin B-12 absorption in healthy adults with adequate vitamin B-12 status. *Am J Clin Nutr* 85:1057, 2007.
337. Kahn SB Williams WS, Barnes LA, et al: Methylmalonic acid excretion: A sensitive indicator of vitamin B12 deficiency. *J Lab Clin Med* 66:75, 1965.
338. Norman E, Morrison J: Screening elderly populations for cobalamin (vitamin B12) deficiency using the urinary methylmalonic acid assay by gas chromatography mass spectrometry. *Am J Med* 94:589, 1993.
339. Norman E, Martelo O, Denton M: Cobalamin (vitamin B12) deficiency detection by urinary methylmalonic acid quantitation. *Blood* 59:1128, 1982.
340. Lindenbaum J, Savage D, Stabler S, Allen R: Diagnosis of cobalamin deficiency: II. Relative sensitivities of serum cobalamin, methylmalonic acid, and total homocysteine concentrations. *Am J Hematol* 34:99, 1990.
341. Green R: Screening for vitamin B12 deficiency: Caveat emptor. *Ann Intern Med* 124:509, 1996.
342. Solomon LR: Cobalamin-responsive disorders in the ambulatory care setting. Unreliability of cobalamin, methylmalonic acid and homocysteine testing. *Blood* 105:978, 2005.
343. Stabler S, Allen R, Barrett R, et al: Cerebrospinal fluid methylmalonic acid levels in normal subjects and patients with cobalamin deficiency. *Neurology* 41:1627, 1991.
344. Fairbanks V, Wahner H, Phyliky R: Tests for pernicious anemia: The "Schilling test." *Mayo Clin Proc* 58:541, 1983.
345. Bor M, Cetin M, Aytac S, et al: Nonradioactive vitamin B12 absorption test evaluated in controls and in patients with inherited malabsorption of vitamin B12. *Clin Chem* 51:2151, 2005.
346. Carkeet C, Dueker S, Lango J, et al: Human vitamin B12 absorption measurement by accelerator mass spectrometry using specifically labeled (14)C-cobalamin. *Proc Natl Acad Sci U S A* 103:5694, 2006.
347. Metz J: The deoxyuridine suppression test. *Crit Rev Clin Lab Sci* 20:205, 1984.
348. Boddy K, King P, Mervyn L, et al: Retention of cyanocobalamin, hydroxocobalamin, and coenzyme B12 after parenteral administration. *Lancet* 2:710, 1968.
349. Coleman D, Donohue D, Finch C, et al: Erythrokinetics in pernicious anemia. *Blood* 11:807, 1956.
350. Hillman R, Adamson J, Burka E: Characteristics of vitamin B12 correction of the abnormal erythropoiesis of pernicious anemia. *Blood* 31:419, 1968.
351. Sumner A, Chin M, Abrahm J, et al: Elevated methylmalonic acid and total homocysteine levels show high prevalence of vitamin B12 deficiency after gastric surgery. *Ann Intern Med* 124:469, 1996.
352. Paulk EJ, Farrar WJ: Diverticulosis of the small intestine and megaloblastic anemia: Intestinal microflora and absorption before and after tetracycline administration. *Am J Med* 37:473, 1964.

353. Kuzminski A, Del Giacco E, Allen R, et al: Effective treatment of cobalamin deficiency with oral cobalamin. *Blood* 92:1191, 1998.
354. Crosby W: Improvisation revisited. Oral cyanocobalamin without intrinsic factor for pernicious anemia. *Arch Intern Med* 140:1582, 1980.
355. Andrès E, Kurtz J, Perrin A, et al: Oral cobalamin therapy for the treatment of patients with food-cobalamin malabsorption. *Am J Med* 111:126, 2001.
356. Lederle F: Oral cobalamin for pernicious anemia: Back from the verge of extinction. *J Am Geriatr Soc* 46:1125, 1998.
357. Amess J, Burman J, Rees G, et al: Megaloblastic haemopoiesis in patients receiving nitrous oxide. *Lancet* 2:339, 1978.
358. Kondo H, Osborne M, Kolhouse J, et al: Nitrous oxide has multiple deleterious effects on cobalamin metabolism and causes decreases in activities of both mammalian cobalamin-dependent enzymes in rats. *J Clin Invest* 67:1270, 1981.
359. Lumb M, Sharer N, Deacon R, et al: Effects of nitrous oxide-induced inactivation of cobalamin on methionine and S-adenosylmethionine metabolism in the rat. *Biochim Biophys Acta* 756:354, 1983.
360. O'Sullivan H, Jennings F, Ward K, et al: Human bone marrow biochemical function and megaloblastic hematopoiesis after nitrous oxide anesthesia. *Anesthesiology* 55:645, 1981.
361. Skacel P, Hewlett A, Lewis J, et al: Studies on the haemopoietic toxicity of nitrous oxide in man. *Br J Haematol* 53:189, 1983.
362. Kano Y, Sakamoto S, Sakuraya K, et al: Effects of leucovorin and methylcobalamin with N_2O anesthesia. *J Lab Clin Med* 104:711, 1984.
363. Layzer R, Fishman R, Schafer J: Neuropathy following abuse of nitrous oxide. *Neurology* 28:504, 1978.
364. Easton D: Severe thrombocytopenia associated with acute folic acid deficiency and severe hemorrhage in two patients. *Can Med Assoc J* 130:418, 1984.
365. Beard M, Hatipov C, Hamer J: Acute onset of folate deficiency in patients under intensive care. *Crit Care Med* 8:500, 1980.
366. Henderson G, Suresh M, Vitols K, Huennekens F: Transport of folate compounds in L1210 cells: Kinetic evidence that folate influx proceeds via the high-affinity transport system for 5-methyltetrahydrofolate and methotrexate. *Cancer Res* 46:1639, 1986.
367. Schoo M, Pristupa Z, Vickers P, Scrimgeour K: Folate analogues as substrates of mammalian folylpolyglutamate synthetase. *Cancer Res* 45:3034, 1985.
368. Huennekens FM, Duffy TH, Pope LE: Biochemistry of methotrexate: Teaching an old drug new tricks, in *Cancer Biology and Therapeutics*, edited by JG Cory, A Szentivanyi, p. 45. Plenum, New York, 1987.
369. Kesavan V, Sur P, Doig M, et al: Effects of methotrexate on folates in Krebs ascites and L1210 murine leukemia cells. *Cancer Lett* 30:55, 1986.
370. Spiegel R, Cooper P, Blum R, et al: Treatment of massive intrathecal methotrexate overdose by ventriculolumbar perfusion. *N Engl J Med* 311:386, 1984.
371. Yarchoan R, Broder S: Development of antiretroviral therapy for the acquired immunodeficiency syndrome and related disorders. A progress report. *N Engl J Med* 316:557, 1987.
372. Richman D, Fischl M, Grieco M, et al: The toxicity of azidothymidine (AZT) in the treatment of patients with AIDS and AIDS-related complex. A double-blind, placebo-controlled trial. *N Engl J Med* 317:192, 1987.
373. Boudes P, Zittoun J, Sobel A: Folate, vitamin B12, and HIV infection. *Lancet* 335:1401, 1990.
374. Krakoff I, Brown N, Reichard P: Inhibition of ribonucleoside diphosphate reductase by hydroxyurea. *Cancer Res* 28:1559, 1968.
375. Termanini B, Gibril F, Sutliff V, et al: Effect of long-term gastric acid suppressive therapy on serum vitamin B12 levels inpatients with Zollinger-Ellison syndrome. *Am J Med* 104:422, 1998.
376. Koop H, Bachem M: Serum iron, ferritin, and vitamin B12 during prolonged omeprazole therapy. *J Clin Gastroenterol* 14:288, 1992.
377. Rosenblatt DS: Inherited disorders of folate and cobalamin transport and metabolism, in *The Metabolic and Molecular bases of Inherited Metabolic Disease*, 8th ed, edited by WA Fenton, p 3897. McGraw-Hill, New York, 2001.
378. Whitehead V: Acquired and inherited disorders of cobalamin and folate in children. *Br J Haematol* 134:125, 2006.
379. Grasbeck R, Gordin R, Kantero I, Kuhlback B: Selective vitamin B12 malabsorption and proteinuria in young people. A syndrome. *Acta Med Scand* 167:289, 1960.
380. Zimran A, Hershko C: The changing pattern of megaloblastic anemia: Megaloblastic anemia in Israel. *Am J Clin Nutr* 37:855, 1983.
381. Aminoff M, Carter J, Chadwick R, et al: Mutations in CUBN, encoding the intrinsic factor-vitamin B12 receptor, cubilin, cause hereditary megaloblastic anaemia 1. *Nat Genet* 21:309, 1999.
382. He Q, Madsen M, Kilkenney A, et al: Amnionless function is required for cubilin brush-border expression and intrinsic factor-cobalamin (vitamin B12) absorption *in vivo*. *Blood* 106:1447, 2005.
383. Carmel R: Gastric juice in congenital pernicious anemia contains no immunoreactive intrinsic factor molecule: Study of three kindreds with variable ages at presentation, including a patient first diagnosed in adulthood. *Am J Hum Genet* 35:67, 1983.
384. Cooper B, Rosenblatt D: Inherited defects of vitamin B12 metabolism. *Annu Rev Nutr* 7:291, 1987.
385. Miller D, Bloom G, Streiff R, et al: Juvenile "congenital" pernicious anemia. Clinical and immunologic studies. *N Engl J Med* 275:978, 1966.
386. Cooper BA: Megaloblastic anaemia and disorders affecting utilisation of vitamin B12 and folate in childhood. *Clin Haematol* 5:631, 1976.
387. Thomas P, Hoffbrand A, Smith I: Neurological involvement in hereditary transcobalamin II deficiency. *J Neurol Neurosurg Psychiatry* 45:74, 1982.
388. Carmel R, Green R, Rosenblatt D, Watkins D: Update on cobalamin, folate, and homocysteine. *Hematology Am Soc Hematol Educ Program* 62, 2003.
389. Barshop B, Wolff J, Nyhan W, et al: Transcobalamin II deficiency presenting with methylmalonic aciduria and homocystinuria and abnormal absorption of cobalamin. *Am J Med Genet* 35:222, 1990.
390. Rosenblatt D, Hosack A, Matiaszuk N: Expression of transcobalamin II by amniocytes. *Prenat Diagn* 7:35, 1987.
391. Namour F, Olivier J, Abdelmouttaleb I, et al: Transcobalamin codon 259 polymorphism in HT-29 and Caco-2 cells and in Caucasians: Relation to transcobalamin and homocysteine concentration in blood. *Blood* 97:1092, 2001.
392. Miller JW, Ramos MI, Garrod MG, et al: Transcobalamin II 775G>C polymorphism and indices of vitamin B12 status in healthy older adults. *Blood* 100:718, 2002.
393. Mcintyre O, Sullivan L, Jeffries G, Silver R: Pernicious anemia in childhood. *N Engl J Med* 272:981, 1965.
394. Fowler B: Genetic defects of folate and cobalamin metabolism. *Eur J Pediatr* 157 Suppl 2:S60, 1998.
395. Watkins D, Matiaszuk N, Rosenblatt D: Complementation studies in the cblA class of inborn error of cobalamin metabolism: Evidence for interallelic complementation and for a new complementation class (cblH). *J Med Genet* 37:510, 2000.
396. Rosenblatt D, Cooper B, Pottier A, et al: Altered vitamin B12 metabolism in fibroblasts from a patient with megaloblastic anemia and homocystinuria due to a new defect in methionine biosynthesis. *J Clin Invest* 74:2149, 1984.
397. Leclerc D, Campeau E, Goyette P, et al: Human methionine synthase: CDNA cloning and identification of mutations in patients of the cblG complementation group of folate/cobalamin disorders. *Hum Mol Genet* 5:1867, 1996.
398. Gulati S, Chen Z, Brody L, et al: Defects in auxiliary redox proteins lead to functional methionine synthase deficiency. *J Biol Chem* 272:19171, 1997.
399. Watkins D, Rosenblatt DS: Failure of lysosomal release of vitamin B12: A new complementation group causing methylmalonic aciduria (cblF). *Am J Hum Genet* 39:404, 1986.
400. van der Meer S, Spaapen L, Fowler B, et al: Prenatal treatment of a patient with vitamin B12-responsive methylmalonic acidemia. *J Pediatr* 117:923, 1990.
401. Erbe R: Inborn errors of folate metabolism (second of two parts). *N Engl J Med* 293:807, 1975.
402. Min S, Oh S, Karp G, et al: The clinical course and genetic defect in the PCFT gene in a 27-year-old woman with hereditary folate malabsorption. *J Pediatr* 153:435, 2008.
403. Zittoun J: Congenital errors of folate metabolism. *Baillieres Clin Haematol* 8:603, 1995.
404. Arakawa T, Narisawa K, Tanno K, et al: Megaloblastic anemia and mental retardation associated with hyperfolic-acidemia: Probably due to N5 methyltetrahydrofolate transferase deficiency. *Tohoku J Exp Med* 93:1, 1967.
405. Fox R, Wood M, Royse-Smith D, O'Sullivan W: Hereditary orotic aciduria: Types I and II. *Am J Med* 55:791, 1973.
406. van der Zee S, Schretlen E, Monnens L: Megaloblastic anaemia in the Lesch-Nyhan syndrome. *Lancet* 1:1427, 1968.
407. Bazarbachi A, Muakkit S, Ayas M, et al: Thiamine-responsive myelodysplasia. *Br J Haematol* 102:1098, 1998.
408. Boros L, Steinkamp M, Fleming J, et al: Defective RNA ribose synthesis in fibroblasts from patients with thiamine-responsive megaloblastic anemia (TRMA). *Blood* 102:3556, 2003.
409. Zdebska E, Mendek-Czajkowska E, Ploski R, et al: Heterozygosity of CDAN II (HEMPAS) gene may be detected by the analysis of erythrocyte membrane glycoconjugates from healthy carriers. *Haematologica* 87:126, 2002.
410. Maeda K, Saeed S, Rebuck J, Monto R: Type I dyserythropoietic anemia. A 30-year follow-up. *Am J Clin Pathol* 73:433, 1980.
411. Wickramasinghe S, Parry T, Williams C, et al: A new case of congenital dyserythropoietic anaemia, type III: Studies of the cell cycle distribution and ultrastructure of erythroblasts and of nucleic acid synthesis in marrow cells. *J Clin Pathol* 35:1103, 1982.
412. Najfeld V, McArthur J, Shashaty G: Monosomy 7 in a patient with pancytopenia and abnormal erythropoiesis. *Acta Haematol* 66:12, 1981.
413. Camaschella C: Recent advances in the understanding of inherited sideroblastic anaemia. *Br J Haematol* 143:27, 2008.
414. Roggli V, Saleem A: Erythroleukemia: A study of 15 cases and literature review. *Cancer* 49:101, 1982.
415. Matherly LH, Barlowe CK, Phillips VM, Goldman ID: The effect of 4-aminoantifolates on 5-formyltetrahydrofolate metabolism. *J Biol Chem* 262:710, 1987.
416. Magee F, O'Sullivan H, McCann SR: Megaloblastosis and low-dose trimethoprim sulfamethoxazole [letter]. *Ann Intern Med* 95:657, 1981.
417. Swinson CM, Perry J, Lumb M, Levi AJ: Role of sulphasalazine in the aetiology of folate deficiency in ulcerative colitis. *Gut* 22:456, 1981.
418. Boots M, Phillips M, Curtis JR: Megaloblastic anemia and pancytopenia due to proguanil in patients with chronic renal failure. *Clin Nephrol* 18:106, 1981.
419. Fossella FV: Pemetrexed for treatment of advanced non-small cell lung cancer. *Semin Oncol* 31:100, 2004.
420. Bethell FH, Thompson DS: Treatment of leukemia and related disorders with 6-mercaptopurine. *Ann N Y Acad Sci* 60:436, 1954.
421. Cristoph R, Pisnay D, Hartl W: Megaloblastic anaemia following treatment of rheumatoid arthritis with Imuran. *Med Welt* 46:1824, 1971.
422. Klippel JH, Decker JL: Relative macrocytosis in cyclophosphamide and azathioprine therapy. *JAMA* 229:180, 1974.

423. Amos RJ, Amess JA: Megaloblastic haemopoiesis due to acyclovir [letter]. *Lancet* 1:242, 1983.
424. Reyes P, Heidelberger C: Fluorinated pyrimidines. *Mol Pharmacol* 1:14, 1963.
425. Cornell RC, Milstein HG, Fox CM: Anemia of azaribine in the treatment of psoriasis. *Arch Dermatol* 112:1717, 1976.
426. Frenkel EP, Arthur C: Induced ribotide reductive conversion by hydroxyurea and its relationship to megaloblastosis. *Cancer Res* 27:1016, 1967.
427. Papac RJ: Clinical and hematologic studies with 1-b-D-arabinosylcytosine. *J Natl Cancer Inst* 40:997, 1968.
428. Druskin MS, Wallen MH, Bonagura L: Anticonvulsant-associated anemia. *N Engl J Med* 267:483, 1962.
429. Gerson CD, Hepner GW, Brown N, et al: Inhibition of diphenylhydantoin of folic acid absorption in man. *Gastroenterology* 63:246, 1972.
430. Carl GF, Smith ML, Furman GM, et al: Phenytoin treatment and folate supplementation affect folate concentrations and methylation capacity in rats. *J Nutr* 121:1214, 1991.
431. Isojarvi FI, Pakarinen AJ, Myllyla VV: Basic haematological parameters, serum gamma-glutamyl-transferase activity, and erythrocyte folate and serum vitamin B_{12} levels during carbamazepine and oxcarbazepine therapy. *Seizure* 6:207, 1997.
432. Lindenbaum J, Whitehead N, Reyner F: Oral contraceptive hormones, folate metabolism and cervical epithelium. *Am J Clin Nutr* 28:346, 1975.
433. Hainivaara O, Palva IP: Malabsorption and deficiency of vitamin B_{12} caused by treatment with para-aminosalicylic acid. *Acta Med Scand* 177:337, 1965.
434. Callaghan TS, Hadden DR, Tomkin GH: Megaloblastic anaemia due to vitamin B_{12} malabsorption associated with long-term metformin treatment. *Br Med J* 280:1214, 1980.
435. Webb DI, Chodos RB, Mahar CQ, Faloon WW: Mechanism of vitamin B_{12} malabsorption in patients receiving colchicine. *N Engl J Med* 279:845, 1968.
436. Dobbins WO, Herrero BA, Mansbach CM: Morphological alterations associated with neomycin induced malabsorption. *Am J Med Sci* 255:63, 1968.
437. Lerman BB, Ali N, Green D: Megaloblastic, dyserythropoietic anemia following arsenic ingestion. *Ann Clin Lab Sci* 10:515, 1980.

CHAPTER 42
DISORDERS OF IRON METABOLISM

Ernest Beutler

SUMMARY

Iron is a component of all living organisms. It plays an important metabolic role, particularly in electron transfer reactions. Much of the iron in the human body is in circulating red cells, which contain 1 mg of iron per 1 mL of packed cells. Iron is stored in the form of ferritin or hemosiderin. Smaller amounts of iron are present in myoglobin and in many enzymes. Because little iron is lost from the body under normal circumstances, the iron content of the body is regulated by modulating iron absorption. Separate pathways exist for the absorption of heme and inorganic iron. The process appears to involve a ferrireductase, a divalent iron transporter DMT-1, hephaestin, and ferroportin. Iron absorption increases in the presence of iron deficiency and it decreases when there is iron overload. The central regulator or iron homeostasis is the hepatic antimicrobial peptide hepcidin. Ferroportin serves as the receptor for hepcidin and is destroyed when the complex is formed. This impairs transport from intestinal mucosal cells and from macrophages into the plasma, and serves to lower iron absorption and plasma iron levels and to increase macrophage iron. Once ferric iron enters the plasma, it is bound by transferrin, which after forming a complex with the transferrin receptor, transports the metal into cells. The transferrin receptor is internalized together with bound transferrin and iron, and the iron is released inside the cell into an acidified vacuole. The transferrin receptor then recycles to the cell surface.

Many of the proteins involved in iron homeostasis are regulated by the abundance of iron through binding of one of the iron-regulatory proteins (IRPs) to iron-responsive elements (IREs) located within stem loop structures of the corresponding messenger ribonucleic acids (mRNAs). IRP-1 is cytoplasmic aconitase that binds to the IRE when it is not complexed with iron and does not bind when iron is present; IRP-2, a closely related protein, is destabilized by the presence of iron. When IRPs bind to IREs at the 5′ end of the mRNA, they prevent translation; when they bind at the 3′ end, they stabilize the message.

Iron deficiency and iron-deficiency anemia are common nutritional and hematologic disorders. In infants and young children iron deficiency is most commonly caused by insufficient dietary iron. Rarely, it can result from mutations in *TMPRSS6*, a gene encoding a membrane protease that serves normally as a downregulator of hepcidin transcription. In young women, iron deficiency is most often the result of blood loss in menstruation or as a result of loss during pregnancy and childbirth. In older adults, bleeding may be from the gastrointestinal tract, as from hemorrhoids, peptic ulcer, hiatus hernia, colon cancer, or angiodysplasia. It may result from uterine leiomyomas or carcinoma, or a renal tumor. Pulmonary blood loss may be etiologic through chronic hemoptysis caused by infection or malignancy, or as a result of idiopathic pulmonary hemosiderosis. However, bloody sputum may be swallowed, and pulmonary bleeding may be mistaken for gastrointestinal bleeding. Iron deficiency has adverse effects on activity of numerous enzymes, and in infants can result in impairment of growth and intellectual development. The hematologic features of iron deficiency are nonspecific and too often confused with other causes of microcytic anemia such as thalassemias, chronic inflammation, and renal neoplasms. A low serum ferritin concentration is a good indicator of iron deficiency, but ferritin levels are elevated by inflammation and can be particularly high in cancer, which lessens their sensitivity for the detection of iron deficiency coexisting with the anemia of chronic inflammation. The plasma iron is decreased and the iron-binding capacity increased in severe iron deficiency, but these alterations are not uniformly present in mild iron deficiency, and low plasma iron levels are also characteristic of the anemia of chronic inflammation. Other laboratory tests that are useful include assays for serum transferrin receptor, erythrocyte ferritin concentration, reticulocyte hemoglobin content, and erythrocyte zinc protoporphyrin. Diagnosis of iron deficiency, particularly in an adult, obliges the clinician to determine the site and cause of blood loss, and to rectify it whenever possible. Treatment of iron deficiency with ferrous salts, in doses of 100 to 200 mg of elemental iron daily, is superior to, much safer, and far less costly than parenteral therapy. Enteric-coated and prolonged-release preparations should be avoided. Complete correction of anemia is expected in 8 to 12 weeks, depending on patient's age. If this response is not achieved, the patient and the diagnosis require reevaluation. Administration of iron should be continued for 12 months after correction of anemia, or for as long as bleeding continues. Parenteral iron is used in patients with gastrointestinal disease, noncompliant patients, and patients undergoing renal dialysis. Iron sucrose and iron gluconate complexes are preferred to iron dextran because they are less likely to cause serious adverse events.

Increased body iron stores have the capacity to produce tissue damage. Iron storage disease (hemochromatosis) can be the result of mutations of genes that are involved in regulation of iron homeostasis or transport. Included are the genes encoding HFE, transferrin receptor 2, ferroportin, hemojuvelin, and hepcidin. Alternatively, iron overload can be the result of iron given in the form of red blood cell transfusions, particularly in individuals with ineffective erythropoiesis, a disorder that seems to facilitate iron absorption. Among the most common causes of secondary hemochromatosis are thalassemia major, myelodysplastic anemias, dyserythropoietic anemias, and pyruvate kinase deficiency.

The diagnosis of hemochromatosis depends, in large part, upon increased serum ferritin levels, which tend to reflect increased iron stores. However, ferritin levels are also increased in patients with chronic inflammation or neoplasia or with the hyperferritinemia cataract syndrome, a disorder caused by mutations in the IRE of the ferritin light chain. The transferrin saturation is usually increased in patients with hereditary hemochromatosis even when the ferritin level is normal.

Full-blown hemochromatosis is characterized by cirrhosis of the liver, darkening of the skin, diabetes, cardiomyopathies, and possibly by arthropathies. Iron deposition is primarily in hepatocytes, with macrophages and intestinal mucosal cells being relatively iron poor. The most common causes of genetic hemochromatosis are mutations of the *HFE* gene. Two mutations are involved: the c.854G→A (C282Y) and c.187C→G (H63D) substitutions. Increased transferrin saturation values, serum ferritin levels, and iron stores were found in a majority of homozygotes for the C282Y mutation and in many compound heterozygotes for C282Y/H63D or homozygotes for H63D. However, clinical manifestations even among homozygotes for the C282Y mutation are rare, in

Acronyms and abbreviations that appear in this chapter include: ALA synthase, aminolevulinic acid synthase; AST, aspartate aminotransferase; BMP, bone morphogenetic protein; dcytb, duodenal cytochrome b; DMT, divalent metal transporter; GRACILE syndrome, growth retardation, aminoaciduria, cholestasis, iron overload, lactic acidosis, early death syndrome; Hgb, hemoglobin; HLA, human leukocyte antigen; IL, interleukin; IRE, iron-responsive element; IRP, iron-regulatory protein; MAO, monoamine oxidase; MCHC, mean corpuscular hemoglobin concentration; MCV, mean corpuscular volume; MRI, magnetic resonance imaging; RDA, recommended daily allowance; RDW, red cell distribution width; STEAP3, six-transmembrane epithelial antigen of prostate 3; TfR, transferrin receptor; TIBC, total iron-binding capacity; TS, transferrin saturation; UIBC, unsaturated iron-binding capacity.

contrast to biochemical and/or histologic manifestations of the increased iron levels, which are common. The penetrance of the C282Y homozygous state with respect to clinical manifestations is approximately 1 percent and that of the other HFE genotypes is probably the order of 0.01 percent. An earlier onset and more severe type of hemochromatosis with high penetrance, juvenile hemochromatosis, is the result of mutations of the hemojuvelin or the hepcidin gene. Ferroportin mutations produced two types of autosomal dominant iron overload. In one of these the iron is deposited chiefly in macrophages; the other is similar to hereditary hemochromatosis because of HFE mutations.

Iron can be removed from patients with hereditary hemochromatosis by serial phlebotomy, but in patients with impaired erythropoiesis, iron chelation therapy with either desferoxamine or the oral chelators deferiprone or deferasirox is required.

Iron is a key element in the metabolism of all living organisms. Iron is a component of heme, which is the active site of electron transport in cytochromes and cytochrome oxygenase, essential coenzymes in the Krebs cycle. The heme moiety of hemoglobin and myoglobin binds O_2, providing the means to transfer O_2 from the lungs to tissues. In the root nodules of legumes, hemoglobin catalyzes the fixation of atmospheric N_2 by symbiotic bacteria. Heme is also the active site of peroxidases that protect cells from oxidative injury by reducing peroxides to water. In plants, iron-containing ferredoxins are essential for an early step of photosynthesis. DNA synthesis requires the enzyme ribonucleotide reductase to convert ribonucleotides to deoxyribonucleotides. Neither bacteria nor nucleated cells proliferate when the supply of iron is insufficient.

DISTRIBUTION OF IRON

The most important iron compartments are summarized in Table 42–1.

HEMOGLOBIN

Hemoglobin, which is 0.34 percent iron by weight, contains approximately 2 g of body iron in men and 1.5 g in women. One milliliter of packed erythrocytes contains approximately 1 mg of iron.

STORAGE COMPARTMENT

Iron is stored either as ferritin or as hemosiderin. The former is water-soluble; the latter is water-insoluble. The protein shell apoferritin is composed of 24 similar or identical subunits arranged as 12 dimers forming a dodecahedron that approximates a hollow sphere (Fig. 42–1).[1–3] The apoferritin monomers are of H (heavy) or L (light) type. L monomers have 15 hydrophilic residues that may bind iron, thereby promoting its retention and serving as sites for ferrihydrite crystal growth. H monomers have fewer hydrophilic residues, but contribute an iron-binding histidyl to the intermonomeric pore (where iron atoms enter or exit). H monomers have ferroxidase activity, thereby enabling apoferritin to take up or release iron quite rapidly. Apoferritin that is rich in H monomers takes up iron more readily, but retains it less avidly than does ferritin composed predominantly of L monomers. Much of the storage iron in liver and spleen is in ferritin containing mostly L monomers.

Ferritin is found in virtually all cells of the body and also in tissue fluids. In blood plasma ferritin is present in minute concentrations. It is glycosylated and largely composed of L subunits. The plasma (serum) ferritin concentration usually correlates roughly with total-body iron stores, making measurement of serum ferritin levels important in the diagnosis of disorders of iron metabolism.

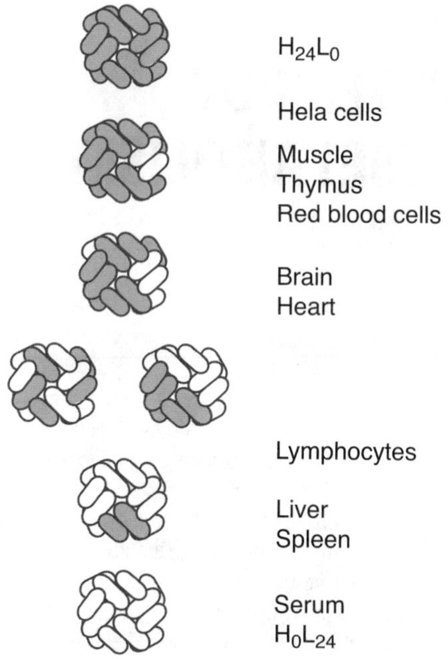

FIGURE 42–1. Schematic of human "isoferritins" of different subunit compositions. Each ferritin subunit is depicted as a "sausage" and subunits are packed in a symmetrical shell. Twelve of the 24 subunits are visible. Mammalian ferritins are composed of two subunits of different primary structures, known as H and L. In the diagram *shaded* subunits represent human H chains and plain subunits, L chains. H-chain and L-chain homopolymers are shown respectively at the *top* and *bottom* of the figure, and heteropolymers of descending H content are placed between the homopolymers. Coassembly of the two subunit types is possible because many of the inter-subunit contact residues are conserved. The sources of various ferritins are listed in the *right-hand column*, such that their average subunit compositions are indicated (e.g., muscle ferritin about 20 H 4 L, liver ferritin about 2–3 H: 22–21 L). Most of the data were obtained by immunoassay using H- or L-chain specific antisera. The composition of human brain ferritin was measured after subunit separation by gel electrophoresis. The pair of molecules in the *fourth position* indicates that subunits may be clustered differently in molecules of the same composition. *In vitro* assembly experiments indicate that dimers are a first assembly intermediate and it is likely that these dimers are antiparallel pairs formed by association of subunits along their axes as shown here. It may be supposed that H chains (or L chains) forming on their polysomes would associate into homodimers before coassembly into heteropolymers, although there is no evidence for this. *(From Harrison PM, Arosio P,[3] with permission from Elsevier.)*

TABLE 42–1. Iron Compartments in Normal Man*

Compartment	Iron Content (mg)	Total Body Iron (%)
Hemoglobin iron	2000	67
Storage iron (ferritin, hemosiderin)	1000	27
Myoglobin iron	130	3.5
Labile pool	80	2.2
Other tissue iron	8	0.2
Transport iron	3	0.08

*These values represent estimates for an "average" person, that is, 70 kg (154 lb) in weight and 177 cm (70 inches) in height. The values are derived from data in several sources.

The size of the storage compartment is quite variable. Normally in adult men it amounts to 800 to 1000 mg; in adult women it is a few hundred milligrams. The mobilization of storage iron involves the reduction of Fe^{+++} to Fe^{++}, its release from the core crystal and its diffusion out of the apoferritin shell. As it passes from cytosol to plasma, it must be reoxidized, either by hephaestin in the cell membrane or by ceruloplasmin in plasma, before it binds to transferrin.

Hemosiderin is found predominantly in macrophages. Microscopically, in unstained tissue sections or marrow films it appears as clumps or granules of golden refractile pigment. Hemosiderin contains approximately 25 to 30 percent iron by weight. Under pathologic conditions, it may accumulate in large quantities in almost every tissue of the body. Hemosiderin is heterogeneous and is structurally related to the mineral ferrihydrite.[4]

MYOGLOBIN

Myoglobin is structurally similar to hemoglobin, but it is monomeric: Each myoglobin molecule consists of a heme group nearly surrounded by loops of a long polypeptide chain containing approximately 150 amino acid residues. It is present in small amounts in all skeletal and cardiac muscle cells, where it may serve as an oxygen reservoir to protect against cellular injury during periods of oxygen deprivation.

LABILE IRON POOL

The existence of a labile iron pool was postulated from studies of the rate of clearance of injected ^{59}Fe from plasma.[5,6] Iron leaves the plasma and enters the interstitial and intracellular fluid compartments for a brief time before it is incorporated into heme or storage compounds. Some of the iron reenters plasma, causing a biphasic curve of ^{59}Fe clearance 1 to 2 days after injection. The change in slope defines the size of the labile pool, normally 80 to 90 mg of iron. It is now sometimes considered to be equivalent to the chelatable iron pool,[7] which can be measured as loosely bound iron by flow cytometry.[8]

TISSUE IRON COMPARTMENT

Tissue iron normally amounts to 6 to 8 mg. This includes cytochromes and other iron-containing enzymes. Although a small compartment, it is an extremely vital one and is sensitive to iron deficiency.[9–11]

TRANSPORT COMPARTMENT

From the standpoint of its total iron content, normally about 3 mg, the transport compartment of plasma is the smallest but the most active of the iron compartments: Its iron normally turns over at least 10 times each day. This is a common pathway for interchange of iron between compartments.

Transferrins and Lactoferrins

Transferrins and lactoferrins comprise a group of glycoproteins that transport iron in plasma and in milk, respectively. They are single polypeptide chains with a Mr of approximately 80 kDa. Each molecule has two binding sites for Fe^{+++}. Each is bilobed, and within each lobe the iron-binding site is in a cleft between two domains that are designated N and C (for amino-terminal and carboxy-terminal). Thus, each complete transferrin or lactoferrin molecule has two N domains and two C domains. Within each lobe, Fe^{+++} is bound to both the N and C domains, which fold over and enclose the Fe^{+++}.[12,13] Normally, approximately one-third of the transferrin iron-binding sites are occupied by iron. Approximately 200 mg (2.5 μmol) of transferrin, carrying approximately 100 mcgμ (1.8 μmol) of iron per deciliter is normally present in human plasma. Apotransferrin (transferrin devoid of iron) is synthesized by hepatocytes and by cells of the monocyte-macrophage system.[14,15] At least 30 genetically determined molecular variants of transferrin have been described in humans.[16] In most cases their properties are normal, but there are exceptions,[17] and one relatively common transferrin variant may be a risk factor for iron-deficiency anemia,[18] although its kinetic properties seem to be normal[19] and it does not appear to affect iron absorption.[20]

TABLE 42–2. Minimal Daily Iron Requirements

	Amount That Must Be Absorbed Daily for Hemoglobin Synthesis (mg)	Minimal Amount That Should Be Ingested Daily (mg)
Infants	1	10
Children	0.5	5
Young, nonpregnant women	2	20
Pregnant women	3	30
Men and postmenopausal women	1	10

DIETARY IRON

CONTENT

An average American male ingests 10 to 20 mg of iron daily.[21,22] Table 42–2 shows the age- and sex-specific daily requirements for iron. The amount of iron absorbed by a normal adult male need only balance the small amount that is excreted, mostly in the stool, approximately 0.5 mg per day.[23] A higher iron requirement exists during growth periods or when there is blood loss. In women, iron absorbed must be sufficient to replace that lost through menstruation or diverted to the fetus during pregnancy.

The iron gained by food during cooking or other food processing is in the form of simple inorganic salts iron–amino acid complexes. Heme, as from hemoglobin and myoglobin, normally comprises about one-third of dietary iron.

BIOAVAILABILITY

Oxalates, phytates, and phosphates complex with iron retard iron absorption, whereas simple reducing substances, such as hydroquinone, ascorbate, lactate, pyruvate, succinate, fructose, cysteine, and sorbitol,[24–28] increase iron absorption. The effect of ethanol on iron absorption seems to be relatively minor.[29,30] Red wine, contrary to popular belief, inhibits iron absorption,[31,32] probably because of the presence of polyphenols. Gastric secretion, the transit time, and mucus secretion all play roles in iron absorption.[33] In mice, alcohol suppresses the response of hepcidin to iron, a response that is HFE dependent,[34] and this may contribute to iron loading that is seen in some alcoholic subjects.

IRON ABSORPTION

Iron normally enters the body through the gastrointestinal tract, mostly through the duodenum. The amount of iron absorbed is normally

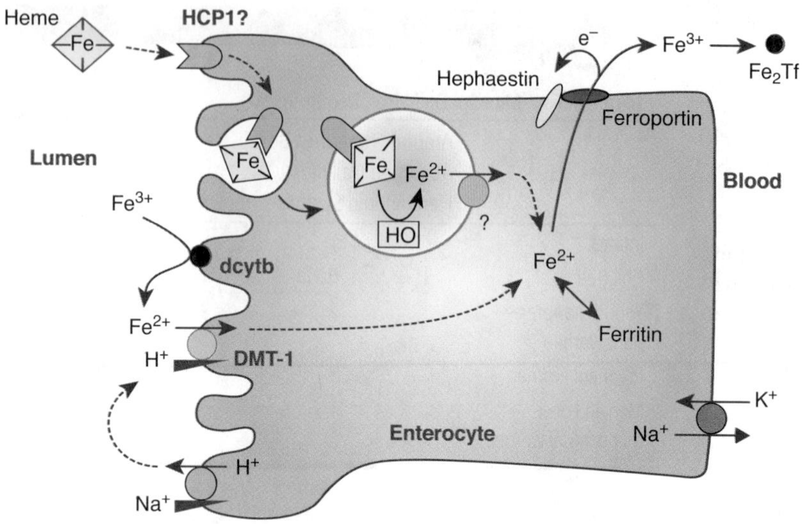

FIGURE 42–2. Schematic of iron uptake from the intestine and transfer to the plasma by an intestinal villus cell. Nonheme dietary iron includes Fe(II) and Fe(III) salts and organic complexes. Fe^{3+} is reduced to Fe^{2+} by ascorbic acid and apical membrane ferrireductases that include duodenal cytochrome b (dcytb). The acid microclimate at the brush border provides an H^+ electrochemical potential gradient to drive transport of Fe^{2+} via the divalent metal-ion transporter (DMT-1) into the enterocyte. DMT-1 may also contribute to the absorption of other nutritionally important metal ions (e.g., Mn^{2+}). Heme can be taken up by endocytosis, and Fe^{2+} is liberated within the endosome/lysosome, but the molecular identity of proteins involved, including heme carrier protein 1 (HCP1), is yet to be elucidated. Basolateral export of Fe^2 may be mediated by ferroportin in association with hephaestin. HO, heme oxygenase; Fe_2Tf, diferric transferrin. *(From Mackenzie B and Garrick,[700] with permission from the American Physiological Society.)*

tightly regulated according to body needs. Active erythropoiesis and/or iron deficiency upregulates absorption; iron overload downregulates absorption.

MECHANISM OF TRANSPORT ACROSS THE INTESTINAL MUCOSA

Heme Iron

Understanding the mechanism of iron absorption has been made more difficult by the fact that the pathways for the absorption of inorganic iron and for heme are different. These pathways seem to merge within the intestinal cell, however, the feeding of heme is not followed by the appearance of heme in the plasma.[35] The existence of an intestinal heme transporter named HCP1 (heme carrier protein 1) has been described.[36] Nevertheless, HCP1 is identical to the proton-coupled folate transporter (PCFT or SLC46A1) and mutations in HCP1/PCFT are associated with familial folate malabsorption and have no heme or iron-deficiency phenotype.[37]

Ferric Iron

Following the reduction of ferric iron to ferrous iron by duodenal cytochrome b (dcytb) reductase,[38,39] ferrous iron is transported into the intestinal villus cell by the divalent metal transporter (DMT)-1. Pulse-chase experiments have demonstrated a pathway in which a β_3-integrin and a protein designated as mobilferrin are involved in transporting iron into the intestinal cell.[40] The partial amino acid sequence of the latter has been found to be that of calreticulin. It has been suggested that β_3-integrin, calreticulin, and DMT-1 form a complex designated as paraferritin (although it contains no ferritin). Basolateral export is mediated by ferroportin in association with hephaestin to export and oxidize iron in the ferric state. Ferric iron is taken up by plasma apotransferrin. Figure 42–2 illustrates some of the steps that are thought to regulate iron transport across the mucosal cell.

MAINTENANCE OF IRON HOMEOSTASIS

The mechanism by which body iron content is regulated by the modulation of iron absorption has been a subject of intense interest for the past 65 years. It was suggested that there was a "mucosal block," implying that the administration of a dose of iron prevents any further absorption for a considerable period of time. This concept was introduced in 1943, but was based on faulty experimental evidence.[41] In reality, no such block exists; for each increment in dose of an inorganic iron compound there is a corresponding increment in the amount of iron absorbed,[42,43] with some evidence of a saturable receptor[44] (Fig. 42–3). However, there is a close relationship between perceived iron need and iron dose, on the one hand, and the amount of iron absorbed, on the other.[41]

A number of genes that encode proteins with demonstrated effects on iron homeostasis have been identified (Table 42–3). To some extent their role can be deduced from the effect of their deletion in human mutations or knockout mice, or from their overproduction. Several models incorporating these proteins in schemes of iron absorption and regulation of absorption have been proposed,[45,46] but their exact role has not yet been definitively assigned. It is postulated that iron is reduced by the duodenal cytochrome b5 and the ferrous iron is then transported into the cell by means of DMT-1. To exit into the plasma from the abluminal surface of the intestinal mucosal cell the iron is reoxidized by hephaestin and transported from the cell by ferroportin.

Hepcidin

Hepcidin, a 25-amino-acid peptide with 4 disulfide bonds,[47] plays a central role regulating the absorption of iron from the intestine mucosal cell and its release from macrophages. It is an antimicrobial peptide

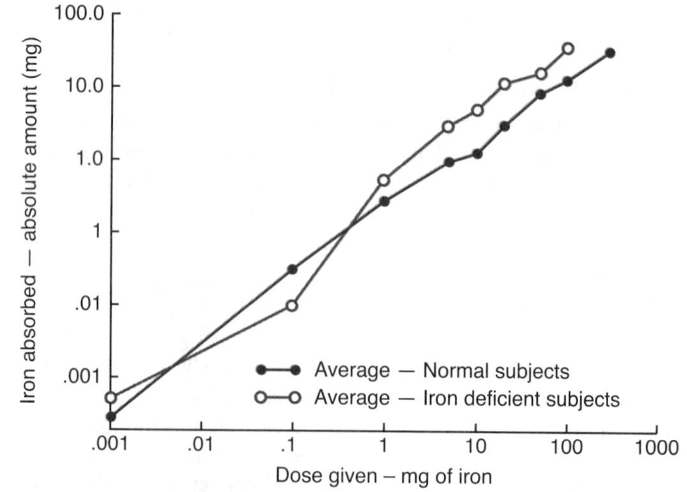

FIGURE 42–3. The relationship between oral iron dosage and amount of iron absorbed in humans. When the logarithm of the dose is plotted against the logarithm of the amount of iron absorbed, a rectilinear relationship is observed. Thus, at all levels, the greater the dose of iron, the more is absorbed, although the percent of the dose that is absorbed progressively declines. *(Drawn from data of Smith and Pannacciuli.[43])*

TABLE 42–3. Proteins That Play a Role in Iron Homeostasis

Proteins That Affect Iron Homeostasis and Man and Mouse	Effect of Deficiency	References to Human Data	References to Murine Data	Comments
HFE	Fe Increased	510	642, 648, 706	Most patients with hereditary hemochromatosis are homozygous for the 845 A→G (C282Y) mutation of this gene
Ferroportin (SLC11A3)	Macrophage Fe increased	707		Autosomal dominant
β_2-microglobulin	Fe increased		708, 709	Believed to function by facilitating transport of *HFE* to membrane
Transferrin	Fe increased	497, 498	710	
Transferrin receptor-1	Lethal; increased CNS Fe	Unknown	628	
Transferrin receptor-2	Increased Fe	611	711	
Hephaestin	Fe deficiency	Unknown	712	Sex-linked gene; deletion of exons is cause of *sla* mouse
Iron-regulatory protein-2 (IRP2)	Fe Increased	Unknown	713	Brain deposition
Ferritin H chain	Fe Increased	714		Dominant IRE mutation
Duodenal cytochrome b (dcytb)	Unknown		38	
Nramp1 (SLC11A1)	Alters iron distribution in macrophages	Unknown	715	Deficiency increases susceptibility to infection in mice
Nramp2 (DMT-1)	Hypochromic microcytic anemia and hepatic siderosis in people; Fe deficiency in rodents	623, 624, 627, 716–719	625, 626	Anemia is ameliorated by erythropoietin therapy in humans; same naturally occurring mutations found in the *mk* mouse and the Belgrade rat
Ceruloplasmin	Fe increased	500	720	Brain accumulation and neurologic disease
Hepcidin	Fe increased	721	722, 723	May be the ultimate regulator of iron homeostasis, both with respect to total body iron and iron in infection
Hemojuvelin	Fe increased	566	Unknown	May be part of signaling pathway to hepcidin
Tmprss6	Fe deficiency	724–726	67, 727	May be part of signaling pathway to hepcidin

that retains weak antimicrobial activity.[48] Presumably in the course of evolution this peptide was selected to modulate iron homeostasis as one of the defenses of the body against microorganisms. Overexpression of hepcidin results in marked iron-deficiency anemia in mice[49] and a refractory anemia resembling the anemia of chronic inflammation in humans,[50] and injection of synthetic hepcidin downregulates iron absorption.[51] Hepcidin exerts its iron-regulatory effect by binding to ferroportin, a transmembrane iron-transport protein expressed both on intestinal mucosal cells and macrophages. Once hepcidin has bound to ferroportin, the ferroportin is internalized and undergoes proteolysis.[52,53] With membrane ferroportin depleted, iron cannot be transported from the mucosal cell or from the macrophage into the plasma. This results in decreased iron absorption from the gastrointestinal tract and a fall in the plasma iron level. Like other antimicrobial peptides, hepcidin production is stimulated by inflammatory cytokines such as interleukin (IL)-1 and IL-6, and it is likely that overproduction of hepcidin is one of the factors in the pathogenesis of the anemia of chronic inflammation (see Chap. 37).

The regulation of hepcidin production seems to be largely or entirely transcriptional. Hepcidin mRNA levels increase with iron-loading, inflammatory stimuli,[54–56] and treatment with bone morphogenetic protein (BMP),[57–59] and is decreased by hypoxia, hypoxia-inducible factor (HIF)-1,[60] and iron withdrawal.[61] For reasons that are not understood, the effect of iron is observed only *in vivo*; isolated hepatocytes do not show consistent stimulation by iron, although minimal effects have been reported when the cells were harvested immediately after sacrifice of an animal.[62]

It is not clear how elevated iron levels are sensed in the intact organism, but clues are provided by hereditary disorders in which hepcidin transcription is dysregulated. As indicated in Table 42–3, impairment of the function of several genes is associated with iron overload in humans and in experimental animals. In addition to those encoding hepcidin itself and its receptor, ferroportin, prominent among these are those encoding HFE, transferrin receptor-2, BMPs, and hemojuvelin. Apparently these proteins represent a part of the system that upregulates the hepcidin transcription system normally to prevent iron overload. It has been suggested that complexes of HFE, transferrin receptor-1, and transferrin receptor-2 are a part of the regulatory cascade that stimulates the transcription of hepcidin and that hemojuvelin serves as a coreceptor for the BMPs.[57,63] A soluble fragment of hemojuvelin acts as an inhibitor of the interaction of BMP with the receptor, and this may represent one regulatory mechanism.[64,65] Regulation of hepcidin transcription itself is complex, involving the formation of a complex of liver-specific and response-specific transcription factors bound to a distal

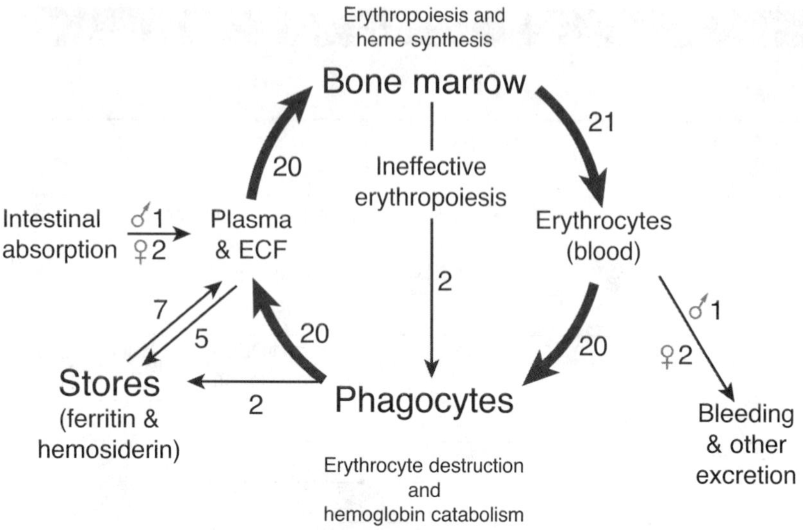

FIGURE 42–4. The iron cycle in humans. Iron is tightly conserved in a nearly closed system in which each iron atom cycles repeatedly from plasma and extracellular fluid (ECF) to the marrow, where it is incorporated into hemoglobin. Then it moves into the blood within erythrocytes and circulates for 4 months. It then travels to phagocytes of the mononuclear phagocyte system, where senescent erythrocytes are engulfed and destroyed, hemoglobin is digested, and iron is released to plasma, where the cycle continues. With each cycle, a small proportion of iron is transferred to storage sites, where it is incorporated into ferritin or hemosiderin, a small proportion of storage iron is released to plasma, a small proportion is lost in urine, sweat, feces, or blood, and an equivalent small amount of iron is absorbed from the intestinal tract. In addition, a small proportion (approximately 10%) of newly formed erythrocytes normally is destroyed within the marrow and its iron released, bypassing the circulating blood part of the cycle (ineffective erythropoiesis). The numbers indicate the approximate amount of iron (in milligrams) that enters and leaves each of these iron compartments every day in healthy adults who do not have bleeding and other blood disorders.

BMP-RE2/bZIP/HNF4α/COUP region and to the proximal BMP-RE1/STAT region of the hepcidin promoter, possibly by physical association of the two regions.[66]

A pathway that inhibits the transcription of hepcidin exists as well. Tmprss6, a membrane serine protease, prevents the upregulation of hepcidin transcription. This function was discovered when random mutagenesis in mice produced an iron-deficient animal with mutagenized Tmprss6.[67] Subsequently, humans with mutations of the tmprss6 ortholog were shown to manifest iron resistant iron deficiency anemia (see "Genetic Factors" below).

TRANSPORT OF IRON

Once an atom of iron enters the body, it is virtually in a closed system (Fig. 42–4) in which it cycles almost endlessly from the plasma to the developing erythroblast (where it is used in hemoglobin synthesis), thence into the circulating blood for approximately 4 months, and then to macrophages. Here it is removed from heme by heme oxygenase and released back into the plasma to repeat the cycle.

The major function of the transport protein transferrin is to move iron from wherever it enters the plasma (intestinal villi, splenic sinusoids) to the erythroblasts of the marrow and to other sites of utilization.

ENDOCYTOSIS OF TRANSFERRIN

Diferric transferrin binds to the transferrin receptor (TfR) on the cell surface and the transferrin-TfR complex forms clusters in pits on the cell membrane.[68] The complex is then internalized by endocytosis (Fig. 42–5). Within the cytosol the transferrin-TfR complex is in a clathrin-coated vesicle. The vesicles fuse with endosomes, in which occur acidification and release of iron from transferrin. Transformation into lysosomes does not occur. Neither transferrin nor TfR is degraded in the process. Within the vesicle, a low pH of approximately pH 5 causes the release of one iron atom. The apotransferrin-TfR complex then returns to the cell membrane, where at neutral pH, apotransferrin is released to the interstitial fluid to reenter plasma and take up more iron.[61]

The transferrin receptor is a protein consisting of two subunits that are linked by disulfide bonds.[69] It is a group II transmembrane protein: its amino-terminus is on the cytoplasmic side of the membrane, and its carboxy-terminus is on the outer surface.[70] Because of the role of TfR in the binding and endocytosis of diferric transferrin, control of TfR biosynthesis is a major mechanism for regulation of iron metabolism. Synthesis of TfR is induced by iron deficiency, or, experimentally, by incubation with an iron-chelating agent such as desferrioxamine. Conversely, synthesis of TfR is inhibited by heme,[71] but this effect can be completely abolished by the addition of the iron chelator desferrioxamine.[72] It is currently believed that iron derived from heme by heme oxygenase causes destabilization of TfR mRNA by a mechanism that involves the IRE/IRP regulatory system (Fig. 42–6).[73] The transferrin receptor binds to HFE,[63] the product of the *HFE* gene involved in hereditary hemochromatosis, but the functional consequences of this interaction are unclear.

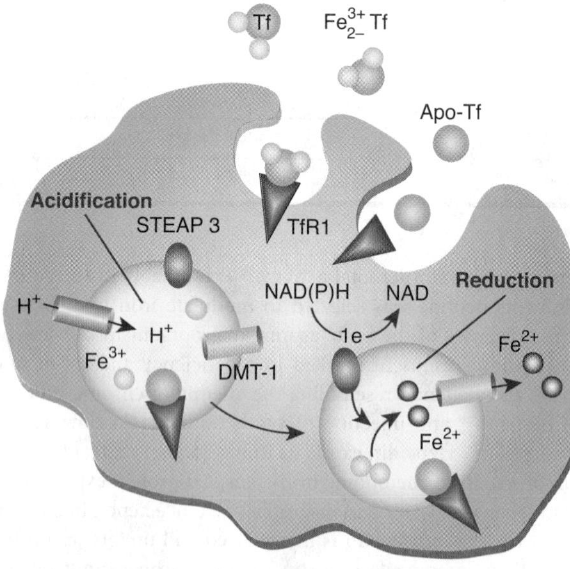

FIGURE 42–5. The transferrin cycle. Holotransferrin (Fe^{3+}_2-Tf) binds to transferrin receptors (TfR1) on the cell surface. The complexes localize to clathrin-coated pits, which invaginate to initiate endocytosis. Specialized endosomes form, and become acidified through the action of a proton pump. Acidification leads to protein conformational changes that release iron from transferrin. STEAP 3 reduces ferric iron to ferrous iron, enabling iron transport out of the endosomes through the activity of the divalent metal transporter 1 protein (DMT-1). Subsequently, Apotransferrin (Apo-Tf) and the transferrin receptor both return to the cell surface, where they dissociate at neutral pH. Both proteins participate in further rounds of iron delivery. In nonerythroid cells, iron is stored as ferritin and hemosiderin. *(From McKie AT,[701] with permission from the Nature Publishing Group.)*

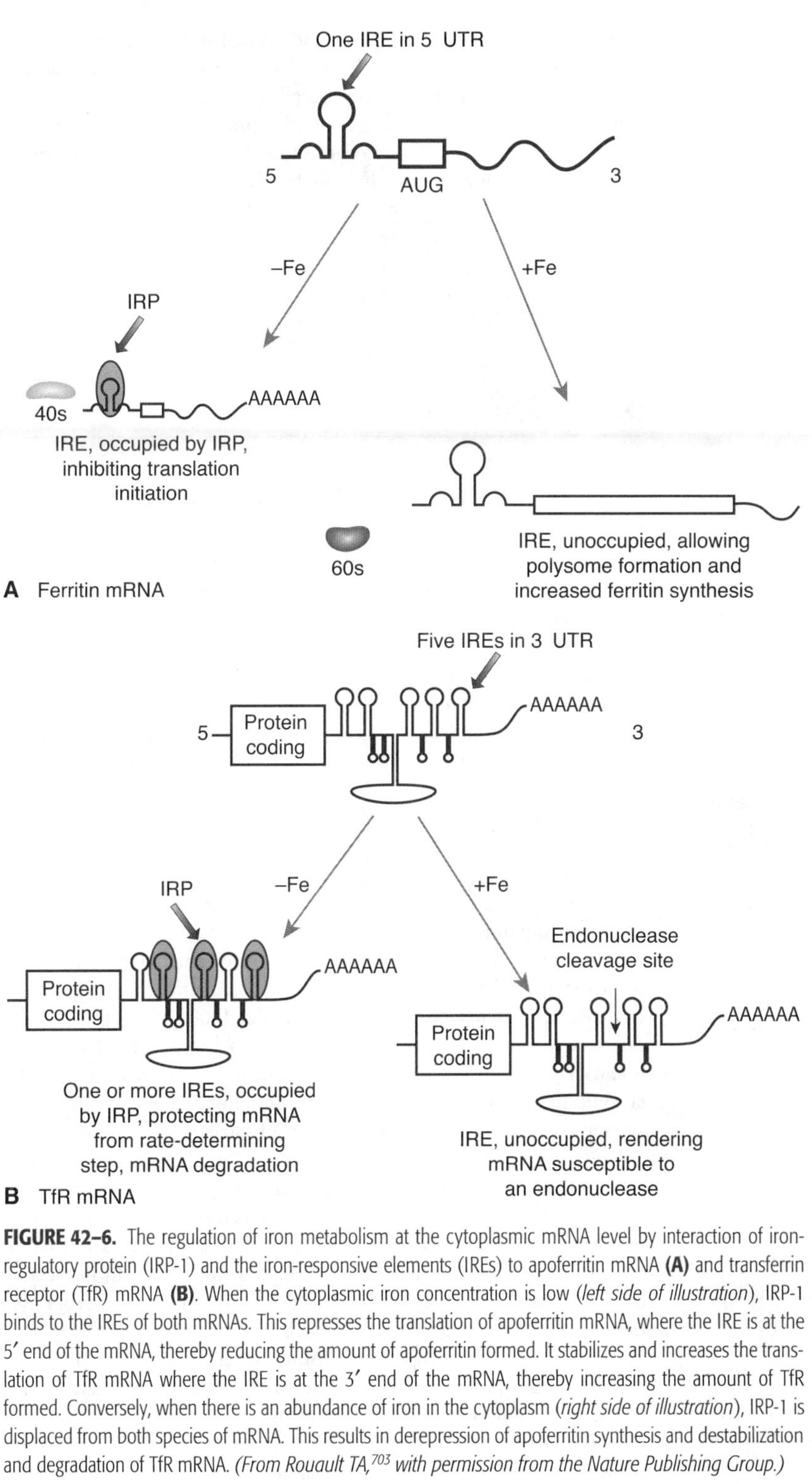

FIGURE 42–6. The regulation of iron metabolism at the cytoplasmic mRNA level by interaction of iron-regulatory protein (IRP-1) and the iron-responsive elements (IREs) to apoferritin mRNA **(A)** and transferrin receptor (TfR) mRNA **(B)**. When the cytoplasmic iron concentration is low (*left side of illustration*), IRP-1 binds to the IREs of both mRNAs. This represses the translation of apoferritin mRNA, where the IRE is at the 5′ end of the mRNA, thereby reducing the amount of apoferritin formed. It stabilizes and increases the translation of TfR mRNA where the IRE is at the 3′ end of the mRNA, thereby increasing the amount of TfR formed. Conversely, when there is an abundance of iron in the cytoplasm (*right side of illustration*), IRP-1 is displaced from both species of mRNA. This results in derepression of apoferritin synthesis and destabilization and degradation of TfR mRNA. *(From Rouault TA,[703] with permission from the Nature Publishing Group.)*

IRON IN THE ERYTHROBLAST

Once within the developing erythroblast, iron must be transported to mitochondria to be incorporated into heme, or taken up by ferritin within siderosomes. Within the vesicle, STEAP3 (six-transmembrane epithelial antigen of prostate 3) effects the reduction of ferric to ferrous iron and another protein DMT-1 (Nramp2) induces the release of Fe^{++} into the cytosol, where it is taken up by mitochondria for heme synthesis.[61]

Within mitochondria, iron is inserted into protoporphyrin by heme synthetase (ferrochelatase). When heme synthesis is impaired, as in lead poisoning or in the sideroblastic anemias (see Chap. 58), the mitochondria accumulate excessive amounts of amorphous iron aggregates. The mitochondria can then be stained by the Prussian blue reaction and are seen by light microscopy as a ring of large blue siderotic granules encircling the erythroblast nucleus (ringed sideroblast). In normal marrow, siderotic granules are also demonstrable in erythroblast cytoplasm. However, these are very small, usually only one to three in number, and randomly distributed in the cytoplasm. These normal siderotic granules are ferritin aggregates located in lysosomal organelles designated siderosomes.[74] Erythroblasts containing these siderotic granules, *sideroblasts*, normally represent 20 to 50 percent of the erythrocyte precursors of the marrow and as visualized by light microscopy. In iron deficiency and in the anemia that accompanies chronic disorders, sideroblasts almost disappear from the marrow. Conversely, in some states of iron overload, they may become more numerous and contain excessive numbers of granules.

Mitochondrial Ferritin

Ring sideroblasts contain a ferritin isoform that is a product of an intronless, IRE-lacking, ferritin gene on chromosome 5q23.1 that is specifically targeted to mitochondria by a 60-amino-acid-leader sequence.[75–77] Mitochondrial ferritin lacks IRE and, thus, is not subject to iron-dependent translational control. Its function appears to be to reduce the labile iron pool and decrease the level of reactive oxygen species.[78] Mitochondrial ferritin has limited tissue expression and is found in high concentrations in the mitochondria of normal testes and in the sideroblasts of patients with sideroblastic anemia.[75,79,80]

THE INTRACELLULAR REGULATION OF IRON METABOLISM

The synthesis of apoferritin, TfR, aminolevulinic acid (ALA) synthase, apotransferrin, aconitase, DMT-1, and ferroportin is regulated posttranscriptionally. The mRNA for each of these proteins contains one or several IREs. If the IRE is located at the 5′ end of the mRNA, it serves to regulate translation; 3′ IREs regulate the stability of the mRNA. Each IRE consists of a stem and loop structure, in which the loop is the nucleotide sequence CAGUG (Fig. 42–7). The apoferritin mRNA has, as its IRE, a single stem-loop structure in the 5′ (upstream) untranslated region. In contrast to the apoferritin IRE, there are as many as 5 stems-loops in the 3′ (downstream) untranslated portion of TfR mRNA.[81] The IREs exert their effect by binding one of the two IRPs. IRP-1 is cytoplasmic aconitase with four iron-sulfur clusters and the ability to bind iron, which is required for its aconitase activity; IRP-2 is highly homologous to IRP-1 but differs by the presence of a 73-amino-acid insertion in the N-terminus and a lack of aconitase activity. In the absence of iron, IRP-1 binds to IREs, but in its presence becomes a cytoplasmic aconitase. IRP-2, on the other hand, is proteolyzed in the presence of iron. Nitric oxide has an effect on the IRE/IRP system. It increases binding of IRP-1 to IREs and enhances degradation of IRP-2, therefore exerting contradictory effects on the

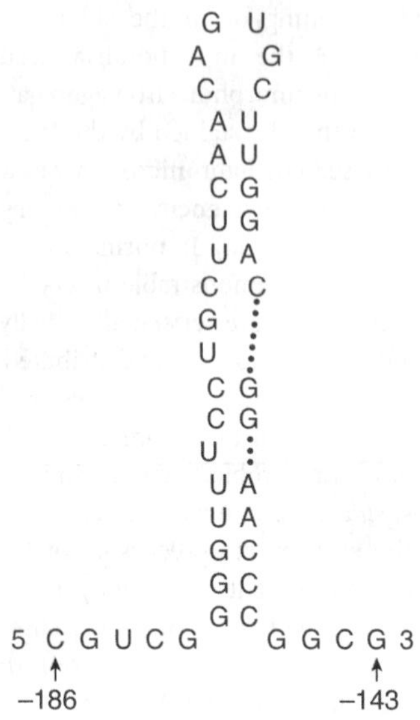

FIGURE 42–7. The stem-loop structure that is the iron-responsive element of apoferritin mRNA. *(Reproduced with permission from Matthias W, et al: A model for the structure and functions of iron-responsive elements,* Gene Dec 72:10(1-2):201–208, 1988.)

regulation of protein synthesis. Moreover, nitric oxide may also destabilize IRP-2.[82–84]

Although the first-discovered IRP-1 has received the most attention, the importance of IRP-2 is emphasized by the fact that targeted disruption of the gene that encodes this protein causes a severe adult-onset neurologic disorder, whereas the disruption of IRP-1 causes no obvious phenotype.[85] Moreover, IRP-1 does not bind efficiently to IREs at normal tissue oxygen tensions.[86] The effect of binding of IRPs to 3′ IREs is to increase the stability of the mRNA and thus to enhance the synthesis of the gene product; conversely, when the iron content of cytosol is high, the displacement of IRPs from these IREs leads to decreased synthesis of these proteins. Figure 42–6 illustrates these relationships for the regulation of synthesis of apoferritin and TfR.

ROLE OF THE MONOCYTE-MACROPHAGE SYSTEM

Destruction of aged erythrocytes and hemoglobin degradation occur within macrophages (see Chap. 32). This proceeds at a rate sufficient to release approximately 20 percent of the hemoglobin iron from the cell to the plasma compartment within a few hours. Approximately 80 percent of this iron is rapidly reincorporated into hemoglobin. Thus, 19 to 69 percent of the hemoglobin iron of nonviable erythrocytes reappears in circulating red cells in 12 days. The remainder of the iron enters the storage pool as ferritin or hemosiderin and then turns over very slowly. In normal subjects, approximately 40 percent of this iron remains in storage after 140 days. When there is an increased iron demand for hemoglobin synthesis, however, storage iron may be mobilized more rapidly.[87] Conversely, in the presence of infection or another inflammatory process or malignancy, iron is much more slowly reused in hemoglobin synthesis.[87–89]

IRON EXCRETION

The body conserves iron with remarkable efficiency. Most iron loss occurs by way of desquamated intestinal cells in the feces and it normally amounts to about 0.5 mg per day,[23] less than one-thousandth of total body iron. Exfoliation of skin and dermal appendages and perspiration result in a much smaller losses. Even in tropical climates, the loss of iron in sweat is minimal.[90] Very small amounts of iron are lost in the urine. Lactation may cause excretion of approximately 1 mg iron daily, thus doubling the overall rate of iron loss. Blood loss by normal menstruation contributes to negative iron balance.

Although total daily iron loss is normally approximately 1 mg for males,[23] it averages approximately 2 mg for menstruating women. Persons with marked iron overload, as in hemochromatosis, may lose as much as 4 mg of iron daily, probably because of the shedding of iron-laden cells, principally macrophages.

IRON DEFICIENCY

DEFINITION AND HISTORY

Iron deficiency is the state in which the content of iron in the body is less than normal. It occurs in varying degrees of severity that merge imperceptibly into one another. Iron depletion is the earliest stage of iron deficiency, in which storage iron is decreased or absent but serum iron concentration, transferrin saturation, and blood hemoglobin levels are normal. Iron deficiency without anemia is a somewhat more advanced stage of iron deficiency, characterized by decreased or absent storage iron, usually low serum iron concentration and transferrin saturation, but without frank anemia. Iron-deficiency anemia is the most advanced stage of iron deficiency. It is characterized by decreased or absent iron stores, low serum iron concentration, low transferrin saturation, and low blood hemoglobin concentration.

In certain rare disorders, such as idiopathic pulmonary hemosiderosis or paroxysmal nocturnal hemoglobinuria (see Chap. 40), iron-deficiency anemia may occur without iron depletion as a result of redistribution of body iron and thus is inaccessible for hemoglobin synthesis.

The clinical manifestations of iron-deficiency anemia appear to have been recognized in earliest times. A disease characterized by pallor, dyspnea, and edema was described in about 1500 B.C. in the *Papyrus Ebers*, a manual of therapeutics believed to be the oldest complete manuscript extant.[91] This ancient disease may have been caused by chronic blood loss from hookworm infestation. Chlorosis, or "green sickness," was well known to European physicians after the middle of the 16th century. In France, by the middle of the 17th century, iron salts and other remedies (including, oddly enough, phlebotomy) were used in its treatment. Not long thereafter, iron was recommended by Sydenham as a specific remedy for chlorosis. For the 100 years preceding 1930, iron was used in the treatment of chlorosis, often in ineffective doses, although the mechanism of action of iron and the appropriateness of its use were highly controversial.

By the beginning of the 20th century, it had been established that chlorosis was characterized by a decrease in the iron content of the blood and by the presence of hypochromic erythrocytes, but it was not until the classic 1932 studies by Heath, Strauss, and Castle[92] that it was shown that the response of anemia to iron was stoichiometrically related to the amount of iron given and that chlorosis was, indeed, iron deficiency. The history of iron deficiency has been reviewed in greater detail elsewhere.[41,93]

EPIDEMIOLOGY

The prevalence of iron-deficiency anemia varies so much between age groups, between the sexes, between economic groups, and by geography, that overall prevalence statistics are almost meaningless. Estimates that suggest that as many as three-quarters of the world's population are iron deficient have been made, but these estimates are undoubtedly

TABLE 42–4. Prevalence of Iron Deficiency and Iron-Deficiency Anemia in Some Selected Populations

Population	Sex	Age Group (years)	Iron Deficiency	Iron-Deficiency Anemia
Chile[728]		Full-term infants	30.7	22.6
Inner City, USA[729]		3rd and 4th graders	2.9	1
Sweden[730]	F	15–16	40	
	M		15	
Norway[731]	F	20–55	32	4.2
USA 1999–2000[732]		1–2	7	2
		2–4	5	
		6–11	4	
	M	12–15	5	
	M	16–69	2	
	M	>70	3	
	F	12–49	12	3
	F	50–69	9	3
	F	>70	6	1
Canada[733]		Infants		4.3
Southern California HFE wt/wt[734]	F	26–49	12.4	3.2
	M	26–95	0.7	0.4
Turkey	F, M	4 months–2 years	21.9	26.2
		2–6	10.2	6.1
		6–12	1.8	4.2
		12–18	2.8	13.9
Colombian school children and adolescents[735]	F, M	6–18	4.9	0.6
Mexican pregnant and adolescents[736]	F	11–17		80
Ethiopian lactating women[737]	F	28.4 ± 6.12		22.3
Iranian children[738]	F, M	6 months–5 years		19.7
Belgian pregnant women[739]	F	15–44		
1st trimester				1.5
3rd trimester				23
New Zealand children[740]	F, M	0.5–2.0	5.6	4.3
South African factory workers[741]	F	18–55	40	27.4
Urban New Zealand[740]	F, M	0.5–2.0	18.6	5.6

extravagant.[94] Table 42–4 provides some data regarding the prevalence in different populations.

ETIOLOGY AND PATHOGENESIS

Etiology

Iron deficiency may occur as a result of chronic blood loss, diversion of iron to fetal and infant erythropoiesis during pregnancy and lactation, inadequate dietary iron intake, malabsorption of iron, intravascular hemolysis with hemoglobinuria, diversion of iron to nonhematopoietic tissues like the lung, genetic factors, or a combination of these factors.

Bleeding Gastrointestinal In men and in postmenopausal women, iron deficiency is most commonly caused by chronic bleeding from the gastrointestinal tract. Table 42–5 lists the causes of such blood loss. In the adult, the most common causes are peptic ulcer, erosion in a hiatal hernia, gastritis (including that caused by alcohol or aspirin ingestion), hemorrhoids, vascular anomalies (such as angiodysplasia), and neoplasms. In one study of 114 outpatients referred to gastroenterologists for investigation of iron deficiency, 45 had upper gastrointestinal and 18 had colonic sources of bleeding.[95] In 100 other patients in whom the site of bleeding could not be established by any means short of laparotomy, a malignancy was found to be the cause in 10 percent.[96] Enteritis after therapeutic irradiation of abdominal viscera[96] may also be a cause of gastrointestinal bleeding leading to iron-deficiency anemia. Colon cancer, colonic diverticula, periampullary tumors, leiomyomas, adenomas, and other malignant or benign neoplasms of the intestine are among the causes of chronic blood loss.[97–101]

Diaphragmatic Hernia Diaphragmatic (hiatal) hernia is often associated with gastrointestinal bleeding. The frequency of anemia ranges from 8 to 38 percent.[102–105] Bleeding is much more likely to occur in patients with paraesophageal or large hernias than in those with sliding hernias or small ones.[102,103,106] It is likely that hemorrhage follows mucosal injury at the neck of the sac, where the herniated stomach rides to and fro over the crus of the diaphragm during respiration.[102,103,105] Mucosal changes cannot always be demonstrated by esophagoscopy or gastroscopy in patients who have had blood loss from hiatus hernia. However, a linear gastric erosion, also called a "Cameron ulcer," commonly occurs on the crests of mucosal folds at the level of the diaphragm, and appears to be the site of bleeding. In a series of 109 cases of large diaphragmatic hernias, a third had such linear erosions; most of these patients were anemic.[106]

Gastritis, Varices, Ulcers, and Inflammation Gastritis as a result of drug ingestion is another common cause of bleeding. Aspirin ingestion is as likely to cause bleeding in patients without preexisting ulcer as in those with peptic ulcer.[107] Other medications (such as glucocorticoids, indomethacin, ibuprofen, or other nonsteroidal antiinflammatory drugs) may also cause bleeding by inducing gastric or duodenal ulcers or colitis.[108] Gastritis caused by alcohol ingestion can also cause significant blood loss.

Chronic blood loss from esophageal or gastric varices can lead to iron-deficiency anemia. Chronic blood loss is often the cause of anemia in rheumatoid arthritis (perhaps a result of the aspirin or glucocorticoid therapy) and inflammatory bowel disease.[109] Hemorrhoidal bleeding may lead to severe iron-deficiency anemia. Chronic blood loss may result from diffuse gastric mucosal hypertrophy (Ménétrier disease).[110] Peptic ulcers of the stomach or duodenum are common causes of iron

TABLE 42–5. Sources of Blood Loss

Respiratory tract
Carcinoma
Epistaxis
Idiopathic pulmonary hemosiderosis
Infections
Telangiectases
Alimentary tract
Esophagus
Varices
Stomach
Angiodysplasia
Antral vascular ectasia
Carcinoma
Gastritis
Hemangioma
Hiatus hernia
Hypergastrinemia
Leiomyoma (Ménétrier disease)
Mucosal hypertrophy
Ulcer
Varices
"Watermelon stomach"
Colon
Amebiasis
Angiodysplasia
Carcinoma
Diverticulum
Hemangioma
Polyp
Telangiectasia
Ulcerative colitis
Biliary tract
Aberrant pancreas
Carcinoma
Cholelithiasis
Intrahepatic bleeding
Ruptured aneurysm
Trauma

deficiency, and an association between infection with *Helicobacter pylori* and iron-deficiency anemia has been documented in numerous studies.[111–113] Surprisingly, it has been found in some studies, one of them controlled,[114] that putative iron-deficient patients infected with *H. pylori* do not respond to oral iron alone but do respond to eradication of *H. pylori*. This has been interpreted as suggesting that the organism itself may sequester iron and render it unavailable for absorption.[111,115] This would require trapping of an enormous amount of iron, and an alternative explanation may be that response to this particular organism results in laboratory findings that simulate iron deficiency, but that this represents a subset of anemia of chronic infection. Indeed, some have considered the evidence of a causal association between *H. pylori* and iron deficiency unproven.[116]

Gastric ulceration and bleeding can also occur in disorders of hypergastrinemia, as in Zollinger-Ellison syndrome and pseudo–Zollinger-Ellison syndrome.[117] Intestinal parasitism, particularly by hookworms, is a major cause of gastrointestinal blood loss in many parts of the world.[118,119] Achlorhydria is common in such patients[120] and may play a role.

Anemia that follows subtotal gastrectomy is usually attributed to reduced absorption of dietary iron[121] (see "Malabsorption of Iron" below), but occult intermittent gastrointestinal bleeding may also be a contributory factor. Of 8 patients whose erythrocytes were labeled with $Na_2{}^{51}CrO_4$ to permit precise quantitation of daily fecal blood loss,[122] 7 were shown to lose from 3.2 to 6.5 mL of blood per day. This is a very slight but significant increase in daily fecal blood loss that over a span of several years could well lead to iron-deficiency anemia. Chemical tests for fecal blood loss are usually insensitive to a daily loss of less than 5 to 10 mL of blood, although this depends to some extent on the site of bleeding within the gastrointestinal tract.

Vascular Anomalies The lesions of angiodysplasia may occur in any part of the gastrointestinal tract, but are most frequent in the cecum or ascending colon.[123] These tiny vascular anomalies may be the cause of significant blood loss. Endoscopy is usually required for diagnosis.[123] Gastric antral vascular ectasia exhibits a characteristic endoscopic appearance ("watermelon stomach"), and is another cause of blood loss.[124,125] Hemorrhage into the gallbladder is a rare cause of chronic iron deficiency anemia.[99]

Tortuous, dilated sublingual venous structures, the cherry hemangiomas commonly seen in the elderly, and the spider telangiectases of chronic liver disease are usually easily distinguished from the lesions of hereditary hemorrhagic telangiectasia. Bleeding from intestinal telangiectases has also been observed in scleroderma[126] and in Turner syndrome,[127] as a manifestation of bleeding from abnormal blood vessels. Cutaneous hemangiomas (blue rubber bleb nevus) may be associated with hemorrhage from intestinal hemangiomas.[128–130]

In hereditary hemorrhagic telangiectasia (see Chap. 123), characteristic lesions commonly occur on fingertips, nasal septum, tongue, lips, margins (helices) of ears, oral and pharyngeal mucosa, palms and soles, and other epithelial and cutaneous surfaces throughout the body. Those lesions that occur in the gastrointestinal tract are particularly likely to bleed and to cause iron deficiency.

Meckel Diverticulum Meckel diverticulum is a very common abnormality representing a vestigial remnant of the omphalomesenteric duct. In children, bleeding from this structure accounts for a small proportion of cases of iron-deficiency anemia.[131]

Bleeding Disorders Hemostatic defects, particularly those related to abnormal platelet function or number may lead to gastrointestinal bleeding. Gastrointestinal bleeding is common in von Willebrand disease (see Chap. 127). Polycythemia vera is typically associated with iron deficiency as a result either of spontaneous gastrointestinal hemorrhage that commonly occurs in this disorder, or phlebotomy therapy, or both mechanisms (Chap. 121).

When a patient with a disorder of hemostasis suffers from gastrointestinal bleeding, one must consider the possibility that the bleeding may not be caused by a hemostatic defect alone, but that an anatomic lesion of the gastrointestinal tract may also be present.

Cow's Milk Anemia Ingestion of whole cow's milk may induce protein-losing enteropathy and gastrointestinal bleeding in infants,[131,132] probably on the basis of hypersensitivity or allergy. In four such cases observed endoscopically, erosive gastritis or gastroduodenitis was demonstrated as the probable source of bleeding.[133] At least during the first year of life, children should not be given whole bovine milk, either raw or pasteurized.[132,134] More protracted heating, as in preparation of infant formulas, eliminates this problem. Intrinsic lesions of the gastrointestinal tract, such as those listed above, may cause bleeding in infants, as well as in older children. In infants or small children, peptic ulcer is an uncommon cause of gastrointestinal bleeding.

Respiratory Tract Persistent recurrent hemoptysis may lead to iron-deficiency anemia. It may be a result of congenital anomalies of the respiratory tract, endobronchial vascular anomalies, chronic infections, neoplasms, or valvular heart disease. Severe iron-deficiency anemia is a manifestation of idiopathic pulmonary hemosiderosis and of Goodpasture syndrome (progressive glomerulonephritis with intrapulmonary hemorrhage).[135] In some of these disorders, hemoptysis may not be observed, but sufficient amounts of blood-laden sputum may be swallowed to result in positive tests for occult blood in the stools. Iron deficiency occurs in a large proportion of patients with cystic fibrosis, and is related to the volume of sputum but not to the degree of pancreatic insufficiency, suggesting that iron loss in sputum may play an important role.[136]

Genitourinary Tract Menstrual bleeding is a very common cause of iron deficiency.[137] The amount of blood lost with menstruation varies markedly from one woman to another and is often difficult to evaluate by questioning the patient. The average menstrual blood loss is approximately 40 mL per cycle. Blood loss exceeds 80 mL (equivalent to approximately 30 mg of iron) per cycle in only 10 percent of women.[138] The volume of blood lost in the course of one menstrual cycle may be as high as 495 mL in apparently healthy, nonanemic women who do not regard their menstrual flow to be excessive. The amount of menstrual blood lost does not seem to vary markedly from one cycle to another for any given individual.[139] Oral contraceptives reduce menstrual blood loss,[140,141] but the use of an intrauterine coil for contraception increases menstrual blood loss,[142] especially during the first year of use. Because the absorption of 1 mg of iron per day requires a dietary intake of between 10 and 20 mg of iron, it is easy to understand why, with an average dietary iron intake of approximately 10 mg per day, iron balance in many menstruating women is precarious.

Excessive bleeding may be caused by uterine fibroids and malignant neoplasms. Neoplasms, stones, or inflammatory disease of the kidney, ureter, or bladder may cause enough chronic blood loss to produce iron deficiency. In one unusual case, urinary iron loss was documented.[143]

Factitious Anemia Factitious anemia as a result of self-inflicted bleeding may present a formidable diagnostic and therapeutic problem. This rare condition has also been called, in literary allusion to a fictitious character, "Lasthénie de Ferjol syndrome" (in Barbey d'Aurevilly's gloomy novel, *Une Histoire Sans Nom*, Lasthénie de Ferjol was a young woman noted for extreme pallor and languor, who habitually and secretly practiced autodesanguination by thrusting needles into her heart). Most patients are women, and patients are often employed in a medical setting. There is often a history of numerous blood transfusions. The anemia is chronic and may be severe, with blood hemoglobin concentration persistently as low as 5 to 6 g/dL. The site of induced blood loss is obscure. Hence, patients are subjected to numerous radiographic and endoscopic examinations, usually to no avail. The patients are usually refractory to medical advice and therapy.[144–146] The patients may be depressed and suicidal; some also suffer anorexia nervosa. Psychiatric care is needed, but often is unsuccessful. Rarely, the outcome of self-bleeding may be fatal.[145]

Nosocomial (Iatrogenic) Anemia In the course of medical care, repetitive blood sampling, especially in intensive care units, may result in removal of a large amount of blood,[147,148] and this iatrogenic phlebotomy can result in iron-deficiency anemia.

The use of extracorporeal dialysis for treatment of chronic renal disease may cause iron deficiency, often superimposed upon the anemia of chronic renal disease. The retention of blood in the dialyzing equipment is a major cause, along with gastrointestinal bleeding, blood sampling and bleeding incident to vascular access.[149,150]

Anemia Incident to Blood Donation Each whole-blood donation removes approximately 200 mg of iron from the body. Lesser amounts of iron are removed in the course of donating platelets or leukocytes. Potential donors are screened in blood banks, so that those with frank anemia are not phlebotomized. Yet, by the time they are excluded from donation, some blood donors are iron depleted and may readily develop iron-deficiency anemia with relatively small additional blood loss.[151,152]

Pregnancy and Parturition

In pregnancy, the average iron loss resulting from diversion of iron to the fetus, blood loss at delivery (equivalent to an average of 150 to 200 mg of iron), and lactation is altogether approximately 900 mg; in terms of iron content, this is equivalent to the loss of more than 2 L of blood. Approximately 30 mg of iron may be expended monthly in lactation. Because most women begin pregnancy with low iron reserves, these additional demands frequently result in iron-deficiency anemia. Iron depletion has been reported in some 85 to 100 percent of pregnant women. The incidence is lower in women who take oral iron supplementation.[153–155] Iron-deficient mothers are likely to have smaller babies with low iron reserves.[156–159] Although some groups have suggested that routine iron supplementation of pregnant women is not indicated,[160] most experts agree that iron supplementation during pregnancy is a desirable, but it is often neglected.[161]

Dietary Iron Deficiency

In infants, iron deficiency is most often a result of the use of unsupplemented milk diets, which contain an inadequate amount of iron. During the first year of life, the full-term infant requires approximately 160 mg and the premature infant approximately 240 mg of iron to meet the needs of an expanding red cell mass. Approximately 50 mg of this need is fulfilled by the destruction of erythrocytes that occurs physiologically during the first week of life. The rest must come from the diet. Milk products are very poor sources of iron, and prolonged breast- or bottle-feeding of infants frequently leads to iron-deficiency anemia unless iron supplementation is implemented. This is especially true of premature infants. Table 42–6 lists the iron content of several widely used infant foods. In recognition of the high prevalence of iron deficiency, and its adverse effects, when infant formula is not iron-supplemented, the American Academy of Pediatrics[162] has urged that all infant formulas be iron-fortified; unfortunately, this practice is not universal in North America. In older children, an iron-poor diet may also contribute to the development of iron-deficiency anemia, particularly during rapid growth periods.

Table 42–7 shows the estimates of average daily iron intake for various segments of the U.S. population. For most persons in the United States, iron intake is approximately 5 to 7 mg/1000 calories. Children and young women are usually in precarious iron balance, their iron intake being less than 80 percent of the recommended daily allowance (RDA).[163] Fortification of bread and cereals with ferrous sulfate or metallic iron[164] is commonplace. When this practice has been suspended because of concern for the possibility of increasing iron storage in patients with the hemochromatosis genotype, the result has been an increased incidence of iron-deficiency anemia.[165]

The scant iron supply of the American diet places young women and children at particular risk of negative iron balance (see Table 42–7). Among men in the 18- to 20-year-old age range, iron deficiency may also be found, presumably because of the iron demands imposed by the recent growth spurt.[166] Because the adult male needs to absorb only approximately 1 mg iron daily from his diet to maintain normal iron balance, iron deficiency in older men is very rarely caused by insufficient

TABLE 42–6. Iron Content of Infant Foods

Liquid Food	Iron Content (mg/L)*
Breast milk	1.1
Evaporated milk	1.8
Evaporated milk, diluted 13:19	0.7
Whole cows' milk	0.7
Similac, "low iron"	1.3
Similac, "with iron"	11.5
Enfamil, "low iron"	0.45
Enfamil, "with iron"	11.5
Semisolid Food	**Iron Content (mg/serving)†**
Cereal, various (Gerber)	6.75
Purees	0–0.60
Vegetables	0.30–1.20
Meat and vegetable mixes	

*For commercially prepared infant formulas, iron content is as stated by manufacturer, in 1999. The brand-name products shown are examples only, and do not imply endorsement by the authors.

†For cereal and puree preparations, iron content was calculated from statement of the manufacturer, ambiguously expressed as "percent of daily amount." Communication with Gerber Products, Inc. indicated that the "daily amount" is 15 mg, i.e., the old RDA (recommended daily allowance) that is 2.5-fold greater than the current RDA for infants. Thus, the many (Gerber) cereal products examined, whether of wheat, rice, or mixed grains, all contain (according to the manufacturer) 6.75 mg of reduced iron per 15 g of dry powder (500 ppm) that is intended to be mixed with water, milk, or formula in volume up to 250 mL, for each serving.

dietary intake alone. Exceptions to this rule are known, such as the case of a man who remained on a nearly iron-free diet for 27 years.[167]

Malabsorption of Iron

Gastric secretion of hydrochloric acid is often reduced in iron deficiency.[168–171] Histamine-fast achlorhydria has been found in as many as 43 percent of patients with iron deficiency.[126,171] Gastric function may improve after correction of the iron deficiency, so that iron deficiency may be both a cause and a result of impairment of gastric iron secretion. However, in persons older than the age of 30 years, the achlorhydria is usually irreversible.[172] Furthermore, when atrophic gastritis coexists with iron deficiency, no improvement in gastric secretory function has followed iron therapy.[173] Autoimmune gastritis often associated with *H. pylori* infection may play an important role in both iron-deficiency anemia and, in later life, in the development of pernicious anemia.[174,175]

Intestinal malabsorption of iron is quite an uncommon cause of iron deficiency except after gastrointestinal surgery and in malabsorption syndromes. Ten to 34 percent of patients who have undergone subtotal gastric resection develop iron-deficiency anemia years later.[121] Many such patients have impaired absorption of food iron, caused in part by more rapid gastrojejunal transit and in part by partially digested food bypassing some of the duodenum as a result of the location of the anastomosis. Fortunately, medicinal iron is well absorbed in post–partial gastrectomy patients. Moreover, gastrointestinal blood loss may also play an important role in anemia following gastric resection (see "Bleeding, Gastrointestinal" above). In malabsorption syndromes, absorption of iron may be so limited that iron-deficiency anemia develops over a period of years. Celiac disease, whether overt or occult, may be associated with iron-deficiency anemia.[121,176]

Intravascular Hemolysis and Hemoglobinuria

Iron-deficiency anemia may occur in paroxysmal nocturnal hemoglobinuria (see Chap. 40) and in hemolysis resulting from mechanical erythrocyte trauma from intracardiac myxomas,[177] valvular prostheses, or patches[178–180] (see Chaps. 32 and 51). In these disorders, iron is lost in the urine as hemosiderin and ferritin in desquamated tubular cells, and as hemoglobin dimers.[180]

Iron deficiency occurs frequently in athletes engaged in a variety of sports (see Chaps. 32 and 51). There may be mild anemia. Increased intravascular hemolysis,[181] presumably with some renal loss of iron, may play a role, but gastrointestinal blood loss has been demonstrated in persons engaged in strenuous athletic pursuits, and this is presumably the major cause of the iron deficiency.[182–185] Hemoglobinuria and hemosiderinuria is also seen in competitive and recreational runners, that is, *march hemoglobinuria* (see Chaps. 32 and 51).

TABLE 42–7. Daily Dietary Iron Intake in the United States, Mean Values for Selected Groups*

Daily (age and sex)	Estimated Fe Intake (mg/day)	Recommended Daily Allowance (mg)	Percent of Recommended Allowance
Infant, 6–11 months	11.9	6	200
Child, 1–2 years	8.4	10	84
Female, 14–30 years	10.5	15	70
Female, pregnant	14	30	47
Female, lactating	14	15	93
Female, 60–65 years	10.2	10	102
Male, 12 and older	>12	12	>100

*Modified from data obtained during the interval 1982–1984 and published in "Mineral Contents of Foods and Total Diets: The Selected Minerals in Foods Survey, 1982–1984,"[22] and from data collected during 1989–90 in the Third National Health and Nutrition Examination Survey (NHANES-III). The data obtained in these two large surveys, that were undertaken 7 years apart, provided nearly identical results; hence, they have been combined in this table. It should be noted that in the latter survey, RDAs (recommended daily allowances) for iron were based on those recommended in 1989, following substantial reduction in the estimated dietary iron requirements for infants, children, and young females. Differences between ethnic groups were negligible. To simplify the table, results for all males age 12 and older were combined, as there were only minimal differences between the age groups. A similar simplification occurred by combining data for all females in the age range 14 to 30 years, exclusive of those who were pregnant or lactating.

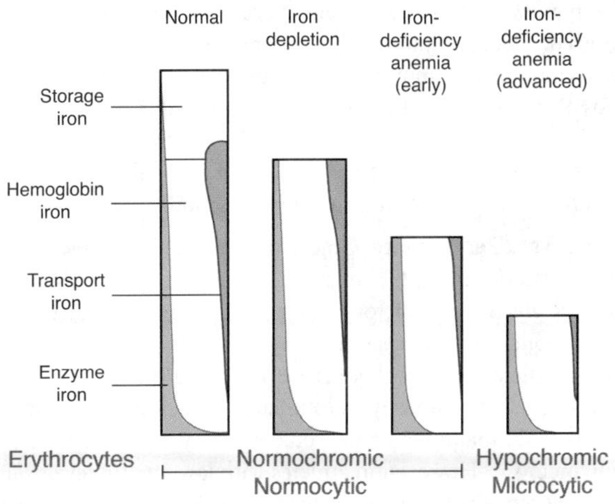

FIGURE 42–8. Stages in the development of iron deficiency. Early iron deficiency (iron depletion) is usually not accompanied by any abnormalities in blood; at this stage, serum iron concentration is occasionally below normal values and storage iron is markedly depleted. As iron deficiency progresses, development of anemia precedes appearance of morphologic changes in blood, although some cells may be smaller and paler than normal; serum iron concentration is usually low at this time, but it may be normal. With advanced iron depletion, classic changes of hypochromic, microcytic, hypoferremic anemia become manifest. *(Used with permission from* Lichtman's Atlas of Hematology, *www.accessmedicine.com.)*

Genetic Factors

Based on twin studies,[186] genetic factors play a role in iron deficiency. A transferrin polymorphism that may increase the risk of developing iron-deficiency anemia,[18] a platelet collagen receptor polymorphism,[187] and mutations of the membrane serine protease tmprss6[67] have been identified as genetic factors that cause or predispose to iron deficiency.

PATHOGENESIS

As iron deficiency develops different compartments are depleted in iron in a sequential, overlapping fashion, as illustrated schematically in Figure 42–8.

Erythrocyte Survival and Ferrokinetics

Slight to moderate shortening of erythrocyte survival is characteristic of iron-deficiency anemia, particularly when it is severe.[188,189] A study of the movement of iron between various iron compartments (e.g., plasma pool, labile pool, and hemoglobin compartment) may be performed by intravenous injection of radioactive iron (^{59}Fe) followed by measurement of the rate of clearance of ^{59}Fe from plasma and of its incorporation into the hemoglobin of circulating erythrocytes. Chapter 31 discusses the principles underlying such "ferrokinetic" studies.

In iron deficiency, plasma iron clearance is rapid and is closely inversely correlated with the serum iron concentration. The plasma iron transport rate may be normal or increased. The percentage of iron utilized in hemoglobin synthesis is normal or increased.[189] There is usually little or no evidence of ineffective erythropoiesis.

Iron-Containing Proteins

As the body becomes depleted of iron, changes occur in many tissues. Hemosiderin and ferritin virtually disappear from marrow and other storage sites. There is a decreased activity of many other important iron proteins: cytochrome c, cytochrome oxidase, succinic dehydrogenase, aconitase,[9,10,190] xanthine oxidase,[191] and myoglobin.[192] Reduced activity has also been reported for some enzymes that do not contain or require iron. Phosphocreatine content is decreased and inorganic phosphorus is increased in skeletal muscle of iron-deficient rats.[193] Many of the affected enzymes are in the oxidative glycolytic (Krebs) cycle of mitochondria. Conversely, the activities of several mitochondrial matrix enzymes are increased in skeletal muscle of iron-deficient animals.[193,194]

In iron deficiency the levels of some of the proteins involved in iron homeostasis—dcytb, hephaestin, DMT-1, and ferroportin—are upregulated.[195]

Muscular Function and Exercise Tolerance

Iron-deficient rats have impaired exercise tolerance and are prone to lactic acidosis when exercised. The activity of α-glycerophosphate dehydrogenase was diminished in the skeletal muscle of iron-deficient rats, and this finding might explain the greater proclivity of iron-deficient rats to lactic acidosis[196] upon exercise. However, in skeletal muscle of iron-deficient guinea pigs, the activity of this enzyme is normal.[197] The brown fat of iron-deficient rats has lower-than-normal activities of the reduced form of nicotinamide adenine dinucleotide and of succinate and α-glycerophosphate oxidases.[198]

Besides these metabolic aberrations of muscle cells in iron deficient rodents, ultrastructural studies show swollen mitochondria with distorted cristae, and there is evidence of mitochondrial DNA damage.[199] Despite these changes, mitochondrial cytochrome c increases adaptively on repetitive electrical stimulus of muscle.[200]

A study of energy transport pathways of submitochondrial particles of rat liver and skeletal muscle showed the latter to be less sensitive to iron depletion than the former.[201] Phosphorus-31 magnetic resonance spectroscopy studies demonstrated increased breakdown of phosphocreatine in muscles of iron-deficient rats,[202] but mitochondrial abnormalities could not be demonstrated in humans.[203]

In human athletes, iron supplementation has been associated with improved performance,[204–206] although earlier studies did not document any aberrations in oxygen consumption in exercising iron-deficient human subjects.[207]

Neurologic Changes

Monoamine oxidase (MAO) activity is low in the liver and platelets of patients with iron deficiency.[208–211] MAO is involved in the synthesis and catabolism of important neurotransmitters such as dopamine, norepinephrine, and serotonin. Furthermore, iron-deficient children and iron-deficient rats excrete substantially more urinary norepinephrine than do iron-replete children or rats, an anomaly that is corrected within a few days of inception of iron therapy.[210,211] The brains of iron-deficient rats exhibit reduction in the number of dopamine D2 receptors that are also important in neurotransmission.[212]

Weanling rats given iron-deficient diets showed poor feeding efficiency, growth retardation, decrease in concentration and greater than normal rates of turnover of norepinephrine in brown fat and heart, hypertrophy of brown fat and heart, reduction in plasma thyroxine and triiodothyronine, low hepatic content of carnitine, and impaired ketogenesis.[213,214] Prolonged iron deficiency in rats also caused abnormal formation of teeth[215] and cochlea,[216] and hearing loss.[217] However, these effects have not been described in humans.

Host Defenses

Iron deficiency affects immune function and the susceptibility to infection.[218,219] Some studies found that iron depletion prevents growth of microorganisms and therefore protects against infections; others observed that iron deficiency impairs host defenses.[220–224] Iron-deficient mice fail to develop autoimmune encephalomyelitis, an animal model of human multiple sclerosis.[225]

Growth and Metabolism

Iron-deficiency anemia is associated with reduction in children's height,[226,227] and treatment promotes growth.[228] Together with zinc deficiency, it has been held responsible for dwarfism.[229] The larger birth weight of infants from iron-supplemented mothers is discussed above (see "Pregnancy and Parturition" above). Impaired thermoregulation has also been demonstrated.[230]

Histologic Findings

Iron deficiency may lead to histologic changes in various organs. The rapidly proliferating cells of the upper part of the alimentary tract seem particularly susceptible to the effect of iron deficiency. There may be atrophy of the mucosa of the tongue and esophagus,[231] stomach,[232,233] and small intestine.[234] The epithelium of the lateral margins of the tongue is reduced in thickness despite increase in the progenitor compartment. This thinning presumably reflects accelerated exfoliation of epithelial cells.[235] Buccal mucosa has shown thinning and keratinization of epithelium and increased mitotic activity.[236,237] However, light microscopic and electron microscopic examination of exfoliated oral mucosal cells showed no aberrations in morphology of nuclei or cytoplasm of the cells of patients with iron-deficiency anemia.[238]

In iron-deficiency anemia resulting from idiopathic pulmonary hemosiderosis, characteristic pathologic changes are found in the lungs, including intense deposition of iron in the littoral cells of the alveoli and interstitial fibrosis.[239]

Widening of diploic spaces of bones, particularly those of the skull and hands,[240,241] may be a consequence of chronic iron deficiency beginning in infancy. In the skull, this is of the same character as in thalassemia, except that in β-thalassemia major there is maxillary hypertrophy, whereas in severe iron-deficiency anemia maxillary growth and pneumatization are normal. The sella turcica may be abnormally small in iron-deficient children, and it has been suggested that this implies reduction in pituitary hormonal secretion in long-standing iron-deficiency anemia.[242]

CLINICAL FEATURES

Clinical Manifestations of Anemia

The anemia in iron-deficient patients can be very severe, with blood hemoglobin levels of <4g/dL being encountered in some patients. Severe iron-deficiency anemia is associated with all of the various symptoms of anemia, resulting from hypoxia and the body's response to hypoxia, as described in Chap. 31. Thus, tachycardia with palpitations and pounding in the ears, headache, light-headedness and even angina pectoris may all occur in patients who are severely anemic.

Clinical Manifestations That May Be Unrelated to Anemia

The clinical features of iron-deficiency encompass those caused by a deficiency of an element essential for life, *viz.* iron, and symptoms caused by the anemia itself. The question of whether these can, at least in some patients, be dissociated is one that is difficult to approach experimentally, and the question of whether or not "iron deficiency without anemia" can cause symptoms cannot be considered definitively settled. Nonetheless, the idea that clinical chlorosis could occur without anemia has been observed clinically for more than a century (see refs. 41 and 243 for reviews), and a number of controlled studies seemed to show that various manifestations of iron-deficiency anemia can occur in individuals whose hemoglobin is within the accepted normal range,[206,243–248] but there also have been a few studies in which no effect could be discerned.[249] In one randomized, double-blind study, patients with iron deficiency had greater symptomatic improvement with iron medication than with placebos[243]; in other studies with a somewhat different experimental design, this was not true.[250,251] However, it is clear from a number of controlled studies, both in infants[252,253] and in adults,[254] that frank anemia is not required for iron deficiency to impair function.

Decreased Work Performance Objective measurements of work performance and studies using O_2 consumption as an index of work performance have given contradictory results, but a comprehensive review[255] led to the conclusion that severe iron deficiency (Hgb <8 g/dL) and mild iron deficiency (Hgb between 8 and 12 g/dL) led to decreased work performance, primarily as estimated by VO_2max measurements, but the evidence that nonanemic iron deficiency had such an effect was less convincing.[255] However, in athletes with low ferritin levels but normal hemoglobin levels, iron-supplemented subjects showed an increased VO_2max without a change in their red cell mass,[245] and in other studies nonanemic subjects treated with iron showed improved performance and/or VO_2max.[205,206,246–248]

Headache Although iron-deficient patients frequently complain of headache,[256–258] headache is a common symptom and the data that have been presented are all anecdotal.

Paresthesia and Other Neurologic Symptoms Paresthesia is thought to be common in iron deficiency,[256] but there are no controlled studies to support this impression. Our investigations show that numbness in the extremities is no more common in iron-deficient than in iron-sufficient patients (Table 42–8). In children, breath-holding spells have been attributed to iron deficiency.[259] Anecdotal reports of intracranial hypertension with papilledema[257,259–262] are buttressed by apparent response to iron therapy. Stroke in children has been associated with iron-deficiency anemia.[259,263] The thrombocytosis that may sometimes accompany iron deficiency may play a pathogenic role.[263,264]

Oral and Nasopharyngeal Symptoms Burning of the tongue[265,266] has also been described anecdotally in many accounts of iron deficiency, and although this symptom has been observed to diminish with treatment, no controlled studies have been performed. The tongue symptoms may be a result of concurrent pyridoxine deficiency.[267] We have had the opportunity of comparing the frequencies of these symptoms in a large population of women attending a health appraisal clinic, and found that none of these symptoms occurred at a higher frequency in an iron-deficient group of women (TS <16%; serum ferritin <20 ng/mL) when compared with a group of iron-sufficient women (TS >20%; serum ferritin >60 ng/mL) (see Table 42–8). Although iron deficiency has been proposed as a cause of atrophic rhinitis,[268,269] the evidence for this is equivocal; perhaps it is a contributory factor.

Dysphagia In the laryngopharynx, mucosal atrophy may lead to web formation in the postcricoid region, thereby giving rise to dysphagia (Paterson-Kelly also known as Plummer-Vinson syndrome).[270] If these alterations are of long duration, they may lead to pharyngeal carcinoma. Although it has been generally thought that these changes are secondary to long-standing iron deficiency, this mechanism is not universally accepted.[266]

The frequency of the condition is considered to have decreased considerably,[270] and its very existence has sometimes been doubted, although cases with the features of this disorder continue to be reported,[271–273] even in children.[273] Abnormal motility of the esophagus has also been documented in iron-deficient patients.[274]

Menstrual Bleeding An increase in the volume of menstrual blood loss has been considered to be both a result and a cause of iron deficiency,[275,276] but this observation has been disputed.[277]

TABLE 42–8. Frequency of Some Findings Commonly Ascribed to Iron Deficiency in White Women Aged 20–49 Attending a Health Appraisal Clinic

Symptom	Iron Deficient (No.)	Iron Nondeficient (No.)	Iron Deficient, Hgb <10 g/dL
Frequent headaches	30.8% (452)	30.7% (685)	40.0% (15)
Mouth, tongue, or jaw problem	18.5% (470)	17.4% (688)	12.5% (16)
Numbness in hands or feet	38.8% (469)	36.6% (687)	62.5% (16)
Tired or decreased energy	41.2% (461)	38.9% (684)	43.8% (16)
Severe fatigue, tiredness, or exhaustion	19.1% (450)	19.7% (678)	33.3% (15)
White blood count (per μL)	6512 ± 1681 (131)	6878 ± 1825 (2499)	6237 ± 930 (16)
Platelet count (per μL)	297,309 (131)	255,731 ± 56,167 (2499)	341,875 ± 100,782 (16)

No. = the number of women responding to the question on the questionnaire.

Pica The craving to eat unusual substances, for example, dirt, clay, ice, laundry starch, salt, cardboard, and hair, is a classic manifestation of iron deficiency and is usually cured promptly by iron therapy.[278,279]

Hair Loss It has been suggested that hair loss may be a consequence of iron deficiency and in one study there were significantly lowered ferritin levels in women with androgenetic alopecia and alopecia areata, but not in those women with telogen effluvium (a form of nonscarring alopecia characterized by diffuse hair shedding) or alopecia areata totalis/universalis,[280] but the validity of a cause-and-effect relationship has been challenged.[281] In a large multivariate analysis, low ferritin levels were a risk factor for hair loss.[282]

Infant and Childhood Development In infants iron deficiency is associated with poor attention span, poor response to sensory stimuli, and retarded behavioral and developmental achievement even in the absence of anemia.[252,253,259,283–288] Although a considerable number of studies with a positive outcome have been reported, many of these have been criticized because of a lack of controls, and the possibility that socioeconomic factors may have a confounding effect.[289]

Hyperactivity Syndromes It has been speculated that there is a relationship between restless legs syndrome, Tourette syndrome, and attention deficit hyperactivity disorder and that iron deficiency contributes to their pathophysiology.[290] Restless legs syndrome, a common nocturnal problem, especially in the elderly, has been associated with iron deficiency and reported to improve on therapy,[291–294] but controlled studies have shown only minor benefit or none at all.[294,295] In children there may be a relationship between iron deficiency and attention deficit hyperactivity disorder.[294]

Physical Findings

The physical findings in iron-deficiency anemia include pallor, glossitis (smooth, red tongue), stomatitis, and angular cheilitis. Koilonychia, once a common finding, is now encountered rarely (Fig. 42–9). Retinal hemorrhages and exudates may be seen in severely anemic patients (e.g., hemoglobin concentration of <5 g/dL). Splenomegaly has occasionally been attributed to iron-deficiency anemia,[166] but when it occurs, it is probably from other causes.[296]

LABORATORY FEATURES

In severe, uncomplicated iron-deficiency anemia, the erythrocytes are hypochromic and microcytic; the plasma iron concentration is diminished; the iron-binding capacity is increased; the serum ferritin concentration is low; the serum transferrin receptor and erythrocyte zinc protoporphyrin concentrations are increased; and the marrow is depleted of stainable iron. Unfortunately, the classic combination of laboratory findings occurs consistently only when iron-deficiency anemia is far advanced, when there are no complicating factors such as infection or malignant neoplasms, and when there has not been previous therapy with transfusions or parenteral iron.

Blood Cells

Erythrocytes Anisocytosis is the earliest recognizable morphologic change of erythrocytes in iron-deficiency anemia (Fig. 42–10).[297,298] The anisocytosis is typically accompanied by mild ovalocytosis. As the iron deficiency worsens, a mild normochromic, normocytic anemia often develops.[297–301] With further progression, hemoglobin concentration,

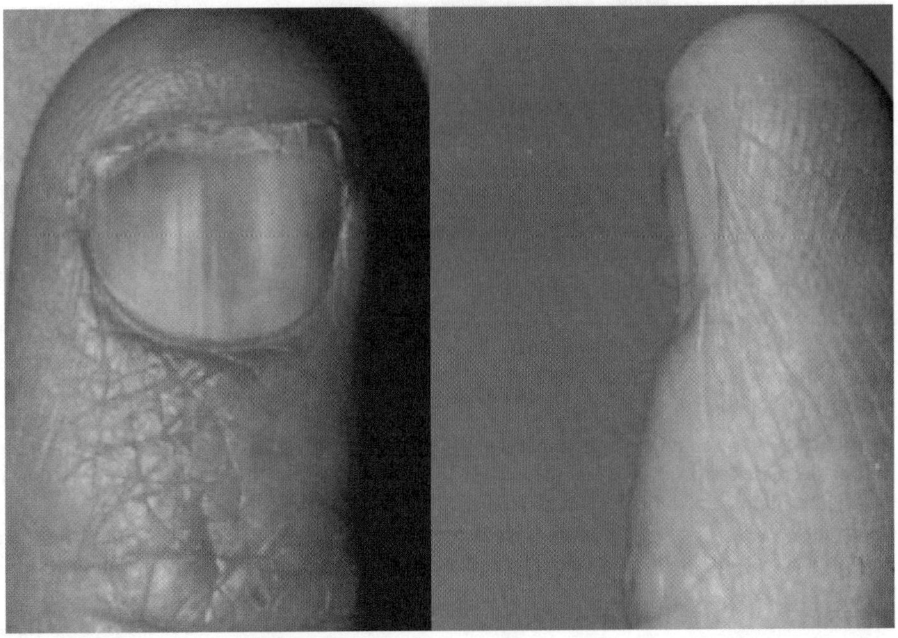

FIGURE 42–9. Koilonychia. Note the ridging, thinning, and spoon-like concavity of the fingernails. *(Used with permission from* Lichtman's Atlas of Hematology, *www.accessmedicine.com.)*

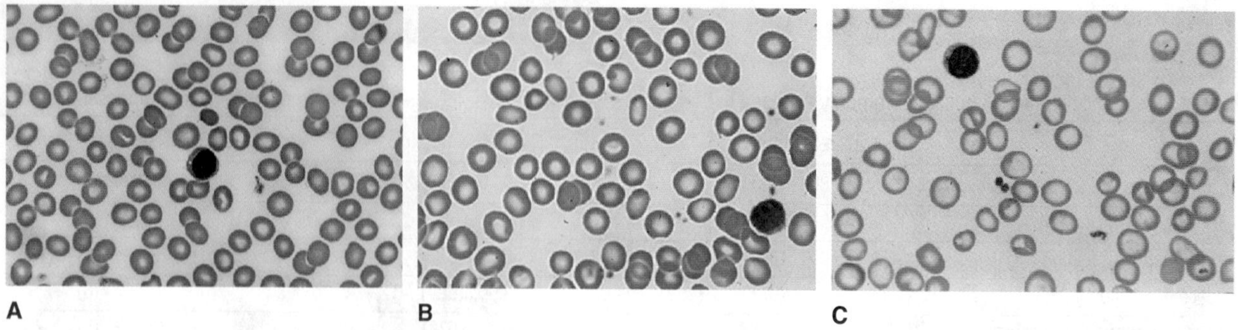

FIGURE 42–10. Variability in morphologic diagnosis of iron-deficiency anemia from blood film. As in all deficiency states leading to anemia, the blood film morphology and blood cell changes are a function of the severity of the deficiency. **A.** Normal blood film. Normocytic-normochromic red cells with normal shape. **B.** Mild iron deficiency. Serum iron, ferritin, and transferring saturation were consistent with mild iron deficiency. Cannot discern if mean red cell size has decreased. There may be a few red cells that have larger central pallor, but arguable. A few cells have oval or elliptical shape. **C.** Severe iron deficiency. Serum iron, ferritin, and transferring saturation were consistent with severe iron deficiency. Note obvious increase in overtly hypochromic cells and higher frequency of microcytes. *(Used with permission from* Lichtman's Atlas of Hematology, *www.accessmedicine.com.)*

erythrocyte count, mean corpuscular volume (MCV), and mean erythrocyte hemoglobin content all decline together. In infants and children, hypochromia may occur earlier in the course of iron deficiency, and erythrocyte counts in excess of 5×10^{12}/L (5,000,000/μL) are sometimes encountered.[302] As the indices change the erythrocytes appear microcytic and hypochromic on stained blood films. Target cells may sometimes be present. Elongated hypochromic elliptocytes may be seen, in which the long sides are nearly parallel. Such cells have been called "pencil cells," although they more nearly resemble cigars in shape.

The red cell indices are consistently abnormal in adults only when iron-deficiency anemia is moderate or severe (e.g., in males with hemoglobin concentrations <12 g/dL or in women with hemoglobin concentrations <10 g/dL) (Fig. 42–11). The distribution of erythrocyte volume (e.g., red cell distribution width [RDW]) is usually increased in established iron-deficiency anemia. The RDW is reported often as the coefficient of variation (in percent) of erythrocyte volume (see "Differential Diagnosis" below). The sensitivity and specificity of erythrocyte indices for iron deficiency may be increased by use of formulae that incorporate MCV, RDW, serum ferritin concentration, and serum transferrin saturation to produce an iron index[303] or combinations of other functions.[304,305]

Leukocytes Leukopenia has been found in some patients with iron-deficiency anemia,[171] but the overall distribution of leukocyte counts in iron-deficient patients seems to be approximately normal.[299]

Platelets Thrombocytopenia and thrombocytosis have both been attributed to iron deficiency. Thrombocytosis has been reported in 50 to 75 percent of adults with classic iron-deficiency anemia caused by chronic blood loss.[299,306] However, thrombocytosis usually occurs only in those patients who are actively bleeding.[307] In infants and children, thrombocytopenia occurs almost as frequently (28%) as does thrombocytosis (35%); thrombocytopenia is associated with more severe anemia.[308,309] Marked thrombocytopenia may also occur in iron-deficient adults, either as the presenting hematologic problem or early during the response to iron therapy for anemia.[310–312]

Reticulocytes It is sometimes stated that the reticulocyte count is normal or decreased in iron deficiency,[166,265] but in series of patients in which the number of reticulocytes is reported, the number is often mildly increased,[234,299,313,314] a finding consistent with the increased erythroid activity of the marrow (see "Marrow" below).

Marrow

Both the degree of cellularity of the marrow and the relative proportion of erythroid to myeloid cells are variable.[315] In severe iron deficiency, erythroblasts of the marrow may be smaller than normal, with narrow, ragged rims of cytoplasm containing little hemoglobin. However, the morphologic changes in the marrow are not sufficiently distinctive to be of diagnostic value.

Decreased or absent hemosiderin in the marrow is characteristic of iron deficiency. Hemosiderin appears in the unstained marrow film as golden refractile granules, but the hemosiderin content of the marrow film is more readily and more reliably evaluated after staining by the simple Prussian blue method. Stored iron in the macrophages of the marrow can be seen in marrow spicules in marrow sections, or in marrow aspirate films. Iron granules, normally found in the cytoplasm of approximately 30 percent of erythroblasts, become rare but may not be entirely absent.

Because most body iron is divided between stores and the red cell mass, and iron is not excreted, most anemias are characterized by increased storage iron. Iron-deficiency anemia is the exception, as iron stores are depleted before the red cell mass is compromised. Thus, evaluation of iron stores should be a sensitive and usually reliable means for the differentiation between iron-deficiency anemia and all other anemias. Clinically, this is most directly achieved by evaluating the amount of iron in marrow macrophages, and this direct assessment of iron stores has long been considered the "gold standard" for the diagnosis of iron deficiency.[316,317] There are, however, technical barriers to the accurate histochemical determination of marrow iron. First, an invasive procedure, marrow aspiration, is required. Second, the differentiation of iron within macrophages from artifacts is no trivial matter, and it takes considerable experience and skill to obtain accurate results. In one study only 74 of 108 cases had been accurately reported.[318] Moreover, misleading results may be obtained in patients who have been transfused or who have been treated with parenteral iron.[317] The marrow of such patients may contain normal, or even increased, quantities of stainable iron in the face of typical iron-responsive iron-deficiency anemia. In such patients, iron that is seen on marrow examination is not readily available for erythropoiesis. Furthermore, the ability of marrow to store iron seems to be impaired in some patients with chronic myelogenous leukemia,[319] and possibly in those with myelofibrosis. In such patients, absence of marrow iron is often observed without other evidence of iron deficiency, and such patients do not respond to iron therapy. For such reasons the primacy of marrow iron estimation has been questioned.[320]

Serum Iron Concentration

The serum iron concentration is usually low in untreated iron-deficiency anemia; however, it may be normal.[301,321,322] The serum iron concentration

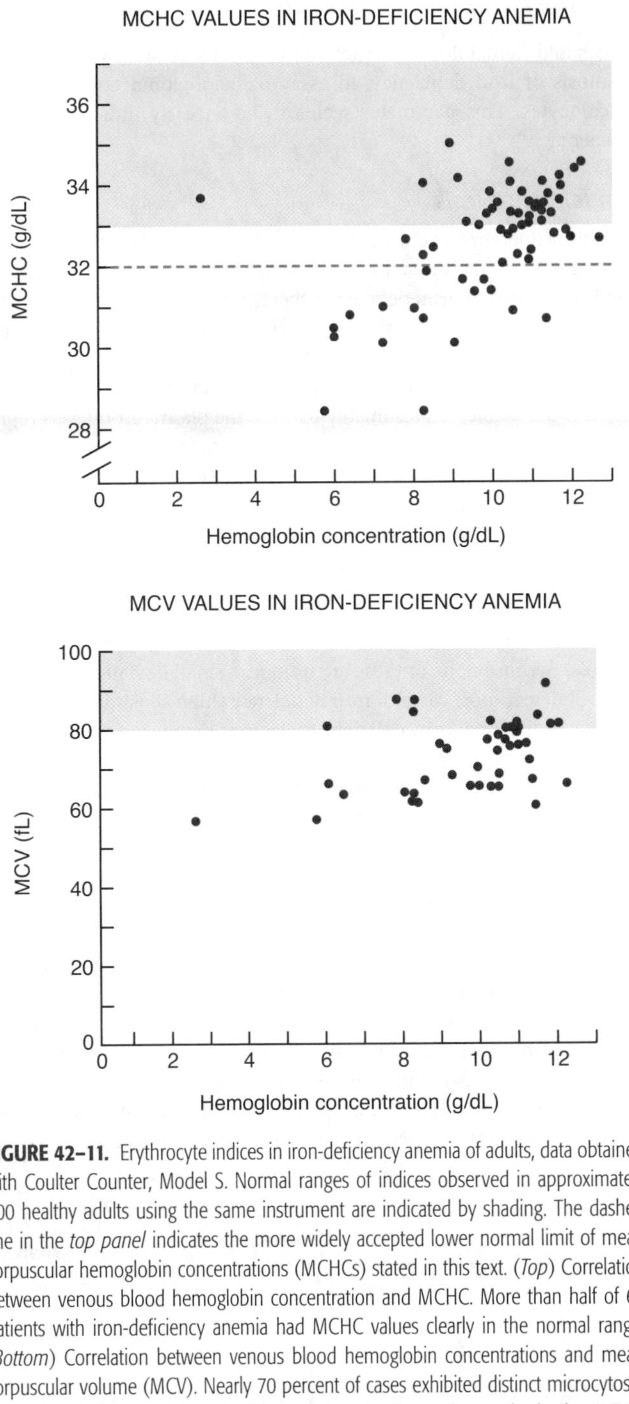

FIGURE 42–11. Erythrocyte indices in iron-deficiency anemia of adults, data obtained with Coulter Counter, Model S. Normal ranges of indices observed in approximately 500 healthy adults using the same instrument are indicated by shading. The dashed line in the *top panel* indicates the more widely accepted lower normal limit of mean corpuscular hemoglobin concentrations (MCHCs) stated in this text. (*Top*) Correlation between venous blood hemoglobin concentration and MCHC. More than half of 62 patients with iron-deficiency anemia had MCHC values clearly in the normal range. (*Bottom*) Correlation between venous blood hemoglobin concentrations and mean corpuscular volume (MCV). Nearly 70 percent of cases exhibited distinct microcytosis. Thus when indices are determined by automated cell-counting methods, the MCV is much more sensitive than is the MCHC in detecting changes of iron deficiency. However, at least 30 percent of cases of iron-deficiency anemia will be misdiagnosed if physicians rely on the erythrocyte indices. *(From Beutler E, Fairbanks VF,[704] with permission from Academic Press.)*

also is influenced by many pathologic and physiologic states. Physiologically, the serum iron concentration has a diurnal rhythm; it decreases in late afternoon and evening, reaching a nadir near 9 PM and increases to its maximum between 7 and 10 AM. Although numerous studies show that diurnal variation occurs,[323–325] it is doubtful whether this is of sufficient clinical importance to require all serum iron values to be drawn in the morning.[326] Serum iron levels decrease at about the time of menstrual bleeding, either when menses are under normal hormonal control[327,328] or when bleeding occurs after withdrawal of oral contraceptive agents.[140,329] The serum iron concentration is reduced in the presence of either acute or chronic inflammatory processes[330,331] or malignancy[332] and following acute myocardial infarction.[333,334] The serum iron concentration under these circumstances may be decreased sufficiently to suggest iron deficiency. Conversely, during chemotherapy of malignancy, the serum iron concentration may be quite elevated. This effect is observed from the third to the seventh day after inception of chemotherapy of a variety of tumors.[335]

Normal or high concentrations of serum iron are commonly observed even in patients with iron-deficiency anemia if such patients receive iron medication before blood is drawn for these measurements. Even multiple vitamin preparations, which commonly contain approximately 18 mg of elemental iron per tablet, can result in this effect. Oral iron medication should be withheld for 24 hours. Parenteral injection of iron dextran may result in a very high serum iron concentration (e.g., 500 to 1000 mcg/dL), at least with some methods,[336] for several weeks. The elevation of serum iron levels after infusion of sodium ferric gluconate or iron sucrose is of much shorter duration[337,338] and is unlikely to interfere with the diagnostic value of the serum iron level.

Iron-Binding Capacity and Transferrin Saturation

The iron-binding capacity is a measure of the amount of transferrin in circulating blood. Normally, there is enough transferrin present in 100 mL serum to bind 4.4 to 8.0 μmol (250 to 450 mcg) of iron; because the normal serum iron concentration is approximately 1.8 μmol/dL (100 mcg/dL), transferrin may be found to be approximately one-third saturated with iron. The unsaturated or latent iron-binding capacity (UIBC) is easily measured with radioactive iron or by spectrophotometric techniques. The sum of the UIBC and the plasma iron represents total iron-binding capacity (TIBC). TIBC may also be measured directly. In iron-deficiency anemia, UIBC and TIBC are often increased; a transferrin saturation of 15 percent or less is usually found. However, exceptions are so common as to detract considerably from the diagnostic value of measuring transferrin saturation in the diagnosis of iron deficiency.[317,339] A normal value for transferrin saturation often accompanies a low serum iron concentration in the anemia of chronic inflammation.

Serum Ferritin

Serum ferritin contains relatively little iron, yet serum ferritin concentration correlates with total-body iron stores,[340,341] although the correlation is not as strong as has sometimes been suggested.[342–344] Serum ferritin concentrations of 10 mcg/L or less are characteristic of iron-deficiency anemia. In iron deficiency without anemia, serum ferritin concentration is typically in the range of 10 to 20 mcg/L. In one series of 73 patients, marrow iron was depleted whenever the serum ferritin level was less than 70 mcg/L.[345] In another study in which patients with iron-deficiency anemia were compared with those with anemia of chronic inflammation, a cutoff point of 32 mcg/L provided a sensitivity of 79.2 percent and a specificity of 96.9 percent.[346] A moderate increase in serum ferritin concentration occurs in inflammatory disorders, such as rheumatoid arthritis, in chronic renal disease, and in malignancies.[347] In Gaucher disease, the serum ferritin concentration is commonly in the range of thousands of mcg/L.[348,349] When one of these conditions coexists with iron deficiency, as they often do, the serum ferritin concentration is commonly in the normal range; interpretation of results of this assay then becomes difficult. In patients with rheumatoid arthritis who are anemic, concomitant iron deficiency may be suspected when the serum ferritin concentration is less than 60 mcg/L.[350] Moderate increases in serum ferritin concentrations are also characteristic of some malignancies and may closely reflect remissions and relapses.[351] Increases in serum ferritin concentration occur in patients with hepatitis[352] and in patients with end-stage renal disease.[353]

Oral or parenteral iron administration also increases serum ferritin concentration.[354] This appears to be particularly a problem in infants given oral iron.[355] In adults with iron-deficiency anemia given oral iron in a dose of 60 mg of elemental iron thrice daily, the serum ferritin concentration remained below 10 mcg/L for 2 to 3 weeks.[354] However, the serum ferritin assay is unreliable in confirming a diagnosis of iron deficiency when iron therapy has been given for more than 3 weeks. Parenteral administration of iron dextran results in a rise in serum ferritin concentration to normal or supranormal values within 24 hours, and this effect persists for at least a month.[354]

Erythrocyte Ferritin

Erythrocyte ferritin concentration is increased in thalassemias and sideroblastic anemias, and decreased in iron deficiency. These changes appear to parallel those of serum ferritin concentration, although it has been suggested that basic red cell ferritin is not influenced by inflammation, and could therefore detect iron deficiency when the erythrocyte ferritin concentration was normal in the elderly.[356] In another study of anemic males, erythrocyte ferritin determinations appeared to have no more value than those of serum ferritin. The combination of both was more effective in the diagnosis of iron deficiency.[357] Erythrocyte ferritin levels are currently rarely used in the diagnosis of iron deficiency.

Erythrocyte Zinc Protoporphyrin

Erythrocyte protoporphyrin, principally zinc protoporphyrin, is increased in disorders of heme synthesis, including iron deficiency, lead poisoning, and sideroblastic anemias, as well as other conditions. This procedure requires small blood samples. It is quite sensitive in the diagnosis of iron deficiency and practical for large-scale screening programs designed to identify children with either iron deficiency or lead poisoning.[358] It does not differentiate between iron deficiency and chronic lead poisoning[359] or the anemia that accompanies inflammatory or malignant processes.[360]

Serum Transferrin Receptor

The role of transferrin receptor in transporting transferrin iron into cells is described earlier (see "Transport of Iron" above). The circulating receptor is a truncated form of the cellular receptor, lacking the transmembrane and cytoplasmic domains of the cellular receptor. It circulates bound to transferrin. Sensitive immunologic methods can detect approximately 5 mg/L of receptor in serum. The levels of circulating transferrin receptor apparently mirror the amount of cellular receptor, and because receptor synthesis is greatly increased when cells lack iron, the amount of the circulating receptor increases in iron deficiency but not in the anemia of chronic inflammation.[361–363] This test for iron deficiency has gradually come into clinical use, but the methodology has not yet been standardized, making laboratory-to-laboratory comparisons difficult. Like the serum ferritin and serum iron, serum transferrin receptor assay results may be confounded by poorly understood variations in patients with malignancies; in patients in whom the serum transferrin receptor concentration is reduced; and in patients with rheumatoid arthritis or thalassemia trait, in whom, in the absence of iron deficiency, it is increased. A method for performing reproducible assays for the soluble transferrin receptor has been standardized.[364] The ratio of serum transferrin receptor to serum ferritin seems to be a useful but not infallible reflection of body iron stores.[365–367] However, several studies show that the soluble transferrin index calculated as a ratio of the sTfR/log ferritin (TfR-F Index) is superior to other means for detection of iron deficiency.[368,369]

Reticulocyte Hemoglobin Content

Automated hematology instruments may offer as a new method for diagnosis of iron deficiency an assay of hemoglobin content within reticulocytes. This parameter seems to be an early indicator of iron deficiency.[370–372]

Iron-Tolerance Tests

In an iron-tolerance test, the patient receives an oral dose of an inorganic iron compound, and the subsequent change in the serum iron concentration is measured. In iron deficiency, there is an increased rate of absorption of the test dose, and this is sometimes reflected in a more rapid increase and a higher plateau than in normal subjects. This procedure was espoused for the diagnosis of iron deficiency 60 years ago.[373] However it is unreliable,[317] presumably because the plasma iron levels represent the balance between absorption rate, which is increased in iron deficiency, and iron clearance, which is also increased. Although occasional attempts have been made from to reintroduce this method,[374] particularly using small doses of iron,[375] it is rarely used today.

DIFFERENTIAL DIAGNOSIS

Iron-deficiency anemia is characterized by many abnormal laboratory features. Because none of these are unique, a small deviation from normal will detect most cases of iron deficiency (high sensitivity), but also falsely identify non–iron-deficient subjects as being iron deficient (low specificity). On the other hand, a large deviation from normal will exclude most nondeficient patients (high specificity), but miss many iron-deficient subjects (low sensitivity). This tradeoff is shown graphically in so-called *receiver operator characteristic curves*. These curves are constructed by plotting the sensitivity against the false positive rate (1-specificity) at various values of the analyte. Figure 42–12 shows receiver operator characteristic curve for some tests for iron deficiency. The situation is complicated in the case of iron deficiency by the fact that the diagnostic problem faced by the physician is not one of differentiating a patient with iron-deficiency anemia from a normal person, but rather from a patient who has an anemia with a different etiology. It is partly for this reason that a simple algorithm for the diagnosis of iron deficiency does not exist. In a severely anemic patient, microcytosis would have very high specificity and high sensitivity compared to nor-

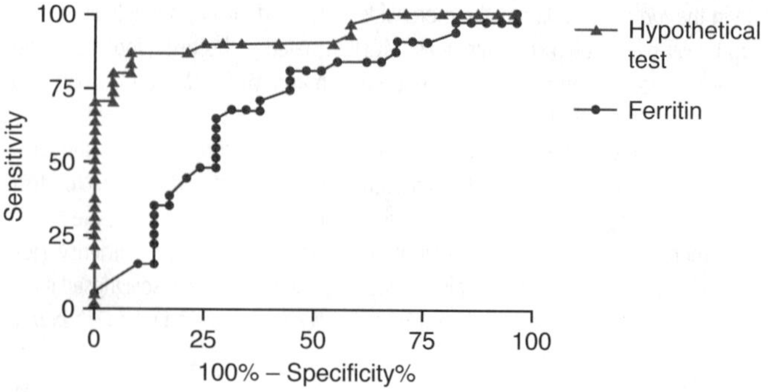

FIGURE 42–12. Two receiver operator curves. As the specificity increases the sensitivity decreases. The receiver-operator properties of serum ferritin are far from ideal. When the specificity is high (to the *left on the abscissa*) the sensitivity is low, only when the specificity is low is the sensitivity adequate. The curve that would be obtained with a nearly ideal test for iron deficiency gives high specificity and high sensitivity. In the curve shown a cutoff value could be found that allows one to identify 75 percent of patients with iron deficiency with a specificity of over 90 percent. Unfortunately, no such test exists.

mal, but compared to a patient with thalassemia the specificity would be very low, indeed. Similarly, a low serum ferritin level is an excellent test in the general population, but it is a relatively little value in patients with chronic renal disease. Another problem that is inherent in evaluating diagnostic tests for iron deficiency is the standard that is applied to decide who is iron deficient and who is not. Marrow iron has served as one "gold standard" but has limitations, as discussed earlier (see "Marrow" above). Alternatively, the response to iron therapy serves as a powerful indicator of whose anemia is actually a result of a deficiency of iron. Here, too, there are limitations, in that some iron-deficient patients may fail to respond adequately because of factors such as infection. Lacking an absolute test for iron deficiency, the ability of the physician to use judgment relevant to the particular patient's circumstances is of paramount importance.

The forms of anemia that must be distinguished from iron-deficiency anemia most frequently include those of thalassemia minor, chronic inflammatory disease, malignancy, chronic liver disease, and chronic renal disease. It is the microcytic anemias that are most likely to be confused with iron deficiency. Table 42–9 summarizes such anemias, and each is discussed elsewhere in this volume. Attention is directed here primarily to laboratory aids for differentiating iron-deficiency anemia from the frequently occurring disorders that may have similar manifestations.

Thalassemia Minor

In many parts of the world, and in many communities of North America, the frequency of β-thalassemia minor is second only to that of iron deficiency as a cause of hypochromic microcytic anemia (see Chap. 47). In African Americans, homozygosity for α-thalassemia-2, that is the state in which only single α-globin gene is present on each chromosome, is a common cause of microcytosis. Approximately 3 percent of African Americans are homozygous for α-thalassemia-2. The condition is associated with only a very modest lowering of the blood hemoglobin level.[376] Heterozygotes may also have microcytosis, although usually they are hematologically normal. Among persons of Mediterranean ancestry both α- and β-thalassemia are very prevalent, particularly the latter. Among Asians, particularly in those from Southeast Asia, α-thalassemia minor, β-thalassemia minor, and hemoglobin E trait, all occur frequently. All are characterized by microcytosis, and none can be distinguished reliably from the others on the basis of erythrocyte morphology or erythrocyte indices alone. In each of these conditions there may be only mild to moderate microcytosis without any other distinctive changes. However, in the majority of patients with α- or β-thalassemia minor, hemoglobin Lepore trait, and hemoglobin E trait, the erythrocyte count is greater than 5×10^{12} per L (5,000,000/μL), despite low hemoglobin concentration.[377,378] Homozygous hemoglobin E is also characterized by marked hypochromia, microcytosis, abundant target cells, and elevated erythrocyte count, but usually not by more than minimal anemia[379] (see Chap. 48).

In contrast to the findings in these hemoglobinopathies, erythrocyte counts of 5×10^{12} per L (5,000,000/μL) or higher are relatively uncommon among adults with iron-deficiency anemia.[380] However, erythrocytosis may be seen in children with iron-deficiency anemia or in polycythemia vera patients who have become iron deficient following hemorrhage or therapeutic phlebotomy.[302] Consequently, while the mean MCV is almost always reduced in α- or β-thalassemia minor and in homozygous hemoglobin E, with values of 60 to 70 fl being the rule, values this low are seen only in severe iron-deficiency anemia. In hemoglobin Lepore trait and hemoglobin E trait, only minimal microcytosis is observed.[377–379] The widespread adoption of the routine measurement of MCV has led to proposals that criteria for differentiation of iron deficiency from thalassemia minor might be based, in part, on the values of the erythrocyte count and the MCV.[381] Some proposed rules[382] could separate iron deficiency from thalassemia minor with 90 percent reliability when groups of iron deficiency and thalassemic patients were of nearly equal numbers. However, in a population in which iron deficiency is more prevalent than thalassemia minor, use of these criteria would result in an excessive number of diagnostic errors. None of these and other proposed rules[383–385] seems completely reliable for distinguishing iron deficiency from thalassemia.

Because anisocytosis is an early morphologic feature of iron deficiency, it has been suggested that measurements of variation in erythrocyte size permit discrimination between iron-deficiency anemia and other microcytic anemias.[383,386] However, hemoglobinopathies and thalassemias[386–388] commonly exhibit increased RDW values, as do some anemias that are a result of chronic inflammation.[310,389,390] Hence, these conditions cannot be differentiated reliably by such measurements.

Mild reticulocytosis, polychromatophilia and basophilic stippling are more likely to be encountered in β-thalassemia minor, $\delta\beta$-thalassemia minor, and hemoglobin Lepore trait than in iron-deficiency anemia, but may be absent in these disorders. The serum iron concentration is usually normal or increased in thalassemic syndromes and is usually low in iron-deficiency anemia. Similarly, examination of marrow iron stores helps to differentiate these disorders. The presence of β-thalassemia trait is substantiated by the demonstration of increased proportions of hemoglobin A_2 and F, or by the presence on electrophoresis of hemoglobin H or Lepore (see Chap. 47). At present, the diagnosis of α-thalassemia minor is usually made on the basis of exclusion of other causes of microcytosis, but it can be confirmed by measuring globin chain synthetic rates or by direct demonstration of mutations in α-globin genes by DNA-based techniques.

Iron deficiency may mask concurrent thalassemia. The amounts of both hemoglobin A_2 and hemoglobin H are diminished disproportion-

TABLE 42–9. Microcytic Disorders That May Be Confused with Iron Deficiency

Thalassemias and hemoglobinopathies (see Chap. 47)
β-Thalassemia major
β-Thalassemia minor
$\delta\beta$-Thalassemia minor
α-Thalassemia-minor
Hemoglobin Lepore trait
Hemoglobin E trait
Homozygous hemoglobin E disease
Hemoglobin H disease
Combination of above (compound heterozygotes)
Blockade of heme synthesis caused by chemicals (see Chaps. 51 and 58)
Lead
Pyrazinamide
Isoniazid
Other disorders
Sideroblastic anemias (see Chap. 58)
Hereditary sex-linked
Idiopathic acquired
Anemia of chronic inflammation (see Chap. 37)
DMT-1 human mutations

ately to the reduction in hemoglobin A in the presence of iron deficiency[391] (see Chap. 46); however, usually the hemoglobin A_2 level remains above the normal range.

Anemia of Chronic Inflammation

The anemia of chronic inflammation (see Chap. 37) is usually normochromic and normocytic, but hypochromic microcytic anemia occurs in 20 to 30 percent of patients with chronic infections or malignancies.[330,331] Thus these disorders cannot be distinguished from iron-deficiency anemia by examination of the blood film. Furthermore, the serum iron concentration is usually decreased in these disorders,[330,331,392] sometimes severely. In iron deficiency, the TIBC is usually increased, whereas in inflammatory and neoplastic diseases it is commonly decreased, but there is considerable overlap among TIBC values of normal subjects, those with iron-deficiency anemia, and those with chronic inflammatory diseases.

In iron-deficiency anemia, the transferrin saturation is usually <16 percent, whereas in chronic inflammation it is usually >16 percent.[331] However, this widely used criterion is actually quite unreliable. Transferrin saturation may be normal in iron-deficiency anemia, and conversely, low saturation is sometimes observed in chronic inflammation.[331] However, circulating soluble transferrin receptors increase in iron deficiency but not in the anemia of chronic inflammation.[347,361–363,393] The serum ferritin level is usually diminished in iron deficiency, but it is generally increased in chronic inflammatory and neoplastic disorders.[345,394] Measurement of the ratio of soluble transferrin receptor to ferritin has been found to be very useful in distinguishing the anemia of chronic inflammation from that of iron deficiency.[393] Examination of the marrow for stainable iron is particularly helpful. The latter is greatly decreased in amount or absent in iron deficiency anemia and normal or increased in the other disorders.

Anemia of Chronic Liver Disease

The erythrocytes in the blood film from patients with chronic liver disease may be normochromic and normocytic, macrocytic, or hypochromic. Target cells are frequently present in large numbers. Because the blood film in iron-deficiency anemia may also display these features, differential diagnosis must be based on other observations. Serum ferritin levels are useful in detecting iron deficiency in the setting of cirrhosis.[395,396] The serum iron concentration, however, does not seem to correlate well with iron stores.[396]

Anemia of Chronic Renal Disease

Iron deficiency is frequent in patients with chronic renal disease (see Chap. 36). Iron-deficiency anemia is particularly difficult to diagnose in patients with chronic renal disease (see Chap. 36). Because the problem is fairly common, and perhaps because of commercial interest in identifying those patients who can benefit from iron therapy, a large number of studies have been done to determine the best way to diagnose iron deficiency in patients undergoing extracorporeal dialysis. The serum iron concentration may be normal or decreased, depending on the cause of the renal disease. In one study,[397] the percentage of hypochromic erythrocytes was the most efficient, with other tests ranking as follows: reticulocyte hemoglobin > soluble transferrin receptor > erythrocyte zinc protoporphyrin > transferrin saturation > ferritin. But in another study[398] the area-under-the-receiver-operating-characteristic curve was largest for serum ferritin and but less for transferrin receptor and erythrocyte ferritin. Other measurements, including the TIBC, transferrin saturation and serum transferrin receptor had even less predictive value. Another comparison showed erythrocyte ferritin to be somewhat less efficient in the diagnosis of iron deficiency than serum ferritin.[398] Still another study[399] averred that the reticulocyte hemoglobin content and reticulocytes in a high-fluorescent-intensity region, a measure of reticulocyte immaturity, were the best methods, particularly if the results of the two tests were combined. Reticulocyte hemoglobin levels have become quite popular in the management of patients in renal failure[372] and may have the advantage of giving results that reflect the current iron status in patients who are being treated.[400]

Anemia of Hemolytic Disease

Hemolytic disease can usually be distinguished from iron-deficiency anemia on the basis of the blood film. The marked poikilocytosis, polychromatophilia, spherocytosis, Heinz bodies, basophilic stippling, and other morphologic features characteristic of various types of hemolysis usually are not seen in iron-deficiency anemia. Furthermore, reticulocytosis is usually marked in hemolytic disorders but minimal or absent in iron-deficiency anemia. However, there are some outstanding exceptions to these generally valid principles.

In unstable hemoglobin disorders, such as hemoglobin H disease or hemoglobin Köln disease, erythrocytic hypochromia may be pronounced. In these disorders, there is moderate reticulocytosis, which helps to differentiate them from iron-deficiency anemia. The serum iron concentration is normal or increased. Chapter 48 discusses the detection of unstable hemoglobins.

When there is chronic intravascular hemolysis, erythrocytes in the blood film may display marked morphologic abnormalities, such as burr cells and schizocytes. Yet, because of loss of iron in the urine, iron deficiency may be the dominant cause of the resulting anemia. Evaluation of iron content in marrow aspirates or measurement of serum iron concentration and TIBC may clarify the diagnosis in this form of anemia.

Hypoplastic and Aplastic Anemia

In their early phases, these disorders cannot reliably be differentiated from mild iron-deficiency anemia on the basis of erythrocyte morphology alone (see Chap. 34). The reticulocyte count is generally less than 0.5 percent in hypoplastic or aplastic anemia. The presence of neutropenia and thrombocytopenia suggests a diagnosis of aplastic anemia, but mild neutropenia may also occur in iron-deficiency anemia.[401] The serum iron concentration is usually increased in aplastic anemia; and the percentage transferrin saturation is then elevated. Marrow aspiration may produce scant material for cytologic study, and marrow biopsy may be necessary. An iron stain usually reveals increased amounts of hemosiderin in aplastic or hypoplastic anemia. However, if chronic bleeding has occurred, for example, as a consequence of thrombocytopenia, iron stores may be depleted.

Myeloproliferative Diseases

In polycythemia vera, erythrocytes may be small and hypochromic (see Chap. 86). Even in the absence of distinctive morphologic changes in erythrocytes, the serum iron concentration is usually decreased, the TIBC is normal or increased, and marrow aspirates show little or no hemosiderin. Ferrokinetic studies show accelerated plasma iron incorporated into the hemoglobin of circulating erythrocytes.[402] These findings simply reflect iron deficiency, which is almost always present in this disease, as a result of marked expansion in total hemoglobin mass, increased gastrointestinal blood loss, and/or therapeutic phlebotomy. The marrow hemosiderin content is often decreased in other myeloproliferative disorders,[319] possibly because of a defect in macrophage storage of iron.

Sideroblastic Anemia

In this heterogeneous group of disorders (see Chap. 58), the blood findings often simulate those of iron-deficiency anemia. Reticulocytosis is usually absent, and the serum iron concentration and serum ferritin is generally normal or increased. Marrow examination shows increased amounts of stainable iron.

Congenital Dyserythropoietic Anemia

In the rare congenital dyserythropoietic anemias (see Chap. 39), erythrocyte morphologic abnormalities may resemble those of iron deficiency or thalassemia (see Chap. 47). In general, in congenital dyserythropoietic anemias, poikilocytosis is very striking and occurs with less reduction in MCV than in iron deficiency or thalassemias. Often, however, such cases are believed to be thalassemic until the marrow is examined.

Megaloblastic Anemia

In pernicious anemia and other types of megaloblastic anemia (see Chap. 41), the blood film usually shows changes sufficiently distinctive that there is little difficulty in differential diagnosis. One potential source of error is the change in serum iron concentration that occurs after therapy. In the patient with pernicious anemia or folic acid deficiency, early after starting treatment, the serum iron concentration decreases markedly as iron is utilized rapidly for hemoglobin synthesis.[403] Thus the finding of a low serum iron concentration in such circumstances should not be taken as evidence of iron deficiency. Iron-deficiency anemia and anemia as a consequence of folic acid or vitamin B_{12} deficiency may coexist. During the course of treatment, with the rapid increase in the number of red cells, the typical manifestations of severe iron deficiency may develop.[404] The mixture of microcytic-hypochromic and normocytic-normochromic cells has been called *dimorphic anemia* (see "Coexisting Microcytic Anemia" in Chaps. 41 and 58).

Anemia of Hypothyroidism

The anemia of severe hypothyroidism (myxedema; see Chap. 38) is usually normochromic and normocytic and may be accompanied by mild-to-moderate depression of serum iron concentration. Ferrokinetic studies may show a decreased rate of plasma iron transport but normal iron utilization. Marrow examination may be required to determine whether iron deficiency is present, especially as iron deficiency often complicates myxedema because of menorrhagia, common in this disorder.

Therapeutic Trial

In the final analysis, the response to iron therapy is the proof of correctness of diagnosis of iron-deficiency anemia. Furthermore, some physicians or patients may not have access to all the techniques described for diagnosis of iron-deficiency anemia. In this event, the patient's response to therapy may become a primary diagnostic measure. Iron administration in such a therapeutic trial should usually be by the oral route only. A therapeutic trial under any circumstances should be followed carefully. If the cause of anemia is iron deficiency, adequate iron therapy should result in reticulocytosis with a peak occurring after 1 to 2 weeks of therapy, although if anemia is mild, the reticulocyte response may be minimal. A significant increase in the hemoglobin concentration of the blood should be evident 3 to 4 weeks later, and the hemoglobin concentration should attain a normal value within 2 to 4 months. Unless there is evidence of continued, substantial blood loss, a malabsorption syndrome, or evidence of *H. pylori* infection, the absence of these changes must be taken as evidence that iron deficiency is not the cause of anemia. Iron therapy should be discontinued and another cause for the anemia sought.

Special Studies to Delineate the Cause of Iron Deficiency

The physician who establishes a diagnosis of iron deficiency resulting from blood loss has the obligation to determine the site and cause of hemorrhage. Examination of the stools for the presence of blood is particularly helpful in determining what additional studies should be carried out. Specimens should be examined on several days, because bleeding may be intermittent. Occasionally, it is helpful to label the patient's erythrocytes with ^{51}Cr sodium chromate and to determine quantitatively the amount of blood lost daily. When there is reason to believe that bleeding is from the gastrointestinal tract, roentgenographic and other imaging studies and endoscopic investigation are indicated. The latter often include gastroscopy, esophagoscopy, and colonoscopy. Numerous clinical studies indicate that intensive investigation of patients, particularly men and postmenopausal women, reveals unexpected bleeding lesions, many of which are curable or treatable.[101,405–408]

Percutaneous retrograde angiography of celiac or mesenteric arteries has proved valuable in localizing sites of active gastrointestinal bleeding, when rate of blood flow into the intestinal lumen is 0.5 mL/min or greater.[97,409] This procedure should be considered for any patient actively bleeding from the gastrointestinal tract, in whom the site of blood loss has not been established by other methods, including endoscopy, and for whom surgery is contemplated. Angiography should be carried out prior to barium contrast studies. The rate of bleeding may be increased following angiography.[409] Diverticula often contain ectopic gastric mucosa, that will concentrate pertechnetate following intravenous injection for scintigraphic study; such scintigrams have been useful in identifying Meckel diverticulum as the cause of gastrointestinal blood loss.[410,411] *H. pylori* infection should be sought, particularly in patients who are iron deficient but who do not seem to respond to therapy.

In some cases, small-bowel endoscopy by laparoscopy may detect bleeding lesions when less invasive methods have failed.[412,413] Rarely, exploratory laparotomy may be warranted, because some adults with unexplained occult bleeding have gastrointestinal malignancies.

An iron stain of sputum may reveal hemosiderin-laden macrophages when there is intrapulmonary bleeding.

THERAPY

Once it has been established that a patient is deficient in iron, replacement therapy should be instituted without further delay.

Iron may be administered in one of several forms: orally, as simple iron salts; parenterally, as an iron-carbohydrate complex; or as a blood transfusion. In general, the oral route is preferred. In most patients, iron-deficiency anemia is a disorder of long duration and slow progression. Precipitous measures to restore a normal hemoglobin concentration by transfusing the patient are never warranted and are, indeed, hazardous. There is usually time to wait for normal mechanisms of erythropoiesis to respond to the body's needs and for gradual adjustment of the cardiovascular system to reexpansion of the total circulating erythrocyte volume.

ORAL IRON THERAPY

Dietary Therapy

The patient should be encouraged to eat a diversified diet supplying all nutritional requirements. Nonetheless, it must be emphasized that neither meat nor any other dietary article contains enough iron to be useful therapeutically. Meat contains small amounts of myoglobin and hemoglobin and insignificant amounts of iron in other proteins. Although heme iron is better absorbed than inorganic iron, the quantity of heme iron in meat is actually quite small. In fact, an average (3-ounce) serving of steak provides only about 3 mg of iron. Provision of sufficient dietary iron to permit a maximal rate or recovery from iron-deficiency anemia might require a daily intake of at least 10 pounds of steak. For these and other reasons, medicinal iron is much superior to dietary iron in the therapy of iron deficiency.

Iron Preparations

The pharmaceutical market is glutted with iron preparations in nearly every conceivable form; each promoted to appeal to physician or patient for one reason or another. The following simple principles may help the physician to find a way through this chaos.

1. Each dose of an inorganic iron preparation for an adult should contain between 30 and 100 mg of elemental iron. Doses of this magnitude cause unpleasant side effects relatively infrequently.[414,415] Smaller doses have been popular in the past, but these may result in a slower recovery of the patient or no recovery at all. Small doses of iron preparations containing some heme have been reported to be effective in correcting iron deficiency in pregnancy.[416,417]
2. The iron should be readily released in acidic or neutral gastric juice or duodenal juice (usually pH 5 to 6), because maximal absorption occurs when iron is presented to the duodenal mucosa. Enteric-coated and prolonged-release preparations dissolve slowly in any of these fluids. Thus with such preparations the iron that eventually is released may be presented to a portion of the intestinal mucosa in which absorption is least efficient. Some patients who have been treated unsuccessfully with enteric-coated or prolonged-release iron preparations respond promptly to the administration of non-enteric-coated ferrous salts (Fig. 42–13).
3. The iron, once released, should be readily absorbed. Iron is absorbed in the ferrous form; consequently, only ferrous salts should be used.
4. Side effects should be infrequent. This seems not to be a particular problem for any of the common commercially available iron compounds. Despite the claims of pharmaceutical companies, there is no convincing evidence that any one effective preparation is superior in this respect to any other.
5. The cost to the patient should be small.
6. The use of preparations containing several therapeutic agents is to be condemned.

Physicians should be aware that if ferrous sulfate is prescribed generically, the choice of preparation is left to the pharmacist who may dispense enteric-coated tablets. It is advisable to specify "nonenteric" or to prescribe by brand name a product that is not enteric-coated.

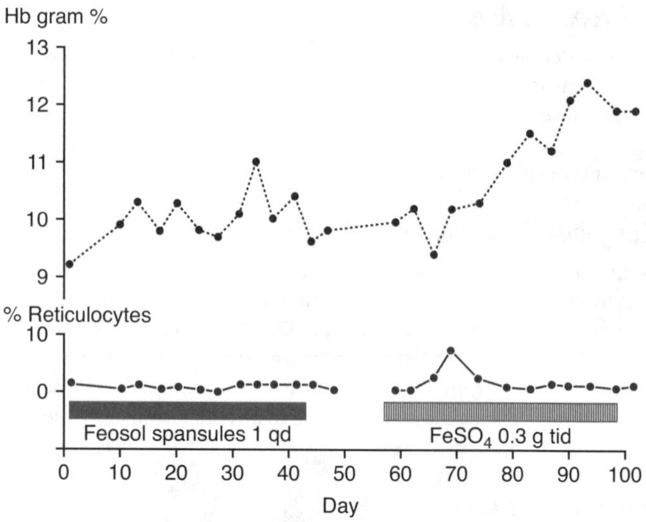

FIGURE 42–13. Rate of response of patient with iron-deficiency anemia to 43 days of treatment with prolonged-release Feosol spansules (containing 325 mg ferrous sulfate), one capsule daily, the dosage recommended by the manufacturer, followed by 43 days of treatment with nonenteric ferrous sulfate (0.3 g three times daily). Clearly, 325 mg of ferrous sulfate daily in prolonged-release form failed to elicit any significant hematopoietic response in this case. The rapid response subsequently elicited with conventional ferrous sulfate may be taken as a typical response to effect therapy in adequate dosage, whether by oral or parenteral route. *(From Beutler E, Meerkreebs G,[705] with permission from the Massachusetts Medical Society.)*

Although substances such as ascorbic acid, succinate, and fructose enhance iron absorption, the gain is offset to a large extent by the increase in frequency of side effects, cost of therapy, or both. There is no convincing evidence to support the use of chelated forms of iron or of iron in combination with wetting agents.

Dosage For the therapy of iron deficiency in adults, the dosage should be sufficient to provide between 150 and 200 mg elemental iron daily. The iron may be taken orally in three or four doses 1 hour before meals. Infants may be given 6 mg/kg[418] daily in divided doses for therapy, or a daily dose of 12.5 mg daily for prophylaxis of iron deficiency (Table 42–10).[419]

Side Effects Mild gastrointestinal side effects occur occasionally in the form of nausea, heartburn, constipation, or looseness of stools. A metallic taste may be experienced. In some patients, these side effects may be psychological in origin.[414] The majority of patients tolerate the usual therapeutic doses of iron without the least side effect. However, there is no doubt that some patients, perhaps 1 or 2 of 10, experience symptoms that may be ascribed to the iron preparation and may be related in part to the size of the dose.[415,420] In such cases, reduction of the frequency of administration to 1 tablet a day for a few days may

TABLE 42–10. Iron Preparations for Pediatric Use

Chemical Designation	mg/mL	Commercial (Proprietary) Designation	Iron Content, Therapeutic Dosage
Ferrous sulfate solution, USP	8		1, 2, or 3 times daily
Ferrous sulfate solution, concentrated	25	Fer-In-Sol	20 drops, 3 or 4 times daily
Ferrous sulfate elixir (5% ethanol)	9	Feosol elixir	1 tsp, 2 or 3 times daily

alleviate the symptoms; later, the patient may be able to tolerate treatment in full dosage. It might also be useful to change to another iron preparation, especially one with a different external appearance.

Carbonyl iron has been proposed as an alternative to iron salts, on the assertion that it can be given in large doses with minimal side effects. This substance is actually metallic iron powder, with a particle size less than 5 μm. Because it is insoluble, it is not absorbed until converted to the ionic form. The bioavailability of carbonyl iron has been estimated to be approximately 70 percent of that of an equivalent amount of ferrous sulfate,[421] but oral doses of 1 to 3 g/day may be required for optimal therapy. Oral doses as high as 600 mg three times daily did not produce toxic effects.[422]

There has been speculation in the medical literature[423] and some data[424] suggesting that iron might be a risk factor for cardiovascular disease. However, the bulk of evidence suggests that no such effect exists,[425–431] nor does it seem that iron supplementation causes an increased frequency of infections.[432] Similarly, it has been claimed that there is association between elevated ferritin levels and diabetes,[433,434] but this is not been the case in most investigations.[435]

Acute Iron Poisoning Acute iron poisoning is usually a consequence of the accidental ingestion by infants or small children of iron-containing medications intended for use by adults. Any potent oral preparation may cause acute iron poisoning, and this serious disorder is not at all rare. For example, in the Los Angeles area alone there were five deaths from iron poisoning among children 11 to 18 months of age in the seven-month period following June 1992.[436]

The earliest manifestation of iron poisoning is vomiting, usually within 1 hour of the ingestion. There may be hematemesis or melena. Restlessness, hypotension, tachypnea, and cyanosis may develop soon thereafter, and may be followed within a few hours by coma and death. So inexorable a course is not the rule, however, and only approximately 1 percent of such poisonings have a fatal outcome.[437] Usually, medical aid is sought early and, with proper treatment, most iron-poisoned children survive. The initial treatment is prompt evacuation of the stomach. In the home, this may be induced by digital stimulation of the pharyngeal gag reflex. Oral administration of a tepid solution of baking soda serves two useful purposes: it may provoke emesis, and the bicarbonate ion complexes with the iron and retards absorption. If a child has ingested more than 60 mg of iron per kg body weight, hospital treatment is indicated.[438] In the emergency room, gastric intubation and lavage should be performed promptly, preferably with a solution containing 4 g sodium bicarbonate (or 3.6 g disodium phosphate and 0.8 g monosodium phosphate) per deciliter. Before the tube is withdrawn, a solution containing 5 to 10 g desferrioxamine, or approximately 60 mL of the bicarbonate or phosphate solution, should be introduced into the stomach. Supportive measures should be used as needed for shock or for metabolic acidosis should these develop. Desferrioxamine is the agent of choice for specific therapy of hyperferremia. It usually should be administered intramuscularly in an initial dose of 1 g, followed by 0.5 g intramuscularly 4 and 8 hours later and thereafter at 12-hour intervals as the clinical status warrants. If the child is hypotensive, the dose may be administered intravenously at a rate not exceeding 15 mg/kg per hour for a total initial dose of 1 g, with repetition of this dosage started every 4 to 12 hours as the clinical status of the patient seems to warrant.[439] Improvement often appears several hours to a few days after onset of iron poisoning. This improvement may be permanent, but it may also be misleading, because pneumonitis or severe hepatic or neurologic decompensation may soon supervene. There may be seizures, coma, hyperreflexia, jaundice, and bilirubinemia. Children who survive for 3 or 4 days usually recover without sequelae. However, gastric strictures and fibrosis or intestinal stenosis may occur as late complications. These have been reported as early as 6 weeks after acute iron poisoning.[438,440–442]

Parenteral Iron Therapy

Indications In view of the significantly greater hazards and cost of parenteral therapy, the choice of this mode of administration must be carefully considered, but occasionally it becomes necessary to administer iron by the parenteral route. The indications are malabsorption, intolerance to iron taken orally, iron need in excess of an amount that can be taken orally, and noncompliance of the patient. Parenteral iron administration, together with erythropoietin, appears to alleviate the anemia that otherwise may complicate long-term dialysis treatment of patients with chronic renal disease. For reasons that are not well understood, these patients do not appear to respond adequately to oral iron therapy.[433,444]

Calculating Dosage It is easy to estimate the amount of iron that needs to be given by merely remembering that 1 mL of red cells contains approximately 1 mg of iron. However, various formulas have been used for estimating total dose required for treatment. Because total blood volume is approximately 65 mL/kg and the iron content of hemoglobin is 0.34 percent by weight, the simplest formula for estimating the total dose required for correction of anemia only is as follows:

$$\text{The dose of iron (mg)} = \text{Whole-blood hemoglobin deficit (g/dL)} \times \text{Body weight (lbs)}$$

Assuming normal mean hemoglobin concentration of 16 g/dL, a male weighing 170 pounds, whose hemoglobin concentration is 7 g/dL, would require $170 \times (16 - 7) = 1530$ mg iron to correct this anemia. To this should be added a sufficient quantity of iron to replete iron stores, approximately 1000 mg for men and approximately 600 mg for women. Thus a 170-pound male with a hemoglobin concentration of 7 g/dL should receive 2530 mg iron.

Preparations **Iron Sucrose** Known under a variety of generic names, iron sucrose (Eisenzucker; ferric hydroxide sucrose; ferric oxide, saccharated; ferrum oxydatum saccharatum; iron (III) hydroxide-sucrose complex; Oxyde de Fer Sucre; saccharated iron oxide; XI-921) is the oldest of the intravenous iron preparations, having been first used in humans in 1947.[445] For many years it was largely replaced by iron dextran, but iron sucrose complexes have enjoyed a renaissance, the newer complexes having the advantage of greater safety.

Iron sucrose is a complex of polynuclear iron ferric hydroxide in sucrose. It has a molecular mass of approximately 34,000 to 60,000 daltons.[446] Sold in the United States as Venofer, it contains 20 mg of iron per milliliter. After intravenous injection iron is cleared from the plasma with an initial half-life of approximately 30 minutes,[446] after which it is removed with a half-life of approximately 6 hours. It is taken up by macrophages, where the iron is released.

The dose recommended by the manufacturer is 5 mL (100 mg of elemental iron), administered no more frequently than three times weekly. However, iron sucrose has been administered to patients with chronic kidney disease at a dosage of 500 mg infused over 3 hours on 2 consecutive days, and considered to be safe and effective[447]; it has also been suggested that high doses may depress neutrophils' intracellular killing function.[448]

Adverse events reported by more than 5 percent of treated patients included hypotension (36%), cramps (23%), nausea, headache, vomiting, and diarrhea. It is not certain to what extent these are actually caused by the iron preparation. Less common adverse effects include headache, fever, chest pain, hypertension, dizziness, dyspnea, cough, pleuritis, and pain at the site of reaction. It is estimated that 20 million doses of iron sucrose administered to more than 1 million patients worldwide resulted in 52 anaphylactoid reactions, of which 22 were considered serious. There were no deaths.[446] Iron sucrose has been administered without adverse event to patients who manifest sensitivity reactions to iron dextran or sodium ferric gluconate.[449,450]

Iron Dextran Iron dextran is a complex of iron and dextran with an average mass equivalent to 165,000 g/mole with a range of approximately ±10 percent daltons. The commercial preparation (INFeD Injection; Watson in the United States) is marketed as a stable, dark brown, slightly acidic (pH 6) solution containing 50 mg elemental iron per milliliter. The manufacturer recommends intravenous test doses of 0.5 mL before therapy is started and that each dose consist of only 2 mL or less. Much larger doses ("total-dose infusion") have also been employed very widely and are generally considered more convenient, safe, and cost-effective,[159,451–456] although an increase in minor reactions has been noted.[457] It may even be argued that a single infusion is less likely to elicit an immune response than multiple injections given over a period of several weeks. If any adverse effect is noted, injection must be terminated at once and appropriate countermeasures taken. A syringe containing a solution of epinephrine should be immediately accessible for treatment of anaphylaxis should this occur.

After intramuscular injection iron dextran is slowly absorbed, approximately 72 hours being required for 50 percent of a dose to move out of the injection site.[458,459] It is slowly cleared from plasma. Peak plasma concentrations of thousands of micrograms of iron per deciliter are found even 10 days after intramuscular injection; the plasma iron concentration decreases slowly, reaching normal values after 3 to 4 weeks.[460] Iron dextran is cleared from plasma by the macrophages, and ultimately the iron is used in hemoglobin synthesis. Mobilization of iron dextran from an intramuscular site is relatively slow and incomplete; 20 to 35 percent of the dose may remain at the injection site 1 month later.[461,462] Furthermore, the rate of incorporation of iron dextran into hemoglobin is somewhat slower than that for simpler ferric hydroxide colloids.[462,463] It appears that the iron dextran complex is only slowly dissociated in macrophages, and iron granules may be seen in marrow macrophages in iron dextran-treated patients even after iron-deficiency anemia has recurred.

Intramuscular administration of iron dextran causes a moderate degree of pain at the injection site and a dark stain in the skin that may remain for as long as 1 to 2 years. "Z-track" and other techniques of injection recommended by the manufacturer reduce, but do not eliminate, the discoloration of the skin. Intravenous administration also may cause local side effects, in the form of thrombophlebitis. This occurs most commonly when iron dextran is diluted with 5 percent glucose solution, less frequently when diluted with isotonic saline solution, and infrequently when iron dextran is injected undiluted. Thrombophlebitis at the injection site appears to be unusual with the technique of total-dose infusion, and other adverse effects appear to be no more frequent than with the intramuscular route.

The frequency of systemic reactions of iron dextran therapy has been markedly variable in different series, ranging from less than 2 percent to more than 25 percent of patients.[464] Dextran is a biologic product the exact structure of which is apparently difficult to control, and the frequency of adverse effects varies, probably due to variations in manufacturing techniques. Arthralgia and fever may be experienced by as many as one-third of patients. Other systemic reactions are infrequent and include hypotension, myalgia, headache, abdominal pain, nausea and vomiting, dizziness, lymphadenopathy, pleural effusion, pruritus, urticaria, seizures, flushing, chills, and phlebitis. Lymphadenopathy[465,466] and allergic purpura[467] have been noted. Several cases have been observed in which iron dextran infusion was followed by an acute febrile illness accompanied by tender lymphadenopathy and splenomegaly lasting 10 to 14 days.[456,468] Pleocytosis of the cerebrospinal fluid has been observed[469] during a febrile reaction to iron dextran; in this case, there was also a blood leukocyte count of 88,000/μL (88×10^9/L). In another patient meningismus without increased leukocytes in the spinal fluid but a high spinal fluid iron concentration was documented.[470] Pancytopenia may follow iron dextran therapy.[471] Acute, severe exacerbation of arthritis has been observed following iron dextran therapy in patients with rheumatoid arthritis[464] or ankylosing spondylitis.[472] Intramuscular deposition of iron dextran has led to malignancy in some experimental animals.[473,474] Fibrosarcoma and undifferentiated pleomorphic sarcoma have developed at the site of injection in several human subjects following repeated or protracted iron dextran therapy.[475–477] This appears to be an extremely rare phenomenon and may in some cases have been coincidental rather than causally related.

The most dangerous complication of iron dextran therapy is anaphylactic reaction. This occurs in less than 1 percent of patients treated by either the intramuscular or intravenous route. It is not dose-dependent and may follow the infusion of only a few drops of diluted iron dextran solution or a fraction of a milliliter of intramuscularly injected iron dextran. This calls into question the usefulness of giving a test dose, and it is doubtful whether such a test dose serves any useful purpose. Characteristically, during the first few minutes of infusion, the patient complains of difficulty breathing, or a choking or smothering sensation, becomes sweaty and anxious, may complain of nausea, and may vomit. Respiratory stridor may be observed, followed by apnea. The blood pressure may drop abruptly; stupor and coma may quickly supervene. At the first evidence of this reaction, the infusion must be terminated, and epinephrine should immediately be injected subcutaneously (0.5 mL of 1:1000 aqueous epinephrine). Other measures to combat shock and anaphylaxis are appropriate. Most patients survive, but 31 fatalities were reported in the United States between 1976 and 1996.[478] Stroke or myocardial infarction may follow anaphylactic shock induced by iron dextran.[479]

Freshly opened vials of iron dextran may contain as much as 100 mg divalent iron per deciliter. Iron dextran causes hypotension when administered intravenously to cats, and the hypotensive effect correlates to some extent with the amount of divalent iron in the solution.[480] Successful administration of iron dextran after pretreatment with methylprednisolone, diphenhydramine, ephedrine, and Promit (very-low-molecular-weight dextran) has been reported in a patient with a previous anaphylactic response,[481] and the use of glucocorticoids to prevent delayed reactions[456] had been advocated, but circumstances would need to be very unusual to justify readministration of iron dextran to a patient who had experienced a severe reaction.

Sodium Ferric Gluconate Complex in Sucrose Injection Sodium ferric gluconate complex, sold in the United States as Ferrlecit, is a stable macromolecular complex of innate and ferric iron, with a molecular weight approximating 289,000 to 440,000 daltons. Each milliliter contains 12.5 mg of elemental iron. The manufacturer recommends administration of doses of 125 mg of elemental iron with the preparation diluted in 100 mL of 0.9 percent sodium chloride and given intravenously over a period of 1 hour.[482] However, doses of as high as 500 mg have been given with apparent safety.[483,484] Adverse reactions include hypotension (29%), cramps (25%), dizziness (13%), dyspnea (11%), paresthesias (6%), coughing (6%), nausea, vomiting, and/or diarrhea (2%), hypertension (0.6%), allergic reaction (0.5%), chest pain (0.5%), pleuritis (0.5%), and back pain (0.4%).[482] It is by no means clear that all of these symptoms were actually related to the drug. Injection-site reactions have been reported by 33 percent of the subjects. Severe life-threatening hypersensitivity reactions are rare but do occur.[478] In contrast to those occurring with iron dextran, such episodes have not been reported to have a fatal outcome with sodium ferric gluconate. Although the number of reactions to these two iron preparations seems to be similar, the more severe reactions, leading to death, seem to be more common with iron dextran.[478,485]

COURSE AND PROGNOSIS

Course

If therapy is adequate, the correction of iron-deficiency anemia is usually gratifying. Symptoms such as headache, fatigue, pica, paresthesias, and burning sensation of the oropharyngeal mucosa may abate within a few days. In the blood, the reticulocyte count begins to increase after a few days, usually reaches a maximum at about 7 to 12 days, and thereafter decreases. When anemia is mild, little or no reticulocytosis may be observed. Little change in hemoglobin concentration or hematocrit value is to be expected for the first 2 weeks, but then the anemia is corrected rapidly. The hemoglobin concentration in the blood may be halfway back to normal after 4 to 5 weeks of therapy. By the end of 2 months of therapy, and often much sooner, the hemoglobin concentration should have reached a normal level. There is little difference in the rate of response whether iron is administered by the oral or the parenteral route,[486] except in patients with intestinal malabsorption.[487] Differences that have been encountered[488] may well be a result of noncompliance of patients given oral iron. If the diagnosis of iron-deficiency anemia is correct, anemia and other manifestations of iron deficiency will respond to adequate therapy. However, the physician is occasionally disappointed in the results of treatment of patients who seem to have iron deficiency anemia. In some cases this apparent failure of therapy is a result of treatment of patients with iron preparations that are virtually insoluble, enteric-coated, or contain iron in only minute amounts. Careful inquiry into the nature, duration, and regularity of iron therapy may reveal a reason for the failure of therapy and permit a gratifying response to be elicited with adequate therapy. Other questions that should be asked in evaluation of such a case are these: (1) Has bleeding been controlled? (2) Has the patient been on iron therapy long enough to show a response? (3) Has the dose of iron been adequate? (4) Are there other factors—inflammatory disease, neoplastic disease, hepatic or renal disease, concomitant deficiencies (vitamin B_{12}, folic acid, thyroid)—that might retard response? Prominent among these are *H. pylori* infection.[111,114,121] It has also been suggested that ingestion of large amounts of black tea[489–491] may prevent the response of an iron-deficient patient to what would otherwise be adequate therapy. (5) Is the diagnosis correct?

Prognosis

When the cause of the iron deficiency is a benign disorder, the prognosis is excellent, provided bleeding is controlled or can be compensated for by continual iron therapy. Too often, therapy is interrupted as soon as anemia has been corrected, and iron stores are not replenished. Such inadequately treated patients are likely to have recurrent anemia.[492,493] For this reason, and because iron therapy brings about replenishment of iron stores very slowly, oral therapy should be continued for at least 12 months after anemia has been corrected. If there is a benign cause of recurrent bleeding that is corrected, such as hiatal hernia, menorrhagia, or hereditary hemorrhagic telangiectasia, oral iron therapy may be continued indefinitely; if the bleeding is especially brisk, supplementation with parenterally administered iron or, rarely, with transfusion may be needed. Continuous iron administration may also be required in patients with iron deficiency secondary to intravascular hemolysis with hemoglobinuria.

IRON STORAGE DISEASE

DEFINITION AND HISTORY

The terms *iron storage disease* and *hemochromatosis* are used to designate an increase of tissue iron resulting in a disease state; *hemosiderosis* denotes an increase of tissue iron stores with or without tissue damage. Classically hemochromatosis has been characterized by bronzing of the skin, cirrhosis, and diabetes, and was once called *bronzed diabetes.* Since the 1970s, usage of the term *hemochromatosis* has expanded well beyond its original meaning. This diagnosis is now commonly applied to persons who have increased body iron as suggested by increased serum ferritin levels, and even to those who merely have the hemochromatosis *HFE* genotype, regardless of the level of their iron stores.

TABLE 42–11. Classification of Hemochromatosis

I. Hereditary Hemochromatosis
   A. Classical hemochromatosis (hereditary hemochromatosis; HFE hemochromatosis) (type 1)
   B. Juvenile hemochromatosis (type 2)
      1. Abnormality in hemojuvelin
      2. Abnormality of hepcidin
   C. Transferrin receptor-2 deficiency (type 3)
   D. Ferroportin deficiency (includes some cases of African iron overload)[609,610,742] (type 4)
   E. Ferritin H-chain IRE mutation[714]
   F. African iron overload
   G. Neonatal hemochromatosis (?)
II. Secondary Hemochromatosis

Hemochromatosis may be divided into genetic forms and acquired forms. The former have sometimes been designated as *primary* and the latter as *secondary* forms. The disorder once designated *idiopathic hemochromatosis* and now as *hereditary hemochromatosis* usually is applied to the common genetic form of the disorder, found principally in those of northern European ancestry, and as a result of mutations in the *HFE* gene. This form of the disease has also been called *type I hemochromatosis*; we prefer to designate it as *classical hemochromatosis.* But there are other forms of hereditary hemochromatosis as well. *Juvenile hemochromatosis* from hemojuvelin and hepicidin muations (type 2), hemochromatosis as a result of transferrin receptor-2 mutations (type 3), hemochromatosis caused by ferroportin mutations (type 4), and *African iron overload* are among these types. Table 42–11 classifies hereditary hemochromatosis. *Secondary hemochromatosis* occurs in patients who receive multiple blood transfusions, particularly when they have ineffective erythropoiesis.

Iron accumulation in localized sites, particularly the brain, occurs in disorders other than hemochromatosis. One of these has been termed *neonatal hemochromatosis*. It is of unknown origin, and characterized by hepatic and extrahepatic iron deposition and fulminant hepatitis.[494] The GRACILE (growth retardation, aminoaciduria, cholestasis, iron overload, lactic acidosis, and early death) syndrome is an autosomal recessive disorder found mostly among Finns, and is caused by a mutation in the BCS1L gene.[495] Neuroferritinopathy is a neurologic disorder caused by a structural mutation near the carboxy end of the ferritin light chain. Clinical features include a dystonic dysarthria with chorea, dystonia, and parkinsonian manifestations being found in some patients.[496] Increased iron deposition is also characteristic of atransferrinemia.[497,498] Hepatic iron is also found in human DMT-1 mutations.[623] Increased quantities of brain iron are characteristic of ceruloplasminemia,[499,500] and are found in Alzheimer's disease, parkinsonism, Friedreich ataxia, Hallervorden-Spatz syndrome, and multiple system atrophy.[501] Because none of these are primarily hematologic disorders, and in most the role of iron deposition is secondary to another underlying pathology, they are not discussed further here.

Hemochromatosis was first described by Trousseau in 1865 (cited in ref. 502). The massive accumulation of iron that occurred in this disease was recognized as its hallmark, but other metals were known to accumulate also, and it was thought by some that the toxic metal might be copper.[503] The ingenious development of serial phlebotomy as treatment for the disease suggested by Finch in 1949,[504] and implemented on a larger scale by Davis and Arrowsmith in 1952,[505] made it clear that iron accumulation was the most important pathogenetic factor. In 1935, Sheldon helped to focus attention on this disease in a classic monograph.[502] He suggested that the disease might be hereditary and addressed the prevalence of hemochromatosis, proposing that although it was not as rare as had been thought, it was a relatively uncommon disorder. Sheldon's view that hemochromatosis might have a genetic basis was strongly contested by MacDonald,[506,507] who considered the disorder to be caused by increased iron intake, particularly in wine. However, the existence of a hereditary factor was firmly established when Simon and colleagues[508] showed that the disease was tightly linked to the human leukocyte antigen (HLA locus). These investigators[509] demonstrated both linkage within families and linkage disequilibrium in populations. They realized that the HLA-A or HLA-B gene products themselves were not involved in the pathogenesis of the disease; rather the gene that did cause hemochromatosis was located nearby. A quarter of a century passed before success attended one of the many attempts to clone the gene responsible for the disease. Surprisingly, the gene proved to be *HFE* (initially named *HLA-H*), one of the many HLA-like genes on chromosome 6.[510] This finding, and the availability of new, powerful animal models for the study of iron homeostasis resulted in the discovery of many new genes involved in the regulation of body iron content (see Table 42–3).

The identification of the *HFE* gene made it possible, for the first time, to assess accurately the gene frequency and penetrance of the *HFE* mutations. This brought about a fusion of the apparently contrasting views of MacDonald and Simon. The penetrance of the homozygous state is so low that it could be considered a risk factor, rather than the major cause of the disease.[511]

EPIDEMIOLOGY

At one time all forms of hemochromatosis were considered to be rare. The male-to-female ratio was 18:1.[256,502] With the widespread availability in the 1970s of means for measuring serum iron, transferrin saturation, and ferritin levels, hereditary hemochromatosis grew to be regarded as a very common disorder with a sex ratio of approximately 1.5:1.[512,513] Indeed, as indicated below (see "Genetics" below), the prevalence of mutations of the *HFE* gene is very high. The most significant of these is the c.845 A→G (C282Y) mutation, and with a gene frequency of approximately 0.07 in the northern European population, approximately 5 in 1000 northern Europeans are homozygous for the mutation. The C282Y and S65C mutations are almost entirely confined to individuals with European ancestry. The H63D mutation is more widespread geographically, but is also most common in Europeans. Within Europe the highest gene frequencies are encountered in the southern British Isles and in northern France.[514] Table 42–12 summarizes the prevalence of these polymorphic mutations. A splicing mutation polymorphism, IVS5+1 G/A, is present among the Vietnamese,[515] but seems to have little or no consequence with respect to iron accumu-

TABLE 42–12. The Prevalence of Common Hemochromatosis Alleles in Different Large-Scale (>1000) Population Surveys

		Gene Frequency			
Population	No. of Subjects	C282Y	S65C	H63D	Reference
African American	1373	0.016	ND	0.032	743
Maine, USA 98.6% white	1001	0.066	ND	0.151	744
New Zealand	1064	0.079	ND	0.130	745
Brittany, France	1000	0.065	ND	ND	746
Europe	1450	0.038	ND	0.136	747
California, USA white	31,227	0.062	0.016*	0.149	748
California, USA black	1501	0.019	0.0068†	0.045	748
California, USA Asian	1815	0.001	0‡	0.036	748
Michigan, USA non-Hispanic white	3532	0.057	ND	0.14	754
Denmark	6020	0.056	0.018	0.128	749
England	6261	0.068	ND	0.141	750
Italy, north	1132	0.032	0.013	0.134	751
Poland, NW	1517	0.340	ND	0.158	752
Madrid, Spain	1000	0.017	ND	0.164	753

ND = Not done.

*Only 7739 persons tested.

†Only 369 persons tested.

‡Only 450 persons tested.

lation. In addition to these relatively common mutations many sporadic mutations confined to single families have been documented.[516–518] Not all patients with hereditary hemochromatosis have mutations of the *HFE* gene. Whereas in northern Europe almost all patients with hemochromatosis have these mutations, iron storage disease in southern Europe,[519,520] India[521] and Turkey[522] is much more likely to be a result of mutations in other genes, mostly unidentified.

Although earlier studies attributed nonspecific symptoms in patients to hemochromatosis,[523–525] large controlled series have shown that most such symptoms are not present in homozygotes for the C282Y mutation at a higher frequency than in controls,[526–529] or a borderline increase, at most, invariably in groups of patients who were aware of their diagnosis when answering questions about symptoms. These findings are consistent with the very low prevalence of hemochromatosis reported in autopsy series[530–532] and in hospital surveys.[533,534] The probable prevalence of symptomatic clinical hemochromatosis in northern European populations is probably only about 5 in 100,000 individuals. If patients with abnormal liver function tests and/or fibrosis on liver biopsy are included, the number of affected may be several-fold higher. The factors that determine whether a patient with the C282Y homozygous genotype develops disease are not well understood. The patient's sex is clearly a modifying factor, with more severe manifestations observed in males.[535] Pregnancy and menstrual losses tend to ameliorate the disease in women. Other genetic factors that might interact with the C282Y homozygous genotype in producing clinically significant iron storage disease have been sought, but not found,[536] except rare instances in which coinheritance of mutations of the hepcidin gene may be responsible.[537,538] An increased proportion of severely affected patients have a large alcohol intake.[539]

The widespread perception that classical hereditary hemochromatosis frequently led to clinical disease resulted in enthusiasm for population-based screening.[540–543] However, the cost–benefit analysis used was based upon the assumptions that life-threatening disease manifestations will occur in 43 percent of males and in 28 percent of females,[540] estimates that were based upon the prevalence of disease in patients, most of whom had been diagnosed clinically with hemochromatosis. With the realization that the clinical penetrance is much lower, interest in screening the general population for hemochromatosis has largely disappeared, and efforts have been made to find high-risk groups in which screening could be justified (Fig. 42–14).[544]

The prevalence of other forms of hemochromatosis, including juvenile hemochromatosis, hemochromatosis as a result of ferroportin deficiency, and atransferrinemia, is much lower than that the prevalence of classical hereditary hemochromatosis. These forms of hemochromatosis are rare diseases.

ETIOLOGY AND PATHOGENESIS

Toxicity of Iron

Accepting and releasing electrons is the main basis of the importance of iron to living organisms. The same capacity to undergo reversible oxidation-reduction reactions appears to be the basis of the harm that excessive amounts of iron can inflict. One of the pathways that is considered to be of greatest importance is the Haber-Weiss reaction:

$$Fe^{++} + H_2O_2 \rightarrow Fe^{+++} + + OH- + \cong HO$$

$$O_2^{-} + Fe^{+++} \rightarrow O_2 + Fe^{++}$$

The sum of these two reactions is the Fenton reaction:

$$O_2^{-} + H_2O_2 \rightarrow O_2 + OH^{-} + \cong HO$$

The hydroxyl radical (≅OH) is second in reactivity only to atomic oxygen and has been implicated in producing damage to polysaccharides, DNA, and enzymes, and in causing lipid peroxidation.[545] Although there is no direct evidence that hydroxyl radical generation is the main pathway of tissue damage in hemochromatosis, this common conjecture seems to be a reasonable one. A possible role of ferryl ions (FeO_2^{+}) in mediating tissue damage also has been suggested.[546]

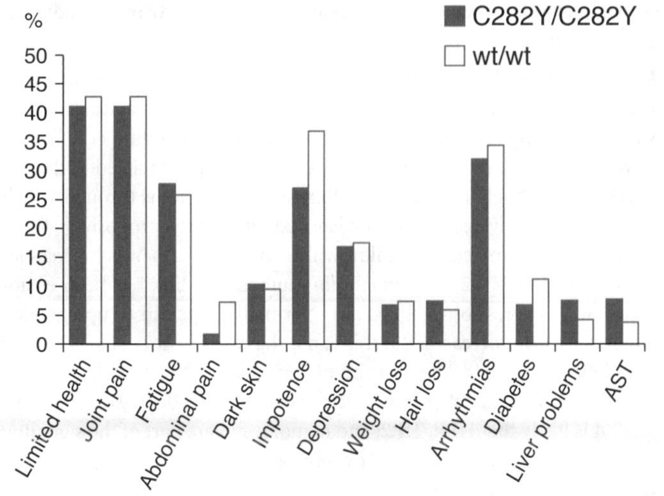

FIGURE 42–14. Penetrance of hemochromatosis in a large outpatient population. Patients were assessed by a questionnaire, laboratory studies, and physical examination before the patient or physician was aware of the results of genotyping for the C282Y or H63D *HFE* mutation. There were 156 homozygotes for the C282Y mutation and more than 19,000 wild-type (wt/wt) controls. The only significant difference was in the aspartate aminotransferase (AST). Only one patient had a typical symptoms and findings of hemochromatosis.

Demonstrating a damaging affect of iron alone on experimental animals has been difficult. Although in some studies, subtle biochemical defects have been documented,[547–549] frank cirrhotic changes have not been found. In iron-loaded gerbils, cirrhosis did not occur if the diet was enriched in vitamin E.[550] Memory and motor-behavior deficits were found in rats treated as pups with large amounts of iron.[551] In rats, iron alone does not cause fibrosis, and alcohol alone causes only minor liver abnormalities. However, administration of both excess iron and alcohol results in fibrosis.[552] These findings in rats are quite consistent with the strong association that has been demonstrated to exist between alcohol ingestion and cirrhosis in patients with the hemochromatosis genotype.[512,539] In a number of species iron overload has been observed in nature, particularly after a diet other than the animal's native diet is fed[553–559] (see "Animal Models" below).

Iron can be stored in ferritin in the cytoplasm of all cells. The multiple isoferritins found in human tissues are composed of variable proportions of two subunits: L-ferritin (light) and H-ferritin (heavy).[79,80] Because free iron is potentially harmful to the cell, it is sequestered and detoxified to the less-soluble ferric form by ferroxidase activity; H-ferritin exerts most of its ferroxidase activity in the cytosol. The mitochondrial ferritin, expressed in the mitochondrial matrix, also has potent ferroxidase activity[77] and is markedly upregulated in sideroblastic anemias.[368] Because the distinction between ferritin and ringed sideroblasts after Prussian blue staining is often difficult, flow cytometry demonstration of mitochondrial ferritin facilitates the distinction between increased erythroid iron such as that seen in thalassemia major and intermedia from sideroblastic anemias' mitochondrial iron.[369]

Causes of Iron Overload

Because body iron content is maintained by regulating absorption, excess body iron can accumulate only when absorption is dysregulated or when iron is injected into the body, either in the form of medicinal iron or as transfused erythrocytes.

Dysregulation of Iron Absorption A variety of mutations are known to cause increased iron absorption in experimental animals and in man, as summarized in Table 42–3. Mutations in the genes encoding HFE, transferrin receptor-2, ferroportin, and hepcidin are all associated with iron overload. Although a number of different model systems through which such mutations dysregulate iron absorption have been proposed,[45,46] the actual mechanism remains unknown. In the case of hemochromatosis caused by *HFE*, *TfR2*, or *hemojuvelin* mutations, a link has been established with expression of hepcidin. Normally, hepcidin is upregulated when body iron increases. But this is not the case in either *Hfe-*, *Tfr2-*, or *Hjv*-deficient mice[560–563] or in the human disease,[564–566] both of which exhibit disproportionately low hepcidin levels for the degree of iron overload. It is likely that HFE, TfR2, and hemojuvelin are part of the signaling pathway that regulates hepcidin expression.

Ineffective Erythropoiesis A strong relationship between ineffective erythropoiesis and total-body iron burden exists.[567] The amount of body iron may greatly exceed the quantity that can be accounted for through blood transfusion.[568] The mechanism by which active erythropoiesis and destruction of red cell precursors in the marrow stimulates iron absorption is unknown, but it is notable that iron storage disease is particularly common in disorders such as thalassemia, hereditary dyserythropoietic anemia, and pyruvate kinase deficiency.

The iron overload commonly observed in thalassemia major patients likely results, at least in part, from inhibition of the iron regulatory protein hepcidin by high levels of growth differentiation factor 15 (GDF15), a member of the transforming growth factor-β (TGF-β) superfamily.[569] GDF15 overexpression was also observed in congenital dyserythropoietic anemia.[570]

An induction of mitochondrial ferritin gene expression in mitochondria in sideroblastic anemias[76,79] is not yet fully elucidated, but it likely plays a protective role against oxygen radicals.[78]

Transfusion or Iron Therapy Iron overload can be iatrogenic in origin. Because erythrocytes contain 1 mg of iron per milliliter, transfusion of 450 mL of whole blood or of 200 mL of red cells adds 200 mg of total iron to the body, iron that will not be excreted. Thus, a patient who requires 2 units of blood monthly will accumulate 4.8 g of iron per year. If the need for transfusion is occasioned by a disorder in which ineffective erythropoiesis plays a prominent role, the accumulation of iron is even greater. Thalassemia is such a circumstance, and iron overload is probably the most important cause of death in patients with this disorder (see Chap. 47).

The homeostatic mechanisms of the body are such that the inappropriate administration of iron by the oral route is very unlikely to produce clinically significant iron overload. Of the few cases that have been described,[571–575] all but one[573] (a child without tissue damage) were documented before the cloning of the *HFE* gene, leaving open the distinct possibility that the patients were merely homozygotes for hemochromatosis whose disease had been accelerated by excess iron intake. Documented iron overload after iron injection is even less common[576] and has not been accompanied by demonstrable tissue damage. Industrial exposure to iron dust (welder siderosis) results in deposition of iron in the lungs, and an increase in ferritin levels has been documented.[577]

Pathology

Affected tissues and organs exhibit a deep brown color. Histologic examination reveals prominent hemosiderin deposition in many tissues and organs.

Liver The liver is often enlarged. After cirrhosis has developed, the organ becomes granular or coarsely nodular. In the liver of patients with classical hemochromatosis, transferrin receptor 2 mutations and in juvenile hemochromatosis, hemosiderin is found primarily in hepatocytes, bile duct epithelium, and, to a lesser degree, Kupffer cells and other mesenchymal cells. Prior to the development of cirrhosis, the hemosiderin accumulates primarily in periportal hepatocytes and is less toward the central veins. The iron of cirrhotic livers is mostly in the periphery of regenerative nodules. Fibrosis begins periportally, then fibrous septa traverse the lobules. Usually, the distortion of the architecture is not as severe or as uniform as in alcoholic cirrhosis.[578] The cirrhosis of hemochromatosis usually has a micronodular appearance. Iron in bile duct epithelium has sometimes been considered a specific marker for hemochromatosis, but is not reliable. The amount of iron in the liver is always greatly increased. This is apparent on inspection of sections stained for iron with the Prussian Blue reaction, and can be quantitated on liver biopsy specimens. An iron concentration of more than 300 μmol/g dry weight is considered strong evidence for hemochromatosis when factors such as transfusions are eliminated as the cause.

In the original description of African iron overload, the liver pathology was deemed to be indistinguishable from that of classical hemochromatosis,[579] but in newer studies[580] it seems that only some of the affected patients manifest iron storage, primarily in the hepatocytes; some have storage primarily in Kupffer cells. In the case of patients with ferroportin mutations that prevent transport of iron, storage of iron takes place mostly in the Kupffer cells, and fibrosis seems to be absent; ferroportin mutations that prevent interaction with hepcidin, on the other hand, are associated with hepatocytes iron overload, as is seen in classical hemochromatosis.[581]

Heart Cardiac iron overload occurs later than hepatic iron overload.[582] The myocardium is thickened and the heart is often enlarged; arrhythmias and myocardial failure follows. Accumulation of cardiac iron is the leading cause of death in transfused patients with β-thalassemia major. Patients with transfusion-dependent anemias, such as congenital dyserythropoietic anemia and Diamond-Blackfan syndrome, also develop iron overload-induced cardiomyopathy. In transfused patients with myelodysplastic syndrome transfusion threshold guidelines of 75 units of blood was suggested as a risk factor of cardiac iron overload,[582] but this is not based on firm data. Direct cardiac iron measurement using magnetic resonance imaging predicts cardiac complications and can stratify the risk of subsequent cardiac dysfunction. This technique measures the half-life, T2*, of cardiac muscle darkening (with respect to echo time) produced by magnetically active stored cardiac iron.[582] Two separate publications, one evaluating cardiac iron overload by cardiac T2* magnetic resonance imaging, the other looking at causes of mortality, showed that deferiprone can unload myocardial iron faster than deferoxamine.[583,584]

Marrow The quantity of iron in the marrow of patients with classical hereditary hemochromatosis is only modestly increased, if increased at all. The iron is characteristically distributed into small, equal-size granules,[585] and these have been found to be located in endothelial lining cells rather than in macrophages.[586] Indeed, in classical hereditary hemochromatosis, both macrophages[587] and intestinal mucosal cells are iron-poor relative to the overall iron burden.

Other Tissues Although more iron than normal is found in intestinal mucosal cells,[588] in relationship to the total iron burden as indicated by the serum ferritin level, the amount of iron is strikingly decreased.[589] The same relationship has been noted in HFE knockout mice.[590] In contrast, in patients with transfusional iron overload, macrophages are heavily laden with iron, presumably derived from transfused red cells.

Testes are often atrophic.

Genetics

Genetic factors play an important role in the etiology of iron storage disease. This is true not only in the primary forms of the disorder, but also in secondary hemochromatosis, where genetic disorders of erythropoiesis are the most common causes. The genetics of these disorders, including the thalassemias, dyserythropoietic anemias, and red cell enzymopathies, are described elsewhere in this text (see Chaps. 39, 46, and 47). Mutations of several genes that play an important role in iron homeostasis have been found to lead to iron storage disease.[516]

***HFE* Mutations** The most common cause of hereditary hemochromatosis is a mutation of the *HFE* gene. This HLA-like gene resides on chromosome 6. Three polymorphic mutations have been identified. These are located at nucleotides 187, 193, and 845 of the cDNA (complementary DNA) and encode the H63D, S65C, and C282Y mutations, respectively. The phenotypic effect of these mutations on iron homeostasis are manifested in the following order: C282Y > H63D > S65C. Hereditary hemochromatosis is essentially an autosomal recessive disorder. Approximately two-thirds of homozygotes for the C282Y and a slightly lower percentage of compound heterozygotes for the C282Y and H63D mutations manifest increased serum transferrin saturations and serum ferritin levels. Individuals heterozygous for either the C282Y or the H63D mutation have, on the average, significantly higher transferrin saturations and serum ferritin levels than do wild-type homozygotes. However, the magnitude of this increase is very low. For example, the average transferrin saturation of man with the wild-type genotype is 26.69 percent and heterozygotes for the C282Y mutation have a transferrin saturation averaging 30.63 percent. The increase in the geometric mean of the serum ferritin is even less, from 118 to 122 ng/mL.[526] The effect of the H63D mutation is even less, and that of the S65C mutation barely perceptible.[591]

In spite of the minimal effect of the heterozygous state for *HFE* mutations on iron homeostasis it has been proposed by a number of investigators that heterozygotes are at increased risk for a variety of disorders. It has been suggested that heterozygosity for the C282Y mutation is associated with more fibrosis in chronic hepatitis,[592,593,593–595] but not in alcoholic liver disease.[596–598] It is also been claimed that the prevalence of the heterozygous state is significantly higher in patients with autoimmune hepatitis.[599] Other studies found an association between the heterozygous state and hepatocellular carcinoma[600] or breast cancer.[601] What has not been taken into account in the studies is the fact that the *HFE* gene is in linkage disequilibrium with many immune-response genes on chromosome 6; consequently, it is not possible to distinguish the minor effects that *HFE* mutations may have on iron homeostasis from variation in the immune response. The suggestion that increased iron levels are a risk factor for cardiovascular disease has been made repeatedly,[602,603] but a number of well-conducted negative studies[426–428,430,604–606] cast serious doubt on this premise.

***HAMP* (Hepcidin) Mutations** Mutations of hepcidin are rare, and are associated with severe juvenile hemochromatosis.[516,607]

***SCL40A1* (Ferroportin) Mutations** Mutations of the gene encoding ferroportin cause an autosomal dominant iron storage disease. Murine studies suggest that the dominant nature of ferroportin disease is a result of a dominant negative effect.[608] In the case of patients with ferroportin mutations that do not localized to the cell surface, preventing transport of iron, storage of iron takes place mostly in the Kupffer cells, and cirrhosis does not occur. Conversely, ferroportin mutations that prevent interaction with hepcidin are associated with hepatocyte iron overload, as is seen in classical hemochromatosis.[581] A triplet deletion that causes the loss of a valine has been encountered repeatedly. A common polymorphism c.744G→T (Gln284His) shows an association with African iron overload, but is clearly not present in all patients who manifest this syndrome.[609,610]

***TfR-2* Mutations** Mutations of *TfR-2* cause an autosomal recessive disorder that is indistinguishable clinically from hereditary hemochromatosis.[611–615]

Hemojuvelin Mutations Several different mutations of a gene designated as *HFE2* and as *HJV* cause juvenile hemochromatosis.[566,616–621] Hemojuvelin belongs to the class of glycosylphosphatidylinositol-anchored repulsive-guidance molecules, and may act as a coreceptor for bone morphogenetic proteins.[622]

DMT-1 Human Mutations DMT-1 human mutations are all associated with hepatic hemosiderosis and most with abnormal liver function tests in addition to microcytic hypochromic anemia.[623,624] This is in contrast to mice and rats with DMT-1 mutations,[625,626] as these DMT-1-deficient rodents are iron deficient. This is likely because humans, unlike rodents, can also absorb heme-containing iron.[627]

Animal Models

Naturally Occurring Models In nature, a number of animal species, such as myna birds,[628,629] the toco toucan,[558,630] Salers cattle,[559] a pony,[631] horses,[632] lemurs,[633] and the browsing rhinoceros, are iron-loaded.[557] The latter two species may represent an interesting paradigm for iron storage in captive species. Although the browsing rhinoceros species are iron loaded, grazing species are not. It seems likely that because iron is not readily available in the leaves eaten by the browsing species, it has evolved to more efficiently take up iron from its diet—more efficiently than needed when fed a zoo diet. Comparison of the *HFE* gene of browsing and grazing rhinoceros species showed numerous differences, but it is not clear whether any of these are related to the hyperabsorption of iron that is observed.[634] Similarly, lemurs subsist on a diet rich in leaves in the wild state, but are fed an iron-rich diet in captivity.[633]

Models Produced by Iron Loading Numerous efforts have been made to create models of hemochromatosis by loading laboratory animals with iron, either by the oral or parenteral route.[635–640] Some of these appear to simulate the human disease in one respect or another. For example, the iron-loaded gerbil[640,641] develops heart disease, features of which resemble the human disease. Moreover, such models have been used for the study of potential chelating agents.

Targeted Disruption Models Targeted disruption of most of the genes involved in iron homeostasis has been achieved. Included are *HFE*,[642,643] transferrin receptor 2,[644] iron-regulatory protein-2,[645] ferroportin,[646] hemojuvelin,[562] and hepcidin.[647] The effect of various combinations of gene knockouts, including *HFE*, β_2-microglobulin, hephaestin, and transferrin receptor, have been documented.[648]

■ CLINICAL FEATURES

Classical Hereditary Hemochromatosis

Onset The clinical features of the most common form of hereditary hemochromatosis are cirrhosis of the liver, darkening of the skin, cardiomyopathies, and diabetes. In contrast to the juvenile form of the disease, in which onset is usually in the second or third decade of life, classical hereditary hemochromatosis associated with mutations of the *HFE* gene generally is diagnosed in the fifth or six decade of life.

General Symptomatology Many symptoms are attributed to hereditary hemochromatosis, including abdominal pain, weakness, lethargy, fatigue, loss of libido, impotence, and arthropathies. However, all of these symptoms are common in an aging population, and epidemiologic studies show that none of them are more common in patients with the HFE hemochromatosis, even those with the biochemical phenotype, than they are in the general population.[526–529,649–651]

Arthropathies The arthralgia of patients with hemochromatosis is claimed to have characteristic features.[652] It is said to tend to begin at the small joints of the hands, especially the second and third metacarpal joints, and that in some cases episodes of acute synovitis may occur as in calcium pyrophosphosphate dehydrate deposition arthropathy (pseudogout; chondrocalcinosis). Radiologically the arthropathy resembles that of osteoarthritis with joint space loss, subchondral cysts, sclerosis, and osteophytosis. The features that have been considered distinctive include the joint distribution, the presence of shape osteophytes emerging from the radial sides of the metacarpal distal epiphysis, and the presence of radiolucent zones in the subchondral area of the femoral head. In one investigation using historical controls, a borderline statistically significant increase in the number of patients with chondrocalcinosis who were homozygous for the C282Y mutation was documented.[653] However, properly blinded, controlled studies have not shown that any form of arthritis is more common in hereditary hemochromatosis than in the general population.[116,528] Arthritis was not mentioned by Sheldon as one of the clinical manifestations of hemochromatosis in his detailed monograph.[502] Moreover, it is generally recognized that arthritis does not respond to phlebotomy therapy; in one study 9.2 percent of patients reported improvement of joint pain with treatment and 34 percent said that it was worse.[654] In fact, in a large survey virtually none of the nonspecific findings reported by patients[654] improved significantly with therapy. The possibility that excess iron does produce joint symptoms does remain open but unproven.[655]

Liver When cirrhosis is present there is a greatly increased risk of the patient developing a hepatoma.[656,657]

Porphyria Cutanea Tarda Porphyria cutanea tarda is a disease that is well known to be associated with mild iron overload and that responds to phlebotomy treatment (see Chap. 57). Numerous studies document that the prevalence of patients with this disorder who also have mutations of the *HFE* gene is considerably increased. Some of these patients are homozygotes; others heterozygotes.[658–660]

Juvenile Hemochromatosis

The penetrance of the rare juvenile form of the disease seems to be high and cardiomyopathies and endocrine deficiencies are the major clinical features.[661,494] Joint manifestations were found to be relatively common in patients with juvenile hemochromatosis.[662]

African Iron Overload

It is not clear to what extent African iron overload is symptomatic. Among the Bantu, where the disorder was originally described, there are many complicating factors, including malnutrition and high alcohol intake. Among African Americans various associated disorders have been noted, but a cause-and-effect relationship is not clear. In one series of 23 patients, 5 had arthropathy, 2 had diabetes mellitus, 2 had hypogonadism, and there were no instances of cirrhosis.[580]

Secondary Hemochromatosis

The clinical findings in patients with hemochromatosis secondary to blood transfusion and/or disorders of erythropoiesis are, in general, indistinguishable from those found in patients with the primary hemochromatosis.[567]

LABORATORY FEATURES

The main laboratory features of hereditary hemochromatosis are an increased transferrin saturation, and increased serum ferritin level. Five to 10 percent of patients with classical HFE hemochromatosis manifest increased liver enzyme levels in the serum. In secondary hemochromatosis anemia and the other manifestations of the underlying disorder are found. Macrocytosis of the erythrocytes is a common feature[663,664]; this finding seems unrelated to liver disease and its cause is unknown.

Differential Diagnosis

A large number of methods have been introduced that allow the amount of storage iron to be estimated.[665] The suspicion that a patient may have primary hemochromatosis is generally raised by an increased serum transferrin saturation, particularly when it is found together with and elevated serum ferritin level. An increased transferrin saturation commonly occurs in patients with chronic liver disease who have no mutations in the *HFE* gene.[666] Ferritin is an acute phase protein and levels are elevated in a variety of disorders. Particularly high levels are encountered in patients with Gaucher disease,[349] in some malignancies,[394,667] and in patients with the hyperferritinemia-cataract syndrome. The latter disorder is an uncommon autosomal dominant defect in which a mutation in the 5′ IRE of the ferritin light chain prevents binding of the IRPs, resulting in unrestrained constitutive production of the ferritin chains.[668,669]

Many clinicians have considered a liver biopsy the "gold standard" for the diagnosis of iron overload. The material obtained at biopsy not only provides the opportunity to assess the histopathology of the liver of the patient, but also to quantitate the amount of nonheme iron in the specimen. Dividing the iron content by the patient's age provides an iron index; a value greater than 2 implies the presence of hemochromatosis.[670] Although in some situations liver biopsy may provide useful information, it is an invasive procedure that, although low-risk, cannot be considered to be free of risk. Enthusiasm for subjecting every patient with potential hemochromatosis to liver biopsy has diminished with the ready availability of genetic analysis. Moreover, a simple way to determine whether a patient is iron overloaded is to institute a program of phlebotomies. This is an essentially harmless way to determine how much storage iron the body contains. Other noninvasive, but less-readily available methods, for determining whether excess iron is present in the liver are the superconducting quantum interference device (SQUID)[671] and magnetic resonance imaging (MRI).[665,672–675] MRI is able to detect increased amounts of iron in the liver, but generally special techniques are required, and accuracy is satisfactory only at relatively high iron levels.[665,672,674]

For detection of cardiac iron overload, T2* magnetic resonance imaging[582] is a superior diagnostic approach.

THERAPY

The treatment of hemochromatosis consists of removing the accumulated iron. In the case of patients who are able to mount an erythropoietin response to phlebotomy, removal of blood is generally the treatment of choice. When the patient has marked impairment of erythropoiesis, as in thalassemia and dyserythropoietic anemia, it is necessary to employ chelating agents to remove iron, although occasionally serial phlebotomy will stimulate sufficient erythropoiesis to make it a viable therapy.[676]

Phlebotomy

Each milliliter of packed red cells contains approximately 1 mg of iron. Thus, the removal of 500 mL of blood with a hematocrit of 40 percent removes approximately 200 mg of iron. As the red cell mass is restored to its prephlebotomy size, iron is mobilized from the stores. When the stores have been exhausted the signs of iron deficiency develop, and this is the endpoint of the initial part of the phlebotomy program. The patient is then followed and a schedule of maintenance phlebotomies is established with the frequency of phlebotomies tailored to maintain the serum ferritin level, the best indicator of body stores, below 100 ng/mL.

The actual volume of blood removed at each phlebotomy depends on the patient's size. Most average-size patients tolerate removal of 500 mL, but patients who weigh 50 kg or less are better treated by the removal of correspondingly smaller volumes of blood. Many patients may complain of symptoms following the first few phlebotomies. Better compliance is achieved if such symptoms are minimized by performing phlebotomies only every 14 days initially, increasing the frequency to weekly phlebotomies once the patient has become accustomed to the procedure and the activity of the marrow has been stimulated so as to replace the lost erythrocytes rapidly. The hematocrit or hemoglobin and the MCV of the red cells should be measured before each phlebotomy is undertaken. If there has been a substantial decrease in the hematocrit or hemoglobin, the phlebotomy should be deferred. The MCV may rise early in the treatment program, but as iron deficiency develops it will fall, signaling that the endpoint has been reached or is near. The transferrin saturation and serum ferritin level should be measured every 2 or 3 months. When the transferrin saturation is less than 10 percent and the serum ferritin less than 10 ng/mL, phlebotomy should be discontinued and the patient monitored every 4 to 8 weeks. When the serum ferritin is in the 50 to 100 ng/mL range, the maintenance phase should be initiated. Some patients may require phlebotomies monthly to maintain a normal ferritin value, whereas others may only require two or three phlebotomies per year.

Chelation Therapy

Chelation therapy instituted in a timely manner can decrease the potential morbidity caused by iron overload and prolong the life of patients with hereditary chronic iron-loading disorders such as thalassemia major. It also has a place in the management of some patients with acquired marrow dysplasias provided that the prognosis of the underlying disorder, and the patient's psychological state, justifies the somewhat cumbersome implementation of parenteral chelation. As oral chelating agents become more readily available, the application of chelation therapy to myelodysplastic states may broaden.

Desferrioxamine

Desferrioxamine is a naturally occurring iron chelating compound elaborated by the microorganism *Streptomyces pilosus*, having evolved to enable the microbe to obtain iron from its environment. One molecule of this chelator binds one atom of iron. Its molecular weight is 560 daltons. The iron complex is excreted into the urine and feces. Urine iron is derived primarily from red cells broken down by macrophages, whereas fecal iron is believed to be from iron chelated in the liver.[677]

Desferrioxamine is poorly absorbed from the gastrointestinal tract and must therefore be given parenterally, either by the subcutaneous or intravenous route. Rapid intravenous or intramuscular injection results in the relatively little iron mobilization; instead, it is necessary to administer desferrioxamine by slow intravenous or subcutaneous infusion over a period of 8 to 10 hours. An alternate method is twice-daily subcutaneous injection,[678] but this is not well tolerated by all patients.[679] Increasing doses of desferrioxamine result in increased iron excretion,[680] and the usual recommended dose is 30 to 50 mL/kg.[677] The administration of 200 mg of ascorbic acid *after* the infusion of desferrioxamine has been started increases the amount of iron excreted, and is therefore recommended. However, it is considered potentially hazardous to administer ascorbic acid to iron overloaded patients in the absence of a powerful chelating agent because the mobilization of iron from tissues has been thought to produce acute cardiac damage.[681] The amount of iron excreted will vary from patient-to-patient and depends to a large extent on the iron burden. Because the treatment is cumbersome and costly, one should be reasonably certain that sufficient good is being accomplished to justify the effort. This can be achieved by measuring urine output of iron after a test desferrioxamine infusion, bearing in mind that urinary excretion may account for only one-third of the iron excreted, fecal excretion accounting for the rest.[682]

Desferrioxamine is usually well tolerated. Minor local reactions such as local pruritus, induration, or pain at the site of infusion are not uncommon. Large doses are associated with hearing loss, night blindness and other visual abnormalities, growth retardation, and skeletal changes. At very high doses occasional cases of kidney and lung abnormalities have been reported.[677]

Oral Chelating Agents

The inconvenience and high cost of therapy with desferrioxamine has stimulated an intensive search for safe, orally active chelating agents. Deferiprone (L-1) is an orally effective agent that is currently available. At the end of 2009 it was licensed in many countries (not including the United States). It is a bidentate chelating agent; three molecules of deferiprone bind one iron atom. Its molecular weight is only 139 daltons and it is excreted almost entirely in the urine. The usual dose is 75 mg/kg per day divided into three doses. Deferiprone administration is associated with a number of toxic effects, including gastrointestinal disturbances, transient increases in the serum levels of liver enzymes, and zinc deficiency. The main concern has centered on the propensity of the drug to produce neutropenia and agranulocytosis. The latter complication occurs in approximately 1 percent of patients. It appears to be idiosyncratic, is more common in females, and appears to be reversible. Neutropenia with a granulocyte level between 0.5 and 1.5×10^9/L (500 and 1500/μL) recurs in an additional 5 percent of patients. Treatment should be stopped at the first sign of a fall in the leukocyte count.[365,677] It has been suggested that deferiprone may be more effective in removing iron from the heart and desferrioxamine more effective with respect to liver iron accumulations.[365] Preliminary investigations suggest that a combination of desferrioxamine and deferiprone may be more effective than either alone.[683,684]

Two studies suggested that deferiprone can unload myocardial iron faster than deferoxamine.[583,584]

Deferasirox (ICL670 or Exjade), a tridented triazole component, is a newer oral iron chelating ageint.[685] At a dose of 30 mg/kg per day, it was found as efficient as desferrioxamine and is generally well tolerated. It has been recommended for patients who are noncompliant with desferrioxamine,[686] but some questions have been raised with respect to safety and efficacy.[687]

COURSE AND PROGNOSIS

A century ago when classical hereditary hemochromatosis was first recognized as a disease entity the average survival after diagnosis was only 18.5 months,[502] most of the deaths being a result of diabetic coma in the preinsulin era. The outlook in this disease has changed in the current century to one in which the life span of patients with hemochromatosis is normal or nearly so. This is largely a result of the change in the definition of the disorder. In the early 20th century, the diagnosis was reserved for the rare patient with full-blown bronzed diabetes. Today, the diagnosis is applied to any person found to be homozygous for the C282Y mutation, or, indeed, anyone with an increased transferrin saturation and elevated serum ferritin level. In reality, patients with a diagnosis of hemochromatosis based on genetic and/or biochemical criteria have a normal life span. Although this has erroneously been attributed to the institution of therapy,[688,689] it applies equally to untreated patients discovered in population surveys. If such untreated patients suffered an early demise in the absence of treatment one would expect their number to diminish in cohorts of increasing age, but this does not appear to be the case, even in very large series.[690] Surprisingly, long-term followup of patients not treated by phlebotomy shows little or no increase of serum ferritin levels, even after a followup of as much as 23 years.[649,691] This is not to suggest that patients do not die of hereditary hemochromatosis; it is simply that the penetrance of the disorder as detected on genetic or biochemical bases is so low that the few deaths that do occur cannot be detected even in very sizable series.

For those patients with classical hereditary hemochromatosis who are clinically affected, it is likely that removal of iron by phlebotomy prevents further complications and prolongs life span. Although controlled studies of the effect of phlebotomy are not ethically feasible, serial observations in patients undergoing phlebotomy suggest that cirrhosis is either stabilized[692] or may, at least in some patients, improve.[505,692–696] Platelet counts improvement a large proportion of patients with cirrhosis undergoing phlebotomy.[697]

The course of untreated juvenile hemochromatosis seems less benign. Cardiac deaths seem to be particularly common,[698] and in a few cases cardiac transplantation has been performed successfully,[494] but there are insufficient data concerning this rare disorder to allow one to provide more precise information about the outlook.

The prognosis in thalassemia major and similar disorders is grim when iron chelation is not performed (see Chap. 47).[699] Death is most frequently a result of cardiac failure. It is estimated that approximately 3000 thalassemia patients die each year as a result of iron overload.[365]

REFERENCES

1. Koorts AM, Viljoen M: Ferritin and ferritin isoforms I: Structure-function relationships, synthesis, degradation and secretion. *Arch Physiol Biochem* 113:30, 2007.
2. Hempstead PD, Yewdall SJ, Fernie AR, et al: Comparison of the three-dimensional structures of recombinant human H and horse L ferritins at high resolution. *J Mol Biol* 268:424, 1997.
3. Harrison PM, Arosio P: The ferritins: Molecular properties, iron storage function and cellular regulation. *Biochim Biophys Acta* 1275:161, 1996.
4. Ward RJ, Legssyer R, Henry C, Crichton RR: Does the haemosiderin iron core determine its potential for chelation and the development of iron-induced tissue damage? *J Inorg Biochem* 79:311, 2000.
5. Pollycove M, Mortimer R: The quantitative determination of iron kinetics and hemoglobin synthesis in human subjects. *J Clin Invest* 40:753, 1961.
6. Hosain F, Marsaglia G, Finch CA: Blood ferrokinetics in normal man. *J Clin Invest* 46:1, 1967.
7. Petrat F, de Groot H, Sustmann R, Rauen U: The chelatable iron pool in living cells: A methodically defined quantity. *Biol Chem* 383:489, 2002.
8. Prus E, Fibach E: Flow cytometry measurement of the labile iron pool in human hematopoietic cells. *Cytometry A* 73:22, 2008.
9. Beutler E: Tissue effects of iron deficiency, in *Iron Metabolism*, edited by F Gross, SR Naegeli, HD Philps, p 256. Springer-Verlag, Berlin, 1963.
10. Dallman PR, Beutler E, Finch CA: Effects of iron deficiency exclusive of anaemia. *Br J Haematol* 40:179, 1978.
11. Lozoff B: Perinatal iron deficiency and the developing brain. *Pediatr Res* 48:137, 2000.
12. Bailey S, Evans RW, Garratt RC, et al: Molecular structure of serum transferrin at 3.3-A resolution. *Biochemistry* 27:5804, 1988.
13. van Haeringen B, de Lange F, van Stokkum IHM, et al: Dynamic structure of human serum transferrin from transient electric birefringence experiments. *Proteins: Structure, Function and Bioinformatics* 23:233, 1998.
14. Haurani FI, Meyer A, O'Brien R: Production of transferrin by the macrophage. *J Reticuloendothel Soc* 14:309, 1973.
15. Thorbecke GJ, Liem HH, Knight S, Cox K, Muller-Eberhard U: Sites of formation of the serum proteins transferrin and hemopexin. *J Clin Invest* 52:725, 1973.
16. Welch S, Langmead L: A comparison of the structure and properties of normal human transferrin and a genetic variant of human transferrin. *Int J Biochem* 22:275, 1990.
17. Young SP, Bomford A, Madden AD, et al: Abnormal in vitro function of a variant human transferrin. *Br J Haematol* 56:581, 1984.
18. Lee PL, Halloran C, Trevino R, et al: Human transferrin G277S mutation: A risk factor for iron deficiency anaemia. *Br J Haematol* 115:329, 2001.
19. Aisen P: The G277S mutation in transferrin does not disturb function. *Br J Haematol* 121:674, 2003.
20. Sarria B, Navas-Carretero S, Lopez-Parra AM, et al: The G277S transferrin mutation does not affect iron absorption in iron deficient women. *Eur J Nutr* 46:57, 2007.
21. Moore CV: Iron nutrition and requirements. *Ser Haematol* 6:1, 1965.
22. Pennington JA, Young BE, Wilson DB, et al: Mineral content of foods and total diets: The Selected Minerals in Foods Survey, 1982 to 1984. *J Am Diet Assoc* 86:876, 1986.
23. Dubach R, Moore CV, Callender S: Studies in iron transportation and metabolism IX. The excretion of iron as measured by the isotope technique. *J Lab Clin Med* 45:599, 1955.
24. Herndon JF, Rice EG, Tucker RG, et al: Iron absorption and metabolism. III. The enhancement of iron absorption in rats by D-sorbitol. *J Nutr* 64:615, 1958.
25. Hallberg L, Sölvell L: Iron absorption studies: [1] Determination of the absorption rate of iron in man. [2] Absorption of a single dose of iron in man. [3] Iron absorption during constant intragastric infusion of iron in man. [4] Effect of iron and transferrin intravenously on iron absorption and turnover in man (Sölvell alone). *Acta Med Scand Suppl* 358:1, 1960.
26. Pollack S, Kaufman RM, Crosby WH: Iron absorption: Effects of sugars and reducing agents. *Blood* 24:577, 1964.
27. Slatkavitz CA, Clydesdale FM: Solubility of inorganic iron as affected by proteolytic digestion. *Am J Clin Nutr* 47:487, 1988.
28. Taylor PG, Martinez-Torres C, Romano EL, Layrisse M: The effect of cysteine-containing peptides released during meat digestion on iron absorption in humans. *Am J Clin Nutr* 43:68, 1986.
29. Charlton RW, Jacobs P, Seftel H, Bothwell TH: Effect of alcohol on iron absorption. *Br Med J* 2:1427, 1964.
30. Celada A, Rudolf H, Donath A: Effect of a single ingestion of alcohol on iron absorption. *Am J Hematol* 5:225, 1978.
31. Bezwoda WR, Torrance JD, Bothwell TH, et al: Iron absorption from red and white wines. *Scand J Haematol* 34:121, 1985.
32. Cook JD, Reddy MB, Hurrell RF: The effect of red and white wines on nonheme-iron absorption in humans. *Am J Clin Nutr* 61:800, 1995.
33. Hankes LV, Jansen CR, Schmaeler M: Ascorbic acid catabolism in Bantu with hemosiderosis (scurvy). *Biochem Med* 9:244, 1974.
34. Flanagan JM, Peng H, Beutler E: Effects of alcohol consumption on iron metabolism in mice with hemochromatosis mutations. *Alcohol Clin Exp Res* 31:138, 2006.
35. Weintraub LR, Weinstein MB, Huser H, Rafal S: Absorption of hemoglobin iron: The role of a heme-splitting substance in the intestinal mucosa. *J Clin Invest* 47:531, 1968.
36. Shayeghi M, Latunde-Dada GO, Oakhill JS, et al: Identification of an intestinal heme transporter. *Cell* 122:789, 2005.
37. Qiu A, Jansen M, Sakaris A, et al: Identification of an intestinal folate transporter and the molecular basis for hereditary folate malabsorption. *Cell* 127:917, 2006.
38. Latunde-Dada GO, Van der Westhuizen J, Vulpe CD, Anderson GJ, et al: Molecular and functional roles of duodenal cytochrome B (dcytb) in iron metabolism. *Blood Cells Mol Dis* 29:356, 2002.
39. McKie AT, Barrow D, Latunde-Dada GO, et al: An iron-regulated ferric reductase associated with the absorption of dietary iron. *Science* 291:1755, 2001.
40. Conrad ME, Umbreit JN: Pathways of iron absorption. *Blood Cells Mol Dis* 29:336, 2002.
41. Beutler E: History of iron in Medicine. *Blood Cells Mol Dis* 29:297, 2002.
42. Beutler E, Kelly BM, Beutler F: The regulation of iron absorption. II. Relationship between iron dosage and iron absorption. *Am J Clin Nutr* 11:559, 1962.
43. Smith MD, Pannacciulli IM: Absorption of inorganic iron from graded doses: Its significance in relation to iron absorption tests and the "mucosal block" theory. *Br J Haematol* 4:428, 1958.
44. Gitlin D, Cruchaud A: On the kinetics of iron absorption in mice. *J Clin Invest* 41:344, 1962.
45. Andrews NC: Forging a field: The golden age of iron biology. *Blood* 112:219, 2008.
46. Lee P, Beutler E: Hepcidin and iron overload. *Annu Rev Pathol* 4:489-415, 2009.
47. Park CH, Valore EV, Waring AJ, Ganz T: Hepcidin, a urinary antimicrobial peptide synthesized in the liver. *J Biol Chem* 276:7806, 2001.
48. Krause A, Neitz S, Magert HJ, et al: LEAP-1, a novel highly disulfide-bonded human peptide, exhibits antimicrobial activity. *FEBS Lett* 480:147, 2000.
49. Nicolas G, Bennoun M, Porteu A, et al: Severe iron deficiency anemia in transgenic mice expressing liver hepcidin. *Proc Natl Acad Sci U S A* 99:4596, 2002.
50. Weinstein DA, Roy CN, Fleming MD, et al: Inappropriate expression of hepcidin is associated with iron refractory anemia: Implications for the anemia of chronic disease. *Blood* 100:3776, 2002.
51. Laftah AH, Ramesh B, Simpson RJ, et al: Effect of hepcidin on intestinal iron absorption in mice. *Blood* 103:3940, 2004.
52. Nemeth E, Tuttle MS, Powelson J, et al: Hepcidin regulates iron efflux by binding to ferroportin and inducing its internalization. *Science* 306:2090, 2004.
53. De Domenico I, Ward DM, Langelier C, et al: The molecular mechanism of hepcidin-mediated ferroportin down-regulation. *Mol Biol Cell* 18:2569, 2007.
54. Nemeth E, Valore EV, Territo M, et al: Hepcidin, a putative mediator of anemia of inflammation, is a type II acute-phase protein. *Blood* 101:2461, 2003.
55. Nicolas G, Viatte L, Bennoun M, et al: Hepcidin, a new iron regulatory peptide. *Blood Cells Mol Dis* 29:327, 2002.
56. Nicolas G, Chauvet C, Viatte L, et al: The gene encoding the iron regulatory peptide hepcidin is regulated by anemia, hypoxia, and inflammation. *J Clin Invest* 110:1037, 2002.
57. Babitt JL, Huang FW, Xia Y,et al: Modulation of bone morphogenetic protein signaling in vivo regulates systemic iron balance. *J Clin Invest* 117:1933, 2007.

58. Truksa J, Peng H, Lee P, Beutler E: Different regulatory elements are required for response of hepcidin to IL-6 and bone morphogenetic proteins BMP 4 and 9. *Br J Haematol* 139:138, 2007.
59. Babitt JL, Huang FW, Wrighting DM, et al: Bone morphogenetic protein signaling by hemojuvelin regulates hepcidin expression. *Nat Genet* 38:531, 2006.
60. Peyssonnaux C, Zinkernagel AS, Schuepbach RA, et al: Regulation of iron homeostasis by the hypoxia-inducible transcription factors (HIFs). *J Clin Invest* 117:1926, 2007.
61. De Domenico I, Vey Ward D, Kaplan J: Regulation of iron acquisition and storage: Consequences for iron-linked disorders. *Nat Rev Mol Cell Biol* 9:72, 2008.
62. Lin L, Nemeth E, Goodnough JB, et al: Iron-transferrin regulates hepcidin synthesis in primary hepatocyte culture through hemojuvelin and BMP2/4. *Blood* 110:2182, 2007.
63. Schmidt PJ, Toran PT, Giannetti AM, et al: The transferrin receptor modulates HFE-dependent regulation of hepcidin expression. *Cell Metab* 7:205, 2008.
64. Lin L, Nemeth E, Goodnough JB, et al: Soluble hemojuvelin is released by proprotein convertase-mediated cleavage at a conserved polybasic RNRR site. *Blood Cells Mol Dis* 40:122, 2008.
65. Silvestri L, Pagani A, Camaschella C: Furin-mediated release of soluble hemojuvelin: A new link between hypoxia and iron homeostasis. *Blood* 111:924, 2008.
66. Truksa J, Lee P, Beutler E: Two BMP responsive elements, STAT, and bZIP/HNF4/COUP motifs located in the distal part of the hepcidin promoter are critical for BMP, SMAD1 and HJV responsiveness. *Blood* 113:688, 2009.
67. Du X, She E, Gelbart T, Truksa J, et al: The serine protease TMPRSS6 is required to sense iron deficiency. *Science* 320:1088, 2008.
68. Dautry-Varsat A: Receptor-mediated endocytosis: The intracellular journey of transferrin and its receptor. *Biochimie* 68:375, 1986.
69. Schneider C, Williams JG: Molecular dissection of the human transferrin receptor. *J Cell Sci* 3(Suppl):139,1985.
70. Zerial M, Melancon P, Schneider C, Garoff H: The transmembrane segment of the human transferrin receptor functions as a signal peptide. *EMBO J* 5:1543, 1986.
71. Ward J H, Jordan I, Kushner, J P, Kaplan, J: Heme regulation of HeLa cell transferrin receptor number. *J Biol Chem* 259:13235, 1984.
72. Rouault T, Rao K, Harford J, et al: Hemin, chelatable iron, and the regulation of transferrin receptor biosynthesis. *J Biol Chem* 260:14862, 1985.
73. Pantopoulos K: Iron metabolism and the IRE/IRP regulatory system: An update. *Ann N Y Acad Sci* 1012:1, 2004.
74. Cartwright GE, Deiss A: Sideroblasts, siderocytes, and sideroblastic anemia. *N Engl J Med* 292:185, 1975.
75. Levi S, Corsi B, Bosisio M, et al: A human mitochondrial ferritin encoded by an intronless gene. *J Biol Chem* 276:24437, 2001.
76. Levi S, Arosio P: Mitochondrial ferritin. *Int J Biochem Cell Biol* 36:1887, 2004.
77. Drysdale J, Arosio P, Invernizzi R, et al: Mitochondrial ferritin: A new player in iron metabolism. *Blood Cells Mol Dis* 29:376, 2002.
78. Campanella A, Rovelli E, Santambrogio P, et al: Mitochondrial ferritin limits oxidative damage regulating mitochondrial iron availability: Hypothesis for a protective role in Friedreich ataxia. *Hum Mol Genet* 18:1, 2009.
79. Cazzola M, Invernizzi R, Bergamaschi G, et al: Mitochondrial ferritin expression in erythroid cells from patients with sideroblastic anemia. *Blood* 101:1996, 2003.
80. Napier I, Ponka P, Richardson DR: Iron trafficking in the mitochondrion: Novel pathways revealed by disease. *Blood* 105:1867, 2005.
81. Cairo G, Pietrangelo A: Iron regulatory proteins in pathobiology. *Biochem J* 352 Pt 2:241, 2000.
82. Bouton C, Drapier JC: Iron regulatory proteins as NO signal transducers. *Sci STKE* 2003:e17, 2003.
83. Kim S, Ponka P: Nitric oxide-mediated modulation of iron regulatory proteins: Implication for cellular iron homeostasis. *Blood Cells Mol Dis* 29:400, 2002.
84. Kim S, Wing SS, Ponka P: S-Nitrosylation of IRP2 regulates its stability via the ubiquitin-proteasome pathway. *Mol Cell Biol* 24:330, 2004.
85. Rouault TA: Post-transcriptional regulation of human iron metabolism by iron regulatory proteins. *Blood Cells Mol Dis* 29:309, 2002.
86. Meyron-Holtz EG, Ghosh MC, Rouault TA: Mammalian tissue oxygen levels modulate iron regulatory protein activities *in vivo*. Science 306:2087, 2004.
87. Noyes WD, Bothwell TH, Finch CA: The role of the reticulo-endothelial cell in iron metabolism. *Br J Haematol* 6:43, 1960.
88. Haurani FI, Burke W, Martinez EJ: Defective reutilization of iron in the anemia of inflammation. *J Lab Clin Med* 65:560, 1965.
89. O'Shea MJ, Kershenobich D, Tavill AS: Effects of inflammation on iron and transferrin metabolism. *Br J Haematol* 25:707, 1973.
90. Green R, Charlton R, Seftel H, et al: Body iron excretion in man: A collaborative study. *Am J Med* 45:336, 1968.
91. Bryan CP: *The Papyrus Ebers*. Appleton-Century-Crofts, New York, 1931.
92. Heath CW, Strauss MB, Castle WB: Quantitative aspects of iron deficiency in hypochromic anemia. *J Clin Invest* 11:1293, 1932.
93. Poskitt EME: Early history of iron deficiency. *Br J Haematol* 122:554, 2003.
94. Stoltzfus R: Defining iron-deficiency anemia in public health terms: A time for reflection. *J Nutr* 131:565S, 2001.
95. McIntyre AS, Long RG: Prospective survey of investigations in outpatients referred with iron deficiency anaemia. *Gut* 34:1102, 1993.
96. Retzlaff JA, Hagedorn AB, Bartholomew LG: Abdominal exploration for gastrointestinal bleeding of obscure origin. *JAMA* 177:104, 1961.
97. Baum S, Nusbaum M, Blakemore WS, Finkelstein AK: The preoperative radiographic demonstration of intra-abdominal bleeding from undetermined sites by percutaneous selective celiac and superior mesenteric arteriography. *Surgery* 58:797, 1965.
98. Prichard PJ, Tjandra JJ: Colorectal cancer. *Med J Aust* 169:493, 1998.
99. Fitzpatrick J: Hemocholecyst: A neglected cause of gastrointestinal hemorrhage. *Ann Intern Med* 55:1008, 1961.
100. Kaminski N, Shaham D, Eliakim R: Primary tumours of the duodenum. *Postgrad Med J* 69:136, 1993.
101. Coban E, Timuragaoglu A, Meric M: Iron deficiency anemia in the elderly: Prevalence and endoscopic evaluation of the gastrointestinal tract in outpatients. *Acta Haematol* 110:25, 2003.
102. Windsor CW, Collis JL: Anaemia and hiatus hernia: Experience in 450 patients. *Thorax* 22:73, 1967.
103. Holt JM, Mayet FG, Warner GT, et al: Iron absorption and blood loss in patients with hiatus hernia. *Br Med J* 3:22, 1968.
104. Moskovitz M, Fadden R, Min T, et al: Large hiatal hernias, anemia, and linear gastric erosion: Studies of etiology and medical therapy. *Am J Gastroenterol* 87:622, 1992.
105. Weston AP: Hiatal hernia with cameron ulcers and erosions. *Gastrointest Endosc Clin N Am* 6:671, 1996.
106. Cameron AJ, Higgins JA: Linear gastric erosion. A lesion associated with large diaphragmatic hernia and chronic blood loss anemia. *Gastroenterology* 91:338, 1986.
107. Roth WL, Valdes-Dapena A, Pieses P, Buchman E: Topical action of salicylates in gastrointestinal erosion and hemorrhage. *Gastroenterology* 44:146, 1963.
108. Faucheron JL, Parc R: Non-steroidal anti-inflammatory drug-induced colitis. *Int J Colorectal Dis* 11:99, 1996.
109. Oldenburg B, Koningsberger JC, Henegouwen GPV, et al: Review article: Iron and inflammatory bowel disease. *Aliment Pharmacol Ther* 15:429, 2001.
110. Singh AK, Cumaraswamy RC, Corrin B: Diffuse hypertrophy of gastric mucosa (Menetrier's disease) and iron-deficiency anaemia. *Gut* 10:735, 1969.
111. Barabino A: Helicobacter pylori-related iron deficiency anemia: A review. *Helicobacter* 7:71, 2002.
112. Perez RF, Castellanos Monedero JJ, Gonzalez CP, et al: Effect of *Helicobacter pylori* eradication on iron deficiency anemia of unknown origin. *Gastroenterol Hepatol* 31:213, 2008.
113. Chen LH, Luo HS: Effects of H pylori therapy on erythrocytic and iron parameters in iron deficiency anemia patients with H pylori-positive chronic gastritis. *World J Gastroenterol* 13:5380, 2007.
114. Choe YH, Kim SK, Son BK, et al: Randomized placebo-controlled trial of *Helicobacter pylori* eradication for iron-deficiency anemia in preadolescent children and adolescents. *Helicobacter* 4:135, 1999.
115. Yokota SI, Konno M, Mino E, et al: Enhanced Fe ion-uptake activity in *Helicobacter pylori* strains isolated from patients with iron-deficiency anemia. *Clin Infect Dis* 46:e31,2008.
116. Bini EJ: *Helicobacter pylori* and iron deficiency anemia: Guilty as charged? *Am J Med* 111:495, 2001.
117. Zaatar R, Younoszai MK, Mitros F: Pseudo-Zollinger-Ellison syndrome in a child presenting with anemia. *Gastroenterology* 92:508, 1987.
118. Crompton DW, Nesheim MC: Nutritional impact of intestinal helminthiasis during the human life cycle. *Annu Rev Nutr* 22:35, 2002.
119. Mahadeva S, Qua CS, Yusoff W, Sulaiman W: Repeat endoscopy for recurrent iron deficiency anemia: An (un)expected finding from southeast Asia. *Dig Dis Sci* 52:523, 2007.
120. Annibale B, Capurso G, Lahner E, et al: Concomitant alterations in intragastric pH and ascorbic acid concentration in patients with *Helicobacter pylori* gastritis and associated iron deficiency anaemia. *Gut* 52:496, 2003.
121. Annibale B, Capurso G, Delle FG: The stomach and iron deficiency anaemia: A forgotten link. *Dig Liver Dis* 35:288, 2003.
122. Kimber C, Patterson JF, Weintraub LR: The pathogenesis of iron deficiency anemia following partial gastrectomy. A study of iron balance. *JAMA* 202:935, 1967.
123. Sorbi D, Conio M, Gostout CJ: Vascular disorders of the small bowel. *Gastrointest Endosc Clin N Am* 9:71, 1999.
124. Toyota M, Hinoda Y, Nakagawa N, et al: Gastric antral vascular ectasia causing severe anemia. *J Gastroenterol* 31:710, 1996.
125. Blanc P, Phelip JM, Bertolino JG, et al: Watermelon stomach: A rare cause of iron deficiency anemia, surgically treatable; a new case with review of the literature. *Ann Chir* 128:462, 2003.
126. Holt JM, Wright R: Anaemia due to blood loss from the telangiectases of scleroderma. *Br Med J* 3:537, 1967.
127. Reinhart WH, Mordasini C, Staubli M, Scheurer U: Abnormalities of gut vessels in Turner's syndrome. *Postgrad Med J* 59:122, 1983.
128. Hagood MF, Gathright JB, Jr.: Hemangiomatosis of the skin and gastrointestinal tract: Report of a case. *Dis Colon Rectum* 18:141, 1975.
129. Ohishi M, Tanaka Y, Higuchi Y, et al: Multiple facial hemangiomas and iron-deficiency anemia: Blue rubber-bleb nevus syndrome. *Head Neck Surg* 7:249, 1985.
130. Morris SJ, Kaplan SR, Ballan K, Tedesco FJ: Blue rubber-bleb nevus syndrome. *JAMA* 239:1887, 1978.
131. Ferrara M, Coppola L, Coppola A, Capozzi L: Iron deficiency in childhood and adolescence: Retrospective review. *Hematology* 11:183, 2006.
132. Male C, Persson LA, Freeman V, et al: Prevalence of iron deficiency in 12-mo-old infants from 11 European areas and influence of dietary factors on iron status (Euro-Growth study). *Acta Paediatr* 90:492, 2001.

133. Coello-Ramirez P, Larrosa-Haro A: Gastrointestinal occult hemorrhage and gastroduodenitis in cow's milk protein intolerance. *J Pediatr Gastroenterol Nutr* 3:215, 1984.
134. Karr MA, Mira M, Alperstein G, et al: Iron deficiency in Australian-born children of Arabic background in central Sydney. *Med J Aust* 174:165, 2001.
135. Hudson BG, Tryggvason K, Sundaramoorthy M, Neilson EG: Alport's syndrome, Goodpasture's syndrome, and type IV collagen. *N Engl J Med* 348:2543, 2003.
136. Reid DW, Withers NJ, Francis L, et al: Iron deficiency in cystic fibrosis: Relationship to lung disease severity and chronic Pseudomonas aeruginosa infection. *Chest* 121:48, 2002.
137. Hallberg L, Hulthen L, Bengtsson C: Iron balance in menstruating women. *Eur J Clin Nutr* 49:200, 1995.
138. Hallberg L, Hogdahl AM, Nilsson L, Rybo G: Menstrual blood loss—A population study. Variation at different ages and attempts to define normality. *Acta Obstet Gynecol Scand* 45:320, 1966.
139. Hallberg L, Nilsson L: Constancy of individual menstrual blood loss. *Acta Obstet Gynecol Scand* 43:352, 1964.
140. Burton JL: Effect of oral contraceptives on haemoglobin, packed-cell volume, serum—Iron, and total iron-binding capacity in healthy women. *Lancet* 1:978, 1967.
141. Escobedo L, Lee NC: Beyond contraception: The health benefits and risks of the pill. *IPPF Med Bull* 22:1, 1988.
142. Kivijarvi A, Timonen H, Rajamaki A, Gronroos M: Iron deficiency in women using modern copper intrauterine devices. *Obstet Gynecol* 67:95, 1986.
143. Kildahl-Andersen O, Dahl IM, Thorstensen K, Sagen E: Iron deficiency anemia in a patient with excessive urinary iron loss. *Eur J Haematol* 64:204, 2000.
144. Fey MF, Radvila A: Long term follow-up of factitious anaemia. *BMJ* 296:1504, 1988.
145. Hirayama Y, Sakamaki S, Tsuji Y, et al: Fatality caused by self-bloodletting in a patient with factitious anemia. *Int J Hematol* 78:146, 2003.
146. Piccillo GA, Miele L, Mondati EG, et al: Eighteen needles to forget . . . an unnamed past. *J Forensic Leg Med* 14:304, 2007.
147. Henry ML, Garner WL, Fabri PJ: Iatrogenic anemia. *Am J Surg* 151:362, 1986.
148. Dale JC, Ruby SG: Specimen collection volumes for laboratory tests. *Arch Pathol Lab Med* 127:162, 2003.
149. Nissenson AR, Strobos J: Iron deficiency in patients with renal failure. *Kidney Int Suppl.* 69:S18, 1999.
150. Kalocheretis P, Vlamis I, Belesi C, et al: Residual blood loss in single use dialyzers: Effect of different membranes and flux. *Int J Artif Organs* 29:286, 2006.
151. Boulton F, Collis D, Inskip H, et al: A study of the iron and HFE status of blood donors, including a group who failed the initial screen for anaemia. *Br J Haematol* 108:434, 2000.
152. Milman N, Byg KE, Ovesen L, et al: Iron status in Danish men 1984–94: A cohort comparison of changes in iron stores and the prevalence of iron deficiency and iron overload. *Eur J Haematol* 68:332, 2002.
153. Makrides M, Crowther CA, Gibson RA, et al: Efficacy and tolerability of low-dose iron supplements during pregnancy: A randomized controlled trial. *Am J Clin Nutr* 78:145, 2003.
154. Bashiri A, Burstein E, Sheiner E, Mazor M: Anemia during pregnancy and treatment with intravenous iron: Review of the literature. *Eur J Obstet Gynecol Reprod Biol* 110:2, 2003.
155. Bayoumeu F, Subiran-Buisset C, et al: Iron therapy in iron deficiency anemia in pregnancy: Intravenous route versus oral route. *Am J Obstet Gynecol* 186:518, 2002.
156. Hercberg S, Galan P, Preziosi P, Aissa M: Consequences of iron deficiency in pregnant women—Current issues. *Clin Drug Investig* 19:1, 2000.
157. Villar J, Merialdi M, Gulmezoglu AM, et al: Nutritional interventions during pregnancy for the prevention or treatment of maternal morbidity and preterm delivery: An overview of randomized controlled trials. *J Nutr* 133:1606S, 2003.
158. Rasmussen KM, Stoltzfus RJ: New evidence that iron supplementation during pregnancy improves birth weight: New scientific questions. *Am J Clin Nutr* 78:673, 2003.
159. Mamula P, Piccoli DA, Peck SN, et al: Total dose intravenous infusion of iron dextran for iron-deficiency anemia in children with inflammatory bowel disease. *J Pediatr Gastroenterol Nutr* 34:286, 2002.
160. Cook JD: Iron-deficiency anaemia. *Baillieres Clin Haematol* 7:787, 1994.
161. Cogswell ME, Kettel-Khan L, Ramakrishnan U: Iron supplement use among women in the United States: Science, policy and practice. *J Nutr* 133:1974S, 2003.
162. Anonymous: Iron fortification of infant formulas. American Academy of Pediatrics. Committee on Nutrition. *Pediatrics* 104:119, 1999.
163. Federation of American Societies for Experimental Biology LSRO: *Third Report on Nutritional Monitoring in the US. Executive Summary.* U.S. Government Printing Office, Washington, DC, 1995.
164. Hurrell R, Bothwell T, Cook JD, et al: The usefulness of elemental iron for cereal flour fortification: A SUSTAIN Task Force report. Sharing United States Technology to Aid in the Improvement of Nutrition. *Nutr Rev* 60:391, 2002.
165. Hallberg L, Hulthen L: Perspectives on iron absorption. *Blood Cells Mol Dis* 29:562, 2002.
166. Leonard BJ: Hypochromic anaemia in R.A.F. recruits. *Lancet* 1:899, 1954.
167. Rosenbaum E, Leonard JW: Nutritional iron deficiency anemia in an adult male. Report of a case. *Ann Intern Med* 60:683, 1964.
168. Shearman DJ, Delamore IW, Gardner DL: Gastric function and structure in iron deficiency. *Lancet* 1:845, 1966.
169. Dagg JH, Goldberg A, Gibbs WN, Anderson JR: Detection of latent pernicious anaemia in iron-deficiency anaemia. *Br Med J* 2:619, 1966.
170. Voigt D, Bruschke G: Gastric mucosa and iron deficiency. *Dtsch Med Wochenschr* 92:1082, 1967.
171. Voigt D, Dieterich WR, Brushke G, Herrmann H: On blood concentrations of leukocytes and thrombocytes in iron deficiency. *Blut* 14:267, 1967.
172. Stone WD: Gastric secretory response to iron therapy. *Gut* 9:99, 1968.
173. Davidson WM, Markson JL: The gastric mucosa in iron-deficiency anaemia. *Lancet* 269:639, 1955.
174. Hershko C: A hematologist's view of unexplained iron deficiency anemia in males: Impact of *Helicobacter pylori* eradication. *Blood Cells Mol Dis* 38:45, 2007.
175. Hershko C, Ronson A, Souroujon M, et al: Variable hematological presentation of autoimmune gastritis: Age-related progression from iron deficiency to cobalamin depletion. *Blood* 107:1673, 2006.
176. Dickey W, McConnell B: Celiac disease presenting as the Paterson-Brown Kelly (Plummer-Vinson) syndrome. *Am J Gastroenterol* 94:527, 1999.
177. Vuopio P, Nikkilä EA: Hemolytic anemia and thrombocytopenia in a case of left atrial myxoma associated with mitral stenosis. *Am J Cardiol* 17:585, 1966.
178. Eyster E, Mayer K, McKenzie S: Traumatic hemolysis with iron deficiency anemia in patients with aortic valve lesions. *Ann Intern Med* 68:995, 1968.
179. Reynolds RD, Coltman CA Jr, Beller BM: Iron treatment in sideropenic intravascular hemolysis due to insufficiency of Starr-Edwards valve prostheses. *Ann Intern Med* 66:659, 1967.
180. Sears DA, Anderson PR, Foy AL, et al: Urinary iron excretion and renal metabolism of hemoglobin in hemolytic diseases. *Blood* 28:708, 1966.
181. Deitrick RW: Intravascular haemolysis in the recreational runner. *Br J Sports Med* 25:183, 1991.
182. Eliakim A, Nemet D, Constantini N: Screening blood tests in members of the Israeli National Olympic team. *J Sports Med Phys Fitness* 42:250, 2002.
183. Wilkinson JG, Martin DT, Adams AA, Liebman M: Iron status in cyclists during high-intensity interval training and recovery. *Int J Sports Med* 23:544, 2002.
184. Nielsen P, Nachtigall D: Iron supplementation in athletes. Current recommendations. *Sports Med* 26:207, 1998.
185. Mechrefe A, Wexler B, Feller E: Sports anemia and gastrointestinal bleeding in endurance athletes. *Med Health R I* 80:216, 1997.
186. Whitfield JB, Treloar S, Zhu G, et al: Relative importance of female-specific and non-female-specific effects on variation in iron stores between women. *Br J Haematol* 120:860, 2003.
187. Carlsson LE, Hempel S, Greinacher A: Iron deficiency anaemia in young women—A hypothesis on the impact of the platelet collagen receptor GPIaIIa polymorphism GPIa-C807T. *Eur J Haematol* 68:341, 2002.
188. Loría A, Sanchez-Medal L, Lisker R, et al: Red cell life span in iron deficiency anaemia. *Br J Haematol* 13:294, 1967.
189. Pollycove M: Iron metabolism and kinetics. *Semin Hematol* 3:235, 1966.
190. Beutler E: Iron enzymes in iron deficiency. *Blut* 6:130, 1960.
191. Srivastava SK, Sanwal GG, Tewari KK: Biochemical alterations in rat tissue in iron deficiency anaemia and repletion with iron. *Indian J Biochem Biophys* 2:257, 1965.
192. Celsing F, Ekblom B, Sylvén C, et al: Effects of chronic iron deficiency anaemia on myoglobin content, enzyme activity, and capillary density in the human skeletal muscle. *Acta Med Scand* 223:451, 1988.
193. Ohira Y, Cartier LJ, Chen M, Holloszy JO: Induction of an increase in mitochondrial matrix enzymes in muscle of iron-deficient rats. *Am J Physiol* 253:C639, 1987.
194. Cartier LJ, Ohira Y, Chen M, et al: Perturbation of mitochondrial composition in muscle by iron deficiency. Implications regarding regulation of mitochondrial assembly. *J Biol Chem* 261:13827, 1986.
195. Zoller H, Theurl I, Koch RO, et al: Duodenal cytochrome B and hephaestin expression in patients with iron deficiency and hemochromatosis. *Gastroenterology* 125:746, 2003.
196. Finch CA, Gollnick PD, Hlastala MP, et al: Lactic acidosis as a result of iron deficiency. *J Clin Invest* 64:129, 1979.
197. MacDonald VW, Charache S, Hathaway PJ: Iron deficiency anemia: Mitochondrial alpha-glycerophosphate dehydrogenase in guinea pig skeletal muscle. *J Lab Clin Med* 105:11, 1985.
198. Mackler B, Person R, Grace R: Iron deficiency in the rat: Effects on energy metabolism in brown adipose tissue. *Pediatr Res* 19:989, 1985.
199. Walter PB, Knutson MD, Paler-Martinez A, et al: Iron deficiency and iron excess damage mitochondria and mitochondrial DNA in rats. *Proc Natl Acad Sci U S A* 99:2264, 2002.
200. Harlan WR, Williams RS: Activity-induced adaptations in skeletal muscles of iron-deficient rabbits. *J Appl Physiol* 65:782, 1988.
201. Evans TC, Mackler B: Effect of iron deficiency on energy conservation in rat liver and skeletal muscle submitochondrial particles. *Biochem Med* 34:93, 1985.
202. Thompson CH, Green YS, Ledingham JG, et al: The effect of iron deficiency on skeletal muscle metabolism of the rat. *Acta Physiol Scand* 147:85, 1993.
203. Thompson CH, Kemp GJ, Taylor DJ, et al: No evidence of mitochondrial abnormality in skeletal muscle of patients with iron-deficient anaemia. *J Intern Med* 234:149, 1993.
204. Hinton PS, Sinclair LM: Iron supplementation maintains ventilatory threshold and improves energetic efficiency in iron-deficient nonanemic athletes. *Eur J Clin Nutr* 61:30, 2007.
205. Brownlie T, Utermohlen V, Hinton PS, Haas JD: Tissue iron deficiency without anemia impairs adaptation in endurance capacity after aerobic training in previously untrained women. *Am J Clin Nutr* 79:437, 2004.

206. Hinton PS, Giordano C, Brownlie T, Haas JD: Iron supplementation improves endurance after training in iron-depleted, nonanemic women. *J Appl Physiol* 88:1103, 2000.
207. Beutler E, Larsh S, Tanzi F: Iron enzymes in iron deficiency: VII. Oxygen consumption measurements in iron-deficient subjects. *Am J Med Sci* 239:759, 1960.
208. Youdim MBH, Green AR: Biogenic monoamine metabolism and functional activity in iron-deficient rats: Behavioural correlates. *Ciba Found Symp* 51:201, 1977.
209. Youdim MB, Green AR: Iron deficiency and neurotransmitter synthesis and function. *Proc Nutr Soc* 37:173, 1978.
210. Beard J, Tobin B, Smith SM: Norepinephrine turnover in iron deficiency at three environmental temperatures. *Am J Physiol* 255:R90-R96,1988.
211. Webb TE, Krill CE, Jr., Oski FA, Tsou KC: Relationship of iron status to urinary norepinephrine excretion in children 7–12 years of age. *J Pediatr Gastroenterol Nutr* 1:207, 1982.
212. Youdim MB, Ben Shachar D: Minimal brain damage induced by early iron deficiency: Modified dopaminergic neurotransmission. *Isr J Med Sci* 23:19, 1987.
213. Bartholmey SJ, Sherman AR: Impaired ketogenesis in iron-deficient rat pups. *J Nutr* 116:2180, 1986.
214. Beard J: Feed efficiency and norepinephrine turnover in iron deficiency. *Proc Soc Exp Biol Med* 184:337, 1987.
215. Prime SS, MacDonald DG, Noble HW, Rennie JS: Effect of prolonged iron deficiency on enamel pigmentation and tooth structure in rat incisors. *Arch Oral Biol* 29:905, 1984.
216. Sun AH, Xiao SZ, Li BS, et al: Iron deficiency and hearing loss. Experimental study in growing rats. *ORL J Otorhinolaryngol Relat Spec* 49:118, 1987.
217. Sun AH, Xiao SZ, Zheng Z, et al: A scanning electron microscopic study of cochlear changes in iron-deficient rats. *Acta Otolaryngol* 104:211, 1987.
218. Beard JL: Iron biology in immune function, muscle metabolism and neuronal functioning. *J Nutr* 131:568S, 2001.
219. Ahluwalia N, Sun J, Krause D, et al: Immune function is impaired in iron-deficient, homebound, older women. *Am J Clin Nutr* 79:516, 2004.
220. Weinberg ED: Iron out-of-balance: A risk factor for acute and chronic diseases. *Hemoglobin* 32:117, 2008.
221. Fischbach MA, Lin H, Liu DR, Walsh CT: How pathogenic bacteria evade mammalian sabotage in the battle for iron. *Nat Chem Biol* 2:132, 2006.
222. Weinberg ED: Iron withholding: A defense against viral infections. *Biometals* 9:393, 1996.
223. Weinberg ED: Iron withholding: A defense against infection and neoplasia. *Physiol Rev* 64:65, 1984.
224. Weinberg ED: Iron and infection. *Microbiol Rev* 42:45, 1978.
225. Grant SM, Wiesinger JA, Beard JL, Cantorna MT: Iron-deficient mice fail to develop autoimmune encephalomyelitis. *J Nutr* 133:2635, 2003.
226. Chwang LC, Soemantri AG, Pollitt E: Iron supplementation and physical growth of rural Indonesian children. *Am J Clin Nutr* 47:496, 1988.
227. Pizarro F, Olivares M, Hertrampf E, Walter T: Growth in terms of length of Chilean infants of low socioeconomic status: 1978–1992. *Arch Latinoam Nutr* 46:107, 1996.
228. Bandhu R, Shankar N, Tandon OP: Effect of iron on growth in iron deficient anemic school going children. *Indian J Physiol Pharmacol* 47:59, 2003.
229. Prasad AS, Halsted JA, Nadimi M: Syndrome of iron deficiency anemia, hepatosplenomegaly, hypogonadism, dwarfism and geophagia. *Am J Med* 31:532, 1961.
230. Rosenzweig PH, Volpe SL: Iron, thermoregulation, and metabolic rate. *Crit Rev Food Sci Nutr* 39:131, 1999.
231. Baird IM, Dodge OG, Palmer FJ, Wawman RJ: The tongue and oesophagus in iron-deficiency anaemia and the effect of iron therapy. *J Clin Pathol* 14:603, 1961.
232. Cheli R, Dodero M, Celle G, Vasalotti M: Gastric biopsy and secretory findings in hypochromic anaemias. *Acta Haematol* 22:1, 1959.
233. Lees F, Rosenthal FD: Gastric mucosal lesions before and after treatment in iron deficiency anaemia. *Q J Med* 27:19, 1958.
234. Naiman JL, Oski FA, Diamond LK, et al: The gastrointestinal effects of iron deficiency anemia. *Pediatrics* 33:83, 1964.
235. Scott J, Valentine JA, St Hill CA, West CR: Morphometric analysis of atrophic changes in human lingual epithelium in iron deficiency anaemia. *J Clin Pathol* 38:1025, 1985.
236. Boddington MM, Spriggs AI: Changes in buccal cells in the anaemias. *J Clin Pathol* 12:222, 1959.
237. Jacobs A: The buccal mucosa in anaemia. *J Clin Pathol* 13:463, 1960.
238. Macleod RI, Hamilton PJ, Soames JV: Quantitative exfoliative oral cytology in iron-deficiency and megaloblastic anemia. *Anal Quant Cytol Histol* 10:176, 1988.
239. Milman N, Pedersen FM: Idiopathic pulmonary haemosiderosis. Epidemiology, pathogenic aspects and diagnosis. *Respir Med* 92:902, 1998.
240. Shahidi NT, Diamond LK: Skull changes in infants with chronic iron-deficiency anemia. *N Engl J Med* 262:137, 1960.
241. Moseley JE: Skeletal changes in the anemias. *Semin Roentgenol* 9:169, 1974.
242. Reimann F, Berker F, Gokmen E, Kucukcakirlar T: Behaviour of the sella turcica in juveniles with severe iron deficiency. *Rofo* 129:598, 1978.
243. Beutler E, Larsh SE, Gurney CW: Iron therapy in chronically fatigued, non-anemic women: A double-blind study. *Ann Intern Med* 52:378, 1960.
244. Halterman JS, Kaczorowski JM, Aligne CA, et al: Iron deficiency and cognitive achievement among school-aged children and adolescents in the United States. *Pediatrics* 107:1381, 2001.
245. Friedmann B, Weller E, Mairbaurl H, Bartsch P: Effects of iron repletion on blood volume and performance capacity in young athletes. *Med Sci Sports Exerc* 33:741, 2001.
246. Zhu YI, Haas JD: Altered metabolic response of iron-depleted nonanemic women during a 15-km time trial. *J Appl Physiol* 84:1768, 1998.
247. Zhu YI, Haas JD: Iron depletion without anemia and physical performance in young women. *Am J Clin Nutr* 66:334, 1997.
248. Rowland TW, Deisroth MB, Green GM, Kelleher JF: The effect of iron therapy on the exercise capacity of nonanemic iron-deficient adolescent runners. *Sports Med* 142:165, 1988.
249. Duport N, Preziosi P, Boutron-Ruault MC, et al: Consequences of iron depletion on health in menstruating women. *Eur J Clin Nutr* 57:1169, 2003.
250. Cochrane AL, Elwood PC: Iron deficiency without anaemia. *Lancet* 1:591, 1968.
251. Cusack RP, Brown WD: Iron deficiency in rats: Changes in body and organ weights, plasma proteins, hemoglobins, myoglobins, and catalase. *J Nutr* 86:383, 1965.
252. Lozoff B, Clark KM, Jing Y, et al: Dose-response relationships between iron deficiency with or without anemia and infant social-emotional behavior. *J Pediatr* 152:696, 2008.
253. Shafir T, Angulo-Barroso R, Jing Y, et al Iron deficiency and infant motor development. *Early Hum Dev* 84:479, 2008.
254. Murray-Kolb LE, Beard JL: Iron treatment normalizes cognitive functioning in young women. *Am J Clin Nutr* 85:778, 2007.
255. Haas JD, Brownlie T: Iron deficiency and reduced work capacity: A critical review of the research to determine a causal relationship. *J Nutr* 131:676S, 2001.
256. De Mulder R: Iron: Metabolism, biochemistry, and clinical physiology—Review of recent literature. *Arch Intern Med* 102:254, 1958.
257. Ikkala E, Laitinen L: Papilloedema due to iron deficiency anaemia. *Acta Haematol* 29:368, 1963.
258. Morrow JJ, Dagg JH, Goldberg A: A controlled trial of iron therapy in sideropenia. *Scott Med J* 13:78, 1968.
259. Yager JY, Hartfield DS: Neurologic manifestations of iron deficiency in childhood. *Pediatr Neurol* 27:85, 2002.
260. Lubeck MJ: Papilledema caused by iron-deficiency anemia. *Trans Am Acad Ophthalmol Otolaryngol* 63:306, 1959.
261. Capriles LF: Intracranial hypertension and iron-deficiency anemia: Report of four cases. *Arch Neurol* 9:147, 1963.
262. Biousse V, Rucker JC, Vignal C, et al: Anemia and papilledema. *Am J Ophthalmol* 135:437, 2003.
263. Maguire JL, deVeber G, Parkin PC: Association between iron-deficiency anemia and stroke in young children. *Pediatrics* 120:1053, 2007.
264. Basak R, Chowdhury AM, Fatmi LE, et al: Stroke in the young: Relationship with iron deficiency anemia and thrombocytosis. *Mymensingh Med J* 17:74, 2008.
265. Stevens AR Jr: The mechanism and treatment of iron-deficiency anemia. *Arch Intern Med* 96:550, 1956.
266. Jacobs A, Kilpatrick GS: The Paterson-Kelly syndromes. *Br Med J* 2:79, 1964.
267. Jacobs A, Cavill I: The oral lesions of iron deficiency anaemia: Pyridoxine and riboflavin status. *Br J Haematol* 24:291, 1968.
268. Bernát I, Valló J: Ozaena: The causes of its familial occurrence. *Acta Med Acad Sci Hung* 20:89, 1964.
269. Akhnoukh S, Saad EF: Iron-deficiency in atrophic rhinitis and scleroma. *Indian J Med Res* 85:576, 1987.
270. Chen TS, Chen PS: Rise and fall of the Plummer-Vinson syndrome. *J Gastroenterol Hepatol* 9:654, 1994.
271. Khan FY, El-Hiday AH, Morad NA: Plummer-Vinson syndrome associated with solid-pseudopapillary tumor of the pancreas. *Chin Med J (Engl)* 120:1553, 2007.
272. Malhotra P, Malhotra N, Jhakhar S: Plummer Vinson syndrome. *J Assoc Physicians India* 55:785, 2007.
273. Ganesh R, Janakiraman L, Sathiyasekaran M: Plummer-Vinson syndrome: An unusual cause of dysphagia. *Ann Trop Paediatr* 28:143, 2008.
274. Miranda AL, Dantas RO: Esophageal contractions and oropharyngeal and esophageal transits in patients with iron deficiency anemia. *Am J Gastroenterol* 98:1000, 2003.
275. Taymor ML, Sturgis SH, Yahia C: The etiological role of chronic iron deficiency in production of menorrhagia. *JAMA* 187:323, 1964.
276. Samuels AJ: Studies in patients with functional menorrhagia. The antihemorrhagic effect of the adequate repletion of iron stores. *Isr J Med Sci* 1:851, 1965.
277. Jacobs A, Butler EB: Menstrual blood-loss in iron-deficiency anaemia. *Lancet* 2:407, 1965.
278. Kathula SK: Craving lemons: Another form of pica in iron deficiency. *Am J Med* 121:e1, 2008.
279. Louw VJ, du PP, Malan A, van DL, van WD, Joubert G: Pica and food craving in adult patients with iron deficiency in Bloemfontein, South Africa. *S Afr Med J* 97:1069, 2007.
280. Kantor J, Kessler LJ, Brooks DG, Cotsarelis G: Decreased serum ferritin is associated with alopecia in women. *J Invest Dermatol* 121:985, 2003.
281. Chamberlain AJ, Dawber RPR: Significance of iron status in hair loss in women. *Br J Dermatol* 149:428, 2003.
282. Deloche C, Bastien P, Chadoutaud S, et al.: Low iron stores: A risk factor for excessive hair loss in non-menopausal women. *Eur J Dermatol* 17:507, 2007.
283. Gordon N: Iron deficiency and the intellect. *Brain Dev* 25:3, 2003.

284. Oner O, Alkar OY, Oner P: Relation of ferritin levels with symptom ratings and cognitive performance in children with attention deficit-hyperactivity disorder. *Pediatr Int* 50:40, 2008.
285. Cankaya H, Oner AF, Egeli E, et al: Auditory brainstem response in children with iron deficiency anemia. *Acta Paediatr Taiwan* 44:21, 2003.
286. Agaoglu L, Torun O, Unuvar E, et al: Effects of iron deficiency anemia on cognitive function in children. *Arzneimittelforschung* 57:426, 2007.
287. Corapci F, Radan AE, Lozoff B: Iron deficiency in infancy and mother-child interaction at 5 years. *J Dev Behav Pediatr* 27:371, 2006.
288. Lozoff B, Georgieff MK: Iron deficiency and brain development. *Semin Pediatr Neurol* 13:158, 2006.
289. Grantham-McGregor S, Ani C: A review of studies on the effect of iron deficiency on cognitive development in children. *J Nutr* 131:649S, 2001.
290. Cortese S, Lecendreux M, Bernardina BD, et al: Attention-deficit/hyperactivity disorder, Tourette's syndrome, and restless legs syndrome: The iron hypothesis. *Med Hypotheses* 70:1128, 2008.
291. Patel S: Restless legs syndrome and periodic limb movements of sleep: Fact, fad, and fiction. *Curr Opin Pulm Med* 8:498, 2002.
292. Earley CJ: Restless legs syndrome. *N Engl J Med* 348:2103, 2003.
293. Silber MH, Richardson JW: Multiple blood donations associated with iron deficiency in patients with restless legs syndrome. *Mayo Clin Proc* 78:52, 2003.
294. Sloand JA, Shelly MA, Feigin A, et al: A double-blind, placebo-controlled trial of intravenous iron dextran therapy in patients with ESRD and restless legs syndrome. *Am J Kidney Dis* 43:663, 2004.
295. Earley CJ, Horska A, Mohamed MA, et al: A randomized, double-blind, placebo-controlled trial of intravenous iron sucrose in restless legs syndrome. *Sleep Med* 10:206, 2009.
296. Aksoy M, Erdem S, Baserer G: On the pathogenesis of the hepatosplenomegaly in chronic iron deficiency anaemia. A study of five patients with a syndrome of chronic iron deficiency anaemia, hepatosplenomegaly, hypogonadism and dwarfism. *Acta Hepatosplenol* 15:241, 1968.
297. Bessman JD, Feinstein DI: Quantitative anisocytosis as a discriminant between iron deficiency and thalassemia minor. *Blood* 53:288, 1979.
298. Fairbanks VF: Is the peripheral blood film reliable for the diagnosis of iron deficiency anemia. *Am J Clin Pathol* 55:447, 1971.
299. Kasper CK, Whissell DYE, Wallerstein RO: Clinical aspects of iron deficiency. *JAMA* 191:359, 1965.
300. Conrad ME, Crosby WH: The natural history of iron deficiency induced by phlebotomy. *Blood* 20:173, 1962.
301. Beutler E: The red cell indices in the diagnosis of iron-deficiency anemia. *Ann Intern Med* 50:313, 1959.
302. Aslan D, Altay C: Incidence of high erythrocyte count in infants and young children with iron deficiency anemia: Re-evaluation of an old parameter. *J Pediatr Hematol Oncol* 25:303, 2003.
303. Charache S, Gittlelsohn AM, Allen H, et al: Noninvasive assessment of tissue iron stores. *Am J Clin Pathol* 88:333, 1987.
304. Witte DL, Kraemer DF, Johnson GF, et al: Prediction of bone marrow iron findings from tests performed on peripheral blood. *Am J Clin Pathol* 85:202, 1986.
305. Beck JR, Cornwell GG, Rawnsley HM: Multivariate approach to predictive diagnosis of bone-marrow iron stores. *Am J Clin Pathol* 70:665, 1978.
306. Kokkinos J, Levine SR: Thrombocytosis secondary to iron deficiency and recurrent cerebral ischemia possibly improved by plateletpheresis. *Cerebrovasc Dis* 3:177, 1993.
307. Dincol K, Aksoy M: On the platelet levels in chronic iron deficiency anemia. *Acta Haematol* 41:135, 1969.
308. Gross S, Keefer V, Newman AJ: The platelets in iron-deficiency anemia. I. The response to oral and parenteral iron. *Pediatrics* 34:315, 1964.
309. Perlman MK, Schwab JG, Nachman JB, Rubin CM: Thrombocytopenia in children with severe iron deficiency. *J Pediatr Hematol Oncol* 24:380, 2002.
310. Marsh WL, Jr., Bishop JW, Darcy TP: Evaluation of red cell volume distribution width (RDW). *Hematol Pathol* 1:117, 1987.
311. Soff GA, Levin J: Thrombocytopenia associated with repletion of iron in iron-deficiency anemia. *Am J Med Sci* 295:35, 1988.
312. Berger M, Brass LF: Severe thrombocytopenia in iron deficiency anemia. *Am J Hematol* 24:425, 1987.
313. de Lima GA, Grotto HZ: Soluble transferrin receptor and immature reticulocytes are not useful for distinguishing iron-deficiency anemia from heterozygous beta-thalassemia. *Sao Paulo Med J* 121:90, 2003.
314. Valentine WN, Tanaka KR: The glyoxalase content of human erythrocytes and leukocytes. *Acta Haematol* 26:303, 1961.
315. Beutler E, Drennan W, Block M: The bone marrow and liver in iron deficiency anemia: A histopathologic study of sections with special reference to the stainable iron content. *J Lab Clin Med* 43:427, 1954.
316. Rath CE, Finch CA: Sternal marrow hemosiderin: A method for the determination of available iron stores in man. *J Lab Clin Med* 33:81, 1948.
317. Beutler E, Robson M, Buttenwieser E: A comparison of the serum iron, iron-binding capacity, sternal marrow iron and other methods in the clinical evaluation of iron stores. *Ann Intern Med* 48:60, 1958.
318. Barron BA, Hoyer JD, Tefferi A: A bone marrow report of absent stainable iron is not diagnostic of iron deficiency. *Ann Hematol* 80:166, 2001.
319. Cervantes F, Rozman C, Piera C, Fernandez M-R: Decreased bone marrow iron in chronic granulocytic leukaemia: A consistent finding not reflecting iron deficiency. *Blut* 53:305, 1986.
320. Cavill IA: Iron status indicators: Hello new, goodbye old? *Blood* 101:372, 2003.
321. Ellis LD, Jensen WN, Westerman MP: Marrow iron. An evaluation of depleted stores in a series of 1,332 needle biopsies. *Ann Intern Med* 61:44, 1964.
322. Garby L, Irnell L, Werner I: Iron deficiency in women of fertile age in a Swedish community. II. Efficiency of several laboratory tests to predict the response of iron supplementation. *Acta Med Scand* 185:107, 1969.
323. Hamilton LD, Gubler CJ, Cartwright GE, Wintrobe MM: Diurnal variation in the plasma iron level of man. *Proc Soc Exp Biol Med* 61:44, 1964.
324. Hoyer K: Physiologic variations in the iron content of human blood serum. I. The variations from week to week, from day to day, and through twenty-four hours. II. Further studies of the intra diem variations. *Acta Med Scand* 119:562, 1944.
325. Speck B: Diurnal variation of serum iron and the latent iron-binding in normal adults. *Helv Med Acta* 34:231, 1968.
326. Dale JC, Burritt MF, Zinsmeister AR: Diurnal variation of serum iron, iron-binding capacity, transferrin saturation, and ferritin levels. *Am J Clin Pathol* 117:802, 2002.
327. Zilva JF, Patston VJ: Variations in serum-iron in healthy women. *Lancet* 1:459, 1966.
328. Fujino M, Dawson EB, Holeman T, McGanity WJ: Interrelationships between estrogenic activity, serum iron and ascorbic acid levels during the menstrual cycle. *Am J Clin Nutr* 18:256, 1966.
329. Mardell M, Zilva JF: Effect of oral contraceptives on the variations in serum-iron during the menstrual cycle. *Lancet* 2:1323, 1967.
330. Cartwright GE: The anemia of chronic disorders. *Semin Hematol* 3:351, 1966.
331. Bainton DF, Finch CA: The diagnosis of iron deficiency anemia. *Am J Med* 37:62, 1964.
332. Banerjee RN, Narang RM: Haematological changes in malignancy. *Br J Haematol* 13:829, 1967.
333. Handjani AM, Banihashemi A, Rafiee R, Tolou H: Serum iron in acute myocardial infarction. *Blut* 23:363, 1971.
334. Syrkis I, Machtey I: Hypoferremia in acute myocardial infarction. *J Am Geriatr Soc* 21:28, 1973.
335. Follezou JY, Bizon M: Cancer chemotherapy induces a transient increase of serum-iron level. *Neoplasma* 33:225, 1986.
336. Seligman PA, Schleicher RB: Comparison of methods used to measure serum iron in the presence of iron gluconate or iron dextran. *Clin Chem* 45:898, 1999.
337. Pai AB, Boyd AV, McQuade CR, et al: Comparison of oxidative stress markers after intravenous administration of iron dextran, sodium ferric gluconate, and iron sucrose in patients undergoing hemodialysis. *Pharmacotherapy* 27:343, 2007.
338. Warady BA, Seligman PA, Dahl NV: Single-dosage pharmacokinetics of sodium ferric gluconate complex in iron-deficient pediatric hemodialysis patients. *Clin J Am Soc Nephrol* 2:1140, 2007.
339. Driggers DA, Reeves JD, Lo EYT, Dallman PR: Iron deficiency in one-year-old infants: Comparison of results of a therapeutic trial in infants with anemia or low-normal hemoglobin values. *J Pediatr* 98:753, 1981.
340. Lipschitz DA, Cook JD, Finch CA: A clinical evaluation of serum ferritin as an index of iron stores. *N Engl J Med* 290:1213, 1974.
341. Mazza P, Giua R, De Marco S, et al: Iron overload in thalassemia: Comparative analysis of magnetic resonance imaging, serum ferritin and iron content of the liver. *Haematologica* 80:398, 1995.
342. Beutler E, Felitti V, Ho N, Gelbart T: Relationship of body iron stores to levels of serum ferritin, serum iron, unsaturated iron binding capacity and transferrin saturation in patients with iron storage disease. *Acta Haematol* 107:145, 2002.
343. Bonkovsky HL, Slaker DP, Bills EB, Wolf DC: Usefulness and limitations of laboratory and hepatic imaging studies in iron-storage disease. *Gastroenterology* 99:1079, 1990.
344. Hallberg L, Hulthen L: High serum ferritin is not identical to high iron stores. *Am J Clin Nutr* 78:1225, 2003.
345. Coenen JLLM, Van Dieijen-Visser MP, Van Pelt J, et al: Measurements of serum ferritin used to predict concentrations of iron in bone marrow in anemia of chronic disease. *Clin Chem* 37:560, 1991.
346. van Tellingen A, Kuenen JC, de Kieviet W, et al: Iron deficiency anaemia in hospitalised patients: Value of various laboratory parameters. Differentiation between IDA and ACD. *Neth J Med* 59:270, 2001.
347. Sears DA: Anemia of chronic disease. *Med Clin North Am* 76:567, 1992.
348. Zimran A, Kay AC, Gelbart T, et al: Gaucher disease: Clinical, laboratory, radiologic and genetic features of 53 patients. *Medicine (Baltimore)* 71:337, 1992.
349. Morgan MAM, Hoffbrand AV, Laulicht M, et al: Serum ferritin concentration in Gaucher's disease. *Br Med J* 286:1864, 1983.
350. Hansen TM, Hansen NE: Serum ferritin as indicator of iron responsive anaemia in patients with rheumatoid arthritis. *Ann Rheum Dis* 45:596, 1986.
351. Matzner Y, Konijn AM, Hershko C: Serum ferritin in hematologic malignancies. *Am J Hematol* 9:13, 1980.
352. Ioannou GN, Tung BY, Kowdley KV: Iron in hepatitis C: Villain or innocent bystander? *Semin Gastrointest Dis* 13:95, 2002.
353. Dennison HA: Limitations of ferritin as a marker of anemia in end stage renal disease. *ANNA J* 26:409, 1999.
354. Wheby MS: Effect of iron therapy on serum ferritin levels in iron-deficiency anemia. *Blood* 56:138, 1980.

355. Siimes MA, Addiego JE Jr, Dallman PR: Ferritin in serum: Diagnosis of iron deficiency and iron overload in infants and children. *Blood* 43:581, 1974.
356. Galàn P, Sangaré N, Preziosi P, et al: Is basic red cell ferritin a more specific indicator than serum ferritin in the assessment of iron stores in the elderly? *Clin Chim Acta* 189:159, 1990.
357. Balaban EP, Sheehan RG, Demian SE, et al: Evaluation of bone marrow iron stores in anemia associated with chronic disease: A comparative study of serum and red cell ferritin. *Am J Hematol* 42:177, 1993.
358. Mei Z, Parvanta I, Cogswell ME, et al: Erythrocyte protoporphyrin or hemoglobin: Which is a better screening test for iron deficiency in children and women? *Am J Clin Nutr* 77:1229, 2003.
359. Fischer AB, Georgieva R, Nikolova V, et al: Health risk for children from lead and cadmium near a non-ferrous smelter in Bulgaria. *Int J Hyg Environ Health* 206:25, 2003.
360. Houston T, Moore M, Porter D, et al: Abnormal haem biosynthesis in the chronic anaemia of rheumatoid arthritis. *Ann Rheum Dis* 53:167, 1994.
361. Cook JD, Skikne BS, Baynes RD: Serum transferrin receptor. *Annu Rev Med* 44:63, 1993.
362. Ahluwalia N: Diagnostic utility of serum transferrin receptors measurement in assessing iron status. *Nutr Rev* 56:133, 1998.
363. Provan D: Mechanisms and management of iron deficiency anaemia. *Br J Haematol* 105 Suppl 1:19, 1999.
364. Pfeiffer CM, Cook JD, Mei Z, et al: Evaluation of an automated soluble transferrin receptor (sTfR) assay on the Roche Hitachi analyzer and its comparison to two ELISA assays. *Clin Chim Acta* 382:112, 2007.
365. Beutler E, Hoffbrand AV, Cook JD: Iron deficiency and overload. *Hematology Am Soc Hematol Educ Program* 40, 2003.
366. Cook JD, Flowers CH, Skikne BS: The quantitative assessment of body iron. *Blood* 101:3359, 2003.
367. Pavai S, Jayaranee S, Sargunan S: Soluble transferrin receptor, ferritin and soluble transferrin receptor—Ferritin index in assessment of anaemia in rhaeumatoid arthritis. *Med J Malaysia* 62:303, 2007.
368. Punnonen K, Irjala K, Rajamäki A: Serum transferrin receptor and its ratio to serum ferritin in the diagnosis of iron deficiency. *Blood* 89:1052, 1997.
369. Suominen P, Punnonen K, Rajamäki A, Irjala K: Serum transferrin receptor and transferrin receptor-ferritin index identify healthy subjects with subclinical iron deficits. *Blood* 92:2934, 1998.
370. Brugnara C, Zurakowski D, DiCanzio J, et al: Reticulocyte hemoglobin content to diagnose iron deficiency in children. *JAMA* 281:2225, 1999.
371. Kaneko Y, Miyazaki S, Hirasawa Y, et al: Transferrin saturation versus reticulocyte hemoglobin content for iron deficiency in Japanese hemodialysis patients. *Kidney Int* 63:1086, 2003.
372. Kim JM, Ihm CH, Kim HJ: Evaluation of reticulocyte haemoglobin content as marker of iron deficiency and predictor of response to intravenous iron in haemodialysis patients. *Int J Lab Hematol* 30:46, 2008.
373. Jasinski B: Eisenresorptionsversuche für die Diagnose und Differential diagnose der Eisenmangelanämien insbesondere für die Erkennung der Eisenmangel- zustande ohne Anämie. *Schweiz Med Wochenschr* 79:291, 1949.
374. Crosby WH, O'Neil-Cutting MA: A small-dose iron tolerance test as an indicator of mild iron deficiency. *JAMA* 251:1986, 1984.
375. Costa A, Liberato LN, Palestra P, Barosi G: Small-dose iron tolerance test and body iron content in normal subjects. *Eur J Haematol* 46:152, 1991.
376. Beutler E, West C: Hematologic differences between African-Americans and whites: The roles of iron deficiency and α-thalassemia on hemoglobin levels and mean corpuscular volume. *Blood* 106:740, 2005.
377. Duma H, Efremov G, Sadikario A, et al: Study of nine families with haemoglobin-Lepore. *Br J Haematol* 15:161, 1968.
378. Fairbanks VF, Gilchrist GS, Brimhall B, et al: Hemoglobin E trait reexamined: A cause of microcytosis and erythrocytosis. *Blood* 52:109, 1979.
379. Fairbanks VF, Oliveros R, Brandabur JH, et al: Homozygous hemoglobin E mimics beta-thalassemia minor without anemia or hemolysis: Hematologic, functional, and biosynthetic studies of first North American cases. *Am J Hematol* 8:109, 1980.
380. Johnson C, Tegos C, Beutler E: Thalassemia minor: Routine erythrocyte measurements and differentiation from iron deficiency. *Am J Clin Pathol* 80:31, 1983.
381. England JM, Walford DM, Waters DA: Re-assessment of the reliability of the haematocrit. *Br J Haematol* 23:247, 1972.
382. Rose MS: Epitaph for the M.C.H.C. *Br Med J* 4:169, 1971.
383. Han P, Fung KP: Discriminant analysis of iron deficiency anaemia and heterozygous thalassaemia traits: A 3-dimensional selection of red cell indices. *Clin Lab Haematol* 13:351, 1991.
384. Lin CK, Lin JS, Chen SY, et al: Comparison of hemoglobin and red blood cell distribution width in the differential diagnosis of microcytic anemia. *Arch Pathol Lab Med* 116:1030, 1992.
385. Junca J, Flores A, Roy C, et al: Red cell distribution width, free erythrocyte protoporphyrin, and England-Fraser index in the differential diagnosis of microcytosis due to iron deficiency or beta-thalassemia trait. A study of 200 cases of microcytic anemia. *Hematol Pathol* 5:33, 1991.
386. McClure S, Custer E, Bessman JD: Improved detection of early iron deficiency in nonanemic subjects. *JAMA* 253:1021, 1985.
387. Aslan D, Gumruk F, Gurgey A, Altay C: Importance of RDW value in differential diagnosis of hypochrome anemias. *Am J Hematol* 69:31, 2002.
388. Flynn MM, Reppun TS, Bhagavan NV: Limitations of red blood cell distribution width (RDW) in evaluation of microcytosis. *Am J Clin Pathol* 85:445, 1986.
389. Wians FH, Jr., Urban JE, Keffer JH, Kroft SH: Discriminating between iron deficiency anemia and anemia of chronic disease using traditional indices of iron status vs transferrin receptor concentration. *Am J Clin Pathol* 115:112, 2001.
390. Thompson WG, Meola T, Lipkin M, Freedman ML: Red cell distribution width, mean corpuscular volume, and transferrin saturation in the diagnosis of iron deficiency. *Arch Intern Med* 148:2128, 1988.
391. Cartei G, Chisesi T, Cazzavillan M, et al: Relationship between Hb and HbA2 concentrations in beta-thalassemia trait and effect of iron deficiency anaemia. *Biomedicine* 25:282, 1976.
392. Meyer CT, Troncale FJ, Galloway S, Sheahan DG: Arteriovenous malformations of the bowel: An analysis of 22 cases and a review of the literature. *Medicine (Baltimore)* 60:36, 1981.
393. Kohgo Y, Torimoto Y, Kato J: Transferrin receptor in tissue and serum: Updated clinical significance of soluble receptor. *Int J Hematol* 76:213, 2002.
394. Matthay KK, Villablanca JG, Seeger RC, et al: Treatment of high-risk neuroblastoma with intensive chemotherapy, radiotherapy, autologous bone marrow transplantation, and 13-*cis*-retinoic acid. *N Engl J Med* 341:1165, 1999.
395. Intragumtornchai T, Rojnukkarin P, Swasdikul D, Israsena S: The role of serum ferritin in the diagnosis of iron deficiency anaemia in patients with liver cirrhosis. *J Intern Med* 243:233, 1998.
396. Prieto J, Barry M, Sherlock S: Serum ferritin in patients with iron overload and with acute and chronic liver diseases. *Gastroenterology* 68:525, 1975.
397. Tessitore N, Solero GP, Lippi G, et al: The role of iron status markers in predicting response to intravenous iron in haemodialysis patients on maintenance erythropoietin. *Nephrol Dial Transplant* 16:1416, 2001.
398. Fernandez-Rodriguez AM, Guindeo-Casasus MC, Molero-Labarta T, et al: Diagnosis of iron deficiency in chronic renal failure. *Am J Kidney Dis* 34:508, 1999.
399. Chuang CL, Liu RS, Wei YH, et al: Early prediction of response to intravenous iron supplementation by reticulocyte haemoglobin content and high-fluorescence reticulocyte count in haemodialysis patients. *Nephrol Dial Transplant* 18:370, 2003.
400. Fishbane S, Shapiro W, Dutka P, et al: A randomized trial of iron deficiency testing strategies in hemodialysis patients. *Kidney Int* 60:2406, 2001.
401. Lima CS, Paula EV, Takahashi T, et al: Causes of incidental neutropenia in adulthood. *Ann Hematol* 85:705, 2006.
402. Ellis LD, Westerman MP, Balcerzak SP: The effect of iron stores on ferrokinetics in polycythaemia. *Br J Haematol* 13:892, 1967.
403. Hilal H, McCurdy PR: A pitfall in the interpretation of serum iron values. *Ann Intern Med* 66:983, 1967.
404. Demiroglu H, Dundar S: Pernicious anaemia patients should be screened for iron deficiency during follow up. *N Z Med J* 110:147, 1997.
405. Annibale B, Capurso G, Chistolini A, D'Ambra G, et al: Gastrointestinal causes of refractory iron deficiency anemia in patients without gastrointestinal symptoms. *Am J Med* 111:439, 2001.
406. Bampton PA, Holloway RH: A prospective study of the gastroenterological causes of iron deficiency anaemia in a General Hospital. *Aust N Z J Med* 26:793, 1996.
407. Kepczyk T, Cremins JE, Long BD, et al: A prospective, multidisciplinary evaluation of premenopausal women with iron-deficiency anemia. *Am J Gastroenterol* 94:109, 1999.
408. Rockey DC, Cello JP: Evaluation of the gastrointestinal tract in patients with iron-deficiency anemia. *N Engl J Med* 329:1691, 1993.
409. Chait A, Dann RH: G-I bleed after angiography. *N Engl J Med* 286:1418, 1972.
410. Al Onaizi I, Al Awadi F, Al Dawood AL: Iron deficiency anaemia: An unusual complication of Meckel's diverticulum. *Med Princ Pract* 11:214, 2002.
411. Berquist TH, Nolan NG, Adson MA, Schutt AJ: Diagnosis of Meckel's diverticulum by radioisotope scanning. *Mayo Clin Proc* 48:98, 1973.
412. Lu CC, Huang FC, Lee SY, Huang HY: Laparoscopy diagnosis and treatment excision of bleeding Meckel's diverticulum in a child: Report of one case. *Acta Paediatr Taiwan* 44:41, 2003.
413. Annibale B, Capurso G, Baccini F, et al: Role of small bowel investigation in iron deficiency anaemia after negative endoscopic/histologic evaluation of the upper and lower gastrointestinal tract. *Dig Liver Dis* 35:784, 2003.
414. Kerr DN, Davidson S: Gastrointestinal intolerance to oral iron preparations. *Lancet* 2:489, 1958.
415. Hallberg L, Ryttinger L, Sölvell L: Side-effects of oral iron therapy. A double-blind study of different iron compounds in tablet form. *Acta Med Scand* 459:3, 1966.
416. Eskeland B, Malterud K, Ulvik RJ, Hunskaar S: Iron supplementation in pregnancy: Is less enough? A randomized, placebo controlled trial of low dose iron supplementation with and without heme iron. *Acta Obstet Gynecol Scand* 76:822, 1997.
417. Fogelholm M, Suominen M, Rita H: Effects of low-dose iron supplementation in women with low serum ferritin concentration. *Eur J Clin Nutr* 48:753, 1994.
418. Leung AK, Chan KW: Iron deficiency anemia. *Adv Pediatr* 48:385, 2001.
419. Allen LH: Iron supplements: Scientific issues concerning efficacy and implications for research and programs. *J Nutr* 132:813S, 2002.
420. O'Sullivan DJ, Higgins PG, Wilkinson JF: Oral iron compounds: A therapeutic comparison. *Lancet* 269:482, 1955.
421. Gordeuk VR, Brittenham GM, Hughes M, et al: High-dose carbonyl iron for iron deficiency anemia: A randomized double-blind trial. *Am J Clin Nutr* 46:1029, 1987.
422. Brittenham GM, Klein HG, Kushner JP, Ajioka RS: Preserving the national blood supply. *Hematology Am Soc Hematol Educ Program* 422, 2001.

423. Sullivan JL: Iron and coronary heart disease. Iron makes myocardium vulnerable to ischaemia. *BMJ* 307:1066, 1993.
424. Tuomainen TP, Kontula K, Nyyssonen K, et al: Increased risk of acute myocardial infarction in carriers of the hemochromatosis gene Cys282Tyr mutation—A prospective cohort study in men in eastern Finland. *Circulation* 100:1274, 1999.
425. Sempos CT, Looker AC, Gillum RF: Iron and heart disease: The epidemiologic data. *Nutr Rev* 54:73, 1996.
426. Waalen J, Felitti V, Gelbart T, et al: Prevalence of coronary heart disease associated with *HFE* mutations in adults attending a health appraisal center. *Am J Med* 113:472, 2002.
427. Knuiman MW, Divitini ML, Olynyk JK, et al: Serum ferritin and cardiovascular disease: A 17-year follow-up study in Busselton, Western Australia. *Am J Epidemiol* 158:144, 2003.
428. Auer J, Rammer M, Berent R, et al: Body iron stores and coronary atherosclerosis assessed by coronary angiography. *Nutr Metab Cardiovasc Dis* 12:285, 2002.
429. Bozzini C, Girelli D, Tinazzi E, et al: Biochemical and genetic markers of iron status and the risk of coronary artery disease: An angiography-based study. *Clin Chem* 48:622, 2002.
430. Claeys D, Walting M, Julmy F, et al: Haemochromatosis mutations and ferritin in myocardial infarction: A case-control study. *Eur J Clin Invest* 32 Suppl 1:3, 2002.
431. Gunn IR, Maxwell FK, Gaffney D, et al: Haemochromatosis gene mutations and risk of coronary heart disease: A west of Scotland coronary prevention study (WOSCOPS) substudy. *Heart* 90:304, 2004.
432. Gera T, Sachdev HP: Effect of iron supplementation on incidence of infectious illness in children: Systematic review. *BMJ* 325:1142, 2002.
433. Jiang R, Manson JE, Meigs JB, et al: Body iron stores in relation to risk of type 2 diabetes in apparently healthy women. *JAMA* 291:711, 2004.
434. Moczulski DK, Grzeszczak W, Gawlik B: Role of hemochromatosis C282Y and H63D mutations in HFE gene in development of type 2 diabetes and diabetic nephropathy. *Diabetes Care* 24:1187, 2001.
435. Halsall DJ, McFarlane I, Luan J, et al: Typical type 2 diabetes mellitus and HFE gene mutations: A population-based case-control study. *Hum Mol Genet* 12:1361, 2003.
436. Toddler deaths resulting from ingestion of iron supplements—Los Angeles, 1992–1993. *MMWR Morb Mortal Wkly Rep* 42:111, 1993.
437. Klein-Schwartz W, Oderda GM, Gorman RL, et al: Assessment of management guidelines. Acute iron ingestion. *Clin Pediatr (Phila)* 29:316, 1990.
438. Walter T, Olivares M, Pizarro F, Munoz C: Iron, anemia, and infection. *Nutr Rev* 55:111, 1997.
439. Westlin WF: Deferoxamine in the treatment of acute iron poisoning. Clinical experiences with 172 children. *Clin Pediatr (Phila)* 5:531, 1966.
440. Greengard J, McEnery JT: Iron poisoning in children. *GP* 37:88, 1968.
441. Whitten CF, Brough AJ: The pathophysiology of acute iron poisoning. *Clin Toxicol* 4:585, 1971.
442. McEnery JT: Hospital management of acute iron ingestion. *Clin Toxicol* 4:603, 1971.
443. Silverberg DS, Iaina A, Peer G, et al: Intravenous iron supplementation for the treatment of the anemia of moderate to severe chronic renal failure patients not receiving dialysis. *Am J Kidney Dis* 27:234, 1996.
444. Nissenson AR, Berns JS, Sakiewicz P, et al: Clinical evaluation of heme iron polypeptide: Sustaining a response to rHuEPO in hemodialysis patients. *Am J Kidney Dis* 42:325, 2003.
445. Nissim JA: Intravenous administration of iron. *Lancet* 2:49, 1947.
446. Yee J, Besarab A: Iron sucrose: The oldest iron therapy becomes new. *Am J Kidney Dis* 40:1111, 2002.
447. Blaustein DA, Schwenk MH, Chattopadhyay J,et al: The safety and efficacy of an accelerated iron sucrose dosing regimen in patients with chronic kidney disease. *Kidney Int* 64:S72-S77,2003.
448. Deicher R, Ziai F, Cohen G, et al: High-dose parenteral iron sucrose depresses neutrophil intracellular killing capacity. *Kidney Int* 64:728, 2003.
449. Van Wyck DB, Cavallo G, Spinowitz BS, et al: Safety and efficacy of iron sucrose in patients sensitive to iron dextran: North American clinical trial. *Am J Kidney Dis* 36:88, 2000.
450. Charytan C, Schwenk MH, Al Saloum MM, Spinowitz BS: Safety of iron sucrose in hemodialysis patients intolerant to other parenteral iron products. *Nephron Clin Pract* 96:C63, 2004.
451. Bhowmik D, Modi G, Ray D, et al: Total dose iron infusion: Safety and efficacy in predialysis patients. *Ren Fail* 22:39, 2000.
452. Sloand JA, Shelly MA, Erenstone AL, et al: Safety and efficacy of total dose iron dextran administration in patients on home renal replacement therapies. *Perit Dial Int* 18:522, 1998.
453. Ahsan N: Infusion of total dose iron versus oral iron supplementation in ambulatory peritoneal dialysis patients: A prospective, cross-over trial. *Adv Perit Dial* 16:80, 2000.
454. Auerbach M, Winchester J, Wahab A, et al: A randomized trial of three iron dextran infusion methods for anemia in EPO-treated dialysis patients. *Am J Kidney Dis* 31:81, 1998.
455. Reynoso-Gomez E, Salinas-Rojas V, Lazo-Langner A: Safety and efficacy of total dose intravenous iron infusion in the treatment of iron-deficiency anemia in adult non-pregnant patients. *Rev Invest Clin* 54:12, 2002.
456. Auerbach M, Witt D, Toler W, et al: Clinical use of the total dose intravenous infusion of iron dextran. *J Lab Clin Med* 111:566, 1988.
457. Khaodhiar L, Keane-Ellison M, Tawa NE, et al: Iron deficiency anemia in patients receiving home total parenteral nutrition. *JPEN J Parenter Enteral Nutr* 26:114, 2002.
458. Muranda M, Rivera H, Ortega F, et al: Experience with the use of iron-dextran labeled with Fe59. *Rev Med Chil* 93:134, 1965.
459. Will G: The absorption, distribution and utilization of intramuscularly administered iron-dextran: A radio-isotope study. *Br J Haematol* 14:395, 1968.
460. Marchasin S, Wallerstein RO: The treatment of iron-deficiency anemia with intravenous iron dextran. *Blood* 23:354, 1964.
461. Grimes AJ, HUTT MS: Metabolism of 59Fe-dextran complex in human subjects. *Br Med J* 33:1074, 1957.
462. Garby L, Sjolin S: Some observations on the distribution kinetics of radioactive colloidal iron (Imferon and ferric hydroxide). *Acta Med Scand* 157:319, 1957.
463. Henderson PA, Hillman RS: Characteristics of iron dextran utilization in man. *Blood* 34:357, 1969.
464. Burns DL, Pomposelli JJ: Toxicity of parenteral iron dextran therapy. *Kidney Int Suppl* 69:S119, 1999.
465. Theodoropoulos G, Makkous A, Constantoulakis M: Lymph node enlargement after a single massive infusion of iron dextran. *J Clin Pathol* 21:492, 1968.
466. Solanki SV, Kabrawala VN: Lymphadenopathy due to parenteral iron therapy. *J Indian Med Assoc* 51:22, 1968.
467. Amitai A, Acker M: Adverse effects of intramuscular iron injection. *Acta Haematol* 68:341, 1982.
468. Hamstra RD, Block MH, Schocket AL: Intravenous iron dextran in clinical medicine. *JAMA* 243:1726, 1980.
469. Forristal T, Witt M: Pleocytosis after iron dextran injection. *Lancet* 1:1428, 1968.
470. Wallerstein RO: Intravenous iron-dextran complex. *Blood* 32:690, 1968.
471. Hurvitz H, Kerem E, Gross-Kieselstein E, Brand A, Branski D: Pancytopenia caused by iron-dextran. *Arch Dis Child* 61:194, 1986.
472. Cantor RI, Downs GE, Abruzzo JL: Acute exacerbation of ankylosing spondylitis after an iron dextran infusion. *Ann Intern Med* 77:933, 1972.
473. Richmond HG: Induction of sarcoma in the rat by iron-dextran complex. *Br Med J* 46:947, 1959.
474. Carter RL, Mitchley BC, Roe FJ: Induction of tumours in mice and rats with ferric sodium gluconate and iron dextran glycerol glycoside. *Br J Cancer* 22:521, 1968.
475. Greenberg G: Sarcoma after intramuscular iron injection. *Br Med J* 1:1508, 1976.
476. MacKinnon AE, Bancewicz J: Sarcoma after injection of intramuscular iron. *Br Med J* 2:277, 1973.
477. Robertson AG, Dick WC: Intramuscular iron and local oncogenesis. *Br Med J* 1:946, 1977.
478. Faich G, Strobos J: Sodium ferric gluconate complex in sucrose: Safer intravenous iron therapy than iron dextrans. *Am J Kidney Dis* 33:464, 1999.
479. Mitchell ABS, Morton GA: Choice of iron therapy. *Practitioner* 213:370, 1974.
480. Cox JS, King RE, Reynolds GF: Valency investigations of iron dextran ("Imferon"). *Nature* 207:1202, 1965.
481. Altman LC, Petersen PE: Successful prevention of an anaphylactoid reaction to iron dextran. *Ann Intern Med* 109:346, 1988.
482. *Physicians' desk reference: PDR.* Medical Economics Co., Oradell, NJ, 2003.
483. Folkert VW, Michael B, Agarwal R, et al: Chronic use of sodium ferric gluconate complex in hemodialysis patients: Safety of higher-dose (> or = 250 mg) administration. *Am J Kidney Dis* 41:651, 2003.
484. Jain AK, Bastani B: Safety profile of a high dose ferric gluconate in patients with severe chronic renal insufficiency. *J Nephrol* 15:681, 2002.
485. Eichbaum Q, Foran S, Dzik S: Is iron gluconate really safer than iron dextran? *Blood* 101:3756, 2003.
486. Pritchard JA, Hunt CF: A comparison of the hematologic responses following the routine prenatal administration of intramuscular and oral iron. *Surg Gynecol Obstet* 106:516, 1958.
487. McCurdy PR: Oral and parenteral iron therapy: A comparison. *JAMA* 191:859, 1965.
488. Komolafe JO, Kuti O, Ijadunola KT, Ogunniyi SO: A comparative study between intramuscular iron dextran and oral ferrous sulphate in the treatment of iron deficiency anaemia in pregnancy. *J Obstet Gynaecol* 23:628, 2003.
489. Gabrielli GB, De Sandre G: Excessive tea consumption can inhibit the efficacy of oral iron treatment in iron-deficiency anemia. *Haematologica* 80:518, 1995.
490. Hurrell RF, Reddy M, Cook JD: Inhibition of non-haem iron absorption in man by polyphenolic-containing beverages. *Br J Nutr* 81:289, 1999.
491. Mahlknecht U, Weidmann E, Seipelt G: The irreplaceable image: Black tea delays recovery from iron-deficiency anemia. *Haematologica* 86:559, 2001.
492. Fry J: Clinical patterns and course of anaemias in general practice. *Br Med J* 2:1732, 1961.
493. Beveridge BR, Bannerman RM, Evanson JM, Witts LJ: Hypochromic anaemia. *Q J Med* 34:145, 1965.
494. Cox TM, Halsall DJ: Hemochromatosis-neonatal and young subjects. *Blood Cells Mol Dis* 29:411, 2002.
495. Fellman V: The GRACILE syndrome, a neonatal lethal metabolic disorder with iron overload. *Blood Cells Mol Dis* 29:444, 2002.
496. Crompton DE, Chinnery PF, Fey C, et al: Neuroferritinopathy: A window on the role of iron in neurodegeneration. *Blood Cells Mol Dis* 29:522, 2002.
497. Asada-Senju M, Maeda T, Sakata T, et al: Molecular analysis of the transferrin gene in a patient with hereditary hypotransferrinemia. *J Hum Genet* 47:355, 2002.
498. Beutler E, Gelbart T, Lee P, et al: Molecular characterization of a case of atransferrinemia. *Blood* 96:4071, 2000.

499. Loreal O, Turlin B, Pigeon C, et al: Aceruloplasminemia: New clinical, pathophysiological and therapeutic insights. *J Hepatol* 36:851, 2002.
500. Nittis T, Gitlin JD: The copper-iron connection: Hereditary aceruloplasminemia. *Semin Hematol* 39:282, 2002.
501. Sipe JC, Lee P, Beutler E: Brain iron metabolism and neurodegenerative disorders. *Dev Neurosci* 24:188, 2002.
502. Sheldon JH: *Haemochromatosis*. Oxford University Press, London, 1935.
503. Mallory FB: Hemochromatosis and chronic poisoning with copper. *Arch Intern Med* 37:336, 1926.
504. Finch C: Iron metabolism in hemochromatosis. *J Clin Invest* 28:780, 1949.
505. Davis WD, Arrowsmith WR: The effect of repeated phlebotomies in hemochromatosis. *J Lab Clin Med* 39:526, 1952.
506. MacDonald RA: Idiopathic hemochromatosis. Genetic or acquired? *Arch Intern Med* 112:82, 1963.
507. MacDonald RA: Primary hemochromatosis: Inherited or acquired? *Prog Hematol* 5:324, 1966.
508. Simon M, Pawlotsky Y, Bourel M, et al: Hémochromatose idiopathique: Maladie associée à l'antigène tissulaire. *Nouv Presse Med* 4:1432, 1975.
509. Simon M, Bourel R, Fauchet R, Genetet B: Association of HLA-A3 and HLA-B14 antigens with idiopathic hemochromatosis. *Gut* 17:332, 1976.
510. Feder JN, Gnirke A, Thomas W, et al: A novel MHC class I-like gene is mutated in patients with hereditary haemochromatosis. *Nat Genet* 13:399, 1996.
511. Beutler E: The *HFE* Cys282Tyr mutation as a necessary but not sufficient cause of hereditary hemochromatosis. *Blood* 101:3347, 2003.
512. Scotet V, Merour MC, Mercier AY, et al: Hereditary hemochromatosis: Effect of excessive alcohol consumption on disease expression in patients homozygous for the C282Y mutation. *Am J Epidemiol* 158:129, 2003.
513. Beutler E, Gelbart T, West C, et al: Mutation analysis in hereditary hemochromatosis. *Blood Cells Mol Dis* 22:187, 1996.
514. Lucotte G, Dieterlen F: A European allele map of the C282Y mutation of hemochromatosis: Celtic versus Viking origin of the mutation? *Blood Cells Mol Dis* 31:262, 2003.
515. Steiner M, Leiendecker-Foster C, McLaren GD, et al: Hemochromatosis (HFE) gene splice site mutation IVS5+1 G/A in North American Vietnamese with and without phenotypic evidence of iron overload. *Transl Res* 149:92, 2007.
516. Beutler L, Beutler E: Hematologically important mutations: Hemochromatosis. *Blood Cells Mol Dis* 33:40, 2004.
517. Cukjati M: A novel homozygous frameshift deletion c.471del of HFE associated with hemochromatosis. *Clin Genet* 71:350, 2007.
518. Dupradeau FY, Pissard S, Coulhon MP, et al: An unusual case of hemochromatosis due to a new compound heterozygosity in HFE (p.[Gly43Asp;His63Asp]+[Cys282Tyr]): Structural implications with respect to binding with transferrin receptor 1. *Hum Mutat* 29:206, 2007.
519. De Marco F, Liguori R, Giardina MG, et al: High prevalence of non-HFE gene-associated haemochromatosis in patients from southern Italy. *Clin Chem Lab Med* 42:17, 2004.
520. Camaschella C, Fargion S, Sampietro M, et al: Inherited HFE-unrelated hemochromatosis in Italian families. *Hepatology* 29:1563, 1999.
521. Shukla P, Julka S, Bhatia E, et al: HFE, hepcidin and ferroportin gene mutations are not present in Indian patients with primary haemochromatosis. *Natl Med J India* 19:20, 2006.
522. Simsek H, Balaban YH, Yilmaz E, et al: Mutations of the HFE gene among Turkish hereditary hemochromatosis patients. *Ann Hematol* 84:646, 2005.
523. Adams P, Brissot P, Powell L: EASL International Consensus Conference on Haemochromatosis—Part II. Expert document. *J Hepatol* 33:487, 2000.
524. Bulaj ZJ, Ajioka RS, Phillips JD, et al: Disease-related conditions in relatives of patients with hemochromatosis. *N Engl J Med* 343:1529, 2000.
525. Olynyk JK, Cullen DJ, Aquilia S, et al: A population-based study of the clinical expression of the hemochromatosis gene. *N Engl J Med* 341:718, 1999.
526. Beutler E, Felitti VJ, Koziol JA, et al: Penetrance of the 845G→A (C282Y) *HFE* hereditary haemochromatosis mutation in the USA. *Lancet* 359:211, 2002.
527. Waalen J, Felitti V, Gelbart T, et al: Prevalence of hemochromatosis-related symptoms in homozygotes for the C282Y mutation of the *HFE* gene. *Mayo Clin Proc* 77:522, 2002.
528. Åsberg A, Hveem K, Kruger O, Bjerve KS: Persons with screening-detected haemochromatosis: As healthy as the general population? *Scand J Gastroenterol* 37:719, 2002.
529. McLaren GD, McLaren CE, Adams PC, et al: Clinical manifestations of hemochromatosis in *HFE* C282Y homozygotes identified by screening. *Can J Gastroenterol* 22:923, 2008.
530. MacDonald RA: Hemochromatosis and cirrhosis in different geographic areas. *Am J Med Sci* 249:36, 1965.
531. MacSween RNM, Scott AR. Hepatic cirrhosis: A clinicopathological review of 520 cases. *J Clin Pathol* 26:936, 1972.
532. Yang Q, McDonnell SM, Khoury MJ, et al: Hemochromatosis-associated mortality in the United States from 1979 to 1992: An analysis of multiple-cause mortality data. *Ann Intern Med* 129:946, 1998.
533. McCune CA, Al Jader LN, May A, et al: Hereditary haemochromatosis: Only 1% of adult HFE C282Y homozygotes in South Wales have a clinical diagnosis of iron overload. *Hum Genet* 111:538, 2002.
534. Finch SC, Finch CA: Idiopathic hemochromatosis, an iron storage disease. A. Iron metabolism in hemochromatosis. *Medicine (Baltimore)* 34:381, 1955.
535. Moirand R, Adams PC, Bicheler V, et al: Clinical features of genetic hemochromatosis in women compared with men. *Ann Intern Med* 127:105, 1997.
536. Lee PL, Gelbart T, West C, et al: Seeking candidate mutations that affect iron homeostasis. *Blood Cells Mol Dis* 29:471, 2002.
537. Merryweather-Clarke AT, Cadet E, Bomford A, et al: Digenic inheritance of mutations in *HAMP* and *HFE* results in different types of haemochromatosis. *Hum Mol Genet* 12:2241, 2003.
538. Jacolot S, Le Gac G, Scotet V, et al: *HAMP* as a modifier gene that increases the phenotypic expression of the *HFE* pC282Y homozygous genotype. *Blood* 103:2835, 2004.
539. Fletcher LM, Powell LW: Hemochromatosis and alcoholic liver disease. *Alcohol* 30:131, 2003.
540. Adams PC, Gregor JC, Kertesz AE, Valberg LS: Screening blood donors for hereditary hemochromatosis: Decision analysis model based on a 30-year database. *Gastroenterology* 109:177, 1995.
541. Kushner JP: Screening for hemochromatosis. *Gastroenterology* 109:315, 1995.
542. Niederau C, Niederau CM, Lange S, et al: Screening for hemochromatosis and iron deficiency in employees and primary care patients in western Germany. *Ann Intern Med* 128:337, 1998.
543. Allen K, Williamson R: Screening for hereditary haemochromatosis should be implemented now. *BMJ* 320:183, 2000.
544. Pinsky LE, Imperatore G, Burke W: Diabetes and HFE mutations: Cause or coincidence? *West J Med* 176:114, 2002.
545. McCord JM: Iron, free radicals, and oxidative injury. *Semin Hematol* 35:5, 1998.
546. Gutteridge JM: Iron and oxygen: A biologically damaging mixture. *Acta Paediatr Scand Suppl* 361:78, 1989.
547. Brown EB, Jr, Durbach R, Smith D, et al: Studies on iron transportation and metabolism. X. Long-term iron overload in dogs. *J Lab Clin Med* 50:862, 1957.
548. Bacon BR, Park CH, Brittenham GM, et al: Hepatic mitochondrial oxidative metabolism in rats with chronic dietary iron overload. *Hepatology* 5:789, 1985.
549. Houglum K, Filip M, Witztum JL, Chojkier M: Malondialdehyde and 4-hydroxynonenal protein adducts in plasma and liver of rats with iron overload. *J Clin Invest* 86:1991, 1990.
550. Pietrangelo A, Gualdi R, Casalgrandi G, et al: Molecular and cellular aspects of iron-induced hepatic cirrhosis in rodents. *J Clin Invest* 95:1824, 1995.
551. Schroder N, Fredriksson A, Vianna MRM, et al: Memory deficits in adult rats following postnatal iron administration. *Behav Brain Res* 124:77, 2001.
552. Tsukamoto H, Horne W, Kamimura S, et al: Experimental liver cirrhosis induced by alcohol and iron. *J Clin Invest* 96:620, 1995.
553. Mete A, Jalving R, van Oost BA, et al: Intestinal over-expression of iron transporters induces iron overload in birds in captivity. *Blood Cells Mol Dis* 34:151, 2005.
554. Norrdin RW, Hoopes KJ, O'Toole D: Skeletal changes in hemochromatosis of salers cattle. *Vet Pathol* 41:612, 2004.
555. Bailey TA, Flach EJ: Disease and mortality among great bustards (Otis tarda) at Whipsnade Wild Animal Park, 1989 to 1999. *Vet Rec* 153:397, 2003.
556. Sergejew T, Forgiarini P, Schnebli HP: Chelator-induced iron excretion in iron-overloaded marmosets. *Br J Haematol* 110:985, 2000.
557. Paglia DE: Dietary iron overloads in browsing rhinoceroses. *News Letter* Zoo Nutrition Center Wildlife Conservation Society, Bronx, NY, Feb 3, 1999.
558. Cornelissen H, Ducatelle R, Roels S: Successful treatment of a channel-billed Toucan (*Ramphastos vitellinus*) with iron storage disease by chelation therapy: Sequential monitoring of the iron content of the liver during the treatment period by quantitative chemical and image analyses. *J Avian Med Surg* 9:131, 1995.
559. House JK, Smith BP, Maas J, et al: Hemochromatosis in Salers cattle. *J Vet Intern Med* 8:105, 1994.
560. Nicolas G, Viatte L, Lou DQ, et al: Constitutive hepcidin expression prevents iron overload in a mouse model of hemochromatosis. *Nat Genet* 34:97, 2003.
561. Ahmad KA, Ahmann JR, Migas MC, et al: Decreased liver hepcidin expression in the hfe knockout mouse. *Blood Cells Mol Dis* 29:361, 2002.
562. Huang FW, Pinkus JL, Pinkus GS, et al: A mouse model of juvenile hemochromatosis. *J Clin Invest* 115:2187, 2005.
563. Kawabata H, Fleming RE, Gui D, et al: Expression of hepcidin is down-regulated in TfR2 mutant mice manifesting a phenotype of hereditary hemochromatosis. *Blood* 105:376, 2005.
564. Ganz T: Hepcidin, a key regulator of iron metabolism and mediator of anemia of inflammation. *Blood* 102:783, 2003.
565. Nemeth E, Roetto A, Garozzo G, et al: Hepcidin is decreased in TFR2 hemochromatosis. *Blood* 105:1803, 2005.
566. Papanikolaou G, Samuels ME, Ludwig EH, et al: Mutations in HFE2 cause iron overload in chromosome 1q-linked juvenile hemochromatosis. *Nat Genet* 36:77, 2004.
567. Bottomley SS: Secondary iron overload disorders. *Semin Hematol* 35:77, 1998.
568. Pippard MJ, Weatherall DJ: Iron absorption in non-transfused iron loading anaemias: Prediction of risk for iron loading, and response to iron chelation treatment, in beta thalassaemia intermedia and congenital sideroblastic anaemias. *Haematologia (Budap)* 17:17, 1984.
569. Tanno T, Bhanu NV, Oneal PA, et al: High levels of GDF15 in Thalassemia suppress expression of iron regulatory protein hepcidin. *Nat Med* 3:1096, 2007.

570. Tamary H, Shalev H, Perez-Avraham G, et al: Elevated growth differentiation factor 15 expression in patients with congenital dyserythropoietic anemia type I. *Blood* 112:5241, 2008.
571. Castleman B, Towne VW: Case records of the Massachusetts General Hospital. Case 38512. *N Engl J Med* 247:992, 1952.
572. Johnson BF: Hemochromatosis resulting from prolonged oral iron therapy. *N Engl J Med* 278:1100, 1968.
573. Pearson HA, Ehrenkranz RA, Rinder HM, Riely CA: Hemosiderosis in a normal child secondary to oral iron medication. *Pediatrics* 105:429, 2000.
574. Turnberg LA: Excessive oral iron therapy causing haemochromatosis. *Br Med J* 1:1360, 1965.
575. Wallerstein RO, Robbins SL: Hemochromatosis after prolonged oral iron therapy in a patient with chronic hemolytic anemia. *Am J Med* 14:256, 1953.
576. Saven A, Beutler E: Iron overload after prolonged intramuscular iron therapy. *N Engl J Med* 321:331, 1989.
577. Doherty MJ, Healy M, Richardson SG, Fisher NC: Total body iron overload in welder's siderosis. *Occup Environ Med* 61:82, 2004.
578. Witte DL, Crosby WH, Edwards CQ, et al: Hereditary hemochromatosis. *Clin Chim Acta* 245:139, 1996.
579. Isaacson C, Seftel HC, Keeley KJ, Bothwell TH: Siderosis in the Bantu: The relationship between iron overload and cirrhosis. *J Lab Clin Med* 58:845, 1961.
580. Barton JC, Acton RT, Rivers CA, et al: Genotypic and phenotypic heterogeneity of primary iron overload in African Americans with primary iron overload. *Blood Cells Mol Dis* 31:310, 2003.
581. De Domenico I, McVey WD, Musci G, Kaplan J: Iron overload due to mutations in ferroportin. *Haematologica* 91:92, 2006.
582. Wood JC: Cardiac iron across different transfusion-dependent diseases. *Blood Rev* 22 Suppl 2:S14, 2008.
583. Borgna-Pignatti C, Cappellini MD, De Stefano P, et al: Cardiac morbidity and mortality in deferoxamine- or deferiprone-treated patients with thalassemia major. *Blood* 107:3733, 2006.
584. Pennell DJ, Berdoukas V, Karagiorga M, et al: Randomized controlled trial of deferiprone or deferoxamine in beta-thalassemia major patients with asymptomatic myocardial siderosis. *Blood* 107:3738, 2006.
585. Beutler E: The clinical evaluation of iron stores. *N Engl J Med* 256:692, 1957.
586. Düllmann J, Wulfhekel U: The diagnostic significance of bone-marrow iron in hereditary hemochromatosis. *Ann N Y Acad Sci* 526:357, 1988.
587. Ross CE, Muir WA, Ng ABP, et al: Hemochromatosis. Pathophysiologic and genetic considerations. *Am J Clin Pathol* 63:179, 1975.
588. Astaldi G, Meardi G, Lisino T: The iron content of jejunal mucosa obtained by Crosby's biopsy in hemochromatosis and hemosiderosis. *Blood* 28:70, 1966.
589. Whittaker P, Skikne BS, Covell AM, et al: Duodenal iron proteins in idiopathic hemochromatosis. *J Clin Invest* 83:261, 1989.
590. Simpson RJ, Debnam ES, Laftah AH, et al: Duodenal non-heme iron content correlates with iron stores in mice, but the relationship is altered by *Hfe* gene knock-out. *Blood* 101:3316, 2003.
591. Beutler E, Felitti VJ, Ho NJ, Gelbart T: Commentary: An *HFE* S65C variant is not associated with increased transferrin saturation in voluntary blood donors by Naveen Arya, Subrata Chakrabrati, Robert A. Hegele, Paul C. Adams. *Blood Cells Mol Dis* 25:358, 1999.
592. Smith BC, Grove J, Guzail MA, et al: Heterozygosity for hereditary hemochromatosis is associated with more fibrosis in chronic hepatitis C. *Hepatology* 27:1695, 1998.
593. Bonkovsky HL, Troy N, McNeal K, et al: Iron and HFE or TfR1 mutations as comorbid factors for development and progression of chronic hepatitis C. *J Hepatol* 37:848, 2002.
594. Gehrke SG, Stremmel W, Mathes I, et al: Hemochromatosis and transferrin receptor gene polymorphisms in chronic hepatitis C: Impact on iron status, liver injury and HCV genotype. *J Mol Med* 81:780, 2003.
595. Martinelli ALC, Franco RF, Villanova MG, et al: Are haemochromatosis mutations related to the severity of liver disease in hepatitis C virus infection? *Acta Haematol* 102:152, 1999.
596. Frenzer A, Rudzki Z, Norton ID, Butler WJ: Heterozygosity of the haemochromatosis mutation, C282Y, does not influence susceptibility to alcoholic cirrhosis. *Scand J Gastroenterol* 33:1324, 1998.
597. Grove J, Daly AK, Burt AD, et al: Heterozygotes for HFE mutations have no increased risk of advanced alcoholic liver disease. *Gut* 43:262, 1998.
598. Aldersley MA, Howdle PD, Wyatt JI, et al: Haemochromatosis gene mutation in liver disease patients. *Lancet* 349:1025, 1997.
599. Hohler T, Leininger S, Kohler HH, et al: Heterozygosity for the hemochromatosis gene in liver diseases—Prevalence and effects on liver histology. *Liver* 20:482, 2000.
600. Fargion S, Stazi MA, Fracanzani AL, et al: Mutations in the HFE gene and their interaction with exogenous risk factors in hepatocellular carcinoma. *Blood Cells Mol Dis* 27:505, 2001.
601. Kallianpur AR, Hall LD, Yadav M, et al: Increased prevalence of the HFE C282Y hemochromatosis allele in women with breast cancer. *Cancer Epidemiol Biomarkers Prev* 13:205, 2004.
602. Yuan XM, Li W: The iron hypothesis of atherosclerosis and its clinical impact. *Ann Med*35:578, 2003.
603. Wolff B, Volzke H, Ludemann J, et al: Association between high serum ferritin levels and carotid atherosclerosis in the Study of Health in Pomerania (SHIP). *Stroke* 35:453, 2004.
604. Candore G, Balistreri CR, Lio D, et al: Association between HFE mutations and acute myocardial infarction: A study in patients from Northern and Southern Italy. *Blood Cells Mol Dis* 31:57, 2003.
605. Heath ALM, Fairweather-Tait SJ: Health implications of iron overload: The role of diet and genotype. *Nutr Rev* 61:45, 2003.
606. Galan P, Noisette N, Estaquio C, et al: Serum ferritin, cardiovascular risk factors and ischaemic heart diseases: A prospective analysis in the SU.VI.MAX (SUpplementation en VItamines et Mineraux AntioXydants) cohort. *Public Health Nutr* 9:70, 2006.
607. Porto G, Roetto A, Daraio F, et al: A Portuguese patient homozygous for the -25G>;A mutation of the HAMP promoter shows evidence of steady-state transcription but fails to up-regulate hepcidin levels by iron. *Blood* 106:2922, 2005.
608. Zohn IE, De D, I, Pollock A, Ward DM, et al: The flatiron mutation in mouse ferroportin acts as a dominant negative to cause ferroportin disease. *Blood* 109:4174, 2007.
609. Beutler E, Barton JC, Felitti VJ, et al: Ferroportin (*SCL40A1*) variant associated with iron overload in African-Americans. *Blood Cells Mol Dis* 31:305, 2003.
610. Gordeuk VR, Caleffi A, Corradini E, et al: Iron overload in Africans and African-Americans and a common mutation in the *SCL40A1* (ferroportin 1) gene. *Blood Cells Mol Dis* 31:299, 2003.
611. Camaschella C, Roetto A, Cali A, et al: The gene TFR2 is mutated in a new type of haemochromatosis mapping to 7q22. *Nat Genet* 25:14, 2000.
612. Girelli D, Bozzini C, Roetto A, Alberti F, et al: Clinical and pathologic findings in hemochromatosis type 3 due to a novel mutation in transferrin receptor 2 gene. *Gastroenterology* 122:1295, 2002.
613. Mattman A, Huntsman D, Lockitch G, et al: Transferrin receptor 2 (TfR2) and HFE mutational analysis in non-C282Y iron overload: Identification of a novel TfR2 mutation. *Blood* 100:1075, 2002.
614. Roetto A, Totaro A, Piperno A, et al: New mutations inactivating transferrin receptor 2 in hemochromatosis type 3. *Blood* 97:2555, 2001.
615. Piperno A, Roetto A, Mariani R, et al: Homozygosity for transferrin receptor-2 Y250X mutation induces early iron overload. *Haematologica* 89:359, 2004.
616. Huang FW, Rubio-Aliaga I, Kushner JP, et al: Identification of a novel mutation (C321X) in HJV. *Blood* 104:2176, 2004.
617. Lanzara C, Roetto A, Daraio F, et al: The spectrum of hemojuvelin gene mutations in 1q-linked juvenile hemochromatosis. *Blood* 103:4317, 2004.
618. Lee PL, Beutler E, Rao SV, Barton JC: Genetic abnormalities and juvenile hemochromatosis mutations of the *HJV* gene encoding hemojuvelin. *Blood* 103:4669, 2004.
619. Pissia M, Polonifi K, Politou M, et al: Prevalence of the G320V mutation of the HJV gene, associated with juvenile hemochromatosis, in Greece. *Haematologica* 89:742, 2004.
620. Janosi A, Andrikovics H, Vas K, et al: Homozygosity for a novel nonsense mutation (G66X) of the HJV gene causes severe juvenile hemochromatosis with fatal cardiomyopathy. *Blood* 105:432, 2005.
621. Aguilar-Martinez P, Lok CY, Cunat S, et al: Juvenile hemochromatosis caused by a novel combination of hemojuvelin G320V/R176C mutations in a 5-year old girl. *Haematologica* 92:421, 2007.
622. Xia Y, Yu PB, Sidis Y, et al: Repulsive guidance molecule RGMa alters utilization of bone morphogenetic protein (BMP) type II receptors by BMP2 and BMP4. *J Biol Chem* 282:18129, 2007.
623. Mims MP, Guan Y, Pospisilova D, et al: Identification of a human mutation of DMT1 in a patient with microcytic anemia and iron overload. *Blood* 105:1337, 2005.
624. Pospisilova D, Mims MP, Nemeth E, et al: DMT1 mutation: Response of anemia to darbepoetin administration and implications for iron homeostasis. *Blood* 108:404, 2006.
625. Fleming MD, Trenor CC3, Su MA, et al: Microcytic anaemia mice have a mutation in Nramp2, a candidate iron transporter gene. *Nat Genet* 16:383, 1997.
626. Fleming MD, Romano MA, Su MA, et al: Nramp2 is mutated in the anemic Belgrade (b) rat: Evidence of a role for nramp2 in endosomal iron transport. *Proc Natl Acad Sci U S A* 95:1148, 1998.
627. Mims MP, Prchal JT: Divalent metal transporter 1. *Hematology* 10:339, 2005.
628. Randell MG, Patnaik AK, Gould WJ: Hepatopathy associated with excessive iron storage in mynah birds. *J Am Vet Med Assoc* 179:1214, 1981.
629. Gosselin SJ, Kramer LW: Pathophysiology of excessive iron storage in mynah birds. *J Am Vet Med Assoc* 183:1238, 1983.
630. Spalding MG, Kollias GV, Mays MB, et al: Hepatic encephalopathy associated with hemochromatosis in a toco toucan. *J Am Vet Med Assoc* 189:1122, 1986.
631. Lavoie JP, Teuscher E: Massive iron overload and liver fibrosis resembling haemochromatosis in a racing pony. *Equine Vet J* 25:552, 1993.
632. Pearson EG, Hedstrom OR, Poppenga RH: Hepatic cirrhosis and hemochromatosis in three horses. *J Am Vet Med Assoc* 204:1053, 1994.
633. Spelman LH, Osborn KG, Anderson MP: Pathogenesis of hemosiderosis in lemurs: Role of dietary iron, tannin, and ascorbic acid. *Zoo Biol* 8:239, 1989.
634. Beutler E, West C, Speir JA, et al: The HFE gene of browsing and grazing rhinoceroses: A possible site of adaptation to a low-iron diet. *Blood Cells Mol Dis* 27:342, 2001.
635. Awai M, Narasaki M, Yamanoi Y, Seno S: Induction of diabetes in animals by parenteral administration of ferric nitrilotriacetate. A model of experimental hemochromatosis. *Am J Pathol* 95:663, 1979.
636. Brighton CT, Bigley EJ, Smolenski BI: Iron-induced arthritis in immature rabbits. *Arthritis Rheum* 13:849, 1970.

637. Carthew P, Dorman BM, Edwards RE, et al: A unique rodent model for both the cardiotoxic and hepatotoxic effects of prolonged iron overload. *Lab Invest* 69:217, 1993.
638. Iancu TC, Ward RJ, Peters TJ: Ultrastructural observations in the carbonyl iron-fed rat, an animal model for hemochromatosis. *Virchows Arch B Cell Pathol Incl Mol Pathol* 53:208, 1987.
639. MacDonald RA, Pechet GS: Experimental hemochromatosis in rats. *Am J Pathol* 46:85, 1965.
640. Yang T, Dong WQ, Kuryshev YA, et al: Bimodal cardiac dysfunction in an animal model of iron overload. *J Lab Clin Med* 140:263, 2002.
641. Hershko C, Link G, Konijn AM, et al: The iron-loaded gerbil model revisited: Effects of deferoxamine and deferiprone treatment. *J Lab Clin Med* 139:50, 2002.
642. Zhou XY, Tomatsu S, Fleming RE, et al: HFE gene knockout produces mouse model of hereditary hemochromatosis. *Proc Natl Acad Sci U S A* 95:2492, 1998.
643. Coppin H, Darnaud V, Kautz L, et al: Gene expression profiling of Hfe-/- liver and duodenum in mouse strains with differing susceptibilities to iron loading: Identification of transcriptional regulatory targets of Hfe and potential hemochromatosis modifiers. *Genome Biol* 8:R221, 2007.
644. Wallace DF, Summerville L, Subramaniam VN: Targeted disruption of the hepatic transferrin receptor 2 gene in mice leads to iron overload. *Gastroenterology* 132:301, 2007.
645. Galy B, Ferring D, Minana B, et al: Altered body iron distribution and microcytosis in mice deficient in iron regulatory protein 2 (IRP2). *Blood* 106:2580, 2005.
646. Gunshin H, Fujiwara Y, Custodio AO, et al: Slc11a2 is required for intestinal iron absorption and erythropoiesis but dispensable in placenta and liver. *J Clin Invest* 115:1258, 2005.
647. Lesbordes-Brion JC, Viatte L, Bennoun M, et al: Targeted disruption of the hepcidin1 gene results in severe hemochromatosis. *Blood* 108:1402, 2006.
648. Levy JE, Montross LK, Andrews NC: Genes that modify the hemochromatosis phenotype in mice. *J Clin Invest* 105:1209, 2000.
649. Andersen RV, Tybjaerg-Hansen A, Appleyard M, et al: Hemochromatosis mutations in the general population: Iron overload progression rate. *Blood* 103:2914, 2004.
650. Waalen J, Felitti VJ, Gelbart T, et al: Penetrance of hemochromatosis. *Blood Cells Mol Dis* 29:418, 2002.
651. Adams PC, Reboussin DM, Barton JC, et al: Hemochromatosis and iron-overload screening in a racially diverse population. *N Engl J Med* 352:1769, 2005.
652. Ines LS, da Silva JAP, Malcata AB, Porto AL: Arthropathy of genetic hemochromatosis: A major and distinctive manifestation of the disease. *Clin Exp Rheumatol* 19:98, 2001.
653. Timms AE, Sathananthan R, Bradbury L, et al: Genetic testing for haemochromatosis in patients with chondrocalcinosis. *Ann Rheum Dis* 61:745, 2002.
654. McDonnell SM, Preston BL, Jewell SA, et al: A survey of 2,851 patients with hemochromatosis: Symptoms and response to treatment. *Am J Med* 106:619, 1999.
655. Jordan JM: Arthritis in hemochromatosis or iron storage disease. *Curr Opin Rheumatol* 16:62, 2004.
656. Beaton M, Adams PC: Prognostic factors and survival in patients with hereditary hemochromatosis and cirrhosis. *Can J Gastroenterol* 20:257, 2006.
657. Willis G, Bardsley V, Fellows IW, et al: Hepatocellular carcinoma and the penetrance of HFE C282Y mutations: A cross sectional study. *BMC Gastroenterol* 5:17, 2005.
658. Kratka K, Talikova-Cimburova M, Michalikova H, et al: High prevalence of HFE gene mutations in patients with porphyria cutanea tarda in the Czech Republic. *Br J Dermatol* 159:585, 2008.
659. Toll A, Celis R, Ozalla M, et al: The prevalence of HFE C282Y gene mutation is increased in Spanish patients with porphyria cutanea tarda without hepatitis C virus infection. *J Eur Acad Dermatol Venereol* 20:1201, 2006.
660. Harper P, Floderus Y, Holmstrom P, et al: Enrichment of HFE mutations in Swedish patients with familial and sporadic form of porphyria cutanea tarda. *J Intern Med* 255:684, 2004.
661. Camaschella C, Roetto A, De Gobbi M: Juvenile hemochromatosis. *Semin Hematol* 39:242, 2002.
662. Vaiopoulos G, Papanikolaou G, Politou M, et al: Arthropathy in juvenile hemochromatosis. *Arthritis Rheum* 48:227, 2003.
663. Barton JC, Bertoli LF, Rothenberg BE: Peripheral blood erythrocyte parameters in hemochromatosis: Evidence for increased erythrocyte hemoglobin content. *J Lab Clin Med* 135:96, 2000.
664. Beutler E, Felitti V, Gelbart T, Ho N: The effect of *HFE* genotypes in patients attending a health appraisal clinic. *Ann Intern Med* 133:329, 2000.
665. Jensen PD: Evaluation of iron overload. *Br J Haematol* 124:697, 2004.
666. Poullis A, Moodie SJ, Ang L, et al: Routine transferrin saturation measurement in liver clinic patients increases detection of hereditary haemochromatosis. *Ann Clin Biochem* 40:521, 2003.
667. Jacobs A: Serum ferritin and malignant tumours. *Med Oncol Tumor Pharmacother* 1:149, 1984.
668. Cazzola M, Skoda RC: Translational pathophysiology: A novel molecular mechanism of human disease. *Blood* 95:3280, 2000.
669. Craig JE, Clark JB, McLeod JL, et al: Hereditary hyperferritinemia-cataract syndrome: Prevalence, lens morphology, spectrum of mutations, and clinical presentations. *Arch Ophthalmol* 121:1753, 2003.
670. Bothwell TH, MacPhail AP: Hereditary hemochromatosis: Etiologic, pathologic, and clinical aspects. *Semin Hematol* 35:55, 1998.
671. Brittenham GM, Sheth S, Allen CJ, Farrell DE: Noninvasive methods for quantitative assessment of transfusional iron overload in sickle cell disease. *Semin Hematol* 38:37, 2001.
672. Wang ZJ, Haselgrove JC, Martin MB, et al: Evaluation of iron overload by single voxel MRS measurement of liver T2. *J Magn Reson Imaging* 15:395, 2002.
673. Pomerantz S, Siegelman ES: MR imaging of iron depositional disease. *Magn Reson Imaging Clin N Am* 10:105, 2002.
674. Bonkovsky HL, Rubin RB, Cable EE, et al: Hepatic iron concentration: Noninvasive estimation by means of MR imaging techniques. *Radiology* 212:227, 1999.
675. Alustiza JM, Artetxe J, Castiella A, et al: MR quantification of hepatic iron concentration. *Radiology* 230:479, 2004.
676. Hofmann WK, Kaltwasser JP, Hoelzer D, et al: Successful treatment of iron overload by phlebotomies in a patient with severe congenital dyserythropoietic anemia type II. *Blood* 89:3068, 1997.
677. Porter JB: Practical management of iron overload. *Br J Haematol* 115:239, 2001.
678. Borgna-Pignatti C, Cohen A: Evaluation of a new method of administration of the iron chelating agent deferoxamine. *J Pediatr* 130:86, 1997.
679. Franchini M, Gandini G, Veneri D, Aprili G: Safety and efficacy of subcutaneous bolus injection of deferoxamine in adult patients with iron overload: An update. *Blood* 103:747, 2004.
680. Blume KG, Beutler E, Chillar RK, et al: Continuous intravenous deferoxamine infusion treatment of secondary hemochromatosis in adults. *JAMA* 239:2149, 1978.
681. Nienhuis AW: Vitamin C and iron. *N Engl J Med* 304:170, 1981.
682. Kruger N, Kijewski H, Konig R, et al: Deferoxamine in hemosiderosis. Fecal iron excretion during continuous subcutaneous infusion. *Dtsch Med Wochenschr* 109:1682, 1984.
683. Gomber S, Saxena R, Madan N: Comparative efficacy of desferrioxamine, deferiprone and in combination on iron chelation in thalassemic children. *Indian Pediatr* 41:21, 2004.
684. Kattamis A, Kassou C, Berdousi H, et al: Combined therapy with desferrioxamine and deferiprone in thalassemic patients: Effect on urinary iron excretion. *Haematologica* 88:1423, 2003.
685. Deugnier Y, Brissot P, Loreal O: Iron and the liver: Update 2008. *J Hepatol* 48 Suppl 1:S113, 2008.
686. Angelucci E, Barosi G, Camaschella C, et al: Italian Society of Hematology practice guidelines for the management of iron overload in thalassemia major and related disorders. *Haematologica* 93:741, 2008.
687. Kontoghiorghes GJ: Ethical issues and risk/benefit assessment of iron chelation therapy: Advances with deferiprone/deferoxamine combinations and concerns about the safety, efficacy and costs of deferasirox. *Hemoglobin* 32:1, 2008.
688. Niederau C, Fischer R, Sonnenberg A, et al: Survival and causes of death in cirrhotic and in noncirrhotic patients with primary hemochromatosis. *N Engl J Med* 313:1256, 1985.
689. Niederau C, Fischer R, Puerschel A, et al: Long-term survival in patients with hereditary hemochromatosis. *Gastroenterology* 110:1107, 1996.
690. Waalen J, Nordestgaard BG, Beutler E: Meta-analysis of survival of homozygotes for the HFE C282Y mutation. Unpublished. 2003.
691. Olynyk JK, Hagan SE, Cullen DJ, et al: Evolution of untreated hereditary hemochromatosis in the Busselton population: A 17-year study. *Mayo Clin Proc* 79:309, 2004.
692. Block M, Moore G, Wasi P, Haiby G: Histogenesis of the hepatic lesion in primary hemochromatosis: With consideration of the pseudo-iron deficient state produced by phlebotomies. *Am J Pathol* 47:89, 1965.
693. Blumberg RS, Chopra S, Ibrahim R: Primary hepatocellular carcinoma in idiopathic hemochromatosis after reversal of cirrhosis. *Gastroenterology* 95:1399, 1988.
694. Knauer CM, Gamble CN, Monroe LS: The reversal of hemochromatotic cirrhosis by multiple phlebotomies. Report of a case. *Gastroenterology* 49:667, 1965.
695. Powell LW, Kerr JF: Reversal of "cirrhosis" in idiopathic haemochromatosis following long-term intensive venesection therapy. *Australas Ann Med* 19:54, 1970.
696. Weintraub LR, Conrad ME, Crosby WH: The treatment of hemochromatosis by phlebotomy. *Med Clin North Am* 50:1579, 1966.
697. Franchini M: Platelet count increase following phlebotomy in iron overloaded patients with liver cirrhosis. *Hematology* 8:259, 2003.
698. De Gobbi M, Roetto A, Piperno A, et al: Natural history of juvenile haemochromatosis. *Br J Haematol* 117:973, 2002.
699. Borgna-Rignatti C, Zurlo MG, DeStefano P, et al: Survival in thalassemia with conventional treatment. *Prog Clin Biol Res* 309:27, 1989.
700. Mackenzie B, Garrick MD: Iron Imports. II. Iron uptake at the apical membrane in the intestine. *Am J Physiol Gastrointest Liver Physiol* 289:G981, 2005.
701. McKie AT: A ferrireductase fills the gap in the transferrin cycle. *Nat Genet* 37:1159, 2005.
702. Hentze MW, Rouault TA, Caughman SW, et al: A cis-acting element is necessary and sufficient for translational regulation of human ferritin expression in response to iron. *Proc Natl Acad Sci U S A* 84:6730, 1987.
703. Rouault TA: The role of iron regulatory proteins in mammalian iron homeostasis and disease. *Nat Chem Biol* 2:406, 2006.
704. Beutler E, Fairbanks VF: The effects of iron deficiency, in *Iron in Biochemistry and Medicine II*, edited by A Jacobs, M Worwood, p 393. Academic Press, New York, 1980.
705. Beutler E, Meerkreebs G: Letter to the editor. *N Engl J Med* 274:1152, 1966.
706. Beutler E: Commentary. Targeted disruption of the *HFE* gene. *Proc Natl Acad Sci U S A* 95:2033, 1998.
707. Njajou OT, Vaessen N, Joosse M, et al: A mutation in SLC11A3 is associated with autosomal dominant hemochromatosis. *Nat Genet* 28:213, 2001.

708. de Sousa M, Reimao R, Lacerda R, et al: Iron overload in beta 2-microglobulin-deficient mice. *Immunol Lett* 39:105, 1994.
709. Rothenberg BE, Voland JR: β2 Knockout mice develop parenchymal iron overload: A putative role for class I genes of the major histocompatibility complex in iron metabolism. *Proc Natl Acad Sci U S A* 93:1529, 1996.
710. Trenor CC, Campagna DR, Sellers VM, et al: The molecular defect in hypotransferrinemic mice. *Blood* 96:1113, 2000.
711. Fleming RE, Ahmann JR, Migas MC, et al: Targeted mutagenesis of the murine transferrin receptor-2 gene produces hemochromatosis. *Proc Natl Acad Sci U S A* 99:10653, 2002.
712. Vulpe CD, Kuo YM, Murphy TL, et al: Hephaestin, a ceruloplasmin homologue implicated in intestinal iron transport, is defective in the sla mouse. *Nat Genet* 21:195, 1999.
713. LaVaute T, Smith S, Cooperman S, et al: Targeted deletion of the gene encoding iron regulatory protein-2 causes misregulation of iron metabolism and neurodegenerative disease in mice. *Nat Genet* 27:209, 2001.
714. Kato J, Fujikawa K, Kanda M, et al: A mutation, in the iron-responsive element of H ferritin mRNA, causing autosomal dominant iron overload. *Am J Hum Genet* 69:191, 2001.
715. Wyllie S, Seu P, Goss JA: The natural resistance-associated macrophage protein 1 Slc11a1 (formerly Nramp1) and iron metabolism in macrophages. *Microbes Infect* 4:351, 2002.
716. Lam-Yuk-Tseung S, Mathieu M, Gros P: Functional characterization of the E399D DMT1/NRAMP2/SLC11A2 protein produced by an exon 12 mutation in a patient with microcytic anemia and iron overload. *Blood Cells Mol Dis* 35:212, 2005.
717. Priwitzerova M, Nie G, Sheftel AD, et al: Functional consequences of the human DMT1 (SLC11A2) mutation on protein expression and iron uptake. *Blood* 106:3985, 2005.
718. Beaumont C, Delaunay J, Hetet G, et al: Two new human DMT1 gene mutations in a patient with microcytic anemia, low ferritinemia, and liver iron overload. *Blood* 107:4168, 2006.
719. Iolascon A, d'Apolito M, Servedio V, et al: Microcytic anemia and hepatic iron overload in a child with compound heterozygous mutations in DMT1 (SCL11A2). *Blood* 107:349, 2006.
720. Harris ZL, Durley AP, Man TK, Gitlin JD: Targeted gene disruption reveals an essential role for ceruloplasmin in cellular iron efflux. *Proc Natl Acad Sci U S A* 96:10812, 1999.
721. Roetto A, Papanikolaou G, Politou M, et al: Mutant antimicrobial peptide hepcidin is associated with severe juvenile hemochromatosis. *Nat Genet* 33:21, 2003.
722. Nicolas G, Bennoun M, Devaux I, et al: Lack of hepcidin gene expression and severe tissue iron overload in upstream stimulatory factor 2 (USF2) knockout mice. *Proc Natl Acad Sci U S A* 98:8780, 2001.
723. Pigeon C, Ilyin G, Courselaud B, et al: A new mouse liver-specific gene, encoding a protein homologous to human antimicrobial peptide hepcidin, is overexpressed during iron overload. *J Biol Chem* 276:7811, 2001.
724. Finberg KE, Heeney MM, Campagna DR, et al: Mutations in TMPRSS6 cause iron-refractory iron deficiency anemia (IRIDA). *Nat Genet* 40:569, 2008.
725. Guillem F, Lawson S, Kannengiesser C, et al: Two nonsense mutations in the TMPRSS6 gene in a patient with microcytic anemia and iron deficiency. *Blood* 112:2089, 2008.
726. Melis MA, Cau M, Congiu R, et al: A mutation in the TMPRSS6 gene, encoding a transmembrane serine protease that suppresses hepcidin production, in familial iron deficiency anemia refractory to oral iron. *Haematologica* 93:1473, 2008.
727. Folgueras AR, Martin de LF, Pendas AM, et al: The membrane-bound serine protease matriptase-2 (Tmprss6) is an essential regulator of iron homeostasis. *Blood* 112:2539, 2008.
728. Lozoff B, De Andraca I, Castillo M, et al: Behavioral and developmental effects of 112(6):2539 preventing iron-deficiency anemia in healthy full-term infants. *Pediatrics* 112:846, 2003.
729. Tershakovec AM, Weller SC: Iron status of inner-city elementary school children: Lack of correlation between anemia and iron deficiency. *Am J Clin Nutr* 54:1071, 1991.
730. Hallberg L, Hultén L, Lindstedt G, et al: Prevalence of iron deficiency in Swedish adolescents. *Pediatr Res* 34:680, 1993.
731. Borch-Iohnsen B, Sandstad B, Asberg A: Iron status among 3005 women aged 20–55 years in Central Norway: The Nord-Trondelag Health Study (the HUNT study). *Scand J Clin Lab Invest* 65:45, 2005.
732. Centers for Disease Control and Prevention: Iron deficiency—United States, 1999–2000. *MMWR Morb Mortal Wkly Rep* 51:897, 2002.
733. Christofides A, Schauer C, Zlotkin SH. Iron deficiency and anemia prevalence and associated etiologic risk factors in First Nations and Inuit communities in Northern Ontario and Nunavut. *Can J Public Health* 96:304, 2005.
734. Beutler E, Felitti V, Gelbart T, Waalen J: Haematological effects of the C282Y HFE mutation in homozygous and heterozygous states among subjects of northern and southern European ancestry. *Br J Haematol* 120:887, 2003.
735. Agudelo GM, Cardona OL, Posada M, et al: Prevalence of iron-deficiency anemia in schoolchildren and adolescents, Medellin, Colombia, 1999. *Rev Panam Salud Publica* 13:376, 2003.
736. Casanueva E, Jimenez J, Meza-Camacho C, et al: Prevalence of nutritional deficiencies in Mexican adolescent women with early and late prenatal care. *Arch Latinoam Nutr* 53:35, 2003.
737. Haidar J, Muroki NM, Omwega AM, Ayana G: Malnutrition and iron deficiency in lactating women in urban slum communities from Addis Ababa, Ethiopia. *East Afr Med J* 80:191, 2003.
738. Kadivar MR, Yarmohammadi H, Mirahmadizadeh AR, et al: Prevalence of iron deficiency anemia in 6 months to 5 years old children in Fars, Southern Iran. *Med Sci Monit* 9:CR100, 2003.
739. Massot C, Vanderpas J: A survey of iron deficiency anaemia during pregnancy in Belgium: Analysis of routine hospital laboratory data in Mons. *Acta Clin Belg* 58:169, 2003.
740. Soh P, Ferguson EL, McKenzie JE, et al: Iron deficiency and risk factors for lower iron stores in 6–24-month-old New Zealanders. *Eur J Clin Nutr* 58:71, 2004.
741. Wolmarans P, Dhansay MA, Mansvelt EP, et al: Iron status of South African women working in a fruit-packing factory. *Public Health Nutr* 6:439, 2003.
742. Pietrangelo A: The ferroportin disease. *Blood Cells Mol Dis* 32:131, 2004.
743. Barton JC, Acton RT: Inheritance of two HFE mutations in African Americans: Cases with hemochromatosis phenotypes and estimates of hemochromatosis phenotype frequency. *Genet Med* 3:294, 2001.
744. Bradley LA, Johnson DD, Palomaki GE, et al: Hereditary haemochromatosis mutation frequencies in the general population. *J Med Screen* 5:34, 1998.
745. Burt MJ, George PM, Upton JD, et al: The significance of haemochromatosis gene mutations in the general population: Implications for screening. *Gut* 43:830, 1998.
746. Jouanolle AM, Fergelot P, Raoul ML, et al: Prevalence of the C282Y mutation in Brittany: Penetrance of genetic hemochromatosis? *Ann Genet* 41:195, 1998.
747. Merryweather-Clarke AT, Pointon JJ, Shearman JD, Robson KJH: Global prevalence of putative haemochromatosis mutations. *J Med Genet* 34:275, 1997.
748. Beutler E, Felitti VJ, Waalen J, et al: Unpublished. 2003.
749. Pedersen P, Milman N: Genetic screening for HFE hemochromatosis in 6,020 Danish men: penetrance of C282Y, H63D, and S65C variants. *Ann Hematol.* 2009 Jan 22. [Epub ahead of print]
750. Chambers V, Sutherland L, Palmer K, et al: Haemochromatosis-associated HFE genotypes in English blood donors: Age-related frequency and biochemical expression. *J Hepatol* 39:925, 2003.
751. Mariani R, Salvioni A, Corengia C, et al: Prevalence of HFE mutations in upper Northern Italy: Study of 1132 unrelated blood donors. *Dig Liver Dis* 35:479, 2003.
752. Raszeja-Wyszomirska J, Kurzawski G, et al: Frequency of mutations related to hereditary haemochromatosis in northwestern Poland. *J Appl Genet* 49:105, 2008.
753. Ropero P, Briceno O, Mateo M, et al: Frequency of the C282Y and H63D mutations of the hemochromatosis gene (HFE) in a cohort of 1,000 neonates in Madrid (Spain). *Ann Hematol* 85:323, 2006.
754. Barry E, Derhammer T, Elsea SH: Prevalence of three hereditary hemochromatosis mutant alleles in the Michigan Caucasian population. *Community Genet* 8:173, 2005.

CHAPTER 43

ANEMIA RESULTING FROM OTHER NUTRITIONAL DEFICIENCIES

Ralph Green*

SUMMARY

The anemia that results from deficiencies of vitamin B_{12}, folic acid (see Chap. 41), or iron (see Chap. 42) are, in general, clearly defined and are relatively common. In contrast, the characteristics of anemia that may occur with deficiencies of micronutrients, such as some of the other vitamins and minerals, are poorly defined and relatively rare in humans. When present, they exist not as isolated deficiencies of one vitamin or one mineral but rather as a combination of deficiencies. In this context, it is difficult to deduce which abnormalities are a result of which deficiency. Studies in experimental animals may not accurately reflect the role of micronutrients in humans. Accordingly, our knowledge of the effect of many micronutrients on hematopoiesis is fragmentary and based on clinical observations and interpretations that may be flawed. The daily requirements of some of the micronutrients are available at http://www.nal.usda.gov/fnic/dga/rda.pdf and the levels normally found in the serum, red cell, and leukocytes are shown in Table 43–1.

VITAMIN-DEFICIENCY ANEMIAS

VITAMIN A DEFICIENCY

Chronic deprivation of vitamin A results in anemia similar to that observed in iron deficiency.[1–4] Mean corpuscular volume (MCV) and mean corpuscular hemoglobin concentration (MCHC) are reduced. Anisocytosis and poikilocytosis may be present, and serum iron levels are low. Unlike iron-deficiency anemia but similar to the anemia of chronic disease, the iron stores in the liver and marrow are increased, the serum transferrin concentration usually is normal or decreased, and administration of medicinal iron does not correct the anemia. The suggestion that vitamin A may facilitate iron absorption[5] has not been confirmed.[6]

Surveys conducted in developing countries suggest that vitamin A deficiency represents a public health problem among schoolchildren.[7,8] The prevalence of vitamin A deficiency closely coincides with the prevalence of iron deficiency in this demographic setting. However, there is no known casual relationship between the two nutrients beyond both occurring in a setting of generalized malnutrition. Although vitamin A deficiency is recognized to occur in the United States, the relationship between it and anemia is not known.

Acronyms and abbreviations that appear in this chapter include: MCV, mean corpuscular volume.

*This chapter was written by Ernest Beutler in previous editions and portions of the chapter in the 7th edition have been retained.

DEFICIENCIES OF MEMBERS OF THE VITAMIN B GROUP

Isolated nutritional deficiencies of members of the vitamin B group, with the exception of folic acid and vitamin B_{12}, are very uncommon in humans. Evidence linking isolated nutritional deficiencies of pyridoxine, riboflavin, pantothenic acid, and niacin to anemia in patients is inconclusive. In animals experimentally induced deficiency states are more commonly associated with hematologic abnormalities.

Vitamin B_6 Deficiency

Vitamin B_6 includes pyridoxal, pyridoxine, and pyridoxamine. These components are converted to pyridoxal 5-phosphate, which acts as a coenzyme in the decarboxylation and transamination of amino acids and in the synthesis of aminolevulinic acid, the porphyrin precursor (see Chap. 57). Vitamin B_6 deficiency induced in infants is associated with a hypochromic microcytic anemia.[9] A malnourished patient with a hypochromic anemia who failed to respond to iron therapy but subsequently responded to administration of vitamin B_6 has been described.[10] Occasionally, patients receiving therapy with antituberculosis agents, such as isoniazid, which interfere with vitamin B_6 metabolism, develop a microcytic anemia that can be corrected with large doses of pyridoxine.[11,12] Pyridoxine is usually prescribed with isoniazid to prevent such an effect. Some patients with sideroblastic anemias (see Chap. 58) respond to the administration of large doses of pyridoxine, but these patients are not deficient in this vitamin. Pyridoxine, because it is involved in a multiplicity of transamination and decarboxylation reactions, can affect many metabolic processes. Derangements in these pathways, sometimes involving anemia, are usually the result of inborn errors affecting the pathways of vitamin B_6 metabolism and specific pyridoxal phosphate-dependent enzymes or the result of inborn errors that lead to accumulation of small molecules that react with pyridoxal phosphate and inactivate it.[13] Other acquired conditions that may influence pyridoxine metabolism include drugs that react with pyridoxal phosphate or that affect the metabolism, malabsorptive states such as celiac disease and renal dialysis, which leads to increased losses of vitamin B_6 vitamers from the circulation as these vitamers are bound to plasma albumin.[14]

Riboflavin Deficiency

Riboflavin deficiency results in a decrease in red cell glutathione reductase activity because this enzyme requires flavin adenine dinucleotide for activation. The glutathione reductase deficiency induced by riboflavin deficiency is not associated with a hemolytic anemia or increased susceptibility to oxidant-induced injury (see Chap. 46).[15] Human volunteers maintained on a semisynthetic riboflavin-deficient diet and fed the riboflavin antagonist galactoflavin develop pure red cell aplasia.[16] Vacuolated erythroid precursors are evident prior to the development of aplasia. This anemia is reversed specifically by administration of riboflavin. Although it has been suggested that riboflavin deficiency causes anemia,[17] possibly by interfering with iron release from ferritin,[16] the relationship between dietary riboflavin deficiency and anemia is not at all clear. Thus, poor riboflavin status may interfere with iron handling and contribute to the etiology of anemia when iron intakes are low. There is also some evidence to suggest that riboflavin may exert its effects secondarily on other nutrients of primary hematologic interest, such as folate and cobalamin.[18]

Pantothenic Acid Deficiency

Pantothenic acid deficiency, when artificially induced in humans, is not associated with anemia.[19]

TABLE 43–1. Blood Vitamin and Mineral Levels (Adult Values)

Vitamin or Mineral	Serum Level	Plasma Level	Red Cell Level	White Cell Level
Copper	11–24 μmol/L		14–24 μmol/L	
Folate	7–45 nmol/L		>320 nmol/L	
Riboflavin (B_2)	110–640 nmol/L		265–1350 nmol/L	
Vitamin A	1–3 μmol/L			
Vitamin B_6		20–122 nmol/L		
Vitamin C		25–85 μmol/L		11–30 attomol/cell
Vitamin E	12–40 μmol/L			
Selenium	1200–2000 nmol/L			
Zinc	11–18 μmol/L			

SOURCE: Modified with permission from Milne D: Trace elements (p 1029) and McCormick DB, Greene HL: Vitamins (p 999), in *Tietz Textbook of Clinical Chemistry*, 3rd ed, edited by CA Burtis, EF Ashwood. WB Saunders, Philadelphia, 1999.

Niacin Deficiency

Pellagra (niacin deficiency) is associated with anemia, which responds to treatment with niacin.[20] However, it is not clear whether the anemia is a direct or an indirect effect of niacin deficiency.

Thiamine Deficiency

Megaloblastic anemia, responsive to thiamine, occurs in a childhood syndrome in association with diabetes and sensorineural deafness. The underlying defect in this condition has been identified as being the result of a defect in the high-affinity thiamine transporter which primarily affects the synthesis of nucleic acid ribose via the nonoxidative branch of the pentose cycle.[21] The decrease in ribose synthesis is a consequence of the thiamine-dependent pentose-cycle enzyme transketolase. Reduced nucleic acid production through impaired transketolase catalysis appears to be the underlying biochemical disturbance that likely induces cell-cycle arrest or apoptosis in marrow cells and leads to the thiamine-responsive megaloblastic anemia syndrome in these patients.

VITAMIN C (ASCORBIC ACID) DEFICIENCY

Although approximately 80 percent of patients with scurvy[22] are anemic, attempts to induce anemia in human volunteers by severely restricting dietary ascorbic acid have been unsuccessful.[23] Anemia observed in subjects with scurvy is not simply the result of a deficiency of ascorbic acid but rather a result of bleeding or a deficiency of folic acid.[22] Human subjects with scurvy and megaloblastic anemia fail to correct their anemia with vitamin C administration if they are maintained on a folic acid–deficient diet. When folic acid is given to these subjects in a dose of 50 mcg/day, a prompt hematologic response is observed.[24]

Ascorbic acid, in common with other compounds that contribute to cellular reducing potential, participates in the maintenance of dihydrofolate reductase in its reduced, or active, form. Impaired dihydrofolate reductase activity results in an inability to form tetrahydrofolic acid, the metabolically active form of folic acid (see Chap. 41). Patients with scurvy and megaloblastic anemia excrete 10-formylfolic acid as the major urinary folate metabolite. Following ascorbic acid therapy, 5-methyltetrahydrofolic acid becomes the major urinary folate metabolite. This observation has led to the suggestion that ascorbic acid prevents the irreversible oxidation of methyltetrahydrofolic acid to formylfolic acid.[25] Failure to synthesize tetrahydrofolic acid or protect it from oxidation ultimately results in megaloblastic anemia. Under these circumstances, ascorbic acid therapy will produce a hematologic response only if enough folic acid is present to interact with the ascorbic acid.[26] Dietary iron deficiency in children often occurs in association with dietary ascorbic acid deficiency. Iron balance may be compromised by ascorbic acid deficiency because this vitamin serves to facilitate intestinal iron absorption by maintaining iron in the more soluble reduced or ferrous (Fe^{2+}) state. Patients with scurvy, particularly children, may require both iron and vitamin C to correct a hypochromic microcytic anemia.[27] Scurvy itself may cause iron deficiency as a consequence of external bleeding. In patients with iron overload from repeated blood transfusions, the level of vitamin C in leukocytes is often decreased because of rapid conversion of ascorbate to oxalate.[28] Deferoxamine (desferrioxamine)-induced iron excretion is diminished when stores of vitamin C are reduced, but excretion returns to expected values with vitamin C supplementation.[29,30] Large doses of ascorbic acid may be harmful in patients with iron overload and should be given only after an infusion of deferoxamine mesylate (Desferal) has been initiated (see Chap. 42). The presence of scurvy in patients with iron overload may protect them from tissue damage.[31] In scorbutic guinea pigs and in Bantu subjects with nutritional vitamin C deficiency and dietary hemosiderosis, iron accumulates in the monocyte-macrophage system rather than in the parenchymal cells of the liver.[32,33]

VITAMIN E DEFICIENCY

Vitamin E, α-tocopherol, is a fat-soluble vitamin that appears to be an antioxidant in humans. It is not an essential cofactor in any recognized reactions. Nutritional deficiency of vitamin E in humans is extremely uncommon because of the widespread occurrence of α-tocopherol in food. The daily requirement of *d*-α-tocopherol for adults ranges from 5 to 7 mg, but the requirement varies with the polyunsaturated fatty acid content of the diet and the content of peroxidizable lipids in tissues. Hematologic manifestations of vitamin E deficiency in humans are limited to the neonatal period and to pathologic states associated with chronic fat malabsorption.

Low-birth-weight infants are born with low serum and tissue concentrations of vitamin E. When these infants are fed a diet unusually rich in polyunsaturated fatty acids and inadequate in vitamin E, a hemolytic anemia often develops by 4 to 6 weeks of age, particularly if iron is also present in the diet.[34] The anemia often is associated with morphologic alterations of the erythrocytes,[35] thrombocytosis, and edema of the dorsum of the feet and pretibial area.[36] Treatment with vitamin E produces a prompt increase in hemoglobin level, a decrease in the elevated reticulocyte count, normalization of the red cell life span, and disappearance of thrombocytosis and edema. Modifications of infant formulas have all but eliminated vitamin E deficiency in preterm infants.[37]

Vitamin E deficiency is common in patients with cystic fibrosis if the patients are not receiving daily supplements of the water-soluble form of the vitamin.[38] Red cell life span in such patients is shortened to an average ^{51}Cr half-life of 19 days (normal: ~30 days). After vitamin E therapy, the red cell half-life increases to 27.5 days.[39] Severe anemia may be present.[38]

Pharmacologic doses of vitamin E have been employed with apparent success in the absence of vitamin deficiency to compensate for genetic defects that limit the erythrocytes' defense against oxidant injury. Chronic administration of vitamin E 400 to 800 U/day lengthened the red cell life span in some,[40,41] but not all,[42] studies of patients with hereditary hemolytic anemias associated with glutathione synthetase deficiency or glucose-6-phosphate dehydrogenase deficiency.

Administration of vitamin E (450 U/day for 6–36 weeks) to patients with sickle cell anemia significantly reduced the number of irreversibly sickled erythrocytes.[43] Adult patients with sickle cell anemia have been reported to have significantly lower serum tocopherol values compared with normal controls,[44,45] and in children with sickle cell anemia, those with vitamin E deficiency have significantly more irreversibly sickled cells than did children without vitamin E deficiency.[46]

TRACE METAL DEFICIENCY

COPPER DEFICIENCY

Copper is present in a number of metalloproteins. Among the cuproenzymes are cytochrome *c* oxidase, dopamine β-hydroxylase, urate oxidase, tyrosine and lysyl oxidase, ascorbic acid oxidase, and superoxide dismutase (erythrocuprein). More than 90 percent of the copper in the blood is carried bound to ceruloplasmin, an α_2-globulin with ferroxidase activity. Copper appears to be required for the absorption and utilization of iron. Copper, in the form of hephaestin,[47] converts iron to the ferric (Fe^{3+}) state for its transport by transferrin.

Copper deficiency has been described in malnourished children[48] and in both infants and adults[49–51] receiving parenteral alimentation. There is increasing recognition of copper deficiency associated with anemia occurring as complication following gastric resection or bariatric gastric reduction surgery.[52] Copper deficiency is characterized by an anemia, often macrocytic, that is unresponsive to iron therapy, hypoferremia, neutropenia, and usually the presence of vacuolated erythroid and granulocytic precursors in the marrow.[50–53] Iron-containing plasma cells, a decrease in granulocyte precursors and ring sideroblasts have also been reported.[53] Consequently, copper deficiency should enter the differential diagnosis in patients with features of myelodysplastic syndrome, particularly if there is a history of previous gastric surgery (see Chap. 88).[53] Neurologic findings, most commonly a result of myeloneuropathy, are frequently present so that copper deficiency should be considered in the differential diagnosis of a patient with anemia and associated myeloneuropathy suspected of having cobalamin deficiency with subacute combined degeneration of the spinal cord.[54]

Radiologic abnormalities generally are present in infants and young children with copper deficiency. These abnormalities include osteoporosis, flaring of the anterior ribs with spontaneous rib fractures, cupping and flaring of long-bone metaphyses with spur formation and submetaphyseal fractures, and epiphyseal separation. These changes have frequently been misinterpreted as signs of scurvy. Copper deficiency with a resultant microcytic anemia can be produced by chronic ingestion of massive quantities of zinc. Dietary zinc in large doses leads to copper deficiency by impairing copper absorption.[55,56]

The diagnosis of copper deficiency can be established by demonstrating a low serum ceruloplasmin or serum copper level, but the copper level is thought to be more reliable because ceruloplasmin behaves as an acute phase protein.[52] Adequate normal values for the first 2 to 3 months have not been well defined and normally are lower than the levels observed later in life. Despite these limitations, a serum copper level less than 70 mcg/dL (11 micromol/L) or a ceruloplasmin level less than 15 mg/dL after age 1 or 2 months can be regarded as evidence of copper deficiency. In later infancy, childhood, and adulthood, serum copper values should normally exceed 70 mcg/dL. Low serum copper values may be observed in hypoproteinemic states, such as exudative enteropathies and nephrosis, and in Wilson disease. In these circumstances, a diagnosis of copper deficiency cannot be established by serum measurements alone but requires analysis of liver copper content or clinical response after a therapeutic trial of copper supplementation.

The anemia and neutropenia are quickly corrected by administration of copper. Treatment of copper-deficient infants consists of administration of approximately 2.5 mg of copper (~80 mcg/kg per day) oral supplementation as a copper sulfate solution.[57] Intravenous bolus injection of copper chloride also has been used.[53]

ZINC DEFICIENCY

Zinc is required for a large number of zinc metalloenzymes, zinc-activated enzymes, and "zinc finger" transcription factors. Zinc deficiency occurs in a variety of pathologic states in humans, including hemolytic anemias such as thalassemia[58] and sickle cell anemia.[59] Zinc deficiency with or without an associated copper deficiency has been described in a patient receiving intensive deferrioxamine therapy[60] and in patients with decreased renal reabsorption of trace minerals.[61]

Although human zinc deficiency may produce growth retardation, impaired wound healing, impaired taste perception, immunologic abnormalities, and acrodermatitis enteropathica, at present there is no evidence that isolated zinc deficiency produces anemia.

SELENIUM DEFICIENCY

Selenium deficiency occurs in patients who live in areas where the selenium content of the soil is very low[62] and has been observed in patients receiving total parenteral nutrition.[63,64] Although this results in a striking decrease in the level of red cell glutathione peroxidase, there do not appear to be any adverse hematologic consequences.

ANEMIA OF STARVATION

Studies conducted during World War II among prisoners of war and conscientious objectors demonstrated that semistarvation for 24 weeks can result in a mild to moderate normocytic normochromic anemia.[65] Marrow cellularity is usually reduced and is accompanied by a decreased erythroid/myeloid ratio. Measurements of red cell volume and plasma volume suggest that dilution is a major factor responsible for the reduction in hemoglobin concentration.

In persons subjected to complete starvation either for experimental purposes or as treatment of severe obesity, anemia was not observed during the first 2 to 9 weeks of fasting.[66] Starvation for 9 to 17 weeks produced a decrease in hemoglobin and marrow hypocellularity.[67] Resumption of a normal diet was accompanied by reticulocytosis and disappearance of anemia. It has been suggested that the anemia of starvation is a response to a hypometabolic state with its attendant decrease in oxygen requirements.[68]

ANEMIA OF PROTEIN DEFICIENCY (KWASHIORKOR)

Even strict vegetarians do not seem to develop hematologic problems related to the absence of animal proteins,[69] except for some vegans who were reported to suffer from vitamin B_{12} deficiency.[70] The deficiency in this situation is caused, however, by cobalamin insufficiency rather than animal protein, and results from the natural occurrence of cobalamin exclusively in foods of animal origin. Kwashiorkor is largely a disease of the underdeveloped world but occasionally is seen even among the children of educated and well-to-do parents when the children are fed an inappropriate diet.[71,72]

In infants and children with protein-calorie malnutrition, the hemoglobin concentration may fall to 8 g/dL of blood,[72,73] but some children with kwashiorkor have normal hemoglobin levels, probably because of a decreased plasma volume. The anemia is normocytic and normochromic, but the size and shape of red cells on the blood film vary considerably. The white blood cells and the platelets usually are normal. The marrow is most often normally cellular or slightly hypocellular, with a reduced erythroid to myeloid ratio. Erythroblastopenia, reticulocytopenia, and a marrow containing a few giant pronormoblasts may be found, particularly if the children have an infection. With treatment of the infection, erythroid precursors may appear in the marrow and the reticulocyte count may rise. When nutrition is improved by giving high-protein diets (powdered milk or essential amino acids), reticulocytosis, a slight fall in hematocrit because of hemodilution, and then a rise in hemoglobin level, hematocrit, and red blood cell count occur. Improvement is very slow, however, and during the third or fourth week, when the children are clinically improved and serum protein levels are approaching normal, another episode of erythroid marrow aplasia may develop. The relapse is not associated with infection, does not respond to antibiotics, and does not remit spontaneously. It does respond to either riboflavin or prednisone. Children who develop this complication may die suddenly unless they are treated with riboflavin or prednisone. It has been suggested that the erythroblastic aplasia is a manifestation of riboflavin deficiency.[74]

Although the plasma volume is reduced to a variable degree in children with kwashiorkor, the total circulating red cell volume decreases in proportion to the decrease in lean body mass as protein deprivation reduces metabolic demands. During repletion, an increase in plasma volume may occur before an increase in red cell volume, and the anemia may seem to become more severe despite reticulocytosis.

From the study of the anemia of protein deficiency in rats, it was deduced that oxygen consumption and therefore erythropoietin production are reduced.[75] Other studies confirmed this observation but related the reduction to calorie deprivation with its associated decrease in the blood levels of triiodothyronine (T_3) and thyroxine (T_4). As a result, erythropoiesis decreases and the reticulocyte count falls. The plasma iron turnover and red cell uptake of radioactive iron are markedly reduced, and the red cell volume gradually declines.[75] Protein deficiency also produces a maturation block at the erythroblast level and a slight decrease in the erythropoietin-sensitive progenitor cell pool.[76] If exogenous erythropoietin is provided, normal erythropoiesis is restored despite protein depletion,[77] an observation that explains the successful use of starved rats in the bioassay for erythropoietin.

ALCOHOLISM

Chronic alcohol ingestion often is associated with anemia. The anemia may result from nutritional deficiencies, chronic gastrointestinal bleeding, hepatic dysfunction, or direct toxic effects of alcohol on erythropoiesis. Quite commonly all these factors work in concert to produce the anemia. Pyridoxal phosphate and folate deficiency are common in alcoholics.[78] Alcohol affects not only the red cells, as described here, but also platelet production (see Chap. 113).[79,80]

Macrocytosis is common in chronic alcoholics[81] and is often associated with a megaloblastic anemia. Among hospitalized malnourished alcoholics it is the most common type of anemia, occurring alone or in combination with ringed sideroblasts in approximately 40 percent of patients.[82,83] In contrast, megaloblastic anemia is rarely observed in nonhospitalized chronic alcoholics or relatively well-nourished subjects admitted to the hospital for alcohol withdrawal.[84] Anemia, when associated with megaloblastic marrow changes in alcoholics, almost always results from folate deficiency. Iron deficiency often is associated with folate deficiency in alcoholics.[84] In patients with both nutritional deficiencies, the blood film is "dimorphic," with macrocytes, hypersegmented neutrophils, and hypochromic microcytes. This is also the case when folate deficiency coexists with a sideroblastic process.[82,83] Consequently, MCV may be normal but because of marked anisopoikilocytosis the red cell distribution width (RDW) is elevated. Although liver disease is frequently present in alcoholics with megaloblastic anemia, it is not responsible for the folate deficiency. Megaloblastic anemia occurs almost exclusively in alcoholics who have been eating poorly. It is seen more commonly in heavy drinkers of wine and whiskey, which contain little or no folate, than in drinkers of beer, which is a rich source of the vitamin. Although decreased dietary folate intake appears to be a necessary factor in the etiology of the megaloblastic anemia, ethanol itself interferes with folate metabolism (see Chap. 41).[85,86]

However, macrocytosis does not always indicate the presence of a megaloblastic anemia,[81] reticulocytosis secondary to hemolysis or bleeding, or liver disease. A so-called macrocytosis of alcoholism is found in as many as 82 to 96 percent of alcoholics.[87] In these patients, the macrocytosis usually is mild, with mean cell volume in the range of 100 to 110 fl, and anemia is usually absent. In the blood film, the macrocytes are typically round rather than oval, and neutrophil hypersegmentation is not present. The macrocytosis persists until the patient abstains from alcohol. Even then, MCV does not become completely normal for periods of 2 to 4 months in view of the life span of erythrocytes.[86]

Alcohol ingestion for 5 to 7 days produces vacuolization of early red cell precursors, and formation of vacuoles can be observed in *in vitro* marrow cell cultures.[83,88] These changes disappear promptly when alcohol ingestion is discontinued. Vacuolization of a similar appearance occurs in subjects who are fed a phenylalanine-deficient diet, patients treated with chloramphenicol or pyrazinamide, patients in hyperosmolar coma, and individuals deficient in copper or riboflavin.[87]

Two relatively uncommon hematologic complication of alcoholism are Zieve syndrome,[89,90] consisting of alcohol-induced liver disease, often hyperlipidemia, jaundice, and transient spherocytic hemolytic anemia and spur cell hemolytic anemia, associated with severe alcohol-induced liver disease, often requiring hepatic transplantation for resolution.[91,92] Chapter 45 discusses these syndromes.

REFERENCES

1. Blackfan KD, Wolbach SB: Vitamin A deficiency in infants, a clinical and pathological study. *J Pediatr* 3:679, 1933.
2. Vitamin A and iron deficiency. *Nutr Rev* 47:119, 1989.
3. Majia LA, Hodges RE, Arroyave G, et al: Vitamin A deficiency and anemia in Central American children. *Am J Clin Nutr* 30:1175, 1977.
4. Hodges RE, Sauberlich HE, Canham JE, et al: Hematopoietic studies in vitamin A deficiency. *Am J Clin Nutr* 31:876, 1978.
5. Kolsteren P, Rahman SR, Hilderbrand K, Diniz A: Treatment for iron deficiency anaemia with a combined supplementation of iron, vitamin A and zinc in women of Dinajpur, Bangladesh. *Eur J Clin Nutr* 53:102, 1999.
6. Walczyk T, Davidsson L, Rossander-Hulthen L, et al: No enhancing effect of vitamin A on iron absorption in humans. *Am J Clin Nutr* 77:144, 2003.
7. Calis JC, Phiri KS, Faragher EB, et al: Severe anemia in Malawian children. *N Engl J Med* 358:888, 2008.
8. Tatala SR, Kihamia CM, Kyungu LH, Svanberg U: Risk factors for anaemia in schoolchildren in Tanga Region, Tanzania. *Tanzan J Health Res* 10:189, 2008.
9. Snyderman SE, Holt LE Jr, Carretero R, Jacobs KG: Pyridoxine deficiency in the human infant. *Am J Clin Nutr* 1:200, 1953.
10. Foy H, Kondi A: Hypochromic anemias of the tropics associated with pyridoxine and nicotinic acid deficiencies. *Blood* 13:1054, 1958.
11. McCurdy PR, Donohoe RF, Magovern M: Reversible sideroblastic anemia caused by pyrazinoic acid (pyrazinamide). *Ann Intern Med* 64:1280, 1966.

12. Frimpter GW: Pyridoxine (B_6) dependency syndromes. *Ann Intern Med* 68:1131, 1968.
13. Clayton PT: B_6-responsive disorders: A model of vitamin dependency. *J Inherit Metab Dis* 29:17, 2006.
14. Anderson BB, Newmark PA, Rawlins M, Green R: Plasma binding of vitamin B_6 compounds. *Nature* 250:502, 1974.
15. Beutler E, Srivastava SK: Relationship between glutathione reductase activity and drug-induced haemolytic anaemia. *Nature* 226:759, 1970.
16. Lane M, Alfrey CP: The anemia of human riboflavin deficiency. *Blood* 22:811, 1963.
17. Foy H, Kondi A: A case of true red cell aplastic anaemia successfully treated with riboflavin. *J Pathol Bacteriol* 65:559, 1953.
18. Powers HJ: Riboflavin (vitamin B-2) and health. *Am J Clin Nutr* 77:1352, 2003.
19. Hodges RE, Bean WB, Ohlson MA, Bleiler RE: Human pantothenic acid deficiency produced by omegamethylpantothenic acid. *J Clin Invest* 38:1421, 1959.
20. Spivak JL, Jackson DL: Pellagra: An analysis of 18 patients and a review of the literature. *Johns Hopkins Med J* 140:295, 1977.
21. Boros LG, Steinkamp MP, Fleming JC, et al: Defective RNA ribose synthesis in fibroblasts from patients with thiamine-responsive megaloblastic anemia (TRMA). *Blood* 102:3556, 2003.
22. Reuler JB, Broudy VC, Cooney TG: Adult scurvy. *JAMA* 253:805, 1985.
23. Hodges RE, Baker EM, Hood J, et al: Experimental scurvy in man. *Am J Clin Nutr* 22:535, 1969.
24. Zalusky R, Herbert V: Megaloblastic anemia in scurvy with response to 50 micrograms of folic acid daily. *N Engl J Med* 265:1033, 1961.
25. Stokes PL, Melikian V, Leeming RL, et al: Folate metabolism in scurvy. *Am J Clin Nutr* 28:126, 1975.
26. Cox EV, Meynell MJ, Northam BE, Cooke WT: The anaemia of scurvy. *Am J Med* 42:220, 1967.
27. Clark NG, Sheard NF, Kelleher JF: Treatment of iron-deficiency anemia complicated by scurvy and folic acid deficiency. *Nutr Rev* 50:134, 1992.
28. Wapnick AA, Lynch SR, Krawitz P, et al: Effects of iron overload on ascorbic acid metabolism. *BMJ* 3:704, 1968.
29. Wapnick AA, Lynch SR, Charlton RW, et al: The effect of ascorbic acid deficiency on desferrioxamine-induced urinary iron excretion. *Br J Haematol* 17:563, 1969.
30. Chapman RW, Hussain MA, Gorman A, et al: Effect of ascorbic acid deficiency on serum ferritin concentration in patients with beta-thalassaemia major and iron overload. *J Clin Pathol* 35:487, 1982.
31. Cohen A, Cohen IJ, Schwartz E: Scurvy and altered iron stores in thalassemia major. *N Engl J Med* 304:158, 1981.
32. Lipschitz DA, Bothwell TH, Seftel HC, et al: The role of ascorbic acid in the metabolism of storage iron. *Br J Haematol* 20:155, 1971.
33. Bothwell TH, Abrahams C, Bradlow BA, Charlton RW: Idiopathic and Bantu hemochromatosis. *Arch Pathol* 79:163, 1965.
34. Williams ML, Shoot RJ, O'Neal PL, Oski FA: Role of dietary iron and fat on vitamin E deficiency anemia of infancy. *N Engl J Med* 292:887, 1975.
35. Oski FA, Barness LA: Hemolytic anemia in vitamin E deficiency. *Am J Clin Nutr* 21:45, 1968.
36. Ritchie JH, Fish MB, McMasters V, Grossman M: Edema and hemolytic anemia in premature infants. A vitamin E deficiency syndrome. *N Engl J Med* 279:1185, 1968.
37. Zipursky A: Vitamin E deficiency anemia in newborn infants. *Clin Perinatol* 11:393, 1984.
38. Wilfond BS, Farrell PM, Laxova A, Mischler E: Severe hemolytic anemia associated with vitamin E deficiency in infants with cystic fibrosis. Implications for neonatal screening. *Clin Pediatr (Phila)* 33:2, 1994.
39. Farrell PM, Bieri JG, Fratantoni JF, et al: The occurrence and effects of human vitamin E deficiency. A study in patients with cystic fibrosis. *J Clin Invest* 60:233, 1977.
40. Corash L, Spielberg S, Bartsocas C, et al: Reduced chronic hemolysis during high-dose vitamin E administration in Mediterranean-type glucose-6-phosphate dehydrogenase deficiency. *N Engl J Med* 303:416, 1980.
41. Eldamhougy S, Elhelw Z, Yamamah G, et al: The vitamin E status among glucose-6 phosphate dehydrogenase deficient patients and effectiveness of oral vitamin E. *Int J Vitam Nutr Res* 58:184, 1988.
42. Johnson GJ, Vatassery GT, Finkel B, Allen DW: High-dose vitamin E does not decrease the rate of chronic hemolysis in glucose-6-phosphate dehydrogenase deficiency. *N Engl J Med* 308:1014, 1983.
43. Natta CL, Machlin LJ, Brin M: A decrease in irreversibly sickled erythrocytes in sickle cell anemia patients given vitamin E. *Am J Clin Nutr* 33:968, 1980.
44. Tangney CC, Phillips G, Bell RA, et al: Selected indices of micronutrient status in adult patients with sickle cell anemia (SCA). *Am J Hematol* 32:161, 1989.
45. Ren H, Ghebremeskel K, Okpala I, et al: Patients with sickle cell disease have reduced blood antioxidant protection. *Int J Vitam Nutr Res* 78:139, 2008.
46. Ndombi IO, Kinoti SN: Serum vitamin E and the sickling status in children with sickle cell anaemia. *East Afr Med J* 67:720, 1990.
47. Anderson GJ, Frazer DM, McKie AT, Vulpe CD: The ceruloplasmin homolog hephaestin and the control of intestinal iron absorption. *Blood Cells Mol Dis* 29:367, 2002.
48. Graham GG, Cordano A: Copper depletion and deficiency in the malnourished infant. *Johns Hopkins Med J* 124:139, 1969.
49. Spiegel JE, Willenbucher RF: Rapid development of severe copper deficiency in a patient with Crohn's disease receiving parenteral nutrition. *JPEN J Parenter Enteral Nutr* 23:169, 1999.
50. Hirase N, Abe Y, Sadamura S, et al: Anemia and neutropenia in a case of copper deficiency: Role of copper in normal hematopoiesis. *Acta Haematol* 87:195, 1992.
51. Fuhrman MP, Herrmann V, Masidonski P, Eby C: Pancytopenia after removal of copper from total parenteral nutrition. *JPEN J Parenter Enteral Nutr* 24:361, 2000.
52. Halfdanarson TR, Kumar N, Li CY, et al: Hematological manifestations of copper deficiency: A retrospective review. *Eur J Haematol* 80:523, 2008.
53. Gregg X, Reddy V, Prchal J: Copper deficiency masquerading as myelodysplastic syndrome. *Blood* 100:1493, 2002.
54. Kumar N, Gross JB, Ahlskog JE: Copper deficiency myelopathy produces a clinical picture like subacute combined degeneration. *Neurology* 63:33, 2004.
55. Hein MS: Copper deficiency anemia and nephrosis in zinc-toxicity: A case report. *S D J Med* 56:143, 2003.
56. Igic PG, Lee E, Harper W, Roach KW: Toxic effects associated with consumption of zinc. *Mayo Clin Proc* 77:713, 2002.
57. Cordano A: Clinical manifestations of nutritional copper deficiency in infants and children. *Am J Clin Nutr* 67:1012S, 1998.
58. Fuchs GJ, Tienboon P, Linpisarn S, et al: Nutritional factors and thalassaemia major. *Arch Dis Child* 74:224, 1996.
59. Prasad AS: Zinc deficiency in patients with sickle cell disease. *Am J Clin Nutr* 75:181, 2002.
60. Yuzbasiyan-Gurkan VA, Brewer GJ, Vander AJ, et al: Net renal tubular reabsorption of zinc in healthy man and impaired handling in sickle cell anemia. *Am J Hematol* 31:87, 1989.
61. De Virgiliis S, Congia M, Turco MP, et al: Depletion of trace elements and acute ocular toxicity induced by desferrioxamine in patients with thalassaemia. *Arch Dis Child* 63:250, 1988.
62. Thomson CD, Rea HM, Doesburg VM, Robinson MF: Selenium concentrations and glutathione peroxidase activities in whole blood of New Zealand residents. *Br J Nutr* 37:457, 1977.
63. Kien CL, Ganther HE: Manifestations of chronic selenium deficiency in a child receiving total parenteral nutrition. *Am J Clin Nutr* 37:319, 1983.
64. Cohen HJ, Brown MR, Hamilton D, et al: Glutathione peroxidase and selenium deficiency in patients receiving home parenteral nutrition: Time course for development of deficiency and repletion of enzyme activity in plasma and blood cells. *Am J Clin Nutr* 49:132, 1989.
65. Keys A, Brozek J, Henschel A, et al: *The Biology of Semistarvation*. University of Minnesota Press, Minneapolis, 1950.
66. Thomson TJ, Runcie J, Miller V: Treatment of obesity by total fasting for up to 249 days. *Lancet* 2:992, 1966.
67. Drenick EJ, Swendseid ME, Blahd WH, Tuttle SG: Prolonged starvation as treatment for severe obesity. *JAMA* 187:100, 1964.
68. Caro J, Silver R, Erslev AJ, et al: Erythropoietin production in fasted rats. Effects of thyroid hormones and glucose supplementation. *J Lab Clin Med* 98:860, 1981.
69. Lowik MR, Schrijver J, Odink J, et al: Long-term effects of a vegetarian diet on the nutritional status of elderly people (Dutch Nutrition Surveillance System). *J Am Coll Nutr* 9:600, 1990.
70. Chanarin I, Malkowska V, O'Hea AM, et al: Megaloblastic anaemia in a vegetarian Hindu community. *Lancet* 2:1168, 1985.
71. Carvalho NF, Kenney RD, Carrington PH, Hall DE: Severe nutritional deficiencies in toddlers resulting from health food milk alternatives. *Pediatrics* 107:E46, 2001.
72. Lunn PG, Morley CJ, Neale G: A case of kwashiorkor in the UK. *Clin Nutr* 17:131, 1998.
73. Adams EB, Scragg JN, Naidoo BT, et al.: Observations on the aetiology and treatment of anaemia in kwashiorkor. *Br Med J* 3:451, 1967.
74. Foy H, Kondi A: Comparison between erythroid aplasia in marasmus and kwashiorkor and the experimentally induced erythroid aplasia in baboons by riboflavin deficiency. *Vitam Horm* 26:653, 1968.
75. Delmonte L, Aschkenasy A, Eyquem A: Studies on the hemolytic nature of protein-deficiency anemia in the rat. *Blood* 24:49, 1964.
76. Naets JP, Wittek M: Effect of starvation on the response to erythropoietin in the rat. *Acta Haematol* 52:141, 1974.
77. Ito K, Reissmann KR: Quantitative and qualitative aspects of steady state erythropoiesis induced in protein-starved rats by long-term erythropoietin injection. *Blood* 27:343, 1966.
78. Gloria L, Cravo M, Camilo ME, et al: Nutritional deficiencies in chronic alcoholics: Relation to dietary intake and alcohol consumption. *Am J Gastroenterol* 92:485, 1997.
79. Savage D, Lindenbaum J: Anemia in alcoholics. *Medicine (Baltimore)* 65:322, 1986.
80. Girard DE, Kumar KL, McAfee JH: Hematologic effects of acute and chronic alcohol abuse. *Hematol Oncol Clin North Am* 1:321, 1987.
81. Fernando OV, Grimsley EW: Prevalence of folate deficiency and macrocytosis in patients with and without alcohol-related illness. *South Med J* 91:721, 1998.
82. Colman N, Herbert V: Hematologic complications of alcoholism: Overview. *Semin Hematol* 17:164, 1980.
83. Sullivan LW, Herbert V: Suppression of hematopoiesis by ethanol. *J Clin Invest* 43:2048, 1964.
84. Eichner ER, Hillman RS: Effect of alcohol on serum folate level. *J Clin Invest* 52:584, 1973.
85. Lindenbaum J: Folate and vitamin B_{12} deficiencies in alcoholism. *Semin Hematol* 17:119, 1980.
86. Seppa K, Laippala P, Saarni M: Macrocytosis as a consequence of alcohol abuse among patients in general practice. *Alcohol Clin Exp Res* 15:871, 1991.

87. McCurdy PR, Rath CE: Vacuolated nucleated bone marrow cells in alcoholism. *Semin Hematol* 17:100, 1980.
88. Yeung KY, Klug PP, Lessin LS: Alcohol-induced vacuolization in bone marrow cells: Ultrastructure and mechanism of formation. *Blood Cells* 13:487, 1988.
89. Zieve L: Jaundice, hyperlipemia and hemolytic anemia: A heretofore unrecognized syndrome associated with alcoholic fatty liver and cirrhosis. *Ann Intern Med* 48:471, 1958.
90. Melrose WD, Bell PA, Jupe DM, Baikie MJ: Alcohol-associated haemolysis in Zieve's syndrome: A clinical and laboratory study of five cases. *Clin Lab Haematol* 12:159, 1990.
91. Chitale AA, Sterling RK, Post AB, et al: Resolution of spur cell anemia with liver transplantation: A case report and review of the literature. *Transplantation* 65:993, 1998.
92. Malik P, Bogetti D, Sileri P, et al: Spur cell anemia in alcoholic cirrhosis: Cure by orthotopic liver transplantation and recurrence after liver graft failure. *Int Surg* 87:201, 2002.

CHAPTER 44

ANEMIA ASSOCIATED WITH MARROW INFILTRATION

Archana M. Agarwal and Josef T. Prchal

SUMMARY

Myelophthisic anemia is an anemia caused by marrow infiltration, typically by metastatic cancer, but also by any nonhematopoietic tissue, for example, granulomatous fibrotic tissues. It can present with an overt leukoerythroblastic picture or with only a few teardrop-shaped red cells on a blood film. These changes may represent an early spread of the tumor (or other nonhematopoietic tissue) to the marrow or may indicate massive replacement of the marrow space. The diagnosis can be made by standard marrow biopsy. Radioisotope scanning and magnetic resonance imaging, although not very sensitive, can be helpful in locating the biopsy site and can also help in estimating the percentage of involvement of the marrow space.

DEFINITION AND HISTORY

Myelophthisic anemia is the term that has been used to describe diverse pathologic processes, including Fanconi anemia,[1] but currently refers to anemia resulting from the presence of spotty to massive marrow infiltration with abnormal cells or tissue components. Strictly speaking, the blasts of acute leukemia, plasma cells of myeloma, and cells of lymphoma, chronic leukemia, and myeloproliferative disorders fit this definition. However, the term *myelophthisic anemia*[2] is best reserved for marrow replacement by nonhematologic tumors and nonhematopoietic tissue. Minimal to moderate involvement usually does not cause symptoms or hematologic changes. Such infiltration is clinically significant, however, because in patients with an established diagnosis of cancer, it indicates metastatic dissemination of the tumor and usually an incurable disorder. Although extensive infiltration may lead to anemia or even pancytopenia, anemia can be frequently accompanied by an elevated leukocyte count, often with immature myeloid cells in the blood. Platelets can be increased, decreased, or normal (megakaryocytic fragments are seen occasionally in the blood). The condition accompanied by teardrop-shaped red cells (dacrocytes), prematurely released nucleated red cells, and immature myeloid cells is referred to as *leukoerythroblastic reaction* (see Chaps. 2 and 29), which generally reflects extramedullary hematopoiesis, predominantly from the spleen.[3]

ETIOLOGY AND PATHOGENESIS

Tumor metastasis results from the complex interactions between the tumor cells and the surrounding microenvironment. Invasion is the primary process of metastasis and occurs often as a result of loss of E-cadherin. E-cadherin is a calcium-dependent cell adhesion molecule that likely plays a role in intercellular adhesion and inhibition of invasion by neoplastic cells. The loss of E-cadherin can be caused by many mechanisms, including mutations and gene silencing.[4] Many members of the family of matrix metalloproteinases can also participate in the process of tumor cell invasion. Stromal cells such as tumor-associated macrophages and growth factors secreted by them such as fibroblast growth factor are also known to promote tumor spread.[5]

Acronyms and abbreviations that appear in this chapter include: MRI, magnetic resonance imaging; ^{99m}Tc, a radioisotope of technetium; ^{99m}Tc sestamibi, a radioisotope of technetium attached to the sestamibi molecule.

Table 44–1 lists the most common causes of extensive cellular infiltration of marrow. In myelofibrotic disorders of both primary and secondary origin, the fibrosis restricts the available marrow space and disrupts marrow architecture (see Chap. 91). The disruption may cause cytopenias with production of deformed red cells, especially poikilocytes and teardrop-shaped cells, and premature release of erythroblasts, myelocytes, and giant platelets. The blood leukocyte count also may be elevated. Similar abnormalities following marrow replacement by calcium oxalate crystals have been reported.[6]

Anemia seen in metastatic cancer most frequently results from cytokine release leading to anemia of chronic inflammation (see Chap. 37), iron deficiency, for example, gastrointestinal or uterine bleeding (see Chap. 42), or other nutritional deficiencies (see Chaps. 41 and 43). However, marrow replacement causing a myelophthisic anemia as the sole cause of anemia also occurs. The marrow microenvironment is susceptible to implantation of bloodborne malignant cells. Almost all cancers can metastasize to the marrow,[7–9] but the most common are cancers of the lung, breast, and prostate. Metastatic foci in the marrow can be found in 20 to 30 percent of patients with small-cell carcinoma of the lung at the time of diagnosis and in more than 50 percent of patients at autopsy.[10] Development of a frank leukoerythroblastic blood picture occurs much less frequently,[7] and its absence is not a reliable indicator that the marrow is not involved.

The characteristic abnormalities observed in patients with myelophthisic anemia may result partly from an attempt for compensatory extramedullary blood formation that generally reflects extramedullary hematopoiesis predominantly from the spleen. A similar picture can be seen when the marrow is replaced by numerous granulomas,[11,12] for example, sarcoidosis, disseminated tuberculosis, fungal infections, or by macrophages containing indigestible lipids, as in Gaucher and Niemann-Pick diseases (see Chap. 73).[13]

Marrow necrosis can be an underlying cause of myelophthisic anemia. The morphologic picture, best observed in hematoxylin-and-eosin–stained biopsy of marrow, consists of cell debris and occasional necrotic cells in a background of marrow fibrosis. Marrow necrosis is generally considered to be very rare, accounting for less than 1 percent of marrow biopsies. Tumors and septicemia are generally the underlying cause,[14] but sickle cell disease[15,16] and arsenic therapy in acute promyelocytic leukemia are other causes.[17] The frequency of the diagnosis of marrow necrosis is a function of the area of marrow that must be involved to draw such a conclusion. The diagnostic frequency increases if a small area of necrotic marrow is considered sufficient to make the diagnosis.[18]

Because myelophthisic anemia is so uncommon, only a few rigorous studies of the pathogenesis of anemia in this entity have been conducted. *In vitro* study of hematopoietic progenitors reveals only a moderate decrease of their proportion and proliferative capacity.[19] Similar reports of erythropoiesis quantitation by ferrokinetic studies reveal only a moderate defect (see Chap. 31).[20] The following confounding factors contribute to anemia: elevated hepcidin (see Chap. 37) and other factors, including hematopoiesis-inhibiting cytokines released from tumor cells (see Chap. 37) and iron (Chap. 42) and folate (Chap. 41) deficiencies. When they are excluded, the finding discussed above suggests that only massive marrow replacement leads to anemia.

TABLE 44–1. Causes of Marrow Infiltration

I. Fibroblasts and Collagen
   A. Primary myelofibrosis (see Chap. 91)
   B. Fibrosis of other myeloproliferative disorders
   C. Fibrosis of hairy cell leukemia (see Chap. 95)
   D. Metastatic malignancies
   E. Sarcoidosis[11,12]
   F. Secondary myelofibrosis with pulmonary hypertension
II. Other Noncellular Material
   A. Oxalosis[6]
III. Tumor Cells
   A. Carcinoma (lung, breast, prostate, kidney, thyroid, and neuroblastoma)[7,9]
   B. Sarcoma[8]
IV. Granulomas (inflammatory cells)[12]
   A. Miliary tuberculosis
   B. Fungal infections
   C. Sarcoidosis
V. Macrophages
   A. Gaucher disease (see Chap. 73)
   B. Niemann-Pick disease[13]
VI. Marrow Necrosis
   A. Sickle cell anemia[15]
   B. Septicemia[14]
   C. Tumors[14]
   D. Arsenic therapy[17]
VII. Failure of Osteoclast Development
   A. Osteopetrosis[27]

CLINICAL FEATURES

Symptoms and signs associated with infiltrative marrow disorders usually are related to the underlying disease. Other symptoms, such as fatigue, may be caused by anemia itself. Some patients are asymptomatic, and the incidental discovery of cytopenias and leukoerythroblastic blood morphology leads to diagnosis of an underlying disorder.

LABORATORY FEATURES

BLOOD

The anemia usually is mild to moderate, but it can be severe. White cell and platelet counts may vary, but the most characteristic feature is the morphologic appearance of red cells on the blood film. These cells may show anisocytosis and poikilocytosis, but the presence of teardrop forms and nucleated red cells is particularly suggestive of marrow infiltration (see Chap. 29). The combination of nucleated red cells and immature myeloid precursors constitutes the leukoerythroblastic picture that is characteristic of marrow infiltration and extramedullary hematopoiesis (Fig. 44–1). The presence of cancer cells on the blood film occurs occasionally and always indicates marrow invasion (Fig. 44–2).[21]

MARROW

Marrow biopsy is the most reliable procedure used to diagnose marrow-infiltrative disease and should be performed in all patients with suspected metastatic carcinoma or hematologic features of myelophthisic anemia (Fig. 44–3). Marrow aspiration[22] does not provide a reliable yield of tumor cells and is particularly difficult in primary or secondary myelofibrosis. The inability to aspirate marrow (dry tap) leads to a high degree of suspicion of marrow replacement and accompanying myelofibrosis. Because the diagnostic marrow yield from biopsies depends on the amount of tissue examined, bilateral posterior iliac crest marrow biopsies may be necessary. In patients with metastatic cancer involving the marrow, the blood CD34-positive cell count can be up to 50 times higher than in patients with metastatic cancer without marrow involvement.[23]

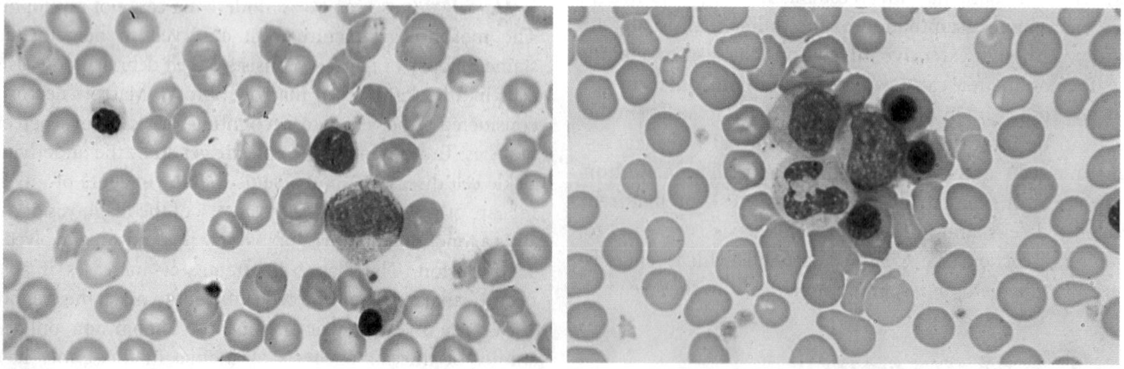

A B

FIGURE 44–1. A. Blood film. Two nucleated red cells and a promyelocyte and a lymphocyte. The red cells show occasional but increased poikilocytosis. The patient had metastatic renal carcinoma to several sites including marrow. **B.** Blood film. White cell concentrate (buffy coat). Three nucleated red cells, two myelocytes, and a segmented neutrophil are evident. Another nucleated red cell can be partially visualized at right margin of field. In this case the blood film did not have evidence of a leukoerythroblastic reaction, but evidence was found in a film of the white cell concentrate. Because the white cell concentrate is the layer between the red cells and plasma in centrifuged blood, the red cells aspirated with the white cells are usually of lower density than average and reticulocyte rich, as evident here. Red cell morphology is not representative of the direct blood film. Patient had carcinoma of the lung metastatic to marrow. In leukoerythroblastic reactions the red cell precursors that escape the marrow are usually orthochromatic erythroblasts, although occasionally earlier precursors may be seen. *(From* Lichtman's Atlas of Hematology, *www.accessmedicine.com. Used with permission.)*

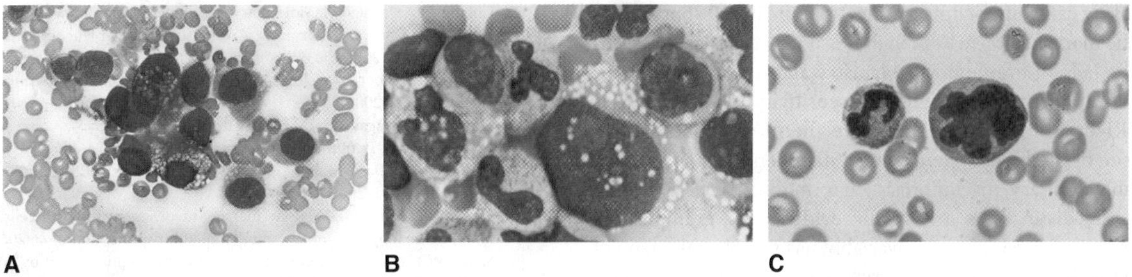

FIGURE 44–2. *Carcinocythemia.* **A.** Blood film. Clump of breast cancer cells in blood of patient with metastatic breast cancer. **B.** Blood film. Large cell with nuclear and cytoplasmic vacuolization in center of field and several smaller surrounding cells with vacuoles are breast cancer cells in this patient's blood. **C.** Blood film. Lung cancer cells in blood. Note very large size and bizarre nuclear abnormality. *(From* Lichtman's Atlas of Hematology, *www.accessmedicine.com. Used with permission.)*

■ ISOTOPE AND IMAGING PROCEDURES

Technetium-99m (^{99m}Tc) sestamibi uptake reliably identifies marrow infiltration by Gaucher cells. Sestamibi is a pharmaceutical agent used in nuclear medicine imaging. Magnetic resonance imaging (MRI) is also helpful for defining the severity of marrow replacement and is being used with increasing frequency. This imaging approach is especially useful for following resolution of marrow infiltration in patients with type 1 Gaucher disease who are treated with enzyme-replacement therapy.[24] An isotopic bone scan or MRI study showing focal accumulation of radioactive tracers can be helpful in locating a suitable site for biopsy,[25] but a negative study of the area does not exclude the possibility of marrow involvement. On MRI, marrow necrosis characteristically has an extensive, diffuse, geographic pattern of signal abnormality consisting of a central area of variable signal intensity surrounded by a distinct peripheral enhancing rim.[16]

DIFFERENTIAL DIAGNOSIS

The cause of a leukoerythroblastic blood picture is known to occur in a patient with metastatic cancer or overt hematologic malignancy. In the

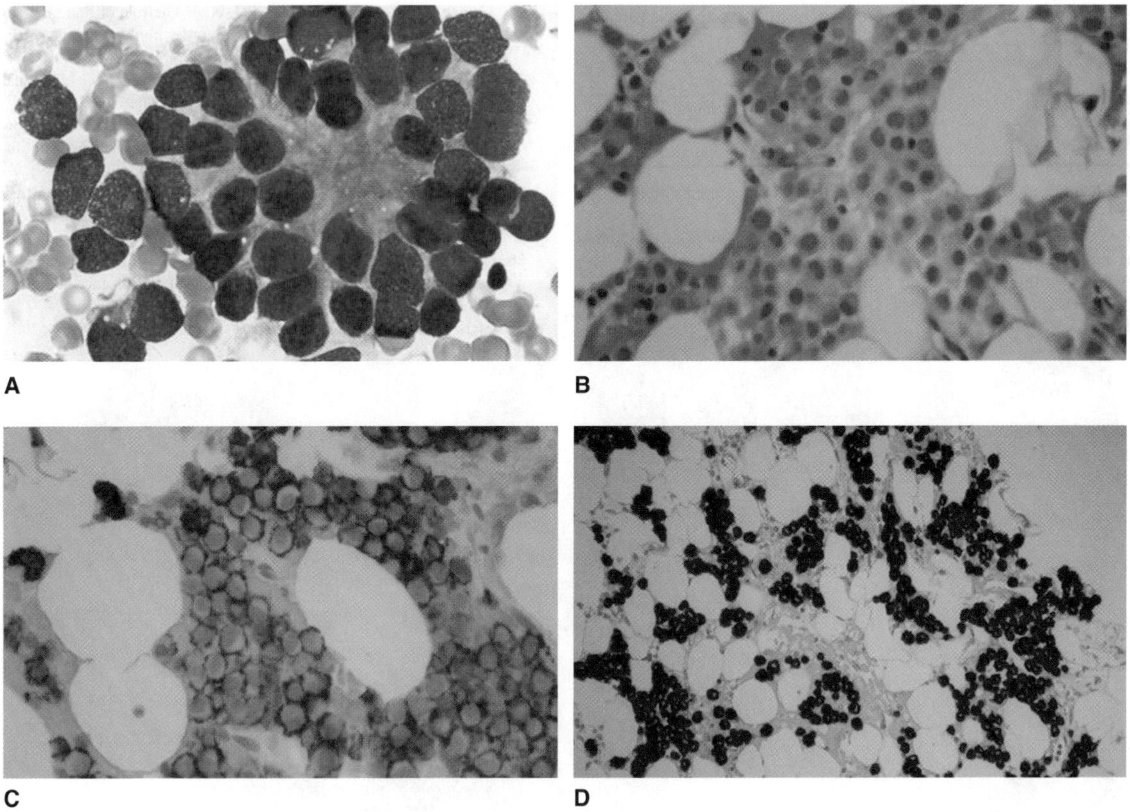

FIGURE 44–3. A. Marrow film. Metastatic neuroblastoma cells. Note characteristic rosette formation of this tumor. **B.** Marrow section. Patient with infiltrating lobular carcinoma of the breast. The marrow is replaced with a monotonous infiltrate of presumptive tumor cells. **C.** Marrow section. Same marrow as in **(B)** but stained with CD138. Note intense staining of cells. This stain can react with carcinoma cells as well as plasma cells. No detectable lambda or kappa light chain staining was present. **D.** Marrow section. Same marrow as in **(B)** and **(C)** with cytokeratin immunohistochemistry. Mixture of high- and low-molecular-weight (AE-1/3 and Cam 5.2) anticytokeratin antibodies were used, stained by standard peroxidase–antiperoxidase technique using 3-amino-9-ethylcarbazole substrate, confirming metastatic (breast) cancer cells. *(From* Lichtman's Atlas of Hematology, *www.accessmedicine.com. Used with permission.)*

absence of a likely cause after clinical evaluation, the initial approach to diagnosis is the marrow biopsy. Although it is not a very sensitive technique, with the help of immunocytochemistry and flow cytometry for tumor-specific antigens, its diagnostic sensitivity and specificity increases. MRI or isotopic scanning before the marrow may aid in locating the site of the biopsy. Hematologic disorders causing marrow fibrosis, notably primary myelofibrosis, may mimic a myelophthisic disorder, but the distinctions are usually evident. For example, the patient with primary myelofibrosis invariably has splenic enlargement and the patient with metastatic cancer nearly always does not (see Chap. 91). If the myelophthisis is the result of a storage disease or other infiltrative cause, the appropriate chemical tests, as well as marrow biopsy, are helpful in diagnosis. Nucleated red cells and leukocytosis can be seen in acute conditions, including overwhelming sepsis, acute severe hypoxia, postcardiac arrest, and chronic conditions such as thalassemia major, congestive heart failure, and severe hemolytic anemia.

THERAPY, COURSE, AND PROGNOSIS

The goal of treatment is managing the underlying disease. Patients with marrow infiltration caused by cancer should be treated appropriately; however, in some instances the presence of marrow infiltration may not adversely affect the outcome. If treatment is successful, not only the malignant cells but also the reactive fibrosis surrounding metastatic foci may completely disappear. In hormone-refractory prostate cancer, the presence of a leukoerythroblastic picture does not seem to influence survival.[26] However, in most patients with cancers metastatic to the marrow, only short-term survival is a rule.

REFERENCES

1. Baumann T: [Constitutional general myelophthisis with multiple degeneration (Fanconi syndrome).] *Ann Paediatr* 177:65, 1951.
2. Rundles RW, Jonsson U: Metastases in bone marrow and myelophthisic anemia from carcinoma of the prostate. *Am J Med Sci* 218:241, 1949.
3. Vaughan J: Leuco-erythroblastic anaemia. *J Pathol Bacteriol* 42:541, 1936.
4. Thiery JP: Epithelial-mesenchymal transitions in tumour progression. *Nat Rev Cancer* 2:442, 2002.
5. Chiang AC, Massague J: Molecular basis of metastasis. *N Engl J Med* 359:2814, 2008.
6. Halil O, Farringdon K: Oxalosis: An unusual cause of leucoerythroblastic anaemia. *Br J Haematol* 122:2, 2003.
7. Makoni SN, Laber DA: Clinical spectrum of myelophthisis in cancer patients. *Am J Hematol* 76:92, 2004.
8. Shinkoda Y, Nagatoshi Y, Fukano R, et al: Rhabdomyosarcoma masquerading as acute leukemia. *Pediatr Blood Cancer* 52:286, 2009.
9. Mohanty SK, Dash S: Bone marrow metastasis in solid tumors. *Indian J Pathol Microbiol* 46:613, 2003.
10. Hirsch FR, Hansen HH: Bone marrow involvement in small cell anaplastic carcinoma of the lung: Prognostic and therapeutic aspects. *Cancer* 46:206, 1980.
11. Saliba WR, Elias MS: Recurrent severe hypercalcemia caused by bone marrow sarcoidosis. *Am J Med Sci* 330:147, 2005.
12. Eid A, Carion W, Nystrom JS: Differential diagnoses of bone marrow granuloma. *West J Med* 164:510, 1996.
13. Hsu YS, Hwu WL, Huang SF, et al: Niemann-Pick disease type C (a cellular cholesterol lipidosis) treated by bone marrow transplantation. *Bone Marrow Transplant* 24:103, 1999.
14. Paydas S, Ergin M, Baslamisli F, et al: Bone marrow necrosis: Clinicopathologic analysis of 20 cases and review of the literature. *Am J Hematol* 70:300, 2002.
15. Conrad ME, Studdard H, Anderson LJ: Aplastic crisis in sickle cell disorders: bone marrow necrosis and human parvovirus infection. *Am J Med Sci* 295:212, 1988.
16. Tang YM, Jeavons S, Stuckey S, et al: MRI features of bone marrow necrosis. *AJR Am J Roentgenol* 188:509, 2007.
17. Chim CS, Lam CC, Wong KF, et al: Atypical blasts and bone marrow necrosis associated with near-triploid relapse of acute promyelocytic leukemia after arsenic trioxide treatment. *Hum Pathol* 33:849, 2002.
18. Conrad ME: Bone marrow necrosis. *J Intensive Care Med* 10:171, 1995.
19. Dainiak N, Kulkarni V, Howard D, et al: Mechanisms of abnormal erythropoiesis in malignancy. *Cancer* 51:1101, 1983.
20. Cazzola M, Bergamaschi G, Huebers HA, et al: Pathophysiological classification of acquired bone marrow failure based on quantitative assessment of erythroid function. *Eur J Haematol* 38:426, 1987.
21. Gallivan MV, Lokich JJ: Carcinocythemia (carcinoma cell leukemia). Report of two cases with English literature review. *Cancer* 53:1100, 1984.
22. Garrett TJ, Gee TS, Lieberman PH, et al: The role of bone marrow aspiration and biopsy in detecting marrow involvement by nonhematologic malignancies. *Cancer* 38:2401, 1976.
23. Ciancia R, Martinelli V, Cosentini E, et al: High number of circulating CD34+ cells in patients with myelophthisis. *Haematologica* 90:976, 2005.
24. Mariani G, Filocamo M, Giona F, et al: Severity of bone marrow involvement in patients with Gaucher's disease evaluated by scintigraphy with ^{99m}Tc-sestamibi. *J Nucl Med* 44:1253, 2003.
25. Terk MR, Dardashti S, Liebman HA: Bone marrow response in treated patients with Gaucher disease: evaluation by T1-weighted magnetic resonance images and correlation with reduction in liver and spleen volume. *Skeletal Radiol* 29:563, 2000.
26. Shamdas GJ, Ahmann FR, Matzner MB, et al: Leukoerythroblastic anemia in metastatic prostate cancer. Clinical and prognostic significance in patients with hormone-refractory disease. *Cancer* 71:3594, 1993.
27. Stark Z, Savarirayan R: Osteopetrosis. *Orphanet J Rare Dis* 4:5, 2009.

CHAPTER 45

THE RED BLOOD CELL MEMBRANE AND ITS DISORDERS: HEREDITARY SPHEROCYTOSIS, ELLIPTOCYTOSIS, AND RELATED DISEASES

Patrick G. Gallagher

SUMMARY

Hereditary spherocytosis is an inherited hemolytic anemia characterized by spherically shaped erythrocytes on the blood film, reticulocytosis, and splenomegaly. The principal cellular defect is the propensity to lose membrane surface area during passage through the splenic circulation, leading to spherical shape and decreased deformability. Splenic destruction of nondeformable spherocytes leads to anemia. Membrane loss results from defects in several membrane proteins, including ankyrin, band 3, α-spectrin, β-spectrin, and protein 4.2. Significant clinical, laboratory, biochemical, and genetic heterogeneity exists among patients with hereditary spherocytosis. *Hereditary elliptocytosis* is characterized by the presence of elliptical erythrocytes on the blood film, often with no or very slight shortening of red cell survival. The principal defect in the erythrocyte is a mechanical weakness caused by abnormalities in the proteins involved in the membrane skeleton, including α-spectrin, β-spectrin, protein 4.1, and glycophorin C. The majority of patients are asymptomatic, and therapy is rarely necessary. *Hereditary pyropoikilocytosis* is a rare cause of severe hemolytic anemia characterized by erythrocyte morphology similar to that seen in thermal burns. *Acanthocytosis* is characterized by the presence of contracted, dense erythrocytes with irregular projections on blood films, which may be seen in patients with severe liver disease, abetalipoproteinemia, after splenectomy, various neurologic disorders, and as a correlate of certain aberrant red cell antigens. Acanthocytes have abnormal red cell membrane lipid composition. The associated hemolysis is mild and rarely requires therapy. *Stomatocytosis* is a condition in which the red blood cells are principally composed of stomatocytes, red cells characterized by a central hemoglobin-free area shaped like a cigar or sausage or a very small circle. Stomatocytosis can be an inherited disorder or can occur in association with several acquired abnormalities. Stomatocytosis frequently is associated with abnormal red cell cation content, hydration, and membrane lipids. Great heterogeneity in the laboratory manifestations and clinical course of the stomatocytosis syndromes is observed. In some cases, abnormalities of band 3 and Rh-associated glycoproteins lead to altered membrane permeability.

Acronyms and abbreviations that appear in this chapter include: α^{LELY}, low-expression Lyon α-spectrin; α^{LEPRA}, low-expression Prague α-spectrin; AQP1, aquaporin-1; ATP, adenosine triphosphate; BPG, bisphosphoglycerate; FP, familial pseudohyperkalemia; GPC, glycophorin C; GPD, glycophorin D; HAc, hereditary acanthocytosis; HE, hereditary elliptocytosis; HPP, hereditary pyropoikilocytosis; HS, hereditary spherocytosis; HSt, hereditary stomatocytosis; LCAT, lecithin-cholesterol acetyltransferase; MAGUK, membrane-associated guanylate kinase; MCHC, mean corpuscular hemoglobin concentration; MCV, mean corpuscular volume; PE, phosphatidylethanolamine; PI, phosphatidylinositol; PS, phosphatidylserine; RhAG, Rh-associated glycoprotein.

THE RED CELL MEMBRANE

The erythrocyte membrane accounts for 1 percent of total weight of the red cell, yet it plays an integral role in the maintenance of erythrocyte integrity. The red cell membrane and its skeleton provide the erythrocyte the flexibility, durability, and tensile strength to undergo large deformations during repeated passages through narrow microcirculatory channels. The red cell membrane maintains a nonreactive exterior so that erythrocytes do not adhere to endothelial cells or aggregate and occlude the microcirculation. The membrane plays an important role in metabolism by selectively and reversibly binding and inactivating glycolytic enzymes. It retains organic phosphates and other vital compounds and permits efflux of metabolic waste. It also sequesters the reductants required to prevent damage by oxygen. During erythropoiesis, the membrane responds to erythropoietin and imports the iron required for hemoglobin synthesis. At the level of the organism, the membrane participates in the maintenance of pH homeostasis by participating in the exchange of chloride and bicarbonate.

The easy accessibility of the human erythrocyte has resulted in the erythrocyte membrane being the most thoroughly studied in cell biology. Erythrocytes are the cells about which the most detailed information concerning the normal structure and function of their membrane and the molecular pathology of disorders caused primarily by abnormal membrane or cytoskeletal structure is available. The erythrocyte membrane remains the paradigm for ongoing studies of other cell types. Although the primary structure (Fig. 45–1) and a number of the important functions of the red cell membrane are known, its study continues to yield important insights into our understanding of membrane structure and function. Genetic investigation of disorders of the erythrocyte membrane has advanced our understanding of the normal structure–function relationships of the membrane and has provided us with an understanding of the inheritance and expression of these disorders.

COMPOSITION OF THE RED CELL MEMBRANE

The erythrocyte membrane is composed of three major structural elements: a lipid bilayer primarily composed of phospholipids and cholesterol that provides a permeability barrier between the external environment and the red cell cytoplasm; integral proteins embedded in the lipid bilayer that span the membrane; and a membrane skeleton on the internal side of the red cell membrane that provides structural integrity to the cell.

■ MEMBRANE LIPIDS

Composition

Lipids comprise 50 to 60 percent of red cell membrane mass. The principal membrane lipids are phospholipids and cholesterol, which are present in nearly equal amounts.[1,2] Small amounts of glycolipids, primarily globoside, are present. The primary phospholipids are phosphatidylcholine ([PC] 28% of total phospholipids), phosphatidylethanolamine ([PE] 27%), sphingomyelin (26%), phosphatidylserine ([PS] 13%), and phosphatidylinositol.

Membrane phosphoinositides are phospholipids that contain phosphatidylinositol (PI) or its phosphorylated forms PI-4-monophosphate

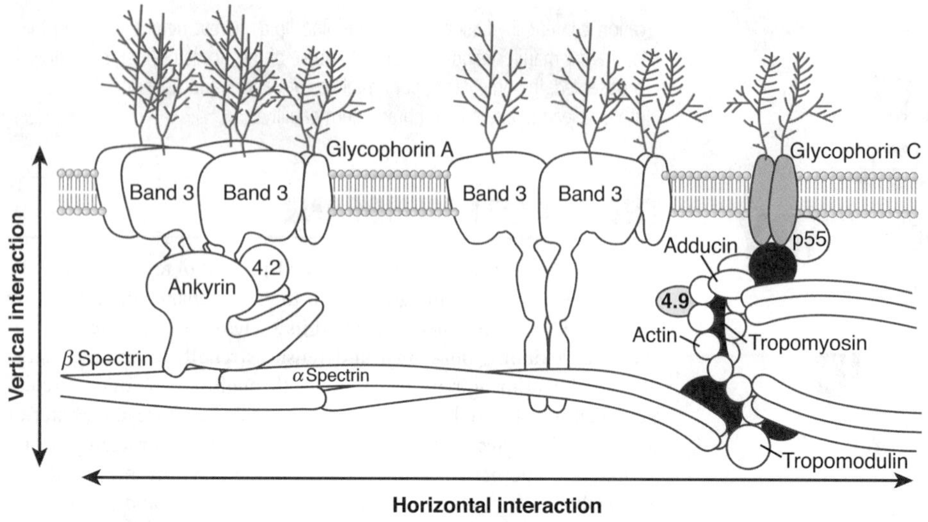

FIGURE 45–1. Schematic illustrating the molecular assembly of the major erythrocyte membrane proteins and a model of the principal molecular defect in hereditary spherocytosis (HS), elliptocytosis (HE), and pyropoikilocytosis (HPP). Membrane protein–protein and protein–lipid associations can be divided into two categories: (1) *vertical interactions*, which are perpendicular to the plane of the membrane and involve spectrin–ankyrin–band 3 interaction, spectrin–protein 4.1–glycophorin C connection, and weak interactions between spectrin and the negatively charged lipids of the inner half of the membrane lipid bilayer; and (2) *horizontal interactions*, which are parallel to the plane of the membrane, and include α-spectrin–β-spectrin and β-spectrin–protein 4.1 interactions. *(From Tse WT, Lux SE: Red blood cell membrane disorders.* Br J Haematol *104:2, 1999, with permission.)*

and PI-4,5-biphosphate. In nucleated cells, phosphoinositides are precursors of important intracellular second messengers such as inositol-1,4,5-triphosphate and diacylglycerol that participate in regulation of many cellular processes. In mature erythrocytes, phosphoinositides represent 2 to 5 percent of total phospholipids, residing largely at the inner membrane surface and undergoing rapid phosphorylation and dephosphorylation. In red cells, they are involved in regulation of calcium transport and interaction of transmembrane and skeletal proteins (e.g., glycophorin C and protein 4.1). They have been proposed to participate in the control of the discocyte-echinocyte shape transformation.

In the erythrocyte, cholesterol is present in a free, unesterified form. It is almost entirely hydrophobic. Its primary role appears to be controlling membrane fluidity even under conditions that might lead to phospholipid crystallization and rigidification of the bilayer.

Membrane Lipid Distribution

Phospholipids are asymmetrically distributed in the red cell membrane with PS and PE primarily in the inner hemileaflet; sphingomyelin and PC are outwardly oriented. This asymmetric distribution of phospholipids is a dynamic system involving a constant exchange ("flip-flop")[3] between the phospholipids of the two bilayer leaflets. Maintenance of this asymmetry appears to be important in the regulation of hemostasis, as PS on the outer leaflet provides a site for prothrombinase binding, causing the red cell surface to become prothrombotic. Phospholipid flipping may contribute to the occurrence of thromboses in a variety of disorders, including sickle cell disease, thalassemia, and diabetes, because exposed phospholipids trigger conversion of prothrombin to thrombin and activate the coagulation cascade.[4] The presence of PS on the outer surface of the red cell is one of the earliest changes in apoptosis. It has been correlated with complement activation and red cell clearance by macrophages and liposomes.

Enzymes called *flippases* actively translocate PS and PE to the inner leaflet. *Floppases* catalyze translocation to the outer leaflet. Asymmetry seems to depend on the fact that flipping occurs at a higher rate than flopping. Flippase activity is mediated, at least in part, by a 130-kDa integral membrane protein that is a member of the Mg^+-dependent, P-glycoprotein adenosine triphosphatase (ATPase) family.[5] Floppase activity in red cell membranes appears to be mediated by the multidrug resistance protein-1 (MRP1).[6]

A *scramblase* activated by elevated intracellular calcium promotes randomization and loss of membrane.[7] Scramblase mediates redistribution of membrane phospholipids in activated, injured, or apoptotic cells.[8] Derangements within the red cell often raise intracellular calcium by direct or indirect damage to ion channels and pumps. Scott syndrome is a congenital bleeding disorder in which red cells and platelets expose subnormal amounts of PS on the outer surface in response to calcium, but the situation does not appear to result from scramblase deficiency.[9,10]

Glycolipids and cholesterol are intercalated between the phospholipids in the bilayer, with their long axes perpendicular to the bilayer plane. Red cell glycolipids are located entirely in the external half of the bilayer, with their carbohydrate moieties extending into the aqueous phase. They carry several important red cell antigens, including A, B, H, and P, and may serve other important functions. The location of membrane cholesterol is less certain, but cholesterol appears to be present in about equal proportions on both sides of the bilayer.

Detergent-resistant membrane domains or lipid rafts are present in erythrocytes.[11] These membrane microdomains contain stomatin, flotillin-1 and flotillin-2, the Duffy receptor, heterotrimeric $G\alpha_S$, CD55, CD58, and CD59. Alterations in erythrocyte calcium lead to shedding of rafts as large vesicles containing stomatin and small vesicles containing synexin and sorcin.[12] Neither of these vesicles contains flotillin. Lipid rafts play an important role in protein recruitment to the malarial parasite vacuole during erythrocyte invasion.[13]

Lipid Synthesis and Renewal

Synthesis and assembly of red cell membrane lipids occurs during erythropoiesis. Mature erythrocytes are unable to synthesize fatty acids, phospholipids, or cholesterol *de novo*. They depend on lipid exchange and fatty acid acylation for phospholipid repair and renewal. These renewal pathways, although limited, permit slow replacement of membrane lipid components.[14]

Lipid exchange rates vary considerably. Exchange of unesterified cholesterol occurs in several hours. Outer bilayer phospholipid PC and sphingomyelin exchange with the phospholipids of plasma lipoproteins occurs over a period of days.[15,16] Because of their inaccessibility, the inner bilayer phospholipids PS and PE are unable to participate in lipid exchange.[15] Unesterified membrane cholesterol exchanges readily with the unesterified cholesterol in plasma lipoproteins, where the unesterified membrane cholesterol is partially converted to esterified cholesterol by lecithin-cholesterol acyltransferase (LCAT). Because the newly formed cholesteryl ester cannot return to the red cell membrane, LCAT catalyzes a unidirectional pathway that depletes the membrane of cholesterol and decreases its surface area. Virtually no esterified cholesterol is present in the membrane. The process is reversed when LCAT is absent or inactive, leading to a net accumulation of free cholesterol in the cells.

In addition to passive exchange, free fatty acids can be incorporated into red cell phospholipids in a two-step reaction requiring lysophospholipid, ATP, magnesium, and coenzyme A.[17] Following acylcoenzyme A formation, the fatty acid is incorporated into the lysophospholipid at the inner bilayer leaflet. This pathway also participates in maintenance of phospholipid asymmetry, as evidenced by rapid outward translocation of the newly synthesized PC.[18] Although this pathway consumes a small amount of energy, it may be important for detoxification of naturally formed lysophosphatides in the cells, as evidenced by their gradual accumulation during ATP depletion.

Lipid Bilayer Fluidity

Under physiologic conditions, the lipid bilayer is in a liquid state, allowing transmembrane proteins and cell surface molecules (such as surface antigens) to move in the plane of the membrane. Lipid bilayer fluidity is influenced by several factors, including (1) temperature, which determines the phase transition between a liquid state and gel state; (2) free cholesterol content, as the rigid sterol ring of cholesterol decreases lipid bilayer fluidity; and (3) the length and degree of phospholipid fatty acid saturation. Saturated fatty acids with a relatively rigid backbone resist motion, whereas unsaturated fatty acids have relatively unrestricted movements, thereby increasing the fluidity of the lipid bilayer. Because of the differences in the composition of phospholipids between the two bilayer halves, the bilayer is asymmetric in terms of the fluidity of the two hemileaflets.[17,18]

MEMBRANE PROTEINS

Several general observations can be made about erythrocyte membrane proteins. Most of these proteins are also present in nonerythroid cells, where they fulfill similar functions. Many of the proteins are members of superfamilies of proteins that are structurally related but genetically distinct. This genetic diversity explains why the clinical expression of many (but not all) red cell membrane protein mutations is confined to the erythroid lineage. Tissue- and developmental stage-specific alternative splicing or use of alternate initiation codons or alternate promoters creates multiple isoforms of many of these proteins. Finally, many are large, multifunctional proteins. As a result, mutations within a given region of the protein may lead to distinct differences in abnormalities of function and clinical phenotype.

Membrane proteins are classified according to the ease with which they can be removed from whole red cell membrane preparations in the laboratory. Integral proteins are firmly embedded into or through the lipid bilayer by hydrophobic domains within their amino acid sequences; only harsh reagents such as detergents can extract them. Peripheral proteins are more loosely associated; they are extracted by high or low salt or by high pH. Peripheral proteins are attached indirectly to the lipid bilayer by covalent or noncovalent binding, usually to the cytoplasmic domains of embedded or anchored proteins. Peripheral proteins typically are associated with the interior or cytoplasmic face, whereas many integral proteins often protrude into both spaces. The affinity with which proteins associate with the membrane is not a static property. Rather, proteins can become more or less tightly bound according to their state of phosphorylation, methylation, glycosylation, or lipid modification (myristoylation, palmitoylation, or farnesylation).

Fairbanks and colleagues[19] assigned names to the proteins extracted from red cell membranes (see Fig. 45–1 and Table 45–1). These designations were based on protein mobility in a sodium dodecyl sulfate-polyacrylamide gel system. The slowest migrating band was band (or protein) 1, the next slowest band was band 2, and so on. Subbands were designated with decimals. After further analysis, some of these proteins, such as bands 1 and 2, were renamed α- and β-spectrin. Other proteins, such as protein 4.1, were never renamed.

INTEGRAL MEMBRANE PROTEINS

Band 3

This protein (anion exchanger-1, SLC4A1) is an abundant (~10^6 copies per cell) transmembrane glycoprotein with a molecular mass of approximately 100 kDa. It serves as a regulator of ion content, red cell deformability, intermediary metabolism, and possibly red cell senescence.[20] The NH_2-terminus of the protein encodes a 43-kDa cytoplasmic domain with COOH-terminus of the protein folded into helices and β sheets to form the membrane-spanning domain. The region between the NH_2-terminus and the first membrane-spanning segment forms an interhinge domain.

Band 3 is the major anion (chloride–bicarbonate) exchanger of the red cell. It regulates metabolic pathways by sequestering key pathway enzymes, such as the glycolytic enzymes glyceraldehyde-3-phosphate dehydrogenase, phosphoglycerate kinase, and aldolase, and carbonic anhydrase II and IV. Band 3 contains important binding sites for interaction with other membrane proteins, including ankyrin, protein 4.1, protein 4.2, and the Rh–Rh-associated glycoprotein (RhAG) complex.[20–23] Binding of the cytoplasmic domain to ankyrin is one of the critical mechanisms for attachment of the membrane skeleton to the plasma membrane and may be a crucial determinant of the flexibility or rigidity of the erythrocyte. Extracellular domain polymorphisms of band 3 are the antigens for several blood groups, including the Diego and Wright blood groups, and several other low-incidence antigens.

Glycophorins

Glycophorins are the most abundant integral membrane glycoproteins in erythrocytes. Because of their high sialic acid content, they account for more than 95 percent of the periodic acid-Schiff–staining capacity of erythrocytes.[24] The glycophorins are *O*-glycosylated. They are composed of a single extracellular hydrophilic NH_2-terminal domain, a single membrane-spanning domain, and a COOH-terminal cytoplasmic tail.[20] Characterization of complementary DNA (cDNA) and genomic clones encoding the glycophorins has revealed that they fall into two distinct subgroups. Glycophorins A and B are homologous to each other and are encoded by two closely linked genes. Glycophorin C (GPC) and glycophorin D (GPD) arise from a single locus bearing no particular homology to the genes for glycophorins A and B. GPD differs from GPC by use of an alternate translation start site created by alternative splicing.

Glycophorins constitute more than 60 percent of the net negative surface charge of red cells; thus, they may modulate red cell–red cell and red cell–endothelial cell interactions. GPC, which participates in a complex with protein 4.1 and p55, plays a critical role in regulating the stability, deformability, and shape of the membrane. GPC deficiency leads to elliptocytic erythrocytes that are less stable and less deformable than normal red cells. Glycophorins serve as receptors for several infectious agents, including *Plasmodium falciparum*. The glycophorins carry a number of blood group antigens, including MN, Ss, Miltenberger V, En(a–), M^KM^k, and Gerbich (see Chap. 137).

Other Integral Membrane Proteins

The red cell membrane contains other integral membrane proteins, including a number involved in clinical immunohematology, such as the Rh proteins (see Chap. 137), the Xk and Kell glycoprotein, and the Kidd, Duffy, and Lutheran glycoproteins. Rh proteins are part of a

TABLE 45–1. Major Red Cell Membrane Proteins

Band	Protein	Mr (gel)	Mr (calc)	Copies Per Cell ($\times 10^3$)	Percentage of Total[a]	Gene Symbol	Chromosomal Localization	Amino Acids	Gene Size (kb)	No. of Exons	Involvement in Hemolytic Anemias
1	α-Spectrin	240	280	240	16	*SPTA1*	1q22-q23	2429	80	52	HE, HS, HPP
2	β-Spectrin	220	246	240	14	*SPTB*	14q23-q24.2	2137	>100	32	HE, HS, HPP
2.1	Ankyrin[b]	210	206	120	4.5	*ANK1*	8p11.2	1881	>100	40	HS
2.9	α-Adducin[c]	103	81	30	2	*ADDA*	4p16.3	737	85	16	N
2.9	β-Adducin[c]	97	80	30	2	*ADDB*	2p13–2p14	726	~100	17	N
3	Anion exchanger-1	90–100	102	1200	27	*EPB3*	17q21-qter	911	17	20	HS, SAO, HAc
4.1	Protein 4.1	80	66	200	5	*EL11*	1p33-p34.2	588[d]	>100	23	HE
4.2	Protein 4.2	72	77	200	5	*EB42*	15q15-q21	691	20	13	HS
4.9	Dematin[e]	48 + 52	43	40[f]	1	*EPB49*	8p21.1	383	–	–	N
4.9	p55[e]	55	53	80	–	*MPP1*	Xq28	466	–	–	N
5	β-Actin	43	42	400–500	5.5	*ACTB*	7pter-q22	375	>4	6	N
5	Tropomodulin	43	41	30	–	*TMOD*	9q22	359	–	–	N
6	G-3P-D[g]	35	37	500	3.5[g]	*GAPD*	12p13.31-p13.1	335	5	9	N
7	Stomatin	31	32	–	2.5	*EPB72*	9q33-q34	288	12	7	HSt
7	Tropomyosin	27 + 29	28	80	1	*TPM3*	1q31	239	–	–	N
PAS-1	Glycophorin A[h]	36	–	500–1000	85	*GYPA*	4q28-q31	131	>40	7	HE
PAS-2	Glycophorin C[h]	32	14	50–100	4	*GYPC*	2q14-q21	128	14	4	HE
PAS-3	Glycophorin B[h]	20	–	100–300	10	*GYPB*	4q28-q31	72	>30	5	N
	Glycophorin D[h]	23	–	20	1	*GYPD*	2q14-q21	107	14	4	N
	Glycophorin E	–	–	–	–	*GYPE*	4q28-q31	59	>30	4	N

–, Information not available; G-3-PD, glyceraldehyde 3-phosphate dehydrogenase; HAc, hereditary acanthocytosis; HE, hereditary elliptocytosis; HPP, hereditary pyropoikilocytosis; HS, hereditary spherocytosis; HSt, hereditary stomatocytosis; N, no hematologic abnormalities reported; SAO, Southeast Asian ovalocytosis.

[a]Quantitation based on scanning of sodium dodecylsulfate polyacrylamide gel electrophoresis of red cell membranes prepared from healthy blood donors. For glycophorins, values indicate the fraction of periodic acid-Schiff–positive material.

[b]Bands 2.1, 2.2, 2.3, and 2.6 are protein isoforms of erythroid ankyrin, at least some of which are produced by alternative splicing of ankyrin messenger RNA.

[c]Because adducin comigrates with band 3, no numerical band designation is available.

[d]Numerous erythroid and nonerythroid isoforms of protein 4.1 produced by alternative splicing have been described. Values correspond to the major erythroid protein 4.1 isoform.

[e]Both dematin and p55 migrate within the 4.9 band.

[f]40,000 of dematin trimers are present in one red cell.

[g]Variable amounts of band 6 are detected in red cell membranes.

[h]Detectable on periodic acid-Schiff–stained gels only.

macromolecular complex composed of two Rh proteins, two RhAGs, CD47, LW glycoprotein, glycophorin B, and protein 4.2.[25,26] The Rh–RhAG complex interacts with ankyrin to link the membrane skeleton to the lipid bilayer via interactions with band 3.[22] Additional integral membrane proteins include stomatin, the LW protein, which may be involved in macrophage–erythroblast interactions during erythropoiesis, and various ion pumps and channels (see below).

PERIPHERAL MEMBRANE PROTEINS

The major proteins of the erythrocyte membrane skeleton are spectrin; ankyrin; actin; proteins 4.1, 4.2, and 4.9; p55; and the adducins. These proteins form an interlocking network that attaches to the inner face of the membrane, primarily by binding to the cytoplasmic domains of band 3 and the glycophorins.

Spectrin

This protein is the most abundant and largest in the erythrocyte membrane skeleton, constituting 75 percent of erythrocyte membrane mass and present at a concentration of approximately 200,000 molecules per cell.[27] Spectrin is composed of two subunits, α and β, which, despite many similarities, are structurally distinct and encoded by separate genes (Fig. 45–2).[28] Both α- and β-spectrin contain homologous 106-amino-acid repeats that are folded into α-helical segments containing three antiparallel helices connected by short nonhelical segments. The presence of spectrin repeats suggests spectrin evolved from duplication of a single ancestral gene.[29]

The fundamental structure of the spectrin molecule is that of $\alpha\beta$ heterodimers that align and intertwine with each other in antiparallel fashion with respect to their NH_2-termini to form flexible, rod-like molecules

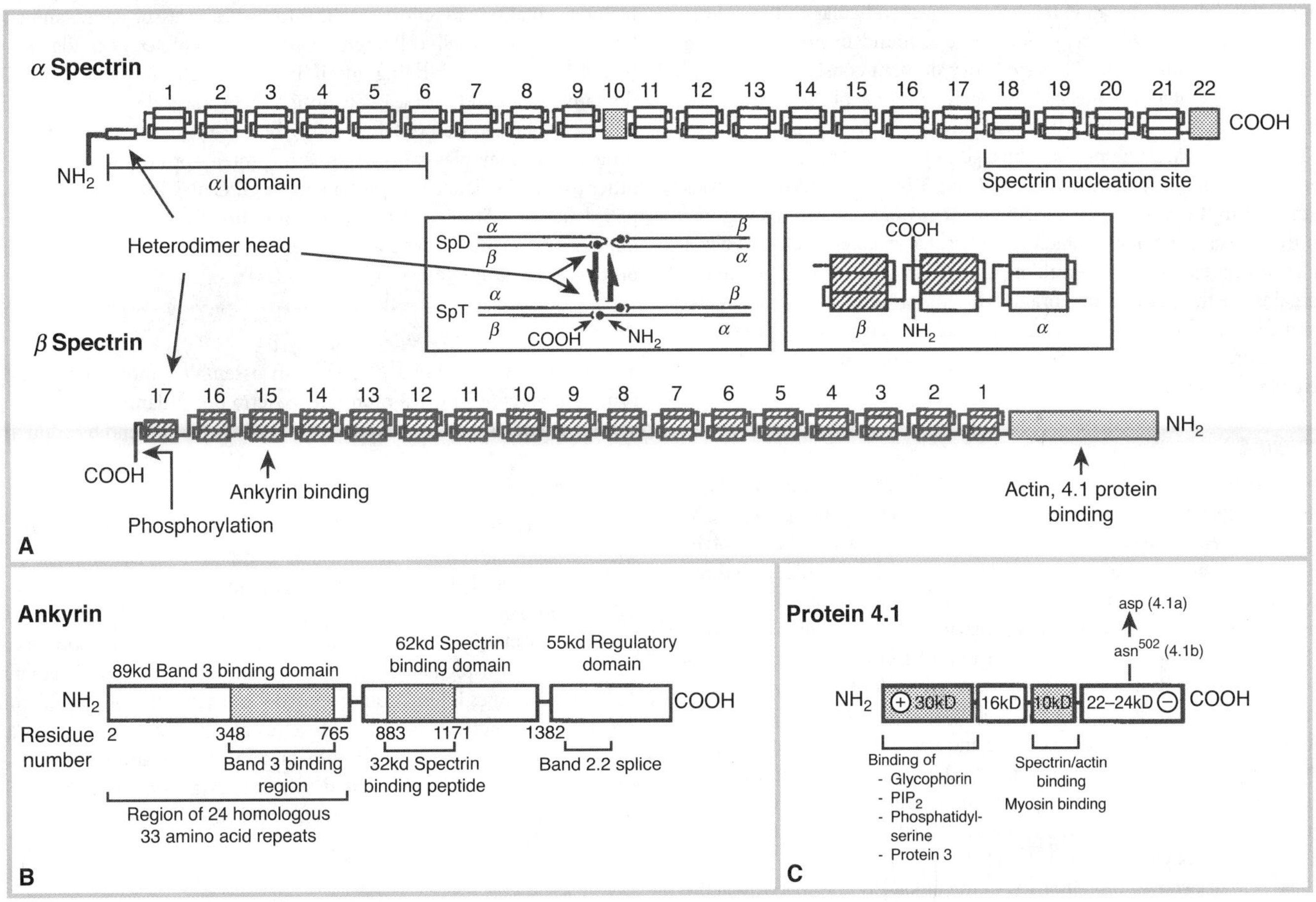

FIGURE 45–2. Spectrin, ankyrin, and protein 4.1. **A.** α-Spectrin and β-spectrin. Both proteins are composed of multiple homologous triple helical repetitive segments, numbered starting from the NH_2-terminus. α-Spectrin and β-spectrin are shown in antiparallel orientation, their configuration in the spectrin heterodimer. *Stippled regions* represent nonhomologous segments. The αI domain (a tryptic peptide of α-spectrin involved in spectrin self-association), the spectrin nucleation site, and the ankyrin, actin, and protein 4.1 protein-binding sites are shown. In the head region of spectrin, α- and β-spectrin interact, forming either a heterodimer (SpD) or tetramer (SpT). The contact site between the α and β chains of a spectrin heterodimer or the opposing α and β chains of the tetramer is formed by a combined αβ triple helical segment (*inset*). **B.** Ankyrin. The three major functional and structural domains, as defined by limited proteolytic digestion, are shown. The band 3 and spectrin-binding regions are *shaded*. The regulatory domain is subject to extensive alternative splicing, including the band 2.2 splice, which produces an activated form of ankyrin. **C.** Protein 4.1. The four major functional and structural domains, as defined by limited proteolytic digestion, are shown. The regions where the 4.1 protein binds to other membrane proteins are *shaded*. The protein 4.1a isoform is derived from the 4.1b isoform by deamidation of asparagine 508.

(see Fig. 45–2).[27] These dimers further self-associate to form tetramers and higher-order oligomers. These tetramers, composed of multiple repeats, provide a strong, elastic, rod-like filament that associates with multimolecular complexes capable of lending shape and resiliency to the overlying plasma membrane via formation of a lattice-like meshwork linked to integral membrane proteins.[30] Direct interactions of a weaker nature also may occur between spectrin filaments and the lipid bilayer itself. The side-to-side assembly of α- and β-spectrin chains in a zipper-like fashion begins at a defined nucleation site composed of four repeats from each chain, α_{19} to α_{22} and β_1 to β_4, respectively.[31] After tight association of complementary nucleation sites, a conformational change is initiated that promotes pairing of the remainder of the two chains. A common α-spectrin variant, α^{lely} (low-expression Lyon), interferes with normal nucleation and decreases the synthesis of functionally competent spectrin chains and may influence clinical expression of spectrin mutations (see "Membrane Biogenesis and Aging" below).[32]

The NH_2-terminus of α-spectrin and the COOH-terminus of β-spectrin are the regions involved in αβ heterodimer self-association.[27] Spectrin also binds to actin and protein 4.1 via the NH_2-terminus of β-spectrin and ankyrin via sites in repeats β_{15} and β_{16} near the COOH-terminus, respectively.[33–35] Other nonrepeat sequences in spectrin provide the recognition sites for binding to other modifiers, including kinases and calmodulin. The functions of spectrin are to maintain cellular shape, regulate the lateral mobility of integral membrane proteins, and provide structural support for the lipid bilayer. Defects in the αβ self-association site are associated with hereditary elliptocytosis (HE) and hereditary pyropoikilocytosis (HPP). Compound heterozygosity or homozygosity for defects that do not influence the αβ self-association site is associated with severe, recessively inherited spherocytosis.

Ankyrin

This asymmetric polar protein can be separated into three functional domains by mild proteolysis: an NH_2-terminal membrane-binding domain that contains sites for band 3 and other ligands, a central domain that contains sites for spectrin binding, and a COOH-terminal "regulatory" domain that influences ankyrin–protein interactions (see Fig. 45–2).[27] The membrane-binding domain contains 24 tandem repeats called *cdc10/ankyrin repeats*, which contain multiple protein-binding sites.[36] Ankyrin repeats are highly conserved, L-shaped structures composed of a pair of α-helices that form an antiparallel coiled-coil, followed by an extended loop perpendicular to the helices and a β hairpin.[37] These repeats have been found in proteins with a wide variety of functions. The regulatory domain consists of multiple isoforms generated by alternative splicing.[36] One of these isoforms (ankyrin 2.2) enhances ankyrin binding to band 3 and spectrin.

Ankyrin provides the primary linkage to the membrane skeleton via spectrin binding, the lipid bilayer via band 3 binding, and interactions with the Rh–RhAG complex. Disruption of any of these linkages significantly decreases membrane stability. Ankyrin also appears to be involved in local segregation of integral membrane proteins within functional domains on the plasma membrane. The importance of ankyrin in the maintenance of membrane stability is underscored by the observation that abnormalities of ankyrin are the most common cause of typical hereditary spherocytosis (HS).

Protein 4.1

This phosphoprotein can be separated by mild chymotryptic digestion into four proteolytic domains: 30 kDa, 16 kDa, 10 kDa, and 22 to 24 kDa (see Fig. 45–2). In red cells, two molecular weight forms are found, protein 4.1a and protein 4.1b, with protein 4.1a predominating in older erythrocytes. Protein 4.1a is derived from protein 4.1b by the gradual deamidation of an asparagine residue in a nonenzymatic, age-dependent manner. Alternative splicing leads to the production of a large number of tissue- and developmental stage-specific protein 4.1 isoforms.[38] For example, alternatively spliced isoforms of the 10-kDa domain contain the spectrin–actin binding site and provide erythroid and stage-specific specificity. Protein 4.1 utilizes two different initiation codons. The upstream initiation codon encodes a protein of 135 kDa found in most nonerythroid cells.[38] The downstream initiation codon encodes the 80-kDa protein found primarily in erythrocytes.

The primary role of protein 4.1 is in the linkage of the spectrin–actin membrane skeleton to the lipid bilayer by facilitating complex formation between spectrin–actin fibers, the cytoplasmic domain of band 3, and p55/GPC (see Fig. 45–1). Qualitative or quantitative defects of protein 4.1 lead to HE, with concomitant GPC and p55 deficiency in some cases.[39] HE-related protein 4.1 mutations include variants that affect protein 4.1 alternative splicing and initiation codon usage. Interestingly, mice with targeted disruption of the protein 4.1 gene demonstrate, in addition to hematologic effects, subtle neurologic abnormalities.[40] The applicability of this observation to humans with defects of protein 4.1 is unknown.

Protein 4.2

Protein 4.2 is a member of the transglutaminase family of proteins.[41] However, protein 4.2 does not possess transglutaminase activity because it lacks a critical residue in the active transglutaminase site. At least four isoforms of protein 4.2 have been created by alternative splicing; the functional significance of the four isoforms is not known. Protein 4.2 binds to several proteins, including band 3, protein 4.1, ankyrin, and ankyrin–protein 3 complexes. The major function of protein 4.2 is to stabilize spectrin–actin–ankyrin association with band 3. It also may protect the membrane skeleton from premature aging by binding calcium and other cofactors that normally activate red cell transglutaminases, as these transglutaminases otherwise would crosslink proteins and lead to their inactivation. Deficiency of protein 4.2 has been associated with recessively inherited HS. Erythrocytes from mice with targeted inactivation of the protein 4.2 gene are dehydrated spherocytes with altered cation content (increased K^+/decreased Na^+).[42]

p55

This molecule is a phosphoprotein member of the membrane-associated guanylate kinase (MAGUK) family of proteins.[43] Homologues of p55 include signal transduction proteins, tumor suppressor genes, and proteins important in cell–cell interactions. The p55 molecule binds to protein 4.1 through a binding motif in the COOH-terminal MAGUK domain and to GPC via a PDZ motif.[43] A primary deficiency state for p55 has not been described, possibly because it is a widely expressed protein. p55 may play a critical role in protein–protein interactions in other tissues. Deficiency of protein 4.1 or GPC may lead to concomitant p55 deficiency. Studies of this interesting protein may shed important light on mechanisms whereby the erythrocyte membrane influences other cellular processes.

Actin

The erythrocyte contains β-type actin assembled into short F-actin protofilaments of 12 to 18 monomers. Actin protofilaments are capped at the pointed end by tropomodulin and at the barbed end by adducin.

Adducin

Adducin, a calcium/calmodulin-binding phosphoprotein located at the spectrin–actin junctional complex, is composed of $\alpha\beta$-adducin heterodimers. α- and β-adducin are structurally similar proteins encoded by separate genes. Adducin contains a myristoylated alanine-rich C-kinase substrate (MARCKS) phosphorylation domain that controls calcium/calmodulin-regulated capping and bundling of actin filaments. Adducin promotes interaction of spectrin and actin and binds and bundles actin filaments. A primary deficiency of adducin in human disease has not been described. Mice with targeted inactivation of α- or β-adducin suffer from compensated spherocytic anemia, suggesting the adducins may be candidate genes for recessively inherited hemolytic anemia.[44,45]

Other Peripheral Membrane Proteins

Dematin (protein 4.9), tropomyosin, proteins related to troponin, myosin, and other proteins associated with actin in nonerythroid cells are found in erythrocytes. The glucose transporter-1 protein is the receptor for adducin and dematin in the erythrocyte membrane, providing a linkage between the junctional complex and the plasma membrane.[46]

FUNCTION OF THE RED CELL MEMBRANE

The roles of the erythrocyte membrane include assembling and organizing proteins of the lipid bilayer and the underlying skeleton, providing the red cell with its unique deformability and stability, participating in membrane biogenesis and aging, and providing a barrier between the erythrocyte cytoplasm and the external environment with selective permeability.

MEMBRANE ASSEMBLY AND ORGANIZATION

Membrane organization arises from interactions between integral membrane proteins and other molecules contacting the hydrophilic faces of the membrane and by protein–protein or protein–lipid interactions within the bilayer or the underlying membrane skeleton. The avidity of these interactions is modulated by posttranslational modifications of the participating proteins. By utilizing the cytoplasmic domains of embedded proteins as attachment points, the membrane skeleton not only affixes itself to the lipid bilayer but also provides a means to order the topologic arrangement of transmembrane proteins.[47] This attachment constrains motion along the transverse plane.

In the intact erythrocyte membrane, the membrane skeleton appears as a lattice-like network, with approximately 60 percent of the lipid bilayer directly laminated to the underlying membrane skeleton.[48] When skeletal preparations are stretched, the individual skeletal proteins can be visualized as a highly ordered lattice of hexagons. The corners of each hexagon are globular structures called the *junctional complex*, composed of complexes of F-actin, dematin, adducin, and protein 4.1.[49] Spectrin tetramers form the arms of the hexagons, cross-bridging individual junctional complexes. Spectrin cross-bridges are largely formed by spectrin tetramers, with occasional double tetramers or hexamers. Each spectrin tetramer is composed of two $\alpha\beta$ heterodimers assembled at their "head" regions into tetramers. At their tails, the tetramers bind to junctional complexes of actin, with the aid of protein 4.1 and adducin. The *horizontal* protein contacts are important in the maintenance of the structural integrity of the cell, accounting for the high tensile strength of the erythrocyte (see Fig. 45–1).

The skeleton is affixed to the integral proteins of the membrane by several protein–protein interactions.[27] Spectrin tetramers are connected to ankyrin, the major skeleton/membrane linkage protein via an interaction site in β-spectrin. Ankyrin links the underlying spectrin skeleton to tetramers of band 3, the major transmembrane protein of the red cell, and the Rh–RhAG complex. At the distal ends of spectrin tetramers, spectrin binds to the membrane via linkage to protein 4.1, which binds GPC and protein p55. In addition, both spectrin and protein 4.1 bind weakly to PS, which preferentially is located at the inner leaflet of the lipid bilayer. These *vertical* protein–protein and protein–lipid interactions are critical in the stabilization of the lipid bilayer, precluding its loss from the cells (see Fig. 45–1).

Hereditary spherocytosis is characterized by defects of *vertical* interactions, which lead to uncoupling of the lipid bilayer from the skeleton and a release of membrane microvesicles. In contrast, the principal defects in HE and pyropoikilocytosis involve *horizontal* interactions of membrane skeletal proteins, for example, interactions between α spectrin and β spectrin that maintain the two-dimensional integrity of the skeleton. Overall, membrane protein interactions are more complex than this model but are a good starting point for understanding the pathophysiologic effects of membrane protein mutations. For instance, spectrin mutations that cause hemolytic anemia and do not directly destabilize spectrin self-association or spectrin–ankyrin binding have been described. These mutations disrupt cooperative interactions between proteins of the membrane skeleton, linkage adaptor proteins, and/or proteins of the lipid bilayer.[50]

Red cell membrane proteins are subject to a variety of posttranslational modifications or other regulatory effects, including phosphorylation, fatty acid acylation, methylation, glycosylation, deamidation, oxidation, and limited proteolytic cleavage. With the exception of membrane protein phosphorylation, such modifications are relatively static and irreversible. In contrast, membrane protein phosphorylation represents a highly dynamic system of multiple protein kinases and phosphatases that constantly phosphorylate and dephosphorylate serine, threonine, and tyrosine residues, often in a manner that is amino acid and protein site specific, thereby tightly regulating association of membrane proteins. Additionally, membrane protein associations are influenced by a variety of intracellular factors, including calcium, calmodulin, phosphoinositides, and polyanions such as 2,3-bisphosphoglycerate (BPG).

The red cell surface is negatively charged, primarily because of a high concentration of neuraminic acid residues. Ninety percent of the residues reside on glycophorin A; the remainder are shared by the other glycophorins and band 3. Alterations in erythrocyte surface charge appear to have deleterious effects on the cell. For example, in sickle red cells, surface charge clustering may play a role in the adhesion of these cells to the surface of endothelial cells.

■ CELLULAR DEFORMABILITY AND MEMBRANE STABILITY

The most important property of red cells required for normal survival is cellular deformability.[51] *Deformability* refers to the ability of the erythrocyte to undergo distortions and deformations and then to resume its normal shape without fragmentation or loss of integrity. This situation is best exemplified in the wall of the splenic sinus, where red cells squeeze through narrow slits among the endothelial cells lining the splenic sinus wall. The cellular deformability of erythrocytes is determined by three factors: (1) cell geometry (biconcave disc shape); (2) cytoplasmic viscosity, principally determined by the properties and the concentration of hemoglobin in the cells; and (3) intrinsic viscoelastic properties of the red cell membrane (or membrane deformability). Among the three factors, cell geometry as determined by the contribution of the surface-to-volume ratio is the most important, as exemplified by the cellular lesion of hereditary spherocytes. On the other hand, the intrinsic viscoelastic properties of the red cell likely have a relatively small effect on red cell survival. Southeast Asian ovalocytes are very rigid, yet they have a normal survival *in vivo*.

The cellular geometry, that is, the biconcave disc shape of red cells, is critical for the cells' survival. This cell surface shape provides a high ratio of surface area to cellular volume. The normal volume of the erythrocyte is approximately 90 μm^3. The minimum surface area that could encase this volume is a sphere of approximately 98 μm^3. The surface area of a biconcave disc enclosing this volume is approximately 140 μm^3. Thus, shape alone provides the red cell with a considerable amount of redundant membrane and cytoskeleton. This feature provides the extra membrane surface area needed when red cells swell. More importantly, this geometric arrangement allows red cells to stretch as they undergo deformation and distortion in response to the mechanical stress of the circulation. Loss of membrane by partial phagocytosis in immune hemolytic anemias or by fragmentation of bits of membrane from the cell in patients with cytoskeletal defects leads to elliptocytic or spherocytic shapes having greatly reduced surface area and, therefore, much less deformability.[52] The consequent reduction in tolerance of these cells to osmotic stress explains why anemias resulting from membrane defects often are accompanied by osmotic fragility, the basis for the clinical laboratory test. Similarly, if erythrocytes are engorged with water, they become macrospherocytic and less deformable.

Thus, the organization of the membrane skeleton and its attachment to the plasma membrane influence the stability and deformability of the red cell. In the resting state, the folded helical segments of spectrin are highly coiled. Membrane deformation is accompanied by a rearrangement of the spectrin–actin-based membrane skeleton network. Some spectrin molecules become uncoiled and extended, whereas others become more compressed and folded, resulting in no net change in surface area. Thus, shape changes but surface area does not. Depending on metabolic energy influx, the membrane exhibits solid-to-fluid transitions with these changes.[53] The extent to which stretching and compression are possible determines the extent of deformability. Mutations or acquired alterations in membrane proteins that influence the spectrin–actin-based lattice of proteins leads to membrane loss with a concomitant decrease in surface area and a change in cell geometry.

Red cell viscosity is largely determined by hemoglobin content.[52] At normal intracellular concentrations (27–35 g/dL), viscosity contributes very little to cellular deformability. When erythrocytes become dehydrated, the effective intracellular hemoglobin concentration rises, and viscosity increases exponentially. Membrane pumps and channels normally maintain intracellular volumes that hold hemoglobin concentrations below the level at which cytoplasmic viscosity has an impact on deformability. Inherited anomalies of pumps or channels (e.g., hereditary xerocytosis) or derangements caused by polymerized or crystallized hemoglobin (e.g., sickle cell anemia or hemoglobin C disease) lead to cellular dehydration and greatly increased red cell viscosity.

■ MEMBRANE MATERIAL PROPERTIES

The material properties of the membrane reflect the properties of the lipid bilayer and the skeleton. During deformation, the membrane undergoes bending, which is restricted by the incompressibility of the lipid bilayer. It has been proposed that such bending is facilitated by rapid translocation of cholesterol from the inner to the outer hemileaflet (Fig. 45–3). Red cells that are suspended in hypotonic solutions, as during osmotic fragility testing (see "Laboratory Features" below), swell. They reach a nearly spherical shape because the bilayer membrane cannot expand its surface area more than 3 to 4 percent. Further lowering of osmotic pressure results in membrane rupture, and intracellular hemoglobin is discharged into the supernatant.

The membrane skeleton determines both the solid and semisolid properties of the membrane. The solid properties are exemplified by an elastic extension of cells that completely restores their normal shape after the applied force is removed. An example is a cell that was deformed when it passed through fenestrations of the splenic sinus wall. The elastic recovery of normal shape is facilitated by the unique molecular anatomy of the skeletal lattice. Here the individual hexagons are in a compact, unextended configuration, with the junctional complexes close to each other and the crosslinking arms of spectrin tetramers folded between them, thus allowing large unidirectional extensions without disruption of the lattice (see Fig. 45–3). The skeleton remains unperturbed during such deformation. On the other hand, application of large or prolonged forces allows the skeletal elements to reorganize into a new configuration, producing a permanent plastic deformation. When the force is excessive, membrane fragmentation ensues. An example is when red cells are trapped by fibrin strands in damaged vessels (see Chap. 50). After release from this site, the erythrocytes either are permanently deformed or are fragmented.

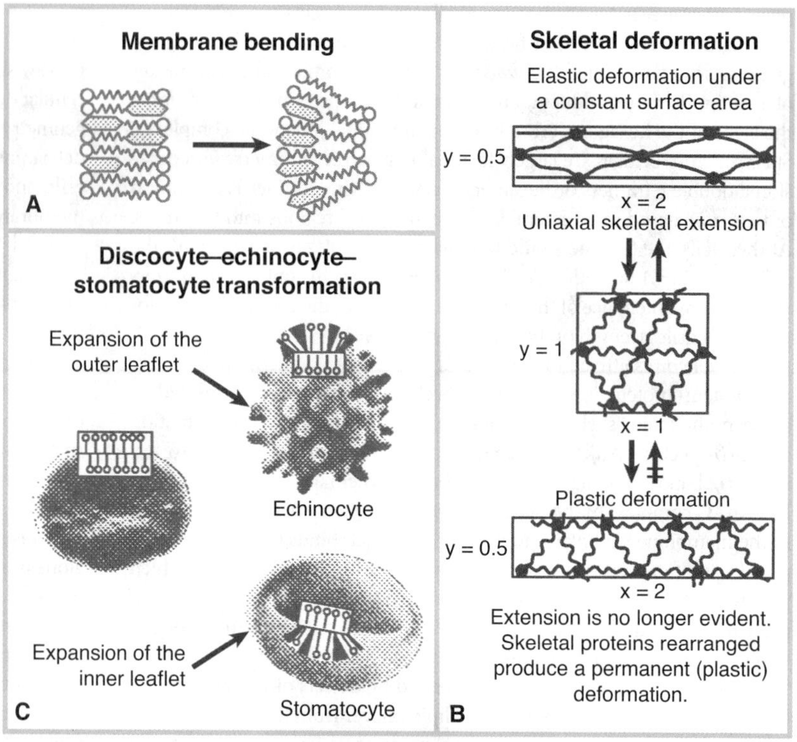

FIGURE 45–3. Material properties of the red cell membrane. **A.** Membrane bending. The degree of membrane bending is restricted by the limited compressibility of the lipid bilayer. Rapid translocation of cholesterol (*shaded diamonds*) from the inner to the outer leaflet reduces compression of the inner bilayer leaflet, thereby facilitating bending. **B.** Skeletal deformation. Although hydrophobicity of the red cell membrane lipid bilayer precludes the increase in its surface area without rupture, the membrane can undergo a large deformation under a constant surface area because of the viscoelastic properties of the membrane skeleton. During uniaxial extension, the skeleton undergoes stretching (*top rectangle*). After cessation of an external force, a surface area is resumed because the protein connections within this elastic skeletal network remain intact. Extensive or prolonged uniaxial extension leads to rearrangement of the skeletal network because of disruption of existing skeletal protein connections and formation of new protein contacts. This process leads to a permanent plastic deformation (*bottom rectangle*). **C.** Bilayer couple hypothesis and stomatocyte–discocyte–echinocyte transformation. Red cell shape reflects the ratio of the surface areas of the two hemileaflets of the lipid bilayer. The compounds (*black triangles*) that preferentially intercalate into the outer hemileaflet of the lipid bilayer produce its expansion, followed by red cell crenation (echinocytosis or acanthocytosis). In contrast, expansion of the inner lipid bilayer leaflet produces a cup shape (stomatocytosis) and surface invaginations.

MEMBRANE BIOGENESIS AND AGING

Membrane protein biosynthesis occurs asynchronously during erythropoiesis. Early in erythroid development, the major proteins of the membrane skeleton (spectrin, ankyrin, and protein 4.1) are synthesized.[54] However, they turn over rapidly and do not assemble into a permanent network. At the proerythroblast stage, synthesis of band 3 is initiated and, with synthesis of protein 4.1, increases up to the late erythroblast stage. During this time, messenger RNA (mRNA) levels and synthesis of spectrin and ankyrin protein decline. In contrast, the fraction of newly assembled spectrin and ankyrin protein on the membrane progressively increases, and the turnover of these proteins on the membrane declines.

Increased recruitment and stabilization of spectrin and ankyrin on the membrane despite declining synthesis of these proteins is temporally related to a progressive increase in the synthesis of band 3 and protein 4.1, the principal bilayer anchors of the membrane skeleton.[54] Early studies suggested the early steps of red cell membrane assembly were controlled by band 3 production where, after insertion into the membrane, band 3 directed the assembly of stable macromolecular complexes from presynthesized pools of other proteins. The role of band 3 in membrane assembly has been questioned by the following findings: (1) the organization of preformed pools of cytoskeletal elements induced by band 3 synthesis is not seen in noncultured cells, and (2) several vertebrate models of erythrocyte band 3 deficiency exhibit normal membrane biogenesis even though their red cell membranes are unstable in the circulation.

Biosynthesis and assembly of spectrin subunits is complex. β-Spectrin biosynthesis exceeds α-spectrin biosynthesis in early erythroblasts derived from both embryonic (yolk sac) and fetal/adult (liver/spleen) origins. This ratio is preserved during later stages of erythropoiesis in embryonic cells, but not in fetal-/adult-derived late erythroblasts and reticulocytes. In reticulocytes, α-spectrin gene expression increases, whereas β-spectrin gene expression remains constant, resulting in a predominance of α-spectrin mRNA and protein during the late stages, when active assembly of the actual membrane occurs most rapidly. $\alpha\beta$-Spectrin subunits are incorporated into the membrane in a 1:1 stoichiometric ratio, regardless of their synthesis rates.[55] This point is important in the analysis of inherited hemolytic anemias. Human α-spectrin synthesis exceeds that of β-spectrin by 2:1 to 4:1 during the later stages of erythropoiesis, when membrane assembly presumably proceeds rapidly. Therefore, the availability of β-spectrin subunits determines the maximum rate and amount of stable spectrin assembly. Thus, mutations reducing steady-state levels of newly synthesized β-spectrin should have a far greater phenotypic impact than mutations causing a comparable decrease in α-spectrin biosynthesis. Analyses of patients with hereditary hemolytic anemias support this prediction.

At the stage of orthochromatic erythroblast, when membrane biogenesis is nearly completed, the cell membrane undergoes a series of critical remodeling steps.[56,57] The membrane surrounding the nucleus contains an actin ring that likely participates in expulsion of the nucleus from the erythroblast. At the same time, the spectrin skeleton segregates into the region of the incipient reticulocyte, while some surface receptors cluster in membrane regions surrounding the extruded nucleus.

Some synthesis of spectrin, band 3, protein 4.1, and GPC continues in the newly enucleated reticulocyte, but most membrane remodeling occurs after translation. The reticulocyte possesses mitochondria, polyribosomes, and numerous membrane proteins that are either absent or much less abundant in mature red cells. In addition, phospholipid composition and inside–outside lipid distribution are different. Reticulocytes are far less deformable and considerably more unstable mechanically than are mature erythrocytes. Maturation begins in the marrow and lasts for 2 or 3 days. It is completed in the circulation and perhaps in the spleen, where it is termed *splenic polishing*. Reticulocytes first become cup shaped before they acquire their final biconcave disc shape. This process involves major reorganization of membrane phospholipids and cytoskeletal and embedded proteins, and loss of lipids and proteins, including receptors for transferrin, insulin, and fibronectin.

RED CELL AGING

Chap. 32 discusses the mechanism of red cell aging.

FETAL RED CELLS

Fetal erythrocytes differ in a number of respects from adult cells, including activity of glycolytic and nonglycolytic enzymes, altered ATP and phosphate metabolism, differences in methemoglobin content and oxygen affinity, and altered storage characteristics.[58] These erythrocytes exhibit increased rigidity, increased mechanical fragility, and decreased life span (average: 45–70 days) compared to adult red cells.

Membranes of fetal and adult erythrocytes differ. ABO and I antigens and the receptors for the adsorbed serum antigens of the Lewis system are incompletely expressed. Fetal membranes are more permeable to monovalent cations and contain less Na^+-K^+ ATPase activity. They contain more phospholipid and cholesterol per cell and, as a consequence, have a larger surface-to-volume ratio and are slightly more osmotically resistant than adult cells. The ratio of sphingomyelin to PC is increased in fetal membranes, and differences in fatty acid composition exist. However, the changes likely balance each other, as membrane fluidity is normal. The protein composition of fetal red cell membrane is quantitatively normal.

MEMBRANE PERMEABILITY

The normal red cell membrane is nearly impermeable to monovalent and divalent cations, thereby maintaining a high potassium, low sodium, and very low calcium content. In contrast, the red cell is highly permeable to water and anions, which are readily exchanged. As a result, erythrocytes behave as nearly perfect osmometers. Water and ion transport pathways in the red cell membrane (Fig. 45–4) include energy-driven membrane pumps, gradient-driven systems, and various channels.[59] An important feature of the normal red cell is its ability to maintain a constant volume. The mechanisms by which red cells "sense" changes in cell volume and activate appropriate volume regulatory pathways are unknown. Glucose is transported without expenditure of energy utilizing a transporter. Larger charged molecules, such as ATP and related compounds, do not cross the normal red cell membrane, although phosphoenolpyruvate is an exception to this rule.[59]

The effects of disruption of the red cell permeability barrier are illustrated by complement-mediated hemolysis. Complete complement activation on the red cell surface leads to formation of the membrane attack complex, which is composed of terminal complement components embedded in the lipid bilayer. This multimolecular complex acts as a cation channel, allowing passive movements of sodium, potassium, and calcium across the membrane according to their concentration gradients. Attracted by fixed anions, such as hemoglobin, ATP, and 2,3-BPG, sodium accumulates in the cell in excess of potassium loss and of the compensatory efforts of the Na^+-K^+ pump. The resulting increase in intracellular monovalent cations and water is followed by cell swelling and, ultimately, colloid osmotic hemolysis.

ENERGY-DRIVEN MEMBRANE PUMPS

In the red cell, two ion-motive ATPase-dependent cation pumps maintain low intracellular sodium and calcium and high potassium.[59] The ouabain-inhibitable Na^+-K^+ ATPase (the sodium pump) extrudes sodium in exchange for potassium in a 3:2 stoichiometry. Ca^{2+} ATPase is a calmodulin-activated pump that extrudes calcium from the red cell and maintains a very low intracellular calcium concentration, thus protecting cells from multiple deleterious effects of calcium. Examples of deleterious effects include echinocytosis, membrane vesiculation, calpain activation, membrane proteolysis, and cellular dehydration. Elevated intracellular calcium plays an important role in the pathophysiology of sickle cell disease, as increased levels of intracellular calcium observed during sickling result from increased Ca^{2+} flux and reduced activity of Ca^{2+} ATPase. The membrane also contains an ATP-driven oxidized glutathione transporter and amino acid transport systems.[59]

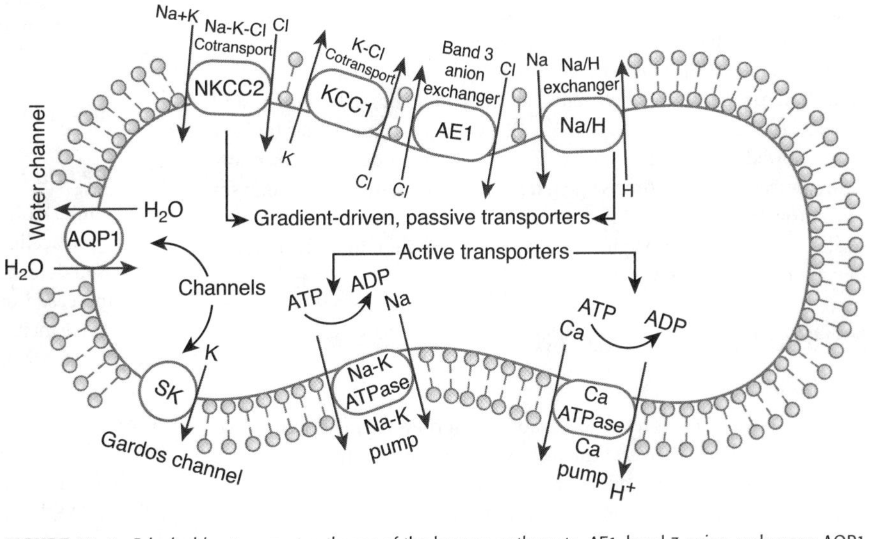

FIGURE 45–4. Principal ion transport pathways of the human erythrocyte. AE1, band 3 anion exchanger; AQP1, water channel aquaporin 1; KCC1, KCl cotransport system of the family of chloride–cation cotransporters; NKCC2, basolateral molecular form of Na-K-Cl cotransport; SK, small conductance potassium channel. *(Reproduced with permission from Brugnara C.[59])*

GRADIENT-DRIVEN SYSTEMS

The Na^+-K^+ gradient established by the sodium pump is used by several passive, gradient-driven systems to move ions across the red cell membrane.[59] The systems include the K^+-Cl^- cotransporter, band 3, the Na^+-K^+-Cl^- cotransporter, and the Na^+-H^+ exchanger. The Na^+-K^+-Cl^- cotransporter plays only a minor role in the red cell. The Na^+-H^+ exchanger appears to play a role primarily in early erythrocyte maturation. The K^+-Cl^- cotransporter is a typical carrier-mediated cotransporter, which is particularly active in reticulocytes.[60] It is activated by cell swelling, acidification, depletion of intracellular magnesium, and thiol oxidation.

CHANNELS

Channels of the red cell include voltage-gated channels (mediated via Na^+-K^+ ATPase), water channels (the aquaporins), and the Ca^{2+}-activated K^+ channel.[59] The Ca^{2+}-activated K^+ channel, also called the *Gardos channel* after its discoverer Dr. George Gardos, causes selective loss of K^+ in response to increased intracellular Ca^{2+}. In sickle cells, increased activity of the Gardos channel and the K^+-Cl^- cotransporter leads to net loss of K^+ and water, leading to cellular dehydration and formation of intermediate and hyperdense erythrocytes.[61] These proteins have been manipulated pharmacologically in attempts to improve cellular hydration of the red cell and ameliorate the clinical course of patients with sickle cell disease.

The aquaporins are membrane channel proteins that serve as selective pores through which water crosses the plasma membrane.[62] Aquaporin-1 (AQP1), which is expressed in many tissues including erythrocytes, contributes to the ability of the red cell to adjust rapidly to changes in osmolality. AQP1 contains the epitope for the Colton blood group system. The genetic basis of the rare Colton-null phenotype has been identified as a mutation of the highly conserved NPA (asparagine-proline-alanine) motif of AQP1 essential for channel function.[63] Colton-null individuals exhibit no obvious clinical phenotype, although mice with targeted inactivation of AQP1 become hyperosmolar after fluid restriction.[63]

RED CELL MEMBRANE DISORDERS

Hemolytic anemias resulting from defects in the erythrocyte membrane comprise an important group of hereditary anemias. HS, HE, and HPP are the most common disorders among this group. Originally classified by their morphologic presentation, detailed studies have demonstrated considerable overlap among these disorders and significant heterogeneity in their clinical, morphologic, laboratory, and molecular characteristics (Table 45–2). Advances in molecular biology have allowed further characterization of these disorders and, in many cases, detection of the precise genetic defect. These molecular analyses have provided additional information on the pathogenesis of these disorders and important insights into the structure–function relationships of erythrocyte membrane proteins.

TABLE 45–2. Erythrocyte Membrane Protein Defects in Inherited Disorders of Red Cell Shape

Protein	Disorder	Comment
Ankyrin	HS	Most common cause of typical dominant HS
Band 3	HS, SAO, NIHF, HAc	"Pincered" HS spherocytes seen on blood film presplenectomy; SAO results from 9 amino acid deletion
β-Spectrin	HS, HE, HPP, NIHF	"Acanthocytic" spherocytes seen on blood film presplenectomy; location of mutation in β-spectrin determines clinical phenotype
α-Spectrin	HS, HE, HPP, NIHF	Location of mutation in α-spectrin determines clinical phenotype; α-spectrin mutations most common cause of typical HE
Protein 4.2	HS	Primarily found in Japanese patients
Protein 4.1	HE	Found in certain European and Arab populations
GPC	HE	Concomitant protein 4.1 deficiency is basis of HE in GPC defects

GPC, glycophorin C; HAc, hereditary acanthocytosis; HE, hereditary elliptocytosis; HPP, hereditary pyropoikilocytosis; HS, hereditary spherocytosis; NIHF, nonimmune hydrops fetalis; SAO, Southeast Asian ovalocytosis.

HEREDITARY SPHEROCYTOSIS

Definition and History

Hereditary spherocytosis refers to a group of disorders characterized by red cells that lose their relatively thin, disk shape and become thicker, tending to a spherical shape. The latter shape abnormality can be mild, retaining some central concavity, or extreme, losing all concavity. These erythrocytes have increased osmotic fragility. HS was first described more than 100 years ago by the two Belgian physicians Vanlair and Masius. Twenty years later, the disease was rediscovered by Wilson and Minkowsky, who reported eight cases of HS in three generations of one family. The description of increased erythrocyte osmotic fragility by Chauffard, reports of correction of anemia and hemolysis by splenectomy, and the studies of Ham and Castle implicating the spleen in the conditioning of hereditary spherocytes followed. Dacie[64] elegantly reviews the early history of HS.

A defect of the erythrocyte membrane was implicated when HS membranes were found to be leaky to sodium and to exhibit a loss of lipids, leading to surface area deficiency. Subsequently, abnormalities of proteins of the erythrocyte membrane were identified as the etiology of the HS defect.

Epidemiology

HS occurs in all racial and ethnic groups. It is the most common inherited anemia in individuals of northern European ancestry, affecting approximately 1 in 2500 individuals in the United States and England. Males and females are affected equally. Clinical, laboratory, biochemical, and genetic heterogeneity characterize the spherocytosis syndromes.

Etiology and Pathogenesis

The hallmark of HS erythrocytes is loss of membrane surface area relative to intracellular volume, accounting for the spheroidal shape and decreased deformability of the red cell.[65] The loss of surface area results from increased membrane fragility caused by defects in proteins of the erythrocyte membrane, including ankyrin, band 3, β-spectrin, α-spectrin, and protein 4.2. Increased fragility leads to membrane vesiculation and surface area loss (Fig. 45–5). Splenic trapping of nondeformable spherocytes, followed by conditioning and destruction of these abnormal erythrocytes, causes the hemolysis experienced by HS patients. Thus, the spleen plays an important role in hemolysis, secondary to the basic defect of the erythrocyte membrane.

Red Cell Membrane Protein Defects

Studies of HS erythrocyte membranes have revealed quantitative abnormalities of several membrane proteins including combined spectrin and

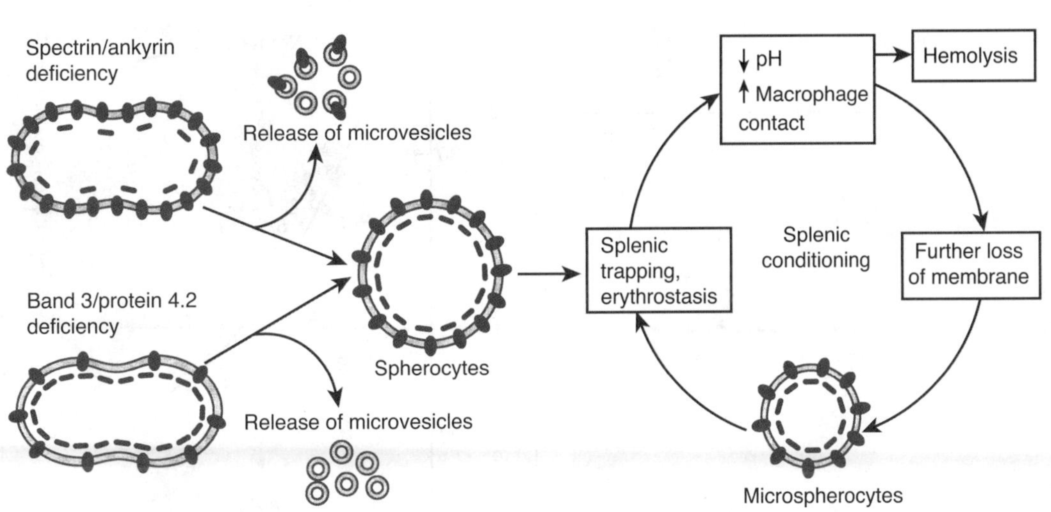

FIGURE 45–5. Pathobiology of HS. The primary defect in HS is a deficiency of membrane surface area, leading to spherocyte formation. Decreased surface area may be produced by two different mechanisms: (1) defects of spectrin and ankyrin lead to reduced density of the membrane skeleton, destabilizing the overlying lipid bilayer and releasing band 3–containing microvesicles; whereas (2) defects of band 3 or protein 4.2 lead to band 3 deficiency and loss of its lipid-stabilizing effect, resulting in loss of band 3–free microvesicles. Both pathways result in membrane loss, decreased surface area, and spherocyte formation with decreased deformability. The abnormal erythrocytes become trapped in the hostile environment of the spleen, where splenic conditioning inflicts further membrane damage, amplifying the cycle of red cell membrane injury. *(From Gallagher PG, Jarolim P: Red cell membrane disorders, in* Hematology: Basis Principles and Practice, *edited by R Hoffman, EJ Benz Jr, SJ Shattil, B Furie, HJ Cohen, LE Silberstein, P McGlave, p 576. WB Saunders, Philadelphia, 2000, with permission.)*

ankyrin deficiency, band 3 deficiency, isolated spectrin deficiency, and protein 4.2 deficiency.[65,66] Multiple genetic loci are involved. The majority of HS mutations are private, that is, each kindred has a unique mutation, implying no selective advantage to mutations.

Ankyrin Concomitant spectrin and ankyrin deficiency is a common finding in HS erythrocyte membranes (Fig. 45–6). Several mechanisms, including decreased synthesis of ankyrin, decreased ankyrin assembly on the membrane, and assembly of an abnormal ankyrin, could lead to decreased assembly of spectrin on the membrane when spectrin-binding sites on ankyrin are decreased, absent, or defective.

Genetic screening has identified a number of ankyrin gene mutations in patients and has demonstrated that ankyrin defects are the most common cause of typical, dominant HS.[66,67] The majority of ankyrin mutations are either frameshift or nonsense mutations that lead to a defective ankyrin molecule, ankyrin deficiency, or both. Missense mutations may disrupt normal ankyrin–protein interactions. One such variant, ankyrin^{Walsrode}, identified in a kindred whose erythrocyte membranes were deficient in band 3, ankyrin, and spectrin, resulted from a mutation in the band 3 binding domain of ankyrin that decreased its affinity for band 3.[68] With one exception, all ankyrin mutations described to date have been private. The exception, ankyrin^{Florianopolis}, is a recurrent frameshift mutation associated with severe dominantly inherited HS. Genetic variants have been identified in the promoter of the ankyrin gene in a number of patients with recessively inherited HS.[66] The functional significance of these mutations on ankyrin gene expression is beginning to be revealed.[69]

Cytogenetic studies have identified a few ankyrin-deficient HS patients with dysmorphic features, psychomotor retardation, and hypogonadism.[70] These patients suffer from a contiguous gene syndrome that includes deletion of the ankyrin gene locus at 8p11.2.

Band 3, the Anion Exchanger A subset of patients with typical dominant HS whose red cells are approximately 20 to 40 percent deficient in band 3 and protein 4.2, but have a normal spectrin content, has been described.[65] These patients generally have mild to moderate HS and pincered spherocytes on blood films.

A variety of band 3 gene mutations associated with HS have been identified, including missense, nonsense, duplication, insertion, deletion, and RNA-processing mutations.[71] The missense mutations include a group of mutations that replace highly conserved arginine residues in the transmembrane domain. The mutant proteins do not fold properly and fail to insert into the endoplasmic reticulum and, ultimately, into the erythrocyte membrane. Nonsense mutations lead to decreased band 3 mRNA accumulation, presumably because of mRNA instability. In HS patients with band 3^{Campinas} and band 3^{Pribram}, which are defects in band 3 mRNA processing, renal tubular acidosis has been observed.[72,73]

Spectrin Erythrocytes from most HS patients, including the dominant and the recessive forms, are spectrin deficient. The degree of spectrin deficiency correlates with the spheroidicity of erythrocytes, their ability to withstand shear stress, the degree of hemolysis, and the response to splenectomy (see Fig. 45–6).[74,75]

In humans, α-spectrin synthesis exceeds β-spectrin synthesis by a ratio of approximately 2:1 to 4:1. Patients heterozygous for an α-spectrin defect should still produce enough normal α-spectrin chains to pair with all, or nearly all, of the β-spectrin chains that are synthesized. Thus, patients with α-spectrin defects are symptomatic only when the defect is found in the homozygous or compound heterozygous state. In a similar manner, deficiency of the limiting β-spectrin chains resulting from β-spectrin defects should be expressed as a dominantly inherited trait.

α-Spectrin The mechanisms of spectrin deficiency in most HS patients with recessively inherited HS are unknown. A number of patients with severe recessively inherited HS and marked spectrin deficiency have a mutant allele, α^{LEPRA} (low-expression Prague α-spectrin). α^{LEPRA} produces approximately one-sixth the correctly spliced α-spectrin transcript as the normal allele because of aberrant mRNA processing. In one patient, the combination of the LEPRA allele with another defect of α-spectrin *in trans*, a truncated α-spectrin chain, α^{Prague}, led to severe spectrin deficiency and severe spherocytic anemia.[76] Whether α^{LEPRA} is the etiology of many cases of α-spectrin–linked HS has not been determined. An amino acid substitution in the αII domain of spectrin, $\alpha^{\text{Bug Hill}}$, has been identified in many patients with spectrin-deficient, recessive HS.[77] Studies suggest $\alpha^{\text{Bug Hill}}$ is not itself responsible for HS but likely is a polymorphic variant that in some, but not all, cases is in linkage disequilibrium with another uncharacterized α-spectrin gene defect that causes HS.

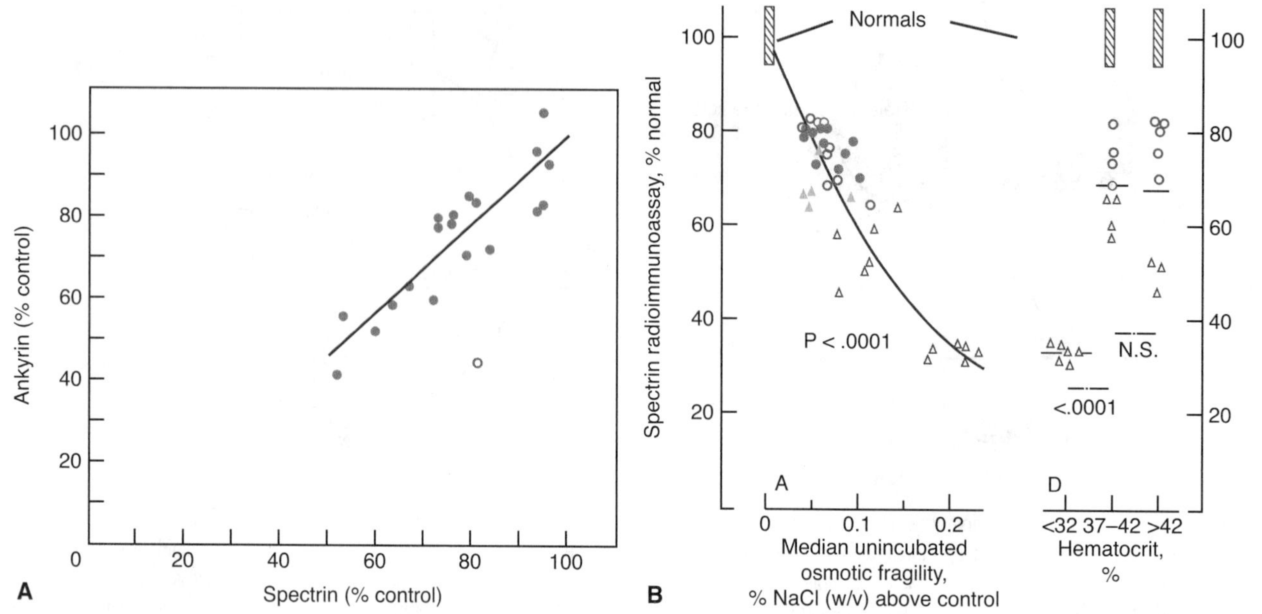

FIGURE 45–6. Role of ankyrin and spectrin in HS. **A.** Correlation of spectrin and ankyrin deficiencies in 20 dominant HS kindreds. Each point, expressed as a percentage of the control (100%), represents the mean value of a kindred for both red cell spectrin and ankyrin levels. Within experimental error, the degree of spectrin and ankyrin deficiency is essentially identical in these families with one exception (*open circle*), an otherwise typical family in which red cells are primarily ankyrin deficient. *(Reproduced with permission from Savvides P, Shalev O, John KM, Lux SE: Combined spectrin and ankyrin deficiency is common in autosomal dominant hereditary spherocytosis.* Blood *82:2953, 1993.)* **B.** Correlation between red cell spectrin deficiency and unincubated osmotic fragility (a measure of spheroidicity) in HS. Spectrin content, as measured by radioimmunoassay, is shown on the *vertical axis*. Osmotic fragility, as measured by NaCl concentration producing 50 percent hemolysis of erythrocytes, is shown on the *horizontal axis*. *Circles* represent patients with typical autosomal dominant HS. *Triangles* represent patients with atypical, nondominant HS. *Open symbols* represent patients who have undergone splenectomy. (*Right panel*) Hematocrit of every patient at least 4 months after splenectomy. Note that markedly spectrin-deficient patients have more spherical red cells and incomplete response to splenectomy. *(Reproduced with permission from Agre P, Asimos A, Casella JF, et al.[74])*

β-Spectrin A group of patients heterozygous for defects in the limiting β-spectrin chain associated with spectrin deficiency and dominant HS have been described.[65] These patients suffer from typical HS with a subpopulation of acanthocytes. The majority of β-spectrin mutations have been associated with null alleles, including frameshift, nonsense, and initiator codon mutations. One frameshift mutation of β-spectrin, caused by a single nucleotide deletion, spectrin^{Houston}, has been found in patients from several unrelated kindreds, suggesting the deletion might be a common β-spectrin mutation associated with HS.[78] Truncated β-spectrin chains caused by genomic deletions, exon skipping, and frameshift mutations have been described. A few missense mutations associated with HS have been reported. One of these missense mutations, spectrin^{Kissimmee}, is an unstable β-spectrin that lacks the ability to bind protein 4.1 and binds poorly to actin because of a point mutation in a highly conserved region of β-spectrin thought to be involved in protein 4.1 binding.[79]

Protein 4.2 Protein 4.2-deficient patients with recessively inherited HS, primarily from Japan, have been described.[71,80] One common variant, protein 4.2^{Nippon}, is caused by a point mutation that presumably affects protein 4.2 mRNA processing.[80] Other variants are caused by homozygosity or compound heterozygosity for frameshift, missense, or mRNA processing mutations of the protein 4.2 gene. Deficiency of protein 4.2 has been observed in patients with mutations in the cytoplasmic domain of band 3.[81,82] These mutations presumably involve the region of band 3–protein 4.2 interactions.

Secondary Membrane Defects

Cation Content and Membrane Permeability Potassium and water content are diminished in HS red cells, particularly those obtained from splenic pulp. The passive permeability of HS red cells to sodium is increased, presumably secondary to the underlying skeletal defect.[83] The excessive sodium influx activates Na^+-K^+ ATPase, the monovalent cation pump, and the accelerated pumping increases ATP turnover and glycolysis. Dehydration of HS red cells likely is caused, at least in part, by the adverse environment of the spleen, given that spherocytes from surgically removed spleens are the most dehydrated.

The pathways causing HS red cell dehydration are not clearly defined. One candidate is increased K-Cl cotransport, which is activated by acid pH. HS red cells, particularly from unsplenectomized subjects, have a low intracellular pH reflecting the low pH of the splenic environment. The K^+-Cl^- cotransport pathway also is activated by oxidative damage, which likely is inflicted by splenic macrophages. Finally, overactivity of Na^+-K^+ ATPase, triggered by increased intracellular sodium, can dehydrate red cells directly, because three sodium ions are extruded in exchange for only two potassium ions, and the loss of monovalent cations is accompanied by water.

Membrane Lipids The principal lipid abnormality of hereditary spherocytes is a symmetrical loss of each species of membrane lipid as part of the overall loss of membrane surface, the hallmark of HS pathobiology. The relative proportions of cholesterol and the various phospholipids are normal, and the phospholipids show the usual transmembrane asymmetry, even in severe cases.

Role of the Spleen

The spleen plays a secondary but important role in the pathophysiology of HS. Splenic destruction of abnormal erythrocytes with decreased deformability is the primary cause of hemolysis. Physical entrapment of spherocytes in the splenic microcirculation and ingestion by phagocytes are proposed mechanisms of destruction.

Splenic Trapping of Nondeformable Spherocytes Because of their diminished deformability, spherocytes are unable to traverse the slits between the endothelial and adventitial cells that form a wall separating the splenic cords of the red pulp from the splenic sinuses (see Chap. 5). The decrease in red cell deformability is primarily related to decreased surface area and secondarily to greater internal viscosity that results from mild cellular dehydration. In addition, the splenic environment is hostile to erythrocytes. Low pH, glucose, and ATP concentrations, and high local concentrations of toxic free radicals produced by adjacent phagocytes all contribute to membrane damage.

Conditioning and Destruction of Spherocytes in the Spleen Impeded spherocyte passage through the sinus wall fenestrations leads to a markedly engorged red pulp and pulp cords with relatively empty venous sinuses.[84] Red cells are "conditioned" in this location, becoming more osmotically fragile and more spherical, with a lower net sodium and potassium content than cells obtained from the systemic circulation.[85] Splenic conditioning is a consequence of multiple episodes of splenic stasis. The estimated residence time of HS erythrocytes in the cords is between 10 and 100 minutes. Only 1 to 10 percent of blood entering the spleen is detained by the congested cords, whereas greater than 90 percent is rapidly shunted into the venous circulation.

Phagocytosis by macrophages in the spleen is the final step in the cycle of spherocyte destruction. The stimulus for phagocytosis by the macrophage is unknown.

Inheritance

The genes responsible for HS include ankyrin, β-spectrin, band 3 protein, α-spectrin, and protein 4.2. In approximately two-thirds to three-fourths of HS patients, inheritance is autosomal dominant. In the remaining patients, dominant inheritance cannot be demonstrated. Inheritance may be autosomal recessive or result from a *de novo* mutation. Cases with autosomal recessive inheritance result from defects in either α-spectrin or protein 4.2. A surprising number of *de novo* mutations have been reported in the HS genes.[79,86,87] A few cases of HS resulting from homozygous or compound heterozygous defects in band 3 or spectrin that result in fetal death or severe hemolytic anemia presenting in the neonatal period have been reported.[88,89] In general, affected individuals of the same kindred experience similar degrees of hemolysis. Rarely, members of the same kindred experience varying degrees of hemolysis. When HS is identified in one or more siblings whose parents have no identifiable abnormalities or great variability exists in the clinical severity of affected HS family members, a number of explanations can be sought. Possible explanations include inheritance of a modifier allele that influences the expression of a membrane protein, leading to the variability in clinical expression; variable penetrance of the genetic defect; a *de novo* mutation; a mild form of recessively inherited HS; or tissue-specific mosaicism of the defect.[90]

Clinical Features

The clinical manifestations of the spherocytosis syndromes vary widely. The typical clinical picture of HS combines evidence of hemolysis (anemia, jaundice, reticulocytosis, gallstones, splenomegaly) with spherocytosis (spherocytes on the blood film and increased osmotic fragility) and a positive family history. Mild, moderate, and severe forms of HS have been defined according to differences in hemoglobin, bilirubin, and reticulocyte counts (Table 45–3), which can be correlated with the degree of compensation for hemolysis. Initial assessment of a patient with suspected HS should include a family history and questions about history of anemia, jaundice, gallstones, and splenectomy. Physical examination should seek signs such as scleral icterus, jaundice, and splenomegaly.

Typical Hereditary Spherocytosis Hereditary spherocytosis typically presents in infancy or childhood but may present at any age. In children, anemia is the most frequent finding (50%), followed by splenomegaly, jaundice, or a positive family history.[65] No comparable data exist for adults. Two-thirds to three-fourths of HS patients have incompletely compensated hemolysis and mild to moderate anemia. The anemia often is asymptomatic, except for fatigue and mild pallor or, with children, nonspecific parental complaints, such as irritability. Jaundice is seen at some time in about half of patients, usually in association with viral infections. When present, jaundice is acholuric, that is, unconjugated hyperbilirubinemia without detectable bilirubinuria. Palpable splenomegaly is detectable in most (75–95%) older children and adults. Typically the spleen is modestly enlarged (2–6 cm below the costal margin), but it may be massive. No proven correlation exists between the spleen size and the severity of HS. However, given the pathophysiology and response of the

TABLE 45–3. Classification of Hereditary Spherocytosis

Laboratory Findings	HS Trait or Carrier	Mild Spherocytosis	Moderate Spherocytosis	Moderately Severe Spherocytosis*	Severe Spherocytosis†
Hemoglobin (g/dL)	Normal	11–15	8–12	6–8	<6
Reticulocytes (%)	1–2	3–8	± 8	≥10	≥10
Bilirubin (mg/dL)	0–1	1–2	± 2	2–3	≥3
Spectrin content (% of normal)‡	100	80–100	50–80	40–80§	20–50
Blood film	Normal	Mild spherocytosis	Spherocytosis	Spherocytosis	Spherocytosis and poikilocytosis
Osmotic fragility					
Fresh blood	Normal	Normal or slightly increased	Distinctly increased	Distinctly increased	Distinctly increased
Incubated blood	Slightly increased	Distinctly increased	Distinctly increased	Distinctly increased	Markedly increased

*Values in untransfused patients.

†By definition, patients with severe spherocytosis are transfusion dependent. Values were obtained immediately prior to transfusion.

‡Normal, $245 \pm 27 \times 10^3$ spectrin dimers per erythrocyte.

§Spectrin content is variable in this group of patients, presumably reflecting heterogeneity of the underlying pathophysiology.

SOURCE: Reproduced with permission from Eber SW, Armbrust R, and Schroter W.[90]

disease to splenectomy, such a correlation probably exists. Typical HS is associated with both dominant and recessive inheritance. Although the recessively inherited forms tend to be more severe, considerable overlap exists.

Compensated Hereditary Spherocytosis Approximately 20 to 30 percent of HS patients have "compensated hemolysis," that is, production and destruction are balanced, and the hemoglobin concentration of the blood is virtually normal.[65,90] Although the erythrocyte life span may only be approximately 20 to 30 days, patients adequately compensate for hemolysis with increased marrow erythropoiesis. Because these patients are not anemic, they usually are asymptomatic. In some cases, diagnosis may be difficult because hemolysis, splenomegaly, and spherocytosis are unusually mild. For example, in this group of patients, reticulocyte counts are generally less than 6 percent, and spherocytes are present on blood film in only approximately 60 percent of patients. Many of these individuals escape detection until adulthood when they are being evaluated for unrelated disorders or when complications related to anemia or chronic hemolysis occur. Hemolysis may become severe with illnesses that cause further splenomegaly, such as infectious mononucleosis, or may be exacerbated by other factors, such as pregnancy or sustained, vigorous exercise. Because of the asymptomatic course of HS in these patients, diagnosis of HS should be considered during evaluation of incidentally noted splenomegaly, gallstones at a young age, or anemia resulting from parvovirus B19 infection or other viral infections.

Moderately Severe and Severe Hereditary Spherocytosis Approximately 5 to 10 percent of HS patients have moderately severe to severe anemia. Patients with "moderately severe" disease typically have a hemoglobin level of 6 to 8 g/dL, reticulocytes approximately 10 percent, bilirubin 2 to 3 mg/dL, and 40 to 80 percent of the normal red cell spectrin content. The category includes patients with both dominant and recessive HS and a variety of molecular defects. Patients with "severe" disease, by definition, have life-threatening anemia and are transfusion dependent. They almost always have recessive HS. Most have isolated, severe spectrin deficiency (<40%), which is thought to result from a defect in α-spectrin.[74,75] Patients with severe HS often have some irregularly contoured or budding spherocytes or bizarre poikilocytes in addition to typical spherocytes on blood film. Such cells are rare prior to splenectomy in patients with moderately severe disease, but some may be seen postsplenectomy. In addition to the risks of recurrent transfusions, patients often suffer from hemolytic and aplastic crises and may develop complications of severe uncompensated anemia, including growth retardation, delayed sexual maturation, and aspects of thalassemic facies.

Asymptomatic Carriers Parents of patients with recessive HS are clinically asymptomatic and do not have anemia, splenomegaly, hyperbilirubinemia, or spherocytosis on the blood films. However, most have subtle laboratory signs of HS, including slight reticulocytosis (~2%), diminished haptoglobin levels, and slightly elevated osmotic fragility. The incubated osmotic fragility test probably is the most sensitive measure of this condition, particularly the 100 percent red cell lysis point, which occurs at a higher sodium chloride concentration in carriers (0.43 ± 0.05 g NaCl/dL) compared to normal subjects (0.23 ± 0.07 g NaCl/dL).[90] However, no single test is sufficient. Carriers can be detected reliably only by considering the results of a battery of tests. At least 1.4 percent of the carrier population is estimated to be silent carriers.

Pregnancy and Hereditary Spherocytosis

Most patients do well during pregnancy.[91] Some patients experience anemia beyond that expected from expanded plasma volume resulting from increased hemolysis. A few patients are symptomatic only during pregnancy. Episodes of hemolytic crisis requiring transfusion and cases of folic acid deficiency have been described in pregnant HS patients.

Hereditary Spherocytosis in Infancy

Anemia is the most common finding in neonates with HS, present in approximately 90 percent of cases. Some infants have required blood transfusion to treat their anemia. Of interest, the degree of anemia seen in the neonatal period does not predict the severity of anemia seen in later life. Jaundice occurs in about half of HS neonates and may be severe enough to require phototherapy or exchange transfusion. Jaundice in neonates with HS may be accentuated by coinheritance of Gilbert syndrome, but this can be attenuated by phenobarbital.[92] Because kernicterus is a risk, exchange transfusions may be necessary, but in most cases the jaundice can be controlled with phototherapy.

Rarely, patients suffer from severe hemolytic anemia presenting *in utero* or shortly after birth, continuing through the first year of life. Patients may require regular blood transfusions and, in some cases, early splenectomy. These severe HS patients usually suffer from significant spectrin deficiency resulting from presumed homozygosity or compound heterozygosity for α-spectrin gene defects. Several cases of hydrops fetalis in HS patients requiring intrauterine transfusion because of severe anemia associated with band 3 or spectrin defects have been reported.

Complications

Gallbladder Disease Chronic hemolysis leads to formation of bilirubinate gallstones, the most frequently reported complication in up to half of HS patients. Coinheritance of Gilbert syndrome uridine diphosphoglucuronate glucuronosyltransferase gene polymorphism markedly increases the risk of gallstone formation.[93] Although gallstones have been detected in infants, most gallstones occur in adolescents, children, and young adults.[65,94] Routine management should include interval ultrasonography to detect gallstones because many patients with cholelithiasis and HS are asymptomatic. Interval ultrasonography allows prompt diagnosis and treatment and prevents complications of symptomatic biliary tract disease, including biliary obstruction, cholecystitis, and cholangitis.

Hemolytic, Aplastic, and Megaloblastic Crises Hemolytic crises usually are associated with viral illnesses and typically occur in childhood. They generally are mild and characterized by jaundice, increased spleen size, decreased hematocrit, and reticulocytosis. Medical intervention rarely is necessary. During severe hemolytic crises, marked jaundice, anemia, lethargy, abdominal pain, and tender splenomegaly occur. Hospitalization and erythrocyte transfusion may be required.

Aplastic crises following virally induced marrow suppression are uncommon but may result in severe anemia with serious complications, including congestive heart failure or even death. The most common etiologic agent in these cases is parvovirus B19, which causes erythema infectiosum. Parvovirus infection typically presents with fever, chills, lethargy, vomiting, diarrhea, myalgia, and a maculopapular rash on the face (slapped cheek syndrome), trunk, and extremities.

Parvovirus B19 selectively infects erythropoietic progenitor cells and inhibits their growth (see Chap. 34).[95] Parvovirus infections frequently are associated with mild neutropenia, thrombocytopenia, or pancytopenia. During the aplastic phase, hematocrit level and reticulocyte count fall, marrow erythroblasts disappear, and, as the plasma iron turnover decreases, plasma iron level increases. Giant pronormoblasts, a hallmark of the cytopathic effects of parvovirus B19, often appear in the marrow. As production of new red cells declines, the remaining cells age, and microspherocytosis and osmotic fragility increase. Bilirubin levels may decrease as the number of abnormal red cells that can be destroyed declines. Return of marrow function is heralded by a fall in serum iron concentration and emergence of granulocytes, platelets, and, finally, reticulocytes.

Virally induced aplastic crisis brings many patients to medical attention, particularly asymptomatic HS patients with normally compensated hemolysis.[96] As expected, because parvovirus may simultaneously infect multiple members of a family, leading to aplastic crises, "epidemics" or "outbreaks" of HS have been reported.[97] Diagnostic confusion may arise during reemergence of marrow function, when the physician may mistake an aplastic crisis for a hemolytic crisis. Because aplastic crises usually last 10 to 14 days (about half the life span of typical HS red cells), the hemoglobin value usually falls to about half its usual level before recovery occurs. In patients with severe HS, the anemia may be profound, requiring hospitalization and transfusion.

Megaloblastic crisis occurs in HS patients with increased folate demands, such as pregnant patients, growing children, or patients recovering from an aplastic crisis. This complication is preventable with appropriate folate supplementation.

Other Complications Dermatologic manifestations of HS, including skin ulceration, gouty tophi, and chronic leg dermatitis, are uncommon.[98] These dermatologic manifestations usually heal rapidly after splenectomy. The pathogenesis of these manifestations is unknown but is proposed to be related to alterations in erythrocyte deformability, as suggested in patients with sickle cell anemia.

Findings attributable to extramedullary hematopoiesis have been described in some HS patients. The findings include poor growth and deformities of the hand and skull. Extramedullary tumors, particularly along the thoracic and lumbar spine or in the kidney hila, have been described in HS patients, including patients with untreated mild to moderate HS.[98,99] Biopsy may be performed because the masses may be mistaken for a malignant tumor. However, the biopsy procedure may be complicated by significant hemorrhage because of the composition of the masses. Magnetic resonance imaging appears to be a reliable and safer alternative diagnostic modality. Postsplenectomy, the masses involute and undergo fatty metamorphosis. However, they do not decrease in size.

HS has been suggested to predispose patients to hematologic malignancies, including myeloproliferative disorders, particularly myeloma.[100] Chronic mononuclear phagocyte stimulation via splenic clearance of abnormal erythrocytes inducing proliferation of lymphocytes, plasma cells, and macrophages has been suggested as a possible pathogenic mechanism. Thrombosis has been reported in several HS patients, usually postsplenectomy.

Iron overload has been described in untransfused HS patients both with coinherited hemochromatosis and in patients without HFE (hemochromatosis gene) mutations. Untreated HS may aggravate underlying heart disease, particularly in the elderly. Progressive anemia resulting from loss of marrow reserve may gradually worsen underlying heart failure. Angioid streaks have been described in the optic fundi of several adult HS patients.

Nonerythroid Manifestations

Clinical manifestations are confined to the erythroid lineage in most patients with HS, but a few exceptions have been observed. Several HS kindred have been reported with cosegregating nonerythroid manifestations, particularly neuromuscular abnormalities including cardiomyopathy, slowly progressive spinocerebellar degenerative disease, spinal cord dysfunction, and movement disorders.

The observation that erythrocyte ankyrin and β-spectrin are also expressed in muscle, brain, and spinal cord raises the possibility that these HS patients suffer from defects of one of these proteins.[65] The hypothesis is further supported by studies of ankyrin-deficient *nb/nb* mice.[101] These mice have almost no detectable ankyrin and suffer from a severe, spherocytic hemolytic anemia and late-onset cerebellar ataxia that parallels a gradual loss of Purkinje cells. A further possibility is that another, yet to be described gene locus is causative. For example, mice that do not express the junctional complex membrane protein β-adducin suffer from a spherocytic anemia and neurologic manifestations.[44]

Heterozygous defects of band 3 have been described in patients with inherited distal renal tubular acidosis and normal erythrocytes. This finding is in contrast to most patients with heterozygous mutations of band 3, who have normal renal acidification and abnormal erythrocytes. Two kindreds with coinherited HS *and* renal acidification defects resulting from band 3 mRNA processing mutations, band 3^{Pribram} and band 3^{Campinas} have been described.[72,73]

Laboratory Features

Like the clinical presentation of HS, laboratory findings in HS are heterogeneous.

Blood Film Erythrocyte morphology in HS is variable. Typical HS patients have blood films with easily identifiable spherocytes lacking central pallor (Fig. 45–7). Less commonly, patients present with only a few spherocytes on the film or, at the other end of the spectrum, with numerous small, dense spherocytes and bizarre erythrocyte morphology with anisocytosis and poikilocytosis. Rarely, spherostomatocytes are seen.

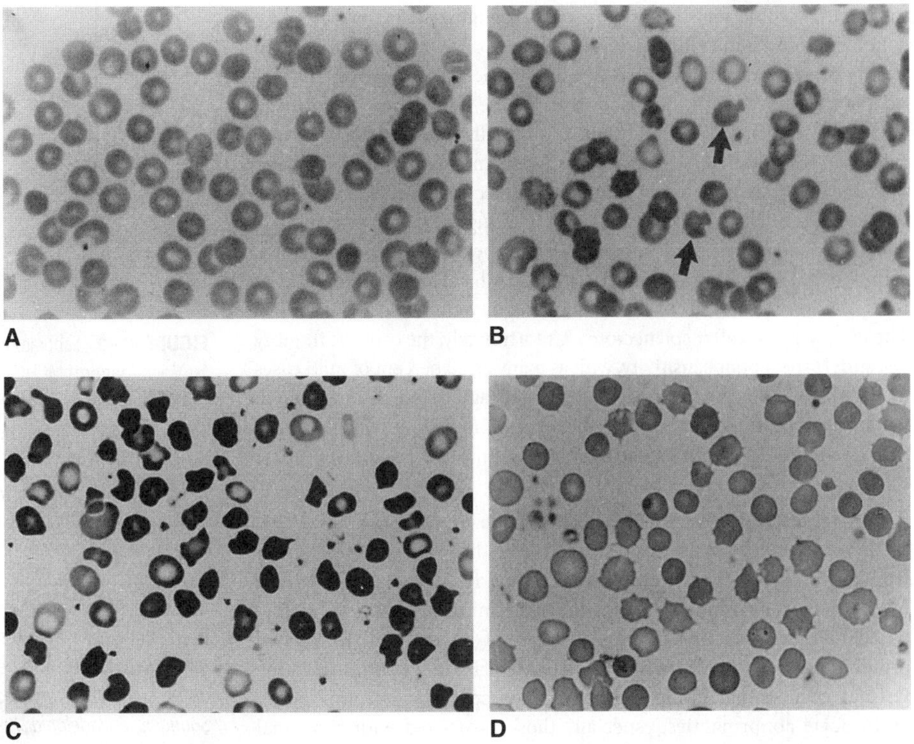

FIGURE 45–7. Blood films from patients with HS of varying severity. **A.** Typical HS with mild deficiency of red cell spectrin and ankyrin. Although many cells have spheroidal shape, some cells retain a central concavity. **B.** HS with pincered red cells (*arrows*), as typically seen in HS associated with band 3 deficiency. Occasionally, spiculated red cells also are present. **C.** Severe atypical HS resulting from severe combined spectrin and ankyrin deficiency. In addition to spherocytes, many cells with irregular contour are present. **D.** HS with isolated spectrin deficiency resulting from β-spectrin mutation. Some spherocytes have prominent surface projections resembling spheroacanthocytes. *(Blood film **D** courtesy of DL Wolfe.)*

Specific morphologic findings have been identified in patients with certain membrane protein defects, such as pincered erythrocytes (band 3) or spherocytic acanthocytes (β-spectrin). When examining blood from a patient with suspected spherocytosis, a high-quality film with the erythrocytes properly separated and some cells with central pallor in the field of examination is important because spherocytes are an artifact.

Erythrocyte Indices Most patients have mild to moderate anemia with hemoglobin in the 9 to 12 g/dL range (see Table 45–3). Mean corpuscular hemoglobin concentration (MCHC) is increased (between 35% and 38%) because of relative cellular dehydration in approximately 50 percent of patients, but all HS patients have some dehydrated cells. In one pediatric study, an MCHC >35.4 g/dL and a red cell distribution (RDW) width >14 had a sensitivity of 63 percent and a specificity of 100 percent for the diagnosis of HS.[102] Laser-based cell counters provide a histogram of hyperdense erythrocytes (MCHC >40 g/dL) that has been used as a screening test and is claimed to be sufficiently accurate to identify nearly all HS patients (Fig. 45–8A).[103] Finally, mean corpuscular volume (MCV) usually is normal except in cases of severe HS, when MCV is slightly decreased. Typically, MCV is relatively low for the age of the cells in most HS patients, reflecting the dehydrated state of the HS erythrocytes.

Osmotic Fragility In the normal erythrocyte, a redundancy of cell membrane gives the cell its characteristic discoid shape and provides it with abundant surface area. Spherocytes have a decreased surface area relative to cell volume, resulting in their abnormal shape. This change is reflected in the increased osmotic fragility found in these cells (see Fig. 45–8B). Osmotic fragility is tested by adding increasingly hypotonic concentrations of saline solution to red cells. The normal erythrocyte is able to increase its volume by swelling, but spherocytes, which already are at maximum volume for surface area, burst at higher than normal saline concentrations. Some HS individuals have a normal osmotic fragility on freshly drawn red blood cells, with the osmotic fragility curve approximating the number of spherocytes seen on the blood film.[104] However, after incubation at 37°C for 24 hours, HS red cells lose membrane surface area more readily than normal because their membranes are leaky and unstable. Thus, incubation accentuates the defect in HS erythrocytes and brings out the defect in osmotic fragility, making incubated osmotic fragility the standard test in diagnosing HS.[104] When the spleen is present, a subpopulation of very fragile erythrocytes that have been conditioned by the spleen form the "tail" of the osmotic fragility curve (see Fig. 45–8B). The tail disappears after splenectomy. Unfortunately, the osmotic fragility test suffers from poor sensitivity, with as many as 20 percent of mild cases of HS missed after incubation. The osmotic fragility test is unreliable in patients having small numbers of spherocytes, including recently transfused patients. The test results are abnormal in other conditions where spherocytes are present.

Additional Testing Other investigations, such as the autohemolysis test, the hypertonic cryohemolysis test, and the acidified glycerol test, suffer from lack of specificity, are cumbersome to perform, and are not widely used. Membrane binding of eosin-5-maleimide, a flow cytometry-based method reflecting relative amounts of band 3 and Rh-related proteins, has been used as a screening test for HS. Like osmotic fragility testing, eosin-5-maleimide binding is not specific, detecting other erythrocyte abnormalities, especially those associated with abnormal band 3, including congenital dyserythropoietic anemia, and abnormalities of erythrocyte hydration and viscosity, including sickle cell disease and cryohydrocytosis.[105] Moreover, samples must be processed quickly, as storage may alter tests results.[106]

Specialized testing is available for studying difficult cases or cases requiring additional information. Useful tests for these purposes include structural and functional studies of erythrocyte membrane proteins, such as protein quantitation, and ion transport. Membrane rigidity and fragility can be examined using an ektacytometer. cDNA and genomic DNA analyses can be performed when a molecular diagnosis is desired.

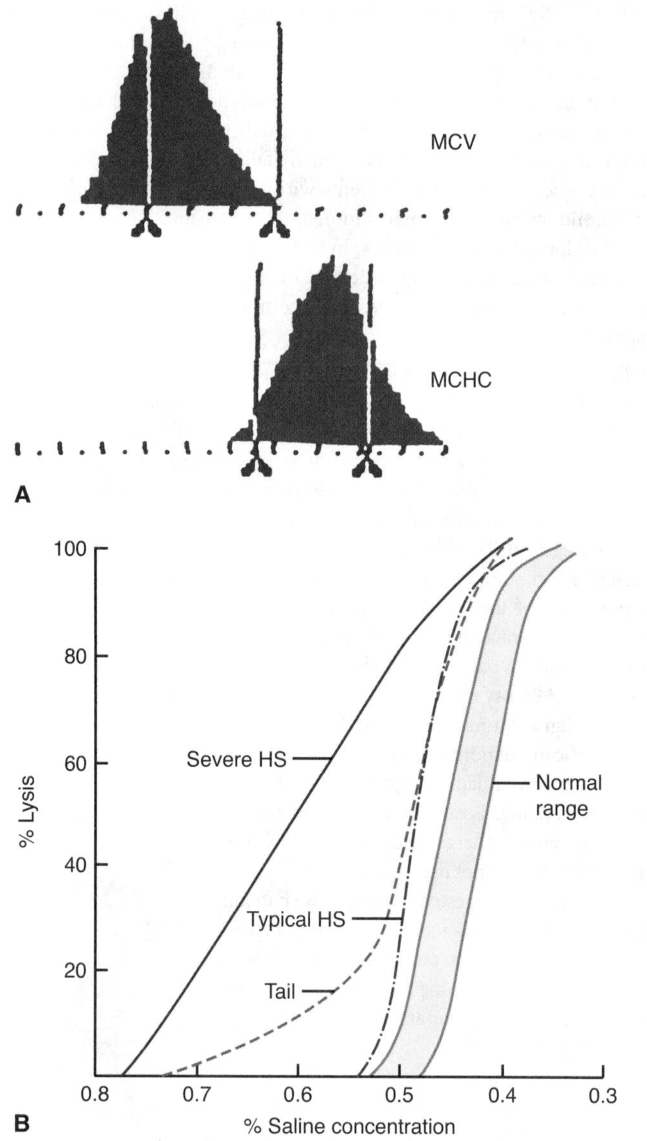

FIGURE 45–8. Laboratory diagnosis of HS. **A.** Histograms of the distribution of (*top*) MCV and (*bottom*) MCHC in red cells of a patient with HS before splenectomy. *Vertical lines* mark the normal limits of the distributions. Data were collected with a Technicon H1 laser-scattering blood counter. The patient has subpopulations of microcytes (low MCV) and dehydrated cells (high MCHC), which presumably represent conditioned microspherocytes. All 21 HS patients in one study had similar subpopulations. *(Reproduced with permission from Pati AR, Patton WN, Harris EI: The use of the Technicon H1 in the diagnosis of hereditary spherocytosis.* Clin Lab Haematol *11:27, 1989.)* **B.** Osmotic fragility testing. The *shaded area* is the normal range. Results representative of both typical and severe spherocytosis are shown. A "tail," representing very fragile erythrocytes that have been conditioned by the spleen, is common in many HS patients prior to splenectomy. *(Reproduced with permission from Gallagher PG, Forget BG, Lux SE: Disorders of the erythrocyte membrane, in* Hematology of Infancy and Childhood, *p 544. WB Saunders, Philadelphia, 1998.)*

Other laboratory manifestations of HS are markers of ongoing hemolysis. Reticulocytosis, increased serum bilirubin, increased lactate dehydrogenase, increased urinary and fecal urobilinogen, and decreased serum haptoglobin reflect increased erythrocyte production or destruction and variable proportions of intravascular and extravascular hemolysis components. In many cases of HS, the reticulocyte count appears to be elevated disproportionately relative to the degree of anemia. This finding has been observed even in HS patients with normal hemoglobin levels.

Differential Diagnosis

Initial laboratory investigation should include a complete blood count with a blood film, reticulocyte count, direct antiglobulin test (Coombs test), and serum bilirubin. An incubated osmotic fragility should be obtained. Rarely, additional specialized testing is required to confirm the diagnosis. In neonates, ABO incompatibility should be considered, but its differentiation from HS becomes clear several months after birth. Other causes of spherocytic hemolytic anemia, such as autoimmune hemolysis, clostridial sepsis, transfusion reactions, severe burns, and bites from snakes, spiders, bees, and wasps, should be viewed in the appropriate clinical context. Occasional spherocytes are seen in patients with a large spleen (e.g., in cirrhosis or myelofibrosis) or in patients with microangiopathic anemias (see Chap. 50), but differentiation of these conditions from HS does not usually present diagnostic difficulties.

HS may be obscured in disorders that increase the surface to volume ratio of erythrocytes, such as obstructive jaundice, iron deficiency, β-thalassemia trait or hemoglobin–sickle cell disease, and vitamin B_{12} or folate deficiency. In obstructive jaundice, spherocytosis can be obscured by accumulation of cholesterol and phospholipids in the membrane that characteristically accompanies this condition. In normal subjects, this process leads to target cell formation. Hereditary spherocytes acquire a discoidal appearance, and their survival in the circulation is improved. Iron deficiency corrects the abnormal shape but does not improve survival of HS erythrocytes.

Therapy and Prognosis

Splenectomy Splenic sequestration is the primary determinant of erythrocyte survival in HS patients. Thus, splenectomy cures or alleviates the anemia in the overwhelming majority of patients, reducing or eliminating the need for red cell transfusions, which has obvious implications for future iron overload and risk of end-organ damage. The incidence of cholelithiasis is decreased. Postsplenectomy, spherocytosis and altered osmotic fragility persist, but the "tail" of the osmotic fragility curve, created by conditioning of a subpopulation of spherocytes by the spleen, disappears. Erythrocyte life span nearly normalizes, and reticulocyte counts fall to normal or near-normal levels. Changes typical of the postsplenectomy state, including Howell-Jolly bodies, target cells, siderocytes, and acanthocytes, become evident on the blood film. Postsplenectomy, patients with the most severe forms of HS still suffer from shortened erythrocyte survival and hemolysis, but their clinical improvement is striking.[74,75]

Complications of Splenectomy Early complications of splenectomy include local infection or bleeding and pancreatitis, presumably resulting from injury to the tail of the pancreas incurred during spleen removal. In general, the morbidity of splenectomy for HS is lower than the morbidity of other hematologic disorders. Chapter 55 discusses the complications of splenectomy.

Indications for Splenectomy In the past, splenectomy, which has a low operative mortality, was considered routine in HS patients. However, the risk of overwhelming postsplenectomy infection and the emergence of penicillin-resistant pneumococci have led to reevaluation of the role of splenectomy in the treatment of HS.[107] Considering the risks and benefits, a reasonable approach is to splenectomize all patients with severe spherocytosis and all patients suffering from significant signs or symptoms of anemia, including growth failure, skeletal changes, leg ulcers, and extramedullary hematopoietic tumors. Other candidates for splenectomy are older HS patients suffering from vascular compromise of vital organs.

Whether patients with moderate HS and compensated, asymptomatic anemia should undergo splenectomy is controversial. Patients with mild HS and compensated hemolysis can be followed and referred for splenectomy if clinically indicated. Treatment of patients with mild to moderate HS and gallstones is debatable, particularly because new treatments for cholelithiasis, including laparoscopic cholecystectomy, and endoscopic sphincterotomy, lower the risk of this complication. If such patients have symptomatic gallstones, a combined cholecystectomy and splenectomy can be performed, particularly if acute cholecystitis or biliary obstruction has occurred. No evidence indicates any benefit to performing cholecystectomy and splenectomy separately, as performed in the past.

Because the risk of postsplenectomy sepsis is very high during infancy and early childhood, splenectomy should be delayed until age 5 to 9 years if possible, and to at least 3 years if feasible, even if chronic transfusions are required in the interim. No evidence indicates further delay is useful. In fact, further delay may be harmful because the risk of cholelithiasis increases dramatically in children older than age 10 years.

When splenectomy is warranted, laparoscopic splenectomy has become the method of choice in centers with surgeons experienced in the technique.[108] If desired, the procedure can be combined with laparoscopic cholecystectomy. Laparoscopic splenectomy results in less postoperative discomfort, a quicker return to preoperative diet and activities, shorter hospitalization, decreased costs, and smaller scars. The risk of bleeding increases during the operation, and approximately 10 percent of laparoscopic operations (for all causes) must be converted to standard splenectomies. Even very large spleens (>600 g) can be removed laparoscopically because the spleen is placed in a large bag, diced, and eliminated via suction catheters.

Partial splenectomy via laparotomy has been advocated for infants and young children with significant anemia associated with erythrocyte membrane disorders.[109] The goals of this procedure are to allow for palliation of hemolysis and anemia while maintaining some residual splenic immune function. Long-term followup data for this procedure have been variable.

Prior to splenectomy, patients should be immunized with vaccines against pneumococcus, *Haemophilus influenzae* type B, and meningococcus, preferably several weeks preoperatively. Use of prophylactic antibiotics postsplenectomy for prevention of pneumococcal sepsis is controversial. Postsplenectomy, prophylactic antibiotics (penicillin V 125 mg orally twice daily for patients younger than age 7 years or 250 mg orally twice daily for those older than age 7 years, including adults) are recommended for at least 5 years postsplenectomy by some and for life by others. The optimal duration of prophylactic antibiotic therapy postsplenectomy is unknown. Presplenectomy and, in severe cases, postsplenectomy, HS patients should take folic acid (1 mg/day orally) to prevent folate deficiency.

Splenectomy Failure Splenectomy failure is uncommon. Failure may result from an accessory spleen missed during splenectomy, from development of splenunculi as a consequence of autotransplantation of splenic tissue during surgery, or from another intrinsic red cell defect, such as pyruvate kinase deficiency. Accessory spleens occur in 15 to 40 percent of patients and must always be sought. Recurrence of hemolytic anemia years or even decades following splenectomy should raise suspicion of an accessory spleen, particularly if Howell-Jolly bodies are no longer found on blood film. Definitive confirmation of ectopic splenic tissue can be achieved by a radiocolloid liver–spleen scan or a scan using ^{51}Cr-labeled, heat-damaged red cells.

Genetic Counseling

After a patient is diagnosed with HS, family members should be examined for the presence of HS. A history, physical examination for splenomegaly, complete blood count, examination of the blood film for spherocytes, and a reticulocyte count should be obtained for parents, children, and siblings, if available.

HEREDITARY ELLIPTOCYTOSIS, PYROPOIKILOCYTOSIS, AND RELATED DISORDERS

Definition and History

HE is characterized by the presence of elliptical or oval erythrocytes on the blood films of affected individuals.[39,110,111] In 1904, Dresbach, a physiologist at Ohio State University in Columbus, Ohio, reported the first description of HE. Dresbach discovered the condition in a medical student during a laboratory exercise in which the students were examining their own blood.[112] The report elicited some controversy because the student died soon thereafter, leading to speculation that the student actually suffered from pernicious anemia. The demonstration of the disease in three generations of one family by Hunter and Adams[113] clearly established the hereditary nature of this disorder. Dacie[110] has reviewed the history of HE.

HPP is a rare cause of anemia first described in three children with severe neonatal anemia with erythrocyte morphology similar to that seen in patients suffering severe burns.[39,114] The erythrocytes from these patients also exhibited increased thermal sensitivity. Subsequently, other patients, mostly of African descent, with similar clinical and laboratory findings have been described.[115–117] A strong relationship exists between HE and HPP. Approximately one-third of parents or siblings of patients with HPP have typical HE, and many of these family members share identical mutations in erythrocyte spectrin. In addition, many patients with HPP proceed to develop typical mild to moderate HE. Patients with HPP tend to experience severe hemolysis and anemia in infancy that gradually improves but then evolves toward typical hemolytic HE later in life. The blood film remains striking.

Epidemiology

The worldwide incidence of HE is estimated to be 1 in 2000 to 1 in 4000 individuals.[39] The true incidence of HE is unknown because its clinical severity is heterogeneous and many patients are asymptomatic. It is common in individuals of African and Mediterranean descent, presumably because elliptocytes confer some resistance to malaria. The incidence of HE is 6 percent in Benin, Africa.[111] Genetic haplotyping studies suggest one HE mutation common in Africa has a "founder effect" with origins in central Africa similar to that attributed to hemoglobin S, Benin-type.[39]

Etiology and Pathogenesis

The principal defect in HE and HPP erythrocytes is mechanical weakness or fragility of the erythrocyte membrane skeleton. As in HS, studies of erythrocyte membrane proteins in these disorders have identified abnormalities of various erythrocyte membrane proteins, including α- and β-spectrin, protein 4.1, and GPC.[39] The majority of defects occur in spectrin, the principal structural protein of the erythrocyte membrane skeleton. Most spectrin defects in HE and HPP impair the ability of spectrin dimers to self-associate into tetramers and oligomers, thereby disrupting the membrane cytoskeleton.[118] Structural and functional defects of protein 4.1 lead to disruption of spectrin–actin attachment to the membrane via GPC, causing changes in cell shape and membrane stability similar to those found in abnormalities of spectrin. The mechanical instability in GPC variants appears to result from secondary protein 4.1 deficiency. In all of these defects, disruption of the membrane skeleton leads to mechanical instability sufficient to cause red cell fragmentation with hemolytic anemia under conditions of normal circulatory shear stress.[51]

The pathobiology of elliptocytic shape is less clear. Red cell precursors in common HE are round. The cells become progressively more elliptical as they age *in vivo*. Elliptocytes and poikilocytes may become permanently stabilized in shape because weakened spectrin heterodimer contacts facilitate skeletal reorganization following axial deformation of cells from prolonged or excessive shear stress. The reorganization likely involves breakage of the unidirectionally stretched protein connections, followed by formation of new protein contacts that preclude recovery of the normal biconcave shape. This process accounts for the permanent deformation of irreversibly sickled cells.

Spectrin in Hereditary Elliptocytosis and Pyropoikilocytosis The abnormalities of either α- or β-spectrin associated with the majority of cases of HE and HPP result from mutations in the spectrin heterodimer self-association site.[118] Figure 45–9 shows diagrammatically the repeats of spectrin involved in self-association and the locations of reported mutations. Most of the mutations are missense mutations at or very near highly conserved residues of α spectrin. The missense mutations are primarily either α helix-breaking mutations that replace the normal residue with a proline or glycine, or charge-shift mutations. In contrast to HS, the elliptocytosis and pyropoikilocytosis syndromes, while also quite heterogeneous, are associated with distinct spectrin mutations in persons of similar genetic backgrounds, suggesting a "founder effect" for the mutations.

HE or HPP phenotype–spectrin mutation genotype correlations are difficult to establish. Great clinical phenotypic heterogeneity exists among individuals with the same spectrin mutation. The heterogeneity exists even among individuals from the same kindred. A few general phenotype–genotype correlations can be made. Mutations at the contact

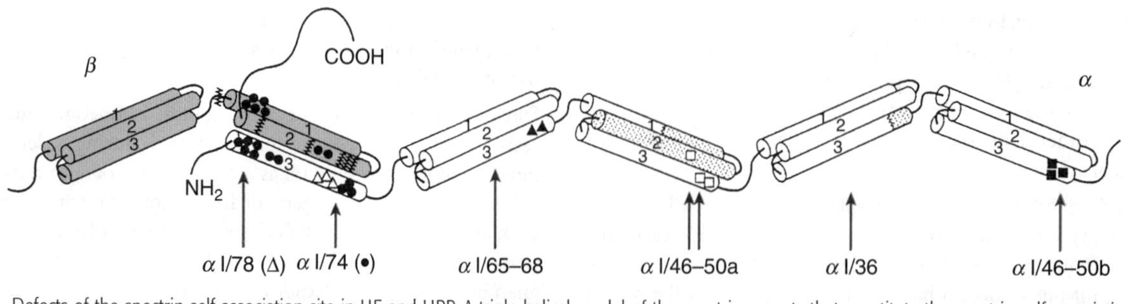

FIGURE 45–9. Defects of the spectrin self-association site in HE and HPP. A triple helical model of the spectrin repeats that constitute the spectrin self-association site is shown. *Symbols* denote positions of various genetic defects identified in patients with HE or HPP. Limited tryptic digestion of spectrin, followed by two-dimensional gel electrophoresis, identifies abnormal cleavage sites (*arrows*) in spectrin associated with various mutations. *(Modified with permission from Gallagher PG, Forget BG, Lux SE: Disorders of the erythrocyte membrane, in* Hematology of Infancy and Childhood, *p 544. WB Saunders, Philadelphia, 1998.)*

sites of α- and β-spectrin in the spectrin self-association site tend to be more severe.[115,116] For example, mutations of codon 28, which is located in this contact site region, are generally associated with phenotypically severe HE or HPP. On the other hand, a common mutation in blacks from West and Central Africa, a leucine insertion at codon 154, is phenotypically very mild, even in the homozygous state.[119] Because of the great phenotypic variability, the presence of low-expression modifier alleles of spectrin has been postulated (see "Molecular Determinants of Clinical Severity" below).

In contrast to α-spectrin mutations, a variety of β-spectrin mutations have been identified in HE and HPP patients, including frameshift and splicing mutations that lead to truncated β-spectrin chains lacking the spectrin self-association site. Three β-spectrin mutations, spectrin^{Providence}, spectrin^{Cagliari}, and spectrin^{Buffalo},[120–122] lead to severe fetal or neonatal anemia and nonimmune hydrops fetalis when inherited in the homozygous state. Five of six homozygotes died; the one survivor remains transfusion dependent.

Protein 4.1 Protein 4.1 defects associated with HE are much less common than spectrin defects. Protein 4.1 is a multifunctional protein that undergoes complex patterns of tissue- and stage-specific alternative splicing. It contains several important functional sites, including a spectrin–actin binding domain and a GPC binding domain. Partial deficiency of protein 4.1 is associated with asymptomatic HE, whereas complete deficiency leads to hemolytic anemia. Homozygous 4.1 (–/–) erythrocytes fragment more rapidly than normal at moderate shear stress, an indication of the intrinsic instability of the erythrocytes (Fig. 45–10). Membrane mechanical stability can be restored by reconstituting the deficient red cells with protein 4.1 or the protein 4.1–spectrin–actin binding site.[123] Homozygous protein 4.1 (–) erythrocytes also lack p55 and have only 30 percent of the normal content of GPC. The 4.1 (–) erythrocytes and GPC (–) Leach erythrocytes (see "Epidemiology" above) demonstrate decreased invasion and growth of *P. falciparum in vitro*.[124]

Most patients with protein 4.1–associated elliptocytosis are from certain European and Arab populations. Protein 4.1 utilizes tissue-specific translation start sites. Several HE mutations involve the downstream initiator codon. In one HE mutant lacking the downstream initiator codon, an erythroid stage-specific switch occurs from the upstream initiator codon to the downstream initiator codon. In affected patients, HE phenotype does not develop until after the developmentally regulated switch has occurred.[125] HE-related protein 4.1 variants as a result of deletion or duplication of the exons involved in spectrin, actin, and protein 4.1 binding have been described.

Glycophorin C Elliptocytes are present on the blood films of patients whose erythrocytes carry the Leach phenotype (i.e., lacking the Gerbich antigens Ge-1, Ge-2, Ge-3, and Ge-4) and lack both GPC and GPD. The Leach phenotype usually results from a 7-kb deletion of genomic DNA that removes exons 3 and 4 from the GPC/GPD locus.[126] A frameshift mutation resulting from a nucleotide deletion has been described as the cause of this phenotype. GPC-deficient subjects also are partially deficient in protein 4.1 and lack p55, presumably because these proteins form a complex and recruit or stabilize each other on the membrane. Protein 4.1 deficiency in Leach erythrocytes is speculated to be the cause of the elliptocytic shape. In contrast to other forms of HE, which are dominantly inherited, heterozygous carriers are asymptomatic, with normal red blood cell morphology, whereas homozygous subjects have no anemia, with only mild elliptocytosis seen on blood film.

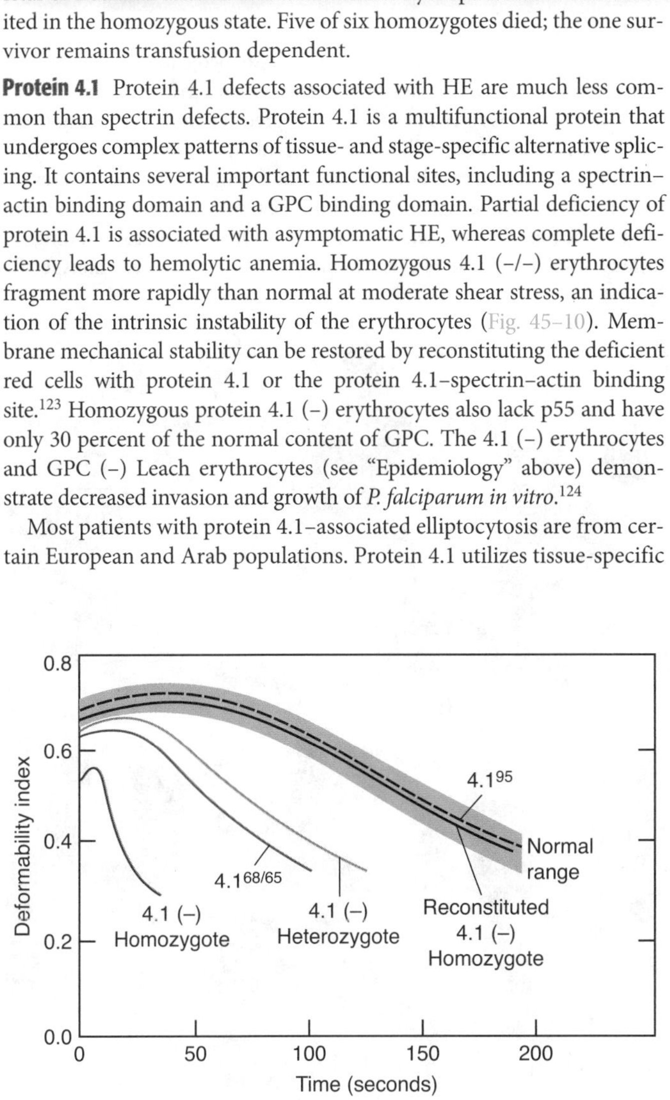

FIGURE 45–10. Stability of erythrocyte membranes with defects in protein 4.1. Red cell membranes were subjected to shear stress in an ektacytometer, and deformability was measured as a function of time. A fall in deformability occurred as the membranes fragmented. Cells completely lacking protein 4.1 (–/–) have very fragile membranes, and normal fragility can be restored by reconstitution with normal protein 4.1. Heterozygous protein 4.1 mutant cells (+/– and the variant 65/68) have intermediate stability. *(Reproduced with permission from Mohandas N, Chasis JA: Red blood cell deformability, membrane material properties and shape: Regulation by transmembrane, skeletal and cytosolic proteins and lipids.* Semin Hematol *30:171, 1993.)*

Molecular Determinants of Clinical Severity

The severity of hemolysis in common HE often varies not only among different kindred but also within a given family. Erythrocyte spectrin content and the percentage of dimeric spectrin in crude spectrin extracts are the principal determinants of hemolysis severity. The percentage of dimeric spectrin in crude spectrin extracts depends on the degree of dysfunction of the mutant spectrin and the gene dose (i.e., heterozygote vs. homozygote or compound heterozygote) or the presence of other genetic defects *in trans*. Mutations in the spectrin self-association contact site produce a more severe defect of spectrin function and clinical phenotype than do other elliptocytogenic mutations.

The low-expression Lyon α-spectrin (α^{LELY}) allele is the best characterized polymorphism affecting spectrin content and clinical severity. The allele is characterized by an amino acid substitution, Leu1857Val, and partial skipping of exon 46.[127] The abnormalities are located in the spectrin heterodimer nucleation site (i.e., where spectrin monomers assemble into heterodimers). The α-spectrin chains lacking exon 46 are poorly assembled into $\alpha\beta$ heterodimers and are rapidly degraded.[128] Alone, the α^{LELY} allele is clinically silent, even when inherited in the homozygous state, because α-spectrin normally is synthesized in threefold to fourfold excess.[54] When the α^{LELY} allele is present *in trans* to an elliptocytogenic α-spectrin mutation, it increases the mutant spectrin concentration and worsens the disease. Conversely, when the α^{LELY} allele is *in cis* to an α-spectrin mutation, it mutes the elliptocytic phenotype.

Certain acquired factors may affect the clinical severity of HE. In neonatal red cells, the weak binding of 2,3-BPG by fetal hemoglobin leads to an increase in free 2,3-BPG, which in turn induces a superimposed destabilization of spectrin–actin–protein 4.1 interaction.[129] Finally, hemolytic anemia can be worsened by several acquired conditions, including those that alter microcirculatory stress to the cells.

Inheritance

HE is inherited as an autosomal dominant disorder in most patients. Clinical severity is highly variable among different kindreds, reflecting heterogeneous molecular lesions, and, to a lesser extent, in a given kindred, presumably because of other genetic or acquired defects that modify disease expression. Rare cases of *de novo* mutation have been described,[130] as has an HE kindred with a contiguous gene deletion syndrome inherited in an X-linked pattern.[131]

Clinical Features

The clinical presentation of HE is heterogenous, ranging from asymptomatic carriers to patients with severe, life-threatening anemia. The overwhelming majority of patients with HE are asymptomatic and are diagnosed incidentally during testing for unrelated conditions.

Asymptomatic carriers who possess the same molecular defect as an affected HE relative but who have normal or near normal blood films have been identified. The erythrocyte life span is normal, and the patients are not anemic. Asymptomatic HE patients may experience hemolysis in association with infections, hypersplenism, vitamin B_{12} deficiency, or microangiopathic hemolysis such as disseminated intravascular coagulation or thrombotic thrombocytopenic purpura. In the latter two conditions, increased hemolysis may result from microcirculatory damage superimposed on the underlying mechanical instability of red cells.

HE patients with chronic hemolysis experience moderate to severe hemolytic anemia with elliptocytes and poikilocytes on blood film. Red cell life span is decreased, and patients may develop complications of chronic hemolysis, such as gallbladder disease. In some kindreds, the hemolytic HE has been transmitted through several generations. In other kindreds, not all HE subjects have chronic hemolysis; some have only mild hemolysis, presumably because another genetic factor modifies disease expression. The blood films of the most severe HE patients with chronic hemolysis exhibit elliptocytes, poikilocytes, and very small microspherocytes. Thus, their clinical presentation is indistinguishable from HPP.

HPP represents a subtype of common HE, as evidenced by the coexistence of HE and HPP in the same family and the presence of the same molecular defect of spectrin.[114,115] Unlike HE subjects carrying the spectrin mutation, red cells of HPP subjects are also partially deficient in spectrin. Typically, one parent of the HPP offspring carries an elliptocytogenic α-spectrin mutation, while the other parent is fully asymptomatic and has no detectable biochemical abnormality. In many patients, the asymptomatic parent carries a silent "thalassemia-like" defect of spectrin synthesis, enhancing the expression of the spectrin mutant and leading to a superimposed spectrin deficiency in HPP offspring.[115] Some HPP subjects inherit two structural variants of α-spectrin. In these HPP patients, spectrin deficiency may result from instability of the mutant spectrin. HPP is seen predominantly in subjects of African descent, but HPP also has been diagnosed in subjects of Arabic and European descent.[39]

Hereditary Elliptocytosis and Pyropoikilocytosis in Infancy

Clinical symptoms of elliptocytosis are uncommon in the neonatal period. Typically, elliptocytes do not appear on the blood film until the patient is 4 to 6 months old. Occasionally, severe forms of HE present in the neonatal period with severe, hemolytic anemia with marked poikilocytosis and jaundice. These patients may require red cell transfusion, phototherapy, or exchange transfusion. Usually, even in severely affected patients, the hemolysis abates between 6 and 12 months of age, and the patient progresses to typical HE with mild anemia. Infrequently, patients remain transfusion dependent beyond the first year of life and require early splenectomy. In cases of suspected neonatal HE or HPP, review of family history and analysis of blood films from the parents usually are of greater diagnostic benefit than other available studies.

A few cases of hydrops fetalis accompanied by fetal or early neonatal death as a result of unusually severe forms of HE have been described.[121] One severely affected hydropic infant salvaged by intrauterine transfusions and early exchange transfusion has remained transfusion dependent for more than 2 years.

Laboratory Features

The hallmark of HE is the presence of cigar-shaped elliptocytes on blood film (Fig. 45–11). These normochromic, normocytic elliptocytes may number from a few to 100 percent. The degree of hemolysis does not correlate with the number of elliptocytes present. Spherocytes, stomatocytes, and fragmented cells may be seen. Osmotic fragility is abnormal in severe HE and in HPP. The reticulocyte count generally is less than 5 percent but may be higher when hemolysis is severe. Other laboratory findings in HE are similar to those of other hemolytic anemias and are nonspecific

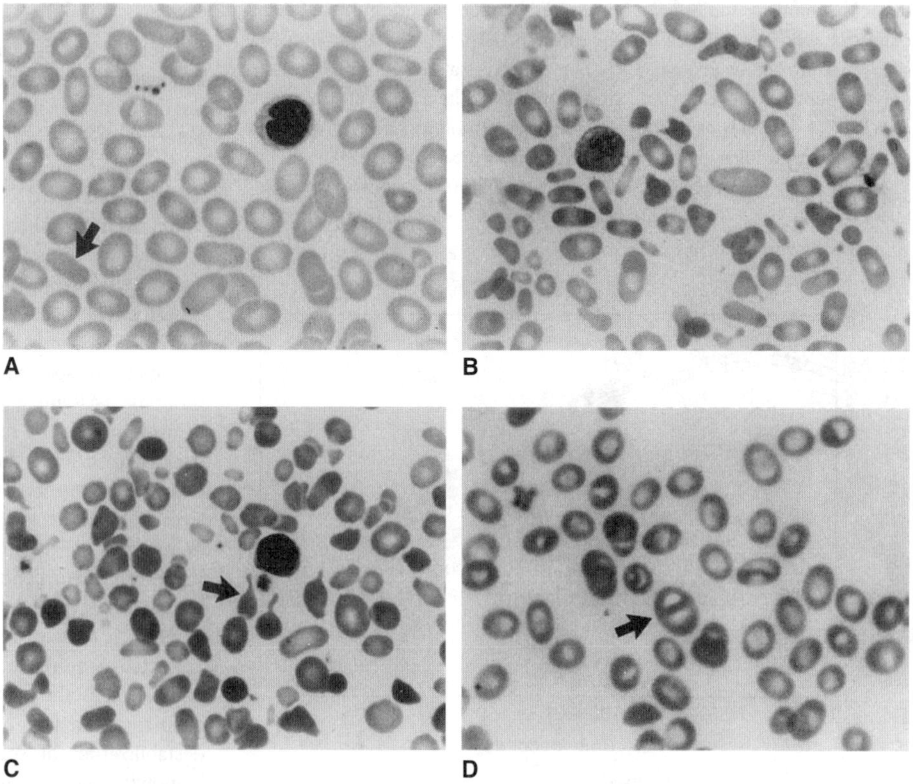

FIGURE 45–11. Blood films from patients with various forms of HE. **A.** Simple heterozygote with mild common HE associated with an elliptocytogenic spectrin mutation. Note the predominant elliptocytosis, with some rod-shaped cells (*arrow*) and the virtual absence of poikilocytes. **B.** Compound heterozygosity for common HE resulting from a double heterozygous state for two spectrin mutations. Both parents have mild HE. Many elliptocytes and numerous fragments and poikilocytes are present. **C.** HPP. The patient is a compound heterozygote for an α-spectrin self-association site mutation and a defect characterized by reduced synthesis of the protein. Note prominent microspherocytosis, micropoikilocytosis, and fragmentation. Only a few elliptocytes are present. Some poikilocytes are in the process of budding (*arrow*). **D.** Southeast Asian (Melanesian) ovalocytosis. The majority of cells are oval. Some cells contain either a longitudinal slit or a transverse ridge (*arrow*).

markers of increased erythrocyte production and destruction. For example, increased serum bilirubin, increased urinary urobilinogen, and decreased serum haptoglobin reflect increased erythrocyte destruction.

In HPP, in addition to the blood film findings seen in HE, many HPP erythrocytes are bizarrely shaped, with fragmentation or budding (see Fig. 45–11C). Microspherocytosis is common, and MCV usually is low (50–70 fl). Pyknocytes are prominent on blood films of neonates with HPP. The thermal instability of erythrocytes, originally reported as diagnostic of HPP, is not unique to this disorder; it is also commonly found in HE erythrocytes.

Specialized testing has been used in difficult cases or cases requiring a molecular diagnosis. Specialized tests include analysis of membrane proteins by one-dimensional gel electrophoresis, limited tryptic digestion of membrane spectrin followed by one- or two-dimensional gel electrophoresis, spectrin dimer self-association assays, ektacytometry, and cDNA and genomic DNA analyses.

Differential Diagnosis

Elliptocytes may be seen in association with several disorders, including megaloblastic anemias, hypochromic microcytic anemias (iron-deficiency anemia and thalassemia), myelodysplastic syndromes, and myelofibrosis. In these conditions, elliptocytosis is acquired and generally represents less than one-quarter of red cells seen on blood film. History and additional laboratory testing usually clarify the diagnosis of these disorders. Pseudoelliptocytosis is an artifact of blood film preparation. Pseudoelliptocytes are found only in certain areas of the film, usually near its tail. The long axes of pseudoelliptocytes are parallel, whereas the axes of true elliptocytes are distributed randomly.

Therapy and Prognosis

Therapy is rarely needed in patients with HE. In rare cases, occasional red blood cell transfusions may be required. In cases of severe HE and HPP, splenectomy has been palliative, as the spleen is the site of erythrocyte sequestration and destruction. The same indications for splenectomy in HS can be applied to patients with symptomatic HE or HPP. Postsplenectomy, patients with HE or HPP exhibit increased hematocrit, decreased reticulocyte counts, and improved clinical symptoms.

Patients should be followed for signs of decompensation during acute illnesses. Interval ultrasonography to detect gallstones should be performed. Patients with significant hemolysis should receive daily folate supplementation.

■ SOUTHEAST ASIAN OVALOCYTOSIS

Southeast Asian ovalocytosis, also known as *Melanesian elliptocytosis* or *stomatocytic elliptocytosis*, is a dominantly inherited trait characterized by the presence of oval red cells, many of which contain one or two transverse ridges or a longitudinal slit (see Fig. 45–11D). The condition is widespread in certain ethnic groups of Malaysia, Papua New Guinea, the Philippines, and Indonesia. Numerous abnormalities of Southeast Asian ovalocytosis erythrocytes have been reported, including increased red cell rigidity, decreased osmotic fragility, increased thermal stability, resistance to shape change by echinocytic agents, and reduced expression of many red cell antigens. Thus, Southeast Asian ovalocytosis red cells are unique among the elliptocytes in that they are rigid and hyperstable rather than unstable.[132] A remarkable feature of Southeast Asian ovalocytosis erythrocytes is their resistance to *in vitro* invasion by several strains of malaria parasites, including *P. falciparum* and *Plasmodium knowlesi*.[133]

The Southeast Asian ovalocytosis phenotype is the result of heterozygosity for two band 3 mutations *in cis*: the deletion of 27-bp encoding amino acids 400 to 408 located at the boundary of the cytoplasmic and membrane domains of band 3 and the amino acid substitution Lys56Glu.[134] The latter is an asymptomatic polymorphism. Homozygosity for Southeast Asian ovalocytosis is hypothesized to lead to embryonic lethality.[135] Southeast Asian ovalocytosis erythrocytes exhibit increased binding of band 3 to ankyrin, increased tyrosine phosphorylation of band 3, inability to transport sulfate anions, and markedly restricted lateral and rotational mobility of the band 3 protein in the membrane.

Clinically, the finding on blood film of at least 30 percent oval-shaped red cells, some containing a central slit or a transverse ridge, and the notable absence of clinical and laboratory evidence of hemolysis in a patient from the above-noted ethnic groups are highly suggestive of the diagnosis. A useful screening test is the demonstration of resistance of ovalocytes or their ghosts to changes in shape resulting from treatments that produce spiculation in normal cells, such as overnight incubation of red cells or exposure of ghosts to salt solutions. Rapid genetic diagnosis can be made by amplifying the region containing the 27-bp deletion from genomic DNA or reticulocyte cDNA and demonstrating a smaller band compared to control after electrophoresis.

In vivo, evidence indicates Southeast Asian ovalocytosis provides some protection against all forms of malaria, particularly against heavy infections and cerebral malaria.[136] The prevalence of Southeast Asian ovalocytosis increases with age in populations challenged by malaria, suggesting a selective advantage. The mechanism of malaria resistance of Southeast Asian ovalocytosis cells is speculative. Band 3 serves as one of the malaria receptors, as evidenced by inhibition of invasion *in vitro* by band 3–specific peptides.[137]

■ ACANTHOCYTOSIS

Spiculated red cells are classified into two types: acanthocytes and echinocytes. *Acanthocytes* are contracted, dense cells with irregular projections from the red cell surface that vary in width and length. *Echinocytes* have small, uniform projections spread evenly over the circumference of the red cell. The differences are clearly seen on scanning electron micrographs,[138] but may be difficult to ascertain on blood films. Acanthocytes almost always are accompanied by echinocytes, but echinocytes may be present alone. Diagnostically, the distinction is not critical, and disorders of spiculated red cells generally are classified together. Normal adults may have up to 3 percent spiculated erythrocytes on blood film, with higher levels in patients with functional or actual splenectomy, in individuals after ingestion of alcohol or certain medications (e.g., indomethacin, salicylates, furosemide), and in premature infants (mean: 5.5%; range: 1–25%). Spiculated cells, particularly echinocytes, are common artifacts of blood film preparation.

Acanthocytes are present on the blood films of patients with severe liver disease, abetalipoproteinemia, certain inherited neurologic disorders without abetalipoproteinemia, and in association with inheritance of certain red cell antigen polymorphisms such as the McLeod phenotype. Abnormal red cell membrane lipid composition and altered lipid distribution between the inner and outer leaflets of the bilayer characterize these conditions. Smaller numbers of acanthocytes (<10%) may be seen in patients with myelodysplasia, hypothyroidism, and anorexia nervosa. Echinocytes may be found on the blood films of patients with severe uremia, glycolytic defects, and microangiopathic hemolytic anemia, and transiently after transfusion of stored red cells.

■ ACANTHOCYTOSIS IN SEVERE LIVER DISEASE

Definition

The anemia in patients with liver disease is of complex etiology.[139] Common causes include blood loss, iron or folate deficiency, hypersplenism, and marrow suppression from alcohol, malnutrition, hepatitis infection, or other factors. Acquired abnormalities of the red cell membrane may contribute to the anemia in these patients; one is a syndrome of hemolysis with acanthocytosis or "spur" cells, so-called spur cell anemia.[140] Although only a small number of patients with end-stage liver disease acquire spur cell anemia, the prevalence of liver disease is so high that these individuals account for the majority of cases of acanthocytosis seen in clinical practice.

Etiology and Pathogenesis

Acanthocyte formation *in vivo* is a two-step process involving accumulation of free (nonesterified) cholesterol in the red cell membrane and remodeling of abnormally shaped red cells by the spleen.[141,142] Acanthocytes result from increased acquisition of free cholesterol from the plasma because of abnormal cholesterol to lipoprotein ratios.[141] In severe liver disease, a very high ratio of free cholesterol to phospholipids is found in lipoproteins. Free cholesterol readily partitions into the membrane, where it preferentially associates with the outer leaflet, making the membrane less fluid. The spleen attempts to remodel the membrane, leading to rigid, spherical erythrocytes with the characteristic spiculated projections (Fig. 45–12).[142] Over time, the poorly deformable cells have difficulty negotiating the narrow sinusoids of the splenic circulation and are hemolyzed (see Chap. 5).

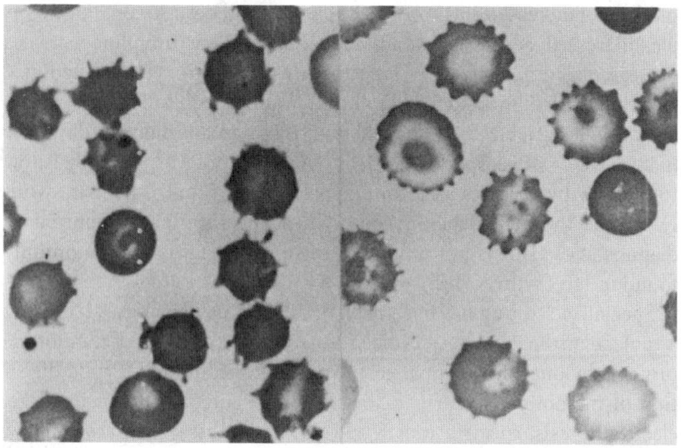

FIGURE 45–12. A. Blood film from a patient with liver cirrhosis and spur cell anemia. **B.** The conditioning effect of the spleen is evidenced by the spheroidal shape of the cells and the remodeling of the spicules. *(Reproduced with permission from Cooper RA, Kimball DB, Durocher JR.[142])*

Clinical Features

Spur cell anemia is characterized by rapidly progressive hemolytic anemia with large numbers of acanthocytes on blood film.[141,143] Splenomegaly and jaundice become more prominent and are accompanied by severe ascites, bleeding diatheses, and hepatic encephalopathy. Spur cell anemia is most common in patients with alcoholic liver disease, but similar clinical syndromes have been described in association with advanced metastatic liver disease, cardiac cirrhosis, Wilson disease, fulminant hepatitis, and infantile cholestatic liver disease.

Laboratory Features

Most patients have moderate anemia with a hematocrit of 20 to 30 percent, marked indirect hyperbilirubinemia, and laboratory evidence of severe hepatocellular disease. Blood films reveal significant acanthocytosis (see Fig. 45–12). Echinocytes, target cells, and microspherocytes, many with very fine spicules, are found in some patients.

Differential Diagnosis

Spur cell hemolytic anemia should be distinguished from other hemolytic syndromes associated with liver disease, including (1) chronic, mild hemolysis with occasional spherocytes seen in patients with congestive splenomegaly, (2) transient hemolysis associated with fatty metamorphosis of the liver and hypertriglyceridemia (which does not appear to have a causal relationship to hemolysis), (3) transient hemolytic anemia with stomatocytosis, and (4) hemolytic anemia with rigid and occasionally spiculated red cells (echinocytes), which has been reported in malnourished alcoholics with severe hypophosphatemia. Spur cell anemia appears to differ from Zieve syndrome, a poorly defined syndrome of hyperlipoproteinemia, jaundice, and spherocytic hemolytic anemia that occurs in alcoholic patients with liver disease.[144]

Therapy, Course, and Prognosis

The anemia of spur cell anemia usually is not a significant clinical problem, but it can aggravate preexisting anemias, for example, resulting from gastrointestinal bleeding, to the point that erythrocyte transfusion is required. The life span of spur cells is markedly decreased because of splenic sequestration, and, as expected, hemolysis abates after splenectomy. However, splenectomy is a dangerous and potentially fatal procedure in these critically ill patients and is generally not recommended. Spur cell anemia is an ominous clinical marker of the terminal stages of liver disease. Prior to the availability of liver transplantation, patients who reached this stage rarely lived for more than a few weeks. Spontaneous resolution of spur cell anemia may occur after orthotopic liver transplantation.

■ ABETALIPOPROTEINEMIA (BASSEN-KORNZWEIG SYNDROME)

Definition

Abetalipoproteinemia is an autosomal recessive disorder characterized by progressive ataxic neurologic disease, dietary fat malabsorption, retinitis pigmentosa, and acanthocytosis found in people of diverse ethnic backgrounds.[145]

Etiology and Pathogenesis

The primary molecular defect in this disorder is a failure to synthesize or secrete lipoproteins containing products of the apolipoprotein B gene.[145] In some patients, the inability results from lack of microsomal transfer protein, which catalyzes the transport of triglyceride, cholesterol ester, and phospholipid from phospholipid surfaces.[146] Microsomal transfer protein, a heterodimer of protein disulfide isomerase and a large 88-kDa subunit, is located in the lumen of hepatic microsomes and intestinal epithelia, the sites of lipoprotein synthesis. Other than apolipoprotein B, microsomal transfer protein is the only tissue-specific component required for secretion of apoprotein B-containing lipoproteins. All lipoproteins that contain apolipoprotein B are absent in plasma. Consequently, preformed triglycerides are not transported from the intestinal mucosa, and plasma triglycerides are nearly absent. Plasma cholesterol and phospholipid levels are markedly decreased, with a relative increase of sphingomyelin at the expense of lecithin.

In this condition, marrow red cell precursors, nucleated red cells, and reticulocytes have normal shape. Acanthocytosis becomes apparent as the red cells mature in the circulation, worsening with increasing red cell age.[147] Incubating normal red cells in abetalipoproteinemic serum does not produce acanthocytes, but normal red cells acquire acanthocytic changes when transfused into an abetalipoproteinemic recipient. Erythrocyte membrane proteins are normal, but lipids are not.[148] The cholesterol to phospholipid ratio is normal or slightly increased, reflecting changes in the distribution of plasma phospholipids and a decrease in LCAT activity. The PC concentration is decreased, and sphingomyelin is correspondingly increased. In abetalipoproteinemic acanthocytes, excess sphingomyelin is suggested to be preferentially confined to the outer membrane bilayer leaflet, causing an expansion of its surface area that may be responsible for the irregularities in cell surface contour.

Clinical Features

The disorder manifests in the first month of life by steatorrhea. Intestinal biopsy typically reveals engorgement of mucosal cells with lipid droplets. Atypical retinitis pigmentosa, which often results in blindness, and progressive neurologic abnormalities characterized by ataxia and intention tremors develop between 5 and 10 years of age and progress to death in the second or third decade.[145]

Laboratory Features

Patients usually have mild anemia with normal red cell indices and normal or slightly increased reticulocyte counts.[145,147] Acanthocytosis is prominent, ranging from approximately 50 to 90 percent of red cells. Despite the lipid abnormalities and frequent concomitant vitamin E deficiency, the hemolysis is mild, especially compared to the hemolysis that occurs with spur cell anemia (see "Acanthocytosis in Severe Liver Disease" above). The enlarged, congested spleen in patients with portal hypertension and spur cell anemia has been suggested to worsen the hemolysis, whereas the spleen is normal in patients with abetalipoproteinemia. Coagulopathy may be observed.[146]

Differential Diagnosis

The related disorders hypobetalipoproteinemia, normotriglyceridemic abetalipoproteinemia, and chylomicron retention disease are associated with partial production of apolipoprotein B-containing lipoproteins or with secretion of lipoproteins containing truncated forms of apolipoprotein B. Patients with these disorders may experience neurologic disease and acanthocytosis, depending on the severity of the underlying defect. Even patients with heterozygous hypobetalipoproteinemia may have acanthocytosis, but typically they do not.[149]

Therapy, Course, and Prognosis

Treatment includes dietary restriction of triglycerides and supplementation with high doses of vitamins A, K, D, and E.[145] Water-soluble forms of vitamin E, such as D-α-tocopherol polyethylene glycol succinate, are available for use. The role of vitamin E in the pathophysiology and clinical symptomatology of abetalipoproteinemia is unknown. Vitamin E deficiency has been suggested to be the primary stimulus for secondary manifestations of the disease, such as neuropathy, based on the observations that vitamin E may stabilize or even improve neuromuscular and retinal abnormalities in these patients and because a similar neuropathy has been observed in patients with chronic cholestasis.

ACANTHOCYTOSIS WITH NEUROLOGIC DISEASE AND NORMAL LIPOPROTEINS

Chorea-Acanthocytosis Syndrome

Chorea-acanthocytosis is a rare autosomal recessive disorder characterized by normolipoproteinemic acanthocytosis and progressive neurodegenerative disease with onset in adolescence or adult life.[150] Chorea-acanthocytosis is characterized by progressive orofacial dyskinesias with tics, limb chorea, lip and tongue biting; neurogenic muscle hypotonia and atrophy; absent or diminished reflexes; and increased serum creatine phosphokinase. Neuroimaging demonstrates abnormalities of the putamen and the head of the caudate.

Patients are not anemic, and red cell survival is only slightly decreased. In some patients, the acanthocytosis may precede the onset of neurologic symptoms. The mechanism of acanthocytosis in chorea-acanthocytosis is unknown. Plasma and erythrocyte membrane lipids and membrane fatty acid composition are normal except for a high content of saturated fatty acids.[151] Red cell membrane fluidity is decreased, and intramembrane particles are unevenly distributed, presumably because of altered lipid fluidity. Increased proteolysis of ankyrin, band 3, and protein 4.2 and increased membrane protein phosphorylation, especially of band 3, may contribute to the cell shape change. A point mutation near the COOH-terminus of band 3 has been identified in one unusual kindred with chorea-acanthocytosis.[152] The chorein gene has been cloned and mutations identified in chorea-acanthocytosis families from diverse ethnic backgrounds.[153–155] Chorein does not belong to any gene family, and no known structural motifs or domains have been identified. In yeast, its homologue is involved in protein sorting and transport.

Inherited neuroacanthocytosis syndromes other than chorea-acanthocytosis have been described.[155] These include (1) McLeod syndrome, which is described below, (2) Huntington disease-like 2, a recessively inherited syndrome with acanthocytosis, tics, parkinsonism, and occasional motor neuron disease caused by mutations in junctophilin-3, and (3) pantothenate kinase-associated neurodegeneration (formerly known as Hallervorden-Spatz syndrome), with features of progressive dementia, dystonia, spasticity, pallidal and retinal degeneration, and its allelic variant HARP syndrome (hypobetalipoproteinemia, acanthocytosis, retinitis pigmentosa, pallidal degeneration), both caused by mutations in pantothenate kinase 2.

ERYTHROCYTE DISORDERS ASSOCIATED WITH ABNORMALITIES OF KELL AND LUTHERAN BLOOD GROUPS

McLeod Syndrome

The McLeod syndrome is an X-linked anomaly of the Kell blood group system characterized by mild compensated hemolytic anemia with variable acanthocytosis and, in some patients, late-onset myopathy or chorea.[156,157] The Kell antigen consists of two major protein components: a 37-kDa protein that carries the Kx antigen, a precursor molecule necessary for the Kell antigen expression, and a 93-kDa protein that carries the Kell blood group antigen. Red cells with the McLeod phenotype have no detectable Kx antigen, and they have a marked deficiency of the 93-kDa protein that carries the Kell antigen. The *XK* gene encodes a novel 444-amino-acid integral membrane transporter. Mutations of the *XK* gene have been identified in McLeod patients.[158] Male hemizygotes who lack Kx have 80 to 85 percent acanthocytes on the blood film and mild, compensated hemolysis. Because of red cell mosaicism-produced X inactivation, female heterozygote carriers may have occasional acanthocytes on blood film,[157] and women with markedly skewed X inactivation may have more severe symptoms.

McLeod red cells should be distinguished from Kell null (K_o) red cells, which have a normal shape. In K_o cells, only the Kell antigen carrying 93-kDa glycoprotein is absent; the cells have twice the amount of the Kx antigen.[159] Patients with McLeod syndrome must be identified because they may develop antibodies that are compatible only with McLeod syndrome red cells if they receive transfusions.

The McLeod phenotype has been described in association with chronic granulomatous disease of childhood, retinitis pigmentosa, and Duchenne muscular dystrophy. These variable manifestations may result from contiguous gene deletion syndromes, as the genetic locus for these disorders is Xp21.[160] This situation may explain the occasional findings of either echinocytes or stomatocytes in Duchenne dystrophy or a choreiform disorder in some subjects with McLeod phenotype. Furthermore, some subjects with the McLeod phenotype exhibit laboratory features of myopathy and, later in life, a neurologic disorder that is first manifested by areflexia and, after the fifth decade, progresses to dystonia and choreiform movements.

Lutheran Blood Group

Approximately 1 in 3000 to 5000 people inherit the dominantly acting inhibitor *In(Lu)*, which suppresses expression of Lu^a and Lu^b, the major antigens of the Lutheran blood group system. Patients with the *In(Lu)* Lu(a–b–) phenotype *may* have abnormally shaped red cells, including poikilocytes and acanthocytes, without evidence of anemia or hemolysis.[161] The osmotic fragility of fresh *In(Lu)* Lu(a–b–) erythrocytes is normal. However, after incubation, the cells lose potassium and become osmotically resistant. Patients with this rare blood group have mutations in the erythroid transcription factor EKLF/KLF1.[162]

■ ACANTHOCYTOSIS IN OTHER CONDITIONS

A small number of acanthocytes are observed in malnutrition resulting from diverse causes, including anorexia nervosa and cystic fibrosis. The red cell shape normalizes after adequate nutritional status is restored. Very mild acanthocytosis (0.5–2%) is common in 20 to 65 percent of patients with hypothyroidism.[163] Because hypothyroidism is much more common than the other disorders that cause spiculated red cells, the finding of acanthocytes on the blood film should prompt consideration of the patient's thyroid function. This association may unmask undiagnosed cases of hypothyroidism.

STOMATOCYTOSIS AND RELATED DISORDERS

Stomatocytes are red cells characterized by a central hemoglobin-free area shaped like a cigar or sausage or a very small circle (Fig. 45–13).[164] No unifying theory explains this morphologic abnormality, which is an artifact resulting from folding of the cells during blood film preparation. Stomatocytosis, the condition in which the red blood cells are principally composed of stomatocytes, can be an inherited disorder or can occur in association with several acquired abnormalities. The latter often are associated with inherited abnormalities in red cell cation permeability that may be associated with abnormal red cell hydration or membrane lipids.[165] Disturbances of erythrocyte hydration range from the extremes of dehydration to overhydration. These variants have been divided into provisional categories based on clinical severity, morphology, cation content, lipid and protein composition, genetics, and response to splenectomy (Table 45–4).[166]

■ DEHYDRATED STOMATOCYTOSIS/ HEREDITARY XEROCYTOSIS

Definition

Dehydrated hereditary stomatocytosis (HSt), also known as *hereditary xerocytosis* or *dessicocytosis*, is the most common form of the HSt syndromes.[164–166] The predominant phenotype associated with this disorder is an autosomal dominant hemolytic anemia with red cell dehydration and decreased osmotic fragility. This phenotype has been extended to include recurrent fetal loss, hydrops fetalis, and pseudohyperkalemia (see "Therapy, Course, and Prognosis" below).

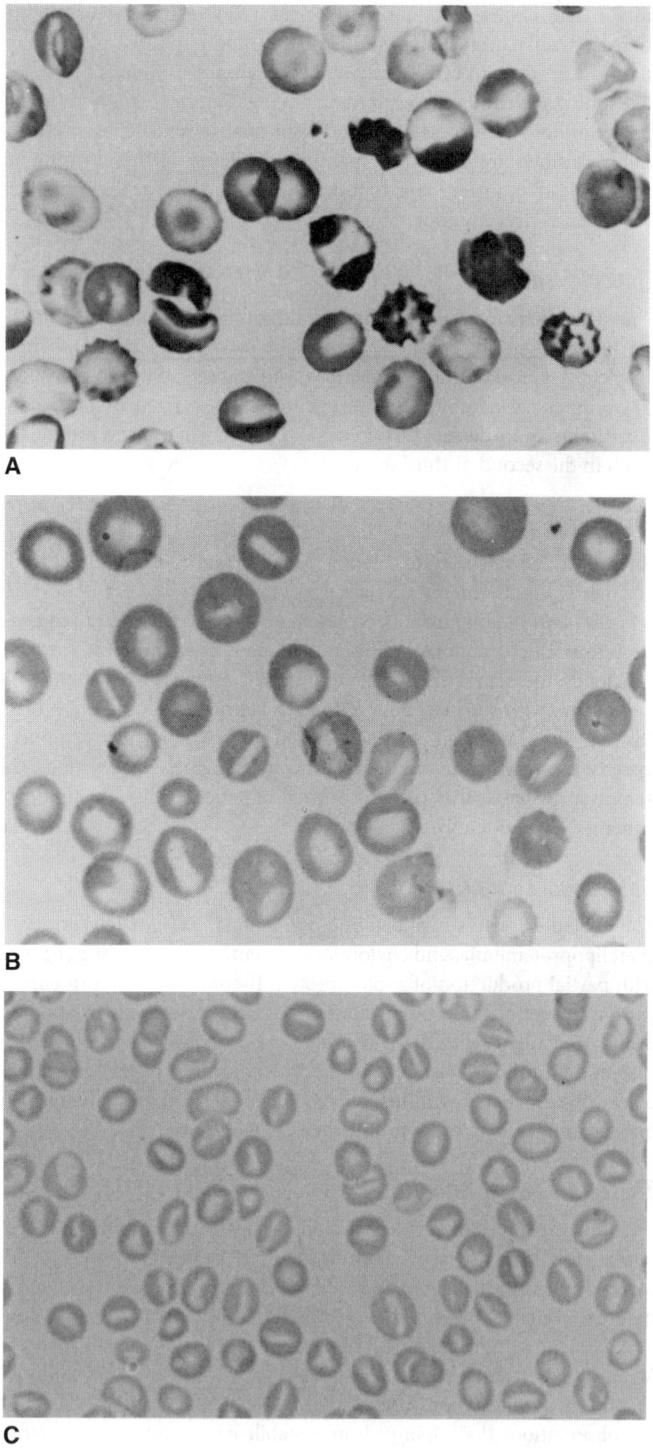

FIGURE 45–13. Stomatocytosis and variants. Blood film from patients with **A.** hereditary xerocytosis (dessicocytosis), **B.** stomatocytosis (hydrocytosis), and **C.** acquired stomatocytosis as a result of alcoholic liver disease. *(**A** and **B** reproduced with permission from Lande WM, Mentzer WC.[164])*

Etiology and Pathogenesis

The underlying permeability defect is complex and involves a net loss of potassium from the red cells (typically approximately 20%) that is not accompanied by a proportional gain of sodium.[165,166] Consequently, the net intracellular cation content and cell water content are

TABLE 45–4. Heterogeneity of the Hereditary Stomatocytosis Syndromes

	Stomatocytosis (Hydrocytosis)		Intermediate Syndromes			
	Severe Hemolysis	Mild Hemolysis	Cryohydrocytosis	Stomatocytic Xerocytosis	Xerocytosis with High Phosphatidylcholine	Xerocytosis
Hemolysis	Severe	Mild–moderate	Moderate	Mild	Moderate	Moderate
Anemia	Severe	Mild–moderate	Mild–moderate	None	Mild	Moderate
Blood film	Stomatocytes	Stomatocytes	Stomatocytes	Stomatocytes	Targets	Targets, echinocytes
MCV (80–100 fl)*	110–150	95–130	90–105	91–98	84–92	100–110
MCHC (32–36%)	24-30	26–29	34–40	33–39	34–38	34–38
Unincubated osmotic fragility	Markedly increased	Increased	Normal	Decreased	Markedly decreased	Markedly decreased
RBC Na^+ (5–12)†	60–100	30–60	40–50	10–20	10–15	10–20
RBC K^+ (90–103)	20–55	40–85	55–65	75–85	75–90	60–80
RBC Na^++K^+ (95–110)	110–140	115–145	100–105	87–103	93–99	75–90
Phosphatidylcholine content	Normal	± Increased	Normal	Normal	Increased	Normal
Cold autohemolysis	No	No	Yes	No	No	?
Effect of splenectomy‡	Good	Good	Fair	?	?	? Poor
Inheritance	Autosomal dominant?, autosomal recessive	Autosomal dominant	Autosomal dominant	Autosomal dominant	Autosomal dominant	Autosomal dominant

MCHC, mean corpuscular hemoglobin concentration; MCV, mean corpuscular volume; RBC, red blood cell.

*Values in parentheses are the normal range.

†Values for sodium, potassium, and sodium + potassium are mEq/L RBC.

‡Splenectomy may be contraindicated in these syndromes; see text for details.

SOURCE: Reproduced with permission from Gallagher PG, Forget BG, Lux SE: Disorders of the erythrocyte membrane, in *Hematology of Infancy and Childhood*, p 544. WB Saunders, Philadelphia, 1998.

decreased. In some cases, erythrocytes have increased membrane lipids, particularly PC, and reduced 2,3-BPG content.[167]

The precise genetic basis of this disorder remains unknown. A locus for some, but not all, cases of dehydrated HSt locus has been mapped to 16q23-qter.[168]

Clinical Features

Patients may present with compensated hemolytic anemia, jaundice, splenomegaly, and gallstones. This syndrome has been extended to include recurrent fetal loss, hydrops fetalis, neonatal hepatitis, and familial pseudohyperkalemia.[165] Individuals with familial pseudohyperkalemia present with asymptomatic hyperkalemia attributable to an altered passive leak of potassium across the red cell membrane *in vitro*, similar to the mechanism considered defective in xerocytosis.[169] Pseudohyperkalemia is observed in approximately one-third of xerocytosis patients. Xerocytosis, hydrops fetalis, and pseudohyperkalemia are linked in several kindreds.[170,171] Variable penetrance appears to present in this disorder, with significant disparity in clinical symptomatology between affected individuals in the same kindred. Genetic linkage analyses have mapped the familial pseudohyperkalemia locus to the same location as xerocytosis, supporting the hypothesis that the syndromes are allelic.[172]

Laboratory Features

The hematologic picture is that of mild to moderate hemolytic anemia (see Table 45–4) with increased MCHC, a reflection of cellular dehydration. Frequently, MCV is mildly increased, an artifact of Coulter-type electronic counters. In these counters, conversion of pulse height (from the resistance of a cell passing through an electric field) to a cellular volume is dependent on cell shape. Xerocytes do not deform to the same degree as normal cells, which causes the MCV to be approximately 10 percent too high. The hematocrit also is affected because the level is calculated from the MCV. Blood films do not always reveal stomatocytes, which are more prominent on wet films, but frequently target cells, dessicocytes, and spiculated cells are seen (see Fig. 45–13A). In some of the cells, hemoglobin is concentrated ("puddled") in discrete areas on the cell periphery. Erythrocyte osmotic fragility is decreased.

Therapy, Course, and Prognosis

Most patients experience only mild anemia, and therapy is not required. The patients should receive folate supplementation and be monitored for complications of hemolysis.

The effects of splenectomy have been variable, with many xerocytosis patients experiencing little or no improvement in anemia. Xerocytes have been suggested to be so functionally compromised that they are detected and eliminated in other areas of the macrophage-monocyte system. Splenectomy should be carefully considered in patients with hereditary xerocytosis. Several patients have developed hypercoagulability after splenectomy, leading to life-threatening thrombotic episodes.[173] Note that all cases of thrombosis have occurred after splenectomy. *In vitro*, stomatocytic erythrocytes from a splenectomized xerocytosis individual demonstrated increased endothelial adherence compared to stomatocytic erythrocytes from unsplenectomized family members without hypercoagulability.[174] In one hypercoagulable xerocytosis patient, pentoxifylline decreased red cell adherence.[174] Fortunately, the majority of HSt patients can maintain an adequate hemoglobin level so that splenectomy is not required. Results of treatment of splenectomized patients with long-term warfarin (Coumadin) have been variable. In a few severe cases, erythrocyte hypertransfusion has been beneficial. Unfortunately, the procedure is complicated by iron overload, a significant problem even in the absence of transfusion.

Neonates with xerocytosis have required phototherapy, red cell transfusion, and, in some cases, exchange transfusion, for treatment of anemia and hyperbilirubinemia. In a few cases, *in utero* transfusion has been required. The presence of hydrops fetalis is not a predictor of the severity of anemia later in life. Some infants experience little or no anemia later in childhood.

HEREDITARY STOMATOCYTOSIS-HYDROCYTOSIS

Definition and History

The overhydrated HSt syndromes, also known as *hereditary hydrocytosis*, are characterized by a dominantly inherited hemolytic anemia with red cell overhydration and macrocytosis. The syndrome was first described by Lock and coworkers[175] in a girl with dominantly inherited hemolytic anemia whose blood film contained red cells with a wide transverse slit, stomatocytes. Later, abnormal cation transport and cellular overhydration—hallmarks of this disorder—were discovered.[176]

Etiology and Pathogenesis

The principal lesion involves a sodium leak leading to increased intracellular sodium and water content and mildly decreased intracellular potassium.[165,177] This action is followed by a compensatory increase in the active transport of sodium and potassium by the Na^+-K^+-ATPase pump, which normally maintains low intracellular sodium and high potassium concentrations, and an ensuing increase in glycolysis. However, pump hyperactivity cannot compensate for the vastly increased sodium leak. In some patients, mutations in the RhAG protein, a component of the Rh-RhAG protein complex, have been described.[178]

The osmotic fragility of hydrocytes is markedly increased because many of the swollen red cells approach their critical hemolytic volume. For unexplained reasons, red cell membrane lipids and, consequently, membrane surface area also are increased, but the increased area is insufficient to correct the osmotic fragility. Red cell deformability is decreased.

The red cells of some patients with overhydrated HSt lack a 31-kDa integral membrane protein called *band 7.2b* or *stomatin* involved in membrane organization and cholesterol-related processes. Varying degrees of stomatin deficiency have been described in erythrocytes from most but not all patients with HSt, with younger erythroid cells demonstrating less deficiency.[179] However, the stomatin cDNA from several HSt patients was normal.[179] These results suggest a stomatin defect is not the primary defect in HSt. Because the interaction of stomatin with the glucose transporter Glut-1 switches Glut-1 from a glucose transporter to an dehydroascorbic acid transporter in human erythrocytes, it has been proposed that it might be beneficial for overhydrated stomatocytes to inhibit this interaction, providing the cells the energy they need, resulting in stomatin loss.[180]

Clinical Features

The hydrocytosis syndromes are much less common than the xerocytosis disorders. Moderate to severe anemia is present.[165] Jaundice and splenomegaly are common, as are complications of chronic hemolysis such as cholelithiasis. A tendency for iron overload, independent of transfusion status or splenectomy, has been described. No other organ system abnormalities have been described. Neonatal anemia and hyperbilirubinemia have been reported.

Laboratory Features

The blood film reveals striking stomatocytosis (see Fig. 45–13B). In addition to the anemia, red cell indices show decreased MCHC and elevated MCV (see Table 45–4). In some patients, the macrocytosis is extreme, with MCV up to 150 fl. Erythrocyte osmotic fragility is markedly increased.

Therapy, Course, and Prognosis

The majority of hydrocytosis patients suffer from significant lifelong anemia. Similar to patients with HS, patients with hydrocytosis should be monitored for complications of hemolysis, such as cholelithiasis and parvovirus infection, and should receive folate supplementation.

The results of splenectomy in this group of disorders have been variable.[166] In some patients, hemolytic anemia is improved, although often not fully corrected, by splenectomy. In other patients, the severity of hemolysis is unchanged. Splenectomy should be carefully considered in patients with the disorder. Like patients with xerocytosis, several patients with hydrocytosis have developed hypercoagulability after splenectomy, leading to catastrophic thrombotic episodes.[173] *In vivo*, venous thromboemboli predominate, sometimes with complicating pulmonary or portal hypertension. The thrombotic risk is independent of postsplenectomy thrombosis, and all cases of thrombosis have occurred in splenectomized patients. Results of treatment of splenectomized patients with long-term warfarin have been variable. In severe cases, erythrocyte hypertransfusion has been beneficial. Unfortunately, the procedure is complicated by iron overload, a significant problem even in the absence of transfusion.

Neonates with hydrocytosis have required phototherapy, red cell transfusion, and, in some cases, exchange transfusion for treatment of anemia and hyperbilirubinemia.

INTERMEDIATE SYNDROMES

Some reported cases of HSt share features of hereditary xerocytosis and hereditary hydrocytosis. These disorders have been characterized as *intermediate syndromes* (see Table 45–4).[166] Characteristically, patients have stomatocytes and/or target cells on blood film. Erythrocyte osmotic fragility is either normal or decreased. Red cell sodium and potassium permeabilities are increased, but the intracellular cation concentration and the red cell volume are either normal or slightly reduced. In a few patients, red cells undergo spontaneous *in vitro* hemolysis after storage at 5°C, hence the designation *cryohydrocytosis*.[181] In some cases of cryohydrocytosis, missense mutations have been found in band 3, between membrane span eight and the last two membrane-spanning domains. *In vitro* studies suggest these mutations convert band 3 from an anion exchanger to a nonselective cation leak channel.[182]

A dominantly inherited hemolytic anemia with stomatocytosis, occasional target cells, spherocytes, and decreased osmotic fragility, in which the main red cell membrane abnormality involved an almost 50 percent increase in PC and a corresponding decrease in PE, has been described.[183] In wet preparations, approximately 30 percent of the cells were stomatocytes. The molecular basis of the syndrome is unclear. Because abnormalities in membrane phospholipid composition have not been systematically investigated, it is unclear whether the disorder represents a distinct disease entity.

Rh Deficiency Syndrome

Rh deficiency syndrome designates rare individuals who have either absent (Rh_{null}) or markedly reduced (Rh_{mod}) Rh antigen expression and reduced or absent proteins of the Rh–RhAG complex, including Rh, RhAG, LW, glycophorin B, CD47, and protein 4.2. Mild to moderate hemolytic anemia associated with the presence of stomatocytes and occasional spherocytes on blood film are observed.[184,185] Chap. 137 reviews the structure, localization, and functions of the Rh antigens.

Although the clinical syndromes are similar, the genetic bases of the Rh deficiency syndrome are heterogeneous, and at least two groups can be defined. The *amorph type* results from mutations of Rh30, RhD, and RhE polypeptides. The *regulatory type* results from mutations of Rh50, a modulator of Rh gene expression. Studies of these rare patients have provided evidence that both the Rh locus and Rh50 are required for the expression and function of Rh as a multimeric complex in the red cell membrane.

Red cells of some Rh_{null} patients have increased osmotic fragility reflecting a markedly reduced membrane surface area. The cells also are dehydrated, as indicated by decreased cell cation and water content and increased cell density. Potassium transport and Na^+-K^+ pump activity are increased, possibly because of reticulocytosis. Hemolytic anemia is improved by splenectomy.

FAMILIAL DEFICIENCY OF HIGH-DENSITY LIPOPROTEINS

Severe deficiency or absence of high-density lipoproteins leads to accumulation of cholesteryl esters in many tissues, leading to clinical findings of large orange tonsils and hepatosplenomegaly. Reported hematologic manifestations include moderately severe hemolytic anemia with stomatocytosis.[186] Membrane lipid analyses have shown a low cholesterol content leading to a decreased ratio of cholesterol to phospholipid and a relative increase in PC at the expense of sphingomyelin.

ACQUIRED STOMATOCYTOSIS

Few stomatocytes (3–5%) are commonly found on blood films of normal subjects. Prospective analysis of films from a large number of hospitalized patients revealed an overall incidence of stomatocytosis (>5% of stomatocytes) of 2.3 percent.[187] Fifty-nine percent of the patients had 5 to 20 percent stomatocytes, 35 percent had 20 to 50 percent stomatocytes, and 6 percent had more than 50 percent stomatocytes. A wide variety of medications and diagnoses, including malignant neoplasms, cardiovascular disease, hepatobiliary disease, and alcoholism, were associated with stomatocytosis. Additional studies are required to determine which associations are specific and reproducible. For instance, acquired stomatocytosis is common in alcoholics, particularly those with acute alcoholism (see Fig. 45–13C).[188] Vinca alkaloids, such as vincristine and vinblastine, may induce hemolysis, with increased sodium permeability and stomatocytosis at the doses used for chemotherapy of leukemias and lymphomas.[189,190] The molecular basis of stomatocytosis in these conditions is unknown. Stomatocytosis is rarely associated with clinically significant hematologic abnormalities.

REFERENCES

1. Jakobik V, Burus I, Decsi T: Fatty acid composition of erythrocyte membrane lipids in healthy subjects from birth to young adulthood. *Eur J Pediatr* 168:141, 2009.
2. Ways P, Hanahan DJ: Characterization and quantification of red cell lipids in normal man. *J Lipid Res* 5:318, 1964.
3. Bevers EM, Comfurius P, Dekkers DW, et al: Lipid translocation across the plasma membrane of mammalian cells. *Biochim Biophys Acta* 1439:317, 1999.
4. Daleke DL: Regulation of phospholipid asymmetry in the erythrocyte membrane. *Curr Opin Hematol* 15:191, 2008.
5. Devaux PF, Herrmann A, Ohlwein N, et al: How lipid flippases can modulate membrane structure. *Biochim Biophys Acta* 1778:1591, 2008.
6. Dekkers DW, Comfurius P, Schroit AJ, et al: Transbilayer movement of NBD-labeled phospholipids in red blood cell membranes: Outward-directed transport by the multidrug resistance protein 1 (MRP1). *Biochemistry* 37:14833, 1998.
7. Sahu SK, Gummadi SN, Manoj N, et al: Phospholipid scramblases: An overview. *Arch Biochem Biophys* 462:103, 2007.
8. Zhao J, Zhou Q, Wiedmer T, et al: Level of expression of phospholipid scramblase regulates induced movement of phosphatidylserine to the cell surface. *J Biol Chem* 273:6603, 1998.
9. Dekkers DW, Comfurius P, Vuist WM, et al: Impaired Ca^{2+}-induced tyrosine phosphorylation and defective lipid scrambling in erythrocytes from a patient with Scott syndrome: A study using an inhibitor for scramblase that mimics the defect in Scott syndrome. *Blood* 91:2133, 1998.
10. Stout JG, Basse F, Luhm RA, et al: Scott syndrome erythrocytes contain a membrane protein capable of mediating Ca^{2+}-dependent transbilayer migration of membrane phospholipids. *J Clin Invest* 99:2232, 1997.
11. Salzer U, Prohaska R: Stomatin, flotillin-1, and flotillin-2 are major integral proteins of erythrocyte lipid rafts. *Blood* 97:1141, 2001.
12. Salzer U, Hinterdorfer P, Hunger U, et al: Ca(++)-dependent vesicle release from erythrocytes involves stomatin-specific lipid rafts, synexin (annexin VII), and sorcin. *Blood* 99:2569, 2002.
13. Murphy SC, Samuel BU, Harrison T, et al: Erythrocyte detergent-resistant membrane proteins: Their characterization and selective uptake during malarial infection. *Blood* 103:1920, 2004.
14. Mulder E, van Deenen LL: Metabolism of red-cell lipids. I. Incorporation *in vitro* of fatty acids into phospholipids from mature erythrocytes. *Biochim Biophys Acta* 106:106, 1965.
15. Reed CF: Incorporation of orthophosphate-^{32}P into erythrocyte phospholipids in normal subjects and in patients with hereditary spherocytosis. *J Clin Invest* 47:2630, 1968.
16. Shohet SB, Nathan DG, Karnovsky ML: Stages in the incorporation of fatty acids into red blood cells. *J Clin Invest* 47:1096, 1968.
17. Renooij W, Van Golde LM: Asymmetry in the renewal of molecular classes of phosphatidylcholine in the rat-erythrocyte membrane. *Biochim Biophys Acta* 558:314, 1979.
18. Shohet SB, Haley JE: Red cell membrane shape and stability: Relation to cell lipid renewal pathways and cell ATP. *Nouv Rev Fr Hematol* 12:761, 1972.
19. Fairbanks G, Steck TL, Wallach DF: Electrophoretic analysis of the major polypeptides of the human erythrocyte membrane. *Biochemistry* 10:2606, 1971.
20. Williamson RC, Toye AM: Glycophorin A: Band 3 aid. *Blood Cells Mol Dis* 41:35, 2008.
21. Stefanovic M, Markham NO, Parry EM, et al: An 11-amino acid beta-hairpin loop in the cytoplasmic domain of band 3 is responsible for ankyrin binding in mouse erythrocytes. *Proc Natl Acad Sci U S A* 104:13972, 2007.
22. Bruce LJ, Beckmann R, Ribeiro ML, et al: A band 3-based macrocomplex of integral and peripheral proteins in the RBC membrane. *Blood* 101:4180, 2003.
23. Zhang D, Kiyatkin A, Bolin JT, et al: Crystallographic structure and functional interpretation of the cytoplasmic domain of erythrocyte membrane band 3. *Blood* 96:2925, 2000.
24. Reid ME, Mohandas N: Red blood cell blood group antigens: Structure and function. *Semin Hematol* 41:93, 2004.
25. Nicolas V, Le Van Kim C, Gane P, et al: Rh-RhAG/ankyrin-R, a new interaction site between the membrane bilayer and the red cell skeleton, is impaired by Rh(null)-associated mutation. *J Biol Chem* 278:25526, 2003.
26. Westhoff CM: The structure and function of the Rh antigen complex. *Semin Hematol* 44:42, 2007.
27. Bennett V, Healy J: Organizing the fluid membrane bilayer: Diseases linked to spectrin and ankyrin. *Trends Mol Med* 14:28, 2008.
28. Gallagher PG, Forget BG: Spectrin genes in health and disease. *Semin Hematol* 30:4, 1993.
29. Thomas GH, Newbern EC, Korte CC, et al: Intragenic duplication and divergence in the spectrin superfamily of proteins. *Mol Biol Evol* 14:1285, 1997.
30. Grum VL, Li D, MacDonald RI, et al: Structures of two repeats of spectrin suggest models of flexibility. *Cell* 98:523, 1999.
31. Li D, Tang HY, Speicher DW: A structural model of the erythrocyte spectrin heterodimer initiation site determined using homology modeling and chemical cross-linking. *J Biol Chem* 283:1553, 2008.
32. Alloisio N, Morle L, Marechal J, et al: Sp alpha V/41: A common spectrin polymorphism at the alpha IV-alpha V domain junction. Relevance to the expression level of hereditary elliptocytosis due to alpha-spectrin variants located in trans. *J Clin Invest* 87:2169, 1991.
33. Becker PS, Schwartz MA, Morrow JS, et al: Radiolabel-transfer cross-linking demonstrates that protein 4.1 binds to the N-terminal region of beta spectrin and to actin in binary interactions. *Eur J Biochem* 193:827, 1990.
34. Ipsaro JJ, Huang L, Mondragon A: Structures of the spectrin-ankyrin interaction binding domains. *Blood* 113:5385, 2009.
35. Stabach PR, Simonovic I, Ranieri MA, et al: The structure of the ankyrin-binding site of beta-spectrin reveals how tandem spectrin-repeats generate unique ligand-binding properties. *Blood* 113:5377, 2009.
36. Gallagher PG, Tse WT, Scarpa AL, et al: Structure and organization of the human ankyrin-1 gene. Basis for complexity of pre-mRNA processing. *J Biol Chem* 272:19220, 1997.
37. Michaely P, Tomchick DR, Machius M, et al: Crystal structure of a 12 ANK repeat stack from human ankyrinR. *EMBO J* 21:6387, 2002.
38. Hou VC, Conboy JG: Regulation of alternative pre-mRNA splicing during erythroid differentiation. *Curr Opin Hematol* 8:74, 2001.

39. Gallagher PG: Hereditary elliptocytosis: Spectrin and protein 4.1R. *Semin Hematol* 41:142, 2004.
40. Shi ZT, Afzal V, Coller B, et al: Protein 4.1R-deficient mice are viable but have erythroid membrane skeleton abnormalities. *J Clin Invest* 103:331, 1999.
41. Satchwell TJ, Shoemark DK, Sessions RB, et al: Protein 4.2: A complex linker. *Blood Cells Mol Dis* 42:201, 2009.
42. Peters LL, Jindel HK, Gwynn B, et al: Mild spherocytosis and altered red cell ion transport in protein 4. 2-null mice. *J Clin Invest* 103:1527, 1999.
43. Chishti AH: Function of p55 and its nonerythroid homologues. *Curr Opin Hematol* 5:116, 1998.
44. Gilligan DM, Lozovatsky L, Gwynn B, et al: Targeted disruption of the beta adducin gene (Add2) causes red blood cell spherocytosis in mice. *Proc Natl Acad Sci U S A* 96:10717, 1999.
45. Robledo RF, Ciciotte SL, Gwynn B, et al: Targeted deletion of alpha-adducin results in absent beta- and gamma-adducin, compensated hemolytic anemia, and lethal hydrocephalus in mice. *Blood* 112:4298, 2008.
46. Khan AA, Hanada T, Mohseni M, et al: Dematin and adducin provide a novel link between the spectrin cytoskeleton and human erythrocyte membrane by directly interacting with glucose transporter-1. *J Biol Chem* 283:14600, 2008.
47. De Matteis MA, Morrow JS: The role of ankyrin and spectrin in membrane transport and domain formation. *Curr Opin Cell Biol* 10:542, 1998.
48. Liu SC, Derick LH, Palek J: Visualization of the hexagonal lattice in the erythrocyte membrane skeleton. *J Cell Biol* 104:527, 1987.
49. Salomao M, Zhang X, Yang Y, et al: Protein 4.1R-dependent multiprotein complex: New insights into the structural organization of the red blood cell membrane. *Proc Natl Acad Sci U S A* 105:8026, 2008.
50. Giorgi M, Cianci CD, Gallagher PG, et al: Spectrin oligomerization is cooperatively coupled to membrane assembly: A linkage targeted by many hereditary hemolytic anemias? *Exp Mol Pathol* 70:215, 2001.
51. Mohandas N, Chasis JA: Red blood cell deformability, membrane material properties and shape: Regulation by transmembrane, skeletal and cytosolic proteins and lipids. *Semin Hematol* 30:171, 1993.
52. Mohandas N, Chasis JA, Shohet SB: The influence of membrane skeleton on red cell deformability, membrane material properties, and shape. *Semin Hematol* 20:225, 1983.
53. Li J, Lykotrafitis G, Dao M, et al: Cytoskeletal dynamics of human erythrocyte. *Proc Natl Acad Sci U S A* 104:4937, 2007.
54. Hanspal M, Palek J: Biogenesis of normal and abnormal red blood cell membrane skeleton. *Semin Hematol* 29:305, 1992.
55. Peters LL, White RA, Birkenmeier CS, et al: Changing patterns in cytoskeletal mRNA expression and protein synthesis during murine erythropoiesis *in vivo*. *Proc Natl Acad Sci U S A* 89:5749, 1992.
56. Chasis JA, Prenant M, Leung A, et al: Membrane assembly and remodeling during reticulocyte maturation. *Blood* 74:1112, 1989.
57. Koury MJ, Bondurant MC, Rana SS: Changes in erythroid membrane proteins during erythropoietin-mediated terminal differentiation. *J Cell Physiol* 133:438, 1987.
58. Gallagher PG: Disorders of erythrocyte metabolism and shape, in *Hematologic Problems in the Neonate*, edited by RD Christensen, p 209. WB Saunders, Philadelphia, 1999.
59. Brugnara C: Erythrocyte membrane transport physiology. *Curr Opin Hematol* 4:122, 1997.
60. Adragna NC, Fulvio MD, Lauf PK: Regulation of K-Cl cotransport: From function to genes. *J Membr Biol* 201:109, 2004.
61. Brugnara C: Sickle cell disease: From membrane pathophysiology to novel therapies for prevention of erythrocyte dehydration. *J Pediatr Hematol Oncol* 25:927, 2003.
62. Carbrey JM, Agre P: Discovery of the aquaporins and development of the field. *Handb Exp Pharmacol* 3, 2009.
63. Chretien S, Catron JP: A single mutation inside the NPA motif of aquaporin-1 found in a Colton- null phenotype. *Blood* 93:4021, 1999.
64. Dacie JV. The life span of the red blood cell and circumstances of its premature death, in *Blood Pure and Eloquent*, edited by MM Wintrobe, p 211. McGraw-Hill, New York, 1980.
65. Perrotta S, Gallagher PG, Mohandas N: Hereditary spherocytosis. *Lancet* 372:1411, 2008.
66. Eber SW, Gonzalez JM, Lux ML, et al: Ankyrin-1 mutations are a major cause of dominant and recessive hereditary spherocytosis. *Nat Genet* 13:214, 1996.
67. Mariani M, Barcellini W, Vercellati C, et al: Clinical and hematologic features of 300 patients affected by hereditary spherocytosis grouped according to the type of the membrane protein defect. *Haematologica* 93:1310, 2008.
68. Eber SW, Pekrun A, Reinhardt D, et al: Hereditary spherocytosis with ankyrin Walsrode, a variant ankyrin with decreased affinity for band 3. *Blood* 84:362a, 1994.
69. Gallagher PG, Sabatino DE, Basseres DS, et al: Erythrocyte ankyrin promoter mutations associated with recessive hereditary spherocytosis cause significant abnormalities in ankyrin expression. *J Biol Chem* 276:41683, 2001.
70. Lux SE, Tse WT, Menninger JC, et al: Hereditary spherocytosis associated with deletion of human erythrocyte ankyrin gene on chromosome 8. *Nature* 345:736, 1990.
71. An X, Mohandas N: Disorders of red cell membrane. *Br J Haematol* 141:367, 2008.
72. Lima PR, Gontijo JA, Lopes de Faria JB, et al: Band 3 Campinas: A novel splicing mutation in the band 3 gene (AE1) associated with hereditary spherocytosis, hyperactivity of Na+/Li+ countertransport and an abnormal renal bicarbonate handling. *Blood* 90:2810, 1997.
73. Rysava R, Tesar V, Jirsa M Jr, et al: Incomplete distal renal tubular acidosis coinherited with a mutation in the band 3 (AE1) gene. *Nephrol Dial Transplant* 12:1869, 1997.
74. Agre P, Asimos A, Casella JF, et al: Inheritance pattern and clinical response to splenectomy as a reflection of erythrocyte spectrin deficiency in hereditary spherocytosis. *N Engl J Med* 315:1579, 1986.
75. Agre P, Casella JF, Zinkham WH, et al: Partial deficiency of erythrocyte spectrin in hereditary spherocytosis. *Nature* 314:380, 1985.
76. Wichterle H, Hanspal M, Palek J, et al: Combination of two mutant alpha spectrin alleles underlies a severe spherocytic hemolytic anemia. *J Clin Invest* 98:2300, 1996.
77. Tse WT, Gallagher PG, Jenkins PB, et al: Amino-acid substitution in alpha-spectrin commonly coinherited with nondominant hereditary spherocytosis. *Am J Hematol* 54:233, 1997.
78. Hassoun H, Vassiliadis JN, Murray J, et al: Characterization of the underlying molecular defect in hereditary spherocytosis associated with spectrin deficiency. *Blood* 90:398, 1997.
79. Becker PS, Tse WT, Lux SE, et al: Beta spectrin Kissimmee: A spectrin variant associated with autosomal dominant hereditary spherocytosis and defective binding to protein 4.1. *J Clin Invest* 92:612, 1993.
80. Bouhassira EE, Schwartz RS, Yawata Y, et al: An alanine-to-threonine substitution in protein 4.2 cDNA is associated with a Japanese form of hereditary hemolytic anemia (protein 4.2NIPPON). *Blood* 79:1846, 1992.
81. Jarolim P, Palek J, Rubin HL, et al: Band 3 Tuscaloosa: Pro327Arg327 substitution in the cytoplasmic domain of erythrocyte band 3 protein associated with spherocytic hemolytic anemia and partial deficiency of protein 4.2. *Blood* 80:523, 1992.
82. Rybicki AC, Qiu JJ, Musto S, et al: Human erythrocyte protein 4.2 deficiency associated with hemolytic anemia and a homozygous 40glutamic acidlysine substitution in the cytoplasmic domain of band 3 (band 3Montefiore). *Blood* 81:2155, 1993.
83. De Franceschi L, Olivieri O, Miraglia del Giudice E, et al: Membrane cation and anion transport activities in erythrocytes of hereditary spherocytosis: Effects of different membrane protein defects. *Am J Hematol* 55:121, 1997.
84. Young LE, Platzer RF, Ervin DM, et al: Hereditary spherocytosis. II. Observations on the role of the spleen. *Blood* 6:1099, 1951.
85. Emerson CP Jr, Shein SC, Ham TH, et al: Studies on the destruction of red blood cells. IX. Quantitative methods for determining the osmotic and mechanical fragility of red cells in the peripheral blood and splenic pulp; the mechanism of increased hemolysis in hereditary spherocytosis (congenital hemolytic jaundice) as related to the functions of the spleen. *AMA Arch Intern Med* 97:1, 1956.
86. Miraglia del Giudice E, Francese M, Nobili B, et al: High frequency of de novo mutations in ankyrin gene (ANK1) in children with hereditary spherocytosis. *J Pediatr* 132:117, 1998.
87. Miraglia del Giudice E, Lombardi C, Francese M, et al: Frequent *de novo* monoallelic expression of beta-spectrin gene (SPTB) in children with hereditary spherocytosis and isolated spectrin deficiency. *Br J Haematol* 101:251, 1998.
88. Perrotta S, Nigro V, Iolascon A, et al: Dominant hereditary spherocytosis due to band 3 Neapolis produces a life-threatening anemia at the homozygous state. *Blood* 92:9a, 1998.
89. Ribeiro ML, Alloisio N, Almeida H, et al: Severe hereditary spherocytosis and distal renal tubular acidosis associated with the total absence of band 3. *Blood* 96:1602, 2000.
90. Eber SW, Armbrust R, Schroter W: Variable clinical severity of hereditary spherocytosis: Relation to erythrocytic spectrin concentration, osmotic fragility, and autohemolysis. *J Pediatr* 117:409, 1990.
91. Pajor A, Lehoczky D, Szakacs Z: Pregnancy and hereditary spherocytosis. Report of 8 patients and a review. *Arch Gynecol Obstet* 253:37, 1993.
92. Delhommeau F, Cynober T, Schischmanoff PO, et al: Natural history of hereditary spherocytosis during the first year of life. *Blood* 95:393, 2000.
93. Iolascon A, Faienza MF, Moretti A, et al: UGT1 promoter polymorphism accounts for increased neonatal appearance of hereditary spherocytosis. *Blood* 91:1093, 1998.
94. Tamary H, Aviner S, Freud E, et al: High incidence of early cholelithiasis detected by ultrasonography in children and young adults with hereditary spherocytosis. *J Pediatr Hematol Oncol* 25:952, 2003.
95. Young NS: Hematologic manifestations and diagnosis of parvovirus B19 infections. *Clin Adv Hematol Oncol* 4:908, 2006.
96. Lefrere JJ, Courouce AM, Girot R, et al: Six cases of hereditary spherocytosis revealed by human parvovirus infection. *Br J Haematol* 62:653, 1986.
97. McLellan NJ, Rutter N: Hereditary spherocytosis in sisters unmasked by parvovirus infection. *Postgrad Med J* 63:49, 1987.
98. Giraldi S, Abbage KT, Marinoni LP, et al: Leg ulcer in hereditary spherocytosis. *Pediatr Dermatol* 20:427, 2003.
99. Sutton CD, Garcea G, Marshall LJ, et al: Pelvic extramedullary haematopoiesis associated with hereditary spherocytosis. *Eur J Haematol* 70:326, 2003.
100. Conti JA, Howard LM: Hereditary spherocytosis and hematologic malignancy. *N J Med* 91:95, 1994.
101. Peters LL, Barker JE. Spontaneous and targeted mutations in erythrocyte membrane skeleton genes: Mouse models of hereditary spherocytosis, in *Hematopoiesis*, edited by LI Zon, p. 582. Oxford University Press, New York, 2001.
102. Michaels LA, Cohen AR, Zhao H, et al: Screening for hereditary spherocytosis by use of automated erythrocyte indexes. *J Pediatr* 130:957, 1997.
103. Pati AR, Patton WN, Harris RI: The use of the Technicon H1 in the diagnosis of hereditary spherocytosis. *Clin Lab Haematol* 11:27, 1989.
104. Young LE, Izzo MJ, Platzer RF: Hereditary spherocytosis. I. Clinical, hematologic and genetic features in 28 cases, with particular reference to the osmotic and mechanical fragility of incubated erythrocytes. *Blood* 6:1073, 1951.

105. King MJ, Smythe JS, Mushens R: Eosin-5-maleimide binding to band 3 and Rh-related proteins forms the basis of a screening test for hereditary spherocytosis. *Br J Haematol* 124:106, 2004.
106. Girodon F, Garcon L, Bergoin E, et al: Usefulness of the eosin-5-maleimide cytometric method as a first-line screening test for the diagnosis of hereditary spherocytosis: Comparison with ektacytometry and protein electrophoresis. *Br J Haematol* 140:468, 2008.
107. Schilling RF: Risks and benefits of splenectomy versus no splenectomy for hereditary spherocytosis—A personal view. *Br J Haematol* 145:728, 2009.
108. Rescorla FJ, West KW, Engum SA, et al: Laparoscopic splenic procedures in children: Experience in 231 children. *Ann Surg* 246:683, 2007.
109. Tracy ET, Rice HE: Partial splenectomy for hereditary spherocytosis. *Pediatr Clin North Am* 55:503, 2008.
110. Dacie JV: Hereditary elliptocytosis (HE), in *The Haemolytic Anaemias,* vol 1, 3rd ed, p 216. Churchill Livingstone, Edinburg, 1985.
111. Glele-Kakai C, Garbarz M, Lecomte MC, et al: Epidemiological studies of spectrin mutations related to hereditary elliptocytosis and spectrin polymorphisms in Benin. *Br J Haematol* 95:57, 1996.
112. Dresbach M: Elliptical human red cell corpuscles. *Science* 19:469, 1904.
113. Hunter WC, Adams RB: Hematologic study of three generations of a white family showing elliptical erythrocytes. *Ann Intern Med* 2:1162, 1929.
114. Zarkowsky HS, Mohandas N, Speaker CB, et al: A congenital haemolytic anaemia with thermal sensitivity of the erythrocyte membrane. *Br J Haematol* 29:537, 1975.
115. Coetzer T, Palek J, Lawler J, et al: Structural and functional heterogeneity of alpha spectrin mutations involving the spectrin heterodimer self-association site: Relationships to hematologic expression of homozygous hereditary elliptocytosis and hereditary pyropoikilocytosis. *Blood* 75:2235, 1990.
116. Coetzer TL, Sahr K, Prchal J, et al: Four different mutations in codon 28 of alpha spectrin are associated with structurally and functionally abnormal spectrin alpha I/74 in hereditary elliptocytosis. *J Clin Invest* 88:743, 1991.
117. Marchesi SL, Letsinger JT, Speicher DW, et al: Mutant forms of spectrin alpha-subunits in hereditary elliptocytosis. *J Clin Invest* 80:191, 1987.
118. Gaetani M, Mootien S, Harper S, et al: Structural and functional effects of hereditary hemolytic anemia-associated point mutations in the alpha spectrin tetramer site. *Blood* 111:5712, 2008.
119. Roux AF, Morle F, Guetarni D, et al: Molecular basis of Sp alpha I/65 hereditary elliptocytosis in North Africa: Insertion of a TTG triplet between codons 147 and 149 in the alpha-spectrin gene from five unrelated families. *Blood* 73:2196, 1989.
120. Gallagher PG, Petruzzi MJ, Weed SA, et al: Mutation of a highly conserved residue of betaI spectrin associated with fatal and near-fatal neonatal hemolytic anemia. *J Clin Invest* 99:267, 1997.
121. Gallagher PG, Weed SA, Tse WT, et al: Recurrent fatal hydrops fetalis associated with a nucleotide substitution in the erythrocyte beta-spectrin gene. *J Clin Invest* 95:1174, 1995.
122. Sahr KE, Coetzer TL, Moy LS, et al: Spectrin Cagliari. An AlaGly substitution in helix 1 of beta spectrin repeat 17 that severely disrupts the structure and self-association of the erythrocyte spectrin heterodimer. *J Biol Chem* 268:22656, 1993.
123. Takakuwa Y, Tchernia G, Rossi M, et al: Restoration of normal membrane stability to unstable protein 4.1-deficient erythrocyte membranes by incorporation of purified protein 4.1. *J Clin Invest* 78:80, 1986.
124. Chishti AH, Palek J, Fisher D, et al: Reduced invasion and growth of *Plasmodium falciparum* into elliptocytic red blood cells with a combined deficiency of protein 4.1, glycophorin C, and p55. *Blood* 87:3462, 1996.
125. Conboy JG, Chasis JA, Winardi R, et al: An isoform-specific mutation in the protein 4.1 gene results in hereditary elliptocytosis and complete deficiency of protein 4.1 in erythrocytes but not in nonerythroid cells. *J Clin Invest* 91:77, 1993.
126. Winardi R, Reid M, Conboy J, et al: Molecular analysis of glycophorin C deficiency in human erythrocytes. *Blood* 81:2799, 1993.
127. Wilmotte R, Marechal J, Morle L, et al: Low expression allele alpha LELY of red cell spectrin is associated with mutations in exon 40 (alpha V/41 polymorphism) and intron 45 and with partial skipping of exon 46. *J Clin Invest* 91:2091, 1993.
128. Wilmotte R, Harper SL, Ursitti JA, et al: The exon 46-encoded sequence is essential for stability of human erythroid alpha-spectrin and heterodimer formation. *Blood* 90:4188, 1997.
129. Mentzer WC, Jr., Iarocci TA, Mohandas N, et al: Modulation of erythrocyte membrane mechanical stability by 2,3-diphosphoglycerate in the neonatal poikilocytosis/elliptocytosis syndrome. *J Clin Invest* 79:943, 1987.
130. Lorenzo F, Miraglia del Giudice E, Alloisio N, et al: Severe poikilocytosis associated with a de novo alpha 28 ArgCys mutation in spectrin. *Br J Haematol* 83:152, 1993.
131. Jonsson JJ, Renieri A, Gallagher PG, et al: Alport syndrome, mental retardation, midface hypoplasia, and elliptocytosis: A new X linked contiguous gene deletion syndrome? *J Med Genet* 35:273, 1998.
132. Mohandas N, Lie-Injo LE, Friedman M, et al: Rigid membranes of Malayan ovalocytes: A likely genetic barrier against malaria. *Blood* 63:1385, 1984.
133. Hadley T, Saul A, Lamont G, et al: Resistance of Melanesian elliptocytes (ovalocytes) to invasion by *Plasmodium knowlesi* and *Plasmodium falciparum* malaria parasites *in vitro*. *J Clin Invest* 71:780, 1983.
134. Jarolim P, Palek J, Amato D, et al: Deletion in erythrocyte band 3 gene in malaria-resistant Southeast Asian ovalocytosis. *Proc Natl Acad Sci U S A* 88:11022, 1991.
135. Liu SC, Jarolim P, Rubin HL, et al: The homozygous state for the band 3 protein mutation in Southeast Asian ovalocytosis may be lethal. *Blood* 84:3590, 1994.
136. Genton B, al-Yaman F, Mgone CS, et al: Ovalocytosis and cerebral malaria. *Nature* 378:564, 1995.
137. Li X, Chen H, Oo TH, et al: A co-ligand complex anchors *Plasmodium falciparum* merozoites to the erythrocyte invasion receptor band 3. *J Biol Chem* 279:5765, 2004.
138. Bessis FA: Red cell shapes: An illustrated classification and its rationale, in *Red Cell Shape: Physiology, Pathology and Ultrastructure,* edited by M Bessis, RI Weed, PF Leblond, p 1. Springer-Verlag, New York, 1973.
139. Colman N, Herbert V: Hematologic complications of alcoholism: Overview. *Semin Hematol* 17:164, 1980.
140. Cooper RA: Hemolytic syndromes and red cell membrane abnormalities in liver disease. *Semin Hematol* 17:103, 1980.
141. Cooper RA, Diloy Puray M, Lando P, et al: An analysis of lipoproteins, bile acids, and red cell membranes associated with target cells and spur cells in patients with liver disease. *J Clin Invest* 51:3182, 1972.
142. Cooper RA, Kimball DB, Durocher JR: Role of the spleen in membrane conditioning and hemolysis of spur cells in liver disease. *N Engl J Med* 290:1279, 1974.
143. Silber R, Amorosi E, Lhowe J, et al: Spur-shaped erythrocytes in Laennec's cirrhosis. *N Engl J Med* 275:639, 1966.
144. Zieve L: Jaundice, hyperlipemia and hemolytic anemia: A heretofore unrecognized syndrome associated with alcoholic fatty liver and cirrhosis. *Ann Intern Med* 48:471, 1958.
145. Kane J, Havel R: Disorders of the biogenesis and secretion of lipoproteins containing the B apolipoproteins, in *The Metabolic and Molecular Bases of Inherited Disease,* edited by C Scriver, A Beaudet, W Sly, DL Valle, p 1853. McGraw-Hill, New York, 1995.
146. Zamel R, Khan R, Pollex RL, et al: Abetalipoproteinemia: Two case reports and literature review. *Orphanet J Rare Dis* 3:19, 2008.
147. Simon ER, Ways P: Incubation hemolysis and red cell metabolism in acanthocytosis. *J Clin Invest* 43:1311, 1964.
148. Jones JW, Ways P: Abnormalities of high density lipoproteins in abetalipoproteinemia. *J Clin Invest* 46:1151, 1967.
149. Ross RS, Gregg RE, Law SW, et al: Homozygous hypobetalipoproteinemia: A disease distinct from abetalipoproteinemia at the molecular level. *J Clin Invest* 81:590, 1988.
150. Hardie RJ, Pullon HW, Harding AE, et al: Neuroacanthocytosis. A clinical, haematological and pathological study of 19 cases. *Brain* 114(Pt 1A):13, 1991.
151. Critchley EM, Clark DB, Wikler A: Acanthocytosis and neurological disorder without betalipoproteinemia. *Arch Neurol* 18:134, 1968.
152. Bruce LJ, Kay MM, Lawrence C, et al: Band 3 HT, a human red-cell variant associated with acanthocytosis and increased anion transport, carries the mutation Pro-868Leu in the membrane domain of band 3. *Biochem J* 293:317, 1993.
153. Rampoldi L, Dobson-Stone C, Rubio JP, et al: A conserved sorting-associated protein is mutant in chorea-acanthocytosis. *Nat Genet* 28:119, 2001.
154. Ueno S, Maruki Y, Nakamura M, et al: The gene encoding a newly discovered protein, chorein, is mutated in chorea-acanthocytosis. *Nat Genet* 28:121, 2001.
155. Walker RH, Jung HH, Dobson-Stone C, et al: Neurologic phenotypes associated with acanthocytosis. *Neurology* 68:92, 2007.
156. Jung HH, Danek A, Frey BM: McLeod syndrome: A neurohaematological disorder. *Vox Sang* 93:112, 2007.
157. Wimer BM, Marsh WL, Taswell HF, et al: Haematological changes associated with the McLeod phenotype of the Kell blood group system. *Br J Haematol* 36:219, 1977.
158. Redman CM, Russo D, Lee S: Kell, Kx and the McLeod syndrome. *Baillieres Best Pract Res Clin Haematol* 12:621, 1999.
159. Redman CM, Marsh WL, Scarborough A, et al: Biochemical studies on McLeod phenotype red cells and isolation of Kx antigen. *Br J Haematol* 68:131, 1988.
160. Peng J, Redman CM, Wu X, et al: Insights into extensive deletions around the XK locus associated with McLeod phenotype and characterization of two novel cases. *Gene* 392:142, 2007.
161. Udden MM, Umeda M, Hirano Y, et al: New abnormalities in the morphology, cell surface receptors, and electrolyte metabolism of In(Lu) erythrocytes. *Blood* 69:52, 1987.
162. Singleton BK, Burton NM, Green C, et al: Mutations in EKLF/KLF1 form the molecular basis of the rare blood group In(Lu) phenotype. *Blood* 112:2081, 2008.
163. Wardrop C, Hutchison HE: Red-cell shape in hypothyroidism. *Lancet* 1:1243, 1969.
164. Lande WM, Mentzer WC: Haemolytic anaemia associated with increased cation permeability. *Clin Haematol* 14:89, 1985.
165. Delaunay J: The hereditary stomatocytoses: Genetic disorders of the red cell membrane permeability to monovalent cations. *Semin Hematol* 41:165, 2004.
166. Gallagher PG, Forget BG, Lux SE: Disorders of the erythrocyte membrane, in *Hematology of Infancy and Childhood,* edited by DG Nathan, SH Orkin, p 544. WB Saunders, Philadelphia, 1998.
167. Clark MR, Shohet SB, Gottfried EL: Hereditary hemolytic disease with increased red blood cell phosphatidylcholine and dehydration: One, two, or many disorders? *Am J Hematol* 42:25, 1993.
168. Carella M, Stewart G, Ajetunmobi JF, et al: Genomewide search for dehydrated hereditary stomatocytosis (hereditary xerocytosis): Mapping of locus to chromosome 16 (16q23-qter). *Am J Hum Genet* 63:810, 1998.
169. Stewart GW, Corrall RJ, Fyffe JA, et al: Familial pseudohyperkalaemia. A new syndrome. *Lancet* 2:175, 1979.

170. Grootenboer S, Schischmanoff PO, Cynober T, et al: A genetic syndrome associating dehydrated hereditary stomatocytosis, pseudohyperkalaemia and perinatal oedema. *Br J Haematol* 103:383, 1998.
171. Grootenboer S, Schischmanoff PO, Laurendeau I, et al: Pleiotropic syndrome of dehydrated hereditary stomatocytosis, pseudohyperkalemia, and perinatal edema maps to 16q23-q24. *Blood* 96:2599, 2000.
172. Iolascon A, Stewart GW, Ajetunmobi JF, et al: Familial pseudohyperkalemia maps to the same locus as dehydrated hereditary stomatocytosis (hereditary xerocytosis). *Blood* 93:3120, 1999.
173. Stewart GW, Amess JAL, Eber SW, et al: Thrombo-embolic disease after splenectomy for hereditary stomatocytosis. *Br J Haematol* 93:303, 1996.
174. Smith BD, Segel GB: Abnormal erythrocyte endothelial adherence in hereditary stomatocytosis. *Blood* 89:3451, 1997.
175. Lock SP, Smith RS, Hardisty RM: Stomatocytosis: A hereditary red cell anomaly associated with haemolytic anaemia. *Br J Haematol* 7:303, 1961.
176. Zarkowsky HS, Oski FA, Sha'afi R, et al: Congenital hemolytic anemia with high sodium, low potassium red cells. I. Studies of membrane permeability. *N Engl J Med* 278:573, 1968.
177. Ellory JC, Gibson JS, Stewart GW: Pathophysiology of abnormal cell volume in human red cells. *Contrib Nephrol* 123:220, 1998.
178. Bruce LJ, Guizouarn H, Burton NM, et al: The monovalent cation leak in overhydrated stomatocytic red blood cells results from amino acid substitutions in the Rh-associated glycoprotein. *Blood* 113:1350, 2009.
179. Fricke B, Argent AC, Chetty MC, et al: The "stomatin" gene and protein in overhydrated hereditary stomatocytosis. *Blood* 102:2268, 2003.
180. Bruce LJ: Hereditary stomatocytosis and cation leaky red cells—Recent developments. *Blood Cells Mol Dis* 42:216, 2009.
181. Fricke B, Jarvis HG, Reid CD, et al: Four new cases of stomatin-deficient hereditary stomatocytosis syndrome: Association of the stomatin-deficient cryohydrocytosis variant with neurological dysfunction. *Br J Haematol* 125:796, 2004.
182. Bruce LJ, Robinson HC, Guizouarn H, et al: Monovalent cation leaks in human red cells caused by single amino-acid substitutions in the transport domain of the band 3 chloride-bicarbonate exchanger, AE1. *Nat Genet* 37:1258, 2005.
183. Lane PA, Kuypers FA, Clark MR, et al: Excess of red cell membrane proteins in hereditary high-phosphatidylcholine hemolytic anemia. *Am J Hematol* 34:186, 1990.
184. Burton NM, Anstee DJ: Structure, function and significance of Rh proteins in red cells. *Curr Opin Hematol* 15:625, 2008.
185. Cartron JP: Rh-deficiency syndrome. *Lancet* 358 Suppl:S57, 2001.
186. Oram JF, Vaughan AM: ATP-Binding cassette cholesterol transporters and cardiovascular disease. *Circ Res* 99:1031, 2006.
187. Davidson RJ, How J, Lessels S: Acquired stomatocytosis: Its prevalence of significance in routine haematology. *Scand J Haematol* 19:47, 1977.
188. Wisloff F, Boman D: Acquired stomatocytosis in alcoholic liver disease. *Scand J Haematol* 23:43, 1979.
189. Neville AJ, Rand CA, Barr RD, et al: Drug-induced stomatocytosis and anemia during consolidation chemotherapy of childhood acute leukemia. *Am J Med Sci* 287:3, 1984.
190. Ohsaka A, Kano Y, Sakamoto S, et al: A transient hemolytic reaction and stomatocytosis following vinca alkaloid administration. *Nippon Ketsueki Gakkai Zasshi* 52:7, 1989.

CHAPTER 46

DISORDERS OF RED CELLS RESULTING FROM ENZYME ABNORMALITIES

Wouter W. van Solinge and Richard van Wijk*

SUMMARY

Red cells possess an active metabolic machinery that provides energy to pump ions against electrochemical gradients, to maintain red cell shape, to keep hemoglobin iron in the reduced form, and to maintain enzyme and hemoglobin sulfhydryl groups. The main source of metabolic energy comes from glucose. Glucose is metabolized through the glycolytic pathway and through the hexose monophosphate shunt. Glycolysis catabolizes glucose to pyruvate and lactate, which represent the end products of glucose metabolism in the erythrocyte, because it lacks the mitochondria required for further oxidation of pyruvate. Adenosine diphosphate (ADP) is phosphorylated to adenosine triphosphate (ATP), and nicotinamide adenine dinucleotide $(NAD)^+$ is reduced to NADH in glycolysis. 2,3-Bisphosphoglycerate, an important regulator of the oxygen affinity of hemoglobin, is generated during glycolysis. The hexose monophosphate shunt oxidizes glucose-6-phosphate, reducing $NADP^+$ to reduced nicotinamide adenine dinucleotide phosphate (NADPH). In addition to glucose, the red cell has the capacity to utilize some other sugars and nucleosides as a source of energy. The red cell lacks the capacity for *de novo* purine synthesis, but has a salvage pathway that permits synthesis of purine nucleotides from purine bases. The red cell contains high concentrations of glutathione, which is maintained almost entirely in the reduced state by NADPH through the catalytic activity of glutathione reductase. Glutathione is synthesized from glycine, cysteine, and glutamic acid in a two-step process that requires ATP as a source of energy. Catalase and glutathione peroxidase serve to protect the red cell from oxidative damage. The maturation of reticulocytes into erythrocytes is associated with a rapid decrease in the activity of several enzymes. However, the decrease in activities of other enzymes occurs much more slowly or not at all with aging.

Erythrocyte enzyme deficiencies may lead to hemolytic anemia; expression of the defect in other cell lines may lead to pathologic changes such as neuromuscular abnormalities. Glucose-6-phosphate dehydrogenase (G-6-PD) deficiency is the most common erythrocyte enzyme defect. In some populations, more than 20 percent of people may be affected by this enzyme deficiency. In the common polymorphic forms, such as G-6-PD A–, G-6-PD Mediterranean, or G-6-PD Canton, hemolysis occurs only during the stress imposed by infection or administration of "oxidative" drugs, and in some individuals upon ingestion of fava beans. Neonatal icterus, which appears largely with the interaction with an independent defect in bilirubin conjugation, is the clinically most serious complication of G-6-PD deficiency. Patients with uncommon, functionally very severe, genetic variants of G-6-PD experience chronic hemolysis, a disorder designated hereditary nonspherocytic hemolytic anemia.

Hereditary nonspherocytic hemolytic anemia also occurs as a consequence of other enzyme deficiencies, the most common of which is pyruvate kinase deficiency. Glucosephosphate isomerase, triosephosphate isomerase, and pyrimidine 5′-nucleotidase deficiency are included among the relatively rare causes of hereditary nonspherocytic hemolytic anemia. In the case of some deficiencies, notably those of glutathione synthetase, triosephosphate isomerase, and phosphoglycerate kinase, the defect is expressed throughout the body, and neurologic and other defects may be a prominent part of the clinical syndrome.

Diagnosis is best achieved by determining red cell enzyme activity either with a quantitative assay or a screening test. Except for the basophilic stippling of erythrocytes that is characteristic of pyrimidine 5′-nucleotidase deficiency, red cell morphology is of little or no help in differentiating one red cell enzyme deficiency from another. A variety of molecular lesions have been defined in most of these enzyme deficiencies. Accurate diagnosis is necessary for genetic counseling and is helpful in recommendations for treatment, as patients with some enzyme deficiencies (e.g., glucosephosphate isomerase deficiency) tend to respond more favorably to splenectomy than do others (e.g., G-6-PD deficiency). Some of the defects, such as pyruvate kinase and glucosephosphate isomerase deficiencies, are transmitted as autosomal recessive disorders, whereas G-6-PD and phosphoglycerate kinase (PGK) deficiencies are X linked.

Acronyms and abbreviations that appear in this chapter include: 2,3-BPG, 2,3-bis phosphoglycerate; ADA, adenosine deaminase; ADP, adenosine diphosphate; AIDS, acquired immunodeficiency syndrome; ATP, adenosine triphosphate; BPG, bisphosphoglycerate; DPG, diphosphoglycerate; EDTA, ethylenediaminetetraacetic acid; EMP, Embden-Meyerhof direct glycolytic pathway; G-6-PD, glucose-6-phosphate dehydrogenase; GPI, glucose phosphate isomerase; GSH, reduced glutathione; GSSG, oxidized glutathione; HNSHA, hereditary nonspherocytic hemolytic anemia; LDH, lactate dehydrogenase; NAD, nicotinamide adenine dinucleotide; NADPH, nicotinamide adenine dinucleotide phosphate (reduced form); nt, nucleotide; PFK, phosphofructose kinase; PGK, phosphoglycerate kinase; PK, pyruvate kinase; UDPG, uridine diphosphoglucose; UDPGT, uridine diphosphoglucuronate glucuronosyltransferase.

*This chapter is based in part on Chapter 45 of the previous edition of this text, which was written by Dr. Ernest Beutler.

DEFINITION AND HISTORY

Deficiencies in the activities of a number of erythrocyte enzymes may lead to shortening of the red cell life span. G-6-PD deficiency was the first of these to be recognized and is the most common.

The recognition of G-6-PD deficiency was the result of investigations of the hemolytic effect of the antimalarial drug primaquine, carried out in the 1950s and described in detail elsewhere.[1,2] These early studies defined G-6-PD deficiency as a hereditary sex-linked enzyme deficiency that affected primarily the erythrocytes, older cells being more severely affected than newly formed ones because of age-dependent decline of mutant enzyme activity. They showed that this enzyme deficiency was very prevalent in individuals of African, Mediterranean, and Asian ethnic origins, but that it could be found in virtually any population. The common (polymorphic) forms of G-6-PD deficiency were found to be associated with anemia only under conditions of stress, such as the administration of oxidative drugs, infection, and the neonatal period.

Chronic hemolysis in the absence of a stress occurs in uncommon, functionally severe forms of G-6-PD deficiency and in patients with a variety of other red cell enzyme deficiencies. Such patients have one type of *hereditary nonspherocytic hemolytic anemia*. Although patients fitting the description of hereditary nonspherocytic hemolytic anemia had been documented earlier, the designation was first introduced by Crosby[3] in 1950. Dacie and colleagues[4] subsequently reported several families in which affected members manifested hemolytic anemia from an early age and in whom the osmotic fragility of the red cells was normal. The latter finding was the main feature that distinguished this disorder from hereditary spherocytosis. Thus, defined essentially by exclusion as a hereditary hemolytic anemia that is not hereditary spherocytosis (or without any major aberration of red cell morphology), it is not at all surprising that hereditary nonspherocytic hemolytic anemia has proven to be extremely heterogeneous both in etiology and in clinical manifestations. Sometimes this disorder is also designated *congenital nonspherocytic hemolytic anemia*, but the name hereditary is more accurate and is therefore preferable. Although hereditary ovalocytosis, pyropoikilocytosis, stomatocytosis (see Chap. 45), and even sickle cell disease and thalassemia major (see Chaps. 47 and 48) are hereditary hemolytic anemias that are also nonspherocytic, they are not included in this category.

Although a deficiency of G-6-PD was found to be responsible for hemolysis in a few patients with hereditary nonspherocytic hemolytic anemia, in the overwhelming majority of cases the cause remained obscure. In 1954, Selwyn and Dacie[5] studied autohemolysis (spontaneous lysis of red cells after sterile incubation for 24–48 hours at 37°C [98.6°F]) in four patients with hereditary nonspherocytic hemolytic anemia and found that in two of them lysis was only slightly increased and was prevented by glucose; these patients were designated as type 1, whereas the others, in whom glucose failed to correct autohemolysis, were classified as type 2. Autohemolysis of the erythrocytes of type 2 patients was modified by the addition of adenosine triphosphate (ATP), a substance that we now recognize does not penetrate the red cell membrane. Instead, its modifying influence was probably exerted chiefly by virtue of its effect on the osmolarity and pH of the suspending solution. However, these findings suggested to DeGruchy and associates[6] that patients with type 2 autohemolysis suffered from a defect in ATP generation. This proposal, born of a misunderstanding of red cell biochemistry, turned out to be correct, as one of the major causes of hereditary nonspherocytic hemolytic anemia proved to be a deficiency of the ATP-generating enzyme pyruvate kinase (PK),[7] but this was only the first of a large number of enzyme defects that have been shown to account for this heterogeneous syndrome.[8,9]

EPIDEMIOLOGY

The most common red cell enzyme abnormality is deficiency of G-6-PD. Its prevalence among white populations ranges from less than 1 in 1000 among northern European populations to 50 percent of the males among Kurdish Jews. G-6-PD deficiency is also found among certain Chinese populations and in Southeast Asia, but it is rare in Japan. G-6-PD deficiency of the A– type is very common in West Africa, and the prevalence among American males of African descent is approximately 11 percent.[10] The distribution of G-6-PD deficiency among various population groups has been presented in detail elsewhere.[11,12] The global prevalence of G-6-PD deficiency is estimated to be 4.9 percent, rendering an estimated 330 million people affected by G-6-PD deficiency worldwide.[13]

The high frequency of G-6-PD–deficient genes in many populations implies that G-6-PD deficiency confers a selective advantage. The suggestion that resistance to malaria could account for the high frequency of G-6-PD deficiency paralleling the worldwide distribution of malaria was examined in numerous epidemiologic studies in Africa and elsewhere.[14,15] Important supporting evidence was obtained from studies in heterozygotes for G-6-PD A– that showed a higher degree of infestation of G-6-PD–sufficient cells than of G-6-PD–deficient cells.[16] Deficient cells infested with malaria parasites may be phagocytosed more efficiently than normal cells.[17] The current understanding is that the uniform state of the A– form of G-6-PD deficiency in hemizygous male children, and possibly homozygous female children, confers significant protection against severe, life-threatening malaria.[18] The nature of protection from the mosaic state of G-6-PD deficiency in heterozygous females remains to be established.[18,19]

A higher prevalence of G-6-PD deficiency in individuals with sickle cell disease than in the general African population reflects a favorable effect of the enzyme deficiency on the clinical course of the sickling disorders.[20,21] However, the increased prevalence of G-6-PD deficiency in patients with sickle disease may merely result from the markedly heterogeneous genetic composition of Americans of African descent; those with more African genes are more likely to inherit sickle hemoglobin and G-6-PD A–.[22] Similar factors may be responsible for the slight excess of G-6-PD deficiency observed among patients with SS hemoglobin in Arab populations.[23]

PK deficiency is the most common cause of hereditary nonspherocytic hemolytic anemia. Estimates of heterozygote frequency performed on a large number of cord blood samples have provided estimates of 1 percent in whites and 2.4 percent in Americans of African descent.[24] Based on large-scale mutation analysis, it has been estimated that the population prevalence of PK deficiency among whites is approximately 50 cases per 1 million population.[25] Estimates of other deficiency alleles, such as those for adenylate kinase, diphosphoglycerate mutase, enolase, triosephosphate isomerase (TPI), and PGK, have also been made on large numbers of cord bloods.[24] A particularly high incidence of heterozygous TPI deficiency (>4%) in Americans of African descent is supported by family studies.[26]

In addition to the common G-6-PD mutations, there are mutations in other enzymes that are repeatedly encountered in the population. In PK, the 1529G→A mutation is the most common mutation in the United States,[27] and in northern and central Europe[28]; the 1456C→T mutation is prevalent in southern Europe[29]; and the 1468C→T mutation in Asia.[30] Similarly, the 315G→C mutation is recurrently encountered in TPI.[31] In phosphofructose kinase (PFK) deficiency, one-third of the reported patients are of Jewish origin and in this population an intronic splice site mutation, IVS5+1G→A,[32] and a single base-pair deletion, 2003delC,[33] are among the most frequently encountered mutations. In each of these instances, the existence of each mutation in the context of the same haplotype implies that there has been a *founder effect*, that is, the mutation occurred only once, and all individuals now carrying it are descendants of the person who sustained the original mutation. The expansion of the mutation could represent a selective advantage for heterozygotes, but also may result from random factors or from a selective advantage provided by one or more tightly linked genes.

ETIOLOGY AND PATHOGENESIS

■ RED CELL METABOLISM

Although the binding, transport, and delivery of oxygen do not require the expenditure of metabolic energy by the red cell, a source of energy is required if the red cell is to perform its function efficiently and to survive in the circulation for its full life span of approximately 120 days. This energy is needed to maintain (1) the iron of hemoglobin in the divalent form, (2) the high potassium and low calcium and sodium levels within the cell against a gradient imposed by the high plasma calcium and sodium and low plasma potassium levels, (3) the sulfhydryl groups of red cell enzymes, hemoglobin, and membranes in the active, reduced form, and (4) the biconcave shape of the cell. If the red cell is deprived of a source of energy, it becomes sodium and calcium logged and potassium depleted, and the red cell shape changes from a flexible biconcave disc. Such a cell is quickly removed from the circulation by the filtering action of the spleen and by a monocyte-macrophage system. Even if it survived, such an energy-deprived cell would gradually turn brown as hemoglobin is oxidized to methemoglobin by the very high concentrations of oxygen within the erythrocyte. The cell would then be unable to perform its function of transporting oxygen and carbon dioxide.

The process of extracting energy from a substrate, such as glucose, and of utilizing this energy is carried out by a large number of enzymes (Table 46–1). Because the red cell loses its nucleus before it enters the circulation and most of its RNA within 1 or 2 days of its release into the circulation, it does not have the capacity to synthesize new proteins to replace those that may become degraded during its life span. The enzymes present in the red cells were formed largely by the nucleated marrow cell and, to a lesser extent, the reticulocyte.

Glucose Metabolism

Glucose is the normal energy source of the red cell. It is metabolized by the erythrocyte along two major routes: the glycolytic pathway and the hexose monophosphate shunt. The steps in these pathways are essentially the same as those found in other tissues and in other organisms, including even relatively simple ones such as *Escherichia coli* and yeast. Unlike most other cells, however, the red cell lacks a citric acid cycle. Only the reticulocytes maintain some capacity for the breakdown of pyruvate to CO_2, with the attendant highly efficient production of ATP. The mature red cell extracts energy from glucose almost solely by anaerobic glycolysis. Before glucose can be metabolized by the red cell, it must pass through the membrane. The membrane contains a carrier[34] that can combine with glucose and other sugars at the cell surface and release them at the interior surface of the membrane. The red cell membrane contains insulin receptors, but the transport of glucose into red cells is independent of insulin.

Pathways of Glucose Metabolism **Direct Glycolytic Pathway** In the Embden-Meyerhof direct glycolytic pathway (EMP; Fig. 46–1), glucose is catabolized anaerobically to pyruvate or lactate. Although 2 moles of high-energy phosphate in the form of ATP are utilized in preparing glucose for its further metabolism, up to 4 moles of adenosine diphosphate (ADP) may be phosphorylated to ATP during the metabolism of each mole of glucose, giving a net yield of 2 moles of ATP per mole of glucose metabolized. The rate of glucose utilization is limited largely by the hexokinase and PFK reactions. Both of the enzymes catalyzing these reactions have a relatively high pH optimum and have very little activity at pH levels lower than 7. For this reason, red cell glycolysis is very pH sensitive, being stimulated by a rise in pH. However, at higher than physiologic pH levels, the stimulation of hexokinase and phosphofructokinase activity merely results in the accumulation of fructose diphosphate and triose phosphates, because the availability of nicotinamide adenine dinucleotide $(NAD)^+$ for the glyceraldehyde phosphate dehydrogenase reaction becomes a limiting factor.

Branching of the metabolic stream after the formation of 1,3-bisphosphoglycerate (1,3-BPG) provides the red cell with flexibility in regard to the amount of ATP formed in the metabolism of each mole of glucose. 1,3-BPG may be metabolized to 2,3-bisphosphoglycerate (2,3-BPG) also known as 2,3-diphosphoglycerate (2,3-DPG), thus "wasting" the high-energy phosphate bond in position 1 of the glycerate. Removing the phosphate group at position 2 by bisphosphoglycerate phosphatase results in the formation of 3-phosphoglycerate. Both reactions in this unique glycolytic bypass, known as the *Rapoport Luebering shunt*, are catalyzed by the erythroid-specific multifunctional enzyme bisphosphoglycerate mutase.[35] Alternatively, 3-phosphoglycerate may be formed directly from 1,3-BPG through the PGK step, resulting in phosphorylation of 1 mole of ADP to ATP. Although metabolism of glucose through the 2,3-BPG step occurs without any net gain of high-energy phosphate bonds in the form of ATP, metabolism through the PGK step results in

TABLE 46–1. Activities of Some Red Cell Enzymes

Enzyme	Activity at 37°C (98.6°F) IU/g Hgb (mean ± SD)	Reference
Acetylcholinesterase	36.93 ± 3.83	452
Adenosine deaminase	1.11 ± 0.23	452
Adenylate kinase	258 ± 29.3	452
Aldolase	3.19 ± 0.86	452
Bisphosphoglyceromutase	4.78 ± 0.65	452
Catalase	153,117 ± 2390	452
Enolase	5.39 ± 0.83	452
Galactokinase	0.0291 ± 0.004	452
Galactose-4-epimerase	0.231 ± 0.061	452
Glucose phosphate isomerase	60.8 ± 11.0	452
Glucose-6-phosphate dehydrogenase	8.34 ± 1.59	452
γ-Glutamylcysteine synthetase	1.05 ± 0.19	454
Glutathione peroxidase*	30.82 ± 4.65	452
Glutathione reductase without FAD	7.18 ± 1.09	452
Glutathione reductase with FAD	10.4 ± 1.50	452
Glutathione-S-transferase	6.66 ± 1.81	452
Glutathione synthetase	0.34 ± 0.06	453
Glyceraldehyde phosphate dehydrogenase	226 ± 41.9	452
Hexokinase	1.78 ± 0.38	452
Lactate dehydrogenase	200 ± 26.5	452
Monophosphoglyceromutase	37.71 ± 5.56	452
NADH-methemoglobin reductase	19.2 ± 3.85(30°)	452
NADPH diaphorase	2.26 ± 0.16	452
Nucleoside phosphorylase	359 ± 32	3
Phosphofructokinase	11.01 ± 2.33	452
Phosphoglucomutase	5.50 ± 0.62	452
Phosphoglycerate kinase	320 ± 36.1	452
Phosphoglycolate phosphatase	1.23 ± 0.10	452
Phosphomannose isomerase	0.054 ± 0.026	4
Pyrimidine 5′-nucleotidase	0.138 ± 0.018	452
Pyruvate kinase	15.0 ± 1.99	452
6-Phosphogluconate dehydrogenase	8.78 ± 0.78	452
6-Phosphogluconolactonase	50.6 ± 5.9	452
Ribosephosphate isomerase	200	452
Superoxide dismutase	2225 ± 303	452
Transaldolase	1.21 ± 0.24	5
Transketolase	0.725 ± 0.17	5
Triose phosphate isomerase	2111 ± 397	452

FAD, flavin adenine dinucleotide; NADH, reduced form of nicotinamide adenine dinucleotide; NADPH, nicotinamide adenine dinucleotide phosphate.

*For U.S. and European subjects.

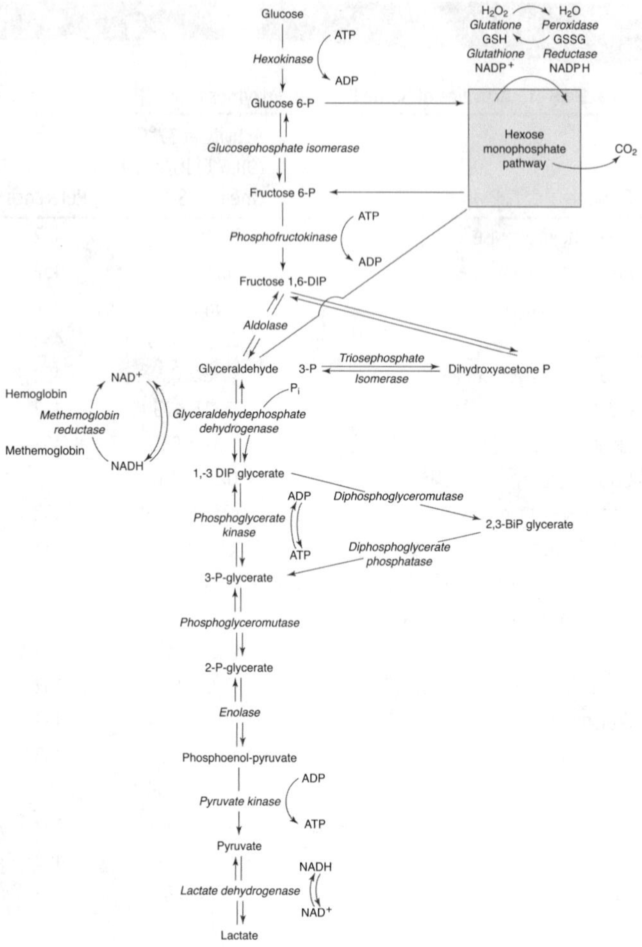

FIGURE 46–1. Glucose metabolism of the erythrocyte. The details of the hexose monophosphate pathway are shown in Figure 46–2.

the formation of two such bonds per mole of glucose metabolized. This portion of the direct glycolytic pathway has been called the *energy clutch*.[36] Regulation of metabolism at this branch point determines not only the rate of ADP phosphorylation to ATP but also the concentration of 2,3-BPG, an important regulator of the oxygen affinity of hemoglobin (see Chaps. 48 and 56). The concentration of 2,3-BPG depends on the balance between its rate of formation and degradation by bisphosphoglycerate mutase. Hydrogen ions inhibit the bisphosphoglycerate mutase reaction and stimulate the phosphatase reaction. Thus, red cell 2,3-BPG levels are exquisitely sensitive to pH: a rise in pH causes a rise in 2,3-BPG levels, whereas acidosis results in 2,3-BPG depletion. It may be that the ratio of oxyhemoglobin to deoxyhemoglobin also influences 2,3-BPG synthesis by virtue of the fact that only deoxyhemoglobin binds this compound, thus affecting the concentration of free 2,3-BPG that is available for feedback inhibition of the enzymes that lead to its formation. However, the available evidence suggests that the pH is the primary controlling factor.

Metabolism of glucose by way of the Embden-Meyerhof pathway may also yield reducing energy in the form of the reduced form of nicotinamide adenine dinucleotide (NADH). The reduction of NAD^+ to NADH occurs in the glyceraldehyde-3-phosphate dehydrogenase step. If NADH is reoxidized in reducing methemoglobin to hemoglobin, the end product of glucose metabolism is pyruvate. If NADH is not reoxidized by methemoglobin, however, pyruvate is reduced in the lactate dehydrogenase (LDH) step, forming lactate as the final end product of glucose metabolism. The lactate or pyruvate formed is transported from the red cell[37] and is metabolized elsewhere in the body. Thus, the erythrocyte has a flexible Embden-Meyerhof pathway that can adjust the amount of ADP phosphorylated per mole of glucose according to the requirement of the cell.

The regulation of red cell glycolytic metabolism is very complex. Products of some reactions may stimulate others. For example, the PK reaction is exquisitely sensitive to fructose 1,6-diphosphate, the product of PFK. Conversely, other metabolic products may serve as strong enzyme inhibitors. Attempts have been made to construct computer models that simulate this network of reactions in normal and pathologic conditions.[38–43]

Hexose Monophosphate Shunt Not all the glucose metabolized by the red cell passes through the direct glycolytic pathway. A direct oxidative pathway of metabolism, the hexose monophosphate shunt, also functions. In this pathway, glucose-6-phosphate is oxidized at position 1, yielding carbon dioxide. In the process of glucose oxidation, $NADP^+$ is reduced to NADPH (reduced nicotinamide adenine dinucleotide phosphate). The pentose phosphate formed when glucose is decarboxylated undergoes a series of molecular rearrangements, eventuating in the formation of a triose, glyceraldehyde-3-phosphate, and a hexose, fructose-6-phosphate (Fig. 46–2). These are normal intermediates in anaerobic glycolysis and thus can rejoin that metabolic stream. Because the glucose phosphate isomerase reaction is freely reversible, allowing fructose-6-phosphate to be converted to glucose-6-phosphate, recycling through the hexose monophosphate pathway is also possible. Unlike the anaerobic glycolytic pathway, the hexose monophosphate pathway does not generate any high-energy phosphate bonds. Its primary function appears to be the reduction of $NADP^+$, and, indeed, the amount of glucose passing through this pathway appears to be regulated by the amount of $NADP^+$ that has been made available by the oxidation of NADPH. NADPH appears to function primarily as a substrate for the reduction of glutathione-containing disulfides in the erythrocyte through mediation of the enzyme glutathione reductase, which catalyzes the conversion of oxidized glutathione (GSSG) to reduced glutathione (GSH) and the

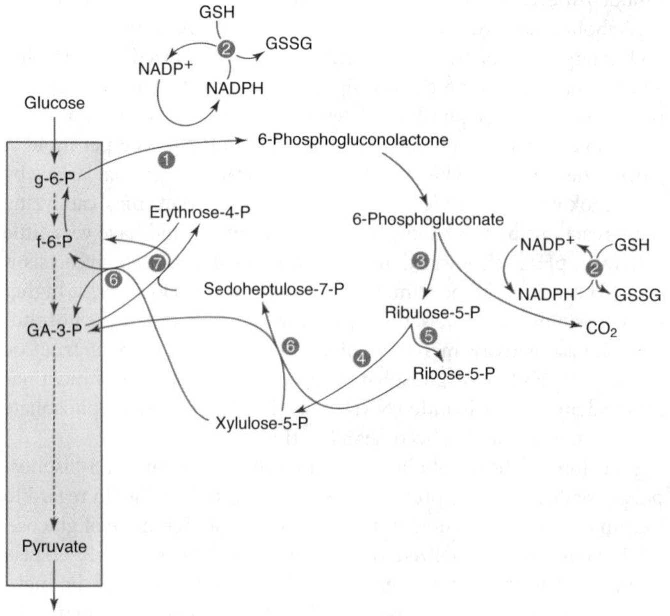

FIGURE 46–2. Hexose monophosphate pathway of the erythrocyte: (1) glucose-6-phosphate dehydrogenase, (2) glutathione reductase, (3) phosphogluconate dehydrogenase, (4) ribulose-phosphate epimerase, (5) ribosephosphate isomerase, (6) transketolase, and (7) transaldolase.

reduction of mixed disulfides of hemoglobin and GSH.[44] $NADP^+$ also strongly binds to catalase and may affect its activity.[45,46]

As in the case of anaerobic glycolysis, efforts have been made to construct a computer model of the hexose monophosphate pathway of red cells.[39,42]

Enzymes of Glucose Metabolism **Hexokinase** Hexokinase catalyzes the phosphorylation of glucose in position 6 by ATP. It thus serves as the first step in the utilization of glucose, whether by the anaerobic or the hexose monophosphate pathway. Mannose or fructose may also serve as a substrate for this enzyme. Red cell hexokinase does not phosphorylate galactose.[47] Reticulocytes have much higher levels of hexokinase activity than do mature red cells.[48,49]

Hexokinase has an absolute requirement for magnesium. It is strongly inhibited by its product, glucose-6-phosphate, and is released from this inhibition by the inorganic phosphate ion[50,51] and by high concentrations of glucose.[52] Inorganic phosphate enhances the rate of glucose utilization by red cells. This effect is not exerted through hexokinase but through stimulation of the PFK reaction, resulting in a lowered glucose-6-phosphate concentration within the cell and thus releasing hexokinase from inhibition.[53] GSSG[54] and other disulfides, as well as 2,3-BPG,[55] inhibit hexokinase. The determination of the structures of the human and rat hexokinase isozymes have provided substantial insight into ligand-binding sites and subsequent modes of interaction of these ligands.[56,57]

The two major fractions of red cell hexokinase have been designated HK_I and HK_R; the latter fraction being unique to erythrocytes and particularly to reticulocytes.[58] Both red cell isozymes are produced from the hexokinase I gene (*HK1*).[59] The gene is localized on chromosome 10q22 and spans more than 100 kb. It encompasses 25 exons,[60] which, by tissue-specific transcription, generate multiple transcripts by alternative use of the 5′ exons.[61] Erythroid-specific transcriptional control results in a unique red blood cell–specific messenger ribonucleic acid (mRNA) that differs from hexokinase-I transcripts at the 5′ end. Consequently, hexokinase-R lacks the porin-binding domain that mediates hexokinase-I binding to mitochondria.[62] Hexokinase deficiency is a rare cause of hereditary nonspherocytic hemolytic anemia.

Glucose Phosphate Isomerase Glucose-6-phosphate isomerase (GPI) catalyzes the interconversion of glucose-6-phosphate and fructose-6-phosphate, the second step of the Embden-Meyerhof pathway. The crystal structure of human GPI has been resolved. The enzyme is a homodimer, composed of two subunits of 63 kDa each. The enzyme's active site is composed of polypeptide chains from both subunits, making the dimeric form essential for catalytic activity.[63] The gene encoding GPI is located on chromosome 19q13.1 and consists of 18 exons, spanning at least 50 kb, with a complementary DNA (cDNA) of 1.9 kb in length.[64] GPI deficiency is one of the causes of hereditary nonspherocytic hemolytic anemia.

Phosphofructokinase PFK catalyses the rate-limiting phosphorylation of fructose-6-phosphate by ATP to fructose-1,6-diphosphate. The enzyme has a molecular mass of around 380 kDa. Red cell phosphofructokinase exists as a series of homo- or heterotetramers comprised of muscle (M) and liver (L) subunits. A platelet (P) subunit has also been identified.[65] The genes for the PFK-M and PFK-L subunits have been cloned. The gene encoding the M subunit (*PFKM*) has been assigned to chromosome 12q13.3 and spans 30 kb. It contains 27 exons and at least three promoter regions.[67] The L-subunit encoding gene (*PFKL*) is located on chromosome 21q22.3, it contains 22 exons and spans more than 28 kb.[68] The enzyme requires magnesium for activity and is stimulated by ADP, inorganic phosphate, ammonia, and fructose-2,6-diphosphate.[66] Deficiency of PFK is associated with mild hemolytic anemia and with type VII glycogen storage disease.

Aldolase Aldolase reversibly cleaves fructose-1,6-diphosphate into two trioses. The "upper" half of the fructose-1,6-diphosphate molecule becomes dihydroxyacetone phosphate and the "lower" half becomes glyceraldehyde-3-phosphate. Aldolase is a homotetrameric enzyme comprised of subunits of 40 kDa each.[69] Three distinct isoenzymes have been identified: aldolase A, B, and C. The 364-amino-acids-long aldolase A subunits are expressed in erythrocytes, but also in muscle and brain.[70] Aldolase activity is markedly influenced by red cell age. The gene for aldolase A (*ALDOA*) is located on chromosome 16q22-24. It spans 7.5 kb and consists of 12 exons. Several transcription-initiation sites were identified and *ALDOA* pre-mRNA is spliced in a tissue-specific manner.[71] Aldolase deficiency is a very rare cause of hereditary nonspherocytic hemolytic anemia.

Triosephosphate Isomerase Triosephosphate isomerase is the enzyme of the anaerobic glycolytic pathway that has the highest activity. Its metabolic role is to catalyze interconversion of the two trioses formed by the action of aldolase: dihydroxyacetone phosphate and glyceraldehyde-3-phosphate. Although equilibrium is in favor of dihydroxyacetone phosphate, glyceraldehyde-3-phosphate undergoes continued oxidation through the action of glyceraldehyde phosphate dehydrogenase and is thus removed from the equilibrium. Triosephosphate isomerase is a dimer consisting of two identical subunits of 248 amino acids.[72] There are no isoenzymes known, but three distinct electrophoretic forms can be distinguished as a result of posttranslational modifications.[73] Red blood cell triosephosphate isomerase activity is not red-cell-age dependent. Triosephosphate isomerase is transcribed from a single gene, located on chromosome 12p13. The gene spans 3.5 kb and contains 7 exons. Three processed pseudogenes have been identified.[74] A deficiency of triosephosphate isomerase has been found in patients with hereditary nonspherocytic hemolytic anemia associated with a severe neuromuscular disorder.

Glyceraldehyde-3-Phosphate Dehydrogenase Glyceraldehyde-3-phosphate dehydrogenase performs the dual functions of oxidizing and phosphorylating glyceraldehyde-3-phosphate, producing 1,3-BPG. In the process, NAD^+ is reduced to NADH. This enzyme is closely associated with the red cell membrane.[75] It interacts with and is stimulated by oxyhemoglobin, an interaction that could have a regulatory role.[76] The crystal structure of human liver glyceraldehyde-3-phosphate dehydrogenase reveals a homotetramer, each subunit of which is bound to a nicotinamide adenine dinucleotide (NAD^+) molecule.[77]

Phosphoglycerate Kinase PGK effects the transfer to ADP of the high-energy phosphate from the 1-carbon of 1,3-DPG to form ATP. The reaction is readily reversible and can be bypassed by the Rapoport-Luebering shunt. The isoenzyme PGK-1 is ubiquitously expressed in all somatic cells and is a 48-kDa monomeric enzyme of 417 amino acids.[78] The gene encoding PGK-1 is located on the long arm of the X-chromosome (Xq13).[79] The gene spans 23 kb and is composed of 11 exons.[80] Deficiency of PGK is a rare cause of nonspherocytic hemolytic anemia, often associated with neuromuscular abnormalities.

Bisphosphoglycerate Mutase The same protein molecule is responsible for both bisphosphoglycerate mutase and bisphosphoglycerate phosphatase activities in the erythrocyte.[35,81] This enzyme is particularly important because it regulates the concentration of 2,3-BPG of erythrocytes. In its role as a bisphosphoglyceromutase, the enzyme competes with PGK for 1,3-BPG as a substrate. It changes 1,3-BPG to 2,3-BPG, thereby dissipating the energy of the high-energy acylphosphate bond.[82] It is inhibited by its product 2,3-BPG and by inorganic phosphate, and it is activated by 2-phosphoglycerate and by increased pH levels. It requires 3-phosphoglycerate for activity. In its role as bisphosphoglycerate phosphatase it catalyzes the removal of the phosphate group from carbon 2 of 2,3-BPG.[82] It is inhibited by its product 3-phosphoglycerate and by sulfhydryl reagents. It is most active at a slightly acid pH and is strongly stimulated by bisulfite and phosphoglycolate. Phosphoglycolate, the most potent activator of phosphatase activity, is present in erythrocytes at very low concentrations,[83] but the source of this substance in red cells is a mystery.[84,85] Phosphoglycolate phosphatase, the enzyme that hydrolyzes phosphoglycolate, has also been identified in erythrocytes.[86]

Bisphosphoglycerate mutase is a homodimer, with 30-kDa subunits consisting of 258 amino acids. The crystal structure of human bisphosphoglycerate mutase has been determined, providing a rationale for the specific residues that are crucial for synthase, mutase, and phosphatase activity.[87] The gene for bisphosphoglycerate mutase (*BPGM*) has been mapped to chromosome 7q31-34 and it consists of 3 exons, spanning more than 22 kb.[88]

A deficiency of bisphosphoglycerate mutase results in a marked decrease in red cell 2,3-BPG levels. The consequent left shift of the oxygen dissociation curve leads to erythrocytosis (see Chap. 56).

Monophosphoglycerate Mutase An equilibrium is established between 3-phosphoglycerate and 2-phosphoglycerate by phosphoglyceromutase.[89] 2,3-BPG acts as an essential cofactor for the transformation. Only one case of monophosphoglycerate mutase deficiency has been characterized at the molecular level.[90] The clinical consequences of this red blood cell enzymopathy remain to be established.

Enolase Enolase is homodimeric enzyme that establishes an equilibrium between 2-phosphoglycerate and phosphoenolpyruvate. The reaction is facilitated by the presence of metal ions.[91] Aside from its enzymatic function in the glycolytic pathway, α-enolase (ENO1)[92] has been implicated in numerous diseases, including metastatic cancer, autoimmune disorders, ischemia, and bacterial infection. The gene for enolase (*ENO1*) is located on chromosome 1p36.[93]

Pyruvate Kinase The transfer of phosphate from phosphoenolpyruvate to ADP, forming ATP and pyruvate, is catalyzed by the allosteric enzyme PK.[94] This is one of the energy-yielding steps of glycolysis. Four PK isoenzymes are present in mammalian tissues: PK-M1 (in skeletal muscle), PK-M2 (in leukocytes, kidney, adipose tissue, and lungs), PK-L (in liver), and PK-R (in red blood cells). The four PK isoenzymes are products of only two genes (*PKLR* and *PKM2*). The PK-M1 and PK-M2 enzymes are formed from the *PKM2* gene by alternative splicing.[95] PK-L (the liver enzyme) and PK-R (the erythrocyte enzyme) are products of the other gene (*PKLR*), transcribed by two different, tissue-specific promoters.[96,97] *PKLR* consists of 12 exons and spans more than 10 kb.[98,99] Exon 2 but not exon 1 is present in the processed liver transcript; in the red cell enzyme exon 1, but not exon 2, is represented.[97] The red blood cell–specific mRNA is 2 kb in length and codes for a PK-R subunit of 574 amino acids.[100] PK-R is a homotetramer, each subunit containing an N domain, A domain, B domain, and C domain (Fig. 46–3).[101] Domain A is the most highly conserved, whereas the B and C domains are more variable.[102] The active site lies in a cleft between the A domain and the flexible B domain. The C domain contains the binding site for fructose-1,6-diphosphate. Both intra- and intersubunit interactions are considered to be key determinants of the allosteric response, which involves switching of the PK tetramer from the low-affinity T-state to the high-affinity R-state.[103–108] Red cell PK manifests sigmoid kinetics with respect to phosphoenolpyruvate in the absence of fructose-1,6-diphosphate. Hyperbolic kinetics are observed in the presence of even minute amounts of fructose-1,6-diphosphate,[109,110] so that at low concentrations of phosphoenolpyruvate the enzyme activity is greatly increased by fructose diphosphate. PK deficiency is the most common cause of hereditary nonspherocytic hemolytic anemia.

Lactate Dehydrogenase LDH catalyzes the reversible reduction of pyruvate to lactate by NADH, the last step in the Embden-Meyerhof pathway. The enzyme is composed of H (heart) and M (muscle) subunits. In red cells, the predominant subunit is H.[111] However, hereditary absence of the H subunit seems to be a benign condition, usually without clinical manifestations,[112] although one case with hemolysis has been reported.[113,114] Absence of the M subunit has been reported as well,[111] and was unaccompanied by hematologic manifestations. Judging from the origin of the reports, LDH deficiency appears to be most common in Japan, where population surveys show a gene frequency of approximately 0.05 for each deficiency,[115] and several mutations have been identified.[115]

Glucose-6-Phosphate Dehydrogenase G-6-PD is the most extensively studied erythrocyte enzyme.[2] It catalyzes the oxidation of glucose-6-phosphate to 6-phosphogluconolactone, which is rapidly hydrolyzed to 6-phosphogluconic acid, the first step in the hexose monophosphate pathway. $NADP^+$ is reduced to NADPH in the reaction, generating 1 mol of NADPH. The molecular weight of the highly purified enzyme has been reported to be 240 kDa,[116] but in its purified form, the molecular weight probably is approximately 105 kDa.[117] In the

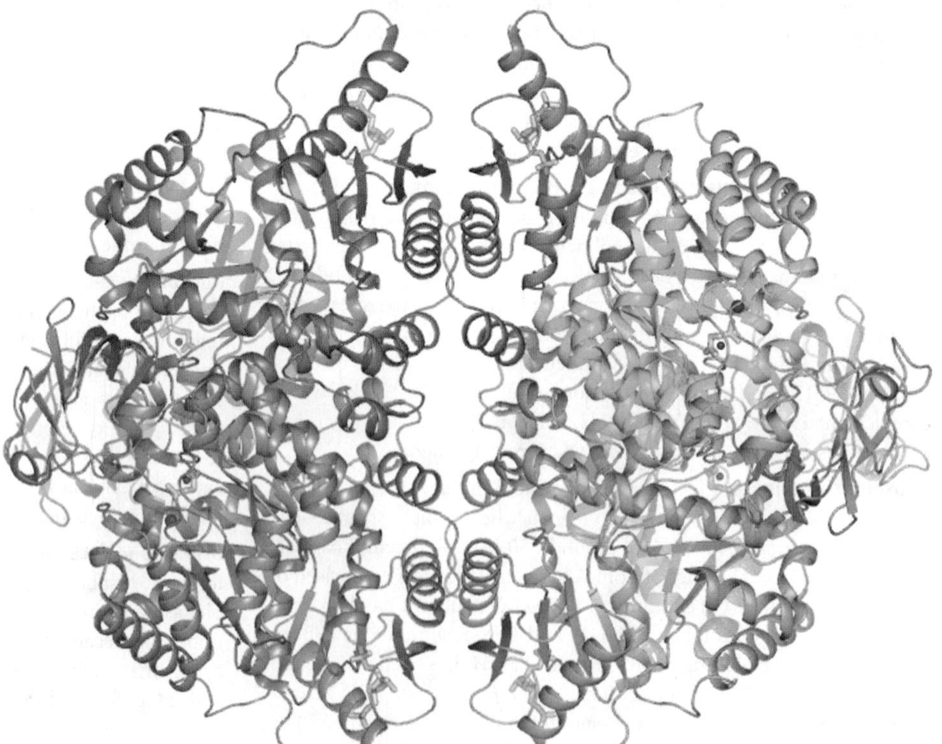

FIGURE 46–3. Ribbon representation of the human erythrocyte pyruvate kinase tetramer. The substrate phosphoglycolate and the allosteric effector fructose-1,6-diphosphate are shown in ball-and-stick representation, and colored yellow and gray, respectively. Metal ions in the active site are shown as blue (potassium) and pink (manganese) spheres. Individual subunits are colored lime, cyan, violet, and orange.

absence of NADP,+ G-6-PD dissociates into inactive subunits. The enzyme is a dimer (predominately; Fig. 46–4) or tetramer (pH dependent) in the active form, comprised of identical subunits 515-amino-acids long of approximately 59 kDa. The three-dimensional model of the crystal structure of human G-6-PD shows that each monomer is built up by two domains. The extensive interface between the two monomers is of crucial importance for enzymatic stability and activity.[118] The gene coding for G-6-PD is located on the X-chromosome (Xq28), spans 18 kb, and consists of 13 exons of which exon 1 is noncoding.[215]

G-6-PD is strongly inhibited by physiologic amounts of NADPH[119] and, to a lesser extent, by physiologic concentrations of ATP.[120] It has much higher enzyme-activity reticulocytes than mature red cells, especially for the mutant forms of the enzyme.[48,49] Many mutations, involving the activity, stability, and kinetic properties of the enzyme, are known.[12,121]

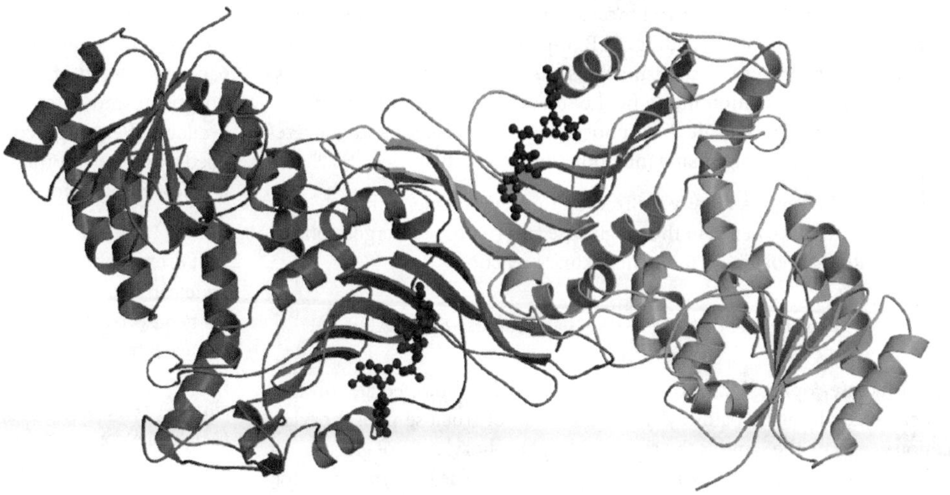

FIGURE 46–4. A dimer of human glucose-6-phosphate dehydrogenase. Subunits A and B are colored red and blue. Structural $NADP^+$ molecules are drawn in ball-and-stick mode and colored dark blue.

Phosphogluconolactonase Although 6-phosphogluconolactone, the direct product of the oxidation of glucose-6-phosphate by G-6-PD, hydrolyzes spontaneously at a relatively rapid rate at a physiologic pH, enzymatic hydrolysis is much more rapid and is required for normal metabolic flow through the stimulated hexose monophosphate pathway.[122,123] Partial deficiency of the enzyme has been observed[124] and is probably benign.[125]

Phosphogluconate Dehydrogenase Phosphogluconate dehydrogenase catalyzes the oxidation of phosphogluconate to ribulose-5-phosphate and CO_2 and the reduction of $NADP^+$ to NADPH. Variability of electrophoretic mobility of the enzyme is common in humans and in several animal species.[126] Deficiency of the enzyme has been observed only rarely and appears to be essentially innocuous or possibly associated with mild hemolysis.[127–129]

Ribosephosphate Isomerase Ribosephosphate isomerase catalyzes the interconversion of ribulose-5-phosphate and ribose-5-phosphate.[130] Deficiency of the enzyme has been described, but was associated with slowly progressive leukoencephalopathy. No dysfunction of red cells was reported.[131]

Ribulose-Phosphate Epimerase Ribulose-phosphate epimerase converts ribulose-5-phosphate to xylulose-5-phosphate.[132] The exact activity of this enzyme in human hemolysates has not been reported but seems to be less than that of ribosephosphate isomerase.

Transketolase Transketolase effects the transfer of two carbon atoms from xylulose-5-phosphate to ribose-5-phosphate, resulting in the formation of the 7-carbon sugar sedoheptulose-7-phosphate and the 3-carbon sugar glyceraldehyde-3-phosphate.[130,132] It can also catalyze the reaction between xylulose-5-phosphate and erythrose-4-phosphate, producing fructose-6-phosphate and glyceraldehyde-3-phosphate. Thiamine pyrophosphate is a coenzyme for transketolase, and the activity of erythrocyte transketolase has been used as an index of the adequacy of thiamine nutrition.[133]

Transaldolase The conversion of seduhepulose-7-phosphate and glyceraldehyde-3-phosphate into erythrose-4-phosphate and fructose-6-phosphate is catalyzed by transaldolase.[132] This is another one in the series of molecular rearrangements that leads in the conversion of the 5-carbon sugar formed in the phosphogluconate dehydrogenase step to metabolic intermediates of the EMP. One patient with transaldolase deficiency has been described, suffering from hepatosplenomegaly. No hemolysis was demonstrated.[134]

L-Hexonate Dehydrogenase Red cells contain L-hexonate dehydrogenase, an enzyme that has the capacity to reduce aldoses such as glucose, galactose, or glyceraldehyde to their corresponding polyol (i.e., glucose to sorbitol, galactose to dulcitol, and glyceraldehyde to glycerol). NADPH serves as a hydrogen donor for this reaction.[135] Aldose reductase,[136] another enzyme that can catalyze this reaction, may also be present in red cells.

Utilization of Substrates Other Than Glucose as Energy Sources

The red cell has the capacity to utilize several other substrates in addition to glucose as a source of energy. Among these are adenosine, inosine, fructose, mannose, galactose, dihydroxyacetone, and lactate. Although in the circulation red cells normally rely on glucose as their energy source, the utilization of other substrates, particularly during blood storage (see Chap. 140) and in certain experimental situations, is of interest.

Adenosine and Inosine Adenosine has been used as an experimental blood preservative, and it may also be metabolized by human red cells *in vivo*.[137] Adenosine is deaminated to inosine by the enzyme adenosine deaminase (ADA)[138]:

$$\text{Adenosine} \xrightarrow{\text{ADA}} \text{Inosine} + NH_3$$

It apparently plays a regulatory role in the concentration of purine nucleotides in the red cell. Deficiency of ADA is associated with severe combined immunodeficiency (see Chap. 82).[139] In this disorder, large quantities of deoxyadenine nucleotides, not normally present in erythrocytes, accumulate. A hereditary increase in activity of this enzyme in the erythrocyte is associated with nonspherocytic hemolytic anemia. For reasons that are not understood, ADA activity also increases in the red cells of AIDS patients[140] and of those with Diamond-Blackfan anemia.[141]

Inosine formed in the ADA reaction or added directly to red cells may enter the erythrocyte and undergo phosphorolysis to form hypoxanthine and ribose-1-phosphate:

$$\text{Inosine} + \text{Pi} \xrightarrow{\text{Nucleoside Phosphorylase}} \text{R-1-P} + \text{Hypoxanthine}$$

This reaction is of particular interest because it results in the introduction of a phosphorylated sugar, R-1-P, into the erythrocyte without the utilization of ATP.[142] The R-1-P may then be further metabolized to yield high-energy phosphate. The nucleoside phosphorylase reaction appears to be the only practical means by which ATP can be formed in the cell without first expending ATP to prepare an unphosphorylated substrate for further metabolism. Consequently, the use of inosine has received much attention in the field of blood banking (see Chap. 140). Deficiency of nucleoside phosphorylase is associated with severe immunodeficiency and many mutations have been identified.[143–145]

Fructose Fructose is readily utilized by the erythrocyte, although at a rate somewhat slower than that of glucose.[146] Fructose undergoes phosphorylation at position 6 in the hexokinase reaction:

$$\text{Fructose} + \text{ATP} \xrightarrow[\text{Mg}^{2+}]{\text{Hexokinase}} \text{Fructose-6-P} + \text{ADP}$$

Fructose-6-phosphate is a normal metabolic intermediate in the anaerobic glycolytic pathway. Thus, the result of fructose phosphorylation is exactly the same as the result of the phosphorylation of glucose.

Fructose may also be metabolized by another red cell enzyme, sorbitol dehydrogenase.[147] This enzyme reduces fructose to its corresponding polyol, sorbitol, with NADH serving as a hydrogen donor. The reaction is reversible, and a pathway therefore exists for the formation of fructose from glucose through L-hexonate dehydrogenase and sorbitol dehydrogenase.

Mannose Mannose is also phosphorylated in the hexokinase reaction[148]:

$$\text{Mannose} + \text{ATP} \xrightarrow[\text{Mg}^{2+}]{\text{Hexokinase}} \text{Mannose-6-P} + \text{ADP}$$

Mannose-6-phosphate must be isomerized to fructose-6-phosphate before it is further metabolized by erythrocytes. This is accomplished by phosphomannose isomerase (PMI)[149]:

$$\text{Mannose-6-P} \xrightleftharpoons{\text{PMI}} \text{Fructose-6-P}$$

Phosphomannose isomerase of red cells has very low activity, even at its pH optimum of 5.9.[148] The rate of mannose utilization is therefore limited by the activity of phosphomannose isomerase. Young red cells have enhanced phosphomannose isomerase activity and can therefore utilize mannose at a more rapid rate than can mature red cells.

Galactose The utilization of galactose by erythrocytes is more complex than that of most other substrates. At low concentrations of galactose, metabolism occurs by way of galactokinase, galactose-1-phosphate uridyltransferase, and phosphoglucomutase.[150] Unlike fructose, mannose, and glucose, galactose is phosphorylated at position 1:

$$\alpha\text{-Galactose} + \text{ATP} \xrightarrow[\text{Mg}^{2+}]{\text{Galactokinase}} \alpha\text{-Galactose-1-P} + \text{ADP}$$

The galactose-1-phosphate formed in the galactokinase reaction exchanges with the glucose-1-phosphate moiety of uridine diphosphoglucose (UDPG) in the galactose-1-phosphate uridyltransferase reaction:

$$\alpha\text{-Galactose-1-P} + \text{UDPG} \xrightleftharpoons{\text{Transferase}} \alpha\text{-Galactose-1-P} + \text{UDPgalactose}$$

The uridine diphosphogalactose (UDPgalactose) formed in this reaction is epimerased to UDPG:

$$\text{UDAgalactose} \xrightleftharpoons[\text{NAD}^+]{\text{Eprimerase}} \text{UDPG}$$

The α-glucose-1-phosphate in the transferase reaction is transformed to α-glucose-6-phosphate in the phosphoglucomutase reaction with glucose-1,6-diphosphate acting as coenzyme:

$$\alpha\text{-Glucose-1-P} \xrightleftharpoons[\text{Glucose-1,6-diP}]{\text{PGM}} \alpha\text{-Glucose-6-P}$$

The α-glucose-6-phosphate formed may join the direct metabolic stream after conversion by phosphoglucose isomerase to fructose-6-phosphate. It may also undergo anomerization to β-glucose-6-phosphate and enter the hexose monophosphate pathway if $NADP^+$ is available. Very high concentrations of galactose appear to be metabolized by way of another pathway, as yet poorly delineated. This pathway is known not to involve galactose-1-phosphate uridyltransferase or to have the capacity to reduce NAD^+.[47]

Dihydroxyacetone and Glyceraldehyde As indicated earlier, glyceraldehyde can be reduced in erythrocytes to glycerol in the L-hexonate dehydrogenase reaction. In addition, glyceraldehyde and dihydroxyacetone can each be phosphorylated by ATP in the presence of the enzyme triokinase.[151] Like other kinases, this enzyme has a requirement for magnesium. A remarkable feature of this enzyme is its extraordinarily low K_m (Michaelis constant) for dihydroxyacetone. It is half-saturated with this substrate at a concentration of only 0.5 μM. The products of the triokinase reaction, dihydroxyacetone phosphate or glyceraldehyde-3-phosphate, are normal metabolic intermediates and can be metabolized in the usual fashion. Because of its capacity to act as an alternate substrate for red cell energy metabolism and 2,3-BPG formation, dihydroxyacetone has been studied as an experimental additive for blood storage.[152]

Glycogen Metabolism

Red cells have the capacity to form and to break down glycogen. They contain the enzymes UDPG-glycogen glucosyltransferase, α-1,4-glucan, and α-1,4-glucan-6-glycosyltransferase (the brancher enzyme) for the formation of glycogen from glucose-1-phosphate. They contain the enzymes phosphorylase and amylo-1,6-glucosidase (the debrancher enzyme) for the breakdown of glycogen.[153] Only very little glycogen is present in normal red cells,[154] and most of what was thought to be in red cells may actually be platelet and leukocyte glycogen.[155] The function of glycogen in red cell metabolism is not understood.

Glutathione Metabolism of the Erythrocyte

The red cell contains a high concentration (approximately 2 mM) of the sulfhydryl-containing tripeptide GSH.[156] Red cell GSH appears to undergo a rapid turnover, with a terminal half-life ($T_{1/2}$) of approximately 4 days.[157] Glutathione biosynthesis occurs in two steps:

$$\text{Glutamate} + \text{Cysteine} + \text{ATP} \rightarrow \gamma\text{-Glutamylcysteine} + \text{ADP} + \text{P}_i$$

$$\gamma\text{-Glutamylcysteine} + \text{Glycine} + \text{ATP} \rightarrow \text{GSH} + \text{ADP} + \text{P}_i$$

The first step is catalyzed by γ-glutamylcysteine synthetase. This enzyme is a heterodimer composed of a catalytic 73-kDa heavy chain and a regulatory 31-kDa light chain.[158] The subunits are encoded by separate genes, located on chromosome 6p12 (*GCLC*)[159] and 1p21 (*GCLM*),[160] respectively. The second step is irreversible and mediated by glutathione synthetase. This enzyme is a homodimer of 52 kDa.[161] The 23-kb gene coding for glutathione synthetase (*GSS*) is located on chromosome 20q11.2.[162]

The red cell requires a system for the synthesis of GSH because of the active transport of GSSG from the erythrocyte.[163] It has also been suggested that a requirement for GSH synthesis comes from the amino-acid-transporting function of the γ-glutamyl cycle.[164] However, this pathway is not present in red cells.[165,166]

One important function of GSH in the erythrocyte is the detoxification of low levels of hydrogen peroxide that may form spontaneously or as a result of drug administration. In either event, the superoxide radical may be formed first and then be converted to H_2O_2 by the action of the copper-containing enzyme superoxide dismutase.[167] Hydrogen peroxide is reduced to water through the mediation of the enzyme glutathione peroxidase.[168] Glutathione peroxidase is a selenium-containing[169] tetrameric enzyme consisting of 21-kDa subunits. A polymorphism affecting the activity of this enzyme, which is most common in persons of Mediterranean descent,[170] has been described. The consequent decreases in enzyme activity are without clinical effect. The genes for several glutathione peroxidases have been cloned, including that of the erythrocyte.[171] Glutathione peroxidase levels are regulated by selenium at two levels: during mRNA formation, and during translation of the mRNA as a result of the regulation of selenocysteine incorporation specified by a unusual use of the UGA codon.[172,173]

GSH also functions in maintaining integrity of the erythrocyte by reducing sulfhydryl groups of hemoglobin membrane.[174] In the process of reducing peroxides or oxidized protein sulfhydryl groups, GSH is converted to GSSG, or may form mixed disulfides. GSSG, like certain other disulfides, has the capacity to inhibit red cell hexokinase,[54,175] although greater than physiologic levels appear to be needed for this effect. It may also complex with hemoglobin A to form hemoglobin A_3.[176]

Glutathione reductase (GSR) provides an efficient mechanism for the reduction of GSSG to GSH in the red cell. A mitochondrial and a cytoplasmic isozyme are both produced from the same mRNA, most likely by alternative initiation of translation.[177] GSR is a homodimer, linked by a disulfide bridge. Each 56-kDa subunit contains four domains, of which domains 1 and 2 bind FAD (flavin adenine dinucleotide) and NADPH, respectively. Domain 4 constitutes the interface.[178] The subunit is encoded by the *GSR* gene, located on chromosome 8p21.1.[179] *GSR* spans 50 kb and contains 13 exons.[177]

Glutathione reductase is a flavin enzyme, and either NADPH or NADH may serve as a hydrogen donor.[180] In the intact cell, only the NADPH system appears to function.[181] The same enzyme system appears to have the capacity to reduce mixed disulfides of GSH and proteins.[44] Although inherited deficiencies of this enzyme exist,[182] the activity of red cell glutathione reductase is strongly influenced by the riboflavin content of the diet.[183] Red cells also contain thioltransferase that can catalyze GSH-dependent reduction of some disulfides.[184]

Oxidized glutathione is actively extruded from the erythrocyte[163,185,186] by a system consisting of at least two GSSG-activated adenosine triphosphatases that serve as an enzymatic basis for this transport process.[187] In addition to transporting GSSG, the system appears to have the capacity to transport thioether conjugates of GSH and electrophiles formed by the action of glutathione-S-transferase.[188,189] Erythrocytes contain a glutathione-S-transferase that is distinct from the predominant liver forms of the enzyme. This enzyme, designated either type III or ρ to distinguish it from the liver enzymes, catalyzes the formation of a thioether bond between GSH and a variety of xenobiotics. The role of glutathione-S-transferase in the erythrocyte has not been established. It may be that it serves to cleanse the blood of xenobiotics to which the red cell membrane is permeable. Glutathione-S-transferase could conjugate such substances to glutathione, and the detoxified product of conjugation would be transported out of the red cell for subsequent disposal. The enzyme has the capacity to reversibly bind heme, and a possible role in heme transport has been postulated.[190] Fairly severe deficiency of this enzyme is associated with hemolytic anemia, but a cause-and-effect relationship has not been established.[191]

GENETICS

The great majority of red cell enzyme deficiencies that cause hemolytic anemia are hereditary. Most are inherited as autosomal recessive disorders, but G-6-PD deficiency and PGK deficiency are X chromosome-linked. The vast majority of the genes encoding for the red cell enzymes have been identified, making the molecular diagnosis of hereditary red cell enzyme deficiency possible. Occasionally, acquired forms of enzyme deficiencies, particularly PK deficiency, have been encountered, usually in patients with hematologic neoplasia.[192–195]

ENZYME DEFICIENCIES—BIOCHEMICAL GENETICS AND MOLECULAR BIOLOGY

Table 46–2 lists the erythrocyte enzyme deficiencies that have been shown to cause hemolytic anemia and other hematologic diseases. Other red cell enzyme deficiencies (Table 46–3) do not appear to cause a functional abnormality of the erythrocyte.[196] For example, acatalasemia, the state in which there is a virtually total absence of red cell catalase, is devoid of hematologic manifestations.[197] Similarly, red cells without cholinesterase[198] survive normally in most cases.

The lack of clinical manifestations is not always clear-cut. In some instances, hemolytic anemia is reported in some individuals with a given deficiency but not in others. For example, most subjects with LDH deficiency have no anemia, but cases with hemolysis have been reported.[114] Such ambiguity could result from differences in environmental and genetic factors or from bias of ascertainment. Erythrocyte enzyme assays are usually carried out on patients with hemolytic anemia. Thus, a benign enzyme defect may be thought, mistakenly, to cause hemolysis because it is found in a patient with hemolytic anemia. Deficiencies of PGK and of glutathione synthetase are usually associated with hereditary nonspherocytic hemolytic anemia, but cases have been reported in which these deficiencies were unassociated with any hematologic manifestations.[199,200] At times it has been suggested that moderate decreases in the activity of glutathione peroxidase causes hemolytic anemia, but the best available evidence indicates that this enzyme is not ordinarily rate limiting in erythrocyte metabolism and not associated with hemolytic anemia.[8] Table 46–3 includes deficiencies that may cause hemolytic anemia but for which a cause-and-effect relationship has not been clearly established, such as those of phosphogluconolactonase,[124] enolase,[201,202] and glutathione-S-transferase.[191]

Patients with unstable hemoglobins (see Chap. 48) may present with the clinical picture of hereditary nonspherocytic hemolytic anemia. Hemolytic anemia resulting from abnormalities in the lipid composition of the red cell membrane, particularly increased phosphatidyl choline, occur rarely (see Chap. 45).

Glucose-6-Phosphate Dehydrogenase

Biochemical Genetics The "normal" or wild-type enzyme is designated as G-6-PD B. Many variants of G-6-PD have been detected all over the world, associated with a wide range of biochemical characteristics and phenotypes. Accordingly, five classes of G-6-PD variants can be distinguished based on enzymatic activity and clinical manifestations (Table 46–4).[203] Before it became possible to characterize G-6-PD variants at the DNA level, they were distinguished from each other on the basis of biochemical characteristics, such as electrophoretic mobility, K_m for NADP and glucose-6-P, ability to utilize substrate analogues, pH activity profile, and thermal stability. To facilitate comparison of variants characterized in different laboratories, international standards for the methodology were established.[204] In the case of the common G-6-PD A– and G-6-PD Mediterranean mutations, the abnormal enzyme may be synthesized at normal or near-normal rates but has decreased stability *in vivo*.[205] The amount of enzyme antigen in the red cells declines concurrently with enzyme activity.[206] This suggests that the mutant protein in these variants is rendered unusually sensitive to proteolysis in the environment of the erythrocyte.[207] Other mutations also result in the formation of enzyme molecules with decreased enzyme activity[206] and with altered kinetic properties,[208] some of which may render them functionally inadequate. Detailed biochemical characteristics of some 400 putatively distinct G-6-PD variants have been tabulated.[209]

TABLE 46–2. Red Cell Enzyme Abnormalities Leading to Hematologic Disease

Enzyme	Clinical Features	Inheritance	Red Cell Morphology	Diagnosis (Reference) Screening Test	Diagnosis (Reference) Assay	Response to Splenectomy*	Approximate Frequency†
Hexokinase	HNSHA	AR	Unremarkable	–	455	+ +	Rare
Glucose phosphate isomerase	HNSHA; neurologic abnormalities (?)	AR	Unremarkable	455	455	+ + +	Unusual
Phosphofructokinase	HNSHA and/or muscle glycogen storage disease	AR	Unremarkable	–	455	0	Rare
Aldolase	HNSHA and mild liver glycogen storage; ? myopathy, mental retardation	AR	Unremarkable	–	455	?	Very rare
Triosephosphate isomerase	HNSHA and severe neuromuscular disease	AR	Unremarkable	455	455		Rare
Phosphoglycerate kinase	HNSHA; myoglobinuria behavioral disturbances	SL	Unremarkable	–	455	+ +	Rare
Bisphosphoglycerate mutase	Erythrocytosis	AR	Unremarkable	–	455		Very rare
Pyruvate kinase	HNSHA	AR	Usually unremarkable; occasionally contracted echinocytes	455	455	+ +	Unusual
Glucose-6-phosphate dehydrogenase	HNSHA; drug- or infection-induced hemolysis; favism	SL	Usually unremarkable; rarely "bite cells"	455	455	±	Very common
Glutathione reductase	Drug-sensitive hemolytic anemia and favism	AR	Unremarkable	455	455	?	Very rare
γ-Glutamylcysteine synthetase	HNSHA, drug- or infection-induced hemolysis, neurologic abnormalities (?)	AR	Unremarkable	521	523	?	Very rare
Glutathione synthetase	HNSHA; drug- or infection-induced hemolysis; neurologic defect and 5-oxoprolinuria in some cases	AR	Usually unremarkable	521	523	0	Rare
Pyrimidine 5′-nucleotidase	HNSHA; ? mental retardation in some cases	AR	Prominent stippling	282	524	0	Rare
Adenylate kinase	HNSHA	AR	Unremarkable	–	455		Rare
Adenosine deaminase (increased activity)	HNSHA	AD	Unremarkable	–	455		Rare
NADH-cytochrome b_5 reductase (see Chap. 49)	Methemoglobinemia; sometimes with mental retardation	AR	Unremarkable	522	455		Unusual

AD, autosomal dominant; AR, autosomal recessive; HNSHA, hereditary nonspherocytic hemolytic anemia; SL, sex linked.

*On a scale of 0 to 4+, where 4+ is a complete response. In many cases, data are meager.

†Very common if incidence is >5%. Unusual if >100 cases reported. Rare if 10–100 cases reported. Very rare if <10 cases reported.

G-6-PD deficiency has been encountered in the rat, dog,[210] mouse,[211] and horse.[212] Targeted deletion in the mouse causes embryonic lethality.[213]

Molecular Biology The gene for G-6-PD is located on the X-chromosome (Xq28). It spans 18 kb, containing 13 exons. The coding sequence begins in exon 2. The intron between exons 2 and 3 spans nearly 10 kb.[214] The promoter shares many features common of other housekeeping genes.[215] Methylation of certain cytidines at the 3′ end is believed to have a regulatory function.[216] The enzyme is composed of 515 amino acids with a calculated molecular weight of approximately 59 kDa. Aggregation of these inactive monomers into catalytically active dimers and higher forms requires the presence of NADP (see Fig. 46–4).[217] Hence, NADP is bound to the enzyme both as a structural component and as one of the substrates of the reaction.[218] Examination of mutants suggested that amino acids 386 and 387 bind one of the phosphates of NADP.[219] This seems to be borne out by crystallographic studies, which

TABLE 46–3. Red Cell Enzyme Abnormalities Not Leading to Hematologic Disease

Enzyme	Clinical Features	Inheritance	Diagnosis Reference Assay	Estimated Frequency*	Reference
6-Phosphogluconate dehydrogenase (complete deficiency)	None	AR	455	Unusual	127–129
6-Phosphogluconolactonase (partial defect)	Probably none	AD	456	Unusual	124, 125
δ-ALA dehydrase	None	AD	457		
Acetylcholinesterase	None	AR	455	Very rare	198
Adenine phosphoribosyl transferase	Kidney stones	AR	458	Rare	459
Adenosine deaminase (decreased activity)	Immunodeficiency	AR	455	Rare	139
AMP deaminase	None	AR	460	Unusual	461
Carbonic anhydrase I	None	AR	462	Rare	463
Carbonic anhydrase II	Osteoporosis	AR		Rare	464
Catalase	Oral ulcers in some types	AR	455	Rare	197
Enolase	HNSHA?	AD?	455	Rare	201, 202
Galactokinase	Cataracts	AR	455	Rare	465
Galactose-1-P-uridyltransferase	Cataracts; mental retardation; liver disease	AR	455	Rare	466
Glutathione peroxidase (partial deficiency)	None	AR and AD[456]	455	Very common	455
Glutathione reductase (partial deficiency)	None	Usually not inherited[456]	455	Very common	8, 467
Glutathione-S-transferase	HNSHA	?	455	Very rare	191
Glyceraldehyde-3-phosphate dehydrogenase (partial defect)	None	AD	455	Unusual	468
Glyoxalase I	None	AR		Rare	469
Hypoxanthine-guanine phosphoribosyl transferase (HGPRT)	Lesch-Nyhan syndrome (neurologic symptoms and gout)	SL	470	Rare	471
Inosine triphosphatase	None	AR	463	Rare	472
Lactate dehydrogenase	None	AR	455	Rare	112
NADPH diaphorase	None	AR	455	Rare	473
Phosphoglucomutase	None	AR	455	Rare	474
Uroporphyrinogen 1 synthase	Acute intermittent porphyria	AD	475	Unusual (common in selected populations)	476

AD, autosomal dominant; ALA, aminolevulinic acid; AMP, adenosine monophosphate; AR, autosomal recessive; HNSHA, hereditary nonspherocytic hemolytic anemia; SL, sex linked.

*Very common if incidence is >5%, common if 1–5%, unusual if 0.01–1%, rare if <0.01%.

show this region to be close to the intersubunit interface where structural NADP is bound.[118] The glucose-6-phosphate binding site has been identified at amino acid 205.[221] The three-dimensional model of the crystal structure of human G-6-PD shows that the G-6-PD monomer is built up by two domains, a N-terminal domain and a large $\beta\alpha$ domain with an antiparallel nine-stranded sheet. The extensive interface between the two monomers is of crucial importance for enzymatic stability and activity.[118]

Under physiologic conditions, the active human enzyme exists in a dimer-tetramer equilibrium. Lowering the pH causes a shift towards the tetrameric form.[220]

African Variants Among persons of African descent, a mutant enzyme G-6-PD A+, with normal activity is polymorphic. It migrates electrophoretically more rapidly than the normal B enzyme, has substitution of Asn to Asp at codon 126, resulting from nucleotide 376A→G.[222] G-6-PD A– is the principal deficient variant found among people of African origin. The red cells contain only 5 to 15 percent of the normal amount of enzyme activity; however because of the instability of the enzyme, the age dependent decline of the activity renders old red cells severely deficient and susceptible to hemolysis. These two electrophoretically rapid variants are common in African populations have in common a nucleotide substitution at cDNA nucleotide 376 that produces the amino acid substitution responsible for the rapid electrophoretic mobility. Most samples with G-6-PD A– manifest an additional mutation at nucleotide 202, which accounts for its *in vivo* instability.[223] Less commonly, the additional mutation is at a different site (see Table 46–4). Thus G-6-PD A– arose in an individual who

TABLE 46–4. Some G-6-PD Variants That Have Been Characterized at the DNA Level*

Variant	Nucleotide Substitution	WHO Class†	Amino Acid Substitution	Reference
Aures	c.143T→C	2	p.Ile48Thr	477
A–				223
Distrito Federal				478
Matera				479
Castilla	c.202G→A	3	p.Val68Met	478
Betica				224
Tepic				478
Ferrara				480
A	c.376A→G	4	p.Asn126Asp	222
Mediterranean				479
Dallas				481
Birmingham	c.563C→T	2	p.Ser188 Phe	481
Sassari				482
Cagliari				482
Panama				E. Beutler (unpublished)
A–	c.680G→T	3	p.Arg227Leu	223
	c.376A→G		p.Asn126Asp	
Seattle				482
Lodi	c.844G→C	2	p.Asp282His	483
Modena				480
				484
A–	c.968T→C	3	p.Leu323 Pro	223
Betica	c.376A→G		p.Asn126Asp	
Selma				
Chatham	c.1003G→A	3	p.Ala335Thr	479
Mt. Sinai	c.1159C→T	1	p.Arg387Cys	485
	c.376A→G		p.Asn126Asp	
Nashville	c.1178G→A	1	p.Arg393His	414
Anaheim				486
Calgary				
Portici				
Alhambra	c.1180G→C	1	p.Val394Leu	487
Utrecht	c.1225C→T	1	p.Pro409Ser	233
Taiwan-Hakka	c.1376G→T	2	p.Arg459Leu	488
Gifu-like				
Agrigento-like				489
Canton				
Cosenza	c.1376G→C	2	p.Arg459Pro	490

*See Beutler E, Vulliamy TJ[491] for tabulation.

†Class 1, severely deficient, associated with nonspherocytic hemolytic anemia; class 2, severe deficiency (1–10% residual activity), associated with acute hemolytic anemia; class 3, moderate deficiency (10–60% residual activity); class 4, not deficient (60–150% activity); class 5, increased activity (>150%).

already had the G-6-PD A+ mutation. However, the ancestral human sequence has been deduced to be that of G-6-PD B, both by showing that this is the sequence of the chimpanzee,[224] our nearest relative, and by analysis of linkage dysequilibrium.[225] The nucleotide 202 mutation results in G-6-PD deficiency,[226] as the 202 mutation has been found in a patient with deficiency without the presence of the nucleotide 376 mutation.[227]

Variants in the Mediterranean Region Among white populations, G-6-PD deficiency is most common in Mediterranean countries. The most common enzyme variant in this region is G-6-PD Mediterranean.[208] The enzyme activity of the red cells of individuals who have inherited this abnormal gene is barely detectable. Other variants are also prevalent in the Mediterranean region, including G-6-PD A– and G-6-PD Seattle (see Table 46–4).

Variants in Asia A great many different variants have been described in Asian populations. Some of these proved to be identical at a molecular level (e.g., G-6-PD Gifu, Agrigento, Canton, and Taiwan-Hakka all have the same mutation at cDNA nucleotide 1376), but DNA analysis has shown that more than 10 different mutations are found in various Asian populations.[228–230]

Variants Producing Hereditary Nonspherocytic Hemolytic Anemia Some mutations of G-6-PD result in chronic hemolysis without, but exacerbated by, precipitating causes. These variants are class I mutants (World Health Organization [WHO] class 1, see also Table 46–4).[203] From a functional point of view, these mutations are more severe than the more commonly occurring polymorphic forms of the enzyme, such as G-6-PD Mediterranean and G-6-PD A–, but the *in vitro* enzyme activity may actually be greater in such variants. It has been suggested that specific biochemical characteristics, such as susceptibility to inhibition by NADPH, might explain the chronic hemolysis that occurs in patients with such variants,[119] but no unifying principle that accounts for the clinical effects of variants has been found. On a molecular level, such variants are often located in exons 10 and 11, encoding the subunit interface,[118,219] or in the region of the glucose-6-phosphate binding site.[232] There are, however, exceptions to this rule.[27,232] The clinical severity of these variants can be quite variable.[233]

Pyruvate Kinase

PK deficiency is the most common cause of nonspherocytic hemolytic anemia because of defective enzyme. Like G-6-PD deficiency, the disease is genetically heterogeneous, with different mutations causing different kinetic changes in the enzyme that is formed. There are even cases in which the activity of PK as measured *in vitro* is higher than normal, but a kinetically abnormal enzyme is responsible for the occurrence of hemolytic anemia.[234] Kinetic characterization and analysis of

PK mutants is considerably more complex than analysis of G-6-PD mutants. Most PK-deficient patients are compound heterozygous for two different (missense) mutations, rather than homozygous for one. Assuming that stable mutant monomers are synthesized, up to seven different tetrameric forms of PK may be present in compound heterozygous individuals, each with distinct structural and kinetic properties. This complicates genotype-to-phenotype correlations in these individuals as it is difficult to infer which mutation is primarily responsible for deficient enzyme function and the clinical phenotype.[235,236] More than 190 mutations in the *PKLR* gene encoding the red cell PK have been identified (www.pklrmutationdatabase.com). Seventy percent of these mutations are missense mutations affecting conserved residues in structurally and functionally important domains of PK. There appears to be no direct relationship between the nature and location of the substituted amino acid and the type of molecular perturbation.[101] Hence, the nature of the mutation has relatively little predictive value with respect to the severity of the clinical course and the phenotypic expression of identical mutations can be strikingly different in patients.[235–239]

Because PK deficiency provides protection against infection and replication of *Plasmodium falciparum* in human erythrocytes, it has been suggested that PK deficiency may confer a protective advantage against malaria in human populations in areas where this disease is endemic.[240,241]

PK deficiency has also been recognized in dogs, cats, and mice.[212] In dogs and mice, the deficiency causes severe anemia and marked reticulocytosis, closely resembling human PK deficiency. Basenji dogs completely lack PK-R enzymatic activity and, instead, only the PK-M2 isozyme is expressed in their red blood cells.[242] PK-deficient mice show delayed switching from PK-M2 to PK-R, resulting in delayed onset of the hemolytic anemia.[243]

Other Enzyme Deficiencies

Hexokinase Deficiency Seventeen families with HK deficiency have been described to date[244] and only three patients have been characterized at the molecular level.[245–247] Two of these patients were homozygous, either for a highly conserved substitution in the enzyme's active site[247] or a lethal out-of-frame deletion of exons 5 to 8 of *HK1*.[246]

In mice, a mutation designated *downeast anemia* causes severe hemolytic anemia with extensive tissue iron deposition and marked reticulocytosis, representing a mouse model of generalized HK deficiency.[248]

Glucosephosphate Isomerase Deficiency Glucosephosphate isomerase deficiency is second to PK deficiency in frequency, with respect to glycolytic enzymopathies. Approximately 50 families with glucosephosphate isomerase deficiency have been described worldwide.[249] Hydrops fetalis appears more common in GPI deficiency than in other enzyme deficiencies.[250] In rare cases, GPI deficiency also affects nonerythroid tissues, causing neurologic symptoms and granulocyte dysfunction.[251] Most mutations in *GPI* are missense mutations.[249] Mapping of these mutations to the crystal structure of the human enzyme and recombinant expression of genetic variants has provided considerable insight in the molecular mechanisms causing hemolytic anemia in this disorder.[63,252] Homozygous GPI-deficient mice exhibit hematologic features resembling that of the human enzymopathy. In addition, other tissues are also affected, indicating a reduced glycolytic capability of the whole organism.[253]

Phosphofructokinase Deficiency Because red cells contain both PFK M- and L-subunits, mutations affecting either gene will lead to decreased red cell enzyme activity in PFK deficiency. In both cases the resulting hemolysis is usually mild. In case of the M subunit being affected, hemolysis is accompanied by myopathy. Fifteen PFK-deficient *PFKM* alleles have been detected and characterized.[254,255] A canine model of PFK-M deficiency characterized by a chronic compensated hemolytic disorder and exertional myopathy has been described in dogs.[256]

Aldolase Deficiency Only six patients with aldolase deficiency have been described. All displayed moderate chronic hemolytic anemia, either by itself[257] or accompanied by myopathy,[258–260] rhabdomyolysis,[261] psychomotor retardation,[259] or mental retardation[258,259]

Triosephosphate Isomerase Deficiency Triosephosphate isomerase deficiency is characterized by hemolytic anemia, often accompanied by neonatal hyperbilirubinemia requiring exchange transfusion. In addition, patients display progressive neurological dysfunction, increased susceptibility to infection, and cardiomyopathy.[262] Most affected individuals die in childhood before the age of 6 years, but there are remarkable exceptions.[263] Fourteen different mutations have been described in *TPI1*.[264] Knowledge of the crystal structure of the human enzyme has provided insight into the probable effect of mutation.[72] Mice models of triosephosphate isomerase deficiency have been developed.[265] These models suggest that homozygosity for triosephosphate isomerase-null alleles may be lethal at an early stage of development.[266]

Phosphoglycerate Kinase Deficiency PGK deficiency is one of the relatively uncommon causes of hereditary nonspherocytic hemolytic anemia. Mutations in this X chromosome-linked disorder may cause chronic hemolysis with or without mental retardation, and they may cause myopathies, often with episodes of myoglobinuria, or a combination of these clinical manifestations. Twenty-six families have been described and in 20 of these families, the mutations are known.[267] The reason for different clinical manifestations of mutations of the same gene remains unknown.

Bisphosphoglycerate Mutase Deficiency Bisphosphoglycerate mutase deficiency is a very rare disorder. Only two affected families have been characterized, suggesting that bisphosphoglycerate mutase deficiency is inherited as an autosomal recessive disorder; however, some heterozygous relatives have had a borderline high hemoglobin concentration.[268,269] Erythrocytosis was the predominant feature of the clinically normal probands, likely resulting from reduced 2,3-BPG levels[270] and, consequently, the increased oxygen affinity of hemoglobin (see Chap. 56).

Glutathione Reductase Deficiency Only two patients with glutathione reductase deficiency have been characterized at the molecular level. The total absence of glutathione reductase in the red cells of members of one family was associated with only rare episodes of hemolysis, possibly caused by fava beans. The patient of the other family presented with severe neonatal jaundice on the second day of life.[182]

γ-Glutamylcysteine Synthetase Deficiency γ-Glutamylcysteine synthetase deficiency is associated with mild hereditary nonspherocytic hemolytic anemia that may be fully compensated. Drug- and infection-induced hemolytic crises may occur. Nine unrelated γ-glutamylcysteine synthetase-deficient families have been described, of which four were characterized at the molecular level.[271–274] In all these cases, the causative mutation affected the heavy subunit of γ-glutamylcysteine synthetase. In approximately half of the patients with γ-glutamylcysteine synthetase deficiency, the hemolytic anemia is associated with progressive neurological manifestations.[274]

Glutathione Synthetase Deficiency Glutathione synthetase deficiency is the most common abnormality of red cell glutathione metabolism. Three distinct clinical forms of glutathione synthetase deficiency can be distinguished, most likely reflecting different mutations or epigenetic modifications in the *GSS* gene.[275] Mild to moderate hemolytic anemia is a predominant feature of the first two types of glutathione synthetase deficiency. The third and most severe type is characterized by massive urinary excretion of 5-oxoproline, metabolic acidosis, hemolytic anemia, and central nervous system damage.[276] Importantly, 5-oxoprolinuria may have other causes.[275] More than 30 mutations have been identified associated with glutathione synthetase deficiency.[277,278]

Pyrimidine 5′-Nucleotidase Deficiency Pyrimidine 5′-nucleotidase deficiency is the most frequent disorder of red cell nucleotide metabolism and a relatively common cause of mild-to-moderate hemolytic anemia.[279] More than 100 patients have been reported, but because of the relatively mild phenotype, many patients may remain undetected. No correlation has been found between residual activity and degree of hemolysis.[280] Pyrimidine 5′-nucleotidase deficiency is the only red cell enzyme deficiency in which red cell morphology is helpful because of prominent and characteristic basophilic stippling on the blood film, together with an accumulation of pyrimidine nucleotides in the red cell.[281] A number of mutations have been reported.[282] No relationship between the genotype and phenotype could be established.

Adenylate Kinase Deficiency Adenylate kinase deficiency has been reported in 12 unrelated families. In all but one case,[283] the deficiency was associated with moderate to severe hemolytic anemia. In some of the patients, mental retardation and psychomotor impairment was also observed.[284,285] Although the possible cause–effect relationship between *AK1* mutations and hemolytic anemia has initially been questioned, increasing evidence supports the existence of a relationship between the enzyme molecular defect and reduced red cell survival.[286–289] It appears that the degree of anemia is correlated with the position and type of mutation within the gene of adenylate kinase rather than the residual enzymatic deficiency.[289]

Adenosine Deaminase Hyperactivity An increased activity of adenosine deaminase is associated with hereditary nonspherocytic hemolytic anemia. It is the only red cell disorder that is inherited in an autosomal dominant disorder.[290] Adenosine deaminase hyperactivity results in depletion of red cell ATP, and hemolysis. Few cases with a 30- to 70-fold increase in activity have been described. The molecular mechanism of this disorder has not been identified but the markedly increased amounts of ADA mRNA in affected individuals indicate that the red blood cell–specific overexpression occurs at the mRNA level,[291] probably as the result of a mutation in the vicinity of the ADA gene.[292]

Cytochrome b_5 reductase deficiency causes recessive congenital methemoglobinemia (see Chap. 49). Two distinct clinical forms can be distinguished. Cyanosis is a prominent feature of both types but the more severe form (type II) is accompanied by neurologic impairment and reduced life expectancy. More than 40 mutations have been described in the *CYB5R3* gene (previously known as *DIA1*). Some of these mutations were identified in patients belonging to either class of recessive congenital methemoglobinemia.[293] Cytochrome b_5 reductase deficiency has also been recognized in dogs and cats.[212]

■ MECHANISM OF HEMOLYSIS

G-6-PD Deficiency and Other Deficiencies of Hexose Monophosphate Shunt Enzymes

The life span of G-6-PD–deficient red cells is shortened under many circumstances, particularly during drug administration and infection. The exact reason for this is not known.

Drug-Induced Hemolysis Drug-induced hemolysis in G-6-PD–deficient cells is generally accompanied by the formation of Heinz bodies, particles of denatured hemoglobin, and stromal protein (see Chap. 48), formed only in the presence of oxygen.[294] The mechanism by which Heinz bodies are formed and become attached to red cell stroma has been the subject of considerable investigation and speculation. Exposure of red cells to certain drugs results in the formation of low levels of hydrogen peroxide as the drug interacts with hemoglobin.[295] In addition, some drugs may form free radicals that oxidize GSH without the formation of peroxide as an intermediate.[296] The formation of free radicals of GSH through the action of peroxide or by the direct action of drugs may be followed either by oxidation of GSH to the disulfide form (GSSG) or complexing of the glutathione with hemoglobin to form a mixed disulfide. Such mixed disulfides are believed to form initially with the sulfhydryl group of the β-93 position of hemoglobin.[297] The mixed disulfide of GSH and hemoglobin is probably unstable and undergoes conformational changes exposing interior sulfhydryl groups to oxidation and mixed disulfide formation. Globin chain separation into free α and β chains also occurs.[298] Phenylhydrazine-like drugs also have been shown to form a hemochromogen directly with hemoglobin, a complex forming between the iron of ferriheme and the nitrogen bound to the benzene ring of the drug.[299] Once such oxidation has occurred, hemoglobin is denatured irreversibly and will precipitate as Heinz bodies. Normal red cells can defend themselves to a considerable extent against such changes by reducing GSSG to GSH and by reducing the mixed disulfides of GSH and hemoglobin through the glutathione reductase reaction.[44] However, the reduction of these disulfide bonds requires a source of NADPH. Because G-6-PD–deficient red cells are unable to reduce $NADP^+$ to NADPH at a normal rate, they are unable to reduce hydrogen peroxide or the mixed disulfides of hemoglobin and GSH. Moreover, because catalase contains tightly bound NADPH[300] that is required for activity, the lack of freely available NADPH generation may, in addition, impede disposal of hydrogen peroxide by the catalase-dependent pathway.[301] When such cells are challenged by drugs, they form Heinz bodies more readily than do normal cells. Cells containing Heinz bodies encounter difficulty in traversing the splenic pulp[302] and are eliminated relatively rapidly from the circulation. Figure 46–5 summarizes the metabolic events that may lead to red cell damage and eventually destruction.

The formation of methemoglobin frequently accompanies the administration of drugs that have the capacity to produce hemolysis of G-6-PD–deficient cells.[303] The heme groups of methemoglobin become detached from the globin more readily than do the heme

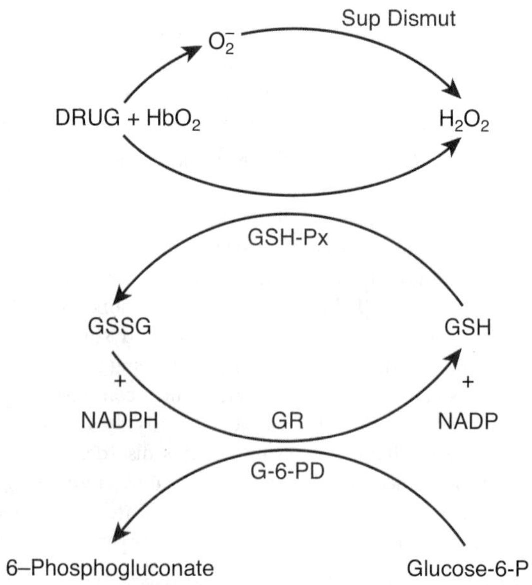

FIGURE 46–5. Reactions through which hydrogen peroxide is generated and detoxified in the erythrocyte. In G-6-PD deficiency and related disorders, inadequate generation of NADPH results in accumulation of GSSG and probably of H_2O_2. The accumulation of these substances leads to hemoglobin denaturation, Heinz body formation, and, consequently, to decreased red cell survival. GR, glutathione reductase; GSH-Px, glutathione peroxidase; GSSG, glutathione disulfide (oxidized glutathione); Sup Dismut, superoxide dismutase.

groups of oxyhemoglobin.[304] It is not clear whether methemoglobin formation plays an important role in the oxidative degradation of hemoglobin to Heinz bodies or whether formation of methemoglobin is merely an incidental side effect of oxidative drugs.[305,306]

Infection-Induced Hemolysis The mechanism of hemolysis induced by infection or occurring spontaneously in G-6-PD–deficient subjects is not well understood. The generation of hydrogen peroxide by phagocytizing leukocytes may play a role in this type of hemolytic reaction.[306]

Favism Substances capable of destroying red cell GSH have been isolated from fava beans.[307] Favism occurs only in G-6-PD–deficient subjects, but not all individuals in a particular family may be sensitive to the hemolytic effect of the beans. Nonetheless, some tendency toward familial occurrence has suggested that an additional genetic factor may be important.[308] The observation of increased excretion of glucaric acid[309] led to the suggestion that a defect in glucuronide formation might be present. An excess of individuals with the acid phosphatase ACP_1 A/C genotype has been found and attributed to a decrease in the *f* isoform of this tyrosine phosphatase.[310] Immunologic factors do not seem to play a role in favism.[311] Increased levels of red cell calcium[312,313] and consequent "cross-bonding" of membranes may occur. Such bonding of the facing inner membrane surfaces[314] may play a role in the destruction of red cells.

Neonatal Jaundice Icterus neonatorum in G-6-PD deficiency probably results principally from inadequate processing of bilirubin by the immature liver of G-6-PD–deficient infants, although shortening of red cell life span may play a role. Anemia does not appear to be present in these infants, and there is only a slight increase in carbon monoxide production, signifying a minimal decrease in red cell life span.[315,316] Severe jaundice resulting from G-6-PD deficiency seems to be limited to infants who have also inherited a mutation of the uridine diphosphoglucuronate glucuronosyltransferase-1 gene (*UGT1A1*) promoter[317] or, in Asia, the c.211G→A coding mutation.[318] In adults, these mutations are associated with Gilbert syndrome. The limited data available on liver G-6-PD in deficient adults[319] suggest that a considerable degree of deficiency may be present. If such a deficiency also is present in infants, it may play a role in impairing the borderline ability of infant livers with the *UGT1A1* promoter defect to catabolize bilirubin. Although an increased incidence of neonatal icterus has been observed in Mediterranean infants with G-6-PD deficiency and among the Chinese,[320] jaundice seems to be less common among neonates with the A– type of enzyme deficiency, although some cases have been reported in G-6-PD–deficient infants, particularly in Africa,[321–323] but also in the United States.[324] The cause of the relatively low incidence of neonatal jaundice in infants with G-6-PD A– mutation is not clear. It could result from the higher residual enzyme activity but does not appear to be related to the incidence of the UGT1A1 promoter mutation, which is actually more common in Africans and less common in Asians than it is in Europeans.[325]

Deficiencies of Other Enzymes of the Hexose Monophosphate Shunt and of Glutathione Metabolism

Deficiencies of γ-glutamylcysteine synthetase[274] and of glutathione synthetase[278] are associated with a decrease in red cell GSH levels, and the mild hemolysis that occurs in these disorders probably has a pathogenesis similar to the hemolysis that occurs in G-6-PD deficiency. The same is probably true for glutathione reductase deficiency.[182] Other defects of the hexose monophosphate shunt and associated metabolic pathways are not associated with hemolysis (see Table 46–3).

Other Enzyme Deficiencies How deficiencies of enzymes other than those of the hexose monophosphate pathway result in shortening of red cell life-span remains unknown, although it has been the object of much experimental work and of speculation. It is often believed that ATP depletion is a common pathway in producing damage to the cell leading to its destruction,[326] but the evidence that this is the case is not always compelling.[327] It is possible that, at least in some cases, alteration of the levels of red cell intermediate metabolites interferes with synthesis of cell components in early stages of development of the cell. In agreement with this observation it has been found that PK deficiency in mice alters not only the survival of red cells but also the maturation of erythroid progenitors, resulting in ineffective erythropoiesis.[328]

CLINICAL FEATURES

■ COMMON FORMS OF G-6-PD DEFICIENCY

Individuals who inherit the common (polymorphic) forms of G-6-PD deficiency, such as G-6-PD A– or G-6-PD Mediterranean, usually have no clinical manifestations. The major clinical consequence of G-6-PD deficiency is hemolytic anemia in adults and neonatal icterus in infants. Usually the anemia is episodic, but some of the unusual variants of G-6-PD may cause nonspherocytic congenital hemolytic disease (see "Variants Producing Hereditary Nonspherocytic Hemolytic Anemia" above). In general, hemolysis is associated with stress, most notably drug administration, infection, and, in certain individuals, exposure to fava beans.

Drug-Induced Hemolytic Anemia

Table 46–5 lists the drugs and other chemicals that may have the capacity to precipitate hemolytic reactions in G-6-PD–deficient individuals. Some drugs, such as chloramphenicol, may induce mild hemolysis in a person with severe, Mediterranean-type G-6-PD deficiency,[329] but not in those with the milder A– or Canton[330] types of deficiency. Drugs that are innocuous when given in normal doses (Table 46–6) may be hemolytic when given in excessive doses. A case in point is ascorbic acid, which does not cause hemolytic anemia in normal doses but which can produce severe, even fatal, hemolysis at doses of 80 g or more intravenously.[331–333] Furthermore, there appears to be a difference in the severity of the reaction to the same drug of different individuals with the same G-6-PD variant. For example, red cells from a

TABLE 46–5. Drugs and Chemicals That Should Be Avoided by Persons with G-6-PD Deficiency*

Acetanilid[294]	Nitrofurantoin (Furadantin)[505]
Dapsone[492]	Phenazopyridine (Pyridium)[506]
Fava beans	Phenylhydrazine[294]
Dimercaptosuccinic acid[493†]	Primaquine[294]
Furazolidone (Furoxone)[494,495]	Sulfacetamide[294]
Glibenclamide[496†]	Toluidine blue[507†]
Isobutyl nitrite[400,497]	Sulfanilamide[294]
Methylene blue[498]	Sulfapyridine[294]
Nalidixic acid (NegGram)[499,500†]	Thiazolesulfone[294]
Naphthalene[501,502]	Trinitrotoluene (TNT)[508]
Niridazole (Ambilhar)[503,504]	Urate oxidase[509]

*Further details may be found in Beutler E.[8]

†Single case reports. Cause and effect not certain.

TABLE 46–6. Drugs That Probably Can Safely Be Given in Normal Therapeutic Doses to G-6-PD–Deficient Subjects without Nonspherocytic Hemolytic Anemia*

Acetaminophen (paracetamol, Tylenol, hydroxyacetanilide)[294,510]
Acetophenetidin (phenacetin)[294]
Acetylsalicylic acid (aspirin)[452,510]
Aminopyrine (Pyramidon, aminopyrine)[511]
Antazoline (Antistine)[452]
Antipyrine[510]
Ascorbic acid (vitamin C)[452]
Benzhexol (Artane)[510]
Chloramphenicol[329,330,510]
Chloroguanide (Proguanil, Paludrine)[510]
Chloroquine[452,510,512]
Colchicine[510]
Diphendydramine (Benadryl)[452]
Isoniazid[510,513]
L-Dopa[510,514]
Menadione sodium bisulfite (Vitamin K3)[515]
p-Aminobenzoic acid[452]
p-Aminosalicylic acid[513]
Phenylbutazone[510]
Phenytoin[510]
Probenecid (Benemid)[510,515]
Procainamide hydrochloride (Pronestyl)[452]
Pyrimethamine (Daraprim)[452,510]
Quinine[515]
Streptomycin[510]
Sulfacytine[516]
Sulfadiazine[452,517]
Sulfaguanidine[517]
Sulfamerazine[452]
Sulfamethoxazole (Gantanol)[334]
Sulfamethoxypyridazine (Kynex)[518,519]
Sulfisoxazole (Gantrisin)[515,516]
Tiaprofenic acid[520]
Trimethoprim[510]
Tripelennamine (Pyribenzamine)[452]
Vitamin K[48]

*Further details may be found in Beutler E.[8]

single G-6-PD–deficient individual were hemolyzed in the circulation of some recipients who were given thiazolsulfone, but their survival was normal in the circulation of others.[294] Sulfamethoxazole, which was clearly hemolytic in experimental studies, does not appear to be a common cause of hemolysis in a clinical setting.[334] Undoubtedly, individual differences in the metabolism and excretion of drugs influence the extent to which G-6-PD–deficient red cells are destroyed.[335,336]

Typically, an episode of drug-induced hemolysis in G-6-PD–deficient individuals begins 1 to 3 days after drug administration is initiated.[337] Heinz bodies appear in the red cells, and the hemoglobin concentration begins to decline rapidly.[338] As hemolysis progresses, Heinz bodies disappear from the circulation, presumably as they or the erythrocytes that contain them are removed by the spleen. In severe cases, abdominal or back pain may occur. The urine may turn dark or even black. Within 4 to 6 days, there is generally an increase in the reticulocyte count, except in instances in which the patient has received the offending drug for treatment of an active infection as infection depresses erythropoiesis (see Chap. 37). Because of the tendency of infections and certain other stressful situations to precipitate hemolysis in G-6-PD–deficient individuals, many drugs have been incorrectly implicated as a cause. Other drugs, such as aspirin, have appeared on many lists of proscribed medications because very large doses could slightly reduce the red cell life span. It is important to recognize that such drugs (see Table 46–6) do not produce clinically significant hemolytic anemia. Advising patients not to ingest these drugs may not only deprive patients of potentially helpful medications, but will also weaken their confidence in the advice that they have received. Most G-6-PD–deficient patients, after all, have taken aspirin without untoward effect and are likely to distrust an advisor who counsels them that the ingestion of aspirin will have catastrophic effects.

In the A– type of G-6-PD deficiency, the hemolytic anemia is self-limited[337] because the young red cells produced in response to hemolysis have nearly normal G-6-PD levels and are relatively resistant to hemolysis.[339] The hemoglobin level may return to normal even while the same dose of drug that initially precipitated hemolysis is administered. In contrast, hemolysis is not self-limited in the more severe Mediterranean type of deficiency.[340]

Hemolytic Anemia Occurring during Infection

Anemia often develops rather suddenly in G-6-PD–deficient individuals within a few days of onset of a febrile illness. The anemia is usually relatively mild, with a decline in the hemoglobin concentration of 3 or 4 g/dL. Hemolysis has been noted particularly in patients suffering from pneumonia and in those with typhoid fever. The fulminating form of the disease occurs particularly frequently among G-6-PD–deficient patients who are infected with Rocky Mountain spotted fever.[341] Jaundice is not a prominent part of the clinical picture, except where hemolysis occurs in association with infectious hepatitis.[342,343] In that case, it can be quite intense. Presumably because of the effect of the infection, reticulocytosis is usually absent, and recovery from the anemia is generally delayed until after the active infection has abated.

Favism

Favism is potentially one of the gravest clinical consequences of G-6-PD deficiency. It occurs much more commonly in children than in adults and occurs almost exclusively in persons who have inherited variants of G-6-PD that cause severe deficiency (most frequently associated with the Mediterranean variant), but rarely the disorder has been noted in patients with G-6-PD A–.[344] The onset of hemolysis may be quite sudden, having been reported to occur within the first hours after exposure to fava beans. More commonly, the onset is gradual, hemolysis being noticed 1 to 2 days after ingestion of the beans.[345] The urine becomes red or quite dark, and in severe cases shock may develop within a short time. Care should be taken to avoid acute renal failure. The oxidative stress causes membrane changes in erythrocytes, leading to extravascular hemolysis (in addition to the intravascular destruction).[12] Sometimes the patient or parent does not realize that fava beans have been ingested, as they may be incorporated into foods such as Yew Dow, eaten by the Chinese,[346] or falafel, eaten in the Middle East. Occasionally ingestion of other foodstuffs, such as unripe peaches[347] or a spiced Nigerian barbecued meat known as red suya,[348] has been reported to precipitate hemolysis. The toxic constituents of the fava beans are transmitted into the milk of breast-feeding mothers, putting affected babies at risk.[349]

Neonatal Icterus

Icterus neonatorum without evidence of immunologic incompatibility occurs in some infants with G-6-PD deficiency.[350] In fact, it has been suggested that approximately 30 percent of all male newborns with neonatal jaundice may have G-6-PD deficiency.[250,351] Jaundice is usually evident by 1–4 days of age, and can be more severe in premature born infants.[352] The jaundice may be quite severe and, if untreated, may result in kernicterus. Thus, G-6-PD deficiency is a preventable cause of mental retardation,[353,354] and this aspect of the disorder has considerable public health significance. Newborn babies with severe neonatal jaundice should be tested for G-6-PD deficiency. The condition is often not associated with severe hemolysis.[355]

Nonspherocytic Hemolytic Anemia

As described, the anemia in G-6-PD deficiency is usually episodic and acute, but some sporadic variants of G-6-PD may cause nonspherocytic congenital hemolytic disease, exacerbated by oxidative stress. Affected individuals have a history of severe neonatal jaundice, and features of chronic hemolysis (see below). The hemolysis is mainly extravascular.

Effects on Other Tissues

In the common variants of G-6-PD, such as G-6-PD A– and Mediterranean, and even in most of the severely deficient variants, there is usually no demonstrated defect in leukocyte number or function.[356] However, there have been reports of isolated instances of leukocyte dysfunction associated with rare, severely deficient variants of G-6-PD.[357–363] Patients with G-6-PD deficiency do not have a bleeding tendency, and studies of platelet function have yielded conflicting results.[364,365] Occasionally, cataracts have been observed in patients with variants of G-6-PD that produce nonspherocytic hemolytic anemia.[366–368] The incidence of senile cataracts may be increased in G-6-PD deficiency,[369,370] but this remains controversial.[371] Although claims have been made that an association exists between various kinds of G-6-PD deficiency and cancer,[372,373] the data are not convincing, and a detailed investigation of hematologic malignancies in patients with G-6-PD Mediterranean shows no effect.[374]

HEREDITARY NONSPHEROCYTIC HEMOLYTIC ANEMIA

Most patients with hereditary nonspherocytic hemolytic anemia manifest only the usual clinical signs and symptoms of chronic hemolysis. The degree of anemia in this group of disorders varies widely. In some cases of very severe PK deficiency, scarcely any deficient cells survive in the circulation, and only transfused cells are found or steady-state hemoglobin levels as low as 5 g/dL are encountered. Other patients with hereditary nonspherocytic hemolytic anemia may manifest compensated hemolysis with a normal steady-state hemoglobin concentration. Chronic jaundice is a common finding, and splenomegaly is often present. Gallstones are common. As in other forms of chronic hemolytic anemia, ankle ulcers may be present.[375,376] Pregnancy has been thought to precipitate hemolysis in patients with PK deficiency, perhaps even in heterozygotes.[377,378] In PK deficiency, the increased 2,3-BPG levels ameliorate the anemia by lowering the oxygen-affinity of hemoglobin. Some PK-deficient patients present with hydrops fetalis.[379]

In the case of some enzyme defects, characteristic nonhematologic systemic manifestations may be present, and these may be the only sign of the enzyme deficiency. For example, patients with PFK deficiency may have type VII muscle glycogen storage disease. In some patients with this defect, hemolysis is present without muscle manifestations, but in others both muscle abnormalities and hemolysis occur.[65] Glutathione synthetase deficiency may be associated with 5-oxoprolinuria and neuromuscular disturbances, and such abnormalities may occur either with[382] or without hematologic abnormalities.[200] On the other hand, some patients with glutathione synthetase deficiency manifest only the hematologic abnormalities.[383] Spinocerebellar degeneration was documented in the first case of γ-glutamylcysteine synthetase described[384,385] but was not present in subsequently investigated patients.[383,386] Patients with TPI deficiency nearly always manifest serious neuromuscular disease, and most of the patients who inherit this abnormality die in the first decade of life,[387–389] but there are exceptions, as only one of two brothers with the same genotype manifested neurologic disease (see below "Genetic Modifiers of the Phenotypes).[390,391] Neurologic symptoms have also been noted in a patient with glucosephosphate isomerase deficiency.[392] This enzyme seems to be identical to neuroleukin, which could explain the existence of neurologic manifestations. Myoglobinuria has been encountered in patients with PGK,[199,393] aldolase,[259] and G-6-PD deficiency.[394] Table 46–2 summarizes the clinical features of enzyme deficiencies causing nonspherocytic hemolytic anemia.

GENETIC MODIFIERS OF THE PHENOTYPES

The clinical phenotype of both acute and chronic hemolysis can be modified by coinherited (although unrelated) other defects of the red cells. Combined deficiencies of, for example, GPI and G-6-PD,[395] of PK and band 3,[396] of PK and α-thalassemia,[397] and of PK and G-6-PD[378] have been documented.

The inheritance of extended polymorphic *UGT1A1* promoter alleles exacerbates the icterus both in neonates and in adults with G-6-PD deficiency (see also "Mechanism of Hemolysis" above).[398]

A striking example of complex interplay defining the differences between the genotype and the phenotype was described in a Hungarian family with TPI deficiency. Two adult germ-line-identical compound heterozygous brothers displayed strikingly different phenotypes. Both had the same severe decrease in TPI activity and congenital hemolytic anemia, but only one suffered from severe neurologic disorder. Studies aimed at the pathogenesis of this differing phenotype indicated functional differences in lipid environment of the red cell membrane proteins influencing the enzyme activities.[390]

The variety of clinical features associated with the various enzymopathies, regardless of the underlying molecular mechanism, do unequivocally demonstrate that the phenotype of hereditary red blood cell enzymopathies is not solely dependent on the molecular properties of mutant proteins but rather reflects a complex interplay between physiologic, environmental, and other (genetic) factors. Putative phenotypic modifiers include differences in genetic background, concomitant functional polymorphisms of other glycolytic enzymes (many enzymes are regulated by their product or other metabolites), posttranslational modification, ineffective erythropoiesis, and different splenic function. As an example, persistent expression of the PK-M2 isozyme has been reported in the red blood cells of patients (and animals) with severe PK deficiency.[237,380] The survival of these patients, though not in all cases, may be enabled by this compensatory increase in PK activity.[381]

LABORATORY FEATURES

Varying degrees of anemia and reticulocytosis are the main hematologic laboratory features of patients with hereditary nonspherocytic hemolytic anemia. Heinz bodies often are found in the erythrocytes of G-6-PD–deficient patients undergoing drug-induced hemolysis. In the absence of hemolysis, the light-microscopic morphology of G-6-PD–deficient red cells appears to be normal. Differences in the texture of the membrane of the cells have, however, been observed under electron microscopy.[399] When a hemolytic drug is administered to a G-6-PD–deficient patient, Heinz bodies (see Chap. 29) develop in the erythrocytes immediately preceding and in the early phases of the hemolytic episode. If the hemolytic anemia is very severe, spherocytosis and red cell fragmentation may be seen in the stained film. Despite the fact that "bite cells" have been noted in the blood of a G-6-PD–deficient patient undergoing drug-induced hemolysis,[400] the association with G-6-PD deficiency is doubtful since such cells are usually lacking in acute hemolytic states of patients with common G-6-PD variants or in G-6PD-deficient patients with chronic hemolysis. Moreover, "bite cells" have been noted in G-6PD nondeficient patients.[401,402]

The presence of small, densely staining cells has often been noted in the blood films of patients with hereditary nonspherocytic hemolytic anemia with defects other than G-6-PD deficiency. Particularly when manifesting an echinocytic appearance, such cells have been thought to be common in PK deficiency. In one reported case,[403] spectacular numbers of such cells were observed. However, cells of this type are seen in many blood films both from patients with glycolytic enzyme deficiencies and from those with other disorders and it is hazardous to attempt to make an enzymatic diagnosis on the basis of such findings. Basophilic stippling of the erythrocytes is prominent in most patients with pyrimidine 5′-nucleotidase deficiency but may not be apparent in blood that has been collected in ethylenediaminetetraacetic acid (EDTA) anticoagulant. Leukopenia occasionally is observed in patients with hereditary nonspherocytic hemolytic anemia, possibly secondary to splenic enlargement. Other laboratory stigmata of increased hemolysis may include increased levels of serum bilirubin, decreased haptoglobin levels, and increased serum LDH activity. Reticulocytosis is frequently observed, which may result in increased mean corpuscular volume of erythrocytes. In PK deficiency, splenectomy increases reticulocyte counts even further because in particular the younger PK-deficient red blood cells are preferentially sequestered by the spleen.[404]

Diagnosis of red cell enzyme deficiencies usually depends on the demonstration of decreased enzyme activity either through a quantitative assay or a screening test.[156,405–407] Assay of most of the enzymes generally is carried out by measuring the rate of reduction or oxidation of nicotinamide adenine nucleotides in an ultraviolet spectrophotometer, and a number of screening tests that depend upon the development or loss of fluorescence have been devised.[156] However, difficulties arise when the patient has been transfused so that the blood drawn represents a mixture of the patient's own cells and those obtained from the blood bank. Under the circumstances, DNA analysis may prove invaluable, because the DNA is extracted from blood leukocytes and transfused leukocytes do not persist in the circulation.

Although detection of G-6-PD deficiency in the healthy, fully affected (hemizygous) male can be achieved readily through either assay or screening tests, difficulties arise when a patient with G-6-PD deficiency of the A– type has undergone a hemolytic episode. As the older, more enzyme-deficient cells are removed from the circulation and are replaced by young cells, the level of the enzyme begins to increase toward normal. Under such circumstances, suspicion that the patient may be G-6-PD deficient should be raised by the fact that enzyme activity is not increased, even though the reticulocyte count is elevated. Centrifugation of the blood followed by testing of the most dense, reticulocyte depleted red cells has been employed as a means for the detection of G-6-PD deficiency in persons with the A– defect who recently have undergone hemolysis.[408,409] It is helpful to carry out family studies or to wait until the circulating red cells have aged sufficiently to betray their lack of enzyme.

Even greater difficulties are encountered in attempting to diagnose heterozygotes for G-6-PD deficiency.[410] Because the gene is X linked, a population of normal red cells coexists with the deficient cells. This may mask the enzyme deficiency when screening tests are used. Even enzyme assays carried out on erythrocytes of heterozygous females frequently may be in the normal range. Here methods that depend upon histochemical demonstration of individual red cell enzyme activity may be useful.[411,412] In addition, the ascorbate cyanide test,[413] in which screening is carried out on a whole-cell population rather than on a lysate, may be more sensitive than the other screening procedures. However, when the nucleotide substitution is known, heterozygotes are easily detected by polymerase chain reaction–based analysis of the mutation.[414] Prenatal diagnosis of G-6-PD deficiency is also possible using this approach.[415]

The laboratory diagnostics of red cells enzyme deficiencies is best done in specialized laboratories. Specimens can be shipped by mail to reference laboratories. As a rule, whole-blood specimens anticoagulated with EDTA are suitable and the specimens can be sent at room temperature. Exceptions are assays for phosphorylated sugar intermediates, 2,3-BPG, and nucleotide intermediates, which are unstable in freshly drawn blood and require immediate deproteinization in perchloric acid. Several aspects should be kept in mind when interpreting test results. First, care must be taken to remove leukocytes and platelets in assays such as for PK, as these cells do contain PK activity, obscuring a deficiency in the red cells. Second, one should be aware of the already mentioned red cell age dependency of, for example, PK, HK, and G-6-PD. The measurement of these enzymes simultaneously can give an idea about red cell age and relative deficiencies. If patients received blood transfusions, interpreting results from red cell enzyme assays is generally not possible because the presence of donor erythrocytes will obscure any deficiencies. Some mutant enzymes display a normal activity *in vitro*, whereas *in vivo* severe hemolysis can occur. More sophisticated assays to measure, for example, heat instability and kinetics, have to be used in those cases.

As for G-6-PD deficiency, molecular diagnosis is now available for most red cell enzyme deficiencies.

DIFFERENTIAL DIAGNOSIS

Drug-induced hemolytic anemia resulting from G-6-PD deficiency is similar in its clinical features and in certain laboratory features to drug-induced hemolytic anemia associated with unstable hemoglobins (see Chap. 48). Other enzyme defects affecting the pentose-phosphate shunt, such as a deficiency of glutathione synthetase, also may mimic G-6-PD deficiency. The diagnosis of hemoglobinopathies can be excluded by performing a stability test and hemoglobin electrophoresis. Both of these are normal in G-6-PD deficiency. Some of the screening tests, particularly the ascorbate cyanide test,[413] may give positive results in the above-named disorders, but a G-6-PD assay or the fluorescent screening test will be positive only in G-6-PD deficiency. In addition, defects of the erythrocyte membrane should be excluded (see Chap. 45), but these cytoskeletal and other membrane defects are associated with characteristic morphologic abnormalities that makes them easy to differentiate from hemolysis because of enzyme defects.

Physicians often attempt to establish the cause of hereditary nonspherocytic hemolytic anemia on the basis of the appearance of red cells on a blood film. In reality, red cell morphology is helpful only in the diagnosis of pyrimidine 5′-nucleotidase deficiency because of the characteristic stippling of the red cells that is observed in that disorder.

The appearance of Heinz bodies suggests the possible presence of an unstable hemoglobin, or defective GSH metabolism. They are more likely to be present after splenectomy.

Because the laboratory diagnosis of these disorders may entail considerable expenditure of time and effort, it is prudent to perform the simplest tests for the most common causes of hereditary nonspherocytic hemolytic anemia first. Accordingly, it is useful to carry out screening tests[156,406] for G-6-PD and PK activity and an isopropanol stability test[416] to detect an unstable hemoglobin. If prominent stippling of erythrocytes is present, examination of the ultraviolet spectrum of a perchloric acid extract of the erythrocytes may help to establish the diagnosis of pyrimidine 5′-nucleotidase deficiency.[417] Beyond these relatively simple procedures it is probably rarely profitable to pick and choose individual enzyme assays on the basis of family history or clinical manifestations. Rather, it is usually appropriate to submit a blood sample to a reference laboratory that has the capability of performing all the enzyme assays listed in Table 46–2. The estimation of the red cell membrane lipid composition and the study of membrane proteins usually are carried out only in research laboratories.

Prenatal diagnosis of some of the defects causing hereditary nonspherocytic hemolytic anemia has been achieved.[418–425] For this purpose, DNA-based diagnosis is usually preferable because it can be carried out earlier in the pregnancy, and although the levels of red cell enzymes in fetal blood have been documented,[426,427] there is relatively little experience in prenatal diagnosis and little knowledge of what variables, such as leukocyte contamination, may affect the results.

THERAPY

G-6-PD DEFICIENCY

G-6-PD–deficient individuals should avoid drugs that might induce hemolytic episodes (see Table 46–5). However, it is important to realize that such patients are able to tolerate most drugs. Unfortunately, in the 1950s and 1960s, a number of case reports incorrectly suggested that some drugs had hemolytic potential that subsequently were shown to be safe. Table 46–6 lists such drugs. Although it is possible that some of these may be hemolytic in some patients or under some circumstances, this is unlikely, and G-6-PD–deficient patients should not be deprived of the possible benefit of these drugs.

If hemolysis occurs as a result of drug ingestion or infection, particularly in the milder A– type of deficiency, transfusion usually is not required. If, however, the rate of hemolysis is very rapid, as may occur, for example, in favism, transfusions of packed cells may be useful. Good urine flow should be maintained in patients with hemoglobinuria to avert renal damage. Infants with neonatal jaundice resulting from G-6-PD deficiency may require phototherapy or exchange transfusion; in areas in which G-6-PD deficiency is prevalent, care must be taken not to give G-6-PD–deficient blood to such newborns.[428] A single dose of Sn-mesoporphyrin, a potent inhibitor of heme oxygenase, has been advocated to eliminate the need for phototherapy.[429] Patients with hereditary nonspherocytic hemolytic anemia resulting from G-6-PD deficiency usually do not require any therapy. Splenectomy is often ineffective, although some improvement has been reported in a number of cases following removal of the spleen.[8,430] In most cases, the anemia is not very severe, but in some instances frequent transfusions have been necessary.[27,431] The antioxidant properties of vitamin E have been tested in G-6-PD–deficient subjects, and a slight but statistically significant reduction in hemolysis was observed.[432,433] These results could not be confirmed in other studies.[434,435] It has been suggested that desferrioxamine decreases hemolysis.[436–438]

OTHER ENZYME DEFICIENCIES

Most patients with hereditary nonspherocytic hemolytic anemia secondary to red cell enzymopathies do not require therapy, other than blood transfusion during hemolytic periods, if the anemia needs clinically to be corrected. There are patients with PK deficiency who need to be transfused continually. Chronic transfusion therapy usually requires iron chelation if of sufficient iron load. Patients with TPI deficiency generally die as children, not because of the severity of the anemia but because of the severe neuromuscular effects of the enzyme deficiency. It has been proposed that the exogenous replacement of TPI might be useful for the treatment of this deficiency,[439] but no clinical trials have been carried out. PK deficiency has been treated successfully by stem cell transplantation,[440] but this is still only very rarely done. Studies are under way to improve gene therapy in pyruvate kinase deficiency.[441,442] In PK deficiency erythroid cells have been treated *ex vivo* with glycolytic intermediates to correct for metabolic dysfunction.[443] The jaundice of glucosephosphate isomerase deficiency has been treated by the administration of phenobarbital.[444]

The principal decision that the physician must make regarding patients with hereditary nonspherocytic hemolytic anemia is whether or not they require a splenectomy. This decision is not made easily as the response is unpredictable, and some patients who fail to respond may develop serious thrombotic complications resulting from postsplenectomy thrombocytosis that is often exaggerated when splenectomy does not ameliorate the hemolysis. The recommendation that is made should be based upon the following considerations: (1) severity of the disease, (2) family history of response to splenectomy, (3) the underlying defect, and (4) perhaps the need for cholecystectomy. Because it is unusual to obtain more than a partial response to splenectomy, this procedure should probably be reserved for patients whose quality of life is impaired by their anemia. The operation needs to be particularly considered for patients who need frequent transfusion and for those who require gallbladder surgery, in which splenectomy might be carried out as part of the same procedure. The best guide to the likely efficacy of splenectomy is probably the response to splenectomy of other affected family members. Unfortunately, such information is only occasionally available. The physician must therefore rely upon the experience of other patients with hereditary nonspherocytic hemolytic anemia of similar etiology to serve as a guide. However, even as the large group of patients with hereditary nonspherocytic hemolytic anemia represents a heterogeneous population, so individuals with a single enzymatic lesion, such as PK deficiency, are heterogeneous. Each family is likely to be afflicted with a distinct mutant enzyme, and the various mutants may differ both with respect to clinical manifestations and with respect to response to splenectomy. Some of the available information regarding response to splenectomy of patients with hereditary nonspherocytic hemolytic anemia has been reviewed[8] and is summarized in Table 46–2. Relatively little is known of the response of patients with unstable hemoglobins to splenectomy (see Chap. 48).

Glucocorticoids are of no known value in this group of disorders. Folic acid is often given, as in other patients with increased marrow activity, but without proven hematologic benefit. In the absence of iron deficiency, iron is contraindicated. Iron overload is not a frequent complication in this group of disorders but has been reported to occur, particularly in connection with PK deficiency.[445,446]

COURSE AND PROGNOSIS

Hemolytic episodes in the A– type of deficiency are usually self-limited, even if drug administration is continued. This is not the case in the more severe Mediterranean type of deficiency.[447] In patients with hereditary nonspherocytic hemolytic anemia resulting from G-6-PD deficiency, gallstones may occur, and the incidence of cholelithiasis may even be increased in patients with polymorphic forms of G-6-PD deficiency in Sardinia.[448] During periods of infections or drug administration, anemia may increase in severity. Otherwise, the hemoglobin level of affected subjects remains relatively stable.

Nearly all patients with drug- or infection-induced hemolysis recover uneventfully. Favism must be considered, by comparison, a relatively dangerous disease. Prior to the institution of modern hospital therapy, fatalities from favism were not uncommon. The other very serious complication of G-6-PD deficiency is neonatal icterus. If not recognized early and properly treated, it can lead to kernicterus. With the shortened period of hospitalization attending parturition, the incidence of this grave complication has increased.[449]

In one large population study, a decreasing incidence of G-6-PD deficiency was noted with increasing age of the population,[450] but no such change was observed in another.[22] Although age stratification might represent evidence of a shorter life span for individuals with the A– deficiency, other factors are more likely explanations. Examination of the health records of more than 65,000 U.S. Veterans Administration males failed to reveal any higher frequency of any illness in G-6-PD–deficient compared to nondeficient subjects.[10] In view of the benign nature of the common types of G-6-PD deficiency, community-based population screening is not recommended. However, screening for G-6-PD deficiency of all patients admitted to the hospital may be useful in anticipating hemolytic reactions and in understanding them if they occur; however, this recommendation has not been submitted to rigorous analysis and is controversial because of low likelihood of any preventable hemolysis. This is particularly prudent if a drug such as dapsone, known to cause hemolysis in G-6-PD–deficient individuals, is to be given. Study of family members of patients with this X chromosome-linked enzyme deficiency can be helpful in providing appropriate counseling to affected individuals.

The diagnosis of hereditary nonspherocytic hemolytic anemia has been made as late as the seventh decade,[196] and the disease can be fatal in the first few years of life. TPI deficiency appears to have the worst prognosis of all of the known defects that cause this disorder. With few exceptions, patients with this deficiency have died by the fifth or sixth year of life, usually of cardiopulmonary failure. PK deficiency, too, can be fatal in early childhood; the gene prevalent among the Amish of Pennsylvania produces particularly severe disease.[451] Unless the affected homozygous children have their spleens removed, the disorder is commonly lethal. In PK deficiency, compound heterozygotes and homozygotes can suffer of major side effects as a result of the chronic hemolysis and the burden of repeated transfusions and iron chelation. In general, however, hereditary nonspherocytic hemolytic anemia is a relatively mild disease and most affected individuals lead a relatively normal life, apparently without much compromise of life span.

REFERENCES

1. Beutler E: G6PD deficiency. *Blood* 84:3613, 1994.
2. Beutler E: Glucose-6-phosphate dehydrogenase deficiency: A historical perspective. *Blood* 111:16, 2008.
3. Crosby WH: Hereditary nonspherocytic hemolytic anemia. *Blood* 5:233, 1950.
4. Dacie JV: The Congenital Anaemias, in *The Haemolytic Anaemias*, p 171. Grune & Stratton, New York, 1960.
5. Selwyn JG, Dacie JV: Autohemolysis and other changes resulting from the incubation in vitro of red cells from patients with congenital hemolytic anemia. *Blood* 9:414, 1954.
6. Robinson MA, Loder PB, DeGruchy GC: Red-cell metabolism in non-spherocytic congenital haemolytic anaemia. *Br J Haematol* 7:327, 1961.
7. Valentine WN, Tanaka KR, Miwa S: A specific erythrocyte glycolytic enzyme defect (pyruvate kinase) in three subjects with congenital non-spherocytic hemolytic anemia. *Trans Assoc Am Physicians* 74:100, 1961.
8. Beutler E: *Hemolytic Anemia in Disorders of Red Cell Metabolism*. Plenum Press, New York, 1978.
9. van Wijk R, van Solinge WW: The energy-less red blood cell is lost: Erythrocyte enzyme abnormalities of glycolysis. *Blood* 106:4034, 2005.
10. Heller P, Best WR, Nelson RB, Becktel J: Clinical implications of sickle-cell trait and glucose-6-phosphate dehydrogenase deficiency in hospitalized black male patients. *N Engl J Med* 300:1001, 1979.
11. Vulliamy TJ, Luzzatto L: Glucose-6-phosphate dehydrogenase deficiency and related disorders, in *Blood Principles and Practice of Hematology*, 2nd ed, edited by RI Handin, SE Lux IV, p 1921. Lippincott Williams & Wilkins, Philadelphia, 2003.
12. Cappellini MD, Fiorelli G: Glucose-6-phosphate dehydrogenase deficiency. *Lancet* 371:64, 2008.
13. Nkhoma ET, Poole C, Vannappagari V, et al: The global prevalence of glucose-6-phosphate dehydrogenase deficiency: A systematic review and meta-analysis. *Blood Cells Mol Dis* 42:267, 2009.
14. Tishkoff SA, Varkonyi R, Cahinhinan N, et al: Haplotype diversity and linkage disequilibrium at human G6PD: Recent origin of alleles that confer malarial resistance. *Science* 293:455, 2001.
15. Tripathy V, Reddy BM: Present status of understanding on the G6PD deficiency and natural selection. *J Postgrad Med* 53:193, 2007.
16. Luzzatto L, Usanga EA, Reddy S: Glucose 6-phosphate dehydrogenase deficient red cells: Resistance to infection by malarial parasites. *Science* 164:839, 1969.
17. Cappadoro M, Giribaldi G, O'Brien E, et al: Early phagocytosis of glucose-6-phosphate dehydrogenase (G6PD)-deficient erythrocytes parasitized by plasmodium falciparum may explain malaria protection in G6PD deficiency. *Blood* 92:2527, 1998.
18. Guindo A, Fairhurst RM, Doumbo OK, et al: X-linked G6PD deficiency protects hemizygous males but not heterozygous females against severe malaria. *PLoS Med* 4:e66, 2007.
19. Ruwende C, Khoo SC, Snow RW, et al: Natural selection of hemi- and heterozygotes for G6PD deficiency in Africa by resistance to severe malaria. *Nature* 376:246, 1995.
20. Lewis RA, Hathorn M: Correlation of S hemoglobin with glucose-6-phosphate dehydrogenase deficiency and its significance. *Blood* 26:176, 1965.
21. Piomelli S, Reindorf CA, Arzanian MT, Corash LM: Clinical and biochemical interactions of glucose-6-phosphate dehydrogenase deficiency and sickle-cell anemia. *N Engl J Med* 287:213, 1972.
22. Steinberg MH, West MS, Gallagher D, et al: Effects of glucose-6-phosphate dehydrogenase deficiency upon sickle cell anemia. *Blood* 71:748, 1988.
23. Warsy AS: Frequency of glucose-6-phosphate dehydrogenase deficiency in sickle-cell disease. *Hum Hered* 35:143, 1985.
24. Mohrenweiser HW: Functional hemizygosity in the human genome: Direct estimate from twelve erythrocyte enzyme loci. *Hum Genet* 77:241, 1987.
25. Beutler E, Gelbart T: Estimating the prevalence of pyruvate kinase deficiency from the gene frequency in the general white population. *Blood* 95:3585, 2000.
26. Watanabe M, Zingg BC, Mohrenweiser HW: Molecular analysis of a series of alleles in humans with reduced activity at the triosephosphate isomerase locus. *Am J Hum Genet* 58:308, 1996.
27. Baronciani L, Tricta F, Beutler E: G6PD "Campinas:" A deficient enzyme with a mutation at the far 3′ end of the gene. *Hum Mutat* 2:77, 1993.
28. Lenzner C, Nürnberg P, Thiele BJ, et al: Mutations in the pyruvate kinase L gene in patients with hereditary hemolytic anemia. *Blood* 83:2817, 1994.
29. Manco L, Abade A: Pyruvate kinase deficiency: Prevalence of the 1456C→T mutation in the Portuguese population. *Clin Genet* 60:472, 2001.
30. Zanella A, Bianchi P: Red cell pyruvate kinase deficiency: From genetics to clinical manifestations. *Baillieres Best Pract Res Clin Haematol* 13:57, 2000.
31. Schneider A, Westwood B, Yim C, et al: The 1591C mutation in triosephosphate isomerase (TPI) deficiency. Tightly linked polymorphisms and a common haplotype in all known families. *Blood Cells Mol Dis* 22:115, 1996.
32. Raben N, Sherman J, Miller F, et al: A 5′ splice junction mutation leading to exon deletion in an Ashkenazic Jewish family with phosphofructokinase deficiency (Tarui disease). *J Biol Chem* 268:4963, 1993.
33. Sherman JB, Raben N, Nicastri C, et al: Common mutations in the phosphofructokinase-M gene in Ashkenazi Jewish patients with glycogenesis VII—And their population frequency. *Am J Hum Genet* 55:305, 1994.
34. Baldwin SA, Lienhard GE: Purification and reconstitution of glucose transporter from human erythrocytes. *Methods Enzymol* 174:39, 1989.
35. Rosa R, Gaillardon J, Rosa J: Diphosphoglycerate mutase and 2,3-diphosphoglycerate phosphatase activities of red cells: Comparative electrophoretic study. *Biochem Biophys Res Commun* 51:536, 1973.
36. Keitt AS, Bennett DC: Pyruvate kinase deficiency and related disorders of red cell glycolysis. *Am J Med* 41:762, 1966.
37. Poole RC, Halestrap AP: Identification and partial purification of the erythrocyte L-lactate transporter. *Biochem J* 283:855, 1992.
38. Wiback SJ, Palsson BO: Extreme pathway analysis of human red blood cell metabolism. *Biophys J* 83:808, 2002.
39. de Atauri P, Ramirez MJ, Kuchel PW, et al: Metabolic homeostasis in the human erythrocyte: In silico analysis. *Biosystems* 83:118, 2006.

40. Kauffman KJ, Pajerowski JD, Jamshidi N, et al: Description and analysis of metabolic connectivity and dynamics in the human red blood cell. *Biophys J* 83:646, 2002.
41. Sun X, Lu ZH: The response of the metabolic network of the red blood cell to pyruvate kinase deficiency. *Conf Proc IEEE Eng Med Biol Soc* 1:913, 2005.
42. Durmus Tekir S, Cakir T, Ulgen KO: Analysis of enzymopathies in the human red blood cells by constraint-based stoichiometric modeling approaches. *Comput Biol Chem* 30:327, 2006.
43. Çakir T, Tacer CS, Ülgen KÖ: Metabolic pathway analysis of enzyme-deficient human red blood cells. *Biosystems* 78:49, 2004.
44. Srivastava SK, Beutler E: Glutathione metabolism of the erythrocyte. The enzymic cleavage of glutathione-haemoglobin preparations by glutathione reductase. *Biochem J* 119:353, 1970.
45. Scott MD, Wagner TC, Chiu DTY: Decreased catalase activity is the underlying mechanism of oxidant susceptibility in glucose-6-phosphate dehydrogenase-deficient erythrocytes. *Biochim Biophys Acta* 1181:163, 1993.
46. Gaetani GF, Ferraris AM, Rolfo M, et al: Predominant role of catalase in the disposal of hydrogen peroxide within human erythrocytes. *Blood* 87:1595, 1996.
47. Beutler E, Mathai CK: Genetic variation in red cell galactose-1-phosphate uridyl transferase, in *Hereditary Disorders of Erythrocyte Metabolism*, edited by E Beutler, p 66. Grune & Stratton, New York, 1968.
48. Zimran A, Torem S, Beutler E: The *in vivo* ageing of red cell enzymes: Direct evidence of biphasic decay from polycythemic rabbits with reticulocytosis. *Br J Haematol* 69:67, 1988.
49. Jansen G, Koenderman L, Rijksen G, et al: Age dependent behaviour of red cell glycolytic enzymes in haematological disorders. *Br J Haematol* 61:51, 1985.
50. Wilson JE: Isozymes of mammalian hexokinase: Structure, subcellular localization and metabolic function. *J Exp Biol* 206:2049, 2003.
51. Cárdenas ML, Cornish-Bowden A, Ureta T: Evolution and regulatory role of the hexokinases. *Biochim Biophys Acta* 1401:242, 1998.
52. Fujii S, Beutler E: High glucose concentrations partially release hexokinase from inhibition by glucose-6-phosphate. *Proc Natl Acad Sci U S A* 82:1552, 1985.
53. Gerber G, Kloppick E, Rapoport S: Öber den Einfluss des Anorganischen Phosphats auf die Glykolyse; seine Unwirksamkeit auf die Hexokinase des Menschenerythrozyten. *Acta Biol Med Ger* 18:305, 1967.
54. Beutler E, Teeple L: The effect of oxidized glutathione (GSSG) on human erythrocyte hexokinase activity. *Acta Biol Med Ger* 22:707, 1969.
55. Beutler E: 2,3-Diphosphoglycerate affects enzymes of glucose metabolism in red blood cells. *Nat New Biol* 232:20, 1971.
56. Mulichak AM, Wilson JE, Padmanabhan K, Garavito RM: The structure of mammalian hexokinase-1. *Nat Struct Biol* 5:555, 1998.
57. Aleshin AE, Fromm HJ, Honzatko RB: Multiple crystal forms of hexokinase I: New insights regarding conformational dynamics, subunit interactions, and membrane association. *FEBS Lett* 434:42, 1998.
58. Murakami K, Blei F, Tilton W, et al: An isozyme of hexokinase specific for the human red blood cell (HK_R). *Blood* 75:770, 1990.
59. Ruzzo A, Andreoni F, Magnani M: Structure of the human hexokinase type I gene and nucleotide sequence of the 5′ flanking region. *Biochem J* 331:607, 1998.
60. Andreoni F, Ruzzo A, Magnani M: Structure of the 5′ region of the human hexokinase type I (HKI) gene and identification of an additional testis-specific HKI mRNA. *Biochim Biophys Acta* 1493:19, 2000.
61. Murakami K, Kanno H, Miwa S, Piomelli S: Human HK_R isozyme: Organization of the hexokinase I gene, the erythroid-specific promoter, and transcription initiation site. *Mol Genet Metab* 67:118, 1999.
62. Murakami K, Piomelli S: Identification of the cDNA for human red blood cell-specific hexokinase isozyme. *Blood* 89:762, 1997.
63. Read J, Pearce J, Li X, et al: The crystal structure of human phosphoglucose isomerase at 1.6 A resolution: Implications for catalytic mechanism, cytokine activity and haemolytic anaemia. *J Mol Biol* 309:447, 2001.
64. Xu W, Lee P, Beutler E: Human glucose phosphate isomerase: Exon mapping and gene structure. *Genomics* 29:732, 1995.
65. Vora S: Isozymes of human phosphofructokinase: Biochemical and genetic aspects, in *Isozymes: Current Topics in Biological and Medical Research*, edited by MC Rattazzi, JG Scandalios, GS Whitt, p 3. Alan R. Liss, New York, 1983.
66. Bosca L, Aragon JJ, Sols A: Modulation of muscle phosphofructokinase at physiological concentration of enzyme. *J Biol Chem* 260:2100, 1985.
67. Yamada S, Nakajima H, Kuehn MR: Novel testis- and embryo-specific isoforms of the phosphofructokinase-1 muscle type gene. *Biochem Biophys Res Commun* 316:580, 2004.
68. Elson A, Levanon D, Brandeis M, et al: The structure of the human liver-type phosphofructokinase gene. *Genomics* 7:47, 1990.
69. Gamblin SJ, Davies GJ, Grimes JM, et al: Activity and specificity of human aldolases. *J Mol Biol* 219:573, 1991.
70. Beutler E, Scott S, Bishop A, et al: Red cell aldolase deficiency and hemolytic anemia: A new syndrome. *Trans Assoc Am Physicians* 86:154, 1973.
71. Izzo P, Costanzo P, Lupo A, et al: Human aldolase A gene. Structural organization and tissue-specific expression by multiple promoters and alternate mRNA processing. *Eur J Biochem* 174:569, 1988.
72. Mande SC, Mainfroid V, Kalk KH, et al: Crystal structure of recombinant human triosephosphate isomerase at 2.8 A resolution. Triosephosphate isomerase-related human genetic disorders and comparison with the trypanosomal enzyme. *Protein Sci* 3:810, 1994.
73. Peters J, Hopkinson DA, Harris H: Genetic and non-genetic variation of triose phosphate isomerase isozymes in human tissues. *Ann Hum Genet* 36:297, 1973.
74. Brown JR, Daar IO, Krug JR, Maquat LE: Characterization of the functional gene and several processed pseudogenes in the human triosephosphate isomerase gene family. *Mol Cell Biol* 5:1694, 1985.
75. Schrier SL: Organization of enzymes in human erythrocyte membranes. *Am J Physiol* 210:139, 1966.
76. Brookes PS, Land JM, Clark JB, Heales SJR: Stimulation of glyceraldehyde-3-phosphate dehydrogenase by oxyhemoglobin. *FEBS Lett* 416:90, 1997.
77. Ismail SA, Park HW: Structural analysis of human liver glyceraldehyde-3-phosphate dehydrogenase. *Acta Crystallogr D Biol Crystallogr* 61:1508, 2005.
78. Huang IY, Welch CD, Yoshida A: Complete amino acid sequence of human phosphoglycerate kinase. Cyanogen bromide peptides and complete amino acid sequence. *J Biol Chem* 255:6412, 1980.
79. Chen SH, Malcolm LA, Yoshida A, Giblett ER: Phosphoglycerate kinase: An X-linked polymorphism in man. *Am J Hum Genet* 23:87, 1971.
80. Michelson AM, Markham AF, Orkin SH: Isolation and DNA sequence of a full-length cDNA clone for human X chromosome-encoded phosphoglycerate kinase. *Proc Natl Acad Sci U S A* 80:472, 1983.
81. Ikura K, Sasaki R, Narita H, et al: Multifunctional enzyme, bisphosphoglyceromutase/2,3-bisphosphoglycerate phosphatase/phosphoglyceromutase from human erythrocytes. *Eur J Biochem* 66:515, 1976.
82. Rose ZB: The enzymology of 2,3-bisphosphoglycerate. *Adv Enzymol Relat Areas Mol Biol* 51:211, 1980.
83. Vora S, Spear D: Demonstration and quantitation of phosphoglycolate in human red cells. *Clin Res* 34:664A, 1986.
84. Fujii S, Beutler E: Where does phosphoglycolate come from in red cells? *Acta Haematol* 73:26, 1985.
85. Sasaki H, Fujii S, Yoshizaki Y, et al: Phosphoglycolate synthesis by human erythrocyte pyruvate kinase. *Acta Haematol* 77:83, 1987.
86. Beutler E, West C: An improved assay and some properties of phosphoglycolate phosphatase. *Anal Biochem* 106:163, 1980.
87. Wang Y, Wei Z, Bian Q, et al: Crystal structure of human bisphosphoglycerate mutase. *J Biol Chem* 279:39132, 2004.
88. Joulin V, Peduzzi J, Romeo PH, et al: Molecular cloning and sequencing of the human erythrocyte 2,3-bisphosphoglycerate mutase cDNA: Revised amino acid sequence. *EMBO J* 5:2275, 1986.
89. Hass LF, Kappel WK, Muller KB, Engle RL: Evidence for structural homology between human red cell phosphoglycerate mutase and 2,3-bisphosphoglycerate synthase. *J Biol Chem* 253:77, 1978.
90. Repiso A, Perez de la Ossa P, Aviles X, et al: Red blood cell phosphosphoglycerate mutase. Description of the first human BB isoenzyme mutation. *Haematologica* 88:ECR07, 2003.
91. Hoorn RKJ, Filkweert JP, Staal GEJ: Purification and properties of enolase of human erythrocytes. *Int J Biochem* 5:845, 1974.
92. Kang HJ, Jung SK, Kim SJ, Chung SJ: Structure of human alpha-enolase (hENO1), a multifunctional glycolytic enzyme. *Acta Crystallogr D Biol Crystallogr* 64:651, 2008.
93. White PS, Jensen SJ, Rajalingam V, et al: Physical mapping of the CA6, ENO1, and SLC2A5 (GLUT5) genes and reassignment of SLC2A5 to 1p36.2. *Cytogenet Cell Genet* 81:60, 1998.
94. Valentine WN, Tanaka KR, Paglia DE: Hemolytic anemias and erythrocyte enzymopathies. *Ann Intern Med* 103:245, 1985.
95. Noguchi T, Inoue H, Tanaka T: The M_1- and M_2-type isozymes of rat pyruvate kinase are produced from the same gene by alternative RNA splicing. *J Biol Chem* 261:13807, 1986.
96. Kanno H, Fujii H, Miwa S: Structural analysis of human pyruvate kinase L-gene and identification of the promoter activity in erythroid cells. *Biochem Biophys Res Commun* 188:516, 1992.
97. Noguchi T, Yamada K, Inoue H, et al: The L- and R-type isozymes of rat pyruvate kinase are produced from a single gene by use of different promoters. *J Biol Chem* 262:14366, 1987.
98. Tani K, Fujii H, Nagata S, Miwa S: Human liver type pyruvate kinase: Complete amino acid sequence and the expression in mammalian cells. *Proc Natl Acad Sci U S A* 85:1792, 1988.
99. Lenzner C, Nürnberg P, Jacobasch G, Thiele B-J: Complete genomic sequence of the human PK-L/R-gene includes four intragenic polymorphisms defining different haplotype backgrounds of normal and mutant PK-genes. *DNA Seq* 8:45, 1997.
100. Kanno H, Fujii H, Hirono A, Miwa S: CDNA cloning of human R-type pyruvate kinase and identification of a single amino acid substitution (Thr^{384}→Met) affecting enzymatic stability in a pyruvate kinase variant (PK Tokyo) associated with hereditary hemolytic anemia. *Proc Natl Acad Sci U S A* 88:8218, 1991.
101. Valentini G, Chiarelli LR, Fortin R, et al: Structure and function of human erythrocyte pyruvate kinase—Molecular basis of nonspherocytic hemolytic anemia. *J Biol Chem* 277:23807, 2002.
102. Enriqueta Muñoz M, Ponce E: Pyruvate kinase: Current status of regulatory and functional properties. *Comp Biochem Physiol B Biochem Mol Biol* 135:197, 2003.
103. Jurica MS, Mesecar A, Heath PJ, et al: The allosteric regulation of pyruvate kinase by fructose-1,6-bisphosphate. *Structure* 6:195, 1998.
104. Mattevi A, Valentini G, Rizzi M, et al: Crystal structure of *Escherichia coli* pyruvate kinase type I: Molecular basis of the allosteric transition. *Structure* 3:729, 1995.

105. Rigden DJ, Phillips SE, Michels PA, Fothergill-Gilmore LA: The structure of pyruvate kinase from *Leishmania mexicana* reveals details of the allosteric transition and unusual effector specificity. *J Mol Biol* 291:615, 1999.
106. Valentini G, Chiarelli L, Fortin R, et al: The allosteric regulation of pyruvate kinase. *J Biol Chem* 275:18145, 2000.
107. Wooll JO, Friesen RHE, White MA, et al: Structural and functional linkages between subunit interfaces in mammalian pyruvate kinase. *J Mol Biol* 312:525, 2001.
108. Fenton AW, Blair JB: Kinetic and allosteric consequences of mutations in the subunit and domain interfaces and the allosteric site of yeast pyruvate kinase. *Arch Biochem Biophys* 397:28, 2002.
109. Kahn A, Marie J, Garreau H, Sprengers ED: The genetic system of the L-type pyruvate kinase forms in man. Subunit structure, interrelation and kinetic characteristics of the pyruvate kinase enzymes from erythrocytes and liver. *Biochim Biophys Acta* 523:59, 1978.
110. Blume KG, Hoffbauer RW, Busch D, et al: Purification and properties of pyruvate kinase in normal and in pyruvate kinase deficient human red blood cells. *Biochim Biophys Acta* 227:364, 1971.
111. Takayasu S, Fujiwara S, Waki T: Hereditary lactate dehydrogenase M-subunit deficiency: Lactate dehydrogenase activity in skin lesions and in hair follicles. *J Am Acad Dermatol* 24:339, 1991.
112. Joukyuu R, Mizuno S, Amakawa T, et al: Hereditary complete deficiency of lactate dehydrogenase H-subunit. *Clin Chem* 35:687, 1989.
113. Takatani T, Takaoka N, Tatsumi M, et al: A novel missense mutation in human lactate dehydrogenase B-subunit gene. *Mol Genet Metab* 73:344, 2001.
114. Wakabayashi H, Tsuchiya M, Yoshino K, et al: Hereditary deficiency of lactate dehydrogenase H-subunit. *Intern Med* 35:550, 1996.
115. Maekawa M, Sudo K, Nagura K, et al: Population screening of lactate dehydrogenase deficiencies in Fukuoka Prefecture in Japan and molecular characterization of three independent mutations in the lactate dehydrogenase-B(H) gene. *Hum Genet* 93:74, 1994.
116. Yoshida A, Stamatoyannopoulos G, Motulsky A: Negro variant of glucose-6-phosphate dehydrogenase deficiency (A–) in man. *Science* 155:97, 1967.
117. Rattazzi MC: Glucose-6-phosphate dehydrogenase from human erythrocytes: Molecular weight determination by gel filtration. *Biochem Biophys Res Commun* 31:16, 1968.
118. Au SWN, Gover S, Lam VMS, Adams MJ: Human glucose-6-phosphate dehydrogenase: The crystal structure reveals a structural NADP(+) molecule and provides insights into enzyme deficiency. *Structure* 8:293, 2000.
119. Yoshida A: Hemolytic anemia and G-6-PD deficiency. *Science* 179:532, 1973.
120. Ben-Bassat I, Beutler E: Inhibition by ATP of erythrocyte glucose-6-phosphate dehydrogenase variants. *Proc Soc Exp Biol Med* 142:410, 1973.
121. Mason PJ, Bautista JM, Gilsanz F: G6PD deficiency: The genotype-phenotype association. *Blood Rev* 21:267, 2007.
122. Beutler E, Kuhl W: Limiting role of 6-phosphogluconolactonase in erythrocyte hexose monophosphate pathway metabolism. *J Lab Clin Med* 106:573, 1985.
123. Rakitzis ET, Papandreou P: Kinetic analysis of 6-phosphogluconolactone hydrolysis in hemolysates. *Biochem Mol Biol Int* 37:747, 1995.
124. Beutler E, Kuhl W, Gelbart T: 6-Phosphogluconolactonase deficiency, a hereditary erythrocyte enzyme deficiency: Possible interaction with glucose-6-phosphate dehydrogenase deficiency. *Proc Natl Acad Sci U S A* 82:3876, 1985.
125. Thorburn DR, Kuchel PW: Computer simulation of the metabolic consequences of the combined deficiency of 6-phosphogluconolactonase and glucose-6-phosphate dehydrogenase in human erythrocytes. *J Lab Clin Med* 110:70, 1987.
126. Shih L, Justice P, Hsia DY: Purification and characterization of genetic variants of 6-phosphogluconate dehydrogenase. *Biochem Genet* 1:359, 1968.
127. Parr CW, Fitch LI: Inherited quantitative variations of human phosphogluconate dehydrogenase. *Ann Hum Genet* 30:339, 1967.
128. Caprari P, Caforio MP, Cianciulli P, et al: 6-Phosphogluconate dehydrogenase deficiency in an Italian family. *Ann Hematol* 80:41, 2001.
129. Vives Corrons JL, Colomer D, Pujades A, et al: Congenital 6-phosphogluconate dehydrogenase (6PGD) deficiency associated with chronic hemolytic anemia in a Spanish family. *Am J Hematol* 53:221, 1996.
130. Dische Z: The pentose phosphate metabolism in red cells, in *The Red Blood Cell*, edited by C Bishop, DM Surgenor, p 189. Academic Press, New York, 1964.
131. Huck JH, Verhoeven NM, Struys EA, et al: Ribose-5-phosphate isomerase deficiency: New inborn error in the pentose phosphate pathway associated with a slowly progressive leukoencephalopathy. *Am J Hum Genet* 74:745, 2004.
132. Brownstone YS, Denstedt OF: The pentose phosphate metabolic pathway in the human erythrocyte. II. The transketolase and transaldolase activity of the human erythrocyte. *Can J Biochem* 39:533, 1961.
133. Nakasaki H, Ohta M, Soeda J, et al: Clinical and biochemical aspects of thiamine treatment for metabolic acidosis during total parenteral nutrition. *Nutrition* 13:110, 1997.
134. Verhoeven NM, Huck JH, Roos B, et al: Transaldolase deficiency: Liver cirrhosis associated with a new inborn error in the pentose phosphate pathway. *Am J Hum Genet* 68:1086, 2001.
135. Beutler E, Guinto E: The reduction of glyceraldehyde by human erythrocytes. L-Hexonate dehydrogenase activity. *J Clin Invest* 53:1258, 1974.
136. Das B, Srivastava SK: Purification and properties of aldose reductase and aldehyde reductase II from human erythrocyte. *Arch Biochem Biophys* 238:670, 1985.
137. Kim HD: Is adenosine a second metabolic substrate for human red blood cells. *Biochim Biophys Acta* 1036:113, 1990.
138. Gabrio BW, Finch CA, Huennekens FM: Erythrocyte preservation: A topic in molecular biochemistry. *Blood* 11:103, 1956.
139. Resta R, Thompson LF: SCID: The role of adenosine deaminase deficiency. *Immunol Today* 18:371, 1997.
140. Casoli C, Lisa A, Magnani G, et al: Prognostic value of adenosine deaminase compared to other markers for progression to acquired immunodeficiency syndrome among intravenous drug users. *J Med Virol* 45:203, 1995.
141. Glader BE, Backer K: Elevated red cell adenosine deaminase activity: A marker of disordered erythropoiesis in Diamond-Blackfan anaemia and other haematologic diseases. *Br J Haematol* 68:165, 1988.
142. Accorsi A, Piacentini MP, Piatti E, Fazi A: Purine nucleoside phosphorylase from human erythrocytes: A kinetic study of the fully separated isoenzymes. *Biochem Int* 24:23, 1991.
143. Parvaneh N, Teimourian S, Jacomelli G, et al: Novel mutations of NP in two patients with purine nucleoside phosphorylase deficiency. *Clin Biochem* 41:350, 2008.
144. Tsuda M, Horinouchi K, Sakiyama T, Owada M: Novel missense mutation in the purine nucleoside phosphorylase gene in a Japanese patient with purine nucleoside phosphorylase deficiency. *Pediatr Int* 44:333, 2002.
145. Markert ML, Finkel BD, McLaughlin TM, et al: Mutations in purine nucleoside phosphorylase deficiency. *Hum Mutat* 9:118, 1997.
146. Valentine WN, Oski FA, Paglia DE, et al: Erythrocyte hexokinase and hereditary hemolytic anemia, in *Hereditary Disorders of Erythrocyte Metabolism*, edited by E Beutler, p 288. Grune & Stratton, New York, 1968.
147. Barretto OCO, Beutler E: The sorbitol oxidizing enzyme of red blood cells. *J Lab Clin Med* 85:645, 1975.
148. Beutler E, Teeple L: Mannose metabolism in the human erythrocyte. *J Clin Invest* 48:461, 1969.
149. Bruns FH, Noltmann E: Phosphomannoisomerase, an SH-dependent metal-enzyme complex. *Nature* 181:1467, 1958.
150. Beutler E: Galactosemia: Screening and diagnosis. *Clin Biochem* 24:293, 1991.
151. Beutler E, Guinto E: Dihydroxyacetone metabolism by human erythrocytes: Demonstration of triokinase activity and its characterization. *Blood* 41:559, 1973.
152. Wood L, Beutler E: The effect of ascorbate and dihydroxyacetone on the 2,3-diphosphoglycerate and ATP levels of stored human red cells. *Transfusion* 14:272, 1974.
153. Moses SW, Chayoth R, Levin S, et al: Glucose and glycogen metabolism in erythrocytes from normal and glycogen storage disease type III subjects. *J Clin Invest* 47:1343, 1968.
154. Sidbury JB Jr, Cornblath M, Fisher J, House E: Glycogen in erythrocytes of patients with glycogen storage disease. *Pediatrics* 27:103, 1961.
155. Bartels H: Untersuchungen zur Frage des Glykogen-Gehaltes von Erythrocyten, in *Metabolism and Membrane Permeability of Erythrocytes and Thrombocytes*, edited by E Deutsch, E Gerlach, K Moser, p 132. Georg Thieme Verlag, Stuttgart, 1968.
156. Beutler E: *Red Cell Metabolism: A Manual of Biochemical Methods*. Grune & Stratton, New York, 1984.
157. Dimant E, Landberg E, London IM: The metabolic behavior of reduced glutathione in human and avian erythrocytes. *J Biol Chem* 213:769, 1955.
158. Gipp JJ, Bailey HH, Mulcahy RT: Cloning and sequencing of the cDNA for the light subunit of human liver gamma-glutamylcysteine synthetase and relative mRNA levels for heavy and light subunits in human normal tissues. *Biochem Biophys Res Commun* 206:584, 1995.
159. Sierra-Rivera E, Summar ML, Dasouki M, et al: Assignment of the gene (GLCLC) that encodes the heavy subunit of gamma-glutamylcysteine synthetase to human chromosome 6. *Cytogenet Cell Genet* 70:278, 1995.
160. Sierra-Rivera E, Dasouki M, Summar ML, et al: Assignment of the human gene (GLCLR) that encodes the regulatory subunit of gamma-glutamylcysteine synthetase to chromosome 1p21. *Cytogenet Cell Genet* 72:252, 1996.
161. Gali RR, Board PG: Sequencing and expression of a cDNA for human glutathione synthetase. *Biochem J* 310(Pt 1):353, 1995.
162. Webb GC, Vaska VL, Gali RR, et al: The gene encoding human glutathione synthetase (GSS) maps to the long arm of chromosome 20 at band 11.2. *Genomics* 30:617, 1995.
163. Lunn G, Dale GL, Beutler E: Transport accounts for glutathione turnover in human erythrocytes. *Blood* 54:238, 1979.
164. Vina JR, Palacin M, Puertes IR, et al: Role of the gamma-glutamyl cycle in the regulation of amino acid translocation. *Am J Physiol* 257:E916, 1989.
165. Young JD, Ellory JC, Wright PC: Evidence against the participation of the gamma-glutamyltransferase-gamma-glutamylcyclotransferase pathway in amino acid transport by rabbit erythrocytes. *Biochem J* 152:713, 1975.
166. Board PG, Smith JE: Erythrocyte gamma-glutamyl transpeptidase. *Blood* 49:667, 1977.
167. Winterbourn CC, Hawkins RE, Brian M, Carrell RW: The estimation of red cell superoxide dismutase activity. *J Lab Clin Med* 85:337, 1975.
168. Cohen G, Hochstein P: Glutathione peroxidase: The primary agent for the elimination of hydrogen peroxide in erythrocytes. *Biochemistry* 2:1420, 1963.
169. Rotruck JT, Pope AL, Ganther HE, et al: Selenium: Biochemical role as a component of glutathione peroxidase. *Science* 179:588, 1973.
170. Beutler E, Matsumoto F: Ethnic variation in red cell glutathione peroxidase activity. *Blood* 46:103, 1975.

171. Burk RF: Molecular biology of selenium with implications for its metabolism. *FASEB J* 5:2274, 1991.
172. Stadtman TC: Selenocysteine. *Annu Rev Biochem* 65:83, 1996.
173. Harrison PR, Plumb M, Frampton J, et al: Regulation of erythroid-specific gene expression. *Biomed Biochim Acta* 49:S5, 1990.
174. Jacob HS, Jandl JH: Effects of sulfhydryl inhibition on red blood cells. I. Mechanism of hemolysis. *J Clin Invest* 41:779, 1962.
175. Magnani M, Stocchi V, Ninfali P, et al: Action of oxidized and reduced glutathione on rabbit red blood cell hexokinase. *Biochim Biophys Acta* 615:113, 1980.
176. Huisman THJ, Dozy AM: Studies on the heterogeneity of hemoglobin. V. Binding of hemoglobin with oxidized glutathione. *J Lab Clin Med* 60:302, 1962.
177. Kelner MJ, Montoya MA: Structural organization of the human glutathione reductase gene: Determination of correct cDNA sequence and identification of a mitochondrial leader sequence. *Biochem Biophys Res Commun* 269:366, 2000.
178. Karplus PA, Schulz GE: Refined structure of glutathione reductase at 1.54 A resolution. *J Mol Biol* 195:701, 1987.
179. Sinet PM, Bresson JL, Couturier J, et al: [Possible localization of the glutathione reductase (EC 1.6.4.2) on the 8p21 band]. *Ann Genet* 20:13, 1977.
180. Wong KK, Blanchard JS: Human erythrocyte glutathione reductase: PH dependence of kinetic parameters. *Biochemistry* 28:3586, 1989.
181. Beutler E, Yeh MKY: Erythrocyte glutathione reductase. *Blood* 21:573, 1963.
182. Kamerbeek NM, van Zwieten R, de Boer M, et al: Molecular basis of glutathione reductase deficiency in human blood cells. *Blood* 109:3560, 2007.
183. Beutler E: Glutathione reductase: Stimulation in normal subjects by riboflavin supplementation. *Science* 165:613, 1969.
184. Mieyal JJ, Starke DW, Gravina SA, Hocevar BA: Thioltransferase in human red blood cells: Kinetics and equilibrium. *Biochemistry* 30:8883, 1991.
185. Srivastava SK, Beutler E: The transport of oxidized glutathione from human erythrocytes. *J Biol Chem* 244:9, 1969.
186. Prchal J, Srivastava SK, Beutler E: Active transport of GSSG from reconstituted erythrocyte ghosts. *Blood* 46:111, 1975.
187. Kondo T, Kawakami Y, Taniguchi N, Beutler E: Glutathione disulfide-stimulated Mg 2+-ATPase of human erythrocyte membranes. *Proc Natl Acad Sci U S A* 84:7373, 1987.
188. Board PG: Transport of glutathione S-conjugate from human erythrocytes. *FEBS Lett* 124:163, 1981.
189. Kondo T, Murao M, Taniguchi N: Glutathione S-conjugate transport using inside-out vesicles from human erythrocytes. *Eur J Biochem* 125:551, 1982.
190. Harvey JW, Beutler E: Binding of heme by glutathione S-transferase: A possible role of the erythrocyte enzyme. *Blood* 60:1227, 1982.
191. Beutler E, Dunning D, Dabe IB, Forman L: Erythrocyte glutathione S-transferase deficiency and hemolytic anemia. *Blood* 72:73, 1988.
192. Abe S: Secondary red cell pyruvate kinase deficiency I. Study of 30 subjects of malignant hematological disorders. *Nippon Ketsueki Gakkai Zasshi* 39:247, 1976.
193. Kornberg A, Goldfarb A: Preleukemia manifested by hemolytic anemia with pyruvate-kinase deficiency. *Arch Intern Med* 146:785, 1986.
194. Boivin P, Galand C, Hakim J, Kahn A: Acquired erythroenzymopathies in blood disorders: Study of 200 cases. *Br J Haematol* 31:531, 1975.
195. Kahn A: Abnormalities of erythrocyte enzymes in dyserythropoiesis and malignancies. *Clin Haematol* 10:123, 1981.
196. Beutler E: Red cell enzyme defects as non-diseases and as diseases. *Blood* 54:1, 1979.
197. Goth L, Rass P, Pay A: Catalase enzyme mutations and their association with diseases. *Mol Diagn* 8:141, 2004.
198. Shinohara K, Tanaka KR: Hereditary deficiency of erythrocyte acetylcholinesterase. *Am J Hematol* 7:313, 1979.
199. Rosa R, George C, Fardeau M, et al: A new case of phosphoglycerate kinase deficiency: PGK Creteil associated with rhabdomyolysis and lacking hemolytic anemia. *Blood* 60:84, 1982.
200. Marstein S, Jellum E, Halpern B, et al: Biochemical studies of erythrocytes in a patient with pyroglutamic acidemia (5-oxoprolinemia). *N Engl J Med* 295:406, 1976.
201. Stefanini M: Chronic hemolytic anemia associated with erythrocyte enolase deficiency exacerbated by ingestion of nitrofurantoin. *Am J Clin Pathol* 58:408, 1972.
202. Boulard-Heitzmann P, Boulard M, Tallineau C, et al: Decreased red cell enolase activity in a 40-year-old woman with compensated haemolysis. *Scand J Haematol* 33:401, 1984.
203. Glucose-6-phosphate dehydrogenase deficiency. WHO Working Group. *Bull World Health Organ* 67:601, 1989.
204. Betke K, Beutler E, Brewer GJ, et al: Standardization of procedures for the study of glucose-6-phosphate dehydrogenase. Report of a WHO scientific group. *World Health Organ Tech Rep Ser* No 366:1967.
205. Piomelli S, Corash LM, Davenport DD, et al: *In vivo* lability of glucose-6-phosphate dehydrogenase in GdA– and Gd Mediterranean deficiency. *J Clin Invest* 47:940, 1968.
206. Kahn A, Cottreau D, Boivin P: Molecular mechanism of glucose-6-phosphate dehydrogenase deficiency. *Humangenetik* 25:101, 1974.
207. Beutler E: Selectivity of proteases as a basis for tissue distribution of enzymes in hereditary deficiencies. *Proc Natl Acad Sci U S A* 80:3767, 1983.
208. Kirkman HN, Schettini F, Pickard BM: Mediterranean variant of glucose-6-phosphate dehydrogenase. *J Lab Clin Med* 63:726, 1964.
209. Beutler E: Genetics of glucose-6-phosphate dehydrogenase deficiency. *Semin Hematol* 27:137, 1990.
210. Smith JE, Ryer K, Wallace L: Glucose-6-phosphate dehydrogenase deficiency in a dog. *Enzyme* 21:379, 1976.
211. Sanders S, Smith DP, Thomas GA, Williams ED: A glucose-6-phosphate dehydrogenase (G6PD) splice site consensus sequence mutation associated with G6PD enzyme deficiency. *Mutat Res* 374:79, 1997.
212. Harvey JW: Pathogenesis, laboratory diagnosis, and clinical implications of erythrocyte enzyme deficiencies in dogs, cats, and horses. *Vet Clin Pathol* 35:144, 2006.
213. Longo L, Vanegas OC, Patel M, et al: Maternally transmitted severe glucose 6-phosphate dehydrogenase deficiency is an embryonic lethal. *EMBO J* 21:4229, 2002.
214. Chen EY, Cheng A, Lee A, et al: Sequence of human glucose-6-phosphate dehydrogenase cloned in plasmids and a yeast artificial chromosome (YAC). *Genomics* 10:792, 1991.
215. Martini G, Toniolo D, Vulliamy T, et al: Structural analysis of the X-linked gene encoding human glucose 6-phosphate dehydrogenase. *EMBO J* 5:1849, 1986.
216. Battistuzzi G, D'Urso M, Toniolo D, et al: Tissue-specific levels of human glucose-6-phosphate dehydrogenase correlate with methylation of specific sites at the 3′ end of the gene. *Proc Natl Acad Sci U S A* 82:1465, 1985.
217. Kirkman HN, Hendrickson EM: Glucose-6-phosphate dehydrogenase from human erythrocytes. II. Subactive states of the enzyme from normal persons. *J Biol Chem* 237:2371, 1962.
218. Canepa L, Ferraris AM, Miglino M, Gaetani GF: Bound and unbound pyridine dinucleotides in normal and glucose-6-phosphate dehydrogenase-deficient erythrocytes. *Biochim Biophys Acta* 1074:101, 1991.
219. Hirono A, Kuhl W, Gelbart T, et al: Identification of the binding domain for NADP + of human glucose-6-phosphate dehydrogenase by sequence analysis of mutants. *Proc Natl Acad Sci U S A* 86:10015, 1989.
220. Cohen P, Rosemeyer MA: Subunit interactions of glucose-6-phosphate dehydrogenase from human erythrocytes. *Eur J Biochem* 8:8, 1969.
221. Camardella L, Caruso C, Rutigliano B, et al: Human erythrocyte glucose-6-phosphate dehydrogenase: Identification of a reactive lysyl residue labelled with pyridoxal 5′-phosphate. *Eur J Biochem* 171:485, 1988.
222. Takizawa T, Yoneyama Y, Miwa S, Yoshida A: A single nucleotide base transition is the basis of the common human glucose-6-phosphate dehydrogenase variant A(+). *Genomics* 1:228, 1987.
223. Hirono A, Beutler E: Molecular cloning and nucleotide sequence of cDNA for human glucose-6-phosphate dehydrogenase variant A(–). *Proc Natl Acad Sci U S A* 85:3951, 1988.
224. Beutler E, Kuhl W, Vives-Corrons JL, Prchal JT: Molecular heterogeneity of G6PD A. *Blood* 74:2550, 1989.
225. Vulliamy TJ, Othman A, Town M, et al: Polymorphic sites in the African population detected by sequence analysis of the glucose-6-phosphate dehydrogenase gene outline the evolution of the variants A and A–. *Proc Natl Acad Sci U S A* 88:8568, 1991.
226. Town M, Bautista JM, Mason PJ, Luzzatto L: Both mutations in G6PD A– are necessary to produce the G6PD deficient phenotype. *Hum Mol Genet* 1:171, 1992.
227. Hirono A, Kawate K, Honda A, et al: A single mutation 202G→A in the human glucose-6-phosphate dehydrogenase gene (G6PD) can cause acute hemolysis by itself. *Blood* 99:1498, 2002.
228. Xu W, Westwood B, Bartsocas CS, et al: Glucose-6 phosphate dehydrogenase mutations and haplotypes in various ethnic groups. *Blood* 85:257, 1995.
229. Ganczakowski M, Town M, Bowden DK, et al: Multiple glucose 6-phosphate dehydrogenase-deficient variants correlate with malaria endemicity in the Vanuatu archipelago (southwestern Pacific). *Am J Hum Genet* 56:294, 1995.
230. Tang TK, Huang CS, Huang MJ, et al: Diverse point mutations result in glucose-6-phosphate dehydrogenase (G6PD) polymorphism in Taiwan. *Blood* 79:2135, 1992.
231. Vulliamy T, Luzzatto L, Hirono A, Beutler E: Hematologically important mutations: Glucose-6-phosphate dehydrogenase. *Blood Cells Mol Dis* 23:302, 1997.
232. MacDonald D, Town M, Mason P, et al: Deficiency in red blood cells. *Nature* 350:115, 1991.
233. van Wijk R, Huizinga EG, Prins I, et al: Distinct phenotypic expression of two *de novo* missense mutations affecting the dimer interface of glucose-6-phosphate dehydrogenase. *Blood Cells Mol Dis* 32:112, 2004.
234. Beutler E, Forman L, Rios-Larrain E: Elevated pyruvate kinase activity in patients with hemolytic anemia due to red cell pyruvate kinase "deficiency." *Am J Med* 83:899, 1987.
235. Zanella A, Fermo E, Bianchi P, et al: Pyruvate kinase deficiency: The genotype-phenotype association. *Blood Rev* 21:217, 2007.
236. Van Wijk R, Huizinga EG, Van Wesel ACW, et al: Fifteen novel mutations in *PKLR* associated with pyruvate kinase (PK) deficiency: Structural implications of amino acid substitutions in PK. *Hum Mutat* 30:446, 2009.
237. Lenzner C, Nurnberg P, Jacobasch G, et al: Molecular analysis of 29 pyruvate kinase-deficient patients from central Europe with hereditary hemolytic anemia. *Blood* 89:1793, 1997.
238. Demina A, Varughese KI, Barbot J, et al: Six previously undescribed pyruvate kinase mutations causing enzyme deficiency. *Blood* 92:647, 1998.
239. van Wijk R, van Solinge WW: Pyruvate kinase deficiency: Genotype to phenotype. *Hematology (EHA Educ Program)* 2:55, 2006.
240. Durand PM, Coetzer TL: Pyruvate kinase deficiency protects against malaria in humans. *Haematologica* 93:939, 2008.
241. Ayi K, Min-Oo G, Serghides L, et al: Pyruvate kinase deficiency and malaria. *N Engl J Med* 358:1805, 2008.

242. Whitney KM, Goodman SA, Bailey EM, Lothrop CD, Jr: The molecular basis of canine pyruvate kinase deficiency. *Exp Hematol* 22:866, 1994.
243. Tsujino K, Kanno H, Hashimoto K, et al: Delayed onset of hemolytic anemia in CBA- Pk-1 slc /Pk-1 slc mice with a point mutation of the gene encoding red blood cell type pyruvate kinase. *Blood* 91:2169, 1998.
244. Kanno H: Hexokinase: Gene structure and mutations. *Baillieres Best Pract Res Clin Haematol* 13:83, 2000.
245. Bianchi M, Magnani M: Hexokinase mutations that produce nonspherocytic hemolytic anemia. *Blood Cells Mol Dis* 21:2, 1995.
246. Kanno H, Murakami K, Hariyama Y, et al: Homozygous intragenic deletion of type I hexokinase gene causes lethal hemolytic anemia of the affected fetus. *Blood* 100:1930, 2002.
247. Van Wijk R, Rijksen G, Huizinga EG, et al: HK Utrecht: Missense mutation in the active site of human hexokinase associated with hexokinase deficiency and severe nonspherocytic hemolytic anemia. *Blood* 101:345, 2003.
248. Peters LL, Lane PW, Andersen SG, et al: Downeast anemia (dea), a new mouse model of severe nonspherocytic hemolytic anemia caused by hexokinase (HKI) deficiency. *Blood Cells Mol Dis* 27:850, 2001.
249. Kugler W, Lakomek M: Glucose-6-phosphate isomerase deficiency. *Baillieres Best Pract Res Clin Haematol* 13:89, 2000.
250. Matthay KK, Mentzer WC: Erythrocyte enzymopathies in the newborn. *Clin Haematol* 10:31, 1981.
251. Schroter W, Eber SW, Bardosi A, et al: Generalised glucosephosphate isomerase (GPI) deficiency causing haemolytic anaemia, neuromuscular symptoms and impairment of granulocytic function: A new syndrome due to a new stable GPI variant with diminished specific activity (GPI Homburg). *Eur J Pediatr* 144:301, 1985.
252. Lin HY, Kao YH, Chen ST, Meng M: Effects of inherited mutations on catalytic activity and structural stability of human glucose-6-phosphate isomerase expressed in Escherichia coli. *Biochim Biophys Acta* 1794:315, 2009.
253. Merkle S, Pretsch W: Glucose-6-phosphate isomerase deficiency associated with nonspherocytic hemolytic anemia in the mouse: An animal model for the human disease. *Blood* 81:206, 1993.
254. Fujii H, Miwa S: Other erythrocyte enzyme deficiencies associated with non-haematological symptoms: Phosphoglycerate kinase and phosphofructokinase deficiency. *Baillieres Best Pract Res Clin Haematol* 13:141, 2000.
255. Nakajima H, Raben N, Hamaguchi T, Yamasaki T: Phosphofructokinase deficiency; past, present and future. *Curr Mol Med* 2:197, 2002.
256. Gerber K, Harvey JW, D'Agorne S, et al: Hemolysis, myopathy, and cardiac disease associated with hereditary phosphofructokinase deficiency in two Whippets. *Vet Clin Pathol* 38:46, 2009.
257. Kishi H, Mukai T, Hirono A, et al: Human aldolase A deficiency associated with a hemolytic anemia: Thermolabile aldolase due to a single base mutation. *Proc Natl Acad Sci U S A* 84:8623, 1987.
258. Beutler E, Scott S, Bishop A, et al: Red cell aldolase deficiency and hemolytic anemia: A new syndrome. *Trans Assoc Am Physicians* 86:154, 1973.
259. Kreuder J, Borkhardt A, Repp R, et al: Brief report: Inherited metabolic myopathy and hemolysis due to a mutation in aldolase A. *N Engl J Med* 334:1100, 1996.
260. Esposito G, Vitagliano L, Costanzo P, et al: Human aldolase A natural mutants: Relationship between flexibility of the C-terminal region and enzyme function. *Biochem J* 380:51, 2004.
261. Yao DC, Tolan DR, Murray MF, et al: Hemolytic anemia and severe rhabdomyolysis caused by compound heterozygous mutations of the gene for erythrocyte/muscle isozyme of aldolase, ALDOA(Arg303X/Cys338Tyr). *Blood* 103:2401, 2004.
262. Schneider AS: Triosephosphate isomerase deficiency: Historical perspectives and molecular aspects. *Baillieres Best Pract Res Clin Haematol* 13:119, 2000.
263. Orosz F, Olah J, Alvarez M, et al: Distinct behavior of mutant triosephosphate isomerase in hemolysate and in isolated form: Molecular basis of enzyme deficiency. *Blood* 98:3106, 2001.
264. Orosz F, Olah J, Ovadi J: Triosephosphate isomerase deficiency: Facts and doubts. *IUBMB Life* 58:703, 2006.
265. Pretsch W: Triosephosphate isomerase activity-deficient mice show haemolytic anaemia in homozygous condition. *Genet Res* 91:1, 2009.
266. Zingg BC, Pretsch W, Mohrenweiser HW: Molecular analysis of four ENU induced triosephosphate isomerase null mutants in Mus musculus. *Mutat Res* 328:163, 1995.
267. Beutler E: PGK deficiency. *Br J Haematol* 136:3, 2007.
268. Lemarchandel V, Joulin V, Valentin C, et al: Compound heterozygosity in a complete erythrocyte bisphosphoglycerate mutase deficiency. *Blood* 80:2643, 1992.
269. Hoyer JD, Allen SL, Beutler E, et al: Erythrocytosis due to biphosphoglycerate mutase deficiency with concurrent glucose-6-phosphate dehydrogenase (G-6-PD) deficiency. *Am J Hematol* 75:205, 2004.
270. Rosa R, Prehu MO, Beuzard Y, Rosa J: The first case of a complete deficiency of diphosphoglycerate mutase in human erythrocytes. *J Clin Invest* 62:907, 1978.
271. Beutler E, Gelbart T, Kondo T, Matsunaga AT: The molecular basis of a case of gamma-glutamylcysteine synthetase deficiency. *Blood* 94:2890, 1999.
272. Ristoff E, Augustson C, Geissler J, et al: A missense mutation in the heavy subunit of gamma-glutamylcysteine synthetase gene causes hemolytic anemia. *Blood* 95:2193, 2000.
273. Hamilton D, Wu JH, Alaoui-Jamali M, Batist G: A novel missense mutation in the gamma-glutamylcysteine synthetase catalytic subunit gene causes both decreased enzymatic activity and glutathione production. *Blood* 102:725, 2003.
274. Manu Pereira M, Gelbart T, Ristoff E, et al: Chronic non-spherocytic hemolytic anemia associated with severe neurological disease due to gamma-glutamylcysteine synthetase deficiency in a patient of Moroccan origin. *Haematologica.* 92:e102, 2007.
275. Ristoff E, Larsson A: Inborn errors in the metabolism of glutathione. *Orphanet J Rare Dis* 2:16, 2007.
276. Shi ZZ, Habib GM, Rhead WJ, et al: Mutations in the glutathione synthetase gene cause 5-oxoprolinuria. *Nat Genet* 14:361, 1996.
277. Dahl N, Pigg M, Ristoff E, et al: Missense mutations in the human glutathione synthetase gene result in severe metabolic acidosis, 5-oxoprolinuria, hemolytic anemia and neurological dysfunction. *Hum Mol Genet* 6:1147, 1997.
278. Njalsson R, Ristoff E, Carlsson K, et al: Genotype, enzyme activity, glutathione level, and clinical phenotype in patients with glutathione synthetase deficiency. *Hum Genet* 116:384, 2005.
279. Vives i Corrons JL: Chronic non-spherocytic haemolytic anaemia due to congenital pyrimidine 5′ nucleotidase deficiency: 25 years later. *Baillieres Best Pract Res Clin Haematol* 13:103, 2000.
280. Chiarelli LR, Fermo E, Zanella A, Valentini G: Hereditary erythrocyte pyrimidine 5′-nucleotidase deficiency: A biochemical, genetic and clinical overview. *Hematology* 11:67, 2006.
281. Valentine WN, Fink K, Paglia DE, et al: Hereditary hemolytic anemia with human erythrocyte pyrimidine 5′-nucleotidase deficiency. *J Clin Invest* 54:866, 1974.
282. Chiarelli LR, Morera SM, Galizzi A, et al: Molecular basis of pyrimidine 5′-nucleotidase deficiency caused by 3 newly identified missense mutations (c.187T→C, c.469G→C and c.740T→C) and a tabulation of known mutations. *Blood Cells Mol Dis* 40:295, 2008.
283. Beutler E, Carson D, Dannawi H, et al: Metabolic compensation for profound erythrocyte adenylate kinase deficiency. *J Clin Invest* 72:648, 1983.
284. Toren A, Brok-Simoni F, Ben-Bassat I, et al: Congenital haemolytic anaemia associated with adenylate kinase deficiency. *Br J Haematol* 87:376, 1994.
285. Bianchi P, Zappa M, Bredi E, et al: A case of complete adenylate kinase deficiency due to a nonsense mutation in AK-1 gene (Arg 107 → Stop, CGA → TGA) associated with chronic haemolytic anaemia. *Br J Haematol* 105:75, 1999.
286. Matsuura S, Igarashi M, Tanizawa Y, et al: Human adenylate kinase deficiency associated with hemolytic anemia. A single base substitution affecting solubility and catalytic activity of the cytosolic adenylate kinase. *J Biol Chem* 264:10148, 1989.
287. Qualtieri A, Pedace V, Bisconte MG, et al: Severe erythrocyte adenylate kinase deficiency due to homozygous A→G substitution at codon 164 of human AK1 gene associated with chronic haemolytic anaemia. *Br J Haematol* 99:770, 1997.
288. Corrons JL, Garcia E, Tusell JJ, et al: Red cell adenylate kinase deficiency: Molecular study of 3 new mutations (118G→A, 190G→A, and GAC deletion) associated with hereditary nonspherocytic hemolytic anemia. *Blood* 102:353, 2003.
289. Abrusci P, Chiarelli LR, Galizzi A, et al: Erythrocyte adenylate kinase deficiency: Characterization of recombinant mutant forms and relationship with nonspherocytic hemolytic anemia. *Exp Hematol* 35:1182, 2007.
290. Valentine WN, Paglia DE, Tartaglia AP, Gilsanz F: Hereditary hemolytic anemia with increased red cell adenosine deaminase (45- to 70-fold) and decreased adenosine triphosphate. *Science* 195:783, 1977.
291. Chottiner EG, Ginsburg D, Tartaglia AP, Mitchell BS: Erythrocyte adenosine deaminase overproduction in hereditary hemolytic anemia. *Blood* 74:448, 1989.
292. Chen EH, Tartaglia AP, Mitchell BS: Hereditary overexpression of adenosine deaminase in erythrocytes: Evidence for a cis-acting mutation. *Am J Hum Genet* 53:889, 1993.
293. Percy MJ, Lappin TR: Recessive congenital methaemoglobinaemia: Cytochrome b(5) reductase deficiency. *Br J Haematol* 141:298, 2008.
294. Dern RJ, Beutler E, Alving AS: The hemolytic effect of primaquine. V. Primaquine sensitivity as a manifestation of a multiple drug sensitivity. *J Lab Clin Med* 45:30, 1955.
295. Cohen G, Hochstein P: Generation of hydrogen peroxide in erythrocytes by hemolytic agents. *Biochemistry* 3:895, 1964.
296. Kosower NS, Song KR, Kosower EM, Correa W: Glutathione. II. Chemical aspects of azo ester procedure for oxidation to disulfide. *Biochim Biophys Acta* 192:8, 1969.
297. Birchmeier W, Tuchschmid PE, Winterhalter H: Comparison of human hemoglobin A carrying glutathione as a mixed disulfide with the naturally occurring human hemoglobin A3. *Biochemistry* 12:3667, 1973.
298. Rachmilewitz EA, Harari E, Winterhalter KH: Separation of alpha- and beta-chains of hemoglobin A by acetylphenylhydrazine. *Biochim Biophys Acta* 371:402, 1974.
299. Itano HA, Hosokawa K, Hirota K: Induction of haemolytic anaemia by substituted phenylhydrazines. *Br J Haematol* 32:99, 1976.
300. Kirkman HN, Gaetani GF: Catalase: A tetrameric enzyme with four tightly bound molecules of NADPH. *Proc Natl Acad Sci U S A* 81:4343, 1984.
301. Gaetani GF, Rolfo M, Arena S, et al: Active involvement of catalase during hemolytic crises of favism. *Blood* 88:1084, 1996.
302. Rifkind RA: Heinz body anemia: An ultrastructural study. II. Red cell sequestration and destruction. *Blood* 26:433, 1965.
303. Bunn HEF, Jandl JH: Exchange of heme among hemoglobin molecules. *Proc Natl Acad Sci U S A* 56:974, 1966.
304. Jandl JH: The Heinz body hemolytic anemias. *Ann Intern Med* 58:702, 1963.
305. Beutler E: Abnormalities of glycolysis (HMP shunt). *Bibl Haematol* 29:146, 1968.
306. Baehner RL, Nathan DG, Castle WB: Oxidant injury of Caucasian glucose-6-phosphate dehydrogenase-deficient red blood cells by phagocytosing leukocytes during infection. *J Clin Invest* 50:2466, 1971.

307. Arese P, De Flora A: Denaturation of normal and abnormal erythrocytes II. Pathophysiology of hemolysis in glucose-6-phosphate dehydrogenase deficiency. *Semin Hematol* 27:1, 1990.
308. Stamatoyannopoulos G, Fraser GR, Motulsky AG, et al: On the familial predisposition to favism. *Am J Hum Genet* 18:253, 1966.
309. Cassimos CHR, Malaka-Zafiriu K, Tsiures J: Urinary d-glucaric acid excretion in normal and G-6-PD deficient children with favism. *J Pediatr* 84:871, 1974.
310. Bottini E, Bottini FG, Borgiani P, Businco L: Association between ACP1 and favism: A possible biochemical mechanism. *Blood* 89:2613, 1997.
311. Fiorelli G, Podda M, Corrias A, Fargion S: The relevance of immune reactions in acute favism. *Acta Haematol* 51:211, 1974.
312. Turrini F, Naitana A, Mannuzzu L, et al: Increased red cell calcium, decreased calcium adenosine triphosphatase, and altered membrane proteins during fava bean hemolysis in glucose-6-phosphate dehydrogenase-deficient (Mediterranean variant) individuals. *Blood* 66:302, 1985.
313. De Flora A, Benatti U, Guida L, et al: Favism: Disordered erythrocyte calcium homeostasis. *Blood* 66:294, 1985.
314. Fischer TM, Meloni T, Pescarmona GP, Arese P: Membrane cross bonding in red cells in favic crisis: A missing link in the mechanism of extravascular haemolysis. *Br J Haematol* 59:159, 1985.
315. Kaplan M, Vreman HJ, Hammerman C, et al: Contribution of haemolysis to jaundice in Sephardic Jewish glucose-6-phosphate dehydrogenase deficient neonates. *Br J Haematol* 93:822, 1996.
316. Kaplan M, Muraca M, Hammerman C, et al: Imbalance between production and conjugation of bilirubin: A fundamental concept in the mechanism of neonatal jaundice. *Pediatrics* 110:e47, 2002.
317. Kaplan M, Renbaum P, Levy-Lahad E, et al: Gilbert syndrome and glucose-6-phosphate dehydrogenase deficiency: A dose-dependent genetic interaction crucial to neonatal hyperbilirubinemia. *Proc Natl Acad Sci U S A* 94:12128, 1997.
318. Huang CS, Chang PF, Huang MJ, et al: Glucose-6-phosphate dehydrogenase deficiency, the UDP-glucuronosyl transferase 1A1 gene, and neonatal hyperbilirubinemia. *Gastroenterology* 123:127, 2002.
319. Oluboyede OA, Esan GJF, Francis TI, Luzzatto L: Genetically determined deficiency of glucose 6-phosphate dehydrogenase (type A-) is expressed in the liver. *J Lab Clin Med* 93:783, 1979.
320. Piomelli S: G6PD-related neonatal jaundice, in *Glucose-6-Phosphate Dehydrogenase*, edited by A Yoshida, E Beutler, p 95. Academic Press, Orlando, FL, 1986.
321. Ifekwunigwe AE, Luzzatto L: Kernicterus in G-6-PD-deficiency. *Lancet* 1:667, 1966.
322. Eshaghpour E, Oski FA, Williams M: The relationship of erythrocyte glucose-6-phosphate dehydrogenase deficiency to hyperbilirubinemia in Negro premature infants. *J Pediatr* 70:595, 1967.
323. Lopez R, Cooperman JM: Glucose-6-phosphate dehydrogenase deficiency and hyperbilirubinemia in the newborn. *Am J Dis Child* 122:66, 1971.
324. Herschel M, Ryan M, Gelbart T, Kaplan M: Hemolysis and hyperbilirubinemia in an African American neonate heterozygous for glucose-6-phosphate dehydrogenase deficiency. *J Perinatol* 22:577, 2002.
325. Beutler E, Gelbart T, Demina A: Racial variability in the UDP-glucuronosyltransferase 1 (UGT1A1) promoter: A balanced polymorphism for regulation of bilirubin metabolism? *Proc Natl Acad Sci U S A* 95:8170, 1998.
326. Valentine WN, Paglia DE: The primary cause of hemolysis in enzymopathies of anaerobic glycolysis: A viewpoint. *Blood Cells* 6:819, 1980.
327. Beutler E: The primary cause of hemolysis in enzymopathies of anaerobic glycolysis: A viewpoint. A commentary. *Blood Cells* 6:827, 1980.
328. Aizawa S, Harada T, Kanbe E, et al: Ineffective erythropoiesis in mutant mice with deficient pyruvate kinase activity. *Exp Hematol* 33:1292, 2005.
329. McCaffrey RP, Halsted CH, Wahab MFA, Robertson RP: Chloramphenicol-induced hemolysis in Caucasian glucose-6-phosphate dehydrogenase deficiency. *Ann Intern Med* 74:722, 1971.
330. Chan TK, Chesterman CN, McFadzean AJS, Todd D: The survival of glucose-6-phosphate dehydrogenase-deficient erythrocytes in patients with typhoid fever on chloramphenicol therapy. *J Lab Clin Med* 77:177, 1971.
331. Mehta JB, Singhal SB, Mehta BC: Ascorbic-acid-induced haemolysis in G-6-PD deficiency. *Lancet* 336:944, 1990.
332. Campbell GD, Jr., Steinberg MH, Bower JD: Ascorbic acid-induced hemolysis in G-6-PD deficiency. *Ann Intern Med* 82:810, 1975.
333. Rees DC, Kelsey H, Richards JDM: Acute haemolysis induced by high dose ascorbic acid in glucose-6-phosphate dehydrogenase deficiency. *BMJ* 306:841, 1993.
334. Markowitz N, Saravolatz LD: Use of trimethoprim-sulfamethoxazole in a glucose-6-phosphate dehydrogenase-deficient population. *Rev Infect Dis* 9(Suppl 2):S218, 1987.
335. Magon AM, Leipzig RM, Zannoni VG, Brewer GJ: Interactions of glucose-6-phosphate dehydrogenase deficiency with drug acetylation and hydroxylation reactions. *J Lab Clin Med* 97:764, 1981.
336. Woolhouse NM, Atu-Taylor LC: Influence of double genetic polymorphism on response to sulfamethazine. *Clin Pharmacol Ther* 31:377, 1982.
337. Dern RJ, Beutler E, Alving AS: The hemolytic effect of primaquine. II. The natural course of the hemolytic anemia and the mechanism of its self-limited character. *J Lab Clin Med* 44:171, 1954.
338. Beutler E, Dern RJ, Alving AS: The hemolytic effect of primaquine. III. A study of primaquine-sensitive erythrocytes. *J Lab Clin Med* 44:177, 1954.
339. Beutler E, Dern RJ, Alving AS: The hemolytic effect of primaquine. IV. The relationship of cell age to hemolysis. *J Lab Clin Med* 44:439, 1954.
340. George JN, Sears DA, McCurdy P, Conrad ME: Primaquine sensitivity in Caucasians: Hemolytic reactions induced by primaquine in G-6-PD deficient subjects. *J Lab Clin Med* 70:80, 1967.
341. Walker DH, Hawkins HK, Hudson P: Fulminant Rocky Mountain spotted fever. *Arch Pathol Lab Med* 107:121, 1983.
342. Huo TI, Wu JC, Chiu CF, Lee SD: Severe hyperbilirubinemia due to acute hepatitis a superimposed on a chronic hepatitis B carrier with glucose-6-phosphate dehydrogenase deficiency. *Am J Gastroenterol* 91:158, 1996.
343. Chau TN, Lai ST, Lai JY, Yuen H: Haemolysis complicating acute viral hepatitis in patients with normal or deficient glucose-6-phosphate dehydrogenase activity. *Scand J Infect Dis* 29:551, 1997.
344. Pietrapertosa A, Palma A, Campanale D, et al: Genotype and phenotype correlation in glucose-6-phosphate dehydrogenase deficiency. *Haematologica* 86:30, 2001.
345. Kattamis CA, Kyriazakou M, Chaidas S: Favism. Clinical and biochemical data. *J Med Genet* 6:34, 1969.
346. Wong WY, Powars D, Williams WD: "Yewdow"-induced anemia. *West J Med* 151:459, 1989.
347. Globerman H, Novak T, Chevion M: Haemolysis in a G6PD-deficient child induced by eating unripe peaches. *Scand J Haematol* 33:337, 1984.
348. Williams CKO, Osotimehin BO, Ogunmola GB, Awotedu AA: Haemolytic anaemia associated with Nigerian barbecued meat (red suya). *Afr J Med Med Sci* 17:71, 1988.
349. Schiliro G, Russo A, Curreri R, et al: Glucose-6-phosphate dehydrogenase deficiency in Sicily. Incidence, biochemical characteristics and clinical implications. *Clin Genet* 15:183, 1979.
350. Kaplan M, Hammerman C: Severe neonatal hyperbilirubinemia. *Clin Perinatol* 25:575, 1998.
351. Kaplan M, Hammerman C, Vreman HJ, et al: Acute hemolysis and severe neonatal hyperbilirubinemia in glucose-6-phosphate dehydrogenase-deficient heterozygotes. *J Pediatr* 139:137, 2001.
352. Lopez R, Cooperman JM: Glucose-6-phosphate dehydrogenase deficiency and hyperbilirubinemia in the newborn. *Am J Dis Child* 122:66, 1971.
353. Fok TF, Lau SP: Glucose-6-phosphate dehydrogenase deficiency: A preventable cause of mental retardation. *Br Med J (Clin Res Ed)* 292:829, 1986.
354. Singh H: Glucose-6-phosphate dehydrogenase deficiency: A preventable cause of mental retardation. *Br Med J (Clin Res Ed)* 292:397, 1986.
355. Kaplan M, Hammerman C: Understanding and preventing severe neonatal hyperbilirubinemia: Is bilirubin neurotoxicity really a concern in the developed world? *Clin Perinatol* 31:555, 2004.
356. Ardati KO, Bajakian KM, Tabbara KS: Effect of glucose-6-phosphate dehydrogenase deficiency on neutrophil function. *Acta Haematol* 97:211, 1997.
357. Van Bruggen R, Bautista JM, Petropoulou T, et al: Deletion of leucine 61 in glucose-6-phosphate dehydrogenase leads to chronic nonspherocytic anemia, granulocyte dysfunction, and increased susceptibility to infections. *Blood* 100:1026, 2002.
358. Cooper MR, DeChatelet LR, McCall CE, et al: Complete deficiency of leukocyte glucose-6-phosphate dehydrogenase with defective bactericidal activity. *J Clin Invest* 51:769, 1972.
359. Gray GR, Klebanoff SJ, Stamatoyannopoulos G, et al: Neutrophil dysfunction, chronic granulomatous disease, and nonspherocytic haemolytic anaemia caused by complete deficiency of glucose-6-phosphate dehydrogenase. *Lancet* 2:530, 1973.
360. Vives-Corrons JL, Feliu E, Pujades MA, et al: Severe glucose-6-phosphate dehydrogenase (G 6 PD) deficiency associated with chronic hemolytic anemia, granulocyte dysfunction and increased susceptibility to infections. Description of a new molecular variant (G 6 PD Barcelona). *Blood* 59:428, 1982.
361. Roos D, van Zwieten R, Wijnen JT, et al: Molecular basis and enzymatic properties of glucose 6-phosphate dehydrogenase Volendam, leading to chronic nonspherocytic anemia, granulocyte dysfunction, and increased susceptibility to infections. *Blood* 94:2955, 1999.
362. Rosa-Borges A, Sampaio MG, Condino Neto A, et al: Glucose 6 phosphate dehydrogenase deficiency with recurrent infections: Case report. *J Pediatr (Rio J)* 77:331, 2001.
363. Chao YC, Huang CS, Lee CN, et al: Higher infection of dengue virus serotype 2 in human monocytes of patients with G6PD deficiency. *PLoS ONE* 3:e1557, 2008.
364. Gray GR, Naiman SC, Robinson GCF: Platelet function and G-6-PD deficiency. *Lancet* 1:997, 1974.
365. Schwartz JP, Cooperberg AA, Rosenberg A: Platelet-function studies in patients with glucose-6-phosphate dehydrogenase deficiency. *Br J Haematol* 27:273, 1974.
366. Westring DW, Pisciotta AV: Anemia, cataracts, and seizures in patient with glucose-6-phosphate dehydrogenase deficiency. *Arch Intern Med* 118:385, 1966.
367. Harley JD, Agar NS, Gruca MA, et al: Cataracts with a glucose-6-phosphate dehydrogenase variant. *Br Med J (Clin Res Ed)* 2:86, 1975.
368. Harley JD, Agar NS, Yoshida A: Glucose-6-phosphate dehydrogenase variants: Gd (+) Alexandra associated with neonatal jaundice and Gd (–) Camperdown in a young man with lamellar cataracts. *J Lab Clin Med* 91:295, 1978.
369. Panich V, Na-Nakorn S: G 6 PD deficiency in senile cataracts. *Hum Genet* 55:123, 1980.
370. Orzalesi N, Sorcinelli R, Guiso G: Increased incidence of cataract in male subjects deficient in glucose-6-phosphate dehydrogenase. *Arch Ophthalmol* 99:69, 1981.
371. Bhatia RPS, Patel R, Dubey B: Senile cataract and glucose-6-phosphate dehydrogenase deficiency in Indians. *Trop Geogr Med* 42:349, 1990.

372. Zampella EJ, Bradley EL, Pretlow TG: Glucose-6-phosphate dehydrogenase: A possible clinical indicator for prostatic carcinoma. *Cancer* 49:384, 1982.
373. Sulis E: G-6-PD deficiency and cancer. *Lancet* 1:1185, 1972.
374. Ferraris AM, Broccia G, Meloni T, et al: Glucose-6-phosphate dehydrogenase deficiency and incidence of hematologic malignancy. *Am J Hum Genet* 42:516, 1988.
375. Mueller-Soyano A, De Roura ET, Duke PR, et al: Pyruvate kinase deficiency and leg ulcers. *Blood* 47:807, 1976.
376. Curiel CD, Velasquez GA, Papa R: Hemolytic anemia and leg ulcers due to pyruvate kinase deficiency. Report of the second Venezuelan family. *Sangre (Barc)* 22:64, 1977.
377. Amankwah KS, Dick BW, Dodge S: Hemolytic anemia and pyruvate kinase deficiency in pregnancy. *Obstet Gynecol* 55(Suppl):42S, 1980.
378. Vives Corrons JL, Garcia AM, Sosa AM, et al: Heterozygous pyruvate kinase deficiency and severe hemolytic anemia in a pregnant woman with concomitant, glucose-6-phosphate dehydrogenase deficiency. *Ann Hematol* 62:190, 1991.
379. Ferreira P, Morais L, Costa R, et al: Hydrops fetalis associated with erythrocyte pyruvate kinase deficiency. *Eur J Pediatr* 159:481, 2000.
380. Kanno H, Wei DC, Chan LC, et al: Hereditary hemolytic anemia caused by diverse point mutations of pyruvate kinase gene found in Japan and Hong Kong. *Blood* 84:3505, 1994.
381. Diez A, Gilsanz F, Martinez J, et al: Life-threatening nonspherocytic hemolytic anemia in a patient with a null mutation in the PKLR gene and no compensatory PKM gene expression. *Blood* 106:1851, 2005.
382. Wellner VP, Sekura R, Meister A, Larsson A: Glutathione synthetase deficiency, an inborn error of metabolism involving the gamma-glutamyl cycle in patients with 5-oxoprolinuria (pyroglutamic aciduria). *Proc Natl Acad Sci U S A* 71:2505, 1974.
383. Hirono A, Iyori H, Sekine I, et al: Three cases of hereditary nonspherocytic hemolytic anemia associated with red blood cell glutathione deficiency. *Blood* 87:2071, 1996.
384. Konrad PN, Richards F, II, Valentine WN, Paglia DE: Gamma-glutamyl-cysteine synthetase deficiency. *N Engl J Med* 286:557, 1972.
385. Richards F, II, Cooper MR, Pearce LA, et al: Familial spinocerebellar degeneration, hemolytic anemia, and glutathione deficiency. *Arch Intern Med* 134:534, 1974.
386. Beutler E, Moroose R, Kramer L, et al: Gamma-glutamylcysteine synthetase deficiency and hemolytic anemia. *Blood* 75:271, 1990.
387. Skala H, Dreyfus JC, Vives-Corrons JL, et al: Triose phosphate isomerase deficiency. *Biochem Med* 18:226, 1977.
388. Valentine WN, Schneider AS, Baughan MA, et al: Hereditary hemolytic anemia with triosephosphate isomerase deficiency. *Am J Med* 41:27, 1966.
389. Schneider AS, Valentine WN, Baughan MA, et al: Triosephosphate isomerase deficiency. A multi-system inherited enzyme disorder: Clinical and genetic aspects, in *Hereditary Disorders of Erythrocyte Metabolism*, edited by E Beutler, p 265. Grune & Stratton, New York, 1968.
390. Hollan S, Magocsi M, Fodor E, et al: Search for the pathogenesis of the differing phenotype in two compound heterozygote Hungarian brothers with the same genotypic triosephosphate isomerase deficiency. *Proc Natl Acad Sci U S A* 94:10362, 1997.
391. Hollan S, Fujii H, Hirono A, et al: Hereditary triosephosphate isomerase (TPI) deficiency: Two severely affected brothers one with and one without neurological symptoms. *Hum Genet* 92:486, 1993.
392. Kugler W, Breme K, Laspe P, et al: Molecular basis of neurological dysfunction coupled with haemolytic anaemia in human glucose-6-phosphate isomerase (GPI) deficiency. *Hum Genet* 103:450, 1998.
393. DiMauro S, Dalakas M, Miranda AF: Phosphoglycerate kinase deficiency: Another cause of recurrent myoglobinuria. *Ann Neurol* 13:11, 1983.
394. Bresolin N, Bet L, Moggio M, et al: Muscle glucose-6-phosphate dehydrogenase deficiency. *J Neurol* 236:193, 1989.
395. Clarke JL, Vulliamy TJ, Roper D, et al: Combined glucose-6-phosphate dehydrogenase and glucosephosphate isomerase deficiency can alter clinical outcome. *Blood Cells Mol Dis* 30:258, 2003.
396. Branca R, Costa E, Rocha S, et al: Coexistence of congenital red cell pyruvate kinase and band 3 deficiency. *Clin Lab Haematol* 26:297, 2004.
397. Beutler E, Forman L: Coexistence of alpha-thalassemia and a new pyruvate kinase variant: PK Fukien. *Acta Haematol* 69:3, 1983.
398. Sampietro M, Lupica L, Perrero L, et al: The expression of uridine diphosphate glucuronosyltransferase gene is a major determinant of bilirubin level in heterozygous beta-thalassaemia and in glucose-6-phosphate dehydrogenase deficiency. *Br J Haematol* 99:437, 1997.
399. Danon D, Sheba C, Ramot B: The morphology of glucose 6 phosphate dehydrogenase deficient erythrocytes: Electron-microscopic studies. *Blood* 17:229, 1961.
400. Beaupre SR, Schiffman FJ: Rush hemolysis. A "bite-cell" hemolytic anemia associated with volatile liquid nitrite use. *Arch Fam Med* 3:545, 1994.
401. Greenberg MS: Heinz body hemolytic anemia. *Arch Intern Med* 136:153, 1976.
402. Nathan DM, Siegel AJ, Bunn HF: Acute methemoglobinemia and hemolytic anemia with phenazopyridine. *Arch Intern Med* 137:1636, 1977.
403. Oski FA, Nathan DG, Sidel VW, Diamond LK: Extreme hemolysis and red-cell distortion in erythrocyte pyruvate kinase deficiency. *N Engl J Med* 270:1023, 1964.
404. Mentzer WC Jr, Baehner RL, Schmidt-Schönbein H, et al: Selective reticulocyte destruction in erythrocyte pyruvate kinase deficiency. *J Clin Invest* 50:688, 1971.
405. Miwa S, Boivin P, Blume KG, et al: Recommended methods for the characterization of red cell pyruvate kinase variants. *Br J Haematol* 43:275, 1979.
406. Beutler E, Blume KG, Kaplan JC, et al: International Committee for Standardization in Haematology: Recommended methods for red-cell enzyme analysis. *Br J Haematol* 35:331, 1977.
407. Beutler E, Blume KG, Kaplan JC, et al: International Committee for Standardization in Haematology: Recommended screening test for glucose-6-phosphate dehydrogenase (G-6-PD) deficiency. *Br J Haematol* 43:465, 1979.
408. Herz F, Kaplan E, Scheye ES: Diagnosis of erythrocyte glucose-6-phosphate dehydrogenase deficiency in the negro male despite hemolytic crisis. *Blood* 35:90, 1970.
409. Ringelhahn B: A simple laboratory procedure for the recognition of A- (African type) G6PD deficiency in acute haemolytic crisis. *Clin Chim Acta* 36:272, 1972.
410. Beutler E: X-inactivation in heterozygous G-6-PD variant females, in *Glucose-6-Phosphate Dehydrogenase*, edited by A Yoshida, E Beutler, p 405. Academic Press, Orlando, FL, 1986.
411. Beutler E: G-6-PD activity of individual erythrocytes and X-chromosomal inactivation, in *Biochemical Methods in Red Cell Genetics*, edited by JJ Yunis, p 95. Academic Press, New York, 1969.
412. Vogels IMC, van Noorden CJF, Wolf BHM, et al: Cytochemical determination of heterozygous glucose-6-phosphate dehydrogenase deficiency in erythrocytes. *Br J Haematol* 63:402, 1986.
413. Jacob H, Jandl JH: A simple visual screening test for G-6-PD deficiency employing ascorbate and cyanide. *N Engl J Med* 274:1162, 1966.
414. Beutler E, Kuhl W, Gelbart T, Forman L: DNA sequence abnormalities of human glucose-6-phosphate dehydrogenase variants. *J Biol Chem* 266:4145, 1991.
415. Beutler E, Kuhl W, Fox M, et al: Prenatal diagnosis of glucose-6-P dehydrogenase (G6PD) deficiency. *Acta Haematol* 87:103, 1992.
416. Carrell RW, Kay R: A simple method for the detection of unstable haemoglobins. *Br J Haematol* 23:615, 1972.
417. Valentine WN, Paglia DE, Fink K, Madokoro G: Lead poisoning. Association with hemolytic anemia, basophilic stippling, erythrocyte pyrimidine 5′-nucleotidase deficiency, and intraerythrocytic accumulation of pyrimidines. *J Clin Invest* 58:926, 1976.
418. Pekrun A, Neubauer BA, Eber SW, et al: Triosephosphate isomerase deficiency: Biochemical and molecular genetic analysis for prenatal diagnosis. *Clin Genet* 47:175, 1995.
419. Beutler E: Red blood enzyme disorders, in *Hematologic Disorders in Maternal–Fetal Medicine*, edited by MM Bern MM, FD Frigoletto Jr, p 199. Wiley-Liss, New York, 1990.
420. Baronciani L, Beutler E: Prenatal diagnosis of pyruvate kinase deficiency. *Blood* 84:2354, 1994.
421. Gupta N, Bianchi P, Fermo E, et al: Prenatal diagnosis for a novel homozygous mutation in PKLR gene in an Indian family. *Prenat Diagn* 27:117, 2007.
422. Kedar PS, Nampoothiri S, Sreedhar S, et al: First-trimester prenatal diagnosis of pyruvate kinase deficiency in an Indian family with the pyruvate kinase-Amish mutation. *Genet Mol Res* 6:470, 2007.
423. Repiso A, Corrons JL, Vulliamy T, et al: New haplotype for the Glu104Asp mutation in triose-phosphate isomerase deficiency and prenatal diagnosis in a Spanish family. *J Inherit Metab Dis* 28:807, 2005.
424. Rouger H, Girodon E, Goossens M, et al: PK Mondor: Prenatal diagnosis of a frameshift mutation in the LR pyruvate kinase gene associated with severe hereditary nonspherocytic haemolytic anaemia. *Prenat Diagn* 16:97, 1996.
425. Arya R, Lalloz MR, Nicolaides KH, et al: Prenatal diagnosis of triosephosphate isomerase deficiency. *Blood* 87:4507, 1996.
426. Dallapiccola B, Novelli G, Ferranti G, et al: First trimester monitoring of a pregnancy at risk for glucose phosphate isomerase deficiency. *Prenat Diagn* 6:101, 1986.
427. Lestas AN, Rodeck CH, White JM: Normal activities of glycolytic enzymes in the fetal erythrocytes. *Br J Haematol* 50:439, 1982.
428. Mimouni F, Shohat S, Reisner SH: G6PD-deficiency donor blood as a cause of hemolysis in two preterm infants. *Isr J Med Sci* 22:120, 1986.
429. Kappas A, Drummond GS, Valaes T: A single dose of Sn-mesoporphyrin prevents development of severe hyperbilirubinemia in glucose-6-phosphate dehydrogenase-deficient newborns. *Pediatrics* 108:25, 2001.
430. Hamilton JW, Jones FG, McMullin MF: Glucose-6-phosphate dehydrogenase Guadalajara—A case of chronic non-spherocytic haemolytic anaemia responding to splenectomy and the role of splenectomy in this disorder. *Hematology* 9:307, 2004.
431. Beutler E, Mathai CK, Smith JE: Biochemical variants of glucose-6-phosphate dehydrogenase giving rise to congenital nonspherocytic hemolytic disease. *Blood* 31:131, 1968.
432. Corash L, Spielberg S, Bartsocas C, et al: Reduced chronic hemolysis during high-dose vitamin E administration in Mediterranean-type glucose-6-phosphate dehydrogenase deficiency. *N Engl J Med* 303:416, 1980.
433. Spielberg SP, Boxer LA, Corash LM, Schulman JD: Improved erythrocyte survival with high dose vitamin E in chronic hemolyzing G6PD and glutathione synthetase deficiencies. *Ann Intern Med* 90:53, 1978.
434. Johnson GJ, Vatassery GT, Finkel B, Allen DW: High-dose vitamin E does not decrease the rate of chronic hemolysis in glucose-6-phosphate dehydrogenase deficiency. *N Engl J Med* 308:1014, 1983.
435. Newman JG, Newman TB, Bowie LJ, Mendelsohn J: An examination of the role of vitamin E in glucose-6-phosphate dehydrogenase deficiency. *Clin Biochem* 12:149, 1979.
436. Al Rimawi HS, Al Sheyyab M, Batieha A, et al: Effect of desferrioxamine in acute haemolytic anaemia of glucose-6-phosphate dehydrogenase deficiency. *Acta Haematol* 101:145, 1999.

437. Ekert H, Rawlinson I: Deferoxamine and favism. *N Engl J Med* 312:1260, 1985.
438. Khalifa AS, El-Alfy MS, Mokhtar G, et al: Effect of desferrioxamine B on hemolysis in glucose-6-phosphate dehydrogenase deficiency. *Acta Haematol* 82:113, 1989.
439. Ationu A, Humphries A, Lalloz MRA, et al: Reversal of metabolic block in glycolysis by enzyme replacement in triosephosphate isomerase-deficient cells. *Blood* 94:3193, 1999.
440. Tanphaichitr VS, Suvatte V, Issaragrisil S, et al: Successful bone marrow transplantation in a child with red blood cell pyruvate kinase deficiency. *Bone Marrow Transplant* 26:689, 2000.
441. Kanno H, Utsugisawa T, Aizawa S, et al: Transgenic rescue of hemolytic anemia due to red blood cell pyruvate kinase deficiency. *Haematologica* 92:731, 2007.
442. Meza NW, Quintana-Bustamante O, Puyet A, et al: *In vitro* and *in vivo* expression of human erythrocyte pyruvate kinase in erythroid cells: A gene therapy approach. *Hum Gene Ther* 18:502, 2007.
443. Kanno H, Aisaki K-I, Hamada T, et al: Ex vivo treatment of erythroid cells with glycolytic intermediates for metabolic correction of pyruvate kinase deficiency. *Blood* 104:3689, 2004.
444. Schroter W: Successful long-term phenobarbital therapy of hyperbilirubinemia in congenital hemolytic anemia due to glucose phosphate isomerase deficiency. *Eur J Pediatr* 135:41, 1980.
445. Zanella A, Bianchi P, Iurlo A, et al: Iron status and HFE genotype in erythrocyte pyruvate kinase deficiency: Study of Italian cases. *Blood Cells Mol Dis* 27:653, 2001.
446. Andersen FD, d'Amore F, Nielsen FC, et al: Unexpectedly high but still asymptomatic iron overload in a patient with pyruvate kinase deficiency. *Hematol J* 5:543, 2004.
447. Pannacciulli I, Tizianello A, Ajmar F, Salvidio E: The course of experimentally-induced hemolytic anemia in a primaquine-sensitive Caucasian. A case study. *Blood* 25:92, 1965.
448. Meloni T, Forteleoni G, Noja G, et al: Increased prevalence of glucose-6-phosphate dehydrogenase deficiency in patients with cholelithiasis. *Acta Haematol* 85:76, 1991.
449. Johnson LH, Bhutani VK, Brown AK: System-based approach to management of neonatal jaundice and prevention of kernicterus. *J Pediatr* 140:396, 2002.
450. Petrakis NL, Wiesenfeld SL, Sams BJ, et al: Prevalence of sickle-cell trait and glucose-6-phosphate dehydrogenase deficiency. *N Engl J Med* 282:767, 1970.
451. Bowman HS, McKusick VA, Dronamraju KR: Pyruvate kinase deficient hemolytic anemia in an Amish isolate. *Am J Hum Genet* 17:1, 1965.
452. Beutler E: The hemolytic effect of primaquine and related compounds. A review. *Blood* 14:103, 1959.
453. Beutler E: The study of glucose-6-phosphate dehydrogenase: History and molecular biology. *Am J Hematol* 42:53, 1993.
454. Newton WA, Jr, Bass JC: Glutathione sensitive chronic non-spherocytic hemolytic anemia. *Am J Dis Child* 96:501, 1958.
455. Beutler E: *Red Cell Metabolism: A Manual of Biochemical Methods*. Grune & Stratton, New York, 1975.
456. Beutler E, Kuhl W, Gelbart T: Blood cell phosphogluconolactonase: Assay and properties. *Br J Haematol* 62:577, 1986.
457. Bird TD, Hamernyik P, Nutter JY, Labbe RF: Inherited deficiency of delta-aminolevulinic acid dehydratase. *Am J Hum Genet* 31:662, 1979.
458. Kamatani N, Hakoda M, Otsuka S, et al: Only three mutations account for almost all defective alleles causing adenine phosphoribosyltransferase deficiency in Japanese patients. *J Clin Invest* 90:130, 1992.
459. Hidaka Y, Palella TD, O'Toole TE, et al: Human adenine phosphoribosyltransferase. Identification of allelic mutations at the nucleotide level as a cause of complete deficiency of the enzyme. *J Clin Invest* 80:1409, 1987.
460. Ogasawara N, Goto H, Yamada Y, Watanabe T: Distribution of AMP-deaminase isozymes in rat tissues. *Eur J Biochem* 87:297, 1978.
461. Yamada Y, Goto H, Wakamatsu N, Ogasawara N: A rare case of complete human erythrocyte AMP deaminase deficiency due to two novel missense mutations in AMPD3. *Hum Mutat* 17:78, 2001.
462. Armstrong JM, Myers DV, Verpoorte JA, Edsall JT: Purification and properties of human erythrocyte carbonic anhydrases. *J Biol Chem* 241:5137, 1966.
463. Kendall AG, Tashian RE: Erythrocyte carbonic anhydrase I: Inherited deficiency in humans. *Science* 197:471, 1977.
464. Roth DE, Venta PJ, Tashian RE, Sly WS: Molecular basis of human carbonic anhydrase II deficiency. *Proc Natl Acad Sci U S A* 89:1804, 1992.
465. Simonelli F, Giovane A, Frunzio S, et al: Galactokinase activity in patients with idiopathic presenile and senile cataract. *Metab Pediatr Syst Ophthalmol* 15:53, 1992.
466. Karas N, Gobec L, Pfeifer V, et al: Mutations in galactose-1-phosphate uridyltransferase gene in patients with idiopathic presenile cataract. *J Inherit Metab Dis* 26:699, 2003.
467. Beutler E: Effect of flavin compounds on glutathione reductase activity: *In vivo* and *in vitro* studies. *J Clin Invest* 48:1957, 1969.
468. McCann SR, Finkel B, Cadman S, Allen DW: Study of a kindred with hereditary spherocytosis and glyceraldehyde-3-phosphate dehydrogenase deficiency. *Blood* 47:171, 1976.
469. Valentine WN, Paglia DE, Neerhout RC, Konrad PN: Erythrocyte glyoxalase II deficiency with coincidental hereditary elliptocytosis. *Blood* 36:797, 1970.
470. Johnson LA, Gordon RB, Emmerson BT: Hypoxanthine-guanine phosphoribosyltransferase: A simple spectrophotometric assay. *Clin Chim Acta* 80:203, 1977.
471. Larovere LE, Romero N, Fairbanks LD, et al: A novel missense mutation, c.584A → C (Y195S), in two unrelated Argentine patients with hypoxanthine-guanine phosphoribosyl-transferase deficiency, neurological variant. *Mol Genet Metab* 81:352, 2004.
472. Sumi S, Marinaki AM, Arenas M, et al: Genetic basis of inosine triphosphate pyrophosphohydrolase deficiency. *Hum Genet* 111:360, 2002.
473. Sass MD, Caruso CJ, Farhangi M: TPNH-methemoglobin reductase deficiency: A new red-cell enzyme defect. *J Lab Clin Med* 70:760, 1967.
474. Ferrell RE, Escallon M, Aguilar L, Bertin T: Erythrocyte phosphoglucomutase: A family study of a PGM1 deficient allele. *Hum Genet* 67:306, 1984.
475. Chamberlain BR, Buttery JE: Reappraisal of the uroporphyrinogen I synthase assay, and a proposed modified method. *Clin Chem* 26:1346, 1980.
476. Strand LJ, Meyer UA, Felsher BF, et al: Decreased red cell uroporphyrinogen I synthetase activity in intermittent acute porphyria. *J Clin Invest* 51:2530, 1972.
477. Nafa K, Reghis A, Osmani N, et al: G6PD Aures: A new mutation (48 Ile→Thr) causing mild G6PD deficiency is associated with favism. *Hum Mol Genet* 2:81, 1993.
478. Beutler E, Kuhl W, Ramirez E, Lisker R: Some Mexican glucose-6-phosphate dehydrogenase (G-6-PD) variants revisited. *Hum Genet* 86:371, 1991.
479. Vulliamy TJ, D'Urso M, Battistuzzi G, et al: Diverse point mutations in the human glucose 6-phosphate dehydrogenase gene cause enzyme deficiency and mild or severe hemolytic anemia. *Proc Natl Acad Sci U S A* 85:5171, 1988.
480. Fiorelli G, Anghinelli L, Carandina G, et al: Point mutations in two G6PD variants previously described in Italy. *Blood* 76(Suppl):7a, 1990.
481. Beutler E, Kuhl W: The NT 1311 polymorphism of G6PD: G6PD Mediterranean mutation may have originated independently in Europe and Asia. *Am J Hum Genet* 47:1008, 1990.
482. De Vita G, Alcalay M, Sampietro M, et al: Two point mutations are responsible for G6PD polymorphism in Sardinia. *Am J Hum Genet* 44:233, 1989.
483. Ninfali P, Bresolin N, Baronciani L, et al: Glucose-6-phosphate dehydrogenase Lodi 844C: A study on its expression in blood cells and muscle. *Enzyme* 45:180, 1991.
484. Demir AY, van Solinge WW, van Oirschot B, et al: Glucose-6-phosphate dehydrogenase deficiency in an elite long-distance runner. *Blood* 113:2118, 2009.
485. Vlachos A, Westwood B, Lipton JM, Beutler E: G6PD Mt. Sinai: A new severe hemolytic variant characterized by dual mutations at nucleotides 376G and 1159T (N126D). *Hum Mutat* Suppl 1:S154, 1998.
486. Filosa S, Calabrï V, Vallone D, et al: Molecular basis of chronic non-spherocytic haemolytic anaemia: A new G6PD variant (393 Arg→His) with abnormal K m GPD and marked instability. *Br J Haematol* 80:111, 1992.
487. Beutler E, Westwood B, Prchal J, et al: New glucose-6-phosphate dehydrogenase mutations from various ethnic groups. *Blood* 80:255, 1992.
488. Zuo L, Chen E, Du CS, et al: Genetic study of Chinese G6PD variants by direct PCR sequencing. *Blood* 76 (Suppl):51a, 1990.
489. Stevens DJ, Wanachiwanawin W, Mason PJ, et al: G6PD Canton a common deficient variant in South East Asia caused by a 459 Arg→Leu mutation. *Nucleic Acids Res* 18:7190, 1990.
490. Calabro V, Mason PJ, Filosa S, et al: Genetic heterogeneity of glucose-6-phosphate dehydrogenase deficiency revealed by single-strand conformation and sequence analysis. *Am J Hum Genet* 52:527, 1993.
491. Beutler E, Vulliamy TJ: Hematologically important mutations: Glucose-6-phosphate dehydrogenase. *Blood Cells Mol Dis* 28:93, 2002.
492. Fanello CI, Karema C, Avellino P, et al: High risk of severe anaemia after chlorproguanil-dapsone+artesunate antimalarial treatment in patients with G6PD (A–) deficiency. *PLoS ONE* 3:e4031, 2008.
493. Gerr F, Frumkin H, Hodgins P: Hemolytic anemia following succimer administration in a glucose-6-phosphate dehydrogenase deficient patient. *J Toxicol Clin Toxicol* 32:569, 1994.
494. Rajkondawar VL, Modi TH, Mishra SN: Drug induced acute haemolytic anaemia in glucose-6-phosphate dehydrogenase deficiency subjects. *J Assoc Physicians India* 16:589, 1968.
495. Omar MES, Wahab MFA: Treatment of typhoid and paratyphoid fever with furazolidone. *J Trop Med Hyg* 70:43, 1967.
496. Meloni G, Meloni T: Glyburide-induced acute haemolysis in a G6PD-deficient patient with NIDDM. *Br J Haematol* 92:159, 1996.
497. Little C, Schacter B: Hemolytic anemia following isobutyl nitrate (IBN) inhalation in a patient with glucose-6-phosphate dehydrogenase (G-6-PD) deficiency. *Blood* 54 (Suppl 1):34A, 1979.
498. Rosen PJ, Johnson C, McGehee WG, Beutler E: Failure of methylene blue treatment in toxic methemoglobinemia. Association with glucose-6-phosphate dehydrogenase deficiency. *Ann Intern Med* 75:83, 1971.
499. Belton EM, Jones RV: Haemolytic anaemia due to nalidixic acid. *Lancet* 2:691, 1965.
500. Mandal BK, Stevenson J: Haemolytic crisis produced by nalidixic acid. *Lancet* 1:614, 1970.
501. Melzer-Lange M, Walsh-Kelly C: Naphthalene-induced hemolysis in a black female toddler deficient in glucose-6-phosphate dehydrogenase. *Pediatr Emerg Care* 5:24, 1989.
502. Todisco V, Lamour J, Finberg L: Hemolysis from exposure to naphthalene mothballs. *N Engl J Med* 325:1660, 1991.
503. Lapierre J, Holler C, Tourte-Schaefer C, et al: [Hemolytic anemia after antibilharzia treatment with niridazole in an Antillean with G6PD deficiency] [letter]. *Nouv Presse Med* 5:147, 1976.
504. Thomas M, Agnus D, Poirot JL, Golvan YJ: Hemolysis induced by niridazole in two patients with deficiency of G-6-PD. *Nouv Presse Med* 5:1537, 1976.
505. Chan TK, Todd D, Tso SC: Drug-induced haemolysis in glucose-6-phosphate dehydrogenase deficiency. *Br Med J (Clin Res Ed)* 2:1227, 1976.

506. Tishler M: Phenazopyridine-induced hemolytic anemia in a patient with G-6-PD deficiency. *Acta Haematol* 70:208, 1983.
507. Teunis BS, Leftwich EI, Pierce LE: Acute methemoglobinemia and hemolytic anemia due to toluidine blue. *Arch Surg* 101:527, 1970.
508. Djerassi LS, Vitany L: Haemolytic episode in G6PD deficient workers exposed to TNT. *Br J Ind Med* 32:54, 1975.
509. Ducros J, Saingra S, Rampal M, et al: Hemolytic anemia due to G6PD deficiency and urate oxidase in a kidney-transplant patient. *Clin Nephrol* 35:89, 1991.
510. Chan TK, Todd D, Tso SC: Red cell survival studies in glucose-6-phosphate dehydrogenase deficiency. *Bull Hong Kong Med Assoc* 26:41, 1974.
511. Herman J, Ben-Meir S: Overt hemolysis in patients with glucose-6-phosphate dehydrogenase deficiency. *Isr J Med Sci* 2:340, 1975.
512. Gaetani GD, Mareni C, Ravazzolo R, Salvidio E: Haemolytic effect of two sulphonamides evaluated by a new method. *Br J Haematol* 32:183, 1976.
513. McCurdy PR, Donohoe RF: Pyridoxine-responsive anemia conditioned by isonicotinic acid hydrazide. *Blood* 27:352, 1966.
514. Gaetani G, Salvidio E, Pannacciulli I, et al: Absence of haemolytic effects of L-DOPA on transfused G6PD-deficient erythrocytes. *Experientia* 26:785, 1970.
515. Zail SS, Charlton RW, Bothwell TH: The haemolytic effect of certain drugs in Bantu subjects with a deficiency of glucose-6-phosphate dehydrogenase. *S Afr J Med Sci* 27:95, 1962.
516. Heinrich RA, Smith TC, Buchanan RA: A pharmacological study of a new sulfonamide in glucose-6-phosphate dehydrogenase deficient subjects. *J Clin Pharmacol* 11:428, 1971.
517. Szeinberg A, Pras M, Sheba C, et al: The hemolytic effect of various sulfonamides on subjects with a deficiency of glucose-6-phosphate dehydrogenase of erythrocytes. *Isr J Med Sci* 18:176, 1959.
518. Kellermeyer RW, Tarlov AR, Brewer GJ, et al: Hemolytic effect of therapeutic drugs. Clinical considerations of the Primaquine-type hemolysis. *JAMA* 180:388, 1962.
519. Kellermeyer RW, Tarlov AR, Schrier SL, Alving AS: Hemolytic effect of commonly used drugs on erythrocytes deficient in glucose-6-phosphate dehydrogenase. *J Lab Clin Med* 52:827, 1958.
520. Mela Q, Perpignano G, Ruggiero V, Longatti S: Tolerability of tiaprofenic acid in patients with glucose-6-phosphate dehydrogenase (G6PD) deficiency. *Drugs* 35:107, 1988.
521. Beutler E, Duron O, Kelly BM: Improved method for the determination of blood glutathione. *J Lab Clin Med* 61:882, 1963.
522. Kaplan J-C, Nicolas A, Hanlickova-Leroux A, Beutler E: A simple spot screening test for fast detection of red cell NADH-diaphorase deficiency. *Blood* 36:330, 1970.
523. Beutler E, Gelbart T: Improved assay of the enzymes of glutathione synthesis: Gamma-glutamylcysteine synthetase and glutathione synthetase. *Clin Chim Acta* 158:115, 1986.
524. Torrance J, West C, Beutler E: A simple rapid radiometric assay for pyrimidine-5′-nucleotidase. *J Lab Clin Med* 90:563, 1977.

CHAPTER 47

THE THALASSEMIAS: DISORDERS OF GLOBIN SYNTHESIS

David J. Weatherall

SUMMARY

The thalassemias are the commonest monogenic diseases in man. They occur at a high gene frequency throughout the Mediterranean populations, the Middle East, the Indian subcontinent, and Myanmar, and in a line stretching from southern China through Thailand and the Malay peninsula into the island populations of the Pacific. They are also seen commonly in countries in which there has been immigration from these high-frequency populations.

There are two main classes of thalassemia, α and β, in which the α- and β-globin genes are involved, and rarer forms caused by abnormalities of other globin genes. These conditions all have in common an imbalanced rate of production of the globin chains of adult hemoglobin, excess α chains in β-thalassemia and excess β chains in α-thalassemia. Several hundred different mutations at the α- and β-globin loci have been defined as the cause of the reduced or absent output of α or β chains. The high frequency and genetic diversity of the thalassemias is related to past or present heterozygote resistance to malaria.

The pathophysiology of the thalassemias can be traced to the deleterious effects of the globin-chain subunits that are produced in excess. In β-thalassemia, excess α chains cause damage to the red cell precursors and red cells and lead to profound anemia. This causes expansion of the ineffective marrow, with severe effects on development, bone formation, and growth. The major cause of morbidity and mortality is the effect of iron deposition in the endocrine organs, liver, and heart, which results from increased intestinal absorption and the effects of blood transfusion. The pathophysiology of the α-thalassemias is different because the excess β chains that result from defective α-chain production form β_4 molecules, or hemoglobin H, which is soluble and does not precipitate in the marrow. However, it is unstable and precipitates in older red cells. Hence, the anemia of α-thalassemia is hemolytic rather than dyserythropoietic.

The clinical pictures of α- and β-thalassemia vary widely, and knowledge is gradually being amassed about some of the genetic and environmental factors that modify these phenotypes.

Because the carrier states for the thalassemias can be identified and affected fetuses can be diagnosed by DNA analysis after the ninth to tenth week of gestation, these conditions are widely amenable to prenatal diagnosis. Currently, marrow transplantation is the only way in which they can be cured.

Symptomatic management is based on regular blood transfusion, iron chelation therapy, and the judicious use of splenectomy. Experimental approaches to their management include the stimulation of fetal hemoglobin synthesis and attempts at somatic cell gene therapy.

Acronyms and abbreviations that appear in this chapter include: ATP, adenosine triphosphate; ATR-16, α-thalassemia chromosome 16-linked mental retardation syndrome; ATR-X, α-thalassemia X-linked mental retardation syndrome; bp, base pairs; DNase I, an enzyme used to detect DNA-protein interaction; EKLF, a transcription factor erythroid Kruppel-like factor; HPFH, hereditary persistence of fetal hemoglobin; HS, hypersensitive site to DNase I treatment; LCR, locus control region; MCS, multispecies conserved sequences; PCR, polymerase chain reaction; PHD region, a DNA region with zinc finger motif commonly deleted in ATR-X α-thalassemia; RFLP, restriction fragment length polymorphism.

DEFINITIONS AND HISTORY

In 1925, Cooley and Lee[1] first described a form of severe anemia that occurred early in life and was associated with splenomegaly and bone changes. In 1932, George H. Whipple and William L. Bradford[2] published a comprehensive account of the pathologic findings in this disease. Whipple coined the phrase *thalassic anemia*[3,4] and condensed it to *thalassemia*, from θαλασσα ("the sea"), because early patients were all of Mediterranean background. The true genetic character of the disorder became fully appreciated after 1940. The disease described by Cooley and Lee is the homozygous state of an autosomal gene for which the heterozygous state is associated with much milder hematologic changes. The severe homozygous condition became known as *thalassemia major*. The heterozygous states, thalassemia trait, were designated according to their severity as *thalassemia minor* or *minima*.[3,5–7] Later, the term *thalassemia intermedia* was used to describe disorders that were milder than the major form but more severe than the traits.

Thalassemia is not a single disease but a group of disorders, each resulting from an inherited abnormality of globin production.[7] The conditions form part of the spectrum of diseases known collectively as the *hemoglobinopathies*, which can be classified broadly into two types. The first subdivision consists of conditions, such as sickle cell anemia, that result from an inherited structural alteration in one of the globin chains. Although such abnormal hemoglobins may be synthesized less efficiently or broken down more rapidly than normal adult hemoglobin, the associated clinical abnormalities result from the physical properties of the abnormal hemoglobin (see Chap. 48). The second major subdivision of the hemoglobinopathies, the thalassemias, consists of inherited defects in the rate of synthesis of one or more of the globin chains. The result is imbalanced globin chain production, ineffective erythropoiesis, hemolysis, and a variable degree of anemia.

Several monographs describe the historical aspects of thalassemia in greater detail.[5,7]

DIFFERENT FORMS OF THALASSEMIA

Thalassemia can be defined as a condition in which a reduced rate of synthesis of one or more of the globin chains leads to imbalanced globin-chain synthesis, defective hemoglobin production, and damage to the red cells or their precursors from the effects of the globin subunits that are produced in relative excess.[7,8] Table 47–1 summarizes the main varieties of thalassemia that have been defined with certainty.

The β-thalassemias are divided into two main varieties. In one form, β^0-thalassemia, there is no β-chain production. In the other form, β^+-thalassemia, there is a partial deficiency of β-chain production. The hallmark of the common forms of β-thalassemia is an elevated level of hemoglobin A_2 in heterozygotes. In a less common class of β-thalassemias, heterozygotes have normal hemoglobin A_2 levels. Other rare forms include varieties of β-thalassemia intermedia that are inherited in a dominant fashion, that is, heterozygotes are severely affected, and there is a variety in which the genetic determinants are not linked to the β-globin gene cluster.[7,9,10]

The $\delta\beta$-thalassemias are heterogeneous. In some cases, no δ or β chains are synthesized. Originally, these disorders were classified according to the structure of the hemoglobin F produced, that is, $^G\gamma^A\gamma(\delta\beta)^0$- and

TABLE 47–1. Thalassemias and Related Disorders

α-Thalassemia
α^0
α^+
Deletion ($-\alpha$)
Nondeletion (α^T)
β-Thalassemia
β^0
β^+
Normal Hgb A_2
Dominant
Unlinked to β-globin genes
$\delta\beta$-Thalassemia
$(\delta\beta)^+$
$(\delta\beta)^0$
$(^A\gamma\,\delta\beta)^0$
γ-Thalassemia
δ-Thalassemia
δ^0
δ^+
$\varepsilon\gamma\delta\beta$-Thalassemia
HPFH
Deletion
$(\delta\beta)^0$, $(^A\gamma\,\delta\beta)^0$
Nondeletion
Linked to β-globin genes
$^G\gamma\beta^+$, $^A\gamma\beta^+$
Unlinked to β-globin genes

$^G\gamma\,(\delta\beta)^0$-thalassemia. This classification is illogical. The conditions are best described by the globin chains that are defectively synthesized, that is, simply $(\delta\beta)$,$^+$ $(\delta\beta)$,^{0} and $(^A\gamma\delta\beta)^0$-thalassemia.[7,10] In the $(\delta\beta)^+$-thalassemias, an abnormal hemoglobin is produced that has normal α chains combined with non-α chains consisting of the N-terminal residues of the δ chain fused to the C-terminal residues of the β chain. These fusion variants, called the *Lepore hemoglobins*, show structural heterogeneity.

The δ-thalassemias[7,10] are characterized by reduced output of δ chains and hence reduced hemoglobin A_2 levels in heterozygotes and an absence of hemoglobin A_2 in homozygotes. They are of no clinical significance except that, when inherited with β-thalassemia trait, the level of hemoglobin A_2 is reduced to the normal range.

A disorder characterized by defective ε-, γ-, δ-, and β-chain synthesis has been defined at the clinical and molecular level.[7,10] The homozygous state for this condition, $\varepsilon\gamma\delta\beta$-thalassemia, presumably is not compatible with fetal survival. It has been observed only in heterozygotes.

Hereditary persistence of fetal hemoglobin (HPFH) is a heterogeneous condition characterized by persistent fetal hemoglobin.[7,9,10] It is classified into deletion and nondeletion forms. The deletion forms of HPFH can be classified, like $\delta\beta$-thalassemia, as $(\delta\beta)^0$ HPFH and then subdivided according to the particular population in which this occurs and its associated molecular defect. In effect, the deletion forms of HPFH are very similar to β-thalassemia except for more efficient γ-chain synthesis and, therefore, less chain imbalance and a milder phenotype. The homozygous state is associated with mild thalassemic changes. In fact, the β-thalassemias and deletion forms of HPFH form a clinical continuum. The nondeletion forms of HPFH also are heterogeneous. In some cases, they are associated with mutations that involve the β-globin gene cluster and in which there is β-chain synthesis *cis* to the HPFH determinant. These conditions are subdivided into $^G\gamma\beta^+$ HPFH and $^A\gamma\beta^+$ HPFH. Again, they often are subclassified according to the population in which they occur, for example, Greek HPFH, British HPFH, and so on. Finally, a heterogeneous group of HPFH determinants is associated with very low levels of persistent fetal hemoglobin, the genetic loci of which, at least in some cases, are not linked to the β-globin gene cluster.

Because α chains are present in both fetal and adult hemoglobins, a deficiency of α-chain production affects hemoglobin synthesis in fetal and in adult life. A reduced rate of α-chain synthesis in fetal life results in an excess of γ chains, which form γ_4 tetramers, or hemoglobin Bart's. In adult life, a deficiency of α chains results in an excess of β chains, which form β_4 tetramers, or hemoglobin H. Because there are two α-globin genes per haploid genome, the genetics of α-thalassemia is more complicated than that of β-thalassemia. There are two main groups of α-thalassemia determinants.[7,10] First, in the α^0-thalassemias (formerly called α-thalassemia 1), no α chains are produced from an affected chromosome; that is, both linked α-globin genes are inactivated. Second, in the α^+-thalassemias (formerly called α-thalassemia 2), the output of one of the linked pair of α-globin genes is defective. The α^+-thalassemias are subdivided into deletion and nondeletion types. Both the α^0-thalassemias and deletion and nondeletion forms of α^+-thalassemia are extremely heterogeneous at the molecular level. There are two major clinical phenotypes of α-thalassemia: the hemoglobin Bart's hydrops syndrome, which usually reflects the homozygous state for α^0-thalassemia, and hemoglobin H disease, which usually results from the compound heterozygous state for α^0- and α^+-thalassemia.

Because the structural hemoglobin variants and the thalassemias occur at a high frequency in some populations, the two types of genetic defect can be found in the same individual. The different genetic varieties of thalassemia and their combinations with the genes for abnormal hemoglobins produce a series of disorders known collectively as the *thalassemia syndromes*.[7]

EPIDEMIOLOGY AND POPULATION GENETICS

The β-thalassemias are distributed widely in Mediterranean populations, the Middle East, parts of India and Pakistan, and throughout Southeast Asia (Fig. 47–1).[7,11,12] The disease is common in Tajikistan, Turkmenistan, Kyrgyzstan, and the People's Republic of China. Because of the extensive migration from areas of high gene frequency such as the Mediterranean region (e.g., Italy, Greece), Africa, and Asia to the Americas, the α- and β-thalassemia genes and clinical disease are relatively common, especially in North, but also South, America. The β-thalassemias are rare in Africa, except for isolated pockets in West Africa, notably Liberia, and in parts of North Africa. However, β-thalassemia occurs sporadically in all racial groups and has been observed in the homozygous state in persons of pure Anglo-Saxon heritage. Thus, a patient's racial background does not preclude the diagnosis.

The $\delta\beta$-thalassemias have been observed sporadically in many racial groups, although no high-frequency populations have been defined. Similarly, the hemoglobin Lepore syndromes have been found in many populations, but, with the possible exceptions of central Italy, Western Europe, and parts of Spain and Portugal, these disorders have not been found to occur at a high frequency in any particular region.

The α-thalassemias occur widely throughout Africa, the Mediterranean countries, the Middle East, and Southeast Asia (Fig. 47–2).[7,11,12]

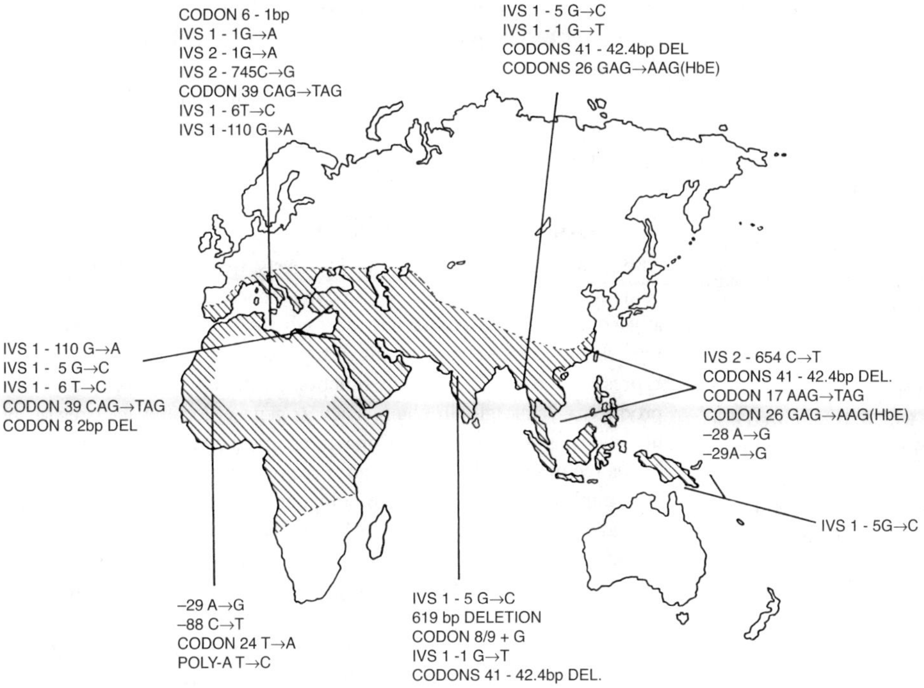

FIGURE 47–1. World distribution of β-thalassemia.

The α^0-thalassemias are found most commonly in Mediterranean and Oriental populations, but are extremely rare in African and Middle Eastern populations. However, the deletion forms of α^+-thalassemia occur at a high frequency throughout West Africa, the Mediterranean, the Middle East, and Southeast Asia. In United States, about 30 percent of Americans of African descent carry the gene α^+-thalassemia. Up to 80 percent of the population of some parts of Papua New Guinea are carriers for the deletion form of α^+-thalassemia. How common the nondeletion forms of α^+-thalassemia are in any particular populations is uncertain, but they have been reported quite frequently in some of the Mediterranean island populations and in the Middle Eastern and Southeast Asian populations. Because the hemoglobin Bart hydrops syndrome and hemoglobin H disease require the action of an α^0-thalassemia determinant, these disorders are found at a high frequency only in Southeast Asia and in parts of the Mediterranean region. The α-chain termination mutants, such as hemoglobin Constant Spring, seem to be particularly common in Southeast Asia. Approximately 4 percent of the population in Thailand are carriers.

In 1949, J.B.S. Haldane[13] suggested that thalassemia had reached its high frequency in tropical regions because heterozygotes are protected against malaria.[13] Although many population studies have tested this hypothesis, elucidation of some of the extremely complex population genetics underlying polymorphic systems such as the thalassemias has been possible only with the advent of recombinant DNA technology.

In each of the high-frequency areas for the β-thalassemias, a few common mutations and varying numbers of rare mutations are seen (see Fig. 47–1). Furthermore, in each of these regions the pattern of mutations is different, usually found in the context of different haplotypes in the associated β-globin gene cluster.[11,14,15] Similar observations have been made in the α-thalassemias (see Fig. 47–2).[7,11] These studies suggest the thalassemias arose independently in different populations and then achieved their high frequency by selection. Although some movement of the thalassemia genes may have resulted from drift, independent mutation and selection undoubtedly provide the overall basis for their world distribution. Early studies in Sardinia showing that β-thalassemia is less common in the mountainous regions where malarial transmission is low supported Haldane's suggestion that β-thalassemia reached its high frequency because of protection against malarial infections.[16] For many years these data remained the only convincing evidence for a protective effect. However, later studies using malaria endemicity data and globin-gene mapping showed a clear altitude-related effect on the frequency of α-thalassemia in Papua New Guinea. In addition, a sharp cline (a gradual change of species phenotype over a geographical area) in the frequency of α-thalassemia has been found in the region stretching south from Papua New Guinea through the island populations of Melanesia to New Caledonia. This is mirrored by a similar gradient in the distribution of malaria.[17] The effect of drift and founder effect in these island populations has been largely excluded by showing that other DNA polymorphisms have a random distribution through the region, with no evidence of a cline similar to that characterizing the distribution of α-thalassemia and malaria.

Firm evidence for protection of individuals with mild forms of α^+-thalassemia against *Plasmodium falciparum* malaria has been provided. In a case control study performed in Papua New Guinea, the homozygous state for α^+-thalassemia offered approximately 60 percent protection against hospital admittance because of serious complications of malaria, notably coma or profound anemia.[18] Similar levels of protection by α-thalassemia against *P. falciparum* malaria have been found in several different African populations.[19] However, it is becoming clear that there are complex genetic epistatic interactions between protective polymorphisms of this kind. For example, while α-thalassemia and the sickle cell trait both offer strong protection against *P. falciparum* malaria, in those who inherit both traits, the protection is cancelled out and they are fully susceptible to the disease.[20] Interactions of this type will have an important effect on the gene frequency of protective polymorphisms in countries in which more than one exists in the same population.

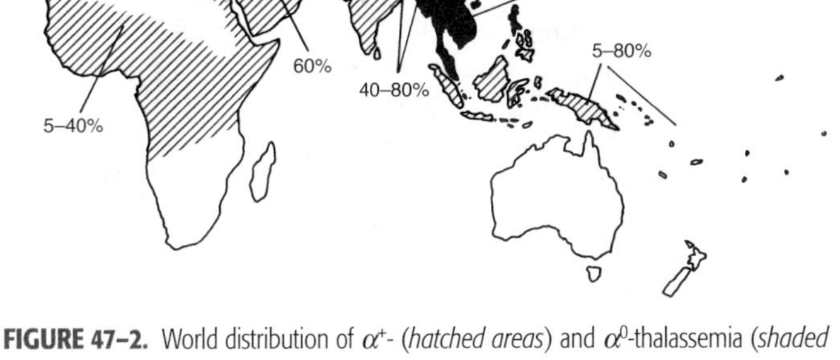

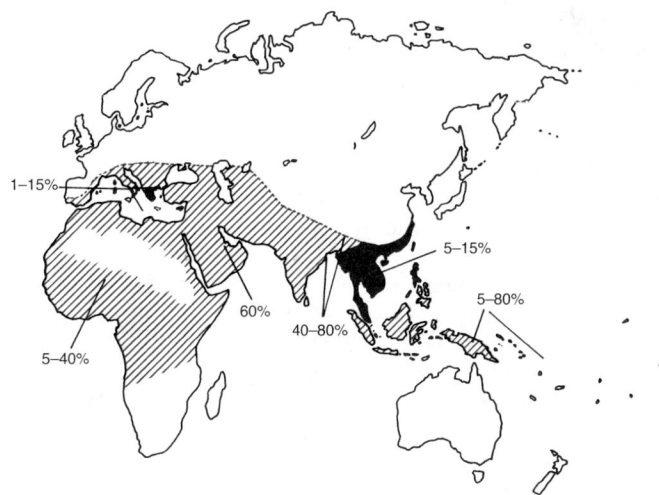

FIGURE 47–2. World distribution of α^+- (*hatched areas*) and α^0-thalassemia (*shaded areas*).

There is growing evidence that both immune and cellular mechanisms may underlie these protective effects of different red cell polymorphisms against malarial infection. Followup studies of cohorts of babies with α-thalassemia suggest that, in the first year of life, they are more prone to *Plasmodium vivax* and *P. falciparum* malaria. Since there is evidence for cross immunization between these two species, it is possible that this effect induces early immunization that may result in babies with α-thalassemia being more resistant to *P. falciparum* malaria later in life.[21] At the cellular level there is no evidence that α-thalassemia has any effect on the rates of parasite invasion and growth in red cells. However, parasitized α-thalassemic red cells are more susceptible to phagocytosis *in vitro*, and are less able than normal cells to form rosettes, an *in vitro* phenomena whereby uninfected cells bind to infected cells that is strongly associated with severity of infection, and express low levels of complement receptor 1, which is required for rosette formation.[22] These highly complex immune and cellular interactions are discussed in detail in recent reviews.[19,23,24] Although there are less data of this kind available for the β-thalassemias, there is strong indirect evidence that their high frequency has also been maintained by protection against *P. falciparum* malaria.

ETIOLOGY AND PATHOGENESIS

GENETIC CONTROL AND SYNTHESIS OF HEMOGLOBIN

The structure and ontogeny of the hemoglobins are reviewed in Chaps. 6 and 48, respectively. Only those aspects with particular relevance to the thalassemia problem are discussed here.

Human adult hemoglobin is a heterogeneous mixture of proteins consisting of the major component hemoglobin A and the minor component hemoglobin A_2, which constitutes approximately 2.5 percent of the total. In intrauterine life, the main hemoglobin is hemoglobin F. The structure of these hemoglobins is similar. Each consists of two separate pairs of identical globin chains. Except for some of the embryonic hemoglobins (see below), all normal human hemoglobins have one pair of α chains. In hemoglobin A, the α chains are combined with β chains ($\alpha_2\beta_2$), in hemoglobin A_2 with δ chains ($\alpha_2\delta_2$), and in hemoglobin F with γ chains ($\alpha_2\gamma_2$).

Human hemoglobin shows further heterogeneity, particularly in fetal life, and this has important implications for understanding the thalassemias and for approaches to their prenatal diagnosis. Hemoglobin F is a mixture of molecular species with the formulas $\alpha_2\gamma_2^{136Gly}$ and $\alpha_2\gamma_2^{136Ala}$. The γ chains containing glycine at position 136 are designated $^G\gamma$ chains. The γ chains containing alanine are called $^A\gamma$ chains. At birth, the ratio of molecules containing $^G\gamma$ chains to those containing $^A\gamma$ chains is approximately 3:1. The ratio varies widely in the trace amounts of hemoglobin F present in normal adults.

Before week 8 of intrauterine life, three embryonic hemoglobins—Gower 1 ($\xi_2\varepsilon_2$), Gower 2 ($\alpha_2\varepsilon_2$), and Portland ($\xi_2\gamma_2$)—are present. The ξ and ε chains are the embryonic counterparts of the adult α and β and γ and δ chains, respectively. ξ-Chain synthesis persists beyond the embryonic stage of development in some of the α-thalassemias. Persistent ε-chain production has not been found in any of the thalassemia syndromes. During fetal development, an orderly switch from ξ- to α-chain and from ε- to γ-chain production occurs, followed by β- and δ-chain production after birth.

Figure 47–3 shows the different human hemoglobins and the arrangements of the α-gene cluster on chromosome 16 and the β-gene cluster on chromosome 11.

GLOBIN GENE CLUSTERS

Although some individual variability exists, the α-gene cluster usually contains one functional ξ gene and two α genes, designated α_2 and α_1. It also contains four pseudogenes: $\psi\xi_1$, $\psi\alpha_1$, $\psi\alpha_2$, and θ_1.[9,10] The latter is remarkably conserved among different species. Although it appears to be expressed early in fetal life, its function is unknown. It likely does not produce a viable globin chain. Each α gene is located in a region of homology approximately 4 kb long, interrupted by two small nonhomologous regions.[25–27] The homologous regions are believed to result from gene duplication, and the nonhomologous segments are believed to arise subsequently by insertion of DNA into the noncoding regions around one of the two genes. The exons of the two α-globin genes have identical sequences. The first intron in each gene is identical. The second intron of α_1 is nine bases longer and differs by three bases from that in the α_2 gene.[27–29] Despite their high degree of homology, the sequences of the two α-globin genes diverge in their 3′ untranslated regions 13 bases beyond the TAA stop codon. These differences provide an opportunity to assess the relative output of the genes, an important part of the analysis of the α-thalassemias.[30,31] Production of α_2 messenger RNA appears to exceed that of α_1 by a factor of 1.5 to 3. $\psi\xi_1$ and ξ_2 genes also are highly homologous. The introns are much larger than those of α-globin genes. In contrast to the latter, IVS-1 is larger than IVS-2. In each ξ gene, IVS-1 contains several copies of a simple repeated 14-base pair (bp) sequence that is similar to sequences located between the two ξ genes and near the human insulin gene. The coding sequence of the first exon of $\psi\xi_1$ contains three base changes, one of which gives rise to a premature stop codon, thus making $\psi\xi_1$ an inactive pseudogene.

The regions separating and surrounding the α-like structural genes have been analyzed in detail. Of particular relevance to thalassemia is the polymorphic nature of this gene cluster.[32] The cluster contains five hypervariable regions: one downstream from the α_1 gene, one between the ξ and $\psi\xi$ genes, one in the first intron of both the ξ and $\psi\xi$ genes, and one 5′ to the cluster. These regions consist of varying numbers of tandem repeats of nucleotide sequences. Taken together with single-base restriction fragment length polymorphisms (RFLPs), the variability of the α-globin gene cluster reaches a heterozygosity level of approximately

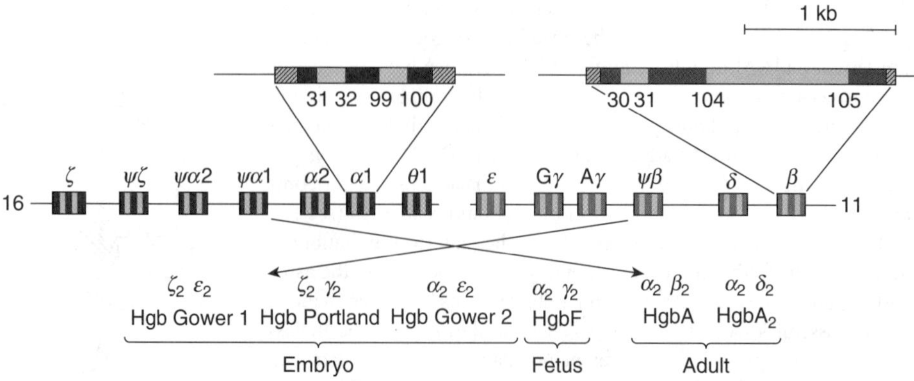

FIGURE 47–3. Genetic control of human hemoglobin. The main globin gene clusters are located on chromosomes 11 and 16. At each stage of development, different genes in these clusters are activated or repressed. The different globin chains directed by individual genes are synthesized independently and combine in random fashion as indicated by the *arrows*.

0.95. Thus, each parental α-globin gene cluster can be identified in the majority of persons. This heterogeneity has important implications for tracing the history of the thalassemia mutations.

Figure 47–3 shows the arrangement of the β-globin gene cluster on the short arm of chromosome 11. Each of the individual genes and their flanking regions have been sequenced.[33–36] Like the α_1 and α_2 gene pairs, the $^{G}\gamma$ and $^{A}\gamma$ genes share a similar sequence. In fact, the $^{G}\gamma$ and $^{A}\gamma$ genes on one chromosome are identical in the region 5′ to the center of the large intron yet show some divergence 3′ to that position. At the boundary between the conserved and divergent regions, a block of simple sequence may be a "hot spot" for initiation of recombination events that lead to unidirectional gene conversion.

Like the α-globin genes, the β-gene cluster contains a series of single-point RFLPs, although in this case no hypervariable regions have been identified.[37,38] The arrangement of RFLPs, or haplotypes, in the β-globin gene cluster falls into two domains. The 5′ side of the β gene, spanning approximately 32 kb from the ε gene to the 3′ end of the ψβ gene, contains three common patterns of RFLPs. The region encompassing about 18 kb to the 3′ side of the β-globin gene also contains three common patterns in different populations. Between these regions is a sequence of about 11 kb in which there is randomization of the 5′ and 3′ domains; hence, a relatively higher frequency of recombination can occur.[38] The β-globin gene haplotypes are similar in most populations but differ markedly in individuals of African origin. These findings suggest the haplotype arrangements were laid down very early during evolution. The findings are consistent with data obtained from mitochondrial DNA polymorphisms pointing to the early emergence of a relatively small population from Africa with subsequent divergence into other racial groups.[39] Again, they are extremely useful for analyzing the population genetics and history of the thalassemia mutations.

The regions flanking the coding regions of the globin genes contain a number of conserved sequences essential for their expression.[28,33] The first conserved sequence is the TATA box, which serves accurately to locate the site of transcription initiation at the CAP site, usually about 30 bases downstream. It also appears to influence the rate of transcription. In addition, two so-called upstream promoter elements are present. A second conserved sequence, the CCAAT box, is located 70 or 80 bp upstream. The third conserved sequence, the CACCC homology box, is located further 5′, approximately 80 to 100 bp from the CAP site. It can be either inverted or duplicated. These promoter sequences also are required for optimal transcription. Mutations in this region of the β-globin gene cause its defective expression. The globin genes also have conserved sequences in their 3′ flanking regions, notably AATAAA, which is the polyadenylation signal site.

Regulation of Globin Gene Clusters

Figure 47–4 summarizes the mechanism of globin gene expression. The primary transcript is an messenger RNA (mRNA) precursor containing both intron and exon sequences. During its stay in the nucleus, it undergoes a good deal of processing that entails capping the 5′ end and polyadenylation of the 3′ end, both of which probably serve to stabilize the transcript (see Chap. 9). The intervening sequences are removed from the mRNA precursor in a complex two-stage process that relies on certain critical sequences at the intron–exon junctions.

The method by which globin gene clusters are regulated is important to understanding the pathogenesis of the thalassemias. Many details remain to be determined, but studies performed over the last few years have provided at least an outline of some of the major mechanisms of globin gene regulation.[7,9,40–42]

Most of the DNA within cells that is not involved in gene transcription is packaged into a compact form that is inaccessible to transcription factors and RNA polymerase. Transcriptional activity is characterized by

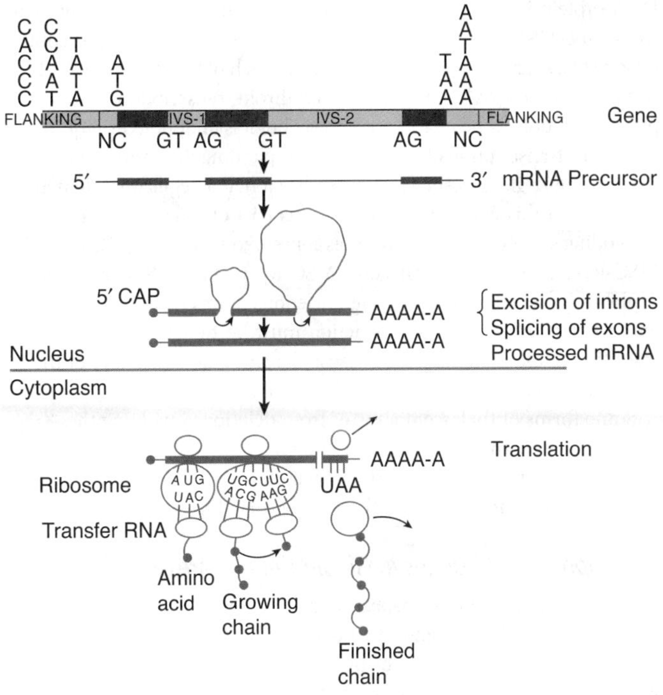

FIGURE 47–4. Expression of a human globin gene.

a major change in the structure of the chromatin surrounding a particular gene. These alterations in chromatin structure can be identified by enhanced sensitivity to exogenous nucleases. Erythroid lineage-specific nuclease-hypersensitive sites are found at several locations in the β-globin gene cluster, which vary during different stages of development. In fetal life, these sites are associated with the promoter regions of all four globin genes. In adult erythroid cells, the sites associated with the γ genes are absent. The methylation state of the genes plays an important role in their ability to be expressed. In human and other animal tissues, the globin genes are extensively methylated in nonerythroid organs and are relatively undermethylated in hematopoietic tissues. Changes in chromatin configuration around the globin genes at different stages of development are reflected by alterations in their methylation state.

In addition to the promoter elements, several other important regulatory sequences have been identified in the globin gene clusters. For example, several enhancer sequences thought to be involved with tissue-specific expression have been identified. Their sequences are similar to the upstream activating sequences of the promoter elements. Both consist of a number of "modules," or motifs, that contain binding sites for transcriptional activators or repressors. The enhancer sequences are thought to act by coming into spatial apposition with the promoter sequences to increase the efficiency of transcription of particular genes. It now is clear that transcriptional regulatory proteins may bind to both the promoter region of a gene and to the enhancer. Some of these transcriptional proteins, GATA-1 and NFE-2, for example, appear to be largely restricted to hematopoietic tissues.[40] These proteins may bring the promoter and the enhancer into close physical proximity, permitting transcription factors bound to the enhancer to interact with the transcriptional complex that forms near the TATA box. At least some of these hematopoietic gene transcription factors likely will be developmental-stage specific.

Another set of erythroid-specific nuclease-hypersensitive sites is located upstream from the embryonic globin genes in both the α- and β-gene clusters. These sites mark the regions of particularly important control elements. In the case of the β-globin gene cluster, the region is marked by five hypersensitive sites to DNase I treatment (an enzyme used to detect

DNA-protein interaction).[40] The most 5′ site (HS5) does not show tissue specificity. HS1 through HS4, which together form the locus control region (LCR), are largely erythroid specific. Each of the regions of the LCR contains a variety of binding sites for erythroid transcription factors. The precise function of the LCR is not known, but it is undoubtedly required to establish a transcriptionally active domain spanning the entire globin gene cluster. The α-globin gene cluster also has a major regulatory element of this kind, in this case HS40.[41] This forms part of four highly conserved noncoding sequences, or multispecies conserved sequences (MCSs), called MSC-R1-R4; of these elements only MSC-R2, that is HS40, is essential for α-globin gene expression. Although deletions of this region inactivate the entire α-globin gene cluster, its action must be fundamentally different from that of the β-globin LCR because the chromatin structure of the α-gene cluster is in an open conformation in all tissues.

Some forms of thalassemia result from deletions involving these regulatory regions. In addition, the phenotypic effects of deletions of these gene clusters are strongly positional, which may reflect the relative distance of particular genes from the LCR and HS40.

Developmental Changes in Globin Gene Expression

One particularly important aspect of human globin genes is regulation of the switch from fetal to adult hemoglobin. Because many of the thalassemias and related disorders of the β-globin gene cluster are associated with persistent γ-chain synthesis, a full understanding of their pathophysiology must include an explanation for this important phenomenon, which plays a considerable role in modifying their phenotypic expression.

The complex topic of hemoglobin switching has been the subject of several extensive reviews.[7,42] β-Globin synthesis commences early during fetal life, at approximately 8 to 10 weeks' gestation. β-Globin synthesis continues at a low level, approximately 10 percent of the total non–α-globin chain production, up to approximately 36 weeks' gestation, after which it is considerably augmented. At the same time, γ-globin chain synthesis starts to decline so that, at birth, approximately equal amounts of γ- and β-globin chains are produced. Over the first year of life, γ-chain synthesis gradually declines. By the end of the first year, γ-chain synthesis amounts to less than 1 percent of the total non–α-globin chain output. In adults the small amount of hemoglobin F is confined to an erythrocyte population called *F cells*.

How this series of developmental switches is regulated is not clear. The process is not organ specific but is synchronized throughout the developing hematopoietic tissues. Although environmental factors may be involved, the bulk of experimental evidence suggests some form of "time clock" is built into the hematopoietic stem cell. At the chromosomal level, regulation appears to occur in a complex manner involving both developmental stage-specific *trans*-activating factors and the relative proximity of the different genes of the β-globin gene cluster to LCR. The elements involved in the stage-specific regulation of human globin genes have not been identified, except for EKLF (erythroid Kruppel-like factor), a developmental stage-enriched protein that activates human β-globin gene expression and is involved in human γ- to β-globin gene switching.[43]

Fetal hemoglobin synthesis can be reactivated at low levels in states of hematopoietic stress and at higher levels in certain hematologic malignancies, notably juvenile myeloid leukemia. However, high levels of hemoglobin F production are seen consistently in adult life only in the hemoglobinopathies.

MOLECULAR BASIS OF THE THALASSEMIAS

Once cloning and sequencing of globin genes from patients with many different forms of thalassemia were possible, the wide spectrum of mutations underlying these conditions became clear. A picture of remarkable heterogeneity has emerged. For more extensive coverage of this topic, the reader is referred to several monographs and reviews.[7,9,10,44–46]

β-THALASSEMIA

β-Thalassemia is extremely heterogeneous at the molecular level.[7] More than 200 different mutations have been found in association with the β-thalassemia phenotype.[7] Broadly, they fall into deletions of the β-globin gene and nondeletional mutations that may affect the transcription, processing, or translation of β-globin messenger (see Table 47–2 and Fig. 47–5). Each major population group has a different set of β-thalassemia mutations, usually consisting of two or three mutations forming the bulk and large numbers of rare mutations. Because of this distribution pattern, only about 20 alleles account for the majority of all β-thalassemia determinants (see Fig. 47–1).

Gene Deletions

At least 17 different deletions affecting only the β genes have been described. With one exception, the deletions are rare and appear to be

TABLE 47–2. Molecular Pathology of the β-Thalassemias

β^0- or β^+-Thalassemia
Transcription
Deletions
Insertions
Promoter
5′ UTR
Processing of mRNA
Junctional
Consensus splicing sequences
Cryptic splice sites in introns
Cryptic splice sites in exons
Poly (A) addition site
Translation
Initiation
Nonsense
Frameshift
Posttranslational stability
Unstable β-chain variants
Normal Hgb A_2 β-Thalassemia
β-Thalassemia and δ-thalassemia, *cis* or *trans*
"Silent" β-thalassemia
Some promoter mutations
CAP +1, CAP +3, etc.
5′ UTR
Some splice mutations
Dominant β-thalassemia
Mainly point mutations or rearrangements in exon 3
Other unstable variants

mRNA, messenger RNA; UTR, untranslated region.

NOTE: A full list of mutations is given in references 7 and 45.

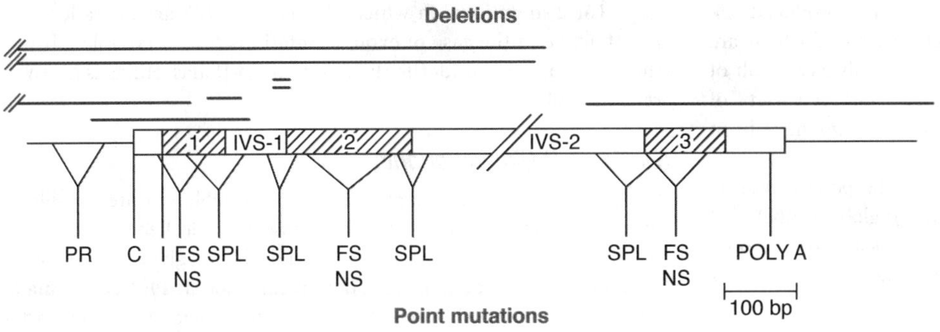

FIGURE 47–5. Classes of mutations that underlie β-thalassemia. PR, promoter; C, CAP site; I, initiation site; FS, frameshift; NS, nonsense mutation; SPL, splicing mutation; POLY A, polyA addition site mutation.

isolated, single events. The 619-bp deletion at the 3′ end of the β gene is more common,[47] but even that is restricted to the Sind and Gujarati populations of Pakistan and India, where it accounts for approximately 50 percent of β-thalassemia alleles.[48] The Indian 619-bp deletion removes the 3′ end of the β gene but leaves the 5′ end intact. Many of the other deletions remove the 5′ end of the gene and leave the δ gene intact.[49–53] Homozygotes for these deletions have β^0-thalassemia. Heterozygotes for the Indian deletion have increased hemoglobin A_2 and F levels identical to those seen in heterozygotes for the other common forms of β-thalassemia. Heterozygotes for the other deletions all have unusually high hemoglobin A_2 levels.[7] Increased δ-chain production results from increased δ-gene transcription in *cis* to the deletion, possibly as a result of reduced competition from the deleted 5′ β gene for transcription factors.

Other Transcriptional Mutations

Several different base substitutions involve the conserved sequences upstream from the β-globin gene.[7] In every case, the phenotype is β^+-thalassemia, although considerable variability exists in the clinical severity associated with different mutations of this type. Several mutations, at positions −88 and −87 relative to the mRNA CAP site, for example,[54,55] are close to the CCAAT box, whereas others lie within the TATA box homology.[56–59]

Some mutations upstream from the β-globin gene are associated with even more subtle alterations in phenotype. For example, a C→T substitution at position −101, which involves one of the upstream promoter elements, is associated with "silent" β-thalassemia, that is, a completely normal ("silent") phenotype that can be identified only by its interaction with more severe forms of β-thalassemia in compound heterozygotes.[60] A single example of an A→C substitution at the CAP site (+1) was described in an Asian Indian who, despite being homozygous for the mutation, appeared to have the phenotype of the β-thalassemia trait.[61]

Upstream regulatory mutations confirm the importance of the role of conserved sequences in this region as regulators of the transcription of the β-globin genes and provide the basis for some of the mildest forms of β-thalassemia, particularly those in African populations, and for some varieties of "silent" β-thalassemia.

RNA-Processing Mutations

One surprise about β-thalassemia has been the remarkable diversity of the single-base mutations that can interfere with the intranuclear processing of mRNA.

The boundaries of exons and introns are marked by invariant dinucleotides, GT at the 5′ (donor) and AG at the 3′ (receptor) sites. Single-base changes that involve either of these splice junctions totally abolish normal RNA splicing and result in the β^0-thalassemia phenotype.[7,62–66]

Highly conserved sequences involved in mRNA processing surround the invariant dinucleotides at the splice junctions. Different varieties of β-thalassemia involve single-base substitutions within the consensus sequence of the IVS-1 donor site.[55,58,63–69] These mutations are particularly interesting because of the remarkable variability in their associated phenotypes. For example, substitution of the G in position 5 of IVS-1 by C or T results in severe β^+-thalassemia.[55] On the other hand, a T→C change at position 6, found commonly in the Mediterranean region,[70] results in a very mild form of β^+-thalassemia. The G→C change at position 5 has also been found in Melanesia and appears to be the most common cause of β-thalassemia in Papua New Guinea.[71]

RNA processing is affected by mutations that create new splice sites within either introns or exons. Again, these lesions are remarkably variable in their phenotypic effect, depending on the degree to which the new site is utilized compared with the normal splice site. For example, the G→A substitution at position 110 of IVS-1, which is one of the most common forms of β-thalassemia in the Mediterranean region, leads to only approximately 10 percent splicing at the normal site and hence results in a severe β^+-thalassemia phenotype.[72,73] Similarly, a mutation that produces a new acceptor site at position 116 in IVS-1 results in little or no β-globin mRNA production and the β^0-thalassemia phenotype.[74] Several mutations that generate new donor sites within IVS-2 of the β-globin gene have been described.[55,68]

Another mechanism for abnormal splicing is activation of donor sites within exons (Fig. 47–6). For example, within exon 1 is a cryptic donor site in the region of codons 24 through 27. This site contains a GT dinucleotide. An adjacent substitution that alters the site so that it more closely resembles the consensus donor splice site results in its activation, even though the normal site is active. Several mutations in this region can activate this site so that it is utilized during RNA processing, with the production of abnormal mRNAs.[75–78] Three of the substitutions—A→G in codon 19, G→A in codon 26, and G→T in codon 27—result in reduced production of β-globin mRNA and an amino acid substitution so that the mRNA that is spliced normally is

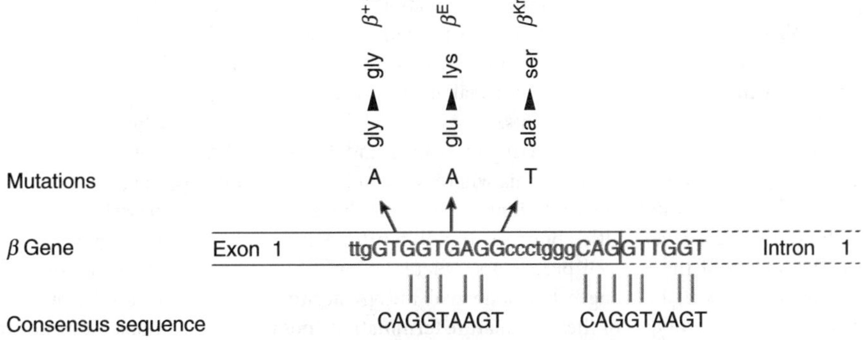

FIGURE 47–6. Activation of cryptic splice sites in exon 1 as the cause of β^+-thalassemia, hemoglobin E, and hemoglobin Knossos. The similarities between the 5′ splice region of intron 1 and the cryptic splice region in exon 1 are shown in *capitals*.

translated into protein. The abnormal hemoglobins produced are hemoglobins Malay, E, and Knossos, respectively, all of which are associated with a β-thalassemia phenotype, presumably as a result of reduced overall output of normal mRNA (Fig. 47–6). A variety of other cryptic splice mutations within introns and exons have been described.[44]

Another class of processing mutations involves the polyadenylation signal site AAUAAA in the 3′ untranslated region of β-globin mRNA.[79–81] For example, a T→C substitution in this sequence leads to only one-tenth the normal amount of β-globin mRNA and hence the severe β^+-thalassemia phenotype.[79]

Mutations Causing Abnormal Translation of Messenger RNA

Base substitutions that change an amino acid codon into a chain termination codon, that is, nonsense mutations, prevent translation of the mRNA and result in β^0-thalassemia. Many substitutions of this type have been described.[7,44] For example, a codon 17 mutation is common in Southeast Asia,[82,83] and a codon 39 mutation occurs at a high frequency in the Mediterranean region.[84,85]

The insertion or deletion of one, two, or four nucleotides in the coding region of the β-globin gene disrupts the normal reading frame and results, upon translation of the mRNA, in the addition of anomalous amino acids until a termination codon is reached in the new reading frame. Several frameshift mutations of this type have been described.[7,44] Two mutations—the insertion of one nucleotide between codons 8 and 9 and a deletion of four nucleotides in codons 41 and 42—are common in Asian Indians.[63] The latter deletions are found frequently in different populations in Southeast Asia.[83]

An unusual β^+-thalassemia was described in a patient from the Czech and Slovak Federated Republic in whom a full-length L1 transposon was inserted into the second intron of β-globin, creating a β^+-thalassemia phenotype by an undefined molecular mechanism.[86]

Dominantly Inherited β-Thalassemia

Families in which a picture indistinguishable from moderately severe β-thalassemia has segregated in Mendelian dominant fashion have been reported sporadically.[87,88] Because this condition often is characterized by the presence of inclusion bodies in the red cell precursors, it has been called *inclusion body β-thalassemia*. However, because all severe forms of β-thalassemia have inclusions in the red cell precursors, the term *dominantly inherited β-thalassemia* is preferred.[7,89] Sequence analysis has shown that these conditions are heterogeneous at the molecular level, but that many involve mutations of exon 3 of the β-globin gene. The mutations include frameshifts, premature chain termination mutations, and complex rearrangements that lead to synthesis of truncated or elongated and highly unstable β-globin gene products.[7,89–93] The most common mutation of this type is a GAA→TAA change at codon 121 that leads to synthesis of a truncated β-globin chain.[94] Although an abnormal β-chain product from loci affected by mutations of this type is unusual, many of these conditions are designated as hemoglobin variants.

The reason why mutations occurring in exons 1 and 2 produce the classic form of recessive β-thalassemia whereas the bulk of the dominant thalassemias result from mutations in exon 3 has become clearer. In the former case, very little abnormal β-globin mRNA is found in the cytoplasm of the red cell precursors, whereas exon 3 mutations are associated with full-length but abnormal mRNA accumulation. The different phenotypes of these premature termination codons have been suggested to reflect a phenomenon called *nonsense-mediated RNA decay*, a surveillance system to prevent transport of mRNA coding for truncated peptides. Presumably this process is active in the case of exon 1or 2 mutations, in which affected mRNAs are degraded, but is not active in the case of exon 3 mutations.[95–97] A complete list of the mutations that underlie the dominant β-thalassemias is given in reference 44.

Unstable β-Globin Variants

Some β-globin chain variants are highly unstable but are capable of forming a viable tetramer. The resulting unstable hemoglobins may precipitate in the red cell precursors or in the blood, giving rise to a spectrum of conditions ranging from dominantly inherited β-thalassemia to a hemolytic anemia similar to the anemia associated with other unstable hemoglobins. The first unstable hemoglobin to be described was hemoglobin Indianapolis.[98] Its structure was characterized by DNA analysis performed on stored autopsy material; however, the original description proved to be incorrect.[99]

Silent β-Thalassemia

A number of extremely mild β-thalassemia alleles are either silent or almost unidentifiable in heterozygotes (see Table 47–2). Some alleles are in the region of the promoter boxes of the β-globin gene, but others involve the CAP sites or the 5′ or 3′ untranslated regions.[7,44] These alleles usually are identified by finding a form of β-thalassemia intermedia in which one parent has a typical thalassemia trait and the other parent appears to be normal but, in fact, is a carrier of one of the mild β-thalassemia alleles.

β-Thalassemia Mutations Unlinked to the β-Globin Gene Cluster

Several family studies have suggested the existence of mutations that result in the β-thalassemia phenotype but do not segregate with the β-globin genes[100]; however, their molecular basis has not been determined. Further evidence for the existence of novel mutations of this type can be found in reference 7.

Variant Forms of β-Thalassemia

In several forms of β-thalassemia, the hemoglobin A_2 level is normal in heterozygotes. Some cases result from "silent" β-thalassemia alleles, whereas others reflect the coinheritance of β- and δ-thalassemia.[7]

■ δβ-THALASSEMIA

The $\delta\beta$-thalassemias are classified into the $(\delta\beta)^+$- and $(\delta\beta)^0$-thalassemias (Table 47–3). The $(\delta\beta)^0$-thalassemias are further divided into $(\delta\beta)^0$-thalassemia, in which both the δ- and β-globin genes are deleted, and $(^A\gamma\delta\beta)^0$-thalassemia, in which the $^G\gamma$, δ, and β genes are deleted. Because many different deletion forms of $\delta\beta$-thalassemia have been described, they are further classified according to the country in which they were first identified (see Table 47–3).

(δβ)⁰- and (ᴬγδβ)⁰-Thalassemia

Nearly all these conditions result from deletions involving varying lengths of the β-globin gene cluster. Many different varieties have been described in different populations (see Table 47–3), although their heterozygous and homozygous phenotypes are very similar.[7] Rare forms of these conditions result from more complex gene rearrangements. For example, one form of $(^A\gamma\delta\beta)^0$-thalassemia, found in Indian populations, does not result from a simple linear deletion but rather from a complex rearrangement with two deletions, one affecting the $^A\gamma$ gene and the other the δ and β genes. The intervening region is intact but inverted.[101] Figure 47–7 illustrates some of these conditions.

TABLE 47–3. $\delta\beta$ **Thalassemias**

($\delta\beta$)+-Thalassemia
Hgb Lepore thalassemia
Hgb Lepore Washington-Boston
Hgb Lepore Hollandia
Hgb Lepore Baltimore
Phenocopies of $(\delta\beta)^+$-thalassemia
Sardinian $\delta\beta$-thalassemia
Corfu $\delta\beta$-thalassemia
Chinese $\delta\beta$-thalassemia
β-Thalassemia with δ-thalassemia
$(\delta\beta)^\circ$-Thalassemia
Sicilian
Indian
Japanese
Spanish
Black
Eastern European
Macedonian
Turkish
Laotian
Thai
$(A\gamma\delta\beta)^\circ$-Thalassemia
Indian
German
Cantonese
Turkish
Malay 2
Belgian
Black
Chinese
Yunnanese
Thai
Italian

NOTE: Details of the molecular pathology of these conditions are given in references 7 and 45.

$(\delta\beta)^+$-Thalassemia

The $(\delta\beta)^+$-thalassemias usually are associated with the production of structural hemoglobin variants called Lepore.[102] Hemoglobin Lepore contains normal α chains and non-α chains that consist of the first 50 to 80 amino acid residues of the δ chains and the last 60 to 90 residues of the normal C-terminal amino acid sequence of the β chains. Thus, the Lepore non-α chain is a β-fusion chain. Several different varieties of hemoglobin Lepore have been described—Washington-Boston, Baltimore, and Hollandia—in which the transition from δ to β sequences occurs at different points.[7] The fusion chains probably arose by nonhomologous crossing over between part of the δ locus on one chromosome and part of the β locus on the complementary chromosome (Fig. 47–8). This event results from misalignment of chromosome pairing during meiosis so that a δ-chain gene pairs with a β-chain gene instead of with its homologous partner.[103] Figure 47–8 shows such a mechanism should give rise to two abnormal chromosomes: the first, the Lepore chromosome, will have no normal δ or β loci but simply a $\delta\beta$ fusion gene. Opposite the homologous pairs of chromosomes should be an anti-Lepore ($\delta\beta$) fusion gene and normal δ and β loci. A variety of anti–Lepore-like hemoglobins have been discovered, including hemoglobins Miyada, P-Congo, Lincoln Park, and P-Nilotic.[7] All the hemoglobin Lepore disorders are characterized by a severe form of $\delta\beta$-thalassemia. The output of the γ-globin genes on the chromosome with the $\delta\beta$ fusion gene is not increased sufficiently to compensate for the low output of the $\delta\beta$ fusion product. The reduced rate of production of the $\delta\beta$ fusion chains of hemoglobin Lepore presumably reflects the fact that its genetic determinant has the δ gene promoter region, which is structurally different from the β-globin gene promoter and is associated with a reduced rate of transcription of its gene product.

$\delta\beta$-Thalassemia-Like Disorders Resulting from Two Mutations in the β-Globin Gene Cluster

A heterogeneous group of nondeletion $\delta\beta$-thalassemias has been described, most resulting from two mutations in the $\varepsilon\gamma\delta\beta$-globin gene cluster (see Table 47–3). Strictly speaking, they are not all $\delta\beta$-thalassemias, but they often appear in the literature under this title because their phenotypes resemble the deletion forms of $(\delta\beta)^0$-thalassemia. In the Sardinian form of $\delta\beta$-thalassemia, the β-globin gene has the common Mediterranean codon 39 nonsense mutation that leads to an absence of β-globin synthesis. The relatively high expression of the $^A\gamma$ gene in *cis* gives this condition the $\delta\beta$-thalassemia phenotype because of a point mutation at position –196 upstream from the $^A\gamma$ gene (see "Hereditary Persistence of Fetal Hemoglobin" below). The phenotypic picture, in which heterozygotes have 15 to 20 percent hemoglobin F and normal hemoglobin A_2 levels, is identical to that of $\delta\beta$-thalassemia.[103] Another condition having the β-thalassemia phenotype, with greater than 20 percent hemoglobin F in heterozygotes, has been described in a Chinese patient in whom defective β-globin chain synthesis appears to result from an A→G change in the ATA sequence in the promoter region of the β-globin gene.[104] The increased γ-chain synthesis, which appears to involve both $^G\gamma$ and $^A\gamma$ *cis* to this mutation, remains unexplained. A disorder originally called $\delta\beta$-thalassemia has been described in the Corfu population.[105,106] The condition results from two mutations in the β-globin gene cluster: first, a 7201-bp deletion that starts in the δ-globin gene, IVS-2, position 818 to 822, and extends upstream to a 5′ breakpoint located 1719 to 1722 bp 3′ to the $\psi\beta$-gene termination codon; and second, a G→A mutation at position 5 in the donor site consensus region of IVS-1 of the β-globin gene. The output from this chromosome consists of relatively high levels of γ chains with very low levels of β chains. The condition resembles $\delta\beta$-thalassemia in the homozygous state, with almost 100 percent hemoglobin F, traces of hemoglobin A, but no hemoglobin A_2. Heterozygotes have only slightly elevated hemoglobin F levels, with a phenotype similar to "normal $A_2\beta$-thalassemia."

■ $\varepsilon\gamma\delta\beta$-THALASSEMIA

These rare conditions[107–113] result from long deletions that begin upstream from the β-gene complex 55 kb or more 5′ to the ε gene and terminate within the cluster (see Fig. 47–7). In two cases, designated Dutch[110,111] and English,[112] the deletions leave the β-globin gene intact, but no β-chain production occurs even though the gene is expressed in heterologous systems.

The molecular basis for inactivation of the β-globin gene *cis* to these deletions was clarified by the discovery of the LCR about 50 kb upstream from the $\varepsilon\gamma\delta\beta$-globin gene cluster (see "Genetic Control and Synthesis of Hemoglobin" above). Removal of this critical regulatory region seems to

Scale (kb): −40 −30 0 10 20 30 40 50 60 70 80 90 100 110 120 130 140 150 160 170 kb

Gene order: ε — $^{G}\gamma$ — $^{A}\gamma$ — $\psi\beta$ — δ — β

β-Thalassemia — *% HgbF in heterozygotes*

	% HgbF in heterozygotes
Small deletions	0.2–6.9
1 Turkish	1.9–2.0
2 Filipino	1.0–9.1
3 UK Asian	3.2–4.7
4 Dutch	4–11
5 Australian	2.5–7.2
6 Southern Italian	9.0

δβ Fusion

7 Hgb Lepore	0.5–6.5

δ-Thalassemia

8 Corfu	1.1–2.8

γβ Fusion

9 Hgb Kenya	5–10

$^{G}\gamma\,^{A}\gamma\,(\delta\beta)°$ Thalassemia

10 Mediterranean	5.9–19.0
11 SE Asian	9.9–20.0
12 E European	13.0–24.0
13 Black	25.0*
14 Macedonian/Turkish	4.2–13.5
15 Indian	16.6
16 Spanish	5.0–13.0
17 Japanese	7.0–8.0

$^{G}\gamma(^{A}\gamma\delta\beta)°$ Thalassemia

18 Black	4.0–16.5
19 Chinese	9.3–23.0
20 Belgian	14.2–23.0
21 Indian	9.7–18.1
22 Yunnanese	9.3–16.7
23 Malaysian 2	
24 German	9.9–12.5
25 Turkish	10.0–13.5
26 SE Asian	17.2–22.9
27 Italian	?

$^{G}\gamma\,^{A}\gamma\,(\delta\beta)°$ HPFH

28 Black	18.6–31.0
29 Ghanaian	22.4–26.6
30 Indian	17.0–25.0
31 Italian 1	14.0–30.0
32 Italian 2	16.0–20.0
33 Vietnamese/SEA	14.1–26.6

$(\varepsilon\,^{G}\gamma\,^{A}\gamma\delta\beta)°$ Thalassemia

34 Anglo-Saxon	
35 Dutch	
36 English	
37 Scottish-Irish	
38 Hispanic	
39 Mexican, Canadian, Yugoslavian	

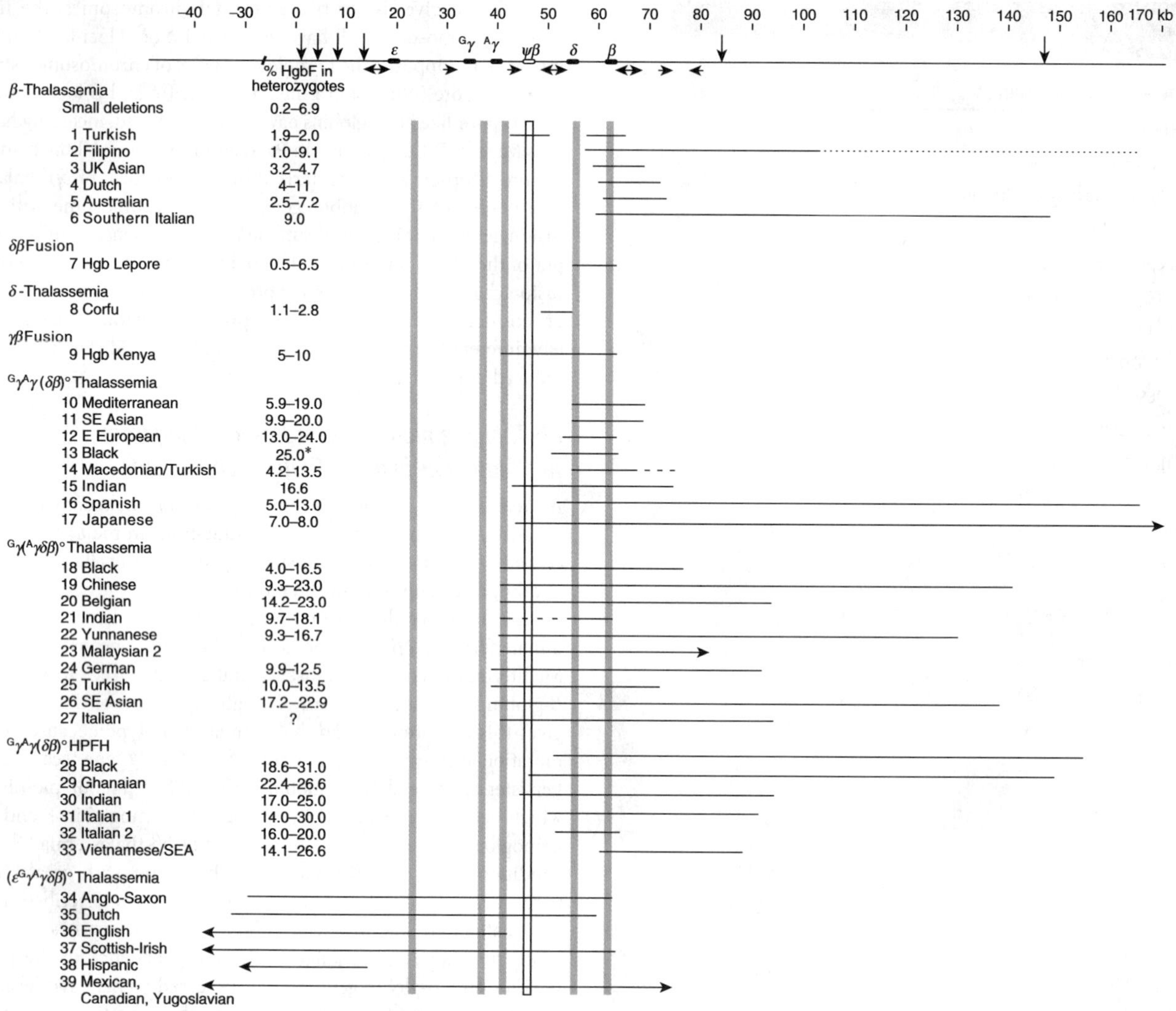

FIGURE 47–7. Some deletions responsible for the β- and $\delta\beta$-thalassemias and hereditary persistence of fetal hemoglobin.

Examples — Crossover region between residues

Anti-Lepore
- Hgb Miyada — β 12 & δ 22
- Hgb P (Congo) — β 22 & δ 87

Lepore
- Hgb Lepore (Hollandia) — δ 22 & β 50
- Hgb Lepore (Baltimore) — δ 50 & β 86
- Hgb Lepore (Boston) — δ 87 & β 116

Kenya — Hgb Kenya — δ 81 & β 86

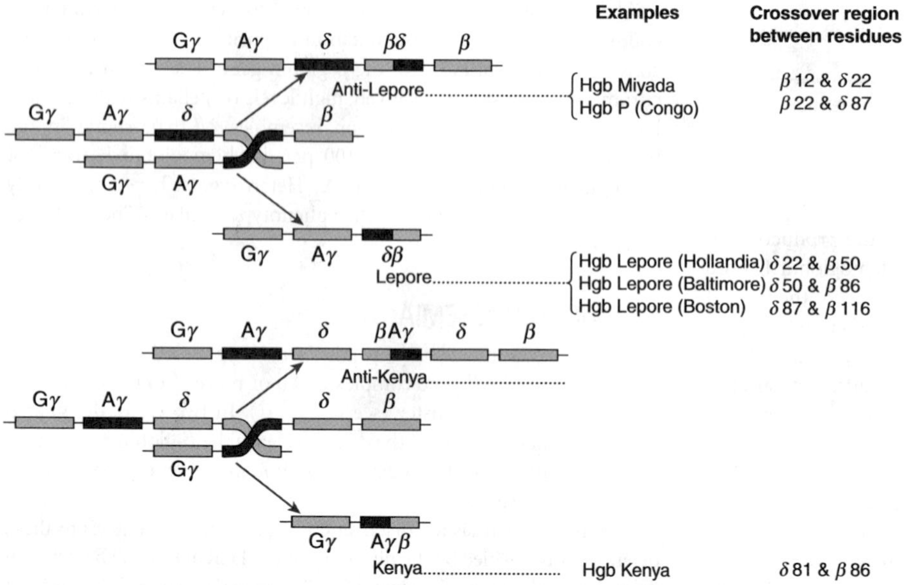

FIGURE 47–8. Mechanisms for the production of the Lepore and anti-Lepore hemoglobins.

completely inactivate the downstream globin gene complex. The Hispanic form of $\varepsilon\gamma\delta\beta$-thalassemia[113] results from a deletion that includes most of the LCR, including four of the five DNase-1-hypersensitive sites. These lesions appear to close down the chromatin domain that usually is open in erythroid tissues and delay replication of the β-globin genes in the cell cycle. Thus, although they are rare, the lesions have been of considerable importance because analysis of the Dutch deletion first pointed to the possibility of a major control region upstream from the β-like-globin gene cluster and ultimately led to the discovery of the β-globin LCR.

◼ HEREDITARY PERSISTENCE OF FETAL HEMOGLOBIN

This heterogeneous group of conditions produces phenotypes very similar to those of the $\delta\beta$-thalassemias, except that defective β-chain production appears to be almost, but in some forms not completely, compensated by persistent γ-chain production. These conditions are best classified into deletion and nondeletion forms (Table 47–4). In the past, the conditions were classified into pancellular and heterocellular varieties, depending on the intercellular distribution of fetal hemoglobin. However, this subdivision now appears to bear little relevance to their molecular basis and probably relates more to the particular level of fetal hemoglobin and how its cellular distribution is determined.[7]

The deletion forms of HPFH are heterogeneous (Fig. 47–7). The two African varieties result from extensive deletions of similar length (<70 kb) but with staggered ends, differing phenotypically only in the proportions of $^{G}\gamma$ and $^{A}\gamma$ chains produced.[114] Another type of HPFH results from misalignment during crossing over between the $^{A}\gamma$- and β-globin genes, resulting in production of $^{A}\gamma\beta$ fusion genes (see Fig. 47–8). The latter give rise to $\delta\beta$ fusion products that combine with α chains to form the hemoglobin variant called hemoglobin Kenya.[115,116] Hemoglobin Kenya is associated with an increased output of hemoglobin F, although at a lower level than in the deletion forms of HPFH. A theory that adequately explains the phenotypic differences between $\delta\beta$-thalassemia and the deletion forms of HPFH has not been developed.[7]

The nondeletion determinants of HPFH can be classified into those that map within the β-globin gene cluster and those that segregate independently. The former are subdivided into $^{G}\gamma\beta^{+}$ and $^{A}\gamma\beta^{+}$ varieties, indicating persistent $^{G}\gamma$- or $^{A}\gamma$-chain synthesis in association with β-globin production directed by the β gene *cis* (on the same chromosome) to the HPFH determinant. Analysis of the overexpressed γ genes revealed in each case a single-base substitution in the region immediately upstream from the transcription start site.[7,117–120] Clustering of these substitutions and lack of similar changes in normal γ genes suggest they are responsible for persistent hemoglobin F production (Fig. 47–9). This region of DNA likely is involved in binding of *trans*-acting proteins involved in the normal developmental repression of γ-gene expression, either by decreasing the affinity for an inhibitory factor normally present in adult life or by increasing the affinity for a factor promoting gene expression. The most common of these conditions are Greek $^{A}\gamma\beta^{+}$ HPFH and a form of $^{G}\gamma\beta^{+}$ HPFH, which has been found in several different African populations. If the upstream point mutations associated with persistent γ-chain production occur on the same chromosome as β-globin genes that carry β^{0}-thalassemia mutations, the clinical phenotype is converted from HPFH to $\delta\beta$-thalassemia, albeit with different hemoglobin A_2 levels.

In some cases, other nondeletional forms of HPFH have been related to small structural changes in the β-globin gene cluster (see Table 47–4). Although strictly speaking not a true form of HPFH, because even in homozygotes it may not be associated with increased hemoglobin F levels, the T→C polymorphism at position –158 to the $^{G}\gamma$-globin gene[121] might be associated with an increased output of hemoglobin F under conditions of erythropoietic stress.

Other forms of HPFH are characterized by the persistence of low levels of fetal hemoglobin production distributed in a heterocellular manner. In all populations studied, a small proportion of individuals have an increased amount of hemoglobin F and F cells, that is, red cells that can be detected when blood films are treated with antibodies against hemoglobin F. Although this condition originally was called the Swiss form of HPFH because it was first recognized in Swiss army recruits,[122] it is observed in every racial group. Using a variety of genetic approaches, it has become clear that a number of genes

TABLE 47–4. Hereditary Persistence of Fetal Hemoglobin

- Deletion (Pancellular*)
  - $(\delta\beta)^{0}$
    - Black (HPFH 1)
    - Ghanaian (HPFH 2)
    - Indian (HPFH 3)
    - Italian (HPFH 4 and 5)
    - Vietnamese (HPFH 6)
  - $^{G}\gamma(^{A}\gamma\beta)^{+}$ (Hgb Kenya)
- Nondeletion
  - Linked to β-globin gene cluster (pancellular*)
    - $^{G}\gamma\beta^{+}$
      - Black $^{G}\gamma$-202 C→G
      - Tunisian $^{G}\gamma$-200+C
      - Black/Sardinian $^{G}\gamma$-175 T→C
      - Japanese $^{G}\gamma$-114 C→T
      - Australian $^{G}\gamma$-114 C→G
    - $^{A}\gamma\beta^{+}$
      - Greek/Sardinian/Black $^{A}\gamma$-117 G→A
      - British $^{A}\gamma$-198 T→C
      - Black $^{A}\gamma$-202 C→T
      - Italian/Chinese $^{A}\gamma$-196 C→T
      - Brazilian $^{A}\gamma$-195 C→G
      - Black $^{A}\gamma$-175 T→C
      - Black $^{a}\gamma$-114 to –102 (del)
      - Georgia $^{A}\gamma$-114 C→T
    - $^{G}\gamma^{A}\gamma\beta^{+}$
  - Linked to β-globin gene cluster (heterocellular*)
    - Atlanta
    - Czech
    - Seattle
    - Others (including some cases of $^{G}\gamma$-158 T→C)
  - Unlinked to β-globin gene cluster (heterocellular*)
    - Chromosome 6
    - Others

*The intercellular distribution of Hgb F is not always reported, and some inconsistencies are present within groups. Complete details are given in reference 7.

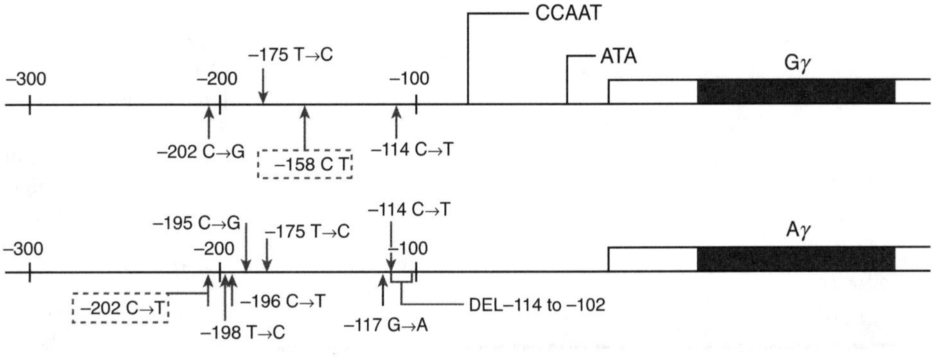

FIGURE 47–9. Some upstream point mutations associated with hereditary persistence of fetal hemoglobin.

may be involved in the generation of heterocellular HPFH, including loci at Xp22.2-p22.3, 6q23, 8q, and 2p15.[123–128] The latter linkage has been identified as the oncogene *BCL11–α*. The mechanism whereby these different loci affect the level of F cells in normal individuals and increase their levels in conditions like thalassemia and sickle cell anemia remain to be determined, but their coinheritance with these conditions may have an extremely beneficial effect of their associated phenotypes.[129]

δ-THALASSEMIA

Several point mutations and deletions that reduce δ-globin synthesis have been described. They are summarized in reference 7.

α-THALASSEMIA

Table 47–5 summarizes the different classes of α-thalassemia mutations. The α-globin gene haplotype can be written αα, indicating the α1 and α2 genes, respectively. A normal individual has the genotype αα/αα. A deletion involving one (–α) or both (– –) α genes can be further classified based on its size, written as a superscript; thus, $-\alpha^{3.7}$ indicates a deletion of 3.7 kb including one α gene. When the sizes of the deletions are not established, a superscript describing their geographic or family origin is useful; thus, $--^{MED}$ describes a deletion of both α genes first identified in individuals of Mediterranean origin. In thalassemia haplotypes in which both genes are intact, that is, nondeletion lesions, the nomenclature $\alpha^{T}\alpha$ is given, with the superscript T indicating the gene is thalassemic. However, when the precise molecular defect is known, as in hemoglobin Constant Spring, for example, $\alpha^{T}\alpha$ can be replaced by the more informative $\alpha^{CS}\alpha$. The molecular pathology and population genetics of the α-thalassemias have been the subject of several extensive reviews.[7,41,45,130,131]

TABLE 47–5. Classes of Mutations That Cause α-Thalassemia

α^0-Thalassemia
Deletions involving both α-globin genes
Deletions downstream from α_2 gene
Truncations of telomeric region of 16p
Deletions of HS40 region
α^+-Thalassemia
Deletions involving α_2 or α_1 genes
Point mutations involving α_2 or α_1 genes
mRNA processing
Splice site
Poly(A) signal
mRNA translation
Initiation
Nonsense, frameshift
Termination
Posttranslational
Unstable α-globin variants
α-Thalassemia Mental Retardation
ATR-16
Deletions or telomeric truncations of 16p
Translocations
ATR-X
Mutations of *ATR-X*
Deletions
Splice site
Missense
Nonsense

NOTE: Complete lists of individual mutations are found in references 7, 10, and 51.

α^0-Thalassemia

To date, 29 deletions that involve both α genes, and therefore abolish α-chain production from the affected chromosome, have been described (Fig. 47–10).[7] Several of the 3′ breakpoints fall within a 6- to 8-kb region at the 3′ end of the α-globin complex, suggesting this represents a breakpoint cluster region with a high level of recombination.[132] In at least five of the deletions, the 5′ breakpoints also appear to cluster. This gives rise to a situation in which the 5′ breakpoints are located approximately the same distance apart and in the same order along a chromosome as their respective 3′ breakpoints. It is possible that such staggered deletions arise from illegitimate recombination events that delete an integral number of chromatin loops as they pass through their nuclear attachment points during replication. This mechanism has also been suggested to underlie some of the deletion forms of HPFH. One of these deletions ($--^{MED}$) involves a more complex rearrangement that introduces a new piece of DNA bridging the two breakpoints in the α-gene cluster. This new sequence originates upstream from the α cluster and appears to have been replicated into the junction in a manner suggesting that the upstream segment of DNA also lies at the base of a replication loop. At least some of these deletions seem to have arisen by recombination events between Alu repeat sequences.

Several other mechanisms for the generation of α^0-thalassemia have been identified. In one case of unusual genetic interest, a long (>18 kb) deletion that removes the α1 gene and the region downstream was identified in which the α2 gene remains intact but is completely inactivated, giving the α^0-thalassemia phenotype. Although the inactive α2 gene retains all its local and remote *cis*-regulatory elements, its expression is completely silenced and its CpG island is completely methylated as a result of transcription of antisense RNA expressed from a locus that had been juxtaposed to the α2 gene because of the large deletion.[133,134] In some cases, this condition results from a terminal truncation of the short arm of chromosome 16 to a site 50 kb distal to the α-globin genes.[135] It is interesting that the telomeric consensus sequence (TTAGGGG)n has been added directly to the site of the break. Because this mutation is stably inherited, telomeric DNA alone appears sufficient to stabilize the broken chromosome end. This observation raises the possibility that other genetic diseases result from chromosomal truncations.

Several deletions have been identified that appear to downregulate α-globin genes by removing the α-globin LCR (HS40).[7,136,137] In each case, the α-globin genes are left intact, although in one the 3′ breakpoint is found between the ξ and ψξ genes, thus removing the ξ gene. These deletions appear to completely inactivate the α-globin gene complex, just as deletions of the β-globin LCR inactivate the entire β-gene complex. Such deletions have not been observed in the homozygous state, presumably because they would be lethal.

α^+-Thalassemia Gene Deletions

The most common forms of α^+-thalassemia ($-\alpha^{3.7}$ and $-\alpha^{4.2}$) involve deletion of one or the other of the duplicated α-globin genes (Figs. 47–10 and 47–11).

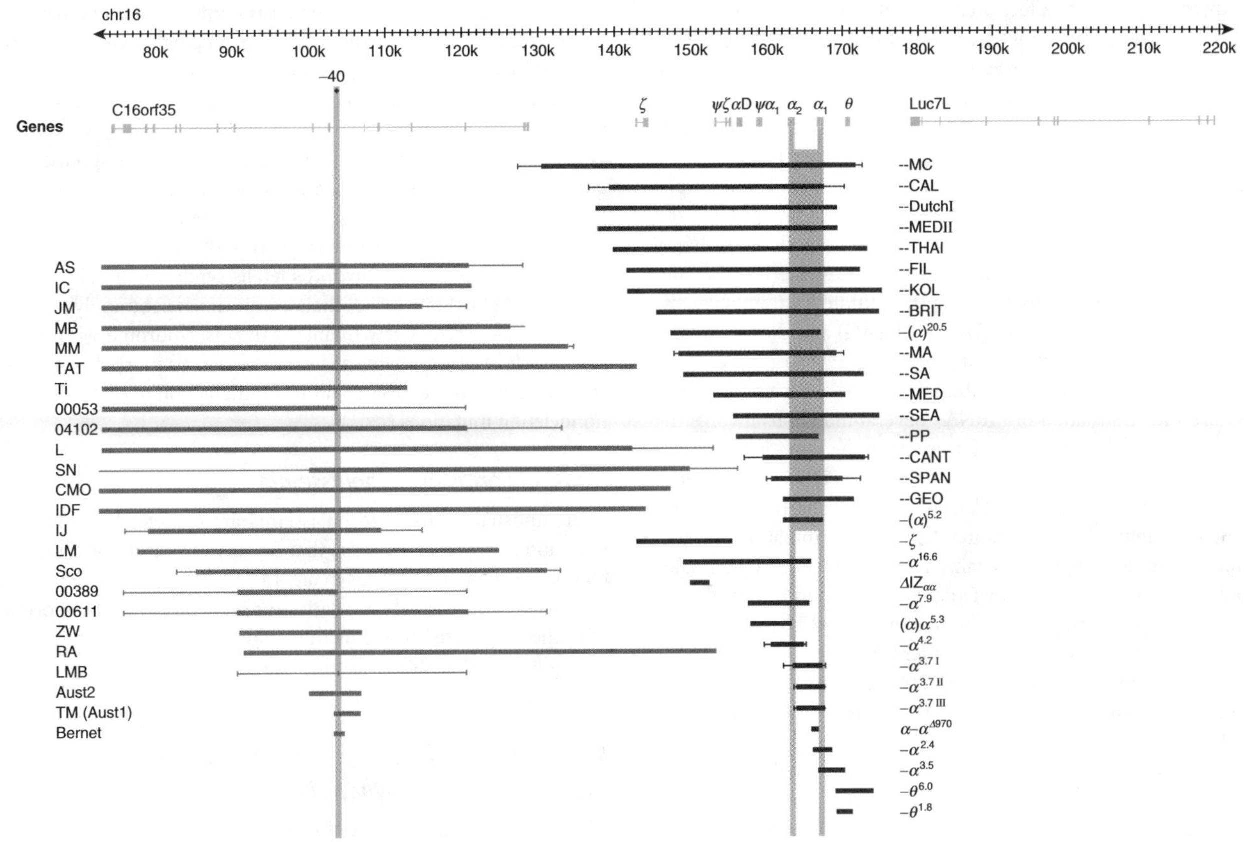

FIGURE 47–10. Some deletions of the α-globin gene cluster responsible for α^0-thalassemia. Deletions: MC, initials of patient; CAL, initials of patient; THAI, Thai; FIL, Filipino; CI, Conway Islands; BRIT, United Kingdom; SA, South Africa; MED, Mediterranean; SEA, Southeast Asian; SPAN, Spanish. The top line indicates the size of the region in kilobases (K). The second line shows the different genes that constitute the α-globin gene cluster, HS40, the major regulatory region of the cluster, and the position of other genes in the region. The lines in blue represent the size of the deletions that have been described in α^0-thalassemia, while those in red below them on the right-hand side of the figure show some of the deletions that have now been reported in different forms of α^+-thalassemia. The lines in yellow on the left side of the figure represent some of the deletions that have been reported upstream from the α-globin gene cluster, which, because they remove the major regulatory region, result in the phenotype of α^0-thalassemia. For a more detailed list of these deletions and references to those marked in this diagram, see reference 45.

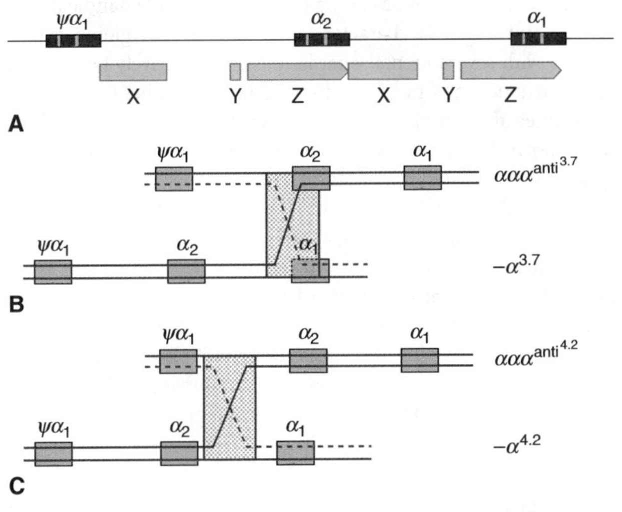

FIGURE 47–11. Mechanisms for production of the common deletion forms of α^+-thalassemia. **A.** Normal α-globin gene cluster showing the homology boxes X, Y, and Z. **B.** Rightward crossover through the Z bones, giving rise to the 3.7-kb deletion and a chromosome with three α-globin genes. **C.** Leftward crossover through the Z boxes, giving rise to a 4.2-kb deletion and a chromosome containing three α genes.

Each α gene is located within a region of homology approximately 4 kb long, interrupted by two nonhomologous regions. The homologous regions are believed to have resulted from an ancient duplication event and to have subsequently subdivided, presumably by insertions and deletions, to give three homologous subsegments referred to as X, Y, and Z (see Fig. 47–11). The duplicated Z boxes are 3.7 kb apart, and the X boxes are 4.2 kb apart. Misalignment and reciprocal crossover between these segments at meiosis can give rise to chromosomes with either single ($-\alpha$) or triplicated ($\alpha\alpha\alpha$) α-globin genes. Such an occurrence between homologous Z boxes deletes 3.7 kb of DNA (rightward deletion). A similar crossover between the two X blocks deletes 4.2 kb of DNA (leftward deletion $-\alpha^{4.2}$).[138] The corresponding triplicated α-gene arrangements are referred to as $\alpha\alpha\alpha^{\text{anti-3.7}}$ and $\alpha^{\text{anti-4.2}}$.[139–141] More detailed analysis of these crossover events indicates they occur more commonly in the Z box. At least three different $-\alpha^{3.7}$ deletions have been found, depending on exactly where the crossover occurred.[142] These deletions are designated $-\alpha^{3.7\text{I}}$, $-\alpha^{3.7\text{II}}$, and $-\alpha^{3.7\text{III}}$, respectively. Other, rarer deletions of a single α gene have been observed.[7]

Nondeletion α-Thalassemia

Because expression of the $\alpha 2$ gene is two to three times greater than expression of the $\alpha 1$ gene, the finding that most of the nondeletion mutants discovered to date affect predominantly $\alpha 2$ gene expression is not surprising. Presumably this is ascertainment bias because of the greater phenotypic effect of these lesions. It also is possible that defective expression of the $\alpha 2$ gene has come under greater selective pressure.

Like the β-thalassemia mutations, α-thalassemia mutations[7] can be classified according to the level of gene expression they affect (see Table 47–5). Several processing mutations have been identified. For example, a pentanucleotide deletion includes the 5′ splice site of IVS-1 of the α_2-globin gene. This mutation involves the invariant GT donor splicing sequence and thus completely inactivates the $\alpha 2$ gene.[143] A second mutant of this type, found commonly in the Middle East, involves the poly-A addition signal site (AATAAA→AATAAG) and downregulates the $\alpha 2$ gene by interfering with 3′ end processing.[144,145]

A second group of nondeletion α-thalassemias results from mutations that interfere with translation of mRNA.[7] Several mutations involve the initiation codon.[146–149] In one case, for example, the initiation codon is inactivated by a T→C transition.[146] In another case, efficiency of initiation is reduced by a dinucleotide deletion in the consensus sequence around the start signal.[149] Five mutations that affect termination of translation and give rise to elongated α chains have been identified: hemoglobins Constant Spring, Icaria, Koya Dora, Seal Rock, and Pakse.[7] Each mutation specifically changes the termination codon TAA so that an amino acid is inserted instead of the chain terminating (Fig. 47–12). This process is followed by read-through of mRNA that is not normally translated until another "in-phase" stop codon is reached. Thus, each of these variants has an elongated α chain. The "read-through" of α-globin mRNA that usually is not utilized likely reduces its stability.[150] Several nonsense mutations occur, for example, one in exon 3 of the α_2-globin gene.[151] Finally, several mutations occur that cause α-thalassemia by producing highly unstable α-globin chains, including hemoglobins Quong Sze,[152] Suan Doc,[153] Petah Tikvah,[154] and Evanston.[155] A complete list of nondeletion α-thalassemia alleles is given in reference 45.

Interactions of α-Thalassemia Haplotypes

Many α-thalassemia haplotypes have been described, and potentially more than 500 interactions are possible![7] Phenotypically, these phenotypes result in four broad categories: (1) normal, (2) conditions characterized by mild hematologic changes but no clinical abnormality, (3) hemoglobin H disease, and (4) hemoglobin Bart's hydrops fetalis syndrome. The heterozygous states for deletion or nondeletion forms of α^+-thalassemia either cause extremely mild hematologic abnormalities or are completely silent.

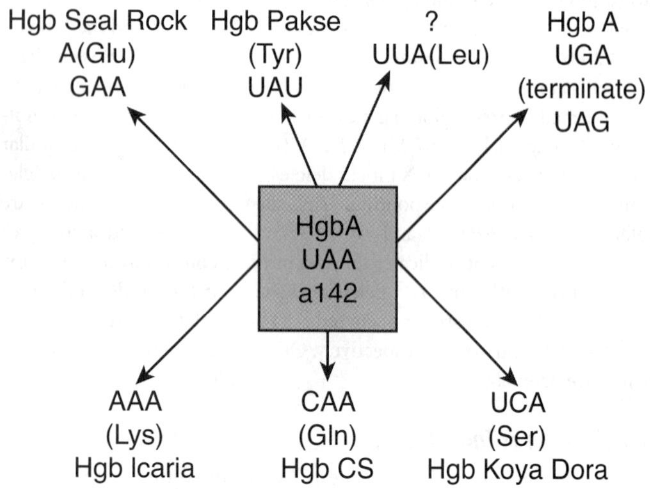

FIGURE 47–12. Point mutations in the α-globin gene termination codon.

In populations where α-thalassemia is common, the homozygous state for α^+-thalassemia ($-\alpha/-\alpha$) can produce a hematologic phenotype identical to that of the heterozygous state for α^0-thalassemia ($--/\alpha\alpha$), that is, mild anemia with reduced mean cell hemoglobin and mean cell volume values.

Hemoglobin H disease usually results from the compound heterozygous state for α^0-thalassemia and either deletion or non-deletion α^+-thalassemia. It occurs most frequently in Southeast Asia ($--^{SEA}/-\alpha^{3.7}$) and the Mediterranean region (usually $--^{MED}/-\alpha^{3.7}$).

The hemoglobin Bart's hydrops fetalis syndrome usually results from the homozygous state for α^0-thalassemia, most commonly $--^{SEA}/--^{SEA}$ or $--^{MED}/--^{MED}$. A few infants with this syndrome who synthesized very low levels of α chains at birth have been reported. Gene-mapping studies suggest these cases result from interaction of α^0-thalassemia with nondeletion mutations ($\alpha\alpha^T$).

Unusual Forms of α-Thalassemia

Some unusual forms of α-thalassemia are completely unrelated to the common forms of the disease that occur in tropical populations. These conditions, which can occur in any racial groups, include α-thalassemia associated with mental retardation or leukemia. Their importance lies with the diagnostic problems they may present and, more importantly, the light that elucidation of the α-thalassemia pathology may shed on broader disease mechanisms.

Molecular Pathology of the α-Thalassemia Mental Retardation Syndrome

The first descriptions of noninherited forms of α-thalassemia associated with mental retardation suggested the lesions involving the α-globin gene locus were acquired in the paternal germ cells and that their molecular pathology might help elucidate the associated developmental changes.[156] Two separate syndromes of this type now are evident. In one group of patients, long deletions involve the α-globin gene cluster and remove at least one megabase.[157] This condition can arise in several ways, including unbalanced translocation involving chromosome 16, truncation of the tip of chromosome 16, and loss of the α-globin gene cluster and parts of its flanking regions by other mechanisms. These findings localize a region of about 1.7 Mb in band 16p13.3 proximal to the α-globin genes as being involved in mental handicap.[41]

The second group is characterized by defective α-globin synthesis associated with severe mental retardation and a relatively homogeneous pattern of dysmorphology.[158] Extensive structural studies have shown no abnormalities of the α-globin genes. These chromosomes direct the synthesis of normal amounts of α globin in mouse erythroleukemia cells, suggesting that α-thalassemia results from deficiency of a *trans*-activating factor involved in regulation of the α-globin genes. This condition is encoded by a locus on the short arm of the X chromosome.[159] *ATR-X*, the gene involved, is a DNA helicase with many features of a DNA-binding protein. Many different mutations of this gene have been identified in different families with the *ATR-X* syndrome.[131,160] Studies have identified a PHD region and an ATPase/helicase domain.[161] Because patients with *ATR-X* show defective methylation of recombinant DNA arrays and related defects, this condition likely is one of a growing list of disorders that result from disordered chromatin remodeling.[162,163]

α-Thalassemia and Myelodysplasia

The hematologic findings of hemoglobin H disease or mild α-thalassemia occasionally are observed in elderly patients with myeloid leukemia or the myelodysplastic syndrome. Earlier studies suggested this finding resulted from an acquired defect of α-globin synthesis in which the α-globin genes were completely inactivated in the neoplastic hemopoietic cell line.[164] The molecular basis for this observation now is known to reside in a variety of different mutations involving *ATR-X*.[41,165] The relationship of these somatic mutations of *ATR-X* to the neoplastic transformation remains to be determined. The molecular defect of other cases of acquired α-thalassemia, such as that seen in variable combined immunodeficiency,[166] remains to be defined.

PATHOPHYSIOLOGY

Almost all the pathophysiologic features of the thalassemias can be related to a primary imbalance of globin-chain synthesis. This phenomenon makes the thalassemias fundamentally different from all the other genetic and acquired disorders of hemoglobin production and, to a large extent, explains their extreme severity in the homozygous and compound heterozygous states (Fig. 47–13).

The anemia of β-thalassemia has three major components. First and most important is ineffective erythropoiesis with intramedullary destruction of a variable proportion of the developing red cell precursors. Second is hemolysis resulting from destruction of mature red cells containing α-chain inclusions. Third are the hypochromic and microcytic red cells that result from the overall reduction in hemoglobin synthesis.

Because the primary defect in β-thalassemia involves β-chain production, synthesis of hemoglobins F and A_2 should be unaffected. Fetal hemoglobin production *in utero* is normal. The clinical manifestations of thalassemia appear only when the neonatal switch from γ- to β-chain production occurs. However, fetal hemoglobin synthesis persists beyond the neonatal period in nearly all forms of β-thalassemia (see "Persistent Fetal Hemoglobin Production and Cellular Heterogeneity" below). β-Thalassemia heterozygotes have an elevated level of hemoglobin A_2. The elevated level appears to reflect not only a relative decrease in hemoglobin A as a result of defective β-chain synthesis but also an absolute increase in the output of δ chains both *cis* and *trans* to the mutant β-globin gene.[7]

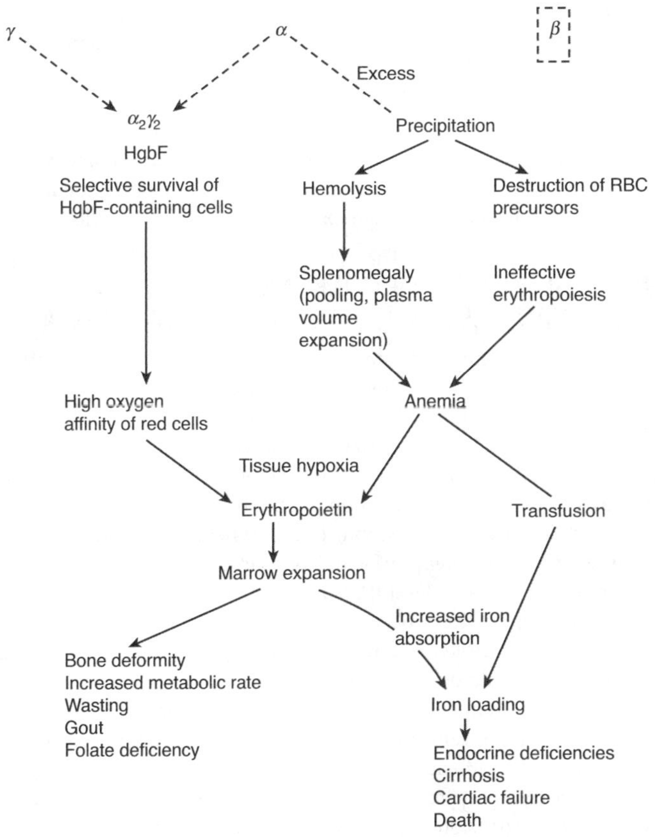

FIGURE 47–13. Pathophysiology of β-thalassemia. RBC, red blood cell.

Because α chains are shared by hemoglobins F, A, and A_2, there is no increase in hemoglobin F in the α-thalassemias. The excess γ and β chains formed as a result of defective α-chain production produce soluble homotetramers (see "Mechanisms and Consequences of Erythroid Precursor Damage and Red Cell Damage" below). Hence there is less ineffective erythropoiesis than in β-thalassemia and the major cause of anemia is hemolysis and poorly hemoglobinized red cells.

IMBALANCED GLOBIN-CHAIN SYNTHESIS

Measurements of *in vitro* globin-chain synthesis in the blood or marrow of patients with different types of thalassemia[167,168] and family studies that allow examination of the action of thalassemia genes in patients who also inherited α- or β-globin structural variants[7,9] provide a clear picture of the action of the thalassemia determinants. In homozygous β-thalassemia, β-globin synthesis is either absent or markedly reduced. The result is excessive production of α-globin chains. α-Globin chains are incapable of forming a viable hemoglobin tetramer, so the chains precipitate in red cell precursors. The resulting inclusion bodies can be demonstrated by both light and electron microscopy.[169,170] In the marrow, precipitation can be seen in the earliest hemoglobinized precursors and throughout the erythroid maturation pathway.[171] These large inclusions are responsible for intramedullary destruction of red cell precursors and hence for the ineffective erythropoiesis characterizing all the β-thalassemias. A large proportion of the developing erythroblasts are destroyed within the marrow in severe cases.[172] Any red cells that are released are prematurely destroyed by mechanisms that are considered below in "Mechanisms and Consequences of Erythroid Precursor and Red Cell Damage." β-Thalassemia heterozygotes also have imbalanced globin-chain synthesis, but the magnitude of α-chain excess is much less and presumably can be resolved by the proteolytic enzymes of the red cell precursors.[173] Notwithstanding, a mild degree of ineffective erythropoiesis occurs.

Although there is marked globin-chain imbalance in the severe α-thalassemias,[7,167] the excess γ and β chains form homotetramers that do not precipitate in the red-cell precursors to the same extent as excess α chains in β-thalassemia. Hence the pathophysiology of anemia is fundamentally different between the two conditions.

MECHANISMS AND CONSEQUENCES OF ERYTHROID PRECURSOR AND RED CELL DAMAGE

Damage to the red cell membrane by the globin-chain precipitation process occurs by two major routes: generation of hemichromes (see Chap. 48) from excess α chains with subsequent structural damage to the red cell membrane, and similar damage mediated through the degradation products of excess α chains.[7,174–176] The degradation products of free α chains—globin, heme, hemin (oxidized heme), and free iron—also play a role in damaging red cell membranes. Excess globin chains bind to different membrane proteins and alter their structure and function. Excess iron, by generating oxygen free radicals, damages several red cell membrane components (including lipids and protein) and intracellular organelles. Heme and its products can catalyze the formation of a variety of reactive oxygen species that can damage the red-cell membrane. These changes are reflected in an increased rate of apoptosis of red cell precursors.[177] The red cells are rigid and underhydrated, leak potassium, and have increased levels of calcium and low, unstable levels of ATP. Damage to the red cells can also be mediated by the presence of rigid inclusion bodies during passage of the red cells through the spleen.

The consequences of excess non–α-chain production in the α-thalassemias are quite different. Because α chains are shared by both fetal and adult hemoglobin (see Chaps. 6 and 48), defective α-chain production is manifest in both fetal and adult life. In the fetus, it leads to excess γ-chain production; in the adult, it leads to an excess of β chains. Excess γ chains form γ_4 homotetramers or hemoglobin Bart's[178]; excess β chains form β_4 homotetramers or hemoglobin H.[179] The fact that γ and β chains form homotetramers is the reason for the fundamental difference in the pathophysiology of α- and β-thalassemia. Because γ_4 and β_4 tetramers are soluble, they do not precipitate to any significant degree in the marrow, and therefore the α-thalassemias are not characterized by severe ineffective erythropoiesis. However, β_4 tetramers precipitate as red cells age, with the formation of inclusion bodies. Thus, the anemia of the more severe forms of α-thalassemia in the adult results from a shortened survival of red cells consequent to their damage in the microvasculature of the spleen as a result of the presence of the inclusions. In addition, because of the defect in hemoglobin synthesis, the cells are hypochromic and microcytic. Hemoglobin Bart's is more stable than hemoglobin H and does not form large inclusions.

Although, as is the case in β-thalassemia, excess globin chains cause damage to the red cell membrane, the mechanisms are different in the two forms of the disease. As described in "Etiology and Pathogenesis" above, in β-thalassemia, excess α chains result in mechanical instability and oxidative damage to a variety of membrane proteins, notably protein 4.1. However, in α-thalassemia, the membranes are hyperstable, and no evidence of oxidation or dysfunction of this protein is present. Furthermore, the state of red cell hydration is different in α-thalassemia. Accumulation of excess β chains results in increased hydration. These differences in the pathophysiology of membrane damage between α- and β-thalassemia are discussed in detail in references 4 and 174 to 176.

Another factor exacerbates the tissue hypoxia of the anemia of the α-thalassemias. Both hemoglobin Bart's and hemoglobin H show no heme–heme interaction and have almost hyperbolic oxygen dissociation curves with very high oxygen affinities. Thus, they are not able to liberate oxygen at physiologic tissue tensions; in effect, they are useless as oxygen carriers.[7]

As a consequence, infants with high levels of hemoglobin Bart's have severe intrauterine hypoxia. This is the major basis for the clinical picture of homozygous α^0-thalassemia, which results in the stillbirth of hydropic infants late in pregnancy or at term. Oxygen deprivation is reflected by the grossly hydropic state of the infant, presumably as a result of increased capillary permeability, and by severe erythroblastosis. Deficient fetal oxygenation probably is responsible for the enormously hypertrophied placentas and possibly for the associated developmental abnormalities that occur with the severe forms of intrauterine α-thalassemia.[7]

PERSISTENT FETAL HEMOGLOBIN PRODUCTION AND CELLULAR HETEROGENEITY

Children with severe thalassemia have an increased level of hemoglobin F that persists into childhood and later.[7,10] In the β^0-thalassemias, hemoglobin F is the only hemoglobin produced, except for small amounts of hemoglobin A_2. Examination of the blood using staining methods specific for hemoglobin F shows that it is heterogeneously distributed among the red cells.[7] Persistent hemoglobin F production is not a major feature of the more severe forms of α-thalassemia.

The mechanism of persistent γ-chain synthesis in the thalassemias is incompletely understood. Normal adults have small quantities of hemoglobin F that are heterogeneously distributed among the red cells. Cells with demonstrable hemoglobin F are called *F cells*. One important mechanism for high hemoglobin F levels in the blood of patients with β-thalassemia is cell selection.[7,180–183] The major cause of ineffective erythropoiesis and shortened red cell survival in β-thalassemia is the deleterious effect of excess α chains on erythroid maturation in the marrow and on the survival of red cells in the blood. Therefore, red cell precursors that produce γ chains are at a selective advantage. Excess α chains combine with γ chains to produce hemoglobin F; therefore, the magnitude of α-chain precipitation is less. Differential centrifugation experiments[181–183] and *in vivo* labeling studies[180] have shown that populations of red cells with relatively large amounts of hemoglobin F are more efficiently produced and survive longer in the blood. The blood of patients with homozygous β-thalassemia shows remarkable cellular heterogeneity with respect to red cell survival, such as populations of cells containing predominantly hemoglobin A that are destroyed very rapidly in the spleen and elsewhere, cells with a much longer survival that contain relatively more hemoglobin F, and populations of intermediate age and hemoglobin constitution.[7,182]

Although cell selection is probably the main reason for the increased levels of hemoglobin F in the red cells in β-thalassemia, other mechanisms may also be involved. In any form of "stress erythropoiesis," that is, rapid erythroid proliferation, there is a tendency for a relative increase in γ-chain production. Furthermore, as discussed in "Hereditary Persistence of Fetal Hemoglobin" above, several genes or chromosomal locations have been defined in which polymorphisms are involved in the increased basal production of γ chains and a relative increase in the number of F cells in the blood. The interaction of these different loci appear to be responsible for high levels of hemoglobin F production in β-thalassemia and sickle cell anemia with the production of milder phenotypes.[125–128,184] However, biosynthesis studies indicate that marrow expansion and the selective survival of F-cell precursors and their progeny are the major factors in hemoglobin F production in hemoglobin E/β-thalassemia.[183]

Because a reciprocal relation exists between γ- and δ-chain synthesis, the red cells of β-thalassemia homozygotes containing large amounts of hemoglobin F have relatively low hemoglobin A_2 levels.[7] Thus, the measured percent hemoglobin A_2 in these individuals is the average of a very heterogeneous cell population. This finding probably accounts for the extreme variability in hemoglobin A_2 levels found in homozygotes for this disorder. A further consequence of the persistence of hemoglobin F in β-thalassemia is the high oxygen affinity of the red cells.

CONSEQUENCES OF COMPENSATORY MECHANISMS FOR THE ANEMIA OF THALASSEMIA

The profound anemia of homozygous β-thalassemia and the relatively high oxygen affinity of hemoglobin F combine to cause severe tissue hypoxia. Because of the high oxygen affinity of hemoglobins Bart's and H, a similar defect in tissue oxygenation occurs in the more severe forms of α-thalassemia. The major adaptive response to hypoxia is increased erythropoietin production. It has been found that in severely anemic children with hemoglobin E β-thalassemia, age and hemoglobin levels are independent variables in erythropoietin response and that for a given hemoglobin level there is a relatively high response in very young children.[185] These observations provide an explanation for the rather unstable phenotype of many intermediate forms of β-thalassemia during early childhood. The major effect of these very high levels of erythropoietin production is expansion of the dyserythropoietic marrow. The results are deformities of the skull and face and porosity of the long bones.[7] Extramedullary hematopoietic tumors may develop in extreme cases. Apart from the production of severe skeletal deformities, marrow expansion may cause pathologic fractures and sinus and middle ear infection as a result of ineffective drainage.

Another important effect of the enormous expansion of the marrow mass is the diversion of calories required for normal development to the ineffective red cell precursors. Thus, patients severely affected by thalassemia show poor development and wasting. The massive turnover of erythroid precursors may result in secondary hyperuricemia and gout and severe folate deficiency.

The effects of gross intrauterine hypoxia in homozygous α^0-thalassemia have been described. In the symptomatic forms of α-thalassemia (e.g., hemoglobin H disease) that are compatible with survival into adult life, bone changes and other consequences of erythroid expansion are seen, although less commonly than in β-thalassemia.

SPLENOMEGALY: DILUTIONAL ANEMIA

Constant exposure of the spleen to red cells with inclusions consisting of precipitated globin chains gives rise to the phenomenon of "work hypertrophy." Progressive splenomegaly occurs in both α- and β-thalassemia and may worsen the anemia.[7,10] A large spleen acts as a sump for red cells, sequestering a considerable proportion of the red cell mass. Furthermore, splenomegaly may cause plasma volume expansion, a complication that can be exacerbated by massive expansion of the erythroid marrow. The combination of pooling of the red cells in the spleen and plasma volume expansion can exacerbate the anemia in both α- and β-thalassemia.

ABNORMAL IRON METABOLISM

β-Thalassemia homozygotes who are anemic manifest increased intestinal iron absorption that is related to the degree of expansion of the red cell precursor population. Iron absorption is decreased by blood transfusion.[7,10] Increased absorption causes a steady accumulation of iron, first in the Kupffer cells of the liver and the macrophages of the spleen and later in the parenchymal cells of the liver (see Chap. 42). Most patients homozygous for β-thalassemia require regular blood transfusion; thus, transfusional siderosis adds to the iron accumulation. Iron accumulates in the endocrine glands,[7,186] particularly in the parathyroids, pituitary, pancreas, liver, and, most important, in the myocardium.[7,187,188] Iron accumulation in the myocardium leads to death by involving the conducting tissues or by causing intractable cardiac failure. Other consequences of iron loading include diabetes, hypoparathyroidism, hypothyroidism, and abnormalities of hypothalamic–pituitary function leading to growth retardation and hypogonadism.[7,186]

Accurate information is available regarding the levels of body iron, as reflected by hepatic iron, at which patients are at risk for serious complications of iron overload.[7,189] These studies, which extrapolate data obtained from patients with genetic hemochromatosis, suggest that patients with hepatic iron levels of approximately 80 μmol of iron per gram of liver, wet weight (~15 mg of iron per gram of liver, dry weight), are at increased risk for hepatic disease and endocrine organ damage. Patients with higher body iron burdens are at particular risk for cardiac disease and early death.

Disordered iron metabolism is less common in the adult forms of α-thalassemia. The reason is not clear, but the milder degree of anemia, fewer transfusions, and the less marked erythroid expansion of the marrow are likely explanations.

The mechanisms whereby iron, and in particular non–transferrin-bound iron mediate tissue damage, and recent evidence about the central role of hepcidin in the abnormal regulation of iron absorption in disorders like thalassemia are discussed in Chap. 42.

INFECTION

All forms of severe thalassemia appear to be associated with an increased susceptibility to bacterial infection.[7] The reason is not known. The relatively high serum iron levels may favor bacterial growth. Another possible mechanism is blockade of the monocyte–macrophage system as a result of the increased rate of destruction of red cells. No consistent defects in white cell or immune function have been reported, and high serum iron levels as an important factor remain to be unequivocally demonstrated. The one exception is infection with *Yersinia enterocolitica*, a normally nonvirulent pathogen that can produce its own siderophore and hence can thrive in iron excess. Transfusion-dependent patients with thalassemia are at particular risk for blood-borne infections including hepatitis B, hepatitis C, HIV/AIDS, and, in some parts of the world, malaria.

COAGULATION DEFECTS

The increasing knowledge about the potential hypercoagulable state in some forms of thalassemia has been reviewed in detail.[174–176,190] Evidence indicates that patients, particularly after splenectomy and with high platelet counts, may develop progressive pulmonary arterial disease as a result of platelet aggregation in the pulmonary circulation. Furthermore, using thalassemic red cells as a source of phospholipids, enhanced thrombin generation has been demonstrated in a prothrombinase assay. The procoagulant effect of thalassemia cells appears to result from increased expression of anionic phospholipids on the red cell surface. Normally, neutral or negatively charged phospholipids are confined to the inner leaflet of the red cell membrane, an effect that is mediated by the action of aminophospholipid translocase, an enzyme sometimes known as flippase. In effect, this enzyme flips aminophospholipids that are diffused to the outer leaflet back to the inner leaflet (see Chap. 45). The current belief is that these aminophospholipids in thalassemic red cells are moved to the outer leaflet, thus providing a surface on which coagulation can be activated. Other nonspecific changes in the coagulation pathway and its antagonists have been observed in patients with different forms of thalassemia.

There is increasing evidence that, as in the case of sickle cell anemia (see Chap. 48), the hemolytic component of the anemia of β-thalassemia is associated with the release of hemoglobin and arginase resulting in impaired nitric oxide availability and endothelial dysfunction with progressive pulmonary hypertension.[191] There may be other contributions to this complication including increased coagulability and local structural damage to the lungs relating to excess iron deposition.

CLINICAL HETEROGENEITY

The pathophysiologic mechanisms described above provide the basis for the remarkably diverse clinical findings in the thalassemia syndromes.[7,192] All the manifestations of β-thalassemia can be related to excess α-chain production. Thus, any mechanism that reduces the excess of α chains should reduce the clinical severity of the disease. Several elegant "experiments of nature" have shown that this reasoning is true and, incidentally, have confirmed that globin-chain imbalance is the major factor determining the severity of the thalassemias.

Coinheritance of α-thalassemia can reduce the severity of the more severe forms of β-thalassemia.[193,194] The effect is much more marked in individuals who are homozygotes or compound heterozygotes for different forms of β^+-thalassemia. β^0-Thalassemia homozygotes who have inherited α-thalassemia seem to be protected little, if at all.

Severe β-thalassemia can be modified by the coinheritance of genetic determinants for enhanced production of γ chains. Several determinants may be involved. For example, inheritance of a particular RFLP haplotype in the region 5′ to the β-globin gene may be an important factor.[195,196] This particular β-globin gene haplotype is associated with a single base change, C→T, at position −158 relative to the $^G\gamma$-globin gene, an alteration that creates a cleavage site for the restriction enzyme Xmn I.[121] An excess of individuals homozygous for T (XmnI+ +) with the phenotype of thalassemia intermedia exist compared with thalassemia major in different populations.[196–198] Whether this polymorphism is the only factor that increases hemoglobin F production in these cases is not absolutely clear. As discussed under "Hereditary Persistence of Fetal Hemoglobin" above, it is now clear that there are loci on chromosomes 2, 6, and 8, and possibly the X chromosome, at which polymorphisms are involved in the elevation of fetal hemoglobin synthesis and that their coinheritance may significantly modify the phenotype of different forms of β-thalassemia.

Some mutations that cause β-thalassemia are associated with a mild phenotype because they result in only modest reduction of β-chain production.[7] For example, mutations at positions −29 and −88 are associated with mild β^+-thalassemia in Africans. Similarly, particularly mild phenotypes are commonly found with a base substitution at position 6 in IVS-1 and at position −87 in the 5′-flanking region of the β-globin gene in Mediterranean populations. The homozygous state for the IVS-1 position 6 mutation usually produces an extremely mild form of β-thalassemia. When these "mild" mutations are coinherited with more severe β-thalassemia determinants, the compound heterozygous states are characterized by a more severe form of thalassemia intermedia. Other forms of thalassemia intermedia are associated with the homozygous state for $\delta\beta$-thalassemia, the various interactions of β-thalassemia with $\delta\beta$-thalassemia, and heterozygous β-thalassemia of the severe variety or in association with triplicated α-gene loci.[7,10,198] These complex interactions are the subject of several extensive reviews.[198–200]

These mechanisms for the phenotypic variability of the β-thalassemias represent only the beginning of our understanding of the genetic diversity of these conditions. Hence, defining a series of genetic modifiers that act at different levels is useful.[192] Primary modifiers represent the diversity of mutations at the β-globin gene locus. Secondary modifiers are those, such as α-thalassemia and increased hemoglobin F production, that directly modify the relative degree of the imbalanced globin chain output. However, an increasing number of tertiary modifiers, that is, genetic diversity, have an important effect on the complications of the disease. These include loci involved in iron, bone, and bilirubin metabolism and in determining resistance of susceptibility to infection. Furthermore, phenotypic diversity may reflect different degrees of adaptation to anemia and the effect of the environment. These complex issues have been reviewed[192] and are illustrated in Figure 47–14. Several extensive reviews of the pathophysiology of the intermediate forms of β-thalassemia in different populations are available.[199,200]

The α-thalassemias, particularly hemoglobin H disease, show considerable clinical diversity. Some of this variability can be related to particular genotypes,[7,41] but the reasons for the heterogeneity of these disorders is not clear.

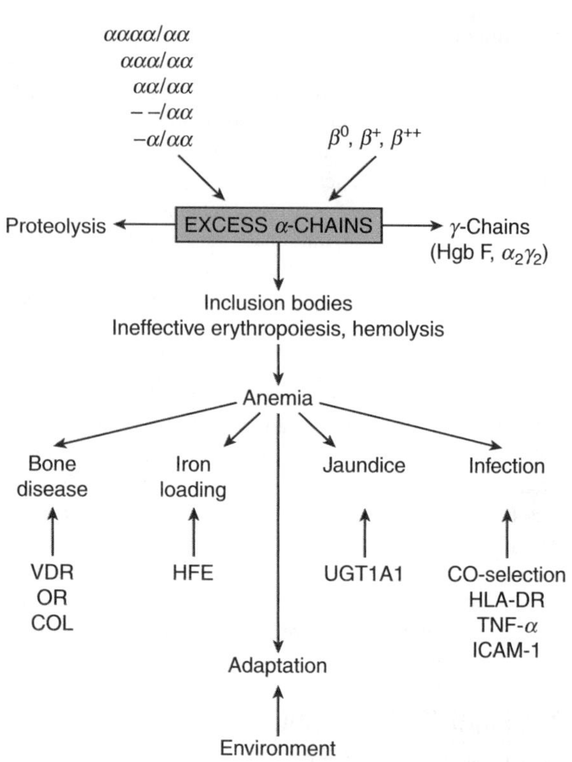

FIGURE 47–14. Different levels of modification of the β-thalassemia phenotype. COL, various genes involved in collagen metabolism; Co-Selection, indicates variable selection of genes involved in susceptibility to infection along with different thalassemia genes; HFE, gene for hereditary hemochromatosis; ICAM, intercellular adhesion molecule; OR, estrogen receptor; TNF, tumor necrosis factor; UGT1A1, uridine diphosphate-glucuronyltransferase; VDR, vitamin D receptor. *(Adapted with permission from Weatherall DJ.[192])*

CLINICAL FEATURES

β- AND δβ-THALASSEMIAS

The most clinically severe form of β-thalassemia is thalassemia major. A milder clinical picture, characterized by a later onset and either no transfusion requirement or at least fewer transfusions than are required to treat the major form of the illnesses, is designated *β-thalassemia intermedia*. *β-Thalassemia minor* is the term used to describe the heterozygous carrier state for β-thalassemia. More extensive accounts of the clinical features of these conditions are given in two monographs.[7,9]

β-THALASSEMIA MAJOR

The homozygous or compound heterozygous state for β-thalassemia, thalassemia major, produces the clinical picture first described by Cooley and Lee[1] in 1925. Affected infants are well at birth. Anemia usually develops during the first few months of life and becomes progressively more severe. The infants fail to thrive and may have feeding problems, bouts of fever, diarrhea, and other gastrointestinal symptoms. The majority of infants who develop transfusion-dependent homozygous β-thalassemia present with these symptoms within the first year of life. A later onset suggests the condition will develop into one of the intermediate forms of β-thalassemia (see "Pathophysiology" above).

The course of the disease in childhood depends almost entirely on whether the child is maintained on an adequate transfusion program.[7,9] The classic textbook picture of Cooley anemia describes the disease as it was seen before these children could be maintained with relatively normal hemoglobin levels by regular blood transfusions. If adequate transfusion is possible, children grow and develop normally and have no abnormal physical signs. Few of the complications of the disorder occur during childhood. The disease presents a problem only when the effects of iron loading resulting from ineffective erythropoiesis and from repeated blood transfusions become apparent at the end of the first decade. Children who are treated with an adequate iron chelation regimen develop normally, although some of them remain short in height.

An inadequately transfused child develops the typical features of Cooley anemia. Growth is stunted. With bossing of the skull and overgrowth of the maxillary region, the face gradually assumes a "mongoloid" appearance. These changes are associated with a characteristic radiologic appearance of the skull, long bones, and hands (Fig. 47–15). The diploe widens, with a "hair on end" or "sun ray" appearance and a lacy trabeculation of the long bones and phalanges. Gross skeletal deformities can occur. The liver and spleen are enlarged, and the

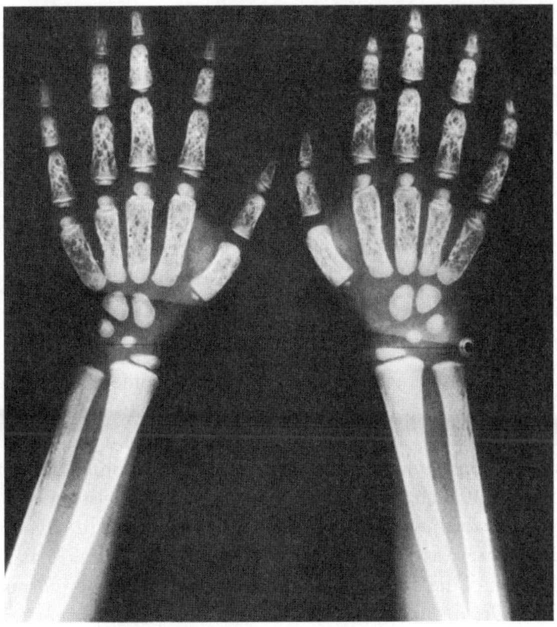

FIGURE 47–15. Radiologic appearances of the hands in homozygous β-thalassemia. The scattered lucent areas in the bones of the fingers reflect the marked expansion of marrow in distal areas.

pigmentation of the skin increases. Many features of a hypermetabolic state, as evidence by fever, wasting, and hyperuricemia, may develop.

The clinical course is characterized by severe anemia with frequent complications. These children are particularly prone to infection, which is a common cause of death. Spontaneous fractures occur commonly as a result of the expansion of the marrow cavities with thinning of the long bones and skull. Maxillary deformities often lead to dental problems from malocclusion. Formation of massive deposits of extramedullary hematopoietic tissue may cause neurologic complications. With the gross splenomegaly that may occur, secondary thrombocytopenia and leukopenia frequently develop, leading to a further tendency to infection and bleeding. Splenectomy is frequently performed to reduce transfusion frequency and severe thrombocytopenia; however, postsplenectomy infections are particularly common.[7] Bleeding tendency may be seen in the absence of thrombocytopenia. Epistaxis is particularly common. These hemostatic problems are associated with poor liver function in some cases. Chronic leg ulceration may occur but is more common in thalassemia intermedia.

Children who have grown and developed normally throughout the first 10 years of life as a result of regular blood transfusion begin to develop the symptoms of iron loading as they enter puberty, particularly if they have not received adequate iron chelation.[7,9] The first indication of iron loading usually is the absence of the pubertal growth spurt and failure of the menarche. Over the succeeding years, a variety of endocrine disturbances may develop, particularly diabetes mellitus, hypogonadotrophic hypogonadism, and growth hormone deficiency. Hypothyroidism and adrenal insufficiency also occur but are less common.[7,186] Toward the end of the second decade, cardiac complications arise, and death usually occurs in the second or third decade as a result of cardiac siderosis.[187–189] Cardiac siderosis may cause an acute cardiac death with arrhythmia, or intractable cardiac failure. Both of these complications can be precipitated by intercurrent infection.

Even the adequately transfused child who has received chelation therapy may suffer a number of complications. Bloodborne infection, notably with hepatitis B or C,[201] HIV,[202] or malaria[203] is extremely common in some populations, although the frequency is decreasing with the use of widespread blood-donor screening programs. Delayed puberty and growth retardation are common and probably reflect hypogonadotrophic hypogonadism and damage to the pituitary gland.[201,204] Osteoporosis is being recognized increasingly and may, at least in part, be a reflection of hypogonadism.[201]

β-THALASSEMIA INTERMEDIA

The clinical phenotype of patients designated as having thalassemia intermedia is more severe than the usual asymptomatic thalassemia trait but milder than transfusion-dependent thalassemia major.[7,199,200] The syndrome encompasses disorders with a wide spectrum of disability. At the severe end, patients present with anemia later than patients with the transfusion-dependent forms of homozygous β-thalassemia and are just able to maintain a hemoglobin level of approximately 6 g/dL without transfusion. However, their growth and development are retarded. The patients become seriously disabled, with marked skeletal deformities, arthritis, and bone pain; progressive splenomegaly; growth retardation; and chronic ulcerations above the ankles. At the other end of the spectrum, patients remain completely asymptomatic until adult life and are transfusion independent, with hemoglobin levels as high as 10 to 12 g/dL. All varieties of intermediate severity are observed. Some patients become disabled simply from the effects of hypersplenism. Intensive studies of the molecular pathology of this condition have provided some guidelines about genotype–phenotype relationships that are useful for genetic counseling (Table 47–6).

Overall, the clinical features of the intermediate forms of β-thalassemia are similar to the features of β-thalassemia major. At the severe end of the spectrum, particularly in cases of growth retardation, patients

TABLE 47–6. Genotypes of Patients with β-Thalassemia Intermedia

Mild forms of β-thalassemia
Homozygosity for mild β^+-thalassemia alleles
Compound heterozygosity for two mild β^+-thalassemia alleles
Compound heterozygosity for a "silent" or mild and more severe β-thalassemia allele
Inheritance of α- and β-thalassemia
β^+-Thalassemia with α^0-thalassemia (– –/αα) or α^+-thalassemia (–α/αα or –α/–α)
β^+-Thalassemia with genotype of Hgb H disease (– –/–α)
β-Thalassemia with elevated γ-chain synthesis
Homozygous β-thalassemia with heterocellular HPFH
Homozygous β-thalassemia with homozygous $^G\gamma$ 158 T→C change (some cases)
Compound heterozygosity for β-thalassemia and deletion forms of HPFH
Compound heterozygosity for β-thalassemia and β-chain variants
Hgb E/β-thalassemia
Other interactions with rare β-chain variants
Heterozygous β-thalassemia with triplicated or quadruplicated α-chain genes (ααα or αααα)
Dominant forms of β-thalassemia
Interactions of β- and $(\delta\beta)^+$- or $(\delta\beta)^0$-thalassemia

HPFH, hereditary persistence of fetal hemoglobin.

should be treated with regular transfusion. However, a number of important complications, including progressive hypersplenism, occur in patients with milder forms. Clinically significant iron loading as a result of increased absorption is seen even in patients with infrequent transfusions (see Chap. 42). Iron overload results in frequent diabetes and endocrine disturbances, typically by fourth decade of life. A high incidence of pigment gallstones, skeletal deformities, bone and joint disease, leg ulcers, and thrombotic tendency, particularly after splenectomy, is observed.[7]

Hematologists should be aware that in patients heterozygous for rare forms of β-thalassemia, a phenotype of thalassemia intermedia that results in the clinical constellation of autosomal dominant thalassemia (discussed in "Pathophysiology" above) is encountered on rare occasions.

■ β-THALASSEMIA MINOR

The heterozygous state for β-thalassemia is usually identified during family studies of patients with more severe forms of β-thalassemia, population surveys, or, most frequently, by the chance finding of the characteristic hematologic changes during a routine study. There is an extensive literature on this condition,[7] some of which suggests that affected individuals may have symptoms of anemia and, not infrequently, splenomegaly, while other studies suggest that the condition is completely symptomless and palpable splenomegaly does not occur. Surprisingly, none of these studies have been controlled. A controlled study reported that individuals with the β-thalassemia trait suffer from fatigue and other symptoms indistinguishable from those with mild anemias from other causes. There was no difference in the frequency of palpable splenomegaly between the thalassemic and control groups.[205] The trait not infrequently causes a moderately severe anemia of pregnancy, in some cases requiring transfusion. Some β-thalassemia carriers have increased iron stores, although this is most often a result of inappropriate iron therapy based on a misdiagnosis. In countries where there is a relatively high frequency of genetic determinants for hemochromatosis, the possibility of their coinheritance should be borne in mind if a patient with β-thalassemia trait with an unusually high plasma iron or serum ferritin level is encountered.

■ α-THALASSEMIAS

Hemoglobin Bart's Hydrops Fetalis Syndrome

This disorder is a frequent cause of stillbirth in Southeast Asia. Infants either are stillborn between 34 and 40 weeks' gestation or are born alive but die within the first few hours.[7,206] Pallor, edema, and hepatosplenomegaly are seen. The clinical picture resembles hydrops fetalis as a result of Rh blood group incompatibility. Massive extramedullary hemopoiesis and enlargement of the placenta are noted at autopsy. A variety of congenital anomalies have been observed.

The rescue of a few infants with this syndrome by prenatal detection and exchange transfusion has been reported. These babies have grown and developed normally, although they are blood-transfusion dependent.[207,208]

This condition is associated with a high incidence of maternal toxemia of pregnancy and difficulties at the time of delivery because of the massive placenta.[206] The reason for placental hypertrophy is unknown, although severe intrauterine hypoxia is suspected because a similar phenomenon is observed in hydrops infants with Rh incompatibility.

Hemoglobin H Disease

Hemoglobin H disease was described independently in the United States and in Greece in 1956.[209,210] The clinical findings are variable. A few patients are affected almost as severely as patients with β-thalassemia major, but most patients have a much milder course.[7,211] Lifelong anemia with variable splenomegaly occurs; bone changes are unusual.

As discussed earlier in "Etiology and Pathogenesis," a few attempts have been made to correlate the genotype with the phenotype of hemoglobin H disease. In general, as expected, patients with a nondeletion form of α-thalassemia affecting the predominant $\alpha 2$ gene interacting with an α^0-thalassemia determinant $\alpha^T\alpha/--$, or $\alpha^{ConstantSpring}\alpha/--$, for example, have higher hemoglobin H levels, a greater degree of anemia, and a more severe clinical course than patients with the $--/-\alpha$ genotype.[212–215]

Milder Forms of α-Thalassemia, Including the Traits $\alpha^T\alpha/--$ or $\alpha^{ConstantSpring}\alpha/--$

Because two α-globin genes exist per haploid genome, a wide spectrum of different conditions with overlapping phenotypes result from their various interactions.[7] The carrier states for the deletion and nondeletion forms of α-thalassemia, $-\alpha/\alpha\alpha$ and $\alpha^T\alpha/\alpha\alpha$, are symptomless. Similarly, the homozygous states for the deletion forms of α^+-thalassemia, $-\alpha/-\alpha$, and the heterozygous state for α^0-thalassemia, $--/\alpha\alpha$, are symptomless, although they are associated with mild anemia and red cell changes. On the other hand, the homozygous states for the nondeletion forms of α-thalassemia, $\alpha^T\alpha/\alpha^T\alpha$, are associated with an extremely diverse series of phenotypes. As mentioned in "Interactions of α-Thalassemia Haplotypes" above in "Etiology and Pathogenesis," they sometimes result in the clinical picture of hemoglobin H disease. In other patients, they are associated with only mild hypochromic anemia.[7] The homozygous states for the chain termination mutants, notably hemoglobin Constant Spring, constitute a special case because they produce a particularly characteristic phenotype. In this case, moderate hemolytic anemia with splenomegaly and characteristic hematologic findings are seen.[7,216,217]

α-Thalassemia and Mental Retardation

The clinical phenotype of these conditions associated with an intact α-globin locus is heterogeneous. In cases associated with chromosomal deletion (tip of chromosome 16; ATR-16), the clinical defects vary with the extent of chromosomal defect; only α-thalassemia and mental retardation are constant.[157]

The clinical phenotype in the second group of these disorders, which are caused by mutations of *ATR-X*, includes skeletal abnormalities, dysmorphic face, neonatal hypotonus, genital abnormalities, and a variety of less constant features, in addition to mental retardation and α-thalassemia.[158]

$\varepsilon\gamma\delta\beta$-Thalassemia

The clinical picture varies with the stage of development.[7] Neonates may be significantly anemic and require transfusions. In contrast, children and adults with this condition are asymptomatic. They have the clinical and laboratory picture of heterozygous β-thalassemia, with the exception of a normal hemoglobin A_2 level. The reason for this discrepancy of developmental differences of the clinical phenotype has not been identified. The homozygous state is assumed to be lethal.

LABORATORY FEATURES

■ β-THALASSEMIA MAJOR

Hemoglobin levels at presentation may range from 2 to 3 g/dL or even lower.[7] The red cells show marked anisopoikilocytosis, with hypochromia, target cell formation, and a variable degree of basophilic stippling (Fig. 47–16). The appearance of the blood film varies, depending on whether the spleen is intact. In nonsplenectomized patients, large poikilocytes are common. After splenectomy, large, flat macrocytes and

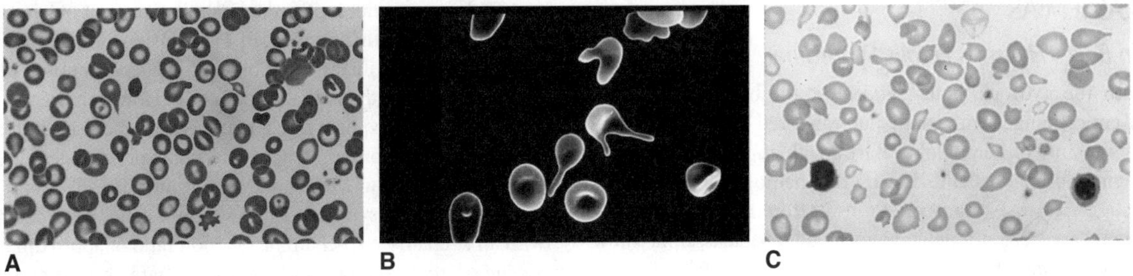

FIGURE 47–16. Blood films in β-thalassemia. **A.** β-Thalassemia minor. Anisocytosis. poikilocytosis. hypochromia. Occasional spherocytes and stomatocytes. **B.** Scanning electron micrograph of cells in **(A)** showing more detail of the poikilocytes. Note the knizocyte (pinch-bottle cell) at the lower right. **C.** β-Thalassemia major. Marked anisocytosis with many microcytes. Marked poikilocytosis. Anisochromia. Nucleated red cell on the right. Small lymphocyte on the left. *(Used with permission from* Lichtman's Atlas of Hematology, *www.accessmedicine.com.)*

small, deformed microcytes are frequently seen. The reticulocyte count is moderately elevated, and nucleated red cells nearly always are present in the blood. These red cell forms may reach very high levels after splenectomy. The white cell and platelet counts are slightly elevated unless secondary hypersplenism occurs. Staining of the blood with methyl violet, particularly in splenectomized subjects, reveals stippling or ragged inclusion bodies in the red cells.[169] These inclusions can nearly always be found in the red cell precursors in the marrow. The marrow usually shows erythroid hyperplasia with morphologic abnormalities of the erythroblasts, such as striking basophilic stippling and increased iron deposition. Iron kinetic studies indicate markedly ineffective erythropoiesis, and red cell survival usually is shortened. Populations of cells with very short survival and longer-lived populations of cells are seen. The latter contain relatively more fetal hemoglobin. An increased level of fetal hemoglobin, ranging from less than 10 percent to greater than 90 percent, is characteristic of homozygous β-thalassemia. No hemoglobin A is produced in β^0-thalassemia. The acid elution test shows that fetal hemoglobin is heterogeneously distributed among the red cells. Hemoglobin A_2 levels in homozygous β-thalassemia may be low, normal, or high. However, expressed as a proportion of hemoglobin A, the hemoglobin A_2 level almost invariably is elevated. Differential centrifugation studies indicate some heterogeneity of hemoglobin F and A_2 distribution among thalassemic red cells, but their level in whole blood gives little indication of their total rates of synthesis.

In vitro hemoglobin synthesis studies using marrow or blood show a marked degree of globin-chain imbalance. Marked excess of α-chain over β- and γ-chain production is always observed. Other aspects of the laboratory findings in this condition, including red cell survival, iron absorption, ferrokinetics, erythrokinetics, and the consequences of iron loading, were discussed earlier (see "Etiology and Pathogenesis" above).

The examination of siblings, parents, and children can be very important in confirming the diagnosis by finding the abnormalities in other family members, and the examining physician should make every effort to obtain a complete blood count in family members. With the exception of higher hemoglobin levels, the hematological changes in β-thalassemia intermedia are similar to those in β-thalassemia major (Fig. 47–17).

β-THALASSEMIA MINOR

Hemoglobin values of patients with β-thalassemia minor usually range from 9 to 11 g/dL. The most consistent finding is small, poorly hemoglobinized red cells (Fig. 47–16), resulting in mean cell hemoglobin (MCH) values of 20 to 22 pg and mean corpuscular volume (MCV) values of 50 to 70 fl. The red cell count is usually normal or elevated and the hemoglobin and hematocrit is usually slightly below normal; however, the red cell indices are particularly useful in screening for heterozygous carriers of thalassemia in population surveys. The marrow in heterozygous β-thalassemia shows slight erythroid hyperplasia with rare red cell inclusions. Megaloblastic transformation as a result of folic acid deficiency occurs occasionally, particularly during pregnancy. A mild degree of ineffective erythropoiesis is noted, but red cell survival is normal or nearly normal. The hemoglobin A_2 level is increased to 3.5 to 7 percent. The level of fetal hemoglobin is elevated in approximately 50 percent of cases, usually to 1 to 3 percent and rarely to greater than 5 percent.

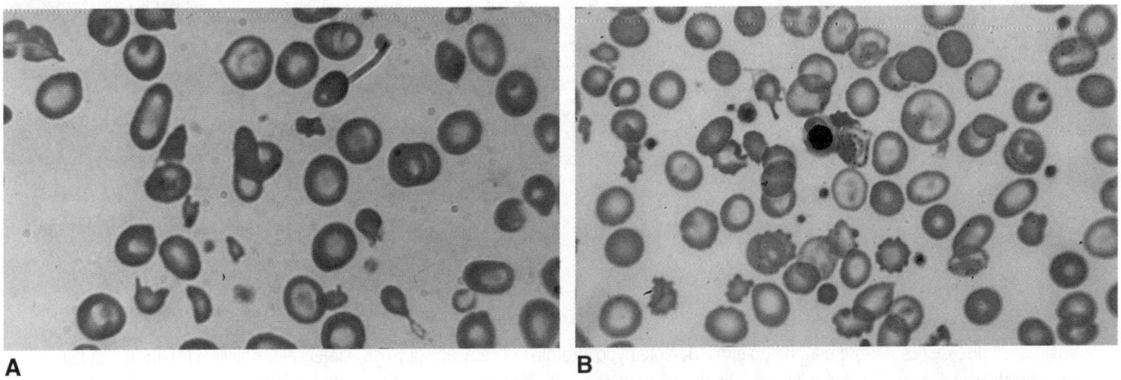

FIGURE 47–17. A. Thalassemia intermedia. Blood films. Marked anisocytosis, poikilocytosis with elliptical, oval, tear-drop-shaped, and fragmented red cells. Target cells. **B.** Postsplenectomy. Morphology similar to that in **(A)** but with a nucleated red cell, coarsely stippled cell in center of field, and large and numerous platelets, indicative of the changes superimposed by splenectomy. *(Used with permission from* Lichtman's Atlas of Hematology, *www.accessmedicine.com.)*

α-THALASSEMIAS

Hemoglobin Bart's Hydrops Fetalis Syndrome

In infants with the hydrops fetalis syndrome, the blood film shows severe thalassemic changes with many nucleated red cells. The hemoglobin consists mainly of hemoglobin Bart's, with approximately 10 to 20 percent hemoglobin Portland. Usually no hemoglobin A or F is present, although rare cases that seem to result from interaction of α^0-thalassemia with a severe nondeletion form of α^+-thalassemia show small amounts of hemoglobin A.

Hemoglobin H Disease

The blood film shows hypochromia and anisopoikilocytosis. The reticulocyte count usually is approximately 5 percent. Incubation of the red cells with brilliant cresyl blue results in ragged inclusion bodies in almost all cells. These bodies form because of precipitation of hemoglobin H *in vitro* as a result of redox action of the dye. After splenectomy, large, single Heinz bodies are observed in some cells (Fig. 47–18). These bodies are formed by *in vitro* precipitation of the unstable hemoglobin H molecule and are seen only after splenectomy. Hemoglobin H constitutes between 5 and 40 percent of the total hemoglobin. Traces of hemoglobin Bart's may be present, and the hemoglobin A_2 level usually is slightly subnormal.

α^0-Thalassemia and α^+-Thalassemia Traits

The α^0-thalassemia trait is characterized by the presence of 5 to 15 percent hemoglobin Bart's at birth.[7] This hemoglobin disappears during maturation and is not replaced by a similar amount of hemoglobin H. An occasional cell with hemoglobin H inclusion bodies may appear after incubation with brilliant cresyl blue. This phenomenon is often used as a diagnostic test for the α-thalassemia trait. However, the test is difficult to standardize and requires much experience to be useful. In adult life, the red cells of heterozygotes have morphologic changes of heterozygous thalassemia with low MCH and MCV values. The electrophoretic pattern is normal. Globin-synthesis studies show a deficit of α-chain production, with an α-chain–to–β-chain production ratio of approximately 0.7.

The α^+-thalassemia trait (–α/αα) is characterized by no or minimal hematologic changes, 1 to 2 percent of hemoglobin Bart's at birth in some but not all cases, and a slightly reduced α-chain–to–β-chain production ratio of approximately 0.8; thus, this genotype often is referred to as *silent carrier*. Extensive studies comparing the level of hemoglobin Bart's at birth with a DNA analyses demonstrated that there is no detectable hemoglobin Bart's in a significant number of newborns who are heterozygous for α^+-thalassemia.[218,219] Globin-gene synthetic ratios can be distinguished from normal only by studying relatively large numbers of samples and comparing the mean α-to-β ratio with that of normal control subjects. This approach is not reliable for diagnosing individual cases of the α^+-thalassemia trait, and, unfortunately, no reliable method of diagnosis is available except for DNA analysis.

Homozygous State for Nondeletion Types of α-Thalassemia

The homozygous state for nondeletion forms of α-thalassemia involving the dominant (α2) globin gene causes a more severe deficit of

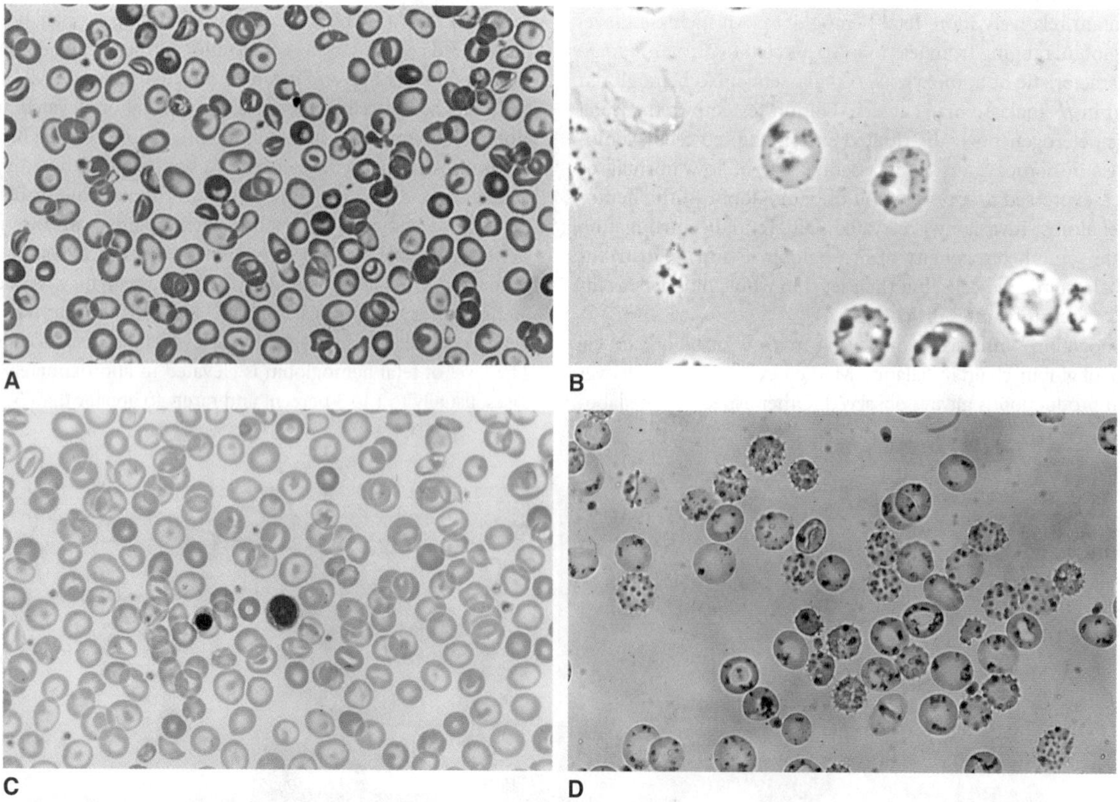

FIGURE 47–18. Hemoglobin H disease (α-thalassemia). Blood films. **A.** Note hypochromic red cells, anisocytosis, target cells, poikilocytes, including tear-drop-shaped red cells. **B.** Wet preparation stained with crystal violet. Inclusions in red cells (Heinz bodies) usually attached to membrane. **C.** Postsplenectomy. Note reduction in poikilocytes and frequency of target cells, a change consistent with hemoglobin H disease and enhanced by postsplenectomy effects. A nucleated red cell is in this field, reflecting an increase in their prevalence in the blood after splenectomy. **D.** Blood incubated for 90 minutes with brilliant cresyl blue. Numerous hemoglobin H intracellular precipitates (precipitates of excess β-globin chains). The frequent crenation is an artifact of the incubation conditions. *(Used with permission from* Lichtman's Atlas of Hematology, *www.accessmedicine.com.)*

α chains than do the deletion forms of α^+-thalassemia. In some cases, the homozygous state produces hemoglobin H disease. The homozygous state for hemoglobin Constant Spring or other chain-termination mutations is associated with moderately severe hemolytic anemia in which, for reasons not explained, no hemoglobin H is present but small amounts of hemoglobin Bart's persist into adult life. The homozygous states for the other nondeletion forms of α^+-thalassemia are associated with hemoglobin H disease.

In the homozygous state for hemoglobin Constant Spring, the blood picture shows mild thalassemic changes with normal-size red cells.[216,217] The hemoglobin consists of approximately 5 to 6 percent hemoglobin Constant Spring, normal hemoglobin A_2 levels, and trace amounts of hemoglobin Bart's. The remainder is hemoglobin A.

The heterozygous state for hemoglobin Constant Spring shows no hematologic abnormality. The hemoglobin pattern is normal except for the presence of approximately 0.5 percent hemoglobin Constant Spring. The latter can be observed on alkaline starch-gel electrophoresis as a faint band migrating between hemoglobin A_2 and the origin. It is best seen on heavily loaded starch gels and is easily missed if other electrophoretic techniques are used (Fig. 47–19). In the newborn, usually 1 to 3 percent hemoglobin Bart's is present in the cord blood.

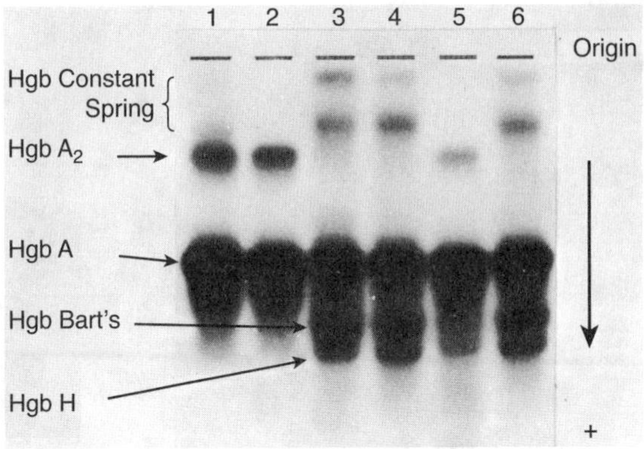

FIGURE 47–19. Hemoglobin Constant Spring. Starch gel electrophoresis of *1,2,* normal adult; *3,4,* compound heterozygotes for hemoglobin Constant Spring and α^0-thalassemia with hemoglobin H disease; *5,* normal adult; and *6,* compound heterozygote for α^0-thalassemia and hemoglobin Constant Spring.

Homozygous State for Deletion Forms of α^+-Thalassemia

The homozygous state for deletion forms of α^+-thalassemia is characterized by a thalassemic blood picture with 5 to 10 percent hemoglobin Bart's at birth and hematologic findings similar to those in α^0-thalassemia heterozygotes in adult life. In general, the $-\alpha^{4.2}$ deletion is associated with a more severe phenotype than is the $-\alpha^{3.7}$ deletion.[7]

DIFFERENTIAL DIAGNOSIS

The clinical and hematologic findings in homozygous β-thalassemia and hemoglobin H disease are so characteristic that the diagnosis usually is not difficult. Figure 47–20 shows a simple flowchart for laboratory investigations of a suspected case.

In early childhood, distinguishing the thalassemias from the congenital sideroblastic anemias may be difficult, but the marrow appearances in the latter are quite characteristic. Because of the high hemoglobin F levels encountered in juvenile chronic myelogenous leukemia, this disorder may superficially resemble β-thalassemia. However, the finding of primitive cells in the marrow, the absence of elevated hemoglobin A_2 levels on hemoglobin electrophoresis, the decrease in carbonic anhydrase in juvenile chronic myelogenous leukemia, and characteristic *in vitro* responses of myeloid progenitors *in vitro* to granulocyte-monocyte colony-stimulating factor (see Chap. 90) readily differentiate this disorder from β-thalassemia.

LESS COMMON FORMS OF THALASSEMIA

$(\delta\beta)^0$-THALASSEMIA

The homozygous state for $\delta\beta$-thalassemia is clinically milder than Cooley anemia and is one form of thalassemia intermedia.[220–222] Only hemoglobin F is present; hemoglobins A and A_2 are not produced. Heterozygous $\delta\beta$-thalassemia is hematologically similar to β-thalassemia minor.[7] The fetal hemoglobin level is higher (range: 5–20%), and the hemoglobin A_2 value is normal or slightly reduced. As in β-thalassemia, the fetal hemoglobin is heterogeneously distributed among the red cells, thus distinguishing this disorder from hereditary persistence of fetal hemoglobin (Fig. 47–21).

Heterozygosity for both β-thalassemia and $\delta\beta$-thalassemia results is a condition clinically similar to but milder than Cooley anemia. The hemoglobin consists largely of hemoglobin F, with a small amount of hemoglobin A_2. This finding is seen because the associated β-thalassemia gene has usually been the β^0 variety. $\delta\beta$-Thalassemia has also been observed in individuals heterozygous for hemoglobin S or C.[7]

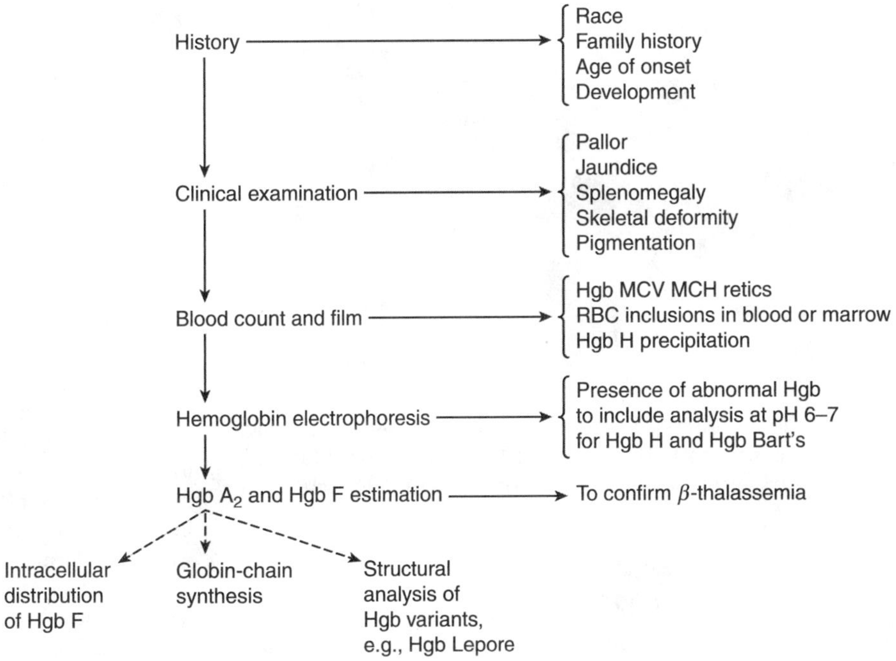

FIGURE 47–20. Flowchart showing an approach to diagnosis of the thalassemia syndromes. MCH, mean cell hemoglobin; MCV, mean corpuscular volume; RBC, red blood cell count.

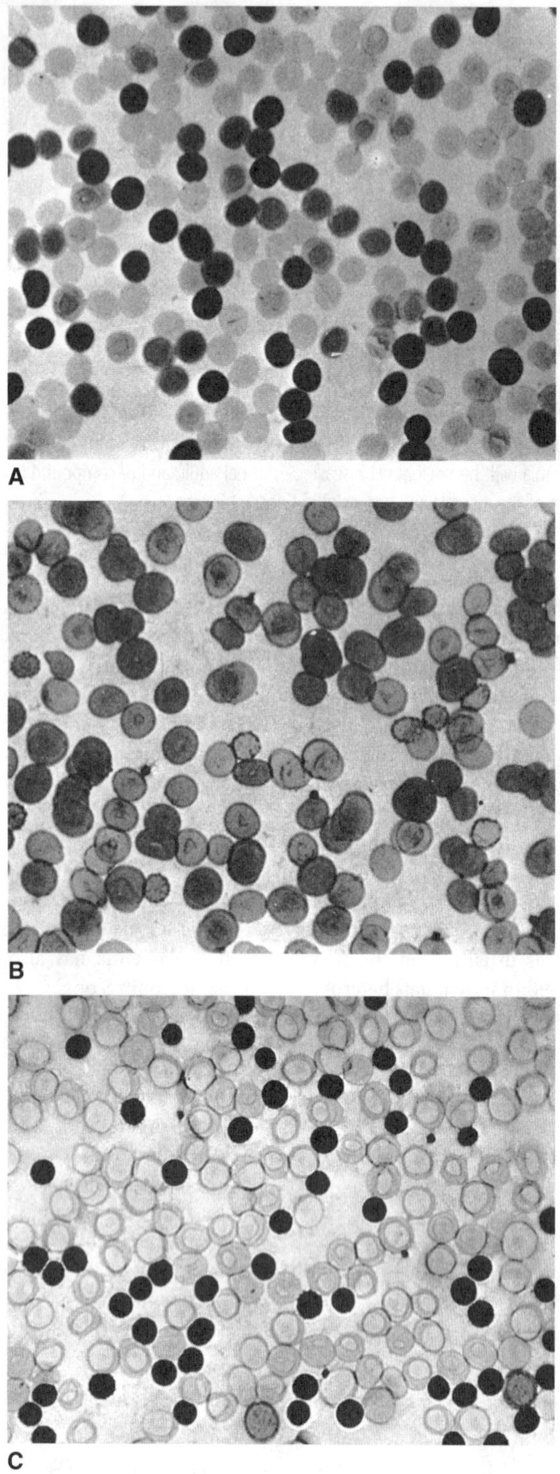

FIGURE 47–21. Acid elution preparations of blood films from **(A)** $\delta\beta$-thalassemia, **(B)** hereditary persistence of fetal hemoglobin, and **(C)** artificial mixture of fetal and adult red cells. The dark cells contain hemoglobin F. Hemoglobin F is resistant to acid elution.

$(\delta\beta)^+$-THALASSEMIA AND HEMOGLOBIN LEPORE DISORDERS

The hemoglobin Lepore disorders have been described in the homozygous state and in the heterozygous state, either alone or in association with β- or $\delta\beta$-thalassemia, hemoglobin S, or hemoglobin C.[7,9,223] In the homozygous state, approximately 20 percent of the hemoglobin is of the Lepore type and 80 percent is fetal hemoglobin. Hemoglobins A and A_2 are absent. The clinical picture is variable. Some cases are identical to transfusion-dependent homozygous β-thalassemia; others are associated with the clinical picture of thalassemia intermedia. In the heterozygous state, the findings are similar to those of β-thalassemia minor. The hemoglobin consists of approximately 10 percent hemoglobin Lepore, with a reduced level of hemoglobin A_2 and a slight but consistent increase in fetal hemoglobin level. The Lepore hemoglobins have been found sporadically in most racial groups. In the majority of cases, chemical analysis has shown that these hemoglobins are identical to hemoglobin Lepore Washington-Boston. Hemoglobin Lepore Hollandia and Lepore Baltimore have been observed in only a few patients.[7,223]

HEREDITARY PERSISTENCE OF FETAL HEMOGLOBIN

The current knowledge about the molecular pathology of HPFH was described earlier in "Etiology and Pathogenesis." Table 47–4 summarizes the currently accepted classification and nomenclature of this complex group of conditions. The different forms of HPFH are of very little clinical importance except that they may interact with thalassemia or the structural hemoglobin variants.

$(\delta\beta)^0$ HPFH

Homozygotes for $(\delta\beta)^0$ HPFH have 100 percent hemoglobin F. Their blood shows mild thalassemic changes, with reduced MCH and MCV values very similar to those observed in heterozygous β-thalassemia. Similarly, they have imbalanced globin chain production, with ratios in the range of those observed in β-thalassemia heterozygotes.[224] Heterozygotes have approximately 20 to 30 percent hemoglobin F, slightly reduced hemoglobin A_2 values, and completely normal blood pictures. Thus, this condition appears to be an extremely well-compensated form of $\delta\beta$-thalassemia in which the output of γ chains almost but not entirely compensates for the complete absence of β and δ chains. The different molecular forms of this condition show no difference in phenotype except in the proportion of $^{G}\gamma$ chains. The African forms of $(\delta\beta)^0$ HPFH have been found in association with hemoglobins S and C or with β-thalassemia (see Chap. 48). These compound heterozygous states are associated with little clinical disability.[7]

Nondeletion Types of HPFH

Many nondeletion forms of HPFH associated with point mutations upstream from the γ-globin genes have been described (see Table 47–4). $^{G}\gamma\beta^+$ HPFH has been found in the heterozygous and compound heterozygous states with β-globin chain variants in African populations. No associated clinical or hematologic findings have been reported. Compound heterozygotes for $^{G}\gamma\beta^+$ HPFH and hemoglobins S or C produce 45 percent of the abnormal hemoglobin, ~30 percent hemoglobin A, and ~20 percent hemoglobin F containing only $^{G}\gamma$ chains.[225,226]

The most common form of nondeletion HPFH is $^{A}\gamma\beta^+$ HPFH, which is found in Greeks.[227–229] In the homozygous state, no clinical or hematologic abnormalities are noted. The hemoglobin findings are characterized by approximately 25 percent fetal hemoglobin and reduced hemoglobin A_2 levels of approximately 0.8 percent.[230] Heterozygotes, who also are hematologically normal, have 10 to 15 percent hemoglobin F, almost all of the $^{A}\gamma$ variety. Compound heterozygotes with β-thalassemia have high hemoglobin F levels and a clinical picture that is only slightly more severe than the β-thalassemia trait.

In the British form of $^{A}\gamma\beta^+$ HPFH,[231] heterozygotes have approximately 5 to 12 percent hemoglobin F, whereas homozygotes have approximately

20 percent. No associated hematologic abnormalities are seen, although surprisingly in this form of nondeletion HPFH the hemoglobin F seems to be unevenly distributed among the red cells.

A heterogeneous group of conditions is associated with persistent production of small amounts of hemoglobin F in adult life. They are categorized under the general heading of *heterocellular HPFH*. Their clinical importance is that, when they are coinherited with different forms of β-thalassemia, they may lead to greater output of hemoglobin F and, hence, to a milder phenotype. This type of interaction should be suspected when one parent of a patient with β-thalassemia intermedia has an unusually high level of hemoglobin F for the β-thalassemia trait. Similarly, unaffected lateral relatives or other family members with slightly elevated hemoglobin F levels may be found.

β-THALASSEMIA ASSOCIATED WITH β-CHAIN STRUCTURAL HEMOGLOBIN VARIANTS

The most clinically important associations of β-thalassemia with β structural hemoglobin variants are sickle cell thalassemia, hemoglobin C thalassemia, and hemoglobin E thalassemia (see Chap. 48). In addition, many interactions of β-thalassemia with rare structural variants have been reported.[7,9,10]

Sickle cell thalassemia[7,232,233] occurs in parts of Africa and in the Mediterranean, particularly Greece and Italy. It also has been observed in the Middle East and parts of India. The clinical consequences of carrying one gene for hemoglobin S and one gene for β-thalassemia depend entirely on the type of β-thalassemia mutation. The interaction between the sickle cell gene and β^0-thalassemia is characterized by a clinical disorder that is very similar to sickle cell anemia. Similarly, the interaction of the sickle cell gene with the more severe forms of β^+-thalassemia associated with marked reduction in β-globin synthesis yields a similar clinical phenotype. On the other hand, the interaction of the sickle cell gene with very mild forms of β^+-thalassemia may be quite innocuous.[233] The latter disorder is characterized by mild anemia associated with splenomegaly and a hemoglobin composition of approximately 60 to 70 percent hemoglobin S, 25 percent hemoglobin A, and an elevated level of hemoglobin A_2. In all these interactions, one parent shows the sickle cell trait, and the other parent shows the β-thalassemia trait.

Hemoglobin C thalassemia is a mild hemolytic disorder associated with splenomegaly.[7,9,10] Again, the hemoglobin pattern varies depending on whether the thalassemia gene is the β^+ or β^0 type. This relatively innocuous condition has been recorded mainly in North Africa, but it also is found in West Africa. It is characterized by a mild hemolytic anemia and splenomegaly with a blood picture showing the numerous target cells characteristic of all the hemoglobin C disorders.

Hemoglobin E thalassemia, which occurs at a high frequency in the eastern half of the Indian subcontinent and throughout Southeast Asia, is one of the most important hemoglobinopathies in the world population.[7,9,10,234–240] As mentioned earlier in "Etiology and Pathogenesis," hemoglobin E is synthesized at a reduced rate and hence produces the clinical phenotype of a mild form of β-thalassemia. Hence, when hemoglobin E is inherited with β-thalassemia—and most often this is a β^0-or severe β^+-thalassemia mutation in Southeast Asia and India—a marked deficit of β-chain production results, with the clinical picture of severe β-thalassemia. Hemoglobin E thalassemia shows a remarkable variability in clinical expression,[234–238] ranging from a mild form of thalassemia intermedia to a transfusion-dependent condition clinically indistinguishable from homozygous β-thalassemia. The reasons for this variability of expression are not understood, although some of the factors involved are identical to those that modify other forms of β-thalassemia.[239,240]

In more severe cases of hemoglobin E thalassemia, severe anemia with growth retardation, leg ulcers, bone deformity, marked tendency to infection, iron loading, and variable splenomegaly and hypersplenism are seen. Large tumor masses composed of extramedullary erythropoietic tissue may cause a variety of compression syndromes, including a clinical picture that closely mimics a cerebral tumor. Another curious picture that seems to be restricted to splenectomized patients is an obliterative occlusion of the pulmonary vasculature that is believed to result from an extremely high platelet count.[241]

The clinical course and complications in transfusion-dependent patients are similar to those observed in homozygous β-thalassemia. In the milder forms, the main complications are progressive hypersplenism, organ damage as a result of progressive iron loading from an increased rate of absorption, extramedullary erythropoietic tumor masses, bone disease, and infection. The blood picture shows a typical thalassemic pattern. The hemoglobin consists of E, F, and A_2. Usually no hemoglobin A is present because the β^0-thalassemias are particularly common in the parts of the world where hemoglobin E is found.

Recent studies have emphasized the complex interactions between genetic factors,[239,240] differences in adaptation to anemia, particularly in early life (see "Pathophysiology" above) and the environment, notably proneness to malarial infection, that underlie the widely differing and unstable phenotypes of patients with hemoglobin E β-thalassemia.[238,239]

β-THALASSEMIA WITH NORMAL HEMOGLOBIN A_2 LEVEL

Rare forms of β-thalassemia are seen in which heterozygotes have normal hemoglobin A_2 levels. Their main clinical importance is that they can be confused with the more severe forms of α-thalassemia in the heterozygous state and therefore may cause difficulties in genetic counseling and prenatal diagnosis. Based on hematologic studies, two main classes of "normal hemoglobin A_2 β-thalassemia"—sometimes called types 1 and 2—are seen.[242] Type 1 is the "silent" form of β-thalassemia. Type 2 is heterogeneous, with many cases representing the compound heterozygous state for β-thalassemia and δ-thalassemia.

"Silent" β-thalassemia[7,243] is characterized by no hematologic changes in heterozygotes. Several mild forms of β-thalassemia that underlie this phenotype are described (see references 44, 45). Although this condition can be partly identified by demonstrating a mild degree of globin-chain imbalance, with α-to-β synthesis ratios of approximately 1.5:1, it can only be diagnosed with certainty by DNA analysis. Compound heterozygotes for this condition and β^0-thalassemia have a mild form of β-thalassemia intermedia.

Normal hemoglobin A_2 β-thalassemia type 2 in heterozygotes is indistinguishable from typical β-thalassemia with elevated hemoglobin A_2 levels.[242] The homozygous state has not been described. The compound heterozygous state for this gene and for β-thalassemia with raised hemoglobin A_2 levels is characterized by a clinical picture of severe transfusion-dependent β-thalassemia. Family data obtained in Italy and Sardinia suggest this condition represents the compound heterozygous state for both β-thalassemia and δ-thalassemia.[244,245] Most of the δ-thalassemias have been observed *trans* to β-thalassemia. However, the form of δ-thalassemia resulting from loss of an A in codon 59 occurs on the same chromosome as the hemoglobin Knossos mutation, which is associated with a mild form of β-thalassemia.[246] This finding explains the normal level of hemoglobin A_2 associated with this condition, which is the most common form of normal hemoglobin A_2 β-thalassemia in the Mediterranean region.

Several other conditions, mentioned earlier in this chapter in "Etiology and Pathogenesis," are associated with a phenotype that is indistinguishable from normal A_2 β-thalassemia. These conditions include the heterozygous states for the Corfu form of $\delta\beta$-thalassemia, and $\varepsilon\gamma\delta\beta$-thalassemia.

OTHER UNUSUAL FORMS OF β-THALASSEMIA

The clinical features of the dominant β-thalassemias resemble the features of thalassemia intermedia.[7] Moderate anemia and splenomegaly are seen, with a blood picture showing thalassemic red cell changes. The marrow shows erythroid hyperplasia with well-marked inclusion bodies in the red cell precursors. The latter may be seen in the blood after splenectomy. Hemoglobin analysis shows hemoglobins A and A_2 are present, and the hemoglobin F level is not usually elevated much higher than that seen in β-thalassemia trait. Hemoglobin A_2 levels are always raised.

Other unusual varieties of β-thalassemia include those categorized by unusually high hemoglobin F or A_2 levels. Most of these conditions result from deletions involving the β-globin gene and its promoter region. For example, the so-called Dutch[247] form of β-thalassemia is associated with unusually high hemoglobin F levels in heterozygotes and high hemoglobin A_2 levels. Several other conditions of this type, which result from different-size deletions, have been reported (see reference 7).

δ^0-THALASSEMIA

δ^0-Thalassemia causes a complete absence of hemoglobin A_2 in homozygotes and a reduced hemoglobin A_2 level in heterozygotes.[248] It is of no clinical significance except for its effect of reducing hemoglobin A_2 levels in β-thalassemia heterozygotes.

$\varepsilon\gamma\delta\beta$-THALASSEMIA

This heterogeneous condition has been observed only in the heterozygous state in a few families.[7,108,109] It is characterized by neonatal hemolysis and, in adult life, by the hematologic picture of heterozygous β-thalassemia with normal hemoglobin A_2 levels.

α-THALASSEMIA IN ASSOCIATION WITH α- AND β-CHAIN HEMOGLOBIN VARIANTS

Several α-globin structural variants are caused by single amino acid substitutions at α-chain loci on chromosomes that carry only a single α-chain gene. Individuals who inherit variants of this type and an α^0-thalassemia determinant have a form of hemoglobin H disease in which the hemoglobin consists of the α-chain variant hemoglobin and hemoglobin H. Well-documented examples include hemoglobin QH disease ($- -/-\alpha^{Q}$),[249,250] hemoglobin G Philadelphia H disease ($- -/-\alpha^{G}$),[251,252] and hemoglobin Hasharon H disease ($- -/-\alpha^{Hash}$).[253] Many examples of the coexistence of the homozygous or heterozygous states for β-chain hemoglobin variants and different α-thalassemia determinants have been reported.[7,9,10] Particularly well-characterized disorders include the various interactions of α^0- and α^+-thalassemia with hemoglobin E[7,234] and hemoglobin S (see Chap. 48).[254,255] Carriers for these hemoglobin variants who also have the α^0- or α^+-thalassemia traits have thalassemic red cell indices and unusually low levels of the abnormal hemoglobin. Individuals with sickle cell anemia who have α-thalassemia show thalassemic red cell changes, more persistent splenomegaly, and lower hemoglobin F values than do patients without the thalassemia genes.

THERAPY, COURSE, AND PROGNOSIS

The only forms of treatment available for thalassemic children are regular blood transfusions, iron chelation therapy in an attempt to prevent iron overload, judicious use of splenectomy in cases complicated by hypersplenism, and a good standard of general pediatric care.[7,9,256] Marrow transplantation has an important role in selected cases (see Chap. 21).

TRANSFUSION

Children with β-thalassemia who are maintained at a hemoglobin level of 9.5 to 14 g/dL grow and develop normally. They do not develop the distressing skeletal complications of thalassemia.[7,256] Maintaining a lower hemoglobin level than this range without any deleterious effects on development and with the added advantage of reducing the level of iron loading may be possible. This regimen maintains a mean pretransfusion level that does not exceed 9.5 g/dL.[257] A transfusion program should not be started too early, and it should be initiated only when the hemoglobin level is too low to be compatible with normal development. If transfusion is started too soon, thalassemia intermedia may be missed, and the child may be transfused unnecessarily. Usually blood transfusions are given every 4 weeks on an outpatient basis. To avoid transfusion reactions, washed, filtered, or frozen red cells should be used so that the majority of the white cells and plasma-protein components are removed (see Chap. 140).

IRON CHELATION

Every child who is maintained on a high-transfusion regimen ultimately develops iron overload and dies of siderosis of the myocardium. Therefore, such children must be started on a program of iron chelation within the first 2 to 3 years of life.[256] Despite extensive searches for an oral chelating agent, deferoxamine (desferrioxamine) is currently the only drug of proven long-term value for treatment of thalassemia. It is best administered by an 8- to 12-hour overnight pump-driven infusion in the subcutaneous tissues of the anterior abdominal wall.[258,259] Chelation therapy should commence by the time the serum ferritin level reaches approximately 1000 mcg/dL. In practice, this level usually is seen after the 12th to 15th transfusion. To prevent toxicity, infants must not be overchelated when the iron burden is still low. The initial dose usually is 20 mg/kg 5 nights per week, with 100 mg of oral vitamin C (200 mg in older children and adults) on the day of infusion, after the infusion has been initiated.[259] Some evidence and widespread opinion indicate ascorbate precipitates myocardiopathy in these patients if it is given before deferoxamine infusion is started.[260,261] In patients who are heavily iron loaded, particularly those patients with cardiac or endocrine complications, the body iron stores can be effectively lowered by continuous intravenous infusion of deferoxamine at a dose of up to 50 mg/kg body weight. The procedure usually entails insertion of an intravenous delivery system.

Extensive experience with the use of deferoxamine and its toxic effects has been reported.[189] No serious complications occur other than local erythema and painful subcutaneous nodules at the site of infusions and extremely rare severe allergic reactions. These reactions can be controlled, at least in part, by including 5 to 10 mg hydrocortisone in the infusion. Probably of greatest concern is neurosensory toxicity, which has been documented in up to 30 percent of cases. Toxicity causes high-frequency hearing loss that may become symptomatic.[262,263] In a few cases, the toxicity did not respond to discontinuation of the drug, and permanent hearing loss resulted. Ocular toxicity has been reported.[262] Symptoms include visual failure, night and color blindness, and field loss. Reversal of symptoms after discontinuation of the drug has been reported. Deferoxamine may cause bone changes and growth retardation, sometimes associated with bone pain. Body measurements characteristically show a reduced crown-pubis–to–pubis-heel ratio.[264] These changes may be associated with radiologic abnormalities of the vertebral column. These complications can be prevented by exercising extreme care in monitoring patients receiving long-term desferrioxamine therapy. Young children or individuals from whom most of the iron has been removed by chelation are at particularly high risk. Formal audiometry and ophthalmologic examinations at 6-month intervals are recommended.

Because of the practical difficulties of a nightly subcutaneous infusion of deferoxamine there has been an intensive search for effective oral chelating drugs. Two of these agents are currently available, deferiprone (Ferriprox, L1) and deferasirox. The extensive literature on these agents has been reviewed.[265–267] Deferiprone is administered at a dosage of 75 mg/kg in three daily doses. Unfortunately there have been limited numbers of long-term trials comparing its efficacy with desferrioxamine, but overall it appears to be less effective than desferrioxamine at maintaining safe body iron levels. Its administration is accompanied by a number of complications, the most important of which is neutropenia and, in some cases, agranulocytosis with some fatalities. Hence it is recommended that patients receiving this agent have a weekly white cell count. It also causes arthritis which varies in severity and between different ethnic groups. However, by virtue of its membrane-crossing capacity it has been suggested that it may be more effective in removing cardiac iron. Unfortunately, to date, all the studies that suggest that it may reduce the frequency of cardiac complications in transfusion-dependent thalassemics have been retrospective and there are no long-term controlled data available. It is currently suggested that it should be used in combination with desferrioxamine, particularly for its cardiac-iron sparing effect; again, long-term prospective data are required to confirm this interesting suggestion.

The initial studies of deferasirox were promising[266] and suggested that this agent in doses of 5 or 10 mg/kg per day, or higher in those who are heavily iron-loaded, was as effective as desferrioxamine in containing adequate hepatic iron levels. Preliminary clinical studies also showed that this agent may be effective for removing excess cardiac iron. Recent followup data have confirmed these early observations.[267] The most frequent adverse reactions to deferasirox included gastrointestinal disturbances, transient rashes, and a nonprogressive increase in serum creatinine. It is still too early to be sure about the overall effectiveness of this agent, however, or to assess its long-term safety.

Because of the extremely well-documented data showing long-term survival or patients adequately treated with deferoxamine,[268–270] this agent is still recommended as the first-line choice for management of transfusion-dependent thalassemia. The true role of combination therapy of deferoxamine and deferiprone, or deferasirox as a single agent, still remain to be determined by careful prospective studies.

Careful monitoring of the degree of iron accumulation during chelation therapy is absolutely vital. The simplest approach, particularly in countries where most sophisticated technology is not available, is a regular estimation of the serum ferritin level, which should be maintained at less than 1500 mcg/L. The value of hepatic iron concentration assessment was discussed earlier in "Abnormal Iron Metabolism." Newer noninvasive approaches to assessing body iron burden have been developed. There is now strong evidence that, with adequate calibration, the measurement and mapping of liver iron concentrations using magnetic resonance imaging (MRI) is an extremely effective approach for the regular assessment of the effectiveness of chelation therapy.[271] Similarly, there have been advances in the noninvasive estimation of myocardial iron using T2* MRI. Evidence obtained using this approach suggests that there may be a variable correlation between hepatic and cardiac iron concentrations.[272] Clearly functional cardiologic studies should be combined with assessment of cardiac iron levels, particularly the ejection fraction, pulmonary artery pressure, and other parameters of cardiac activity. The true value of these new approaches to assessing myocardial iron levels and function require further study by prospective controlled trials.

Increasing evidence indicates children maintained at a high hemoglobin level do not develop hypersplenism.[7] However, enlargement of the spleen with increased transfusion requirements occurs commonly in patients maintained at a lower hemoglobin level. Splenectomy should be performed if transfusion requirements increase dramatically or pain develops because of the size of the spleen. Because of the risk of overwhelming pneumococcal infections, splenectomy should not be performed in children younger than age 5 years. These children should receive a pneumococcal vaccine prior to the procedure. They then should be placed on prophylactic oral penicillin after the operation. *Haemophilus influenzae* type B and meningococcal vaccines also are recommended.

Children with severe thalassemia are still prone to other infections. Presentation with abdominal pain, diarrhea, and vomiting should always suggest an infection with a member of the *Yersinia* class of bacteria. Empirical treatment should start immediately with either an aminoglycoside or a cotrimoxazole. Transfusion-transmitted virus infection is common in some populations. All chronically transfused patients should be tested annually for hepatitis C, hepatitis B, and HIV. Patients with serologic evidence of chronic active hepatitis should be considered for treatment with interferon-α and ribavirin.

As mentioned earlier in "Abnormal Iron Metabolism," subtle endocrine deficiencies are increasingly recognized, particularly those associated with growth retardation and hypogonadism. These patients require expert endocrinologic assessment and replacement therapy when appropriate.

STEM CELL TRANSPLANTATION

By 1997, more than 1000 marrow transplants had been performed at three centers in Italy.[273–276] Based on this experience and on later data,[7] the prognosis evidently depended on the adequacy of iron chelation up to the time of transplantation. Hence, patients were divided into three classes: class I patients had a history of adequate iron chelation and neither liver fibrosis nor hepatomegaly; class II patients had one or two of these characteristics; and class III patients had all three characteristics. Among children in class I who had undergone transplantation early in the course of the disease, disease-free survival was assessed at 90 to 93 percent at 5 years, with a 4 percent risk of mortality related to the procedure. For class II patients, the intermediate-risk group, the survival and disease-free survival rates were 86 percent and 82 percent, respectively. For class III, the high-risk group, the survival and disease-free survival rates were 62 percent and 51 percent, respectively. Apart from the immediate complications of severe infection in the posttransplantation period, most of the problems were related to development of acute or chronic graft-versus-host disease. The overall frequency of mild to severe grades ranges from 27 to 30 percent.[277] Modification of preparative drug regimens has reduced the frequency of drug toxicity. The occurrence of mixed chimerism may be a risk factor for graft-versus-host disease. No case of hematologic malignancy has been observed in the longest followup of patients between 15 and 20 years after transplantation. Recent experience has fully confirmed these pioneering studies.[278] The current status of blood stem cell therapy has been reviewed[278] and is discussed further in Chap. 28.

GENERAL CARE

Management of thalassemia requires a high standard of general pediatric care. Infection should be treated early. If the diet is deficient in folate, supplements should be given. Supplementation probably is unnecessary in children maintained on a high-transfusion regimen. Particular attention should be paid to the ear, nose, and throat because of chronic sinus infection and middle-ear diseases resulting from bone deformity of the skull. Similarly, regular dental surveillance is essential because poorly transfused thalassemic children have a variety of deformities of the maxilla and poorly developed teeth. In the later stages of the illness, when iron loading becomes the major feature, endocrine replacement therapy may be necessary. Symptomatic treatment for metabolic bone disease and cardiac failure also may be needed.

THERAPIES OF SPECIAL TYPES OF THALASSEMIA

Hemoglobin H disease usually requires no specific therapy, although splenectomy may be of value in cases associated with severe anemia and splenomegaly.[7,9,10] Because splenectomy may be followed by a higher incidence of thromboembolic disease than occurs in splenectomized children with β-thalassemia,[7] the spleen should be removed only in cases of extreme anemia and splenomegaly. Oxidant drugs should not be given to patients with hemoglobin H disease. The management of symptomatic sickle cell thalassemia follows the lines described for sickle cell anemia (see Chap. 48).

Thalassemia intermedia presents a particularly complex therapeutic problem. Whether a child with a steady-state hemoglobin level of 6 to 7 g/dL should be transfused is difficult to determine with certainty. Probably the best compromise is to watch such children very closely during the first years of life. If they grow and develop normally and no signs of bone changes are evident, they should be maintained without transfusion. If, however, their early growth pattern is retarded or their activity is limited because of their anemia, they should be placed on a regular transfusion regimen. If hypersplenism plays a role in their anemia as the children grow older, splenectomy should be performed. Because many of these patients have significant iron loading from the gastrointestinal tract, regular estimations of serum iron and ferritin should be obtained and chelation therapy instituted when appropriate.

EXPERIMENTAL APPROACHES TO TREATMENT

Two main experimental approaches are being pursued in the search for more effective therapy of the thalassemias: (1) reactivation or augmentation of fetal hemoglobin production and (2) somatic gene therapy.

The main rationale for employing agents that have been used in attempts to increase hemoglobin F production is based on the observation that patients recovering from cytotoxic drug therapy or during other periods of erythroid expansion may reactivate hemoglobin F synthesis. In addition, the observation that butyrate analogues might have a stimulating effect on hemoglobin F production has led to a number of studies of their potential for management of thalassemia. A number of clinical trials have been performed.[279–282] Agents that have been used include various cytotoxic drugs, erythropoietin, and several different butyrate analogues. Overall, these agents, used alone or in combination, have produced some small effects on fetal hemoglobin production, but the results of these trials have been disappointing. Some notable exceptions were seen, however, particularly several cases of homozygosity or compound heterozygosity for hemoglobin Lepore in which use of either a combination of sodium phenylbutyrate and hydroxyurea or hydroxyurea alone produced a spectacular rise in hemoglobin F production. In the case of two homozygotes for hemoglobin Lepore, the necessity for further transfusion was eliminated.[283] This finding raises the intriguing possibility that certain mutations, possibly deletions of the β-globin gene cluster, are more susceptible to this type of approach.

The other experimental approach involves somatic gene therapy. Currently the therapy is mainly directed at gene transfer into potential hematopoietic stem cells using retroviral vectors.[284] Other approaches also are being taken, including attempts at the restoration of normal splicing in cases of splicing mutations[285] and use of *trans*-splicing ribozymes to correct β-globin gene transcripts.[286] However, studies using murine models with recombinant lentiviral vectors suggest that sustained, high-level globin gene expression may be possible, at least in this experimental system.[287,288] Although there continues to be slow progress toward somatic-cell gene therapy as applied to the hemoglobin disorders,[282,289] and clinical trials are imminent, it is still not clear how long this novel approach will take to reach the clinic.

PROGNOSIS

The prognosis for patients with severe forms of β-thalassemia who are adequately treated by transfusion and chelation has improved dramatically over the years. Three large studies investigated the influence of effective long-term desferrioxamine use on the development of cardiac disease.[268–270] In one study, patients who had maintained sustained reduction of body iron, as estimated by a serum ferritin level less than 2500 mcg/L over 12 years of followup, had an estimated cardiac disease-free survival rate of 91 percent. This finding is in contrast to patients in whom most determinations of serum ferritin level exceeded this value, in whom the estimated cardiac disease-free survival rate was less than 20 percent. In a second study, the relationship between survival and total-body iron burden was measured directly using hepatic storage iron values. Patients who had maintained hepatic iron concentrations of at least 15 mg of iron per gram of liver, dry weight, had a 32 percent probability of survival to age 25 years. No cardiac disease developed in patients who maintained hepatic iron levels below this threshold. These and other studies provide unequivocal evidence that adequate transfusion and chelation are associated with longevity and good quality of life. On the other hand, poor compliance or unavailability of chelating agents still is associated with a poor prospect of survival much beyond the second decade.

PREVENTION

In parts of the world where the incidence of thalassemia is high, the disease places an immense economic burden on society. For example, if all the thalassemic children born in Cyprus were treated by regular blood transfusions and iron chelating therapy, it was estimated that within 15 years the total medical budget of the island would be required to treat this single disease.[290] Clearly, this approach was not feasible, so considerable effort was directed toward developing programs for prevention of the different forms of thalassemia.

The goal of prevention can be achieved in two ways. The first is prospective genetic counseling, that is, screening total populations while the children still are at school and warning carriers about the potential risks of marriage to another carrier. Few data are available about the value of programs of this type; a pilot study in Greece was unsuccessful.[291] Because it is believed this approach will not be successful in many populations, considerable effort has been directed toward developing prenatal diagnosis programs.

Prenatal diagnosis for prevention of thalassemia entails screening mothers at the first prenatal visit, screening the father in cases in which the mother is α-thalassemia carrier, and offering the couple the possibility of prenatal diagnosis and termination of pregnancy if both mother and father are carriers of a gene for a severe form of thalassemia. Currently, these programs are devoted mainly to prenatal diagnosis of the severe transfusion-dependent forms of homozygous β^+ or β^0-thalassemia. Considerable experience has been gained in prenatal diagnosis of mothers at risk for having a fetus with the hemoglobin Bart hydrops syndrome, considering the distress caused by a long and difficult pregnancy and the obstetric problems resulting from the birth of a hydropic infant with a massive placenta.

The first efforts at prenatal detection of β-thalassemia utilized fetal blood sampling and globin-chain synthesis analysis carried out at approximately week 18 of pregnancy. Despite the technical difficulties involved, the method was applied successfully in many countries and resulted in a reduced birth rate of infants with β-thalassemia.[292] The technique is associated with a low maternal morbidity rate, a fetal mortality rate of approximately 3 to 4 percent, and an error rate of 1 to 2 percent. Its main disadvantage is that it must be carried out relatively late in pregnancy. For this reason, efforts turned to first trimester prenatal diagnosis.

DNA technology has enabled diagnosis of important hemoglobin disorders *in utero* by fetal DNA analysis. Although analysis can be carried out on DNA derived from amniotic fluid, the approach has drawbacks because, again, it must be done relatively late in pregnancy, and often amniotic fluid cells must be grown in culture to obtain a sufficient amount of DNA.[293] However, DNA can be obtained as early as week 9 of pregnancy by chorionic villus sampling. Although the safety of this technique remains to be fully evaluated and limb reduction deformities may occur when the procedure is carried out very early in pregnancy (9 or 10 weeks), chorionic villus sampling has become the major method for prenatal diagnosis of the thalassemias based on subsequent experience with the technique.[7,293–297]

Remarkable advances in DNA technology have provided a variety of methods for the direct identification of mutations in fetal DNA.[7] Even in families with extremely rare mutations, rapid DNA sequencing technology allows a diagnosis to be made very rapidly. The error rate using these different approaches varies, mainly depending on the experience of the particular laboratory; low rates, less than 1 percent, are reported from most centers. Potential sources of error include maternal contamination of fetal DNA and nonpaternity.

The application of this new technology has caused a major reduction in the birth rate of infants with thalassemia throughout the Mediterranean region and the Middle East, and in parts of the Indian subcontinent and Southeast Asia. Several approaches continue to be explored in an attempt to avoid the use of invasive procedures like chorion villous sampling. A variety of methods are being used to harvest fetal DNA from fetal cells in maternal blood or from maternal plasma[298,299] and there are increasing numbers of attempts at preimplantation diagnosis of thalassemias.[300,301] There is every expectation that some of these approaches will reach the clinic in the near future.[302]

THALASSEMIA AS A GLOBAL HEALTH PROBLEM

The remarkable advances in the diagnosis, prevention, and treatment of the thalassemias described in this chapter are only relevant to the richer countries of the world. In many developing countries in which there is a very high frequency of thalassemia, there are very limited facilities for their diagnosis and management. Because many of these countries are going through the epidemiologic transition, which involves improvements in nutrition, cleaner water supplies, and better public health services, babies with serious forms of thalassemia who previously would have died of infection or profound anemia are now surviving to present for treatment.

Approaches to the better control and management of the thalassemias in poor countries have been reviewed.[303,304] They include the development of partnerships between centers in the rich and poor countries for training workers in this field, and, once these are developed, for the further evolution of partnerships between those poorer countries where there is knowledge and expertise of the field with those where no knowledge or facilities exist. Without organizations along these lines the thalassemias will continue to cause the premature death of hundreds of thousands of infants worldwide.

REFERENCES

1. Cooley TB, Lee P: A series of cases of splenomegaly in children with anemia and peculiar bone changes. *Trans Am Pediatr Soc* 37:29, 1925.
2. Whipple GH, Bradford WL: Racial or familial anemia of children associated with fundamental disturbances of bone and pigment metabolism (Cooley von Jaksch). *Am J Dis Child* 44:336, 1932.
3. Whipple CH, Bradford WL: Mediterranean disease—Thalassemia (erythroblastic anemia of Cooley): Associated pigment abnormalities simulating hemochromatosis. *J Pediatr* 9:279, 1936.
4. Weatherall DJ: Toward an understanding of the molecular biology of some common inherited anemias: The story of thalassemia, in *Blood, Pure and Eloquent*, edited by MM Wintrobe, p 373. McGraw-Hill, New York, 1980.
5. Bannerman RM: *Thalassemia: A Survey of Some Aspects*. Grune & Stratton, New York, 1961.
6. Chernoff AI: The distribution of the thalassemia gene: A historical review. *Blood* 14:899, 1959.
7. Weatherall DJ, Clegg JB: *The Thalassaemia Syndromes*, 4th ed. Blackwell, Oxford, 2001.
8. Ingram VM, Stretton AOW: Genetic basis of the thalassemia diseases. *Nature* 184:1903, 1959.
9. Steinberg MH, Forget BG, Higgs DR, Weatherall DJ: *Disorders of Hemoglobin*, 2nd ed. Cambridge University Press, Cambridge, UK, 2009.
10. Weatherall DJ, Clegg JB, Higgs DR, Wood WG: The hemoglobinopathies, in *The Metabolic and Molecular Bases of Inherited Disease*, 8th ed, edited by CR Scriver, AL Beauder, WS Sly, D Valle, p 4571. McGraw-Hill, New York, 2001.
11. Weatherall DJ, Clegg JB: Inherited haemoglobin disorders: An increasing global health problem. *Bull World Health Organ* 79:704, 2001.
12. Christianson A, Howson CP, Modell B: *March of Dimes Global Report on Birth Defects*. March of Dimes Birth Defects Foundation, New York, 2006.
13. Haldane JBS: The rate of mutation of human genes. *Hereditas* 35(Suppl):267, 1949.
14. Orkin SH, Kazazian HH: The mutation and polymorphism of the human β-globin gene and its surrounding DNA. *Annu Rev Genet* 18:131, 1984.
15. Orkin SH, Antonarakis SE, Kazazian HH: Polymorphisms and molecular pathology of the human β-globin gene. *Prog Hematol* 13:49, 1983.
16. Siniscalco M, Bernini L, Filippi G, et al: Population genetics of haemoglobin variants, thalassemia and glucose-6-phosphate dehydrogenase deficiency, with particular reference to malaria hypothesis. *Bull World Health Organ* 34:379, 1966.
17. Flint J, Hill AVS, Bowden DK, et al: High frequencies of α thalassemia are the result of natural selection by malaria. *Nature* 321:744, 1986.
18. Allen SJ, O'Donnell A, Alexander NDE, et al: α^+-Thalassemia protects children against disease due to malaria and other infections. *Proc Natl Acad Sci U S A* 94:14736, 1997.
19. Williams TN: Red blood cell defects and malaria. *Mol Biochem Parasitol* 149:121, 2006.
20. Williams TN, Mwangi TW, Wambua S, et al: Negative epistasis between the malaria-protective effects of alpha+-thalassemia and the sickle cell trait. *Nat Genet* 37:1253, 2005.
21. Williams TN, Maitland K, Bennett S, et al: High incidence of malaria in α-thalassemic children. *Nature* 383:522, 1996.
22. Cockburn IA, Mackinnon MJ, O'Donnell A, et al: A human complement receptor 1 polymorphism that reduces *Plasmodium falciparum* rosetting confers protection against severe malaria. *Proc Natl Acad Sci U S A* 101:272, 2004.
23. Weatherall DJ: Genetic variation and susceptibility to infection: the red cell and malaria. *Br J Haematol* 141:276, 2008.
24. Kwiatkowski DP: How malaria has affected the human genome and what human genetics can teach us about malaria. *Am J Hum Genet* 77:171, 2005.
25. Orkin SH: The duplicated human α globin genes lie close together in cellular DNA. *Proc Natl Acad Sci U S A* 75:5950, 1978.
26. Lauer J, Shen C-KJ, Maniatis T: The chromosomal arrangement of human α-like globin genes: Sequence homology and α-globin gene deletions. *Cell* 20:119, 1980.
27. Liebhaber SA, Goossens N, Kan YW: Homology and concerted evolution at the α_1 and α_2 loci of human α-globin. *Nature* 290:26, 1981.
28. Liebhaber SA, Goossens MJ, Kan YW: Cloning and complete nucleotide sequence of human 5′-α-globin gene. *Proc Natl Acad Sci U S A* 77:7054, 1980.
29. Proudfoot NJ, Maniatis T: The structure of a human α-globin pseudo-gene and its relationship to α-globin duplication. *Cell* 21:537, 1980.
30. Liebhaber SA, Kan YW: Differentiation of the mRNA transcripts originating from the α_1- and α_2-globin loci in normals and α-thalassemics. *J Clin Invest* 68:439, 1981.
31. Orkin SH, Goff SC: The duplicated human α-globin genes: Their relative expression as measured by RNA analysis. *Cell* 24:345, 1981.
32. Higgs DR, Wainscoat JS, Flint J, et al: Analysis of the human α globin gene cluster reveals a highly informative genetic locus. *Proc Natl Acad Sci U S A* 83:5156, 1986.
33. Fritsch EF, Lawn RM, Maniatis T: Molecular cloning and characterization of the human β-like globin gene cluster. *Cell* 19:959, 1980.
34. Spritz RA, DeRiel JK, Forget BG, Weissman SM: Complete nucleotide sequence of the human δ-globin gene. *Cell* 21:639, 1980.
35. Baralle FE, Shoulders CC, Proudfoot NJ: The primary structure of the human ε globin gene. *Cell* 21:621, 1980.
36. Slightom JL, Blechl AE, Smithies O: Human $^G\gamma$- and $^A\gamma$-globin genes: Complete nucleotide sequences suggest that DNA can be exchanged between these duplicated genes. *Cell* 21:627, 1980.
37. Jeffrey AJ: DNA sequences in the $^G\gamma$-, $^A\gamma$-, δ-, and β-globin genes of man. *Cell* 18:1, 1979.
38. Antonarakis SE, Boehm CD, Giardina PVJ, Kazazian HH: Nonrandom association of polymorphic restriction sites in the β-globin gene complex. *Proc Natl Acad Sci U S A* 79:137, 1982.
39. Wainscoat JS, Hill AVV, Boyce A, et al: Evolutionary relationships of human populations from an analysis of nuclear DNA polymorphisms. *Nature* 319:491, 1982.

40. Orkin SH: Transcription factors that regulate lineage decisions, in *The Molecular Basis of Blood Disease*, 3rd ed, edited by G Stamatoyannopoulos, PW Majerus, RM Perlmutter, H Varmus, p 80. Saunders, Philadelphia, 1994.
41. Higgs DR, Weatherall DJ: The alpha thalassaemias. *Cell Mol Life Sci* 66:1154, 2008.
42. Bank A: Regulation of human fetal hemoglobin: New players, new complexities. *Blood* 107:435, 2006.
43. Donze D, Townes TM, Bieker JJ: Role of erythroid Kruppel-like factor in human gamma- to beta-globin gene switching. *J Biol Chem* 270:1955, 1995.
44. Thein SL, Wood WG: The molecular basis of β thalassemia, $\delta\beta$ thalassemia, and hereditary persistence of fetal hemoglobin, in *Disorders of Hemoglobin* 2nd ed, edited by MH Steinberg, BG Forget, DR Higgs, DJ Weatherall, p 323. Cambridge University Press, Cambridge, UK, 2009.
45. Higgs DR: The molecular basis of α thalassemia, in *Disorders of Hemoglobin* 2nd ed, edited by MH Steinberg, BG Forget, DR Higgs, DJ Weatherall, p 241. Cambridge University Press, Cambridge, UK, 2009.
46. Giardine B, van Baal S, Kaimakis P, et al: HbVar database of human hemoglobin variants and thalassemia mutations: 2007 Update. *Hum Mutat* 28:206, 2007.
47. Orkin SH, Old JM, Weatherall DJ, Nathan DG: Partial deletion of β-globin gene DNA in certain patients with β^0-thalassemia. *Proc Natl Acad Sci U S A* 76:2400, 1979.
48. Thein SL, Old JM, Wainscoat JS, Weatherall DJ: Population and genetic studies suggest a single origin for the Indian deletion β^0 thalassaemia. *Br J Haematol* 57:271, 1984.
49. Anand R, Boehm CD, Kazazian HH, Vanin EF: Molecular characterization of a β^0-thalassemia resulting from a 1.4-kb deletion. *Blood* 72:636, 1988.
50. Padanilam BJ, Felice AE, Huisman THJ: Partial deletion of the 5′ β globin gene region causes β^0 thalassemia in members of an American Black family. *Blood* 64:941, 1984.
51. Popovich BW, Rosenblatt DS, Kendall AG, Nishioka Y: Molecular characterization of an atypical β thalassemia caused by a large deletion in the 5′ β-globin gene region. *Am J Hum Genet* 39:797, 1986.
52. Diaz-Chico JC, Yang KG, Kutlar A, et al: A 300 bp deletion involving part of the 5′ β-globin gene region is observed in members of a Turkish family with β-thalassemia. *Blood* 70:583, 1987.
53. Aulehla-Scholtz C, Spielberg R, Horst J: A β-thalassemia mutant caused by a 300 bp deletion in the human β-globin gene. *Hum Genet* 81:298, 1989.
54. Orkin SH, Antonarakis SE, Kazazian HH: Base substitution at position −88 in a β-thalassemic globin gene: Further evidence for the role of the distal promoter element ACACCC. *J Biol Chem* 259:8679, 1984.
55. Orkin SH, Kazazian HH, Antonarakis SE, et al: Linkage of β-thalassemia mutations and β-globin gene polymorphisms with DNA polymorphisms in human globin gene cluster. *Nature* 296:267, 1982.
56. Poncz M, Ballantine M, Solowiejczyk D, et al: β-Thalassemia in a Kurdish Jew. *J Biol Chem* 257:5994, 1983.
57. Orkin SH, Sexton JP, Cheng TC, et al: TATA box transcription mutation in β-thalassemia. *Nucleic Acids Res* 11:4727, 1983.
58. Antonarakis SE, Orkin SH, Cheng T-C, et al: B-Thalassemia in American Blacks: Novel mutations in the TATA box and IVS-2 acceptor splice site. *Proc Natl Acad Sci U S A* 81:1154, 1984.
59. Surrey S, Delgrosso K, Malladi P, Schwartz E: Functional analysis of a β-globin gene containing a TATA box mutation from a Kurdish Jew with β-thalassemia. *J Biol Chem* 260:6507, 1985.
60. Gonzalez-Redondo JH, Stoming TA, Kutlar A, et al: A C→T substitution at nt −101 in a conserved DNA sequence of the promoter region of the β-globin gene is associated with "silent" β-thalassemia. *Blood* 73:1705, 1989.
61. Wong C, Dowling CE, Saiki RK, et al: Characterization of beta-thalassemia mutations using direct genomic sequencing of amplified single copy DNA. *Nature* 330:384, 1987.
62. Treisman R, Orkin SH, Maniatis T: Specific transcription and RNA splicing defects in five cloned β-thalassemia genes. *Nature* 302:591, 1983.
63. Kazazian HH, Orkin SH, Antonarakis SE, et al: Molecular characterization of seven β-thalassaemia mutations in Asian Indians. *EMBO J* 3:593, 1984.
64. Padanilam BJ, Huisman THJ: The β^0-thalassemia in an American Black family is due to a single nucleotide substitution in the acceptor splice junction of the second intervening sequence. *Am J Hematol* 22:259, 1986.
65. Atweh GF, Anagnou NP, Shearin J, et al: B-Thalassemia resulting from a single nucleotide substitution in an acceptor splice site. *Nucleic Acids Res* 13:777, 1985.
66. Orkin SH, Sexton JP, Goff SC, Kazazian HH: Inactivation of an acceptor splice site by a short deletion in β-thalassemia. *J Biol Chem* 258:7249, 1983.
67. Atweh GF, Wong C, Reed R, et al: A new mutation in IVS-1 of the human β globin gene causing β thalassemia due to abnormal splicing. *Blood* 70:147, 1987.
68. Cheng T, Orkin SH, Antonarakis SE, et al: B-Thalassemia in Chinese: Use of *in vivo* RNA analysis and oligonucleotide hybridization in systematic characterization of molecular defects. *Proc Natl Acad Sci U S A* 81:2821, 1984.
69. Gonzalez-Redondo JH, Stoming TA, Lanclos KD, et al: Clinical and genetic heterogeneity in Black patients with homozygous β-thalassemia from the southeastern United States. *Blood* 72:1007, 1988.
70. Tamagnini GP, Lopes MC, Castanheira ME, et al: β^+ Thalassaemia—Portuguese type: Clinical, haematological and molecular studies of a newly defined form of β thalassaemia. *Br J Haematol* 54:189, 1983.
71. Hill AVS, Bowden DK, O'Shaughnessy DF, et al: β-Thalassemia in Melanesia: Association with malaria and characterization of a common variant. *Blood* 72:9, 1988.
72. Spritz RA, Jagadeeswaran P, Choudary PV, et al: Base substitution in an intervening sequence of a β^+ thalassemic human globin gene. *Proc Natl Acad Sci U S A* 78:2455, 1981.
73. Busslinger M, Moschanas N, Flavell RA: B^+ Thalassemia: Aberrant splicing results from a single point mutation in an intron. *Cell* 27:289, 1981.
74. Metherall JE, Collins RS, Pan J, et al: B^0 thalassaemia caused by a base substitution that creates an alternative splice acceptor site in an intron. *EMBO J* 5:2551, 1986.
75. Orkin HH, Kazazian HH, Antonarakis SE, et al: Abnormal RNA processing due to the exon mutation of β^E-globin gene. *Nature* 300:768, 1982.
76. Goldsmith ME, Humphries RK, Bey T, et al: "Silent" nucleotide substitution in β^+ thalassemia globin gene activated splice site in coding sequence RNA. *Proc Natl Acad Sci U S A* 88:2318, 1983.
77. Orkin SH, Antonarakis SE, Loukopoulos D: Abnormal processing of β Knossos RNA. *Blood* 64:311, 1984.
78. Yang KG, Kutlar F, George E, et al: Molecular characterization of β-globin gene mutations in Malay patients with Hb E–β-thalassaemia major. *Br J Haematol* 72:73, 1989.
79. Orkin SH, Cheng T-C, Antonarakis SE, Kazazian HH: Thalassaemia due to a mutation in the cleavage-polyadenylation signal of the human β-globin gene. *EMBO J* 4:453, 1985.
80. Jankovic L, Efremov GD, Petkov G, et al: Three novel mutations leading to β thalassemia. *Blood* 74:226, 1989.
81. Rund D, Filon D, Rachmilewitz EA, et al: Molecular analysis of β-thalassemia in Kurdish Jews: Novel mutations and expression studies. *Blood* 74:821, 1989.
82. Chang JC, Kan YW: β-Thalassemia: A nonsense mutation in man. *Proc Natl Acad Sci U S A* 76:2886, 1979.
83. Kazazian HH, Dowling CE, Waber PG, et al: The spectrum of β-thalassemia genes in China and Southeast Asia. *Blood* 68:964, 1986.
84. Trecartin RF, Liebhaber SA, Chang JC, et al: B Thalassemia in Sardinia is caused by a nonsense mutation. *J Clin Invest* 68:1012, 1981.
85. Rosatelli C, Leoni GB, Tuveri T, et al: B Thalassaemia mutations in Sardinians: Implications for prenatal diagnosis. *J Med Genet* 24:97, 1987.
86. Kimberland ML, Divoky V, Prchal J, et al: Full-length human L1 insertions retain the capacity for high frequency retrotransposition in cultured cells. *Hum Mol Genet* 8:1557, 1999.
87. Weatherall DJ, Clegg JB, Knox-Macaulay HHM, et al: A genetically determined disorder with features both of thalassaemia and congenital dyserythropoietic anaemia. *Br J Haematol* 24:681, 1973.
88. Stamatoyannopoulos G, Woodson R, Papayannopoulou T, et al: Inclusion-body β-thalassemia trait: A form of β thalassemia producing clinical manifestations in simple heterozygotes. *N Engl J Med* 290:939, 1974.
89. Thein SL: Dominant β thalassaemia: Molecular basis and pathophysiology. *Br J Haematol* 80:273,1992.
90. Thein SL, Hesketh C, Taylor P, et al: Molecular basis for dominantly inherited inclusion body β thalassemia. *Proc Natl Acad Sci U S A* 87:3924, 1990.
91. Beris RP, Miescher PA, Diaz-Chico JC, et al: Inclusion body β-thalassemia trait in a Swiss family is caused by an abnormal hemoglobin (Geneva) with an altered and extended β chain carboxy-terminus due to a modification in codon 114. *Blood* 72:801, 1988.
92. Kazazian HH, Dowling CE, Hurwitz RL, et al: Thalassemia mutations in exon 3 of the β-globin gene often cause a dominant form of thalassemia and show no predilection for malarial-endemic regions of the world. *Am J Hum Genet* 45:A242, 1989.
93. Fei YJ, Stoming TA, Kutlar A, et al: One form of inclusion body β thalassemia is due to a GAAÆTAA mutation at codon 121 of the β chain. *Blood* 73:1075, 1989.
94. Kazazian HH, Orkin SH, Boehm CD, et al: Characterization of a spontaneous mutation to a β-thalassemia allele. *Am J Hum Genet* 38:860, 1986.
95. Sachs AB: Messenger RNA degradation in eukaryotes. *Cell* 74:413, 1993.
96. Thermann R, Neu-Yilkins J, Deters A, et al: Binary specification of nonsense codons by splicing and cytoplasmic translation. *EMBO J* 17:3484, 1998.
97. Thein SL: Is it dominantly inherited β thalassaemia or just a β-chain variant that is highly unstable? *Br J Haematol* 107:12, 1999.
98. Adams JG, Steinberg MH, Boxer LA, et al: The structure of hemoglobin Indianapolis [(β112 (G14) arginine]: An unstable variant detectable only by isotopic labeling. *J Biol Chem* 254:3479, 1979.
99. Coleman MB, Steinberg MH, Adams JGI: Hemoglobin Terre Haute [β106 (G8) Arginine]: A posthumous correction to the original structure of Hb Indianapolis. *Blood* 76:57, 1990.
100. Thein SL, Wood WG, Wickramasinghe SN, Galvin MC: B-Thalassemia unlinked to the β-globin gene in an English family. *Blood* 82:961, 1993.
101. Jones RW, Old JM, Trent RJ, et al: Major rearrangement in the human β-globin gene cluster. *Nature* 291:39, 1981.
102. Baglioni C: The fusion of two peptide chains in hemoglobin Lepore and its interpretation as a genetic deletion. *Proc Natl Acad Sci U S A* 48:1880, 1962.
103. Ottolenghi S, Giglioni B, Pulazzini A, et al: Sardinian $\delta\beta^0$-thalassemia: A further example of a C to T substitution at position −196 of the $^A\gamma$ globin gene promoter. *Blood* 69:1058, 1987.
104. Atweh GF, Zhu X-X, Brickner HW, et al: The β-globin gene on the Chinese $\delta\beta$-thalassemia chromosome carries a promoter mutation. *Blood* 70:1470, 1987.
105. Wainscoat JS, Thein SL, Wood WG, et al: A novel deletion in the β globin gene complex. *Ann N Y Acad Sci* 445:20, 1985.
106. Kulozik A, Yarwood N, Jones RW: The Corfu $\delta\beta^0$ thalassemia: A small deletion acts at a distance to selectively β globin gene expression. *Blood* 71:457, 1988.
107. Fritsch EF, Lawn RM, Maniatis T: Characterization of deletions which affect the expression of fetal globin genes in man. *Nature* 279:598, 1979.

108. Orkin SH, Goff SC, Nathan DG: Heterogeneity of DNA deletion in $\gamma\delta\beta$-thalassemia. *J Clin Invest* 67:878, 1981.
109. Pirastu M, Kan YW, Lin CC, et al: Hemolytic disease of the newborn caused by a new deletion of the entire β-globin cluster. *J Clin Invest* 72:602, 1983.
110. Fearon EF, Kazazian HH, Waber PG, et al: The entire β-globin gene cluster is deleted in a form of $\gamma\delta\beta$-thalassemia. *Blood* 61:1269, 1983.
111. Van Der Ploeg LHT, Konings A, Cort M, et al: $\gamma\beta$-Thalassaemia studies showing that deletion of the γ- and δ-genes influence β-globin gene expression in man. *Nature* 283:637, 1980.
112. Curtin P, Pirastu M, Kan YW, et al: A distant gene deletion affects β-globin gene function in an $\gamma\delta\beta$-thalassemia. *J Clin Invest* 76:1554, 1985.
113. Driscoll MC, Dobkin CS, Alter BP: $\gamma\delta\beta$-Thalassemia due to a de novo mutation deleting the 5′ β-globin gene activation-region hypersensitive sites. *Proc Natl Acad Sci U S A* 86:7470, 1989.
114. Tuan D, Feingold E, Newman M, et al: Different 3′ end points of deletions causing $\delta\beta$-thalassemia and hereditary persistence of fetal hemoglobin: Implications for the control of γ-globin gene expression in man. *Proc Natl Acad Sci U S A* 80:6937, 1983.
115. Kendall AG, Ojwang PJ, Schroeder WA, Huisman THJ: Hemoglobin Kenya, the product of a $\gamma\beta$ fusion gene: Studies of the family. *Am J Hum Genet* 25:548, 1973.
116. Smith DH, Clegg JB, Weatherall DJ, Gilles HM: Hereditary persistence of foetal haemoglobin associated with a $\gamma\beta$ fusion variant, haemoglobin Kenya. *Nat New Biol* 246:184, 1973.
117. Collins FS, Stoeckert CJ, Serjeant GR, et al: $^{G}\gamma\beta^{+}$ hereditary persistence of fetal hemoglobin: Cosmid cloning and identification of a specific mutation 5′to the $^{G}\gamma$ gene. *Proc Natl Acad Sci U S A* 81:4894, 1984.
118. Giglioni B, Casini C, Mantovani R, et al: A molecular study of a family with Greek hereditary persistence of fetal hemoglobin and β-thalassemia. *EMBO J* 3:2641, 1984.
119. Gelinas R, Endlich B, Pfeiffer C, et al: G to A substitution in the distal CCAAT box of the $^{A}\gamma$-globin gene in Greek hereditary persistence of fetal haemoglobin. *Nature* 313:323, 1985.
120. Tate VE, Wood WG, Weatherall DJ: The British form of hereditary persistence of fetal haemoglobin results from a single base mutation adjacent to an S1 hypersensitive site 5′ to the $^{A}\gamma$globin gene. *Blood* 68:1389, 1986.
121. Gilman JG, Huisman THJ: DNA sequence variation associated with elevated fetal $^{G}\gamma$ globin production. *Blood* 66:783, 1985.
122. Marti HR: *Normale und Abnormale Menschliche Haemoglobin*. Springer-Verlag, Berlin, 1963.
123. Dover GJ, Smith KD, Chang YC, et al: Fetal hemoglobin levels in sickle cell disease and normal individuals are partially controlled by an X-linked gene located at Xp22.2. *Blood* 80:816, 1992.
124. Craig JE, Rochette J, Fisher CA, et al: Dissecting the loci controlling fetal haemoglobin production on chromosomes 11p and 6q by the regressive approach. *Nat Genet* 12:58, 1996.
125. Garner C, Silver N, Best S, et al: Quantitative trait loci on chromosome 8q influences the switch from fetal to adult hemoglobin. *Blood* 104:2184, 2004.
126. Menzel S, Garner C, Gut I, et al: A QTL influencing F cell production maps to a gene encoding a zinc-finger protein on chromosome 2p15.*Nat Genet* 39:1197, 2007.
127. Uda M, Galanello R, Sanna S, et al: Genome-wide association study shows *BCL11A* associated with persistent fetal hemoglobin and amelioration of the phenotype of β-thalassemia. *Proc Natl Acad Sci U S A* 105:1620, 2008.
128. Menzel S, Thein SL: Genetic architecture of hemoglobin F control. *Curr Opin Hematol* 16:179, 2009.
129. Wood WG, Weatherall DJ, Clegg JB: Interaction of heterocellular hereditary persistence of foetal haemoglobin with β thalassaemia and sickle cell anaemia. *Nature* 264:247, 1976.
130. Gibbons RJ, Wada T: ATRX and X-linked (alpha)-thalassemia mental retardation syndrome, in *Inborn Errors of Development*, edited by CJ Epstein, RP Erickson, A Wynshaw-Boris, p 747. Oxford University Press, Oxford, UK, 2004.
131. Gibbons RJ, Wada T, Fisher CA, et al: Mutations in the chromatin-associated protein ATRX. *Hum Mutat* 29:796, 2008.
132. Nicholls RB, Fischel-Ghodsian N, Higgs DR: Recombination at the human α globin gene cluster: Sequence features and topological constraints. *Cell* 49:369, 1987.
133. Barbour VM, Tufarelli C, Sharpe JA, et al: α-thalassemia resulting from a negative chromosomal position effect. *Blood* 96:800, 2000.
134. Tufarelli C, Stanley JA, Garrick D, et al: Transcription of antisense RNA leading to gene silencing and methylation as a novel cause of human genetic disease. *Nat Genet* 34:157, 2003.
135. Wilkie AOM, Lamb J, Harris PC, et al: A truncated human chromosome 16 associated with α thalassaemia is stabilized by addition of telomeric repeat (TTAGGG). *Nature* 346:868, 1990.
136. Hatton CSR, Wilkie AOM, Drysdale HC, et al: Alpha thalassemia caused by a large (62 kb) deletion upstream of the human α globin gene cluster. *Blood* 76:221, 1990.
137. Liebhaber SA, Griese E-U, Cash FE, et al: Inactivation of human α-globin gene expression by a de novo deletion located upstream of the α-globin gene cluster. *Proc Natl Acad Sci U S A* 81:9431, 1990.
138. Embury SH, Miller JA, Dozy AM, et al: Two different molecular organizations account for the single α-globin gene of the α-thalassemia-2 genotype. *J Clin Invest* 66:1319, 1980.
139. Higgs DR, Old JM, Pressley L, et al: A novel α-globin gene arrangement in man. *Nature* 284:632, 1980.
140. Goossens M, Dozy AM, Embury SH, et al: Triplicated α-globin loci in humans. *Proc Natl Acad Sci U S A* 77:518, 1980.
141. Trent RJ, Higgs DR, Clegg JB, Weatherall DJ: A new triplicated α-globin gene arrangement in man. *Br J Haematol* 49:149, 1981.
142. Higgs DR, Hill AVS, Bowden DK, Weatherall DJ: Independent recombination events between duplicated human α globin genes: Implications for their concerted evolution. *Nucleic Acids Res* 12:6965, 1984.
143. Orkin SH, Goff SC, Hechtman RL: Mutation in an intervening sequence splice junction in man. *Proc Natl Acad Sci U S A* 78:5041, 1981.
144. Higgs DR, Goodbourn SEY, Lamb J, et al: α-Thalassaemia caused by a polyadenylation signal mutation. *Nature* 306:398, 1983.
145. Thein SL, Wallace RB, Pressley L, et al: The polyadenylation site mutation in the α-globin gene cluster. *Blood* 71:313, 1988.
146. Pirastu M, Saglio G, Chang JC, et al: Initiation codon mutation as a cause of α thalassemia. *J Biol Chem* 259:12315, 1984.
147. Olivieri NF, Chang LS, Poon AO, et al: An α-globin gene initiation codon mutation in a Black family with Hb H disease. *Blood* 70:729, 1987.
148. Paglietti E, Galanello R, Moi P, et al: Molecular pathology of haemoglobin H disease in Sardinians. *Br J Haematol* 63:485, 1986.
149. Morle F, Lopez B, Henni T, Godet J: α-Thalassaemia associated with the deletion of two nucleotides at position –2 and –3 preceding the AUG codon. *EMBO J* 4:1245, 1985.
150. Weatherall DJ, Clegg JB: The α-chain termination mutants and their relationship to the α thalassaemias. *Philos Trans R Soc London B Biol Sci* 271:411, 1975.
151. Liebhaber SA, Coleman MB, Adams JG, et al: Molecular basis for non-deletion α thalassemia in American Blacks $\alpha_2^{116GAG\rightarrow UAG}$. *J Clin Invest* 80:154, 1987.
152. Liebhaber SA, Kan YW: A Thalassemia caused by an unstable α-globin mutant. *J Clin Invest* 71:461, 1983.
153. Sanguansermsri T, Matrogoon S, Changlosh L, Fletz G: Hemoglobin Suan-Dok ($\alpha_2^{109(G16)LEU\rightarrow ARG}\beta_2$): An unstable variant associated with α thalassemia. *Hemoglobin* 3:161, 1979.
154. Honig GR, Shamsuddin M, Zaizov R, et al: Hemoglobin Petah Tikvah (α_{110} Ala→Asp): A new unstable variant with α-thalassemia-like expression. *Blood* 57:705, 1981.
155. Honig GR, Shamsuddin M, Vida LN, et al: Hemoglobin Evanston (α_{14} Trp→Arg): An unstable α-chain variant expressed as α-thalassemia. *J Clin Invest* 73:1740, 1984.
156. Weatherall DJ, Higgs DR, Bunch C, et al: Hemoglobin H disease and mental retardation: A new syndrome or a remarkable coincidence? *N Engl J Med* 305:607, 1981.
157. Wilkie AOM, Buckle VJ, Harris PC, et al: Clinical features and molecular analysis of the α thalassemia/mental retardation syndromes: I. Cases due to deletions involving chromosome band 16p13.3. *Am J Hum Genet* 46:1112, 1990.
158. Wilkie AOM, Zeitlin HC, Lindenbaum RH, et al: Clinical features and molecular analysis of the α-thalassemia/mental retardation syndromes: II. Cases without detectable abnormality of the α globin complex. *Am J Hum Genet* 46:1127, 1990.
159. Gibbons RJ, Suthers GK, Wilkie AOM, et al: X-linked α thalassemia/ mental retardation (ATR-X) syndrome: Localization to Xq12–21.31 by X-inactivation and linkage analysis. *Am J Hum Genet* 51:1136, 1992.
160. Gibbons RJ, Picketts DJ, Villard L, Higgs DR: Mutations in a putative global transcriptional regulator cause X-linked mental retardation with α-thalassemia (ATR-X syndrome). *Cell* 80:837, 1995.
161. Gibbons RJ, Bachoo S, Picketts DJ, et al: Mutations in transcriptional regulator *ATRX* establish the functional significance of a PHD-like domain. *Nat Genet* 17:146, 1997.
162. Ausió J, Levin DB, De Amorim GV, et al: Syndromes of disordered chromatin remodeling. *Clin Genet* 64:83, 2003.
163. Gibbons RJ, McDowell TL, Raman S, et al: Mutations in ATRX, encoding a SWI/SNF-like protein, cause diverse changes in the pattern of DNA methylation. *Nat Genet* 24:368, 2000.
164. Weatherall DJ, Old J, Longley J, et al: Acquired haemoglobin H disease in leukaemia: Pathophysiology and molecular basis. *Br J Haematol* 38:305, 1978.
165. Gibbons RJ, Pellagatti A, Garrick D, et al: Identification of acquired somatic mutations in the gene encoding chromatin-remodeling factor ATRX in the alpha-thalassemia myelodysplasia syndrome (ATMDS). *Nat Genet* 34:446, 2003.
166. Belickova M, Schroeder HW, Guan YL, et al: Clonal hematopoiesis and acquired thalassemia in common variable immunodeficiency. *Mol Med* 1:56, 1995.
167. Weatherall DJ, Clegg JB, Naughton MA: Globin synthesis in thalassemia: An in vitro study. *Nature* 208:1061, 1965.
168. Weatherall DJ, Clegg JB, Na-Nakorn S, Wasi P: The pattern of disordered haemoglobin synthesis in homozygous and heterozygous β-thalassaemia. *Br J Haematol* 16:251, 1969.
169. Fessas P: Inclusions of hemoglobin in erythroblasts and erythrocytes of thalassemia. *Blood* 21:21, 1963.
170. Wickramasinghe SN, Hughes M: Some features of bone marrow macrophages in patients with β-thalassaemia. *Br J Haematol* 38:23, 1978.
171. Yataganas X, Fessas P: The pattern of hemoglobin precipitation in thalassemia and its significance. *Ann N Y Acad Sci* 165:270, 1969.
172. Finch CA, Deubelbeiss K, Cook JD, et al: Ferrokinetics in man. *Medicine (Baltimore)* 49:17, 1970.
173. Chalavelakis G, Clegg JB, Weatherall DJ: Imbalanced globin chain synthesis in heterozygous β-thalassemic bone marrow. *Proc Natl Acad Sci U S A* 72:3853, 1975.
174. Rund D, Rachmilewitz E: Advances in the pathophysiology and treatment of thalassemia. *Crit Rev Oncol Hematol* 20:237, 1995.
175. Schrier SL: Pathobiology of thalassemic erythrocytes. *Curr Opin Hematol* 4:75, 1997.

176. Fibach E, Rachmilewitz E: The role of oxidative stress in hemolytic anemia. *Curr Mol Med* 8:609, 2008.
177. Yuan J, Angelucci E, Lucarelli G, et al: Accelerated programmed cell death (apoptosis) in erythroid precursors of patients with severe beta-thalassemia (Cooley's anemia). *Blood* 82:374, 1993.
178. Ager JAM, Lehmann H: Observations in some "fast" haemoglobins: K, J, N, and "Bart's." *Br Med J* 1:929, 1958.
179. Rigas DA, Kohler RD, Osgood EE: New hemoglobin possessing a higher electrophoretic mobility than normal adult hemoglobin. *Science* 121:372, 1955.
180. Gabuzda TG, Nathan DG, Gardner FH: The turnover of hemoglobins A F and A_2 in the peripheral blood of three patients with thalassemia. *J Clin Invest* 42:1678, 1963.
181. Loukopoulos D, Fessas P: The distribution of hemoglobin types in thalassemic erythrocyte. *J Clin Invest* 44:231, 1965.
182. Nathan DG, Gunn RB: Thalassemia: The consequences of unbalanced hemoglobin synthesis. *Am J Med* 41:815, 1966.
183. Rees DC, Porter JB, Clegg JB, Weatherall DJ: Why are hemoglobin F levels increased in Hb E/β thalassemia? *Blood* 94:3199, 1999.
184. Thein SL, Weatherall DJ: A non-deletion hereditary persistence of fetal hemoglobin (HPFH) determinant not linked to the β-globin gene complex, in *Hemoglobin Switching, Part B: Cellular and Molecular Mechanisms*, edited by G Stamatoyannopoulos, AW Nienhuis, p 97. Alan R. Liss, New York, 1989.
185. O'Donnell A, Premawardhena A, Arambepola M, et al: Age-related changes in adaptation to severe anemia in childhood in developing countries. *Proc Natl Acad Sci U S A* 104:9440, 2007.
186. Multicentre study on prevalence of endocrine complications in thalassemia major. Italian Working Group on Endocrine Complications in Non-endocrine Diseases. *Clin Endocrinol (Oxf)* 42:581, 1995.
187. Jessup M, Manno CS: Diagnosis and management of iron-induced heart disease in Cooley's anemia. *Ann N Y Acad Sci* 850:242, 1998.
188. Wood JC, Enriquez C, Ghugre N, et al: Physiology and pathophysiology of iron cardiomyopathy in thalassemia. *Ann N Y Acad Sci* 1054:386, 2005.
189. Olivieri NF, Brittenham GM: Iron-chelating therapy and the treatment of thalassemia. *Blood* 89:739, 1997.
190. Singer ST, Ataga KI: Hypercoagulability in sickle cell disease and beta-thalassemia. *Curr Mol Med* 8:639, 2008.
191. Morris CR, Kuypers FA, Kato GJ, et al: Hemolysis-associated pulmonary hypertension in thalassemia. *Ann N Y Acad Sci* 1054:481, 2005.
192. Weatherall DJ: Phenotype-genotype relationships in monogenic disease: Lessons from the thalassaemias. *Nat Rev Genet* 2:245, 2001.
193. Weatherall DJ, Pressley L, Wood WG, et al: The molecular basis for mild forms of homozygous β thalassaemia. *Lancet* 1:527, 1981.
194. Wainscoat JS, Old JM, Weatherall DJ, Orkin SH: The molecular basis for the clinical diversity of β thalassaemia in Cypriots. *Lancet* 1:1235, 1983.
195. Labie D, Pagnier J, Lapoumeroulie C, et al: Common haplotype dependency of high $^{G}\gamma$-globin gene expression and high Hb F levels in β-thalassemia and sickle cell anemia patients. *Proc Natl Acad Sci U S A* 82:2111, 1985.
196. Thein SL, Sampietro M, Old JM, et al: Association of thalassaemia intermedia with a beta-globin gene haplotype. *Br J Haematol* 65:370, 1987.
197. Thein SL, Hesketh C, Wallace RB, Weatherall DJ: The molecular basis of thalassaemia major and thalassaemia intermedia in Asian Indians: Application to prenatal diagnosis. *Br J Haematol* 70:225, 1988.
198. Ho PJ, Hall GW, Luo LY, et al: Beta thalassaemia intermedia: Is it possible to predict phenotype from genotype? *Br J Haematol* 100:70, 1998.
199. Rund D, Oron-Karni V, Filon D, et al: Genetic analysis of β-thalassemia intermedia in Israel: Diversity of mechanisms and unpredictability of phenotype. *Am J Hematol* 54:16, 1997.
200. Rund D, Fucharoen S: Genetic modifiers in hemoglobinopathies. *Curr Mol Med* 8:600, 2008.
201. Wonke B, Hoffbrand AV, Bouloux P, et al: New approaches to the management of hepatitis and endocrine disorders in Cooley's anemia. *Ann N Y Acad Sci* 850:232, 1998.
202. Girot R, Lefrére JJ, Schettini F, et al: HIV infection and AIDS in thalassemia, in *Thalassemia 1990: 5th Annual Meeting of the COOLEY-CARE Group*, edited by P Rebulla, P Fessas, p 69. Centro Trasfusionale Ospedale Maggiore Policlinico Dio Milano, Athens, 1991.
203. Choudhury NV, Dubey ML, Jolly JG, et al: Post-transfusion malaria in thalassaemia patients. *Blut* 61:314, 1990.
204. Chatterjee R, Katz M, Cox TF, Porter JB: Prospective study of the hypothalmic-pituitary axis in thalassaemic patients who developed secondary amenorrhoea. *Clin Endocrinol (Oxf)* 39:287, 1993.
205. Premawardhena A, Arambepola M, Katugaha N, et al: Is the beta thalassaemia trait of clinical importance? *Br J Haematol* 141:407, 2008.
206. Liang ST, Wong VCW, So WWK, et al: Homozygous α-thalassaemia: Clinical presentation, diagnosis and management: A review of 46 cases. *Br J Obstet Gynaecol* 92:680, 1985.
207. Beaudry MA, Ferguson DJ, Pearse K, et al: Survival of a hydropic infant with homozygous α-thalassemia-1. *J Pediatr* 108:713, 1986.
208. Bianchi DW, Beyer EC, Stark AR, et al: Normal long-term survival with α thalassemia. *J Pediatr* 108:716, 1986.
209. Gouttas A, Fessas P, Tsevrenis H, Xefteri E: Description d'une nouvelle variete d'anemie hemolytique congenitale. *Sang* 26:911, 1955.
210. Rigas DA, Koler RD, Osgood EE: Hemoglobin H: Clinical, laboratory, and genetic studies of a family with a previously undescribed hemoglobin. *J Lab Clin Med* 47:51, 1956.
211. Wasi P: Hemoglobinopathies in Southeast Asia, in *Distribution and Evolution of the Hemoglobin and Globin Loci*, edited by JE Bowman, p 179. Elsevier, New York, 1983.
212. Kattamis C, Tzotzos S, Kanavakis E, et al: Correlation of clinical phenotype to genotype in haemoglobin H disease. *Lancet* 1:442, 1988.
213. Galanello R, Pirastu M, Melis MA, et al: Phenotype-genotype correlation in haemoglobin H disease in childhood. *J Med Genet* 20:425, 1983.
214. Fuchareon S, Winichagoon P, Pootrakul P, et al: Differences between two types of Hb H disease, α-thalassemia 1/α-thalassemia 2 and α-thalassemia 1/Hb Constant Spring. *Birth Defects Orig Artic Ser* 23:309, 1988.
215. Styles L, Foote DH, Kleman KM, et al: Hemoglobin H-Constant Spring disease: An under recognized, severe form of α thalassemia. *Int J Pediatr Hematol Oncol* 4:69, 1977.
216. Lie-Injo LE, Ganesan J, Clegg JB, Weatherall DJ: Homozygous state for Hb Constant Spring (slow-moving Hb X components). *Blood* 43:251, 1974.
217. Derry S, Wood WG, Pippard MJ, et al: Hematologic and biosynthetic studies in homozygous hemoglobin Constant Spring. *J Clin Invest* 73:1673, 1984.
218. Higgs DR, Pressley L, Clegg JB, et al: Detection of α-thalassaemia in negro infants. *Br J Haematol* 46:39, 1980.
219. Higgs DR, Lamb J, Aldridge BE, et al: Inadequacy of Hb Bart's as an indicator of α-thalassaemia. *Br J Haematol* 48:177, 1982.
220. Silvestroni E, Bianco I, Reitano G: Three cases of homozygous $\delta\beta$-thalassemia (or microcythemia) with high haemoglobin F in a Sicilian family. *Acta Haematol* 40:220, 1968.
221. Ramot BN, Ben-Bassat I, Gafni D, Zaanoon R: A family with three $\delta\beta$-thalassemia homozygotes. *Blood* 35:158, 1970.
222. Tsistrakis GA, Amarantos SP, Konkouris LL: Homozygous $\beta\delta$-thalassaemia. *Acta Haematol* 51:185, 1974.
223. Efremov GD: Hemoglobins Lepore and anti-Lepore. *Hemoglobin* 2:197, 1978.
224. Charache S, Clegg JB, Weatherall DJ: The Negro variety of hereditary persistence of fetal haemoglobin is a mild form of thalassaemia. *Br J Haematol* 34:527, 1976.
225. Huisman THJ, Miller A, Schroeder WA: A $^{G}\gamma$ type of hereditary persistence of fetal hemoglobin with β chain production in *cis*. *Am J Hum Genet* 27:765, 1975.
226. Higgs DR, Clegg JB, Wood WG, Weatherall DJ: $^{G}\gamma\delta\beta^{+}$-Type of hereditary persistence of fetal haemoglobin in association with Hb C. *J Med Genet* 16:288, 1979.
227. Fessas P, Stamatoyannopoulos G: Hereditary persistence of fetal hemoglobin in Greece: A study and a comparison. *Blood* 24:223, 1964.
228. Sofroniadou K, Wood WG, Nute PE, Stamatoyannopoulos G: Globin chain synthesis in Greek type ($^{A}\gamma$) of hereditary persistence of fetal haemoglobin. *Br J Haematol* 29:137, 1975.
229. Clegg JB, Metaxatou-Mavromati A, Kattamis C, et al: Occurrence of $^{G}\gamma$ Hb F in Greek HPFH: Analysis of heterozygotes and compound heterozygotes with β thalassaemia. *Br J Haematol* 43:521, 1979.
230. Camaschella C, Oggiano L, Sampietro M, et al: The homozygous state of G to A—117 $^{A}\gamma$hereditary persistence of fetal hemoglobin. *Blood* 73:1999, 1989.
231. Weatherall DJ, Cartner R, Clegg JB, et al: A form of hereditary persistence of fetal haemoglobin characterized by uneven cellular distribution of haemoglobin F and the production of haemoglobins A and A_2 in homozygotes. *Br J Haematol* 29:205, 1975.
232. Silvestroni E, Bianco I: *La Malattia Microdrepanocitica*. Il Pensiero Scientifico, Rome, 1955.
233. Serjeant GR: *Sickle Cell Disease*, 3rd ed. Oxford University Press, New York, 2001.
234. Fucharoen S, Winichagoon P: Hemoglobinopathies in Southeast Asia: Molecular biology and clinical medicine. *Hemoglobin* 21:299, 1997.
235. Agarwal S, Gulati R, Singh K: Hemoglobin E-beta thalassemia in Uttar Pradesh. *Indian Pediatr* 34:287, 1997.
236. Khanh NC, Thu LT, Truc DB, et al: Beta-thalassemia/haemoglobin E disease in Vietnam. *J Trop Pediatr* 36:43, 1990.
237. De Silva S, Fisher CA, Members of the Sri Lanka Thalassaemia Study, et al: Thalassaemia in Sri Lanka: Implications for the future health burden of Asian populations. *Lancet* 355:786, 2000.
238. Olivieri NF, Muraca GM, O'Donnell A, et al: Studies in haemoglobin E beta-thalassaemia. *Br J Haematol* 141:388, 2008.
239. Premawardhena A, Fisher CA, Olivieri NF, et al: Haemoglobin E β thalassaemia in Sri Lanka. *Lancet* 366:1467, 2005.
240. Fisher CA, Premawardhena A, De Silva S, et al: The molecular basis for the thalassaemias in Sri Lanka. *Br J Haematol* 121:1, 2003.
241. Sonakul D, Suwanagool P, Sirivaidyapong P, Fucharoen S: Distribution of pulmonary thromboembolic lesions in thalassemic patients, in *Thalassemia: Pathophysiology and Management*, Part A, edited by S Fucharoen, PT Rowley, NW Paul, p 375. Alan R. Liss, New York, 1988.
242. Kattamis C, Metaxatou-Mavromati A, Wood WG, et al: The heterogeneity of normal Hb A_2-β thalassaemia in Greece. *Br J Haematol* 42: 109, 1979.
243. Schwartz E: The silent carrier of beta thalassemia. *N Engl J Med* 281:1327, 1969.
244. Bianco I, Graziani B, Carboni C: Genetic patterns in thalassemia inter-media (constitutional microcytic anemia): Familial, hematologic and biosynthetic studies. *Hum Hered* 27:257, 1977.
245. Pirastu M, Ristaldi MS, Loudianos G, et al: Molecular analysis of atypical β-thalassemia heterozygotes. *Ann N Y Acad Sci* 612:90, 1990.
246. Olds RJ, Sura T, Jackson B, et al: A novel δ^{0} mutation in *cis* with Hb Knossos: A study of different interactions in three Egyptian families. *Br J Haematol* 78:430, 1991.

247. Schokker RC, Went LN, Bok J: A new genetic variant of β-thalassaemia. *Nature* 209:44, 1966.
248. Ohta Y, Yamaoka K, Sumida I, et al: Homozygous delta-thalassemia first discovered in Japanese family with hereditary persistence of fetal hemoglobin. *Blood* 37:706, 1971.
249. Vella F, Wells RMC, Ager JAM: A haemoglobinopathy involving haemoglobin H and a new (Q) haemoglobin. *Br J Haematol* 1:752, 1958.
250. Lie-Injo LE, Pillay RP, Thuraisingham V: Further cases of Hb-Q-H disease (Hb Q-α-thalassemia). *Blood* 28:830, 1966.
251. Milner PF, Huisman THJ: Studies on the proportion and synthesis of haemoglobin G Philadelphia in red cells of heterozygotes, a homozygote, and a heterozygote for both haemoglobin G and α thalassaemia. *Br J Haematol* 34:207, 1976.
252. Rieder RF, Woodbury DH, Rucknagel DL: The interaction of α-thalassaemia and haemoglobin G Philadelphia. *Br J Haematol* 32:159, 1976.
253. Pich P, Saglio G, Camaschella C, et al: Interaction between Hb Hasharon and α thalassemia: An approach to the problem of the number of human α loci. *Blood* 51:339, 1978.
254. Higgs DR, Aldridge BE, Lamb J, et al: The interaction of alpha-thalassemia and homozygous sickle cell disease. *N Engl J Med* 306:1441, 1982.
255. Embury SH, Dozy AM, Miller J, et al: Concurrent sickle-cell anemia and α-thalassemia. *N Engl J Med* 306:270, 1982.
256. Olivieri N, Weatherall DJ: Clinical aspects of β thalassemia and related disorders, in *Disorders of Hemoglobin*, 2nd ed, edited by MH Steinberg, BG Forget, DR Higgs, DJ Weatherall, p 357. Cambridge University Press, Cambridge, UK, 2009.
257. Cazzola M, Borgna-Pignatti C, Locatelli F, et al: A moderate transfusion regimen may reduce iron loading in β-thalassemia major without producing excessive expansion of erythropoiesis. *Transfusion* 37:135, 1997.
258. Propper RD, Cooper B, Rufo RR, et al: Continuous subcutaneous administration of deferoxamine in patients with iron overload. *N Engl J Med* 297:418, 1977.
259. Pippard MJ, Callender ST, Letsky EA, Weatherall DJ: Prevention of iron loading in transfusion-dependent thalassaemia. *Lancet* 1:1178, 1978.
260. Pippard MJ, Callender ST, Weatherall DJ: Intensive iron-chelation therapy with desferrioxamine in iron loading patients. *Clin Sci Mol Med* 54:99, 1978.
261. Nienhuis AW: Safety of intensive chelation therapy. *N Engl J Med* 296:114, 1977.
262. Olivieri NF, Bunic JR, Chew E, et al: Visual and auditory neurotoxicity in patients receiving subcutaneous deferoxamine infusions. *N Engl J Med* 314:869, 1986.
263. Porter JB, Jawson MS, Huehns ER, et al: Desferrioxamine ototoxicity: Evaluation of risk factors in thalassaemia patients and guidelines for safe dosage. *Br J Haematol* 73:403, 1989.
264. Olivieri NF, Basran RK, Talbot AL, et al: Abnormal growth in thalassemia major associated with deferoxamine-induced destruction of spinal cartilage and compromise of sitting height. *Blood* 86:482a, 1995.
265. Porter JB: Practical management of iron overload. *Br J Haematol* 115:239, 2001.
266. Nisbet-Brown E, Olivieri NF, Giardina PJ, et al: Effectiveness and safety of ICL670 in iron-loaded patients with thalassaemia: A randomized, double-blind, placebo-controlled dose-escalation trial. *Lancet* 361:1597, 2003.
267. Cappellini MD, Piga A: Current status in iron chelation in hemoglobinopathies. *Curr Mol Med* 8:663, 2008.
268. Olivieri NF, Nathan DG, MacMillan JH, et al: Survival in medically treated patients with homozygous β-thalassemia. *N Engl J Med* 331:574, 1994.
269. Brittenham GM, Griffith PM, Nienhuis AW, et al: Efficacy of deferoxamine in preventing complications of iron overload in patients with thalassemia major *N Engl J Med* 331:567, 1994.
270. Borgna-Pignatti C, Rugolotto S, De Stefano P, et al: Survival and complications in patients with thalassemia major treated with transfusion and deferoxamine. *Haematologica* 89:1187, 2004.
271. St Pierre TG, Clark PR, Chua-Anusorn W: Measurement and mapping of liver iron concentrations using magnetic resonance imaging. *Ann N Y Acad Sci* 1054:379, 2005.
272. Pennell DJ: T2* magnetic resonance and myocardial iron in thalassemia. *Ann N Y Acad Sci* 1054:373, 2005.
273. Lucarelli G, Giardini C, Baronciani D: Bone marrow transplantation in β-thalassemia. *Semin Hematol* 32:297, 1995.
274. Lucarelli G, Giardini C, Baronciani D: Bone marrow transplantation in thalassemia. *Semin Hematol* 32:297, Review, 1995.
275. Di Bartolomeo P, Di Girolamo G, Olioso P, et al: The Pescara experience of allogenic bone marrow transplantation in thalassemia. *Bone Marrow Transplant* 19(Suppl 2):48, 1997.
276. Argiolu F, Sanna MA, Addari MC, et al: Bone marrow transplantation in thalassemia: The experience of Cagliari. *Bone Marrow Transplant* 19(Suppl 2):65, 1997.
277. Gaziev D, Polchi P, Galimberti M, et al: Graft-versus-host disease following bone marrow transplantation for thalassemia: An analysis of incidence and risk factors. *Transplantation* 63:854, 1997.
278. Michlitsch JG, Walters MC: Recent advances in bone marrow transplantation in hemoglobinopathies. *Curr Mol Med* 8:675, 2008.
279. Olivieri NF, Weatherall DJ: The therapeutic reactivation of fetal haemoglobin. *Hum Mol Genet* 7:1655, 1998.
280. Swank RA, Stamatoyannopoulos G: Fetal gene reactivation. *Curr Opin Genet Dev* 8:366, 1998.
281. Weatherall DJ: Pharmacological treatment of monogenic disease. *Pharmacogenomics J* 3:264, 2003.
282. Quek L, Thein SL: Molecular therapies in beta-thalassaemia. *Br J Haematol* 136:353, 2007.
283. Olivieri NF, Rees DC, Ginder GD, et al: Treatment of thalassaemia major with phenylbutyrate and hydroxyurea. *Lancet* 350:491, 1997.
284. Sadelain M: Genetic treatment of the haemoglobinopathies: Recombinations and new combinations. *Br J Haematol* 98:247, 1997.
285. Dominski Z, Kole R: Restoration of correct splicing in thalassemic pre-mRNA by antisense oligonucleotides. *Proc Natl Acad Sci U S A* 90:8673, 1993.
286. Lan N, Howrey RP, Lee S-W, et al: Ribozyme-mediated repair of sickle β-globin mRNAs in erythrocyte precursors. *Science* 280:1593, 1998.
287. Rivella S, Sadelain M: Therapeutic globin gene delivery using lentiviral vectors. *Curr Opin Mol Ther* 4:505, 2002.
288. Persons DA, Nienhuis AW: Gene therapy for the hemoglobin disorders. *Curr Hematol Rep* 2:348, 2003.
289. Sadelain M, Boulad F, Lisowki L, et al: Stem cell engineering for the treatment of severe hemoglobinopathies. *Curr Mol Med* 8:690, 2008.
290. WHO Working Group: Hereditary anemias: Genetic basis, clinical features, diagnosis and treatment. *Bull World Health Organ* 60:543, 1982.
291. Stamatoyannopoulos G: Problems of screening and counseling in the hemoglobinopathies, in *Proceedings of the IV International Conference on Birth Defects*, p 268. Exerpta Medica, Vienna, 1974.
292. Alter BP: Antenatal diagnosis: Summary of results. *Ann N Y Acad Sci* 612:237, 1990.
293. Kazazian HH, Phillips JAI, Boehm CD, et al: Prenatal diagnosis of β-thalassemia by amniocentesis: Linkage analysis of multiple polymorphic restriction endonuclease sites. *Blood* 56:926, 1980.
294. Old JM, Ward RHT, Petrou M, et al: First trimester diagnosis for haemoglobinopathies: A report of 3 cases. *Lancet* 2:1413, 1982.
295. Old JM, Fitches A, Heath C, et al: First trimester fetal diagnosis for haemoglobinopathies: Report on 200 cases. *Lancet* 2:763, 1986.
296. Cao A, Galanello R, Rosatelli MC: Prenatal diagnosis and screening of the haemoglobinopathies. *Clin Haematol* 11:215, 1998.
297. Modell B, Petrou M, Layton M, et al: Audit of prenatal diagnosis for haemoglobin disorders in the United Kingdom: The first 20 years. *BMJ* 315:779, 1997.
298. Cheung M-C, Goldberg JD, Kan YW: Prenatal diagnosis of sickle cell anemia and thalassemia by analysis of fetal cells in maternal blood. *Nat Genet* 14:264, 1996.
299. Hung ECW, Chiu RWK, Lo YMD. Detection of circulating fetal nucleic acids: A review of methods and applications. *J Clin Pathol* 62:308, 2009.
300. Kuliev A, Rechitsky S, Verlinsky O, et al: Preimplantation diagnosis of thalassemias. *J Assist Reprod Genet* 15:219, 1998.
301. Kuliev A, Rechitsky S, Verlinsky O, et al: Birth of healthy children after preimplantation diagnosis of thalassemia. *J Assist Reprod Genet* 16:201, 1999.
302. Qureshi N, Foote D, Walters MC, et al: Outcomes of preimplantation genetic diagnosis therapy in treatment of beta-thalassemia: A retrospective analysis. *Ann N Y Acad Sci* 1054:500, 2005.
303. World Health Organization (WHO): *Genomics and World Health*. WHO, Geneva, 2002.
304. Weatherall DJ, Akinyanju O, Fucharoen S, et al: Inherited disorders of hemoglobin, in *Disease Control Priorities in Developing Countries* 2nd ed, edited by DT Jamison, JG Breman, AR Measham, G Alleyne, M Claeson, DB Evans, P Jha, A Mills, P Musgrove, p 663. Oxford University Press and the World Bank, New York, 2006.

CHAPTER 48

DISORDERS OF HEMOGLOBIN STRUCTURE: SICKLE CELL ANEMIA AND RELATED ABNORMALITIES

Kavita Natarajan, Tim M. Townes, and Abdullah Kutlar

SUMMARY

Hemoglobinopathies are the most common inherited red cell disorders worldwide. Among these disorders, sickle cell syndromes and thalassemias constitute major public health problems. A glutamic acid to valine substitution at the 6th amino acid of the β-globin chain of human adult hemoglobin (Hb A) results in formation of sickle hemoglobin. Sickle cell disease results from homozygosity for this mutation or from a compound heterozygosity for sickle hemoglobin and β-thalassemia or another β-globin variant such as hemoglobin C, D, E, or O-Arab. The sickle mutation renders the hemoglobin molecule insoluble upon deoxygenation; thus red cells containing deoxy Hb S polymer are rigid and have impaired rheologic properties. The downstream effects of the sickling process include red cell membrane changes leading to potassium loss and cellular dehydration, interaction with vascular endothelium and neutrophils and monocytes, hemolysis, nitric oxide depletion, activation of inflammatory markers, and a prothrombotic tendency. These processes lead to hemolytic anemia, an inflammatory state, painful vasoocclusive episodes, and damage to multiple organ systems with a resultant shortened life expectancy. There is considerable heterogeneity in the severity of sickle cell disease; the best known modifier of the disease is an elevated level of hemoglobin F, which exerts a potent antisickling effect. Concomitant α-thalassemia is also a modifier of sickling, which leads to a decrease in hemolysis. In recent years, there has been an interest in nonglobin genetic modifiers of sickle cell disease. Genome-wide association studies may be expected to shed light on genetic modulation of disease severity. Over the past three decades, advances in supportive care and implementation of disease-modifying therapies have led to an increase in life expectancy. Hydroxyurea has emerged as an effective disease-modifying agent that has been approved by the FDA for use in adult patients with sickle cell disease. Although its main mechanism of action is to enhance hemoglobin F production, other effects such as a decrease in neutrophils, platelets, and decreased expression of adhesion molecules contribute to its efficacy. Novel agents, most notably, DNA methyltransferase 1 inhibitors (5′-azacytidine and decitabine) and histone deacetylase inhibitors (butyrate derivates and others), are now in clinical trials. Evolving therapies include Gardos channel inhibitors to improve red cell hydration and antiadhesive therapies to prevent interaction of blood cells with microvascular endothelium. To date, the only curative therapy is stem cell transplantation.

Sickle trait, the heterozygous state for sickle hemoglobin, affects approximately 8 percent of Americans of African descent, and with rare exceptions is asymptomatic. Hb C is associated with target cells and spherocytes in the blood film and splenomegaly. Hb D disease is essentially asymptomatic. Hb E is very common in Southeast Asia, and because of large population movements from this area, it has also become a prevalent hemoglobinopathy in other regions of the world. Hb E is a thalassemic variant, and its coinheritance with β^0-thalassemia mutations can result in severe transfusion-dependent thalassemia major. Unstable hemoglobin variants appear as rare, sporadic cases and are characterized by a Heinz body hemolytic anemia. Variants that alter the oxygen affinity of the hemoglobin molecule either lead to erythrocytosis (high oxygen-affinity variants) or anemia (low oxygen-affinity variants) and are diagnosed as rare causes of these syndromes.

Acronyms and abbreviations that appear in this chapter include: ACS, acute chest syndrome; CSSCD, Cooperative Study of Sickle Cell Disease; GFR, glomerular filtration rate; Hb, hemoglobin; iPS, induced pluripotential stem; LDH, lactate dehydrogenase; PCV7, polyvalent conjugate 7 of pneumococcal vaccine; SCD, sickle cell disease; SCT, stem cell transplantation; $sPLA_2$, secretory phospholipase A_2; STOP, Stroke Prevention Trial in Sickle Cell Disease; TCD, transcranial Doppler.

HISTORY OF SICKLE CELL DISEASE: THE FIRST "MOLECULAR DISEASE"

The first case of sickle cell disease (SCD), reported in 1910, was that of a dental student from Grenada, Walter Clement-Noel, studying in Chicago. Dr. James Herrick and his intern, Dr. Ernest Irons, were in charge of Mr. Noel's care between 1904 and 1907, during which time he had several bouts of fever and cough and a history of leg ulcers, jaundice, and exercise intolerance. Herrick and Irons made astute clinical observations and prepared blood films and photomicrographs of nucleated red blood cells and of red cells having a "slender sickle shape" (Fig. 48–1).[1] During the next decade, two more cases of this unusual anemia were reported. In 1915, Cook and Meyer raised the question of a genetic basis for the disorder based on the family history of the third reported case. In 1917, Victor Emmel used *in vitro* culture to show that sickled red cells represented a physical alteration of morphologically normal-appearing red cells and were not released from the marrow as sickle cells.[2] He also demonstrated that the morphologically normal red cells of the father of a patient became sickle-shaped after *in vitro* culture. The patient's mother was not alive. Vernon Mason, who reported the fourth case in 1922, coined the term *sickle cell anemia* after observing similarities between all the cases reported up to that time. In 1923, Sydenstricker and Huck noted "latent-sicklers" among relatives of the diagnosed patients, confirming and expanding on Emmel's findings. In 1927, Hahn and Gillespie showed that sickling was related to low oxygen tension and low pH.[3] In 1933, Diggs distinguished the difference of symptomatic cases, called sickle cell anemia, from asymptomatic cases that were termed *sickle cell trait*, and he found that approximately 8 percent of Americans of African descent had the sickle cell trait.[4] Irving Sherman, while a medical student at Johns Hopkins, showed that sickled red cells were birefringent under a polarizing microscope and that this finding was reversible with oxygenation of the cells. This observation ultimately led Linus Pauling to study sickle hemoglobin after being advised of this property of sickle cells by William Castle, a noted research hematologist. Indeed, in 1949, Pauling and his colleagues demonstrated electrophoretic differences between hemoglobins from normal, sickle cell trait, and sickle cell anemia subjects and hypothesized that there must be chemical differences, thus establishing sickle cell anemia as the first molecular disease described. In the late 1950s, Hunt and Ingram sequenced the globin peptide and linked the abnormality to a change in the amino acid composition of the β-globin chain: the replacement of glutamic acid by valine at residue 6. Marotta and coworkers showed in 1977 that the corresponding change in codon 6 of the β-globin gene was GAG→GTG.

The history of sickle cell anemia serves as an inspiring reminder of the power of clinical and laboratory observations, and in an era of

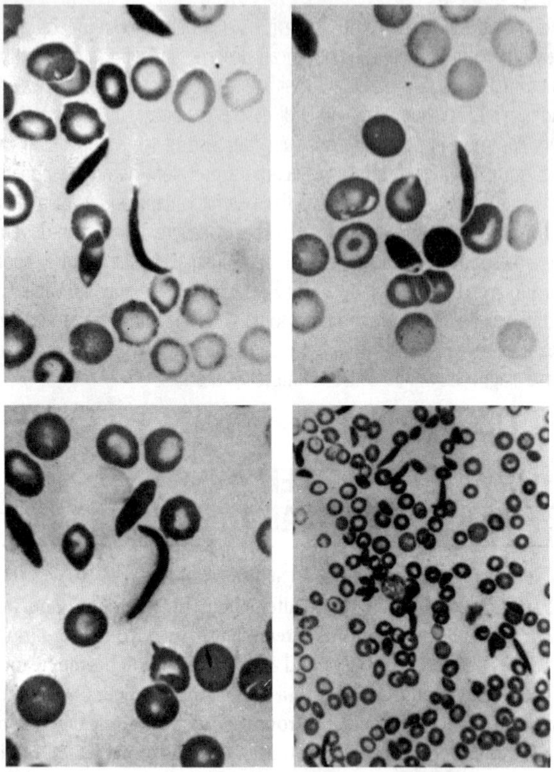

FIGURE 48–1. Peculiar elongated and sickle-shaped red cells from the first report of sickle cell anemia with depiction of sickle cells. *(Reproduced from Herrick JB,[1] with permission.)*

mechanistic basic science research serves to highlight the importance of bedside to bench and bench to bedside research integration.[5–8]

EPIDEMIOLOGY OF SICKLE CELL DISEASE

The observation that sickle cell trait may have a survival advantage against some environmental factors was first suggested by Dr. Alan Raper in East Africa in 1949. Drs. Mackey and Vivarelli suggested that the environmental influence might be malaria. It was subsequently noted that blood from sickle cell trait persons contained less malarial parasites and that the sickle trait conferred some protection against malaria in early childhood. The mechanism of such protection has been the matter of much debate. Plausible mechanisms include selective sickling of parasitized red cells resulting in more effective removal by the monocyte-macrophage system, an inhibitory effect on parasite growth by increased red cell potassium loss, decreased red cell pH, and increased endothelial adherence of parasitized sickle red cells.

Thus, the prevalence of sickle cell anemia closely mirrors the worldwide distribution of falciparum malaria; however, as a result of migration of peoples to the industrialized Western countries sickle cell disease has become prevalent in areas where malaria is not endemic.

The World Health Organization (WHO) estimates in 2006 stated that 5 percent of the world population carries a gene for hemoglobinopathies. Sickle cell anemia is highly prevalent in sub-Saharan and equatorial Africa with lesser but significant prevalence in the Middle East, India, and the Mediterranean region. Incidence of SCD in sub-Saharan African countries ranges between 1 and 2 percent, which translates into approximately 500,000 cases per year.

In the United States, the Centers for Disease Control and Prevention estimates that sickle cell anemia is present in 1 in 500 African American live births; 1 in 12 African Americans have the trait, and approximately 100,000 Americans, largely of African descent, live with the disease. In Hispanic Americans, the rate of sickle cell disease is 1 in 36,000 live births. As of 2002, in the United States, more than $1 billion is spent per year on hospitalizations for SCD.[9]

Previously, speculation existed as to whether the sickle mutation arose once and gained worldwide distribution or whether the mutation had arisen independently in different regions of the world. The nonrandom association of restriction endonuclease polymorphisms in the β-globin cluster define the β-globin haplotype. The β-globin gene cluster yields five distinct haplotypes associated with sickle cell mutations (see Chap. 9).[10–12] Four of the five patterns occur in Africa and are designated as the Senegal, Benin, Bantu, and Cameroon haplotypes, whereas the fifth arose on the Indian subcontinent.[13] These findings indicate that the sickle mutation arose independently at five different times.

NOMENCLATURE OF ABNORMAL HEMOGLOBINS

Following the molecular characterization of Hb S by Ingram and colleagues in 1956, there has been a rapid and exponential increase in the number of variant or "abnormal" hemoglobins.[14] This number now exceeds 1000. A detailed description of variant hemoglobins, their chemical and functional properties, and population distribution can be found on the Globin Gene Server website (http://globin.cse.psu.edu/). Initially, newly described variants were designated by letters of the alphabet (e.g., Hb C, D, E, J, etc.). When the letters of the alphabet were exhausted, the practice of naming the variant hemoglobins after the geographic location where they originated from was adapted (e.g., Hb Koln, Hb Zurich, etc.). Variants with electrophoretic or functional properties similar to previously described abnormal hemoglobins were designated with the letter and the geographic location: for example, Hb D-Punjab, Hb E-Saskatoon, Hb M-Hyde Park, and so forth. Some alphabetic designations were also used to indicate electrophoretic properties of certain variants; for example, there are a number of Hb Ds (D-Punjab, D-Iran, D-Ibadan). All of these variants share the electrophoretic properties of Hb S-like mobility on alkaline (cellulose acetate) electrophoresis, whereas they move with Hb A at acidic pH (citrate agar electrophoresis). Similarly, Hb Es have Hb C-like mobility on alkaline electrophoresis and move with Hb A on citrate agar electrophoresis.

The vast majority of hemoglobin variants arise as a result of single nucleotide mutations, leading to an amino acid change in either α-, β-, δ-, or γ-globin subunits of the hemoglobin tetramer resulting in variants of Hb A (α or β), Hb A_2 (δ), or Hb F (γ). Other mechanisms include small deletions or insertions, elongated chains, and fusions (for a detailed description of hemoglobin variants and associated clinical syndromes, see "Other Abnormal Hemoglobins" below.

The coinheritance of Hb S with some other variant hemoglobins or β-thalassemia mutations results in a number of sickling syndromes. In the United States, the most common sickling disorder is homozygous Hb S (Hb SS, sickle cell anemia), which is now commonly referred to as SCD. This is followed by sickle cell-Hb C disease (Hb SC), sickle cell β^+ thalassemia (Hb Sβ^+-thal), and sickle cell-β^0-thalassemia (Hb Sβ^0-thal). Other rarer forms include Hb SD-Punjab, Hb SO-Arab, and Hb SE diseases. Coinheritance of a large number of β-chain variants with Hb S does not result in a symptomatic sickling disorder; rather, they are clinically and hematologically indistinguishable from sickle cell trait (Hb AS).

Hb C is found in 17 to 28 percent of West Africans, particularly east of the Niger River in the vicinity of North Ghana. The selective factors that account for this high prevalence are unknown at present but Hb C probably confers some resistance to infection with malaria. The prevalence of Hb C among Americans of African descent is 2 to 3 percent. Sporadic cases also have been reported in other populations, including Italians and Afrikaners.

Hb D Punjab, now recognized to be identical with Hb D Los Angeles because both have the structure $\alpha_2\beta_2$121 Glu→Gln, also interacts with Hb S in forming aggregates in the deoxy conformation. Hb D has been found in many parts of the world, including Africa, northern Europe, and India.

Hb E is so prevalent that it may be the most common abnormal hemoglobin or second in prevalence only to hemoglobin S. Hb E is found principally in Burma, Thailand, Laos, Cambodia, Malaysia, and Indonesia. In some areas, Hb E is found with a carrier rate of 30 percent. On the other hand, it is not prevalent among the Chinese. Studies of restriction length polymorphisms in the β-globin cluster indicate the Hb E mutation has arisen several times independently. It, too, probably confers some resistance to infection with malaria.

THE STRUCTURE AND FUNCTION OF NORMAL HEMOGLOBIN

The red protein hemoglobin serves to transport oxygen from the lungs to the tissues and CO_2 from the tissues back to the lungs. Hemoglobin also destroys the physiologically important nitric oxide (NO) molecule. It has evolved to perform its gas transport functions in a highly efficient manner. The oxygen affinity of hemoglobin permits nearly complete saturation with oxygen in the lungs, as well as efficient oxygen unloading in the tissues because of its sigmoid oxygen dissociation curve. This curve results from the fact that hemoglobin is an allosteric molecule; its conformation, and hence the oxygen affinity, changes as each successive molecule of oxygen is bound. Hemoglobin also plays an important role in acid–base balance: deoxyhemoglobin binds protons and oxyhemoglobin releases protons.

Regulation of the oxygen dissociation curve to meet the needs of the body is remarkable. Hypoxic tissues become acidotic acutely, and the protons released produce a shift in the oxygen dissociation curve that enables more oxygen to be delivered to the tissue. However, longer-term acidosis or alkalosis (as occurs at high altitudes) is counteracted by modulation of red cell 2,3-bisphosphoglycerate (2,3-BPG), serving to decrease hemoglobin-oxygen affinity (see Chap. 46).

Normal mammalian hemoglobins contain two pairs of unlike polypeptide chains: one chain of each pair is α or α-like and the other is non-α (β, γ, or δ). The α-chains of all human hemoglobins encountered after early embryogenesis are the same. The non-α chains include the β-chain of normal adult hemoglobin (Hb A [$\alpha_2\beta_2$]), the γ-chain of fetal hemoglobin (Hb F [$\alpha_2\gamma_2$]), and the δ-chain of Hb A_2 (Hb A_2 [$\alpha_2\delta_2$]), the minor component, which accounts for 2.5 percent of the hemoglobin of normal adults. Chap. 47 discusses the regulation of production of the globin chains.

Certain residues in the amino acid sequence of each polypeptide chain appear to be critical to stability and function. Such residues are usually the same (invariant) in α or β chains. The NH_2-terminal valines of the β chains are important in 2,3-BPG interactions. The C-terminal residues are important in the salt bridges that characterize the unliganded molecules. Areas of contact between chains and between heme and globin tend to contain invariant residues.

The non-α (β, γ, δ, or ε) chains are all 146 amino acids in length; the β-chain begins with valine and histidine. The C-terminal residues are Tyr β145 and His β146. The δ-chain (of Hb A_2) differs from the β-chain (of Hb A) in only 10 residues. The first eight residues and the C-terminal residues 127–146 are the same in δ- and β-chains.

The γ-chain of fetal hemoglobin (Hb F) differs from the β-chain by 39 residues. The N-terminal residues of the γ-chain and β-chain are glycine and valine, respectively, whereas the C-terminal residues Tyr β145 and His β146 are the same as in γ and β chains. In addition to the different N-terminal residues, several other differences in primary structure between the γ and β chains are noteworthy. The γ-chain contains isoleucine, whereas the β chains do not. The γ genes are duplicated: one codes for glycine ($^G\gamma$) and the other for alanine ($^A\gamma$)[7] at residue 136, giving rise to two kinds of γ chains. In addition, a common polymorphism, the substitution of threonine for isoleucine, is frequently found at residue 75 of the $^A\gamma$-chain.

Approximately 75 percent of the amino acids in α or β chains are in a helical arrangement. All hemoglobins studied have a similar helical content (Fig. 48–2A). Eight helical areas, lettered A to H, occur in the β chains. Hemoglobin nomenclature specifies that amino acids within helices are designated by the amino acid number and the helix letter, whereas amino acids between helices bear the number of the amino acid and the letters of the two helices. Thus, residue EF3 is the third residue of the segment connecting the E and F helices, whereas residue F8 is the eighth residue of the F helix. Alignment according to helical designation makes homology evident: Residue F8 is the proximal heme-linked histidine, and the histidine on the distal side of the heme is E7.

Figures 48–2B and C shows the tertiary structure of the α and β chains. The prosthetic group of hemoglobin is ferroprotoporphyrin IX; Figure 48–3A shows its structure. The heme group is located in a crevice between the E and F helices in each chain (Fig. 48–3B). The highly polar propionate side chains of the heme are on the surface of the molecule and are ionized at physiologic pH. The rest of the heme is inside the molecule, surrounded by nonpolar residues except for two histidines. The iron atom is linked by a coordinate bond to the imidazole nitrogen (N) of histidine F8. The E7 *distal* histidine, on the other side of the heme plane, is not bonded to the iron atom but is very close to the ligand-binding site.

The sigmoid oxygen dissociation curve is a function of the change of the conformation of the molecule from the liganded to the unliganded state (Table 48–1). In the deoxy state, the hemoglobin tetramer is held together by intersubunit salt bonds (Fig. 48–4) and intersubunit hydrophobic contacts (see Fig. 48–2B), in addition to a certain number of hydrogen bonds. In deoxyhemoglobin, 2,3-BPG is situated in the central cavity between the two β chains (see Fig. 48–2B). The change in conformation of the hemoglobin molecule is brought about by a complex, coordinated series of changes in the structure of the molecule as heme binds oxygen. The oxygen dissociation curve can be linearized by a transformation known as the Hill plot:

$$\log[y/(1-y)] = \log K + n \log pO_2$$

where K is an empiric overall constant without physicochemical basis. The slope n is taken as a convenient measure of cooperativity. Values of n in noninteracting hemoglobins that exhibit hyperbolic, not sigmoid, oxygen dissociation curves (e.g., myoglobin and Hg Hb) are approximately 1. In a normal tetrameric hemoglobin with four oxygen-reactive sites, the maximum value for n is 4.0; however, n values of 2.7 to 3.0 are found in normal hemoglobin.

The point at which the hemoglobin is one-half saturated with oxygen (P_{50}) is the usual measurement of oxygen affinity. It depends upon pH (the Bohr effect), temperature, and 2,3-BPG concentration. In common practice, P_{50} is standardized at 37°C and pH 7.20. P_{50} of freshly drawn blood is approximately 26.7 torr under standard conditions, but the partial pressure of oxygen (P_{O2}) of hemoglobin from which 2,3-BPG has been removed is only approximately 13 torr. Although fetal and newborn red cells have 2,3-BPG levels similar to those of adults, their oxygen dissociation curve is left shifted (increased oxygen affinity) with a P_{50} of approximately 23 torr because fetal hemoglobin does not react as strongly with 2,3-BPG as does adult hemoglobin.

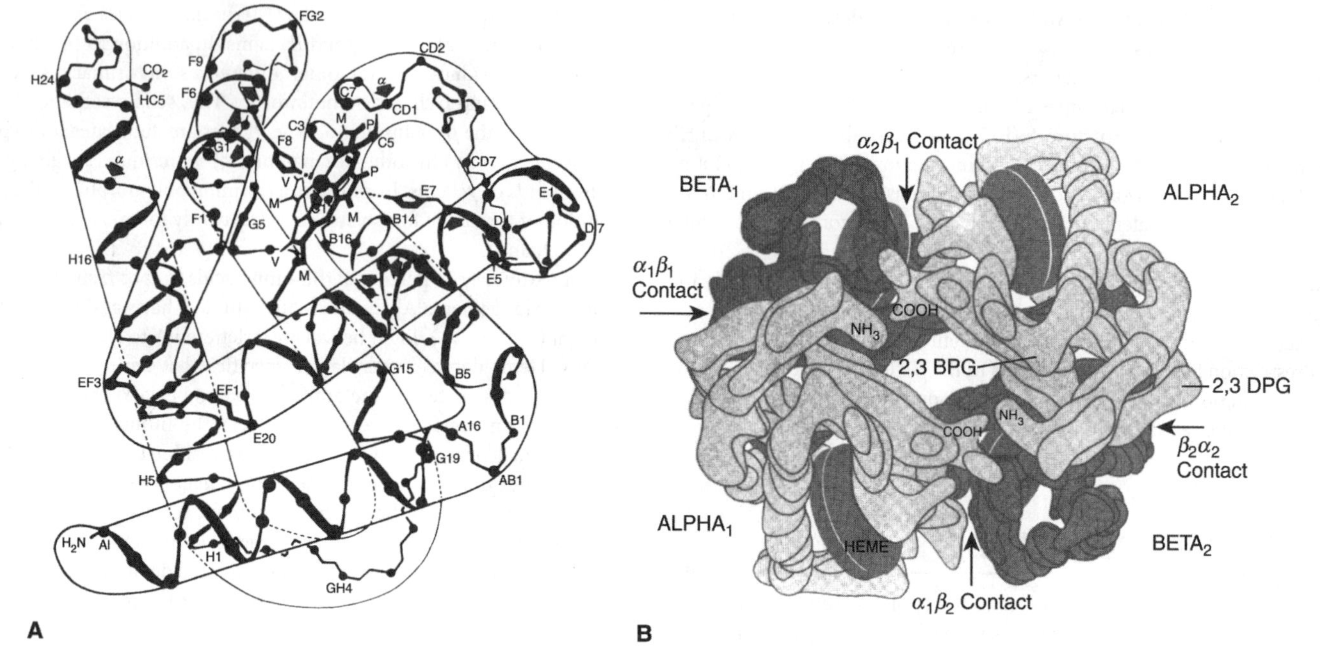

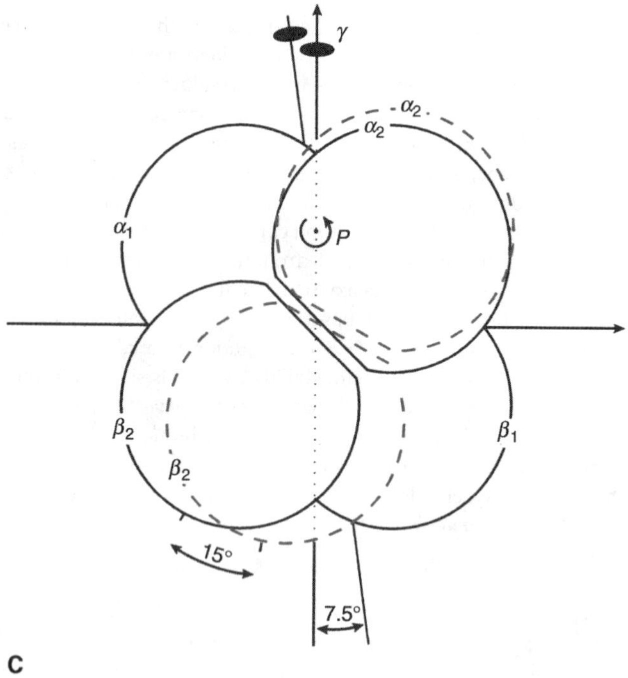

FIGURE 48–2. **A.** Representation of the structure of β chains. *Arrows* indicate sites of substitutions in a number of unstable hemoglobins. **B.** The hemoglobin molecule, as deduced from x-ray diffraction studies, shown from above. The molecule is composed of four subunits: two identical α chains (*light blocks*) and two identical β chains (*dark blocks*). 2,3-BPG binds to the two β chains in the deoxyhemoglobin molecule. **C.** Schematic of rotation of $\alpha_2\beta_2$ dimer relative to $\alpha_1\beta_1$ in quaternary structure change from deoxyhemoglobin (*solid lines*) to carboxyhemoglobin (*dashed lines*). *(Modified from Baldwin J, Chothia C: Haemoglobin: The structural changes related to ligand binding and its allosteric mechanism.* J Mol Biol *129:196, 1979, by permission of authors and publisher, Academic Press Ltd, London.)*

Although oxygen is the major physiologic ligand of the heme group of hemoglobin, the binding of carbon monoxide (CO) and NO by heme is of great importance (see Chap. 49). CO binds to hemoglobin with approximately 400 times the affinity of oxygen. As a result, relatively low ambient concentrations of CO may result in displacement of a large proportion of the oxygen from hemoglobin. To make matters worse from a clinical point of view, CO has a pronounced effect of the oxygen dissociation curve, shifting it to the left. Thus, the clinical effect of CO poisoning is appreciably greater than that which can be accounted for on the basis of displacement of oxygen alone. When NO is bound by hemoglobin, the hemoglobin is oxidized to methemoglobin in the reaction:

$$HbO_2 + NO \rightarrow MetHb + NO_3^-$$

Removal of NO by hemoglobin may play an important physiologic role and account for the esophageal pain sometimes encountered in paroxysmal nocturnal hemoglobinuria (see Chap. 40) and for the hypertension occurring after infusion of some experimental hemoglobin solutions.

PATHOPHYSIOLOGY OF SICKLE CELL ANEMIA

■ PATHWAYS INVOLVED

The sine qua non of sickle cell anemia is a Glu→Val substitution in the sixth amino acid of the β-globin gene. However, the pathophysiologic processes that result in the clinical phenotype extend beyond the red

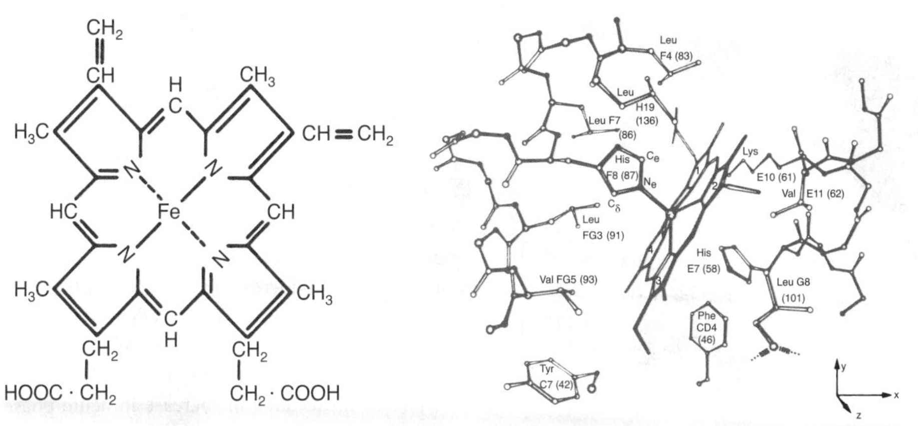

A B

FIGURE 48–3. **A.** Structure of heme (ferroprotoporphyrin IX). **B.** Heme group and its environment in the unliganded α-chain. Only selected side chains are shown; the heme 4-propionate is omitted. *(Reproduced from Gelin BR, Lee AW, Karplus M: Hemoglobin tertiary structural change on ligand binding.* J Mol Biol *171:489, 1983, with permission.)*

cell (Fig. 48–5). There is tremendous clinical heterogeneity from one patient to another and in the same patient over time. The heterogeneity for the same genotypic abnormality therefore implies that a multitude of other factors must contribute to the pathology of sickle cell anemia. The pathology is now far removed from the simplistic theory of hypoxia induced microvascular occlusion. Sickle cell anemia is a chronic inflammatory state punctuated by acute increase in inflammation wherein the endothelium, white blood cells, notably neutrophils and monocytes, platelets, coagulation pathways, several plasma proteins, adhesion molecules, and derangements in nitric oxide metabolism participate in addition to the abnormality in hemoglobin polymerization described several decades ago (Fig. 48–6). Added to that are the complex differences in tissue-specific vascular beds and differences in various parts of the vasculature in the same organ. Also, variation in several genes other than the β-globin gene that modify the milieu in which organ damage occurs may play a role. The pathophysiology of sickle cell anemia is described in separate sections; however, because no single, dominant pathway explains the multitude of manifestations, no single therapeutic modality serves to abrogate all of the pathology. Most experiments are in isolation in animal models or relatively simplistic experimental conditions with few *in vivo* studies in humans and, thus, do not replicate the complexity of this disorder.

HEMOGLOBIN POLYMERIZATION

Aggregation of deoxy Hb S molecules into polymers occurs when aggregates reach a thermodynamically critical size. This process is termed *homogenous nucleation*, and the smallest aggregate formed that favors polymer growth is called the critical nucleus.[15–20] Addition of subsequent deoxy Hb S molecules to already formed polymers is termed heterogenous nucleation, which results in polymer branching (see Fig. 48–6). Polymer growth is, therefore, an exponential process wherein there is a delay time between presence of deoxy Hb S molecules and polymer formation. This delay time is inversely proportional to the concentration of Hb S molecules. Polymer formation alters the rheologic properties of the red cell.

The quaternary structure of oxy Hb S cannot maintain axial and lateral hydrophobic contacts unlike that in the deoxygenated state, thus explaining the unsickling phenomenon upon reoxygenation.[21–24] The sickling process which is initially reversible with oxygenation of deoxy Hb S eventually leads to the formation of sickle-shaped red cells that fail to return to their normal discoid shape with oxygenation due to membrane damage imparted by repeated cycles of sickling and unsickling in the circulation. These cells are then termed *irreversibly sickled cells*. The rate and extent of polymerization is dependent on several factors including intracellular hemoglobin concentration, presence of hemoglobins other than Hb S, blood oxygen saturation, pH, temperature, and 2,3-BPG levels.[25] Microvascular occlusion by sickle red cells containing polymers is favored by prolonged transit times through the microcirculation, rapid deoxygenation and increased numbers of dense sickle red cells that contain polymers even at O_2 saturation levels found in the arterial circulation.[25–28] Arguments against Hb S polymerization as the major determinant of sickle cell pathophysiology include lack of clinically significant events despite constant sickling of red cells, the association of neutrophilia with vasoocclusive crises, and clinical features that imply macrovascular rather than microvascular perturbation, for example, large-vessel stroke.[29]

TABLE 48–1. Nomenclature of Hemoglobin Quaternary Structures

Liganded (Oxygen Bound)	Unliganded (Reduced)
Oxy	Deoxy
R-state	T-state
Relaxed	Tense
High affinity	Low affinity

CELLULAR DEHYDRATION

Membrane injury in Hb SS red cells results in impaired cation homeostasis. Sickle red cells have a decreased capacity to maintain intracellular

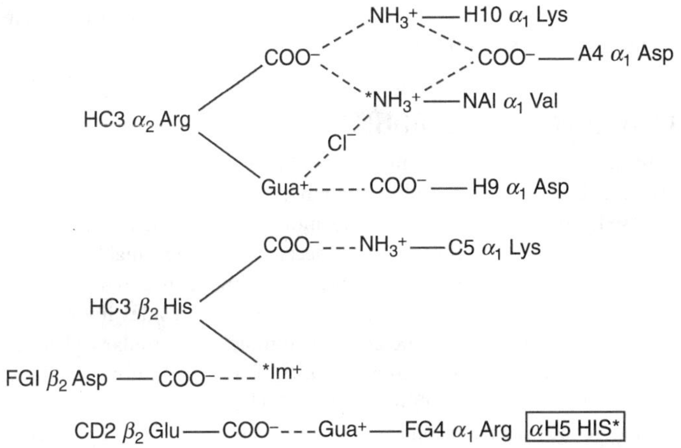

FIGURE 48–4. Salt bridges in deoxyhemoglobin (* = ionizable group less protonated at pH 9.0 than at pH 7.0). These groups account for 60% of the alkaline Bohr effect. The remainder is due to αH5 His. *(Reproduced from Perutz MF, Wilkinson AJ, Paoli M, Dodson GG: The stereochemical effects in hemoglobin revisited.* Biophys Biomol Struct *27:1, 1998, with permission.)*

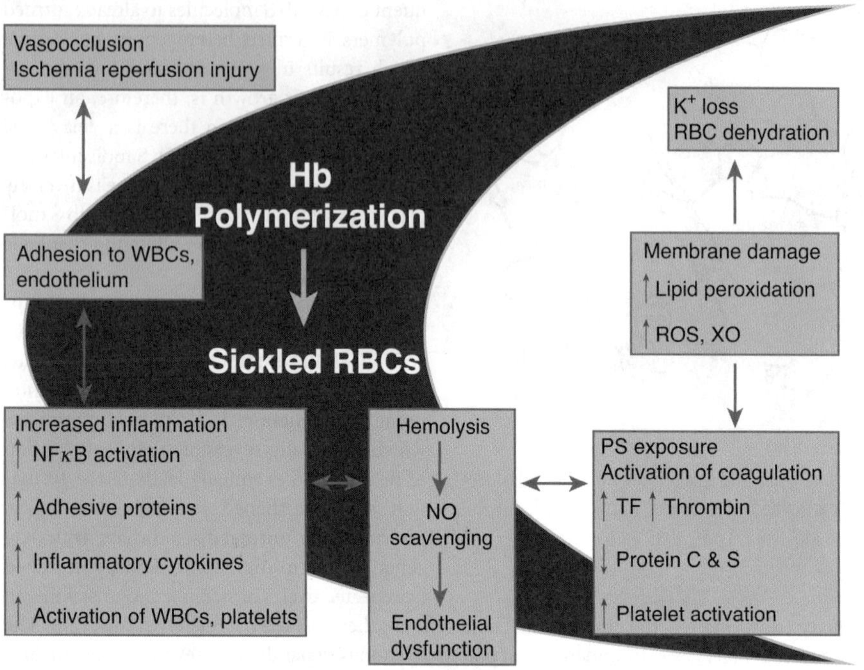

FIGURE 48–5. Schema summarizing the pathophysiology of sickle cell anemia. See text section "Pathophysiology" for further discussion. K$^+$, potassium; NO, nitric oxide; PS, phosphatidylserine; RBC, red blood cell; ROS, reactive oxygen species; TF, tissue factor; WBC, white blood cell; XO, xanthine oxidase.

potassium as a result of the activation of the calcium-activated potassium channel (Gardos channel), and the potassium-chloride cotransport channel. The net result is loss of intracellular potassium and water resulting in cellular dehydration.[30–35] This effectively increases the red cell hemoglobin concentration, favoring sickling.

■ NITRIC OXIDE SCAVENGING

NO is a key component of the vascular endothelium that has vasodilatory, antiinflammatory, and antiplatelet properties.[36] NO is a soluble gas synthesized from L-arginine by endothelial NOS (eNOS).[37] Decreased NO production and substrate levels, that is, L-arginine, have been documented in SCD especially during vasoocclusive crisis.[38–42] Chronic hemolysis with release of plasma free hemoglobin results in scavenging of NO with consequent endothelial dysfunction, which may favor sickle cell adherence.[43,44]

■ ABNORMAL CELL ADHESIVENESS

Seminal work by several groups showed that sickle red cells adhere to stimulated endothelium unlike their normal counterparts.[45,46] Newly released red cells, reticulocytes, are more adherent than dense sickle red cells.[47,48] It is thought that this is because more deformable red cells adhere to the endothelium behind which the dense red cells are trapped, leading to microvascular occlusion.[25] Molecules involved in sickle red cell adhesion to the endothelium include vascular cell adhesion molecule (VCAM)-1, integrin $\alpha_V\beta_3$, P-selectin, Lutheran blood group antigen, and thrombospondin.[49–54] The site of adhesion is purported to be the postcapillary venule at which site sickle red cells appear to interact with white cells adherent to the endothelium rather than engaging the endothelium directly.[27]

High neutrophil counts are an adverse prognostic factor in sickle cell anemia. Because of their larger size, adherent leukocytes cause greater decrease in vessel caliber than red cells. Diapedesis occurs in postcapillary venules, a site of vasoocclusion in sickle cell anemia.[27,55–57] Increased levels of the neutrophil adhesion molecules, L-selectin, and $\alpha_M\beta_2$ integrins are associated with a severe clinical phenotype.[55,58]

■ INFLAMMATION

Sickle cell anemia is characterized by chronic leukocytosis, abnormal activation of neutrophils and monocytes, and an increase in several proinflammatory mediators like tumor necrosis factor (TNF)-α, interleukin (IL)-6, and IL-1β. Several adhesion molecules are upregulated, for example, VCAM, selectins, and integrins, and an increase in acute phase reactants, such as C-reactive protein, secretory phospholipase A_2 (sPLA$_2$), and activation of the coagulation sequence occur.[58–70] It is an open question whether inflammation is caused by abnormally adhesive red cells to the vascular endothelium or whether inflammation causes abnormal red cell adhesiveness. Both are probably true given that red cell adhesiveness incites endothelial activity and infections with resultant inflammation precipitate clinically significant vascular events in patients.

■ ISCHEMIA–REPERFUSION INJURY

Akin to other disease states, for example, myocardial infarction, resolution of vasoocclusion results in reperfusion injury characterized by generation of oxidant stress, lipid peroxidation, and upregulation of nuclear factor-κB, a key player in the inflammatory process.[58,71,72]

■ ACTIVATION OF THE COAGULATION SYSTEM

The initiator of coagulation, tissue factor, is elevated in patients with sickle cell anemia.[36,68,73–75] Tissue-factor-bearing microparticles from monocytes and macrophages and circulating endothelial cells are seen.[58,68,74] Phosphatidylserine exposure on the surface of red cells provides an impetus for the coagulation process.[76] Heightened thrombin generation, platelet activation, and fibrinolysis can result in favoring a procoagulant state.[63,77,78]

■ CHRONIC VASCULOPATHY

Several vascular beds in sickle cell anemia display changes akin to atherosclerotic vascular disease: large vessel intima hyperplasia and smooth muscle proliferation.[79,80] However, the characteristic lipid laden plaques of atherosclerotic vascular disease are not present.[58]

Inflammatory stimuli lead to both neutrophil, monocyte, and endothelial activation with increased white cell-red cell adhesion resulting in increased vasoocclusion. Antiinflammatory agents decrease these effects.[81] Clinically, amelioration of the inflammatory phenotype by glucocorticoids is followed by a rebound effect after cessation of the drugs.[81,82]

■ SICKLE CELL TRAIT

Inheritance of only one Hb S allele is termed *sickle cell trait* (Hb AS). It is present in approximately 8 percent of Americans of African descent with a higher prevalence in regions of Africa. An estimated 300 million people carry the trait worldwide.[83] The percentage of Hb A is always higher (~60%) than Hb S (~40%) in sickle cell trait.

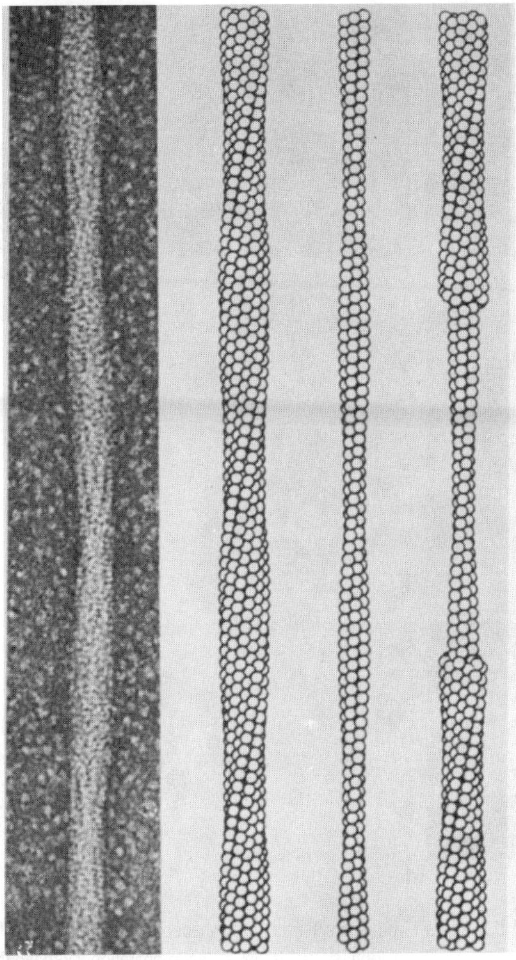

FIGURE 48–6. Electron micrograph of negatively stained fiber of Hg S and the structure deduced by three-dimensional image reconstruction. The reconstructed fiber is presented as ball models, with each ball representing a Hg S tetramer. The models are presented as the outer sheath (*left*), the inner core (*center*), and a combination of both inner and outer filaments (*right*). *(Reproduced from Edelstein SJ: Structures of the fibers of hemoglobin S.* Texas Rep Biol Med *81:221, 1980, with permission.)*

Hb AS is considered a generally asymptomatic state with few problems for the individual over a lifetime. Hb AS cells sickle at O_2 tension of approximately 15 torr.[84]

Plasma myeloperoxidase and red cell sickling have been reported to increase during exercise with fluid restriction in Hb AS subjects.[85] Plasma levels of VCAM-1 are higher in Hb AS subjects and remain elevated following exercise compared to normal controls or Hb AS subjects with concomitant α-thalassemia, which is suggestive of subtle microcirculatory dysfunction in this population.[86]

Hb A in the cell prevents sickling except in the most unusual circumstances. Clinically, Hb AS subjects can have microscopic infarction of the renal medulla, leading to a concentrating defect and hyposthenuria.[87] Renal papillary infarctions can also occur. The medullary environment is characterized by anoxia, hyperosmolarity, and low pH, which predisposes to sickling. Rarely, gross hematuria is observed. Renal neoplasm or stones should be excluded in those with persistent gross hematuria. Risk of urinary tract infection is higher in females with Hb AS, especially during pregnancy. End-stage renal disease occurs at an earlier age for Hb AS patients with polycystic kidney disease.[88]

Splenic infarction occurs under extreme environmental conditions in persons with Hb AS; most resolve spontaneously.[89,90] Caution and immediate intervention is also warranted in those Hb AS individuals who develop traumatic hyphema.[91] There is an increased association with venous thromboembolism in persons with Hb AS compared to Hb AA individuals.[92] Hb AS patients do not have increased perioperative morbidity or mortality. The life span of patients with Hb AS is normal.[93]

LABORATORY FEATURES

Sickle cell anemia is characterized by a laboratory profile of evidence of hemolytic anemia with increases in lactate dehydrogenase (LDH), indirect bilirubin, reticulocyte count, and a decrease in serum haptoglobin. Anemia is usually normochromic, normocytic with a steady-state hemoglobin level between 5 and 11 g/dL.[14,94] Sickle cells are often evident on the blood film (Fig. 48–7). The red cell density is increased with a normal mean cell hemoglobin concentration (MCHC).[95] Serum erythropoietin level is decreased relative to the degree of anemia.[96] Elevated neutrophil and platelet counts are observed even in asymptomatic patients reflective of persistent low-grade inflammation.[97–99]

Elevations in immunoglobulins, especially immunoglobulin (Ig) A are seen.[100] Plasma tocopherol and zinc levels are low.[101–103] Serum ferritin is increased, especially in iron overloaded patients. Elevated brain natriuretic peptide is seen in patients with pulmonary hypertension and congestive heart failure. Morphologically, classic sickle red cells are seen on blood film examination, and the marrow shows erythroid hyperplasia.

■ DIAGNOSIS

Sickle cell anemia can be accurately diagnosed with high-performance liquid chromatography (HPLC) and isoelectric focusing.[104] Rapid methods like solubility testing and sickling of red cells using sodium metabisulfite are less reliable tests.[105] Polymerase chain reaction is the method of choice for prenatal diagnosis.[106] No Hb A is found in patients with Hb SS, Hb SC, or Hb Sβ^0 diseases. Varying amounts of Hb A (depending on the severity of the β-thalassemia mutation) are found in Hb Sβ^+-thalassemia subjects.

COURSE AND PROGNOSIS

Study of mortality trends in the United States between 1968 and 1992 revealed a decrease in mortality of 41, 47, and 53 percent in subjects between ages 1 and 4 years, 5 and 9 years, and 10 and 14 years, respectively.[107] Penicillin prophylaxis was a key factor in the decline in mortality during this period. Data on mortality trends between 1983 and 2002 showed a significant decrease in mortality between ages 0 and 3 years for the periods 1995 to 1998 and 1999 to 2002.[108] The decline in mortality coincided with the introduction of pneumococcal polyvalent conjugate 7 (PCV7) vaccine. No decrease in mortality was noted in older age groups.[108] Average life expectancy of patients with Hb SS disease in the United States is 42 and 48 years for males and females, respectively.[109] As the sickle cell population ages, it is likely that causes of death will change from an infectious etiology to those related to end-organ damage.

CLINICAL FEATURES AND MANAGEMENT

The reader is referred to the National Institutes of Health, National Heart, Lung and Blood Institute's guidelines from 2002 for an extensive review on the topic.[110] General approaches to SCD management and pain management are described separately (Table 48–2).

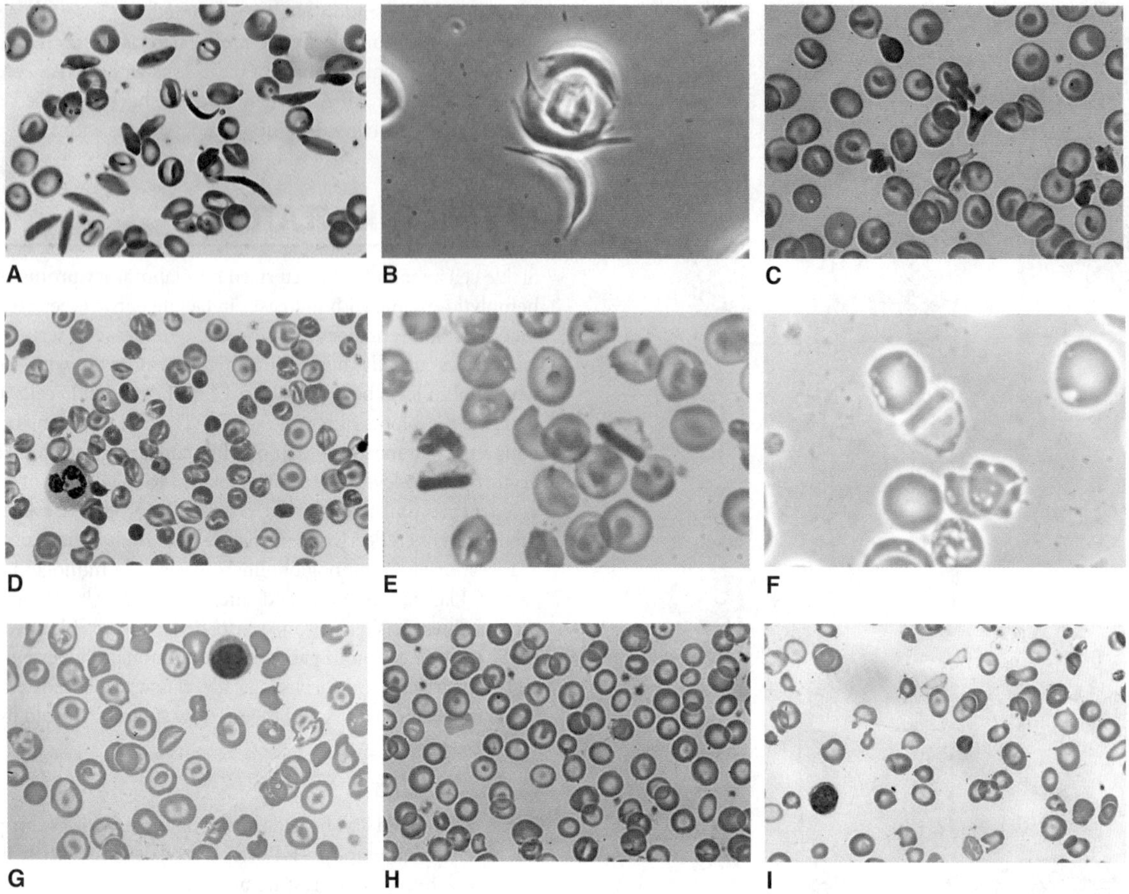

FIGURE 48–7. Blood cell morphology in patients with structural hemoglobinopathies. **A.** Blood film. Hb SS disease with characteristic sickle-shaped cells and extreme elliptocytes with dense central hemoglobin staining. Both shapes are characteristic of sickled cells. Occasional target cells. **B.** Phase contrast microscopy of wet preparation. Note the three sickled cells with terminal fine-pointed projections as a result of tactoid formation and occasional target cells. **C.** Hb SC disease. Blood film. Note high frequency of target cells characteristic of Hb C and the small dense, irregular, contracted cells reflective of their content of Hb S. **D.** Hb CC disease. Blood film. Characteristic combination of numerous target cells and a population of dense (hyperchromatic) microspherocytes. Of the nonspherocytic cells, virtually all are target cells. **E.** Hb CC disease postsplenectomy. Blood film. Note the rod-like inclusions in two cells as a result of Hb C para-crystalinization. These cells are virtually all removed in patients with spleens. **F.** Hb CC disease postsplenectomy. Phase contrast microscopy of wet preparation. Note the Hb C crystalline rod in a cell. **G.** Hb DD disease. Blood film. Note Frequent target cells admixed with population of small spherocytes, poikilocytes, and tiny red cell fragments. **H.** Hb EE disease. Blood film. Hypochromia, anisocytosis, and target cells. **I.** Hb E thalassemia. Blood film. Marked anisocytosis (primarily microcytes) and poikilocytosis. Hypochromia. *(Used with permission from* Lichtman's Atlas of Hematology, *www.accessmedicine.com.)*

■ CRISES

The typical course for a sickle cell patient is that of periods of relatively normal functioning despite the chronic anemia, punctuated by periods of either pain in various anatomic sites, for example, the abdomen, chest, or extremities, a further decline in blood hemoglobin concentration, or other manifestations termed "a crisis." Crises have typically been classified as vasoocclusive painful crisis, aplastic crisis, sequestration crisis, and hemolytic crisis.

Vasoocclusive Crisis

The hallmark of sickle cell disease is the vasoocclusive pain crisis. It is the most common clinical manifestation but can occur with varying frequency in different individuals. It results from the complex interplay between sickled red cells, neutrophils, endothelium, and plasma factors as outlined in the section on pathophysiology. The end result is that of tissue hypoxia leading to tissue death and accompanying pain. Crisis may affect any tissue, but patients typically complain of pain in the chest, lower back, and extremities. Abdominal pain occurs and may mimic acute abdomen from other causes. Fever is often present, even in the absence of infection. Episodes may be precipitated by dehydration, infection, and cold weather, although in about half of the cases no precipitating factor is found.[111] Repeated splenic infarctions in childhood typically result in "autosplenectomy" and loss of splenic function by age 6 to 8 years.[112]

Phases of vasoocclusive episodes have been described in children and adults.[113,114] These include a prodromal phase characterized by low intensity pain, paresthesias, decreased red cell deformability, and an increase in irreversibly sickled cells (see "Hemoglobin Polymerization" above) followed by an initial, evolving phase characterized by increasing pain and worsening of hematologic parameters. This is then followed by an established (inflammatory) phase with steady, severe pain, increased hemolysis, increased neutrophils, and increased acute phase reactants, at which time patients typically seek medical care. Physical signs may include fever, joint swelling, and effusion. The final phase is that of resolution and recovery, wherein all of the above clinical and laboratory abnormalities gradually revert to baseline.

The characterization of phases has implications for clinical research, especially in pain management, when interventions early in the course of a crisis could result in better outcomes for patients.

TABLE 48–2. Pathophysiologic Mechanisms and Potential Therapeutic Targets in SCD

Pathophysiology/Complication	Therapeutic Interventions
Hb S polymerization	Hb F induction
Cellular dehydration	Gardos channel inhibition
	Potassium-chloride cotransport channel inhibition
Adhesion to endothelium	
Red cells	Antiselectin
	Antiintegrin
Neutrophils	Antiselectin
	Intravenous immunoglobulin
	Hydroxyurea
Inflammation	NF-κB inhibition
	Immunomodulatory drugs
	Hydroxyurea
	Statins
NO scavenging	Nitric oxide donor (NO, HU, BH4)
	Prostaglandin E_5 inhibition
	Modulation of hemolysis
Coagulation	Tissue factor inhibition
	Antiplatelet therapy
	Anticoagulation
Hyposplenism/Infection	Penicillin prophylaxis
Ischemia-reperfusion	Xanthine oxidase inhibition
	Myeloperoxidase inhibition
Iron overload	Iron chelation

Aplastic Crisis

Aplastic crisis in sickle cell anemia is akin to that seen in other hematologic disorders where there is a cessation in red cell production in the face of ongoing hemolysis resulting in an acute, severe drop in hemoglobin levels. The characteristic laboratory finding is a decrease in reticulocyte count to less than 1 percent. It is usually associated with infections. The most common causative agent is parvovirus B19, which attaches to the P antigen receptor on erythroid progenitor cells, causing a temporary arrest in red cell production (see Chap. 35).[115,116] Recurrent aplastic crises by parvovirus B19 is rare because of the development of protective antibodies. Although classically responsible for decreased red cell production, pancytopenia may occur. Other rare complications associated with parvovirus B19 include acute splenic sequestration, hepatic sequestration, acute chest syndrome, marrow necrosis, and renal dysfunction.[115,117–122] Most cases of parvovirus B19 infection resolve within 2 weeks. However, patients with severe symptomatic anemia need red cell transfusion.[123] Siblings of SCD patients with parvovirus infections should be monitored closely for aplastic crisis given high secondary attack rates (>50%).

Sequestration Crisis

This type of crisis is characterized by sudden, massive pooling of red cells, especially in the spleen, which may result in hypovolemic shock and cardiovascular collapse.[124] It is typically seen in infants and children (usually <5 years of age) prior to autoinfarction of the spleen but can be seen in adults with Hb SC disease or Hb Sβ-thalassemia with persisting splenomegaly.[125–127] Hepatic sequestration can also occur. A minor sequestration episode is usually accompanied by a hemoglobin of more than 7 g/dL, and a major episode usually is one in which the hemoglobin is less than 7 g/dL or the hemoglobin has decreased by 3 g/dL from baseline.[128]

Acute splenic sequestration crisis and hepatic sequestration crisis can present with rapidly enlarging spleen or liver, pain, hypoxemia, and hypovolemic shock. Treatment consists of either red cell transfusion or exchange transfusion. Transfusion carries the risk of hyperviscosity when the sequestration crisis resolves and the sequestered red cells are returned to the general circulation. Acute splenic sequestration crisis can be recurrent, especially in children.[129] Long-term treatment to prevent recurrence is debated. Some report chronic exchange transfusion as a means of delaying splenectomy until the child is older while others did not see any benefit to this treatment. Splenectomy is recommended for those with life-threatening splenic sequestration crisis or chronic hypersplenism. Patients younger than 2 years of age can be placed on chronic transfusion until they are older, at which time splenectomy should be considered. Partial splenectomy is probably best avoided in most cases. Parental education is of importance in early recognition of the problem in order to seek medical care promptly.[124,129,130]

Hyperhemolytic Crisis

This is a term used to describe the occurrence of episodes of accelerated hemolysis characterized by decreased blood hemoglobin, increasing reticulocytes, and other markers of hemolysis (hyperbilirubinemia, increased LDH). Episodes of hyperhemolysis are known to occur in certain conditions; resolution phase of a vasoocclusive crisis during which irreversibly sickled red cells and dense red cells trapped in the microcirculation are rapidly destroyed is one such example. Delayed hemolytic transfusion reactions, which can be seen in multiply transfused, alloimmunized patients is another condition associated with hyperhemolysis.[131,132] The existence of "hyperhemolytic crises" in other circumstances, particularly related to concurrent glucose-6-phosphate dehydrogenase deficiency, is questionable.

■ MANAGEMENT OF PAIN

Patients with SCD have acute pain, chronic pain, or both. As a symptom, pain is often underrated in its intensity and undertreated by caregivers, especially inexperienced physicians. Patients are often perceived as drug seekers or drug addicts, when in fact less than 10 percent of patients are addicted, a number comparable to other disease states. Nonsatisfactory relief of pain drives patients to behaviors that appear to healthcare givers as signs of addiction—a state termed "pseudoaddiction." A study comparing sickle cell anemia patients who use the emergency department frequently or infrequently found significant impairment in quality of life and increased markers of disease severity in those who use the emergency department frequently, dispelling the myth that frequent emergency department use indicates narcotic-addicted individuals when in fact they have more severe disease.[133–138]

Acute pain is managed with opioids, nonsteroidal antiinflammatory drugs (NSAIDs), acetaminophen, or a combination of these medications. Immediate pain assessment and frequent reassessment with appropriate application of medications until pain relief is obtained is important. For adults and children weighing more than 50 kg, morphine can be started at a dose of 0.1 to 0.15 mg/kg. The hydromorphone dose should be 0.015 to 0.02 mg/kg intravenously. These are recommended doses for opioid-naïve patients and are at the lower end of the dosing range.[110,139,140] The use of meperidine is controversial. Many hospitals have discontinued its use given the neurologic side effects, especially in patients with renal failure and at risk for the serotonin syndrome in conjunction with use of other medications.[141–143] The syndrome is a potentially life-threatening adverse drug reaction that may occur following therapeutic drug use or inadvertent interactions between drugs. It is a consequence of excess serotonergic activity in the central nervous system and peripheral serotonin receptors. The excess serotonin activity produces a spectrum of specific symptoms including cognitive (e.g., mental confusion, headache, agitation, coma), autonomic (e.g., sweating, shivering, hyperthermia, elevated blood pressure, tachycardia, nausea), and somatic effects (e.g., tremor, muscle twitching, hyperreflexia). The symptoms may range from barely perceptible to fatal. Numerous drugs and drug combinations have been reported to produce the syndrome. However, the use of morphine is not benign and concerns of increased association of acute chest syndrome, dysphoria, and neuroexcitatory side effects have been raised.[144–148] Prior use of opioid therapy should be taken into consideration when deciding on initial opioid doses as patients may be tolerant and require higher doses. Caution should be exercised with NSAIDs and acetaminophen if there is renal or hepatic dysfunction. Patients with acute pain are better managed in a setting dedicated to sickle cell patients.[149] A multidisciplinary approach is needed for pain management, especially if chronic pain is present.[150,151] Opioid side effects should be anticipated and managed. Antidepressants, anticonvulsants, and clonidine can be used for neuropathic pain. Occasionally, severe, unrelenting pain may require red cell transfusion to decrease sickle cells below 30 percent in the blood.[152]

■ PULMONARY MANIFESTATIONS

Acute Chest Syndrome

The acute chest syndrome (ACS) is a constellation of signs and symptoms in patients with SCD that includes a new infiltrate on chest radiograph defined by alveolar consolidation but not atelectasis, chest pain, fever, tachypnea, wheezing, or cough, and hypoxia (Fig. 48–8).[153] It is the leading cause of mortality in patients with SCD.[109] A large multicenter study of ACS showed that the etiology varied depending on age; while infections with viruses and bacteria were found to be the leading cause in the pediatric age-group, a large number of adults developed ACS as a result of pulmonary fat microembolization, derived from marrow necrosis, usually during the course of a vasoocclusive crisis.[154] Asthma also is associated with ACS.[155] Regardless of the triggering factor, the pathogenesis of ACS involves increased intrapulmonary sickling, intrapulmonary inflammation with increased microvascular permeability, and alveolar consolidation. The clinical severity of the syndrome is variable; in some patients the syndrome rapidly evolves with bilateral infiltrates and consolidation leading to acute respiratory failure requiring intubation and ventilatory assistance.

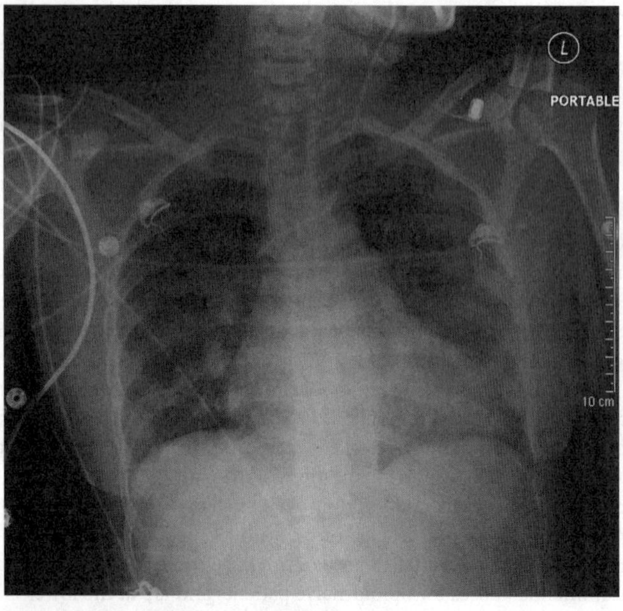

FIGURE 48–8. Anteroposterior view of chest radiograph depicting bilateral, patchy, lung infiltrates in a 30-year-old female with SCD and evolving acute chest syndrome.

An age greater than 20 years, a platelet count greater than 200,000/μL, multilobar lung involvement, and a history of cardiac disease are independent risk factors for respiratory failure.[154] Thrombocytopenia is an independent predictor of neurologic complications during hospitalization, which was seen in 22 percent of adult patients in the National Acute Chest Syndrome study.

The treatment of acute chest syndrome includes oxygenation, incentive spirometry, adequate pain control to avoid chest splinting, antimicrobial therapy that covers atypical bacteria, avoidance of overhydration, application of bronchodilators and red cell transfusion to decrease intrapulmonary sickling.[154,156–161] $sPLA_2$ has been recognized as a predictor of ACS in patients with SCD with a vasoocclusive crisis.[162–166] An anti-$sPLA_2$ agent is being studied as treatment for ACS. A current SCD clinical research network protocol is looking at the role of early transfusion in patients with vasoocclusion and increased $sPLA_2$ in the prevention of ACS.

Pulmonary Hypertension

Approximately one-third of adult SCD patients have pulmonary hypertension as defined by a tricuspid regurgitant jet velocity of ≥2.5 m/sec on echocardiography (pulmonary artery systolic pressure of >25 torr).[167,168] Although a lower threshold jet velocity is used for diagnosis of pulmonary hypertension in patients with SCD (2.5 vs. 3.0 m/s), this threshold still translates into an increased risk of death in this population.[153,167–169] Median survival for patients with pulmonary hypertension determined by right-heart catheterization was 25.6 months.[170] It is unclear whether elevations in pulmonary artery pressure is a direct cause of increased mortality or just serves as a marker of a more severe disease phenotype.

Some of the principal proposed mechanisms of pulmonary hypertension include nitric oxide scavenging through reactions with plasma hemoglobin, increased reactive oxygen species, increased arginase activity resulting in substrate reduction for nitric oxide synthesis, and increased platelet activation.[44,153,171–182] Other causes include parenchymal lung disease with chronic hypoxemia from repeated episodes of ACS, thromboembolism, and chronic liver disease with portal-pulmonary hypertension.[183] Left-ventricular diastolic dysfunction with resultant pulmonary venous hypertension may also be a contributing factor.[167,184]

Clinical symptoms of pulmonary hypertension include fatigue, dizziness, and dyspnea on exertion, chest pain, and syncope. These may be unrecognized as being related to pulmonary hypertension as pulmonary hypertension is often undiagnosed in patients with sickle cell disease.

Few data exist on effective treatment of pulmonary hypertension in SCD. Small studies have shown tolerability and efficacy of sildenafil, a phosphodiesterase 5 inhibitor, in patients with pulmonary hypertension. However, the number of subjects studied has been too small to draw firm conclusions. Results of randomized trials should be forthcoming. In the interim, pulmonary hypertension may be treated following guidelines set for the treatment of primary pulmonary hypertension unrelated to SCD.

Asthma, Abnormal Pulmonary Function Tests, and Airway Hyperreactivity

Asthma is a common comorbidity in SCD. Several reports suggest a higher than average prevalence in patients with SCD.[185–194] Inflammation, hypoxemia, and increased oxidative stress associated with asthma may contribute to the vasculopathy of SCD.[155] Increased awareness, recognition, and treatment can result in decreased pulmonary morbidity.

Pulmonary function tests collected as part of the Cooperative Study of Sickle Cell Disease (CSSCD) revealed abnormalities in 90 percent of the 310 patients.[195] Approximately 50 to 75 percent of the cohort had restrictive lung disease and another 13 percent showed isolated decline in lung diffusion capacity. The prevalence of obstructive lung disease was low, probably a reflection of the cross-sectional nature of the study and a lack of data on maneuvers that test for airway hyperreactivity.

Asthma treatment follows general treatment guidelines as in the non-SCD populations.

CARDIAC MANIFESTATIONS

The hemodynamic burden of anemia in SCD results in an elevated cardiac output. There is minimal increase in heart rate as a result of successful adaptation with increasing stroke volume contributing to the increase in cardiac output.[196,197]

Clinical manifestations are those of a hyperdynamic circulation that includes a forceful precordial apical impulse and systolic and diastolic flow murmurs. Striking tachycardia may occur during periods of increased hemodynamic stress as with infection. Systolic and diastolic cardiac abnormalities can begin early in childhood.[198] Diastolic left ventricular dysfunction is an independent risk factor for death, and patients having both left ventricular dysfunction and pulmonary hypertension carry a poor prognosis.[199] Cardiac autonomic dysfunction is prevalent in SCD and may contribute to the sudden death seen in the patient population.[200–208] Fat embolization or vasoocclusion of coronary arteries leading to myocardial ischemia has also been reported.[204] Although chest pain is common in SCD and coronary occlusion is not, patients with chest pain should be evaluated for ischemic heart disease.

Blood pressure in patients with SCD is significantly lower than age-, sex-, and race-matched controls partly secondary to anemia.[198] Mild hypertension is associated with end-organ damage. Careful monitoring of blood pressure and judicious intervention is indicated. Diuretics may be used keeping in mind that SCD patients may have obligate hyposthenuria.

CENTRAL NERVOUS SYSTEM

Originally thought to be a small-vessel disease, stroke in SCD is a macrovascular phenomenon with devastating consequences that affects approximately 11 percent of patients younger than 20 years of age.[209,210] Risk is highest in the first decade of life followed by a second smaller peak after age 29 years. Ischemic stroke is most common in children and older adults, whereas hemorrhagic stroke predominates in the third decade of life.[210] Recurrent stroke is most common in the first 2 years following the primary event.[211]

Cerebral blood flow is significantly increased in SCD because of chronic anemia and hypoxemia. Cerebral vasculature is unable to vasodilate further in response to increased hypoxic stress thereby causing ischemia.[212,213] Stenosis of large vessels, chronic hemolysis with its attendant complications, deranged nitric oxide metabolism, red cell endothelial interactions, perfusion–reperfusion injury, and a hypercoagulable state are contributing factors.[213] Other uncommon causes include fat embolization after marrow infarction and venous sinus thrombosis. Cardioembolic disease is rare despite the increased prevalence of cardiomegaly in this patient population.[214,215] Moyamoya type fragile collaterals have been reported in more than one-fifth of patients with prior stroke, possibly leading to hemorrhagic stroke in later life.[214,216–220] An increased frequency of intracranial aneurysms and occurrence of subarachnoid hemorrhage has also been reported.

Risk factors for ischemic stroke include transient ischemic attack, recent or recurrent acute chest syndrome, hypertension, and neutrophilia, whereas anemia and neutrophilia are independent risk factors for hemorrhagic stroke.[210] Patients with nocturnal hypoxemia and silent brain infarcts detected on magnetic resonance imaging also have an increased stroke risk.[221–225] Sickle cell genotypes other than Hb SS carry a lower risk as do patients with Hb Sα-thalassemia.[210,226,227] The best predictor of stroke risk, however, is an increased blood flow velocity in major intracranial arteries on transcranial Doppler (TCD) ultrasonography.[227] Blood flow velocities less than 170 cm/s are considered normal. Velocities between 170 and 200 cm/s are termed conditional, and velocities of greater than 200 cm/s are considered high and are associated with a 10-fold increase in ischemic stroke in children 2 to 16 years of age.

There is an increased frequency of stroke among siblings of patients with SCD than would be expected by chance alone, raising the possibility of other modifier genes contributing to stroke risk.[214] The TNF (−308) G/A promoter polymorphism is associated with increased large-vessel stroke risk. The interleukin-4 receptor gene 503 S/P variant is also associated with increased risk, albeit not reaching statistical significance in the population studied. The leukotriene C_4 synthase (−444) C variant may be protective.[228] The clinical features of stroke in sickle cell disease encompasses the classic findings of stroke in other disorders including but not limited to hemiparesis, seizures, coma, paresthesia, headaches, and cranial nerve palsies. Neurocognitive deficits in attention and functions, such as memory and language have been described.[229] Impairment may begin early in infancy. Apart from subjects with overt stroke, those with "silent" infarcts, characterized by abnormal magnetic resonance imaging findings without overt neurologic manifestations of classic stroke also have neurocognitive sequelae.

Imaging approaches for acute stroke are the same as those for non-SCD patients. Magnetic resonance imaging (MRI) and magnetic resonance angiography (MRA) should be performed when stroke is suspected.

Prevention of Primary Stroke

Based on the results from the Stroke Prevention in Sickle Cell Disease (STOP) Study, it is recommended that asymptomatic children with Hb SS disease who are older than 2 years of age should be screened for stroke risk using TCD.[227] Those persons with two abnormal readings—defined as TCD velocities greater than 200 cm/s should be offered a chronic red cell transfusion program for primary stroke prevention. Repeat TCD screenings should be done every 3 to 12 months even in patients who have normal or conditional baseline velocities, because they can evolve into a higher risk category. Children with other risk factors for stroke or velocities closer to 200 cm/s should be screened more frequently. More data are needed to clearly define frequency of repeat screenings. Despite obstacles to TCD screening, clinical practice changes based on the STOP Study translated into declining stroke rates since 1991.[230,231]

Prevention of Secondary Stroke

Patients with SCD who present with a stroke and are not on chronic transfusion should be on a transfusion program to prevent secondary strokes. Exchange transfusion may be preferable to periodic red cell transfusion. In a retrospective study, children who received a periodic transfusion had a fivefold higher relative risk of a recurrent stroke compared to those on an exchange transfusion regimen.[232] Despite chronic transfusions, patients may have a recurrent stroke. One study showed that 5 of 6 cerebral infarctions and 7 of 16 transient ischemic attacks occurred in patients with Hb S greater than 30 percent.[233] Therefore, patients who have had a stroke while on chronic transfusion should have Hb S monitored, and if greater than 30 percent, should have their transfusion regimen optimized. A decreased stroke risk was demonstrated in patients who were transitioned to hydroxyurea from chronic transfusions.[234] Overlapping transfusion until adequate hydroxyurea dose was reached resulted in recurrence rates comparable to that of chronic transfusion only, while abrupt discontinuation of transfusion prior to starting hydroxyurea had a negative impact. Hydroxyurea was shown to decrease high and conditional TCD velocities in more than 90 percent of patients studied.[235]

Standard therapies for ischemic stroke in the non-SCD population, like tissue-type plasminogen activator, have not been studied in patients with SCD and, therefore, no recommendations can be made for or against such interventions. Treatment guidelines for intracranial hemorrhage are as those for non–SCD-related intracranial hemorrhage; role of transfusion is less clear in SCD especially when cause of intracranial hemorrhage is unclear. Patients with moyamoya disease who have a particularly poor outcome may benefit from revascularization using encephaloduroarteriosynangiosis.[236,237]

GENITOURINARY

Renal Failure

The acidic, hypoxic, and hypertonic environment of the renal medulla promotes sickling of Hb SS erythrocytes, leading to ischemia of the renal microcirculation.[238] Collateral vessel formation interferes with the countercurrent exchange mechanism ultimately leading to loss of medullary function.[239]

Paracrine effects of prostaglandin may cause glomerular hyperfiltration. Papillary necrosis as a result of renal infarction and glomerulopathy characterized by glomerulomegaly, focal, and segmental glomerulosclerosis are characteristically seen in sickle cell nephropathy (Fig. 48–9).

The incidence of renal failure varies between 4 and 20 percent.[240–243] However, it is increasingly recognized that renal pathology may be more prevalent given the imprecision of the conventional markers of glomerular filtration rate (GFR) estimation and increased longevity of sickle cell patients. More than two-thirds of patients older than age 40 years will have increased albumin excretion reflecting glomerular damage.[244,245] Glomerular hyperfiltration, microalbuminuria, and macroalbuminuria occur sequentially in SCD patients starting at a relatively early age and increasing in frequency with advancing age.[245] Isosthenuria is prevalent in patients with SCD, which may increase the risk of dehydration. It is irreversible without transfusion beyond the age of 15 years.[246]

Angiotensin-converting enzyme inhibitors decrease proteinuria and may reverse pathologic changes such as focal segmental glomerulosclerosis. However, large-scale studies are needed to characterize the true magnitude of the benefit. Effective blood pressure control, avoidance of nephrotoxic agents, and treatment of urinary tract infection are the cornerstones of treatment. Relative decrease in serum erythropoietin levels in relation to anemia is observed. Patients may benefit from erythropoietin treatment. Care should be taken to avoid inducing hyperviscosity.[96,242,247–249]

Hematuria

Hematuria, usually painless, can result from papillary necrosis, rupture of collateral vessels, and, rarely, from neoplasm. Patients with repeated or protracted hematuria should be evaluated for a renal neoplasm or other causes of hematuria. There is a preponderance of bleeding from

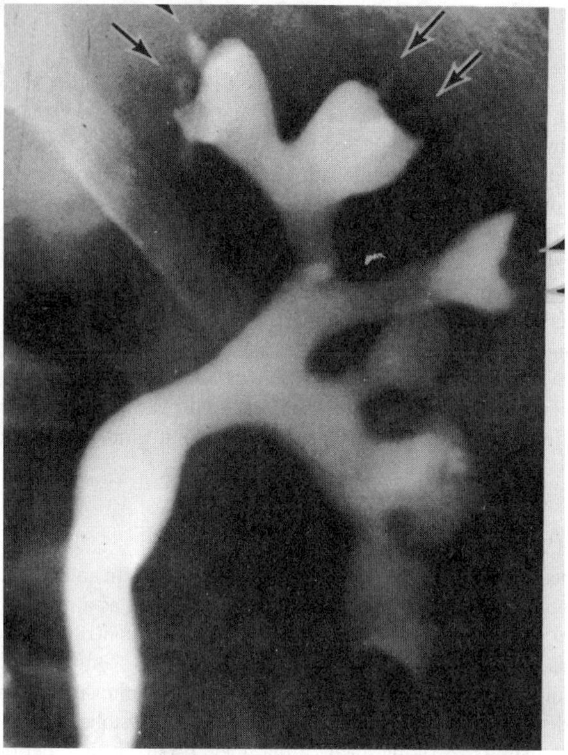

FIGURE 48–9. Renal papillary necrosis in a patient with sickle cell trait. Note the small medullary cavities in the upper three calyces of the left kidney (*arrows*). *(Reproduced from Harrow BR, Sloane JA, Liebman NC: Roentgenographic demonstration of papillary necrosis in sickle-cell trait.* N Engl J Med *268:969, 1963, with permission.)*

the left kidney as a result of the "nutcracker" phenomenon, in which the longer right renal vein is compressed between the aorta and superior mesenteric artery, resulting in increased venous pressure.[246,250]

Proteinuria and Renal Tubular Acidosis

In addition to the hyperfiltration, proteinuria, and glomerulopathy described earlier, distal renal tubular acidosis is often present but clinical metabolic acidosis is rare.

The focus of research has been to detect nephropathy at earlier stages in the hope of slowing or preventing disease progression. Glomerular hyperfiltration and tubular secretion give falsely normal results for serum creatinine. By the time serum creatinine is in the conventional range of renal failure, GFR is already less than 30 to 40 mL/min per 1.73 m^2.[251,252] Serum cystatin C, an inhibitor of cysteine proteases, correlates closely with GFR. It circumvents the problems associated with serum creatinine measurements as it is not affected by muscle mass, protein intake, drugs, inflammatory stimuli, or substances interfering with assay performance.[252] It is a more reliable marker of renal dysfunction in this population. *N*-acetyl-β-D-glucosaminidase was found to be a useful marker for tubular damage in Hb Sβ-thalassemia patients.[244]

Priapism

Priapism occurs in as many as 45 percent of patients with SCD with often devastating psychological consequences.[253–255] It presents with engorgement of the corpora cavernosa, sparing the corpora spongiosum and glans penis, and can be continuous or "stuttering." "Stuttering" priapism is a term used for episodes that last less than 3 hours but are repetitive.[256,257] Priapism in SCD is described as a "low flow" state with sickling of red cells in the sinusoids of corpora cavernosa causing venous stasis and setting up a vicious cycle of factors that favor "sickling." Repeated episodes cause corporeal fibrosis resulting in impotence in 36 to 86 percent of patients.[258] Resolution in 12 hours portends a more favorable prognosis.[250,259]

Aspiration of the corpus cavernosa followed by epinephrine injections, exchange transfusion, and α and β agonists have all been used, but data regarding efficacy are sparse. In recalcitrant cases, a shunt is performed but results in permanent impotence. Prophylaxis has been attempted with pseudoephedrine and gonadotropin-releasing hormone analogues to suppress testosterone, but, again, solid data are lacking.[253,260–264]

Nocturnal Enuresis

Nocturnal enuresis is prevalent in 25 to 33 percent of the pediatric sickle cell population, which is higher compared to that of age-matched controls.[265–267] It tends to decrease with age but is still prevalent in adults. Social and environmental factors, decreased functional bladder capacity, and decreased arousal during sleep appear to be contributing factors.

MUSCULOSKELETAL SYSTEM

Vasoocclusive crisis described previously is commonly manifested by marrow infarction causing musculoskeletal pain, swelling at involved sites, fever, and leukocytosis. Marrow hypercellularity is thought to predispose to this phenomenon by causing a decrease in local blood flow and oxygenation.

Dactylitis

Dactylitis is a term used to describe painful swelling of digits of hands and feet ("hand-foot syndrome"; Fig. 48–10). It occurs early in infancy as hematopoietic marrow is still present in these bones at this age. Most episodes resolve within 2 weeks.[268–271] Epiphyseal infarction can result in joint pain and swelling mimicking septic arthritis. Vertebral body infarctions with subsequent collapse causes the classic "fish mouth" appearance on plain radiographs.

Osteomyelitis and Bone Infarction

Impaired cellular and humoral immunity together with infarction of bone contribute to this complication with an estimated prevalence of 12 percent (Fig. 48–11). Nontypical serotypes of Salmonella, *Staphylococcus aureus*, and Gram-negative bacilli are the principal infectious offenders. No single lab test or imaging reliably differentiates osteomyelitis from infarction.[268,270,272–276]

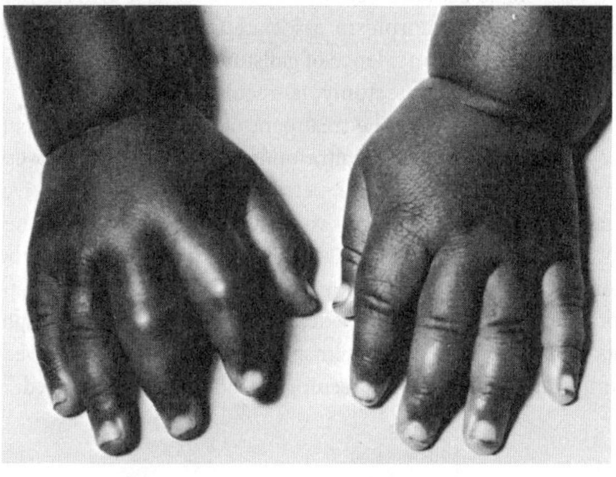

FIGURE 48–10. Sickle cell dactylitis (hand-foot syndrome). Note the swelling of the right hand involving the thumb and first and second fingers. *(Reproduced from Diggs LW: Sickle cell crisis.* Am J Clin Pathol *44:1, 1965, with permission).*

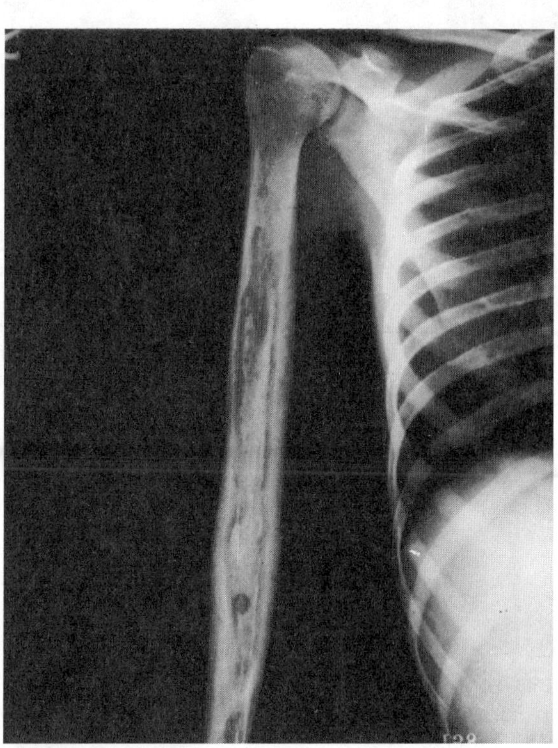

FIGURE 48–11. *Salmonella typhimurium* osteomyelitis in a patient with Hb SC disease. *(Reproduced from River GL, Robbins AB, Schwartz SO: SC hemoglobin: A clinical study.* Blood *18:385, 1961, with permission.)*

Osteopenia and Osteoporosis

Osteopenia and osteoporosis is very prevalent in Hb SS disease, especially given the young age of the patients. The lumbar spine appears to be the most affected. Low body mass index is a consistent correlate of decreased bone density.

A vast majority of children with SS disease will show decline in growth compared to normal peers. Puberty is delayed on an average by 12 to 24 months, as is skeletal age. Some factors such as nutritional status could be modified and decrease the effect on growth.

Avascular Necrosis

Vasoocclusion resulting in infarction of articular surfaces of long bone occurs most commonly in the femur followed by the humerus. It is a complication more prevalent than previously believed as more sensitive imaging studies have been used. It was previously thought to occur with increased frequency in Hb SC disease as opposed to Hb SS. However, with increased longevity of Hb SS patients, its prevalence is greatest in patients with Hb SS disease.[277–279] As per CSSCD estimates, 50 percent of patients by age 33 years will have avascular necrosis of the femoral head (Fig. 48–12). The presence of concurrent deletional α-thalassemia ($-\alpha^{3}$·7) and a history of frequent vasoocclusive crises are classic risk factors for femoral avascular necrosis. Studies have shown that polymorphisms in *BMP6*, annexin A_2, and Klotho genes are risk factors for avascular necrosis.[280] Other musculoskeletal complications of Hb SS disease include decreased bone mineral density, growth retardation, and delayed skeletal maturation in children.[281,282]

Patients present with chronic joint pain with progressive decrease in range of motion of affected joints. Multiple joints are commonly involved.[283] The vast majority of untreated patients will progress to femoral head collapse within 5 years.[284]

The natural history of asymptomatic avascular necrosis of the hip has been elucidated.[285] The seminal findings of the study were that symptoms

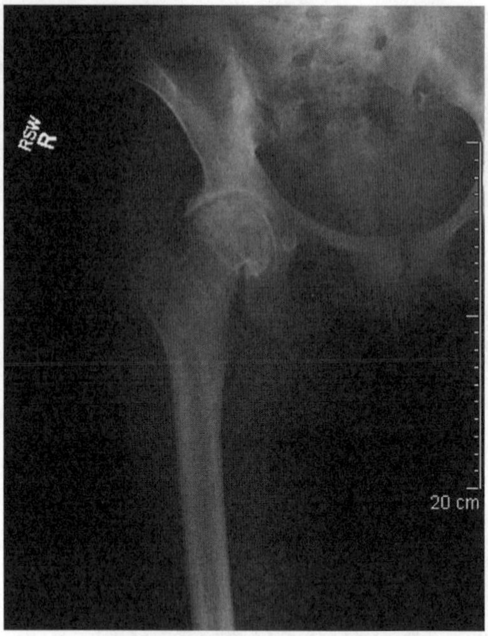

FIGURE 48–12. Avascular necrosis of the right hip in a 31-year-old female with SCD depicting a patchy lucency and sclerosis and irregular contour of the femoral head and loss of the joint space.

always preceded hip collapse. The duration to collapse was shorter with more advanced stages at study onset and the majority of patients progress to symptomatic avascular necrosis requiring intervention.

Avascular necrosis has been treated with a number of modalities including core decompression, osteotomy, bone grafting, surface arthroplasty, and joint replacement. The only randomized trial in avascular necrosis compared core decompression and physical therapy versus physical therapy alone and did not show a difference in outcome between the two arms; however, followup was short and a significant number of stage III hips were included.[286] In our experience, core decompression is a useful option in early stage avascular necrosis. Several studies associate total hip replacement in SCD with a higher rate of orthopedic and medical complications. However, other studies show a lower rate of orthopedic complications. Structural bone diseases in SCD make joint replacement challenging.[287–289]

LEG ULCERS

Skin ulcers are seen in several chronic hemolytic states. Leg ulcers occur in 2 to 40 percent of cases with sickle cell disease. There appears to be a geographic predilection with the highest rate being reported in Jamaica.[14,290] In the United States, leg ulcers are seen in 4 to 6 percent of patients with SCD.[291] They are most common in patients older than 10 years of age. They typically occur on the lower extremities, especially on the malleoli, and cause chronic pain and disability. Venous stasis is a predisposing factor. There appears to be association with occurrence of priapism and pulmonary hypertension, possibly reflective of a "hemolytic phenotype."[290,292,293] Once established, the ulcers are recalcitrant and significantly impair quality of life.[292]

Concomitant α-thalassemia appears to have a protective effect. The relationship between hydroxyurea use and increased occurrence of leg ulcers has not been established. Occasionally, osteomyelitis may be complicated by secondary skin breakdown.

Polymorphisms in Klotho, *TEK*, and several other genes in the transforming growth factor(TGF)-β and bone morphogenic protein (BMP) pathway are associated with leg ulcers.[280]

Treatment of leg ulcers is largely empiric, based on sparse, if any, evidence. Leg elevation, bed rest when practical and feasible, wet-to-dry dressings, gentle debridement, Unna boots, and treatment of infection and topical or systemic antibiotics are commonly used. The peptide encoding integrin-interaction site of many extracellular matrix proteins (RGD peptide) enhanced healing of the ulcers in preliminary studies, but, unfortunately, it never came to clinical practice because of nonmedical reasons.[294]

Induction of fetal hemoglobin may enhance ulcer resolution, although hydroxyurea has been reported to induce leg ulcers (see Chap. 86).[295,296]

HEPATOBILIARY

Chronic liver abnormalities in SCD are frequent and are reflective of different etiologies of liver dysfunction that include vasoocclusion, transfusion, iron overload, pigment gallstones with bile duct obstruction, acute or chronic cholecystitis, viral hepatitis, and cholestasis.[297,298] A quarter of patients in one study had sickling as the sole explanation for liver abnormalities, with the remainder of patients having viral hepatitis, cholelithiasis, hemosiderosis, alcohol abuse, or diabetes mellitus as underlying causes.[297,299] Bilirubin levels are usually not above 4 mg/dL and the direct fraction contributes less than 10 percent of the total bilirubin.[300] Vasoocclusion involves the hepatic sinusoids in as many as 39 percent of patients and results in a mixed hepatocellular-cholestatic or a purely cholestatic picture.[301] Severe hepatic cholestasis with serum bilirubin levels as high as 100 mg/dL is a catastrophic situation needing exchange transfusion for resolution. A lesser degree of cholestasis may resolve with more conservative measures.[301] Mild and progressive cholestatic syndromes have been described. In the former there is increase in bilirubin with modest increase in alkaline phosphatase and an increase in serum transaminases with no impairment of hepatic synthetic function. Patients may have pruritus in addition to jaundice. The biochemical abnormalities usually resolve without treatment in a few months. Progressive cholestasis, on the other hand, results in impaired liver synthetic function and a striking increase in alkaline phosphatase in addition to bilirubin. Multiorgan dysfunction and right upper quadrant pain are seen and chronic transfusion is recommended to reverse the process. Both of the above syndromes are caused by intrasinusoidal sickling and Kupffer cell hyperplasia.[302–304]

Sequestration crises characterized by a painful, enlarging liver have been described.[299] Chronic hemolysis produces an increased burden on the heme catabolic pathway leading to increased unconjugated bilirubin and formation of pigment gallstones. The incidence of gallstones increases with age, with a reported prevalence of 50 percent at 22 years of age.[305–307]

Coinherited α-thalassemia (see Chap. 47) decreases bilirubin levels in patients with sickle cell disease, and the number of UGT1A1 promoter (TA) repeats (the polymorphism associated with Gilbert syndrome) is strongly associated with incidence of gallstones and bilirubin levels.[308]

Laparoscopic cholecystectomy is recommended in symptomatic patients with cholelithiasis. The treatment of asymptomatic patients with positive findings on abdominal ultrasonography is more controversial. In the Jamaican cohort study, only 7 percent of patients with positive ultrasonograms had symptoms suggestive of biliary tract disease and needed a cholecystectomy. However, patients in the United States appear to be more symptomatic and the majority of gallbladders taken after only a positive ultrasonogram have pathologic evidence of cholecystitis.[305] Asymptomatic patients with negative screening ultrasonograms should be observed; however, timing and frequency of screening has not been standardized.

EYE

The microvasculature of the retina with relative hypoxemia facilitates "sickling" akin to several other vascular beds. Microcirculatory obstruction occurs followed by neovascularization and arteriovenous aneurysms. Hemorrhage, scarring, and retinal detachment leading to blindness are the sequelae. Changes occur at the periphery, thereby sparing central vision at earlier stages. The term *sickle cell retinopathy* encompasses nonproliferative and proliferative changes. It has been postulated that microcirculatory changes easily accessible for inspection as in the conjunctiva could serve as a "window" to the severity of vasculopathy in SCD.

Nonproliferative changes include "salmon-patch" hemorrhages, peripheral retinal lesions termed "black sunbursts," and iridescent spots, whereas neovascularization is characteristic of proliferative changes, giving a pattern of vascular lesions resembling a marine invertebrate and is termed "sea fans."[309]

Increased levels of plasma and intraocular vascular endothelial growth factor have been documented in proliferative sickle cell retinopathy, as have angiopoietin 1 and 2 and von Willebrand factor. Pigment epithelium derived factor, an angiogenesis inhibitor, is increased as well, especially in nonviable "sea fans."[310–312]

Proliferative sickle cell retinopathy may differ from other proliferative retinopathies in that spontaneous regression of neovascularization can occur in up to 60 percent of cases.[313,314] The Jamaican cohort study reported an annual incidence of 0.5 cases per 100 Hb SS subjects versus 2.5 cases per 100 Hb SC subjects. Prevalence was greater in Hb SC subjects as well, with a 43 percent rate in the third decade versus 14 percent for those with Hb SS. However, there was a 32 percent incidence of spontaneous regression. Irreversible visual loss occurred only in 2 percent of Hb SC subjects up to 26 years of age observed at time of the study.[313]

Central retinal artery occlusion is rare in Hb SS disease.[315] Conjunctival vascularity is decreased in SCD patients compared to controls with further decreased vascularity and decreased conjunctival red cell velocities during vasoocclusion.[316–319]

An orbital compression syndrome characterized by fever, headache, orbital swelling, and visual impairment secondary to optic nerve dysfunction has been reported in SCD. Orbital marrow infarction is a common cause.[320]

All patients with sickle hemoglobinopathies should have a yearly ophthalmology examination beginning in childhood. The examination should be carried out by an ophthalmologist and should include slit-lamp examination of the anterior chamber and detailed retinal visualization including a fluorescein angiography in addition to visual acuity.

The evaluation of treatment of proliferative sickle retinopathy is complicated by the fact that spontaneous regression may occur. Laser photocoagulation remains the most commonly performed procedure for this finding. Traumatic hyphema needs urgent optical referral since increased sickle red cells can cause obstruction of outflow channels, resulting in acute glaucoma. This may cause decrease in retinal and optic nerve perfusion causing further visual problems. Unresolved vitreous hemorrhage and retinal detachment may need surgical intervention. Exchange transfusion to keep Hb A at more than 50 percent is recommended. Central retinal artery occlusion needs urgent exchange transfusion and ophthalmology referral.[313,321–323]

SPLEEN

Functional asplenia defined as impaired mononuclear phagocyte system functions of the spleen occurs early in the course of patients with SCD. It is defined by the presence of Howell-Jolly bodies in the blood and absence of ^{99m}Tc splenic uptake even in the presence of a palpable spleen. Slow blood flow in the red pulp of the spleen sets the stage for increased red cell sickling. Repeated splenic infarctions lead to "autosplenectomy." As a consequence, patients are prone to microbial infections, especially with encapsulated microorganisms such as Streptococcus pneumoniae. Hypertransfusion early in childhood, prior to age 7 years, may lead to reversal of functional asplenia. Marrow transplantation and hydroxyurea have resulted in reversal of functional asplenia in some older subjects. Splenic sequestration occurs in young children.[324–331]

PREGNANCY

In a study of obstetric outcomes among 284 women with SCD, 190 women (66.9%) had a total of 410 pregnancies. This accounts for a rate of 2.15 pregnancies per woman among those who had at least one pregnancy. The overall rate of pregnancy in this cohort was 1.4 per woman.[332] A third of patients will have adverse obstetric outcomes as defined by miscarriages, stillbirths, or ectopic implantation with rates of livebirths significantly lower than average.[332] Preterm delivery occurs in 30 to 50 percent of pregnant SCD patients and 20 percent of newborns have low birth weight.[333,334] A fivefold risk of venous thromboembolism is present during pregnancy.[335]

Other significant findings included higher rates of cesarean section, infection, gestational hypertension, preeclampsia or eclampsia, intrauterine growth retardation, and asymptomatic bacteriuria.[336]

Pulmonary hypertension and cardiomyopathy are more likely to occur at delivery. The mortality rate for SCD patients during pregnancy is 72.4 deaths/100,000 deliveries compared to 12.7 deaths/100,000 deliveries in those without SCD.

The role of prophylactic red cell transfusions in pregnancy is not clear. Two studies found no benefit, whereas one showed improvement. Most experts prefer not to transfuse a patient during an uncomplicated pregnancy unless adverse clinical events warrant use of red cell transfusion.[337–339]

Contraception advice is similar as for women without SCD, although some studies in SCD suggest increased venous thromboembolism risk with oral contraceptives.[92]

INFECTION

Patients with SCD are predisposed to infections for a variety of reasons, including functional asplenia and defective neutrophil responses.[340–344] In a landmark paper published by E. Barrett-Connor in 1971, the magnitude of this problem was highlighted.[344] Functional asplenia results in susceptibility to encapsulated microorganisms, particularly *S. pneumoniae*, especially in children younger than 5 years of age. The CSSCD data reported a 7.98 per 100 patient years rate of invasive bacterial infection in children younger than 3 years of age.[345]

Given the high incidence of infection, especially in childhood, infection prevention and rapid diagnosis of established infections is of paramount importance.[346,347] The pneumococcal vaccine PCV7 can be administered in infancy with effective immunologic response prior to 2 years of age. The American Academy of Pediatrics recommends a total of four doses in a schedule at ages 2, 4, 8, and 12 to 15 months. The PCV7 vaccine decreases invasive pneumococcal disease by as much as 80 to 90 percent.[348] The pneumococcal polysaccharide vaccine (PPV23) covers more serotypes but is not immunogenic prior to age 24 months and response lasts for 3 years. The first dose is recommended at 24 months with additional doses 3 to 5 years later.[347,349–352]

Oral penicillin prophylaxis is still recommended at a dose of 125 mg twice a day for children between ages 0 and 3 years and at 250 mg twice a day between ages 3 and 5 years.[353] Penicillin prophylaxis beyond 5 years is recommended only for patients with recurrent pneumococcal infections or who have had a surgical splenectomy. Patients allergic to penicillin are offered erythromycin.

Meningococcal vaccination although recommended by the American Academy of Pediatrics is not routinely offered because of a lack of efficacy data.

Standard pediatric immunizations protecting against *Haemophilus influenzae* and hepatitis B virus should be given. Influenza virus vaccine should be given annually.

Parents and caregivers of children should be educated to recognize infections and to seek medical attention early. Diagnosis of established infections varies by site and offending agent. For invasive pneumococcal disease, ceftriaxone remains the drug of choice despite concerns of immune-mediated hemolysis. Organisms seen more typically in patients with SCD, for example, *Salmonella* osteomyelitis, atypical bacteria such as *Mycoplasma pneumoniae*, and *Chlamydia* isolated in acute chest syndrome, should be treated with appropriate antibiotics. Local antibiotic resistance patterns influence decision of empiric antibiotic treatment.

The spectrum of infectious complications in adults may be different. One study reported data on blood infections in adults.[340] Pneumococcal infections were rare. *S. aureus* was the predominant organism. Patients with *S. aureus* had a predilection for bone–joint infection. Those with indwelling venous catheters and a severe disease course appeared to have a high risk for bloodstream infections.

ANESTHESIA AND SURGERY

Patients with SCD should have careful monitoring of hemoglobin concentration, hydration, oxygen, and metabolic studies in the perioperative period. Transfusion to keep hemoglobin levels around 10 g/dL is recommended; no increased benefit is seen with more aggressive transfusion regimens.[233] Care should be taken to avoid transfusion-induced hyperviscosity. All surgical procedures deserve special attention.[354–356]

Acute chest syndrome and vasoocclusive crisis occur with higher frequency in the perioperative period. Increased age is associated with increased complications.

MODIFIERS OF DISEASE SEVERITY

Variation in the clinical severity and some laboratory findings of SCD are well known. Some patients have a rather mild course with few problems related to SCD and survive into the sixth or seventh decade. In contrast, some patients have a difficult course with multiple complications, frequent hospitalizations, severe organ damage, and a significantly shortened life expectancy.[357,358] Two well-known genetic modifiers of disease severity are concomitant α-thalassemia and high red cell Hb F content. However, these two factors do not account for the vast clinical diversity of SCD. This observation and the completion of the human genome project have provided the impetus to study polymorphisms in candidate genes as potential modifiers of disease severity. Association of polymorphisms in candidate genes and different features of SCD such as stroke,[228,359,360] acute chest syndrome,[361] bilirubin levels and cholelithiasis,[362–365] avascular necrosis,[280] priapism,[366] and leg ulcers,[290] as well as Hb F levels[367–372] and Hb F response to hydroxyurea,[373] have been studied in different groups of patients. Polymorphisms in the TGF-β–BMP pathway, a ubiquitous signaling pathway that is involved in many cellular processes, have emerged as recurrent findings in many of these studies. Some of the associations have functional consequences; the association of bilirubin levels with polymorphisms in the UGT1A1 promoter is such an example. The 7TA repeat in the promoter leads to a decreased activity of this enzyme and hence a decrease in glucuronidation of bilirubin. Thus, the association of this polymorphism with higher bilirubin levels can easily be understood. On the other hand, the mechanisms by which polymorphisms in the ubiquitous TGF-β–BMP pathway are associated with various complications of SCD are unknown, and thus a causal relationship cannot yet be established. Functional studies of these variants and genome wide association studies are expected to provide a better insight into genetic modulation of the phenotype of SCD.

As a result of these association studies, it has been proposed that SCD encompasses two distinct subphenotypes with different complications of the disease clustering into one or the other.[374] One of these subphenotypes is termed hemolysis-endothelial dysfunction; patients with brisk hemolysis (elevated LDH, bilirubin, high reticulocyte counts) are grouped under this subphenotype. Elevated levels of cell-free hemoglobin in plasma leads to NO depletion; in turn, this results in increased microvascular tone, increased cell adhesion to the endothelium, activation of the endothelium, and an inflammatory state. The disease complications associated with this phenotype include pulmonary hypertension, leg ulcers, priapism, and possibly stroke. At the other end of the spectrum is the viscosity-vasoocclusion subphenotype; patients in this subgroup do not have brisk hemolysis. They have higher hemoglobin and hematocrit levels and hence higher blood viscosity as a result. Clinical features of this subphenotype include acute chest syndrome, frequent pain episodes, avascular necrosis, and retinopathy. Factors that ameliorate hemolysis and lead to a higher hemoglobin and hematocrit (such as concomitant α-thalassemia and relatively high levels of Hb F) shift the subphenotype toward viscosity-vasoocclusion. Although this classification provides an interesting and useful conceptual framework in understanding the basic pathophysiologic mechanisms and in designing therapies targeting these mechanisms, this distinction of subphenotypes is not absolute and significant overlap exists.

GENERAL MANAGEMENT OF SICKLE CELL DISEASE

PHARMACOTHERAPEUTICS TO INCREASE FETAL HEMOGLOBIN LEVELS

Recognition of the fact that Hb F results in ameliorating the phenotype of SCD lead to research focused on Hb F modulation as a therapy for SCD. The γ-chains of Hb F are excluded from the deoxy Hb S polymer; thus the presence of Hb F in sickle red cells exerts a potent antisickling effect. This effect has also been supported by clinical observations; the manifestations of SCD do not become apparent in the first few months of life until the switch from γ-chain production to β-chain production is almost complete in the postnatal period. Additionally, the phenotypes of some compound heterozygous states with Hb S and other inherited globin disorders that lead to increased expression of Hb F in the adult life ($\delta\beta$-thalassemias, hereditary persistence of fetal hemoglobin) are very mild (see Chap. 47). In fact, compound heterozygotes for Hb S and deletional hereditary persistence of fetal hemoglobin, in which there is continued high levels of Hb F expression (30–35%) uniformly distributed in all red cells (pancellular), are clinically asymptomatic and hematologically normal. In the late 1970s, further evidence in support of the ameliorating effect of high Hb F came from the observation of Saudi Arabian sickle cell anemia patients who had few, if any, symptoms of SCD, had mild anemia, and were not diagnosed until adult age.[375] These individuals had Hb F levels in the 20 to 25 percent range as opposed to the African or African American patients, the majority of whom had Hb F levels of approximately 5 percent. Similar patients were reported from India, and this genetic propensity for high Hb F production in SCD patients was linked to a unique β-globin gene cluster haplotype (Saudi Arabian-Indian) that is distinct from those found in Africa. These observations paved the way for intense investigations on the cellular and molecular mechanisms of the fetal to adult (γ to β) switch during the perinatal period and the search for "antiswitching" agents, agents that would facilitate retaining elevated Hb F

TABLE 48–3. Antiswitching Therapies

Drug	Mechanism
Hydroxyurea	Myelosuppression Antiinflammatory Nitric oxide donor Increased cyclic guanosine monophosphate
Decitabine	DNA methyltransferase 1 inhibition, i.e., hypomethylation
5′-Azacitidine	DNA methyltransferase 1 inhibition, i.e., hypomethylation
Butyrate derivatives	Histone deacetylase inhibition
Histone deacetylase inhibitors	Histone deacetylase inhibition
Immunomodulatory drugs	P38 mitogen-activated protein kinase pathway

levels. The observation that there is a transient increase in Hb F production during recovery from marrow aplasia or suppression provided the rationale for the use of myelosuppressive agents as *antiswitching* therapy (Table 48–3). Antiswitching indicates a mechanism to prevent the switch from γ-globin chains to β-globin chains.

Hydroxyurea

Although many myelosuppressive agents have been studied in primates and some have been used in a small number of patients, only one of these, hydroxyurea, was used in large-scale clinical trials starting in the early 1980s. This is largely attributable to its excellent oral bioavailability, relatively short half-life (important from the standpoint of rapid reversibility of toxicity), no evidence that its use led to increase cancer prevalence, and few side effects.

Hydroxyurea is the only FDA-approved agent for the treatment of SCD. It is a ribonucleotide reductase inhibitor and is S-phase specific in the cell cycle. The mechanism whereby hydroxyurea increases Hb F synthesis is not fully understood; it has been postulated that the myelosuppressive effect leads to the recruitment of early erythroid progenitors which have retained their fetal (γ) globin synthesis capability, giving rise to the production of RBCs with a higher Hb F content. Some studies have shown that HU acts as a NO donor, and increases Hb F synthesis via cGMP pathway. [376] It has several other actions that explain its efficacy in SCD other than increasing Hb F. These include decrease in white blood cells, platelets, and reticulocytes, improvement in red cell hydration, and a decrease in red cell adhesiveness to the vascular endothelium (Fig. 48–13).[377–379]

In the landmark Multicenter Study of Hydroxyurea, hydroxyurea was shown to decrease frequency of painful crises, acute chest syndrome, hospitalizations, and blood transfusions. Followup showed a 40 percent decrease in mortality in patients randomized to the drug.[161,380] Hydroxyurea is recommended in patients with three or more vasoocclusive episodes or history of acute chest syndrome. It can be started at a dose of 15 mg/kg given as a single daily dose and escalated until toxicity or a maximum dose of 35 mg/kg is reached. Periodic monitoring of blood cell counts and serum chemistries, especially in the first year of treatment is important. The dose should be decreased in renal failure. Although not proven to have teratogenic or leukemogenic potential in SCD patients, it is recommended that it not to be used in pregnant or breast-feeding patients. Concerns about detrimental effect on spermatogenesis have also been raised based on studies in mice.[381–384]

Patients receiving hydroxyurea who die while on treatment are likely to be older when therapy is initiated, more anemic, likely to have Bantu or Cameron haplotypes, and have impaired renal function.[357]

One clinical trial and several observational studies have been published on the use of hydroxyurea in children. Therapy is well tolerated with improved growth rates, preservation of organ function, and the additional benefits seen in adults.[385–395] There are ongoing trials investigating the use of the drug in infants.

Other Hb F–Inducing Agents

Although significant advances have been made in understanding the basic mechanism(s) of the perinatal switch from γ- to β-globin synthesis, this knowledge is far from complete. Certain epigenetic mechanisms (histone deacetylation and DNA methylation) are involved in the silencing of the γ-globin genes postnatally. This has led to the utilization of agents that target the two common epigenetic silencing mechanisms, that is, histone deacetylase inhibitors and DNA methyltransferase 1 inhibitors.

The histone deacetylase inhibitors that have been most widely used in early phase small clinical trials in SCD and in some patients with β-thalassemia are butyrate derivatives (arginine butyrate, sodium phenyl butyrate, isobutyramide). Arginine butyrate has to be administered by intravenous infusion; earlier studies suggested that continuous daily infusions of arginine butyrate were not very effective in leading to a sustained increase in Hb F.[295] Later, it was shown that daily continuous infusion induced tachyphylaxis and failed to cause a sustained Hb F response. An intermittent schedule of administration (4 days, given every 4 weeks) was efficacious in increasing Hb F.[396] Although orally administered sodium phenyl butyrate was effective in increasing Hb F, the daily doses required for maintaining a Hb F response required the administration of a large number of tablets and was impractical.[397] Newer, more effective oral butyrate derivatives are being evaluated in clinical trials. A number of new histone deacetylase inhibitors increase Hb F synthesis in cell culture systems and in animal studies, but have not yet been studied in clinical trials.

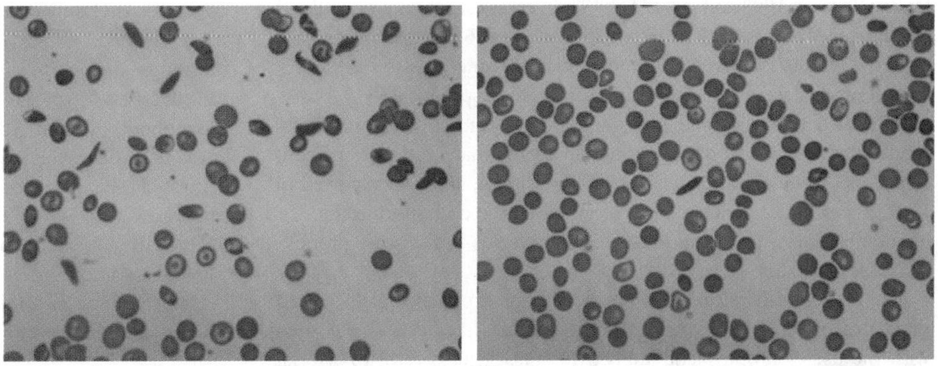

A B

FIGURE 48–13. Blood film from SCD patients: effect of hydroxyurea therapy. **A.** Blood film before therapy. Note frequent sickled cells. **B.** Marked decrease in sickle cells with therapy. *(Courtesy of Dr. Scott Drury and Dr. Elizabeth Manaloor, Department of Pathology, Medical College of Georgia.)*

The two DNA methyl transferase inhibitors with antiswitching activity are 5-azacytidine and decitabine (5-aza-2-deoxycytidine). Both of these agents are myelosuppressive when used in higher doses; however, in low dose, they are potent inhibitors of DNA methyltransferase 1 and have been shown to increase Hb F synthesis in baboons and in patients with sickle cell disease.[398–405] Unlike 5-azacytidine, which incorporates into both DNA and RNA, decitabine incorporates only in DNA and is believed to have a better genotoxicity profile. It has been effective in increasing Hb F and ameliorating the disease severity in patients with SCD who have been refractory to hydroxyurea.[400]

Immunomodulatory agents (thalidomide and its derivatives) increase Hb F synthesis in erythroid colonies from SCD patients. These agents are currently in early phase clinical trials. [406]

HEMATOPOIETIC STEM CELL TRANSPLANTATION

Because sickle cell disease is an inherited defect in the hematopoietic stem cell, stem cell transplantation (SCT) is an attractive option to permanently cure the disease rather than managing its sequelae piecemeal. However, the tremendous phenotypic variability that characterizes the disorder combined with lack of an accurate model to foretell which patients are likely to have a catastrophic disease course make selecting patients for SCT challenging. SCT ideally should be done in patients who are likely to have a severe disease course but instituted early, prior to end-organ damage. The risk-to-benefit ratio of the morbidity and mortality associated with allogeneic SCT has to be weighed against the disease severity of a nonmalignant hematologic disorder. Lack of a matched sibling donor for the majority of SCD patients and prior transfusions resulting in increased recipient exposure to donor antigens are some of the other major impediments to transplantation.[407]

Most of the transplantations done in SCD are in children and are myeloablative with a matched-sibling donor, and the results are encouraging (see Chap. 21). Marrow has been the predominant source of stem cells used in these transplantations. The majority of patients were transplanted for cerebral vasculopathy or history of acute chest syndrome or recurrent vasoocclusive episodes. Safety of using Hb AS donors has been established. Two decades of experience by the French group was reported in 2007. The conditioning regimen was busulfan and cyclophosphamide with antithymocyte globulin added in 1992. The rejection rate was significantly reduced with addition of antithymocyte globulin (decreased from 22.6% to 3%). Overall survival and event-free survival were 93.1 and 86.1 percent with a median of 6 years of followup.[408] Two patients with cord blood transplants (see Chap. 21) did not develop graft-versus-host disease.[408] The French study resulted in overall survival and event-free survival similar to those of two prior series published from Belgium and the United States in 1998 and 2000.[408–410] The Center for International Blood & Marrow Transplant Research experience of 67 patients was also reported in 2007.[411] Five-year probabilities of being disease free and of overall survival were 85 percent and 97 percent, respectively.[409,410] Transplant-related mortality and infections are the leading cause of death. Acute graft versus host disease occurs in approximately 10 to 15 percent of patients while chronic graft-versus-host disease has been reported in 12 to 20 percent of patients. Most series have used cyclosporine alone or in combination with methotrexate for graft-versus-host disease prophylaxis (see Chap. 21).

The rate of graft rejection is very low. Prior experience of increased incidence of seizures following transplantation has been ameliorated with the use of prophylactic anticonvulsants. Strict control of arterial hypertension, correction of hypomagnesemia, penicillin prophylaxis posttransplantation, maintenance of hemoglobin ≥10 g/dL, and platelets >50,000/μL during transplantation are important. Reversible posterior leukoencephalopathy has been reported, especially after cyclosporine use. Long-term toxicity still remains a concern especially in relation to growth, reproduction, and secondary malignancies. Gonadal dysfunction occurs, especially when transplantation is done in the immediate prepubertal period.

In an attempt to decrease morbidity and mortality from marrow transplantation, nonmyeloablative regimens have been used. However, loss of stable donor engraftment after tapering of immunosuppression in the majority of patients has been a problem.[412–414]

TRANSFUSION

Red cell transfusion is used frequently in SCD on an acute or chronic basis. The rationale for transfusion in SCD is twofold. Besides increasing hemoglobin concentration and thereby increasing oxygen carrying capacity of the blood, transfusion also decreases the percentage of circulating Hb S-containing red cells. Hemoglobin level alone should not constitute an indication to transfusion as patients adapt to their level, and it is important to know the patient's baseline hemoglobin concentration. It is also important to calculate whether the reticulocyte count, a surrogate for marrow function, is adequate or not.

Indications for acute red cell transfusion include symptomatic anemia, acute chest syndrome, stroke, aplastic and sequestration crises, other major organ damage secondary to vasoocclusion, and occurrence of unrelenting priapism. Transfusion is also considered prior to major surgery or surgery involving critical organs. The best established indication for chronic transfusion is stroke and an abnormal TCD velocity. Patients with other chronic or recurrent events are sometimes placed on chronic transfusion as well. Inappropriate indications for transfusion include chronic steady-state anemia, uncomplicated vasoocclusive episode, pregnancy, minor surgeries, infection, and avascular necrosis.

One can use red cell transfusion or an exchange transfusion.[415] Transfusion is easier to perform and is generally associated with fewer complications compared to exchange transfusion. Exchange transfusion, however, has the advantage of not raising total hemoglobin, and thereby total viscosity, while decreasing the percent of Hb SS cells. It also does not result in iron overload.

Patients with Hb SS transport less oxygen to their tissues beyond a hematocrit of 30 percent as a result of increased blood viscosity.[416–418]

Alloimmunization occurs in 18 to 36 percent of transfused SCD patients.[419–422] Many alloantibodies are transient and therefore the magnitude of the problem may be greater. In the United States the majority of blood donors are of European descent, and the majority of SCD patients are of African descent. This results in blood group antigenic disparity, and antibodies to E, C, K, Jkb, S, and Fyb are common. Extended antigen phenotyping (Kell, Duffy, Kidd, Lewis, Lutheran, P, and M&S) in addition to the usual ABO and D antigens and leukodepletion of blood products is recommended.[415,423,424] Delayed hemolytic transfusion reaction complicates approximately 3 percent of transfusions in SCD and may present as a painful crises. It typically occurs a week after transfusion and is caused by alloantibodies to non-ABO antigens. It can cause the hemoglobin to fall lower than the prior pretransfusion level and can be associated with a depressed reticulocyte count and autoantibodies. Serial hemoglobin electrophoresis will reveal a rapid decrease in the percent of Hb A as opposed to Hb S. Patients should be transfused only if symptomatic under such circumstances since further transfusion can exacerbate the problem.

Iron overload and its attendant complications and infection transmission remain the other major complications of transfusion.

MANAGEMENT OF IRON OVERLOAD

Iron overload (see Chap. 42) in SCD is similar to other chronically transfused populations.[425–427] The multicenter study of iron overload research group have published preliminary data on a observational cohort of transfusional iron-overloaded patients with thalassemia and SCD compared to nontransfused patients with SCD.[428]

Diagnosing significant iron overload accurately and early can be difficult. Serum ferritin is an easy, widely employed method, but is unreliable in SCD as it is an acute-phase reactant. Its measurements can result in over- or underestimation and is poorly correlated to liver iron content.[429] A serum ferritin value of greater than 1000 mg/mL in the steady state has been used as an indication of iron overload. Liver iron content is the current accepted standard and a value of 7.7 mg/g dry weight is used as indication for treatment.[430] However, noninvasive methods of assessment of iron overload like SQUID or MRI T2* (see Chap. 42) are becoming standard. Transfusion of a total of 120 mL of red blood cells/kg of body weight can also be used as a chelation trigger.[423]

Chelation (see Chap. 42) was typically carried out with desferoxamine at a dose of 25 to 40 mg/kg per day given over 8 hours subcutaneously.[431] Desferoxamine can reverse cardiac iron overload. A once-daily oral iron chelator, deferasirox, is now approved and available for use in the United States. It is a tridentate ligand that binds iron with a high affinity in a 2:1 ratio. It has a half-life of 8 to16 hours and is metabolized by glucuronidation and excreted in the feces. In an open-label phase II trial of deferasirox versus desferoxamine in a 2:1 randomization, safety and tolerability were established. Nausea and vomiting, abdominal pain, rash, reversible increase in liver function tests, and stable increases in serum creatinine were reported. Rare cases of anaphylaxis occurring mostly in the first month of starting treatment have also been reported. Postmarketing reports suggest an increased incidence of renal failure, and caution is to be exercised in a patient population where renal insufficiency may not be readily appreciated prior to starting treatment. Postmarketing experience has also reported cases of fatal hepatotoxicity and agranulocytosis. Auditory and ophthalmic side effects occur in less than 1 percent of patients; however, annual eye and auditory examinations are recommended for deferasirox as they are for desferoxamine. Recommended daily dose is 20 mg/kg body weight; dose may be adjusted every 3 to 5 months in increments of 5 to 10 mg/kg if therapeutic goal is not achieved. Dose should not exceed 40 mg/kg. Safety in combination with other iron chelators has not been established.[432]

EVOLVING THERAPIES

Gardos Channel Inhibitors

Dehydration of sickle red cells results in increased intracellular concentration of Hb S, thereby increasing Hb S polymer formation. Dehydration appears to be a consequence of increased potassium egress via the potassium-chloride cotransport pathway and the calcium activated potassium efflux pathway (Gardos channel).

Senicapoc (ICA-17043), a potent oral Gardos channel inhibitor, was studied in a randomized, placebo-controlled, double-blind trial with changes in hemoglobin from baseline as the primary endpoint. Patients in the high-dose arm at 10 mg per day showed significant increase in hemoglobin from baseline, decreased hemolysis, and a decrease in dense red cells and reticulocytes when compared to placebo. No decrease in number of painful crises was noted, but patients in the trial did not have frequent vasoocclusive crises at study entry.[433] The safety profile was excellent with occasional nausea, diarrhea, and increased γ-glutamyl transferase levels as the main adverse events. Failure of the drug to decrease painful crises in a phase III study should not eliminate this agent from further study, as a decrease in hemolysis can decrease the pathologic effects of the disease.

DNA Hypomethylation

The γ-globin gene promoter is hypomethylated during fetal development but is hypermethylated in embryonic and adult life, suggesting that hypomethylation of the γ promoter is important in hemoglobin production; consequently, DNA hypomethylation is appealing as a strategy to keep high levels of Hb F in adults. However, the exact mechanism by which the two hypomethylating agents, 5-azacytidine and decitabine, act remains to be elucidated. Early studies in humans showed increased Hb F but concerns over myelotoxicity, carcinogenesis, and mutagenesis resulted in hydroxyurea being developed for treatment of SCD.

Because not all patients with SCD benefit from hydroxyurea, there has been a resurgence of interest in developing other treatment strategies for SCD. Decitabine, a hypomethylating agent incorporated only into DNA as opposed to 5-azacytidine, which is incorporated into both DNA and RNA, has been studied in three small clinical trials in patients with SCD. Doses used were much lower than the typical myelotoxic doses used previously in SCD and those that are currently used in myelodysplastic syndrome. Both intravenous and subcutaneous routes have been used and have shown substantial increases in Hb F, decreased hemolysis, and decrease in markers of inflammation and coagulation. Neutrophil nadirs were transient and coincided with increase in platelet counts. Marrow hematopoietic differentiation favoring megakaryocytic and erythroid differentiation over granulocyte and monocyte lineage differentiation could explain this. Although long-term toxicity data are still not available, several studies have suggested cancer chemoprotective effects of decitabine rather than carcinogenic effects.

OTHER ABNORMAL HEMOGLOBINS

The number of hemoglobin variants discovered to date totals 1018. Fortunately, the vast majority of these variants does not cause any clinical or hematologic problems, and therefore are of interest to geneticists and biochemists (http://globin.cse.psu.edu). Most of the hemoglobin variants are missense mutations in the globin genes (α, β, γ, or δ) resulting from single nucleotide substitutions. Other uncommon mechanisms include deletion or insertion of one or more nucleotides altering the reading frame and fusion of globin genes with deletion of intergenic DNA sequences ($\gamma\beta$ fusion in Hb Kenya and $\delta\beta$ fusion in Hb Lepore), mutations of the termination codon leading to the production of elongated globin chains.

Hemoglobin variants that significantly alter the structure, stability, synthesis, or function of the molecule have hematologic and/or clinical consequences. These can be classified in certain categories (Table 48–4). Hb S and Hb C are two examples of mutations on the surface of the hemoglobin molecule that alter both the charge and the physical/chemical properties of the molecule with polymer formation in the case of deoxyhemoglobin S and crystallization in Hb C with profound effects on the function, morphology, rheology, and life span of the red cells. Several mechanisms account for the pathogenesis of unstable hemoglobin variants. The common mechanism involves the precipitation of the unstable hemoglobin molecule within the red cell with attachment to the inner layer of the red cell membrane ("Heinz body" formation); red cells containing membrane-attached Heinz bodies (see Chap. 29, Fig. 29–12) have impaired deformability and filterability leading to their premature destruction (congenital Heinz body hemolytic anemia). Mutations in certain residues alter the oxygen affinity of the hemoglobin molecule; a stabilization of the R (relaxed, oxy) state will result in high O_2 affinity variants and erythrocytosis. Conversely, a stabilization of the T (tense, deoxy) configuration will result in a variant with low O_2 affinity with enhanced unloading of O_2 to the tissues with resultant cyanosis and anemia in certain cases (because of the suppression of the O_2-sensing pathway) (see Chap. 49). Mutations of the heme binding site, particularly those affecting the conserved proximal (F8) and distal (E7) histidine residues, lead to the oxidation of the iron atom in heme from ferrous (Fe^{2+})

TABLE 48–4. Clinically Significant Hemoglobin Variants

I. Altered physical/chemical properties
  A. Hb S (deoxyhemoglobin S polymerization): sickle syndromes
  B. Hb C (crystallization): hemolytic anemia; microcytosis
II. Unstable hemoglobin variants
  A. Congenital Heinz body hemolytic anemia (N = 135)
III. Variants with altered oxygen affinity
  A. High-affinity variants: erythrocytosis (N = 92)
  B. Low-affinity variants: anemia, cyanosis
IV. M hemoglobins
  A. Methemoglobinemia, cyanosis (N = 9)
V. Variants causing a thalassemic phenotype (N = 50)
  A. β-Thalassemia
    1. Hb Lepore ($\delta\beta$) fusion (N = 3)
    2. Aberrant RNA processing (Hb E, Hb Knossos, Hb Malay)
    3. Hyperunstable globins (Hb Geneva, Hb Westdale, etc.)
  B. α-Thalassemia
    1. Chain-termination mutants (Hb Constant Spring)
    2. Hyperunstable variants (Hb Quong Sze)

SOURCE: Modified and updated from Bunn HF, Forget BG: *Hemoglobin: Molecular, Genetic, and Clinical Aspects*. WB Saunders, Philadelphia, 1986

to ferric (Fe^{3+}) state with resultant methemoglobinemia (M hemoglobins) and cyanosis (see Chap. 49). A group of mutations alter both the structure and the synthetic rate of the globin chain leading to a "thalassemic" phenotype (see Chap. 47). These include fusion hemoglobins (e.g., Hb Lepore, where the 5′ δ-globin sequences are fused to 3′ β-globin sequences with deletion of the intergenic DNA; this puts the $\delta\beta$-fusion gene under the transcriptional control of the inefficient δ-globin promoter with low expression of the fusion globin and hence the thalassemic phenotype), mutations that cause both a missense mutation and create an aberrant splice site (e.g. Hb E, Hb Knossos, and Hb Malay), and "hyperunstable" globins where the nascent globin chains are highly unstable, undergo rapid proteolytic degradation, and result in a reduction in the affected globin.

Except for the commonly occurring variants (Hb S, C, E, and D-Los Angeles), very few abnormal hemoglobins have been observed in the homozygous state. Variant hemoglobins are usually found in the heterozygous state. Although γ-chain variants are expressed in fetal life and their level gradually decreases as the γ to β (fetal to adult) globin switch progresses during the postnatal period, β- and α-chain variants are expressed throughout life. δ-Globin variants are expressed at very low levels and can be detected only after the switch to adult globin synthesis is complete. Because α-globin chains are present in all of the hemoglobins expressed after the embryonic stage (Hb F-$\alpha_2\gamma_2$; Hb A-$\alpha_2\beta_2$, and HbA$_2$-$\alpha_2\delta_2$), α-chain variants are associated with the production of variant Hb F ($\alpha_2^x\gamma_2$) and HbA$_2$ ($\alpha_2^x\delta_2$) as well. In heterozygous states, β-chain variants constitute 40 to 50 percent of the hemoglobin in red cells; it should, however, be kept in mind that certain factors affect the amount of variant β chains in carriers. These include the stability of the variant, the surface charge of the variant β-chain, and the presence of concomitant α- or β-thalassemia (see Chap. 47). The more unstable the variant, the lower the quantity. Surface charge of the variant also plays a role in determining the quantity in red cells; this is because the formation of the $\alpha\beta$-dimers ($\alpha_1\beta_1$ and $\alpha_2\beta_2$ contacts) is the critical first step in hemoglobin tetramer formation, and this step is primarily driven by electrostatic interactions between α and β chains. Because the α-globin chains have a relatively positive surface charge, they interact more readily with relatively negatively charged β-globin variants to form $\alpha\beta$ dimers. This is reflected in the higher percentage of negatively charged β-globin variants such as Hb N-Baltimore (β95Lys→Glu), which is found in approximately 50 percent in heterozygotes compared to β-globin variants with a positive surface charge, Hb S (β6Glu→Val) or Hb C (β6Glu→Lys) whose quantity in the heterozygote is 40 to 45 percent. In the presence of α-thalassemia, negatively charged β-globin variants compete more favorably for the available α-chains; this phenomenon is reflected in even lower percentages of Hb S and Hb C in heterozygous carriers of these variants in the presence of common deletional forms of α-thalassemia (Hb S of 30–35% in individuals with heterozygous α^+-thalassemia, $-\alpha/\alpha\alpha$; and 25–30% in homozygous α^+-thalassemia, $-\alpha/-\alpha$).[434,435] Conversely, the amount of a β-globin variant will increase if there is a β-thalassemia allele in *trans*; the percentage of the variant will be inversely proportional to the output of the β-thalassemia allele; thus, the higher the variant the lower the output of the β^+-thalassemia allele. In the case of a β^0-thalassemia allele in *trans*, the variant will amount to 90 percent or more of the hemoglobin in red cells, with Hb A$_2$ and Hb F constituting the remainder. The quantity of α-globin variants is also variable, depending on the α-globin gene involved, and the presence of concomitant α- or β-thalassemia. Because there are normally four α-globin loci ($\alpha\alpha/\alpha\alpha$) and the 5′$\alpha$-globin genes ($\alpha_2$) are expressed at a higher level, some of the variation in the level of α-globin variants depends on which α-globin gene carries the mutation; α_2 globin mutations are usually present at 20 to 25 percent of the total hemoglobin, whereas α_1-globin variants are expressed at a lower level (15–20%). Concomitant α-thalassemia results in a higher level of expression of α-globin variants. Observations on the different levels of expression of the common α-globin variant, Hb G-Philadelphia (α68Asn→Lys), is a case in point.[436] Although this variant is found in approximately 25 percent of northern Italians, its percentages in Americans of African descent can be either 33 or approximately 50 percent. This is clearly related to the different genotypes found in these two distinct populations: In northern Italy and Sardinia, the genotype is $\alpha^G\alpha/\alpha\alpha$, with an expression level of 25 percent, whereas in Americans of African descent, the G-Philadelphia mutation is commonly found on a hybrid $\alpha_2\alpha_1$ gene associated with the common 3.7-kb α^+-thalassemia deletion ($-\alpha^G/\alpha\alpha$) with approximately 33 percent expression. When there is an α^+-thalassemia deletion in *trans* ($-\alpha^G/-\alpha$ genotype), as expected, the level of Hb G-Philadelphia will be approximately 50 percent. Coinheritance of α-chain variants with β-thalassemia results in the reduction of the α-chain variant.

Hb C DISEASE

Definition and History

Hb C was the second hemoglobin variant described after Hb S.[437] Homozygous Hb C was described by Spaet and colleagues[438] and Ranney and colleagues.[439] Hb C trait is found in 2 percent of Americans of African descent, and approximately 1 in 6000 have homozygous Hb C.[440] Coinheritance of Hb C with Hb S results in Hb SC disease, which is the second most common form of SCD in the United States. There are also rare cases of Hb C-β^+ and Hb C-β^0-thalassemia. Hb C is thought to have originated in Central West Africa; in parts of West Africa, the prevalence of Hb C can reach 12.5 percent. The Hb C gene was found on three distinct β-globin cluster haplotypes, termed CI, CII, and CIII; the most common is CI, accounting for 70 percent or more of the chromosomes studied.[441]

Etiology and Pathogenesis

Hb C is the result of a GAG→AAG transition in codon 6 of the β-globin gene, which changes the amino acid residue at this position from glutamic acid to lysine (Glu→Lys). The resultant positively charged hemoglobin variant can easily be distinguished from Hb A and Hb S by electrophoresis and chromatography, including HPLC. Hb C does not differ from Hb A in terms of its solubility; however, purified solutions of Hb C are found to form tetragonal crystals in high molarity phosphate buffer. Red cells from homozygous Hb C individuals are also found to form crystals when incubated with hypertonic saline; Hb C crystals are also observed *in vivo*, particularly in the red cells of splenectomized Hb CC patients (see Fig. 48–7). Crystal-containing Hb CC red cells have impaired deformability and filterability. Another interesting characteristic of Hb CC red cells is their propensity for K^+ loss, which is followed by water loss; unlike in sickle red cells, this K^+ leak does not appear to be mediated through either the K-Cl cotransport or the Ca^{2+} activated K^+ efflux (Gardos channel); this is thought to be a volume-stimulated K^+ efflux.[440] The consequence of this K^+ loss is dehydrated, often spherocytic, red cells with increased MCHC, and decreased osmotic fragility. These changes result in impaired rheologic properties of Hb CC red cells; their life span is reduced to 40 days.

Clinical Features

Mild to moderate splenomegaly is a common feature of homozygous Hb C. Like many other chronic hemolytic states, cholelithiasis may be present. Hb CC individuals do not suffer from vasoocclusion or episodic pain. Occasionally, abdominal pain may be present and can be a result of splenomegaly and/or cholelithiasis. Pregnancy does not pose an increased risk to women with Hb CC. Life expectancy of Hb CC individuals is comparable to non–Hb C Americans of African descent.

Laboratory Features

Hb CC individuals have a mild to moderate hemolytic anemia. Blood hemoglobin is usually in the 10 to 11 g/dL range. There is associated reticulocytosis usually in the 3 to 4 percent range. There usually is mild microcytosis (mean corpuscular volume [MCV]: 70–75 fl). Blood film shows an abundance of target cells, occasional microspherocytes, and Hb C crystals especially in splenectomized patients (see Fig. 48–7). Indirect bilirubin may be mildly elevated. White cell and platelet counts are normal in the absence of hypersplenism.

Differential Diagnosis

The diagnosis is usually made by hemoglobin electrophoresis. Hb C moves to a cathodic position, comigrating with Hb A_2, Hb E, and Hb O-Arab in alkaline pH (cellulose acetate) electrophoresis. The distinction from these hemoglobins can be made by electrophoresis on citrate agar in acid pH where Hb E and Hb A_2 comigrate with Hb A; Hb O-Arab has a Hb S-like mobility, and Hb C has a unique migration pattern. Alternatively, newer diagnostic methods can be used; these include isoelectric focusing, where Hb C can be distinguished from other hemoglobins with similar mobility on cellulose acetate electrophoresis. In cation exchange HPLC and capillary electrophoresis, Hb C has a distinct elution pattern and can be distinguished from Hb E and Hb O-Arab; these latter methods also have the advantage of separating and quantifying Hb A_2 in Hb C homozygotes and in Hb C trait. This confers the advantage of readily differentiating between Hb CC and rare cases of Hb C-β^0-thalassemia (where Hb A_2 is significantly higher, ~5%).

Therapy

The vast majority of Hb CC individuals do not require any therapeutic intervention. Cholecystectomy may be required in individuals who have symptomatic gallstones. Few patients with Hb CC develop hypersplenism with a reduction in white cell and platelet counts, and occasionally worsening of anemia. In such instances, splenectomy should be considered. Another indication for splenectomy is pain associated with an enlarged spleen. It is important to apply the usual precautions in patients considered for splenectomy (appropriate vaccinations, prophylactic antibiotic use, and delaying splenectomy in young children). Folic acid supplementation, as usually done in many chronic hemolytic states, is of no proven value.

Hb E DISEASE

Definition and History

Hb E (β26Glu→Lys) was the fourth abnormal hemoglobin described.[442] It is most commonly found in Southeast Asia; in some areas (in the border between Thailand, Laos, and Cambodia, the so-called Hb E triangle) the reported gene frequency may reach as high as 0.50.[443] This high frequency is thought to be the result of a protective effect against malaria. Hb E is also found in other malaria-endemic areas such as Bangladesh, India, and Madagascar. Hb E now has a wide distribution as a result of the large population movements from Southeast and South Asia to Western Europe and North America, and may now be the most common Hb variant worldwide.

Etiology and Pathogenesis

The GAG→AAG mutation in codon 26 of the β-globin gene not only leads to a missense mutation (Glu→Lys) at this position, but also activates a cryptic donor splice site at the boundary of exon 1 and intron 1 by increasing the sequence similarity of this site to a consensus splice sequence. The resultant aberrant splicing through this alternate site leads to a decrease in the correctly spliced messenger RNA and hence a β^+-thalassemic phenotype. This is reflected in the fact that heterozygotes for Hb E have 25 to 30 percent of the variant; in the presence of concomitant α-thalassemia, this quantity decreases even further. The coinheritance of Hb E with a host of other globin mutants (α and β thalassemias, other hemoglobin variants), which are also common in the populations where Hb E is prevalent, results in a wide spectrum of hemoglobinopathies with varying degrees of severity (Hb E disorders or Hb E syndromes). The most significant of these is Hb E-β-thalassemia syndromes. Hb E has also been reported in combination with Hb S (Hb SE disease).

Clinical Features

Individuals with homozygous Hb E are asymptomatic. Most patients do not have hepatosplenomegaly or jaundice. They are usually diagnosed during screening programs or family studies of individuals with severe Hb E disorders. Hb E-β-thalassemia is a rather heterogeneous group of disorders varying from a mild thalassemia intermedia like phenotype to severe transfusion dependent thalassemia major (see Chap. 47). Part of this heterogeneity results from the type of coinherited β-thalassemia mutation. Patients who are compound heterozygotes for Hb E and one of the mild β^+-thalassemia mutations (such as the mild promoter mutation, −28A→G) have a mild to moderate anemia, whereas patients with compound heterozygosity for Hb E and one of the more severe β^+-thalassemia mutations (such as IVS I nucleotide 5 or IVS II nucleotide 654 mutations) do have a more severe phenotype with severe anemia and transfusion dependency. There is also a large heterogeneity among patients with Hb E-β^0-thalassemia; these patients do not produce any Hb A and have only Hb E and varying amounts of Hb F. Known factors that influence the phenotype include the ability to produce Hb F and the presence of concomitant α-thalassemia. Individuals who have the propensity to synthesize significant amounts of Hb F (such as those who have the Xmn I C→T mutation in the Gγ-globin promoter) are able to ameliorate the globin-chain imbalance and thus have a milder phenotype. Concomitant α-thalassemia also mitigates the course of the disease by decreasing globin-chain imbalance. In some cases, there may be nonglobin modifiers that impact on the phenotype. Patients with severe forms of Hb E-β^0-thalassemia have clinical features very similar to β-thalassemia major; they develop complications such as hypersplenism, iron overload, increased susceptibility to infections, thromboembolic complications, and heart failure, and have a shortened life expectancy.[443]

Laboratory Features

Hb E trait individuals have a borderline microcytosis (MCV in the lower 80s). Homozygotes for Hb E are usually not significantly anemic (hemoglobin: 11–13 g/dL), but they are microcytic (MCV: ~70 fl). Blood film shows target cells, hypochromia, and microcytosis (see Fig. 48–7). Osmotic fragility of the red cells is decreased. Hemoglobin electrophoresis shows 90 percent or greater Hb E and 5 to 10 percent Hb F. Certain chromatography techniques that can separate Hb E from Hb A_2 reveal elevated levels of Hb A_2. Patients with mild forms of Hb E-β^+-thalassemia have hemoglobin levels in the 9.0 to 9.5 g/dL range, whereas those with severe Hb E-β^+-thalassemia are more severely anemic (hemoglobin: 6.5–8.0 g/dL). Individuals with Hb E-β^0-thalassemia have varying degrees of anemia, depending on their ability to produce Hb F; these patients have Hb E in the 40 to 60 percent range with the remainder being Hb F. Patients with higher Hb F values are less anemic.

Therapy

Hb E homozygotes do not require any therapy. Patients with severe Hb E-β^0-thalassemia are similar to thalassemia intermedia or major; most of the latter patients should be on a chronic transfusion regimen aiming at hemoglobin levels of approximately 10 g/dL; iron chelation should be a part of standard therapy. Splenectomy should be considered when hypersplenism develops. Patients with a thalassemia intermedia-like phenotype may require sporadic transfusions. Hydroxyurea can increase Hb F levels and decrease ineffective erythropoiesis in Hb E-β-thalassemia.[444] SCT (including umbilical cord blood-derived stem cells in one patient) has also been used in Hb E-β-thalassemia.

Course and Prognosis

The prognosis is dependent upon the clinical phenotype. Patients with milder phenotypes tend to do well. Severe Hb E-β-thalassemia patients require chronic red cell transfusion and iron chelation therapy; this obviously will place a great burden on the economies of countries where this disease is prevalent. SCT, although potentially curative, will not be available for the vast majority of these patients. Prenatal diagnosis and neonatal screening should be an important part of the strategies to decrease the disease burden and improve care. Long-term use of hydroxyurea and other novel Hb F-inducing agents as modifiers of disease (histone deacetylase inhibitors and DNA methyltransferase 1 inhibitors) can be an important addition to therapy.

Hb D DISEASE

Hb D is the third variant hemoglobin identified.[445] The substitution in Hb D is a glutamic acid to glutamine at the 121st amino acid of the β-globin chain (β121Glu→Gln). Hb D has an S-like mobility on alkaline electrophoresis but comigrates with Hb A on acid pH. Subsequently, a number of other hemoglobin variants with the same electrophoretic properties were discovered and named Hb D (Hb D-Ibadan, Hb D-Gainesville, etc). The most common Hb D is Hb D-Los Angeles (β121Glu→Gln), the originally discovered Hb D, which is identical to Hb D-Punjab. It is most commonly found in Punjab, India. Two to 3 percent of the population of this region carries the Hb D gene. Subsequently, it has also been found in a number of other populations including Europeans, Mediterranean region, and Americans of African descent.[446]

Hb D heterozygotes are completely asymptomatic, are not anemic, and have normal red cell indices. Homozygotes for Hb D-Los Angeles are asymptomatic and are hematologically normal with normal red cell indices. Blood films may show target cells (see Fig. 48–7). Osmotic fragility may be decreased. Compound heterozygotes for Hb D-Los Angeles and a β^0-thalassemia mutation have mild microcytic anemia and show minimal hemolysis. Coinheritance of Hb D-Los Angeles with Hb S results in a severe sickle cell disease phenotype not different from homozygous Hb S.

Hb D-Los Angeles should be distinguished from Hb S. This can be done by a combination of routine alkaline and acid Hb electrophoretic methods. Techniques such as isoelectric focusing, HPLC, and capillary electrophoresis readily provide this distinction. Such methods allow accurate diagnosis of SCD because of compound heterozygosity for Hb S and Hb D-Los Angeles.

UNSTABLE HEMOGLOBINS

Unstable hemoglobins form an important group of clinically significant variants. Several different mechanisms lead to the generation of unstable variants, which result in a congenital hemolytic anemia with inclusion bodies in red cells (Heinz bodies), hence the term *congenital Heinz body hemolytic anemia*.

Definition and History

Cathie reported a 10-month-old child with hemolytic anemia, jaundice, and splenomegaly in 1952.[447] Splenectomy did not result in improvement. The patient's red cells had large Heinz bodies (see Chap. 29). Similar cases were reported from around the world, and the observation that these cases were characterized by the precipitation of their hemolysate upon exposure to heat, suggested an hemoglobin abnormality as the cause. Subsequently, nearly all of similar cases were found to have a variant hemoglobin, and Cathie's case was found to have Hb Bristol (β67Val→Asp). To date, 135 unstable variants have been reported; the vast majority are sporadic cases reported only once. Few have been observed repeatedly in different populations.

Etiology and Pathogenesis

Several different mechanisms lead to the instability of the globin molecule with precipitation in the red cell leading to hemolysis. These are summarized below.

Substitutions Near the Heme Pocket Heme is inserted into a hydrophobic pocket in each globin molecule where it is in contact with a number of invariant nonpolar amino acid residues (see Fig. 48–3). Substitution of these invariant nonpolar residues will decrease the stability of heme-globin association and ultimately lead to the instability of the globin moiety. Hb Zurich (β63His→Arg), Koln (β98Val→Met), and Hammersmith (β42Phe→Ser) are examples of this group.

Disruption of Secondary Structure (α Helix) The secondary structure of globin chains is 75 percent in the conformation of an α helix (see Fig. 48–2). Proline residues cannot participate in an α helical conformation. Thus, the substitution of a proline residue for any other amino acid except for the first three residues of an α helix will disrupt the secondary structure and lead to the disruption and precipitation of the mutant globin chain.

Mutations in $\alpha_1\beta_1$ Interface The first step in the assembly of the hemoglobin tetramer is the formation of an αβ dimer. This structure is stabilized by a secondary structure that exposes the charged amino acids (glutamic acid, aspartic acid, lysine, and arginine) on the surface of the molecule in contact with water and stabilizes the interior of the molecule ($\alpha_1\beta_1$ interface) with hydrophobic interactions. Substitution of a charged (polar) residue for a nonpolar amino acid involved in $\alpha_1\beta_1$ contact will disrupt and destabilize this dimer formation and lead to the precipitation of the hemoglobin molecule.

Amino Acid Deletions Deletion of one or more amino acid residues is expected to disrupt the secondary structure of the globin chains and may lead to instability of the mutant chain. Mutant globins with deletion of one or more residues have been reported. Examples of this type include Hb Leiden (β6 or β7Glu→0), Hb Gun Hill (β91–95→0), and Hb Freiburg (β23Val→0).

Elongated Globin Chains Some variants result from either a mutation in the termination codon or a frameshift leading to the synthesis of longer than normal globin chains. These variants tend to be unstable because of the presence of a nonfunctional fragment. Examples include Hb Cranston and Hb Tak.

Whatever the underlying mechanism may be, unstable hemoglobin variants precipitate within developing red cell precursors forming hemichromes (intermediate substances in hemoglobin denaturation) and ultimately aggregates that attach to the inner layer of red cell membrane (Heinz bodies). Heinz bodies can be visualized with supravital stains, such as brilliant cresyl blue. Red cells with Heinz bodies have impaired rheologic properties (deformability and filterability) and are trapped in the splenic circulation (see Chaps. 5, 33, and 55) with pitting of the membrane-attached bodies. Hemolysis ultimately ensues. The degree of hemolysis is proportionate to the quantity and the instability of the variant.

Clinical Features

Patients with unstable hemoglobin variants have varying degrees of hemolytic anemia. This can range from a compensated, asymptomatic hemolytic state to severe, life-threatening hemolysis. Generally, hemolytic anemia is mild to moderate and does not require therapeutic intervention. Typically, hemolysis is exacerbated by increased oxidant stress such as infections and the use of oxidant drugs. Patients may have jaundice and splenomegaly. As is the case with other chronic hemolytic states, gallstones may develop. Hypersplenism can be a problem in some cases. Many unstable hemoglobin variants that are associated with mild, compensated hemolysis are diagnosed fortuitously or during population screening for hemoglobinopathies. Unstable variants are inherited in a mendelian pattern; they are usually manifest in the heterozygous state. There are instances of *de novo* mutations without evidence of the variant in parents of an affected individual. Many of the 135 known unstable variants are found in one case or in a limited number of instances. However, some unstable variants like Hb Koln (β98Val→Met) and Hb Zurich (β67His→Arg) have been found in many populations around the world. In terms of the clinical phenotype, unstable β-globin variants are generally more symptomatic because of the higher level of expression.

Laboratory Features

Patients with unstable hemoglobin variants may have varying degrees of anemia. Generally, the anemia is mild and does not require therapeutic intervention. However, exacerbation of anemia during exposure to oxidant stress (such as infections and the use of oxidant drugs) is a common feature. Features of a hemolytic state (reticulocytosis, indirect hyperbilirubinemia, elevated lactate dehydrogenase, decreased or undetectable haptoglobin) are present. Red cell morphology shows polychromasia, anisocytosis, poikilocytosis, and occasionally basophilic stippling. A typical feature of this disorder is the presence of Heinz bodies best visualized with supravital staining with brilliant cresyl blue as membrane attached inclusion bodies in red cells. Hemoglobin electrophoresis reveals the presence of an additional abnormal hemoglobin band. The quantity of the variant Hb is variable and inversely proportional to the degree of instability of the abnormal hemoglobin (e.g., the more unstable the variant, the less the quantity). More accurate quantification can be achieved with cation exchange or reversed phase HPLC. The presence of an unstable variant in the hemolysate can be demonstrated by simple tests of stability. The most commonly used tests are heat denaturation and isopropanol precipitation. The heat denaturation test is more cumbersome and time consuming and is seldom used in practice. The isopropanol precipitation test is a simple screening test for unstable variants and involves the incubation of the hemolysate with a 17 percent solution of isopropanol; hemolysates containing unstable hemoglobin variants will form a precipitate, whereas a normal hemolysate will remain clear.

HEMOGLOBIN M AND ALTERED-AFFINITY HEMOGLOBINS

M hemoglobins result from mutations around the heme pocket that disrupt the hydrophobic nature of this structure with resultant oxidation of the iron in the heme moiety from ferrous (Fe^{2+}) to ferric (Fe^{3+}) state and cause methemoglobinemia (see Chap. 49, "Variants with Altered Oxygen Affinity").

Mutations in certain critical areas of the globin molecule alter the affinity of the globin for oxygen. In general, mutations that stabilize the molecule in the T (tense, deoxy) state lead to low oxygen affinity variants, which can clinically manifest as cyanosis or mild anemia (see Chap. 49). Mutations that stabilize the R (relaxed, oxy) state or destabilize the T state result in high O_2 affinity variants. These variants will cause secondary polycythemia (see Chap. 56). The mutations that affect the ligand binding affinity of the hemoglobin molecule are mostly in the $\alpha_1\beta_2$ interface. Rarely, mutations in the $\alpha_1\beta_1$ interface lead to altered O_2 affinity. Another mechanism in the generation of high O_2 affinity mutants involves mutations that alter the binding of 2,3-BPG.

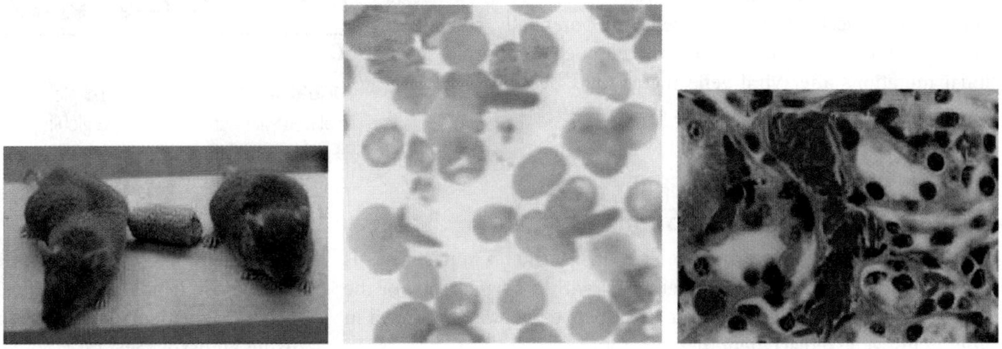
A B C

FIGURE 48–14. A. Transgenic/knockout sickle mice. The mouse α- and β-globin genes are deleted and the human α-, γ-, and β-globin genes are present as transgenes containing locus control regions (LCR sequences). The LCR γ-βS transgene in these animals was designed to switch hemoglobins 1–3 weeks after birth. The transgenic/knockout mice are relatively healthy at birth and then develop severe anemia and typical organ pathology when the switch to Hb S is completed at approximately 3 weeks of age. **B.** Blood film from sickle mice. **C.** Occluded vessel in the medulla of the kidney of a sickle mouse. These lesions result in the inability to concentrate urine.

MOUSE MODELS OF SICKLE CELL DISEASE

During the first few months after birth, sickle cell disease is normally a relatively benign disorder because Hb F has potent antisickling properties. Hb F, which comprises approximately 70 percent of total hemoglobin at birth, is gradually replaced by Hb S. Rising Hb S levels result in the onset of disease between 3 and 6 months of age. A knockout/transgenic mouse model that mimics this switch from Hb F to Hb S has been produced.[448] The locus control region (LCR) γ-βS transgene in these animals was designed to switch hemoglobins after birth,[448–450] rather than before birth,[451–456] as observed in animals produced with cosmid, bacterial artificial chromosome (BAC) or yeast artificial chromosome (YAC) transgenes. The LCR γ-βS transgenic animals are relatively healthy at birth and then develop severe anemia and typical organ pathology (see Fig. 48–14 on previous page) when the switch to Hb S is completed at approximately 3 weeks of age.[457] The same γ-βS configuration was used to produce a knockin mouse model of sickle cell disease. Mouse β-globin genes were replaced with human γ- and βS-globin genes and mouse α-globin genes were replaced with human α-globin genes (Fig. 48–15). These animals switch human hemoglobins (Hb F to Hb S) after birth and develop the same severe anemia as the knockout/transgenic mice at approximately 3 weeks of age.

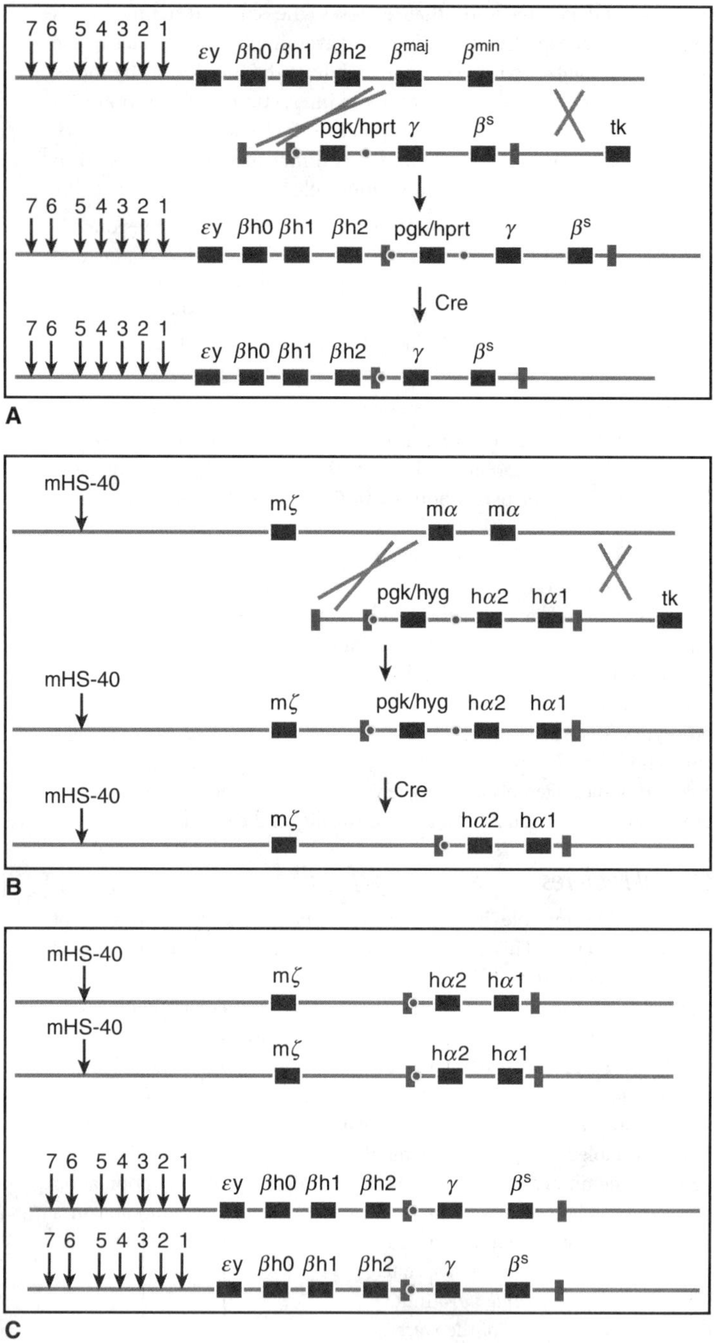

FIGURE 48–15. **A.** Human γ-βS globin gene knockin scheme. Mouse β-globin genes are replaced with human γ- and βS-globin genes. **B.** Human α-globin knockin scheme. Mouse β-globin genes are replaced with human α-globin genes. **C.** Globin locus genotype of homozygous knockin sickle mice.

GENE ADDITION THERAPY IN HEMATOPOIETIC STEM CELLS

Two groups have corrected SCD in mouse models by transduction of hematopoietic stem cells with lentiviral vectors containing antisickling globin genes followed by transplantation of these cells into syngeneic recipients (Fig. 48–16).[458,459] Although self-inactivating lentiviral vectors with or without insulator elements should provide a safe and effective treatment for hemoglobinopathies,[460] some concerns about insertional mutagenesis persist.[461] If viral integration inhibits a tumor suppressor gene or activates an oncogene, leukemia can result. Although relatively few insertional mutations have been observed in viral gene therapy studies, the severe combined immunodeficiency gene therapy trials in France demonstrated that leukemic cell clones can arise from insertional activation of LMO-2,[462] and experiments in nonhuman primates suggested that insertional inactivation of BCL-2A1 can result in acute myelogenous leukemia.[463] The risk of mutagenesis is a consequence of random insertion of one or more copies of the viral vector in a large number of cells. If 2 to 3 million CD34+ cells per kilogram of body weight are transduced and transplanted, a 50-kg patient would receive 100 million cells and, potentially, 100 million different viral insertions. Although the number of reported, insertional mutations after viral gene therapy has been low, the large number of insertion sites remains a concern.

GENE REPLACEMENT THERAPY IN INDUCED PLURIPOTENT STEM CELLS

An approach that bypasses the problem of insertional mutagenesis is replacement of the sickle globin gene (βS) with a normal copy of the gene (βA). The knockin sickle mice described above were produced in order to test gene replacement therapies for the disease.[457] Figure 48–17 illustrates correction of anemia and organ pathology by gene replacement in embryonic stem (ES) cells. In August 2006, Yamanaka's group published their landmark results demonstrating that primary skin fibroblasts of mice could be reprogrammed into ES-like cells termed *induced pluripotent stem* (iPS) cells.[464] Amazingly, the delivery of only four transcription factors (Oct4, Sox2, Klf4, and c-Myc) were required to reprogram skin fibroblasts to pluripotential stem cells that could form most, if not all, cell types. These results pioneered a method for producing patient-specific, ES-like cells without the ethical concerns of using embryos. Several laboratories quickly reproduced and extended these results,[465–469] and gene replacement was successfully performed in the knockin sickle iPS cells; one βS allele was replaced with a βA allele.[470] This experiment demonstrated that the enzymatic machinery for homologous recombination was functional in iPS cells. The corrected iPS cells were differentiated into hematopoietic progenitors in vitro, and these cells were transplanted into irradiated sickle recipients.

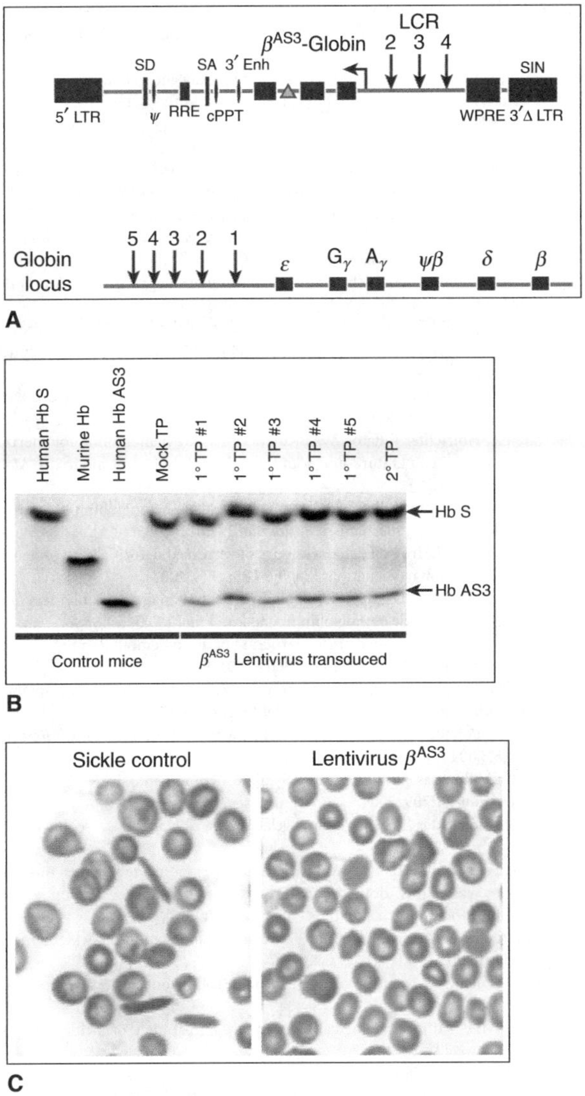

FIGURE 48–16. A. Antisickling β-globin lentiviral vector and human β-globin locus. **B.** Purified hematopoietic stem cells were transduced with the βAS3 lentiviral vector and transplanted into myeloablated recipients. Four months after primary transplant (1°TP) or 4 months after secondary transplant (2°TP; total of 8 months), erythroid cell lysates were analyzed by isoelectric focusing. Approximately 25% of total hemoglobin was human $\alpha_2\beta$AS3. **C.** Blood films of sickle control and lentivirus βAS3 transduced mice.

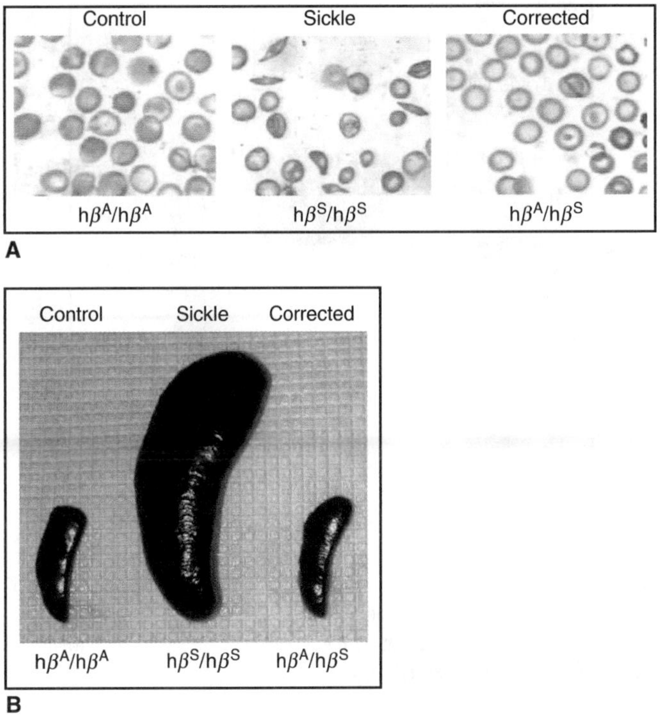

FIGURE 48–17. Blood films **(A)** and spleens **(B)** of humanized sickle mice before (hβS/hβS) and after (hβA/hβS) gene replacement therapy.

Erythroid cells derived from these progenitors synthesized high levels of human Hb A and corrected the hemolytic anemia and organ pathology that characterize sickle cell disease in humans.[470]

GENE REPLACEMENT IN HUMAN iPS CELLS?

In the fall of 2007, human iPS cells were derived from primary skin fibroblasts.[471–474] These cells are similar to human ES cells and can be differentiated into cells derived from all three germ layers. Based on these initial results, it is reasonable to expect that protocols used to differentiate human ES cells into transplantable progenitors of many cell types will soon be possible.[475] Homologous recombination in human ES cells has been reported[476]; however, pure colonies of genetically modified cells are more difficult to obtain than pure colonies of mouse ES or iPS cells because the cells must be subcultured as clumps. One approach to circumvent this problem is to perform homologous recombination in primary somatic cells before reprogramming into iPS cells. One endogenous βS gene has been replaced with a βA gene in human sickle skin fibroblasts (Wu, Sun, Pawlik, and Townes, unpublished). After conversion to iPS cells, corrected hematopoietic progenitors can be derived for transplantation.

PROSPECTS FOR GENE REPLACEMENT THERAPY IN HUMANS

Figure 48–18 illustrates an iPS cell approach for therapy in human sickle patients. As mentioned above, gene replacement therapy avoids the problem of insertional mutagenesis that can result from gene addition therapy. However, the production of human iPS cells for clinical application must avoid stable, long-term insertion of reprogramming genes in the genome. Alternative methods also have been developed to transiently deliver the reprogramming factors to somatic cells with "hit and run" vectors,[477–481] nonintegrating viral vectors,[481] or recombinant proteins.[482,483] The efficiency of production of fully reprogrammed iPS cells by these methods varies tremendously, and the ultimate method of choice will require additional experimentation.

Another challenge is the efficient differentiation of human iPS cells into transplantable hematopoietic stem cells (HSCs). Presently, murine iPS cells are induced to form embryoid bodies, and overexpression of HoxB4 in mesodermal cells is required for efficient differentiation into HSCs. However, HoxB4-directed differentiation of mesodermal progenitors into HSCs is not as effective in human cells; therefore, additional factors will be required for efficient human iPS to HSC differentiation. These factors must also be delivered transiently to cells before clinical trials can be initiated.

Because differentiation of iPS cells into HSCs will never be 100 percent efficient, purification of HSCs from undifferentiated iPS cells before transplantation is essential for the prevention of teratomas. Fluorescent activated cell sorting for HSC markers and against iPS cell

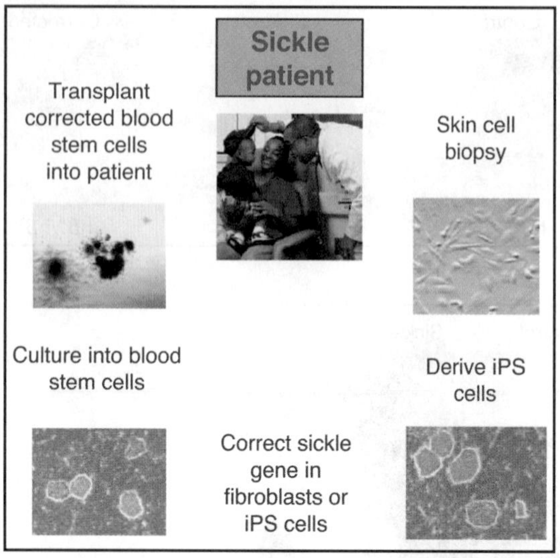

FIGURE 48–18. Approach for gene replacement therapy in human sickle patients. Skin fibroblasts or keratinocytes are reprogrammed into iPS cells, and one of the *β*S genes is replaced with a *β*A gene. These corrected iPS cells are differentiated into corrected hematopoietic stem cells that are transplanted into the patient from whom the skin biopsy was originally obtained.

antigens is one option. Clinical grade sorters are now available, and these instruments will be important for the successful translation of this technology to humans.

Some myeloablative conditioning of patients may be required to "create space" in the marrow for transplanted cells. Although the corrected HSCs are genetically identical to the patient, except for the correction of the sickle mutation, the conditions for efficient engraftment of HSCs derived in culture may be slightly different from HSCs derived from marrow. Therefore, clinical studies will be required to determine whether conditioning is necessary and, if so, to determine the dose and intensity of an optimal regimen.

The correction of sickle cell disease in a humanized mouse model by gene replacement therapy in iPS cells[470] and the derivation of human iPS cells that can be differentiated into erythroid cells[471–474] suggest that an effective patient-specific cell therapy for this disease can be developed in the next several years. These results also provide a foundation for the development of effective gene replacement therapies for other heritable and acquired diseases.

REFERENCES

1. Herrick JB: Peculiar elongated and sickle-shaped red corpuscles in a case of severe anemia. *Arch Intern Med*6:517, 1910.
2. Emmel VE: A study of the erythrocytes in a case of severe anemia with elongated and sickle-shaped red blood corpuscles. *Arch Intern Med* 20:586, 1917.
3. Hanh EV, Gillespie EB: Report of a case greatly improved by splenectomy: Experimental study of sickle cell formation. *Arch Intern Med* 39:233, 1927.
4. Diggs LW, Ahmann CF, Bibb J: The incidence and significance of the sickle cell trait. *Ann Intern Med* 7:769, 1933.
5. Gormley M: The first "molecular disease": A story of Linus Pauling, the intellectual patron. *Endeavour* 31:71, 2007.
6. Haller JO, Berdon WE, Franke H: Sickle cell anemia: The legacy of the patient (Walter Clement Noel), the interne (Ernest Irons), and the attending physician (James Herrick) and the facts of its discovery. *Pediatr Radiol* 31:889, 2001.
7. Serjeant GR: The emerging understanding of sickle cell disease. *Br J Haematol* 112:3, 2001.
8. Williams VL: Pathways of innovation: A history of the first effective treatment for sickle cell anemia. *Perspect Biol Med* 47:552, 2004.
9. Okumura MJ, Campbell AD, Nasr SZ, Davis MM: Inpatient health care use among adult survivors of chronic childhood illnesses in the United States. *Arch Pediatr Adolesc Med*160:1054, 2006.
10. Kan YW, Dozy AM: Polymorphism of DNA sequence adjacent to human beta-globin structural gene: Relationship to sickle mutation. *Proc Natl Acad Sci U S A* 75:5631, 1978.
11. Nagel RL, Fabry ME, Pagnier J, et al: Hematologically and genetically distinct forms of sickle cell anemia in Africa. The Senegal type and the Benin type. *N Engl J Med* 312:880, 1985.
12. Pagnier J, Mears JG, Dunda-Belkhodja O, et al: Evidence for the multicentric origin of the sickle cell hemoglobin gene in Africa. *Proc Natl Acad Sci U S A* 81:1771, 1984.
13. Powars DR: Sickle cell anemia: Beta s-gene-cluster haplotypes as prognostic indicators of vital organ failure. *Semin Hematol* 28:202, 1991.
14. Beutler E (ed): *Disorders of Hemoglobin Structure: Sickle Cell Anemia and Related Abnormalities.* McGraw-Hill, New York, 2003.
15. Dykes GW, Crepeau RH, Edelstein SJ: Three-dimensional reconstruction of the 14-filament fibers of hemoglobin S. *J Mol Biol* 130:451, 1979.
16. Fronticelli C, Gold R: Conformational relevance of the beta6Glu replaced by Val mutation in the beta subunits and in the beta(1–55) and beta(1–30) peptides of hemoglobin S. *J Biol Chem* 251:4968, 1976.
17. Wishner BC, Ward KB, Lattman EE, Love WE: Crystal structure of sickle-cell deoxyhemoglobin at 5 A resolution. *J Mol Biol* 98:179, 1975.
18. Ferrone FA, Hofrichter J, Eaton WA: Kinetics of sickle hemoglobin polymerization. I. Studies using temperature-jump and laser photolysis techniques. *J Mol Biol* 183:591, 1985.
19. Ferrone FA, Hofrichter J, Eaton WA: Kinetics of sickle hemoglobin polymerization. II. A double nucleation mechanism. *J Mol Biol* 183:611, 1985.
20. Huang Z, Hearne L, Irby CE, et al: Kinetics of increased deformability of deoxygenated sickle cells upon oxygenation. *Biophys J* 85:2374, 2003.
21. Carragher B, Bluemke DA, Gabriel B, et al: Structural analysis of polymers of sickle cell hemoglobin. I. Sickle hemoglobin fibers. *J Mol Biol* 199:315, 1988.
22. Padlan EA, Love WE: Refined crystal structure of deoxyhemoglobin S. II. Molecular interactions in the crystal. *J Biol Chem* 260:8280, 1985.
23. Vekilov PG: Sickle-cell haemoglobin polymerization: Is it the primary pathogenic event of sickle-cell anaemia? *Br J Haematol* 139:173, 2007.
24. Ferrone FA: Polymerization and sickle cell disease: A molecular view. *Microcirculation* 11:115, 2004.
25. Ballas SK, Mohandas N: Sickle red cell microrheology and sickle blood rheology. *Microcirculation* 11:209, 2004.
26. Eaton WA, Hofrichter J: Hemoglobin S gelation and sickle cell disease. *Blood* 70:1245, 1987.
27. Kaul DK, Fabry ME, Nagel RL: Microvascular sites and characteristics of sickle cell adhesion to vascular endothelium in shear flow conditions: Pathophysiological implications. *Proc Natl Acad Sci U S A* 86:3356, 1989.
28. Noguchi CT, Schechter AN: The intracellular polymerization of sickle hemoglobin and its relevance to sickle cell disease. *Blood* 58:1057, 1981.
29. Embury SH: The not-so-simple process of sickle cell vasoocclusion. *Microcirculation* 11:101, 2004.
30. Steinberg MH: Pathophysiologically based drug treatment of sickle cell disease. *Trends Pharmacol Sci* 27:204, 2006.
31. Stuart MJ, Nagel RL: Sickle-cell disease. *Lancet* 364:1343, 2004.
32. Brugnara C: Sickle cell disease: From membrane pathophysiology to novel therapies for prevention of erythrocyte dehydration. *J Pediatr Hematol Oncol* 25:927, 2003.
33. Stocker JW, De Franceschi L, McNaughton-Smith GA, et al: ICA-17043, a novel Gardos channel blocker, prevents sickled red blood cell dehydration in vitro and in vivo in SAD mice. *Blood* 101:2412, 2003.
34. Bennekou P, Pedersen O, Moller A, Christophersen P: Volume control in sickle cells is facilitated by the novel anion conductance inhibitor NS1652. *Blood* 95:1842, 2000.
35. Joiner CH, Jiang M, Claussen WJ, et al: Dipyridamole inhibits sickling-induced cation fluxes in sickle red blood cells. *Blood* 97:3976, 2001.
36. Aslan M, Freeman BA: Redox-dependent impairment of vascular function in sickle cell disease. *Free Radic Biol Med* 43:1469, 2007.
37. Gladwin MT, Schechter AN: Nitric oxide therapy in sickle cell disease. *Semin Hematol* 38:333, 2001.
38. Enwonwu CO, Xu XX, Turner E: Nitrogen metabolism in sickle cell anemia: Free amino acids in plasma and urine. *Am J Med Sci* 300:366, 1990.
39. Lopez BL, Barnett J, Ballas SK, et al: Nitric oxide metabolite levels in acute vaso-occlusive sickle-cell crisis. *Acad Emerg Med* 3:1098, 1996.
40. Lopez BL, Davis-Moon L, Ballas SK, Ma XL: Sequential nitric oxide measurements during the emergency department treatment of acute vasoocclusive sickle cell crisis. *Am J Hematol* 64:15, 2000.
41. Morris CR, Kuypers FA, Larkin S, et al: Arginine therapy: A novel strategy to induce nitric oxide production in sickle cell disease. *Br J Haematol* 111:498, 2000.
42. Morris CR, Kuypers FA, Larkin S, et al: Patterns of arginine and nitric oxide in patients with sickle cell disease with vaso-occlusive crisis and acute chest syndrome. *J Pediatr Hematol Oncol* 22:515, 2000.
43. Frenette PS, Atweh GF: Sickle cell disease: Old discoveries, new concepts, and future promise. *J Clin Invest* 117:850, 2007.
44. Reiter CD, Wang X, Tanus-Santos JE, et al: Cell-free hemoglobin limits nitric oxide bioavailability in sickle-cell disease. *Nat Med* 8:1383, 2002.
45. Hebbel RP, Yamada O, Moldow CF, et al: Abnormal adherence of sickle erythrocytes to cultured vascular endothelium: Possible mechanism for microvascular occlusion in sickle cell disease. *J Clin Invest* 65:154, 1980.

46. Hoover R, Rubin R, Wise G, Warren R: Adhesion of normal and sickle erythrocytes to endothelial monolayer cultures. *Blood* 54:872, 1979.
47. Barabino GA, McIntire LV, Eskin SG, et al: Rheological studies of erythrocyte-endothelial cell interactions in sickle cell disease. *Prog Clin Biol Res* 240:113, 1987.
48. Mohandas N, Evans E: Sickle erythrocyte adherence to vascular endothelium. Morphologic correlates and the requirement for divalent cations and collagen-binding plasma proteins. *J Clin Invest* 76:1605, 1985.
49. Kaul DK, Tsai HM, Liu XD, et al: Monoclonal antibodies to alphaVbeta3 (7E3 and LM609) inhibit sickle red blood cell-endothelium interactions induced by platelet-activating factor. *Blood* 95:368, 2000.
50. Frenette PS: Sickle cell vaso-occlusion: Multistep and multicellular paradigm. *Curr Opin Hematol* 9:101, 2002.
51. Gee BE, Platt OS: Sickle reticulocytes adhere to VCAM-1. *Blood* 85:268, 1995.
52. Parsons SF, Lee G, Spring FA, et al: Lutheran blood group glycoprotein and its newly characterized mouse homologue specifically bind alpha5 chain-containing human laminin with high affinity. *Blood* 97:312, 2001.
53. Swerlick RA, Eckman JR, Kumar A, et al: Alpha 4 beta 1-integrin expression on sickle reticulocytes: Vascular cell adhesion molecule-1-dependent binding to endothelium. *Blood* 82:1891, 1993.
54. Udani M, Zen Q, Cottman M, et al: Basal cell adhesion molecule/lutheran protein. The receptor critical for sickle cell adhesion to laminin. *J Clin Invest* 101:2550, 1998.
55. Okpala I: The intriguing contribution of white blood cells to sickle cell disease—A red cell disorder. *Blood Rev* 18:65, 2004.
56. Okpala I: Leukocyte adhesion and the pathophysiology of sickle cell disease. *Curr Opin Hematol* 13:40, 2006.
57. Tan P, Luscinskas FW, Homer-Vanniasinkam S: Cellular and molecular mechanisms of inflammation and thrombosis. *Eur J Vasc Endovasc Surg* 17:373, 1999.
58. Hebbel RP, Osarogiagbon R, Kaul D: The endothelial biology of sickle cell disease: Inflammation and a chronic vasculopathy. *Microcirculation* 11:129, 2004.
59. Steinberg MH, Mohandas N (eds): *Laboratory Values*. Raven, New York, 1994.
60. Belcher JD, Marker PH, Weber JP, et al: Activated monocytes in sickle cell disease: Potential role in the activation of vascular endothelium and vaso-occlusion. *Blood* 96:2451, 2000.
61. Benkerrou M, Delarche C, Brahimi L, et al: Hydroxyurea corrects the dysregulated L-selectin expression and increased H(2)O(2) production of polymorphonuclear neutrophils from patients with sickle cell anemia. *Blood* 99:2297, 2002.
62. Fadlon E, Vordermeier S, Pearson TC, et al: Blood polymorphonuclear leukocytes from the majority of sickle cell patients in the crisis phase of the disease show enhanced adhesion to vascular endothelium and increased expression of CD64. *Blood* 91:266, 1998.
63. Francis R Jr, Hebbel RP (eds): *Hemostasis*. Raven, New York, 1994.
64. Hofstra TC, Kalra VK, Meiselman HJ, Coates TD: Sickle erythrocytes adhere to polymorphonuclear neutrophils and activate the neutrophil respiratory burst. *Blood* 87:4440, 1996.
65. Inwald DP, Kirkham FJ, Peters MJ, et al: Platelet and leucocyte activation in childhood sickle cell disease: Association with nocturnal hypoxaemia. *Br J Haematol* 111:474, 2000.
66. Lard LR, Mul FP, de Haas M, et al: Neutrophil activation in sickle cell disease. *J Leukoc Biol* 66:411, 1999.
67. Nath KA, Grande JP, Haggard JJ, et al: Oxidative stress and induction of heme oxygenase-1 in the kidney in sickle cell disease. *Am J Pathol* 158:893, 2001.
68. Solovey A, Gui L, Key NS, Hebbel RP: Tissue factor expression by endothelial cells in sickle cell anemia. *J Clin Invest* 101:1899, 1998.
69. Solovey A, Lin Y, Browne P, et al: Circulating activated endothelial cells in sickle cell anemia. *N Engl J Med* 337:1584, 1997.
70. Wun T, Cordoba M, Rangaswami A, et al: Activated monocytes and platelet-monocyte aggregates in patients with sickle cell disease. *Clin Lab Haematol* 24:81, 2002.
71. Granger DN, Korthuis RJ: Physiologic mechanisms of postischemic tissue injury. *Annu Rev Physiol* 57:311, 1995.
72. Grisham MB, Granger DN, Lefer DJ: Modulation of leukocyte-endothelial interactions by reactive metabolites of oxygen and nitrogen: Relevance to ischemic heart disease. *Free Radic Biol Med* 25:404, 1998.
73. Eilertsen KE, Osterud B: Tissue factor: (patho)physiology and cellular biology. *Blood Coagul Fibrinolysis* 15:521, 2004.
74. Key NS, Slungaard A, Dandelet L, et al: Whole blood tissue factor procoagulant activity is elevated in patients with sickle cell disease. *Blood* 91:4216, 1998.
75. Krishnaswamy S: The interaction of human factor VIIa with tissue factor. *J Biol Chem* 267:23696, 1992.
76. Setty BN, Kulkarni S, Dampier CD, Stuart MJ: Fetal hemoglobin in sickle cell anemia: Relationship to erythrocyte adhesion markers and adhesion. *Blood* 97:2568, 2001.
77. Kurantsin-Mills J, Ofosu FA, Safa TK, et al: Plasma factor VII and thrombin-antithrombin III levels indicate increased tissue factor activity in sickle cell patients. *Br J Haematol* 81:539, 1992.
78. Tomer A, Harker LA, Kasey S, Eckman JR: Thrombogenesis in sickle cell disease. *J Lab Clin Med* 137:398, 2001.
79. Hillery CA, Panepinto JA: Pathophysiology of stroke in sickle cell disease. *Microcirculation* 11:195, 2004.
80. Prengler M, Pavlakis SG, Prohovnik I, Adams RJ: Sickle cell disease: The neurological complications. *Ann Neurol* 51:543, 2002.
81. Kaul DK, Liu XD, Choong S, et al: Anti-inflammatory therapy ameliorates leukocyte adhesion and microvascular flow abnormalities in transgenic sickle mice. *Am J Physiol* 287:H293, 2004.
82. Griffin TC, McIntire D, Buchanan GR: High-dose intravenous methylprednisolone therapy for pain in children and adolescents with sickle cell disease. *N Engl J Med* 330:733, 1994.
83. Tsaras G, Owusu-Ansah A, Boateng FO, Amoateng-Adjepong Y: Complications associated with sickle cell trait: A brief narrative review. *Am J Med* 122:507, 2009.
84. Harris JW, Brewster HH, Ham TH, Castle WB: Studies on the destruction of red blood cells. X. The biophysics and biology of sickle-cell disease. *AMA Arch Intern Med* 97:145, 1956.
85. Bergeron MF, Cannon JG, Hall EL, Kutlar A: Erythrocyte sickling during exercise and thermal stress. *Clin J Sport Med* 14:354, 2004.
86. Monchanin G, Serpero LD, Connes P, et al: Effects of progressive and maximal exercise on plasma levels of adhesion molecules in athletes with sickle cell trait with or without alpha-thalassemia. *J Appl Physiol* 102:169, 2007.
87. Gupta AK, Kirchner KA, Nicholson R, et al: Effects of alpha-thalassemia and sickle polymerization tendency on the urine-concentrating defect of individuals with sickle cell trait. *J Clin Invest* 88:1963, 1991.
88. Yium J, Gabow P, Johnson A, et al: Autosomal dominant polycystic kidney disease in blacks: Clinical course and effects of sickle-cell hemoglobin. *J Am Soc Nephrol* 4:1670, 1994.
89. Kark JA, Ward FT: Exercise and hemoglobin S. *Semin Hematol* 31:181, 1994.
90. Austin H, Key NS, Benson JM, et al: Sickle cell trait and the risk of venous thromboembolism among blacks. *Blood* 110:908, 2007.
91. Pastore LM, Savitz DA, Thorp JM Jr: Predictors of urinary tract infection at the first prenatal visit. *Epidemiology* 10:282, 1999.
92. Austin H, Lally C, Benson JM, et al: Hormonal contraception, sickle cell trait, and risk for venous thromboembolism among African American women. *Am J Obstet Gynecol* 200:620.e1, 2009.
93. Heller P, Best WR, Nelson RB, Becktel J: Clinical implications of sickle-cell trait and glucose-6-phosphate dehydrogenase deficiency in hospitalized black male patients. *N Engl J Med* 300:1001, 1979.
94. Glader BE, Propper RD, Buchanan GR: Microcytosis associated with sickle cell anemia. *Am J Clin Pathol* 72:63, 1979.
95. Mohandas N, Johnson A, Wyatt J, et al: Automated quantitation of cell density distribution and hyperdense cell fraction in RBC disorders. *Blood* 74:442, 1989.
96. Sherwood JB, Goldwasser E, Chilcote R, et al: Sickle cell anemia patients have low erythropoietin levels for their degree of anemia. *Blood* 67:46, 1986.
97. Boggs DR, Hyde F, Srodes C: An unusual pattern of neutrophil kinetics in sickle cell anemia. *Blood* 41:59, 1973.
98. Buchanan GR, Glader BE: Leukocyte counts in children with sickle cell disease. Comparative values in the steady state, vaso-occlusive crisis, and bacterial infection. *Am J Dis Child* 132:396, 1978.
99. Corvelli AI, Binder RA, Kales A: Disseminated intravascular coagulation in sickle cell crisis. *South Med J* 72:505, 1979.
100. Ballas SK, Burka ER, Lewis CN, Krasnow SH: Serum immunoglobulin levels in patients having sickle cell syndromes. *Am J Clin Pathol* 73:394, 1980.
101. Karayalcin G, Lanzkowsky P, Kazi AB: Zinc deficiency in children with sickle cell disease. *Am J Pediatr Hematol Oncol* 1:283, 1979.
102. Natta C, Machlin L: Plasma levels of tocopherol in sickle cell anemia subjects. *The Am J Clin Nutr* 32:1359, 1979.
103. Niell HB, Leach BE, Kraus AP: Zinc metabolism in sickle cell anemia. *JAMA* 242:2686, 1979.
104. Mario N, Baudin B, Aussel C, Giboudeau J: Capillary isoelectric focusing and high-performance cation-exchange chromatography compared for qualitative and quantitative analysis of hemoglobin variants. *Clin Chem* 43:2137, 1997.
105. Partington MD, Aronyk KE, Byrd SE: Sickle cell trait and stroke in children. *Pediatr Neurosurg* 20:148, 1994.
106. Steinberg MH: DNA diagnosis for the detection of sickle hemoglobinopathies. *Am J Hematol* 43:110, 1993.
107. Davis H, Schoendorf KC, Gergen PJ, Moore RM Jr: National trends in the mortality of children with sickle cell disease, 1968 through 1992. *Am J Public Health* 87:1317, 1997.
108. Yanni E, Grosse SD, Yang Q, Olney RS: Trends in pediatric sickle cell disease-related mortality in the United States, 1983–2002. *J Pediatr* 154:541, 2009.
109. Platt OS, Brambilla DJ, Rosse WF, et al: Mortality in sickle cell disease. Life expectancy and risk factors for early death. *N Engl J Med* 330:1639, 1994.
110. National Heart, Lung, and Blood Institute: *The Management of Sickle Cell Disease*, p 59. National Institutes of Health, NIH Publication #02-2117, 2002.
111. Yale SH, Nagib N, Guthrie T: Approach to the vaso-occlusive crisis in adults with sickle cell disease. *Am Fam Physician* 61:1349, 2000.
112. Powars DR: Natural history of sickle cell disease—The first ten years. *Semin Hematol* 12:267, 1975.
113. Jacob E, Beyer JE, Miaskowski C, et al: Are there phases to the vaso-occlusive painful episode in sickle cell disease? *J Pain Symptom Manage* 29:392, 2005.
114. Ballas SK: The sickle cell painful crisis in adults: Phases and objective signs. *Hemoglobin* 19:323, 1995.
115. Smith-Whitley K, Zhao H, Hodinka RL, et al: Epidemiology of human parvovirus B19 in children with sickle cell disease. *Blood* 103:422, 2004.

116. Godeau B, Galacteros F, Schaeffer A, et al: Aplastic crisis due to extensive bone marrow necrosis and human parvovirus infection in sickle cell disease. *Am J Med* 91:557, 1991.
117. Eichhorn RF, Buurke EJ, Blok P, et al: Sickle cell-like crisis and bone marrow necrosis associated with parvovirus B19 infection and heterozygosity for haemoglobins S and E. *J Intern Med* 245:103, 1999.
118. Tolaymat A, Al Mousily F, MacWilliam K, et al: Parvovirus glomerulonephritis in a patient with sickle cell disease. *Pediatr Nephrol* 13:340, 1999.
119. Balkaran B, Char G, Morris JS, et al: Stroke in a cohort of patients with homozygous sickle cell disease. *J Pediatr* 120:360, 1992.
120. Lowenthal EA, Wells A, Emanuel PD, et al: Sickle cell acute chest syndrome associated with parvovirus B19 infection: Case series and review. *Am J Hematol* 51:207, 1996.
121. Mallouh AA, Qudah A: Acute splenic sequestration together with aplastic crisis caused by human parvovirus B19 in patients with sickle cell disease. *J Pediatr* 122:593, 1993.
122. Koduri PR, Patel AR, Pinar H: Acute hepatic sequestration caused by parvovirus B19 infection in a patient with sickle cell anemia. *Am J Hematol* 47:250, 1994.
123. Brown KE, Young NS, Alving BM, Barbosa LH: Parvovirus B19: Implications for transfusion medicine. Summary of a workshop. *Transfusion* 41:130, 2001.
124. Kinney TR, Ware RE, Schultz WH, Filston HC: Long-term management of splenic sequestration in children with sickle cell disease. *J Pediatr* 117:194, 1990.
125. Solanki DL, Kletter GG, Castro O: Acute splenic sequestration crises in adults with sickle cell disease. *Am J Med* 80:985, 1986.
126. Bowcock SJ, Nwabueze ED, Cook AE, et al: Fatal splenic sequestration in adult sickle cell disease. *Clin Lab Haematol* 10:95, 1988.
127. Koduri PR, Agbemadzo B, Nathan S: Hemoglobin S-C disease revisited: Clinical study of 106 adults. *Am J Hematol* 68:298, 2001.
128. Vichinsky E, Lubin BH: Suggested guidelines for the treatment of children with sickle cell anemia. *Hematol Oncol Clin North Am* 1:483, 1987.
129. Powell RW, Levine GL, Yang YM, Mankad VN: Acute splenic sequestration crisis in sickle cell disease: Early detection and treatment. *J Pediatr Surg* 27:215, 1992.
130. Rao S, Gooden S: Splenic sequestration in sickle cell disease: Role of transfusion therapy. *Am J Pediatr Hematol Oncol* 7:298, 1985.
131. Talano JA, Hillery CA, Gottschall JL, et al: Delayed hemolytic transfusion reaction/hyperhemolysis syndrome in children with sickle cell disease. *Pediatrics* 111:e661, 2003.
132. King KE, Shirey RS, Lankiewicz MW, et al: Delayed hemolytic transfusion reactions in sickle cell disease: Simultaneous destruction of recipients' red cells. *Transfusion* 37:376, 1997.
133. Solomon LR: Treatment and prevention of pain due to vaso-occlusive crises in adults with sickle cell disease: An educational void. *Blood* 111:997, 2008.
134. Grahmann PH, Jackson KC 2nd, Lipman AG: Clinician beliefs about opioid use and barriers in chronic nonmalignant pain. *J Pain Palliat Care Pharmacother* 18:7, 2004.
135. Labbe E, Herbert D, Haynes J: Physicians' attitude and practices in sickle cell disease pain management. *J Palliat Care* 21:246, 2005.
136. Elander J, Lusher J, Bevan D, et al: Understanding the causes of problematic pain management in sickle cell disease: Evidence that pseudoaddiction plays a more important role than genuine analgesic dependence. *J Pain Symptom Manage* 27:156, 2004.
137. Ballas SK: Ethical issues in the management of sickle cell pain. *Am J Hematol* 68:127, 2001.
138. Aisiku IP, Smith WR, McClish DK, et al: Comparisons of high versus low emergency department utilizers in sickle cell disease. *Ann Emerg Med* 53:587, 2009.
139. Rees DC, Olujohungbe AD, Parker NE, et al: Guidelines for the management of the acute painful crisis in sickle cell disease. *Br J Haematol* 120:744, 2003.
140. Benjamin L, Dampier, CD, Jacox, A, et al: *Guideline for Management of Acute Pain in Sickle-Cel Disease.* No.1, American Pain Society, Glenview, IL, 1999.
141. Ballas SK: Meperidine for acute sickle cell pain in the emergency department: Revisited controversy. *Ann Emerg Med* 51:217, 2008.
142. Howland MA, Goldfrank LR: Why meperidine should not make a comeback in treating patients with sickle cell disease. *Ann Emerg Med* 51:203, 2008.
143. Morgan MT: Use of meperidine as the analgesic of choice in treating pain from acute painful sickle cell crisis. *Ann Emerg Med* 51:202, 2008.
144. Smith MT: Neuroexcitatory effects of morphine and hydromorphone: Evidence implicating the 3-glucuronide metabolites. *Clin Exp Pharmacol Physiol* 27:524, 2000.
145. Nadvi SZ, Sarnaik S, Ravindranath Y: Low frequency of meperidine-associated seizures in sickle cell disease. *Clin Pediatr (Phila)* 38:459, 1999.
146. Seifert CF, Kennedy S: Meperidine is alive and well in the new millennium: Evaluation of meperidine usage patterns and frequency of adverse drug reactions. *Pharmacotherapy* 24:776, 2004.
147. Buchanan ID, Woodward M, Reed GW: Opioid selection during sickle cell pain crisis and its impact on the development of acute chest syndrome. *Pediatr Blood Cancer* 45:716, 2005.
148. Kopecky EA, Jacobson S, Joshi P, Koren G: Systemic exposure to morphine and the risk of acute chest syndrome in sickle cell disease. *Clin Pharmacol Ther* 75:140, 2004.
149. Benjamin LJ, Swinson GI, Nagel RL: Sickle cell anemia day hospital: An approach for the management of uncomplicated painful crises. *Blood* 95:1130, 2000.
150. Platt OS, Thorington BD, Brambilla DJ, et al: Pain in sickle cell disease. Rates and risk factors. *N Engl J Med* 325:11, 1991.
151. Vichinsky EP, Johnson R, Lubin BH: Multidisciplinary approach to pain management in sickle cell disease. *Am J Pediatr Hematol Oncol* 4:328, 1982.
152. Styles LA, Vichinsky E: Effects of a long-term transfusion regimen on sickle cell-related illnesses. *J Pediatr* 125:909, 1994.
153. Gladwin MT, Vichinsky E: Pulmonary complications of sickle cell disease. *N Engl J Med* 359:2254, 2008.
154. Vichinsky EP, Neumayr LD, Earles AN, et al: Causes and outcomes of the acute chest syndrome in sickle cell disease. National Acute Chest Syndrome Study Group. *N Engl J Med* 342:1855, 2000.
155. Morris CR: Asthma management: Reinventing the wheel in sickle cell disease. *Am J Hematol* 84:234, 2009.
156. Emre U, Miller ST, Gutierez M, et al: Effect of transfusion in acute chest syndrome of sickle cell disease. *The J Pediatr* 127:901, 1995.
157. Emre U, Miller ST, Rao SP, Rao M: Alveolar-arterial oxygen gradient in acute chest syndrome of sickle cell disease. *J Pediatr* 123:272, 1993.
158. Bellet PS, Kalinyak KA, Shukla R, et al: Incentive spirometry to prevent acute pulmonary complications in sickle cell diseases. *N Engl J Med* 333:699, 1995.
159. Uchida K, Rackoff WR, Ohene-Frempong K, et al: Effect of erythrocytapheresis on arterial oxygen saturation and hemoglobin oxygen affinity in patients with sickle cell disease. *Am J Hematol* 59:5, 1998.
160. Bernini JC, Rogers ZR, Sandler ES, et al: Beneficial effect of intravenous dexamethasone in children with mild to moderately severe acute chest syndrome complicating sickle cell disease. *Blood* 92:3082, 1998.
161. Charache S, Terrin ML, Moore RD, et al: Effect of hydroxyurea on the frequency of painful crises in sickle cell anemia. Investigators of the Multicenter Study of Hydroxyurea in Sickle Cell Anemia. *N Engl J Med* 332:1317, 1995.
162. Ballas SK, Files B, Luchtman-Jones L, et al: Secretory phospholipase A2 levels in patients with sickle cell disease and acute chest syndrome. *Hemoglobin* 30:165, 2006.
163. Bargoma EM, Mitsuyoshi JK, Larkin SK, et al: Serum C-reactive protein parallels secretory phospholipase A2 in sickle cell disease patients with vasoocclusive crisis or acute chest syndrome. *Blood* 105:3384, 2005.
164. Kuypers FA, Styles LA: The role of secretory phospholipase A2 in acute chest syndrome. *Cell Mol Biol (Noisy-le-grand)* 50:87, 2004.
165. Styles LA, Aarsman AJ, Vichinsky EP, Kuypers FA: Secretory phospholipase A(2) predicts impending acute chest syndrome in sickle cell disease. *Blood* 96:3276, 2000.
166. Styles LA, Schalkwijk CG, Aarsman AJ, et al: Phospholipase A2 levels in acute chest syndrome of sickle cell disease. *Blood* 87:2573, 1996.
167. Gladwin MT, Sachdev V, Jison ML, et al: Pulmonary hypertension as a risk factor for death in patients with sickle cell disease. *N Engl J Med* 350:886, 2004.
168. Ataga KI, Moore CG, Jones S, et al: Pulmonary hypertension in patients with sickle cell disease: A longitudinal study. *Br J Haematol* 134:109, 2006.
169. De Castro LM, Jonassaint JC, Graham FL, et al: Pulmonary hypertension associated with sickle cell disease: Clinical and laboratory endpoints and disease outcomes. *Am J Hematol* 83:19, 2008.
170. Castro O, Hoque M, Brown BD: Pulmonary hypertension in sickle cell disease: Cardiac catheterization results and survival. *Blood* 101:1257, 2003.
171. Repka T, Hebbel RP: Hydroxyl radical formation by sickle erythrocyte membranes: Role of pathologic iron deposits and cytoplasmic reducing agents. *Blood* 78:2753, 1991.
172. Kristiansen M, Graversen JH, Jacobsen C, et al: Identification of the haemoglobin scavenger receptor. *Nature* 409:198, 2001.
173. Ryter SW, Otterbein LE, Morse D, Choi AM: Heme oxygenase/carbon monoxide signaling pathways: Regulation and functional significance. *Mol Cell Biochem* 234–235:249, 2002.
174. Baranano DE, Rao M, Ferris CD, Snyder SH: Biliverdin reductase: A major physiologic cryoprotectant. *Proc Natl Acad Sci U S A* 99:16093, 2002.
175. Hebbel RP: Auto-oxidation and a membrane-associated "Fenton reagent": A possible explanation for development of membrane lesions in sickle erythrocytes. *Clin Haematol* 14:129, 1985.
176. Reiter CD, Gladwin MT: An emerging role for nitric oxide in sickle cell disease vascular homeostasis and therapy. *Curr Opin Hematol* 10:99, 2003.
177. Morris CR, Kato GJ, Poljakovic M, et al: Dysregulated arginine metabolism, hemolysis-associated pulmonary hypertension, and mortality in sickle cell disease. *JAMA* 294:81, 2005.
178. Villagra J, Shiva S, Hunter LA, et al: Platelet activation in patients with sickle disease, hemolysis-associated pulmonary hypertension, and nitric oxide scavenging by cell-free hemoglobin. *Blood* 110:2166, 2007.
179. Raghavachari N, Xu X, Harris A, et al: Amplified expression profiling of platelet transcriptome reveals changes in arginine metabolic pathways in patients with sickle cell disease. *Circulation* 115:1551, 2007.
180. Ataga KI, Moore CG, Hillery CA, et al: Coagulation activation and inflammation in sickle cell disease-associated pulmonary hypertension. *Haematologica* 93:20, 2008.
181. van Beers EJ, Spronk HM, Ten Cate H, et al: No association of the hypercoagulable state with sickle cell disease related pulmonary hypertension. *Haematologica* 93:e42, 2008.
182. Westerman M, Pizzey A, Hirschman J, et al: Microvesicles in haemoglobinopathies offer insights into mechanisms of hypercoagulability, haemolysis and the effects of therapy. *Br J Haematol* 142:126, 2008.
183. Benza RL: Pulmonary hypertension associated with sickle cell disease: Pathophysiology and rationale for treatment. *Lung* 186:247, 2008.
184. Anthi A, Machado RF, Jison ML, et al: Hemodynamic and functional assessment of patients with sickle cell disease and pulmonary hypertension. *Am J Respir Crit Care Med* 175:1272, 2007.
185. Koumbourlis AC, Zar HJ, Hurlet-Jensen A, Goldberg MR: Prevalence and reversibility of lower airway obstruction in children with sickle cell disease. *J Pediatr* 138:188, 2001.

186. Morris C, Kuypers, FA, Lavrisha, L, et al: Elevated arginase activity and limited arginine bioavailability: A common feature of asthma and sickle cell disease [abstract 2819]. *Blood* 102:764a, 2003.
187. Boyd JH, Moinuddin A, Strunk RC, DeBaun MR: Asthma and acute chest in sickle-cell disease. *Pediatr Pulmonol* 38:229, 2004.
188. Bryant R: Asthma in the pediatric sickle cell patient with acute chest syndrome. *J Pediatr Health Care* 19:157, 2005.
189. Knight-Madden JM, Forrester TS, Lewis NA, Greenough A: Asthma in children with sickle cell disease and its association with acute chest syndrome. *Thorax* 60:206, 2005.
190. Nordness ME, Lynn J, Zacharisen MC, et al: Asthma is a risk factor for acute chest syndrome and cerebral vascular accidents in children with sickle cell disease. *Clin Mol Allergy* 3:2, 2005.
191. Boyd JH, Macklin EA, Strunk RC, DeBaun MR: Asthma is associated with acute chest syndrome and pain in children with sickle cell anemia. *Blood* 108:2923, 2006.
192. Sylvester KP, Patey RA, Broughton S, et al: Temporal relationship of asthma to acute chest syndrome in sickle cell disease. *Pediatr Pulmonol* 42:103, 2007.
193. Boyd JH, Macklin EA, Strunk RC, DeBaun MR: Asthma is associated with increased mortality in individuals with sickle cell anemia. *Haematologica* 92:1115, 2007.
194. Hagar RW, Michlitsch JG, Gardner J, et al: Clinical differences between children and adults with pulmonary hypertension and sickle cell disease. *Br J Haematol* 140:104, 2008.
195. Klings ES, Wyszynski DF, Nolan VG, Steinberg MH: Abnormal pulmonary function in adults with sickle cell anemia. *Am J Respir Crit Care Med* 173:1264, 2006.
196. Varat MA, Adolph RJ, Fowler NO: Cardiovascular effects of anemia. *Am Heart J* 83:415, 1972.
197. Balfour IC, Covitz W, Davis H, et al: Cardiac size and function in children with sickle cell anemia. *Am Heart J* 108:345, 1984.
198. Pegelow CH, Colangelo L, Steinberg M, et al: Natural history of blood pressure in sickle cell disease: Risks for stroke and death associated with relative hypertension in sickle cell anemia. *Am J Med* 102:171, 1997.
199. Caldas MC, Meira ZA, Barbosa MM: Evaluation of 107 patients with sickle cell anemia through tissue Doppler and myocardial performance index. *J Am Soc Echocardiogr* 21:1163, 2008.
200. Braden DS, Covitz W, Milner PF: Cardiovascular function during rest and exercise in patients with sickle-cell anemia and coexisting alpha thalassemia-2. *Am J Hematol* 52:96, 1996.
201. Covitz W: Cardiac Disease in *Sickle Cell Disease: Basic Principles and Clinical Approaches,* Chapter 49, pp. 725-734, edited by S Embury. Raven Press, New York, 1994.
202. Covitz W, Espeland M, Gallagher D, et al: The heart in sickle cell anemia. The Cooperative Study of Sickle Cell Disease (CSSCD). *Chest* 108:1214, 1995.
203. Dang NC, Johnson C, Eslami-Farsani M, Haywood LJ: Myocardial injury or infarction associated with fat embolism in sickle cell disease: A report of three cases with survival. *Am J Hematol* 80:133, 2005.
204. James TN, Riddick L, Massing GK: Sickle cells and sudden death: Morphologic abnormalities of the cardiac conduction system. *J Lab Clin Med* 124:507, 1994.
205. Leight L, Snider TH, Clifford GO, Hellems HK: Hemodynamic studies in sickle cell anemia. *Circulation* 10:653, 1954.
206. Martin CR, Johnson CS, Cobb C, et al: Myocardial infarction in sickle cell disease. *J Natl Med Assoc* 88:428, 1996.
207. Rodgers GP, Walker EC, Podgor MJ: Is "relative" hypertension a risk factor for vaso-occlusive complications in sickle cell disease? *Am J Med Sci* 305:150, 1993.
208. Sachdev V, Machado RF, Shizukuda Y, et al: Diastolic dysfunction is an independent risk factor for death in patients with sickle cell disease. *J Am Coll Cardiol* 49:472, 2007.
209. Stockman JA, Nigro MA, Mishkin MM, Oski FA: Occlusion of large cerebral vessels in sickle-cell anemia. *N Engl J Med* 287:846, 1972.
210. Ohene-Frempong K, Weiner SJ, Sleeper LA, et al: Cerebrovascular accidents in sickle cell disease: Rates and risk factors. *Blood* 91:288, 1998.
211. Steen RG, Xiong X, Langston JW, Helton KJ: Brain injury in children with sickle cell disease: Prevalence and etiology. *Ann Neurol* 54:564, 2003.
212. Prohovnik I, Pavlakis SG, Piomelli S, et al: Cerebral hyperemia, stroke, and transfusion in sickle cell disease. *Neurology* 39:344, 1989.
213. Wang WC: The pathophysiology, prevention, and treatment of stroke in sickle cell disease. *Curr Opin Hematol* 14:191, 2007.
214. Switzer JA, Hess DC, Nichols FT, Adams RJ: Pathophysiology and treatment of stroke in sickle-cell disease: Present and future. *Lancet Neurol* 5:501, 2006.
215. Rothman SM, Fulling KH, Nelson JS: Sickle cell anemia and central nervous system infarction: A neuropathological study. *Ann Neurol* 20:684, 1986.
216. Powars D, Adams RJ, Nichols FT, et al: Delayed intracranial hemorrhage following cerebral infarction in sickle cell anemia. *J Assoc Acad Minor Phys* 1:79, 1990.
217. Diggs LW, Brookoff D: Multiple cerebral aneurysms in patients with sickle cell disease. *South Med J* 86:377, 1993.
218. Anson JA, Koshy M, Ferguson L, Crowell RM: Subarachnoid hemorrhage in sickle-cell disease. *J Neurosurg* 75:552, 1991.
219. Oyesiku NM, Barrow DL, Eckman JR, et al: Intracranial aneurysms in sickle-cell anemia: Clinical features and pathogenesis. *J Neurosurg* 75:356, 1991.
220. Preul MC, Cendes F, Just N, Mohr G: Intracranial aneurysms and sickle cell anemia: Multiplicity and propensity for the vertebrobasilar territory. *Neurosurgery* 42:971, 1998.
221. Miller ST, Macklin EA, Pegelow CH, et al: Silent infarction as a risk factor for overt stroke in children with sickle cell anemia: A report from the Cooperative Study of Sickle Cell Disease. *J Pediatr* 139:385, 2001.
222. Pegelow CH, Macklin EA, Moser FG, et al: Longitudinal changes in brain magnetic resonance imaging findings in children with sickle cell disease. *Blood* 99:3014, 2002.
223. Kirkham FJ, Hewes DK, Prengler M, et al: Nocturnal hypoxaemia and central-nervous-system events in sickle-cell disease. *Lancet* 357:1656, 2001.
224. Kinney TR, Sleeper LA, Wang WC, et al: Silent cerebral infarcts in sickle cell anemia: A risk factor analysis. The Cooperative Study of Sickle Cell Disease. *Pediatrics* 103:640, 1999.
225. Moser FG, Miller ST, Bello JA, et al: The spectrum of brain MR abnormalities in sickle-cell disease: A report from the Cooperative Study of Sickle Cell Disease. *AJNR Am J Neuroradiol* 17:965, 1996.
226. Adams RJ, Kutlar A, McKie V, et al: Alpha thalassemia and stroke risk in sickle cell anemia. *Am J Hematol* 45:279, 1994.
227. Adams R, McKie V, Nichols F, et al: The use of transcranial ultrasonography to predict stroke in sickle cell disease. *N Engl J Med* 326:605, 1992.
228. Hoppe C, Klitz W, Cheng S, et al: Gene interactions and stroke risk in children with sickle cell anemia. *Blood* 103:2391, 2004.
229. Berkelhammer LD, Williamson AL, Sanford SD, et al: Neurocognitive sequelae of pediatric sickle cell disease: A review of the literature. *Child Neuropsychol* 13:120, 2007.
230. Fullerton HJ, Gardner M, Adams RJ, et al: Obstacles to primary stroke prevention in children with sickle cell disease. *Neurology* 67:1098, 2006.
231. Fullerton HJ, Adams RJ, Zhao S, Johnston SC: Declining stroke rates in Californian children with sickle cell disease. *Blood* 104:336, 2004.
232. Hulbert ML, Scothorn DJ, Panepinto JA, et al: Exchange blood transfusion compared with simple transfusion for first overt stroke is associated with a lower risk of subsequent stroke: A retrospective cohort study of 137 children with sickle cell anemia. *J Pediatr* 149:710, 2006.
233. Vichinsky EP, Haberkern CM, Neumayr L, et al: A comparison of conservative and aggressive transfusion regimens in the perioperative management of sickle cell disease. The Preoperative Transfusion in Sickle Cell Disease Study Group. *N Engl J Med* 333:206, 1995.
234. Ware RE, Zimmerman SA, Sylvestre PB, et al: Prevention of secondary stroke and resolution of transfusional iron overload in children with sickle cell anemia using hydroxyurea and phlebotomy. *J Pediatr* 145:346, 2004.
235. Zimmerman SA, Schultz WH, Burgett S, et al: Hydroxyurea therapy lowers transcranial Doppler flow velocities in children with sickle cell anemia. *Blood* 110:1043, 2007.
236. Dobson SR, Holden KR, Nietert PJ, et al: Moyamoya syndrome in childhood sickle cell disease: A predictive factor for recurrent cerebrovascular events. *Blood* 99:3144, 2002.
237. Hankinson TC, Bohman LE, Heyer G, et al: Surgical treatment of moyamoya syndrome in patients with sickle cell anemia: Outcome following encephaloduroarteriosynangiosis. *J Neurosurg Pediatr* 1:211, 2008.
238. Saborio P, Scheinman JI: Sickle cell nephropathy. *J Am Soc Nephrol* 10:187, 1999.
239. Van Eps L, de Jong PE (eds): *Sickle Cell Disease.* Little, Brown, Boston, 1997.
240. Sklar AH, Campbell H, Caruana RJ, et al: A population study of renal function in sickle cell anemia. *Int J Artif Organs* 13:231, 1990.
241. Falk RJ, Scheinman J, Phillips G, et al: Prevalence and pathologic features of sickle cell nephropathy and response to inhibition of angiotensin-converting enzyme. *N Engl J Med* 326:910, 1992.
242. Powars DR, Elliott-Mills DD, Chan L, et al: Chronic renal failure in sickle cell disease: Risk factors, clinical course, and mortality. *Ann Intern Med* 115:614, 1991.
243. Powars DR, Chan LS, Hiti A, et al: Outcome of sickle cell anemia: A 4-decade observational study of 1056 patients. *Medicine (Baltimore)* 84:363, 2005.
244. Guasch A, Navarrete J, Nass K, Zayas CF: Glomerular involvement in adults with sickle cell hemoglobinopathies: Prevalence and clinical correlates of progressive renal failure. *J Am Soc Nephrol* 17:2228, 2006.
245. McKie KT, Hanevold CD, Hernandez C, et al: Prevalence, prevention, and treatment of microalbuminuria and proteinuria in children with sickle cell disease. *J Pediatr Hematol Oncol* 29:140, 2007.
246. Scheinman J: *Sickle Cell Nephropathy in Pediatric Nephrology,* pp. 908-919, edited by M Holliday, TM Barratt, ED Avner. Williams & Wilkins, Boston, 1994.
247. Foucan L, Bourhis V, Bangou J, et al: A randomized trial of captopril for microalbuminuria in normotensive adults with sickle cell anemia. *Am J Med* 104:339, 1998.
248. Steinberg MH: Erythropoietin for anemia of renal failure in sickle cell disease. *N Engl J Med* 324:1369, 1991.
249. Little JA, McGowan VR, Kato GJ, et al: Combination erythropoietin-hydroxyurea therapy in sickle cell disease: Experience from the National Institutes of Health and a literature review. *Haematologica* 91:1076, 2006.
250. Bruno D, Wigfall DR, Zimmerman SA, et al: Genitourinary complications of sickle cell disease. *J Urol* 166:803, 2001.
251. Guasch A, Cua M, Mitch WE: Early detection and the course of glomerular injury in patients with sickle cell anemia. *Kidney Int* 49:786, 1996.
252. Alvarez O, Zilleruelo G, Wright D, et al: Serum cystatin C levels in children with sickle cell disease. *Pediatr Nephrol* 21:533, 2006.
253. Mantadakis E, Cavender JD, Rogers ZR, et al: Prevalence of priapism in children and adolescents with sickle cell anemia. *J Pediatr Hematol Oncol* 21:518, 1999.
254. Fowler JE Jr, Koshy M, Strub M, Chinn SK: Priapism associated with the sickle cell hemoglobinopathies: Prevalence, natural history and sequelae. *J Urol* 145:65, 1991.
255. Emond AM, Holman R, Hayes RJ, Serjeant GR: Priapism and impotence in homozygous sickle cell disease. *Arch Intern Med* 140:1434, 1980.

256. Hamre MR, Harmon EP, Kirkpatrick DV, et al: Priapism as a complication of sickle cell disease. *J Urol* 145:1, 1991.
257. Larocque MA, Cosgrove MD: Priapism: A review of 46 cases. *J Urol* 112:770, 1974.
258. Miller ST, Rao SP, Dunn EK, Glassberg KI: Priapism in children with sickle cell disease. *J Urol* 154:844, 1995.
259. Powars DR, Johnson CS: Priapism. *Hematol Oncol Clin North Am* 10:1363, 1996.
260. Douglas L, Fletcher H, Serjeant GR: Penile prostheses in the management of impotence in sickle cell disease. *Br J UrolJ Urol* 65:533, 1990.
261. Levine LA, Guss SP: Gonadotropin-releasing hormone analogues in the treatment of sickle cell anemia-associated priapism. *J Urol* 150:475, 1993.
262. Lowe FC, Jarow JP: Placebo-controlled study of oral terbutaline and pseudoephedrine in management of prostaglandin E1-induced prolonged erections. *Urology* 42:51, 1993.
263. Walker EM Jr, Mitchum EN, Rous SN, et al: Automated erythrocytapheresis for relief of priapism in sickle cell hemoglobinopathies. *J Urol* 130:912, 1983.
264. Winter CC: Priapism cured by creation of fistulas between glans penis and corpora cavernosa. *J Urol* 119:227, 1978.
265. Field JJ, Austin PF, An P, et al: Enuresis is a common and persistent problem among children and young adults with sickle cell anemia. *Urology* 72:81, 2008.
266. Jordan SS, Hilker KA, Stoppelbein L, et al: Nocturnal enuresis and psychosocial problems in pediatric sickle cell disease and sibling controls. *J Dev Behav Pediatr* 26:404, 2005.
267. Barakat LP, Smith-Whitley K, Schulman S, et al: Nocturnal enuresis in pediatric sickle cell disease. *J Dev Behav Pediatr* 22:300, 2001.
268. Almeida A, Roberts I: Bone involvement in sickle cell disease. *Br J Haematol* 129:482, 2005.
269. Kim SK, Miller JH: Natural history and distribution of bone and bone marrow infarction in sickle hemoglobinopathies. *J Nucl Med* 43:896, 2002.
270. Lonergan G, Cline, DB, Abbondanzo, SL: Sickle cell anemia. *Radiographics* 21:971, 2001.
271. Smith J: Bone disorders in sickle cell disease. *Hematol Oncol Clin North Am* 10:1345, 1996.
272. Atkins BL, Price EH, Tillyer L, et al: Salmonella osteomyelitis in sickle cell disease children in the east end of London. *J Infect* 34:133, 1997.
273. Burnett MW, Bass JW, Cook BA: Etiology of osteomyelitis complicating sickle cell disease. *Pediatrics* 101:296, 1998.
274. William R, Hussein SS, Jeans WD, et al: A prospective study of soft-tissue ultrasonography in sickle cell disease patients with suspected osteomyelitis. *Clin Radiol* 55:307, 2000.
275. Umans H, Haramati N, Flusser G: The diagnostic role of gadolinium enhanced MRI in distinguishing between acute medullary bone infarct and osteomyelitis. *Magn Reson Imaging* 18:255, 2000.
276. Neonato M, Guilloud-Bataille M, Beauvais P, et al: Acute clinical events in 299 homozygous sickle cell patients living in France. French study group on sickle cell disease. *Eur J Haematol* 65:155, 2000.
277. Milner P, Kraus AP, Sebes JJ, et al: Sickle cell disease as a cause of osteonecrosis of the femoral head. *N Engl J Med* 325:1479, 1991.
278. Ware H, Brooks AP, Toye R, Berney SI: Sickle cell disease and silent avascular necrosis of the hip. *J Bone Joint Surg* 73:947, 1991.
279. Adekile AD, Gupta R, Yacoub F, et al: Avascular necrosis of the hip in children with sickle cell disease and high Hb F: Magnetic resonance imaging findings and influence of alpha-thalassemia trait. *Acta Haematol* 105:27, 2001.
280. Baldwin C, Nolan VG, Wyszynski DF, et al: Association of klotho, bone morphogenic protein 6, and annexin A2 polymorphisms with sickle cell osteonecrosis. *Blood* 106:372, 2005.
281. Claster S, Vichinsky EP: Managing sickle cell disease. *BMJ* 327:1151, 2003.
282. Collett-Solberg PF, Ware RE, O'Hara SM: Asymmetrical closure of epiphyses in a patient with sickle cell anemia. *J Pediatr Endocrinol Metab* 15:1207, 2002.
283. Milner P, Kraus AP, Sebes JJ, et al: Osteonecrosis of the humeral head in sickle cell disease. *Clin Orthop Relat Res* 289:136, 1993.
284. Hernigou P, Bachir D, Galacteros F: The natural history of symptomatic osteonecrosis in adults with sickle-cell disease. *J Bone Joint Surg* 85A:500, 2003.
285. Hernigou P, Habibi A, Bachir D, Galacteros F: The natural history of asymptomatic osteonecrosis of the femoral head in adults with sickle cell disease. *J Bone Joint Surg* 88:2565, 2006.
286. Neumayr LD, Aguilar C, Earles AN, et al: Physical therapy alone compared with core decompression and physical therapy for femoral head osteonecrosis in sickle cell disease. Results of a multicenter study at a mean of three years after treatment. *J Bone Joint Surg* 88:2573, 2006.
287. Hernigou P, Zilber S, Filippini P, et al: Total THA in adult osteonecrosis related to sickle cell disease. *Clin Orthop Relat Res* 466:300, 2008.
288. Moran MC, Huo MH, Garvin KL, et al: Total hip arthroplasty in sickle cell hemoglobinopathy. *Clin Orthop Relat Res* 294:140, 1993.
289. Acurio MT, Friedman RJ: Hip arthroplasty in patients with sickle-cell haemoglobinopathy. *J Bone Joint Surg Br* 74:367, 1992.
290. Nolan VG, Adewoye A, Baldwin C, et al: Sickle cell leg ulcers: Associations with haemolysis and SNPs in Klotho, TEK and genes of the TGF-beta/BMP pathway. *Br J Haematol* 133:570, 2006.
291. Koshy M, Entsuah R, Koranda A, et al: Leg ulcers in patients with sickle cell disease. *Blood* 74:1403, 1989.
292. Halabi-Tawil M, Lionnet F, Girot R, et al: Sickle cell leg ulcers: A frequently disabling complication and a marker of severity. *Br J Dermatol* 158:339, 2008.
293. Kato GJ, McGowan V, Machado RF, et al: Lactate dehydrogenase as a biomarker of hemolysis-associated nitric oxide resistance, priapism, leg ulceration, pulmonary hypertension, and death in patients with sickle cell disease. *Blood* 107:2279, 2006.
294. Wethers DL, Ramirez GM, Koshy M, et al: Accelerated healing of chronic sickle-cell leg ulcers treated with RGD peptide matrix. RGD Study Group. *Blood* 84:1775, 1994.
295. Sher GD, Olivieri NF: Rapid healing of chronic leg ulcers during arginine butyrate therapy in patients with sickle cell disease and thalassemia. *Blood* 84:2378, 1994.
296. Best PJ, Daoud MS, Pittelkow MR, Petitt RM: Hydroxyurea-induced leg ulceration in 14 patients. *Ann Intern Med* 128:29, 1998.
297. Traina F, Jorge SG, Yamanaka A, et al: Chronic liver abnormalities in sickle cell disease: A clinicopathological study in 70 living patients. *Acta Haematol* 118:129, 2007.
298. Banerjee S, Owen C, Chopra S: Sickle cell hepatopathy. *Hepatology* 33:1021, 2001.
299. Koskinas J, Manesis EK, Zacharakis GH, et al: Liver involvement in acute vaso-occlusive crisis of sickle cell disease: Prevalence and predisposing factors. *Scand J Gastroenterol* 42:499, 2007.
300. West MS, Wethers D, Smith J, Steinberg M: Laboratory profile of sickle cell disease: A cross-sectional analysis. The Cooperative Study of Sickle Cell Disease. *J Clin Epidemiol* 45:893, 1992.
301. Ahn H, Li CS, Wang W: Sickle cell hepatopathy: Clinical presentation, treatment, and outcome in pediatric and adult patients. *Pediatr Blood Cancer* 45:184, 2005.
302. Buchanan GR, Glader BE: Benign course of extreme hyperbilirubinemia in sickle cell anemia: Analysis of six cases. *J Pediatr* 91:21, 1977.
303. Johnson CS, Omata M, Tong MJ, et al: Liver involvement in sickle cell disease. *Medicine (Baltimore)* 64:349, 1985.
304. Shao SH, Orringer EP: Sickle cell intrahepatic cholestasis: Approach to a difficult problem. *Am J Gastroenterol* 90:2048, 1995.
305. Suell MN, Horton TM, Dishop MK, et al: Outcomes for children with gallbladder abnormalities and sickle cell disease. *J Pediatr* 145:617, 2004.
306. Rennels MB, Dunne MG, Grossman NJ, Schwartz AD: Cholelithiasis in patients with major sickle hemoglobinopathies. *Am J Dis Child* 138:66, 1984.
307. Bond LR, Hatty SR, Horn ME, et al: Gall stones in sickle cell disease in the United Kingdom. *Br Med J (Clin Res Ed)* 295:234, 1987.
308. Vasavda N, Menzel S, Kondaveeti S, et al: The linear effects of alpha-thalassaemia, the UGT1A1 and HMOX1 polymorphisms on cholelithiasis in sickle cell disease. *Br J Haematol* 138:263, 2007.
309. To KW, Nadel AJ: Ophthalmologic complications in hemoglobinopathies. *Hematol Oncol Clin North Am* 5:535, 1991.
310. Mohan JS, Lip PL, Blann AD, et al: The angiopoietin/Tie-2 system in proliferative sickle retinopathy: Relation to vascular endothelial growth factor, its soluble receptor Flt-1 and von Willebrand factor, and to the effects of laser treatment. *Br J Ophthalmol* 89:815, 2005.
311. Aiello LP, Avery RL, Arrigg PG, et al: Vascular endothelial growth factor in ocular fluid of patients with diabetic retinopathy and other retinal disorders. *N Engl J Med* 331:1480, 1994.
312. Aiello LP, Northrup JM, Keyt BA, et al: Hypoxic regulation of vascular endothelial growth factor in retinal cells. *Arch Ophthalmol* 113:1538, 1995.
313. Downes SM, Hambleton IR, Chuang EL, et al: Incidence and natural history of proliferative sickle cell retinopathy: Observations from a cohort study. *Ophthalmology* 112:1869, 2005.
314. Condon PI, Serjeant GR: Behaviour of untreated proliferative sickle retinopathy. *Br J Ophthalmol* 64:404, 1980.
315. Liem RI, Calamaras DM, Chhabra MS, et al: Sudden-onset blindness in sickle cell disease due to retinal artery occlusion. *Pediatr Blood Cancer* 50:624, 2008.
316. Paton D: The conjunctival sign of sickle-cell disease. *Arch Ophthalmol* 66:90, 1961.
317. Paton D: The conjunctival sign ox sickle-cell disease. Further observations. *Arch Ophthalmol* 68:627, 1962.
318. Cheung AT, Chen PC, Larkin EC, et al: Microvascular abnormalities in sickle cell disease: A computer-assisted intravital microscopy study. *Blood* 99:3999, 2002.
319. Knisely MH, Bloch EH, Eliot TS, Warner L: Sludged blood. *Science* 106:431, 1947.
320. Curran EL, Fleming JC, Rice K, Wang WC: Orbital compression syndrome in sickle cell disease. *Ophthalmology* 104:1610, 1997.
321. Sayag D, Binaghi M, Souied EH, et al: Retinal photocoagulation for proliferative sickle cell retinopathy: A prospective clinical trial with new sea fan classification. *Eur J Ophthalmol* 18:248, 2008.
322. Fox PD, Minninger K, Forshaw ML, et al: Laser photocoagulation for proliferative retinopathy in sickle haemoglobin C disease. *Eye* 7(Pt 5):703, 1993.
323. Fox PD, Vessey SJ, Forshaw ML, Serjeant GR: Influence of genotype on the natural history of untreated proliferative sickle retinopathy—An angiographic study. *Br J Ophthalmol* 75:229, 1991.
324. O'Brien RT, McIntosh S, Aspnes GT, Pearson HA: Prospective study of sickle cell anemia in infancy. *J Pediatr* 89:205, 1976.
325. Seeler RA, Metzger W, Mufson MA: Diplococcus pneumoniae infections in children with sickle cell anemia. *Am J Dis Child* 123:8, 1972.
326. Pearson HA, Spencer RP, Cornelius EA: Functional asplenia in sickle-cell anemia. *N Engl J Med* 281:923, 1969.
327. Ferster A, Bujan W, Corazza F, et al: Bone marrow transplantation corrects the splenic reticuloendothelial dysfunction in sickle cell anemia. *Blood* 81:1102, 1993.

328. Buchanan GR, McKie V, Jackson EA, et al: Splenic phagocytic function in children with sickle cell anemia receiving long-term hypertransfusion therapy. *J Pediatr* 115:568, 1989.
329. Pearson HA, Gallagher D, Chilcote R, et al: Developmental pattern of splenic dysfunction in sickle cell disorders. *Pediatrics* 76:392, 1985.
330. Claster S, Vichinsky E: First report of reversal of organ dysfunction in sickle cell anemia by the use of hydroxyurea: Splenic regeneration. *Blood* 88:1951, 1996.
331. Ozsoylu S: Splenic function in sickle cell disease. *J Pediatr* 106:530, 1985.
332. Adam S, Jonassaint J, Kruger H, et al: Surgical and obstetric outcomes in adults with sickle cell disease. *Am J Med* 121:916, 2008.
333. Smith JA, Espeland M, Bellevue R, et al: Pregnancy in sickle cell disease: Experience of the Cooperative Study of Sickle Cell Disease. *Obstet Gynecol* 87:199, 1996.
334. Sun PM, Wilburn W, Raynor BD, Jamieson D: Sickle cell disease in pregnancy: Twenty years of experience at Grady Memorial Hospital, Atlanta, Georgia. *Am J Obstet Gynecol* 184:1127, 2001.
335. James AH, Jamison MG, Brancazio LR, Myers ER: Venous thromboembolism during pregnancy and the postpartum period: Incidence, risk factors, and mortality. *Am J Obstet Gynecol* 194:1311, 2006.
336. Villers MS, Jamison MG, De Castro LM, James AH: Morbidity associated with sickle cell disease in pregnancy. *Am J Obstet Gynecol* 199:125 e1, 2008.
337. Koshy M, Burd L, Wallace D, et al: Prophylactic red-cell transfusions in pregnant patients with sickle cell disease. A randomized cooperative study. *N Engl J Med* 319:1447, 1988.
338. Tuck SM, James CE, Brewster EM, et al: Prophylactic blood transfusion in maternal sickle cell syndromes. *Br J Obstet Gynaecol* 94:121, 1987.
339. Koshy M, Chisum D, Burd L, et al: Management of sickle cell anemia and pregnancy. *J Clin Apher* 6:230, 1991.
340. Zarrouk V, Habibi A, Zahar JR, et al: Bloodstream infection in adults with sickle cell disease: Association with venous catheters, Staphylococcus aureus, and bone-joint infections. *Medicine (Baltimore)* 85:43, 2006.
341. Mollapour E, Porter JB, Kaczmarski R, et al: Raised neutrophil phospholipase A2 activity and defective priming of NADPH oxidase and phospholipase A2 in sickle cell disease. *Blood* 91:3423, 1998.
342. Overturf GD: Infections and immunizations of children with sickle cell disease. *Adv Pediatr Infect Dis* 14:191, 1999.
343. Sullivan JL, Ochs HD, Schiffman G, et al: Immune response after splenectomy. *Lancet* 1:178, 1978.
344. Barrett-Connor E: Bacterial infection and sickle cell anemia. An analysis of 250 infections in 166 patients and a review of the literature. *Medicine (Baltimore)* 50:97, 1971.
345. Zarkowsky HS, Gallagher D, Gill FM, et al: Bacteremia in sickle hemoglobinopathies. *J Pediatr* 109:579, 1986.
346. Leikin SL, Gallagher D, Kinney TR, et al: Mortality in children and adolescents with sickle cell disease. Cooperative Study of Sickle Cell Disease. *Pediatrics* 84:500, 1989.
347. Adamkiewicz TV, Sarnaik S, Buchanan GR, et al: Invasive pneumococcal infections in children with sickle cell disease in the era of penicillin prophylaxis, antibiotic resistance, and 23-valent pneumococcal polysaccharide vaccination. *J Pediatr* 143:438, 2003.
348. Gaston MH, Verter JI, Woods G, et al: Prophylaxis with oral penicillin in children with sickle cell anemia. A randomized trial. *N Engl J Med* 314:1593, 1986.
349. Halasa NB, Shankar SM, Talbot TR, et al: Incidence of invasive pneumococcal disease among individuals with sickle cell disease before and after the introduction of the pneumococcal conjugate vaccine. *Clin Infect Dis* 44:1428, 2007.
350. Kyaw MH, Lynfield R, Schaffner W, et al: Effect of introduction of the pneumococcal conjugate vaccine on drug-resistant Streptococcus pneumoniae. *N Engl J Med* 354:1455, 2006.
351. American Academy of Pediatrics, Section on Hematology/Oncology Committee on Genetics: Health supervision for children with sickle cell disease. *Pediatrics* 109:526, 2002.
352. Adamkiewicz TV, Silk BJ, Howgate J, et al: Effectiveness of the 7-valent pneumococcal conjugate vaccine in children with sickle cell disease in the first decade of life. *Pediatrics* 121:562, 2008.
353. Falletta JM, Woods GM, Verter JI, et al: Discontinuing penicillin prophylaxis in children with sickle cell anemia. Prophylactic Penicillin Study II. *J Pediatr* 127:685, 1995.
354. Koshy M, Weiner SJ, Miller ST, et al: Surgery and anesthesia in sickle cell disease. Cooperative Study of Sickle Cell Diseases. *Blood* 86:3676, 1995.
355. Firth PG, Head CA: Sickle cell disease and anesthesia. *Anesthesiology* 101:766, 2004.
356. Griffin TC, Buchanan GR: Elective surgery in children with sickle cell disease without preoperative blood transfusion. *J Pediatr Surg* 28:681, 1993.
357. Kutlar A: Sickle cell disease: A multigenic perspective of a single gene disorder. *Hemoglobin* 31:209, 2007.
358. Steinberg MH: Predicting clinical severity in sickle cell anaemia. *Br J Haematol* 129:465, 2005.
359. Sebastiani P, Ramoni MF, Nolan V, et al: Genetic dissection and prognostic modeling of overt stroke in sickle cell anemia. *Nat Genet* 37:435, 2005.
360. Taylor JGt, Tang DC, Savage SA, et al: Variants in the VCAM1 gene and risk for symptomatic stroke in sickle cell disease. *Blood* 100:4303, 2002.
361. Sharan K, Surrey S, Ballas S, et al: Association of T-786C eNOS gene polymorphism with increased susceptibility to acute chest syndrome in females with sickle cell disease. *Br J Haematol* 124:240, 2004.
362. Adekile A, Kutlar F, McKie K, et al: The influence of uridine diphosphate glucuronosyltransferase 1A promoter polymorphisms, beta-globin gene haplotype, co-inherited alpha-thalassemia trait and Hb F on steady-state serum bilirubin levels in sickle cell anemia. *Eur J Haematol* 75:150, 2005.
363. Fertrin KY, Melo MB, Assis AM, et al: UDP-glucuronosyltransferase 1 gene promoter polymorphism is associated with increased serum bilirubin levels and cholecystectomy in patients with sickle cell anemia. *Clin Genet* 64:160, 2003.
364. Haverfield EV, McKenzie CA, Forrester T, et al: UGT1A1 variation and gallstone formation in sickle cell disease. *Blood* 105:968, 2005.
365. Passon RG, Howard TA, Zimmerman SA, et al: Influence of bilirubin uridine diphosphate-glucuronosyltransferase 1A promoter polymorphisms on serum bilirubin levels and cholelithiasis in children with sickle cell anemia. *J Pediatr Hematol Oncol* 23:448, 2001.
366. Nolan VG, Baldwin C, Ma Q, et al: Association of single nucleotide polymorphisms in Klotho with priapism in sickle cell anaemia. *Br J Haematol* 128:266, 2005.
367. Close J, Game L, Clark B, et al: Genome annotation of a 1.5 Mb region of human chromosome 6q23 encompassing a quantitative trait locus for fetal hemoglobin expression in adults. *BMC Genomics* 5:33, 2004.
368. Garner CP, Tatu T, Best S, et al: Evidence of genetic interaction between the beta-globin complex and chromosome 8q in the expression of fetal hemoglobin. *Am J Hum Genet* 70:793, 2002.
369. Lettre G, Sankaran VG, Bezerra MA, et al: DNA polymorphisms at the BCL11A, HBS1L-MYB, and beta-globin loci associate with fetal hemoglobin levels and pain crises in sickle cell disease. *Proc Natl Acad Sci U S A* 105:11869, 2008.
370. Thein SL, Menzel S: Discovering the genetics underlying foetal haemoglobin production in adults. *Br J Haematol* 145:455, 2009.
371. Uda M, Galanello R, Sanna S, et al: Genome-wide association study shows BCL11A associated with persistent fetal hemoglobin and amelioration of the phenotype of beta-thalassemia. *Proc Natl Acad Sci U S A* 105:1620, 2008.
372. Wyszynski DF, Baldwin CT, Cleves MA, et al: Polymorphisms near a chromosome 6q QTL area are associated with modulation of fetal hemoglobin levels in sickle cell anemia. *Cell Mol Biol (Noisy-le-grand)* 50:23, 2004.
373. Wyszynski DF, Baldwin CT, Cleves MA, et al: Genetic polymorphisms associated with fetal hemoglobin response to hydroxyurea in patients with sickle cell anemia. *Blood Coagul Fibrinolysis* 104(Suppl):34a, 2004.
374. Kato GJ, Gladwin MT, Steinberg MH: Deconstructing sickle cell disease: Reappraisal of the role of hemolysis in the development of clinical subphenotypes. *Blood Rev* 21:37, 2007.
375. Pembrey ME, Wood WG, Weatherall DJ, Perrine RP: Fetal haemoglobin production and the sickle gene in the oases of Eastern Saudi Arabia. *Br J Haematol* 40:415, 1978.
376. Platt OS: Hydroxyurea for the treatment of sickle cell anemia. *N Engl J Med* 358:1362, 2008.
377. Gladwin MT, Shelhamer JH, Ognibene FP, et al: Nitric oxide donor properties of hydroxyurea in patients with sickle cell disease. *Br J Haematol* 116:436, 2002.
378. Hillery CA, Du MC, Wang WC, Scott JP: Hydroxyurea therapy decreases the in vitro adhesion of sickle erythrocytes to thrombospondin and laminin. *Br J Haematol* 109:322, 2000.
379. Orringer EP, Blythe DS, Johnson AE, et al: Effects of hydroxyurea on hemoglobin F and water content in the red blood cells of dogs and of patients with sickle cell anemia. *Blood* 78:212, 1991.
380. Steinberg MH, Barton F, Castro O, et al: Effect of hydroxyurea on mortality and morbidity in adult sickle cell anemia: Risks and benefits up to 9 years of treatment. *JAMA* 289:1645, 2003.
381. Brawley OW, Cornelius LJ, Edwards LR, et al: National Institutes of Health Consensus Development Conference statement: Hydroxyurea treatment for sickle cell disease. *Ann Intern Med* 148:932, 2008.
382. Lanzkron S, Strouse JJ, Wilson R, et al: Systematic review: Hydroxyurea for the treatment of adults with sickle cell disease. *Ann Intern Med* 148:939, 2008.
383. Shelby MD: National Toxicology Program Center for the Evaluation of Risks to Human Reproduction: Guidelines for CERHR expert panel members. *Birth Defects Res B Dev Reprod Toxicol* 74:9, 2005.
384. Shelby MD: NTP-CERHR Expert Panel Report on the Reproductive and Developmental Toxicity of Hydroxyurea in *Center for the Evaluation of Risks to Human Reproduction*. US Department of Health and Human Services, January 2007.
385. Ferster A, Tahriri P, Vermylen C, et al: Five years of experience with hydroxyurea in children and young adults with sickle cell disease. *Blood* 97:3628, 2001.
386. Ferster A, Vermylen C, Cornu G, et al: Hydroxyurea for treatment of severe sickle cell anemia: A pediatric clinical trial. *Blood* 88:1960, 1996.
387. Hoppe C, Vichinsky E, Quirolo K, et al: Use of hydroxyurea in children ages 2 to 5 years with sickle cell disease. *J Pediatr Hematol Oncol* 22:330, 2000.
388. Jayabose S, Tugal O, Sandoval C, et al: Clinical and hematologic effects of hydroxyurea in children with sickle cell anemia. *J Pediatr* 129:559, 1996.
389. Scott JP, Hillery CA, Brown ER, et al: Hydroxyurea therapy in children severely affected with sickle cell disease. *J Pediatr* 128:820, 1996.
390. Zimmerman SA, Schultz WH, Davis JS, et al: Sustained long-term hematologic efficacy of hydroxyurea at maximum tolerated dose in children with sickle cell disease. *Blood* 103:2039, 2004.
391. Gulbis B, Haberman D, Dufour D, et al: Hydroxyurea for sickle cell disease in children and for prevention of cerebrovascular events: The Belgian experience. *Blood* 105:2685, 2005.
392. Hankins JS, Ware RE, Rogers ZR, et al: Long-term hydroxyurea therapy for infants with sickle cell anemia: The HUSOFT extension study. *Blood* 106:2269, 2005.

393. Kinney TR, Helms RW, O'Branski EE, et al: Safety of hydroxyurea in children with sickle cell anemia: Results of the HUG-KIDS study, a phase I/II trial. Pediatric Hydroxyurea Group. *Blood* 94:1550, 1999.
394. Strouse JJ, Lanzkron S, Beach MC, et al: Hydroxyurea for sickle cell disease: A systematic review for efficacy and toxicity in children. *Pediatrics* 122:1332, 2008.
395. Wang WC, Wynn LW, Rogers ZR, et al: A two-year pilot trial of hydroxyurea in very young children with sickle-cell anemia. *J Pediatr* 139:790, 2001.
396. Atweh GF, Sutton M, Nassif I, et al: Sustained induction of fetal hemoglobin by pulse butyrate therapy in sickle cell disease. *Blood* 93:1790, 1999.
397. Dover GJ, Brusilow S, Charache S: Induction of fetal hemoglobin production in subjects with sickle cell anemia by oral sodium phenylbutyrate. *Blood* 84:339, 1994.
398. DeSimone J, Heller P, Schimenti JC, Duncan CH: Fetal hemoglobin production in adult baboons by 5-azacytidine or by phenylhydrazine-induced hemolysis is associated with hypomethylation of globin gene DNA. *Prog Clin Biol Res* 134:489, 1983.
399. Saunthararajah Y, Hillery CA, Lavelle D, et al: Effects of 5-aza-2′-deoxycytidine on fetal hemoglobin levels, red cell adhesion, and hematopoietic differentiation in patients with sickle cell disease. *Blood* 102:3865, 2003.
400. Saunthararajah Y, Molokie R, Saraf S, et al: Clinical effectiveness of decitabine in severe sickle cell disease. *Br J Haematol* 141:126, 2008.
401. Charache S, Dover G, Smith K, et al: Treatment of sickle cell anemia with 5-azacytidine results in increased fetal hemoglobin production and is associated with nonrandom hypomethylation of DNA around the gamma-delta-beta-globin gene complex. *Proc Natl Acad Sci U S A* 80:4842, 1983.
402. DeSimone J, Heller P, Hall L, Zwiers D: 5-Azacytidine stimulates fetal hemoglobin synthesis in anemic baboons. *Proc Natl Acad Sci U S A* 79:4428, 1982.
403. Ley TJ, DeSimone J, Noguchi CT, et al: 5-Azacytidine increases gamma-globin synthesis and reduces the proportion of dense cells in patients with sickle cell anemia. *Blood* 62:370, 1983.
404. Lowrey CH, Nienhuis AW: Brief report: Treatment with azacitidine of patients with end-stage beta-thalassemia. *N Engl J Med* 329:845, 1993.
405. Mavilio F, Giampaolo A, Care A, et al: Molecular mechanisms of human hemoglobin switching: Selective undermethylation and expression of globin genes in embryonic, fetal, and adult erythroblasts. *Proc Natl Acad Sci U S A* 80:6907, 1983.
406. Moutouh-de Parseval LA, Verhelle D, Glezer E, et al: Pomalidomide and lenalidomide regulate erythropoiesis and fetal hemoglobin production in human CD34+ cells. *J Clin Invest* 118:248, 2008.
407. Walters MC, Patience M, Leisenring W, et al: Barriers to bone marrow transplantation for sickle cell anemia. *Biol Blood Marrow Transplant* 2:100, 1996.
408. Bernaudin F, Socie G, Kuentz M, et al: Long-term results of related myeloablative stem-cell transplantation to cure sickle cell disease. *Blood* 110:2749, 2007.
409. Vermylen C, Cornu G, Ferster A, et al: Haematopoietic stem cell transplantation for sickle cell anaemia: The first 50 patients transplanted in Belgium. *Bone Marrow Transplant* 22:1, 1998.
410. Walters MC, Storb R, Patience M, et al: Impact of bone marrow transplantation for symptomatic sickle cell disease: An interim report. Multicenter investigation of bone marrow transplantation for sickle cell disease. *Blood* 95:1918, 2000.
411. Panepinto JA, Walters MC, Carreras J, et al: Matched-related donor transplantation for sickle cell disease: Report from the Center for International Blood and Transplant Research. *Br J Haematol* 137:479, 2007.
412. Bhatia M, Walters MC: Hematopoietic cell transplantation for thalassemia and sickle cell disease: Past, present and future. *Bone Marrow Transplant* 41:109, 2008.
413. Horan JT, Liesveld JL, Fenton P, et al: Hematopoietic stem cell transplantation for multiply transfused patients with sickle cell disease and thalassemia after low-dose total body irradiation, fludarabine, and rabbit anti-thymocyte globulin. *Bone Marrow Transplant* 35:171, 2005.
414. Iannone R, Casella JF, Fuchs EJ, et al: Results of minimally toxic nonmyeloablative transplantation in patients with sickle cell anemia and beta-thalassemia. *Biol Blood Marrow Transplant* 9:519, 2003.
415. Telen MJ: Principles and problems of transfusion in sickle cell disease. *Semin Hematol* 38:315, 2001.
416. Chien S, Usami S, Bertles JF: Abnormal rheology of oxygenated blood in sickle cell anemia. *J Clin Invest* 49:623, 1970.
417. Morris CL, Gruppo RA, Shukla R, Rucknagel DL: Influence of plasma and red cell factors on the rheologic properties of oxygenated sickle blood during clinical steady state. *J Lab Clin Med* 118:332, 1991.
418. Schmalzer EA, Lee JO, Brown AK, et al: Viscosity of mixtures of sickle and normal red cells at varying hematocrit levels. Implications for transfusion. *Transfusion* 27:228, 1987.
419. Davies SC, McWilliam AC, Hewitt PE, et al: Red cell alloimmunization in sickle cell disease. *Br J Haematol* 63:241, 1986.
420. Orlina AR, Unger PJ, Koshy M: Post-transfusion alloimmunization in patients with sickle cell disease. *Am J Hematol* 5:101, 1978.
421. Rosse WF, Gallagher D, Kinney TR, et al: Transfusion and alloimmunization in sickle cell disease. The Cooperative Study of Sickle Cell Disease. *Blood* 76:1431, 1990.
422. Sarnaik S, Schornack J, Lusher JM: The incidence of development of irregular red cell antibodies in patients with sickle cell anemia. *Transfusion* 26:249, 1986.
423. Vichinsky EP: Current issues with blood transfusions in sickle cell disease. *Semin Hematol* 38:14, 2001.
424. Wahl S, Quirolo KC: Current issues in blood transfusion for sickle cell disease. *Curr Opin Pediatr* 21:15, 2009.
425. Ballas SK: Iron overload is a determinant of morbidity and mortality in adult patients with sickle cell disease. *Semin Hematol* 38:30, 2001.
426. Manci EA, Culberson DE, Yang YM, et al: Causes of death in sickle cell disease: An autopsy study. *Br J Haematol* 123:359, 2003.
427. Vichinsky E, Butensky E, Fung E, et al: Comparison of organ dysfunction in transfused patients with SCD or beta thalassemia. *Am J Hematol* 80:70, 2005.
428. Fung EB, Harmatz P, Milet M, et al: Morbidity and mortality in chronically transfused subjects with thalassemia and sickle cell disease: A report from the multi-center study of iron overload. *Am J Hematol* 82:255, 2007.
429. Brittenham GM, Cohen AR, McLaren CE, et al: Hepatic iron stores and plasma ferritin concentration in patients with sickle cell anemia and thalassemia major. *Am J Hematol* 42:81, 1993.
430. Olivieri NF: Progression of iron overload in sickle cell disease. *Semin Hematol* 38:57, 2001.
431. Silliman CC, Peterson VM, Mellman DL, et al: Iron chelation by deferoxamine in sickle cell patients with severe transfusion-induced hemosiderosis: A randomized, double-blind study of the dose-response relationship. *J Lab Clin Med* 122:48, 1993.
432. Vichinsky E, Onyekwere O, Porter J, et al: A randomised comparison of deferasirox versus deferoxamine for the treatment of transfusional iron overload in sickle cell disease. *Br J Haematol* 136:501, 2007.
433. Ataga KI, Smith WR, De Castro LM, et al: Efficacy and safety of the Gardos channel blocker, senicapoc (ICA-17043), in patients with sickle cell anemia. *Blood* 111:3991, 2008.
434. Steinberg MH, Adams JG 3rd, Dreiling BJ: Alpha thalassaemia in adults with sickle-cell trait. *Br J Haematol* 30:31, 1975.
435. Wong SC, Ali MA, Boyadjian SE: Sickle cell traits in Canada. Trimodal distribution of Hb S as a result of interaction with alpha-thalassaemia gene. *Acta Haematol* 65:157, 1981.
436. Sciarratta GV, Sansone G, Ivaldi G, et al: Alternate organization of alpha G-Philadelphia globin genes among U.S. black and Italian Caucasian heterozygotes. *Hemoglobin* 8:537, 1984.
437. Itano HA, Neel JV: A new inherited abnormality of human hemoglobin. *Proc Natl Acad Sci U S A* 36:613, 1950.
438. Spaet TH, Alway RH, Ward G: Homozygous type c hemoglobin. *Pediatrics* 12:483, 1953.
439. Ranney HM, Larson DL, McCormack GH Jr: Some clinical, biochemical and genetic observations on hemoglobin C. *J Clin Invest* 32:1277, 1953.
440. Nagel R, Steinberg MH: Hb SC disease and Hb C disorder, in *Disorders of Hemoglobin: Genetics, Pathophysiology, and Clinical Management*, edited by MH Steinberg, BG Forget, DR Higgs, RL Nagel, pp 765–785. Cambridge University Press, Cambridge, UK, 2001.
441. Boehm CD, Dowling CE, Antonarakis SE, et al: Evidence supporting a single origin of the beta(C)-globin gene in blacks. *Am J Hum Genet* 37:771, 1985.
442. Itano HA, Bergren WR, Sturgeon P: Identification of fourth abnormal human hemoglobin. *J Am Chem Soc* 76:2278, 1954.
443. Fucharoen S: Hb E disorders, in *Disorders of Hemoglobin: Genetics, Pathophysiology, and Clinical Management*, edited by MH Steinberg, BG Forget, DR Higgs, RL Nagel, pp 1139–1154. Cambridge University Press, Cambridge, UK, 2001.
444. Fucharoen S, Siritanaratkul N, Winichagoon P, et al: Hydroxyurea increases hemoglobin F levels and improves the effectiveness of erythropoiesis in beta-thalassemia/hemoglobin E disease. *Blood* 87:887, 1996.
445. Itano HA: A third abnormal hemoglobin associated with hereditary hemolytic anemia. *Proc Natl Acad Sci U S A* 37:775, 1951.
446. Huisman THJ, Carver MFH, Efremov GD: *A Syllabus of Human Hemoglobin Variants.* Sickle Cell Anemia Foundation, Augusta, GA, 1998.
447. Cathie IAB: Apparent idiopathic Heinz body anaemia. *Great Ormond St J* 3:343, 1952.
448. Ryan TM, Ciavatta DJ, Townes TM: Knockout-transgenic mouse model of sickle cell disease. *Science* 278:873, 1997.
449. Behringer RR, Ryan TM, Palmiter RD, et al: Human gamma- to beta-globin gene switching in transgenic mice. *Genes Dev* 4:380, 1990.
450. Ryan TM, Townes TM, Reilly MP, et al: Human sickle hemoglobin in transgenic mice. *Science* 247:566, 1990.
451. Gaensler KM, Kitamura M, Kan YW: Germ-line transmission and developmental regulation of a 150-kb yeast artificial chromosome containing the human beta-globin locus in transgenic mice. *Proc Natl Acad Sci U S A* 90:11381, 1993.
452. Greaves DR, Fraser P, Vidal MA, et al: A transgenic mouse model of sickle cell disorder. *Nature* 343:183, 1990.
453. Kaufman RM, Pham CT, Ley TJ: Transgenic analysis of a 100-kb human beta-globin cluster-containing DNA fragment propagated as a bacterial artificial chromosome. *Blood* 94:3178, 1999.
454. Paszty C, Brion CM, Manci E, et al: Transgenic knockout mice with exclusively human sickle hemoglobin and sickle cell disease. *Science* 278:876, 1997.
455. Peterson KR, Clegg CH, Huxley C, et al: Transgenic mice containing a 248-kb yeast artificial chromosome carrying the human beta-globin locus display proper developmental control of human globin genes. *Proc Natl Acad Sci U S A* 90:7593, 1993.
456. Strouboulis J, Dillon N, Grosveld F: Developmental regulation of a complete 70-kb human beta-globin locus in transgenic mice. *Genes Dev* 6:1857, 1992.
457. Wu LC, Sun CW, Ryan TM, et al: Correction of sickle cell disease by homologous recombination in embryonic stem cells. *Blood* 108:1183, 2006.

458. Levasseur DN, Ryan TM, Pawlik KM, Townes TM: Correction of a mouse model of sickle cell disease: Lentiviral/antisickling beta-globin gene transduction of unmobilized, purified hematopoietic stem cells. *Blood* 102:4312, 2003.
459. Pawliuk R, Westerman KA, Fabry ME, et al: Correction of sickle cell disease in transgenic mouse models by gene therapy. *Science* 294:2368, 2001.
460. Puthenveetil G, Scholes J, Carbonell D, et al: Successful correction of the human beta-thalassemia major phenotype using a lentiviral vector. *Blood* 104:3445, 2004.
461. Imren S, Fabry ME, Westerman KA, et al: High-level beta-globin expression and preferred intragenic integration after lentiviral transduction of human cord blood stem cells. *J Clin Invest* 114:953, 2004.
462. Hacein-Bey-Abina S, Von Kalle C, Schmidt M, et al: LMO2-associated clonal T cell proliferation in two patients after gene therapy for SCID-X1. *Science* 302:415, 2003.
463. Seggewiss R, Pittaluga S, Adler RL, et al: Acute myeloid leukemia associated with retroviral gene transfer to hematopoietic progenitor cells of a rhesus macaque. *Blood* 107:3865, 2006.
464. Takahashi K, Yamanaka S: Induction of pluripotent stem cells from mouse embryonic and adult fibroblast cultures by defined factors. *Cell* 126:663, 2006.
465. Blelloch R, Venere M, Yen J, Ramalho-Santos M: Generation of induced pluripotent stem cells in the absence of drug selection. *Cell Stem Cell* 1:245, 2007.
466. Maherali N, Sridharan R, Xie W, et al: Directly reprogrammed fibroblasts show global epigenetic remodeling and widespread tissue contribution. *Cell Stem Cell* 1:55, 2007.
467. Meissner A, Wernig M, Jaenisch R: Direct reprogramming of genetically unmodified fibroblasts into pluripotent stem cells. *Nat Biotechnol* 25:1177, 2007.
468. Okita K, Ichisaka T, Yamanaka S: Generation of germline-competent induced pluripotent stem cells. *Nature* 448:313, 2007.
469. Wernig M, Meissner A, Foreman R, et al: *In vitro* reprogramming of fibroblasts into a pluripotent ES-cell-like state. *Nature* 448:318, 2007.
470. Hanna J, Wernig M, Markoulaki S, et al: Treatment of sickle cell anemia mouse model with iPS cells generated from autologous skin. *Science* 318:1920, 2007.
471. Takahashi K, Tanabe K, Ohnuki M, et al: Induction of pluripotent stem cells from adult human fibroblasts by defined factors. *Cell* 131:861, 2007.
472. Yu J, Vodyanik MA, Smuga-Otto K, et al: Induced pluripotent stem cell lines derived from human somatic cells. *Science* 318:1917, 2007.
473. Park IH, Zhao R, West JA, et al: Reprogramming of human somatic cells to pluripotency with defined factors. *Nature* 451:141, 2008.
474. Lowry WE, Richter L, Yachechko R, et al: Generation of human induced pluripotent stem cells from dermal fibroblasts. *Proc Natl Acad Sci U S A* 105:2883, 2008.
475. Murry CE, Keller G: Differentiation of embryonic stem cells to clinically relevant populations: Lessons from embryonic development. *Cell* 132:661, 2008.
476. Zwaka TP, Thomson JA: Homologous recombination in human embryonic stem cells. *Nat Biotechnol* 21:319, 2003.
477. Chang CW, Lai YS, Pawlik KM, et al: Polycistronic lentiviral vector for "hit and run" reprogramming of adult skin fibroblasts to induced pluripotent stem cells. *Stem Cells* 27:1042, 2009.
478. Ivics Z, Li MA, Mates L, et al: Transposon-mediated genome manipulation in vertebrates. *Nat Methods* 6:415, 2009.
479. Soldner F, Hockemeyer D, Beard C, et al: Parkinson's disease patient-derived induced pluripotent stem cells free of viral reprogramming factors. *Cell* 136:964, 2009.
480. Woltjen K, Michael IP, Mohseni P, et al: piggyBac transposition reprograms fibroblasts to induced pluripotent stem cells. *Nature* 458:766, 2009.
481. Yu J, Hu K, Smuga-Otto K, et al: Human induced pluripotent stem cells free of vector and transgene sequences. *Science* 324:797, 2009.
482. Kim SY, Mocanu C, McLeod DS, et al: Expression of pigment epithelium-derived factor (PEDF) and vascular endothelial growth factor (VEGF) in sickle cell retina and choroid. *Exp Eye Res* 77:433, 2003.
483. Zhou H, Wu S, Joo JY, et al: Generation of induced pluripotent stem cells using recombinant proteins. *Cell Stem Cell* 4:381, 2009.

CHAPTER 49
METHEMOGLOBINEMIA AND OTHER DYSHEMOGLOBINEMIAS

Neeraj Agarwal and Josef T. Prchal

SUMMARY

Normal hemoglobin can be oxidized to methemoglobin. Methemoglobinemia occurs because of either increased production of oxidized hemoglobin because of exposure to environmental agents or diminished reduction of oxidized hemoglobin because of underlying germ line mutations. Hemoglobin can also bind gases such as carbon monoxide (CO) and nitric oxide (NO), resulting in the formation of carboxyhemoglobin (COHb) and nitrosohemoglobin. Sulfhemoglobinemia only occurs because of increased production secondary to occupational exposure to sulphur compounds or exposure to oxidant medications. These modified hemoglobins, also known as dyshemoglobins, depending upon the severity and individual predisposition, can result in varying degree of clinical manifestations. Prompt diagnosis is the key to effective and timely treatment.

METHEMOGLOBINEMIA

DEFINITION AND HISTORY

A bluish discoloration of the skin and mucous membrane, designated *cyanosis*, has been recognized since antiquity as a manifestation of lung or heart disease. Cyanosis resulting from drug administration has also been recognized since before 1890.[1] Toxic methemoglobinemia occurs when various drugs or toxic substances either oxidize hemoglobin directly in the circulation or facilitate its oxidation by molecular oxygen.

In 1912, Sloss and Wybauw[2] reported a case of a patient with idiopathic methemoglobinemia. Later Hitzenberger[3] suggested that a hereditary form of methemoglobinemia might exist, and subsequently, numerous such cases were reported.[4] In 1948, Hörlein and Weber[5] described a family in which eight members over four generations manifested cyanosis. The absorption spectrum of methemoglobin was abnormal. They demonstrated that the defect must reside in the globin portion of the molecule. Subsequently, Singer[6] proposed that such abnormal hemoglobins be given the designation hemoglobin M. The cause of another form of methemoglobinemia that occurs independently of drug administration and without the existence of any abnormality of the globin portion of hemoglobin was first explained by Gibson,[7] who clearly pointed to the site of the enzyme defect, nicotinamide adenine dinucleotide (reduced form; NADH) diaphorase, also designated as methemoglobin reductase, and currently cytochrome b_5 reductase. More than 50 years after Gibson's insightful studies, the genetic disorder that he had predicted was verified at the DNA level.[8]

The existence of abnormal hemoglobins that cause cyanosis through quite another mechanism was first recognized in 1968 with the description of hemoglobin Kansas.[9] Here the cyanosis resulted not from methemoglobin, as occurs in hemoglobin M, but rather from an abnormally low oxygen affinity of the mutant hemoglobin. Thus, at normal oxygen tensions, a large amount of deoxygenated hemoglobin is present in the blood.

Acronyms and abbreviations that appear in this chapter include: AOP2, antioxidant protein 2; 2,3-BPG, 2,3-bisphosphoglycerate; cGMP, cyclic guanosine monophosphate; cNOS, constitutive nitric oxide synthase; CO, carbon monoxide; COHb, carboxyhemoglobin; eNOS, endothelial NO synthase; GSH, reduced glutathione; Hgb, hemoglobin; iNOS, inducible nitric oxide synthase; NADH, nicotinamide adenine dinucleotide (reduced form); NADPH, nicotinamide adenine dinucleotide phosphate (reduced form); NO, nitric oxide; NOS, nitric oxide synthase; SNO-Hgb, S-nitroso hemoglobin; SpCO, arterial carboxyhemoglobin concentration; SpMet, arterial methemoglobin concentration; SpO_2, arterial oxygen saturation.

EPIDEMIOLOGY

Methemoglobinemia occurring as a result of cytochrome b_5 reductase deficiency is more common among Native Americans, both in Alaska and in the continental United States, and among the Yakuts of Russian Siberia than in other ethnic groups.[10–12] Methemoglobinemia resulting from hemoglobins M is sporadic, as is the occurrence of toxic methemoglobinemia, although the latter is related to industrial exposure, and is, therefore, most common among workers in the chemical industry.

ETIOLOGY AND PATHOGENESIS

Methemoglobinemia decreases the oxygen-carrying capacity of blood because the oxidized iron cannot reversibly bind oxygen. Moreover, when one or more iron atoms have been oxidized, the conformation of hemoglobin is changed so as to increase the oxygen affinity of the remaining ferrous heme groups. In this way methemoglobinemia exerts a dual effect in impairing the supply of oxygen to tissues.[13]

Toxic Methemoglobinemia

Hemoglobin is continuously oxidized *in vivo* from the ferrous to the ferric state. The rate of such oxidation is accelerated by many drugs and toxic chemicals, including sulfonamides, lidocaine and other aniline derivatives, and nitrites. A vast number of chemical substances may cause methemoglobinemia.[14–16] Table 49–1 lists some of the agents that are responsible for clinically significant methemoglobinemia in clinical practice.

The most common offenders include benzocaine and lidocaine.[17–26] In some cases, the patients have been unaware that they have been ingesting one of the drugs known to produce methemoglobinemia; dapsone is apparently used in some "street drugs."[27,28] Nitrates and the nitrites contaminating water supplies or used as preservatives in foods are also common offending agents.[29–37]

Cytochrome b_5 Reductase Deficiency

Cytochrome b_5 reductase, catalyzes a step in the major pathway for methemoglobin reduction. Cytochrome b_5 reductase , also known as reduced nicotinamide adenine dinucleotide (NADH) diaphorase, reduces cytochrome b_5, using NADH as a hydrogen donor. The reduced cytochrome b_5 reduces, in turn, methemoglobin to hemoglobin. A steady-state methemoglobin level is achieved when the rate of methemoglobin formation equals the rate of methemoglobin reduction either through the cytochrome b_5 reductase or through a relatively minor auxiliary mechanism such as direct chemical reduction by ascorbate and reduced glutathione. A reduced nicotinamide adenine dinucleotide phosphate (NADPH)-linked enzyme, NADPH diaphorase does not play a role in methemoglobin reduction except when a linking dye such as methylene blue is supplied (see "Therapy, Course, and Prognosis" below). A marked diminution in the activity of cytochrome b_5 reductase will result in the accumulation of the brown pigment in circulating erythrocytes.

TABLE 49–1. Some Drugs That Cause Methemoglobinemia

Phenazopyridine (Pyridium)[182–184]
Sulfamethoxazole[185]
Dapsone[27,28,186]
Aniline[111,112]
Paraquat/monolinuron[187–189]
Nitrate[29–31,104]
Nitroglycerin[182,190]
Amyl nitrite[191]
Isobutyl nitrite[192]
Sodium nitrite[30,105]
Benzocaine[17–19]
Prilocaine[193–195]
Methyleneblue[110]
Chloramine[189,196]

A balance to methemoglobin formation is antioxidant protein 2 (AOP2), which is present in high concentrations in human and mouse red cells. This member of the peroxiredoxin protein family binds to hemoglobin and prevents spontaneous, as well as oxidant-induced, methemoglobin formation.[38] Mutations of this gene or its acquired deficiency are theoretical candidates responsible for congenital and acquired methemoglobinemia. Cyanosis resulting from abnormal M and low-oxygen-affinity hemoglobins is inherited as an autosomal dominant disorder. In contrast, hereditary methemoglobinemia resulting from cytochrome b_5 reductase deficiency is inherited in an autosomal recessive fashion.

Accordingly, hereditary deficiency of the enzyme that reduces cytochrome b_5, cytochrome b_5 reductase, is one cause of methemoglobinemia. Many mutations of cytochrome b_5 reductase have been identified at the nucleotide level,[8,39–52] and the functional effect of some of these have been deduced from the structure of the enzyme.[43,50,53] Although most of the mutants have been found in whites, five unique mutations were found in Chinese,[54] at least three in Thai,[45,55] two in African Americans,[56] and one in an Asian Indian.[57] In addition, a common polymorphism (allele frequency = 0.023) has been identified in Americans of African descent; it does not appear to impair the activity of the enzyme.[58] Most of the patients with cytochrome b_5 reductase deficiency merely have methemoglobinemia, and these have been classified as having type I disease. Type II disease deficiency also exists in nonerythroid cells, such as fibroblasts and lymphocytes.[59] Patients with this form of disease are afflicted, in addition to methemoglobinemia, with a progressive encephalopathy and mental retardation. The finding that fatty acid elongation is defective in the platelets and leukocytes of such patients[60] may provide a clue to the type of defect that could occur in the central nervous system, where fatty acid elongation plays an important role in myelination. It was reported that rare patients with deficiency of cytochrome b_5 reductase in nonerythroid cells do not suffer any neurologic disorder, and it has been suggested that they be designated as having type III disease,[61,62] however, existence of such an entity has been challenged and type III disease likely does not exist.[63]

Heterozygosity for Cytochrome b_5 Reductase Deficiency

Heterozygotes for cytochrome b_5 reductase deficiency are not usually clinically methemoglobinemic. However, under the stress of administration of drugs that normally induce only slight, clinically unimportant, methemoglobinemia, such persons have been reported to become severely cyanotic because of methemoglobinemia.[64] Although, in this report, the affected patients were Ashkenazi Jews, prevalence of cytochrome b_5 reductase deficiency in 500 unselected Jewish subjects was found to be low.[65] In addition, predisposition to acute toxic methemoglobinemia in heterozygous subjects for cytochrome b_5 reductase deficiency seems to be quite uncommon.[63]

Animal models of cytochrome b_5 reductase deficiency have been described in dogs, cats, and horses.[66,67]

Infant Susceptibility

A combination of both increased hemoglobin oxidation and decreased methemoglobin reduction also may occur. Because the activity of cytochrome b_5 reductase is normally low in newborn infants,[68] they are particularly susceptible to the development of methemoglobinemia. Thus, serious degrees of methemoglobinemia have been observed in infants as a result of toxic materials, such as aniline dyes used on diapers,[69] and the ingestion of nitrate-contaminated water[31,37] and even of beets.[70] Bacterial action in the intestinal tract may reduce nitrates to nitrites, which, in turn, cause methemoglobinemia. In rural areas, fatal methemoglobinuria in infants caused by drinking water from wells contaminated with nitrates still occurs.[71]

Methemoglobinemia occurring in acidotic infants with diarrhea is a syndrome that may have a fatal outcome.[72–76] Such infants have normal red cell cytochrome b_5 reductase activity, and the mechanism by which methemoglobinemia occurs is unknown. However, the syndrome seems most common when soy formula is being fed[77] and breast-feeding appears to be protective.[71]

Cytochrome b_5 Deficiency

Rarely, the defect leading to methemoglobinemia may not be in the cytochrome b_5 reductase that transfers hydrogen to the cytochrome b_5, but rather to a deficiency in the cytochrome b_5 itself.[78–80]

Hemoglobin M

Structural Alterations The molecular mechanisms by which hemoglobin binds oxygen and releases it are discussed in Chap. 48. Heme is held in a hydrophobic "heme pocket" between the E and F α helices of each of the four globin chains. The iron atom in the heme forms four bonds with the pyrrole nitrogen atoms of the porphyrin ring and a fifth covalent bond with the imidazole nitrogen of a histidine residue in the nearby F α helix (Fig. 49–1).[81] This histidine, residue 87 in the α chain and 92 in the β chain, is designated as the proximal histidine. On the opposite side of the porphyrin ring the iron atom lies adjacent to another histidine residue to which, however, it is not covalently bonded. This distal histidine occupies position 58 in the α chain and position 63 in the β chain. Under normal circumstances oxygen is occasionally discharged from the heme pocket as a superoxide anion, removing an electron from the iron and leaving it in the ferric state. The enzymatic machinery of the red cell efficiently reduces the iron to the divalent form, converting the methemoglobin to hemoglobin (see Chap. 46).

In most of the hemoglobins M, tyrosine has been substituted for either the proximal or the distal histidine. Tyrosine can form an iron-phenolate complex that resists reduction to the divalent state by the normal metabolic systems of the erythrocyte. Four hemoglobins M are a consequence of substitution of tyrosine for histidine in the proximal and distal sites of the α and β chains. As Table 49–2 shows, these four hemoglobins M have been designated by the geographic names Boston, Saskatoon, Iwate, and Hyde Park.

Analogous His→Tyr substitutions in the γ chain of fetal hemoglobin have also been documented and have been designated hemoglobin FM_{Osaka}[82] and $FM_{Fort\ Ripley}$.[83]

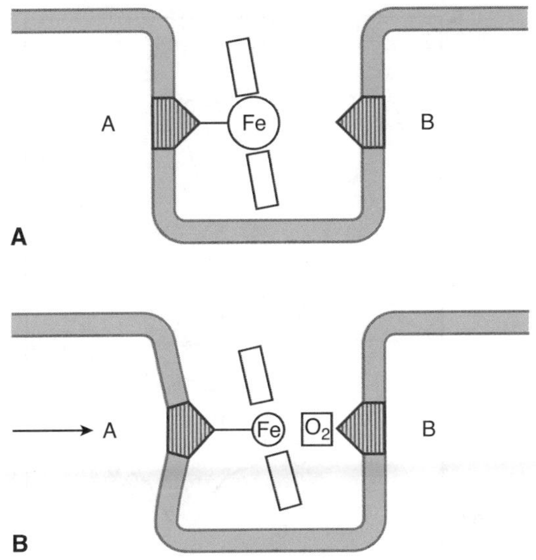

FIGURE 49–1. Diagrammatic representation of the heme group inserted into the heme pocket. **A**, proximal histidine; **B**, distal histidine. **A.** In the deoxygenated form, the larger ferrous atom lies out of the place of the porphyrin ring. **B.** In the oxygenated form, the now smaller "ferric-like" atom can slip into the plane of the porphyrin ring. As a result, the proximal histidine, and helix F into which it is incorporated, are displaced. *(From Lehmann H and Huntsman RG,[81] with permission.)*

Another hemoglobin M, Hgb $M_{Milwaukee}$, is formed by substitution of glutamic acid for valine in the 67th residue of the β chain, rather than substitution of tyrosine for histidine. The glutamic acid side chain points toward the heme group and its γ-carboxyl group interacts with the iron atom, stabilizing it in the ferric state.

It is rare for methemoglobinemia to occur as a result of hemoglobinopathies other than hemoglobin M, but $Hemoglobin_{Chile}$ (β28 Leu→Met) is such a hemoglobin. Producing hemolysis only with drug administration, this unstable hemoglobin is characterized clinically by chronic methemoglobinemia.[84]

CLINICAL FEATURES

Drug Ingestion

Methemoglobinemia may be chronic or acute. Severe acute methemoglobinemia, usually the consequence of drug ingestion or toxic exposure, can produce symptoms of anemia, as methemoglobin lacks the capacity to transport oxygen. Symptoms may include shortness of breath, palpitations, and vascular collapse. Chemicals that induce methemoglobinemia are often also capable of causing hemolysis, and a combination of hemolytic anemia and methemoglobinemia may occur. Chronic methemoglobinemia, whether a result of exposure to drugs or toxins or to hereditary causes, is usually asymptomatic. Cyanosis, even if present, may not be discernible in African American subjects.[85] In instances when the methemoglobin levels are very high (>20% of the total pigment), mild erythrocytosis is occasionally noted (see Chap. 56).

M Hemoglobin

Patients with hemoglobin M also manifest cyanosis. In the case of α-globin variants, the dusky color of the infants will be noted at birth, but the clinical manifestations of β-globin variants become apparent only after β chains have largely replaced the fetal γ chains at 6 to 9 months of age. In spite of the impaired hemoglobin function, no cardiopulmonary symptoms are observed and there is no clubbing. In the case of Hgb $M_{Saskatoon}$ and Hgb $M_{Hyde\ Park}$, hemolytic anemia with jaundice may be present. The hemolytic state may be exacerbated by administration of sulfonamides.[86]

TABLE 49–2. Properties of Hemoglobins M

Hemoglobin	Amino Acid Substitution	Oxygen Dissociation and Other Properties	Clinical Effect	Reference
Hgb M_{Boston}	α58 (E7)His→Tyr	Very low O_2 affinity, almost nonexistent heme–heme interaction, no Bohr effect	Cyanosis resulting from formation of methemoglobin	197
Hgb $M_{Saskatoon}$	β63 (E7)His→Tyr	Increased O_2 affinity, reduced heme–heme interaction, normal Bohr effect, slightly unstable	Cyanosis resulting from methemoglobin formation, mild hemolytic anemia exacerbated by ingestion of sulfonamides	197, 198
Hgb $M_{I\ wate}$	α87 (F8)His→Tyr	Low O_2 affinity, negligible heme–heme interaction, no Bohr effect	Cyanosis resulting from formation of methemoglobin	197, 199
Hgb $M_{Kankakee}$				
Hgb $M_{Oldenburg}$				
Hgb M_{Sendai}				
Hgb $M_{Hyde\ Park}$	β92 (F8)His→Tyr	Increased O_2 affinity, reduced heme interaction, normal Bohr effect, slightly unstable	Cyanosis resulting from formation of methemoglobin, mild hemolytic anemia	102
Hgb Milwaukee 2				
Hgb M_{Akita}				
Hgb $M_{Milwaukee}$	β67 (E11)Val →Glu	Low O_2 affinity, reduced heme–heme interaction, normal Bohr effect, slightly unstable	Cyanosis resulting from methemoglobin formation	200
Hgb FM_{Osaka}	$^G\gamma$63His→Tyr	Low O_2 affinity, increased Bohr effect. Methemoglobinemia	Cyanosis at birth	82
Hgb $FM_{Fort\ Ripley}$	$^G\gamma$92His→Tyr	Slightly increased O_2 affinity	Cyanosis at birth	201

Cytochrome b_5 Reductase Deficiency

Hereditary methemoglobinemia resulting from cytochrome b_5 reductase deficiency may, as noted above, be associated with mental retardation. In one case, skeletal anomalies also were documented.[87]

LABORATORY FEATURES

Toxic Methemoglobinemia

In toxic methemoglobinemia, an elevated level of methemoglobin is found, but the activity of cytochrome b_5 reductase is normal. Methemoglobin levels are best measured using the change of absorbance of methemoglobin at 630 nm that occurs when cyanide is added, converting the methemoglobin to cyanmethemoglobin.[88,89] Errors in diagnosis are frequently made when automated instruments designed to estimate levels of reduced hemoglobin, oxygenated hemoglobin, methemoglobin, and carboxyhemoglobin are used. Most automated instruments do not properly make this distinction.[90,91]

Clinical incidence of methemoglobinemia can be overestimated by cooximeter measurements compared to the more specific Evelyn-Malloy method.[92] This method involves direct spectrophotometric analysis and should be used when methemoglobinemia is suspected. This is achieved by lysing the blood in a slightly acid buffer and measuring the optical density at 630 nm before and after adding a small amount of neutralized cyanide. The absorption of methemoglobin at this wavelength disappears when it is converted to cyanmethemoglobin. Although this method was described in 1938,[88] it remains the most accurate technique for the estimation of methemoglobin in the blood. Details of its performance can be found in an earlier edition of this text[93] and elsewhere.[86]

An eight-wavelength pulse oximeter, Masimo Rad-57 (the Rainbow-SET Rad-57 Pulse CO-Oximeter, Masimo Inc, Irvine, CA), has been approved by the U.S. Food and Drug Administration for the measurement of both carboxyhemoglobin and methemoglobin. The Rad-57 uses eight wavelengths of light instead of the usual two, and is thereby able to measure more than two species of human hemoglobin.[94] In addition to the usual arterial oxygen saturation (SpO_2) value, the Rad-57 displays the pulse oximeter's estimates of arterial carboxyhemoglobin concentration (SpCO) and arterial methemoglobin concentration (SpMet). In a study on healthy human volunteers in whom controlled levels of methemoglobin and carboxyhemoglobin were induced, the Rad-57 measured carboxyhemoglobin with an uncertainty of ±2 percent within the range of 0 to 15 percent, and measured methemoglobin with an uncertainty of 0.5 percent within the range of 0 to 12 percent.[94]

Cytochrome b_5 Reductase Deficiency

In hereditary methemoglobinemia resulting from cytochrome b_5 reductase deficiency, between 8 and 40 percent of the hemoglobin is in the oxidized (methemoglobin) form. The blood may have a chocolate-brown color. Cytochrome b_5 reductase activity is best measured using ferricyanide as a receptor, measuring the rate of oxidation of NADH.[95,96] The residual level of enzyme activity is usually less than 20 percent of normal in patients with methemoglobinemia resulting from deficiency of this enzyme. An immunoassay has been described,[97] but such an assay would not detect mutants in which enzyme molecules with impaired catalytic activity are present. For unknown reasons, glutathione reductase activity is usually also diminished.[98]

Cytochrome b_5 Deficiency

Cytochrome b_5 assays may be useful if cytochrome b_5 reductase activity is normal.[99]

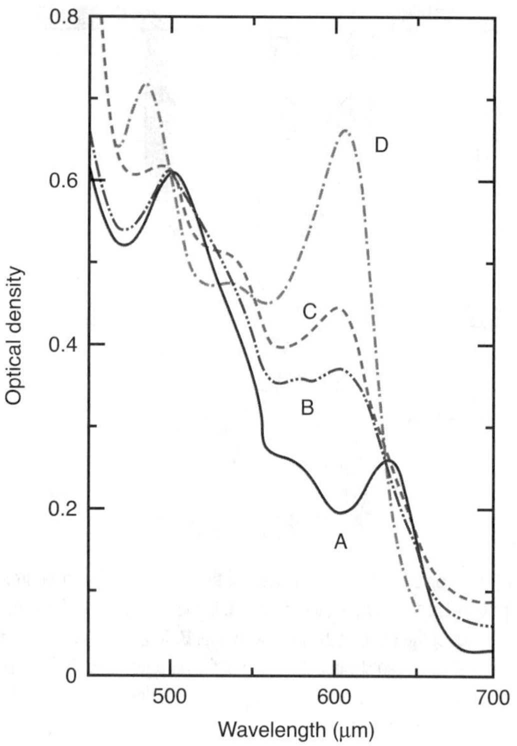

FIGURE 49–2. Absorption spectra at pH 7.0. **A**, methemoglobin A; **B**, methemoglobin M_{Boston}; **C**, methemoglobin $M_{Saskatoon}$; **D**, methemoglobin A fluoride complex. For purposes of comparison, all the optical densities have been made equal to 0.61 at 500 nm. *(From Gerald PS and George P,[100] with permission of the American Association for the Advancement of Science.)*

M Hemoglobin

Optical Spectrum Figure 49–2 illustrates the spectrum of normal methemoglobin A at pH 7.0.[100] Hemoglobin M can be differentiated from methemoglobin formed from hemoglobin A by its absorption spectrum in the range of 450 to 750 nm. Because only some 20 to 35 percent of the total hemoglobin will ordinarily be the hemoglobin M, the mixed spectra of methemoglobin A and the hemoglobin M may be difficult to interpret. Therefore, it is preferable to perform these spectral studies on purified hemoglobin M isolated by electrophoretic or chromatographic means.[81]

Electrophoresis All hemoglobin M samples should be converted to methemoglobin so that any difference found in electrophoresis will be the result of the amino acid substitution and not the different charge of the iron atom. Electrophoresis at pH 7.1 is most useful for separation of hemoglobins M because the imidazole groups of histidine have a net positive charge at this pH, whereas at higher pH levels the histidines and the substituting tyrosines are both neutral.

Other Biochemical Methods The hemoglobins M differ in their reactivity to cyanide and to azide ions.[101] This property may help to identify the subunit affected because the iron-phenolate bonds are stronger in the α-chain variants than in the β-chain variants. However, definitive identification of the variant requires peptide or DNA analysis. Hemoglobins that cause cyanosis because of a diminished oxygen affinity may be detected by determining the oxygen dissociation curve of blood, being certain that the 2,3-bisphosphoglycerate (2,3-BPG) level is normal, or by estimating the oxygen dissociation curve of hemoglobin, which has been stripped of 2,3-BPG by extensive dialysis against an appropriate buffer. Many of the hemoglobins with decreased oxygen affinity are unstable (see Chap. 48) and will precipitate in the isopropanol stability test.[101] In many laboratories it may be easier to analyze the coding sequence of the globin chains at the DNA level than to attempt to determine the properties of the hemoglobin.[102]

■ TREATMENT AND COURSE

Toxic Methemoglobinemia

Acute toxic methemoglobinemia may represent a serious medical emergency. Because of the loss of oxygen-carrying capacity of the blood and because of the left shift in the oxygen dissociation curve that occurs when methemoglobin is present in high concentration,[103] acute methemoglobinemia may be life-threatening when the level of the pigment exceeds half of the total circulating hemoglobin. Levels of methemoglobin exceeding 60 to 70 percent of the total pigment may be associated with vascular collapse, coma, and death,[104,105] but recovery was documented in one patient with a level as high as 81.5 percent of the total pigment.[106]

Methylene blue[107] is an effective treatment for patients with methemoglobinemia because NADPH formed in the hexose monophosphate pathway can rapidly reduce this dye to leukomethylene blue in a reaction catalyzed by NADPH diaphorase. Leukomethylene blue, in turn, nonenzymatically reduces methemoglobin to hemoglobin.[108] An exception to the efficacy of this treatment exists in those patients who are glucose-6-phosphate dehydrogenase deficient (see Chap. 46). In these subjects, methylene blue would not only fail to give the desired effect on methemoglobin levels, but might compound the patient's difficulty by inducing an acute hemolytic episode[109] or by increasing the level of methemoglobin.[110]

In patients with acute toxic methemoglobinemia who are symptomatic or whose methemoglobin level is rising rapidly, the intravenous administration of 1 or 2 mg methylene blue per kilogram body weight over a period of 5 minutes is the preferred treatment because of its very rapid action.[111] Use of excessive amounts of methylene blue should be avoided: The administration of repeated doses of 2 mg methylene blue per kilogram body weight has produced acute hemolysis even in patients with normal glucose-6-phosphate dehydrogenase levels.[112]

The response to treatment is so rapid, with marked lowering or normalization of methemoglobin levels within an hour or two that no other treatment is usually needed, but the patient should be observed carefully, because continued absorption of a toxic substance from the gastrointestinal tract may cause recurrence of the methemoglobinemia. In patients who are in shock, blood transfusion may be helpful. Cimetidine, used as a selective inhibitor of N-hydroxylation, may decrease the methemoglobinemia produced by dapsone in patients with dermatitis herpetiformis.[113]

Hereditary Methemoglobinemia

The course of hereditary methemoglobinemia is benign, but patients with this disorder should be shielded from exposure to aniline derivatives, nitrites, and other agents that may, even in normal persons, induce methemoglobinemia.

Hereditary methemoglobinemia resulting from cytochrome b_5 reductase deficiency is readily treated by the administration of ascorbic acid, 300 to 600 mg orally daily divided into three or four doses. Although intravenously administered methylene blue is very effective in correcting this type of methemoglobinemia, it is not suitable for the long-term therapy that needs to be given if the state is to be treated at all. Riboflavin administration seems to benefit some patients[114] but not others.[115]

The iron phenolate complex that exists in the hemoglobins M prevents the reduction of ferric to ferrous iron. For this reason the methemoglobinemia does not respond to administration of ascorbic acid or of methylene blue. No effective treatment exists for the cyanosis that is present in patients with abnormal hemoglobins with reduced oxygen affinity.

SULFHEMOGLOBIN

■ DEFINITION AND HISTORY

Sulfhemoglobinemia refers to the presence in the blood of hemoglobin derivatives that are defined by their characteristic absorption of light at 620 nm which, unlike methemoglobin, is not abolished by the addition of cyanide. Sulfhemoglobin derives its name from the fact that it can be produced *in vitro* from the action of hydrogen sulfide on hemoglobin[116] and that the feeding of dogs with elemental sulfur has been associated with sulfhemoglobinemia.[117]

■ ETIOLOGY AND PATHOGENESIS

Sulfhemoglobin may contain one excess sulfur atom. The sulfur atom appears to be bound to a β-pyrrole carbon atom at the periphery of the porphyrin ring.[118–120] Sulfhemoglobinemia is associated with the ingestion of various drugs, particularly sulfonamides, phenacetin, acetanilid, and phenazopyridine.[90,121] It also occurs independently of drug use, and is thought to be related to chronic constipation or to purging.[122] Some patients with sulfhemoglobinemia or a past history of this disorder appear to have increased levels of red blood cell reduced glutathione (GSH).[123] The reason for this and its relationship to sulfhemoglobinemia is not clearly understood, but it may be of significance that some of the types of drugs that are associated with sulfhemoglobinemia cause an elevation of red cell GSH levels, probably by activating the enzyme glutathione synthase[124] or by increasing intracellular glutamate levels.[125]

Evidence for the occurrence of hereditary sulfhemoglobinemia is not convincing,[126] and it is likely that the single family reported represents a hemoglobin M hemoglobinopathy.

■ CLINICAL FEATURES

Sulfhemoglobinemia is characterized by cyanosis. Drugs that cause sulfhemoglobinemia often have the capacity to produce accelerated red cell destruction as well. Thus, mild hemolysis is sometimes observed in patients with sulfhemoglobinemia.

■ LABORATORY FEATURES

Sulfhemoglobin is detected in the lysate of blood treated with ferricyanide, cyanide, and ammonia by comparing the optical density at 620 nm with that at 540 nm.[88,89]

■ TREATMENT AND COURSE

Sulfhemoglobinemia is almost always a benign disorder. Unlike methemoglobin, sulfhemoglobin does not produce a left shift in the oxygen dissociation curve but rather decreases the affinity of hemoglobin for oxygen.[121] The disorder tends to recur in the same persons after exposure to drugs but does not generally appear to affect their overall health. Unlike methemoglobin, sulfhemoglobin cannot be converted to hemoglobin. Thus, once sulfhemoglobinemia occurs, it will persist until the erythrocytes carrying the abnormal pigment reach the end of their life span.

TABLE 49–3. Some Abnormal Hemoglobins Associated with Low Oxygen Affinity

Hemoglobin	Amino Acid Substitution	Oxygen Dissociation and Other Properties	Clinical Effect	Reference
$Hgb_{Seattle}$	β70 (E14)Ala→Asp	Decreased O_2 affinity normal heme-heme interaction	Mild chronic anemia associated with reduced urinary erythropoietin; physiologic adaptation to more efficient oxygen release to tissues	126
Hgb_{Kansas}	β102 (G4)Asn→Thr	Very low O_2 affinity, low heme-heme interaction, dissociates into dimers in ligand form	Cyanosis resulting from deoxyhemoglobin, mild anemia	202

LOW-OXYGEN AFFINITY HEMOGLOBINS: A CAUSE OF CYANOSIS

ETIOLOGY AND PATHOGENESIS

In some hemoglobin variants the deoxy conformation of the hemoglobin molecule is favored because the angle of the heme is altered from that found normally in deoxyhemoglobin. Such changes occur in $Hgb_{Hammersmith}$, $Hgb_{Bucuresti}$, Hgb_{Torino}, and $Hgb_{Peterborough}$. In other instances the quaternary conformation is changed by mutations involving the $\alpha_1\beta_2$ contact (Hgb_{Kansas}, $Hgb_{Titusville}$, and $Hgb_{Yoshizuka}$). Table 49–3 summarizes properties of abnormal hemoglobins associated with low oxygen affinity.

CLINICAL FEATURES

In response to the improved tissue oxygen supply brought about by a right-shifted oxygen dissociation curve, the "oxygen sensor" of the body decreases the output of erythropoietin.[126] As a result, the steady-state level of hemoglobin is diminished; mild anemia is characteristic of patients with hemoglobins with a decreased oxygen affinity.

LABORATORY FEATURES

Affinity of Hgb with oxygen is expressed as the P50, which is the partial pressure of oxygen in blood at which 50 percent of the Hgb is saturated with oxygen. The venous P50 can be measured directly using a cooximeter which is no longer easily available in routine and even reference laboratories. Lichtman and colleagues have reported a mathematical formula which can be used to calculate P50 reliably.[127] Calculating P50 using this formula requires the following venous gas parameters: partial pressure of oxygen (venous P_{O2}), venous pH and venous oxygen saturation, and uses antilog mathematical function that many clinicians find difficult to use for calculation. An electronic version (in Microsoft Excel program) of this mathematical formula is available for rapid calculation of P50 from venous blood gases.[128] The P50 of a healthy person with normal Hgb is 26 ± 1.3 mm Hg. An abnormally low P50 reflects an increased affinity of hemoglobin for oxygen and vice versa. Measurement of P50 is especially useful for detecting those high affinity hemoglobin mutants associated with polycythemia (see Chap. 56).

DIFFERENTIAL DIAGNOSIS

Cyanosis resulting from methemoglobinemia or sulfhemoglobinemia should be differentiated from cyanosis resulting from cardiac or pulmonary disease particularly when right-to-left shunting is present. In the latter instances the arterial oxygen tension will be low, while in methemoglobinemia and sulfhemoglobinemia it should be normal. One should be certain, however, that the oxygen tension was measured directly and not deduced from the percent saturation of hemoglobin. Blood from a patient with cyanosis because of arterial oxygen desaturation promptly becomes bright red upon being shaken with air. In addition, these causes of cyanosis are readily differentiated by carrying out quantitative blood methemoglobin and sulfhemoglobin levels. Because of the potential lethal nature of high levels of methemoglobin and because prompt treatment may be lifesaving, a high index of suspicion is important. A patient with cyanosis whose arterial blood is brown with a P_{O2} that is found to be normal on blood gas examination is likely to have methemoglobinemia. One should not rely on the readings of a pulse oximeter, as false readings may be obtained in the presence of methemoglobin. Rapid examination of a blood sample using an automatic analyzer such as a cooximeter is the first step in confirming the diagnosis. Treatment should not be delayed, but, as pointed out above in "Laboratory Features," direct spectrophotometric analysis should be carried out on the pretreatment sample as soon as possible to distinguish between methemoglobinemia and sulfhemoglobinemia.

A family history is usually helpful in differentiating hereditary methemoglobinemia as a result of cytochrome b_5 reductase deficiency from hemoglobin M disease. The former has a recessive mode of inheritance, the latter a dominant mode. Thus, cyanosis in successive generations suggests the presence of hemoglobin M; normal parents but possibly affected siblings implies the presence of cytochrome b_5 reductase. Consanguinity is more common in cytochrome b_5 reductase deficiency. In cytochrome b_5 reductase deficiency, incubation of the blood with small amounts of methylene blue will result in rapid reduction of the methemoglobin; in hemoglobin M disease, such reduction does not take place. The absorption spectra of methemoglobin and its derivatives are normal in cytochrome b_5 reductase deficiency; they are abnormal in hemoglobin M disease. In the case of toxic methemoglobinemia, cyanosis is generally of relatively recent origin, and a history of exposure to drug or toxin may usually be obtained; in hereditary methemoglobinemia a history of lifelong cyanosis may usually be elicited.

OTHER DYSHEMOGLOBINS

CARBON MONOXIDE AND CARBOXYHEMOGLOBIN

CO is a toxic, odorless, colorless, and tasteless gas. It can be unknowingly inhaled to dangerous levels when present in the high concentration in the atmosphere with serious clinical implications.[129]

Epidemiology

Acute CO intoxication is one of the most common causes of morbidity as a result of poisoning in the United States. In the United States, CO poisoning results in approximately 40,000 emergency department visits per year.[130,131] Approximately 500 accidental deaths because of CO poisoning occur annually, with the number of intentional CO-related deaths being 5 to 10 times higher.[132,133] Primary sources of CO are home appliances, and the majority of exposures occurred during the fall and winter months. During warmer months, boating activities are another source of exposure.[134] Death rate is highest among elderly and can be attributed to delayed diagnosis because symptoms often resemble those of associated comorbidities.[135,136] The exhaust produced by the typical home-use 5.5-kW generator contains as much CO as that of six idling automobiles.[137]

Chronic CO intoxication is commonly caused by cigarette smoking which can increase the carboxyhemoglobin (COHb) level to 15 percent. Houses with defective heating exhaust systems and vehicles that leak CO into the passenger compartment, either because of mechanical failure or driving with the rear hatch-door open, are the second most common cause of chronic CO exposure. Occupations that involve a high risk for CO intoxication include garage work with improper ventilation, toll-booth attendants, tunnel workers, fire fighters, and workers exposed to paint remover, aerosol propellant, and organic solvents containing dichloromethane.[138]

Etiology and Pathogenesis

CO binds with high affinity with the heme of hemoglobin—and with lesser affinities to myoglobin and cytochromes—at the iron core, a site that it shares with O_2.[139]

At equilibrium in physiologic conditions, CO affinity for hemoglobin is approximately 240 times greater than that of O_2. This very high equilibrium constant is the result of reaction kinetics. Contrary to popular belief, CO reacts more slowly than O_2 with the heme of hemoglobin. Once CO is bound to heme, its "off" rate is only 0.015 mol/L per second in contrast to 35 mol/L per second for O_2.[139] This extraordinarily slow-release process produces a very high affinity constant of CO for heme and a life-threatening danger for individuals exposed to high levels of CO. Once two molecules of CO are bound to hemoglobin, the hemoglobin switches to the relaxed (R) state, which increases the affinity of Hgb for oxygen. As a consequence of this phenomenon, called the Darling-Roughton effect,[103] the hemoglobin O_2 affinity increases in parallel with increasing CO levels making tissue delivery of oxygen more difficult.

In the absence of environmental CO, the blood of adults contains approximately 1 to 2 percent COHb. This represents approximately 80 percent of the total body CO, the remainder probably sequestered in myoglobin and other heme-binding proteins. This CO is endogenously produced,[140] originating from the degradation of heme by the rate-limiting heme oxygenase–cytochrome P450 complex, which produces CO and biliverdin. Caloric restriction, dehydration, infancy, and the genetic variations reported in Japanese and Native Americans generate higher endogenous levels of CO. Hemolytic anemia, hematomas, and infection tend to increase CO production up to threefold. Fetuses and newborns have double the normal adult levels of COHb. Drugs such as diphenylhydantoin and phenobarbital, by inducing the cytochrome P450 complex, increase CO production. Normal adult level of COHb is less than 1 to 2 percent. Hemolysis can produce COHb levels of more than 2 percent. Levels more than 3 percent must have an exogenous origin, except for rare conditions as occur in carriers of abnormal hemoglobins such as Hgb_{Zurich}. The affinity of Hgb_{Zurich} for CO is approximately 65 times that of normal hemoglobin.[141]

Pregnant women and fetuses are particularly at risk,[142] because they already have higher levels of COHb. CO readily crosses the placenta and half-life of CO in the fetus is as much as five times longer than it is in the mother.[143] The O_2 affinity of Hgb F is shifted to the left[144,145] as a result of its lack of 2,3-BPG binding, making the Darling-Roughton effect particularly pernicious. This is one reason why cigarette smoking during pregnancy is hazardous to the fetus.

Clinical and Laboratory Features

CO poisoning is a clinical diagnosis that is confirmed by laboratory testing. Signs and symptoms consistent with CO poisoning in certain circumstances should raise the suspicion of CO intoxication. A higher index of suspicion should attend the simultaneous presentation of multiple patients from the same family or housing complex. The eight-wavelength pulse oximeter (Masimo Rad-57) has been reported to be accurate in measuring carboxyhemoglobin concentration in normal healthy volunteers,[94] as well as in emergency room patients.[146]

Acute intoxication with CO rapidly affects the central and peripheral nervous systems and cardiopulmonary functions. Cerebral edema is common, as is impaired peripheral nervous system. CO induces increased capillary permeability in the lung resulting in acute pulmonary edema. Cardiac arrhythmias, generalized hypoxemia, and respiratory failure are the common causes of CO-related death. In survivors, considerable neurologic deficits might remain. Acute CO intoxication in children[147] sometimes has unique symptomatology resembling gastroenteritis. Surviving children are more likely to have severe sequelae such as leukoencephalopathy, white matter destruction, and severe myocardial ischemia.[148]

Chronic intoxication in adults might result in irritability, nausea, lethargy, headaches, and sometimes a flu-like condition. Higher COHb levels produce somnolence, palpitations, cardiomegaly, and hypertension and could contribute to atherosclerosis. Chronic CO poisoning can produce erythrocytosis, the magnitude of which varies with the level of COHb. By increasing red cell production, chronic CO poisoning can mask the mild anemia of acquired or congenital hemolytic disorders.

Therapy, Course, and Prognosis

The most important step in the treatment for CO poisoning is prompt removal of patients from the source of CO followed by administering 100 percent supplemental O_2 via a tight-fitting mask. The serum elimination half-life of CO is 5 hours when breathing room air, and 30 minutes with O_2 therapy (100 percent O_2 at 3 atm).[143]

For mild to moderate cases of CO poisoning, which more often happens with chronic intoxication, removing the patient from the source of environmental CO is usually curative. If the COHb level is high, breathing 100 percent O_2 will increase the rate of CO removal.

In severe cases of CO poisoning, which more often occur with acute intoxication, after identification and removal of the source of CO, 100 percent O_2 should be administered with cardiac monitoring. Endotracheal intubation should be done in any patient with impaired mental status and other interventions should be dictated by the symptomatology.

Because of conflicting evidence, there is no absolute indication for the use of hyperbaric O_2 treatment for patients with CO poisoning. Hyperbaric O_2 might be indicated in patients who have obvious neurologic abnormalities, have cardiac dysfunction, have persistent symptoms despite normobaric O_2, or have metabolic acidosis.[149] Hyperbaric O_2, has complications of its own, such as bronchial irritation and pulmonary edema, and should be reserved for exceptional cases of CO intoxication. Locations of hyperbaric chambers throughout the world and in the United States can be found at the Undersea and Hyperbaric Medical Society website, www.uhms.org, under "chamber directory."

Pregnant women exposed to CO are at particularly high risk. CO poisoning is especially dangerous to the fetus because CO readily crosses the placenta and half-life of CO in the fetus is as much as five times longer than it is in the mother. For these reasons, treatment with hyperbaric O_2

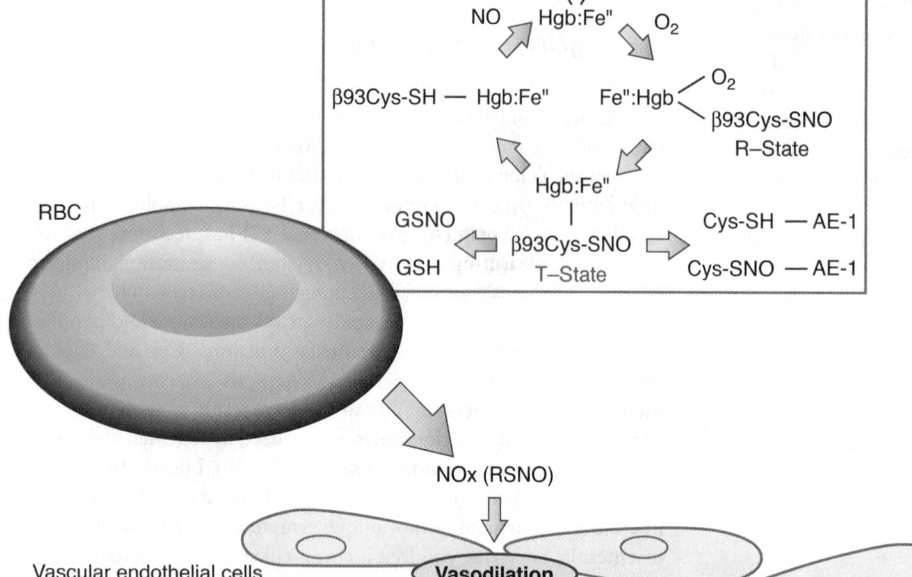

FIGURE 49–3. S-nitrosylated hemoglobin (SNO-Hgb) and hypoxic vasodilation. *(From Parker C: Is SNO-HB a snow job? The Hematologist: ASH News and Reports 6(1):12, 2009. Copyright American Society of Hematology, used with permission.)*

should be carried during pregnancy when the COHb levels exceed 15 percent. In a limited number of studies done on pregnant patients, hyperbaric O_2 does not seem to adversely affect the fetus.[150,151]

■ NITRIC OXIDE AND NO-HEMOGLOBINS

Physiology and Chemistry

Nitric oxide (NO), a soluble gas, is continuously synthesized in endothelial cells by isoforms of the NO synthase (NOS) enzyme. A functional NOS transfers electrons from NADPH to its heme center, where L-arginine is oxidized to L-citrulline and NO.[152] Vasodilation is caused by diffusion of NO into the smooth muscle cells wherein NO binds avidly to the heme of soluble guanylyl cyclase producing cyclic guanosine monophosphate (cGMP), which activates cGMP-dependent protein kinases, and ultimately produces smooth muscle relaxation.[152]

Blood NO levels are set by the balance between the production of NO by NOS and the binding or scavenging of NO by the heme groups of erythrocyte hemoglobin. The half-life of NO in whole blood (5×10^9 red blood cells [RBCs]/mL) is estimated to be 1.8 milliseconds.[153] The short half-life of NO greatly limits its diffusional distance in blood and only maintains NO as a paracrine vasoregulator.[154,155] This does not explain how hemoglobin is capable of transducing NO bioactivity far from their location of formation.

A dynamic cycle is reported to exist, in which hemoglobin is S-nitrosylated in the lung when red blood cells are oxygenated, and the NO group is released during arterial-venous transit in the hypoxic tissues.[156,157] These activities of hemoglobin are mediated by S-nitroso hemoglobin (SNO-Hgb). According to the SNO-Hgb hypothesis, this vasodilator function is carried by a micropopulation of hemoglobins that have undergone the addition of NO to a critical cysteine (cys*β*93) via S-nitrosylation, forming SNO-Hgb.[158] In this model, the allosterically controlled equilibrium of NO groups between hemes and cysteine thiols enables erythrocytes to convert oxygen gradients into a graded signal for vasodilatation, thereby enhancing perfusion sufficiency (Fig. 49–3). When hemoglobin is oxygenated (and undergoes a tense [T] to relaxed [R] transition) in lungs, some of the NO on the heme is transferred to the cysteine to form SNO-Hgb. Upon deoxygenation, SNO-Hgb is destabilized and some of the NO (in the form of NO^+) on the cysteine is transferred back to heme and some is exported out by the red blood cell in to the vascular lumen mediating vasodilation.[156,158,159] However, this model has been challenged by careful studies of transgenic animals with and without mutant cys*β*93 hemoglobin.[160–162] According to SNO-Hgb hypothesis, NO is transported by red blood cells from lungs to the hypoxic tissues in protected form as SNO-Hgb, and is delivered in the hypoxic microvasculature at the same time as oxygen, coupling hemoglobin deoxygenation to vasodilation. Another mechanism by which hemoglobin may transduce NO bioactivity is by functioning as nitrite reductase.[163,164] Deoxygenated hemoglobin reacts with nitrite to form NO and methemoglobin and causes vasodilation along the physiologic oxygen gradient. Although this reaction is experimentally associated with NO generation, kinetic analysis suggests that NO should not be able to escape inactivation in the erythrocyte.[165] This inactivation or scavenging of NO is avoided by the formation of an intermediate species, that is, dinitrogen trioxide (N_2O_3). Products of the nitrite-hemoglobin reaction generate N_2O_3 via a novel reaction of NO and nitrite-bound methemoglobin.[166] N_2O_3 diffuses out of the red cell, later forms NO, and effects vasodilation and/or forms nitrosothiols (SNO) (Fig. 49–4).

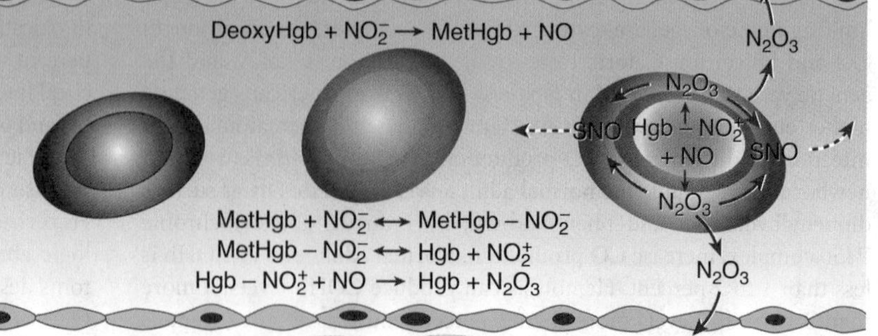

FIGURE 49–4. Hemoglobin deoxygenation occurs in capillaries. Nitrite reacts with deoxyHgb that is oxidized to MetHgb and NO. The NO binds to hemes of deoxyHgb, and also undergoes dioxygenation to form nitrate and MetHgb from oxyHgb. MetHgb binds nitrite to form an adduct with some Fe(II)-NO_2, that is, Hgb-NO. This species reacts quickly with NO to form N_2O_3, which can diffuse out of the red cell, forming NO and effecting vasodilation and/or forming nitrosothiols (SNOs). *(With permission from Nature Publishing.)*

According to this paradigm, nitrite, previously thought to be an inert end product of endogenous nitric oxide metabolism, is the main stable NO reservoir in blood and tissues.[167,168] Nitrite is formed during normoxic condition and then reduced to NO and N_2O_3 along the physiologic oxygen and pH gradient by the heme globins.[166]

Pathophysiology and Potential Therapeutic Applications

NO was long considered highly toxic. Exogenous administration of nitric oxide by inhalation activates cytosolic guanylate cyclase, increasing intracellular levels of cGMP, resulting in relaxation of the smooth muscles in the pulmonary arteries.

Based on this observation, inhaled NO (iNO) has been used to manage the acute pulmonary hypertension seen in adult respiratory distress syndrome, sickle cell disease, and primary or secondary pulmonary hypertension. Even though NO lowers the pulmonary artery pressure and improves oxygenation in acute respiratory distress syndrome in both adults and children, it has not consistently resulted in an improvement in mortality.

At present, prolonged administration of iNO is not considered as first-line therapy for pulmonary artery hypertension; instead, it is used only for vasoreactivity testing in these patients.[169] Inhaled NO does have beneficial effects in animal models and in preliminary human trials of acute vasoocclusive crisis and chest syndrome associated with sickle cell disease.[170–172] Preliminary animal data suggesting beneficial effects of iNO therapy in the setting of ischemia–reperfusion injury (lung, heart, and intestine) are reported.[173] However, iNO also is associated with multiple side effects, such as methemoglobinemia,[174] left-heart failure,[175] renal insufficiency,[176] and a "rebound" increase in pulmonary artery pressure upon discontinuation of iNO that may result in cardiovascular collapse.[177]

Direct repletion of S-nitrosothiol in the lung and blood has the potential to avoid toxicities related to iNO. In a porcine model of acute lung injury, inhaled ethyl nitrite, but not iNO, efficiently repleted lung SNOs, lowered pulmonary vascular resistance, improved oxygenation dose-dependently, and had a protective effect against a decline in cardiac output.[178]

In humans, newborns with persistent pulmonary hypertension improved oxygenation and hemodynamics following ethyl nitrite inhalation.[179] Use of cell-free hemoglobin is associated with vasoconstriction and subsequent development of hypertension. Increased vascular resistance and vasoconstriction is mediated mainly by the scavenging of NO as a result of high affinity of free hemoglobin for NO.[180,181]

REFERENCES

1. Hsieh H, Jaffe ER: The metabolism of methemoglobin in human erythrocytes, in *The Red Blood Cell*, edited by DM Surgenor, p 799. Academic Press, New York. 1975.
2. Sloss A, Wybauw R: Un Cas de methemoglobinemie idiopathique. *Ann Soc R Sci Med Nat Bruxettes* 70:206, 1912.
3. Hitzenberger K: Autotoxic cyanosis due to intraglobular methemoglobinemia. *Wien Arch Med* 23:85, 1932.
4. Jaffe E: Hereditary methemoglobinemias associated with abnormalities in the metabolism of erythrocytes. *Am J Med* 41:786, 1966.
5. Horlein H, Weber G: Über Chronische familiare Methämoglobinamie und eine neue Modification des Methämoglobins. *Dtsch Med Wochenschr* 73:476, 1948.
6. Singer K: Hereditary hemolytic disorders associated with abnormal hemoglobins. *Am J Med* 18:633, 1955.
7. Gibson QH: The reduction of methaemoglobin in red blood cells and studies on the cause of idiopathic methaemoglobinaemia. *Biochem J* 42:13, 1948.
8. Percy M, Gillespie M, Savage G, et al: Familial idiopathic mutations in NADH-cytochrome b5 reductase. *Blood* 100:3447, 2002.
9. Bonaventura J, Riggs A: Hemoglobin Kansas, a human hemoglobin with a neutral amino acid substitution and an abnormal oxygen equilibrium. *J Biol Chem* 243:980, 1968.
10. Scott E, Hoskins D: Hereditary methemoglobinemia in Alaskan Eskimos and Indians. *Blood* 13:795, 1958.
11. Balsamo P, Hardy W, Scott E: Hereditary methemoglobinemia due to diaphorase deficiency in Navajo Indians. *J Pediatr* 65:928, 1964.
12. Nazarenko LP, Sazhenova EA, Nazarenko SA, Banshchikova ES: [A search for mutations in the DIA1 gene in case of hereditary methemoglobinemia type I in the iakut population]. *Genetika* 39:858, 2003.
13. Sorensen PR: The influence of pH, pCO_2 and concentrations of dyshemoglobins on the oxygen dissociation curve (ODC) of human blood determined by non-linear least squares regression analysis. *Scand J Clin Lab Invest Suppl* 203:163, 1990.
14. Bodansky O: Methemoglobinemia and methemoglobin-producing compounds. *Pharmacol Rev* 3:144, 1951.
15. Kiese M: The biochemical production of ferrihemoglobin-forming derivatives from aromatic amines and mechanisms of ferrihemoglobin formation. *Pharmacol Rev* 18:1091, 1966.
16. Dean BS, Lopez G, Krenzelok EP: Environmentally-induced methemoglobinemia in an infant. *J Toxicol Clin Toxicol* 30:127, 1992.
17. Kuschner WG, Chitkara RK, Canfield J Jr, et al: Benzocaine-associated methemoglobinemia following bronchoscopy in a healthy research participant. *Respir Care* 45:953, 2000.
18. Abdallah HY, Shah SA: Methemoglobinemia induced by topical benzocaine: A warning for the endoscopist. *Endoscopy* 34:730, 2002.
19. Novaro G, Aronow H, Militello M, et al: Benzocaine-induced methemoglobinemia: Experience from a high-volume transesophageal echocardiography laboratory. *J Am Soc Echocardiogr* 16:170, 2003.
20. Collins JF: Methemoglobinemia as a complication of 20% benzocaine spray for endoscopy. *Gastroenterology* 98:211, 1990.
21. Cooper HA: Methemoglobinemia caused by benzocaine topical spray. *South Med J* 90:946, 1997.
22. Guerriero SE: Methemoglobinemia caused by topical benzocaine. *Pharmacotherapy* 17:1038, 1997.
23. Klein SL, Nustad RA, Feinberg SE, Fonseca RJ: Acute toxic methemoglobinemia caused by a topical anesthetic. *Pediatr Dent* 5:107, 1983.
24. McGuigan MA: Benzocaine-induced methemoglobinemia. *Can Med Assoc J* 125:816, 1981.
25. O'Donohue WJ Jr, Moss LM, Angelillo VA: Acute methemoglobinemia induced by topical benzocaine and lidocaine. *Arch Intern Med* 140:1508, 1980.
26. McKinney CD, Postiglione KF, Herold DA: Benzocaine-adultered street cocaine in association with methemoglobinemia. *Clin Chem* 38:596, 1992.
27. Falkenhahn M, Kannan S, O'Kane M: Unexplained acute severe methaemoglobinaemia in a young adult. *Br J Anaesth* 86:278, 2001.
28. Lee SW, Lee JY, Lee KJ, Kim M, Kim MJ: A case of methemoglobinemia after ingestion of an aphrodisiac, later proven as dapsone. *Yonsei Med J* 40:388, 1999.
29. Johnson CJ, Kross BC: Continuing importance of nitrate contamination of groundwater and wells in rural areas. *Am J Ind Med* 18:449, 1990.
30. Chan TY: Food-borne nitrates and nitrites as a cause of methemoglobinemia. *Southeast Asian J Trop Med Public Health* 27:189, 1996.
31. Knobeloch L, Proctor M: Eight blue babies. *WMJ* 100:43, 2001.
32. Askew GL, Finelli L, Genese CA, et al: Boilerbaisse: An outbreak of methemoglobinemia in New Jersey in 1992. *Pediatrics* 94:381, 1994.
33. Bakshi SP, Fahey JL, Pierce LE: Brief recording: Sausage cyanosis—Acquired methemoglobinemic nitrite poisoning. *N Engl J Med* 277:1072, 1967.
34. Bradberry SM, Whittington RM, Parry DA, Vale JA: Fatal methemoglobinemia due to inhalation of isobutyl nitrite. *J Toxicol Clin Toxicol* 32:179, 1994.
35. Bradberry SM, Gazzard B, Vale JA: Methemoglobinemia caused by the accidental contamination of drinking water with sodium nitrite. *J Toxicol Clin Toxicol* 32:173, 1994.
36. Harris JC, Rumack BH, Peterson RG, McGuire BM: Methemoglobinemia resulting from absorption of nitrates. *JAMA* 242:2869, 1979.
37. Lukens JN: Landmark perspective: The legacy of well-water methemoglobinemia. *JAMA* 257:2793, 1987.
38. Stuhlmeier K, Kao, JJ, Wallbrandt, P, et al: Antioxidant protein 2 prevents methemoglobin formation in erythrocyte hemolysates. *Eur J Biochem*270:334, 2003.
39. Percy MJ, McFerran NV, Lappin TR: Disorders of oxidised haemoglobin. *Blood Rev* 19:61, 2005.
40. Percy MJ, Oren H, Savage G, Irken G: Congenital methaemoglobinaemia type I in a Turkish infant due to a novel mutation, Pro144Ser, in NADH-cytochrome b5 reductase. *Hematol J* 5:367, 2004.
41. Percy MJ, Crowley LJ, Davis CA, et al: Recessive congenital methaemoglobinaemia: Functional characterization of the novel D239G mutation in the NADH-binding lobe of cytochrome b5 reductase. *Br J Haematol* 129:847, 2005.
42. Percy MJ, Crowley LJ, Boudreaux J, Barber MJ: Expression of a novel P275L variant of NADH:cytochrome b5 reductase gives functional insight into the conserved motif important for pyridine nucleotide binding. *Arch Biochem Biophys* 447:59, 2006.
43. Dekker J, Eppink, M, van Zwieten, R, et al: Seven new nucleotides in the nicotinamide adenine dinucleotide reduced-cytochrome b(5) reductase gene leading to methemoglobinemia type I. *Blood* 97:1106, 2001.
44. Grabowska D, Plochocka D, Jablonska-Skwiecinska E, et al: Compound heterozygosity of two missense mutations in the NADH-cytochrome b5 reductase gene of a Polish patient with type I recessive congenital methaemoglobinaemia. *Eur J Haematol* 70:404, 2003.
45. Higasa K, Manabe, J, Yubisui, T, et al: Molecular basis of hereditary methaemoglobinaemia, types I and II: Two novel mutations in the NADH-cytochrome b5 reductase gene. *Br J Haematol* 103:922, 1998.

46. Wu YS, Huang CH, Wan Y, et al: Identification of a novel point mutation (Leu72Pro) in the NADH-cytochrome b5 reductase gene of a patient with hereditary methaemoglobinaemia type I. *Br J Haematol* 102:575, 1998.
47. Manabe J, Arya, R, Sumimoto, H, et al: Two novel mutations in the reduced nicotinamide adenine dinucleotide (NADH)-cytochrome b5 reductase gene of a patient with generalized type, hereditary methemoglobinemia. *Blood* 88:3208, 1996.
48. Vieira L, Kaplan JC, Kahn A, et al: Four new mutations in the NADH-cytochrome b5 reductase gene from patients with recessive congenital methemoglobinemia type II. *Blood* 85:2254, 1995.
49. Shirabe K, Fujimoto, Y, Yubisui, T, et al: An in-frame deletion of codon 298 of the NADH-cytochrome b5 reductase gene results in hereditary methemoglobinemia type II (generalized type). A functional implication for the role of the COOH-terminal region of the enzyme. *J Biol Chem* 269:5952, 1994.
50. Kugler W, Pekrun A, Laspe P, et al: Molecular basis of recessive congenital methemoglobinemia, types I and II: Exon skipping and three novel missense mutations in the NADH-cytochrome b5 reductase (diaporase 1) gene. *Hum Mutat* 17:348, 2001.
51. Kedar PS, Colah RB, Ghosh K, Mohanty D: Congenital methemoglobinemia due to NADH-methemoglobin reductase deficiency in three Indian families. *Haematologia (Budap)* 32:543, 2002.
52. Percy MJ, Aslan D: NADH-cytochrome b5 reductase in a Turkish family with recessive congenital methaemoglobinaemia type I. *J Clin Pathol* 61:1122, 2008.
53. Bewley M, Marohnic, C, Barber, M. The structure and biochemistry of NADH-dependent cytochrome b5 reductase are now consistent. *Biochemistry* 40:13574, 2001.
54. Wang Y, Wu, Y, Zheng P, et al: A novel mutation in the NADH-cytochrome b5 reductase gene of a Chinese patient with recessive congenital methemoglobinemia. *Blood* 95:3250, 2000.
55. Shotelersuk V, Tosukhowong, P, Chotivitayatarakorn, P, et al: A Thai boy with hereditary enzymopenic methemoglobinemia type II. *J Med Assoc Thai* 83:1380, 2000.
56. Jenkins M, Prchal J: A novel mutation found in the 3 domain of NADH-cytochrome b5 reductase in an African-American family with type I congenital methemoglobinemia. *Blood* 87:2993, 1996.
57. Nussenzveig R, Lingam HB, Gaikwad A, et al: A novel mutation of the cytochrome-b5 reductase gene in an Indian patient: The molecular basis of type I methemoglobinemia. *Haematologica* 91:1542, 2006.
58. Jenkins M, Prchal J: A high frequency polymorphism of NADH-cytochrome b5 reductase in African-Americans. *Hum Genet* 99:248, 1997.
59. Leroux A, Junien C, Kaplan J, Bamberger J. Generalised deficiency of cytochrome b5 reductase in congenital methaemoglobinaemia with mental retardation. Nature 258:619, 1975.
60. Takeshita M, Tamura M, Kugi M, et al: Decrease of palmitoyl-CoA elongation in platelets and leukocytes in the patient of hereditary methemoglobinemia associated with mental retardation. *Biochem Biophys Res Commun* 148:384, 1987.
61. Tanishima K, Tanimoto K, Tomoda A, et al: Hereditary methemoglobinemia due to cytochrome b5 reductase deficiency in blood cells without associated neurologic and mental disorders. *Blood* 66:1288, 1985.
62. Katsube T, Sakamoto N, Kobayashi Y, et al: Exonic point mutations in NADH-cytochrome b5 reductase genes of homozygotes for hereditary methemoglobinemia, types I and III: Putative mechanisms of tissue-dependent enzyme deficiency. *Am J Hum Genet* 48:799, 1991.
63. Maran J, Guan Y, Ou CN, et al: Heterogeneity of the molecular biology of methemoglobinemia: A study of eight consecutive patients. *Haematologica* 90:687, 2005.
64. Cohen R, Sachs J, Wicker D, et al: Methemoglobinemia provoked by malarial chemoprophylaxis in Vietnam. *N Engl J Med* 279:1127, 1968.
65. Moore MR, Conrad ME, Bradley EL Jr, Prchal JT: Studies of nicotinamide adenine dinucleotide methemoglobin reductase activity in a Jewish population. *Am J Hematol* 12:13, 1982.
66. Fine DM, Eyster GE, Anderson LK, Smitley A: Cyanosis and congenital methemoglobinemia in a puppy. *J Am Anim Hosp Assoc* 35:33, 1999.
67. Harvey JW, Ling GV, Kaneko JJ: Methemoglobin reductase deficiency in a dog. *J Am Vet Med Assoc* 164:1030, 1974.
68. Lo SC, Agar NS: NADH-methemoglobin reductase activity in the erythrocytes of newborn and adult mammals. *Experientia* 42:1264, 1986.
69. Graubarth J, Bloom CJ, Coleman FC, Solomon HN: Dye poisoning in the nursery: A review of seventeen cases. *JAMA* 128:1155, 1945.
70. Sanchez-Echaniz J, Benito-Fernandez J, Mintegui-Raso S: Methemoglobinemia and consumption of vegetables in infants. *Pediatrics* 107:1024, 2001.
71. Hanukoglu A, Danon PN: Endogenous methemoglobinemia associated with diarrheal disease in infancy. *J Pediatr Gastroenterol Nutr* 23:1, 1996.
72. Yano S, Danish E, Hsia Y: Transient methemoglobinemia with acidosis in infants. *J Pediatr* 100:415, 1982.
73. Bricker T, Jefferson LS, Mintz AA: Methemoglobinemia in infants with enteritis. *J Pediatr* 102:161, 1983.
74. Hanukoglu A, Fried D, Bodner D: Methemoglobinemia in infants with enteritis [editorial correspondence]. *J Pediatr* 102:161, 1983.
75. Seeler R: Methemoglobinemia in infants with enteritis [editorial correspondence]. *J Pediatr* 102:162, 1983.
76. Danish E: Methemoglobinemia in infants with enteritis [reply]. *J Pediatr* 102:162, 1983.
77. Murray KF, Christie DL: Dietary protein intolerance in infants with transient methemoglobinemia and diarrhea. *J Pediatr* 122:90, 1993.
78. Hegesh E, Hegesh J, Kaftory A: Congenital methemoglobinemia with a deficiency of cytochrome b5. *N Engl J Med* 314:757, 1986.
79. Mansouri A, McClellan JL: Congenital methemoglobinemia with cytochrome b5 deficiency. *N Engl J Med* 315:893, 1986.
80. Tauber A, Blanchard RA: Congenital methemoglobinemia with cytochrome b_5 deficiency. *N Engl J Med* 315:894, 1986.
81. Lehmann H, Huntsman RG: *Man's Haemoglobins* p 213. Lippincott, Philadelphia, 1974.
82. Hayashi A, Fujita T, Fujimura M, Titani K: A new abnormal fetal hemoglobin, Hb FM-Osaka (alpha 2 gamma 2 63His replaced by Tyr). *Hemoglobin* 4:447, 1980.
83. Priest JR, Watterson J, Jones RT, et al: Mutant fetal hemoglobin causing cyanosis in a newborn. *Pediatrics* 83:734, 1989.
84. Hojas-Bernal R, McNab-Martin P, Fairbanks VF, et al: Hb Chile [beta28(B10)Leu→Met]: An unstable hemoglobin associated with chronic methemoglobinemia and sulfonamide or methylene blue-induced hemolytic anemia. *Hemoglobin* 23:125, 1999.
85. Prchal J, Borgese N, Moore M, et al: Congenital methemoglobinemia due to methemoglobin reductase deficiency in two unrelated American black families. *Am J Med* 89:516, 1990.
86. Dacie J, Lewis SM: Chemical and physico-chemical methods of haematological importance, in *Practical Haematology*, p 476. Grune & Stratton, New York, 1998.
87. Yawata Y, Ding L, Tanishima K, Tomoda A: New variant of cytochrome b5 reductase deficiency (b5RKurashiki) in red cells, platelets, lymphocytes, and cultured fibroblasts with congenital methemoglobinemia, mental and neurological retardation, and skeletal anomalies. *Am J Hematol* 40:299, 1992.
88. Evelyn K, Malloy H: Microdetermination of oxyhemoglobin, methemoglobin, and sulfhemoglobin in a single sample of blood. *J Biol Chem* 126:655, 1938.
89. Beutler E: Carboxyhemoglobin, methemoglobin, and sulfhemoglobin determinations, in *Hematology*, 5th ed, edited by E Beutler, MA Lichtman, BS Coller, TJ Kipps, p L50. McGraw-Hill, New York, 1995.
90. Halvorsen SM, Dull WL: Phenazopyridine-induced sulfhemoglobinemia: Inadvertent rechallenge. *Am J Med* 91:315, 1991.
91. Watcha MF, Connor MT, Hing AV: Pulse oximetry in methemoglobinemia. *Am J Dis Child* 143:845, 1989.
92. Molthrop D, Wheeler R, Hall K, et al: Evaluation of the methemoglobinemia associated with sulofenur. *Invest New Drugs* 12:99, 1994.
93. Beutler E, Gelbart T: Carboxyhemoglobin, methemoglobin, and sulf-hemoglobin determinations, in *Hematology*, 4th ed, edited by WJ Williams, E Beutler, AJ Erslev, MA Lichtman, p 1732. McGraw-Hill, New York 1990.
94. Barker S, Curry J, Redford D, et al: Measurement of carboxyhemoglobin and methemoglobin by pulse oximetry: A human volunteer study. *Anesthesiology* 105:892, 2006.
95. Beutler E: *Red Cell Metabolism: A Manual of Biochemical Methods*. Grune & Stratton, New York, 1984.
96. Board P: NADH-ferricyanide reductase, a convenient approach to the evaluation of NADH-methaemoglobin reductase in human erythrocytes. *Clin Chim Acta* 109:233, 1981.
97. Lan FH, Tang YC, Huang CH, et al: Antibody-based spot test for NADH-cytochrome b5 reductase activity for the laboratory diagnosis of congenital methemoglobinemia. *Clin Chim Acta* 273:13, 1998.
98. Das Gupta A, Vaidya MS, Bapat JP, et al: Associated red cell enzyme deficiencies and their significance in a case of congenital enzymopenic methemoglobinemia. *Acta Haematol* 64:285, 1980.
99. Kaftory A, Hegesh E: Improved determination of cytochrome b5 in human erythrocytes. *Clin Chem* 30:1344, 1984.
100. Gerald PS, George P: Second spectroscopically abnormal methemoglobin associated with hereditary cyanosis. *Science* 129:393, 1959.
101. Carrell RW, Kay R: A simple method for the detection of unstable haemoglobins. *Br J Haematol* 23:615, 1972.
102. Hutt PJ, Pisciotta AV, Fairbanks VF, et al: DNA sequence analysis proves Hb M-Milwaukee-2 is due to beta-globin gene codon 92 (CAC→TAC), the presumed mutation of Hb M-Hyde Park and Hb M-Akita. *Hemoglobin* 22:1, 1998.
103. Darling R, Roughton F: The effect of methemoglobin on the equilibrium between oxygen and hemoglobin. *Am J Physiol* 137:56, 1942.
104. Johnson CJ, Bonrud PA, Dosch TL, et al: Fatal outcome of methemoglobinemia in an infant. *JAMA* 257:2796, 1987.
105. Ellis M, Hiss Y, Shenkman L: Fatal methemoglobinemia caused by inadvertent contamination of a laxative solution with sodium nitrite. *Isr J Med Sci* 28:289, 1992.
106. Caudill L, Walbridge J, Kuhn G: Methemoglobinemia as a cause of coma. *Ann Emerg Med* 19:677, 1990.
107. Clifton J 2nd, Leikin JB: Methylene blue. *Am J Ther* 10:289, 2003.
108. Beutler E, Baluda MC: Methemoglobin reduction. Studies of the interaction between cell populations and of the role of methylene blue. *Blood* 22:323, 1963.
109. Rosen P, Johnson C, McGehee WG, et al: Failure of methylene blue treatment in toxic methemoglobinemia: Associations with glucose-6-phosphate dehydrogenase deficiency. *Ann Intern Med* 75:83, 1971.
110. Bilgin H, Ozcan B, Bilgin T: Methemoglobinemia induced by methylene blue perturbation during laparoscopy. *Acta Anaesthesiol Scand* 42:594, 1998.
111. Kearney TE, Manoguerra AS, Dunford JV Jr: Chemically induced methemoglobinemia from aniline poisoning. *West J Med* 140:282, 1984.
112. Harvey J, Keitt A: Studies of the efficacy and potential hazards of methylene blue therapy in aniline-induced methemoglobinemia. *Br J Haematol* 54:29, 1983.

113. Coleman M, Rhodes LE, Scott AK, et al: The use of cimetidine to reduce dapsone-dependent methaemoglobinaemia in dermatitis herpetiformis patients. *Br J Clin Pharmacol* 34:244, 1992.
114. Kaplan J, Chirouze M: Therapy of recessive congenital methaemoglobinemia by oral riboflavin. *Lancet* 2:1043, 1978.
115. Beutler E: Important recent advances in the field of red cell metabolism: Practical implications, in *Erythrocytes, Thrombocytes, Leukocytes*, edited by E Gerlach, K Moser, E Deutsch, W Wilmanns, p 123. George Thieme Verlag, Stuttgart, 1973.
116. Lemberg R, Legge JW: *Hematin Compounds and Bile Pigments*. Inter-science Publishers, New York, 1949.
117. Harrop GJ, Waterfield RL: Sulphemoglobinemia. *JAMA* 95:647, 1930.
118. Nichol A, Hendry I, Movell DB, et al: Mechanism of formation of sulfhemoglobin. *Biochim Biophys Acta* 156:97, 1968.
119. Berzofsky JA, Peisach J, Horecker BL: Sulfheme proteins. IV. The stoichiometry of sulfur incorporation and the isolation of sulfhemin, the prosthetic group of sulfmyoglobin. *J Biol Chem* 247:3783, 1972.
120. Berzofsky J, Peisach J, Blumberg WE: Sulfheme proteins. II. The reversible oxygenation of ferrous sulfmyoglobin. *J Biol Chem* 246:7366, 1971.
121. Park CM, Nagel RL: Sulfhemoglobinemia. Clinical and molecular aspects. *N Engl J Med* 310:1579, 1984.
122. Discombe G: Sulphaemoglobinaemia and glutathione. *Lancet* 2:371, 1960.
123. McCutcheon A: Sulphaemoglobinaemia and glutathione. *Lancet* 2:290, 1960.
124. Paniker NV, Beutler E: The effect of methylene blue and diaminodiphenysulfone on red cell reduced glutathione synthesis. *J Lab Clin Med* 80:481, 1972.
125. Smith JE, Mahaffey E, Lee M: Effect of methylene blue on glutamate and reduced glutathione of rabbit erythrocytes. *Biochem J* 168:587, 1977.
126. Stamatoyannopoulos G, Parer JT, Finch CA: Physiologic implications of a hemoglobin with decreased oxygen affinity (hemoglobin Seattle). *N Engl J Med* 281:916, 1969.
127. Lichtman MA, Murphy MS, Adamson JW: Detection of mutant hemoglobins with altered affinity for oxygen. A simplified technique. *Ann Intern Med* 84:517, 1976.
128. Agarwal N, Mojica-Henshaw MP, Simmons ED, et al: Familial polycythemia caused by a novel mutation in the beta globin gene: Essential role of P50 in evaluation of familial polycythemia. *Int J Med Sci* 4:232, 2007.
129. Vreman H, Mahoney JJ, Stevenson DK: Carbon monoxide and carboxyhemoglobin. *Adv Pediatr* 42:303, 1995.
130. Hampson N: Emergency department visits for carbon monoxide poisoning in the pacific northwest. *J Emerg Med* 16:695, 1998.
131. Weaver L: Carbon monoxide poisoning. *Crit Care Clin* 15:297, 1999.
132. Ernst A, Zibrak JD: Carbon monoxide poisoning. *N Engl J Med* 339:1603, 1998.
133. Centers for Disease Control and Prevention: Carbon monoxide poisoning from hurricane-associated use of portable generators—Florida 2004. *MMWR Morb Mortal Wkly Rep* 54:697, 2005.
134. Centers for Disease Control and Prevention: Unintentional non-fire-related carbon monoxide exposures—United States, 2001–2003. *MMWR Morb Mortal Wkly Rep* 54:36, 2005.
135. Mott J, Wolfe MI, Alverson CJ, et al: National vehicle emissions policies and practices and declining US carbon monoxide-related mortality. *JAMA* 288:988, 2002.
136. Harper A, Croft-Baker J: Carbon monoxide poisoning: Undetected by both patients and their doctors. *Age Ageing* 33:105, 2004.
137. US Environmental Protection Agency: Emission facts: Idling vehicle emissions. Publication EPA420-F-98-014. US Environmental Protection Agency, Washington, DC, 1998.
138. Stewart R, Fisher TN, Hosko MJ, et al: Carboxyhemoglobin elevation after exposure to dichloromethane. *Science* 176:295, 1972.
139. Antonini E, Brunori M: Frontiers of Biology, in Neuberger A, Taum EL (eds): Hemoglobin and myoglobin in their reactions with ligands. Vol. 21. Amsterdam, The Netherlands, North Holland, 1971, p 19.
140. Sjostrand T: Endogenous formation of carbon monoxide in man. *Nature* 164:580, 1949.
141. Giacometti G, Brunori M, Antonini E, et al: The reaction of hemoglobin Zurich with oxygen and carbon monoxide. *J Biol Chem* 255:6160, 1980.
142. Balster R, Ekelund LG, Grover RF: Evaluation of subpopulations potentially at risk to carbon monoxide exposure, in *EPA 600/8-90/045F: Air Quality Criteria for Carbon Monoxide*, pp 12–11 to 12–23. Environmental Criteria and Assessment Office, Office of Health and Environmental Assessment, Office of Research and Development, US Environmental Protection Agency, Research Triangle Park, NC, 1991.
143. Hampson N, Dunford RG, Kramer CC, et al: Selection criteria utilized for hyperbaric oxygen treatment of carbon monoxide poisoning. *J Emerg Med* 13:227, 1995.
144. Benesch R, Maeda N, Benesch R: 2,3-Diphosphoglycerate and the relative affinity of adult and fetal hemoglobin for oxygen and carbon dioxide. *Biochim Biophys Acta* 257:178, 1972.
145. Engel R, Rodkey FL, O'Neal JD, et al: Relative affinity of human fetal hemoglobin for CO and O_2. *Blood* 33:37, 1969.
146. Suner S, Partridge R, Sucov A, et al: Non-invasive screening for carbon monoxide toxicity in the emergency department is valuable. *Ann Emerg Med* 49:718; author reply 719, 2007.
147. Gemelli F, Cattani R: Carbon monoxide poisoning in childhood. *Br Med J (Clin Res Ed)* 291:1197, 1985.
148. Lacey D: Neurologic sequellae of acute carbon monoxide intoxication. *Am J Dis Child* 135:145, 1981.
149. Kao L, Nanagas KA: Carbon monoxide poisoning. *Emerg Med Clin North Am* 22:985, 2004.
150. Elkharrat D, Raphael JC, Korach JM, et al: Acute carbon monoxide intoxication and hyperbaric oxygen in pregnancy. *Intensive Care Med* 17:289, 1991.
151. Koren G, Sharav T, Pastuszak A, et al: A multicenter, prospective study of fetal outcome following accidental carbon monoxide poisoning in pregnancy. 5:397, 1991.
152. Ignarro LJ: Nitric oxide. A novel signal transduction mechanism for transcellular communication. *Hypertension* 16:477, 1990.
153. Liu X, Miller MJ, Joshi MS, et al: Diffusion-limited reaction of free nitric oxide with erythrocytes. *J Biol Chem* 273:18709, 1998.
154. Azarov I, Huang KT, Basu S, Gladwin MT, et al: Nitric oxide scavenging by red blood cells as a function of hematocrit and oxygenation. *J Biol Chem* 280:39024, 2005.
155. Kim-Shapiro D, Schechter AN, Gladwin MT. Unraveling the reactions of nitric oxide, nitrite, and hemoglobin in physiology and therapeutics. *Arterioscler Thromb Vasc Biol* 26:697, 2006.
156. Jia L, Bonaventura C, Bonaventura J, et al: S-nitrosohaemoglobin: A dynamic activity of blood involved in vascular control. *Nature* 380:221, 1996.
157. Stamler J, Jia L, Eu JP, et al: Blood flow regulation by S-nitrosohemoglobin in the physiological oxygen gradient. *Science* 276:2034, 1997.
158. Singel D, Stamler JS: Chemical physiology of blood flow regulation by red blood cells: Role of nitric oxide and S-nitrosohemoglobin. *Annu Rev Physiol* 67:99, 2005.
159. Gow A, Stamler JS: Reactions between nitric oxide and haemoglobin under physiological conditions. *Nature* 391:169, 1998.
160. Gladwin MT, Wang X, Reiter CD, et al: S-Nitrosohemoglobin is unstable in the reductive erythrocyte environment and lacks O_2/NO-linked allosteric function. *J Biol Chem* 277:27818, 2002.
161. Isbell TS, Sun CW, Wu LC, et al: SNO-hemoglobin is not essential for red blood cell-dependent hypoxic vasodilation. *Nat Med* 14:773, 2008.
162. Parker C: Is SNO-Hgb a snow job? I still can't decide. *The Hematologist* 6:12, 2009.
163. Cosby K, Partovi KS, Crawford JH, et al: Nitrite reduction to nitric oxide by deoxyhemoglobin vasodilates the human circulation. *Nat Med* 9:1498, 2003.
164. Gladwin MT, Kim-Shapiro DB: The functional nitrite reductase activity of the heme-globins. *Blood* 112:2636, 2008.
165. Gladwin MT, Schechter AN, Kim-Shapiro DB, et al: The emerging biology of the nitrite anion. *Nat Chem Biol* 1:308, 2005.
166. Basu S, Grubina R, Huang J, et al: Catalytic generation of N_2O_3 by the concerted nitrite reductase and anhydrase activity of hemoglobin. *Nat Chem Biol* 3:785, 2007.
167. Lauer T, Preik M, Rassaf T, et al: Plasma nitrite rather than nitrate reflects regional endothelial nitric oxide synthase activity but lacks intrinsic vasodilator action. *Proc Natl Acad Sci U S A* 98:12814, 2001.
168. Shiva S, Wang X, Ringwood LA, et al: Ceruloplasmin is a NO oxidase and nitrite synthase that determines endocrine NO homeostasis. *Nat Chem Biol* 2:486, 2006.
169. Badesch D, Abman, SH, Ahearn, GS, et al: Medical therapy for pulmonary arterial hypertension: ACCP evidence-based clinical practice guidelines. *Chest* 126(1 Suppl):35S, 2004.
170. Martinez-Ruiz R, Montero-Huerta P, Hromi J, et al: Inhaled nitric oxide improves survival rates during hypoxia in a sickle cell (SAD) mouse model. *Anesthesiology* 94:1113, 2001.
171. Weiner D, Hibberd PL, Betit P, et al: Preliminary assessment of inhaled nitric oxide for acute vaso-occlusive crisis in pediatric patients with sickle cell disease. *JAMA* 289:1136, 2003.
172. Sullivan K, Goodwin SR, Evangelist J, et al: Nitric oxide successfully used to treat acute chest syndrome of sickle cell disease in a young adolescent. *Crit Care Med* 27:2563, 1999.
173. McMahon T, Doctor A: Extrapulmonary effects of inhaled nitric oxide: Role of reversible S-nitrosylation of erythrocytic hemoglobin. *Proc Am Thorac Soc* 3:153, 2006.
174. Young J, Dyar O, Xiong L, et al: Methaemoglobin production in normal adults inhaling low concentrations of nitric oxide. *Intensive Care Med* 20:581, 1994.
175. Loh E, Stamler JS, Hare JM, et al: Cardiovascular effects of inhaled nitric oxide in patients with left ventricular dysfunction. *Circulation* 90:2780, 1994.
176. Lundin S, Mang H, Smithies M, et al: Inhalation of nitric oxide in acute lung injury: Results of a European multicentre study. The European Study Group of Inhaled Nitric Oxide. *Intensive Care Med* 25:911, 1999.
177. Christenson J, Lavoie A, O'Connor M, et al: The incidence and pathogenesis of cardiopulmonary deterioration after abrupt withdrawal of inhaled nitric oxide. *Am J Respir Crit Care Med* 161:1443, 2000.
178. Moya M, Gow AJ, McMahon TJ, et al: S-nitrosothiol repletion by an inhaled gas regulates pulmonary function. *Proc Natl Acad Sci U S A* 98:5792, 2001.
179. Moya M, Gow AJ, Califf RM, et al: Inhaled ethyl nitrite gas for persistent pulmonary hypertension of the newborn. *Lancet* 360:141, 2002.
180. Gulati A, Sen AP, Sharma AC, et al: Role of ET and NO in resuscitative effect of diaspirin cross-linked hemoglobin after hemorrhage in rat. *Am J Physiol* 273:H827, 1997.
181. Gibson J, Maxwell RA, Schweitzer JB, et al: Resuscitation from severe hemorrhagic shock after traumatic brain injury using saline, shed blood, or a blood substitute. *Shock* 17:234, 2002.
182. Paris PM, Kaplan RM, Stewart RD, Weiss LD: Methemoglobin levels following sublingual nitroglycerin in human volunteers. *Ann Emerg Med* 15:171, 1986.
183. Gavish D, Knobler H, Gottehrer N, et al: Methemoglobinemia, muscle damage and renal failure complicating phenazopyridine overdose. *Isr J Med Sci* 22:45, 1986.

184. Christensen CM, Farrar HC, Kearns GL: Protracted methemoglobinemia after phenazopyridine overdose in an infant. *J Clin Pharmacol* 36:112, 1996.
185. Damergis JA, Stoker JM, Abadie JL: Methemoglobinemia after sulfamethoxazole and trimethoprim. *JAMA* 249:590, 1983.
186. Wagner A, Marosi C, Binder M, et al: Fatal poisoning due to dapsone in a patient with grossly elevated methaemoglobin levels. *Br J Dermatol* 133:816, 1995.
187. Ng LL, Nai KR, Polak A: Paraquat ingestion with methaemoglobinaemia treated with methylene blue. *Br Med J (Clin Res Ed)* 284:1445, 1982.
188. Proudfoot AT: Methaemoglobinaemia due to monolinuron-not paraquat. *Br Med J (Clin Res Ed)* 285:812, 1982.
189. de Torres JP, Strom JA, Jaber BL, Hendra KP: Hemodialysis-associated methemoglobinemia in acute renal failure. *Am J Kidney Dis* 39:1307, 2002.
190. Gibson GR, Hunter JB, Raabe DS Jr, et al: Methemoglobinemia produced by high-dose intravenous nitroglycerin. *Ann Intern Med* 96:615, 1982.
191. Forsyth RJ, Moulden A: Methaemoglobinaemia after ingestion of amyl nitrite. *Arch Dis Child* 66:152, 1991.
192. Guss DA, Normann SA, Manoguerra AS: Clinically significant methemoglobinemia from inhalation of isobutyl nitrite. *Am J Emerg Med* 3:46, 1985.
193. Nilsson A, Engberg G, Henneberg S, et al: Inverse relationship between age-dependent erythrocyte activity of methaemoglobin reductase and prilocaine-induced methaemoglobinaemia during infancy. *Br J Anaesth* 64:72, 1990.
194. Duncan PG, Kobrinsky N: Prilocaine-induced methemoglobinemia in a newborn infant. *Anesthesiology* 59:75, 1983.
195. Lloyd CJ: Chemically induced methaemoglobinaemia in a neonate. *Br J Oral Maxillofac Surg* 30:63, 1992.
196. Davidovits M, Barak A, Cleper R, et al: Methaemoglobinaemia and haemolysis associated with hydrogen peroxide in a paediatric haemodialysis centre: A warning note. *Nephrol Dial Transplant* 18:2354, 2003.
197. Gerald PS, Efron ML: Chemical studies of several varieties of Hb M. *Proc Natl Acad Sci U S A* 47:1758, 1961.
198. Stavem P, Stromme J, Lorkin PA, Lehmann H: Haemoglobin M Saskatoon with slight constant haemolysis, markedly increased by sulphonamides. *Scand J Haematol* 9:566, 1972.
199. Hayashi N, Motokawa Y, Kikuchi G: Studies on relationships between structure and function of hemoglobin M-Iwate. *J Biol Chem* 241:79, 1966.
200. Horst J, Schafer R, Kleihauer E, Kohne E: Analysis of the Hb M Milwaukee mutation at the DNA level. *Br J Haematol* 54:643, 1983.
201. Hain RD, Chitayat D, Cooper R, et al: Hb FM-Fort Ripley: Confirmation of autosomal dominant inheritance and diagnosis by PCR and direct nucleotide sequencing. *Hum Mutat* 3:239, 1994.
202. Reissmann KR, Ruth WE, Nomura T: A human hemoglobin with lowered oxygen affinity and impaired heme-heme interactions. *J Clin Invest* 40:1826, 1961.

CHAPTER 50
HEMOLYTIC ANEMIA RESULTING FROM PHYSICAL INJURY TO RED CELLS

Kelty R. Baker and Joel Moake

SUMMARY

Erythrocyte fragmentation and hemolysis occur when red cells are forced at high shear stress through partial vascular occlusions or over abnormal vascular surfaces. "Split" red cells, or schistocytes, are prominent on blood films under these conditions, and considerable quantities of lactate dehydrogenase are released into the blood from traumatized red cells. In the high-flow (high-shear) microvascular (arteriolar/capillary) or arterial circulation, partial vascular obstructions are caused by platelet aggregates in the systemic microvasculature during episodes of thrombotic thrombocytopenic purpura by platelet-fibrin thrombi in the renal microvasculature in the hemolytic-uremic syndrome; and by malfunction of a cardiac prosthetic valve in valve-related hemolysis. Less-extensive red cell fragmentation, hemolysis, and schistocytosis occur under conditions of more moderate vascular occlusion or endothelial surface abnormalities, sometimes under conditions of lower shear stress. These latter entities include excessive platelet aggregation, fibrin polymer formation, and secondary fibrinolysis in the arterial or venous microcirculation (disseminated intravascular coagulation); in the placental vasculature in preeclampsia/eclampsia and the syndrome of hemolysis, elevated liver enzymes and low platelets (HELLP) in march hemoglobinuria; and in giant cavernous hemangiomas (the Kasabach-Merritt phenomenon).

PREECLAMPSIA/ECLAMPSIA AND HELLP SYNDROME

■ DEFINITION AND HISTORY

A life-threatening condition of pregnancy denoted by eclampsia, hemolysis, and thrombocytopenia was first noted in the German literature by Stahnke in 1922.[1] Subsequently, Pritchard and coworkers described three cases in English and suggested that an immunologic process might account for both the preeclampsia or eclampsia and the hematologic abnormalities.[2] Although initially known as edema-proteinuria-hypertension gestosis type B,[3] a catchier phrase, HELLP syndrome (H for hemolysis, EL for elevated liver function tests, and LP for low platelet counts), was later applied by Louis Weinstein in 1982.[4]

Acronyms and abbreviations that appear in this chapter include: ADA, antidiuretic hormone; ADAMTS13, a disintegrin and metalloproteinase with thrombospondin domain 13; ALT, alanine transaminase; aPTT, activated partial thromboplastin time; AST, aspartate transaminase; AT, antithrombin; DIC, disseminated intravascular coagulation; HELLP, hemolysis, elevated liver enzymes, and low platelet count; LDH, lactate dehydrogenase; MAHA, microangiopathic hemolytic anemia; PGF, placental growth factor; PGI_2, prostaglandin I_2; PT, prothrombin time; PTT, partial thromboplastin time; sEng, soluble endoglin; sFlt-1, soluble form of fms-like tyrosine kinase 1; sVEGFR-1, soluble vascular endothelial growth factor receptor-1; TGF-β, transforming growth factor-β; TTP, thrombotic thrombocytopenic purpura; VEGF, vascular endothelial growth factor; VWF, von Willebrand factor.

■ EPIDEMIOLOGY

HELLP syndrome occurs in approximately 0.5 percent of pregnancies overall,[5] in 4 to 12 percent of those complicated by preeclampsia (hypertension + proteinuria), and in 30 to 50 percent of those complicated by eclampsia (hypertension + proteinuria + seizures). Approximately 15 percent of patients ultimately diagnosed with HELLP syndrome present with neither hypertension nor proteinuria.[6] Two-thirds of HELLP patients are diagnosed antepartum, usually between 27 and 37 weeks. The remaining one-third are diagnosed in the postpartum period, usually from a few to 48 hours following delivery (occasionally as long as 6 days).[7,8] Additional risk factors for HELLP syndrome include persons of European descent, multiparity, and older maternal age (older than age 34 years).[5] Although the presence of homozygosity for the 677 (C→T) polymorphism of the methylenetetrahydrofolate reductase gene may be a modest risk factor for the development of preeclampsia, this weak association does not exist for HELLP syndrome.[9] Whether or not the factor V Leiden or prothrombin 20210 gene mutations are risk factors for HELLP syndrome remains controversial.[10–12]

■ ETIOLOGY AND PATHOGENESIS

To survive, a developing embryo must acquire a supply of maternal blood. During a normal pregnancy, the first wave of trophoblastic invasion into the decidua occurs at 10 to 12 days. This is followed by a second wave at 16 to 22 weeks, when these specialized placental epithelial cells replace the endothelium of the uterine spiral arteries and intercalate within the muscular tunica, increasing the vessels' diameters and decreasing their resistance. As a result, the spiral arteries are remodeled into unique hybrid vessels composed of fetal and maternal cells, and the vasculature is converted into a high flow-low resistance system resistant to vasoconstrictors circulating in the maternal blood.[13] In a preeclamptic pregnancy, this second wave fails to penetrate adequately the spiral arteries of the uterus, perhaps as a result of reduced placental expression of syncytin and subsequent altered cell fusion processes during placentogenesis.[14] The resultant poorly perfused hypoxic placenta then releases the extracellular domain (soluble) form of fms-like tyrosine kinase 1 (sFLT-1), also known as soluble vascular endothelial growth factor receptor-1 (sVEGF receptor-1, or sVEGFR-1). sVEGFR-1 functions as an antiangiogenic protein because it binds to vascular endothelial growth factor (VEGF) and placental growth factor (PGF), and prevents their interaction with endothelial cell receptors. The result is glomerular endothelial cell and placental dysfunction.[15–17] Direct and indirect sequelae include increased vascular tone, hypertension, proteinuria, enhanced platelet activation and aggregation, and (possibly) decreased levels of the vasodilators prostaglandin I_2 (PGI_2) and nitrous oxide (NO).[5,17] Concurrent activation of the coagulation cascade results in platelet-fibrin deposition in the capillaries, multiorgan microvascular injury, microangiopathic hemolytic anemia, elevated liver enzymes because of hepatic necrosis, and thrombocytopenia because of peripheral consumption.[5]

Another antiangiogenic molecule, a soluble form of endoglin, also increases in patient serum during early and severe preeclampsia.[18] Endoglin is part of the transforming growth factor-β (TGF-β) complex, and is expressed on vascular endothelial cells and syncytiotrophoblasts.

The shed extracellular domain of endoglin, soluble endoglin (sEng), is capable of binding to and inactivating the proangiogenic growth factors, TGF-β_1 and TGF-β_3. The presence of elevated serum levels of both sFLT-1 (sVEGFR-1) and sEng may be associated with the progression of preeclampsia to HELLP.[17,18]

CLINICAL FEATURES

Ninety percent of patients with HELLP syndrome will present with malaise and right upper quadrant or epigastric pain. Between 45 and 86 percent will have nausea or vomiting, 55 to 67 percent will have edema, 31 to 50 percent will have headache, and a smaller percentage may complain of visual changes. Fever is not typically seen. Whereas hypertension is found in 85 percent, 15 percent of those with HELLP syndrome will not present with either hypertension or proteinuria.[6]

LABORATORY FEATURES

In 54 to 86 percent of patients, the blood film has schistocytes, helmet cells, and burr cells consistent with microangiopathic hemolytic anemia. Reticulocytosis can be present. Low haptoglobin levels are both sensitive (83%) and specific (96%) for confirming the presence of hemolysis caused by HELLP, and returned to normal within 24 to 30 hours postpartum.[6]

Lactate dehydrogenase (LDH) levels are usually above normal. It has been suggested that the ratio of LDH 5 (an isoenzyme found specifically in the liver) to total LDH is elevated in proportion to the severity of HELLP. The high LDH seen in HELLP is most likely the result, principally, of liver damage rather than hemolysis. Serum levels of aspartic acid transaminase (AST) and alanine transaminase (ALT) can be more than 100 times normal, whereas alkaline phosphatase values are typically only about twice normal and total bilirubin ranges between 1.2 and 5 mg/dL. Liver enzymes usually return to baseline within 3 to 5 days postpartum.[6]

The degree of thrombocytopenia has been utilized in a classification system to predict maternal morbidity and mortality, the rapidity of postpartum recovery, the risk of disease recurrence, and perinatal outcome. This "Mississippi triple class system" places those patients with platelet counts less than 50,000/μL in class 1 (~13% incidence of bleeding); those with platelet counts between 50,000 and 100,000/μL in class 2 (~8% incidence of bleeding); and those with a platelet count greater than 100,000/μL in class 3 (no increased bleeding risk). Not surprisingly, patients with class 1 HELLP syndrome suffer the highest incidence of perinatal morbidity and mortality, and have the most protracted recovery periods postpartum.[19] There is a direct correlation between the extent of thrombocytopenia and serum measurements of liver function,[20] but the same cannot be said for the severity of associated hepatic histopathologic changes.[21] If a marrow aspiration and biopsy are performed, abundant megakaryocytes are found consistent with a consumptive thrombocytopenia and reduction of the normal platelet life span of approximately 10 days to 3 to 5 days.[19] The platelet count nadir occurs 23 to 29 hours postpartum, with subsequent normalization within 6 to 11 days.[7]

The prothrombin time (PT) and activated partial thromboplastin time (aPTT) are usually within normal limits, although some have reported that a prolonged aPTT can be found in 50 percent of patients.[22] Although low fibrinogen levels are inconsistently found, other measures of increased coagulation and secondary fibrinolysis may be present. These include decreased protein C and antithrombin III (AT III) levels, and increased D-dimer and thrombin-AT III values. von Willebrand factor (VWF) antigen levels increase in proportion to the severity of the disease, reflecting the extent of endothelial damage; however, no unusually large VWF multimers are present in plasma[23] and ADAMTS13 (a disintegrin and metalloproteinase with thrombospondin domains-13) levels are within a broad normal range (ADAMTS13 normally declines moderately during pregnancy).[24,25] This is in contrast to the severe deficiency of ADAMTS13 in familial and autoantibody-mediated types of thrombotic thrombocytopenic purpura (TTP).[26] Unlike TTP, the thrombi found in organs affected by HELLP contain increased amounts of fibrin and low levels of VWF.[23]

In patients with severe liver involvement, hepatic ultrasonography shows large, irregular, well-demarcated (or "geographical") areas of increased echogenicity.[27] Liver biopsy shows periportal or focal necrosis, platelet-fibrin deposits in the sinusoids, and vascular microthrombi. As the disease progresses, large areas of necrosis can coalesce and dissect into the liver capsule. This produces a subcapsular hematoma and the risk of hepatic rupture.[5]

DIFFERENTIAL DIAGNOSIS

Other complications of pregnancy that can be confused with HELLP include TTP[28] and the hemolytic-uremic syndrome, sepsis, disseminated intravascular coagulation (DIC), connective tissue disease, antiphospholipid antibody syndrome, and acute fatty liver of pregnancy. This latter entity is also seen in the last trimester or postpartum and presents with thrombocytopenia and right upper quadrant pain, but the levels of AST and ALT only rise to 1 to 5 times normal and the PT and PTT are both prolonged. Oil-red-O staining of liver biopsies demonstrates fat in the cytoplasm of centrilobular hepatocytes, and routine stains show inflammation and patchy hepatocellular necrosis. Because it causes right upper quadrant pain and nausea, HELLP has also been misdiagnosed as viral hepatitis, biliary colic, esophageal reflux, cholecystitis, and gastric cancer. Conversely, other conditions misdiagnosed as HELLP syndrome include cardiomyopathy, dissecting aortic aneurysm, acute cocaine intoxication, essential hypertension and renal disease, and alcoholic liver disease.[19]

THERAPY

Supportive care of HELLP includes intravenous administration of magnesium sulfate to control hypertension and prevent eclamptic seizures, management of fluids and electrolytes, judicious transfusion of blood products, stimulation of fetal lung maturation with beclomethasone, and delivery of the fetus as soon as possible.[19] Indications for delivery include a severe disease presentation, maternal DIC, fetal distress, and a gestational age greater than 32 weeks with evidence of lung maturity.[6] Cesarean section under general anesthesia is used in 60 to 97 percent of cases, but vaginal delivery after induction can be attempted if the fetus is older than 32 weeks of age and the mother's cervical anatomy is favorable. Postpartum curettage is helpful in lowering the mean arterial pressure and increasing the urine output and platelet count. Transfusion therapy with packed red cells, platelets, or fresh-frozen plasma is indicated in cases complicated by severe anemia or bleeding because of coagulopathy.

Adjunctive therapy for HELLP consists of administration of dexamethasone and plasma exchange. Dexamethasone 10 mg intravenously every 12 hours results in increased urine output and platelet counts, decreased AST and LDH levels, and a trend toward reduced neonatal morbidity and mortality.[29] It does not affect the rate of infection or maternal recovery postpartum, and should be continued for at least 2 days following recovery so as to prevent a "rebound" of elevated liver enzymes (including LDH), thrombocytopenia, and oliguria. Plasma exchange cannot arrest or reverse HELLP syndrome when utilized antepartum, but may minimize hemorrhage and morbidity when used peripartum. It can also be tried postpartum in the 5 percent of patients who fail to improve within 72 to 96 hours of delivery. These women are more likely to be younger than 20 years of age or nulliparous.[7] Whether or not plasma exchange can effectively lower circulating levels of sVEGF and/or sEng is not known. Liver transplantation may be necessary in occasional patients with HELLP complicated by large hematomas or total hepatic necrosis.[30] It is not yet known if replacement with some (possibly modified) form of VEGF and/or TGF-β may have future therapeutic use in preeclampsia or HELLP.

■ COURSE AND PROGNOSIS

Most patients stabilize within 24 to 48 hours following delivery; however, maternal death occurs in 3 to 5 percent. Mortality rates as high as 25 percent were reported prior to 1980. Events leading to maternal death include cerebral hemorrhage, cardiopulmonary arrest, DIC, adult respiratory distress syndrome, and hypoxic ischemic encephalopathy.[5] Other complications include infection, placenta abruptio, postpartum hemorrhage, intraabdominal bleeding, and subcapsular liver hematomas with resultant rupture (a fatal event in 50 percent of those in whom it occurs).[6] The latter patients complain of right-sided shoulder pain and are found to be in shock with ascites or pleural effusions. The hematoma is usually present in the anterior superior portion of the right lobe of the liver.[5] If the liver remains intact when discovered, abdominal palpation, seizures, and emesis should be avoided or prevented. Emergency surgery is required for hepatic artery embolization or ligation, hepatic lobectomy, or even liver transplantation in patients with total hepatic necrosis.[5,19]

Renal complications of HELLP include acute renal failure, hyponatremia, and nephrogenic diabetes insipidus as a result of impaired hepatic metabolism of vasopressinase and resultant "resistance to vasopressin" (antidiuretic hormone). Pulmonary complications of HELLP consist of pleural effusions, pulmonary edema, and adult respiratory distress syndrome. Neurologic sequelae of HELLP not mentioned above include retinal detachment, postictal cortical blindness, and hypoglycemic coma.[31]

Fetal morbidity and mortality are approximately 9 to 24 percent.[6] Complications are usually a result of prematurity, placental abruption, and intrauterine asphyxia. Intrauterine growth retardation is seen in 39 percent of infants. One-third of all babies born to mothers with HELLP have thrombocytopenia, but intraventricular hemorrhage is seen in only approximately 4 percent of thrombocytopenic infants.[32]

HELLP syndrome complicates 2 to 5 percent of all pregnancies,[5] and can recur in as many as 27 percent of those affected during subsequent pregnancies.[33] Other hypertensive disorders of pregnancy (preeclampsia or pregnancy-induced hypertension) are also relatively common in future pregnancies (27% of second and subsequent pregnancies).[34] Women who recover from preeclampsia/HELLP may also be more likely to develop subsequent hypertension and cardiovascular disorders, possibly because of some persistent abnormal balance between proangiogenic and antiangiogenic factors.[17]

DISSEMINATED MALIGNANCY

■ DEFINITION AND HISTORY

The association between widespread malignancy and hemolytic anemia associated with pathologic changes in small blood vessels was first noted by Brain and colleagues in 1962.[35]

■ EPIDEMIOLOGY

Cancer-associated microangiopathic hemolytic anemia (MAHA) has been described in a wide variety of malignancies (Table 50–1). MAHA is more likely to be associated with metastatic malignant disease than with localized cancers or benign tumors.[36] Approximately 80 percent of the tumors are mucinous adenocarcinomas of either the stomach (55%), breast (13%), or lung (10%). The median age at diagnosis is 50 years, with a slight male predominance.[37]

TABLE 50–1. Cancers Associated with Microangiopathic Hemolytic Anemia

Gastric (55%)[37,40]
Breast (13%)[129]
Lung (10%)[35]
Other Adenocarcinomas
Unknown primary[38]
Prostate[35]
Colon[38]
Gallbladder
Pancreas
Ovary
Other Malignancies
Hemangiopericytoma[36]
Hepatoma
Melanoma
Small cell cancer of the lung[130]
Testicular cancer
Squamous cell cancer of the oropharynx
Thymoma
Erythroleukemia[131]

■ ETIOLOGY AND PATHOGENESIS

MAHA as a result of malignancy can be caused by either of two distinct mechanisms: (1) DIC with intravascular occlusions (often partial) of small vessels by platelet-fibrin thrombi; or (2) intravascular tumor emboli.[35,38] In the first mechanism,[1] intravascular activation of coagulation may occur from excessive exposure of tissue factor on phagocytes, activated endothelial cells, or tumor cells. Alternatively, a protease in the mucin secreted by adenocarcinomas may directly activate factor X.[39] Subsequent activation of coagulation factors, thrombin generation, fibrin polymer deposition, and platelet aggregation result in the formation of intravascular platelet-fibrin thrombi, and the shearing of red cells attempting to maneuver past the partial platelet-fibrin occlusions in the high-flow microvasculature. Finally, circulating carcinoma mucins may interact with leukocyte L-selectin and platelet P-selectin, causing the rapid generation of platelet-rich microthrombi.[40] In the second mechanism,[2] intravascular tumor emboli partially occlude small vessels, mechanically or chemically disrupt the endothelium and promote platelet adherence to exposed subendothelium, coagulation activation and fibrin polymer formation, intimal hyperplasia, and vascular hypertrophy.[35,37,38]

■ LABORATORY FEATURES

Patients with cancer-associated DIC/MAHA present with moderate-to-severe anemia. The peripheral smear reveals schistocytes (accounting for approximately 5–21% of the red cells), burr cells, microspherocytes, reticulocytes/polychromasia, and nucleated red cells.[38] Although the reticulocyte count may be high, it is an unreliable measure of hemolysis because extensive replacement of the marrow by metastatic tumor (see Chap. 44) may prevent the reticulocytosis expected with MAHA. Other indicators of hemolysis that may be more reliable include increased levels of serum unconjugated bilirubin and LDH, the presence of plasma hemoglobin, and elevated urine urobilinogen and free hemoglobin (as $\alpha\beta$ dimers).[37] Absent or low levels of haptoglobin may also be found; however, haptoglobin is an acute phase reactant that may be increased in malignancy.[38] The direct Coombs test is negative.[37,41]

Additional findings in MAHA include thrombocytopenia, with mean platelet counts of approximately 50,000/μL (range: 3–225/μL),[37] caused by a shortened platelet life span without demonstrable sequestration of platelets in the liver or spleen. Some patients with malignant tumors, however, may have preexisting thrombocytosis, and so superimposed MAHA may reduce the platelet count only toward "normal" values.[38] A normal-to-high white blood cell count with immature myeloid precursors may also be seen.[37,38,41] Leukoerythroblastosis caused by marrow invasion (see Chap. 44), along with MAHA, is highly suggestive of metastatic malignancy.[38] Marrow aspiration and biopsy will demonstrate erythroid hyperplasia, normal-to-high numbers of megakaryocytes, and (in approximately 55% of patients) cancer cells.[41]

Additional laboratory evidence of DIC has been reported in approximately 50 percent of patients with MAHA secondary to malignancy. Findings include reduced levels of fibrinogen (mean: 177 g/dL; range: 8–490 mg/dL), increased levels of D-dimers (or fibrin degradation products), and prolonged prothrombin and thrombin times.[37] In the early phase of DIC, aPTTs may be shortened (e.g., to < 23 seconds).[42–45] It is not known if shortened aPTT values reflect the presence of activated coagulation factors in the plasma, consumption of coagulation inhibitor proteins faster than their production by hepatic cells (e.g., protein C, protein S, antithrombin, tissue factor pathway inhibitor), or the presence in plasma of a cysteine protease capable of directly activating factor X.[39] Cancer-related DIC has been reported to be associated with a deficiency of the VWF-cleaving protease, ADAMTS13.[46] Although this was disputed by some investigators,[47] ADAMTS13 levels gradually decrease in DIC patients with poor survival rates,[48] perhaps as a result of ADAMTS13 consumption onto the long VWF multimeric strings released from cytokine-stimulated endothelial cells.[49]

In comparison, there is an unequivocal decline in plasma ADAMTS13 values during sepsis-induced DIC.[50–53] In this entity, microbial[54] and/or neutrophil[55] proteases may cleave and inactivate circulating ADAMTS13. Levels of ADAMTS13 below approximately 20 to 50 percent of normal[50,51] may be insufficient to cleave the storm of long VWF strings secreted from microvascular endothelial cells stimulated by inflammatory cytokines (interleukins 6 and 8, tumor necrosis factor-α).[49,51,52,56] If plasma ADAMTS13 values fall below approximately 20% of normal, microvascular thrombi and multiorgan failure are more likely.[50] In sepsis/DIC, Gram-negative bacterial proteases may also cleave and inactivate the normally circulating endogenous anticoagulant, tissue factor pathway inhibitor. This latter effect may cause, or contribute to, the overactivation of coagulation in Gram-negative sepsis.[57]

DIFFERENTIAL DIAGNOSIS

The most common cause of anemia in malignancy is anemia of chronic inflammation (see Chap. 37). Other diagnostic considerations include blood loss, myelophthisis as a result of disease metastatic to the marrow (see Chap. 44), DIC/MAHA (see Chap. 130), and autoimmune hemolytic anemia (see Chap. 53). The latter is more often found with lymphoproliferative disease (see Chaps. 97 and 98) but is occasionally seen with carcinoma of the stomach, colon, breast, and cervix.[58] The treatment of cancer can also induce anemia by causing myelosuppression, oxidative hemolysis (doxorubicin, pentostatin), autoimmune hemolysis (cisplatin, chlorambucil, cyclophosphamide, melphalan, teniposide, methotrexate), or thrombotic microangiopathic anemia (mitomycin C, cisplatin, gemcitabine).

THERAPY

Heparin, glucocorticoids, dipyridamole, indomethacin, and ε-aminocaproic acid have all been tried without success for malignancy-associated DIC/MAHA. Plasma infusion and platelet transfusions, sometimes with additional cryoprecipitate containing fibrinogen, may be useful during bleeding episodes associated with prolonged prothrombin and aPTT times, low fibrinogen levels, and thrombocytopenia. Control of the underlying metastatic malignancy, if achievable, may also be beneficial.

COURSE AND PROGNOSIS

MAHA caused by cancer is usually a preterminal event. Life expectancy following diagnosis is 2 to 150 days, with a mean of 21 days.[37,38]

HEART VALVE HEMOLYSIS

DEFINITION AND HISTORY

Anemia arising after cardiac valve replacement was first described in 1954,[59] soon after corrective valvular surgery became possible. This anemia was subsequently shown to be caused by erythrocyte shearing and fragmentation as the red cells traversed the turbulent flow through or around the prosthetic valve.[60] Since then, prevention of irreversible red cell injury has been a goal when designing new prostheses; as a result, the incidence of significant valve-associated hemolysis has declined from 5 to 15 percent in the 1960s and 1970s[61,62] to less than 1 percent with newer-generation prostheses.[63] However, compensated hemolysis can occur with any type of valve prosthesis and can be detected in almost every patient when assayed using appropriate methods.[61,64,65] Additionally, intravascular hemolysis can be seen following mitral valve repair[66] and in unoperated patients with native valvular disease.[61,67]

EPIDEMIOLOGY

A variety of factors can increase the chance of valvular hemolysis: the presence of central or paravalvular regurgitation,[62,68] placement of small valve prostheses with resultant high transvalvular pressure gradients,[62] and regurgitation because of bioprosthetic valve failure, seen especially once the valve is more than 10 to 15 years old.[68] Patients with ball-and-cage valves,[64] bileaflet valves versus tilting disc valves,[69] mechanical valve prostheses versus xenograft tissue prostheses,[70] and double-valve as compared to single-valve replacement,[69] are more likely to experience clinically significant hemolysis. Some studies have found no difference in the degree of hemolysis when comparing aortic and mitral valve prostheses,[65,69] whereas others have found that the aortic location is associated with slightly greater hemolysis than the mitral location.[71–73]

ETIOLOGY AND PATHOGENESIS

Valve-related hemolysis occurs when red cells are exposed to the shearing stresses created by turbulent blood flow through and around a valve prosthesis, impaction against foreign surfaces or cardiac structures such as the wall of the atrial appendage,[68] or large pressure fluctuations between cardiac chambers. A transvalvular pressure gradient of more than 50 torr can generate shearing forces exceeding 4000 dynes/cm^2, more than the 3000 dynes/cm^2 usually needed to cause red cell fragmentation.[74] In a study looking at malfunctioning mitral valve prostheses, sophisticated computer modeling using transesophageal echocardiography demonstrated a maximal shear value of 6000 dynes/cm^2 when the regurgitant jet was divided by a solid structure such as a loose suture or dehisced annuloplasty ring. A maximal shear rate of 4500 dynes/cm^2 was found when the regurgitant jet was suddenly decelerated by a solid structure like the left atrial appendage, or when the blood was regurgitated through a small orifice (< 2 mm in diameter) such as a leaflet perforation or a paravalvular leak.[68] Lack of endothelialization of the prosthetic ring may contribute to the severity of hemolysis following valve repair or replacement, but it is unclear if this is primary or secondary to the high-velocity jet of blood preventing fibrous incorporation of the prosthetic materials.[68,75] Similarly, lack of endothelialization of the Teflon patch can result in clinically significant hemolysis necessitating reoperation following repair of a ventricular septal defect.[76] These sorts of surface interactions appear to be more important at lower shear-stress values (< 1500 dynes/cm^2) when the amount of hemolysis depends more directly on the area of the contact surface and the time of exposure.[77] Additionally, excessive wear of the cloth that covers caged-ball prostheses, such as the Starr-Edwards valve, can cause ballooning of the material into the blood jet, with resultant turbulence and hemolysis.[78] A modified Blalock-Taussig shunt also has been reported to cause hemolytic anemia.[79]

CLINICAL FEATURES

Patients with valve-induced hemolysis can present with symptoms caused by anemia or congestive heart failure, pallor, icterus, and dark urine (described variously as red, brown, or black). Urine excreted during periods of physical activity may be darker than that excreted at rest.[80] Similarly, hemolysis can be exacerbated by supraventricular tachycardia or other tachyarrhythmias and regress once normal sinus rhythm is restored.[81] Valve dysfunction should be suggested by a change in the intensity or quality of a previously audible sound, the appearance of a new murmur, or a change in the characteristics of a preexisting murmur.[82]

LABORATORY FEATURES

Helpful laboratory studies include review of the blood film, which will reveal moderate poikilocytosis, schistocytosis, and polychromasia. The red cells are usually normochromic and normocytic but can occasionally be hypochromic and microcytic as a result of long-standing urinary iron loss[61] and increased erythropoiesis caused by ongoing hemolysis.[62] The reticulocyte count, urine hemosiderin, plasma hemoglobin, and serum levels of total and indirect bilirubin, and LDH can be elevated, whereas the serum haptoglobin will be depressed. Both the number of schistocytes in the blood[61,64] and the elevation of LDH[64,65,83,84] correlate with the severity of hemolysis. Hemoglobinuria is usually seen only in those with particularly severe hemolysis and high LDH levels. There is no correlation between the severity of hemolysis and bilirubin levels, however, and whether the reticulocyte count is helpful in assessing the severity of hemolysis is controversial.[64,65] The aforementioned laboratory tests can be used as a means to determine the degree of hemolysis and to help guide management (Table 50–2).[64]

Red cell labeling studies demonstrate that erythrocyte life span is markedly shortened to between 6 and 9 days.[76,80] Measurement of erythrocyte creatine, a relatively simple but not yet widely available assay, can be performed in lieu of red cell labeling studies. Young erythrocytes contain much higher levels of creatine than older cells. Thus, an increase in erythrocyte creatine represents shortened red cell survival and is significantly correlated with total peak flow velocity across the valve and the severity of any associated hemolysis.[85] When performed, marrow aspiration will be remarkable for erythroid hyperplasia.[75,80] As a result of hemosiderin deposition, magnetic resonance imaging of the kidneys will reveal reduced signal intensity of the renal cortex compared with the medulla on T1- and T2-weighted images, both with and without gadolinium enhancement.[86]

TABLE 50–2. Severity of Prosthetic Valve Hemolysis

	Mild	Moderate	Severe
Hemosiderinuria	Present	Present	Marked
Hemoglobinuria	Absent	Absent	Absent
Schistocytosis	<1%	>1%	>>1%
Reticulocytosis	<5%	>5%	>>5%
Haptoglobin	Decreased	Absent	Absent
LDH	<500 Units/L	>500 Units/L	>>500 Units/L

Adapted from Eyster E, Rothchild J, Mychajliw O.[64]

DIFFERENTIAL DIAGNOSIS

Factors that can promote valve-associated hemolysis or worsen the resultant anemia include iron deficiency (see Chap. 42), because anemia increases cardiac output and shear stress and iron-poor red cells are more fragile than normal; folate deficiency (see Chap. 41) arising from increased erythropoiesis; anemia of chronic disease because of endocarditis; anticoagulant-induced gastrointestinal hemorrhage (see Chaps. 37, 134, and 135); and increased cardiac output as a consequence of strenuous physical exertion.[82]

THERAPY

Appropriate therapy for hemolytic anemia arising from valvular dysfunction consists of iron and folate replacement (if deficient) and surgical repair or replacement of the malfunctioning prosthesis (if indicated).[87] Poor surgical candidates with perivalvular leaks may benefit from percutaneous closure with an Amplatzer occluder device.[88] Adjunctive measures to be tried include β-blockade to slow the velocity of the circulation,[89] erythropoietin therapy to stimulate erythropoiesis further,[90] and pentoxifylline therapy to increase the deformability of red cells.[91]

Although some authors have not found the use of pentoxifylline to be beneficial,[92] several case reports have described amelioration of valve-related hemolysis and resultant decreased need for red cell transfusion in patients receiving pentoxifylline.[93–95] A prospective study of 40 individuals with double (mitral and aortic) valve replacements randomized patients to receive either no treatment or pentoxifylline 400 mg orally three times daily for 120 days. The group who received pentoxifylline had significantly higher hemoglobin and haptoglobin levels, and significantly lower LDH, total and indirect bilirubin, and corrected reticulocyte levels, after 4 months of treatment. Of the nine patients with severe hemolysis (LDH >1500 U/L), six individuals had amelioration or complete resolution of their disease, while three patients' hemolysis persisted unchecked, suggesting that pentoxifylline therapy is beneficial in more than 60 percent of those with valve-related hemolysis.[96]

Between 15 and 30 percent of patients will develop black pigment gallstones following valve surgery, the majority occurring within 6 months of the procedure. Whether this is a result of acute hemolysis associated with use of the heart-lung machine[97] or chronic hemolysis because of the valve replacement itself[98,99] is uncertain; however, therapy with ursodeoxycholic acid 600 mg daily beginning 1 week before surgery significantly decreases the incidence of gallstone formation from approximately 29 percent in those who were left untreated to approximately 8 percent ($P < 0.01$).[100]

COURSE AND PROGNOSIS

Evidence of hemolysis can be seen within days[60] or weeks[64,76,80] following valve surgery. If reoperation is required, reported mortality rates range between 0 and 6 percent,[75,101] and hemolytic anemia can occasionally recur.[60,101]

OTHER CAUSES OF NONIMMUNE HEMOLYSIS

MARCH HEMOGLOBINURIA

In 1881, Fleischer described a German soldier in whom hemoglobinuria was brought on by marching.[102] Although usually reported in young males, no doubt explained by their more frequent participation in severe and prolonged exertion, it can also be seen in women.[103,104] The presenting complaint is passage of dark urine immediately following physical exertion in the upright position, occasionally accompanied by nausea, abdominal cramps, aching in the back or legs, a "stitch in the side," or a burning feeling in the soles of the feet. Physical examination is usually unrevealing, although hepatosplenomegaly and transient jaundice have been rarely reported.[105]

Davidson proved definitively in 1969 that march hemoglobinuria is caused by red cell trauma within the vessels of the soles of the feet, and its severity is influenced by the hardness of the running surface, the distance run, the heaviness of the athlete's stride, and the protective adequacy of his footwear.[105] He also showed that the condition could be prevented by using padded insoles, a finding later substantiated by other authors.[106,107] Hemoglobinuria has also been seen following other types of trauma in activities as diverse as repetitive slapping of the forehead,[108] karate exercises,[109] basketball followed by congo drum playing,[110] and kendo (a Japanese martial art where heavily padded combatants strike each other repeatedly with bamboo swords).[103]

Because the estimated quantity of blood hemolyzed in an average paroxysm is only 6 to 40 mL, anemia is uncommon and if present is usually mild[105]; however repeated episodes can cause iron deficiency, which may lead to or accentuate anemia (see Chap. 42). Morphologic evidence of red cell damage is not seen, although one patient was found to have poikilocytes and occasional "four-leaf clover" cells after exercise.[111] Renal damage is not commonly seen, but cases of acute tubular necrosis and resultant acute renal insufficiency have been described.[112–115]

KASABACH-MERRITT PHENOMENON

First described in 1940,[116] the Kasabach-Merritt phenomenon is a syndrome that usually develops in early childhood, and is characterized by thrombocytopenia, microangiopathic hemolytic anemia, consumptive coagulopathy, and hypofibrinogenemia caused by an enlarging kaposiform hemangioendothelioma or tufted angioma.[117] Kaposiform hemangioendotheliomas are highly aggressive, vascular tumors that occur equally in males and females, and show little tendency to resolve spontaneously. They can be locally invasive but have never been reported to metastasize.[118] Complications can include hemothorax or pericardial effusion.[118,119] It is postulated that endothelial cell abnormalities and vascular stasis lead to activation of platelets and the coagulation cascade within the tumor's vessels, with subsequent depletion of both platelets and clotting factors. Microangiopathic hemolytic anemia results from mechanical trauma sustained by the erythrocytes traversing the tumor's abnormal, partially thrombosed vascular channels.[120]

Although numerous therapies are used, the mortality rate of Kasabach-Merritt phenomenon can be as high as 30 percent.[121] Even though surgical resection is always followed by normalization of hematologic parameters, many lesions are too large to be resected without severe disfigurement. Other treatments include glucocorticoids, interferon-α, antifibrinolytic agents, and the antiplatelet agents ticlopidine and aspirin, low-molecular-weight heparin, embolization, radiation, laser therapy, and chemotherapy utilizing vincristine, cyclophosphamide, actinomycin D, or methotrexate.[117,118,120,122,123]

MISCELLANEOUS

Microangiopathic hemolytic anemia has also been seen in malignant systemic hypertension, pulmonary hypertension, giant cavernous hemangiomas of the liver,[124] and various vasculitides, including Wegener granulomatosis[125,126] and giant cell arteritis.[127] Osmotically induced hemolysis has occurred when distilled water is used as an irrigant during transurethral resection of the prostate.[128]

REFERENCES

1. Stahnke E: Über das Verhalten der Blutplättchen bei Eklampsie. *Zentralbl Gynakol* 46:391, 1922.
2. Pritchard JA, Weisman R Jr, Ratnoff OD, Vosburgh GJ: Intravascular hemolysis, thrombocytopenia and other hematologic abnormalities associated with severe toxemia of pregnancy. *N Engl J Med* 250:89, 1954.
3. Goodlin RC, Cotton DB, Haesslein HC: Severe edema-proteinuria-hypertension gestosis. *Am J Obstet Gynecol* 132:595, 1978.
4. Weinstein L: Syndrome of hemolysis, elevated liver enzymes, and low platelet count: A severe consequence of hypertension in pregnancy. *Am J Obstet Gynecol* 142:159, 1982.
5. Rahman TM, Wendon J: Severe hepatic dysfunction in pregnancy. *Q J Med* 95:343, 2002.
6. Rath W, Faridi A, Dudenhausen JW: HELLP syndrome. *J Perinat Med* 28:249, 2000.
7. Martin JN Jr, Magann EF, Blake PG, et al: Analysis of 454 pregnancies with severe preeclampsia/eclampsia HELLP syndrome using the 3-class system of classification. *Am J Obstet Gynecol* 68:386, 1993.
8. Sibai BM, Ramadan MK, Usta I, et al: Maternal morbidity and mortality in 442 pregnancies with hemolysis, elevated liver enzymes, and low platelets (HELLP syndrome). *Am J Obstet Gynecol* 169:1000, 1993.
9. Zusterzeel PLM, Visser W, Blom HJ, et al: Methylenetetrahydrofolate reductase polymorphisms in preeclampsia and the HELLP syndrome. *Hypertens Pregnancy* 19:299, 2000.
10. Krauss T, Augustin HG, Osmers R, et al: Activated protein C resistance and factor V Leiden in patients with haemolysis, elevated liver enzymes, low platelets syndrome. *Obstet Gynecol* 92:457, 1998.
11. Bozzo M, Carpani G, Leo L, et al: HELLP syndrome and factor V Leiden. *Eur J Obstet Gynecol Reprod Biol* 95:55, 2001.
12. Benedetto C, Marozio L, Salton L, et al: Factor V Leiden and factor II G20210A in preeclampsia and HELLP syndrome. *Acta Obstet Gynecol Scand* 81:1095, 2002.
13. Zhou Y, McMaster M, Woo K, et al: Vascular endothelial growth factor ligands and receptors that regulate human cytotrophoblast survival are dysregulated in severe preeclampsia and hemolysis, elevated liver enzymes, and low platelets syndrome. *Am J Pathol* 160:1405, 2002.
14. Knerr I, Beinder E, Rascher W: Syncytin, a novel human endogenous retroviral gene in human placenta: Evidence for its dysregulation in preeclampsia and HELLP syndrome. *Am J Obstet Gynecol* 186:210, 2002.
15. Levine RJ, Maynard SE, Qian C, et al: Circulating angiogenic factors and the risk of preeclampsia. *N Engl J Med* 350:672, 2004.
16. Widmer M, Villar J, Beniani A, et al: Mapping the theories of preeclampsia and the role of angiogenic factors: A systematic review. *Obstet Gynecol* 109:168, 2007.
17. Mutter WP, Karumanchi SA: Molecular mechanisms of preeclampsia. *Microvasc Res* 75:1, 2008.
18. Kim YN, Lee DS, Jeong DH, et al: The relationship of the level of circulating antiangiogenic factors to the clinical manifestations of preeclampsia. *Prenat Diagn* 29:464, 2009.
19. Magann EF, Martin JN Jr: Twelve steps to optimal management of HELLP syndrome. *Clin Obstet Gynecol* 42:532, 1999.
20. Thiagarajah S, Bourgeois FJ, Harbert GM, Caudle MR: Thrombocytopenia in preeclampsia: Associated abnormalities and management principles. *Am J Obstet Gynecol* 150:1, 1984.
21. Barton JR, Riely CA, Adamed TA, et al: Hepatic histopathologic condition does not correlate with laboratory abnormalities in HELLP syndrome (hemolysis, elevated liver enzymes, and low platelet count). *Am J Obstet Gynecol* 167:1538, 1992.
22. De Boer K, Büller HR, Ten Cate JW, Treffers PE: Coagulation studies in the syndrome of haemolysis, elevated liver enzymes and low platelets. *Br J Obstet Gynaecol* 98:42, 1991.

23. Thorp JM Jr, Gilbert GC II, Moake JL, Bowes WA Jr: von Willebrand factor multimeric levels and patterns in patients with severe preeclampsia. *Obstet Gynecol* 75:163, 1990.
24. Lattuada A, Rossi E, Calzarossa C, et al: Mild to moderate reduction of a von Willebrand factor cleaving protease (ADAMTS13) in pregnant women with HELLP microangiopathic syndrome. *Haematologica* 88:1029, 2003.
25. Molvarec A, Rigo J, Boze T, et al: Increased plasma von Willebrand factor antigen levels but normal von Willebrand factor cleaving protease (ADAMTS13) activity in preeclampsia. *Thromb Haemost* 101:305, 2009.
26. Moake JL: Thrombotic microangiopathies. *N Engl J Med* 347:589, 2002.
27. Thomas EA, Copplestone JA, Dubbins PA, Friend JR: The radiologist cries "HELLP"! *Br J Radiol* 64:964, 1991.
28. Rehberg JF, Briery CM, Hudson WT, et al: Thrombotic thrombocytopenic purpura masquerading as hemolysis, elevated liver enzymes, low platelets (HELLP) syndrome in late pregnancy. *Obstet Gynecol* 108:817, 2006.
29. Magann EF, Bass D, Chauhan SP, et al: Antepartum corticosteroids: Disease stabilization in patients with the syndrome of hemolysis, elevated liver enzymes, and low platelets (HELLP). *Am J Obstet Gynecol* 171:1148, 1994.
30. Erhard J, Lange R, Niebel W, et al: Acute liver necrosis in the HELLP syndrome: Successful outcome after orthotopic liver transplantation. A case report. *Transpl Int* 6:179, 1993.
31. Reubinoff BE, Schenker JG: HELLP syndrome—a syndrome of hemolysis, elevated liver enzymes and low platelet count—complicating preeclampsia-eclampsia. *Int J Gynaecol Obstet* 36:95, 1991.
32. Harms K, Rath W, Herting E, Kuhn W: Maternal hemolysis, elevated liver enzymes, low platelet count, and neonatal outcome. *Am J Perinatol* 12:1, 1995.
33. Sullivan CA, Magann EF, Perry KG Jr, et al: The recurrence risk of the syndrome of hemolysis, elevated liver enzymes, and low platelets: Subsequent pregnancy outcome and long term prognosis. *Am J Obstet Gynecol* 172:125, 1995.
34. van Pampus MG, Wolf H, Mayruhu G, et al: Long-term follow-up in patients with a history of (H)ELLP syndrome. *Hypertens Pregnancy* 20:15, 2001.
35. Brain MC, Dacie JV, Hourihane DO: Microangiopathic haemolytic anemia: The possible role of vascular lesions in pathogenesis. *Br J Haematol* 8:358, 1962.
36. Kupers EC, Friedman NB, Lee S, Wolfstein RS: Metastatic hemangiopericytoma associated with microangiopathic hemolytic anemia: Review and report of a case. *J Am Geriatr Soc* 23:411, 1975.
37. Antman KH, Skarin AT, Mayer RJ, et al: Microangiopathic hemolytic anemia and cancer: A review. *Medicine (Baltimore)* 58:377, 1979.
38. Lohrmann H-P, Adam W, Heymer B, Kubanek B: Microangiopathic hemolytic anemia in metastatic carcinoma. Report of eight cases. *Ann Intern Med* 79:368, 1973.
39. Gordon SG, Cross BA: A factor X-activating cysteine protease from malignant tissue. *J Clin Invest* 67:1665, 1981.
40. Wahrenbrock M, Borsig L, Le D, et al: Selectin-mucin interactions as a probable molecular explanation for the association of Trousseau syndrome with mucinous adenocarcinomas. *J Clin Invest* 112:853, 2003.
41. Lynch EC, Bakken CL, Casey TH, Alfrey CP Jr: Microangiopathic hemolytic anemia in carcinoma of the stomach. *Gastroenterology* 52:88, 1967.
42. Moake JL: Disseminated intravascular coagulation, in *Conn's Current Therapy*, edited by RE Rakel, p 338. WB Saunders, Philadelphia, 1989.
43. Reddy NM, Hall SW, MacKintosh R: Partial thromboplastin time: Prediction of adverse events and poor prognosis by low abnormal values. *Arch Intern Med* 159:2706, 1999.
44. Tripodi A, Chantarangkul V, Martinelli I, et al: A shortened activated partial thromboplastin time is associated with the risk of venous thromboembolism. *Blood* 104:3631, 2004.
45. Lippi G, Favaloro EJ: Activated partial thromboplastin time: New tricks for an old dogma. *Semin Thromb Hemost* 34:604, 2008.
46. Oleksowicz L, Bhagwati N, DeLeon-Fernandez M: Deficient activity of von Willebrand's factor-cleaving protease in patients with disseminated malignancies. *Cancer Res* 59:2244, 1999.
47. Fontana S, Gerritsen HE, Hovinga JK, et al: Microangiopathic haemolytic anaemia in metastasizing malignant tumours is not associated with a severe deficiency of the von Willebrand factor-cleaving protease. *Br J Haematol* 113:100, 2001.
48. Hyun J, Kim HK, Kim JE, et al: Correlation between plasma activity of ADAMTS13 and coagulopathy, and prognosis in disseminated intravascular coagulation. *Thromb Res* 124:75, 2009.
49. Bernardo A, Ball C, Nolasco L, et al: Effects of inflammatory cytokines on the release and cleavage of the endothelial cell-derived ultra-large von Willebrand factor multimers under flow. *Blood* 104:100, 2004.
50. Ono T, Mimuro J, Madoiwa S, et al: Severe secondary deficiency of von Willebrand factor-cleaving protease (ADAMTS13) in patients with sepsis-induced disseminated intravascular coagulation: Its correlation with development of renal failure. *Blood* 107:528, 2006.
51. Nguyen TC, Liu A, Liu L, et al: Acquired ADAMTS13 deficiency in pediatric patients with severe sepsis. *Haematologica* 92:121, 2007.
52. Martin K, Borgel D, Lerolle N, et al: Decreased ADAMTS13 (a disintegrin-like and metalloprotease with thrombospondin type 1 repeats) is associated with a poor prognosis in sepsis-induced organ failure. *Crit Care Med* 35:2375, 2007.
53. Lerolle N, Dunois-Larde C, Badirou I, et al: Von Willebrand factor is a major determinant of ADAMTS13 decrease during mouse sepsis induced by cecum ligation and puncture. *J Thromb Haemost* 7:843, 2009.
54. Chung MC, Popova TG, Jorgensen SC, et al: Degradation of circulating von Willebrand factor and its regulator ADAMTS13 implicated secreted *Bacillus anthracis* metalloproteases in anthrax consumptive coagulopathy. *J Biol Chem* 283:9531, 2008.
55. Song SH, Kim HK, Park MH, Cho HI: Neutrophil CD64 expression is associated with severity and progress of disseminated intravascular coagulation. *Thromb Res* 121:499, 2007.
56. de Mast O, Groot E, Lenting PJ, et al: Hemolysis after mitral valve repair: A report of five cases and literature review. *J Heart Valve Dis* 17:24, 2008.
57. Yun TH, Cott JE, Tapping RI, et al: Proteolytic inactivation of tissue factor pathway inhibitor by bacterial omptins. *Blood* 113:1139, 2009.
58. Ellis LD, Westerman MP: Autoimmune hemolytic anemia and cancer. *JAMA* 193:962, 1965.
59. Rose JC, Hufnagel CA, Fries ED, et al: The hemodynamic alterations produced by plastic valvular prosthesis for severe aortic insufficiency in man. *J Clin Invest* 33:891, 1954.
60. Rodgers BM, Sabiston DC Jr: Hemolytic anemia following prosthetic valve replacement. *Circulation* 39:155, 1969.
61. Marsh GW, Lewis SM: Cardiac haemolytic anaemia. *Semin Hematol* 6:133, 1969.
62. Kloster FE: Diagnosis and management of complications of prosthetic heart valves. *Am J Cardiol* 35:872, 1975.
63. Iguro Y, Moriyama Y, Yamaoka A, et al: Clinical experience of 473 patients with the Omnicarbon prosthetic heart valve. *J Heart Valve Dis* 8:674, 1999.
64. Eyster E, Rothchild J, Mychajliw O: Chronic intravascular hemolysis after aortic valve replacement. *Circulation* 44:657, 1971.
65. Crexells C, Aerichide N, Bonny Y, et al: Factors influencing hemolysis in valve prosthesis. *Am Heart J* 84:161, 1972.
66. Demirsoy E, Yilmaz O, Sirin G, et al: Hemolysis after mitral valve repair; a report of five cases and literature review. *J Heart Valve Dis* 17:24, 2008.
67. Kawase I, Matsuo T, Sasayama K, et al: Hemolytic anemia with aortic stenosis resolved by urgent aortic valve replacement. *Ann Thorac Surg* 86:645, 2008.
68. Garcia MJ, Vandervoort P, Stewart WJ, et al: Mechanisms of hemolysis with mitral prosthetic regurgitation. *J Am Coll Cardiol* 27:399, 1996.
69. Skoularigis J, Essop MR, Skudicky D, et al: Frequency and severity of intravascular hemolysis after left-sided cardiac valve replacement with Medtronic Hall and St. Jude Medical prostheses, and influence of prosthetic type, position, size and number. *Am J Cardiol* 71:587, 1993.
70. Chang H, Lin FY, Hung CR, Chu SH: Chronic intravascular hemolysis after valvular surgery. *J Formos Med Assoc* 89:880, 1990.
71. Yacoub MH, Keeling DH: Chronic haemolysis following insertion of ball valve prostheses. *Br Heart J* 30:676, 1968.
72. Falk RH, Mackinnon J, Wainscoat J, et al: Intravascular haemolysis after valve replacement: Comparative study between Starr-Edwards (ball valve) and Bjork-Shiley (disc valve) prosthesis. *Thorax* 34:746, 1979.
73. Febres-Roman PR, Bourg WC, Crone RA, et al: Chronic intravascular hemolysis after aortic valve replacement with Ionescu-Shiley xenograft: Comparative study with Bjork-Shiley prosthesis. *Am J Cardiol* 46:735, 1980.
74. Nevaril CG, Lynch EC, Alfrey CP, et al: Erythrocyte damage and destruction induced by shearing stress. *J Lab Clin Med* 71:784, 1968.
75. Cerfolio RJ, Orszulak TA, Daly RC, Schaff HV: Reoperation for hemolytic anaemia complicating mitral valve repair. *Eur J Cardiothorac Surg* 11:479, 1997.
76. Sayed HM, Dacie JV, Handley DA, et al: Haemolytic anaemia of mechanical origin after open heart surgery. *Thorax* 16:356, 1961.
77. Leverett LB, Hellums JD, Alfrey CP, Lynch EC: Red blood cell damage by shear stress. *Biophys J* 12:257, 1972.
78. Murakami M, Tanaka H, Watanabe M, et al: Severe hemolysis due to cloth wear 23 years after aortic valve replacement on a Starr-Edwards ball valve model 2320. *Cardiovasc Surg* 10:284, 2002.
79. Ryerson LM, Wechsler SB, Ohye RG: Hemolytic anemia secondary to modified Blalock-Taussig shunt. *Pediatr Cardiol* 28:238, 2007.
80. Sears DA, Crosby WH: Intravascular hemolysis due to intracardiac prosthetic devices. *Am J Med* 39:341, 1965.
81. Papadogiannakis A, Xydakis D, Sfakianaki M, et al: An unusual cause of severe hyperkalemia in a dialysis patient. *J Cardiovasc Med (Hagerstown)* 8:541, 2007.
82. Maraj R, Jacobs LE, Ioli A, Kotler MN: Evaluation of hemolysis in patients with prosthetic heart valves. *Clin Cardiol* 21:387, 1998.
83. Myhre E, Rasmussen K, Andersen A: Serum lactic dehydrogenase activity in patients with prosthetic heart valves: A parameter of intravascular hemolysis. *Am Heart J* 80:463, 1970.
84. Thompson ME, Lewis JH, Prokolab FL, et al: Indexes of intravascular hemolysis quantification of coagulation factors, and platelet survival in patients with porcine heterograft valves. *Am J Cardiol* 51:489, 1983.
85. Okumiya T, Ishikawa-Nishi M, Doi T, et al: Evaluation of intravascular hemolysis with erythrocyte creatine in patients with cardiac valve prostheses. *Chest* 125:2115, 2004.
86. Lee JW, Kim SH, Yoon CJ: Hemosiderin deposition on the renal cortex by mechanical hemolysis due to malfunctioning prosthetic cardiac valve: Report of MR findings in two cases. *J Comput Assist Tomogr* 23:445, 1999.
87. Amidon TM, Chou TM, Rankin JS, Ports TA: Mitral and aortic paravalvular leaks with hemolytic anemia. *Am Heart J* 125:122, 1993.
88. Shapira Y, Hirsch R, Kornowski R, et al: Percutaneous closure of perivalvular leaks with Amplatzer occluders: Feasibility, safety, and short-term results. *J Heart Valve Dis* 16:305, 2007.

89. Okita Y, Miki S, Kusuhara K, et al: Propranolol for intractable hemolysis after open heart operation. *Ann Thorac Surg* 52:1158, 1991.
90. Shapira Y, Bairey O, Vatury M, et al: Erythropoietin can obviate the need for repeated heart valve replacement in high-risk patients with severe mechanical hemolytic anemia: Case reports and literature review. *J Heart Valve Dis* 10:431, 2001.
91. Ward A, Clissold SP: Pentoxifylline: A review of its pharmacodynamic and pharmacokinetic properties, and its therapeutic efficacy. *Drugs* 34:50, 1987.
92. Okita Y, Miki S: Reply to the editor. *Ann Thorac Surg* 54:7, 1992.
93. Jim RT: New therapy for cardiac valve prosthesis caused by microangiopathic hemolytic anemia: A case report. *Hawaii Med J* 47:285, 1988.
94. Golino A, Stassano P, Spampinato N: Hemolysis after open heart operations [letter]. *Ann Thorac Surg* 54:1246, 1992.
95. Geller S, Gelber R: Pentoxifylline treatment for microangiopathic hemolytic anemia caused by mechanical heart valves. *Md Med J* 48:173, 1999.
96. Golbasi I, Turkay C, Timuragaoglu A, et al: The effect of pentoxifylline on haemolysis in patients with double cardiac prosthetic valves. *Acta Cardiol* 58:379, 2003.
97. Azemoto R, Tsuchiya Y, Ai T, et al: Does gallstone formation after open cardiac surgery result only from latent hemolysis by replaced valves? *Am J Gastroenterol* 91:2185, 1996.
98. Merendino KA. Manhas DR: Man-made gallstones: A new entity following cardiac valve replacement. *Ann Surg* 177:694, 1973.
99. Harrison EC, Roschke EJ, Meyers HI, et al: Cholelithiasis: A frequent complication of artificial heart valve replacement. *Am Heart J* 95:483, 1978.
100. Ai T, Azemoto R, Saisho H: Prevention of gallstones by ursodeoxycholic acid after cardiac surgery. *J Gastroenterol* 38:1071, 2003.
101. Lam BK, Cosgrove DM, Bhudia SK, Gillinov AM: Hemolysis after mitral valve repair: Mechanisms and treatment. *Ann Thorac Surg* 77:191, 2004.
102. Fleischer R: Ueber eine neue Form von Haemoglobinurie beim Menschen. *Berl Klin Wschr* 18:691, 1881.
103. Urabe M, Hara Y, Hokama A, et al: A female case of march hemoglobinuria induced by kendo (Japanese fencing) exercise. *Nippon Naika Gakkai Zasshi* 75:1657, 1986.
104. Gilligan A: March hemoglobinuria in a woman. *N Engl J Med* 243:944, 1950.
105. Davidson RJL: March or exertional haemoglobinuria. *Semin Hematol* 6:150, 1969.
106. Buckle RM: Exertional (march) haemoglobinuria: Reduction of haemolytic episodes by use of Sorbo-rubber insoles in shoes. *Lancet* 68:1136, 1965.
107. Sagov SE: March hemoglobinuria treated with rubber insoles: Two case reports. *J Am Coll Health Assoc* 19:146, 1970.
108. Ensor CW, Barrett JOW: Paroxysmal haemoglobinuria of traumatic origin. *Medico-Chirurgical Trans* 86:165, 1903.
109. Streeton JA: Traumatic haemoglobinuria caused by karate exercises. *Lancet* 2:191, 1967.
110. Schwartz KA, Flessa HC: March hemoglobinuria. Report of a case after basketball and congo drum playing. *Ohio State Med J* 69:448, 1973.
111. Watson EM, Fischer LC: Paroxysmal "march" haemoglobinuria with a report of a case. *Am J Clin Pathol* 5:151, 1935.
112. Pollard TD, Weiss IW: Acute tubular necrosis in a patient with march hemoglobinuria. *N Engl J Med* 283:803, 1970.
113. Susa S, Dumovic B, Pantovic R: March hemoglobinuria associated with acute renal failure. *Vojnosanit Pregl* 29:407, 1972.
114. Ciko Z, Radojicic B, Lazic D: Pathogenesis of acute renal insufficiency in march hemoglobinuria. *Vojnosanit Pregl* 30:198, 1973.
115. Yashpal M, Abdulkader TA, Chatterji JC: Acute tubular necrosis in march haemoglobinuria. *J Assoc Physicians India* 28:145, 1980.
116. Kasabach HH, Merritt KK: Capillary hemangioma with extensive purpura: Report of a case. *Am J Dis Child* 59:1063, 1940.
117. Haisley-Royster C, Enjolras O, Frieden IJ, et al: Kasabach-Merritt phenomenon: A retrospective study of treatment with vincristine. *J Pediatr Hematol Oncol* 24:459, 2002.
118. San Miguel FL, Spurbeck W, Budding C, Horton J: Kaposiform hemangioendothelioma: A rare cause of spontaneous hemothorax in infancy. Review of the literature. *J Pediatr Surg* 43:E37, 2008.
119. Walsh MA, Carcao M, Pope E, Lee K-J: Kaposiform hemangioendothelioma presenting antenatally with a pericardial effusion. *J Pediatr Hematol Oncol* 30:761, 2008.
120. Ortel TL, Onorato JJ, Bedrosian CL, Kaufman RE: Antifibrinolytic therapy in the management of the Kasabach Merritt syndrome. *Am J Hematol* 29:44, 1988.
121. Esterly NB: Kasabach-Merritt syndrome in infants. *J Am Acad Dermatol* 8:504, 1983.
122. Hall GW: Kasabach-Merritt syndrome: Pathogenesis and management. *Br J Haematol* 112:851, 2001.
123. Hauer J, Graubner U, Konstantopoulos N, et al: Effective treatment of kaposiform hemangioendotheliomas associated with Kasabach-Merritt phenomenon using four-drug regimen. *Pediatr Blood Cancer* 49:852, 2006.
124. Shimizu M, Miura J, Itoh H, Saitoh Y: Hepatic giant cavernous hemangioma with microangiopathic hemolytic anemia and consumption coagulopathy. *Am J Gastroenterol* 85:1411, 1990.
125. Crummy CS, Perlin E, Moquin RB: Microangiopathic hemolytic anemia in Wegener's granulomatosis. *Am J Med* 51:544, 1971.
126. Jordan JM, Manning M, Allen NB: Multiple unusual manifestations of Wegener's granulomatosis: Breast mass, microangiopathic hemolytic anemia, consumptive coagulopathy, and low erythrocyte sedimentation rate. *Arthritis Rheum* 29:1527, 1986.
127. Zauber NP, Echikson AB: Giant cell arteritis and microangiopathic hemolytic anemia. *Am J Med* 73:928, 1982.
128. Chen SS, Lin AT, Chen KK, Chang LS: Hemolysis in transurethral resection of the prostate using distilled water as the irrigant. *J Chin Med Assoc* 69:270, 2006.
129. Stratford EC, Tanaka KR: Microangiopathic hemolytic anemia in metastatic carcinoma. Report of a case and biochemical studies. *Arch Intern Med* 116:346, 1965.
130. Davis S, Rambotti P, Grignani F, Steinhouse K: Microangiopathic hemolytic anemia and pulmonary small-cell carcinoma [letter]. *Ann Intern Med* 103:638, 1985.
131. Atkins JN, Muss HB: Case report: Schistocytes in erythroleukemia. *Am J Med Sci* 289:110, 1985.

CHAPTER 51

HEMOLYTIC ANEMIA RESULTING FROM CHEMICAL AND PHYSICAL AGENTS

Brian S. Bull and Paul C. Herrmann

SUMMARY

Circulating erythrocyte numbers may be decreased by intravascular hemolysis or by sequestration of red cells followed by their destruction within the mononuclear phagocytic system. The mechanisms of intravascular hemolysis from physical or chemical agents include hypotonic lysis, pore formation within the erythrocyte membrane by a broad range of biotoxins, and heat damage to the spectrin skeleton.

Extravascular sequestration and destruction are initiated by oxidizing agents such as oxygen, arsine gas, and chlorates. Allied mechanisms appear to be responsible for erythrocytolysis and for neocytolysis, the selective destruction of young red cells, a phenomenon unique to microgravity.

In addition, hemolysis can be induced by other agents, although their mechanism of action has not been defined. Table 51–1 lists some of these agents. Descriptions of erythrocyte damage caused by lead, copper, and radiation are also included in the text.

MECHANISMS OF HEMOLYSIS

There are two principle means by which circulating red cells may be removed other than by bleeding (see Chap. 32). The first is intravascular hemolysis. The second is red cell sequestration and destruction by the mononuclear phagocytic system.

Chaps. 46 and 48 discuss the hemolysis that results when certain drugs are administered to patients deficient in glucose-6-phosphate dehydrogenase (G-6-PD) or with unstable hemoglobins. Immune mechanisms may also play a role in drug- or toxin-induced hemolytic anemias, and are discussed in Chap. 53. Microangiopathic hemolytic anemias (see Chap. 50) can also be caused by drugs such as mitomycin. The present chapter deals with drugs, toxins, and other physical agents that can cause red cell destruction, which are not discussed in other chapters.

HEMOLYSIS CAUSED BY INTRAVASCULAR MECHANISMS

HYPOTONIC LYSIS

When large amounts of distilled water gain access to the systemic circulation, either by intravenous injection or when used as an irrigating solution during surgery, hemolysis will occur.[1] Severe hemolysis may also result from water inhalation in near-drowning.[2] Another rare, but not insignificant, example is hypotonic lysis secondary to water intoxication which occurs from polydipsia in the setting of psychiatric illness or hazing rituals.[3]

PORE FORMATION WITHIN THE RED BLOOD CELL MEMBRANE

Bee[4,5] and wasp[6–8] stings are associated with severe hemolysis, and spider or scorpion bites occasionally are followed by hemolytic anemia and hemoglobinuria.[9–14] Sometimes this may occur without a discernible skin lesion.[15] The spiders usually responsible are *Loxosceles laeta* and *L. recluse* with sphingomyelinase D as the causative toxin. The venom preferentially hydrolyzes band 3 of the red cell membrane protein.[16] It is unclear why some people are susceptible to hemolysis when exposed to such venom, whereas other individuals are not. Regardless, the hemolysis is mediated by complement through the direct association of C1q with the erythrocyte membrane.[17]

One of the most intriguing mechanisms of hemolysis is that induced by a class of pore forming cytotoxins. A bacterial source (*Bacillus cereus*)[18] is responsible for most human cases. Toxins resulting in similar mechanisms of hemolysis are found in a number of marine organisms such as sea cucumbers (*Cucumaria echinata*)[19] and sea anemones (*Stichodactyla helianthus*).[20] X-ray crystallography reveals these toxins to be composed of a number of associated proteins that span the erythrocyte membrane forming an ion permeable pore.[19] The ensuing hemolysis affects aged cells to a greater extent than young cells.

DAMAGE TO SKELETAL OR STRUCTURAL PROTEINS

It has been known for more than 100 years that heating blood to temperatures above 47°C rapidly produces visible damage to erythrocytes (Fig. 51–1A). The sequence of events has been defined in detail.[21] Cells damaged by heating show morphologic changes and increases in osmotic and mechanical fragility.[22] These observations explain the severe hemolytic anemia that occurs in patients with extensive burns. Spherocytosis and increased osmotic fragility are found in many patients, and blood films may show fragmentation, budding, spherocytosis, and severe microspherocytosis. These changes are particularly evident if films are made promptly after the burn occurs. Alterations of red cell lipids have been documented,[23] but it is not clear whether these play any physiologic role in erythrocyte survival. Gross hemoglobinemia was observed in 11 of 40 patients with second- and third-degree burns involving 15 to 65 percent of the body surface area.[24] It seems likely that the acute hemolytic anemia occurring within the first 24 hours following a burn results from the direct effect of heat on circulating erythrocytes. However, splenic sequestration may also play a role as suggested by the fact that heat-damaged, but intact, cells are rapidly removed when reinjected into the circulation.[22] Hemolysis occurring more than 24 hours after the burn may result from the infusion of isoagglutinins (particularly anti-A) in pooled plasma, when patients receive plasma for therapeutic reasons.[25] Alternatively, the hemolysis may be the result of the septicemia or disseminated intravascular coagulation that are common complications of extensive burn injury.

In addition to acute lytic damage, heat can shorten the erythrocyte's normal survival time. When heated, the spectrin comprising the erythrocyte skeleton melts and spectrin's molecular architecture becomes randomized. Upon cooling, the randomized architecture becomes rigid.[26] This rigidity prevents the membrane from rotating around the cell contents.[27] A normal erythrocyte in a flowing fluid behaves physically as a drop of fluid[28] because the flexible membrane allows the surface of the cell to rotate around the intracellular contents. Because of

Acronyms and abbreviations that appear in this chapter include: AsH_3, arsenic hydride (arsine gas); EDTA, ethylenediaminetetraacetic acid; G-6-PD, glucose-6-phosphate dehydrogenase; HFE, hemochromatosis gene; NADPH, reduced nicotinamide adenine dinucleotide phosphate.

TABLE 51–1. Drugs and Chemicals That Have Been Reported to Cause Hemolytic Anemia

Chemicals	Drugs
Aniline[95]	Amyl nitrite[103,104]
Apiol[96]	Mephenesin[105]
Dichlorprop (herbicide)[97]	Methylene blue[106,107]
Formaldehyde[49]	Omeprazole[108]
Hydroxylamines[98]	Pentachlorophenol[109]
Lysol[99]	Phenazopyridine (Pyridium)[110,111]
Mineral spirits[100]	Salicylazosulfapyridine (Azulfidine)[112,113]
Nitrobenzene[101]	Tacrolimus[114]
Resorcin[102]	

the normal erythrocyte's fluid-like properties, collisional kinetic energy is coupled to the viscous hemoglobin solution within the cell allowing large amounts of collisional energy to be dissipated through the entire cell. This protects the membrane from the damage that would ensue from undissipated energy localized only to the membrane. The rigidity of a previously heated red cell membrane prevents this coupling of kinetic energy to the intracellular contents, forcing the membrane to absorb it in total. Repeated assault by such concentrated kinetic energy results in serious membrane damage, shortening the red cell life span.

Although snake venom may cause hemolysis *in vitro* by converting lecithin to lysolecithin (see Chap. 45), hemolysis rarely results from a snake bite,[29] and when it does occur, it may represent microangiopathic hemolytic anemia associated with coagulation abnormalities induced by the venom.[30]

HEMOLYSIS CAUSED BY EXTRAVASCULAR SEQUESTRATION AND DESTRUCTION MECHANISMS

■ OXIDANT DAMAGE

Oxygen is a powerful oxidizing agent. Fortunately, biologic membranes are protected from spontaneous oxidation as a result of a reaction barrier imposed by subtle quantum mechanical properties of the oxygen molecule.[31] The binding interaction of oxygen with hemoglobin involves a significant change in the quantum properties of the oxygen molecule[32] and consequently an exceptionally reactive superoxide molecule occasionally escapes, leaving behind oxidized hemoglobin. A number of enzyme systems are present within the red cell to protect the cell from superoxide, without which it is estimated that 2 to 3 percent of the total hemoglobin would be oxidized daily.[33,34] These enzyme systems include superoxide dismutase which converts superoxide to hydrogen peroxide. Catalase, glutathione peroxidase and peroxiredoxins detoxify the hydrogen peroxide by dismutation, coupling to glutathione and the reduced form of nicotinamide adenine dinucleotide phosphate (NADPH) respectively. Although the hemolysis that occurs when these systems are overwhelmed by a high oxidant load or decreased enzyme capacity is largely dealt with elsewhere (see Chap. 46), a few subtle and often overlooked examples are briefly described below.

Oxygen Gas (O_2)

Hemolytic anemia can occur in settings in which ambient oxygen concentration is increased markedly. In astronauts exposed to 100 percent oxygen, hemolytic anemia has been observed.[35] Also, in at least one patient, hyperbaric oxygenation was associated with acute hemolysis.[36] Hemolysis in this instance may have resulted from abnormal peroxidation of lipids in the erythrocytes, but evidence supporting this view was indirect and equivocal. Ozone, which has been widely used in some countries for a variety of therapeutic purposes, had no effect on red cell enzymes and intermediates at the 30 mcg/mL concentration commonly infused, but did produce some *in vitro* hemolysis at that concentration.[37]

Arsenic Hydride

Arsenic exposure is a major cause of anemia in regions of the world with high environmental contamination. Examples include Bangladesh's tainted water supply,[38] as well as areas of China where coal containing high concentrations of arsenic is burned as fuel. The most erythrotoxic form of arsenic appears to be arsine gas. The inhalation of arsine gas (arsenic hydride, AsH_3) is a well-recognized cause of hemolytic anemia (see Fig. 51–1B).[39–41] Arsine is formed during many industrial processes. Most commonly, it results from the reaction of hydrogen, which has been generated by the action of acid on metal, with available arsenic compounds. The arsenic is usually present as a contaminant of either the acid or the metal, so that the contact with arsenic compounds

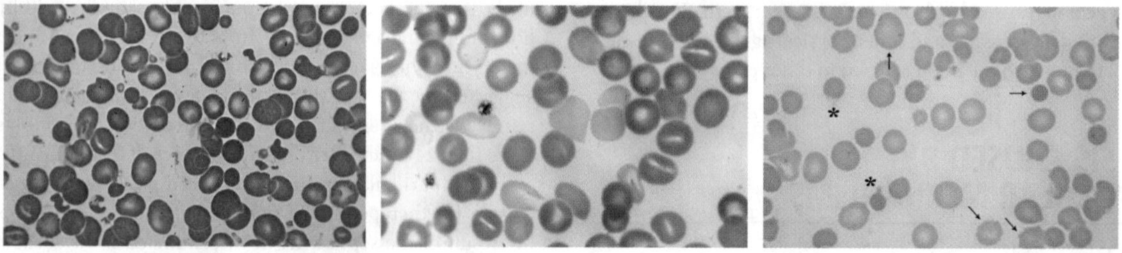

A B C

FIGURE 51–1. A. Blood film prepared at admission from a patient who had suffered severe burn injury involving a large percentage of the body surface. Note the presence of normal erythrocytes (apparently from vessels not exposed to heat damage) along with populations of normocytic and microcytic spherocytes. In addition, there are numerous red cell fragments, some smaller than platelets. **B.** Blood film prepared from a patient exposed to arsenic hydride. Note the very pale red cells resulting from partial hemoglobin loss secondary to membrane damage. An extreme example, represented by the virtual ghost thinly rimmed with scant residual hemoglobin, can be found in the upper left-hand corner. **C.** Wilson disease. In this image from a patient with Wilson disease, there are numerous visible sequelae of oxidative damage caused by excess copper. The striking microspherocytosis indicates damage to the membrane. Damage to hemoglobin is demonstrated by the Heinz bodies projecting from red cells (*asterisks* show two examples). The *horizontal arrow* points to one of several spherocytes. The *vertical arrow* points to a macrocyte (reticulocyte). An occasional cell shows damage to both membrane and hemoglobin. The presence of echinocytes (*oblique arrows* show two examples) suggests that the liver is also affected. *(Used with permission from* Lichtman's Atlas of Hematology, *www.accessmedicine.com. Image* **C** *was kindly provided for the* Atlas *by Barbara J. Bain, Imperial College, London, UK.)*

may not be apparent from the history. Exposure to sufficient amounts of the gas will lead to severe anemia, jaundice, and hemoglobinuria. The mechanism of hemolysis appears to occur via oxidation of sulfhydryl groups in the erythrocyte membrane and associated cytoskeleton as the effect can be inhibited *in vitro* with compounds that reduce dithiols.[42,43] Additional evidence for an oxidative mechanism is the demonstration of decreased levels of reduced glutathione in erythrocytes exposed to AsH_3.[44]

Chlorates

Sodium and potassium chlorate are oxidative drugs that produce methemoglobinemia, Heinz bodies, and hemolytic anemia.[45] While it has been presumed that the mechanism of hemolysis is similar to that resulting from other oxidative drugs, enigmatically, no cases have been observed in patients deficient in G-6-PD. The rare instances of chlorate poisoning that have been reported usually resulted from prescription errors in which sodium chlorate was dispensed instead of sodium chloride.[46] Hemolytic anemia with Heinz body formation has also occurred in patients undergoing dialysis when the water contained a substantial amount of chloramines. Oxidative damage to the red cells of these patients was demonstrated by the presence of Heinz bodies, a positive ascorbate-cyanide test, and methemoglobinemia.[47,48] Leaching of formaldehyde from plastic used in water filters employed for hemodialysis is also a cause of hemolytic anemia. The effect of the low levels of formaldehyde found in the water was not mediated through a fixative effect but rather by inducing metabolic changes in the red cells.[49]

ERYTHROCYTOLYSIS: CELL SUICIDE

Chap. 29 provides a detailed description of erythrocytolysis (eryptosis). Briefly, eryptosis causes opsonization of damaged erythrocytes for ingestion and destruction by macrophages. In addition to global environmental insults such as osmotic shock and oxidative stress, certain toxic ions, including gold and aluminum, may act through eryptosis.[50,51]

Neocytolysis

Astronauts experience significant anemia after space flight even in the presence of normal ambient oxygen concentration. The mechanism depends on central pooling of blood in microgravity with an associated decrease in erythropoietin. Radiolabeling studies of erythrocytes indicated that the anemia was caused by selective hemolysis of young erythrocytes less than 12 days old. Further investigation and speculation suggest that decreased erythropoietin concentration is responsible for the hemolysis. Because erythropoietin inhibits eryptosis, and eryptosis is a mechanism predominantly affecting young cells, eryptosis may be the mechanism underlying the neocytolysis phenomenon. In addition to space flight, neocytolysis is related to the anemia associated with renal failure or which results when high-altitude dwellers relocate to sea level.[52,53]

UNKNOWN AND MISCELLANEOUS MECHANISMS

CHEMICAL AND PHYSICAL AGENTS NOT PREVIOUSLY CLASSIFIED

A variety of chemical and physical agents cause hemolytic anemia through unknown or not well-characterized mechanisms. There are isolated reports of hemolytic anemia occurring after the administration of a variety of chemical substances (Table 51–1). Hemolytic anemia produced by phenazopyridine is often associated with "bite cells" and "blister cells".[54] In addition to the list in Table 51–1, the salient features of anemia associated with lead, copper, and radiation exposure are briefly described below.

Lead

Lead poisoning (plumbism) has been recognized since antiquity. The ingestion of beverages containing lead leached from highly soluble lead glazes or earthenware containers has been blamed for the decline and fall of the Roman aristocracy and is even now an occasional cause of lead intoxication.[55] The distillation of alcohol in leaded flasks is another rare cause of plumbism in certain areas, although the practice was prohibited in 1723 by the Massachusetts Bay Colony after it was noticed that consumption of rum so distilled resulted in abdominal pain known as the "dry gripes."[55] Among the earliest published descriptions of lead poisoning is a letter written in 1786 by Benjamin Franklin,[56,57] who had learned as a printer that working over small furnaces with melted lead or drying racks of wet lead type in front of a fire might cause pain in the hands.

Today, lead intoxication in children generally results from ingestion of flaking lead paint or from chewing lead-painted articles. In 1998, 8 percent of U.S. children were affected. By 2004, the latest date for which data are available, this had dropped to 1 percent.[58] Lead poisoning tends to be more severe in iron-deficient children, even when appropriate corrections are made for differing exposure.[59] Conversely a negative influence of *HFE* mutations on blood lead levels has been found.[60] In adults, lead poisoning occurs primarily as the result of inhalation of lead compounds used or produced in industrial processes[61] such as battery manufacture,[62] or as a result of leaching from pottery or dishes that come in contact with food.[63,64] Restoring tapestries and producing pottery and tiles[65,66] also can cause lead poisoning.

Modest shortening of red cell life span is a relatively constant feature of the disorder.[67,68] *In vitro* treatment of red cells with lead produces membrane damage. Lead interferes with the cation pump,[69,70] possibly inhibiting membrane adenosine triphosphatase.[71,72] It is not at all clear, however, that the hemolysis observed in lead poisoning is caused by these changes. A mechanism involving free radicals and Fenton type chemistry around the iron atoms of hemoglobin has been proposed.[73] In some children with lead poisoning, an electrophoretically fast moving hemoglobin indistinguishable from hemoglobin A_3 comprises approximately 15 percent of the total pigment.[74]

Generally, the anemia of lead intoxication is not primarily a result of hemolysis. Lead interferes with the normal production of erythrocytes, probably through a combination of mechanisms. Inhibition of activity of the hexose monophosphate shunt has been documented. However, it is suggested that hemolysis may play some role in the anemia associated with lead intoxication.[75]

Examination of the blood often provides the key diagnostic clue to lead poisoning, and thus the hematologic findings are of special interest. Remarkably complete observations of the acute hematologic changes occurring after the intravenous injection of lead in an attempt to treat malignant disease were published in 1928.[76] Distortion of red cells was observed both in blood films and in wet preparations made immediately after infusion of lead. The anemia of chronic lead poisoning is usually mild in the adult, but is frequently more severe in children. A relatively close relationship exists between blood lead levels and the hematocrit.[77] The red cells are normocytic and slightly hypochromic. The hypochromia may result from coexisting iron deficiency.[78] Basophilic stippling of the erythrocytes may be fine or coarse, and the number of granules seen in each cell may be quite variable. When blood is collected in ethylenediaminetetraacetic acid (EDTA; "purple top" tube), as is commonly done, the stippling may disappear.[79] Young polychromatophilic cells are most likely to be stippled. Electron microscopic studies have demonstrated that the basophilic granules represent abnormally aggregated ribosomes.[80] Ringed sideroblasts are frequently found in the marrow (see Chaps. 29 and 58). Iron-laden mitochondria are present[80] but do not appear to contribute to the basophilic stippling that is observed on light microscopy.

Meso-2,3-dimercaptosuccinic acid, an orally administered chelating agent, has been used to treat lead poisoning.[81,82]

Copper

Hemolysis has also resulted from ingestion of copper sulfate in suicide attempts and from accumulation of toxic amounts from hemodialysis fluid contaminated by copper pipes.[83,84] Hemolysis in Wilson disease has been attributed to the elevated plasma copper levels characteristic of that disorder.[85–87] Spherocytic hemolytic anemia with a hematocrit below 25 percent may be the presenting symptom (see Fig. 51–1C).[88] The pathogenesis of this hemolytic anemia may be related to oxidation of intracellular glutathione, hemoglobin, and NADPH, along with inhibition of G-6-PD by copper.[89] However, the amount of copper required to inhibit G-6-PD is large, and copper in much lower concentrations inhibits pyruvate kinase,[90] hexokinase, phosphogluconate dehydrogenase, phosphofructokinase, and phosphoglycerate kinase activities, suggesting the hemolysis may result from global metabolic insult.[91] Plasma exchange has been used successfully to treat the hemolytic anemia of Wilson disease.[92]

Radiation

Although decreased red cell survival is part of the complex series of events occurring after administration of large doses of total body radiation,[93] erythrocytes appear to be very resistant to the direct effects of radiation.[94] Such shortened red cell survival as may occur after radiation is probably related largely to red cell loss through internal bleeding and to various secondary events such as infection.

REFERENCES

1. Landsteiner EK, Finch CA: Hemoglobinemia accompanying transurethral resection of the prostate. *N Engl J Med* 237:310, 1947.
2. Rath CE: Drowning hemoglobinuria. *Blood* 8:1099, 1953.
3. Farrell DJ, Bower L: Fatal water intoxication. *J Clin Pathol* 56:803, 2003.
4. Bresolin NL, Carvalho FLC, Goes JEC, et al: Acute renal failure following massive attack by Africanized bee stings. *Pediatr Nephrol* 17:625, 2002.
5. Dacie JV: *The Hæmolytic Anæmias: Congenital and Acquired*, 2d ed. Grune & Stratton, New York, 1960.
6. Monzon C, Miles J: Hemolytic-anemia following a wasp sting. *J Pediatr* 96:1039, 1980.
7. Schulte KL, Kochen MM: Hemolytic-anemia in an adult after a wasp sting. *Lancet* 2:478, 1981.
8. Vachvanichsanong P, Dissaneewate P, Mitarnun W: Non-fatal acute renal failure due to wasp stings in children. *Pediatr Nephrol* 11:734, 1997.
9. Barretto OC, Cardoso JL, Decillo D: Viscerocutaneous form of loxoscelism and erythrocyte glucose-6-phosphate deficiency. *Rev Inst Med Trop Sao Paulo* 27:264, 1985.
10. Chadha JS, Leviav A: Hemolysis, renal-failure, and local necrosis following scorpion sting. *JAMA* 241:1038, 1979.
11. Madrigal GC, Wenzl JE, Ercolani RL: Toxicity from a bite of brown spider (*Loxosceles reclusus*)—Skin necrosis, hemolytic anemia, and hemoglobinuria in a 9-year-old child. *Clin Pediatr (Phila)* 11:641, 1972.
12. Nance WE: Hemolytic anemia of necrotic arachnidism. *Am J Med* 31:801, 1961.
13. Wasserman GS, Siegel C: Loxoscelism (brown recluse spider bites)—Review of the literature. *Clin Toxicol* 14:353, 1979.
14. Wright SW, Wrenn KD, Murray L, Seger D: Clinical presentation and outcome of brown recluse spider bite. *Ann Emerg Med* 30:28, 1997.
15. Hostetler MA, Dribben W, Wilson DB, Grossman WJ: Sudden unexplained hemolysis occurring in an infant due to presumed *Loxosceles* envenomation. *J Emerg Med* 25:277, 2003.
16. Barretto OC, Satake M, Nonoyama K, Cardoso JLC: The calcium-dependent protease of *Loxosceles* gaucho venom acts preferentially upon red cell band 3 transmembrane protein. *Braz J Med Biol Res* 36:309, 2003.
17. Tambourgi DV, Pedrosa MF, de Andrade RM, et al: Sphingomyelinases D induce direct association of C1q to the erythrocyte membrane causing complement mediated autologous haemolysis. *Mol Immunol* 44:576, 2007.
18. Fagerlund A, Lindback T, Storset AK, et al: *Bacillus cereus* Nhe is a pore-forming toxin with structural and functional properties similar to the ClyA (HlyE, SheA) family of haemolysins, able to induce osmotic lysis in epithelia. *Microbiology* 154:693, 2008.
19. Uchida T, Yamasaki T, Eto S, et al: Crystal structure of the hemolytic lectin CEL-III isolated from the marine invertebrate *Cucumaria echinata*: Implications of domain structure for its membrane pore-formation mechanism. *J Biol Chem* 279:37133, 2004.
20. Celedon G, Gonzalez G, Barrientos D, et al: Stycholysin II, a cytolysin from the sea anemone *Stichodactyla helianthus* promotes higher hemolysis in aged red blood cells. *Toxicon* 51:1383, 2008.
21. Ham TH, Shen SC, et al: Studies on the destruction of red blood cells; thermal injury; action of heat in causing increased spheroidicity, osmotic and mechanical fragilities and hemolysis of erythrocytes; observations on the mechanisms of destruction of such erythrocytes in dogs and in a patient with a fatal thermal burn. *Blood* 3:373, 1948.
22. Wagner HN, Gaertner RA, Feagin OT, et al: Removal of erythrocytes from circulation. *Arch Intern Med* 110:90, 1962.
23. Pratt VC, Tredget EE, Clandinin MT, Field CJ: Fatty acid content of plasma lipids and erythrocyte phospholipids are altered following burn injury. *Lipids* 36:675, 2001.
24. Shen SC, Ham TH, Fleming EM: Studies on the destruction of red blood cells. III. Mechanism and complications of hemoglobinuria in patients with thermal burns: Spherocytosis and increased osmotic fragility of red blood cells. *N Engl J Med* 229:701, 1943.
25. Topley E, Bull JP, Maycock WD, et al: The relation of the isoagglutinins in pooled plasma to the haemolytic anaemia of burns. *J Clin Pathol* 16:79, 1963.
26. Bull BS, Brailsford JD: Red-cell membrane deformability—New data. *Blood* 48:663, 1976.
27. Bull B: Red-cell biconcavity and deformability—Macromodel based on flow chamber observations. *Nouv Rev Fr Hematol* 12:835, 1972.
28. Schmid-Schonbein H, Wells R: Fluid drop-like transition of erythrocytes under shear. *Science* 165:288, 1969.
29. Reid HA: Cobra bites. *Br Med J* 2:540, 1964.
30. Gillissen A, Theakston RDG, Barth J, et al: Neurotoxicity, hemostatic disturbances and hemolytic-anemia after a bite by a Tunisian saw-scaled or carpet viper (*Echis pyramidum-complex*)—Failure of antivenom treatment. *Toxicon* 32:937, 1994.
31. Taube H: Mechanisms of oxidation with oxygen. *J Gen Physiol* 49:29, 1965.
32. Collman JP, Hermann PC, Fu L, et al: Aza-crown capped porphyrin models of myoglobin: Studies of the steric interactions of gas binding. *J Am Chem Soc* 119:3481, 1997.
33. Harris JW, Kellermeyer RW: *The Red Cell: Production, Metabolism, Destruction: Normal and Abnormal*. Rev. ed. Harvard University Press, Cambridge, MA, 1970.
34. Bunn HF, Forget BG: *Hemoglobin—Molecular, Genetic, and Clinical Aspects*. WB Saunders, Philadelphia, 1986.
35. Tavassoli M: Anemia of spaceflight. *Blood* 60:1059, 1982.
36. Mengel CE, Kann HE Jr, Heyman A, Metz E: Effects of *in vivo* hyperoxia on erythrocytes. II. Hemolysis in a human after exposure to oxygen under high pressure. *Blood* 25:822, 1965.
37. Zimran A, Wasser G, Forman L, et al: Effect of ozone on red blood cell enzymes and intermediates. *Acta Haematol* 102:148, 1999.
38. Biswas D, Banerjee M, Sen G, et al: Mechanism of erythrocyte death in human population exposed to arsenic through drinking water. *Toxicol Appl Pharmacol* 230:57, 2008.
39. Mahmud H, Foller M, Lang F: Arsenic-induced suicidal erythrocyte death. *Arch Toxicol* 83:107, 2009.
40. Phoon WH, Chan MO, Goh CH, et al: Five cases of arsine poisoning. *Ann Acad Med Singapore* 13:394, 1984.
41. Romeo L, Apostoli P, Kovacic M, et al: Acute arsine intoxication as a consequence of metal burnishing operations. *Am J Ind Med* 32:211, 1997.
42. Rael LT, Ayala-Fierro F, Carter DE: The effects of sulfur, thiol, and thiol inhibitor compounds on arsine-induced toxicity in the human erythrocyte membrane. *Toxicol Sci* 55:468, 2000.
43. Winski SL, Barber DS, Rael LT, Carter DE: Sequence of toxic events in arsine-induced hemolysis in vitro: Implications for the mechanism of toxicity in human erythrocytes. *Fundam Appl Toxicol* 38:123, 1997.
44. Blair PC, Thompson MB, Bechtold M, et al: Evidence for oxidative damage to red blood cells in mice induced by arsine gas. *Toxicology* 63:25, 1990.
45. Eysseric H, Vincent F, Peoc'h M, et al: A fatal case of chlorate poisoning: Confirmation by ion chromatography of body fluids. *J Forensic Sci* 45:474, 2000.
46. Jackson RC, Mcdonnell H, Elder WJ: Sodium-chlorate poisoning—Complicated by acute renal failure. *Lancet* 2:1381, 1961.
47. Caterson RJ, Savdie E, Raik E, et al: Heinz-body hemolysis in hemodialyzed patients caused by chloramines in Sydney tap water. *Med J Aust* 2:367, 1982.
48. Eaton JW, Kolpin CF, Swofford HS, et al: Chlorinated urban water—Cause of dialysis-induced hemolytic-anemia. *Science* 181:463, 1973.
49. Orringer EP, Mattern WD: Formaldehyde-induced hemolysis during chronic-hemodialysis. *N Engl J Med* 294:1416, 1976.

50. Niemoeller OM, Kiedaisch V, Dreischer P, et al: Stimulation of eryptosis by aluminium ions. *Toxicol Appl Pharmacol* 217:168, 2006.
51. Sopjani M, Foller M, Lang F: Gold stimulates Ca^{2+} entry into and subsequent suicidal death of erythrocytes. *Toxicology* 244:271, 2008.
52. Rice L, Alfrey CP: Modulation of red cell mass by neocytolysis in space and on Earth. *Pflugers Arch* 441:R91, 2000.
53. Rice L, Alfrey CP: The negative regulation of red cell mass by neocytolysis: Physiologic and pathophysiologic manifestations. *Cell Physiol Biochem* 15:245, 2005.
54. Yoo D, Lessin LS: Drug-associated "bite cell" hemolytic anemia. *Am J Med* 92:243, 1992.
55. Klein M, Namer R, Harpur E, Corbin R: Earthenware containers as a source of fatal lead poisoning—Case study and public-health considerations. *N Engl J Med* 283:669, 1970.
56. Andreasen NJ: Benjamin Franklin: Physicus et medicus. *JAMA* 236:57, 1976.
57. Bigelow J: *The Complete Works of Benjamin Franklin.* GP Putnam's Sons, New York, 1888.
58. Jones RL, Homa DM, Meyer PA, et al: Trends in blood lead levels and blood lead testing among U.S. children aged 1 to 5 years, 1988–2004. *Pediatrics* 123:e376, 2009.
59. Bradman A, Eskenazi B, Sutton P, et al: Iron deficiency associated with higher blood lead in children living in contaminated environments. *Environ Health Perspect* 109:1079, 2001.
60. Wright RO, Silverman EK, Schwartz J, et al: Association between hemochromatosis genotype and lead exposure among elderly men: The normative aging study. *Environ Health Perspect* 112:746, 2004.
61. Staudinger KC, Roth VS: Occupational lead poisoning. *Am Fam Physician* 57:719, 1998.
62. Froom P, Kristal-Boneh E, Benbassat J, et al: Predictive value of determinations of zinc protoporphyrin for increased blood lead concentrations. *Clin Chem* 44:1283, 1998.
63. Autenrieth T, Schmidt T, Habscheid W: Lead poisoning caused by a Greek ceramic cup. *Dtsch Med Wochenschr* 123:353, 1998.
64. Kakosy T, Hudak A, Naray M: Lead intoxication epidemic caused by ingestion of contaminated ground paprika. *J Toxicol Clin Toxicol* 34:507, 1996.
65. Fischbein A, Wallace J, Sassa S, et al: Lead poisoning from art restoration and pottery work: Unusual exposure source and household risk. *J Environ Pathol Toxicol Oncol* 11:7, 1992.
66. Vahter M, Counter SA, Laurell G, et al: Extensive lead exposure in children living in an area with production of lead-glazed tiles in the Ecuadorian Andes. *Int Arch Occup Environ Health* 70:282, 1997.
67. Waldron HA: The anaemia of lead poisoning: A review. *Br J Ind Med* 23:83, 1966.
68. Westerman MP, Pfitzer E, Ellis LD, Jensen WN: Concentrations of lead in bone in plumbism. *N Engl J Med* 273:1246, 1965.
69. Khalil-Manesh F, Tartaglia-Erler J, Gonick HC: Experimental model of lead nephropathy. IV. Correlation between renal functional changes and hematological indices of lead toxicity. *J Trace Elem Electrolytes Health Dis* 8:13, 1994.
70. Vincent PC, Blackburn CRB: The effects of heavy metal ions on the human erythrocyte. I Comparisons of the action of several heavy metals. *Aust J Exp Biol Med Sci* 36:471, 1958.
71. Hasan J, Vihko V, Hernberg S: Deficient red cell membrane/Na^+ + K^+/-ATPase in lead poisoning. *Arch Environ Health* 14:313, 1967.
72. Hernberg S, Nikkanen J: Enzyme inhibition by lead under normal urban conditions. *Lancet* 1:63, 1970.
73. Casado MF, Cecchini AL, Simao AN, et al: Free radical-mediated pre-hemolytic injury in human red blood cells subjected to lead acetate as evaluated by chemiluminescence. *Food Chem Toxicol* 45:945, 2007.
74. Charache S, Weatherall DJ: Fast hemoglobin in lead poisoning. *Blood* 28:377, 1966.
75. Lachant NA, Tomoda A, Tanaka KR: Inhibition of the pentose-phosphate shunt by lead—A potential mechanism for hemolysis in lead-poisoning. *Blood* 63:518, 1984.
76. Brookfield RW: Blood changes occurring during the course of treatment of malignant disease by lead, with special reference to punctate basophilia and the platelets. *J Pathol* 31:277, 1928.
77. Schwartz J, Landrigan PJ, Baker EL Jr, et al: Lead-induced anemia: Dose-response relationships and evidence for a threshold. *Am J Public Health* 80:165, 1990.
78. Clark M, Royal J, Seeler R: Interaction of iron deficiency and lead and the hematologic findings in children with severe lead poisoning. *Pediatrics* 81:247, 1988.
79. White JM, Selhi HS: Lead and Red-Cell. *Br J Haematol* 30:133, 1975.
80. Jensen WN, Moreno GD, Bessis MC: An electron microscopic description of basophilic stippling in red cells. *Blood* 25:933, 1965.
81. Berlin CM Jr: Lead poisoning in children. *Curr Opin Pediatr* 9:173, 1997.
82. Miller AL: Dimercaptosuccinic acid (DMSA), a non-toxic, water-soluble treatment for heavy metal toxicity. *Altern Med Rev* 3:199, 1998.
83. Klein WJ Jr, Metz EN, Price AR: Acute copper intoxication. A hazard of hemodialysis. *Arch Intern Med* 129:578, 1972.
84. Manzler AD, Schreiner AW: Copper-induced acute hemolytic anemia. A new complication of hemodialysis. *Ann Intern Med* 73:409, 1970.
85. Deiss A, Lee GR, Cartwright GE: Hemolytic anemia in Wilson's disease. *Ann Intern Med* 73:413, 1970.
86. Hansen PB: Wilson's disease presenting with severe hemolytic anemia. *Ugeskr Laeger* 150:1229, 1988.
87. McIntyre N, Clink HM, Levi AJ, et al: Hemolytic anemia in Wilson's disease. *N Engl J Med* 276:439, 1967.
88. Grudeva-Popova JG, Spasova MI, Chepileva KG, Zaprianov ZH: Acute hemolytic anemia as an initial clinical manifestation of Wilson's disease. *Folia Med (Plovdiv)* 42:42, 2000.
89. Fairbanks VF: Copper sulfate-induced hemolytic anemia. Inhibition of glucose-6-phosphate dehydrogenase and other possible etiologic mechanisms. *Arch Intern Med* 120:428, 1967.
90. Blume KG, Hoffbauer RW, Lohr GW, Rudiger HW: Genetische und biochemische Aspekte der Pyruvatkinase menschlicher Erythrozyten. *Verh Dtsch Ges Inn Med* 75:450, 1969.
91. Boulard M, Beutler E, Blume KG: Effect of copper on red-cell enzyme-activities. *J Clin Invest* 51:459, 1972.
92. Kiss JE, Berman D, Van Thiel D: Effective removal of copper by plasma exchange in fulminant Wilson's disease. *Transfusion* 38:327, 1998.
93. Stohlman F Jr, Brecher G, Schneiderman M, Cronkite EP: The hemolytic effect of ionizing radiations and its relationship to the hemorrhagic phase of radiation injury. *Blood* 12:1061, 1957.
94. Jin YS, Anderson G, Mintz PD: Effects of gamma irradiation on red cells from donors with sickle cell trait. *Transfusion* 37:804, 1997.
95. Lubash GD, Phillips RE, Bonsnes RW, Shields JD: Acute aniline poisoning treated by hemodialysis—Report of case. *Arch Intern Med* 114:530, 1964.
96. Lowenstein L, Ballew DH: Fatal acute haemolytic anaemia, thrombocytopenic purpura, nephrosis and hepatitis resulting from ingestion of a compound containing apiol. *Can Med Assoc J* 78:195, 1958.
97. Schroder C, Kruger E, Abel J: Acute poisoning caused by the herbicide dichlorprop (preparation SYS 67 PROP). *Kinderarztl Prax* 59:81, 1991.
98. Martin H, Woerner W, Rittmeister B: Hemolytic anemia by inhalation of hydroxylamines, with a contribution to the problem of Heinz body formation. *Klin Wochenschr* 42:725, 1964.
99. Fisher B: The significance of Heinz bodies in anemias of obscure etiology. *Am J Med Sci* 230:143, 1955.
100. Nierenberg DW, Horowitz MB, Harris KM, James DH: Mineral spirits inhalation associated with hemolysis, pulmonary edema, and ventricular fibrillation. *Arch Intern Med* 151:1437, 1991.
101. Hunter D: Industrial toxicology. *QJM* 12:185, 1943.
102. Gasser C: Perakute hämolytische Innenkörperanämie mit Methämoglobinämie nach Behandlung eines Säuglingsekzems mit Resorcin. *Helv Paediatr Acta* 9:285, 1954.
103. Brandes JC, Bufill JA, Pisciotta AV: Amyl nitrite-induced hemolytic-anemia. *Am J Med* 86:252, 1989.
104. Graves TD, Mitchell S: Acute haemolytic anaemia after inhalation of amyl nitrite. *J R Soc Med* 96:594, 2003.
105. Pugh JI, Enderby GEH: Haemoglobinuria after intravenous myanesin. *Lancet* 2:387, 1947.
106. Poinsot J, Guillois B, Margis D, et al: Neonatal hemolytic anemia after intra-amniotic injection of methylene blue. *Arch Fr Pediatr* 45:657, 1988.
107. Sills MR, Zinkham WH: Methylene blue-induced Heinz body hemolytic anemia. *Arch Pediatr Adolesc Med* 148:306, 1994.
108. Davidson S, Seldon M, Jones B: Omeprazole and Heinz-body haemolytic anaemia. *Aust N Z J Med* 27:441, 1997.
109. Hassan AB, Seligmann H, Bassan HM: Intravascular haemolysis induced by pentachlorophenol. *Br Med J (Clin Res Ed)* 291:21, 1985.
110. Adams JG, Heller P, Abramson RK, Vaithianathan T: Sulfonamide-induced hemolytic anemia and hemoglobin Hasharon. *Arch Intern Med* 137:1449, 1977.
111. Greenberg MS: Heinz body hemolytic anemia. "Bite cells"—A clue to diagnosis. *Arch Intern Med* 136:153, 1976.
112. Kaplinsky N, Frankl O: Salicylazosulphapyridine-induced Heinz body anemia. *Acta Haematol* 59:310, 1978.
113. Ward PC, Schwartz BS, White JG: Heinz-body anemia: "Bite cell" variant—A light and electron microscopic study. *Am J Hematol* 15:135, 1983.
114. Lin CC, King KL, Chao YW, et al: Tacrolimus-associated hemolytic uremic syndrome: A case analysis. *J Nephrol* 16:580, 2003.

CHAPTER 52

HEMOLYTIC ANEMIA RESULTING FROM INFECTIONS WITH MICROORGANISMS

Marshall A. Lichtman*

SUMMARY

Hemolytic anemia is a prominent part of the clinical presentation of patients infected with organisms such as the malaria parasites, *Babesia*, and *Bartonella*, which directly invade the erythrocyte. Malaria is probably the most common cause of hemolytic anemia on a worldwide basis, and much has been learned about how the parasite enters the erythrocyte and the mechanism of anemia. Falciparum malaria, in particular, can cause severe and sometimes fatal hemolysis (blackwater fever). Other organisms cause hemolytic anemia by producing a hemolysin (e.g., *Clostridium perfringens*), by stimulating an immune response (e.g., *Mycoplasma pneumoniae*), by enhancing macrophage recognition and hemophagocytosis, or by as yet unknown mechanisms. The many different infections that have been associated with hemolytic anemia are tabulated and references to the original studies provided.

Shortening of erythrocyte life span occurs commonly in the course of inflammatory and infectious diseases. This may occur particularly in patients with glucose-6-phosphate dehydrogenase (G-6-PD) deficiency (see Chap. 46), splenomegaly (see Chap. 55), and in the microvascular fragmentation syndrome (see Chap. 50). In some infections, however, rapid destruction of erythrocytes represents a prominent part of the overall clinical picture (Table 52–1).[1–49] This chapter deals only with the latter states.

Several distinct mechanisms may lead to hemolysis during infections.[49] These include direct invasion of or injury to the erythrocytes by the infecting organism, as in malaria, babesiosis, and bartonellosis; elaboration of hemolytic toxins, as by *Clostridium perfringens*; and development of antibodies, either autoantibodies against red cell antigens or deposition of microbial antigens or immune complexes on erythrocytes.[50]

MALARIA

EPIDEMIOLOGY

Known since antiquity, malaria is the world's most common cause of hemolytic anemia.[36] Human malaria is caused by one of four species of a protozoan, *Plasmodium*. In 2000, more than 500 million annual episodes of malaria occurred worldwide and nearly 20 percent of all childhood deaths (representing 800,000 children per year) in sub-Saharan Africa were attributed to malaria.[51] Severe malarial anemia is most commonly seen in young children and pregnant women.[52]

Malaria transmission depends on geography, rainfall patterns, and the breeding sites of the *Anopheles* mosquito, the specific vector. Some regions have conditions that make malaria common throughout the year, so-called endemic areas, whereas in other places there are seasonal peaks, usually the rainy season when mosquito breeding is enhanced. Persons in Africa, Asia, the Middle East, and parts of Europe may be at risk. Travelers to such places are at high risk because of lack of immunity and because when they return home, the diagnosis might not be considered promptly. Malaria may also be transmitted by blood transfusion or organ donation from an infected donor.

LIFE CYCLE

Sporozoites enter the circulation while the female *Anopheles* mosquito takes a blood meal. They invade and multiply in hepatocytes. The latter cells rupture when engorged and release merozoites that invade the red cell. In the red cell, the merozoites also cycle through these stages: trophozoites (ring-forms), which then can convert to schizonts. Mature schizonts burst the red cells and release merozoites that invade other red cells. The bursting and release coincides with the abrupt rises in temperature and related signs and symptoms seen in malaria. A small fraction of merozoites in red cells convert to male and female gametes that are ingested when the mosquito bites. In the mosquito, they fuse and form an oocyst that divides asexually into numerous sporozoites. The sporozoites migrate to the mosquito's salivary glands from where they reenter a victim's blood upon the next bite, initiating a malarial infection. *Plasmodium vivax* and *Plasmodium ovale* can persist in the liver in a dormant stage (hypnozoites) and produce relapses months or years later.

ALTERATIONS IN THE INFECTED RED CELL

After the host is bitten by an infected female *Anopheles* mosquito, the sporozoites invade the liver and possibly other internal organs in the asymptomatic tissue stage of malaria. Merozoites, emerging at first from the tissues and later from previously parasitized red cells, bind to glycophorins A and B by means of a 175-kDa protein that has been designated the erythrocyte-binding antigen (EBA-175).[53–55] A complex series of events, not yet fully understood, eventuates in invasion of the interior of the red cell by the parasite.[35,51] Having entered the erythrocyte, the parasite grows intracellularly, nourished by the cell's contents, facilitated by the 80pS red cell anion channel.[56]

Erythrocytes infected with *Plasmodium falciparum* develop surface knobs[57,58] that contain rceeptors, especially the *P. falciparum* erythrocyte membrane protein-1 (PfEMP-1), for endothelial proteins. All parasites bind to CD36 antigen (platelet glycoprotein IV) and thrombospondin found on endothelial surfaces, whereas some bind to the intercellular adhesion molecule-1 (ICAM-1), and a few bind to the vascular cell adhesion molecule (VCAM)[59–63] and mediate the adherence of parasitized cells to endothelium. Rosetting of parasitized cells with unparasitized cells also occurs through another mechanism mediated by complement receptor-1 (CR1) on uninfected erythrocytes.[64] One of the membrane proteins of *P. falciparum* binds specifically to the spectrin on the inner surface of the red cell membrane.[65] The anemia of falciparum malaria is characteristically normocytic-normochromic anemia with a paucity of reticulocytes (see "Pathogenesis of the Anemia" below). If microcytosis is present, the concomitant presence of α- or β-thalassemia or iron deficiency should be considered.[66] A large number of genetic polymorphisms that interfere with invasion of erythrocytes by parasites and their

Acronyms and abbreviations that appear in this chapter include: CR1, complement receptor 1; EBA, erythrocyte-binding antigen; G-6-PD, glucose-6-phosphate dehydrogenase; ICAM, intercellular adhesion molecule; PfEMP, *Plasmodium falciparum* erythrocyte membrane protein; RSP-2, ring surface protein 2; VCAM, vascular cell adhesion molecule.

*This chapter was written by Ernest Beutler in previous editions and portions of the chapter in the 7th edition have been retained.

TABLE 52–1. Organisms Causing Hemolytic Anemia

Aspergillus[1]
Bacillus anthracis[2]
Babesia microti and *Babesia divergens*[3]
Bartonella bacilliformis[4,5]
Campylobacter jejuni[6,7]
Clostridium perfringens(Welchii)[8,9]
Coxsackie virus[10]
Cytomegalovirus[11]
Diplococcus pneumoniae[12]
Epstein-Barr virus[13,14]
Escherichia coli[15,16]
Fusobacterium necrophorum[17]
Haemophilus influenzae[12,23]
Hepatitis A[18–20]
Hepatitis B[19,21]
Hepatitis C[22]
Herpes simplex virus[10]
Human immunodeficiency virus[24–26] (see Chap. 83)
Influenza A virus[27,28]
Leishmania donovani[30]
Leptospira interrogans serovar *ballum* and/or *Leptospira kirschneri* serovar *butembo*[29]
Mumps virus[31]
Mycobacterium tuberculosis[12,32]
Mycoplasma pneumoniae[33]
Neisseria intracellularis[12]
Parvovirus B19[34]
Plasmodium falciparum[35]
Plasmodium malariae[35]
Plasmodium vivax[36]
Rubella virus[37,38]
Rubeola virus[10]
Salmonella[12,39]
Shigella[40,41]
Streptococcus[12,42–45]
Toxoplasma[12]
Trypanosoma brucei[46]
Varicella virus[10,47]
Vibrio cholerae[12]
Yersinia enterocolitica[48]

proliferation have developed in areas where malaria has been a leading cause of death for many generations.[64,67–69] These include G-6-PD deficiency, Southeast Asian ovalocytosis, CR1 deficiency, the thalassemias, sickle cell anemia (Chaps. 46–48), and other hemoglobinopathies.

PLASMODIUM SPECIES AND SEVERITY OF ANEMIA

There are four plasmodial species that cause human malaria: *P. falciparum, P. vivax, P. malariae,* and *P. ovale*. The first two cause the most cases worldwide and are principally associated with hemolytic anemia. *P. vivax* invades only young red cells, whereas *P. falciparum* attacks both young and old cells. Thus, anemia tends to be more severe in the latter form of malaria and is the most deadly type.[35]

PATHOGENESIS OF THE ANEMIA

Hemolytic Mechanisms

Destruction of parasitized red cells appears to occur largely in the spleen, and splenomegaly typically is present in chronic malarial infection. The "pitting" of parasites from infected erythrocytes may also occur in the spleen.[70] The degree of parasitemia, in part, determines the destruction of infected erythrocytes. Low rates of red cell parasitemia may have little effect on the development of anemia, whereas high rates, for example, 10 percent, may have very significant effects.[71] The degree to which anemia develops often seems to be disproportionate to the number of cells infected with the parasite. It is estimated that 10 times the number of uninfected red cells are removed for each infected red cell, dramatically magnifying the hemolytic rate. Osmotic fragility is increased in nonparasitized cells, as well as in cells containing plasmodia.[72] The erythrocyte cation permeability is altered in monkeys with malaria.[73] Hemin accumulation facilitates hemolytic cell loss via a process of programmed cell death, referred to as eryptosis. This suicidal death pathway is mediated by increased cell calcium, increased annexin-V binding, and ceramide formation.[74] It has been suggested that oxidative damage to red cell lipids occurs[75,76] and that there is an abnormality in the phosphorylation of membranes of parasitized red cells.[77] *P. falciparum*-infected red cells have a highly irregular surface. This may be produced by the intracellular growth of the plasmodium, or it could represent the site of parasite entry. Nonparasitized cells often have similar surface defects,[78] suggesting a phenomenon known to occur in simian malaria,[79] the "pitting" of parasites from an infected cell.

Activation of hepatosplenic macrophages enhance red cell clearance supported by red cell surface changes in both parasitized and unparasitized cells that foster recognition and erythrophagocytosis by macrophages. Both marked loss of red cell deformability and deposition of immunoglobulin (IgG) and complement (C3d), sometimes resulting in a positive direct antiglobulin reaction, may enhance red cell removal by macrophages.[80,81] Parasite products are part of the immune complexes on the red cell surface. The *P. falciparum* ring surface protein 2 (RSP-2) mediates adhesion of infected red cells to endothelial cells and is deposited on uninfected cells, undoubtedly providing a mechanism for removal of these cells by mediating complement-dependent phagocytosis.[66] Splenomegaly further enhances red cell removal from the circulation.

Decrease in Erythropoiesis

P. falciparum also decreases the erythropoietin response, results in less erythropoiesis than expected for the degree of anemia, reticulocytopenia, and coincidentally striking dyserythropoiesis with stippling, cytoplasmic vacuolization, nuclear fragmentation and multinuclearity.[66] The inhibition of the erythroid response (anemia of chronic disease) is secondary to release of the cytokines interferon-γ and tumor necrosis factor-α, and the interleukin-10-to-tumor-necrosis-factor ratio, which when low correlates with severe malarial anemia in children (see Chap. 37).[66]

BLACKWATER FEVER

The fever associated with malaria, accompanied by rigors, headache, abdominal pain, nausea and vomiting, and extreme fatigue, is characteristically cyclic, varying in frequency according to the malaria type. Although classic periodicity is often absent, febrile paroxysms of *P. vivax* malaria tend to occur every 48 hours; those of *P. malariae* infection

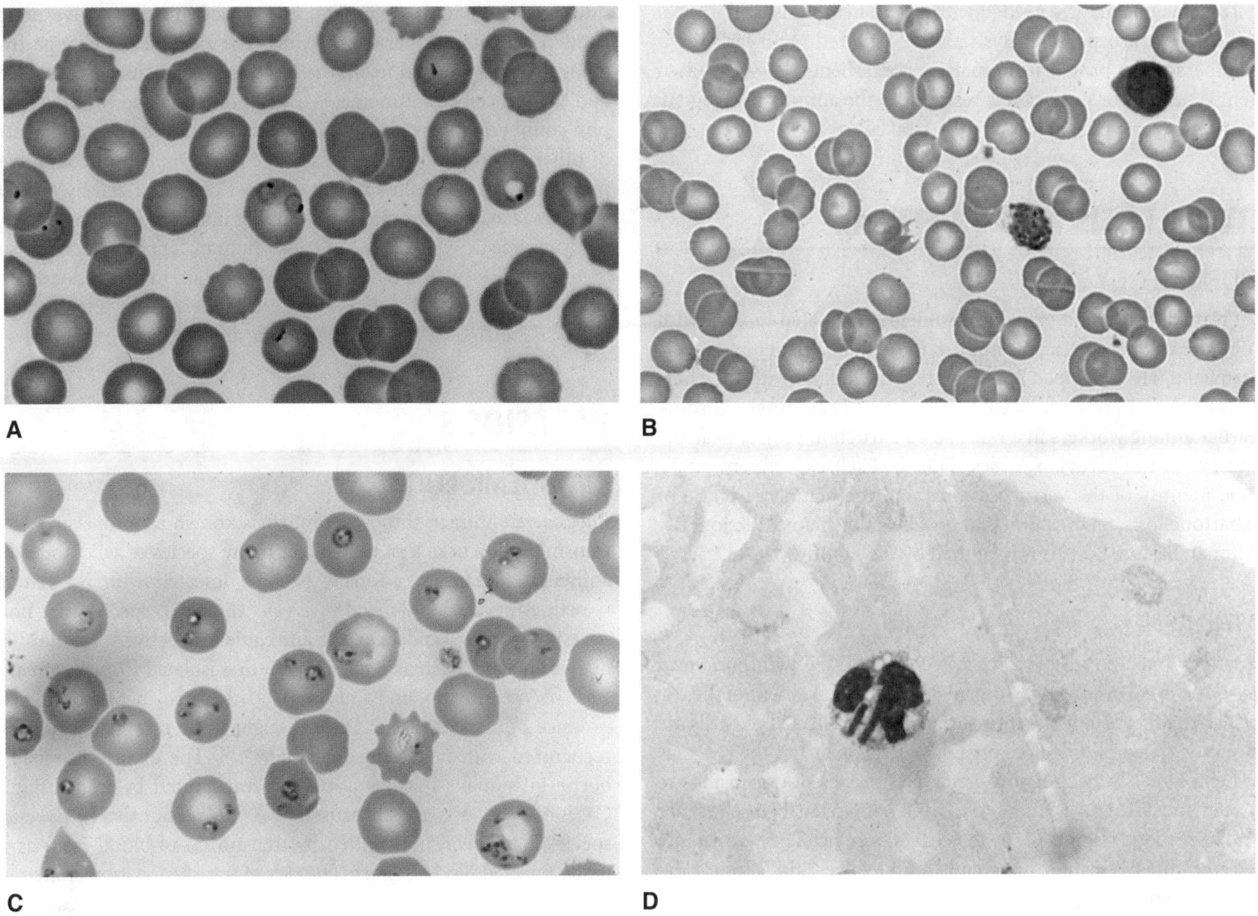

FIGURE 52–1. A. Blood film from a patient with malaria caused by *Plasmodium falciparum*. Several red cells contain ring forms. Note red cell with double ring form in center of the field, characteristic of *P. falciparum* infection. Note the ring form with double dots at the left edge of figure, suggestive of *P. falciparum* infection. Note also high rate of parasitemia (~10% of red cells in this field) characteristic of *P. falciparum* infection. **B.** Blood film from a patient with malaria caused by *Plasmodium vivax*. Note mature schizont. **C.** Blood film from a patient with *Babesia microti* infection. The heavy parasitemia is characteristic of babesiosis (about two-thirds of red cells infected). **D.** Blood film from a patient with *Clostridium perfringens* septicemia. Few red cells evident as a result of intense erythrolysis. Neutrophil with two bacilli (*C. perfringens*). *(Used with permission from* Lichtman's Atlas of Hematology, *www.accessmedicine.com.)*

occur each 72 hours; and those of *P. falciparum* malaria, daily. In the latter cases, the periodicity is the result the synchronization of schizogony with schizont rupture occurring at regular intervals. It is schizont rupture that accounts for the fever and associated symptoms. Falciparum malaria is occasionally associated with particularly severe hemolysis, hemoglobinemia, hemoglobinuria, and the passage of dark, almost black, urine. This disorder, also called *blackwater fever*, is no longer common. At one time it was seen frequently among Europeans in Africa and in India, usually after quinine was given to treat malaria. The event seems to be related to the intermittent use of antimalarials.[82]

DIAGNOSTIC METHODS

Diagnosis of malaria depends upon demonstration of the parasites on the blood film[83] or demonstration of the appropriate DNA sequences in the blood.[84,85] The morphologic differentiation of *P. falciparum* from other forms of malaria, principally *P. vivax*, is clinically important as *P. falciparum* infection may constitute a clinical emergency. If more than 5 percent of the red cells infected contain parasites, the infection is almost certainly with *P. falciparum*. In an infection with this organism, rings are practically the only form of parasite evident on the blood film. The finding of two or more rings within the same red cells is regarded as pathognomic of *P. falciparum* (Fig. 52–1A and B).[85] In nonimmune patients, examination of the blood film for malarial parasites should be made for at least 3 days after onset of symptoms because parasitemia may not reach detectable levels for several days. The sensitivity of the blood film for the detection of intracellular malarial forms can be enhanced by treating the blood with saponin.[86]

TREATMENT

Early treatment is important. The spread of antimalarial therapy has resulted in major problems with drug resistance. Eradication of blood forms can be achieved with individual agents or combinations of antimalarials. Artemisinins are the most effective agents for *P. falciparum*. Numerous studies are in progress to determine the best single agent or combination of agents to be used in the treatment of malaria in different regions.[87] Many such drugs are capable of producing severe hemolysis in patients with G-6-PD deficiency, which is relevant in areas with endemic malaria[88] (see Chap. 46).

COURSE AND PROGNOSIS

When acute, unusually severe hemolysis occurs in the course of falciparum malaria (blackwater fever), the physician should be certain that a hemolytic drug is not being administered to a G-6-PD–deficient individual. Transfusions may be needed with severe hemolysis, and if renal failure occurs, extracorporeal dialysis may be required. With early institution of therapy the prognosis in malaria is excellent. However, when treatment is delayed or the strain is resistant to the administered agent, *P. falciparum* malaria may follow a rapid, fatal course.

BARTONELLOSIS (OROYA FEVER)

EPIDEMIOLOGY

In 1885, Daniel A. Carrión, a medical student, inoculated himself with blood obtained from a verrucous node of the skin of a patient with verruca peruviana. He developed a fatal hemolytic anemia with the characteristics of Oroya fever, a disease that had first been observed some years earlier among workers in a railroad construction project near the city of Oroya in the Peruvian Andes. This fatal self-experiment established the identity of the verrucosa form and the hemolytic phase of human bartonellosis, an infection that now bears the name Carrión disease.[5] Human bartonellosis is transmitted by the sandfly.

PATHOGENESIS

After a sandfly bite, the red blood cells become infected with *Bartonella bacilliformis*. It is believed that the organism does not grow within the red cell, but rather adheres to its exterior surface: When infected red cells are washed with citrated plasma, free organisms are found but the red cells are not hemolyzed. In hanging-drop cultures, masses of organisms are clearly seen outside the erythrocytes, while the cells themselves are intact.[89] The osmotic fragility of the red cells is normal.[5] They are rapidly removed from the circulation, apparently both by liver and spleen. Normal red cells transfused into patients with bartonellosis meet a similar fate.[4] A 130-kDa *Bartonella* protein that causes erythrocytes to acquire trenches, indentations, and invaginations has been purified from culture broths and has been called *deformin*.[90] In addition, two *B. bacilliformis* genes, designated *ialA* and *ialB*, predicted to encode polypeptides of 170 amino acids (20.1 kDa) and of 186 amino acids (19.9 kDa), respectively, greatly enhance the ability of *Escherichia coli* to invade erythrocytes.[91]

CLINICAL FINDINGS

As demonstrated by Carrión's experiment, bartonellosis has two clinical stages. The acute hemolytic anemia, *Oroya fever*, represents the early, invasive stage of a chronic granulomatous disorder, the late stage of which is designated *verruca peruviana*. Most patients manifest no clinical symptoms during the Oroya fever phase, but when anemia does occur, its onset is dramatic. Red counts as low as 750,000/μL (0.750×10^{12}/L) have been documented.[92] In addition to symptoms of anemia, patients manifest thirst, anorexia, sweating, and generalized lymphadenopathy. Spleen and liver enlargement are unusual. Large numbers of nucleated red cells appear in the blood film, and reticulocytosis is often striking. The white cell count is variable. Diagnosis is established by demonstrating the presence of the organism *B. bacilliformis* on the erythrocytes. Giemsa-stained blood films reveal red-violet rods varying in length from 1 to 3 μm and in width from 0.25 to 0.2 μm. Although molecular methods for diagnosis of *Bartonella* species are available,[93] in a person with the clinical picture, the examination of the blood film can be accomplished and therapy initiated, rapidly.

TREATMENT AND COURSE

Oroya fever responds well to treatment with penicillin, streptomycin, chloramphenicol, and the tetracyclines. The mortality rate among untreated patients is very high, but those who do survive undergo a sudden transitional period in which the *Bartonellae* change from an elongated to a coccoid form, the number of parasitized cells decreases, and the red cell count increases. Lymphocytosis and improved neutrophil count are observed with disappearance of the fever and abatement of other symptoms. The second stage of *Bartonella* infection, verruca peruviana, is a nonhematologic disorder characterized by an eruption over the face and extremities developing into bleeding warty tumors.

Other species of *Bartonella* cause human febrile infections such as "cat-scratch fever," or "trench fever," or can infect individuals with acquired immunodeficiency disease, but these disorders are not ordinarily associated with severe hemolytic anemia.[94–96]

BABESIOSIS

EPIDEMIOLOGY

Babesiae are intraerythrocytic protozoas known as piroplasms. They are transmitted by ticks that may infect many species of wild and domestic animals. Humans occasionally become infected with *Babesia microti* (North America) or *Babesia divergens* (Europe), species that normally parasitize rodents, and, deer, elk, and cattle, respectively.[97] Other *Babesia*-like piroplasms, such as *Babesia WA1*, first isolated from a patient in the state of Washington, and *Babesia MO1*, isolated in Missouri, may also produce human disease.[98] Once thought to be rare, babesiosis is being recognized with increasing frequency.[99,100] The disease is usually tick-borne in humans but has also been transmitted by transfusion.[101–106] Cases of babesiosis, mostly caused by *B. microti* but also by *Babesia WA1* species, have been transmitted by transfusion of blood from asymptomatic infected blood donors. The risk of transfusion-transmitted babesiosis is higher than generally appreciated and in endemic areas represents a threat to the blood supply. Presumably because of the distribution of the vector in the United States, the disease is most common in the northeastern coastal and Great Lakes regions where it became known as "Nantucket fever," but has also been encountered in the Midwest.[107] Infections with *B. divergens* usually occur in splenectomized patients, but this is not the case with *B. microti* infections.[3]

CLINICAL FINDINGS

The symptoms are prompted by reproduction of the organisms in the red cell and subsequent cell lysis. The clinical expression is broad, reflecting the degree of parasitemia. The incubation period ranges from 1 week to 3 months but usually is about 3 weeks. The disease generally has a gradual onset with malaise, anorexia, and fatigue, followed by fever (sometimes as high as 40°C [104°F]), chills, sweats, and muscle and joint pains. The onset, occasionally, may be fulminant. Hepatic and splenic enlargement may be evident.[108]

A moderate degree of hemolytic anemia is usually present; on occasion it has been sufficiently severe to cause hypotension,[109] and transfusion has occasionally been required.[97] The hemolysis may last a few days, but in asplenic, elderly, or otherwise immunocompromised patients, it can go on for months. Elevation in serum transaminases, lactic dehydrogenase, unconjugated bilirubin, and alkaline phosphatase is correlated with the severity of the parasitemia. Thrombocytopenia and leukopenia may occur, which may be the result of inflammatory cytokine release.[108]

DIAGNOSIS

The history may indicate exposure to a tick-infested area, recent blood transfusion, or asplenia. Parasites can be seen in the red cells in Giemsa-stained thin blood films. They appear as darkly stained ring forms with light blue cytoplasm. Merozoites may also be visible. Infrequently, the classical Maltese cross tetrad can be found. This intraerythrocytic structure consists of four daughter cells of *Babesia* connected by cytoplasmic bridges, resembling a Maltese cross. The parasitemia can be very high, affecting more than 75 percent of red cells (Fig. 52–1C).[108] Immunofluorescent tests for antibodies to *Babesia* are available and polymerase chain reaction-based diagnostic tests are the test of choice for confirmation of an active infection in an individual bearing antibodies to *Babesia* and for following the response to therapy.[108]

The onset of fever and hemolytic anemia after transfusion should lead to the consideration of babesiosis.

TREATMENT AND COURSE

Most mild *B. microti* infections respond without treatment. The infection has responded to drug therapy with clindamycin and quinine,[110] but failure to respond to antibiotics has also been encountered.[102] The two-drug combination can increase rate of clearance of parasites, but they have consequential side effects. A combination of atovaquone and azithromycin has also been proposed as treatment.[98,111] Whole-blood or red cell exchange can result in marked improvement in recalcitrant cases.[111,108]

COINFECTION

In endemic areas two or more parasites may coinfect an individual by a tick bite. *B. microti and Babesia burgdorferi* (Lyme disease) may both enter the human circulation as a result of the *Ixodes* tick bite, as can several other parasites (e.g., human granulocytic ehrlichiosis). Initial signs and symptoms may be similar. Successful early treatment for Lyme disease may leave a residual *B. microti* infection because antibiotic therapy for the former will not eradicate the latter.[108]

CLOSTRIDIUM PERFRINGENS SEPTICEMIA

EPIDEMIOLOGY

C. perfringens (formerly *C. welchii*) sepsis is most likely to occur in patients who have undergone septic abortion. It has also been observed following acute cholecystitis,[112] as a result of an intrahepatic abscess,[9] and, rarely, after amniocentesis.[113]

PATHOGENESIS

C. perfringens are gram-positive, encapsulated, spore-forming, anaerobic bacilli. The organism causes gas gangrene in soft tissues. The α toxin of *C. perfringens* is a lecithinase C that reacts with lipoprotein complexes at cell surfaces, liberating potent hemolytic substances, lysolecithins. This toxin is the agent that causes intravascular hemolysis and its subsequent effects. It has also been suggested that erythrocyte membrane proteolysis plays an important role in hemolysis.[114]

CLINICAL FEATURES

Severe, often fatal hemolysis occurs in patients with *C. perfringens* septicemia. Striking hemoglobinemia and hemoglobinuria occur. The serum may become a brilliant red, and the urine is a dark-brown mahogany color. The lysis of red cells (decreasing packed red cell volume) and the high plasma hemoglobin can produce a marked dissociation between the blood hemoglobin and hematocrit level. For example, hematocrits approaching zero with blood hemoglobins of perhaps 8 g/dL can occur. Dehemoglobinized red cell "ghosts" may be evident on the blood film (Fig. 52–1D). Microspherocytes are prominent (see Chap. 45), and leukocytosis with a left shift as well as thrombocytopenia are often present. Acute renal and hepatic failure usually develops, and the prognosis is grave; more than half of the patients die, even with appropriate treatment (see Chap. 130).[8,115]

THERAPY AND COURSE

Therapy consists of antibiotic therapy, fluid support, red cell transfusion, and where appropriate surgical debridement.[116] The infection is often of abrupt onset and overwhelming, and the profundity of the hemolysis and secondary organ damage (e.g., renal) results in a high mortality rate.

OTHER INFECTIONS

A variety of other infections occasionally have been associated with hemolytic anemia. The mechanisms involved vary. Some organisms, among them such common pathogens as *Haemophilus influenzae, E. coli*, and *Salmonella* species, can produce red cell agglutination *in vitro*, but it is not known whether this phenomenon is important in initiating *in vivo* hemolysis.[117] Bacteria may also produce destruction of red cells indirectly when bacterial polysaccharides are adsorbed onto erythrocytes. Action of an antibody directed against the antigen-coated cells results in their agglutination[118] or in complement-mediated lysis.[23] The unmasking of T-type antigens by bacteria renders the cell polyagglutinable. This may be a rare cause of hemolysis occurring in the course of bacterial infections.[119,120]

Many different types of microorganisms may play a role in precipitating autoimmune hemolytic disease (see Chap. 53). In one study of 234 patients,[10] 55 were found to have an antecedent bacterial infection, 18 of these exhibiting an "unequivocal etiologic relationship" of infection to anemia. However, the principal evidence for such a relationship was a temporal one. A number of viral agents, including measles, cytomegalovirus, varicella, herpes simplex, influenza A and B, Epstein-Barr, human immunodeficiency virus[24–26] (see Chap. 83), and coxsackievirus have also been associated with immune hemolytic disease.[10,121] Various mechanisms have been postulated, including absorption of immune complexes and complement, cross-reacting antigen, and a true autoimmune state with possible loss of tolerance secondary to the infectious organism.[10] Histopathologic and sometimes virologic evidence of infection with cytomegalovirus has been reported in a high percentage of children with lymphadenopathy and hemolytic anemia.[122] A positive antiglobulin reaction was demonstrated in some of these patients, and it has been suggested that some cases of "idiopathic autoimmune hemolytic anemia" are in reality caused by cytomegalovirus infection.[122]

The high cold agglutinin titer that sometimes develops in the course of *Mycoplasma pneumoniae* pneumonia (see Chap. 53) may occasionally result in hemolytic anemia[1,33] or compensated hemolysis, although most patients with high cold agglutinin titers do not become anemic. The red cells of a number of patients with kala azar were found to be agglutinated with anticomplement and anti-non–γ-globulin serum.[30] Both splenic and hepatic sequestration of red cells appears to occur in this disease.[13]

Microangiopathic hemolytic anemia is discussed in detail in Chaps. 50 and 130. This disorder may be triggered by a variety of infections, some of which are caused by well-characterized organisms such as species of *Shigella*,[123,124] *Campylobacter*,[125] and *Aspergillus*.[1]

REFERENCES

1. Robboy SJ, Salisbury K, Ragsdale B, et al: Mechanism of aspergillus-induced microangiopathic hemolytic anemia. *Arch Intern Med* 128:790, 1971.

2. Freedman A, Afonja O, Chang MW, et al: Cutaneous anthrax associated with microangiopathic hemolytic anemia and coagulopathy in a 7-month-old infant. *JAMA* 287:869, 2002.
3. Pruthi RK, Marshall WF, Wiltsie JC, Persing DH: Human babesiosis. *Mayo Clin Proc* 70:853, 1995.
4. Reynafarje C, Ramos J: The hemolytic anemia of human bartonellosis. *Blood* 17:562, 1961.
5. Ricketts WE: *Bartonella bacilliformis* anemia (Oroya fever). A study of thirty cases. *Blood* 3:1025, 1948.
6. Smith MA, Shah NR, Lobel JS, Hamilton W: Methemoglobinemia and hemolytic anemia associated with *Campylobacter jejuni* enteritis. *Am J Pediatr Hematol Oncol* 10:35, 1988.
7. Damani NN, Humphrey CA, Bell B: Haemolytic anaemia in *Campylobacter* enteritis. *J Infect* 26:109, 1993.
8. Rogstad B, Ritland S, Lunde S, Hagen AG: *Clostridium perfringens* septicemia with massive hemolysis. *Infection* 21:54, 1993.
9. Kreidl KO, Green GR, Wren SM: Intravascular hemolysis from a *Clostridium perfringens* liver abscess. *J Am Coll Surg* 194:387, 2002.
10. Pirofsky B: Infectious disease and autoimmune hemolytic anemia, in *Autoimmunization and the Autoimmune Hemolytic Anemias*, p 147. Waverly Press, Baltimore, 1969.
11. van Spronsen DJ, Breed WP: Cytomegalovirus-induced thrombocytopenia and haemolysis in an immunocompetent adult. *Br J Haematol* 92:218, 1996.
12. Dacie JV: Secondary or symptomatic hemolytic anemias, in *The Haemolytic Anaemias, Part III*, edited by JV Dacie, p 908. Grune & Stratton, New York, 1967.
13. Tonkin AM, Mond HG, Alford FP, Hurley TH: Severe acute haemolytic anaemia complicating infectious mononucleosis. *Med J Aust* 2:1048, 1973.
14. Whitelaw F, Brook MG, Kennedy N, Weir WR: Haemolytic anaemia complicating Epstein-Barr virus infection. *Br J Clin Pract* 49:212, 1995.
15. Ludwig K, Ruder H, Bitzan M, et al: Outbreak of *Escherichia coli* O157: H7 infection in a large family. *Eur J Clin Microbiol Infect Dis* 16:238, 1997.
16. Pennings CM, Seitz RC, Karch H, Lenard HG: Haemolytic anaemia in association with *Escherichia coli* O157 infection in two sisters. *Eur J Pediatr* 153:656, 1994.
17. Chand DH, Brady RC, Bissler JJ: Hemolytic uremic syndrome in an adolescent with Fusobacterium necrophorum bacteremia. *Am J Kidney Dis* 37:E22, 2001.
18. Gundersen SG, Bjoerneklett A, Bruun JN: Severe erythroblastopenia and hemolytic anemia during a hepatitis A infection. *Scand J Infect Dis* 21:225, 1989.
19. Kanematsu T, Nomura T, Higashi K, Ito M: Hemolytic anemia in association with viral hepatitis. *Nippon Rinsho* 54:2539, 1996.
20. Urganci N, Akyildiz B, Yildirmak Y, Ozbay G: A case of autoimmune hepatitis and autoimmune hemolytic anemia following hepatitis A infection. *Turk J Gastroenterol* 14:204, 2003.
21. Gurgey A, Yuce A, Ozbek N, Kocak N: Acute hemolysis in association with hepatitis B infection in a child with beta-thalassemia trait. *Turk J Pediatr* 36:259, 1994.
22. Etienne A, Gayet S, Vidal F, et al: Severe hemolytic anemia due to cold agglutinin complicating untreated chronic hepatitis C: Efficacy and safety of anti-CD20 (rituximab) treatment. *Am J Hematol* 75:243, 2004.
23. Shurin SB, Anderson P, Zollinger J, Rathbun RK: Pathophysiology of hemolysis in infections with *Haemophilus influenzae* type B. *J Clin Invest* 77:1340, 1986.
24. Rheingold SR, Burnham JM, Rutstein R, Manno CS: HIV infection presenting as severe autoimmune hemolytic anemia with disseminated intravascular coagulation in an infant. *J Pediatr Hematol Oncol* 26:9, 2004.
25. Koduri PR, Singa P, Nikolinakos P: Autoimmune hemolytic anemia in patients infected with human immunodeficiency virus-1. *Am J Hematol* 70:174, 2002.
26. Saif MW: HIV-associated autoimmune hemolytic anemia: An update. *AIDS Patient Care STDS* 15:217, 2001.
27. Watanabe T: Hemolytic uremic syndrome associated with influenza A virus infection. *Nephron* 89:359, 2001.
28. Asaka M, Ishikawa I, Nakazawa T, et al: Hemolytic uremic syndrome associated with influenza A virus infection in an adult renal allograft recipient: Case report and review of the literature. *Nephron* 84:258, 2000.
29. Trowbridge AA, Green JB III, Bonnett JD, et al: Hemolytic anemia associated with leptospirosis. Morphologic and lipid studies. *Am J Clin Pathol* 76:493, 1981.
30. Woodruff AW, Topley E, Knight R, Downie CGB: The anaemia of kala azar. *Br J Haematol* 22:319, 1972.
31. Ozen S, Damarguc I, Besbas N, et al: A case of mumps associated with acute hemolytic crisis resulting in hemoglobinuria and acute renal failure. *J Med* 25:255, 1994.
32. Kuo PH, Yang PC, Kuo SS, Luh KT: Severe immune hemolytic anemia in disseminated tuberculosis with response to antituberculosis therapy. *Chest* 119:1961, 2001.
33. Fiala M, Myhre BA, Chinh LT, et al: Pathogenesis of anemia associated with *Mycoplasma pneumoniae*. *Acta Haematol* 51:297, 1974.
34. Chambers LA, Rauck AM: Acute transient hemolytic anemia with a positive Donath-Landsteiner test following parvovirus B19 infection. *J Pediatr Hematol Oncol* 18:178, 1996.
35. Weatherall DJ, Miller LH, Baruch DI, et al: Malaria and the red cell. *Hematology Am Soc Hematol Educ Program* 35, 2002.
36. White NJ: The treatment of malaria. *N Engl J Med* 335:800, 1996.
37. Moriuchi H, Yamasaki S, Mori K, et al: A rubella epidemic in Sasebo, Japan in 1987, with various complications. *Acta Paediatr Jpn* 32:67, 1990.
38. Yoneda S, Yoshikawa M, Yamane Y, et al: A case of rubella complicated by hemolytic anemia. *Kansenshogaku Zasshi* 74:724, 2000.
39. Albaqali A, Ghuloom A, Al Arrayed A, et al: Hemolytic uremic syndrome in association with typhoid fever. *Am J Kidney Dis* 41:709, 2003.
40. Houdouin V, Doit C, Mariani P, et al: A pediatric cluster of Shigella dysenteriae serotype 1 diarrhea with hemolytic uremic syndrome in 2 families from France. *Clin Infect Dis* 38:e96, 2004.
41. Kavaliotis J, Karyda S, Konstantoula T, et al: Shigellosis of childhood in northern Greece: Epidemiological, clinical and laboratory data of hospitalized patients during the period 1971–1996. *Scand J Infect Dis* 32:207, 2000.
42. Shepherd AB, Palmer AL, Bigler SA, Baliga R: Hemolytic uremic syndrome associated with group A beta-hemolytic streptococcus. *Pediatr Nephrol* 18:949, 2003.
43. Apilanez UM, Areses TR, Ruiz Benito MA, et al: Hemolytic uremic syndrome secondary to Streptococcus pneumoniae pulmonary infection. *An Esp Pediatr* 57:378, 2002.
44. Reynolds E, Espinoza M, Monckeberg G, Graf J: Hemolytic-uremic syndrome and *Streptococcus pneumoniae*. *Rev Med Chil* 130:677, 2002.
45. Brandt J, Wong C, Mihm S, et al: Invasive pneumococcal disease and hemolytic uremic syndrome. *Pediatrics* 110:371, 2002.
46. Wéry M, Mulumba PM, Lambert PH, Kazyumba L: Hematologic manifestations, diagnosis, and immunopathology of African trypanosomiasis. *Semin Hematol* 19:83, 1982.
47. Papalia MA, Schwarer AP: Paroxysmal cold haemoglobinuria in an adult with chicken pox. *Br J Haematol* 109:328, 2000.
48. Von Knorring J, Pettersson T: Haemolytic anaemia complicating *Yersinia enterocolitica* infection. Report of a case. *Scand J Haematol* 9:149, 1972.
49. Berkowitz FE: Hemolysis and infection: Categories and mechanisms of their interrelationship. *Rev Infect Dis* 13:1151, 1991.
50. Seitz RC, Buschermohle G, Dubberke G, et al: The acute infection-associated hemolytic anemia of childhood: Immunofluorescent detection of microbial antigens altering the erythrocyte membrane. *Ann Hematol* 67:191, 1993.
51. Rowe AK, Rowe SY, Snow RW, et al: The burden of malaria mortality among African children in the year 2000. *Int J Epidemiol* 35:691, 2006.
52. Greenwood BM: The epidemiology of malaria. *Ann Trop Med Parasitol* 91:763, 1997.
53. Pasvol G, Clough B, Carlsson J: Malaria and the red cell membrane. *Blood Rev* 6:183, 1992.
54. Orlandi PA, Klotz FW, Haynes JD: A malaria invasion receptor, the 175-kilodalton erythrocyte binding antigen of *Plasmodium falciparum* recognizes the terminal Neu5Ac(alpha 2–3)Gal-sequences of glycophorin A. *J Cell Biol* 116:901, 1992.
55. Sim BKL, Chitnis CE, Wasniowska K, et al: Receptor and ligand domains for invasion of erythrocytes by *Plasmodium falciparum*. *Science* 264:1941, 1994.
56. Huber SM, Lang C, Lang F, Duranton C: Organic osmolyte channels in malaria-infected erythrocytes. *Biochem Biophys Res Commun* 376:514, 2008.
57. Nakamura K, Hasler T, Morehead K, et al: *Plasmodium falciparum*-infected erythrocyte receptor(s) for CD36 and thrombospondin are restricted to knobs on the erythrocyte surface. *J Histochem Cytochem* 40:1419, 1992.
58. Aikawa M, Kamanura K, Shiraishi S, et al: Membrane knobs of unfixed *Plasmodium falciparum* infected erythrocytes: New findings as revealed by atomic force microscopy and surface potential spectroscopy. *Exp Parasitol* 84:339, 1996.
59. Newbold C, Warn P, Black G, et al: Receptor-specific adhesion and clinical disease in *Plasmodium falciparum*. *Am J Trop Med Hyg* 57:389, 1997.
60. Baruch DI, Ma XC, Singh HB, et al: Identification of a region of PfEMP1 that mediates adherence of *Plasmodium falciparum* infected erythrocytes to CD36: Conserved function with variant sequence. *Blood* 90:3766, 1997.
61. Pasloske BL, Howard RJ: Malaria, the red cell, and the endothelium. *Annu Rev Med* 45:283, 1994.
62. Udomsangpetch R, Taylor BJ, Looareesuwan S, et al: Receptor specificity of clinical *Plasmodium falciparum* isolates: Nonadherence to cell-bound E-selectin and vascular cell adhesion molecule-1. *Blood* 88:2754, 1996.
63. McCormick CJ, Craig A, Roberts D, et al: Intercellular adhesion molecule-1 and CD36 synergize to mediate adherence of *Plasmodium falciparum*-infected erythrocytes to cultured human microvascular endothelial cells. *J Clin Invest* 100:2521, 1997.
64. Cockburn IA, MacKinnon MJ, O'Donnell A, et al: A human complement receptor 1 polymorphism that reduces *Plasmodium falciparum* rosetting confers protection against severe malaria. *Proc Natl Acad Sci U S A* 101:272, 2004.
65. Herrera S, Rudin W, Herrera M, et al: A conserved region of the MSP-1 surface protein of *Plasmodium falciparum* contains a recognition sequence for erythrocyte spectrin. *EMBO J* 12:1607, 1993.
66. Lamikanra AA, Brown D, Potocnik A, et al: Malarial anemia: Of mice and men. *Blood* 110:18, 2007.
67. Mombo LE, Ntoumi F, Bisseye C, et al: Human genetic polymorphisms and asymptomatic *Plasmodium falciparum* malaria in Gabonese school-children. *Am J Trop Med Hyg* 68:186, 2003.
68. Clegg JB, Weatherall DJ: Thalassemia and malaria: New insights into an old problem. *Proc Assoc Am Physicians* 111:278, 1999.
69. Zimmerman PA, Patel SS, Maier AG, et al: Erythrocyte polymorphisms and malaria parasite invasion in Papua New Guinea. *Trends Parasitol* 19:250, 2003.
70. Angus BJ, Chotivanich K, Udomsangpetch R, White NJ: In vivo removal of malaria parasites from red blood cells without their destruction in acute falciparum malaria. *Blood* 90:2037, 1997.

71. Jakeman GN, Saul A, Hogarth WL, Collins WE: Anaemia of acute malaria infections in non-immune patients primarily results from destruction of uninfected erythrocytes. *Parasitology* 119(Pt 2):127, 1999.
72. George JN, Wicker DJ, Fogel BJ, et al: Erythrocytic abnormalities in experimental malaria. *Proc Soc Exp Biol Med* 124:1086, 1967.
73. Overman RR: Reversible cellular permeability alterations in disease. In vivo studies on sodium, potassium and chloride concentrations in erythrocytes of the malarious monkey. *Am J Physiol* 152:113, 1948.
74. Gatidis S, Föller M, Lang F: Hemin-induced suicidal erythrocyte death. *Ann Hematol* 2009.
75. Clark IA, Hunt NH: Evidence for reactive oxygen intermediates causing hemolysis and parasite death in malaria. *Infect Immun* 39:1, 1983.
76. Stocker R, Cowden WB, Tellan RL, et al: Lipids from *Plasmodium vinckei*-infected erythrocytes and their susceptibility to oxidative damage. *Lipids* 22:51, 1987.
77. Yuthavong Y, Limpaiboon T: The relationship of phosphorylation of membrane proteins with the osmotic fragility and filterability of *Plasmodium berghei*-infected mouse erythrocytes. *Biochim Biophys Acta* 929:278, 1987.
78. Balcerzak SP, Arnold JD, Martin DC: Anatomy of red cell damage by *Plasmodium falciparum* in man. *Blood* 40:98, 1972.
79. Conrad ME: Pathophysiology of malaria. Hematologic observations in human and animal studies. *Ann Intern Med* 70:134, 1969.
80. Jenkins NE, Chakravorty SJ, Urban BC, et al: The effect of *Plasmodium falciparum* infection on expression of monocyte surface molecules. *Trans R Soc Trop Med Hyg* 100:1007, 2006.
81. Helegbe GK, Goka BQ, Kurtzhals JA, et al: Complement activation in Ghanaian children with severe Plasmodium falciparum malaria. Malar J. 6:165, 2007.
82. Price R, van Vugt M, Phaipun L, et al: Adverse effects in patients with acute falciparum malaria treated with artemisinin derivatives. *Am J Trop Med Hyg* 60:547, 1999.
83. Anthony RL, Bangs MJ, Anthony JM, Purnomo: On-site diagnosis of *Plasmodium falciparum, P. vivax*, and *P. malariae* by using the quantitative buffy coat system. *J Parasitol* 78:994, 1992.
84. Weiss JB: DNA probes and PCR for diagnosis of parasitic infections. *Clin Microbiol Rev* 8:113, 1995.
85. Oliveira DA, Holloway BP, Durigon EL, et al: Polymerase chain reaction and a liquid-phase, nonisotopic hybridization for species-specific and sensitive detection of malaria infection. *Am J Trop Med Hyg* 52:139, 1995.
86. Orjih AU: Requirements for maximal enrichment of viable intraerythrocytic Plasmodium falciparum rings by saponin hemolysis. *Exp Biol Med (Maywood)* 233:1359, 2008.
87. Orimadegun AE, Amodu OK, Olumese PE, et al: Early home treatment of childhood fevers with ineffective antimalarials is deleterious in the outcome of severe malaria. *Malar J* 7:143, 2008.
88. Beutler E, Duparc S, G6PD Deficiency Working Group: Glucose-6-phosphate dehydrogenase deficiency and antimalarial drug development. *Am J Trop Med Hyg* 77:779, 2007.
89. Aldana L: Bacteriologia de la enfermedad de carrion. *Cronica Med* 46:235, 1929.
90. Xu YH, Lu ZY, Ihler GM: Purification of deformin, an extracellular protein synthesized by *Bartonella bacilliformis* which causes deformation of erythrocyte membranes. *Biochim Biophys Acta* 1234:173, 1995.
91. Mitchell SJ, Minnick MF: Characterization of a two-gene locus from *Bartonella bacilliformis* associated with the ability to invade human erythrocytes. *Infect Immun* 63:1552, 1995.
92. Weinman D: Human *Bartonella* infection and African sleeping sickness. *Bull N Y Acad Med* 22:647, 1946.
93. García-Esteban C, Gil H, Rodríguez-Vargas M, et al: Molecular method for *Bartonella* species identification in clinical and environmental samples. *J Clin Microbiol* 46:776, 2008.
94. Dalton MJ, Robinson LE, Cooper J, et al: Use of *Bartonella* antigens for serologic diagnosis of cat-scratch disease at a national referral center. *Arch Intern Med* 155:1670, 1995.
95. Eremeeva ME, Gerns HL, Lydy SL, et al: Bacteremia, fever, and splenomegaly caused by a newly recognized *Bartonella* species. *N Engl J Med* 356:2381, 2007.
96. Koehler JE, Sanchez MA, Tye S, et al: Prevalence of *Bartonella* infection among human immunodeficiency virus-infected patients with fever. *Clin Infect Dis* 37:559, 2003.
97. Reubush TK II, Cassaday PB, Marsh HJ, et al: Human babesiosis on Nantucket Island. *Ann Intern Med* 86:6, 1977.
98. Krause PJ: Babesiosis. *Med Clin North Am* 86:361, 2002.
99. Krause PJ, McKay K, Gadbaw J, et al: Increasing health burden of human babesiosis in endemic sites. *Am J Trop Med Hyg* 68:431, 2003.
100. Herwaldt BL, McGovern PC, Gerwel MP, et al: Endemic babesiosis in another eastern state: New Jersey. *Emerg Infect Dis* 9:184, 2003.
101. Jacoby GA, Hunt JV, Kosinski KS, et al: Treatment of transfusion-transmitted babesiosis by exchange transfusion. *N Engl J Med* 303:1098, 1980.
102. Smith RP, Evans AT, Popovsky M, et al: Transfusion-acquired babesiosis and failure of antibiotic treatment. *JAMA* 256:2726, 1986.
103. Herwaldt BL, Kjemtrup AM, Conrad PA, et al: Transfusion-transmitted babesiosis in Washington State: First reported case caused by a WA1-type parasite. *J Infect Dis* 175:1259, 1997.
104. Nelson R: Blood on demand. *Am Heritage Invention Technol* 19:24, 2004.
105. Dobroszycki J, Herwaldt BL, Boctor F, et al: A cluster of transfusion-associated babesiosis cases traced to a single asymptomatic donor. *JAMA* 281:927, 1999.
106. Kjemtrup AM, Lee B, Fritz CL, et al: Investigation of transfusion transmission of a WA1-type babesial parasite to a premature infant in California. *Transfusion* 42:1482, 2002.
107. Steketee RW, Eckman MR, Burgess EC, et al: Babesiosis in Wisconsin. A new focus of disease transmission. *JAMA* 253:2675, 1985.
108. Homer MJ, Aguilar-Delfin I, Telford SR 3rd, et al: Babesiosis. *Clin Microbiol Rev* 13:451, 2000.
109. Cheng D, Yakobi-Shvilli R, Fernandez J: Life-threatening hypotension from babesiosis hemolysis. *Am J Emerg Med* 20:367, 2002.
110. Wittner M, Rowin KS, Tanowitz HB, et al: Successful chemotherapy of transfusion babesiosis. *Ann Intern Med* 96:601, 1982.
111. Weiss LM: Babesiosis in humans: A treatment review. *Expert Opin Pharmacotherapy* 3:1109, 2002.
112. Clancy MT, OBriain S: Fatal *Clostridium welchii* septicaemia following acute cholecystitis. *Br J Surg* 62:518, 1975.
113. Hamoda H, Chamberlain PF: *Clostridium welchii* infection following amniocentesis: a case report and review of the literature. *Prenat Diagn* 22:783, 2002.
114. Simpkins H, Kahlenberg A, Rosenberg A, et al: Structural and compositional changes in the red cell membrane during *Clostridium welchii* infection. *Br J Haematol* 21:173, 1971.
115. Mahn HE, Dantuono LM: Postabortal septicotoxemia due to *Clostridium welchii. Am J Obstet Gynecol* 70:604, 1955.
116. Moustoukas NM, Nichols RL, Voros D: Clostridial sepsis: Unusual clinical presentations. *South Med J* 78:440, 1985.
117. Neter E: Bacterial hemagglutination and hemolysis. *Bacteriol Rev* 20:166, 1956.
118. Ceppellini R, De Gregorio M: Crisi emolitica in animali batterio-immuni transfusi con sangue omologo sensibilizzato in vitro mediante l'antigene batterico specifico. *Boll Ist Sieroter Milan* 32:445, 1953.
119. Dausset J, Moullec J, Bernard J: Acquired hemolytic anemia with polyagglutinability of red blood cells due to a new factor. *Blood* 14:1079, 1959.
120. Klein PJ, Vierbuchen M, Roth B, et al: Hemolytic anemia in infections caused by neuraminidase-producing bacteria. *Verh Dtsch Ges Pathol* 67:415, 1983.
121. McGinniss MH, Macher AM, Rook AH, Alter HJ: Red cell autoantibodies in patients with acquired immune deficiency syndrome. *Transfusion* 26:405, 1986.
122. Zuelzer WW, Stulberg CS, Page RH, et al: The Emily Cooley lecture. Etiology and pathogenesis of acquired hemolytic anemia. *Transfusion* 6:438, 1966.
123. Ullis KC, Rosenblatt RM: *Shiga* bacillus dysentery complicated by bacteremia and disseminated intravascular coagulation. *J Pediatr* 83:90, 1973.
124. Chesney R, Kaplan BS: Hemolytic-uremic syndrome with shigellosis. *J Pediatr* 84:312, 1974.
125. Dickgiesser A: Campylobacter infection and the hemolytic-uremic syndrome. *Immun Infekt* 11:71, 1983.

CHAPTER 53
HEMOLYTIC ANEMIA RESULTING FROM IMMUNE INJURY

Charles H. Packman

SUMMARY

Autoimmune hemolytic anemia (AHA) is characterized by shortened red blood cell (RBC) survival and the presence of autoantibodies directed against autologous RBCs. A positive direct antiglobulin test (DAT, also known as the Coombs test) is essential for diagnosis. Most patients with AHA (80%) exhibit warm-reactive antibodies of the immunoglobulin (Ig) G isotype on their red cells. Most of the remainder of patients exhibit cold-reactive autoantibodies. Two types of cold-reactive autoantibodies to RBCs are recognized: cold agglutinins and cold hemolysins. Cold agglutinins are generally of IgM isotype, whereas cold hemolysins usually are of IgG isotype. The DAT may detect IgG, proteolytic fragments of complement (mainly C3), or both on the RBCs of patients with warm-antibody AHA. In cold-antibody AHA, only complement is detected because the antibody dissociates from the RBCs during washing of the cells. About half of patients with AHA have no underlying associated disease; these cases are termed primary or idiopathic. Secondary cases are associated with underlying autoimmune, malignant, or infectious diseases or with ingestion of certain drugs.

Although most patients do not require transfusion of RBCs, transfusion should not be withheld from those with symptomatic anemia. In warm-antibody AHA, glucocorticoids are effective in slowing the rate of hemolysis. Splenectomy is indicated for patients who require an unacceptably high maintenance dose or prolonged administration of glucocorticoids. Intravenous immunoglobulin may provide short-term control of hemolysis. Immunosuppressive drugs and danazol have been used successfully in refractory cases. In cold agglutinin- and cold hemolysin-mediated hemolysis, keeping the patient warm and treating underlying lymphoproliferative disorders usually are effective. Rituximab has been effective in reported cases of both warm and cold AHA. Drug-immune hemolytic anemia usually is ameliorated by discontinuation of the offending drug.

DEFINITION AND HISTORY

The two main features of immune red blood cell (RBC) injury are (1) shortened RBC survival *in vivo* and (2) evidence of host antibodies reactive with autologous RBCs, most frequently demonstrated by a positive direct antiglobulin test (DAT), also known as the Coombs test. Most cases in adults are mediated by warm-reactive autoantibodies. A smaller proportion of patients exhibit cold-reactive autoantibodies or drug-related antibodies.

By the early 20th century, reticulocytes, spherocytes, and osmotic fragility of RBCs had been described. Clinicians could diagnose hemolytic anemia, but the distinction between congenital and acquired forms was imprecise. Some clinicians even doubted the existence of acquired hemolytic anemia.[1] The sera of some patients with hemolytic anemia directly agglutinated saline suspensions of normal or autologous human RBCs. These serum factors, later shown to be specific antibodies (largely of the immunoglobulin [Ig] M class), were termed *direct* or *saline agglutinins*. In a smaller proportion of cases, the patients' sera could mediate lysis of the test RBCs in the presence of fresh serum as a complement source. The heat-stable factors (antibodies) necessary for *in vitro* complement-mediated lysis were called *hemolysins*. However, in the majority of cases of hemolytic anemia, neither direct agglutinins nor hemolysins could be demonstrated. In 1945, Coombs and colleagues[2] reported that RBCs coated with nonagglutinating Rh antibodies (now known to be of the IgG isotype) could be agglutinated by rabbit antiserum to human γ-globulin. That is, the rabbit antiglobulin serum cross-linked IgG antibody-coated RBCs to produce visible agglutination. Addition of rabbit antiglobulin serum to a suspension of washed RBCs isolated from patients with suspected autoimmune hemolytic anemia (AHA) produced agglutination in many cases, including those patients lacking saline agglutinins or hemolysins. RBCs from patients with congenital hemolytic anemia did not agglutinate.[3,4] This procedure now is termed the *direct antiglobulin (Coombs) test*. Subsequent studies established that positive direct antiglobulin reactions in AHA are attributable to coating of the RBCs with immunoglobulins (mainly IgG) and/or complement proteins. When the RBCs are coated chiefly with complement proteins, a positive DAT depends upon the presence of anticomplement (principally anti-C3) in the antiglobulin reagent.

Cryopathic hemolytic syndromes are caused by autoantibodies that bind RBCs optimally at temperatures less than 37°C and usually less than 31°C. Two major types of "cold antibody" may produce AHA. Cold agglutinins, which directly agglutinate RBCs, mediate cold agglutinin disease. The Donath-Landsteiner autoantibody, which is not an agglutinin but a potent hemolysin, mediates paroxysmal cold hemoglobinuria. In both cryopathic syndromes, the complement system plays a major role in RBC injury (see Chap. 17); as such, much greater potential exists for direct intravascular hemolysis than in warm-antibody–mediated AHA.

Cold agglutinins were first described by Landsteiner[5] in 1903. However, recognition of the connection among cold agglutinins, hemolytic anemia, and Raynaud-like peripheral vascular phenomena evolved slowly. In 1918, Clough and Richter[6] detected cold agglutinins in a patient with pneumonia. In 1925 and 1926, Iwai and MeiSai[7,8] reported two patients with cold agglutinins and Raynaud phenomenon and showed that flow of blood through capillary tubes *in vitro* or in superficial capillaries *in vivo* was impeded at low temperatures. During the late 1940s and early 1950s, the observations of many workers gradually established the pathogenic importance of cold agglutinins in RBC injury. Schubothe[9] introduced the term *cold agglutinin disease* in 1953 and clearly distinguished the disorder from other acquired hemolytic syndromes.

In current usage, cold agglutinin disease pertains to patients with chronic AHA in which the autoantibody directly agglutinates human RBCs at temperatures below body temperature, maximally at 0 to 5°C. Fixation of complement to a patient's RBCs by cold agglutinins *in vivo* occurs at higher temperatures but generally less than 37°C. Cold agglutinins typically are IgM, although occasionally they may be immunoglobulins of other isotypes. The cold agglutinins in chronic cold agglutinin disease generally are monoclonal. Most cold agglutinins have specificity for oligosaccharide antigens (I or i) of the RBC (see "Origin of Cold Agglutinins" below).

Acronyms and abbreviations that appear in this chapter include: AHA, autoimmune hemolytic anemia; CLL, chronic lymphocytic leukemia; DAF, decay accelerating factor; DAT, direct antiglobulin test; HLA, human leukocyte antigen; HRF, homologous restriction factor; HS, hereditary spherocytosis; IAT, indirect antiglobulin test; Ig, immunoglobulin; IGHV, immunoglobulin heavy chain variable region; PNH, paroxysmal nocturnal hemoglobinuria; RBC, red blood cell; SLE, systemic lupus erythematosus.

Donath and Landsteiner first described the cold hemolysin that bears their name in 1904. The Donath-Landsteiner antibody is responsible for complement-mediated hemolysis in paroxysmal cold hemoglobinuria, a rare form of AHA in adults. The disorder is characterized by recurrent episodes of massive hemolysis following cold exposure.[10,11] A related form of hemolytic anemia occurs much more commonly in children (or young adults) as an acute, self-limited hemolytic process following several types of viral syndromes.[10–16] The disease was recognized during the latter half of the 19th century, when the disease was more common because of its association with congenital or tertiary syphilis. With the advent of effective therapy for syphilis, this cause of paroxysmal cold hemoglobinuria has almost disappeared. Now, recurrent paroxysmal cold hemoglobinuria occurs very rarely in a chronic idiopathic form.[10,11] An increasing proportion of Donath-Landsteiner autoantibody-mediated hemolytic anemias occurs as a single postviral episode in children, without recurrent attacks (paroxysms). The prognosis for such cases is excellent. Thus, rather than paroxysmal cold hemoglobinuria, a proposed term for this latter entity is *Donath-Landsteiner hemolytic* anemia.[13,14]

The first example of drug-related immune blood cell destruction was Ackroyd's description of sedormid purpura in 1949.[17] In 1953, Snapper and coworkers[18] described a case of immune hemolysis and pancytopenia in a patient treated with mephenytoin (Mesantoin). Hemolysis ceased upon withdrawal of the drug. In 1956, Harris[19] reported what are now classic studies of a patient who developed immune hemolytic anemia during a second course of stibophen administered for treatment of schistosomiasis. Since then, many drugs have been implicated in the production of positive DATs and accelerated RBC destruction.

CLASSIFICATION

Warm-Reactive versus Cold-Reactive Red Cell Antibody

AHA can be classified in two complementary ways (Table 53–1). The majority of cases (80–90% in adults) are mediated by warm-reactive autoantibodies[10,11,20] or antibodies displaying optimal reactivity with human RBCs at 37°C. A smaller proportion of cases is attributable to cold-reactive autoantibodies exhibiting greater affinity for RBCs at temperatures less than 37°C. The distinction is important, not only because of differences in the pathophysiology of RBC injury but also in the therapeutic approaches required. An even smaller proportion of patients with AHA exhibit both cold-reactive and warm-reactive autoantibodies,[21,22] which apparently recognize different antigens on the RBC membrane.[23] RBC destruction is generally more severe in mixed cases.

Absence or Presence of an Associated Disease

Classification of AHA based on the presence or absence of underlying diseases also is useful (see Table 53–1). When no recognizable underlying disease is present, the AHA is termed *primary* or *idiopathic*. When AHA appears to be a manifestation or complication of an underlying disorder, the term *secondary AHA* is applied. Lymphocytic malignancies, particularly chronic lymphocytic leukemia (CLL) and lymphomas, account for about half of all secondary AHA cases and for the majority of AHA cases mediated by cold agglutinins.[24] Systemic lupus erythematosus (SLE) and other autoimmune diseases account for a lesser but considerable proportion of secondary AHA cases. A large proportion of patients with mixed cold and warm autoantibodies have SLE.[21,22] Infectious mononucleosis and *Mycoplasma pneumoniae* occasionally are associated with cryopathic AHA. Despite the frequent occurrence of immune thrombocytopenia and positive DATs in patients infected with HIV, AHA is relatively rare in these patients.[25–27] Table 53–1 lists other associated diseases that are less commonly reported. The etiologic and pathogenic significance of these associations is poorly understood, but most of the associated diseases involve components of the immune system, either by neoplasia or by aberrant immunopathologic responses.

TABLE 53–1. Classification of Hemolytic Anemia as a Result of Immune Injury

I. Warm-Autoantibody Type: Autoantibody Maximally Active at Body Temperature (37°C)
  A. Primary or idiopathic warm AHA
  B. Secondary warm AHA
    1. Associated with lymphoproliferative disorders (e.g., Hodgkin lymphoma)
    2. Associated with the rheumatic disorders, particularly systemic lupus erythematosus (SLE)
    3. Associated with certain nonlymphoid neoplasms (e.g., ovarian tumors)
    4. Associated with certain chronic inflammatory diseases (e.g., ulcerative colitis)
    5. Associated with ingestion of certain drugs (e.g., α-methyldopa)

II. Cold-Autoantibody Type: Autoantibody Optimally Active at Temperatures <37°C
  A. Mediated by cold agglutinins
    1. Idiopathic (primary) chronic cold agglutinin disease (usually associated with clonal B-lymphocyte proliferation)
    2. Secondary cold agglutinin hemolytic anemia
      a. Postinfectious (e.g., *Mycoplasma pneumoniae* or infectious mononucleosis)
      b. Associated with malignant B-cell lymphoproliferative disorder
  B. Mediated by cold hemolysins
    1. Idiopathic (primary) paroxysmal cold hemoglobinuria (very rare)
    2. Secondary
      a. Donath-Landsteiner hemolytic anemia, usually associated with an acute viral syndrome in children (relatively common)
      b. Congenital or tertiary syphilis in adults (very rare)

III. Mixed Cold and Warm Autoantibodies
  A. Primary or idiopathic mixed AHA
  B. Secondary mixed AHA
    1. Associated with the rheumatic disorders, particularly SLE

IV. Drug-Immune Hemolytic Anemia
  A. Hapten or drug adsorption mechanism
  B. Ternary (immune) complex mechanism
  C. True autoantibody mechanism

Drug-Mediated Cases

Certain drugs also mediate immune injury to RBCs, and three general mechanisms are recognized (see Table 53–1 and Fig. 53–1). This classification is based on the effector mechanism of RBC injury, because the induction mechanism for formation of drug-related RBC antibodies is unknown. Two of the mechanisms, hapten-drug adsorption and ternary complex formation, involve drug-dependent antibodies. In the third mechanism, the drugs in question appear to induce formation of true autoantibodies capable of reacting with human RBCs in the

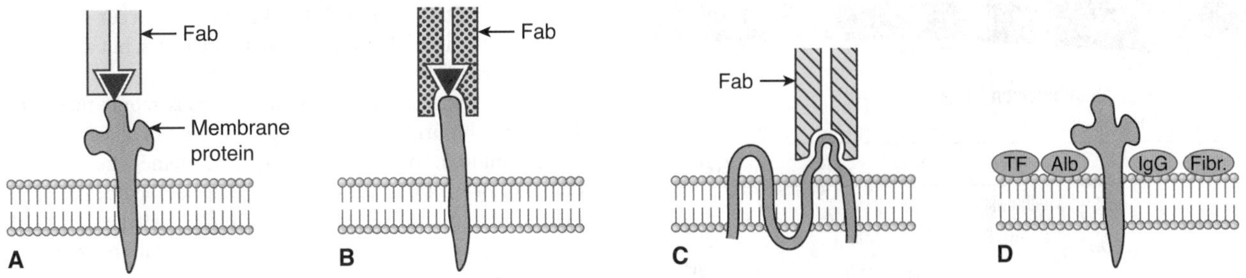

FIGURE 53–1. Effector mechanisms by which drugs mediate a positive direct antiglobulin test. Relationships of drug, antibody-combining site, and red blood cell membrane protein are shown. Panels *A, B,* and *C* show only a single immunoglobulin Fab region (bearing one combining site). **A.** Drug adsorption/hapten mechanism. The drug (▼) binds avidly to an unknown red blood cell membrane protein *in vivo*. Antidrug antibody (usually IgG) binds to the protein-bound drug. The membrane protein is not known to be part of the epitope recognized by the antidrug antibody. The direct antiglobulin test (with anti-IgG) detects IgG antidrug antibody on the patient's circulating (drug-coated) red blood cells. The indirect antiglobulin test detects antibody in the patient's serum only when the test red blood cells have been previously coated with the drug by incubation *in vitro.* **B.** Ternary complex mechanism. Drug binds loosely or in undetectable amounts to red blood cell membrane. However, in the presence of appropriate antidrug antibody, a stable trimolecular (ternary) complex is formed by drug, red blood cell membrane protein, and antibody. In general, the antibody-combining site (Fab) recognizes both drug and membrane protein components but binds only weakly to either drug or protein unless both are present in the reaction mixture. In this mechanism, the direct antiglobulin test typically detects only red blood cell–bound complement components (e.g., C3 fragments) that are bound covalently and in large number to the patient's red blood cells *in vivo*. The antibody itself escapes detection, possibly because of its low concentration but also because washing of the red cells (in the antiglobulin test procedure) apparently dissociates antibody and drug from the cells, leaving only the covalently bound C3 fragments. The indirect antiglobulin test also detects complement proteins on the test red blood cells when both antibody (patient serum) and a complement source (fresh patient serum or fresh normal serum) are present in the reaction mixture together with the drug. **C.** Autoantibody induction. Some drug-induced antibodies can bind avidly to red blood cell membrane proteins (usually Rh proteins) in the absence of the inducing drug and are indistinguishable from the autoantibodies of patients with autoimmune hemolytic anemia. The direct antiglobulin test detects the IgG antibody on the patient's red blood cells. The indirect antiglobulin test usually detects antibody in the serum of patients with active hemolysis. **D.** Drug-induced nonimmunologic protein adsorption. Certain drugs cause plasma proteins to attach nonspecifically to the red blood cell membrane. The direct antiglobulin test detects nonspecifically bound IgG and complement components. If special antiglobulin reagents are used, other plasma proteins, such as transferrin, albumin, and fibrinogen, also may be detected. In contrast to the other mechanisms of drug-induced red blood cell injury, this mechanism does not shorten red blood cell survival *in vivo*.

absence of the inciting drug. These types of drug-mediated immune injury to RBCs often are referred to collectively as *drug-immune hemolytic anemia* to distinguish them from *de novo* AHA. Distinguishing among the mechanisms is not always possible, and some cases involve a combination of mechanisms. In addition, drug-related nonimmunologic protein adsorption by RBCs may result in a positive DAT without actual RBC injury. This phenomenon should be distinguished from the three forms of drug-immune RBC injury. Table 53–2 lists drugs documented to cause either immune injury or a positive DAT.

EPIDEMIOLOGY

The annual incidence of warm-antibody AHA is 1 per 75,000 to 80,000 population.[11] Estimates of the frequency of primary (idiopathic) AHA vary from 20 to 80 percent of all types of AHA, depending on the referral patterns of the reporting center.[11,20,111] In general, AHA is considered secondary (1) when AHA and the underlying disease occur together with greater frequency than can be accounted for by chance alone; (2) when the AHA reverses simultaneously with correction of the associated disease; or (3) when AHA and the associated disease are related by evidence of immunologic aberration.[11] Using these criteria, the frequency of primary warm-antibody AHA probably is closer to 50 percent of all cases. Careful followup of patients with primary AHA is essential, because hemolytic anemia may be the presenting finding in a patient who subsequently develops overt evidence of an underlying disorder. For example, in one series, 18 of 107 patients with AHA developed a malignant lymphoproliferative disorder at a median of 26.5 months after diagnosis of the AHA.[112]

Warm-antibody AHA has been diagnosed in people of all ages, from infants to the elderly. The majority of patients are older than 40 years of age, with peak incidence around the seventh decade. This age distribution probably reflects, in part, the increased frequency of lymphoproliferative malignancies in the elderly, resulting in an age-related increase in the frequency of secondary AHA. Although multiple cases are occasionally observed in families,[113–115] most cases of primary AHA arise sporadically. Development of AHA does not have an apparent association with any particular human leukocyte antigen (HLA) haplotype or other genetic factor.

Cold agglutinin disease is less common than warm-antibody AHA, with a prevalence of approximately 14 per million,[24] accounting for only 10 to 20 percent of all cases of AHA.[10,11,116] Women are affected more commonly than men.[10,11] No genetic or racial factors are known to contribute to the pathogenesis of this disease.

Secondary cold agglutinin disease is seen most commonly in adolescents or young adults as a self-limited process associated with *M. pneumoniae* infections or infectious mononucleosis and, rarely, in children with chickenpox. The term also has been used to describe a chronic disorder occurring in older patients with known malignant lymphoproliferative diseases. On the other hand, idiopathic (primary) chronic cold agglutinin disease has its peak incidence after age 50 years. This disorder, with its characteristic monoclonal IgM cold agglutinins, may be considered a special form of monoclonal gammopathy (see Chap. 108). Nearly all of these patients exhibit clonal B lymphocyte proliferation.[24] As with other "essential" or idiopathic monoclonal gammopathies, some patients in this group gradually develop features of a B-cell lymphoproliferative disorder resembling Waldenström macroglobulinemia. Thus, the distinction between primary and secondary types of chronic cold agglutinin disease is not absolute.

Although the majority of patients with mycoplasma pneumonia have significant cold agglutinin titers, they only infrequently develop clinical hemolytic anemia.[117–119] However, subclinical RBC injury may occur. In *M. pneumoniae* infections, weakly positive direct antiglobulin reactions and/or mild reticulocytosis are often noted in the absence of anemia in a

TABLE 53–2. Association between Drugs and Positive Direct Antiglobulin Tests

Drug	Reference	Drug	Reference
Hapten or Drug Adsorption Mechanism			
Penicillins	28–34	Carbromal	43
Cephalosporins	35–39	Tolbutamide	44, 45
Tetracycline	40, 41	Cianidanol	46
6-Mercaptopurine	42	Hydrocortisone	47
		Oxaliplatin	48
Ternary Complex Mechanism			
Stibophen	19	Probenecid	59
Quinine	49	Nomifensine	60–62
Quinidine	50, 51	Cephalosporins	37–39, 63
Chlorpropamide	52, 53	Diethylstilbestrol	64
Rifampicin	55	Amphotericin B	65
Antazoline	56	Doxepin	66
Thiopental	57	Diclofenac	67, 68
Tolmetin	58	Etodolac	69
Metformin	54	Hydrocortisone	47
		Oxaliplatin	48
		Pemetrexed	70
Autoantibody Mechanism			
Cephalosporins	39	Cianidanol	46
Tolmetin	58	Latamoxef	82
Nomifensine	60	Glafenine	82
α-Methyldopa	71–74	Procainamide	83
L-Dopa	75–79	Diclofenac	67, 84
Mefenamic acid	80, 81	Pentostatin	85
Teniposide	82	Fludarabine	86
Oxaliplatin	48	Cladribine	87
Efalizumab	88	Lenalidomide	89
Nonimmunologic Protein Adsorption			
Cephalosporins	90, 91	Cisplatin	48, 92
Oxaliplatin	48		
Carboplatin	48		
Uncertain Mechanism of Immune Injury			
Mesantoin	18	Streptomycin	100
Phenacetin	49	Ibuprofen	101
Insecticides	93	Triamterene	102
Chlorpromazine	94	Erythromycin	103
Melphalan	95	5-Fluorouracil	104
Isoniazid	96	Nalidixic acid	105
p-Aminosalicylic acid	97	Sulindac	106
Acetaminophen	98	Omeprazole	107
Thiazides	99	Temafloxacin	108
Efavirenz	110	Carboplatin	109

substantial number of cases.[117] Cold agglutinins occur in more than 60 percent of patients with infectious mononucleosis, but again, hemolytic anemia is rare.[120–122]

Medical centers that receive many referrals report that paroxysmal cold hemoglobinuria constitutes 2 to 5 percent of all cases of AHA.[10,11] Among children, however, Donath-Landsteiner hemolytic anemia accounted for 32.4 percent of 68 immune hemolytic syndromes diagnosed over a 4-year period.[15] Commonly, the diagnosis is missed because of lack of physicians' awareness or failure to perform the proper serologic studies (see "Serologic Features" below).[12,15] Thus, the true incidence may be higher. Although familial occurrence has been reported, no racial or genetic risk factors are known.[10] As noted, most childhood cases follow either specific viral infections or upper respiratory infections of undefined etiology.[10–15]

Older series report that drug-immune hemolytic anemia accounts for 12 to 18 percent of immune hemolytic anemias.[11] The disorder is much less common now that α-methyldopa and megaunit doses of penicillin rarely are used. The current incidence of drug-immune hemolytic anemia is estimated at 1 per 1 million population, approximately 88 percent of which result from the second- and third-generation cephalosporins, cefotetan, and ceftriaxone.[123]

ETIOLOGY AND PATHOGENESIS

ETIOLOGY

Warm-Antibody Autoimmune Hemolytic Anemia

The etiology of AHA is unknown. In warm-antibody AHA, the autoantibodies that mediate RBC destruction are predominantly (but not exclusively) IgG globulins possessing relatively high binding affinity for human RBCs at 37°C. As a result, the major share of plasma autoantibody is bound to the patient's circulating RBCs. Eluates prepared from the patient's washed, autoantibody-coated RBCs constitute an important source of purified autoantibody for investigation of specificity, immunoglobulin structure, or other properties. In addition, sera from patients with warm AHA often are used in blood banks for cross-matching and for general screening of antibody specificity. The quantity of such autoantibody in serum may be low and in some cases may not reflect the full spectrum of anti-RBC specificity revealed in concurrently prepared RBC eluates.[124]

In patients with primary AHA, erythrocyte autoantibodies are the only recognizable immunologic aberration. Furthermore, the autoantibodies of any one patient often are specific for only a single RBC membrane protein (see "Serologic Features" below). The narrow spectrum of autoreactivity suggests the mechanism underlying AHA development in such patients is not secondary to a generalized defect in immune regulation. Rather, these patients may develop warm-antibody AHA through an aberrant immune response to a self-antigen or to an immunogen that mimics a self-antigen.

In patients with secondary AHA, the disease may be associated with a fundamental disturbance in the immune system, for example, when in the setting of lymphoma, CLL, SLE, primary agammaglobulinemia (common variable immunodeficiency), or hyper-IgM immunodeficiency syndrome. In these settings, warm-antibody AHA most likely arises through an underlying defect in immune regulation, although the contribution of an aberrant immune response to self-antigen cannot be excluded. AHA seems especially frequent in patients with low-grade lymphoma or CLL treated with fludarabine[86] or 2-chlorodeoxyadenosine (cladribine).[87] The T-lymphocytopenia induced by these drugs may exacerbate the preexisting tendency of patients to form autoantibodies.

A long-recognized but poorly understood phenomenon, the development of AHA or a positive DAT following RBC transfusion, has received renewed interest lately.[125,126] Although generally transient, the positive DAT may persist for up to 300 days in some transfusion recipients, long after any transfused RBCs have disappeared.[127,128] It is not clear whether this represents true autoimmunity or some other mechanism, for example, microchimerism resulting from temporary engraftment of passenger memory lymphocytes from the RBC donor.[125]

A still unexplained observation is that certain drugs, such as α-methyldopa, can induce warm-reacting IgG anti-RBC autoantibodies in otherwise normal persons. The autoantibodies induced by α-methyldopa have Rh-related serologic and immunochemical[129] specificity similar to that of autoantibodies arising in many patients with "spontaneous" AHA. A critical difference is that the drug-associated autoantibodies subside when the drug is discontinued, suggesting that (1) the latent potential to form this type of anti-RBC autoantibody is present in many immunologically normal individuals, and (2) the steps required to generate such autoantibodies do not necessarily create a sustained autoimmune state. On the other hand, maintenance of chronic idiopathic AHA may be either secondary to a continuing (but unknown) stimulus or induced by a short stimulus to which the patient continues to respond.

Normal subjects sometimes have a positive DAT when they volunteer to donate blood.[130,131] The positive DAT in these normal donors often results from warm-reacting IgG autoantibodies, similar in serologic specificity[124] and in IgG subclass[130] to the autoantibodies occurring in AHA. Although many of these donors remain Coombs positive without developing overt hemolytic anemia, a few have been documented to develop AHA.[130,131] The prevalence of positive DATs in normal blood donors is approximately 1 in 10,000.[130,132] Because blood donation *per se* likely does not contribute to an increased risk of developing autoantibodies, the 1 in 10,000 proportion likely is the approximate frequency of positive DATs in the entire population. A proportion of patients who present with clinically overt primary AHA may come from a subset of asymptomatic individuals who are DAT positive, but this notion is not established.

Several concepts have been developed to explain immunologic tolerance to self-antigens.[133–136] Relevant to warm-antibody AHA, membrane-bound antigens expressed in a multivalent array at high concentration may induce tolerance by effecting clonal deletion of autoreactive B cells.[137] Both the Rh-related and the non-Rh types of RBC antigens targeted by AHA autoantibodies (see "Serologic Features" below) are expressed normally by human fetal erythrocytes, as early as 10 to 12 weeks of life.[138] However, because new B cells develop daily in the marrow throughout life and because B cells may somatically mutate their Ig receptors, self-tolerance in the B cell compartment is never assured. Analogy to observations in NZB mice[139,140] suggests the peritoneal cavity is a privileged compartment that shelters autoreactive B cells from host RBCs, allowing them to escape deletion, later to produce anti-RBC autoantibodies with appropriate T-cell help. The strong predominance of IgG antibodies in AHA suggests B-cell isotype switching, which is consistent with the idea of an antigen-driven process. Moreover, because T-cell help is necessary for inducing B-cell isotype switching, the pathway(s) to autoantibody induction in AHA also may involve an abnormal or unique mode of antigen presentation to T cells.[141]

Origin of Cold Agglutinins

A high proportion of monoclonal IgM cold agglutinins with either anti-I or anti-i specificity have heavy-chain variable regions encoded by IGHV (immunoglobulin heavy chain variable region)4–34, formerly designated IGHV4.21.[136,142–144] This V_H gene encodes a distinct idiotype identified by the rat monoclonal antibody 9G4. This idiotype is expressed both by the cold agglutinins themselves and on the surface immunoglobulin of B cells synthesizing cold agglutinins or related immunoglobulins possessing IGHV4–34 sequences.[145] Using the 9G4 monoclonal antibody as a probe, this idiotype was found not only in a very high proportion of circulating B cells and marrow lymphoplasmacytoid cells of patients with lymphoma-associated chronic cold agglutinin disease, but also in a smaller proportion of B cells in the blood and lymphoid tissues of normal adult donors and in the spleens of 15-week human fetuses.[145] These data suggest B cells expressing the IGHV4–34 gene (or a closely related sequence) are present throughout ontogeny. Therefore, chronic cold agglutinin disease may represent a marked, unregulated expansion of a subset (clone) of such B cells.

Light-chain V-region gene use in anti-I cold agglutinins is highly selective. A strong bias toward use of the κIII variable region subgroup (Vκ-III) is observed.[143–146] Light-chain selection among anti-i cold agglutinins, however, is much more variable and includes the λ type.[143–147]

Observations that pathologic cold agglutinins are synthesized with distinct and highly selected V-region sequences must be viewed against the background of two other subsequent observations. First, IGHV4–34 or related IGHV genes also may encode the heavy-chain variable regions of other types of antibodies, such as rheumatoid factor autoantibodies and alloantibodies to a variety of blood group antigens, including polypeptide determinants such as Rh.[148] Second, normal human antibodies to an exogenous carbohydrate antigen, *Haemophilus influenzae* type b capsular polysaccharide, also are encoded by a restricted set of IGHV genes[149] and Ig light-chain V genes.[150] Thus, regulation of Ig gene use for production of anti-I or anti-i cold agglutinins may not differ fundamentally from normal antibody formation to other carbohydrate antigens.

In the setting of B-cell lymphoma or Waldenström macroglobulinemia, cold agglutinins may be produced by the malignant clone itself. Two patients with lymphoma and monoclonal cold agglutinin were identified as having a karyotypically abnormal B-cell clone that produced a cold agglutinin identical to that found in their sera.[151,152] Trisomy 3 has been the most frequently observed karyotypic abnormality in patients with non-Hodgkin lymphoma and cold agglutinins.[151,153]

Normal human sera generally have naturally occurring cold agglutinins in low titer (usually 1/32 or less). Otherwise healthy persons may develop elevated titers of cold agglutinins specific for I/i antigens during certain infections (e.g., *M. pneumoniae*, Epstein-Barr virus, cytomegalovirus). In contrast to other forms of cold agglutinin disease, hyperproduction of these postinfectious cold agglutinins is transient. Some evidence indicates postinfectious cold agglutinins may be less clonally restricted than those occurring in chronic cold agglutinin disease,[154] but this finding is not universal.[155] Whether IGHV4–34 also encodes most heavy-chain variable regions of all naturally occurring or postinfectious cold agglutinins remains to be determined.

The increased production of cold agglutinins in response to infection with *M. pneumoniae* may be secondary to the fact that the oligosaccharide antigens of the I/i type serve as specific *Mycoplasma* receptors.[156] This process may lead to altered antigen presentation involving a complex between a self-antigen (I/i) and a non–self-antigen *(Mycoplasma)*. Alternatively, the anti-i cold agglutinins may arise as a consequence of polyclonal B cell activation, as occurs in infectious mononucleosis (see Chap. 84).

The mechanism(s) whereby dissimilar infectious agents (e.g., spirochetes and several types of virus) induce the immune system to produce Donath-Landsteiner antibodies with specificity for the human P blood group antigen (see "Serologic Features" below) is not known.

PATHOGENESIS

Pathogenic Effects of Warm Antibodies

Warm autoantibodies to RBCs in AHA are pathogenic. In contrast to autologous RBCs, labeled RBCs lacking the antigen targeted by the autoantibodies may survive normally in patients with warm-antibody AHA.[10,157,158] Furthermore, transplacental passage of IgG anti-RBC autoantibodies from a mother with AHA to the fetus can induce intrauterine or neonatal hemolytic anemia.[159] Finally, despite notable exceptions and differences related to IgG subclass of the autoantibody, in general, an inverse relationship between the quantity of RBC-bound IgG antibody and RBC survival is noted in serial studies performed on animals and patients.[160–165]

In warm-antibody AHA, the patient's RBCs typically are coated with IgG autoantibodies with or without complement proteins. Autoantibody-coated RBCs are trapped by macrophages in the Billroth cords of the spleen and, to a lesser extent, by Kupffer cells in the liver (see Chap. 68).[157,160,161,163–167] The process leads to generation of spherocytes and fragmentation and ingestion of antibody-coated RBCs.[168,169] The macrophage has surface receptors for the Fc region of IgG, with preference for the IgG_1 and IgG_3 subclasses[170,171] and surface receptors for opsonic fragments of C3 (C3b and C3bi) and C4b.[172–174] When present together on the RBC surface, IgG and C3b/ C3bi appear to act cooperatively as opsonins to enhance trapping and phagocytosis.[163,164,173–177] Although RBC sequestration in warm-antibody AHA occurs primarily in the spleen,[157,164–166] very large quantities of RBC-bound IgG[160,161,167] or the concurrent presence of C3b on the RBCs[160,163,164] may favor trapping in the liver.

Interaction of a trapped RBC with splenic macrophages may result in phagocytosis of the entire cell. More commonly, a type of partial phagocytosis results in spherocyte formation. As RBCs adhere to macrophages via the Fc receptors, portions of RBC membrane are internalized by the macrophage. Because membrane is lost in excess of contents, the noningested portion of the RBC assumes a spherical shape, the shape with the lowest ratio of surface area to volume.[168,169,178] Spherical RBCs are more rigid and less deformable than normal RBCs. As such, spherical RBCs are fragmented further and eventually destroyed in future passages through the spleen. Spherocytosis is a consistent and diagnostically important hallmark of AHA,[179] and the degree of spherocytosis correlates well with the severity of hemolysis.[10]

Direct complement-mediated hemolysis with hemoglobinuria is unusual in warm-antibody AHA, even though many warm autoantibodies fix complement. The failure of C3b-coated RBCs to be hemolyzed by the terminal complement cascade (C5–C9) has been attributed, at least in part, to the ability of complement regulatory proteins (factors I and H) in plasma and C3b receptors on the RBC surface to alter the hemolytic function of cell-bound C3b and C4b.[180] Glycosylphosphatidylinositol-linked erythrocyte membrane proteins, such as decay accelerating factor (DAF; CD55) and homologous restriction factor (HRF; CD59), may limit the action of autologous complement on autoantibody-coated RBCs.[181–183] DAF inhibits the formation and function of cell-bound C3-converting enzyme,[181] thus, indirectly limiting formation of C5-converting enzyme. HRF, on the other hand, impedes C9 binding and formation of the C5b–9 membrane attack complex.[182]

Cytotoxic activities of macrophages and lymphocytes also may play a role in the destruction of RBCs in warm-antibody AHA. Monocytes can lyse IgG-coated RBCs *in vitro* independently of phagocytosis.[184,185] Cell-bound complement is neither necessary nor sufficient for such cytotoxicity, but bound C3b/C3d can potentiate the effects of IgG.[185] In one study, cytotoxicity, but not phagocytosis, was inhibited by hydrocortisone *in vitro*.[184] Lymphocytes also can lyse IgG antibody-coated RBCs *in vitro*.[186–188] The relative contribution of antibody-dependent monocyte- and lymphocyte-mediated cytotoxicity to RBC destruction in patients with warm-antibody AHA is not known.

Pathogenic Effects of Cold Agglutinins and Hemolysins

Most cold agglutinins are unable to agglutinate RBCs at temperatures higher than 30°C. The highest temperature at which these antibodies cause detectable agglutination is termed the *thermal amplitude*. The value varies considerably among patients. Generally, patients with cold agglutinins with higher thermal amplitudes have a greater risk for cold agglutinin disease.[9] For example, active hemolytic anemia has been observed in patients with cold agglutinins of modest titer (e.g., 1:256) and high thermal amplitudes.[189]

The pathogenicity of a cold agglutinin depends upon its ability to bind host RBCs and to activate complement.[10,175,190,191] This process is called *complement fixation*. Although *in vitro* agglutination of the RBCs may be maximal at 0 to 5°C, complement fixation by these antibodies may occur optimally at 20 to 25°C and may be significant at even higher physiologic temperatures.[10,189,190] Agglutination is not required for the process. The great preponderance of cold agglutinin molecules are IgM pentamers, but small numbers of IgM hexamers with cold agglutinin activity are found in patients with cold agglutinin disease. Hexamers fix complement and lyse RBCs more efficiently than do pentamers, suggesting that hexameric IgM plays a role in the pathogenesis of hemolysis in these patients.[192]

Cold agglutinins may bind to RBCs in superficial vessels of the extremities, where the temperature generally ranges between 28 and 31°C, depending upon ambient temperature.[193] Cold agglutinins of high thermal amplitude may cause RBCs to aggregate at this temperature, thereby impeding RBC flow and producing acrocyanosis. In addition, the RBC-bound cold agglutinin may activate complement via the classic pathway. Once activated complement proteins are deposited onto the RBC surface, the cold agglutinin need not remain bound to the RBCs for hemolysis to occur. Instead, the cold agglutinin may dissociate from the RBCs at the higher temperatures in the body core and again be capable of binding other RBCs at the lower temperatures in the superficial vessels. As a result, patients with cold agglutinins of high thermal amplitude tend toward a sustained hemolytic process and acrocyanosis.[194] In contrast, patients with antibodies of lower thermal amplitude require significant chilling to initiate complement-mediated injury of RBCs. This sequence may result in a burst of hemolysis with hemoglobinuria.[194] Combinations of these clinical patterns also occur. Cold agglutinins of the IgA isotype, an isotype that does not fix complement, may cause acrocyanosis but not hemolysis.[195] Thus, the relative degree of hemolysis or impeded RBC flow is influenced significantly by the properties and quantity of the cold agglutinins in a given patient.

Complement fixation by cold agglutinins may effect RBC injury by two major mechanisms: (1) direct lysis and (2) opsonization for hepatic and splenic macrophages. Both mechanisms probably operate to varying degrees in any patient. Direct lysis requires propagation of the full C1 to C9 sequence on the RBC membrane. If this process occurs to a significant degree, the patient may experience intravascular hemolysis leading to hemoglobinemia and hemoglobinuria. Intravascular hemolysis of this severity is relatively rare because phosphatidylinositol-linked RBC membrane proteins (DAF and HRF) protect against injury by autologous complement components. Thus, the complement sequence on many RBCs is completed only through the early steps, leaving opsonic fragments of C3 (C3b/C3bi) and C4 (C4b) on the cell surface. The fragments provide only a weak stimulus for phagocytosis by monocytes *in vitro*.[177,196] However, activated macrophages may ingest C3b-coated particles avidly.[197] Accordingly, RBCs heavily coated with C3b (and/or C3bi) may be removed from the circulation by macrophages either in the liver or, to a lesser extent, the spleen.[164,190,198,199] The trapped RBCs may be ingested entirely or released back into the circulation as spherocytes after losing plasma membrane.

In vivo studies of the fate of ^{51}Cr-labeled C3b-coated RBCs[163,190,198,199] indicate many of the erythrocytes trapped in the liver or spleen gradually may reenter the circulation. The released cells generally are coated

TABLE 53–3. Major Mechanisms of Drug-Related Hemolytic Anemia and Positive Direct Antiglobulin Tests

	Hapten/Drug Adsorption	Ternary Complex Formation	Autoantibody Binding	Nonimmunologic Protein Adsorption
Prototype drug	Penicillin	Quinidine	α-Methyldopa	Cephalothin
Role of drug	Binds to red cell membrane	Forms ternary complex with antibody and red cell membrane component	Induces formation of antibody to native red cell antigen	Possibly alters red cell membrane
Drug affinity to cell	Strong	Weak	None demonstrated to intact red cell but binding to membranes reported	Strong
Antibody to drug	Present	Present	Absent	Absent
Antibody class predominating	IgG	IgM or IgG	IgG	None
Proteins detected by direct antiglobulin test	IgG, rarely complement	Complement	IgG, rarely complement	Multiple plasma proteins
Dose of drug associated with positive antiglobulin test	High	Low	High	High
Presence of drug required for indirect antiglobulin test	Yes (coating test red cells)	Yes (added to test medium)	No	Yes (added to test medium)
Mechanism of red cell destruction	Splenic sequestration of IgG-coated red cells	Direct lysis by complement plus splenic–hepatic clearance of C3b-coated red cells	Splenic sequestration	None

with the opsonically inactive C3 fragment C3dg. Conversion of cell-bound C3b or C3bi to C3dg results from the action of the naturally occurring complement inhibitor factor I in concert with factor H or CR1 receptors.[174] The surviving C3dg-coated RBCs circulate with a near-normal life span[163,190,198,199] and are resistant to further uptake of cold agglutinins or complement.[190,198,200] However, C3dg-coated RBCs also may react *in vitro* with anticomplement (anti-C3) serum in the DAT. In fact, most of the antiglobulin-positive RBCs of patients with cold agglutinin disease are coated with C3dg.

In paroxysmal cold hemoglobinuria, the mechanism of hemolysis probably parallels *in vitro* events (see "Serologic Features" below). During severe chilling, blood flowing through skin capillaries is exposed to low temperatures. The Donath-Landsteiner antibody and early acting complement components presumably bind to RBCs at the lowered temperatures. Upon return of the cells to 37°C in the central circulation, the cells are lysed by propagation of the terminal complement sequence through C9. The Donath-Landsteiner antibody itself dissociates from the RBCs at 37°C. Erythrocyte membrane proteins that restrict C5b–9 assembly (e.g., HRFs) may be less effective in controlling Donath-Landsteiner antibody-initiated complement activation than that initiated by cold agglutinins.

Pathogenesis of Drug-Mediated Immune Injury

Table 53–3 summarizes the three mechanisms of drug-mediated immune injury to RBCs. Drugs also may mediate protein adsorption to RBCs by nonimmune mechanisms, but RBC injury does not occur.

Hapten or Drug Adsorption Mechanism This mechanism applies to drugs that can bind firmly to proteins, including RBC membrane proteins. The classic setting is very-high-dose penicillin therapy,[28–34] which is encountered less commonly today than in previous decades.

Most individuals who receive penicillin develop IgM antibodies directed against the benzylpenicilloyl determinant of penicillin, but this antibody plays no role in penicillin-related immune injury to RBCs. The antibody responsible for hemolytic anemia is of the IgG class, occurs less frequently than the IgM antibody, and may be directed against the benzylpenicilloyl,[31] or, more commonly, nonbenzylpenicilloyl determinants.[28–30,32] Other manifestations of penicillin sensitivity usually are not present.

All patients receiving high doses of penicillin develop substantial coating of RBCs with penicillin. The penicillin coating itself is not injurious. If the penicillin dose is very high ($10–30 \times 10^6$ units per day, or less in the setting of renal failure) and promotes cell coating and if the patient has an IgG antipenicillin antibody, the antibody binds to the RBC-bound penicillin molecules and the DAT with anti-IgG becomes positive (see Fig. 53–1A).[29,31,32,50,201] Antibodies eluted from patients' RBCs or present in their sera react in the indirect antiglobulin test (IAT) only against penicillin-coated RBCs. This step is critical in distinguishing these drug-dependent antibodies from true autoantibodies.

Not all patients receiving high-dose penicillin develop a positive DAT reaction or hemolytic anemia because only a small proportion of such individuals produce the requisite antibody. Destruction of RBCs coated with penicillin and IgG antipenicillin antibody occurs mainly through sequestration by splenic macrophages.[30,202] In some patients with penicillin-induced immune hemolytic anemia, blood monocytes and presumably splenic macrophages may lyse the IgG-coated RBCs without phagocytosis.[203] Hemolytic anemia resulting from penicillin typically occurs only after the patient has received the drug for 7 to 10 days and ceases a few days to 2 weeks after the patient discontinues taking the drug.

Low-molecular-weight substances, such as drugs, generally are not immunogenic in their own right. Induction of antidrug antibody is thought to require firm chemical coupling of the drug (as a hapten) to a protein carrier. In the case of penicillin, the carrier protein involved in antibody induction need not be the same as the erythrocyte membrane protein to which penicillin is coupled in the effector phase, that is, when the IgG antipenicillin antibodies bind to penicillin-coated RBCs. In contrast to evidence on the ternary complex mechanism, no evidence indicates the drug-dependent antibodies responsible for RBC injury in this hapten/drug adsorption mechanism also recognize native erythrocyte membrane structures.

Cephalosporins have antigenic cross-reactivity with penicillin[204–206] and bind firmly to RBC membranes, as do semisynthetic penicillins.[33,34] Hemolytic anemia similar to that seen with penicillin has been ascribed to cephalosporins[35–39] and some semisynthetic penicillins.[33,34] Tetracycline[40,41] and tolbutamide[44,45] also may cause hemolysis by this mechanism. Carbromal causes positive IgG antiglobulin reactions by a similar mechanism,[43] but hemolytic anemia has not been described.

Ternary Complex Mechanism: Drug–Antibody–Target Cell Interaction Many drugs can induce immune injury not only of RBCs but also of platelets or granulocytes by a process that differs in several ways from the mechanism of hapten/drug adsorption (see Table 53–3). First, drugs in this group (see Table 53–2) exhibit only weak direct binding to blood cell membranes. Second, a relatively small dose of drug is capable of triggering destruction of blood cells. Third, cellular injury appears to be mediated chiefly by complement activation at the cell surface. The cytopathic process induced by such drugs previously has been termed the *innocent bystander* or *immune complex mechanism*. The terminology reflected the prevailing notion that, *in vivo*, drug–antibody complexes formed first (immune complexes) and then became secondarily bound to target blood cells as "innocent bystanders," either nonspecifically or possibly via membrane receptors (e.g., Fcγ receptors on platelets or C3b receptors on red cells), with the potential for subsequent activation of complement by bound complexes.

The "immune complex" and "innocent bystander" terminology now seems less appropriate because of models developed from research on analogous drug-dependent platelet injury[207–209] (see Chap. 119) and a series of relevant serologic observations on drug-mediated immune hemolytic anemia. These studies suggest blood cell injury is mediated by a cooperative interaction among three reactants to generate a ternary complex (see Fig. 53–1B) involving (1) the drug (or drug metabolite in some cases), (2) a drug-binding membrane site on the target cell, and (3) antibody. For example, several patients possess drug-dependent antibodies that exhibited specificity for RBCs bearing defined alloantigens such as those of the Rh, Kell, or Kidd blood groups. That is, even in the presence of drug, the antibodies were selectively nonreactive with human RBCs lacking the alloantigen in question.[57,82,210–212] In each case, high-affinity drug binding to cell membrane could not be demonstrated. The drug-dependent antibody is thought to bind, through its Fab domain, to a compound neoantigen consisting of loosely bound drug and a blood group antigen intrinsic to the red cell membrane. Elegant studies on quinidine- or quinine-induced immune thrombocytopenia have demonstrated the IgG antibodies implicated in this disorder bind through their Fab domains, not by their Fc domains to platelet Fcγreceptors.[213,214]

The data elucidate how one patient with quinidine sensitivity may have selective destruction of platelets and another may have selective destruction of RBCs. This process occurs because the pathogenic antibody recognizes the drug only in combination with a particular membrane structure of the RBC (e.g., a known alloantigen) or of the platelet (e.g., α domain of the glycoprotein Ib complex). Therefore, at least in these cases, the target cell does not appear to be purely an innocent bystander. Binding of the drug itself to the target cell membrane is weak until the attachment of the antibody to *both* drug and cell membrane is stabilized. Yet the binding of the antibody is drug dependent. Such a three-reactant interdependent "troika" is unique to this mechanism of immune cytopenia.

The foregoing discussion depicting drugs as creating a "self + nonself" neoantigen on the target cell applies to the effector phase as opposed to the induction phase of the process. However, the same drug-binding membrane protein appears to be involved in forming the immunogen that induces the antibody, as evidenced by drug-dependent antibodies exhibiting selective reactivity with defined red cell alloantigens (carrier specificity).[57,82,210–212] How this process is accomplished in the absence of evidence for strong, covalent binding of the drugs in this group to a host membrane protein remains to be elucidated.

RBC destruction by this mechanism may occur intravascularly after completion of the whole complement sequence, resulting in hemoglobinemia and hemoglobinuria. Some destruction of intact C3b-coated RBCs may be mediated by splenic and liver sequestration via the C3b/C3bi receptors on macrophages. The DAT is positive usually only with anticomplement reagents, but exceptions occur. Sometimes, however, the drug-dependent antibody itself can be detected on the RBCs if the offending drug (or its metabolites) is included in all steps of the antiglobulin test, including washing.[215]

Autoantibody Mechanism A variety of drugs induce the formation of autoantibodies reactive with autologous (or homologous) RBCs in the absence of the instigating drug (see Tables 53–2 and 53–3). The most studied drug in this category has been α-methyldopa, an antihypertensive agent that no longer is commonly used.[71–74] Levodopa and several unrelated drugs also have been implicated.[39,46,58,60,67,75–84] Patients with CLL treated with pentostatin,[85] fludarabine,[86] or cladribine[87] are particularly predisposed to autoimmune hemolysis, which usually is severe and sometimes fatal.

Positive DAT reactions (with anti-IgG reagents) in patients taking α-methyldopa vary in frequency from 8 to 36 percent. Patients taking higher doses of the drug develop positive reactions with greater frequency.[71,73,74] A lag period of 3 to 6 months exists between the start of therapy and development of a positive antiglobulin test. The delay is not shortened when the drug is administered to patients who previously had positive antiglobulin tests while taking α-methyldopa.[73]

In contrast to the frequent observation of positive antiglobulin reactions, less than 1 percent of patients taking α-methyldopa exhibit hemolytic anemia.[72] Development of hemolytic anemia does not depend on drug dose. The hemolysis usually is mild to moderate and occurs chiefly by splenic sequestration of IgG-coated RBCs. α-Methyldopa has been proposed to suppress splenic macrophage function in some patients, and normal survival of antibody-coated RBCs in such patients may be related, in part, to this effect of the drug.[216]

The DAT reaction usually is positive only for IgG.[11] Occasionally, weak anticomplement reactions also are encountered.[11] Patients with immune hemolytic anemia resulting from α-methyldopa therapy typically exhibit strongly positive DAT reactions and serum antibody, evidenced by the IAT reaction.[11] Antibodies in the serum or eluted from RBC membranes react optimally at 37°C with unaltered autologous or homologous RBCs in the absence of drug (see Fig. 53–1C).[72,74,217] Frequently the autoantibodies are reactive with determinants of the Rh complex,[72,74,217] and at least some appear to target the same 34-kDa Rh-related polypeptide targeted by the autoantibodies in many cases of "spontaneously arising" AHA.[129] Thus, distinguishing these drug-induced antibodies from similar warm-reacting autoantibodies in idiopathic AHA currently is not possible.

The mechanism by which a drug induces formation of an autoantibody is unknown. Radiolabeled α-methyldopa does not react directly with the membranes of intact human RBCs.[74,218] However, both α-methyldopa and levodopa reportedly bind to isolated RBC membranes. Binding of the drug to membranes of intact RBCs is inhibited by RBC superoxide dismutase and probably by hemoglobin.[218,219] Although not formally demonstrated, these drugs probably bind to membrane antigens of cells that are relatively hemoglobin free, for example, cells at the early proerythroblast stage or RBC stroma. In any case, the resulting altered membrane antigens then may induce autoantibodies. The concept that a drug–membrane compound neoantigen could lead to production of an autoantibody is supported by studies of patients receiving drugs unrelated to α-methyldopa. Patients simultaneously developed a drug-dependent antibody and an autoantibody, both of which showed specificity for the same RBC alloantigen.[82] Another hypothesis is that α-methyldopa interacts with human T lymphocytes, resulting in loss of suppressor cell function.[220] Subsequent studies, however, have failed to demonstrate any evidence for such a mechanism.[221]

Uncommonly, patients with CLL treated with the purine analogues fludarabine[86,222,223] or cladribine[87] develop AHA. Risk factors for hemolysis include previous therapy with a purine analogue, high β_2-microglobulin, a positive DAT prior to therapy, and hypogammaglobulinemia. Purine analogues are potent suppressors of T lymphocytes. These drugs may accelerate the preexisting T-cell immune suppression that normally occurs during progression of CLL, exacerbating the underlying tendency to autoimmunity in CLL. However, the degree of depletion of T-cell subsets is similar in patients who develop hemolysis and in patients who do not.

Nonimmunologic Protein Adsorption Less than 5 percent of patients receiving cephalosporin antibiotics develop positive antiglobulin reactions[11] as a result of nonspecific adsorption of plasma proteins to their RBC membranes.[90,91,224] This process may occur within 1 to 2 days after the drug is instituted. Multiple plasma proteins, including immunoglobulins, complement, albumin, fibrinogen, and others, may be detected on RBC membranes in such cases.[224,225] Hemolytic anemia resulting from this mechanism has not been reported. The clinical importance of this phenomenon is its potential to complicate crossmatch procedures unless the drug history is considered. Cephalosporin antibiotics also may induce RBC injury by the hapten mechanism, by the ternary complex mechanism, and by the autoantibody mechanism. The latter reactions are more serious but apparently occur less frequently than nonimmunologic protein adsorption.

CLINICAL FEATURES

WARM-ANTIBODY AUTOIMMUNE HEMOLYTIC ANEMIA

Presenting complaints of warm-antibody AHA usually are referable to the anemia itself, although occasionally jaundice is the immediate cause for the patient to seek medical advice. Symptom onset usually is slow and insidious over several months, but occasionally a patient has sudden onset of symptoms of severe anemia and jaundice over a period of a few days. In secondary AHA, the symptoms and signs of the underlying disease may overshadow the hemolytic anemia and associated features.

In idiopathic AHA with only mild anemia, results of physical examination may be normal. Even patients with relatively severe hemolytic anemia may have only modest splenomegaly. However, in very severe cases, particularly those of acute onset, patients may present with fever, pallor, jaundice, hepatosplenomegaly, hyperpnea, tachycardia, angina, or heart failure.

Clinical warm-antibody AHA may be aggravated or first become apparent during pregnancy.[159,226,227] Most cases are mild, however, and the prognosis for the fetus is generally good, provided the mother is treated early.[226]

COLD-ANTIBODY AUTOIMMUNE HEMOLYTIC ANEMIA

Most patients with cold agglutinin hemolytic anemia have chronic hemolytic anemia with or without jaundice. In other patients, the principal feature is episodic, acute hemolysis with hemoglobinuria induced by chilling (see discussion of thermal amplitude in "Pathogenic Effects of Cold Agglutinins and Hemolysins" above). Combinations of these clinical features may occur. Acrocyanosis and other cold-mediated vasoocclusive phenomena affecting the fingers, toes, nose, and ears are associated with sludging of RBCs in the cutaneous microvasculature. Skin ulceration and necrosis are distinctly unusual. Hemolysis occurring in *M. pneumoniae* infections is acute in onset, typically appearing as the patient is recovering from pneumonia and coincident with peak titers of cold agglutinins. The hemolysis is self-limited, lasting 1 to 3 weeks.[11] Hemolytic anemia in infectious mononucleosis develops either at the onset of symptoms or within the first 3 weeks of illness.[121]

Other physical findings are variable, depending upon the presence of an underlying disease. Splenomegaly, a characteristic finding in lymphoproliferative diseases or infectious mononucleosis, may be observed in idiopathic cold agglutinin disease.

In paroxysmal cold hemoglobinuria, constitutional symptoms are prominent during a paroxysm. A few minutes to several hours after cold exposure, the patient develops aching pains in the back or legs, abdominal cramps, and perhaps headaches. Chills and fever usually follow. The first urine passed after onset of symptoms typically contains hemoglobin. The constitutional symptoms and hemoglobinuria generally last a few hours. Raynaud phenomenon and cold urticaria sometimes occur during an attack; jaundice may follow.

DRUG-IMMUNE HEMOLYTIC ANEMIA

A careful history of drug exposure should be obtained from all patients with hemolytic anemia and/or a positive DAT. As in idiopathic AHA, the clinical picture in drug-immune hemolytic anemia is quite variable. The severity of symptoms largely depends upon the rate of hemolysis. In general, patients with hapten/drug adsorption (e.g., penicillin) and autoimmune (e.g., α-methyldopa) types of drug-induced hemolytic anemia exhibit mild to moderate hemolysis, with insidious onset of symptoms developing over a period of days to weeks. In contrast, the ternary complex mechanism (e.g., cephalosporins or quinidine) often causes sudden, severe hemolysis with hemoglobinuria. In the latter setting, hemolysis can occur after only one dose of the drug in a patient previously exposed to the drug. Acute renal failure may accompany severe hemolysis by the ternary complex mechanism.[39,55,57,61,62,84] Several reports indicate that second- and third-generation cephalosporins may cause severe, even fatal, hemolysis by the ternary complex mechanism.[37–39,63]

LABORATORY FEATURES

GENERAL FEATURES

By definition, patients with AHA present with anemia, the severity of which ranges from life-threatening to very mild. Patients with warm antibody AHA may present with hematocrit levels less than 10 percent or may have compensated hemolytic anemia and a near-normal hematocrit. For the latter patients, the predominant laboratory features are an increased reticulocyte count and a positive DAT. Occasionally, the patient has leukopenia and neutropenia.[10,228] Platelet counts typically are normal. Rarely, severe immune thrombocytopenia is associated with warm-antibody AHA. This constellation is termed *Evans syndrome*.[229] In this syndrome, the RBC and platelet antibodies are apparently distinct.[230]

Patients with classic chronic cold agglutinin disease exhibit mild to moderate, fairly stable anemia, with hematocrit levels only occasionally as low as 15 to 20 percent. In contrast, patients with paroxysmal cold hemoglobinuria have hematocrit levels that decrease rapidly during a paroxysm. During a paroxysm, leukopenia is noted early, followed by leukocytosis. Complement titers frequently are depressed because of consumption of complement proteins during hemolysis.

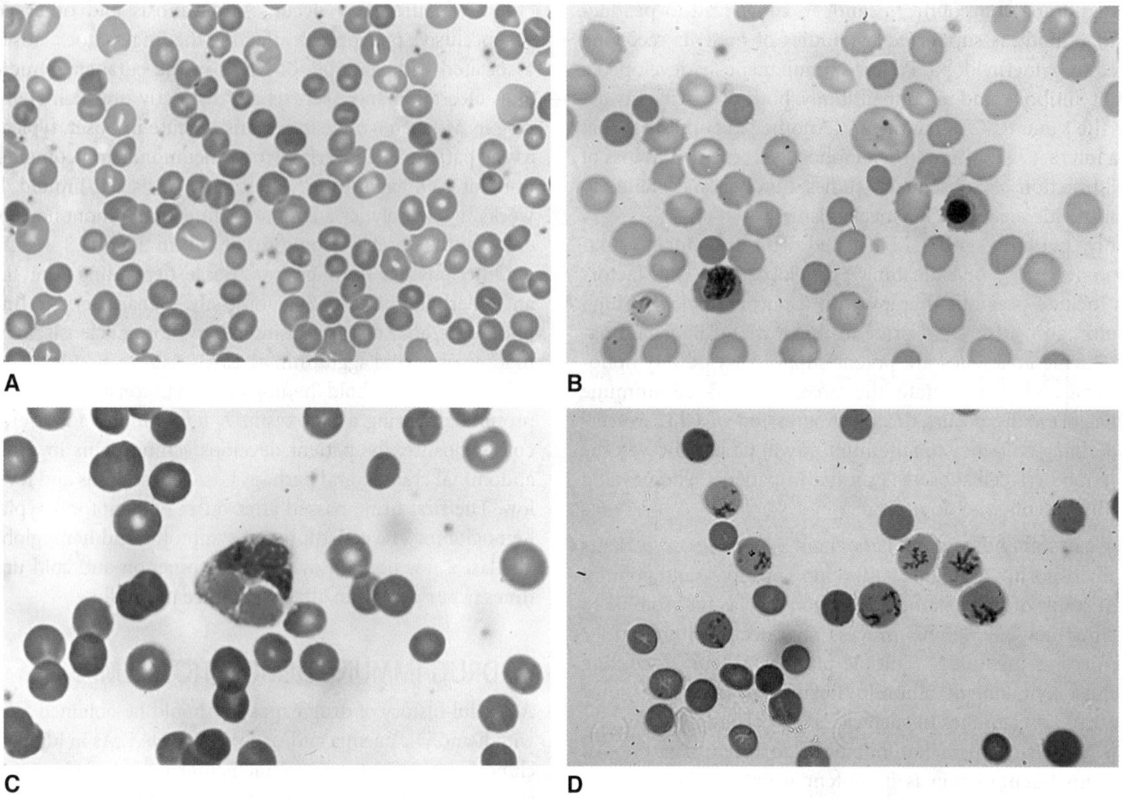

FIGURE 53–2. A. Blood film. Autoimmune hemolytic anemia. Moderately severe. Note high frequency of microspherocytes (small hyperchromatic RBCs) and the high frequency of macrocytes (putative reticulocytes). **B.** Blood film. Autoimmune hemolytic anemia. Severe. Note the low density of red cells on the film (profound anemia), high frequency of microspherocytes (hyperchromatic), and the large red cells (putative reticulocytes). Note the two nucleated RBCs and the Howell-Jolly body (nuclear remnant) in the macrocyte. Nucleated RBCs and Howell-Jolly bodies may be seen in autoimmune hemolytic anemia with severe hemolysis or after splenectomy. **C.** Blood film. Autoimmune hemolytic anemia. Severe. Monocyte engulfing two red cells (erythrophagocytosis). Note frequent microspherocytes and scant red cell density. **D.** Reticulocyte preparation. Autoimmune hemolytic anemia. Note high frequency of reticulocytes, the large cells with precipitated ribosomes. Remaining cells are microspherocytes. *(Used with permission from* Lichtman's Atlas of Hematology, *www.accessmedicine.com.)*

In drug-immune hemolytic anemia of the hapten/drug adsorption and true autoantibody types, the hematologic findings are similar to those described for spontaneously occurring warm-antibody AHA. Most patients exhibit anemia and reticulocytosis. Leukopenia and thrombocytopenia may be noted in cases of ternary complex-mediated hemolysis.

Evaluation of the blood film can reveal several features related to all types of AHA (Fig. 53–2). Polychromasia indicates a reticulocytosis, reflecting an increased rate of reticulocyte egress from the marrow. Spherocytes are seen in patients with moderate to severe hemolytic anemia. Unless hereditary spherocytosis cannot be excluded, this finding suggests an immune hemolytic process. RBC fragments, nucleated RBCs, and occasionally erythrophagocytosis by monocytes may be seen in severe cases (Fig. 53–2). Most patients have mild leukocytosis and neutrophilia. Additionally, patients with cold-antibody AHA may exhibit RBC autoagglutination in the blood film and in chilled anticoagulated blood (Fig. 53–3).

The reticulocyte count usually is elevated. Nevertheless, early in the course of the disease, more than one-third of all patients may have transient reticulocytopenia despite a normal or hyperplastic erythroid marrow.[231–234] The mechanism is unknown, but autoantibodies reactive against antigens on reticulocytes are speculated to lead to their selective destruction.[232] One unusual patient with warm-antibody AHA, reticulocytopenia, and marrow erythroid aplasia had a serum autoantibody that inhibited erythroid colony formation *in vitro*.[235] The aplastic crisis remitted after the serum IgG level was lowered by immunoadsorption. Reticulocytopenia also may be seen in patients with marrow function compromised by an underlying disease, parvovirus infection, toxic chemicals, or nutritional deficiency. Marrow examination usually reveals erythroid hyperplasia and may provide evidence of an underlying lymphoproliferative disorder.

Hyperbilirubinemia (chiefly unconjugated) is highly suggestive of hemolytic anemia, although its absence does not exclude the diagnosis. Total bilirubin is only modestly increased (up to 5 mg/dL) and, with rare exceptions, the conjugated (direct) fraction constitutes less than 15 percent of the total. Urinary urobilinogen is increased regularly, but bile is not detected in the urine unless serum conjugated bilirubin is increased. Usually, serum haptoglobin levels are low, and lactate dehydrogenase levels are elevated. Hemoglobinuria is encountered in rare patients with warm-antibody AHA and hyperacute hemolysis, more commonly in patients with cold agglutinin disease, and characteristically in patients with paroxysmal cold hemoglobinuria and with drug-immune hemolytic anemia mediated by the ternary complex mechanism.

Direct Antiglobulin Test Pattern

Diagnosis of AHA or drug-immune hemolytic anemia requires demonstration of immunoglobulin and/or complement bound to the patient's RBCs. As a screening procedure, use of a "broad-spectrum" antiglobulin (Coombs) reagent—that is, one that contains antibodies directed against human immunoglobulin and complement components (principally C3)—is customary. If agglutination is noted with a broad-spectrum

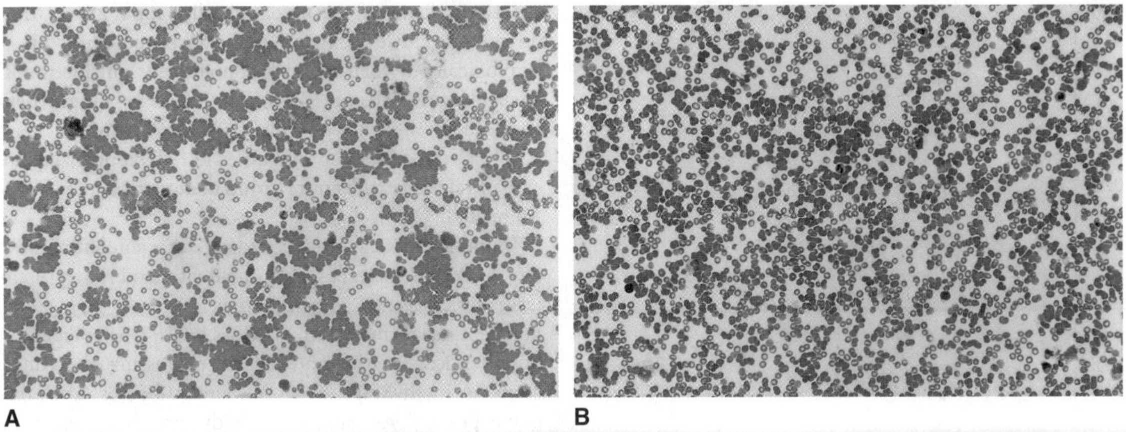

FIGURE 53–3. Blood films. **A.** Cold-reactive (IgM) antibody. Red cell agglutination at room temperature. **B.** Same blood examined at 37°C. Note marked reduction in agglutination. *(Used with permission from* Lichtman's Atlas of Hematology, *www.accessmedicine.com.)*

reagent, antisera reacting selectively with IgG (the "gamma" Coombs) or with C3 (the "nongamma" Coombs) are used to define the specific pattern of RBC sensitization. Monospecific antisera to IgM or IgA also have been used in selected cases.

Three possible *major* patterns of direct antiglobulin reaction in AHA and drug-immune hemolytic anemia exist: (1) RBCs coated with only IgG, (2) RBCs coated with IgG and complement components, and (3) RBCs coated with complement components without detectable immunoglobulin.[10,116,236,237] In patterns 2 and 3, the complement components most readily detected are C3 fragments (mainly C3dg). Each pattern is associated with accelerated RBC destruction. Positive antiglobulin reactions with anti-IgA or anti-IgM are encountered less commonly, often in association with bound IgG and/or complement.[238–244] Table 53–4 summarizes the diagnostic significance of each of these major patterns (see "Serologic Features" below).

TABLE 53–4. Major Reaction Patterns of the Direct Antiglobulin Test and Associated Types of Immune Injury

Reaction Pattern	Type of Immune Injury
IgG alone	Warm-antibody autoimmune hemolytic anemia
	Drug-immune hemolytic anemia: hapten drug adsorption type or autoantibody type
Complement alone	Warm-antibody autoimmune hemolytic anemia with subthreshold IgG deposition
	Cold-agglutinin disease
	Paroxysmal cold hemoglobinuria
	Drug-immune hemolytic anemia: ternary complex type
IgG plus complement	Warm-antibody autoimmune hemolytic anemia
	Drug-immune hemolytic anemia: autoantibody type (rare)

SEROLOGIC FEATURES

Warm-Antibody Autoimmune Hemolytic Anemia

Free versus Bound Autoantibody The autoantibody molecules in patients with warm-antibody AHA exist in a reversible, dynamic equilibrium between RBCs and plasma.[245,246] In addition to the major portion of autoantibody bound to the patient's RBCs (detected by the DAT), "free" autoantibody may be detected in the plasma or serum of these patients by the IAT. In the IAT, the patient's serum or plasma is incubated with normal donor erythrocytes at the appropriate temperature (in this case, 37°C). The cells are washed, suspended in saline solution, and then tested for agglutination by antiglobulin serum. The presence of unbound autoantibody in plasma depends upon the total amount of antibody being produced and the binding affinity of the antibody for RBC antigens. In general, patients whose RBCs are heavily coated with IgG more likely exhibit plasma autoantibody. Protease-modified RBCs are more sensitive than native RBCs in detecting plasma autoantibody, but such data must be interpreted with caution, because alloantibodies, naturally occurring antibodies to cryptic antigens, and other serum components may interact with enzyme-modified RBCs. Patients with a positive IAT as a result of a warm-reactive autoantibody should also have a positive DAT. A patient with a serum anti-RBC antibody (positive IAT) and a negative DAT probably does not have an autoimmune process but rather an alloantibody stimulated by prior transfusion or pregnancy.

Quantity of RBC-Bound Autoantibody Figure 53–4 relates the intensity of the direct antiglobulin reaction, using specific anti-IgG serum, to the number of IgG molecules bound per RBC. The latter was determined by a sensitive antibody-consumption method.[247] A trace-positive antiglobulin reaction (read macroscopically) detects 300 to 400 molecules of IgG per cell.[247,248] In another laboratory, a trace-positive antiglobulin reaction with anti-C3 was obtained with 60 to 115 molecules C3 per cell.[175]

More sensitive methods for quantifying RBC-bound IgG allow identification of AHA patients having all the usual hallmarks of warm-antibody AHA but a negative DAT with antiimmunoglobulin and anticomplement reagents.[247–249] In many patients, the RBCs are coated with quantities of IgG autoantibody that are too low to give a positive DAT (subthreshold IgG). However, the specialized methods (e.g., anti-IgG consumption assays, automated enhanced agglutination techniques, enzyme-linked immunoassays, radioimmunoassays) detect very small quantities of cell-bound IgG. In such cases, studies with highly concentrated RBC eluates confirm these IgG molecules are warm-reacting anti-RBC autoantibodies.[247] Patients generally have relatively mild hemolysis and often respond favorably to glucocorticoid therapy. By these specialized methods, subthreshold IgG also may be detected in a significant number of patients exhibiting the "complement alone" pattern of direct antiglobulin reaction in the absence of drug sensitivity or cold agglutinins. In such cases, studies with concentrated RBC eluates

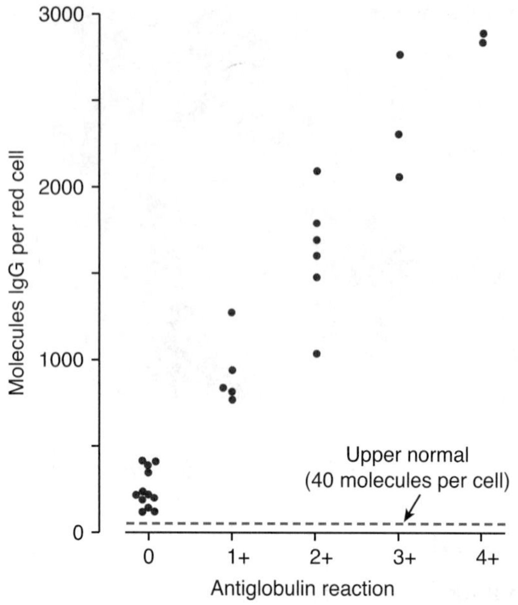

FIGURE 53–4. Comparison of direct antiglobulin reactions (with anti-IgG serum) with molecules of red blood cell–bound IgG determined by a quantitative antibody consumption assay (method described by Gilliland BC, Leddy JP, Vaughan JH[247]). The two assays were conducted concurrently on the same blood specimen. The antiglobulin reactions were performed manually and read macroscopically.

suggest subthreshold quantities of bound IgG antibodies are capable of fixing much larger quantities of C3 to the cell membrane.[247]

Nature of the Autoantibodies and RBC Target Antigens In any series of warm-antibody AHA patients, the correlation between the strength of the antiglobulin reaction (IgG molecules per RBC) and the rate of RBC destruction is variable. The IgG subclass of warm autoantibodies influences the degree to which these antibodies shorten RBC survival. IgG_1 is the most commonly encountered subclass, either alone or in combination with other IgG subclasses.[238,250] IgG_1 and IgG_3 autoantibodies appear to be more effective in decreasing RBC life span than do those of the IgG_2 or IgG_4 subclass.[238,251]

The difference may result from the greater affinity of macrophage Fc receptors for IgG_1 and IgG_3[170,171] and the higher complement-fixing activity of IgG_1 or IgG_3 antibodies relative to the activity of IgG_2 or IgG_4 antibodies.[180]

Autoantibodies eluted from patients' RBCs or present in their plasma typically bind to all the common types of human RBCs represented in test panels used by blood banks and thus might appear to be nonspecific. However, the antibodies of any one patient typically recognize one or more antigenic determinants (epitopes) that are common to almost all human RBCs, that is, "public" antigens. These antibodies have been useful for evaluating RBC membrane structures and for identifying rare RBC phenotypes, namely, RBCs that lack a common blood group antigen(s). Nearly half of all AHA patients have autoantibodies specific for epitopes on Rh proteins.[10,11,124,252–254] The autoantibodies of such patients commonly do not react with human Rh_{null} RBCs, which lack expression of the Rh complex. Occasionally, the anti-Rh autoantibodies have anti-e, anti-E, or anti-c (or, more rarely, anti-D) specificity. Patients who have autoantibodies with selective specificity (e.g., anti-e) nearly always have other autoantibodies reactive with all human RBCs, except Rh_{null}. Autoantibodies with such specificity are designated collectively as Rh related.[129,254]

The remaining patients with warm-antibody AHA have IgG autoantibodies that are fully reactive with Rh_{null} RBCs.[10,11,124,252–254] The exact specificity of the autoantibodies for many of these patients is undefined. However, in other instances, autoantibody specificity for serologically defined blood group antigens outside the Rh system has been identified (using RBCs of appropriate antigen-deficient phenotype) including anti-Wr^b,[124] anti-En^a,[255] anti-LW,[256] anti-U,[257] anti-Ge,[243,258] anti-Sc1,[259] or antibodies to Kell blood group antigens.[260] For ease of reference, the entire group of autoantibodies is designated non-Rh related.[129,254]

Immunochemical studies indicate the autoantibodies from almost any AHA patient react with individual membrane proteins. The major target of Rh-related autoantibodies is a 32- to 34-kDa nonglycosylated polypeptide lacking on Rh_{null} RBCs.[129,261] This polypeptide is similar, if not identical, to the polypeptide expressing the Rh(e) alloantigen. Many α-methyldopa–induced autoantibodies also react with this polypeptide.[129] Autoantibodies with non-Rh serologic specificity react with the band 3 anion transporter[129,262] or with both band 3 and glycophorin A.[129] The latter autoantibodies may react with an epitope formed through the interaction of these two proteins on the RBC membrane.[263] It is interesting to note that anti-RBC autoantibodies in NZB mice exhibit anti–band 3 specificity.[264] Furthermore, naturally occurring anti–band 3 IgG autoantibodies are found in almost all humans.[265,266] These autoantibodies may play a role in the clearance of senescent RBCs by reacting with neoantigens formed on these cells by proteolytic alteration[265] or aggregation[266] of band 3 proteins. Such neoantigens are not found on younger RBCs. An important but unanswered question concerns the possible relationship between naturally occurring and pathologic anti–band 3 autoantibodies.

Cold-Antibody Hemolytic Anemia

Cold agglutinins are distinguished by their ability to directly agglutinate saline-suspended human RBCs at low temperature, maximally at 0 to 5°C. The reaction is reversible by warming. In chronic cold agglutinin disease, serum titers are commonly 1:10,000 or higher and may reach 1:1,000,000 or more. Cold agglutinins are characteristically IgM. IgA or IgG cold agglutinins have been reported,[11,195,267] sometimes in combination with IgM.[268] In mixed warm- and cold-antibody AHA, warm-reactive IgG autoantibodies are found in association with IgM cold agglutinins.[21]

The DAT result is positive with anticomplement reagents. The antibody itself, however, is not detected by the DAT because the cold agglutinins readily dissociate from the RBCs both *in vivo* and during the washing steps of the standard antiglobulin procedure. In contrast, C4b and C3b are covalently bound to target RBCs via thioester linkages. In one unusual case, a low-titer IgG cold agglutinin could be detected by washing the patient's RBCs in ice-cold saline solution and performing the DAT at 4°C.[267]

The majority of cold agglutinins are reactive with oligosaccharide antigens of the I/i system, which are precursors of the ABH and Lewis blood group substances.[269–271] The I/i determinants are bound to erythrocyte membrane glycoprotein (band 3 anion transporter) or to glycolipids.[270,271] Anti-I and anti-i reportedly bind solubilized RBC glycoproteins at 37°C, suggesting the temperature dependence of cold agglutination of intact RBCs may be a function of temperature-induced conformational effects on the cell surface.[272,273]

I antigens are expressed strongly on adult RBCs but weakly on neonatal (cord) RBCs. The converse is true of i antigens, indicating I/i antigen expression is developmentally regulated.[270] The differences between adult and cord blood RBCs allow evaluation of the serologic specificity of cold agglutinins.[10,11,195] I/i antigens, or structurally related analogues, occur in human saliva, milk, amniotic fluid, and hydatid cyst fluid,[195] and are expressed on human lymphocytes, neutrophils, and monocytes.[274]

Anti-I is the predominant specificity of cold agglutinins in idiopathic cold agglutinin disease, in patients with *M. pneumoniae*, and in some cases of lymphoma. Cold agglutinins with anti-i specificity are found in patients with infectious mononucleosis and in some patients with lymphoma. A small percentage of cold agglutinin-containing sera react equally well with adult and neonatal RBCs. These antibodies recognize antigens outside the I/i system, including Pr antigens, consisting of carbohydrate epitopes of glycophorins that are inactivated by protease treatment[195] and, less commonly, the M or P blood group antigens.[275,276] Most cold agglutinins associated with chickenpox exhibit anti-Pr specificity. A single case with anti-I specificity has been observed.[277] Hemolysis resulting from a cold agglutinin with anti-Pr specificity occurred following an allogeneic marrow transplant.[278]

In hemolytic anemia associated with infectious mononucleosis, the patient's serum may contain IgM anti-i cold agglutinins or cold-reactive nonagglutinating IgG anti-i with IgM cold-reactive anti-IgG antibodies ("rheumatoid factors") that may cross-link the IgG-coated RBCs to produce agglutination.[279]

In paroxysmal cold hemoglobinuria, the direct antiglobulin reaction usually is positive during and briefly following an acute attack because of the coating of surviving RBCs with complement, primarily C3dg fragments. The Donath-Landsteiner antibody is responsible for complement deposition on the cells; it is a nonagglutinating IgG that binds RBCs only in the cold. It readily dissociates from the RBCs at room temperature. In adults subject to recurring episodes in association with cold exposure, the DAT result remains negative between attacks. The antibody is detected by the biphasic Donath-Landsteiner test, in which the patient's fresh serum is incubated with RBCs initially at 4°C and the mixture is then warmed to 37°C.[11] Intense hemolysis occurs. Addition of fresh guinea pig serum or ABO-compatible human serum may be necessary to serve as a source of fresh complement if the patient's serum has been stored or is complement depleted. Antibody titers rarely exceed 1:16. The Donath-Landsteiner antibody typically has specificity for the P blood group antigen, a glycosphingolipid structure.[271] The P antigen also occurs on lymphocytes and skin fibroblasts.[16] The latter finding might be related in some way to the occurrence of cold urticaria in paroxysmal cold hemoglobinuria, a phenomenon that may be transferred passively by serum to normal skin.[10] Antibody specificities for RBC antigens other than the P blood group have been noted.[280]

Drug-Immune Hemolytic Anemia

In the hapten/drug adsorption mechanism of immune injury associated with cephalosporins or penicillin, the patient's drug-coated RBCs bind drug-specific IgG antibody and exhibit positive DAT reactions with anti-IgG. Rarely, both anti-IgG and anti-C3d antisera produce positive DAT reactions. Such cases could have superficial resemblance to warm-antibody AHA. The key serologic difference is that, in this form of drug-immune hemolytic anemia, the antibodies in the patient's serum or eluted from the patient's RBCs react *only* with drug-coated RBCs. In contrast, the IgG antibodies in warm-type AHA react with unmodified human RBCs and may show preference for certain known blood groups (e.g., within the Rh complex). Such serologic distinction and the history of exposure to high blood levels of penicillin or a cephalosporin should be instructive.

In hemolysis mediated by the ternary complex mechanism, the DAT is positive with anticomplement serum. Immunoglobulins are only rarely detectable on the patient's RBCs. This pattern is similar to that encountered in AHA mediated by cold agglutinins. Moreover, the brisk type of hemolysis in the ternary complex mechanism also is seen in certain cases of cold-antibody AHA. In the drug-induced cases, however, the cold agglutinin titer and the Donath-Landsteiner test result are normal, and demonstration of serum antibody acting on human RBCs depends upon the presence of the drug in the test system. Thus, the IAT reaction with anticomplement serum may be positive only if the incubation mixture permits interaction of (1) normal RBCs; (2) antidrug antibody from the patient's serum; (3) the relevant drug, either still in the patient's serum or added *in vitro* in appropriate concentration; and (4) a source of complement, that is, fresh normal serum or the patient's own serum if freshly obtained. A negative result does not necessarily absolve the suspected drug because the critical determinant may be a metabolite of the drug in question. In some cases, use of urine or serum (of the patient or a volunteer taking the drug) as a source of drug metabolite has permitted successful demonstration of a drug-dependent mechanism.[60,211,215,281]

In patients with true autoantibodies as a result of α-methyldopa, the DAT reaction is strongly positive for IgG, but complement only rarely is detected on the patient's RBCs. Autoantibody to RBCs is regularly present in the serum of patients and mediates a positive IAT reaction with unmodified human RBCs, often showing specificity related to the Rh complex. No presently available specific serologic test can separate idiopathic warm-reacting IgG autoantibodies with Rh-related specificities from those induced by α-methyldopa administration. The evidence must be circumstantial, with the helpful knowledge that discontinuation of α-methyldopa, without any form of immunosuppressive therapy, consistently permits a slow recovery from anemia and a gradual disappearance of anti-RBC antibodies.

Drugs now not known to cause immune RBC injury will be implicated in the future. In any patient with a clinical picture compatible with drug-related immune hemolysis, a reasonable approach is stopping any drug that is suspect while serologic studies are being performed. The patient should be monitored for improvement in hematocrit level, decrease in reticulocytosis, and gradual disappearance of the positive DAT. Repeat challenge with the suspected drug may confirm the diagnosis, but this measure is seldom necessary in patient management and may be unsafe. Therefore, rechallenge to exclude a drug-immune hemolytic anemia should be undertaken only for compelling reasons, such as the need to use the specific drug for the patient's illness.

DIFFERENTIAL DIAGNOSIS

Several nonautoimmune diseases may result in spherocytic anemia, such as hereditary spherocytosis (HS), Zieve syndrome, clostridial sepsis, and the hemolytic anemia preceding Wilson disease. Among the hereditary hemolytic anemias, HS can resemble acquired AHA most closely because the spherocytic anemia associated with HS may be detected first in adulthood (see Chap. 45). In addition, splenomegaly may be prominent in both HS and AHA. Family studies of patients with HS, however, usually can identify other affected individuals. Most important, in hereditary hemolytic anemia the DAT is negative.

In hemolytic anemia accompanied by a positive DAT, serologic characterization of the autoantibody may distinguish warm-antibody AHA from cold-reacting autoantibody syndromes. Diagnosis of a drug-immune hemolytic anemia depends upon a history of appropriate drug intake supported by compatible serologic findings. In patients who recently received a transfusion, a positive DAT reaction may reflect the binding of a newly formed alloantibody to donor RBCs in the patient's circulation (delayed transfusion reaction; see Chap. 140). This findi[ng] could lead to a false impression of an autoimmune process.

Recent recipients of allogeneic blood stem cell transplants o[r] organ transplants may develop autoimmune hemolysis.[282] [...] former, antibodies are produced by the stem cell graft agai[nst] also produced by the stem cell graft; that is, both antibodies and RBCs are of donor origin. In the case of solid organ transplants, the recipient's own lymphocytes make antibody against recipient RBCs. In both situations, the autoimmunity is thought to arise from immunosuppressive therapy causing delayed reconstitution or dysfunction of T-cell immunity, leading to development of antibodies autologous to the offended immune system.

Recipients of transplants may also develop an *allo*immune hemolytic anemia that mimics warm-antibody AHA. The problem is seen in kidney, liver, or hematopoietic stem cell transplants and usually occurs when an organ from a blood group O donor is transplanted into a blood group A or B recipient. B lymphocytes present in the donated organ or stem cell product form alloantibodies against recipient RBCs.[283–287] Patients of blood group O who receive a stem cell transplant from a donor of blood group A or B may develop a transiently positive DAT and hemolysis of RBCs made by the marrow graft because of temporary persistence of previously synthesized host anti-A or anti-B.[288] Furthermore, some group O stem cell transplant recipients exhibit mixed hematopoietic chimerism with persistence of host B lymphocytes that can make alloantibodies directed against RBCs made by the stem cell graft.[288] In these settings, the findings of hemolysis and a positive DAT as a result of anti-A and anti-B probably are diagnostic of an alloimmune process, because *auto*antibodies directed against the major blood group antigens A and B are extremely rare.

Other acquired types of hemolytic anemia are less easily confused with either warm- or cold-antibody AHA because spherocytes are not prominent on the blood film and the DAT is negative. Patients with paroxysmal nocturnal hemoglobinuria (PNH) may complain of dark urine (hemoglobinuria). This finding is unusual in patients with warm-antibody AHA but can occur in patients with the cold-antibody syndromes. Decreased levels of CD55 and CD59 on blood cells, detected by flow analysis, are characteristic of PNH but not AHA (see Chap. 40). Microangiopathic hemolytic disorders, such as thrombotic thrombocytopenic purpura and hemolytic uremic syndrome, can be distinguished from AHA by examining the blood film. In the microangiopathic hemolytic diseases, the blood film displays marked RBC fragmentation and minimal spherocytosis. In addition, microangiopathic hemolytic anemias more frequently are associated with thrombocytopenia than is either warm- or cold-antibody AHA.

The clinical and laboratory features of chronic cold agglutinin disease are sufficiently distinctive so that the diagnostic possibilities are limited. In general, a high-titer cold agglutinin (>1:10,000) and a positive DAT with anticomplement serum (but not with anti-IgG) are consistent with cold agglutinin disease. In many instances of drug-immune hemolytic anemia, the DAT result also is positive only for complement. The drug history and a low (or absent) cold agglutinin titer, however, help to distinguish drug-immune hemolytic anemia from cold agglutinin disease. If the patient has an elevated cold agglutinin level and a positive DAT result with both anti-IgG and anti-C3, then the patient may have a mixed-type AHA. Warm-antibody AHA, hereditary hemolytic disorders, and PNH should be excluded in cases exhibiting primarily a chronic hemolytic anemia. The pattern of antiglobulin reaction, family history, the result of analysis of CD55/CD59 on blood cells provide additional help in difficult ...ses. When the hemolysis is episodic, paroxysmal cold hemoglobinuria, ...hemoglobinuria, and PNH also should be considered. When cold- ...ipheral vasoocclusive symptoms are predominant, the ...osis should include cryoglobulinemia and Raynaud ...without an associated rheumatic disease. Infec- ... *pneumoniae* infection, and lymphoma can be ...e clinical settings.

...emoglobinuria must be distinguished from the ...ronic cold agglutinin disease manifesting episodic hemolysis and hemoglobinuria. This distinction is made primarily in the laboratory. In general, patients with paroxysmal cold hemoglobinuria lack high titers of cold agglutinins. Furthermore, the Donath-Landsteiner antibody is a potent *in vitro* hemolysin, in contrast to most cold agglutinins, which are weak hemolysins. Warm-antibody AHA, march hemoglobinuria, myoglobinuria, and PNH can be distinguished through the history and appropriate laboratory studies.

Immune hemolysis caused by drugs should be distinguished from (1) the warm- or cold-antibody types of idiopathic AHA, (2) congenital hemolytic anemias such as hereditary spherocytosis, and (3) drug-mediated hemolysis resulting from disorders of red cell metabolism, such as glucose-6-phosphate dehydrogenase deficiency. Patients with drug-immune hemolytic anemia have a positive DAT that distinguishes this group from patients with inherited RBC defects.

THERAPY

GENERAL

Transfusion

The clinical consequences of AHA or drug-immune hemolytic anemia are related to the severity of the anemia and acuity of its onset. Many patients develop anemia over a period sufficient to allow for cardiovascular compensation and hence do not require RBC transfusions. However, RBC transfusions may be necessary and should not be withheld from a patient with an underlying disease complicating the anemia, such as symptomatic coronary artery disease, or a patient who rapidly develops severe anemia with signs and/or symptoms of circulatory failure, as in paroxysmal cold hemoglobinuria or ternary complex drug-immune hemolysis.

Transfusion of RBCs in immune hemolytic anemia presents two difficulties: (1) cross-matching and (2) the short half-life of the transfused RBCs (see Chap. 140). Finding truly serocompatible donor blood is nearly always impossible except in rare cases when the autoantibody is specific for a defined blood group antigen (see "Serologic Features" above).

It is most important to identify the patient's ABO type so as to avoid a hemolytic transfusion reaction mediated by anti-A or anti-B. This part of the matching process allows for selection of either ABO-identical or -compatible blood for transfusion. With respect to compatibility, the more difficult technical issue relates to the detection of RBC alloantibodies which may be masked by the presence of the autoantibody.

Clinicians often speak of "least incompatible" blood for transfusion, but this term has lately fallen into disrepute because it lacks a precise definition.[289,290] In fact all units will be serologically incompatible but units that are incompatible because of the presence of autoantibody are less dangerous to transfuse than those units that are incompatible because of an alloantibody.

Before transfusing an incompatible unit, the patient's serum must be tested carefully for an alloantibody that could cause a severe hemolytic transfusion reaction against donor RBCs, especially in patients with a history of pregnancy, abortion or prior transfusion.[254,291–293] Patients who have neither been pregnant nor transfused with blood products are unlikely to harbor an alloantibody. Early consultation between the clinician and the blood bank physician is essential. An understanding of the basic aspects of blood compatibility testing, coupled with the knowledge of a patient's pregnancy and transfusion history allow for informed discussion and confident transfusion of mismatched blood if the situation demands.

Once selected, the packed RBCs should be administered slowly. During the transfusion, the patient should be monitored for signs of a hemolytic transfusion reaction (see Chap. 140). The transfused cells may be destroyed as fast as or perhaps even faster than the patient's own cells. However, the increased oxygen-carrying capacity provided by the transfused cells may be sufficient to maintain the patient during the acute interval required for other modes of therapy to become effective.

For patients with AHA who require chronic transfusion support, use of prophylactic antigen-matched donor RBCs for transfusion has been proposed as a means of preventing alloimmunization.[294] This process is feasible only in institutions with access to a good selection of phenotyped RBC units and a reference laboratory.[295]

THERAPY OF WARM-ANTIBODY AUTOIMMUNE HEMOLYTIC ANEMIA

Glucocorticoids

Therapy with glucocorticoids has reduced the mortality associated with severe idiopathic warm-antibody AHA. Glucocorticoids were first used for this disorder almost 60 years ago.[296] Glucocorticoids can cause dramatic cessation or marked slowing of hemolysis in about two-thirds of patients.[10,11,116,297,298] Approximately 20 percent of treated patients with warm-antibody AHA achieve complete remission. Approximately 10 percent show minimal or no response to glucocorticoids. The best responses are seen in idiopathic cases or in those related to SLE.

Most patients should be treated with oral prednisone at an initial daily dose of 60 to 100 mg. Critically ill patients with rapid hemolysis may receive intravenous methylprednisolone 100 to 200 mg in divided doses over the first 24 hours. High doses of prednisone may be required for 10 to 14 days. When the hematocrit stabilizes or begins to increase, the prednisone dose can be decreased in rapid-step dose reductions to approximately 30 mg/day. With continued improvement, the prednisone dose can be further decreased at a rate of 5 mg/day every week, to a dose of 15 to 20 mg/day. These doses should be administered for 2 to 3 months after the acute hemolytic episode has subsided, after which the patient can be weaned from the drug over 1 to 2 months or treatment switched to an alternate-day therapy schedule (e.g., 20–40 mg every other day). Alternate-day therapy reduces glucocorticoid side effects but should be attempted only after the patient has achieved stable remission on daily prednisone in the range from 15 to 20 mg/day. Therapy should not be stopped until the DAT becomes negative. Although many patients achieve full remission of their first hemolytic episode, relapses may occur after the glucocorticoids are discontinued. Therefore, patients should be followed for at least several years after treatment. A relapse may require repeat glucocorticoid therapy, splenectomy, or immunosuppression.

Occasionally, patients who present with only a positive DAT, minimal hemolysis, and stable hematocrit require no treatment. However, these patients should be observed for clinical deterioration because the rate of RBC destruction may increase spontaneously.

Glucocorticoids may influence hemolysis in warm-antibody AHA by several mechanisms. Earlier investigators noted that hematologic improvement was often, but not always, accompanied by reduction in the strength of the DAT.[10] The subsequent observation of a decrease in cell-bound and/or free serum autoantibody during stable glucocorticoid-induced remission suggested improved RBC survival following treatment with glucocorticoids resulted from a decrease in synthesis of anti-RBC autoantibodies.[162,245] However, this finding cannot explain why glucocorticoid-treated patients often improve within 24 to 72 hours, a time much shorter than the half-life of anti-RBC autoantibody. Rather, glucocorticoids may suppress RBC sequestration by splenic macrophages.[164,165,176,299] A quantitative decrease in one of the three known classes of Fcγ receptors[170,171] has been observed in the blood monocytes of AHA patients during glucocorticoid therapy.[300]

Splenectomy

Nearly one-third of patients with warm-antibody AHA require prednisone chronically in doses greater than 15 mg/day to maintain an acceptable hemoglobin concentration. These patients are candidates for laparoscopic splenectomy.

Splenectomy removes the primary site of RBC trapping. Investigations in human[162] and animal[164] subjects confirm that maintenance of a given rate of RBC destruction requires 6 to 10 times more RBC-bound IgG in splenectomized subjects than in nonsplenectomized subjects. Continuation of hemolysis after splenectomy is partly related to persisting high levels of autoantibody, favoring RBC destruction in the liver by hepatic Kupffer cells.[162,164,167]

Several investigators noted the amount of RBC-bound autoantibody decreased in AHA patients following splenectomy.[10,297,301] However, a significant proportion of patients show no change in cell-bound autoantibody following splenectomy. The processes determining the rate of autoantibody production are poorly understood. The beneficial effect of splenectomy may be related to several factors interacting in complex fashion.[302]

A patient's clinical data currently constitute the best selection criteria for splenectomy. Attempts to select potential responders by ^{51}Cr RBC sequestration studies have been disappointing.[10,297,303] In most cases, a reasonable approach is to continue glucocorticoids for 1 to 2 months while waiting for a maximal response. However, if no response is noted within 3 weeks, the patient's condition deteriorates, or the anemia is very severe, splenectomy should be performed sooner.

Results of splenectomy are variable. Approximately two-thirds of AHA patients have a partial or complete remission following splenectomy.[297,302] However, the relapse rate is disappointingly high. Many patients require further glucocorticoid therapy to maintain acceptable hemoglobin levels, although often at a lower dose than required prior to splenectomy.[10,116,297] Alternate-day therapy is preferable to daily therapy in these cases if adequate control of the anemia can be achieved.

The immediate mortality and morbidity from splenectomy depend upon the presence of underlying disease and the preoperative clinical status but generally are quite low.[304] Following splenectomy, children, more than adults, have an increased risk for developing sepsis as a result of encapsulated organisms.[305] Vaccination against *H. influenzae* type b and pneumococcal and meningococcal organisms is recommended at least 2 weeks prior to surgery.[306]

Rituximab

Rituximab is a monoclonal antibody directed against the CD20 antigen expressed on B lymphocytes and is used for treatment of B-cell lymphoma. Its use for treatment of AHA is based on the antibody's ability to eliminate B lymphocytes, including presumably those making autoantibodies to RBCs. However, the mechanism of action is more complex than that, as the effect of rituximab can occur very early, before the autoantibodies can recede. In fact, sometimes in responding patients, autoantibody levels are not significantly affected.[307,308] Opsonized B lymphocytes may decoy effector monocytes and macrophages from autoantibody complexes and normalize autoreactive T lymphocyte responses.[307]

In a large prospective series,[309] 13 of 15 children with warm-antibody AHA responded to rituximab 375 mg/m^2 weekly for 2 to 4 weeks. Many other case series support the use of rituximab in adults, with response rates ranging from 40 to 100 percent.[308,310]

Other Immunosuppressive Drugs

Cytotoxic drugs such as cyclophosphamide, 6-mercaptopurine, azathioprine, and 6-thioguanine have been given to patients with AHA to suppress synthesis of autoantibody. Direct evidence of such an effect is lacking. Although immunosuppressive therapy is not universally accepted, beneficial responses to immunosuppressive drugs have been observed in some patients who did not respond to glucocorticoids.[11,311] Importantly, the majority of patients with warm-antibody AHA respond to glucocorticoids and/or splenectomy and usually are not candidates for immunosuppressive therapy. At present, immunosuppressive therapy should be reserved primarily for patients who do not respond to glucocorticoids and splenectomy or for patients who are poor surgical risks.[311]

The most successful approach used high-dose cyclophosphamide 50 mg/kg ideal body weight per day for 4 consecutive days, with granulocyte colony-stimulating factor support.[312] Of 9 patients, 8 of whom had warm autoantibodies, all became transfusion independent. All patients had prolonged severe cytopenias and required hospitalization for a median of 21 days. Cyclophosphamide may cause severe hemorrhagic cystitis.

For patients who may not tolerate prolonged cytopenias, the drugs of choice are cyclophosphamide 60 mg/m^2 or azathioprine 80 mg/m^2 given daily. If the patient tolerates the drug, continue treatment for up to 6 months while waiting for a response. When response occurs, the patient can be weaned slowly from the drug. If no response is observed, the alternative drug can be tried. Because cyclophosphamide and azathioprine suppress hematopoiesis, blood counts, including reticulocyte count, must be monitored with extra care during therapy. Treatment with either agent increases the risk of subsequent neoplasia.

Patients with refractory AHA have been treated effectively with the purine analogue 2-chlorodeoxyadenosine (cladribine)[313] and with mycophenolate mofetil.[314,315] Alemtuzumab was successfully used to treat 5 patients with refractory AHA associated with CLL.[316]

Other Therapies

For patients with chronic compensated hemolysis, treatment with folate at 1 mg/day is recommended to satisfy the increased demands for the vitamin because of increased red cell production. Plasma exchange or plasmapheresis has been used in patients with warm-antibody AHA. Improvement has been reported in a few cases, but use of the method is controversial.[317,318] Thymectomy has been reported useful in a few children who were refractory to glucocorticoids and splenectomy.[311] Selective injury to splenic macrophages by administration of vinblastine-loaded, IgG-sensitized platelets reportedly was successful in a few patients.[319] Several anecdotal reports and a case series indicate short-term successful treatment of patients with AHA using high-dose intravenous γ-globulin.[320–324] Uncontrolled studies indicate danazol, a nonvirilizing androgen, may be useful in patients with AHA.[325,326] Danazol may eliminate the need for splenectomy when combined with prednisone and may allow for a shorter duration of prednisone therapy.[326] Some patients with ulcerative colitis and AHA unresponsive to glucocorticoids and splenectomy may respond to colectomy.[327] In patients with AHA associated with an ovarian dermoid cyst, cyst removal produces remission of the hemolysis.[328]

THERAPY OF COLD-ANTIBODY HEMOLYTIC ANEMIA

Keeping the patient warm, particularly the patient's extremities, is moderately effective in providing symptomatic relief. This action may be the only measure required in patients with mild chronic hemolysis. In symptomatic patients, rituximab is effective and well tolerated. In two prospective trials, approximately half the patients responded to rituximab 375 mg/m^2 weekly for 4 weeks.[329,330] Patients who relapsed responded to a second course of rituximab at about the same rate. Chlorambucil or cyclophosphamide may be helpful for patients with symptomatic chronic cold agglutinin disease.[9–11,331,332] Results of splenectomy[10,11,333] or use of glucocorticoids[10,11] generally have been disappointing, although exceptions have been reported,[10,189,267,268] particularly in atypical cases. Experimental[164] and clinical[189] bases exist for considering very high doses of glucocorticoids in seriously ill patients. RBC transfusions generally are reserved for patients with severe anemia of rapid onset who are in danger of cardiorespiratory complications. Washed RBCs often are used to avoid replenishing depleted complement components and reactivating the hemolytic process. In critically ill patients, plasma exchange (with replacement by albumin-containing saline solution) may provide transient amelioration of hemolysis.[334–336]

Most contemporary cases of paroxysmal cold hemoglobinuria are self-limited. Acute attacks in both chronic and transient forms of paroxysmal cold hemoglobinuria may be prevented by avoiding cold exposure. Glucocorticoid therapy and splenectomy have not been useful. When paroxysmal cold hemoglobinuria is associated with syphilis, effective treatment of the infection may result in complete remission. Antihistaminic and adrenergic agents may relieve symptoms of cold urticaria.

THERAPY OF DRUG-IMMUNE HEMOLYTIC ANEMIA

Discontinuation of the offending drug often is the only treatment needed. This measure is essential and may be lifesaving in patients with severe hemolysis mediated by the ternary complex mechanism.

In the past, high-dose penicillin was not necessarily discontinued because of a positive DAT alone. A change in therapy was considered mainly in the presence of overt hemolytic anemia. For example, lowering the penicillin dose and coadministering other antibiotics sometimes allowed continuation of the drug, particularly if hemolysis was not severe. For other drugs causing only mild hemolysis by the hapten-drug adsorption mechanism, in the unlikely event that no alternatives are available, a similar approach may be effective.

In patients taking α-methyldopa in the absence of hemolysis, a positive DAT has not necessarily been an indication for stopping the drug. However, given all the choices available, considering alternative antihypertensive therapy is prudent. Because less information on the natural history of autoantibodies induced by drugs other than α-methyldopa is available, discontinuation of the offending drug is advisable unless no suitable alternative exists.

Glucocorticoids are generally unnecessary, and their efficacy is questionable. However, prednisone is effective in patients with CLL and autoimmune hemolysis caused by purine analogues,[86,87] as are cyclosporine, rituximab, and intravenous immunoglobulin.[223] For treatment of CLL, combination of cyclophosphamide with fludarabine, with or without rituximab, seems to reduce the frequency of fludarabine-induced AHA.[222,223] Transfusions should be given in the unusual circumstance of severe, life-threatening anemia. Problems with cross-matching, similar to those encountered in warm-antibody AHA, may occur in patients with a strongly positive IAT, for example, in α-methyldopa–related cases. Patients with hemolytic anemia resulting from the hapten/drug adsorption mechanism should have a compatible cross-match because the serum antibody reacts only with drug-coated cells. However, if therapy with the offending drug is still in progress, transfused cells may be destroyed at an increased rate as they become coated with drug *in vivo*. Patients with ternary complex mediated hemolysis will also hemolyze transfused RBCs until the offending drug clears from the plasma.

Several cases of transfusion-associated graft-versus-host disease as a result of purine analogues have been reported in CLL patients transfused for hemolysis.[87,337,338] Such patients, who have an immunodeficiency state secondary to CLL, impairing their ability to eliminate the transfused lymphocytes, should receive irradiated blood products.

COURSE AND PROGNOSIS

Patients with idiopathic warm-antibody AHA have unpredictable clinical courses characterized by relapses and remissions. No particular feature of the illness has been a consistent predictor of outcome. Despite a rather high initial rate of response to glucocorticoids and splenectomy, the overall mortality rate was significant (up to 46%) in several older series, but much lower in more recent studies.[10,11,297,339,340] The actuarial survival at 10 years reportedly is 73 percent.[339] Pulmonary emboli, infection, and cardiovascular collapse are causes of death. Thromboembolic episodes in the form of deep vein thrombosis or splenic infarcts are relatively common during active phases of the disease.[297,340] In one series, 8 of 30 patients with AHA developed venous thromboembolism; 19 of the patients had antiphospholipid antibodies, including 6 of the 8 patients with thromboembolism.[341] In another retrospective analysis of 36 exacerbations of severe AHA in 28 patients, only 6 of whom were tested and found negative for antiphospholipid antibodies, venous thromboembolism occurred in 5 of 15 exacerbations without anticoagulation and in 1 of 21 with anticoagulation.[342] The contribution of antiphospholipid antibodies to morbidity and mortality in AHA is not clear from these data. However, it seems prudent to consider prophylactic anticoagulation for patients with AHA and antiphospholipid antibodies or other risk factors for venous thromboembolism.

The prognosis in secondary warm-antibody AHA largely depends upon the course of the underlying disease.

In children, warm-antibody AHA frequently follows an acute infection or immunization.[301,343,344] Most of these patients exhibit a self-limited course and respond rapidly to glucocorticoids. Children with chronic AHA tend to be older.[344,345] Those who recover from the initial hemolytic episode have a good prognosis and are unlikely to relapse, although exceptions are known. The overall mortality rate is lower than in adults, ranging from 10 to 30 percent,[301,343–347] with higher mortality rates in those with chronic AHA[301,347] and associated autoimmune thrombocytopenia (Evans syndrome).[348]

Patients with idiopathic cold agglutinin disease often have a relatively benign course and survive for many years.[9–11,332] Occasionally, death results from infection or severe anemia or, not uncommonly, from an underlying lymphoproliferative process.

The postinfectious forms of cold agglutinin disease typically are self-limited. Recovery generally occurs in a few weeks. A few cases with massive hemoglobinuria have been complicated by acute renal failure, requiring temporary hemodialysis.

Postinfectious forms of paroxysmal cold hemoglobinuria terminate spontaneously within a few days to weeks after onset,[12–15] although the Donath-Landsteiner antibody may persist in low titer for several years.[10] Most patients with chronic idiopathic paroxysmal cold hemoglobinuria survive for many years despite occasional paroxysms of hemolysis.

Immune hemolysis in response to drugs usually is mild, and the prognosis is good. Occasional episodes of exceptionally severe hemolysis with renal failure or death have been reported, usually because of drugs operating through the ternary complex mechanism or purine analogues in patients with CLL.[39,55,57,61–64,66,84,86,105,106] In hemolysis resulting from ternary complex or hapten/drug adsorption mechanisms, the DAT becomes negative shortly after the drug is discontinued, that is, soon after the drug clears from the circulation. In addition, the hemolysis associated with α-methyldopa–induced autoantibodies ceases promptly after drug cessation. However, a positive DAT of gradually diminishing intensity may remain for weeks or months.

REFERENCES

1. Packman C: Historical review: The spherocytic haemolytic anaemias. *Br J Haematol* 112:888, 2001.
2. Coombs RRA, Mourant AE, Race EE: A new test for the detection of weak and incomplete Rh agglutinins. *Br J Exp Pathol* 26:255, 1945.
3. Boorman KE, Dodd BE, Loutit JF: Haemolytic icterus (acholuric jaundice), congenital and acquired. *Lancet* 1:812, 1946.
4. Loutit JF, Mollison PL: Haemolytic icterus (acholuric jaundice), congenital and acquired. *J Pathol Bacteriol* 58:711, 1946.
5. Landsteiner K: Uber Beziehungen zwischen dem Blutserum und den Körperzeller. *Munch Med Wochenschr* 50:1812, 1903.
6. Clough MC, Richter IM: A study of an autoagglutinin occurring in a human serum. *Bull Johns Hopkins Hosp* 29:86, 1918.
7. Iwai S, Mei-Sai N: Etiology of Raynaud's disease: A preliminary report. *Jpn Med World* 5:119, 1925.
8. Iwai S, Mei-Sai N: Etiology of Raynaud's disease. *Jpn Med World* 6:345, 1926.
9. Schubothe H: The cold hemagglutinin disease. *Semin Hematol* 3:27, 1966.
10. Dacie JV: *The Haemolytic Anaemias*, vol 3, *The Autoimmune Haemolytic Anaemias*, 3d ed. Churchill Livingstone, New York, 1992.
11. Petz LD, Garratty G: *Immune Hemolytic Anemias*. Churchill Livingstone, Philadelphia, 2004.
12. Nordhagen R, Stensvold K, Winsnes A, et al: Paroxysmal cold hemoglobinuria. The most frequent autoimmune hemolytic anemia in children? *Acta Paediatr Scand* 73:258, 1984.
13. Wolach B, Heddle N, Barr RD, et al: Transient Donath-Landsteiner hemolytic anemia. *Br J Haematol* 48:425, 1981.
14. Sokol RJ, Hewitt S, Stamps BK: Autoimmune hemolysis associated with Donath-Landsteiner antibodies. *Acta Haematol* 68:268, 1982.
15. Gottsche B, Salama A, Mueller-Eckhardt C: Donath-Landsteiner autoimmune hemolytic anemia in children: A study of 22 cases. *Vox Sang* 58:281, 1990.
16. Fellous M, Gerbal A, Tessier C, et al: Studies on the biosynthetic pathway of human P erythrocyte antigens using somatic cells in culture. *Vox Sang* 26:518, 1974.
17. Ackroyd JF: The pathogenesis of thrombocytopenic purpura due to hypersensitivity to sedormid. *Clin Sci (Lond)* 7:249, 1949.
18. Snapper I, Marks D, Schwartz L, Hollander L: Hemolytic anemia secondary to Mesantoin. *Ann Intern Med* 39:619, 1953.
19. Harris JW: Studies on the mechanism of drug-induced hemolytic anemia. *J Lab Clin Med* 47:760, 1956.
20. Sokol RJ, Hewitt S, Stamps BK: Autoimmune haemolysis: An 18-year study of 865 cases referred to a regional transfusion centre. *Br Med J* 282:2023, 1981.
21. Sokol RJ, Hewitt S, Stamps BK: Autoimmune haemolysis: Mixed warm and cold antibody type. *Acta Haematol* 69:266, 1983.
22. Shulman IA, Branch DR, Nelson JM, et al: Autoimmune hemolytic anemias with both cold and warm autoantibodies. *JAMA* 253:1746, 1985.
23. Kajii E, Miura Y, Ikemoto S: Characterization of autoantibodies in mixed-type autoimmune hemolytical anemia. *Vox Sang* 60:45, 1991.
24. Berentsen S, Bo K, Shammas F, et al: Chronic cold agglutinin disease of the "idiopathic" type is a premalignant or low-grade malignant lymphoproliferative disease. *APMIS* 105:354, 1997.
25. Telen MJ, Roberts KB, Bartlett JA: HIV-associated autoimmune hemolytic anemia: Report of a case and review of the literature. *J Acquir Immune Defic Syndr* 3:933, 1990.
26. Rapoport AP, Rowe JM, McMican A: Life-threatening autoimmune hemolytic anemia in patient with acquired immune deficiency syndrome. *Transfusion* 28:190, 1988.
27. Saif M: HIV Associated autoimmune hemolytic anemia: An update. *AIDS Patient Care* 15:217, 2001.
28. VanArsdel PP Jr, Gilliland BC: Anemia secondary to penicillin treatment: Studies on two patients with non-allergic serum hemagglutinins. *J Lab Clin Med* 65:277, 1965.
29. Petz LD, Fudenberg HH: Coombs-positive hemolytic anemia caused by penicillin administration. *N Engl J Med* 274:171, 1966.
30. Swanson MA, Chanmougan D, Schwartz RS: Immuno-hemolytic anemia due to antipenicillin antibodies. *N Engl J Med* 274:178, 1966.
31. Levine B, Redmond A: Immunochemical mechanisms of penicillin-induced Coombs positivity and hemolytic anemia in man. *Int Arch Allergy Appl Immunol* 1:594, 1967.
32. White JM, Brown DL, Hepner GW, Worlledge SM: Penicillin-induced hemolytic anaemia. *Br Med J* 3:26, 1968.
33. Seldon MR, Bain B, Johnson CA, Lennox CS: Ticarcillin-induced immune haemolytic anaemia. *Scand J Haematol* 28:459, 1982.
34. Tuffs L, Manoharan A: Flucloxacillin-induced haemolytic anaemia. *Med J Aust* 144:559, 1986.
35. Gralnick HR, McGinnis MH, Elton W, McCurdy P: Hemolytic anemia associated with cephalothin. *JAMA* 217:1193, 1971.
36. Branch DR, Berkowitz LR, Becker RL, et al: Extravascular hemolysis following the administration of cefamandole. *Am J Hematol* 18:213, 1985.
37. Chambers LA, Donovan BA, Kruskall MS: Ceftazidime-induced hemolysis patient with drug-dependent antibodies reactive by immune complex and drug adsorption mechanisms. *Am J Clin Pathol* 95:393, 1991.
38. Gallagher NI, Schergen AK, Sokol-Anderson ML, et al: Severe immune-mediated hemolytic anemia secondary to treatment with cefotetan. *Transfusion* 32:266, 1992.
39. Garratty G, Nance S, Lloyd M, Domen R: Fatal immune hemolytic anemia due to cefotetan. *Transfusion* 32:269, 1992.
40. Wenz B, Klein RL, Lalezari P: Tetracycline-induced immune hemolytic anemia. *Transfusion* 14:265, 1974.

41. Simpson MB, Pryzbylik J, Innis B, Denham MA: Hemolytic anemia after tetracycline therapy. *N Engl J Med* 312:840, 1985.
42. Pujol M, Fernandez F, Sancho JM, et al: Immune hemolytic anemia induced by 6-mercaptopurine. *Transfusion* 40:75, 2000.
43. Steanini M, Johnson NL: Positive antihuman globulin test in patients receiving carbromal. *Am J Med Sci* 259:49, 1970.
44. Bird GWG, Ecles GH, Litchfield JA, et al: Haemolytic anaemia associated with antibodies to tolbutamide and phenacetin. *Br Med J* 1:728, 1972.
45. Malacarne P, Castaldi G, Bertusi M, Zavagli G: Tolbutamide-induced hemolytic anemia. *Diabetes* 26:156, 1977.
46. Salama A, Mueller-Eckhardt C: Cianidanol and its metabolites bind tightly to red cells and are responsible for the production of auto- and/or drug-dependent antibodies against these cells. *Br J Haematol* 66:263, 1987.
47. Martinengo M, Ardenghi DF, Tripodi G, Reali G: The first case of drug-induced immune hemolytic anemia due to hydrocortisone. *Transfusion* 48:1925, 2008.
48. Arndt P, Garratty G, Isaak E, et al: Positive direct and indirect antiglobulin tests associated with oxaliplatin can be due to drug antibody and or drug-induced nonimmunologic protein adsorption. *Transfusion* 49:711, 2009.
49. Muirhead EE, Halden ER, Groves M: Drug-dependent Coombs (antiglobulin) test and anemia: Observations on quinine and acetophenetidin (phenacetin). *Arch Intern Med* 101:827, 1958.
50. Croft JD Jr, Swisher SN, Gilliland BC, et al: Coombs test positivity induced by drugs: Mechanisms of immunologic reactions and red cell destruction. *Ann Intern Med* 68:176, 1968.
51. Freedman AL, Barr PS, Brody E: Hemolytic anemia due to quinidine: Observations on its mechanism. *Am J Med* 20:806, 1956.
52. Logue GL, Boyd AE, Rosse WF: Chlorpropamide-induced immune hemolytic anemia. *N Engl J Med* 283:900, 1970.
53. Kopicky JA, Packman CH: The mechanisms of sulfonylurea-induced immune hemolysis. Case report and review of the literature. *Am J Hematol* 23:283, 1986.
54. Kashyap AS, Kashyap S: Hemolytic anemia due to metformin. *Postgrad Med J* 76:125, 2000.
55. Pereira A, Sanz C, Cervantes F, Castillo R: Immune hemolytic anemia and renal failure associated with rifampicin-dependent antibodies with anti-I specificity. *Ann Hematol* 63:56, 1991.
56. Bengtsson U, Staffan A, Aurell M, Kaijser B: Antazoline-induced immune hemolytic anemia, hemoglobinuria and acute renal failure. *Acta Med Scand* 198:223, 1975.
57. Habibi B, Basty R, Chodez S, Prunat A: Thiopental-related immune hemolytic anemia and renal failure. *N Engl J Med* 312:353, 1985.
58. Squires JE, Mintz PD, Clark S: Tolmetin-induced hemolysis. *Transfusion* 25:410, 1985.
59. Sosler SD, Behzad V, Garratty G, et al: Immune hemolytic anemia associated with probenecid. *Am J Clin Pathol* 84:391, 1985.
60. Salama A, Mueller-Eckhardt C: Two types of nomifensine-induced immune haemolytic anaemias: Drug-dependent sensitization and/or auto-immunization. *Br J Haematol* 64:613, 1986.
61. Habibi B, Cartron JP, Bretagne M, et al: Anti-nomifensine antibody causing immune hemolytic anemia and renal failure. *Vox Sang* 40:79, 1981.
62. Fulton JD, Briggs JD, Dominiczak AF, et al: Intravascular haemolysis and acute renal failure induced by nomifensine. *Scott Med J* 31:242, 1986.
63. Garratty G, Postoway N, Schwellenbach J, McMahill PC: A fatal case of ceftriaxone (Rocephin)-induced hemolytic anemia associated with intravascular immune hemolysis. *Transfusion* 31:176, 1991.
64. Rosenfeld CS, Winters SJ, Tedrow HE: Diethylstilbestrol-associated hemolytic anemia with a positive direct antiglobulin test result. *Am J Med* 86:617, 1989.
65. Salama A, Burger M, Mueller-Eckhardt C: Acute immune hemolysis induced by a degradation product of amphotericin B. *Blut* 58:59, 1989.
66. Wolf B, Conradty M, Grohmann R, et al: A case of immune complex hemolytic anemia, thrombocytopenia, and acute renal failure associated with doxepin use. *J Clin Psychiatry* 50:99, 1989.
67. Salama A, Kroll H, Wittmann G, Mueller-Eckhardt C: Diclofenac-induced immune haemolytic anaemia: Simultaneous occurrence of red blood cell autoantibodies and drug-dependent antibodies. *Br J Haematol* 95:640, 1996.
68. Bougie D, Johnson ST, Weitekamp LA, Aster RH: Sensitivity to metabolite of diclofenac as a cause of acute immune hemolytic anemia. *Blood* 90:407, 1997.
69. Cunha PD, Lord RS, Johnson ST, et al: Immune hemolytic anemia caused by sensitivity to a metabolite of etodolac, a nonsteroidal anti-inflammatory drug. *Transfusion* 40:663, 2000.
70. Park GM, Han KS, Chang YH, et al: Immune hemolytic anemia after treatment with pemetrexed for lung cancer. *J Thorac Oncol* 3:196 2008.
71. Carstairs KC, Breckenridge A, Dollery CT, Worlledge SM: Incidence of a positive direct Coombs test in patients on alpha-methyldopa. *Lancet* 2:133, 1966.
72. Worlledge SM, Carstairs KC, Dacie JV: Autoimmune haemolytic anaemia associated with α-methyldopa therapy. *Lancet* 2:135, 1966.
73. Breckenridge A, Dollery CT, Worlledge SM, et al: Positive direct Coombs tests and antinuclear factors in patients treated with methyldopa. *Lancet* 2:1265, 1967.
74. Lo Buglio AF, Jandl JH: The nature of alpha-methyldopa red cell antibody. *N Engl J Med* 276:658, 1967.
75. Cotzias GC, Papavasiliou PS: Autoimmunity in patients treated with levodopa. *JAMA* 207:1353, 1969.
76. Henry RE, Goldberg LS, Sturgeon P, Ansel RD: Serologic abnormalities associated with L-dopa therapy. *Vox Sang* 20:306, 1971.
77. Joseph C: Occurrence of positive Coombs test in patients treated with levodopa. *N Engl J Med* 286:1400, 1972.
78. Gabor EP, Goldberg LS: Levodopa-induced Coombs positive haemolytic anaemia. *Scand J Haematol* 11:201, 1973.
79. Territo MC, Peters RW, Tanaka KR: Autoimmune hemolytic anemia due to levodopa therapy. *JAMA* 226:1347, 1973.
80. Scott GL, Myles AB, Bacon PA: Autoimmune haemolytic anaemia and mefenamic acid therapy. *Br Med J* 3:543, 1968.
81. Robertson JH, Kennedy CC, Hill CM: Haemolytic anaemia associated with mefenamic acid. *Ir J Med Sci* 140:226, 1971.
82. Habibi B: Drug-induced red blood cell autoantibodies co-developed with drug-specific antibodies causing a hemolytic anaemia. *Br J Haematol* 61:139, 1985.
83. Kleinman S, Nelson R, Smith L, Goldfinger D: Positive direct antiglobulin tests and immune hemolytic anemia in patients receiving procainamide. *N Engl J Med* 311:809, 1984.
84. Kramer MR, Levene C, Hershko C: Severe reversible autoimmune haemolytic anaemia and thrombocytopenia associated with diclofenac therapy. *Scand J Haematol* 36:118, 1986.
85. Byrd JC, Hertler AA, Weiss RB, et al: Fatal recurrence of autoimmune hemolytic anemia following pentostatin therapy in a patient with a history of fludarabine-associated hemolytic anemia. *Ann Oncol* 6:300, 1995.
86. Weiss R, Freiman J, Kweder S, et al: Hemolytic anemia after fludarabine therapy for chronic lymphocytic leukemia. *J Clin Oncol* 16:1885, 1998.
87. Chasty RC, Myint H, Oscier DG, et al: Autoimmune haemolysis in patients with B-CLL treated with chlorodeoxyadenosine (CDA). *Leuk Lymphoma* 29:391, 1998.
88. Kwan JM, Reese AM, Trafeli JP: Delayed autoimmune hemolytic anemia in efalizumab-treated psoriasis. *J Am Acad Dermatol* 58:1053, 2008.
89. Darabi K, Kantamnei S, Weirnik PH: Lenalidomide-induced warm autoimmune hemolytic anemia. *J Clin Oncol* 24:e59, 2006.
90. Gralnick HR, Wright LD, McGinnis MH: Coombs' positive reactions associated with sodium cephalothin therapy. *JAMA* 199:725, 1967.
91. Molthan L, Reidenberg MM, Eichman MF: Positive direct Coombs' tests due to cephalothin. *N Engl J Med* 277:123, 1967.
92. Zeger G, Smith L, McQuiston D, Goldfinger D: Cisplatin-induced nonimmunologic adsorption of immunoglobulin by red cells. *Transfusion* 28:493, 1988.
93. Muirhead EE, Groves M, Guy R, et al: Acquired hemolytic anemia, exposures to insecticides and positive Coombs' test dependent on insecticide preparations. *Vox Sang* 4:277, 1959.
94. Lindberg LG, Norden A: Severe hemolytic reaction to chlorpromazine. *Acta Med Scand* 170:195, 1961.
95. Eyster ME: Melphalan (Alkeran) erythrocyte agglutinin and hemolytic anemia. *Ann Intern Med* 66:573, 1967.
96. Robinson MG, Foadi M: Hemolytic anemia with positive Coombs' test. Association with isoniazid therapy. *JAMA* 208:656, 1969.
97. Mueller-Eckhardt C, Kretschmer V, Coburg KH: Allergic, immunohemolytic anemia due to para-aminosalicylic acid (PAS). Immunohematologic studies of three cases. *Dtsch Med Wochenschr* 97:234, 1972.
98. Manor E, Marmor A, Kaufman S, Leiba H: Massive hemolysis caused by acetaminophen. *JAMA* 236:2777, 1976.
99. Vilal JM, Blum L, Dosik H: Thiazide-induced immune hemolytic anemia. *JAMA* 236:1723, 1976.
100. Letona JM-L, Barbolla L, Frieyro E, et al: Immune haemolytic anaemia and renal failure induced by streptomycin. *Br J Haematol* 35:561, 1977.
101. Korsager S, Sorensen H, Jensen OH, Falk JV: Antiglobulin tests for determination of autoimmunohaemolytic anaemia during long-term treatment with ibuprofen. *Scand J Rheumatol* 10:174, 1981.
102. Takahashi H, Tsukada T: Triamterene-induced immune hemolytic anemia with acute intravascular hemolysis and acute renal failure. *Scand J Haematol* 23:169, 1979.
103. Wong KY, Boose GM, Issitt CH: Erythromycin-induced hemolytic anemia. *J Pediatr* 98:647, 1981.
104. Sandvei P, Nordhagen R, Michaelsen TE, Wolthuis K: Fluorouracil (5-FU) induced acute immune haemolytic anaemia. *Br J Haematol* 65:357, 1987.
105. Tafani O, Mazzoli M, Landini G, Alterini B: Fatal acute immune haemolytic anaemia caused by nalidixic acid. *Br Med J* 285:936, 1982.
106. Angeles ML, Reid ME, Yacob UA, et al: Sulindac-induced immune hemolytic anemia. *Transfusion* 34:255, 1994.
107. Marks DR, Joy JV, Bonheim NA: Hemolytic anemia associated with the use of omeprazole. *Am J Gastroenterol* 86:217, 1991.
108. Blum MD, Graham DJ, McCloskey CA: Temafloxacin syndrome: Review of 95 cases. *Clin Infect Dis* 18:946, 1994.
109. Marani TM, Trich MB, Armstrong KS, et al: Carboplatin-induced immune hemolytic anemia. *Transfusion* 36:1016, 1996.
110. Freercks RJ, Mehta U, Stead DF, Meintjes GA: Haemolytic anaemia associated with efavirenz. *AIDS* 20:1212, 2006.
111. Chaplin H, Avioli LV: Autoimmune hemolytic anemia. *Arch Intern Med* 137:346, 1977.
112. Sallah S, Wan J, Hanrahan L: Future development of lymphoproliferative disorders in patients with autoimmune hemolytic anemia. *Clin Cancer Res* 7:791, 2001.

113. Pirofsky B: Hereditary aspects of autoimmune hemolytic anemia: A retrospective analysis. *Vox Sang* 14:334, 1968.
114. Dobbs CE: Familial auto-immune hemolytic anemia. *Arch Intern Med* 116:273, 1965.
115. Cordova MS, Baez-Villasenor J, Mendez JJ, Campos E: Acquired hemolytic anemia with positive antiglobulin (Coombs' test) in mother and daughter. *Arch Intern Med* 117:692, 1966.
116. Eyster ME, Jenkins DE Jr: Erythrocyte coating substances in patients with positive direct antiglobulin reactions: Correlation of gamma-G globulin and complement coating with underlying diseases, overt hemolysis and response to therapy. *Am J Med* 46:360, 1969.
117. Feizi T: Cold agglutinins, the direct Coombs' test and serum immunoglobulins in *Mycoplasma pneumoniae* infection. *Ann N Y Acad Sci* 143:801, 1967.
118. Jacobson LB, Longstreth GF, Edington TS: Clinical and immunologic features of transient cold agglutinin hemolytic anemia. *Am J Med* 54:514, 1973.
119. Murray HW, Masur H, Senterfit LB, Roberts RB: The protean manifestations of *Mycoplasma pneumoniae* infection in adults. *Am J Med* 58:229, 1975.
120. Rosenfield RE, Schmidt PJ, Calvo RC, McGinniss MH: Anti-i, a frequent cold agglutinin in infectious mononucleosis. *Vox Sang* 10:631, 1965.
121. Worlledge SM, Dacie JV: Haemolytic and other anaemias in infectious mononucleosis, in *Infectious Mononucleosis*, edited by RL Carter, HG Penman, p 82. Blackwell Science, Oxford, 1969.
122. Hossaini AA: Anti-i in infectious mononucleosis. *Am J Clin Pathol* 53:198, 1970.
123. Arndt P, Garratty G: Cross-reactivity of cefotetan and ceftriaxone antibodies, associated with hemolytic anemia, with other cephalosporins and penicillin. *Am J Clin Pathol* 118:256, 2002.
124. Issitt PD, Pavone BG, Goldfinger D, et al: Anti-Wr^b and other autoantibodies responsible for positive direct antiglobulin test in 150 individuals. *Br J Haematol* 34:5, 1976.
125. Garratty G: Autoantibodies induced by blood transfusions. *Transfusion* 44:5, 2004.
126. Young PP, Uzieblo A, Trulock E, et al: Autoantibody formation after alloimmunization: Are blood transfusions a risk factor for autoimmune hemolytic anemia? *Transfusion* 44:67, 2004.
127. Salama A, Mueller-Eckhardt C: Delayed hemolytic transfusion reactions: Evidence for complement activation involving allogeneic and autologous red cells. *Transfusion* 24:188, 1984.
128. Ness PM, Shirey RS, Thoman SK, Buck SA: The differentiation of delayed serologic and delayed hemolytic transfusion reactions: Incidence, long-term serologic findings and clinical significance. *Transfusion* 30:688, 1990.
129. Leddy JP, Falany JL, Kissel GE, et al: Erythrocyte membrane proteins reactive with human (warm-reacting) anti-red cell autoantibodies. *J Clin Invest* 91:1672, 1993.
130. Gorst DW, Rawlinson VI, Merry AH, Stratton F: Positive direct anti-globulin test in normal individuals. *Vox Sang* 38:99, 1980.
131. Bareford D, Langster G, Gilks L, Demick-Torey LA: Follow-up of normal individuals with a positive antiglobulin test. *Scand J Haematol* 35:348, 1985.
132. Worlledge SM: The interpretation of a positive direct antiglobulin test. *Br J Haematol* 39:157, 1978.
133. Nossal GJV: B-cell selection and tolerance. *Curr Opin Immunol* 3:193, 1991.
134. Basten A, Brink R, Peake P, et al: Self-tolerance in the B-cell repertoire. *Immunol Rev* 122:5, 1991.
135. Kroemer G, Martinez-A C: Mechanisms of self-tolerance. *Immunol Today* 13:401, 1992.
136. Leddy JP: Immune hemolytic anemia, in *Clinical Immunology: Principles and Practice*, edited by RR Rich, TA Fleisher, BD Schwartz, WT Shearer, W Strober, p 1273. Mosby, St. Louis, 1996.
137. Hartley SB, Crosbie J, Brink R, et al: Elimination from peripheral lymphoid tissue of self-reactive B lymphocytes recognizing membrane bound antigens. *Nature* 353:765, 1991.
138. Leddy JP: Reactivity of human gamma-G erythrocyte autoantibodies with fetal, autologous and maternal red cells. *Vox Sang* 17:525, 1969.
139. Okamoto M, Murakami M, Shimizu A, et al: A transgenic model of autoimmune hemolytic anemia. *J Exp Med* 175:71, 1992.
140. Murakami M, Tsubata T, Okamoto M, et al: Antigen-induced apoptotic death of Ly-1 B cells responsible for autoimmune disease in transgenic mice. *Nature* 357:77, 1992.
141. Lin RH, Mamula MJ, Hardin JA, Janeway CA: Induction of autoreactive B cells allows priming of autoreactive T cells. *J Exp Med* 173:1433, 1991.
142. Silverman GJ, Carson DA: Structural characterization of human monoclonal cold agglutinins: Evidence for a distinct primary sequence-defined V_H4 idiotype. *Eur J Immunol* 20:351, 1990.
143. Silberstein LE, Jefferies LC, Goldman J, et al: Variable region gene analysis of pathologic human autoantibodies to the related i and I red blood cell antigens. *Blood* 78:2372, 1991.
144. Pascual V, Victor K, Spellerberg M, et al: V_H restriction among human cold agglutinins: The V_H4–21 gene segment is required to encode anti-I and anti-i specificities. *J Immunol* 149:2337, 1992.
145. Stevenson FK, Smith GJ, North J, et al: Identification of normal B-cell counterparts of neoplastic cells which secrete cold agglutinins of anti-I and anti-i specificity. *Br J Haematol* 72:9, 1989.
146. Silverman GJ, Chen PP, Carson DA: Cold agglutinins: Specificity, idiotype and structural analysis, in *Idiotypes in Biology and Medicine: Chemistry and Immunology*, vol 48, edited by DA Carson, PP Chen, TJ Kipps, p 109. Karger, Basel, 1990.
147. Feizi T: Lambda chains in cold agglutinins. *Science* 156:111, 1987.
148. Thompson KM, Sutherland J, Barden G, et al: Human monoclonal antibodies against blood group antigens preferentially express a V_H4–21 variable region gene-associated epitope. *Scand J Immunol* 34:509, 1991.
149. Adderson EE, Shackelford PG, Quinn A, et al: Restricted immunoglobulin VH usage and VDJ combinations in the human response to *Haemophilus influenzae* type b capsular polysaccharide: Nucleotide sequences of monospecific anti-*Haemophilus* antibodies and polyspecific antibodies cross-reacting with self-antigens. *J Clin Invest* 91:2734, 1993.
150. Adderson EE, Shackelford PG, Insel RA, et al: Immunoglobulin light chain variable region gene sequences for human antibodies to *Haemophilus influenzae* type b capsular polysaccharide are dominated by a limited number of V kappa and V lambda segments and VJ combinations. *J Clin Invest* 89:729, 1992.
151. Silberstein LE, Robertson GA, Hannam-Harris AC, et al: Etiologic aspects of cold agglutinin disease: Evidence of cytogenetically defined clones of lymphoid cells and the demonstration that an anti-Pr cold autoantibody is derived from an aberrant B cell clone. *Blood* 67:1705, 1986.
152. Gordon J, Silberstein LE, Moreau L, Nowell PC: Trisomy 3 in cold agglutinin disease. *Cancer Genet Cytogenet* 46:89, 1990.
153. Michaux L, Dierlamm J, Wlodarska I, et al: Trisomy 3q11-q29 is recurrently observed in B-cell non-Hodgkin's lymphomas associated with cold agglutinin syndrome. *Ann Hematol* 76:201, 1998.
154. Harboe M, Lind K: Light chain types of transiently occurring cold haemagglutinins. *Scand J Haematol* 3:269, 1966.
155. Feizi T: Monotypic cold agglutinins in infection by *Mycoplasma pneumoniae*. *Nature* 215:540, 1967.
156. Feizi T, Loveless W: Carbohydrate recognition by *Mycoplasma pneumoniae* and pathologic consequences. *Am J Respir Crit Care Med* 154:S133, 1996.
157. Mollison PL: Measurement of survival and destruction of red cells in haemolytic syndromes. *Br Med Bull* 15:59, 1959.
158. Hollander L: Erythrocyte survival time in a case of acquired haemolytic anaemia. *Vox Sang* 4:164, 1954.
159. Chaplin H, Cohen R, Bloomberg G, et al: Pregnancy and idiopathic autoimmune haemolytic anaemia: A prospective study during 6 months gestation and 3 months "post-partum." *Br J Haematol* 24:219, 1973.
160. Mollison PL, Crome P, Hughes-Jones NC, Rochna E: Rate of removal from the circulation of red cells sensitized with different amounts of antibody. *Br J Haematol* 11:461, 1965.
161. Mollison PL, Hughes-Jones NC: Clearance of Rh-positive red cells by low concentration of Rh antibody. *Immunology* 12:63, 1967.
162. Rosse WF: Quantitative immunology of immune hemolytic anemia: II. The relationship of cell-bound antibody to hemolysis and the effect of treatment. *J Clin Invest* 50:734, 1971.
163. Schreiber AD, Frank MM: Role of antibody and complement in the immune clearance and destruction of erythrocytes: I. *In vivo* effects of IgG and IgM complement-fixing sites. *J Clin Invest* 51:575, 1972.
164. Atkinson JP, Schreiber AD, Frank MM: Effects of corticosteroids and splenectomy on the immune clearance and destruction of erythrocytes. *J Clin Invest* 52:1509, 1973.
165. Atkinson JP, Frank MM: Complement independent clearance of IgG sensitized erythrocytes: Inhibition by cortisone. *Blood* 44:629, 1974.
166. Jandl JH, Richardson-Jones A, Castle WB: The destruction of red cells by antibodies in man: I. Observations on the sequestration and lysis of red cells altered by immune mechanisms. *J Clin Invest* 36:1428, 1957.
167. Jandl JH, Kaplan ME: The destruction of red cells by antibodies in man: III. Quantitative factors influencing the pattern of hemolysis *in vivo*. *J Clin Invest* 39:1145, 1960.
168. Abramson N, LoBuglio AF, Jandl JH, Cotran RS: The interaction between human monocytes and red cells: Binding characteristics. *J Exp Med* 132:1191, 1970.
169. LoBuglio AF, Cotran RS, Jandl JH: Red cells coated with immunoglobulin G: Binding and sphering by mononuclear cells in man. *Science* 158:1582, 1967.
170. Anderson CL, Looney RJ: Human leukocyte IgG Fc receptors. *Immunol Today* 7:264, 1986.
171. Ravetch JV, Kinet J-P: Fc receptors. *Annu Rev Immunol* 9:457, 1991.
172. Gigli I, Nelson RA: Complement-dependent immune phagocytosis: I. Requirements of C1, C4, C2, C3. *Exp Cell Res* 51:45, 1968.
173. Lay WF, Nussenzweig V: Receptors for complement on leukocytes. *J Exp Med* 128:991, 1968.
174. Ross GD: Opsonization and membrane complement receptors, in *Immunobiology of the Complement System*, edited by GD Ross, p 87. Academic Press, Orlando, 1986.
175. Fischer JT, Petz LD, Garratty G, Cooper NR: Correlations between quantitative assay of red cell bound C3, serologic reactions, and hemolytic anemia. *Blood* 44:359, 1974.
176. Schreiber AD, Parsons J, McDermott P, Cooper RA: Effect of corticosteroids on the human monocyte IgG and complement receptors. *J Clin Invest* 56:1189, 1975.
177. Ehlenberger AG, Nussenzweig V: The role of membrane receptors for C3b and C3d in phagocytosis. *J Exp Med* 145:357, 1977.
178. Rosse WF, De Boisfleury A, Bessis M: The interaction of phagocytic cells and red cells modified by immune reactions: Comparison of antibody and complement coated red cells. *Blood Cells* 1:345, 1975.
179. Dameshek W, Schwartz SO: Acute hemolytic anemia (acquired hemolytic icterus, acute type). *Medicine (Baltimore)* 19:231, 1940.

180. Leddy JP, Rosenfeld SI: Role of complement in hemolytic anemia and thrombocytopenia, in *Immunobiology of the Complement System*, edited by GD Ross, p 213. Academic Press, Orlando, 1986.
181. Nicholson-Weller A, Burge J, Fearon DT, et al: Isolation of a human erythrocyte membrane glycoprotein with decay-accelerating activity for C3 convertases of the complement system. *J Immunol* 129:184, 1982.
182. Lachmann PJ: The control of homologous lysis. *Immunol Today* 12:312, 1991.
183. Packman CH: Pathogenesis and management of paroxysmal nocturnal hemoglobinuria. *Blood Rev* 12:1, 1998.
184. Fleer A, Van Schaik MLJ, Von dem Borne AEG Kr, Engelfriet CP: Destruction of sensitized erythrocytes by human monocytes *in vitro*: Effects of cytochalasin B, hydrocortisone and colchicine. *Scand J Immunol* 8:515, 1978.
185. Kurlander RJ, Rosse WF, Logue WL: Quantitative influence of antibody and complement coating of red cells on monocyte-mediated cell lysis. *J Clin Invest* 61:1309, 1978.
186. Urbaniak SJ: Lymphoid cell dependent (K-cell) lysis of human erythrocytes sensitized with rhesus alloantibodies. *Br J Haematol* 33:409, 1976.
187. Handwerger BS, Kay NW, Douglas SD: Lymphocyte-mediated antibody-dependent cytolysis: Role in immune hemolysis. *Vox Sang* 34:276, 1978.
188. Milgrom H, Shore SL: Lysis of antibody-coated human red cells by peripheral blood mononuclear cells: Altered effector cell profile after treatment of target cells with enzymes. *Cell Immunol* 39:178, 1978.
189. Schreiber AD, Herskovitz BS, Goldwein M: Low-titer cold-hemagglutinin disease. *N Engl J Med* 296:1490, 1977.
190. Evans RS, Turner E, Bingham M, Woods R: Chronic hemolytic anemia due to cold agglutinins: II. The role of C in red cell destruction. *J Clin Invest* 47:691, 1968.
191. Atkinson JP, Frank MM: Studies on *in vivo* effects of antibody: Interaction of IgM antibody and complement in the immune clearance and destruction of erythrocytes in man. *J Clin Invest* 54:339, 1974.
192. Hughey CT, Brewer JW, Colosia AD, et al: Production of IgM hexamers by normal and autoimmune B cells: Implications for the physiologic role of hexameric IgM. *J Immunol* 161:4091, 1998.
193. Logue GL, Rosse WF, Gockerman JP: Measurement of the third component of complement bound to red blood cells in patients with the cold agglutinin syndrome. *J Clin Invest* 52:493, 1973.
194. Evans RS, Turner E, Bingham M: Studies with radioiodinated cold agglutinins of ten patients. *Am J Med* 38:378, 1965.
195. Roelcke D: Cold agglutination: Antibodies and antigens. *Clin Immunol Immunopathol* 2:266, 1974.
196. Mantovani B, Rabinovitch M, Nussenzweig V: Phagocytosis of immune complexes by macrophages: Different roles of the macrophage receptor sites for complement (C3) and for immunoglobulin (IgG). *J Exp Med* 135:780, 1972.
197. Silverstein SC, Steinman RM, Cohn ZA: Endocytosis. *Annu Rev Biochem* 46:669, 1977.
198. Jaffe CH, Atkinson JP, Frank MM: The role of complement in the clearance of cold agglutinin-sensitized erythrocytes in man. *J Clin Invest* 58:942, 1976.
199. Brown DL, Nelson DA: Surface microfragmentation of red cells as a mechanism for complement-mediated immune spherocytosis. *Br J Haematol* 24:301, 1973.
200. Evans RS, Turner E, Bingham M: Chronic hemolytic anemia due to cold agglutinins: I. The mechanism of resistance of red cells to C hemolysis by cold agglutinins. *J Clin Invest* 46:1461, 1967.
201. Kerr RO, Cardamone J, Dalmasso AP, Kaplan ME: Two mechanisms of erythrocyte destruction in penicillin-induced hemolytic anemia. *N Engl J Med* 287:1322, 1972.
202. Nesmith LW, Davis JW: Hemolytic anemia caused by penicillin. *JAMA* 203:27, 1968.
203. Yust I, Frisch B, Goldsher N: Simultaneous detection of two mechanisms of immune destruction of penicillin-treated human red blood cells. *Am J Hematol* 13:53, 1982.
204. Brandriss MW, Smith JW, Steinman HG: Common antigenic determinants of penicillin G, cephalothin and 6-aminopenicillanic acid in rabbits. *J Immunol* 94:696, 1965.
205. Abraham GN, Petz LD, Fudenberg HH: Immuno-hematological cross-allergenicity between penicillin and cephalothin in humans. *Clin Exp Immunol* 3:343, 1968.
206. Petz LD: Immunologic cross reactivity between penicillins and cephalosporins: A review. *J Infect Dis* 137:S74, 1978.
207. Kunicki TJ, Russell N, Nurten AT, et al: Further studies of the human platelet receptor for quinine- and quinidine-dependent antibodies. *J Immunol* 126:398, 1981.
208. Christie DJ, Aster RH: Drug-antibody-platelet interaction in quinine-and quinidine-induced thrombocytopenia. *J Clin Invest* 70:989, 1982.
209. Berndt MC, Chong BH, Bull HA, et al: Molecular characterization of quinine/quinidine drug-dependent antibody platelet interaction using monoclonal antisera. *Blood* 66:1292, 1985.
210. Sosler SD, Behzad O, Garratty G, et al: Acute hemolytic anemia associated with a chlorpropamide-induced apparent auto-anti-Jk_a. *Transfusion* 24:206, 1984.
211. Salama A, Mueller-Eckhardt C: Rh blood group-specific antibodies in immune hemolytic anemia induced by nomifensine. *Blood* 68:1285, 1986.
212. Salama A, Mueller-Eckhardt C: On the mechanisms of sensitization and attachment of antibodies to RBC in drug-induced immune hemolytic anemia. *Blood* 69:1006, 1987.
213. Christie DJ, Mullen PC, Aster RH: Fab-mediated binding of drug-dependent antibodies to platelets in quinidine- and quinine-induced thrombocytopenia. *J Clin Invest* 75:310, 1985.
214. Smith ME, Reid DM, Jones CE, et al: Binding of quinine- and quinidine-dependent drug antibodies to platelets is mediated by the Fab domain of immunoglobulin G and is not Fc dependent. *J Clin Invest* 29:912, 1987.
215. Salama A, Mueller-Eckhardt C: The role of metabolite-specific antibodies in nomifensine-dependent immune hemolytic anemia. *N Engl J Med* 313:469, 1985.
216. Kelton JG: Impaired reticuloendothelial function in patients treated with methyldopa. *N Engl J Med* 313:596, 1985.
217. Bakemeier RF, Leddy JP: Erythrocyte autoantibody associated with alpha-methyldopa: Heterogeneity of structure and specificity. *Blood* 32:1, 1968.
218. Green FA, Jung CY, Rampal A, Lorusso DJ: Alpha-methyldopa and the erythrocyte membrane. *Clin Exp Immunol* 40:554, 1980.
219. Green Fa, Jung CY, Hui H: Modulation of alpha-methyldopa binding to the erythrocyte membrane by superoxide dismutase. *Biochem Biophys Res Commun* 95:1037, 1980.
220. Kirtland HH III, Mohler DN, Horwitz DA: Methyldopa inhibition of suppressor-lymphocyte function. A proposed cause of autoimmune hemolytic anemia. *N Engl J Med* 302:825, 1980.
221. Garratty G, Arndt P, Prince HE, Schulman IA: The effect of methyldopa and procainamide on suppressor cell activity in relation to red cell autoantibody production. *Br J Haematol* 84:310, 1993.
222. Dearden C, Wade R, Else M, et al: The prognostic significance of a positive direct antiglobulin test in chronic lymphocytic leukemia: A beneficial effect of the combination of fludarabine and cyclophosphamide on the incidence of hemolytic anemia. *Blood* 111:1820, 2008.
223. Borthakur G, O'Brien S, Wierda WG, et al: Immune anaemias in patients with chronic lymphocytic leukaemia treated with fludarabine, cyclophosphamide and rituximab-incidence and predictors. *Br J Haematol* 136:800, 2007.
224. Spath P, Garratty G, Petz LD: Studies on the immune response to penicillin and cephalothin in humans: II. Immunohematologic reactions to cephalothin administration. *J Immunol* 107:860, 1971.
225. Garratty G, Petz L: Drug-induced hemolytic anemia. *Am J Med* 58:398, 1975.
226. Sokol RJ, Hewitt S, Stamps BK: Erythrocyte autoantibodies, autoimmune haemolysis and pregnancy. *Vox Sang* 43:169, 1982.
227. Issaragrisil S, Kruatrachue M: An association of pregnancy and auto-immune haemolytic anaemia. *Scand J Haematol* 31:63, 1983.
228. Evans RS, Duane RT: Acquired hemolytic anemia: I. The relation of erythrocyte antibody production to activity of the disease: II. The significance of thrombocytopenia and leukopenia. *Blood* 4:1196, 1949.
229. Evans RS, Takahashi K, Duane RT, et al: Primary thrombocytopenic purpura and acquired hemolytic anemia: Evidence for a common etiology. *Arch Intern Med* 87:48, 1951.
230. Pegels JG, Helmerhorst FM, vanLeeuwen EF, et al: The Evans syndrome: Characterization of the responsible autoantibodies. *Br J Haematol* 51:445, 1982.
231. Liesveld JL, Rowe JM, Lichtman MA: Variability of the erythropoietic response in autoimmune hemolytic anemia: Analysis of 109 cases. *Blood* 69:820, 1987.
232. Hegde UM, Gordon-Smith EC, Worlledge SM: Reticulocytopenia and absence of red cell autoantibodies in immune haemolytic anaemia. *Br Med J* 2:1444, 1977.
233. Conley CL, Lippman SM, Ness P: Autoimmune hemolytic anemia with reticulocytopenia: A medical emergency. *JAMA* 244:1688, 1980.
234. Greenberg J, Curtis-Cohen M, Gill FM, Cohen A: Prolonged reticulocytopenia in autoimmune hemolytic anemia of childhood. *J Pediatr* 97:784, 1980.
235. Mangan KF, Besa EC, Shadduck RK, et al: Demonstration of two distinct antibodies in autoimmune hemolytic anemia with reticulocytopenia and red cell aplasia. *Exp Hematol* 12:788, 1984.
236. Leddy JP: Immunological aspects of red cell injury in man. *Semin Hematol* 3:48, 1966.
237. Engelfriet CP, Borne AE vd, Giessen M vd, et al: Autoimmune haemolytic anaemias: I. Serological studies with pure anti-immunoglobulin reagents. *Clin Exp Immunol* 3:605, 1968.
238. Engelfriet CP, Borne AE, Beckers D, van Loghem JJ: Autoimmune haemolytic anaemia: Serological and immunochemical characteristics of the autoantibodies: Mechanisms of cell destruction. *Ser Haematol* 7:328, 1974.
239. Suzuki S, Amano T, Mitsunaga M, et al: Autoimmune hemolytic anemia associated with IgA autoantibody. *Clin Immunol Immunopathol* 21:247, 1981.
240. Wolf CF, Wolf DJ, Peterson P: Autoimmune hemolytic anemia with predominance of IgA autoantibody. *Transfusion* 22:238, 1982.
241. Szymanski IO, Teno R, Rybak ME: Hemolytic anemia due to a mixture of low-titer IgG lambda and IgM lambda agglutinins reacting optimally at 22°C. *Vox Sang* 51:112, 1986.
242. Reusser P, Osterwalder B, Burri H, Speck B: Autoimmune hemolytic anemia associated with IgA: Diagnostic and therapeutic aspects in a case with long-term follow-up. *Acta Haematol* 77:53, 1987.
243. Göttsche B, Salama A, Mueller-Eckhardt C: Autoimmune hemolytic anemia associated with an IgA autoanti-Gerbich. *Vox Sang* 58:211, 1990.
244. Arndt P, Leger RM, Garratty G: Serologic findings in autoimmune hemolytic anemia associated with immunoglobulin M warm autoantibodies. *Transfusion* 49:235, 2009.
245. Evans RS, Bingham M, Boehni P: Autoimmune hemolytic disease: Antibody dissociation and activity. *Arch Intern Med* 108:338, 1961.
246. Evans RS, Bingham M, Turner E: Autoimmune hemolytic disease: Observations of serological reactions and disease activity. *Ann N Y Acad Sci* 124:422, 1965.

247. Gilliland BC, Leddy JP, Vaughan JH: The detection of cell-bound antibody on complement-coated human red cells. *J Clin Invest* 49:898, 1970.
248. Gilliland BC, Baxter E, Evans RS: Red cell antibodies in acquired hemolytic anemia with negative antiglobulin serum tests. *N Engl J Med* 285:252, 1971.
249. Gilliland BC: Coombs-negative immune hemolytic anemia. *Semin Hematol* 13:267, 1976.
250. Sokol RJ, Hewitt S, Booker DJ, Bailey A: Erythrocyte autoantibodies, subclasses of IgG and autoimmune haemolysis. *Autoimmun Rev* 6:99, 1990.
251. von dem Borne AE, Beckers D, van der Meulen FW, Engelfriet CP: IgG_4 autoantibodies against erythrocytes, without increased hemolysis: A case report. *Br J Haematol* 37:137, 1977.
252. Weiner W, Vos GH: Serology of acquired hemolytic anemia. *Blood* 22:606, 1963.
253. Vos GH, Petz L, Funenberg HH: Specificity of acquired haemolytic anaemia autoantibodies and their serological characteristics. *Br J Haematol* 19:57, 1970.
254. Leddy JP, Peterson P, Yeaw MA, Bakemeier RF: Patterns of serologic specificity of human gamma-G erythrocyte autoantibodies. *J Immunol* 105:677, 1970.
255. Bell CA, Zwicker H: Further studies on the relationship of anti-En^a and anti-Wr^b in warm autoimmune hemolytic anemia. *Transfusion* 18:572, 1978.
256. Celano MJ, Levine P: Anti-LW specificity in autoimmune acquired hemolytic anemia. *Transfusion* 7:265, 1967.
257. Marsh WL, Reid ME, Scott EP: Autoantibodies of U blood group specificity in autoimmune haemolytic anaemia. *Br J Haematol* 22:625, 1972.
258. Shulman IA, Vengelen-Tyler V, Thompson JC, et al: Autoanti-Ge associated with severe autoimmune hemolytic anemia. *Vox Sang* 59:232, 1990.
259. Owen I, Chowdhury V, Reid ME, et al: Autoimmune hemolytic anemia associated with anti-Sc 1.*Transfusion* 32:173, 1992.
260. Marsh WL, Oyen R, Alicea E, et al: Autoimmune hemolytic anemia and the Kell blood groups. *Am J Hematol* 7:155, 1979.
261. Barker RN, Casswell KM, Reid ME, et al: Identification of autoantigens in autoimmune haemolytic anaemia by a non-radioisotope immunoprecipitation method. *Br J Haematol* 82:126, 1992.
262. Victoria EJ, Pierce SW, Branks MJ, Masouredis SP: IgG red blood cell autoantibodies in autoimmune hemolytic anemia bind to epitopes on red blood cell membrane band 3 glycoprotein. *J Lab Clin Med* 115:74, 1990.
263. Telen MJ, Chasis JA: Relationship of the human erythrocyte Wr^b antigen to an interaction between glycophorin A and band 3. *Blood* 76:842, 1990.
264. Barker RN, De la Sa Oliveira GG, Elson CJ, et al: Pathogenic autoantibodies in the NZB mouse are specific for erythrocyte band 3 protein. *Eur J Immunol* 23:1723, 1993.
265. Kay MMB, Marchalonis JJ, Hughes J, et al: Definition of a physiologic aging autoantigen by using synthetic peptides of membrane protein band 3: Localization of the active antigenic sites. *Proc Natl Acad Sci U S A* 87:5734, 1990.
266. Turrini F, Mannu F, Arese P, et al: Characterization of autologous antibodies that opsonize erythrocytes with clustered integral membrane proteins. *Blood* 181:3146, 1993.
267. Curtis BR, Lamon J, Roelcke D, Chaplin H: Life-threatening, antiglobulin test-negative, acute autoimmune hemolytic anemia due to a non-complement-activating IgG 1k cold antibody with Pr_a specificity. *Transfusion* 30:838, 1990.
268. Silberstein LE, Berkman EM, Schreiber AD: Cold hemagglutinin disease associated with IgG cold reactive antibody. *Ann Intern Med* 106:238, 1987.
269. Feizi T, Kabat EA, Vicari G, et al: Immunochemical studies on blood groups: XLVII. The I antigen complex precursors in the A, B, H, Le^a, and Le^b blood group system: Hemagglutination inhibition studies. *J Exp Med* 133:39, 1971.
270. Hakomori S: Blood group ABH and Ii antigens of human erythrocytes: Chemistry, polymorphism, and their developmental change. *Semin Hematol* 18:39, 1981.
271. Marcus DM: A review of the immunogenic and immunomodulatory properties of glycosphingolipids. *Mol Immunol* 21:1083, 1984.
272. Rosse WF, Lauf PK: Reaction of cold agglutinins with I antigen solubilized from human red cells. *Blood* 36:777, 1970.
273. Lauf PK, Rosse WF: The reactivity of red blood cell membrane glycophorin with "cold-reacting" antibodies. *Clin Immunol Immunopathol* 4:1, 1975.
274. Pruzanski W, Shumak KH: Biologic activity of cold-reacting autoantibodies. *N Engl J Med* 297:583, 1977.
275. Chapman J, Murphy MF, Waters AH: Chronic cold hemagglutinin disease due to an anti-M-like autoantibody. *Vox Sang* 42:272, 1982.
276. von dem Borne AEG, Mol JJ, Joustra-Maas N, et al: Autoimmune hemolytic anemia with monoclonal IgM (kappa) anti-P cold autohemolysins. *Br J Haematol* 50:345, 1982.
277. Terada K, Tanaka H, Mori R, et al: Hemolytic anemia associated with cold agglutinin during chickenpox and a review of the literature. *J Pediatr Hematol Oncol* 20:149, 1998.
278. Tamura T, Kanamori H, Yamazaki E, et al: Cold agglutinin disease following allogeneic bone marrow transplantation. *Bone Marrow Transplant* 13:321, 1994.
279. Capra JD, Dowling P, Cook S, Kunkel HG: An incomplete cold-reactive gamma G antibody with i specificity in infectious mononucleosis. *Vox Sang* 16:10, 1969.
280. Shirey RS, Park K, Ness PM, et al: An anti-i biphasic hemolysin in chronic paroxysmal cold hemoglobinuria. *Transfusion* 26:62, 1986.
281. Salama A, Santoso S, Mueller-Eckhardt C: Antigenic determinants responsible for the reactions of drug-dependent antibodies with blood cells. *Br J Haematol* 78:535, 1991.
282. Sokol R, Stamps R, Booker D, et al: Posttransplant immune-mediated hemolysis. *Transfusion* 42:198, 2002.
283. Lundgren G, Asaba H, Bergström J, et al: Fulminating anti-A autoimmune hemolysis with anuria in a renal transplant recipient: A therapeutic role of plasma exchange. *Clin Nephrol* 16:211, 1981.
284. Ramsey G, Nusbacher J, Starzl TE, Lindsay GD: Isohemagglutinins of graft origin after ABO-unmatched liver transplantation. *N Engl J Med* 311:1167, 1984.
285. Mangal AK, Growe GH, Sinclair M, et al: Acquired hemolytic anemia due to "auto"-anti-a or "auto"-anti-b induced by group O homograft in renal transplant recipients. *Transfusion* 24:201, 1984.
286. Hazlehurst GR, Brenner MK, Wimperis JZ, et al: Haemolysis after T-cell depleted bone marrow transplantation involving minor ABO incompatibility. *Scand J Haematol* 37:1, 1986.
287. Solheim BG, Albrechtsen D, Egeland T, et al: Auto-antibodies against erythrocytes in transplant patients produced by donor lymphocytes. *Transplant Proc* 6:4520, 1987.
288. Sniecinski IJ, Oien L, Petz LD, Blume KG: Immunohematologic consequences of major ABO-mismatched bone marrow transplantation. *Transplantation* 45:530, 1988.
289. Petz LD: "Least incompatible" units for transfusion in autoimmune hemolytic anemia: Should we eliminate this meaningless term? A commentary for clinicians and transfusion medicine professionals. *Transfusion* 42:1503, 2003.
290. Ness PM: How do I encourage clinicians to transfuse mismatched blood to patients with autoimmune hemolytic anemia in urgent situations? *Transfusion* 46:1859, 2006.
291. Issitt PD: Autoimmune hemolytic anemia and cold hemagglutinin disease: Clinical disease and laboratory findings. *Prog Clin Pathol* 7:137, 1978.
292. Wallhermfechtel MA, Pohl BA, Chaplin H: Alloimmunization in patients with warm autoantibodies: A retrospective study employing three donor alloabsorptions to aid in antibody detection. *Transfusion* 24:482, 1984.
293. Branch DR, Petz LD: Detecting alloantibodies in patients with autoantibodies. *Transfusion* 39:6, 1999.
294. Shirey RS, Boyd JS, Parwani AV, et al: Prophylactic antigen matched donor blood for patients with warm autoantibodies: An algorithm for transfusion management. *Transfusion* 42:1435, 2002.
295. Garratty G, Petz LD: Approaches to selecting blood for transfusion to patients with autoimmune hemolytic anemia. *Transfusion* 42:1390, 2002.
296. Dameshek W, Rosenthal MC, Schwartz SO: The treatment of acquired hemolytic anemia with adrenocorticotrophic hormone (ACTH). *N Engl J Med* 244:117, 1951.
297. Allgood JW, Chaplin H Jr: Idiopathic acquired autoimmune hemolytic anemia: A review of forty-seven cases treated from 1955 to 1965. *Am J Med* 43:254, 1967.
298. Meyer O, Stahl D, Beckhove P, et al: Pulsed high-dose dexamethasone in chronic autoimmune haemolytic anaemia of warm type. *Br J Haematol* 98:860, 1997.
299. Greendyke RM, Bradley EB, Swisher SN: Studies of the effects of administration of ACTH and adrenal corticosteroids on erythrophagocytosis. *J Clin Invest* 44:746, 1965.
300. Fries LF, Brickman CM, Frank MM: Monocyte receptors for the Fc portion of IgG increase in number in autoimmune hemolytic anemia and other hemolytic states and are decreased by glucocorticoid therapy. *J Immunol* 131:1240, 1983.
301. Habibi B, Homberg JC, Schaison G, Salmon C: Autoimmune hemolytic anemia in children: A review of 80 cases. *Am J Med* 56:61, 1974.
302. Christensen BE: The pattern of erythrocyte sequestration in immunohaemolysis: Effects of prednisone treatment and splenectomy. *Scand J Haematol* 10:120, 1973.
303. Parker AC, MacPherson AIS, Richmond J: Value of radiochromium investigation in autoimmune haemolytic anemia. *Br Med J* 1:208, 1977.
304. Schwartz SI, Bernard RP, Adams JT, Bauman AW: Splenectomy for hematologic disorders. *Arch Surg* 101:338, 1970.
305. Eichner ER: Splenic function: Normal, too much and too little. *Am J Med* 66:311, 1979.
306. Centers for Disease Control and Prevention: Recommended adult immunization schedule—United States 2003–2004. *MMWR Morb Mortal Wkly Rep* 52:965, 2003.
307. Taylor RP, Lindorfer MA: Drug insight: The mechanism of action of rituximab in autoimmune disease—The immune complex decoy hypothesis. *Nat Clin Pract Rheumatol* 3:86, 2007.
308. Garvey B: Rituximab in the treatment of autoimmune haematological disorders. *Br J Haematol* 141:149, 2008.
309. Zecca M, Nobili B, Ramenghi U, et al: Rituximab for the treatment of refractory autoimmune hemolytic anemia in children. *Blood* 101:3857, 2003.
310. Bussone G, Ribeiro E, Dechartres A, et al: Efficacy and safety of rituximab in adults' warm antibody autoimmune hemolytic anemia: Retrospective analysis of 27 cases. *Am J Hematol* 84:153, 2009.
311. Murphy S, LoBuglio AF: Drug therapy of autoimmune hemolytic anemia. *Semin Hematol* 13:323, 1976.
312. Moyo VM, Smith D, Brodsky I, et al: High-dose cyclophosphamide for refractory autoimmune hemolytic anemia. *Blood* 100:704, 2002.
313. Beutler E: New chemotherapeutic agent: 2-Chlorodeoxyadenosine. *Semin Hematol* 31:40, 1994.
314. Kotb R, Pinganaud C, Trichet C, et al: Efficacy of mycophenolate mofetil in adult refractory auto-immune cytopenias: A single center preliminary study. *Eur J Haematol* 75:60, 2005.
315. Howard J, Hoffbrand AV, Prentice HG, Mehta A: Mycophenolate mofetil for the treatment of refractory auto-immune haemolytic anaemia and auto-immune thrombocytopenic purpura. *Br J Haematol* 117:712, 2002.

316. Karlsson C, Hansson L, Celsing F, Lundin J. Treatment of severe refractory autoimmune hemolytic anemia in B-cell chronic lymphocytic leukemia with alemtuzumab (humanized CD52 monoclonal antibody). *Leukemia* 21:511, 2007.
317. Shumak KH, Rock GA: Therapeutic plasma exchange. *N Engl J Med* 310:762, 1984.
318. Council Report: Current status of therapeutic plasmapheresis and related techniques. *JAMA* 253:819, 1985.
319. Ahn YS, Harrington WJ, Byrnes JJ, et al: Treatment of autoimmune hemolytic anemia with vinca-loaded platelets. *JAMA* 249:2189, 1983.
320. Leickly FE, Buckley RH: Successful treatment of autoimmune hemolytic anemia in common variable immunodeficiency with high-dose intravenous gamma globulin. *Am J Med* 82:159, 1987.
321. Oda H, Honda A, Sugita K, et al: High-dose intravenous intact IgG infusion in refractory autoimmune hemolytic anemia (Evans syndrome). *J Pediatr* 107:744, 1985.
322. Bussel JB, Cunningham-Rundles C, Abraham C: Intravenous treatment of autoimmune hemolytic anemia with very high dose gammaglobulin. *Vox Sang* 41:264, 1986.
323. Besa EC: Rapid transient reversal of anemia and long-term effects of maintenance intravenous immunoglobulin for autoimmune hemolytic anemia in patients with lymphoproliferative disorders. *Am J Med* 84:691, 1988.
324. Flores G, Cunningham-Rundles C, Newland AC, Bussel JB: Efficacy of intravenous immunoglobulin in the treatment of autoimmune hemolytic anemia: Results in 73 patients. *Am J Hematol* 44:237, 1993.
325. Ahn YS, Harrington WJ, Mylvaganam R, et al: Danazol therapy for autoimmune hemolytic anemia. *Ann Intern Med* 102:298, 1985.
326. Pignon J-M, Poirson E, Rochant H: Danazol in autoimmune haemolytic anaemia. *Br J Haematol* 83:343, 1993.
327. Giannadaki E, Potamianos S, Roussomoustakaki M, et al: Autoimmune hemolytic anemia and positive Coombs' test associated with ulcerative colitis. *Am J Gastroenterol* 92:1872, 1997.
328. Cobo F, Pereira A, Nomdedeu B, et al: Ovarian dermoid cyst-associated autoimmune hemolytic anemia. *Am J Clin Pathol* 105:567, 1996.
329. Berentsen S, Ulvestad E, Gjertsen BT, et al: Rituximab for primary cold agglutinin disease: A prospective study of 37 courses of therapy in 27 patients. *Blood* 103:2925, 2004.
330. Schollkopf, C, Kjeldsen L, Bjerrum OW, et al: Rituximab in chronic cold agglutinin disease: A prospective study of 20 patients. *Leuk Lymphoma* 47:253, 2006.
331. Hippe E, Jensen KB, Olesen H, et al: Chlorambucil treatment of patients with cold agglutinin syndrome. *Blood* 35:68, 1970.
332. Evans RS, Baxter E, Gilliland BC: Chronic hemolytic anemia due to cold agglutinins: A 20-year history of benign gammopathy with response to chlorambucil. *Blood* 42:463, 1973.
333. Bell CA, Zwicker H, Sacks HJ: Autoimmune hemolytic anemia. *Am J Clin Pathol* 60:903, 1973.
334. Taft EG, Propp RP, Sullivan SA: Plasma exchange for cold agglutinin hemolytic anemia. *Transfusion* 17:173, 1977.
335. Brooks BD, Steane EA, Sheehan RG, Frenkel EP: Therapeutic plasma exchange in the immune hemolytic anemias and immunologic thrombocytopenic purpura. *Prog Clin Biol Res* 106:317, 1982.
336. Silberstein LE, Berkman EM: Plasma exchange in autoimmune hemolytic anemia (AIHA). *J Clin Apher* 1:238, 1983.
337. Zulian GB, Roux E, Tiercy J-M, et al: Transfusion-associated graft-versus-host disease in a patient treated with cladribine (2-chlorodeoxyadenosine): Demonstration of exogenous DNA in various tissue extracts by PCR analysis. *Br J Haematol* 89:83, 1995.
338. Briz M, Cabrera R, Sanjuan I: Diagnosis of transfusion-associated graft-versus-host disease by polymerase chain reaction fludarabine-treated B-chronic lymphocytic leukaemia. *Br J Haematol* 91:409, 1995.
339. Silverstein MN, Gomes MR, Elveback LR, et al: Idiopathic acquired hemolytic anemia: Survival in 117 cases. *Arch Intern Med* 129:85, 1972.
340. Dausset J, Colombani J: The serology and the prognosis of 128 cases of autoimmune hemolytic anemia. *Blood* 14:1280, 1959.
341. Pullarkat V, Ngo M, Iqbal S, et al: Detection of lupus anticoagulant identifies patients with autoimmune haemolytic anaemia at increased risk of venous thromboembolism. *Br J Haematol* 118:1166, 2002.
342. Hendrick AM: Auto-immune haemolytic anaemia—A high-risk disorder for thromboembolism? *Hematology* 8:53, 2003.
343. Buchanan GR, Boxer LA, Nathan DG: The acute and transient nature of idiopathic immune hemolytic anemia in childhood. *J Pediatr* 88:780, 1976.
344. Zupanska B, Lawkowicz W, Gorska B, et al: Autoimmune haemolytic anemia in children. *Br J Haematol* 34:511, 1976.
345. Heisel MA, Ortega JA: Factors influencing prognosis in childhood autoimmune hemolytic anemia. *Am J Pediatr Hematol Oncol* 5:147, 1983.
346. Carapella de Luca E, Casadei AM, DiPero G, et al: Autoimmune haemolytic anemia in childhood: Follow-up in 29 cases. *Vox Sang* 36:13, 1979.
347. Sokol RJ, Hewitt S, Stamps BK, Hitchen PA: Autoimmune haemolysis in childhood and adolescence. *Acta Haematol* 72:245, 1984.
348. Wang WC: Evans syndrome in childhood: Pathophysiology, clinical course, and treatment. *Am J Pediatr Hematol Oncol* 10:330, 1988.

CHAPTER 54

ALLOIMMUNE HEMOLYTIC DISEASE OF THE FETUS AND NEWBORN

Jayashree Ramasethu and Naomi L. C. Luban

SUMMARY

Alloimmune hemolytic disease of the fetus and newborn is caused by the action of transplacentally transmitted maternal immunoglobulin (Ig) G antibodies on paternally inherited antigens present on fetal red cells but absent on the maternal red cells. Maternal IgG antibodies bind to fetal red cells, causing hemolysis. As a consequence of the hemolytic process, anemia, extramedullary hematopoiesis, and neonatal hyperbilirubinemia sometimes result in fetal loss or neonatal death or disability. Collaboration among maternal–fetal medicine specialists, hematologists, radiologists, and neonatologists has substantially reduced perinatal mortality and morbidity resulting from this condition. Antenatal diagnostic methods identify fetuses at risk for developing hemolysis and assess disease severity in affected fetuses. After birth, phototherapy and exchange transfusions prevent serum bilirubin from rising to levels that could produce bilirubin encephalopathy and resultant brain damage (kernicterus). Severely affected fetuses who in the past died before birth, secondary to severe anemia and hydrops, now are saved by vigilant antenatal monitoring and intrauterine transfusions. Antibody against D antigen prophylaxis protocols have successfully prevented alloimmune hemolytic disease resulting from rhesus D sensitization, but alloimmune hemolytic disease resulting from other red cell antibodies still occurs. Advances in immunohematology and molecular biology may offer new avenues for prevention and treatment in the future.

DEFINITION AND HISTORY

Alloimmune hemolytic disease of the fetus and newborn (HDFN) is a disorder in which the life span of fetal and/or neonatal red cells is shortened as a result of binding of transplacentally transferred maternal immunoglobulin (Ig) G antibodies on fetal red cell antigens foreign to the mother, inherited by the fetus from the father. The resulting hemolysis may cause fetal and neonatal anemia and significant neonatal jaundice. There are three main classes of alloimmune HDFN, based on the antigen(s) involved: Rh (rhesus), ABO, and other red cell antigens.

Prior to the development of medical interventions in the 1950s, almost half of all newborn infants with Rh HDFN died or were severely handicapped. Although the clinical condition was described in newborn infants as early as the 1600s, it was only in the 1930s and 1940s that the pathophysiology of Rh HDFN was uncovered. In 1932, Diamond and colleagues[1] recognized that the clinical syndromes of stillbirth with unusual erythroblastic activity in the extramedullary sites and blood, fetal hydrops, anemia in the newborn, and "icterus gravis neonatorum" were closely related and likely had the same pathophysiology in the hematopoietic system. In 1938, Ruth Darrow, a pathologist who lost a baby to kernicterus, postulated that hemolysis of fetal red blood cells was a result of maternal antibody produced in response to fetal hemoglobin.[2] The discovery of the Rh factor by Landsteiner and Weiner led to elucidation of Rh HDN by Levine and colleagues who established that erythroblastosis fetalis was caused by immunization of an Rh-negative mother by the red cells from an Rh-positive fetus.[3] Antibodies produced by the sensitized mother crossed the placenta in the next pregnancy and coated the fetal Rh-positive cells, leading to hemolysis, anemia, hydrops, and severe neonatal jaundice.

Acronyms and abbreviations that appear in this chapter include: anti-D, antibody against D antigen; DAT, direct antiglobulin test; ΔOD_{450}, change in optical density at 450 nm; FMH, fetal–maternal hemorrhage; HDFN, alloimmune hemolytic disease of the fetus and newborn; Ig, immunoglobulin; IUT, intrauterine transfusion; IVIg, intravenous immunoglobulin G; RBC, red blood cell; Rh, rhesus.

Neonatal mortality from Rh HDFN decreased considerably with the development of exchange transfusion techniques for correction of severe anemia and hyperbilirubinemia.[4] However, severely affected fetuses continued to die *in utero* before 34 weeks' gestation. In 1961, Liley demonstrated the prognostic value of amniotic fluid spectrophotometry in identifying fetuses at risk and then showed that intrauterine transfusions could prevent fetal deaths.[5] The most dramatic reduction in the incidence of Rh HDFN was achieved in the 1960s and 1970s with the development of postpartum and antepartum antibody against D antigen (anti-D) prophylaxis to prevent Rh sensitization.[6]

Despite these advances, Rh HDFN has not disappeared, and cases of hemolytic disease of the newborn resulting from red cell antibodies directed toward antigens other than the Rh blood group system are being increasingly recognized.[8–12] The lessons learned from management of the fetus and newborn with Rh HDFN have been applied with considerable success to all forms of HDFN, with significant decreases in mortality and morbidity in the past century. The 21st century has seen further improvements in both diagnostic methods and therapeutic strategies.

ETIOLOGY AND PATHOGENESIS

CAUSAL ANTIBODIES

The epidemiology of HDFN varies in different ethnic and racial groups; the frequency of specific blood group alleles in a given population determines the probability of blood group incompatibility and maternal alloimmunization. Approximately 16 percent of Americans of European descent are RhD negative, compared to 7 to 8 percent of African Americans, 5 percent of Indians, and 0.3 percent of Chinese people.[13–15]

Antigen-negative women may have naturally occurring antibodies to certain red cell antigens (anti-A or anti-B) or may develop antibodies as a result of exposure to foreign red cell antigens through blood transfusion or, more often, by silent fetomaternal hemorrhage during pregnancy or at delivery. More than 50 different red cell antigens are associated with maternal alloimmunization[7–12] and with HDFN of varying severity (Table 54–1).

Antibodies that cause HDFN can be categorized into three main classes: (1) antibodies directed against the D antigen in the Rh blood group system, (2) antibodies directed against the A and B antigens, and (3) antibodies directed against the remaining red cell antigens. Antenatal screening programs detect clinically significant antibodies in 0.01 to 0.4 percent of pregnant women.[7–12] Screening programs generally do not include testing O group mothers for high titers of anti-A or anti-B antibodies, as they do not predict neonatal ABO disease with accuracy. Despite the success of Rh prophylaxis, anti-D antibodies still constitute a large proportion of antibodies detected in Europe and the United States. When D is excluded, non-D Rh antibodies (c, C, e, E, cc, and Ce) and

TABLE 54–1. RBC Antibodies Associated with HDFN

Blood Group	Frequently Associated with Severe HDFN	Occasionally Associated with Severe HDFN	Usually Associated with Mild HDFN	Not a Cause of HDFN
Rh	D, c	C, E, f, Ce, Cw, Cx, Ew, G, Hro, Rh29, Rh32, Rh42, Goa, Bea, Evans, Tar, Sec, JAL, STEM	E, e, f, Cx, Dw, Rh29, Riv, LOCR	
Kell	K	K, Kpa, Kpb, Ku, Jsa, Jsb, Ula, K11, K22	Ku, Jsa, K11	K23, K24
Duffy		Fya	Fyb, Fy3	
Kidd		Jka	Jkb, Jk3	
MNS		M, S, s, U, Mia, Vw, Mur, Mta, Hut, Hil, Mv, Far, sD, Ena, MUT	M, S, s, U, Mta, Mit	N
Lutheran			Lua, Lub	
Lewis				Lea, Leb
Other		JFV, Jones, Kg, MAM, REIT, Rd, Vel, Dia, Wra, Co3, PPIPk	Dib, Sc3, Ge2,Ge3, Ge4, LSa, Lan, JFV, HOFM	P1, Wrb, Yta, Ytb, Sc1, Sc2, CROM, CH/RG, KN, JMH

SOURCE: Adapted from Moise KJ[7] and Eder AF.[52]

antibodies belonging to the Kell, Duffy, Kidd, and MNS systems, are most frequently involved.[7,8] In one tertiary center in the United States, the frequencies of specific alloimmunizations were anti-D 18.4 percent, anti-E 14 percent, anti-c 5.8 percent, anti-C 4.7 percent, Kell group 22 percent, anti-MNS 4.7 percent, anti-Fya (Duffy) 5.4 percent, and anti-Jka 1.5 percent.[9] In Sweden, alloimmunization during pregnancy was detected in 0.4 percent of 78,145 pregnancies, with significant alloimmunization (defined as titer level of 8 or more) in 0.16 percent. Anti-D immunizations were responsible for 60 percent of significant immunizations, followed by anti-Fya in 10 percent, anti-c in 7 percent, and anti-K in 4 percent.[10] In the Netherlands, the prevalence of confirmed positive antibody screens at first trimester screening was 1232 in 100,000 antibody screens, with the prevalence of alloantibodies other than anti-D being 328 per 100,000. Of these, only 191 per 100,000 antibody screens implied a risk for occurrence of HDFN because the father carried the antigen. Anti-E and anti-D were the most frequent, followed by anti-K and anti-c.[11] In Asia, antibodies of different specificities are responsible for HDFN. A retrospective review of antenatal testing results in 28,303 women in Hong Kong, China, revealed clinically significant antibodies in 0.27 percent of ethnic Chinese women, with the most common antibodies being anti-Mi (57.6%), anti-E (19.7%), anti-S (10.6%), and anti-c (7.6%).[12]

The mere presence of antibodies on screening tests may not be clinically significant, because of the unique characteristics of some antibodies. For example, IgM antibodies do not cross the placenta. Alternatively, Lewis and Chido antigens are poorly expressed on fetal and neonatal red cells and therefore are not susceptible to destruction by maternal antibodies. Only IgG antibodies capable of crossing the placenta have the potential to affect the fetus and only if the fetus is antigen positive for the specific antibody. The clinical severity of HDFN may be affected by the class and subclass of IgG antibody, the concentration of antibody in the maternal circulation, and the rate of transplacental transfer. Fetal factors having a significant impact on the severity of hemolysis in the presence of maternal alloantibodies include the presence and concentration of antigens on the surface of fetal red cells, the competing effect of similar antigens present in fetal tissues other than fetal red cells, and the competency of the fetal mononuclear phagocyte system.

Rh HDFN is discussed first because it is archetypal of this condition. The distinguishing features of the other classes of alloimmune HDFN are highlighted.

■ RHD HEMOLYTIC DISEASE

Genetics and Molecular Basis of D Polymorphisms

The antigens of the Rh system are encoded by a pair of genes, *RHD* and *RHCE,* on the short arm of chromosome 1. The genes each have 10 exons, share 94 percent sequence identity, and are closely linked in opposite orientation (5′*RHD* 3′- 3′ *RHCE* 5′) with the sense strand of *RHD* becoming the antisense strand of *RHCE*. The Rh genes produce nonglycosylated, palmitoylated proteins of around 417 amino acids, which traverse the red cell membrane and exhibit 6 extracellular loops which define their antigenic activity. Anti-D antibody molecules recognize the epitopes on the external loops of RhD protein (see Chap. 137).

RhD-positive individuals may have one or two copies of *RHD* (heterozygous or homozygous RhD-positive, respectively). More than 150 alleles have been defined for *RHD* and more are likely to be revealed as population studies expand.[16] A number of *RHD* alleles responsible for RhD protein variants with altered D antigen expression have been classified according to their phenotype and molecular variation as partial D, weak D, and DEL. Amino acid substitutions located in an extracellular loop could result in different forms of partial D. Carriers of partial D may produce anti-D upon exposure to normal D antigen. Amino acid substitutions located in the transmembrane or intracellular segments of the RhD protein result in a weak D phenotype. The expressed D antigen is reduced quantitatively but not qualitatively, so carriers are not usually susceptible to anti-D immunization. However, weak D type 15, weak D type 4.2 or DAR, and weak D type 7 may produce anti-D. DEL is a very weakly expressed D antigen found in 30 percent of D-"negative" blood donors in East Asia.

In white populations, all D-negative individuals are homozygous for deletion of *RHD,* which encompasses the whole of *RHD* and part of each of the flanking Rh boxes. The resultant RhD-negative phenotype is characterized by the absence of the whole RhD protein from the red cell membrane, although the RhCcEe protein is usually present. Only 18 percent of D-negative black Africans are homozygous for *RHD* deletion. The majority (66%) of D-negative black Africans have an inactive RHD gene RHψ, while 15 percent have a hybrid gene RHD-CE-D^s, neither of which produces epitopes of D.

Pregnant women with the frequent weak D type 1 to type 3 may be transfused with D-positive blood and are not susceptible to alloimmunization. Women with DVI, and DNB, both partial D variants, may produce anti-D when exposed to normal D antigen.[16,17]

Fetomaternal Hemorrhage and Anti-D Alloimmunization

Asymptomatic transplacental passage of fetal red cells occurs in 75 percent of pregnant women at some time during pregnancy or during labor and delivery.[18] The incidence of fetomaternal transfusion increases with advancing gestation: from 3 percent in the first trimester, to 12 percent in the second trimester, to 45 percent in the third trimester, to 64 percent at delivery. The average volume of fetal blood in the maternal circulation after delivery is approximately 0.1 mL in most women and less than 1 mL in 96 percent of women.[19] Intrapartum fetomaternal hemorrhage of more than 30 mL may occur in up to 1 percent of deliveries.[20] Massive fetomaternal hemorrhage may present with decreased fetal movement and sinusoidal heart rhythm (undulating wave form alternating with a flat or smooth baseline fetal heart rate); however, it also may be clinically silent, with no clinical signs differentiating such deliveries from those with minimal fetomaternal hemorrhage.[20,21] Fetomaternal transfusion can also result from obstetric procedures such as chorionic villus sampling, amniocentesis, funipuncture, therapeutic abortion, external cephalic version, cesarean section, and manual removal of the placenta, and from pathologic conditions such as abdominal trauma, spontaneous abortion, or ectopic pregnancy.[19,22–24]

The potential for immunization of the mother is determined by the extent of fetomaternal hemorrhage and by the presence of maternal–fetal blood group incompatibility. The presence of D-positive red cells in a D-negative mother initially provokes a weak and slow primary immune response, which takes up to 4 weeks and consists of transient elevation of IgM antibodies. Subsequently, approximately 5 to 15 weeks after exposure to the D-positive red cells, anti-D IgG antibodies capable of crossing the placenta are produced. The D antigen is the most immunogenic of the Rh antigens and, indeed, of all red cell antigens (after ABO).[25] The D protein differs from the CcEe protein by 35 amino acids, and is processed by antigen-processing cells in the spleen and lymphoid tissue of D-negative individuals into multiple short allogeneic linear peptides, which stimulate helper T cells, which then activate B cells to produce IgM and later IgG antibodies. Memory T and B cells that are generated following the initial immune response are long lived, and exposure to the antigen even years later results in an accelerated antibody response as a result of rapid proliferation of antigen-specific clones. Repeated exposure to D-positive fetal red blood cells, as in a second D-positive pregnancy in a sensitized D-negative woman, produces a brisk secondary immune response marked by rapid production of large amounts of anti-D IgG antibody by maternal memory B lymphocytes.

In the absence of RhIg prophylaxis, sensitization occurs in 7 to 16 percent of women at risk, within 6 months after delivery of the first Rh-positive ABO-compatible fetus. The relatively low rate of 16 percent of primary alloimmunization in Rh-negative women at risk may be a result of the low volume of fetomaternal hemorrhage (FMH) in most women. Repetitive exposure to minuscule amounts of D-positive red cells in D-negative women who abuse intravenous drugs and share needles with RhD-positive partners has been reported to lead to severe Rh sensitization.[26] Fetomaternal ABO incompatibility offers some protection against primary Rh immunization because incompatible fetal red cells are destroyed rapidly by maternal anti-A and anti-B antibodies, reducing maternal exposure to RhD antigenic sites. Primary Rh immunization occurs in 2 percent of women at risk after delivery of an ABO-incompatible fetus.[27] ABO incompatibility confers no protection against the secondary immune response once sensitization has occurred.[27]

Hemolysis

Binding of transplacentally transferred maternal anti-D IgG antibodies to D-antigen sites on the fetal red cell membrane is followed by adherence of the coated red cells to the Fcγ receptors of macrophages with rosette formation, leading to extravascular noncomplement-mediated phagocytosis and lysis, predominantly in the spleen.[28,29] Although Rh antigens are found on fetal cells as early as week 7 of gestation, active transport of IgG across the placenta is slow until 20 to 24 weeks of gestation. The degree of hemolysis may be influenced by the functional immaturity of the fetal mononuclear phagocyte system prior to 20 weeks of gestation, maternal IgG levels, the IgG subclass, and the rate of transplacental transfer.[30,31] Although IgG anti-D consists mainly of IgG_1 and IgG_3 subclasses, the relative contribution of each of these subclasses to the severity of hemolytic disease in the newborn remains controversial.[28–31] Occasionally, women who are severely alloimmunized deliver babies with unexpectedly mild hemolysis. Protection from severe hemolytic disease in the fetuses of such women may result from inhibitory anti-human leukocyte antigen (HLA) antibodies with specificity for allogeneic monocytes, which block Fcγ receptors on mononuclear phagocytic cells.[32,33]

Fetal anemia secondary to hemolysis results in compensatory extramedullary hematopoiesis in the liver, spleen, kidneys, and adrenal glands, associated with an outpouring of immature nucleated red blood cells in the fetal circulation. Increased fetal plasma erythropoietin levels have been reported with severe fetal anemia.[34] The marked increase in erythropoiesis may be accompanied by down-modulation of platelet and neutrophil production.[35] Severe fetal thrombocytopenia (platelet count $< 50 \times 10^9$/L) was found in 3 percent of all fetal blood samplings and in 23 percent of severely hydropic fetuses in one center, when fetal platelet counts were measured prior to intrauterine transfusions in RhD alloimmunized pregnancies.[36] Extensive extramedullary hemopoiesis in the liver and spleen may cause portal and umbilical venous hypertension, leading to ascites, pleural effusions, and consequent pulmonary hypoplasia.[37] Trophoblastic hypertrophy and placental edema cause impaired placental function. Hypoproteinemia as a result of liver dysfunction leads to generalized edema. "Hydrops fetalis" (Fig. 54–1), a state of anasarca, is the end result of a combination of anemia, hypoproteinemia, cardiac failure, elevated venous pressures, increased capillary permeability, and impaired lymphatic clearance. Prior to the institution of intrauterine transfusions, most of these fetuses died *in utero* or soon after birth.

Although fetal bilirubin levels are elevated secondary to hemolysis, the placenta effectively transports most of the lipid-soluble unconjugated fetal bilirubin, so the baby is not clinically jaundiced at birth. Some of the fetal bilirubin is excreted into the amniotic fluid, and bilirubin concentrations in amniotic fluid reflect bilirubin concentrations in fetal blood and are related to albumin concentrations in fetal blood and in the amniotic fluid.[38] The mechanism of entry of bilirubin into the amniotic fluid

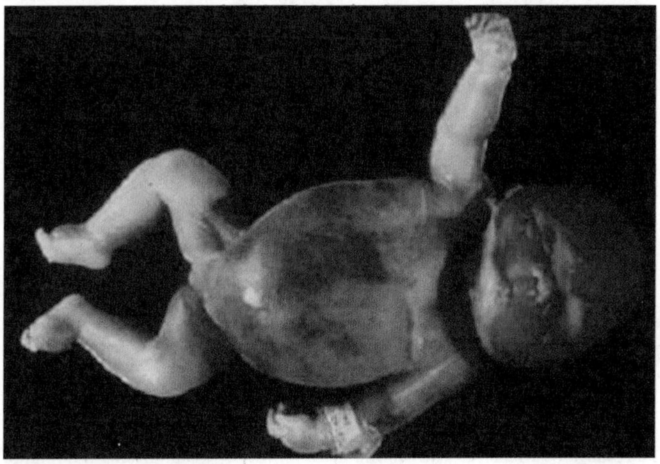

FIGURE 54–1. Hydrops fetalis.

compartment has been debated, but of the five possible pathways (excretion through the fetal kidneys, meconium, skin, fetal lung secretions, and transmembranous), transmembranous appears to be most likely.[39] At birth, the newborn infant's immature liver is incapable of handling the large bilirubin load that results from the ongoing destruction of antibody-coated neonatal red cells, and unconjugated bilirubin levels rise.

After birth, the quantity of maternal antibodies in the neonatal circulation decreases over the next 12 weeks, with a half-life of approximately 25 days. Infants with moderate to severe hemolytic disease may develop significant anemia beyond the immediate neonatal period lasting up to age 8 to 12 weeks. Delayed anemia is related to continuing hemolysis because of persistence of maternal antibodies and a hyporegenerative component with decreased red cell production, associated with low serum concentrations of erythropoietin.[40–42]

ABO HEMOLYTIC DISEASE

ABO hemolytic disease of the newborn (HDN) occurs almost exclusively in infants with blood group A or B who are born to group O mothers, although there are rare case reports of HDN in group B infants born to group A mothers and in AB infants born to O group mothers.[43,44] ABO incompatibility is present in approximately 15 percent of O group pregnancies, but ABO hemolytic disease is estimated to occur in only 1 to 3 percent of births, almost certainly because most anti-A and anti-B antibodies are of the IgM type, which is incapable of crossing the placenta, and only a small proportion of group O individuals produce anti-A and anti-B IgG antibodies that may be transferred across the placenta. A significant component of anti-A and anti-B antibody is IgG_2, which is transported less readily across the placenta than is IgG_1 or IgG_3 and is a less-efficient mediator of macrophage-induced red cell clearance.[13,45] Antenatal testing of anti-A and anti-B levels in group O mothers has little value in predicting ABO hemolytic disease in the newborn infant. This is partly as a consequence of the small number of fully developed A or B antigen sites on fetal red blood cells and the fact that the effect of anti-A and anti-B antibodies on red cells is further diluted by other fetal tissues bearing these surface antigens. Hemolysis occurs by noncomplement-mediated phagocytosis of Ig-coated red cells, similar to Rh HDFN. The blood film in ABO hemolytic disease of the newborn is marked by the presence of microspherocytes, a feature not usually seen in Rh hemolytic disease of the newborn. Microspherocytosis is attributed to loss of membrane surface area when the spleen removes antigen–antibody complexes from the affected cell (see Chap. 53).

ABO hemolytic disease of the newborn usually results in early neonatal jaundice requiring phototherapy and, rarely, exchange transfusions.[46] A higher incidence and greater severity of jaundice is reported in southeast Asians, Hispanics, Arabs, and South African and American blacks.[47–49] The increased incidence and severity of hyperbilirubinemia in certain populations may result from the presence of a variant uridine diphosphate glucuronyltransferase gene promoter.[50] Severe fetal anemia with hydrops has been rarely reported.[49] Unlike Rh disease, ABO hemolytic disease of the newborn may affect the first-born ABO-incompatible infant because anti-A and anti-B IgG antibodies may be present normally in group O adults. A recurrence rate of 88 percent has been reported in siblings having the same blood type as the affected index baby, with two-thirds of the affected siblings requiring therapy.[51] Table 54–2 lists the differences between Rh and ABO hemolytic disease of the newborn.

TABLE 54–2. Comparison of Rh and ABO Hemolytic Disease of the Newborn

	Rh	ABO
Blood groups		
Mother	Negative	O
Infant	Positive	A or B
Type of antibody	IgG_1 and /or IgG_3	IgG_2
Clinical aspects		
Occurrence in first-born	5%	40–50%
Predictable severity in subsequent pregnancies	Usually	No
Stillbirth and/or hydrops	Frequent	Rare
Severe anemia	Frequent	Rare
Degree of jaundice	+++	+ to ++
Hepatosplenomegaly	+++	+
Laboratory findings		
Maternal antibodies	Always present	Not clear-cut
Direct antiglobulin test (infant)	+	+ or –
Microspherocytes	0	+
Treatment		
Antenatal measures	Yes	No
Exchange transfusion frequency	Approx. 2/3	Occasional
Donor blood type	Rh-negative, group specific when possible	Group O only
Incidence of late anemia	Common	Rare

HEMOLYTIC DISEASE CAUSED BY OTHER RED CELL ANTIBODIES

A review of the fetal and neonatal outcome of pregnancies associated with alloimmunization to non-D antigens shows that although many antibodies reportedly cause hemolysis, case reports in the literature appear to be biased toward the more severe cases.[7] Table 54–1 lists the antibodies frequently associated with HDFN.[7,52] There is considerable variability in the clinical spectrum of hemolytic disease produced by the different antibodies, so some overlap may be noted between different categories, but anti-RhD, anti-Rhc, and anti-Kell are often associated with severe HDFN. The prevalence of anti-Kell antibodies surpassed anti-D antibodies in one series of alloimmunized pregnant women in the United States.[9]

Kell

The Kell blood group system consists of at least 28 discrete antigens, of which 8 are associated with HDFN. The *KEL* gene is located on chromosome 7q34. Kell antigens are located on the red cell membrane glycoprotein CD238. Kell is unique in that it spans the red blood cell (RBC) membrane once; it has a short N terminal domain of 47 amino acids in the cytosol and a large C terminal domain (665 amino acids) outside the membrane. Kell glycoprotein is linked to the integral membrane protein XK, a membrane transporter. The absence of the Kx antigen on XK and the weakened expression of Kell antigens define the McLeod phenotype: acanthocytic RBCs and a neuromuscular and neurodegenerative disease. The most common of the K antigens, K and K1, are expressed by erythroid progenitor cells and mature erythroid cell. Only 9 percent of people of European ancestry and 1 to 2 percent of people of African ancestry express K or K1, and almost all K-positive individuals are heterozygous.[53] Like RhD, there are many different mutations and amino acid substitutions that result in five sets of high- and low-prevalence antigens, including K null and K mod. Approximately 30 to 50 percent of alloimmunization in Kell-negative women results from blood transfusion rather than sensitization by fetomaternal hemorrhage from a Kell-positive fetus.[54,55] Kell hemolytic disease is uncommon even in alloimmunized pregnancies because fetal anemia resulting from transplacentally transmitted antibodies can occur only in a Kell-positive fetus. The partner of a Kell-negative woman is likely to be Kell-positive in less than 10 percent of pregnancies, and only half of these pregnancies are incompatible because of paternal heterozygosity. Published results on the outcome of maternal Kell alloimmunization indicate between 2.5 and 10 percent of Kell-immunized pregnancies end in the delivery of affected infants, but approximately half the infants require intervention, with fetal hydrops and severe anemia being common presentations.[55–57] Unlike RhD hemolytic disease, fetal anemia in anti-Kell alloimmunization does not result solely from hemolysis but also is secondary to suppression of fetal erythropoiesis. Clinical observations of inappropriately low levels of circulating reticulocytes and normoblasts for the degree of anemia in affected fetuses have long been noted, and suppression of erythropoiesis has been established by *in vitro* studies showing that growth of Kell-positive erythroid progenitor cells is inhibited by monoclonal IgG and IgM anti-Kell antibodies.[58] Anti-Kell antibodies are also postulated to cause fetal anemia by promoting the immune destruction of early erythroid K-positive progenitor cells by macrophages in the fetal liver.[59] Furthermore, anti-Kell antibodies have been associated with suppression of megakaryocyte and granulocyte colony-forming units with resultant fetal and neonatal thrombocytopenia and pancytopenia.[60,61]

CLINICAL FEATURES OF HDFN

Anemia, jaundice, and hepatosplenomegaly are the hallmarks of hemolytic disease of the newborn. The clinical spectrum of affected infants is highly variable. In Rh hemolytic disease of the newborn, half of the infants have mild disease and do not require intervention. One-fourth of affected infants are born at term with moderate anemia and develop severe jaundice. In the days prior to intrauterine intervention, hydrops developed *in utero* in the remaining one-fourth of infants; half became hydropic prior to 34 weeks' gestation. Hydrops recurs in 90 percent of affected pregnancies, often at an earlier gestation. In Kell hemolytic disease of the newborn, the clinical spectrum of hemolytic disease of the newborn is less predictable, ranging from mild anemia or hyperbilirubinemia to frank hydrops. Jaundice is the predominant feature of ABO hemolytic disease, but anemia and mild hepatosplenomegaly may also be seen. Severe fetal anemia and hydrops is unusual in this condition.[49]

ANEMIA

Infants with mild hemolytic disease of the newborn may have cord blood hemoglobin concentrations only slightly lower than the age-related normal range. Hemoglobin values usually continue to fall after birth in all affected infants. Hemolysis continues until all incompatible red cells and/or circulating maternal alloantibody are eliminated from the circulation. Physical examination in infants having moderate to severe anemia reveals pallor, tachypnea, and tachycardia. Signs of cardiovascular collapse and tissue hypoxemia appear with severe anemia (hemoglobin <4 g/dL, hematocrit <15%).

NEONATAL JAUNDICE

Most infants with hemolytic disease are not jaundiced at birth, although the umbilical cord and vernix caseosa may be stained with bilirubin from the amniotic fluid in severely affected infants. Clinical jaundice usually develops during the first day of life, often in the first few hours of life in severely affected infants. The jaundice progresses in a cephalopedal direction with rising bilirubin levels. In patients with mild disease, the serum indirect bilirubin peaks by the fourth or fifth day and then declines slowly. Premature infants may have higher levels of serum bilirubin for a longer duration because of lower hepatic glucuronyl transferase activity. Conjugated hyperbilirubinemia at birth is sometimes noted in infants who received multiple intrauterine transfusions.

KERNICTERUS

An important complication of elevated serum levels of indirect bilirubin in the neonate is the development of bilirubin encephalopathy.[62] This disorder, also termed *kernicterus*, is caused by bilirubin pigment deposition in the basal ganglia and brainstem nuclei, leading to neuronal necrosis. Acute bilirubin encephalopathy is initially marked by lethargy, poor feeding, and hypotonia. With increasing severity, the infant develops a high-pitched cry, fever, hypertonia progressing to frank opisthotonos, and irregular respiration. Hypertonia becomes less pronounced gradually. The infants then develop any or all of the classic sequelae of kernicterus: choreoathetoid cerebral palsy, gaze abnormalities, especially in upward gaze, sensorineural hearing loss, and cognitive deficits. The clinical presentation of bilirubin encephalopathy in preterm infants may be less distinctive. Abnormal or absent brainstem auditory evoked potentials and magnetic resonance imaging scans demonstrating the characteristic bilateral lesions of the globus pallidus help confirm the clinical diagnosis of kernicterus.

Infants with HDFN are at higher risk for kernicterus than are other infants with the same bilirubin level from other causes.[63] Heme pigments produced during active hemolysis are hypothesized to inhibit bilirubin–albumin binding. Alternatively, many conditions that potentially compromise the blood–brain barrier, such as prematurity, acidosis, hypoxemia, hypothermia, and hypoglycemia, are present in severely affected infants, making them more vulnerable to bilirubin encephalopathy.

OTHER CLINICAL FEATURES

Hepatosplenomegaly is usually present. Marked enlargement is seen in newborn infants with hydrops. Hydropic babies also have generalized edema, and they may have ascites, and pleural and pericardial effusions. Respiratory distress may be present as a result of pulmonary hypoplasia, pleural and/or pericardial effusions, or surfactant deficiency. Purpura associated with thrombocytopenia is sometimes seen in severely affected infants and may be a bad prognostic sign. The placenta is thickened, enlarged, and pale.

Babies who received intrauterine transfusions may still have hepatosplenomegaly and anemia at birth and may develop significant hyperbilirubinemia.[64]

OBSTETRIC HISTORY

The course and outcome of prior pregnancies are of vital importance in the initial evaluation of an alloimmunized pregnancy. The history of early fetal deaths or hydrops is ominous. In Rh alloimmunization, the severity of hemolytic disease of the newborn either remains the same or worsens in subsequent affected pregnancies. Hydrops recurs in 90 percent of affected pregnancies, often at an earlier gestation. Alloimmunized women who report previous neonatal deaths, neonatal exchange transfusions, or intrauterine transfusions should receive closer fetal surveillance.[65] Jaundice as a result of hemolysis often recurs to the same degree of severity in subsequent affected siblings. The history of prior blood transfusions may be obtained in women sensitized to antigens other than D, especially if Kell alloimmunization is detected. Establishment of paternity for each pregnancy is particularly relevant in both Rh and Kell alloimmunization, because the fetus is at risk only if the father is positive for the antigen in question. ABO hemolytic disease of the newborn may affect the first-born ABO-incompatible infant. Although rare, severe ABO hemolytic disease of the newborn may recur in subsequent ABO-incompatible pregnancies.[51]

LABORATORY INVESTIGATIONS

The evaluation and management of HDFN require close collaboration between obstetricians, maternal fetal medicine specialists, radiologists, hematologists, and neonatologists. Figure 54–2 is an algorithm for the clinical management of an alloimmunized pregnancy.

MATERNAL IMMUNOHEMATOLOGIC TESTING

The aims of antenatal serologic testing are to identify Rh-negative women and to detect maternal alloimmunization. The practice guidelines and recommendations for prenatal and perinatal immunohematologic and molecular testing have been established in the United States by the American Association of Blood Banks.[53]

Every obstetrical patient should have samples obtained between 10 and 16 weeks' gestation and tested for ABO and RhD typing and for screening for the presence of red cell alloantibodies. Whether the pregnant

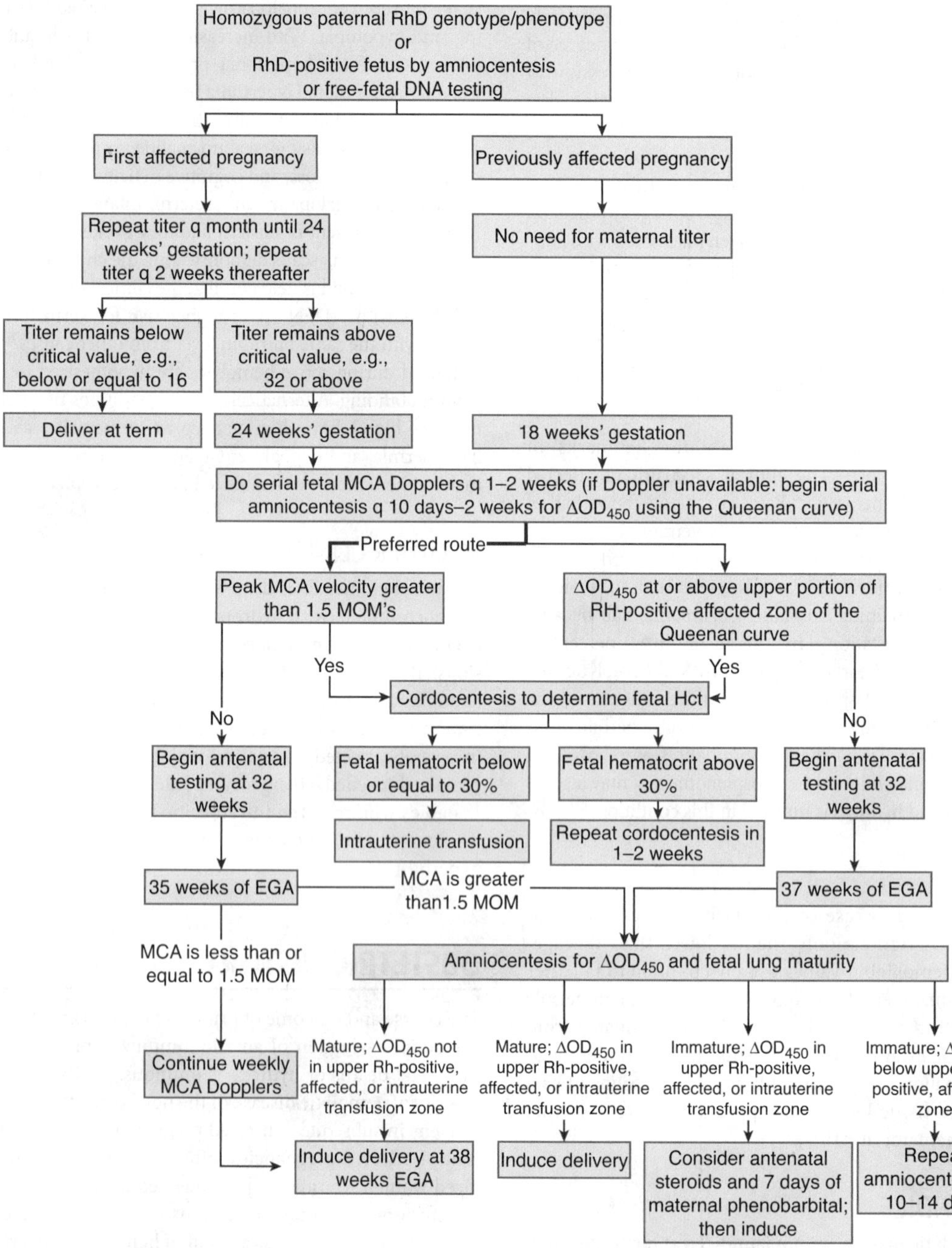

FIGURE 54–2. Algorithm for clinical management of Rh alloimmunized pregnancy. ΔOD, deviation in amniotic fluid optical density; EGA, estimated gestational age; Hct, hematocrit; MCA, middle cerebral artery; MOM, multiples of the median for gestational age; Rh, rhesus. *(Reproduced with permission from Moise KJ.[68])*

woman is D-positive or -negative, a second sample should be obtained at 28 weeks' gestation to confirm the ABO and D, and to further evaluate the pregnant mother for other red cell alloantibodies. D typing discrepancies must always be investigated and resolved, and may require use of different manufacturer's reagents, as the monoclonal reagents may have different reactivities.

Further routine blood grouping or screening in the third trimester or at delivery is unnecessary, as studies document that the incidence of clinically significant antibodies detected for the first time during delivery is low and neonatal complications are nonexistent.[66,67] Third trimester testing should be performed if there is a history of significant antibodies, blood transfusion, or traumatic delivery.

If an unexpected antibody is identified anytime during pregnancy, the specificity, concentration, origin, and likelihood of HDFN must be determined. The indirect antiglobulin test using reagent red cells suspended in low ionic strength solution or polyethylene glycol is recommended; enzyme enhancement techniques provide no added benefit. The reagent cells used for antibody screening should express C, c, D, E, e, K, k, Fy^a, Fy^b, Jk^a, Jk^b, S, s, M, N, Le^a. Screening cells with low-frequency antigens is not required (see Chap. 137).

Blood samples from women with immune anti-D should be tested monthly until 28 weeks' gestation and every 2 weeks thereafter.[68] Antibody titers are reported as the reciprocal of the highest dilution step at which agglutination is observed. A difference of two dilutions is considered a significant change. Testing is performed in parallel with previously frozen samples to minimize the possibility that changes in the titer result from differences in technique or reagent red cell selection.[53] A critical titer is defined as the titer associated with significant risk of fetal anemia or hydrops, and is the threshold at which the fetus will need monitoring. Once the critical titer is reached and a decision is made to monitor the fetus by ultrasonography or amniocentesis, further antibody titration plays no role in assessment of fetal status. Antibody titration is not useful for monitoring pregnancies after the first affected pregnancy.

The critical titer varies from 8 to 32 in different laboratories in the United States.[68] In the United Kingdom and Europe, the level of anti-D is compared to an international standard and reported in IU/mL. Anti-D levels of 4 IU/mL or greater prompt referral to a specialist fetomaternal unit for further monitoring; at levels of 4 to 15 IU/ mL, there is a potential risk of moderate HDFN; levels greater than 15 IU/mL imply a risk of severe HDN.[69] In the Netherlands, the critical titer is defined as 16 or greater.[8]

When RhIg has been administered during pregnancy, a positive antibody titer may be detected (generally 2–4) which does not correlate with either the effectiveness of the RhIg and/or the extent of FMH. Specific laboratory techniques may be used, if required, to distinguish between passive RhIg and active alloimmunization to D. In the actively alloimmunized mother, anti-D can be detected in saline phase and blocked by 2-mercapto ethanol or dithiothreitol (DTT) treatment of the maternal red cells, while RhIg anti-D will not be blocked.

The significance of titer levels for antibodies other than D have not been defined. Maternal anti-Kell titers, in particular, correlate poorly with fetal outcome.[58] In a review of 156 anti–Kell-positive pregnancies over 37 years, McKenna and colleagues found that all severely affected fetuses had a titer of at least 1:32.[56] Bowman and colleagues also noted that a titer of 1:32 or greater was present in 16 of 17 severely affected pregnancies, but 1 patient with a titer of 1:8 had a grossly hydropic fetus at 23 weeks' gestation.[57] In the Netherlands, anti-Kell titers as low as 1:2 prompt referral to a perinatal center.[55] Some authors recommend further testing of the fetus if a critical titer of 1:8 is attained and paternal red cell typing is K+.[7] In a case series of women with anti-c isoimmunization, a titer of 1:32 or greater was invariably associated with severe fetal or neonatal disease.[67]

The imperfect predictive value of serologic tests has led to the development of functional cellular assays that measure the ability of maternal antibodies to cause red cell destruction, thus providing better noninvasive differentiation of pregnancies at increased risk of fetal anemia. In these assays, red blood cells sensitized with maternal antibodies are incubated with effector cells carrying Fcγreceptors, such as lymphocytes or monocytes, to measure cellular interaction, such as binding, phagocytosis, or cytotoxic lysis.[29] Many authors have reported on the superiority of the monocyte monolayer assay, the chemiluminescence test, and the antibody-dependent cell-mediated cytotoxicity assay, compared to serologic tests, in predicting severity of hemolytic disease in the fetus and newborn. However, these tests are complex, difficult to standardize, and have not gained wide acceptance in the United States.

DETERMINATION OF PATERNAL ZYGOSITY AND FETAL BLOOD TYPE

When a clinically significant alloantibody is identified, or if there is a history of a previous fetus or neonate affected by HDFN, the next step is to determine if the fetus is at risk because he/she carries the corresponding antigen. If the father is homozygous for the corresponding antigen the fetus is at definite risk for HDFN. The child of an antigen negative mother and a heterozygous antigen positive father has a 50 percent chance of being antigen negative and thus being unaffected by prior maternal alloimmunization. When the father is heterozygous or paternal zygosity is unknown, determination of fetal blood type early in pregnancy allows early institution of monitoring and therapy in antigen positive fetuses who are at risk and forestalling invasive and potentially risky procedures in antigen negative fetuses.

Paternal zygosity is determined using serology for all common blood group antigens implicated in HDFN except for D. The probable RhD zygosity in RhD-positive persons may be inferred, but not definitively, from serologic phenotyping studies, based on gene frequencies in certain populations, and the fact that the C/c and E/e antigens are closely linked to the RhD locus.[13,52] Elucidation of the genetic structure of the prevalent RhD locus and the deletion responsible for RhD-negative phenotypes in whites has led to the development of more direct and robust methods of determination of RhD zygosity by polymerase chain reaction (PCR) tests.[16] Using PCR to amplify the 9-kb sequence of D outside of the flanking Rhesus box improves the reliability of assigning zygosity.[71]

If paternal heterozygosity is suspected or confirmed, determination of fetal blood type is helpful in planning further management. There are several sources of fetal tissue for fetal blood group genotyping. These include blood obtained by cordocentesis, chorionic villus sampling and cervical tissue obtained by transvaginal lavage; each has risks to the fetus and issues related to quality of sample. Cordocentesis, amniocentesis, and chorionic villus sampling for fetal genetic typing carry a significant risk of fetomaternal hemorrhage with increased risk of augmenting maternal sensitization and of fetal loss.[22,23] The advent of noninvasive methods of prenatal diagnosis using fetal DNA extracted from maternal plasma as early as the first trimester of pregnancy has obviated those concerns and has dramatically improved the ability to perform molecular testing on fetal tissue.[72]

Fetal DNA in maternal plasma can be identified as early as 5 weeks' gestation and is derived from apoptotic syncytiotrophoblasts; fetal DNA disappears within hours of parturition. Fetal DNA used for typing is extracted using real-time quantitative polymerase chain reaction (RT-PCR) using methods which distinguish fetal from maternal DNA. Most protocols amplify two or three exons or more which include *RHD* exons 4 to 7 and 10 to avoid false positives when the fetus has *RHD*ψ.[73] Confirmation of detection of nonmaternal markers is required and can be accomplished by testing for the presence of the Y chromosome in male fetuses and/or housekeeping genes such as hemoglobin β chain, β actin, albumin, or chemokine receptor 5. A recent meta-analysis reviewed 37 publications describing 44 protocols reporting noninvasive Rh genotyping using fetal DNA obtained from more than 3000 maternal blood samples; an accuracy rate of 94.8 percent was reported.[74] Very high accuracy rates (>96%) have been reported for noninvasive fetal RhCE genotyping from maternal blood.[75] Several commercial companies are in process of developing diagnostic fetal DNA testing kits that will improve testing and accuracy. K antigen typing presents its own challenges and some success has been obtained in fetal K detection using matrix-assisted laser desorption/ionization time-of-flight mass spectrometry-based single-allele-based extension reaction.[76]

AMNIOTIC FLUID SPECTROPHOTOMETRY

In 1961, the spectrophotometric analysis of amniotic fluid for bilirubin, an indirect indicator of the degree of fetal hemolysis, was shown to be useful in predicting the severity of fetal anemia.[77] Elevations of optical density at 450 nm (ΔOD_{450}) reflect the concentration of amniotic fluid bilirubin, which is derived from the fetus.[34,35] The change in optical density is quantified by measuring the elevation of the optical density at 450 nm above a line connecting the optical density values obtained at 375 and 550 nm and then plotting it against gestational age. The original Liley chart, from 27 weeks to term, defined three zones: readings in zone 3, the upper zone, indicate severe fetal disease with hydrops or impending fetal death; readings in zone 1, the lowest zone, indicate mild or no hemolytic disease with a 10 percent risk of needing a postnatal exchange transfusion; and readings in zone 2 indicate moderate disease.[77] The Liley chart was later modified by Queenan to include data from 14 to 40 weeks gestation and had 4 zones, with the lowest zone representing unaffected fetuses and the highest zone associated with increased risk of intrauterine death (Fig. 54–3).[78] The Queenan chart has been found to be slightly more accurate than the Liley chart.[79] However, amniocentesis for the measurement of amniotic fluid ΔOD_{450} carries the risks of membrane rupture, infection, worsening of sensitization and fetal loss. It is also unreliable for detection of fetal anemia caused by Kell antibodies, because Kell HDFN is largely a result of suppression of fetal erythropoiesis rather than hemolysis. For these reasons, amniotic fluid spectrophotometry is being replaced by noninvasive, middle cerebral artery Doppler ultrasound monitoring for fetal anemia.[68,80]

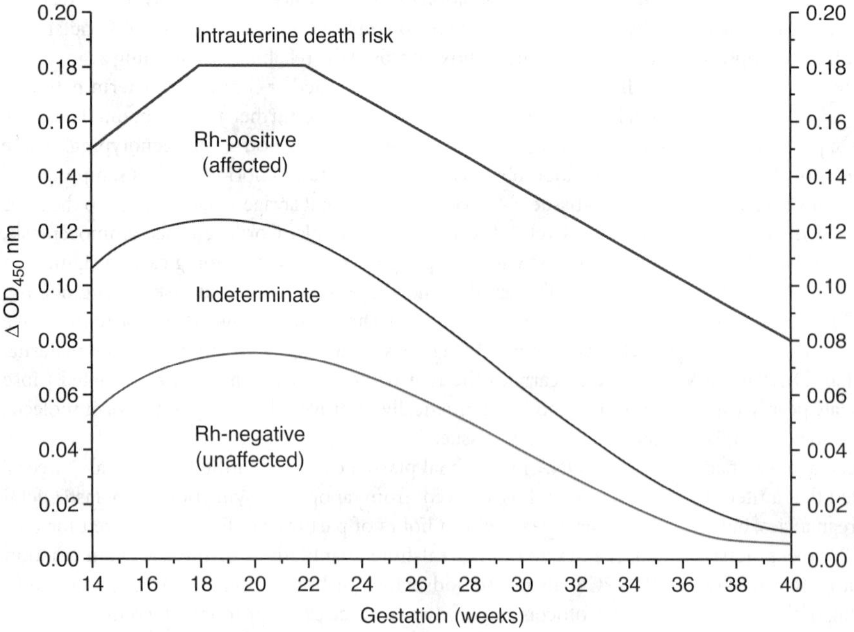

FIGURE 54–3. Queenan curve for ΔOD_{450} values from 14 to 40 weeks' gestation. *(Reproduced with permission from Queenan JT, Tomai TP, Ural SH, King JC.[78])*

ULTRASONOGRAPHY

Ultrasonography is noninvasive, can be performed serially, and can be combined with other diagnostic studies to assess the fetal condition, estimate the need for further aggressive management, and obtain a biophysical profile of the fetus to determine fetal well-being. As hydrops develops in the anemic fetus, a consistent pattern may be noted on ultrasonography. Polyhydramnios appears first, followed by placental enlargement, hepatomegaly, pericardial effusion, ascites, scalp edema, and pleural effusions in succession. Nevertheless, in the absence of overt hydrops, ultrasonographic parameters, such as intrahepatic and extrahepatic vein diameters, abdominal and head circumference, head-to-abdominal-circumference ratio, intraperitoneal volume, splenic size, and liver length have not been reliable in distinguishing mild from severe fetal anemia.[81] In the anemic fetus, decreased viscosity of the blood and increased cardiovascular output lead to a hyperdynamic circulation. Cerebral blood flow increases further in response to hypoxemia, resulting in increased blood flow velocity. Values greater than 1.5 multiples of the median for gestational age correlate highly with moderate or severe fetal anemia (Fig. 54–4).[80] Doppler measurement of peak velocity of systolic blood flow in the middle cerebral artery has been found to be more sensitive and accurate for detecting severe fetal anemia than measurement of amniotic fluid ΔOD_{450}.[79] Measurements may be initiated as early as 18 weeks of gestation and repeated at 1- to 2-week intervals until 35 weeks gestation. After 38 weeks, a higher false-positive rate in the detection of fetal anemia necessitates amniocentesis for ΔOD_{450} and fetal lung maturity testing if elevated levels are noted.[68]

FETAL BLOOD SAMPLING

Fetal blood sampling (also called *percutaneous umbilical blood sampling* or *cordocentesis*) allows direct measurement of blood indices to specifically evaluate the degree of severity of fetal hemolytic disease as early as 17 to 18 weeks' gestation.[82] Indications for fetal blood sampling in alloimmunized pregnancies include fetal blood typing, confirmation of severe fetal anemia suspected based on amniocentesis with ΔOD_{450} measurements in Liley zone 3 or in the "intrauterine death zone" in the Queenan graph, elevated peak middle cerebral artery Doppler velocities, or ultrasonographic evidence of early or frank hydrops.[68,78,81] The procedure is performed under local anesthesia. A 20- to 22-gauge spinal needle is inserted into the umbilical vein at the level of cord insertion into the placenta, under ultrasonographic guidance (Fig. 54–5). Specimens of fetal blood are obtained for direct measurement of complete blood count, reticulocyte count, red cell antigen phenotyping, direct antiglobulin test (DAT), bilirubin, blood gases, and lactate to assess acid–base status. Blood should be available for immediate intrauterine transfusion when the procedure is being performed for suspected severe fetal anemia. Complications of fetal blood sampling include fetal loss, with procedure-related rates ranging from 0 to 4.9 percent, umbilical cord bleeding, chorioamnionitis, and significant risk of fetomaternal hemorrhage with anamnestic maternal sensitization.[83,84]

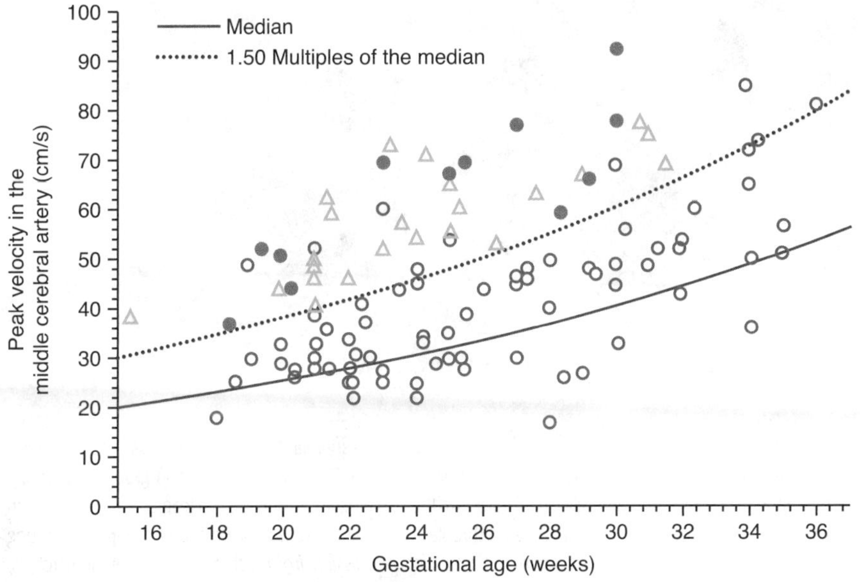

FIGURE 54–4. Peak velocity of systolic blood flow in the middle cerebral artery in 111 fetuses at risk for anemia as a result of maternal alloimmunization. *Open circles*, fetuses with either mild or no anemia; *solid circles*, fetuses with hydrops; *triangles*, fetuses with moderate or severe anemia. *(Reproduced with permission from Mari G, Deter RL, Carpenter RL, et al.[81])*

LABORATORY TESTS IN THE NEONATE

A sample of cord blood should be collected from all newborns at the time of delivery. However, specific testing of cord blood samples is performed only if the mother is Rh negative, if the maternal serum contains red cell alloantibodies of potential clinical significance, or if the neonate develops signs of hemolytic disease. Tests should include ABO and Rh typing and a DAT. Many birth hospitals routinely test cord blood for the infant's blood type and DAT if the mother is O Rh-positive in order to detect ABO alloimmunization before the infant is discharged home.

In severe Rh alloimmunization, high titers of maternal antibody may block Rh-antigenic sites on the neonatal red cells, leading to false-negative Rh typing. Antepartum RhIg given to the mother may cause a weakly positive DAT result in the infant at birth. Contamination of the cord blood sample with Wharton jelly during collection can also result in a false-positive DAT result. Although the DAT usually is positive in all forms of alloimmune HDFN, the test cannot predict reliably the degree of clinical severity.[85,86] This is especially true for cases resulting from ABO sensitization. When fetomaternal ABO incompatibility is present, the presence of maternally derived IgG anti-A or anti-B in the infant's serum may be demonstrated by the indirect antiglobulin test to support the diagnosis of ABO hemolytic disease. On the other hand, it is important to bear in mind that hemolysis in ABO-incompatible, DAT-negative infants may result from hematologic causes other than alloimmunization or from red cell membrane defects (see Chap. 45).[87] Elution of maternal antibody from the infant's red cells, followed by tests to determine the specificity of the antibody in the eluate, may be useful, particularly when several antibodies are present in the maternal serum or when the maternal antibody screen is negative.[53]

Measurement of end-tidal carbon monoxide, corrected for ambient carbon monoxide levels, provides a direct measurement of heme catabolism to confirm a hemolytic process, but this test is not widely available.[88]

Cord blood hemoglobin and indirect bilirubin determinations more closely reflect disease severity. Most infants with cord hemoglobin levels within the age-adjusted normal range do not require exchange transfusion. Usually, a cord hemoglobin level less than 11 g/dL in a term newborn and/or a cord-indirect bilirubin level greater than 4.5 to 5 mg/dL indicates severe hemolysis and often warrants early exchange transfusion. Early exchange transfusion also may be indicated if the rate of rise of bilirubin, measured every 4 to 6 hours, exceeds 0.5 mg/dL per hour. The reticulocyte count usually is greater than 6 percent and may approach 30 to 40 percent in severe Rh disease. The blood film in Rh disease is characterized by increased nucleated red blood cell counts, polychromasia, and anisocytosis. Severely affected infants have thrombocytopenia with platelet counts less than 30,000/mL. Microspherocytosis is seen primarily in ABO hemolytic disease (Fig. 54–6). Low reticulocyte counts disproportionate to the low hematocrit may be noted in Kell hemolytic disease of the newborn. Severely affected infants may have hypoglycemia, secondary to hyperinsulinemia. Arterial blood gas analysis may reveal metabolic acidosis and/or respiratory decompensation. Hypoalbuminemia is often present.

Infants who received intrauterine transfusions may have mild or moderate anemia with little reticulocytosis. Because most of their circulating red cells are transfused antigen-negative cells, the DAT result may be negative, but the indirect antiglobulin test result will be strongly positive.

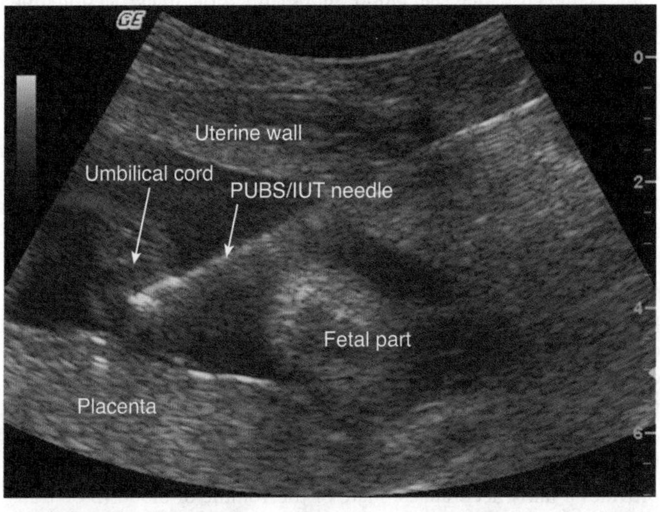

FIGURE 54–5. Ultrasound-guided fetal blood sampling and intravascular transfusion. *(Courtesy of Kerry Lewis, MD, Division of Maternal-Fetal Medicine, Howard University Hospital, Washington, DC.)*

DIFFERENTIAL DIAGNOSIS

Hydrops fetalis may be secondary to cardiac anomalies or arrhythmias, fetal genetic or metabolic disorders including α-thalassemia (see Chap. 47), intrauterine infections such as syphilis or toxoplasmosis, or any of a multitude of causes that lead to severe derangements in fetal homeostasis. These disorders are classified as nonimmune hydrops and are differentiated from anasarca secondary to HDFN by the absence of any clinically significant red cell alloantibodies in the mother's blood. Parvovirus B19 infection of the mother at any time during gestation can cause nonimmune hydrops, profound fetal anemia, and death.

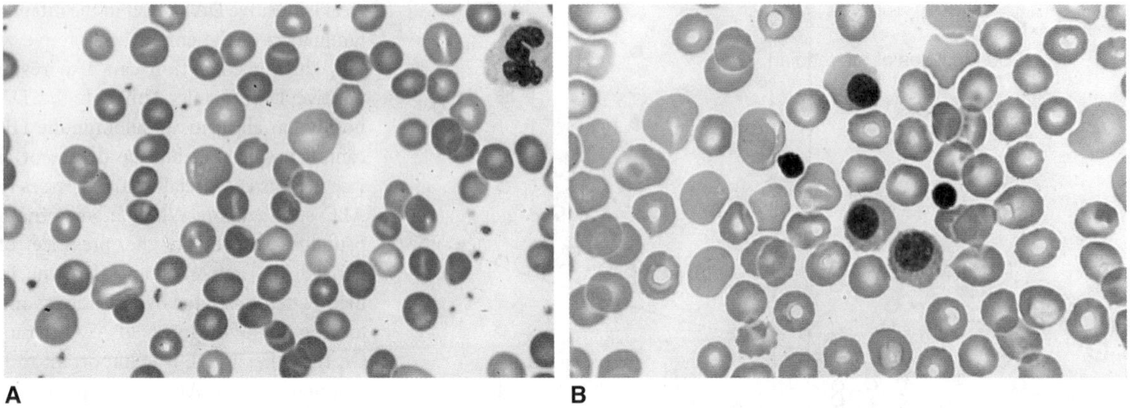

FIGURE 54–6. Alloimmune hemolytic disease of the newborn. Blood films. **A.** Infant with ABO blood group alloimmune hemolytic anemia. Note the high prevalence of spherocytes and the large polychromatophilic cells, indicative of reticulocytosis, both findings reflecting the alloimmune hemolytic anemia. **B.** Infant with Rh blood group alloimmune hemolytic anemia. Note spherocytes (many appear as stomatocytes); the many large polychromatophilic cells, reflecting the reticulocytosis; and the nucleated red cells (three in this field). Two bare red cell nuclei are present from erythroblast nuclear ejection in the blood. The intense erythroblastosis is characteristic of Rh blood group alloimmune hemolytic anemia and is less frequent and less prominent in ABO blood group alloimmune hemolytic anemia. *(Used with permission from* Lichtman's Atlas of Hematology, *www.accessmedicine.com.)*

Neonatal anemia caused by intrinsic red cell defects such as hereditary spherocytosis (see Chap. 45), red cell enzyme deficiencies (see Chap. 46), and specific hemoglobinopathies (see Chap. 48) can give a similar clinical picture to hemolytic disease of the newborn.[89] The absence of maternal red cell alloantibodies, a negative DAT result, and detection of the specific defect determining the disorder clarify the diagnosis.

Disorders of bilirubin metabolism usually are not associated with anemia. Hepatitis or obstructive biliary diseases present with direct hyperbilirubinemia, most often after the first week of life.

THERAPY

■ INTRAUTERINE FETAL TRANSFUSION

Intrauterine transfusions correct fetal anemia and reduce the risk of congestive heart failure and hydrops fetalis. Fetal bilirubin is cleared very efficiently by the placenta and the mother, so bilirubin removal is not necessary until after birth. Percutaneous intraperitoneal fetal transfusion pioneered by Liley in the 1960s[5] has been largely replaced by ultrasound-guided direct intravascular transfusion into the umbilical vein, either in the intrahepatic portion or into the umbilical cord at the insertion site in the placenta (see Fig. 54–4).[82,90] The intravascular technique offers precise diagnostic evaluation of the fetal status (see "Fetal Blood Sampling" above) and is effective, even in hydropic fetuses, by circumventing the problem of erratic and often poor absorption of red blood cells from the peritoneal cavity in such fetuses. Intraperitoneal transfusions may be necessary when intravascular access is difficult, as in early pregnancy when the umbilical vessels are narrow or later when increased fetal size prevents access to the umbilical cord.[91,92] The relative merits of direct simple intravascular transfusion versus intravascular exchange transfusion have been debated, but the shorter procedure time associated with direct simple intrauterine intravascular transfusion has made it the procedure of choice at most centers.[90] The first fetal blood sampling with transfusion ideally is performed when the fetus is anemic but before hydrops develops. Transfusions are given at fetal hematocrit levels of 25 to 30 percent or less, or if the fetal hemoglobin is 4 to 6 standard deviations below the mean for gestational age. Generally, the hematocrit drops by 1 to 2 percent per day in the transfused hydropic fetus. The fall in hematocrit is rapid in fetuses with severe hemolytic disease, often necessitating a second transfusion within 7 to 14 days. The interval between subsequent transfusions usually is 21 to 28 days. The nonhydropic fetus can tolerate rapid blood infusions of 5 to 7 mL/min because of the capacitance of the placenta. The hydropic fetus requires slower transfusion rates and can tolerate only smaller, more frequent transfusions. Very low pretransfusion fetal hematocrit levels, rapid large increases in posttransfusion hematocrit level, and increases in umbilical venous pressure during intrauterine transfusions are associated with fetal death after transfusion.[93,94]

Red cells for intrauterine transfusions should be fresh, O-negative red blood cells that are antigen-negative for any other identified antibody, cytomegalovirus seronegative or leukocyte depleted, irradiated, and cross-matched against the mother's blood.[95,96] Fetuses are at risk for both posttransfusion cytomegalovirus and graft-versus-host disease. Red cell units 7 days old or less are preferred. Many centers also use blood that is negative for sickle hemoglobin to prevent sickling in the fetus at low oxygen tension. A rare donor registry may be needed in cases of unusual or combination antibodies. In this circumstance, frozen, deglycerolized red blood cells may be the only available product. Some centers use maternal blood, supporting serial maternal donations with iron and folate therapy.[97] Rigorous testing for infectious markers must be performed and red cells should be washed free of maternal serum. Maternal red blood cells have the potential advantage of decreasing the risk of sensitization to new red cell antigens associated with exposure to donor units[98] and are postulated to last longer than random donor red cells because of the reticulocytosis produced by repeated donations, but a significant difference has not been shown between maternal red cell and donor red cell transfusions.[98,99]

Blood is transfused to increase the fetal hematocrit to between 40 and 45 percent. The blood is often washed free of additive solutions, and packed to a hematocrit of 70 to 85 percent in a volume calculation based on estimated fetal placental blood volume, fetal hematocrit, and hematocrit of donor blood. Various nomograms and formulas for the calculation of donor blood volume have been published.[100,101] If the hematocrit of the donor unit is approximately 75 percent, multiplying the estimated fetal weight in grams (estimated by ultrasonography) by a factor of 0.02 provides a fairly accurate estimate of the volume of blood to be transfused to achieve a fetal hematocrit increment of 10 percent.[102]

Complications of intrauterine transfusion (IUT) are rare in centers with experience. Van Kamp and colleagues estimated procedure-related complication rates of 2.9 percent in the absence of hydrops and 3.9 percent in the presence of hydrops in a cohort study of 254 fetuses treated with 740 IUTs in a single center.[103] The most common problem was transient fetal heart rate abnormalities, which occurred in 8 percent of procedures. The procedure-related pregnancy loss rate was calculated to be 1.6 percent per procedure. Fetal distress during or after the procedure may compel emergency cesarean section. Cord accidents such as hemorrhage from the puncture site or rupture of the cord are rare.

DELIVERY

The decision regarding the appropriate time to deliver the baby is based on gestational age, fetal weight and lung maturity, fetal response to the intrauterine transfusions, ease of performing the transfusions, and antenatal ultrasonography and Doppler studies for fetal anemia. Transfusions usually are provided up to 35 weeks so as to prolong gestation safely until the risks of preterm birth and its attendant complications are minimized.[68] Amniocentesis may be repeated late in gestation, at approximately 37 weeks, to study ΔOD_{450} values and assess fetal lung maturity prior to delivery.

IMMUNOMODULATION

In women with severe alloimmunization and with fetal losses or hydrops very early in pregnancy, a variety of methods have been used to suppress the antibody response and prolong survival of the fetus until intrauterine transfusions become technically feasible. Attempts to induce immunologic tolerance in the mother by the administration of oral D+ RBC stroma were found to be ineffective. Administrations of intravenous IgG (IVIg), serial plasmapheresis, or plasmapheresis combined with IVIg have been successful in some cases.[92,104,105] IVIg may cause nonspecific Fc blockade of the fetal reticuloendothelial system. Another interesting development is the design of recombinant mutant D specific antibodies which lack destructive activity towards red cells, but, following administration to the mother, have the potential to cross the placenta and block the binding of hemolytic maternal anti-D to fetal red cells.[106] In addition, the observation that alloimmunized women with offspring who exhibit mild hemolytic disease have significantly higher incidence of anti-HLA A, anti-B, anti-C, and anti-DR antibodies than mothers of children with severe hemolytic disease has given rise to the hypothesis that severe hemolytic disease can be prevented in women lacking anti-HLA antibodies by injecting them with the father's leukocytes before or at the beginning of a new pregnancy to provoke anti-HLA antibody production, thus providing another avenue of immunomodulation.[32,33,107]

TREATMENT OF THE AFFECTED NEONATE

Results of antenatal monitoring and obstetric interventions during pregnancy and the history of the outcome of previous pregnancies allow the neonatal team to anticipate the needs of the infant born with hemolytic disease. In infants with severe hemolytic disease without the benefit of intrauterine transfusions, severe anemia and hydrops are the immediate life-threatening concerns and often are accompanied by perinatal asphyxia, surfactant deficiency, hypoglycemia, acidosis, and thrombocytopenia. The next imperative is preventing bilirubin encephalopathy resulting from severe unconjugated hyperbilirubinemia. Exchange transfusions and phototherapy are the mainstays of treatment.

Resuscitation and stabilization of hydropic infants is challenging. Endotracheal intubation and positive-pressure ventilation with oxygen is usually necessary. Drainage of pleural effusions and ascites may be required to facilitate gas exchange. Metabolic acidosis and hypoglycemia require correction. A partial exchange transfusion may be performed using packed red cells to improve hemoglobin levels and oxygenation. A double-volume exchange transfusion is considered only after the initial stabilization.

In a study of 191 infants born alive after intrauterine transfusions between 1988 and 1999, the hematocrit at birth ranged from 13 to 51 percent.[108] Endotracheal ventilation was required more often in babies who had been severely hydropic *in utero*, but the requirements for exchange transfusion or simple transfusion did not differ between babies who had been hydropic *in utero* and those without evidence of hydrops. Although some centers report no difference in the frequency of exchange transfusions in babies who have had IUTs compared with babies who have not had IUTs,[108,109] other centers report that infants who received multiple intrauterine transfusions are usually born closer to term and often require less phototherapy and fewer exchange transfusions in the neonatal period.[64,110] Nonetheless, many infants with severe HDFN require additional packed red cell transfusions for severe and prolonged hyporegenerative anemia secondary to suppression of fetal erythropoiesis.[41,42,109] Approximately three-quarters of term and near-term infants who had received IUT for Rh HDFN required transfusion within 6 months of age, compared with 26 percent of infants with Rh HDFN who had not received an IUT.[109]

Exchange Transfusion

Exchange transfusion corrects anemia, removes bilirubin and free maternal antibody in the plasma, and replaces the infant's blood with antigen-negative red blood cells that should have normal *in vivo* survival. A double-blood-volume exchange (calculated as 2×80 mL/kg in a term infant or 2×100 mL/kg in a preterm infant) replaces approximately 85 percent of the infant's blood volume with antigen-negative red blood cells. A single-blood-volume exchange transfusion replaces only 65 percent of the infant's blood volume. A double-blood-volume exchange should eliminate more than 50 percent of the intravascular bilirubin. However, the amount of bilirubin reduction often is less, reflecting the equilibrating tissue-bound pool. Infusion of albumin prior to the exchange transfusion may help bilirubin binding, thus increasing the amount of bilirubin removed. Equilibration of extravascular and intravascular bilirubin and continued breakdown of red cells by persisting maternal antibodies result in a rebound of bilirubin following initial exchange transfusion, sometimes requiring repeated exchange transfusions in severe hemolytic disease.

The indications for early exchange transfusions performed within 9 to 12 hours of birth are debated but have remained essentially unchanged over the last 40 years, with minor modifications. Cord hemoglobin levels 110 g/L or less, cord bilirubin levels 5.5 mg/dL or greater, and rapidly rising bilirubin levels 0.5 mg/dL per hour or greater despite phototherapy are commonly used criteria for early exchange transfusions. Early exchange transfusion has the advantage of replacing sensitized red cells with normal cells, thereby removing not only bilirubin but also the source of future bilirubin. Because bilirubin is distributed in the extracellular fluids, efficiency is enhanced by removing sensitized cells early in the process.

"Late" exchange transfusions are performed when serum bilirubin levels threaten to exceed approximately 20 to 22 mg/dL in term infants. The American Academy of Pediatrics Subcommittee on Hyperbilirubinemia provided revised guidelines for exchange transfusion in infants 35 or more weeks' gestation.[111] In view of the fact that bilirubin levels rise steadily from birth and peak at approximately 72 to 96 hours of age, exchange transfusion should be considered if serum bilirubin levels reach 15 mg/dL in an infant of 35 weeks' gestation or 17 mg/dL in an infant of 38 weeks' gestation despite intensive phototherapy. Immediate exchange transfusion is recommended in infants showing signs of acute bilirubin encephalopathy, even if bilirubin levels are falling.[111]

Conjugated or direct bilirubin values are not subtracted from total bilirubin levels when considering levels for exchange transfusions. Exchange transfusions are performed at lower bilirubin levels in premature infants, particularly those with hypoxemia, acidosis, and hypothermia, but little data are available to guide intervention in these infants. In infants with birth weights of at least 1500 g, exchange transfusions usually are performed at bilirubin levels of 13 to 16 mg/dL but may be considered even at levels as low as 8 to 9 mg/dL in sick babies of 24 weeks' gestation.[112] The bilirubin-to-albumin ratio (total serum bilirubin mg/dL to albumin g/dL), considered to be a surrogate measure of free bilirubin, may provide additional data in determining the need for exchange transfusion in both term and preterm neonates.[111,113]

Blood chosen for the exchange transfusion should be ABO and Rh compatible, (Rh-negative in Rh HDN), negative for the antigen(s) responsible for the hemolytic disease, and cross-matched against the mother's blood. Plasma-reduced whole blood (if available) or packed red cells reconstituted with plasma, with a packed cell volume adjusted to 0.5 to 0.6 is suitable for correction of anemia and hyperbilirubinemia. Blood may be anticoagulated with citrate phosphate dextrose; heparin has been used in some countries. Additive anticoagulant solutions are usually avoided. If only red blood cells stored in additive solutions are available, the additive solution can be removed by washing or by centrifugation and removal of the supernatant solution, prior to reconstitution of the red cells with plasma. The blood should be as fresh as possible (<7 days) to maximize the *in vivo* survival of the transfused red cells, irradiated and leukocyte depleted.[95]

Exchange transfusions can be performed by the traditional push–pull method with a single vascular access, usually the umbilical vein, or by isovolumetric techniques utilizing two access sites (umbilical artery and vein or peripheral artery and vein) for simultaneous removal of the infant's blood and administration of new blood (Fig. 54–7).[114] Aliquots of 5 to 20 mL, with a maximum of 5 mL/kg, are withdrawn or infused in the discontinuous method at a rate not exceeding 5 mL/kg every 3 minutes to prevent rapid fluctuations in arterial pressure, which are accompanied by changes in intracranial pressure. During an isovolumetric exchange, volumes to be removed or reinfused should not exceed 2 mL/kg per minute. The exchange usually lasts 1 to 2 hours.

Potential complications of exchange transfusion include hypocalcemia, hyperglycemia, hypoglycemia, thrombocytopenia, dilutional coagulopathy, neutropenia, disseminated intravascular coagulation, umbilical venous and/or arterial thrombosis, necrotizing enterocolitis, and infection (see Chap. 140). Thrombocytopenia and hypocalcemia are reported to be the most common complications (incidence ranging from 29–47%).[115,116] The risk of death or permanent serious sequelae has been reported to be as high as 12 percent in sick infants, compared with less than 1 percent in healthy infants, in a retrospective review of exchange transfusions performed in two neonatal intensive care units between 1981 and 1995.[117] Another center reported no increase in the number of complications and no exchange transfusion–related deaths over a 21-year period, even though there was a decline in the frequency of exchange transfusions performed over the years.[116] Careful clinical judgment is required to balance the potential risk of adverse events from exchange transfusion with the risk of bilirubin encephalopathy in neonates who are premature, sick, or both.

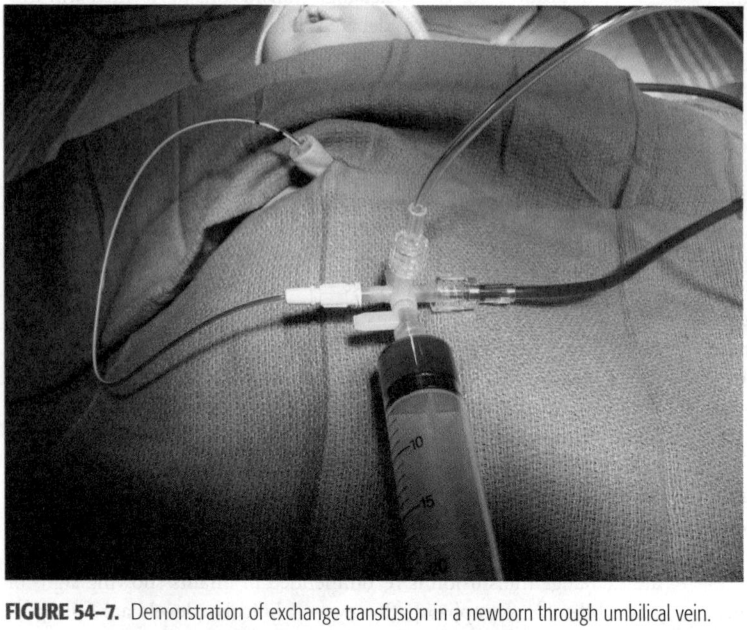

FIGURE 54–7. Demonstration of exchange transfusion in a newborn through umbilical vein.

Phototherapy

Phototherapy is the mainstay of treatment for unconjugated hyperbilirubinemia; the objective of treatment is preventing bilirubin neurotoxicity. Exposure of bilirubin to light results in structural and configurational isomerization of bilirubin to less toxic and less lipophilic products that are excreted efficiently without hepatic conjugation. The effectiveness of phototherapy is influenced by the wavelength and irradiance of light, the surface area of exposed skin, and the duration of exposure. Intensive phototherapy involves the use of high levels of irradiance ($\geq$30 μW/cm^2) in the 430- to 490-nm band, delivered to as much of the infant's surface area as possible. Intensive phototherapy effectively reduces bilirubin levels and decreases the need for exchange transfusions for hyperbilirubinemia in ABO and Rh hemolytic disease of the newborn.[118,119] Earlier protocols called for early institution of phototherapy in all infants with hemolytic disease, resulting in the unnecessary, albeit usually benign, treatment of large numbers of infants with mild hemolytic disease whose bilirubin levels would not have risen to nonphysiologic levels even without treatment. Nonetheless, early and intensive phototherapy should be initiated in infants with moderate or severe hemolysis or in infants with rapidly rising bilirubin levels (>0.5 mg/dL per hour). In full-term infants (at least 38 weeks' gestation) with HDFN, intensive phototherapy should be initiated if total bilirubin levels are 5 mg/dL or greater at birth, 10 mg/dL at 24 hours after birth, or approximately 13 to 15 mg/ dL at 48 to 72 hours after birth.[111] Phototherapy is recommended at lower levels for preterm or sick infants. Therapy often is initiated at bilirubin levels less than 5 mg/dL in preterm infants with HDFN so as to avoid potentially risky exchange transfusions.[111,112]

Other Treatments

Intravenous Immunoglobulin Administration of high-dose intravenous immunoglobulin, as soon as possible after the diagnosis of HDFN is made, decreases the need for phototherapy and exchange transfusions.[120,121] The decreased bilirubin levels in infants treated with intravenous immunoglobulin is attributed to reduction in hemolysis secondary to blockade of mononuclear phagocyte Fc receptors. Administration of 0.5 to 1 g/kg over 2 hours is recommended if total serum bilirubin levels continue to rise despite intensive phototherapy or the total serum bilirubin level is within 2 to 3 mg/dL of the exchange transfusion level. The dose can be repeated in 12 hours if necessary.[111]

Metalloporphyrins Synthetic heme analogues suppress bilirubin production by competitively inhibiting the activity of heme oxygenase, the rate-limiting enzyme in the catabolism of heme to biliverdin. Sn-protoporphyrin, a potent heme oxygenase inhibitor, blunts the postnatal rise and peak bilirubin levels in term newborns with ABO hemolytic disease.[122] In a meta-analysis of randomized controlled trials of metalloporphyrins for treatment of unconjugated jaundice in term and preterm infants, metalloporphyrin-treated infants appeared to have short-term benefits compared to controls, including lower maximum bilirubin levels in one study, lower frequency of severe hyperbilirubinemia in one study, decreased need for phototherapy, and a shorter duration of hospitalization. However, there are insufficient data to support or refute the possibility that treatment with a metalloporphyrin decreases the risk of neonatal kernicterus or long-term neurodevelopmental impairment as a result of bilirubin encephalopathy.[123] In addition, metalloporphyrins are photochemically active, and a transient erythematous rash in some tin mesoporphyrin-treated infants who received phototherapy has been reported. Further documentation of safety and effectiveness of heme analogues is required, particularly because the alternative option of phototherapy for treatment of jaundice is widely accepted and usually safe.

Recombinant Human Erythropoietin Recombinant human erythropoietin decreases the need for postnatal transfusions in infants with late hyporegenerative anemia of Rh hemolytic disease and in neonates with Kell hemolytic disease.[41,124,125] In 103 patients with Rh hemolytic disease, administration of 200 U/kg of recombinant erythropoietin subcutaneously, three times per week for 6 weeks, reportedly reduced the number of erythrocyte transfusions to a mean of 1.5, and 55 percent of patients did not require any transfusions.[126]

OUTCOME

Perinatal survival rates greater than 90 percent have been achieved with intrauterine transfusions in nonhydropic fetuses with severe HDFN.[103,108] The overall survival rate for hydropic fetuses is lower (78–89%) despite intrauterine transfusions.[108,110] An 11-year study from 1988 to 1999 examined 80 fetuses with immune hydrops. The survival rate for fetuses with mild hydrops was 98 percent, with intrauterine reversal of hydrops in 88 percent of the fetuses. The outcome in severe fetal hydrops was poor, with reversal of hydrops in 39 percent of cases. The survival rate for fetuses with persistent hydrops was only 26 percent.[108] This study underscores the importance of early diagnosis and treatment of fetal anemia, before hydrops develops. Implementation of a nationwide first trimester screening program for red cell antibodies in the Netherlands in 1998 was associated with increased referrals for suspected fetal anemia, more timely referrals and an increase in perinatal survival in Kell HDFN from 61 percent to 100 percent.[55]

The neurodevelopmental outcome for infants saved by intrauterine transfusion has generally been excellent, with almost 90 percent of survivors being free of disability, even when they have been profoundly anemic *in utero*.[64,110] Cerebral palsy and hearing disabilities have been noted in survivors.[110,127]

It is estimated that kernicterus, secondary to bilirubin encephalopathy, is associated with at least 10 percent mortality and at least 70 percent long-term morbidity.[128] Although the preponderance of kernicterus cases occurred in infants with bilirubin levels higher than 20 mg/dL, it has been shown that when treated promptly with phototherapy or exchange transfusion, peak bilirubin levels in the range of 25 and 29.9 mg/dL were not associated with adverse neurodevelopmental outcomes in term or near-term infants.[128,129] However, there was an adverse association with IQ among infants with a positive DAT and a total serum bilirubin level of 25 mg/dL or more, supporting the American Academy of Pediatrics recommendations to initiate treatment at lower levels for jaundiced infants if they have a positive DAT.[63,111,129] The association of elevated bilirubin levels with lower IQ scores is surprising, because the neuropathology of bilirubin toxicity involves neuronal injury in the basal ganglia and brainstem auditory and oculomotor nuclei, with resultant choreoathetoid cerebral palsy and hearing loss.[62] Preterm infants may be more vulnerable to brain injury from elevated bilirubin levels.[130]

PREVENTION

TRANSFUSION GUIDELINES

Transfusion of blood phenotypically matched for D, other Rh, and for Kell antigens has been advocated for premenopausal women to prevent alloimmunization.[7,8] Despite Rh and K-matching, 25 percent (53/212) of women treated with IUT formed new antibodies, 53 percent of which were directed against non-Rh and -K antigens, suggesting the need for broader RBC antigen matching.[98]

Rh IMMUNOGLOBULIN

Use of RhIg is the standard of care for the prevention of maternal D immunization. Prophylaxis similar to RhIg does not exist for alloimmunization to antigens other than D. Postpartum administration of RhIg to all nonsensitized Rh-negative women who deliver an Rh-positive infant decreases the incidence of Rh isoimmunization from 12 percent to approximately 2 percent.[6] However approximately 1.8 percent of Rh-negative women apparently are sensitized from small asymptomatic transplacental hemorrhages during pregnancy. Further reduction in the incidence of Rh-isoimmunization to 0.1 percent has been achieved by antepartum RhIg prophylaxis at 28 weeks' gestation. This is the current standard recommendation in the United States.[131] In the United Kingdom, routine antenatal anti-D prophylaxis can be given as two doses of anti-D immunoglobulin of 500 IU (one at 28 weeks' and one at 34 weeks' gestation), as two doses of anti-D immunoglobulin of 1000 to 1650 IU (one at 28 weeks' and one at 34 weeks' gestation), or as a single dose of 1500 IU at 28 weeks' gestation.[132]

The mechanism by which RhIg prevents sensitization to the D antigen is not understood. Some of the proposed mechanisms are accelerated clearance and destruction of D-positive red cells from the circulation, antibody-mediated immune suppression, and the production of immunomodulatory cytokines.[28]

RhIg is prepared from plasma pools of screened, sensitized human donors; the plasma is tested using PCR and serologic methods for all known transfusion transmitted organisms. Several physicochemical inactivation steps are used to further inactivate potential infectious organisms and include solvent-detergent treatment, ion exchange chromatography and nanofiltration; viral inactivation processes have the potential to decrease the biologic activity. Both high-dose (300 mcg) and minidose (50 mcg) vials are available. There are currently four formulations, including two preparations which may be administered intravenously.[133]

The standard dose of 300 mcg RhIg (1500 IU) affords protection against a fetomaternal transfusion of 15 mL of Rh-positive red blood cells or 30 mL of Rh-positive whole blood. However, fetomaternal hemorrhage in excess of 30 mL may occur in women without predisposing risk factors.[19,20] The blood of all Rh-negative nonimmunized women should be tested for fetomaternal hemorrhage approximately 1 hour after delivery of an Rh-positive baby.[53,131] During the antenatal period, testing is indicated after 20 weeks' gestation if clinical circumstances suggest the possibility of excessive transplacental hemorrhage (e.g., abdominal trauma or abruptio placentae). Screening for fetomaternal hemorrhage can be performed by the rosette test, which detects as little as 2.5 mL of whole blood. If the rosette test result is positive, the number

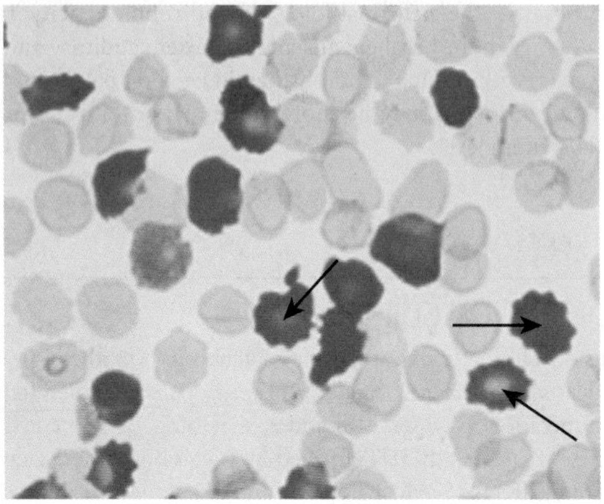

FIGURE 54–8. Kleihauer-Betke test. Maternal red blood cells appear as pale "ghost cells," whereas fetal red blood cells containing hemoglobin F are resistant to acid denaturation. Crenated red cells (*arrows*) are an artifact of the drying in preparation of the slide. *(Reproduced from Lazarchick J, ASH Image bank 2004–100983, with permission.)*

of fetal red cells in the maternal circulation is quantified more accurately by the Kleihauer-Betke test, which is based on the resistance of fetal hemoglobin to acid elution, unlike adult hemoglobin (Fig. 54–8).[134] False-positive results can be obtained in maternal conditions associated with increased fetal hemoglobin, such as hereditary persistence of fetal hemoglobin, sickle cell disease, or sickle cell trait (see Chaps. 47 and 48). Flow cytometric methods are used in some laboratories for both screening and quantification of fetal red cells.

The recommended dose of RhIg should be administered as soon as possible, within 72 hours of delivery of an Rh-positive baby. If RhIg is accidentally omitted, some protection still can be obtained with administration up to 13 days and possibly up to 28 days after delivery. RhIg is ineffective once alloimmunization to RhD antigen has occurred. RhIg is also indicated following pregnancy termination, miscarriage, amniocentesis, chorionic villus sampling, or other manipulation during pregnancy. A smaller 50-mcg dose is adequate if pregnancy is terminated at less than 12 weeks' gestation.[131] No definite evidence-based recommendations are available regarding administration of RhIg to women with threatened abortion and a live fetus or embryo at or before 12 weeks' gestation. If therapeutic or spontaneous abortion occurs after the first trimester, the standard 300-mcg dose is recommended.[131]

If a woman was exposed to more than 30 mL of D-positive blood, either secondary to fetomaternal hemorrhage or as a result of inadvertent transfusion of D-positive cells, the dose of RhIg should be calculated to cover the volume of D-positive cells to prevent immunization (20 mcg of RhIg for 1 mL of D+ red blood cells or 2 mL of whole blood).[53,133,135] Multiple doses of RhIg, calculated to cover the volume of exposure, can be given intramuscularly every 12 hours until the total dose is administered.[6] Intravenous preparations of RhIg, can be administered with much less discomfort to the patient, following the package insert recommendations.[133] When large volumes of D mismatched erythrocytes are transfused (>20% of circulating D+ RBCs) an exchange transfusion with D-negative blood may help to decrease the dose of RhIg required.[133] For D-mismatched platelet transfusions, a standard dose of RhIg is usually sufficient; use of apheresis platelets with minimal RBC contamination should be preferentially selected whenever possible.

RhD alloimmunization occurs despite recommended prophylaxis in 0.1 percent of pregnancies, but many cases of preventable Rh alloimmunization continue to occur because of failure to implement immunoprophylaxis protocols.

MONOCLONAL ANTIBODY

RhIg currently is produced from the plasma of D-negative male volunteers injected with D-positive red blood cells. Although polyclonal RhIg is extremely safe, concerns regarding potential transmission of infectious agents and a possible shortage of this specialized human-derived plasma have motivated a search for alternative prophylactic agents. Anti-D monoclonal and recombinant antibodies have been produced from human immunoglobulin genes or B cells using human B-cell lines, Chinese hamster ovary cells, mouse human heterohybridomas, and rat myelomas and are being evaluated for their potential to replace polyclonal RhIg for RhD prophylaxis.[136,137] Several of these products have undergone early clinical studies to determine safety and efficacy, as yet without success, likely because of significant heterogeneity in antibody efficacy and bioavailability. Some antibodies from rodent cell lines resulted in enhancing the immune response to D-positive red cells rather than preventing it, and these undesirable *in vivo* responses appeared to be related to the species specific glycosylation of IgG. Further developments and trials are necessary before monoclonal anti-D antibodies will be available for therapeutic use.

REFERENCES

1. Diamond LK, Blackfan KD, Baty JM: Erythroblastosis fetalis and its association with universal edema of the fetus, icterus gravis neonatorum and anemia of the newborn. *J Pediatr* 1:269, 1932.
2. Darrow RR: Icterus gravis (erythroblastosis neonatorum, examination of etiologic considerations). *Arch Pathol* 25:378, 1938.
3. Levine P, Katzin EM, Burnham L: Isoimmunization in pregnancy: Its possible bearing on the etiology of erythroblastosis fetalis. *JAMA* 116:825, 1941.
4. Diamond LK, Allen FH Jr, Thomas WO Jr: Erythroblastosis fetalis: VII. Treatment with exchange transfusion. *N Engl J Med* 244:39, 1951.
5. Liley AW: The use of amniocentesis and fetal transfusion in erythroblastosis fetalis. *Pediatrics* 35:836, 1965.
6. Bowman J: Thirty five years of Rh prophylaxis. *Transfusion* 43:1661, 2003.
7. Moise KJ: Fetal anemia due to nonrhesus D red cell alloimmunization. *Semin Fetal Neonatal Med* 13:207, 2008.
8. Poole J, Daniels G: Blood group antibodies and their significance in transfusion medicine. *Transfus Med Rev* 21:58, 2007.
9. Geifman-Holtzman O, Wojtowycz M, Kosmas E, Artal R: Female alloimmunization with antibodies known to cause hemolytic disease. *Obstet Gynecol* 89:272, 997.
10. Gottvall T, Filbey D: Alloimmunization in pregnancy during the years 1992–2005 in the central west region of Sweden. *Acta Obstet Gynecol Scand* 87:843, 2008.
11. Koelewijn JM, Vrijkotte TG, van der Schoot CE, et al: Effect of screening for red cell antibodies, other than anti-D, to detect hemolytic disease of the fetus and newborn: A population study in the Netherlands. *Transfusion* 48:941, 2008.
12. Lee CK, Ma ESK, Tang M, et al: Prevalence and specificity of clinically significant red cell alloantibodies in Chinese women during pregnancy—A review of cases from 1997 to 2001. *Transfus Med* 13:227, 2003.
13. Garratty G, Glynn SA, McEntire R, et al: for the Retrovirus Epidemiology Donor Study: ABO and Rh(D) phenotype frequencies of different racial/ethnic groups in the United States. *Transfusion* 44:703, 2004.
14. Joseph KS: Controlling Rh haemolytic disease of the newborn in India. *Br J Obstet Gynaecol* 98:369, 1991.
15. Mak KH, Yan KF, Cheng SS, Yuen MY: Rh phenotypes of Chinese blood donors in Hong Kong, with special reference to weak D antigens. *Transfusion* 33:348, 1993.
16. Flegel WA: Molecular genetics of RH and its clinical application. *Transfus Clin Biol* 13:4, 2006.
17. Denomme GA, Wagner FF, Fernandes BJ, et al: Partial D, weak D types and novel RHD alleles among 33,864 multiethnic patients: Implications for anti-D alloimmunization and prevention. *Transfusion* 45:1554, 2005.
18. Bowman JM, Pollack JM, Penston LE: Fetomaternal transplacental hemorrhage during pregnancy and after delivery. *Vox Sang* 51:117, 1986.
19. Sebring ES, Polesky HF: Fetomaternal hemorrhage: Incidence, risk factors, time of occurrence, and clinical effects. *Transfusion* 30:344, 1990.
20. Ness PM, Baldwin ML, Niebyl JR: Clinical high-risk designation does not predict excess fetomaternal hemorrhage. *Am J Obstet Gynecol* 156:154, 1987.
21. Pourbak S, Rund CR, Crookston KP: Three cases of massive fetomaternal hemorrhage presenting without clinical suspicion. *Arch Pathol Lab Med* 128:463, 2004.
22. Jansen MWJC, Brandenburg H, Wildshut HIJ, et al: The effect of chorionic villus sampling on the number of fetal cells isolated from maternal blood and on maternal serum alpha-fetoprotein levels. *Prenat Diagn* 17:953, 1997.

23. Bowman JM, Pollack JM: Transplacental fetal hemorrhage after amniocentesis. *Obstet Gynecol* 66:749, 1985.
24. Bowman JM, Pollock JM, Peterson LE, et al: Fetomaternal hemorrhage following funipuncture: Increase in severity of maternal red-cell alloimmunization. *Obstet Gynecol* 84:839, 1994.
25. Urbaniak SJ. Alloimmunity to RhD in humans. *Transfus Clin Biol* 13:19, 2006.
26. Bowman J, Harman C, Manning F, et al: Intravenous drug abuse causes Rh immunization. *Vox Sang* 61:96, 1991.
27. Bowman JM: Fetomaternal ABO incompatibility and erythroblastosis fetalis. *Vox Sang* 50:104, 1986.
28. Kumpel BM: On the immunologic basis of Rh immunoglobulin (anti-D) prophylaxis. *Transfusion* 46:1652, 2006.
29. Hadley AG: Laboratory assays for predicting the severity of haemolytic disease of the fetus and newborn. *Transpl Immunol* 10:191, 2002.
30. Palfi M, Hilden J, Gottval T, Selbing A: Placental transport of maternal immunoglobulin G in pregnancies at risk of Rh(D) hemolytic disease of the newborn. *Am J Reprod Immunol* 39;323, 1998.
31. Lambin P, Debbia M, Puillandre P, Brossard Y: IgG1 and IgG3 in maternal serum and on the RBCs of infants suffering from HDFN: Relationship with the severity of the disease. *Transfusion* 42:1537, 2002.
32. Neppert J, v Witzleben-Schürholz E, Zupanska B, et al: High incidence of maternal HLA A B and C antibodies associated with a mild course of haemolytic disease of the newborn. Group for the Study of Protective Maternal HLA Antibodies in the Clinical Course of HDFN. *Eur J Haematol* 63:120, 1999.
33. Shepard SL, Noble AL, Filbey D, Hadley AG: Inhibition of monocyte chemiluminescent response to anti-D sensitized red cells by Fc gamma RI-blocking antibodies which ameliorate the severity of haemolytic disease of the newborn. *Vox Sang* 70:157, 1996.
34. Thilaganathan B, Salvesan D, Abbas A, et al: Fetal plasma erythropoietin concentration in red blood cell-isoimmunized pregnancies. *Am J Obstet Gynecol* 167:1292, 1992.
35. Koenig JM, Christensen RD: Neutropenia and thrombocytopenia in infants with Rh hemolytic disease. *J Pediatr* 114:625, 1989.
36. Smits-Wintjens VEHJ, Walther FJ, Lopriore E: Rhesus haemolytic disease of the newborn: Postnatal management, associated morbidity and long-term outcome. *Semin Fetal Neonatal Med* 13:265, 2008.
37. Nicolaides KH: Studies in fetal physiology and pathophysiology in Rhesus disease. *Semin Perinatol* 13:328, 1989.
38. Sikkel E, Passman SA, Oepkes D: On the origin of amniotic fluid bilirubin. *Placenta* 25:463, 2004.
39. Passman SA, Sikkel E, Le Cessie S, et al: Bilirubin/albumin ratios in fetal blood and in amniotic fluid in Rhesus immunization. *Obstet Gynecol* 111:1083, 2008.
40. Hayde M, Widness JA, Pollack A, et al: Rhesus isoimmunization: Increased hemolysis during early infancy. *Pediatr Res* 41:716, 1997.
41. Al-Alaiyan S, Al Omran A: Late hyporegenerative anemia in neonates with rhesus hemolytic disease. *J Perinat Med* 27:112, 1999.
42. Pessler F, Hart D: Hyporegenerative anemia associated with Rh hemolytic disease: Treatment failure of recombinant erythropoietin. *J Pediatr Hematol Oncol* 24:689, 2002.
43. Wang M: Hemolytic disease of the newborn caused by a high titer anti-group B IgG from a group A mother. *Pediatr Blood Cancer* 45:861, 2005.
44. Deng ZH, Seltsam A, Ye YW, et al: Haemolytic disease of fetus and newborn caused by ABO antibodies in a cis AB offspring. *Transfus Apher Sci* 39:123, 2008.
45. Kaplan M, Na'amad M, Kenan A, et al: Failure to predict hemolysis and hyperbilirubinemia by IgG subclass in blood group A or B infants born to group O mothers. *Pediatrics* 123:e132, 2009.
46. Sarici SU, Yurdakok M, Serdar MA, et al: An early (sixth hour) serum bilirubin measurement is useful in predicting the development of significant hyperbilirubinemia and severe ABO hemolytic disease in a selective high risk population of newborns with ABO incompatibility. *Pediatrics* 109:e53, 2002.
47. Lin M, Broadberry RE: ABO Hemolytic disease of the newborn is more severe in Taiwan than in white populations. *Vox Sang* 68:136, 1995.
48. Miqdad AM, Abdelbasit OB, Shaheed MM, et al: Intravenous immunoglobulin G (IVIG) for significant hyperbilirubinemia in ABO hemolytic disease of the newborn. *J Matern Fetal Neonatal Med* 16:163, 2004.
49. Ziprin JH, Payne E, Hamidi L, et al: ABO incompatibility due to immunoglobulin G anti-B antibodies presenting with severe fetal anemia. *Transfus Med* 15:57, 2005.
50. Kaplan M, Hammerman C, Renbaum P, et al: Gilbert's syndrome and hyperbilirubinemia in ABO incompatible neonates. *Lancet* 356:652, 2000.
51. Katz MA, Kanto WP, Korotkin JH: Recurrence rate of ABO hemolytic disease of the newborn. *Obstet Gynecol* 59:611, 1982.
52. Eder AF: Update on HDFN: New information on long-standing controversies. *Immunohematol* 22:188, 2006.
53. Kennedy MS: Perinatal issues in transfusion practice, in *Technical Manual.* 16th ed, edited by JD Roback, MR Combs, BJ Grossman, CD Hillyer, p 625. AABB Press, Bethesda, MD, 2008.
54. Grant SR, Kilby MD, Meer L, et al: The outcome of pregnancy in Kell immunization. *BJOG* 107:481, 2000.
55. Kamphuis MM, Lindenburg I, van Kamp IL, et al: Implementation of routine screening for Kell antibodies: Does it improve perinatal survival? *Transfusion* 48:953, 2008.
56. McKenna DS, Nagaraja HN, O'Shaughnessy R: Management of pregnancies complicated by anti-Kell isoimmunization. *Obstet Gynecol* 93:667, 1999.
57. Bowman JM, Pollack JM, Manning FA, et al: Maternal Kell blood group alloimmunization. *Obstet Gynecol* 79:239, 1992.
58. Vaughan JI, Manning M, Warwick RM, et al: Inhibition of erythroid progenitor cells by anti-Kell antibodies in fetal alloimmune anemia. *N Engl J Med* 338:798, 1998.
59. Daniels G, Hadley A, Green CA: Causes of fetal anemia in hemolytic disease due to anti-K. *Transfusion* 43:115, 2003.
60. Wagner T, Bernaschek G, Geissler K: Inhibition of megakaryopoiesis by Kell related antibodies. *N Engl J Med* 343:72, 2000.
61. Wagner T: Pancytopenia due to suppressed hematopoiesis in a case of fatal hemolytic disease of the newborn associated with anti-K supported by molecular K1 typing. *J Pediatr Hematol Oncol* 26:13, 2004.
62. Shapiro SM: Definition of the clinical spectrum of kernicterus and bilirubin induced neurologic dysfunction. *J Perinatol* 25:54, 2005.
63. Kuzniewicz M, Newman TB: Interaction of hemolysis and hyperbilirubinemia on neurodevelopmental outcomes in the Collaborative Perinatal Project. *Pediatrics* 123:1045, 2009.
64. Janssens HM, deHaan MJJ, van Kamp IL, et al: Outcome for children treated with fetal intravascular transfusions because of severe blood group antagonism. *J Pediatr* 131:373, 1997.
65. Lobato G: Relationship between obstetric history and rh(D) alloimmunization severity. *Arch Gynecol Obstet* 277:245, 2008.
66. Andersen AS, Praetorius L, Jorgensen HL, et al: Prognostic value of screening for irregular antibodies late in pregnancy in rhesus positive women. *Acta Obstet Gynecol Scand* 81:407, 2002.
67. Adeniji AA, Fuller I, Dale T, Lindow SW: Should we continue to screen rhesus D positive women for the development of atypical antibodies in late pregnancy. *J Matern Fetal Neonatal Med* 20:59, 2007.
68. Moise KJ: Management of rhesus alloimmunization in pregnancy. *Obstet Gynecol* 112:164, 2008.
69. British Committee for Standards in Haematology Blood Transfusion Task Force: Guideline for blood grouping and antibody testing in pregnancy. *Transfus Med* 17:252, 2007.
70. Hackney DN, Knudtson EJ, Rossi KQ, et al: Management of pregnancies complicated by anti-c isoimmunization. *Obstet Gynecol* 103:24, 2004.
71. Denomme GA, Fernandes BJ: Fetal blood group genotyping. *Transfusion* 47:64S, 2007.
72. Lo YMD, Bowell PJ, Selinger M, et al: Prenatal determination of fetal Rh-D status by analysis of peripheral blood of Rhesus negative mothers. *Lancet* 341:1147, 1993.
73. Geiffman Holtzman O, Grotegut CA, Gaughan JP: Diagnostic accuracy of noninvasive fetal Rh genotyping from maternal blood—A metaanalysis. *Am J Obstet Gynecol* 195:1163, 2006.
74. Geiffman Holtzman O, Grotegut CA, Gaughan JP, et al: Non-invasive fetal RhCE genotyping from maternal blood. *BJOG* 116:144, 2009.
75. Daniels G, Finning K, Martin P, Massey E: Noninvasive prenatal diagnosis of fetal blood group phenotypes: Current practice and future prospects. *Prenat Diagn* 29:101, 2009.
76. Li Y, Finning K, Daniels G, et al: Noninvasive genotyping fetal Kell blood group (*KEL1*) using cell free fetal DNA in maternal plasma by MALDI-TOF mass spectrometry. *Prenat Diagn* 28:203, 2008.
77. Liley AW: Liquor amnii analysis in the management of the pregnancy complicated by Rhesus sensitization. *Am J Obstet Gynecol* 82:1359, 1961.
78. Queenan JT, Tomai TP, Ural SH, King JC: Deviation in amniotic fluid optical density at a wavelength of 450 nm in Rh-immunized pregnancies from 14 to 40 weeks' gestation: A proposal for clinical management. *Am J Obstet Gynecol* 168:1370, 1993.
79. Oepkes D: Doppler ultrasonography versus amniocentesis to predict fetal anemia. *N Engl J Med* 355:156, 2006.
80. Mari G, Deter RL, Carpenter RL, et al: for the Collaborative Group for Doppler Assessment of the Blood Velocity in Anemic Fetuses: Noninvasive diagnosis by Doppler ultrasonography of fetal anemia due to maternal red cell alloimmunization. *N Engl J Med* 342:9, 2000.
81. Dukler D, Oepkes D, Seaward G, et al: Noninvasive tests to predict fetal anemia: A study comparing Doppler and ultrasound parameters. *Am J Obstet Gynecol* 188:1310, 2003.
82. Daffos F, Capella-Pavlovsky M, Forestier F: Fetal blood sampling during pregnancy with use of a needle guided by ultrasound: A study of 606 consecutive cases. *Am J Obstet Gynecol* 153:655, 1985.
83. Buscaglia M, Ghisoni L, Bellotti M, et al: Percutaneous umbilical blood sampling: Indication changes and procedure loss rate in a nine years' experience. *Fetal Diagn Ther* 11:106, 1996.
84. Ghidini A, Sepulveda W, Lockwood CJ, Romero R: Complications of fetal blood sampling. *Am J Obstet Gynecol* 168:1339, 1993.
85. Dinesh D: Review of positive direct antiglobulin tests found on cord blood sampling. *J Paediatr Child Health* 41:504, 2005.
86. Heddle NM, Wentworth P, Anderson DR, et al: Three examples of Rh haemolytic disease of the newborn with a negative direct antiglobulin test. *Transfus Med* 5:113, 1995.
87. Herschel M, Karrison T, Wen M, et al: Isoimmunization is unlikely to be the cause of hemolysis in ABO incompatible but direct antiglobulin test negative neonates. *Pediatrics* 110:127, 2002.

88. Herschel M, Karrison T, Wen M, et al: Evaluation of the direct antiglobulin (Coombs') test for identifying newborns at risk for hemolysis as determined by end tidal carbon monoxide concentration ($ETCO_c$); and comparison of the Coombs' test with $ETCO_c$ for detecting significant jaundice. *J Perinatol* 22:341, 2002.
89. Ramasethu J: Hemolytic disease of the newborn, in *Handbook of Pediatric Transfusion Medicine*, edited by CD Hillyer, RG Strauss, NLC Luban, p 191. Elsevier Academic, New York, 2004.
90. Oepkes D, Adama van Scheltema P: Intrauterine transfusions in the management of fetal anemia and fetal thrombocytopenia. *Semin Fetal Neonatal Med* 12:432, 2007.
91. Howe DT, Michailides CD: Intraperitoneal transfusion in severe early onset Rh isoimmunization. *Obstet Gynecol* 110:880, 2007.
92. Fox C: Early intraperitoneal transfusion and adjuvant maternal immunoglobulin therapy in the treatment of severe red cell alloimmunization prior to fetal intravascular transfusion. *Fetal Diagn Ther* 23:159, 2008.
93. Radunovic N, Lockwood CJ, Alvarez M, et al: The severely anemic and hydropic isoimmune fetus: Changes in fetal hematocrit associated with intrauterine death. *Obstet Gynecol* 79:390, 1992.
94. Hallak M, Moise KJ, Hesketh DE, et al: Intravascular transfusion of fetuses with Rhesus incompatibility: Prediction of fetal outcome by changes in umbilical venous pressure. *Obstet Gynecol* 80:286, 1992.
95. Wong ECC, Luban NLC: Intrauterine, neonatal and pediatric transfusion, in *Transfusion Therapy: Clinical Principles and Practice*, 2nd ed, edited by PD Mintz, p 159. AABB Press, Bethesda, MD, 2005.
96. Gibson BE, Todd A, Roberts I, et al: British Committee for Standards in Haematology Transfusion Task Force: Writing Group. Transfusion guidelines for neonates and older children. *Br J Haematol* 124:433, 2004.
97. Gonsoulin WJ, Moise KJ Jr, Milam JD, et al: Serial maternal blood donations for intrauterine transfusions. *Obstet Gynecol* 75:158, 1990.
98. Schonewille H, Klumper FJ, van de Watering LM, et al: High additional maternal red cell alloimmunization after Rhesus- and K-matched intrauterine intravascular transfusions for hemolytic disease of the fetus. *Am J Obstet Gynecol* 196:143.e1, 2007.
99. el-Azeem SA, Samuels P, Rose RL, et al: The effect of the source of transfused blood on the rate of consumption of transfused red blood cells in pregnancies affected by red blood cell alloimmunization. *Am J Obstet Gynecol* 177:753, 1997.
100. Nicolaides KH, Clewell WH, Rodeck CH: Measurement of human fetoplacental blood volume in erythroblastosis fetalis. *Am J Obstet Gynecol* 157:50, 1987.
101. Hoogeven M, Meerman RH, Pasman S, Egberts J: A new method to determine the fetoplacental volume based on dilution of fetal hemoglobin and an estimation of plasma fluid loss after intrauterine intravascular transfusion. *BJOG* 109:1132, 2002.
102. Giannina G, Moise KJ Jr, Dorman K: A simple method to estimate the volume for fetal intrauterine transfusion. *Fetal Diagn Ther* 13:94, 1998.
103. Van Kamp IL, Klumper FJ, Oepkes D, et al: Complications of intrauterine intravascular transfusion for fetal anemia due to maternal red cell alloimmunization. *Am J Obstet Gynecol* 192:171, 2005.
104. Ruma MS: Combined plasmapheresis and intravenous immune globulin for the treatment of severe maternal red cell alloimmunization. *Obstet Gynecol* 196:e1, 2007.
105. Collinet P, Subtil D, Puech F, Vaast P: Successful treatment of extremely severe fetal anemia due to Kell isoimmunization. *Obstet Gynecol* 100:1102, 2002.
106. Nielsen LK, Green TH, Sandlie I, et al: *In vitro* assessment of recombinant, mutant immunoglobulin G anti-D devoid of hemolytic activity for treatment of ongoing hemolytic disease of the fetus and newborn. *Transfusion* 48:12, 2008.
107. Whitecar PW, Farb R, Subramanyam L, et al: Paternal leukocyte alloimmunization as a treatment for hemolytic disease of the newborn in a rabbit model. *Am J Obstet Gynecol* 187:977, 2002.
108. Van Kamp IL, Klumper FJCM, Bakkum RSLA, et al: The severity of immune fetal hydrops is predictive of fetal outcome after intrauterine treatment. *Am J Obstet Gynecol* 185:668, 2001.
109. De Boer IP, Zeestraten ECM, Lopriore E, et al: Pediatric outcome in Rhesus hemolytic disease treated with and without intrauterine transfusion. *Am J Obstet Gynecol* 198:E1, 2008.
110. Harper DC, Swingle HM, Weiner CP, et al: Long-term neurodevelopmental outcome and brain volume after treatment for hydrops fetalis by *in utero* intravascular transfusion. Am J Obstet Gynecol 195:192, 2006.
111. American Academy of Pediatrics: Clinical Practice Guideline. Subcommittee on Hyperbilirubinemia. Management of hyperbilirubinemia in the newborn infant 35 or more weeks gestation. *Pediatrics* 114:297, 2004.
112. Maisels MJ, Watchko JF: Treatment of jaundice in low birth weight infants. *Arch Dis Child Fetal Neonatal Ed* 88:F459, 2003.
113. Hulzebos CV, van Imhoff DE, Bos AF, et al: Usefulness of the bilirubin albumin ratio for predicting bilirubin induced neurotoxicity in premature infants. *Arch Dis Child Fetal Neonatal Ed* 93:F384, 2008.
114. Ramasethu J: Exchange transfusions, in *Atlas of Procedures in Neonatology*, 4th ed, edited by MG MacDonald, J Ramasethu, p 329. Lippincott, Williams & Wilkins, Philadelphia, 2007.
115. Patra K, Storfer-Isser A, Siner B, et al: Adverse events associated with neonatal exchange transfusion in the 1990s. *J Pediatr* 144:626, 2004.
116. Steiner LA, Bizzarro MJ, Ehrenkranz RA, Gallagher PG: A decline in the frequency of exchange transfusions and its effect on exchange related mortality and morbidity. *Pediatrics* 120:27, 2007.
117. Jackson JC: Adverse events associated with exchange transfusion in healthy and healthy and ill newborns. *Pediatrics* 99:e7, 1997.
118. Tan KL, Lim GC, Boey KW: Phototherapy for ABO haemolytic hyperbilirubinemia. *Biol Neonate* 61:358, 1992.
119. Ebbesen F: Evaluation of the indications for early exchange transfusion in Rhesus haemolytic disease during phototherapy. *Eur J Pediatr* 133:37, 1980.
120. Gottstein R, Cooke RWI: Systematic review of intravenous immunoglobulin in haemolytic disease of the Newborn. *Arch Dis Child Fetal Neonatal Ed* 88:F6, 2003.
121. Alcock GS, Liley H: Immunoglobulin infusion for isoimmune haemolytic disease in neonates. *Cochrane Database Syst Rev* 3:CD003313, 2002.
122. Kappas A, Drummond GS, Manola T, et al: Sn-protoporphyrin use in the management of hyperbilirubinemia in term newborns with direct Coombs-positive ABO incompatibility. *Pediatrics* 81:485, 1988.
123. Suresh GK, Martin CL, Soll RF: Metalloporphyrins for treatment of unconjugated hyperbilirubinemia in neonates. *Cochrane Database Syst Rev* 2:CD004207, 2003.
124. Ovaly F, Samancy N, Dagoglu T: Management of late anemia in rhesus hemolytic disease: Use of recombinant human erythropoietin (a pilot study). *Pediatr Res* 39:831, 1996.
125. Dhodapkar KM, Blei F: Treatment of hemolytic disease of the newborn caused by anti-Kell antibody with recombinant erythropoietin. *J Pediatr Hematol Oncol* 23:69, 2003.
126. Ovaly F: Late anemia in Rh haemolytic disease. *Arch Dis Child Fetal Neonatal Ed* 88:F444, 2003.
127. Hudon L, Moise KJ Jr, Hegemier SE, et al: Long-term neurodevelopmental outcome after intrauterine transfusion for the treatment of fetal hemolytic disease. *Am J Obstet Gynecol* 179:858, 1998.
128. Ip S, Chung M, Kulig J, et al: An evidence based review of important issues concerning neonatal hyperbilirubinemia. *Pediatrics* 114:e130, 2004.
129. Newman TB, Liljestrand P, Jeremy RJ, et al: Outcomes among newborns with total serum bilirubin levels of 25 mg per deciliter or more. *N Engl J Med* 354:1889, 2006.
130. Gkoltsiou K, Tzoufi M, Counsell S, et al: Serial brain MRI and ultrasound findings: Relation to gestational age, bilirubin level, neonatal neurologic status and neurodevelopmental outcome in infants at risk of kernicterus. *Early Hum Dev* 84:829, 2008.
131. American College of Obstetrics and Gynecology: *ACOG Practice Bulletin. Prevention of RhD alloimmunization, number 4 (replaces educational bulletin number 14, October 1990).* Clinical Management Guidelines for Obstetricians and Gynecologists, 1999.
132. National Institute for Health and Clinical Excellence: *Pregnancy (Rhesus Negative Women) Routine Anti-D Review: Final Appraisal Determination*, 2008. Available at www.nice.org.uk/guidance/index.jsp?action=download&o=40807.
133. Ayache S: Prevention of D sensitization after mismatched transfusion of blood components: Toward optimal use of RhIG. *Transfusion* 48:1990, 2008.
134. Kleihauer E, Braun H, Betki K: Demonstration von fetalem Hämoglobin in den Erythrocyten eines Blutausstrichs. *Klin Wochenschr* 35:637, 1957.
135. Ramsey G, College of American Pathologists Transfusion Medicine Resource Committee: Inaccurate doses of R immune globulin after rh-incompatible fetomaternal hemorrhage: Survey of laboratory practice. *Arch Pathol Lab Med* 133:465, 2009.
136. Kumpel BM: Efficacy of RhD monoclonal antibodies in clinical rials as replacement therapy for prophylactic anti-D immunoglobulin: More questions than answers. *Vox Sang* 93:99, 2007.
137. Kumpel BM: Lessons learned from many years of experience using anti-D in humans for prevention of RhD immunization and haemolytic disease of the fetus and newborn. *Clin Exp Immunol* 154:1, 2008.

CHAPTER 55

HYPERSPLENISM AND HYPOSPLENISM

Jaime Caro and Ubaldo Martinez Outschoorn

SUMMARY

The spleen culls aged and abnormal cells from the blood; removes intraerythrocytic inclusions through a process called *pitting*; sequesters approximately one-third of the normal intravascular platelet pool; removes bacteria, foreign particles, and tumor cells from the blood; and by virtue of the T and B lymphocytes and macrophages in the white pulp, plays a role in immune surveillance and antibody formation. Splenomegaly can occur as a result of vascular engorgement or cellular infiltration, and it is frequently associated with a combination of neutropenia, thrombocytopenia, and anemia. Hypersplenism is defined as one or more blood cytopenias in the setting of splenomegaly. Hypersplenism can occur with moderate or minimal splenic enlargement as a result of exaggerated removal of physically abnormal (e.g., hereditary spherocytosis) or antibody-coated blood cells (e.g., autoimmune hemolytic anemia). The presence of splenomegaly in a patient with blood cytopenias is useful to narrow the etiology, although trapping in the enlarged spleen may not be the cause of the blood cytopenias. Thrombocytopenia in the setting of cirrhosis and splenomegaly is because of pooling in the enlarged spleen and a relative decrease in thrombopoietin. Anemia and neutropenia in cirrhosis with splenomegaly are poorly understood, but a relative reduction in erythropoietin levels and decreased marrow myeloid progenitor cells have been described. Splenectomy has been used in cases of severe thrombocytopenia requiring chronic platelet transfusions or leading to bleeding, although its efficacy is uncertain. Thrombopoietin receptor agonists are another option in the management of thrombocytopenia, and nonpeptide thrombopoietin receptor agonists have been shown to increase platelet counts in patients with thrombocytopenia associated with hepatitis C virus-related cirrhosis. Splenectomy may be justified in the case of massive splenomegaly, infarction, or disabling symptoms of pain and compression of neighboring structures. In some circumstances, benefit can be achieved by partial destruction of splenic tissue by embolization using intraarterial infusion of gel microparticles. Hyposplenism can result from agenesis, atrophy, surgical removal of the spleen, or reduction of splenic function by disease. In the latter case, disturbance in splenic circulation disrupts the specific architecture required for the spleen's culling, phagocytic, and pitting functions. Hyposplenism may be suspected by alterations in red cell morphology, such as target cells or acanthocytes; red cell inclusions, such as Howell-Jolly and Pappenheimer bodies (siderotic granules highlighted with polychrome stains); pitted red cells; or an elevated platelet count. The presence of pitted red cells identified by interference-contrast microscopy is perhaps the most specific blood finding of hyposplenism, followed by Howell-Jolly bodies. The most devastating consequence of hyposplenism is sudden overwhelming sepsis by encapsulated bacteria. Immunizations and prophylactic antibiotics can decrease the risk of sepsis. A high awareness and prompt antibiotic treatment of febrile episodes are warranted.

Acronyms and abbreviations that appear in this chapter include: G-CSF, granulocyte colony-stimulating factor; Ig, immunoglobulin; PEGrHuMGDF, pegylated human recombinant megakaryocyte growth and development factor.

HYPERSPLENISM

HISTORY

The spleen has intrigued physicians and philosophers since ancient times.[1] The spleen has been assigned mysterious powers, but its association with destruction of blood cells was not elucidated until the turn of the 20th century. The exaggerated and unfounded worry about somatic complaints often reflected by the sense of pain in the spleen (left hypochondrium) led to the term *hypochondriac.* In 1899, Chauffard proposed that increased splenic activity causes hemolysis.[2] This proposal provided the impetus for therapeutic splenectomy, which was performed first in 1910 by Sutherland and Burghard[3] in a patient with splenic anemia (hereditary spherocytosis) and subsequently by Kaznelson[4] in a patient with essential thrombocytopenia (immune thrombocytopenic purpura) in 1916.

DEFINITION

Hypersplenism is defined as blood cytopenias in the setting of splenomegaly. Splenomegaly can occur as a result of vascular congestion associated with elevated venous pressures, histiophagocytic hyperplasia, other cellular infiltration, or because of the inability of physically abnormal red cells, such as sickle cells, or antibody-coated cells, such as in autoimmune hemolytic anemia, to navigate the circulation or avoid engulfment by the mononuclear phagocyte population of the normal spleen.[5] The blood cytopenias are not generally corrected by relief of portal hypertension.[6,7]

ONTOGENY

The embryonic spleen appears in the first trimester of gestation as a multiply lobulated condensation of highly vascular mesenchymal cell aggregate interposed in the arterial circulation in the dorsal mesogastrium. The full scope of the molecular basis of splenic organogenesis is not known. The *Hox11 and WT1* genes are essential for its formation, and defects in their expression result in hyposplenia or asplenia.[8–10]

The lymphoid compartment, the white pulp, begins its development early in the second trimester of gestation, when mature T cells, principally CD4+, form a continuous layer along the length of the vessels (periarteriolar sheaths). CD8+ cells reside in splenic cords and a specialized subset of $\gamma\delta$T cells homes to the pulp (see Chap. 5). Immunoglobulin (Ig) D+ and IgG+ B lymphocytes form localized deposits, the primary lymph follicles. Secondary follicles arise later in life, after exposure to immunologic stimuli, and have a distinctive structure that includes a germinal center, a mantle zone, and a marginal zone containing IgM+ and IgG+ B lymphocytes.[11,12]

STRUCTURE AND FUNCTIONAL ORGANIZATION

The normal adult spleen weighs 135 ± 30 g and has a blood flow that is approximately 4 to 5 percent of the cardiac output. The spleen's principal structure is organized around an arborizing array of arterioles that branch and narrow until they terminate in either (1) the stroma of cords, forming the open circulation, or (2) the sinusoids, forming the closed circulation of the spleen (see Chap. 5). The cordal elements include histiocytes, antigen-presenting cells, pericytes, fibroblasts, and other cells necessary to maintain the discontinuous basal lamina that separates cords from lumen.[13] Lymphatic tissue is inconspicuous and found in T-cell-rich zones in the periarteriolar lymphoid sheaths.

The arterial vascular tree, which is lined by conventional CD31+ and CD34+ endothelial cells, branches into arterioles that terminate abruptly in caps of cordal macrophages. Blood cells must pass clusters of macrophages to enter the sinusoids.[13] The sinusoids, the origin of the venous circulation, are lined by specialized cells having combined phagocytic and endothelial activities and a distinctive CD31+, CD34–, CD68+, CD8+ phenotype. A principal function of the spleen is to serve as a filter removing aged or defective red cells and foreign particles by its content of mononuclear phagocytes. This function is accomplished by diverting part of the splenic blood supply into the red pulp, where the blood slowly percolates through the nonendothelialized mesh studded with macrophages. The blood then reenters the circulation through narrow slits, measuring 1 to 3 μm, in the endothelium of the venous sinuses. The bulk of the blood is rapidly channeled through vessels that link the arterioles with the venous sinuses. This blood is not filtered or modified.[14]

About one third of platelets are normally sequestered in the spleen.[15] In many animals, such as dogs and horses, the red pulp is a reservoir for red cells, and splenic contraction provides the red cell volume with a functionally important boost.[16] In humans, however, the splenic capsule is poorly contractile, and the spleen does not store red cells to any significant degree.[17] Although margination of neutrophils occurs in the spleen, it is unclear to what degree it occurs.[18] Granulocyte colony-stimulating factor (G-CSF) was administered to cirrhotic patients, causing a rise in the blood neutrophil count, then Indium white blood cell scans of the spleen were performed, which did not show significant uptake.[19]

The slow transit of blood through the red pulp permits macrophages to recognize and destroy antibody- or complement-coated cells and microorganisms and to ingest poorly deformable cells or particles retained mechanically by the narrow exit slits in the venous sinuses.

PATHOPHYSIOLOGY

Filtration and elimination of defective cells occur notably in hereditary abnormalities of the red cell membranes, such as spherocytosis, elliptocytosis, or stomatocytosis (see Chap. 45), or with antibody-coated red cells (see Chap. 53), neutrophils (see Chap. 65), or platelets (see Chap. 119). In these circumstances, cytopenias of varying severity may ensue. The spleen not only removes antibody-coated cells, but also produces antibodies, especially antiplatelet antibodies.[20] Thus, the benefits of splenectomy in immune thrombocytopenic purpura is a result of both the decreased production of antiplatelet antibodies as well as decreased clearance by macrophages of antibody-coated platelets through the Fc recognition function of its large macrophage population.

Splenomegaly increases the proportion of blood channeled through the red pulp.[13,21] Spleen enlargement may result from expansion of the red pulp compartment with increased blood flow; extramedullary hematopoiesis, notably in primary myelofibrosis; hyperplasia or neoplasia involving the white pulp, such as in infectious mononucleosis or lymphoma; or histiophagocytic hyperplasia.

The increased size of the filtering bed is more pronounced when the splenomegaly is caused by congestion as in portal hypertension than when it is caused by cellular infiltration as in leukemias, extramedullary hematopoiesis, or amyloidosis. Even in space-occupying disorders such as Gaucher disease (see Chap. 73) and myelofibrosis (see Chap. 91), splenomegaly may be associated with hypersplenic sequestration of normal cells.

Splenomegaly increases the vascular surface area and thereby the marginated neutrophil pool.[18,19] Platelets are especially likely to be sequestered in an enlarged spleen. However, sequestered white cells and platelets survive in the spleen and may be available when increased demand requires neutrophils or platelets, although their release may be slow.[22]

Some patients with anemia and splenomegaly have a relative erythropoietin deficiency.[23] In one study of cirrhotic patients, 30 percent had a blunted erythropoietin response to anemia.[24] Dilution of red cells in an expanded plasma volume is another commonly cited cause of anemia,[25] although some studies do not demonstrate hemodilution.[26] Iron deficiency associated with chronic blood loss, folic acid and vitamin B_{12} deficiency, and increased red cell destruction are frequently investigated although rarely found in patients with liver disease.[27] Red cells are destroyed prematurely in the red pulp in the setting of splenomegaly, but only rarely does this explain the anemia.[28]

Varying amounts of erythrophagocytosis are present, reflecting the normal culling of senescent red cells. Erythrophagocytosis increases as a result of hemolytic anemia and viral infections, and in alloimmunized transfusion recipients. Macrophages within the sinusoids contain red cell fragments. When the process is pronounced, the littoral cells become cuboidal and stand out on the basement membrane ("hobnails"). Sickle cell disease and red cell membrane disorders such as hereditary spherocytosis lead to sequestration of the poorly deformed red cells in the cords but little extrasinusoidal erythrophagocytosis is seen, in contrast to immune hemolytic anemia where macrophage erythrophagocytosis is prominent.[13]

The increased blood flow from an enlarged spleen expands the splenic and portal veins. A significant increase in portal venous pressure may occur when hepatic vessel compliance is decreased, as in cirrhosis or myelofibrosis (see Chap. 91). This process initiates a vicious cycle in which portal hypertension contributes to splenomegaly and organ enlargement leads to increased arterial flow which in turn increases portal pressure.

Table 55–1 lists causes of splenomegaly, and Table 55–2 lists causes of massive splenic enlargement.

CLINICAL FEATURES

Slight to moderate enlargement of the spleen usually does not produce local symptoms. Even massive splenomegaly can be well tolerated. However, not infrequently, the patient complains of a sagging feeling or other types of abdominal discomfort, early satiety from gastric encroachment, and trouble sleeping on one side. Pleuritic-like pain in the left upper quadrant or referred to the left shoulder may accompany splenic infarcts, which may be recurrent.

In children with sickle cell anemia or patients with malaria, the spleen may become acutely enlarged and painful as a result of a sudden increase in red cell pooling and sequestration. These sequestration crises are characterized by sudden aggravation of the anemia. Splenic rupture is uncommon but can occur spontaneously with most causes of splenic enlargement or after blunt trauma. Rupture related to the splenic enlargement in infectious mononucleosis is a classic example.

The volume of an enlarged spleen is difficult to assess by palpation and percussion. Children and thin patients with low diaphragms may have a palpable spleen tip without splenomegaly.[29] Generally, a palpable spleen signifies splenomegaly and is measured by the number of centimeters the spleen extends below the left costal margin. Splenic size is most accurately measured with abdominal ultrasound or computed tomographic scans (see Chap. 1, Figs. 1–1 and 1–2). Magnetic resonance imaging is used primarily to identify cysts, abscesses, and infarcts.[30]

SPLENOPTOSIS

A wandering spleen (splenoptosis) is an uncommon phenomenon in which the spleen hangs by a long pedicle of mesentery. The condition may present in three ways: (1) an asymptomatic mass in the pelvis, (2) intermittent abdominal pain with or without gastrointestinal symptoms, or (3) less often, an acute abdomen resulting from torsion. The diagnosis of splenoptosis may be made coincidentally on an imaging study.[31] The condition may be accompanied by signs of hypersplenism,

TABLE 55–1. Classification and Most Common Causes of Splenomegaly

I. Congestive
- A. Right-sided congestive heart failure
- B. Budd-Chiari syndrome (inferior vena cava and hepatic vein thrombosis)
- C. Cirrhosis with portal hypertension
- D. Portal or splenic vein thrombosis

II. Immunologic
- A. Viral infection
  1. Acute HIV infection/chronic infection
  2. Acute mononucleosis
  3. Dengue fever
  4. Rubella (rare except newborns)
  5. Cytomegalovirus infection (rare except newborns)
  6. Herpes simplex (rare except newborns)
- B. Bacterial infection
  1. Subacute bacterial endocarditis
  2. Brucellosis
  3. Tularemia
  4. Melioidosis
  5. Listeriosis
  6. Plague
  7. Secondary syphilis
  8. Relapsing fever
  9. Psittacosis
  10. Ehrlichiosis
  11. Rickettsial diseases (scrub typhus, Rocky Mountain spotted fever, Q fever)
  12. Tuberculosis
  13. Splenic abscess (most common organisms are *Enterobacteriaceae*, *Staphylococcus aureus*, streptococcus group D, and anaerobic organisms as part of mixed flora infections)
- C. Fungal Infection
  1. Blastomycosis
  2. Histoplasmosis
  3. Systemic candidiasis and hepatosplenic candidiasis
- D. Parasitic infection
  1. Malaria
  2. Kala-azar
  3. Leishmaniasis
  4. Schistosomiasis
  5. Babesiosis
  6. Coccidioidomycosis
  7. Paracoccidioidomycosis
  8. Trypanosomiasis (cruzi, brucei)
  9. Toxoplasmosis (rare except newborns)
  10. Echinococcosis
  11. Cysticercosis
  12. Visceral larva migrans (*Toxocara* infection)
- E. Inflammatory/autoimmune
  1. Systemic lupus erythematosus (SLE)
  2. Felty syndrome
  3. Juvenile rheumatoid arthritis
  4. Autoimmune lymphoproliferative syndrome (ALP syndrome)
  5. Hemophagocytic syndrome
  6. Common variable immunodeficiency
  7. Anti-D immunoglobulin administration

III. Associated with hemolysis
- A. Thalassemia major and intermedia
- B. Pyruvate kinase deficiency
- C. Hereditary spherocytosis
- D. Autoimmune hemolytic anemia (rare)
- E. Sickle cell disease, more common in early childhood (splenic sequestration), hemoglobin C disease, and some other hemoglobinopathies

IV. Infiltrative
- A. Nonmalignant
  1. Splenic hematoma (splenic cysts are usually a late complication of a hematoma)
  2. Littoral cell angioma
  3. Disorders of sphingolipid metabolism
     - a. Gaucher disease
     - b. Niemann-Pick disease
  4. Cystinosis
  5. Amyloidosis (light-chain amyloid and amyloid A protein)
  6. Multicentric Castleman disease
  7. Mastocytosis
  8. Hypereosinophilic syndrome
  9. Sarcoidosis
- B. Extramedullary hematopoiesis
  1. Primary myelofibrosis
  2. Osteopetrosis (childhood)
  3. Thalassemia major
- C. Malignant
  1. Hematologic
     - a. Chronic lymphocytic leukemia (especially prolymphocytic variant)
     - b. Chronic myeloid leukemia
     - c. Polycythemia vera
     - d. Hairy cell leukemia
     - e. Heavy chain disease
     - f. Hepatosplenic lymphoma
     - g. Acute leukemia (acute lymphoblastic leukemia/acute myeloid leukemia)
     - h. Hodgkin and other lymphomas
  2. Nonhematologic
     - a. Metastatic carcinoma (rare)
     - b. Neuroblastoma
     - c. Wilms tumor
     - d. Leiomyosarcoma
     - e. Fibrosarcoma
     - f. Malignant fibrous histiocytoma
     - g. Kaposi sarcoma
     - h. Hemangiosarcoma
     - i. Lymphangiosarcoma
     - j. Hemangioendothelial sarcoma

V. Iatrogenic
- A. Granulocyte colony-stimulating factor administration
- B. Erythropoietin administration

TABLE 55–2. Causes of Massive Splenomegaly

I.	Myeloproliferative disorders
	A. Primary myelofibrosis
	B. Chronic myeloid leukemia
II.	Lymphomas
	A. Hairy cell leukemia
	B. Chronic lymphocytic leukemia (especially prolymphocytic variant)
III.	Infectious
	A. Malaria
	B. Leishmaniasis (kala azar)
IV.	Extramedullary hematopoiesis
	A. Thalassemia major
V.	Infiltrative
	A. Gaucher disease

hyposplenism, and often, when developing slowly, is initially mistaken for a pelvic or lower abdominal tumor.

LABORATORY FEATURES

The characteristic features of hypersplenism are splenomegaly, blood cytopenias, and exclusion of other causes of cytopenias (e.g., anemia caused by bleeding). The blood cell morphology usually is normal, although a few spherocytes may result from metabolic conditioning of red cells during repeated slow transits through the expanded red pulp. Tests, such as epinephrine mobilization, were used in the past to try to distinguish sequestration from ineffective cellular production, but results are difficult to interpret as epinephrine also releases platelets and neutrophils from marginal pools.[32]

Thrombocytopenia is a common finding in patients with hepatic cirrhosis and portal hypertension. In a retrospective study, 64 percent of patients with nonalcoholic cirrhosis had thrombocytopenia.[33] Other studies have found that about one-third of patients with cirrhosis develop severe thrombocytopenia or neutropenia.[34,35] Decompensated liver disease and history of alcohol consumption are independent risk factors for hypersplenism,[36] but why some patients develop marked blood cytopenias is not clear, although folate deficiency is a factor in some instances. The presence of thrombocytopenia or leukopenia in patients with chronic liver disease is associated with increased mortality.[37]

Ultrasound-guided fine-needle biopsy of the spleen can be useful in circumstances in which the spleen holds the tissue required for diagnosis, such as splenic lymphoma. However, fine-needle aspiration is rarely a definitive diagnostic tool but can indicate monoclonality of splenic lymphocytes, which is helpful and forces further diagnostic evaluation. Aspiration cytology and core biopsy can be obtained with relative safety in experienced hands using image-guided fine needles.[38]

The response to transfusion of blood products, especially platelets, may be significantly impaired in patients with massive splenomegaly.[39]

THERAPY, COURSE, AND PROGNOSIS

Total Splenectomy

Splenectomy is indicated as an emergency procedure after abdominal trauma and partial rupture of the spleen. It also may be indicated when splenic size or infarcts causes sustained left upper abdominal pain or discomfort. Splenectomy has been used for the treatment of functionally significant blood cytopenias.[39] In such circumstances, case reports have described dramatic restoration of blood counts to normal levels within days to weeks after splenectomy; however, the only controlled trial evaluating relief of cytopenias showed no improvement.[6] Orthotopic liver transplant corrects the cytopenias in the majority of patients with cirrhosis.[40]

Hereditary spherocytosis, immune thrombocytopenic purpura, and immune hemolytic anemia are the most common indications for splenectomy. Splenectomy exerts its effect in autoimmune cytopenias by improving cell survival and also by decreasing autoantibody production. In thalassemia major, an improvement in the anemia is well described after splenectomy. In such cases, splenectomy may improve the response to transfusion. Some children with sickle cell anemia may benefit from splenectomy if repeated sequestration crises with abdominal pain occur before autosplenectomy renders the spleen inactive.[41]

Splenectomy in patients with a massive spleen size (>1500 g), especially in primary myelofibrosis, is accompanied by higher morbidity and mortality than is removal of the spleen for immune blood cytopenia.[42] Possible postoperative complications include extensive adhesions with collateral blood vessels, hepatic or portal vein thrombosis, injury to the tail of the pancreas, operative site infections, and subdiaphragmatic abscesses.

Laparoscopic splenectomy performed by experienced surgeons for suitable hematologic conditions can result in less abdominal trauma and pain, shorter hospital stays, and smaller abdominal scars.[43] An advantage of open splenectomy in hematologic conditions such as the treatment of immune thrombocytopenic purpura is the increased ease of searching assiduously for accessory spleens.

Partial Splenectomy

Partial splenectomy has been explored because it may minimize the risks of immediate postsplenectomy thrombocytosis and overwhelming sepsis that may result from a complete absence of protective splenic filtering.[44] However, the degree of thrombocytosis after splenectomy wanes to some degree with time postsplenectomy. Reduction of the splenic volume has been performed with ligation of some of the splenic arteries or the intraarterial infusion of Gelfoam particles causing embolization.[45–48] These procedures induce large splenic infarcts and reduce the active splenic mass. Arterial embolization can be performed percutaneously or intravascularly, but the patients must be observed closely for a number of days to weeks to detect signs of intraabdominal rupture of the splenic infarcts. The long-term results of embolization have been encouraging.[46–48] Treatment with partial arterial embolization for recurrent thrombocytopenia in children temporarily improved the platelet count in approximately 70 percent of patients.[49]

Splenic Radiation

Splenic radiation for treatment of an enlarged spleen is used sparingly. The procedure may be associated with severe cytopenias and especially thrombocytopenia (abscopal effect). It can be used in patients with an absolute contraindication to splenectomy who might benefit symptomatically from reduction of a massively enlarged spleen.[50]

Liver Transplantation

Thrombopoietin synthesis and secretion are impaired in liver failure and this is corrected after liver transplantation.[51,52] However, thrombocytopenia may not be corrected after liver transplant if the splenomegaly persists.

Thrombopoietic Growth Factors

After thrombopoietin was cloned[53,54] several thrombopoietin mimetic drugs have been developed and tested. A phase II study reported that the nonpeptide thrombopoietin mimetic drug eltrombopag increases platelet counts in patients with thrombocytopenia as a result of hepatitis C virus-related cirrhosis.[55]

First-generation thrombopoietic drugs such as recombinant human thrombopoietin and pegylated human recombinant megakaryocyte growth and development factor (PEGrHuMGDF) are no longer being used as some patients had increased thrombocytopenia. Autoantibodies formed against PEGrHuMGDF cross-reacted with and neutralized endogenous thrombopoietin, producing thrombocytopenia in healthy human subjects.[56,57]

Erythropoietin and Granulocyte Colony-Stimulating Factor

There are minimal data to support the use of erythropoietic or myeloid growth factors in patients with splenomegaly and blood cytopenias. Patients with cirrhosis who have inappropriately low serum erythropoietin levels may benefit from treatment with exogenous erythropoietin; however, it may increase spleen size. Two reports documented the use of erythropoietin before and after liver transplantation to amplify marrow erythropoiesis in patients who refused blood transfusions for religious reasons.[58,59] These reports demonstrated that liver transplantation in the setting of advanced cirrhosis can be successfully undertaken without the use of blood products.

A rise in the neutrophil count after G-CSF administration was described. In one report, in patients with cirrhosis and leukopenia, the mean absolute neutrophil count increased from 1300 ± 200/μL to 4100 ± 200/μL following subcutaneous administration of G-CSF for 7 days.[19] However, the clinical benefit of such treatment is not clear.

HYPOSPLENISM

DEFINITION

Hyposplenism is the designation for decreased splenic function resulting from diseases that impair function or from the absence of splenic tissue because of agenesis, atrophy (e.g., autoinfarction of sickle cell disease), or splenectomy. Splenic hypofunction may be associated with a normal spleen size. In some cases, engorgement of ingested materials impairs the macrophage-dependent functions of the spleen. Impaired filtering function may cause a mild thrombocytosis. Functional or anatomical asplenia, especially after surgical removal in infants and children, increases the risk of an overwhelming bacterial infection. Table 55–3 lists conditions associated with hyposplenism.

TABLE 55–3. Conditions Associated with Hyposplenism

Miscellaneous
Surgical splenectomy
Splenic irradiation
Sickle hemoglobinopathies
Congenital asplenia
Thrombosis of splenic artery or vein
Normal infants
Gastrointestinal and hepatic diseases
Celiac disease
Dermatitis herpetiformis
Inflammatory bowel disease
Cirrhosis
Autoimmune disorders
Systemic lupus erythematosus
Rheumatoid arthritis
Vasculitis
Glomerulonephritis
Hashimoto thyroiditis
Sarcoidosis
Hematologic and neoplastic disorders
Graft-versus-host disease
Chronic lymphocytic leukemia
Non-Hodgkin lymphoma
Hodgkin lymphoma
Amyloidosis
Advanced breast cancer
Hemangiosarcoma
Sepsis/infectious diseases
Malaria
Disseminated meningococcemia

CLINICAL FEATURES

The normal neonate and the elderly adult may have findings suggestive of impaired splenic function.[60] These include the presence of Howell-Jolly bodies and erythrocyte pits (see "Laboratory Features" below). However, the clinical significance of functional hyposplenism is uncertain.[61–63]

Sickle cell anemia and surgical splenectomy are the most common causes of hyposplenism. In sickle cell anemia, hyposplenism may be functional in young children with enlarged spleens and disordered circulation and may be the result of atrophy after repeated infarcts have destroyed splenic tissue in older children and adults. Although the presence of an enlarged spleen usually suggests hypersplenism, spleen size is not a reliable index of splenic function. Complete splenic replacement by cysts, neoplastic tissue, or amyloid is an example of hyposplenic splenomegaly.[64] Acute sequestration crises in children with sickle hemoglobinopathies, and occasionally in patients with malaria, may clog the red cell pulp with cellular debris and lead to hyposplenism.[65,66]

Congenital asplenia may be found in infants with situs inversus and other developmental abnormalities.[38] Autoimmune disorders, such as glomerulonephritis,[67] systemic lupus erythematosus,[68,69] and rheumatoid arthritis,[70] are occasionally associated with laboratory evidence and clinical manifestations (overwhelming sepsis with encapsulated bacteria) of functional hyposplenism. Hyposplenism also occurs in chronic graft-versus-host disease,[71,72] sarcoidosis,[73] alcoholic liver cirrhosis,[74,75] hepatic amyloidosis,[76,77] celiac disease,[78,79] and in inflammatory bowel disease.[80,81] The mechanisms for these associations are unknown.

Splenic replacement by neoplastic cells, as in lymphomas and leukemias, usually does not cause hyper- or hyposplenism. Splenic irradiation[82] and vascular obstruction[83] may also lead to functional hyposplenism.

OVERWHELMING SEPSIS

Absence of a functional spleen may lead to life-threatening infections by removal of an efficient filtering bed in which opsonized organisms are destroyed by splenic macrophages. The responsible organism is typically an encapsulated bacteria, such as *Streptococcus pneumoniae*, *Neisseria meningitidis*, or *Haemophilus influenzae*. Unrestrained *in vivo* proliferation of such microorganisms may cause fatal septicemia.[84–86] The risk is greatest among infants whose general immunologic system has not matured enough to counteract bacterial infections, although the risk is present regardless of the patient's age. For this reason, splenectomy in children should be deferred until 5 years of age if possible. The risk of sepsis varies depending on the reason for the splenectomy. In a child with an underlying immune disorder, such as Wiskott-Aldrich syndrome, the risk is very high. The infectious risk is higher in children with thalassemia than in those with hereditary spherocytosis and lowest in those with splenectomy for splenic trauma. The risk is reduced by the use of pneumococcal and *H. influenzae* vaccines prior to splenectomy and prophylactic penicillin therapy.[87]

Because the spleen is a major component of the mononuclear phagocyte system and has substantial lymphatic tissue in the white pulp, hyposplenism or splenectomy can also reduce antibody synthesis that may be beneficial in autoimmune disorders.

LABORATORY FEATURES

The reduction or absence of normal splenic function is accompanied by a slight to moderate increase in white cell and platelet counts. Howell-Jolly bodies, target cells, Pappenheimer bodies, and occasional acanthocytes often are present in the blood film (see Chap. 29) but the finding of pitted erythrocytes in wet preparations is the most specific of all the blood findings.[88] Target cells reflecting an increased red cell surface[89] are almost always present in the asplenic state, but only 1:100 to 1:1000 red cells is affected. A sensitive indication of hyposplenism is the appearance of pits or pocks on the cell surface.[90] These pits consist of submembranous vacuoles and can be seen only in wet preparations of red cells using direct interference-contrast microscopy. Intracellular vesiculation containing hemoglobin is a normal occurrence during aging of the red cell in the circulation. This process is intensified in the last half of the erythrocyte life span and leads to a decreased mean cell hemoglobin level as the vesicles are removed (pitted) by the spleen. In asplenic individuals the vesicles are more numerous and enlarge, forming vacuoles that are evident by interference-phase microscopy.[88] This finding is the most specific evidence of hyposplenism, followed by the presence of DNA inclusions in circulating red cells (Howell-Jolly bodies; Fig. 55–1).

Oxidative drugs may produce Heinz bodies even in normal individuals, but the spleen effectively removes these red cell inclusions, as well as Pappenheimer bodies (see Chap. 29). Heinz bodies may be observed in supravitally stained blood films after splenectomy. Nucleated red cells rarely are seen on blood films after splenectomy, except in patients with hemolytic disorders in whom the number of nucleated red cells may increase dramatically. The reticulocyte count remains within normal values, and the life span of red cells is unchanged as other organs take up the function of removing senescent erythrocytes.

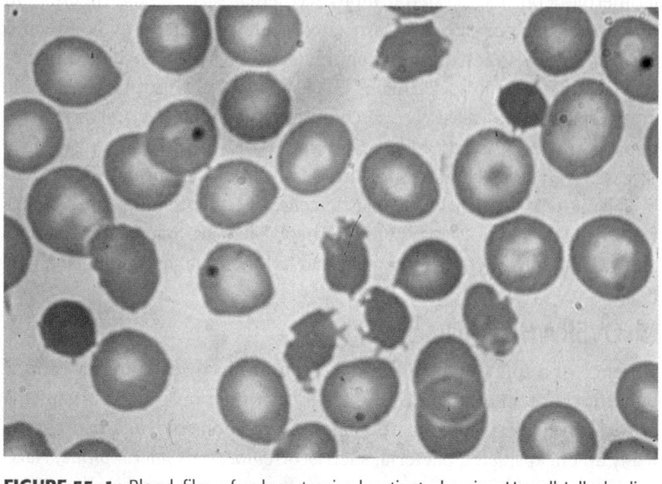

FIGURE 55–1. Blood film of splenectomized patient showing Howell-Jolly bodies. Note also the acanthocytes and occasional target cell. These also are characteristic postsplenectomy red cell changes. *(Used with permission from* Lichtman's Atlas of Hematology, *www.accessmedicine.com.)*

Technetium-99m sulfur-colloid particles are used for spleen scanning, a reliable measure of the capacity of the spleen to clear particulate matter from the bloodstream.[91]

THERAPY, COURSE, AND PROGNOSIS

Vaccination against *H. influenzae*, *N. meningitidis*, and *S. pneumoniae* is recommended in previously unvaccinated individuals prior to splenectomy.[92] Prophylactic immunization has significantly reduced, but not eliminated, the risk of overwhelming infection.[87,93–95] Oral penicillin or a macrolide as prophylaxis for asplenic patients is recommended based on publicized guidelines despite problems with compliance and resistance.[96,97] Physicians should advise all asplenic patients that any febrile episode (>38°C) should be considered an emergency requiring immediate medical attention. A febrile asplenic patient must have blood and urine cultures drawn, followed by antibiotic treatment. Patients should be given written information about asplenia and carry a card or medical alert bracelet to alert health professionals of the risk of overwhelming infection.[96,97] Dental work, especially tooth extraction, should be preceded by broad spectrum antibiotics, such as amoxicillin, if the patient is not taking prophylactic antibiotics. Patients should be educated about risks of travel, including risk of malaria infection or animal bites, which could be deadly unless promptly treated.[96,97]

REFERENCES

1. Crosby WH: The spleen, in *Blood, Pure and Eloquent*, edited by MM Wintrobe, p 96. McGraw-Hill, New York, 1980.
2. Chauffard AME: Des hepatites d'origine splenique. *Semin Med* 19:177, 1899.
3. Sutherland GA, Burghard FF: The treatment of splenic anaemia by splenectomy. *Lancet* 2:1819, 1910.
4. Kaznelson P: Verschwinden der hamorrhagischen Diathesis bei einen falle von "Essentieller Thrombopenia." *Wien Klin Wochenschr* 29:1451, 1916.
5. Crosby WH: Hypersplenism. *Annu Rev Med* 13:127, 1962.
6. Mutchnick MG, Lerner E, Conn HO: Effect of portacaval anastomosis on hypersplenism. *Dig Dis Sci* 25:929, 1980.
7. Jabbour N, Zajko A, Orons P, et al: Does transjugular intrahepatic portosystemic shunt (TIPS) resolve thrombocytopenia associated with cirrhosis? *Dig Dis Sci* 43:2459, 1998.
8. Roberts CW, Shutter JR, Korsmeyer SJ: Hox11 controls the genesis of the spleen. *Nature* 368:747, 1994.
9. Dear TN, Colledge WH, Carlton MB, et al: The Hox11 gene is essential for cell survival during spleen development. *Development* 121:2909, 1995.
10. Roberts CW, Sonder AM, Lumsden A, et al: Developmental expression of HOV11 and specification of splenic cell fate. *Am J Pathol* 146:1089, 1995.
11. Steininger B, Barth P, Herbst B, et al: The species-specific structure of microanatomical compartments in the human spleen. *Immunology* 92:307, 1997.
12. Bourdessoule D, Gaulard P, Mason DY: Preferential localization of human lymphocytes bearing −/− T cell receptors to the red pulp of the spleen. *J Clin Pathol* 43:461, 1990.
13. Kraus MD: Splenic histology and histopathology: An update. *Semin Diagn Pathol* 20:84, 2003.
14. Rosse WF: The spleen as a filter [editorial]. *N Engl J Med* 317:704, 1987.
15. Bowdler AJ: Splenomegaly and hypersplenism. *Clin Haematol* 12:467, 1983.
16. Areas Elenas N, Ewald R, Crosby WH: The reservoir function of the spleen and its relation to postsplenectomy anemia of the dog. *Blood* 24:299, 1964.
17. Wadenvik H, Kutti J: The spleen and pooling of blood cells. *Eur J Haematol* 41:1, 1988.
18. Aster RH: Pooling of platelets in the spleen: Role in the pathogenesis of "hypersplenic thrombocytopenia." *J Clin Invest* 45:645, 1966.
19. Gurakar A, Fagiuoli S, Gavaler JS, et al: The use of granulocyte-macrophage colony-stimulating factor to enhance hematologic parameters of patients with cirrhosis and hypersplenism. *J Hepatol* 21:582, 1994.
20. Karpatkin S: The spleen and thrombocytopenia. *Clin Haematol* 12:591, 1983.
21. Zwiebel WJ, Mountford RA, Halliwell MJ, Wells PN: Splanchnic blood flow in patients with cirrhosis and portal hypertension: Investigation with duplex Doppler US. *Radiology* 194:807, 1995.
22. Brubaker LH, Johnson CA: Correlation of splenomegaly and abnormal neutrophil pooling (margination). *J Lab Clin Med* 92:508, 1978.
23. Siciliano M, Tomasello D, Milani A, et al: Reduced serum levels of immunoreactive erythropoietin in patients with cirrhosis and chronic anemia. *Hepatology* 22:1132, 1995.

24. Vasilopoulos S, Hally R, Caro J, et al: Erythropoietin response to post-liver transplantation anemia. *Liver Transpl* 6:349, 2000.
25. Hess CE, Ayers CR, Sandusky WR, et al: Mechanism of dilutional anemia in massive splenomegaly. *Blood* 47:629, 1976.
26. Zhang B, Lewis SM: Splenic hematocrit and the splenic plasma pool. *Br J Haematol* 66:97, 1987.
27. Jandl JH: The anemia of liver disease: Observations on its mechanism. *J Clin Invest* 34:390, 1955.
28. Christensen BE: Quantitative determination of splenic red cell blood destruction in patients with splenomegaly. *Scand J Haematol* 14:295, 1975.
29. McIntyre OR, Ebaugh FA: Palpable spleens in college freshmen. *Ann Intern Med* 66:301, 1967.
30. Sty JR, Wells RG: Imaging the spleen, in *Disorders of the Spleen: Pathophysiology and Management*, edited by C Pochedly, RH Sills, AD Schwartz, p 355. Marcel Dekker, New York, 1989.
31. Buehner M, Baker MS: The wandering spleen. *Surg Gynecol Obstet* 175:373, 1992.
32. Joyce RA, Boggs DR, Hasiba U, Srodes CH: Marginal neutrophil in the pool size in normal subjects as measured by epinephrine infusion. *J Lab Clin Med* 88:614, 1976.
33. Alvarez OA, Lopera GA, Patel V, et al: Improvement of thrombocytopenia due to hypersplenism after transjugular intrahepatic portosystemic shunt placement in cirrhotic patients. *Am J Gastroenterol* 91:134, 1996.
34. Peck-Radosavljevic M: Hypersplenism. *Eur J Gastroenterol Hepatol* 13:317, 2001.
35. Bashour FN, Teran JC, Mullen KD: Prevalence of peripheral blood cytopenias (hypersplenism) in patients with nonalcoholic chronic liver disease. *Am J Gastroenterol* 95:2936, 2000.
36. Liangpunsakul S, Ulmer BJ, Chalasani N: Predictors and implications of severe hypersplenism in patients with cirrhosis. *Am J Med Sci* 326:111, 2003.
37. Qamar A, Grace N, Groszmann R, et al: Incidence, prevalence and clinical significance of abnormal hematological indices in compensated cirrhosis. *Clin Gastroenterol Hepatol* 7:689, 2009.
38. Civardi G, Vallisa D, Berte R, et al: Ultrasound guided fine needle biopsy of the spleen: High clinical efficacy and low risk in a multicenter Italian study. *Am J Hematol* 67:93, 2001.
39. Pochedly C, Sills RH, Schwartz A: *Disorders of the Spleen: Pathophysiology and Management*. Marcel Dekker, New York, 1989.
40. Yanaga K, Tzakis A, Shimade M, Campbell W, et al: Reversal of hypersplenism following orthotopic liver transplantation *Ann Surg* 210:180, 1989.
41. Al-Salem AH, Qaisaruddin S, Nasserallah Z, et al: Splenectomy in patients with sickle-cell disease. *Am J Surg* 172:254, 1996.
42. Mohren M, Markman I, Dworschak U, et al: Thromboembolic complications after splenectomy for hematologic diseases. *Am J Hematol* 76:143, 2004.
43. Caprotti R, Porta G, Franciosi C, et al: Laparoscopic splenectomy for hematological disorders. *Int Surg* 83:303, 1998.
44. Bar-Moor JA: Partial splenectomy in Gaucher's disease. *J Pediatr Surg* 28:686, 1993.
45. Banani SA: Partial dearterialization of the spleen in thalassemia major. *J Pediatr Surg* 33:449, 1998.
46. Stanley P, Shen TC: Partial embolization of the spleen in patients with thalassemia. *J Vasc Interv Radiol* 6:137, 1995.
47. Palsson B, Hallen M, Forsberg AM, Alwmark A: Partial splenic embolization: Long-term outcome. *Langenbecks Arch Surg* 387:421, 2003.
48. Petersons A, Volrats O, Bernsteins A: The first experience with nonoperative treatment of hypersplenism in children with portal hypertension. *Eur J Pediatr Surg* 12:299, 2002.
49. Watanabe Y, Todani T, Noda T: Changes in splenic volume after partial splenic embolization in children. *J Pediatr Surg* 31:241, 1996.
50. Paulino AC, Reddy AC: Splenic irradiation in the palliation of patients with lymphoproliferative and myeloproliferative disorders. *Am J Hosp Palliat Care* 13:32, 1996.
51. Peck-Radosavljevic M, Wichlas M, Zacherl J, et al: Thrombopoietin induces rapid resolution of thrombocytopenia after orthotopic liver transplantation through increased platelet production. *Blood* 95:795, 2000.
52 Rios R, Sangro B, Herrero I, et al: The role of thrombopoietin in the thrombocytopenia of patients with liver cirrhosis. *Am J Gastroenterol* 100:1311, 2005.
53. Lok S, Kaushansky K, Holly RD, et al: Cloning and expression of murine thrombopoietin cDNA and stimulation of platelet production *in vivo*. *Nature* 369:565, 1994.
54. de Sauvage FJ, Hass PE, Spencer SD, et al: Stimulation of megakaryocytopoiesis and thrombopoiesis by the c-Mpl ligand. *Nature* 369:533, 1994.
55. McHutchinson JG, Dusheiko G, Shiffman ML, et al: Eltrombopag in patients with cirrosis associated with hepatitis C. *N Engl J Med* 357:2227, 2007.
56. Li J, Yang C, Xia Y, et al: Thrombocytopenia caused by the development of antibodies to thrombopoietin. *Blood* 98:3241, 2001.
57. Basser RL, O'Flaherty E, Green M, et al: Development of pancytopenia with neutralizing antibodies to thrombopoietin after multicycle chemotherapy supported by megakaryocyte growth and development factor. *Blood* 99:2599, 2002.
58. Ramos H, Todo S, Kang Y, et al: Liver transplantation without the use of blood products. *Arch Surg* 129:528, 1994.
59. Snook NJ, O'Beirne HA, Enright S, et al: Use of recombinant human erythropoietin to facilitate liver transplantation in a Jehovah's Witness. *Br J Anaesth* 76:740,1996.
60. Freedman RM, Johnston D, Mahoney MJ, et al: Development of splenic reticuloendothelial function in neonates. *J Pediatr* 96:466, 1980.
61. Padmanabhan J, Risemberg HM, Rome RD: Howell-Jolly bodies in the peripheral blood of full-term and premature neonates. *Johns Hopkins Med J* 132:146, 1973.
62. Markus HS, Toghill PJ: Impaired splenic function in elderly people. *Age Ageing* 20:287, 1991.
63. Ravaglia G, Forti P, Biagi F, et al: Splenic function in old age. *Gerontology* 44:91, 1998.
64. Steinberg MH, Gatling RR, Tavassoli M: Evidence of hyposplenism in the presence of splenomegaly. *Scand J Haematol* 31:437, 1983.
65. Looareesuwan S, Ho M, Wallanagoon Y, et al: Dynamic alteration in splenic function during acute falciparum malaria. *N Engl J Med* 317: 675, 1987.
66. Emond AM, Callis R, Darvill D, et al: Acute splenic sequestration in homozygous sickle cell disease: Natural history and management. *J Pediatr* 107:201, 1985.
67. Lawrence SE, Pussell BA, Charlesworth JA: Splenic function in primary glomerulonephritis. *Adv Exp Med Biol* 641:1, 1982.
68. Webster J, Williams BD, Smith AP, et al: Systemic lupus erythematosus presenting as pneumococcal septicemia and septic arthritis. *Ann Rheum Dis* 49:181, 1990.
69. Liote F, Angle J, Gilmore N, Osterland CK: Asplenism and systemic lupus erythematosus. *Clin Rheumatol* 14:220, 1995.
70. Jarolim DR: Asplenia and rheumatoid arthritis [letter]. *Ann Intern Med* 97:61, 1982.
71. Kalhs P, Panzer S, Kletter K, et al: Functional asplenia after bone marrow transplantation. *Ann Intern Med* 109:461, 1988.
72. Cuthbert RJ, Iqbal A, Gates A, et al: Functional hyposplenism following allogeneic bone marrow transplantation. *J Clin Pathol* 48:257, 1995.
73. Stone RW, McDaniel WR, Armstrong EM, et al: Acquired functional asplenia in sarcoidosis. *J Natl Med Assoc* 77:930, 1985.
74. Muller AF, Toghill PJ: Splenic function in alcoholic liver disease. *Gut* 33:1386, 1992.
75. Muller AF, Toghill PJ: Functional hyposplenism in alcoholic liver disease: A toxic effect of alcohol? *Gut* 35:679, 1994.
76. Gertz MA, Kyle RA: Hepatic amyloidosis (primary [AL], immunoglobulin light chain): The natural history in 80 patients. *Am J Med* 85:73, 1988.
77. Powsner RA, Simms RW, Chudnovsky A, et al: Scintigraphic functional hyposplenism in amyloidosis. *J Nucl Med* 39:221, 1998.
78. Robinson PJ, Bullen AW, Hall R, et al: Splenic size and functions in adult coeliac disease. *Br J Radiol* 53:532, 1980.
79. O'Grady JG, Stevens FM, Harding B, et al: Hyposplenism and gluten sensitive enteropathy. *Gastroenterology* 87:1316, 1984.
80. Palmer KR, Sherriff SB, Holdsworth CD, et al: Further experience of hyposplenism in inflammatory bowel disease. *Q J Med* 50:461, 1981.
81. Muller AF, Toghill PJ: Hyposplenism in gastrointestinal disease. *Gut* 36:165, 1995.
82. Dailey MO, Coleman CN, Kaplan HS: Radiation-induced splenic atrophy in patients with Hodgkin disease and non-Hodgkin lymphoma. *N Engl J Med* 302:215, 1990.
83. Spencer RP, Sziklas JJ, Turner JW: Functional obstruction of splenic blood vessel in adults: A radiocolloid study. *Int J Nucl Med Biol* 9:208, 1982.
84. Torres J, Bisno AL: Hyposplenism and pneumococcemia. *Am J Med* 55:851, 1973.
85. Cavenagh JD, Joseph AE, Dilly S, Bevan DH: Splenic sepsis in sickle cell disease. *Br J Haematol* 86:187, 1994.
86. Gopal V, Bisno AL: Fulminant pneumococcal infections in "normal" asplenic hosts. *Arch Intern Med* 137:1526, 1977.
87. Konradsen HB, Henrichsen J: Pneumococcal infections in splenectomized children are preventable. *Acta Paediatr Scand* 80:423, 1991.
88. Corazza GR, Ginaldi L, Zoli G, et al: Howell-Jolly body counting as a measure of splenic function: A reassessment. *Clin Lab Haematol* 12:269, 1990.
89. Holroyde CP, Oski FA, Gardner FH: The "pocked" erythrocytes. *N Engl J Med* 281:516, 1969.
90. Reinhart WH, Chien S: Red cell vacuoles: Their size and distribution under normal conditions and after splenectomy. *Am J Hematol* 27:265, 1988.
91. Rutland MD: Correlation of splenic function with the splenic uptake rate of Tc-colloids. *Nucl Med Commun* 13:843, 1992.
92. Kobel DE, Friedl A, Cerny T, et al: Pneumococcal vaccine in patients with absent or dysfunctional spleen. *Mayo Clin Proc* 75:749, 2000.
93. Ward KM, Celebi JT, Gmyrek R, Grossman ME: Acute infectious purpura fulminans associated with asplenism or hyposplenism. *J Am Acad Dermatol* 47:493, 2002.
94. Sumaraju V, Smith LG, Smith SM: Infectious complications in asplenic hosts. *Infect Dis Clin North Am* 15:551, 2001.
95. Castagnola E, Fioredda F: Prevention of life-threatening infections due to encapsulated bacteria in children with hyposplenia or asplenia: A brief review of current recommendations for practical purposes. *Eur J Haematol* 71:319, 2003.
96. Guidelines for the prevention and treatment of infection in patients with an absent or dysfunctional spleen. *BMJ* 312:430, 1996.
97. Davies JM, Barnes R, Milligan D: Update of guidelines for the prevention and treatment of infection in patients with an absent or dysfunctional spleen. *Clin Med* 2:440, 2002.

CHAPTER 56
PRIMARY AND SECONDARY POLYCYTHEMIAS (ERYTHROCYTOSIS)

Josef T. Prchal

SUMMARY

Polycythemia is characterized by an increased red cell volume. Primary polycythemias are caused by acquired or inherited mutations causing changes within hematopoietic stem cells or erythroid progenitors, leading to an accumulation of red cells. The most common primary polycythemia, polycythemia rubra vera, which is a clonal disorder, is discussed in Chap. 86, but other inherited polycythemias, such as mutations in the von Hippel-Lindau (*VHL*) gene or in the erythropoietin receptor (*EPOR*) gene are discussed herein. In contrast, secondary polycythemias are caused by either an appropriate or inappropriate increase in the red cell mass as a result of augmented levels of erythropoietin; these polycythemias can also be either acquired or hereditary. Although the clinical presentations of primary and secondary polycythemias may be quite similar, distinguishing among them is important for accurate diagnoses and proper management.

For example, many secondary polycythemic states represent an appropriate physiologic compensation to tissue hypoxia, and it is unwise to treat these by phlebotomies. There is no solid evidence that either congenital or acquired primary or secondary polycythemias benefit from phlebotomies; however, an occasional patient may experience hyperviscosity symptoms and may benefit from isovolemic reduction of hematocrit. Enalapril controls post-renal transplantation erythrocytosis, and resection of erythropoietin-secreting tumors typically corrects the associated polycythemia.

DEFINITION AND HISTORY

The term *polycythemia,* denoting an increased amount of blood, has traditionally been applied to those conditions in which the mass of erythrocytes is increased. Erythrocytosis is an alternative term that has been applied to an increase in red cell mass. Although this usage has much to recommend it, no consensus about terminology has been reached. Many physicians use erythrocytosis interchangeably with polycythemia. In some instances, however, time-honored terms such as post-renal transplantation erythrocytosis will be used. A classification of the polycythemias is presented in Chap. 33 in Table 33–2.

Acronyms and abbreviations used in this chapter include: *AR*, human androgen-receptor gene; 2,3-BPG, 2,3-bisphosphoglycerate; COPD, chronic obstructive pulmonary disease; EPOR, erythropoietin receptor (protein); *EPOR*, erythropoietin receptor (gene); HIF-1, hypoxia-inducible factor; JAK, Janus-type tyrosine kinase; PAI-1, plasminogen activator inhibitor; PFCP, primary familial and congenital polycythemia; PHD2, proline hydroxylase 2; STAT, signal transducer and activator of transcription; VEGF, vascular endothelial growth factor; VHL, von Hippel-Lindau syndrome.

PRIMARY POLYCYTHEMIAS

Polycythemia vera (see Chap. 86) and *primary familial and congenital polycythemia* (PFCP) are primary polycythemic disorders with erythroid progenitors that are hypersensitive to erythropoietin.[1–3] These are a result of somatic (polycythemia vera) or germ-line (PFCP) mutations that are intrinsic to erythropoietic progenitors and result in an augmented response to erythropoietin. Some congenital polycythemias, as best described in Chuvash polycythemia, have erythroid progenitors that are hypersensitive to erythropoietin but also may have normal or even increased erythropoietin levels despite the increased red cell volume.[4,5] Thus, these rare, inherited polycythemias share features of both primary and secondary polycythemias.[6]

SECONDARY POLYCYTHEMIAS

The term *secondary polycythemias,* more appropriately *secondary erythrocytosis,* refers to those conditions in which only erythrocytes are increased in number and volume. Although the term *secondary erythrocytosis* is more descriptive of this group of disorders, secondary polycythemia is a time-honored name and is used interchangeably with secondary erythrocytosis. *Secondary polycythemia* is a term that describes a group of disorders characterized by an increased red cell mass brought about by enhanced stimulation of red cell production by a physiologic mediator such as erythropoietin. Secondary polycythemia may be subdivided into *appropriate polycythemia* responding normally to tissue hypoxia (i.e., high-altitude polycythemia and hemoglobins with increased affinity for oxygen affinity), and *inappropriate polycythemia* in which erythropoiesis is being stimulated by the aberrant production of erythropoietin-secreting tumors or in response to erythropoietin or other stimulators of erythropoiesis (i.e., post-renal transplantation erythrocytosis).[6]

In his important monograph on barometric pressure published in 1878, Paul Bert showed that physiologic impairment observed at high altitude was caused by a reduction in the oxygen content of the air.[7] A few years earlier, his friend and mentor Dennis Jourdanet had observed an increase in the number of red corpuscles in the blood of the highlanders of Mexico,[8] and Bert recognized that such an increase would tend to ameliorate the effect of atmospheric hypoxia. However, neither Bert nor Jourdanet suspected a cause-and-effect relationship. It was not until 1890, when Viault[9] observed a prompt increase in the number of his own red corpuscles after having traveled from Lima, Peru, at sea level, to Morococha, at 4570 m (15,000 ft) above sea level, that altitude erythrocytosis was accepted as a compensatory adaptation to hypoxia.[10] At about the same time, it was observed that many patients with cyanosis were also polycythemic. Both *cardiacos negros* (Ayerza syndrome),[11] with severe pulmonary failure and arterial oxygen desaturation, and children with *morbus caeruleus,* or right-to-left shunt through a congenital cardiac malformation, were found to have increased red cell counts.[12] Mechanical or neurogenic hypoventilation as a cause of cyanosis and polycythemia was first popularized in 1956 with the classic description of the pickwickian syndrome by Burwell and associates[13] Polycythemia associated with carboxyhemoglobinuria resulting in hypoxemia because of smoking, and with tissue hypoxia as a result of inherited abnormal hemoglobins with high oxygen binding to hemoglobin, was recognized more recently.[14] Erythrocytosis associated with abnormal hemoglobins with an increased affinity to oxygen also represents an appropriate response to hypoxia first noted by Charache and colleagues[14] in 1966 when they described hemoglobin Chesapeake.

In addition to appropriate and inappropriate secondary polycythemias, the cause of relative erythrocytosis is often known, that is, diuretic use, dehydration from excessive sweating, and so forth. However, there are some patients with mild erythrocytosis in which neither the cause nor the clinical significance is clear. These patients do not have an increased red cell mass, and their erythrocytosis is the result of decreased plasma volume. Consequently, the disorder is not a true polycythemia and is designated *apparent, spurious,* or *relative polycythemia.* In 1905, Gaisbock reported that a number of hypertensive patients had plethora and an elevated red cell count but no splenomegaly, a condition he termed *polycythemia hypertonica,* sometimes called *Gaisbock syndrome.*[15] In 1952, direct measurement of blood volume in patients with polycythemia led Lawrence and Berlin to identify a subgroup of patients with a normal red cell volume but reduced plasma volume. Although some members of this group were hypertensive, the authors were more impressed by their tense and anxious behavior and coined the term *stress polycythemia.*[16]

EPIDEMIOLOGY

PRIMARY POLYCYTHEMIAS

Primary Familial and Congenital Polycythemia

This autosomal dominant disorder (designated PFCP) is uncommon. However, they are more prevalent than is generally appreciated, as many affected subjects are initially misdiagnosed as having polycythemia vera. By this estimate, its prevalence is similar to congenital polycythemias caused by high oxygen affinity hemoglobin mutants and more common than 2,3-biphosphoglycerate deficiency.[17]

SECONDARY POLYCYTHEMIAS

Inappropriate Tissue Elaboration of Erythropoietin

The prevalence of the various types of secondary polycythemia is a function of the underlying cause, such as the geographical location of the patient or the presence of a causative neoplasm. Approximately 1 to 3 percent of all patients with pheochromocytoma/paraganglioma have erythrocytosis.[18] Rare patients with congenital erythrocytosis will develop pheochromocytoma or paraganglioma.[19] While uterine leiomyomas in premenopausal women are very common, having been estimated at 20 to 40 percent, the occurrence of erythrocytosis ranges from 0.02 to 0.5 percent of cases of leiomyoma.[20] Isolated instances of polycythemia have been attributed to a myxoma of the atrium,[21] hamartoma of the liver,[22] and focal hyperplasia of the liver.[23] Erythrocytosis and inappropriate secretions of erythropoietin may be found in approximately 15 percent of patients with cerebellar hemangiomas.[24,25]

Post-Renal Transplantation Erythrocytosis

This syndrome, defined as a persistent elevation of the hematocrit over 51 percent, is a relatively common condition found in approximately 5 to 10 percent of renal allograft recipients.[26,27] Post-renal transplantation erythrocytosis usually develops within 8 to 24 months after transplantation, despite persistently good function of the allograft, and resolves spontaneously within 2 years in approximately 25 percent of patients.[28] Factors that increase the likelihood of its development are lack of erythropoietin therapy prior to transplantation, a history of smoking, diabetes mellitus, renal artery stenosis, low serum ferritin levels, and normal or higher pretransplantation erythropoietin levels. Post-renal transplantation erythrocytosis is also more frequent in patients who are not undergoing graft rejection.

Chuvash Polycythemia

A Russian hematologist, Lydia A. Polyakova, described polycythemia in the Chuvash population (an ethnic isolate in the mid–Volga River region of Russia of Asian descent) in the early 1960s,[29] and by 1974, 103 cases from 81 families had been described.[29] Since then, more cases have come to light; hundreds of children and adults suffer from this condition, indicating that Chuvash polycythemia is the only known endemic congenital polycythemia in the world.[30] Outside of Chuvashia, Chuvash polycythemia (CP) has also been found sporadically in diverse ethnic and racial groups,[31,32] and a high prevalence of this disorder has been reported on the Italian island of Ischia.[33]

ETIOLOGY AND PATHOGENESIS

PRIMARY POLYCYTHEMIAS

Primary Familial and Congenital Polycythemia

In contrast to polycythemia vera, PFCP is caused by germ-line rather than somatic mutations. It is congenital and manifests autosomal dominant inheritance[3] and, less frequently, sporadic occurrence. Like polycythemia vera (see Chap. 86), it is primary in that the defect is in the erythroid progenitor and erythropoietin levels are low.

To date, 12 mutations of the erythropoietin receptor (*EPOR*) gene associated with PFCP have been described (Table 56–1). Nine of the 12 result in truncation of the EPOR cytoplasmic carboxyl-terminal, and are the only mutations convincingly linked with PFCP. Such truncations lead to a loss in the negative regulatory domain of the EPOR (see Chaps. 31 and 33). Three missense *EPOR* mutations have also been described, but these have not been linked to PFCP or any other disease phenotype (Table 56–1).

Erythropoietin-mediated activation of erythropoiesis involves several steps (also see Chap. 31). First, erythropoietin activates its receptor by inducing conformational changes of its dimers. These changes lead to initiation of an erythroid-specific cascade of events. The first signal is initiated by conformation change induced activation of Janus-type

TABLE 56–1. Summary of Erythropoietin Receptor Gene Mutations

Type of Mutation	Mutation	Structural Defect	Association with PFCP	Reference
Deletion (7bp)	Del5985–5991	Frameshift > ter truncation	Yes	136, 163
Duplication (8bp)	5968–5975	Frameshift > ter truncation	Yes	193
Nonsense	G6002	Trp439 > ter truncation	Yes	194
Nonsense	5986 *C*→*T*	Gln435 > ter truncation	Yes	195
Nonsense	5964*C*→*G*	Tyr426 > ter truncation	Yes	135
Nonsense	5881*C*→*T*	Glu399 > ter truncation	Yes	196
Nonsense	5959*G*→*T*	Glu425 > ter truncation	Yes	197
Insertion (G)	5974insG	Frameshift > ter truncation	Yes	198
Insertion (T)	5967insT	Frameshift > ter truncation	Yes	199
Substitution	6148*C*→*T*	Pro 488 > Ser	No	163, 200
Substitution	6146*A*→*G*	Asn487 > Ser	No	201
Substitution	2706*A*→*T*	Unknown	No	197

Ter, termination codon.

SOURCE: Adapted with permission from Kralovics R, Indrak K, Stopka T, et al.[163]

tyrosine kinase (JAK) 2 and its phosphorylation and activation of a transcription factor, signal transducer and activator of transcription (STAT) 5, which regulates erythroid-specific genes. This "on" signal is negated by dephosphorylation of the EPOR by the hematopoietic phosphatase (also known as SHP1), that is, the "off" signal. EPOR truncations lead to a loss of the negative regulatory domain of the EPOR, a binding site for hematopoietic cell phosphatase, leading to a gain-of-function mutation of the *EPOR* (Fig. 56–1).

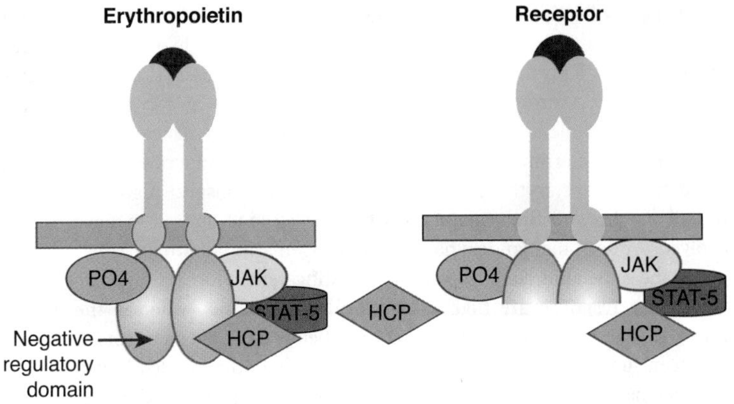

FIGURE 56–1. *Left panel:* Erythropoietin binding to a normal erythropoietin receptor results in interaction of a protein kinase (JAK) with the receptor. The interaction leads to phosphorylation of the receptor and initiates a cascade of signaling that ultimately results in erythroid progenitor proliferation and differentiation. This process is self-regulatory. Activated signal transduction molecules, hematopoietic cell phosphatase binds to the C-terminal of the EPOR, which is a negative regulatory domain. This interaction dephosphorylates the receptor and turns off the signaling resulting in cessation of erythroid progenitor proliferation. *Right panel:* Patients with mutated gain-of-function *EPOR* gene lack the C-terminal portion of the receptor that contains the negative regulatory domain. Erythropoietin binds and the signal transduction pathway is activated by change of configuration of erythropoietin receptor dimer, but because there is no structure for hematopoietic cell phosphatase to bind on the activated erythropoietin receptor dimer, the receptor is left in the activated position, resulting in unbridled erythroid proliferation and an elevated red cell mass.

SECONDARY POLYCYTHEMIAS

The morbidity of polycythemia vera (discussed in Chap. 86) is largely a result of increased activated neutrophils and perhaps attendant pathologic platelet–endothelial interactions, whereas in secondary polycythemias, it is presumably related to the increase in blood viscosity.[34] However, the effect of blood viscosity on oxygen delivery is often oversimplified, and the emphasis on the hematocrit alone may lead to ill-advised therapeutic interventions. In the normovolemic state, the viscosity increases in a log-linear fashion as hematocrit increases and the effect is particularly pronounced when the hematocrit rises above 50 percent. Absolute polycythemia is not a normovolemic state, however, but is accompanied by an increase in blood volume, which, in turn, enlarges the vascular bed and decreases the peripheral resistance (see Chap. 33). Thus hypervolemia can increase oxygen transport, and the optimum for oxygen transport occurs at higher hematocrit values than in normovolemic states. Consequently, despite the attendant increase in viscosity, an increase in hematocrit may generally be of benefit in appropriate secondary polycythemias. However, at some point, the high viscosity causes an increase in the work of the heart and a reduction in blood flow to most tissues and may be responsible for cerebral and cardiovascular impairment.

Appropriate Polycythemias

High-Altitude Polycythemia Adaptive adjustments of humans living at high altitude involve a series of steps that reduce the steepness of the oxygen gradient between the atmosphere and the mitochondria (Fig. 56–2).[35] The initial oxygen gradient between atmospheric and alveolar air can be reduced by an increase in respiratory rate and volume. Because dead space and water vapor pressure are constant and acclimatized individuals do not ventilate excessively, the normal sea level gradient of about 60 torr is only reduced to about 40 torr at Morococha at 4540 m (14,900 ft) above sea level.[35] Further reduction can be achieved, and at the top of Mount Everest, extreme hyperventilation reduces the gradient to less than 10 torr. A shift in the oxygen dissociation curve to the right, which represents decreased affinity of hemoglobin for oxygen, may be of benefit for short-term high-altitude acclimatization,[36] but its usefulness for chronic acclimatization has probably been exaggerated.[37] In the unacclimatized subject exposed acutely to high altitude, hyperventilation alkalosis leads initially to a shift of the oxygen dissociation curve to the left, representing an increased affinity of hemoglobin for oxygen, and to additional tissue hypoxia. The alkalosis and the hypoxia will in turn promote red cell synthesis of 2,3-bisphosphoglycerate (2,3-BPG) and cause the oxygen dissociation curve to shift back to a normal or even a right-shifted position (Chap. 48). In chronic acclimatization, the blood pH is slightly increased, and when this is taken into account the dissociation curve is shifted approximately to normal.[38] It seems questionable if a shift to the right would be to the advantage of high-altitude dwellers.[39] There is a relationship between higher altitude and hemoglobin concentration response, best studied among Andean highlanders, and Europeans in the United States; hemoglobin concentration is almost 10 percent higher in those Andean highlanders living at 5500 m than in those living at 4355 m. Furthermore, Andean high-altitude native dwellers have a gradual increase in their hemoglobin levels with age[40] and with body weight.[41]

In a subset of Andean high-altitude native dwellers, Quechua and Ayamara Indians, polycythemia becomes excessive and, in some cases, results in chronic mountain sickness with its associated constitutional symptoms and pulmonary hypertension.[40,42] This excessive erythrocytosis, called Monge disease or chronic mountain sickness,[42,43] is also described in Han Chinese living in Tibet[44] and occurs in whites living in high altitudes.[45]

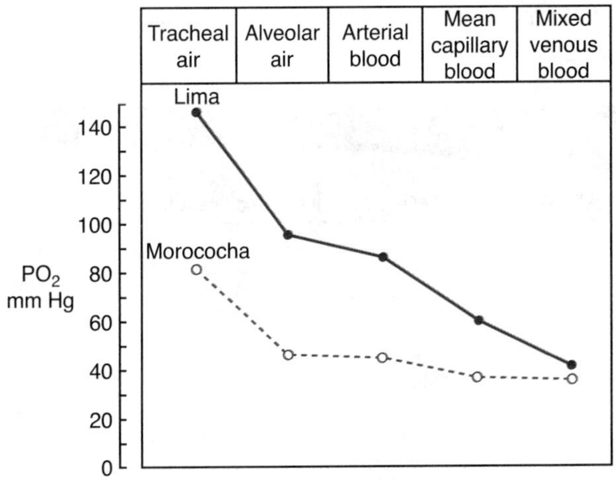

FIGURE 56–2. The oxygen gradient from atmospheric air to the tissues in individuals living at sea level and in Morococha, Peru, at 4540 m (14,900 ft) above sea level.

The polycythemia encountered by high-altitude dwellers is often considered to be a universal, uniform adaptation process to hypoxia that would arise in all normal individuals. However, in reality there is marked variability in erythropoietin levels and the subsequent polycythemic response to chronic hypoxia,[40] suggesting that some of these factors may be genetically determined. The same degree of hypoxia induces substantial differences in erythropoietin production in response to high altitude.[46–48] Three distinct adaptations to high altitude appear to have evolved. Andean highlanders have higher oxygen saturation than Tibetans at the same altitude.[46] Tibetan mean resting ventilation and hypoxic ventilatory response are higher than Andean Aymaras, whereas the mean Tibetan hemoglobin concentration is below the Andean means. It has been suggested that high levels of nitric oxide in the exhaled breath of Tibetans may improve oxygen delivery by inducing vasodilation and increasing blood flow to tissues, thus making the compensatory increased red cell volume unnecessary.[49–51] Another distinct successful pattern of human adaptation in high-altitude dwellers that contrasts with both the Andean "classic" (arterial hypoxemia with polycythemia) and the Tibetan (arterial hypoxemia with normal venous hemoglobin concentration) patterns evolved in Ethiopia. Although Ethiopian high dwellers have normal average hemoglobin concentration (15.9 and 15.0 g/dL for males and females, respectively), they have yet unexplained surprisingly high oxygen saturation of hemoglobin of 95.3 percent despite their hypoxic environment (reviewed in reference 46). Their cerebral circulation is increased but is insensitive to hypoxia, unlike Peruvian high-altitude dwellers.[52] Thus, Ethiopian highlanders maintain venous hemoglobin concentrations and arterial oxygen saturation within the ranges of sea level populations, despite the decrease in the ambient oxygen tension at high altitude.[53] It is likely that this individual variability is a function of genetic differences in hypoxia sensing and hypoxia response pathways (see Chaps. 31 and 33); the exact mechanism remains to be identified.[41,46,48,54] Tibetans and Ethiopians have lived as mountain dwellers much longer than the Quechua or Ayamara Indians (and Han Chinese moving to Tibet and whites moving to high altitudes), suggesting that extreme elevation of the red cell mass is a maladaptation that Tibetans avoided by evolving a more efficient, or less detrimental, compensatory mechanism than that which causes Monge disease.

Understanding the etiology of polycythemia of high altitude is made more complex by a study of inhabitants of the Peruvian mining community of Cerro de Pasco (altitude 4280 m) with excessive erythrocytosis (mean hematocrit: 76%; range: 66–91%). About half of those with a hematocrit greater than 75 percent had toxic serum cobalt levels,[55] suggesting that other erythropoiesis promoting factors such as cobalt[56] can augment hypoxia induction of erythropoietin causing the extreme polycythemias (see Chap. 31). Most high-altitude dwellers, however, do not have measurable levels or a history of exposure to cobalt or other heavy metals.[57]

Pulmonary and Cardiac Disease Degrees of arterial hypoxia comparable to those observed in individuals at high altitudes are observed in patients with right-to-left shunting because of cardiac or intrapulmonary shunts or to ventilation defects, as in chronic obstructive pulmonary disease (COPD). Patients with right-to-left shunting develop a degree of erythrocytosis that is comparable to that observed with similar degrees of desaturation at high altitudes,[58] but many patients with COPD with severe cyanosis are not polycythemic. This has been attributed to the infections and inflammation often present in the lungs, resulting in the anemia of chronic inflammation, and to an increase in plasma volume; however, why some patients with lung disease and congenital heart disease develop polycythemia, while others do not, is not clear. Eisenmenger syndrome, characterized by elevated pulmonary vascular resistance and right-to-left shunting of blood, is usually accompanied by polycythemia.[59]

Sleep Apnea-Induced Syndrome In the colorful pickwickian syndrome,[60] now more widely known as sleep apnea syndrome, the polycythemia is characterized by association with extreme obesity and somnolence. The sleep apnea syndrome[61] can, if severe, cause arterial hypoxemia and hypercapnia, somnolence, and secondary polycythemia.[62] Although the evidence is largely anecdotal,[63] secondary polycythemia is a widely recognized complication of long-standing sleep apnea, reported to be found in 5 to 10 percent of those with nocturnal apnea and hypopnea.[64] However, in a study of 263 (189 men and 74 women), patients with severe sleep apnea had significantly higher hematocrit values than did patients with mild to moderate sleep apnea or nonapneic controls ($p < 0.01$). However, only one patient had a hematocrit in the range of clinical polycythemia.[65]

Smoker's Polycythemia Heavy smoking will result in the formation of carboxyhemoglobin, which does not transport oxygen (reviewed in reference 66), and also causes an increase in oxygen affinity of the remaining normal hemoglobin. The carboxyhemoglobin increases in relationship to number of cigarettes or cigars smoked each day (Table 56–2). This leads to tissue hypoxia, erythropoietin production, and stimulation of red cell production.[67] Smoking may also cause a reduction in plasma volume,[68] and either the augmentation of the red cell mass or the shrinkage of plasma volume could easily explain the rise in the hematocrit. Chronic carbon monoxide poisoning is an important but generally unappreciated cause of mild polycythemia.[69] The increased carboxyhemoglobin is also related to density of traffic in urban areas, that is, traffic policemen have elevated levels. Vehicle exhausts are an important source although unlikely to cause measurable polycythemia.

TABLE 56–2. Blood Oxygen Capacity in Smokers with Polycythemia

Subject	Hemoglobin (Hgb) (g/dL)	Carboxyhemoglobin (COHb) (g/dL)	Hgb-COHb (g/dL)	Affinity Correction (g/dL)	Adjusted Hgb (g/dL)
Healthy male nonsmokers	16 (14–18)	0.16 (0.08–0.25)	15.8 (14–18)	0	16 (14–18)
Male smokers with increased hemoglobin concentration	20 (17–23)	2 (1–3)	18 (16–21)	1.5 (0.5–2.0)	16.5 (15–19)

The male smokers include 10 consecutive subjects studied with elevated hematocrit and no evidence for polycythemia vera. The hemoglobin available for O_2 binding in blood is the Hgb-COHb. COHb also influences the residual hemoglobin to bind oxygen more tightly, making it less accessible to tissues. A correction for this effect has been calculated and is labeled *affinity correction*. The adjusted hemoglobin indicates the blood concentrations that would be present in the subjects in the absence of excess carbon monoxide. Thus, the blood hemoglobin in this group of smokers was increased by 3.5 g/dL on the average (from 16.5 [last column] to 20 [first column]) as a result of smoking-induced carboxyhemoglobinemia.

SOURCE: Data provided by Marshall A. Lichtman, MD.

Polycythemia Secondary to Mutant (High-Affinity) Hemoglobins Hemoglobins with certain amino acid substitutions manifest an increased affinity for oxygen, producing tissue hypoxia and a compensatory erythrocytosis (see Chap. 48). Mutations affecting the amino acids of the $\alpha_1\beta_2$-globin chain contact affect normal rotation within the molecule and impair the rate of deoxygenation. Changes in the carboxy-terminal and penultimate amino acids also impair intramolecular motions and tend to keep the molecules in a high-affinity state. Alterations in the amino acids lining the central cavity of hemoglobin destabilize the binding of 2,3-BPG in this cavity and lead to increased oxygen affinity (reviewed in reference 66). Finally, some heme pocket mutations interfere with deoxygenation; however, most hemoglobins with mutations involving amino acids in the heme pocket are unstable and associated with hemolytic anemia and cyanosis. The inheritance of these disorders is autosomal dominant. An up-to-date listing that includes such hemoglobin variants may be found at www.ncbi.nlm.nih.gov/entrez/dispomim.cgi?id=141900 and www.ncbi.nlm.nih.gov/entrez/dispomim.cgi?id=141850.

Polycythemia Secondary to Red Cell Enzyme Deficiencies Deficiencies of red cell enzymes in early steps of glycolysis sometimes cause marked decreases in the levels of 2,3-BPG (see Chap. 46). This results in an increased oxygen affinity of hemoglobin and, in some cases, polycythemia (reviewed in references 6 and 70). Polycythemia is particularly likely to occur in bisphosphoglyceromutase deficiency.[71] Occasionally, mild polycythemia occurs in patients with methemoglobinemia caused by cytochrome b_5 reductase (methemoglobin reductase) deficiency (reviewed in references 6 and 70; see Chap. 49).

Chemically Induced Tissue Hypoxia A number of chemicals have been suspected of causing histotoxic anoxia and secondary polycythemia, but the only chemical with a predictable capacity to cause erythrocytosis is cobalt.[56] Cobalt administration increases erythropoietin production by increasing hypoxia-inducible factor (HIF)-1 (see below and Chap. 31).[72]

Inappropriate Polycythemias: Congenital Disorders of Hypoxia Sensing

Chuvash Polycythemia Chuvash polycythemia is the only known endemic congenital polycythemia. Chuvash polycythemia is caused by an abnormality in the oxygen-sensing pathway. The condition causes thrombotic and hemorrhagic vascular complications, which lead to early mortality; survival beyond the age of 60 years is uncommon.[29,73] The inheritance is autosomal recessive, and affected patients tend to have normal blood gases, normal calculated P_{50} (normal hemoglobin oxygen affinity), normal to increased erythropoietin levels, absence of genetic linkage to *erythropoietin* and *EPOR* loci, and no evidence of abnormal hemoglobin.[73] In a study of five multiplex Chuvash families with CP, a homozygous mutation of the von Hippel-Lindau (*VHL*) gene (598C→T) was found in the affected individuals. This mutation impairs the interaction of pVHL (protein von Hippel-Lindau) with both HIF-1α and HIF-2α, thus reducing the rate of ubiquitin-mediated destruction of HIF-1α and HIF-2α (see Chap. 31). As a result, the level of HIF-1 and HIF-2 heterodimers increases and leads to an increased expression of target genes, including erythropoietin, vascular endothelial growth factor *(VEGF)*, and plasminogen activator inhibitor *(PAI)*-1, among others.[4,5] Figure 56–3 depicts the effect of this mutation on hypoxic sensing. The role of circulating erythropoietin in the Chuvash polycythemia phenotype is indisputable; however, there must be other factors associated with the Chuvash polycythemia VHL mutation that contribute to the polycythemic phenotype as the erythroid progenitors of Chuvash polycythemia patients are hypersensitive *in vitro* to extrinsic erythropoietin; the mechanism of this observation remains unexplained.[4,5] Despite increased expression of HIF-1α and HIF-2α and VEGF in normoxia, CP patients do not display a predisposition to tumor formation. Imaging studies of 33 CP patients revealed unsuspected cerebral ischemic lesions in 45 percent but no tumors characteristic of VHL syndrome.[74] A high prevalence of this disorder on the Italian island of Ischia has been reported.[33] The Chuvash VHL598C→T mutation has also been described in whites in the United States and Europe and in people of Punjabi/Bangladeshi Asian ancestry.[75] Some patients with congenital polycythemia have proved to be compound heterozygotes for the Chuvash *VHL* 598C→T mutation and other *VHL* mutations, including 562C→G, *VHL* 598C→T and 574C→T, and *VHL* 598C→T and 388C→G (see Table 56–3). Additionally, a Croatian boy was homozygous for *VHL* 571C→G, the first example of a homozygous *VHL* germline mutation other than *VHL* 598C→T causing polycythemia.[32,76–81]

A small number of cases of congenital polycythemia that appear to have mutation of only one *VHL* allele confound an obvious pathophysiologic explanation. In an Ukrainian family, two children with polycythemia were heterozygotes for *VHL* 376G→T (D126Y) but the father with the same mutation was not polycythemic.[82] An English patient was a heterozygote for *VHL* 598C→T[83]; however, the inheritance of deletion of a *VHL* allele, or null *VHL* allele, in a trans position was not excluded. Subsequently, two polycythemic *VHL* heterozygous patients were described in whom a null VHL allele was more rigorously excluded[76,77]; the molecular mechanism of their polycythemic phenotype remains to be elucidated.

To address the question of whether the *VHL* 598C→T substitution occurred in a single founder or resulted from recurrent mutational events, haplotype analysis of 8 highly informative single nucleotide polymorphic markers covering 340 kb spanning the *VHL* gene was performed on 101 subjects bearing the *VHL* 598C→T mutation and 447 normal unrelated individuals from Chuvash, Southeast Asian, white, Hispanic and African American ethnic groups.[30] Polymorphism of the *VHL* locus in normal controls (having a wild *VHL 598C* allele) and subjects bearing Chuvash polycythemia *VHL 598T* were in strong linkage disequilibrium. These studies indicated that in most individuals, the *VHL* 598C→T mutation arose in a single ancestor between 51,000 and 12,000 years ago. However, this is not the case for a Turkish

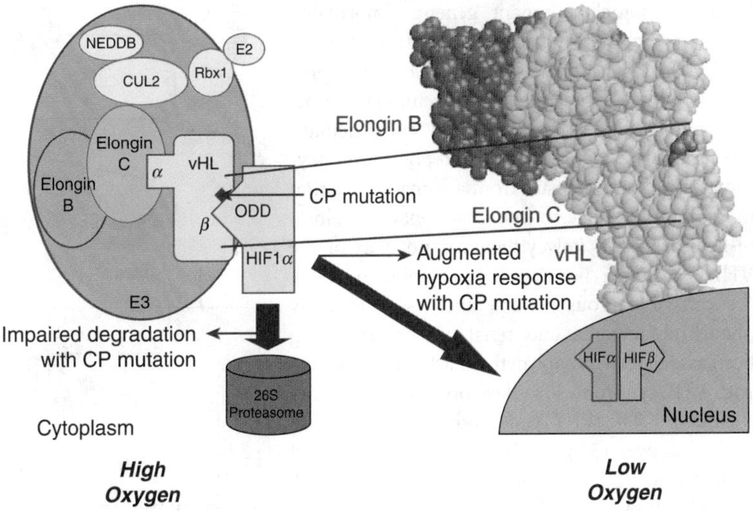

FIGURE 56–3. Elongins B, C, and proteins Rbx1, Cul2 E2, NEDD 8 are interacting proteins that facilitate VHL function. Interaction of mutated VHL protein with HIF-1α. The Chuvash VHL mutation leads to the impaired interaction with HIF-1α, which results in impaired degradation in 26S proteasome and augmented hypoxia sensing.

TABLE 56–3. VHL Mutations Associated with Congenital Polycythemia

VHL Genotype	Ethnicities	Reference	Clinical Features
235C→T/586C→G	White	76	
598C→T/598C→T	Chuvash, Danish, U.S. (white), Bangladeshi, Pakistani, Russian, Turkish	76, 77, 80, 81, 202	Frequent thrombotic complications
598C→T/574C→T	U.S. (white)	80	
598C→T/562C→G	U.S. (white)	80	
598C→T/388G→C	U.S. (white)	81	
571C→G/571C→G	Croatian	80	
311G→T/wild-type	German (?)	77	
376G→T/wild-type	Ukrainian	81	?VHL syndrome
598C→T/wild-type	English, German	77	
523A→G/wild-type	Portuguese	76	A-T patient

A-T, ataxia-telangiectasia.

polycythemic family with a *VHL* 598C→T mutation wherein the *VHL* 598C→T mutation occurred independently.[77]

Chuvash polycythemia homozygotes have a decreased survival because of thrombotic complications, mostly venous,[74] and thus are under negative selection pressure. The high frequency of the mutation in some areas may be a result of random factors ("drift"), but it is also possible that the propagation of the *VHL* 598C→T mutation is the result of a survival advantage for heterozygotes. Such an advantage might be related to subtle improvement of iron metabolism, erythropoiesis, embryonic development, energy metabolism[84] or some other as yet unknown effect. A potential protective role of a mildly augmented hypoxic response is improved protection against bacterial infections, as the hypoxia-mediated response was reported to be essential for the bactericidal action of neutrophils.[85]

Classic von Hippel-Lindau Syndrome VHL syndrome is an autosomal dominant genetic abnormality affecting the post-translational control of HIF-1α.[86–88] The syndrome is characterized by a propensity for developing renal cell carcinomas, retinal hemangioblastomas, cerebellar and spinal hemangioblastomas, pancreatic cysts, and pheochromocytomas. The tumors result from a somatic mutation in addition to the germ-line mutation, that is, loss-of-heterozygosity. Polycythemia is not part of the VHL syndrome; however, hemangioblastomas of the central nervous system, and less commonly pheochromocytoma and renal cancer, have long been associated with polycythemia.[88] Other patients with VHL syndrome also develop acquired polycythemia.[74,88] The *VHL* gene codes for 213 amino acids, and over 130 germ-line mutations associated with classic VHL syndrome have been identified, virtually all of them 5′ to the codon 200 position that is mutated in Chuvash polycythemia.[89] Figure 56–4 depicts schematically the effect of the Chuvash polycythemia mutation in context of other previously found *VHL* mutations.

Other Congenital Disorders of Hypoxia Sensing

Proline Hydroxylase Deficiency A family with a proline hydroxylase domain protein 2 (PHD2) mutation (950C→G) has been described in which heterozygotes for this mutation have mild or borderline polycythemia.[90] Since their description, four additional patients with unexplained polycythemia who are heterozygote carriers of different mutations in PHD2 have been reported (two frameshift mutations, 606delG and 840_841insA, both located in exon 1, and two nonsense mutations, 1112G→A and 1129C→T, in exon 3).[91,92] One of these patients had a major thrombotic event (thrombosis of the sagittal sinus). In both cases, heterozygotes for this mutation had a mild or borderline polycythemia that the authors referred to as erythrocytosis. Testing for erythropoietin hypersensitivity of erythroid progenitors was not reported. Because of the small family size, the possibility of a non-erythroid etiology for the erythrocytosis could not be excluded, but this work further supports the concept that abnormalities in factors involved in the regulation of HIF signaling can result in polycythemia.

HIF-2α Gain-of-Function Mutations A family was described in which members with polycythemia were heterozygous carriers of a HIF-2α Gly537Trp mutation which served to stabilize the HIF-2α protein.[70,93] The same group subsequently reported four additional polycythemic patients with heterozygous Met535Val or Gly537Arg mutations in the HIF-2α gene.[94] The patients tend to present at a young age with elevated erythropoietin. These findings support the importance of the proline hydroxylase, HIF-2α, VHL axis in human erythropoietin regulation and in the pathogenesis of familial polycythemias caused by abnormal hypoxia sensing. Discoverers of this mutation concluded that HIF-2α may be central to regulating erythropoietin levels.[93] Although it is clear that HIF-2 is the transcription factor that regulates hepatic erythropoietin production, the kidney is the major site of erythropoietin synthesis. HIF-1α was identified by its binding to a 3′ *hypoxia responsive element* of kidney erythropoietin.[95] In contrast, the liver erythropoietin gene is regulated by upstream nucleotide sequences,[96] and only approximately 10 to 20 percent of erythropoietin is produced by the liver.[97] A potential alternative explanation for the phenotype described is that it may result

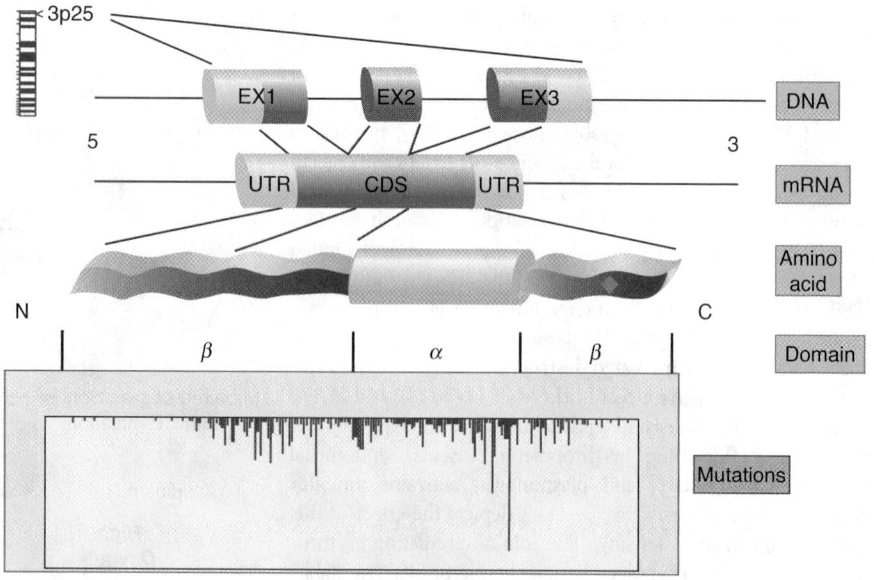

FIGURE 56–4. VHL gene structure and mutation Three exons of VHL genes are depicted encoding for UTR (untranslated portion of messenger RNA [mRNA]), and coding sequences (CDs). VHL domains βαβ are shown. The relative number of reported VHL gene mutations are depicted in *vertical lines*. The location of CP mutation is depicted by the *diamond*.

predominantly from autonomous liver-generated erythropoietin (possibly with suppressed renal erythropoietin production). This conclusion is supported by experimental evidence.[98]

Unexplained Congenital Polycythemias with Elevated or Inappropriately Normal Levels of Erythropoietin

The majority of patients with congenital polycythemias with inappropriately normal or elevated erythropoietin levels do not have *VHL* mutations, *PHD2* and *HIF-2α* mutations, hemoglobinopathies, or 2,3-BPG deficiency, and the molecular basis of polycythemia in these cases remains to be elucidated. However, some such families show dominant inheritance,[99] while in others it is recessive, and in some it is sporadic. It is unclear why, in some families with the same mutation, the phenotype differs. Lesions in genes linked to hypoxia independent regulation of HIF, as well as oxygen-dependent gene regulation pathways, are leading candidates for mutation screening in polycythemic patients with normal or elevated erythropoietin without *VHL* or proline hydroxylase mutations.

Renal Polycythemia and Post-Renal Transplant Erythrocytosis

Absolute erythrocytosis has been observed in a considerable number of patients with solitary renal cysts, polycystic renal disease, or hydronephrosis.[100] In most of these cases erythropoietin assays on cyst fluid, serum, or urine have disclosed the presence of erythropoietin.[101] Patients with polycystic disease have a hematocrit value slightly higher than normal and definitely higher than would have been expected of patients with uremia. In some patients on prolonged dialysis treatment, cystic transformation occurs in the native kidneys. This acquired cystic disease is occasionally associated with marked erythrocytosis.[82] In patients with pheochromocytoma/paraganglioma and erythrocytosis, erythropoietin assays of serum and urine have disclosed higher-than-normal levels, and the erythrocytosis is most likely caused by excessive erythropoietin secretion by the tumor. This assumption has been supported by the presence of erythropoietin messenger RNA (mRNA) in tumor cells.[102] Wilms tumors[103] and paraganglioma[104] are also occasionally associated with an erythrocytosis. However, many of these cases may have a somatic VHL gene mutation that, in combination with a germ-line mutation of another allele, may constitute an unrecognized VHL syndrome. A patient with congenial erythrocytosis and recurrent paraganglioma with a PHD2 mutation was described. Tumor tissue exhibited a loss of heterozygosity of PHD2 in the tumor, suggesting that PHD2 could be a tumor-suppressor gene.[19]

Partial obstruction of the renal artery would be expected to cause renal tissue hypoxia and a physiologic stimulation of erythropoietin production. Nevertheless, it has proved quite difficult to induce erythrocytosis in laboratory animals by placing a Goldblatt clamp on the renal arteries.[105] Only a few of the many patients who have arteriosclerotic narrowing of the renal arteries have been reported to have been polycythemic.[106]

Post-Renal Transplantation Erythrocytosis Although the full molecular basis of post-renal transplantation erythrocytosis remains unknown, angiotensin II (see Chaps. 31 and 33) plays an important role in its pathogenesis.[83] There is growing evidence that increased activity of angiotensin II-angiotensin receptor 1 pathway makes the erythroid progenitors hypersensitive to angiotensin II.[107,108] Furthermore, angiotensin II can modulate release of erythropoiesis stimulatory factors (see Chap. 31) including erythropoietin and insulin-like growth factor-1.[109,110] Studies of venous effluents have determined that the native rather than the transplanted kidneys are the source of the inappropriate production of erythropoietin[111] and in some patients removal of the native kidneys has led to rapid restoration of normal hematocrit values.[112] The condition is rarely seen in patients with nonrenal solid-organ allografts. The role of angiotensin II in augmenting erythropoiesis was confirmed by anemia in angiotensin-converting enzyme knockout mice.[113] Prior to the late 1990s when the use of angiotensin-converting enzyme inhibitors increased as a means to reduce proteinuria, the incidence of erythrocytosis in renal transplantation patients was approximately 8 to 10 percent within the first 2 years after engraftment.

Polycythemia with Connective Tissue Tumors

Occasionally, there is an association of erythrocytosis with large uterine myomas.[20] Usually, the tumor has been huge and extirpation has routinely been followed by a hematologic "cure." The suggestion that the tumor interferes with pulmonary ventilation, has not been supported by the normal arterial gas findings in the few patients so studied. Another possible mechanism is that the large abdominal mass causes mechanical interference with the blood supply to the kidneys, resulting in renal hypoxia and erythropoietin production. Inappropriate erythropoietin secretion by smooth muscle cells has been demonstrated both in uterine myomas and in one case of cutaneous leiomyoma.[20,114] Rare cases of polycythemia attributed to a myxoma of the atrium,[21] hamartoma of the liver,[22] and focal hyperplasia of the liver[23] have been documented.

Brain Tumors

In adequately studied patients with erythrocytosis and cerebellar hemangiomas, the arterial gas tensions have been normal. That the tumors are directly responsible for the polycythemia can be surmised from the identification of erythropoietin in cyst fluid and stromal cells and from a case in which erythropoietin mRNA was present in the tumor.[115] Although in these cases a mutation of VHL gene was not sought, it is likely that these tumors were a manifestation of an underlying VHL syndrome as cerebellar hemangiomas are an integral feature of VHL syndrome.

Hepatoma

In 1958, McFadzean and coworkers reported that almost 10 percent of patients in Hong Kong with hepatocarcinoma developed erythrocytosis.[116] Since then, this association has been recognized as an important clinical clue in the diagnostic consideration of patients with liver disease.[117] The cause of erythrocytosis is probably inappropriate production of erythropoietin by the neoplastic cells.[118] Normal hepatocytes and to a lesser degree nonparenchymal liver cells produce small amounts of erythropoietin both constitutively and in response to hypoxia.

Endocrine Disorders

Pheochromocytomas,[119] aldosterone-producing adenomas,[120] Bartter syndrome,[121] and dermoid cyst of the ovary[122] have been described in association with erythrocytosis. Erythropoietin levels were found elevated in the serum and returned to normal after extirpation of the tumors. A number of pathogenetic mechanisms have been suggested (see Chaps. 31 and 38), including decreased plasma volume, mechanical interference with renal blood supply; hypertensive damage to renal parenchyma; functional interaction between aldosterone, renin, and erythropoietin; and inappropriate secretion of erythropoietin by the tumors. Mild polycythemia may be present in patients with Cushing syndrome; however, its pathophysiologic basis is not entirely clear.

The erythropoietic effect of androgens is of considerable practical importance.[123] For many years, it was assumed that the higher red cell count in males was caused by androgens because the hemoglobin levels of boys and girls were identical up until the time of puberty. It was not until pharmacologic doses of testosterone were administered to women with carcinoma of the breast that the full erythropoietic potency of androgens was appreciated.[124] Since then, various androgen preparations

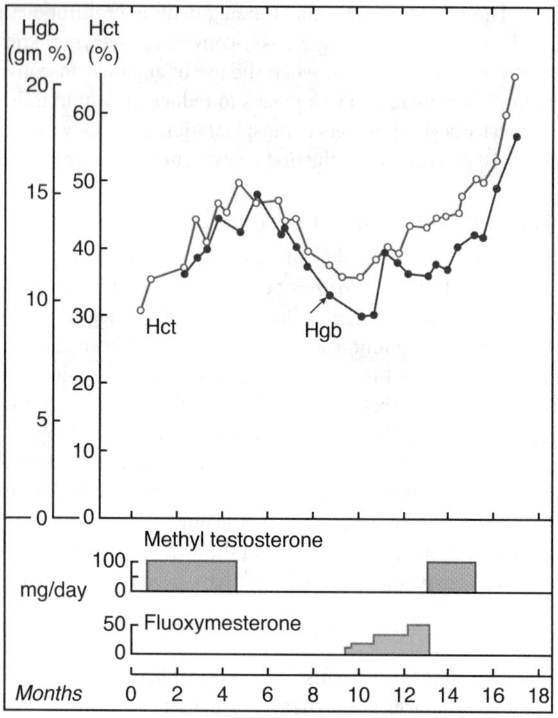

FIGURE 56–5. Erythropoietic response to testosterone derivatives in a patient with myelofibrosis.

have been used in the treatment of refractory anemias, occasionally causing dramatic overshoots into the polycythemic range (Fig. 56–5).

The erythropoietic effect of androgens appears to be caused both by their capacity to stimulate erythropoietin production[125] and by their capacity to induce differentiation of marrow stem cells directly.[123] These two effects have specific structural requirements. Androgens with the 5α-H configuration stimulate renal and extrarenal erythropoietin production, whereas androgens with the 5β-H configuration enhance the differentiation of stem cells.[125]

Neonatal Polycythemia

Polycythemia at birth is a normal physiologic response to intrauterine hypoxia and to the high oxygen affinity of red cells containing hemoglobin F (see Chap. 6). However, it may become excessive and even symptomatic, especially in infants of diabetic mothers, or if the clamping of the cord is delayed, permitting placental blood to boost the blood volume of the infant.[126] Because it is difficult to recognize symptoms of hyperviscosity in the neonate, many pediatricians perform a partial exchange transfusion if the venous hematocrit is above 65 percent at birth.[127]

Apparent (Relative) Polycythemia

Some believe that apparent polycythemia is merely a mild absolute polycythemia accentuated by a compensatory reduction in plasma volume. Others suggest that it is caused by a primary reduction in plasma volume and have associated it with hypertension, obesity, and stress. When the red cell volume is documented to be normal, spurious polycythemia is also an appropriate term. Its clinical significance has also been disputed. The high hematocrit with its associated high viscosity is believed by some to be a risk factor heralding cerebral and cardiac complications, whereas others believe it is merely a well-tolerated blemish. Because the designation *apparent polycythemia*[128] is noncommittal, it is used here.

The main clinical associations with apparent polycythemia are obesity, hypertension, and smoking. In obese patients the finding of a normal red cell volume may be spurious, because if the volume is expressed in terms of lean body weight, some of these patients would have a significant increase in red cell mass. In hypertensive patients, there is no adequate explanation for the apparent increase in red cell production or decrease in plasma volume. Sleep apnea (common in patients with congestive failure), excessive production of atrial natriuretic factor, increased adrenal activation, decreased aldosterone secretion, and hypoxic vasoconstriction are all factors that have been invoked,[129–131] but with little enthusiasm. Chronic administration of diuretics to treat hypertension may be a more likely cause.[131]

CLINICAL FEATURES

PRIMARY FAMILIAL AND CONGENITAL POLYCYTHEMIA

Although PFCP is uncommon, it is frequently misdiagnosed.[17] Unlike those with polycythemia vera, patients with PFCP lack splenomegaly, neutrophilia, basophilia, thrombocytosis and JAK2 mutation. Unless exposed to alkylating agents or radioactive phosphorus, as many have been, do not progress to acute leukemia or myelodysplastic syndrome.[132] Generally thought to be benign, it is likely that this condition, caused by chronic augmented erythropoietin signaling in all tissues bearing *EPOR*, predisposes patients to severe cardiovascular problems.[133] An increased incidence of cardiovascular disease was observed in affected members of PFCP families.[134] Erythrocytosis may be very severe with hemoglobin levels that typically exceed 20 g/dL in men and 18 g/dL in women. Headaches are commonly present. Hypertension, coronary artery disease, and strokes have been reported to occur, but do not appear to be clearly related to an elevated hematocrit as they also occur in aggressively phlebotomized patients with normal hematocrit[135]; however, these are not a constant feature of the disorder.[136]

CHUVASH POLYCYTHEMIA

The recessive polycythemia that is endemic in Chuvashia (Autonomous Republic of the Russian Federation) is characterized by elevations of the hemoglobin level to a mean of 22.6 with a standard deviation of 1.4 g/L.[73] Some patients are symptomatic with headache and fatigue and with signs including clubbing, thrombosis, and peptic ulcer. Chuvash polycythemia is associated with a history of thrombosis, relatively low blood pressure (also seen in heterozygotes), and varicose veins.[4,73,74] As of yet, no significant association of thrombosis and elevated hematocrit and history of phlebotomies has been found.[74] A matched cohort study of 96 patients diagnosed in 1977 (65 spouses and 79 unaffected community members of the same age, sex, and village of birth) found that homozygosity for VHL 598C→T was associated with polycythemia, varicose veins, lower blood pressures, elevated serum VEGF and PAI-1 levels, and premature mortality related to cerebral vascular events and both venous and arterial thrombotic events.[74]

Because Chuvash polycythemia is characterized by a germ-line mutation in the *VHL* gene, it was expected that homozygotes for this mutation might develop certain vascular tumors similar to those associated with classic VHL syndrome. Tumors typical of classic VHL syndrome, such as spinocerebellar hemangioblastomas, renal carcinomas, and pheochromocytomas/paragangliomas, were not found, indicating that increased expression of HIF-1α and VEGF is not sufficient for tumorigenesis. Benign vertebral body hemangiomas (a distinct entity from hemangioblastoma) were found in significantly more patients with CP compared to controls (55% vs. 21%). Imaging studies of 33 CP patients revealed unsuspected cerebral ischemic lesions in 45 percent patients.[74] Affected patients have a significant risk to develop pulmonary hypertension.[137–139]

OTHER CONGENITAL DISORDERS OF HYPOXIA SENSING

Because of their only recent discovery and their apparent rarity, reliable clinical information is lacking. However, these disorders, in view of their global deregulation of hypoxia sensing, are expected to also have an extraerythroid manifestation. One subject with a sporadic gain-of-function of HIF-2α mutation also had hypersensitive erythroid progenitors to erythropoietin, suggesting that this entity, similar to Chuvash polycythemia, shares features of primary and secondary polycythemic disorders.

SECONDARY ACQUIRED POLYCYTHEMIA

Tolerance to high altitudes varies greatly, but most normal individuals have no discomfort at altitudes of up to 2130 m (7000 ft). Above this altitude, and especially if the ascent is rapid, some manifestations of cerebral hypoxia are common. Headaches, sleeplessness, and palpitations are frequently encountered, and weakness, nausea, vomiting, and mental dullness may be present. More severe manifestations include pulmonary and cerebral edema, which may lead to death. Cheyne-Stokes respiration commonly occurs, especially during sleep. These symptoms constitute the syndrome of *acute mountain sickness*.[140]

Ruddy cyanosis and physiologic emphysema are the two characteristic features of some humans living at high altitudes. Venous and capillary engorgement can be observed readily in the conjunctiva, mucous membranes, and skin and may contribute to the remarkable capacity of Tibetan Sherpas to walk barefoot and sleep on ice and snow.[141] Asymptomatic retinal hemorrhages are seen frequently at high altitudes but rarely at altitudes of 3000 m (9000 ft) or less.[142] Splenomegaly and jaundice are unusual, although the sustained erythrocytosis is associated with an increased rate of red cell destruction and bilirubin generation. It has been stated that Monge disease includes low fertility[42,45]; however, this may not be universally so. High-altitude native-resident Tibetans exhibit two distinct genotypes for increased oxygen affinity of hemoglobin. Women with genotypes for high oxygen saturation have more surviving children.[143] This finding suggests that high-altitude hypoxia is acting as an agent of natural selection on the locus for oxygen saturation of hemoglobin by the mechanism of higher infant survival of Tibetan women with high oxygen-saturation genotypes.[53,143–146]

The polycythemia associated with smoking is generally asymptomatic, but there may be an increase in thrombotic events; however, this may be a result of smoking rather than polycythemia.

Large studies of patients with Eisenmenger syndrome[59] and other patients with cyanotic heart disease[147] caution against routine phlebotomy for asymptomatic elevation of the hematocrit; in fact, thrombotic complications were not observed in these studies. Animal studies support these recommendations; transgenic mice with extreme polycythemia (hematocrit 85%) because of constitutive overexpression of erythropoietin did not develop the expected thrombotic complications.[148] Adults with cyanotic congenital heart disease are at risk of having cerebrovascular events. This risk is increased in the presence of hypertension, atrial fibrillation, history of phlebotomy, and microcytosis, the latter condition having the strongest significance ($p < 0.005$). The authors of these findings endorsed a more conservative approach toward phlebotomy and more aggressive approach toward treating microcytosis in adults with cyanotic congenital heart disease.[149]

In a prospective cohort of stable COPD U.S. Veterans Administration outpatients (n = 683), polycythemia prevalence was low and, unlike anemia, had no association with worsened outcomes.[150]

Renal Polycythemia and Post-Renal Transplantation Erythrocytosis

The erythrocytosis of renal disease and of the post-renal transplantation state can be very severe. Erythrocyte counts may be as high as 8×10^{12}/L and be associated with hypertension and congestive failure.[151] At higher hematocrit levels (usually >60%), thrombotic events may complicate the clinical course[27,28,152]; however, frequent comorbidities that are associated or causative of renal failure are frequently also factors predisposing to thrombosis, and the risk of erythrocytosis associated thrombosis have not been submitted to multivariate rigorous statistical analyses.

Tumors

The erythrocytosis that occurs with tumors is generally mild,[115] and the predominating clinical manifestations are those of the tumor itself. Even moderate elevations to a hematocrit of 64 percent have been encountered without symptoms referable to the polycythemia.[23] Resection of erythropoietin tumor cures associated polycythemia.[81]

Neonatal Polycythemia

Of 55 infants with neonatal polycythemia, 85 percent had signs and symptoms attributed to this disorder. These included "feeding problems" (21.8%), plethora (20.0%), lethargy (14.5%), cyanosis (14.5%), respiratory distress (9.1%), jitteriness (7.3%), and hypotonia (7.3%). Other findings included hypoglycemia (40.0%) and hyperbilirubinemia (21.8%). In a larger group of nearly 1000 infants, 6 had an intracranial hemorrhage.[126]

LABORATORY FEATURES

PRIMARY FAMILIAL AND CONGENITAL POLYCYTHEMIA

Characteristic laboratory findings of PFCP are: (1) an increased red blood cell mass without increased leukocyte or platelet counts; (2) a normal hemoglobin–oxygen dissociation curve; (3) invariably low serum erythropoietin levels; and (4) *in vitro* hypersensitivity of erythroid progenitors to erythropoietin.[5] PFCP is often misdiagnosed as polycythemia vera. Whereas, the leukocytes are typically normal, platelet counts are often mildly decreased, presumably by dilution of the normal platelet mass by an often dramatic increase of red cell and whole-blood volumes. Some patients come to attention because of concurrent medical problems that may cause leukocytosis and secondary thrombocytosis, falsely suggesting phenotype of polycythemia vera.

Chuvash Polycythemia

Blood profiling in patients with Chuvash polycythemia indicates increased hemoglobin and hematocrit and lower white blood cell and platelet counts than in controls. Erythropoietin ranges from normal (but never close to the lower limits of normal) to elevated, at times exceeding 10 times the mean normal value. In larger studies, their hemoglobin-adjusted serum erythropoietin concentrations were approximately 10-fold higher in *VHL* 598C→T homozygotes than in controls.[4,5,74]

Affected subjects have lower CD4 counts, elevated levels of both proinflammatory and antiinflammatory cytokines, and altered plasma thiol levels, with elevated homocysteine and glutathione and low cysteine concentrations.[137,153,154] Their PAI-1 and serum VEGF levels are also increased.[4,73,74] The serum ferritin, as well as circulating transferrin receptor levels, are higher in Chuvash polycythemia homozygotes as compared to their unaffected relatives and spouses.[4,5,74] The ferritin-adjusted transferrin receptor concentration was approximately threefold higher in *VHL* 598C→T homozygotes than in unaffected participants (p <0.0005), which is consistent with upregulation by HIF-1. This indicates that storage iron is similar between *VHL* 598C→T homozygotes and unaffected controls despite the dramatically higher hemoglobin concentrations and phlebotomy therapy in the Chuvash polycythemia patients.

Chuvash polycythemia is a recently described disorder; thus, additional laboratory findings because of augmentation of hypoxia sensing are expected to be described.

Other Congenital Polycythemias from Augmented Hypoxia Sensing

At present, the paucity of data precludes any reliable description of other congenital polycythemias from augmented hypoxia sensing. However some affected subjects have unexpectedly low normal erythropoietin levels.

■ SECONDARY POLYCYTHEMIA

Characteristically, only the numbers of erythrocytes in the blood are increased in secondary polycythemia. An increase in the leukocyte count and splenomegaly may be present as another feature of the underlying disease, for example, the pulmonary infection in chronic obstructive lung disease with *cor pulmonale*; or as seen in Monge disease among Andean high dwellers and patients inheriting high-affinity hemoglobin that is also unstable (see Chaps. 33 and 48). In patients with appropriate polycythemia, the underlying defect is usually demonstrable. Arterial hypoxia can be demonstrated in most cases. However, some obese patients who, like Mr. Wardle's proverbial boy, Joe, characters in *The Pickwick Papers* by Charles Dickens, are always half asleep, will be very much awake when exposed to arterial punctures and ventilatory testing, and their apprehensive hyperventilation will result in the disappearance of all the abnormalities in arterial oxygen tension. As soon as they return to bed, however, they will go to sleep again and display the characteristic somnolent cyanosis. In inappropriate polycythemia, the laboratory findings will be those of the underlying defect.

DIFFERENTIAL DIAGNOSIS

Also refer to Chap. 33 and Figure 56–6.

Distinguishing between polycythemia vera and other polycythemic disorders can be very challenging. The diagnosis of polycythemia vera may be straightforward if patients have the classic criteria as defined by the most recent World Health Organization criteria[155] and the JAK2 mutation; often, however, patients with either polycythemia vera or other polycythemic disorders present with an incomplete phenotype. Some of the clinical and laboratory features that can be helpful for differential diagnosis are summarized in Table 33–2 and in Figure 56–6.

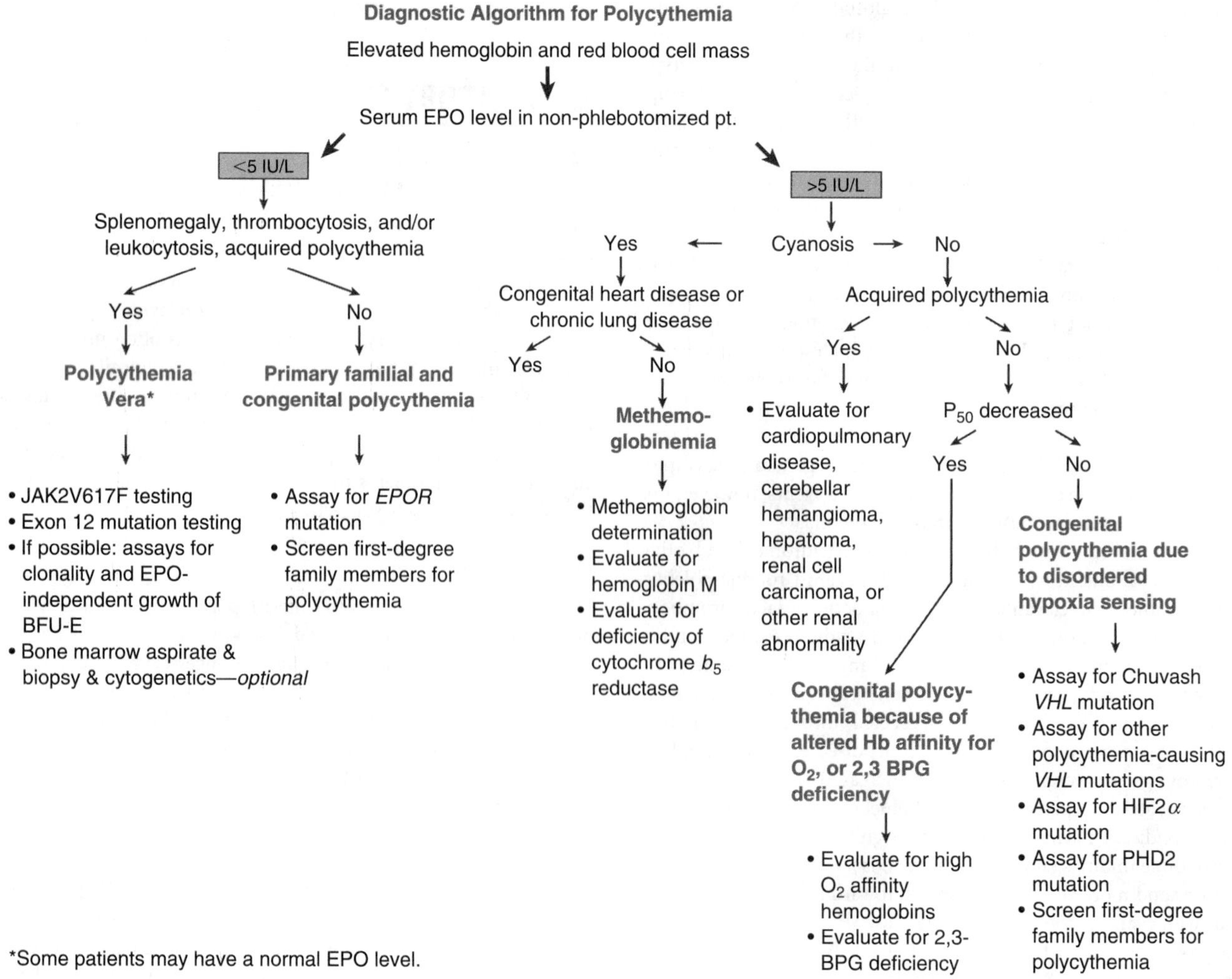

FIGURE 56–6. Diagnostic algorithm for polycythemia based on erythropoietin level. BFU–E, burst-forming unit–erythroid.

RED CELL MASS DETERMINATION

Determination of red cell mass is invaluable for differentiation of apparent (spurious) polycythemia from true polycythemic states. Unfortunately, the determination of the red cell mass is expensive and, when performed by the inexperienced, often inaccurate.[156] It is not useful in distinguishing polycythemia vera from secondary polycythemia, the differentiation that is usually needed, because it is increased in both disorders. Ideally, the red cell volume and plasma volume should be measured separately. Unfortunately, the ^{131}I-labeled albumin necessary to measure the plasma volume is often unavailable. Fortunately, in most cases, the diagnosis of polycythemia vera and other true polycythemic states can be established with confidence without measuring the red cell volume.

ERYTHROID COLONY CULTURES

In vitro assays of erythroid progenitor cells permit the study of their responsiveness to erythropoietin. This can be applied to polycythemia vera and erythroid progenitor growth without added erythropoietin,[157] referred to as "endogenous erythroid colonies." Detection of endogenous erythroid colonies in cultures of marrow or blood may be the most specific test for polycythemia vera.[31,158,159] In one study, all patients with polycythemia vera, but none with secondary or other causes of polycythemia, had endogenous erythroid colonies.[160] Rare endogenous erythroid colonies may at times be observed in PFCP and in Chuvash polycythemia and in a single studied subject with the HIF-2α mutation,[161] but unlike the endogenous erythroid colonies of polycythemia vera, these are abrogated by pretreatment with erythropoietin and erythropoietin receptor-blocking antibodies.[162,163]

In experienced hands, endogenous erythroid colonies is a specific and sensitive means for detecting polycythemia vera and may be useful in diagnosing patients with unusual presentations of polycythemia vera, such as Budd-Chiari syndrome[164–167] or isolated thrombocytosis.[168] However, this test has not been standardized, is expensive and laborious, and technical variations make interlaboratory results difficult to compare.

ERYTHROPOIETIN LEVELS

All patients with PFCP we have encountered[79] have erythropoietin below normal levels or below levels of detection. Thus, a low erythropoietin level is not pathognomonic of polycythemia vera as patients with PFCP have as low or lower erythropoietin levels.[17]

Because polycythemia vera is distinguished by the fact that erythroid cells proliferate even in the absence of substantial levels of erythropoietin, one would expect that at high hematocrit levels the production of erythropoietin would be inhibited and the serum levels consequently reduced. Older erythropoietin assays were too insensitive to detect subnormal levels of erythropoietin, but using improved technology, several studies have documented serum erythropoietin levels below the normal reference range in patients with polycythemia vera.[169–171] Erythropoietin levels remain low even after phlebotomy,[169] which increases erythropoietin levels in normal individuals. However, erythropoietin levels in Budd-Chiari syndrome may be normal or even increased.[172]

Patients with secondary polycythemia usually have normal to elevated erythropoietin levels, although considerable overlap exists in the range of erythropoietin levels between some patients with polycythemia vera and those with secondary polycythemia.[170,173]

CLONALITY IN FEMALE SUBJECTS USING ASSAYS EMPLOYING X-CHROMOSOME–BASED POLYMORPHISM ASSAYS

The principal role of the clonality assay is to differentiate polycythemia vera with an incomplete phenotype or atypical presentation from idiopathic or yet undiagnosed polycythemia/erythrocytosis. Polycythemia vera results from an acquired mutation in a pluripotential hematopoietic progenitor cell. Clonality studies based on the phenomenon of X-chromosome inactivation[174] show that red cells, granulocytes, platelets, monocytes, and B lymphocytes are all part of the clone.[175,176] The majority of T lymphocytes and natural killer cells are polyclonal, but a small proportion of these cells are also derived from the polycythemia vera clone[177]; this is presumed to be a result of the presence of long-lived normal T cells that preceded the development of the clone. Unfortunately, interpretation of publications on the applicability of X-chromosome inactivation for differential diagnosis of polycythemia vera is hampered by the many methodologic and conceptual differences that have drawn conflicting conclusions.[178] Some discrepancies are a result of the fact that two different approaches, which are not comparable, are used to distinguish the active from the inactive X-chromosome; one uses X-chromosome differential methylation,[179] typically using the polymorphic CAG repeat in the human androgen-receptor gene (*AR*),[180] versus the more biologically sound but more technically demanding transcriptional analysis of the active X-chromosome.[179,181] Furthermore, the wide range of skewing of the X-chromosome allelic usage that is normally present[182] is often misinterpreted as clonality, and the potentially clonal myeloid cells are not compared to the polyclonal control cells of the same origin.[31] In about 100 female polycythemia vera patients, the reticulocytes, platelets and granulocytes were always clonal, with the exception of a few patients who converted to polyclonal hematopoiesis after therapy with interferon-α.[31] Although it was previously reported that clonality assays based on X-chromosome inactivation are not suitable for studies of older women using the *AR* assay,[183–185] that was not confirmed by studies using quantitative transcriptional analysis of active X-chromosomes.[186]

OTHER POLYCYTHEMIAS

The clinical history is of the utmost importance for the differential diagnosis of polycythemic states. The differentiation of an acquired from congenital disorder, and a distinction between sporadic versus familial occurrence of polycythemia, when possible, will streamline the diagnosis. Thus, an autosomal dominant disorder is likely caused by polycythemia from a gain-of-function erythropoietin receptor gene or PHD2 mutations, or a high-affinity hemoglobin. Recessively inherited conditions may be caused by VHL gene mutations. Although rare patients with polycythemia vera may have a history of other affected family members, the polycythemia vera is virtually always an acquired condition. Many familial polycythemias are the result of yet-to-be-discovered genetic events.

Patients with a low level of erythropoietin and autosomal dominant inheritance should have sequence analysis of the erythropoietin receptor. This will define the defect in some patients with PFCP; if the polycythemia is acquired and present in multiple relatives, a diagnosis of familial polycythemia vera should be pursued. Patients with secondary polycythemia have a genuine increase in the number of circulating erythrocytes and of the red cell mass. Such patients do not typically have the increase in the platelet count and leukocyte count or the splenomegaly that is characteristic of polycythemia vera. The lack of involvement of other formed elements in hematopoietic proliferation should arouse suspicion that the patient may have a polycythemia other than polycythemia vera. However, reactive thrombocytosis, leukocytosis, and splenomegaly may occasionally also be present in secondary polycythemia, which then renders the distinction from polycythemia vera more difficult. In patients in whom secondary polycythemia is caused by lung or cardiac disease, clubbing is often present. In some cases, determining the arterial oxygen saturation will clarify the diagnosis, but modest arterial oxygen desaturation may also be present in polycythemia vera.[58,187] Imaging of the kidneys may reveal a neoplasm or cyst in some patients. Determining the oxygen dissociation curve, or estimation of P_{50} from venous blood[188] will detect abnormalities related to increased oxygen affinity either because of inheritance of a high affinity hemoglobin (see Chap. 48), or because of very rare 2,3-BPG depletion, as in phosphoglyceromutase deficiency (see Chap. 46). The mild polycythemia associated with hereditary methemoglobinemia (see Chap. 49) is readily diagnosed because of coexistent cyanosis.

In patients with elevated erythropoietin or erythropoietin levels inappropriately normal for the degree of hemoglobin elevation, analysis of *VHL*, *PHD2*, and *HIF-2α* genes may be in order; some of these patients may have a history of autosomal recessive inheritance and they have a typical history of congenital polycythemia. It may also be useful to determine the carboxyhemoglobin level of the blood if smoker's polycythemia is suspected.

SPURIOUS POLYCYTHEMIA

The erythrocytosis observed in patients with spurious polycythemia (apparent polycythemia, stress polycythemia) is a consequence of a decrease in the plasma volume.[128] The erythrocytosis that is observed does not represent a true increase in the red cell mass. Usually the increase in the hematocrit is very modest. Such patients do not have an increased white blood count, thrombocytosis, or splenomegaly. The arterial oxygen saturation is normal. The estimation of the red cell mass and plasma volume is required to establishing a diagnosis of spurious polycythemia, but it should be recognized that during the natural history of patients who develop primary or secondary polycythemia, their red cell mass is, at some point, within the normal range while it is rising to abnormal values. However, because of the significant error rate of red cell volume measurement, it is recommended that both red cell volume and plasma volume are measured simultaneously.

THERAPY

POLYCYTHEMIAS OTHER THAN POLYCYTHEMIA VERA

Treatment of patients with post-renal transplantation erythrocytosis with drugs that suppress the renal–angiotensin system has virtually eliminated the need for therapeutic phlebotomy. The maximal reduction of hemoglobin and hematocrit levels usually manifests by 6 months after starting therapy with either angiotensin-converting enzyme inhibitor, enalapril, or angiotensin II receptor type 1 blocker, losartan.[83] Some patients are exquisitely sensitive and may become severely anemic.

High-altitude polycythemia is also associated with pulmonary hypertension, proteinuria, and elevated blood pressure. A prospective randomized trial of enalapril reported decreased hemoglobin concentration, proteinuria and beneficial effect on elevated blood pressure.[189]

When erythrocytosis is secondary to a renal tumor or cyst, pheochromocytoma, myoma, or brain tumor, removal of the neoplasm has usually resulted in disappearance of the erythrocytosis.

No specific therapy is currently available for polycythemic subjects with *EPOR*, *VHL*, *PHD2*, and *HIF-2α* mutations.

Lowering the hematocrit to a normal or near-normal level by phlebotomy is the usual but empiric treatment of secondary polycythemia,[190,191] but should be always viewed in the context of a particular polycythemic subject.[59,147] The appropriate level is that at which the patient becomes asymptomatic. Although cytotoxic agents are sometimes used for this purpose, phlebotomy is preferred, if indeed needed, because of the leukemogenic risk of the agents that are used in polycythemia vera. This author favors, in most instances, a benign neglect unless specific therapy such as that seen in erythropoietin-secreting tumors or post-renal transplantation erythrocytosis is available. One should phlebotomize only those patients who are symptomatic from the elevated red cell mass, and continue to do so cautiously only if symptoms respond promptly to phlebotomy.

COURSE AND PROGNOSIS

CHUVASH POLYCYTHEMIA

In a study of 96 patients with Chuvash polycythemia diagnosed before 1977 (65 spouses, and 79 community members of the same age, sex, and village of birth), the estimated survival to 65 years was ≤31 percent for Chuvash polycythemia patients versus ≥67 percent for spouses and community members ($p \leq 0.002$).[74]

OTHER POLYCYTHEMIAS

The clinical course of secondary polycythemia is largely a function of the underlying disorder. In patients with PFCP secondary to mutations of the erythropoietin receptor gene, coronary artery disease and strokes have been reported,[135] although not in all series.[136] However the rarity of PFCP secondary to mutations of the erythropoietin receptor, *VHL*, *PHD2*, and *HIF-2α* gene mutations, and polycythemias from globin mutations and or red cell enzyme deficiencies precludes any meaningful prognostic evaluation; however, the effect of gain-of-function of erythropoietin receptor mutation is currently being evaluated in animal models of this disorder.[192]

REFERENCES

1. Juvonen E, Ikkala E, Fyhrquist F, et al: Autosomal dominant erythrocytosis caused by increased sensitivity to erythropoietin. *Blood* 78:3066, 1991.
2. Perrine GM, Prchal JT, Prchal JF: Study of a polycythemic family. *Blood* 50:134, 1977.
3. Prchal JT, Crist WM, Goldwasser E, et al: Autosomal dominant polycythemia. *Blood* 66:1208, 1985.
4. Ang SO, Chen H, Gordeuk VR, et al: Endemic polycythemia in Russia: Mutation in the VHL gene. *Blood Cells Mol Dis* 28:57, 2002.
5. Ang SO, Chen H, Hirota K, et al: Disruption of oxygen homeostasis underlies congenital Chuvash polycythemia. *Nat Genet* 32:614, 2002.
6. Prchal JT, Gregg XT: Erythropoiesis—Genetic abnormalities, in *Erythropoietins and Erythropoiesis*, 2nd ed, edited by M Graham, MA Foote, SG Elliott, p 61. Birkhäuer-Verlag AG, Basel, Switzerland, 2009.
7. Bert P: *La Pression Barometrique*. Bailliere, Paris, 1878.
8. Jourdanet D: *De l'Anemie des Altitudes et de l'Anemie en General dans ses Rapports Avec la Pression l'Atmorphere*. Bailliere, Paris, 1863.
9. Viault F: Sur l'augmentation considerable du nombre des globules rouges dans le sang chez les habitants des hauts plateaux de l'Amerique du Sud. *CR Acad Sci* 111:917, 1890.
10. Erslev AJ: Blood and mountains, in *Blood, Pure and Eloquent*, edited by MM Wintrobe, p 257. McGraw-Hill, New York, 1980.
11. Leopold SS: The etiology of pulmonary arteriosclerosis (Ayerza's syndrome). *Am J Med* 219:152, 1950.
12. Abbott ME: *Atlas of Congenital Heart Disease*. American Heart Association, New York, 1936.
13. Burwell CS, Robin, ED Whaley, RD, Bickelman, AG: Extreme obesity associated with alveolar hypoventilation: A pickwickian syndrome. *Am J Med* 21:811, 1956.
14. Charache S, Weatherall DJ, Clegg JB: Polycythemia associated with a hemoglobinopathy. *J Clin Invest* 45:813, 1966.
15. Fairbanks VF, Klee GG, Wiseman GA, et al: Measurement of blood volume and red cell mass: Re-examination of ^{51}Cr and ^{125}I methods. *Blood Cells Mol Dis* 22:169, 1996.
16. Lawrence JH, Berlin NI: Relative polycythemia—The polycythemia of stress. *Yale J Biol Med* 24:498, 1952.
17. Prchal JT: Classification and molecular biology of polycythemias (erythrocytoses) and thrombocytosis. *Hematol Oncol Clin North Am* 17:1151, 2003.
18. Thorling EB: Paraneoplastic erythrocytosis and inappropriate erythropoietin production. A review. *Scand J Haematol* 17:1, 1972.
19. Ladroue C, Carcenac R, Leporrier M, et al: PHD2 mutation and congenital erythrocytosis with paraganglioma. *N Engl J Med* 359:2685, 2008.
20. LevGur M, Levie MD: The myomatous erythrocytosis syndrome: A review. *Obstet Gynecol* 86:1026, 1995.

21. Levinson JP, Kincaid OW: Myxoma of the right atrium associated with polycythemia. Report of successful excision. *N Engl J Med* 264:1187, 1961.
22. Josephs BN, Robbins G, Levine A: Polycythemia secondary to hamartoma of the liver. *JAMA* 179:867, 1961.
23. Sandler A, Rivlin L, Filler R, et al: Polycythemia secondary to focal nodular hyperplasia. *J Pediatr Surg* 32:1386, 1997.
24. Constans JP, Meder F, Maiuri F, et al: Posterior fossa hemangioblastomas. *Surg Neurol* 25:269, 1986.
25. Sharma RR, Cast IP, O'Brien C: Supratentorial haemangioblastoma not associated with von Hippel-Lindau complex or polycythaemia: Case report and literature review. *Br J Neurosurg* 9:81, 1995.
26. Dagher FJ, Ramos E, Erslev AJ, et al: Are the native kidneys responsible for erythrocytosis in renal allorecipients? *Transplantation* 28:496, 1979.
27. Kessler M, Hestin D, Mayeux D, et al: Factors predisposing to post-renal transplant erythrocytosis. A prospective matched-pair control study. *Clin Nephrol* 45:83, 1996.
28. Gaston RS, Julian BA, Curtis JJ: Posttransplant erythrocytosis: An enigma revisited. *Am J Kidney Dis* 24:1, 1994.
29. Polyakova LA: Familial erythrocytosis among inhabitants of the Chuvash ASSR. *Probl Gematol Pereliv Krovi* 10:30, 1974.
30. Liu E, Percy MJ, Amos CI, et al: The worldwide distribution of the VHL 598C→T mutation indicates a single founding event. *Blood* 103:1937, 2004.
31. Liu E, Jelinek J, Pastore YD, et al: Discrimination of polycythemias and thrombocytoses by novel, simple, accurate clonality assays and comparison with PRV-1 expression and BFU–E response to erythropoietin. *Blood* 101:3294, 2003.
32. Percy MJ, Beard ME, Carter C, et al: Erythrocytosis and the Chuvash von Hippel-Lindau mutation. *Br J Haematol* 123:371, 2003.
33. Perrotta S, Nobili B, Ferraro M, et al: von Hippel-Lindau-dependent polycythemia is endemic on the island of Ischia: Identification of a novel cluster. *Blood* 107:514, 2006.
34. Chetty KG, Light RW, Stansbury DW, et al: Exercise performance of polycythemic chronic obstructive pulmonary disease patients. Effect of phlebotomies. *Chest* 98:1073, 1990.
35. Hurtado A: Acclimatization of high altitudes, in *Physiological Effects of High Altitude*, edited by WH Weihe, p 1. Macmillan, New York, 1964.
36. Moore LG, Brewer GJ: Beneficial effect of rightward hemoglobin-oxygen dissociation curve shift for short-term high-altitude adaptation. *J Lab Clin Med* 98:145, 1981.
37. Finch CA, Lenfant C: Oxygen transport in man. *N Engl J Med* 286:407, 1972.
38. Winslow RM, Monge CC, Statham NJ, et al: Variability of oxygen affinity of blood: Human subjects native to high altitude. *J Appl Physiol* 51:1411, 1981.
39. Eaton JW, Skelton TD, Berger E: Survival at extreme altitude: Protective effect of increased hemoglobin-oxygen affinity. *Science* 183:743, 1974.
40. Leon-Velarde F, Gamboa A, Chuquiza JA, et al: Hematological parameters in high altitude residents living at 4,355, 4,660, and 5,500 meters above sea level. *High Alt Med Biol* 1:97, 2000.
41. Mejia OM, Prchal JT, Leon-Velarde F, et al: Genetic association analysis of chronic mountain sickness in an Andean high-altitude population. *Haematologica* 90:13, 2005.
42. Monge CC: Life in the Andes and chronic mountain sickness. *Science* 95:79, 1942.
43. Maignan M, Rivera-Ch M, Privat C, et al: Pulmonary pressure and cardiac function in chronic mountain sickness patients. *Chest* 135:499, 2009.
44. Wu TY, Ding SQ, Liu JL, et al: Who should not go high: Chronic disease and work at altitude during construction of the Qinghai-Tibet railroad. *High Alt Med Biol* 8:88, 2007.
45. Winslow RM, Monge CC: *Hypoxia, Polycythemia and Chronic Mountain Sickness.* Johns Hopkins University Press, Baltimore, MD, 1987.
46. Beall CM: Two routes to functional adaptation: Tibetan and Andean high-altitude natives. *Proc Natl Acad Sci U S A* 104 Suppl 1:8655, 2007.
47. Winslow RM, Chapman KW, Gibson CC, et al: Different hematologic responses to hypoxia in Sherpas and Quechua Indians. *J Appl Physiol* 66:1561, 1989.
48. Zhou ZN, Zhuang JG, Wu XF, et al: Tibetans retained innate ability resistance to acute hypoxia after long period of residing at sea level. *J Physiol Sci* 58:167, 2008.
49. Beall CM, Laskowski D, Strohl KP, et al: Pulmonary nitric oxide in mountain dwellers. *Nature* 414:411, 2001.
50. Erzurum SC, Ghosh S, Janocha AJ, et al: Higher blood flow and circulating NO products offset high-altitude hypoxia among Tibetans. *Proc Natl Acad Sci U S A* 104:17593, 2007.
51. Schwab M, Jayet PY, Stuber T, et al: Pulmonary-artery pressure and exhaled nitric oxide in Bolivian and Caucasian high altitude dwellers. *High Alt Med Biol* 9:295, 2008.
52. Claydon VE, Gulli G, Slessarev M, et al: Cerebrovascular responses to hypoxia and hypocapnia in Ethiopian high altitude dwellers. *Stroke* 39:336, 2008.
53. Beall CM: High-altitude adaptations. *Lancet* 362 Suppl:s14, 2003.
54. Jedlickova K, Stockton DW, Chen H, et al: Search for genetic determinants of individual variability of the erythropoietin response to high altitude. *Blood Cells Mol Dis* 31:175, 2003.
55. Jefferson JA, Escudero E, Hurtado ME, et al: Excessive erythrocytosis, chronic mountain sickness, and serum cobalt levels. *Lancet* 359:407, 2002.
56. Goldwasser E, Jacobson LO, Fried W, et al: Mechanism of the erythropoietic effect of cobalt. *Science* 125:1085, 1957.
57. Bernardi L, Roach RC, Keyl C, et al: Ventilation, autonomic function, sleep and erythropoietin. Chronic mountain sickness of Andean natives. *Adv Exp Med Biol* 543:161, 2003.
58. Murray JF: Classification of polycythemic disorders. With comments on the diagnostic value of arterial blood oxygen analysis. *Ann Intern Med* 64:892, 1966.
59. Vongpatanasin W, Brickner ME, Hillis LD, et al: The Eisenmenger syndrome in adults. *Ann Intern Med* 128:745, 1998.
60. Kuhl W: History of clinical research on the sleep apnea syndrome. The early days of polysomnography. *Respiration* 64 Suppl 1:5, 1997.
61. Block AJ, Boysen PG, Wynne JW, et al: Sleep apnea, hypopnea and oxygen desaturation in normal subjects. A strong male predominance. *N Engl J Med* 300:513, 1979.
62. Moore-Gillon JC, Treacher DF, Gaminara EJ, et al: Intermittent hypoxia in patients with unexplained polycythaemia. *Br Med J (Clin Res Ed)* 293:588, 1986.
63. Hoffstein V, Mateika S: Differences in abdominal and neck circumferences in patients with and without obstructive sleep apnoea. *Eur Respir J* 5:377, 1992.
64. Carlson JT, Hedner J, Fagerberg B, et al: Secondary polycythaemia associated with nocturnal apnoea—A relationship not mediated by erythropoietin? *J Intern Med* 231:381, 1992.
65. Choi JB, Loredo JS, Norman D, et al: Does obstructive sleep apnea increase hematocrit? *Sleep Breath* 10:155, 2006.
66. Agarwal N, Nagel RL, Prchal JT: Dyshemoglobinemias, in *Disorders of Hemoglobin: Genetics, Pathophysiology, and Clinical Management*, 2nd ed, edited by MH Steinberg, p 607. Cambridge University Press, Cambridge, UK, 2009.
67. Smith JR, Landaw SA: Smokers' polycythemia. *N Engl J Med* 298:6, 1978.
68. Stonesifer LD: How carbon monoxide reduces plasma volume. *N Engl J Med* 299:311, 1978.
69. Aitchison R, Russell N: Smoking—A major cause of polycythaemia. *J R Soc Med* 81:89, 1988.
70. Agarwal N, Gordeuk RV, Prchal JT: Genetic mechanisms underlying regulation of hemoglobin mass. *Adv Exp Med Biol* 618:195, 2007.
71. Galacteros F, Rosa R, Prehu MO, et al: [Diphosphoglyceromutase deficiency: New cases associated with erythrocytosis]. *Nouv Rev Fr Hematol* 26:69, 1984.
72. Xia M, Huang R, Sun Y, et al: Identification of chemical compounds that induce HIF-1 alpha activity. *Toxicol Sci* 112:153, 2009
73. Sergeyeva A, Gordeuk VR, Tokarev YN, et al: Congenital polycythemia in Chuvashia. *Blood* 89:2148, 1997.
74. Gordeuk VR, Sergueeva AI, Miasnikova GY, et al: Congenital disorder of oxygen sensing: Association of the homozygous Chuvash polycythemia VHL mutation with thrombosis and vascular abnormalities but not tumors. *Blood* 103:3924, 2004.
75. Percy MJ, McMullin MF, Jowitt SN, et al: Chuvash-type congenital polycythemia in 4 families of Asian and Western European ancestry. *Blood* 102:1097, 2003.
76. Bento MC, Chang KT, Guan Y, et al: Congenital polycythemia with homozygous and heterozygous mutations of von Hippel-Lindau gene: Five new Caucasian patients. *Haematologica* 90:128, 2005.
77. Cario H, Schwarz K, Jorch N, et al: Mutations in the von Hippel-Lindau (VHL) tumor suppressor gene and VHL-haplotype analysis in patients with presumable congenital erythrocytosis. *Haematologica* 90:19, 2005.
78. Collins TS, Arcasoy MO: Iron overload due to X-linked sideroblastic anemia in an African American man. *Am J Med* 116:501, 2004.
79. Gordeuk VR, Stockton DW, Prchal JT: Congenital polycythemias/erythrocytoses. *Haematologica* 90:109, 2005.
80. Pastore Y, Jedlickova K, Guan Y, et al: Mutations of von Hippel-Lindau tumor-suppressor gene and congenital polycythemia. *Am J Hum Genet* 73:412, 2003.
81. Pastore YD, Jelinek J, Ang S, et al: Mutations in the VHL gene in sporadic apparently congenital polycythemia. *Blood* 101:1591, 2003.
82. Navarro J, Aguilera A, Liano F, et al: Phlebotomy for polycythemia associated with acquired cystic renal disease in a patient on hemodialysis. *Nephron* 62:110, 1992.
83. Mrug M, Julian BA, Prchal JT: Angiotensin II receptor type 1 expression in erythroid progenitors: Implications for the pathogenesis of postrenal transplant erythrocytosis. *Semin Nephrol* 24:120, 2004.
84. Semenza GL: HIF-1 and mechanisms of hypoxia sensing. *Curr Opin Cell Biol* 13:167, 2001.
85. Cramer T, Yamanishi Y, Clausen BE, et al: HIF-1alpha is essential for myeloid cell-mediated inflammation. *Cell* 112:645, 2003.
86. Friedrich CA: von Hippel-Lindau syndrome. A pleomorphic condition. *Cancer* 86:2478, 1999.
87. Haase VH, Glickman JN, Socolovsky M, et al: Vascular tumors in livers with targeted inactivation of the von Hippel-Lindau tumor suppressor. *Proc Natl Acad Sci U S A* 98:1583, 2001.
88. Krieg M, Marti HH, Plate KH: Coexpression of erythropoietin and vascular endothelial growth factor in nervous system tumors associated with von Hippel-Lindau tumor suppressor gene loss of function. *Blood* 92:3388, 1998.
89. Richards FM: Molecular pathology of von HippelLindau disease and the VHL tumour suppressor gene. *Expert Rev Mol Med* 2001:1, 2001.
90. Percy MJ, Zhao Q, Flores A, et al: A family with erythrocytosis establishes a role for prolyl hydroxylase domain protein 2 in oxygen homeostasis. *Proc Natl Acad Sci U S A* 103:654, 2006.
91. Al-Sheikh M, Moradkhani K, Lopez M, et al: Disturbance in the HIF-1alpha pathway associated with erythrocytosis: Further evidences brought by frameshift and nonsense mutations in the prolyl hydroxylase domain protein 2 (PHD2) gene. *Blood Cells Mol Dis* 40:160, 2008.
92. Percy MJ, Furlow PW, Beer PA, et al: A novel erythrocytosis-associated PHD2 mutation suggests the location of a HIF binding groove. *Blood* 110:2193, 2007.
93. Percy MJ, Furlow PW, Lucas GS, et al: A gain-of-function mutation in the HIF2A gene in familial erythrocytosis. *N Engl J Med* 358:162, 2008.

94. Percy MJ, Beer PA, Campbell G, et al: Novel exon 12 mutations in the HIF2A gene associated with erythrocytosis. *Blood* 111:5400, 2008.
95. Hirota K, Semenza GL: Regulation of angiogenesis by hypoxia-inducible factor 1. *Crit Rev Oncol Hematol* 59:15, 2006.
96. Semenza GL, Koury ST, Nejfelt MK, et al: Cell-type-specific and hypoxia-inducible expression of the human erythropoietin gene in transgenic mice. *Proc Natl Acad Sci U S A* 88:8725, 1991.
97. Prchal JT, Gordeuk VR: The HIF2A gene in familial erythrocytosis. *N Engl J Med* 358:1966; author reply 1966, 2008.
98. Boutin AT, Weidemann A, Fu Z, et al: Epidermal sensing of oxygen is essential for systemic hypoxic response. *Cell* 133:223, 2008.
99. Maran J, Jedlickova K, Stockton D, Prchal JT: Finding the novel molecular defect in a family with high erythropoietin autosomal dominant polycythemia. *Blood* 102:162b, 2003.
100. Bailey RR, Shand BI, Walker RJ: Reversible erythrocytosis in a patient with a hydronephrotic horseshoe kidney. *Nephron* 70:104, 1995.
101. Hammond D, Winnick S: Paraneoplastic erythrocytosis and ectopic erythropoietins. *Ann N Y Acad Sci* 230:219, 1974.
102. Da Silva JL, Lacombe C, Bruneval P, et al: Tumor cells are the site of erythropoietin synthesis in human renal cancers associated with polycythemia. *Blood* 75:577, 1990.
103. Lal A, Rice A, al Mahr M, et al: Wilms tumor associated with polycythemia: Case report and review of the literature. *J Pediatr Hematol Oncol* 19:263, 1997.
104. Grignon DJ, Eble JN: Papillary and metanephric adenomas of the kidney. *Semin Diagn Pathol* 15:41, 1998.
105. Fisher JW, Samuels AI: Relationship between renal blood flow and erythropoietin production in dogs. *Proc Soc Exp Biol Med* 125:482, 1967.
106. Beebe HG, Chesebro K, Merchant F, et al: Results of renal artery balloon angioplasty limit its indications. *J Vasc Surg* 8:300, 1988.
107. Danovitch GM, Jamgotchian NJ, Eggena PH, et al: Angiotensin-converting enzyme inhibition in the treatment of renal transplant erythrocytosis. Clinical experience and observation of mechanism. *Transplantation* 60:132, 1995.
108. Mrug M, Stopka T, Julian BA, et al: Angiotensin II stimulates proliferation of normal early erythroid progenitors. *J Clin Invest* 100:2310, 1997.
109. Glicklich D, Burris L, Urban A, et al: Angiotensin-converting enzyme inhibition induces apoptosis in erythroid precursors and affects insulin-like growth factor-1 in posttransplantation erythrocytosis. *J Am Soc Nephrol* 12:1958, 2001.
110. Gossmann J, Burkhardt R, Harder S, et al: Angiotensin II infusion increases plasma erythropoietin levels via an angiotensin II type 1 receptor-dependent pathway. *Kidney Int* 60:83, 2001.
111. Thevenod F, Radtke HW, Grutzmacher P, et al: Deficient feedback regulation of erythropoiesis in kidney transplant patients with polycythemia. *Kidney Int* 24:227, 1983.
112. Friman S, Nyberg G, Blohme I: Erythrocytosis after renal transplantation; treatment by removal of the native kidneys. *Nephrol Dial Transplant* 5:969, 1990.
113. Cole J, Ertoy D, Lin H, et al: Lack of angiotensin II-facilitated erythropoiesis causes anemia in angiotensin-converting enzyme-deficient mice. *J Clin Invest* 106:1391, 2000.
114. Venencie PY, Puissant A, Boffa GA, et al: Multiple cutaneous leiomyomata and erythrocytosis with demonstration of erythropoietic activity in the cutaneous leiomyomata. *Br J Dermatol* 107:483, 1982.
115. Trimble M, Caro J, Talalla A, et al: Secondary erythrocytosis due to a cerebellar hemangioblastoma: Demonstration of erythropoietin mRNA in the tumor. *Blood* 78:599, 1991.
116. McFadzean AJS, Todd D, Tsang, KC: Polycythemia in primary carcinoma of the liver. *Blood* 13:427, 1958.
117. Davidson CS: Hepatocellular carcinoma and erythrocytosis. *Semin Hematol* 13:115, 1976.
118. Muta H, Funakoshi A, Baba T, et al: Gene expression of erythropoietin in hepatocellular carcinoma. *Intern Med* 33:427, 1994.
119. Shulkin BL, Shapiro B, Sisson JC: Pheochromocytoma, polycythemia, and venous thrombosis. *Am J Med* 83:773, 1987.
120. Mann DL, Gallagher NI, Donati RM: Erythrocytosis and primary aldosteronism. *Ann Intern Med* 66:335, 1967.
121. Erkelens DW, Statius van Eps LW: Bartter's syndrome and erythrocytosis. *Am J Med* 55:711, 1973.
122. Ghio R, Haupt E, Ratti M, et al: Erythrocytosis associated with a dermoid cyst of the ovary and erythropoietic activity of the tumour fluid. *Scand J Haematol* 27:70, 1981.
123. Shahani S, Braga-Basaria M, Maggio M, et al: Androgens and erythropoiesis: A review. *J Endocrinol Invest* 32:704, 2009.
124. Gardner FH, Nathan DG, Piomelli S, et al: The erythrocythaemic effects of androgen. *Br J Haematol* 14:611, 1968.
125. Besa EC: Hematologic effects of androgens revisited: An alternative therapy in various hematologic conditions. *Semin Hematol* 31:134, 1994.
126. Wiswell TE, Cornish JD, Northam RS: Neonatal polycythemia: Frequency of clinical manifestations and other associated findings. *Pediatrics* 78:26, 1986.
127. Black VD, Lubchenco LO, Koops BL, et al: Neonatal hyperviscosity: Randomized study of effect of partial plasma exchange transfusion on long-term outcome. *Pediatrics* 75:1048, 1985.
128. Pearson TC: Apparent polycythaemia. *Blood Rev* 5:205, 1991.
129. Chrysant SG, Frohlich ED, Adamopoulos PN, et al: Pathophysiologic significance of "stress" or relative polycythemia in essential hypertension. *Am J Cardiol* 37:1069, 1976.
130. Isbister JP: The contracted plasma volume syndromes (relative polycythaemias) and their haemorheological significance. *Baillieres Clin Haematol* 1:665, 1987.
131. Leth A: Changes in plasma and extracellular fluid volumes in patients with essential hypertension during long-term treatment with hydrochlorothiazide. *Circulation* 42:479, 1970.
132. Prchal JT: Personal communication and direct experience with about 100 affected subjects. 2009.
133. Queisser W, Heim ME, Schmitz JM, et al: [Idiopathic familial erythrocytosis. Report on a family with autosomal dominant inheritance]. *Dtsch Med Wochenschr* 113:851, 1988.
134. Prchal JT, Semenza GL, Prchal J, et al: Familial polycythemia. *Science* 268:1831, 1995.
135. Kralovics R, Sokol L, Prchal JT: Absence of polycythemia in a child with a unique erythropoietin receptor mutation in a family with autosomal dominant primary polycythemia. *J Clin Invest* 102:124, 1998.
136. Arcasoy MO, Degar BA, Harris KW, et al: Familial erythrocytosis associated with a short deletion in the erythropoietin receptor gene. *Blood* 89:4628, 1997.
137. Bushuev VI, Miasnikova GY, Sergueeva AI, et al: Endothelin-1, vascular endothelial growth factor and systolic pulmonary artery pressure in patients with Chuvash polycythemia. *Haematologica* 91:744, 2006.
138. Gladwin MT: Polycythemia, HIF-1alpha and pulmonary hypertension in Chuvash. *Haematologica* 91:722, 2006.
139. Smith TG, Brooks JT, Balanos GM, et al: Mutation of von Hippel-Lindau tumour suppressor and human cardiopulmonary physiology. *PLoS Med* 3:e290, 2006.
140. Zafren K, Honigman B: High-altitude medicine. *Emerg Med Clin North Am* 15:191, 1997.
141. Bishop BC: Wintering in the high Himalayas. *Natl Geogr Mag* 122:503, 1962.
142. Botella de Maglia J, Martinez-Costa R: [High altitude retinal hemorrhages in the expeditions to 8,000 meter peaks. A study of 10 cases]. *Med Clin (Barc)* 110:457, 1998.
143. Beall CM, Song K, Elston RC, et al: Higher offspring survival among Tibetan women with high oxygen saturation genotypes residing at 4,000 m. *Proc Natl Acad Sci U S A* 101:14300, 2004.
144. Beall CM: Oxygen saturation increases during childhood and decreases during adulthood among high altitude native Tibetans residing at 3,800–4,200m. *High Alt Med Biol* 1:25, 2000.
145. Beall CM: Tibetan and Andean contrasts in adaptation to high-altitude hypoxia. *Adv Exp Med Biol* 475:63, 2000.
146. Beall CM, Decker MJ, Brittenham GM, et al: An Ethiopian pattern of human adaptation to high-altitude hypoxia. *Proc Natl Acad Sci U S A* 99:17215, 2002.
147. Thorne SA: Management of polycythaemia in adults with cyanotic congenital heart disease. *Heart* 79:315, 1998.
148. Shibata J, Hasegawa J, Siemens HJ, et al: Hemostasis and coagulation at a hematocrit level of 0.85: Functional consequences of erythrocytosis. *Blood* 101:4416, 2003.
149. Ammash N, Warnes CA: Cerebrovascular events in adult patients with cyanotic congenital heart disease. *J Am Coll Cardiol* 28:768, 1996.
150. Cote C, Zilberberg MD, Mody SH, et al: Haemoglobin level and its clinical impact in a cohort of patients with COPD. *Eur Respir J* 29:923, 2007.
151. Stefenelli T, Silberbauer K, Ulrich W, et al: Cardial decompensation caused by hypertension and polyglobulia associated with multiple renal oncocytomas. *Clin Nephrol* 23:307, 1985.
152. Lezaic V, Biljanovic-Paunovic L, Pavlovic-Kentera V, et al: Erythropoiesis after kidney transplantation: The role of erythropoietin, burst promoting activity and early erythroid progenitor cells. *Eur J Med Res* 6:27, 2001.
153. Niu X, Miasnikova GY, Sergueeva AI, et al: Altered cytokine profiles in patients with Chuvash polycythemia. *Am J Hematol* 84:74, 2009.
154. Sergueeva AI, Miasnikova GY, Okhotin DJ, et al: Elevated homocysteine, glutathione and cysteinylglycine concentrations in patients homozygous for the Chuvash polycythemia VHL mutation. *Haematologica* 93:279, 2008.
155. Tefferi A, Thiele J, Vardiman JW: The 2008 World Health Organization classification system for myeloproliferative neoplasms: Order out of chaos. *Cancer* 115:3842, 2009.
156. Beutler E: Polycythemia. *Med Grand Rounds* 3:142, 1984.
157. Prchal JF, Axelrad AA: Bone-marrow responses in polycythemia vera [letter]. *N Engl J Med* 290:1382, 1974.
158. Kralovics R, Buser AS, Teo SS, et al: Comparison of molecular markers in a cohort of patients with chronic myeloproliferative disorders. *Blood* 102:1869, 2003.
159. Weinberg RS: *In vitro* erythropoiesis in polycythemia vera and other myeloproliferative disorders. *Semin Hematol* 34:64, 1997.
160. Shih LY, Lee CT, See LC, et al: *In vitro* culture growth of erythroid progenitors and serum erythropoietin assay in the differential diagnosis of polycythaemia. *Eur J Clin Invest* 28:569, 1998.
161. Prchal JT: Personal communication. 2009.
162. Fisher MJ, Prchal JF, Prchal JT, et al: Anti-erythropoietin (EPO) receptor monoclonal antibodies distinguish EPO-dependent and EPO-independent erythroid progenitors in polycythemia vera. *Blood* 84:1982, 1994.
163. Kralovics R, Indrak K, Stopka T, et al: Two new EPO receptor mutations: Truncated EPO receptors are most frequently associated with primary familial and congenital polycythemias. *Blood* 90:2057, 1997.
164. Acharya J, Westwood NB, Sawyer BM, et al: Identification of latent myeloproliferative disease in patients with Budd-Chiari syndrome using X-chromosome inactivation patterns and in vitro erythroid colony formation. *Eur J Haematol* 55:315, 1995.
165. De Stefano V, Teofili L, Leone G, et al: Spontaneous erythroid colony formation as the clue to an underlying myeloproliferative disorder in patients with Budd-Chiari syndrome or portal vein thrombosis. *Semin Thromb Hemost* 23:411, 1997.

166. Pagliuca A, Mufti GJ, Janossa-Tahernia M, et al: *In vitro* colony culture and chromosomal studies in hepatic and portal vein thrombosis—Possible evidence of an occult myeloproliferative state. *Q J Med* 76:981, 1990.
167. Valla D, Casadevall N, Lacombe C, et al: Primary myeloproliferative disorder and hepatic vein thrombosis. A prospective study of erythroid colony formation *in vitro* in 20 patients with Budd-Chiari syndrome. *Ann Intern Med* 103:329, 1985.
168. Shih LY, Lee CT: Identification of masked polycythemia vera from patients with idiopathic marked thrombocytosis by endogenous erythroid colony assay. *Blood* 83:744, 1994.
169. Birgegard G, Wide L: Serum erythropoietin in the diagnosis of polycythaemia and after phlebotomy treatment. *Br J Haematol* 81:603, 1992.
170. Messinezy M, Westwood NB, El-Hemaidi I, et al: Serum erythropoietin values in erythrocytoses and in primary thrombocythaemia. *Br J Haematol* 117:47, 2002.
171. Mossuz P, Girodon F, Donnard M, et al: Diagnostic value of serum erythropoietin level in patients with absolute erythrocytosis. *Haematologica* 89:1194, 2004.
172. Thurmes PJ, Steensma DP: Elevated serum erythropoietin levels in patients with Budd-Chiari syndrome secondary to polycythemia vera: Clinical implications for the role of JAK2 mutation analysis. *Eur J Haematol* 77:57, 2006.
173. Remacha AF, Montserrat I, Santamaria A, et al: Serum erythropoietin in the diagnosis of polycythemia vera. A follow-up study. *Haematologica* 82:406, 1997.
174. Beutler E, Yeh M, Fairbanks VF: The normal human female as a mosaic of X-chromosome activity: Studies using the gene for C-6-PD-deficiency as a marker. *Proc Natl Acad Sci U S A* 48:9, 1962.
175. Adamson JW, Fialkow PJ, Murphy S, et al: Polycythemia vera: Stem-cell and probable clonal origin of the disease. *N Engl J Med* 295:913, 1976.
176. Prchal JT: Pathogenetic mechanisms of polycythemia vera and congenital polycythemic disorders. *Semin Hematol* 38:10, 2001.
177. Kralovics R, Guan Y, Prchal JT: Acquired uniparental disomy of chromosome 9p is a frequent stem cell defect in polycythemia vera. *Exp Hematol* 30:229, 2002.
178. Chen GL, Prchal JT: X-linked clonality testing: Interpretation and limitations. *Blood* 110:1411, 2007.
179. Curnutte JT, Hopkins PJ, Kuhl W, et al: Studying X inactivation. *Lancet* 339:749, 1992.
180. Allen RC, Zoghbi HY, Moseley AB, et al: Methylation of HpaII and HhaI sites near the polymorphic CAG repeat in the human androgen-receptor gene correlates with X chromosome inactivation. *Am J Hum Genet* 51:1229, 1992.
181. Prchal JT, Guan YL, Prchal JF, et al: Transcriptional analysis of the active X-chromosome in normal and clonal hematopoiesis. *Blood* 81:269, 1993.
182. Prchal JT, Prchal JF, Belickova M, et al: Clonal stability of blood cell lineages indicated by X-chromosomal transcriptional polymorphism. *J Exp Med* 183:561, 1996.
183. Busque L, Mio R, Mattioli J, et al: Nonrandom X-inactivation patterns in normal females: Lyonization ratios vary with age. *Blood* 88:59, 1996.
184. Champion KM, Gilbert JG, Asimakopoulos FA, et al: Clonal haemopoiesis in normal elderly women: Implications for the myeloproliferative disorders and myelodysplastic syndromes. *Br J Haematol* 97:920, 1997.
185. Gale RE, Fielding AK, Harrison CN, et al: Acquired skewing of X-chromosome inactivation patterns in myeloid cells of the elderly suggests stochastic clonal loss with age. *Br J Haematol* 98:512, 1997.
186. Swierczek SI, Agarwal N, Nussenzveig RH, et al: Hematopoiesis is not clonal in healthy elderly women. *Blood* 112:3186, 2008.
187. Lertzman M, Frome BM, Israels LG, et al: Hypoxia in polycythemia vera. *Ann Intern Med* 60:409, 1964.
188. Lichtman MA, Murphy MS, Adamson JW: Detection of mutant hemoglobins with altered affinity for oxygen. A simplified technique. *Ann Intern Med* 84:517, 1976.
189. Plata R, Cornejo A, Arratia C, et al: Angiotensin-converting-enzyme inhibition therapy in altitude polycythaemia: A prospective randomised trial. *Lancet* 359:663, 2002.
190. Manglani MV, DeGroff CG, Dukes PP, et al: Congenital erythrocytosis with elevated erythropoietin level: An incorrectly set "erythrostat"? *J Pediatr Hematol Oncol* 20:560, 1998.
191. Piccirillo G, Fimognari FL, Valdivia JL, et al: Effects of phlebotomy on a patient with secondary polycythemia and angina pectoris. *Int J Cardiol* 44:175, 1994.
192. Divoky V, Prchal JT: Mouse surviving solely on human erythropoietin receptor (EPOR): Model of human EPOR-linked disease. *Blood* 99:3873, 2002.
193. Watowich SS, Xie X, Klingmuller U, et al: Erythropoietin receptor mutations associated with familial erythrocytosis cause hypersensitivity to erythropoietin in the heterozygous state. *Blood* 94:2530, 1999.
194. de la Chapelle A, Traskelin AL, Juvonen E: Truncated erythropoietin receptor causes dominantly inherited benign human erythrocytosis. *Proc Natl Acad Sci U S A* 90:4495, 1993.
195. Furukawa T, Narita M, Sakaue M, et al: Primary familial polycythaemia associated with a novel point mutation in the erythropoietin receptor. *Br J Haematol* 99:222, 1997.
196. Arcasoy MO, Harris KW, Forget BG: A human erythropoietin receptor gene mutant causing familial erythrocytosis is associated with deregulation of the rates of Jak2 and Stat5 inactivation. *Exp Hematol* 27:63, 1999.
197. Kralovics R, Prchal JT: Genetic heterogeneity of primary familial and congenital polycythemia. *Am J Hematol* 68:115, 2001.
198. Sokol L, Luhovy M, Guan Y, et al: Primary familial polycythemia: A frameshift mutation in the erythropoietin receptor gene and increased sensitivity of erythroid progenitors to erythropoietin. *Blood* 86:15, 1995.
199. Kralovics R, Sokol L, Broxson EH Jr, et al: The erythropoietin receptor gene is not linked with the polycythemia phenotype in a family with autosomal dominant primary polycythemia. *Proc Assoc Am Physicians* 109:580, 1997.
200. Sokol L, Prchal JF, D'Andrea A, et al: Mutation in the negative regulatory element of the erythropoietin receptor gene in a case of sporadic primary polycythemia. *Exp Hematol* 22:447, 1994.
201. Le Couedic JP, Mitjavila MT, Villeval JL, et al: Missense mutation of the erythropoietin receptor is a rare event in human erythroid malignancies. *Blood* 87:1502, 1996.
202. Hultberg B, Sjoblad S, Ockerman PA: Properties of five acid hydrolases in human skin fibroblast cultures. Possible use in the diagnosis of inborn lysosomal diseases. *Acta Paediatr Scand* 62:474, 1973.

CHAPTER 57
THE PORPHYRIAS

John D. Phillips and Karl E. Anderson

SUMMARY

Porphyrias are diseases that result from derangements of specific enzymes in the heme biosynthetic pathway that lead to overproduction and accumulation of pathway intermediates and cause neurologic symptoms, photocutaneous symptoms, or both. Multiple inherited mutations have been identified in all the porphyrias. However, porphyria cutanea tarda (PCT), which is caused by a primarily acquired deficiency of the fifth enzyme in the heme biosynthetic pathway, specifically in the liver, is usually not associated with a mutation of this enzyme.

Porphyrias can be classified as either hepatic or erythropoietic, depending on the principal site of initial accumulation of excess pathway intermediates. Erythropoietic porphyrias are characterized by childhood onset and a generally stable clinical course. Hepatic porphyrias almost always develop during adult life, and are more variable because of multiple influences of drugs, hormones, and nutritional factors on the heme biosynthetic pathway in the liver.

Porphyrias are also classified as acute or cutaneous. The four acute porphyrias are associated with neurologic manifestations that usually occur as acute attacks. δ-Aminolevulinate dehydratase porphyria (ADP) is an autosomal recessive disorder caused by a deficiency of the second enzyme in the pathway and is the most rare type of porphyria. ADP has been classified as hepatic, but also has erythropoietic features. The three other acute porphyrias, namely acute intermittent porphyria (AIP), hereditary coproporphyria (HCP), and variegate porphyria (VP), are autosomal dominant hepatic porphyrias, and result from deficiencies of the third, sixth, and seventh enzymes in the pathway, respectively. HCP and VP are also classified as cutaneous, because photocutaneous lesions may develop, especially in VP. AIP is the most common acute porphyria and the second most common porphyria. Disease expression is highly variable, and the great majority of individuals who inherit deficiencies of these enzymes remain latent through all or most of their lives. Attacks are produced by factors that increase hepatic heme synthesis, including certain drugs, some steroid hormones and their metabolites, and restriction of dietary calories and carbohydrate. Treatment of acute porphyrias includes glucose loading and hemin infusions, which repress δ-aminolevulinic acid synthase, the rate-limiting enzyme of the heme biosynthetic pathway in the liver.

Cutaneous porphyrias are associated with either blistering skin lesions or, in erythropoietic protoporphyria (EPP), with acute nonblistering photosensitivity. Blistering skin manifestations are identical in PCT, HCP and VP. Similar lesions in congenital erythropoietic porphyria (CEP) are much more severe and often associated with loss of digits and facial mutilation. CEP results from a severe deficiency of the fourth enzyme in the pathway and is inherited in an autosomal recessive fashion. Hemolytic anemia is common, and severe cases may be transfusion dependent, and may even present *in utero* with fetal hydrops. Hematopoietic stem cell transplantation in early childhood is the most effective treatment.

EPP is the third most common porphyria and the most common in children. It is usually caused by a deficiency of the final enzyme in the pathway. In most families, inheritance of EPP is autosomal dominant, and a severe ferrochelatase mutation is inherited from one parent. However, the pattern is unusual, because a low-expression normal allele, which by itself does not cause disease, is also required, and is inherited from the other parent. Autosomal recessive inheritance has been documented in a few families, with inheritance of two disease-causing mutations. Protoporphyrin-containing gallstones may develop in EPP. An uncommon but potentially life-threatening complication is protoporphyric hepatopathy, which is a result of the cholestatic effects of protoporphyrin, and may require liver transplantation. Sequential marrow transplantation can prevent recurrent hepatopathy in the transplanted liver.

PCT is an iron-related hepatic porphyria that usually begins in middle or late adult life. Hepatic uroporphyrinogen decarboxylase (UROD) is reduced in the presence of iron to approximately 20 percent of normal in PCT. Iron does not directly inhibit UROD. Multiple susceptibility factors, including use of alcohol, smoking, estrogens, hepatitis C, and HIV contribute to generation of a UROD inhibitor. HFE (hemochromatosis gene) mutations that cause excess iron absorption are common in PCT. A minority of patients are heterozygous for UROD mutations and are said to have familial PCT. Polyhalogenated aromatic hydrocarbons cause PCT in laboratory animals and occasionally in humans. PCT responds well to treatment by repeated phlebotomy, which reduces hepatic iron, or low-dose hydroxychloroquine or chloroquine, which mobilizes accumulated hepatic porphyrins. Hepatoerythropoietic porphyria is the homozygous form of familial PCT, and is usually a severe disorder that starts in childhood and resembles CEP clinically.

Acronyms and abbreviations that appear in this chapter include: ADP, δ-aminolevulinate dehydratase deficiency porphyria; AIP, acute intermittent porphyria; ALA, δ-aminolevulinic acid; ALAD, δ-aminolevulinic acid dehydratase; ALAS, δ-aminolevulinic acid synthase; ALAS1, δ-aminolevulinic acid synthase, housekeeping form; ALAS2, δ-aminolevulinic acid synthase, erythroid specific form; CEP, congenital erythropoietic porphyria; CPO, coproporphyrinogen oxidase; CPRE, coproporphyrinogen oxidase gene promoter regulatory element; CRIM, cross-reactive immunologic material; CYP, cytochrome P450; EC, enzyme commission; EPP, erythropoietic protoporphyria; FECH, ferrochelatase; HCP, hereditary coproporphyria; HEP, hepatoerythropoietic porphyria; HFE, hemochromatosis gene; HMB, hydroxymethylbilane; PBG, porphobilinogen; PBGD, porphobilinogen deaminase; PCT, porphyria cutanea tarda; PGC-1α, peroxisomal proliferator-activated cofactor 1α; PPO, protoporphyrinogen oxidase; PXR, pregnane X receptor; SCS-βA, β subunit of ATP specific succinyl coenzyme A synthetase; UROD, uroporphyrinogen decarboxylase; VP, variegate porphyria; XLSA, X-linked sideroblastic anemia.

DEFINITION AND HISTORY

The porphyrias are a group of metabolic diseases resulting from derangements, usually of a genetic nature, in the activity of specific enzymes in the heme biosynthetic pathway, leading to overproduction and accumulation of pathway intermediates. Symptoms of these diseases can be neurologic, photocutaneous, or both. The intermediates that accumulate include porphyrins and the porphyrin precursors δ-aminolevulinic acid (ALA) and porphobilinogen (PBG) and their derivatives, which are excreted in urine and feces. Patterns of these substances in plasma, erythrocytes, urine, and feces are characteristic for each porphyria, and are the basis for screening tests and more comprehensive biochemical characterization.

Porphyrias are classified as either *erythropoietic* or *hepatic*, depending on the principal site of accumulation of pathway intermediates. The erythropoietic porphyrias are congenital erythropoietic porphyria (CEP), which is very rare, and erythropoietic protoporphyria (EPP), which is the third most common porphyria and the most common in children. Hepatic porphyrias include the acute porphyrias, which cause acute attacks of neurologic symptoms, and porphyria cutanea tarda (PCT), which is the most common of the porphyrias, and causes chronic blistering lesions on sun-exposed areas of the skin. The acute porphyrias include ALA dehydratase deficiency porphyria, acute intermittent porphyria (AIP), hereditary coproporphyria (HCP), and variegate porphyria (VP). VP and less commonly HCP, can also cause skin manifestations identical to those in PCT.

A type of porphyria has been associated with each of the eight enzymes in the heme biosynthetic pathway (Table 57–1 and Fig. 57–1). Mutations affecting the erythroid form of ALA synthase (ALAS2) are associated with X-linked sideroblastic anemia (see Chap. 58). Gain-of-function mutations of ALAS2 also are associated with a variant form of EPP. Table 57–2 summarizes the major clinical and laboratory features of the porphyrias.

A case of CEP reported by Schultz in 1874 was the first description of porphyria in the literature. This case was a 33-year-old man with photosensitivity since age 3 months, anemia, splenomegaly, red-wine-colored urine as a result of a pigment resembling hematoporphyrin, and brown-colored bones at autopsy.[1,2] In 1898, T. McCall Anderson described two brothers (ages 23 and 26 years) who most likely had CEP,[3] and suffered from *hydroa aestivale*, with red urine, pruritus, and blistering of sun-exposed skin, especially in summer, leading to extensive scarring and mutilation or ears and nose (Fig. 57–2). Using available methods, their urine was also demonstrated to contain a substance related to hematoporphyrin.[4] In 1889, Stokvis first described a case of acute porphyria in an elderly woman who developed dark-red urine and later died after taking sulphonal, a drug related to the barbiturates.[5]

Hans Günther[6] published a monograph on porphyrins in 1911 and classified porphyrias into four groups: (1) those that have an acute onset without association with drug ingestion, (2) those that are caused by sulphonal or trional, (3) hematoporphyria congenita, and (4) chronic hematoporphyria. The first two groups correspond to the acute porphyrias, which may present with attacks sometimes related to ingestion of certain drugs, the second group to CEP and hepatoerythropoietic porphyria (HEP), and the fourth to PCT. In 1923, Archibald Garrod proposed the term *inborn errors of metabolism* for a number of inherited metabolic disorders, including the porphyrias.[7]

Sachs noted an Ehrlich-positive chromogen that was not urobilinogen in urine of patients with acute porphyria in 1931.[8] In 1937, Waldenström noted that excretion of this chromogen was an autosomal dominant trait in AIP families, which he identified as PBG in 1939.[9,10] The classification of porphyrias as erythropoietic and hepatic was proposed in 1954 by Schmid, Schwartz, and Watson.[11] An epidemic of hexachlorobenzene-induced PCT in eastern Turkey in 1957[12,13] provided the foundation for the development of animal models of this disorder using this and other halogenated polyaromatic hydrocarbons.[14–17] Strand and coworkers described the enzyme deficiency in AIP for the first time in 1970,[18] and Bonkovsky and coworkers first reported treatment of a porphyria patient with hemin in 1971.[19] In the past 30 years, the enzymes of the heme biosynthetic pathway have been defined in terms of their amino acid composition, genomic and complementary DNA (cDNA) sequences, and crystal structures. Erythroid-specific and housekeeping transcripts have been described for at least four enzymes in the pathway, and progress made in understanding the regulation of heme synthesis in specific tissues, especially the marrow and liver. Multiple mutations have been described in each of the human porphyrias, and some specific treatments introduced.

ETIOLOGY AND PATHOGENESIS

HEME

Heme (iron protoporphyrin IX, Fig. 57–3) is essential for all cells and functions as the prosthetic group of numerous hemoproteins such as

TABLE 57–1. Human Porphyrias: Specific Enzymes Affected by Mutations, Modes of Inheritance, Classification, and Major Types of Clinical Features of Each of the Human Porphyrias

Porphyria*	Affected Enzyme	Known Mutations	Inheritance	Classification	Principal Clinical Features
Erythropoietic protoporphyria (EPP)—variant form	δ-Aminolevulinic acid (ALA) synthase erythroid-specific form (ALAS2)	2 (gain of function)	Sex-linked recessive	Erythropoietic	Nonblistering photosensitivity
δ-Aminolevulinic acid dehydratase porphyria (ADP)	ALA dehydratase (ALAD)	11	Autosomal recessive	Hepatic†	Neurovisceral
Acute intermittent porphyria (AIP)	PBG deaminase (PBGD)	273	Autosomal dominant	Hepatic	Neurovisceral
Congenital erythropoietic porphyria (CEP)	Uroporphyrinogen III synthase (UROS)	36	Autosomal recessive	Erythropoietic	Neurovisceral
Porphyria cutanea tarda (PCT)	Uroporphyrinogen decarboxylase (UROD)	70 (includes HEP)	Autosomal dominant‡	Hepatic	Blistering photosensitivity
Hepatoerythropoietic porphyria (HEP)	UROD	–	Autosomal recessive	Hepatic†	Blistering photosensitivity
Hereditary coproporphyria (HCP)	Coproporphyrinogen oxidase (CPO)	42	Autosomal dominant	Hepatic	Neurovisceral; blistering photosensitivity (uncommon)
Variegate porphyria (VP)	Protoporphyrinogen oxidase (PPO)	130	Autosomal dominant	Hepatic	Neurovisceral; blistering photosensitivity (common)
EPP—classic form	Ferrochelatase (FECH)	90	Autosomal dominant	Erythropoietic	Nonblistering photosensitivity

*Porphyrias are listed in the order of the affected enzyme in the heme biosynthetic pathway.

†These porphyrias also have erythropoietic features, including increases in erythrocyte zinc protoporphyrin.

‡UROD inhibition in PCT is mostly acquired, but an inherited deficiency of the enzyme predisposes in familial (type 2) disease.

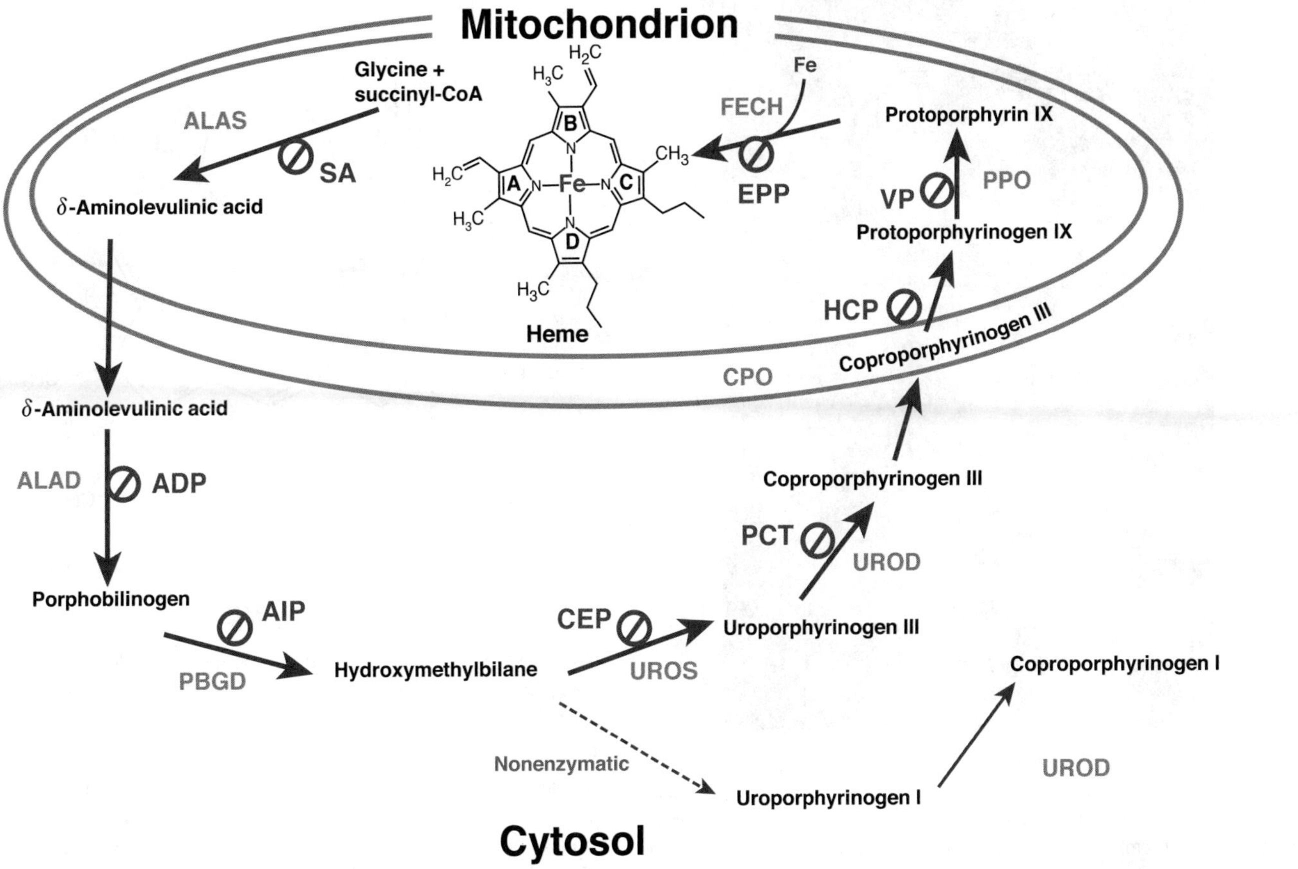

FIGURE 57–1. Enzymes and intermediates in the heme biosynthetic pathway and the type of porphyria associated with a deficiency of each enzyme (indicated by ⊘). Gain-of-function mutation of the erythroid form of ALA synthase is not shown. Abbreviations: ADP, ALA dehydratase porphyria; AIP, acute intermittent porphyria; ALA, δ-aminolevulinic acid; ALAD, δ-aminolevulinic acid dehydratase; ALAS, δ-aminolevulinic acid synthase; CEP, congenital erythropoietic porphyria; CPO, coproporphyrinogen oxidase; EPP, erythropoietic protoporphyria; HCP, hereditary coproporphyria; PBG, porphobilinogen; PBGD, porphobilinogen deaminase; PCT, porphyria cutanea tarda; PPO, protoporphyrinogen oxidase; UROD, uroporphyrinogen decarboxylase; UROS, uroporphyrinogen III synthase; VP, variegate porphyria.

TABLE 57–2. Biochemical Findings Including Major Increases in Porphyrins and Porphyrin Precursors in the Human Porphyrias*

Porphyria	Erythrocytes	Plasma	Urine	Stool
ADP*	Zinc protoporphyrin	ALA†	ALA, coproporphyrin III	†
AIP	Decreased PBGD activity (most cases)†	ALA, PBG† (~620 nm)‡	ALA, PBG, uroporphyrin	†
CEP	Uroporphyrin I; coproporphyrin I	Uroporphyrin I, coproporphyrin I (~620 nm)‡	Uroporphyrin I; coproporphyrin I	Coproporphyrin I
PCT and HEP	Zinc protoporphyrin (in HEP)	Uroporphyrin, heptacarboxyl porphyrin (~620 nm)‡	Uroporphyrin, heptacarboxyl porphyrin	Heptacarboxyl porphyrin, isocopro-porphyrins
HCP	†	§ (~620 nm)‡	ALA, PBG, coproporphyrin III	Coproporphyrin III
VP	†	Protoporphyrin (~628 nm)‡	ALA, PBG, coproporphyrin III	Coproporphyrin III, protoporphyrin
EPP	Free protoporphyrin	Protoporphyrin¶ (~634 nm)‡	**	Protoporphyrin†

*Abbreviations as in Table 57–1.

†Porphyrin levels normal or slightly increased.

‡Fluorescence emission peak of diluted plasma at neutral pH.

§Plasma porphyrins usually normal, but increased when blistering skin lesions develop.

¶Zinc protoporphyrin ≤5% of total in classic EPP, but 15–50% in variant form.

**Urine porphyrins (especially coproporphyrin) increase only with hepatopathy.

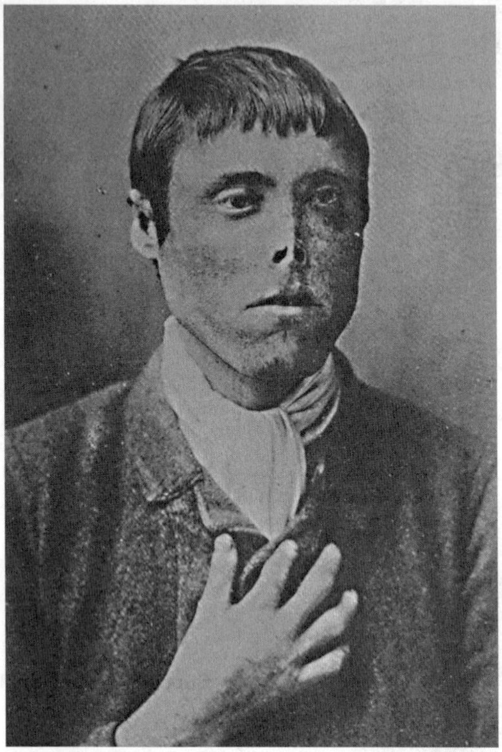

FIGURE 57–2. A 23-year-old Scottish fisherman with congenital erythropoietic porphyria and scarring and mutilation of the face, ears, and digits as a consequence of repeated sun exposure. He was described in 1898 as having red urine containing excess porphyrins and "hydroa aestivale," because the symptoms, which began at age 3 years, worsened in early summer. A 26-year-old brother was similarly affected. *(Reproduced from Anderson TM,[3] with permission.)*

hemoglobin, myoglobin, respiratory cytochromes, cytochromes P450 (CYPs), catalase, peroxidase, tryptophan pyrrolase, and nitric oxide synthase. Approximately 85 percent of heme is synthesized in the marrow to meet the requirement for hemoglobin formation; the remainder is synthesized largely in the liver.[20] Most heme synthesized in the liver is required for CYPs, which are located primarily in the endoplasmic reticulum, where they turn over rapidly and oxidize a variety of chemicals, including drugs, environmental carcinogens, endogenous steroids, vitamins, fatty acids, and prostaglandins.[21]

The term *heme* may refer more specifically to ferrous protoporphyrin IX, and is readily oxidized *in vitro* to hemin, that is, ferric protoporphyrin IX. Hemin has one residual positive charge and is usually isolated as a halide, most commonly as the chloride. In alkaline solution the halide is replaced by a hydroxyl ion to form hematin (Fig. 57–4). Heme can form further hexacoordinated complexes with nitrogenous bases to form a *hemochrome* or *hemochromogen*; for example, pyridine hemochromogen is useful for identification and quantification of heme and hemoproteins. In medicine, hemin is also a generic term for heme preparations used as intravenous therapies for acute porphyrias, such as lyophilized hematin and heme arginate.

The ferrous iron atom (Fe^{2+}) in heme has six electron pairs, of which four are bound to the pyrrolic nitrogens of the porphyrin macrocycle, leaving two unoccupied electron pairs, one above and the other below the plane of the porphyrin ring. In hemoglobin, one of these pairs is coordinated with a histidine residue of the globin chain. The other coordination site in deoxyhemoglobin is protected from oxidation by the nonpolar environment of surrounding amino acid residues, and is available to bind molecular oxygen for transport from the lung to other tissues. To reversibly bind oxygen, the iron in hemoglobin must be in the ferrous state. Methemoglobin (oxidized hemoglobin) that is generated in erythrocytes is continuously reduced to ferrous hemoglobin by the reduced form of nicotinamide adenine dinucleotide–cytochrome b_5 reductase–cytochrome b_5 system (see Chap. 49).

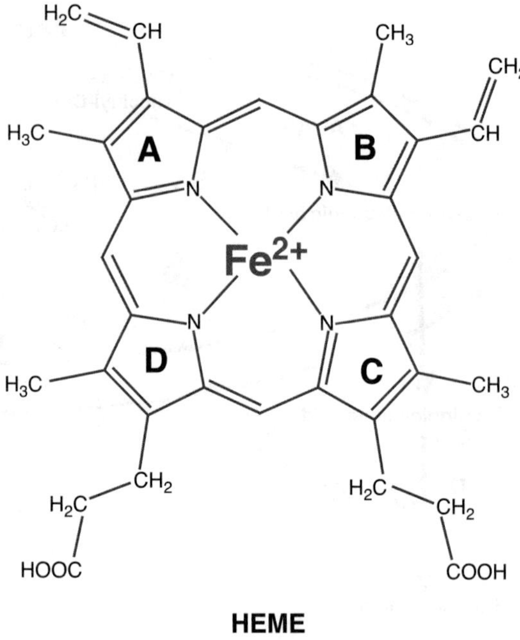

FIGURE 57–3. Structure of heme. The pyrrole rings are labeled A through D, according to the nomenclature of Hans Fischer.

Heme Biosynthesis

Figure 57–5 shows the enzymatic steps involved in heme biosynthesis in eukaryotic cells. The first and last three enzymes are mitochondrial and the intermediate four are cytosolic. Erythroid heme synthesis occurs in marrow erythroblasts and reticulocytes, which contain mitochondria. Circulating erythrocytes lack mitochondria and no longer synthesize heme. They contain residual cytosolic enzymes of the heme biosynthetic pathway and zinc protoporphyrin. Activity of these enzymes declines during the life span of erythrocytes in the circulation.

δ-Aminolevulinate Synthase (Succinyl CoA: Glycine C-Succinyl Transferase, Decarboxylating; Enzyme Commission (EC) 2.3.1.37) The first enzyme in the heme biosynthetic pathway catalyzes the condensation of glycine and

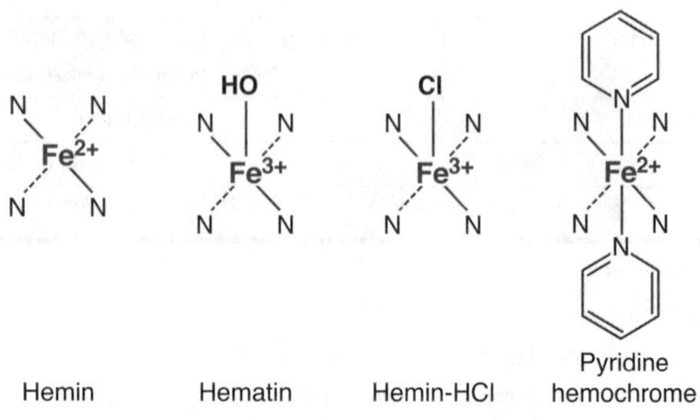

FIGURE 57–4. Forms of iron protoporphyrin IX. The porphyrin macrocycle is represented only by its pyrrole nitrogen atoms.

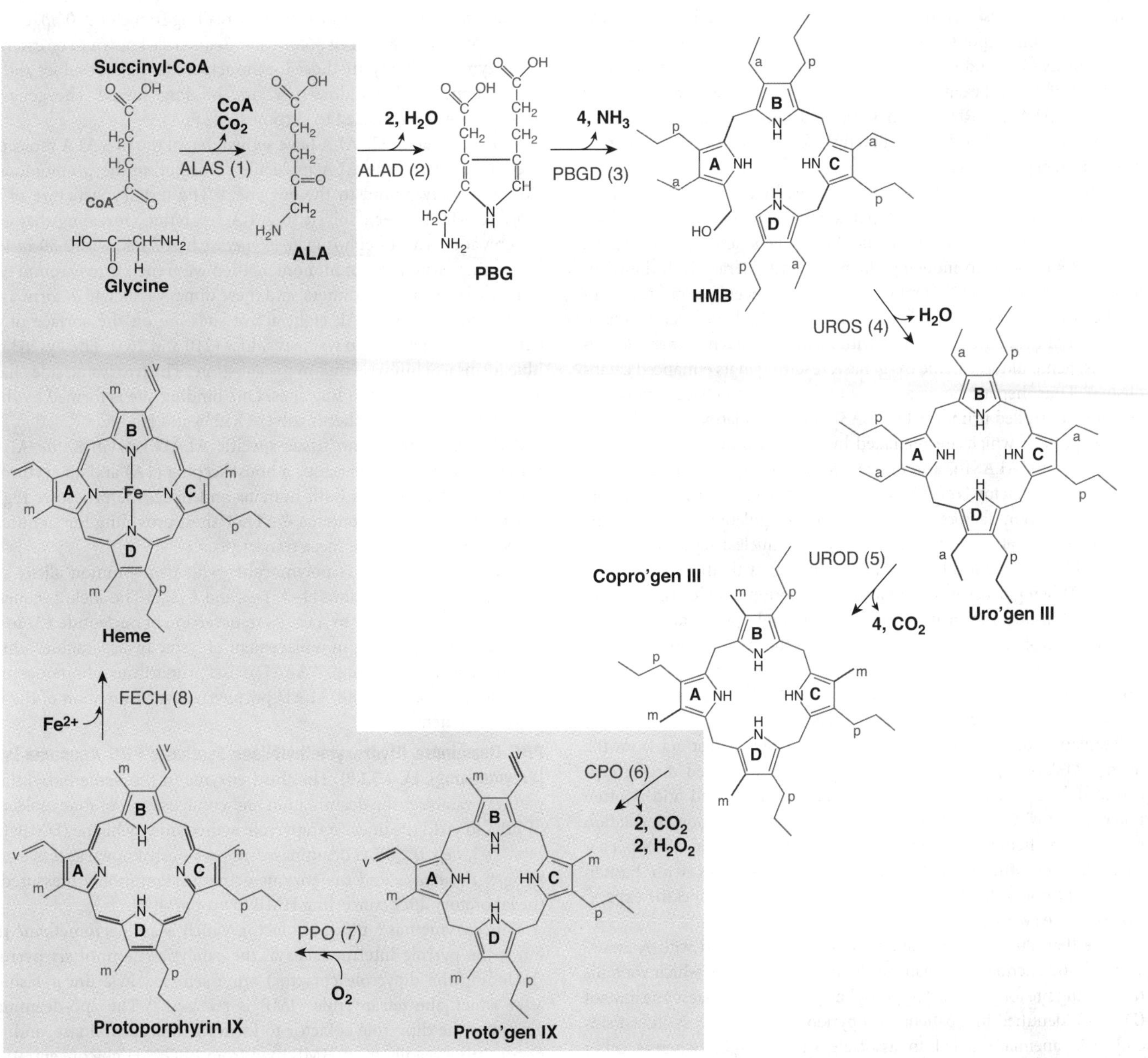

FIGURE 57–5. The heme biosynthesis pathway. The subcellular distribution of the eight enzymes and their substrates and intermediates are shown; enzymes within the light blue shading are located in the mitochondrion, and the others in the cytosol. The substrate positions that are changed are shown in blue, bold lines. ALA, δ-aminolevulinic acid; Copro'gen, coproporphyrinogen; HMB, hydroxymethylbilane; PBG, porphobilinogen; Proto, protoporphyrin; Proto'gen, protoporphyrinogen; Uro'gen, uroporphyrinogen. a, $-CH_2COOH$; p, $-CH_2-CH_2-COOH$; m, $-CH_3$; v, $-CH=CH_2$; carbon groups shown in red, carbon atom derived from the α-carbon of glycine; *, location of the α-carbon atom from glycine in the pyrrole ring that undergoes reversion. Step 1, ALA synthase; step 2, ALA dehydratase; step 3, PBG deaminase; step 4, Uro'gen III cosynthase; step 5, Uro'gen decarboxylase; step 6, Copro'gen oxidase; step 7, Proto'gen oxidase; step 8, ferrochelatase.

succinyl coenzyme A (CoA) to form ALA (see Fig. 57–5, *step 1*), and requires pyridoxal 5′-phosphate as a cofactor. ALAS in mammalian cells is localized to the mitochondrial matrix.[22] The enzyme is synthesized as a precursor protein in the cytosol and transported into mitochondria. Two separate ALAS genes encode housekeeping (tissue nonspecific) and erythroid-specific forms of the enzyme (ALAS1 and ALAS2, respectively).[23,24] The gene locus for human ALAS1 is at 3p.21, and for ALAS2 it is at Xp11.2.[24] The human ALAS2 gene encodes a precursor of 587 amino acids, with an Mr of 64,600. Nucleotide sequences for the ALAS2 and the ALAS1 isoforms are approximately 60 percent similar. No homology is observed between the aminoterminal regions, whereas high homology (~73%) is seen after residue 197 of the nonspecific form.[25] The two human ALAS genes appear to have evolved by duplication of a common ancestral gene that encoded a primitive catalytic site. Subsequently, the DNA sequences were modified to encode gene-specific regulatory regions, functioning mostly at the amino termini.[26]

The promoter in the human ALAS2 gene contains several putative erythroid-specific *cis*-acting elements including both a GATA-1 and an NF-E2 binding site.[26,27] Both GATA-1 and NF-E2 are erythroid transcription factors that also bind other DNA sites, such as the promoters of the human β-globin, porphobilinogen deaminase (PBGD), and uroporphyrinogen synthase (UROS) genes.[28] Thus, ALAS2 gene expression is under the regulatory influence of erythroid transcription factors such as GATA-1 and is coordinated with expression of other genes involved in hemoglobin synthesis. Additionally, ALAS2 messenger RNA (mRNA) contains an iron-responsive element in its 5′-untranslated region,[27] similar to mRNAs encoding ferritin[27] and the transferrin receptor (see Chap. 42).[29] Gel retardation analysis showed that the iron-responsive element in ALAS2 mRNA is functional and suggests that translation of the erythroid-specific mRNA is directly linked to the availability of iron, or heme, in erythroid cells.[30]

In the liver, synthesis of ALAS1 is induced by a variety of chemicals including drugs and steroids that increase the demand for hepatic CYPs. Upstream enhancer elements in the ALAS1 gene and certain hepatic CYP genes respond to inducing chemicals and interact with the pregnane X receptor (PXR).[31] Hemin, even at low concentrations, represses synthesis of ALAS1 in liver,[32] accounting for the beneficial effects of treatment of the acute porphyrias with hemin. At much higher concentrations, heme induces heme oxygenase, resulting in its enhanced catabolism.[33] Thus, hepatic heme availability is balanced between synthesis, which is controlled primarily by ALAS1, and degradation by heme oxygenase, both of which are regulated by heme at different intracellular concentrations. ALAS1 is also upregulated by the peroxisomal proliferator-activated cofactor 1α (PGC-1α),[34] a coactivator of nuclear receptors and transcription factors.[35] Transcriptional regulation of ALAS1 by PGC-1α is mediated by interaction of NRF-1 (nuclear regulatory factor 1) and FOXO-1 (a forkhead family member) with the ALAS1 promoter.[36] When glucose levels are low, transcription of PGC-1α is upregulated,[37,38] in turn increasing ALAS1, which might precipitate an attack of acute porphyria in an individual with the appropriate inherited enzyme deficiency. Thus, upregulation of PGC-1α provides an explanation for the induction of acute attacks of porphyria with fasting, as well as the therapeutic value of glucose loading.[39,40]

Regulation of heme synthesis in erythroid cells is distinct from the liver.[41] ALAS2 expression in erythroid cells is increased during erythroid differentiation when heme synthesis is increased and is often upregulated by heme treatment.[42,43] This contrasts with downregulation of ALAS1 by heme in the liver. The β subunit of human ATP-specific succinyl coenzyme A synthetase (SCS-βA) associates with human ALAS2 but not with ALAS1, contributing to erythroid-specific expression of heme synthesis.[44]

More than 20 ALAS2 mutations have been associated with X-linked sideroblastic anemia (see Chap. 58); many are in exon 9, which contains the binding site for pyridoxal 5′-phosphate (K391). But at least one mutant (D190V) identified in a patient with pyridoxine-refractory X-linked sideroblastic anemia,[45] failed to associate with SCS-βA, whereas other ALAS2 mutants did not have this property. The mature D190V mutant protein, but not its precursor protein, underwent abnormal processing; indicating that appropriate association of SCS-βA and ALAS2 is necessary for functioning of ALAS2 in mitochondria.[44] Gain-of-function mutations of ALAS2 have been identified in patients with a variant form of EPP.[46]

δ-Aminolevulinate Dehydratase (PBG Synthase; δ-Aminolevulinate Hydrolase; EC 4.2.1.24) ALA dehydratase (ALAD) is a cytosolic enzyme that catalyzes the condensation of two molecules of ALA to form the monopyrrole PBG, with removal of two molecules of water (see Fig. 57–5, *step 2*). The enzyme functions as a homooctamer, and requires an intact sulfhydryl group and zinc for activity. ALAD activity is inhibited by sulfhydryl reagents[47] and by lead, which displaces zinc.[48] In lead poisoning (see Chap. 51), erythrocyte ALAD activity is markedly inhibited, urinary ALA and coproporphyrin excretion increased, erythrocyte zinc protoporphyrin elevated, and neurologic symptoms resemble those seen in acute porphyrias.[49] 4,6-Dioxoheptanoic acid (succinylacetone) is a substrate analogue and potent inhibitor of ALAD,[50,51] and is a byproduct of the enzyme deficiency in hereditary tyrosinemia type I. This substance is found in urine and blood of patients with this disease, who may also have increased ALA and symptoms resembling acute porphyrias.[52,53]

Human ALAD mRNA has an open-reading frame of 990 bp, encoding a protein with an Mr of 36,274.[54,55] Sequences known to be essential for enzymatic activity are those for the active site lysine residues and for the cysteine- and histidine-rich zinc binding sites.[54] The gene for human ALAD is localized to chromosome 9p34.[56]

Studies using [^{14}-C]-ALA have shown that of the two ALA molecules used as substrate, the ALA molecule contributing the propionic acid side is initially bound to the enzyme.[38] The tertiary structure of the yeast ALAD has been solved to 2.3-Å resolution, revealing that each subunit adopts a triosephosphate isomerase barrel fold with a 39-residue N-terminal arm. Pairs of monomers then wrap their arms around each other to form compact dimers, and these dimers associate to form a 422 symmetric octamer.[57] All eight active sites are on the surface of the octamer and possess two lysine residues (210 and 263). The Lys263 residue forms a Schiff base link to the substrate. The two lysine side chains are close to two zinc binding sites. One binding site is formed by three cysteine residues; the other involves Cys234 and His142.

Although there are no tissue-specific ALAD isozymes, the ALAD mRNA has two splice variants, a housekeeping (1A) and an erythroid-specific (1B) form.[56] In both humans and mice, the promoter region upstream of exon 1B contains GATA-1 sites, providing for significant tissue-specific control of these transcripts.[58]

The human enzyme is polymorphic with two common alleles that occur in three combinations (1–1, 1–2, and 2–2).[55] The allele 2 sequence differs from allele 1 only by a G→C transversion of nucleotide 177 in the coding region, resulting in replacement of lysine by asparagine, a more electronegative amino acid.[59] ALAD exists primarily as a homooctamer. Mutations associated with ALAD porphyria favor formation of the less active hexamer.[60–62]

PBG Deaminase (Hydroxymethylbilane Synthase; PBG Ammonia-Lyase [Polymerizing], EC 4.3.1.8) The third enzyme in the heme biosynthetic pathway catalyzes the deamination and condensation of four molecules of PBG to yield the linear tetrapyrrole hydroxymethylbilane (HMB; (see Fig. 57–5, *step 3*).[63] PBG deaminase was previously known as *uroporphyrinogen I synthase*, and the enzyme activity is commonly measured in the laboratory after converting HMB to uroporphyrin I.

This enzyme has a unique cofactor, which is a dipyrromethane that binds the pyrrole intermediates at the catalytic site until six pyrroles (including the dipyrrole cofactor) are assembled in a linear fashion, after which the tetrapyrrole HMB is released.[64] The apo-deaminase generates the dipyrrole cofactor to form the holo-deaminase, and this occurs more readily from HMB than from PBG.[65] High concentrations of PBG may inhibit formation of the holo-deaminase.

The gene encoding human PBG deaminase maps to chromosome 11q23→11qter,[66] and consists of 15 exons spread over 10 kb of DNA.[67] Distinct erythroid-specific and housekeeping isoforms are produced through alternative splicing of two distinct primary mRNA transcripts arising from two promoters.[68,69] The housekeeping promoter is upstream of exon 1 and is active in all tissues, while the erythroid-specific promoter, which is upstream of exon 2, is active only in erythroid cells. The human housekeeping and erythroid-specific enzymes isoforms contain 361 and 344 amino acid residues, respectively.[70] Of the additional 17 residues at the N-terminal end of the housekeeping form, 11 are encoded by exon 1, and 6 by a short segment of exon 3 that immediately precedes a methionine codon that initiates translation of the erythroid isoform. Erythroid-specific *trans*-acting factors, such as GATA-1 and NF-E2, recognize sequences in the erythroid promoter.[71] A 1320-bp stretch of perfect identity is present between the erythroid and the nonerythroid PBG deaminase, but with a mismatch in the first exon at their 5′ extremities. An additional inframe AUG codon present 51 bp upstream from the initiating codon of the erythroid cDNA accounts for the additional 17 amino acid residues at the N-terminus of the housekeeping isoform.

Accordingly, a splice site mutation at the last position of exon 1, or a base transition in intron 1, in certain patients with AIP results in decreased PBG deaminase expression in nonerythroid tissues including the liver, but not in erythroid cells, because transcription of the gene in erythroid cells starts downstream of the site of the genetic lesion.[72]

Uroporphyrinogen III Synthase (Uroporphyrinogen III Cosynthase; EC 4.2.1.75) UROS, a cytosolic enzyme, catalyzes the formation of uroporphyrinogen III from hydroxymethylbilane. The process involves an intramolecular rearrangement that affects only ring D of the porphyrin macrocycle (see Fig. 57–5, *step 4*).[63] In the absence of this enzyme, HMB spontaneously forms the ring structure uroporphyrinogen I, which like the III isomer is a substrate for uroporphyrinogen decarboxylase (UROD). However, because coproporphyrinogen I is not a substrate for coproporphyrinogen oxidase (CPO) the type I porphyrinogen isomers are not further metabolized, and only the type III isomers are precursors of heme.

The UROS cDNA has an open-reading frame of 798 bp, and the predicted protein product consists of 263 amino acid residues, with an Mr of 28,607.[24] The amino acid compositions of the hepatic and the purified erythrocyte enzyme are essentially identical, and no tissue-specific isoforms have been described.

The interspecies homology for the UROS proteins is below 10 percent, depending on the number and divergence of the species being compared. However, the crystal structures of uroporphyrinogen III cosynthase from human and *Thermus thermophilus* have been solved and are very similar.[73,74] The structure supports a mechanism that includes the formation of a spirolactam intermediate by positioning the A and D rings such that the noncatalytic closure, to form uroporphyrinogen I, is not possible.[74]

Uroporphyrinogen Decarboxylase (EC 4.1.1.37) UROD is a cytosolic enzyme that catalyzes the sequential removal of the four carboxylic groups of the carboxymethyl side chains in uroporphyrinogen to yield coproporphyrinogen (see Fig. 57–5, *step 5*). The four successive decarboxylation reactions yield 7-, 6-, 5-, and 4-carboxylated porphyrinogens. Increased amounts of these intermediates can be identified as the corresponding oxidized porphyrins in liver, plasma, urine and stool in human PCT and in laboratory animal models in which hepatic UROD is inhibited. An inhibitor of UROD activity, a partially oxidized substrate molecule,[75] is produced in liver of experimental animals in response to halogenated polycyclic aromatic hydrocarbons such as hexachlorobenzene, dioxin, and polychlorinated biphenyls, and other compounds able to activate the Ah receptor,[76] and is believed to explain UROD inhibition in human PCT.[75] Human UROD is a 42-kDa polypeptide encoded by a single gene containing 10 exons spread over 3 kb and functions as a homodimer.[77] The gene has been mapped to chromosome 1p34.[78]

Although the UROD gene contains two initiation sites, both sites are used with the same frequencies in all tissues, and the gene is transcribed into a unique mRNA.[79] Recombinant human UROD purified to homogeneity has been crystallized, and its crystal structure was determined at 1.60-Å resolution.[80] The purified protein is a dimer with a dissociation constant of 0.1 μM.[81] The 40.8-kDa polypeptide forms a single domain with a distorted $(\beta/\alpha)_8$-barrel fold, and a distinctive deep cleft for the enzyme's active site is formed by loops at the C-terminal ends of the barrel strands. The protein forms a homodimer with one active-site cleft per monomer located adjacent to its neighbor in the dimer. The structure creates a single extended cleft that is large enough to accommodate two substrate molecules in close proximity. Although both uroporphyrinogen I and III are metabolized by UROD, only the III isomer is further metabolized to heme.[82]

Coproporphyrinogen Oxidase (EC 4.1.1.37) CPO is located in the inner membrane space of the mitochondria in mammalian cells. The enzyme catalyzes the removal of the carboxyl group and two hydrogens from the propionic groups of pyrrole rings A and B, forming vinyl groups at these positions (see Fig. 57–5, *step 6*). The enzyme is isomer specific for coproporphyrinogen III, yielding protoporphyrinogen IX (see Fig. 57–5, *step 6*). The gene for human CPO has been assigned to chromosome 3q12, spans approximately 14 kb, and consists of seven exons and six introns.[83] cDNA cloning for this enzyme was first reported in mouse erythroleukemia cells.[84] The predicted protein comprises 354 amino acid residues (Mr = 40,647), with a putative leader sequence of 31 amino acid residues. The result is a mature protein consisting of 323 amino acid residues (Mr = 37,225).[84] Potential regulatory elements exist in the GC-rich promoter region of the gene, such as six Sp1, four GATA-1, one CACCC site, and the *CPO* gene promoter regulatory element (CPRE).[85] CPRE binds specifically to a CPRE-binding protein, which has a leucine-zipper-like structure and serves as a DNA sequence-specific transcription factor that regulates gene expression.[85] Tissue-specific expression of CPO is significant. For example, binding proteins to the Spl-like element, CPRE and GATA-1, cooperatively function in *CPO* gene expression in erythroid cells. The CPRE-binding protein by itself plays a principal role in basal expression of CPO in nonerythroid cells.[86] *CPO* mRNA increases during erythroid cell differentiation.[87,88] Newly synthesized human CPO contains a 110-amino-acid N-terminal signal peptide,[87,88] which is removed during transport into the intermembrane space of mitochondria, yielding a mature protein of 354 amino acid residues (Mr = 36,842). A five-base insertional mutation in the middle of this presequence has been described in one patient with HCP.[89]

Protoporphyrinogen Oxidase (EC 1.3.3.4) The penultimate step in heme biosynthesis is the oxidation of protoporphyrinogen IX to protoporphyrin IX, with removal of six hydrogen atoms. This reaction is mediated by the mitochondrial enzyme protoporphyrinogen oxidase (PPO; see Fig. 57–5, *step 7*). Human PPO cDNA has been cloned.[90] The gene is present as a single copy per haploid genome, at chromosome 1q22.[91] PPO consists of 477 amino acids with an Mr of 50,800. The deduced protein exhibits a high degree of homology over its entire length to the amino acid sequence of PPO encoded by the *HEMY* gene of *Bacillus subtilis*. PPO has been crystallized and the structure shows that the enzyme is a homodimer.[92] Sequences required for import into the mitochondria have been identified.[93,94] Expression of PPO is upregulated, approximately fourfold, in the developing erythron from two GATA-1 binding sites located in exon 1.[95]

Ferrochelatase (Protoheme-Ferrolyase; EC 4.99.1.1) The final step of heme biosynthesis is the insertion of iron into protoporphyrin IX. This reaction is catalyzed by the mitochondrial enzyme ferrochelatase (FECH; see Fig. 57–5, *step 8*). The enzyme utilizes protoporphyrin IX, rather than its reduced form, as substrate, but requires the reduced ferrous form of iron.[96] The gene encoding human ferrochelatase has been assigned to chromosome 18q.[97,98] Two ferrochelatase mRNA species, approximately 2.5 kb and approximately 1.6 kb in size, are derived from the utilization of two alternative polyadenylation sites in the mRNA. The human ferrochelatase gene contains a total of 11 exons and has a minimum size of approximately 45 kb.[97] A major site of transcription initiation is at an adenine, 89 bp upstream from the translation-initiating ATG. The promoter region contains a potential binding site for several transcription factors, Sp1, NF-E2, and GATA-1, but not a typical TATA or CAAT sequence. The transcripts are identical in all tissues examined.

The crystal structure of *B. subtilis* ferrochelatase has been determined at 1.9-Å resolution.[99] Subsequently the structure of human ferrochelatase was solved and the location of the substrate binding site determined. The enzyme functions as a homodimer and associates with the inside of the inner mitochondrial membrane.[99] The mechanism of catalysis has not been identified nor has a function been assigned to the ^2Fe-^2S cluster that is present in human ferrochelatase. Lead inhibits ferrochelatase, and a structure of the protein-lead complex has been solved, indicating a critical role for the pi helix in catalysis.[100] Ferrochelatase seems to have a structurally conserved core region that is common to the enzyme from bacteria, plants, and mammals.

Control of Heme Synthesis in the Liver and Erythroid Cells

Tissue-specific aspects of heme synthesis have been studied mostly in erythroid cells and hepatocytes, as the marrow and liver have the greatest requirements for heme. The rate of heme synthesis in the liver is largely regulated by ALAS1 activity. The synthesis of ALAS1, in turn, is under feedback control by heme, which regulates ALAS1 at the levels of transcription, translation, and transfer into mitochondria. Many chemicals, hormones, and drugs increase the synthesis of hepatic CYPs, which increases the demand for heme and leads to induction of ALAS1. In addition, the ALAS1 gene contains upstream enhancer elements that are responsive to inducing chemicals and interact with the PXR. Therefore, ALAS1 and CYPs are subject to direct induction by xenobiotics and glucocorticoid hormones.[31] Chemical exposures that induce hepatic heme oxygenase and accelerate the destruction of hepatic heme, or inhibit heme formation, can also induce hepatic ALAS1.

ALAS2 is not inducible in erythroid cells by drugs that induce ALAS1 in hepatocytes.[101] The synthesis of ALAS2 is uninfluenced, or often upregulated, by hemin, at both the transcriptional and the translational levels.[30,43,102] Hemin treatment of marrow cultures increases erythroid colony-forming units,[103] whereas hemin treatment of hepatocytes inhibits synthesis of ALAS1 and CYPs. An additional distinct difference in these ALAS isoforms is that SCS-βA associates with ALAS2[44] but not with ALAS1, suggesting a tissue-specific difference in mitochondrial transport of these isoforms.

ERYTHROPOIETIC PORPHYRIAS

There are two major erythropoietic porphyrias in humans. CEP is one of the least-common porphyrias, but is well known as a result of its long history and the severe photomutilation of exposed areas such as the face and fingers that is a dramatic feature in many cases (Fig. 57–2). EPP is the third most common porphyria, and the most common in children, but was not well described until 1965. Characteristics in most patients with erythropoietic porphyrias that are distinct from the hepatic porphyrias include childhood onset, stable symptoms and levels of porphyrins over time, and severity largely determined by genotype rather than factors such as drugs and glucocorticoid hormones that affect the heme pathway, primarily in the liver. An erythropoietic component may be important in ALAD deficiency porphyria (ADP) and homozygous forms of other hepatic porphyrias, such as HEP (the homozygous form of familial PCT), AIP, HCP, and VP, as indicated by substantial increases in erythrocyte zinc protoporphyrin.

■ CONGENITAL ERYTHROPOIETIC PORPHYRIA

Definition and History

CEP is caused by a deficiency of UROS (see Fig. 57–5, *step 4*), is an autosomal recessive condition, and is also known as Günther disease. It results in accumulation and excretion of type I porphyrins, especially uroporphyrin I and coproporphyrin I (see Table 57–1 and Fig. 57–1). Characteristic manifestations of CEP include chronic, severe photosensitivity and hemolytic anemia evident in early childhood. Atypical presentations include milder disease that resembles PCT, and onset during adult life in association with a myeloproliferative disorder.[104] Early case descriptions of CEP appeared in 1874 and 1898,[3] and approximately 130 cases were reported up to 1997.[105] However, some of these patients may have had HEP, which has very similar clinical features. Perhaps the most well-known patient was Mathias Petry, who survived until age 34, and beginning in 1915, worked with the porphyrin chemist Hans Fisher, providing samples for early studies of porphyrin chemistry.[106]

Pathophysiology

The uroporphyrinogen III synthase defects in CEP are remarkably heterogeneous at the molecular level, with at least 36 different mutations of the UROS gene, and one GATA-1 mutation reported to date.[107,108] The UROS mutations include deletions, insertions, rearrangements, splicing abnormalities, and both missense and nonsense mutations. Twenty-three of the mutations are missense mutations that are well distributed throughout the gene. Of the 12 single-base substitutions, 4 (T228M, G225S, A66V, A104V) were hotspot mutations, occurring at CpG dinucleotides.[109] The identification of a mutation that altered the penultimate nucleotide in exon 4, resulting in an E81D mutation, also produced exon skipping on approximately 85 percent of the transcripts from that allele.[110] With the exception of V82F, all CEP missense mutations occurred in amino acid residues that are conserved in both the mouse and the human enzyme.

Genotype–phenotype comparison of the UROS mutations in CEP was studied by prokaryotic expression of mutant cDNAs. Mean activities of the mutant enzymes expressed in *Escherichia coli* ranged from 0 to 36 percent of the activity expressed by the normal cDNA. The majority of the mutant cDNAs expressed polypeptides with no enzymatic activity. However, V82F, E81D, A66V, A104V, and V99A showed 36, 30, 15, 8, and 6 percent enzyme activity, respectively, compared with the normal control. A66V and V82F were thermodynamically unstable mutants.[109,110] Homoallelism for C73R, the most common mutation, was found in five patients and was associated clinically with the most severe phenotypes, such as hydrops fetalis and transfusion dependency from birth.

Pathogenesis of the Clinical Findings

Porphyrins in their oxidized state are reddish, fluorescent, and photosensitizing, whereas porphyrin precursors and the reduced porphyrinogens are colorless and nonfluorescent. Most marrow normoblasts in CEP display marked fluorescence as a result of porphyrin accumulation, principally in the nuclei.[111] Much of the excess production and excretion of porphyrins is accounted for by ineffective erythropoiesis in the marrow. Porphyrin concentrations are also increased in circulating erythrocytes, and hemolysis may result from exposure to light in the dermal capillaries, causing cell damage and leading to intravascular lysis or uptake by the spleen. Splenomegaly is very common in CEP and is presumed to be secondary to the hemolytic process. The excess porphyrins that are produced by the marrow or released by hemolysis are transported in plasma to the skin, leading to photosensitivity.

Clinical Features

Severe cutaneous photosensitivity is noted soon after birth in most cases. The disease may be recognized even earlier as a cause of hydrops fetalis. Phototherapy for hyperbilirubinemia may cause severe cutaneous burns and scarring in patients with unrecognized CEP. Brown staining of the teeth by porphyrins (erythrodontia) is evident when the teeth erupt. The cutaneous lesions in CEP resemble those found in PCT, but are usually much more severe, reflecting the much higher porphyrin levels in CEP. Some cases are relatively mild, and may resemble PCT in terms of the severity of photosensitivity. Late-onset cases are associated with myeloproliferative disorders, with expansion of a clone of erythroid cells bearing a somatic mutation and displaying UROS deficiency.[104]

Subepidermal bullous lesions are characteristic, and progress to crusted erosions that heal with scarring and areas of hyper- and hypopigmentation. Also common is hypertrichosis, which is sometimes severe, and alopecia. Loss of facial features and digits is common and results from recurrent blisters, infection, and scarring. Fingers may be shortened and tapered as a consequence of scarring and contraction of the skin. Erythrodontia, with brown staining and red fluorescence of the teeth under long-wave ultraviolet light is characteristic, and results from deposition of porphyrins in the developing deciduous and permanent teeth *in utero*. Porphyrins are also deposited in bone. The skeleton is also affected by expansion of the marrow, leading to pathologic fractures, vertebral compression, short stature, and osteolytic and sclerotic lesions. Vitamin D deficiency resulting from avoiding sunlight might also contribute.

Anemia may be severe and lead to transfusion dependence in the more severe cases. Uncorrected anemia can increase erythropoiesis, which in turn is a stimulus to porphyrin production by the abnormal erythropoietic cells in the marrow. Erythrocytes exhibit polychromasia, poikilocytosis, anisocytosis, and basophilic stippling, and reticulocytes and nucleated red blood cells are increased.[108]

Diagnosis

CEP may be suspected even before birth if a sibling is known to have CEP. However, the family history is often negative. CEP should be suspected as a cause of hydrops fetalis, as the disease can be diagnosed and treated *in utero*. Aspirated amniotic fluid is dark brown in color and contains large amounts of porphyrins. The diagnosis of CEP is often made after birth when pink to dark-brown staining of the diapers, with red fluorescence under long-wave ultraviolet light, is noted. Cutaneous vesicles and bullae on sun-exposed areas may be severe, with scarring.

Urinary porphyrin excretion is markedly increased, and often in the range of 50 to 100 mg/day (normal: up to ~0.3 mg/day). Uroporphyrin I and coproporphyrin I account for most of the increase, although the III isomers and hepta-, hexa-, pentacarboxylate porphyrins are also increased. Fecal porphyrins are increased, and are predominantly coproporphyrin I. Plasma total porphyrins are markedly increased as well, with a pattern of individual porphyrins similar to that in urine. Markedly increased erythrocyte porphyrins are predominantly uroporphyrin I and coproporphyrin I, although protoporphyrin IX may predominate especially in milder cases.

CEP must be distinguished by biochemical testing from other causes of blistering skin lesions. HEP can present with photosensitivity in early childhood. Mild cases of CEP may be misdiagnosed as PCT.

The diagnosis should be confirmed in all cases by DNA studies, which can identify causative mutations in almost all cases. This is especially important for genetic counseling and for prenatal diagnosis in subsequent pregnancies. Demonstration of a GATA-1 mutation in one case, illustrates that on occasion a genetic defect outside the heme biosynthetic pathway can cause CEP.[108]

Therapy

Patients should be advised that it is essential to avoid sunlight, trauma to the skin, and infections, so as to avoid severe scarring and loss of facial features and digits. Topical sunscreens that block long-wave ultraviolet light (ultraviolet A light) and oral treatment with β-carotene are somewhat helpful,[112] but are marginally beneficial in most cases. Erythrocyte transfusions are essential in patients with severe anemia.[113] Transfusions to maintain the hematocrit above 35 percent, with an iron chelator to avoid iron overload, has been beneficial in some cases.[114] Hydroxyurea to reduce erythropoiesis and porphyrin production may also be considered.[115] Splenectomy has provided short-term benefit. Oral charcoal reportedly was quite effective in one patient,[116] and ascorbic acid and α-tocopherol improved anemia in another.[105] Successful pregnancy and delivery of a healthy, unaffected infant with erythrodontia as a result of exposure to maternal porphyrins before birth has been reported.[117]

Hematopoietic stem cell transplantation is the treatment of choice when a suitable donor is available, especially for young patients.[118] When transplantation is successful, there is marked clinical improvement and reduction in porphyrin levels, even if these are not completely normalized. Gene therapy is being explored using retroviral and lentiviral vectors and hematopoietic stem cells from patients with CEP.[119,120]

ERYTHROPOIETIC PROTOPORPHYRIA

Definition and History

In most cases, EPP is caused by a partial deficiency of FECH (Fig. 57–5, *step 8*) activity, which results in the accumulation of the substrate protoporphyrin in the marrow. A biochemically variant form of the disease was shown to be a result of ALAS2 gain-of-function mutations (ALAS; see Fig. 57–1).[46] EPP is characterized by onset of nonblistering cutaneous photosensitivity in early childhood. EPP is the most common porphyria in children and the third most common in adults. Reported prevalence varies between 5 and 15 cases per 1 million individuals.[121–123] Protoporphyric hepatopathy is a potentially fatal complication estimated to occur in less than 5 percent of patients.

Pathophysiology

In most families, EPP is an autosomal dominant disease with variable penetrance, in which a severe ferrochelatase mutation is inherited from one parent. More than 75 different mutations, including nonsense, missense, splice-site mutations, nonsense mutations, and deletions, insertions, and rearrangements have been described. Splicing mutations are most common. Recombinant human ferrochelatase, when engineered to have individual exon skipping for exons 3 through 11, lacks significant enzyme activity when expressed in *E. coli*, and almost all such variants lacked the [^{2}Fe-^{2}S] cluster.[124]

It was noted, however, that EPP patients have only 30 percent or less of normal ferrochelatase activity, rather than 50 percent, which would be expected in an autosomal dominant condition. It was shown that a low-expression (hypomorphic) intronic polymorphism (a –23C→T transition) is found in the wild-type allele of patients with EPP, which was inherited from the other parent.[125–127] This polymorphism favors the use of a cryptic acceptor splice site 63 bases upstream of the normal splice site. The aberrantly spliced mRNA contains a premature stop codon and is degraded by a nonsense-mediated decay mechanism.[127] The result is a lower steady-state level of wild-type *FECH* mRNA. Coinheritance of the hypomorphic allele in *trans* to a loss-of-function mutant allele was found in 98 percent of French cases with EPP,[128] and with a similar frequency in South African patients.[122] The frequency of the IVS 3–48C hypomorphic allele is common in the white population, and by itself has no phenotype. Its frequency varies widely in different populations and relates to the observed differences in the prevalence of EPP.[121–123]

Other underlying genetic mechanisms must be considered in newly identified EPP families. In a few families, true autosomal recessive inheritance, with a *FECH* mutation inherited from each parent has been described. Interestingly, autosomal recessive EPP is sometimes associated with seasonal palmar keratoderma. Other features in some patients with this unexplained association include neurologic symptoms, less-than-expected increases in erythrocyte protoporphyrin and absence of liver dysfunction.[129]

Patterns in families with a variant form of EPP in which FECH mutations were not found suggested sex-linked inheritance, and this led to discovery of gain-of-function mutations of ALAS2 (the only heme pathway enzyme found on the X chromosome).[46] This was the first demonstration that a mutation of ALAS, the first enzyme in the pathway, can be associated with a type of porphyria.

EPP can develop late in life in patients with clonal hematological disorders and expansion of a clone of hematopoietic cells with deletion of one *FECH* allele.[130,131] For example, a patient with a myeloproliferative disorder later developed severe EPP because of clonal expansion of a cell of erythropoietic lineage with a *FECH* deletion and the IVS3–48C/T polymorphism, and died of EPP-induced liver disease.[132]

Pathogenesis of the Clinical Findings

Marrow reticulocytes are thought to be the primary source of the excess protoporphyrin in EPP.[133–135] Most of the excess erythrocyte protoporphyrin in circulating erythrocytes is found in a small percentage of younger cells as free protoporphyrin, which is not complexed with zinc, in contrast to other conditions associated with increased erythrocyte protoporphyrin content. Free protoporphyrin in these cells declines much more rapidly with red cell age than it does in conditions associated with increased erythrocyte zinc protoporphyrin.[133,135] Free protoporphyrin, but not zinc protoporphyrin, is released from erythrocytes following irradiation, which may explain why lead intoxication and iron deficiency, which are associated with elevated erythrocyte zinc protoporphyrin levels, are not associated with photosensitivity.[136] Excess protoporphyrin is taken up from plasma by hepatocytes and excreted in bile and feces, and may undergo enterohepatic recirculation. Hepatocytes may also provide a limited additional source of excess protoporphyrin in this disease.

Light-excited porphyrins generate free radicals and singlet oxygen,[137] which in EPP can lead to peroxidation of lipids[138] and crosslinking of membrane proteins.[139] Skin irradiation in EPP patients leads to complement activation and polymorphonuclear chemotaxis, which contributes to the development of skin pathology.[140] Skin histopathology is not specific, but may include thickened capillary walls in the papillary dermis surrounded by amorphous hyaline-like deposits, immunoglobulin, complement, and periodic acid-Schiff–positive mucopolysaccharides.[141] Basement membrane abnormalities are less marked than in other forms of porphyria.[142]

Protoporphyric hepatopathy is a feared complication that develops in less than 5 percent of patients, and is attributed to the cholestatic effects of excess protoporphyrin presented to the liver. This complication may begin with chronic abnormalities in liver function tests and then progress rapidly as a vicious cycle of increasing protoporphyrin levels in plasma and erythrocytes and worsening liver function and photosensitivity. Hepatopathy is sometimes precipitated by another cause of liver dysfunction such as viral or alcoholic hepatitis. Protoporphyrin is cholestatic, and can form crystalline structures in hepatocytes and impair mitochondrial function, leading to decreased hepatic bile formation and flow.[143,144] Accumulated protoporphyrin may appear as brown pigment in hepatocytes, Kupffer cells, and biliary canaliculi and doubly refractive with a Maltese cross appearance under polarizing microscopy.[145] Significant changes in expression of several genes involved in wound-healing, organic anion transport, and oxidative stress were found in DNA microarray studies in explanted livers of patients who underwent liver transplantation for this complication.[146]

Clinical Features

Photosensitivity is present from early childhood in almost all cases, but may not be recognized until parents observe that an affected infant cries and develops skin swelling and erythema when exposed to sunlight. Indeed, EPP is the most common porphyria in children.

Cutaneous photosensitivity in EPP is acute and nonblistering, which is distinctly different from the more chronic, blistering skin manifestations of the other cutaneous porphyrias. Symptoms in a series of 32 patients with EPP are tabulated in Table 57–3. Skin symptoms are usually worse during spring and summer and affect light-exposed areas, especially of the face and hands. Characteristically, stinging or burning pain develops within 1 hour of sunlight exposure, and is followed by erythema and edema—described as solar urticaria, sometimes as petechiae, and less commonly as purpura. Patients with a history of these symptoms may display no objective cutaneous signs. Artificial lights may contribute to photosensitivity.[147] Over time, chronic changes may include leathery hyperkeratotic skin especially on the dorsa of the hands and finger joints, mild scarring, and separation of the nail plate (onycholysis). Bullae, skin fragility, hypertrichosis, hyperpigmentation, severe scarring, and mutilation are very unusual.

Mild anemia has been reported in 20 to 50 percent of cases of EPP, but the pathogenesis is not understood. Microcytosis, hypochromia, and reticulocytosis are sometimes noted,[133,148,149] but there is little evidence for impaired erythropoiesis or abnormal iron metabolism,[150,151] and hemolysis is absent or very mild. Iron accumulation in erythroblasts and ring sideroblasts have been noted in marrow in some patients.[152] Although decreased transferrin saturation may suggest iron deficiency, serum ferritin and soluble transferrin receptor are usually normal.[153] Because iron deficiency may be detrimental and further limit heme synthesis and increase protoporphyrin accumulation, iron status should be carefully evaluated in EPP patients, keeping in mind that serum ferritin in the lower part of the normal range, especially in women, may be indicative of depleted iron stores.

Precipitating factors that are important in the hepatic porphyrias do not appear to play an important role in EPP. Although more long-term followup studies are needed, porphyrin levels and symptoms typically do not change over time, unless liver dysfunction develops. Concurrent iron deficiency or other marrow problems might also lead to further increases in porphyrin levels and photosensitivity. Pregnancy is reported to lower erythrocyte protoporphyrin levels somewhat and increase tolerance to sunlight.[154]

Neurovisceral manifestations are absent in uncomplicated EPP. Patients with severe protoporphyric hepatopathy may develop a severe motor neuropathy similar to that seen in the acute porphyrias.[155]

TABLE 57–3. Common Clinical Features of Erythropoietic Protoporphyria from a Series of 32 Cases[146]

Symptoms and Signs	Incidence (% of Total)
Burning	97
Edema	94
Itching	88
Erythema	69
Scarring	19
Vesicles	3
Anemia	27
Cholelithiasis	12
Abnormal liver function results	4

Autosomal recessive EPP associated with palmar keratoderma has also been associated with unexplained neurological symptoms.[129]

Gallstones containing large amounts of protoporphyrin are common, and may require cholecystectomy at an unusually early age.[156] Liver function and liver protoporphyrin content are usually normal in EPP. However, protoporphyric hepatopathy, which is the most life-threatening complication of EPP, develops in 1 to 5 percent of patients. This complication results from the cholestatic effects of protoporphyrin presented in excess amounts to the liver. It is sometimes the major presenting feature of EPP,[157] and may be chronic or progress rapidly to death from liver failure. Unnecessary surgery for suspected biliary obstruction can be detrimental and should be avoided.[144] Operating room lights during liver transplantation or other surgery, especially in patients with hepatopathy, can cause marked photosensitivity with extensive burns of the skin and peritoneum and photodamage of circulating erythrocytes.[158]

Diagnosis

Painful, nonblistering photosensitivity suggests the diagnosis. A substantial elevation of erythrocyte protoporphyrin is expected, but is not specific, since erythrocyte zinc protoporphyrin is predominantly increased in conditions such as homozygous porphyrias (other than most cases of CEP), iron deficiency, lead poisoning, anemia of chronic disease,[159] hemolytic conditions,[160] and many other erythrocyte disorders. A unique finding in EPP is increased erythrocyte protoporphyrin with a predominance of free rather than zinc protoporphyrin. This occurs because FECH, which can utilize metals in addition to iron, catalyzes the formation of zinc protoporphyrin, and this activity is deficient in most cases of EPP. Because FECH is not deficient in variant cases with gain-of-function mutations of ALAS2, erythrocytes contain increased amounts of both zinc and free protoporphyrin, although the latter still predominates.

Consequently, the diagnosis of EPP requires demonstration of an increase in free protoporphyrin in red cells, which can be measured by an ethanol extraction or high-performance liquid chromatography method. There is confusion about terminology used by different laboratories. For example, testing for what in the past was termed "free erythrocyte protoporphyrin" (especially in screening for lead poisoning) in fact measured zinc protoporphyrin.

The plasma porphyrin concentration is almost always at least mildly increased in EPP, but often less than in other cutaneous porphyrias, and may be normal in mild cases. Plasma porphyrins in EPP are particularly subject to photodegradation during sample processing unless great care is taken to shield the sample from natural or fluorescent light.[161] For these reasons, measurement of erythrocyte rather than plasma porphyrin should be the primary screening test for EPP.

Fecal porphyrins are increased in most cases, and consist mostly of protoporphyrin. Urine porphyrins are normal, except after hepatopathy develops, which causes increases in urinary coproporphyrin as is typical for other forms of liver diseases.

Therapy

Avoidance of sunlight exposure is important, and often requires changes in lifestyle and the working environment. Topical sunscreens that absorb ultraviolet A and sunblocks containing zinc oxide or titanium dioxide may be helpful. Orally administered β-carotene, which probably quenches activated oxygen radicals,[162] is the most studied treatment for EPP.[163] It may afford some protection after 1 to 3 months of therapy, but results are variable. A daily dose of 120 to 180 mg or higher is recommended to achieve a serum β-carotene level of 600 to 800 mcg/dL.[147] Oral cysteine may also quench excited oxygen species and increase tolerance to sunlight in EPP.[164] Other treatments that aim to either increase skin pigmentation or scavenge activated oxygen species have been reviewed[163] and include dihydroxyacetone/Lawsone, vitamin C and narrow-wave ultraviolet B phototherapy to increase melanin.[165] Afamelanotide, an α-melanocyte-stimulating hormone analogue that increases skin melanin, is in clinical trials as a treatment for EPP.[166]

It is advisable to monitor liver function tests at least yearly, avoid iron deficiency as assessed by serum ferritin, and avoid severe caloric restriction and drugs or hormone preparations that impair hepatic excretory function.[167,168] Because sunlight exposure is limited, vitamin D supplementation is recommended.

Management of protoporphyric liver disease is difficult. The condition may resolve spontaneously, especially if another reversible cause of liver dysfunction, such as viral hepatitis or alcohol, is contributing.[142,169] Cholestyramine,[144,170,171] ursodeoxycholic acid,[172] vitamin E, red blood cell transfusions,[173] plasma exchange, and intravenous hemin may be given to bridge patients until liver transplantation or there is spontaneous improvement.[174] Success of liver transplantation is comparable to that in other liver diseases, even though protoporphyric hepatopathy may recur in the new liver.[175] Acute motor neuropathy has developed in some patients with protoporphyric liver disease after transfusion[176] or liver transplantation,[155,177] and is sometimes reversible.[178]

Marrow transplantation can achieve remission in human EPP,[179] as well in murine models of protoporphyria.[180] Sequential liver and marrow transplantation can correct the overproduction of protoporphyrin by the marrow and prevent recurrence of liver disease.[181] Promising studies in murine models suggest a future role for gene therapy in human EPP.[182,183]

■ ACUTE PORPHYRIAS

The acute porphyrias are comprised of four disorders caused by different enzyme deficiencies, and are distinctive for intermittent neurologic symptoms that usually occur as acute exacerbations during adult life. Similar symptoms occur in lead poisoning, hereditary tyrosinemia type I, and in some reported cases of porphyria with dual enzyme deficiencies.

ALA Dehydratase Porphyria

Definition and History δ-Aminolevulinate dehydratase (deficiency) porphyria (ADP) is an autosomal recessive disorder resulting from severe deficiency of ALA dehydratase activity (see Table 57–1 and Fig. 57–1). This is the rarest of the porphyrias, with only six cases documented at the molecular level.[57,182–186]

Pathophysiology The molecular defect in five cases was compound heterozygosity for two distinct ALA dehydratase mutations (see Fig. 57–5, *step 2*).[60,184] Four were males (three in Germany and one in the United States) with onset of symptoms in their teens, whereas one Swedish case developed severe symptoms in infancy.[185] The sixth patient was a Belgian male who developed ADP at age 63 years and was found to have two inherited base transitions in one allele, and was therefore heterozygous for ALA dehydratase deficiency.[186,187] He also developed polycythemia vera and his erythrocyte ALAD activity was less than 1 percent of normal, while lymphocyte ALAD activity was greater than 20 percent of normal. Heterozygous ALAD deficiency was apparently clinically silent in this patient until there was expansion of a clone of erythroid cells that carried the mutant ALAD allele.[187]

Thus ADP is highly heterogeneous at the molecular level, with a total of 11 mutant alleles identified in these 6 patients.[60] An additional mutation was found in a healthy Swedish girl with markedly decreased ALAD activity (12% of normal), which was detected by ALAD measurement during neonatal screening for hereditary tyrosinemia.[188] The same mutation was found in a U.S. male patient with acute porphyria who also had a *CPO* mutation and an unusual pattern of porphyrin precursors and porphyrins reflecting dual enzyme deficiencies.[189] Thus, heterozygous ALAD deficiency may rarely be combined with another enzyme deficiency, or may itself cause porphyria if a marrow disorder leads to clonal expansion of the mutant *ALAD* allele.

Human ALAD consists of eight identical oligomers, each with two zinc-binding sites. Lead can bind at least one of these sites and impair enzyme activity. Some mutations found in ADP may affect zinc binding, or favor formation of a hexameric enzyme with decreased activity rather than the fully active octamer. Thus ADP has been described as a conformational disease.[62]

ADP is classified as one of the hepatic porphyrias because it closely resembles the other acute porphyrias. However, the site of overproduction of ALA is not established, and the Swedish infant with severe, early onset disease did not benefit from liver transplantation.[190] Substantial increase in erythrocyte zinc protoporphyrin also suggests an erythroid component. The excess urinary coproporphyrin III in ADP may originate from metabolism of ALA to porphyrinogens in a tissue other than the site of ALA overproduction. Indeed, ALA loading in normal subjects was shown to cause substantial coproporphyrinuria.[191] The pathogenesis of the neurologic symptoms is poorly understood, as in other acute porphyrias.

Clinical Features The four adolescent males had intermittent symptoms resembling other acute porphyrias, including abdominal pain, vomiting, extremity pain, and motor neuropathy, although exacerbating factors were less evident.[60,192] Two German cases had initial acute attacks and then remained well during 20 years of followup.[193] The third German case[194] and the U.S. case[60] have had further attacks and have been maintained on prophylactic hemin infusions. The Swedish infant had more severe neurologic disease, including failure to thrive, and died after liver transplantation.[195] The 63-year-old man in Belgium developed an acute motor polyneuropathy concurrently with a myeloproliferative disorder.[104,186,196]

Diagnosis A biochemical diagnosis of ADP includes demonstration of markedly deficient erythrocyte ALAD activity, marked elevation in urinary ALA and coproporphyrin III and erythrocyte zinc protoporphyrin, with little or no increase in urinary PBG. Erythrocyte ALAD activity is approximately half-normal in both parents. Lead poisoning is differentiated by increased blood lead and restoration of ALAD activity *in vitro* by reduced glutathione or dithiothreitol.[184,197] Although biochemical measurements can strongly suggest ADP, the diagnosis must be confirmed by DNA studies.

Patients with hereditary tyrosinemia type I may also have ALAD inhibition and increased excretion of ALA.[52] Succinylacetone (4,6-dioxoheptanoic acid), a structural analogue of ALA and a potent ALAD inhibitor, accumulates as a result of an inherited deficiency of fumarylacetoacetate hydrolase in these patients. A diagnosis of tyrosinemia can be made by demonstrating succinylacetone in urine by measuring ALAD activity in normal blood after addition of a patient's urine. ALA dehydratase protein is not reduced in this disease.[198]

Therapy Because few cases have been documented, treatment recommendations are based on limited experience. Hemin was beneficial in the four male patients, but there was little or no response to glucose. A long-term preventive hemin regimen was effective in two of these patients. The Swedish infant did not respond to glucose or hemin, and did not improve greatly after liver transplantation.[190] Whether transplantation would benefit less severe cases is unknown. Hemin produced a biochemical response but no clinical improvement in the late-onset case in Belgium, who had a peripheral neuropathy but no acute attacks.[196]

Acute Intermittent Porphyria

Definition and History AIP is an autosomal dominant disorder caused by a partial deficiency of PBG deaminase (see Table 57–1 and Fig. 57–1). Symptoms usually occur as acute attacks and are neurologic in origin. In most countries this is the most common acute porphyria and the second most common porphyria. Most individuals who inherit the enzyme deficiency (probably more than 90 percent) never develop symptoms, but are at some risk to develop symptoms after puberty. The first case of acute porphyria was described in 1889 by Stokvis[5] who noted a relationship of the symptoms to the drug Sulfonal, which is related to the barbiturates.

The prevalence of AIP was estimated to be 1 to 2 per 100,000 in Europe,[199] and 2.4 per 100,000 in Finland.[200] Up to 300 PBGD mutations have been described in AIP. Many *PBGD* mutations are found in only one or a few families.[201,202] The disease occurs in all races, but clusters as a result of founder effects occur in some countries. A notable cluster because of a prevalent founder mutation in northern Sweden is associated with a disease prevalence of 1 per 1500.[203] The prevalence of low PBG deaminase activity, which includes latent gene carriers of AIP, is as high as 1 per 500 in the general population of Finland.[204] Based on DNA studies, the minimal prevalence of the AIP-associated genes in France has been calculated to be 1 per 1675.[205]

Pathophysiology PBG deaminase is also known as HMB synthase. The term uroporphyrinogen I synthase is obsolete, because HMB is the product of the enzyme. *PBGD* mutations have been classified based in part on the presence or absence of cross-reactive immunologic material (CRIM), which indicates the presence of inactive enzyme protein. *Type I* mutations are CRIM-negative, with reduction of both enzyme activity and protein to approximately 50 percent of normal in heterozygotes. *Type II* mutations are associated with reduced PBGD activity only in nonerythroid tissue. These patients with "variant AIP" comprise less than 5 percent of AIP patients, and have normal erythrocyte PBGD activity and decreased hepatic activity because, as explained earlier, transcription of the gene to form the erythroid-specific enzyme starts downstream of the site of the mutation. *Type III* are CRIM-positive mutations that result in decreased activity with structurally abnormal enzyme protein.[206] *Type IIIa* are mutations associated with moderately increased CRIM,[207] and *type IIIb* with markedly increased CRIM.[208] These mutation types have not been convincingly related to differences in clinical expression, which is understandable because the residual approximately 50 percent of normal enzyme activity in AIP is primarily a product of the normal PBGD allele.

Pathogenesis of the Clinical Findings A partial deficiency of PBGD is not sufficient to cause clinical expression of AIP, and most individuals who inherit this enzyme deficiency remain healthy with normal porphyrin precursor excretion throughout life. Most of the heme synthesized in the liver is utilized for CYP enzymes, which are abundant in liver and turn over more rapidly than most other cellular hemoproteins. Therefore, many drugs and hormones are inducers of ALAS because they are inducers of CYP enzymes and increase the demand for heme synthesis.[209]

The partial enzyme deficiency in AIP apparently impairs heme synthesis sufficiently, especially when heme synthesis is stimulated, to compromise feedback regulation of the rate-limiting enzyme ALAS1 by a regulatory heme pool. In addition, ALAS and CYP genes share upstream enhancer elements that respond to inducing chemicals and interact with PXR.[31] Therefore, half-normal PBGD activity can become limiting when there is exposure to drugs or hormones that induce ALAS1 and CYPs.

It is generally accepted, although not proven, that hepatic PBGD remains constant at approximately 50 percent of normal activity during exacerbations and remissions of AIP, as in erythrocytes. An early report suggested that the enzyme activity is considerably less than half-normal in liver during an acute attack,[18] but additional data is lacking. It has been suggested that once the disease becomes activated, excess PBG may interfere with assembly of the dipyrromethane cofactor for this enzyme.

The following potential mechanisms have been proposed to explain neurologic dysfunction in the acute porphyrias: (1) Heme pathway intermediates or products derived from them may be neurotoxic. This hypothesis is most favored, although the evidence is not conclusive. (2) PBG deaminase deficiency in the nervous system tissues may limit heme synthesis and formation of important hemoproteins. Regulation of heme and hemoprotein synthesis in nervous tissue is difficult to study, and there is little direct evidence for this hypothesis. (3) Impaired hepatic heme synthesis during an attack may lead to decreased activity of hepatic tryptophan pyrrolase, which might increase levels of tryptophan in plasma and brain, leading to increased synthesis of the neurotransmitter 5-hydroxytryptamine. (4) Vasospasm might result from decreased production of nitrous oxide by the hemoprotein enzyme nitrous oxide synthase, and account for cerebral manifestations of AIP,[210,211] and possibly compromise intestinal blood flow.[212]

ALA is increased in a number of disorders with similar neurologic manifestations, including all four of the acute porphyrias, lead poisoning, and hereditary tyrosinemia type I, which favors a neuropathic role for this porphyrin precursor or perhaps a derivative. ALA can enter cells readily and be converted to porphyrins, which, in turn, may have toxic potential.[213] ALA is also structurally similar to γ-aminobutyric acid and can interact with γ-aminobutyric acid receptors.[214,215] However, studies of ALA loading have not shown adverse effects.[216]

Impaired motor function and ataxia develop in mice with PBGD deficiency induced by gene targeting.[217,218] Induction of hepatic CYPs is impaired in these animals and corrected by heme.[219] But motor neuropathy can develop even with normal or only slightly increased ALA in plasma and urine in these mice, which suggests a primary role for heme deficiency in porphyric neuropathy.[220]

Clinical improvement and normalization of porphyrin precursor excretion after liver transplantation in patients with severe AIP is a clear indication that the liver plays an essential role in neuropathic processes in the acute porphyrias.[221]

Precipitating Factors Acute attacks are precipitated in some heterozygotes by various endogenous or exogenous factors. These factors are additive, and additional unknown genetic factors are also likely to contribute. Some individuals remain susceptible to repeated attacks even after avoidance of known precipitants. Many precipitating factors cause *induction of hepatic ALAS1*, which is closely associated with induction of CYPs and leads to overproduction of ALA and other pathway intermediates. The partially deficient activity of PBGD then becomes rate limiting.

Drugs and Other Exogenous Chemicals Most drugs that are harmful in AIP and other acute porphyrias are known inducers of hepatic CYPs. These drugs increase *de novo* heme synthesis, thereby derepressing hepatic ALAS1, and may also directly induce this rate-limiting enzyme.[31] Table 57–4 lists some drugs known to be harmful and safe. Information regarding safety of many drugs in clinical practice is uncertain or lacking. More extensive drug safety databases are available at the websites of the American Porphyria Foundation (www.porphyriafoundation.com) and the European Porphyria Initiative (www.porphyria-europe.com). Ethanol and other alcohols are inducers of ALAS and some CYPs.[222,223] Smoking is known to increase CYPs in humans, probably from exposure to polycyclic aromatic hydrocarbons, and has been associated with more frequent symptoms of acute porphyria.[224]

Endocrine Factors Rarity of symptoms before puberty and more common clinical expression in women point to hormonal factors as important contributors in AIP. Although estrogens are considered harmful, it is likely that progesterone is mostly responsible for cyclic premenstrual attacks that occur in some women. Progesterone, certain metabolites of testosterone, and synthetic progestins are potent inducers of ALAS1. Thus administration of progestational agents should be avoided. Diabetes mellitus is not known to precipitate attacks of porphyria, and has been observed to decrease the frequency of attacks and lower porphyrin precursor levels, possibly in relation to high circulating glucose levels.[225]

TABLE 57–4. A Partial List of Drugs Known to Be Unsafe or Safe in the Acute Porphyrias

Unsafe		Safe
Alcohol	Methyprylon	Acetaminophen
Barbiturates*	Metoclopramide*	Aspirin
Carbamazepine*	Phenytoin*	Atropine
Carisoprodol*	Primidone*	Bromides
Clonazepam (high doses)	Progesterone and synthetic progestins*	Cimetidine
Danazol*	Pyrazinamide*	Erythropoietin*†
Diclofenac* and possibly other NSAIDs	Pyrazolones (aminopyrine, antipyrine)	Gabapentin
Ergots	Rifampin*	Glucocorticoids
Estrogens*‡	Succinimides (ethosuximide, methsuximide)	Insulin
Ethchlorvynol*	Sulfonamide antibiotics*	Narcotic analgesics
Glutethimide*	Valproic acid*	Penicillin and derivatives
Griseofulvin*		Phenothiazines
Mephenytoin		Ranitidine*†
Meprobamate* (also mebutamate*, tybamate*)		Streptomycin
		Vigabatrin

NSAIDs, nonsteroidal antiinflammatory drugs.

*Porphyria is listed as a contraindication, warning, precaution, or adverse effect in U.S. labeling for these drugs.

†Although porphyria is listed as a precaution in U.S. labeling, these drugs are regarded as safe by other sources.

‡Estrogens are unsafe for porphyria cutanea tarda, but can be used with caution in the acute porphyrias.

NOTE: More complete sources, such as the websites of the American Porphyria Foundation (www.porphyriafoundation.com) and the European Porphyria Initiative (www.porphyria-europe.com), should be consulted before using drugs not listed here.

SOURCE: Modified from Anderson et al.[40]

Pregnancy Pregnancy is usually well tolerated.[210] Attacks during pregnancy are sometimes a result of harmful drugs or reduced caloric intake. Metoclopramide, a contraindicated drug, is associated with exacerbation of the disease when used to treat hyperemesis gravidarum.[226,227] But for reasons that are not clear, some women experience attacks during pregnancy even when harmful factors are avoided.

Nutrition Reduced intake of calories and carbohydrate can exacerbate acute porphyrias. This may occur from efforts to lose weight, or during an illness or surgery. Under these conditions, upregulation of PGC-1α can lead to induction of ALAS1, increases in ALA and PBG, and symptoms of acute porphyria, and these effects are reversed by administration of carbohydrate.[34,228] Starvation, may also induce hepatic heme oxygenase,[229] which may deplete hepatic heme and contribute to ALAS1 induction.

Stress Various forms of physical or psychological stress may exacerbate acute porphyrias, although the mechanisms are not well defined. Medical illnesses, fever, infections, alcoholic excess, and surgery may decrease food intake and contribute to induction of hepatic ALAS1 and heme oxygenase. Psychological stress may also lead to decreased food intake and have other metabolic effects.

Clinical Features Symptoms are almost never seen before puberty, and most commonly develop in women in the third or fourth decade of life. Acute attacks are life-threatening but rarely fatal if promptly recognized and treated. Frequently recurring attacks and chronic symptoms can be disabling in a minority of patients. Although the most prominent symptoms are a result of effects on the nervous system, liver and kidney damage may be important in the long term. In very rare homozygous cases, severe neurologic manifestations are seen early in childhood, and acute attacks are not prominent.[230–232]

Symptoms and signs are nonspecific and highly variable. Abdominal pain is the most common symptom, occurring in 85 to 95 percent of cases.[199,233,234] It is usually severe, steady, and poorly localized, but may be cramping, and is often accompanied by nausea, vomiting, constipation, and abdominal distention because of ileus. Pain in the chest and extremities are also common. Tachycardia is the most common physical sign, occurring in up to 80 percent of acute attacks,[233] and often accompanied by hypertension, sweating, tremors, and other effects of sympathetic overactivity and excess catecholamine production. There is little or no abdominal tenderness, fever, or leukocytosis because inflammation is not prominent. Bowel sounds are usually decreased, but are sometimes increased with diarrhea. The urine is often dark (because of porphobilin, a degradation product of PBG) or reddish (because of porphyrins, including uroporphyrin formed nonenzymatically from PBG). Urinary hesitancy and dysuria may occur as a consequence of bladder dysfunction. Acute mental symptoms may include insomnia, anxiety, restlessness, disorientation, paranoia, and hallucinations.

Paresis because of peripheral motor neuropathy usually occurs with prolonged, severe attacks, but is sometimes an early or even initial manifestation.[235,236] Porphyric neuropathy is primarily motor and results from axonal degeneration, which may be followed by demyelinization.[237] Muscle weakness may not be detected until it is quite advanced, because it usually begins in the proximal muscles of the upper extremities. Paresis is usually symmetrical, but may be asymmetrical or focal. Course tremors, clonus, and increased reflexes are sometimes prominent. Sensory loss may develop, especially in the distal extremities. Cranial nerve involvement and cortical blindness have been described.

Motor neuropathy may progress to respiratory and bulbar paralysis and death, especially if diagnosis and treatment are delayed and harmful drugs continued. Death may result from respiratory arrest or cardiac arrhythmia.[237,238] Most attacks treated promptly resolve within days or even hours. Advanced neuropathy because of a severe attack is potentially completely reversible, with improvement continuing for up to 1 to 2 years.[239]

Hyponatremia is common during severe attacks and is sometimes a result of the syndrome of inappropriate antidiuretic hormone secretion, resulting from hypothalamic involvement. However, hyponatremia may be accompanied by reductions in blood volume,[240] indicating that increased antidiuretic hormone secretion in this setting is an appropriate physiologic response.[238] For example, hyponatremia may sometimes result from gastrointestinal loss, poor intake, and excess renal sodium loss.[238,241,242] A possible nephrotoxic effect of ALA may explain renal tubular sodium loss and impaired renal function in some patients.[241] Other electrolyte abnormalities may include hypomagnesemia and hypercalcemia.[243] Seizures may result from hyponatremia or represent a neurologic effect of acute porphyria.

Chronic mental symptoms, such as depression, are difficult to attribute to AIP. Chronic pain accompanied by depression develops in some patients after frequent exacerbations, and risk for suicide is increased. The disease also predisposes to chronic arterial hypertension and impaired renal function.[210,244,245] The latter may progress and require renal transplantation.[246,247]

Mild abnormalities in serum transaminases are common in AIP.[248] More advanced liver disease may develop and the risk of hepatocellular carcinoma is greatly increased (60–70-fold) in AIP, and is not related to specific *PBGD* mutations.[249–257] Serum α-fetoprotein was not increased and the uninvolved liver was not cirrhotic in most acute porphyria cases with liver cancer reported to date. Increased serum thyroxin levels because of increased thyroxin-binding globulin occurs in some patients with AIP, and occasionally hyperthyroidism and porphyria occur together.[258] Elevated low-density lipoprotein cholesterol is apparently less commonly observed in this disorder than in the past.[259]

Diagnosis A high index of suspicion is required for *initial diagnosis* of the acute porphyrias. Because the disease so often remains latent, there is often no family history of porphyria. Acute porphyria should be considered in patients with unexplained abdominal pain or other characteristic symptoms when initial evaluation does not suggest another more common explanation, and ruled in or out by rapid assessment of urinary PBG, which is both sensitive and specific. A substantial increase in PBG, which can be determined rapidly by a commercial kit,[260] establishes that a patient has either AIP, HCP, or VP. Consensus recommendations are that all major medical centers should retain the capacity for rapid urinary PBG testing on single-void urine specimens, as collection of 24-hour urines and reliance on outside laboratories for screening can greatly delay diagnosis and treatment. The urine specimen should be saved for later quantitative measurement of PBG, ALA, and total porphyrin levels. If PBG is substantially increased, samples of plasma, erythrocytes and feces should also be obtained prior to treatment with hemin. This approach provides for rapid initial diagnosis of AIP, HCP, and VP, subsequent biochemical differentiation of these conditions and diagnosis of ADP. In patients with renal failure, PBG can be measured in serum by a specialized laboratory.[40] Figure 57–6 presents a diagnostic flow chart for use when acute porphyria is suspected.

PBG excretion is generally 50 to 200 mg/day (normal range: 0 to ~4 mg/day) during acute attacks of AIP. Excretion of ALA is usually about half that of PBG (expressed as mg/day). Increases in ALA and PBG can persist for prolonged periods between attacks of acute porphyria, especially in AIP. Increases in ALA and PBG are less striking during acute attacks of HCP and VP and often decrease more rapidly.

The *diagnosis of an acute attack* is largely clinical, and is not based on a specific level of ALA or PBG. Levels of ALA and PBG during an acute attack may be increased compared to baseline levels, which fluctuate considerably and can be difficult to establish between attacks. Intravenous hemin causes dramatic, rapid but often transient decreases in these levels.

Urinary porphyrins are increased in AIP, are predominantly uroporphyrin, and account for reddish urine (ALA and PBG are colorless). Uroporphyrin can form nonenzymatically from PBG in urine prior to excretion. However, there is evidence that porphyrins in this condition are predominantly type III, which may be formed enzymatically,[261] perhaps from ALA transported to tissues other than the liver.[213] Total fecal porphyrins and plasma porphyrins are normal or slightly increased in AIP, and erythrocyte zinc protoporphyrin concentrations may be nonspecifically increased.

Erythrocyte PBGD activity is approximately half-normal in most (70–80%) patients with AIP. However, this measurement is not definitive for confirming or excluding the diagnosis. As described earlier, some PBGD mutations cause the enzyme to be deficient only in nonerythroid tissues. Moreover, the ranges of activity for normals and AIP are wide and overlapping, and the erythrocyte enzyme is highly age-dependent,[160] such that an increase in the proportion of younger cells in the circulation can

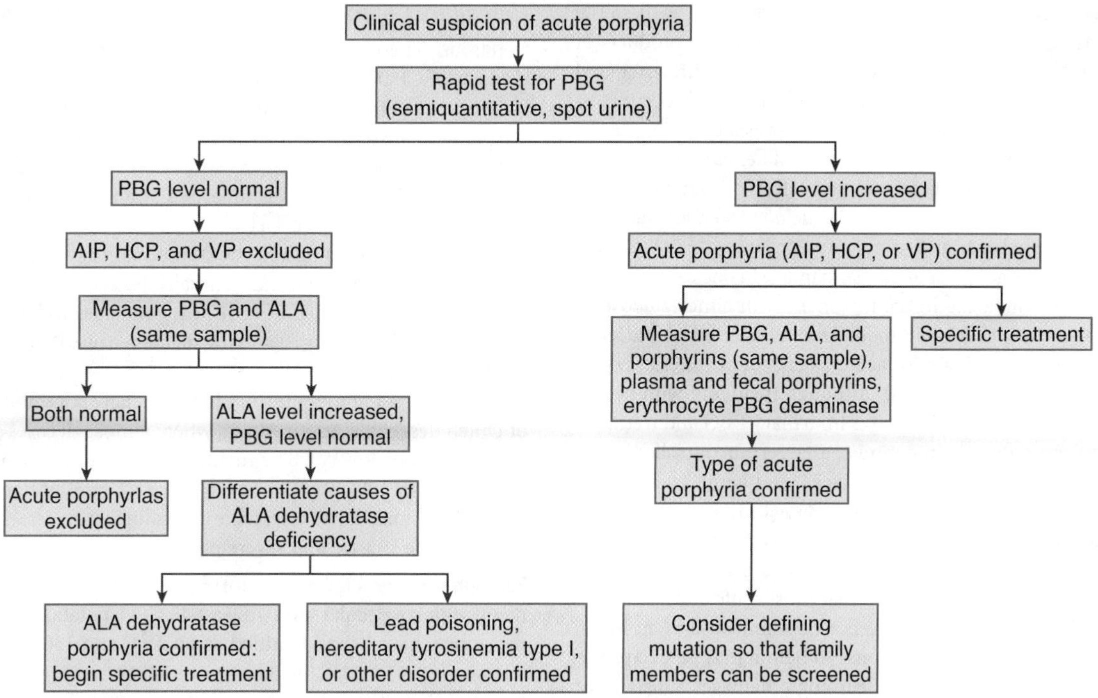

FIGURE 57–6. Recommended laboratory evaluation of patients with concurrent symptoms suggesting an acute porphyria, indicating how the diagnosis is established or excluded by biochemical testing and when specific therapy should be initiated. This schema is not applicable to patients who have been recently treated with hemin or who have recovered from past symptoms suggestive of porphyria. Levels of δ-aminolevulinic acid (*ALA*) and porphobilinogen (*PBG*) may be less increased in hereditary coproporphyria (*HCP*) and variegate porphyria (*VP*) and decrease more quickly with recovery than in acute intermittent porphyria (*AIP*). Mutation detection provides confirmation and greatly facilitates detection of relatives with latent porphyria.

raise the activity into the normal range in AIP patients with a concurrent condition such as hemolytic anemia or hepatic disease.[262,263] This measurement also does not distinguish between latent and active disease. For these reasons, and because it does not detect other acute porphyrias, erythrocyte PBGD measurement is not useful for initial diagnosis of ill patients. However, it is useful for confirming a diagnosis of AIP and for screening of asymptomatic family members.

Once the diagnosis of AIP is established by biochemical methods, it is useful to identify the underlying *PBGD* mutation. This confirms the diagnosis and, most importantly, enables reliable and definitive identification of other gene carriers by DNA testing. PBGD deficiency can be documented in the fetus by measuring the enzyme activity or by identifying the maternal or paternal mutation in amniotic fluid cells. However, prenatal diagnosis is usually not indicated because the great majority of heterozygous carriers of PBGD mutations have a good prognosis.

Therapy Hospitalization is usually required for treatment of attacks, although well-characterized patients with frequently recurring mild attacks that respond rapidly to treatment are sometimes managed as outpatients. Hospitalization facilitates treatment of severe symptoms; intravenous therapies; and monitoring of respiration, electrolytes, and nutritional status. Admission to intensive care is warranted if the vital capacity is impaired. Harmful drugs should be discontinued whenever possible. Pain, nausea, and vomiting are generally severe and require narcotic analgesics, chlorpromazine or another phenothiazine, or ondansetron. Low doses of short-acting benzodiazepines are probably safe for anxiety and insomnia.[40] β-Adrenergic blocking agents may be useful to control tachycardia and hypertension, but may be hazardous in patients with hypovolemia or incipient cardiac failure.[264] Seizures are treated by correcting hyponatremia, if present. Almost all anticonvulsant drugs have at least some potential for exacerbating acute porphyrias. Clonazepam may be less harmful than phenytoin, barbiturates, or valproic acid.[265,266] Bromides, gabapentin, and vigabatrin are safe.

Carbohydrate Loading Glucose and other carbohydrates repress hepatic ALAS1 and reduce porphyrin precursor excretion, but the effects are weak compared to those of hemin. Attacks with mild pain and without severe manifestations such as paresis and hyponatremia may be treated with carbohydrate loading.[40] Oral glucose polymer solutions may be given if tolerated. Intravenous treatment with 300 to 500 g of intravenous glucose, usually administered as a 10 percent solution, is recommended.[40] However, the dilutional effects of a large volume of free water may increase risk of hyponatremia. A more complete parenteral nutrition regimen may be needed if oral or enteral feeding is not possible.

Intravenous Hemin Hemin is much more potent in reducing levels of ALA and PBG compared to glucose. Although controlled clinical trials are lacking for all current therapies for acute attacks of porphyria, consensus recommendations are that the clinical benefits of hemin are superior to other available therapies.[40,267,268] Hemin is available in the United States as a lyophilized hematin preparation (Panhematin, Lundbeck, Deerfield, IL), and was the first drug approved under the Orphan Drug Act. Heme arginate (Normosang, Orphan Europe, Paris, France), which is a stable preparation of heme and arginine, is available in Europe and South Africa.[268,269] Hemin, when infused intravenously as hematin, heme albumin, or heme arginate, becomes bound to circulating hemopexin and albumin and is then taken up primarily by hepatocytes. It then enters and reconstitutes the regulatory heme pool and represses the synthesis of hepatic ALAS1. This results in a dramatic reduction in porphyrin precursor excretion. The standard regimen for treatment of acute attacks is 3 to 4 mg/kg daily for 4 days. Treatment may be extended if a response is not observed within this time. Hemin has been administered safely during pregnancy.[40,268,269]

Product labeling recommends reconstitution of hematin with sterile water. But it was subsequently discovered that degradation products of hematin begin to form immediately upon reconstitution with water, and these are responsible for phlebitis at the site of infusion, which occurs frequently and can lead to loss of venous access with repeated dosing, and a transient anticoagulant effect.[270,271] Stabilization of hematin with 25 percent human albumin can prevent these adverse effects,[272] and is currently recommended.[40,273] Uncommon side effects include fever, aching, malaise, hemolysis, anaphylaxis, and circulatory collapse.[274,275] Excessive dosing caused reversible acute renal tubular damage in one case.[276]

Controlled trials comparing initial treatment with either glucose or hemin are lacking, except for one randomized, double-blind, placebo-controlled trial of heme arginate for acute attacks of porphyria, which was underpowered (only 12 patients). Although treatment with hemin was delayed for 2 days, striking decreases in urinary PBG and trends in clinical benefit were noted.[277] In contrast, a larger uncontrolled study enrolled 22 patients who had 51 acute attacks, and heme arginate was initiated within 24 hours of admission in 37 attacks (73%); all patients responded and hospitalization was less than 7 days in 90 percent of cases.[268] Therefore, based on this and numerous other uncontrolled clinical studies, it is now recommended that most acute attacks of porphyria be treated promptly with intravenous hemin, without an initial trial of intravenous glucose.[40,268] Response to hemin may be delayed or incomplete when there is advanced neurologic damage. Subacute or chronic symptoms are unlikely to respond.

Liver Transplantation Liver transplantation has been highly effective in several patients who were disabled by recurrent attacks of AIP.[221] This may be an option for severely affected patients.

Other Therapies Cimetidine has been recommended for human acute porphyrias based on uncontrolled observations in small numbers of patients.[278,279] This drug inhibits hepatic CYPs, and can prevent experimental forms of porphyria induced by agents such as allylisopropylacetamide that undergo activation by these enzymes.[280] However, these mechanisms are not immediately relevant to inherited porphyrias in humans. Therefore, cimetidine cannot be recommended as an alternative to hemin.

Prevention of Acute Attacks Multiple inciting factors must be avoided especially in patients who continue to have repeated attacks. Consultation with a dietitian may be useful to identify dietary indiscretions, and to help maintain a well-balanced diet somewhat high in carbohydrate (60–70% of total calories). There is little evidence that additional dietary carbohydrate helps further in preventing attacks. Iron deficiency, if present, should be corrected. Patients who wish to lose excess weight should do so gradually and when they are clinically stable.

Gonadotropin-releasing hormone analogues can prevent repeated attacks that are confined to the luteal phase of the menstrual cycle,[281–283] but are less effective in patients with attacks partially associated with the cycle. If treatment is effective after several months, low-dose estradiol, preferably by the transdermal route, or a bisphosphonate may be added to prevent bone loss and other side effects, or treatment changed to a low-dose oral contraceptive. Hemin administered once or twice weekly can prevent frequent, noncyclic attacks of porphyria in some patients.[284]

Long-Term Monitoring Patients with acute porphyrias are at risk for renal damage and hepatocellular carcinoma. Renal function should be monitored, hypertension controlled, and nephrotoxic drugs avoided. Current recommendations are that patients with acute porphyrias who are older than age 50 years, and especially those with continued elevations of ALA and PBG, be screened at least annually by ultrasonogram or an alternative imaging method to detect hepatocellular carcinoma at an early stage.[40]

Hereditary Coproporphyria and Variegate Porphyria

Definition These closely related hepatic porphyrias are caused by deficiencies of CPO and PPO, the sixth and seventh enzymes of the heme biosynthetic pathway. They present with neurovisceral symptoms, as in AIP, or with blistering skin lesions identical to those seen in PCT. Cutaneous manifestations are much more common in VP than in HCP. The enzyme deficiency in each is inherited as an autosomal dominant trait with variable penetrance (see Table 57–1 and Fig. 57–1). As in AIP, most individuals who inherit the trait remain asymptomatic. Both disorders are less common and generally less severe than AIP in most countries. The incidence of HCP was estimated to be 2 per 1,000,000 population in Denmark,[285] and the incidence of VP in Finland reported at 1.3 per 100,000.[286]

Because of a founder effect, VP is especially common among whites of Dutch descent in South Africa, where almost all cases share the same PPO mutation (R59W). The incidence of VP in that country was estimated at 3 per 1000 population.[287] Very rare cases of homozygous HCP and VP are manifested by severe neurologic impairment early in life, but not acute attacks, and severe photosensitivity.[288]

Pathophysiology Like other porphyrias, HCP and VP are heterogeneous at the molecular level. At least 43 *CPO* mutations, mostly missense mutations, have been identified in HCP,[289] and 130 *PPO* mutations in VP (see Table 57–1). Clinical expression is variable and onset of neurologic manifestations are influenced by the same factors that are important in AIP.

CPO catalyzes the two-step decarboxylation of coproporphyrinogen III to yield protoporphyrinogen IX, with intermediate formation of harderoporphyrinogen, a tricarboxyl porphyrinogen. A single active site carries out both decarboxylations, and most of the harderoporphyrinogen formed is not released before being further decarboxylated to protoporphyrinogen IX. However, a variant form of HCP termed *harderoporphyria* is a result of *CPO* mutations that favor premature release of harderoporphyrinogen from the enzyme.[290]

Clinical Features Neurovisceral manifestations are identical to those in other acute porphyrias. Although both HCP and VP are generally less severe than AIP, attacks may be life-threatening. Blistering skin lesions may be seen, and are much more common in VP than in HCP. Factors that contribute to attacks, including drugs, hormones, and dietary factors, are also the same as in AIP. Oral contraceptives may precipitate cutaneous manifestations of VP. Risk of chronic hypertension, renal disease, and hepatocellular carcinoma are increased, as in AIP.

Diagnosis Urinary PBG is elevated during acute attacks, and usually is the basis for diagnosis of these acute porphyrias. However, increases in PBG may be less than in AIP, and more transient. Levels of coproporphyrin III are markedly increased in urine and feces, whereas in AIP fecal porphyrins are normal or only slightly increased. Fecal porphyrins in HCP are almost entirely coproporphyrin III, whereas in VP both coproporphyrin III and protoporphyrin are approximately equally increased. The fecal coproporphyrin III:I ratio is sensitive for diagnosis of HCP, even in asymptomatic stages of the disease.[291] Plasma porphyrin concentration is commonly increased in VP, seldom increased in HCP unless there are cutaneous manifestations, and are normal or only slightly increased in AIP. A characteristic plasma porphyrin fluorescence maximum observed at neutral pH is a very specific marker for VP, and is believed to represent protoporphyrin bound covalently to plasma proteins.[292] The fluorescence maximum as at approximately 626 nm in VP, approximately 634 in EPP, and approximately 620 in other porphyrias. This fluorometric method is more effective than examination of fecal porphyrins for detecting asymptomatic VP,[293] and is useful for rapidly differentiating VP and PCT. Erythrocyte PBG deaminase activity is normal in HCP and VP, and usually deficient in AIP. Assays for CPO and PPO are not widely available. DNA studies are most reliable for identifying asymptomatic carriers, once the mutation affecting the family is identified.

Harderoporphyria is a variant form of HCP that results from a homozygous defect of a structurally altered CPO, such that harderoporphyrinogen is released prematurely from the enzyme. This variant is identified by finding a predominance of harderoporphyrin in urine and feces. Neonatal hemolytic anemia is a distinctive feature of this condition.[294] Increases in porphyrin precursors and porphyrins may be more severe in homozygous HCP and VP, with substantial increases in erythrocyte zinc protoporphyrin.

Therapy The identification and avoidance of precipitating factors is essential. Treatment of acute attacks is the same as in AIP. Treatment of the phototoxic manifestations is not satisfactory. Although the lesions are identical to the blistering skin lesions seen in PCT, there is no response in HCP and VP to phlebotomies or low-dose chloroquine or hydroxychloroquine. Therefore, avoidance of sunlight and use of protective clothing is most important. Yearly screening for hepatocellular carcinoma by imaging is recommended after age 50 years, especially in individuals with persistent increases in porphyrin precursors or porphyrins.

Porphyria Cutanea Tarda and Hepatoerythropoietic Porphyria

Definition PCT is caused by a deficiency of hepatic UROD activity and is manifested by the development of chronic, blistering skin lesions on the dorsal aspects of the hands and other sun-exposed areas of skin in middle or late life. This iron-related disorder is the most common and readily treated form of porphyria (see Table 57–1 and Fig. 57–1). The enzyme deficiency develops specifically in the liver in the presence of multiple susceptibility factors most of which are believed to contribute to generation of a UROD inhibitor. The disease has been classified as types 1 to 3, based on the presence or absence of heterozygous UROD mutations and other unknown inherited factors. Patients with familial (type 2) PCT are heterozygous for UROD mutations, which are inherited as an autosomal dominant trait with low penetrance. HEP is the homozygous (or compound heterozygous) form of familial (type 2) PCT, which usually presents in childhood and resembles CEP clinically. Rarely, hepatocellular carcinomas may secrete porphyrins and simulate PCT; however the enzyme defect was not established in such cases.[295]

PCT must be differentiated from other porphyrias that cause identical blistering skin lesions and from pseudoporphyria (also known as pseudo-PCT). The latter is a poorly understood condition that presents with lesions that closely resemble PCT, but with plasma porphyrins that are not significantly increased. Potentially photosensitizing drugs, such as nonsteroidal antiinflammatory agents, are sometimes implicated.

Pathophysiology UROD sequentially decarboxylates uroporphyrinogen (which has eight carboxyl side chains) to yield coproporphyrinogen (with four carboxyl groups). When hepatic UROD is profoundly inhibited, the substrate and the intermediate and final products of the reaction accumulate as the oxidized porphyrins in the liver (mostly uroporphyrin and heptacarboxylporphyrin), and then appear in plasma and urine. Photosensitivity results from activation of porphyrins in the skin by long wave ultraviolet light and generation of reactive oxygen species.

Hepatic UROD activity is inhibited to less than approximately 20 percent of normal in all patients with PCT. Types 1, 2, and 3 are not fundamentally different or clinically distinguished from each other. Patients with type 1 or "sporadic" PCT have no UROD mutations and no family history of PCT. Approximately 80 percent of patients fall into this category. Type 2 or "familial" PCT comprises approximately 20 percent of cases who are heterozygous for UROD mutations; but because the penetrance of this trait is low there are usually no other documented cases in the family. In families with type 3, which is rare, more than one member has PCT, but there is no UROD mutation; these familial cases presumably share other inherited or environmental susceptibility factors.

Although hepatic UROD activity must be reduced to approximately 20 percent of normal in order for PCT to be manifest, the amount of enzyme protein, when measured immunochemically in liver, remains at its genetically determined level, which in type 2 cases is approximately 50 percent of normal.[296,297] Mice heterozygous for mutant UROD alleles are much more sensitive to porphyrinogenic stimuli than wild-type animals.[298] In heterozygous mice that display porphyric phenotypes, hepatic UROD protein is half-normal, but the catalytic activity of the enzyme is reduced to approximately 20 percent, suggesting the existence of an inhibitor of hepatic UROD.[298,299]

Although iron does not directly inhibit UROD, there is considerable evidence that PCT is an iron-related disease, with hepatic siderosis seen in almost all cases. This explains why *HFE* (hemochromatosis gene) mutations that lead to increased intestinal iron absorption predispose to development of PCT (see Chap. 42). Individuals who inherit a UROD mutation have approximately 50 percent of normal enzyme activity from birth, such that a UROD inhibitor can more readily reduce enzyme activity to less than approximately 20 percent of normal. How iron and other known or suspected susceptibility factors such as alcohol, smoking, estrogens, hepatitis C, HIV, hepatic steatosis, and other suspected factors contribute to the development of PCT is less-well understood, but these may act in part by increasing oxidative stress in hepatocytes. A deficiency of ascorbic acid[300–302] and perhaps other antioxidants[303] may play a role in some patients. Smoking may also act by inducing hepatic CYPs, including CYP1A2, which is essential for causing uroporphyria in rodent models,[304,305] and may produce a UROD inhibitor, which has been characterized as a uroporphomethene. This substance is a product of partial oxidation of uroporphyrinogen, and is found in the liver of mice that are heterozygous for a UROD mutation, homozygous for an *HFE* mutation (C282Y), and develop uroporphyria spontaneously.[75] Other potential mechanisms for lowering of hepatic UROD activity in PCT, such as oxidative damage to UROD active site residues, are less favored but have not been excluded.[306]

Patients with familial (type 2) PCT are heterozygous for mutations that reduce UROD activity and immunoreactivity to approximately 50 percent of normal in all tissues. At least 70 different mutations of the UROD gene have been identified in type 2 PCT and HEP (see Table 57–1). Most are missense mutations, with each occurring in one or a few families. Homozygosity for a null UROD mutation is lethal in early neonatal life. Therefore, in HEP at least one of the mutant UROD alleles must preserve at least some catalytic activity. Knowledge of the crystal structure of UROD allows mapping of specific mutations and prediction of their impact on enzyme structure and function. Expression studies in eukaryotic cells suggest that some mutations may destabilize the enzyme protein in a tissue-specific manner.[307]

Pathogenesis of the Clinical Findings A distinctive feature of PCT is massive accumulation of porphyrins in the liver. As a result, fresh hepatic tissue shows strong red fluorescence on exposure to long-wave ultraviolet light. Microscopic, birefringent, needle-like inclusions are found in lysosomes, and paracrystalline inclusions in mitochondria. Increased stainable iron is very common. Other nonspecific hepatic findings are probably partly a result of the disease itself, although the effects of associated factors such as alcohol and hepatitis C are difficult to differentiate. Liver histopathology includes hepatocyte necrosis, inflammation, increased iron, and increased fat. Mild abnormalities in liver function tests, especially serum transaminases and γ-glutamyltranspeptidase, are present in almost all cases, but cirrhosis is unusual. The risk of hepatocellular carcinoma is increased, especially in those with more prolonged disease, cirrhosis, or other risk factors such as hepatitis C or alcoholic liver disease.[308–310]

Excess porphyrins are transported in plasma from the liver to the skin. Skin histopathology includes subepidermal blistering and deposition of periodic acid-Schiff–positive material around blood vessels and fine fibrillar material in the upper dermis and at the dermoepithelial junction. Immunoglobulin G, other immunoglobulins, and complement are deposited around dermal blood vessels and at the dermoepithelial junction. Splits in the lamina lucida of the basement membrane lead to formation of fluid-containing bullae.[311] These histologic changes are found in other cutaneous porphyrias as well as pseudoporphyria and are not diagnostic for PCT. Activation of the complement system after irradiation has been demonstrated in PCT patients both *in vivo* and *in vitro* in sera,[312] and is thought to result from generation of reactive oxygen species.

Susceptibility Factors PCT is a highly heterogeneous disease, with multiple susceptibility factors expected in the individual patient.[313] Multiple factors are important in familial as well as sporadic PCT, because heterozygosity for a UROD mutation is a susceptibility factor that does not of itself reduce hepatic enzyme activity sufficiently to cause the disease. The environmental, infectious, and inherited factors discussed below, none of which is invariably present, are known or suspected to play an important role. Their prevalence may show considerable geographic variation in PCT patients as well as healthy subjects.

Alcohol PCT has long been associated with excess alcohol use. Alcohol and its metabolites may induce ALAS1 and CYP2E1, generate active oxygen species that contribute to oxidative damage, cause mitochondrial injury, deplete reduced glutathione and other antioxidant defenses, increase production of endotoxin, activate Kupffer cells, and increase iron absorption.

Smoking and Cytochrome P450 Enzymes Smoking is less extensively studied as a risk factor but is commonly associated with alcohol use in PCT.[313] Smoking may increase oxidative stress in hepatocytes, and induces CYP1A2, which is essential to the development of uroporphyria in rodent models. CYP levels have been found to be increased in liver in human PCT,[314] but it is not clear which CYP might be important in pathogenesis of the human disease. A study of caffeine metabolism did not find evidence for increased CYP1A2 activity *in vivo* in PCT, even when smokers and nonsmokers were analyzed separately.[315] However, a more inducible polymorphism of CYP1A2 has been found to be more common in PCT than in normal subjects.[316]

Estrogens Estrogen use is very common in women with PCT.[313,317,318] In the past, some men developed the disease after treatment of prostate cancer with estrogens.[317] Female rats or males treated with estrogens are more susceptible to development of chemically induced uroporphyria than untreated males.[319] The mechanism is not established, although estrogens can generate reactive oxygen species in some experimental systems.[306,320]

Hepatitis C Reported prevalence of hepatitis C in PCT has ranged from 21 to 92 percent in various countries, and greatly exceeds the prevalence of this viral infection in healthy subjects, which shows considerable geographic variation. Hepatitis C is associated with excess fat, some iron accumulation, mitochondrial dysfunction, and oxidative stress in hepatocytes, which may contribute to the development of PCT. Dysregulation of the iron regulatory hormone hepcidin may contribute to iron accumulation in hepatitis C.[321,322]

Human Immunodeficiency Virus PCT is less commonly associated with HIV infection than with hepatitis C.[323] Occasionally PCT is the initial manifestation of this infection. The mechanism is unknown.

Iron and HFE Mutations Mild to moderate iron overload is found in most patients with PCT, and iron deficiency is protective. The importance of iron has been confirmed in animal models, such as rodents treated with hexachlorobenzene and other halogenated polyaromatic hydrocarbons.[306] Mice with disruption of one UROD allele (UROD[+/−]) and two disrupted HFE alleles (HFE[−/−]) develop uroporphyria without administration of exogenous chemicals.[298] Prevalence of the C282Y mutation of the *HFE* gene, which is the major cause of hemochromatosis in whites, is increased in both sporadic and familial PCT, and 10 to 20 percent of patients may be C282Y homozygotes (see Chap. 42).[324] In southern Europe, where the C282Y is less prevalent, the H63D mutation is more commonly associated with PCT.[325] Excess iron may contribute to UROD inhibition by providing an oxidative environment that is apparently needed for generation of a UROD inhibitor. Hepatic hepcidin expression is reduced in hemochromatosis, and is further reduced in PCT compared to patients without PCT and comparable iron overload, suggesting that reduced expression of this hormone is important in causing hepatic siderosis in PCT.[326]

Antioxidants Substantial reductions in plasma levels of ascorbate and carotenoids have been noted in some patients with PCT.[301–303] Ascorbate deficiency in rodents enhances susceptibility to development or uroporphyria, and ascorbate decreases uroporphyrin accumulation except in animals treated with large amounts of iron.[300]

Polyhalogenated Aromatic Hydrocarbons A large outbreak of PCT occurred during a period of food shortage in a population in eastern Turkey in the 1950s from consumption of seed wheat treated with the fungicide hexachlorobenzene.[13] Smaller outbreaks and individual cases have occurred after exposures to other chemicals such as 2,3,7,8-tetrachlorodibenzo-*p*-dioxin (TCDD, dioxin).[327] Such exposures are rarely identified in PCT patients in clinical practice. These chemicals were subsequently shown to cause hepatic UROD deficiency and biochemical features resembling PCT in laboratory animals, and many studies that followed have greatly increased our understanding of this acquired enzyme deficiency.[306,328]

Clinical Features Disease onset is usually in the fourth or fifth decade of life, and is more common in men. Onset may occur earlier in familial (type 2) disease or in cases with the C282Y/C282Y *HFE* genotype.[329] Fluid-filled vesicles develop most commonly on the backs of the hands (Fig. 57–7A). Skin friability is increased and blisters often follow minor trauma. These also occur on the forearms, face, ears, neck, legs, and feet. The blisters often rupture, crust over, and are prone to infection before healing slowly. Milia may precede or follow vesicle formation. Facial hypertrichosis and hyperpigmentation are particularly noticed by female patients (see Fig. 57–7B). Severe thickening of affected areas of skin is termed *pseudoscleroderma* and resembles systemic scleroderma.

Blistering skin lesions in VP and HCP are identical to those in PCT. Those in CEP and HEP resemble PCT but are usually much more severe and mutilating. Mild or moderate erythrocytosis is common in PCT, and is not well explained. Chronic lung disease from smoking may contribute.

Drugs that exacerbate the acute porphyrias are only occasionally reported to play a role in PCT.[330] PCT may occur with other conditions predisposing to iron overload such as myelofibrosis[331,332] and end-stage renal disease,[333] and with diabetes mellitus[310] and cutaneous and systemic lupus erythematosus. PCT associated with end-stage renal disease is usually more severe, sometimes with severe mutilation. Lack of urinary porphyrin excretion in these patients leads to much higher concentrations of porphyrins in plasma, and the excess porphyrins are poorly dialyzable.[333] The disease occasionally develops during pregnancy, perhaps related to effects of estrogen.

The clinical manifestations of HEP usually resemble CEP, with onset of blistering skin lesions, hypertrichosis, scarring, and red urine in infancy or childhood. Sclerodermoid skin changes are sometimes prominent. Excess porphyrins originate mostly from the liver in this condition. Unusually mild cases have been described.[334]

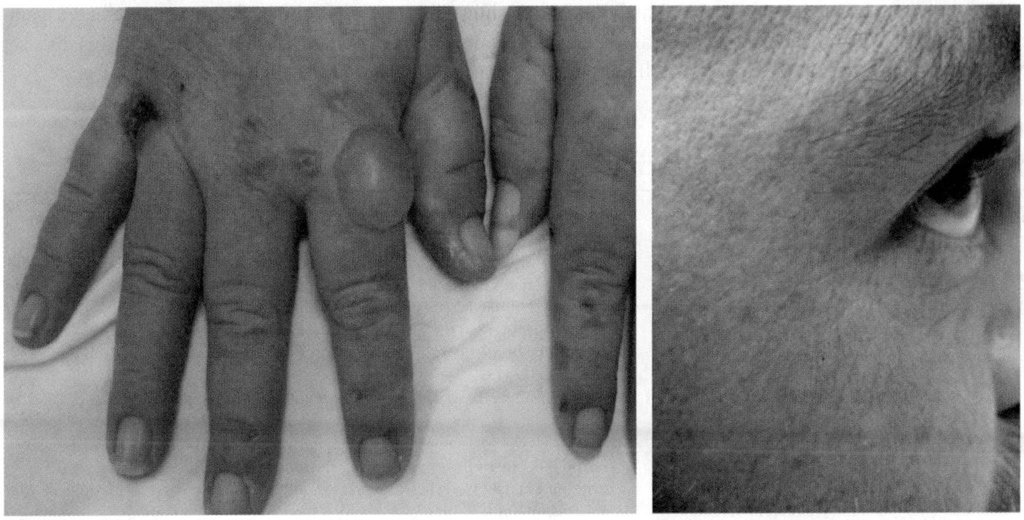
A B

FIGURE 57–7. Cutaneous findings in porphyria cutanea tarda include **(A)** bullous lesions most commonly on the dorsal aspects of the hands and fingers, which rupture and crust over, and **(B)** facial hirsutism most noticeable on the upper cheeks.

Diagnosis A diagnosis of PCT is established by finding a substantial elevation of porphyrins in urine or plasma, with a predominance of uroporphyrin and heptacarboxylporphyrin. Hexa- and pentacarboxylporphyrins and coproporphyrin are also increased. Levels of PBG are normal, and urinary ALA is normal or slightly increased. The pattern of porphyrins in feces is complex, and includes heptacarboxyl porphyrin and isocoproporphyrins. The latter are overproduced in the presence of UROD deficiency because pentacarboxylporphyrinogen is a substrate for CPO, leading to formation of dehydroisocoproporphyrinogen, which is excreted in bile and undergoes oxidation by intestinal bacteria to isocoproporphyrins.[335]

Measurement of plasma porphyrins and determination of the fluorescence emission peak at neutral pH is especially useful for screening patients with blistering skin lesions. A substantial increase with a peak at approximately 620 nm is most commonly caused by PCT, and excludes VP and pseudoporphyria, which are the most common conditions that mimic PCT clinically.[336] Plasma porphyrin measurements are essential for diagnosis of PCT in patients with advanced renal disease; the reference range is higher in patients with renal failure than in normals.[337]

Erythrocyte porphyrins are substantially increased in CEP and HEP, but are normal or only modestly increased in PCT. Rare cases of HCP with blistering lesions are identified by a predominance of coproporphyrin III in urine and especially feces. Familial (type 2) cases are identified by half-normal erythrocyte UROD activity or preferably by DNA studies to identify a UROD mutation. Erythrocyte UROD activity is 5 to 30 percent of normal in HEP, and DNA studies reveal that a UROD mutation is inherited from each parent.

Biochemical findings in HEP resemble PCT, with predominant accumulation and excretion of uroporphyrin, heptacarboxyl porphyrin and isocoproporphyrins. However, in contrast to PCT, erythrocyte zinc protoporphyrin is substantially increased. At least one genotype may be associated with predominant excretion of pentacarboxylporphyrin.[334]

Therapy Treatment is highly effective but specific in both sporadic and familial PCT, and therefore should be initiated only after the diagnosis is well established. It is sometimes reasonable to start treatment after a plasma porphyrin screen is consistent with PCT and excludes VP and pseudoporphyria (see above, "Diagnosis"). Patients should be questioned and tested for all known susceptibility factors, including use of alcohol, tobacco, and estrogens, hepatitis C, HIV, *HFE* mutations, and inherited UROD deficiency (erythrocyte UROD activity or preferably UROD mutations), because their presence influences management. Serum ferritin should be measured before starting treatment. Patients are advised to stop drinking and smoking and to discontinue estrogens. A nutritionally adequate intake of ascorbic acid and other nutrients should be assured, but treatment with this vitamin should not be used as primary therapy.

Improvement may occur after removing one or more susceptibility factors, but without phlebotomy or low-dose hydroxychloroquine recovery is unpredictable or slow.[338] Repeated phlebotomy is the preferred treatment at most centers. The original rationale proposed by Ippen in 1961 was to decrease the commonly associated mild or moderately increased hemoglobin, stimulate erythropoiesis, and perhaps channel excess heme pathway intermediates to hemoglobin synthesis.[339] However the oxidized porphyrins that accumulate in PCT cannot reenter the heme biosynthetic pathway and be converted to heme, and it is now understood that phlebotomy is effective by reducing body iron stores and liver iron content. Treatment with an iron chelator such as desferrioxamine is less efficient than phlebotomies in reducing iron, but may be tried when the latter are contraindicated.[340]

Approximately 450 mL of blood is removed, usually at 2-week intervals. In one series an average of 5.4 phlebotomies was required for remission, but many more are needed in some patients with coexisting hemochromatosis and marked increases in serum ferritin levels. Hemoglobin or hematocrit levels are followed as safety (not therapeutic) targets, to prevent symptomatic anemia. Usually, the hemoglobin should not fall below 10 to 11 g/dL, but the baseline value and the age and clinical condition of the patient are also considered. The therapeutic target is a serum ferritin near 15 ng/mL, which is close to the lower limit of normal and associated with tissue iron depletion but usually not anemia. Additional iron depletion is not beneficial, and causes anemia. Treatment is also guided by plasma (or serum) porphyrin levels, which are more convenient to measure repeatedly than urine porphyrins, and fall more slowly than the serum ferritin. Plasma porphyrins usually decline from initial levels of 10 to 25 mcg/dL during treatment, and fall below the upper limit of normal (~1 mcg/dL) within weeks after phlebotomies are completed.[341,342] New skin lesions are generally decreased at the end of treatment, but some may occur for a few weeks after plasma porphyrin levels become normal. Severe sclerodermatous changes and liver function abnormalities can also improve.

After a remission is obtained, continued phlebotomies are generally not needed. However, relapses may occur, especially in patients who resume use of alcohol, and are treated by another course of phlebotomies. For patients with the C282Y/C282Y or C282Y/H63D *HFE* genotypes, management guidelines for hemochromatosis should be followed. Continued phlebotomies as needed to maintain a serum ferritin below approximately 50 ng/mL may also be beneficial in patients who have experienced recurrences of PCT, although published experience is limited. It is also advisable to follow porphyrin levels and reinstitute phlebotomies promptly if porphyrin levels begin to rise. Liver imaging and a serum α-fetoprotein determination should be repeated as screening for hepatocellular carcinoma. After remission, transdermal estrogen can be resumed in women, if needed, with little risk for recurrence of PCT.[315]

A low-dose regimen of hydroxychloroquine or chloroquine is also effective,[306,343–348] and most appropriate when phlebotomy is contraindicated or poorly tolerated, if iron overload is not severe. However, this treatment is preferred at some centers because it is more convenient and much less expensive. These 4-aminoquinoline antimalarials do not appear to deplete hepatic iron, and the mechanism for their effects in PCT are not fully understood. Full therapeutic doses of these drugs exacerbate photosensitivity in PCT, induce fever, malaise, and nausea, markedly increase urinary and plasma porphyrins, and increase serum transaminases, other liver function tests, and ferritin. This reaction can even unmask previously unrecognized PCT.[349] Although these adverse effects are followed by complete remission,[350] they should be avoided by a low-dose treatment regimen (hydroxychloroquine 100 mg or chloroquine 125 mg—one-half of a standard tablet—twice weekly) at least until plasma or urine porphyrins are normalized.[343,346,347] However, some patients may respond poorly and require later treatment with larger doses, or phlebotomy.[350] There is a small risk of retinopathy,[351] which may be lower with hydroxychloroquine. Prospective studies comparing different treatment approaches in PCT are lacking. In a retrospective study low-dose chloroquine was ineffective in patients homozygous for the *C282Y* mutation of the *HFE* gene,[352] which suggests that the degree of excess hepatic iron may influence response to this treatment.

These 4-aminoquinolines are not effective in other porphyrias, and do not mobilize all types of porphyrins from liver and other tissues.[353] Chloroquine may form complexes with a variety of porphyrins, which might promote their mobilization from liver,[354,355] but this does not appear to explain their effects in PCT. These drugs may colocalize with excess porphyrins in lysosomes and other intracellular organelles and promote their release by a process that involves transient cell damage. It was suggested that mobilization of hepatic iron may be important,[347,356,357] but serum ferritin concentrations do not change significantly during treatment.

PCT may improve after treatment of coexisting hepatitis C. However, for several reasons PCT should be treated first and hepatitis C later in most cases. First, PCT is usually more symptomatic and can be treated more quickly and effectively. Second, there is some evidence that treatment of hepatitis C may be more effective after iron reduction. Third, interferon and ribavirin commonly cause anemia, which usually precludes phlebotomy for PCT. Hydroxychloroquine may be an option during treatment with interferon and ribavirin, but initial worsening of liver function tests, even with a low-dose regimen, may cause concern. It is reasonable to consider continued low-dose hydroxychloroquine after PCT is in remission to avoid a recurrence of PCT during treatment of hepatitis C, but there is little experience with this approach. Reports that PCT patients are often resistant to treatment of hepatitis C,[358,359] contrast with reports of successful treatment, and prospective studies are needed.

Treatment of PCT associated with end-stage renal disease is more difficult, as phlebotomy is often contraindicated by anemia. Erythropoietin administration can correct anemia, mobilize iron, and support phlebotomy in many cases.[333,360,361] High-flux hemodialysis may remove porphyrins from plasma and provide some benefit.[362] PCT is not a contraindication to renal transplantation, which is likely to lead to remission[363] partly because of resumption of endogenous erythropoietin production. The level of plasma porphyrins are often especially high in these patients, and should be assessed prior to surgery, because there may be some risk of skin and peritoneal burns from exposure to operating room lights.

Management of HEP emphasizes avoiding sunlight, as in CEP. Oral charcoal was helpful in a severe case associated with dyserythropoiesis.[116] Phlebotomy has shown little or no benefit. Retrovirus-mediated gene transfer can correct porphyria in cell lines from patients with this disease, which suggests that gene therapy may be applicable in the future.[364]

REFERENCES

1. Moore MR, McColl KE: *Disorders of Porphyrin Metabolism.* Plenum, New York, 1987.
2. Schultz JH: Ein fall von pemphigus, kompliziert durch lepra visceralis. Thesis for medical degree. Greifswald University, Greifswald, 1874.
3. Anderson TM: Hydroa aestivale in two brothers, complicated with the presence of haematoporphyrin in the urine. *Br J Dermatol* 10:1, 1898.
4. Harris DF: Haematoporphyrinuria and its relations to the source of urobilin. *J Anat Physiol* 31:383, 1897.
5. Stokvis BJ: Over Twee Zeldsame Kleuerstoffen in Urine van Zicken. *Ned Tijdschr Geneeskd* 13:409, 1889.
6. Günther H: Die haematoporphyrie. *Dtsch Arch Klin Med* 105:89, 1911.
7. Garrod AE: *Inborn Errors of Metabolism.* Hodder & Stoughton, London, 1923.
8. Sachs P: Ein fall von akuter porphyrie mit hochgradiger muskelatrophied. *Klin Wochenschr* 10:1123, 1931.
9. Waldenström J: Studien über Porphyrie. *Acta Med Scand Suppl* 82:1, 1937.
10. Waldenström J, Vahlquist BC: Studien uber die entstehung der roten harnpigmente (uroporphyrin und porphobilin) bein der akuten porphyrie aus iher farblosen vorstufe (porphobilinogen). *Hoppe Seylers Z Physiol Chem* 260:189, 1939.
11. Schmid R, Schwartz S, Watson CJ: Porphyrin content of bone marrow and liver in the various forms of porphyria. *Arch Intern Med* 93:167, 1954.
12. Cam C, Nigogosyan G: Acquired toxic porphyria cutanea tarda due to hexachlorobenzene. *JAMA* 183:90, 1963.
13. Schmid R: Cutaneous porphyria in Turkey. *N Engl J Med* 263:397, 1960.
14. Ockner RK, Schmid R: Acquired porphyria in man and rat due to hexachlorobenzene intoxication. *Nature* 189:499, 1961.
15. Rimington C, Ziegler G: Experimental porphyria in rats induced by chlorinated benzenes. *Biochem Pharmacol* 12:1387, 1963.
16. Schmid R: Hepatotoxic drugs causing porphyria in man and animals. *S Afr J Lab Clin Med* 14:212, 1963.
17. Schmid R: Acquired porphyria. *JAMA* 183:133, 1963.
18. Strand LJ, Felsher BF, Redeker AG, Marver HS: Heme biosynthesis in intermittent acute porphyria: Decreased hepatic conversion of porphobilinogen to porphyrins and increased delta-aminolevulinic acid synthetase activity. *Proc Natl Acad Sci U S A* 67:1315, 1970.
19. Bonkowsky HL, Tschudy DP, Collins A, et al: Repression of the overproduction of porphyrin precursors in acute intermittent porphyria by intravenous infusions of hematin. *Proc Natl Acad Sci U S A* 68:2725, 1971.
20. Granick S, Sassa S: δ-Aminolevulinic acid synthase and the control of heme and chlorophyll synthesis, in *Metabolic Regulation,* edited by HJ Vogel, p 77. Academic Press, New York, 1971.
21. Sassa S, Kappas A: Genetic, metabolic and biochemical aspects of the porphyrias. *Adv Hum Genet* 11:121, 1981.
22. McKay R, Druyan R, Getz GS, Rabinowitz M: Intramitochondrial localization of delta-aminolaevulate synthetase and ferrochelatase in rat liver. *Biochem J* 114:455, 1969.
23. Riddle RD, Yamamoto M, Engel JD: Expression of delta-aminolevulinate synthase in avian cells: Separate genes encode erythroid-specific and nonspecific isozymes. *Proc Natl Acad Sci U S A* 86:792, 1989.
24. Tsai SF, Bishop DF, Desnick RJ: Human uroporphyrinogen III synthase: Molecular cloning, nucleotide sequence, and expression of a full-length cDNA. *Proc Natl Acad Sci U S A* 85:7049, 1988.
25. Bishop DF: Two different genes encode delta-aminolevulinate synthase in humans: Nucleotide sequences of cDNAs for the housekeeping and erythroid genes. *Nucleic Acids Res* 18:7187, 1990.
26. Cox TC, Bawden MJ, Martin A, May BK: Human erythroid 5-aminolevulinate synthase: Promoter analysis and identification of an iron-responsive element in the mRNA. *EMBO J* 10:1891, 1991.
27. Aziz N, Munro HN: Iron regulates ferritin mRNA translation through a segment of its 5′ untranslated region. *Proc Natl Acad Sci U S A* 84:8478, 1987.
28. Lowry JA, Mackay JP: GATA-1: One protein, many partners. *Int J Biochem Cell Biol* 38:6, 2006.
29. Casey JL, Di Jeso B, Rao K, et al: The promoter region of the human transferrin receptor gene. *Ann N Y Acad Sci* 526:54, 1988.
30. Melefors O, Goossen B, Johansson HE, et al: Translational control of 5-aminolevulinate synthase mRNA by iron-responsive elements in erythroid cells. *J Biol Chem* 268:5974, 1993.
31. Podvinec M, Handschin C, Looser R, Meyer UA: Identification of the xenosensors regulating human 5-aminolevulinate synthase. *Proc Natl Acad Sci U S A* 101:9127, 2004.
32. Elferink CJ, Srivastava G, Maguire DJ, et al: A unique gene for 5-aminolevulinate synthase in chickens. Evidence for expression of an identical messenger RNA in hepatic and erythroid tissues. *J Biol Chem* 262:3988, 1987.

33. Kitchin KT: Regulation of rat hepatic delta-aminolevulinic acid synthetase and heme oxygenase activities: Evidence for control by heme and against mediation by prosthetic iron. *Int J Biochem* 15:479, 1983.
34. Handschin C, Lin J, Rhee J, et al: Nutritional regulation of hepatic heme biosynthesis and porphyria through PGC-1alpha. *Cell* 122:505, 2005.
35. Wu Z, Puigserver P, Andersson U, et al: Mechanisms controlling mitochondrial biogenesis and respiration through the thermogenic coactivator PGC-1. *Cell* 98:115, 1999.
36. Virbasius JV, Scarpulla RC: Activation of the human mitochondrial transcription factor A gene by nuclear respiratory factors: A potential regulatory link between nuclear and mitochondrial gene expression in organelle biogenesis. *Proc Natl Acad Sci U S A* 91:1309, 1994.
37. Scassa ME, Guberman AS, Ceruti JM, Canepa ET: Hepatic nuclear factor 3 and nuclear factor 1 regulate 5-aminolevulinate synthase gene expression and are involved in insulin repression. *J Biol Chem* 279:28082, 2004.
38. Scassa ME, Guberman AS, Varone CL, Canepa ET: Phosphatidylinositol 3-kinase and Ras/mitogen-activated protein kinase signaling pathways are required for the regulation of 5-aminolevulinate synthase gene expression by insulin. *Exp Cell Res* 271:201, 2001.
39. Phillips JD, Kushner JP: Fast track to the porphyrias. *Nat Med* 11:1049, 2005.
40. Anderson KE, Bloomer JR, Bonkovsky HL, et al: Recommendations for the diagnosis and treatment of the acute porphyrias. *Ann Intern Med* 142:439, 2005.
41. Sassa S: Heme stimulation of cellular growth and differentiation. *Semin Hematol* 25:312, 1988.
42. Dandekar T, Stripecke R, Gray NK, et al: Identification of a novel iron-responsive element in murine and human erythroid delta-aminolevulinic acid synthase mRNA. *EMBO J* 10:1903, 1991.
43. Fujita H, Yamamoto M, Yamagami T, et al: Erythroleukemia differentiation. Distinctive responses of the erythroid-specific and the nonspecific delta-aminolevulinate synthase mRNA. *J Biol Chem* 266:17494, 1991.
44. Furuyama K, Sassa S: Interaction between succinyl CoA synthetase and the heme-biosynthetic enzyme ALAS-E is disrupted in sideroblastic anemia. *J Clin Invest* 105:757, 2000.
45. Furuyama K, Fujita H, Nagai T, et al: Pyridoxine refractory X-linked sideroblastic anemia caused by a point mutation in the erythroid 5-aminolevulinate synthase gene. *Blood* 90:822, 1997.
46. Whatley SD, Ducamp S, Gouya L, et al: C-terminal deletions in the ALAS2 gene lead to gain of function and cause X-linked dominant protoporphyria without anemia or iron overload. *Am J Hum Genet* 83:408, 2008.
47. Sassa S: Delta-aminolevulinic acid dehydratase assay *Enzyme* 28:133, 1982.
48. Tsukamoto I, Yoshinaga T, Sano S: The role of zinc with special reference to the essential thiol groups in delta-aminolevulinic acid dehydratase of bovine liver. *Biochim Biophys Acta* 570:167, 1979.
49. Granick JL, Sassa S, Kappas A: Some biochemical and clinical aspects of lead intoxication. *Adv Clin Chem* 20:287, 1978.
50. Sassa S, Kappas A: Hereditary tyrosinemia and the heme biosynthetic pathway. Profound inhibition of delta-aminolevulinic acid dehydratase activity by succinylacetone. *J Clin Invest* 71:625, 1983.
51. Tschudy DP, Hess RA, Frykholm BC: Inhibition of delta-aminolevulinic acid dehydrase by 4,6-dioxoheptanoic acid. *J Biol Chem* 256:9915, 1981.
52. Lindblad B, Lindstedt S, Steen G: On the enzymic defects in hereditary tyrosinemia. *Proc Natl Acad Sci U S A* 74:4641, 1977.
53. Wetmur JG, Bishop DF, Ostasiewicz L, Desnick RJ: Molecular cloning of a cDNA for human delta-aminolevulinate dehydratase. *Gene* 43:123, 1986.
54. Bishop TR, Cohen PJ, Boyer SH, et al: Isolation of a rat liver delta-aminolevulinate dehydrase (ALAD) cDNA clone: Evidence for unequal ALAD gene dosage among inbred mouse strains. *Proc Natl Acad Sci U S A* 83:5568, 1986.
55. Wetmur JG, Bishop DF, Cantelmo C, Desnick RJ: Human delta-aminolevulinate dehydratase: Nucleotide sequence of a full-length cDNA clone. *Proc Natl Acad Sci U S A* 83:7703, 1986.
56. Potluri VR, Astrin KH, Wetmur JG, et al: Human delta-aminolevulinate dehydratase: Chromosomal localization to 9q34 by *in situ* hybridization. *Hum Genet* 76:236, 1987.
57. Erskine PT, Senior N, Awan S, et al: X-ray structure of 5-aminolaevulinate dehydratase, a hybrid aldolase. *Nat Struct Biol* 4:1025, 1997.
58. Bishop TR, Miller MW, Beall J, et al: Genetic regulation of delta-aminolevulinate dehydratase during erythropoiesis. *Nucleic Acids Res* 24:2511, 1996.
59. Wetmur JG, Kaya AH, Plewinska M, Desnick RJ: Molecular characterization of the human delta-aminolevulinate dehydratase 2 (ALAD2) allele: Implications for molecular screening of individuals for genetic susceptibility to lead poisoning. *Am J Hum Genet* 49:757, 1991.
60. Akagi R, Kato N, Inoue R, et al: δ-Aminolevulinate dehydratase (ALAD) porphyria: The first case in North America with two novel ALAD mutations. *Mol Genet Metab* 87:329, 2006.
61. Inoue R, Akagi R: Co-synthesis of human delta-aminolevulinate dehydratase (ALAD) mutants with the wild-type enzyme in cell-free system—Critical importance of conformation on enzyme activity. *J Clin Biochem Nutr* 43:143, 2008.
62. Jaffe EK, Stith L: ALAD porphyria is a conformational disease. *Am J Hum Genet* 80:329, 2007.
63. Battersby AR, Fookes CJ, Matcham GW, McDonald E: Biosynthesis of the pigments of life: Formation of the macrocycle. *Nature* 285:17, 1980.
64. Jordan PM: The biosynthesis of 5-aminolevulinic acid and its transformation into coproporphyrinogen in animals and bacteria, in *Biosynthesis of Heme and Chlorophylls,* edited by HA Dailey, p 55. McGraw-Hill, New York, 1990.
65. Awan SJ, Siligardi G, Shoolingin-Jordan PM, Warren MJ: Reconstitution of the holoenzyme form of Escherichia coli porphobilinogen deaminase from apoenzyme with porphobilinogen and preuroporphyrinogen: A study using circular dichroism spectroscopy. *Biochemistry (Mosc)* 36:9273, 1997.
66. Wang AL, Arredondo-Vega FX, Giampietro PF, et al: Regional gene assignment of human porphobilinogen deaminase and esterase A4 to chromosome 11q23 leads to 11qter. *Proc Natl Acad Sci U S A* 78:5734, 1981.
67. Chretien S, Dubart A, Beaupain D, et al: Alternative transcription and splicing of the human porphobilinogen deaminase gene result either in tissue-specific or in housekeeping expression. *Proc Natl Acad Sci U S A* 85:6, 1988.
68. Grandchamp B, Beaumont C, de Verneuil H, et al: Genetic expression of porphobilinogen deaminase and UROD during the erythroid differentiation of mouse erythroleukemic cells, in *Porphyrins and Porphyrias,* edited by Y Nordmann, p 35. John Libbey, London, 1986.
69. Grandchamp B, De Verneuil H, Beaumont C, et al: Tissue specific expression of porphobilinogen deaminase. Two isoenzymes from a single gene. *Eur J Biochem* 162:105, 1987.
70. Raich N, Romeo PH, Dubart A, et al: Molecular cloning and complete primary sequence of human erythrocyte porphobilinogen deaminase. *Nucleic Acids Res* 14:5955, 1986.
71. Mignotte V, Eleouet JF, Raich N, Romeo PH: *Cis-* and *trans-*acting elements involved in the regulation of the erythroid promoter of the human porphobilinogen deaminase gene. *Proc Natl Acad Sci U S A* 86:6548, 1989.
72. Grandchamp B, Picat C, De Rooij FWM, et al: Molecular analysis of acute intermittent porphyria in a Finnish family with normal erythrocyte porphobilinogen deaminase. *Eur J Clin Invest* 19:415, 1989.
73. Mathews MA, Schubert HL, Whitby FG, et al: Crystal structure of human uroporphyrinogen III synthase. *EMBO J* 20:5832, 2001.
74. Schubert HL, Phillips JD, Heroux A, Hill CP: Structure and mechanistic implications of a uroporphyrinogen III synthase-product complex. *Biochemistry (Mosc)* 47:8648, 2008.
75. Phillips JD, Bergonia HA, Reilly CA, et al: A porphomethene inhibitor of uroporphyrinogen decarboxylase causes porphyria cutanea tarda. *Proc Natl Acad Sci U S A* 104:5079, 2007.
76. Smith AG, Clothier B, Robinson S, et al: Interaction between iron metabolism and 2,3,7,8-tetrachlorodibenzo-p-dioxin in mice with variants of the Ahr gene: A hepatic oxidative mechanism. *Mol Pharmacol* 53:52, 1998.
77. Romana M, Dubart A, Beaupain D, et al: Structure of the gene for human uroporphyrinogen decarboxylase. *Nucleic Acids Res* 15:7343, 1987.
78. de Verneuil H, Grandchamp B, Foubert C, et al: Assignment of the gene for uroporphyrinogen decarboxylase to human chromosome 1 by somatic cell hybridization and specific enzyme immunoassay. *Hum Genet* 66:202, 1984.
79. Romeo PH, Raich N, Dubart A, et al: Molecular cloning and nucleotide sequence of a complete human uroporphyrinogen decarboxylase cDNA. *J Biol Chem* 261:9825, 1986.
80. Whitby FG, Phillips JD, Kushner JP, Hill CP: Crystal structure of human uroporphyrinogen decarboxylase. *EMBO J* 17:2463, 1998.
81. Phillips JD, Whitby FG, Kushner JP, Hill CP: Characterization and crystallization of human uroporphyrinogen decarboxylase. *Protein Sci* 6:1343, 1997.
82. Phillips JD, Whitby FG, Kushner JP, Hill CP: Structural basis for tetrapyrrole coordination by uroporphyrinogen decarboxylase. *EMBO J* 22:6225, 2003.
83. Cacheux V, Martasek P, Fougerousse F, et al: Localization of the human coproporphyrinogen oxidase gene to chromosome band 3q12. *Hum Genet* 94:557, 1994.
84. Kohno H, Furukawa T, Yoshinaga T, et al: Coproporphyrinogen oxidase. Purification, molecular cloning, and induction of mRNA during erythroid differentiation. *J Biol Chem* 268:21359, 1993.
85. Takahashi S, Furuyama K, Kobayashi A, et al: Cloning of a coproporphyrinogen oxidase promoter regulatory element binding protein. *Biochem Biophys Res Commun* 273:596, 2000.
86. Takahashi S, Taketani S, Akasaka JE, et al: Differential regulation of coproporphyrinogen oxidase gene between erythroid and nonerythroid cells *Blood* 92:3436, 1998.
87. Conder LH, Woodard SI, Dailey HA: Multiple mechanisms for the regulation of haem synthesis during erythroid cell differentiation. Possible role for coproporphyrinogen oxidase. *Biochem J* 275(Pt 2):321, 1991.
88. Taketani S, Yoshinaga T, Furukawa T, et al: Induction of terminal enzymes for heme biosynthesis during differentiation of mouse erythroleukemia cells. *Eur J Biochem* 230:760, 1995.
89. Lamoril J, Deybach JC, Puy H, et al: Three novel mutations in the coproporphyrinogen oxidase gene. *Hum Mutat* 9:78, 1997.
90. Nishimura K, Taketani S, Inokuchi H: Cloning of a human cDNA for protoporphyrinogen oxidase by complementation *in vivo* of a hemG mutant of *Escherichia coli. J Biol Chem* 270:8076, 1995.
91. Taketani S, Inazawa J, Abe T, et al: The human protoporphyrinogen oxidase gene (PPOX): Organization and location to chromosome 1. *Genomics* 29:698, 1995.
92. Koch M, Breithaupt C, Kiefersauer R, et al: Crystal structure of protoporphyrinogen IX oxidase: A key enzyme in haem and chlorophyll biosynthesis. *EMBO J* 23:1720, 2004.
93. Morgan RR, Errington R, Elder GH: Identification of sequences required for the import of human protoporphyrinogen oxidase to mitochondria. *Biochem J* 377:281, 2004.
94. von und zu Fraunberg M, Nyroen T, Kauppinen R: Mitochondrial targeting of normal and mutant protoporphyrinogen oxidase. *J Biol Chem* 278:13376, 2003.
95. de Vooght KM, van Wijk R, van Solinge WW: GATA-1 binding sites in exon 1 direct erythroid-specific transcription of PPOX. *Gene* 409:83, 2008.

96. Porra RJ, Jones OT: Studies on ferrochelatase. 1. Assay and properties of ferrochelatase from a pig-liver mitochondrial extract. *Biochem J* 87:181, 1963.
97. Taketani S, Inazawa J, Nakahashi Y, et al: Structure of the human ferrochelatase gene. Exon/intron gene organization and location of the gene to chromosome 18. *Eur J Biochem* 205:217, 1992.
98. Whitcombe DM, Carter NP, Albertson DG, et al: Assignment of the human ferrochelatase gene (FECH) and a locus for protoporphyria to chromosome 18q22. *Genomics* 11:1152, 1991.
99. Medlock A, Swartz L, Dailey TA, et al: Substrate interactions with human ferrochelatase. *Proc Natl Acad Sci U S A* 104:1789, 2007.
100. Medlock AE, Dailey TA, Ross TA, et al: A pi-helix switch selective for porphyrin deprotonation and product release in human ferrochelatase. *J Mol Biol* 373:1006, 2007.
101. Wada O, Sassa S, Takaku F, et al: Different responses of the hepatic and erythropoietic delta-aminolevulinic acid synthetase of mice. *Biochim Biophys Acta* 148:585, 1967.
102. Ross J, Sautner D: Induction of globin mRNA accumulation by hemin in cultured erythroleukemic cells *Cell* 8:513, 1976.
103. Sassa S, Nagai T: The role of heme in gene expression. *Int J Hematol* 63:167, 1996.
104. Sassa S, Akagi R, Nishitani C, et al: Late-onset porphyrias: What are they? *Cell Mol Biol (Noisy-le-grand)* 48:97, 2002.
105. Fritsch C, Bolsen K, Ruzicka T, Goerz G: Congenital erythropoietic porphyria. *J Am Acad Dermatol* 36:594, 1997.
106. Günther H: in *Handbuch der Krankheiten der Blutes und der Blutbildenden Organe,* edited by A Schittenhelm. Springer-Verlag, Berlin, volume 2, 1925.
107. Ged C, Moreau-Gaudry F, Richard E, et al: Congenital erythropoietic porphyria: Mutation update and correlations between genotype and phenotype. *Cell Mol Biol (Noisy-le-grand)* 55:53, 2009.
108. Phillips JD, Steensma DP, Pulsipher MA, et al: Congenital erythropoietic porphyria due to a mutation in GATA1: The first *trans*-acting mutation causative for a human porphyria. *Blood* 109:2618, 2007.
109. Desnick RJ, Glass IA, Xu W, et al: Molecular genetics of congenital erythropoietic porphyria. *Semin Liver Dis* 18:77, 1998.
110. Shady AA, Colby BR, Cunha LF, et al: Congenital erythropoietic porphyria: Identification and expression of eight novel mutations in the uroporphyrinogen III synthase gene. *Br J Haematol* 117:980, 2002.
111. Watson CJ, Perman V, Spurrell FA, et al: Some studies of the comparative biology of human and bovine porphyria erythropoietica. *Trans Assoc Am Physicians* 71:196, 1958.
112. Seip M, Thune PO, Eriksen L: Treatment of photosensitivity in congenital erythropoietic porphyria (CEP) with beta-carotene. *Acta Derm Venereol* 54:239, 1974.
113. Haining RG, Cowger ML, Labbe RF, Finch CA: Congenital erythropoietic porphyria. II. The effects of induced polycythemia. *Blood* 36:297, 1970.
114. Piomelli S, Poh-Fitzpatrick MB, Seaman C, et al: Complete suppression of the symptoms of congenital erythropoietic porphyria by long-term treatment with high-level transfusions. *N Engl J Med* 314:1029, 1986.
115. Guarini L, Piomelli S, Poh-Fitzpatrick MB: Hydroxyurea in congenital erythropoietic porphyria [letter]. *N Engl J Med* 330:1091, 1994.
116. Pimstone NR, Gandhi SN, Mukerji SK: Therapeutic efficacy of oral charcoal in congenital erythropoietic porphyria. *N Engl J Med* 316:390, 1987.
117. Hallai N, Anstey A, Mendelsohn S, et al: Pregnancy in a patient with congenital erythropoietic porphyria. *N Engl J Med* 357:622, 2007.
118. Dupuis-Girod S, Akkari V, Ged C, et al: Successful match-unrelated donor bone marrow transplantation for congenital erythropoietic porphyria (Günther disease). *Eur J Pediatr* 164:104, 2005.
119. Geronimi F, Richard E, Lamrissi-Garcia I, et al: Lentivirus-mediated gene transfer of uroporphyrinogen III synthase fully corrects the porphyric phenotype in human cells. *J Mol Med* 81:310, 2003.
120. Kauppinen R, Glass IA, Aizencang G, et al: Congenital erythropoietic porphyria: Prolonged high-level expression and correction of the heme biosynthetic defect by retroviral-mediated gene transfer into porphyric and erythroid cells. *Mol Genet Metab* 65:10, 1998.
121. Marko PB, Miljkovic J, Gorenjak M, et al: Erythropoietic protoporphyria patients in Slovenia. *Acta Dermatovenerol Alp Panonica Adriat* 16:99, 2007.
122. Parker M, Corrigall AV, Hift RJ, Meissner PN: Molecular characterization of erythropoietic protoporphyria in South Africa. *Br J Dermatol* 159:182, 2008.
123. Holme SA, Anstey AV, Finlay AY, et al: Erythropoietic protoporphyria in the UK: Clinical features and effect on quality of life. *Br J Dermatol* 155:574, 2006.
124. Nakahashi Y, Fujita H, Taketani S, et al: The molecular defect of ferrochelatase in a patient with erythropoietic protoporphyria. *Proc Natl Acad Sci U S A* 89:281, 1992.
125. Gouya L, Deybach JC, Lamoril J, et al: Modulation of the phenotype in dominant erythropoietic protoporphyria by a low expression of the normal ferrochelatase allele. *Am J Hum Genet* 58:292, 1996.
126. Gouya L, Puy H, Lamoril J, et al: Inheritance in erythropoietic protoporphyria: A common wild-type ferrochelatase allelic variant with low expression accounts for clinical manifestation *Blood* 93:2105, 1999.
127. Gouya L, Puy H, Robreau AM, et al: The penetrance of dominant erythropoietic protoporphyria is modulated by expression of wildtype FECH. *Nat Genet* 30:27, 2002.
128. Gouya L, Martin-Schmitt C, Robreau AM, et al: Contribution of a common single-nucleotide polymorphism to the genetic predisposition for erythropoietic protoporphyria. *Am J Hum Genet* 78:2, 2006.
129. Holme SA, Whatley SD, Roberts AG, et al: Seasonal palmar keratoderma in erythropoietic protoporphyria indicates autosomal recessive inheritance. *J Invest Dermatol* 129:599, 2009.
130. Aplin C, Whatley SD, Thompson P, et al: Late-onset erythropoietic porphyria caused by a chromosome 18q deletion in erythroid cells. *J Invest Dermatol* 117:1647, 2001.
131. Shirota T, Yamamoto H, Hayashi S, et al: Myelodysplastic syndrome terminating in erythropoietic protoporphyria after 15 years of aplastic anemia. *Int J Hematol* 72:44, 2000.
132. Goodwin RG, Kell WJ, Laidler P, et al: Photosensitivity and acute liver injury in myeloproliferative disorder secondary to late-onset protoporphyria caused by deletion of a ferrochelatase gene in hematopoietic cells. *Blood* 107:60, 2006.
133. Bottomley SS, Tanaka M, Everett MA: Diminished erythroid ferrochelatase activity in protoporphyria. *J Lab Clin Med* 86:126, 1975.
134. Clark KGA, Nicholson DC: Erythrocyte protoporphyrin and iron uptake in erythropoietic protoporphyria. *Clin Sci* 41:363, 1971.
135. Piomelli S, Lamola AA, Poh-Fitzpatrick MF, et al: Erythropoietic protoporphyria and lead intoxication: The molecular basis for difference in cutaneous photosensitivity. I. Different rates of disappearance of protoporphyrin from the erythrocytes, both *in vivo* and *in vitro*. *J Clin Invest* 56:1519, 1975.
136. Sandberg S, Brun A, Hovding G, et al: Effect of zinc on protoporphyrin induced photohaemolysis. *Scand J Clin Lab Invest* 40:185, 1980.
137. Spikes JD: Porphyrins and related compounds as photodynamic sensitizers. *Ann N Y Acad Sci* 244:496, 1975.
138. Goldstein BD, Harber LC: Erythropoietic protoporphyria: Lipid peroxidation and red cell membrane damage associated with photohemolysis. *J Clin Invest* 51:892, 1972.
139. Schothorst AA, van Steveninck J, Went LN, Suurmond D: Photodynamic damage of the erythrocyte membrane caused by protoporphyrin in protoporphyria and in normal red blood cells. *Clin Chim Acta* 39:161, 1972.
140. Lim HW, Poh-Fitzpatrick MB, Gigli I: Activation of the complement system in patients with porphyrias after irradiation *in vivo*. *J Clin Invest* 74:1961, 1984.
141. Ryan EA: Histochemistry of the skin in erythropoietic protoporphyria. *Br J Dermatol* 78:501, 1966.
142. Poh-Fitzpatrick MB: The erythropoietic porphyrias. *Dermatol Clin* 4:291, 1986.
143. Berenson MM, Kimura R, Samowitz W, Bjorkman D: Protoporphyrin overload in unrestrained rats: Biochemical and histopathologic characterization of a new model of protoporphyric hepatopathy. *Int J Exp Pathol* 73:665, 1992.
144. Bloomer JR: The liver in protoporphyria. *Hepatology* 8:402, 1988.
145. Bloomer JR, Enriquez R: Evidence that hepatic crystalline deposits in a patient with protoporphyria are composed of protoporphyrin. *Gastroenterology* 82:569, 1982.
146. Bloomer J, Wang Y, Singhal A, Risheg H: Molecular studies of liver disease in erythropoietic protoporphyria. *J Clin Gastroenterol* 39:S167, 2005.
147. Mathews-Roth MM: Systemic photoprotection. *Dermatol Clin* 4:335, 1986.
148. DeLeo VA, Poh-Fitzpatrick M, Mathews-Roth M, Harber LC: Erythropoietic protoporphyria. 10 years experience. *Am J Med* 60:8, 1976.
149. Suurmond D: Some aspects of erythropoietic protoporphyria in the Netherlands. *Dermatologica* 138:303, 1969.
150. Risheg H, Chen FP, Bloomer JR: Genotypic determinants of phenotype in North American patients with erythropoietic protoporphyria. *Mol Genet Metab* 80:196, 2003.
151. Turnbull A, Baker H, Vernon-Roberts B, Magnus IA: Iron metabolism in porphyria cutanea tarda and in erythropoietic protoporphyria. *Q J Med* 42:341, 1973.
152. Rademakers LHPM, Koningsberger JC, Sorber CWJ, et al: Accumulation of iron in erythroblasts of patients with erythropoietic protoporphyria. *Eur J Clin Invest* 23:130, 1993.
153. Delaby C, Lyoumi S, Ducamp S, et al: Excessive erythrocyte PPIX influences the hematologic status and iron metabolism in patients with dominant erythropoietic protoporphyria. *Cell Mol Biol (Noisy-le-grand)* 55:45, 2009.
154. Poh-Fitzpatrick MB: Human protoporphyria: Reduced cutaneous photosensitivity and lower erythrocyte porphyrin levels during pregnancy. *J Am Acad Dermatol* 36:40, 1997.
155. Rank JM, Carithers R, Bloomer J: Evidence for neurological dysfunction in end-stage protoporphyric liver disease. *Hepatology* 18:1404, 1993.
156. Doss MO, Frank M: Hepatobiliary implications and complications in protoporphyria, a 20-year study. *Clin Biochem* 22:223, 1989.
157. Singer JA, Plaut AG, Kaplan MM: Hepatic failure and death from erythropoietic protoporphyria. *Gastroenterology* 74:588, 1978.
158. Key NS, Rank JM, Freese D, et al: Hemolytic anemia in protoporphyria: Possible precipitating role of liver failure and photic stress. *Am J Hematol* 39:202, 1992.
159. Hastka J, Lasserre JJ, Schwarzbeck A, et al: Zinc protoporphyrin in anemia of chronic disorders. *Blood* 81:1200, 1993.
160. Anderson KE, Sassa S, Peterson CM, Kappas A: Increased erythrocyte uroporphyrinogen-I-synthetase, δ-aminolevulinic acid dehydratase and protoporphyrin in hemolytic anemias. *Am J Med* 63:359, 1977.
161. Poh-Fitzpatrick MB, DeLeo VA: Rates of plasma porphyrin disappearance in fluorescent vs. red incandescent light exposure. *J Invest Dermatol* 69:510, 1977.
162. Mathews-Roth MM, Pathak MA, Fitzpatrick TB, et al: Beta carotene therapy for erythropoietic protoporphyria and other photosensitivity diseases. *Arch Dermatol* 113:1229, 1977.
163. Minder EI, Schneider-Yin X, Steurer J, Bachmann LM: A systematic review of treatment options for dermal photosensitivity in erythropoietic protoporphyria. *Cell Mol Biol (Noisy-le-grand)* 55:84, 2009.

164. Mathews-Roth MM, Rosner B: Long-term treatment of erythropoietic protoporphyria with cysteine. *Photodermatol Photoimmunol Photomed* 18:307, 2002.
165. Warren LJ, George S: Erythropoietic protoporphyria treated with narrow-band (TL-01) UVB phototherapy. *Australas J Dermatol* 39:179, 1998.
166. Harms J, Lautenschlager S, Minder CE, Minder EI: An alpha-melanocyte-stimulating hormone analogue in erythropoietic protoporphyria. *N Engl J Med* 360:306, 2009.
167. Gordeuk VR, Brittenham GM, Hawkins CW, et al: Iron therapy for hepatic dysfunction in erythropoietic protoporphyria. *Ann Intern Med* 105:27, 1986.
168. Mercurio MG, Prince G, Weber FL, et al: Terminal hepatic failure in erythropoietic protoporphyria. *J Am Acad Dermatol* 29:829, 1993.
169. Bonkovsky HL, Schned AR: Fatal liver failure in protoporphyria: Synergism between ethanol excess and the genetic defect *Gastroenterology* 90:191, 1986.
170. Bloomer JR: Pathogenesis and therapy of liver disease in protoporphyria. *Yale J Biol Med* 52:39, 1979.
171. Kniffen JC: Protoporphyrin removal in intrahepatic porphyrastasis. *Gastroenterology* 58:1027, 1970.
172. Gross U, Frank M, Doss MO: Hepatic complications of erythropoietic protoporphyria. *Photodermatol Photoimmunol Photomed* 14:52, 1998.
173. Bechtel MA, Bertolone SJ, Hodge SJ: Transfusion therapy in a patient with erythropoietic protoporphyria. *Arch Dermatol* 117:99, 1981.
174. Van Wijk HJ, Van Hattum J, Delafaille HB, et al: Blood exchange and transfusion therapy for acute cholestasis in protoporphyria. *Dig Dis Sci* 33:1621, 1988.
175. McGuire BM, Bonkovsky HL, Carithers RL Jr, et al: Liver transplantation for erythropoietic protoporphyria liver disease. *Liver Transpl* 11:1590, 2005.
176. Todd DJ, Callender ME, Mayne EE, et al: Erythropoietic protoporphyria, transfusion therapy and liver disease. *Br J Dermatol* 127:534, 1992.
177. Nordmann Y: Erythropoietic protoporphyria and hepatic complications. *J Hepatol* 16:4, 1992.
178. Muley SA, Midani HA, Rank JM, et al: Neuropathy in erythropoietic protoporphyrias *Neurology* 51:262, 1998.
179. Poh-Fitzpatrick MB, Wang X, Anderson KE, et al: Erythropoietic protoporphyria: Altered phenotype after bone marrow transplantation for myelogenous leukemia in a patient heteroallelic for ferrochelatase gene mutations. *J Am Acad Dermatol* 46:861, 2002.
180. Fontanellas A, Mazurier F, Landry M, et al: Reversion of hepatobiliary alterations by bone marrow transplantation in a murine model of erythropoietic protoporphyria. *Hepatology* 32:73, 2000.
181. Rand EB, Bunin N, Cochran W, et al: Sequential liver and bone marrow transplantation for treatment of erythropoietic protoporphyria. *Pediatrics* 118:e1896, 2006.
182. Pawliuk R, Tighe R, Wise RJ, et al: Prevention of murine erythropoietic protoporphyria-associated skin photosensitivity and liver disease by dermal and hepatic ferrochelatase. *J Invest Dermatol* 124:256, 2005.
183. Richard E, Robert E, Cario-Andre M, et al: Hematopoietic stem cell gene therapy of murine protoporphyria by methylguanine-DNA-methyltransferase-mediated in vivo drug selection. *Gene Ther* 11:1638, 2004.
184. Sassa S: ALAD porphyria. *Semin Liver Dis* 18:95, 1998.
185. Plewinska M, Thunell S, Holmberg L, et al: Delta-Aminolevulinate dehydratase deficient porphyria: Identification of the molecular lesions in a severely affected homozygote. *Am J Hum Genet* 49:167, 1991.
186. Hassoun A, Verstraeten L, Mercelis R, Martin JJ: Biochemical diagnosis of an hereditary aminolaevulinate dehydratase deficiency in a 63-year-old man. *J Clin Chem Clin Biochem* 27:781, 1989.
187. Akagi R, Nishitani C, Harigae H, et al: Molecular analysis of delta-aminolevulinate dehydratase deficiency in a patient with an unusual late-onset porphyria. *Blood* 96:3618, 2000.
188. Akagi R, Yasui Y, Harper P, Sassa S: A novel mutation of delta-aminolaevulinate dehydratase in a healthy child with 12% erythrocyte enzyme activity. *Br J Haematol* 106:931, 1999.
189. Akagi R, Inoue R, Muranaka S, et al: Dual gene defects involving δ-aminolaevulinate dehydratase and coproporphyrinogen oxidase in a porphyria patient. *Br J Haematol* 132:237, 2006.
190. Thunell S, Henrichson A, Floderus Y, et al: Liver transplantation in a boy with acute porphyria due to aminolaevulinate dehydratase deficiency. *Eur J Clin Chem Clin Biochem* 30:599, 1992.
191. Shimizu Y, Ida S, Naruto H, Urata G: Excretion of porphyrins in urine and bile after the administration of delta-aminolevulinic acid. *J Lab Clin Med* 92:795, 1978.
192. Doss M, von Tiepermann R, Schneider J, Schmid H: New type of hepatic porphyria with porphobilinogen synthase defect and intermittent acute clinical manifestation. *Klin Wochenschr* 57:1123, 1979.
193. Gross U, Sassa S, Jacob K, et al: 5-Aminolevulinic acid dehydratase deficiency porphyria: A twenty-year clinical and biochemical follow-up. *Clin Chem* 44:1892, 1998.
194. Doss MO, Stauch T, Gross U, et al: The third case of Doss porphyria (delta-aminolevulinic acid dehydratase deficiency) in Germany. *J Inherit Metab Dis* 27:529, 2004.
195. Thunell S, Holmberg L, Lundgren J: Aminolaevulinate dehydratase porphyria in infancy. A clinical and biochemical study. *J Clin Chem Clin Biochem* 25:5, 1987.
196. Mercelis R, Hassoun A, Verstraeten L, et al: Porphyric neuropathy and hereditary δ-aminolevulinic acid dehydratase deficiency in an adult. *J Neurol Sci* 95:39, 1990.
197. Fujita H, Sato K, Sano S: Increase in the amount of erythrocyte delta-aminolevulinic acid dehydratase in workers with moderate lead exposure. *Int Arch Occup Environ Health* 50:287, 1982.
198. Sassa S, Fujita H, Kappas A: Succinylacetone and delta-aminolevulinic acid dehydratase in hereditary tyrosinemia: Immunochemical study of the enzyme *Pediatrics* 86:84, 1990.
199. Goldberg A, Moore MR, McColl KEL, Brodie MJ: Porphyrin metabolism and the porphyrias, in *Oxford Textbook of Medicine,* edited by DA Ledingham, DA Warrell, DJ Wetherall, p 9136. Oxford University Press, Oxford, 1987.
200. Mustajoki P, Koskelo P: Hereditary hepatic porphyrias in Finland. *Acta Med Scand* 200:171, 1976.
201. Kauppinen R, von und zu Fraunberg M: Molecular and biochemical studies of acute intermittent porphyria in 196 patients and their families. *Clin Chem* 48:1891, 2002.
202. Grandchamp B: Acute intermittent porphyria. *Semin Liver Dis* 18:17, 1998.
203. Wetterberg L: *A Neuropsychiatric and Genetical Investigation of Acute Intermittent Porphyria*. Scandinavian University Books, Stockholm, 1967.
204. Mustajoki P, Kauppinen R, Lannfelt L, et al: Frequency of low erythrocyte porphobilinogen deaminase activity in Finland. *J Intern Med* 231:389, 1992.
205. Nordmann Y, Puy H, Da Silva V, et al: Acute intermittent porphyria: Prevalence of mutations in the porphobilinogen deaminase gene in blood donors in France. *J Intern Med* 242:213, 1997.
206. Grandchamp B, Picat C, de Rooij F, et al: A point mutation G→A in exon 12 of the porphobilinogen deaminase gene results in exon skipping and is responsible for acute intermittent porphyria. *Nucleic Acids Res* 17:6637, 1989.
207. Desnick RJ, Ostasiewicz LT, Tishler PA, Mustajoki P: Acute intermittent porphyria: Characterization of a novel mutation in the structural gene for porphobilinogen deaminase. Demonstration of noncatalytic enzyme intermediates stabilized by bound substrate. *J Clin Invest* 76:865, 1985.
208. Wilson JH, De Rooy FW, Te Velde K: Acute intermittent porphyria in The Netherlands. Heterogeneity of the enzyme porphobilinogen deaminase. *Neth J Med* 29:393, 1986.
209. Anderson KE, Freddara U, Kappas A: Induction of hepatic cytochrome P-450 by natural steroids: Relationships to the induction of δ-aminolevulinate synthase and porphyrin accumulation in the avian embryo. *Arch Biochem Biophys* 217:597, 1982.
210. Kauppinen R: Prognosis of acute porphyrias and molecular genetics of acute intermittent porphyria in Finland [thesis]. University of Helsinki, Helsinki, Finland, 1992.
211. Sze G: Cortical brain lesions in acute intermittent porphyria. *Ann Intern Med* 125:422, 1996.
212. Lithner F: Could attacks of abdominal pain in cases of acute intermittent porphyria be due to intestinal angina? *J Intern Med* 247:407, 2000.
213. Anderson KE, Drummond GS, Freddara U, et al: Porphyrogenic effects and induction of heme oxygenase in vivo by δ-aminolevulinic acid. *Biochim Biophys Acta* 676:289, 1981.
214. Brennan MJW, Cantrill RC: δ-Aminolaevulinic acid is a potent agonist for GABA autoreceptors *Nature* 280:514, 1979.
215. Müller WE, Snyder SH: δ-Aminolevulinic acid: Influences on synaptic GABA receptor binding may explain CNS symptoms of porphyria. *Ann Neurol* 2:340, 1977.
216. Mustajoki P, Timonen K, Gorchein A, et al: Sustained high plasma 5-aminolaevulinic acid concentration in a volunteer: No porphyric symptoms. *Eur J Clin Invest* 22:407, 1992.
217. Lindberg RL, Porcher C, Grandchamp B, et al: Porphobilinogen deaminase deficiency in mice causes a neuropathy resembling that of human hepatic porphyria. *Nat Genet* 12:195, 1996.
218. Meyer UA, Schuurmans MM, Lindberg RLP: Acute porphyrias: Pathogenesis of neurological manifestations. *Semin Liver Dis* 18:43, 1998.
219. Jover R, Hoffmann F, Scheffler-Koch V, Lindberg RL: Limited heme synthesis in porphobilinogen deaminase-deficient mice impairs transcriptional activation of specific cytochrome P450 genes by phenobarbital. *Eur J Biochem* 267:7128, 2000.
220. Lindberg RL, Martini R, Baumgartner M, et al: Motor neuropathy in porphobilinogen deaminase-deficient mice imitates the peripheral neuropathy of human acute porphyria. *J Clin Invest* 103:1127, 1999.
221. Soonawalla ZF, Orug T, Badminton MN, et al: Liver transplantation as a cure for acute intermittent porphyria. *Lancet* 363:705, 2004.
222. Louis CA, Sinclair JF, Wood SG, et al: Synergistic induction of cytochrome-P450 by ethanol and isopentanol in cultures of chick embryo and rat hepatocytes. *Toxicol Appl Pharmacol* 118:169, 1993.
223. Thunell S, Floderus Y, Henrichson A, et al: Alcoholic beverages in acute porphyria. *J Stud Alcohol* 53:272, 1992.
224. Lip GYH, McColl KEL, Goldberg A, Moore MR: Smoking and recurrent attacks of acute intermittent porphyria. *BMJ* 302:507, 1991.
225. Andersson C, Bylesjo I, Lithner F: Effects of diabetes mellitus on patients with acute intermittent porphyria. *J Intern Med* 245:193, 1999.
226. Milo R, Neuman M, Klein C, Caspi E, Arlazoroff A: Acute intermittent porphyria in pregnancy. *Obstet Gynecol* 73:450, 1989.
227. Shenhav S, Gemer O, Sassoon E, Segal S: Acute intermittent porphyria precipitated by hyperemesis and metoclopramide treatment in pregnancy. *Acta Obstet Gynecol Scand* 76:484, 1997.
228. Welland FH, Hellman ES, Gaddis EM, et al: Factors affecting the excretion of porphyrin precursors by patients with acute intermittent porphyria. I. The effect of diet. *Metabolism* 13:232, 1964.
229. Thaler MM, Dawber NH: Stimulation of bilirubin formation in liver of newborn rats by fasting and glucagon. *Gastroenterology* 72:312, 1977.
230. Beukeveld GJJ, Wolthers BG, Nordmann Y, et al: A retrospective study of a patient with homozygous form of acute intermittent porphyria. *J Inherit Metab Dis* 13:673, 1990.

231. Picat C, Delfau MH, De Rooij FWM, et al: Identification of the mutations in the parents of a patient with a putative compound heterozygosity for acute intermittent porphyria. *J Inherit Metab Dis* 13:684, 1990.
232. Solis C, Martinez-Bermejo A, Naidich TP, et al: Acute intermittent porphyria: Studies of the severe homozygous dominant disease provides insights into the neurologic attacks in acute porphyrias. *Arch Neurol* 61:1764, 2004.
233. Stein JA, Tschudy DP: Acute intermittent porphyria. A clinical and biochemical study of 46 patients. *Medicine (Baltimore)* 49:1, 1970.
234. Waldenstrom J: The porphyrias as inborn errors of metabolism. *Am J Med* 22:758, 1957.
235. Barohn RJ, Sanchez JE, Anderson KE: Acute peripheral neuropathy due to hereditary coproporphyria. *Muscle Nerve* 17:793, 1994.
236. Greenspan GH, Block AJ: Respiratory insufficiency associated with acute intermittent porphyria. *South Med J* 74:954, 1981.
237. Ridley A: Porphyric neuropathy, in *Peripheral Neuropathy*, edited by PJ Dyck, PK Thomas, EH Lambert, R Bunge, p 1704. WB Saunders, Philadelphia, 1984.
238. Stein JA, Curl FD, Valsamis M, Tschudy DP: Abnormal iron and water metabolism in acute intermittent porphyria with new morphologic findings. *Am J Med* 53:784, 1972.
239. Goldberg A: Acute intermittent porphyria. A study of 50 cases. *Q J Med* 28:183, 1959.
240. Bloomer JR, Berk PD, Bonkowsky HL, et al: Blood volume and bilirubin production in acute intermittent porphyria. *N Engl J Med* 284:17, 1971.
241. Eales L, Dowdle EB, Sweeney GD: The electrolyte disorder of the acute porphyric attack and the possible role of delta-aminolaevulic acid [special issue]. *S Afr J Lab Clin Med* 17:89, 1971.
242. Tschudy DP, Lamon JM: Porphyrin metabolism and the porphyrias, in *Duncan's Diseases of Metabolism*, 8th ed, edited by PK Bondy, LE Rosenberg, p 939. WB Saunders, Philadelphia, 1980.
243. Tschudy DP, Valsamis M, Magnussen CR: Acute intermittent porphyria: Clinical and selected research aspects. *Ann Intern Med* 83:851, 1975.
244. Andersson C, Wikberg A, Stegmayr B, Lithner F: Renal symptomatology in patients with acute intermittent porphyria. A population-based study. *J Intern Med* 248:319, 2000.
245. Church SE, McColl KE, Moore MR, Youngs GR: Hypertension and renal impairment as complications of acute porphyria. *Nephrol Dial Transplant* 7:986, 1992.
246. Barone GW, Gurley BJ, Anderson KE, et al: The tolerability of newer immunosuppressive medications in a patient with acute intermittent porphyria. *J Clin Pharmacol* 41:113, 2001.
247. Nunez DJ, Williams PF, Herrick AL, et al: Renal transplantation for chronic renal failure in acute porphyria. *Nephrol Dial Transplant* 2:271, 1987.
248. Ostrowski J, Kostrzewska E, Michalak T, et al: Abnormalities in liver function and morphology and impaired aminopyrine metabolism in hereditary hepatic porphyrias. *Gastroenterology* 85:1131, 1983.
249. Andant C, Puy H, Bogard C, et al: Hepatocellular carcinoma in patients with acute hepatic porphyria: Frequency of occurrence and related factors. *J Hepatol* 32:933, 2000.
250. Andant C, Puy H, Faivre J, Deybach JC: Acute hepatic porphyrias and primary liver cancer [letter]. *N Engl J Med* 338:1853, 1998.
251. Andersson C, Bjersing L, Lithner F: The epidemiology of hepatocellular carcinoma in patients with acute intermittent porphyria. *J Intern Med* 240:195, 1996.
252. Bengtsson NO, Hardell L: Porphyrias, porphyrins and hepatocellular cancer. *Br J Cancer* 54:115, 1986.
253. Gubler JG, Bargetzi MJ, Meyer UA: Primary liver carcinoma in two sisters with acute intermittent porphyria. *Am J Med* 89:540, 1990.
254. Hardell L, Bengtsson NO, Jonsson U, et al: Aetiological aspects on primary liver cancer with special regard to alcohol, organic solvents and acute intermittent porphyria—An epidemiological investigation. *Br J Cancer* 50:389, 1984.
255. Kauppinen R, Mustajoki P: Acute hepatic porphyria and hepatocellular carcinoma. *Br J Cancer* 57:117, 1987.
256. Linet MS, Gridley G, Nyren O, et al: Primary liver cancer, other malignancies, and mortality risks following porphyria: A cohort study in Denmark and Sweden. *Am J Epidemiol* 149:1010, 1999.
257. Lithner F, Wetterberg L: Hepatocellular carcinoma in patients with acute intermittent porphyria. *Acta Med Scand* 215:271, 1984.
258. Hollander CS, Scott RL, Tschudy DP, et al: Increased protein bound iodine and thyroxine binding globulin in acute intermittent porphyria. *N Engl J Med* 277:995, 1967.
259. Mustajoki P, Nikkila EA: Serum lipoproteins in asymptomatic acute porphyria: No evidence for hyperbetalipoproteinemia. *Metabolism* 33:266, 1984.
260. Deacon AC, Peters TJ: Identification of acute porphyria: Evaluation of a commercial screening test for urinary porphobilinogen. *Ann Clin Biochem* 35:726, 1998.
261. Minder EI: Coproporphyrin isomers in acute-intermittent porphyria. *Scand J Clin Lab Invest* 53:87, 1993.
262. Blum M, Koehl C, Abecassis J: Variations in erythrocyte uroporphyrinogen I synthetase activity in nonporphyrias. *Clin Chim Acta* 87:119, 1978.
263. Kostrzewska E, Gregor A: Increased activity of porphobilinogen deaminase in erythrocytes during attacks of acute intermittent porphyria. *Ann Clin Res* 18:195, 1986.
264. Bonkowsky HL, Tschudy DP: Hazard of propranolol in treatment of acute porphyria [letter]. *Br Med J* 4:47, 1974.
265. Bonkowsky HL, Sinclair PR, Emery S, Sinclair JF: Seizure management in acute hepatic porphyria: Risks of valproate and clonazepam. *Neurology* 30:588, 1980.
266. Larson AW, Wasserstrom WR, Felsher BF, Shih JC: Posttraumatic epilepsy and acute intermittent porphyria: Effects of phenytoin, carbamazepine, and clonazepam. *Neurology* 28:824, 1978.
267. Harper P, Wahlin S: Treatment options in acute porphyria, porphyria cutanea tarda, and erythropoietic protoporphyria. *Curr Treat Options Gastroenterol* 10:444, 2007.
268. Mustajoki P, Nordmann Y: Early administration of heme arginate for acute porphyric attacks. *Arch Intern Med* 153:2004, 1993.
269. Tenhunen R, Mustajoki P: Acute porphyria: Treatment with heme. *Semin Liver Dis* 18:53, 1998.
270. Green D, Reynolds N, Klein J, et al: The inactivation of hemostatic factors by hematin. *J Lab Clin Med* 102:361, 1983.
271. Jones RL: Hematin-derived anticoagulant. Generation *in vitro* and *in vivo*. *J Exp Med* 163:724, 1986.
272. Bonkovsky HL, Healey JF, Lourie AN, Gerron GG: Intravenous heme-albumin in acute intermittent porphyria: Evidence for repletion of hepatic hemoproteins and regulatory heme pools. *Am J Gastroenterol* 86:1050, 1991.
273. Anderson KE, Bonkovsky HL, Bloomer JR, Shedlofsky SI: Reconstitution of hematin for intravenous infusion. *Ann Intern Med* 144:537, 2006.
274. Daimon M, Susa S, Igarashi M, et al: Administration of heme arginate, but not hematin, caused anaphylactic shock. *Am J Med* 110:240, 2001.
275. Khanderia U: Circulatory collapse associated with hemin therapy for acute intermittent porphyria. *Clin Pharm* 5:690, 1986.
276. Jeelani Dhar G, Bossenmaier I, Cardinal R, et al: Transitory renal failure following rapid administration of a relatively large amount of hematin in a patient with acute intermittent porphyria in clinical remission. *Acta Med Scand* 203:437, 1978.
277. Herrick AL, McColl KEL, Moore MR, et al: Controlled trial of haem arginate in acute hepatic porphyria. *Lancet* 1:1295, 1989.
278. Cherem JH, Malagon J, Nellen H: Cimetidine and acute intermittent porphyria. *Ann Intern Med* 143:694, 2005.
279. Horie Y, Tanaka K, Okano J, et al: Cimetidine in the treatment of porphyria cutanea tarda. *Intern Med* 35:717, 1996.
280. Marcus DL, Nadel H, Lew G, Freedman ML: Cimetidine suppresses chemically induced experimental hepatic porphyria. *Am J Med Sci* 300:214, 1990.
281. Anderson KE, Spitz IM, Bardin CW, Kappas A: A GnRH analogue prevents cyclical attacks of porphyria. *Arch Intern Med* 150:1469, 1990.
282. De Block CE, Leeuw IH, Gaal LF: Premenstrual attacks of acute intermittent porphyria: Hormonal and metabolic aspects—A case report. *Eur J Endocrinol* 141:50, 1999.
283. Yamamori I, Asai M, Tanaka F, et al: Prevention of premenstrual exacerbation of hereditary coproporphyria by gonadotropin-releasing hormone analogue. *Intern Med* 38:365, 1999.
284. Anderson KE, Egger NG, Goeger DE: Heme arginate for prevention of acute porphyric attacks [abstract]. *Acta Haematol* 98(Suppl 1):120, 1997.
285. With TK: Hereditary coproporphyria and variegate porphyria in Denmark. *Dan Med Bull* 30:106, 1983.
286. Mustajoki P: Variegate porphyria. Twelve years' experience in Finland. *Q J Med* 49:191, 1980.
287. Eales L, Day RS, Blekkenhorst GH: The clinical and biochemical features of variegate porphyria: An analysis of 300 cases studied at Groote Schuur Hospital, Cape Town. *Int J Biochem* 12:837, 1980.
288. Grandchamp B, Phung N, Nordmann Y: Homozygous case of hereditary coproporphyria. *Lancet* 2:1348, 1977.
289. To-Figueras J, Badenas C, Enriquez MT, et al: Biochemical and genetic characterization of four cases of hereditary coproporphyria in Spain. *Mol Genet Metab* 85:160, 2005.
290. Nordmann Y, Grandchamp B, De Verneuil H, et al: Harderoporphyria: A variant hereditary coproporphyria. *J Clin Invest* 72:1139, 1983.
291. Blake D, McManus J, Cronin V, Ratnaike S: Fecal coproporphyrin isomers in hereditary coproporphyria. *Clin Chem* 38:96, 1992.
292. Longas MO, Poh-Fitzpatrick MB: A tightly bound protein-porphyrin complex isolated from the plasma of a patient with variegate porphyria. *Clin Chim Acta* 118:219, 1982.
293. Hift RJ, Davidson BP, van der Hooft C, et al: Plasma fluorescence scanning and fecal porphyrin analysis for the diagnosis of variegate porphyria: Precise determination of sensitivity and specificity with detection of protoporphyrinogen oxidase mutations as a reference standard. *Clin Chem* 50:915, 2004.
294. Lamoril J, Puy H, Gouya L, et al: Neonatal hemolytic anemia due to inherited harderoporphyria: Clinical characteristics and molecular basis *Blood* 91:1453, 1998.
295. Tio TH, Leijnse B, Jarrett A, Rimington C: Acquired porphyria from a liver tumor. *Clin Sci Mol Med* 16:517, 1959.
296. Elder GH, Urquhart AJ, de Salamanca RE, et al: Immunoreactive uroporphyrinogen decarboxylase in the liver in porphyria cutanea tarda. *Lancet* 2:229, 1985.
297. Moran MJ, Fontanellas A, Brudieux E, et al: Hepatic uroporphyrinogen decarboxylase activity in porphyria cutanea tarda patients: The influence of virus C infection. *Hepatology* 27:584, 1998.
298. Phillips JD, Jackson LK, Bunting M, et al: A mouse model of familial porphyria cutanea tarda. *Proc Natl Acad Sci U S A* 98:259, 2001.
299. Elder GH, Lee GB, Tovey JA: Decreased activity of hepatic uroporphyrinogen decarboxylase in sporadic porphyria cutanea tarda. *N Engl J Med* 299:274, 1978.
300. Gorman N, Zaharia A, Trask HS, et al: Effect of iron and ascorbate on uroporphyria in ascorbate-requiring mice as a model for porphyria cutanea tarda. *Hepatology* 45:187, 2007.
301. Percy VA, Naidoo D, Joubert SM, Pegoraro RJ: Ascorbate status of patients with porphyria cutanea tarda symptomatica and its effect on porphyrin metabolism. *S Afr J Med Sci* 40:185, 1975.

302. Sinclair PR, Gorman G, Shedlofsky SI, et al: Ascorbic acid deficiency in porphyria cutanea tarda. *J Lab Clin Med* 130:197, 1997.
303. Rocchi E, Casalgrandi G, Masini A, et al: Circulating pro- and antioxidant factors in iron and porphyrin metabolism disorders. *Ital J Gastroenterol Hepatol* 31:861, 1999.
304. Sinclair PR, Gorman N, Walton HS, et al: CYP1A2 is essential in murine uroporphyria caused by hexachlorobenzene and iron. *Toxicol Appl Pharmacol* 162:60, 2000.
305. Smith AG, Clothier B, Carthew P, et al: Protection of the Cyp1A2(−/−) null mouse against uroporphyria and hepatic injury following exposure to 2,3,7,8-tetrachlorodibenzo-*p*-dioxin. *Toxicol Appl Pharmacol* 173:89, 2001.
306. Elder GH: Porphyria cutanea tarda and related disorders, in *Porphyrin Handbook, Part II,* edited by KM Kadish, K Smith, R Guilard, p 67. Academic Press, San Diego, 2003.
307. Phillips JD, Parker TL, Schubert HL, et al: Functional consequences of naturally occurring mutations in human uroporphyrinogen decarboxylase. *Blood* 98:3179, 2001.
308. Cassiman D, Vannoote J, Roelandts R, et al: Porphyria cutanea tarda and liver disease. A retrospective analysis of 17 cases from a single centre and review of the literature. *Acta Gastroenterol Belg* 71:237, 2008.
309. Gisbert JP, Garcia-Buey L, Alonso A, et al: Hepatocellular carcinoma risk in patients with porphyria cutanea tarda. *Eur J Gastroenterol Hepatol* 16:689, 2004.
310. Rossmann-Ringdahl I, Olsson R: Porphyria cutanea tarda in a Swedish population: Risk factors and complications. *Acta Derm Venereol* 85:337, 2005.
311. Dabski C, Beutner EH: Studies of laminin and type IV collagen in blisters of porphyria cutanea tarda and drug-induced pseudoporphyria. *J Am Acad Dermatol* 25:28, 1991.
312. Pigatto PD, Polenghi MM, Altomare GF, et al: Complement cleavage products in the phototoxic reaction of porphyria cutanea tarda. *Br J Dermatol* 114:567, 1986.
313. Egger NG, Goeger DE, Payne DA, et al: Porphyria cutanea tarda: Multiplicity of risk factors including HFE mutations, hepatitis C, and inherited uroporphyrinogen decarboxylase deficiency. *Dig Dis Sci* 47:419, 2002.
314. Blekkenhorst GH, Eales L, Pimstone NR: Activation of uroporphyrinogen decarboxylase by ferrous iron in porphyria cutanea tarda. *S Afr Med J* 56:918, 1979.
315. Bulaj ZJ, Franklin MR, Phillips JD, et al: Transdermal estrogen replacement therapy in postmenopausal women previously treated for porphyria cutanea tarda. *J Lab Clin Med* 136:482, 2000.
316. Christiansen L, Bygum A, Jensen A, et al: Association between CYP1A2 polymorphism and susceptibility to porphyria cutanea tarda. *Hum Genet* 107:612, 2000.
317. Grossman ME, Bickers DR, Poh-Fitzpatrick MB, et al: Porphyria cutanea tarda. Clinical features and laboratory findings in 40 patients. *Am J Med* 67:277, 1979.
318. Sixel-Dietrich F, Doss M: Hereditary uroporphyrinogen-decarboxylase deficiency predisposing porphyria cutanea tarda (chronic hepatic porphyria) in females after oral contraceptive medication. *Arch Dermatol Res* 278:13, 1985.
319. Legault N, Sabik H, Cooper SF, Charbonneau M: Effect of estradiol on the induction of porphyria by hexachlorobenzene in the rat. *Biochem Pharmacol* 54:19, 1997.
320. Liehr JG: Vitamin C reduces the incidence and severity of renal tumors induced by estradiol or diethylstilbestrol. *Am J Clin Nutr* 54:S1256, 1991.
321. Fujita N, Sugimoto R, Motonishi S, et al: Patients with chronic hepatitis C achieving a sustained virological response to peginterferon and ribavirin therapy recover from impaired hepcidin secretion. *J Hepatol* 49:702, 2008.
322. Nishina S, Hino K, Korenaga M, et al: Hepatitis C virus-induced reactive oxygen species raise hepatic iron level in mice by reducing hepcidin transcription. *Gastroenterology* 134:226, 2008.
323. Wissel PS, Sordillo P, Anderson KE, et al: Porphyria cutanea tarda associated with the acquired immune deficiency syndrome. *Am J Hematol* 25:107, 1987.
324. Roberts AG, Whatley SD, Nicklin S, et al: The frequency of hemochromatosis-associated alleles is increased in British patients with sporadic porphyria cutanea tarda. *Hepatology* 25:159, 1997.
325. Dereure O, Aguilar-Martinez P, Bessis D, et al: HFE mutations and transferrin receptor polymorphism analysis in porphyria cutanea tarda: A prospective study of 36 cases from southern France. *Br J Dermatol* 144:533, 2001.
326. Ajioka RS, Phillips JD, Weiss RB, et al: Down-regulation of hepcidin in porphyria cutanea tarda. *Blood* 112:4723, 2008.
327. Calvert GM, Sweeney MH, Fingerhut MA, et al: Evaluation of porphyria cutanea tarda in U.S. workers exposed to 2,3,7,8-tetrachlorodibenzo-p-dioxin. *Am J Ind Med* 25:559, 1994.
328. Smith A: Porphyria caused by chlorinated AH receptor ligands and associated mechanisms of liver injury and cancer, in *Porphyrin Handbook, Part II,* edited by KM Kadish, K Smith, R Guilard, p 169. Academic Press, San Diego, 2003.
329. Brady JJ, Jackson HA, Roberts AG, et al: Co-inheritance of mutations in the uroporphyrinogen decarboxylase and hemochromatosis genes accelerates the onset of porphyria cutanea tarda. *J Invest Dermatol* 115:868, 2000.
330. Barzilay D, Orion E, Brenner S: Porphyria cutanea tarda triggered by a combination of three predisposing factors. *Dermatology* 203:195, 2001.
331. Au WY, Tam SC, Ho KM, et al: Hypertrichosis due to porphyria cutanea tarda associated with blastic transformation of myelofibrosis. *Br J Dermatol* 141:932, 1999.
332. Lee SC, Yun SJ, Lee JB, et al: A case of porphyria cutanea tarda in association with idiopathic myelofibrosis and CREST syndrome. *Br J Dermatol* 144:182, 2001.
333. Anderson KE, Goeger DE, Carson RW, et al: Erythropoietin for the treatment of porphyria cutanea tarda in a patient on long-term hemodialysis. *N Engl J Med* 322:315, 1990.
334. Armstrong DK, Sharpe PC, Chambers CR, et al: Hepatoerythropoietic porphyria: A missense mutation in the UROD gene is associated with mild disease and an unusual porphyrin excretion pattern. *Br J Dermatol* 151:920, 2004.
335. Elder GH: The metabolism of porphyrins of the isocoproporphyrin series. *Enzyme* 17:61, 1974.
336. Poh-Fitzpatrick MB, Lamola AA: Direct spectrophotometry of diluted erythrocytes and plasma: A rapid diagnostic method in primary and secondary porphyrinemias. *J Lab Clin Med* 87:362, 1976.
337. Poh-Fitzpatrick MB, Sosin AE, Bemis J: Porphyrin levels in plasma and erythrocytes of chronic hemodialysis patients. *J Am Acad Dermatol* 7:100, 1982.
338. Topi GC, Amantea A, Griso D: Recovery from porphyria cutanea tarda with no specific therapy other than avoidance of hepatic toxins. *Br J Dermatol* 3:75, 1984.
339. Ippen H: Treatment of porphyria cutanea tarda by phlebotomy. *Semin Hematol* 14:253, 1977.
340. Rocchi E, Cassanelli M, Ventura E: High weekly intravenous doses of desferrioxamine in porphyria cutanea tarda. *Br J Dermatol* 117:393, 1987.
341. Ratnaike S, Blake D, Campbell D, et al: Plasma ferritin levels as a guide to the treatment of porphyria cutanea tarda by venesection. *Australas J Dermatol* 29:3, 1988.
342. Rocchi E, Gibertini P, Cassanelli M, et al: Serum ferritin in the assessment of liver iron overload and iron removal therapy in porphyria cutanea tarda. *J Lab Clin Med* 107:36, 1986.
343. Ashton RE, Hawk JLM, Magnus IA: Low-dose oral chloroquine in the treatment of porphyria cutanea tarda. *Br J Dermatol* 3:609, 1984.
344. Bruce AJ, Ahmed I: Childhood-onset porphyria cutanea tarda: Successful therapy with low-dose hydroxychloroquine (Plaquenil). *J Am Acad Dermatol* 38:810, 1998.
345. Freesemann A, Frank M, Sieg I, Doss MO: Treatment of porphyria cutanea tarda by the effect of chloroquine on the liver. *Skin Pharmacol* 8:156, 1995.
346. Kordac V, Semradova M: Treatment of porphyria cutanea tarda with chloroquine. *Br J Dermatol* 90:95, 1974.
347. Taljaard JJF, Shanley BC, Stewart-Wynne EG, et al: Studies on low dose chloroquine therapy and the action of chloroquine in symptomatic porphyria. *Br J Dermatol* 87:261, 1972.
348. Timonen K, Niemi KM, Mustajoki P: Skin morphology in porphyria cutanea tarda does not improve despite clinical remission. *Clin Exp Dermatol* 16:355, 1991.
349. Thornsvard MAJCT, Guider BA, Kimball DB: An unusual reaction to chloroquine-primaquine. *JAMA* 235:1719, 1976.
350. Sweeney GD, Jones KG: Porphyria cutanea tarda: Clinical and laboratory features. *Can Med Assoc J* 120:803, 1979.
351. Malkinson FD, Levitt L: Hydroxychloroquine treatment of porphyria cutanea tarda. *Arch Dermatol* 116:1147, 1980.
352. Stolzel U, Kostler E, Schuppan D, et al: Hemochromatosis (HFE) gene mutations and response to chloroquine in porphyria cutanea tarda. *Arch Dermatol* 139:309, 2003.
353. Egger NG, Goeger DE, Anderson KE: Effects of chloroquine in hematoporphyrin-treated animals. *Chem Biol Interact* 102:69, 1996.
354. Cohen SN, Phifer KO, Yielding KL: Complex formation between chloroquine and ferrihaemic acid *in vitro*, and its effect on the antimalarial action of chloroquine. *Nature* 202:805, 1964.
355. Scholnick PL, Epstein J, Marver HS: The molecular basis of the action of chloroquine in porphyria cutanea tarda. *J Invest Dermatol* 61:226, 1973.
356. Chlumska A, Chlumsky J, Malina L: Liver changes in porphyria cutanea tarda patients treated with chloroquine. *Br J Dermatol* 102:261, 1980.
357. Vizethum W, Dahlmann D, Bolsen K, Goerz G: Influence of chloroquine (Resochin) on hexachlorobenzene (HCB) induced porphyria of the rat. *Arch Dermatol Res* 264:125, 1979.
358. Fernandez I, Castellano G, de Salamanca RE, et al: Porphyria cutanea tarda as a predictor of poor response to interferon alfa therapy in chronic hepatitis C. *Scand J Gastroenterol* 38:314, 2003.
359. Rossini A, Contessi GB, Leali C, et al: Efficacy of iron depletion and antiviral therapy in patients with porphyria cutanea tarda (PCT) and hepatitis C virus (HCV) chronic infection [abstract]. *Hepatology* 40(Suppl 1):320A, 2004.
360. Shieh S, Cohen JL, Lim HW: Management of porphyria cutanea tarda in the setting of chronic renal failure: A case report and review. *J Am Acad Dermatol* 42:645, 2000.
361. Yaqoob M, Smyth J, Ahmad R, et al: Haemodialysis-related porphyria cutanea tarda and treatment by recombinant human erythropoietin. *Nephron* 60:428, 1992.
362. Carson RW, Dunnigan EJ, DuBose TDJ, et al: Removal of plasma porphyrins with high-flux hemodialysis in porphyria cutanea tarda associated with end-stage renal disease. *J Am Soc Nephrol* 2:1445, 1992.
363. Stevens BR, Fleischer AB, Piering F, Crosby DL: Porphyria cutanea tarda in the setting of renal failure: Response to renal transplantation. *Arch Dermatol* 129:337, 1993.
364. Fontanellas A, Mazurier F, Moreau-Gaudry F, et al: Correction of uroporphyrinogen decarboxylase deficiency (hepatoerythropoietic porphyria) in Epstein-Barr virus-transformed B-cell lines by retrovirus-mediated gene transfer: Fluorescence-based selection of transduced cells. *Blood* 94:465, 1999.

CHAPTER 58
HEREDITARY AND ACQUIRED SIDEROBLASTIC ANEMIAS

Prem Ponka and Josef T. Prchal

SUMMARY

Sideroblastic anemias are characterized by the presence of ring sideroblasts in the marrow. These cells are erythroid precursors that have accumulated abnormal amounts of mitochondrial iron. A variety of abnormalities of porphyrin metabolism in affected erythroid cells have been documented. Hereditary sideroblastic anemias are usually X linked, as the result of mutations in the erythroid form of 5-aminolevulinic acid (ALA) synthase. Inherited autosomal and mitochondrial forms are also occasionally seen. Acquired sideroblastic anemias can occur as a result of the ingestion of drugs, alcohol, or toxins such as lead or zinc. A separate entity of an acquired sideroblastic anemia is being recognized in growing number of patients with sideroblastic macrocytic anemia and variable degrees thrombocytopenia and leukopenia caused by copper deficiency; the hematologic abnormalities typically resolve after copper replacement. Ring sideroblasts are also a feature of myelodysplastic states, which are discussed in Chap. 88. Some patients with sideroblastic anemia may respond to pharmacologic doses of pyridoxine. Iron loading is common in the sideroblastic anemias and can be treated by phlebotomy when the anemia is mild or with iron chelators (see Chap. 42) when it is more severe.

DEFINITION AND HISTORY

Sideroblastic anemias are a heterogeneous group of disorders that have as common features the presence of large numbers of ringed sideroblasts in the marrow, ineffective erythropoiesis, increased levels of tissue iron, and varying proportions of hypochromic erythrocytes in the blood. They may be acquired or hereditary (Table 58–1).

Acquired sideroblastic anemia may be a neoplastic disease, that is, a clonal disorder that can progress to acute leukemia. This subject is considered in Chap. 88, in which clonal preleukemic disorders are discussed. Sideroblastic anemia may also develop as a result of the administration of certain drugs, exposure to toxins, or coincident to neoplastic or inflammatory disease. Hereditary sideroblastic anemias include X-linked, autosomal, and mitochondrial entities. Occasionally a patient with apparently familial disease has developed a myelodysplastic syndrome later,[1,2] but with these rare exceptions, disorders are distinct and do not coexist or evolve one from the other.

Acronyms and abbreviations that appear in this chapter include: ALA, 5-aminolevulinic acid; *ALAS2*, gene encoding ALA synthase 2; ATP, adenosine triphosphate; Fe-S, iron-sulfur cluster; GLRX5, glutaredoxin 5; MLASA, mitochondrial myopathy and sideroblastic anemia; *PUS1,* pseudouridine synthase 1 gene; STEAP 3, six-transmembrane epithelial antigen of prostate 3-ferric reductase; tRNA, mitochondrial transfer RNA; XLSA/A, X-linked sideroblastic anemia associated with ataxia.

Although the perinuclear distribution of siderotic granules in the nucleated red cells of patients with various types of anemia was described in 1947,[3,4] the concept of sideroblastic anemia as a generic designation was not generally accepted until the publications of Björkman,[5] Dacie and colleagues,[6] Heilmeyer and associates,[7,8] Bernard and colleagues,[9] and Mollin.[10] After description of the primary adult form of refractory sideroblastic anemia,[5,6] similarity to the morphologic and erythrokinetic changes in hereditary (sex-linked) hypochromic anemia was recognized. Cooley[11] described a patient with an anemia with ovalocytosis who was shortly thereafter shown to have inherited a hereditary sex-linked disorder[12] that we now know resulted from an aminolevulinic acid (ALA) synthase mutation.[13] Autosomally inherited cases were also described,[14] and prominent sideroblastic changes of the marrow were found in Pearson marrow-pancreas syndrome (see Chap. 35), a disorder that is associated with mutations of the mitochondrial DNA.[15–19] Subsequently, it became evident that similar abnormalities were associated with a wide variety of diseases,[20] therapy with antituberculosis drugs,[21,22] and lead intoxication.[23–26] In some patients, the anemia responded to large doses of pyridoxine and was designated "pyridoxine-responsive anemia."[10,27–29] These "secondary" acquired disorders were then incorporated into the classification.

EPIDEMIOLOGY

All of the hereditary forms are rare, and no particular ethnic predilection is known. Drug-induced forms occur sporadically among subjects taking the drugs listed in Table 58–1.

ETIOLOGY AND PATHOGENESIS

■ MORPHOLOGIC ASPECTS: THE SIDEROBLASTS

Sideroblasts are erythroblasts containing aggregates of nonheme iron appearing as one or more Prussian blue-positive granules on light microscopy.[30] Chap. 29 discusses the morphology of these cells in normal and abnormal states in detail. In normal subjects, 30 to 50 percent of marrow erythroblasts contain such granules, which, when viewed by electron microscopy, are seen to be neither within mitochondria nor associated with other cytoplasmic organelles.[31] In contrast to the normal cytoplasmic location of siderotic granules, the pathologic sideroblasts in the sideroblastic anemias exhibit large amounts of iron deposited as dust or plaque-like ferruginous micelles between the cristae of mitochondria (see Chap. 29, Fig. 29–10).[32] The iron-loaded mitochondria are distorted and swollen, their cristae are indistinct, and the identification of mitochondria may itself be difficult. In humans, the mitochondria of the erythroblast are distributed perinuclearly,[23] which accounts for the distinctive "ringed" sideroblast identified by Prussian blue staining when mitochondrial iron overload is present (see Fig. 58–1). The morphologic features that characterize pathologic sideroblasts in various disorders have been summarized.[33]

■ PATHOGENESIS

The pathogenesis of most of the sideroblastic anemias is not well understood.[34,35] It is not clear whether the basic mechanism by which abnormal accumulations of intramitochondrial iron occur is the same in inherited and acquired forms of the disease. However, it seems appropriate, given the present state of knowledge, to discuss both forms together. The pathogenesis of the disorder may be viewed from two standpoints: the underlying biochemical lesions and the mechanism(s) of the anemia itself.

TABLE 58–1. Classification of Sideroblastic Anemias

I. Acquired
- A. Primary sideroblastic anemia (myelodysplastic syndromes; see Chap. 88)
  1. Subunit 1 of the mitochondrial cytochrome oxidase[54,55]
- B. Sideroblastic anemia secondary to
  1. Isoniazid[22,115,116,118]
  2. Pyrazinamide[21,116]
  3. Cycloserine[21,116]
  4. Chloramphenicol[21]
  5. Ethanol[21,39]
  6. Lead[23–26]
  7. Chronic neoplastic and inflammatory disease (see Chap. 88)
  8. Zinc[123,124]

II. Hereditary
- A. X chromosome linked
  1. *ALAS2* deficiency[34]
  2. Hereditary sideroblastic anemia with ataxia: mitochondrial ATP binding cassette (*ABCB7*) mutations[48–53,93]
- B. Autosomal
  1. Mitochondrial myopathy and sideroblastic anemia (*PSU1* mutations)[57,107,108]
- C. Mitochondrial
  1. Pearson marrow-pancreas syndrome[15–19]

Biochemical Lesions and Genetics

In the search for the biochemical lesions responsible for the development of sideroblastic anemia, attention has been focused upon an intramitochondrial defect in heme synthesis and on possible disturbances in pyridoxine metabolism.

Defects of Heme Synthesis The possible role of defects in heme biosynthesis have occupied central stage since the early studies of Garby and colleagues,[36] who postulated that such a defect might exist and demonstrated that the level of free erythrocyte protoporphyrin was decreased and that of coproporphyrin was increased. Subsequently, a variety of abnormalities of the levels of precursors and of their rate of incorporation into heme was documented.[37–42] However, the findings have not all been consistent, since levels of free erythrocyte protoporphyrin have often been increased,[43,44] not diminished. The role of mitochondria in the etiology of sideroblastic anemia gained further credence when mutations of the mitochondrial genome were found in patients with Pearson syndrome.[15–19]

Sideroblastic anemia with deficiency of ALA synthase (ALAS) of marrow erythroid cells has been documented in subjects both with the congenital disorder and the acquired disease.[45–47] Identification of the defect at the DNA level in the X-linked gene for erythroid-specific ALA synthase *(ALAS2)* establishes that hereditary X-linked cases result from loss-of-function mutations in this enzyme.[34] Hereditary sideroblastic anemia with spinocerebellar degeneration with ataxia is an X-linked syndrome that appears to be distinct from the other forms of sideroblastic anemia.[48–51] An X-linked adenosine triphosphate (ATP)-binding cassette has been identified as a likely cause for this rare disorder.[48,52,53]

Heteroplasmic point mutations in subunit 1 of the mitochondrial cytochrome oxidase have been documented in two patients with sideroblastic anemia.[54–56]

Rare autosomal forms of inherited sideroblastic anemia have been reported.[57,58] In rare additional patients with sideroblastic anemia, a deficiency of uroporphyrinogen decarboxylase[59,60] and ferrochelatase,[37,42,61–63] enzymes also necessary for the synthesis of heme (see Chap. 57), have been identified, but the defect in heme synthetase could simply result from the inhibitory effect of mitochondrial iron overload on enzyme activity.[42] The suggestion[36] that a defect in coproporphyrinogen oxidase might be responsible for sideroblast formation could not be confirmed by direct measurement.[64] Increased levels of uroporphyrinogen 1 synthase are commonly encountered in the patients with sideroblastic anemias.[40] Alcohol, a common cause of secondary sideroblastic anemia, inhibits heme synthesis at several steps.[39] However, in many instances, no abnormalities in the protoporphyrin synthetic pathway have been demonstrable.[65]

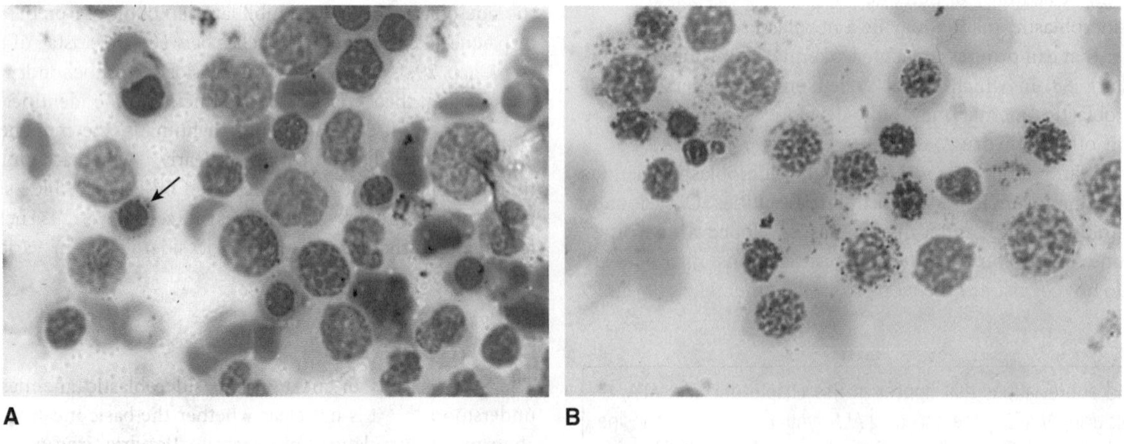

FIGURE 58–1. Marrow films. **A.** Normal marrow stained with Prussian blue. Note several erythroblasts without apparent siderotic (blue-stained) granules. The *arrow* indicates erythroblast with several very small cytoplasmic blue-stained granules. It is very difficult to see siderosomes in most erythroblasts in normal marrow because they are often below the resolution of the light microscope. **B.** Sideroblastic anemia. Note the florid increase in Prussian blue staining granules in the erythroblasts, most with circumnuclear locations. These are classical examples of ringed sideroblast, which are by definition pathological changes in the red cell precursors. In some cases, cytoplasmic iron granules are also increased in size and number, also a pathological change. *(Used with permission from* Lichtman's Atlas of Hematology, *www.accessmedicine.com.)*

Pyridoxine Metabolism A role for pyridoxine has been fostered by the demonstration that pyridoxine deficiency in animals is a prototype of sideroblastic anemia.[32] Sideroblastic anemia can be induced by drugs that reduce the level of pyridoxal phosphate in blood and decrease the ALA synthetase activity in normoblasts.[22,37,41] Moreover, certain sideroblastic disorders, although clearly not a result of pyridoxine deficiency, are nonetheless responsive to pharmacologic doses of pyridoxine.[47,66–68] Pyridoxal phosphate is a necessary coenzyme for the initial reaction of protoporphyrin synthesis, the condensation of glycine and succinyl coenzyme A to form ALA, a reaction mediated by ALA synthetase (see Chap. 57). Furthermore, pyridoxal phosphate is a factor in the enzymatic conversion of serine to glycine (see Chap. 41.) This reaction generates a form of folate coenzyme necessary for the formation of thymidylate, an important step in DNA synthesis. Pyridoxal 5′-phosphate, the active form of the coenzyme, must itself be enzymatically synthesized from pyridoxine. Deficiencies in its biosynthesis have also been invoked as the possible cause of certain sideroblastic anemias,[27,69] but direct measurements of pyridoxal kinase failed to confirm that the postulated lesion was present.[70] There are additional abnormalities that are difficult to rationalize in terms of defects in heme synthesis or abnormalities of pyridoxine metabolism. Sideroblastic anemia has been found in a patient with apparent antibody-mediated red cell aplasia.[71] Dramatically altered activity ratios of a wide diversity of enzymes have been described.[72,73] There are alterations in red cell antigen patterns frequently with an increase of i and a loss of A_1 (see Chap. 137).[74] Similar findings occur in certain hereditary and acquired refractory anemias with cellular marrows but without ringed sideroblasts.[73] Such dyscrasias are also characterized by ineffective erythropoiesis and, except for the lack of ringed sideroblasts, in some instances may be virtually indistinguishable from their sideroblastic counterparts.[75]

Pathogenesis of Ring Sideroblast Formation Iron accumulation within mitochondria is an unusual pathologic phenomenon occurring only in erythroblasts of patients with sideroblastic anemias and, to a much lesser degree, in cardiomyocytes of patients with Friedreich ataxia.[76,77] To our knowledge, a mitochondrial iron accumulation has not been demonstrated in patients with either primary or secondary iron overload. The pathophysiology of ring sideroblast formation in patients with *ALAS2* defects and those caused by inhibitors of porphyrin biosynthesis (see Table 58–1) is likely because of the unique aspects of the regulation of iron metabolism and heme synthesis in erythroid cells.[78] These differences can account for the accumulation of nonheme iron in erythroid mitochondria of sideroblastic anemia patients. In hemoglobin-synthesizing cells, iron is specifically targeted towards mitochondria that avidly take up iron even when the synthesis of protoporphyrin IX is suppressed (see Chap. 57).[79–82] In contrast, nonerythroid cells store iron in excess of metabolic needs within ferritin.[83] Hence, erythroid-specific mechanisms and controls are involved in the transport of iron into mitochondria in erythroid cells, but the nature of these processes, including the role of mitoferrin 1 (see Chap. 42), an inner mitochondrial membrane protein that presumably provides Fe^{2+} to ferrochelatase,[84] is poorly understood. The transferrin-bound iron is used for hemoglobin synthesis[78,82] with a high degree of efficiency and is targeted into erythroid mitochondria, and because no intermediate for cytoplasmic iron transport has ever been identified in erythroid cells, a following hypothesis of intracellular iron trafficking in developing red blood cells has been proposed (Fig. 58–2). This model postulates that iron released from transferrin in the endosome is passed directly from protein to protein until it reaches ferrochelatase, which incorporates Fe^{2+} into protoporphyrin IX[85] in the mitochondria. Such a transfer bypasses the cytosol, as the movement of iron between proteins could be mediated by a direct interaction of the endosome with the mitochondria.[78,86] The results of supporting experiments revealed that (1) iron, delivered to mitochondria via the transferrin-transferrin receptor pathway, is unavailable to cytoplasmic chelators;[87,88] (2) transferrin-containing endosomes move to and contact mitochondria in erythroid cells; and (3) endosomal movement is required for iron delivery to mitochondria.[87] These studies also revealed that cytoplasmic iron not bound to transferrin is inefficiently utilized for heme biosynthesis and that the endosome–mitochondria interaction increases chelatable mitochondrial iron.[87]

An important distinction between erythroid and nonerythroid cells is the presence of a feedback mechanism in which "uncommitted" heme inhibits iron acquisition from transferrin.[89–92] Although it is still unresolved whether heme inhibits transferrin endocytosis[89,90] or iron release from transferrin,[92] the lack of heme as a negative feedback regulator plays an important role in mitochondrial iron accumulation. Additionally, it has been reported that nonheme iron, which accumulates in erythroid mitochondria, cannot be released from the organelle unless it is inserted into heme.[82] This suggests that mitochondria can release iron only when the metal is in a proper chemical form, in this case, inserted into protoporphyrin IX. These considerations provide framework to the pathogenesis of mitochondrial iron accumulation in erythroblasts of patients with sideroblastic anemia caused by *ALAS2* defects, as well as those caused by agents inhibiting porphyrin biosynthesis (see Table 58–1).

A distinct form of X-linked sideroblastic anemia associated with ataxia (XLSA/A) was described in several families with putative mutations mapped to chromosome region Xq13.[50] In contrast to ALAS2-linked disease, the XLSA/A syndrome is associated with elevated erythrocyte protoporphyrin IX levels. It was demonstrated that mutations of *ABCB7* gene is responsible for XLSA/A,[48] and this was confirmed by subsequent reports.[52,93] The ABCB7 protein is thought to transfer iron-sulfur ([Fe-S]) clusters from mitochondria to the cytosol (see Chap. 42).[76,94,95] How the disruption of [Fe-S] cluster export might impede heme biosynthesis, however, is not clear, but the accumulation of erythrocyte zinc-protoporphyrin IX is found in XLSA/A.[48,50,52] Additionally, mouse erythrocytes with mutated (E433K) ABCB7 have an increase in zinc-protoporphyrin IX/heme ratios.[96] Because the formation of zinc-protoporphyrin IX requires ferrochelatase, ABCB7 mutations cannot interfere with the activity of this enzyme. Instead, the loss of function of ABCB7 might somehow diminish the availability of Fe^{2+} (reduced iron, the physiologic substrate for ferrochelatase) required for the assembly of heme from protoporphyrin IX. In X-linked sideroblastic anemia, as in *ALAS2*-associated sideroblastic anemia, decreased levels of heme likely contribute to the pathogenesis of ring sideroblast formation.

Another type of hereditary hypochromic anemia was described in *shiraz* (*sir*) zebrafish mutants.[97] These mutants have a deficiency of glutaredoxin 5 encoded by a gene (*GLRX5*) whose product is required for [Fe-S] cluster assembly. This study demonstrated that the loss of the [Fe-S] cluster in the iron-regulatory protein 1 (IRP1) blocked ALAS2 translation by binding to the iron-responsive element (IRE) located in the 5′-untranslated region of ALAS2 messenger RNA (mRNA). Subsequently, a case of GLRX5 deficiency in an anemic male with iron overload and a low number of ringed sideroblasts was reported.[98] As in zebra fish *shiraz* mutants, ferritin levels were low and transferrin receptor levels were high in the patient's cells; this can be explained by increased IRP1 binding to IREs in mRNAs of these two proteins. However, erythroblasts from zebra fish *shiraz* mutants were not found to contain iron-loaded mitochondria.

The pathophysiology of acquired idiopathic sideroblastic anemias associated with myelodysplastic syndromes is distinct from the above discussed X-linked sideroblastic anemias. In patients with refractory anemias with ring sideroblasts, there is no evidence for a decrease in the formation protoporphyrin IX levels; instead, the amount of protoporphyrin

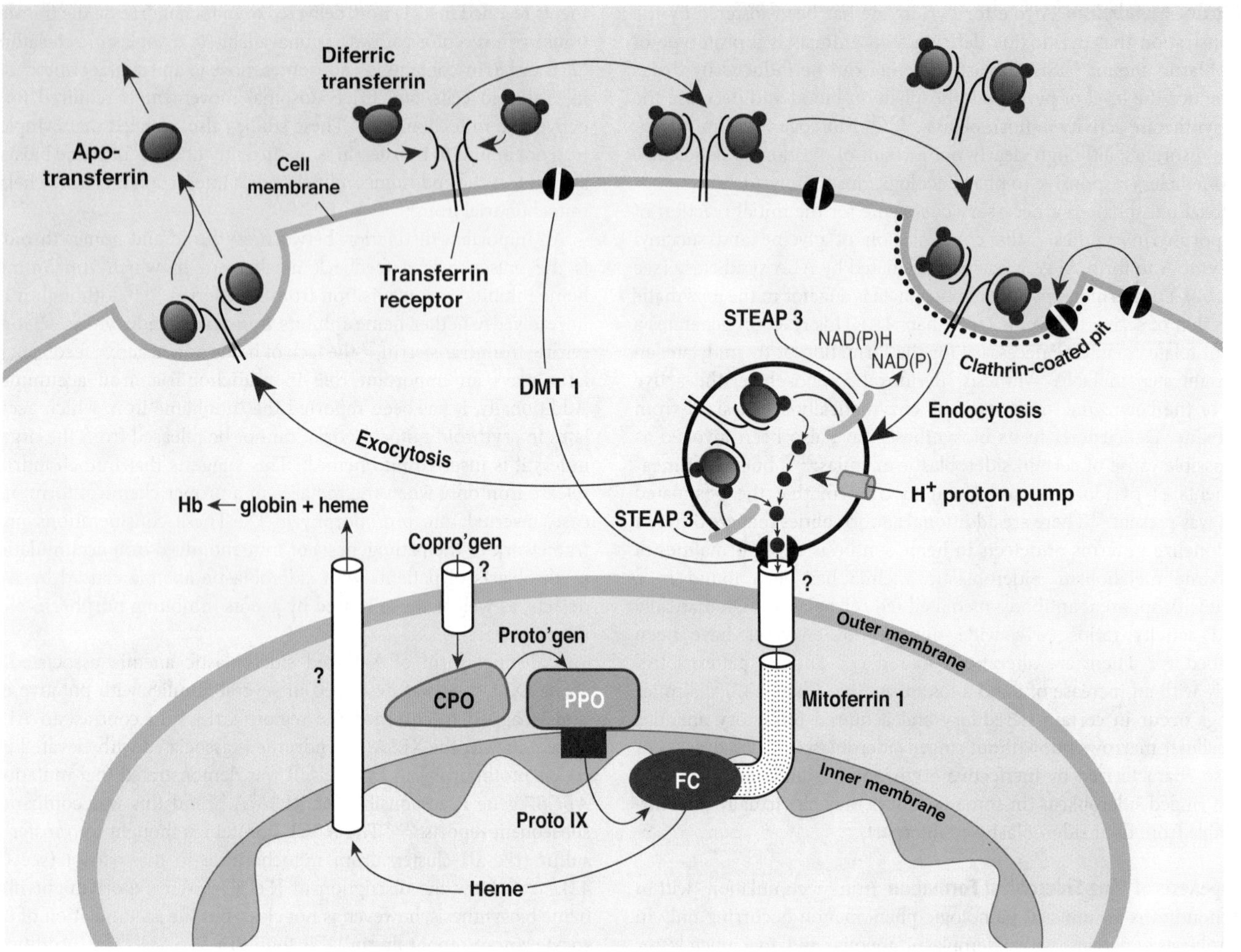

FIGURE 58–2. Schematic representation of iron uptake from transferrin and its delivery to the hemoglobin (Hb) molecule. Extracellular differic transferrin is bound by the membrane-bound transferrin receptor and internalized *via* receptor-mediated endocytosis into an endosome. Iron is released from transferrin by a decrease in pH (~pH 5.5), reduced by STEAP 3, following which the metal is transported through the endosomal membrane by DMT1. In erythroid cells, more than 90% of iron must enter mitochondria wherein ferrochelatase (FC), the enzyme that inserts Fe^{2+} into protoporphyrin IX, resides on the inner leaflet of the inner mitochondrial membrane. The transport of coproporphyrinogen (Copro'gen) into mitochondria is not fully understood. Neither mechanisms nor the regulation of the transport of heme from mitochondria to globin polypeptides are known; however, it has been proposed that a carrier protein, heme binding protein 1 (gene: *HEBP1*), is involved in this process. CPO, coproporphyrinogen oxidase; PPO, protoporphyrinogen oxidase.

IX is moderately increased.[44] It is conceivable that impaired iron reduction could cause intramitochondrial iron accumulation in patients with myelodysplastic syndromes. The discovered ferric reductase, STEAP 3, is involved in the reduction of Fe^{3+} to Fe^{2+} in endosomes (see Fig. 58–2).[99] Based on the model of the direct interorganellar transfer of iron, it can be assumed that there is only one reduction step during the path of iron from endosomes to ferrochelatase. However, the efficient insertion of ferrous ions into protoporphyrin IX may still require a reducing environment in mitochondria that would be provided by an uninterrupted respiratory chain. This proposal is compatible with the fact that sideroblastic anemia accompanying Pearson marrow-pancreas syndrome[100] is caused by deletions of mitochondrial DNA genes whose products are involved in electron transport.[101] Indeed, there are at least some myelodysplasia-associated sideroblastic anemia patients described caused by acquired mutations in cytochrome oxidase, encoded by mitochondrial DNA.[54,55,102–104] However, a rigorous study failed to find cytochrome oxidase mutations in 10 patients with myelodysplasia-associated sideroblastic anemia.[105] Alternatively, another report provided some evidence that *ABCB7* (see the above discussion on XLSA/A) could be a possible candidate gene for refractory anemia with ring sideroblasts.[106]

There are some similarities and some dissimilarities between Pearson marrow-pancreas syndrome and patients with mitochondrial myopathy and sideroblastic anemia (MLASA).[57,107,108] In both cases, there are defects in mitochondrial electron transport chain, likely generating an environment that retards iron access to ferrochelase in the reduced form. Both disorders are hereditary, but Pearson syndrome is caused by large deletions of mitochondrial DNA, whereas MLASA results from a homozygous missense mutation in the nucleus encoded gene, pseudouridine synthase 1 (*PUS1*). It has been proposed that deficient pseudouridylation of mitochondrial transfer RNAs is an etiology of MLASA.[107]

A mitochondrial ferritin is ferritin isoform with ferroxidase activity that is expressed only in mitochondria (see Chap. 42). This protein is encoded by an intronless nuclear gene and can store iron within a shell of homopolymers.[109–111] Although the function and regulation of expression of this protein is not yet understood, it has been demonstrated that the induction of mitochondrial ferritin causes the transfer of iron from cytosolic ferritin to mitochondrial ferritin.[112] The mitochondrial ferritin has a very low expression in all tissues except testis.[109,111] Although mitochondrial ferritin is not expressed in normal erythroblasts, it is expressed in ring sideroblasts of patients with sideroblastic anemias,[113] caused by

ALAS2 defects, as well as those associated with myelodysplastic syndromes. In both, iron is sequestered within mitochondrial ferritin.[113] Further research is needed to explain the mechanism of mitochondrial ferritin induction in erythroblasts of patients with sideroblastic anemias, both hereditary and acquired. Whether the mitochondrial ferritin also accumulates iron in ring sideroblasts of patients with XLSA/A has not yet been studied.

Mechanism of Anemia[114]

The dominant anemia determining factor is ineffective erythropoiesis; the rate of red cell destruction is usually near normal or only moderately accelerated to levels for which a normally functioning marrow could easily compensate. The half-time of disappearance of intravenously injected tracer doses of radioactive iron may be normal, but it usually is rapid (25–50 minutes; normal mean: 90–100 minutes). The plasma iron turnover tends to be increased (1.5–5.9 mg per deciliter of whole blood per day; normal: approximately 0.30–0.70 mg), but incorporation of radioactive iron into heme and its delivery to the blood as newly synthesized hemoglobin are depressed (15–30% of tracer dose; normal: 70–90%). Red cell survival, as determined by the ^{51}Cr technique, varies from a half-time of 15 days to normal, corresponding to a mean erythrocyte life span of approximately 40 to 120 days. As in other kinds of anemia characterized by ineffective erythropoiesis, the fecal stercobilin excreted per day may be greater than can be accounted for by the daily catabolism of circulating hemoglobin.

CLINICAL AND LABORATORY FEATURES

PRIMARY ACQUIRED SIDEROBLASTIC ANEMIA

Chap. 88 describes the features of primary acquired sideroblastic anemia.

SECONDARY ACQUIRED SIDEROBLASTIC ANEMIA

The administration of certain drugs and the ingestion of alcohol may cause sideroblastic anemia (see Table 58–1). The drugs that are most commonly associated with this type of anemia are isonicotinic acid hydrazide,[115] pyrazinamide,[21,22,116] cycloserine,[21,22,116] and all pyridoxine antagonists. Although plasma pyridoxal phosphate levels are often low in alcoholic patients, there is no correlation between these levels and the appearance of ringed sideroblasts in the marrow.[117]

Anemia secondary to drugs may be quite severe, even necessitating transfusion,[22] but characteristically the anemia improves rapidly when the patient is given pyridoxine and/or when administration of the offending drug is discontinued. The red cells are hypochromic, and commonly a dimorphic appearance of the erythrocytes in the blood film, that is, two populations of red cells, can be distinguished. The reticulocyte count is low or normal.[118] In rare instances, a sideroblastic anemia first observed during the course of drug administration has progressed in the face of discontinuing the putative offending drug. In such cases, the patient presumably was suffering from an underlying myelodysplastic disorder.

Copper Deficiency

In 1974, Dunlop and colleagues described two patients with copper deficiency who had extensive bowel surgery and received long-term parenteral hyperalimentation; one was also neutropenic.[119] Gregg and colleagues, in 2002, described a female who several years after gastroduodenal bypass (Billroth II surgery) developed progressive macrocytic anemia, thrombocytopenia, and leukopenia with numerous ring sideroblasts in the marrow, mimicking refractory anemia with ringed sideroblasts. This patient also had optic neuritis and other neurologic abnormalities.[120] The hematologic abnormalities, but not neurologic defects, resolved fully with copper therapy. Since that time numerous similar cases, with and without neurologic abnormalities, have been reported.[121,122] A similar hematologic picture can be seen with zinc-induced copper deficiency.[123,124]

HEREDITARY SIDEROBLASTIC ANEMIA

Hereditary sideroblastic anemia is very uncommon. More instances of the X-chromosome linked varieties than of apparently autosomally inherited cases have been documented.[125] The disorder is heterogeneous. In some of the cases of hereditary iron-loading anemia that are cited below, either the presence of the sideroblasts in the marrow or the hereditary nature of the disorder is presumed; it has not been clearly documented in each case.

Anemia is usually apparent during the first few months[126] or years[36,38] of life; it may even occur prenatally.[102] However, there are patients in whom microcytic anemia first became evident in the eighth and ninth decade of life and were found to have a microcytic, pyridoxine response anemia apparently related to inherited mutations of the *ALAS2* gene.[127,128]

Pallor is the most prominent physical finding; splenomegaly may be present,[46] but not universally so.[36,126] The anemia is characteristically microcytic and hypochromic, and prominent dimorphism of the red cell population has been noted in carrier females of the sex-linked form of the anemia.[12,126,129] This has been regarded as evidence of X-inactivation affecting the locus responsible for this disorder,[38,126,129,130] but it is notable that marked dimorphism sometimes is seen in the red cells of affected males as well[12,36] and in autosomal forms of the disease.[131] The degree of anisocytosis and poikilocytosis is usually striking. Sometimes the anemia can be macrocytic,[2,131,132] especially in mitochondrial forms of the disease. The red cells show marked heterogeneity with respect to resistance to osmotic lysis: a flattened curve indicates that cells with both increased and decreased resistance to lysis are present.[36,133] The white cell count is usually normal or slightly decreased, unless splenectomy has been performed. Then it may be greatly elevated.[134] Splenomegaly is present in most cases.[134] In one family, a platelet function abnormality resembling a storage pool defect was noted,[135] but this could have been an independently inherited disorder.

Pearson marrow-pancreas syndrome is a refractory sideroblastic anemia with vacuolization of marrow precursors and exocrine pancreatic dysfunction occurring during infancy (see Chap. 35).[56,136] Most patients die in infancy, although there is considerable phenotypic variation, presumably depending upon the number of mitochondria affected and their tissue distribution.

TREATMENT

Many patients with hereditary sideroblastic anemia have some response to treatment with pyridoxine in doses of 50 to 200 mg/day,[12,126,129,134,137–139] but failures have also been observed.[8,36,43] Some patients have responded to doses as low as 2.5 mg/day.[134] An additional effect may be achieved by the administration of folic acid.[126] Very rarely patients have been reported to respond to a crude liver extract, and it has been suggested that tryptophan may be an active principle, enhancing the effect of pyridoxine.[140,141] Responses to pyridoxine may result in an increase in the steady-state hemoglobin level of the blood or a decrease in the transfusion requirement, but normalization of the hemoglobin level does not usually occur and the anemia relapses when pyridoxine administration is discontinued.

Iron overloading regularly accompanies this disorder and may be the cause of death (see Chap. 42).[42] Iron storage may be enhanced when the mutations of hereditary hemochromatosis are coinherited.[142] If the anemia is not too severe or if it can be partially corrected by the administration of pyridoxine, phlebotomy may be used to diminish the iron burden.[143,144] Otherwise it may be advisable to attempt to decrease the amount of body iron by the use of chelators (see Chap. 42).

Marrow transplantation, both ablative[145] and nonmyeloblative,[146] has been used on rare occasions to treat hereditary sideroblastic anemia.

REFERENCES

1. Kardos G, Veerman AJ, de Waal FC, et al: Familial sideroblastic anemia with emergence of monosomy 5 and myelodysplastic syndrome. *Med Pediatr Oncol* 26:54, 1996.
2. Tuckfield A, Ratnaike S, Hussein S, et al: A novel form of hereditary sideroblastic anaemia with macrocytosis. *Br J Haematol* 97:279, 1997.
3. Dacie JV, Doniach I: The basophilic property of the iron-containing granules in siderocytes. *J Pathol Bacteriol* 59:684, 1947.
4. McFadzean AJS, Davis LJ: Iron-staining erythrocyte inclusions with special reference to acquired haemolytic anaemia. *Glasgow Med J* 28: 237, 1947.
5. Bjorkman SE: Chronic refractory anemia with sideroblastic bone marrow; a study of four cases. *Blood* 11:250, 1956.
6. Dacie JV, Smith MD, White JC, et al: Refractory normoblastic anaemia: A clinical and haematological study of seven cases. *Br J Haematol* 5:56, 1959.
7. Heilmeyer L, Emmrich J, Hennemann HH, et al: [Chronic hypochromic anemia in two siblings based on iron metabolism disorders (anemia hypochromica sideroachrestica hereditaria).]. *Folia Haematol (Frankf)* 2:61, 1958.
8. Heilmeyer L, Keiderling W, Bilger R, et al: [Chronic refractory anemia with sideroblastic bone marrow (Anemia refractoria sideroblastica)]. *Folia Haematol (Frankf)* 2:49, 1958.
9. Bernard J, Lortholary P, Levy JP, et al: [Primary sideroblastic normochromic anemia]. *Nouv Rev Fr Hematol* 71:723, 1963.
10. Mollin DL: Sideroblasts and sideroblastic anaemia. *Br J Haematol* 11:41, 1965.
11. Cooley TB: A severe type of hereditary anemia with elliptocytosis. Interesting sequence of splenectomy. *Am J Med Sci* 209:561, 1945.
12. Rundles R: Hereditary (sex-linked) anemia. *Am J Med Sci* 211:641, 1946.
13. Cotter PD, Rucknagel DL, Bishop DF: X-linked sideroblastic anemia: Identification of the mutation in the erythroid-specific delta-aminolevulinate synthase gene (ALAS2) in the original family described by Cooley. *Blood* 84:3915, 1994.
14. Kasturi J, Basha HM, Smeda SH, et al: Hereditary sideroblastic anaemia in 4 siblings of a Libyan family—Autosomal inheritance. *Acta Haematol* 68:321, 1982.
15. Cormier V, Rotig A, Quartino AR, et al: Widespread multi-tissue deletions of the mitochondrial genome in the Pearson marrow-pancreas syndrome. *J Pediatr* 117:599, 1990.
16. Danse PW, Jakobs C, Rotig A, et al: [Pearson's syndrome: A multi-system disorder based on a mt-DNA deletion]. *Tijdschr Kindergeneeskd* 59:196, 1991.
17. Gurgey A, Rotig A, Gumruk F, et al: Pearson's marrow-pancreas syndrome in 2 Turkish children. *Acta Haematol* 87:206, 1992.
18. McShane MA, Hammans SR, Sweeney M, et al: Pearson syndrome and mitochondrial encephalomyopathy in a patient with a deletion of mtDNA. *Am J Hum Genet* 48:39, 1991.
19. Rotig A, Cormier V, Blanche S, et al: Pearson's marrow-pancreas syndrome. A multisystem mitochondrial disorder in infancy. *J Clin Invest* 86:1601, 1990.
20. Macgibbon BH, Mollin DL: Sideroblastic anaemia in man: Observations on seventy cases. *Br J Haematol* 11:59, 1965.
21. Hines JD, Grasso JA: The sideroblastic anemias. *Semin Hematol* 7:86, 1970.
22. Verwilghen R, Reybrouck G, Callens L, et al: Antituberculous drugs and sideroblastic anaemia. *Br J Haematol* 11:92, 1965.
23. Bessis MC, Jensen WN: Sideroblastic anaemia, mitochondria and erythroblastic iron. *Br J Haematol* 11:49, 1965.
24. Griggs RC: Lead poisoning: Hematologic aspects. *Prog Hematol* 4:117, 1964.
25. Jensen WN, Moreno G: [The ribosomes and basophilic granulations of erythrocytes in lead poisoning]. *C R Hebd Seances Acad Sci* 258:3596, 1964.
26. Jensen WN, Moreno GD, Bessis MC: An electron microscopic description of basophilic stippling in red cells. *Blood* 25:933, 1965.
27. Gehrmann G: Pyridoxine-responsive anaemias. *Br J Haematol* 11:86, 1965.
28. Harris JW, Whittington RM, Weisman R Jr, et al: Pyridoxine responsive anemia in the human adult. *Proc Soc Exp Biol Med* 91:427, 1956.
29. Horrigan DL, Harris JW: Pyridoxine-responsive anemias in man. *Vitam Horm* 26:549, 1968.
30. Cartwright GE, Deiss A: Sideroblasts, siderocytes, and sideroblastic anemia. *N Engl J Med* 292:185, 1975.
31. Bessis MC: *Living Blood Cells and Their Ultrastructure.* Springer-Verlag, New York, 1973.
32. Hammond E, Deiss A, Carnes WH, et al: Ultrastructural characteristics of siderocytes in swine. *Lab Invest* 21:292, 1969.
33. Koc S, Harris JW: Sideroblastic anemias: Variations on imprecision in diagnostic criteria, proposal for an extended classification of sideroblastic anemias. *Am J Hematol* 57:1, 1998.
34. Fleming MD: The genetics of inherited sideroblastic anemias. *Semin Hematol* 39:270, 2002.
35. Furuyama K, Sassa S: Multiple mechanisms for hereditary sideroblastic anemia. *Cell Mol Biol (Noisy-le-grand)* 48:5, 2002.
36. Garby L, Sjolin S, Vahlquist B: Chronic refractory hypochromic anaemia with disturbed haem-metabolism. *Br J Haematol* 3:55, 1957.
37. Konopka L, Hoffbrand AV: Haem synthesis in sideroblastic anaemia. *Br J Haematol* 42:73, 1979.
38. Lee GR, MacDiarmid WD, Cartwright GE, et al: Hereditary, X-linked, sideroachrestic anemia. The isolation of two erythrocyte populations differing in Xga blood type and porphyrin content. *Blood* 32:59, 1968.
39. McColl KE, Thompson GG, Moore MR, et al: Acute ethanol ingestion and haem biosynthesis in healthy subjects. *Eur J Clin Invest* 10:107, 1980.
40. Pasanen AV, Vuopio P, Borgstrom GH, et al: Haem biosynthesis in refractory sideroblastic anaemia associated with the preleukaemic syndrome. *Scand J Haematol* 27:35, 1981.
41. Tanaka M, Bottomley SS: Bone marrow delta-aminolevulinic acid synthetase activity in experimental sideroblastic anemia. *J Lab Clin Med* 84:92, 1974.
42. Vogler WR, Mingioli ES: Porphyrin synthesis and heme synthetase activity in pyridoxine-responsive anemia. *Blood* 32:979, 1968.
43. Heilmeyer L: *Disturbances in Heme Synthesis.* Charles C. Thomas, Springfield, IL, 1966.
44. Kushner JP, Lee GR, Wintrobe MM, et al: Idiopathic refractory sideroblastic anemia: Clinical and laboratory investigation of 17 patients and review of the literature. *Medicine (Baltimore)* 50:139, 1971.
45. Aoki Y, Urata G, Wada O, et al: Measurement of delta-aminolevulinic acid synthetase activity in human erythroblasts. *J Clin Invest* 53:1326, 1974.
46. Buchanan GR, Bottomley SS, Nitschke R: Bone marrow delta-aminolaevulinate synthase deficiency in a female with congenital sideroblastic anemia. *Blood* 55:109, 1980.
47. Cotter PD, Baumann M, Bishop DF: Enzymatic defect in "X-linked" sideroblastic anemia: Molecular evidence for erythroid delta-aminolevulinate synthase deficiency. *Proc Natl Acad Sci U S A* 89:4028, 1992.
48. Allikmets R, Raskind WH, Hutchinson A, et al: Mutation of a putative mitochondrial iron transporter gene (ABC7) in X-linked sideroblastic anemia and ataxia (XLSA/A). *Hum Mol Genet* 8:743, 1999.
49. Hellier KD, Hatchwell E, Duncombe AS, et al: X-linked sideroblastic anaemia with ataxia: Another mitochondrial disease? *J Neurol Neurosurg Psychiatry* 70:65, 2001.
50. Pagon RA, Bird TD, Detter JC, et al: Hereditary sideroblastic anaemia and ataxia: An X linked recessive disorder. *J Med Genet* 22:267, 1985.
51. Raskind WH, Wijsman E, Pagon RA, et al: X-linked sideroblastic anemia and ataxia: Linkage to phosphoglycerate kinase at Xq13. *Am J Hum Genet* 48:335, 1991.
52. Maguire A, Hellier K, Hammans S, et al: X-linked cerebellar ataxia and sideroblastic anaemia associated with a missense mutation in the ABC7 gene predicting V411L. *Br J Haematol* 115:910, 2001.
53. Shimada Y, Okuno S, Kawai A, et al: Cloning and chromosomal mapping of a novel ABC transporter gene (hABC7), a candidate for X-linked sideroblastic anemia with spinocerebellar ataxia. *J Hum Genet* 43:115, 1998.
54. Broker S, Meunier B, Rich P, et al: MtDNA mutations associated with sideroblastic anaemia cause a defect of mitochondrial cytochrome c oxidase. *Eur J Biochem* 258:132, 1998.
55. Gattermann N, Retzlaff S, Wang YL, et al: Heteroplasmic point mutations of mitochondrial DNA affecting subunit I of cytochrome c oxidase in two patients with acquired idiopathic sideroblastic anemia. *Blood* 90:4961, 1997.
56. Seneca S, De Meirleir L, De Schepper J, et al: Pearson marrow pancreas syndrome: A molecular study and clinical management. *Clin Genet* 51:338, 1997.
57. Casas K, Bykhovskaya Y, Mengesha E, et al: Gene responsible for mitochondrial myopathy and sideroblastic anemia (MSA) maps to chromosome 12q24.33. *Am J Med Genet* 127A:44, 2004.
58. Jardine PE, Cotter PD, Johnson SA, et al: Pyridoxine-refractory congenital sideroblastic anaemia with evidence for autosomal inheritance: Exclusion of linkage to ALAS2 at Xp11.21 by polymorphism analysis. *J Med Genet* 31:213, 1994.
59. Goodman JR, Hall SG: Accumulation of iron in mitochondria of erythroblasts. *Br J Haematol* 13:335, 1967.
60. Kushner J P BA: Decreased activity of hepatic uroporphyrinogen decarboxylase (Urodecarb) in porphyria cutanea tarda (PCT). *Clin Res* 22:1974.
61. Chauhan MS, Dakshinamurti K: Fluorometric assay of B6 vitamers in biological material. *Clin Chim Acta* 109:159, 1981.
62. Lee GR, Cartwright GE, Wintrobe MM: The response of free erythrocyte protoporphyrin to pyridoxine therapy in a patient with sideroachrestic (sideroblastic) anemia. *Blood* 27:557, 1966.
63. Pasanen AV, Salmi M, Vuopio P, et al: Heme biosynthesis in sideroblastic anemia. *Int J Biochem* 12:969, 1980.
64. Pasanen AV, Eklof M, Tenhunen R: Coproporphyrinogen oxidase activity and porphyrin concentrations in peripheral red blood cells in hereditary sideroblastic anaemia. *Scand J Haematol* 34:235, 1985.
65. Vavra JD, Poff SA: Heme and porphyrin synthesis in sideroblastic anemia. *J Lab Clin Med* 69:904, 1967.
66. Barton JR, Shaver DC, Sibai BM: Successive pregnancies complicated by idiopathic sideroblastic anemia. *Am J Obstet Gynecol* 166:576, 1992.
67. Pignon JM, Breton-Gorius J, Bachir D, Rochant H. Congenital sideroblastic anemia without clinical iron overload. A case report. *Nouv Rev Fr Hematol* 32:281, 1990.

68. Murakami R, Takumi T, Gouji J, et al: Sideroblastic anemia showing unique response to pyridoxine. *Am J Pediatr Hematol Oncol* 13:345, 1991.
69. Mason DY, Emerson PM: Primary acquired sideroblastic anaemia: Response to treatment with pyridoxal-5-phosphate. *Br Med J* 1:389, 1973.
70. Chillar RK, Johnson CS, Beutler E: Erythrocyte pyridoxine kinase levels in patients with sideroblastic anemia. *N Engl J Med* 295:881, 1976.
71. Ritchey AK, Hoffman R, Dainiak N, et al: Antibody-mediated acquired sideroblastic anemia: Response to cytotoxic therapy. *Blood* 54:734, 1979.
72. Nishibe H, Yamagata K, Goto H: A case of sideroblastic anaemia associated with marked elevation of erythrocytic arginase activity. *Scand J Haematol* 15:17, 1975.
73. Valentine WN, Konrad PN, Paglia DE: Dyserythropoiesis, refractory anemia, and "preleukemia": Metabolic features of the erythrocytes. *Blood* 41:857, 1973.
74. Rochant H DB, Bouguerra M, Hoi T-H: Hypothesis: Refractory anemias, preleukemic conditions, and fetal erythropoiesis. *Blood* 39:792, 1972.
75. Geschke W, Beutler E: Refractory sideroblastic and nonsideroblastic anemia: A review of 27 cases. *West J Med* 127:85, 1977.
76. Napier I, Ponka P, Richardson DR: Iron trafficking in the mitochondrion: Novel pathways revealed by disease. *Blood* 105:1867, 2005.
77. Pandolfo M: Frataxin deficiency and mitochondrial dysfunction. *Mitochondrion* 2:87, 2002.
78. Ponka P: Tissue-specific regulation of iron metabolism and heme synthesis: Distinct control mechanisms in erythroid cells. *Blood* 89:1, 1997.
79. Adams ML, Ostapiuk I, Grasso JA: The effects of inhibition of heme synthesis on the intracellular localization of iron in rat reticulocytes. *Biochim Biophys Acta* 1012:243, 1989.
80. Borova J, Ponka P, Neuwirt J: Study of intracellular iron distribution in rabbit reticulocytes with normal and inhibited heme synthesis. *Biochim Biophys Acta* 320:143, 1973.
81. Ponka P, Wilczynska A, Schulman HM: Iron utilization in rabbit reticulocytes. A study using succinylacetone as an inhibitor or heme synthesis. *Biochim Biophys Acta* 720:96, 1982.
82. Richardson DR, Ponka P, Vyoral D: Distribution of iron in reticulocytes after inhibition of heme synthesis with succinylacetone: Examination of the intermediates involved in iron metabolism. *Blood* 87:3477, 1996.
83. Harrison PM, Arosio P: The ferritins: Molecular properties, iron storage function and cellular regulation. *Biochim Biophys Acta* 1275:161, 1996.
84. Shaw GC, Cope JJ, Li L, et al: Mitoferrin is essential for erythroid iron assimilation. *Nature* 440:96, 2006.
85. Ajioka RS, Phillips JD, Kushner JP: Biosynthesis of heme in mammals. *Biochim Biophys Acta* 1763:723, 2006.
86. Ponka P, Sheftel AD, Zhang AS: Iron targeting to mitochondria in erythroid cells. *Biochem Soc Trans* 30:735, 2002.
87. Sheftel AD, Zhang AS, Brown C, et al: Direct interorganellar transfer of iron from endosome to mitochondrion. *Blood* 110:125, 2007.
88. Zhang AS, Sheftel AD, Ponka P: Intracellular kinetics of iron in reticulocytes: Evidence for endosome involvement in iron targeting to mitochondria. *Blood* 105:368, 2005.
89. Cox TM, O'Donnell MW, Aisen P, et al: Hemin inhibits internalization of transferrin by reticulocytes and promotes phosphorylation of the membrane transferrin receptor. *Proc Natl Acad Sci U S A* 82:5170, 1985.
90. Iacopetta B, Morgan E: Heme inhibits transferrin endocytosis in immature erythroid cells. *Biochim Biophys Acta* 805:211, 1984.
91. Ponka P, Neuwirt J: Regulation of iron entry into reticulocytes. I. Feedback inhibitory effect of heme on iron entry into reticulocytes and on heme synthesis. *Blood* 33:690, 1969.
92. Ponka P, Schulman HM, Martinez-Medellin J: Haem inhibits iron uptake subsequent to endocytosis of transferrin in reticulocytes. *Biochem J* 251:105, 1988.
93. Bekri S, Kispal G, Lange H, et al: Human ABC7 transporter: Gene structure and mutation causing X-linked sideroblastic anemia with ataxia with disruption of cytosolic iron-sulfur protein maturation. *Blood* 96:3256, 2000.
94. Csere P, Lill R, Kispal G: Identification of a human mitochondrial ABC transporter, the functional orthologue of yeast Atm1p. *FEBS Lett* 441:266, 1998.
95. Lill R, Muhlenhoff U: Iron-sulfur protein biogenesis in eukaryotes: Components and mechanisms. *Annu Rev Cell Dev Biol* 22:457, 2006.
96. Pondarre C, Campagna DR, Antiochos B, et al: Abcb7, the gene responsible for X-linked sideroblastic anemia with ataxia, is essential for hematopoiesis. *Blood* 109:3567, 2007.
97. Wingert RA, Galloway JL, Barut B, et al: Deficiency of glutaredoxin 5 reveals Fe-S clusters are required for vertebrate haem synthesis. *Nature* 436:1035, 2005.
98. Camaschella C, Campanella A, De Falco L, et al: The human counterpart of zebrafish shiraz shows sideroblastic-like microcytic anemia and iron overload. *Blood* 110:1353, 2007.
99. Ohgami RS, Campagna DR, Greer EL, et al: Identification of a ferrireductase required for efficient transferrin-dependent iron uptake in erythroid cells. *Nat Genet* 37:1264, 2005.
100. Pearson HA, Lobel JS, Kocoshis SA, et al: A new syndrome of refractory sideroblastic anemia with vacuolization of marrow precursors and exocrine pancreatic dysfunction. *J Pediatr* 95:976, 1979.
101. Fontenay M, Cathelin S, Amiot M, et al: Mitochondria in hematopoiesis and hematological diseases. *Oncogene* 25:4757, 2006.
102. Andersen K, Kaad PH: Congenital sideroblastic anaemia with intrauterine symptoms and early lethal outcome. *Acta Paediatr* 81:652, 1992.
103. Gattermann N: From sideroblastic anemia to the role of mitochondrial DNA mutations in myelodysplastic syndromes. *Leuk Res* 24:141, 2000.
104. Inoue S, Yokota M, Nakada K, et al: Pathogenic mitochondrial DNA-induced respiration defects in hematopoietic cells result in anemia by suppressing erythroid differentiation. *FEBS Lett* 581:1910, 2007.
105. Shin MG, Kajigaya S, Levin BC, et al: Mitochondrial DNA mutations in patients with myelodysplastic syndromes. *Blood* 101:3118, 2003.
106. Boultwood J, Pellagatti A, Nikpour M, et al: The role of the iron transporter ABCB7 in refractory anemia with ring sideroblasts. *PLoS ONE* 3:e1970, 2008.
107. Bykhovskaya Y, Casas K, Mengesha E, et al: Missense mutation in pseudouridine synthase 1 (PUS1) causes mitochondrial myopathy and sideroblastic anemia (MLASA). *Am J Hum Genet* 74:1303, 2004.
108. Casas KA, Fischel-Ghodsian N: Mitochondrial myopathy and sideroblastic anemia. *Am J Med Genet* 125A:201, 2004.
109. Drysdale J, Arosio P, Invernizzi R, et al: Mitochondrial ferritin: A new player in iron metabolism. *Blood Cells Mol Dis* 29:376, 2002.
110. Levi S, Arosio P: Mitochondrial ferritin. *Int J Biochem Cell Biol* 36:1887, 2004.
111. Levi S, Corsi B, Bosisio M, et al: A human mitochondrial ferritin encoded by an intronless gene. *J Biol Chem* 276:24437, 2001.
112. Nie G, Sheftel AD, Kim SF, et al: Overexpression of mitochondrial ferritin causes cytosolic iron depletion and changes cellular iron homeostasis. *Blood* 105:2161, 2005.
113. Cazzola M, Invernizzi R, Bergamaschi G, et al: Mitochondrial ferritin expression in erythroid cells from patients with sideroblastic anemia. *Blood* 101:1996, 2003.
114. Singh AK, Shinton NK, Williams JD: Ferrokinetic abnormalities and their significance in patients with sideroblastic anaemia. *Br J Haematol* 18:67, 1970.
115. Sharp RA, Lowe JG, Johnston RN: Anti-tuberculous drugs and sideroblastic anaemia. *Br J Clin Pract* 44:706, 1990.
116. Harriss EB, Macgibbon BH, Mollin DL: Experimental sideroblastic anaemia. *Br J Haematol* 11:99, 1965.
117. Pierce HI, McGuffin RG, Hillman RS: Clinical studies in alcoholic sideroblastosis. *Arch Intern Med* 136:283, 1976.
118. McCurdy PR, Donohoe RF: Pyridoxine-responsive anemia conditioned by isonicotinic acid hydrazide. *Blood* 27:352, 1966.
119. Dunlap WM, James GW 3rd, Hume DM: Anemia and neutropenia caused by copper deficiency. *Ann Intern Med* 80:470, 1974.
120. Gregg XT, Reddy V, Prchal JT: Copper deficiency masquerading as myelodysplastic syndrome. *Blood* 100:1493, 2002.
121. Fong T, Vij R, Vijayan A, et al: Copper deficiency: An important consideration in the differential diagnosis of myelodysplastic syndrome. *Haematologica* 92:1429, 2007.
122. Kumar N, Elliott MA, Hoyer JD, et al: "Myelodysplasia," myeloneuropathy, and copper deficiency. *Mayo Clin Proc* 80:943, 2005.
123. Broun ER, Greist A, Tricot G, et al: Excessive zinc ingestion. A reversible cause of sideroblastic anemia and bone marrow depression. *JAMA* 264:1441, 1990.
124. Patterson WP, Winkelmann M, Perry MC: Zinc-induced copper deficiency: Megamineral sideroblastic anemia. *Ann Intern Med* 103:385, 1985.
125. Nusbaum NJ: Concise review: Genetic bases for sideroblastic anemia. *Am J Hematol* 37:41, 1991.
126. Weatherall DJ, Pembrey ME, Hall EG, et al: Familial sideroblastic anaemia: Problem of Xg and X chromosome inactivation. *Lancet* 2:744, 1970.
127. Cotter PD, May A, Fitzsimons EJ, et al: Late-onset X-linked sideroblastic anemia. Missense mutations in the erythroid delta-aminolevulinate synthase (ALAS2) gene in two pyridoxine-responsive patients initially diagnosed with acquired refractory anemia and ringed sideroblasts. *J Clin Invest* 96:2090, 1995.
128. Furuyama K, Harigae H, Kinoshita C, et al: Late-onset X-linked sideroblastic anemia following hemodialysis. *Blood* 101:4623, 2003.
129. Prasad AS, Tranchida L, Konno ET, et al: Hereditary sideroblastic anemia and glucose-6-phosphate dehydrogenase deficiency in a Negro family. *J Clin Invest* 47:1415, 1968.
130. Beutler E: The distribution of gene products among populations of cells in heterozygous humans. *Cold Spring Harb Symp Quant Biol* 29:1964.
131. van Waveren Hogervorst GD, van Roermund HP, Snijders PJ: Hereditary sideroblastic anaemia and autosomal inheritance of erythrocyte dimorphism in a Dutch family. *Eur J Haematol* 38:405, 1987.
132. Fitzsimons EJ, May A: The molecular basis of the sideroblastic anemias. *Curr Opin Hematol* 3:167, 1996.
133. Seip M, Gjessing LR, Lie SO: Congenital sideroblastic anaemia in a girl. *Scand J Haematol* 8:505, 1971.
134. Horrigan DL, Harris JW: Pyridoxine-responsive anemia: Analysis of 62 Cases. *Adv Intern Med* 12:103, 1964.
135. Soslau G, Brodsky I: Hereditary sideroblastic anemia with associated platelet abnormalities. *Am J Hematol* 32:298, 1989.
136. Smith OP, Hann IM, Woodward CE, et al: Pearson's marrow/pancreas syndrome: Haematological features associated with deletion and duplication of mitochondrial DNA. *Br J Haematol* 90:469, 1995.
137. Bishop RC, Bethell FH: Hereditary hypochromic anemia with transfusion hemosiderosis treated with pyridoxine: Report of a case. *N Engl J Med* 261:486, 1959.
138. Harris JW, Horrigan DL: Pyridoxine-responsive anemia—Prototype and variations on the theme. *Vitam Horm* 22:721, 1964.
139. Vogler WR, Mingioli ES: Heme synthesis in pyridoxine-responsive anemia. *N Engl J Med* 273:347, 1965.

140. Albahary C, Boiron M: [Primary refractory anemia with medullary and hepatic hypersiderosis of blood in a woman]. *Acta Med Scand* 163:429, 1959.
141. Horrigan DL: Pyridoxine-responsive anemia: Influence of tryptophan on pyridoxine responsiveness. *Blood* 42:187, 1973.
142. Yaouanq J, Grosbois B, Jouanolle AM, et al: Haemochromatosis Cys282Tyr mutation in pyridoxine-responsive sideroblastic anaemia. *Lancet* 349:1475, 1997.
143. French TJ, Jacobs P: Sideroblastic anaemia associated with iron overload treated by repeated phlebotomy. *S Afr Med J* 50:594, 1976.
144. Weintraub LR, Conrad ME, Crosby WH: Iron-loading anemia. Treatment with repeated phlebotomies and pyridoxine. *N Engl J Med* 275:169, 1966.
145. Urban C, Binder B, Hauer C, et al: Congenital sideroblastic anemia successfully treated by allogeneic bone marrow transplantation. *Bone Marrow Transplant* 10:373, 1992.
146. Medeiros BC, Kolhouse JF, Cagnoni PJ, et al: Nonmyeloablative allogeneic hematopoietic stem cell transplantation for congenital sideroblastic anemia. *Bone Marrow Transplant* 31:1053, 2003.

PART VII

Neutrophils, Eosinophils, Basophils, and Mast Cells

CHAPTER 59

MORPHOLOGY OF NEUTROPHILS, EOSINOPHILS, AND BASOPHILS

C. Wayne Smith

SUMMARY

Early in precursor development in the marrow, cells destined to be leukocytes of the granulocytic series, neutrophils, eosinophils, and basophils, synthesize proteins and store them as cytoplasmic granules. The synthesis of primary or azurophilic granules defines the conversion of the myeloblast, a virtually agranular, primitive cell that is the earliest granulocyte precursor identifiable by light microscopy into the promyelocyte, which is rich in azurophilic granules. Synthesis and accumulation of secondary or specific granules follows. The appearance of specific granules marks the progression of the promyelocyte to neutrophilic, eosinophilic, or basophilic myelocytes. Thereafter, the cell continues maturation into an amitotic cell with a segmented nucleus, capable of ameboid motility, phagocytosis, and microbial killing. The mature granulocytes also develop cytoplasmic and surface structures that permit them to attach to and penetrate the wall of venules. The mature granulocytes enter the blood from the marrow, circulate briefly, and move to the tissues to carry out their major function of host defense.

In the normal adult human, the life of granulocytes is spent in three environments: marrow, blood, and tissues. Marrow is the site of differentiation of hematopoietic stem cells into granulocyte progenitors and of proliferation and terminal maturation (Fig. 59–1). Precursor cell proliferation, which consists of approximately five divisions, occurs only during the first three stages of maturation (blast, promyelocyte, and myelocyte). After the myelocyte stage, the cells are no longer capable of mitosis and enter a large marrow storage pool from which they are released into the blood where they circulate for a few hours before entering tissues.

NEUTROPHILS

■ LIGHT MICROSCOPY AND ELECTRON MICROSCOPY

The Myeloblast

The myeloblast is an immature cell with a large, oval nucleus, sizable nucleoli, and few or no granules. As the earliest morphologically recognizable precursor in the evolution of the neutrophil from the colony-forming cell, it is an immature cell with a large nucleus and multiple nucleoli (Fig. 59–2). The nucleolus is the site of assembly of ribosomal proteins and ribosomal RNA and is a prominent feature of early maturing cells. The scant cytoplasm contains reaction product for peroxidase within the rough-surfaced endoplasmic reticulum and Golgi cisternae and, sometimes, in early developing azurophilic granules. The dense product of the peroxidase reaction serves as a marker of azurophilic granules in human marrow and blood cells for electron and for light microscopy.[1–4]

Acronyms and abbreviations that appear in this chapter include: C3a, serum complement fragment 3a; C5a, serum complement fragment 5a; ECP, eosinophil cationic protein; EDN, eosinophil-derived neurotoxin; EPO, eosinophil peroxidase; Ig, immunoglobulin; IL, interleukin; MBP, major basic protein; PMN, polymorphonuclear neutrophil.

The Promyelocyte

In the promyelocyte stage, the azurophilic or primary granules, large peroxidase-positive granules that stain metachromatically (reddish-purple) with a polychromatic stain such as Wright stain, are formed (see Fig. 59–2). Figure 59–3 shows that the promyelocyte produces and accumulates a large population of peroxidase-positive granules. Most of the granules are spherical and have a diameter of 500 nm, but ellipsoid, crystalline forms and small granules connected by filaments also are present.[5] As with other secretory cells, peroxidase is present throughout the secretory apparatus of the promyelocyte, for example, in cisternae of the rough endoplasmic reticulum, in all Golgi cisternae, in some vesicles, and in all developing granules.[2]

The Neutrophilic Myelocyte

During the myelocyte stage of maturation, the specific or secondary granules, which are peroxidase negative, are formed (see Fig. 59–2). At the end of the promyelocyte stage, peroxidase abruptly disappears from rough endoplasmic reticulum and Golgi cisternae, and the production of azurophilic granules ceases. The myelocyte stage begins with production of peroxidase-negative specific granules.[2]

Figure 59–4 shows that the only peroxidase-positive elements at this stage are the azurophilic granules. The specific granules are formed by the Golgi complex. The granules vary in size and shape but typically are spherical (approximately 200 nm) or rod shaped (130×1000 nm). Figure 59–5 shows the cell also labeled with immunogold particles to illustrate the presence of lactoferrin, a specific granule marker. Approximately three cell divisions occur at this stage of maturation under normal conditions. Additional cell divisions can be inserted between the myeloblast and myelocyte stages of development, when the need for additional granulocytes arises as signaled by increased levels of granulocyte colony-stimulating factor. Mitoses can be observed (Fig. 59–6), and the two types of granules, azurophilic and specific, are distributed to the daughter cells in fairly equal numbers.

Metamyelocyte, Band, and Mature Neutrophil

The metamyelocyte and band neutrophils are nonproliferating cells that precede the development of the mature neutrophil (see Fig. 59–2). The mature, segmented neutrophilic cells contain primary, peroxidase-positive granules and specific peroxidase-negative granules in a 1:2 ratio. The nucleus of the circulating neutrophil is segmented, usually into two to four interconnected lobes. The late stages of maturation consist of nondividing cells that can be distinguished by their nuclear morphology, mixed granule populations, small Golgi regions, and accumulations of glycogen particles. On average, an electron micrograph of a neutrophil displays 200 to 300 granules, and approximately one-third are peroxidase positive (Fig. 59–7).

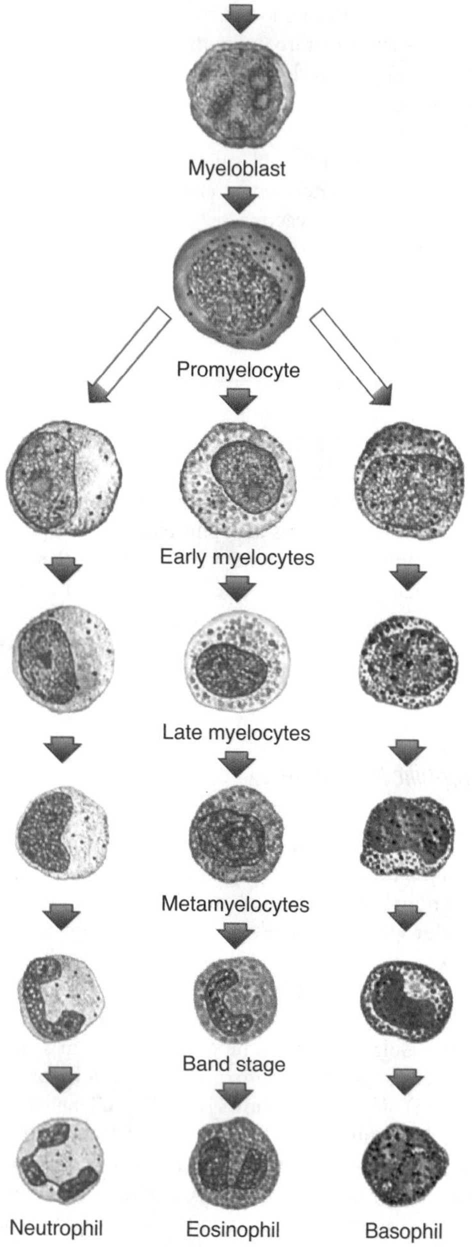

FIGURE 59–1. Diagrammatic representation of the stages of maturation of marrow granulocytes (see text for discussion). Of every 100 nucleated cells in marrow, 0.5% are myeloblasts, 5% are promyelocytes, 12% are neutrophilic myelocytes, 23% are neutrophilic metamyelocytes and bands, and 30% are mature neutrophilic cells, yielding a total of approximately 65% of cells representing developing neutrophils in normal human marrow. A similar pattern of maturation occurs in the eosinophil and basophil lineage although the number of these cell types are fewer. There are about 2.0 % eosinophils and 0.1% basophils in normal marrow (see Chap. 3). *(Used with permission from* Lichtman's Atlas of Hematology, *www.accessmedicine.com.)*

The violet-colored granules seen with light microscopy in mature neutrophils on Wright-stained blood films are azurophilic granules, which staining characteristics are altered during maturation (Fig. 59–8). The azurophilic granules become unapparent in mature neutrophils when exposed to polychrome stains (e.g., Wright stain) and examined by light microscopy. Therefore, the most reliable method to identify azurophilic granules on blood films is staining the cells for peroxidase.

The size of most of the peroxidase-negative, specific granules (approximately 200 nm) is at the limit of resolution of the light microscope. The granules cannot be distinguished individually but are responsible for the pink background color of neutrophil cytoplasm during and after the myelocyte stage.

Peroxidase-negative granules are more numerous than peroxidase-positive granules during the myelocyte stage because peroxidase granule formation ceases after the promyelocyte stage, the number of peroxidase-positive granules per cell is reduced by mitoses, and peroxidase-negative granules continue to be produced during each myelocyte generation. [1]

The purpose of nuclear segmentation is not known. Fluorescence *in situ* hybridization with chromosome-specific probes has shown that chromosomes are randomly distributed among the nuclear lobes.[6] Some mature neutrophils in women have drumstick- or club-shaped nuclear appendages. These appendages contain the inactivated X chromosome. An X chromosome-specific nucleic acid probe has confirmed the position of the X chromosomes in the drumstick structure of leukocyte nuclei by *in situ* hybridization.[7]

EOSINOPHILS

LIGHT MICROSCOPY OF EOSINOPHILS IN MARROW AND BLOOD FILMS

The earliest morphologically identifiable form of an eosinophilic leukocyte is as a late myeloblast or early promyelocyte (see Fig. 59–1). This cell is approximately 15 μm in diameter and has a large nucleus with nucleoli and a few blue or azurophilic granules in intensely basophilic cytoplasm. The later eosinophilic promyelocyte and myelocyte contain mostly acidophilic granules. A lineage-committed eosinophil progenitor has been identified that expresses high levels of interleukin (IL)-5 receptor and is negative for myeloperoxidase.[8] The fully mature eosinophilic leukocyte has a bilobed nucleus (see Fig. 59–8), and its cytoplasm is filled with large eosinophilic granules, the rim of which stains with peroxidase and Sudan black. Multilobed nuclei, comparable to those of neutrophils, are rare. Eosinophils are susceptible to mechanical damage during preparation of blood films.

ELECTRON MICROSCOPY AND CYTOCHEMISTRY

Eosinophils of the promyelocyte and myelocyte stages stain positively for peroxidase in all cisternae of the rough-surfaced endoplasmic reticulum, including transitional elements and the perinuclear cisterna; clusters of smooth vesicles at the periphery of the Golgi complex; all cisternae of the Golgi complex; and all immature and mature specific granules.[4,9] Mature granules are completely filled with peroxidase except in areas occupied by centrally located crystals.

In the later stages of development, after granule formation has ceased, the eosinophils contain few of the organelles associated with the synthesis and packaging of secretory proteins. The endoplasmic reticulum is sparse or virtually nonexistent. The Golgi complex is small and inconspicuous. The cytoplasm of the mature eosinophil (Fig. 59–9) primarily contains granules and glycogen. Most of the granules are specific granules with crystals, which usually are centrally located. After the myelocyte stage, peroxidase can no longer be detected in the endoplasmic reticulum or Golgi elements of the eosinophil by any of the enzyme procedures; however, peroxidase can be found in the matrix of granules.[1,9]

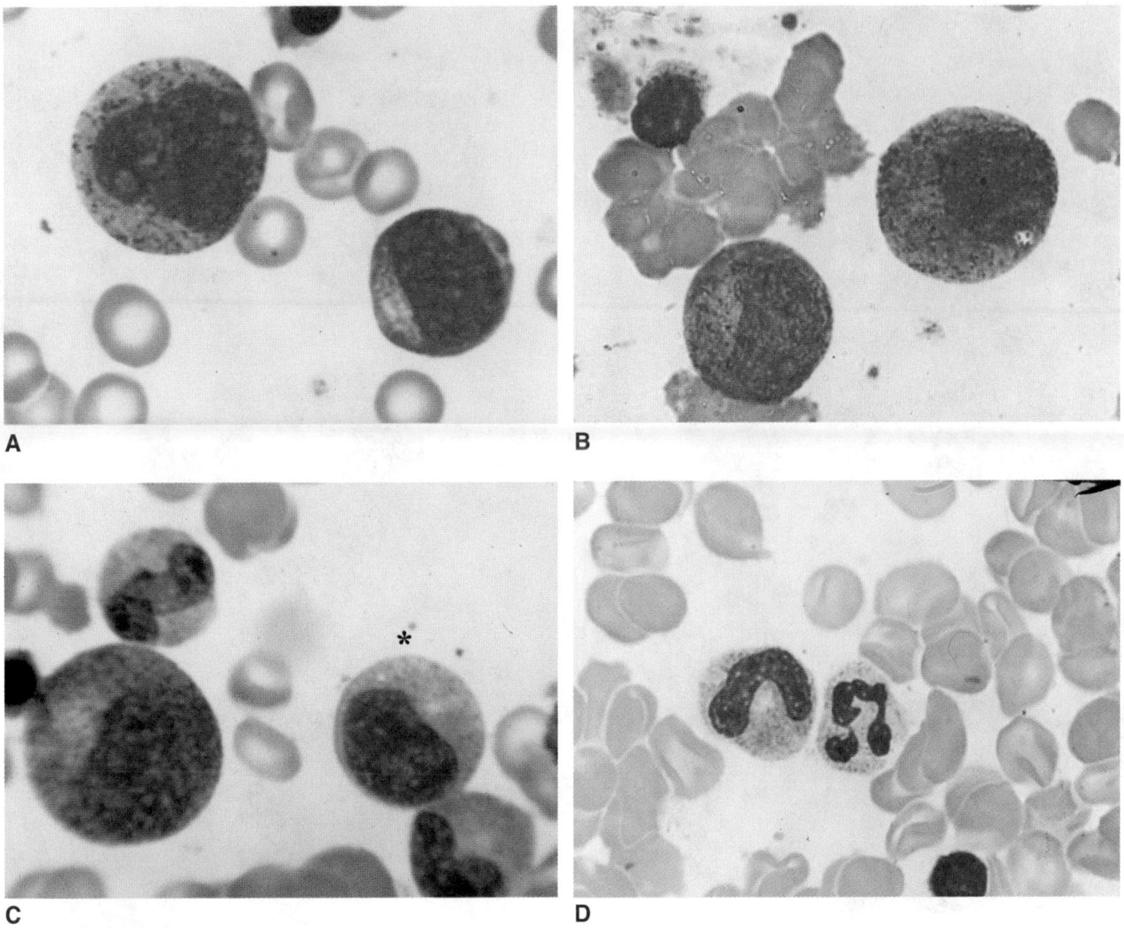

FIGURE 59–2. Marrow films. **A.** Myeloblast is the smaller cell to the lower right. It is the first recognizable precursor in the granulocytic series. It has a high nuclear-to-cytoplasmic ratio. Note the myeloblast contains nucleoli and an agranular cytoplasm. A promyelocyte is in the upper left of the field. This cell is the largest granulocyte precursor in the marrow. It often has overt nucleoli, usually more cytoplasm than the myeloblast, and azurophilic (primary) granules scattered throughout the cytoplasm and overlying the nucleus. **B.** Two very early neutrophilic myelocytes. They are very similar to the promyelocyte in appearance with nucleoli and scattered azurophilic granules throughout the cytoplasm. The distinguishing feature is the burst of tan coloring at the site of the Golgi zone, indicating the initial synthesis of neutrophilic granules. **C.** Large cell to the left is an early neutrophilic myelocyte with more neutrophilic granules evident spreading from the Golgi zone at the hilus of the nucleus. It still has some features of the promyelocyte. The cell beneath the asterisk is a late neutrophilic myelocyte. The cell has decreased in size, the nuclear chromatin has condensed. Nucleoli are not evident and the cytoplasm is nearly filled with neutrophilic granules. Below the neutrophilic myelocyte is a neutrophilic metamyelocyte, characterized by its reniform nucleus and cytoplasm filled with neutrophilic granules. The cell above the large early myelocyte on the left is a band neutrophil. The nucleus has reached the shape of a sausage and is about equal in diameter through its length. **D.** A band neutrophil (*left*) and a segmented neutrophil (*right*). Neutrophilic granules, because of their small size, are not resolvable by the light microscope and are inferred by the characteristic tan staining quality of the cytoplasm. *(Used with permission from* Lichtman's Atlas of Hematology, *www.accessmedicine.com.)*

■ GRANULES

Contents

As with neutrophils, eosinophils contain distinct granular organelles: primary granules, crystalloid granules, small granules, and secretory vesicles.[10] The crystalloid granules (see Fig. 59–9) are the largest, 0.5 to 0.8 μm in diameter, and contain much of the granular protein. The proteins packaged in these granules are highly basic proteins, with the crystalline core being mostly major basic protein (MBP).[11,12] The granule matrix contains eosinophil peroxidase (EPO), eosinophil cationic protein (ECP), and eosinophil-derived neurotoxin (EDN). The primary granules contain Charcot-Leyden crystals. Charcot-Leyden crystals are bipyramidal crystals observed in fluids in association with eosinophilic inflammatory reactions. They possess lysophospholipase activity and comprise 7 to 10 percent of total eosinophil protein.[13,14] The ultrastructural localization of this protein is in a large, crystal-free granule and supports the presence of a distinct primary granule population in mature eosinophils.[4,14,15] MBP consists of two homologues and is an abundant granular protein, 5 to 10 pg per cell. Mature eosinophils can no longer express this protein so all MBP is stored during development.[16] EPO is an abundant heme-containing protein (approximately 15 pg per cell) that catalyzes the peroxidation of halides together with hydrogen peroxide forming bactericidal hypohalous acids.[17,18] ECP is a bactericidal protein that exists in two isoforms (ECP-1 and ECP-2) with activity toward helminthic parasites. EDN shares high sequence homology with ECP and is abundant, approximately 10 pg per cell. Other granule-stored proteins include several enzymes of potential importance in inflammation, including acid phosphatase, collagenase, matrix metalloproteases, histaminase, catalase, and phospholipase D.[19–22] Chapter 62 discusses

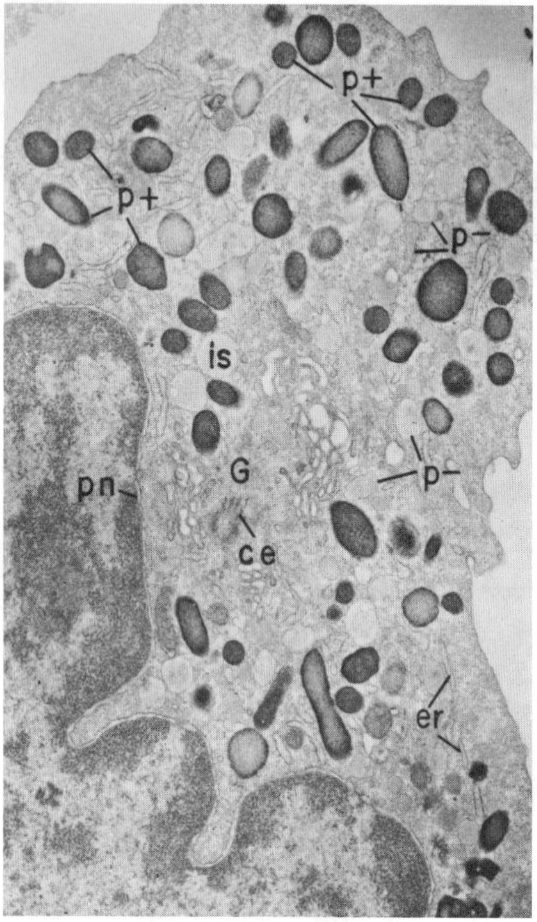

FIGURE 59–3. Electron micrograph of a neutrophilic promyelocyte from normal human marrow stained for peroxidase. This cell is the largest of the neutrophilic series. It has a sizable, slightly indented nucleus with a nucleolus (*nu*), a prominent Golgi region (*G*), and cytoplasm packed with dense peroxidase-positive (*p*+) azurophilic granules of varying shapes and sizes. Peroxidase reaction product is visible in less concentrated form within all compartments of the secretory apparatus–endoplasmic reticulum (*er*), perinuclear cisterna, and Golgi cisternae (*G*). No reaction product is apparent in the cytoplasmic matrix or mitochondria (*m*) (×8000).

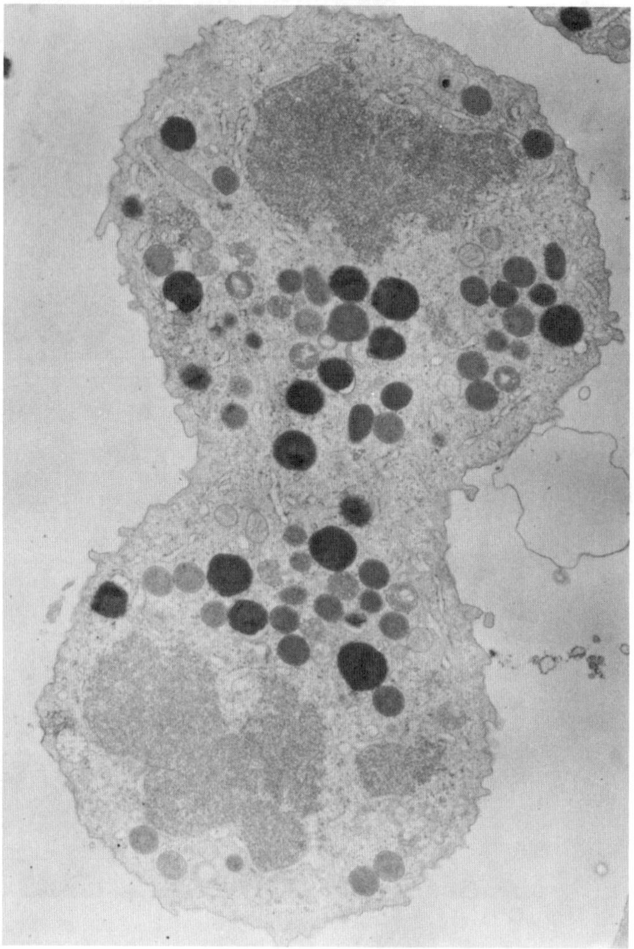

FIGURE 59–5. Portion of cytoplasm stained for peroxidase to mark the azurophil granules and then immunolabeled with gold particles to detect lactoferrin. The peroxidase-positive (p+) azurophil granules contain dense reaction product, whereas the lighter specific granules are peroxidase negative. Many of the peroxidase-negative granules (*arrows*) have gold label within their matrix (×70,000).

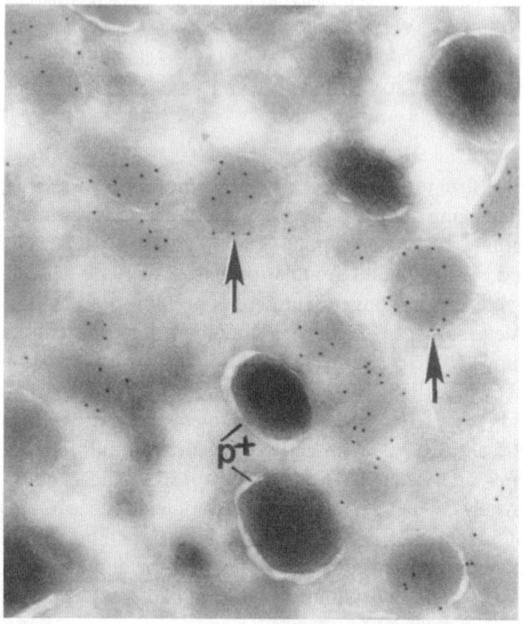

FIGURE 59–4. Neutrophilic myelocyte reacted for peroxidase. At this stage, the cell is smaller than the promyelocyte, the nucleus is more indented, and the cytoplasm contains two different types of granules: (1) large, peroxidase-positive azurophilic granules (*p*+) and (2) generally smaller specific granules (*p*–), which do not stain for peroxidase. A number of immature specific granules that are larger, less compact, and more irregular in contour than mature granules appear in the Golgi region (*G*). Note that peroxidase reaction product is present only in azurophilic granules and not in the rough-surfaced endoplasmic reticulum (*er*), perinuclear cisterna (*pn*), or Golgi cisternae (*G*). This finding is in keeping with the fact that azurophilic granule production has ceased and only peroxidase-negative specific granules are produced during the myelocyte stage (×20,000). ce, Centriole.

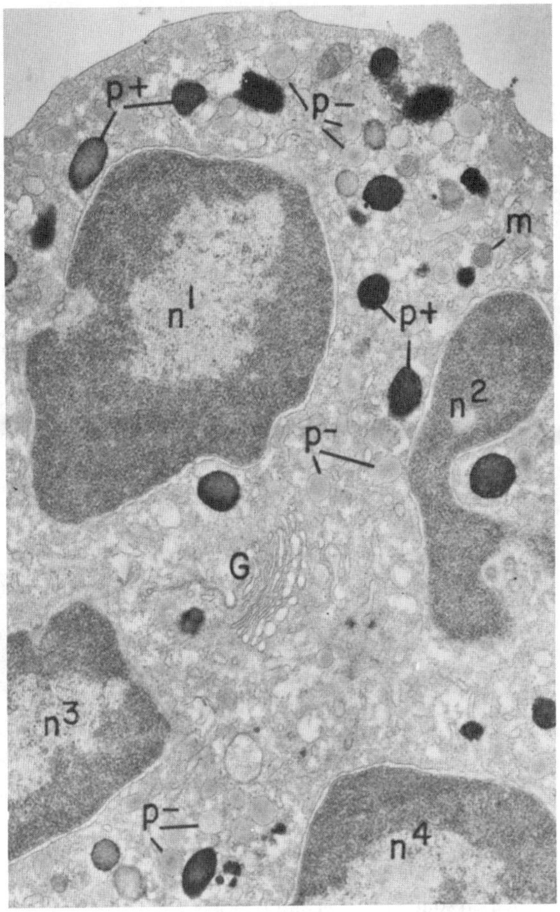

FIGURE 59–6. Myelocyte from rabbit marrow in the late stage of mitosis. This myelocyte is in telophase. Note that the granules are relatively equally distributed to the daughter cells (×15,000).

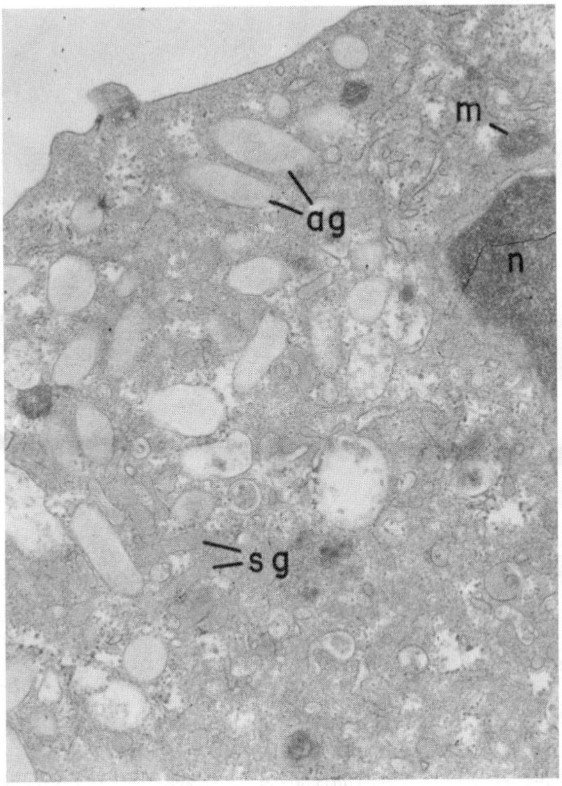

FIGURE 59–7. Mature neutrophil from normal human marrow reacted for peroxidase. The cytoplasm is filled with granules of the two basic types: (1) the smaller, pale, peroxidase-negative granules (p−) and (2) the large, dense, peroxidase-positive granules (p+). The nucleus is condensed and lobulated (n^1–n^4), the Golgi region (G) is small and without any forming granules, the endoplasmic reticulum is scant, and mitochondria (m) are few (×21,000).

the functional aspects of these granular proteins. In addition, mature eosinophils retain the ability to synthesize a diverse array of proteins including cytokines and chemokines,[23,24] adhesion molecules,[25–28] receptors for cytokines, complement components, lipid mediators, and immunoglobulins.[29–34]

■ BASOPHILS AND MAST CELLS

Basophils (see Fig. 59–8) and mast cells (see Chap. 63) are derived from progenitors in the marrow. Mast cells exit the marrow as immature precursors and terminally differentiate in tissues and basophils mature in the marrow before entering the circulation.[35–38] The granules of the two cell types stain metachromatically but are distinct when examined by electron microscopy (Figs. 59–10 and 59–11). Identification of basophils in tissue at the light microscopic level is difficult without the use of cell specific antibodies.[39] Basophils and mast cells express the Fc Receptor 1. The cells can phagocytose sensitized red cells but are less active phagocytes than the other granulocytes. They lack significant amounts of antibacterial or lysosomal enzymes. Basophils are found in small numbers in blood (0.5% of total leukocytes) and can be seen in tissues in which inflammation resulting from hypersensitivity to proteins,

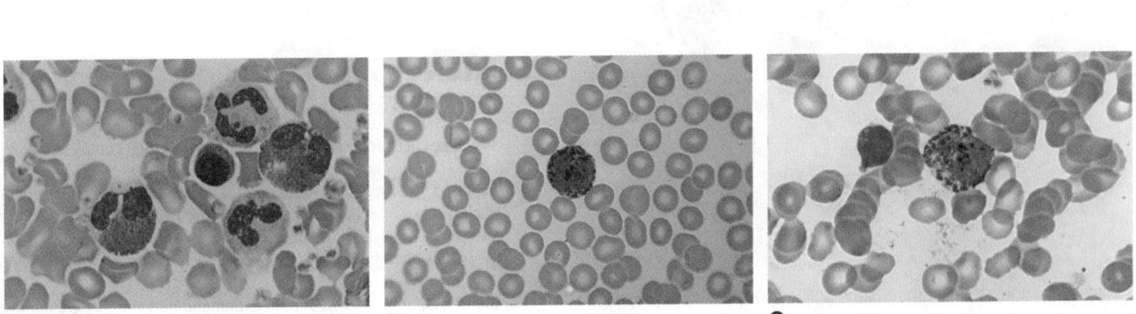

A B C

FIGURE 59–8. Images of granulocytes in blood films. **A.** Image shows two neutrophils, two eosinophils with bilobed nuclei, and a single small lymphocyte. **B.** and **C.** Images are of basophils showing densely stained metachromatic cytoplasmic granules. *(Used with permission from* Lichtman's Atlas of Hematology, *www.accessmedicine.com.)*

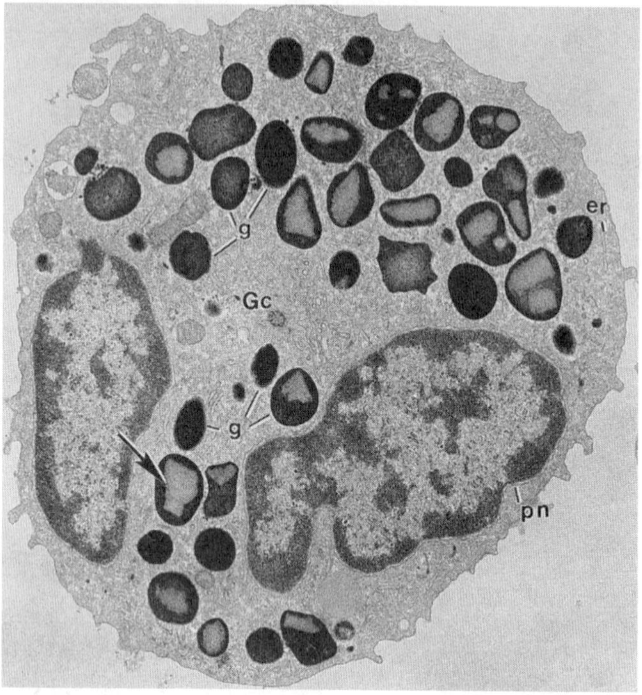

FIGURE 59–9. Human mature eosinophil incubated for peroxidase. Reaction product is present only in granules (*g*). The rough endoplasmic reticulum (*er*), including the perinuclear cisterna (*pn*) and the Golgi cisternae (*Gc*), does not contain reaction product. Most of the granules (*arrow*) contain the distinctive crystalline bar (×8000).

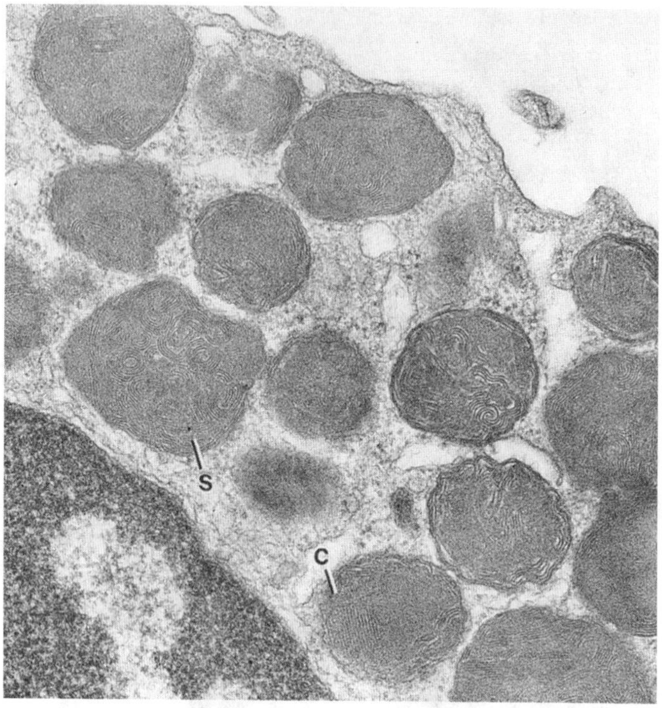

FIGURE 59–11. Portion of a mast cell from human marrow. Note the granules are filled with scroll-like (*s*) and crystal (*c*) images and are distinct from human basophil granules (see Fig. 59–10) in fine structural morphology (×50,000).

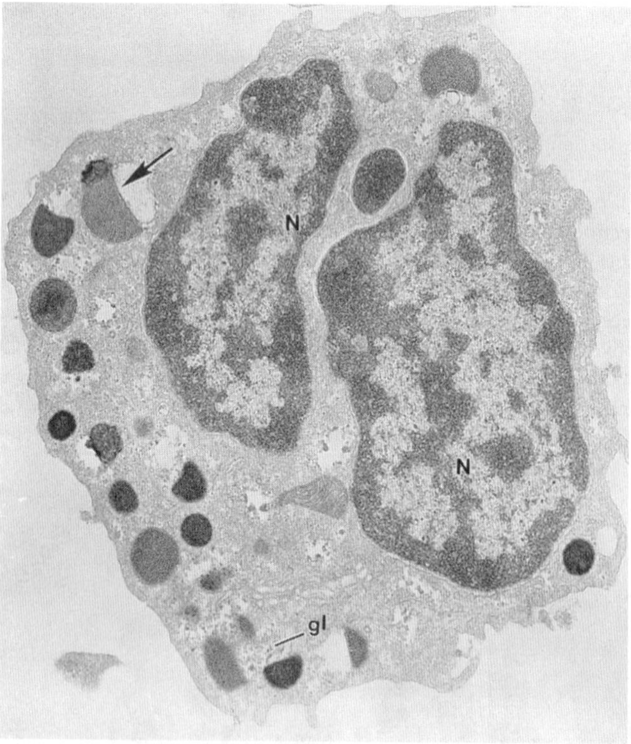

FIGURE 59–10. Mature basophil from human blood stained for peroxidase activity. Note unusually large nucleus (*N*) and scattered glycogen particles (*gl*). Human basophil granules contain peroxidase, as illustrated by their density (as a result of the presence of reaction product) in this type of preparation. They usually are spherical, difficult to fix, and may be speckled in appearance (*arrow*) (×17,000).

contact allergy, or skin allograft rejection is present. They have been shown to be rich sources of IL-4 and IL-13.[35,36,40]

Mast cells are normal residents of connective tissue throughout the body. Mast cell granules contain various substances, including several preformed biologically active substances such as histamine, which causes increased vascular permeability; eosinophil chemotactic factor of anaphylaxis; and heparin, which has antithrombin activity.[41–44] This accounts for the metachromatic staining quality of the granules. The generation of anaphylatoxin (C3a, C5a) or the interaction of allergen with immunoglobulin (Ig) E receptors of plasma membrane can stimulate extracellular release of these granule contents and of several newly formed substances, such as slow-reacting substance of anaphylaxis, a leukotriene that causes contraction of human bronchioles and increased vascular permeability, and platelet-activating factor, which causes platelet aggregation and the subsequent release of serotonin. This phenomenon is called IgE-mediated mast cell degranulation.[42] Mast cells also have been implicated in various diseases that are accompanied by neovascularization (see Chap. 63).

REFERENCES

1. Bainton DF Farquhar MG: Origin of granules in polymorphonuclear leukocytes. Two types derived from opposite faces of the Golgi complex in developing granulocytes. *J Cell Biol* 28:277, 1966.
2. Bainton DF, Ullyot JL, Farquhar MG: The development of neutrophilic polymorphonuclear leukocytes in human bone marrow. *J Exp Med* 134:907, 1971.
3. Bainton DF: Distinct granule populations in human neutrophils and lysosomal organelles identified by immuno-electron microscopy. *J Immunol Methods* 232:153, 1999.
4. Bainton DF, Farquhar MG: Segregation and packaging of granule enzymes in eosinophilic leukocytes. *J Cell Biol* 45:54, 1970.
5. Pryzwansky KB, Breton-Gorius J: Identification of a subpopulation of primary granules in human neutrophils based upon maturation and distribution. Study by transmission electron microscopy cytochemistry and high voltage electron microscopy of whole cell preparations. *Lab Invest* 53:664, 1985.

6. Aquiles, Sanchez J, Karni RJ, Wangh LJ: Fluorescent *in situ* hybridization (FISH) analysis of the relationship between chromosome location and nuclear morphology in human neutrophils. *Chromosoma* 106:168, 1997.
7. Hochstenbach PF, Scheres JM, Hustinx TW, et al: Demonstration of X chromatin in drumstick-like nuclear appendages of leukocytes by in situ hybridization on blood smears. *Histochemistry* 84:383, 1986.
8. Mori Y, Iwasaki H, Kohno K, et al: Identification of the human eosinophil lineage-committed progenitor: Revision of phenotypic definition of the human common myeloid progenitor. *J Exp Med* 206:183, 2009.
9. Bainton DF: Developmental biology of neutrophils and eosinophils, in *Inflammation: Basic Principles and Clinical Correlates*, 2nd ed, edited by JI Gallin, R Goldstein, R Snyderman, p 13. Raven Press, New York, 1992.
10. Hogan SP, Rosenberg HF, Moqbel R, et al: Eosinophils: Biological properties and role in health and disease. *Clin Exp Allergy* 38:709, 2008.
11. Gleich GJ, Loegering DA, Maldonado JE: Identification of a major basic protein in guinea pig eosinophil granules. *J Exp Med* 137:1459, 1973.
12. Melo RC, Spencer LA, Perez SA, et al: Vesicle-mediated secretion of human eosinophil granule-derived major basic protein. *Lab Invest* 89:769, 2009.
13. Calafat J, Janssen H, Knol EF, et al: Ultrastructural localization of Charcot-Leyden crystal protein in human eosinophils and basophils. *Eur J Haematol* 58:56, 1997.
14. Holtsberg FW, Ozgur LE, Garsetti DE, et al: Presence in human eosinophils of a lysophospholipase similar to that found in the pancreas. *Biochem J* 309:141, 1995.
15. Dvorak AM, Letourneau L, Login GR, et al: Ultrastructural localization of the Charcot-Leyden crystal protein (lysophospholipase) to a distinct crystalloid-free granule population in mature human eosinophils. *Blood* 72:150, 1988.
16. Popken-Harris P, Checkel J, Loegering D, et al: Regulation and processing of a precursor form of eosinophil granule major basic protein (ProMBP) in differentiating eosinophils. *Blood* 92:623, 1998.
17. Ten RM, Pease LR, McKean DJ, et al: Molecular cloning of the human eosinophil peroxidase. Evidence for the existence of a peroxidase multigene family. *J Exp Med* 169:1757, 1989.
18. Weiss SJ, Test ST, Eckmann CM, et al: Brominating oxidants generated by human eosinophils. *Science* 234:200, 1986.
19. Human Eosinophils: Biological and Clinical Aspects, edited by Gianni Marone. *Chemical Immunology* Vol.76, 2000. Karger AG, Basel, Switzerland. p 1–56.
20. Ohno I, Ohtani H, Nitta Y, et al: Eosinophils as a source of matrix metalloproteinase-9 in asthmatic airway inflammation. *Am J Respir Cell Mol Biol* 16:212, 1997.
21. Gauthier MC, Racine C, Ferland C, et al: Expression of membrane type-4 matrix metalloproteinase (metalloproteinase-17) by human eosinophils. *Int J Biochem Cell Biol* 35:1667, 2003.
22. Wiehler S, Cuvelier SL, Chakrabarti S, et al: P38 MAP kinase regulates rapid matrix metalloproteinase-9 release from eosinophils. *Biochem Biophys Res Commun* 315:463, 2004.
23. Lacy P, Moqbel, R: Eosinophil cytokines. *Chem Immunol* 76:134, 2000.
24. Moqbel R, Lacy P: Eosinophil cytokines, in *Inflammatory Mechanisms in Asthma*, edited by WW Busse, ST Holgate, p 227. Marcel Dekker, New York, 1998.
25. Georas SN, McIntyre BW, Ebisawa M, et al: Expression of a functional laminin receptor (alpha 6 beta 1, very late activation antigen-6) on human eosinophils. *Blood* 82:2872, 1993.
26. Grayson MH, Van der Vieren M, Sterbinsky SA, et al: $\alpha d\beta 2$ integrin is expressed on human eosinophils and functions as an alternative ligand for vascular cell adhesion molecule 1 (VCAM-1). *J Exp Med* 188:2187, 1998.
27. Tachimoto H, Bochner BS: The surface phenotype of human eosinophils. *Chem Immunol* 76:45, 2000.
28. Bochner BS, Busse WW: Allergy and asthma. *J Allergy Clin Immunol* 115:953, 2005.
29. Phillips RM, Stubbs VE, Henson MR, et al: Variations in eosinophil chemokine responses: An investigation of CCR1 and CCR3 function, expression in atopy, and identification of a functional CCR1 promoter. *J Immunol* 170:6190, 2003.
30. Elsner J, Dulkys Y, Gupta S, et al: Differential pattern of CCR1 internalization in human eosinophils: Prolonged internalization by CCL5 in contrast to CCL3. *Allergy* 60:1386, 2005.
31. Ponath PD, Qin S, Post TW, et al: Molecular cloning and characterization of a human eotaxin receptor expressed selectively on eosinophils. *J Exp Med* 183:2437, 1996.
32. Lee JH, Chang HS, Kim JH, et al: Genetic effect of CCR3 and IL5RA gene polymorphisms on eosinophilia in asthmatic patients. *J Allergy Clin Immunol* 120:1110, 2007.
33. Takatsu K, Kouro T, Nagai Y: Interleukin 5 in the link between the innate and acquired immune response. *Adv Immunol* 101:191, 2009.
34. DiScipio RG, Schraufstatter IU: The role of the complement anaphylatoxins in the recruitment of eosinophils. *Int Immunopharmacol* 7:1909, 2007.
35. Sullivan BM, Locksley RM: Basophils: A nonredundant contributor to host immunity. *Immunity* 30:12, 2009.
36. Gurish MF, Boyce JA: Mast cells: Ontogeny, homing, and recruitment of a unique innate effector cell. *J Allergy Clin Immunol* 117:1285, 2006.
37. Arinobu Y, Iwasaki H, Gurish MF, et al: Developmental checkpoints of the basophil/mast cell lineages in adult murine hematopoiesis. *Proc Natl Acad Sci U S A* 102:18105, 2005.
38. Arinobu Y, Iwasaki H, Akashi K: Origin of basophils and mast cells. *Allergol Int* 58:21, 2009.
39. Falcone FH, Haas H, Gibbs BF: The human basophil: A new appreciation of its role in immune responses. *Blood* 96:4028, 2000.
40. Gessner A, Mohrs K, Mohrs M: Mast cells, basophils, and eosinophils acquire constitutive IL-4 and IL-13 transcripts during lineage differentiation that are sufficient for rapid cytokine production. *J Immunol* 174:1063, 2005.
41. Dvorak AM: Cell biology of the basophil. *Int Rev Cytol* 180:87, 1998.
42. Wedemeyer J, Tsai M, Galli SJ: Roles of mast cells and basophils in innate and acquired immunity. *Curr Opin Immunol* 12:624, 2000.
43. Marone G, Galli SJ, Kitamura Y: Probing the roles of mast cells and basophils in natural and acquired immunity, physiology and disease. *Trends Immunol* 23:425, 2002.
44. Dvorak AM: Histamine content and secretion in basophils and mast cells. *Prog Histochem Cytochem* 33:III, 1998.

CHAPTER 60
COMPOSITION OF NEUTROPHILS

C. Wayne Smith

SUMMARY

Neutrophils are differentiated, relatively short-lived cells with an extensive array of surface receptors for response to inflammatory and phagocytic stimuli. A prominent feature of these cells is the presence of four distinguishable classes of cytoplasmic granules that contain a remarkable number of factors active in inflammation, tissue repair, and resistance to microbial infection. Blood neutrophils are not end-stage cells but exhibit the capacity for changes in phenotypic characteristics and life span, depending on the stimulating milieu of cytokines and chemokines. Gene expression profiling studies indicate the neutrophil is a transcriptionally active cell, responsive to environmental stimuli, and capable of a complex series of early and late changes in gene expression.

Circulating neutrophils are not the terminally differentiated short-lived cells without transcriptional activities of earlier conceptualizations. Consideration of the "composition" of the neutrophil should include (1) the prepackaged components of the cell that are released on acute stimulation (i.e., the classic attributes of the neutrophil) and (2) the phenotypic changes in various physiologic and pathologic environments that have functional significance. In addition, considerations of cell composition are most effectively expressed in the context of pathways leading to significant physiologic and pathologic functions.

Acronyms and abbreviations that appear in this chapter include: ADP, adenosine diphosphate; AML1–3, transcription factor for various hematologic lineages; AMP, adenosine monophosphate; ATP, adenosine triphosphate; BPI, bactericidal/permeability-increasing protein; C5a, chemotactic fragment of complement component C5; CAP37, cationic protein of molecular weight 37; CCR, C-C chemokine receptor; C/EBPε, regulating factor of gene expression; CR3, complement receptor 3, also called CD11b/CD18, Mac-1, or integrin $\alpha_m\beta_2$; CR4, complement receptor 4, also called CD11c/CD18 or integrin $\alpha_x\beta_2$; CXC, chemokine IL-8; FcαR, receptor I for the Fc region of IgA; FcεRI, receptor I for the Fc region of IgE; FcγRI, receptor I for the Fc region of IgG; FcγRIIA, receptor IIA for the Fc region of IgG; FcγRIIIB, receptor IIIB for the Fc region of IgG; GATA-1, lineage-specific transcription factor; G-CSF, granulocyte colony-stimulating factor; GM-CSF, granulocyte-monocyte colony-stimulating factor; hCAP, human cationic peptide; HNP, human neutrophil peptide; ICAM, intercellular adhesion molecule; Ig, immunoglobulin; IL, interleukin; IL-1RA, interleukin-1 receptor antagonist; JAK2, Janus-associated kinase 2; LFA-1, lymphocyte function antigen-1, also called CD11a/CD18 or integrin $\alpha_1\beta_2$; LPS, lipopolysaccharide; LTB_4, leukotriene B_4; MMP-8, metalloproteinase-8, also called collagenase; MMP-9, metalloproteinase-9, also called gelatinase B; NAD, nicotinamide adenine dinucleotide; NADH, reduced form of nicotinamide adenine dinucleotide; NADP, nicotinamide adenine dinucleotide phosphate; NADPH, reduced form of nicotinamide adenine dinucleotide phosphate; NFκB1/p50, transcription factor; PAF, platelet-activating factor; PSGL, P-selectin glycoprotein ligand; PU.1, lineage-specific transcription factor; SNAP, soluble NSF (N-ethylmaleimide-sensitive factor)-attachment protein; TGF, transforming growth factor; TNF, tumor necrosis factor; uPAR, urokinase-plasminogen activator receptor; VAMP, vesicle-associated membrane protein; VEGF, vascular endothelial growth factor.

NEUTROPHIL GRANULES

A prominent characteristic of neutrophils is the abundance of cytoplasmic granules, the features of which are only partially defined. Cell fractionation and ultrastructural studies have revealed many of the contents of the four subsets of granules in mature neutrophils. Table 60–1 lists some of the components and illustrates the compartmentalization of diverse functionally significant receptors, enzymes, membrane constituents, and antimicrobial proteins. The granules function as intracellular stores of both membrane proteins and soluble proteins that may be incorporated into the plasma membrane or released, thereby assisting the neutrophil in diverse functionally important activities such as adhesion, migration, phagocytosis, and killing of microorganisms. Segregation of the proteins into different subpopulations of granules allows neutrophils to contain prestored proteins that could not exist in the same compartment, and the contents of the different granules are important at different times and places in the life of the cell.

The diversity of neutrophil granules appears to be linked to the timing of biosynthesis during myelopoiesis. The hypothesis is that the different subsets of granules are the result of differences in the biosynthetic windows of the various granule proteins during maturation[1] and not the result of specific sorting between individual granule subsets (see Chap. 66). The control of biosynthesis is exerted by transcription factors that control the expression of the genes for the various granule proteins. Several transcription factors have been identified as relevant in the timing of granule protein synthesis, including the lineage-specific transcription factor GATA-1, the lineage-specific transcription factor PU.1, transcription factor for various hematologic lineages (AML1–3), and regulating factor of gene expression C/EBPε.[1–3] The importance of C/EBPε has been emphasized by the recognition of mutations in this protein in patients with the rare syndrome called "specific granule deficiency,"[4–6] a condition that leads to increased susceptibility to bacterial infections. In neutrophils from these patients, total cellular content and release of the secondary and tertiary granule markers (e.g., lactoferrin, B_{12}-binding protein, and lysozyme) are diminished, although levels of primary granule constituents (e.g., myeloperoxidase, β-glucuronidase) generally are normal.

The granular constituents are released from the membrane-enclosed granules into phagosomes or transported to the cell surface by a process of exocytosis following stimulation of the neutrophil.[7] The signal cascade following stimulation of specific receptors on the cytoplasmic membrane results in elevated intracellular Ca^{2+}, lipid remodeling, and protein kinase activation, which culminate in fusion of granules with phagosomes or the cell-surface membrane. The process is rapid, highly efficient, and involves families of docking proteins related to those found in neurons (e.g., vesicle-associated membrane protein [VAMP]-2, syntaxin-4, and soluble NSF [*N*-ethylmaleimide-sensitive factor]-attachment protein [SNAP]-23).[8]

The granule subsets appear to have a significant differential sensitivity to undergo exocytosis, ranging from secretory vesicles to tertiary, secondary, and primary granules, with primary granules being most resistant. The significance of this differential release is incompletely understood, but some aspects are apparent in the functions of the constituents within the granules and granular membranes. For example, secretory vesicles and tertiary granules contain receptors, such as CD11b/CD18 (adhesion molecule, Mac-1), formyl peptide receptor (chemotactic receptor), FcγRIIIB (Fc receptor), and gelatinase

TABLE 60–1. Neutrophil Granules

Granules	Membrane Markers	NADPH Oxidase	Receptors	Antimicrobial	Enzymes	Other Factors
Primary (azurophilic)	CD63 CD68 V-type H^+-ATPase			BPI-protein Defensins (HNP 1–4) CAP37 Myeloperoxidase Lysozyme	Elastase Cathepsin G Proteinase 3 α-Mannosidase β-Glucuronidase β-Glycerophosphatase Sialidase *N*-Acetyl-β-glucosaminidase	Acid mucopolysaccharide α_1-Antitrypsin
Secondary (specific)	CD15 CD66 CD67 CD11b/CD18	gp91phox p22phox Rap1A Rap2	Formyl peptide R CR3 (CD11b/CD18) Fibronectin R G-protein α-subunit Laminin R Thrombospondin R TNF R uPAR VAMP-2 Vitronectin R	Lactoferrin Lysozyme hCAP-18	Gelatinase B (MMP-9) Histaminase Sialidase Collagenase (MMP-8) Heparinase	β_2-Microglobulin Vitamin B_{12}-binding protein Plasminogen activator NGAL (lipocalin)
Tertiary	CD11b/CD18 V-type H^+-ATPase	gp91phox p22phox Rap1A	Formyl peptide R CR3 (CD11b/CD18) u-PAR VAMP-2	Lysozyme	Gelatinase B (MMP-9) Acetyltransferase Diacylglycerol-deacylating enzyme	β_2-Microglobulin Oncostatin M
Secretory vesicles	CD11b/CD18 CD10 CD13 CD45 CD35 CD14	gp91phox p22phox Rap1A	Formyl peptide R CR1 (CD35) CR3 (CD11b/CD18) CR4 (CD11c/CD18) C1qR FcγRIIIB (CD16) u-PAR	CAP37	Proteinase 3	Plasma proteins (e.g., albumin) Decay accelerating factor

SOURCE: Data regarding antimicrobial factors from references 1 and 9–35. Data regarding enzymes from references 1 and 36–50.

(metalloproteinase [MMP]-9), which potentially enhance extracellular interactions of the neutrophil. Primary granules contain microbicidal proteins and acid hydrolases, and the acidic environment of the phagolysosome creates an optimal pH for these enzymes.

BIOACTIVE FACTORS IN GRANULES

Neutrophil granules are particularly rich in factors with antimicrobial activity. Some (e.g., myeloperoxidase) function in conjunction with the reduced form of nicotinamide adenine dinucleotide phosphate (NADPH) oxidase, whereas others (e.g., defensins) exhibit activity independent of the oxidative burst. Others are proteolytic enzymes, surface opsonin receptors, and adhesion molecules. Chaps. 59 and 66 provide detailed discussions of these factors. Tables 60–1 through 60–5 list and categorize factors found within the neutrophils and on their surfaces and are provided as summaries of the prominent components of mature neutrophils.

WATER AND ELECTROLYTES

Approximately 82 percent of the leukocyte weight is water.[82] Early studies[82] performed on mixed leukocytes found an average of 2610 mg (113 mmol) sodium, 889 mg (22.7 mmol) potassium, 72 mg (1.8 mmol) calcium, 10.3 mg (0.18 mmol) iron, 2487 mg (70.2 mmol) chloride, and 299 mg (9.65 mmol) inorganic phosphate per liter of leukocytes. The copper content of neutrophils has been reported to average 4.69 nmol/10^9 cells,[83] zinc 109.2 nmol/10^9 cells[83] and 50.16 nmol/10^9 cells,[84] and magnesium 3.11 fmol/cell.[85] Little selenium is present in neutrophils; the median concentration reported is less than 0.0075

TABLE 60–2. Opsonic Receptors on Neutrophils

Receptor	Characteristics	Ligand
FcγRI (CD64)	72 kDa, transmembrane, induced by IFN-γ	IgG_1, high affinity
FcγRIIA (CD32)	40 kDa, transmembrane, constitutive, A isoform associates with CR3	$IgG_3 > IgG_1$, low affinity, binds polymeric IgG
FcγRIIIB (CD16)	50 kDa, GPI-linked, constitutive, associates with CR3	IgG_1, low affinity, binds polymeric IgG
FcαR (CD89)	60 kDa, transmembrane, constitutive	IgA, polymeric (e.g., sIgA
CR1 (CD35)	160–250 kDa, transmembrane, constitutive	C3b, C4b
CR3 (CD11b/CD18)	165/90 kDa, transmembrane, heterodimer, storage pool in granules	iC3b
CR4 (CD11c/CD18)	145/90 kDa transmembrane, heterodimer	iC3b

GPI, glycosyl phosphatidylinositol; IFN, interferon; sIgA, secretory immunoglobulin A. For other abbreviations and acronyms, see beginning of chapter.

SOURCE: References 51–62.

μmol/10^9 cells.[86] Otherwise, electrolyte determinations on human leukocytes appear to have been limited to leukemic cells and to pus.[85]

CARBOHYDRATES, LIPIDS, AMINO ACIDS, PEPTIDES, PROTEINS, NUCLEOTIDES AND NUCLEIC ACIDS, VITAMINS, AND COFACTORS

The neutrophil is particularly rich in glycogen. The concentration of this complex polysaccharide has been reported to average 7.36 mg/10^9 cells.[87–89] The rate of glucose metabolism by neutrophils is affected by insulin in diabetics but not in normal subjects.[90,91] Inflammatory activation of normal subject neutrophils has been shown to stimulate glucose uptake. The plasma membrane and the membranes of the intracellular organelles are rich in lipids. Five percent of the wet weight of neutrophils is lipid, which is distributed among various classes, as shown in Table 60–5.[92–96] The rare polyphosphoinositides are of special interest as sources of inositol 1,4,5-trisphosphate (a calcium-releasing mediator) and diacylglycerol (which activates protein kinase C).[97,98] The main glycolipid of neutrophils is lactosylceramide.[99]

Table 60–6 summarizes the amino acid concentration in neutrophils. The reduced glutathione content of neutrophils is 9.8 nmol/10^7 cells.[100] The protein content of the neutrophil is 74.2 ± 3.1 (mean ± 1 SE) mg/10^9 cells.[102] These proteins include those of the structural matrix of the neutrophil; proteins required for its locomotion, chemotactic properties, and adhesiveness; and the many granule proteins with bactericidal, hydrolytic, and inflammatory functions.

Table 60–7 summarizes the levels of nucleotides in the neutrophils.[103, 106] Neutrophils contain all the forms of RNA needed for protein synthesis.[107,108] The DNA content of neutrophils is identical to that of all other haploid cells, at 0.7 pg DNA phosphorus per cell.[109]

The average folic acid content of packed leukocytes of normal subjects was 0.1 mcg/mL of packed leukocytes. Approximately 20 percent of the folic acid was free and the remainder conjugated.[110] The cocarboxylate content is 340 mcg/10^{11} cells,[111] pyridoxal phosphate 0.24 to 0.38 ng/10^6 cells,[112] thiamine 67.5 ± 4.1 mcg/100 mL,[113] ascorbic acid 16.5 ± 5.1 mg/100 mL,[113] and folate 92 ng/mL.[114]

TABLE 60–3. Neutrophil Adhesion Molecules

Neutrophil Receptor	Classification	Ligands
L-selectin (CD62L)	Selectin family	PSGL-1, E-selectin
PSGL-1 (CD162)	Mucin family	E-selectin, P-selectin
sLe^X glycoproteins	Various glycoproteins	E-selectin
LFA-1 (CD11a/CD18)	$\alpha_L\beta_2$-Integrin	ICAM-1, ICAM-3
Mac-1 (CD11b/CD18)	$\alpha_M\beta_2$-Integrin	ICAM-1, GPIbα, factor X, fibrinogen, iC3b
CR4 (CD11c/CD18)	$\alpha_X\beta_2$-Integrin	Fibrinogen, iC3b
VLA-2 (CD49b/CD29)	$\alpha_2\beta_1$-Integrin	Collagen, laminin
VLA-3 (CD49c/CD29)	$\alpha_3\beta_1$-Integrin	Collagen, laminin, fibronectin, tenascin
VLA-4 (CD49d/CD29)	$\alpha_4\beta_1$-Integrin	VCAM-1, fibronectin
VLA-5 (CD49e/CD29)	$\alpha_5\beta_1$-Integrin	Fibronectin
VLA-6 (CD49f/CD29)	$\alpha_6\beta_1$-Integrin	Laminin
VLA-9	$\alpha_9\beta_1$-Integrin	VCAM-1, tenascin
$\alpha_V\beta_3$ (CD51/CD61)	β_3-Integrin	Vitronectin

GPIbα, glycoprotein Ibα; sLe^X, sialyl Lewis X; VCAM-1, vascular cell adhesion molecule-1; VLA, very-late antigen. For other abbreviations and acronyms, see beginning of chapter.

SOURCE: References 56 and 63–72.

TABLE 60–4. Chemotactic Receptors on Human Neutrophils

Receptor	Ligands
Formyl peptide receptor (FPR) (high affinity)	f-met-leu-phe (fMLP), other f-met peptides of bacterial origin
Formyl peptide receptor-like 1 (FPRL-1) (low affinity)	f-met peptides, LXA_4, SAA, HIV envelope domains
C5aR (high affinity)	C5a complement fragment
CXCR1 (high affinity)	IL-8 (CXCL8)
CXCR2 (high affinity)	GRO-α (CXCL1), GRO-β (CXCL2), ENA-78 (CXCL5)
CXCR4 in marrow (high affinity)	SDF-1α (CXCL12)
CCR2 (induced; high affinity)	MCP-1 (CCL2)
CCR6 (induced; high affinity)	LARC (CCL20), β-defensin
Platelet-activating factor R (low and high affinity)	Platelet-activating factor
BLT1 (high affinity)	LTB_4
BLT2 (low affinity)	LTB_4, other eicosanoids

SOURCE: References 73–81.

TABLE 60–5. Lipid Composition of Neutrophils

Lipid	Content (%)
Phospholipid	35
Phosphatidylcholine	12
Phosphatidylethanolamine	12
Sphingomyelin	6.5
Phosphatidylserine	1.5
Phosphatidylinositol	1.5
Phosphatidic acid	1.5
Triglyceride	20
Glycolipid	16
Cholesterol	10

Percentages refer to total lipid and the percentages that could be specifically defined, thus does not add up to 100%.

SOURCE: Gottfried.[92]

METABOLISM OF NEUTROPHILS

■ CARBOHYDRATE METABOLISM

Glycolysis

Glycolytic (Embden-Meyerhof) Pathway The main energy-producing pathway in the neutrophil is glycolysis, resulting in the conversion of glucose to lactate.[115–117] When intact or homogenized leukocytes are incubated with glucose uniformly labeled with ^{14}C, approximately 80 percent of the radioactivity is recovered in lactic acid. Glycolysis is inhibited by cortisol. Table 60–8 summarizes the activities of the glycolytic enzymes of neutrophils.[119,120] In some cases, the conditions under which the neutrophils are disrupted have a significant effect on the activities measured.[121] Hexokinase is the rate-limiting enzyme of glycolysis in normal neutrophils.[116] The rate of glycolysis is not altered during phagocytosis,[117] but adenosine triphosphate (ATP) levels, normally 1.9 nmol/10^6 cells, fall to 0.8 nmol/10^6 cells. Both the glycogen stores of neutrophils and the glucose of the plasma can serve as the source of glucose. Galactose, mannose, and fructose can also be metabolized by leukocytes.[122]

Hexose Monophosphate Shunt Pathway Neutrophils also metabolize glucose by way of the hexose monophosphate shunt,[123–125] thus accounting for some of the oxygen consumption of the cells. In resting cells, the amount of glucose metabolized via this route amounts to only 2 to 3 percent of the total glucose consumed by the cell.[124–126] The operation of the hexose monophosphate shunt, however, is of special importance to the neutrophil, because this pathway provides the NADPH needed for generation of microbicidal oxidants.

Glycogen Metabolism Neutrophils contain a large quantity of glycogen arising mostly from glucose. Little net synthesis from substrates occurs at the triose phosphate level. Glycogen turnover increases when these cells are deprived of glucose, especially if they are engaged in phagocytosis, but resynthesis occurs when adequate glucose is added.[87,117,127] During phagocytosis by glucose-starved cells, glycogen phosphorylase activity rises, but phosphorylase kinase and glycogen synthase levels remain unchanged.[127] Glycogen first appears in myelocytes and increases with cell maturation.[128]

TABLE 60–6. Bound Amino Acid Concentrations in Leukocytes (Lymphocytes Included)

Amino Acid	μmol/kg Water*
Alanine	2881 ± 256
Arginine	<290
Ergothioneine	<300
Ethanolamine	<250
Glutamic acid	2745 ± 251
Glutamine	2650 ± 251
Histidine	762 ± 70
Leucine plus isoleucine	1999 ± 195
Lysine	2111 ± 216
Methionine	391 ± 54
O-phosphoethanolamine	2651 ± 389
Ornithine	1767 ± 113
Phenylalanine	647 ± 105
Proline	862 ± 79
Serine plus glycine	13,021 ± 1480
Taurine	28,683 ± 2726
Threonine	2345 ± 174
Tryptophan	222 ± 31
Tyrosine	480 ± 97
Valine	1335 ± 132

Mean ± 1 SD.

SOURCE: McMenamy RH, Lund CC, Neville GJ, et al.[101]

■ PROTEIN SYNTHESIS BY MATURE NEUTROPHILS

Mature neutrophils have been classically viewed as terminally differentiated cells without the ability to synthesize proteins. This view has changed as a result of numerous investigations *in vitro* and *in vivo* showing that neutrophils can synthesize numerous proteins (e.g., cytokines, chemokines, growth factors, interferons) potentially important to the inflammatory process and the regulation of immune reactions. Table

TABLE 60–7. Nucleotides in Leukocytes (Lymphocytes Included)

Nucleotide	nmol/10^9 Cells (Mean ± SE)
NAD	32 ± 2.0*
NADH	25 ± 2.3*
NADP	8 ± 1.5*
NADPH	24 ± 39†
ATP	8800‡
ADP	1600‡
AMP	6100‡

SOURCE: *Silber R, Gabrio BW, Huennekens FM,[103] †Noyes BE, Mevarech M, Stein R, et al.,[104] ‡Löhr GW, Waller HD.[105]

TABLE 60–8. Glycolytic and Related Enzyme Activities in Neutrophils

Enzyme	Activity at 37°C in Neutrophils*	Activity at 30°C in Neutrophils†	Activity at 25°C in Mixed Leukocytes‡
Hexokinase	78 ± 14	39.6 ± 27.3	–
Phosphofructokinase	36 ±2	–	–
Aldolase	76 ± 7	118.7 ± 27.4	123
Glucosephosphate isomerase	4930 ± 716	–	–
Triosephosphate isomerase	7853 ± 323	–	2189
Glyceraldehyde dehydrogenase	3683 ± 124	–	242
Monophosphoglycerate mutase	508 ± 35	–	–
Phosphoglycerate kinase	3744 ± 197	–	890
Enolase	136 ± 17	–	734
Pyruvate kinase	173 ± 11	4125 ± 549	976
Lactate dehydrogenase	1128 ± 51	2981 ± 893	1165
Glucose-6-phosphate dehydrogenase	517 ± 11	596 ± 116.6	176
6-Phosphogluconate dehydrogenase	287 ± 5	–	–
Glutathione reductase	63 ± 7	–	–
Glutathione peroxidase	17 ± 3	–	–
Glutamic oxaloacetic transaminase	25 ± 2	–	43
Adenylate kinase	32 ± 2	163 ± 9.9	149
α-Glycerophosphate dehydrogenase	–	–	23
Isocitric dehydrogenase	–	–	47
Fructose 1,6-diphosphatase	–	0.76 ± 0.18	–
Isocitrate dehydrogenase	–	44.1 ± 6.4	–
Citrate synthase	–	32.0 ± 5.4	–
Malate dehydrogenase	–	482 ± 62.6	–
Transketolase	–	0.99 ± 0.27	–
Phosphorylase A	–	9.60 ± 2.66	–
Lipoamide dehydrogenase	–	29.7 ± 13.8	–
Ca^{2+} ATPase	–	–	28
Mg^{2+} ATPase	–	–	30

*IU/mg protein.[118]

†IU/L.[119]

‡Calculated as units/10^{11} leukocytes,[105] assuming a protein content of 7.4 mg/10^{11} leukocytes.

60–9 lists some of the factors expressed by mature neutrophils. The database for these observations has been extensively reviewed,[129,130] and some concepts are discussed here. As is evident from this list, the diversity is impressive, but the extent of production of each protein by individual neutrophils is limited when compared to mononuclear cells. However, because neutrophils make up the majority of blood mononuclear cells early in an acute inflammatory process, often emigrating in massive numbers, their aggregate synthetic ability may be significant to the course of the inflammatory or healing response. *In vitro*, an array of stimuli have been used to induce protein expression, including lipopolysaccharide (LPS), cytokines, chemotactic factors, adhesive ligands, opsonized particles, and modulatory cytokines such as interleukin (IL)-10 and IL-4.

The signaling pathways leading to new protein synthesis are subjects of extensive studies and are briefly described here. Granulocyte colony-stimulating factor (G-CSF), granulocyte-monocyte colony-stimulating factor (GM-CSF), and IL-10 have the ability to activate signal transducer and activator of transcription (STAT) proteins in neutrophils. Both STAT-1 and STAT-3 and the upstream kinase Janus-associated kinase 2 (JAK2) are rapidly tyrosine phosphorylated.[131,132] Neutrophils express NFκB1/p50, p65/RelA, and c-Rel. Tumor necrosis factor-alpha (TNF-α), IL-1β, and IL-15 cause the rapid loss of IκBα and the concomitant nuclear accumulation of NFκB/Rel proteins. This pathway is not activated by G-CSF, GM-CSF, IL-8, or IL-10. PU.1 (lineage-specific transcription factor) is expressed in mature neutrophils and constitutively binds to DNA, and the adaptor protein (AP)-1 transcription factor. Several of the inflammatory mediators produced by mature neutrophils are AP1 driven (e.g., TNF, IL-1, IL-8, intercellular adhesion molecule [ICAM]).[132] Production of CXC (chemokine IL-8) by neutrophils has been extensively studied, and a wide range of stimuli can induce its expression.[78] Cytokines such as TNF-α, IL-15, IL-1β, and GM-CSF; chemotactic factors such as C5a, platelet-activating factor (PAF), and leukotriene B_4 (LTB_4); particles such as monosodium urate crystals; microbial products such as LPS and zymosan; interaction with antibody and complement-opsonized bacteria and yeasts; and interactions with extracellular matrix molecules such as laminin and fibronectin have been shown to induce synthesis of IL-8 by neutrophils. In most studies, release of significant amounts of protein from the neutrophils and synthesis of messenger RNA have been demonstrated. Immunocytochemistry and *in situ* hybridization studies provide evidence of IL-8 production in neutrophils infiltrating inflammatory sites.

Some of the stimuli that induce expression of IL-8 also stimulate production by mature neutrophils of other proinflammatory agents, such as growth-related oncogene (GRO)-α, TNF-α, IL-1β, oncostatin M, and C-C chemokines. In addition, neutrophils may produce antiinflammatory agents such as IL-1 receptor antagonist (IL-1RA) and transforming growth factor (TGF)-β. Of interest is the observation that cytokines such as IL-10 may have some selectivity with regard to induction of antiinflammatory factors in neutrophils. Thus, considerable evidence exists for protein synthesis capability in neutrophils, but because this field of study is relatively new, much work remains to define the importance of the various proteins to inflammation, immune reactions and healing, the selectivity of the conditions, and disease states linked to the synthetic activities of neutrophils.

PHENOTYPIC CHANGES

Phenotypic changes occur in neutrophils under specific conditions.[133,134] Degranulation results in marked changes in surface expression of an array of proteins arriving at the surface from the storage pools of granules (e.g., CD11b/CD18, CD66, some β_1 integrins). These phenomena can be seen in degrees in circulating neutrophils. Exposure of neutrophils to activating factors results in surface and functional changes as a result of new synthesis (e.g., FcgRI following elevations in interferon [IFN]-g) or shedding (e.g., loss of L-selectin), also seen in circulating

TABLE 60–9. Proteins Synthesized by Neutrophils

Cytokines	Receptors	Chemokines	Growth Factors	Miscellaneous
TNF-α	IL-1 receptor antagonist (IL-1RA)	IL-8	G-CSF	Fas ligand
IL-1β		GRO-α	M-CSF	CD40
IL-12	TGF-β	GRO-β	GM-CSF	CD83
IFN-α		IP-10	IL-3	CCR6
IL-6		MIP-1α	VEGF	CCR2
Oncostatin M		MIP-1β	TGF-β	HLA-DR
		MCP-1		

CCR, C-C chemokine receptor; CD, cluster of differentiation; G-CSF, granulocyte colony-stimulating factor; GM-CSF, granulocyte-monocyte colony-stimulating factor; GRO, growth-related oncogene; HLA-DR, human leukocyte antigen-D related; IFN, interferon; IL, interleukin; IP, interferon-inducible protein; MCP, membrane cofactor protein; M-CSF, monocyte colony-stimulating factor; MIP, macrophage inflammatory protein; TGF, transforming growth factor; TNF, tumor necrosis factor; VEGF, vascular endothelial growth factor.

neutrophils. Cytokines (e.g., IL-15, IL-1, TNF) induce *de novo* synthesis of proteins (as noted in Table 60–9) to various degrees in blood neutrophils. Substantial changes occur once the neutrophil leaves the vasculature, increasing its expression of β_1-integrins, C-C chemokine receptors (CCRs), and protein synthesis.

Evidence indicates that in response to specific combinations of cytokines (e.g., GM-CSF, TNF-α, IFN-γ), neutrophils can acquire phenotypic and functional characteristics of immature dendritic antigen-presenting cells.[133] Thus, any consideration of the "composition" of neutrophils requires a detailed understanding of the stage of development and the environment to which the neutrophil is exposed *in vivo*. The neutrophil is a remarkably versatile cell.

Gene expression profiling has provided rich insights into the capacity of the mature neutrophil to change in response to environmental stimuli. Following exposure to 10 ng/mL *Escherichia coli* LPS, 307 genes are activated or repressed.[135] These changes include transcription factors, cytokines, chemokines, interleukins, surface antigens, toll-like receptors, and members of immune mediator gene families. Major changes in gene expression occur following LPS,[136] migration in wounds,[137] activation by phagocytosis,[138] or during the processes of apoptosis.[139] These findings indicate that the neutrophil is a transcriptionally active cell responsive to environmental stimuli and capable of a complex series of both early and late changes in gene expression.

REFERENCES

1. Borregaard N, Sorensen OE, Theilgaard-Monch K: Neutrophil granules: A library of innate immunity proteins. *Trends Immunol* 28:340, 2007.
2. Gombart AF, Kwok SH, Anderson KL, et al: Regulation of neutrophil and eosinophil secondary granule gene expression by transcription factors C/EBP epsilon and PU.1. *Blood* 101:3265, 2003.
3. Lekstrom-Himes JA: The role of C/EBP(epsilon) in the terminal stages of granulocyte differentiation. *Stem Cells* 19:125, 2001.
4. Shiohara M, Gombart AF, Sekiguchi Y, et al: Phenotypic and functional alterations of peripheral blood monocytes in neutrophil-specific granule deficiency. *J Leukoc Biol* 75:190, 2004.
5. Lekstrom-Himes JA, Dorman SE, Kopar P, et al: Neutrophil-specific granule deficiency results from a novel mutation with loss of function of the transcription factor CCAAT/enhancer binding protein epsilon. *J Exp Med* 189:1847, 1999.
6. Gallin JI: Neutrophil specific granule deficiency. *Annu Rev Med* 36:263, 1985.
7. Brumell JH, Volchuk A, Sengelov H, et al: Subcellular distribution of docking/fusion proteins in neutrophils, secretory cells with multiple exocytic compartments. *J Immunol* 155:5750, 1995.
8. Mollinedo F, Calafat J, Janssen H, et al: Combinatorial SNARE complexes modulate the secretion of cytoplasmic granules in human neutrophils. *J Immunol* 177:2831, 2006.
9. Soehnlein O, Lindbom L: Neutrophil-derived azurocidin alarms the immune system. *J Leukoc Biol* 85:344, 2009.
10. Dalli J, Norling LV, Renshaw D, et al: Annexin 1 mediates the rapid anti-inflammatory effects of neutrophil-derived microparticles. *Blood* 112:2512, 2008.
11. Cocucci E, Racchetti G, Meldolesi J: Shedding microvesicles: Artefacts no more. *Trends Cell Biol* 19:43, 2009.
12. Rocha-Pereira P, Santos-Silva A, Rebelo I, et al: The inflammatory response in mild and in severe psoriasis. *Br J Dermatol* 150:917, 2004.
13. Levy O: Impaired innate immunity at birth: Deficiency of bactericidal/permeability-increasing protein (BPI) in the neutrophils of newborns. *Pediatr Res* 51:667, 2002.
14. Nupponen I, Turunen R, Nevalainen T, et al: Extracellular release of bactericidal/permeability-increasing protein in newborn infants. *Pediatr Res* 51:670, 2002.
15. Schultz H, Weiss J, Carroll SF, et al: The endotoxin-binding bactericidal/permeability-increasing protein (BPI): A target antigen of autoantibodies. *J Leukoc Biol* 69:505, 2001.
16. Watorek W: Azurocidin—Inactive serine proteinase homolog acting as a multifunctional inflammatory mediator. *Acta Biochim Pol* 50:743, 2003.
17. Gonzalez ML, Ruan X, Kumar P, et al: Functional modulation of smooth muscle cells by the inflammatory mediator CAP37. *Microvasc Res* 67:168, 2004.
18. Lee TD, Gonzalez ML, Kumar P, et al: CAP37, a neutrophil-derived inflammatory mediator, augments leukocyte adhesion to endothelial monolayers. *Microvasc Res* 66:38, 2003.
19. Tapper H, Karlsson A, Morgelin M, et al: Secretion of heparin-binding protein from human neutrophils is determined by its localization in azurophilic granules and secretory vesicles. *Blood* 99:1785, 2002.
20. Gray PW, Flaggs G, Leong SR, et al: Cloning of the cDNA of a human neutrophil bactericidal protein. Structural and functional correlations. *J Biol Chem* 264:9505, 1989.
21. Boman HG: Antibacterial peptides: Basic facts and emerging concepts. *J Intern Med* 254:197, 2003.
22. Niyonsaba F, Ogawa H, Nagaoka I: Human beta-defensin-2 functions as a chemotactic agent for tumour necrosis factor-alpha-treated human neutrophils. *Immunology* 111:273, 2004.
23. Oppenheim JJ, Biragyn A, Kwak LW, et al: Roles of antimicrobial peptides such as defensins in innate and adaptive immunity. *Ann Rheum Dis* 62 Suppl 2:ii17, 2003.
24. Nizet V, Gallo RL: Cathelicidins and innate defense against invasive bacterial infection. *Scand J Infect Dis* 35:670, 2003.
25. Zanetti M: Cathelicidins, multifunctional peptides of the innate immunity. *J Leukoc Biol* 75:39, 2004.
26. Murakami M, Lopez-Garcia B, Braff M, et al: Postsecretory processing generates multiple cathelicidins for enhanced topical antimicrobial defense. *J Immunol* 172:3070, 2004.
27. Elssner A, Duncan M, Gavrilin M, et al: A novel P2X7 receptor activator, the human cathelicidin-derived peptide LL37, induces IL-1 beta processing and release. *J Immunol* 172:4987, 2004.
28. Davidson DJ, Currie AJ, Reid GS, et al: The cationic antimicrobial peptide LL-37 modulates dendritic cell differentiation and dendritic cell-induced T cell polarization. *J Immunol* 172:1146, 2004.
29. Ibrahim HR, Aoki T, Pellegrini A: Strategies for new antimicrobial proteins and peptides: Lysozyme and aprotinin as model molecules. *Curr Pharm Des* 8:671, 2002.
30. Ganz T, Gabayan V, Liao HI, et al: Increased inflammation in lysozyme M-deficient mice in response to *Micrococcus luteus* and its peptidoglycan. *Blood* 101:2388, 2003.
31. Ganz T: Antimicrobial polypeptides. *J Leukoc Biol* 75:34, 2004.
32. Quinn MT, Gauss KA: Structure and regulation of the neutrophil respiratory burst oxidase: Comparison with nonphagocyte oxidases. *J Leukoc Biol* 76:760, 2004.
33. Klebanoff SJ: Myeloperoxidase. *Proc Assoc Am Physicians* 111:383, 1999.
34. Hampton MB, Kettle AJ, Winterbourn CC: Inside the neutrophil phagosome: Oxidants, myeloperoxidase, and bacterial killing. *Blood* 92:3007, 1998.
35. Wheeler MA, Smith SD, Garcia-Cardena G, et al: Bacterial infection induces nitric oxide synthase in human neutrophils. *J Clin Invest* 99:110, 1997.
36. Pham CT: Neutrophil serine proteases fine-tune the inflammatory response. *Int J Biochem Cell Biol* 40:1317, 2008.
37. Kawabata K, Hagio T, Matsuoka S: The role of neutrophil elastase in acute lung injury. *Eur J Pharmacol* 451:1, 2002.
38. Aprikyan AA, Liles WC, Boxer LA, et al: Mutant elastase in pathogenesis of cyclic and severe congenital neutropenia. *J Pediatr Hematol Oncol* 24:784, 2002.
39. Horwitz M, Benson KF, Duan Z, et al: Role of neutrophil elastase in bone marrow failure syndromes: Molecular genetic revival of the chalone hypothesis. *Curr Opin Hematol* 10:49, 2003.
40. Belaaouaj A: Neutrophil elastase-mediated killing of bacteria: Lessons from targeted mutagenesis. *Microbes Infect* 4:1259, 2002.
41. Hirche TO, Atkinson JJ, Bahr S, et al: Deficiency in neutrophil elastase does not impair neutrophil recruitment to inflamed sites. *Am J Respir Cell Mol Biol* 30:576, 2004.

42. Sennstrom MB, Brauner A, Bystrom B, et al: Matrix metalloproteinase-8 correlates with the cervical ripening process in humans. *Acta Obstet Gynecol Scand* 82:904, 2003.
43. Balbin M, Fueyo A, Tester AM, et al: Loss of collagenase-2 confers increased skin tumor susceptibility to male mice. *Nat Genet* 35:252, 2003.
44. Opdenakker G, Van den Steen PE, Dubois B, et al: Gelatinase B functions as regulator and effector in leukocyte biology. *J Leukoc Biol* 69:851, 2001.
45. Schonbeck U, Mach F, Libby P: Generation of biologically active IL-1 beta by matrix metalloproteinases: A novel caspase-1-independent pathway of IL-1 beta processing. *J Immunol* 161:3340, 1998.
46. Peppin GJ, Weiss SJ: Activation of the endogenous metalloproteinase, gelatinase, by triggered human neutrophils. *Proc Natl Acad Sci U S A* 83:4322, 1986.
47. Ogata Y, Enghild JJ, Nagase H: Matrix metalloproteinase 3 (stromelysin) activates the precursor for the human matrix metalloproteinase 9. *J Biol Chem* 267:3581, 1992.
48. Van den Steen PE, Husson SJ, Proost P, et al: Carboxyterminal cleavage of the chemokines MIG and IP-10 by gelatinase B and neutrophil collagenase. *Biochem Biophys Res Commun* 310:889, 2003.
49. Van den Steen PE, Wuyts A, Husson SJ, et al: Gelatinase B/MMP-9 and neutrophil collagenase/MMP-8 process the chemokines human GCP-2/CXCL6, ENA-78/CXCL5 and mouse GCP-2/LIX and modulate their physiological activities. *Eur J Biochem* 270:3739, 2003.
50. Pelus LM, Bian H, King AG, et al: Neutrophil-derived MMP-9 mediates synergistic mobilization of hematopoietic stem and progenitor cells by the combination of G-CSF and the chemokines GRObeta/CXCL2 and GRObetaT/CXCL2delta4. *Blood* 103:110, 2004.
51. Kwiatkowska K, Sobota A: Signaling pathways in phagocytosis. *Bioessays* 21:422, 1999.
52. Lee WL, Harrison RE, Grinstein S: Phagocytosis by neutrophils. *Microbes Infect* 5:1299, 2003.
53. Hogarth PM: Fc receptors are major mediators of antibody based inflammation in autoimmunity. *Curr Opin Immunol* 14:798, 2002.
54. Amigorena S, Bonnerot C: Fc receptor signaling and trafficking: A connection for antigen processing. *Immunol Rev* 172:279, 1999.
55. Chuang FY, Sassaroli M, Unkeless JC: Convergence of Fc gamma receptor IIA and Fc gamma receptor IIIB signaling pathways in human neutrophils. *J Immunol* 164:350, 2000.
56. Petty HR, Worth RG, Todd RF, III: Interactions of integrins with their partner proteins in leukocyte membranes. *Immunol Res* 25:75, 2002.
57. Hamre R, Farstad IN, Brandtzaeg P, et al: Expression and modulation of the human immunoglobulin A Fc receptor (CD89) and the FcR gamma chain on myeloid cells in blood and tissue. *Scand J Immunol* 57:506, 2003.
58. Hoffmeyer F, Witte K, Schmidt RE: The high-affinity Fc gamma RI on PMN: Regulation of expression and signal transduction. *Immunology* 92:544, 1997.
59. Kakinoki Y, Kubota H, Yamamoto Y: CD64 surface expression on neutrophils and monocytes is significantly up-regulated after stimulation with granulocyte colony-stimulating factor during CHOP chemotherapy for patients with non-Hodgkin's lymphoma. *Int J Hematol* 79:55, 2004.
60. Pangburn MK, Rawal N: Structure and function of complement C5 convertase enzymes. *Biochem Soc Trans* 30:1006, 2002.
61. Sambandam T, Chatham WW: Ligation of CR1 attenuates Fc receptor-mediated myeloperoxidase release and HOCl production by neutrophils. *J Leukoc Biol* 63:477, 1998.
62. Ross GD: Role of the lectin domain of Mac-1/CR3 (CD11b/CD18) in regulating intercellular adhesion. *Immunol Res* 25:219, 2002.
63. Lindbom L, Werr J: Integrin-dependent neutrophil migration in extravascular tissue. *Semin Immunol* 14:115, 2002.
64. Takagi J, Springer TA: Integrin activation and structural rearrangement. *Immunol Rev* 186:141, 2002.
65. Hogg N, Henderson R, Leitinger B, et al: Mechanisms contributing to the activity of integrins on leukocytes. *Immunol Rev* 186:164, 2002.
66. McDowall A, Leitinger B, Stanley P, et al: The I domain of integrin leukocyte function-associated antigen-1 is involved in a conformational change leading to high affinity binding to ligand intercellular adhesion molecule 1 (ICAM-1). *J Biol Chem* 273:27396, 1998.
67. Grayson MH, Van der Vieren M, Sterbinsky SA, et al: Adb2 Integrin is expressed on human eosinophils and functions as an alternative ligand for vascular cell adhesion molecule 1 (VCAM-1). *J Exp Med* 188:2187, 1998.
68. Ortiz-Stern A, Rosales C: Cross-talk between Fc receptors and integrins. *Immunol Lett* 90:137, 2003.
69. Gonzalez-Amaro R, Sanchez-Madrid F: Cell adhesion molecules: Selectins and integrins. *Crit Rev Immunol* 19:389, 1999.
70. McEver RP, Cummings RD: Perspectives Series: Cell adhesion in vascular biology. Role of PSGL-1 binding to selectins in leukocyte recruitment. *J Clin Invest* 100:485, 1997.
71. Urzainqui A, Serrador JM, Viedma F, et al: ITAM-based interaction of ERM proteins with Syk mediates signaling by the leukocyte adhesion receptor PSGL-1. *Immunity* 17:401, 2002.
72. van Buul JD, Mul FP, Van der Schoot CE, et al: ICAM-3 activation modulates cell-cell contacts of human bone marrow endothelial cells. *J Vasc Res* 41:28, 2004.
73. Cicchetti G, Allen PG, Glogauer M: Chemotactic signaling pathways in neutrophils: From receptor to actin assembly. *Crit Rev Oral Biol Med* 13:220, 2002.
74. Paclet MH, Davis C, Kotsonis P, et al: *N*-Formyl peptide receptor subtypes in human neutrophils activate L-plastin phosphorylation through different signal transduction intermediates. *Biochem J* 377:469, 2004.
75. Bae YS, Yi HJ, Lee HY, et al: Differential activation of formyl peptide receptor-like 1 by peptide ligands. *J Immunol* 171:6807, 2003.
76. Bae YS, Park JC, He R, et al: Differential signaling of formyl peptide receptor-like 1 by Trp-Lys-Tyr-Met-Val-Met-CONH2 or lipoxin A4 in human neutrophils. *Mol Pharmacol* 64:721, 2003.
77. Wetsel RA: Structure, function and cellular expression of complement anaphylatoxin receptors. *Curr Opin Immunol* 7:48, 1995.
78. Cheng SS, Kunkel SL: The evolving role of the neutrophil in chemokine networks. *Chem Immunol Allergy* 83:81, 2003.
79. Ishii I, Izumi T, Tsukamoto H, et al: Alanine exchanges of polar amino acids in the transmembrane domains of a platelet-activating factor receptor generate both constitutively active and inactive mutants. *J Biol Chem* 272:7846, 1997.
80. Tager AM, Luster AD: BLT1 and BLT2: The leukotriene B(4) receptors. *Prostaglandins Leukot Essent Fatty Acids* 69:123, 2003.
81. Foxman EF, Kunkel EJ, Butcher EC: Integrating conflicting chemotactic signals. The role of memory in leukocyte navigation. *J Cell Biol* 147:577, 1999.
82. Endres G, Hegert L: Mineralzusammensetzung der bluplättchen und weissen blukörperchen. *Z Biol* 88:451, 1929.
83. Williams NR, Rajput-Williams J, West JA, et al: Plasma, granulocyte and mononuclear cell copper and zinc in patients with diabetes mellitus. *Analyst* 120:887, 1995.
84. Prasad AS, Mantzoros CS, Beck FW, et al: Zinc status and serum testosterone levels of healthy adults. *Nutrition* 12:344, 1996.
85. Loun B, Astles R, Copeland KR, et al: Intracellular magnesium content of mononuclear blood cells and granulocytes isolated from leukemic, infected, and granulocyte colony-stimulating factor-treated patients. *Clin Chem* 41:1768, 1995.
86. Rukgauer M, Zeyfang A, Uhland K, et al: Isolation of corpuscular components of whole blood for the determination of selenium in blood cells. *J Trace Elem Med Biol* 9:130, 1995.
87. Scott RB: Glycogen in human peripheral blood leukocytes. I. Characteristics of the synthesis and turnover of glycogen *in vitro*. *J Clin Invest* 47:344, 1968.
88. Scott RB, Still WJ: Glycogen in human peripheral blood leukocytes. II. The macromolecular state of leukocyte glycogen. *J Clin Invest* 47:353, 1968.
89. Esman V: The glycogen content of WBC from diabetic and nondiabetic subjects. *Scand J Clin Lab Invest* 13:134, 1961.
90. Rauch HC, Loomis ME, Johnson ME, et al: *In vitro* suppression of polymorphonuclear leukocyte and lymphocyte glycolysis by cortisol. *Endocrinology* 68:375, 1961.
91. Martin SP, McKinney GR, Green R, et al: The influence of glucose, fructose, and insulin on the metabolism of leukocytes of healthy and diabetic subjects. *J Clin Invest* 32:1171, 1953.
92. Gottfried EL: Lipids of human leukocytes: Relation to cell type. *J Lipid Res* 8:321, 1967.
93. Gottfried EL: Lipid patterns of leukocytes in health and disease. *Semin Hematol* 9:241, 1972.
94. Boyd EM: The lipid content of the white blood cells in normal young women. *J Biol Chem* 101:623, 1933.
95. Boyd EM, Stephens DJ: A comparison of lipid composition with differential count of the white blood cells. *Proc Soc Exp Biol Med* 33:558, 1936.
96. Kidson C: Relation of leucocyte lipid metabolism to cell age: Studies in infective leucocytosis. *Br J Exp Pathol* 42:597, 1961.
97. Nishizuka Y: Studies and perspectives of protein kinase C. *Science* 233:305, 1986.
98. Berridge MJ, Irvine RF: Inositol trisphosphate, a novel second messenger in cellular signal transduction. *Nature* 312:315, 1984.
99. Symington FW, Murray WA, Bearman SI, et al: Intracellular localization of lactosylceramide, the major human neutrophil glycosphingolipid. *J Biol Chem* 262:11356, 1987.
100. Thornalley PJ, Bellavite P: Modification of the glyoxalase system during the functional activation of human neutrophils. *Biochim Biophys Acta* 931:120, 1987.
101. McMenamy RH, Lund CC, Neville GJ, et al: Studies of unbound amino acid distributions in plasma, erythrocytes, leukocytes and urine of normal human subjects. *J Clin Invest* 39:1675, 1960.
102. Beutler E, Kuhl W. 1991. (Unpublished work)
103. Silber R, Gabrio BW, Huennekens FM: Studies on normal and leukemic leukocytes. III. Pyridine nucleotides. *J Clin Invest* 41:230, 1962.
104. Noyes BE, Mevarech M, Stein R, et al: Detection and partial sequence analysis of gastrin mRNA by using an oligodeoxynucleotide probe. *Proc Natl Acad Sci U S A* 76:1770, 1979.
105. Lohr GW, Waller HD: Zellstoffwechsel und zellaterung. *Klin Wochenschr* 37:833, 1959.
106. Willoughby HW, Waisman HA: Nucleic acid precursors and nucleotides in normal and leukemic blood. I. comparison of formic acid chromatograms. *Cancer Res* 17:942, 1957.
107. Silber R, Unger KW, Ellman L: RNA metabolism in normal and leukaemic leucocytes: Further studies on RNA synthesis. *Br J Haematol* 14:261, 1968.
108. Tryfiates GP, Laszlo J: Human leukemic polyribosomes. *Proc Soc Exp Biol Med* 124:1125, 1967.
109. Garcia AM, Iorio R: Studies on DNA in leukocytes and related cells of mammals. V. The fast green-histone and the Feulgen-DNA content of rat leukocytes. *Acta Cytol* 12:46, 1968.
110. Swendseid ME, Bethell FH, Bird OD: The concentration of folic acid in leukocytes; observations on normal subjects and persons with leukemia. *Cancer Res* 11:864, 1951.
111. Smits G, Florijn E: The aneurinpyrophosphate content of red and white blood corpuscles in the rat and in man, in various states of aneurin provision and in disease. *Biochim Biophys Acta* 3:44, 1949.

112. Boxer GE, Pruss MP, Goodhart RS: Pyridoxal-5-phosphoric acid in whole blood and isolated leukocytes of man and animals. *J Nutr* 63:623, 1957.
113. Barkhan P, Howard AN: Distribution of ascorbic acid in normal and leukaemic human blood. *Biochem J* 70:163, 1958.
114. Hoffbrand AV, Newcombe BF: Leucocyte folate in vitamin B12 and folate deficiency and in leukaemia. *Br J Haematol* 13:954, 1967.
115. Beck WS, Valentine WN: The aerobic carbohydrate metabolism of leukocytes in health and leukemia. I. Glycolysis and respiration. *Cancer Res* 12:818, 1952.
116. Beck WS: A kinetic analysis of the glycolytic rate and certain glycolytic enzymes in normal and leucemic leucocytes. *J Biol Chem* 216:333, 1955.
117. Borregaard N, Herlin T: Energy metabolism of human neutrophils during phagocytosis. *J Clin Invest* 70:550, 1982.
118. Beutler E, West C. 1993. (Unpublished work)
119. Fauth U, Schlechtriemen T, Heinrichs W, et al: The measurement of enzyme activities in the resting human polymorphonuclear leukocyte—Critical estimate of a method. *Eur J Clin Chem Clin Biochem* 31:5, 1993.
120. Lane TA, Beutler E, West C, et al: Glycolytic enzymes of stored granulocytes. *Transfusion* 24:153, 1984.
121. McKinney GR, Martin SP, Rundles RW, et al: Respiratory and glycolytic activities of human leukocytes *in vitro*. *J Appl Physiol* 5:335, 1953.
122. Stjernholm RL, Burns CP, Hohnadel JH: Carbohydrate metabolism by leukocytes. *Enzyme* 13:7, 1972.
123. Sbarra AJ, Karnovsky ML: The biochemical basis of phagocytosis. I. Metabolic changes during the ingestion of particles by polymorphonuclear leukocytes. *J Biol Chem* 234:1355, 1959.
124. Beck WS: Occurrence and control of the phosphogluconate oxidation pathway in normal and leukemic leukocytes. *J Biol Chem* 232:271, 1958.
125. Stjernholm RL, Manak RC: Carbohydrate metabolism in leukocytes. XIV. Regulation of pentose cycle activity and glycogen metabolism during phagocytosis. *J Reticuloendothel Soc* 8:550, 1970.
126. Wood HG, Katz J, Landau BR: Estimation of pathways of carbohydrate metabolism. *Biochem Z* 338:809, 1963.
127. Borregaard N, Juhl H: Activation of the glycogenolytic cascade in human polymorphonuclear leucocytes by different phagocytic stimuli. *Eur J Clin Invest* 11:257, 1981.
128. Wachstein M: The distribution of histochemically demonstrable glycogen in human blood and bone marrow cells. *Blood* 4:54, 1949.
129. Cassatella MA: Neutrophil-derived proteins: Selling cytokines by the pound. *Adv Immunol* 73:369, 1999.
130. Scapini P, Lapinet-Vera JA, Gasperini S, et al: The neutrophil as a cellular source of chemokines. *Immunol Rev* 177:195, 2000.
131. Boneberg EM, Hartung T: Molecular aspects of anti-inflammatory action of G-CSF. *Inflamm Res* 51:119, 2002.
132. Cloutier A, McDonald PP: Transcription factor activation in human neutrophils. *Chem Immunol Allergy* 83:1, 2003.
133. Gonzalez AL, El Bjeirami W, West JL, et al: Transendothelial migration enhances integrin-dependent human neutrophil chemokinesis. *J Leukoc Biol* 81:686, 2007.
134. Girard D: Phenotypic and functional change of neutrophils activated by cytokines utilizing the common cytokine receptor gamma chain. *Chem Immunol Allergy* 83:64, 2003.
135. Tsukahara Y, Lian Z, Zhang X, et al: Gene expression in human neutrophils during activation and priming by bacterial lipopolysaccharide. *J Cell Biochem* 89:848, 2003.
136. Malcolm KC, Arndt PG, Manos EJ, et al: Microarray analysis of lipopolysaccharide-treated human neutrophils. *Am J Physiol Lung Cell Mol Physiol* 284:L663, 2003.
137. Theilgaard-Monch K, Knudsen S, Follin P, et al: The transcriptional activation program of human neutrophils in skin lesions supports their important role in wound healing. *J Immunol* 172:7684, 2004.
138. Kobayashi SD, Voyich JM, Braughton KR, et al: Gene expression profiling provides insight into the pathophysiology of chronic granulomatous disease. *J Immunol* 172:636, 2004.
139. Kobayashi SD, Voyich JM, Braughton KR, et al: Down-regulation of proinflammatory capacity during apoptosis in human polymorphonuclear leukocytes. *J Immunol* 170:3357, 2003.

CHAPTER 61
PRODUCTION, DISTRIBUTION, AND FATE OF NEUTROPHILS

C. Wayne Smith

SUMMARY

Blood neutrophil levels are maintained in a normal steady state by neutropoiesis in the marrow, the distribution of neutrophils between the marginated pool in the microvasculature and the freely circulating pool in the blood, and the rate of egress from blood to tissues. Marrow production of neutrophils is regulated by three principal glycoprotein hormones, or cytokines: interleukin-3, granulocyte-monocyte colony-stimulating factor, and granulocyte colony-stimulating factor. The latter two cytokines are available as recombinant pharmaceutical products that can be administered therapeutically to ameliorate certain causes of neutropenia. Neutrophil interaction with endothelium is mediated by selectins, glycoproteins with sugar-binding sites that support shear-dependent rolling on endothelium, and by integrins on the neutrophil binding to ligands on the endothelial cells, permitting firm attachment to endothelium and emigration into tissues. Neutrophils have a short life span in blood, with a disappearance half-time of approximately 7 hours. The process can be accelerated when inflammation is present and highlights the need for a sustained rate of production to maintain a normal blood neutrophil count. The pathogenesis of neutropenia is more complex to analyze kinetically than anemia or thrombocytopenia because at least four compartments are involved: marrow storage pool, circulating pool, marginated pool, and tissue pool. The latter is particularly difficult to assay. Measurements can be further complicated in the nonsteady state, when dramatic increases in turnover rates and distribution among the four principal pools are in disequilibrium, as occurs during acute inflammatory states.

DEFINITION AND HISTORY

Neutrophils are produced in the marrow, where they arise from progenitor and precursor cells by a process of cellular proliferation and maturation. They differentiate from the pluripotential stem cell[1,2] through a series of progressively more committed progenitor or colony-forming units, including the granulocyte-monocyte colony-forming unit and the granulocyte colony-forming unit, which give rise to neutrophils.[3,4] The early progenitor cells cannot be recognized under the microscope but can be identified by marrow culture (see Chaps. 4 and 16). The earliest microscopically recognizable neutrophil precursor is the myeloblast. From there, the formal sequence of precursor development is myeloblast → promyelocyte → myelocyte → metamyelocyte → band neutrophil → segmented neutrophil (see Chap. 59). The term *granulocyte* often is loosely used to refer to neutrophils, but strictly speaking includes eosinophils and basophils. Eosinophilic (see Chap. 62) and basophilic (see Chap. 63) granulocytes develop from progenitors in a manner analogous to the neutrophils, although commitment to neutrophilic, eosinophilic, or basophilic development probably is established at an early progenitor stage.

Acronyms and abbreviations that appear in this chapter include: β_2-integrin, a member of family of receptors that mediate attachment between a cell and the tissues surrounding it; C5a, chemotactic fragment of complement component C5; CD, one of the cluster of differentiation antigens; CNP, circulating neutrophil pool; CSF, colony-stimulating factor; DF^{32}P, diisopropyl fluorophosphate; G-CSF, granulocyte colony-stimulating factor; GM-CSF, granulocyte-monocyte colony-stimulating factor; IL, interleukin; L-selectin (and other selectins), a member of selectin family of proteins, which are leukocyte cell adhesion molecules; MB, myeloblasts; MNP, marginal neutrophil pool; Mr, relative molecular mass; NTR, neutrophil turnover rate; PMN, polymorphonuclear neutrophils; $T_{1/2}$, half-time; TBNP, total blood neutrophil pool; TNF-α, tumor necrosis factor-α.

The normal human neutrophil production rate is 0.85 to 1.6×10^9 cells/kg per day. Mature neutrophils are stored in the marrow before they are released into the blood. They leave the circulation randomly, with a half-disappearance time of approximately 7 hours. The cells then enter the tissues and probably function for 1 or 2 days before their death or loss into the gastrointestinal tract through mucosal surfaces.

The neutropoietic system has a high production volume, yet it is finely modulated in the steady state and has a great capacity to increase production in response to inflammatory stimuli. This chapter outlines current concepts of neutrophil production, distribution, and survival. For detailed data and methods, the reader is referred to original articles and reviews on neutropoiesis and neutrophil kinetics.[5–17]

REGULATION OF NEUTROPHILIC GRANULOPOIESIS

Although the primary cellular manifestation of commitment is the expression of receptors for lineage-specific hematopoietins, the "decision" for a stem cell to self-renew or differentiate may be partly a random or stochastic event.[1,18] On the other hand, stromal elements, collectively referred to as the *hematopoietic microenvironment*, release short-range signals that regulate the process of commitment from multipotential stem cell pools (see Chap. 4). Although many details of hematopoietic stem cell regulation (see Chap. 16) remain to be elucidated, much is known regarding the interaction of hematopoietic cytokines with their receptors and actions on the committed granulocyte progenitor cells and their mature progeny.[19–24]

HUMORAL REGULATORS

The humoral regulators involved in granulopoiesis have been defined by *in vitro* culture systems.[20,21] Originally identified by their ability to stimulate colony formation from marrow progenitor cells, the hemopoietins (cytokines) came to be called *colony-stimulating factors* (CSF).[25] With regard to neutrophil production, at least four human CSFs have been defined. Granulocyte-monocyte colony-stimulating factor (GM-CSF) is a 22,000 relative molecular mass (Mr) glycoprotein that stimulates the production of neutrophils, monocytes, and eosinophils. Granulocyte colony-stimulating factor (G-CSF) has an Mr of 20,000 and stimulates only the production of neutrophils. Interleukin-3 (IL-3), or multi-CSF, also has an Mr of 20,000 and acts relatively early in hematopoiesis, affecting pluripotential stem cells. Finally, stem cell factor (also known as c-*kit* ligand or steel factor), with an Mr of 28,000, acts in combination with IL-3 and/or GM-CSF to stimulate the proliferation of the early hematopoietic progenitor cells. In addition to their effects on neutrophil precursors, G-CSF and GM-CSF act directly on the neutrophil, enhancing its function. These cytokines regulate the production, survival, and functional activity of neutrophils.[21,22,26–28] The mature neutrophil lacks IL-3 receptors and, thus, is not affected by IL-3. However, IL-3 receptors are present on mature eosinophils and monocytes. IL-3 is produced by activated T lymphocytes and thus is expected to have a physiologic role in circumstances of cell-mediated immunity. GM-CSF also is produced by activated lymphocytes. However, like G-CSF, it also is elaborated by mononuclear phagocytes and endothelial and mesenchymal cells when these cell types are stimulated by certain cytokines, including IL-1, tumor necrosis factor, and bacterial products, such as endotoxin.[29–31] Stem cell factor is secreted by a variety of cells, including marrow stromal cells,[32,33] and affects the development of several kinds of tissues.[32,34]

The activities of exogenously administered biosynthetic (recombinant) human G-CSF and GM-CSF in humans are well documented.[22,27,35–37] G-CSF administration rapidly induces neutrophilia, whereas GM-CSF causes an increase in neutrophils, eosinophils, and monocytes. Because GM-CSF cannot be detected easily in normal plasma, its role as a day-to-day, long-range modulator of neutrophil production is uncertain. Mice in which the GM-CSF gene is "knocked out" have generally normal hematopoiesis but show macrophage abnormalities, pulmonary alveolar proteinosis, and decreased resistance to microbial challenge.[38–41] However, G-CSF appears to be a critical regulator of neutrophil development, as giving an animal an antibody to G-CSF leads to profound neutropenia.[42] The G-CSF knockout mouse shows severe neutropenia.[43] Neutropenia that results from a production disturbance, such as exposure to cytotoxic drugs, is associated with high circulating serum concentrations of G-CSF.[44]

NEUTROPHIL KINETICS

Methods used to study granulocyte kinetics can be categorized as follows: (1) neutrophil depletion or destruction to determine the size and rate of mobilization of reserves and the level of compensatory neutropoiesis; (2) use of radioactive tracers to study neutrophil distribution, production rates, and survival times; (3) mitotic indices of marrow granulocytic cells to assess proliferative activity and cell-cycle times; and (4) induced inflammatory lesions to study cell movement into the tissues. Of these categories, the most popular has been the use of radioactive tracers.

Neutrophil production and neutrophil kinetics usually are analyzed by describing neutrophil movement through a number of interconnected compartments. These compartments can be arranged into three major groups: the marrow, the blood, and the tissue (Fig. 61–1).

THE MARROW

Marrow neutrophils can be divided into the mitotic, or proliferative, compartment (see Fig. 61–1) and the maturation storage compartment. Myeloblasts, promyelocytes, and myelocytes are capable of replication and constitute the mitotic compartment. Earlier progenitor cells are few in number, not morphologically identifiable, and usually neglected in kinetic studies. Metamyelocytes, bands, and mature neutrophils, none of which replicate, constitute the maturation storage compartment.

The number of cell divisions from the myeloblast to the myelocyte stage in the proliferative compartment is estimated to be between four and five.[45] Data obtained using radioactive diisopropyl fluorophosphate ($DF^{32}P$) suggest the existence of three divisions at the myelocyte stage, but the number of cell divisions at each step may not be constant. The major increase in neutrophil number probably occurs at the myelocyte level, because the myelocyte pool is at least four times the size of the promyelocyte pool. Because of the difficulties in measuring human intramarrow neutrophil kinetics, a precise model of the dynamics of the mitotic compartment is not available.

Table 61–1 lists the estimated sizes of the marrow neutrophil compartments and the transit times and cell-cycle stages of the cells in the various compartments. Precise studies have measured a postmitotic pool of $(5.59 \pm 0.9) \times 10^9$ cells/kg and a mitotic pool (promyelocytes and myelocytes) of $(2.11 \pm 0.36) \times 10^9$ cells/kg. These studies led to a calculated normal marrow neutrophil production of 0.85×10^9 cells/kg per day. Radioautographic studies with [^{3}H]thymidine support the concept of an orderly progression from metamyelocytes to mature neutrophils within the maturation storage compartment. These studies also suggest a "first in, first out" pattern for cells leaving this compartment and entering the blood. Several labeling techniques indicate the myelocyte-to-blood transit time is 5 to 7 days.[12,46] Previous studies with $DF^{32}P$ reported a range from 8 to 14 days.[9,45] During infections, however, the myelocyte-to-blood transit time may be as short as 48 hours.[47]

Whether the production of neutrophils in the mitotic compartment exactly equals the neutrophil turnover rate (NTR) is not known with certainty. Studies in dogs suggest some immature neutrophils die in the marrow ("ineffective granulopoiesis").[48] Ineffective granulopoiesis has not been shown in normal humans,[14,49] although ineffective granulopoiesis occurs in some pathologic states. In the myelodysplastic syndromes,[50] substantial intramedullary cell death (see Chap. 88) probably occurs, as may occur in myelofibrosis (see Chap. 91) and some of the idiopathic neutropenic disorders (see Chap. 65). At present, however, no convenient means of quantitating ineffective granulopoiesis is available.

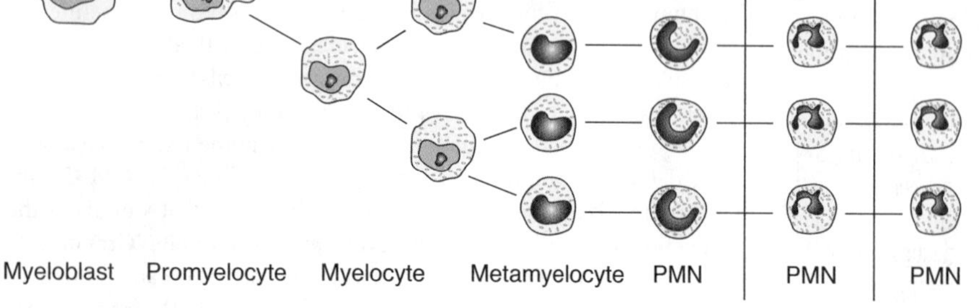

FIGURE 61–1. Scheme of maturation of neutrophil precursor cells. The myeloblast is the first recognizable precursor of neutrophils. Myeloblasts undergo division and maturation into promyelocytes and thereafter into neutrophilic myelocytes, after which stage mitotic capability is lost. The major compartments of precursor proliferation and distribution are indicated across the top of the figure: marrow, blood, and tissues. The marrow precursor compartment is made up of the proliferating compartment (myeloblasts through myelocytes) and the maturation and storage compartment (metamyelocytes) to mature polymorphonuclear neutrophils (PMN). Under normal conditions, cells do not return from the tissue compartment to the blood or marrow.

TABLE 61–1. Marrow Neutrophil Kinetics

	Fraction in Mitosis (Mitotic Index)	Fraction in DNA Synthesis (S Phase)	Transit Time Range (h)	Total Cells (× 10^9/kg)
Mitotic compartment				
Myeloblast	0.025	0.85	23	0.14
Promyelocyte	0.015	0.65	26–78	0.51
Myelocyte	0.011	0.33	17–126	1.95
Maturation storage compartment				
Metamyelocyte			8–108	2.7
Band			12–96	3.6
Polymorphonuclear neutrophil			0–120	2.5

On completion of maturation, the neutrophils are stored in the marrow and are referred to as the *mature neutrophil reserve.* The reserve contains many more cells than are normally circulating in the blood. Table 61–2 lists comparative data on the characteristics of the maturation storage compartment. Under stress, maturation time may be shortened, divisions may be skipped, and release into the blood may occur prematurely.

THE BLOOD

The total blood neutrophil pool (TBNP) consists of all the neutrophils in the vascular spaces. Some of these neutrophils are free in the circulation (the circulating pool), while others roll along the endothelium of small vessels or are temporarily sequestered in the alveolar capillaries of the lung (the marginated pool).[51,52] Cells in the two pools are freely exchangeable. When neutrophils labeled with $DF^{32}P$ are injected into normal subjects, approximately half can be accounted for in the circulating pool; the remainder enters the marginated pool.[5–7] Neutrophils shift from the marginated to the circulating pool with exercise, epinephrine injection, or stress, but eventually the neutrophils leave the blood and enter the tissues. Once the neutrophils enter the tissues, they do not normally return to the blood. The flow of cells is unidirectional.

Rate of Neutrophil Disappearance

$DF^{32}P$-labeled neutrophils disappear from the circulation with a half-time ($T_{1/2}$) of 6.7 hours.[7,53,54] These data are supported by the finding that more than half of Pelger-Huët cells infused into a normal individual disappeared after 6 to 8 hours.[55] Data obtained with ^{51}Cr-labeled neutrophils give substantially longer half-times.[56] The exponential disappearance of cells from the blood suggests the cells leave in a random manner. Thus, neutrophils newly released from the marrow are as likely to leave the blood as are neutrophils that have been circulating for several hours. Neutrophils also are eliminated by programmed cell death and disposed of by the macrophage system.[47,57–59]

Direct observations of blood vessels have revealed some degree of leukocyte rolling along the endothelium (first observed many years ago by Atherton and Born). Although the observation has been clearly confirmed by numerous laboratories in different species of animals, the extent to which this phenomenon contributes to the marginated pool of neutrophils is uncertain.

TABLE 61–2. Comparative Data on Marrow Maturation Storage Compartment

Size (Cells × 10^9 kg)	Transit Time (Days)	Measurement Technique	Reference
6.5–13	4–8	[^{3}H]thymidine, *in vitro* $DF^{32}P$	5
3–23	8–14	*In vivo* and *in vitro* $DF^{32}P$	45
5.6	6.6	^{59}Fe and neutrophil-to-erythroid ratio	14

The Marginated Pool

A more compelling concept of the marginated pool is derived from investigations of the vascular bed of the lung. A distinctive characteristic of this tissue is the complex interconnecting network of short capillary segments where the path from arteriole to venule crosses several alveolar walls (often >8) and often contains more than 50 capillary segments.[60–64] Compared to blood in the large vessels of most vascular beds, the blood in this complex network contains approximately 50-fold more neutrophils and even more lymphocytes and monocytes.[65] Videomicroscopic study of these vessels in animal models has revealed the transit of neutrophils through this network required a median time of 26 seconds and mean time of 6.1 seconds.[66,67] In contrast, the transit times of red blood cells ranges from 1.4 to 4.2 seconds. The increased transit time results primarily from the time neutrophils are stopped within this vascular network. The longer time required for the neutrophils to pass through this bed apparently accounts for their increased concentration.

Recruitment of neutrophils into the lungs through the alveolar capillary network contrasts with the recruitment of neutrophils through postcapillary venules at sites of inflammation. The tethering mechanisms required to capture neutrophils from flowing blood in larger vessels apparently are not necessary in the alveolar capillary bed. The diameters of spherical neutrophils (6–8 μm) are larger than the diameters of many capillary segments (2–15 μm). Approximately 50 percent of the capillary segments would require neutrophils to change their shape in order to pass through.[67–70] Given the large number of capillary segments through which a neutrophil must pass (often >50), most neutrophils must change shape during transit from arteriole to venule. Morphometric analysis of neutrophils in the alveolar capillary beds has revealed significant deviation from spherical shape.[67,68] Computational models of the capillary bed describing flow, hematocrit, pressure gradients, and the effects of deformation on the capillary transit times of neutrophils support the concept that the structure of the capillary bed and the deformation of neutrophils are critical under normal conditions. Thus, the enormous lung vascular bed contains a substantial number of neutrophils that can be mobilized into the systemic circulation with stimuli such as epinephrine or exercise.

During inflammation, much of the sequestration and infiltration occur through vessels so narrow that physical tapping is sufficient to stop the flowing neutrophil.[63,67,71,72] Binding of mediators such as chemotactic factors (e.g., C5a, the chemotactic fragment of complement component C5) to neutrophil receptors induces a transient resistance of the cells to deformation.[73–78] Because neutrophils must deform to pass through the capillary bed, leukocyte activation by inflammatory mediators could affect further concentration of neutrophils at the alveolar walls.[60,71] The role of mechanical factors in the initial sequestration of neutrophils in the alveolar capillaries is supported by evidence that neither L-selectin nor β_2 integrins are required.[71,79,80] In contrast, both selectins and β_2 integrins are required for localization of neutrophils in postcapillary venules at sites of inflammation.

The events following the initial sequestration of neutrophils within alveolar capillary beds apparently are influenced by adhesion molecules. For example, simple systemic activation of neutrophils by intravenous injection of chemotactic factors (e.g., IL-8 or C5a) results in rapid (<1 minute) neutropenia with massive sequestration of neutrophils within alveolar capillaries. This event is not dependent on L-selectin or β_2 integrins, but the retention times within this capillary bed are influenced by these adhesion molecules.[71,80] Adhesion likely is an interaction of leukocyte adhesion molecules and endothelial adhesion molecules. Blockade of the adhesive mechanism (e.g., using blocking monoclonal antibodies) results in release of neutrophils from the lungs.[71,79,81–83] Mediator-induced decreases in deformability are temporally correlated with upregulation of β_2 integrins (e.g., both occurring within approximately 1 minute of exposure to IL-8). This allows both physical trapping and sticking to the vascular wall within the alveolar capillary bed. A similar phenomenon occurs in the liver where sequestration is the result of physical trapping and liver injury is heavily dependent on adhesion of leukocytes through the β_2 integrins.[84]

Neutrophil Turnover Rate

Assuming a random loss of neutrophils from the blood, NTR can be calculated from $T_{1/2}$ and TBNP: NTR = 0.693 × TBNP/$T_{1/2}$. In the steady state, NTR measures the rate of effective neutrophil production. Table 61–3 lists the definitions and calculations related to blood neutrophil kinetics. Table 61–4 lists data for normal human blood neutrophil kinetics. The high production rate of neutrophils under normal conditions is remarkable, especially given that the rate may increase several fold in response to inflammatory stimuli.

Effect of Glucocorticoids and Epinephrine

Glucocorticoids increase TBNP by increasing influx from the marrow and decreasing efflux from the circulation. Five hours after a pharmacologic dose of glucocorticoid, the neutrophil count increases by approximately 4000/μL because of release from the marrow, demargination, and prolongation of $T_{1/2}$ to approximately 10 hours.[85–87] Consistent with the increase in $T_{1/2}$, prednisone reduces the accumulation of neutrophils at induced sites of skin inflammation.[70] With alternate-day, single-dose prednisone, neutrophil counts and kinetics are normal 24 hours after administration and during the day off.[88] Endotoxin causes a prompt neutropenia as a result of cell margination and sequestration, followed in 2 to 4 hours by a rebound neutrophilia as a result of cell release from the marrow. The size of the neutrophilic response correlates with the functional marrow reserves.[89–92] After epinephrine administration, a peak leukocytosis occurs in 5 to 10 minutes and rarely lasts more than 20 minutes. This finding reflects a shift of cells from the marginated to the circulating pool.

TABLE 61–3. Definitions and Calculations Relating to Blood Neutrophil Kinetics

Circulating neutrophil pool (CNP)	Blood neutrophil concentration × blood volume
Total blood neutrophil pool (TBNP)	All neutrophils in the circulation
Marginal neutrophil pool (MNP)	Total blood neutrophil pool less circulating pool (MNP = TBNP – CNP)
Blood clearance half-time ($T_{1/2}$)	Disappearance time of half the labeled neutrophils from circulation
Neutrophil turnover rate (NTR)	$\frac{0.693 \times \text{TBNP}}{T_{1/2}}$

TABLE 61–4. Data for Human Blood Neutrophil Kinetics

Pool	Mean Pool Size × 10^7 kg	95% Limits
TBNP	70	14–160
CNP	31	11–46
MNP	39	0–85
	Mean Value	**95% Limits**
Blood clearance $T_{1/2}$	6.7 h	4–10 h
NTR	63 × 10^7 kg/day	50–340 × 10^7 kg/day

MIGRATION OF NEUTROPHILS INTO TISSUES

The migration of neutrophils from blood into tissue at sites of inflammation involves a series of sequential adhesive steps proceeding from tethering (rolling adhesion) on endothelium under shear conditions in postcapillary venules.[93] This model has been investigated in a variety of vascular beds[94] and *in vitro* with monolayers of endothelial cells in parallel plate flow chambers.[93] The tethering event in this model depends on adhesion molecules in the selectin family, E-selectin and P-selectin on the endothelium, L-selectin on the neutrophil, and ligands for the selectins expressed on both cell types. These adhesion molecules are necessary to efficiently initiate the cascade of adhesive steps ultimately leading to firm attachment of the neutrophils to endothelium. The cascade appears to be necessary for neutrophils to move from blood to tissues because the unstimulated neutrophil is not adhesive to endothelium.[93,95] The integrins necessary for firm adhesion and cell locomotion require stimulation to promote sufficient increases in avidity or affinity to support these functions.

LIFE SPAN OF NEUTROPHILS

After emigrating into tissue, the life span of neutrophils can be significantly prolonged (24–48 hours).[96] Programmed cell death (apoptosis) accounts for significant removal of tissue neutrophils through phagocytosis by macrophages. The constitutive rate of apoptosis of neutrophils is altered by inflammatory cytokines and chemokines. For example, tumor necrosis factor-α (TNF-α) accelerates the rate, but endotoxin, G-CSF, GM-CSF, IL-15, and IL-3 inhibit the rate of apoptosis. The balance of these effects at specific inflammatory sites is poorly understood, but the functional life of neutrophils in tissue appears to be controlled by the rate of apoptosis. Apoptotic neutrophils lose the ability to release granular enzymes in response to external stimuli (see below), and marked changes in cell surface proteins occur (e.g., CD16, CD43, CD62L are greatly reduced). Although the loss of responsiveness may contribute to resolution of the inflammatory process, evidence indicates macrophages also are altered by the phagocytosis of apoptotic neutrophils. In contrast to the macrophage response to phagocytosis of microbes, where secretion of proinflammatory cytokines (e.g., IL-1β) and chemokines (e.g., IL-8) is stimulated, phagocytosis of apoptotic neutrophils fails to provoke secretion of proinflammatory factors; instead, phagocytosis stimulates release of factors that may suppress inflammatory responses (e.g., transforming growth factor-β and prostaglandin E_2). Macrophage recognition of apoptotic neutrophils is partially understood to involve the vitronectin receptor $\alpha_V\beta_3$ and the thrombospondin receptor CD36 on the macrophage surface. In addition, phosphatidylserine residues on the neutrophil are involved.

As Chap. 60 noted, neutrophils are capable of phenotypic changes depending on the tissue and cytokine/chemokine milieu at the time of their migration into tissue. Because our understanding of neutrophil physiology is relatively new, knowing the extent of this phenomenon on neutrophil life span in tissues is not possible at present.

EVALUATION OF ADEQUACY OF NEUTROPHIL RESERVES

WHITE CELL COUNT AND MARROW CELLULARITY

White cell and absolute neutrophil counts are the most widely used guides to the status of neutrophil production. They are useful in evaluating the effects of cytotoxic chemotherapy, although they do not provide quantitative information on the rate of neutrophil production or destruction, the status of marrow reserves, or the presence of abnormalities in cell distribution.

Gauging neutrophil production by the appearance of marrow films, clot sections, or biopsies suffers from the limitations of sampling error and relatively poor correlation with kinetics, as measured by other techniques.[63] For example, the morphologic findings in the marrow of a "maturation arrest," with little neutrophil development beyond the promyelocyte or myelocyte stage, does not distinguish between a defect in precursor cell maturation and rapid mobilization of postmitotic cells from the marrow. Similarly, distinguishing by purely morphologic means neutropenic conditions resulting from ineffective neutropoiesis from conditions caused by peripheral destruction of neutrophils often is difficult. However, despite these limitations, when the absolute neutrophil count and marrow cellularity are used together, they provide a useful guide in most clinical settings. If the absolute neutrophil count is less than 1000/μL (1.0×10^9/L) and multiple marrow aspirations and/or biopsies are hypocellular, the patient almost invariably has impaired production of marrow neutrophils. Very low neutrophil counts predispose to infections by bacteria and certain fungi (e.g., *Candida* and *Aspergillus*). Such infections become especially troublesome as the neutrophil count falls below 500/μL (0.5×10^9/L). Unfortunately, the converse is not true. The finding of cellular marrow and neutrophil count greater than 1000/μL ($>1.0 \times 10^9$/L) does not mean production is normal. Nevertheless, when marrow cellularity and absolute neutrophil count are considered together, they provide the most clinically useful assessment of neutrophil production.

FUNCTIONAL EVALUATION

Several agents that increase neutrophil numbers in circulation, including glucocorticoids, endotoxin, and etiocholanolone, have been used to evaluate neutrophil reserves in a clinical setting. These agents have been supplanted by recombinant human G-CSF, a remarkably nontoxic cytokine that, when given in therapeutic doses (5–8 mcg/kg), increases the blood neutrophil count by stimulating neutropoiesis and accelerating neutrophil release from the marrow storage compartment (see Chap. 16). The increase in neutropoiesis results from a threefold increase in the number of cell divisions in the mitotic compartment and shortening of the maturation time from myelocyte to neutrophil from 4 to 5 days to less than 1 day.[97,98] Thus, as a byproduct of its therapeutic action, G-CSF administration directly tests an individual's capacity to produce neutrophils. This effect of G-CSF makes obsolete most of the older methods for evaluating neutrophil compartments.

G-CSF does not test the distribution of neutrophils between the marginated and circulating pools. On the rare occasions when such information is desirable, epinephrine stimulation can be used to assess the distribution. For this purpose, epinephrine 0.1 mg is infused intravenously over 5 minutes, and blood for white counts is obtained before and 1, 3, and 5 minutes after completion of the epinephrine infusion. Normally the neutrophils increase by approximately 50 percent after epinephrine infusion.[99]

REFERENCES

1. Kondo M, Wagers AJ, Manz MG, et al: Biology of hematopoietic stem cells and progenitors: Implications for clinical application. *Annu Rev Immunol* 21:759, 2003.
2. Spangrude GJ: When is a stem cell really a stem cell? *Bone Marrow Transplant* 32 Suppl 1:S7, 2003.
3. Smaaland R, Sothern RB, Laerum OD, et al: Rhythms in human bone marrow and blood cells. *Chronobiol Int* 19:101, 2002.
4. Metcalf D: Hematopoietic stem cells: Old and new. *Biomed Pharmacother* 55:75, 2001.
5. Athens JW: Neutrophilic granulocyte kinetics and granulopoiesis, in *Regulation of Hematopoiesis*, edited by AS Gordon, p 1143. Appleton-Century-Crofts, New York, 1961.
6. Athens JW, Raab SO, Haab OP, et al: Leukokinetic studies. III. The distribution of granulocytes in the blood of normal subjects. *J Clin Invest* 40:159, 1961.
7. Athens JW, Haab OP, Raab SO, et al: Leukokinetic studies. IV. The total blood, circulating and marginal granulocyte pools and the granulocyte turnover rate in normal subjects. *J Clin Invest* 40:989, 1961.
8. Boggs DR: The kinetics of neutrophilic leukocytes in health and in disease. *Semin Hematol* 4:359, 1967.
9. Cartwright GE, Athens JW, Boggs DR, et al: The kinetics of granulopoiesis in normal man. *Ser Haematol* 1:1, 1965.
10. Cronkite EP: Kinetics of granulocytopoiesis. *Clin Haematol* 8:351, 1979.
11. Cronkite EP, Fliedner TM: Granulocytopoiesis. *N Engl J Med* 270:1347, 1964.
12. Vincent PC: The measurement of granulocyte kinetics. *Br J Haematol* 36:1, 1977.
13. Donohue DM, Gabrio BW, Finch CA: Quantitative measurement of hematopoietic cells of the marrow. *J Clin Invest* 37:1564, 1958.
14. Dancey JT, Deubelbeiss KA, Harker LA, et al: Neutrophil kinetics in man. *J Clin Invest* 58:705, 1976.
15. Friedman AD: Transcriptional regulation of granulocyte and monocyte development. *Oncogene* 21:3377, 2002.
16. Simon HU: Neutrophil apoptosis pathways and their modifications in inflammation. *Immunol Rev* 193:101, 2003.
17. Kuijpers TW: Clinical symptoms and neutropenia: The balance of neutrophil development, functional activity, and cell death. *Eur J Pediatr* 161(Suppl 1):S75, 2002.
18. Ogawa M: Changing phenotypes of hematopoietic stem cells. *Exp Hematol* 30:3, 2002.
19. Friedman AD: Transcriptional regulation of myelopoiesis. *Int J Hematol* 75:466, 2002.
20. Eash KJ, Means JM, White DW, et al: CXCR4 is a key regulator of neutrophil release from the bone marrow under basal and stress granulopoiesis conditions. *Blood* 113:4711, 2009.
21. Skokowa J, Welte K: LEF-1 is a decisive transcription factor in neutrophil granulopoiesis. *Ann N Y Acad Sci* 1106:143, 2007.
22. Fievez L, Desmet C, Henry E, et al: STAT5 is an ambivalent regulator of neutrophil homeostasis. *PLoS ONE* 2:e727, 2007.
23. Velu CS, Baktula AM, Grimes HL: Gfi1 regulates miR-21 and miR-196b to control myelopoiesis. *Blood* 113:4720, 2009.
24. Ai J, Druhan LJ, Loveland MJ, et al: G-CSFR ubiquitination critically regulates myeloid cell survival and proliferation. *PLoS ONE* 3:e3422, 2008.
25. Barreda DR, Hanington PC, Belosevic M: Regulation of myeloid development and function by colony stimulating factors. *Dev Comp Immunol* 28:509, 2004.
26. Panopoulos AD, Watowich SS: Granulocyte colony-stimulating factor: Molecular mechanisms of action during steady state and "emergency" hematopoiesis. *Cytokine* 42:277, 2008.
27. von Vietinghoff S, Ley K: Homeostatic regulation of blood neutrophil counts. *J Immunol* 181:5183, 2008.
28. Touw IP, van de Geijn GJ: Granulocyte colony-stimulating factor and its receptor in normal myeloid cell development, leukemia and related blood cell disorders. *Front Biosci* 12:800, 2007.

29. McGettrick AF, O'Neill LA: Toll-like receptors: Key activators of leucocytes and regulator of haematopoiesis. *Br J Haematol* 139:185, 2007.
30. Zucali JR, Dinarello CA, Oblon DJ, et al: Interleukin 1 stimulates fibroblasts to produce granulocyte-macrophage colony-stimulating activity and prostaglandin E_2. *J Clin Invest* 77:1857, 1986.
31. Metcalf D, Nicola NA, Mifsud S, et al: Receptor clearance obscures the magnitude of granulocyte-macrophage colony-stimulating factor responses in mice to endotoxin or local infections. *Blood* 93:1579, 1999.
32. Akin C, Metcalfe DD: The biology of Kit in disease and the application of pharmacogenetics. *J Allergy Clin Immunol* 114:13, 2004.
33. Heissig B, Werb Z, Rafii S, et al: Role of c-kit/Kit ligand signaling in regulating vasculogenesis. *Thromb Haemost* 90:570, 2003.
34. Wehrle-Haller B: The role of Kit-ligand in melanocyte development and epidermal homeostasis. *Pigment Cell Res* 16:287, 2003.
35. Lalami Y, Paesmans M, Aoun M, et al: A prospective randomised evaluation of G-CSF or G-CSF plus oral antibiotics in chemotherapy-treated patients at high risk of developing febrile neutropenia. *Support Care Cancer* 12:725, 2004.
36. De Waele M, Renmans W, Asosingh K, et al: Growth factor receptor profile of CD34 cells in normal bone marrow, cord blood and mobilized peripheral blood. *Eur J Haematol* 72:193, 2004.
37. Crawford J: Neutrophil growth factors. *Curr Hematol Rep* 1:95, 2002.
38. LeVine AM, Reed JA, Kurak KE, et al: GM-CSF-deficient mice are susceptible to pulmonary group B streptococcal infection. *J Clin Invest* 103:563, 1999.
39. Dranoff G, Crawford AD, Sadelain M, et al: Involvement of granulocyte-macrophage colony-stimulating factor in pulmonary homeostasis. *Science* 264:713, 1994.
40. Stanley E, Lieschke GJ, Grail D, et al: Granulocyte/macrophage colony-stimulating factor-deficient mice show no major perturbation of hematopoiesis but develop a characteristic pulmonary pathology. *Proc Natl Acad Sci U S A* 91:5592, 1994.
41. Huffman JA, Hull WM, Dranoff G, et al: Pulmonary epithelial cell expression of GM-CSF corrects the alveolar proteinosis in GM-CSF–deficient mice. *J Clin Invest* 97:649, 1996.
42. Hammond WP, Csiba E, Canin A, et al: Chronic neutropenia. A new canine model induced by human granulocyte colony-stimulating factor. *J Clin Invest* 87:704, 1991.
43. Lieschke GJ, Grail D, Hodgson G, et al: Mice lacking granulocyte colony-stimulating factor have chronic neutropenia, granulocyte and macrophage progenitor cell deficiency, and impaired neutrophil mobilization. *Blood* 84:1737, 1994.
44. Mempel K, Pietsch T, Menzel T, et al: Increased serum levels of granulocyte colony-stimulating factor in patients with severe congenital neutropenia. *Blood* 77:1919, 1991.
45. Warner HR, Athens JW: An analysis of granulocyte kinetics in blood and bone marrow. *Ann N Y Acad Sci* 113:523, 1964.
46. Dresch C, Faille A, Bauchet J, et al: Granulopoiesis: Comparison of different methods for studying maturation time and bone marrow storage. *Nouv Rev Fr Hematol* 13:5, 1973.
47. Fliedner TM, Cronkite EP, Robertson JS: Granulocytopoiesis. I. Senescence and random loss of neutrophilic granulocytes in human beings. *Blood* 24:402, 1964.
48. Patt HM, Maloney MA: Kinetics of neutrophil balance, in *The Kinetics of Cellular Proliferation*, edited by F Stohlman, p 201. Grune and Stratton, New York, 1959.
49. Cronkite EP: Enigmas underlying the study of hemopoietic cell proliferation. *Fed Proc* 23:649, 1964.
50. Koeffler HP, Golde DW: Human preleukemia. *Ann Intern Med* 93:347, 1980.
51. Doerschuk CM: Mechanisms of leukocyte sequestration in inflamed lungs. *Microcirculation* 8:71, 2001.
52. Schwab AJ, Salamand A, Merhi Y, et al: Kinetic analysis of pulmonary neutrophil retention *in vivo* using the multiple-indicator-dilution technique. *J Appl Physiol* 95:279, 2003.
53. Mauer AM, Athens JW, Ashenbrucker H, et al: Leukokinetic studies: II. A method for labeling granulocytes in vitro with radioactive diisopropylfluorophosphate (DFP32). *J Clin Invest* 39:1481, 1960.
54. Bishop CR, Rothstein G, Ashenbrucker HE, et al: Leukokinetic studies. XIV. Blood neutrophil kinetics in chronic, steady-state neutropenia. *J Clin Invest* 50:1678, 1971.
55. Rosse WF, Gurney CW: The Pelger-Huet anomaly in three families and its use in determining the disappearance of transfused neutrophils from the peripheral blood. *Blood* 14:170, 1959.
56. Dresch C, Najean Y, Bauchet J: Kinetic studies of 51Cr and DF32P labelled granulocytes. *Br J Haematol* 29:67, 1975.
57. Luo HR, Loison F: Constitutive neutrophil apoptosis: Mechanisms and regulation. *Am J Hematol* 83:288, 2008.
58. Edwards SW, Moulding DA, Derouet M, et al: Regulation of neutrophil apoptosis, in *The Neutrophil: An Emerging Regulator of Inflammatory and Immune Response*, edited by MA Cassatella, p 204. Karger, Verona, Italy, 2003.
59. Fadeel B, Kagan VE: Apoptosis and macrophage clearance of neutrophils: Regulation by reactive oxygen species. *Redox Rep* 8:143, 2003.
60. Hogg JC: Neutrophil kinetics and lung injury. *Physiol Rev* 67:1249, 1987.
61. Staub NC, Schultz EL: Pulmonary capillary length in dogs, cat and rabbit. *Respir Physiol* 5:371, 1968.
62. Ambrus CM, Ambrus JL, Johnson GC, et al: Role of the lungs in regulation of the white blood cell level. *Am J Physiol* 178:33, 1954.
63. Doerschuk CM, Allard MF, Martin BA, et al: Marginated pool of neutrophils in rabbit lungs. *J Appl Physiol* 63:1806, 1987.
64. Lien DC, Wagner WW Jr, Capen RL, et al: Physiological neutrophil sequestration in the lung: Visual evidence for localization in capillaries. *J Appl Physiol* 62:1236, 1987.
65. Doerschuk CM, Downey GP, Doherty DE, et al: Leukocyte and platelet margination within microvasculature of rabbit lungs. *J Appl Physiol* 68:1956, 1990.
66. Presson RG Jr, Graham JA, Hanger CC, et al: Distribution of pulmonary capillary red blood cell transit times. *J Appl Physiol* 79:382, 1995.
67. Gebb SA, Graham JA, Hanger CC, et al: Sites of leukocyte sequestration in the pulmonary microcirculation. *J Appl Physiol* 79:493, 1995.
68. Doerschuk CM, Beyers N, Coxson HO, et al: Comparison of neutrophil and capillary diameters and their relation to neutrophil sequestration in the lung. *J Appl Physiol* 74:3040, 1993.
69. Martin BA, Wright JL, Thommasen H, et al: Effect of pulmonary blood flow on the exchange between the circulating and marginating pool of polymorphonuclear leukocytes in dog lungs. *J Clin Invest* 69:1277, 1982.
70. Hogg JC, McLean T, Martin BA, et al: Erythrocyte transit and neutrophil concentration in the dog lung. *J Appl Physiol* 65:1217, 1988.
71. Doerschuk CM: The role of CD18-mediated adhesion in neutrophil sequestration induced by infusion of activated plasma in rabbits. *Am J Respir Cell Mol Biol* 7:140, 1992.
72. Downey GP, Worthen GS, Henson PM, et al: Neutrophil sequestration and migration in localized pulmonary inflammation. Capillary localization and migration across the interalveolar septum. *Am Rev Respir Dis* 147:168, 1993.
73. Brown GM, Brown DM, Donaldson K, et al: Neutrophil sequestration in rat lungs. *Thorax* 50:661, 1995.
74. Buttrum SM, Drost EM, MacNee W, et al: Rheological response of neutrophils to different types of stimulation. *J Appl Physiol* 77:1801, 1994.
75. Downey GP, Doherty DE, Schwab B III, et al: Retention of leukocytes in capillaries: Role of cell size and deformability. *J Appl Physiol* 69:1767, 1990.
76. Downey GP, Worthen GS: Neutrophil retention in model capillaries: Deformability, geometry, and hydrodynamic forces. *J Appl Physiol* 65:1861, 1988.
77. Erzurum SC, Downey GP, Doherty DE, et al: Mechanisms of lipopolysaccharide-induced neutrophil retention. Relative contributions of adhesive and cellular mechanical properties. *J Immunol* 149:154, 1992.
78. Worthen GS, Schwab III B, Elson EL, et al: Mechanics of stimulated neutrophils: Cell stiffening induces retention of capillaries. *Science* 245:183, 1989.
79. Doyle NA, Bhagwan SD, Meek BB, et al: Neutrophil margination, sequestration, and emigration in the lungs of L-selectin–deficient mice. *J Clin Invest* 99:526, 1997.
80. Kubo H, Doyle NA, Graham L, et al: L- and P-selectin and CD11/CD18 in intracapillary neutrophil sequestration in rabbit lungs. *Am J Respir Crit Care Med* 159:267, 1999.
81. Doerschuk CM, Mizgerd JP, Kubo H, et al: Adhesion molecules and cellular biomechanical changes in acute lung injury: Giles F. Filley Lecture. *Chest* 116:37S, 1999.
82. Doerschuk CM, Quinlan WM, Doyle NA, et al: The role of P-selectin and ICAM-1 in acute lung injury as determined using blocking antibodies and mutant mice. *J Immunol* 157:4609, 1996.
83. Gamble JR, Skinner MP, Berndt MC, et al: Prevention of activated neutrophil adhesion to endothelium by soluble adhesion protein GMP140. *Science* 249:414, 1990.
84. Jaeschke H, Farhood A, Fisher MA, et al: Sequestration of neutrophils in the hepatic vasculature during endotoxemia is independent of β_2 integrins and intercellular adhesion molecule-1. *Shock* 6:351, 1996.
85. Bishop CR, Athens JW, Boggs DR, et al: Leukokinetic studies. 13. A non–steady-state kinetic evaluation of the mechanism of cortisone-induced granulocytosis. *J Clin Invest* 47:249, 1968.
86. Dale DC, Fauci AS, Guerry D, IV, et al: Comparison of agents producing a neutrophilic leukocytosis in man. Hydrocortisone, prednisone, endotoxin, and etiocholanolone. *J Clin Invest* 56:808, 1975.
87. Stausz I, Barcsak J, Kekes E, et al: Prednisone-induced acute changes in circulating neutrophil granulocytes: I. In cases of normal granulocyte reserves. *Haematologia (Budap)* 1:319, 1993.
88. Dale DC, Fauci AS, Wolff SM: Alternate-day prednisone. Leukocyte kinetics and susceptibility to infections. *N Engl J Med* 291:1154, 1974.
89. Craddock CG Jr, Perry S, Ventzke LE, et al: Evaluation of marrow granulocytic reserves in normal and disease states. *Blood* 15:840, 1960.
90. Marsh JC, Perry S: The granulocyte response to endotoxin in patients with hematologic disorders. *Blood* 23:581, 1964.
91. DeConti RC, Kaplan SR, Calabresi P: Endotoxin stimulation in patients with lymphoma: Correlation with the myelosuppressive effects of alkylating agents. *Blood* 39:602, 1972.
92. Korbitz BC, Toren FA, Davis HL Jr, et al: The Piromen test: A useful assay of bone marrow granulocyte reserves. *Curr Ther Res Clin Exp* 11:491, 1969.
93. Ley K, Laudanna C, Cybulsky MI, et al: Getting to the site of inflammation: The leukocyte adhesion cascade updated. *Nat Rev Immunol* 7:678, 2007.
94. Zarbock A, Ley K: Neutrophil adhesion and activation under flow. *Microcirculation* 16:31, 2009.
95. von Hundelshausen P, Koenen RR, Weber C: Platelet-mediated enhancement of leukocyte adhesion. *Microcirculation* 16:84, 2009.
96. Haslett C: Granulocyte apoptosis and its role in the resolution and control of lung inflammation. *Am J Respir Crit Care* 160:S5, 1999.
97. Buescher ES, Gallin JI: Leukocyte transfusions in chronic granulomatous disease: Persistence of transfused leukocytes in sputum. *N Engl J Med* 307:800, 1982.
98. Lord BI, Gurney H, Chang J, et al: Haemopoietic cell kinetics in humans treated with rGM-CSF. *Int J Cancer* 50:26, 1992.
99. Buchanan MR, Crowley CA, Rosin RE, et al: Studies on the interaction between GP-180 deficient neutrophils and vascular endothelium. *Blood* 60:160, 1982.

CHAPTER 62

EOSINOPHILS AND THEIR DISORDERS

Andrew J. Wardlaw

SUMMARY

Eosinophils have received considerable attention from the research community in the last decade, in large part, as a result of their potential role in asthma. The concept of the eosinophil as a cell that has protective effects against helminthic parasite infection but can cause tissue damage when inappropriately activated remains intact, although the evidence for both these roles is circumstantial. Eosinophil production and function are profoundly influenced by interleukin-5 (IL-5), and thus eosinophilia is associated with diseases characterized by T-helper (Th) 2-mediated immune responses, fostering B-lymphocyte function, including infections by helminthic parasites and extrinsic asthma. However, eosinophilia also occurs in diseases not obviously associated with Th2 dominance such as intrinsic asthma, the hypereosinophilic syndrome (HES), and inflammatory bowel disease. Thus, IL-5 and other eosinophil mediators can be generated in various types of inflammatory response.

The eosinophil, like other leukocytes, can generate proinflammatory mediators. Eosinophil-specific granule proteins are toxic for a range of mammalian cells and parasitic larvae. Eosinophils, like mast cells, produce sulfidopeptide leukotrienes, as well as other lipid mediators, such as platelet-activating factor (PAF). Cytokine production by eosinophils broadens their potential functions, for example in wound healing through the generation of transforming growth factor (TGF)-α. Synthesis of TGF-β may explain the propensity of eosinophils to be associated with fibrotic reactions such as endomyocardial fibrosis, characteristic of HES, and fibrosing alveolitis.

Considerable effort has gone into trying to unravel the molecular basis of eosinophil tissue recruitment. The selective accumulation of eosinophils is the result of a concerted and integrated series of events involving their production in the marrow and egress therefrom, adhesion to endothelium, selective chemotaxis, and prolonged survival in tissues. These events are controlled, either directly or indirectly, by production of IL-4, IL-5, and IL-13.

The discovery that a proportion of patients with HES have either a clonal abnormality resulting from the creation of a constitutively active novel tyrosine kinase (FIP1L1-PDGFRα) or a T-cell lymphoproliferative disease causing a reactive eosinophilia has offered the prospect of new and more effective treatments for this condition as well as giving dramatic new insights into the control of eosinophil production. There has long been a debate about the extent to which eosinophils cause tissue damage, are innocent bystanders, or even help to ameliorate the condition. This is now being resolved with data showing that specific reduction in eosinophils using anti-IL-5 monoclonal antibody is beneficial in eosinophilic airway disease and hypereosinophilic syndromes.

Acronyms and abbreviations that appear in this chapter include: ABPA, allergic bronchopulmonary aspergillosis; CCR, chemokine receptor; CEL, chronic eosinophilic leukemia; CMPD, chronic myeloproliferative disease; ECF-A, eosinophil chemotactic factor of anaphylaxis; ECP, eosinophil cationic protein; EDN, eosinophil-derived neurotoxin; EPO, eosinophil peroxidase; GM-CSF, granulocyte-monocyte colony-stimulating growth factor; HES, hypereosinophilic syndrome; HLA, human leukocyte antigen; ICAM, intercellular adhesion molecule; IL, interleukin; LAMP, lysosome-associated membrane protein; LIMP, lysosome integral membrane protein; mAb, monoclonal antibody; MBP, major basic protein; PAF, platelet-activating factor; PSGL, P-selectin glycoprotein ligand; SNARE, soluble *N*-ethylmaleimide-sensitive factor attachment protein receptor complex; TGF, transforming growth factor; TRAIL, tumor necrosis factor-related apoptosis-inducing ligand; T_{reg}, T-regulatory cell; VCAM, vascular cell adhesion molecule; VLA, very-late antigen.

EOSINOPHIL MORPHOLOGY AND RECEPTORS

Eosinophils are spherical cells approximately 8 microns in diameter, that are end-stage, nondividing granular leukocytes derived from the marrow.[1] *In vitro*, granulocyte-monocyte colony-stimulating factor (GM-CSF), interleukin (IL)-3, and IL-5 stimulate eosinophil colony growth; additionally, IL-5 is a critical eosinopoietic factor *in vivo*. The electron microscopic morphology of the mature eosinophil has been well described (Fig. 62–1).[2,3] The relatively specific features that distinguish the eosinophil from other leukocytes are a bilobed nucleus, the relatively large eosinophilic specific granules with an electron-dense core, the paucity of mitochondria (approximately 20 per cell) and endoplasmic reticulum, and the dense network of cytoplasmic tubulovesicular structures or secretory vesicles that contain albumin and cytochrome b_{558} and are, therefore, thought to be involved in superoxide production. Eosinophils also contain several lipid bodies that are the major site of eicosanoid synthesis, primary granules, and small granules. Small granules are particularly prominent in tissue eosinophils and contain arylsulfatase B, acid phosphatase, and catalase. They may be derived from specific granules and act as a lysosomal compartment, especially as specific granules do express lysosome-associated membrane proteins 1 and 2 (LAMP1/2) as well as lysosome integral membrane protein 1 (LIMP-1:CD63).[4] Eosinophils also contain multilaminar bodies that contain transforming growth factor (TGF)-α. Eosinophil precursors (eosinophilic myelocytes) derived from cord blood can be first identified morphologically when specific granules (core-containing) appear, although expression of Charcot-Leyden crystal protein and the basic granules proteins can be detected by immunohistochemistry or messenger RNA (mRNA) expression at the promyelocyte stage, at which time they are found in the endoplasmic reticulum, Golgi apparatus, and large, round, coreless granules, most of which develop into specific granules. Transmission electron microscopy can distinguish activated from resting blood eosinophils by the increased number of lipid bodies, primary and small granules, secretory vesicles, and endoplasmic reticulum. Cytoplasmic crystals of Charcot-Leyden protein may also be present. Activated eosinophils are also often less dense than resting cells, although with the advent of immunomagnetic selection rather than density gradients to purify eosinophils density is less often used as a marker of activation.[5] Eosinophils are thought to be relatively poorly phagocytic although they can ingest opsonized zymosan, which is taken up into phagolysosomes formed in part by fusion with specific granules. The eosinophil also degranulates onto large opsonized surfaces such as a Sephadex beads or parasitic larvae in a process called *frustrated phagocytosis*.

The ultrastructure of *in vitro*-activated and tissue-infiltrating eosinophils has suggested three potential mechanisms of degranulation: necrosis or cytolytic degranulation, exocytosis or "classical degranulation," and piecemeal degranulation.[6] Cytolytic degranulation is associated with loss of eosinophil plasma membrane integrity and results in the release of clusters of free membrane-bound granules (termed *Cfegs*), This is commonly observed in eosinophilic inflammation being particularly marked in severe disease, such as fatal attacks of asthma, in which large quantities of basic proteins can be detected in the tissue by immunohistochemistry, often with relatively few intact eosinophils.[7] This type of degranulation is also a feature of milder disease such as allergic

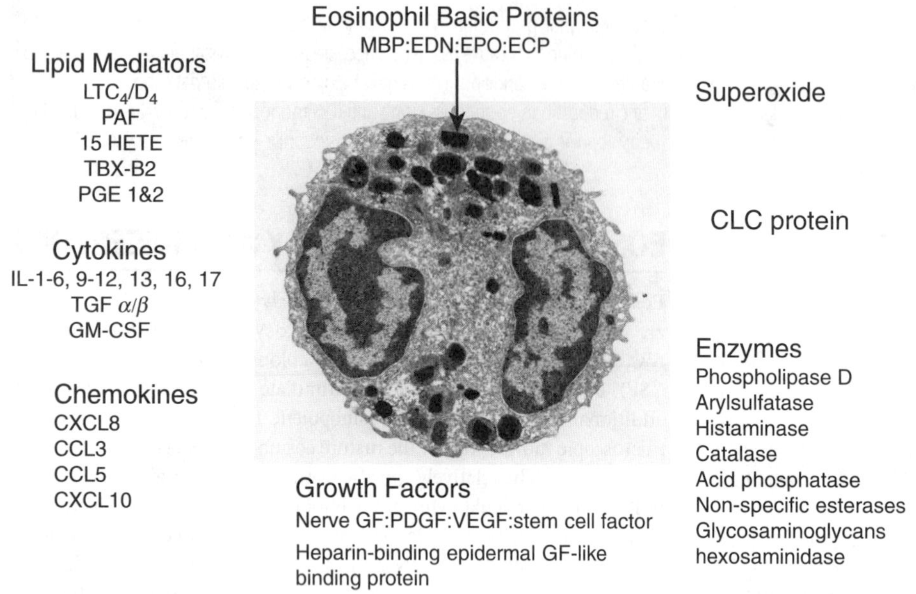

FIGURE 62–1. Transmission electron micrograph (×10,000) of an eosinophil showing the characteristic binucleate cell with specific granules containing an electron dense core. The major contents of the cell are listed. *(Courtesy of Dr. A. Dewar, National Heart and Lung Institute.)* CLC, Charcot Leyden crystal; ECP, eosinophil cationic protein; EDN, eosinophil-derived neurotoxin; EPO, eosinophil peroxidase; GF, growth factor; GM-CSF, granulocyte-monocyte colony-stimulating growth factor; HETE, hydroxyeicosatetraenoic acid; LT, leukotriene; MBP, major basic protein; PAF, platelet-activating factor; PDGF, platelet-derived growth factor; PG, prostaglandin; PSGL, P-selectin glycoprotein ligand; TBX, thromboxane; TGF-β, transforming growth factor-β; VEGF, vascular endothelial growth factor.

rhinitis[8,9] as well as Fc-mediated degranulation *in vitro*.[10] Exocytosis or classical degranulation occurs in mast cells and basophils after crosslinking of immunoglobulin (Ig) E receptors. It describes a process by which granules migrate to the plasma membrane and fuse with it leading to the extrusion of membrane free granule contents. This has been described for eosinophils in the gut, but not the airway mucosa. Piecemeal degranulation was described in cord-blood-derived eosinophils.[11] This term describes the appearance of empty or partially empty granules that retain their structure together with small granule protein-containing vesicles in the cytoplasm, which transport the granule proteins to the cell surface where they are released.[12] These appearances are common in tissue eosinophils in asthma and other allergic diseases.

Many studies have used a model of a mouse challenged with ovalbumin to generate eosinophilia in the lung and increased airway hyperresponsiveness. An interesting and striking feature of this model is that the lung eosinophils do not have the appearance of having undergone degranulation either by cytolysis or piecemeal degranulation.[13] Immunostaining of the mouse lung locates all the basic proteins within intact eosinophils and bronchioalveolar lavage contains no free major basic protein (MBP).[14,15] This is quite unlike human disease where the cell-free basic proteins can be readily detected in both tissue and bronchioalveolar lavage. Consistent with this observation, mice in which the gene for eosinophil peroxide (EPO) or MBP has been deleted had the same phenotype as wild-type mice.[16] However some degranulation may be seen in the lumen.[17] Mice have been genetically modified using two approaches to completely delete eosinophils, one by inserting an eosinophil toxic gene (*PHIL*) into the lineage and one by deleting a high-affinity binding site in the *GATA-1* promoter.[18,19] The GATA-1 promotor-deleted mice still develop airway hyperreactivity and mucus secretion but not airway remodeling, which is consistent with evidence for their role in asthma. In contrast the knock-in *PHIL* mouse did not develop airway hyperresponsiveness and mucus hypersecretion after airway challenge. This discrepancy has not been resolved but both studies point to an important role for eosinophils in this model. Apoptotic eosinophils are small cells with shrunken nuclei and condensed chromatin but an intact plasma membrane.[20] They are readily identifiable in aged cell populations *in vitro* and in cells from the airway lumen such as sputum, but are more difficult to identify in tissues. This has led some investigators to argue that the majority of airway eosinophils, at least in asthma and rhinitis, are removed through luminal entry rather than by undergoing apoptosis in tissue.[6]

Like all granulocytic leukocytes, eosinophils express a large number of membrane receptors that allow them to interact with the extracellular environment (Tables 62–1 and 62–2). These include receptors required for locomotion, activation, growth, and mediator release. Most of the receptors are shared to some extent with other granulocytes but some have a degree of specificity in terms of level of expression and function. An important feature of tissue eosinophils is that they express a different pattern of receptors than do blood eosinophils, consistent with a more activated phenotype. This includes CD69, intercellular adhesion molecule (ICAM)-1 and FcγR1 and increased expression of human leukocyte antigen (HLA)-DR and Mac-1. Changes in expression can be induced *in vitro* by culture with cytokines such as IL-5, but also occur to some extent as the result of transmigration through endothelium.[21]

TABLE 62–1. Eosinophil Adhesion Receptors

	Ligand	
Receptor	**Endothelial**	**Matrix Protein**
Integrins		
$\alpha_4\beta_1$ (VLA-4)	VCAM-1	Fibronectin
$\alpha_4\beta_6$		Laminin
$\alpha_4\beta_7$	MAdCAM-1	Fibronectin
$\alpha_L\beta_2$ (LFA-1)	ICAM-1–3	
$\alpha_M\beta_2$ (Mac-1)	ICAM-1	
$\alpha_x\beta_2$ (P150,95)		
$\alpha_d\beta_2$	VCAM-1 (ICAM-3?)	
Selectins and ligands		
PSGL-1	P-selectin (E-selectin)	
L-selectin	Gly-CAM-1, CD34, Podocalyxin	
Other		
CD44		Hyaluronate
ICAM-3		
PECAM	PECAM	

ICAM, intercellular cell adhesion molecule; MAdCAM, mucosal addressin cell adhesion molecule; PECAM, platelet endothelial cell adhesion molecule; PSGL-1, P-selectin glycoprotein 1; VCAM, vascular cell adhesion molecule.

TABLE 62–2. Some Important Eosinophil Receptors

Immunoglobulin receptors: FcγR11 (CD32); FcαR
Receptors for mediators: CCR3*; CCR1; PAF-R; LTC4/D4/E4-R; LTB4-R; C5aR; C3aR; IL-5R*; IL-3R; IL-4R; IL-13R; CRTh2
Receptors induced by cytokine stimulation: FcγRIII (CD16); FcγR1; CD69; HLA-DR; ICAM-1; CD25; CD4
Well-expressed miscellaneous receptors: CD9; CD45; CR1; CD154 (CD40 ligand); CD95 (Fas); Siglec 8*

CCR, chemokine receptor, HLA, human leukocyte antigen; ICAM, intercellular adhesion molecule; IL, interleukin; LT, leukotriene; PAF, platelet-activating factor.
*Relatively selectively expressed by eosinophils.

A major difference between eosinophils and neutrophils, exploited to purify eosinophils by immunomagnetic selectin, is the expression of CD16 by neutrophils but not eosinophils. Another important difference discussed below is the expression of very-late antigen (VLA)-4 by eosinophils, but not to any great extent by neutrophils. Siglec 8 has been identified as a receptor expressed only by eosinophils, mast cells, and basophils.[22–24] Siglecs are sialic acid-recognizing animal lectins of the immunoglobulin superfamily. Eosinophils, as well as monocytes and a subset of dendritic cells, also express Siglec 10.[25] In contrast, neutrophils express Siglec 9.[26] The function of the Siglec 8 on eosinophils remains uncertain but may be involved in triggering apoptosis.[27,28] Eosinophils express both CD48 and its ligand CD244 (2B4), both members of the Ig superfamily. Crosslinking of CD48 causes eosinophil degranulation.[29] Eosinophils also express a number of inhibitory receptors whose function remains uncertain.[30]

EOSINOPHIL PRODUCTION

Eosinophils are nondividing, end-stage cells that, like other leukocytes, differentiate from the hematopoietic stem cell in the marrow. They share an intermediate stage progenitor with basophils. GATA-1 is a particularly important transcription factor for eosinophil development with deletion of the high affinity binding site in GATA-1 resulting in specific loss of the eosinophil lineage.[31] The *FIP1L1-PDGFRα* receptor mutation, which is responsible for a myeloproliferative form of hypereosinophilic syndrome (HES), chronic eosinophilic leukemia, works through cEBP-α, GATA-2, and GATA-1, showing that these transcription factors are also important in eosinophil development.[32] Eosinophils migrate into the blood, where they circulate with a half-life of approximately 18 hours before entering the tissues. Eosinophils are primarily tissue-dwelling cells, and it has been estimated that there are approximately 100 tissue eosinophils for each eosinophil in the blood, although relatively few studies have been performed on eosinophil kinetics and even fewer have compared eosinophil turnover in health and disease.[33] Approximately 3 percent of cells in normal human adult marrow are eosinophils, of which one-third are mature and two-thirds are precursors.

It has been known for many years that eosinophilia is often T-cell dependant. Characterization of T-cell-derived supernatants led to the characterization of IL-5 and an awareness of the pivotal role that this cytokine plays in eosinophil development.[34,35] IL-3 and GM-CSF are also important in eosinophil development. The three cytokines bind to receptors that share a common β chain but have distinct α chains. IL-5 seems to be a rate-limiting step for eosinophil production in that administration of IL-5 either exogenously or through transgenic manipulation in mice results in a marked eosinophilia[36] and anti–IL-5 in humans dramatically diminishes the blood eosinophil count in asthma.[37] Increased eosinophilopoiesis as a result of increased IL-5 synthesis is a feature of a number of diseases including parasitic and allergic diseases. For example pulmonary eosinophilia caused by *Necator americanus* infection in mice is IL-5 dependent[38] and both the eosinophilia and host defense to filariasis and *Trichinella spiralis* is markedly impaired in IL-5 deficient mice.[39] In asthma, IL-5 mRNA can be detected in increased amounts in the airways as well as the plasma of glucocorticoid-dependent asthmatics.[40,41] However, IL-5 gene-deleted mice still have a baseline eosinophilia and can develop pulmonary eosinophilia after infection with paramyxovirus, demonstrating that cytokines other than IL-5 can cause late differentiation of eosinophils.[42] It is, therefore, an accepted paradigm that a blood and tissue eosinophilia in IgE-mediated diseases, such as atopic asthma and helminthic parasite infections, are caused by antigen-dependent activation of T-helper (Th) 2 cells leading to IL-5 production, increased eosinophilopoiesis, and tissue recruitment of eosinophils. The control of Th2 and Th1 cell development may relate to the cytokine milieu at the time of sensitization, genetically regulated transcriptional control of IL-4, or the route of sensitization and the way in which the antigen is presented.[43,44] The nature of the antigen may also be important. Many allergens have now been purified and sequenced. No common structural features have been established that can explain their allergenicity although many are proteases, which could influence their immunogenicity.[45] The HLA haplotype of individuals responsive to certain allergens has also been investigated. A degree of restriction has been observed, particularly to more simple allergens, with, for example, the phenotype DR2.2 being overrepresented in individuals atopic to the ragweed allergen Amb a V. However, with the majority of allergens, no clear pattern has emerged. While HLA haplotypes may influence responses to individual allergens, it is unlikely to provide a universal explanation for Th2 type responsiveness.

Many eosinophilic diseases including many cases of pulmonary eosinophilia are not associated with atopy and IgE production and therefore do not entirely fit with the Th2-driven eosinophilic paradigm. Although intrinsic asthma is generally assumed to be associated with IL-5 producing T cells, the evidence for this is limited. One model for non-IgE associated eosinophilic disease is those cases of eosinophilic esophagitis caused by a defined food allergen in which there is no specific IgE.[46] In some of these cases the patients are patch test–positive to the food allergen concerned, which raises the possibility of a Th2 type of type IV cell-mediated immunity, but this is still unexplored.

There is increasing interest in the role of T-regulatory (T_{reg}) cells in controlling inappropriate immune responses including those associated with Th2 cell activation.[47] T_{reg} cells were first identified as mediating some aspects of immune tolerance and were then found to play an important role in suppressing immune-mediated inflammatory bowel disease in mice. Three types of T_{reg} cells have been identified: CD4+CD25+ cells that require direct contact to mediate their immune suppressive effects; T_{reg} cells producing TGF-β; and T_{reg} cells producing IL-10.[48–50] A current idea is that the increase in allergic disease that is also paralleled by an increase in autoimmune disease is not the result of a Th1 to Th2 switch but of a failure to develop T_{reg} cell responses, which leads to enhancement of both Th1 and Th2 immunity.[51–53] IL-10-producingT_{reg} cells are of particular interest in the context of pulmonary eosinophilia because of evidence that immunotherapy works by inducing expansion of antigen specific IL-10–producing T_{reg} cells.[54] In addition T_{reg} cells are able to suppress ovalbumin induced pulmonary eosinophilia in mice.[55,56]

EOSINOPHIL HETEROGENEITY

Blood eosinophils from normal individuals are relatively dense cells that can be separated from other leukocytes by density-gradient centrifugation. For many years these differences were the basis for the standard method of purifying eosinophils. This has now been largely superseded by negative immunomagnetic selection based on the expression of the low affinity (FcγRIII, CD16) IgG receptor by neutrophils but not eosinophils. This latter technique has the advantage of improved purity and cell yields as well as enabling purification of eosinophils from individuals with low eosinophil counts.[57] A proportion of eosinophils from individuals with elevated eosinophil counts are less dense than eosinophils from normal subjects. So called hypodense eosinophils appear to be vacuolated and contain smaller granules, although in equal numbers to normal-density eosinophils.[58] The mechanism for this heterogeneity is unclear, although a correlation with eosinophil activation has been a favored hypothesis but the evidence to support this supposition is contradictory.[5]

EOSINOPHIL TRAFFICKING, TISSUE ACCUMULATION, AND APOPTOSIS

Eosinophils are not normally found in tissues other than the gut, and the appearance of increased numbers of these cells can be a notable feature of the pathology of a number of diseases. The normal pattern of gut homing of eosinophils is mediated by eotaxin, which is constitutively expressed in the gut, and the integrin $\alpha_4\beta_7$ binding to mucosal addressin cell adhesion molecule (MAdCAM)-1, which is selectively expressed in the intestine.[59] Although an eosinophilia can accompany a general inflammatory response, as for example in idiopathic pulmonary fibrosis in which increased numbers of eosinophils and neutrophils can be seen in bronchoalveolar lavage fluid, it often occurs without a marked increase in other leukocytes, raising the question of the mechanism behind their specific tissue accumulation. Selective eosinophil accumulation occurs as a result of the coordinated effect of a number of adhesion, chemotactic, and growth or survival orientated signals at each stage in the life cycle of the cell. Generally speaking these events are controlled by mediators released by Th2 cells, in particular the cytokines IL-4, IL-5, IL-13, and possibly IL-9 and IL-25. IL-25 acts through an intermediate cell type to produce IL-5– and IL-13–dependent effects.[60]

Eosinophil trafficking has been extensively investigated,[61–63] and is concisely reviewed here. As well as being crucial for differentiation, IL-5 is also important in promoting emigration of eosinophils from the marrow. In particular, it acts as a priming factor for specific chemoattractants such as eotaxin.[64] Eosinophil emigration from the marrow in guinea pigs is inhibited by blocking anti-CD18 antibodies, but IL-5–dependent emigration was promoted by blocking anti–VLA-4 antibodies.[65] One explanation for this finding is that VLA-4 and vascular cell adhesion molecule (VCAM)-1 are responsible for eosinophil precursors binding to marrow stromal cells, as has been shown for a range of cell types, although it has not been formally demonstrated for eosinophils. The observation that eotaxin decreased adhesion of eosinophils to VCAM-1 while increasing their adhesion to the CD18 ligand bovine serum albumin may be a mechanism for promoting egress from the marrow.[66] A localized inflammatory responses can cause systemic effects has been demonstrated after allergen challenge in mice in which IL-5 producing cells (both T cells and non-T cells), increased in the marrow.[67,68]

Accumulation of leukocytes in tissue is a highly regulated process with the aim of being able to respond effectively to noxious insults without causing an inappropriate inflammatory response. An obligate step in the migration of all leukocytes from the systemic circulation into tissue is their capture by endothelium as they flow at high shear rates through the postcapillary endothelium. A key receptor mediating eosinophil capture is P-selectin. Its low-level surface expression is selectively induced on endothelium by IL-4 and IL-13. Eosinophils express higher levels of P-selectin glycoprotein ligand-1 (PSGL-1), the primary receptor for P-selectin, than other leukocytes, which results in increased avidity for P-selectin compared to neutrophils, especially at the low levels of expression induced by Th2 cytokines.[69] Increased expression of PSGL-1 leading to enhanced recruitment of eosinophils also occurs in allergic disease.[70] IL-4 and IL-13 can also induce low levels of VCAM-1 expression that can bind eosinophils through VLA-4 and also capture flowing cells albeit at lower shear stresses. VLA-4/VCAM-1 and PSGL-1/P-selectin cooperate as a major endothelial control point for selective eosinophil migration.[71] Once captured, eosinophils roll along the surface of the blood vessel until they are activated, which allows the CD18 integrins binding to ICAM-1 and ICAM-2 to nonselectively promote transmigration, although VLA-4/VCAM-1 can also exert selective pressure at this stage. The activation step mediated by chemoattractants expressed on the endothelial surface is another potential point of eosinophil selection as shown by the effect of exogenously added chemoattractants, such as eotaxin, but the identity of the endogenous chemoattractant involved and the extent to which it is selectively expressed in eosinophilic inflammatory sites remains to be resolved.[72]

Once the eosinophil has transmigrated through the endothelium it has to migrate through the basement membrane and into the tissue. Chemokines, as well as other eosinophil chemoattractants, are likely to be central to this process (Table 62–3). Many eosinophil active chemokines bind to chemokine receptor (CCR)-3 and deletion of its coding gene severely impairs eosinophil migration into the lung in the mouse asthma model. In one study, using *CCR3* gene-deleted mice, the cells appeared to be able to migrate through the endothelium, suggesting that CCR3-binding chemokines such as eotaxin were not essential for the activation step, but not through the basement membrane either because they lacked a chemotactic signal or were unable to digest the extracellular matrix.[73] The three specific eosinophil chemokines, eotaxin 1 through 3, play overlapping roles in eosinophil migration into the lung in mice.[74]

Apoptosis is the universal mechanism by which cells undergo cell senescence in a manner that allows them to be efficiently removed by macrophages without inducing an inflammatory response. Morphologic observations have substantiated that eosinophil apoptosis is an unusual event in tissue and that most eosinophils either die by cytolysis or migrate into the lumen where they do become apoptotic.[6,75] A slow

TABLE 62–3. Eosinophil Chemokine Receptors and Their Ligands

Receptor	Chemokine
CCR1*	CCL3 (MIP-1a); CCL5 (RANTES)
CCR3	CCL11 (Eotaxin1); CCL24 (Eotaxin 2); CCL26 (Eotaxin 3) CCL7, 8, 13 (MCP2–4); CCL5
CXCR1 & 2	CXCL8 (IL-8†)

CC, chemokine; IL, interleukin; MCP, monocyte chemotactic protein; MIP, macrophage inhibitory protein; R, receptor; RANTES, regulated on activation, normal T-cell expressed and secreted.

*Only expressed on eosinophils from some donors.

†Only active on *in vivo* activated or cytokine-primed eosinophils (may be indirect effect via neutrophils).

rate of apoptosis in tissues is consistent with the survival signals delivered to eosinophils by the extracellular matrix as part of normal homeostasis as well as increased production of eosinophil growth factors during Th2-mediated inflammation.[76,77] The importance of prolonged survival of eosinophils in tissue as a mechanism for selective accumulation has been supported by studies using anti–IL-5, which effectively inhibits blood and sputum eosinophil numbers but has a much less marked effect on tissue eosinophils.[78] Glucocorticoids directly enhance the rate of eosinophil apoptosis through an unknown mechanism, unlike neutrophils for which they prolong survival.[79] It is tempting to suggest that the dramatic effect of glucocorticoids in resolving eosinophilic inflammation, for example, in simple pulmonary eosinophilia, is a consequence of this direct effect. However, glucocorticoids only induce eosinophil apoptosis at high concentrations and the effect is modest over and above the spontaneous rate of apoptosis. It is more likely that they work by inhibiting the production of eosinophil growth factors such as IL-5, IL-3, and GM-CSF generated both in an autocrine fashion by eosinophils in response to matrix signals and as part of the inflammatory process.[80] Tumor necrosis factor (TNF)-related apoptosis-inducing ligand, another survival modulating mediator related to TNF, prolongs eosinophil survival *in vitro* and *ex vivo* after allergen challenge.[81]

The biochemical mechanisms by which growth factors mediate eosinophil survival is dependent on both new protein synthesis and phosphorylation events. The survival effects of IL-5 are dependent on activation of the RAS-RAF-MEK pathway and the JAK2-STAT1-STAT5 pathway and involve LYN kinase, which binds to the IL5-Rα chain.[82] The roles of p38 and PI3 kinase are less clear. Wortmannin, which blocks PI3 kinase, has no effect on eosinophil apoptosis, although it does inhibit IL-5 enhancement of adhesion to fibrinogen. Eosinophils express significant amounts of the proapoptotic protein BAX and the antiapoptotic BCL-xl, but very little BAD or BCL-2.[83] As in other cell types both spontaneous and FAS-induced eosinophil apoptosis is associated with the migration of BAX into the mitochondria. This leads to loss of mitochondrial membrane potential, cytochrome c release, and activation of downstream caspases. These events are inhibited by IL-5, demonstrating that IL-5 works by blocking BAX translocation.[84,85] Inhibition of BAX activation prevents eosinophil apoptosis even in the absence of cytokines. Treatment of eosinophils with dexamethasone also leads to loss of mitochondrial permeability.[86] GM-CSF–activated Erk1/2 phosphorylates BAX at Thr167, and facilitates interaction with the prolyl isomerase Pin1. If interaction with Pin1 is prevented, BAX is activated and translocated to the mitochondria resulting in apoptosis. Therefore, eosinophil growth factors exert their antiapoptotic effects by fostering the Pin1–BAX interaction.[87]

Another potential mechanism involved in eosinophil tissue accumulation is *in situ* differentiation from eosinophil precursors. Eosinophil precursors can be identified in an IL-5Rα+CD34+ population in blood and are increased after allergen challenge and in atopic disease. These cells have also been found in asthmatic airways.[88]

Of equal importance as endothelial interactions to the kinetics of eosinophil migration are the factors controlling the fate of the eosinophil once it enters the tissue. There are three possible outcomes. The eosinophil can remain in the tissue interacting with matrix proteins, other leukocytes or structural cells such as, in the bronchial mucosa, the epithelium, airway smooth muscle, mucus glands and nerves; alternatively the cell can migrate into the lumen of the gut or airway where it is likely to undergo apoptosis; or it can return to the circulation via the lymphatics. There is limited evidence that eosinophils can recirculate although they have been reported to be present in lymph nodes where it has been speculated that they are involved in antigen presentation.[89] The length of time that eosinophils remain in tissue before migrating into the lumen of gut or bronchus is unclear as there are virtually no studies of the kinetics of eosinophil migration in humans. Anti–IL-5 completely inhibits migration into the lumen, which suggests that transepithelial migration is IL-5 dependent. However, IL-5 only inhibited tissue numbers by at most 50 percent, indicating that other factors are also at play.[78] In a mouse model of asthma, eosinophil migration into the lumen did not occur in the matrix metalloprotease *MMP-2* gene-deleted mouse, which caused the animals to be asphyxiated.[90] Thus, IL-5 may be important in activating the eosinophils to digest the epithelial basement membrane in a MMP-2–dependent manner.[91] As has been shown with senescent neutrophils, when tissue eosinophils become senescent they start to alter their receptor phenotype in a way that inhibits tissue retention and promotes migration into the lumen.[92] The factors controlling the retention and survival of eosinophils in tissue are likely to involve the integration of chemoattractant, adhesive, and survival signals delivered by interactions with matrix proteins and structural cells. Studies modelling eosinophil migration in tissue using collagen gels have shown a different pattern to standard Boyden chamber assays with a much greater, albeit random, migratory response to growth factors than to chemoattractants.[93] This suggests that migration into the lumen requires both a growth factor and a chemotactic stimulus.

ANIMAL MODELS OF EOSINOPHILIC DISEASE

Animal models, particularly the mouse model of ovalbumin challenge that results in a selective and marked pulmonary eosinophilia, have been used extensively to analyze the molecular basis of eosinophil trafficking to the lung and the pathologic consequences of this. The combination of transgenic, gene-deletion and antibody-based manipulations in the mouse are a powerful tool for analyzing the biology of eosinophil migration, although the relevance of the findings to human disease must always be treated with caution. Generally speaking, these studies have supported the concept of eosinophil migration resulting from a series of interlinked and obligate steps requiring that IL-5 provide a pool of circulating eosinophils, prime eosinophils for chemotactic responsiveness, and prolong eosinophil survival, and that IL-4 and IL-13 control adhesion-related events in the endothelium and enhance the release of eosinophil chemoattractants, particularly CCR3-binding chemokines from mesenchymal cells within the airway.[94,95] However, there are other studies of the immune response that challenge this neat concept, in particular by showing potential roles for innate immunity as well as other inflammatory mediators in the process.[96–98]

EOSINOPHIL FUNCTIONS

INACTVATION OF HELMINTHS

The eosinophil exerts its effects largely through its mediators (see Fig. 62–1). These are either newly generated, as is the case with leukotrienes and other lipid mediators, or stored preformed in various compartments within the cytoplasm and released when the eosinophil receives a stimulus to degranulate. The eosinophil is biosynthetically inactive and, although new protein synthesis does occur, the majority of its protein mediators are stored. Although the eosinophil can phagocytose particles, its interactions with larval forms of helminthic parasites serve as a model by which eosinophil function. In this situation, the eosinophil adheres tightly to the organism and releases its granule contents onto the surface of the helminth in a process described as frustrated phagocytosis. The paradigm of eosinophil effector function in host defense was developed from the observation that the basic granule proteins, in particular, were highly toxic for larval parasites and was extended to include a proinflammatory role when they were also shown to be toxic for bronchial epithelium and, therefore, associated with epithelial desquamation, which is a well-established feature of severe asthma. Eosinophils are not thought to play a major role in bacterial host defense and, indeed, bacterial sepsis causes an eosinopenia. However, eosinophils can release mitochondrial DNA, which has antibacterial properties.[99] Eosinophils can also release a plethora of cytokines and chemokines. Many of these chemicals are generated in low amounts compared to other cells, and the extent to which they are important in eosinophil function is not clear.[100]

ROLE IN IMMUNOREGULATION

The eosinophil has also been shown to have the capacity to present antigen to T cells and there is increasing evidence for an immunoregulatory role for eosinophils.[89,101,102]

MEDIATOR RELEASE

Eosinophils can release a number of lipid mediators and are one of the relatively few sources of sulfidopeptide leukotrienes, although per cell they release about 10-fold less than mast cells and basophils.[103] This role contrasts with neutrophils, which produce large amounts of leukotriene (LT) B_4 but little, if any, LTC_4. Sulfidopeptide leukotriene generation by human eosinophils occurs after stimulation with opsonized zymosan and beads coated with IgG. Eosinophils can generate substantial quantities of 15-hydroxyeicosatetraenoic acid via 15-lipoxygenase. Eosinophils also generate platelet activating factor after stimulation with either a calcium ionophore or IgG-coated beads.[104] Eosinophils can generate mediators of the cyclooxygenase pathway, including prostaglandins E_1 and E_2, and thromboxane B_2. The principal sites of eicosanoid formation in eosinophils are the lipid bodies, which contain large amounts of arachidonic acid and enzymes required for eicosanoid synthesis, including 5-lipoxygenase, LTC_4 synthase, and cyclooxygenase.[105] Eosinophils release significant amounts of TGF-β and TGF-α, which has stimulated interest in a potential role in causing structural changes in the lung that come under the heading of airway remodelling. There is evidence that TGF-β released by eosinophils can promote the generation of fibromyocytes and anti–IL-5 reduced the amount of tenascin in the reticular subepithelial membrane.[106,107] Thickening of this membrane is closely associated with eosinophilic airway inflammation, although not with airway hyperresponsiveness or airflow obstruction.[108]

EOSINOPHILIC GRANULE RELEASE

A specific and important feature of eosinophils are the large amounts of basic constituents they contain within their specific granules. These are MBP, eosinophil cationic protein, EPO, and eosinophil-derived neurotoxin. MBP has a molecular mass of 13.8 kDa and a isoelectric point (pI) of 10.9. Its 17 arginine residues account for its alkalinity. It is initially synthesized as an acidic proprotein, which is stored in the eosinophil granule[109]; MBP becomes toxic only after it is released and converted into its final form. Purified MBP is cytotoxic for the schistosomula of *Schistosoma mansoni*, and adherence of eosinophils to IgG-coated schistosomula results in the secretion of MBP onto the tegument of the larvae, resulting in loss of their viability.[110] MBP at concentrations as low as 10 mcg/mL has also been shown to be toxic for both guinea pig and human respiratory epithelial cells, as well as for rat and human pneumocytes.[111] The mechanism of action of MBP on epithelial cells appears to be mediated through its inhibition of adenosine triphosphatase activity. MBP and EPO are strong agonists for platelet activation as well as the activation of mast cells, basophils, and neutrophils.[112] The mechanisms of action of MBP is likely to be related to its hydrophobicity and strong charge. Basophils also contain MBP but only approximately 2 percent of that of eosinophils (see Fig. 62–2).

Eosinophil peroxidase is a heme-containing protein that is synthesized as a single protein and then cleaved into 14- and 58-kDa subunits.[113] The molecule shares a 68 percent identity in amino acid sequence with human neutrophil myeloperoxidase as well as other peroxidase enzymes. The substance is toxic for parasites, respiratory epithelium, and pneumocytes, either alone, or (more potently) when combined with H_2O_2 and halide, the preferred ion *in vivo* being bromide. Eosinophil cationic protein (ECP) is an arginine-rich protein. The complementary DNA encodes for a 27-amino-acid leader sequence and a 133-amino-acid mature polypeptide with a molecular mass of 15.6 kDa. ECP has 66 percent amino acid sequence homology with eosinophil-derived neurotoxin (EDN) and 31 percent homology with human pancreatic ribonuclease, but it has low ribonuclease activity compared to EDN.[114] ECP is toxic for helminthic parasites, isolated myocardial cells, and guinea pig tracheal epithelium. ECP also inhibits lymphocyte proliferation *in vitro*. Both ECP and EDN produce neurotoxicity (the Gordon phenomenon) when injected into the cerebrospinal fluid of experimental animals. ECP may damage cells by a colloid osmotic process, as it can induce non–ion-selective pores in both cellular and synthetic membranes.[115]

EDN, also called *EPX*, is a 16-kDa, glycosylated protein possessing marked ribonuclease activity. The complementary DNA predicts a 134-amino-acid mature polypeptide that is identical to human urinary ribonuclease. Like ECP, it is a member of a ribonuclease multigene family.[116] EDN expression is not restricted to eosinophils, as it is found in mononuclear cells and possibly neutrophils. It is also probably secreted by the liver. It does not appear to be toxic to parasites or mammalian cells, and its only known effect, other than its ribonuclease activity, is neurotoxicity (see Fig. 62–2).

A major constituent of the eosinophil is Charcot-Leyden protein, which is a lysophospholipase. It constitutes up to 10 percent of eosinophil protein and is also found in large quantities in basophils. It was thought to possess lysophospholipase activity but this is not the case. It is a member of the galectin family (galectin 10).[117] Its precise function is unknown.

Vasoactive intestinal peptide has been detected in eosinophils in granulomas from mice infected with schistosomes and the eosinophil contains a number of granule-stored enzymes, which roles in eosinophil function are not clear. These enzymes include acid phosphatase, collagenase, arylsulfatase B, histaminase, phospholipase D, catalase, nonspecific esterases, vitamin B_{12}-binding proteins, and glycosaminoglycans. Eosinophils can undergo a respiratory burst with release of superoxide anion and H_2O_2 in response to stimulation with both particulate stimuli, such as opsonized zymosan, and soluble mediators, such as leukotriene and phorbol myristate acetate. Eosinophils upon equivalent stimulation are twice as chemoluminescent as neutrophils.

EOSINOPHIL SECRETION AND ACTIVATION

A striking feature of eosinophil-rich inflammatory reactions is the high concentration of granule proteins, often in the presence of relatively small numbers of intact eosinophils. Mediator secretion can be triggered physiologically by engagement of immunoglobulin Fc receptors, especially after eosinophil activation has been primed with soluble mediators such as platelet-activating factor and IL-5.[118] The eosinophil expresses receptors for IgG, IgA, and IgD. The eosinophil also binds IgE, and eosinophils can undertake a number of IgE-dependent functions, including killing of schistosomes opsonized with specific IgE. The receptor involved is unclear as the accumulated evidence now suggests that eosinophils do not express either the low-affinity (FcεRII) or high-affinity (FcεRI) IgE receptor to any degree, although they do express high intracellular levels of the α chain of FcεRI.[119]

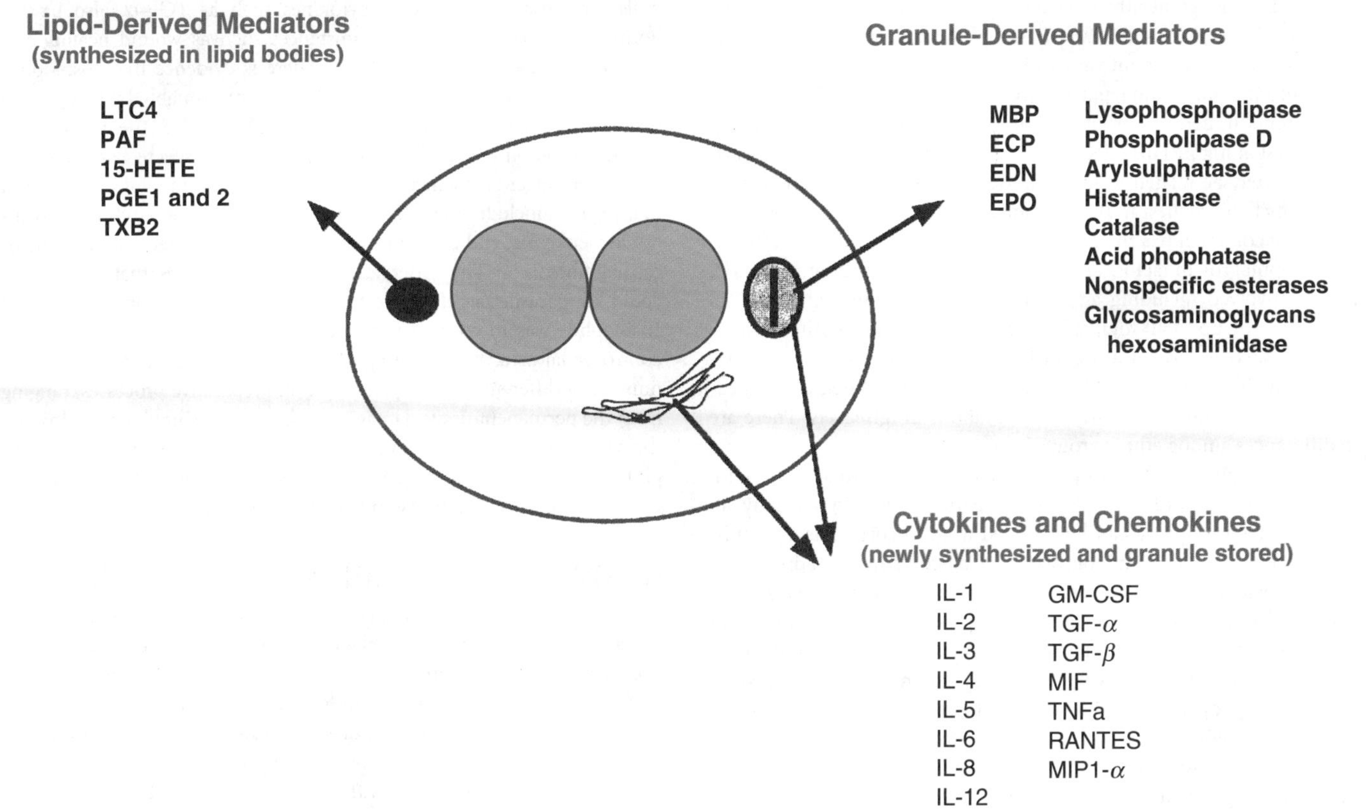

FIGURE 62–2. Representation of eosinophil-derived mediators. ECP, eosinophil cationic protein; EDN, eosinophil-derived neurotoxin; EPO, eosinophil-derived peroxidase; GM-CSF, granulocyte-monocyte colony stimulating factor; HETE, hydroxyeicosatetraenoic acid; LTC, leukotriene C; MBP, major basic protein; MIF, macrophage inhibition factor; MIP, macrophage inhibitory protein; PAF, platelet activating factor; PGE, prostaglandin E; TGF, transforming growth factor; TNF, tumor necrosis factor; TXB, thromboxane B.

Three receptors for IgG have been described: the high-affinity receptor FcγR1 (CD64), and two low-affinity receptors FcγRII (CDw32) and FcγRIII (CD16). CD16 is expressed both as a transmembrane form and a form with a phosphatidylinositol anchor, transcribed from two distinct genes. Only FcγRII is constitutively expressed by eosinophils to any significant degree. A number of eosinophil functions are mediated via this receptor, including schistosomula killing, phagocytosis, secretion of granule proteins, and generation of newly formed, membrane-derived lipid mediators such as platelet-activating factor and LTC_4. After stimulation for 2 days *in vitro* with interferon-γ, eosinophils express CD16 and CD64 as well as CD32.[120] Perhaps the most potent stimulus for eosinophil degranulation is crosslinking of IgA receptors, especially when the cells have been primed with growth factors.[121] Consistent with the preference of eosinophils to secrete their mediators onto a large surface, Fc-mediated degranulation is enhanced if the eosinophils are adherent to a protein-coated surface via the integrin $\alpha_M\beta_2$.[122]

The killing of schistosomula opsonized with nonimmune serum is presumed to be mediated via the complement receptors, CR1, and CR3. Incubation of eosinophils with serum-coated beads results in the release of 15 percent of ECP. Similarly, opsonized zymosan interacts with eosinophils, causing generation of hydrogen peroxide and the phagocytosis of the zymosan. Soluble mediators such as platelet-activating factor, LTB_4, and 5-oxo-eicosatetraenoate can elicit the direct secretion of both granule proteins and lipid mediators, although only with highly activated eosinophils or when used in conjunction with cytochalasin B, which inhibits microtubule assembly (see Fig. 62–2). Eosinophils release their granule components by exocytosis, with individual granules fusing with the plasma membrane. This process involves a guanosine triphosphate-binding protein and is modulated by the intracellular calcium concentration.[123] Like other secretory cells, degranulation of eosinophils is controlled by SNAP (soluble *N*-ethylmaleimide-sensitive factor attachment protein) receptor complex (SNARE) proteins that guide the granules to the cell surface. Vesicular SNAREs expressed on granules bind to target SNAREs expressed on the plasma membrane. The SNARE proteins vesicle-associated membrane protein 2 and 7 appear to be particularly important in eosinophil secretion from granules.[124]

EOSINOPHILS IN DISEASE

■ MEASUREMENT OF EOSINOPHILS IN THE BLOOD

Eosinophils can be enumerated in the blood either by "wet counts" in modified Neubauer chambers, differential counts on dried blood films, or by automated cell counting by flow cytometry.[125] Automated counting that uses detection of eosinophil peroxidase is the most accurate method, followed by counting in a cell chamber. Counting on films is least accurate because of the tendency for eosinophils to congregate at the margins of the slide. Common wet stains for eosinophils include eosin in acetone, phloxine, and Kimura stain, which was originally developed to stain basophils.[126] Many stains, including May-Grünwald-Giemsa, Romanowsky stain, chromotrope 2R, and Biebrich scarlet, identify eosinophils in blood films, cytospin preparations, or tissues.

The eosinophil count should be evaluated in absolute numbers rather than as a percentage of white cells, as the latter will depend on the total cell count. The normal eosinophil count is generally taken as less than

0.4×10^9/L, although healthy medical students in the United States had a range of 0.015 to 0.65×10^9/L.[127] Eosinophil counts are higher in neonates. The eosinophil count varies with age, time of day, exercise status, and environmental stimuli, particularly allergen exposure. Blood eosinophil counts undergo diurnal variation, being lowest in the morning and highest at night. This effect results in a greater than 40 percent variation and may be related to the reciprocal diurnal variation in cortisol levels, which are highest in the morning. The factors that control blood eosinophil counts in health are imperfectly understood. Concentrations of eosinophil growth factors are likely to be important, but other factors may be involved including an element of genetic control.[128] Normal counts vary by up to 40-fold, and, in populations where eosinophilia is common, such as endemically parasitized areas, there are marked variations in the blood eosinophil level, independent of the degree of infection. This variation is comparable to variations in IgE levels. There are no differences among ethnic groups in eosinophil counts.

The eosinophil count in hospitalized patients is less than 10 cells/μL (0.01×10^9/L) in only 0.1 percent of patients, and in virtually all patients the eosinopenia can be ascribed to glucocorticoids, epinephrine, or acute infection. In contrast, beta blockers inhibit adrenaline-induced eosinopenia and can cause a rise in the eosinophil count.

There have been several isolated case reports of patients with absent eosinophils in the blood and marrow.[129] Several patients without eosinophils were reported as having allergic symptoms.[130] In one case, it occurred after drug-induced agranulocytosis[131] and in another there was a serum inhibitor of eosinophil colony formation.[132] A rare disorder, eosinophil peroxidase deficiency, may be brought to light by automatic counting that uses detection of EPO to count eosinophils. EPO deficiency does not have any adverse clinical consequences.[133]

CAUSES OF EOSINOPHILIA

An eosinophilia accompanies a discrete number of diseases, and a high eosinophil count is always a clinically notable observation that should be explained, although an explanation is not always found.[134] The causes of eosinophilia can be classified according to the degree and frequency of occurrence (Table 62–4). The classification of the magnitude of eosinophil counts is arbitrary, but a mild eosinophilia could be regarded as less than 1.0×10^9/L, a moderate elevation as 1.0 to 5.0×10^9/L, and a high eosinophil count as greater than 5.0×10^9/L. The most common cause of an eosinophilia worldwide is infection with helminthic parasites, which can often result in a very high eosinophil count. The most common cause of an eosinophilia in industrialized countries is the atopic allergic diseases, seasonal and perennial rhinitis, atopic dermatitis, and asthma. Allergic disease generally results in only a mild increase in eosinophil counts. A moderate or high eosinophil count in asthma especially outside a severe exacerbation raises the possibility of a complication such as Churg-Strauss syndrome, allergic bronchopulmonary aspergillosis, or eosinophilic pneumonia.[135] Organ-specific diseases such as eosinophilic cellulitis and esophagitis should be considered, although it could be argued that these are part of the HES spectrum. Drug allergy is not always straightforward to diagnose as a cause of an eosinophilia and less common causes include Addison disease (although the eosinophilia is not usually marked).

THE ROLE OF EOSINOPHILS

For years eosinophils were thought to ameliorate inflammatory responses, then through the 1980s and 1990s they were believed to cause tissue damage in some situations. The use of anti–IL-5 and tyrosine kinase inhibitors to inhibit eosinophil production has suggested a complex interaction between eosinophilic inflammation and target organ damage.[136] Eosinophils may, through release of cytokines such as TGF-α, also have a homeostatic role in certain circumstances such as wound healing and mammary gland development.[137,138] There is evidence that eosinophils slow the rate of progression of solid tumors, presumably by being cytotoxic to tumor cells,[139] although other studies have raised the possibility of a tumor promoting role.[140] Eosinophils can cause severe tissue damage under certain circumstances. Chronically high eosinophil counts from many causes including drug reactions, parasitic infections, chronic eosinophilic leukemia, and other forms of HES, are associated with endomyocardial fibrosis.[141] The observation in the mid-1970s that eosinophils could kill parasite targets led to the hypothesis that the principal role of eosinophils was to counter parasitic infection, although this remains a controversial area.[142,143] Consequently, eosinophils are associated with a number of different types of pathologic and reparative processes, ranging from the permanent tissue damage seen in hypereosinophilic syndromes, the partly reversible tissue damage seen in asthma and pulmonary eosinophilia, and tissue repair characteristic of wound healing. The factors that determine which role the eosinophil adopts are unclear.

EOSINOPHILS AND ASTHMA

The relationship between airway inflammation and asthma is complex. In particular, there is no close relationship between the severity of eosinophilic airway inflammation and either the severity of symptoms, airway hyperreactivity, or abnormalities in forced expiratory volume in one second.[144,145] A large number of studies have examined this relationship of eosinophilia in endobronchial biopsies, sputum, and bronchoalveolar lavage and bronchial washings with airway reactivity, and the results show at best a weak correlation. For example, sputum eosinophilia measured in more than 200 outpatients with a diagnosis of asthma (ranging from mild to severe) had a very weak correlation with airway reactivity in atopic subjects and no correlation at all in patients with nonatopic disease.[146] A caveat is that the level of activation of leukocytes such as T cells and eosinophils may be more important than cell numbers, although eosinophil counts usually correlate well with concentrations of eosinophil-specific mediators in the bronchial lavage. There was a reasonable correlation between changes in sputum eosinophils and airway hyperreactivity after allergen challenge as well as in a study of treatment with inhaled glucocorticoids.[147,148] However, even if there was a better correlation between eosinophilic inflammation and severity of asthma *within* an individual it would still mean that there was considerable variability in the sensitivity to airway inflammation between individuals. The potential dissociation between an airway dysfunction phenotype, which leads to many of the symptoms and physiologic abnormalities in asthma and an eosinophilic inflammation predominant phenotype more closely associated with severe exacerbations was demonstrated in an examination of asthma heterogeneity using cluster analysis techniques.[149] This dissociation was further illustrated by clinical trials of an anti–IL-5 monoclonal antibody (mAb; mepolizumab), which markedly reduced eosinophils in the blood and sputum but had no effect on either airway hyperreactivity or lung function in patients with mild asthma, or on the late response to allergen challenge.[37] The interpretation of this study and others using the anti–IL-5 antibody is complicated by the observation that anti–IL-5 only partially depletes the tissue eosinophilia.[78] A dissociation between airway reactivity and the eosinophilia has also been seen in animal models of allergen challenge. For example anti–VLA-4 mAb was able to block ovalbumin induced airway hyperreactivity, but not airway eosinophilia when given by aerosol to mice.[150] In eosinophilic bronchitis in which patients have an eosinophilic airway inflammation but no evidence of asthma (no airway hyperresponsiveness or variable airflow obstruction) the asthma phenotype correlated with the number of mast cells in the airway smooth muscle and the tissue eosinophilia did not differ between the asthmatic

TABLE 62–4. Causes of an Eosinophilia

Disease	Frequency	Usual Degree of Eosinophilia	Comment
Infections			
Parasitic	Common worldwide	Moderate to high	
Bacterial	Rare		Usually cause eosinopenia, although serum ECP levels may be raised, suggesting eosinophil involvement in tissue.
Mycobacterial	Rare		More often secondary to drug therapy.
Invasive fungal	Rare		Apart from allergic reactions, which are common, and coccidioidomycosis, in which as many as 88% of patients have an eosinophilia.
Rickettsial infections	Rare		
Fungi	Rare		Cryptococcus reported as causing CSF eosinophilia.
Viral infections	Rare		There are occasional case reports of an eosinophilia in a variety of viral infections, including herpes and HIV infection.
Allergic diseases			
Allergic rhinitis	Common worldwide	Mild	
Atopic dermatitis	Common especially children	Mild	
Urticaria/angioedema	Common	Variable	Eosinophilia seen in skin even with normal blood count.
Asthma	Common	Mild	Syndrome of intrinsic asthma, nasal polyps, and aspirin intolerance are associated with higher-than-usual eosinophil counts.
Drug reactions			
Many drugs	Uncommon	Mild to high	Antibiotics, NSAIDs, and antipsychotics are the most common groups; count usually returns to normal on stopping drug.
Neoplasms			
Acute eosinophilic leukemia (see Chap. 89)	Rare	High	
Acute myelogenous leukemia with marrow eosinophilia (see Chap. 89)	Uncommon		Often associated with chromosome 16 abnormalities.
Chronic eosinophilic leukemia (see Chap. 90)	Rare	High	See text on HES.
Chronic myelogenous leukemia (see Chap. 90)	Uncommon	Moderate to high	Raised eosinophil counts can be seen uncommonly in chronic myelogenous leukemia.
Lymphomas (see Chap. 106)	Uncommon	Moderate	Often intense tissue eosinophilia with moderately elevated blood eosinophil count; Hodgkin lymphoma most common type. T-cell lymphomas elaborating IL-5 or other eosinopoietic cytokines.
Langerhans cell histiocytosis (see Chap. 72)	Uncommon	Mild	Intense tissue eosinophilia in granulomata but blood eosinophilia unusual.
Solid tumors	Uncommon	Mild to high	Many different tumors reported.
Musculoskeletal disorders			
Rheumatoid arthritis	Uncommon	Mild to high	Occasional case reports. More usually secondary to therapy.
Eosinophilic fasciitis (see Chap. 88)	Rare	High	
Gastrointestinal disorders			
Eosinophilic gastroenteritis	Rare	Mild to moderate	As with many GI diseases there is often a marked tissue eosinophilia with only a mild or no blood eosinophilia.
Eosinophilic esophagitis	Increasingly recognized	Mild	Marked tissue eosinophilia with mild blood eosinophilia.
Celiac disease	Uncommon	None	Tissue eosinophilia.
Inflammatory bowel disease			Eosinophils seen in biopsies in both Crohn disease and ulcerative colitis, but blood eosinophilia unusual.
Allergic gastroenteritis	Uncommon	Mild to high	Young children.

(continued)

TABLE 62–4. Causes of an Eosinophilia (Continued)

Disease	Frequency	Usual Degree of Eosinophilia	Comment
Respiratory tract (for *asthma* see *allergic diseases*)			
Churg-Strauss syndrome	Rare	Moderate to high	Syndrome of eosinophilic vasculitis and asthma.
Pulmonary eosinophilia including eosinophilic pneumonia	Uncommon	Mild to high	Syndrome of eosinophilia and pulmonary infiltrates. Apart from ABPA usually of unknown cause.
Bronchiectasis; cystic fibrosis	Common	Mild	Often associated with asthma or ABPA.
Skin diseases (for *atopic dermatitis* see *allergic diseases*)			
Bullous pemphigoid	Uncommon	Moderate	
Eosinophilic cellulitis	Uncommon	Moderate to high	High eosinophil count distinguishes from bacterial cause.
Miscellaneous causes			
IL-2 therapy	Rare	Moderate to high	For renal cell carcinoma or melanoma.
Hypereosinophilic syndrome	Uncommon	High	
Endomyocardial fibrosis	Uncommon	High	Secondary to any cause of a high eosinophil count.
Hyper IgE syndrome	Uncommon	Moderate to high	
Eosinophilia-myalgia syndrome and toxic oil syndrome	Rare	High	Two related conditions, one caused by poisoning with contaminated cooking oil in Spain and the other by a batch of contaminated tryptophan.

ABPA, Allergic bronchopulmonary aspergillosis; CSF, cerebral spinal fluid; GI, gastrointestinal; HES, hypereosinophilic syndrome; NSAID, nonsteroidal antiinflammatory drug.

and eosinophilic bronchitis groups.[108] Large numbers of eosinophils and mononuclear cells are found in and around the bronchi of patients who have died of asthma, and their bronchial tissue contains large amounts of MBP.[7] The pathology of asthma deaths is at the extreme end of the pathology of asthma exacerbations. There is increasing evidence that an airway eosinophilia is closely associated with the risk of having exacerbations. In one study treatment targeted at reducing the chronic airway eosinophilia resulted in a considerable drop in the number of exacerbations compared to standard management.[151] There is now definitive evidence from two studies using mepolizumab that eosinophils are associated with severe exacerbations of airway disease. Asthmatics with documented eosinophil airway inflammation were treated for up to a year with mepolizumab with the primary outcome of a reduction in sputum eosinophilia in one study and in glucocorticoid dose in another. Both demonstrated that mepolizumab was an effective form of treatment with response correlating with the effect on reducing eosinophils.[152,153]

EOSINOPHILS AND THE SKIN

A large number of skin conditions are associated with infiltration by eosinophils.[154] The normal skin contains few eosinophils so their presence is usually associated with pathology. The most common cause of eosinophilic infiltration of the skin is atopic dermatitis where, as with asthma, the relationship to pathogenesis remains contentious.[155] The skin is one of the most commonly effected organs in hypereosinophilic syndrome, with pruritus being the commonest symptom, although ulceration also occurs.[156]

EOSINOPHILS AND THE GASTROINTESTINAL TRACT

Eosinophils are present in the normal gastrointestinal tract as a result of constitutive expression of eotaxin and MAdCAM-1 the receptor for integrin $\alpha_4\beta_7$ which is expressed by eosinophils.[59] A number of diseases are associated with a gastrointestinal eosinophilia including eosinophilic esophagitis, eosinophilic gastroenteritis, and inflammatory bowel disease.[157] Eosinophilic esophagitis is an increasingly recognized condition in both children and adults. It is associated with food allergy, often in the absence of specific IgE.[158,159] There are case reports of successful treatment of this condition with anti–IL-5, suggesting a proinflammatory role for eosinophils in the disease.[160]

EOSINOPHILS AND PARASITIC DISEASE

The role of eosinophils in parasitic disease is complex and still incompletely understood.[143] The most common helminthic causes of an eosinophilia are summarized in Table 62–5 and a review.[161] Eosinophils can kill a number of opsonized parasites including newborn larvae of *T. spiralis*, larvae of *Nippostrongylus brasiliensis*, a gut parasite in the rat, and larvae of *Fasciola hepatica*, as well as schistosomula of *S. mansoni*. *In vivo*, parasite larvae become opsonized with both specific IgG and IgE antibodies and components of the complement cascade such as C3bi, which can promote adhesion and activation of eosinophils. Dead larvae of *Schistosoma haematobium* and other parasites have been detected in the skin surrounded by eosinophils and eosinophil granule products. Adult worms, both *in vitro* and *in vivo*, appear resistant to eosinophil-mediated damage. Despite the circumstantial evidence of eosinophils being involved in host defense against parasites, there remains some doubt about their role. Except for schistosomiasis there is no obvious correlation between the degree of eosinophilia and protection against infection or reinfection.[162] A number of experiments have been carried out in animal models of helminthic infection using IL-5 gene deletion, IL-5 transgenics, and anti–IL-5 antibodies to ablate the tissue eosinophilia. These studies have suggested that eosinophils may have a protective role in *Strongyloides* and

TABLE 62–5. Helminthic Causes of an Eosinophilia

Parasite (Disease)	Comment
Nematodes	
Ascaris (Ascariasis)	Ascariasis results in higher eosinophil counts in children. Larvae migrate from intestine to lungs where they cause Loeffler syndrome, a form of pulmonary eosinophilia.
Toxocara canis (Toxocariasis)	Infective eggs are present in feces of puppies and pregnant bitches. Larvae in hosts such as chicken. Eosinophilia seen mainly in children younger than age 9 years. Can migrate to eye and cause blindness. Serologic evidence suggests infection not uncommon in industrialized countries.
Loa loa (Filariasis, Loaiasis); *Wuchereria bancrofti* (Filariasis, Elephantiasis); *Brugia malayi* (Filariasis, Elephantiasis); *Onchocerca volvulus* (Filariasis, River Blindness)	Common. Invariably result in marked eosinophilia, especially Loa Loa filariasis infection. Filariasis is the cause of tropical pulmonary eosinophilia caused by migration of adult worms to lung, elephantiasis caused by involvement of lymphatics *(Wuchereria bancrofti* and *Brugia malayi)* and river blindness *(Onchocerca volvulus).* Treatment can result in systemic reaction called *Mazzotti reaction,* possibly as a result of massive eosinophil degranulation.
Ancylostomaduodenale (Ancylostomiasis, Old World Hookworm) and *Necator americanus* (New World Hookworm)	Hookworm infection. *Ancylostoma duodenale* and *Necator americanus.* One of the main causes of eosinophilia in patients returning from tropical countries. Eosinophil counts in region of $2000 \times 10^6/\mu L$.
Strongyloides stercoralis (Strongyloidiasis)	Subclinical infection can persist for more than 20 years. Stool examinations often negative. Cause of eosinophilia in ex-servicemen who spent time in tropics. If *Strongyloides* infection is not considered and these patients are given glucocorticoids for suspected hypereosinophilic syndrome or as trial of therapy, they can develop disseminated disease.
Trichinella spiralis (Trichinosis)	Trichinosis is caused by ingestion of encysted muscle larvae of *Trichinella spiralis.* Most prominent eosinophilia seen during early stages of infection when larvae migrating into striated muscle via the blood. Fatal cases reported of which only 20% were noted to have an eosinophilia.
Others	Other nematodes that can cause eosinophilia include *Trichuris trichiura* (Trichuriasis), *Capillaria philippinensis* (Capillariasis), and *Gnathostoma spinigerum* (Gnathostomiasis). The thread worm, *Enterobius vermicularis* (Pinworm), occasionally causes an eosinophilia when they invade tissues.
Trematodes	
Schistosoma mansoni, S. hematobium, S. japonicum (Schistosomiasis, Bilharzia)	Infection with one of the *Schistosoma* (blood flukes), *S. mansoni, S. haematobium,* or *S. japonicum,* is perhaps the commonest causes of a moderate to high eosinophilia worldwide with 200 million people infected. Infection is nearly always associated with an eosinophilia.
Fasciola	Adult worms of *Fasciola hepatica* reside in the bile ducts, where they are associated with abnormal liver function tests and an eosinophilia.
Cestodes	
Echinococcus	Eosinophilia occurs in 25–50% of patients with hydatid disease.

Filaria but not in *Schistosoma*, *Nippostrongylus*, and *Trichuris* infections. For example, treatment of mice infected with *N. brasiliensis* or *S. mansoni* with neutralizing anti–IL-5 mAbs abolished the eosinophilia without modulating the disease process.[163] In contrast, adding eosinophils in diffusion chambers was shown to kill the larvae of *Strongyloides stercoralis*.[164] The mechanism of eosinophilia in parasitic disease is thought to be similar to allergic disease, because it generates a Th2-type response to helminthic antigens. This effect results in increased production of eosinophil growth factors, in particular IL-5.[165]

HYPEREOSINOPHILIC SYNDROMES

Hypereosinophilic Syndrome

Definition and History HES is an uncommon and potentially fatal group of disorders first described as a distinct entity by Hardy and Anderson in 1968[166] and defined as an eosinophilia of greater than 1.5×10^9 cells/L for more than 6 months with, at that time, no other explanation and evidence of organ damage.[167] Patient series consistently show that the major target organs for tissue damage are the skin, heart, lung, and nervous system.[168,169] The definition and classification of HES is unsatisfactory as conditions such as Churg-Strauss syndrome, eosinophilic pneumonia, eosinophilic gastroenteritis, and other specific conditions are arbitrarily excluded. Attempts are being made to create a more comprehensive and less arbitrary system, but this requires new data on the specific etiology of these diseases.[170]

The World Health Organization considers that all myeloproliferative variants of HES are neoplastic (clonal) disorders (leukemias). Where there is no defined genotypic abnormality the condition has been termed chronic eosinophilic leukemia (CEL)- not otherwise specified (NOS), and where there is a defined mutation such as *FIP1LI-PDGFRα* they fall into a new category of their own.[171] In part, these distinctions are drawn because the cases with a translocation involving a tyrosine kinase (e.g PDGF-R) may be treated with a tyrosine kinase inhibitor.

Epidemiology HES is an uncommon group of disorders with an estimated prevalence (although there is limited data on this), in the region of 1 in 50,000 persons. It occurs sporadically, and there appear to be no significant geographic or environmental influences. For unknown reasons, the myeloproliferative form has a strong male incidence.

Differential Diagnosis A marked blood eosinophilia is a relatively unusual event, and it is found in a restricted range of conditions worldwide (see Tables 62–4 and 62–5).

Etiology and Pathogenesis New insights into both the pathophysiology and management of HES have been offered by the use of anti–IL-5 and the tyrosine kinase inhibitor imatinib mesylate to treat the disease. HES is composed of a heterogenous group of diseases: A minority of patients have a T-cell lymphoproliferative disorder in which the lymphoma cells overproduce IL-5 resulting in reactive eosinophilia and a majority of cases result from somatic mutations in a hematopoietic progenitor cell leading to chronic eosinophilic leukemia, within which group are cases with constitutively active tyrosine kinases. These findings have led to the proposal that there are two broad variants of HES: myeloid and lymphoid.[172]

The myeloid variant is a myeloproliferative disorder that includes marked blood and marrow eosinophilia, in some cases immature cells including blast cells in the marrow and blood, high serum vitamin B_{12}, and serum tryptase, elevated alkaline phosphatase, chromosomal abnormalities, anemia and thrombocytopenia, and splenomegaly. The cardiac and neurologic involvement that is a poor prognostic factor in HES is found mainly, but not exclusively, in this group of patients. A small proportion of these patients go on to develop acute myelogenous leukemia. Demonstration of eosinophil clonality is difficult unless a fusion oncogene is present, leading to constitutive activation of growth factor associated tyrosine kinases. For example, an interstitial deletion on 4q12 results in a fusion protein consisting of the product of the *FIP1L1-PDGFRα* fusion gene, which has constitutive tyrosine kinase activity. This oncogene was shown to be present in 8 of 15 patients with what was thought to be idiopathic HES, all of whom responded to treatment with the tyrosine kinase inhibitor imatinib.[173] This mutation causes the Ba/F3 cell line to become IL-3 independent and is found in the EOL-1 cell line derived from a patient with chronic eosinophilic leukemia.[174] The presence of this mutation and the good response to treatment with imatinib has been confirmed by other groups and is now recognized as the commonest clonal abnormality in myeloid HES (chronic eosinophilic leukemia).[175] Imatinib has also been effective in other patients with apparently idiopathic HES without this particular mutation[173,176] and a number of other uncommon mutated tyrosine kinases have been shown to cause the condition, including the *JAK2 V617F* point mutation usually associated with polycythemia vera,[177] other partners for the *PDGFRα or* the *PDGFRβ* genes, and rearrangements in the *FGFR1* gene on chromosome 8p11 in which most patients progress to an aggressive leukemia or lymphoma.[171,175] Cytogenetic analysis identifies several mutations but not the *FIP1L1-PDGFRa* mutation. Serum tryptase is a good marker of this form of HES, indicating that mast cells are also effected, since tryptase is specific for mast cells (see Chap. 63).[178] It is, however, distinct from systemic mastocytosis.[178]

The lymphoid variant of HES generally follows a more benign course than the myeloid variants, and the former occurs in women more frequently than the myeloid variant. Patients with lymphoid variant of HES tend to respond well to glucocorticoids and do not develop the cardiac fibrosis and other severe complications of the myeloid variant. This difference is probably accounted for by the eosinophils being part of the neoplastic clone in the myeloid variant. The lymphoid variant is usually related to the overproduction of eosinophil-related growth factors, often IL-5, by aberrant T cells. Thus, the eosinophilia is reactive, unlike the myeloid variant. A number of different patterns of T-cell lymphoproliferation have been found in association with HES, the most common being a CD3–CD4+CD5+ subset of T cells.[179–183] In many cases these clones have been shown to secrete increased amounts of eosinophil-related cytokines, such as IL-5, IL-4, and IL-3. Clonality of the phenotypically aberrant T cells has been demonstrated in many cases and some cases progress to progressive malignancy. This variant of the HES is discussed further in Chap. 106.

Clinical Features HES has a heterogeneous presentation with a marked and persistent blood and marrow eosinophilia being the hallmark.[172,183,184] It is a chronic disease that usually presents in the third or fourth decade but can present at any age, including, occasionally, in childhood. It varies from being relatively asymptomatic to an aggressive disease leading to death within a few years if left untreated. The more severe complications are generally found in the myeloproliferative variant of the disease. HES can present with nonspecific symptoms such as general malaise, weight loss, aches and pains, and bouts of sweating or with the organ-specific features involving lung, skin, heart or nervous system. Cardiac complications are common in the chronic myeloproliferative variant of the disease, in particular endomyocardial fibrosis, which leads to a restrictive cardiomyopathy and left ventricular failure. Mitral or tricuspid valve incompetence can occur. Thromboembolic complications of large and small vessels are common in more severe disease, some of which originate from an endomyocardial clot. Some of the central nervous system manifestations are embolic in origin. Respiratory symptoms include cough, usually productive of only small amounts of sputum, and breathlessness. Although airflow obstruction occurs, there is a limited response to bronchodilators and airway hyperresponsiveness is often absent. Wheezing is not a prominent symptom. Pulmonary infiltrates, including alveolar involvement, and nodules may be present. Skin symptoms are particularly common and includes pruritus, sometimes associated with erythematous papules and urticaria.

A variant of HES is referred to as Gleich syndrome, in which patients get recurrent episodes of angioedema. Eosinophilic cellulitis may also be a feature.[185] In addition to embolic events, HES can be associated with confusion, loss of memory and ataxia. In the peripheral nervous system patients can develop mononeuritis multiplex, sensorimotor neuropathy, multifocal neuropathy, and radiculopathy. The differential diagnosis with Churg-Strauss (see "Eosinophilia, Angiitis, and Asthma" below) syndrome can be difficult and may be semantic. Patients can develop mucosal ulcerations. There may be renal system involvement but severe complications are not usually prominent.

Laboratory Features The characteristic laboratory finding is blood and marrow eosinophilia. The blood eosinophilia exceeds 1.5×10^9 cells/L. The eosinophils are principally mature in appearance with segmented nuclei although there may be three segments in some nuclei, not characteristic of normal blood eosinophils. Eosinophilic myelocytes may be present in small numbers. Some cells may be degranulated or larger or smaller than the typical eosinophils. Vacuoles may be present. These morphologic variations are not too dissimilar from benign eosinophilias. Mild anemia and mild thrombocytopenia may be present at diagnosis. Neutrophilia may also occur, occasionally. The marrow is markedly infiltrated with eosinophilic myelocytes and eosinophils, roughly proportional to the height of the blood eosinophil count (see Fig. 62–3). An increase in blast cells is unusual but may occur and may harbinger a more rapid course. Charcot-Leyden crystals may be observed in the marrow as may be the case in any tissue biopsy. Mast cells may also be found. Type III, collagen (argentophilic, reticulin) fibers may be increased as judged with silver stain.

Marrow cytogentic findings may include one of several translocations involving chromosome 5, including t(1;5)(q21;q33), t(5;12)(q31-33;q24), and occasionally other translocation variants, usually involving the *PDGFR* gene on chromosome 5 at bands 31 to 33.

Approach to the Diagnosis Initially, investigations to exclude a reactive cause for the eosinophilia should be undertaken (see "Differential Diagnosis" below). A scheme for investigation of patients with HES has been proposed.[183] This approach is aimed at determining if there is evidence of myeloid clonality, or an abnormal T-cell clone. They include full blood count with examination of a blood film. Measurement of serum immunoglobulins, serum vitamin B_{12}, and serum tryptase; examination of a marrow aspirate and biopsy with marrow cell cytogenetic studies; lymphocyte immunophenotyping and, if available, analysis of IL-5 levels, T-cell receptor gene rearrangement, and analysis of the presence of the *FIP1L1-PDGFRα* fusion by reverse transcription polymerase chain reaction or fluorescence *in situ* hybridization analysis. A chest radiograph, spirometry, biochemical profile, troponin, cortisol, echocardiogram, and cardiac and abdominal ultrasonography should also be undertaken, as well as neurologic investigations, such as nerve conduction or electromyographic studies of involved neuromuscular areas. Depending on

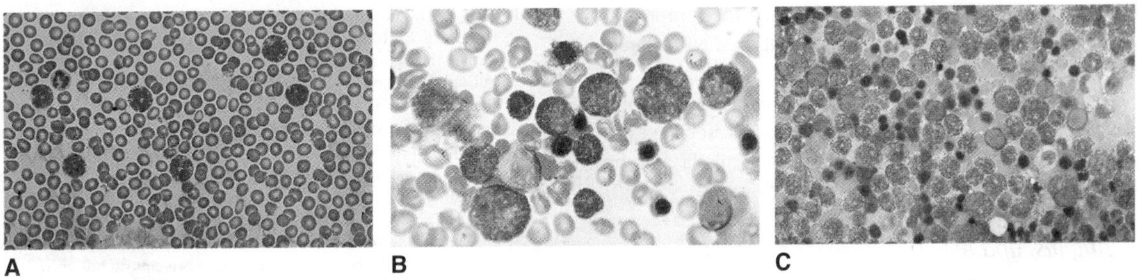

FIGURE 62–3. Chronic eosinophilic leukemia. **A.** Blood film. Marked eosinophilia. Six eosinophils in the low-power field and one segmented neutrophil. **B.** Marrow film. Marked increase in eosinophils. Segmented eosinophils and eosinophilic myelocytes. Five orthochromatic erythroblasts are also in this field. An occasional neutrophilic myelocyte is evident. **C.** Marrow section. Early and late eosinophilic myelocytes dominate granulopoiesis; Segmented eosinophils and erythroblasts are notable. A few neutrophilic precursors are present. *(Used with permission from* Lichtman's Atlas of Hematology, *www.accessmedicine.com.)*

the major site of organ damage, more detailed organ specific investigations such as cardiac magnetic resonance imaging, chest computed tomography, full lung function tests, and gastrointestinal endoscopy may be required. Examination of stools for parasites in patients with chronic eosinophilia is an insensitive investigation and serology, although a more sensitive approach, is only available for common helminthic disorders such as strongyloides, schistosomiasis, and filariasis, so empirical treatment with broad-spectrum antihelminthics can sometimes be justified if there is high clinical suspicion in endemic areas.

Differential Diagnosis The reactive causes of a marked eosinophilia listed in Table 62–4 should be excluded with appropriate investigations. Once these have been excluded the differential diagnosis includes familial eosinophilia, a rare condition that has been mapped to a region of chromosome 5q31-q33,[186] acute eosinophilic leukemia, eosinophilia secondary to malignancy, Churg-Strauss syndrome, and chronic eosinophilic pneumonia. Evidence of end organ damage is unusual in acute eosinophilic leukemia (see Chap. 89). Some patients also appear to have a raised eosinophil count without any evidence of organ damage, so called benign eosinophilia.

Treatment The low incidence of HES means that there are few clinical trials and most agents are used on the basis of anecdotal experience or experience with related diseases. However the use of imatinib for some patients with the myeloproliferative variant and the use of anti–IL-5 for T-cell–driven eosinophilia offer new promise to patients with HES.[187] The mainstay of treatment has been a glucocorticoid, which in many cases, particularly in patients without myeloproliferative disease, is effective at controlling either the eosinophil count or the target organ damage, but risks long-term side effects of those agents. In patients with myeloproliferative features the eosinophil count is not completely controlled with glucocorticoids, although these drugs can still limit organ damage. In patients where glucocorticoids are insufficiently effective, hydroxyurea can be a useful agent to lower the eosinophil count. Other cytotoxic drugs, such as vincristine and cyclophosphamide, are less commonly used. Interferon-α has been used with some success, although it is expensive and has significant side effects, especially in older patients.[188] Imatinib has resulted in remission is patients with the *FIP1L1-PDGFR*α mutation. In the absence of the *FIP1L1-PDGFR*α mutation in patients with myeloproliferative features, a trial of imatinib is indicated as occasional patients without the fusion gene have responded.[189,190] Response to imatinib at a dose of 400 mg/day should be rapid (within 3 weeks) and result in a return of the eosinophil count to within the normal range, if the cause of the eosinophilia is an imatinib-responsive tyrosine kinase mutation. Resistance to treatment has emerged in some cases, as it does with the use of imatinib in chronic myelogenous leukemia.[191] In one patient who developed resistance an alternative tyrosine kinase inhibitor (second generation) was effective.[192] (See Chap. 90 for detail of tyrosine kinase inhibitor use.) Treatment with imatinib has caused acute left ventricular failure in some cases and cardiac troponin has been suggested to monitor therapy.[193] Another approach to treatment has been the use of anti–IL-5 monoclonal antibody. This approach has also shown a response in some patients, even in the absence of raised serum IL-5 concentrations.[160,194] In a double-blind, placebo-controlled trial of *FIP1L1-PDGFR*α–negative HES patients requiring 20 mg or more of prednisolone, mepolizumab, a humanized monoclonal antibody that binds IL-5, allowed a reduction in prednisolone to 10 mg/day in 84 percent of patients (twice the rate of those given placebo) without any increase in the activity of the HES.

Course and Prognosis A series of HES patients reported in 1973 had a 3-year survival of 12 percent; cardiac failure accounted for much of the morbidity and mortality.[167] In a later report, the outlook had improved with a survival of 80 percent at 5 years.[195] The new approaches to treatment outlined above should result in a further improvement in outcome.

Toxic Oil Syndrome

In 1981, more than 20,000 cases of a syndrome manifested by fever, cough, dyspnea and leukocytosis, neutrophilia, and an eosinophil count greater than 750 × $10^6/\mu L$ were reported in Spain.[196] Occasionally, the eosinophil count rose above normal only after the onset of the pulmonary symptoms. Eosinophil degranulation was seen in the effected tissues.[197] Pulmonary infiltrates were evident on radiographs of the chest. Pleural effusion was common, and hypoxemia was frequent. There were 1500 deaths in the cohort. About half the patients went on to a chronic course that mimicked the eosinophilia-myalgia syndrome, with myalgia, eosinophilia, peripheral neuritis, scleroderma-like skin lesions, hair loss, and a sicca syndrome. Other patients improved from the acute or chronic symptoms and signs, but some residual nerve, muscle, or skin damage persisted. Endothelial cell proliferation, mononuclear cell infiltrates around blood vessels (vasculitis), and perineural inflammatory infiltrates were identified histopathologically. Glucocorticoid therapy decreased the pulmonary symptomatology. The disease was thought to be a response to an unlabeled food oil, aniline-denatured rapeseed oil, marketed as pure olive oil.

Reactive Hypereosinophilia and Neoplasms

Exaggerated eosinophilia has been reported in association with a variety of lymphoid and solid tumors, particularly Hodgkin lymphoma.[198] In these cases, the eosinophilia is thought to be the result of an increase of

IL-5 and other cytokines or chemokines elaborated by the tumor cells, although the expression by eosinophils of receptors of the TNF-α family suggest that they could influence tumor growth. The eosinophilia may precede the clinical diagnosis of the tumor, but usually occurs concomitantly. In some cases, successful treatment of the tumor is associated with amelioration of the eosinophilia. Angiolymphoid hyperplasia also has been associated with eosinophilia.[199]

Eosinophilia, Angiitis, and Asthma

A group of related diseases, including polyarthritis nodosa and allergic granulomatosis (Churg-Strauss angiitis), is associated with a prominent eosinophilia.[200] In a review of subjects with asthma and necrotizing angiitis, all patients had anemia and hypereosinophilia, with a mean blood eosinophil count over $8000 \times 10^6/\mu L$.[201] Remission occurs in approximately 90 percent of patients; approximately 10 percent of patients die of the vasculitis.[202] A number of case reports have suggested a link to leukotriene antagonists, although this relationship continues to be debated.[203,204] In subjects with asthma and exaggerated eosinophilia, the development of multiorgan signs (skin, nervous system, kidney, joints, lung, heart, gastrointestinal tract) should lead to consideration of this disorder.

Eosinophilic Fasciitis

This syndrome may occur at any age in both sexes and is characterized by stiffness, pain, and swelling of the arms, forearms, thighs, legs, hands, and feet in descending order of frequency. Malaise, fever, weakness, and weight loss also occur.[205] Eosinophilia greater than 1000 cells/μL is present in most patients but may be intermittent. A biopsy of an affected area, usually required for the diagnosis, shows inflammation, edema, thickening, and fibrosis of the fascia. Synovial tissue may show similar changes. Aplastic anemia, pernicious anemia, isolated cytopenias, and acute leukemia have been associated with eosinophilic fasciitis.

Eosinophiluria and Eosinophilorrachia

The urinary excretion of eosinophils is seen in several inflammatory disorders of the kidney but most often in urinary tract infection or acute interstitial nephritis.[206] Hansel stain is superior to Wright stain in identifying eosinophils in a urinary sediment. Cerebrospinal fluid eosinophilia may occur with infection, shunts, and allergic reactions involving the meninges.[207]

REFERENCES

1. Hogan, SP, Rosenberg HF, Moqbel R, et al: Eosinophils: Biological properties and role in health and disease. *Clin Exp Allergy* 38:709, 2008.
2. Egesten A, Calafat J, Janssen H, et al: Granules of human eosinophilic leucocytes and their mobilization. *Clin Exp Allergy* 31:1173, 2001.
3. Dvorak AM, Weller PF: Ultrastructural analysis of human eosinophils. *Chem Immunol* 76:1, 2000.
4. Persson T, Calafat J, Janssen H, et al: Specific granules of human eosinophils have lysosomal characteristics: Presence of lysosome-associated membrane proteins and acidification upon cellular activation. *Biochem Biophys Res Commun* 291:844, 2002.
5. Wardlaw A: Eosinophil density: What does it mean? *Clin Exp Allergy* 25:1145, 1995.
6. Erjefalt JS, Persson CG: New aspects of degranulation and fates of airway mucosal eosinophils. *Am J Respir Crit Care Med* 161:2074, 2000.
7. Filley WV, Holley KE, Kephart GM, Gleich GJ: Identification by immunofluorescence of eosinophil granule major basic protein in lung tissues of patients with bronchial asthma. *Lancet* 2:11, 1982.
8. Erjefalt JS, Greiff L, Andersson M, et al: Degranulation patterns of eosinophil granulocytes as determinants of eosinophil driven disease. *Thorax* 56:341, 2001.
9. Erjefalt JS, Greiff L, Andersson M, et al: Allergen-induced eosinophil cytolysis is a primary mechanism for granule protein release in human upper airways. *Am J Respir Crit Care Med* 160:304, 1999.
10. Weiler CR, Kita H, Hukee M, Gleich GJ: Eosinophil viability during immunoglobulin-induced degranulation. *J Leukoc Biol* 60:493, 1996.
11. Dvorak AM, Furitsu T, Letourneau L, et al: Mature eosinophils stimulated to develop in human cord blood mononuclear cell cultures supplemented with recombinant human interleukin-5. Part I. Piecemeal degranulation of specific granules and distribution of Charcot-Leyden crystal protein. *Am J Pathol* 138:69, 1991.
12. Duffy SM, Lawley WJ, Kaur D, et al: Inhibition of human mast cell proliferation and survival by tamoxifen in association with ion channel modulation. *J Allergy Clin Immunol* 112:965, 2003.
13. Malm-Erjefalt M, Persson CG, Erjefalt JS: Degranulation status of airway tissue eosinophils in mouse models of allergic airway inflammation. *Am J Respir Cell Mol Biol* 24:352, 2001.
14. Denzler KL, Borchers MT, Crosby JR, et al: Extensive eosinophil degranulation and peroxidase-mediated oxidation of airway proteins do not occur in a mouse ovalbumin-challenge model of pulmonary inflammation. *J Immunol* 167:1672, 2001.
15. Stelts D, Egan RW, Falcone A, et al. Eosinophils retain their granule major basic protein in a murine model of allergic pulmonary inflammation. *Am J Respir Cell Mol Biol* 18:463, 1998.
16. Denzler KL, Farmer SC, Crosby JR, et al: Eosinophil major basic protein-1, does not contribute to allergen-induced airway pathologies in mouse models of asthma. *J Immunol* 165:5509, 2000.
17. Clark K, Simson L, Newcombe N, et al: Eosinophil degranulation in the allergic lung of mice primarily occurs in the airway lumen. *J Leukoc Biol* 75:1001, 2001.
18. Humbles AA, Lloyd CM, McMillan SJ, et al: A critical role for eosinophils in allergic airways remodeling. *Science* 305:1776, 2004.
19. Lee JJ, Dimina D, Macias MP, et al: Defining a link with asthma in mice congenitally deficient in eosinophils. *Science* 305:1773, 2004.
20. Dvorak AM: Images in clinical medicine. An apoptotic eosinophil. *N Engl J Med* 340:437, 1999.
21. Yamamoto H, Sedgwick JB, Vrtis RF, Busse WW: The effect of transendothelial migration on eosinophil function. *Am J Respir Cell Mol Biol* 23:379, 2000.
22. Floyd H, Ni J, Cornish AL, et al: Siglec-8. A novel eosinophil-specific member of the immunoglobulin superfamily. *J Biol Chem* 275(2):861, 2000.
23. Kikly KK, Bochner BS, Freeman SD, et al: Identification of SAF-2, a novel siglec expressed on eosinophils, mast cells, and basophils. *J Allergy Clin Immunol* 105:1093, 2000.
24. Aizawa H, Plitt J, Bochner BS: Human eosinophils express two Siglec-8, splice variants. *J Allergy Clin Immunol* 109:176, 2002.
25. Munday J, Kerr S, Ni J, et al: Identification, characterization and leucocyte expression of Siglec-10, a novel human sialic acid-binding receptor. *Biochem J* 355:489, 2001.
26. Swystun VA, Gordon JR, Davis EB, et al: Mast cell tryptase release and asthmatic responses to allergen increase with regular use of salbutamol. *J Allergy Clin Immunol* 106:57, 2000.
27. Bochner BS: Siglec-8, on human eosinophils and mast cells, and Siglec-F on murine eosinophils, are functionally related inhibitory receptors. *Clin Exp Allergy* 39:317, 2009.
28. Nutku E, Aizawa H, Hudson SA, Bochner BS: Ligation of Siglec-8: A selective mechanism for induction of human eosinophil apoptosis. *Blood* 101:5014, 2003.
29. Munitz A, Bachelet I, Finkelman FD, et al: CD48, is critically involved in allergic eosinophilic airway inflammation. *Am J Respir Crit Care Med* 175:911, 2007.
30. Munitz A, Levi-Schaffer F: Inhibitory receptors on eosinophils: A direct hit to a possible Achilles heel? *J Allergy Clin Immunol* 119:1382, 2007.
31. Yu C, Cantor AB, Yang H, et al: Targeted deletion of a high-affinity GATA-binding site in the GATA-1, promoter leads to selective loss of the eosinophil lineage *in vivo*. *J Exp Med* 195:1387, 2002.
32. Fukushima K, Matsumura I, Ezoe S, et al: FIP1L1-PDGFRalpha imposes eosinophil lineage commitment on hematopoietic stem/progenitor cells. *J Biol Chem* 284:7719, 2009.
33. Spry CJF: The natural history of eosinophils, in *The Immunopharmacology of Eosinophils*, edited by H Smith, RM Cook, p 1. Academic Press, London, 1993.
34. Sanderson CJ: Interleukin-5, eosinophils, and disease. *Blood* 79:3101, 1992.
35. Takatsu K, Kouro T, Nagai T: Interleukin 5, in the link between the innate and acquired immune response. *Adv Immunol* 101:191, 2009.
36. van Rensen EL, Stirling RG, Scheerens J, et al: Evidence for systemic rather than pulmonary effects of interleukin-5, administration in asthma. *Thorax* 56:935, 2001.
37. Leckie MJ, ten Brinke A, Khan J, et al: Effects of an interleukin-5, blocking monoclonal antibody on eosinophils, airway hyper-responsiveness, and the late asthmatic response. *Lancet* 356:2144, 2000.
38. Culley FJ, Brown A, Girod N, et al: Innate and cognate mechanisms of pulmonary eosinophilia in helminth infection. *Eur J Immunol* 32:1376, 2002.
39. Martin C, Al-Qaoud KM, Ungeheuer MN, et al: IL-5, is essential for vaccine-induced protection and for resolution of primary infection in murine filariasis. *Med Microbiol Immunol* 189:67, 2000.
40. Humbert M, Corrigan CJ, Kimmitt P, et al: Relationship between IL-4, and IL-5, mRNA expression and disease severity in atopic asthma. *Am J Respir Crit Care Med* 156:704, 1997.
41. Alexander AG, Barkans J, Moqbel R, et al: Serum interleukin 5, concentrations in atopic and non-atopic patients with glucocorticoid-dependent chronic severe asthma. *Thorax* 49:1231, 1994.
42. Domachowske JB, Bonville CA, Easton AJ, Rosenberg HF: Pulmonary eosinophilia in mice devoid of interleukin-5. *J Leukoc Biol* 71:966, 2002.
43. Finotto S, Neurath MF, Glickman JN, et al: Development of spontaneous airway changes consistent with human asthma in mice lacking T-bet. *Science* 295:336, 2002.
44. Neurath MF, Finotto S, Glimcher LH: The role of Th1/Th2, polarization in mucosal immunity. *Nat Med* 8:567, 2002.

45. Hewitt CR, Horton H, Jones RM, Pritchard DI: Heterogeneous proteolytic specificity and activity of the house dust mite proteinase allergen Der p I. *Clin Exp Allergy* 27:201, 1997.
46. Rothenberg ME, Mishra A, Collins MH, Putnam PE: Pathogenesis and clinical features of eosinophilic esophagitis. *J Allergy Clin Immunol* 108:891, 2001.
47. Ozdemir C, Akdis M, Akdis CA: T regulatory cells and their counterparts: Masters of immune regulation. *Clin Exp Allergy* 39:626, 2009.
48. McHugh RS, Shevach EM: The role of suppressor T cells in regulation of immune responses. *J Allergy Clin Immunol* 110:693, 2002.
49. Levings MK, Sangregorio R, Sartirana C, et al: Human CD25(+)CD4(+) T suppressor cell clones produce transforming growth factor beta, but not interleukin 10, and are distinct from type 1, T regulatory cells. *J Exp Med* 196:1335, 2002.
50. Curotto de Lafaille MA, Lafaille JJ: CD4(+) regulatory T cells in autoimmunity and allergy. *Curr Opin Immunol* 14:771, 2002.
51. Yazdanbakhsh M, Kremsner PG, van Ree R: Allergy, parasites, and the hygiene hypothesis. *Science* 296:490, 2002.
52. Wills-Karp M, Santeliz J, Karp CL: The germless theory of allergic disease: Revisiting the hygiene hypothesis. *Nat Rev Immunol* 1:69, 2001.
53. Umetsu DT, Akbari O, Dekruyff RH: Regulatory T cells control the development of allergic disease and asthma. *J Allergy Clin Immunol* 112:480, 2003.
54. Akdis CA, Blaser K: Mechanisms of interleukin-10-mediated immune suppression. *Immunology* 103:131, 2001.
55. Zuany-Amorim C, Sawicka E, Manlius C, et al: Suppression of airway eosinophilia by killed Mycobacterium vaccae-induced allergen-specific regulatory T-cells. *Nat Med* 8:625, 2002.
56. Suto A, Nakajima H, Kagami SI, et al: Role of CD4(+) CD25(+) regulatory T cells in T helper 2, cell-mediated allergic inflammation in the airways. *Am J Respir Crit Care Med* 164:680, 2001.
57. Hansel TT, De Vries IJ, Iff T, et al: An improved immunomagnetic procedure for the isolation of highly purified human blood eosinophils. *J Immunol Methods* 145:105, 1991.
58. Caulfield JP, Hein A, Rothenberg ME, et al: A morphometric study of normodense and hypodense human eosinophils that are derived in vivo and in vitro. *Am J Pathol* 137:27, 1990.
59. Mishra A, Hogan SP, Brandt EB, et al: Enterocyte expression of the eotaxin and interleukin-5, transgenes induces compartmentalized dysregulation of eosinophil trafficking. *J Biol Chem* 277:4406, 2002.
60. Hurst SD, Muchamuel T, Gorman DM, et al: New IL-17, family members promote Th1, or Th2, responses in the lung: *In vivo* function of the novel cytokine IL-25. *J Immunol* 169:443, 2002.
61. Bochner BS: Road signs guiding leukocytes along the inflammation superhighway. *J Allergy Clin Immunol* 106:817, 2000.
62. Wardlaw AJ: Molecular basis for selective eosinophil trafficking in asthma: A multistep paradigm. *J Allergy Clin Immunol* 104:917, 1999.
63. Rothenberg ME: Eosinophilia. *N Engl J Med* 338:1592, 1998.
64. Palframan RT, Collins PD, Williams TJ, Rankin SM: Eotaxin induces a rapid release of eosinophils and their progenitors from the bone marrow. *Blood* 91:2240, 1998.
65. Palframan RT, Collins PD, Severs NJ, et al: Mechanisms of acute eosinophil mobilization from the bone marrow stimulated by interleukin 5: The role of specific adhesion molecules and phosphatidylinositol 3-kinase. *J Exp Med* 188:1621, 1998.
66. Tachimoto H, Burdick MM, Hudson SA, et al: CCR3-active chemokines promote rapid detachment of eosinophils from VCAM-1, *in vitro*. *J Immunol* 165:2748, 2000.
67. Tomaki M, Zhao LL, Lundahl J, et al: Eosinophilopoiesis in a murine model of allergic airway eosinophilia: Involvement of bone marrow IL-5, and IL-5, receptor alpha. *J Immunol* 165:4040, 2000.
68. Inman MD: Bone marrow events in animal models of allergic inflammation and hyperresponsiveness. *J Allergy Clin Immunol* 106:S235, 2000.
69. Edwards BS, Curry MS, Tsuji H, et al: Expression of P-selectin at low site density promotes selective attachment of eosinophils over neutrophils. *J Immunol* 165:404, 2000.
70. Dang B, Wiehler S, Patel KD: Increased PSGL-1, expression on granulocytes from allergic-asthmatic subjects results in enhanced leukocyte recruitment under flow conditions. *J Leukoc Biol* 72:702, 2002.
71. Woltmann G, McNulty CA, Dewson G, et al: Interleukin-13, induces PSGL-1/P-selectin-dependent adhesion of eosinophils, but not neutrophils, to human umbilical vein endothelial cells under flow. *Blood* 95:3146, 2000.
72. Kitayama J, Mackay CR, Ponath PD, Springer TA: The C-C chemokine receptor CCR3, participates in stimulation of eosinophil arrest on inflammatory endothelium in shear flow. *J Clin Invest* 101:2017, 1998.
73. Humbles AA, Lu B, Friend DS, et al: The murine CCR3, receptor regulates both the role of eosinophils and mast cells in allergen-induced airway inflammation and hyperresponsiveness. *Proc Natl Acad Sci U S A* 99:1479, 2002.
74. Pope SM, Zimmermann N, Stringer KF, et al: The eotaxin chemokines and CCR3, are fundamental regulators of allergen-induced pulmonary eosinophilia. *J Immunol* 175:5341, 2005.
75. Woolley KL, Gibson PG, Carty K, et al: Eosinophil apoptosis and the resolution of airway inflammation in asthma. *Am J Respir Crit Care Med* 154:237, 1996.
76. Simon HU, Yousefi S, Schranz C, et al: Direct demonstration of delayed eosinophil apoptosis as a mechanism causing tissue eosinophilia. *J Immunol* 158:3902, 1997.
77. Anwar AR, Moqbel R, Walsh GM, et al: Adhesion to fibronectin prolongs eosinophil survival. *J Exp Med* 177:839, 1993.
78. Flood-Page PT, Menzies-Gow AN, Kay AB, Robinson DS: Eosinophil's role remains uncertain as anti-interleukin-5, only partially depletes numbers in asthmatic airway. *Am J Respir Crit Care Med* 167:199, 2003.
79. Meagher LC, Cousin JM, Seckl JR, Haslett C: Opposing effects of glucocorticoids on the rate of apoptosis in neutrophilic and eosinophilic granulocytes. *J Immunol* 156:4422, 1996.
80. Walsh GM, Wardlaw AJ: Dexamethasone inhibits prolonged survival and autocrine granulocyte-macrophage colony-stimulating factor production by human eosinophils cultured on laminin or tissue fibronectin. *J Allergy Clin Immunol* 100:208, 1997.
81. Robertson NM, Zangrilli JG, Steplewski A, et al: Differential expression of TRAIL and TRAIL receptors in allergic asthmatics following segmental antigen challenge: Evidence for a role of TRAIL in eosinophil survival. *J Immunol* 169:5986, 2002.
82. Adachi T, Alam R: The mechanism of IL-5, signal transduction. *Am J Physiol* 275:C623, 1998.
83. Dewson G, Walsh GM, Wardlaw AJ: Expression of Bcl-2, and its homologues in human eosinophils. Modulation by interleukin-5. *Am J Respir Cell Mol Biol* 20:720, 1999.
84. Dewson G, Cohen GM, Wardlaw AJ: Interleukin-5, inhibits translocation of Bax to the mitochondria, cytochrome c release, and activation of caspases in human eosinophils. *Blood* 98:2239, 2001.
85. Letuve S, Druilhe A, Grandsaigne M, et al: Involvement of caspases and of mitochondria in Fas ligation-induced eosinophil apoptosis: Modulation by interleukin-5, and interferon-gamma. *J Leukoc Biol* 70:767, 2001.
86. Letuve S, Druilhe A, Grandsaigne M, et al: Critical role of mitochondria, but not caspases, during glucocorticosteroid-induced human eosinophil apoptosis. *Am J Respir Cell Mol Biol* 26:565, 2002.
87. Shen ZJ, Esnault S, Schinzel A, et al: The peptidyl-prolyl isomerase Pin1, facilitates cytokine-induced survival of eosinophils by suppressing Bax activation. *Nat Immunol* 10:257, 2009.
88. Robinson DS, Damia R, Zeibecoglou K, et al: CD34(+)/interleukin-5Ralpha messenger RNA+ cells in the bronchial mucosa in asthma: Potential airway eosinophil progenitors. *Am J Respir Cell Mol Biol* 20:9, 1999.
89. Shi HZ, Humbles A, Gerard C, et al: Lymph node trafficking and antigen presentation by endobronchial eosinophils. *J Clin Invest* 105:945, 2000.
90. Corry DB, Rishi K, Kanellis J, et al: Decreased allergic lung inflammatory cell egression and increased susceptibility to asphyxiation in MMP2-deficiency. *Nat Immunol* 3:347, 2002.
91. Okada S, Kita H, George TJ, et al: Transmigration of eosinophils through basement membrane components in vitro: Synergistic effects of platelet-activating factor and eosinophil-active cytokines. *Am J Respir Cell Mol Biol* 16:455, 1997.
92. Martin C, Burdon PC, Bridger G, et al: Chemokines acting via CXCR2, and CXCR4, control the release of neutrophils from the bone marrow and their return following senescence. *Immunity* 19:583, 2003.
93. Muessel MJ, Scott KS, Friedl P, et al: CCL11, and GM-CSF differentially use the Rho GTPase pathway to regulate motility of human eosinophils in a three-dimensional microenvironment. *J Immunol* 180:8354, 2008.
94. Foster PS, Mould AW, Yang M, et al: Elemental signals regulating eosinophil accumulation in the lung. *Immunol Rev* 179:173, 2001.
95. Rosenberg HF, Phipps S, Foster PS: Eosinophil trafficking in allergy and asthma. *J Allergy Clin Immunol* 119:1303, 2007.
96. Gwinn WM, Damsker JM, Falahati R, et al: Novel approach to inhibit asthma-mediated lung inflammation using anti-CD147, intervention. *J Immunol* 177: 4870, 2006.
97. Uller L, Mathiesen JM, Alenmyr L, et al: Antagonism of the prostaglandin D2, receptor CRTH2, attenuates asthma pathology in mouse eosinophilic airway inflammation. *Respir Res* 8:16, 2007.
98. Sturm EM, Schratl P, Schuligoi R, et al: Prostaglandin E2, inhibits eosinophil trafficking through E-prostanoid 2, receptors. *J Immunol* 181:7273, 2008.
99. Yousefi S, Gold JA, Andina N, et al: Catapult-like release of mitochondrial DNA by eosinophils contributes to antibacterial defense. *Nat Med* 14:949, 2008.
100. Lacy P, Moqbel R: Eosinophil cytokines. *Chem Immunol* 76:134, 2000.
101. Akuthota P, Wang HB, Spencer LA, Weller PF: Immunoregulatory roles of eosinophils: A new look at a familiar cell. *Clin Exp Allergy* 38:1254, 2008.
102. Jacobsen EA, Ochkur SI, Pero RS, et al: Allergic pulmonary inflammation in mice is dependent on eosinophil-induced recruitment of effector T cells. *J Exp Med* 205:699, 2008.
103. Bandeira-Melo C, Weller PF: Eosinophils and cysteinyl leukotrienes. *Prostaglandins Leukot Essent Fatty Acids* 69:135, 2003.
104. Cromwell O, Wardlaw AJ, Champion A, et al: IgG-dependent generation of platelet-activating factor by normal and low density human eosinophils. *J Immunol* 145:3862, 1990.
105. Bozza PT, Yu W, Penrose JF, Morgan ES, et al: Eosinophil lipid bodies: Specific, inducible intracellular sites for enhanced eicosanoid formation. *J Exp Med* 186:909, 1997.
106. Flood-Page P, Menzies-Gow A, Phipps S, et al: Anti-IL-5, treatment reduces deposition of ECM proteins in the bronchial subepithelial basement membrane of mild atopic asthmatics. *J Clin Invest* 112:1029, 2003.
107. Phipps S, Ying S, Wangoo A, Ong YE, et al: The relationship between allergen-induced tissue eosinophilia and markers of repair and remodeling in human atopic skin. *J Immunol* 169:4604, 2002.
108. Brightling CE, Bradding P, Symon FA, et al: Mast-cell infiltration of airway smooth muscle in asthma. *N Engl J Med* 346:1699, 2002.

109. Barker RL, Gleich GJ, Pease LR: Acidic precursor revealed in human eosinophil granule major basic protein cDNA. *J Exp Med* 168:1493, 1988.
110. Butterworth AE, Sturrock RF, Houba V, et al: Eosinophils as mediators of antibody-dependent damage to schistosomula. *Nature* 256:727, 1975.
111. Gleich GJ: Mechanisms of eosinophil-associated inflammation. *J Allergy Clin Immunol* 105:651, 2000.
112. Rohrbach MS, Wheatley CL, Slifman NR, Gleich GJ: Activation of platelets by eosinophil granule proteins. *J Exp Med* 172:1271, 1990.
113. Ten RM, Pease LR, McKean DJ, et al: Molecular cloning of the human eosinophil peroxidase. Evidence for the existence of a peroxidase multigene family. *J Exp Med* 169:1757, 1989.
114. Rosenberg HF, Ackerman SJ, Tenen DG: Human eosinophil cationic protein. Molecular cloning of a cytotoxin and helminthotoxin with ribonuclease activity. *J Exp Med* 170:163, 1989.
115. Young JD, Peterson CG, Venge P, Cohn ZA: Mechanism of membrane damage mediated by human eosinophil cationic protein. *Nature* 321:613, 1986.
116. Rosenberg HF, Tenen DG, Ackerman SJ: Molecular cloning of the human eosinophil-derived neurotoxin: A member of the ribonuclease gene family. *Proc Natl Acad Sci U S A* 86:4460, 1989.
117. Ackerman SJ, Liu L, Kwatia MA, et al: Charcot-Leyden crystal protein (galectin-10) is not a dual function galectin with lysophospholipase activity but binds a lysophospholipase inhibitor in a novel structural fashion. *J Biol Chem* 277:14859, 2002.
118. Kita H, Weiler DA, Abu-Ghazaleh R, et al: Release of granule proteins from eosinophils cultured with IL-5. *J Immunol* 149:629, 1992.
119. Seminario MC, Saini SS, MacGlashan DW Jr, Bochner BS: Intracellular expression and release of Fc epsilon RI alpha by human eosinophils. *J Immunol* 162:6893, 1999.
120. Hartnell A, Kay AB, Wardlaw AJ: IFN-gamma induces expression of Fc gamma RIII (CD16) on human eosinophils. *J Immunol* 148:1471, 1992.
121. Abu-Ghazaleh RI, Fujisawa T, Mestecky J, et al: IgA-induced eosinophil degranulation. *J Immunol* 142:2393, 1989.
122. Kaneko M, Horie S, Kato M, et al: A crucial role for beta 2, integrin in the activation of eosinophils stimulated by IgG. *J Immunol* 155:2631, 1995.
123. Nusse O, Lindau M, Cromwell O, et al: Intracellular application of guanosine-5-*O*-(3-thiotriphosphate) induces exocytotic granule fusion in guinea pig eosinophils. *J Exp Med* 171:775, 1990.
124. Moqbel R, Coughlin JJ: Differential secretion of cytokines. *Sci STKE* 338:26, 2006.
125. Lavigne S, Bosse M, Boulet LP, Laviolette M: Identification and analysis of eosinophils by flow cytometry using the depolarized side scatter-saponin method. *Cytometry* 29:197, 1997.
126. Kimura I, Moritani Y, Tanizaki Y: Basophils in bronchial asthma with reference to reagin-type allergy. *Clin Allergy* 3:195, 1973.
127. Krause JR, Boggs DR: Search for eosinopenia in hospitalized patients with normal blood leukocyte concentration. *Am J Hematol* 24:55, 1987.
128. Gudbjartsson DF, Bjornsdottir US, Halapi E, et al: Sequence variants affecting eosinophil numbers associate with asthma and myocardial infarction. *Nat Genet* 41:342, 2009.
129. Juhlin L, Michaelsson G: A new syndrome characterized by absence of eosinophils and basophils. *Lancet* 1:1233, 1977.
130. Juhlin L, Venge P: Total absence of eosinophils in a patient with chronic urticaria and vitiligo. *Eur J Haematol* 40:368, 1988.
131. Telerman A, Amson RB, Delforge A, et al: A case of chronic aneosinocytosis. *Am J Hematol* 12:187, 1982.
132. Nakahata T, Spicer SS, Leary AG, et al: Circulating eosinophil colony-forming cells in pure eosinophil aplasia. *Ann Intern Med* 101:321, 1984.
133. Joshua H, Zucker A, Presentey B: Peroxidase and phospholipid deficiency in eosinophilic granulocytes among Arabs of the Nazareth district. *Isr J Med Sci* 12:71, 1976.
134. Sade K, Mysels A, Levo Y, Kivity S: Eosinophilia: A study of 100, hospitalized patients. *Eur J Intern Med* 18:196, 2007.
135. Wechsler ME: Pulmonary eosinophilic syndromes. *Immunol Allergy Clin North Am* 27:477, 2007.
136. Bochner BS: Verdict in the case of therapies versus eosinophils: The jury is still out. *J Allergy Clin Immunol* 113:3, quiz 10, 2004.
137. Todd R, Donoff BR, Chiang T, et al: The eosinophil as a cellular source of transforming growth factor alpha in healing cutaneous wounds. *Am J Pathol* 138:1307, 1991.
138. Gouon-Evans V, Rothenberg ME, Pollard JW: Postnatal mammary gland development requires macrophages and eosinophils. *Development* 127:2269, 2000.
139. Munitz A, Levi-Schaffer F: Eosinophils: "New" roles for "old" cells. *Allergy* 59:268, 2004.
140. Wong DT, Bowen SM, Elovic A, et al: Eosinophil ablation and tumor development. *Oral Oncol* 35:496, 1999.
141. Weller PF: The idiopathic hypereosinophilic syndrome. *Arch Dermatol* 132:583, 1996.
142. Fabre V, Beiting DP, Bliss SK, et al: Eosinophil deficiency compromises parasite survival in chronic nematode infection. *J Immunol* 182:1577, 2009.
143. Klion AD, Nutman TB: The role of eosinophils in host defense against helminth parasites. *J Allergy Clin Immunol* 113:30, 2004.
144. Chapman ID, Foster A, Morley J: The relationship between inflammation and hyperreactivity of the airways in asthma. *Clin Exp Allergy* 23:168, 1993.
145. Wardlaw AJ, Brightling C, Green R, et al: Eosinophils in asthma and other allergic diseases. *Br Med Bull* 56:985, 2000.
146. Green RH, Brightling CE, Woltmann G, et al: Analysis of induced sputum in adults with asthma: Identification of subgroup with isolated sputum neutrophilia and poor response to inhaled corticosteroids. *Thorax* 57:875, 2002.
147. Pin I, Freitag AP, O'Byrne PM, et al: Changes in the cellular profile of induced sputum after allergen-induced asthmatic responses. *Am Rev Respir Dis* 145:1265, 1992.
148. Pavord ID, Brightling CE, Woltmann G, Wardlaw AJ: Non-eosinophilic corticosteroid unresponsive asthma [letter]. *Lancet* 353:2213, 1999.
149. Haldar P, Pavord ID, Shaw DE, et al: Cluster analysis and clinical asthma phenotypes. *Am J Respir Crit Care Med* 178:218, 2008.
150. Henderson WR Jr, Chi EY, Albert RK, et al: Blockade of CD49d (alpha4, integrin) on intrapulmonary but not circulating leukocytes inhibits airway inflammation and hyperresponsiveness in a mouse model of asthma. *J Clin Invest* 100:3083, 1997.
151. Green RH, Brightling CE, McKenna S, et al: Asthma exacerbations and sputum eosinophil counts: A randomized controlled trial. *Lancet* 360:1715, 2002.
152. Nair P, Pizzichini MM, Kjarsgaard M, et al: Mepolizumab for prednisone-dependent asthma with sputum eosinophilia. *N Engl J Med* 360:985, 2009.
153. Haldar P, Brightling CE, Hargadon B, et al: Mepolizumab (anti-IL 5) and exacerbation frequency in refractory eosinophilic asthma. *N Engl J Med* 360:973, 2009.
154. Leiferman KM, Gleich GJ: Hypereosinophilic syndrome: Case presentation and update. *J Allergy Clin Immunol* 113:50, 2004.
155. Simon D, Braathen LR, Simon HU: Eosinophils and atopic dermatitis. *Allergy* 59:561, 2004.
156. Leiferman KM, Gleich GJ, Peters MS: Dermatologic manifestations of the hypereosinophilic syndromes. *Immunol Allergy Clin North Am* 27:415, 2007.
157. Rothenberg ME: Eosinophilic gastrointestinal disorders (EGID). *J Allergy Clin Immunol* 113:11, quiz 29, 2004.
158. Straumann A, Spichtin HP, Grize L, et al: Natural history of primary eosinophilic esophagitis: A follow-up of 30 adult patients for up to 11.5 years. *Gastroenterology* 125:1660, 2003.
159. Putnam PE, Rothenberg MD: Eosinophilic esophagitis: Concepts, controversies, and evidence. *Curr Gastroenterol Rep* 11:220, 2009.
160. Garrett JK, Jameson SC, Thomson B, et al: Anti-interleukin-5, (mepolizumab) therapy for hypereosinophilic syndromes. *J Allergy Clin Immunol* 113:115, 2004.
161. Chitkara RK, Krishna G: Parasitic pulmonary eosinophilia. *Semin Respir Crit Care Med* 27:171, 2006.
162. Hagan P, Wilkins HA, Blumenthal UJ, et al: Eosinophilia and resistance to Schistosoma haematobium in man. *Parasite Immunol* 7:625, 1985.
163. Sher A, Coffman RL, Hieny S, Cheever AW: Ablation of eosinophil and IgE responses with anti-IL-5, or anti-IL-4, antibodies fails to affect immunity against Schistosoma mansoni in the mouse. *J Immunol* 145:3911, 1990.
164. Herbert DR, Lee JJ, Lee NA, et al: Role of IL-5, in innate and adaptive immunity to larval Strongyloides stercoralis in mice. *J Immunol* 165:4544, 2000.
165. Limaye AP, Abrams JS, Silver JE, et al: Regulation of parasite-induced eosinophilia: Selectively increased interleukin 5, production in helminth-infected patients. *J Exp Med* 172:399, 1990.
166. Hardy WR, Anderson RE: The hypereosinophilic syndromes. *Ann Intern Med* 68:1220, 1968.
167. Chusid MJ, Dale DC, West BC, Wolff SM: The hypereosinophilic syndrome: Analysis of fourteen cases with review of the literature. *Medicine (Baltimore)* 54:1, 1975.
168. Weller PF, Bubley GJ: The idiopathic hypereosinophilic syndrome. *Blood* 83:2759, 1994.
169. Fauci AS, Harley JB, Roberts WC, et al: The idiopathic hypereosinophilic syndrome. Clinical, pathophysiologic, and therapeutic considerations. *Ann Intern Med* 97:78, 1982.
170. Simon D, Simon HU: Eosinophilic disorders. *J Allergy Clin Immunol* 119:1291, 2007.
171. Vardiman JW, Thiele J, Arber DA, et al: The 2008, revision of the WHO classification of myeloid neoplasms and acute leukemia: Rationale and important changes. *Blood* 114:937, 2009.
172. Sheikh J, Weller PF: Advances in diagnosis and treatment of eosinophilia. *Curr Opin Hematol* 16:3, 2009.
173. Cools J, DeAngelo DJ, Gotlib J, et al: A tyrosine kinase created by fusion of the PDGFRA and FIP1L1, genes as a therapeutic target of imatinib in idiopathic hypereosinophilic syndrome. *N Engl J Med* 348:1201, 2003.
174. Griffin JH, Leung J, Bruner RJ, et al: Discovery of a fusion kinase in EOL-1, cells and idiopathic hypereosinophilic syndrome. *Proc Natl Acad Sci U S A* 100:7830, 2003.
175. Fletcher S, Bain B: Diagnosis and treatment of hypereosinophilic syndromes. *Curr Opin Hematol* 14:37, 2007.
176. Musto P, Perla G, Minervini MM, et al: Imatinib-mesylate for all patients with hypereosinophilic syndrome? *Leuk Res* 28:773, 2004.
177. Helbig G, Stella-Holowiecka B, Majewski M, et al: Interferon alpha induces a good molecular response in a patient with chronic eosinophilic leukemia (CEL) carrying the JAK2V617F point mutation. *Haematologica* 92:e118, 2007.
178. Klion AD, Noel P, Akin C, et al: Elevated serum tryptase levels identify a subset of patients with a myeloproliferative variant of idiopathic hypereosinophilic syndrome associated with tissue fibrosis, poor prognosis, and imatinib responsiveness. *Blood* 101:4660, 2003.
179. Roufosse F, Cogan E, Goldman M: Lymphocytic variant hypereosinophilic syndromes. *Immunol Allergy Clin North Am* 27:389, 2007.
180. Cogan E, Schandene L, Crusiaux A, et al: Brief report: Clonal proliferation of type 2, helper T cells in a man with the hypereosinophilic syndrome. *N Engl J Med* 330:535, 1994.
181. Simon HU, Plotz SG, Dummer R, Blaser K: Abnormal clones of T cells producing interleukin-5, in idiopathic eosinophilia. *N Engl J Med* 341:1112, 1999.

182. Roufosse F, Schandene L, Sibille C, et al: Clonal Th2, lymphocytes in patients with the idiopathic hypereosinophilic syndrome. *Br J Haematol* 109:540, 2000.
183. Roufosse F, Cogan E, Goldman M: Recent advances in pathogenesis and management of hypereosinophilic syndromes. *Allergy* 59:673, 2004.
184. Spry CJF: The idiopathic hypereosinophilic syndrome, in *Eosinophils, Biological and Clinical Aspects*, edited by S Makino, T Fukuda, p 403. CRC Press, Boca Raton, FL, 1991.
185. Davis RF, Dusanjh P, Majid A, et al: Eosinophilic cellulitis as a presenting feature of chronic eosinophilic leukaemia, secondary to a deletion on chromosome 4q12, creating the FIP1L1-PDGFRA fusion gene. *Br J Dermatol* 155:1087, 2006.
186. Klion AD, Law MA, Riemenschneider W, et al: Familial eosinophilia: A benign disorder? *Blood* 103:4050, 2004.
187. Gleich GJ, Leiferman KM: The hypereosinophilic syndromes: Current concepts and treatments. *Br J Haematol* 145:271, 2009.
188. Butterfield JH, Gleich GJ: Response of six patients with idiopathic hypereosinophilic syndrome to interferon alfa. *J Allergy Clin Immunol* 94:1318, 1994.
189. Metzgeroth G, Walz C, Erben P, et al: Safety and efficacy of imatinib in chronic eosinophilic leukaemia and hypereosinophilic syndrome: A phase-II study. *Br J Haematol* 143:707, 2008.
190. Jain N, Cortes J, Quintás-Cardama A, et al: Imatinib has limited therapeutic activity for hypereosinophilic syndrome patients with unknown or negative PDGFRalpha mutation status. *Leuk Res* 33:837, 2009.
191. Salemi S, Yousefi S, Simon D, et al: A novel FIP1L1-PDGFRA mutant destabilizing the inactive conformation of the kinase domain in chronic eosinophilic leukemia/hypereosinophilic syndrome. *Allergy* 64:913, 2009.
192. Cools J, Stover EH, Boulton CL, et al: PKC412, overcomes resistance to imatinib in a murine model of FIP1L1-PDGFRalpha-induced myeloproliferative disease. *Cancer Cell* 3:459, 2003.
193. Pitini V, Arrigo C, Azzarello D, et al: Serum concentration of cardiac troponin T in patients with hypereosinophilic syndrome treated with imatinib is predictive of adverse outcomes. *Blood* 102:3456, 2003.
194. Klion AD, Law MA, Noel P, et al: Safety and efficacy of the monoclonal anti-interleukin-5, antibody SCH55700, in the treatment of patients with hypereosinophilic syndrome. *Blood* 103:2939, 2004.
195. Gotlib J, Cools J, Malone JM 3rd, et al: The FIP1L1-PDGFRalpha fusion tyrosine kinase in hypereosinophilic syndrome and chronic eosinophilic leukemia: Implications for diagnosis, classification, and management. *Blood* 103:2879, 2004.
196. Posada de la Paz M, Philen RM, Borda AI: Toxic oil syndrome: The perspective after 20 years. *Epidemiol Rev* 23:231, 2001.
197. Ten RM, Kephart GM, Posada M, et al: Participation of eosinophils in the toxic oil syndrome. *Clin Exp Immunol* 82:313, 1990.
198. Di Biagio E, Sanchez-Borges M, Desenne JJ, et al: Eosinophilia in Hodgkin disease: A role for interleukin 5. *Int Arch Allergy Immunol* 110:244, 1996.
199. Hallam LA, Mackinlay GA, Wright AM: Angiolymphoid hyperplasia with eosinophilia: Possible aetiological role for immunization. *J Clin Pathol* 42:944, 1989.
200. Hellmich B, Ehlers S, Csernok E, Gross WL: Update on the pathogenesis of Churg-Strauss syndrome. *Clin Exp Rheumatol* 21:S69, 2003.
201. Guillevin L, Guittard T, Bletry O, et al: Systemic necrotizing angiitis with asthma: Causes and precipitating factors in 43 cases. *Lung* 165:165, 1987.
202. Guillevin L, Cohen P, Gayraud M, et al: Churg-Strauss syndrome. Clinical study and long-term follow-up of 96 patients. *Medicine (Baltimore)* 78:26, 1999.
203. Nathani N, Little MA, Kunst H, et al: Churg-Strauss syndrome and leukotriene antagonist use: A respiratory perspective. *Thorax* 63:883, 2008.
204. Guilpain P, Viallard JF, Lagarde P, et al: Churg-Strauss syndrome in two patients receiving montelukast. *Rheumatology (Oxford)* 41:535, 2002.
205. Lakhanpal S, Ginsburg WW, Michet CJ, Doyle JA, Moore SB: Eosinophilic fasciitis: Clinical spectrum and therapeutic response in 52 cases. *Semin Arthritis Rheum* 17:221, 1988.
206. Corwin HL, Bray RA, Haber MH: The detection and interpretation of urinary eosinophils. *Arch Pathol Lab Med* 113:1256, 1989.
207. Hughes PA, Magnet AD, Fishbain JT: Eosinophilic meningitis: A case series report and review of the literature. *Mil Med* 168:817, 2003.

CHAPTER 63
BASOPHILS AND MAST CELLS AND THEIR DISORDERS

Stephen J. Galli, Dean D. Metcalfe,
Daniel A. Arber, and Ann M. Dvorak

SUMMARY

Although basophils and mast cells share biochemical and functional characteristics, they are not identical. In humans, basophils are the least frequent of the three granulocytes, typically accounting for less than 0.5 percent of blood leukocytes. Basophils circulate as mature cells and can be recruited into tissues, particularly at sites of immunologic or inflammatory responses, but they ordinarily do not reside in tissues. By contrast, mast cells typically are derived from blood precursors that lack many of the characteristic features of the mature cells and complete their maturation in the tissues. The mature mast cells can reside in tissues for long periods of time. Mast cells are particularly abundant near blood vessels and nerves and in connective tissues beneath surfaces that are exposed to the external environment, such as the skin, gastrointestinal and urogenital tracts, and respiratory system. Tissue mast cell numbers can increase at sites of parasite infection or in association with certain chronic allergic diseases or other forms of pathology, by recruitment and local maturation of blood precursors and by proliferation of resident mast cells.

Mast cells and basophils express the high-affinity receptor for immunoglobulin (Ig) E (FcεRI) on their surface. Both cell types can be triggered to release potent mediators in response to activation via FcεRI, for example, when their cell-bound IgE recognizes bivalent or multivalent allergens. Accordingly, mast cells and basophils have long been regarded as important effector cells in asthma, hay fever, and other allergic disorders. It is thought that the cells' cytoplasmic granule-associated preformed mediators, including histamine and certain proteases, their lipid mediators (such as prostaglandin D_2 and leukotriene C_4), which are generated upon activation of the cells, and their cytokines, growth factors, and chemokines contribute to many of the characteristic signs and symptoms of these diseases. However, several lines of evidence indicate mast cells and basophils also contribute to protective host responses associated with IgE production, especially those directed against parasites. In mice, mast cells also can contribute to host defense in innate immune responses to certain bacterial infections and to pathology in certain T-cell–associated immunologic disorders not thought to involve IgE, including some autoimmune diseases. Mast cells and basophils also may express immunoregulatory functions through cytokine production and other mechanisms.

Although a variety of systemic disorders have been associated with changes in the numbers of blood basophils and many pathologic processes can be associated with changes in the numbers of tissue mast cells, patients with primary deficiencies in basophils appear to be exceedingly rare (if they exist at all). Patients with a primary deficiency of tissue mast cells have not been reported. By contrast, neoplastic processes can affect both of the lineages. Increased numbers of basophils may be present in association with myeloproliferative neoplasms and several forms of myeloid leukemia. Increased numbers of basophils, sometimes to levels of 20 to 90 percent of blood leukocytes, occur in virtually all patients with chronic myelogenous leukemia. The basophils associated both chronic myelogenous and acute myelogenous leukemias are themselves part of the neoplastic clone. The management of patients with "basophilic leukemia" can be complicated by shock as a result of massive release of histamine and other mediators in association with acute cytolysis.

Disorders of mast cell hyperplasia/neoplasia include solitary mastocytomas, the pathogenesis of which is uncertain, the spectrum of disorders encompassed in the term *mastocytosis*, in which significantly increased numbers of mast cells occur in the skin and/or other organs, and mast cell leukemia. The most common form of mastocytosis, indolent systemic mastocytosis, typically presents with urticaria pigmentosa involving the skin, although other organs may be involved. Patients with indolent systemic mastocytosis have the best prognosis and can expect a normal life span. The prognosis of systemic mastocytosis with associated clonal, hematologic non–mast cell lineage disease depends on the course of the associated disease. Patients with aggressive systemic mastocytosis have a guarded prognosis because of complications arising from rapid increases in tissue mast cell numbers. Patients with mast cell leukemia, who often present with large numbers of immature mast cells in the blood at the time of diagnosis, have a fulminant and rapidly fatal course. Most adult patients with mastocytosis have gain-of-function mutations affecting *KIT*, which encodes the receptor for the major mast cell growth factor stem cell factor (also known as *kit ligand* and *mast cell growth factor*). Some pediatric patients with mastocytosis reportedly have the same Asp816Val gain-of-function *KIT* mutation observed in most adult patients. Some pediatric patients have a dominant inactivating *KIT* mutation, whereas others lack *KIT* mutations entirely.

Acronyms and abbreviations that appear in this chapter include: AML, acute myeloid leukemia; ASM, aggressive systemic mastocytosis; CML, chronic myelogenous leukemia; gp120, glycoprotein 120; H&E, hematoxylin and eosin; IL, interleukin; MCL, mast cell leukemia; MCP, mast cell-committed progenitor; PUVA, psoralen ultraviolet A; SCF, stem cell factor; SCT, stem cell transplantation; SM-AHNMD, systemic mastocytosis with associated clonal hematologic non–mast-cell-lineage disease; TLR, toll-like receptor; TNF, tumor necrosis factor; UP, urticaria pigmentosa.

DISTINGUISHING FEATURES OF BASOPHILS AND MAST CELLS

BASOPHILS

Despite certain striking similarities in biochemistry and function, mammalian basophils and mast cells are not identical (Fig. 63–1).[1–5] The distinction was appreciated by Paul Ehrlich, who described the histochemical staining characteristics of both of these cells in the late 19th century. Many lines of evidence indicate basophils share a common precursor with other granulocytes and monocytes.[1–5] Basophils have a short life span[6] and retain granulocytic features even after emigrating into tissues (Fig. 63–1C).[7]

The human basophil is the least common granulocyte in blood, with a prevalence of approximately 0.5 to 0.6 percent of total leukocytes and approximately 0.3 percent of nucleated marrow cells.[8,9] Although the basophil's prominent metachromatic cytoplasmic granules allow unmistakable identification in Wright-Giemsa–stained films of blood (see Fig. 63–1B) or marrow, accurate basophil determinations require absolute counting methods.[9,10] Differential counts of blood films yield valid results only if the percentage of basophils is substantially elevated or if many thousands of leukocytes are counted.

Interleukin (IL)-3 promotes the production and survival of human basophils *in vitro*[4,11] and can induce basophilia *in vivo*.[12] Findings in IL-3–/– mice indicate IL-3 is not necessary for the development of normal numbers of marrow or blood basophils but is important for the

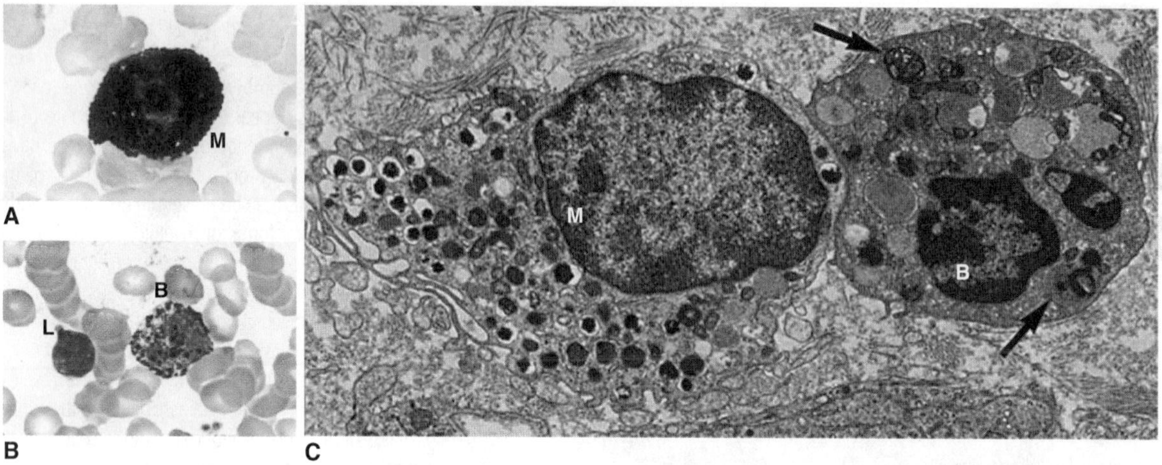

FIGURE 63–1. **A.** Mast cell (*M*) in a Wright-Giemsa-stained marrow aspirate. **B.** A basophil (*B*) and lymphocyte (*L*) in a Wright-Giemsa-stained film prepared from the buffy coat of blood from a normal donor. **C.** Transmission electron micrograph illustrating a mast cell (*M*) and basophil (*B*) in the ileal submucosa of a patient with Crohn disease. The mast cell is a larger, mononuclear cell with a more complex plasma membrane surface and cytoplasmic granules that are smaller and more numerous than those of the basophil. In this section plane, the basophil exhibits two nuclear lobes. Several basophil cytoplasmic granules contain whorls of membranes (*arrows*). Osmium collidine uranyl *en bloc* processing. *(Reproduced with permission from Dvorak AM, Monahan RA, Osage JE, et al.[7])*

marrow and blood basophilia associated with certain T-helper (Th) 2 cell-associated immunologic responses.[13,14] Basophils also express receptors for several other cytokines (Table 63–1).[15–17] IL-3 and many of the other cytokines for which basophils have receptors, including IL-33, can modulate basophil function, for example, by inducing mediator release directly and/or by augmenting the cells' ability to release mediators in response to immunoglobulin (Ig) E-dependent challenge.[4,12,17–19]

MAST CELLS

Mast cells normally reside in the connective tissue, particularly beneath epithelial surfaces and around blood vessels and, in some species, in serous cavities.[1–3,5,20,21] Mast cells are derived from hematopoietic precursors.[20,22,23] Except for a numerically minor population of mast cells that resides in the marrow (Fig. 63–1A),[8] this lineage completes its program of maturation in the tissues.[1–3,20–23] Unlike basophils, mast cells are long-lived. At least some mast cells can locally proliferate in the tissues during a variety of inflammatory or reparative processes.[1–3,20,21] Studies in murine rodents, nonhuman primates, and humans indicate many aspects of mast cell development are critically regulated by stem cell factor (SCF), the ligand for the KIT receptor tyrosine kinase.[13,21,22,24,25] SCF is produced in membrane-associated and in soluble forms, both of which are biologically active.[21,26] In addition to promoting the migration, survival, proliferation, and maturation of cells in the mast cell lineage, SCF can directly promote mast cell mediator release[25,27–29] and, at even lower concentrations, can augment mast cell mediator release in response to stimulation by IgE and antigen.[27,28] Abnormalities affecting *KIT* are involved in the pathogenesis of certain types of mastocytosis (see "Disorders Affecting Mast Cells" below). Moreover, alterations in the production of SCF by fibroblasts and other cells likely contribute to the changes in mast cell numbers that occur during many chronic inflammatory conditions and other pathologic responses.[21,24,30]

MAST CELL AND BASOPHIL HETEROGENEITY

Variation in the morphologic, biochemical, and/or functional characteristics of mast cells from different anatomic locations or from the same organ or site has been reported in several mammalian species, including humans.[1,3,5,20,21,31–33] This phenomenon, often referred to as *mast cell heterogeneity*, raises the possibility that mast cells of different phenotype express different functions in health or disease and may exhibit different sensitivities to pharmacologic manipulation. At least four mechanisms may account for phenotypic variation in mast cell populations: (1) factors promoting branching within the mast cell lineage; (2) factors influencing differentiation and maturation (within single pathways or, if they occur, within multiple pathways); (3) factors modulating mast cell function; and (4) factors influencing local concentrations of exogenous substances not derived from mast cells but taken up and stored in mast cell granules. Of these four mechanisms, experimental evidence has been obtained for all but the first.[33] Basophils can exhibit some variation in phenotypic characteristics, such as immunoreactivity for tryptase, chymase, and carboxypeptidase A,[15] or levels of expression of surface structures, including HLA-DR, CD32 (FcγRII), and receptors for cytokines.[34] Such variation in basophil mediator content and/or cell surface phenotype may reflect individual differences among different subjects and/or the effects of disease processes[15] or the consequences of immunotherapy.[34]

RELATIONSHIP BETWEEN BASOPHILS AND MAST CELLS

Mature basophils and mast cells differ in morphology, natural history, tissue distribution, mediator production, cell surface phenotype, growth factor requirements, and responses to drugs (see Fig. 63–1 and Table 63–1).[1–5] Nevertheless, the two cells do exhibit a number of striking similarities. These similarities, taken together with evidence from rodents indicating that tissue mast cells are derived from circulating marrow-derived precursors,[20,22] had suggested to some investigators that basophils represent the circulating precursor of mast cells. However, current evidence strongly favors the view that mature basophils represent terminally differentiated granulocytes and not circulating mast cell precursors. In addition to the morphologic evidence discussed below, the latter position is supported by the following observations: (1) no evidence has been presented, in any species, indicating that mature circulating basophils are capable of either mitosis or differentiation into mast cells; (2) rare reports of patients with hereditary or acquired abnormalities affecting basophil numbers or morphology indicate that eosinophils also may be affected in these disorders but not mast cells[35–37]; (3) morphologically identifiable

TABLE 63–1. Natural History, Major Mediators, and Surface Membrane Structures of Human Mast Cells and Basophils

Characteristics	Basophils	Mast Cells
Natural History		
Origin of precursor cells	Marrow	Marrow
Site of maturation	Marrow	Connective tissue (a few in marrow)
Mature cells in circulation	Yes (usually <1% of blood leukocytes)	No
Mature cells recruited into tissues from circulation	Yes (during immunologic, inflammatory responses)	No
Mature cells normally residing in connective tissues	No (not detectable by microscopy)	Yes
Proliferative ability of morphologically mature cells	None reported	Yes (limited; under certain circumstances)
Life span	Days (like other granulocytes)	Weeks to months (according to studies in rodents)
Major growth factor	IL-3	SCF
Mediators		
Major mediators stored performed in cytoplasmic granules	Histamine, chondroitin sulfates, tryptase,* chymase,* carboxypeptidase A,* neutral protease with bradykinin-generating activity, β-glucuronidase, elastase, cathepsin G-like enzyme, major basic protein, Charcot-Leyden crystal protein	Histamine, heparin,* chondroitin sulfates,* chymase,* tryptase,* cathepsin G,* carboxypeptidases, major basic protein, acid hydrolases, peroxidase, phospholipases
Major lipid mediators produced on appropriate activation	Leukotriene C_4	Leukotriene B_4, prostaglandin D_2, leukotriene C_4, platelet-activating factor
Cytokines released on appropriate activation	IL-4, IL-13, GM-CSF, VEGF-A, leptin	TNF, TGF-β, IFN-α, VEGF-A–D, IL-6, IL-11, IL-13, IL-16, IL-18, GM-CSF, NGF, PDGF (mouse and human mast cells can secrete many more; see text)
Chemokines	IL-8 (CXCL-8), MIP-1α (CCL3), Eotaxin (CCL-11), MIP-5 (CCL15)	IL-8 (CXCL-8), I-309 (CCL-1), MCP-1 (CCL2), MIP-1α (CCL3), MIP-1β (CCL-4), MCP-3 (CCL-7), RANTES (CCL-5), Eotaxin (CCL-11)
Surface Structures		
Ig receptors	FcεRI, FcγRII (CDw32)	FcεRI, FcγRI (after IFNγ exposure), FcγRII
Cytokine or growth factor receptors for:	IL-1, IL-2 (CD25), IL-3, IL-4, IL-5, IL-6, and IL-8; chemokines (CCR1, -2, -3, -5; CXCR1, -2, -4); and interferons; SCF (basophils express variable numbers of the SCF receptor, Kit)	SCF (ligand for Kit), IFN-γ, IL-4, IL-5, IL-6, IL-9; chemokines (CCR1, -3, -4, -5, -7; CXCR1, -2, -3, -4, -6); thrombopoietin receptor (CD110), GM-CSF, NGF
TLRs	TLR-2 & -4 (but lack CD14)	TLR-1, -2, -3, -4, -5, -6, -7, & -9

IFN, interferon; Ig, immunoglobulin; IL, interleukin; GM-CSF, granulocyte-macrophage colony-stimulating factor; MCP, monocyte chemotactic protein; MIP, macrophage inflammatory protein; NGF, nerve growth factor; PDGF, platelet-derived growth factor; RANTES, regulated on activation, normal T-cell expressed, presumed secreted; SCF, stem cell factor; TNF, tumor necrosis factor; TGF, transforming growth factor; TLR, toll-like receptor; VEGF, vascular endothelial growth factor.

*Basophil and mast cell content of these (and perhaps other) mediators vary, for example, in different subjects and tissues; and/or in association with certain inflammatory diseases.[15]

NOTE: Expression of these and other surface structures, including chemokine receptors, and production of individual cytokines and chemokines, can vary in different *in vitro* or *in vivo* derived basophil or mast cell populations.

SOURCE: Modified from Galli SJ, Dvorak AM, Dvorak HF[1] with permission; data regarding CD antigens are from analyses of blood basophils and lung or uterine mast cells[4]; data regarding chemokine receptors are from references 16 and 17.

human tissue mast cells can exhibit mitotic activity,[38] indicating this cell lineage is capable of replication independent of a stage resembling that of circulating basophils, and (4) in mice, recent evidence indicates that a mast cell-committed progenitor (MCP) present in the marrow arises developmenatally earlier in hematopoiesis than does the granulocyte-macrophage lineage.[23]

MORPHOLOGY OF BASOPHILS AND MAST CELLS

Routine methods of tissue fixation and processing are poorly suited for demonstration of basophils and mast cells. Optimal visualization is achieved in appropriately prepared 1-μm sections or with an ultrastructural approach.[1,2] Ultrastructurally, human basophils are 5 to 7 μm in spherical diameter, exhibit a segmented or, in some cases, unsegmented nucleus with marked condensation of nuclear chromatin, and contain round or oval cytoplasmic granules. The granules are surrounded by a membrane and contain a substructure of dense particles, less dense matrix, and, in some granules, membrane whorls and Charcot-Leyden crystals (see Fig. 63–1C).[1,2] A second, minor population of small, uniform granules is characteristically located close to the nucleus.[39] The cytoplasm of mature human basophils also contains glycogen particles, mitochondria, free ribosomes, and small membrane-bound vesicles. Lipid bodies are rarely present. Other organelles are inconspicuous.

In tissue sections, mast cells typically appear as either round or elongated cells, usually with a nonsegmented nucleus with moderate condensation of nuclear chromatin, and contain prominent cytoplasmic granules. Mast cell granules are smaller, more numerous, and generally more variable in appearance than in basophils and contain scroll-like structures, particles, and crystals, alone or in combination.[1,2] In contrast to the irregularly spaced blunt surface projections of basophils, mast cells are covered by uniformly distributed thin surface processes. Mast cells also differ from basophils in that they have many more cytoplasmic filaments and lack cytoplasmic glycogen deposits. Human mast cells can contain numerous cytoplasmic lipid bodies. Figure 63–1C shows an electron micrograph of a human basophil adjacent to a human mast cell in the same tissue, the ileal submucosa.

BIOCHEMISTRY AND ROLE IN IgE-ASSOCIATED IMMUNE RESPONSES

MEDIATORS

The cytoplasmic granules of basophils and mast cells contain proteoglycans, consisting of sulfated glycosaminoglycans covalently linked to a protein core.[40] Under appropriate conditions, these substances stain metachromatically with basic dyes (see Fig. 63–1A, B). In humans and murine species, individual mast cell populations can contain variable mixtures of heparin and chondroitin sulfate proteoglycans.[20,33,40] Although the sulfated glycosaminoglycans of normal human blood basophils have not yet been characterized, two studies of the proteoglycans synthesized by blood leukocytes (containing 10–75% basophils) of five patients with myeloid leukemia indicate that such cells may produce solely chondroitin sulfates[41] or a mixture of chondroitin sulfates (50–84%) and heparin (8–43%).[42] Normal guinea pig basophils synthesize predominantly (85%) chondroitin sulfates; the remainder is characterized as heparan sulfate rather than heparin.[43] Although the biologic functions of basophil and mast cell proteoglycans are not fully understood, in mice, heparin is required for normal packaging of certain neutral proteases in mast cell cytoplasmic granules.[44,45] Both human mast cells and basophils synthesize and store histamine.[1,40] Basophils represent the source of most (if not all) of the histamine present in normal human blood.[46] Although macrophages,[47] neutrophils,[48] and platelets,[49] as well as basophils,[46] can be induced to produce histamine, mast cells represent the source of virtually all the histamine stored in normal tissues in mice, with the notable exceptions of the glandular stomach and parts of the central nervous system.[50]

In addition to proteoglycans and histamine, basophils and mast cells generate many other products that can influence the course of inflammatory processes (see Table 63–1).[1,3–5,40,51–59] These substances are either preformed and granule associated (e.g., histamine, neutral proteases, proteoglycans) or produced during activation of the cell (e.g., prostaglandin D_2, leukotrienes and other metabolites of arachidonic acid, and platelet-activating factor). Appropriately stimulated mouse or human mast cells can release the cytokine tumor necrosis factor (TNF),[3,5,60,61] and many other cytokines, chemokines and growth factors with effects on inflammation, immunity, hematopoiesis, tissue remodeling, and many other biologic processes.[52–55,57,59,62,63] By contrast, the spectrum of basophil-derived cytokines appears to be more limited but includes IL-4 and IL-13, vascular endothelial growth factor (VEGF)-A,[62] certain chemokines[19] and, at least in mice, IL-6, TNF, and thymic stromal lymphopoietin (TSLP).[5,63–69]

ROLE IN ACUTE REACTIONS

Basophils and mast cells have specific, high-affinity plasma membrane receptors for the Fc region of IgE.[70–74] When IgE antibodies bound to the basophil or mast cell surface are bridged by specific divalent or multivalent antigens, anaphylactic degranulation is triggered.[5,70–74] The critical signal in this event is the bridging of IgE receptors (FcεRI) on the plasma membrane.[70] Morphologically, anaphylactic degranulation involves the fusion of plasma membranes with the membranes delimiting individual cytoplasmic granules or with groups of granules whose membranes have undergone fusion, leading to rapid noncytolytic release of granule contents, such as histamine and other preformed mediators.[1,2] The complex sequence of biochemical events associated with anaphylactic degranulation, the signaling mechanisms that provide positive and negative regulation of this response, and the rationale for the pharmacologic manipulation of these processes have been reviewed.[70–74]

The sudden, massive release of mediators from basophils and mast cells is thought to provoke many of the clinical manifestations of acute immediate hypersensitivity reactions in disorders such as certain forms of bronchial asthma (including fatal asthma, in which basophils can be prominent[75]); urticaria; allergic rhinitis; and anaphylaxis to foods, drugs, insect stings, and other antigens.[1,3,40,55,56,59,66,68,69] Other diverse stimuli, including certain complement fragments (anaphylatoxins), neutrophil lysosomal proteins, a variety of basic peptides and peptide hormones, components of insect or reptile venoms, radiocontrast solutions, cold, calcium ionophores, and certain drugs such as narcotics and muscle relaxants, also may initiate rapid release of mediators from basophils and mast cells, independently of IgE.[1,5,40,55,56,59] The clinical reactions provoked by these agents can closely mimic those of immediate hypersensitivity. Certain agents, including protein Fv, a sialoprotein found in normal liver and released into the intestinal tract in patients with viral hepatitis, or the HIV glycoprotein 120 (gp120), can interact with the V_H3 domain of IgE and thereby induce release of histamine, IL-4, and IL-3 from human basophils and mast cells *in vitro*.[76] The extent to which such proposed "endogenous superallergen" functions of protein Fv or gp120 are important in host defense or in the pathogenesis of viral infections remains to be determined.[76,77] Basophils activated via FcεRI or other mechanisms can exhibit increased surface levels of CD63, CD69, and CD203c, and the clinical value of using such finding to monitor basophil activation *in vivo* is under investigation.[17,78]

ROLE IN LATE-PHASE REACTIONS

In addition to their roles in classic acute immediate hypersensitivity responses, such as anaphylaxis, mast cells and basophils can contribute to late-phase reactions. Late-phase reactions occur when antigen challenge is followed, hours after initial IgE-dependent mast cell activation, by recurrence of signs (e.g., cutaneous edema) and symptoms (e.g., bronchoconstriction).[55,56,79] Much of the morbidity associated with chronic allergic conditions, such as allergic asthma, is widely believed to reflect the actions of leukocytes that are recruited to sites of late-phase reactions.[55,56,79] Studies in mast cell knockin mice (genetically mast cell-deficient mice that have been selectively repaired of their mast cell deficiency) indicate mast cells are responsible for virtually all of the vascular permeability changes and leukocyte infiltration associated with IgE-dependent cutaneous late-phase reactions[80,81] and that TNF importantly contributes to these responses.[80] The extent to which mast cells (or TNF) contribute to late-phase reactions in humans, in which such reactions may have components that are both IgE and T-cell dependent (and in which it has been suggested that certain IgE-dependent mechanisms may not involve mast cells[82]), is not yet clear.[5,55,56,61,79,82,83] However, the lymphocytes, basophils, eosinophils, and other leukocytes that are recruited to these reactions likely produce cytokines and other mediators that regulate further development and, ultimately, resolution of these reactions.[5,55,56,79]

ROLE IN CHRONIC CHANGES ASSOCIATED WITH ALLERGIC DISORDERS

Studies in mast cell knockin mice (see "Other Functions and Mast Cell Knockin Mice" below) indicate that mast cells can contribute importantly to many of the features of chronic asthma, as observed in mouse models of allergic inflammation involving the lungs. The features include the development of airway hyperreactivity to immunologically nonspecific agonists of bronchoconstriction such as methacholine[56,84–87]; infiltration of the airways and lung interstitium with inflammatory cells, including eosinophils, neutrophils, and T cells[56,85–87]; increased deposition of collagen in the lungs and hyperplasia and/or hypertrophy of airway smooth muscle[86]; and induction of increased numbers of mucus-producing goblet cells in the large airways.[86] Thus, such mouse models indicate mast cells and their products can promote the development of much of the pathology and pathophysiologic changes observed in long-standing asthma in humans.[56] Analyses of biopsies of patients with asthma suggest the development of increased numbers of mast cells within the airway smooth muscle layer may be especially important in placing mast cells and their products in proximity to a major target cell in asthma, the bronchial smooth muscle cell.[16,88] Studies in mice indicate that basophils also can enhance the development of IgE-dependent chronic inflammation, even in the absence of mast cells or T cells.[68,81]

IgE-DEPENDENT UPREGULATION OF FcεRI EXPRESSION AND FcεRI-DEPENDENT FUNCTION

Notably, as plasma levels of IgE increase (as typically occurs in subjects with allergic diseases or parasite infections), levels of FcεRI expression on the surface of basophils and mast cells also increase.[89,90] Compared with cells with low "baseline" levels of FcεRI expression, such cells can bind more IgE, release mediators in response to lower concentrations of allergens, and produce significantly larger amounts of preformed and lipid mediators and cytokines.[89–92] Thus, basophils and mast cells in subjects with high levels of IgE may have significantly enhanced ability to express IgE-dependent and/or immunoregulatory functions.[55,71] Exposure of mouse mast cells to certain monoclonal IgE antibodies, in the absence of exposure to the antigen for which the IgE is known to have specificity, can enhance the survival of the cells and, in some cases, induce the cells to release all three classes of mediators (preformed, lipid, cytokines).[93–95] Exposure to IgE in the absence of known antigen also can induce enhanced survival and cytokine and chemokine release *in vitro* derived human mast cells.[96] Although the mechanisms responsible for these intriguing findings are not fully understood, some types of IgE antibodies appear to induce aggregation of FcεRI in the absence of known antigen.[71,95] In some cases, this action may reflect the ability of the antigen-binding portion of the IgE to exist in at least two distinct isomeric forms, one binds the "known" antigen and the other binds an "unknown" antigen that may differ from the known antigen structurally and chemically.[97] The clinical implications of these findings, if any, remain to be defined. However, the observations raise the possibility that high levels of IgE *per se* may have biologic consequences, such as enhanced mast cell survival or mast cell mediator release, which can occur even in the absence of exposure to the antigens to which the patient is known to be allergic.

ROLES IN T-CELL–DEPENDENT RESPONSES NOT INVOLVING IgE

Mast cell activation and/or infiltration of affected tissues with circulating basophils can occur during a variety of T-cell–dependent immunologic responses in both humans and experimental animals.[1,55,59,66–69,98]

Moreover, studies in mast cell knockin mice (see "Other Functions and Mast Cell Knockin Mice" below) show that mast cells can contribute to the expression of mouse models of certain T-cell–associated disorders that are not thought to involve IgE, including experimental autoimmune encephalomyelitis (a mouse model of multiple sclerosis)[99,100] and an antibody-dependent form of destructive arthritis (a model of rheumatoid arthritis).[101] In such settings, mast cell function may partly reflect the activation of these cells via IgG_1 antibodies that recognize the experimental autoantigen, as mouse mast cells can be activated via aggregation of FcγRIII receptors (which bind immune complexes containing IgG_1 antibodies) and via IgE bound to FcγRI.[102–104]

Several groups have shown that mast cell-deficient mice can exhibit reduced expression of some models of T-cell immunity, as in certain examples of contact hypersensitivity or delayed hypersensitivity.[105,106] However, in other, apparently quite similar, models of contact hypersensitivity, genetically mast cell-deficient mice can express apparently unimpaired responses.[107] Whether or not mast cells are required for optimal expression of such hypersensitivity in the particular model tested appears to depend on factors such as the type and dose of hapten and the vehicle used to administer the hapten;[108,109] the conditions of antigen sensitization and challenge, including whether or not artificial adjuvants are used during sensitization and challenge, may also influence the extent to which mast cells contribute to T-cell-associated responses in the lungs.[84–87] In certain settings, mast cells appear to be able to enhance the *development* of acquired immune responses in response to allergen exposure.[57,58,108,110–112] It is hypothesized that they perform this function by expressing roles (such as enhancing dendritic cell migration) that are distinct from the effector functions they may exhibit upon later reexposure to the antigen, when antigen-specific reactions are elicited in subjects who already are sensitized to the antigen of interest. In mice, mast cells also can function to limit the extent and duration of severe contact hypersensitivity responses, including to urushiol, the hapten-containing sap of poison ivy and poison oak; the ability of mast cells to produce the antiinflammatory cytokine IL-10 contributes substantially to the mast cell's antiinflammatory role in this setting.[113]

BIOLOGIC FUNCTIONS OF BASOPHILS AND MAST CELLS

ROLES IN HOST DEFENSE

Basophils and mast cells may have critical roles in the expression of host resistance to certain parasites. Whether the basophil or the mast cell represents the major effector cell type in these responses appears to vary according to factors such as species of parasite, species of host, and site of infection. Thus, in the guinea pig, basophils appear to be required for expression of immune resistance to infestation of the skin by larval ixodid *Amblyomma americanum* ticks,[98,114] whereas expression of IgE-dependent immune resistance to the cutaneous infestation of larval *Haemaphysalis longicornis* ticks in mice is dependent on mast cells.[115] Such findings support the notion that basophils and mast cells express similar or complementary functions as effector cells in host defense against parasites and other agents. Studies in mice[57,58,66–69,108,110–112] and guinea pigs[116] provide evidence that basophils[66–69] and mast cells[57,58,108,110–112] also can have functions that contribute to the positive or negative (in the case of mast cells[57] and perhaps basophils[116]) regulation of adaptive immune responses in several different settings. Whether mast cells and basophils have similar immunoregulatory roles in humans is not clear.

Studies in "mast cell knockin mice"[117–119] (see "Other Functions and Mast Cell Knockin Mice" below) or in mice that lack TNF[120] or certain mast cell-associated proteases[121,122] show that mast cells can contribute to "innate immunity" to host defense against some experimental bacterial infections. Depending on the model system tested, the protective role of the mast cell in such models of "natural immunity" in mice partly results from complement-dependent,[123] toll-like receptor (TLR) 4-dependent,[124] endothelin-1–dependent,[125] or neurotensin-dependent[126] activation of mast cells, inducing the release of mast cell-derived mediators, which, in turn, can contribute to enhanced local recruitment or activation of neutrophils and enhanced clearance of bacteria. Studies in mice indicate mast cells can phagocytose bacteria,[127] and mouse and human mast cells can produce antimicrobial peptides (cathelicidin LL-37 in humans).[128] However, mast cells also may contribute to survival during bacterial infection in mice by additional mechanisms, such as protease-dependent degradation of endothelin-1,[125,129] neurotensin,[126] and perhaps other endogenous peptides that are produced during infections and which contribute to the pathology associated with the disorders. On the other hand, some mast cell functions that may be expressed during bacterial infections in mice, such as the ability of mast cells to degrade IL-6 via dipeptidyl peptidase I[121] or to exhibit mast cell–IL-15–dependent transcriptional downregulation of mast cell protease-2,[130] may have detrimental consequences. Thus, mast cells may have complex roles in innate immune responses, with some actions promoting host defense and survival and others enhancing the pathology associated with the response.

Mast cells and basophils have been implicated in certain viral infections. Mast cell progenitors[131–133] and basophils[134] can become infected with "M tropic" strains of HIV. Although mature mast cells appear to be resistant to such infection, mast cells which matured from infected progenitors while harboring latent infection exhibited enhanced viral replication upon stimulatation with ligands for TLR2, TLR4, or TLR9,[132,133] or via an IgE-dependent mechanism.[133] At least one HIV-derived protein, gp120, can induce mast cell or basophil mediator release (histamine and, in basophils, IL-4 and IL-13) by binding to and crosslinking cell-surface-bound IgE.[76] Many patients infected with HIV develop high levels of IgE and can exhibit exacerbation of the symptoms and signs of their allergic disorders.[76] However, whether the infection of basophils or mast cells or their precursors with HIV, or the activation of these cells in response to antigen- or gp120-induced IgE-dependent stimuli, play important roles in the progression of disease in HIV-infected patients remain to be determined. Many potential secreted products of mast cells or basophils may have effects that enhance (or suppress) host responses to a variety of viruses or contribute to the pathology associated with the infections. Moreover, exposure of *in vitro* derived human mast cells to live dengue virus together with virus-specific antibody induces the cells to release chemokines.[135] However, the extent to which mast cells contribute to host defense or pathology during viral infections is not clear.

OTHER FUNCTIONS AND MAST CELL KNOCKIN MICE

Factors capable of inducing basophil infiltration, mast cell proliferation, and/or basophil or mast cell degranulation are generated during a wide variety of immunologic or pathologic processes and immune responses to parasites.[1,13,20,33,55–57,66,68,69,98,119] As a result, speculation is considerable that basophils and mast cells express critical roles in diverse biologic responses. On the other hand, the precise functions of basophils and mast cells in most of the biologic responses in which the cells have been implicated are obscure. Studies of basophil function in guinea pigs[114,116] and mice[66–69] have employed antibodies to deplete this cell type, and such approaches also have been used to deplete mast cells in mice[136]; however, the antibodies used may also influence other cell types. In the mouse, mutant animals virtually devoid of mast cells (but which have other abnormalities as well) and congenic normal mice can be used to define and quantify the contributions of mast cells to many different biologic responses.[20,50,55,57,58,119,137] A particularly useful approach is transferring cultured mast cells derived from the marrow of normal WBB6F$_1$-*Kit*$^{+/+}$ or C57BL/6-*Kit*$^{+/+}$ mice (or mast cells derived from hematopoietic precursors or embryonic stem cells with spontaneous or targeted mutations that affect mast cell development or function) into the skin, peritoneal cavity or other tissues of WBB6F$_1$-*Kit*$^{W/W\text{-}v}$ or C57BL/6-*Kit*$^{W\text{-}sh/W\text{-}sh}$ mice, which lack mast cells because of mutations at or upstream of the *W/KIT* locus.[55,57,58,119,125,137,138] After sufficient time has been allowed to permit the transferred mast cells to acquire phenotypic characteristics appropriate for their anatomical location, one can compare the features of biologic responses elicited in WBB6F$_1$-*Kit*$^{W/W\text{-}v}$ or C57BL/6-*Kit*$^{W\text{-}sh/W\text{-}sh}$ mice at sites where the mast cell deficiency has been selectively "repaired" (locally or systemically) and at corresponding ("control") mast cell-deficient sites.

Studies using such mast cell knockin mice have provided evidence that mast cells are essential for certain IgE-dependent acute- or late-phase reactions in the skin,[80] gastrointestinal tract,[139] or respiratory system[140]; they also can enhance the expression of certain IgE-independent immunologic responses to exogenous[102] or autoantigens[99,101]; they can significantly augment innate immunity to certain bacterial infections,[119] or to the venom of certain snakes or the honeybee[129,141]; they can contribute to pathology in a model of atherosclerosis[142]; and they can contribute to certain other immunologically nonspecific acute inflammatory reactions.[3,55] Evidence regarding mast cell functions in the mouse can also be obtained in studies of mice in which specific mast cell-associated mediators have been eliminated[122,143,144] or altered to ablate their function.[129] The results of experiments in which C57BL/6-*Kit*$^{W\text{-}sh/W\text{-}sh}$ mice have been crossed with mice carrying mutations influencing tumor development have suggested that mast cells can either enhance or suppress the development or progression of tumors, but such approaches do not rule out potential contributions of phenotypic abnormalities in *Kit*$^{W\text{-}sh/W\text{-}sh}$ mice other than their mast cell deficiency.[58] However, no human patients devoid of mast cells have yet been identified. In addition, the clinical findings in the rare patients who express a deficiency of basophils are not easy to interpret. One patient with a profound basopenia experienced persistent and severe infestation with scabies,[35] a finding that might be viewed as consistent with the role of basophils in resisting ectoparasites in humans. However, that patient also had eosinopenia, IgA deficiency, and multiple other clinical problems.[35] A second basophil-deficient patient had a history of recurrent bacterial and viral infections.[37] However, this patient also had a deficiency of eosinophils, hypogammaglobulinemia, abnormal suppressor T-cell function *in vitro*, and a thymoma.[37]

BLOOD BASOPHIL COUNT

The normal blood basophil count is difficult to define precisely, but several studies place the normal range between approximately 14 to 20 and 80 to 90/μL (approximately 0.014–0.020 and 0.080–0.090 × 10^9/L).[8–10,51,145] The blood basophil count reportedly varies by age,[146] gender (in one study[146] but not in another[9]), and season.[147]

BASOPHILOPENIA

Because numbers of blood basophils can be very low even in apparently normal individuals,[8–10,51,145] determining whether examples of

TABLE 63–2. Conditions Associated with Alterations in Numbers of Blood Basophils

I. Decreased Numbers (Basopenia)
A. Hereditary absence of basophils (very rare)
B. Elevated levels of glucocorticoids
C. Hyperthyroidism or treatment with thyroid hormones
D. Ovulation
E. Hypersensitivity reactions
1. Urticaria
2. Anaphylaxis
3. Drug-induced reactions
F. Leukocytosis (in association with diverse disorders)
II. Increased Numbers (Basophilia)
A. Allergy or inflammation
1. Ulcerative colitis
2. Drug, food, inhalant hypersensitivity
3. Erythroderma, urticaria
4. Juvenile rheumatoid arthritis
B. Endocrinopathy
1. Diabetes mellitus
2. Estrogen administration
3. Hypothyroidism (myxedema)
C. Infection
1. Chicken pox
2. Influenza
3. Smallpox
4. Tuberculosis
D. Iron deficiency
E. Exposure to ionizing radiation
F. Neoplasia
1. "Basophilic leukemia" (see text)
G. Myeloproliferative neoplasms (especially chronic myelogenous leukemia; also polycythemia vera, primary myelofibrosis, essential thrombocythemia)
H. Carcinoma

basophilopenia reflect pathologic processes as opposed to normal variation can be difficult. Nevertheless, reduced numbers of circulating basophils have been reported in several disorders (Table 63–2). Basophilopenia has been recorded in association with urticaria and anaphylaxis,[148,149] but the extent to which the latter finding represents a loss of metachromatic staining of circulating degranulated cells rather than a true decrease in the number of cells is undetermined. Basophilopenia occurs in conditions that also are associated with eosinophilopenia. These conditions often are associated with increased secretion of adrenal glucocorticoids.[51,145,150,151] Basophil counts may diminish, sometimes markedly, during leukocytosis accompanying infection, inflammatory states, immunologic reactions, neoplasia, or hemorrhage.[150] Basophil counts also are diminished in thyrotoxicosis or after pharmacologic administration of thyroid hormones. Conversely, basophil counts may be increased in myxedema or after ablation of thyroid function.[51,150] A rapid and significant drop in blood basophil levels of up to 50 percent has been documented at ovulation.[152] A few patients with an apparent total lack of basophils have been reported.[35,37]

A morphologic abnormality expressed in the majority of eosinophils and basophils but not in other leukocytes or mast cells has been described as an autosomal dominant condition affecting four members of a family.[36] Cytoplasmic inclusions and crystals in basophils resembling the May-Hegglin anomaly have occurred in healthy individuals.

BASOPHILIA

Table 63–2 lists conditions associated with increased numbers of blood basophils *(basophilia)*.

Inflammatory and Immunologic Responses

An increased number of basophils is commonly associated with chronic, IgE-associated hypersensitivity disorders. These disorders often are accompanied by increased levels of IgE. Although serum IgE levels and basophil numbers are not directly related,[153] increased IgE levels are associated with increased expression of FcεRI on the surfaces of both basophils and mast cells.[89,90,154] Moreover, basophils can be recruited into tissues at sites of IgE-associated and other immunologic responses.[1,5,66,68,69,98] Basophil levels may be elevated in ulcerative colitis[155] and juvenile rheumatoid arthritis,[156] whereas many inflammatory conditions that cause a leukocytosis are associated with basophilopenia. Basophilia can occur in subjects exposed to ionizing radiation.[157]

Clonal Myeloid Diseases

Myeloproliferative Neoplasms The concentration of blood basophils is slightly increased in many patients with polycythemia vera (see Chap. 86), primary myelofibrosis (see Chap. 91), and essential thrombocythemia (see Chap. 87). A slight increase in the absolute basophil count may be a useful early sign of a myeloproliferative neoplasm. An increased absolute basophil count occurs in virtually all patients with chronic myelogenous leukemia (CML).[158–160] In some patients, basophils can represent 20 to 90 percent of blood leukocytes (see Chap. 90). Exaggerated basophilia of this type is a poor prognostic sign and may herald transformation to the accelerated phase of CML.[161] The basophil in myeloproliferative neoplasms is derived from the malignant clone and in CML can contain the Ph chromosome[162] and, thus, also the breakpoint cluster gene rearrangement on chromosome 22. The basophils in CML exhibit a variety of ultrastructural and biochemical abnormalities.[163,164] In some cases, the abnormalities obscure the typical distinctions between basophils and mast cells.[165–168] Release of basophil-associated histamine can lead to episodes of flushing, pruritus, and hypotension in occasional patients with basophilic CML.[169,170] Severe peptic ulcer of the stomach and duodenum can occur in association with hypersecretion of gastric acid and pepsin.[171,172] Ph chromosome-positive acute basophilic leukemia may be a presenting manifestation of CML.[173]

Basophilic Leukemias The basis for designating some cases as basophilic leukemias as opposed to examples of myelogenous leukemia with an associated pronounced basophilia is not always clear. Accordingly, we refer to these conditions herein as *leukemias associated with basophilia*. Table 63–3 lists the leukemias associated with basophilia. In addition to extreme basophilia in the chronic phase CML or as a manifestation of the accelerated phase of CML, acute basophilic leukemia can rarely occur *de novo*.[174–180] Thus, acute basophilic leukemia is included in the recent World Health Organization classification of acute myelogenous leukemias (AMLs),[181] but the entity is poorly defined, with no recurring cytogenetic or molecular genetic abnormality described.[179,180,182] Some cases are recognized only by electron microscopy, a procedure not used routinely in the diagnosis or classification of leukemias. One report

TABLE 63–3. Leukemias Associated with Basophilia

Chronic myelogenous leukemia with exaggerated basophilia[162,169–172]
Blast transformation, including acute basophilic transformation, of chronic myelogenous leukemia[169,179]
Acute myelogenous leukemia with t(9;22), t(6;9), t(3;6) or 12p abnormalities and marrow basophilia[179,184–185,189–191]
Acute promyelocytic leukemia with basophilic maturation (see text)[192–194]
"Acute basophilic leukemia"[173–183]

suggests that the detection of a CD123-positive, CD203c-positive, and CD117-negative blast cell immunophenotype may be useful in making a diagnosis of acute basophilic leukemia.[183]

Other types of acute myeloid leukemia that have an associated increase in basophils are more prevalent than acute basophilic leukemia. Such acute leukemias most commonly have t(9;22), t(6;9), t(3;6), or 12p abnormalities.[184–187] The t(9;22) AMLs have features similar to blast crisis of CML and distinguishing *de novo* t(9;22) AML from transformed CML can be difficult.[188] The t(6;9) AML often is associated with erythroid hyperplasia and dysplasia, a high frequency of *FLT3* mutations and poor prognosis.[189–191]

Rare cases of acute promyelocytic leukemia have been described with associated basophils,[192–194] but the so-called hyperbasophilic microgranular variant of this disease refers to cytoplasmic basophilia rather than the presence of basophilic granules,[195] which are unusual in this disease. Similarly, AML with inv(16) or t(16;16) are characteristically associated with cells having large basophilic granules, but the cells containing these granules are generally thought to represent abnormal eosinophils rather than basophils.[196]

Although the clinical and pathologic features of acute basophilic leukemia are largely similar to the features of acute myeloid leukemia, affected patients occasionally exhibit symptoms that result from release of mediators (especially histamine) derived from degranulating or dying basophils.[51,169,170,176,197] Remission induction therapy is similar to the therapy used for other types of AML, but management can be complicated by shock resulting from massive release of histamine and other mediators associated with acute cytolysis.

Chapter 89 provides further details on the acute leukemias associated with basophilia.

DISORDERS AFFECTING MAST CELLS

NORMAL MAST CELL LEVELS

Mast cells cannot be identified in the blood of healthy individuals using standard techniques. However, mast cells can be observed in the blood of monkeys that have been treated chronically with large amounts of the *KIT* ligand SCF[24] and in the blood of some patients with systemic mastocytosis.[198] Increases in tissue mast cells can occur by a combination of enhanced progenitor influx and proliferation of resident mast cells in tissues.[20,199] Human mast cells have been classified according to their content of neutral proteases as MC_T, because the granules contain tryptase but not detectable chymase, and MC_{TC}, whose secretory granules contain both enzymes.[32] The former mast cell type ordinarily predominates in lung and gastrointestinal mucosal tissues, and the latter type in dermis and submucosal tissues.[200–202] Mast cells that express chymase but little or no tryptase (MC_C) also have been described.[203]

SECONDARY CHANGES IN MAST CELL NUMBERS

Although long-term treatment with glucocorticoids (particularly topical treatment of the skin) can result in diminished mast cell numbers,[204] no clinical disorder whose primary feature is a reduction in levels of tissue mast cells has been reported. Studies of small numbers of patients indicate that certain mast cell populations, namely, the MC_T mast cells in the gastrointestinal mucosa, can be strikingly reduced in numbers in subjects with genetically determined or acquired (HIV-induced) immunodeficiency.[205] Human mast cell precursors can be infected *in vitro* with so-called M tropic strains of HIV[131,132,134]; and *in vivo* may comprise a long-lived inducible reservoir of persistent HIV.[133] Whether mast cell infection with HIV contributes to the reduction in gastrointestinal mast cells observed in some subjects with HIV infection remains to be determined.

A number of disorders are associated with small to up to severalfold increases in mast cell numbers in or near the tissues affected by the disorder (Table 63–4). Tissues at sites of recurrent allergic reactions often exhibit increases in mast cell numbers, to levels as high as approximately fourfold normal.[200,206] Small increases in mast cell numbers have been observed at sites of pathology in rheumatoid arthritis, psoriatic arthritis,

TABLE 63–4. Conditions Associated with Secondary Changes in Mast Cell Numbers

I. Decreased Numbers
   A. Long-term treatment with glucocorticoids
   B. Primary or acquired immunodeficiency disorders (certain mast cell populations; see text and reference 205)
II. Increased Numbers
   A. IgE-associated disorders
      1. Allergic rhinitis
      2. Asthma
      3. Urticaria
   B. Connective tissue disorders
      1. Rheumatoid arthritis
      2. Psoriatic arthritis
      3. Scleroderma
      4. Systemic lupus erythematosus
   C. Infectious diseases
      1. Tuberculosis
      2. Syphilis
      3. Parasitic diseases
   D. Neoplastic disorders
      1. Lymphoproliferative diseases* (lymphoplasmacytic lymphoma/Waldenström macroglobulinemia, lymphoma, chronic lymphocytic leukemia)
      2. Hematopoietic stem cell diseases* (acute or chronic myelogenous leukemias, myelodysplastic syndromes, idiopathic refractory sideroblastic anemia)
   E. Lymph nodes draining areas of tumor growth
   F. Osteoporosis*
   G. Chronic liver disease*
   H. Chronic renal disease*

*Can include increases in numbers of mast cells in the marrow.

scleroderma, and systemic lupus erythematosus.[200,206–208] Mast cells are reported to be increased in osteoporosis,[209] but the extent to which this increase reflects decreases in other cell types and/or a decrease in bone matrix is unclear. Numbers of marrow mast cells can be increased in patients with chronic liver or renal diseases.[210] Increases in mast cells also have been documented in infectious diseases, particularly at sites of infection with parasites such as *Strongyloides*, in which a greater than fourfold increase in mast cell numbers can occur.[211] In such settings, mast cell numbers can return toward normal upon resolution of the infection. Finally, mast cell numbers can be increased several-fold in lymph nodes draining areas of tumor growth[210,212] and in subjects with stem cell diseases and lymphoproliferative diseases, including lymphoma in the marrow and in association with CML.[210,213–215]

DISORDERS OF MAST CELLS: HYPERPLASIA AND NEOPLASIA

DEFINITION AND HISTORY

A group of systemic disorders associated with significant increases in mast cell numbers in the skin and internal organs have been brought together under the term *mastocytosis*. The first report of a primary mast cell disorder probably was that of Unna[216] in 1887. Unna found that the skin lesions of urticaria pigmentosa (UP)[217,218] contained numerous mast cells. However, it was not until 1949 that Ellis[219] recognized the systemic nature of the disorder. In addition to the systemic disorders classified as mastocytosis, localized cutaneous aggregates of mast cells, ranging from *mast cell nevuses* and *mastocytomas* in infants and children to multiple nodules in older children, may occur.[220,221] Solitary mastocytomas generally present before age 6 months and usually involute spontaneously, although in rare cases they are followed by UP.[221] The pathogenesis of such lesions has not been elucidated. Accordingly, the remainder of this section focuses on mastocytosis.

The clinical pattern of disease in mastocytosis and its prognosis can vary substantially among patients (see "Course and Prognosis" below). A consensus classification for mastocytosis has been developed to address the issue and to provide guidelines regarding prognosis and treatment (Table 63–5).[222] Patients with indolent disease, who compose the great majority of subjects with mastocytosis, can expect a normal life span. Patients with systemic mastocytosis with associated clonal, hematologic non–mast-cell-lineage disease (SM-AHNMD) have a prognosis determined by the associated hematologic disorder. Patients with aggressive systemic mastocytosis (ASM) generally have a 3- to 5-year survival. Mast cell leukemia (MCL) usually is rapidly fatal.

TABLE 63–5. World Health Organization Classification of Systemic Mastocytosis

Cutaneous mastocytosis (CM)
Urticaria pigmentosa (UP)/Maculopapular cutaneous mastocytosis (MPCM)
Diffuse cutaneous mastocytosis
Solitary mastocytoma of skin
Indolent systemic mastocytosis (ISM)
Systemic mastocytosis with associated clonal, hematologic non–mast-cell-lineage disease (SM-AHNMD)
Aggressive systemic mastocytosis (ASM)
Mast cell leukemia (MCL)
Mast cell sarcoma (MCS)
Extracutaneous mastocytoma

SOURCE: Modified from Horney HP, Metcalfe DD, Bennett JM, et al.[222]

ETIOLOGY AND PATHOGENESIS

Activating mutations in *KIT*, which encodes the SCF receptor, have been documented in patients with mastocytosis. Several lines of evidence indicate such mutations can be involved in the pathogenesis of the disease. The most common of these mutations (Asp816Val), which results in ligand-independent activation of the *KIT* receptor, was first identified in a long-term cell line derived from a patient with mast cell leukemia.[223] It then was detected in mononuclear cells in the blood of patients with mastocytosis who had an associated hematologic disorder,[224] as a somatic mutation in lesional tissue obtained from one patient with an aggressive form of mastocytosis and from a second patient with an indolent form of UP,[225] and in the skin, but not the marrow and blood, of an 11-month-old child with mastocytosis.[226]

Together these findings suggest the mutation occurs initially in a mast cell progenitor and that, as the clone expands, it first becomes detectable in mastocytosis skin lesions. In patients with more severe disease and thus with a larger clonal expansion, it also can be identified in circulating cells. The Asp816Val mutation, or similar 816 activating mutations that result in the substitution of phenylalanine or tyrosine for aspartate, now are believed to occur in almost all adult patients with mastocytosis, in whom the mutation can be readily identified in the skin lesions of UP.[227] Mutations at codon 816 (valine, tyrosine, or phenylalanine for aspartate) have been identified in a subset of pediatric patients, whereas other pediatric patients exhibit a dominant inactivating *KIT* mutation, in which lysine is substituted for glutamic acid in position 839, the site of a potential salt bridge.[227]

The extent to which the presence of various *KIT* mutations, and the anatomical distribution of the affected cells, can be used to predict prognosis or disease severity in patients with mastocytosis largely remains to be determined. Notably, some pediatric patients with mastocytosis appear to lack any *KIT* mutations.[227] Moreover, additional "gain-of-function" mutations of *KIT* in human subjects with mastocytosis may yet remain to be characterized. For example, a novel form of mastocytosis with a transmembrane *KIT* mutation (Phe522Cys) has been described.[228] In a second example, a *PRKG2-PDGFRB* fusion was identified in a patient presenting with increased numbers of mast cells and peripheral basophilia.[229] This case falls within the new World Health Organization category of myeloid neoplasms with *PDGFRB* rearrangements, rather than being categorized as a subvariant of mastocytosis. Gain-of-function mutations of *KIT* also have been reported in gastrointestinal stromal tumors[230] and in one pedigree as a germ-line mutation.[231]

CLINICAL FEATURES

The organs most frequently involved in systemic mastocytosis are the skin, lymph nodes, liver, spleen, marrow, and gastrointestinal tract.

The Skin

The usual presenting lesion of cutaneous mast cell disease is UP/maculopapular cutaneous mastocytosis. UP lesions appear as small yellowish-tan to reddish-brown macules or slightly raised papules (Fig. 63–2), which can exhibit the Darier sign, that is, urticaria after mild friction of the skin.[220,232] The palms, soles, face, and scalp generally remain free of lesions. In many cases, UP develops before age 2 years and subsides by puberty. In adults with UP, extracutaneous involvement by mastocytosis is common.[59,198,232,233] However, some patients, particularly those

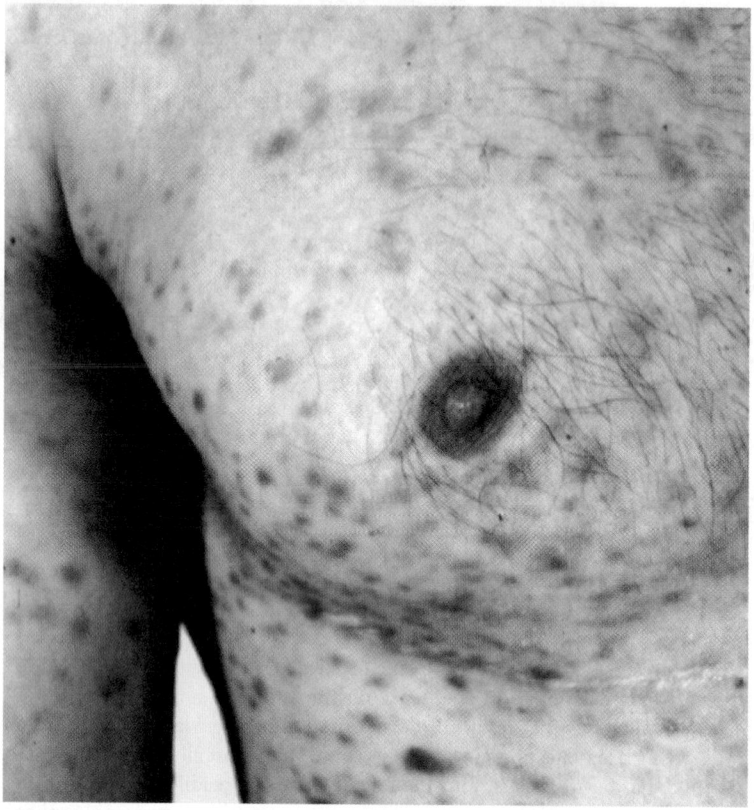

FIGURE 63–2. Urticaria pigmentosa in an adult man with indolent systemic mastocytosis. Multiple pigmented macules are present. If local pressure is applied to the skin, individual lesions show urtication and become raised, pruritic, and erythematous.

with SM-AHNMD, ASM, or MCL, entirely lack cutaneous lesions. In such cases, other organs must be biopsied to make the diagnosis. Diffuse cutaneous mastocytosis is an unusual manifestation of mastocytosis.[221,233] The skin appears yellowish-brown and is thickened. Young children with cutaneous disease may have bullous eruptions with hemorrhage.[221] Some adult patients develop prominent vascularity in association with the skin lesions, a condition termed *telangiectasia macularis eruptiva perstans*.[221]

Lymph Nodes

In one series, peripheral lymphadenopathy occurred in 26 percent and central lymphadenopathy in 19 percent of patients at diagnosis.[234] Lymphadenopathy tends to be most prominent in patients with SM-AHNMD or ASM. Mast cell infiltrates are observed in the node's paracortex, follicles, medullary cords, and sinuses. Additional findings include infiltrates of eosinophils, blood vessel proliferation in association with mast cells in the paracortical areas, and extramedullary hematopoiesis. In hematoxylin and eosin (H&E) stained sections, mast cell infiltrates in the lymph nodes may resemble T-cell lymphomas in their pericortical distribution, the clear cytoplasm that is sometimes exhibited by the mast cells, and the associated vascular proliferation and eosinophilia.[234] Alternatively, when mast cells replace lymphoid follicles, the pattern may resemble follicular hyperplasia or follicular lymphoma.[234] Fibrosis may be observed in lymph nodes involved by mast cell infiltrates.

Liver

Patients frequently exhibit infiltration of the liver with mast cells. Many of these individuals have some associated liver pathology, but severe liver disease is uncommon. When severe liver disease does occur, it typically affects patients with SM-AHNMD or ASM. In one series of 41 patients, 61 percent had some liver disease.[235] Elevated alkaline phosphatase, aminotransaminases, 5′ nucleotidase, or γ-glutamyl transpeptidase was detected in the serum of approximately half of the patients. Hepatomegaly, prominent infiltration of the liver with mast cells, and hepatic fibrosis are positively correlated with elevated levels of alkaline phosphatase and were observed more frequently in patients with aggressive disease; ascites or portal hypertension occurred in some of these individuals. Portal fibrosis was observed in 68 percent and was positively correlated with hepatic inflammation and mast cell infiltrates. Venopathy and associated venoocclusive disease was observed in four patients, all of whom had an associated hematologic disorder.

Spleen

Splenic involvement at diagnosis has been reported in approximately half of patients with systemic disease.[234,236] Mast cells most commonly occurred in a paratrabecular distribution, followed by perifollicular, follicular, and diffuse infiltrates. Trabecular and capsular fibrosis and eosinophilic infiltration also were observed, and extramedullary hematopoiesis was present in the majority of cases. On H&E stained sections, the infiltrates of mast cells produced lesions that may resemble those of T-cell lymphoma, follicular hyperplasia, follicular lymphoma, Kaposi sarcoma, myeloproliferative neoplasms, hairy cell leukemia, or a granulomatous process. Splenomegaly also occurred in the absence of infiltration of the spleen by mast cells.[237] Increased splenic weights greater than 700 g generally occurred in patients within unfavorable categories of mastocytosis.

Marrow

More than 90 percent of adults with systemic mast cell disease have focal mast cell lesions in the marrow,[236,238–241] which typically appear as foci of spindle-shaped mast cells in a fibrotic background (Fig. 63–3), sometimes with associated eosinophils and T and B lymphocytes. The focal mast cell lesions constitute the major criterion in the diagnosis of systemic mastocytosis (Table 63–6).[222] Reticulin staining may be increased, and Masson trichome staining may reveal collagen deposition. In specimens extensively involved by mast cell lesions, the bony trabeculae may be moderately to markedly thickened. Aggressive variants of mastocytosis, such as MCL, should be considered if the percentage of mast cells in the marrow aspirate film exceeds 20 percent of all nucleated cells. In typical MCL, mast cells account for 10 percent or more of blood leukocytes.[222]

In H&E stained sections, the mast cells typically exhibit a spindle-shaped or oval nucleus (see Fig. 63–3A, B), and fine eosinophilic granules are apparent in the cytoplasm at high-power magnification (see Fig. 63–3B). Mast cells with bilobed nuclei may be seen in these lesions and is a finding associated with a poor prognosis.[236] Mast cells stain positively for chloracetate esterase and aminocaproate esterase and, in suitably processed specimens, for mast cell tryptase by immunohistochemistry (see Fig. 63–3D). This is the procedure of choice for visualizing mast cells. Mast cells exhibit immunoreactivity for a variety of paraffin section markers.[242,243] Although they do not express specific B- or T-cell-lineage antigens, mast cells are positive for CD43 and CD68, which may cause confusion with histiocytes, T lymphocytes, or even blast cells. However, the lack of T-cell antigens other than CD2, more specific histiocyte markers, or myeloperoxidase help to exclude

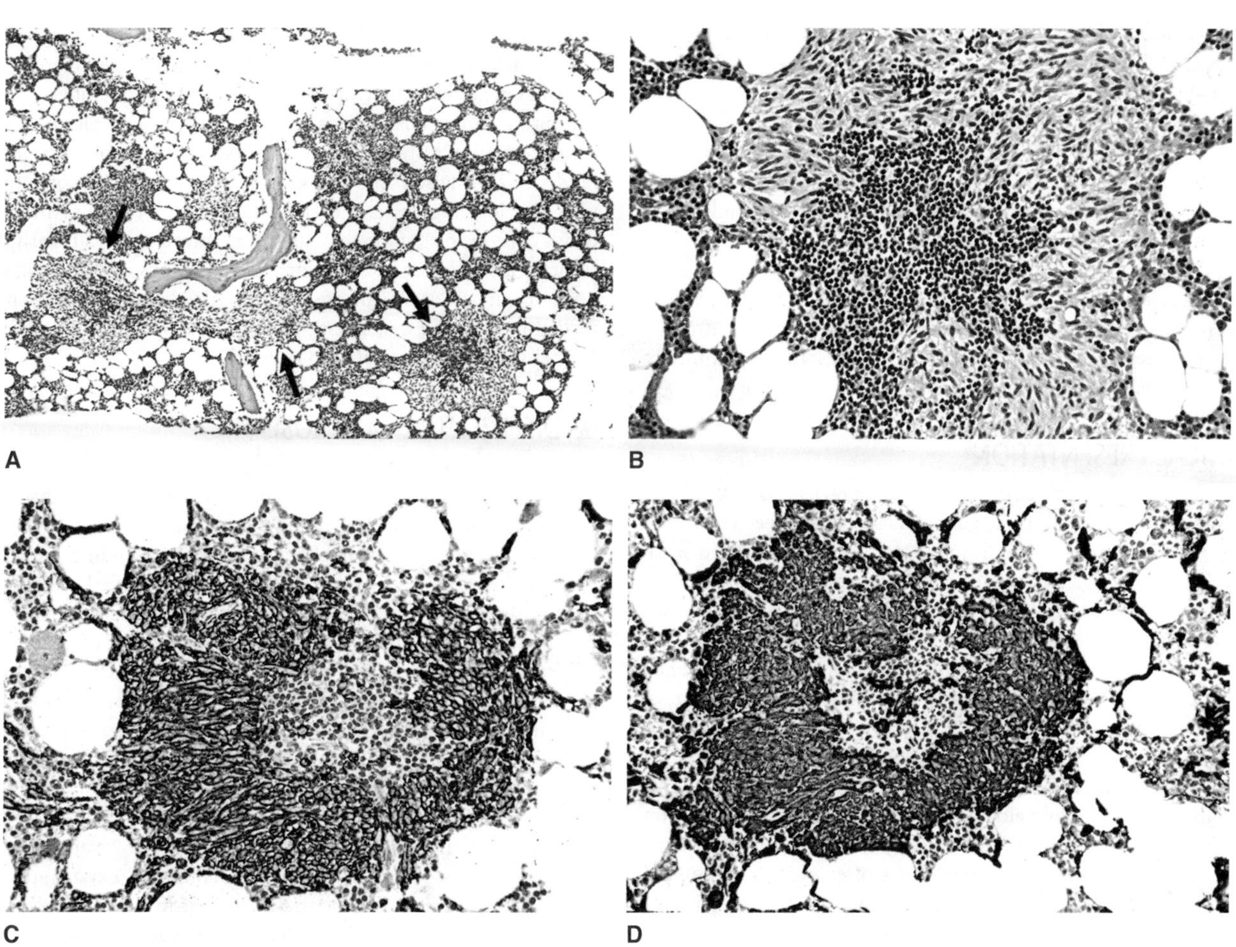

FIGURE 63–3. Marrow sections. Marrow biopsy from an adult with indolent systemic mastocytosis showing characteristic focal aggregates of mast cells, some of which are spindle-shaped, with admixed eosinophils and numerous small lymphocytes; different areas of the specimen were stained by H&E (**A**, **B**; ×40 and ×200, respectively) or with an antibody to human CD117 (**C**; ×200) or tryptase (**D**; ×200). Areas that contain many mast cells are depicted with *arrows* in **A**.

TABLE 63–6. Diagnostic Criteria for Systemic Mastocytosis

Major Criteria
Multifocal, dense infiltrates of mast cells (≥15 mast cells in an aggregate) detected in sections of marrow and/or other extracutaneous organ(s)
Minor Criteria
a. In biopsy sections of marrow or other extracutaneous organs, >25% of the mast cells in the infiltrate are spindle shaped or have atypical morphology, or, of all mast cells in marrow aspirate smears, >25% are immature or atypical mast cells
b. Detection of a point mutation in *KIT* at codon 816 in marrow, blood, or other extracutaneous organ
c. Mast cells in marrow, blood, or other extracutaneous organs that coexpress CD117 with CD2 and/or CD25
d. Serum total tryptase persistently >20 ng/mL (if there is an associated myeloid disorder, this criterion is not valid)
The diagnosis of systemic mastocytosis can be made if one major and one minor criterion are present or if three minor criteria are met.

those cell types. The more specific mast cell markers in paraffin tissues are CD117 (see Fig. 63–3C) and mast cell tryptase (see Fig. 63–3D). Strong CD117 membrane staining is equally sensitive as tryptase for mast cells but is less specific. A subset of marrow myeloblasts gives strong membrane staining for CD117, but this cell type usually can be identified based on positive staining for myeloperoxidase.

Films of marrow aspirates or clot sections alone cannot be used to diagnose mast cell disease in the marrow. Although increased numbers of mast cells may be present in marrow aspirate films of patients with systemic mast cell diseases, similar findings have been reported in patients without mast cell disorders or in patients with a reactive increase in marrow mast cells. However, mast cells in reactive lesions usually are not spindle shaped, nor do they typically exhibit evidence of degranulation. On marrow films, a normal mast cell has a round or oval shape, a round and centrally located, nonlobated nucleus, and a fully granulated cytoplasm. Mast cells from patients with mastocytosis may exhibit phenotypic aberrations, such as a spindle shape, cytoplasmic projections, and hypogranulation. A multilobular and/or eccentrically located nucleus may be observed.[222,244] If at least 25 percent of all mast cells on aspirate smears have aberrant morphology, the findings are considered to support the diagnosis of systemic mastocytosis (minor criterion).[222,244] An aberrant mast cell phenotype also may be detected on flow cytometric analysis of the marrow aspirate. In patients with mastocytosis, mast cells may express CD2, CD25 (minor criterion), and CD33.[244]

Marrow involvement appears to be much less common in children. In a study of 17 children with cutaneous or disseminated mast cell disease, small focal mast cell lesions were observed in marrow biopsies in 10 individuals, and increased mast cells in marrow aspirate films were noted in 5.[240] The focal lesions found in children were uniformly small and perivascular.

Progression of marrow involvement in systemic mast cell disease is variable. Many adults with indolent disease appear to have stable, or even decreasing, marrow involvement over time.[59,236] In contrast, a progressive increase in focal mast cell lesions is more commonly observed in patients with more aggressive patterns of disease.

CLINICAL PRESENTATION

Even though individuals differ in the specific pathogenesis of their disease, all patients within a given category of mastocytosis (see Table 63–5) generally exhibit similar clinical features. Manifestations of the disease largely reflect the local and systemic consequences of mediator release from tissue mast cells. Effects caused by disruption of normal structures by local collections of mast cells also may be seen.

At presentation, patients with mastocytosis may complain of vague and nonspecific constitutional symptoms, such as fatigue, weakness, flushing, and musculoskeletal pain. Some patients experience fever and/or weight loss.[198,233] A subset of patients may present with recurrent episodes of unexplained hypotension.[245] However, most patients with mastocytosis and a hematologic disorder are diagnosed based on marrow biopsy findings, during the investigation of their hematologic disease.[233,236] Patients with aggressive disease often present with unexplained lymphadenopathy and splenomegaly and/or hepatomegaly.

Gastrointestinal disease and associated symptoms are commonly associated with systemic mastocytosis, either at presentation or as the disease progresses.[233,246] Findings include nausea, vomiting, abdominal pain, and diarrhea. Peptic ulcer disease, which is thought to reflect, at least in part, the promotion of gastric acid secretion by elevated histamine levels, occurs in up to 50 percent of patients with systemic disease.[246] With progressive disease, patients may develop mild malabsorption.[246]

If systemic involvement is advanced at the time of diagnosis, patients may exhibit lymphadenopathy, hepatomegaly, and splenomegaly during the initial evaluation.[198,233] Because osteoporosis may accompany systemic disease, pathologic fractures may occur.[247]

LABORATORY FEATURES

When mastocytosis is suspected following the history and results of physical examination, an evaluation in adults should consist of a gross and microscopic examination of the skin, marrow biopsy, and aspirate[198,222,233] and serum for total tryptase.[248] A total serum tryptase persistently greater than 20 ng/mL is a minor criterion in the diagnosis of systemic mastocytosis (see Table 63–6). Additional studies, as suggested by the need to assess the extent of disease or to evaluate pain, may include a bone scan and a skeletal survey. Gastrointestinal evaluation, involving radiographic studies of the upper gastrointestinal tract and small intestines, computed tomographic scan of the abdomen, and endoscopy, also may be justified. In skin biopsies of sites that lack other causes of increased numbers of mast cells, such as chronic inflammatory processes, a 10-fold increase in mast cells numbers is generally considered diagnostic of cutaneous mastocytosis.[206,221,233] In patients with advanced SM-AHNMD or ASM disease, mast cells may be detectable in the blood. Patients with mast cell leukemia have significant numbers of mast cells in the blood.[210,233,236,249–251]

Plasma or urinary histamine levels frequently are increased in systemic mastocytosis.[252] However, the isolated findings of increased levels of histamine or histamine metabolites may reflect a number of other situations, including anaphylaxis. Furthermore, the accuracy of laboratory measurement of histamine depends on the assay used. Urine histamine levels may be falsely elevated as a result of bacterial contamination, pharmacologic agents and their metabolites excreted in the urine, or diets rich in histamine or histamine precursors. Similarly, serum tryptase may be elevated after anaphylaxis. Thus, no single laboratory test is diagnostic of mastocytosis. Rather, the demonstration of mast cell mediators in blood or urine should prompt the clinician to investigate further for the presence of mastocytosis.

DIFFERENTIAL DIAGNOSIS

The differential diagnosis of systemic mastocytosis includes allergic diseases; hereditary or acquired angioneurotic edema; idiopathic flushing, urticaria, or anaphylaxis; carcinoid tumor; and idiopathic capillary leak syndrome. When episodic hypertension is a major finding, pheochromocytoma should be considered. Significant unexplained gastroduodenal ulcer disease requires that Zollinger-Ellison gastrinoma syndrome be ruled out. *Helicobacter pylori* infection should be considered in all patients with ulcer disease, even in patients diagnosed with mastocytosis.

Some diseases have hematologic findings that overlap with those of systemic mastocytosis. The findings include tryptase-positive acute myeloid leukemia, chronic myelogenous leukemia with accumulation of tryptase-positive cells, primary myelofibrosis with mast cell accumulation, and acute or chronic basophilic leukemia.

A somatic mutation in *KIT* at codon 816 (most commonly Asp816Val) is associated especially with adult-onset systemic mastocytosis. Demonstration of a codon 816 gain-of-function mutation, where the most sensitive approach is to look for its presence in sorted marrow-derived mast cells, is a minor criterion in the diagnosis of mastocytosis (see Table 63–6).

THERAPY

Mastocytosis currently has no cure.[253] In addition, no evidence indicates symptomatic therapy significantly alters the course of the underlying disease. [253]

Avoiding Triggers

Management of mastocytosis includes instructing the patient on the avoidance of factors that may trigger symptoms (presumably by direct or indirect activation of mast cell mediator production). The factors can include temperature extremes, physical exertion, or, in some unusual cases, ingestion of ethanol, nonsteroidal antiinflammatory drugs, or opiate analgesics.[233,253]

Epinephrine and H_1 or H_2 Antihistamines

Anaphylaxis may follow insect stings, even in the absence of evidence of allergic sensitivity.[245] Epinephrine-filled syringes and instructions on their use can be given to patients considered at risk for such a reaction. Patients with mast cell disease and a history of anaphylaxis should be advised to carry epinephrine-filled syringes, instructed on their use, and taught to self-medicate, if necessary. These patients also may benefit from the concurrent use of H_1 and H_2 antihistamines prophylactically. Patients may experience severe reactions to iodinated contrast materials. Thus, consideration should be given to premedicating mastocytosis patients with H_1 and H_2 antihistamines and prednisone. Nonsedative H_1 antihistamines decrease skin irritability and pruritus.[233,253–255] More potent H_1 blockers, such as hydroxyzine and doxepin,[256] may be useful in more severe cases. Pruritus may be relieved by approaches that maintain skin hydration. H_2 antihistamines, including ranitidine and famotidine, are used to treat the gastritis and peptic ulcer disease associated with mastocytosis.[233,253,255] H_2 antihistamines may be titrated based on symptom control or to a particular level of gastric secretion. Proton pump inhibitors (omeprazole) are useful for management of gastric hypersecretion.[233,253,255]

OTHER DRUG THERAPY

Disodium Cromoglycate

Oral administration of disodium cromoglycate may be useful for treatment of gastrointestinal cramping and diarrhea.[222,254,257] The agent has been beneficial in cutaneous mast cell disease in children and infants.[258] Other symptoms, including headache, have improved with administration of cromolyn sodium.

Ketotifen

Ketotifen reportedly has been effective in relieving pruritus and wheal formation in cutaneous mastocytosis[259] and improving osteoporosis.[260] By contrast, one pediatric study found ketotifen was no more effective than hydroxyzine.[261] Similarly, in another study, azelastine offered only minimal benefit over chlorpheniramine.[262] Diphosphonates reportedly have been useful for treatment of osteopenia associated with mastocytosis.[263]

Nonsteroidal Antiinflammatory Agents

Nonsteroidal antiinflammatory agents have been useful in some patients whose primary manifestations are recurrent episodes of flushing, syncope, or both.[253] However, these agents may exacerbate ulcer disease. Patients with a history of aspirin sensitivity should not be placed on this therapy unless they first undergo desensitization.

Glucocorticoids or Methoxypsoralen

Cutaneous lesions have been treated with either glucocorticoids[264] or 8-methoxypsoralen plus ultraviolet A (PUVA),[265,266] largely to reduce pruritus or for cosmetic improvement. No evidence indicates such approaches alter the progression of systemic disease. Relapses 3 to 6 months after cessation of PUVA therapy are common. Patients may experience a decrease in the intensity of lesions after exposure to natural sunlight. Repeated or extensive application of glucocorticoids may result in cutaneous atrophy or adrenocortical suppression.[264]

Systemic glucocorticoids are used to decrease significant malabsorption and ascites[267] in patients with advanced disease. In adults, oral prednisone (40–60 mg/day) usually results in decreased symptoms over a 2- to 3-week period. After initial improvement, steroids usually can be tapered to an alternate-day regimen. However, with time, the ascites frequently recurs. Such patients reportedly can benefit from a portacaval shunt.[267]

Patients with more advanced categories of systemic mastocytosis may be candidates for approaches directed at reducing the mast cell burden. None of these approaches has consistently resulted in cure of the disease. The most experience has been reported for interferon alpha (IFN-α).[255,268] It is presumed to act by restricting the proliferation of hematopoietic progenitor cells. Studies with IFN-α, often in combination with glucocorticoids, have reported variable success, with unchanged or modest reductions in marrow infiltration with mast cells, and in tryptase levels.[244] Many patients do report symptomatic benefits. Resolutions of ascites and increased bone remineralization also have been reported. Use of IFN-α is often limited by side effects such as fever, fatigue, and cytopenias. Its use is not routinely recommended for patients with indolent systemic disease, unless there is concomitant severe osteoporosis.

Cladribine

Cladribine (2-chlorodeoxyadenosine), a nucleoside analogue, reportedly induced major clinical and histopathologic response in one patient with systemic mastocytosis.[269] This drug does not require cells in active cell cycle to exert its cytotoxic activity and may be beneficial in slowly progressing neoplastic processes. The drug has myelosuppressive and immunosuppressive properties and thus cannot be recommended for patients with indolent disease.[253]

Hematopoietic Stem Cell Transplantation

Allogeneic stem cell transplantation (SCT) is under study as a treatment option for patients with advanced categories of mastocytosis associated with poor survival. SCT has been used to treat a hematologic disorder associated with mastocytosis in only a few cases.[270–272] Although these studies reported favorable responses of the associated hematologic disorders, complete remission of the mast cell disease was reported in only one study, which used non–T-cell-depleted blood SCT in a patient with an associated myeloproliferative neoplasm.[272] The value of allogeneic SCT in mastocytosis may result from the immunotherapeutic effects of the donor marrow rather than the myeloablative conditioning regimen. Importantly, a protocol utilizing nonmyeloablative blood SCT for treatment of advanced systemic mastocytosis in three patients with advanced mastocytosis reported no effect on mastocytosis progression despite the induction of a graft-versus-mast cell response.[273] Perhaps performing cytoreductive treatment before transplantation may prove more successful.

Tyrosine Kinase Inhibitors

The availability of small-molecular-weight inhibitors of tyrosine kinase suggested the mutated *KIT* tyrosine kinases in mastocytosis as a therapeutic target. Imatinib mesylate (Gleevec; Novartis, Basel, Switzerland) currently is the only such drug available. It has a specific inhibition profile that includes *ABL1*, *KIT*, and *PDGFR* tyrosine kinases.[274–276] Although the drug inhibits wild-type *KIT* and *KIT*-bearing juxtamembrane activating mutations similar to those found in gastrointestinal stromal tumors, it does not inhibit *KIT* bearing codon 816 mutations associated with most common forms of systemic mastocytosis.[277,278] This finding is attributed to a conformational change in *KIT* bearing the codon 816 mutation, which interferes with the association of the drug with the ATP-binding domains of the receptor. Consistent with these observations, imatinib mesylate showed a strong *in vitro* cytotoxic effect on mast cells bearing wild-type *KIT*. Mast cells bearing a codon 816 mutation isolated from marrow of patients with mastocytosis were fairly resistant to the drug.[279] These studies suggest imatinib mesylate is unlikely to be an effective therapy for patients who carry codon 816 mutations. However, the drug appears to be of value in the unusual presentations of mastocytosis that are not associated with codon 816 mutations. For example, a patient with an unusual form of systemic mastocytosis associated with a *KIT* mutation (Phe522Cys) affecting the transmembrane region of the receptor responded to treatment with imatinib.[228] Accordingly, a careful mutational analysis of a sample enriched for lesional mast cells appears to be essential in patients with mastocytosis before contemplating imatinib therapy. Other tyrosine kinase inhibitors that decrease the activity of *KIT* with codon 816 mutations are in clinical trials.[273,280,281]

Some patients with a variant of chronic eosinophilic leukemia (clonal hypereosinophilic syndrome) and *FIPIL1-PDGFRA* fusions exhibit elevated serum tryptase levels, increased numbers of mast cells in the marrow, some of which can appear atypical and spindle shaped, tissue fibrosis, and, like other patients who have the *FIP1L1-PDGFRA* fusion gene, are responsive to imatinib mesylate.[282,283] Such cases are now considered to be within the new World Health Organization category of myeloid and lymphoid neoplasms with eosinophilia and abnormalities of *PDGFRA*, *PDGFRB*, or *FGFR1* (see Chap. 90). Although such patients have laboratory findings that may appear to fulfill the diagnostic criteria for systemic mastocytosis, they exhibit clinical features that differ from the findings in patients with systemic mastocytosis related to gain-of-function mutations of *KIT*. For example, patients with systemic mastocytosis typically present with signs and symptoms related to mast cell infiltration of tissues and histamine release, and marrow mast cells from most patients coexpress CD2 and CD25.[283] By contrast, patients with hypereosinophilia and elevated serum tryptase typically develop end-organ damage associated with eosinophil infiltration of tissues including endomyocardial fibrosis and mucosal ulcerations (see Chap. 62). Such tissues typically do not show evidence of increased numbers of mast cells histologically but do exhibit eosinophil granule deposition in some instances. CD2 was not detected on their marrow mast cells.[283] The extent to which the findings involving mast cells in this subset of hypereosinophilic patients, including the elevations of serum tryptase, reflect consequences of eosinophilia as opposed to intrinsic effects of the *FIPIL1-PDGFRA* fusion gene on the mast cell lineage remains to be determined.

Splenectomy

Splenectomy has been performed on patients with severe aggressive mastocytosis in an attempt to improve their limiting cytopenias.[284] Based on comparisons to historical controls, splenectomy increased survival by an average of 12 months. Patients who had undergone splenectomy appeared to be better able to tolerate chemotherapy. Splenectomy is of no value in the management of indolent mast cell disease.[284]

COURSE AND PROGNOSIS

The prognosis of adult patients with mast cell disorders is related to the disease category. The vast majority of patients who present with UP and indolent systemic mastocytosis (ISM) have a chronic protracted course that responds to symptomatic medical management. A normal life span is expected. Few of these patients progress to more severe forms of the disease; some patients may even experience a diminution in the severity of skin lesions in later years, while their marrow findings remain unchanged.[285] However, elevated serum lactate dehydrogenase levels, a late age of onset, and, in patients with SM-AHNMD, presence of a significant hematologic abnormality (such as a myeloproliferative or myelodysplastic disorder or, more rarely, overt leukemia) are indicators of a poor prognosis and shortened survival.[236] The prognosis for patients with SM-AHNMD depends on the course of the associated hematologic disorder.[236] Patients with ASM have a guarded prognosis because of complications arising from rapid and profound increases in mast cell numbers. These patients usually have a 3- to 5-year survival.[211] Patients with mast cell leukemia also have a short survival.[250]

Mast Cell Leukemia

This disorder develops in a small minority of patients with ISM or SM-AHNMD[249–251,286] but also can be the initial clinical presentation of the mast cell disorder.[222,287–289] Patients with mast cell leukemia may have fever, anorexia, weight loss, fatigue, severe abdominal cramping, nausea, vomiting, diarrhea, flushing, hypotension, pruritus, or bone pain. Peptic ulcer and gastrointestinal bleeding, hepatomegaly, splenomegaly, and lymph node enlargement are frequent findings. Anemia is a constant feature, and thrombocytopenia is nearly always present. The total leukocyte count varies from 10,000 to 150,000/μL (10 to 150 $\times$ 10^9/L), and mast cells compose 10 to 90 percent of leukocytes. Marrow biopsy invariably shows a striking increase in mast cells, sometimes up to 90 percent of marrow cells, although the leukemic mast cells often are hypogranular or agranular. Leukemic mast cells are stained with Sudan black and Alcian blue. They are positive for chloracetate esterase and acid phosphatase and are negative in the peroxidase and α-naphthyl esterase reactions.[250,287]

Mast Cell Sarcoma

This is an exceedingly rare tumor, characterized by nodules at various cutaneous and mucosal sites.[210,222]

REFERENCES

1. Galli SJ, Dvorak AM, Dvorak HF: Basophils and mast cells: Morphologic insights into their biology, secretory patterns, and function. *Prog Allergy* 34:1, 1984.
2. Dvorak AM: *Basophil and Mast Cell Degranulation and Recovery*. Plenum, New York, 1991. *Blood Cell Biochemistry*, vol 4.
3. Galli SJ: New concepts about the mast cell. *N Engl J Med* 328:257, 1993.
4. Valent P: Immunophenotypic characterization of human basophils and mast cells. *Chem Immunol* 61:34, 1995.
5. Metz M, Brockow K, Metcalfe DD, et al: Mast cells, basophils and mastocytosis, in *Clinical Immunology: Principles and Practice,* edited by RR Rich, TA Fleisher, WT Shearer, HW Schroeder III, AJ Frew, CM Weyand, p 345. Mosby Elsevier, London, 2008.
6. Murakami I, Ogawa M, Amo H, et al: Studies on kinetics of human leucocytes in vivo with ^{3}H-thymidine autoradiography. II. Eosinophils and basophils. *Nippon Ketsueki Gakkai Zasshi* 32:384, 1969.
7. Dvorak AM, Monahan RA, Osage JE, et al: Crohn's disease: Transmission electron microscopic studies. II. Immunologic inflammatory response. Alterations of mast cells, basophils, eosinophils, and the microvasculature. *Hum Pathol* 11:606, 1980.
8. Juhlin L: Basophil leukocyte differential in blood and bone marrow. *Acta Haematol* 29:89, 1963.
9. Ducrest S, Meier F, Tschopp C, et al: Flow cytometric analysis of basophil counts in human blood and inaccuracy of hematology analyzers. *Allergy* 60:1446, 2005.
10. Gilbert HS, Ornstein L: Basophil counting with a new staining method using Alcian blue. *Blood* 46:279, 1975.
11. Ishizaka T, Dvorak AM, Conrad DH, et al: Morphologic and immunologic characterization of human basophils developed in cultures of cord blood mononuclear cells. *J Immunol* 134:532, 1985.
12. Ganser A, Lindemann A, Seipelt G, et al: Effects of recombinant human interleukin-3 in patients with normal hematopoiesis and in patients with bone marrow failure. *Blood* 76:666, 1990.
13. Lantz CS, Boesiger J, Song CH, et al: Role for interleukin-3 in mast-cell and basophil development and in immunity to parasites. *Nature* 392:90, 1998.
14. Lantz CS, Min B, Tsai M, et al: IL-3 is required for increases in blood basophils in nematode infection in mice and can enhance IgE-dependent IL-4 production by basophils *in vitro*. *Lab Invest* 88:1134, 2008.
15. Li L, Li Y, Reddel SW, et al: Identification of basophilic cells that express mast cell granule proteases in the peripheral blood of asthma, allergy, and drug-reactive patients. *J Immunol* 161:5079, 1998.
16. Scott K, Bradding P: Human mast cell chemokines receptors: Implications for mast cell tissue localization in asthma. *Clin Exp Allergy* 35:693, 2005.
17. Yamaguchi M, Koketsu R, Suzukawa M, et al: Human basophils and cytokines/chemokines. *Allergol Int* 58:1, 2009.
18. Miura K, Saini SS, Gauvreau G, et al: Differences in functional consequences and signal transduction induced by IL-3, IL-5, and nerve growth factor in human basophils. *J Immunol* 167:2282, 2001.
19. Gilmartin L, Tarleton CA, Schuyler M, et al: A comparison of inflammatory mediators released by basophils of asthmatic and control subjects in response to high-affinity IgE receptor aggregation. *Int Arch Allergy Immunol* 145:182, 2008.
20. Kitamura Y: Heterogeneity of mast cells and phenotypic change between subpopulations. *Annu Rev Immunol* 7:59, 1989.
21. Galli SJ, Zsebo KM, Geissler EN: The kit ligand, stem cell factor. *Adv Immunol* 55:1, 1994.
22. Rodewald HR, Dessing M, Dvorak AM, et al: Identification of a committed precursor for the mast cell lineage. *Science* 271:818, 1996.
23. Chen CC, Grimbaldeston MA, Tsai M, et al: Identification of mast cell progenitors in adult mice. *Proc Natl Acad Sci U S A* 102:11408, 2005.
24. Galli SJ, Iemura A, Garlick DS, et al: Reversible expansion of primate mast cell populations *in vivo* by stem cell factor. *J Clin Invest* 91:148, 1993.
25. Costa JJ, Demetri GD, Harrist TJ, et al: Recombinant human stem cell factor (kit ligand) promotes human mast cell and melanocyte hyperplasia and functional activation *in vivo*. *J Exp Med* 183:2681, 1996.
26. Smith MA, Court EL, Smith JG: Stem cell factor: Laboratory and clinical aspects. *Blood Rev* 15:191, 2001.
27. Bischoff SC, Dahinden CA: C-kit ligand: A unique potentiator of mediator release by human lung mast cells. *J Exp Med* 175:237, 1992.

28. Columbo M, Horowitz EM, Botana LM, et al: The human recombinant c-kit receptor ligand, rhSCF, induces mediator release from human cutaneous mast cells and enhances IgE-dependent mediator release from both skin mast cells and peripheral blood basophils. *J Immunol* 149:599, 1992.
29. Wershil BK, Tsai M, Geissler EN, et al: The rat c-kit ligand, stem cell factor, induces c-kit receptor-dependent mouse mast cell activation *in vivo*. Evidence that signaling through the c-kit receptor can induce expression of cellular function. *J Exp Med* 175:245, 1992.
30. Finotto S, Mekori YA, Metcalfe DD: Glucocorticoids decrease tissue mast cell number by reducing the production of the c-kit ligand, stem cell factor, by resident cells: *In vitro* and *in vivo* evidence in murine systems. *J Clin Invest* 99:1721, 1997.
31. Enerback L: Mast cell heterogeneity: The evolution of the concept of a specific mucosal mast cell, in *Mast Cell Differentiation and Heterogeneity*, edited by AD Befus, J Bienenstock, JA Denburg, p 1. Raven, New York, 1986.
32. Irani AA, Schechter NM, Craig SS, et al: Two types of human mast cells that have distinct neutral protease compositions. *Proc Natl Acad Sci U S A* 83:4464, 1986.
33. Galli SJ: New insights into "the riddle of the mast cells": Microenvironmental regulation of mast cell development and phenotypic heterogeneity. *Lab Invest* 62:5, 1990.
34. Siegmund R, Vogelsang H, Machnik A, et al: Surface membrane antigen alteration on blood basophils in patients with Hymenoptera venom allergy under immunotherapy. *J Allergy Clin Immunol* 106:1190, 2000.
35. Juhlin L, Michaelsson G: A new syndrome characterised by absence of eosinophils and basophils. *Lancet* 1:1233, 1977.
36. Tracey R, Smith H: An inherited anomaly of human eosinophils and basophils. *Blood Cells* 4:291, 1978.
37. Mitchell EB, Platts-Mills TA, Pereira RS, et al: Basophil and eosinophil deficiency in a patient with hypogammaglobulinemia associated with thymoma. *Birth Defects Orig Artic Ser* 19:331, 1983.
38. Dvorak AM, Mihm MC Jr, Dvorak HF: Morphology of delayed-type hypersensitivity reactions in man. II. Ultrastructural alterations affecting the microvasculature and the tissue mast cells. *Lab Invest* 34:179, 1976.
39. Hastie R: A study of the ultrastructure of human basophil leukocytes. *Lab Invest* 31:223, 1974.
40. Schwartz LB, Austen KF: Structure and function of the chemical mediators of mast cells. *Prog Allergy* 34:271, 1984.
41. Metcalfe DD, Bland CE, Wasserman SI: Biochemical and functional characterization of proteoglycans isolated from basophils of patients with chronic myelogenous leukemia. *J Immunol* 132:1943, 1984.
42. Rothenberg ME, Caulfield JP, Austen KF, et al: Biochemical and morphological characterization of basophilic leukocytes from two patients with myelogenous leukemia. *J Immunol* 138:2616, 1987.
43. Orenstein NS, Galli SJ, Dvorak AM, et al: Sulfated glycosaminoglycans of guinea pig basophilic leukocytes. *J Immunol* 121:586, 1978.
44. Forsberg E, Pejler G, Ringvall M, et al: Abnormal mast cells in mice deficient in a heparin-synthesizing enzyme. *Nature* 400:773, 1999.
45. Humphries DE, Wong GW, Friend DS, et al: Heparin is essential for the storage of specific granule proteases in mast cells. *Nature* 400:769, 1999.
46. Porter JF, Mitchell RG: Distribution of histamine in human blood. *Physiol Rev* 52:361, 1972.
47. Oh C, Suzuki S, Nakashima I, et al: Histamine synthesis by non-mast cells through mitogen-dependent induction of histidine decarboxylase. *Immunology* 65:143, 1988.
48. Xu X, Zhang D, Zhang H, et al: Neutrophil histamine contributes to inflammation in mycoplasma pneumonia. *J Exp Med* 203:2907, 2006.
49. Saxena SP, Brandes LJ, Becker AB, et al: Histamine is an intracellular messenger mediating platelet aggregation. *Science* 243:1596, 1989.
50. Galli SJ, Kitamura Y: Genetically mast-cell-deficient W/W^v and Sl/Sl^d mice. Their value for the analysis of the roles of mast cells in biologic responses in vivo. *Am J Pathol* 127:191, 1987.
51. Parwaresch M: *The Human Blood Basophil*. Springer-Verlag, New York, 1976.
52. Nakajima T, Inagaki N, Tanaka H, et al: Marked increase in CC chemokine gene expression in both human and mouse mast cell transcriptomes following Fcepsilon receptor I cross-linking: An interspecies comparison. *Blood* 100:3861, 2002.
53. Sayama K, Diehn M, Matsuda K, et al: Transcriptional response of human mast cells stimulated via the Fc(epsilon)RI and identification of mast cells as a source of IL-11. *BMC Immunol* 3:5, 2002.
54. Okumura S, Kashiwakura J, Tomita H, et al: Identification of specific gene expression profiles in human mast cells mediated by Toll-like receptor 4 and FcepsilonRI. *Blood* 102:2547, 2003.
55. Galli SJ, Kalesnikoff J, Grimbaldeston MA, et al: Mast cells as "tunable" effector and immunoregulatory cells: Recent advances. *Annu Rev Immunol* 23:749, 2005.
56. Galli SJ, Tsai M, Piliponsky AM: The development of allergic inflammation. *Nature* 454:445, 2008.
57. Galli SJ, Grimbaldeston M, Tsai M: Immunomodulatory mast cells: Negative, as well as positive, regulators of immunity. *Nat Rev Immunol* 8:478, 2008.
58. Kalesnikoff J, Galli SJ: New developments in mast cell biology. *Nat Immunol* 9:1215, 2008.
59. Metcalfe DD: Mast cells and mastocytosis. *Blood* 112:946, 2008.
60. Gordon JR, Galli SJ: Mast cells as a source of both preformed and immunologically inducible TNF-alpha/cachectin. *Nature* 346:274, 1990.
61. Walsh LJ, Trinchieri G, Waldorf HA, et al: Human dermal mast cells contain and release tumor necrosis factor alpha, which induces endothelial leukocyte adhesion molecule 1. *Proc Natl Acad Sci U S A* 88:4220, 1991.
62. de Paulis A, Prevete N, Fiorentino I, et al: Expression and functions of the vascular endothelial growth factors and their receptors in human basophils. *J Immunol* 177:7322, 2006.
63. Liu SM, Xavier R, Good KL, et al: Immune cell transcriptome datasets reveal novel leukocyte subset-specific genes and genes associated with allergic processes. *J Allergy Clin Immunol* 118:496, 2006.
64. Brunner T, Heusser CH, Dahinden CA: Human peripheral blood basophils primed by interleukin 3 (IL-3) produce IL-4 in response to immunoglobulin E receptor stimulation. *J Exp Med* 177:605, 1993.
65. Li H, Sim TC, Alam R: IL-13 released by and localized in human basophils. *J Immunol* 156:4833, 1996.
66. Min B: Basophils: What they "can do" versus what they "actually do." *Nat Immunol* 9:1333, 2008.
67. Sokol CL, Barton GM, Farr AG, et al: A mechanism for the initiation of allergen-induced T-helper type 2 responses. *Nat Immunol* 9:310, 2008.
68. Karasuyama H, Mukai K, Tsujimura Y, et al: Newly discovered roles for basophils: A neglected minority gains new respect. *Nat Rev Immunol* 9:9, 2009.
69. Sullivan BM, Locksley RM: Basophils: A nonredundant contributor to host immunity. *Immunity* 30:12, 2009.
70. Beaven MA, Metzger H: Signal transduction by Fc receptors: The Fc epsilon RI case. *Immunol Today* 14:222, 1993.
71. Kawakami T, Galli SJ: Regulation of mast-cell and basophil function and survival by IgE. *Nat Rev Immunol* 2:773, 2002.
72. Gilfillan AM, Tkaczyk C: Integrated signalling pathways for mast-cell activation. *Nat Rev Immunol* 6:218, 2006.
73. Rivera J, Gilfillan AM: Molecular regulation of mast cell activation. *J Allergy Clin Immunol* 117:1214, 2006.
74. Kraft S, Kinet JP: New developments in FcepsilonRI regulation, function and inhibition. *Nat Rev Immunol* 7:365, 2007.
75. Koshino T, Teshima S, Fukushima N, et al: Identification of basophils by immunohistochemistry in the airways of post-mortem cases of fatal asthma. *Clin Exp Allergy* 23:919, 1993.
76. Marone G, Florio G, Petraroli A, et al: Role of human FcepsilonRI+ cells in HIV-1 infection. *Immunol Rev* 179:128, 2001.
77. Marone G, Galli SJ, Kitamura Y: Probing the roles of mast cells and basophils in natural and acquired immunity, physiology and disease. *Trends Immunol* 23:425, 2002.
78. Boumiza R, Monneret G, Forissier MF, et al: Marked improvement of the basophil activation test by detecting CD203c instead of CD63. *Clin Exp Allergy* 33:259, 2003.
79. Kay AB: Allergy and allergic diseases. First of two parts. *N Engl J Med* 344:30, 2001.
80. Wershil BK, Wang ZS, Gordon JR, et al: Recruitment of neutrophils during IgE-dependent cutaneous late phase reactions in the mouse is mast cell-dependent. Partial inhibition of the reaction with antiserum against tumor necrosis factor-alpha. *J Clin Invest* 87:446, 1991.
81. Mukai K, Matsuoka K, Taya C, et al: Basophils play a critical role in the development of IgE-mediated chronic allergic inflammation independently of T cells and mast cells. *Immunity* 23:191, 2005.
82. Ong YE, Menzies-Gow A, Barkans J, et al: Anti-IgE (omalizumab) inhibits late-phase reactions and inflammatory cells after repeat skin allergen challenge. *J Allergy Clin Immunol* 116:558, 2005.
83. Conner E, Bochner BS, Brummet M, et al: The effect of etanercept on the human cutaneous allergic response. *J Allergy Clin Immunol* 121:258, 2008.
84. Kobayashi T, Miura T, Haba T, et al: An essential role of mast cells in the development of airway hyperresponsiveness in a murine asthma model. *J Immunol* 164:3855, 2000.
85. Williams CM, Galli SJ: Mast cells can amplify airway reactivity and features of chronic inflammation in an asthma model in mice. *J Exp Med* 192:455, 2000.
86. Yu M, Tsai M, Tam SY, et al: Mast cells can promote the development of multiple features of chronic asthma in mice. *J Clin Invest* 116:1633, 2006.
87. Nakae S, Ho LH, Yu M, et al: Mast cell-derived TNF contributes to airway hyperreactivity, inflammation, and T_H2 cytokine production in an asthma model in mice. *J Allergy Clin Immunol* 120:48, 2007.
88. Brightling CE, Bradding P, Symon FA, et al: Mast-cell infiltration of airway smooth muscle in asthma. *N Engl J Med* 346:1699, 2002.
89. MacGlashan DW Jr, Bochner BS, Adelman DC, et al: Down-regulation of Fc(epsilon)RI expression on human basophils during in vivo treatment of atopic patients with anti-IgE antibody. *J Immunol* 158:1438, 1997.
90. Yamaguchi M, Lantz CS, Oettgen HC, et al: IgE enhances mouse mast cell Fc(epsilon)RI expression in vitro and in vivo: Evidence for a novel amplification mechanism in IgE-dependent reactions. *J Exp Med* 185:663, 1997.
91. Boesiger J, Tsai M, Maurer M, et al: Mast cells can secrete vascular permeability factor/vascular endothelial cell growth factor and exhibit enhanced release after immunoglobulin E-dependent upregulation of Fc epsilon receptor I expression. *J Exp Med* 188:1135, 1998.
92. Yamaguchi M, Sayama K, Yano K, et al: IgE enhances Fc epsilon receptor I expression and IgE-dependent release of histamine and lipid mediators from human umbilical cord blood-derived mast cells: Synergistic effect of IL-4 and IgE on human mast cell Fc epsilon receptor I expression and mediator release. *J Immunol* 162:5455, 1999.
93. Asai K, Kitaura J, Kawakami Y, et al: Regulation of mast cell survival by IgE. *Immunity* 14:791, 2001.

94. Kalesnikoff J, Huber M, Lam V, et al: Monomeric IgE stimulates signaling pathways in mast cells that lead to cytokine production and cell survival. *Immunity* 14:801, 2001.
95. Kitaura J, Song J, Tsai M, et al: Evidence that IgE molecules mediate a spectrum of effects on mast cell survival and activation via aggregation of the FcepsilonRI. *Proc Natl Acad Sci U S A* 100:12911, 2003.
96. Matsuda K, Piliponsky AM, Iikura M, et al: Monomeric IgE enhances human mast cell chemokine production: IL-4 augments and dexamethasone suppresses the response. *J Allergy Clin Immunol* 116:1357, 2005.
97. James LC, Roversi P, Tawfik DS: Antibody multispecificity mediated by conformational diversity. *Science* 299:1362, 2003.
98. Galli SJ, Askenase PW: Cutaneous basophil hypersensitivity, in *The Reticuloendothelial System: A Comprehensive Treatise,* edited by P Abramoff, SM Phillips, NR Escobar, p 321. Plenum, New York, 1986.
99. Secor VH, Secor WE, Gutekunst CA, et al: Mast cells are essential for early onset and severe disease in a murine model of multiple sclerosis. *J Exp Med* 191:813, 2000.
100. Sayed BA, Christy A, Quirion MR, et al: The master switch: The role of mast cells in autoimmunity and tolerance. *Annu Rev Immunol* 26:705, 2008.
101. Lee DM, Friend DS, Gurish MF, et al: Mast cells: A cellular link between autoantibodies and inflammatory arthritis. *Science* 297:1689, 2002.
102. Miyajima I, Dombrowicz D, Martin TR, et al: Systemic anaphylaxis in the mouse can be mediated largely through IgG1 and FcgammaRIII. Assessment of the cardiopulmonary changes, mast cell degranulation, and death associated with active or IgE- or IgG1-dependent passive anaphylaxis. *J Clin Invest* 99:901, 1997.
103. Strait RT, Morris SC, Yang M, et al: Pathways of anaphylaxis in the mouse. *J Allergy Clin Immunol* 109:658, 2002.
104. Pedotti R, De Voss JJ, Steinman L, et al: Involvement of both "allergic" and "autoimmune" mechanisms in EAE, MS and other autoimmune diseases. *Trends Immunol* 24:479, 2003.
105. Askenase PW, Van Loveren H, Kraeuter-Kops S, et al: Defective elicitation of delayed-type hypersensitivity in *W/W^v* and *SI/SI^d* mast cell-deficient mice. *J Immunol* 131:2687, 1983.
106. Biedermann T, Kneilling M, Mailhammer R, et al: Mast cells control neutrophil recruitment during T cell-mediated delayed-type hypersensitivity reactions through tumor necrosis factor and macrophage inflammatory protein 2. *J Exp Med* 192:1441, 2000.
107. Galli SJ, Hammel I: Unequivocal delayed hypersensitivity in mast cell-deficient and beige mice. *Science* 226:710, 1984.
108. Bryce PJ, Miller ML, Miyajima I, et al: Immune sensitization in the skin is enhanced by antigen-independent effects of IgE. *Immunity* 20:381, 2004.
109. Norman MU, Hwang J, Hulliger S, et al: Mast cells regulate the magnitude and the cytokine microenvironment of the contact hypersensitivity response. *Am J Pathol* 172:1638, 2008.
110. Galli SJ, Nakae S, Tsai M: Mast cells in the development of adaptive immune responses. *Nat Immunol* 6:135, 2005.
111. Jawdat DM, Rowden G, Marshall JS: Mast cells have a pivotal role in TNF-independent lymph node hypertrophy and the mobilization of Langerhans cells in response to bacterial peptidoglycan. *J Immunol* 177:1755, 2006.
112. McLachlan JB, Shelburne CP, Hart JP, et al: Mast cell activators: A new class of highly effective vaccine adjuvants. *Nat Med* 14:536, 2008.
113. Grimbaldeston MA, Nakae S, Kalesnikoff J, et al: Mast cell-derived interleukin 10 limits skin pathology in contact dermatitis and chronic irradiation with ultraviolet B. *Nat Immunol* 8:1095, 2007.
114. Brown SJ, Galli SJ, Gleich GJ, et al: Ablation of immunity to *Amblyomma americanum* by anti-basophil serum: Cooperation between basophils and eosinophils in expression of immunity to ectoparasites (ticks) in guinea pigs. *J Immunol* 129:790, 1982.
115. Matsuda H, Watanabe N, Kiso Y, et al: Necessity of IgE antibodies and mast cells for manifestation of resistance against larval *Haemaphysalis longicornis* ticks in mice. *J Immunol* 144:259, 1990.
116. Galli SJ, Colvin RB, Verderber E, et al: Preparation of a rabbit anti-guinea pig basophil serum: *In vitro* and *in vivo* characterization. *J Immunol* 121:1157, 1978.
117. Echtenacher B, Mannel DN, Hultner L: Critical protective role of mast cells in a model of acute septic peritonitis. *Nature* 381:75, 1996.
118. Malaviya R, Ikeda T, Ross E, et al: Mast cell modulation of neutrophil influx and bacterial clearance at sites of infection through TNF-alpha. *Nature* 381:77, 1996.
119. Galli SJ, Chatterjea D, Tsai M: Roles of mast cells and basophils in innate immunity, in *The Innate Immune Response to Infection,* edited by SHE Kauffmann, R Medzhitov, S Gordon, p 111. ASM Press, Berlin, 2004.
120. Maurer M, Echtenacher B, Hultner L, et al: The c-kit ligand, stem cell factor, can enhance innate immunity through effects on mast cells. *J Exp Med* 188:2343, 1998.
121. Mallen-St Clair J, Pham CT, Villalta SA, et al: Mast cell dipeptidyl peptidase I mediates survival from sepsis. *J Clin Invest* 113:628, 2004.
122. Thakurdas SM, Melicoff E, Sansores-Garcia L, et al: The mast cell-restricted tryptase mMCP-6 has a critical immunoprotective role in bacterial infections. *J Biol Chem* 282:20809, 2007.
123. Prodeus AP, Zhou X, Maurer M, et al: Impaired mast cell-dependent natural immunity in complement C3-deficient mice. *Nature* 390:172, 1997.
124. Supajatura V, Ushio H, Nakao A, et al: Differential responses of mast cell Toll-like receptors 2 and 4 in allergy and innate immunity. *J Clin Invest* 109:1351, 2002.
125. Maurer M, Wedemeyer J, Metz M, et al: Mast cells promote homeostasis by limiting endothelin-1-induced toxicity. *Nature* 432:512, 2004.
126. Piliponsky AM, Chen CC, Nishimura T, et al: Neurotensin increases mortality and mast cells reduce neurotensin levels in a mouse model of sepsis. *Nat Med* 14:392, 2008.
127. Malaviya R, Twesten NJ, Ross EA, et al: Mast cells process bacterial Ags through a phagocytic route for class I MHC presentation to T cells. *J Immunol* 156:1490, 1996.
128. Di Nardo A, Vitiello A, Gallo RL: Cutting edge: Mast cell antimicrobial activity is mediated by expression of cathelicidin antimicrobial peptide. *J Immunol* 170:2274, 2003.
129. Schneider LA, Schlenner SM, Feyerabend TB, et al: Molecular mechanism of mast cell mediated innate defense against endothelin and snake venom sarafotoxin. *J Exp Med* 204:2629, 2007.
130. Orinska Z, Maurer M, Mirghomizadeh F, et al: IL-15 constrains mast cell-dependent antibacterial defenses by suppressing chymase activities. *Nat Med* 13:927, 2007.
131. Bannert N, Farzan M, Friend DS, et al: Human mast cell progenitors can be infected by macrophage tropic human immunodeficiency virus type 1 and retain virus with maturation *in vitro*. *J Virol* 75:10808, 2001.
132. Sundstrom JB, Little DM, Villinger F, et al: Signaling through toll-like receptors triggers HIV-1 replication in latently infected mast cells. *J Immunol* 172:4391, 2004.
133. Sundstrom JB, Ellis JE, Hair GA, et al: Human tissue mast cells are an inducible reservoir of persistent HIV infection. *Blood* 109:5293, 2007.
134. Li Y, Li L, Wadley R, et al: Mast cells/basophils in the peripheral blood of allergic individuals who are HIV-1 susceptible due to their surface expression of CD4 and the chemokine receptors CCR3, CCR5, and CXCR4. *Blood* 97:3484, 2001.
135. King CA, Anderson R, Marshall JS: Dengue virus selectively induces human mast cell chemokine production. *J Virol* 76:8408, 2002.
136. Brandt EB, Strait RT, Hershko D, et al: Mast cells are required for experimental oral allergen-induced diarrhea. *J Clin Invest* 112:1666, 2003.
137. Nakano T, Sonoda T, Hayashi C, et al: Fate of bone marrow-derived cultured mast cells after intracutaneous, intraperitoneal, and intravenous transfer into genetically mast cell-deficient *W/W^v* mice. Evidence that cultured mast cells can give rise to both connective tissue type and mucosal mast cells. *J Exp Med* 162:1025, 1985.
138. Nigrovic PA, Gray DH, Jones T, et al: Genetic inversion in mast cell-deficient W^{sh} mice interrupts *corin* and manifests as hematopoietic and cardiac aberrancy. *Am J Pathol* 173:1693, 2008.
139. Wershil BK, Furuta GT, Wang ZS, et al: Mast cell-dependent neutrophil and mononuclear cell recruitment in immunoglobulin E-induced gastric reactions in mice. *Gastroenterology* 110:1482, 1996.
140. Martin TR, Takeishi T, Katz HR, et al: Mast cell activation enhances airway responsiveness to methacholine in the mouse. *J Clin Invest* 91:1176, 1993.
141. Metz M, Piliponsky AM, Chen CC, et al: Mast cells can enhance resistance to snake and honeybee venoms. *Science* 313:526, 2006.
142. Sun J, Sukhova GK, Wolters PJ, et al: Mast cells promote atherosclerosis by releasing proinflammatory cytokines. *Nat Med* 13:719, 2007.
143. Knight PA, Wright SH, Lawrence CE, et al: Delayed expulsion of the nematode *Trichinella spiralis* in mice lacking the mucosal mast cell-specific granule chymase, mouse mast cell protease-1. *J Exp Med* 192:1849, 2000.
144. Tchougounova E, Pejler G, Abrink M: The chymase, mouse mast cell protease 4, constitutes the major chymotrypsin-like activity in peritoneum and ear tissue. A role for mouse mast cell protease 4 in thrombin regulation and fibronectin turnover. *J Exp Med* 198:423, 2003.
145. Shelley WB, Parnes HM: The absolute basophil count. *JAMA* 192:368, 1965.
146. Thonnard-Neumann E: Studies of basophils, variations with age and sex. *Acta Haematol* 30:221, 1963.
147. Chavance M, Herbeth B, Kauffmann F: Seasonal patterns of circulating basophils. *Int Arch Allergy Appl Immunol* 86:462, 1988.
148. Shelley WB, Juhlin L: New test for detecting anaphylactic sensitivity: Basophil reaction. *Nature* 191:1056, 1961.
149. Grattan CE, Dawn G, Gibbs S, et al: Blood basophil numbers in chronic ordinary urticaria and healthy controls: Diurnal variation, influence of loratadine and prednisolone and relationship to disease activity. *Clin Exp Allergy* 33:337, 2003.
150. Juhlin L: Basophil and eosinophil leukocytes in various internal disorders. *Acta Med Scand* 174:249, 1963.
151. Juhlin L: The effect of corticotrophin and corticosteroids on the basophil and eosinophil granulocytes. *Acta Haematol* 29:157, 1963.
152. Mettler L, Shirwani D: Direct basophil count for timing ovulation. *Fertil Steril* 25:718, 1974.
153. Malveaux FJ, Conroy MC, Adkinson NF Jr, et al: IgE receptors on human basophils. Relationship to serum IgE concentration. *J Clin Invest* 62:176, 1978.
154. Lantz CS, Yamaguchi M, Oettgen HC, et al: IgE regulates mouse basophil Fc epsilon RI expression in vivo. *J Immunol* 158:2517, 1997.
155. Juhlin L: Basophil leukocytes in ulcerative colitis. *Acta Med Scand* 173:351, 1963.
156. Athreya BH, Moser G, Raghavan TE: Increased circulating basophils in juvenile rheumatoid arthritis. A preliminary report. *Am J Dis Child* 129:935, 1975.
157. Fredericks RE, Moloney WC: The basophilic granulocyte. *Blood* 14:571, 1959.
158. Spiers AS, Bain BJ, Turner JE: The peripheral blood in chronic granulocytic leukaemia. Study of 50 untreated Philadelphia-positive cases. *Scand J Haematol* 18:25, 1977.
159. Kamada N, Uchino H: Chronologic sequence in appearance of clinical and laboratory findings characteristic of chronic myelocytic leukemia. *Blood* 51:843, 1978.

160. Drewinko B, Bollinger P, Brailas C, et al: Flow cytochemical patterns of white blood cells in human haematopoietic malignancies. II. Chronic leukaemias. *Br J Haematol* 67:157, 1987.
161. Denburg JA, Browman G: Prognostic implications of basophil differentiation in chronic myeloid leukemia. *Am J Hematol* 27:110, 1988.
162. Goh KO, Anderson FW: Cytogenetic studies in basophilic chronic myelocytic leukemia. *Arch Pathol Lab Med* 103:288, 1979.
163. Denburg JA, Wilson WE, Goodacre R, et al: Chronic myeloid leukaemia: Evidence for basophil differentiation and histamine synthesis from cultured peripheral blood cells. *Br J Haematol* 45:13, 1980.
164. Parkin JL, McKenna RW, Brunning RD: Philadelphia chromosome-positive blastic leukaemia: Ultrastructural and ultracytochemical evidence of basophil and mast cell differentiation. *Br J Haematol* 52:663, 1982.
165. Zucker-Franklin D: Ultrastructural evidence for the common origin of human mast cells and basophils. *Blood* 56:534, 1980.
166. Soler J, O'Brien M, de Castro JT, et al: Blast crisis of chronic granulocytic leukemia with mast cell and basophilic precursors. *Am J Clin Pathol* 83:254, 1985.
167. Weil SC, Hrisinko MA: A hybrid eosinophilic-basophilic granulocyte in chronic granulocytic leukemia. *Am J Clin Pathol* 87:66, 1987.
168. Gabriel LC, Escribano LM, Marie JP, et al: Peroxidase activity in circulating mast cells in blast crisis of chronic granulocytic leukemia. Comparative studies with basophils and cutaneous mast cells. *Am J Clin Pathol* 86:212, 1986.
169. Youman JD, Taddeini L, Cooper T: Histamine excess symptoms in basophilic chronic granulocytic leukemia. *Arch Intern Med* 131:560, 1973.
170. Rosenthal S, Schwartz JH, Canellos GP: Basophilic chronic granulocytic leukaemia with hyperhistaminaemia. *Br J Haematol* 36:367, 1977.
171. Valimaki M, Vuopio P, Salaspuro M: Plasma histamine and serum pepsinogen I concentrations in chronic myelogenous leukaemia. *Acta Med Scand* 217:89, 1985.
172. Anderson W, Helman CA, Hirschowitz BI: Basophilic leukemia and the hypersecretion of gastric acid and pepsin. *Gastroenterology* 95:195, 1988.
173. Xue YQ, Guo Y, Lu DR, et al: A case of basophilic leukemia bearing simultaneous translocations t(8;21) and t(9;22). *Cancer Genet Cytogenet* 51:215, 1991.
174. Cecio A, Dini E, Quattrin N: [Initial electron microscopy studies in 2 cases of acute basophilic leukemia]. *Boll Soc Ital Biol Sper* 46:459, 1970.
175. Dvorak AM, Dickersin GR, Connell A, et al: Degranulation mechanisms in human leukemic basophils. *Clin Immunol Immunopathol* 5:235, 1976.
176. Quattrin N: Follow-up of sixty two cases of acute basophilic leukemia. *Biomedicine* 28:72, 1978.
177. Wick MR, Li CY, Pierre RV: Acute nonlymphocytic leukemia with basophilic differentiation. *Blood* 60:38, 1982.
178. Lertprasertsuke N, Tsutsumi Y: An unusual form of chronic myeloproliferative disorder. Aleukemic basophilic leukemia. *Acta Pathol Jpn* 41:73, 1991.
179. Peterson LC, Parkin JL, Arthur DC, et al: Acute basophilic leukemia. A clinical, morphologic, and cytogenetic study of eight cases. *Am J Clin Pathol* 96:160, 1991.
180. Shvidel L, Shaft D, Stark B, et al: Acute basophilic leukaemia: Eight unsuspected new cases diagnosed by electron microscopy. *Br J Haematol* 120:774, 2003.
181. Arber DA, Brunning RD, Orazi A, et al: Acute myeloid leukaemia, not otherwise specified, in *WHO Classification of Tumours of Haematopoietic and Lymphoid Tissues,* edited by SH Swerdlow, E Campo, NL Harris, ES Jaffe, SA Pileri, H Stein, J Thiele, JW Vardiman, p 130. IARC Press, Lyon, 2008.
182. Staal-Viliare A, Latger-Cannard V, Rault JP, et al: A case of de novo acute basophilic leukaemia: Diagnostic criteria and review of the literature. *Ann Biol Clin (Paris)* 64:361, 2006.
183. Staal-Viliare A, Latger-Cannard V, Didion J, et al: CD203c /CD117-, an useful phenotype profile for acute basophilic leukaemia diagnosis in cases of undifferentiated blasts. *Leuk Lymphoma* 48:439, 2007.
184. Pearson MG, Vardiman JW, Le Beau MM, et al: Increased numbers of marrow basophils may be associated with a t(6;9) in ANLL. *Am J Hematol* 18:393, 1985.
185. Horsman DE, Kalousek DK: Acute myelomonocytic leukemia (AML-M4) and translocation t(6;9)(p23);q34): Two additional patients with prominent myelodysplasia. *Am J Hematol* 26:77, 1987.
186. Matsuura Y, Sato N, Kimura F, et al: An increase in basophils in a case of acute myelomonocytic leukaemia associated with marrow eosinophilia and inversion of chromosome 16. *Eur J Haematol* 39:457, 1987.
187. Hoyle CF, Sherrington P, Hayhoe FG: Translocation (3;6)(q21;p21) in acute myeloid leukemia with abnormal thrombopoiesis and basophilia. *Cancer Genet Cytogenet* 30:261, 1988.
188. Soupir CP, Vergilio JA, Dal Cin P, et al: Philadelphia chromosome-positive acute myeloid leukemia: A rare aggressive leukemia with clinicopathologic features distinct from chronic myeloid leukemia in myeloid blast crisis. *Am J Clin Pathol* 127:642, 2007.
189. Alsabeh R, Brynes RK, Slovak ML, et al: Acute myeloid leukemia with t(6;9) (p23;q34): Association with myelodysplasia, basophilia, and initial CD34 negative immunophenotype. *Am J Clin Pathol* 107:430, 1997.
190. Slovak ML, Gundacker H, Bloomfield CD, et al: A retrospective study of 69 patients with t(6;9)(p23;q34) AML emphasizes the need for a prospective, multicenter initiative for rare "poor prognosis" myeloid malignancies. *Leukemia* 20:1295, 2006.
191. Oyarzo MP, Lin P, Glassman A, et al: Acute myeloid leukemia with t(6;9)(p23;q34) is associated with dysplasia and a high frequency of flt3 gene mutations. *Am J Clin Pathol* 122:348, 2004.
192. Moir DJ, Pearson J, Buckle VJ: Acute promyelocytic transformation in a case of acute myelomonocytic leukemia. *Cancer Genet Cytogenet* 12:359, 1984.
193. Umeda M, Nojima Z, Yamaguchi R, et al: [Two cases of acute promyelocytic leukemia with marked basophilia—A variant type of APL with the capability of differentiating into basophils]. *Rinsho Ketsueki* 28:2004, 1987.
194. Gotoh H, Murakami S, Oku N, et al: Translocations t(15;17) and t(9;14)(q34;q22) in a case of acute promyelocytic leukemia with increased number of basophils. *Cancer Genet Cytogenet* 36:103, 1988.
195. McKenna RW, Parkin J, Bloomfield CD, et al: Acute promyelocytic leukaemia: A study of 39 cases with identification of a hyperbasophilic microgranular variant. *Br J Haematol* 50:201, 1982.
196. Le Beau MM, Larson RA, Bitter MA, et al: Association of an inversion of chromosome 16 with abnormal marrow eosinophils in acute myelomonocytic leukemia. A unique cytogenetic-clinicopathological association. *N Engl J Med* 309:630, 1983.
197. Lewis RA, Goetzl EJ, Wasserman SI, et al: The release of four mediators of immediate hypersensitivity from human leukemic basophils. *J Immunol* 114:87, 1975.
198. Travis WD, Li CY, Bergstralh EJ, et al: Systemic mast cell disease. Analysis of 58 cases and literature review. *Medicine (Baltimore)* 67:345, 1988.
199. Tsai M, Shih LS, Newlands GF, et al: The rat c-kit ligand, stem cell factor, induces the development of connective tissue-type and mucosal mast cells in vivo. Analysis by anatomical distribution, histochemistry, and protease phenotype. *J Exp Med* 174:125, 1991.
200. Irani AA, Garriga MM, Metcalfe DD, et al: Mast cells in cutaneous mastocytosis: Accumulation of the MCTC type. *Clin Exp Allergy* 20:53, 1990.
201. Schwartz LB, Metcalfe DD, Miller JS, et al: Tryptase levels as an indicator of mast-cell activation in systemic anaphylaxis and mastocytosis. *N Engl J Med* 316:1622, 1987.
202. Weidner N, Horan RF, Austen KF: Mast-cell phenotype in indolent forms of mastocytosis. Ultrastructural features, fluorescence detection of avidin binding, and immunofluorescent determination of chymase, tryptase, and carboxypeptidase. *Am J Pathol* 140:847, 1992.
203. Weidner N, Austen KF: Heterogeneity of mast cells at multiple body sites. Fluorescent determination of avidin binding and immunofluorescent determination of chymase, tryptase, and carboxypeptidase content. *Pathol Res Pract* 189:156, 1993.
204. Lavker RM, Schechter NM: Cutaneous mast cell depletion results from topical corticosteroid usage. *J Immunol* 135:2368, 1985.
205. Irani AM, Craig SS, DeBlois G, et al: Deficiency of the tryptase-positive, chymase-negative mast cell type in gastrointestinal mucosa of patients with defective T lymphocyte function. *J Immunol* 138:4381, 1987.
206. Garriga MM, Friedman MM, Metcalfe DD: A survey of the number and distribution of mast cells in the skin of patients with mast cell disorders. *J Allergy Clin Immunol* 82:425, 1988.
207. Malone DG, Irani AM, Schwartz LB, et al: Mast cell numbers and histamine levels in synovial fluids from patients with diverse arthritides. *Arthritis Rheum* 29:956, 1986.
208. Malone DG, Wilder RL, Saavedra-Delgado AM, et al: Mast cell numbers in rheumatoid synovial tissues. Correlations with quantitative measures of lymphocytic infiltration and modulation by antiinflammatory therapy. *Arthritis Rheum* 30:130, 1987.
209. Frame B, Nixon RK: Bone-marrow mast cells in osteoporosis of aging. *N Engl J Med* 279:626, 1968.
210. Lennert K, Parwaresch MR: Mast cells and mast cell neoplasia: A review. *Histopathology* 3:349, 1979.
211. Barrett KE, Neva FA, Gam AA, et al: The immune response to nematode parasites: Modulation of mast cell numbers and function during *Strongyloides stercoralis* infections in nonhuman primates. *Am J Trop Med Hyg* 38:574, 1988.
212. Bowers HM Jr, Mahapatro RC, Kennedy JW: Numbers of mast cells in the axillary lymph nodes of breast cancer patients. *Cancer* 43:568, 1979.
213. Yoo D, Lessin LS, Jensen WN: Bone-marrow mast cells in lymphoproliferative disorders. *Ann Intern Med* 88:753, 1978.
214. Yoo D, Lessin LS: Bone marrow mast cell content in preleukemic syndrome. *Am J Med* 73:539, 1982.
215. Fohlmeister I, Reber T, Fischer R: Bone marrow mast cell reaction in preleukaemic myelodysplasia and in aplastic anaemia. *Virchows Arch A Pathol Anat Histopathol* 405:503, 1985.
216. Unna P: Beitrage zur anatomic und pathogenese der urticaria simplex und pigmentosa. *Mscch Prakt Dermatol Suppl Dermatol Stud* 3:9, 1887.
217. Nettleship E, Tay W: Rare forms of urticaria. *Br Med J* 2:323, 1869.
218. Sangster A: An anomalous mottled rash, accompanied by pruritus, factious urticaria and pigmentation, "urticaria pigmentosa (?)." *Trans Clin Soc Lond* 11:161, 1878.
219. Ellis JM: Urticaria pigmentosa: A report of a case with autopsy. *Arch Pathol (Chic)* 48:426, 1949.
220. Fine J: Mastocytosis. *Int J Dermatol* 19:117, 1980.
221. Soter NA: Mastocytosis and the skin. *Hematol Oncol Clin North Am* 14:537, 2000.
222. Horny HP, Metcalfe DD, Bennett JM, et al: Mastocytosis, in *WHO Classification of Tumours of Haematopoietic and Lymphoid Tissues,* edited by SH Swerdlow, E Campo, NL Harris, ES Jaffe, SA Pileri, H Stein, J Thiele, JW Vardiman, p 54. IARC Press, Lyon, 2008.
223. Furitsu T, Tsujimura T, Tono T, et al: Identification of mutations in the coding sequence of the proto-oncogene c-kit in a human mast cell leukemia cell line causing ligand-independent activation of c-kit product. *J Clin Invest* 92:1736, 1993.
224. Nagata H, Worobec AS, Oh CK, et al: Identification of a point mutation in the catalytic domain of the protooncogene c-kit in peripheral blood mononuclear cells of

patients who have mastocytosis with an associated hematologic disorder. *Proc Natl Acad Sci U S A* 92:10560, 1995.
225. Longley BJ, Tyrrell L, Lu SZ, et al: Somatic c-KIT activating mutation in urticaria pigmentosa and aggressive mastocytosis: Establishment of clonality in a human mast cell neoplasm. *Nat Genet* 12:312, 1996.
226. Nagata H, Okada T, Worobec AS, et al: C-kit mutation in a population of patients with mastocytosis. *Int Arch Allergy Immunol* 113:184, 1997.
227. Longley BJ Jr, Metcalfe DD, Tharp M, et al: Activating and dominant inactivating c-KIT catalytic domain mutations in distinct clinical forms of human mastocytosis. *Proc Natl Acad Sci U S A* 96:1609, 1999.
228. Akin C, Fumo G, Yavuz AS, et al: A novel form of mastocytosis associated with a transmembrane c-kit mutation and response to imatinib. *Blood* 103:3222, 2004.
229. Lahortiga I, Akin C, Cools J, et al: Activity of imatinib in systemic mastocytosis with chronic basophilic leukemia and a PRKG2-PDGFRB fusion. *Haematologica* 93:49, 2008.
230. Hirota S, Isozaki K, Moriyama Y, et al: Gain-of-function mutations of c-kit in human gastrointestinal stromal tumors. *Science* 279:577, 1998.
231. Nishida T, Hirota S, Taniguchi M, et al: Familial gastrointestinal stromal tumours with germline mutation of the KIT gene. *Nat Genet* 19:323, 1998.
232. Czarnetzki BM, Behrendt H: Urticaria pigmentosa: Clinical picture and response to oral disodium cromoglycate. *Br J Dermatol* 105:563, 1981.
233. Hartmann K, Metcalfe DD: Pediatric mastocytosis. *Hematol Oncol Clin North Am* 14:625, 2000.
234. Travis WD, Li CY: Pathology of the lymph node and spleen in systemic mast cell disease. *Mod Pathol* 1:4, 1988.
235. Mican JM, Di Bisceglie AM, Fong TL, et al: Hepatic involvement in mastocytosis: Clinicopathologic correlations in 41 cases. *Hepatology* 22:1163, 1995.
236. Lawrence JB, Friedman BS, Travis WD, et al: Hematologic manifestations of systemic mast cell disease: A prospective study of laboratory and morphologic features and their relation to prognosis. *Am J Med* 91:612, 1991.
237. Horny HP, Ruck MT, Kaiserling E: Spleen findings in generalized mastocytosis. A clinicopathologic study. *Cancer* 70:459, 1992.
238. Horny HP, Parwaresch MR, Lennert K: Bone marrow findings in systemic mastocytosis. *Hum Pathol* 16:808, 1985.
239. Ridell B, Olafsson JH, Roupe G, et al: The bone marrow in urticaria pigmentosa and systemic mastocytosis. Cell composition and mast cell density in relation to urinary excretion of tele-methylimidazoleacetic acid. *Arch Dermatol* 122:422, 1986.
240. Kettelhut BV, Parker RI, Travis WD, et al: Hematopathology of the bone marrow in pediatric cutaneous mastocytosis. A study of 17 patients. *Am J Clin Pathol* 91:558, 1989.
241. Parker RI: Hematologic aspects of systemic mastocytosis. *Hematol Oncol Clin North Am* 14:557, 2000.
242. Natkunam Y, Rouse RV: Utility of paraffin section immunohistochemistry for C-KIT (CD117) in the differential diagnosis of systemic mast cell disease involving the bone marrow. *Am J Surg Pathol* 24:81, 2000.
243. Yang F, Tran TA, Carlson JA, et al: Paraffin section immunophenotype of cutaneous and extracutaneous mast cell disease: Comparison to other hematopoietic neoplasms. *Am J Surg Pathol* 24:703, 2000.
244. Valent P, Akin C, Escribano L, et al: Standards and standardization in mastocytosis: Consensus statements on diagnostics, treatment recommendations and response criteria. *Eur J Clin Invest* 37:435, 2007.
245. Brockow K, Jofer C, Behrendt H, et al: Anaphylaxis in patients with mastocytosis: A study on history, clinical features and risk factors in 120 patients. *Allergy* 63:226, 2008.
246. Cherner JA, Jensen RT, Dubois A, et al: Gastrointestinal dysfunction in systemic mastocytosis. A prospective study. *Gastroenterology* 95:657, 1988.
247. Rafii M, Firooznia H, Golimbu C, Balthazar E: Pathologic fracture in systemic mastocytosis. Radiographic spectrum and review of the literature. *Clin Orthop Relat Res* 260, 1983.
248. Akin C, Soto D, Brittain E, et al: Tryptase haplotype in mastocytosis: Relationship to disease variant and diagnostic utility of total tryptase levels. *Clin Immunol* 123:268, 2007.
249. Joachim G: Über mastzellenleukamie. *Dtsch Arch Klin Med* 87:437, 1906.
250. Travis WD, Li CY, Hoagland HC, et al: Mast cell leukemia: Report of a case and review of the literature. *Mayo Clin Proc* 61:957, 1986.
251. Torrey E, Simpson K, Wilbur S, et al: Malignant mastocytosis with circulating mast cells. *Am J Hematol* 34:283, 1990.
252. Friedman BS, Steinberg SC, Meggs WJ, et al: Analysis of plasma histamine levels in patients with mast cell disorders. *Am J Med* 87:649, 1989.
253. Wilson TM, Metcalfe DD, Robyn J: Treatment of systemic mastocytosis. *Immunol Allergy Clin North Am* 26:549, 2006.
254. Frieri M, Alling DW, Metcalfe DD: Comparison of the therapeutic efficacy of cromolyn sodium with that of combined chlorpheniramine and cimetidine in systemic mastocytosis. Results of a double-blind clinical trial. *Am J Med* 78:9, 1985.
255. Robyn J, Metcalfe DD: Systemic mastocytosis. *Adv Immunol* 89:169, 2006.
256. Sullivan TJ: Pharmacologic modulation of the whealing response to histamine in human skin: Identification of doxepin as a potent *in vivo* inhibitor. *J Allergy Clin Immunol* 69:260, 1982.
257. Soter NA, Austen KF, Wasserman SI: Oral disodium cromoglycate in the treatment of systemic mastocytosis. *N Engl J Med* 301:465, 1979.
258. Welch EA, Alper JC, Bogaars H, et al: Treatment of bullous mastocytosis with disodium cromoglycate. *J Am Acad Dermatol* 9:349, 1983.
259. Czarnetzki BM: A double-blind cross-over study of the effect of ketotifen in urticaria pigmentosa. *Dermatologica* 166:44, 1983.
260. Graves L 3rd, Stechschulte DJ, Morris DC, et al: Inhibition of mediator release in systemic mastocytosis is associated with reversal of bone changes. *J Bone Miner Res* 5:1113, 1990.
261. Kettelhut BV, Berkebile C, Bradley D, et al: A double-blind, placebo-controlled, crossover trial of ketotifen versus hydroxyzine in the treatment of pediatric mastocytosis. *J Allergy Clin Immunol* 83:866, 1989.
262. Friedman BS, Santiago ML, Berkebile C, et al: Comparison of azelastine and chlorpheniramine in the treatment of mastocytosis. *J Allergy Clin Immunol* 92:520, 1993.
263. Cundy T, Beneton MN, Darby AJ, et al: Osteopenia in systemic mastocytosis: Natural history and responses to treatment with inhibitors of bone resorption. *Bone* 8:149, 1987.
264. Barton J, Lavker RM, Schechter NM, et al: Treatment of urticaria pigmentosa with corticosteroids. *Arch Dermatol* 121:1516, 1985.
265. Kolde G, Frosch PJ, Czarnetzki BM: Response of cutaneous mast cells to PUVA in patients with urticaria pigmentosa: Histomorphometric, ultrastructural, and biochemical investigations. *J Invest Dermatol* 83:175, 1984.
266. Czarnetzki BM, Rosenbach T, Kolde G, et al: Phototherapy of urticaria pigmentosa: Clinical response and changes of cutaneous reactivity, histamine and chemotactic leukotrienes. *Arch Dermatol Res* 277:105, 1985.
267. Reisberg IR, Oyakawa S: Mastocytosis with malabsorption, myelofibrosis, and massive ascites. *Am J Gastroenterol* 82:54, 1987.
268. Kluin-Nelemans HC, Jansen JH, Breukelman H, et al: Response to interferon alfa-2b in a patient with systemic mastocytosis. *N Engl J Med* 326:619, 1992.
269. Tefferi A, Li CY, Butterfield JH, et al: Treatment of systemic mast-cell disease with cladribine. *N Engl J Med* 344:307, 2001.
270. Ronnov-Jessen AD, Nielsen PL: [Mastocytosis]. *Ugeskr Laeger* 153:3131, 1991.
271. Fodinger M, Fritsch G, Winkler K, et al: Origin of human mast cells: Development from transplanted hematopoietic stem cells after allogeneic bone marrow transplantation. *Blood* 84:2954, 1994.
272. Przepiorka D, Giralt S, Khouri I, et al: Allogeneic marrow transplantation for myeloproliferative disorders other than chronic myelogenous leukemia: Review of forty cases. *Am J Hematol* 57:24, 1998.
273. Nakamura R, Chakrabarti S, Akin C, et al: A pilot study of nonmyeloablative allogeneic hematopoietic stem cell transplant for advanced systemic mastocytosis. *Bone Marrow Transplant* 37:353, 2006.
274. Buchdunger E, Cioffi CL, Law N, et al: Abl protein-tyrosine kinase inhibitor STI571 inhibits *in vitro* signal transduction mediated by c-kit and platelet-derived growth factor receptors. *J Pharmacol Exp Ther* 295:139, 2000.
275. Buchdunger E, Zimmermann J, Mett H, et al: Inhibition of the Abl protein-tyrosine kinase *in vitro* and *in vivo* by a 2-phenylaminopyrimidine derivative. *Cancer Res* 56:100, 1996.
276. Druker BJ, Tamura S, Buchdunger E, et al: Effects of a selective inhibitor of the Abl tyrosine kinase on the growth of Bcr-Abl positive cells. *Nat Med* 2:561, 1996.
277. Ma Y, Zeng S, Metcalfe DD, et al: The c-KIT mutation causing human mastocytosis is resistant to STI571 and other KIT kinase inhibitors; kinases with enzymatic site mutations show different inhibitor sensitivity profiles than wild-type kinases and those with regulatory-type mutations. *Blood* 99:1741, 2002.
278. Zermati Y, De Sepulveda P, Feger F, et al: Effect of tyrosine kinase inhibitor STI571 on the kinase activity of wild-type and various mutated c-kit receptors found in mast cell neoplasms. *Oncogene* 22:660, 2003.
279. Akin C, Brockow K, D'Ambrosio C, et al: Effects of tyrosine kinase inhibitor STI571 on human mast cells bearing wild-type or mutated c-kit. *Exp Hematol* 31:686, 2003.
280. Gotlib J, Berube C, Growney JD, et al: Activity of the tyrosine kinase inhibitor PKC412 in a patient with mast cell leukemia with the D816V KIT mutation. *Blood* 106:2865, 2005.
281. Valent P, Akin C, Sperr WR, et al: Mastocytosis: Pathology, genetics, and current options for therapy. *Leuk Lymphoma* 46:35, 2005.
282. Klion AD, Noel P, Akin C, et al: Elevated serum tryptase levels identify a subset of patients with a myeloproliferative variant of idiopathic hypereosinophilic syndrome associated with tissue fibrosis, poor prognosis, and imatinib responsiveness. *Blood* 101:4660, 2003.
283. Maric I, Robyn J, Metcalfe DD, et al: KIT D816V-associated systemic mastocytosis with eosinophilia and FIP1L1/PDGFRA-associated chronic eosinophilic leukemia are distinct entities. *J Allergy Clin Immunol* 120:680, 2007.
284. Friedman B, Darling G, Norton J, et al: Splenectomy in the management of systemic mast cell disease. *Surgery* 107:94, 1990.
285. Brockow K, Scott LM, Worobec AS, et al: Regression of urticaria pigmentosa in adult patients with systemic mastocytosis: Correlation with clinical patterns of disease. *Arch Dermatol* 138:785, 2002.
286. Lennert K, Koster E, Martin H: Über die mastzellen-leukaemie. *Acta Haematol* 16:255, 1956.
287. Coser P, Quaglino D, De Pasquale A, et al: Cytobiological and clinical aspects of tissue mast cell leukaemia. *Br J Haematol* 45:5, 1980.
288. Dalton R, Chan L, Batten E, et al: Mast cell leukaemia: Evidence for bone marrow origin of the pathological clone. *Br J Haematol* 64:397, 1986.
289. Valentini CG, Rondoni M, Pogliani EM, et al: Mast cell leukemia: A report of ten cases. *Ann Hematol* 87:505, 2008.

CHAPTER 64

CLASSIFICATION AND CLINICAL MANIFESTATIONS OF NEUTROPHIL DISORDERS

Marshall A. Lichtman

SUMMARY

Neutrophil disorders can be grouped into deficiencies, or neutropenia, excesses, or neutrophilia, and qualitative abnormalities. Neutropenia can have the severe consequence of predisposing to infection, whereas neutrophilia usually is a manifestation of an underlying inflammatory or neoplastic disease: the neutrophilia, per se, having no specific consequences. Qualitative disorders of neutrophils may lead to infection as a result of defective cell translocation to an inflammatory site or defective microbial killing. Neutropenia may reflect an inherited disease that is evident in childhood (such as congenital severe neutropenia [Kostmann syndrome]), but more often it is acquired. A common cause of neutropenia is the adverse effect of a drug. Some cases of neutropenia have no evident cause. The health consequence of neutropenia is a function of the mechanism of the neutropenia, the severity of the decrease in the blood neutrophil count, and the abruptness and duration of the decrease. Neutrophils have also been identified as mediators of vascular or tissue injury. Table 64–1 provides a comprehensive categorization of quantitative and qualitative neutrophil disorders.

CLASSIFICATION

Table 64–1 lists disorders that result from a primary deficiency in neutrophil numbers or function. Neutropenia or neutrophilia also occurs as part of a disorder that affects multiple blood cell lineages, as in infiltrative diseases of the marrow, or intrinsic disorders of multipotential marrow cells, or consumption of several blood cell types in the circulation. These diseases are not included in this classification and are discussed in other parts of this text. In this classification and in this chapter, we consider disorders in which the neutrophil either is the only cell type affected or the dominant cell type affected.

A pathophysiologic classification of neutrophil disorders has proved elusive. Techniques for measuring mechanisms of (1) impaired production resulting from hypoplasia or exaggerated apoptosis of marrow precursors or (2) accelerated destruction of neutrophils are more difficult and complex than the techniques used for red cells or platelets. The low concentration of blood neutrophils, accentuated in neutropenic states, makes radioactive labeling techniques for studying the kinetics of autologous cells in neutropenic subjects difficult if not impossible. The two compartments of neutrophils in the blood (cells marginated along vascular beds as distinct from cells circulating and counted in the blood neutrophil count [see Chap. 65]), the random disappearance of neutrophils from the circulation, the short circulation time of neutrophils, the absence of practical techniques for measuring the size of the tissue neutrophil compartment, and the disappearance of neutrophils by apoptosis or excretion from the tissue compartment also make multicompartmental kinetic analysis difficult. Also, neutropenic disorders are uncommon, and few laboratories are able, or prepared, to undertake the studies necessary to define the mechanisms of their development in sporadic cases. Therefore, efforts to understand the pathophysiology of neutropenia have been of more limited success than that of red cells or platelets. Hence, the classification of neutrophil disorders is partly pathophysiologic and partly descriptive (see Table 64–1). Classification, although imperfect, does provide a language for communication and a basis for rectification as knowledge of the cause and mechanism of each entity advances.

The classification is self-explanatory except in two areas. First, certain childhood (congenital or hereditary) syndromes listed under decreased neutrophilic granulopoiesis could have been listed under chronic hypoplastic neutropenia or chronic idiopathic neutropenia; however, they seem to hold a special interest. Their unique status and their pathogenesis have become further clarified as the mutations linked to each are identified. Three childhood syndromes that are associated with neutropenia are omitted because the neutropenia is part of a more global suppression of hematopoiesis: Pearson syndrome,[1,2] Fanconi syndrome,[3,4] and dyskeratosis congenita (see Chap. 34).[5,6]

A second area requiring explanation is the chronic idiopathic neutropenias. This group includes (1) cases with normocellular marrows but an inadequate compensatory increase in granulopoiesis for the degree of neutropenia and (2) cases with hyperplastic granulopoiesis that apparently is ineffective as a result of apoptosis of marrow neutrophils and late precursors. Unlike hypoplastic neutropenia in which the granulocyte precursors are markedly reduced or absent, precursors are present in the marrow in the idiopathic neutropenias, but the extent of effective granulopoiesis probably is low. A variety of mutations have been discovered that are causal for inherited or sporadic neutropenia syndromes. For example, mutation of the serine protease neutrophil elastase 2 gene (*ELA2*) is found in severe congenital neutropenia (Kostmann syndrome) and cyclic neutropenia. There is evidence that these mutations result in apoptotic loss of marrow neutrophil precursors as a result of downregulation of the BCL-2 family of antiapoptotic proteins, the upregulation of the proapoptotic FAS receptor, or other apoptosis-enhancing pathways, described more fully in Chap. 65.

Qualitative disorders of neutrophils affect their ability to enter the circulation, to leave the circulation, enter inflammatory exudates, or to ingest or kill microorganisms. Chap. 66 describes these in more detail.

CLINICAL MANIFESTATIONS

The clinical manifestations of decreased concentrations or abnormal function of neutrophils principally result from infection. The combined deficit of neutrophils and monocytes characteristic of aplastic anemia, hairy cell leukemia, and cytotoxic therapy leads to susceptibility to a broader spectrum of infectious agents. Increased concentrations of normal neutrophils per se are not associated with clinical manifestations, although increased concentrations of leukemic neutrophil precursors can produce clinical manifestations of microcirculatory leukostasis (see Chap. 85). Neutrophils also play a role in deleterious vascular or tissue effects, as noted in the last entries in Table 64–1 (see "Neutrophilia" below).

NEUTROPENIA

The lower limit of the normal neutrophil count is approximately 1800/μL (1.8×10^9/L) in subjects of European descent and 1400/μL (1.4×10^9/L)

Acronyms and abbreviations that appear in this chapter include: CD, cluster of differentiation; G-CSF, granulocyte colony-stimulating factor; HLA-DR, human leukocyte antigen-D related; Ig, immunoglobulin; WHIM, warts, hypogammaglobulinemia, infection, myelokathexis.

TABLE 64–1. Classification of Neutrophil Disorders

I. Quantitative Disorders of Neutrophils
- A. Neutropenia
  - 1. Decreased neutrophilic granulopoiesis
    - a. Congenital severe neutropenias (Kostmann syndrome and related disorders)[7,8]
    - b. Reticular dysgenesis (congenital aleukocytosis)[9,10]
    - c. Neutropenia and exocrine pancreas dysfunction (Shwachman-Diamond syndrome)[11]
    - d. Neutropenia and immunoglobulin abnormality (e.g., hyper-IgM syndrome)[12–14]
    - e. Neutropenia and disordered cellular immunity (cartilage hair hypoplasia)[15,16]
    - f. Mental retardation, anomalies, and neutropenia (Cohen syndrome)[17,18]
    - g. X-linked cardioskeletal myopathy and neutropenia (Barth syndrome)[19,20]
    - h. Myelokathexis[21,22]
    - i. Warts, hypogammaglobulinemia, infection, myelokathexis (WHIM) syndrome[23,24]
    - j. Neonatal neutropenia and maternal hypertension[25,26]
    - k. Griscelli syndrome[27]
    - l. Glycogen storage disease 1b[28]
    - m. Hermansky-Pudlak syndrome 2[29,30]
    - n. Wiskott-Aldrich syndrome[31]
    - o. Chronic hypoplastic neutropenia
      - (1) Drug-induced[32–35]
      - (2) Cyclic[36,37]
      - (3) Branched-chain aminoacidemia[38]
    - p. Acute hypoplastic neutropenia
      - (1) Drug-induced[32,39,40]
      - (2) Infectious[41]
    - q. Chronic idiopathic neutropenia
      - (1) Benign
        - (a) Familial[42]
        - (b) Sporadic[43]
      - (2) Symptomatic[44–46]
  - 2. Accelerated neutrophil destruction
    - a. Alloimmune neonatal neutropenia[47–49]
    - b. Autoimmune neutropenia[50–52]
      - (1) Idiopathic[52]
      - (2) Drug-induced[52,53]
      - (3) Felty syndrome[54–56]
      - (4) Systemic lupus erythematosus[57,58]
      - (5) Other autoimmune diseases[59–64]
      - (6) Complement activation-induced neutropenia[65]
      - (7) Pure white cell aplasia[64,66–68]
  - 3. Maldistribution of neutrophils
    - a. Pseudoneutropenia[69–71]
- B. Neutrophilia
  - 1. Increased neutrophilic granulopoiesis
    - a. Hereditary neutrophilia[72]
    - b. Trisomy 13 or 18[73]
    - c. Chronic idiopathic neutrophilia[74]
      - (1) Asplenia[75]
    - d. Neutrophilia or neutrophilic leukemoid reactions
      - (1) Inflammation[76,77]
      - (2) Infection[76,77]
      - (3) Acute hemolysis or acute hemorrhage[76]
      - (4) Cancer, including granulocyte colony-stimulating factor (G-CSF)-secreting tumors[76,77,79–82]
      - (5) Drugs (e.g., glucocorticoids, lithium, granulocyte- or granulocyte-monocyte colony-stimulating factor, tumor necrosis factor-α)[76,83–87]
      - (6) Ethylene glycol exposure[76]
      - (7) Exercise[88,89]
    - e. Sweet syndrome[90,91]
    - f. Cigarette smoking[92,93]
    - g. Cardiopulmonary bypass[94]
  - 2. Decreased neutrophil circulatory egress
    - a. Drugs (e.g., glucocorticoids)[95]
  - 3. Maldistribution of neutrophils
    - a. Pseudoneutrophilia[96]

II. Qualitative Disorders of Neutrophils
- A. Defective adhesion of neutrophils
  - 1. Leukocyte adhesion deficiency[97,98]
  - 2. Drug-induced[99]
- B. Defective locomotion and chemotaxis
  - 1. Actin polymerization abnormalities[100–103]
  - 2. Neonatal neutrophils[104]
  - 3. Interleukin-2 administration[105]
  - 4. Cardiopulmonary bypass[94]
- C. Defective microbial killing
  - 1. Chronic granulomatous disease[106,107]
  - 2. RAC-2 deficiency[108,109]
  - 3. Myeloperoxidase deficiency[110,111]
  - 4. Hyperimmunoglobulin E (Job) syndrome[112,113]
  - 5. Glucose-6-phosphate dehydrogenase deficiency[114,115]
  - 6. Extensive burns[116,117]
  - 7. Glycogen storage disease Ib[118,119]
  - 8. Ethanol toxicity[120,121]
  - 9. End-stage renal disease[122]
  - 10. Diabetes mellitus[123]
- D. Abnormal structure of the nucleus or of an organelle
  - 1. Hereditary macropolycytes[124]
  - 2. Hereditary hypersegmentation[125]
  - 3. Specific granule deficiency[126–128]
  - 4. Pelger-Huët anomaly[129,130]
  - 5. Alder-Reilly anomaly[131]
  - 6. May-Hegglin anomaly[132–134]
  - 7. Chédiak-Higashi disease[135,136]

III. Neutrophil-Induced Vascular or Tissue Damage[137–139]
- A. Pulmonary disease[140–145]
- B. Transfusion-related lung injury[146]
- C. Renal disease[147,148]
- D. Arterial occlusion[149,150]
- E. Venous occlussion[151]
- F. Myocardial infarction[152–156]
- G. Ventricular function[153–157]
- H. Stroke[158]
- I. Neoplasia[159–161]

in subjects of African descent.[162–165] An additional small proportion (~5.0 percent) of persons of African descent have neutrophil counts between 1400 and 1000/μL (1.0×10^9/L) without evidence of associated abnormalities and this finding also may represent "ethnic neutropenia." These findings have not been explained by exaggerated margination of neutrophils.[164] Neutropenia is especially striking in Yemenite Jews, another ethnic group with very low "normal" neutrophil counts,[166] and has been reported in West Africans, Caribbean inhabitants of African descent, Ethiopians, and some Arab groups.[164,165] Persons of African descent do not have the increase in neutrophil count seen in Europeans who smoke or are administered glucocorticoids. Americans of Mexican descent have a slightly elevated neutrophil count.[164] A decrement in neutrophil concentration to 1000/μL (1.0×10^9/L) usually poses little threat in the individual with an intact immune system. If the neutrophil count drops farther, the risk of infection may increase, if the decrease reflects a decrease in flux rate into the tissues. Subjects who are chronically neutropenic, as a result of severe marrow cell production abnormalities, with counts less than 500 neutrophils/μL (0.5×10^9/L) may be at heightened risk for developing recurrent infections.[167]

The relationship of frequency or type of infection to neutrophil concentration is imperfect. The cause of the neutropenia, the coincidence of monocytopenia or lymphopenia, concurrent use of alcohol or glucocorticoids, exposure to nosocomial infections, and other factors influence the likelihood of infection.

Infections in neutropenic subjects who are not otherwise compromised usually result from gram-positive cocci and usually are superficial, involving skin, oropharynx, bronchi, anal canal, or vagina. However, any site can become infected, with gram-negative organisms, viruses, or opportunistic organisms possibly involved.

A decrease in neutrophil count can occur abruptly or gradually (see Chap. 65). One type of drug-induced neutropenia is distinguished by the rapidity of onset. Abrupt-onset neutropenia more likely is severe and leads to symptoms. If the neutrophil count approaches zero (agranulocytosis), high fever; chills; necrotizing, painful oral ulcers (agranulocytic angina), and prostration may occur, presumably as a result of sepsis.[157–159] As the disease progresses, headache, stupor, and rash may develop. In the preantibiotic era, persistent agranulocytosis had a fatality rate approaching 100 percent. Even with bactericidal, broad-spectrum antibiotics, severe, sustained neutropenia or agranulocytosis is a serious illness with a high fatality rate.

Pus formation decreases in patients with severe neutropenia.[168] The failure to suppurate can mislead the clinician and delay identification of the infection site because minimal physical or radiographic findings develop. For example, lack of pneumonic consolidation is characteristic of pneumonia in granulocytopenic subjects. An exudate, swelling, heat, and regional adenopathy are much less prevalent in granulocytopenic patients. Fever is common, and local pain, tenderness, and erythema nearly always are present despite a marked reduction in neutrophils.[169]

The mechanism of neutropenia and the severity of the deficiency of cells play roles in clinical manifestations. Chronic idiopathic (benign) neutropenia is associated with apparent normal granulopoiesis in the marrow and is asymptomatic even when the neutropenia has been present for prolonged periods, sometimes in the face of neutrophil counts approaching zero.[43] Presumably the delivery of neutrophils from marrow to tissues is sufficient to prevent infection despite the low blood pool size. Monocyte counts are normal, which may aid in host defenses because monocytes are effective phagocytes.

Chronic idiopathic (symptomatic) neutropenia often is associated with pyoderma and otitis media in children. The former usually is caused by *Staphylococcus aureus, Escherichia coli*, and *Pseudomonas* species, and the latter usually results from infection by pneumococci or *Pseudomonas aeruginosa*. Unexplained chronic gingivitis may be a manifestation of chronic neutropenia. Pneumonia, lung abscesses, stomatitis, hepatic abscesses, or infections in other sites can occur.

Chronic cyclic neutropenia is characterized by periodic oscillations in the number of neutrophils, with the nadir occurring at approximately 3-week intervals.[36] During a period of neutropenia, patients develop malaise; fever; buccal, labial, or lingual ulcers; and cervical adenopathy. Furuncles, carbuncles, cellulitis, infected cuts with lymphangitis, chronic gingivitis, and abscesses of the axilla or groin may occur. Although severe infections may be fatal, life-threatening complications are uncommon. The cycling involves other hematopoietic cells as well, but the neutropenia is the most consequential functionally (see Chap. 65).

Some individuals have neutropenia because a larger proportion of their blood neutrophils is in the marginal rather than the circulating pool. The total blood neutrophil pool is normal, and infections do not result from this atypical distribution of neutrophils. This alteration has been called *pseudoneutropenia*.[69–71]

■ NEUTROPHILIA

An increased neutrophil count can accompany virtually any cause of inflammation, especially inflammation caused by bacterial or fungal organisms, and a variety of cancers, especially if metastatic. Certain drugs, such as glucocorticoids or hematopoietic growth factors and minocycline, can induce neutrophilia, as can ethylene glycol intoxication (see Table 64–1). Acute hemolysis or acute hemorrhage may also result in neutrophilia. A notable cause of neutrophilia is cancers that elaborate granulocyte-colony stimulating factor (G-CSF). Numerous cancers have been associated with neutrophilia and in many cases, elaboration of very high concentrations of G-CSF has been documented. In these cases, neutrophil counts exceeding 100,000 μL (100×10^9/L) are common. Neutrophilia exceeding 50,000 neutrophils/μL (50×10^9/L) has been designated a "leukemoid reaction" and reflects an underlying inflammatory, infectious, or neoplastic cause. A leukemoid reaction can mimic rare types of chronic myelogenous or chronic neutrophilic leukemia. The leukemoid reaction classically (1) is composed largely of mature neutrophils with a low proportion of bands and myelocytes, (2) has increased leukocyte alkaline phosphatase reaction in neutrophils, (3) has increased granulopoiesis with normal maturation and morphology of cells in the marrow, (4) has normal cytogenetics of marrow cells, (5) has polyclonal derived cells in women in whom such studies can be conducted (inactivation of the human androgen receptor gene assay), and (6) has cytometric analysis of neutrophils indicating a cluster of differentiation (CD) 13 and CD15 phenotype with absent expression of human leukocyte antigen-D related (HLA-DR) and CD34.

QUALITATIVE NEUTROPHIL ABNORMALITIES

Neutrophil function depends on the ability of neutrophils to exit the marrow, adhere to endothelium, move, respond to chemotactic gradients, ingest microorganisms, and kill ingested pathogens. Loss of any of these functions can predispose to infection (see Chap. 66). Defects in each step of the neutrophil's participation in the inflammatory response have been identified.[170] Defects in adhesion molecules, cytoplasmic contractile proteins, granule synthesis or contents, or intracellular enzymes may underlie a movement, ingestion, or killing defect. These defects may be inherited or acquired. Chronic granulomatous disease[106,107] and Chédiak Higashi disease[135,136] are two examples of inherited defects. Among the acquired disorders are those extrinsic to the cell, as in the movement, chemotactic, or phagocytic defects of diabetes mellitus, the effects of alcohol abuse, or glucocorticoid excess. Acquired intrinsic disorders usually are manifestations of clonal hematopoietic (myeloid) disorders such as acute myelogenous leukemia (see Chap. 85).

Severe defects in bacterial killing, as occur in chronic granulomatous disease, result in *S. aureus, Klebsiella-Aerobacter, E. coli*, and other catalase-positive bacterial infections. Suppurative lymphadenitis, pneumonia, dermatitis, hepatic abscesses, osteomyelitis, and stomatitis occur, and chronic granulomatous reactions in these sites give the disease its name. Fatality rates have been high. Functional disorders may be severe, as in chronic granulomatous disease. Mild functional disorders predispose to infections that occur infrequently and respond readily to antibiotics. Severe functional disorders result in suppurative lesions because neutrophil influx into inflammatory foci is not impaired, whereas agranulocytosis is associated with nonsuppurative lesions.

NEUTROPHILIA

An overabundance of neutrophils does not result in specific clinical manifestations. Neutrophils, however, can transiently occlude capillaries, as determined by supravital microscopy, and such occlusions may reduce local blood flow transiently and contribute to the development of ischemia. Impairment of reperfusion of the coronary microcirculation has been thought to be dependent, in part, on neutrophil plugging of myocardial capillaries, but these effects can occur at normal neutrophil concentrations. An elevated neutrophil count is a feature of sickle cell disease and is a prognostic variable, increasing the likelihood of vasocclusive events.[171] In patients with ischemic vascular disease, an increased neutrophil count is associated with an increased probability of acute thrombotic episodes and the severity of chronic atherosclerosis.[172]

NEUTROPHIL-INDUCED VASCULAR OR TISSUE DAMAGE

Neutrophil products may contribute to the pathogenesis of inflammatory skin, bowel, synovial, glomerular, and bronchial and interstitial pulmonary diseases (see Table 64–1). Diabetic retinopathy has been ascribed in part to the effects of hyperadhesive neutrophils on retinal capillaries. These products may act as mediators of tissue injury in myocardial infarction. Highly reactive oxygen products of neutrophils may be mutagens that increase the risk of neoplasia. This action may explain, for example, the development of carcinoma of the bowel in patients with chronic ulcerative colitis and the relationship between elevated leukocyte count and the occurrence of lung cancer, independent of the effect of cigarette usage. The oxidants, especially hypochlorous acid and chloramines, released by the neutrophil are extremely short lived and may play a role in tissue injury by inactivating several protease inhibitors in tissue fluids, permitting proteases, especially elastase, collagenase, and gelatinase, to cause tissue injury. Thrombogenesis also has been ascribed to leukocyte products.

REFERENCES

1. Pearson HA, Lobel JS, Kocoshis SA, et al: A new syndrome of refractory sideroblastic anemia with vacuolization of marrow precursors and exocrine pancreatic dysfunction. *J Pediatr* 95:976, 1979.
2. Jacobs LJ, Jongbloed RJ, Wijburg FA, et al: Pearson syndrome and the role of deletion dimers and duplications in the mtDNA. *J Inherit Metab Dis* 27:47, 2004.
3. Bagby GC Jr: Genetic basis of Fanconi anemia. *Curr Opin Hematol* 10:68, 2003.
4. Taniguchi T, D'Andrea AD: Molecular pathogenesis of Fanconi anemia: Recent progress. *Blood* 107:4223, 2006.
5. Srinavin C, Trowbridge A: Dyskeratosis congenita: Clinical features and genetic aspects. *J Med Genet* 12:339, 1975.
6. Walne AJ, Dokal I: Dyskeratosis Congenita: A historical perspective. *Mech Ageing Dev* 129:48, 2008.
7. Ward AC, Dale DC: Genetic and molecular diagnosis of severe congenital neutropenia. *Curr Opin Hematol* 16:9, 2009.
8. Ishikawa N, Okada S, Miki M, et al: Neurodevelopmental abnormalities associated with severe congenital neutropenia due to the R86X mutation in the HAX1 gene. *J Med Genet* 45:802, 2008.
9. Levinsky RJ, Tiedman K: Successful bone-marrow transplantation for reticular dysgenesis. *Lancet* 1:671, 1983.
10. Calhoun DA, Christensen RD: Recent advances in the pathogenesis and treatment of nonimmune neutropenias in the neonate. *Curr Opin Hematol* 5:37, 1998.
11. Shimamura A: Shwachman-Diamond syndrome. *Semin Hematol* 43:178, 2006.
12. Lonsdale D, Doedhar SD, Mercer RD: Familial granulocytopenia associated with immunoglobulin abnormality. *J Pediatr* 71:760, 1967.
13. Kozlowski C, Evans DIK: Neutropenia associated with X-linked agammaglobulinemia. *J Clin Pathol* 44:388, 1991.
14. Lougaris V, Badolato R, Ferrari S, Plebani A: Hyper immunoglobulin M syndrome due to CD40 deficiency: Clinical, molecular, and immunological features. *Immunol Rev* 203:48, 2005.
15. Lux SE, Johnston RB Jr, August CS, et al: Chronic neutropenia and abnormal cellular immunity in cartilage-hair hypoplasia. *N Engl J Med* 282:231, 1970.
16. Trojak JE, Polmar SH, Winkelstein JA: Immunologic studies of cartilage-hair hypoplasia in the Amish. *Johns Hopkins Med J* 148:157, 1981.
17. Olivieri O, Lombardi S, Russo C, Corrocher R: Increased neutrophil adhesive capability in Cohen syndrome, an autosomal recessive disorder associated with granulocytopenia. *Haematologica* 83:778, 1998.
18. Kolehmainen J, Black GC, Saarinen A, et al: Cohen syndrome is caused by mutations in a novel gene, COH1, encoding a transmembrane protein with a presumed role in vesicle-mediated sorting and intracellular protein transport. *Am J Hum Genet* 72:1359, 2003.
19. Barth PG, Scholte HR, Berden JA, et al: An X-linked mitochondrial disease affecting cardiac muscle, skeletal muscle and neutrophil leukocytes. *J Neurol Sci* 62:327, 1983.
20. Yen TY, Hwu WL, Chien YH, et al: Acute metabolic decompensation and sudden death in Barth syndrome: Report of a family and a literature review. *Eur J Pediatr* 167:941, 2008.
21. Bassan R, Viero P, Minetti B, et al: Myelokathexis: A rare form of chronic benign neutropenia. *Br J Haematol* 58:115, 1984.
22. Wetzler M, Talpaz M, Kellagher MJ, et al: Myelokathexis. *JAMA* 267:2179, 1992.
23. Gulino AV: WHIM syndrome: A genetic disorder of leukocyte trafficking. *Curr Opin Allergy Clin Immunol* 3:443, 2003.
24. Balabanian K, Levoye A, Klemm L, et al: Leukocyte analysis from WHIM syndrome patients reveals a pivotal role for GRK3 in CXCR4 signaling. *J Clin Invest* 118:1074, 2008.
25. Koenig JM, Christensen RD: Incidence, neutrophil kinetics and natural history of neonatal neutropenia associated with maternal hypertension. *N Engl J Med* 321:557, 1989.
26. Tsao PN, Teng RJ, Tang JR, Yau KI: Granulocyte colony-stimulating factor in the cord blood of premature neonates born to mothers with pregnancy-induced hypertension. *J Pediatr* 135:56, 1999.
27. Menasche G, Fischer A, de Saint Basile G: Griscelli syndrome types 1 and 2. *Am J Hum Genet* 71:1237, 2002.
28. Kuijpers TW, Maianski NA, Tool AT, et al: Apoptotic neutrophils in the circulation of patients with glycogen storage disease type 1b (GSD1b). *Blood* 101:5021, 2003.
29. Shotelersuk V, Dell'Angelica EC, Hartnell L, et al: A new variant of Hermansky-Pudlak syndrome due to mutations in a gene responsible for vesicle formation. *Am J Med* 108:423, 2000.
30. Huizing M, Scher CD, Strovel E, et al: Nonsense mutations in ADTB3A cause complete deficiency of the beta3A subunit of adaptor complex-3 and severe Hermansky-Pudlak syndrome type 2. *Pediatr Res* 51:150, 2002.
31. Devriendt K, Kim AS, Mathijs G, et al: Constitutively activating mutation in WASP causes X-linked severe congenital neutropenia. *Nat Genet* 27:313, 2001..
32. Vial T, Gallant C, Choqu-Kastylevsky G, Descotes J: Treatment of drug-induced agranulocytosis with haematopoietic growth factors: A review of the clinical experience. *BioDrugs* 11:185, 1999.
33. Andersohn F, Konzen C, Garbe E: Systematic review: Agranulocytosis induced by nonchemotherapy drugs. *Ann Intern Med*146:657, 2007.
34. Crawford J, Dale DC, Kuderer NM, et al: Risk and timing of neutropenic events in adult cancer patients receiving chemotherapy: The results of a prospective nationwide study of oncology practice. *J Natl Compr Canc Netw* 6:109, 2008.
35. Flanagan RJ, Dunk L: Haematological toxicity of drugs used in psychiatry. *Hum Psychopharmacol* 23(Suppl 1):27, 2008.
36. Dale DC, Hammond WP: Cyclic neutropenia: A clinical review. *Blood Rev* 2:178, 1988.
37. Horwitz MS, Duan Z, Korkmaz B, et al: Neutrophil elastase in cyclic and severe congenital neutropenia. *Blood* 109:1817, 2007.
38. Hutchinson R, Bunnell K, Thorne J: Suppression of granulopoietic progenitor cell proliferation by metabolites of the branched-chain amino acids. *J Pediatr* 106:62, 1985.
39. Andrès E, Maloisel F: Idiosyncratic drug-induced agranulocytosis or acute neutropenia. *Curr Opin Hematol* 15:15, 2008.
40. Andrès E, Federici L, Weitten T, et al: Recognition and management of drug-induced blood cytopenias: The example of drug-induced acute neutropenia and agranulocytosis. *Expert Opin Drug Saf* 7:481, 2008.
41. Chuang VW, Wong TY, Leung YH, et al: Review of dengue fever cases in Hong Kong during 1998 to 2005. *Hong Kong Med J* 14:170, 2008.
42. Cutting HO, Lange JE: Familial-benign chronic neutropenia. *Ann Intern Med* 61:876, 1964.
43. Kyle RA: Natural history of chronic idiopathic neutropenia. *N Engl J Med* 302:908, 1970.
44. Yilmaz D, Ritchey AK: Severe neutropenia in children: A single institutional experience. *J Pediatr Hematol Oncol* 29:513, 2007.
45. Vlacha V, Feketea G: The clinical significance of non-malignant neutropenia in hospitalized children. *Ann Hematol* 86:865, 2007.
46. Wlodarski MW, Nearman Z, Jiang Y, et al: Clonal predominance of CD8(+) T cells in patients with unexplained neutropenia. *Exp Hematol* 36:293, 2008.
47. Maheshwari A, Christensen RD, Calhoun DA: Immune neutropenia in the neonate. *Adv Pediatr* 49:317, 2002.

48. Williams BA, Fung YL: Alloimmune neonatal neutropenia: can we afford the consequences of a missed diagnosis? *J Paediatr Child Health* 42:59, 2006.
49. Bux J: Human neutrophil alloantigens. *Vox Sang* 94:277, 2008.
50. Marmont AM: The autoimmune myelopathies. *Semin Hematol* 28:269, 1991.
51. Bux J, Behrens G, Jaeger G, Welte K: Diagnosis and clinical course of autoimmune neutropenia in infancy: Analysis of 240 cases. *Blood* 91:181, 1998.
52. Capsoni F, Sarzi-Puttini P, Zanella A: Primary and secondary autoimmune neutropenia. *Arthritis Res Ther* 7:208, 2005.
53. Winkelstein A, Kiss JE: Immunohematologic disorders. *JAMA* 278:1982, 1997.
54. Bowman SJ: Hematological manifestations of rheumatoid arthritis. *Scand J Rheumatol* 31:251, 2002.
55. Burks EJ, Loughran TP Jr: Pathogenesis of neutropenia in large granular lymphocyte leukemia and Felty syndrome. *Blood Rev* 20:245, 2006.
56. Prochorec-Sobieszek M, Rymkiewicz G, Makuch-asica H, et al: Characteristics of T-cell large granular lymphocyte proliferations associated with neutropenia and inflammatory arthropathy. *Arthritis Res Ther* 10:R55, 2008.
57. Beyan E, Beyan C, Turan M: Hematological presentation in systemic lupus erythematosus and its relationship with disease activity. *Hematology* 12:257, 2007.
58. Chen M, Zhao MH, Zhang Y, Wang H: Antineutrophil autoantibodies and their target antigens in systemic lupus erythematosus. *Lupus* 13:584, 2004.
59. Mathieson PW, O'Neill JH, Durrant STS, et al: Antibody-mediated pure neutrophil aplasia, recurrent myasthenia gravis and previous thymoma. *Q J Med* 74:57, 1990.
60. Brito-Zerón P, Soria N, Muñoz in S, et al: Prevalence and clinical relevance of autoimmune neutropenia in patients with primary Sjögren's syndrome. *Semin Arthritis Rheum* 38:389, 2009.
61. Cuadrado A, Aresti S, Cortés MA, et al: Autoimmune hepatitis and agranulocytosis. *Dig Liver Dis* 41:e14, 2009.
62. Stevens C, Peppercorn MA, Grand RJ: Crohn's disease associated with autoimmune neutropenia. *J Clin Gastroenterol* 13:328, 1991.
63. Ogershok PR, Hogan MB, Welch JE, et al: Spectrum of illness in pediatric common variable immunodeficiency. *Ann Allergy Asthma Immunol* 97:653, 2006.
64. Tamura H, Okamoto M, Yamashita T, et al: Pure white cell aplasia: report of the first case associated with primary biliary cirrhosis. *Int J Hematol* 85:97, 2007.
65. Zachee P, Daeleans R, Pollaris P, et al: Neutrophil adhesion molecules in chronic hemodialysis patients. *Nephron* 68:192, 1994.
66. Levitt LJ, Ries CA, Greenberg PL: Pure white-cell aplasia. Antibody-mediated autoimmune inhibition of granulopoiesis. *N Engl J Med* 308:1141, 1983.
67. Chakupurakal G, Murrin RJ, Neilson JR: Prolonged remission of pure white cell aplasia (PWCA), in a patient with CLL, induced by rituximab and maintained by continuous oral cyclosporin. *Eur J Haematol* 79:271, 2007.
68. Marmont AM, Dominietto A, Gualandi F, et al: Pure white cell aplasia (PWCA) relapsing after allogeneic BMT and successfully treated with nine DLIs. *Biol Blood Marrow Transplant* 12:987, 2006.
69. Joyce RA, Boggs DR, Hasiba U, Srodes CH: Marginal neutrophil pool size in normal subjects and neutropenic patients as measured by epinephrine infusion. *J Lab Clin Med* 88:614, 1976.
70. Carr ME, Whitehead J, Carlson P, et al: Case report: immunoglobulin M-mediated, temperature-dependent neutrophil agglutination as a cause of pseudoneutropenia. *Am J Med Sci* 311:92,1996.
71. Esposito D, Chouinard G, Hardy P, Corruble E: Successful initiation of clozapine treatment despite morning pseudoneutropenia. *Int J Neuropsychopharmacol* 9:489, 2006.
72. Herring WB, Smith LG, Walker RI, Herion JC: Hereditary neutrophilia. *Am J Med* 56:729, 1974.
73. Wiedmeier SE, Henry E, Christensen RD: Hematological abnormalities during the first week of life among neonates with trisomy 18 and trisomy 13: Data from a multihospital healthcare system. *Am J Med Genet A* 146:312, 2008.
74. Ward HN, Reinhard EH: Chronic idiopathic leukocytosis. *Ann Intern Med* 75:193, 1971.
75. Joyce RA, O'Donnell J, Sanghvi J, Westerman MP: Asplenia and abnormal neutrophil kinetics in chronic idiopathic neutrophilia. *Am J Med* 69:633, 1980.
76. Sakka V, Tsiodras S, Giamarellos-Bourboulis EJ, Giamarellou H: An update on the etiology and diagnostic evaluation of a leukemoid reaction. *Eur J Intern Med* 17:394, 2006.
77. Reding MT, Hibbs JR, Morrison VA, et al: Diagnosis and outcome of 100 consecutive patients with extreme granulocytic leukocytosis. *Am J Med* 104:12, 1998.
78. Marsh JC, Boggs DR, Cartwright GE, Wintrobe MM: Neutrophil kinetics in acute infection. *J Clin Invest* 46:1943, 1967.
79. Jardin F, Vasse M, Debled M, et al: Intense paraneoplastic neutrophilic leukemoid reaction related to a G-CSF-secreting lung sarcoma. *Am J Hematol* 80:243, 2005.
80. Nara T, Hayakawa A, Ikeuchi A, et al: Granulocyte colony-stimulating factor-producing cutaneous angiosarcoma with leukaemoid reaction arising on a burn scar. *Br J Dermatol* 149:1273, 2003.
81. Sato T, Omura M, Saito J, et al: Neutrophilia associated with anaplastic carcinoma of the thyroid. *Thyroid* 10:1113, 2000.
82. Sevastos N, Theodossiades G, Malaktari S, Archimandritis AJ: Persistent neutrophilia as a preceding symptom of pheochromocytoma. *J Clin Endocrinol Metab* 90:2472, 2005.
83. Bishop CR: Leukokinetic studies: XIII. A non-steady state kinetic evaluation of the mechanism of cortisone-induced granulocytosis. *J Clin Invest* 47:249, 1968.
84. Crockard AD, Boylan MT, Droogan AG, et al: Methylprednisolone-induced neutrophil leukocytosis-down-modulation of neutrophil L-selectin and Mac-1 expression and induction of colony-stimulating factor. *Int J Clin Lab Res* 28:110, 1998.
85. Murphy DL, Goodwin FK, Bunney WE: Leukocytosis during lithium treatment. *Am J Psychiatry* 127:135, 1971.
86. Salloum E, Stoessel KM, Cooper DL: Hyperleukocytosis and retinal hemorrhages after chemotherapy and filgrastim administration for peripheral blood progenitor cell mobilization. *Bone Marrow Transplant* 21:835, 1998.
87. de Oliveira JP, Levy A, Morel P, Guibal F: Severe neutrophilia induced by infliximab for psoriasis. *Br J Dermatol* 158:200, 2008.
88. Kratz A, Lewandrowski KB, Siegel AJ: Effect of marathon running on hematologic and biochemical laboratory parameters, including cardiac markers. *Am J Clin Pathol* 118:856, 2002.
89. Laing SJ, Jackson AR, Walters R, et al: Human blood neutrophil responses to prolonged exercise with and without a thermal clamp. *J Appl Physiol* 104:20, 2008.
90. Cohen PR: Sweet's syndrome—A comprehensive review of an acute febrile neutrophilic dermatosis. *Orphanet J Rare Dis* 2:34, 2007.
91. Ratzinger G, Burgdorf W, Zelger BG, Zelger B: Acute febrile neutrophilic dermatosis: A histopathologic study of 31 cases with review of literature. *Am J Dermatopathol* 29:125, 2007.
92. Petitti DB, Kipp H: The leukocyte count: Association with intensity of smoking and persistence of effect after quitting. *Am J Epidemiol* 123:89, 1986.
93. Iho S, Tanaka Y, Takauji R, et al: Nicotine induces human neutrophils to produce IL-8 through the generation of peroxynitrate and subsequent activation of NF-kappaB. *J Leukoc Biol* 74:942, 2003.
94. Fung YL, Silliman CC, Minchinton RM, et al: Cardiopulmonary bypass induces enduring alterations to host neutrophil physiology: A single-centre longitudinal observational study. *Shock* 30:642, 2008 .
95. Bishop CR, Athens JW, Boggs DR, et al: Leukokinetic studies XIII. A non-steady-state kinetic evaluation of the mechanism of cortisone-induced granulocytosis. *J Clin Invest* 47:249, 1968.
96. Athens JW, Haab OP, Raab SO, et al: Leukokinetic studies: IV. The total blood, circulating and marginal granulocyte pools and the granulocyte turnover rate in normal subjects. *J Clin Invest* 40:989, 1961.
97. Kuijpers TW, Van Lier RA, Hamann D, et al: Leukocyte adhesion deficiency type 1 (LAD-1)/variant. A novel immunodeficiency syndrome characterized by dysfunctional beta2 integrins. *J Clin Invest* 100:1725, 1997.
98. Etzioni A, Tonetti M: Leukocyte adhesion deficiency II—From A to almost Z. *Immunol Rev* 178:138, 2000.
99. MacGregor RR, Spagnulo PJ, Lentnek AL: Inhibition of granulocyte adherence by ethanol, prednisone, and aspirin, measured with an assay system. *N Engl J Med* 291:642, 1974.
100. Boxer LA, Hedley-White ET, Stossel TP: Neutrophil actin dysfunction and abnormal neutrophil behavior. *N Engl J Med* 291:1043, 1974.
101. Coates TD, Torkildson JC, Torres M, et al: An inherited defect of neutrophil motility and microfilamentous cytoskeleton associated with abnormalities in 47-Kd and 89-Kd proteins. *Blood* 78:1338, 1991.
102. Nunoi H, Yamazaki T, Kanegasaki S: Neutrophil cytoskeletal disease. *Int J Hematol* 74:119, 2001.
103. Hill HR, Augustine NH, Jaffe HS: Human recombinant interferon gamma enhances neonatal PMN activation and movement increases free intracellular calcium. *J Exp Med* 173:767, 1991.
104. Al-Hertani W, Yan SR, Byers DM, Bortolussi R: Human newborn polymorphonuclear neutrophils exhibit decreased levels of MyD88 and attenuated p38 phosphorylation in response to lipopolysaccharide. *Clin Invest Med* 30:E44, 2007.
105. Klempner MS, Noring R, Meir JW, Atkins MB: An acquired chemo-tactic defect in neutrophils from patients receiving interleukin-2 immunotherapy. *N Engl J Med* 322:959, 1990.
106. Kannengiesser C, Gérard B, El Benna J, et al: Molecular epidemiology of chronic granulomatous disease in a series of 80 kindreds: Identification of 31 novel mutations. *Hum Mutat* 29:E132, 2008.
107. Stasia MJ, Li XJ: Genetics and immunopathology of chronic granulomatous disease. *Semin Immunopathol* 30:209, 2008.
108. Gu Y, Williams DA: RAC2 GTPase deficiency and myeloid cell dysfunction in human and mouse. *J Pediatr Hematol Oncol* 24:791, 2002.
109. Williams DA, Tao W, Yang F, et al: Dominant negative mutation of the hematopoietic-specific Rho GTPase, Rac2, is associated with a human phagocyte immunodeficiency. *Blood* 96:1646, 2000.
110. Nauseef WM. Diagnostic assays for myeloperoxidase deficiency. *Methods Mol Biol* 412:525, 2007.
111. Goedken M, McCormick S, Leidal KG, et al: Impact of two novel mutations on the structure and function of human myeloperoxidase. *J Biol Chem* 282:27994, 2007.
112. Minegishi Y, Karasuyama H: Hyperimmunoglobulin E syndrome and tyrosine kinase 2 deficiency. *Curr Opin Allergy Clin Immunol* 7:506, 2007.
113. Holland SM, DeLeo FR, Elloumi HZ, et al: STAT3 mutations in the hyper-IgE syndrome. *N Engl J Med* 357:1608, 2007.
114. Cooper MR, DeChatelet LR, McCall CE, et al: Complete deficiency of leukocyte glucose-6-phosphate dehydrogenase with defective bactericidal activity. *J Clin Invest* 51:769, 1972.
115. Vives Corrons JL, Feliu E, Pujades MA, et al: Severe-glucose-6-phosphate dehydrogenase (G6PD) deficiency associated with chronic hemolytic anemia, granulocyte dysfunction, and increased susceptibility to infections: description of a new molecular variant (G6PD Barcelona). *Blood* 59:428, 1982.

116. Arturson G: Neutrophil granulocyte functions in severely burned patients. *Burns Incl Therm Inj* 11:309, 1985.
117. Ahmed S el-D, el-Shahat AS, Saad SO: Assessment of certain neutrophil receptors, opsonophagocytosis and soluble intercellular adhesion molecule-1 (ICAM-1) following thermal injury. *Burns* 25:395, 1999.
118. Lesma E, Riva E, Giovannini M, et al: Amelioration of neutrophil membrane function underlies granulocyte-colony stimulating factor action in glycogen storage disease 1b. *Int J Immunopathol Pharmacol* 18:297, 2005.
119. Kim SY, Jun HS, Mead PA, et al: Neutrophil stress and apoptosis underlie myeloid dysfunction in glycogen storage disease type Ib. *Blood* 111:5704, 2008.
120. Tamura DY, Moore EE, Patrick DA, et al: Clinically relevant concentrations of ethanol attenuate primed neutrophil bacteriocidal activity. *J Trauma* 44:320, 1998.
121. Breitmeier D, Becker N, Weilbach C, et al: Ethanol-induced malfunction of neutrophils respiratory burst on patients suffering from alcohol dependence. *Alcohol Clin Exp Res* 2008.
122. Porter CJ, Burden RP, Morgan AG, et al: Impaired bacterial killing and hydrogen peroxide production by polymorphonuclear neutrophils in end-stage renal failure. *Nephron* 77:479, 1997.
123. Hopps E, Camera A, Caimi G: Polimorphonuclear leukocytes and diabetes mellitus. *Minerva Med* 99:197, 2008.
124. Davidson WM, Milner RDG, Lawlor SD: Giant neutrophil leukocytes: An inherited anomaly. *Br J Haematol* 6:339, 1960.
125. Undritz VE: Eine neue Sippe mit Erblich—Konstitutioneller Hochsegmentierung der Neutrophilenkerne. *Schweiz Med Wochenschr* 94:1365, 1964.
126. Uzel G, Holland SM: White blood cell defects: Molecular discoveries and clinical management. *Curr Allergy Asthma Rep* 2:385, 2002.
127. Lekstrom-Himes, J. A., Dorman, S. E., Kopar, et al: Neutrophil-specific granule deficiency results from a novel mutation with loss of function of the transcription factor CCAAT/enhancer binding protein. *J Exp Med* 189:1847, 1999.
128. Gombart AF, Koeffler HP: Neutrophil specific granule deficiency and mutations in the gene encoding transcription factor C/EBP (epsilon). *Curr Opin Hematol* 9:36, 2002.
129. Hoffmann K, Dreger CK, Olins AL, et al: Mutations in the gene encoding the lamin B receptor produce an altered nuclear morphology in granulocytes (Pelger-Hüet anomaly). *Nat Genet* 31:410, 2002.
130. Worman HJ, Bonne G: "Laminopathies": A wide spectrum of human diseases. *Exp Cell Res* 313:2121, 2007.
131. Brunning RD: Morphologic alterations in nucleated blood and marrow cells in genetic disorders. *Hum Pathol* 1:99, 1970.
132. Oski FA, Naiman JL, Allen DM, Diamond LK: Leukocytic inclusions—Döhle bodies-associated with platelet abnormality (the May-Hegglin anomaly): Report of a family and review of the literature. *Blood* 20:657, 1962.
133. Pecci A, Panza E, Pujol-Moix N, et al: Position of nonmuscle myosin heavy chain IIA (NMMHC-IIA) mutations predicts the natural history of MYH9-related disease. *Hum Mutat* 29:409, 2008.
134. Seri M, Pecci A, Di Bari F, et al: MYH9-related disease: May-Hegglin anomaly, Sebastian syndrome, Fechtner syndrome, and Epstein syndrome are not distinct entities but represent a variable expression of a single illness. *Medicine (Baltimore)* 82:203, 2003.
135. Westbroek W, Adams D, Huizing M, et al: Cellular defects in Chediak-Higashi syndrome correlate with the molecular genotype and clinical phenotype. *J Invest Dermatol* 127:2674, 2007.
136. Lazarchick J, McRae B: Chediak-Higashi syndrome. *Blood* 105:4162, 2005.
137. Schmid-Schönbein GN: Leukocyte kinetics in the microcirculation. *Biorheology* 24:139, 1987.
138. Smedly LA, Tonnesen MG, Sandhaus RA, et al: Neutrophil-mediated injury to endothelial cells: Enhancement by endotoxin and essential role of neutrophil elastase. *J Clin Invest* 77:1233, 1986.
139. Weiss SJ: Tissue destruction by neutrophils. *N Engl J Med* 320:365, 1989.
140. Swank DW, Moore SB: Roles of the neutrophil and other mediators in adult respiratory distress syndrome. *Mayo Clin Proc* 64:1118, 1989.
141. MacNee W, Wiggs B, Balzberg AS, Hogg JC: The effect of cigarette smoking on neutrophil kinetics in human lungs. *N Engl J Med* 321:924, 1989.
142. Martin TR, Pistorese BP, Hudson LD, Maunder RJ: The function of lung and blood neutrophils in patients with the adult respiratory distress syndrome. Implication for the pathogenesis of lung infections. *Am Rev Respir Dis* 144:254, 1991.
143. Godek JE: Adverse effects of neutrophils on the lung. *Am J Med* 92(Suppl 6A):27S, 1992.
144. Palmgren MS, deShazo RO, Cater RM, et al: Mechanisms of neutrophil damage to human alveolar extracellular matrix: The role of serine and metalloproteases. *J Allergy Clin Immunol* 89:905, 1992.
145. Weiss ST, Segal MR, Sparrow D, Wager C: Relation of FEV1 and peripheral blood leukocyte count to total mortality. *Am J Epidemiol* 142:493, 1995.
146. Fung YL, Goodison KA, Wong JK, Minchinton RM: Investigating transfusion-related acute lung injury (TRALI). *Intern Med J* 33:286, 2003.
147. Boventre JV, Colvin RB: Adhesion molecules in renal disease. *Curr Opin Nephrol Hypertens* 5:254, 1996.
148. Kitching AR, Holdsworth SR, Hickey MJ: Targeting leukocytes in immune glomerular diseases. *Curr Med Chem* 15:448, 2008.
149. Chibber R, Ben-Mahmud BM, Chibber S, Kohner EM: Leukocytes in diabetic retinopathy. *Curr Diabetes Rev* 3:3, 2007.
150. Fadlon E, Vordermeier S, Pearson TC, et al: Blood polymorphonuclear leukocytes from the majority of sickle cell patients in the crisis phase of the disease show adhesion to vascular endothelium and increased expression of CD64. *Blood* 91:266, 1998.
151. Schaub RG, Yamashita A, Simmons CA, et al: Leukocyte-mediated large vein injury and thrombosis: Pharmacologic intervention with lipoxygenase inhibitors, in *Leukocyte Emigration and Its Sequelae*, edited by HZ Morat, p 62. Karger, Basel, 1987.
152. Ranjadayalan K, Umachandran V, Daviews SW, et al: Thrombolytic treatment in acute myocardial infarction: Neutrophil activation, peripheral leucocyte responses, and myocardial injury. *Br Heart J* 66:10, 1991.
153. Welbourn CRB, Goldman G, Paterson IS, et al: Pathophysiology of ischaemia reperfusion injury: Central role of the neutrophil. *Br J Surg* 78:651, 1991.
154. Kassirer M, Zeltser D, Gluzman B, et al: The appearance of L-selectin (low) polymorphonuclear leukocytes in the circulating pool of peripheral blood during myocardial infarction correlates with neutrophilia and the size of the infarct. *Clin Cardiol* 22:721, 1999.
155. Takahashi T, Hiasa Y, Ohara Y, et al: Relationship of admission neutrophil count to microvascular injury, left ventricular dilation, and long-term outcome in patients treated with primary angioplasty for acute myocardial infarction. *Circ J* 72:867, 2008.
156. Takahashi T, Hiasa Y, Ohara Y, et al: Relation between neutrophil counts on admission, microvascular injury, and left ventricular functional recovery in patients with an anterior wall first acute myocardial infarction treated with primary coronary angioplasty. *Am J Cardiol* 100:35, 2007.
157. Kyne L, Hausdorff JM, Knight E, et al: Neutrophilia and congestive heart failure after acute myocardial infarction. *Am Heart J* 139:32, 2000.
158. Buck BH, Liebeskind DS, Saver JL, et al: Early neutrophilia is associated with volume of ischemic tissue in acute stroke. *Stroke* 39:355, 2008.
159. Trush MA, Seed JL, Kensler TW: Oxidant-dependent metabolic activation of polycyclic aromatic hydrocarbons by phorbol ester-stimulated human polymorphonuclear leukocytes: Possible link between inflammation and cancer. *Proc Natl Acad Sci U S A* 82:5194, 1985.
160. Weitzman SA, Weitburg AB, Clark EP, Stossel TP: Phagocytes as carcinogens: Malignant transformation produced by human neutrophil. *Science* 227:1231, 1985.
161. Phillips AN, Neaton JD, Cook DG, et al: The leukocyte count and risk of lung cancer. *Cancer* 69:680, 1992.
162. Reed WW, Diehl LF: Leukopenia, neutropenia, and reduced hemoglobin levels in healthy American Blacks. *Arch Intern Med* 151:501, 1991.
163. Beutler E, West C: Hematologic differences between African-Americans and whites: The roles of iron deficiency and alpha-thalassemia on hemoglobin levels and mean corpuscular volume. *Blood* 106:740, 2005.
164. Hsieh MM, Everhart JE, Byrd-Holt DD, et al: Prevalence of neutropenia in the U.S. population: Age, sex, smoking status, and ethnic differences. *Ann Intern Med* 146:486, 2007.
165. Grann VR, Bowman N, Joseph C, et al: Neutropenia in six ethnic groups from the Caribbean and the U.S. *Cancer* 113:854, 2008.
166. Berliner S, Shapira I, Toker S, et al: Benign hereditary leukopenia-neutropenia does not result from lack of low grade inflammation. A new look in the era of microinflammation. *Blood Cells Mol Dis* 34:135, 2005.
167. Bodey GP, Buckley M, Sathe YS: Quantitative relationships between circulating leukocytes and infection in patients with acute leukemia. *Ann Intern Med* 64:328, 1966.
168. Dale DC, Wolff SM: Skin window studies of the acute inflammatory responses of neutropenic patients. *Blood* 38:138, 1971.
169. Sickles EA, Green WH, Wiernick PH: Clinical presentation of infection in granulocytopenic patients. *Arch Intern Med* 135:715, 1975.
170. Dinauer MC: Disorders of neutrophil function: An overview. *Methods Mol Biol* 412:489, 2007.
171. Wun T: The role of inflammation and leukocytes in the pathogenesis of sickle cell disease. *Hematology* 5:403, 2001.
172. Coller B: Leukocytosis and ischemic vascular disease morbidity and mortality. Is it time to intervene? *Atheroscler Thromb Vasc Biol* 25:658, 2005.

CHAPTER 65
NEUTROPENIA AND NEUTROPHILIA

David C. Dale

SUMMARY

Neutropenia designates a blood absolute neutrophil count that is less than two standard deviations below the normal population mean. Neutropenia can be inherited or acquired. It usually results from decreased production of neutrophil precursor cells in the marrow. Neutropenia also can result from a shift of neutrophils from the circulating into the marginated cell pools in the circulation. Less commonly, neutropenia results from accelerated destruction of neutrophils or increased egress of neutrophil from the circulation into the tissues. Neutropenia can occur with anemia, thrombocytopenia, or both, in which case the condition is a bicytopenia or pancytopenia. When neutropenia is the sole or dominant abnormality, the condition is called "selective" or isolated" neutropenia, such as chronic idiopathic neutropenia or drug-induced neutropenia. In some diseases, several cell lineages are mildly affected but the reduction in neutrophil is the most severe, such as Felty syndrome. Neutropenia may be an indicator of an underlying systemic disease, such as early vitamin B_{12} deficiency. Neutropenia, particularly severe neutropenia (counts <500 neutrophils/μL [0.5×10^9/L]), increases susceptibility to bacterial or fungal infections and impairs the resolution of these infections. Therapy with granulocyte colony-stimulating factor is helpful in increasing blood neutrophil counts for many types of neutropenia. Neutrophilia is an increase in the absolute neutrophil count to a concentration greater than two standard deviations above the normal population mean value. Neutrophilia contributes to the inflammatory response and to resolution of infections. Inflammatory and infectious diseases are the most frequent causes of neutrophilia. Bacterial infections usually produce neutrophilia, whereas viral infections may not produce neutrophilia or may raise the neutrophil count only slightly. Solid tumors occasionally engender striking neutrophilia. When the neutrophil count is very high, it may be referred to as a leukemoid reaction. The rare neutrophilic variants of chronic myeloid leukemia and chronic neutrophilic leukemia may result in striking neutrophilia. Demargination of neutrophils or rapid release of neutrophils from a large marrow pool may transiently increase the blood neutrophil count. Sustained increased require increased production of these cells.

NEUTROPENIA

Neutropenia refers to an absolute blood neutrophil count (total leukocyte count per microliter × percent of neutrophils) that is less than two standard deviations below the normal mean of the population. The terms *leukopenia*, a reduced total white blood cell count, and *granulocytopenia*, reduced numbers of blood granulocytes (neutrophils, eosinophils, and basophils), sometimes are imprecisely used as synonyms for neutropenia. *Agranulocytosis* literally means a complete absence of blood granulocytes, but this term often is used to indicate severe neutropenia, that is, counts less than $0.5 \times 10^3/\mu L$ (0.5×10^9/L).

Acronyms and abbreviations that appear in this chapter include: ANA, antinuclear antibody; G-CSF, granulocyte colony-stimulating factor; GM-CSF, granulocyte-macrophage colony-stimulating factor; Ig, immunoglobulin; IL, interleukin; SDF-1, stromal cell-derived factor-1.

The concentration of neutrophils in blood is influenced by age, activity, and genetic and environmental factors (see Chap. 2). For children from 1 month to 10 years old, neutropenia is defined as a blood neutrophil count less than $1.5 \times 10^3/\mu L$ (1.5×10^9/L). For individuals older than age 10 years, neutropenia is defined as a count less than approximately $1.8 \times 10^3/\mu L$(1.8×10^9/L; see Chap. 6 regarding levels in newborns). Healthy older persons have the same blood neutrophil counts as younger individuals (see Chap. 8). Some racial and ethnic groups, such as Africans, African Americans, and Yemenite Jews, have lower mean neutrophil counts than persons of Asian or European ancestry (see Chap. 2, Table 2–2). The mean differences in neutrophils are modest and have no recognized health consequences.[1,2]

Severe neutropenia is a predisposing factor for infections. The organisms normally are found on the skin, in the nasopharynx, and as part of the intestinal flora. The risk of infections is inversely related to the severity of the neutropenia (see Chap. 22). Individuals with neutrophil counts of 1.0 to $1.8 \times 10^3/\mu L$ ($1.0–1.8 \times 10^9$/L) are at little risk of infection. In general, neutrophil counts between $0.5 \times 10^3/\mu L$ and $1.0 \times 10^3/\mu L$ ($0.5–1.0 \times 10^9$/L) are associated with only slight risk of infection unless other contributing factors are present. Individuals with neutrophil counts less than $0.5 \times 10^3/\mu L$ (0.5×10^9/L) are at substantially greater risk, but the frequency of infections varies considerably, depending on the cause and duration of neutropenia. Severe acute neutropenia (i.e., developing over a few hours or days) usually is associated with greater risk of infection than severe chronic neutropenia (usually present for months or years). Neutropenia resulting from disorders of production that affect early hematopoietic precursor cells (e.g., aplastic anemia, severe congenital neutropenia) leads to greater susceptibility to infections than do conditions with adequate neutrophil precursors in the marrow and neutropenia attributed to accelerated turnover in the blood (e.g., rheumatoid arthritis, Felty syndrome, autoimmune neutropenia). For patients made severely neutropenic by cancer chemotherapy, the risk is greater when the neutrophils are decreasing than with similar counts when neutrophils are increasing. Neutropenia accompanied by monocytopenia, lymphocytopenia, or hypogammaglobulinemia is more serious than isolated neutropenia. Other factors, such as the integrity of the skin and mucous membranes, the vascular supply to tissues, and the nutritional status of the patient, also influence the risk of infections.

PATHOPHYSIOLOGIC MECHANISMS

General Mechanisms

Neutropenia occurs because of (1) hypoplastic neutropoiesis, (2) ineffective neutropoiesis (resulting from exaggerated apoptosis of late precursors), (3) accelerated removal or utilization of circulating neutrophils, (4) shifts of cells from the circulating to the marginal blood pools, or (5) a combination of these mechanisms (Fig. 65–1). Some production disorders are caused by intrinsic abnormalities of hematopoietic progenitor cells (see Chap. 85). Other disorders in cell production are caused by extrinsic factors, including changes in the marrow environment, such as tumor infiltration, fibrosis, or irradiation (see Chap. 44). Myelotoxic chemotherapeutic drugs commonly cause neutropenia because of the high proliferative activity of neutrophil precursors in the marrow and short half-life of neutrophils in the blood. Production of neutrophils is defined as ineffective when, under a steady state of hematopoiesis, a relative abundance of early neutrophil precursors, a paucity of late-maturing cells, and neutropenia occur. This condition has often been referred to as "maturation arrest," but it is almost always explained by either the apoptotic loss of late precursors in the marrow as an intrinsic

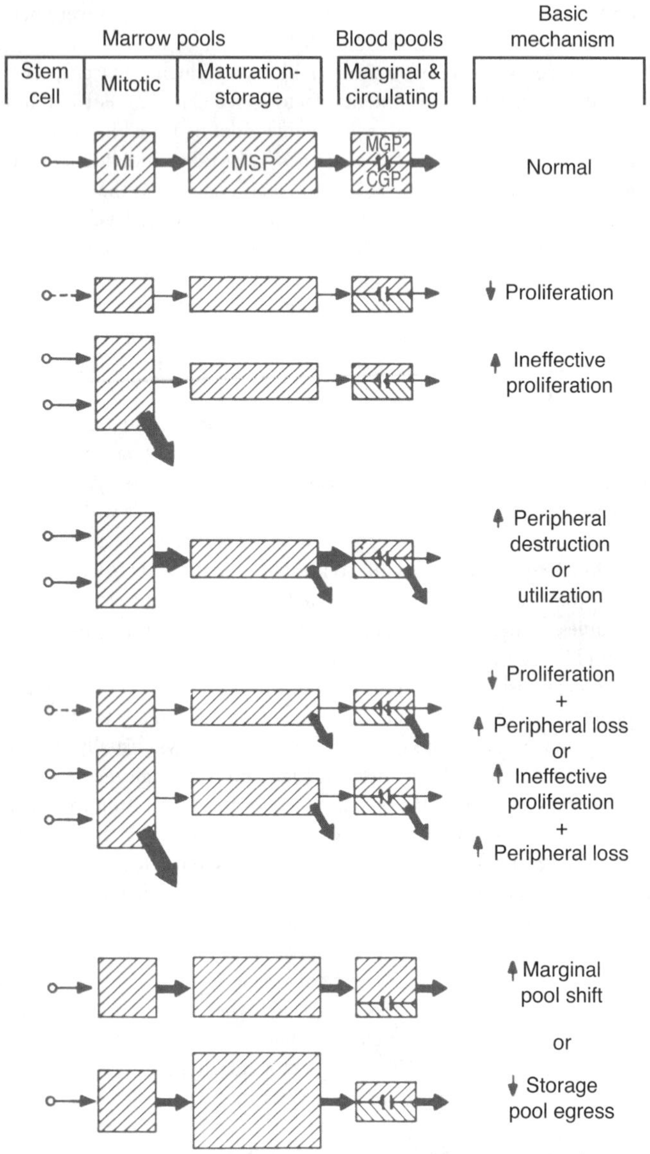

FIGURE 65–1. Mechanisms of neutropenia are shown schematically. The size of each pool is represented by the size of the *cross-hatched areas*. The rate of flow of cells through each compartment is represented by the size of the *arrows*. CGP, circulating granulocyte (neutrophil) pool; MGP, marginated granulocyte (neutrophil) pool; Mi, mitotic; MSP, maturation (marrow storage) pool.

defect in cell maturation or rapid release of segmented neutrophils because of exaggerated peripheral tissue demands.

Accelerated neutrophil utilization occurs with autoimmune neutropenia and acute bacterial infections. When rapid neutrophil utilization and impaired production occur, acute severe neutropenia often develops. The condition is illustrated by the abrupt and sustained fall in neutrophils when an alcoholic patient develops pneumococcal pneumonia. Alcohol suppresses the marrow, and the infection consumes the available neutrophil supply. After myelotoxic cancer chemotherapy, the abrupt fall in blood neutrophils at the onset of infections reflects a similar mechanism: high demand and limited supply. With idiosyncratic drug-induced neutropenia, the counts may fall abruptly because both blood and marrow cells are simultaneously damaged. Acute neutropenia that develops because of a shift of blood neutrophils from the circulating to the marginal blood pools, that is, increased margination (e.g., after injection of endotoxin, with exposure of blood to dialysis membranes, or after intravenous granulocyte colony stimulating factor [G-CSF] or granulocyte-macrophage colony-stimulating factor [GM-CSF]) usually is a transient event. The marginated cells reenter the circulating pool, and the blood supply of neutrophils is rapidly restored from the large reserves of marrow neutrophils entering the blood.

Cellular and Molecular Mechanisms of Neutropenia

Our understanding of the mechanisms of neutropenia at the cellular and molecular levels is increasing rapidly because of advances in molecular genetics and cell biology. For many inherited forms of neutropenia, the genetic mutations causing these diseases are now known, and the mutant protein products have been identified. Some mutations and acquired defects shorten the survival of the precursor cells, that is, they accelerate apoptosis. This form of cell loss now is thought to be the mechanism for "maturation arrest" in several diseases. Examples of increased apoptosis causing neutropenia include vitamin B_{12} deficiency,[3] clonal cytopenias (myelodysplasia),[4] myelokathexis,[5] congenital and cyclic neutropenia,[6,7] and the Shwachman-Diamond syndrome.[8] Neutrophils also can be depleted from the blood and the marrow as a result of extrinsic factors such antineutrophil antibodies and toxic cytokines generated by other cells.[9,10] Some disorders that cause neutropenia also perturb neutrophil function, such as glycogen storage disease type 1b,[11] Chédiak-Higashi syndrome,[12] and HIV infection.[13] Susceptibility to infection in these conditions relates to the combination of defects.

■ CAUSES OF NEUTROPENIA

Causes of neutropenia are classified physiologically as disorders of production, distribution, or turnover. Not every condition fits neatly into this scheme, but it provides a framework for understanding these diverse disorders.

Disorders of Production

Cytotoxic drugs given for cancer chemotherapy and as immunosuppressive agents regularly cause neutropenia by decreasing cell production (see Chap. 20). These drugs now are probably the most frequent cause of neutropenia in the United States. Neutropenia as a result of impaired production is a common feature of several diseases affecting hematopoietic stem cells, such as acute leukemia (see Chaps. 89 and 93), the myelodysplastic syndromes (see Chap. 88), and aplastic anemia (see Chap. 34). The selective causes of impaired production, progressing from disorders of early precursors to disorders presumed to involve defective maturation (ineffective production), are described briefly as follows.

Congenital Disorders **Kostmann Syndrome and Related Disorders** In 1956, Kostmann described congenital neutropenia (agranulocytosis) as an autosomal recessive disease occurring in an extended family in northern Sweden.[14] Phenotypically similar sporadic cases and families with autosomal dominant congenital neutropenia have been reported.[15,16] In severe congenital neutropenia, symptoms and signs of otitis, gingivitis, pneumonia, enteritis, peritonitis, and bacteremia usually begin in the first months of life. At diagnosis, the neutrophil count usually is less than $0.2 \times 10^3/\mu L$ ($0.2 \times 10^9/L$).[17] Monocytosis, mild anemia, thrombocytosis, and splenomegaly frequently are present. Characteristically, the marrow shows early neutrophil precursors (myeloblasts, promyelocytes) but few or no myelocytes or mature neutrophils. Marrow eosinophilia is common. *In vitro* marrow culture studies show poor growth in response to various growth factors and with reduced numbers of marrow neutrophil and monocyte progenitor cell colonies.[18] Usually blood lymphocyte numbers are normal, immunoglobulin levels are normal or increased, and lymphocyte functions are intact.

The majority of patients with sporadic or autosomal dominant severe congenital neutropenia have heterozygous mutations of the gene for neutrophil elastase (also called *ELA-2*). Its product is a protease found normally in the neutrophil's primary granules.[15,19] A variety of mutations in exons 2 through 5 are the cause of this disease.[20,21] In the original Kostmann family, and some other families with autosomal recessive disease, neutropenia is caused by mutations in the *HAX-1* gene.[23] HAX-1 is a mitochondrial protein, and the mutations lead to accelerated apoptosis of myeloid cells, as well as neurologic abnormalities. Mutations in the gene for glucose-6-phosphatase catalytic subunit 3 (*G6PC3*) also cause severe neutropenia as a result of apoptosis of neutrophil precursors, as well as congenital cardiac and urogenital abnormalities.[24]

Mutations in the gene for the receptor for G-CSF also occur in patients with severe congenital neutropenia[25]; however, most of these receptor mutations have caused truncations of the distal portion of the cytoplasmic domain of the receptor, an abnormality associated with altered sensitivity to G-CSF. G-CSF receptor mutations and *RAS* mutations are part of the evolution to myelodysplasia or acute myelogenous leukemia and are not the primary cause of this neutropenia. An exception may be a patient identified with a mutation in the external domain of the G-CSF receptor who responded to treatment with G-CSF and glucocorticoids and has not developed leukemia over several years of observation.[26]

G-CSF is a very effective therapy for all of the recognized subtypes of severe congenital neutropenia, increasing the neutrophil counts and reducing recurrent fevers and infections.[27] Approximately 5 percent of patients do not respond to G-CSF. Hematopoietic transplantation is the only other therapy known to improve the clinical course for these patients.[28] Untreated patients and patients treated with G-CSF are at risk for developing acute myelogenous leukemia. The risk increases with time on treatment with G-CSF, particularly in poorly responsive patients.[29,30]

Congenital Immunodeficiency Diseases Neutropenia is a feature of the congenital immunodeficiency diseases and a contributing factor to their susceptibility to infections (see Chap. 82). In most of these conditions, neutropenia is attributed to a production disorder based largely on histologic examination of the marrow. In X-linked agammaglobulinemia, which is attributed to defective B-cell development and a mutation in a cytoplasmic (Bruton) tyrosine kinase *(BTK)*, severe neutropenia is present in approximately 25 percent of patients.[31] Children with common variable immunodeficiency often have neutropenia associated with thrombocytopenia and hemolytic anemia.[31] Neutropenia occurs in almost half of patients with the X-linked hyperimmunoglobulin-M syndrome, a disorder caused by a mutation in the gene encoding the CD40 ligand.[32] In severe combined immunodeficiency, neutropenia is not always present. The neutropenia varies over time in individual patients. Neutropenia is particularly prominent in the rare immunodeficiency state, reticular dysgenesis.[31] Neutropenia is a less common feature of adenosine deaminase deficiency, the T–B+, T–B–, Wiskott-Aldrich, and Omenn syndromes.[31,33] Neutropenia also occurs on an autoimmune basis in some cases of the Wiskott-Aldrich sundrome.[34] Mutations in the genes for growth factor independent protein-1 (*GFI 1*) can also cause neutropenia.[35]

G-CSF therapy is effective in most patients with neutropenia associated with these immunodeficiency syndromes.

Cartilage Hair Hypoplasia Syndrome This rare autosomal recessive disorder is characterized by short-limbed dwarfism, hyperextensible digits, very fine hair, neutropenia, lymphopenia, and recurrent infections.[31] The genetic locus is at 9p13 and affects a gene coding for an endoribonuclease. The degree of neutropenia is variable, with blood counts ranging from 0.1 to $2.0 \times 10^3/\mu L$ ($0.1–2.0 \times 10^9/L$). An accompanying defect in T-cell proliferation results from an abnormality in the transition from the G_0 to the G_1 phase of the mitotic cycle. Patients have frequent bacterial and viral respiratory infections. Hematopoietic stem cell transplantation can correct the neutropenia and immune deficiency.[36,37]

Shwachman-Diamond Syndrome This autosomal recessive disorder combines short stature, pancreatic exocrine deficiency, and marrow failure with neutropenia beginning early in the neonatal period.[41] Thrombocytopenia and anemia may be severe (see Chap. 34). The chromosomal locus of the mutation is at 7qll, and the mutation affects the *SBDS* gene.[38] The mutation causes a proliferative defect and increased apoptosis of early myeloid progenitor cells.[39] A chemotactic defect also occurs in mature neutrophils.[40] The patients are malnourished, but the neutropenia is not corrected by improving the patients' nutritional status. Treatment with G-CSF raises blood neutrophil levels, and hematopoietic stem cell transplantation corrects the hematologic abnormalities.[41] Without transplantation, the risk of evolution to myelodysplastic syndrome and acute myelogenous leukemia is 20 percent or greater.[41]

Diamond-Blackfan Syndrome Neutropenia is a rare complication of hereditary hypoplastic anemia.[42] Other features include congenital anomalies of the head and upper limbs. Two genetic loci have been identified: 19q13.2 and 8p23.[43,44] The varying severity of neutropenia may reflect genetic heterogeneity among patients with this diagnosis (see Chap. 35).

Griscelli Syndrome This rare autosomal recessive disorder is characterized by pigmentary dilution and variable degrees of cellular immunodeficiency. The syndrome consists of three types. Neutropenia is a feature of type 2 but not types 1 or 3. In type 2, the neutropenia is relatively mild and associated with pancytopenia. These hematologic abnormalities are attributable to a mutation located at 15q21 affecting the *RAB27a* gene.[45] The gene product is a guanosine triphosphatase (GTPase). The mutation also causes abnormal release of granule proteins and hematophagocytosis.[46] As in the Chédiak-Higashi syndrome (see Chap. 66), type 2 patients may develop an acute phase of uncontrolled lymphocyte and macrophage activation leading rapidly to death.[47] Hematopoietic stem cell transplantation can correct the hematologic features. Evolution to myelodysplasia has been reported.[48]

Chédiak-Higashi Syndrome This rare autosomal recessive disorder is characterized by partial oculocutaneous albinism, giant granules in many cells (including granulocytes, monocytes, and lymphocytes), neutropenia, and recurrent infections (see Chap. 66). This syndrome now is attributable to a chromosomal mutation at 1q43 affecting the *LYST* gene.[49] The product of this gene regulates lysosomal trafficking. In Chédiak-Higashi syndrome, the neutropenia usually is mild, and susceptibility to infection is attributed to neutropenia and defective microbicidal activity of the phagocytes.[50]

Myelokathexis, WHIM, and Related Syndromes Myelokathexis is a rare autosomal dominant or sporadically occurring disorder in which patients have severe neutropenia and lymphocytopenia, with total white cell counts often less than $1.0 \times 10^3/\mu L$ ($1.0 \times 10^9/L$).[51] WHIM syndrome, characterized by *w*arts, *h*ypogammaglobulinemia, *i*nfections, and *m*yelokathexis, now is attributable to a mutation in the gene encoding the receptor for stromal cell-derived factor-1 (SDF-1), called *CXCR-4*.[52,53] The ligand-receptor pair SDF-1/CXCR-4 is important for regulating the trafficking of all type of cells, including hematopoietic stem cells, from the marrow to the blood and tissues. In these syndromes, the marrow usually shows abundant precursors and developing neutrophils. Neutrophils in the marrow and the blood show hypersegmentation with pyknotic nuclei and cytoplasmic vacuoles. These morphologic changes and some molecular studies suggest cell loss in the marrow and blood caused by accelerated apoptosis. Favorable responses to G-CSF and GM-CSF occur, as does evolution to the myelodysplastic syndrome. A myelokathexis-like variant of myelodysplastic syndrome has been reported.[54]

Cohen Syndrome Cohen syndrome is another rare cause of neutropenia. Mental retardation, postnatal microcephaly, facial dysmorphism, pigmentary retinopathy, myopia, and intermittent neutropenia are characteristic features. Patients with Cohen syndrome of diverse origins have mutations in the *COH1* gene.[55] Current studies suggest that *COH1* plays a role in vesicle-mediated sorting and transport of proteins within many types of cells.

Lazy Leukocyte Syndrome In the 1970s, a condition called the lazy leukocyte syndrome was described in which the neutrophils also appeared to accumulate in the marrow. The neutrophils were morphologically normal. The neutropenia was attributed to defective chemotaxis of cells from the marrow to the blood.[56] No genetic or molecular mechanism has been identified.

Glycogen Storage Diseases These autosomal recessive disorders are characterized by hypoglycemia, hepatosplenomegaly, seizures, and failure to thrive in infants. Only type 1b is associated with neutropenia.[57] The genetic defect in type 1b maps to chromosome 11q23 and is attributed to a defect in an intracellular transport protein for glucose.[58] The marrow appears normal despite severely reduced blood neutrophils. The neutrophils have a reduced oxidative burst when stimulated and defective chemotaxis.[59] Treatment with G-CSF is effective for correcting the neutropenia and improving the associated inflammatory bowel disease, but has been associated with evolution to acute myelogenous leukemia.[60]

Cyclic Neutropenia Cyclic neutropenia is an autosomal dominant or sporadically occurring disease characterized by regularly recurring episodes of severe neutropenia, usually every 21 days.[61] Regular oscillations of other white cells, reticulocytes, and platelets are sometimes observed. Cyclic neutropenia now is attributable to mutations in the gene for neutrophil elastase (*ELA-2*) at locus 19q3. Most mutations in the *ELA-2* gene are in the regions of exons 4 and 5.[62] The diagnosis usually is made in the first year of life, especially in the presence of a family history of the condition.[63] The neutropenic periods last for 3 to 6 days and often are accompanied by fever, malaise, anorexia, mouth ulcers, and cervical lymphadenopathy. A few cases of acquired cyclic neutropenia in adults, some of whom have an associated clonal proliferation of large granular lymphocytes (see Chap. 96), have been reported.[64]

The diagnosis of cyclic neutropenia can be made only by serial differential white cell counts, at least two or three times per week for a minimum of 6 weeks. Sequencing of the gene may be helpful in confirming the diagnosis.[65] Most affected children survive to adulthood, with symptoms often milder after puberty. Fatal clostridial bacteremia has been reported in several cases, and careful observation is warranted with each neutropenic period in untreated patients. Treatment with G-CSF is very effective.[66] G-CSF does not abolish cycling, but it shortens the neutropenic periods sufficiently to prevent symptoms and infections.

Other Inherited Neutropenia Neutropenia caused by genetic defects of folate, cobalamin, and transcobalamin II A varieties of congenital disorders lead to disturbed function of methylmalonyl coenzyme A mutase and methionine synthetase, the two cobalamin-requiring enzymes. Each of these disorders causes neutropenia, anemia, and thrombocytopenia as a result of ineffective hematopoiesis (see Chap. 41).[67,68]

Several disorders, currently with only descriptive names, may be genetically determined forms of neutropenia. These cases often are called familial (benign) neutropenia and probably are autosomal dominant disorders.[69–71] Some cases of chronic benign neutropenia of childhood (usually a negative family history) may represent new mutations, and patients with chronic idiopathic neutropenia of adulthood may be childhood cases escaping early detection. Until better information is available, these conditions probably are best referred to as "idiopathic neutropenias."

Acquired Disorders Neutropenia in Neonates of Hypertensive Mothers Hypertensive women often have low-birth-weight infants with low neutrophil counts, attributed to decreased production.[71] The neutropenia often is severe with a high risk of infection, particularly during the first few weeks of life. The neutropenia usually resolves within a few weeks. G-CSF elevates the neutrophil count in this form of neonatal neutropenia, but the clinical benefit of treatment remains to be determined.[72]

Neutropenia Resulting from Nutritional Deficiencies Neutropenia is an early and consistent feature of megaloblastic anemias resulting from vitamin B_{12} or folate deficiency. When present it usually is accompanied by macrocytic anemia and mild thrombocytopenia (see Chap. 41). Copper deficiency can cause neutropenia in patients on total parenteral nutrition, with a history of gastrectomy, and in malnourished children[73–75] and the bicytopenia or tricytopenias with a marrow showing dysplastic precursors can masquerade as myelodysplastic syndrome.

Neutropenia Resulting from Immune Suppression of Production Pure white cell aplasia is a rare acquired disorder causing severe selective neutropenia. The marrow is devoid or nearly devoid of neutrophils and their precursors.[76] Ibuprofen, chlorpropamide, excessive zinc, and various infectious and inflammatory diseases are considered possible causes of this syndrome. Differential diagnosis includes aplastic anemia, myelodysplasia, hairy cell leukemia, and neutropenia associated with the large granular lymphocyte syndrome. Immunosuppressive therapy with antithymocyte globulin, glucocorticoids, and cyclosporine has been used in individual cases.

Chronic Idiopathic Neutropenia in Adults This is a distinct syndrome predominantly affecting young adult women aged 18 to 35 years; the female-to-male ratio is approximately 8:1.[69,77] The medical history (lack of episodes of fever, gingivitis, mouth sores, or other infections) and previous blood counts suggest the condition is acquired in most cases. Erythrocyte, reticulocyte, and platelet counts usually are normal. Mild leukopenia and lymphocytopenia may be present, and the spleen is normal or only minimally enlarged. The patients have no chromosomal abnormalities or other evidence of myelodysplasia.[78,79] Marrow examinations show a spectrum of abnormalities, ranging from normal cellularity to selective hypoplasia of the neutrophilic series. In most cases, quantitative marrow studies show the ratio of immature to mature cells is increased, suggesting loss of cells during the maturation process, that is, ineffective granulocytopoiesis.[80] Antineutrophil antibodies, autoantibodies, including antinuclear or antimitochondrial antibodies, are absent.[81] Chronic idiopathic neutropenia in adults is the result of accelerated apoptosis of neutrophils and their precursors mediated via the Fas ligand or interferon-γ.[82] The disease mechanism, that is, activation of the extracellular apoptotic pathway, is similar to the mechanism described for patients with systemic lupus erythematosus.[83]

For most patients, the clinical course can be predicted from the level of blood neutrophils, marrow examination, and prior history of fevers and infections. In general, patients with the lowest levels of blood and marrow neutrophils have the most frequent problems. Long-term observations have shown, however, that some patients have very low blood neutrophil levels for long periods with few or no infections. Evolution to acute leukemia or aplastic anemia generally does not occur. G-CSF increases neutrophils in most patients and is a useful therapy for patients with recurrent fever and infections.[27,84]

DISORDERS AFFECTING NEUTROPHIL UTILIZATION AND TURNOVER

Mechanisms of Immune Neutropenia

Immune disorders primarily alter the distribution of neutrophils in the blood and accelerate neutrophil turnover. Antineutrophil antibodies cause transfusion reactions, alloimmune neonatal neutropenia, and autoimmune neutropenia. Antigen–antibody complexes, autoantibodies, and cytokine-mediated cellular injury are possible contributors to neutropenia of systemic lupus erythematosus and Felty syndrome. The association of neutropenia with increased numbers of circulating large granular lymphocytes demonstrates that cellular and humoral immune mechanisms can cause neutropenia (see Chap. 96).

Neutrophils share surface antigens with other tissues including the i-I antigens and HLA antigens. They also have some specific antigens, including NA-1, NA-2 (now recognized as isotypes of FcγRIII or CD16), NB-1, NC-1, and 9a.[85–87] A number of other antigens can be identified on neutrophils and neutrophil precursors with monoclonal antibodies. The clearest associations of autoantibodies and neutropenia are with NA-1 and NA-2.[88]

Several tests are available for detecting antineutrophil antibodies, including agglutination and microagglutination, cytotoxicity, direct and indirect immunofluorescence, direct and indirect antiglobulin assays, and tests involving the binding of staphylococcal protein A to immunoglobulins on the surface of cells.[88] The agglutination tests are the oldest methods and depend on the propensity of immunoglobulin-coated cells to aggregate. Immunofluorescence tests utilize antihuman γ-globulin tagged with a fluorescein label. These tests can be adapted for quantitative studies with fluorescence-activated cell sorting. Immunofluorescence and staphylococcal protein A-binding tests also can be adapted for examining immunoglobulins bound to single cells, including marrow cells. Direct methods are used to detect the antibodies on the patient's neutrophils. Indirect methods are used to test the patient's plasma or serum against panels of normal cells. Use of paraformaldehyde to expose antigens and to preserve the neutrophils for multiple tests has been especially helpful. Appropriate controls are essential for proper interpretation of these studies. Measurements of apoptosis and cytokine-mediated cellular injury are done through research laboratories.

Causes of Immune-Mediated Neutropenia

Alloimmune Neonatal Neutropenia Newborn infants may have neutropenia for a variety of reasons.[89] In some cases, the disorder results from transplacental passage of maternal immunoglobulin (Ig) G antibodies that bind to the infant's neutrophil-specific antigens, usually the FcγRIIIb (HNA1 or CD16b) isotype inherited from the infant's father.[90,91] Other antigens, such as NB1 glycoprotein (NB1 or CD177), HNA-3a(5b), HLA antigens, and unknown antigens, also may be involved.[88] Overall, this disorder occurs in approximately 1 in 2000 neonates. The disorder usually lasts 2 to 4 months until the passively acquired antibody is lost.

Immune neonatal neutropenia may be severe or relatively mild. It often is not recognized until bacterial infections occur in an otherwise healthy infant. The hematologic picture usually consists of severe neutropenia with normal to increased lymphocytes and normal monocytes, erythrocytes, and platelets. Marrow cellularity is normal or increased, with reduced numbers of mature neutrophils. Alloimmune neonatal neutropenia may be confused with neonatal sepsis because the latter condition also causes severe neutropenia. The diagnosis of alloimmune neutropenia usually is made using neutrophil agglutination or immunofluorescence tests. Treatment should be conservative; antibiotics are used only when necessary. Exchange transfusions to decrease antibody titers or neutrophil transfusions from the patient's mother are rarely needed.

Autoimmune Neutropenia Neutrophil autoantibodies can decrease neutrophil survival and impair neutrophil production. From a clinical perspective, however, distinguishing autoimmune neutropenia from chronic idiopathic neutropenia often is difficult.[92] Patients diagnosed with autoimmune neutropenia have one or more positive tests for antineutrophil antibodies. Their cytopenia is selective; other blood cell counts are normal or near normal. Marrow morphology, colony forming cells, and other tests, including antinuclear antibody tests, are normal. In general, therapy should be conservative and expectant. Intravenous γ-globulin may transiently increase neutrophils, but the therapy is expensive and relatively ineffective. The response to glucocorticoid therapy is unpredictable. Daily or alternate-day G-CSF is effective but should be reserved for patients with recurrent infections. Spontaneous remissions appear to occur much more commonly in children than adults.[93,94]

Systemic Lupus Erythematosus Total leukocyte counts usually are between 2 and $5 \times 10^3/\mu L$ ($2–5 \times 10^9/L$) and neutrophils are less than $1.8 \times 10^9/L$ in approximately 50 percent of patients with systemic lupus erythematosus.[95–98] Mild neutropenia often is accompanied by monocytopenia and lymphocytopenia, anemia, thrombocytopenia, and mild degrees of splenomegaly. Marrow cellularity and maturation of cells usually are normal. An increased amount of IgG is present on the surface of neutrophils, and immune complexes are increased within the neutrophils.[97] Fas and tumor necrosis factor-related apoptosis-inducing ligand (TRAIL) mediate many of the clinical features of autoimmune diseases, including apoptosis of neutrophils in systemic lupus erythematosus. Glucocorticoids, G-CSF, and GM-CSF elevate neutrophils in most patients with lupus, including patients on immunosuppressive therapies, but the mild neutropenia of these patients usually does not require treatment.[97]

Rheumatoid Arthritis, Sjögren Syndrome, and Felty Syndrome Leukopenia in association with rheumatoid arthritis is unusual, occurring in less than 3 percent of large series of patients.[99] Approximately 1 percent of patients with rheumatoid arthritis develop additional features of Felty syndrome (splenomegaly, deforming rheumatoid arthritis, and leukopenia). Usually, these patients have had active, deforming arthritis and very high rheumatoid factor titers. The neutropenia may be moderate to severe; occasionally patients are seen with no circulating neutrophils. The marrow usually is normal or hypercellular but occasionally is hypocellular. Granulopoiesis usually is marked by sufficient precursors but few band or segmented neutrophils. No clear relationship between spleen size and the neutrophil count is evident.

The incidence of bacterial infections in patients with Felty syndrome is low until the neutrophil count is less than $0.2 \times 10^3/\mu L$ ($0.2\times 10^9/L$), which has long suggested that neutrophils are made but that their blood kinetics are altered. The altered kinetics may result from high levels of circulating and intracellular immune complexes and IgG on the surface of neutrophils. Cellular injury via Fas-mediated apoptosis is an additional mechanism for cell loss from the marrow and blood.[100]

In Sjögren syndrome, approximately 30 percent of patients have moderate leukopenia. The total leukocyte count usually is 2 to $5 \times 10^3/\mu L$ ($2–5 \times 10^9/L$) with a normal differential count.[101,102] Rarely, severe neutropenia occurs in association with recurrent bacterial infections.

Therapeutic options for management of neutropenia in these autoimmune disorders include methotrexate, glucocorticoids, G-CSF, GM-CSF, splenectomy, and biologic agents such as rituximab and tocilizumab.[103,104] Results with these therapies are unpredictable.[105,106] Many specialists prefer weekly methotrexate because of its ease of administration, efficacy, and low toxicity.[107] G-CSF or GM-CSF can increase neutrophils but may exacerbate arthralgias.[108] Combinations of these agents is another good alternative. Splenectomy is followed by a rapid increase in counts in approximately two-thirds of cases, but approximately two-thirds of patients who respond to splenectomy have recurrence of neutropenia.[109] A subset of patients with Felty syndrome have a high blood concentration of large granular lymphocytes with a phenotype characteristic of immature natural killer cells.[110] These patients tend to respond poorly to therapies directed toward increasing neutrophil levels but may respond to combinations of methotrexate and G-CSF. Several factors in addition to neutropenia predispose these patients to infections, including monocytopenia, hypocomplementemia, circulating immune complexes, and treatment with glucocorticoids or cytotoxic drugs. In general, treatments to correct neutropenia should be reserved for patients with documented infections.

Other Causes of Neutropenia Associated with Splenomegaly In 1942, Wiseman and Doan[105] described a disorder they called primary splenic neutropenia. Since then, a variety of diseases have been recognized as also possibly causing this type of neutropenia, or pseudoneutropenia. Diseases associated with splenomegaly and neutropenia include sarcoidosis, lymphoma, tuberculosis, malaria, kala azar, and Gaucher disease. Usually thrombocytopenia and anemia are present as well. Immune mechanisms in patients with inflammatory diseases are similar to the mechanisms observed in patients with lupus erythematosus and Felty syndrome may be operative. In other patients, sluggish blood flow through the spleen with passive trapping of neutrophils in the congested red pulp probably is the primary cause. For the most part, the neutropenia in these patients is not sufficiently severe to be of clinical consequence. Removal of the spleen to raise the neutrophil count is rarely indicated.

DRUG-INDUCED NEUTROPENIA

Idiosyncratic drug reactions cause neutropenia with an estimated annual frequency of 3 to 12 cases per 1 million population.[111–113] In 1922, Schultz[114] reported six cases of severe sore throat and prostration with absent blood neutrophils, which led rapidly to sepsis and death. A few years later, this syndrome was associated with the coal tar–derived drug aminopyrine.[106] Over the past 50 years, scores of other drugs have been recognized to cause this syndrome.

Two main types of idiosyncratic drug-induced neutropenia are recognized.[115,116] One type is a dose-related toxicity resulting from interference of the drug with protein synthesis or cell replication. This effect often is nonselective. It can involve the pluripotential hematopoietic stem cells and highly proliferative cells in other organs, such as the epithelial cells of the gastrointestinal tract. Prototype drugs for this type of reaction include phenothiazines, antithyroid drugs, chloramphenicol, and clozapine.[117] Similar effects on marrow cells may be mediated through free radicals and drug metabolites. Patients receiving multiple drugs and patients having high plasma concentration of drugs as a result of the dose administered, slow metabolism, or renal excretory impairment are more prone to these reactions.[118]

A second type of drug-induced neutropenia may not be dose related. The neutropenia is thought to be allergic or immunologic in origin, similar to drug-induced skin reactions and drug-initiated, antibody-mediated erythrocyte destruction. Many drugs can trigger this form of neutropenia.[111, 112] Women are affected more often than men. Older patients are affected more frequently than younger patients. Patients with a history of allergies, including allergies to other drugs, are affected more often than individuals without allergies. Neutropenia may occur at any time but tends to occur relatively early in the course of treatment with drugs to which the patient has been previously exposed.

Our basic understanding of drug-induced neutropenia is limited, partly because of the unpredictable occurrence of cases, the myriad agents involved, and the lack of good animal models for research. Clinical studies suggest the rate of recovery can be roughly predicted from the degree of marrow hypoplasia present when neutropenia is discovered. In patients with sparse marrow neutrophils but normal-appearing precursor cells (promyelocytes and myelocytes), neutrophils reappear in the blood approximately 4 to 7 days after the offending drug is stopped. Often an increase in the blood monocyte count heralds marrow recovery, and an "overshoot" with marked neutrophilia follows. When early precursor cells are severely depleted, recovery may require considerably more time.

Symptomatic patients with drug-induced neutropenia usually present with fever, myalgia, and sore throat, but usually no rash or evidence of allergy elsewhere. Blood examination shows few or absent neutrophils. Mild lymphopenia may be observed, but other cell counts usually are normal. A high level of suspicion and careful clinical history are critical to identifying the offending drug. Differential diagnosis includes acute viral infections, particularly infectious mononucleosis and infectious hepatitis, and acute bacterial sepsis. If other hematologic abnormalities also are present, acute leukemia and aplastic anemia should be considered. Treatment usually consists of supportive care, including broad-spectrum antibiotics for febrile patients. Hematopoietic growth factors may be beneficial, but their use in this setting has not been established in randomized trials.[113]

Table 65–1 lists some of the drugs frequently implicated in neutropenia. Given the rapidity of introduction of new agents, consult the manufacturer, a drug information center, or a poison control center when questions arise to learn if a drug can cause neutropenia.

NEUTROPENIA WITH INFECTIOUS DISEASES

Neutropenia can result from acute or chronic bacterial, viral, parasitic, or rickettsial diseases. Several mechanisms are involved. Certain viral infections, such as infectious mononucleosis, infectious hepatitis, Kawasaki disease, and HIV infection, may cause severe or protracted neutropenia and pancytopenia resulting from infection of hematopoietic precursor cells. Other agents, such as *Rickettsia* and *Bartonella*, can infect endothelial cells. These agents may cause leukopenia, neutropenia, thrombocytopenia, and anemia as part of a generalized vasculitic process. Increased neutrophil adherence to altered endothelial cells may occur in dengue, measles, and other viral infections. With severe Gram-negative bacterial infections, neutropenia probably results from increased adherence to the endothelium and increased utilization at the site of infection. Some chronic infections causing splenomegaly, such as tuberculosis, brucellosis, typhoid fever, malaria, and kala azar, probably cause neutropenia because of splenic sequestration and marrow suppression.

CLINICAL APPROACH TO THE PATIENT PRESENTING WITH NEUTROPENIA

Ordinarily, patients with acute onset of severe neutropenia present with fever, sore throat, and evidence of inflammation beneath the skin or mucous membranes. New respiratory or abdominal symptoms should heighten concern of an urgent clinical situation. Immediate investigation should include a careful history with particular attention to drugs. The physical examination should give careful attention to the oropharynx, sinuses, chest, abdomen, bones for evidence of tenderness, and size of the lymph nodes and spleen. Prompt blood counts and microbial cultures, institution of intravenous fluids, antibiotics, and other supportive measures may be lifesaving. In this situation, fever and infections usually result from surface bacteria sensitive to numerous broad-spectrum agents, unless the patient has been treated recently with antibiotics. A complete blood count should be obtained and a marrow examination considered, particularly if the cause of acute neutropenia is not known. The marrow may reveal fibrosis, selective or nonselective hypoplasia of marrow precursors, excessive blasts, or atypical cells. With this information in hand and supportive care started, further diagnostic tests can be considered.

Chronic neutropenia often is discovered as a chance finding at a routine examination or during the course of investigation of a patient with recurrent fevers and infections. Determining if the neutropenia is

TABLE 65–1. Classification of Widely Used Drugs Associated with Idiosyncratic Neutropenia

Analgesics and Antiinflammatory Agents	Antimalarials
Indomethacin*	Amodiaquine
Gold salts	Chloroquine
Pentazocine	Dapsone
Para-aminophenol derivatives*	Pyrimethamine
Acetaminophen	Quinine
Phenacetin	Antithyroid Drugs*
Pyrazolone derivatives*	Carbimazole
Aminopyrine	Methimazole
Dipyrone	Propylthiouracil
Oxyphenbutazone	Cardiovascular Drugs
Phenylbutazone	Captopril
Antibiotics	Disopyramide
Cephalosporins	Hydralazine
Chloramphenicol*	Methyldopa
Clindamycin	Procainamide
Gentamicin	Propranolol
Isoniazid	Quinidine
Para-aminosalicylic acid	Tocainide
Penicillins and semisynthetic penicillins*	Diuretics
Rifampin	Acetazolamide
Streptomycin	Chlorthalidone
Sulfonamides*	Chlorothiazide
Tetracyclines	Ethacrynic acid
Trimethoprim-sulfamethoxazole	Hydrochlorothiazide
Vancomycin	Hypoglycemic Agents
Anticonvulsants	Chlorpropamide
Carbamazepine	Tolbutamide
Mephenytoin	Hypnotics and Sedatives
Phenytoin	Chlordiazepoxide and other benzodiazepines
Antidepressants	
Amitriptyline	Meprobamate
Amoxapine	Phenothiazines*
Desipramine	Chlorpromazine
Doxepin	Phenothiazines
Imipramine	Other Drugs
Antihistamines–H_2 Blockers	Allopurinol
Cimetidine	Clozapine
Ranitidine	Levamisole
	Penicillamine
	Ticlopidine

*More frequently reported to cause neutropenia in epidemiologic studies.

NOTE: Documentation of the role of specific drugs in the causation of neutropenia is dependent on (1) the frequency of the occurrence among patients, (2) the timing of the event in relationship to drug use, (3) the absence of alternative explanations, or (4) the inadvertent or intentional reuse of the drug (rechallenges) with a similar response. Readers who require supplementary lists of putative drugs involved in the development of neutropenia or wish to read original references for these interactions are referred to references 111 to 113.

chronic or cyclic and the mean level of blood cell counts when the patient is afebrile and relatively well is useful. Other important hematologic and immunologic data include the absolute monocyte, lymphocyte, eosinophil, and platelet counts; hematocrit or hemoglobin determination; and immunoglobulin levels. Patients with hypergammaglobulinemia usually have chronic and recurrent inflammation; patients with hypogammaglobulinemia and neutropenia usually are very susceptible to recurrent infections. Morphologic examination of the blood and marrow can identify some causes of benign neutropenia in children, the Chédiak-Higashi syndrome, and myelokathexis. The marrow examination is most useful for ruling out leukemia and myelodysplastic disorders and assessing the severity of the marrow defect.

In patients with chronic neutropenia, measurement of antinuclear antibodies (ANA) and rheumatoid factor titers and other serologic tests for autoimmune diseases may be useful. Usually, neutropenia associated with these disorders occurs in patients with obvious and severe disease, but occasionally patients are seen with occult splenomegaly, high ANA and rheumatoid factor titers, and a few other symptoms. Examination of the blood and marrow for large granular lymphocytes may be helpful. Infectious and nutritional causes of chronic neutropenia are rare and usually are evident at the time of patient evaluation. In adults, differentiation between chronic idiopathic neutropenia and the myelodysplastic syndromes may be the most difficult. Abnormalities in other cell lines (e.g., anemia with poikilocytosis, anisocytosis, basophilic stippling, and thrombocytopenia, pseudo–Pelger-Huët cells), low proportions of blast cells in the marrow, dysmorphic granulocyte and erythroid precursors, and clonal chromosomal abnormalities indicate myelodysplasia, particularly in older patients. Investigations of the mechanism of neutropenia with marrow and blood kinetic studies, *in vitro* marrow cultures, measurements of marrow granulocyte reserves, and indirect measurements of marrow proliferative activity may be useful in defining mechanisms of neutropenia but are not widely available.

NEUTROPHILIA

Neutrophilia is defined as an increase in the absolute blood neutrophil count to a level greater than two standard deviations above the mean value for normal individuals. For children 1 month or older and adults of all ages, this level is approximately $7.5 \times 10^3/\mu L$ ($7.5 \times 10^9/L$) combining bands and mature neutrophils (see Chap. 2). At birth the mean neutrophil count is $12 \times 10^3/\mu L$ ($12 \times 10^9/L$), and counts as high as 26×10^3 μL ($26 \times 10^9/L$) are regarded as normal (see Chap. 6).

Several terms are used almost synonymously with neutrophilia, including *neutrophilic leukocytosis, polymorphonuclear leukocytosis*, and *granulocytosis. Leukocytosis* is used because an elevated number of neutrophils is the most frequent cause of an increased total white cell count. *Granulocytosis* is less specific than neutrophilia, because granulocytes include eosinophils and basophils as well as neutrophils. Extreme neutrophilia often is referred to as a *leukemoid reaction* because the height of the white cell count may suggest leukemia. This exaggerated reaction may be the result of segmented neutrophils or may be associated with band neutrophils, metamyelocytes, and myelocytes in smaller proportions.

In normal individuals, the neutrophil count follows a diurnal pattern of variation, with peak counts in the late afternoon. Neutrophil counts also rise slightly after meals, with erect posture, and with emotional stimuli. Ordinarily these changes are not sufficient to cause neutrophilia.[119]

■ MECHANISMS OF NEUTROPHILIA

Under normal circumstances, neutrophils follow an orderly progression from the marrow through the blood to tissue sites of utilization.[120] Mild neutrophilia may occur by several mechanisms: increased cell production, accelerated release of cells from the marrow into the blood, shift within the circulation from the marginal to the circulating pool, reduced egress of neutrophils from the blood to tissues, or a combination of these mechanisms. The time required for these events varies substantially. Shifts between the marginal and circulating pools take only a few minutes. Shifts of neutrophils from the marrow to the blood occur within a few hours. Increases in the production of neutrophils, even with intense stimulation, may take at least a few days (Fig. 65–2). With sustained moderate to marked neutrophilia the cause is virtually always increased production of neutrophils.

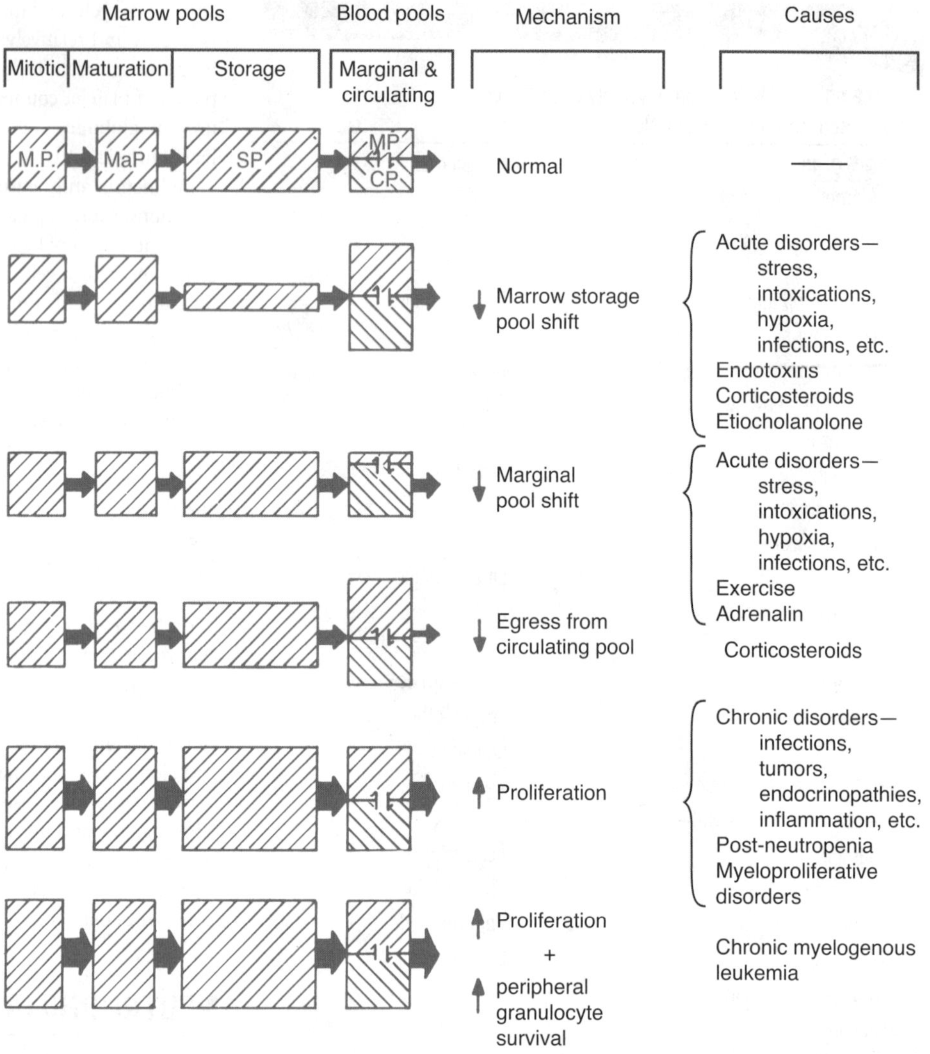

FIGURE 65–2. Mechanisms of neutrophilia are shown schematically. The rate of flow of cells through each compartment is represented by the size of the *arrows*. CP, circulating neutrophil pool; MaP, maturation (postmitotic) pool; M.P., mitotic pool; MP, marginated neutrophil pool; SP, storage pool (marrow reserves).

Acute Neutrophilia

Pseudoneutrophilia (Demargination) Vigorous exercise and acute physical and emotional stress can increase the number of blood neutrophils within a few minutes.[121] The response is mimicked by infusion of epinephrine and other catecholamines that increase heart rate and cardiac output.[122] The response is caused by a shift of cells from the marginal to the circulating pool; hence, it frequently is referred to as *demargination*. This response in humans is dependent partially on release of neutrophils from the spleen,[123] but redistribution from other vascular beds, particularly the pulmonary capillaries, is quantitatively more important. This mechanism can account for about a doubling in neutrophil count. Greater elevations in neutrophils can not be ascribed solely to this mechanism. The increase in lymphocytes, monocytes, and neutrophils that occurs with demargination may be helpful in distinguishing this type of neutrophilia from the response to infections, protracted stress, or glucocorticoid administration. With these conditions, neutrophil counts are elevated, but lymphocyte and monocyte counts generally are depressed.

Marrow Storage Pool Shift Acute neutrophilia occurs as a consequence of release of neutrophils from the marrow storage pool, the *marrow neutrophil reserves*.[124] This mechanism produces acute neutrophilia in response to inflammation and infections. The marrow reserve pool consists principally of segmented neutrophils and bands. Metamyelocytes are not released to the blood except under extreme circumstances. The postmitotic marrow neutrophil pool is approximately 10 times the size of the blood neutrophil pool, and approximately half of these cells are band and segmented neutrophils.[120] In neutrophil production disorders, chronic inflammatory diseases, and malignancies, and with cancer chemotherapy, the size of this pool is reduced and the capacity to develop neutrophilia is impaired. Exposure of blood to foreign surfaces, such as hemodialysis membranes, activates the complement system and causes transient neutropenia, followed by neutrophilia resulting from release of marrow neutrophils. Colony-stimulating factors (G-CSF and GM-CSF) cause acute and chronic neutrophilia by mobilizing cells from the marrow reserves and stimulating neutrophil production.[125,126]

Chronic Neutrophilia

Chronic neutrophilia follows a prolonged stimulus to proliferation of neutrophil precursors. It can be studied experimentally with repeated doses of endotoxin, glucocorticoids, or colony-stimulating factors. Although the details of the mediators and mechanisms for the development of chronic neutrophilia are not understood fully, a general scheme for this response is now widely accepted (see Fig. 65–2). Expansion of cell production follows stimulation of cell divisions within the mitotic precursor pool, that is, divisions of promyelocytes and myelocytes. Subsequently, the size of the postmitotic pool increases. The changes cause an increase in the marrow granulocytic to erythroid ratio. In humans, the neutrophil production rate increases several-fold with chronic infections. Even greater increases may occur in polycythemia vera, chronic myelogenous leukemia, and leukemoid reactions in response to nonhematologic malignancies[127] and to exogenously administered hematopoietic growth factors such as G-CSF,[125,126] with a maximum response taking at least 1 week to develop.

Neutrophilia resulting from decreased egress from the vascular compartment occurs infrequently. A prototype disorder illustrating this mechanism occurs in patients with the neutrophil cell membrane defect CD11a/CD18 deficiency.[128] The neutrophils do not adhere to the capillary endothelium normally, but cell production and marrow release apparently are normal. Because these patients cannot mobilize neutrophils to sites of inflammation when they develop infections, extreme neutrophilia is observed (see Chap. 66). Glucocorticoids may produce a functionally similar state, with neutrophils accumulating in the blood, at least transiently, after each dose is administered.[129] In patients recovering from infections, as the "tissue demand" for neutrophils diminishes, the persistence of neutrophilia may be attributed to this same mechanism. In chronic myelogenous leukemia, accumulation of neutrophils with a longer than normal half-life in the blood partially explains the extreme neutrophilia.[130]

DISORDERS ASSOCIATED WITH NEUTROPHILIA

Neutrophilia in Response to Inflammation and Stress

Table 65–2 lists the categories and causes of acute and chronic neutrophilia. Probably the most frequent causes of acute neutrophilia are exercise, emotional stress, or any other circumstance that raises endogenous epinephrine, norepinephrine, or cortisol levels. Acute neutrophilia occurs in pregnant patients and may be especially notable at the time of entering labor. Acute neutrophilia occurs with induction of general or epidural anesthesia, with all types of surgery, and with other acute events such as seizures, gastrointestinal hemorrhage, subarachnoid hemorrhage, or other internal bleeding.

Neutrophilia occurs with many acute bacterial infections. It occurs less predictably with infections caused by viruses, fungi, and parasites. Many aspects of the complex interactions of microbes with the infected host are not fully understood. Most patients with Gram-positive infections, such as pneumococcal pneumonia, staphylococcal abscesses, and streptococcal pharyngitis, have neutrophilia. Infections caused by Gram-negative bacteria, particularly those resulting in bacteremia or septic shock, may cause neutropenia or extreme neutrophilia.[131] Increased circulating levels of activated complement components, G-CSF, tumor necrosis factor, and interleukin (IL) -1, IL-6, and IL-8 may cause this response. Bacterial infections that have an insidious onset and cause splenomegaly, such as typhoid fever and brucellosis, characteristically do not show neutrophilia except in the initial or disseminated phase. Miliary tuberculosis is an important cause of leukemoid reactions. Neutrophilia is far less common with viral infections. In general, neutrophilia is seen in infections producing substantial tissue injury, evoked by toxins produced by the infecting organisms. Damage to host tissues also is the presumed mechanism of neutrophilia in thermal burns, electric shock, myocardial infarction, pulmonary embolism, sickle cell crisis, and systemic vasculitis.

Many chronic noninfectious conditions cause neutrophilia. Probably the most frequent cause is cigarette smoking.[132,133] Neutrophil counts of smokers are increased in proportion to the amount of exposure. Neutrophil counts of smokers inhaling two packs of cigarettes per day average twice the normal levels. Chronic inflammatory diseases, including dermatitis, bronchitis, rheumatoid arthritis, osteomyelitis, ulcerative colitis, and gout, may cause a persistent neutrophilia. Sweet syndrome is an unusual dermatologic condition manifested as intense neutrophil accumulation in the skin and persistent neutrophilia.[134]

Neutrophilia in Association with Cancer or Heart Disease

Neutrophilia is associated with many nonhematologic malignancies, such as lung and gastrointestinal malignancies, particularly when they metastasize to the liver and lung.[127,135] In some cases, tumor cells produce colony-stimulating factors that presumably cause the neutrophilia by direct marrow stimulation. Tumor necrosis and superinfections are other possible mechanisms. Neutrophilia is unusual in brain tumors, melanoma, prostate cancer, and lymphocytic malignancies.

Neutrophilia is a marker for the occurrence and severity of a variety of illnesses. Neutrophilia is associated with an increased incidence and

TABLE 65–2. Major Causes of Neutrophilia

Acute Neutrophilia	Chronic Neutrophilia
Physical stimuli	Infections
Cold, heat, exercise, convulsions, pain, labor, anesthesia, surgery	Persistence of infections that cause acute neutrophilia
Emotional stimuli	Inflammation
Panic, rage, severe stress, depression	Most acute inflammatory reactions, such as colitis, dermatitis, drug-sensitivity reactions, gout, hepatitis, myositis, nephritis, pancreatitis, periodontitis, rheumatic fever, rheumatoid arthritis, vasculitis, thyroiditis, Sweet syndrome
Infections	Tumors
Many localized and systemic acute bacterial, mycotic, rickettsial, spirochetal, and certain viral infections	Gastric, bronchogenic, breast, renal, hepatic, pancreatic, uterine, and squamous cell cancers; rarely Hodgkin lymphoma, lymphoma, brain tumors, melanoma, and multiple myeloma
Inflammation or tissue necrosis	Drugs, hormones, and toxins
Burns, electric shock, trauma, infarction, gout, vasculitis, antigen-antibody complexes, complement activation	Continued exposure to many substances that produce acute neutrophilia, lithium; rarely as a reaction to other drugs
Drugs, hormones, and toxins	Metabolic and endocrinologic disorders
Colony-stimulating factors, epinephrine, etiocholanolone, endotoxin, glucocorticoids, smoking tobacco, vaccines, venoms	Eclampsia, thyroid storm, overproduction of adrenocorticotropic hormone
	Hematologic disorders
	Rebound from agranulocytosis or therapy of megaloblastic anemia, chronic hemolysis or hemorrhage, asplenia, myeloproliferative disorders, chronic idiopathic leukocytosis
	Hereditary and congenital disorders
	Down syndrome, congenital

severity of coronary heart disease, independent of smoking status.[136,137] Similarly, elevated white cell counts have been associated with increased cancer mortality, independent of smoking history. In patients with cancer, subarachnoid hemorrhage, and other serious inflammatory conditions, neutrophilia portends a less favorable prognosis.

Neutrophilia as a Manifestation of a Hematologic Disorder

In addition to the myeloproliferative syndromes including chronic neutrophilic leukemia and neutrophilic chronic myelogenous leukemia (see Chap. 90), several unusual hematologic conditions may be associated with neutrophilia. The mechanisms for most of these disorders remain obscure. In Down syndrome, transient neonatal leukemoid reactions resembling chronic myelogenous leukemia may occur.[138] This type of neutrophilia may be related to a defect in regulation of neutrophil production caused by chromosome 21 trisomy, but the precise mechanism is unknown. Idiopathic neutrophilic leukocytosis with a negative family history and a similar condition of hereditary neutrophilia with an autosomal dominant pattern of inheritance have been reported[139,140] but are very rare. Careful clinical examination and follow-up almost always reveal the cause of the neutrophilia.

Neutrophilia Associated with Drugs

Many drugs cause neutropenia, but neutrophilia in response to drugs is uncommon except for the well-known effects of epinephrine, other catecholamines, and glucocorticoids. Lithium salts cause sustained neutrophilia.[141] The counts return to normal when the drug is discontinued. The drug increases levels of colony-stimulating factor. Cases of neutrophilia have been reported with ranitidine and quinidine therapy, but such reactions are very uncommon.

CLINICAL APPROACH TO PATIENTS WITH NEUTROPHILIA

In most instances, the finding of neutrophilia, band neutrophils, and toxic granules in the mature cells can be related to an obvious ongoing inflammatory condition. Often the finding of neutrophilia helps confirm the diagnosis of appendicitis, cholecystitis, or bacterial pharyngitis. When the cause of neutrophilia is not readily apparent, especially if the neutrophilia is associated with fever or other signs of inflammation, more subtle infections such as tuberculosis or osteomyelitis should be considered. In addition, a history of smoking and evidence for a chronic anxiety state or an occult malignancy should be sought. If neutrophilia is accompanied by myelocytes and promyelocytes, increased basophils, and unexplained splenomegaly, the diagnosis of a myeloproliferative disease (e.g., chronic myelogenous leukemia, idiopathic myelofibrosis, or polycythemia vera) should be considered. Measurement of leukocyte alkaline phosphatase activity can be a useful screening test in cases of moderate neutrophilia ($15–25 \times 10^3$ neutrophils/μL [$15–25 \times 10^9$ neutrophils/L]). Ordinarily the values are elevated with inflammation of any cause and in subjects receiving glucocorticoid therapy. The values are low in chronic myelogenous leukemia and variable with other myeloproliferative disorders. Serum vitamin B_{12} levels and B_{12}-binding proteins are elevated in both benign neutrophilia and chronic myelogenous leukemia. In unexplained neutrophilia, testing for the cytogenetic alterations and the *BCR* gene rearrangement (see Chap. 90) and *JAK2* gene mutations (see Chap. 91) are important in the diagnostic evaluation. Chap. 90 discusses the diagnosis of chronic myelogenous leukemia and other chronic myelogenous leukemic disorders with prominent neutrophilia.

Epidemiologic studies show an association of neutrophilia with adverse effects of smoking, obesity, coronary artery disease, cerebral vascular disease and malignancies.[142–146] In myeloproliferative disorders, neutrophilia is a predictor of thrombotic events.[147–149] In patients with sickle cell disease, neutrophilia correlates with increased complications and severity of the disease.[150,151] In these patients, treatment with hydroxyurea lowers the blood neutrophil counts and prevents some of these complications. In some inflammatory diseases, glucocorticoids, which raise blood neutrophils, and immunosuppressive therapies, which lower blood neutrophils, are used to reduce inflammation; this is because both of these classes of drugs reduce the deployment of neutrophils and other leukocytes to tissue sites of inflammation. For instance, glucocorticoids usually suppress the inflammation of the skin in Sweet syndrome. In most clinical settings, therapies to reduce the neutrophil count are generally not indicated.

REFERENCES

1. Haddy TB, Rana SR, Castro O: Benign ethnic neutropenia: What is a normal absolute neutrophil count? *J Lab Clin Med* 133:15, 1999.
2. Denic S, Showqi S, Klein C, et al: Prevalence, phenotype and inheritance of benign neutropenia in Arabs. *BMC Blood Disord* 9:3, 2009.
3. Koury MJ, Price JO, Hicks GG: Apoptosis in megaloblastic anemia occurs during DNA synthesis by a p53-independent, nucleoside-reversible mechanism. *Blood* 96:3249, 2000.
4. Kerbauy DB, Deeg HJ: Apoptosis and antiapoptotic mechanisms in the progression of myelodysplastic syndrome. *Exp Hematol* 35:1739, 2007.
5. Kawai T, Malech HL: WHIM syndrome: Congenital immune deficiency disease. *Curr Opin Hematol* 16:20, 2009.
6. Aprikyan AA, Liles WC, Rodger E, et al: Impaired survival of bone marrow hematopoietic progenitor cells in cyclic neutropenia. *Blood* 97:147, 2001.
7. Ward AC, Dale DC: Genetic and molecular diagnosis of severe congenital neutropenia. *Curr Opin Hematol* 16:9, 2009.
8. Watanabe K, Ambekar C, Wang H, et al: SBDS-deficiency results in specific hypersensitivity to Fas stimulation and accumulation of Fas at the plasma membrane. *Apoptosis* 14:77, 2009.
9. Bux J: Molecular nature of antigens implicated in immune neutropenias. *Int J Hematol* 76:399, 2002.
10. Palmblad J, Papdaki HA: Chronic idiopathic neutropenias and severe congenital neutropenia. *Curr Opin Hematol* 15:8, 2008.
11. Melis D, Fulceri R, Parenti G, et al: Genotype/phenotype correlation in glycogen storage disease type 1b: A multicentre study and review of the literature. *Eur J Pediatr* 164:501, 2005.
12. Kaplan J, De Domenico I, Ward DM: Chediak-Higashi syndrome. *Curr Opin Hematol* 15:22, 2008.
13. Kaul D, Coffey MJ, Phare SM, Kazanjian PH: Capacity of neutrophils and monocytes from human immunodeficiency virus-infected patients and healthy controls to inhibit growth of *Mycobacterium bovis*. *J Lab Clin Med* 141:330, 2003.
14. Kostmann R: Infantile genetic agranulocytosis; agranulocytosis infantilis hereditaria. *Acta Paediatr* 45:1, 1956.
15. Dale DC, Link DC: The many causes of severe congenital neutropenia. *N Engl J Med* 360:3, 2009.
16. Bellanne-Chantelot C, Clauin S, Leblanc T, et al: Mutations in the ELA2 gene correlate with more severe expression of neutropenia: A study of 81 patients from the French Neutropenia Register. *Blood* 103:4119, 2004.
17. Welte K, Zeidler C, Dale DC: Severe congenital neutropenia. *Semin Hematol* 43:189, 2006.
18. Konishi N, Kobayashi M, Miyagawa S: Defective proliferation of primitive myeloid progenitor cells in patients with severe congenital neutropenia. *Blood* 94:4077, 1999.
19. Zeidler C, Germeshausen M, Klein C: Clinical implications of ELA2-, HAX1- and G-CSF-receptor (CSF3R) mutations in severe congenital neutropenia. *Br J Haematol* 144:459, 2009.
20. Dale DC, Person RE, Bolyard AA, et al: Mutations in the gene encoding neutrophil elastase in congenital and cyclic neutropenia. *Blood* 96:2317, 2000.
21. Ancliff PJ: Congenital neutropenia. *Blood Rev* 17:209, 2003.
22. Köllner I, Sodeik B, Schreek S, et al: Mutations in neutrophil elastase causing congenital neutropenia lead to cytoplasmic protein accumulation and induction of the unfolded protein response. *Blood* 108:493, 2006.
23. Klein C, Grudzien M, Appaswamy G, et al: HAX1 deficiency causes autosomal recessive severe congenital neutropenia (Kostmann disease). *Nat Genet* 39:86,2007.
24. Boztug K, Appaswamy G, Ashikov A, et al: A syndrome with congenital neutropenia and mutations in G6PC3. *N Engl J Med* 360:32, 2009.
25. Germeshausen M, Skokowa J, Balimaier M, et al: G-CSF receptor mutations in patients with congenital neutropenia. *Curr Opin Hematol* 15:332, 2008.
26. Dror Y, Ward AC, Touw IP, Freedman MH: Combined corticosteroid/granulocyte colony-stimulating factor (G-CSF) therapy in the treatment of severe congenital

neutropenia unresponsive to G-CSF: Activated glucocorticoid receptors synergize with G-CSF signals. *Exp Hematol* 28:1381, 2000.
27. Dale DC, Bolyard AA, Schwinzer BG, et al: The Severe Chronic Neutropenia International Registry: 10-Year Follow-up Report. *Support Cancer Ther* 3:220, 2006.
28. Choi SW, Boxer LA, Pulsipher MA, et al: Stem cell transplantation in patients with severe congenital neutropenia with evidence of leukemic transformation. *Bone Marrow Transplant* 35:473, 2005.
29. Rosenberg PS, Alter BP, Bolyard AA, et al: The incidence of leukemia and mortality from sepsis in patients with severe congenital neutropenia receiving long-term G-CSF therapy. *Blood* 107:4628, 2006.
30. Rosenburg PS, Alter BP, Link DC, et al: Neutrophil elastase mutations and risk of leukaemia in severe congenital neutropenia. *Br J Haematol* 140:210, 2008.
31. Cham B, Bonilla MA, Winkelstein J: Neutropenia associated with primary immunodeficiency syndromes. *Semin Hematol* 39:107, 2002.
32. Rezael N, Aghamohammadi A, Ramyar A, et al: Severe congenital neutropenia or hyper-IgM syndrome? A novel mutation of CD40 ligand in a patient with severe neutropenia. *Int Arch Allergy Immunol* 147:255, 2008.
33. Ochs HD, Filipovich AH, Veys P, et al: Wiskott-Aldrich syndrome: Diagnosis, clinical and laboratory manifestations, and treatment. *Biol Blood Marrow Transplant* 15(Suppl 1):84, 2008.
34. Dupuis-Girod S, Medioni J, Haddad E, et al: Autoimmunity in Wiskott-Aldrich syndrome: Risk factors, clinical features, and outcome in a single-center cohort of 55 patients. *Pediatrics* 111:e622, 2003.
35. Horman SR, Velu CS, Chaubey A, et al: Gfi1 integrates progenitor versus granulocytic transcriptional programming. *Blood* 113:5466, 2009.
36. Berthet F, Siegrist CA, Ozsahin H, et al: Bone marrow transplantation in cartilage-hair hypoplasia: Correction of the immunodeficiency but not of the chondrodysplasia. *Eur J Pediatr* 155:286, 1996.
37. Ammann RA, Duppenthaler A, Bux J, et al: Granulocyte colony-stimulating factor-responsive chronic neutropenia in cartilage-hair hypoplasia. *J Pediatr Hematol Oncol* 26:379, 2004.
38. Boocock GR, Morrison JA, Popovic M, et al: Mutations in SBDS are associated with Shwachman-Diamond syndrome. *Nat Genet* 33:97, 2003.
39. Dror Y, Freedman MH: Shwachman-Diamond syndrome marrow cells show abnormally increased apoptosis mediated through the Fas pathway. *Blood* 97:3011, 2001.
40. Orelio C, Kujpers TW: Shwachman-Diamond syndrome neutrophils have altered chemoattractant-induced F-actin polymerization and polarization characteristics. *Haematologica* 94:409, 2009.
41. Shimamura A: Shwachman-Diamond syndrome. *Semin Hematol* 43:178, 2006.
42. Willig TN, Gazda H, Sieff CA: Diamond-Blackfan anemia. *Curr Opin Hematol* 7:85, 2000.
43. Orfali KA, Ohene-Abuakwa Y, Ball SE: Diamond Blackfan anaemia in the UK: Clinical and genetic heterogeneity. *Br J Haematol* 125:243, 2004.
44. Campagnoli MF, Garelli E, Quarello P, et al: Molecular basis of Diamond-Blackfan anemia: New findings from the Italian registry and a review of the literature. *Haematologica* 89:480, 2004.
45. Griscelli C, Durandy A, Guy-Grand D, et al: A syndrome associating partial albinism and immunodeficiency. *Am J Med* 65:691, 1978.
46. Menasche G, Pastural E, Feldmann J, et al: Mutations in RAB27A cause Griscelli syndrome associated with haemophagocytic syndrome. *Nat Genet* 25:173, 2000.
47. Sanal O, Ersoy F, Tezcan I, et al: Griscelli disease: Genotype-phenotype correlation in an array of clinical heterogeneity. *J Clin Immunol* 22:237, 2002.
48. Baumeister FA, Stachel D, Schuster F, et al: Accelerated phase in partial albinism with immunodeficiency (Griscelli syndrome): Genetics and stem cell transplantation in a 2-month-old girl. *Eur J Pediatr* 159:74, 2000.
49. Barbosa MD, Nguyen QA, Tchernev VT, et al: Identification of the homologous beige and Chediak-Higashi syndrome genes. *Nature* 382:262, 1996.
50. Introne W, Boissy RE, Gahl WA: Clinical, molecular, and cell biological aspects of Chediak-Higashi syndrome. *Mol Genet Metab* 68:283, 1999.
51. Kawai T, Malech HL: WHIM syndrome: Congenital immune deficiency disease. *Curr Opin Hematol* 16:20, 2009.
52. Gorlin RJ, Gelb B, Diaz GA, et al: WHIM syndrome, an autosomal dominant disorder: Clinical, hematological, and molecular studies. *Am J Med Genet* 91:368, 2000.
53. Hernandez PA, Gorlin RJ, Lukens JN, et al: Mutations in the chemokine receptor gene CXCR4 are associated with WHIM syndrome, a combined immunodeficiency disease. *Nat Genet* 34:70, 2003.
54. Rassam SM, Roderick P, al-Hakim I, Hoffrand AV: A myelokathexis-like variant of myelodysplasia. *Eur J Haematol* 42:99, 1989.
55. Seifert W, Holder-Espinasse M, Kühnisch J, et al: Expanded mutational spectrum in Cohen syndrome, tissue expression, and transcript variants of COH1. *Hum Mutat* 30:E404, 2009.
56. Patrone F, Dallegri F, Rebora A, Sacchetti C: Lazy leukocyte syndrome. *Blut* 39:265, 1979.
57. Kannourakis G: Glycogen storage disease. *Semin Hematol* 39:103, 2002.
58. Annabi B, Hiraiwa H, Mansfield BC, et al: The gene for glycogen-storage disease type 1b maps to chromosome 11q23. *Am J Hum Genet* 62:400, 1998.
59. Visser G, Rake JP, Fernandes J, et al: Neutropenia, neutrophil dysfunction, and inflammatory bowel disease in glycogen storage disease type Ib: Results of the European Study on Glycogen Storage Disease type I. *J Pediatr* 13:187, 2000.
60. Schroeder T, Hildebrandt B, Mayatepek E, et al: A patient with glycogen storage disease type Ib presenting with acute myeloid leukemia (AML) bearing monosomy 7 and translocation t(3;8)(q26;q24) after 14 years of treatment with granulocyte colony-stimulating factor (G-CSF): A case report. *J Med Case Reports* 2:319, 2008.
61. Dale DC, Bolyard AA, Aprikyan A: Cyclic neutropenia. *Semin Hematol* 39:89, 2002.
62. Horwitz M, Benson KF, Person RE, et al: Mutations in ELA2, encoding neutrophil elastase, define a 21-day biological clock in cyclic haematopoiesis. *Nat Genet* 23:433, 1999.
63. Palmer SE, Stephens K, Dale DC: Genetics, phenotype, and natural history of autosomal dominant cyclic hematopoiesis. *Am J Med Genet* 66:413, 1996.
64. Dale DC, Hammond WP IV: Cyclic neutropenia: A clinical review. *Blood Rev* 2:178, 1998.
65. Dale DC: ELA2-related neutropenia, in *GeneReviews: Genetic Disease Online Reviews at GeneTests-GeneClinics* [database online]. Copyright, University of Washington, Seattle. Available at www.geneclinics.org. Last accessed June 5, 2009.
66. Hammond WP IV, Price TH, Souza LM, Dale DC: Treatment of cyclic neutropenia with granulocyte colony-stimulating factor. *N Engl J Med* 320:1306, 1989.
67. Fowler B: Genetic defects of folate and cobalamin metabolism. *Eur J Pediatr* 157:S60, 1998.
68. Monagle PT, Tauro GP: Long-term follow up of patients with transcobalamin II deficiency. *Arch Dis Child* 72:237, 1995.
69. Dale DC, Guerry D 4th, Wewerka JR, et al: Chronic neutropenia. *Medicine (Baltimore)* 58:128, 1979.
70. Juul SE, Haynes JW, McPherson RJ: Evaluation of neutropenia and neutrophilia in hospitalized preterm infants. *J Perinatol* 24:150, 2004.
71. James RM, Kinsey SE: The investigation and management of chronic neutropenia in children. *Arch Dis Child* 91:852, 2006.
72. Juul SE, Christensen RD: Effect of recombinant granulocyte colony-stimulating factor on blood neutrophil concentrations among patients with "idiopathic neonatal neutropenia": A randomized, placebo-controlled trial. *J Perinatol* 23:493, 2003.
73. Percival SS: Neutropenia caused by copper deficiency: Possible mechanisms of action. *Nutr Rev* 53:59, 1999.
74. Olivares M, Uauy R: Copper as an essential nutrient. *Am J Clin Nutr* 63:791S 1996.
75. Gregg XT, Reddy V, Prchal JT: Copper deficiency masquerading as myelodysplastic syndrome. *Blood* 100:1493, 2002.
76. Levitt LJ: Chlorpropamide-induced pure white cell aplasia. *Blood* 69:394, 1987.
77. Kyle RA: Natural history of chronic idiopathic neutropenia. *N Engl J Med* 302:908, 1980.
78. Palmblad JE, von dem Borne AE: Idiopathic, immune, infectious, and idiosyncratic neutropenias. *Semin Hematol* 39:113, 2002.
79. Papadaki HA, Palmblad J, Eliopoulos GD: Non-immune chronic idiopathic neutropenia of adult: An overview. *Eur J Haematol* 67:35, 2001.
80. Price TH, Lee MY, Dale DC, Finch CA: Neutrophil kinetics in chronic neutropenia. *Blood* 54:581, 1979.
81. Logue GL, Shastri KA, Laughlin M, et al: Idiopathic neutropenia: Antineutrophil antibodies and clinical correlations. *Am J Med* 90:211, 1991.
82. Palmblad J, Papadaki HA: Chronic idiopathic neutropenias and severe congenital neutropenia. *Curr Opin Hematol* 15:8, 2008.
83. Matsuyama W, Yamamoto M, Higashimoto I, et al: TNF-related apoptosis-inducing ligand is involved in neutropenia of systemic lupus erythematosus. *Blood* 104:184, 2004.
84. Dale DC, Bonilla MA, Davis MW, et al: A randomized controlled phase III trial of recombinant human granulocyte colony-stimulating factor (filgrastim) for treatment of severe chronic neutropenia. *Blood* 81:2496, 1993.
85. Lalezari P, Radel E: Neutrophil-specific antigens: Immunology and clinical significance. *Semin Hematol* 11:281, 1974.
86. Bux J: Molecular nature of antigens implicated in immune neutropenias. *Int J Hematol* 76(Suppl 1):399, 2002.
87. Stroncek D: Neutrophil alloantigens. *Transfus Med Rev* 16:67, 2002.
88. Bux J: Human neutrophil alloantigens. *Vox Sang* 94:277, 2008.
89. Maheshwari A, Christensen RD, Calhoun DA: Immune neutropenia in the neonate. *Adv Pediatr* 49:317, 2002.
90. Puig N, de Haas M, Kleijer M, et al: Isoimmune neonatal neutropenia caused by Fc gamma RIIIb antibodies in a Spanish child. *Transfusion* 35:683, 1995.
91. Maslanka K, Guz K, Uhrynowska M, Zupanska B: Isoimmune neonatal neutropenia due to anti-Fc(gamma) RIIIb antibody in a mother with an Fc(gamma) RIIIb deficiency. *Transfus Med* 11:111, 2001.
92. Maheshwari A, Christensen RD, Calhoun DA: Immune-mediated neutropenia in the neonate. *Acta Paediatr Suppl* 91:98, 2002.
93. Taniuchi S, Masuda M, Hasui M, et al: Differential diagnosis and clinical course of autoimmune neutropenia in infancy: Comparison with congenital neutropenia. *Acta Paediatr* 91:1179, 2002.
94. Smith MA, Smith JG: Clinical experience with the use of rhG-CSF in secondary autoimmune neutropenia. *Clin Lab Haematol* 24:93, 2002.
95. Nossent JC, Swaak AJ: Prevalence and significance of haematological abnormalities in patients with systemic lupus erythematosus. *Q J Med* 80:605, 1991.
96. Bowman SJ: Hematological manifestations of rheumatoid arthritis. *Scand J Rheumatol* 31:251, 2002.
97. Starkebaum G: Chronic neutropenia associated with autoimmune disease. *Semin Hematol* 39:121, 2002.
98. Martinez-Baños D, Crispin JC, Lazo-Langner A, Sánchez-Guerror J: Moderate and severe neutropenia in patients with systemic lupus erythematosus. *Rheumatology* 45:994, 2006.

99. Campion G, Maddison PJ, Goulding N, et al: The Felty syndrome: A case-matched study of clinical manifestations and outcome, serologic features, and immunogenetic associations. *Medicine (Baltimore)* 69:69, 1990.
100. Liu JH, Wei S, Lamy T, Epling-Burnette PK, et al: Chronic neutropenia mediated by fas ligand. *Blood* 95:3219, 2000.
101. Starkebaum G, Dancey JT, Arend WP: Chronic neutropenia: Possible association with Sjogren's syndrome. *J Rheumatol* 8:679, 1981.
102. Coppo P, Sibilia J, Maloisel F, et al: Primary Sjögren's syndrome associated agranulocytosis: A benign disorder? *Ann Rheum Dis* 62:476, 2003.
103. Chandra PA, Margulis Y, Schiff C: Rituximab is useful in the treatment of Felty's syndrome. *Am J Ther* 15:321, 2008.
104. Patel AM, Moreland LW: Tocilizumab versus methotrexate in moderate to severe rheumatoid arthritis. *Curr Rheumatol Rep* 11:313, 2009.
105. Wiseman BK, Doan CA: A newly recognized granulopenic syndrome caused by excessive splenic leukolysis and successfully treated by splenectomy. *Ann Intern Med* 16:1097, 1942.
106. Kracke RR: Relation of drug therapy to neutropenic states. *JAMA* 111:1255, 1938.
107. Wassenberg S, Herborn G, Rau R: Methotrexate treatment in Felty's syndrome. *Br J Rheumatol* 37:908, 1998.
108. Hellmich B, Schnabel A, Gross WL: Treatment of severe neutropenia due to Felty's syndrome or systemic lupus erythematosus with granulocyte colony-stimulating factor. *Semin Arthritis Rheum* 29:82, 1999.
109. Rashba EJ, Rowe JM, Packman CH: Treatment of the neutropenia of Felty syndrome. *Blood Rev* 10:177, 1996.
110. Bowman SJ, Geddes GC, Corrigall V, et al: Large granular lymphocyte expansions in Felty's syndrome have an unusual phenotype of activated CD45RA+ cells. *Br J Rheumatol* 35:1252, 1996.
111. van Staa TP, Boulton F, Cooper C, et al: Neutropenia and agranulocytosis in England and Wales: Incidence and risk factors. *Am J Hematol* 72:248, 2003.
112. Andres E, Noel E, Kurtz JE, et al: Life-threatening idiosyncratic drug-induced agranulocytosis in elderly patients. *Drugs Aging* 21:427, 2004.
113. Andrès E, Maloisel F: Idiosyncratic drug-induced agranulocytosis or acute neutropenia. *Curr Opin Hematol* 15:15, 2008.
114. Schulz W: Ueber digenartige Halserkrankungen. *Dtsch Med Wochenschr* 48:1495, 1922.
115. Uetreicht JP: Reactive metabolites and agranulocytosis. *Eur J Haematol Suppl* 60:33, 1996.
116. Claas FH: Immune mechanisms leading to drug-induced blood dyscrasias. *Eur J Haematol Suppl* 60:64, 1996.
117. Carey PJ: Drug-induced myelosuppression: Diagnosis and management. *Drug Saf* 26:691, 2003.
118. Mauri MC, Rudelli R, Bravin S, et al: Clozapine metabolism rate as a possible index of drug induced granulocytopenia. *Psychopharmacology (Berl)* 35:459, 1998.
119. Garrey WE, Bryan WR: Variations in white blood cell counts. *Physiol Rev* 15:597, 1935.
120. Dancey JT, Deubelbeiss KA, Harker LA, Finch CA: Neutrophil kinetics in man. *J Clin Invest* 58:705, 1976.
121. Quindry JC, Stone WL, King J, Broeder CE: The effects of acute exercise on neutrophils and plasma oxidative stress. *Med Sci Sports Exerc* 35:1139, 2003.
122. Benschop RJ, Rodriquez-Feuerhahn M, Schedlowski M: Catecholamine-induced leukocytosis: Early observations, current research, and future directions. *Brain Behav Immun* 10:77, 1996.
123. Toft P, Helbo-Hansen HS, Tonnesen E, et al: Redistribution of granulocytes during adrenaline infusion and following administration of cortisol in healthy volunteers. *Acta Anaesthesiol Scand* 38:254, 1994.
124. Dale DC, Fauci, AS, Gerry D IV, Wolff SM: Comparison of agents producing neutrophilic leukocytosis in man. *J Clin Invest* 56:808, 1975.
125. Price TH, Chatta GS, Dale DC: The effect of recombinant granulocyte-colony stimulating factor on neutrophil kinetics in normal young and elderly humans. *Blood* 88:335, 1996.
126. Dale DC, Liles WC, Llewellyn C, Price TH: The effects of granulocyte macrophage colony stimulating factor (GM-CSF) on neutrophil kinetics and function in normal human volunteers. *Am J Hematol* 57:7, 1998.
127. Reding MT, Hibbs JR, Morrison VA, et al: Diagnosis and outcome of 100 consecutive patients with extreme granulocytic leukocytosis. *Am J Med* 104:12, 1998.
128. Etzioni A, Tonetti M: Leukocyte adhesion deficiency II—From A to almost Z. *Immunol Rev* 178:138, 2000.
129. Bishop CR, Athens JW, Boggs DR, et al: Leukokinetic studies: XIII. A non-steady state kinetic evaluation of the mechanism of cortisone-induced granulocytosis. *J Clin Invest* 47:249, 1968.
130. Cartwright GE, Athens JW, Haab OP, et al: Blood granulocyte kinetics in conditions associated with granulocytosis. *Ann N Y Acad Sci* 11:963, 1964.
131. Alves-Filho JC, de Freitas A, Spiller F, et al: The role of neutrophils in severe sepsis. *Shock* 30 Suppl 1:3, 2008.
132. Parry H, Cohen S, Schlarb JE, et al: Smoking, alcohol consumption, and leukocyte counts. *Am J Clin Pathol* 107:64, 1997.
133. Miki K, Miki M, Nakamura Y, et al: Early-phase neutrophilia in cigarette smoke-induced acute eosinophilic pneumonia. *Intern Med* 42:839, 2003.
134. Weenig RH, Bruce AJ, McEvoy MT, et al: Neutrophilic dermatosis of the hands: Four new cases and review of the literature. *Int J Dermatol* 43:95, 2004.
135. Shoenfeld Y, Tal A, Berliner S, Pinkhas J: Leukocytosis in nonhematological malignancies—A possible tumor-associated marker. *J Cancer Res Clin Oncol* 111:54, 1986.
136. Zalokar JB, Richard JL, Claude JR: Leukocyte count, smoking, and myocardial infarction. *N Engl J Med* 304:465, 1981.
137. Kirtane AJ, Bui A, Murphy SA, et al: Association of peripheral neutrophilia with adverse angiographic outcomes in ST-elevation myocardial infarction. *Am J Cardiol* 93:532, 2004.
138. Al-Kasim F, Doyle JJ, Massey GV, et al: Incidence and treatment of potentially lethal diseases in transient leukemia of Down syndrome: Pediatric Oncology Group Study. *J Pediatr Hematol Oncol* 24:9, 2002.
139. Ward HN, Reinhard EH: Chronic idiopathic leukocytosis. *Ann Intern Med* 75:193, 1971.
140. Herring WB, Smith LB, Walker R, Herion JC: Hereditary neutrophilia. *Am J Med* 56:729, 1974.
141. Focosi D, Azzarà A, Kast RE, et al: Lithium and hematology: Established and proposed uses. *J Leukoc Biol* 85:20, 2009.
142. Herishanu Y, Rogowski O, Polliack A, Marilus R: Leukocytosis in obese individuals: Possible link in patients with unexplained persistent neutrophilia. *Eur J Haematol* 76:516, 2006.
143. Loimaala A, Rontu R, Vuori I, et al: Blood leukocyte count is a risk factor for intima-media thickening and subclinical carotid atherosclerosis in middle-aged men. *Atherosclerosis* 188:363, 2006.
144. Prasad A, Stone GW, Stuckey TD, et al: Relation between leucocyte count, myonecrosis, myocardial perfusion, and outcomes following primary angioplasty. *Am J Cardiol* 99:1067, 2007.
145. Kruk M, Przyuski J, Kaliczuk L, et al: Hemoglobin, leukocytosis and clinical outcomes of ST-elevation myocardial infarction treated with primary angioplasty: ANIN Myocardial Infarction Registry. *Circ J* 73:323, 2009.
146. Brown DW, Ford ES, Giles WH, et al: Associations between white blood cell count and risk for cerebrovascular disease mortality: NHANES II Mortality Study, 1976–1992. *Ann Epidemiol* 14:425, 2004.
147. Landolfi R, Di Gennaro L, Barbui T, et al: European Collaboration on Low-Dose Aspirin in Polycythemia Vera (ECLAP). Leukocytosis as a major thrombotic risk factor in patients with polycythemia vera. *Blood* 109:2446, 2007.
148. Caramazza D, Caracciolo C, Barone R, et al: Correlation between leukocytosis and thrombosis in Philadelphia-negative chronic myeloproliferative neoplasms. *Ann Hematol* 2009.
149. Marchetti M, Falanga A: Leukocytosis, JAK2V617F mutation, and hemostasis in myeloproliferative disorders. *Pathophysiol Haemost Thromb* 36:148, 2009.
150. Quinn CT, Lee NJ, Shull EP, et al: Prediction of adverse outcomes in children with sickle cell anemia: A study of the Dallas Newborn Cohort. *Blood* 111:544, 2008.
151. Litos M, Sarris I, Bewley S, et al: White blood cell count as a predictor of the severity of sickle cell disease during pregnancy. *Eur J Obstet Gynecol Reprod Biol* 133:169, 2007.

CHAPTER 66
DISORDERS OF NEUTROPHIL FUNCTION

Niels Borregaard and Laurence A. Boxer

SUMMARY

The neutrophil circulates in blood as a quiescent cell. Its main function as a phagocytic and bactericidal cell is performed outside the circulation in tissues where microbial invasion takes place. Neutrophil function is traditionally viewed as chemotaxis, phagocytosis, and bacterial killing. Although these conventionally represent distinct entities, they are functionally related, and rely to a large extent on the same intracellular signal transduction mechanisms that result in localized rises in intracellular Ca^{2+}, changes in organization of the cytoskeleton, assembly of the nicotinamide adenine dinucleotide phosphate (NADPH) oxidase from its cytosolic and membrane integrated subunits, and fusion of granules with the phagosome or neutrophil plasma membrane. Clinical disorders of the neutrophil may arise from impaired function of these normal functions. The clinical presentation of a patient who has a qualitative neutrophil abnormality may be similar to that of one who has an antibody, complement, or toll receptor disorder. In general, evaluation for phagocyte cell disorders should be initiated among those patients who have at least one of the following clinical features: (1) two or more systemic bacterial infections in a relatively short time period; (2) frequent, serious respiratory infections, such a pneumonia or sinusitis, or otitis media, or lymphadenitis; (3) infections present at unusual sites (liver or brain abscess); and (4) infections associated with unusual pathogens (e.g., *Aspergillus* pneumonia, disseminated candidiasis, or infections with *Serratia marcescens*, *Nocardia* species, and *Burkholderia cepacia*).

Acronyms and abbreviations that appear in this chapter include: ADP, adenosine diphosphate; ARF, ADP-ribosylation factor; ASC, apoptosis-associated speck-like protein with a caspase recruitment domain; ATP, adenosine triphosphate; ATPase, adenosine triphosphatase; BPI, bacterial permeability-increasing protein; cAMP, cyclic adenosine monophosphate; cANCA, cytoplasmic antineutrophil cytoplasmic antibody; CARD, caspase recruitment domain; c/EBP, CCAAT/enhancer binding protein; CGD, chronic granulomatous disease; CHS, Chédiak-Higashi syndrome; DAG, diacylglycerol; FAD, flavin prosthetic group; FMF, familial Mediterranean fever; fMLP, formyl-methionyl-leucyl-phenylalanine; G-6-PD, glucose-6-phosphate dehydrogenase; GDP, glucose diphosphate; GPI, glycosylphosphatidylinositol; GTP, guanosine triphosphate; GTPase, guanosine triphosphatase; H_2O_2, hydrogen peroxide; HBP, heparin-binding protein; HETE, hydroxyeicosatetraenoic acid; HLA, human leukocyte antigen; HNP, human neutrophil peptide (synonym: defensin); ICAM, intercellular adhesion molecule; IFN, interferon; Ig, immunoglobulin; IL, interleukin; IP_3, inositol triphosphate; ITAM, immunoreceptor tyrosine-based activation motif; LAD, leukocyte adhesion deficiency; LFA-1, leukocyte function-associated antigen-1; LPS, lipopolysaccharide; LSP-1, lymphocyte-specific protein-1; LTB_4, leukotriene B_4; Mal/TIRAP, MyD88-adaptor-like/toll/interleukin-1 receptor domain containing adaptor protein; MAPK, microtubule-associated protein kinase; MBL, mannose-binding lectin; MMP, matrix metalloproteinase; MPO, myeloperoxidase; MyD88, myeloid differentiation factor 88; NADPH, nicotinamide adenine dinucleotide phosphate (reduced form); NBT, nitroblue tetrazolium; NEM, *N*-ethyl maleimide; NET, neutrophil extracellular trap; NF-κB, nuclear factor-κB; NGAL, neutrophil gelatinase-associated lipocalin; NK, natural killer; NSF, *N*-ethylmaleimide-sensitive fusion protein; PA, phosphatidic acid; PAF, platelet-activating factor; PCR, polymerase chain reaction; PECAM, platelet endothelial adhesion molecule; phox, phagocyte oxidase; PI3K, phosphatidylinositol 3′-kinase; PIP_1, phosphatidylinositol-4-monophosphate; PIP_2, phosphatidylinositol-4,5-bisphosphate; PKC, protein kinase C; PLC, phospholipase C; PLD, phospholipase D; PSGL, P-selectin ligand; SGD, specific granule deficiency; SH3, Src homology 3; sLe^x, sialyl Lewis X; SNAP, soluble NSF attachment protein; SNARE, SNAP receptor; TIR, toll/interleukin-1 receptor; TLR, toll-like receptors; TNF, tumor necrosis factor; TRAM, TRIF-related adaptor molecule; TRAPS, tumor necrosis factor receptor-associated periodic syndrome; TRIF, TIR domain-containing adaptor inducing interferon-β; VAMP-2, vesicle-associated membrane protein-2.

NEUTROPHIL STRUCTURE AND FUNCTION

CHEMOTAXIS AND MOTILITY

The similarity between neutrophil locomotion and that of amebas was noted long ago.[1] Neutrophils can respond to spatial gradients of chemotaxins with differences in concentration of chemotaxin of as little as 1 percent across the cell,[2] although there has been contention as to whether chemotaxis also requires temporal, as well as spatial, sensing.[3] Even with populations of cells as "homogenous" as neutrophils, a broad range of responsiveness is found.[4] During locomotion towards a chemotactic source, neutrophils acquire a characteristic asymmetric shape (Fig. 66–1). In the front of the cell is a pseudopodium, referred to as the *lamellipodium* that advances before the body of the cell containing the nucleus and the cytoplasmic granules. At the rear of the moving cell is a knob-like tail. The lamellipodium undulates or "ruffles" as the neutrophil moves, at a rate of up to 50 μm/min. The membrane lipids also flow during locomotion,[5] and enhanced cytosolic Ca^{2+} is observed along the membrane margin.[6] The lamellipodium, which is very thin, forms immediately when the cell encounters a gradient of chemotactic factor. As the cell moves, the cytoplasm behind the lamellipodium streams forward, almost obliterating it. At this point, some granules appear to contact the cell periphery and release granule contents in response to chemotactic agents. The lamellipodium extends again and the process repeats itself. A flow of cortical materials, composed particularly of actin filaments, has been proposed to account for chemotaxis as well as other cellular movements.[7] This may also account for changes in cell viscosity.

INGESTION

When a neutrophil comes in contact with a particle, the pseudopodium flows around the particle, its extensions fuse, and it thereby encompasses the particle within the phagosome.[1] The ingestion phase can be said to extend from recognition to the end of pseudopodium fusion. The particle thus becomes enclosed within a phagosome into which granules are rapidly discharged, as illustrated in Figure 66–1. As with locomotion, phagocytosis results in Ca^{2+} being released in the vicinity of the active membranes.[6] The number of ingested particles may be eventually limited by the availability of plasma membrane.[7] Locomotion is not a prerequisite for ingestion: If neutrophils collide with a particle not secreting a chemotactic substance, pseudopodia form abruptly at the contact point and envelop the particle. Ingested particles gradually move toward the cell interior, where they tumble about with the nucleus and cytoplasmic granules as the cell moves off. A small number of the phagocytosed particles are actually expelled.[8]

The formation of a lamellipodium is essential for neutrophil locomotion. The interior cytoplasm is squeezed in the direction of the

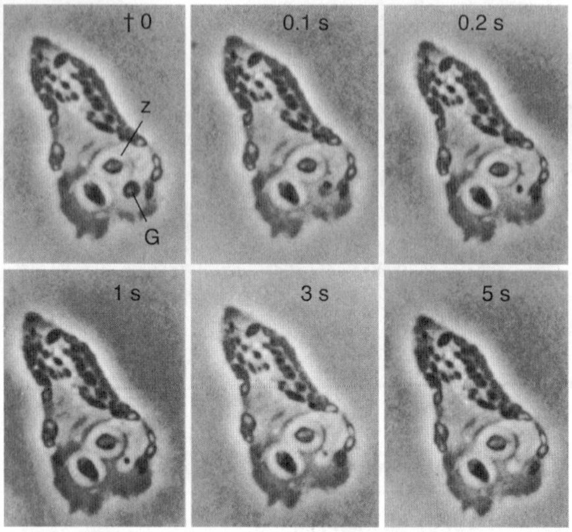

FIGURE 66–1. Cinemicrophotographic observation of granule lysis of a chicken neutrophil following phagocytosis of zymosan particles. Note the lysis of the cytoplasmic granule (G) against one of two ingested zymosan particles (Z). The dense body of the granule disappears from view in the interval of 5 s (original magnification ×1200). *(From Hirsch JG: Cinemicrophotographic observations on granule lysis in polymorphonuclear leucocytes during phagocytosis.* J Exp Med *116:827, 1962, with permission.)*

lamellipodium, possibly by the peripheral cytoplasm in the rear of the cell. The lamellipodium is also required for ingestion. When dissolution of the lamellipodium occurs, the interior contents of the cell are allowed to contact the cell membrane. Granule discharge may occur. Fusion of membranes is a common feature of (1) ingestion, where pseudopodia fuse; (2) degranulation, where granules fuse with the phagosome; and possibly (3) locomotion, where some granules may fuse with the plasma membrane. Pseudopodia form whether neutrophils are suspended in liquid medium or are attached to a surface, but the cell can only move translationally when fixed to a surface; thus it crawls but does not swim. Such "stickiness" is also a phase of ingestion.[7] The neutrophil membrane adheres firmly to particles they ingest, presumably to provide the frictional force needed to move pseudopodia around the particles. Thus, the formation of pseudopodia, membrane fusion, and membrane adhesiveness are all characteristics associated with the functional responses of neutrophils.

ADHESION

The dual neutrophil functions of immune surveillance and *in situ* elimination of microorganisms or cellular debris require rapid transition between a circulating nonadherent state to an adherent state allowing the cells to migrate into tissues when necessary. Initially neutrophils appear at sites on the endothelium adjacent to the site of inflammation. New adhesion molecules on endothelium are induced by inflammatory mediators released by damaged tissues, which result in local extravasation of the neutrophil. In postcapillary venules or in pulmonary capillaries the slow rate, further reduced by vessel dilatation at sites of inflammation, permits a loose and somewhat transient adhesion referred to as "tethering," and results in the rolling of the neutrophil along the endothelium.[9] During this tethering step, neutrophils respond to ligands, primarily chemokines dispatched on the endothelial surface by a signaling event that acts to reorganize the neutrophil surface membrane exposing adhesion molecules, which, in turn, lead to sustained adhesion and spreading (see Chap. 17).

NEUTROPHIL MICROVILLI AND THEIR DYNAMICS

Circulating neutrophils contain surface microvilli of a diameter of 0.3 μm.[10] Moesin, ezrin, and p205 radixin are actin-binding proteins associated with neutrophil plasma membranes and are likely responsible for organization of microvilli on the surface of the cell.[11] These actin binding proteins tether the primary adhesion proteins exposed on the microvilli; e.g., L-selectin and P-selectin ligand 1 (PSGL-1) to the tips of the microvilli.[12] L-selectin is a filamentous glycosylated protein protruding from the tips of the microvilli. L-selectin has a short transmembrane segment and cytosolic component, which can activate the mitogen-activated protein kinase (MAPK) pathway.[13] L-selection, like the other selectins, including P-selectin, which is expressed on platelets and endothelial Weibel-Palade bodies, and E-selectin expressed in endothelial cells, bind with a variable affinity to sialyl fucosylated oligosaccharides including sialyl Lewis X (sLe^x), which is present on multiple specific glycolipids and glycoproteins on leukocytes and inflamed endothelial cells.[14] P-selectin is localized to the membrane of Weibel-Palade bodies and is mobilized to the endothelial cell luminal surface during inflammation. Following expression on the endothelial cells surface, P-selectin makes contact with its major ligand, PSGL-1 on circulating neutrophils. PSGL-1, like L-selectin, is located to the tips of microvilli on neutrophils. It is a heavily O-glycosylated protein with a short transmembrane segment and an intracellular domain that likely transmits signals via the actin binding proteins that tether it to the tip of the microvillus and to Syk protein kinase to initiate cell activation.[15]

ROLLING AND TETHERING

P-selectin is mobilized rapidly to the endothelial cell surface following stimulation by thrombin, histamine, or oxygen radicals and interacts with neutrophil PSGL-1 to initiate neutrophil rolling.[14] Rolling subsequently involves newly expressed E-selectin, which appears on endothelial cells 1 to 2 hours after cell stimulation by interleukin-1 (IL-1), tumor necrosis factor α (TNF-α), or lipopolysaccharide (LPS). E-selectin counterreceptors include PSGL-1 and E-selectin-ligand 1, which is also located on neutrophil microvilli.[16] Both P- and L-selectin contribute sequentially to leukocyte rolling, but L-selectin is involved in the prolonged neutrophil sequestration on inflamed microvasculature. L-selectin is constitutively present on neutrophils and its binding capacity is rapid and transiently increased after neutrophil activation, possibly via receptor oligomerization. Thus far only one inducible L-selectin counterreceptor has been identified on inflamed endothelium. In addition to its binding to endothelial ligands, neutrophil PSGL-1 is a counterreceptor for L-selectin, which permits previously adherent neutrophils to recruit other neutrophils to inflamed endothelium (see Chap. 17).[9,14]

NEUTROPHIL ADHESION AND SPREADING

Figure 66–2 shows a sequence of molecular and biophysical events leading to neutrophil activation and increased adherence during acute inflammatory response *in vivo*. The inflamed endothelium produces chemoattractants such as platelet-activating factor (PAF), leukotriene B_4 (LTB_4), and various chemokines, immobilized by proteoglycans on the luminal surface of endothelial cells.[17] Among these chemokines, IL-8 specifically attracts neutrophils. IL-8 is synthesized by endothelial cells in response to IL-1 or LPS, and is stored in Weibel-Palade bodies; IL-8 then can be released by histamine or thrombin.[18] Additionally, IL-8 can be internalized by endothelial cells and transcytosed from the abluminal surface via vesicular caveolae, and presented to the tips of microvilli of the endothelial cell luminal surface.[19] The binding of signaling molecules such as PAF and IL-8 to surface receptors on the leukocytes activate them in a juxtacrine fashion and triggers changes in affinity or

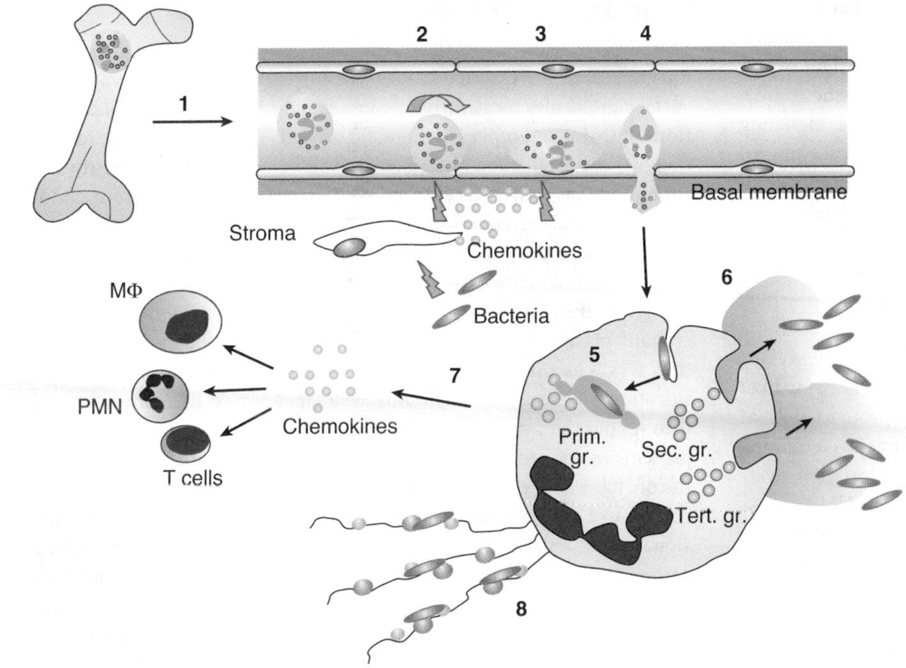

FIGURE 66–2. Neutrophil-mediated inflammatory response. (1) Egress of mature neutrophils from marrow to circulation. (2) Initial tethering and rolling are dominantly mediated by selectins present both on neutrophils and endothelial cells and their ligands. Invasion by bacteria stimulates tissues macrophages to secrete inflammatory cytokines, IL-1 and TNF, which, in turn, activate endothelial cells to express E- and P-selectin and IL-8. E- and P-selectin serve as counterreceptors for the neutrophil P-selectin glycoprotein ligand-1. (3) Activated endothelial cells express intercellular adhesion molecule (ICAM)-1 and ICAM-2, which serve as ligands for the neutrophil β_2 integrins. The β_2 integrins mediate tight adhesion and arrest of the leukocytes in cooperation with the selectins. Localized activation of neutrophils by juxtacrine signaling molecules or chemoattractants that bind to surface receptors is critical for inside-out signaling of β_2 integrins, making them adhesive for the ICAM ligands on the endothelium. (4) Neutrophil invasion through the vascular basement membrane with release of proteases and reactive oxidative intermediates that cause local destruction of the extracellular matrix which allows for migration of the neutrophils into tissues. (5, 6) Uptake of microorganisms into the phagocytic vacuole with concomitant degranulation both into the phagocytic vacuole (azurophil granules and specific granules) and to the exterior (specific granules and gelatinase granules). (7) A burst of transcriptional activity is initiated during diapedesis of neutrophils and during phagocytosis, which results in generation of chemokines such as IL-8, monocyte chemoattractant protein (MCP)-1, macrophage inflammatory protein (MIP)-1α, and IL-1β that may recruit additional cells of the immune system.[27] (8) Formation of neutrophil extracellular traps by extrusion of chromatin and cationic bactericidal granule proteins.[222] MΦ, macrophages; PMN, polymorphonuclear neutrophil.

avidity of β_2 integrins (CD11/CD18) that become incorporated in the neutrophil plasma membrane from secretory vesicles.[9,14,20] β_2 Integrins are recognized by counterligands on endothelial cells, including members of the intercellular adhesion molecule (ICAM) family such as ICAM-1 and ICAM-2. The ICAM glycoproteins are induced by cytokines that include TNF and IL-1. The relative affinity of the β_2 integrins for ICAM is increased by exposure of neutrophils to numerous stimuli, including C5a, N-formylated bacterial peptides, IL-8, and LTB_4. Regulation of the β_2-integrin avidity involves interactions of both α and β chains by their cytoplasmic tails with the cytoskeleton and the subsequent "outside-in signaling."[14] Neutrophils integrate the signals of integrin engagement and those delivered simultaneously by inflammatory cytokines or chemoattractants to activate a cascade of intracellular events resulting in cell spreading (Fig. 66–2).

TRANSENDOTHELIAL MIGRATION

Neutrophil transmigration occurs predominately at the borders of endothelial cells. P-selectin has been shown to be concentrated along endothelial borders and may facilitate neutrophil adhesion. Extravasation requires discontinuation of endothelial cell-to-cell adherent junctions. Cellular activation by IL-8 reduces neutrophil tethering rates to P-selection under flow conditions. The precise molecular mechanisms remain undefined.[14] Tight adhesion mediated by β_2 integrins is also modified for a successful emigration which may involve RhoA kinase modulation of the cytoskeletal-dependent spreading.[21] At the endothelial-type junctions, sequential molecular interactions occur after leukocyte transmigration from the apical surface has been initiated. Platelet-endothelial adhesion molecule-1 (PECAM-1) is localized at junctions of tightly apposed endothelial cells and is involved in the transmigration of neutrophils. PECAM-1 is also expressed at the neutrophil surface and it has been suggested that PECAM-1/PECAM-1 homophilic interaction in a "zipper" model mediates in part the transmigration of leukocytes into the tissues.[9,14] Subsequently, the direction of neutrophil movement in the tissues is guided by the steepest local chemoattractant gradient and then regulated by successive receptor desensitization and attraction by secondary distant agonists. Finally, targeted attractants such as formyl-methionyl-leucyl-phenylalanine (fMLP) and C5a are dominant and override regulatory cell-derived attractants such as LTB_4 or IL-8.[22] This permits the leukocytes recruited by endothelial chemoattractants to migrate away from the endothelial agonist source toward the final microbial target within tissue. Neutrophil migration through the extracellular matrix is mediated by β_2 integrins in concert with β_1 integrins.[17] Neutrophil migration requires the continuous formation of new adhesive contacts at the cell front while the cell rear detaches from the adhesive substrate.

The CD11b/CD18 integrin (MAC-1) is known to interact in cis fashion with glycosylphosphatidylinositol (GPI)-anchored membrane proteins such as FcγRIIIB (CD16), the LPS receptor CD14, and the urokinase plasminogen activator receptor (uPAR; CD87). Integrins behave as transducers mediating signals transferred by these GPI-linked receptors.[23] For instance, FcγRIIIB interaction with CD11b/CD18 promotes antibody-dependent phagocytosis, whereas CD14 interaction with CD11b/CD18 occurs in the presence of LPS and LPS-binding protein to generate proinflammatory mediators, and uPAR interaction with CD11b/CD18 mediates neutrophil migration by recruiting and activating the urokinase-type plasminogen activator.[17]

OTHER NEUTROPHIL SURFACE PROTEINS

Several proteins associated with the surface of the neutrophil function in the normal housekeeping activities such as Na^+/K^+ adenosine triphosphatase (ATPase), but others serve specific functions such as L-selectin, PSGL-1, and integrins. The surface of neutrophils is highly dynamic as a result of the incorporation of membrane from intracellular vesicles and granules, a process that is known to add significantly to the total cell surface measured by an increase in electric capacitance.[24] A number of membrane-bound receptors are localized to secretory vesicles and incorporated into the surface membrane when secretory vesicles fuse with the plasma membrane, as occurs during diapedesis. This enhances the ability of neutrophils to respond to the signals presented by endothelial cells or present in the extravascular tissue.

Toll-like receptors (TLRs) are type-1 transmembrane signaling receptors that interact with specific structures characteristic for microorganisms and generate signals that result in release of chemokines. All 10 TLRs, except TLR3, are expressed in human leukocytes. They recognize different pathogen-associated molecular patterns and share a conserved leucine-rich extracellular domain and a cytoplasmic domain. Toll-like receptors in general transmit signals after dimerization, which leads to recruitment of one of four intracellular adaptor proteins to the TIR (toll/interleukin-1 receptor) domain of the TLR. These are MyD88 (myeloid differentiation factor 88), Mal/TIRAP (MyD88-adaptor-like/toll-interleukin 1 receptor domain containing adaptor protein), TRAM (TRIF-related adaptor molecule), and TRIF (TIR domain-containing adaptor inducing interferon-β). While TLRs (5, 7, 8, and 9) exclusively use MyD88, TLR2 requires both Mal and MyD88 and TLR4 can use either Mal and MyD88 or TRAM and TRIF to signal to NF-κB (nuclear factor-κB) or interferon regulatory factor (IRF)-3.[25,26]

A variety of chemokine receptors are associated with the neutrophil. These are in general G-protein-coupled receptors. Other G-protein-coupled receptors on neutrophils are the purine receptors for adenosine diphosphate (ADP) and adenosine triphosphate (ATP), the PAF receptor C5a, and fMLP receptors. Receptors not belonging to the G-protein-coupled receptor family include receptors for IL-1, IL-10, and TNF-α, and the growth factors receptors for granulocyte colony-stimulating factor (G-CSF) and granulocyte-macrophage colony-stimulating factor (GM-CSF). Both growth factor receptors are important for myeloid development, but may also play an important role in enhancing neutrophil function and gene transcription in mature neutrophils. A burst of transcriptional activity is associated with the diapedesis of neutrophils into tissues, which results in downregulation of proapoptotic genes and upregulation of genes coding for antiapoptotic proteins, upregulation of genes coding for chemokines and cytokines that may recruit macrophages, T cells and additional neutrophils, and downregulation of genes coding for chemokine receptors.[27]

SURFACE COMPONENTS FOR PHAGOCYTOSIS

Neutrophils express the Fcα receptor (CD89) for immunoglobulin (Ig)A and IgG receptors, FcγRIIA (CD32), and FcγRIII (CD16). Neutrophils also express receptors for the complement components, including CD1qR, CR1 (CD35), CR3 (CD11/CD18), and CR4. CR1 binds CD3b, C4b, and C3bi with decreasing of affinity. CR3 recognizes C3bi (a proteolytic fragment of C3b). Of particular importance is that both Fcγ receptors and GPI-coupled receptors appear to be localized to lipid rafts. Lipid rafts are important, but elusive structures that facilitate signal transduction leading to phagocytosis by promoting several membrane protein interactions. Initially the rafts were conceptionally associated with caveolae, which are structures identified on endothelial cells and thought to be important for transendothelial cell traffic. The caveolae were identified by their high content of cholesterol lipids and the presence of the structural protein, caveolin. Rafts were subsequently identified on neutrophils, but these cells are devoid of caveolin.[28] Rafts are perhaps best viewed as patches of surface membrane that attract many hydrophobic proteins including signaling molecules such as tyrosine kinases and phosphatases. Other membrane protein receptors that are not normally associated with rafts may change their conformation and subsequently associate with rafts upon binding their ligands. This is particularly true for the Fcγ and GPI-coupled receptors.

SECRETORY VESICLES

Secretory vesicles are small intracellular vesicles that were discovered during search for the structural basis for upregulation of a variety of surface molecules on neutrophils in response to nanomolar concentrations of fMLP and other chemotactic stimuli. They were initially identified by "latent" alkaline phosphatase.[29] Secretory vesicles of neutrophils should not be confused with the vesicles that carry cargo from endoplasmic reticulum and Golgi in the constitutive secretory pathway of other cells and that are sometimes also named secretory vesicles. Secretory vesicles of neutrophils are specialized endocytosis vesicles that are formed in the latest part of neutrophil maturation in the marrow. They contain plasma proteins, seemingly without any selectivity. Albumin thus serves as a marker for secretory vesicles and has allowed the identification of these as small intracellular vesicles that are scattered throughout the cytoplasm of neutrophils just like granules. The plasma proteins inside secretory vesicles show no sign of degradation, thus no fusion takes place with lysosomal structures.[30] The secretory vesicles behave like the traditional neutrophil granules. They require a specific signal for mobilization.[31] Secretory vesicles are not important for their cargo (plasma proteins), but for their membrane which becomes fully incorporated into the plasma membrane of the neutrophil upon stimulation.[30,32–35] Secretory vesicles host most of the neutrophil chemotactic and GPI-coupled receptors, toll-like receptors, and one of the early acting downstream effectors, phospholipase D.[36] They enrich the plasma membrane with receptors for adhesion and signaling, and can be seen as the structural basis for transition of neutrophils from circulating quiescent cells that do not respond well to stimuli such as chemoattractants and objects to be phagocytosed, to highly responsive cells capable of establishing firm contact with endothelium. The signals generated by tethering of selectins or PSGL1 to the endothelium are sufficient to mobilize secretory vesicles. Secretory vesicles are completely mobilized *in vivo* during neutrophil diapedesis.[14,35]

The first identified marker of secretory vesicles, latent alkaline phosphatase, is known to be elevated in chronic myeloproliferative disorders except for chronic myelogenous leukemia (CML), but the content of secretory vesicles in neutrophils from patients with chronic myeloproliferative disorders is not different from normal neutrophils.[37–39] The best marker for secretory vesicles is CD35 because this, in contrast to alkaline phosphatase, is absent from the plasma membrane of unstimulated neutrophils, and because it is absent from granules (in contrast to $\alpha_M\beta_2$).[20,34,40] It is not known whether secretory vesicles contain lipid rafts, but most GPI-linked proteins are raft associated[41] and, as alluded to above, are localized to secretory vesicles in neutrophils.

GRANULES

Nomenclature of Neutrophil Granules

The neutrophil is known for its granules. When Paul Ehrlich introduced aniline dyes in histochemistry and discovered the different subsets of leukocytes, the neutrophil granules were divided into those that took up the azure dye, the azurophilic granules, and the others, the specific granules.[42,43] When the peroxidase reaction was introduced, the azurophil granules were found to be peroxidase positive as a result of the presence of the major myeloid cell protein, myeloperoxidase (MPO), and the specific granules were thus named peroxidase-negative granules.[44,45] Because the azurophil granules are formed first, in the promyelocyte, and the specific granules later, in the myelocyte, these are also termed primary and secondary granules, respectively. From the study of rabbit neutrophils a third granule subset, termed tertiary granules, was identified in subcellular fractions.[46] Using the same technology, a tertiary granule subset was identified in human neutrophils and shown to contain gelatinase,[47] but the ultrastructure was not determined until the issue of the neutrophil gelatinase (matrix metalloproteinase [MMP]-9) as a possible complex with neutrophil gelatinase-associated lipocalin (NGAL) was identified.[48,49]

Granules were initially viewed of as small bags that emptied their content of bactericidal substances onto the ingested microorganisms when granules fuse with the phagocytic vacuole during phagocytosis, but it later became clear that granules are not only important for their cargo, which may be emptied into the phagocytic vacuole or extracellularly, but also for their membranes, as these contain proteins that become incorporated into the membrane of the phagocytic vacuole and into the surface membrane when the granules are mobilized.[50,51] If granules were classified by their content, both of matrix proteins and membrane proteins, the number of different granule subsets that exists in neutrophils would be meaninglessly high. Yet nature has provided a beautiful setting that allows the neutrophil to fine tune its response to a specific task. *A priori*, there would be two reasons for having different subsets of granules: One would be to ensure that proteins, which cannot coexist, are segregated, that is, protease-sensitive proteins are separated from proteases. The other reason would be to have proteins whose service is needed at one time separated from proteins whose service is needed at a different time.

Heterogeneity of Neutrophil Granules

Among the peroxidase-positive granules, subsets can be identified that are rich in defensins as well as some that are not.[52,53] Functionally, no difference has been identified in terms of the regulation of exocytosis of these peroxidase-positive granule subsets.[54] Other constituents include the serine proteases elastase, cathepsin G, and proteinase 3, and the inactive serine protease azurocidin (or CAP 37), the antimicrobial proteins BPI, lysozyme, and the α-defensins, which are the dominating species.[50] Defensins are also named HNPs (human neutrophil peptides). The membrane of the azurophil granules contains CD63 (granulophysin) and CD67, but their role in neutrophil function remains unclear.[55,56] It is characteristic that many of the proteins present in peroxidase granules are proteolytically processed both at the N-terminus and the C-terminus to the active mature forms, which are stored in the granule matrix. The processing seems to take place in the trans Golgi. N-terminal processing is mediated by cathepsin C, lack of which is characteristic of the Papillon-Lefèvre syndrome.[57–60]

Peroxidase-negative granules can be divided into three subsets based on the distribution of the two marker proteins lactoferrin and gelatinase: granules that contain lactoferrin, but no gelatinase (15% of peroxidase negative granules), granules that contain both proteins (60%), and granules that are rich in gelatinase, but low (or absent) in lactoferrin (25%).[61] The latter are named gelatinase granules or tertiary granules, whereas those that contain lactoferrin are called specific or secondary granules. The specific granules can be further subdivided onto those that contain CRISP3 and those that do not.[62] It is a characteristic of peroxidase-negative granules that the proteins present in their matrix are not proteolytically processed. The matrix metalloproteinases of peroxidase-negative granules are stored as a proform,[63] as is the major bactericidal protein hCAP18.[64,65] No major differences have been identified in the content of membrane proteins of the peroxidase-negative granule subsets. All contain the flavocytochrome $p47^{phox}/gp91^{phox}$ complex that is part of the nicotinamide adenine dinucleotide phosphate (NADPH) oxidase, and all contain the major β_2-integrin $\alpha_M\beta_2$—and these are even shared with the membrane of secretory vesicles.[20,66,67] The divalent cation transporter Nramp1 is localized only to gelatinase granules,[68] and the membrane matrix metalloproteinase leukolysin (MMP-25)[69] is shared between gelatinase granules and secretory vesicles. However, the subsets differ markedly in their propensity for exocytosis. Following neutrophil stimulation, gelatinase granules are exocytosed to a larger extent than granules containing both lactoferrin and gelatinase, and these are more readily mobilized than granules containing lactoferrin but lacking gelatinase. These, in turn, are mobilized more readily than peroxidase-positive granules.[31,35,48,61,70] This organization of granule subsets with different content and differently setpoints to trigger exocytosis allows the neutrophil to mobilize matrix metalloproteinases and integrins necessary for movement through the basal membrane and tissue before the bactericidal peptides and serine protease are called to play, but it puts an enormous task on the organization of the biosynthetic apparatus to secure that the right granule proteins are targeted to the granules with a given trigger for exocytosis.

Targeting by Biosynthetic Timing

The extreme heterogeneity of neutrophil granules and their individual control of exocytosis can be explained simply by timing of their biosynthesis. Granule proteins are synthesized during myelopoiesis from myeloblasts to band cells and segmented neutrophils in the marrow.[44,45,71] The window of biosynthesis of each granule protein is highly individually controlled by combinations of transcription factors that change as the cells differentiate and mature.[72,73] If all granule proteins are targeted to granules during synthesis, the content of newly formed granules would change as the cell matures because the profile of biosynthesis changes. A global view of the change in transcriptional activity of neutrophil precursors during maturation in the marrow confirmed the association between granule localization and transcriptional activity.[74] This simple mechanism largely explains the heterogeneity of granules[75] and their contents, but it does not account for the differences in exocytotic rates among individualized subsets. By timing the biosynthesis of the proteins essential for fusion[76,77] to granules membranes during maturation, it is possible to regulate the rates of exocytosis. Indeed the v-SNARE, vesicle-associated membrane protein (VAMP)-2 is present in a higher density on gelatinase granules than on specific granules and is most highly expressed on secretory vesicles,[78,79] which correlates with the ease of releasing granule subsets from the neutrophil following activation.

Sorting Between the Constitutive and Regulated Exocytotic Pathway

Although the sorting by timing can explain the granule heterogeneity of neutrophil granules, it does not provide any clues to the mechanisms responsible for diverting newly synthesized proteins to granules as opposed to immediate (constitutive) secretion. Not all granule proteins are equally efficiently directed to granules. Lysozyme is poorly retained during biosynthesis.[80] This explains the high concentration of lysozyme in plasma.[81] MPO is efficiently retained and the plasma level of MPO is consequently very low. A particular interesting observation pertains to α-defensins. These are localized exclusively to azurophil granules, but their window of biosynthesis is very similar to that of lactoferrin,[80,73] and defensins and lactoferrin are both controlled by the transcription factor C/EBPε (CCAAT/enhancer binding protein ε), which is absolutely required for biosynthesis of specific granule proteins.[82,83] The absence of defensins from specific granules, despite an active biosynthesis when other specific granule proteins are formed, is explained by a complete lack of sorting of defensins to granules in myelocytes.[72,73,80] Only defensins synthesized at the late promyelocytic stage are routed to granules, whereas defensins synthesized at the myelocyte stage are secreted from cells after biosynthesis.[80] The defensins that are targeted to granules are processed to mature defensins, whereas the defensins that are secreted remain unprocessed. Because the processing of defensins removes a charge neutralizing propiece, it may be that sorting of defensins and other granule proteins to granules depends on their ability to interact with negatively charged proteoglycans that are present in the matrix of granules.[84,85] Serglycin, an intracellular proteoglycan is present in Golgi and immature granules of promyelocytes and disappears as the cells mature.[86] Serglycin is absolutely critical for confining a variety of mast cell proteins to the mast cell granules.[87] Granulocytes from mice with a targeted disruption of the serglycin gene are morphologically normal and contain normal levels of granule proteins except elastase.[88] CD63 was demonstrated to be involved in sorting of elastase to azurophil granules,[89] but this may be indirectly via serglycin. An N-terminal sorting domain has been identified in serglycin and was shown to be essential for routing of serglycin to mast cell granules.[90] No common denominator has been identified that can fully explain why neutrophil proteins are sorted to granules. Perhaps the lack of efficient sorting to granules may not solely be taken as inefficiency, but may be a way to secure a desirable level of antibiotic protein such as lysozyme in plasma,[81] which renders the myeloid cells of the marrow a major secretory organ.

Control of Neutrophil Granule Protein Expression

The biosynthesis of neutrophil granule proteins is controlled at the transcriptional and not the translational level as there is complete congruence between protein biosynthesis and messenger ribonucleic acid (mRNA) levels during myelopoiesis where this has been investigated (Fig. 66–3).[71–73] Not all transcription factors that are responsible for biosynthesis of granule protein have been identified, and the role of an individual transcription factor may be difficult to identify from gene knockout studies as transcription factors may work at multiple stages during myelopoiesis. The transcription factor PU.1 is essential for myelopoiesis because knockout mice do not form myeloid progenitors beyond myeloblasts[91,92]; but this does not preclude PU.1 from regulating transcription of individual granule proteins at a later stage of development.[93–96] Figure 66–3 shows the profile of important myeloid transcription factors during maturation of normal myeloid cells in the marrow *in vivo*. RUNX1 (AML-1), c-myb, CASP, C/EBPα, C/EBPγ, GATA-1, and Elf-1 gene products are all strongly expressed in the myeloblast and promyelocyte, and some of these have been shown to be required for azurophil granule protein expression. Then c-myb, AML-1, GATA-1, and ELF-1 gene products are downregulated as the cells enter the myelocyte stage, heralded by a brisk and transient upregulation of C/EBPε to initiate expression of peroxidase-negative granule proteins[72] in agreement with the lack of specific granules in C/EBPε –/– mice and with the observation of a C/EBPε mutation in patients with the rare specific granule deficiency.[82,83,97,98] PU.1, C/EBPβ, and C/EBPδ also appear at the promyelocyte myelocyte transition, but in contrast to C/EBPε, continue to increase as the cells mature to neutrophils. ELF-1 reappears at the metamyelocyte stage followed by C/EBP-ξ, c-jun, and c-fos that are expressed at the band cell stage and increase in content as the cells mature.[72] Expression of the myeloid specific microRNA-223 increases during maturation of neutrophils in the marrow, and even once released into the circulating. One of the targets of miR-223 is the *Mef2c* transcription factor. Mice that lack miR-223 expand granulopoiesis and the mature neutrophils mount an enhanced respiratory burst in response to phorbol myristate acetate (PMA), indicating that miR-223 acts as a negative regulator of granulopoiesis and neutrophil activation.[99]

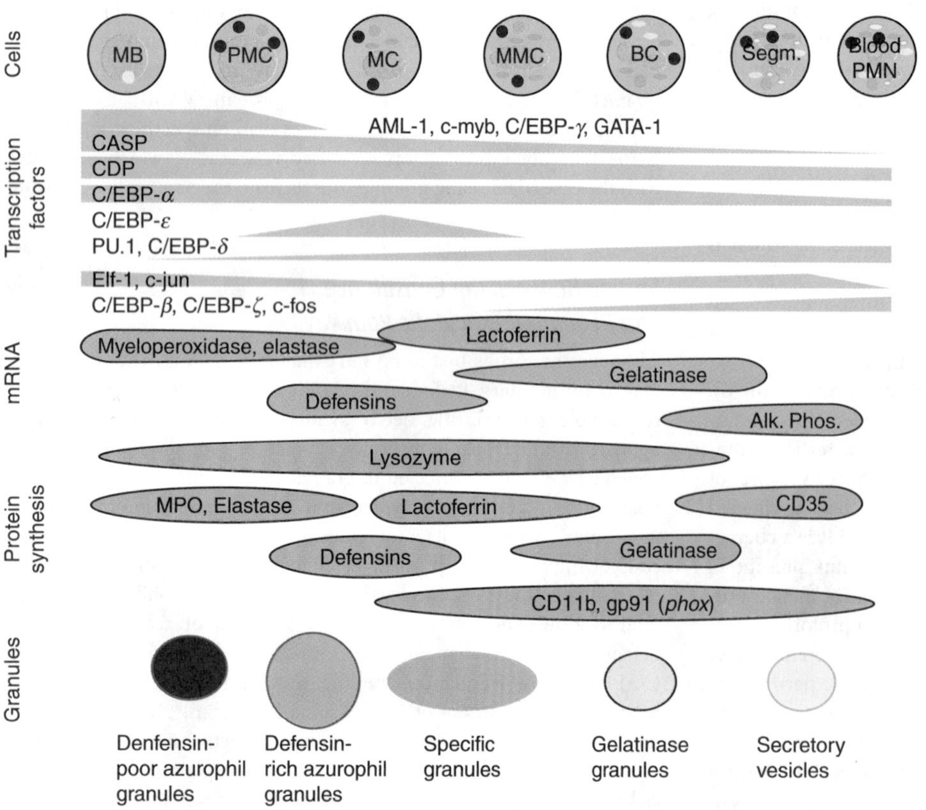

FIGURE 66–3. Formation of granule subsets during myelopoiesis and regulation of granule protein transcription. Difference in the appearance and disappearance of transcription factors regulate the individual window of granule protein gene transcription and translation into protein that is targeted to forming granules, explaining the heterogeneity of neutrophil granules.

FUNCTION OF INDIVIDUAL GRANULE PROTEINS AND THEIR ROLE IN OXIDATIVE AND NONODIXATIVE MICROBIAL KILLING

Proteins of Azurophil Granules

Table 66–1 lists the physical-chemical and functional properties of neutrophil granules.

The protein MPO is a marker of azurophil granules. It is formed as a 90-kDa precursor with an internal disulphide bridge that forms a link between the 57- and the 13.5-kDa subunits that are generated by the proteolytic processing that takes place during routing to granules. The heme group, which is necessary for the redox functions of MPO, associates with the 90-kDa subunit.[100] This seems to be a necessary prerequisite for subsequent processing.[101] MPO reacts with H_2O_2, formed by the NADPH oxidase, and increases the toxic potential of this oxidant. Through oxidation of chloride, tyrosine, and nitrite, the H_2O_2-MPO system induces formation of hypochlorous acid (HOCl), other chlorination products, tyrosine radicals, and reactive nitrogen intermediates, all of which can attack the surface membrane of microorganisms.[102,103]

MPO may be found on endothelial cells during inflammation and can inactivate

TABLE 66–1. Physical-Chemical and Functional Properties of Neutrophil Granules

Granule Protein	Localization	Physicochemical Properties	Function
Myeloperoxidase	Azurophil granule (AG)	Heme protein, 90 kDa proform with an internal disulphide bond between the 57- and the 13.5-kDa subunits, generated by proteolytic processing that takes place during routing to granules	The MPO-halide-H_2O_2 system generates hypochlorous acid (HOCl), other chlorination products, tyrosine radicals, and reactive nitrogen intermediates, all off which can attack the surface membrane of microorganisms
Bacterial permeability-increasing (BPI) protein	AG	55-kDa protein with high homology to the LPS-binding protein of plasma	BPI is organized into two largely symmetrical subdomains one of which is responsible for the binding of LPS and for the antimicrobial activity against Gram-negative microorganisms
Defensins: three α-defensins HNP 1–3	AG	7-kDa proforms processed by proteolytic cleavage to mature 3-kDa defensins that share a characteristic three disulfide bond motif: 1–6, 2–4, 3–5	Defensins are small, amphipathic, pore-forming, anti-bacterial cationic peptides with a broad spectrum of antibacterial activity
Serine proteases of azurophil granules: elastase, cathepsin G, and proteinase 3; azurocidin (CAP37 or heparin-binding protein [HBP]) is enzymatically inactive	AG	28-kDa proforms, processed to active proteases en route to azurophil granules	Serine proteases, but both elastase and cathepsin G have direct antibacterial activities that are not dependent on their enzymatic activity; proteinase 3 liberates the anti-bacterial peptide LL37 from hCAP18; HBP is chemotactic for monocytes; HBP may open endothelial cell tight junctions
Lysozyme	AG ~30%; specific granules (SG) ~50%; gelatinase granules (GG) ~20%	Cationic antimicrobial peptide of 14 kDa; in contrast to many neutrophil granule proteins, lysozyme is inefficiently targeted to granules and circulates free in plasma in a substantial quantity that reflects the normal myelopoietic activity	Lysozyme cleaves peptidoglycan-polymers of bacterial cell walls and displays bactericidal activity towards the nonpathogenic Gram-positive bacteria *Bacillus subtilis*; a particular high serum level is characteristic for the myelomonocytic leukemias
Lactoferrin	SG	78-kDa iron chelator; member of the transferrin protein family with a high affinity for iron and similar iron-binding characteristics as ferritin	The antibacterial activity of lactoferrin does not depend exclusively on its ability to sequester iron. Proteolytic fragments, some of which are known as lactoferricin, are directly bactericidal
Neutrophil-gelatinase-associated lipocalin (NGAL) or siderochelin	SG	25-kDa N-glycosylated member of the lipocalin protein family	NGAL is the first known siderophore-binding eukaryotic protein; NGAL binds enterochelin/enterobactin with high affinity, and blocks growth of *Escherichia coli* by sequestering siderophore-iron complexes
hCAP18	SG	18 kDa; only human member of the cathelicidin protein family	Stored and released intact; binds endotoxin; C-terminal antibactericidal peptide, LL-37 released by proteinase 3; active mainly against Gram-positive bacteria, is chemotactic for T cells, monocytes, and neutrophils and has angiogenetic properties
Neutrophil collagenase	SG	75-kDa matrix metalloproteinase 8 (MMP-8); like other MMPs, MMP-8 is stored inactive and must be N-terminally trimmed to remove the inhibitory peptide	Active against types I, II, and III collagen
Gelatinase	GG	92-kDa matrix metalloproteinase 9 (MMP-9); stored inactive	Active against type IV collagen
Leukolysin, which is distributed among of resting neutrophils	SG ~10%; GG ~40%; secretory vesicles (SV) ~30%; plasma membranes (PM) ~20%	Leukolysin is a 56-kDa GPI-anchored membrane-bound matrix metalloproteinase (MT6-MMP/MMP-25)	Active against fibronectin, chondroitin sulfate proteoglycan, dermatan sulfate proteoglycan
Cytochrome b_{558}, ($gp91^{phox}$, $p22^{phox}$)	SG ~60%; GG ~25%; SV ~15%	Heterodimeric flavoheme protein; 91-kDa glycoprotein subunit (heme-flavin binding); 22 kDa protein subunit, possibly heme binding	Together with $p47^{phox}$, $p67^{phox}$, and $p40^{phox}$, cytochrome b_{558} constitutes the superoxide generating NADPH oxidase of phagocytes

(*continued*)

TABLE 66–1. Physical-Chemical and Functional Properties of Neutrophil Granules (Continued)

Granule Protein	Localization	Physicochemical Properties	Function
CD11b/CD18 (Mac-1, Mo1, CR3, $\alpha_M\beta_2$)	SG ~60%; GG ~25%; SV ~15%	Most prominent β_2-integrin in neutrophils; CD11B = α_M is a glycoprotein of 170 kDa; CD18 = β_2 is a glycoprotein of 95 kDa	Multifunctional integrin that functions as an adhesion receptor binding to members of the immunoglobulin family ICAM-1, to fibronectin, collagen; is important in mediating firm adhesion to vascular endothelial cells; functions as a phagocytosis receptor for C3bi-coated particles
Pentraxin-3	SG	Pentamer of 47-kDa subunits	Binds complement C1q, selected microorganisms
Ficolin-1	GG	Multimer of 32-kDa subunits	Binds acetylated carbohydrates on microorganisms; may activate mannose-binding lectin-associated serine proteases.
Arginase 1	GG	37-kDa glycoprotein	Degrades arginine, the substrate for NO synthase

NO.[104] In addition to the activities of MPO itself, MPO is known for the anti-MPO autoantibodies that are characteristic of the pANCA (perinuclear antineutrophil cytoplasmic antibodies) that are found in vasculitides, in particular those that primarily affect kidneys.[105,106]

Bacterial permeability-increasing protein (BPI) is a 55-kDa protein with high homology to the LPS-binding protein of plasma. It is organized into two largely symmetrical subdomains one of which is responsible for the binding of LPS and for the antimicrobial activity against Gram-negative microorganisms. In contrast to LPS-binding protein, which presents endotoxin to CD14 and elicits a proinflammatory response, BPI binds LPS independent of CD14 and neutralizes the effects of LPS.[107] A transgene expressing high levels of BPI has enhanced resistance against endotoxin.[108]

Defensins are small antibacterial cationic peptides with a broad spectrum of antibacterial activity.[109] They share a characteristic three-disulfide-bond motif.[52,110,111] Based on this, mammalian defensins are divided into α defensins, β defensins, and the cyclical θ defensins.[112] Only α defensins are found in human neutrophils, and reside exclusively in azurophil granules. They are by far the dominating proteins of azurophil granules, yet are only expressed in a subset of granules that are formed late in the promyelocyte stage.[53,73,80] Three defensins have been isolated from azurophil granules, HNP 1 to 3.[52]

The serine proteases of azurophil granules include three major serine proteases present in azurophil granules, elastase, cathepsin G, and proteinase-3. Azurocidin, which is also named CAP37 or heparin-binding protein (HBP), is a fourth but enzymatically inactive serine protease.[113–117] Both elastase and cathepsin G have direct antibacterial activities that are not dependent on their enzymatic activity. Proteinase 3 expression leads to autoantibodies against itself in Wegener granulomatosis, which is known as cANCA (cytoplasmic antineutrophil cytoplasmic antibody).[118] Proteinase 3 is also bound to the surface of circulating neutrophils at levels that vary considerably amongst individuals but are highly constant throughout life in a given individual. The binding is mediated by the NB1 antigen.[119,120] A secreted precursor of proteinase 3 has been suggested to inhibit normal myelopoiesis[121] and to play a role in regulation of myelopoiesis. So far, the only specific substrate of proteinase 3 identified is the cathelicidin of specific granules hCAP18. Proteinase 3 activates hCAP18 by removing the cathelicidin part, and unleashing the antibacterial activity of the C-terminal LL37 peptide.[65]

The membrane of azurophil granules contains CD63 (granulophysin), which is implicated in transmembrane signaling with the β_2 integrins in the activated neutrophil.[55,56,122] Also, the CD68 antigen[73,123] and presenilin appear localized exclusively to the membrane of azurophil granules,[124] whereas stromatin is found in the membrane of all granules,[125] and the vacuolar-type H^+-ATPase is shared between azurophil, gelatinase granules and secretory vesicles.[126] These membrane proteins will translocate to the phagocytic vacuole or to the plasma membrane when neutrophils are activated and engaged in phagocytosis.

Proteins of Peroxidase-Negative Granules

See Table 66–1.

Lactoferrin is the dominating protein of specific granules.[127] It is a 78-kDa iron-chelator, member of the transferrin protein family with a high affinity for iron and similar binding characteristics as ferritin.[128,129] The antibacterial activity of lactoferrin does not depend exclusively on its ability to sequester iron because proteolytic fragments of lactoferrin, some of which are known as lactoferricin, are directly bactericidal.[130,131]

NGAL, or siderocalin, is a 25-kDa N-glycosylated member of the lipocalin protein family.[49] Lipocalins are transport proteins that bind small and often lipophilic substances in their canonical lipocalin pocket.[132] Some NGAL is associated with gelatinase (MMP-9) in a subset of specific granules,[133] but the majority is present either as a monomer or as a homodimer in specific granules. NGAL interferes with the activation and stability of matrix metalloproteinases,[134] but the major activity of NGAL is its binding of siderophores. NGAL binds enterochelin/enterobactin with high affinity, and blocks growth of *Escherichia coli* by sequestering siderophore-iron complexes,[135] which might not be only a neutrophil-specific antibacterial defense because NGAL can be induced in a variety of epithelial cells during inflammation by IL-1.[136]

Nramp1, the cation transporter, was initially identified first in macrophages as an essential resistance factor against mycobacterial infection. It is present in membranes of both specific and gelatinase granules.[68,137]

Lysozyme is a cationic antimicrobial peptide of 14 kDa.[138] In agreement with its biosynthetic profile, lysozyme is present in all granule subsets, with peak concentrations in specific granules.[73,81] Lysozyme cleaves peptidoglycan polymers of bacterial cell walls and displays bactericidal activity towards the nonpathogenic Gram-positive bacteria *Bacillus subtilis*.[139] Lysozyme also binds LPS[140] and reduces cytokine production and mortality caused by LPS in a murine model system of septic shock.[141] In contrast to many neutrophil granule proteins, lysozyme is inefficiently targeted to granules and circulates free in plasma in a substantial quantity that reflects the normal granulopoietic activity.[80,81] Lysozyme is also secreted from activated macrophages,[142] and a particular elevated serum level is characteristic of the leukemias with a large proportion of monocytes.[143]

hCAP18,[64] also known as LL37[144] or CAMP, is the only human member of a family of antimicrobial peptides known as cathelicidins. Cathelicidins are typically found in peroxidase-negative granules of mammalian neutrophils.[145] hCAP18 is a prominent protein of neutrophil specific granules present in equimolar concentrations with lactoferrin.[146] It is also present in plasma at a substantial concentration bound to lipoproteins.[147] In general, cathelicidins are proantibiotic peptides that share a common and highly conserved 14-kDa N-terminal region known as the cathelin region; whereas, the C-terminal regions vary extensively among the different cathelicidins. The C-terminal peptides must be liberated from the cathelin part by proteolysis to become antibacterial. In most species this is carried out by elastase, but in human neutrophils this is done by proteinase 3 from azurophil granules. The liberated C-terminal peptide is known as LL37.[65,144] Like several other neutrophil proteins, hCAP18 is formed by cells in other tissues, and in particular epithelial cells.[65,148–150] It is constitutively expressed in the testis and present in semen. The activating protease is gastricin, a prostate protease that is active at low pH. This cleaves hCAP18 to ALL38, which has the same antibacterial spectrum as LL37.[151] The cathelin part, which is released has some protease inhibitory activity by itself.[152] The LL37 has been shown to stimulate neutrophil, monocyte, and T-cell chemotaxis via the formyl peptide receptor-like-1.[153] In addition, hCAP18/LL37 has angiogenic[154] and endotoxin-neutralizing properties.[155]

Three MMPs have been identified in neutrophils: neutrophil collagenase (MMP-8,75 kDa), which is located to specific granules,[156] gelatinase (MMP-9, 92 kDa), which resides predominantly in gelatinase granules,[157,48] and leukolysin (MT6-MMP/MMP-25, 56 kDa), which is distributed among specific granules (~10%), gelatinase granules (~40%), secretory vesicles (~30%), and the plasma membrane (~20%) of resting neutrophils.[69,158] The MMPs are stored as inactive proforms that are proteolytically activated following exocytosis. Together, the MMPs are capable of degrading major structural components of the extracellular matrix, including collagens, fibronectin, proteoglycans, and laminin, and they are believed to be of central importance for the degradation of vascular basal membranes and interstitial structures during neutrophil extravasation and migration.

CRISP-3 is a novel cysteine-rich protein identified in peroxidase negative granules; it is located in a subset of granules that contain both lactoferrin and gelatinase. So far, no function has been ascribed to CRISP-3.[62]

Two pattern-recognition molecules are found in specific granules and gelatinase granules respectively: pentraxin 3 and ficolin1. Pentraxin 3, a member of the long pentraxins family, is synthesized in myelocytes and metamyelocytes and stored in specific granules of neutrophils. Pentraxin-3 binds the complement component C1q and mediates activation of the classical complement cascade. In addition, pentraxin-3 binds *Klebsiella pneumoniae* outer membrane protein A (KpOmpA) from Gram-negative bacteria especially the *Enterobacteriaceae* species, and binds *Aspergillus fumigatus* conidia. Pentraxin-3 was shown to play a major role in uptake and killing of *A. fumigatus* conidia by neutrophils in a mouse model.[159,160]

Ficolin-1 is present in gelatinase granules. Ficolin-1 binds acetylated carbohydrate structures on Gram-positive bacteria and can recruit mannose-binding lectin-associated serine proteases (MASPs) and activate the lectin complement cascade.[161]

Arginase-1 is a constituent of gelatinase granules[162] and may participate in regulation of T-cell activities by removing arginine, the essential substrate for inducible nitrous oxide synthase. The product proline is essential for collagen synthesis and arginase-1 from neutrophils may thus support wound healing.[163]

Membrane proteins of peroxidase-negative granules are shared among the subsets of peroxidase-negative granules that can be distinguished based on their matrix proteins; that is, specific and azurophil granules. Two exceptions are Nramp1 and MMP-25, which are both present, predominantly in the membrane of gelatinase granules and secretory vesicles.[68,69] Cytochrome b_{558}, which is comprised of gp91*phox* and p22*phox*, forms the membrane component of the NADPH oxidase and is a prominent membrane protein of peroxidase-negative granules.[51,164] It codistributes with the major β_2-integrin of neutrophils CD11b/CD18, with the major part in specific granules, some in gelatinase granules, and some in secretory vesicles. It should be kept in mind that secretory vesicles are rapidly mobilized, and even though only 15 percent of the total cytochrome b_{588} and CD11b localizes to secretory vesicles, this is the fraction that is primarily translocated to the plasma membrane during neutrophil diapesis.[35,20] The CD66 antigens found in the membrane of specific granules may play a role as bacterial receptors (galectin receptors) and generate signals to activate the NADPH oxidase.[165,166]

STIMULUS-RESPONSE COUPLING BY NEUTROPHILS

Stimulus-response coupling by neutrophils has been the subject of intense research for many years. This work has been fruitful in illuminating some of the underlying causes of defects in cell activation. Studies of neutrophil degranulation and oxidative metabolism have also revealed transduction mechanisms common to a wide variety of other important secretory cell types, thereby greatly expanding the relevance of this work. This chapter considers next our current understanding of the activation process, which is shown schematically in Figure 66–4.

The G-protein $\beta\gamma$ subunits may also activate phosphatidyl inositol kinase-γ(PI3-Kγ), which can phosphorylate $PtdInsP_2$ to phosphatidylinositol trisphosphate ($PtdInsP_3$). $PtdInsP_3$ can also trigger the activation of protein kinases, for example, recruit and activate protein kinase B/Akt and PKCδ and ζ. Downstream signaling by PI3-K is generally considered to be mediated by molecules with a pleckstrin homology (PH) domain, which serves as a binding domain for polyphosphorylated phosphoinositides.

Ligation of integrins or Fc-receptors with their ligand leads to activation of proteins tyrosine kinases (PTK) of which *Syk* is prominent. In turn, *Syk* may further activate PI3-K and the immunoreceptor tyrosine-base motifs (ITAMs) located on the cytoplasmic domain of Fc receptors. $PtdInsP_3$ can activate VAV, a guaine-nucleotide-exchange factor (GEF). VAV could then activate the guanosine triphosphatases (GTPases) such as Rac or CDC42. Rac-2 is involved in NADPH activation, whereas, Rac-1 is involved in chemotaxis and degranulation. Growth factor receptors (GFRs) signal through Janus kinases (JAKs), which bind to and phosphorylate tyrosine kinases, which, in turn, activate the transcription factors STAT, leading to further activation of pathways mediated by the son of sevenless (SOS).

Activation of receptors often result in movement of these into detergent in soluble phospholipid domains (RAFT) and further enhance signal transduction. This appears to be especially important for FcR, which upon activation employs the RAF, RAS, and mitogen-activated protein kinase (MAPK) pathways to initiate phagosome formation.

RECEPTOR-LIGAND INTERACTIONS

Formyl Peptide Receptor

Neutrophil responses can be evoked by a variety of particulate and soluble stimuli. Opsonized particles, immune complexes, chemokine and chemotactic factors produced during the inflammatory process activate

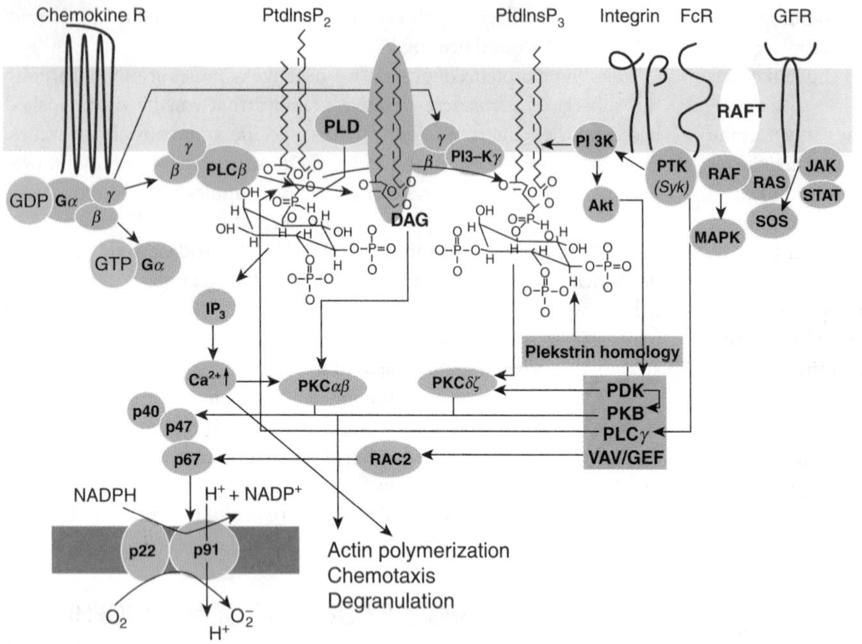

FIGURE 66–4. Signal transduction in neutrophils. G protein-coupled receptors are seven transmembrane receptors that couple to heterotrimeric guanosine triphosphate (GTP)-binding (G) proteins. Agonist binding to the receptor triggers exchange of guanine diphosphate (GDP) for guanine triphosphate (GTP) on the Gα-subunit of the G-protein, and consequently, the disassociation of the *a* subunit for the *βg*-dimer. Both subunits can regulate the activity of multiple effectors such as phospholipase *Cβ* (PLC*β*). PLC*β* cleaves an endogenous lipid, namely phosphatidylinositol bisphosphate ($PtdInsP_2$), yielding diacylglycerol (DAG) and inositol trisphosphate (IP_3). IP_3 is known to liberate calcium from bound intracellular stores leading to a rise in intracellular-free calcium (Ca^{2+})i. The increase in intracellular Ca^{2+} is augmented by an influx of Ca^{2+} from the extracellular space. Increased DAG, in concert with elevated Ca^{2+} can activate protein kinase isozymes *α* and *β* (PKC*αβ*) leading to their translocation to membranous sites. Phospholipase D (PLD) can be activated by PKC converting phosphatidylcholine to phosphatidic (PA) acid. Elevations in PA can mobilize the cytosolic proteins, p47, p67*phox*, and p40*phox* to bind to the membrane-bound proteins gp91*phox* and p22*phox*, which then reduces O_2 to O_{2^-} in the presence of NADPH.

neutrophils by binding to specific cell surface receptors. Of the neutrophil chemotactic receptors, the *N*-formyl peptide receptor is the best characterized. *N*-formyl peptide, the synthetic analogues of bacterial *N*-formyl peptide products, induces a variety of neutrophil responses and has been extensively employed as activating stimuli. Specific receptors for the chemotactic peptide, *N*-formyl-methionyl-leucyl-phenylalanine (fMet-Leu-Phe), have been identified on the neutrophil surface,[167] and binding of the formyl peptide to its receptor correlates with its ability to induce chemotaxis and degranulation.[168] The formyl peptide receptor has been cloned and sequenced[169] and belongs to a family of seven membrane-spanning domain proteins typical of G-protein-coupled receptors. The receptor occurs in several forms, is physically associated with guanine nucleotide binding proteins (G proteins), and the cytoskeleton (see ref. 170 for review). The receptor is highly glycosylated and has a Mr of 50 to 70 kDa. It has been identified on the membranes of gelatinase granules and secretory vesicles, and shown to be mobilized to the cell surface following stimulation.[171]

C5a Receptor

Activation of the complement system generates C5a, a derivative of C5 and the most potent of the chemotactic proteins. C5a induces neutrophil chemotaxis, degranulation, and superoxide generation.[172] Responses to C5a result from interactions with specific receptors on the cell surface.[173] The receptor was identified as a single polypeptide in the plasma membrane with an apparent mass of 40 to 48 kDa.[174] Binding studies show that there are 50,000 to 113,000 receptor sites per cell with a dissociation constant (Kd) of 2×10^{-9} M. The C5a receptor has been isolated and cloned, and is a member of the seven membrane-spanning class of G-protein-coupled receptors.[175]

C3 Receptors

Neutrophils also express receptors for the complement-derived chemotactic factors C3b and C3bi. Receptors for C3b and C3bi (also known as CR1 and CR3, respectively) are sparse on resting neutrophils, but increase significantly in numbers following activation with several stimuli because of incorporation from secretory vesicles (CR1 and CR3) and gelatinase and specific granules (CR3).[20,40] The C3b receptor (CR1) is a glycoprotein with a molecular weight of 205 kDa and is located in secretory vesicles.[40,34]

Integrins

CD11/CD18 integrins also play an important role in cell signaling. The adhesion of cells to surfaces or to other cells can either activate neutrophils directly or "prime" them for an enhanced response to other stimuli. For example, the oxidative burst of neutrophils is very different in cells that are suspended versus those that are adherent to surfaces.[176] H_2O_2 production in response to chemotaxins is influenced by monoclonal antibodies to CD11b, but not CD11a.[177]

Fc Receptors

Neutrophils possess three different receptors for immunoglobulins. Unstimulated cells express FcγRIIA and FcγRIII, also known as CD32 and CD16, respectively. Functionally, the most important of the two is the FcγRIII for clearing immune complexes,[178] and it is attached to the membrane by a GPI linkage.[178] The linkage is relatively labile, so the amount of FcγRIII on the membrane reflects a balance between shedding and mobilization from intracellular stores. FcγRIIA is a conventional protein that spans the plasma membrane.[179] The signal transduction pathways initiated by FcγRIII can crosstalk with the formyl peptide receptor, with CR3, and even with each other. A direct physical linkage between CD11b and FcγRIIIB has been demonstrated by experiments in which capping of one receptor results in co-capping a substantial fraction of the other receptor. CD11b can also interact with the transmembrane FcγRII, and both of these molecules can modify each other's signals.[180]

The SH2-domain containing tyrosine kinase (*Syk*), plays a critical role in the phagocytic pathway mediated by FcγRIIA.[181] A cytoplasmic amino acid motif, known as immunoreceptor tyrosine-based activation motif (ITAM), is present on FcγRIIA and FcγRI/γ(a receptor found on interferon-γ-stimulated myeloid cells) and is essential for the phagocytic response during crosslinking of these two Fc receptors. Binding of Src family protein tyrosine kinases to the ITAM leads to activation of Src family protein tyrosine kinases and ITAM tyrosine phosphorylation. This serves to recruit phosphatidylinositol-3 kinase and *Syk*, which when activated phosphorylates multiple substrates including neighboring ITAMs. *Syk* is recruited from the cytosolic pool. The essential role for *Syk*-affecting signal transduction is reflected by ITAM-dependent activation of actin assembly. Other tyrosine kinases, including Src kinases, especially Lyn, facilitate the formation of the phagosome.[182] Once active microfilaments are formed, they enhance the activity of phospholipase D (PLD) to generate phosphatidic acid (PA), a necessary phospholipid for phagocytosis to ensue.[183,184]

Other Receptors

Three other important G-protein-coupled receptors are for PAF, IL-8, and LTB_4. PAF and IL-8 receptors have been cloned.[185,186] Their intracellular stores and signal transduction mechanisms are largely similar to those used by other G-protein-coupled receptors (e.g., fMLP).[185] IL-8 has two related receptors, for which slightly different signal transduction pathways have been detected.[187]

Toll-Like Receptors

TLRs in general bind pathogen-associated molecular patterns; that is, structures that are "relatively" unique to pathogens and shared among groups of pathogens such as lipopolysaccharide of Gram-negative bacteria. As mentioned previously, TLRs are activated by dimerization induced by ligand binding. The TLRs may dimerize both as homodimers and heterodimers. TLR2 recognizes lipoproteins and lipopeptides in association with either TLR1 or TLR6. TLR4 binds LPS. CD14 is known as an LPS-binding protein but is not itself able to signal and probably presents LPS to TLR4.[188] TLR5 binds flagellin. TLR3 (not present in neutrophils) recognizes double-stranded RNA. TLR7/8 bind viral single-stranded RNA,[189] TLR9 binds unmethylated GpC regions on DNA,[190] and TLR11 binds profilin-like proteins of protozoa.[191] TLR10 does not exist.

G Proteins

The receptors for the chemotactic stimuli, fMet-Leu-Phe, C5a, LTB_4, and PAF are all coupled to cellular responses through a guanine-nucleotide-binding protein similar to the inhibitory protein, Gi, of the adenylate cyclase system. Evidence linking a G protein to these receptors has been provided by studies demonstrating that guanine nucleotides can regulate receptor affinity.[192] A high-affinity guanosine triphosphatase (GTPase) located in neutrophil plasma membranes is stimulated by these same receptor-mediated stimuli.[193] This enzymatic activity is likely to be involved in terminating the activation of the guanine-nucleotide-binding protein. Also, direct linkages between receptors and G proteins have been observed.[169]

Studies using pertussis toxin have proven instrumental in the understanding of G protein involvement in the proposed stimulus–response coupling pathway. Pertussis toxin ADP ribosylates the α subunit of Gi of the adenylate cyclase system and also a 40- to 41-kDa protein in neutrophil plasma membranes.[194] Initial studies demonstrated a strong correlation between the ability of the toxin to catalyze the ADP ribosylation of the membrane protein and its ability to affect cellular responses initiated by surface receptors. Further characterization of a guanine-nucleotide-binding protein in neutrophils indicate that this protein differs both structurally and immunochemically from previously reported guanine-nucleotide-binding proteins.[195] Not only can neutrophil responses be abolished by pertussis toxin, but stable guanine nucleotides can directly stimulate permeabilized neutrophils.[196] In other cells, heterotrimeric G proteins may also play a tonic inhibitory role in degranulation.[197] Although pertussis toxin inhibits fMet-Leu-Phe–induced secretion from intact cells, it does not inhibit degranulation in response to phorbol myristate acetate (PMA), Ca^{2+}, and guanine nucleotides in the permeabilized cell system, suggesting that a second G-protein is involved at distal sites in secretion.[196] Potential candidates in this role are the family of small G proteins (with a Mr of 20 to 30 kDa) that has been reported in neutrophils. Some of these proteins include the RhoA and ADP-ribosylation factor (ARF)-1 among others that are probably involved in vesicular traffic and have been reported to translocate from cytosol to granules following neutrophil stimulation.[198]

Phospolipid Metabolism and Tyrosine Kinase Activation

The next step in signal transduction can be attributed to interactions of receptor-activated G proteins or through FcγRIIA and tyrosine kinases with phospholipases.[199,200] For instance, a membrane-associated phosphoinositide-specific phospholipase is activated upon stimulation with chemotactic stimuli. In particular, phospholipase C hydrolyzes phosphatidylinositol-4,5-bisphosphate (PIP_2) and phosphatidyl inositol-4-monophosphate (PIP_1) to the putative second-messenger products inositol 1,4,5-trisphosphate (IP_3) and 1,2-diacylglycerol (DAG).[201] In permeabilized neutrophils, IP_3 interacts with a specific intracellular receptor and stimulates the release of Ca^{2+}, as well as opens Ca^{2+} channels on the plasma membrane, resulting in rises in intracellular Ca^{2+}.[202] Activation of the small guanosine triphosphate (GTP)-binding proteins of the Rac, Rho, and Cdc42 families regulates actin-dependent processes such as membrane ruffling, formation of pseudopodia, and stress fibers leading to cell adhesion and motility, and appears critical in neutrophil function,[203,204] while working in concert with the phospholipases.

Even in the absence of phospholipase C metabolism, there is a significant increase in DAG and Ca^{2+} intracellularly that accompanies phagocytosis.[205] Ca^{2+} is necessary for granule phagosome fusion and DAG has been linked to both particle ingestion and degranulation.[206] Both can be formed by the activation of PLD, which hydrolyzes phosphatidylcholine to produce PA and choline. Activation of PLD is mediated by Rho and/or ARF.[198] Diacylglycerol is then generated by phosphatidic acid phosphohydrolase, which catalyzes the dephosphorylation of PA. The hallmark of the phosphatidylcholine-derived DAG is the presence of 1-0-alkyl linkages. During PA formation by the action of PLD on phosphatidylcholine, PA can act as a Ca^{2+} ionophore, thereby initiating fusogenic activity.[207] Thus, the phosphatidylcholine acid generated during phagocytosis may promote fusion of neutrophil granules with newly formed phagosomes.

Another downstream target of DAG in phagocytosis is the activation of protein kinase C (PKC), particularly PKCδ, a Ca^{2+}-independent isozyme of PKC found in neutrophils.[183] PKCδ is one of four PKC isozymes that translocate to the plasma membrane during phagocytosis. During phagocytosis, PKCδ is translocated from the cytosol to the plasma membrane. Accompanying the translocation of PKCδ to the membrane, RAF-1 translocation is promoted. Following translocation of these two key components, mitogen-activated kinase (MEK) activation occurs, which is followed by activation of mitogen-activated protein (MAP) kinase/ERK2 and then myosin light-chain kinase.[200] Following phosphorylation of myosin, reorganization of the actin cytoskeletal occurs leading to phagocytosis. Concomitant with the activation of PLD, ceramide is generated by a neutral sphingomyelinase activity found in the plasma membrane of neutrophils and it is most likely important in attenuating the activity of the cells through inhibition of PLD.[205] Following engagement of the Fc receptors and *Syk* activation in the neutrophil, phosphatidylinositol 3'-kinase (PI3K) is also activated. Inhibition of PI3K activity impedes phagocytosis.[183]

Arachidonate Metabolism In addition to their participation as putative second-messenger products in the stimulus–response coupling pathway, many lipid metabolites may be released from stimulated neutrophils, and in turn modulate cell function by interacting with receptors on other neutrophils. Phospholipase A_2, present on both the granules and plasma membranes of neutrophils,[208] as well as the cytosol,[209] is activated during neutrophil stimulation, yielding arachidonic acid as one of the major end products. Arachidonic acid is not only released from stimulated neutrophils, but also serves as a regulator of phospholipase A_2 (PLA_2)

activity and as a stimulus for these cells.[210] Sensitivity of the cells to other stimuli can be enhanced with arachidonic acid and other long-chain fatty acids.[211]

Arachidonic acid can also be metabolized by the lipoxygenase pathway to produce hydroxyeicosatetraenoic acids (HETEs), including 5-HETE, 12-HETE, and 5,12-diHETE.[212] These compounds have also been shown to induce several neutrophil responses.[213] Stimulated neutrophils also produce the diHETE LTB_4 through the lipoxygenase pathway. LTB_4 and other leukotrienes can be released in response to a variety of stimuli.[214] Receptors for LTB_4 have been partially purified, and their activation serves as a potent stimulus for chemotaxis and adherence.[215]

Another potent mediator of inflammation produced by stimulated neutrophils is 1-*O*-alkyl-2-acetyl-sn-glyceryl-3-phosphoryl choline, also as known PAF.[14] Not only is PAF synthesized by neutrophils and activated endothelial cells, but it induces degranulation, aggregation, and superoxide generation.[17] Inflamed endothelium generates PAF, which serves to immobilize neutrophils on the luminal surface of the endothelial cells, thereby facilitating the interaction of the neutrophil integrin receptors with the ICAM ligands on the endothelial cells.

Degranulation and Membrane Fusion

In stimulated cells the signal transduction cascade activates G proteins, followed by enhanced intracellular Ca^{2+}, lipid remodeling, and protein kinase activation. These events culminate in secretion. This ultimate event—the fusion of granule membranes with phagosomes or the plasma membrane—occurs rapidly and is highly efficient.

Fusion Proteins Over the past 20 years the SNARE (soluble *N*-ethylmaleimide-sensitive factor attachment protein receptor) hypothesis has become the reigning paradigm for fusion of biomembranes.[77,216] The hypothesis is centered around the protein that is sensitive to *N*-ethylmaleimide (designated *NEM-sensitive fusion protein* or *NSF*) and several SNAREs on the participating membranes. The SNAREs are termed the v-SNAREs, being found on *v*esicles or granules, and t-SNAREs, being found on the target plasma membranes. The SNARE hypothesis has proven to have great predictive value as the constellation of fusion proteins and their interactions appears in almost all species and tissues. Initial docking of granules with the membrane to which they fuse is likely mediated by Rab-GTPases. Once docking is obtained, SNAREs are recruited to both membranes and interact and mediate actual fusion assisted by SNARE-interacting proteins such as sSec1/Munc18 proteins and a local rise in Ca^{2+}. Disassembly of the fusion complex is mediated by NSF in an ATP-dependent process. [217] The t-SNARE VAMP-2 (vesicle-associated membrane protein-2) is localized to the membranes of specific and gelatinase granule and secretory vesicles in resting human neutrophils,[78,79] and the t-SNARE syntaxin 4 is associated with the plasma membrane as shown by immunoelectron microscopy. Munc18-3 may interact with syntaxin 4 and regulate fusion of secondary and gelatinase granules. VAMP-7 has been associated with azurophil granule fusion and Munc18-2 may interact with syntaxin 3 and regulate azurophil granule fusion[218,219]

Neutrophil Extracellular Traps

What previously was considered pus was identified by Zychlinsky and coworkers as a highly bactericidal structure composed of strands of chromatin and bactericidal neutrophil granule proteins attached.[220,221] These neutrophil extracellular traps (NETs) are extruded from neutrophils in a process called *netosis* and represent one of three death programs of neutrophils: apoptosis, necrosis, and netosis. Neutrophils only undergo netosis if they have mounted a respiratory burst.[222] Thus, the NADPH oxidase activity of stimulated neutrophils serves two purposes, namely to generate reactive oxygen species for microbial killing and to induce formation of the bactericidal NETs after the intact neutrophil has ceased to function. This, in turn, means that patients with defective NADPH oxidase assembly (patients with chronic granulomatous disease) lack both the ability to generate microbicidal oxygen species and the ability to form the NETs.

CLINICAL DISORDERS OF NEUTROPHIL FUNCTION

CLASSIFICATION

Neutrophil dysfunction may arise from (1) the absence of antibodies or complement components required to opsonize microorganisms, an interaction that provides a chemotactic signal; (2) the abnormalities of cytoplasmic and granule movement that alter the chemotactic response or that result in abnormalities of the plasma membrane affecting the cells in terms of capability to modulate movement; and (3) defective microbicidal capability. Comprehensive reviews of these syndromes are available to the interested reader.[223–225]

ABNORMALITIES OF THE SIGNAL MECHANISM AS A RESULT OF ANTIBODY AND COMPLEMENT DEFECTS OR IMPAIRMENT OF PATTERN RECEPTOR RECOGNITION

Because the synergistic action of immunoglobulins and complement proteins creates the opsonins that coat microorganisms and stimulate the development of chemotactic factors, a deficiency of either one may result in impaired neutrophil function. The most profound disturbances arise from abnormalities in C3, because this protein is the focal point for generation of opsonins and chemotactic factors (see Chap. 17).[226–228] Opsonins such as C3b, generated from cleavage of C3, serve to coat bacteria. Opsonization in general refers to the coating of pathogens by serum proteins such that they are more likely to be ingested. Activation of C3 can occur in the absence of an antibody or the classical complement components C1, C2, and C4; thus, disorders of these latter molecules result in less-severe clinical conditions. C3 deficiency is inherited as an autosomal recessive disorder. Homozygotes have undetectable serum levels of C3 and suffer from recurrent severe pyrogenic infections, whereas asymptomatic heterozygotes have half the normal values.

A functional deficiency of C3 protease resulting in severe pyrogenic infections also is seen in patients with a deficiency in C3b inactivator, a protein inhibitor of the alternative complement pathway. Unchecked activation of this pathway leads to hypercatabolism of C3 and factor B.[229] Properidin deficiency also results in a functional deficiency in C3.[230] Properidin is a serum protein that belongs to the alternative complement pathway; it is involved in the stabilization of the enzyme complex C3bBb. The protein is a multimeric glycoprotein with a subunit Mr of 56,000, the gene of which has been cloned.[231] Absence of properidin is associated with severe, often fatal, pyrogenic infections, often with meningococci.

Approximately 5 percent of the population have low serum levels of mannose-binding lectin (MBL),[232] a serum lectin secreted by the liver that binds mannose sugars present and on the surface of bacteria, fungi, and some viruses. MBL is one of the collectin-soluble effector proteins that contribute to the basic armamentarium of innate immunity. MBL can function as an opsonin when bound to the surfaces by activating the complement cascade. A deficiency of MBL has been reported in infants with frequent unexplained infection, chronic diarrhea, and otitis media.[232] Other studies have identified an increased susceptibility to infection by specific pathogens in MBL-deficient individuals, including human immunodeficiency virus, *Plasmodium falciparum*, *Cryptosporidium parvum*, and *Neisseria. meningitides*.[233] The deficiency in MBL largely results from three relatively common single-point mutations in exon 1 of the gene, which leads to the failure of MBL to activate complement.[234] In addition, the protein also modulates disease severity, at least in part through complex, dose-dependent influences on cytokine production.

Phagocytes, including neutrophils, express a large number of cell surface proteins that play crucial functional roles in their biology. Microbial pattern recognition receptors are an essential component of innate immunity, in which they recognize and detect pathogen-associated molecular patterns, resulting in activation of neutrophils and other phagocytes. The mammalian TLR family comprises an important class of pattern-recognition receptors, which recognize a wide range of microbial pathogens and pathogen-related products. At least 12 different TLRs that can be found on mononuclear phagocytes have been described.[235] The neutrophil expresses both TLR2 and TLR4, which permit recognition of peptidoglycan and endotoxin, respectively, and TLR8, which allows recognition of RNA ligands.[236] TLRs signal via MyD88, an adapter protein. MyD88 deficiency in humans can lead to recurrent infections with both Gram-positive and Gram-negative infections, thereby indicating a role for both mononuclear cells and neutrophils in host defense in the MyD88-deficient state.[237]

Because a large number of chemoattractants are generated during inflammation, it is difficult to establish the relative significance of a given individual component. Furthermore, chemotactive factors and opsonins are involved in the activity of both neutrophils and mononuclear phagocytes. Therefore, it is not clear whether the clinical consequences of disorders involving these substances are unique to one or the other of these phagocytic cells. Patients with antibody- or complement-deficient syndromes suffer mainly from infections with encapsulated pathogens such as *Haemophilus influenzae*, pneumococci, streptococci, and meningococci.[238] Furthermore, splenectomized individuals deprived of an organ rich in mononuclear phagocytes have a small, but finite risk of sepsis because of the same microorganisms. Encapsulated pathogens characteristically are not associated with neutropenic states. Antibody coating of encapsulated organisms facilitates their ingestion by mononuclear phagocytes, but may be less important for their ingestion by neutrophils.

ABNORMALITIES OF THE CELLULAR RESPONSES AS THE RESULTS OF DEFECTS IN CYTOPLASMIC MOVEMENT

Degranulaton Abnormalities

Chédiak-Higashi Syndrome **Definition and History** This rare autosomal recessive disease was initially recognized as one in which neutrophils, monocytes, and lymphocytes contained giant cytoplasmic granules.[239] Chédiak-Higashi syndrome (CHS) is now recognized as a disorder of generalized cellular dysfunction characterized by increased fusion of cytoplasmic granules.[240] Pigmentary dilution affecting the hair, skin, and ocular fundi results from pathologic aggregation of melanosomes and is associated with a decreased failure of decussation of the optic and auditory nerves (Table 66–2).[241] Patients with this syndrome exhibit an increased susceptibility to infection, which begins in infancy. Infections most commonly involve the skin and respiratory systems. The susceptibility to infection can be explained in part through defects in neutrophil chemotaxis, degranulation, and bactericidal activity.[239] The presence of giant granules in the neutrophil interferes with their ability to traverse narrow passages between endothelial cells. Other features of the disease include neutropenia,[241] thrombocytopathy,[242] natural killer cell abnormalities[239,243] and peripheral neuropathies.[244] Similar genetic syndromes have been described in mice, mink, cats, rats, cattle, and killer whales.[244]

Although CHS carries the names of Moises Chédiak and Ototaka Higashi, the disorder was first described by Béguez César, a Cuban pediatrician in 1943.[245] Initially characterized by neutropenia and abnormal granules in leukocytes, the syndrome was further delineated in 1948 by Steinbrinck's description of a second case.[246] In 1952, Chédiak reported the hematologic characteristics of the disorder,[247] and in 1953 Higashi emphasized the giant peroxidase-containing granules within patients' neutrophils.[248] Besides the susceptibility of infections, patients often suffer a fatal lymphohistiocytic infiltration known as the accelerated phase occurring months from birth to several years later.[249]

Epidemiology By 2008, 300 cases worldwide had been described, with concentrations in the United States, Japan, northern Europe, and Latin America.[244] Patients of African descent have also been described.

Etiology and Pathogenesis CHS is caused by a fundamental defect in granule morphogenesis that results in abnormally large granules in multiple tissues.[240,250] Giant granules are seen in Schwann cells, leukocytes, and macrophages of the liver and spleen, and certain cells of the pancreas, gastric mucosa, kidney, adrenal gland, and pituitary gland.[244] Giant melanosomes form and prevent the even distribution of melanin, which results in pigmentary dilution of the hair, skin, iris, and optic fundus. Although the giant lysosomes are the primary morphologic feature of the disorder, only cells relying on the secretion by these lysosomes manifest pathological defects. In the early stages of myelopoiesis some of the normal-size azurophil granules coalesce to form giant granules that result in large secondary lysosomes that contain reduced content of hydrolytic enzymes, including proteinases, elastase, and cathepsin G.[239] Many of the myeloid precursors die in the marrow, resulting in a moderate neutropenia, with white cell counts of about 2.5×10^9/L and absolute neutrophil counts ranging from 0.5 to 2.0×10^9/L.[249] The marrow itself appears normal to hypercellular. In spite of the normal ingestion of particles and active oxygen metabolism, these neutrophils kill microorganisms relatively slowly. This delay reflects a slow and inconsistent delivery of diluted amounts of hydrolytic enzymes from the giant granules into the phagosomes, which may predispose the host to bacterial infection.[250,251] In this syndrome, monocytes have the same functional derangements as neutrophils,[239] and in an analogous fashion perforin-deficient natural killer (NK) cells show profoundly impaired cytotoxic activity and are unable to kill many targets.[252]

The CHS blood cell membranes are more fluid than cells of normal individuals,[239,253] and the altered membrane structure could lead to defective regulation of membrane activation, as well as promoting fusion of neutrophil azurophilic granules with each other. Conceivably, changes in membrane fluidity may affect cell function by reducing expression of Mac-1 (CD11b/CD18). The altered membrane fluidity could result in elevated levels of intracellular cyclic adenosine monophosphate, which appears in this disorder and is reflected in the reduced chemotactic responses.[239]

The gene that is mutated in CHS is *CHS1* (syn. *LYST*) found on chromosome 1q, and its size indicates a protein of more than 400 kDa is encoded.[254] During early development, granule biogenesis is normal; and perforin in NK cells, and granule enzymes in myeloid cells are synthesized and routed correctly to the granules. However, once formed the granules fuse to form giant organelles.[255] Several studies led to the suggestion that the enlarged lysosomes found in CHS cells are the results of abnormalities in membrane fusion, which could occur during the biogenesis of the lysosomes. It has been hypothesized that this CHS1 protein interacts with attachment proteins on lysosomes

TABLE 66–2. Clinical Disorders of Neutrophil Function

Disorder	Etiology	Impaired Function	Clinical Consequence
Degranulation abnormalities:			
Chédiak-Higashi syndrome	Autosomal recessive; disordered coalescence of lysosomal granules; responsible gene is CHSI/LYST which encodes a protein hypothesized to regulate granule fusion	Decreased neutrophil chemotaxis; degranulation and bactericidal activity; platelet storage pool defect; impaired NK function, failure to disperse melanosomes	Neutropenia; recurrent pyogenic infections, propensity to develop marked hepatosplenomegaly as a manifestation of the hemophagocytic syndrome
Specific granule deficiency	Autosomal recessive, functional loss of myeloid transcription factor arising from a mutation or arising from reduced expression of Gfi-1 or C/EBPε, which regulates specific granule formation	Impaired chemotaxis and bactericidal activity; bilobed nuclei in neutrophils; defensins, gelatinase, collagenase, vitamin B_{12}-binding protein, and lactoferrin	Recurrent deep-seated abscesses
Adhesion abnormalities:			
Leukocyte adhesion deficiency I	Autosomal recessive; absence of CD11/CD18 surface adhesive glycoproteins (β_2 integrins) on leukocyte membranes most commonly arising from failure to express CD18 mRNA	Decreased binding of C3bi to neutrophils and impaired adhesion to ICAM-1 and ICAM-2	Neutrophilia; recurrent bacterial infection associated with a lack of pus formation
Leukocyte adhesion deficiency II	Autosomal recessive; loss of fucosylation of ligands for selectins and other glycol conjugates arising from mutations of the GDP-fucose transporter	Decreased adhesion to activated endothelium expressing ELAM	Neutrophilia; recurrent bacterial infection without pus
Leukocyte adhesion deficiency III (LAD-1 variant syndrome)	Autosomal recessive; impaired integrin function arising from mutations of FERMT3 which encodes kindlin-3 in hematopoietic cells; kindlin-3 binds to β-integrin and thereby transmits integrin activation	Impaired neutrophil adhesion and platelet activation	Recurrent infections, neutropenia, bleeding tendency
Disorders of cell motility:			
Enhanced motile responses; FMF	Autosomal recessive gene responsible for FMF on chromosome 16, which encodes for a protein called "pyrin"; pyrin regulates caspase-1 and thereby IL-1β secretion; mutated pyrin may lead to heightened sensitivity to endotoxin, excessive IL-1β production, and impaired monocyte apoptosis	Excessive accumulation of neutrophils at inflamed sites which may be the result of excessive IL-1β production	Recurrent fever, peritonitis, pleuritis, arthritis, and amyloidosis
Depressed motile responses:			
Defects in the generation of chemotactic signals	IgG deficiencies; C3 and properdin deficiency can arise from genetic or acquired abnormalities; mannose-binding protein deficiency predominantly in neonates	Deficiency of serum chemotaxis and opsonic activities	Recurrent pyogenic infections
Intrinsic defects of the neutrophil, e.g., leukocyte adhesion deficiency, Chédiak-Higashi syndrome, specific granule deficiency, neutrophil actin dysfunction, neonatal neutrophils; direct inhibition of neutrophil mobility, e.g., drugs	In the neonatal neutrophil there is diminished ability to express β2 integrins and there is a qualitative impairment in β2-integrin function; ethanol, glucocorticoids, cyclic AMP	Diminished chemotaxis; impaired locomotion and ingestion; impaired adherence	Propensity to develop pyogenic infections; possible cause for frequent infections; neutrophilia seen with epinephrine arises from cyclic AMP release from endothelium
Immune complexes	Bind to Fc receptors on neutrophils in patients with rheumatoid arthritis, systemic lupus erythematosus, and other inflammatory states	Impaired chemotaxis	Recurrent pyogenic infections

(continued)

TABLE 66–2. Clinical Disorders of Neutrophil Function (Continued)

Disorder	Etiology	Impaired Function	Clinical Consequence
Hyperimmunoglobulin-E syndrome	Autosomal dominant; responsible gene is Stat 3	Impaired chemotaxis at times; impaired regulation of cytokine production	Recurrent skin and sinopulmonary infections, eczema, mucocutaneous candidiasis, eosinophilia, retained primary teeth, minimal trauma fractures, scoliosis, and characteristic facies
Hyperimmunoglobulin-E syndrome	Autosomal recessive; more then one gene likely contributes to its etiology	High IgE levels, impaired lymphocyte activation to staphylococcal antigens	Recurrent pneumonia without pneumatoceles sepsis, enzyme, boils, mucocutaneous candidiasis, neurologic symptoms, eosinophilia
Microbicidal activity:			
Chronic granulomatous disease	X-linked and autosomal recessive; failure to express functional gp91*phox* in the phagocyte membrane in p22*phox* (autosomal recessive); other autosomal recessive forms of CGD arise from failure to express protein p47*phox* or p67*phox*	Failure to activate neutrophil respiratory burst leading to failure to kill catalase-positive microbes	Recurrent pyogenic infections with catalase-positive microorganisms
G-6-PD deficiency	Less than 5% of normal activity of G-6-PD	Failure to activate NADPH-dependent oxidase, and hemolytic anemia	Infections with catalase-positive microorganisms
Myeloperoxidase deficiency	Autosomal recessive; failure to process modified precursor protein arising from missense mutation.	H_2O_2-dependent antimicrobial activity not potentiated by myeloperoxidase	None
Rac-2 deficiency	Autosomal dominant; dominant negative inhibition by mutant protein of Rac-2 mediated functions	Failure of membrane receptor-mediated O_2 generation and chemotaxis	Neutrophilia, recurrent bacterial infections
Deficiencies of glutathione reductase and glutathione synthetase	Autosomal recessive; failure to detoxify H_2O_2	Excessive formation of H_2O_2	Minimal problems with recurrent pyogenic infections

AMP, adenosine monophosphate; C, complement; CD, cluster designation; CGD, chronic granulomatous disease; G-6-PD, glucose-6-phosphate dehydrogenase; GDP, glucose diphosphate; ELAM, endothelial-leukocyte adhesion molecule; FMF, familial Mediterranean fever; ICAM, intracellular adhesion molecule; Ig, immunoglobulin; IL, interleukin; LAD, leukocyte adhesion deficiency; NADPH, nicotinamide adenine dinucleotide phosphate; NK, natural killer.

SOURCE: Modified from Curnutte JT, Boxer LA: Clinically significant phagocytic cell defects, in *Current Clinical Topics in Infectious Disease*, 6th ed, edited by JS Remington, MN Swartz, p 144. McGraw-Hill, New York, 1985.

(v-SNAREs) and that this mutated protein leads to indiscriminate interactions with v-SNARE to yield uncontrolled fusion of lysosomes with each other.[256]

Clinical Features Characteristically patients with CHS have light skin and silvery hair. They frequently complain of solar sensitivity and photophobia. Other eye findings can include horizontal or rotatory nystagmus. Infections are common and involve the mucous membranes, skin, and respiratory tract. They are susceptible to both Gram-positive and Gram-negative bacteria, as well as fungi, with *Staphylococcus aureus* being the most common infecting organism.[223] Attenuated NK function probably contributes to the increased susceptibility to infection as well. Neurologic signs and symptoms are variable in CHS and may include a peripheral and cranial neuropathy, autonomic dysfunction, weakness, and sensory deficit; and ataxia may also be a prominent feature.

Patients with CHS have prolonged bleeding times with normal platelet counts, resulting from impaired platelet aggregation associated with a deficiency of the storage pools of adenosine diphosphate and serotonin.[242] Electron micrographs reveal normal numbers of α granules in platelets, but decreased numbers of platelet dense bodies.[244]

The accelerated phase of CHS is characterized by lymphocytic proliferation in the liver, spleen, marrow, and central nervous system. The accelerated phase may occur at any age and is now recognized as a genetic form of hemophagocytic lymphohistiocytosis (HLH).[257] Typically, the patient develops hepatosplenomegaly and high fever in the absence of bacterial sepsis. The pancytopenia becomes worse at this stage, producing hemorrhage and an increased susceptibility to infection. The onset of the accelerated phase may be related to the inability of these patients to contain and control the Epstein-Barr virus (EBV) leading to HLH (see Chap. 72). The lymphocyte expansion into the tissue is associated with excessive cytokine production and massive tissue necrosis and organ failure leading to the propensity to recurrent bacterial and viral infections, fever and prostration usually resulting in death.[257] At autopsy, the lymphohistiocytic infiltrates in the liver, spleen, and lymph nodes are extensive, but not neoplastic by histopathologic criteria.[257]

Laboratory Features Currently the only laboratory test diagnostic for CHS is examination of granular cell morphology. The pathognomonic feature is giant peroxidase-positive granules that can be seen in neutrophils.[248] A microscopic examination of hair shafts reveal large, speckled pigment clumps as opposed to the normal pattern of finally divided pigment of melanin spread along the length of the shaft.[244] Similar giant granules can occasionally be present in chronic myelogenous leukemia and acute myelocytic leukemia.[244] Molecular diagnosis of CHS remains difficult and is not commercially available. Heterozygotes for CHS are considered completely normal and cannot be detected clinically or biochemically.

Differential Diagnosis The diagnosis of CHS should be considered in individuals with partial albinism, exaggerated bleeding, and recurrent infections. Patients with CHS must be distinguished from those patients with Griscelli syndrome (GS) and Hermansky-Pudlak syndrome (HPS).

GS is a rare disorder, arising from mutations in the RAB27A gene, and is defined by partial ocular and cutaneous albinism, variable cellular and humeral immunodeficiency, variable neurologic involvement, and the development of the accelerated phase. Individuals with GS lack giant granules in neutrophils and have large pigment clumps in hair shafts.[244] HPS is a disorder of ocular and cutaneous albinism, bleeding diathesis arising from platelet dysfunction, and deposition of ceroid lipofuscin in various organs (see Chap. 121). In contrast to CHS, HPS cells lack giant granules and the patients are not predisposed to recurrent infections.[244]

Therapy, Course, and Prognosis High-dose ascorbic acid (200 mg/day for infants, 2 g/day for adults) has been found to improve the clinical status of some patients in the stable phase.[239] Although there is controversy regarding the efficacy of ascorbic acid, given the safety of the vitamin,[244] it is reasonable to administer it to all patients. The CHS presents a therapeutic dilemma, particularly when the accelerated phase begins. Prophylactic antibiotics do not prevent infections. The only potential for curative therapy for preventing the accelerated phase is marrow transplantation from an human leukocyte antigen (HLA)-compatible donor or an unrelated donor compatible at the D locus.[258] Marrow transplantation reconstitutes normal hematopoietic and immunologic function and corrects the natural killer deficiency in patients before entering the accelerated phase.[258] On the other hand, if the patient is actively in the accelerated phase, stem cell transplantation from a matched unrelated donor is associated with a poor prognosis.[258] Ocular and cutaneous albinism are not corrected after transplantation, nor does transplantation prevent progressive neuropathies from occurring.[259]

Specific Granule Deficiency Specific granule deficiency (SGD) has been described in 5 patients of both sexes and is inherited as an autosomal recessive disorder (see Table 66–2).[239] Besides the absence of specific granules, the nuclei of the neutrophils are bilobed. Patients are afflicted with recurrent infections primarily involving the skin and lungs. *S. aureus* and *Pseudomonas aeruginosa* have been the most commonly observed pathogens, although *Candida albicans* also has been isolated. Specific granule-deficient neutrophils lack gelatinolytic activity in the tertiary granules; vitamin B_{12}-binding protein, lactoferrin, and collagenase in the specific granules; and defensins in the primary granules.[260–262] This disorder also extends to eosinophils that lack the characteristic eosinophil granule proteins; major basic protein, eosinophilic cationic protein, and eosinophil-derived neurotoxin (see Chap. 62).[263] Thus, the disorder is a global defect in phagocytic granules rather than limited to specific granules, as suggested by its name. Neutrophils from these patients are defective in chemotaxis, possibly related to the absence of the intracellular pool of leukocyte adhesion molecules that normally reside in the tertiary and specific granules, and exhibit a mild defect in bactericidal activity, possibly related to the deficiency of the granule constituents, lactoferrin and defensins.[260,264] The impairment in granule protein synthesis affecting the granulocytic cells appears secondary to the functional loss of the myeloid transcription factor, C/EBPε, which was identified in two patients.[265,82] In another case of SGD, the expression of the transcription factor growth factor independence-1 (Gfi-1) was markedly reduced along with a heterozygous mutation of C/EBPε gene.[266] It was suggested that the combined abnormalities blocked specific granule expression leading to the expression of the SGD phenotype. The defect is restricted to blood cells, as normal lactoferrin secretion has been demonstrated in the nasal secretions of an SGD patient despite the abnormality demonstrated in his neutrophils.[261] The diagnosis of SGD is suggested by the presence of neutrophils devoid of specific granules but containing azurophilic granules on the blood film.[239] The diagnosis can be confirmed by demonstrating a severe deficiency in either lactoferrin or vitamin B_{12}-binding protein. An acquired form of SGD can be observed in thermally injured patients or in individuals with myelodysplasia.[239,267] Treatment of SGD is symptomatic, with the administration of parenteral antibiotics for acute infections and surgical drainage of refractory infections. With aggressive medical management, patients may survive into their adult years.

Adhesion Abnormalities

Leukocyte Adhesion Deficiency **Definition and History** Leukocyte adhesion deficiency type I (LAD-1) is a rare autosomal recessive disorder of leukocyte function (see Table 66–2). More than 100 cases have been reported worldwide. The disease is characterized clinically by recurrent soft-tissue infections, delayed wound healing, and severely impaired pus formation despite striking blood neutrophilia.[268] Individuals with this disorder have decreased or absent expression of a family of structurally and functionally related leukocyte surface glycoproteins designated CD11/CD18 complex (also referred to as the β_2-integrin family of leukocyte adhesive proteins; Table 66–3). These proteins include LFA-1 (CD11a/CD18), Mo-1 or Mac-1 (CD11b/CD18), p150,95 (CD11c/CD18), and p160,95 (CD11d/CD18).[268] The CD11 subunits are integral membrane glycoproteins, each spanning the plasma membrane only once. They are approximately 40 percent homologous, suggesting that they arise from a common primordial gene.[268] The three distinct genes encoding the α subunits occur in a cluster on chromosome 16, whereas the gene for the β subunit is located on chromosome 21.[269]

The initial clinical description in 1979 described six children and two families with findings of delayed separation of the umbilical cord and delayed healing at the site of detachment of the cord, recurrent infections despite neutrophilia, neutrophilia persisting during infection-free periods, and impaired neutrophil chemotaxis.[270] The molecular basis for LAD-1 was first suggested by Crowley and colleagues who found that neutrophils from a patient with the disorder lacked a high-molecular-weight membrane glycoprotein.[271] They suggested that the lack of the membrane protein impaired the neutrophil's functional responses. In 1982, Arnaout and coworkers evaluated another patient and confirmed that the membrane glycoprotein with a molecular weight of 150 kDa was missing.[272] They determined that the clinically normal parents and siblings of the proband exhibited intermediate quantities of the glycoprotein, which suggested the existence of a heterozygous carrier state. The disorder then became known as leukocyte adhesion deficiency. Subsequently, in 1984, Dana and colleagues identified glycoprotein 150 as one subunit of a glycoprotein that had two subunits that served as a receptor for a plasma complement component.[273] This was followed by other investigators who found that two other related leukocyte membrane glycoproteins also were deficient. Each of the three glycoproteins was then determined to be heterodimers with one common subunit and one subunit unique to each glycoprotein.[274] Springer and colleagues established that synthesis of a defective subunit common to the three glycoproteins of CD11/CD18 complex resulted in loss of expression of

TABLE 66–3. Biologic and Clinical Features of Leukocyte Adherence Deficiencies 1 and 2

	Genetic Defect	Leukocyte Functional Abnormalities	Clinical Features	Diagnosis
LAD-1	Molecular mutations affecting expression of the β_2-integrin CD18	Neutrophils; adherence spreading, homotypic aggregation, chemotaxis receptor CR3 activities: C3bi binding affecting phagocytosis, respiratory burst, and degranulation in response to C3bi-coated particles*	Autosomal recessive; delayed umbilical cord separation; neutrophilia; defective neutrophil migration into tissue; recurrent bacterial infections; impaired wound healing	Flow cytometry for expression of CD11b/CD18 (Mac-1)
		Monocytes; adherence, CR3 activities		
		Lymphocytes; cytotoxic		
		T-lymphocyte activities; NK cytotoxic activities; blastogenesis		
LAD-2 (CDG–IIc)	Mutations affecting function of GDP-fucose transporter 1 resulting in defective glycosylation expression at the α1,3-position of selectin ligands including sLe^x and other fucosylated proteins requiring fucosylation	Neutrophils; rolling mediated by sLe^x to endothelium; neutrophilia†	Autosomal recessive; recurrent bacterial infections, periodontitis; growth retardation; developmental retardation; Bombay red cell phenotype	Flow cytometry for leukocyte sLe^x (CD15)

*These functional abnormalities and clinical features are a consequence of lack of the CD11b/CD18, which includes CD11a, CD11b, CD11c, and CD11d markers of four different α chains and the common B2 chain CD18 of molecular mass 95 kDa.

†These functional abnormalities and clinical features are a consequence of lack of sLe^x expression on leukocytes.

all three heterodimers.[275] The mutant gene led to expression of a defective subunit common to each of the three glycoproteins in the complex yielding a deficiency of the entire complex. This observation provided the molecular explanation for the cellular defect. In 1985, Anderson and coworkers correlated the extent of clinical severity and magnitude of the cellular abnormalities with the degree of CD11/CD18 deficiency, thereby laying the groundwork for the direct relationship between the glycoprotein deficiency and the clinical presentation.[274]

Etiology and Pathogenesis Each of these molecules contains an α and a β subunit noncovalently associated in an $\alpha\beta$ structure. They all have the same β subunit and are distinguished by their α subunits, which have different isoelectric points, molecular weights, and cell distribution (see Table 66–3).[274] The structure of CD11/CD18 has been deduced from molecular cloning of the various subunits.[274] The x-ray crystal structure and nuclear magnetic resonance analysis have also revealed that activation signals lead to the separation of the α and β subunit cytoplasma tails, thereby converting the bent conformation of each integrin with its headpiece near the plasma membrane into fully extended high-affinity structures in a switchblade-like movement.[276] These studies established that CD11/CD18 are members of a large gene family involved in cell–cell and cell–matrix adhesion (integrins). Several subfamilies of integrins have been described and classified according to the type of their highly homologous β subunits. The α subunits are also homologous to each other, but to a lesser degree than are the associated β subunits. Within each subfamily, a single β subunit usually is shared by several α subunits. Certain α subunits often share more than one β subunit, which alters their specificity for various ligands.[274] The molecular defect involves all three members of the CD11 integrin subfamily. In the patients with LAD-1 who have been evaluated at the molecular level, absent, diminished, or structurally abnormal β subunits (CD18) have been identified.[274] A heterogeneous group of mutations that are confined to the gene on chromosome 21q22.3 have been identified.[274] Many patients have point mutations that result in single amino acid substitutions in CD18, which predominantly reside between amino acids 111 and 361.[274] This peptide domain is highly conserved among all β subunits and appears to be important for interaction with the α subunit. Several affected individuals are compound heterozygotes for two different mutant alleles, whereas others are homozygotes for a single mutant allele. Messenger RNA splicing abnormalities described in two kindreds can result in either deletion or insertion of amino acids in the conserved extracellular domain of CD18. Small deletions within the coding sequences of the CD18 gene disrupting the reading frame or a nucleotide substitution resulting in a premature termination signal has been described. Mutations in CD18 disrupt the association in the $\alpha\beta$ subunits so that maturation, intracellular transport, and all cell surface assembly of functionally active $\alpha\beta$ molecules fail to occur.[274] Approximately half of patients exhibit a low level of CD11/CD18 cell surface molecules and moderate disease, with the remainder having totally absent surface expression of these proteins, which accounts for a profound impairment of neutrophil and monocyte adherence and adhesion-dependent functions *in vitro*, including cell migration, phagocytosis, and complement- or antibody-dependent cytotoxicity.[274,275]

Besides the requirement for surface expression of the CD11/CD18, the molecules must undergo posttranslational modification during leukocyte activation.[277] Two compound heterozygotes with mutation that cause impaired expression and dysfunction of the β_2 gene have been reported to cause variant LAD-1.[278,279] The levels of β_2 integrins were approximately 60 percent of control in each case, which was sufficient for normal adhesive function.[274] Transfection studies indicated that each subject had one mutation that did not support surface expression in β_2 heterodimers, accounting for the reduced levels on the membrane of leukocytes, and a second allele that resulted in surface expression of heterodimers that did not bind ligands. Changes in confirmation in the function of the I-like domain of β_2, which is critical for ligand recognition, probably accounts for the adhesion defect.[9,277]

The bulk of the neutrophil, Mac-1 glycoprotein, is stored inside the cell in the membrane of neutrophil specific and gelatinase granules and in secretory vesicles.[20,280] Exposure of neutrophils to degranulating stimuli results in a 5- to 10-fold increase in the number of Mac-1 molecules on the cell surface, which parallels the fusion of granules to the plasma membrane.[280] Neutrophils from these patients fail to augment their surface adhesive glycoproteins, as the defect in β-subunit synthesis affects both membrane and granule pools of Mac-1.[281] In contrast to Mac-1 and p150,95, leukocyte function-associated antigen 1 (LFA-1) is predominantly confined to the neutrophil plasma membrane. Consequently, the cell surface levels of LFA-1 are not enhanced by neutrophil degranulation.

Lymphocytes deficient in CD11/CD18 are able to adhere to endothelial surfaces via the expression on lymphocytes of very-late antigen-4 (VLA-4) integrin (synonym: integrin $\alpha_4\beta_1$) receptors, which bind to the vascular cell adhesion molecule 1 (VCAM-1), found on the endothelial cells,[282] this residual adhesion may account for the paucity of clinical symptoms related to lymphocyte function. The patients are not unusually susceptible to viral infection although three patients had one or more episodes of aseptic meningitis.[274]

The failure of the LAD-1 neutrophils to migrate to the sites of inflammation outside of the lung and peritoneum arises from their inability to adhere firmly to surfaces and undergo transendothelial migration from venules.[283–285] Failure of LAD-1–deficient neutrophils to undergo transendothelial migration occurs because β_2 integrins bind to intercellular adhesion molecules 1 and 2 (CD54 and ICAM-2) expressed on inflamed endothelial cells.[268,286] LAD-1 neutrophils are able to accumulate in the lung, perhaps through a process of movement mediated by chimneying, which does not require functional integrins.[287] Chemotaxis that occurs despite blockade of CD11/CD18 under special *in vitro* conditions has been dubbed "chimneying." The neutrophils that do arrive at inflammatory sites in the inflamed lung by CD11/CD18-independent processes fail to recognize microorganisms coated with the opsonic complement fragment C3bi (an important stable opsonin formed by the cleavage of C3b by C3b inactivator).[268,288] Other neutrophil functions, such as degranulation and oxidative metabolism, normally triggered by C3bi binding are also diminished and markedly compromised in neutrophils from LAD-1.[268] Similarly, the urokinase-plasminogen activator-receptor and the FcγRIII receptors, both phosphatidylinositol-linked proteins, are defective in their functions because these receptors transduce their signals through CD11/CD18.[180,289] Monocyte function is also impaired. Monocytes of affected individuals have poor fibrinogen-binding function, an activity promoted by the CD11/CD18 complex,[268,290] consequently, such cells are not able to participate effectively in wound healing. Thus, impairment in neutrophil function underlies the propensity to recurrent infections, which is the clinical expression of this disease. Similar genetic syndromes have been discovered in Irish Setter dogs and Holstein cattle.[274] A CD11/CD18-deficient mouse with 2 to 6 percent of normal β_2-integrin expression has been produced by gene targeting.[283,291]

Clinical Features Activated leukocytes of patients with the most severe clinical form express less than 0.3 percent of the normal amount of the β_2 integrins, with those of patients with the moderate phenotype may express 2 to 7 percent of normal numbers of β_2-integrin molecules.[268] The severely affected patients suffer from recurrent and chronic or even gangrenous soft-tissue infections (subcutaneous tissues or mucous membranes), generally by bacterial or fungal microorganisms such as *S. aureus*, *Pseudomonas* spp. and other gram-negative enteric rods, or *Candida* spp. Patients with the moderate phenotype have fewer and less severe infections. Infectious susceptibility and impaired wound healing are related to diminished or delayed infiltration of neutrophils and monocytes into extravascular inflammatory sites. In all patients surviving infancy, severe progressive generalized periodontitis is present. Individuals who are clinically well, but who are heterozygous carriers of LAD have been identified. Their stimulated neutrophils express approximately 50 percent of the normal amount of the Mac-1 α subunit and the common β subunit.[268] The diagnosis of LAD-1 should be considered in infants with a paucity of neutrophils at sites of infection despite blood neutrophilia and have a history of delayed separation of the umbilical cord.

Laboratory Features The diagnosis is made most readily by flow cytometric measurement of surface CD11b in stimulated and unstimulated neutrophils using monoclonal antibodies directed against CD11b (Fig. 66–5). Assessment of neutrophil and monocyte adherence, aggregation, chemotaxis, C3bi-mediated phagocytosis, and cytotoxicity generally demonstrates striking abnormalities that are directly related to the molecular deficiency. Delayed-type hypersensitivity reactions are normal, and most individuals have normal specific antibody synthesis. The ability of lymphocytes to generate specific antibodies explains the self-limited course of varicella or viral respiratory infections. However, some patients have impaired T-lymphocyte–dependent antibody responses, for example, to repeat vaccination with tetanus toxoid, diphtheria toxoid, and polio virus.

Patients with LAD-1 usually have blood neutrophil counts of 15 to 60 × 10^9/L. However, during infectious episodes, they commonly have neutrophil counts in excess of 100 × 10^9/L and sometimes as high as 160 × 10^9/L. Granulocytic hyperplasia is a feature of the marrow examination which may relate to excessive production of IL-17 and granulocyte colony-stimulating factor.[281] Despite elevated blood counts, there is a paucity of neutrophils in inflammatory skin windows and biopsies of infected tissues.

Differential Diagnosis Several patients (4 Arab, 2 Turkish, 1 Pakistani, 1 Brazilian) who had neutrophilia, recurrent bacterial infections, and an inability to form pus have been described.[9,292,293] The patients also had the Bombay blood phenotype (deficiency in H blood group integrins) severe mental retardation, unusual facial appearance, microcephaly, cortical atrophy, seizures, hypotonia, and short stature (see Table 66–2). Functionally, the neutrophils were unable to adhere to E-selectin or cytokine-activated endothelial cells and exhibited impaired chemotaxis and an inability to roll on postcapillary venules *in vivo*. The patients are now classified as having LAD-2 or congenital disorder of glycosylation type 11c (CDG-11c).[294] In contrast to LAD-1, the patients' natural killer cell activity are normal. The LAD-2 neutrophils express normal levels of CD18 integrins, but are deficient in the carbohydrate structure sialyl Lewis X, which renders the cells unable to roll on activated endothelial cells expressing E-selectin (see Table 66–3). Thus, the neutrophils from the patients categorized as having a LAD-2 phenotype are unable to tether to inflamed venules, which is necessary for subsequent activation (see Chap. 17). The LAD-2 can be explained by a congenital disorder of fucosylation of ligands for selectins and other glycoconjugates. Each of the three selectins binds with variable affinity to sialylated and fucosylated oligosaccharides, including sLe^x, which is present on multiple specific glycolipids and glycoproteins on leukocytes and activated endothelial cells.[9] Neutrophils from LAD-2 subjects lack sLe^x, which leads to impaired neutrophil rolling on endothelial cells. Other fucosylated determinants, including the H, Lewis, and secretor blood group antigens are lacking as well, suggesting a global defect in fucosylation. The diminished fucosylation arises from impaired transport of glucose diphosphate (GDP)-fucose from the cytoplasm to the Golgi lumen.[292] A human GDP-fucose transporter (GFTP) that localizes to the Golgi apparatus has been demonstrated to be defective secondary to distinct mutations in the gene encoding the transporter.[9] When fibroblasts and lymphoblastoid cells derived from a LAD-2 patient were grown in the presence millimolar concentrations of fucose, cell-surface fucosylation could be restored. Following this observation oral admin-

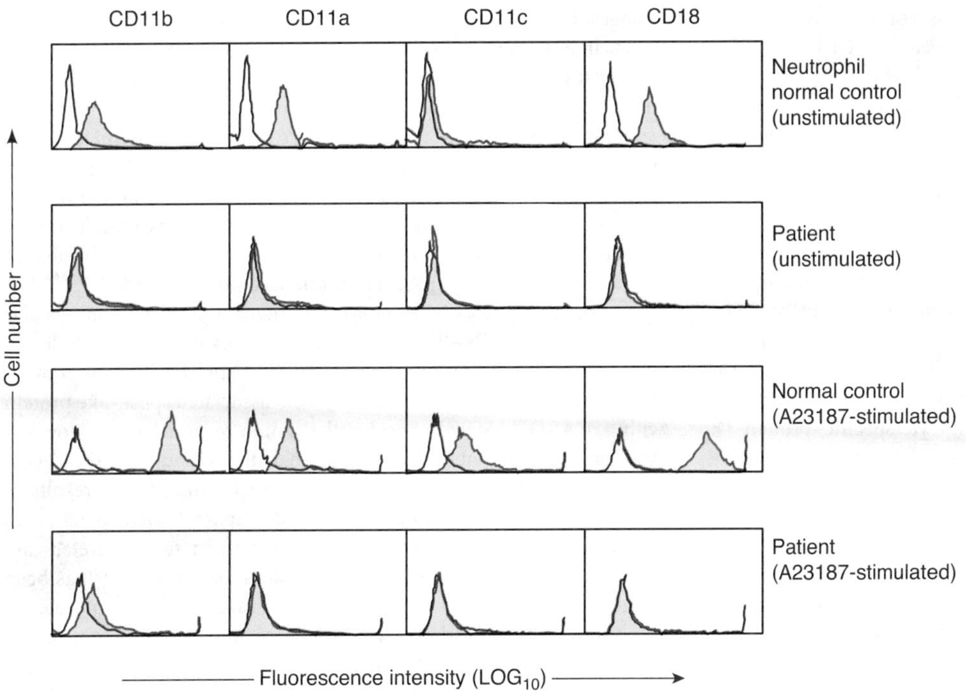

FIGURE 66–5. Specific diagnosis of CD11/CD18 glycoprotein deficiency by indirect immunofluorescence flow cytometric analysis. Blood neutrophils of a pediatric patient suspected of having CD11/CD18 glycoprotein deficiency and those of an abnormal individual were subjected to immunofluorescence staining for the expression of the CD11b, CD11a, CD11c, and CD18 epitope (*cross-hatched histograms*) as compared with the background immunofluorescence staining by isotype-identical negative-control antibodies (*open histograms*). Neutrophils were either stained immediately after purification by Ficoll-Hypaque density centrifugation (unstimulated) or after exposure to calcium ionophore A23187 (1 m*M*) for 15 min at 37°C (98.6°F; A23187-stimulated). A23187 stimulation causes significant increase in CD11b and CD18 epitope staining (surface MO1 expression) by normal neutrophils as compared with unstimulated normal cells. A23187 stimulation also causes a small increase in the CD11b-epitope expression of patient cells (the CD11b cross-hatched histogram becomes distinguishable from background staining after A23187 stimulation), suggesting that this patient has a "moderate" form of the disorder (capable of expressing small but detectable quantities of CD11/CD18 glycoproteins). Flow cytometric analysis was performed on a Coulter Electronics EPICS F C Flow Cytometer with a logarithmic amplifier. *(From Todd R, Freyer DR: The CD11/CD18 leukocyte glycoprotein deficiency.* Hematol Oncol Clin North Am *2:13, 1988, with permission.)*

istration of L-fucose to two Turkish patients led to normalization of neutrophil counts and functional E- and P-selectin ligands on myeloid cells accompanied by abatement of fevers and infections.[9] Two Arab patients, in contrast to the Turkish patients who have different mutations of the gene encoding the putative GDP-fucose transporter, did not respond to oral fucose.[293] A Brazilian LAD-2 patient, like the Turkish patients, initially benefited from oral fucose; but, following expression of sialyl Lewis X on the myeloid cells, the patient developed autoimmune neutropenia.[295] The diagnosis of LAD-3 can be made by flow cytometry analysis of CD15s (sLe^x) expression.

Leukocyte adhesion deficiency type III (LAD-3) also known as LAD-1 variant syndrome compromises two major hallmarks: a moderate LAD-1-like syndrome and severe Glanzmann-like bleeding diathesis (see Chap. 121). Four patients have been described in whom the inheritance appears to be autosomal recessive and is associated with functional defects of the leukocyte and platelet integrins arising from intracellular signaling.[296] The disease initially presents in early childhood and consists of the inability to form pus at sites of microbial infections, as well as a severe bleeding tendency. The neutrophils from the patients display defective adhesion and chemotaxis and are unable to undergo the respiratory burst when triggered by unopsonized zymosan. The molecular basis for LAD-3 arises from mutations in FERMT3, which encodes kindlin-3 in hematopoietic cells. Kindlin-3 binds to regions of the β-integrin tails and constitutes an essential element for integrin activation.[297] Marrow transplantation can be curative.

Another rare cause of neutrophilia and an inability to form pus was observed in a patient with a mutation in the Rac2 GTPase, which is discussed below. The neutrophils from the patient had defects in both adhesion and chemotaxis (see Table 66–2).

Therapy, Course, and Prognosis Treatment of LAD-1 is largely supportive.[268,274] Patients with a history of recurrent infections can be maintained on prophylactic trimethoprim-sulfamethoxazole. Marrow transplantation with HLA-compatible siblings or parental donors has resulted in engraftment and restoration of neutrophil function and remains the treatment of choice for patients with a severe phenotype.[298]

The restoration of CD11/CD18 expression in CD34 peripheral stem cells from LAD-1 following transduction with a retrovirus bearing CD18 and induced to differentiate into neutrophils with growth factors indicates that LAD-1 is caused by a defective CD18 gene and provides a basis for somatic gene therapy, which was accomplished in a dog model.[299,300] Not only did the neutrophils express the integrins, but the cells demonstrated improvement in their functional responses, such as adhesion and the respiratory burst when challenged with ligands for CD11/CD18. These results indicate that *ex vivo* of the transfer gene for CD18 into LAD-1 CD34+ cells followed by reinfusion of the transfused cells may represent a therapeutic approach for LAD.

The severity of infectious complications correlates with the degree of β_2 deficiency. Patients with severe deficiency may die in infancy, and those surviving infancy have a susceptibility to severe, life-threatening, systemic infections. In patients with moderate deficiency, life-threatening infections are infrequent and survival relatively long.[281] Prenatal diagnosis of LAD-1 can be established in families in which the mutations of the two CD18 alleles are known.[301] Chorionic villus DNA can be analyzed. Alternatively, fetal blood neutrophils can be assessed by flow cytometry for expression of Mac-1 at 20 weeks' gestation.

Neutrophil Actin Dysfunction

These patients, like patients with LAD, have recurrent pyogenic infections from birth as a result of defective chemotactic and phagocytic response (see Table 66–2). In one patient, actin isolated from blood and neutrophils could not polymerize under conditions that fully polymerized the actin of neutrophils from normal individuals.[302] Subsequent studies on the index patient's family confirmed that partial actin dysfunction was present in the parents and one sister.[303] One of the parents was found to be a heterozygote for LAD, and the other was not, but further studies established that LAD was not generally associated with defective actin filament assembly.[304,305] The basis of the defective polymerization of actin in the index patient remains unknown, but this disorder of phagocytes is distinct from LAD.

Defective actin polymerization has been described in a 2-month-old infant with severe recurrent bacterial infections associated with impaired chemotaxis and phagocytic response.[306] The patient's neutrophils showed increased expression of CD11b, distinguishing the patient's clinical problem from LAD-1. Morphologically the neutrophils displayed thin, filamentous projections of membrane with an underlying abnormal cytoskeletal structure. Subsequently, a 47-kDa protein was purified that inhibited actin polymerization *in vitro*.[307] Further biochemical studies revealed a markedly defective actin polymerization in the patient's neutrophils along with a severe deficiency of an 89-kDa protein and an elevated level of the 47-kDa protein. The 47-kDa protein has been identified as LSP-1 (lymphocyte-specific protein-1), which is an actin-binding protein present in normal neutrophils. Overexpression of LSP-1 has resulted in bundling of actin in cells, leading to an abnormal cytoskeletal structure and motility defects.[308] Neutrophils from the patient's parents revealed a partial defect in actin polymerization accompanied by intermediate levels of LSP-1 and the 89-kDa protein. These observations suggest that the neutrophil actin dysfunction (NAD) known as NAD47/89 is an autosomal recessive disorder. Because actin dysfunction is lethal, treatment requires restoration of normal neutrophil function by marrow replacement from a normal donor. Marrow transplantation was attempted in both infants. In the first infant, it was unsuccessful, whereas, in the patient with the neutrophil actin dysfunction associated with overexpression of the 47-kDa protein, marrow transplantation was successful.[306,309]

DISORDERS OF NEUTROPHIL MOTILITY

Familial Mediterranean Fever

Definition and History Familial Mediterranean fever (FMF) is an autosomal recessive disease that primarily affects populations surrounding the Mediterranean basin. The disease is characterized by acute limited attacks of fever often accompanied by pleuritis, peritonitis, arthritis, pericarditis, inflammation of the tunica vaginalis of the testes, and erysipelas-like skin disease (see Table 66–2). The initial description occurred in 1908, identifying a Jewish girl who had episodic abdominal pain and fever.[310] Subsequently additional cases were identified,[311] but it took nearly a half century to establish this disorder as familial Mediterranean fever.[312]

Epidemiology More than 10,000 patients worldwide are affected with FMF. It occurs predominantly in Sephardic Jews, Arabs, Turks, Italians, and Armenians.[310] The disorder can occur in other populations, but it is unusual. The frequency of the susceptibility gene varies widely; it is very high among Armenians (ratio of persons with the gene to those without it is 1:7) and Sephardic Jews (1:5 to 1:16), but is lower in Ashkenazi Jews (1:135).

Etiology and Pathogenesis The pathologic findings in FMF are those of nonspecific acute inflammation affecting serosal tissues such as the pleura, peritoneum, and synovium. Neutrophilic infiltration predominates in the affected tissues. Physical and emotional stress, menstruation, and a high-fat diet may trigger the attacks.[313]

The gene responsible for FMF has been identified to be located on chromosome 16. It encodes for a 781-amino-acid protein called *pyrin* or *marenostrin*.[314,315] The gene (MEFV) is predominantly expressed in neutrophils, eosinophils, monocytes, dendritic cells, and synovial and peritoneal fibroblasts, and its expression is upregulated by interferon-γ and tumor necrosis factor, and by the process of myeloid differentiation itself.[316] Nearly all the 50 mutations in the MEFV gene are missense changes, most of which are clustered in on exon 2 and 10.[317] Founder effects in FMF have been established, and it has been suggested that the two most common mutations, V726A and M694V, originated in common ancestors who lived about 2500 years ago in the Middle East.[314]

Although the precise function of pyrin remains ill defined, it has been suggested that PYRIN, one of the four domains of pyrin, bears homology to a number of proteins involved in apoptosis and in inflammation, and is similar to a member of the six-helix-bundle death-domain superfamily that includes death domains and death effector domains known as caspase recruitment domains (CARDs).[318] The pyrin domain appears to allow for the interaction of macromolecular complexes by PYRIN–PYRIN interactions. This interaction has led to the identification of pyrin's ability to interact specifically with another PYRIN-domain protein termed apoptosis-associated speck-like protein with a CARD (ASC).[319] Besides the amino-terminal pyrin domain, ASC has a C-terminal CARD domain that allows binding to the CARD of procaspase-1 (interleukin-1β-converting enzyme), which results in procaspase-1 autoactivation.[318] Activated caspase-1 then metabolizes prointerleukin-1β to interleukin-1β, which is, in turn, secreted and interacts with the IL-1 receptor to mediate inflammation. It has been suggested that pyrin may act as an antiinflammatory molecule by inhibiting ASC-induced interleukin-1 processing, which, in turn, could be defective in FMF. This hypothesis is supported by observing increased IL-1 processing and heightened sensitivity to lipopolysaccharide and impaired apoptosis in peritoneal macrophages from pyrin knockout mice. The puzzle, however, remains as to why serosal tissues are the main targets of inflammation in FMF. Might it be possible that aberrant functioning macrophages are responsible for recruiting neutrophils to the serosal tissue?

Clinical Features Febrile episodes in FMF may begin in infancy, but by age 20 years, 90 percent of patients have had their first attack. The duration and frequency of attacks may vary considerably, even in the same patient.[313] Acute attacks frequently last 24 to 48 hours and recur once or twice a month. In some patients, attacks may recur as frequently as several times a week, or as infrequently as once a year, and symptoms may persist as long as a week during individual episodes. Some patients experience spontaneous remission that persists for years, followed by recurrence of frequent attacks. Peritonitis caused by FMF may resemble an acute abdomen, thereby leading to potential uncertainties about the clinical management of the acute abdominal episode. Attacks of pleuritic pain occur in approximately 25 to 80 percent of patients. Symptoms of pleuritis may sometimes precede abdominal pain, and some patients experience pleuritic attacks without abdominal symptoms. Recurrent pericarditis has been reported, rarely. The course of peritonitis in FMF is similar to attacks at other serosal sites; however, it tends to appear at a late stage of the disease. Mild arthralgia is a common feature of febrile attacks, and monoarticular or oligoarticular arthritis may occur. Arthritis usually affects large joints, the knees in particular, and effusions are common. As many as one-third of the patients experience transient erysipelas-like skin lesions that appear typically on the lower leg, ankle, or dorsum of the foot. These lesions are circumscribed, painful, erythematous areas of swelling, which usually subsides within 24 to 48 hours.

In approximately 25 percent of affected patients a form of renal amyloidosis develops in which the amyloid derives from a normal serum protein called serum amyloid A (amyloidosis of the AA type; see Chap. 110). The amyloidosis progresses over a period of years to renal failure in almost all cases, and the cause of death in patients with FMF is usually attributed to this complication. It appears that polymorphisms in the gene for serum amyloid A increase the susceptibility to renal amyloidosis and that polymorphisms in a gene for the major histocompatibility complex class 1α chain influence the severity of the disease.[312]

Laboratory Features Laboratory findings in FMF are nonspecific. Nonspecific findings include increases in inflammatory mediators such as amyloid A, fibrinogen, and C-reactive protein during febrile attacks.[312] Proteinuria greater than 0.5 g of protein per 24 hours in patients with FMF may suggest amyloidosis.

The cloning of the FMF gene now allows a reliable diagnostic test. By employing a set of polymerase chain reaction (PCR) primers, it is possible to identify the mutations responsible for the disease. Five founder mutations account for 74 percent of FMF carrier chromosomes from typical populations known to harbor the disease.[320] Carrier rates for FMF mutations may be as high as 1:3 in some populations, suggesting that the disease is often underdiagnosed. Some amino acids that cause human disease are often present in wild-type in primates.[321]

Differential Diagnosis The tumor necrosis factor receptor-associated periodic syndrome (TRAPS) was first described in 1982 in a large Irish family.[322] The affected family members had recurrent fever with localized myalgia and painful erythema. Differentiating this disorder from FMF was its response to corticosteroids and the autosomal dominant inheritance of the disorder. Affected patients can have attacks that last for at least 1 or 2 days, but prolonged attacks lasting longer than a week are common. Localized pain and tightness in one muscle group and a migratory pattern of the symptoms are prominent features. The disorder may be associated with colicky abdominal pain, diarrhea or constipation, nausea, and or vomiting. Painful conjunctivitis, periorbital edema, or both are common as well as chest pain secondary to sterile pleuritis.[312] During febrile attacks, painless skin lesions may develop on the trunk or extremities and may migrate distally. Missense mutations in the gene for the type-1 TNF 55-kDa cell membrane receptor, which is required for diagnosis, have been identified. Patients with TRAPS respond dramatically to high doses of oral prednisone (>20 mg). In time, however, the responses wane, requiring higher doses of corticosteroids. Standard doses of a p75:Fc fusion protein, etanercept, administrated subcutaneously twice weekly decreases the frequency, duration, and severity of attacks; thus, etanercept may provide a safer, more effective alternative then corticosteroids in controlling the disease.

Therapy, Course, and Prognosis Colchicine treatment is effective in FMF and may prevent the development of amyloidosis.[313] Prophylactic colchicine, 0.6 mg orally, two to three times a day, prevents or substantially reduces the acute attacks of FMF in most patients. Some patients can abort attack with intermittent doses of colchicine beginning at the onset of attacks (0.6 mg orally every hour for 4 hours, then every 2 hours for four doses, and then every 12 hours for 2 days). In general, patients who benefit from intermittent colchicine therapy are those who experience a recognizable prodrome before developing fever and clear-cut acute symptoms.

The prognosis for normal longevity for patients has been excellent since the recognition that colchicine is an effective treatment of this disease. Most patients can be maintained almost entirely symptom free. However, if amyloidosis develops, it may be followed by the nephrotic syndrome or uremia. Unless the patient receives a renal transplant, the likelihood of eventual death from renal failure is high.

Other Disorders of Neutrophil Motility

The directed migration of neutrophils from the circulation to an inflammatory site is a consequence of chemotaxis and leads to the accumulation of an exudate. For normal chemotaxis to occur, a complex series of events must be coordinated. Chemotactic factors must be generated in sufficient quantities to establish a chemotactic gradient. The neutrophils must have receptors for the chemotactic agents and mechanisms for discerning the direction of the chemotactic gradient. Depressed neutrophil chemotaxis has been observed in a wide variety of clinical conditions (see Table 66–2).[323] These can be stratified as follows: (1) defects in the generation of chemotactic signals; (2) intrinsic defects of the neutrophil; and (3) direct inhibitors of neutrophil motility in response to chemotactic factors.

Older patients with chemotactic disorders may be infected by a variety of microorganisms, including fungi and Gram-positive or Gram-negative bacteria. *S. aureus* is the most frequent bacterial offender. Typically, the skin, gingival mucosa, and regional lymph nodes are involved. Respiratory tract infections are frequent, but sepsis is rare. Delayed or inappropriate signs and symptoms of inflammation are common. Although the cells move slowly in Boyden chambers or other chemotactic assays, they do accumulate in sufficient numbers in inflammatory sites to produce pus. However, detection of patients with neutrophils that have profound defects in chemotaxis usually is accomplished through other phagocytic assays.

Patients with the hereditary deficiency of complement factors C3, C5, or properidin exhibit an increased incidence of bacterial infections because they are unable to form the chemotactic peptide C5a.[324] The degree to which defective chemotaxis plays a role in C3 deficiency is unclear because opsonization and ingestion rates also are abnormal in these disorders. Frequently, chemotactic disorders are associated with other impaired neutrophil functions. For instance, both glycogen storage disease type 1b[325] and Shwachman-Diamond syndrome[326] are chemotactic disorders frequently associated with an absolute neutrophil count below 0.5×10^9/L. Following restoration of a normal neutrophil count with granulocyte colony-stimulating factor, the patients no longer are predisposed to recurrent bacterial infections in spite of a persistent chemotactic defect. Thus, a chemotactic defect observed *in vitro* does not correlate invariably with decreased resistance to bacterial infections *in vivo*.

Among the impaired defense mechanisms of the neonate is neutrophil adherence and chemotaxis, as demonstrated by the *in vitro* response of neonatal neutrophils to a variety of chemotactic factors.[284] The impaired motility of the neonatal neutrophils in part arises from the diminished ability to mobilize neutrophil β_2 integrins following neutrophil activation.[327] Additionally, the neonatal neutrophil may have a qualitative defect in β_2-integrin function, resulting in impaired neutrophil transendothelial migration for up to 1 month after birth.

Drugs and Extrinsic Agents That Impair Neutrophil Motility

Although many pharmacologic agents can influence neutrophil function, few drugs used in clinical medicine affect neutrophil behavior *in vivo*. Ethanol, an inhibitor of phospholipase D, in concentrations that occur in human blood can inhibit neutrophil locomotion and ingestion.[328] Glucocorticoids, especially at high and sustained doses, inhibit neutrophil locomotion, ingestion, and degranulation.[329] Administration of glucocorticoids on alternate days does not interfere with neutrophil movement.[330] Epinephrine does not have a direct affect on neutrophil adhesion but cyclic adenosine monophosphate (cAMP), which is released from endothelial cells following exposure to epinephrine, can depress neutrophil adherence.[331] Similarly, elevated cAMP levels following epinephrine administration may impair neutrophil adherence, leading to diminished neutrophil margination and apparent neutrophilia. Immune complexes, as seen in patients with rheumatoid arthritis or other autoimmune diseases, also can inhibit neutrophil movement by binding to neutrophil Fc receptors.

Hyperimmunoglobulin E Syndrome

Definition and History Autosomal dominant hyperimmunoglobulin E syndrome (HIES) is a disorder characterized by markedly elevated serum IgE levels, chronic dermatitis, and serious recurrent bacterial infections.[332] The skin infections in these patients are remarkable for their absence of surrounding erythema, leading to the formation of "cold abscesses." The neutrophils and monocytes from patients with this syndrome exhibit a variable, but at times profound, chemotactic defect that appears extrinsic to the neutrophil (see Table 66–2).[333]

The syndrome was originally described in 1966 in two red-headed, fair-skinned females who had "cold abscesses" and hyperextensible joints, which led to the appellation "Job's syndrome."[332] Subsequently Buckley and coworkers documented the association of levels of immunoglobulin E with undue susceptibility to infection.[334]

Epidemiology Reports of more than 200 cases have been documented.[334,335] HIES occurs in persons from diverse ethnic backgrounds and does not seem to be more common in any specific population.

Etiology and Pathogenesis Both males and females have been affected, as well as members of succeeding generations, indicating that the disorder is autosomal dominant with an incomplete penetrance form of inheritance.[332] STAT 3 mutations cause most, if not all cases of autosomal dominant HIES. All mutations have been missense mutations or in-frame deletions, leading to the formation of full-length mutant STAT 3 protein, which exerts a dominant negative effect. STAT 3 is a major transduction protein affecting pathways involving wound healing angiogenesis, immunity, and cancer.

The mechanism of the immune deficiencies in HIES remains clouded. Several reports with limited numbers of patients have conflicted results as to whether a chemotactic defect exists and whether there is a T-helper 1/T-helper 2 cytokine imbalance.

Clinical Features HIES may begin as early as day 1 of life.[334] The syndrome is characterized by chronic eczematoid rashes, which are typically papular and pruritic. The rash generally involves the face and extensor surfaces of arms and legs; skin lesions are frequently sharply demarcated and usually lack surrounding erythema. By 5 years of age all patients have had a history of recurrent skin abscess formation with recurrent pneumonias, along with chronic otitis media and sinusitis. Patients may also develop septic arthritis, cellulitis, or osteomyelitis. The major offending pathogen is generally *S. aureus*. Other pathogens commonly infecting patients are *C. albicans, Haemophilus influenzae,* and pneumococci. Other associated features include coarse facial features, including a prominent forehead, deep set eyes, a broad nasal bridge, a wide fleshly nasal tip, mild prognathism facial asymmetry, and hemihypertrophy.[332] There is a high incidence of scoliosis, hyperextensible joints, and delayed shedding of the primary teeth.[332] Occasionally unexplained osteopenia presents, which is often complicated by recurrent bone fractures. Additionally, there is an increased risk of both Hodgkin and non-Hodgkin lymphoma.

Laboratory Features Blood and sputum eosinophilia have been a consistent finding in all patients.[332] Patient serum IgE levels range from 3 to 80 times the upper limit of normal. The serum IgE usually rises above 2000 IU/mL and often is elevated at birth. Upon reaching adulthood the IgE may decline over years, despite the clinical abnormalities of STAT 3 deficiency. Usually patients have normal concentrations of IgG, IgA, and IgM, and may have elevated levels of IgD. Patients often have abnormally low anamnestic antibody response and poor antibody and cell-mediated responses to neoantigens. At times the neutrophils and monocytes of patients have a profound chemotactic defect.

Differential Diagnosis Autosomal recessive-HIES (AR-HIES) is a distinct clinical entity manifested by elevated IgE ligands, and recurrent skin and cutaneous viral infections, but lack the connective tissue and skeletal findings STAT 3 deficiency.[332]

Fatal sepsis occurs in AR-HIES from both Gram-positive and Gram-negative bacteria. Patients with AR-HIES have more symptomatic neurologic disease than STAT 3 deficiency. Autoimmune hemolytic anemia may occur, but neutrophil chemotaxis is normal. The genetic mutation underlying AR-HIES remain unclear. Therapy remains supportive.

Therapy, Course, and Prognosis No known therapy is curative, and management decisions are based on the clinical findings. Prophylactic trimethoprim-sulfamethoxazole is effective in reducing infections with *S. aureus*.[332] Type and route of antibiotic therapy are dictated by the results of the Gram stain and culture in patients with acute bacterial infections. Incision and drainage are essential for the management of abscesses, including superinfected pneumatoceles. Eczematoid dermatitis can be controlled with topical glucocorticoids to reduce inflammation and antihistamines to control pruritus. Intravenous immunoglobulin may decrease the number of infections for some patients. Attention needs to be paid to the scoliosis, fractures and degenerative joints by orthopedists. Retention of primary teeth requires dental expertise.

If the hyperimmunoglobulin IgE is recognized early in life and the patient is maintained on chronic anti-*Staphylococcal* antibiotic therapy, the prognosis remains good. Many such patients have reached maturity, indicating that the syndrome is compatible with prolonged survival. Conversely, if the diagnosis is delayed and the patient develops infected giant pneumatoceles, secondary fungal infections may occur, leading to a morbid state.[332]

DEFECTS IN MICROBICIDAL ACTIVITY

Chronic Granulomatous Disease

Definition and History Chronic granulomatous disease (CGD) is a genetic disorder affecting the function of neutrophils and monocytes. These phagocytic cells are able to ingest, but not kill catalase-positive microorganisms because of an inability to generate antimicrobial oxygen metabolites (see Table 66–2). It is caused by mutations involving one of several genes encoding a component of the NADPH oxidase.[336]

In 1957, two pediatric groups caring for six male infants reported a clinical disorder of chronic suppurative lymphadenitis and recurrent fevers leading to premature deaths in the children.[337,338] In the same time period, three observations assisted in providing the framework to understand the defect in the phagocytes of patients with CGD. Scientists described first that a striking increase in oxygen consumption was found upon particle ingestion by phagocytes, which was not related to mitochondrial oxygen metabolism.[339] Next, it was found that the process of phagocytosis was accompanied by the formation of large quantities of hydrogen peroxide in the cell.[340] Subsequently, it was reported that homogenates of phagocytes consume oxygen when incubated with pyridine nucleotides.[341] These observations indicated that an oxidase enzyme or enzymes in the phagocytes were activated during phagocytosis to convert molecular oxygen into hydrogen peroxide. It was then established that phagocytes from patients with CGD could ingest, but could not kill, the catalase-positive organisms.[341] Building on previous studies that a neutrophil oxidase mediates the increase in oxygen consumption, a pyridine-dependent oxidase was found to be deficient in neutrophils of patients with CGD, which led to their inability to reduce the dye nitroblue tetrazolium (NBT) during phagocytosis of particles.[342] Collectively, these studies laid the groundwork for subsequent studies to unravel the biochemical and genetic defects in CGD.

Epidemiology The incidence of CGD in the United States is 1 per 200,000 births, based on data from the National Institutes of Allergy and Infectious Disease Registry.[343] Data from the Registry indicates that 86 percent of patients are male and 14 percent female; 80 percent are classified as white, 11 percent as black patients, and 3 percent Asians or mixed-race patients. Of the 340 patients in the Registry with adequate information for determination genetic transmission, 70 percent had the X-linked recessive form of the disease.

TABLE 66–4. Diagnostic Classification of Chronic Granulomatous Disease

Affected Component	Inheritance	Subtype	Membrane Bound Cytochrome b558*	Cytosol p47*phox**	Cytosol p67*phox**
gp91*phox*	X	X91^0	Not detectable	Normal	Normal
		X91$^+$	Normal quantity, but nonfunctional	Normal	Normal
		X91$^-$	Defective gp91*phox*, which is poorly functional or expressed in a small fraction of phagocytes	Normal	Normal
p22*phox*	A	A22^0	Not detectable	Normal	Normal
		A22$^+$	Normal quantity, but nonfunctional	Normal	Normal
p47*phox*	A	A47^0	Normal quantity	Not detectable	Normal
p67*phox*		A67^0	Normal	Normal	Not detectable

*Detected by spectral analysis or immunoblotting. In this nomenclature, the first letter represents the mode of inheritance (-linked [X] or autosomal recessive [A]). The number indicates the phox component, which is genetically affected. The superscript symbols indicate whether the level of protein of the affected component is undetectable (0), diminished (–), or normal (+) as measured by immunoblot or spectral analysis.

Etiology and Pathogenesis Several laboratory tests are used to classify forms of CGD and aid in understanding its pathogenesis (Table 66–4). The diagnosis of CGD is based on a compatible clinical history and demonstration of a defective respiratory burst. Several methods detect the production of reactive oxidants. The NBT method relies on the intracellular reduction of NBT by superoxide anion to a blue formazan precipitate that can be seen microscopically.[336] More sensitive methods rely on the reaction of oxidants with specific chemiluminescent and fluorescent probes. The patients with CGD may have heterogeneous array of regular symptoms and severity, depending on which subunit is defective and on the nature of the genetic mutation.

NADPH-Oxidase Function Engulfment of microbes by phagocytic cells is associated with a burst of oxygen consumption that is important for microbicidal killing and digestion. The respiratory burst is accompanied, not by mitochondrial respiration, but by a unique electron transport chain called the NADPH oxidase. Prior to stimulation, the components of the oxidase are physically separated into two major subcellular locations (Fig. 66–6). The membrane-bound portion of the NADPH oxidase contains a heterodimeric cytochrome b_{558} composed of a large, heavily glycosylated subunit with a Mr of 91 kDa, known as a gp91*phox* (91-kDa glycoprotein of the phagocyte oxidase), and a 22-kDa protein known as p22*phox*.[336,344] Eighty to 90 percent of the cytochrome b_{558} is found in specific and gelatinase granules and secretory vesicles of the neutrophil and following neutrophil activation translocates to the plasma membrane.[280,345] The low-molecular-weight GTP-binding protein Rap1A is tightly bound with cytochrome b_{558} and serves to enhance function of the NADPH oxidase. The liberation from cytochrome of Rap1A b_{558} occurs upon phosphorylation of Rap1A.[346] The heavy chain of cytochrome b contains sites for heme binding, flavin adenine dinucleotide (FAD) groups, and NADPH binding.[347–350] The three-dimensional structure of cytochrome b_{558} indicates that the carboxyl-terminal half of the peptide contains sequences for flavin and NADPH binding.[351] There are heme groups, amino-linked glycosylation sites, and a proton conduction channel within the amino-terminus of gp91*phox*.[352] The amino-half of the molecule is hydrophobic and contains the histidines that coordinate heme binding.[353] The p22*phox* also contains a site for heme binding.[347] The synthesis of the p22*phox* peptide is absolutely required for stability of gp91*phox* and for oxidase activity in the membrane.[336] The p22*phox* also contains proline-rich regions that display consensus protein-protein interactions that provide a binding site for p47*phox*.[354] Three other proteins vital to the function of this oxidase system reside in the cytosol of the resting phagocyte. Upon stimulation, translocation of p47*phox* takes place. Phosphorylated p47*phox* together with two other cytoplasmic components of the oxidase, p67*phox* and a low-molecular-weight guanosine triphosphate Rac-2, translocate to the membrane, where they interact with cytoplasmic domains of the transmembrane cytochrome b_{558} to form the active oxidase.[354,355] Both p47*phox* and p67*phox* contain SH3 (Src homology 3) domains that may participate in intramolecular and intermolecular binding with consensus proline-rich regions in p47*phox*.[355] Phosphorylation, which occurs on serines in the cationic C-terminal region of p47*phox*, serves to disrupt this intermolecular interaction, making the SH3 regions available for binding to p22*phox*. Another cytoplasmic component with homology to p47*phox* has been identified to be p40*phox*, which interacts with p67*phox* before and during oxidase assembly.[356] The p40*phox* component stabilizes the preactivation cytoplasmic complexes of p67*phox* and p47*phox*, and may protect p67*phox* from degradation. Its binding of phosphatidylinositol also potentiates superoxide production upon neutrophil activation.[357] Based on the redox properties of cytochrome b_{558}, it is postulated that the cytochrome transfers electrons from NADPH to O_2 during the respiratory burst.

NADPH	flavin	heme	O_2	
→	→	→	→	O^-_2
–330 mV	–256 mV	–245 mV	–160mV	

Cytochrome b_{558} spans the membrane, permitting NADPH to be oxidized at the cytoplasmic surface and oxygen to be reduced to form O_2 on the outer surface of the plasma membrane or on the inner surface of the phagosomal membrane.[358]

A cell-free system for activating the oxidase has permitted the dissection of the enzyme system into its components and the evaluation of the function of each unit.[359–365] Both cytosolic and membrane proteins are required for oxidase activation, and all patients with CGD have defects involving cytochrome b or the cytosolic components p47*phox* or p67*phox*.[336] The membrane and cytosol interaction for oxidase activation in the cell-free system defines the genetic heterogeneity of CGD.[336] Table 66–4 illustrates this point. The neutrophil membrane fractions from patients with XO (-linked, cytochrome b-negative) and AO (autosomal recessive, cytochrome b-negative) CGD do not support oxidase activation even upon addition of normal cytosol, whereas the corresponding patient's cytosol functions normally.[366] The membrane defect in both these types

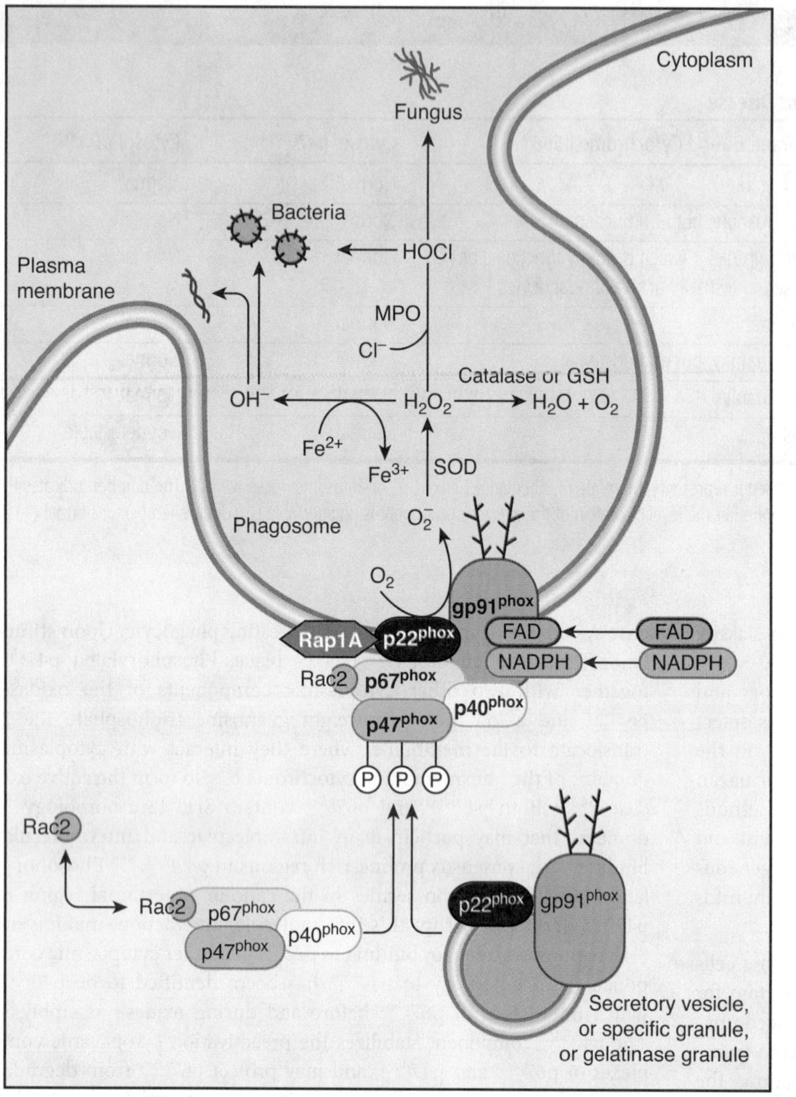

FIGURE 66–6. Possible mechanisms for the production of superoxide anion in neutrophils. Oxygen is reduced to superoxide (O_2^-) by an NADPH oxidase. The oxidase is a composite of (1) a 47-kDa cytosolic protein (p47); (2) a 67-kDa cytosolic protein (p67); (3) a 40-kDa cytosolic protein (p40); (4) a low-molecular-weight cytosolic G-protein, Rac2; and (5) a membrane-bound cytochrome b_{558}. Cytochrome b consists of a 22-kDa protein subunit and a 91-kDa glycoprotein subunit, both of which contain heme. The gp91 subunit is an FAD-dependent flavoprotein that contains the NADPH binding site and ultimately shuttles electrons to molecular oxygen, forming O_2^-, and (6) Rap1A, which serves to enhance the function of the NADPH oxidase. The cytosol components translocate to the membrane and may serve to alter the tertiary structure of cytochrome b, to permit the flow of electrons from NADPH to O_2. The p47 subunit is phosphorylated upon activation of the neutrophil. The p40*phox* component stabilizes the preactivation complex of p67*phox*. The unstable superoxide anion (O_2^-) is converted to hydrogen peroxide (H_2O_2), either spontaneously or by the enzyme superoxide dismutase. H_2O_2 in the presence of myeloperoxidase converts H_2O_2 to hypochlorous acid. Both H_2O_2 and O_2^- can be transformed into hydroxyl radical (OH^-). Hydrogen peroxide can be reduced to H_2O and O_2 by the enzyme catalase or by glutathione (GSH), a product of the hexose-monophosphate shunt. These reactive oxygen species are responsible for microbial killing. Normal oxidative function of the NADPH complex requires fully functional individual components.

of CGD is a result of the absence of cytochrome b. In the case of A+ CGD (autosomal recessive, cytochrome b-positive), the membrane fraction is normal, whereas the cytosol is severely defective.

Genetic Alterations Affecting Cytochrome b The most frequent form of CGD occurs in 70 percent of patients and is caused by mutations in the gp91*phox* gene, termed CYBB, which is located on chromosome Xp21.1.[336,367] These mutations lead to the X-linked form of the disease. Large interstitial deletions causing other X-linked disorders such as retinitis pigmentosa, Duchenne muscular dystrophy, McLeod hemolytic anemia, and ornithine transcarbamylase deficiency, have been reported in a few patients with X-linked CGD.[343,368–370] Mutation analysis of the gene encoding gp91 and a large group of X-linked CGD kindreds has documented many distinct defects, including point mutations, inversions, deletions, or insertions that disrupt the reading frame and nonsense mutations that create a premature stop codon.[367] Some splice site defects have also been identified. In this situation, short deletions in gp91*phox* mRNA are caused by point mutations that produce partial or complete exon skipping during mRNA splicing.[371] This abnormality is a common cause of X-linked CGD. In the remaining patients, point mutations have been identified that generate either premature stop codons or amino acid substitutions that apparently disrupt protein stability or function and lead to a complete lack of detectable cytochrome b_{558} protein in phagocytic cells in most patients with X-linked CGD.[372] In some situations, low levels of functional cytochrome b are present, whereas in others, normal levels of dysfunctional cytochrome b_{558} occur.[372] In the latter situation there is some clustering of defects in regions of known function, such as the NADPH- or flavin-binding consensus regions.[373] Approximately 10 to 15 percent of X-linked CGD arises from new germ line mutations.[374]

A similar array of mutations has been identified in the 5 percent of CGD patients who have abnormalities in the p22*phox* gene, termed CYBA, which is located on chromosome 16q24.[336,373,375] In this autosomal disorder, mutations in the p22*phox* gene result in deletions, frameshifts, and/or missense mutations. Patients with a defective p22*phox* gene do not express the other cytoplasmic unit polypeptide. In one patient, p22*phox* peptide was associated with normal amounts of cytochrome b with normal heme spectrum, but p47*phox* translocation membrane did not occur and there was no oxidase activation because the mutation affected a proline-rich region thought to mediate binding to one of the SH3 domains of p47*phox*. In gp91*phox*-deficient patients, p22*phox* mRNA is present, but it is not translated, which is consistent with the notion that either cytochrome subunit polypeptide is dependent upon the stable expression of the other subunit.[336]

Genetic Alterations Affecting Cytosolic Proteins Two other proteins have been identified as being vital to the function of the NADPH-oxidase system. Their absence results in the syndrome of CGD.[376] These proteins have molecular masses of 47 kDa and 67 kDa, respectively, and are located in the cytosol of resting cells. Defects in the genes for p47*phox*, termed NCF1, which is found on chromosome 7q11, are responsible for the majority of all cases of autosomal recessive CGD, whereas inherited defects for the gene for neutrophil p67*phox*, termed NCF2, account for a small subgroup of autosomal recessive CGD.[336] The function of p47*phox* and p67*phox* in regulating the respiratory burst oxidase is thought to involve activation of the electron transport function of cytochrome b_{558}. The mutation analysis in patients with p47*phox*-deficient forms of CGD reveals an unusual pattern, in that more than 90 percent of mutant alleles have guanine-thymine dinucleotide deletion at the start of exon 2, resulting in frameshift and premature stop.[373,377] The truncated protein is unstable in that it cannot be detected immunologically. The majority of patients appear to be homozygous for this mutation without any history of consanguinity. The $p47^{phox}$ gene occurs in an area of chromosome 7 that has a high degree of evolutionary duplication in normal individuals because a pseudogene highly homologous to the normal $p47^{phox}$ gene exists in the normal genome in this region of duplication. The pseudogene contains the same GT deletion associated with most cases of $p47^{phox}$ CGD. This implies that recombination of the normal gene and pseudogene with conversion of the normal gene to partial pseudotype sequence in that region may be responsible for the high relative rate of this specific mutation in diverse racial groups, which proved to be the case.[378]

A second rare form of CGD is caused by mutations in the gene for the $p67^{phox}$ cytosolic component.[372] The $p67^{phox}$ gene, which has been mapped to the long arm of chromosome 1, spans 37 kb and contains 16 exons. The mutations identified in $p67^{phox}$-deficiency CGD have included missense mutations and spliced junction mutations affecting mRNA processing, which led to nondetectable $p67^{phox}$ protein by immunologic means.[373]

Predisposition to Infection As indicated above, mutations in the gene for cytochrome b_{558} or the cytosolic factors involved in activating the cytochrome are associated with the CGD phenotype. Figure 66–7 shows schematically the manner in which the metabolic deficiency of the CGD neutrophil predisposes the host to infection. Normal neutrophils accumulate hydrogen peroxide and other oxygen metabolites in the phagosomes containing ingested microorganisms. MPO is delivered to the phagosome by degranulation and in this setting hydrogen peroxide acts as a substrate for myeloperoxidase to oxidize halide to hypochlorous acid and chloramines, which kill the microbes. The quantity of hydrogen peroxide produced by the normal neutrophils is sufficient to exceed the capacity of catalase, a hydrogen peroxide-catabolizing enzyme produced by many aerobic microorganisms, including *S. aureus*, most Gram-negative enteric bacteria, *C. albicans*, and *Aspergillus* spp. In contrast, hydrogen peroxide is not produced by CGD neutrophils, and any generated by the microbes themselves may be destroyed by their own catalase. Thus, catalase-positive microbes can multiply inside CGD neutrophils, where they are protected from most circulating antibiotics, and can be transported to distant sites and released to establish new foci of infection.[376] Activation of the oxidase also has a pronounced effect on the pH within the phagocytic vacuole. It is controversial whether activation of the respiratory burst is associated with an alkaline phase, but the pH of the phagocytic vacuole becomes much more acidic in CGD patients than in normal patients.[379,380] The alkaline phase may be important for the antimicrobial and digestive functions of the neutral hydrolases released from the cytoplasmic granules into the vacuole upon phagocytosis. In CGD, the phagocytic vacuoles remain acidic and the bacteria are not digested properly.[381] The impairment in the respiratory burst by CGD neutrophils leads to delayed neutrophil apoptosis and subsequent impaired clearance of degenerating neutrophils by CGD macrophages, which, in turn, predisposes the host to enhanced inflammation.[382] The CGD macrophage is unable to clear CGD neutrophils because of a deficiency of intrinsic IL-4 production, which occurs because of defective phosphatidylserine exposure on CGD neutrophils, that is a necessary requirement to engage CGD macrophage phosphatidylserine membrane receptors and subsequent macrophage activation.[382] In hematoxylin-and-eosin-stained sections from patients, macrophages eventually may contain a golden pigment, which reflects the abnormal accumulation of ingested material and also contributes to the diffuse granulomata that give CGD its descriptive name.[383] On the other hand, when CGD neutrophils ingest pneumococci or streptococci, these organisms generate enough hydrogen peroxide to result in a microbicidal effect.

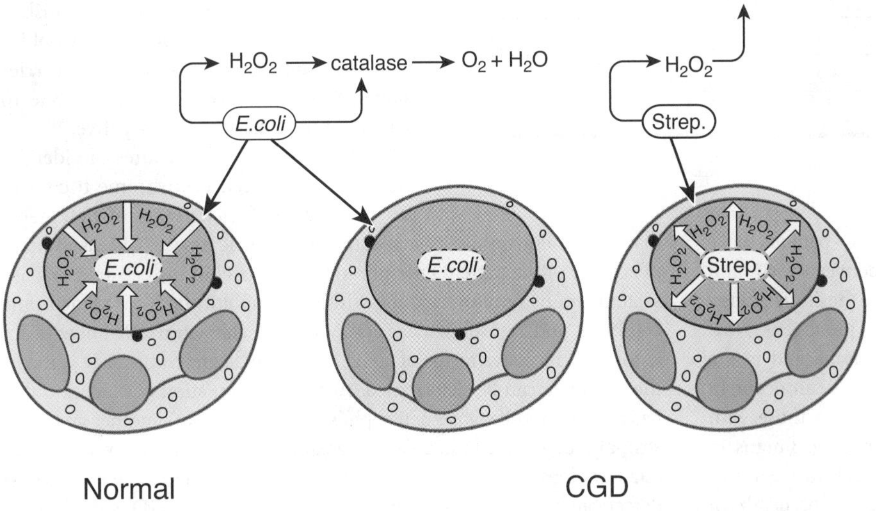

FIGURE 66–7. The pathogenesis of chronic granulomatous disease. The manner in which the metabolic deficiency of the CGD neutrophil predisposes the host to infection is shown schematically. Normal neutrophils accumulate hydrogen peroxide in the phagosome containing ingested *E. coli*. Myeloperoxidase is delivered to the phagosome by degranulation, as indicated by the closed circles, and in this setting, hydrogen peroxide acts as a substrate for myeloperoxidase to oxidize halide to hypochlorous acid and chloramines, which kill the microbes. The quantity of hydrogen peroxide produced by the normal neutrophils is sufficient to exceed the capacity of catalase, a hydrogen peroxide-catabolizing enzyme of many aerobic microorganisms, including most Gram-negative enteric bacteria, *S. aureus*, *C. albicans*, and *Aspergillus* spp. When organisms such as *E. coli* gain entry into the CGD neutrophils, they are not exposed to hydrogen peroxide because the neutrophils do not produce it, and the hydrogen peroxide generated by microbes themselves is destroyed by their own catalase. When CGD neutrophils ingest streptococci or pneumococci, these organisms generate enough hydrogen peroxide to result in a microbicidal effect. On the other hand, as indicated in the middle figure, catalase-positive microbes, such as *E. coli*, can survive within the phagosome of the CGD neutrophil.

Clinical Features Although the clinical presentation is variable, several clinical features suggest the diagnosis of CGD.[336] Any patient with recurrent lymphadenitis should be considered to have CGD. Additionally, patients with bacterial hepatic abscesses, osteomyelitis at multiple sites or in the small bones of the hands and feet, a family history of recurrent infections, or unusual catalase-positive microbial infections all require clinical evaluation for this disorder. Table 66–5 lists the most common clinical infections that afflict CGD patients and Table 66–6 cites their prevalence.

Among the various infections, only perirectal abscess, suppurative adenitis, and bacteremia/fungemia differ significantly in prevalence in the X-linked recessive and autosomal recessive CGD patients.[343] Each of these conditions was twice as common in the X-linked form.

The onset of clinical signs and symptoms may occur from early infancy to young adulthood. Although the majority of patients with CGD (76%) are diagnosed before the age of 5 years, approximately 10 percent are not diagnosed until the second decade of life, and on rare occasions, until the

TABLE 66–5. Common Infecting Organisms Isolated from Chronic Granulomatous Disease Patients

Infection Type	Organism	X-Linked Recessive (%)	Autosomal Recessive (%)
Pneumonia	*Aspergillus* spp.	41	29
	Staphylococcus spp.	11	13
	Burkholderia cepacia	7	11
	Nocardia spp.	6	13
	Serratia spp.	4	5
Abscess			
Subcutaneous	*Staphylococcus* spp.	28	21
	Serratia spp.	19	9
	Aspergillus spp.	7	0
Liver	*Staphylococcus* spp.	52	52
	Serratia spp.	6	4
	Candida spp.	12	0
Lung	*Aspergillus* spp.	27	18
Perirectal	*Staphylococcus* spp.	9	15
Brain	*Aspergillus* spp.	75	25
Suppurative adenitis	*Staphylococcus* spp.	29	12
	Serratia spp.	9	15
	Candida spp.	7	4
Osteomyelitis	*Serratia* spp.	32	12
	Aspergillus spp.	25	18
Bacteremia/fungemia	*Salmonella* spp.	20	13
	Burkholderia cepacia	13	0
	Candida spp.	9	25
	Staphylococcus spp.	11	0

Data adapted from Segal BH, Leto TL, Gallin JI et al.[336]

third decade or later.[343] The organisms infecting CGD patients have changed considerably from those initially reported between 1957 and 1976. *Staphylococcus* caused most of the infections in the initial cases; *Klebsiella* and *E. coli* were then the next most common pathogens. Now *Aspergillus* is the prominent organism causing pneumonia and is the leading cause of death in patients.[336] Invasive aspergillosis can occur in the first few months of life in healthy infants as well as in those with CGD. Although aspergillosis is the most common infecting fungus in CGD, *Candida* and several other fungal strains have been invasive in this disorder. *Burkholderia cepacia* is another leading cause of death in patients with CGD. *Serratia marcescens* is the third leading organism that commonly infects patients with CGD. Infections are characterized by microabscesses and granuloma formation. The presence of pigmented histiocytes is helpful in establishing the diagnosis. Patients may suffer from the consequences of chronic infections including the anemia of chronic disease, lymphadenopathy, hepatosplenomegaly, chronic purulent dermatitis, restrictive lung disease, gingivitis, hydronephrosis, and gastroenteric narrowing.[343] Patients with CGD are also at risk for developing colitis and chorioretinitis, and discoid lupus erythematosus.[343]

Several mothers of patients in whom X-linked inheritance was established had an illness resembling systemic lupus erythematosus.[343] Both X-linked and autosomal recessive patients with CGD also have a similar disorder.[384] It may be that these mothers' and patients' cells are unable to clear immune complexes sufficiently, which is a characteristic feature of CGD cells *in vitro*.[385] Variant alleles of mannose-binding lectin and FcγRIIA especially in combination have been associated with rheumatologic disorders in patients with CGD.[386]

Laboratory Features The defect in the respiratory burst is best determined by measuring superoxide or hydrogen peroxide production in response to both soluble and particulate stimuli.[387] A test that is being employed is the use of flow cytometry using dihydrorhodamine-123 fluorescence.[388] Dihydrorhodamine-123 fluorescence detects oxidant production because it increases fluorescence upon oxidation.[388] In most cases there is no detectable superoxide or hydrogen peroxide generation with either type of stimulus. In the variant form of CGD, however, superoxide may be produced at rates between 0.5 and 10 percent of control.[389]

An alternative method for measuring respiratory burst activity is the NBT test. This assay is performed by microscopically assessing the ability of individual cells to reduce NBT to purple formazan crystals following stimulation. Commonly there is no NBT reduction with most forms of CGD. In some of the variant forms, however, a high percentage of cells may contain some formazan, a finding indicative of a greatly diminished respiratory burst in most of the neutrophils. This test also permits detection of the carrier state in X-linked CGD when as few as 5 to 10 percent of the cells are NBT-negative.[390]

Most sophisticated procedures can identify the molecular defect. Cytochrome b content can be measured in extracts of detergent-disrupted neutrophils by a spectrophotometric assay.[390] Measurement of activity of the patient's membrane and cytosol in the cell-free oxidase system can be employed along with immunoblotting for a cytochrome b subunit and cytosol oxidase component to characterize X-linked from autosomal recessive forms of CGD. Once the diagnosis of CGD is made, the genotype can be determined. A mosaic population of oxidation that has positive and negative neutrophils in a male patient's mother and sister strongly suggests X-linked CGD. Lack of a mosaic pattern among female relatives does not rule out the X-linked mode of inheritance because the defect can arise spontaneously. Prenatal diagnosis of CGD is established by performing analysis of DNA neutrophil oxidant production from umbilical blood samples obtained by fetoscopy.[391] Alternatively, DNA can be analyzed from amniocytes or chorionic villus samples. Restriction fragment length polymorphisms have been successful for diagnosing gp91^{phox} and p67^{phox} deficiency in informative families.[392] In other families PCR technology can be employed to analyze fetal DNA if a family's specific mutation is known.

Differential Diagnosis Leukocytes from patients with CGD have normal glucose-6-phosphate dehydrogenase (G-6-PD) activity. However, a few individuals with apparent CGD have been described that have neutrophils that lack or are almost lacking in G-6-PD activity.[393,394] The erythrocytes of these patients also lack the enzyme, and the patients

TABLE 66–6. Prevalence of Infection Complication of Chronic Granulomatous Disease Patients

Infection Type	X-Linked Recessive (%)	Autosomal Recessive (%)
Pneumonia	80	77
Abscess (all)	68	70
Subcutaneous	43	42
Liver	26	33
Lung	16	14
Brain	3	5
Perirectal	17	7
Suppurative adenitis	59	32
Osteomyelitis	27	21
Bacteremia/fungemia	21	10
Cellulitis	7	5

Data adapted from Segal BH, Leto TL, Gallin JI et al.[336]

have chronic hemolysis. In the cases of severe neutrophil G-6-PD deficiency, an attenuated respiratory burst progressively decreases as a result of the depletion of intracellular NADPH, the primary substrate for the respiratory burst oxidase. CGD and G-6-PD deficiency can be distinguished from each other by the hemolytic anemia seen in the latter disorder and by the fact that erythrocyte G-6-PD activity is normal in CGD and markedly reduced in G-6-PD deficiency.[372]

A variety of studies indicate that the small GTPase Rac-2 plays an essential role in activity of the NADPH and the actin cytoskeleton in human neutrophils.[343] A toddler has been described who presented with a perirectal abscess at 5 weeks of age. This patient subsequently had necrosis of the periumbilical skin and fascia, and his surgical wounds did not heal properly. Functionally his neutrophils had multiple defective components; for example, adhesion to ligands for sialyl Lewis X, chemotaxis, release of primary azurophil granules upon stimulation with chemotactic peptide, and failure to undergo the respiratory burst using the same stimulus.[395,396] Molecular analysis identified the asparagine for aspartic acid mutation at amino acid 57 of one allele of the Rac-2 gene.[395,396] Mutant Rac-2 did not bind GTP and it inhibited and behaved as a dominant negative to impair Rac-2–mediated activation of the respiratory burst.[396] Fortunately, the youngster was successfully transplanted with marrow from a HLA-identical older brother.[396]

Therapy, Course, and Prognosis Because marrow transplantation is the only known recognized cure for CGD, vigorous supportive care along with the use of recombinant interferon continues to be the foundation of treatment.[336] Cultures must be obtained as soon as infection is suspected, as unusual organisms are commonly the source of infection and may grow promptly *in vitro*. Most abscesses require surgical drainage for therapeutic and diagnostic purposes, and prolonged use of antibiotics is often required. If fever occurs, it is advisable to obtain certain studies that aid in the management of septic episodes. These include roentgenograms of the chest and skeleton and a computed tomography (CT) scan of the liver because of the frequency of pneumonia, osteomyelitis, and liver abscesses.[343] Arrangements should be made for prompt medical attention at the first signs of infection. With early intervention, many lesions can be managed by conservative medical means. For example, enlarging lymph nodes often regress when treated with local heat and orally administered antistaphylococcal antibiotics. It is particularly important to obtain a microbiologic diagnosis, and fine-needle aspiration may be helpful in this regard. In general, antibiotic therapy for the offending organisms is indicated and purulent masses should be drained. The cause of fever and prostration cannot always be established, and empiric treatment with broad-spectrum parenteral antibiotics is required. Often it is necessary to treat with antibiotics for a prolonged time until the initially elevated sedimentation rate approaches normal values. *Aspergillus* spp. infection requires treatment with amphotericin B or, in refractory cases, with granulocyte transfusions.[336] Glucocorticoids also may be useful in the treatment of patients with antral and urethral obstruction. The risk of *Aspergillus* infection can be reduced by avoiding marijuana smoke and decaying plant material, such as mulch and hay, both of which contain numerous fungal spores.[397] Long-term oral prophylaxis with trimethoprim-sulfamethoxazole (5 mg/kg per day of trimethoprim) is an accepted practice in the management of patients with CGD.[336] Patients have prolonged infection-free periods, which result from the prevention of infections caused by *S. aureus*, without increasing the incidence of fungal infections. The use of itraconazole prophylactically has reduced the development of fungal infections.[398,399]

Interferon (IFN)-γ(50 mcg/m^2, three times per week) can reduce the number of serious bacterial and fungal infections.[398,400] IFN-γ–enhanced neutrophil function *in vitro* has not been correlated with improvement in the activity of the neutrophil respiratory burst in patients totally lacking the ability to generate superoxide. On the other hand, its use increases the neutrophil expression of the high-affinity Fcγ receptor 1, as well as monocyte expression of FcγRI, FcγRII, FcγRIII, CD11/CD18, and HLA-DR.[401] The IFN-γ protective effect in patients with CGD may involve improved microbial clearance, as suggested by the enhanced phagocytic activity by neutrophils of opsonized *S. aureus*. In rare, X-linked CGD patients able to generate some superoxide, IFN-γ programs granulocyte cells to increase their expression of cytochrome b, which results in normal superoxide generation.[402] With the use of current prophylactic treatments, the mortality in CGD has been reduced to 2 patient deaths per year per 100 patients followed.[336]

CGD patients with mutations that result in 5 to 10 percent of normal-functioning amounts of NADPH have a mild phenotype and better clinical prognosis than do patients with complete absence of any NADPH-oxidase activity.[403,404] Similarly, female carriers of X-linked CGD who have only 3 to 5 percent oxidase-normal neutrophils rarely get serious infections suggestive of the CGD clinical phenotype.[405] Thus, even low levels or partial correction by gene therapy of CGD is likely to provide clinical benefits. In support of that hypothesis, mouse models of X-linked and p47^{phox}-deficient CGD have been developed by gene targeting.[406,407] Studies in the gp91^{phox}- and the p47^{phox}-deficient mouse models of CGD show that retrovirus-mediated gene-therapy-targeting of marrow progenitor cells *ex vivo* can result in the correction of defects in oxidant production *in vivo* in blood neutrophils after radiation conditioning and transplantation of marrow stem cells.[408,409] Protection from infection challenge occurred even when the oxidase-corrected cells comprised less than 10 percent of circulating neutrophils. These promising results suggest that somatic gene therapy can be employed to correct defective phagocyte oxidase function in selected patients with CGD. In a phase I clinical trial, gene therapy for p47^{phox}-deficiency CGD, five adult patients received intravenous infusions of autologous blood stem cells that were *ex vivo* transduced using a retrovirus encoding normal p47^{phox}.[410] Although conditioning therapy was not given prior to the stem cell infusion, functionally corrected neutrophils were detectable in blood for several months.[300] In another study, long-term high-level clinical beneficial correction in *ex vivo* gene therapy of X-linked CGD occurred in two adult patients.[411] Nonablative busulfan conditioning was used to augment gene therapy correction. There needs to be caution regarding the long-term stability and safety of gene therapy. For instance, there are concerns about gene insertion rendering patients vulnerable to developing acute myelogenous leukemia.

Myeloperoxidase Deficiency

The functional and immunochemical absence of the enzyme MPO from granules of neutrophils and monocytes, but not eosinophils, is inherited as an autosomal recessive trait, with a prevalence of 1:2000.[412] MPO, an enzyme that catalyzes the production of hypochlorous acid in the phagosome, causes microbicidal deficiency of the neutrophils early after ingestion of microorganisms (see Table 66–2). However, normal microbicidal activity is observed in approximately 1 hour after a variety of organisms are ingested.[412] Thus, the MPO-deficient neutrophil uses a MPO-independent system for killing bacteria that is slower than the MPO–hydrogen peroxide–halide system, but that is eventually effective in eliminating bacteria. MPO-deficient neutrophils accumulate more hydrogen peroxide than do normal neutrophils; the higher peroxide concentration improves the bactericidal activity of the affected neutrophils. In contrast to the retardation of bactericidal activity, candidacidal activity in MPO-deficient neutrophils is absent.[412] The most significant clinical manifestation in a few patients with diabetes mellitus and MPO deficiency has been severe infection with *C. albicans*. Because this is such a common disorder of phagocytes, it is important to note that the vast majority of patients with this genetic disorder have not been unusually susceptible to pyogenic infections and do not require therapy.

The complementary DNA encoding human MPO has been cloned and the gene structure, including promoter and regulatory elements, delineated.[412] The gene consists of 12 exons and 11 introns and is located on the long arm of chromosome 17, and its expression is finely coordinated with expression of genes encoding other lysosomal proteins. Expression of genes for human neutrophil elastase and myeloperoxidase is very similar; it is low in myeloblasts, peaks during the promyelocyte stage, and eventually drops to low levels in myelocytes. MPO is a symmetric molecule composed of four peptides, where each half consists of a heavy- and a light-chain heterodimer.[412] Each heavy- and light-chain heterodimer starts as a single peptide that is cleaved during the post-translational process to yield the heavy and light chains that form half of the mature molecules. The two halves of the molecule are associated by a disulfide linkage between heavy-subunit residues at their residue C319.

The primary translation product of the gene is a single-chain peptide of 80 kDa that undergoes cotranslational glycosylation at several asparagine residues, followed by a series of modifications of these oligosaccharides. The apopromyeloperoxidase exists for a prolonged time in the endoplasmic reticulum, where it associates reversibly with several endoplasmic reticulum–resident proteins known as molecular chaperones.[412] Subsequent to heme insertion, the enzymatically active promyeloperoxidase undergoes proteolytic cleavage of the pro region. Then, in a prelysosomal compartment, the single peptide is cleaved into the heavy and light subunits, which remain linked. During final sorting within the azurophil lysosome compartment, there is dimerization of half-molecules to form the mature MPO.

Most patients with MPO deficiency have a missense mutation in the gene that results in replacement of arginine 569 with tryptophan.[412] The mutation results in a precursor that associates with molecular chaperones, but does not incorporate heme, resulting in a maturational arrest during processing at the stage of an inactive enzymatic apopromyeloperoxidase. Other patients are heterozygotes with one allele bearing the common mutation and the other being normal, resulting in a partial deficiency.[413] To date, four genotypes have been reported to cause inherited MPO deficiency, each of which results in missense mutations. In the genotype Y173C, a missense mutation results in replacement of a tyrosine at codon 173 with a cysteine residue resulting in the mutant precursor being retained in the endoplasmic reticulum by virtue of its prolonged interaction with the chaperone calnexin, and eventually undergoing degradation in a proteosome.[412] In this way, the quality control system operating in the endoplasmic reticulum retrieves malfolded MPO precursors from the biosynthetic pathway and creates the biochemical phenotype of MPO deficiency. In another patient, a missense mutation resulted in an intact MPO molecule that acquired heme but failed to undergo proteolytic processing to a mature molecule.

Acquired disorders are associated with MPO deficiency. Reported states include lead intoxication, ceroid lipofuscinosis, myelodysplastic syndromes, and acute myelogenous leukemia.[414] One-half of untreated patients with acute myelogenous leukemia and 20 percent of patients with chronic myelogenous leukemia may have MPO deficiency.[414]

Deficiencies of Glutathione Reductase and Glutathione Synthetase

Neutrophils contain enzymes capable of inactivating potentially damaging reduced oxygen byproducts. Disposal of superoxide anion is accomplished through superoxide dismutase, a soluble enzyme that converts superoxide to a hydrogen peroxide. Hydrogen peroxide is detoxified by catalase and by the glutathione peroxidase–glutathione reductase system, which converts hydrogen peroxide to water and oxygen.[415] In addition to the soluble enzymes, cellular vitamin E serves as an antioxidant to prevent damage to the surface of activated neutrophils when releasing hydrogen peroxide.[415] Single cases of profound deficiencies in glutathione reductase[416] and glutathione synthetase[415] have been associated with impaired neutrophil bactericidal activity (see Table 66–2). Both deficiencies are associated with hemolysis under conditions of oxidative stress (see Chap. 46). Glutathione synthetase deficiency also has been associated with intermittent neutropenia during times of mild infection. Vitamin E has been employed to ameliorate the hemolysis and improve neutrophil function in a patient with glutathione synthetase deficiency.[417] Like patients with myeloperoxidase-deficient neutrophils, the patients with glutathione reductase deficiency and glutathione synthetase deficiency are not unusually susceptible to bacterial infections.

DIAGNOSTIC APPROACH TO THE PATIENT WITH SUSPECTED NEUTROPHIL DYSFUNCTION

An increased susceptibility to pyogenic infections must be viewed in light of a number of factors: (1) adequacy of host defense; (2) the microbes to which the host is exposed; and (3) the conditions of the exposure. It is not always easy to establish a diagnosis of a specific neutrophil dysfunction on clinical grounds alone. Patients with recurrent pyogenic infections often yield no clues as to why they are afflicted, and patients with established deficiency of a defense mechanism may have an unimpressive clinical history. On the other hand, patients may be suspected of having a neutrophil dysfunction if they have a history of frequent bacterial or severe infections. Recurrent pulmonary infections, hepatic abscesses, and perirectal abscesses also should alert the clinician to consider further diagnostic evaluation of neutrophil function. For example, the identification of unusual catalase-positive bacteria and fungi, such as *B. cepacia*, *S. marcescens*, *Nocardia*, and *Aspergillus*, could be indicative of CGD.

Because many of the tests of neutrophil function are bioassays with great variability, the results of the tests must be interpreted in light of the patient's clinical condition. For instance, isolated chemotactic defects usually do not explain the propensity for a patient to have recurrent severe infections. Furthermore, variation in bioassays is often intensified by inflammation or infection. Figure 66–8 is an algorithm for evaluation of the patient with recurrent infection.

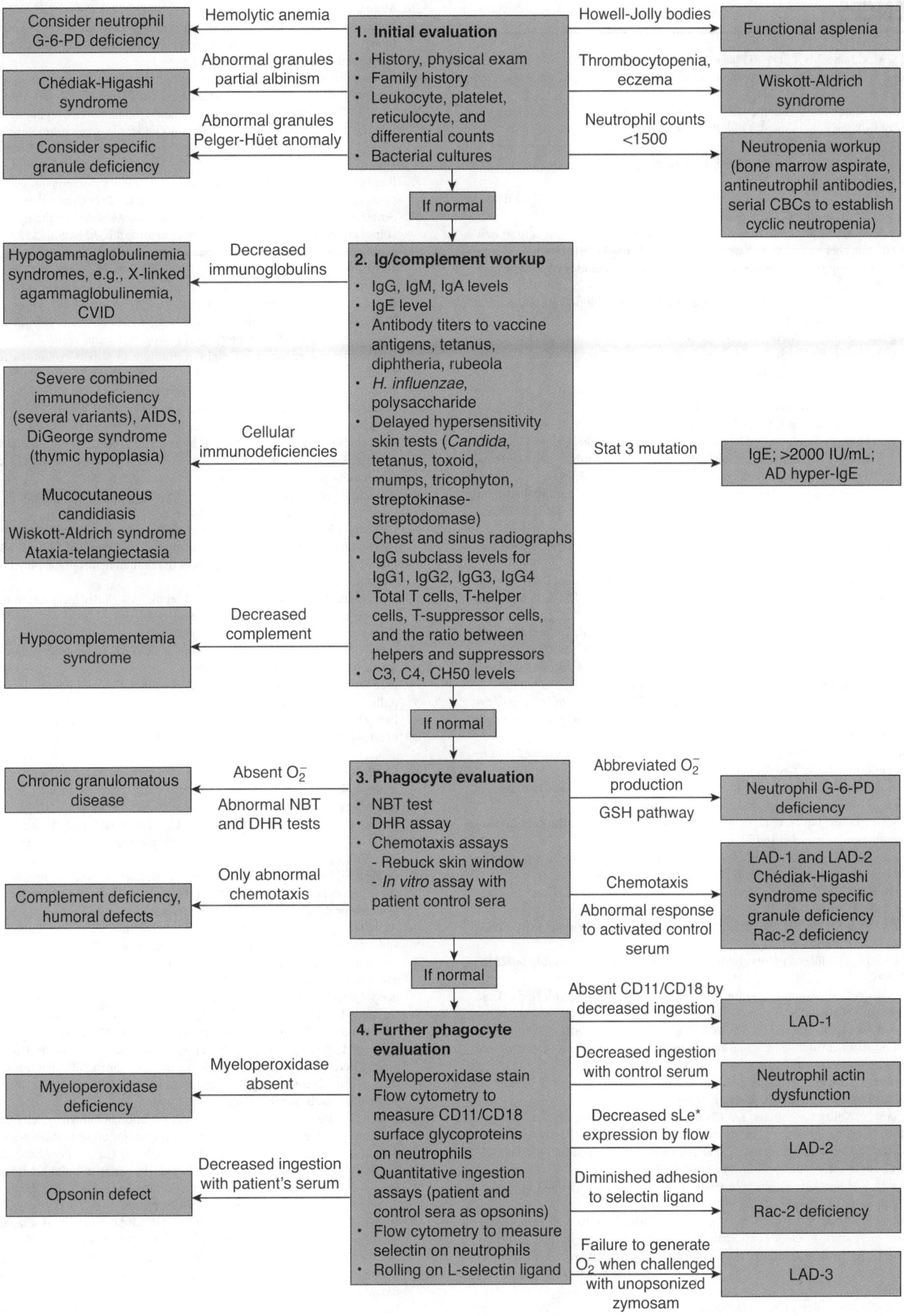

FIGURE 66–8. Algorithm for the workup of patients with recurrent infections. Abbreviations: AD, autosomal dominant; CBC, complete blood count; CVID, common variable immunodeficiency; DHR, delayed hypersensitivity reaction; G-6-PD, glucose-6-phosphate dehydrogenase; GSH, glutathione; Ig, immunoglobulin, LAD, leukocyte adhesion deficiency; NBT, nitroblue tetrazolium.

REFERENCES

1. Mudd S, McCutcheon S, Lucke B: Phagocytosis. *Physiol Rev* 14:210, 1934.
2. Zigmond SH: Ability of polymorphonuclear leukocytes to orient in gradients of chemotactic factors. *J Cell Biol* 75:606, 1977.
3. Foxman EF, Campbell JJ, Butcher EC: Multistep navigation and the combinatorial control of leukocyte chemotaxis. *J Cell Biol* 139:1349, 1997.
4. Quitt M, Torres M, McGuire W, et al: Neutrophil chemotactic heterogeneity to N-formyl-methionyl-leucyl-phenylalanine detected by the under-agarose assay. *J Lab Clin Med* 115:159, 1990.
5. Lee J, Gustafsson M, Magnusson KE, et al: The direction of membrane lipid flow in locomoting polymorphonuclear leukocytes. *Science* 247:1229, 1990.
6. Marks PW, Maxfield FR: Local and global changes in cytosolic free calcium in neutrophils during chemotaxis and phagocytosis. *Cell Calcium* 11:181, 1990.
7. Stossel TP, Hartwig JH, Janmey PA, et al: Cell crawling two decades after Abercrombie. *Biochem Soc Symp* 65:267, 1999.
8. Berlin RD, Fera JP, Pfeiffer JR: Reversible phagocytosis in rabbit polymorphonuclear leukocytes. *J Clin Invest* 63:1137, 1979.
9. Bunting M, Harris ES, McIntyre TM, et al: Leukocyte adhesion deficiency syndromes: Adhesion and tethering defects involving beta 2 integrins and selectin ligands. *Curr Opin Hematol* 9:30, 2002.
10. Shao JY, TingBeall HP, Hochmuth RM: Static and dynamic lengths of neutrophil microvilli. *Proc Natl Acad Sci U S A* 95:6797, 1998.
11. Pestonjamasp K, Amieva MR, Strassel CP, et al: Moesin, ezrin, and p205 are actin-binding proteins associated with neutrophil plasma membranes. *Mol Biol Cell* 6:247, 1995.
12. Bruehl RE, Moore KL, Lorant DE, et al: Leukocyte activation induces surface redistribution of P-selectin glycoprotein ligand-1. *J Leukoc Biol* 61:489, 1997.
13. Green CE, Pearson DN, Christensen NB, et al: Topographic requirements and dynamics of signaling via L-selectin on neutrophils. *Am J Physiol Cell Physiol* 284:C705, 2003.
14. McIntyre TM, Prescott SM, Weyrich AS, et al: Cell-cell interactions: Leukocyte-endothelial interactions. *Curr Opin Hematol* 10:150, 2003.
15. Urzainqui A, Serrador JM, Viedma F, et al: ITAM-based interaction of ERM proteins with Syk mediates signaling by the leukocyte adhesion receptor PSGL-1. *Immunity* 17:401, 2002.
16. Steegmaier M, Borges E, Berger J, et al: The E-selectin-ligand ESL-1 is located in the Golgi as well as on microvilli on the cell surface. *J Cell Sci* 110:687, 1997.
17. Witko-Sarsat V, Rieu P, Descamps-Latscha B, et al: Neutrophils: Molecules, functions and pathophysiological aspects. *Lab Invest* 80:617, 2000.
18. Wolff B, Burns AR, Middleton J, et al: Endothelial cell "memory" of inflammatory stimulation: Human venular endothelial cells store interleukin 8 in Weibel-Palade bodies. *J Exp Med* 188:1757, 1998.
19. Middleton J, Neil S, Wintle J, et al: Transcytosis and surface presentation of IL-8 by venular endothelial cells. *Cell* 91:385, 1997.
20. Sengeløv H, Kjeldsen L, Diamond MS, et al: Subcellular localization and dynamics of Mac-1 ($\alpha_m\beta_2$) in human neutrophils. *J Clin Invest* 92:1467, 1993.
21. Liu L, Schwartz BR, Lin N, et al: Requirement for RhoA kinase activation in leukocyte de-adhesion. *J Immunol* 169:2330, 2002.
22. Foxman EF, Kunkel EJ, Butcher EC: Integrating conflicting chemotactic signals. The role of memory in leukocyte navigation. *J Cell Biol* 147:577, 1999.
23. Petty HR, Todd RF: Integrins as promiscuous signal transduction devices. *Immunol Today* 17:209, 1996.
24. Booth JW, Trimble WS, Grinstein S: Membrane dynamics in phagocytosis. *Semin Immunol* 13:357, 2001.
25. Akira S, Sato S: Toll-like receptors and their signaling mechanisms. *Scand J Infect Dis* 35:555, 2003.
26. Gay NJ, Gangloff M: Structure and function of toll receptors and their ligands. *Annu Rev Biochem* 76:141, 2007.
27. Theilgaard-Monch K, Knudsen S, Follin P, et al: The transcriptional activation program of human neutrophils in skin lesions supports their important role in wound healing. *J Immunol* 172:7684, 2004.
28. Sengeløv H, Voldstedlund M, Vinthen J, et al: Human neutrophils are devoid of the integral membrane protein caveolin. *J Leukoc Biol* 63:563, 1998.
29. Borregaard N, Miller L, Springer TA: Chemoattractant-regulated mobilization of a novel intracellular compartment in human neutrophils. *Science* 237:1204, 1987.
30. Borregaard N, Kjeldsen L, Rygaard K, et al: Stimulus-dependent secretion of plasma proteins from human neutrophils. *J Clin Invest* 90:86, 1992.
31. Sengeløv H, Kjeldsen L, Borregaard N: Control of exocytosis in early neutrophil activation. *J Immunol* 150:1535, 1993.
32. Chaudhuri S, Kumar A, Berger M: Association of ARF and Rabs with complement receptor type-1 storage vesicles in human neutrophils. *J Leukoc Biol* 70:669, 2001.
33. Dahlgren C, Karlsson A, Sendo F: Neutrophil secretory vesicles are the intracellular reservoir for GPI- 80, a protein with adhesion-regulating potential. *J Leukoc Biol* 69:57, 2001.
34. Kumar A, Wetzler E, Berger M: Isolation and characterization of complement receptor type 1 (CR1) storage vesicles from human neutrophils using antibodies to the cytoplasmic tail of CR1. *Blood* 89:4555, 1997.
35. Sengeløv H, Follin P, Kjeldsen L, et al: Mobilization of granules and secretory vesicles during in vivo exudation of human neutrophils. *J Immunol* 154:4157, 1995.
36. Morgan CP, Sengelov H, Whatmore J, et al: ADP-ribosylation-factor-regulated phospholipase D activity localizes to secretory vesicles and mobilizes to the plasma membrane following N-formylmethionyl-leucyl-phenylalanine stimulation of human neutrophils. *Biochem J* 325:581, 1997.
37. Borregaard N, Kjeldsen L, Sengeløv H: Mobilization of granules in neutrophils from patients with myeloproliferative disorders. *Eur J Haematol* 50:189, 1993.
38. Dotti G, Garattini E, Borleri G, et al: Leucocyte alkaline phosphatase identifies terminally differentiated normal neutrophils and its lack in chronic myelogenous leukaemia is not dependent on p210 tyrosine kinase activity. *Br J Haematol* 105:163, 1999.
39. Rambaldi A, Masuhara K, Borleri GM, et al: Flow cytometry of leucocyte alkaline phosphatase in normal and pathologic leucocytes. *Br J Haematol* 96:815, 1997.
40. Sengeløv H, Kjeldsen L, Kroeze W, et al: Secretory vesicles are the intracellular reservoir of complement receptor 1 in human neutrophils. *J Immunol* 153:804, 1994.
41. Muniz M, Riezman H: Intracellular transport of GPI-anchored proteins. *EMBO J* 19:10, 2000.
42. Ehrlich P: Beiträge zur kenntniss der anilinfärbunden and ihrer verwendung in der mikroskopizchen technik. *Archiv für Mikrosk Anatomie* 13:263, 1878.
43. Ehrlich P: Über die specifischen granulationen des blutes. *Archiv für anatomie und physiologie, Physiologische abteilung* 571 Supplementum, 1879.
44. Bainton DF, Farquhar MG: Origin of granules in polymorphonuclear leukocytes. *J Cell Biol* 28:277, 1966.
45. Bainton DF, Ullyot JL, Farquhar M: The development of neutrophilic polymorphonuclear leukocytes in human bone marrow. *J Exp Med* 143:907, 1971.
46. Baggiolini M, Hirsch JG, de Duve C: Resolution of granules from rabbit heterophil leukocytes into distinct populations by zonal sedimentation. *J Cell Biol* 40:529, 1969.
47. Dewald B, Bretz U, Baggiolini M: Release of gelatinase from a novel secretory compartment of human neutrophils. *J Clin Invest* 70:518, 1982.
48. Kjeldsen L, Sengeløv H, Lollike K, et al: Isolation and characterization of gelatinase granules from human neutrophils. *Blood* 83:1640, 1994.
49. Kjeldsen L, Johnsen AH, Sengeløv H, et al: Isolation and primary structure of NGAL, a novel protein associated with human neutrophil gelatinase. *J Biol Chem* 268:10425, 1993.
50. Borregaard N, Cowland JB: Granules of the human neutrophilic polymorphonuclear leukocyte. *Blood* 89:3503, 1997.
51. Borregaard N, Heiple JM, Simons ER, et al: Subcellular localization of the b-cytochrome component of the human neutrophil microbicidal oxidase: Translocation during activation. *J Cell Biol* 97:52, 1983.
52. Ganz T, Selsted M, Szklarek D, et al: Defensins. Natural peptide antibiotics of human neutrophils. *J Clin Invest* 76:1427, 1985.
53. Rice WG, Ganz T, Kinkade JM, et al: Defensin-rich dense granules of human neutrophils. *Blood* 70:757, 1987.
54. Faurschou M, Sorensen OE, Johnsen AH, et al: Defensin-rich granules of human neutrophils: Characterization of secretory properties. *Biochim Biophys Acta* 1591:29, 2002.
55. Cham BP, Gerrard JM, Bainton DF: Granulophysin is located in the membrane of azurophilic granules in human neutrophils and mobilizes to the plasma membrane following cell stimulation. *Am J Pathol* 144:1369, 1994.
56. Skubitz KM, Campbell KD, Iida J, et al: CD63 associates with tyrosine kinase activity and CD11/CD18, and transmits an activation signal in neutrophils. *J Immunol* 157:3617, 1996.
57. de Haar SF, Jansen DC, Schoenmaker T, et al: Loss-of-function mutations in cathepsin C in two families with Papillon-Lefèvre syndrome are associated with deficiency of serine proteinases in PMNs. *Hum Mutat* 23:524, 2004.
58. Andersson E, Hellman L, Gullberg U, et al: The role of the propeptide for processing and sorting of human myeloperoxidase. *J Biol Chem* 273:4747, 1998.
59. Bulow E, Gullberg U, Olsson I: Structural requirements for intracellular processing and sorting of bactericidal/permeability-increasing protein (BPI): Comparison with lipopolysaccharide-binding protein. *J Leukoc Biol* 68:669, 2000.
60. Gullberg U, Bengtsson N, Bulow E, et al: Processing and targeting of granule proteins in human neutrophils. *J Immunol Method* 232:201, 1999.
61. Kjeldsen L, Bainton DF, Sengeløv H, et al: Structural and functional heterogeneity among peroxidase-negative granules in human neutrophils: Identification of a distinct gelatinase containing granule subset by combined immunocytochemistry and subcellular fractionation. *Blood* 82:3183, 1993.
62. Udby L, Calafat J, Sorensen OE, et al: Identification of human cysteine-rich secretory protein 3 (CRISP-3) as a matrix protein in a subset of peroxidase-negative granules of neutrophils and in the granules of eosinophils. *J Leukoc Biol* 72:462, 2002.
63. Kjeldsen L, Bjerrum OW, Hovgaard D, et al: Human neutrophil gelatinase: A marker for circulating blood neutrophils. Purification and quantitation by enzyme linked immunosorbent assay. *Eur J Haematol* 49:180, 1992.
64. Cowland JB, Johnsen AH, Borregaard N: HCAP-18, a cathelin/bactenecin-like protein of human neutrophil specific granules. *FEBS Lett* 368:173, 1995.
65. Sorensen OE, Follin P, Johnsen AH, et al: Human cathelicidin, hCAP-18, is processed to the antimicrobial peptide LL-37 by extracellular cleavage with proteinase 3. *Blood* 97:3951, 2001.
66. Borregaard N, Kjeldsen L, Sengeløv H, et al: Changes in the subcellular localization and surface expression of L-selectin, alkaline phosphatase, and Mac-1 in human neutrophils during stimulation with inflammatory mediators. *J Leukoc Biol* 56:80, 1994.
67. Borregaard N, Lollike K, Kjeldsen L, et al: Human neutrophil granules and secretory vesicles. *Eur J Haematol* 51:187, 1993.

68. Canonne-Hergaux F, Calafat J, Richer E, et al: Expression and subcellular localization of NRAMP1 in human neutrophil granules. *Blood* 100:268, 2002.
69. Kang T, Yi J, Guo A, et al: Subcellular distribution and cytokine- and chemokine-regulated secretion of leukolysin/MT6-MMP/MMP-25 in neutrophils. *J Biol Chem* 276:21960, 2001.
70. Kjeldsen L, Bjerrum OW, Askaa J, et al: Subcellular localization and release of human neutrophil gelatinase, confirming the existence of separate gelatinase-containing granules. *Biochem J* 287:603, 1992.
71. Borregaard N, Sehested M, Nielsen BS, et al: Biosynthesis of granule proteins in normal human bone marrow cells. Gelatinase is a marker of terminal neutrophil differentiation. *Blood* 85:812, 1995.
72. Bjerregaard MD, Jurlander J, Klausen P, et al: The *in vivo* profile of transcription factors during neutrophil differentiation in human bone marrow. *Blood* 101:4322, 2003.
73. Cowland JB, Borregaard N: The individual regulation of granule protein mRNA levels during neutrophil maturation explains the heterogeneity of neutrophil granules. *J Leukoc Biol* 66:989, 1999.
74. Theilgaard-Monch K, Jacobsen LC, Borup R, et al: The transcriptional program of terminal granulocytic differentiation. *Blood* 105:1785, 2005.
75. Le Cabec V, Cowland JB, Calafat J, et al: Targeting of proteins to granule subsets determined by timing not by sorting: The specific granule protein NGAL is localized to azurophil granules when expressed in HL-60 cells. *Proc Natl Acad Sci U S A* 93:6454, 1996.
76. Goda Y: SNAREs and regulated vesicle exocytosis. *Proc Natl Acad Sci U S A* 94:769, 1997.
77. Rothman JE: *Molecular and Cellular Mechanisms of Neurotransmitter Release*, edited by L Stjärne, P Greengard, S Grillner, T Hökfelt, D Ottoson, p 81. Raven Press, New York, 1994.
78. Brumell JH, Volchuk A, Sengelov H, et al: Subcellular distribution of docking/fusion proteins in neutrophils, secretory cells with multiple exocytic compartments. *J Immunol* 155:5750, 1995.
79. Mollinedo F, Martin-Martin B, Calafat J, et al: Role of vesicle-associated membrane protein-2, through q-soluble N-ethylmaleimide-sensitive factor attachment protein receptor/r-soluble N-ethylmaleimide-sensitive factor attachment protein receptor interaction, in the exocytosis of specific and tertiary granules of human neutrophils. *J Immunol* 170:1034, 2003.
80. Arnljots K, Sorensen O, Lollike K, et al: Timing targeting and sorting of azurophil granule proteins in human myeloid cells. *Leukemia* 12:1789, 1998.
81. Lollike K, Kjeldsen L, Sengeløv H, et al: Lysozyme in human neutrophils and plasma. A parameter of myelopoietic activity. *Leukemia* 9:159, 1995.
82. Gombart AF, Shiohara M, Kwok SH, et al: Neutrophil-specific granule deficiency: Homozygous recessive inheritance of a frameshift mutation in the gene encoding transcription factor CCAAT/enhancer binding protein-epsilon. *Blood* 97:2561, 2001.
83. Verbeek W, Wachter M, LekstromHimes J, et al: C/EBP epsilon –/– mice: Increased rate of myeloid proliferation and apoptosis. *Leukemia* 15:103, 2001.
84. Liu L, Ganz T: The pro region of human neutrophil defensin contains a motif that is essential for normal subcellular sorting. *Blood* 85:1095, 1995.
85. Lemansky P, Gerecitano-Schmidek M, Das RC, et al: Targeting myeloperoxidase to azurophilic granules in HL-60 cells. *J Leukoc Biol* 74:542, 2003.
86. Niemann CU, Cowland JB, Klausen P, et al: Localization of serglycin in human neutrophil granulocytes and their precursors. *J Leukoc Biol* 76:406, 2004.
87. Abrink M, Grujic M, Pejler G: Serglycin is essential for maturation of mast cell secretory granule. *J Biol Chem* 279:40897, 2004.
88. Niemann CU, Abrink M, Pejler G, et al: Neutrophil elastase depends on serglycin proteoglycan for localization in granules. *Blood* 109:4478, 2007.
89. Kallquist L, Hansson M, Persson AM, et al: The tetraspanin CD63 is involved in granule targeting of neutrophil elastase. *Blood* 112:3444, 2008.
90. Braga T, Ringvall M, Tveit H, et al: Reduction with dithiothreitol causes serglycin-specific defects in secretory granule integrity of bone marrow derived mast cells. *Mol Immunol* 46:422, 2009.
91. Anderson KL, Smith KA, Conners K, et al: Myeloid development is selectively disrupted in PU.1 null mice. *Blood* 91:3702, 1998.
92. Fisher RC, Lovelock JD, Scott EW: A critical role for PU.1 in homing and long-term engraftment by hematopoietic stem cells in the bone marrow. *Blood* 94:1283, 1999.
93. Eklund EA, Jalava A, Kakar R: PU.1, interferon regulatory factor 1, and interferon consensus sequence-binding protein cooperate to increase gp91(phox) expression. *J Biol Chem* 273:13957, 1998.
94. Gombart AF, Kwok SH, Anderson KL, et al: Regulation of neutrophil and eosinophil secondary granule gene expression by transcription factors C/EBP epsilon and PU.1. *Blood* 101:3265, 2003.
95. Oelgeschlager M, Nuchprayoon I, Luscher B, et al: C/EBP, c-Myb, and PU.1 cooperate to regulate the neutrophil elastase promoter. *Mol Cell Biol* 16:4717, 1996.
96. Simon MC, Olson M, Scott E, et al: Terminal myeloid gene expression and differentiation requires the transcription factor PU.1. *Curr Top Microbiol Immunol* 211:113, 1996.
97. Yamanaka R, Barlow C, Lekstrom-Himes J, et al: Impaired granulopoiesis, myelodysplasia, and early lethality in CCAAT/enhancer binding protein epsilon-deficient mice. *Proc Natl Acad Sci U S A* 94:13187, 1997.
98. Morosetti R, Park DJ, Chumakov AM, et al: A novel, myeloid transcription factor, C/EBP epsilon, is upregulated during granulocytic, but not monocytic, differentiation. *Blood* 90:2591, 1997.
99. Johnnidis JB, Harris MH, Wheeler RT, et al: Regulation of progenitor cell proliferation and granulocyte function by microRNA-223. *Nature* 451:1125, 2008.
100. Arnljots K, Olsson I: Myeloperoxidase precursors incorporate heme. *J Biol Chem* 262:10430, 1987.
101. Nauseef WM, McCormick S, Yi H: Roles of heme insertion and the mannose-6-phosphate receptor in processing of the human myeloid lysosomal enzyme, myeloperoxidase. *Blood* 80:2622, 1992.
102. Klebanoff SJ: Myeloperoxidase. *Proc Assoc Am Physicians* 111:383, 1999.
103. Klebanoff SJ, Nathan CF: Nitrite production by stimulated human polymorphonuclear leukocytes supplemented with azide and catalase. *Biochem Biophys Res Commun* 197:192, 1993.
104. Eiserich JP, Baldus S, Brennan ML, et al: Myeloperoxidase, a leukocyte-derived vascular NO oxidase. *Science* 296:2391, 2002.
105. Savige J, Davies D, Falk RJ, et al: Antineutrophil cytoplasmic antibodies and associated diseases: A review of the clinical and laboratory features. *Kidney Int* 57:846, 2000.
106. Tervaert JW, Goldschmeding R, Elema JD, et al: Association of autoantibodies to myeloperoxidase with different forms of vasculitis. *Arthritis Rheum* 33:1264, 1990.
107. Levy O, Elsbach P: Bactericidal/permeability-increasing protein in host defense and its efficacy in the treatment of bacterial sepsis. *Curr Infect Dis Rep* 3:407, 2001.
108. Alexander S, Bramson J, Foley R, et al: Protection from endotoxemia by adenoviral-mediated gene transfer of human bactericidal/permeability-increasing protein. *Blood* 2003.
109. Ganz T: Defensins: Antimicrobial peptides of innate immunity. *Nat Rev Immunol* 3:710, 2003.
110. Selsted ME, Harwig SSL, Ganz T, et al: Primary structures of three human neutrophil defensins. *J Clin Invest* 76:1436, 1985.
111. Selsted ME, Tang Y-Q, Morris WL, et al: Purification, primary structures, and antibacterial activities of β-defensins, a new family of antimicrobial peptides from bovine neutrophils. *J Biol Chem* 268:6641, 1993.
112. Tang YQ, Yuan J, Ösapay G, et al: A cyclic antimicrobial peptide produced in primate leukocytes by the ligation of two truncated α-defensins. *Science* 286:498, 1999.
113. Almeida RP, Vanet A, Witkosarsat V, et al: Azurocidin, a natural antibiotic from human neutrophils: Expression, antimicrobial activity, and secretion. *Protein Expr Purif* 7:355, 1996.
114. Campanelli D, Detmers PA, Nathan CF, et al: Azurocidin and a homologous serine protease from neutrophils. Differential antimicrobial and proteolytic properties. *J Clin Invest* 85:904, 1990.
115. Flodgaard H, Østergaard E, Bayne S, et al: Covalent structure of two novel neutrophile leucocyte-derived proteins of porcine and human origin. Neutrophile elastase homologues with strong monocyte and fibroblast chemotactic activities. *Eur J Biochem* 197:535, 1991.
116. Gautam N, Olofsson AM, Herwald H, et al: Heparin-binding protein (HBP/CAP37): A missing link in neutrophil-evoked alteration of vascular permeability. *Nat Med* 7:1123, 2001.
117. Tapper H, Karlsson A, Morgelin M, et al: Secretion of heparin-binding protein from human neutrophils is determined by its localization in azurophilic granules and secretory vesicles. *Blood* 99:1785, 2002.
118. Goldschmeding R, Tervaert JW, Dolman KM, et al: ANCA: A class of vasculitis-associated autoantibodies against myeloid granule proteins: Clinical and laboratory aspects and possible pathogenetic implications. *Adv Exp Med Biol* 297:129, 1991.
119. von VS, Tunnemann G, Eulenberg C, et al: NB1 mediates surface expression of the ANCA antigen proteinase 3 on human neutrophils. *Blood* 109:4487, 2007.
120. von VS, Eulenberg C, Wellner M, et al: Neutrophil surface presentation of the antineutrophil cytoplasmic antibody-antigen proteinase 3 depends on N-terminal processing. *Clin Exp Immunol* 152:508, 2008.
121. Skold S, Rosberg B, Gullberg U, et al: A secreted proform of neutrophil proteinase 3 regulates the proliferation of granulopoietic progenitor cells. *Blood* 93:849, 1999.
122. Skubitz KM, Campbell KD, Skubitz APN: CD63 associates with CD11/CD18 in large detergent- resistant complexes after translocation to the cell surface in human neutrophils. *FEBS Lett* 469:52, 2000.
123. Saito N, Pulford KAF, Breton-Gorius J, et al: Ultrastructural localization of the CD68 macrophage-associated antigen in human blood neutrophils and monocytes. *Am J Pathol* 139:1053, 1991.
124. Mirinics ZK, Calafat J, Udby L, et al: Identification of the presenilins in hematopoietic cells with localization of presenilin 1 to neutrophil and platelet granules. *Blood Cells Mol Dis* 28:28, 2002.
125. Feuk-Lagerstedt E, Samuelsson M, Mosgoeller W, et al: The presence of stomatin in detergent-insoluble domains of neutrophil granule membranes. *J Leukoc Biol* 72:970, 2002.
126. Nanda A, Brumell JH, Nordstrom T, et al: Activation of proton pumping in human neutrophils occurs by exocytosis of vesicles bearing vacuolar-type H+-ATPases. *J Biol Chem* 271:15963, 1996.
127. Masson PL, Heremans JF, Schonne E: Lactoferrin, an iron-binding protein in neutrophilic leukocytes. *J Exp Med* 130:643, 1969.
128. Baveye S, Elass E, Mazurier J, et al: Lactoferrin: A multifunctional glycoprotein involved in the modulation of the inflammatory process. *Clin Chem Lab Med* 37:281, 1999.
129. Farnaud S, Evans RW: Lactoferrin-a multifunctional protein with antimicrobial properties. *Mol Immunol* 40:395, 2003.

130. Aguilera O, Ostolaza H, Quiros LM, et al: Permeabilizing action of an antimicrobial lactoferricin-derived peptide on bacterial and artificial membranes. *FEBS Lett* 462:273, 1999.
131. Nibbering PH, Ravensbergen E, Welling MM, et al: Human lactoferrin and peptides derived from its N terminus are highly effective against infections with antibiotic-resistant bacteria. *Infec Immun* 69:1469, 2001.
132. Flower DR: The lipocalin protein family: Structure and function. *Biochem J* 318:1, 1996.
133. Kjeldsen L, Bainton DF, Sengeløv H, et al: Identification of neutrophil gelatinase-associated lipocalin as a novel matrix protein of specific granules in human neutrophils. *Blood* 83:799, 1994.
134. Yan L, Borregaard N, Kjeldsen L, et al: The high molecular weight urinary matrix metalloproteinase (MMP) activity is a complex of gelatinase B/MMP-9 and neutrophil gelatinase-associated lipocalin (NGAL). Modulation of MMP-9 activity by NGAL. *J Biol Chem* 276:37258, 2001.
135. Goetz DH, Holmes MA, Borregaard N, et al: The neutrophil lipocalin NGAL is a bacteriostatic agent that interferes with siderophore-mediated iron acquisition. *Mol Cell* 10:1033, 2002.
136. Cowland JB, Sorensen OE, Sehested M, et al: Neutrophil gelatinase-associated lipocalin is up-regulated in human epithelial cells by IL-1beta, but not by TNF-alpha. *J Immunol* 171:6630, 2003.
137. Cellier M, Govoni G, Vidal S, et al: Human natural resistance-associated macrophage protein: CDNA cloning, chromosomal mapping, genomic organization, and tissue-specific expression. *J Exp Med* 180:1741, 1994.
138. Fleming A: On a remarkable bacteriolytic element found in tissues and excretions. *Proc Roy Soc* 93:306, 1922.
139. Selsted ME, Martinez RJ: Lysozyme: Primary bactericidin in human plasma serum active against Bacillus subtilis. *Infect Immun* 20:782, 1978.
140. Tanida N, Onho N, Adachi Y, et al: Binding of lysozyme to synthetic monosaccharide lipid A analogue, GLA60. *Biol Pharm Bull* 16:288, 1993.
141. Takada K, Ohno N, Yadomae T: Binding of lysozyme to lipopolysaccharide suppresses tumor necrosis factor production in vivo. *Infect Immun* 62:1171, 1994.
142. Keshav S, Chung P, Milon G, et al: Lysozyme is an inducible marker of macrophage activation in murine tissues as demonstrated by in situ hybridization. *J Exp Med* 174:1049, 1991.
143. Sexton C, Buss D, Powell B, et al: Usefulness and limitations of serum and urine lysozyme levels in the classification of acute myeloid leukemia: An analysis of 208 cases. *Leuk Res* 20:467, 1996.
144. Gudmundsson GH, Agerberth B, Odeberg J, et al: The human gene FALL39 and processing of the cathelin precursor to the antibacterial peptide LL-37 in granulocytes. *Eur J Biochem* 238:325, 1996.
145. Zanetti M: Cathelicidins, multifunctional peptides of the innate immunity. *J Leukoc Biol* 75:39, 2004.
146. Sorensen O, Arnljots K, Cowland JB, et al: The human antibacterial cathelicidin, hCAP-18, is synthesized in myelocytes and metamyelocytes and localized to specific granules in neutrophils. *Blood* 90:2796, 1997.
147. Sorensen O, Bratt T, Johnsen AH, et al: The human antibacterial cathelicidin, hCAP-18, is bound to lipoproteins in plasma. *J Biol Chem* 274:22445, 1999.
148. Frohm-Nilsson M., Sandstedt B, Sorensen O, et al: The human cationic antimicrobial protein (hCAP18), a peptide antibiotic, is widely expressed in human squamous epithelia and colocalizes with interleukin-6. *Infect Immun* 67:2561, 1999.
149. Heilborn JD, Nilsson MF, Kratz G, et al: The cathelicidin anti-microbial peptide LL-37 is involved in re-epithelialization of human skin wounds and is lacking in chronic ulcer epithelium. *J Invest Dermatol* 120:379, 2003.
150. Sorensen OE, Cowland JB, Theilgaard-Monch K, et al: Wound healing and expression of antimicrobial peptides/polypeptides in human keratinocytes, a consequence of common growth factors. *J Immunol* 170:5583, 2003.
151. Sorensen OE, Gram L, Johnsen AH, et al: Processing of seminal plasma hCAP-18 to ALL-38 by gastricsin: A novel mechanism of generating antimicrobial peptides in vagina. *J Biol Chem* 278:28540, 2003.
152. Zaiou M, Nizet V, Gallo RL: Antimicrobial and protease inhibitory functions of the human cathelicidin (hCAP18/LL-37) prosequence. *J Invest Dermatol* 120:810, 2003.
153. Yang D, Chen Q, Schmidt AP, et al: LL-37, the neutrophil granule- and epithelial cell-derived cathelicidin, utilizes formyl peptide receptor-like 1 (FPRL1) as a receptor to chemoattract human peripheral blood neutrophils, monocytes, and T cells. *J Exp Med* 192:1069, 2000.
154. Koczulla R, von Degenfeld G, Kupatt C, et al: An angiogenic role for the human peptide antibiotic LL-37/hCAP-18. *J Clin Invest* 111:1665, 2003.
155. Scott MG, Davidson DJ, Gold MR, et al: The human antimicrobial peptide LL-37 is a multifunctional modulator of innate immune responses. *J Immunol* 169:3883, 2002.
156. Murphy G, Reynolds JJ, Bretz U, et al: Collagenase is a component of the specific granules of human neutrophil leucocytes. *Biochem J* 162:195, 1977.
157. Murphy G, Bretz U, Baggiolini M, et al: The latent collagenase and gelatinase of human polymorphonuclear neutrophil leucocytes. *Biochem J* 192:517, 1980.
158. Pei D: Leukolysin/MMP25/MT6-MMP: A novel matrix metalloproteinase specifically expressed in the leukocyte lineage. *Cell Res* 9:291, 1999.
159. Jaillon S, Peri G, Delneste Y, et al: The humoral pattern recognition receptor PTX3 is stored in neutrophil granules and localizes in extracellular traps. *J Exp Med* 204:793, 2007.
160. Mantovani A, Garlanda C, Doni A, et al: Pentraxins in innate immunity: From C-reactive protein to the long pentraxin PTX3. *J Clin Immunol* 28:1, 2008.
161. Aoyagi Y, Adderson EE, Rubens CE, et al: L-Ficolin/mannose-binding lectin-associated serine protease complexes bind to group B streptococci primarily through N-acetylneuraminic acid of capsular polysaccharide and activate the complement pathway. *Infect Immun* 76:179, 2008.
162. Jacobsen LC, Theilgaard-Monch K, Christensen EI, et al: Arginase 1 is expressed in myelocytes/metamyelocytes and localized in gelatinase granules of human neutrophils. *Blood* 109:3084, 2007.
163. Munder M, Schneider H, Luckner C, et al: Suppression of T-cell functions by human granulocyte arginase. *Blood* 108:1627, 2006.
164. Ginsel LA, Onderwater JJM, Fransen JAM, et al: Localization of the low-M_r subunit of cytochrome b_{558} in human blood phagocytes by immunoelectron microscopy. *Blood* 76:2105, 1990.
165. Feuk-Lagerstedt E, Jordan ET, Leffler H, et al: Identification of CD66a and CD66b as the major galectin-3 receptor candidates in human neutrophils. *J Immunol* 163:5592, 1999.
166. Karlsson A, Follin P, Leffler H, et al: Galectin-3 activates the NADPH-oxidase in exudated but not peripheral blood neutrophils. *Blood* 91:3430, 1998.
167. Williams LT, Snyderman R, Pike MC, et al: Specific receptor sites for chemotactic peptides on human polymorphonuclear leukocytes. *Proc Natl Acad Sci U S A* 74:1204, 1977.
168. Schiffmann E, Aswanikumar S, Venkatasubramanian K, et al: Some characteristics of the neutrophil receptor for chemotactic peptides. *FEBS Lett* 117:1, 1980.
169. Boulay F, Tardif M, Brouchon L, et al: The human N-formylpeptide receptor. Characterization of two cDNA isolates and evidence for a new subfamily of G-protein-coupled receptors. *Biochemistry* 29:11123, 1990.
170. Prossnitz ER, Ye RD: The N-formyl peptide receptor: A model for the study of chemoattractant receptor structure and function. *Pharmacol Ther* 74:73, 1997.
171. Sengeløv H, Boulay F, Kjeldsen L, et al: Subcellular localization and translocation of the receptor for N-formyl-methionyl-leucyl-phenylalanine in human neutrophils. *Biochem J* 299:473, 1994.
172. Hugli TE: Structure and function of the anaphylatoxins. *Springer Semin Immunopathol* 7:193, 1984.
173. Chenoweth DE, Hugli TE: Demonstration of specific C5a receptor on intact human polymorphonuclear leukocytes. *Proc Natl Acad Sci U S A* 75:3943, 1978.
174. Rollins TE, Springer MS: Identification of the polymorphonuclear leukocyte C5a receptor. *J Biol Chem* 260:7157, 1985.
175. Boulay F, Mery L, Tardif M, et al: Expression cloning of a receptor for C5a anaphylatoxin on differentiated HL-60 cells. *Biochemistry* 30:2993, 1991.
176. Nathan CF: Neutrophil activation on biological surfaces. Massive secretion of hydrogen peroxide in response to products of macrophages and lymphocytes. *J Clin Invest* 80:1550, 1987.
177. Shappell SB, Toman C, Anderson DC, et al: Mac-1 (CD11b/CD18) mediates adherence-dependent hydrogen peroxide production by human and canine neutrophils. *J Immunol* 144:2702, 1990.
178. Kew RR, Grimaldi CM, Furie MB, et al: Human neutrophil Fc gamma RIIIB and formyl peptide receptors are functionally linked during formyl-methionyl-leucyl-phenylalanine-induced chemotaxis. *J Immunol* 149:989, 1992.
179. Leeuwenberg JF, Van De Winkel JG, Jeunhomme TM, et al: Functional polymorphism of IgG FcRII (CD32) on human neutrophils. *Immunology* 71:301, 1990.
180. Sehgal G, Zhang K, Todd RF, III, et al: Lectin-like inhibition of immune complex receptor-mediated stimulation of neutrophils. Effects on cytosolic calcium release and superoxide production. *J Immunol* 150:4571, 1993.
181. Indik ZK, Park JG, Hunter S, et al: The molecular dissection of Fc gamma receptor mediated phagocytosis. *Blood* 86:4389, 1995.
182. Strzelecka-Kiliszek A, Kwiatkowska K, Sobota A: Lyn and Syk kinases are sequentially engaged in phagocytosis mediated by Fc gamma R. *J Immunol* 169:6787, 2002.
183. Raeder EM, Mansfield PJ, Hinkovska-Galcheva V, et al: Syk activation initiates downstream signaling events during human polymorphonuclear leukocyte phagocytosis. *J Immunol* 163:6785, 1999.
184. Kusner DJ, Barton JA, Wen KK, et al: Regulation of phospholipase D activity by actin. Actin exerts bidirectional modulation of Mammalian phospholipase D activity in a polymerization-dependent, isoform-specific manner. *J Biol Chem* 277:50683, 2002.
185. Didsbury JR, Uhing RJ, Tomhave E, et al: Receptor class desensitization of leukocyte chemoattractant receptors. *Proc Natl Acad Sci U S A* 88:11564, 1991.
186. Nakamura M, Honda Z, Izumi T, et al: Molecular cloning and expression of platelet-activating factor receptor from human leukocytes. *J Biol Chem* 266:20400, 1991.
187. Jones SA, Wolf M, Qin SX, et al: Different functions for the interleukin 8 receptors (IL- 8R) of human neutrophil leukocytes: NADPH oxidase and phospholipase D are activated through IL-8R1 but not IL- 8R2. *Proc Natl Acad Sci U S A* 93:6682, 1996.
188. Jin MS, Lee JO: Structures of the toll-like receptor family and its ligand complexes. *Immunity* 29:182, 2008.
189. Diebold SS: Recognition of viral single-stranded RNA by toll-like receptors. *Adv Drug Deliv Rev* 60:813, 2008.
190. Kindrachuk J, Potter J, Wilson HL, et al: Activation and regulation of toll-like receptor 9: CpGs and beyond. *Mini Rev Med Chem* 8:590, 2008.
191. West AP, Koblansky AA, Ghosh S: Recognition and signaling by toll-like receptors. *Annu Rev Cell Dev Biol* 22:409, 2006.
192. Sklar LA, Bokoch GM, Button D, et al: Regulation of ligand-receptor dynamics by guanine nucleotides. Real-time analysis of interconverting states for the neutrophil formyl peptide receptor. *J Biol Chem* 262:135, 1987.

193. Pelz C, Matsumoto T, Molski TF, et al: Characterization of the membrane-associated GTPase activity: Effects of chemotactic factors and toxins. *J Cell Biochem* 39:197, 1989.
194. Bokoch GM, Bickford K, Bohl BP: Subcellular localization and quantitation of the major neutrophil pertussis toxin substrate, G_n. *J Cell Biol* 106:1927, 1988.
195. Kanaho Y, Kanoh H, Nozawa Y: Activation of phospholipase D in rabbit neutrophils by fMet-Leu-Phe is mediated by a pertussis toxin-sensitive GTP-binding protein that may be distinct from a phospholipase C-regulating protein. *FEBS Lett* 279:249, 1991.
196. Barrowman MM, Cockcroft S, Gomperts BD: Two roles for guanine nucleotides in the stimulus-secretion sequence of neutrophils. *Nature* 319:504, 1986.
197. Ohnishi H, Ernst SA, Yule DI, et al: Heterotrimeric G-protein Gq/11 localized on pancreatic zymogen granules is involved in calcium-regulated amylase secretion. *J Biol Chem* 272:16056, 1997.
198. Mansfield PJ, Carey SS, Hinkovska-Galcheva V, et al: Ceramide inhibition of phospholipase D and its relationship to RhoA and ARF1 translocation in GTP gamma S-stimulated polymorphonuclear leukocytes. *Blood* 103:2363, 2004.
199. Dusi S, Donini M, Dellabianca V, et al: Tyrosine phosphorylation of phospholipase C-gamma 2 is involved in the activation of phosphoinositide hydrolysis by Fc receptors in human neutrophils. *Biochem Biophys Res Commun* 201:1100, 1994.
200. Mansfield PJ, Shayman JA, Boxer LA: Regulation of polymorphonuclear leukocyte phagocytosis by myosin light chain kinase after activation of mitogen-activated protein kinase. *Blood* 95:2407, 2000.
201. Cockcroft S, Baldwin JM, Allan D: The Ca2+-activated polyphosphoinositide phosphodiesterase of human and rabbit neutrophil membranes. *Biochem J* 221:477, 1984.
202. Favre CJ, Lew DP, Krause KH: Rapid heparin-sensitive Ca2+ release following Ca(2+)-ATPase inhibition in intact HL-60 granulocytes. Evidence for Ins(1,4,5)P3-dependent Ca2+ cycling across the membrane of Ca2+ stores. *Biochem J* 302 (Pt 1):155, 1994.
203. Cox D, Chang P, Zhang Q, et al: Requirements for both Rac1 and Cdc42 in membrane ruffling and phagocytosis in leukocytes. *J Exp Med* 186:1487, 1997.
204. Roberts AW, Kim C, Zhen L, et al: Deficiency of the hematopoietic cell-specific Rho family GTPase Rac2 is characterized by abnormalities in neutrophil function and host defense. *Immunity* 10:183, 1999.
205. Mansfield PJ, Hinkovska-Galcheva V, Carey SS, et al: Regulation of polymorphonuclear leukocyte degranulation and oxidant production by ceramide through inhibition of phospholipase D. *Blood* 99:1434, 2002.
206. Blackwood RA, Smolen JE, Transue A, et al: Phospholipase D activity facilitates Ca2+-induced aggregation and fusion of complex liposomes. *Am J Physiol* 272:C1279, 1997.
207. English D, Cui Y, Siddiqui RA: Messenger functions of phosphatidic acid. *Chem Phys Lipids* 80:117, 1996.
208. Diez E, Balsinde J, Mollinedo F: Subcellular distribution of fatty acids, phospholipids and phospholipase A2 in human neutrophils. *Biochim Biophys Acta* 1047:83, 1990.
209. Pessach I, Leto TL, Malech HL, et al: Essential requirement of cytosolic phospholipase A(2) for stimulation of NADPH oxidase-associated diaphorase activity in granulocyte-like cells. *J Biol Chem* 276:33495, 2001.
210. Naccache PH, Showell HJ, Becker EL, et al: Arachidonic acid induced degranulation of rabbit peritoneal neutrophils. *Biochem Biophys Res Commun* 87:292, 1979.
211. Hardy SJ, Robinson BS, Ferrante A, et al: Polyenoic very-long-chain fatty acids mobilize intracellular calcium from a thapsigargin-insensitive pool in human neutrophils. The relationship between Ca2+ mobilization and superoxide production induced by long- and very-long-chain fatty acids. *Biochem J* 311(Pt 2):689, 1995.
212. Borgeat P, Hamberg M, Samuelsson B: Transformation of arachidonic acid and homo-gamma-linolenic acid by rabbit polymorphonuclear leukocytes. Monohydroxy acids from novel lipoxygenases. *J Biol Chem* 251:7816, 1976.
213. Naccache PH, Sha'afi RI, Borgeat P, et al: Mono- and dihydroxyeicosatetraenoic acids alter calcium homeostasis in rabbit neutrophils. *J Clin Invest* 67:1584, 1981.
214. Palmer RM, Salmon JA: Release of leukotriene B4 from human neutrophils and its relationship to degranulation induced by N-formyl-methionyl-leucyl-phenylalanine, serum-treated zymosan and the ionophore A23187. *Immunology* 50:65, 1983.
215. Palmblad J, Malmsten CL, Uden AM, et al: Leukotriene B4 is a potent and stereospecific stimulator of neutrophil chemotaxis and adherence. *Blood* 58:658, 1981.
216. Rothman JE: Mechanisms of intracellular protein transport. *Nature* 372:55, 1994.
217. Wickner W, Schekman R: Membrane fusion. *Nat Struct Mol Biol* 15:658, 2008.
218. Brochetta C, Vita F, Tiwari N, et al: Involvement of Munc18 isoforms in the regulation of granule exocytosis in neutrophils. *Biochim Biophys Acta* 1783:1781, 2008.
219. Logan MR, Lacy P, Odemuyiwa SO, et al: A critical role for vesicle-associated membrane protein-7 in exocytosis from human eosinophils and neutrophils. *Allergy* 61:777, 2006.
220. Brinkmann V, Reichard U, Goosmann C, et al: Neutrophil extracellular traps kill bacteria. *Science* 303:1532, 2004.
221. Brinkmann V, Zychlinsky A: Beneficial suicide: Why neutrophils die to make NETs. *Nat Rev Microbiol* 5:577, 2007.
222. Fuchs TA, Abed U, Goosmann C, et al: Novel cell death program leads to neutrophil extracellular traps. *J Cell Biol* 176:231, 2007.
223. Lekstrom-Himes JA, Gallin JI: Immunodeficiency diseases caused by defects in phagocytes. *N Engl J Med* 343:1703, 2000.
224. Dinauer MC: Disorders of neutrophil function: An overview. *Methods Mol Biol* 412:489, 2007.
225. Dale DC, Boxer L, Liles WC: The phagocytes: Neutrophils and monocytes. *Blood* 112:935, 2008.
226. Mollnes TE, Jokiranta TS, Truedsson L, et al: Complement analysis in the 21st century. *Mol Immunol* 44:3838, 2007.
227. Botto M, Fong KY, So AK, et al: Molecular basis of hereditary C3 deficiency. *J Clin Invest* 86:1158, 1990.
228. Frank MM: Complement deficiencies. *Pediatr Clin North Am* 47:1339, 2000.
229. Alper CA, Abramson N, Johnston RB Jr, et al: Studies *in vivo* and *in vitro* on an abnormality in the metabolism of C3 in a patient with increased susceptibility to infection. *J Clin Invest* 49:1975, 1970.
230. Densen P, Weiler JM, Griffiss JM, et al: Familial properdin deficiency and fatal meningococcemia. Correction of the bactericidal defect by vaccination. *N Engl J Med* 316:922, 1987.
231. Nolan KF, Schwaeble W, Kaluz S, et al: Molecular cloning of the cDNA coding for properdin, a positive regulator of the alternative pathway of human complement. *Eur J Immunol* 21:771, 1991.
232. Super M, Thiel S, Lu J, et al: Association of low levels of mannan-binding protein with a common defect of opsonisation. *Lancet* 2:1236, 1989.
233. Jack DL, Klein NJ, Turner MW: Mannose-binding lectin: Targeting the microbial world for complement attack and opsonophagocytosis. *Immunol Rev* 180:86, 2001.
234. Turner MW: The role of mannose-binding lectin in health and disease. *Mol Immunol* 40:423, 2003.
235. Trinchieri G, Sher A: Cooperation of toll-like receptor signals in innate immune defence. *Nat Rev Immunol* 7:179, 2007.
236. Sabroe I, Prince LR, Jones EC, et al: Selective roles for toll-like receptor (TLR)2 and TLR4 in the regulation of neutrophil activation and life span. *J Immunol* 170:5268, 2003.
237. von Bernuth H, Picard C, Jin Z, et al: Pyogenic bacterial infections in humans with MyD88 deficiency. *Science* 321:691, 2008.
238. Buckley RH: Immunodeficiency diseases. *JAMA* 268:2797, 1992.
239. Boxer LA, Smolen JE: Neutrophil granule constituents and their release in health and disease. *Hematol Oncol Clin North Am* 2:101, 1988.
240. Ward DM, Shiflett SL, Kaplan J: Chédiak-Higashi syndrome: A clinical and molecular view of a rare lysosomal storage disorder. *Curr Mol Med* 2:469, 2002.
241. Creel D, Boxer LA, Fauci AS: Visual and auditory anomalies in Chédiak-Higashi syndrome. *Electroencephalogr Clin Neurophysiol* 55:252, 1983.
242. Boxer GJ, Holmsen H, Robkin L, et al: Abnormal platelet function in Chédiak-Higashi syndrome. *Br J Haematol* 35:521, 1977.
243. Abo T, Roder JC, Abo W, et al: Natural killer (HNK-1+) cells in Chédiak-Higashi patients are present in normal numbers but are abnormal in function and morphology. *J Clin Invest* 70:193, 1982.
244. Introne W, Boissy RE, Gahl WA: Clinical, molecular, and cell biological aspects of Chédiak-Higashi syndrome. *Mol Genet Metab* 68:283, 1999.
245. Beguez-Cesar A: Neutropeneia cronica maligna familiar con granulacioundes atipicas de los leucocitos. *Boletin de la Sociedad Cubana Pediatr* 15:900, 1943.
246. Steinbrinck W: Über ene neue granulations anomalie der leukocyten. *Dtsch Arch Klin Med* 193:577, 1948.
247. Chediak MM: New leukocyte anomaly of constitutional and familial character. *Rev Hematol* 7:362, 1952.
248. Higashi O: Congenital gigantism of peroxidase granules; the first case ever reported of qualitative abnormity of peroxidase. *Tohoku J Exp Med* 59:315, 1954.
249. Blume RS, Bennett JM, Yankee RA, et al: Defective granulocyte regulation in the Chédiak-Higashi syndrome. *N Engl J Med* 279:1009, 1968.
250. White JG, Clawson CC: The Chédiak-Higashi syndrome; the nature of the giant neutrophil granules and their interactions with cytoplasm and foreign particulates. *Am J Pathol* 98:151, 1980.
251. Andrews T, Sullivan KE: Infections in patients with inherited defects in phagocytic function. *Clin Microbiol Rev* 16:597, 2003.
252. Trambas CM, Griffiths GM: Delivering the kiss of death. *Nat Immunol* 4:399, 2003.
253. Ingraham LM, Burns CP, Boxer LA, et al: Fluidity properties and liquid composition of erythrocyte membranes in Chédiak-Higashi syndrome. *J Cell Biol* 89:510, 1981.
254. Barbosa MD, Barrat FJ, Tchernev VT, et al: Identification of mutations in two major mRNA isoforms of the Chédiak-Higashi syndrome gene in human and mouse. *Hum Mol Genet* 6:1091, 1997.
255. Stinchcombe JC, Page LJ, Griffiths GM: Secretory lysosome biogenesis in cytotoxic T lymphocytes from normal and Chédiak-Higashi syndrome patients. *Traffic* 1:435, 2000.
256. Tchernev VT, Mansfield TA, Giot L, et al: The Chédiak-Higashi protein interacts with SNARE complex and signal transduction proteins. *Mol Med* 8:56, 2002.
257. Filipovich AH: Hemophagocytic lymphohistiocytosis and related disorders. *Curr Opin Allergy Clin Immunol* 6:410, 2006.
258. Eapen M, DeLaat CA, Baker KS, et al: Hematopoietic cell transplantation for Chédiak-Higashi syndrome. *Bone Marrow Transplant* 39:411, 2007.
259. Tardieu M, Lacroix C, Neven B, et al: Progressive neurologic dysfunctions 20 years after allogeneic bone marrow transplantation for Chédiak-Higashi syndrome. *Blood* 106:40, 2005.
260. Ganz T, Metcalf JA, Gallin JI, et al: Microbicidal/cytotoxic proteins of neutrophils are deficient in two disorders: Chédiak-Higashi syndrome and "specific" granule deficiency. *J Clin Invest* 82:552, 1988.
261. Lomax KJ, Gallin JI, Rotrosen D, et al: Selective defect in myeloid cell lactoferrin gene expression in neutrophil specific granule deficiency. *J Clin Invest* 83:514, 1989.
262. Johnston JJ, Boxer LA, Berliner N: Correlation of messenger RNA levels with protein defects in specific granule deficiency. *Blood* 80:2088, 1992.

263. Rosenberg HF, Gallin JI: Neutrophil-specific granule deficiency includes eosinophils. *Blood* 82:268, 1993.
264. Gallin JI, Fletcher MP, Seligmann BE, et al: Human neutrophil-specific granule deficiency: A model to assess the role of neutrophil-specific granules in the evolution of the inflammatory response. *Blood* 59:1317, 1982.
265. Lekstrom-Himes JA, Dorman SE, Kopar P, et al: Neutrophil-specific granule deficiency results from a novel mutation with loss of function of the transcription factor CCAAT enhancer binding protein epsilon. *J Exp Med* 189:1847, 1999.
266. Khanna-Gupta A, Sun H, Zibello T, et al: Growth factor independence-1 (Gfi-1) plays a role in mediating specific granule deficiency (SGD) in a patient lacking a gene-inactivating mutation in the C/EBPepsilon gene. *Blood* 109:4181, 2007.
267. Kuriyama K, Tomonaga M, Matsuo T, et al: Diagnostic significance of detecting pseudo-Pelger-Huet anomalies and micro-megakaryocytes in myelodysplastic syndrome. *Br J Haematol* 63:665, 1986.
268. Arnaout MA: Leukocyte adhesion molecules deficiency: Its structural basis, pathophysiology and implications for modulating the inflammatory response. *Immunol Rev* 114:145, 1990.
269. Corbi AL, Larson RS, Kishimoto TK, et al: Chromosomal location of the genes encoding the leukocyte adhesion receptors LFA-1, Mac-1 and p150,95. Identification of a gene cluster involved in cell adhesion. *J Exp Med* 167:1597, 1988.
270. Hayward AR, Harvey BA, Leonard J, et al: Delayed separation of the umbilical cord, widespread infections, and defective neutrophil mobility. *Lancet* 1:1099, 1979.
271. Crowley CA, Curnutte JT, Rosin RE, et al: An inherited abnormality of neutrophil adhesion. Its genetic transmission and its association with a missing protein. *N Engl J Med* 302:1163, 1980.
272. Arnaout MA, Pitt J, Cohen HJ, et al: Deficiency of a granulocyte-membrane glycoprotein (gp150) in a boy with recurrent bacterial infections. *N Engl J Med* 306:693, 1982.
273. Dana N, Todd RF, III, Pitt P, et al: Deficiency of a surface membrane glycoprotein (Mo1) in man. *J Clin Invest* 73:153, 1984.
274. Anderson DC, Smith CW: Leukocyte adhesion deficiencies, in *The Metabolic and Molecular Basis of Inherited Disease*, 8th ed, edited by C Scriver, A Beaudet, W Sly, D Valle, B Childs, K Kinzler, B Vogelstein, p 4829. McGraw-Hill, New York, 2001.
275. Springer TA, Thompson WS, Miller LJ, et al: Inherited deficiency of the Mac-1, LFA-1, p150,95 glycoprotein family and its molecular basis. *J Exp Med* 160:1901, 1984.
276. Wagner DD, Frenette PS: The vessel wall and its interactions. *Blood* 111:5271, 2008.
277. Larson RS, Springer TA: Structure and function of leukocyte integrins. *Immunol Rev* 114:181, 1990.
278. Hogg N, Stewart MP, Scarth SL, et al: A novel leukocyte adhesion deficiency caused by expressed but nonfunctional beta2 integrins Mac-1 and LFA-1. *J Clin Invest* 103:97, 1999.
279. Mathew EC, Shaw JM, Bonilla FA, et al: A novel point mutation in CD18 causing the expression of dysfunctional CD11/CD18 leucocyte integrins in a patient with leucocyte adhesion deficiency (LAD). *Clin Exp Immunol* 121:133, 2000.
280. Petrequin PR, Todd RF, III, Devall LJ, et al: Association between gelatinase release and increased plasma membrane expression of the Mo1 glycoprotein. *Blood* 69:605, 1987.
281. Anderson DC, Springer TA: Leukocyte adhesion deficiency: An inherited defect in the Mac-1, LFA-1, and p150,95 glycoproteins. *Annu Rev Med* 38:175, 1987.
282. Schwartz BR, Wayner EA, Carlos TM, et al: Identification of surface proteins mediating adherence of CD11/CD18-deficient lymphoblastoid cells to cultured human endothelium. *J Clin Invest* 85:2019, 1990.
283. Mizgerd JP, Kubo H, Kutkoski GJ, et al: Neutrophil emigration in the skin, lungs, and peritoneum: Different requirements for CD11/CD18 revealed by CD18-deficient mice. *J Exp Med* 186:1357, 1997.
284. Anderson DC, Rothlein R, Marlin SD, et al: Impaired transendothelial migration by neonatal neutrophils: Abnormalities of Mac-1 (CD11b/CD18)-dependent adherence reactions. *Blood* 76:2613, 1990.
285. Mulligan MS, Varani J, Dame MK, et al: Role of endothelial-leukocyte adhesion molecule 1 (ELAM-1) in neutrophil-mediated lung injury in rats. *J Clin Invest* 88:1396, 1991.
286. Wertheimer SJ, Myers CL, Wallace RW, et al: Intercellular adhesion molecule-1 gene expression in human endothelial cells. Differential regulation by tumor necrosis factor-alpha and phorbol myristate acetate. *J Biol Chem* 267:12030, 1992.
287. Malawista SE, de Boisfleury CA, Boxer LA: Random locomotion and chemotaxis of human blood polymorphonuclear leukocytes from a patient with leukocyte adhesion deficiency-1: Normal displacement in close quarters via chimneying. *Cell Motil Cytoskeleton* 46:183, 2000.
288. Arnaout MA: Structure and function of the leukocyte adhesion molecules CD11/CD18. *Blood* 75:1037, 1990.
289. Cao D, Mizukami IF, Garni-Wagner BA, et al: Human urokinase-type plasminogen activator primes neutrophils for superoxide anion release. Possible roles of complement receptor type 3 and calcium. *J Immunol* 154:1817, 1995.
290. Altieri DC, Bader R, Mannucci PM, et al: Oligospecificity of the cellular adhesion receptor Mac-1 encompasses an inducible recognition specificity for fibrinogen. *J Cell Biol* 107:1893, 1988.
291. Wilson RW, Ballantyne CM, Smith CW, et al: Gene targeting yields a CD18-mutant mouse for study of inflammation. *J Immunol* 151:1571, 1993.
292. Yakubenia S, Wild MK: Leukocyte adhesion deficiency II. Advances and open questions. *FEBS J* 273:4390, 2006.
293. Helmus Y, Denecke J, Yakubenia S, et al: Leukocyte adhesion deficiency II patients with a dual defect of the GDP-fucose transporter. *Blood* 107:3959, 2006.
294. Aebi M, Helenius A, Schenk B, et al: Carbohydrate-deficient glycoprotein syndromes become congenital disorders of glycosylation: An updated nomenclature for CDG. First International Workshop on CDGS. *Glycoconj J* 16:669, 1999.
295. Hidalgo A, Ma S, Peired AJ, et al: Insights into leukocyte adhesion deficiency type 2 from a novel mutation in the GDP-fucose transporter gene. *Blood* 101:1705, 2003.
296. Kuijpers TW, van Bruggen R, Kamerbeek N, et al: Natural history and early diagnosis of LAD-1/variant syndrome. *Blood* 109:3529, 2007.
297. Kuijpers TW, van de Vijver E, Weterman MA, et al: LAD-1/variant syndrome is caused by mutations in FERMT3. *Blood* 113:4740, 2009.
298. Fischer A, Lisowska-Grospierre B, Anderson DC, et al: Leukocyte adhesion deficiency: Molecular basis and functional consequences. *Immunodefic Rev* 1:39, 1988.
299. Bauer TR Jr, Hickstein DD: Gene therapy for leukocyte adhesion deficiency. *Curr Opin Mol Ther* 2:383, 2000.
300. Malech HL, Hickstein DD: Genetics, biology and clinical management of myeloid cell primary immune deficiencies: Chronic granulomatous disease and leukocyte adhesion deficiency. *Curr Opin Hematol* 14:29, 2007.
301. Kral V, Bartunkova J, Svorc K, et al: [The first case of leukocyte integrin deficiency syndrome in the Czech Republic and successful prenatal diagnosis in the affected family]. *Cas Lek Cesk* 135:154, 1996.
302. Boxer LA, Hedley-Whyte ET, Stossel TP: Neutrophil actin dysfunction and abnormal neutrophil behavior. *N Engl J Med* 291:1093, 1974.
303. Southwick FS, Dabiri GA, Stosse TP: Neutrophil actin dysfunction is a genetic disorder associated with partial impairment of neutrophil actin assembly in three family members. *J Clin Invest* 82:1525, 1988.
304. Malech HL, Gallin JI: Current concepts: Immunology neutrophils in human diseases. *N Engl J Med* 317:687, 1987.
305. Southwick FS, Howard TH, Holbrook T, et al: The relationship between CR3 deficiency and neutrophil actin assembly. *Blood* 73:1973, 1989.
306. Coates TD, Torkildson JC, Torres M, et al: An inherited defect of neutrophil motility and microfilamentous cytoskeleton associated with abnormalities in 47-Kd and 89-Kd proteins. *Blood* 78:1338, 1991.
307. Howard T, Li Y, Torres M, et al: The 47-kD protein increased in neutrophil actin dysfunction with 47-and 89-kD protein abnormalities is lymphocyte-specific protein. *Blood* 83:231, 1994.
308. Howard TH, Hartwig J, Cunningham C: Lymphocyte-specific protein 1 expression in eukaryotic cells reproduces the morphologic and motile abnormality of NAD 47/89 neutrophils. *Blood* 91:4786, 1998.
309. Camitta BM, Quesenberry PJ, Parkman R, et al: Bone marrow transplantation for an infant with neutrophil dysfunction. *Exp Hematol* 5:109, 1977.
310. Samuels J, Aksentijevich I, Torosyan Y, et al: Familial Mediterranean fever at the millennium. Clinical spectrum, ancient mutations, and a survey of 100 American referrals to the National Institutes of Health. *Medicine (Baltimore)* 77:268, 1998.
311. Siegal S: Benign paroxysural peritonitis. *Ann Intern Med* 23:1, 1945.
312. Drenth JP, van der Meer JW: Hereditary periodic fever. *N Engl J Med* 345:1748, 2001.
313. Ben Chetrit E, Levy M: Familial Mediterranean fever. *Lancet* 351:659, 1998.
314. Ancient missense mutations in a new member of the RoRet gene family are likely to cause familial Mediterranean fever. The International FMF Consortium. *Cell* 90:797, 1997.
315. A candidate gene for familial Mediterranean fever. The French FMF Consortium. *Nat Genet* 17:25, 1997.
316. Centola M, Wood G, Frucht DM, et al: The gene for familial Mediterranean fever, MEFV, is expressed in early leukocyte development and is regulated in response to inflammatory mediators. *Blood* 95:3223, 2000.
317. Ryan JG, Kastner DL: Fevers, genes, and innate immunity. *Curr Top Microbiol Immunol* 321:169, 2008.
318. Hull KM, Shoham N, Chae JJ, et al: The expanding spectrum of systemic autoinflammatory disorders and their rheumatic manifestations. *Curr Opin Rheumatol* 15:61, 2003.
319. Richards N, Schaner P, Diaz A, et al: Interaction between pyrin and the apoptotic speck protein (ASC) modulates ASC-induced apoptosis. *J Biol Chem* 276:39320, 2001.
320. Touitou I: The spectrum of Familial Mediterranean Fever (FMF) mutations. *Eur J Hum Genet* 9:473, 2001.
321. Schaner P, Richards N, Wadhwa A, et al: Episodic evolution of pyrin in primates: Human mutations recapitulate ancestral amino acid states. *Nat Genet* 27:318, 2001.
322. Williamson LM, Hull D, Mehta R, et al: Familial Hibernian fever. *Q J Med* 51:469, 1982.
323. Lakshman R, Finn A: Neutrophil disorders and their management. *J Clin Pathol* 54:7, 2001.
324. Perlmutter DH, Colten HR: Molecular basis of complement deficiencies. *Immunodefic Rev* 1:105, 1989.
325. Kannourakis G: Glycogen storage disease. *Semin Hematol* 39:103, 2002.
326. Smith OP: Shwachman-Diamond syndrome. *Semin Hematol* 39:95, 2002.
327. Jones DH, Schmalstieg FC, Dempsey K, et al: Subcellular distribution and mobilization of MAC-1 (CD11b/CD18) in neonatal neutrophils. *Blood* 75:488, 1990.
328. Brayton RG, Stokes PE, Schwartz MS, et al: Effect of alcohol and various diseases on leukocyte mobilization, phagocytosis and intracellular bacterial killing. *N Engl J Med* 282:123, 1970.
329. Oseas RS, Allen J, Yang HH, et al: Mechanism of dexamethasone inhibition of chemotactic factor induced granulocyte aggregation. *Blood* 59:265, 1982.

330. Dale DC, Fauci AS, Wolff SM: Alternate-day prednisone. Leukocyte kinetics and susceptibility to infections. *N Engl J Med* 291:1154, 1974.
331. Boxer LA, Allen JM, Baehner RL: Diminished polymorphonuclear leukocyte adherence. Function dependent on release of cyclic AMP by endothelial cells after stimulation of beta-receptors by epinephrine. *J Clin Invest* 66:268, 1980.
332. Freeman AF, Holland SM: The hyper-IgE syndromes. *Immunol Allergy Clin North Am* 28:277, 2008.
333. Engelich G, Wright DG, Hartshorn KL: Acquired disorders of phagocyte function complicating medical and surgical illnesses. *Clin Infect Dis* 33:2040, 2001.
334. Buckley RH: The hyper-IgE syndrome. *Clin Rev Allergy Immunol* 20:139, 2001.
335. Grimbacher B, Holland SM, Gallin JI, et al: Hyper-IgE syndrome with recurrent infections—An autosomal dominant multisystem disorder. *N Engl J Med* 340:692, 1999.
336. Segal BH, Leto TL, Gallin JI, et al: Genetic, biochemical, and clinical features of chronic granulomatous disease. *Medicine (Baltimore)* 79:170, 2000.
337. Berendes H, Bridges RA, Good RA: A fatal granulomatosus of childhood: The clinical study of a new syndrome. *Minn Med* 40:309, 1957.
338. Landing BH, Shirkey HS: A syndrome of recurrent infection and infiltration of viscera by pigmented lipid histiocytes. *Pediatrics* 20:431, 1957.
339. Sbarra AJ, Karnovsky ML: The biochemical basis of phagocytosis. I. Metabolic changes during the ingestion of particles by polymorphonuclear leukocytes. *J Biol Chem* 234:1355, 1959.
340. Iyer GY, Quastel JH: Biochemical aspects of phagocytosis. *Nature* 192:535, 1961.
341. Iyer GY, Quastel JH: NADPH and NADH oxidation by guinea pig polymorphonuclear leucocytes. *Can J Biochem Physiol* 41:427, 1963.
342. Baehner RL, Nathan DG: Quantitative nitroblue tetrazolium test in chronic granulomatous disease. *N Engl J Med* 278:971, 1968.
343. Winkelstein JA, Marino MC, Johnston RB Jr, et al: Chronic granulomatous disease. Report on a national registry of 368 patients. *Medicine (Baltimore)* 79:155, 2000.
344. Parkos CA, Allen RA, Cochrane CG, et al: Purified cytochrome b from human granulocyte plasma membrane is comprised of two polypeptides with relative molecular weights of 91,000 and 22,000. *J Clin Invest* 80:732, 1987.
345. Sengelov H, Follin P, Kjeldsen L, et al: Mobilization of granules and secretory vesicles during in vivo exudation of human neutrophils. *J Immunol* 154:4157, 1995.
346. Abo A, Pick E: Purification and characterization of a third cytosolic component of the superoxide-generating NADPH oxidase of macrophages. *J Biol Chem* 266:23577, 1991.
347. Quinn MT, Mullen ML, Jesaitis AJ: Human neutrophil cytochrome b contains multiple hemes. Evidence for heme associated with both subunits. *J Biol Chem* 267:7303, 1992.
348. Rotrosen D, Yeung CL, Leto TL, et al: Cytochrome b_{558}: The flavin-binding component of the phagocyte NADPH oxidase. *Science* 256:1459, 1992.
349. Segal AW, West I, Wientjes F, et al: Cytochrome b-245 is a flavocytochrome containing FAD and the NADPH-binding site of the microbicidal oxidase of phagocytes. *Biochem J* 284:781, 1992.
350. Sumimoto H, Sakamoto N, Nozaki M, et al: Cytochrome b558, a component of the phagocyte NADPH oxidase, is a flavoprotein. *Biochem Biophys Res Commun* 186:1368, 1992.
351. Zhen L, Yu L, Dinauer MC: Probing the role of the carboxyl terminus of the gp91phox subunit of neutrophil flavocytochrome b558 using site-directed mutagenesis. *J Biol Chem* 273:6575, 1998.
352. Henderson LM, Thomas S, Banting G, et al: The arachidonate-activatable, NADPH oxidase-associated H+ channel is contained within the multi-membrane-spanning N- terminal region of gp91-phox. *Biochem J* 325:701, 1997.
353. Shatwell KP, Dancis A, Cross AR, et al: The FRE1 ferric reductase of Saccharomyces cerevisiae is a cytochrome b similar to that of NADPH oxidase. *J Biol Chem* 271:14240, 1996.
354. Deleo FR, Quinn MT: Assembly of the phagocyte NADPH oxidase: Molecular interaction of oxidase proteins. *J Leukoc Biol* 60:677, 1996.
355. Segal AW: The NADPH oxidase and chronic granulomatous disease. *Mol Med Today* 2:129, 1996.
356. Wientjes FB, Hsuan JJ, Totty NF, et al: $P40^{phox}$, a third cytosolic component of the activation complex of the NADPH oxidase to contain SRC homology 3 domains. *Biochem J* 296:557, 1993.
357. Chen J, He R, Minshall RD, et al: Characterization of a mutation in the Phox homology domain of the NADPH oxidase component p40phox identifies a mechanism for negative regulation of superoxide production. *J Biol Chem* 282:30273, 2007.
358. Cross AR, Jones OT: Enzymic mechanisms of superoxide production. *Biochim Biophys Acta* 1057:281, 1991.
359. Abo A, Boyhan A, West I, et al: Reconstitution of neutrophil NADPH oxidase activity in the cell-free system by four components: p67-phox, p47-phox, p21rac1, and cytochrome b-245. *J Biol Chem* 267:16767, 1992.
360. Clark RA, Volpp BD, Leidal KG, et al: Two cytosolic components of the human neutrophil respiratory burst oxidase translocate to the plasma membrane during cell activation. *J Clin Invest* 85:714, 1990.
361. Heyworth PG, Curnutte JT, Nauseef WM, et al: Neutrophil nicotinamide adenine dinucleotide phosphate oxidase assembly. Translocation of p47-phox and p67-phox requires interaction between p47-phox and cytochrome b_{558}. *J Clin Invest* 87:352, 1991.
362. Knaus UG, Morris S, Dong HJ, et al: Regulation of human leukocyte p21-activated kinases through g protein-coupled receptors. *Science* 269:221, 1995.
363. Bromberg Y, Pick E: Unsaturated fatty acids stimulate NADPH-dependent superoxide production by cell-free system derived from macrophages. *Cell Immunol* 88:213, 1984.
364. Curnutte JT: Activation of human neutrophil nicotinamide adenine dinucleotide phosphate, reduced (triphosphopyridine nucleotide, reduced) oxidase by arachidonic acid in a cell-free system. *J Clin Invest* 75:1740, 1985.
365. McPhail LC, Shirley PS, Clayton CC, et al: Activation of the respiratory burst enzyme from human neutrophils in a cell-free system. Evidence for a soluble cofactor. *J Clin Invest* 75:1735, 1985.
366. Curnutte JT: Molecular basis of the autosomal recessive forms of chronic granulomatous disease. *Immunodefic Rev* 3:149, 1992.
367. Heyworth PG, Curnutte JT, Rae J, et al: Hematologically important mutations: X-linked chronic granulomatous disease (second update). *Blood Cells Mol Dis* 27:16, 2001.
368. Francke U, Ochs HD, de Martinville B, et al: Minor Xp21 chromosome deletion in a male associated with expression of Duchenne muscular dystrophy, chronic granulomatous disease, retinitis pigmentosa, and McLeod syndrome. *Am J Hum Genet* 37:250, 1985.
369. Royer-Pokora B, Kunkel LM, Monaco AP, et al: Cloning the gene for an inherited human disorder-chronic granulomatous disease-on the basis of its chromosomal location. *Nature* 322:32, 1986.
370. Frey D, Mächler M, Seger R, et al: Gene deletion in a patient with chronic granulomatous disease and McLeod syndrome: Fine mapping of the Xk gene locus. *Blood* 71:252, 1988.
371. de Boer M, Bolscher BG, Dinauer MC, et al: Splice site mutations are a common cause of X-linked chronic granulomatous disease. *Blood* 80:1553, 1992.
372. Curnutte JT, Orkin S, Dinauer MC: Genetic disorders of phagocyte function, in *The Molecular Basis of Blood Diseases*, 2nd ed, edited by G Stammatoyannopoulos, p 493. Saunders, Philadelphia, 1994.
373. Roos D, Deboer M, Kuribayashi F, et al: Mutations in the x-linked and autosomal recessive forms of chronic granulomatous disease. *Blood* 87:1663, 1996.
374. Rae J, Newburger PE, Dinauer MC, et al: X-Linked chronic granulomatous disease: Mutations in the CYBB gene encoding the gp91-phox component of respiratory-burst oxidase. *Am J Hum Genet* 62:1320, 1998.
375. Dinauer MC, Pierce EA, Bruns GAP, et al: Human neutrophil cytochrome b light chain (p22-phox). Gene structure, chromosomal location, and mutations in cytochrome-negative autosomal recessive chronic granulomatous disease. *J Clin Invest* 86:1729, 1990.
376. Segal AW: Biochemistry and molecular biology of chronic granulomatous disease. *J Inherit Metab Dis* 15:683, 1992.
377. Casimir CM, Bu-Ghanim HN, Rodaway AR, et al: Autosomal recessive chronic granulomatous disease caused by deletion at a dinucleotide repeat. *Proc Natl Acad Sci U S A* 88:2753, 1991.
378. Roos D: X-CGDbase: A database of X-CGD-causing mutations. *Immunol Today* 17:517, 1996.
379. Jankowski A, Scott CC, Grinstein S: Determinants of the phagosomal pH in neutrophils. *J Biol Chem* 277:6059, 2002.
380. Segal AW: How neutrophils kill microbes. *Annu Rev Immunol* 23:197, 2005.
381. Reeves EP, Lu H, Jacobs HL, et al: Killing activity of neutrophils is mediated through activation of proteases by K+ flux. *Nature* 416:291, 2002.
382. Fernandez-Boyanapalli RF, Frasch SC, McPhillips K, et al: Impaired apoptotic cell clearance in CGD due to altered macrophage programming is reversed by phosphatidylserine-dependent production of IL-4. *Blood* 2009.
383. Johnston RB Jr, Baehner RL: Chronic granulomatous disease: Correlation between pathogenesis and clinical findings. *Pediatrics* 48:730, 1971.
384. Johnston RB Jr: Clinical aspects of chronic granulomatous disease. *Curr Opin Hematol* 8:17, 2001.
385. Petty HR, Francis JW, Boxer LA: Deficiency in immune complex uptake by chronic granulomatous disease neutrophils. *J Cell Sci* 90:425, 1988.
386. Foster CB, Lehrnbecher T, Mol F, et al: Host defense molecule polymorphisms influence the risk for immune-mediated complications in chronic granulomatous disease. *J Clin Invest* 102:2146, 1998.
387. Wolach B, Scharf Y, Gavrieli R, et al: Unusual late presentation of X-linked chronic granulomatous disease in an adult female with a somatic mosaic for a novel mutation in CYBB. *Blood* 105:61, 2005.
388. Crockard AD, Thompson JM, Boyd NA, et al: Diagnosis and carrier detection of chronic granulomatous disease in five families by flow cytometry. *Int Arch Allergy Immunol* 114:144, 1997.
389. Newburger PE, Luscinskas FW, Ryan T, et al: Variant chronic granulomatous disease: Modulation of the neutrophil defect by severe infection. *Blood* 68:914, 1986.
390. Curnutte JT: Chronic granulomatous disease: The solving of clinical riddle at the molecular level. *Clin Immunol Immunopathol* 67:S2, 1993.
391. Newburger PE, Cohen HJ, Rothchild SB, et al: Prenatal diagnosis of chronic granulomatous disease. *N Engl J Med* 300:178, 1979.
392. Pelham A, O'Reilly MA, Malcolm S, et al: RFLP and deletion analysis for X-linked chronic granulomatous disease using the cDNA probe: Potential for improved prenatal diagnosis and carrier determination. *Blood* 76:820, 1990.
393. Cooper MR, DeChatelet LR, McCall CE, et al: Complete deficiency of leukocyte glucose-6-phosphate dehydrogenase with defective bactericidal activity. *J Clin Invest* 51:769, 1972.

394. Vives Corrons JL, Feliu E, Pujades MA, et al: Severe-glucose-6-phosphate dehydrogenase (G6PD) deficiency associated with chronic hemolytic anemia, granulocyte dysfunction, and increased susceptibility to infections: Description of a new molecular variant (G6PD Barcelona). *Blood* 59:428, 1982.
395. Ambruso DR, Knall C, Abell AN, et al: Human neutrophil immunodeficiency syndrome is associated with an inhibitory Rac2 mutation. *Proc Natl Acad Sci U S A* 97:4654, 2000.
396. Williams DA, Tao W, Yang FC, et al: Dominant negative mutation of the hematopoietic-specific Rho GTPase, Rac2, is associated with a human phagocyte immunodeficiency. *Blood* 96:1646, 2000.
397. Chusid MJ, Gelfand JA, Nutter C, et al: Letter: Pulmonary aspergillosis, inhalation of contaminated marijuana smoke, chronic granulomatous disease. *Ann Intern Med* 82:682, 1975.
398. Seger RA: Modern management of chronic granulomatous disease. *Br J Haematol* 140:255, 2008.
399. Gallin JI, Alling DW, Malech HL, et al: Itraconazole to prevent fungal infections in chronic granulomatous disease. *N Engl J Med* 348:2416, 2003.
400. A controlled trial of interferon gamma to prevent infection in chronic granulomatous disease. The International Chronic Granulomatous Disease Cooperative Study Group. *N Engl J Med* 324:509, 1991.
401. Schiff DE, Rae J, Martin TR, et al: Increased phagocyte Fc gammaRI expression and improved Fc gamma-receptor-mediated phagocytosis after in vivo recombinant human interferon-gamma treatment of normal human subjects. *Blood* 90:3187, 1997.
402. Woodman RC, Erickson RW, Rae J, et al: Prolonged recombinant interferon-gamma therapy in chronic granulomatous disease: Evidence against enhanced neutrophil oxidase activity. *Blood* 79:1558, 1992.
403. Seger RA, Tiefenauer L, Matsunaga T, et al: Chronic granulomatous disease due to granulocytes with abnormal NADPH oxidase activity and deficient cytochrome-b. *Blood* 61:423, 1983.
404. Styrt B, Klempner MS: Late-presenting variant of chronic granulomatous disease. *Pediatr Infect Dis* 3:556, 1984.
405. Malech HL, Bauer TR, Hickstein DD: Prospects for gene therapy of neutrophil defects. *Semin Hematol* 34:355, 1997.
406. Pollock JD, Williams DA, Gifford MAC, et al: Mouse model of x-linked chronic granulomatous disease, an inherited defect in phagocyte superoxide production. *Nat Genet* 9:202, 1995.
407. Jackson SH, Gallin JI, Holland SM: The p47(phox) mouse knock-out model of chronic granulomatous disease. *J Exp Med* 182:751, 1995.
408. Mardiney M, III, Jackson SH, Spratt SK, et al: Enhanced host defense after gene transfer in the murine p47phox-deficient model of chronic granulomatous disease. *Blood* 89:2268, 1997.
409. Bjorgvinsdottir H, Ding CJ, Pech N, et al: Retroviral-mediated gene transfer of gp91(phox) into bone marrow cells rescues defect in host defense against Aspergillus fumigatus in murine X-linked chronic granulomatous disease. *Blood* 89:41, 1997.
410. Malech HL, Maples PB, Whiting-Theobald N, et al: Prolonged production of NADPH oxidase-corrected granulocytes after gene therapy of chronic granulomatous disease. *Proc Natl Acad Sci U S A* 94:12133, 1997.
411. Ott MG, Schmidt M, Schwarzwaelder K, et al: Correction of X-linked chronic granulomatous disease by gene therapy, augmented by insertional activation of MDS1-EVI1, PRDM16 or SETBP1. *Nat Med* 12:401, 2006.
412. Hansson M, Olsson I, Nauseef WM: Biosynthesis, processing, and sorting of human myeloperoxidase. *Arch Biochem Biophys* 445:214, 2006.
413. Nauseef WM: Insights into myeloperoxidase biosynthesis from its inherited deficiency. *J Mol Med* 76:661, 1998.
414. Nauseef WM: Myeloperoxidase deficiency. *Hematol Pathol* 4:165, 1990.
415. Boxer, L. A.: The role of antioxidants in modulating neutrophil functional responses, in *Advances in Experimental Medicine*, edited by A Bendich, M Philip, P Tengedy, p 19. Plenum Press, New York, 1990.
416. Roos D, Weening RS, Voetman AA, et al: Protection of phagocytic leukocytes by endogenous glutathione: Studies in a family with glutathione reductase deficiency. *Blood* 53:851, 1979.
417. Boxer LA, Oliver JM, Spielberg SP, et al: Protection of granulocytes by vitamin E in glutathione synthetase deficiency. *N Engl J Med* 301:901, 1979.

PART VIII

Monocytes and Macrophages

CHAPTER 67
MORPHOLOGY OF MONOCYTES AND MACROPHAGES

Steven D. Douglas and Florin Tuluc

SUMMARY

The monocyte is a spherical cell with prominent surface ruffles and blebs when examined by scanning electron microscopy. When reconstructed from sections examined under transmission electron microscopy, the monocyte has a reni form nucleus containing a small nucleolus. The cytoplasm has many mitochondria, microtubules, and microfilaments. The Golgi apparatus is well developed and has neighboring centrioles. Numerous microvilli and microcytotic vesicles are evident at or near the cell surface. The cytoplasm contains scattered granules, akin to lysosomes. The granule contents share features with the primary granules of neutrophils, although, in contrast to the neutrophil, the monocyte granule is characterized by fluoride-inhibitable esterases. As the monocyte enters the tissue and differentiates into a macrophage, the cell volume and number of cytoplasmic granules increase. Cell shape varies, depending on the tissue type in which the macrophage resides (e.g., lung, liver, spleen, brain). A characteristic feature of macrophages is their prominent electron-dense membrane-bound lysosomes, which can be seen fusing with phagosomes to form secondary lysosomes. The latter contain ingested cellular and noncellular material in different stages of degradation. A broad range of surface receptors for many ligands, including the Fc portion of immunoglobulin, complement proteins, cytokines, chemokines, lipoproteins, and others, are on the cell surface. Macrophages differ in appearance, biochemistry, and function based on the environment in which they mature from monocytes. These differences are exemplified by the diversity among dendritic cells of lymph nodes, histiocytes of connective tissue, osteoclasts of bone, Kupffer cells of liver, microglia of the central nervous system, and macrophages of the serosal surfaces, each fashioned to meet the local needs of the mononuclear phagocyte system, which plays a role in inflammation and host defense against microbes.

MONONUCLEAR PHAGOCYTE SYSTEM

Modern study of mammalian phagocytes began with Metchnikoff in the 19th century. An understanding of the ontogeny, kinetics, and function of phagocytic cells in animals led to the concept of the mononuclear phagocyte system.[1,2] The system consists of marrow monoblasts and promonocytes, blood monocytes, and both free and fixed-tissue macrophages. Vascular endothelium, reticular cells, and dendritic cells of lymphoid germinal centers usually are not included in the mononuclear phagocyte system, although the now obsolete term *reticuloendothelial system*[3] denoted these cells as playing some complementary part with mononuclear phagocytes. Monocytes can differentiate into dendritic cells *in vitro*.[4] Monocytes and macrophages comprise the functional system formerly thought to be the reticuloendothelial system. Tissue macrophages share many functional characteristics, such as phagocytic and microbial killing capabilities and adherence to glass or plastic surfaces *in vitro*. Kinetic studies indicate macrophages are transformed monocytes and that the monocyte is derived from differentiation of the hematopoietic stem cell (see Chap. 16).

Acronyms and abbreviations that appear in this chapter include: CR1, complement receptor 1; CR3, complement receptor 3; CSF, colony-stimulating factor; FcR, Fc receptor; GM-CSF, granulocyte-monocyte colony-stimulating factor; HIV, human immunodeficiency virus; HLA, human leukocyte antigen; IgG, immunoglobulin G; IL-4, interleukin-4; IMP, intramembrane particle; LPS, lipopolysaccharide; M-CSF, macrophage colony-stimulating factor; MHC, major histocompatibility complex; TLR, toll-like receptor.

The blood monocyte is a medium to large motile cell that can marginate along vessel walls and has a propensity for adherence to surfaces. Monocytes respond to inflammation and chemotactic stimuli by active diapedesis across vessel walls into inflammatory foci, where they can mature into macrophages, with greater phagocytic capacity and increased content of hydrolytic enzymes. Free macrophages also are present in mammary glands, alveolar spaces, pleura, peritoneum, and synovia. The somewhat less-motile fixed-tissue macrophages are found in different tissues and serous cavities (Table 67–1). The functions of mononuclear phagocytes include phagocytosis and digestion of microorganisms, particulate material, or tissue debris; secretion of chemical mediators and regulators of the inflammatory response; interaction with antigen and lymphocytes in the generation of the immune response; cytotoxicity, such as killing of some tumor cells; and other functions specific for macrophages of particular tissues.

The development of techniques to isolate monocytes from blood of adult subjects led to the discovery that monocytes are heterogeneous with regard to cell volumes. Isolation of purified monocytes by adherence to glass substrates or to gelatin-coated flasks or by centrifugal elutriation reveals distinct populations of monocytes.[1,2] In addition to the usual 12- to 15-μm diameter (when measured on a dried blood film) monocyte, so-called "regular monocytes," a somewhat smaller cell that is less active than its larger, more mature counterpart has been identified. This cell is referred to as a *small immature monocyte*, but its functional significance is not clear.

Monocytes continuously emigrate from the blood into peripheral tissue, with a half-life in the blood of approximately 1 day in mice.[5] Nondividing monocytes can be induced to differentiate into dendritic like cells *in vitro*. However, this process requires culture of the cells for 7 to 10 days with exogenous cytokines, typically interleukin-4 (IL-4) and granulocyte-monocyte colony-stimulating factor (GM-CSF).[6] In the presence of endothelial cells grown on an extracellular matrix, monocytes differentiate along two distinct pathways: toward dendritic cells or macrophages. Monocytes that migrate across endothelium in an abluminal to luminal direction differentiate into dendritic cells. In contrast, monocytes that remain in the subendothelial matrix differentiate into macrophages.

MORPHOLOGY OF MONOCYTE PRECURSORS

Monoblasts and promonocytes are the precursors of monocytes, bearing finely dispersed nuclear chromatin and nucleoli when observed in the stained film of the blood or marrow. The monoblast is a very low prevalence marrow cell, indistinguishable by light microscopy from the myeloblast. Promonocytes are 12 to 18 μm in diameter (as measured on dried blood films) and have characteristic deeply indented, irregularly shaped nuclei with condensed chromatin, and numerous cytoplasmic microfilaments.

In animal studies, a small percentage of marrow cells are phagocytic, synthesize DNA, adhere to glass surfaces, and contain nonspecific esterases.[7] These cells have been referred to as *promonocytes* and are

TABLE 67–1. Distribution of Mononuclear Phagocytes

Marrow	Tissues
Monoblasts	Liver (Kupffer cells)
Promonocytes	Lung (alveolar macrophages)
Monocytes	Connective tissue (histiocytes)
Macrophages	Spleen (red pulp macrophages)
Blood	Lymph nodes
Monocytes	Thymus
Body cavities	Bone (osteoclasts)
Pleural macrophages	Synovium (type A cells)
Peritoneal macrophages	Mucosa-associated lymphoid tissue
Inflammatory tissues	Gastrointestinal tract
Epithelioid cells	Genitourinary tract
Exudate macrophages	Endocrine organs
Multinucleate giant cells	Central nervous system (microglia)
	Skin (histiocyte/dendritic cells)

SOURCE: Adapted from Angen and Ross, in Lewis CE, McGee JO'D.[2] Refer to references 7, 69, 70.

considered as intermediate between monoblasts and the monocytes of the blood.[7] Cytochemical studies identify the promonocyte in normal human marrow. These cells have deeply indented and irregularly shaped nuclei and bundled and scattered single filaments in the cytoplasm. These morphologic features distinguish the promonocyte from the progranulocyte.[8,9] Peroxidase is present throughout the cell secretory apparatus in all cisternae of the rough-surfaced endoplasmic reticulum, the Golgi complex, associated vesicles, and all immature and mature granules. Cytochemical reaction products for acid phosphatase and arylsulfatase also are deposited throughout the secretory apparatus of the promonocyte.

MORPHOLOGY OF MONOCYTES

LIGHT MICROSCOPY

The morphology of monocytes has been investigated by light and phase-contrast optics,[10] scanning and transmission electron microscopy, and freeze-fracture and freeze-etch procedures.[11]

On the stained blood film the monocyte has a diameter of 12 to 15 μm (Fig. 67–1). The monocyte nucleus occupies approximately half the area of the cell and usually is eccentrically placed. The nucleus most often is reniform, but may be round or irregular. It contains a characteristic chromatin net with fine strands bridging small chromatin clumps. Chromatin aggregates are arranged along the internal side of the nuclear membrane. The cytoplasm is spread out, stains grayish-blue with Wright stain, and contains a variable number of fine, pink-purple granules, which at times are sufficiently numerous to give the entire cytoplasm a pink hue. Clear cytoplasmic vacuoles and a variable number of larger azurophilic granulations often are encountered in these cells.

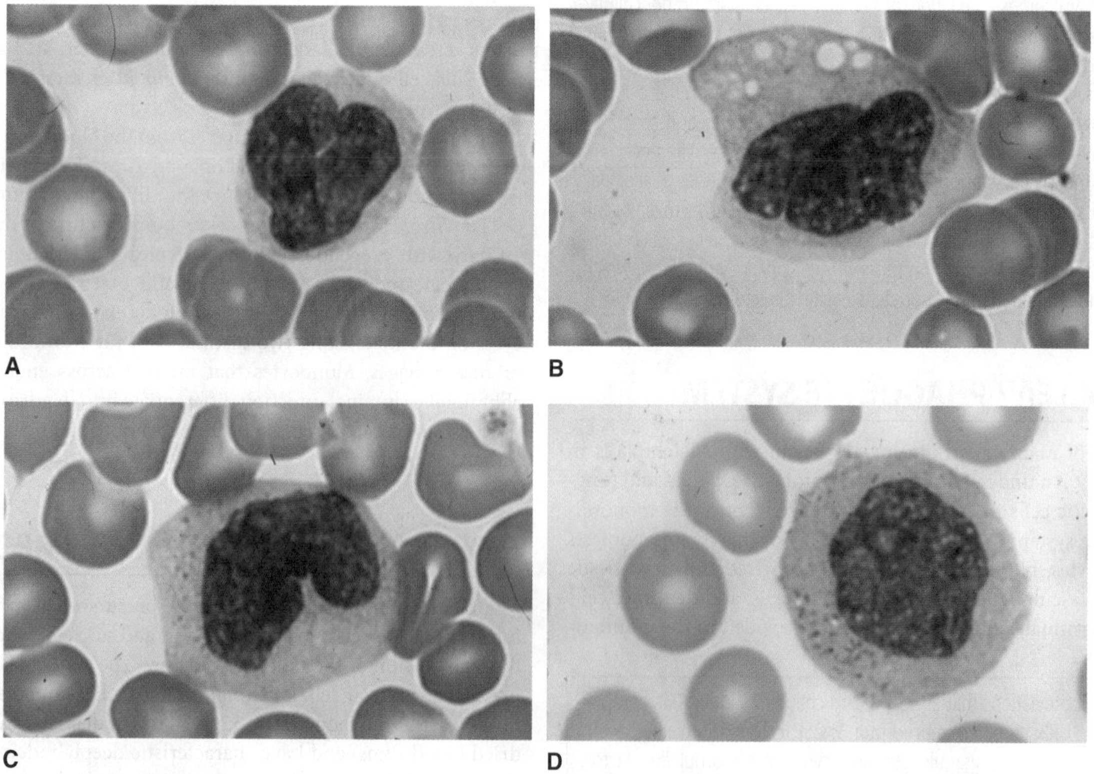

FIGURE 67–1. Blood films. This composite shows four examples of normal monocytes with different nuclear configurations. **A.** In this case the nucleus is contorted on itself and the nucleus:cytoplasmic ratio a bit higher than the average case. **B.** Another contorted nucleus with a lower nucleus:cytoplasmic ratio. Scattered vacuoles are common in monocytes collected in EDTA-anticoagulated blood before film preparation. **C.** Characteristic reniform nuclear shape. **D.** Circular nuclear shape. Azurophilic granules are evident in the cytoplasm of monocytes. *(Used with permission from* Lichtman's Atlas of Hematology, *www.accessmedicine.com.)*

PHASE MICROSCOPY

The monocyte nucleus has a distinct chromatin pattern on a cloudy background when examined by phase-contrast microscopy. The cytoplasm is clear gray. Mitochondria are extremely fine and occasionally form a small, juxtanuclear rosette surrounding the centrosome. The phase-dense cytoplasmic granules, varying in number, are generally at the limit of resolution of light microscopy and appear as fine intracytoplasmic dust. Monocytes contain several types of cytoplasmic vacuoles. The reniform nucleus with a juxtanuclear depression filled by a centrosome and its active undulating movement similar to that of other leukocytes are characteristic of the monocyte. The locomotion of the monocyte has the same pattern of undulating cytoplasmic veils seen in macrophages. The monocyte generally assumes a triangular shape as it moves, with one point trailing behind and the other two points advancing before the cell. Blood monocytes undergo adherence and cytoplasmic spreading following attachment to glass surfaces.[12] The extent of spreading increases in the presence of antigen–antibody complexes, certain divalent metals, and proteolytic enzymes.[12,13] The spread form of the monocyte reveals that the nucleus and granules are located centrally and the abundant hyaloplasm is in the periphery of the cell, terminating in a fringed border that displays undulating movement. The small monocyte may be difficult to distinguish from the large lymphocyte when examined by phase-contrast microscopy.

A striking feature on phase-contrast microscopy is the ruffled plasma membrane that forms prominent phase-dense folds at the cell surface and edges. Some cells have a dense thickening at the edge of the cytoplasm, with microextensions on the thickened edge.

SCANNING ELECTRON MICROSCOPY

The monocyte surface has very prominent ruffles and small surface blebs.[14,15] Extensive ruffling on the monocyte plasma membrane is of functional significance. The monocyte is both motile and phagocytic, and these functions require physical contact with particles or cell surfaces. Reduction in the radius of curvature of the cell surface by formation of ruffles or microvilli may reduce repulsive forces when surface negative-charge groups on the cell approach and contact a negatively charged substratum or cell. In addition, redundancy of the cell membrane may provide reserve membrane required for locomotion and phagocytosis.

TRANSMISSION ELECTRON MICROSCOPY

The nucleus of the monocyte contains one or two small nucleoli surrounded by nucleolar-associated chromatin (Fig. 67–2).[16] The cytoplasm contains a relatively small quantity of endoplasmic reticulum and a variable quantity of ribosomes and polysomes. The mitochondria are numerous, small, and elongated. The Golgi complex is well developed and is situated about the centrosome within the nuclear indentation. Centrioles and filamentous centriolar satellites are often visualized in this region. Microtubules are numerous, and microfibrils are found in bundles surrounding the nucleus. In cultured macrophages, collections of microfilaments are present underneath the plasma membrane near sites of cell attachment either to a substratum or to phagocytosable particles.[17] The cell surface is characterized by numerous microvilli and vesicles of micropinocytosis. The cytoplasmic granules resemble the small granules found in the granulocytic series, measuring approximately 0.05 to 0.2 μm in diameter. They are dense and homogeneous and are surrounded by a limiting membrane. These granules, as with the lysosomal granules of other leukocytes, are packaged by the Golgi apparatus after their enzymatic content has been produced by the ribosomal complex of the cell.[7,8,18] These cytoplasmic granules contain acid phosphatase and arylsulfatase and therefore are primary lysosomes. After endocytosis, lysosomes fuse with the phagosome, forming secondary lysosomes. Some monocyte granules stain positive for peroxidase, whereas others are peroxidase negative.[7,8]

FREEZE-FRACTURE MICROSCOPY

In this technique, a cell suspension is frozen, placed in a high-vacuum chamber, and struck with a blunt edge, thus producing a fracture that propagates through the frozen specimen. The utility of the procedure comes from the remarkable finding that when the fracture encounters a cell, the fracture tends to propagate along the interior of the plasma membrane and thus split the lipid bilayer into its two constituent layers. After fracture, the specimen is coated with platinum, which is electron dense when viewed with transmission electron microscopy. All cell types examined thus far by the freeze-fracture technique reveal intramembrane particles (IMPs) as the predominant topographic feature of the interior of the bilayer. Studies of the erythrocyte have shown that at least some particles contain intercalated membrane proteins, and this has been assumed to be the case for nucleated cells as well. The distribution of IMPs is dramatically altered in a number of cell systems by physiologic stimuli, for example, hormonal stimulation.

Profound changes in the distribution of IMPs on mononuclear phagocytes occur following binding of antibody-coated erythrocytes.[11] Because redistribution of IMPs also occurs in some nonphagocyte Fc receptor (FcR)-bearing cells[11] and after exposure to aggregated immunoglobulin (Ig) G, this alteration in IMPs presumably reflects interaction with FcR. Freeze-etch electron micrographs of the monocyte show nuclear pores traversing both lamellae of the nuclear membrane and contours of cytoplasmic lysosomes and mitochondria (Fig. 67–3).

HISTOCHEMISTRY OF MONOCYTES

Table 67–2 compares the hydrolytic enzyme contents of monocytes, neutrophils, and lymphocytes. Monocytes also give a weak but positive periodic acid-Schiff reaction (for polysaccharides) and Sudan black B reaction (for lipids).

Nonspecific esterase[19–21] is frequently used as a marker for monocytes. Monocyte esterases are inhibited by sodium fluoride, whereas the esterases of the granulocytic series are not. The nonspecific esterase reaction is positive in promyelocytes and myelocytes; therefore, analysis of fluoride inhibition is necessary to distinguish marrow monocytes from early myelocytes. Monocyte granules, although heterogeneous in size (0.3–0.6 μm), are not separable into populations by routine electron microscopic criteria (except in the rat).[22] Identification of monocyte granule populations has depended on subcellular localization of monocyte enzymes by electron microscopic cytochemistry.[8] Human marrow promonocytes and blood monocytes contain granules that comprise two functionally distinct populations.[8,9] One population contains the enzymes acid phosphatase, arylsulfatase, and, in the human (but not in the rabbit), peroxidase. These granules are modified primary lysosomes and are analogous to the azurophil granules of the neutrophil. The monocyte azurophil granule population is heterogeneous in cytochemical reactivity for peroxidase, acid phosphatase, and arylsulfatase.[23,24] Moreover, primary granules that are morphologically identical with other vesicles can be identified as lysosomes cytochemically. The content of the other population of monocyte granules is unknown; however, they lack alkaline phosphatase[23] and hence are not strictly analogous to the specific granules of neutrophils. The lysosomes have a digestive function, whereas the function of the second population is unknown.

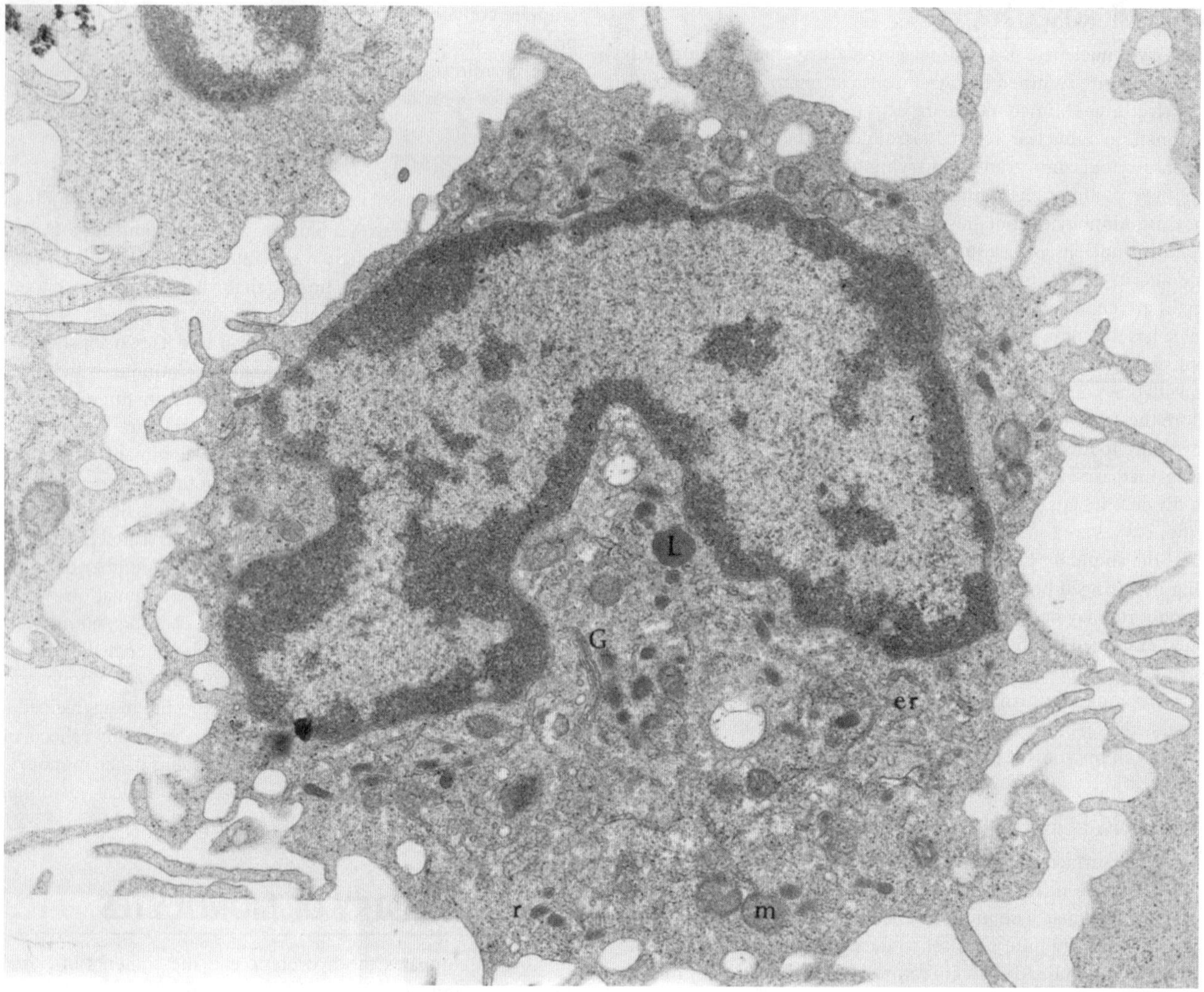

FIGURE 67–2. Transmission electron micrograph of a monocyte. The eccentric reniform nucleus has a thinly dispersed chromatin pattern. The Golgi complex (G) is in a juxtanuclear position. Small electron-dense granules can be seen evolving in the Golgi complex. Small amounts of rough endoplasmic reticulum (er) and polyribosomes (r) are present, particularly about the cell periphery. Mitochondria (m) are concentrated in the region of the Golgi apparatus; they also are scattered in the cell periphery. Lysosomes (L) are small, electron-dense granules surrounded by a limiting membrane. The irregular ruffled cell margin is apparent with numerous microprojections (×24,000).

Approximately 10 percent of granules in normal human blood monocytes stain with reagents that identify complex acid carbohydrates, or "acid mucosubstances."[25] These substances are found in leukemic monocyte granules and in granules of normal neutrophils. Their function is unknown.

MONOCYTE/MACROPHAGE MATURATION AND DIFFERENTIATION

The classic studies of Lewis and Lewis[26] in 1926, Maximow[27] in 1932, and Ebert and Florey[28] in 1939, showed that monocytes transform into macrophages and multinucleated giant cells *in vitro*. Macrophages can be produced from monocytes or hematopoietic progenitor cells culture in cytokines, such as granulocyte-macrophage colony-stimulating factor (GM-CSF) or macrophage-CSF (M-CSF).[29]

The alterations of ultrastructure during transformation into macrophages, epithelioid cells, and giant cells have been described using purified populations of monocytes and *in vitro* culture techniques.[16] As the monocyte matures into the macrophage, the cell enlarges in size, and the lysosomal content and the amount of hydrolytic enzymes within the lysosomes (e.g., phosphatases, esterases, β-glucuronidase, lysozyme, arylsulfatase) increase. At the time, the size and number of mitochondria increase, their energy metabolism increases concomitantly. Production of lactate also increases. The Golgi complex, which packages lysosomes, increases in size and vesicle complexity (Fig. 67–2). Several stimuli (e.g., phorbol myristate acetate) induce formation of multinucleated giant cells from monocytes.[30]

MORPHOLOGY OF MACROPHAGES

Macrophage characteristics are heralded by a significant increase in cell size, increase in the number of cytoplasmic granules, increase in the heterogeneity of cell size and shape, and increase in the number of cytoplasmic clear vacuoles.

■ MOTILITY

An effective monocyte response to infection is predicated upon the ability to migrate and accumulate at sites of inflammation and infection.

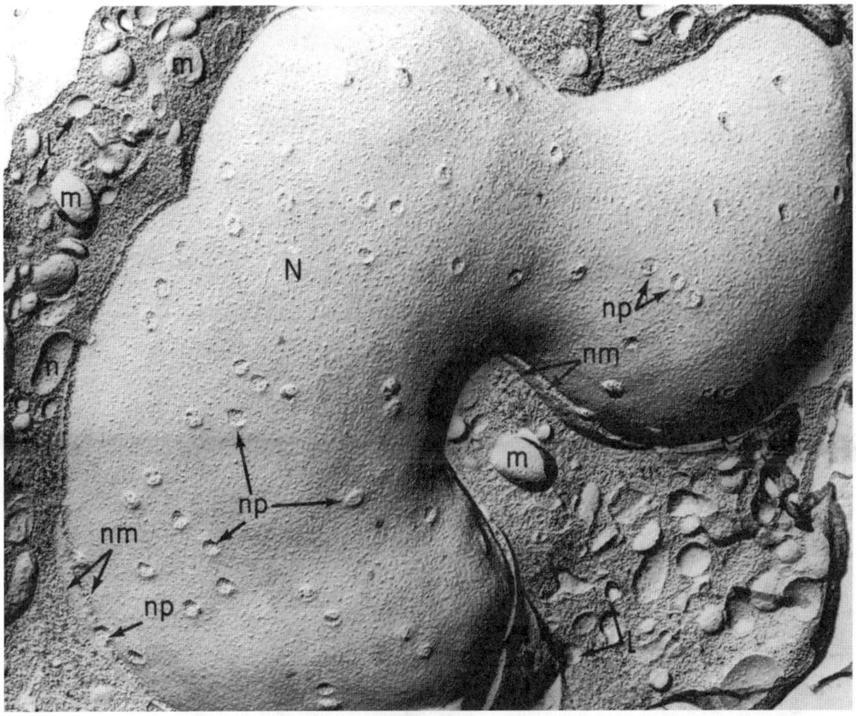

FIGURE 67–3. Freeze-etch electron micrograph of a monocyte. Fracture plane displays the large nucleus (N), with multiple nuclear pores (np) and the two lamellae of the fractured nuclear membrane (nm) evident in some regions. Membrane and cleaved surfaces of mitochondria (m) and lysosomal granules (L) can be identified in the cytoplasm.

Monocytes are capable of both random and directed movement. Random migration is nondirected movement that occurs in the absence of attracting substances. Directed movement, as a result of chemotaxis, refers to monocyte migration that occurs in response to soluble factors or stimuli and that is mediated by different types of receptors on phagocyte cell surfaces.[31] A number of different methods have been used to study macrophage movement both *in vivo*[32] and *in vitro*.[33]

TABLE 67–2. Cytochemical Reactions of Leukocyte Enzymes

Chemical	Monocytes	Neutrophils	Lymphocytes
Acid phosphatase	+ +	+	+
β-Glucuronidase	+ +	+	0 to +
Sulfatase	+	+	0
N-Acetylglucosaminidase	+ +	+ +	0
Lysozyme*	++	+ +	0
Naphthylamidase	+ +	+	0 to +
α-Naphthylbutyrate esterase†	+ +	0 to +	0
Naphthol AS-D chloroacetate esterase	0 to +	+ +	0
Peroxidase	+	+ +	0
Alkaline phosphatase	0	0 to +	0

*Most lysozyme produced by mononuclear phagocytes is secreted rather than stored intracellularly.

†α-Naphthyl acetate and α-naphthyl butyrate esterase activities may appear in human T lymphocytes under certain conditions.

SOURCE: Modified from Braunsteiner H, Schmalzl F,[20] and Li CY, Lam KW, Yam LT.[21]

LIGHT AND PHASE-CONTRAST MICROSCOPY

In vitro culture of monocytes purified from adult human blood has provided an opportunity to observe the maturation of these cells into mature macrophages.

The macrophages of the pulmonary alveoli, peritoneal and pleural cavities, and inflammatory exudates are hypermature cells that have undergone *in vivo* stimulation and maturation. This process results in enhanced bactericidal activity[1,2] because of augmentation of lysosome number and acid hydrolase content.

Macrophages display attributes of morphologic specialization specific to their location and function. The fixed macrophages of the spleen (littoral cells) are involved in the sequestration and destruction of effete or abnormal red cells and exhibit stages of erythrophagocytosis and intracytoplasmic aggregates of ferritin (see Chap. 5). The macrophages of the marrow, the "nurse cells" of the erythroblastic island, play a similar role in erythrophagocytosis and iron storage and transfer (see Chaps. 4 and 29). Hepatic macrophages (Kupffer cells), found in liver sinusoids, also phagocytize red cells and other cellular elements and are important sites of iron storage. Macrophages of the pulmonary alveoli, the lamina propria of the gastrointestinal tract, and the peritoneal and pleural fluids reflect in their morphology a specific function of phagocytosis of microorganisms, cells, and cellular and noncellular debris, characteristic of the specific organ location.

Most macrophages are 25 to 50 μm in diameter on Wright or hematoxylin-and-eosin stained films. (Fig. 67–4) They have an eccentrically placed reniform or fusiform nucleus with one or two distinct nucleoli and finely dispersed, loosely stranded nuclear chromatin that tend to clump in the nuclear interior and along the internal aspect of the nuclear membrane (see Fig. 67–5A). A juxtanuclear clear zone (Golgi complex) is well defined when the Wright stain is used. The cytoplasm shows fine granules and multiple pink-purple, large azurophil granules. The cytoplasmic borders are irregularly serrated. Cytoplasmic vacuoles are present near the cell periphery, reflecting the active pinocytosis in these cells. The surface antigen CD68, also known as *macrosialin*, is commonly used as a macrophage marker. Figure 67–5B shows an immunohistochemistry micrograph of a macrophage in a lymph node. The cytoplasm of the macrophage is intensely positive for CD68, while the surrounding lymphocytes are negative.

On phase-contrast microscopy, living macrophages are large cells with a propensity to adhere to and spread on glass surfaces. Thus, the cell organelles are concentrated within the central portion of the cell and clear veils of hyaloplasm spread about the cell, with intense ruffling of the membrane borders. Vesicles and contractile vacuoles are seen about the cell periphery and in the cell interior. The juxtanuclear clear zone bearing the centrosome and the Golgi complex is particularly dynamic and displays an undulating motion.

ELECTRON MICROSCOPY

Figure 67–6 shows scanning electron micrographs of macrophages adherent to glass surface. Macrophages show a variable degree of differ-

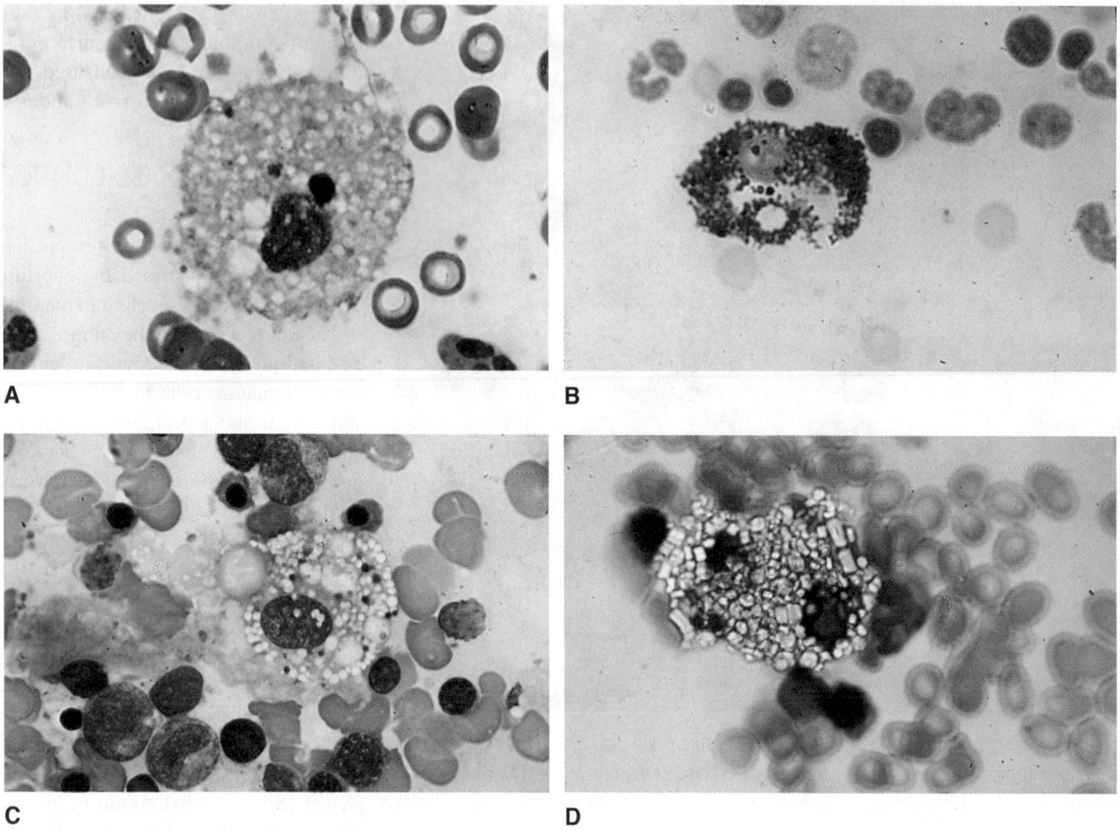

FIGURE 67–4. Marrow Films. Macrophages. These cells characteristically have a circular, sometimes centrally placed and sometimes eccentrically placed nucleus dwarfed by a very large expanse of cytoplasm. **A.** Activated macrophage, full of cytoplasmic vacuoles and some residual ingested cellular debris. **B.** Macrophage stained with Prussian blue showing cytoplasmic iron granules. **C.** Macrophage with erythrophagocytosis. Note pale red cells (partially dehemoglobinized) undergoing hemolysis and destruction. The highly vacolated cytoplasm is presumably the site of red cell degradation. **D.** Macrophage in a patient with cystinosis engorged with cystine crystals. *(Used with permission from* Lichtman's Atlas of Hematology, *www.accessmedicine.com.)*

entiation, nuclear "maturity," ribosomes, mitochondria, and lysosome content. In thin sections, the nucleus varies from horseshoe-shaped to fusiform. The heterochromatin is disposed in fine clumps in the interior of the nucleus and along the internal aspect of the nuclear membrane. Clear spaces between membrane-fixed chromatin aggregates mark the sites of nuclear pores that are relatively abundant on freeze-etch electron micrographs of macrophages and monocytes (see Fig. 67–3). Polyribosomes and scant smooth and rough endoplasmic reticulum are seen about the cell periphery. A well-developed Golgi complex is in a juxtanuclear location. It often is multicentric and contains a concentration of ves-

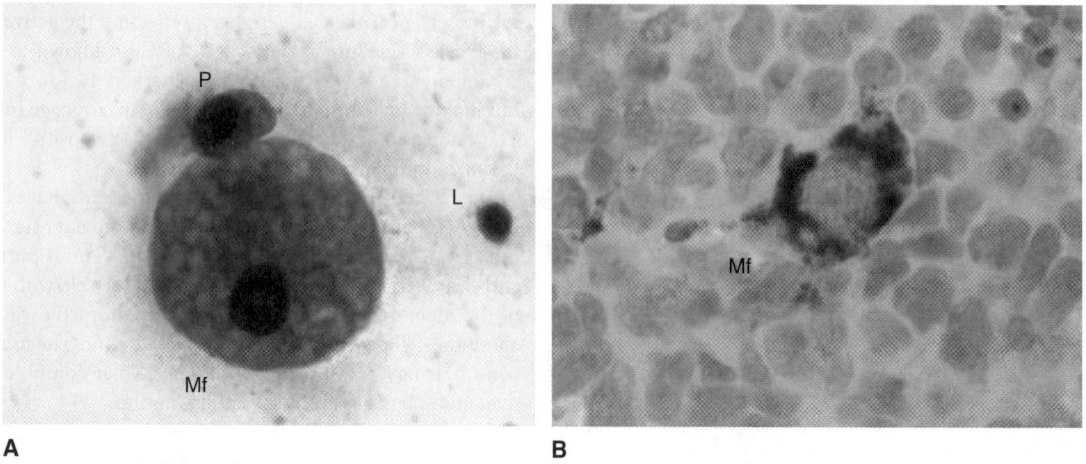

FIGURE 67–5. Micrographs of macrophages (Mf). **A.** Hematoxylin and eosin stain of cytology smear (×400) showing a macrophage, a plasma cell (P), and a lymphocyte (L). **B.** Immunohistochemistry stain for the macrophage marker CD68 of a lymph node (×400). Numerous lymphocytes with blue nuclei surround a macrophage with brown-red cytoplasm. *(Images were provided by Dr. Madalina Tuluc, Thomas Jefferson University Hospital, Philadelphia, PA.)*

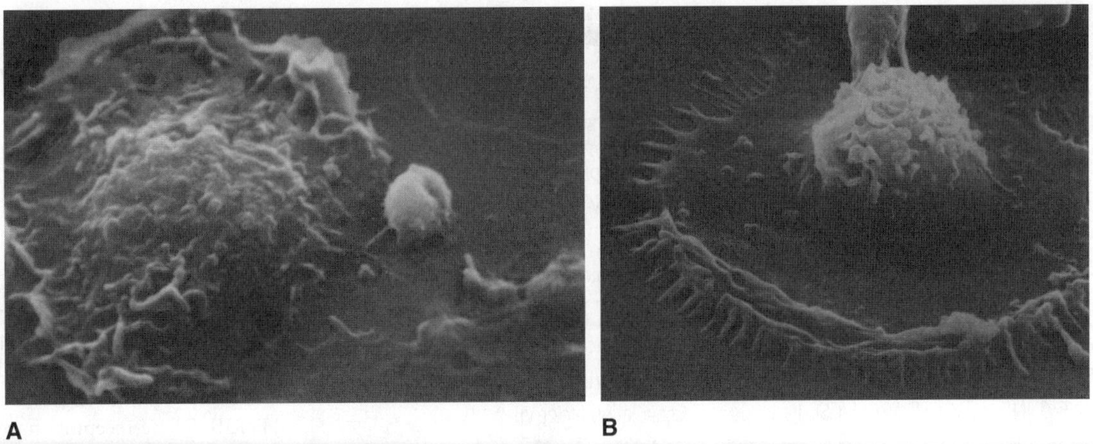

FIGURE 67–6. Scanning electron micrograph of cultured macrophages on coverglasses coated with **(A)** bovine serum albumin (BSA) or **(B)** with immune complexes (BSA- anti-BSA). The macrophage develops prominent peripheral membrane ruffling and numerous microadhesion points to the surface coated with immune complexes.

icles, some with dense inclusions that mark them as early lysosomes. (Fig. 67–7) A relatively constant feature of cells engaged in endocytosis is the large number of microvilli at the cell surface, forming the equivalent of a "brush border." The degree of development of this surface adaptation is related to the phagocytic activity of the cell and its rate of pinocytosis.

The number and size of mitochondria vary with the phagocytic and hence metabolic activity of the cell. Mitochondria tend to be grouped about the region of the Golgi complex, although several usually are seen dispersed about the cell periphery, presumably supplying energy for the active endocytic processes occurring there.

The most constant and characteristic ultrastructural features of macrophages are the electron-dense membrane-bound lysosomes that often can be seen fusing with phagosomes to form secondary lysosomes. Within the secondary lysosomes, ingested cellular, bacterial, and noncellular material

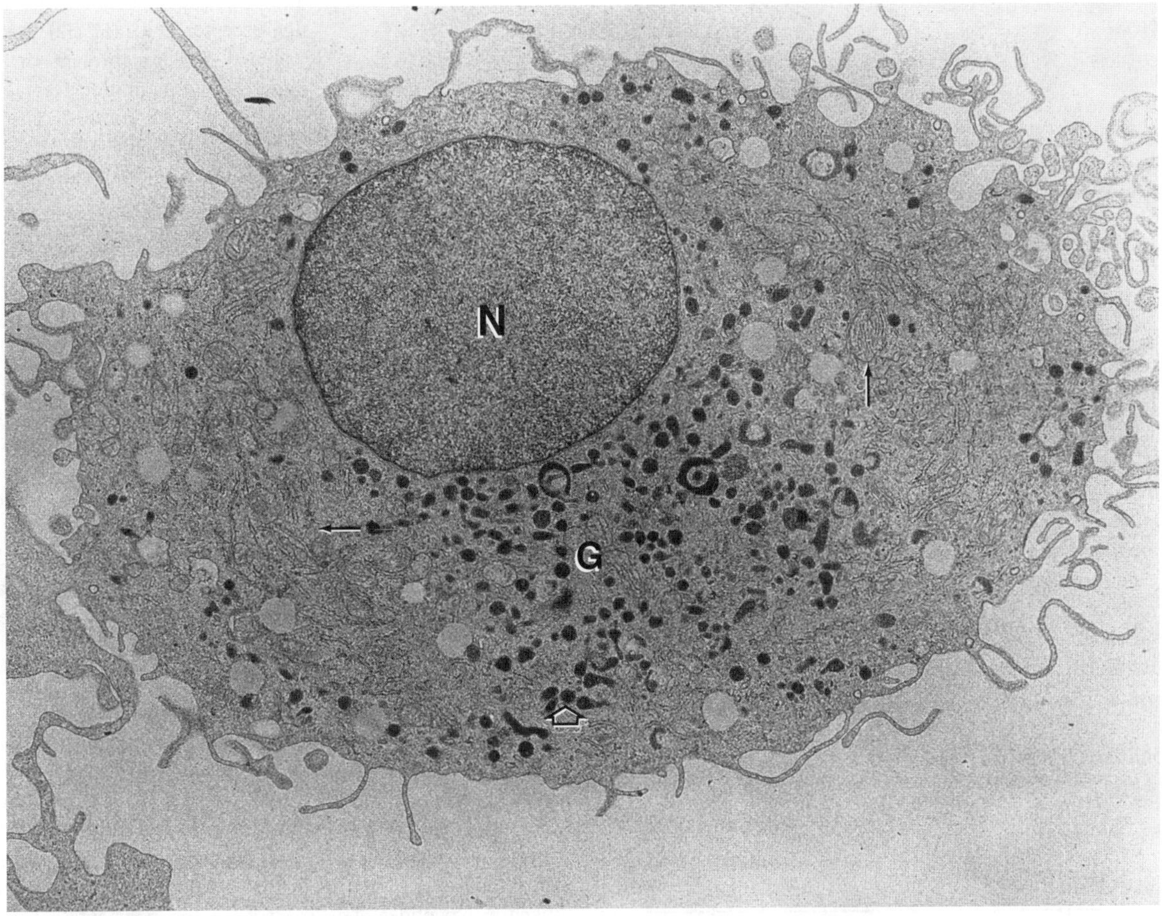

FIGURE 67–7. Electron micrograph of monocyte-derived macrophage cultured *in vitro* for 9 days. G, Golgi zone; N, nucleus. *Arrow on right* indicates endoplasmic reticulum; *arrow on left* indicates mitochondria; *open arrow* indicates lysosomes (×7600).

TABLE 67–3. Surface Receptors of Monocytes and Macrophages

Fc receptors	Transferrin and lactoferrin receptors
IgG_{2a}, IgG_{2b}/IgG_1, IgG_3, IgA, IgE	Lipoprotein lipid receptors
Complement receptors	Anionic low-density lipoproteins
C3b, C3bi, C5a, C1q	PGE_2, LTB_4, LTC_4, PAG
LPS receptors	Apolipoproteins B and E (chylomicron remnants, VLDL)
CD14	Receptors for coagulants and anticoagulants
Cytokine receptors	Fibrinogen/fibrin
MIF, MAF, LIF, CF, MFF, TNF-α, IL-1, IL-2, IL-3, IL-4, IL-10, IL-18, INF-α, INF-β, INF-γ, GM-CSF, M-CSF/CSF-1	Coagulation factor VII
Chemokine receptors	α_1-Antithrombin
CCR1, CCR2A, CCR2B, CCR3, CXCR4, CCR5	Heparin
Macrophage growth factor receptors	Integrins (CD11b, CD18)
M-CSF, GM-CSF	Fibronectin receptors
Receptors for peptides and small molecules	Laminin receptors
Neurokinin-1	Mannosyl, fucosyl, galactosyl residue
H_1, H_2, 5-HT	α_2-Macroglobulin-proteinase complex receptors
1,2,5-Dihydroxy vitamin D_3	Toll-like receptors
N-formylated peptides	TLR2, TLR4, TLR5, TLR9
Enkephalins/endorphins	Others
Substance P	Cholinergic agonists
Hemokinin-1	α_1-Adrenergic agonists
Arg-vasopressin	β_2-Adrenergic agonists
Hormone receptors	
Insulin	
Glucocorticoids	
Angiotensin	

C, complement; GM, granulocyte macrophage; H_1, histamine; 5-HT, 5-hydroxytryptamine; Ig, immunoglobulin; IL, interleukin; INF, interferon; LIF, leukocyte migration inhibition factor; LT, leukotriene; MAF, macrophage-activating factor; MFF, macrophage fusion factor; MIF, macrophage inhibitory factor; PAG, platelet-activating factor; PG, prostaglandin; TNF, tumor necrosis factor; VLDL, very low density lipoprotein.

SOURCE: Adapted from Angen and Ross, in Lewis CE, McGee JO'D.[2] Refer to references 71 to 77.

can be seen in various stages of degradation, often recognizable as degenerating mitochondria or nuclear material. These secondary lysosomes also contain partially degraded material from the late stages of the endocytic process, often appearing as multilamellar lipid bodies.

Microtubules and microfilaments are prominent in macrophages. Actin- and myosin-like proteins have been isolated from monocytes and partially characterized.

Resting macrophages have irregular cell borders and pseudopodia pushed out in all directions. Their cytoplasm has rough endoplasmic reticulum and Golgi complex in the perinuclear area. Lipid globules, primary lysosomes, and mitochondria are characteristically prominent. Activated monocytes/macrophages are motile cells that extend a leading pseudopod as they move forward.[34]

MONOCYTE/MACROPHAGE SURFACE RECEPTORS

Monocyte/macrophage cells have surface receptors that have been characterized by their binding to specific monoclonal antibodies. These receptors (Table 67–3) are markers for origin, growth, differentiation,[35] activation, recognition, migration, and function of the monocyte/macrophage.

RECEPTORS FOR PEPTIDES AND SMALL MOLECULES

Fc Receptors

FcRs for IgG are expressed on the surface of mononuclear cells, macrophages, granulocytes, and platelets.[36,37] FcRs are divided into three distinct classes: FcRI, FcRII, and FcRIII. These receptors have broad ranges of expression on different cells. The first IgG receptor, FcRI (CD64), is a receptor found on monocytes, macrophages, and activated neutrophils. This receptor binds monomeric IgG through the Fc portion of the molecule. This immunoglobulin receptor has increased expression on activated monocytes and macrophages. CD64 allows for receptor-mediated endocytosis of IgG–antigen complexes for presentation to T cells, can trigger the release of cytokines and reactive oxygen intermediates, and can play a role in granulocyte-mediated antibody-dependent cytotoxicity. The second IgG receptor, FcRII (CD32), is a widely distributed receptor present on many cell types, including monocytes, platelets, neutrophils, B cells, some T cells, and some capillary endothelium. This receptor can bind complexed IgG rather than monomeric IgG. This FcR regulates B cell function when coengaged with the B-cell receptor for antigen, namely, surface Ig. It also can induce mediator release from myeloid cells and phagocytosis of Ig-coated particles *in vitro*. Finally, this FcR also can target antigen into presenting pathways. The third IgG receptor, FcRIII (CD16), is expressed by neutrophils, natural killer cells, and tissue macrophages.[38] This receptor can bind Ig in immune complexes and Ig bound to cell surface membranes. It is the main FcR responsible for antibody-dependent cellular cytotoxicity. All three FcRs specifically bind the human IgG subclasses IgG_1 and IgG_3 (see Chap. 77). The interaction of FcR on macrophages with immune complexes results in cell "activation," with an increase in phagocytosis, superoxide production, and prostaglandin and leukotriene release.

Complement Receptors

Activation of the complement system results in liberation of numerous ligands that bind to specific receptors on mononuclear phagocytes. Four receptors that bind fragments of the complement component C3 have been identified.[39] Complement receptor 1 (CR1 or CD35) binds dimeric C3bi and is found on both monocytes and macrophages. Complement receptor 3 (CR3 or CD11b) binds the complement fragment C3b. CR3 is a heterodimeric glycoprotein that is composed of two noncovalently linked polypeptides. The α chain of the polypeptide has an Mr of 185,000, and the β subunit has an Mr of 95,000. This receptor and the leukocyte antigens lymphocyte function-associated antigen (CD11a) and alpha-X integrin chain (CD11c) compose a family of heterodimers that share a common β subunit (CD18).[40] This family is designated the *leukocyte integrin (β_2)* subfamily.[41] These heterodimers are involved in cell–cell interactions, including leukocyte trafficking into the tissues, binding of opsonized particles and plasma proteins, and attachment to various substrates. They also may modulate intercellular adhesion. Elimination of the integrin β_2 subunit causes leukocyte adhesion deficiency.[42]

Toll-Like Receptors

Toll-like receptors (TLRs), identified on macrophages in mammals, are a type of pattern-recognition receptors that recognize structurally conserved molecules derived from microorganisms, including endotoxins (lipopolysaccharide [LPS]) and viral nucleic acids. Toll-like receptors are now considered key molecules responsible for alerting the immune system to the presence of microbial infections. For example, TLR4 is part of a recognition couple for LPS. Pathogen recognition by TLRs activates the innate immune system through the signaling pathway and provokes inflammatory responses, such as cytokine production.[43]

MONOCYTE/MACROPHAGE SURFACE ANTIGENS

Human Leukocyte Antigen Class II Receptors

Monocytes and macrophages serve an important function as antigen-presenting cells. They bear the class II glycoproteins of the major histocompatibility gene complex, human leukocyte antigen (HLA)-DR, HLA-DP, and HLA-DQ. Expression of major histocompatibility complex (MHC) class II antigens on macrophages from different tissues varies widely. Splenic macrophages contain a high percentage of HLA-DR–positive cells (50%), whereas peritoneal macrophages have relatively few (10–20%).[44] The proportion of Ia-positive alveolar macrophages is only approximately 5 percent.[45] Lymphokines, primarily interferon-γ, can induce macrophages to express higher levels of MHC class II antigens,[46] whereas prostaglandin E, α-fetoprotein, and glucocorticoids[47] downregulate HLA-DR antigen expression on macrophages.

CD11

CD11 defines a family of three accessory adhesion surface glycoproteins: CD11a, CD11b, and CD11c. These proteins are distinct α subunits for three heterodimeric surface glycoproteins, each sharing a common β subunit, designated CD18. The α subunits have different isoelectric points, molecular weights, and cell distribution (see Chap. 15).[48] Whereas CD11a is expressed on all leukocytes, CD11b and CD11c are expressed predominantly on monocytes and macrophages, a minor subset of B lymphocytes, and most polymorphonuclear leukocytes. CD11b is expressed on greater than 95 percent of fresh human monocytes and macrophages but declines rapidly on cells maintained *in vitro*. Antibodies specific for CD11b, such as OKM1 or Mo1, may block this complement receptor's ability to bind to CD3bi.[49] Accordingly, these antibodies strongly inhibit complement receptor-mediated rosetting of erythrocyte-IgM antibody–complement complexes.

CD14, CD16, and CD68

The CD14 molecule is one of the most characteristic surface antigens of the monocyte lineage. It is a polypeptide of 356 amino acids that is anchored to the plasma membrane by a phosphoinositol linkage.[50] It is expressed strongly on the surface of monocytes and weakly on the surface of granulocytes and most tissue macrophages. It can be detected on some nonmyeloid cells (e.g., hepatocytes and some epithelial cells). CD14 functions as a receptor for endotoxin (LPS). LPS binds to a serum protein, LPS-binding protein, which facilitates the binding of LPS to CD14. The coreceptor MD2 and TLR4 also are vital in this process. When LPS binds to CD14/MD-2/TLR4 expressed by monocytes or neutrophils, the cells become activated and release cytokines such as tumor necrosis factor and upregulate cell surface molecules, including adhesion molecules. *In vitro*, soluble CD14 binds to LPS, and the complex stimulates cells that do not express CD14 to secrete cytokines and coregulate adhesion molecules.[51]

A subset of human blood monocytes that express low levels of CD14 molecules and high levels of the Fcγ receptor III (FcγR III) CD16 has been identified.[52–54] These CD14+CD16+ monocytes resemble alveolar but not peripheral macrophages. CD14+CD16+ monocytes represent 5 to 10 percent of blood monocytes in normal individuals and can be dramatically expanded in pathologic conditions, such as sepsis, HIV infection, and cancer. CD16+ monocytes produce high levels of proinflammatory cytokines and may represent dendritic cell precursors *in vivo*, because CD16+ monocytes preferentially differentiate into dendritic cells.[55,56] The mechanisms of CD16+ monocyte recruitment into tissues remains unknown.[57]

The CD68 antigen is a specific marker of monocytes and macrophages. Antibodies against the antigen label macrophages and other members of the mononuclear phagocyte lineage in routinely processed tissue sections and have been used to stain a range of lymphoid, histiocytic, and myelomonocytic proliferation.[58]

CD4

T lymphocytes express several surface receptors. The surface antigen CD4 is expressed exclusively in T-helper lymphocytes (see Chap. 78). CD4 and its corresponding messenger ribonucleic acid have been demonstrated on monocytes, macrophages, and the monocyte-like cell line U-937.[59] Although CD4 is present at low concentrations in blood monocytes, the proportion of cells that display this plasma membrane determinant ranges from less than 5 percent to 90 percent. Several monoclonal antibodies that react with different epitopes of the CD4 antigen have been described.[60] The CD4 molecule is involved in induction of T-lymphocyte helper functions (T_4) and T proliferative responses to antigen stimulation; however, its role in the function of monocyte/macrophages has not been determined. An important aspect of the monocyte/macrophage phenotype is the presence of CD4 molecules on the surface of monocytes that can act as receptors for HIV type 1 (HIV-1). HIV-1 uses the CD4 receptors as an entry pathway for infection of monocyte/macrophages.[61]

CHEMOKINE RECEPTORS

Chemokines mediate their activities by binding to target cell surface chemokine receptors that belong to a large family of G-protein coupled, seven transmembrane domain receptors. Human monocytes/macrophages express several chemokine receptors (see Table 67–3). The chemokine receptor CCR5 has been implicated in HIV infection of monocytes/macrophages.[62–66] CCR5 is a major coreceptor on monocytes/macrophages for M-tropic HIV infection. A 32-nucleotide deletion within the CCR5 gene has a highly protective role against acquisition of HIV.[67,68]

REFERENCES

1. van Furth R: *Mononuclear Phagocytes: Characteristics, Physiology and Function*. Martinus Nijhoff, Dordrecht, 1985.
2. Lewis CE, McGee JO'D: *The Macrophage*. Oxford University Press, New York, 1992.
3. Aschoff L: Das reticulo-endotheliale System. *Ergeb Inn Med Kinderheilkd* 26:1, 1924.
4. Randolph GJ, Beaulieu S, Lebecque S, et al: Differentiation of monocytes into dendritic cells in a model of transendothelial trafficking. *Science* 282:480, 1998.
5. van Furth R, Cohn ZA: The origin and kinetics of mononuclear phagocytes. *J Exp Med* 128:415, 1968.
6. Sallusto F, Lanzavecchia A: Efficient presentation of soluble antigen by cultured human dendritic cells is maintained by granulocyte/macrophage colony-stimulating

factor plus interleukin 4 and downregulated by tumor necrosis factor-α. *J Exp Med* 179:1109, 1994.
7. van Furth R: Phagocytic cells: Development and distribution of mono-nuclear phagocytes in normal steady state and inflammation, in *Inflammation: Basic Principles and Clinical Correlates*, 2nd ed, edited by JI Gallin, R Snyderman, p 325. Raven, New York, 1992.
8. Nichols BA, Bainton DF, Farquahr MG: Differentiation of monocytes: Origin, nature and fate of their azurophil granules. *J Cell Biol* 50:498, 1971.
9. Nichols BA, Bainton DF: Differentiation of human monocytes in bone marrow and blood: Sequential formation of two granule populations. *Lab Invest* 29:27, 1973.
10. Ploem JS: Reflection contrast microscopy as a tool in investigations of the attachment of living cells to a glass surface, in *Mononuclear Phagocytes in Immunity, Infection, and Pathology*, edited by R van Furth, p 405. Blackwell, Oxford, 1975.
11. Douglas SD: Alterations in intramembrane particle distribution during interaction of erythrocyte-bound ligands with immunoprotein receptors. *J Immunol* 120:151, 1978.
12. Rabinovitch M, DeStefano MJ: Macrophage spreading in vitro: I. Inducers of spreading. *Exp Cell Res* 77:323, 1973.
13. Douglas SD: Human monocyte spreading *in vitro*: Inducers and effects on Fc and C3 receptors. *Cell Immunol* 21:344, 1976.
14. Ackerman SK, Douglas SD: Purification of human monocytes on microexudate-coated surfaces. *J Immunol* 120:1372, 1978.
15. Zuckerman SH, Ackerman SK, Douglas SD: Long-term peripheral blood monocyte cultures: Establishment and morphology of primary human monocyte-macrophage cell culture. *Immunology* 38:401, 1979.
16. Sutton JS, Weiss L: Transformation of monocytes in tissue culture into macrophages, epithelioid cells and multinucleated giant cells. *J Cell Biol* 29:303, 1966.
17. Reaven EP, Axline SG: Subplasmalemmal microfilaments and micro-tubules in resting and phagocytizing cultivated macrophages. *J Cell Biol* 29:303, 1966.
18. Cohn ZA, Benson B: The differentiation of mononuclear phagocytes: Morphology, cytochemistry, and biochemistry. *J Exp Med* 121:153, 1965.
19. Wachstein M, Wolf G: The histochemical demonstration of esterase activity in human blood and bone marrow smears. *J Histochem Cytochem* 6:457, 1958.
20. Braunsteiner H, Schmalzl F: Cytochemistry of monocytes and macrophages, in *Mononuclear Phagocytes*, edited by R van Furth, p 62. Blackwell, Oxford, 1970.
21. Li CY, Lam KW, Yam LT: Esterases in human leukocytes. *J Histochem Cytochem* 21:1, 1973.
22. van der Rhee HJ, de Winter CPM, Daems WT: Fine structure and peroxidative activity of rat blood monocytes. *Cell Tissue Res* 185:1, 1977.
23. Bodel PT, Nichols BA, Bainton DF: Appearance of peroxidase reactivity within the rough ER of blood monocytes after surface adherence. *J Exp Med* 145:264, 1977.
24. Nichols BA, Bainton DF: Ultrastructure and cytochemistry of mono-nuclear phagocytes, in *Mononuclear Phagocytes in Immunity, Infection and Pathology*, edited by R van Furth, p 17. Blackwell, Oxford, 1975.
25. Parmley RT, Spicer SS, O'Dell RF: Ultrastructural identification of acid complex carbohydrate in cytoplasmic granules of normal and leukemic human monocytes. *Br J Haematol* 39:33, 1978.
26. Lewis MR, Lewis WH: Transformation of mononuclear blood-cells into macrophages, epithelioid cells, and giant cells in hanging-drop blood-cultures from lower vertebrates. Carnegie Institute of Washington, Pub 96. *Contrib Embryol* 18:95, 1926.
27. Maximow AA: The macrophages or histiocytes, in *Special Cytology: The Form and Functions of the Cell in Health and Disease*, vol II, 2nd ed, edited by EV Cowdry, p 711. Hoeber-Harper, New York, 1932.
28. Ebert RH, Florey HW: The extravascular development of the monocyte observed in vitro. *Br J Exp Pathol* 20:341, 1939.
29. Unanue ER: Macrophages, antigen-presenting cells, and the phenomena of antigen handling and presentation, in *Fundamental Immunology* 3rd ed, edited by WE Paul, p 111. Raven Press, New York, 1993.
30. Hassan NF, Kamani N, Messaros M, Douglas SD: Induction of multi-nucleated giant cell formation from human blood-derived monocytes by phorbol myristate acetate in *in vitro* culture. *J Immunol* 143:2179, 1989.
31. Snyderman R, Pike MC: Structure and function of monocytes and macrophages, in *Arthritis and Allied Conditions*, edited by DJ McCarty, p 306. Lea & Febiger, Philadelphia, 1989.
32. Rebuck JW, Crowley JH: A method of studying leukocytic functions *in vivo*. *Ann N Y Acad Sci* 59:757, 1955.
33. Boyden S: The chemotactic effect of mixtures of antibody and antigen on polymorphonuclear leukocytes. *J Exp Med* 115:453, 1962.
34. Fawcett DW, Raviola E: *Bloom and Fawcett: A Textbook of Histology*. Chapman and Hall, New York, 1994.
35. Russell SW, Gordon S: *Macrophage Biology and Activation*. Springer-Verlag, New York, 1992.
36. Metzger H: *Fc Receptors and the Action of Antibodies*. American Society for Microbiology, Washington, DC, 1990.
37. Anderson CL, Guyre PM, Whitin JC, et al: Monoclonal antibodies to Fc receptors for IgG on human mononuclear phagocytes. *J Biol Chem* 261:12856, 1986.
38. Looney RJ, Abraham GN, Anderson CL: Human monocytes and U-937 cells bear two distinct Fc receptors for IgG. *J Immunol* 136:1641, 1986.
39. Wright SD, Griffin FM Jr: Activation of phagocytic cells' C3 receptors for phagocytosis. *J Leukoc Biol* 38:327, 1985.
40. Kishimoto TK, Hollander N, Roberts TM, et al: Heterogenous mutations in the β subunit common to the LFA-1, Mac-1, and p150,95 glycoproteins cause leukocyte adhesion deficiency. *Cell* 50:193, 1987.
41. Hynes RO: Integrins: A family of cell surface receptors. *Cell* 48:549, 1987.
42. Etzioni A, Doerschuk CM, Harlan JM: Of man and mouse: Leukocyte and endothelial adhesion molecule deficiencies. *Blood* 94:3281, 1999.
43. Athman R, Philpott D: Innate immunity via Toll-like receptors and Nod proteins. *Curr Opin Microbiol* 7:25, 2004.
44. Cowing C, Schwartz BD, Dickler HB: Macrophage Ia antigens: I. Macrophage populations differ in their expression on Ia antigens. *J Immunol* 120:378, 1978.
45. Unanue ER, Allen PM: The basis for the immunoregulatory role of macrophages and other accessory cells. *Science* 236:551, 1987.
46. Belle ID: Functional significance of the regulation of macrophage Ia expression. *Eur J Immunol* 14:138, 1984.
47. Snider DD, Ulnae ER: Corticosteroids inhibit murine macrophages, Ia expression and interleukin-1 production. *J Immunol* 129:1803, 1982.
48. Sanchez-Madrid F, Nagy JA, Robbins E, et al: A human leukocyte differentiation antigen family with distinct alpha subunits and a common beta subunit: The lymphocyte-function associated antigen (LFA-1). The C3bi complement receptor (OKM1/Mac) and the p150,95 molecule. *J Exp Med* 158:1785, 1983.
49. Beller DI, Springer TA, Schreiber RD: Anti-Mac-1 selectively inhibits the mouse and human type three complement receptor. *J Exp Med* 156:1000, 1982.
50. Kazazi F, Mathijs J-M, Foley P, Cunningham AL: Variations in CD4 expression by human monocytes and macrophages and their relationship to infection with the human immunodeficiency virus. *J Gen Virol* 70:2661, 1989.
51. Yu B, Hailman E, Wright SD: Lipopolysaccharide binding protein and soluble CD14 catalyze exchange of phospholipid. *J Clin Invest* 99:315, 1997.
52. Passlick B, Flieger D, Ziegler-Heitbrock HW: Identification and characterization of a novel monocyte subpopulation in human peripheral blood. *Blood* 74:2527, 1989.
53. Ziegler-Heitbrock HW, Fingerle G, Strobel M, et al: The novel subset of CD14+/CD16+ monocytes exhibits features of tissue macrophages. *Eur J Immunol* 23:2053, 1993.
54. Ziegler-Heitbrock HW: Heterogeneity of human blood monocytes: The CD14+CD16+ subpopulation. *Immunol Today* 17:424, 1996.
55. Grage-Griebenow E, Flad HD, Ernst M: Heterogeneity of human peripheral blood monocyte subsets. *J Leukoc Biol* 69:11, 2001.
56. Randolph GJ, Sanchez-Schmitz G, Liebman RM, Schakel K: The CD16+ (Fc RIII+) subset of human monocytes preferentially becomes migratory dendritic cells in a model tissue setting. *J Exp Med* 196:517, 2002.
57. Ancuta P, Rao R, Moses A, et al: Fractalkine preferentially mediates arrest and migration of CD16+ monocytes. *J Exp Med* 197:1701, 2003.
58. Collman R, Godfrey B, Cutilli J, et al: Macrophage-tropic strains of human immunodeficiency virus type 1 utilize the CD4 receptor. *J Virol* 64:4468, 1990.
59. Haziot A, Chen S, Ferrero E, et al: The monocyte differentiation antigen, CD14, is anchored to the cell membrane by a phosphatidylinositol linkage. *J Immunol* 141:547, 1988.
60. Schneider EM, Lorenz I, Kogler G, Wernet P: Modulation of monocyte function by CD14-specific antibodies in vitro, in *Leukocyte Typing*, vol IV, edited by W Knapp, B Dörken, WR Gilks, E.P. Rieber, R.E. Schmidt, H. Stein, A.E.G. Kr. von dem Borne, p 794. Oxford University Press, New York, 1989.
61. Warnke RA, Pulford KAF, Pallensen G, et al: Diagnosis of myelomonocytic and macrophage neoplasms in routinely processed tissue biopsies with monoclonal antibody KP1. *Am J Pathol* 135:1089, 1989.
62. Alkhatib G, Combadiere C, Broder CC, et al: CC CKR5: A RANTES, MIP-1alpha, MIP-1beta receptor as a fusion cofactor for macrophage-tropic HIV-1. *Science* 272:1955, 1996.
63. Hill CM, Littman DR: Natural resistance to HIV. *Nature* 382:668, 1996.
64. Deng HK, Liu F, Ellmeier W, et al: Identification of a major co-receptor for primary isolates of HIV. *Nature* 381:661, 1996.
65. Huang Y: The role of a mutant CCR5 allele in HIV transmission and disease progression. *Nat Med* 2:1240, 1996.
66. Dragic T, Litwin V, Allaway GP, et al: HIV entry into CD4 cells is mediated by the chemokine receptor CC-CKR-5. *Nature* 381:667, 1996.
67. Samson M, Libert F, Doranz BJ, et al: Resistance to HIV infection in Caucasian individuals bearing mutant alleles of the CCR-5 chemokine receptor gene. *Nature* 382:722, 1996.
68. Liu R, Paxton WA, Choe S, et al: Homozygous defect in HIV-1 co-receptor accounts for resistance of some multiply-exposed individuals to HIV-1 infection. *Cell* 86:367, 1996.
69. Gordon S, Fraser I, Nath D, et al: Macrophages in tissues and *in vitro*. *Curr Opin Immunol* 4:25, 1992.
70. Lasser AP: The mononuclear phagocyte system: A review. *Hum Pathol* 14:1080, 1983.
71. Fogelman AM, van Lenten BJ, Warden C, et al: Macrophage lipoprotein receptors. *J Cell Sci* 9(Suppl):135, 1988.
72. Adams DO, Hamilton TA: Phagocytic cells. Cytotoxic activities of macrophages, in *Inflammation. Basic Principles and Clinical Correlates*, 2nd ed, edited by JI Galin, IM Goldstein, R Snyderman, p 471. Raven Press, New York, 1992.
73. Werb Z, Goldstein IM: Phagocytic cells: Chemotactic and effector functions of macrophages and granulocytes, in *Basic and Clinical Immunology*, 7th ed, edited by DP Stites, AI Terr, p 96. Appleton and Lange, Norwalk, 1991.
74. Papadimitriou JM, Ashman RB: Macrophages: Current views on their differentiation, structure and function. *Ultrastruct Pathol* 13:343, 1989.
75. Gordon S, Perry H, Rabinowitz S, et al: Plasma membrane receptors of the mononuclear phagocyte system. *J Cell Sci* 9(Suppl):1, 1988.
76. Law SKA: C3 receptors on macrophages. *J Cell Sci* 9(Suppl):67, 1988.
77. Hume DA, Ross IL, Himes SR, et al: The mononuclear phagocyte system revisited. *J Leukoc Biol* 72:621, 2002.

CHAPTER 68
BIOCHEMISTRY AND FUNCTIONS OF MONOCYTES AND MACROPHAGES

Annette Plüddemann and Siamon Gordon

SUMMARY

From the earliest observations by Elie Metchnikoff on phagocytosis and intracellular digestion of microbes and damaged cells by macrophages of invertebrates and higher organisms, their scavenging and host defense functions have been of major interest. In the 1960s Cohn and his colleagues introduced modern cell biologic methods to refine our knowledge of surface receptors, endocytosis, and lysosomal degradation, with emphasis on membrane flow and secretion.[1] These pioneering studies culminated in the discovery of dendritic cells (DCs) as potent, specialized antigen-presenting cells (APCs).[2–3] Subsequent development of monoclonal antibodies[4] and molecular cloning of surface proteins and cytokines, followed by microarray analysis and genomics, provided the sensitive and specific tools to analyze macrophage functions *in vitro* and *in vivo*. These studies have brought insights into macrophage cytotoxic and antimicrobial activities and, to a lesser extent, their trophic, homeostatic functions in the body. Macrophages play a major role in innate as well as adaptive immunity. An important issue is that of heterogeneity among and within monocyte and macrophage populations, as discussed in Chap. 69, which also deals with their growth and differentiation.[5] This chapter focuses on the molecular and cellular properties that bear on the versatile functions of monocytes and macrophages, overlapping in part with the specialized functions of DCs and osteoclasts. General and selected references are provided in recent volumes,[6–8] including Chap. 69.

Abbreviations and acronyms that appear in this chapter include: Ag, antigen; APC, antigen-presenting cell; CD, cluster of differentiation; CR, complement receptor; DC, dendritic cell; EGF, epidermal growth factor; EGF-TM7, epidermal growth factor-seven transmembrane; EMR2, epidermal growth factor-like module containing mucin-like hormone receptor-like 2; ER, endoplasmic reticulum; FcR, Fc receptor; GPCR, G-protein-coupled receptor; IBD, inflammatory bowel disease; ICE, interleukin 1-converting enzyme; IFN, interferon; IFN-αR, IFN-α receptor; IFN-γR, IFN-γ receptor; Ig, immunoglobulin; IL, interleukin; IPAF, ICE-protease activating factor; IRAK, interleukin receptor-associated kinase; IRF, IFN regulatory factor; JAK, Janus kinase; LFA, lymphocyte function-associated antigen; LPS, lipopolysaccharide; MARCO, macrophage receptor with collagenous structure; MPO, myeloperoxidase; MR, mannose receptor; NACHT, domain present in NAIP, CIITA, HET-E, and TP-1; NAIP, neuronal apoptosis inhibitor protein; NALP, NACHT leucine-rich repeat protein; NF, nuclear factor; NLR, NOD-like receptor; NOD, nucleotide-binding oligomerization domain; PI, phosphatidylinositol; PIP_3, phosphatidylinositol 3,4,5 phosphate; PI3K, phosphatidylinositol 3 kinase; PS, phosphatidylserine; SH2, Src homology 2 domain; SR, scavenger receptor; STAT, signal transducers and activator of transcription; TAP, transporter for antigen processing; TLR, toll-like receptor; WASP, Wiskott-Aldrich syndrome protein.

MONOCYTES

This section describes specifically monocytic functions and those expressed in common with their differentiated progeny, macrophages, also covering properties of surface molecules with a clear intravascular function. Their immunomodulatory functions can be expressed directly, or after differentiation of precursors to dendritic cells (DCs). Monocytes respond to activating signals, for example, chemokines, through chemokine receptors, setting in motion a series of adhesion and migration events associated with diapedesis.[9] They play a direct role in sepsis and in more poorly defined changes associated with intravascular coagulation and platelet activation. Their phagocytic potential is mainly expressed after adherence to the vascular endothelium. Monocytes are relatively resistant to virus infection, compared with more differentiated macrophages. Evidence for a Trojan horse function in pathogen dissemination by circulating monocytes is not strong. A major property is their selective adherence to lipid- and platelet-activated endothelium, a precursor to atherogenesis, as demonstrated by Ross' *in vivo* studies with primates.[10] Although metabolic, microbial, or environmental stimuli are normally required to induce monocyte activation, once activated monocytes express a greater potential for cytotoxicity and antimicrobial functions than resident tissue macrophages.

Figure 68–1 shows schematically selected surface receptors implicated in monocytic functions. These include chemokine recognition, adhesion and immunoregulatory molecules. Receptors involved in microbial recognition and innate immunity (e.g., cluster of differentiation [CD]14),[11] phagocytosis (e.g., Fc receptor [FcR], complement receptor), secretory, and killing mechanisms are described below, as are cytokine production and responses. Intracellular granule contents of monocytes include myeloperoxidase (MPO) and lysozyme, although these are less studied than in neutrophils.

ADHESION AND MIGRATION OF MONOCYTES

Monocytes and macrophages are unusual among hematopoietic cells in that they are motile, migratory, ameboid cells, yet capable of sessile, "fixed" life in tissues as resident and more newly recruited cells. Although not as motile as neutrophils, and more difficult to study in physiologically relevant assays *in vitro*, they display lineage-specific, as well as shared, yet distinct properties with DCs, which can be considered as more motile, less-adherent cells specialized for antigen capture and delivery to naïve and primed lymphocytes.[12] They also share receptors and cytoskeletal properties with fibroblasts. Apart from diapedesis in response to endothelial and extravascular signals, monocytes and their progeny display polarization and specialized adhesion structures, most evident in the tight seal of osteoclasts to bone surfaces, so as to localize secretion of powerful catabolic products.

Adhesion is a defining event in the differentiation of monocytes, profoundly influencing the organization of the cell, its plasma membrane, cytoplasm, and nuclear transcription machinery, as well as regulating posttranslational modification of the proteome. Monocytes express diverse integrins, implicated in outside-in as well as inside-out signaling.[13] Particularly important are the β_2-integrin heterodimers, restricted to myeloid cells, as opposed to β_1 and β_3 integrins shared with mesenchymal and other cells. The β_2 integrins, lymphocyte function-associated antigen (LFA)-1 (CD11a/CD18), type 3 complement receptor (CR3, CD11b/CD18) and CD11c/CD18, have been of great value in studies of monocyte/macrophage adhesion. Inhibitory and stimulatory monoclonal antibodies have been generated, and rare inborn errors of metabolism, such as the leukocyte adhesion deficiency syndrome, caused by a genetic deficiency of the

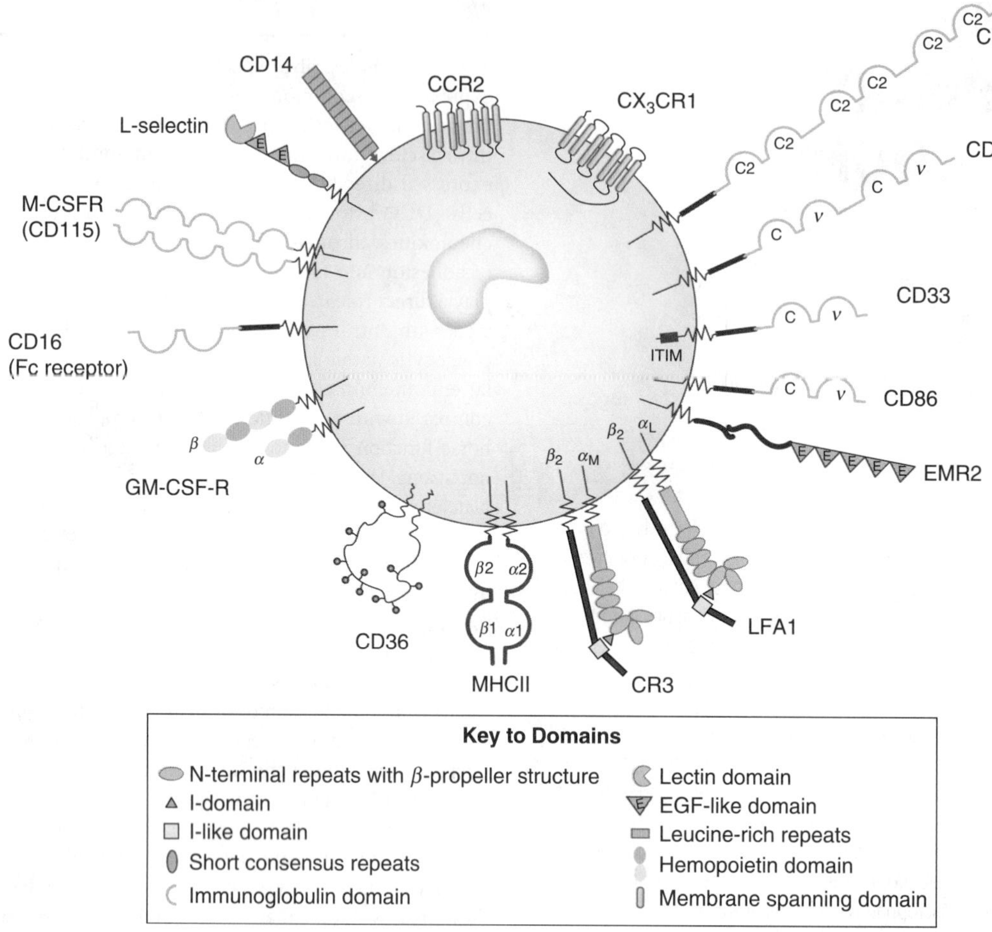

FIGURE 68–1. Schematic representation of selected molecules of varied structure and functions of monocyte receptors and surface antigens.

common β_2 chain, result in defective myeloid cell recruitment to inflammatory stimuli.

The well-known sequence paradigm of rolling (mediated by L-selectin), more stable adhesion (mediated by β_2 integrins), and diapedesis has been extensively studied in neutrophils, and is thought to be similar for monocyte recruitment in response to chemokines, as described in Chap. 69. Monocyte-specific and constitutive migration through different tissue compartments (marrow, blood, tissues) are still poorly understood. An unresolved question is whether circulating monocytes are already "bar coded" for entry to special tissues, such as the CNS, or whether cells enter tissues stochastically from blood. Studies with fractalkine receptor knock-in tracers are bringing new insights into this basic question.[14]

The control of monocyte motility in relation to chemotaxis is not well defined.[15] In particular, the energetics and role of mitochondria in aerobic and hypoxic conditions deserve further study. Mitochondria are prominent in DCs and play a wider role than anticipated in innate resistance to viral infection and in cytosolic stress. Several well known G-protein-coupled receptors (GPCRs), including the array of selective, shared, even redundant chemokine receptors, β-adrenergic receptors, and others contribute to the regulation of directed migration and other cellular functions (Table 68–1).[16,17] In addition, a newly defined family of GPCR with large extracellular domains, includes myeloid-restricted members of the epidermal growth factor-seven transmembrane (EGF-TM7) subfamily with multiple EGF repeats. EMR2 (epidermal growth factor-like module containing mucin-like hormone receptor-like 2) and CD97, structurally related to the F4/80 antigen marker discussed in Chap. 69, likely support additional important monocyte functions.[17] Their ligands include complement regulatory molecules (CD55, associated with paroxysmal nocturnal hemoglobinuria) and chondroitin sulphate B, a matrix component. EMR2 expression on myeloid cells is upregulated by septic shock, its ligation on neutrophils potentiates a range of cellular responses.

The roles of phosphoinositide metabolism, diacylglycerol generation, calcium fluxes, and phosphorylation/dephosphorylation in regulating actin assembly have been studied in human and mouse cells, using mainly neutrophils as a prototype.[15] Genetic models of value for macrophage studies include src kinase knockout animals and the Wiskott-Aldrich syndrome. Small guanosine triphosphatases (GTPases; rac, rho, cdc42) have been implicated in diverse myeloid functions including cell spreading and membrane ruffling. Specialized adhesion structures that deserve further study in macrophages include focal adhesion, podocyte formation (particularly prominent in osteoclasts) and possible participation in tight junctions; hemiconnexons have been reported in macrophages in marrow stroma. CR3 contributes to divalent cation-dependent adhesion of monocytes and macrophages to artificial, serum-coated substrates such as bacteriologic plastic,[18] and the class A scavenger receptor[19] and macrophage receptor with collagenous structure (MARCO; see "Nonopsonic, Non-TLR Receptors" below), which mediate divalent cation-independent adhesion to serum-coated tissue culture plastic *in vitro*. However, the basis of the remarkable, even unique, protease-resistant adhesion of macrophages to foreign materials

TABLE 68–1. Selected GPCR Implicated in Functions of Monocytes and Macrophages

Chemotaxis	Adhesion/Cell–Cell Contact	Activation and Resolution of Inflammation	Alternative Activation	Survival
Chemokine receptors	EGF-TM7 receptors	BAI-1 (brain-specific angiogenesis inhibitor 1)	Purinergic receptors GPR86, GPR105, P2Y8, P2Y11, and P2Y12	Sphingosine-1-phosphate receptors
C5a receptor	Sphingosine-1-phosphate receptors	Formyl peptide receptors	Chemokine receptors	
Leukotriene B_4 receptor	CX_3CR1	Chemokine receptors		
Formyl peptide receptors		C5a receptor		
Platelet-activating factor receptor		EMR2		
EMR2		Protease-activated receptors		
Neuropeptide Y receptor		Platelet-activating factor receptor		
		Leukotriene B_4 receptor		
		Neurokinin receptors		
		Neuropeptide Y receptor		
		Vasoactive intestine peptide receptor		
		Prostaglandin receptors		
		Resolvin		

SOURCE: Table kindly compiled and provided by M. Stacey from references 16, 17, and 116.

remains mysterious. Improved imaging studies, combined with genetic manipulations, will bring further insights into the regulation of monocyte/macrophage adhesion and migration *in vivo*.

INTERACTION OF MONOCYTES AND MACROPHAGES WITH PLATELETS, COAGULATION, AND FIBRINOLYTIC CASCADES

This topic has not received the attention it deserves. Monocytes and resident macrophages line the sinusoids of liver (Kupffer cells) and spleen and readily recognize activated platelets, binding them for clearance and destruction. In addition, monocytes produce potent procoagulants, such as tissue factor, initiating a clotting cascade which, if dysregulated, can lead to diffuse intravascular coagulation during septic shock. Following injury and inflammation, monocytes/macrophages produce urokinase, to generate plasmin, in concert with endothelial cell-derived tissue plasminogen activator.[20] Macrophage production of urokinase is regulated by phagocytic and other stimuli, and the active enzyme can bind to receptors (urokinase plasminogen activator receptor) on the cell surface in a complex interaction with protease–antiprotease complexes, thus localizing fibrinolysis, which is important in wound repair.

The nature and source of the lipid tissue factor produced by monocytes is not well characterized. The cells also produce a complex mix of lipid metabolites, consisting of labile prostaglandins, leukotrienes, and thromboxanes, by utilization of arachidonate-derived precursors and substrates for phospholipase and cyclooxygenase-processing enzymes, among others. The use of lipidomics to characterize such products and study their role in the initiation and resolution of inflammation holds great promise.[21]

RECOGNITION AND CLEARANCE: GENERAL ASPECTS

Resident macrophages of the liver and marrow, as well as in lung and other nonhematopoietic tissues, play a major role in the recognition, phagocytosis, and endocytosis of foreign particles and macromolecules, as well as of modified host components. Clearance can be silent, even suppressing inflammation, mediated by transforming growth factor-β generation, as observed after the uptake of apoptotic cells by macrophages.[22] Production of hematopoietic cells is balanced by their programmed senescence and increased destruction, which can be enhanced in response to microbial and other toxic substances. Macrophages initiate and perpetuate inflammation, both acute and chronic, as a result of their biosynthetic and secretory responses to injurious particles. Uptake and vacuole formation sequester the membrane-enclosed contents for digestion and possible antigen processing and presentation, a specialized property of DCs after their further differentiation from active endocytic to antigen-presenting cells (APCs).[23] In addition, interest has grown explosively in cytosolic recognition systems, designed to protect the cell from various infectious and lytic agents.[24–26] The process of autophagy shares aspects with both membrane-bound and cytoplasmic organelle injury, and has become of great current interest because of its contribution to pathogenesis of infectious, malignant, and inflammatory syndromes.[27]

RECEPTORS FOR UPTAKE: ENDOCYTOSIS AND PHAGOCYTOSIS

Macrophages are proficient at endocytosis (both fluid phase and receptor-mediated) and are highly professional phagocytes of particulates of all kinds of origin, organic (cellular, microbial) as well as inorganic foreign materials.[28] DCs lose their uptake capacity as they mature into APCs, inducing an adaptive immune response or tolerance; immature DCs display active macropinocytosis, a process in which membrane ruffling accompanies formation of a vacuole, as well as capturing exogenous materials for cross-presentation.[23] It is convenient to classify plasma membrane uptake receptors as opsonic and nonopsonic toll-like receptors (TLRs) and non-TLR dependent. The latter category includes a range of scavenger receptors[29–31] and a family of lectin-like, carbohydrate recognition molecules.[4,32] These receptors can cooperate with one another, given the complex ligands presented on the surface of

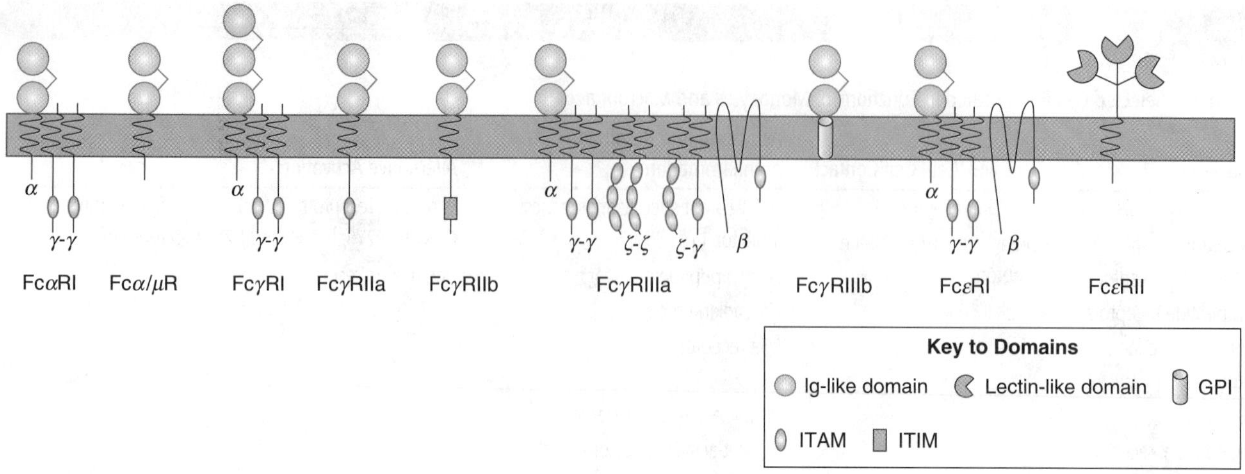

FIGURE 68–2. Human Fc receptors. Myeloid cells express a range of classical Fc receptors that initiate a variety of cellular responses, including phagocytosis, antibody-dependent cell-mediated toxicity, antigen presentation, respiratory burst, and release of inflammatory mediators. Immunoglobulin (Ig) subclasses are bound by extracellular domains; signaling via cytoplasmic immunoreceptor tyrosine-based activation motif (ITAM) or immunoreceptor tyrosine-based inhibition motif (ITIM) is mediated by associated membrane-spanning polypeptides. Activation and inhibitory receptors are usually coexpressed on the cell surface and function in concert, determining the magnitude of effector cell responses.

microorganisms and damaged host cells, or generated within the vacuolar system after uptake.

Opsonic Receptors

The classical opsonins, which promote the uptake of particles, are antibody, immunoglobulin (Ig) G complexed with antigens, and complement, activated by the classical pathway (antibody-dependent IgM or IgG) or recognized directly via the lectin-carbohydrate–stimulated alternative pathway. Fc and complement receptors are heterogeneous in structure, expression, and function, activating or inhibiting macrophage responses,[33,34] as illustrated in Figures 68–2 and 68–3. Other opsonins include fibronectin and milk fat globulin.[35]

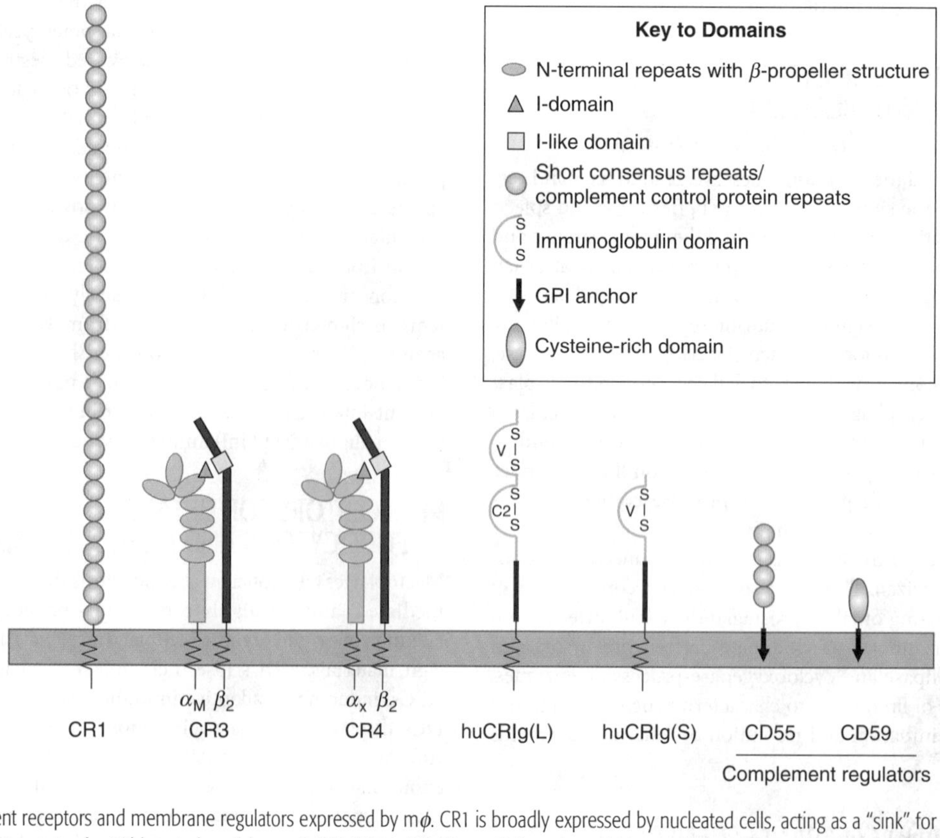

FIGURE 68–3. Complement receptors and membrane regulators expressed by mϕ. CR1 is broadly expressed by nucleated cells, acting as a "sink" for activated complement. CR3 (CD11b/CD18), a phagocytic receptor for C3bi-coated particles, and CR4 (CD11c/CD18) are β_2 integrins, which, together with LFA-1 (CD11a/CD18), mediate adhesion of myeloid cells to endothelium and extracellular matrix and migration. huCRIg (L and S) are long and short forms of a newly described complement-binding receptor on Kupffer cells that mediate uptake of opsonized bacteria. CD55 and CD59 are glycosyl phosphatidylinositol (GPI)-anchored regulators of complement activation.

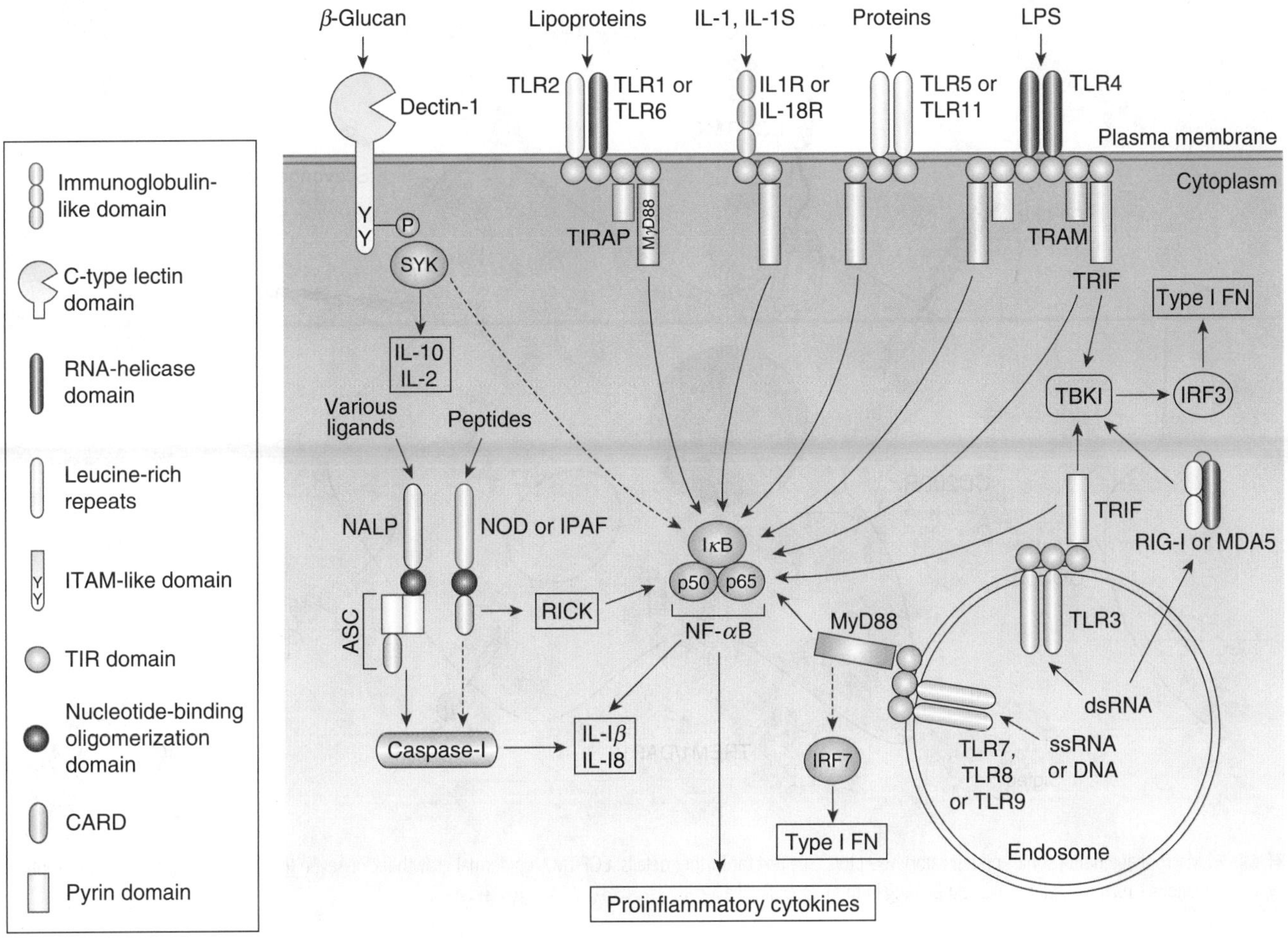

FIGURE 68–4. The main toll-like receptor (TLR) signaling pathways and adaptor molecules. The pathways that are activated by the different receptors are multiple and complex. For example, TLR signaling involves not only nuclear factor-κB (NF-κB) activation, but also mitogen-activated protein kinases, phosphatidylinositol 3-kinase, and several other pathways that markedly affect the overall biologic response to the activation of TLRs. Dectin-1 (a β-glucan receptor) is shown as an example of various signaling-competent cell-surface pattern-recognition receptors. ASC, apoptosis-associated speck-like protein containing a caspase activation and recruitment domain; CARD, caspase activation and recruitment domain; ds, double-stranded; IFN, interferon; IκB, inhibitor of NF-κB; IL, interleukin; IPAF, interleukin-1β–converting enzyme-protease activating factor; IRF, IFN-regulatory factor; LPS, lipopolysaccharide; MDA5, melanoma differentiation-associated gene 5; MyD88, myeloid differentiation primary response gene 88; NACHT, domain present in NAIP, CIITA, HET-E, and TP-1; NALP, NACHT leucine-rich repeat and pyrin-domain-containing protein; NOD, nucleotide-binding oligomerization domain; RICK, receptor-interacting serine/threonine kinase; RIG-I, retinoic acid-inducible gene I; ss, single-stranded; TBK1, TANK-binding kinase 1; TIRAP, toll/IL-1R (TIR) domain-containing adaptor protein; TRAM, TRIF-related adaptor molecule; TRIF, TIR domain-containing adaptor protein inducing IFN-β; SYK, spleen tyrosine kinase. See text for further details. *(Reproduced from Trinchieri G, Sher A,[45] by permission from Macmillan Publishers Ltd,* Nature Reviews Immunology. *Copyright 2007.)*

Through their expression of various opsonic receptors, monocytes, macrophages, and DCs perform versatile roles in innate and adaptive immunity,[36] in antigen clearance and destruction, in autoimmunity, and in pathogenesis of a range of inflammatory and infectious disorders. Genetic polymorphisms influence the expression and functions of FcRs in homeostasis and disease. Although prominent in host protection, invading microorganisms may be able to exploit, even subvert these receptors to facilitate their entry and survival.[37] Opsonic receptors play an important role in clearance of hematopoietic cells, for example, antibody-coated platelets, giving rise to thrombocytopenia, and in therapeutic antibody treatment, for example, to facilitate engraftment. Antibody engineering has provided novel therapeutic agents to minimize undesirable consequences, such as cell activation. The initiation or avoidance of complement activation in particular controls an important effector pathway in tissue injury and repair.

Nonopsonic Receptors: Toll-Like Receptors

These are shown schematically in Figure 68–4 to illustrate their diverse structures and signaling pathways. The discovery of TLR has transformed the study of innate immunity, inflammation and adjuvant actions on APC.[38–40] Receptor structures, heterogeneity of expression, microbial and endogenous ligands, and signaling have been defined, and knowledge of their regulation has begun to offer agents to manipulate TLR signaling in humans. The discovery of inborn errors such as the interleukin receptor-associated kinase (IRAK)-4 deficiency[41] and the role of toll-interleukin receptor adaptor protein (TIRAP) function in *Plasmodium falciparum* infection,[42] for example, have illustrated their role in human

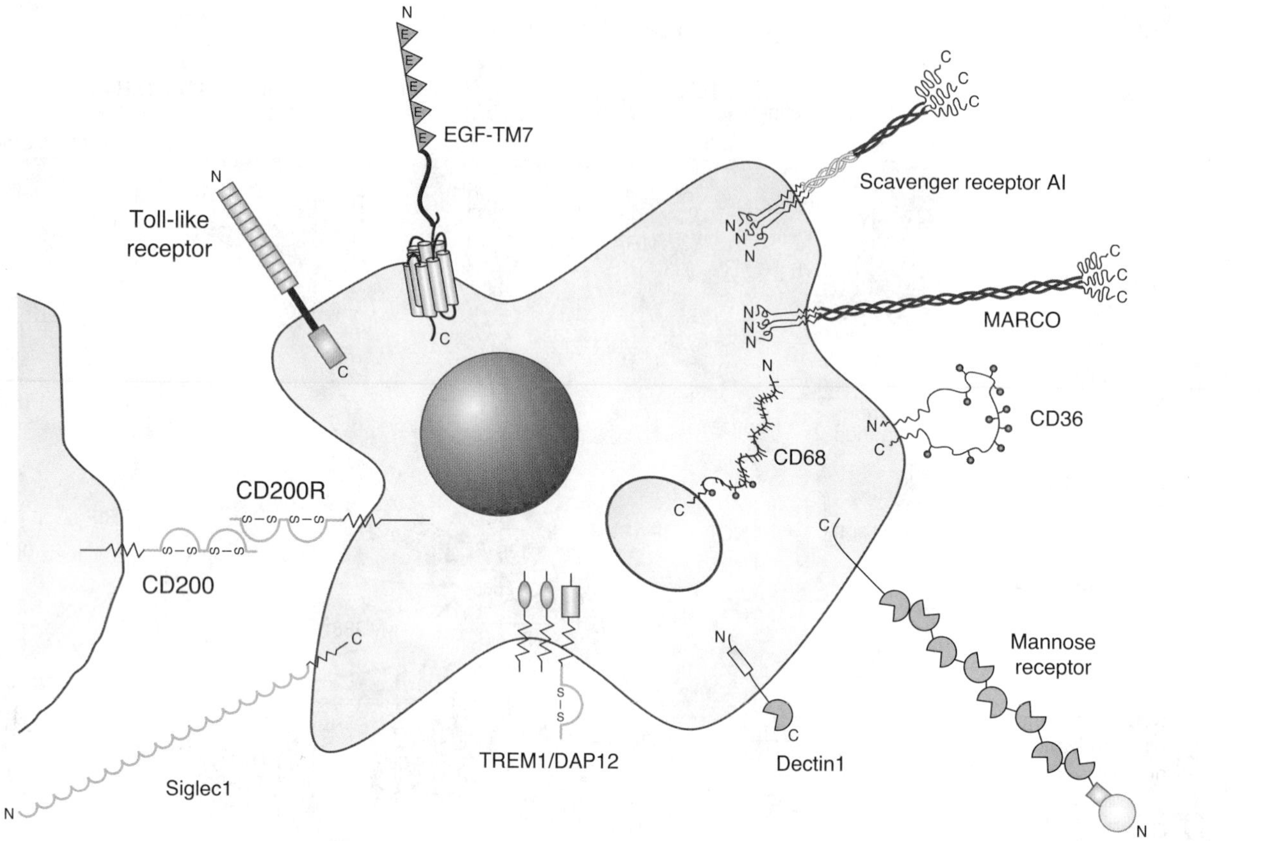

FIGURE 68–5. Macrophage nonopsonic and regulatory receptors. See text for further details. EGF-TM7, epidermal growth factor-seven transmembrane; MARCO, macrophage receptor with collagenous structure; Siglec, sialic acid-binding immunoglobulin-like lectin.

disease. Several concepts have emerged. From the original studies on lipopolysaccharide (LPS) recognition and signaling by the multiprotein complex formed by CD14, LPS binding protein and MD2, and the clarification of the distinct adaptor pathways (MyD88 [myeloid differentiation factor 88], TIRAP/MAL [MyD88 adaptor-like], TRIF [TIR domain-containing adaptor inducing interferon-β], and TRAM [TRIF-related adaptor molecule]), the recognition and sensing of TLR ligands have become clear. The tertiary structure of TLR4 has been reported.[43] TLRs are expressed either on the plasma membrane of myeloid and other cells, or within the vacuole, especially in the case of TLRs 3, 7, and 9, which are implicated in viral nucleic acid recognition. Crosstalk among nuclear factor (NF) κB, interferon (IFN), and mitogen activated protein kinase (MAP) kinase pathways has also become apparent.[44] TLRs have been shown to collaborate with other recognition receptors,[45] such as dectin-1. More controversially, a role has been proposed for TLR signaling in nontranscriptional activities, such as the kinetics of phagosome maturation in macrophages.[46,47]

Mouse knockout and cell biologic studies have been of great value in dissecting the role, processing, transport, and interactions of different components of TLR signaling and function.[38] Random chemically induced mutagenesis has validated the effects of more limited deficiency, compared with whole-gene deletion.[48] The possible value of polymorphisms in human TLR genes and their partner molecules is beginning to be documented.[49]

Nonopsonic, Non-TLR Receptors

The study of lectins and scavenger receptors (SRs) has lagged behind that of the above receptors, but is gaining ground, documenting receptor expression and ligands, mainly in mouse models of inflammation and infection.[29,50,51] Broadly, these receptors are present on macrophages and DCs, and variably on monocytes and neutrophils. They are implicated in the recognition and uptake of microbial and host ligands, and vary in their ability to activate host defense functions. A few highlights of these receptor systems that serve to illustrate their wider functional attributes are shown in Figure 68–5 and Table 68–2. The mannose receptor is mainly involved in endocytosis, with a predominant intracellular localization.[52,53] The mannose receptor is a multilectin, with a dual function that contributes to the clearance of mannose-terminal lysosomal hydrolases and of neutrophil granule glycoproteins such as MPO, as well as of hormones (e.g., thyroglobulin) and exocrine secretion products (e.g., amylase). It plays a role in the capture and transport of mannose-terminal glycoproteins to targets in spleen (marginal metallophilic macrophages) and in lymph nodes (subcapsular sinus macrophages) that express sulfated receptors for its cysteine-rich domain. The outcome of such targeting is either silent disposal or, if combined with TLR stimulation, induction of an immune response.[54] In common with several other nonopsonic receptors, it can play dual, even opposing actions in host protection or in pathogenesis, as shown by ongoing studies in mice.

Dectin-1 is a lectin-like receptor that is widely expressed on myeloid cells, with a single immunoreceptor tyrosine-based activation motif (ITAM)-like motif in its cytoplasmic tail.[55] It recognizes β glucans, abundant in fungal walls, including bioactive zymosan particles, and has been implicated in innate resistance to fungal infection. Dectin-1 activates syk and caspase-recruitment domain (CARD)-9, regulating various effector

TABLE 68–2. Ligands for Selected Nonopsonic, Non–Toll-Like Receptors

Class	Receptor	Microbial Ligands	Endogenous Ligands	Function
Scavenger receptors	SR-A I/II	Gram+/– bacteria Lipoteichoic acid Lipid A *Neisserial* surface proteins	Apoptotic cells Modified low- and high-density lipoproteins (LDL, HDL, apolipoprotein A_1, apolipoprotein E) AGE-modified proteins β-Amyloid	Phagocytosis Endocytosis Foam cell formation Adhesion
	MARCO	Gram+/– bacteria Trehalose dimycolate *Neisserial* surface proteins	Marginal zone B lymphocytes Uteroglobin-related protein	Adhesion Phagocytosis Innate activation
	CD36	Diacylated lipopeptide from Gram+ bacteria *Plasmodium falciparum*-parasitized erythrocytes	Apoptotic cells (with thrombospondin and vitronectin receptor) High-density lipoprotein (HDL) Outer rod segments	Uptake, exchange of lipids, adhesion
Lectins	Dectin-1 DC-SIGN	β-Glucan Mannosyl/fucosyl glycoconjugates viruses (e.g., HIV-1, Dengue)	T lymphocytes (noncarbohydrate) ICAM 2/3 T lymphocytes	Fungal uptake and immunomodulation Adhesion Endocytosis
	Mannose receptor: C-type lectin domains Cysteine-rich domain Fibronectin type II domain	Mannosyl/fucosyl Glycoconjugates on bacteria, viruses, fungi, parasites	Lysosomal hydrolases Thyroglobulin Ribonuclease B Amylase Sulfated carbohydrates in marginal zone (spleen) and subcapsular sinus (lymph node) Collagens	Endocytosis Adhesion Antigen targeting Adhesion

AGE, advanced glycation end product; DC-SIGN, dendritic cell-specific intercellular adhesion molecule-3–grabbing nonintegrin; ICAM, intercellular adhesion molecule; MARCO, macrophage receptor with collagenous structure; SR, scavenger receptor.

SOURCE: Data from references 30, 32, 53, and 55.

pathways such as tumor necrosis factor (TNF)-α, leukotriene production, and Th17 cell activation, with heterogeneity in responses by macrophages and DCs. Dectin-1 collaborates with TLR 2/6 in the response to zymosan. Other lectins expressed by macrophages include sialic acid recognition molecules, Siglec-1 (Sialoadhesin),[56] an extended Ig superfamily plasma membrane protein implicated in cell–cell interactions (see Chap. 69 for a possible role in the hematopoietic system).

SRs are a diverse family of structurally unrelated, promiscuous receptors, with a predilection for polyanionic ligands, expressed by diverse microorganisms, apoptotic cells, and modified host lipoproteins.[30] SR-A I/II and MARCO (class A SR) are collagenous transmembrane receptors that mediate endocytosis, phagocytosis, and cell adhesion. SR-A I/II is upregulated by CSF-1, MARCO by TLR and MyD88-dependent microbial ligands, triggers of innate immune activation.[57] A number of naturally occurring ligands for SR-A have been identified, including apolipoprotein A_1 (C. Neyen and S. Gordon, submitted) and *Neisserial* outer surface proteins,[58] as well as previously described lipid A, lipoteichoic acid, and modified (acetylated) low-density lipoproteins, among others. After initial interest primarily in its role in atherogenesis, attention has also focused on innate immune functions in bacterial infection.

Class B SRs such as CD36 and SR-BI have distinct structures and have been implicated in mycobacterial recognition as well as in the uptake and exchange of lipids.[59–61] CD36, together with thrombospondin, plays a role in apoptotic cell uptake[35] and has been implicated in macrophage fusion. Other SRs, expressed on a variety of cells as well as macrophages, have similar roles in clearance.

APOPTOTIC CELL RECOGNITION

Macrophages take up large numbers of naturally dying cells, hematopoietic and others, through a complex mechanism involving multiple, often redundant nonopsonic receptors.[22,35] A possible role for complement has also been proposed. Figure 68–6 illustrates receptors and ligands that have been implicated. Apart from the SRs already discussed, they include receptors for opsonins such as pentraxin 3[62] and for milk fat globulin, as well as for the vitronectin receptor. Phosphatidylserine (PS) expressed on the outer leaflet of apoptotic cells, contributes to apoptotic cell recognition, but its role is probably more complex as apparently healthy cells can express patches of PS on their surface and PS recognition plays a role in CD36-dependent macrophage–macrophage fusion.[63] The recognition mechanisms for uptake

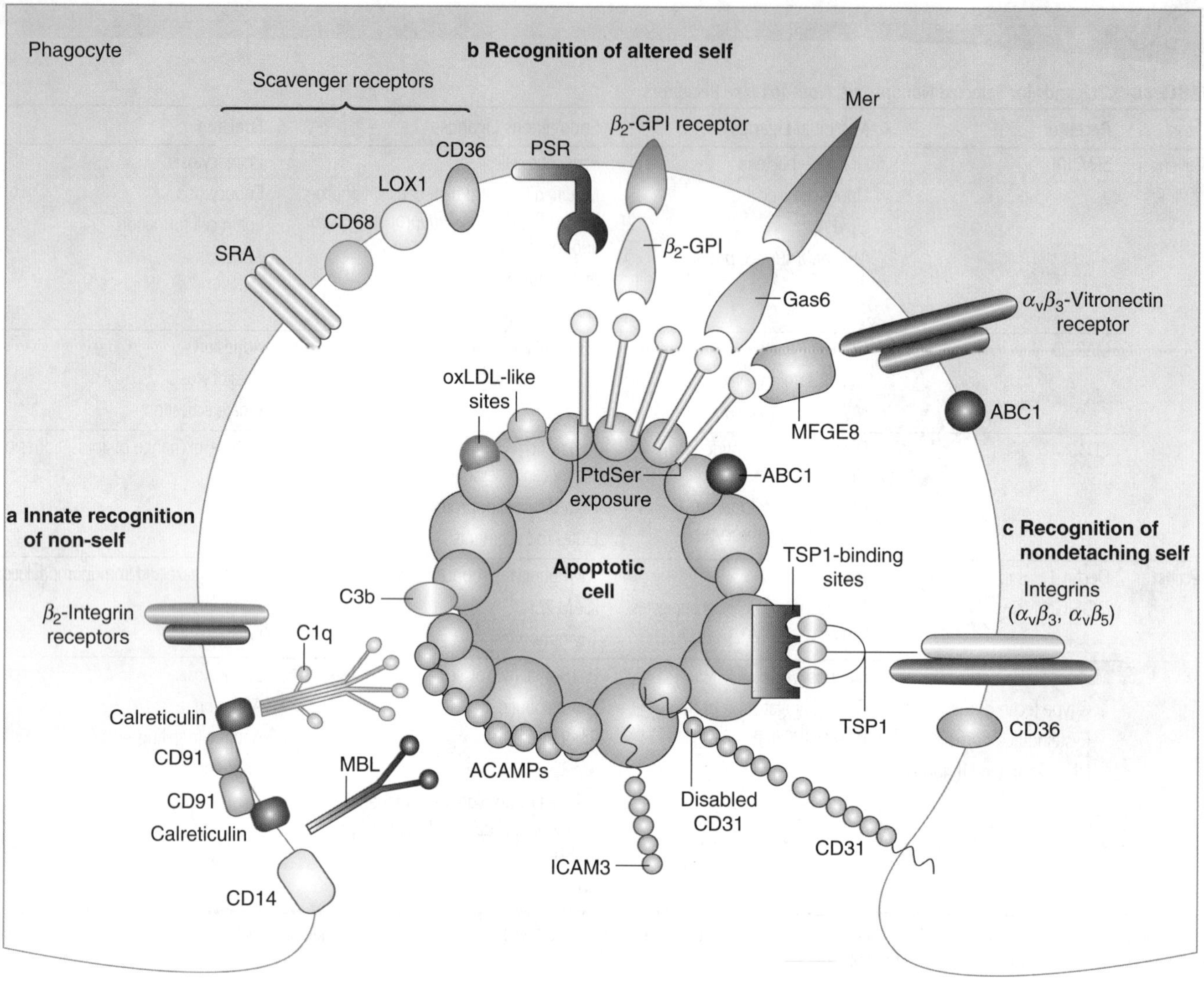

FIGURE 68–6. Phagocytic receptors for apoptotic cell phagocytosis. Macrophages and immature myeloid dendritic cells (DCs) are the main immune cells involved in the clearance of apoptotic cells. They express broadly similar multiple receptors which can bind directly or via opsonic-soluble proteins, for example, mannose-binding lectins (MBLs) to ligands. Phosphatidylserine (PS) becomes exposed on the outer surface of the apoptotic cell and a receptor for this ligand has been long sought. A new receptor (TIM4, and related TIM1) was discovered on resident mϕ, with specificity for PS. Other mϕ populations utilize MFGE8 (a milk fat globulin protein secreted by mϕ) as an opsonin. Discrimination of non- and altered self may involve combinations of different phagocyte receptors. Apoptotic cell uptake results in an antiinflammatory response by mϕ (e.g., release of transforming growth factor-β and prostaglandin E_2), but has also been implicated in cross-presentation by DCs. For further details see Savill J, Dransfield I, Gregory C, Haslett C.[35] *(Reprinted from Savill J, Dransfield I, Gregory C, Haslett C[35] by permission of Macmillan Publishers Ltd,* Nature Reviews Immunology. *Copyright 2002.)*

of necrotic cells and enucleated erythroblast nuclei by macrophages are not clear.

ENDOCYTOSIS AND PHAGOCYTOSIS

Apart from the above ligands, macrophages express receptors for endocytosis of growth factors, cytokines, peptides, and lipids. Macrophages express a functional folate receptor that is induced during activation and can be used to target drugs or tracers to macrophages *in situ*.[64] Hemoglobin–haptoglobin complexes are internalized by CD163, a glucocorticoid-regulated receptor with a remarkable SR-cysteine extracellular domain structure.[65]

The cell biology of endocytosis and of phagocytosis is illustrated in Figures 68–7 to 68–9. Apart from size, and resultant involvement of the cytoskeleton, they have much in common; vesicle/phagosome formation, falling pH and initial digestion, fusion with secretory vesicles derived from the Golgi, and maturation to form secondary lysosomes/phagolysosomes with a more acidic pH, and further digestion.[66–71] Apart from selective fusion with intracellular vesicles, there is extensive membrane flow, recycling, and fusion. Vesicular trafficking in macrophages and other immune cells has been reviewed.[72] Small GTPases play an important role in the control of membrane traffic.[73] Early estimates revealed that a substantial fraction of surface membrane is internalized constitutively by endocytosis; the selectivity or otherwise of membrane protein internalization has also been of interest. Pathways leading to induction of adaptive immune functions are under intense study.[74]

Elegant studies in the mid-1970s utilized opsonic receptors to study the uptake mechanism of antibody-coated erythrocytes.[75] This work gave

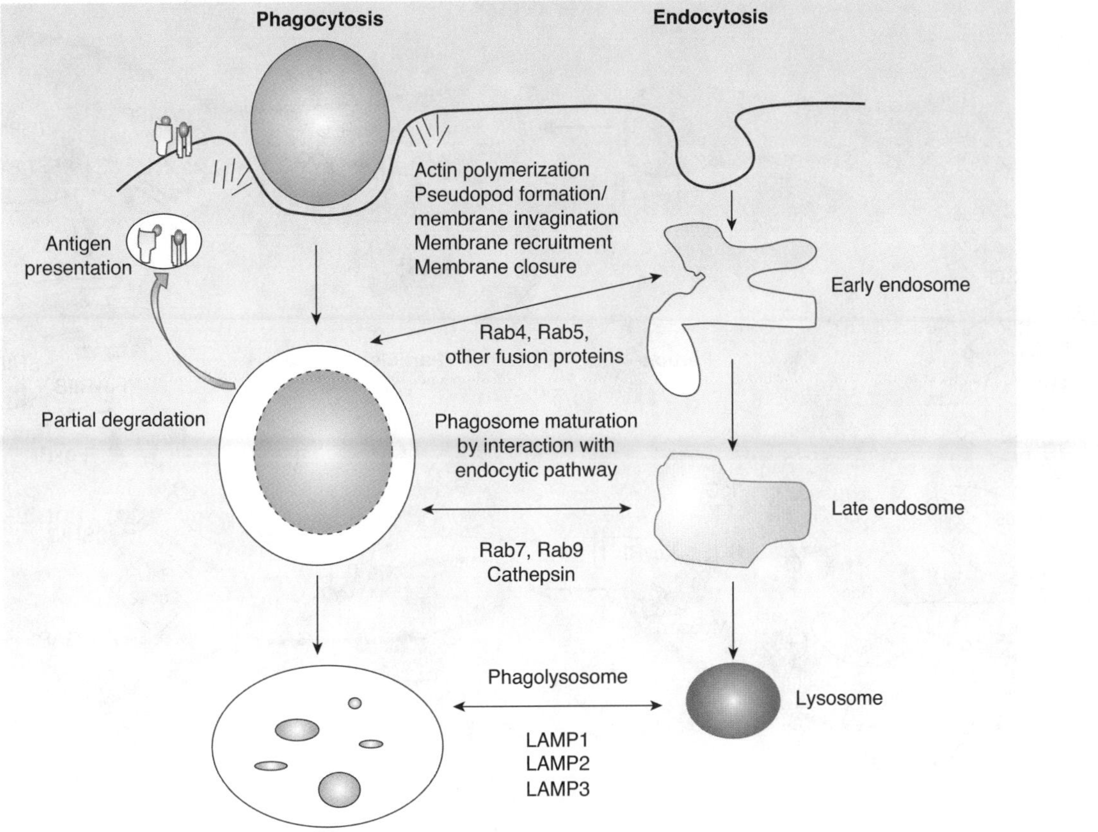

FIGURE 68–7. Phagocytosis and endocytosis pathways. Particulates are taken up by actin-dependent sequential maturation processes, involving membrane fusion and fission, which intersect with the endocytic pathway at several stages. Cytosolic small guanosine triphosphatases (rabs) determine organelle-specific interactions. Membrane is recycled to the plasma membrane, with processed antigen. Progressive acidification and delivery of lysosomal hydrolases result in terminal degradation. Compartment membranes express marker proteins such as LAMP1; the pan-macrophage CD68 antigen is associated with late endosomes and lysosomes.

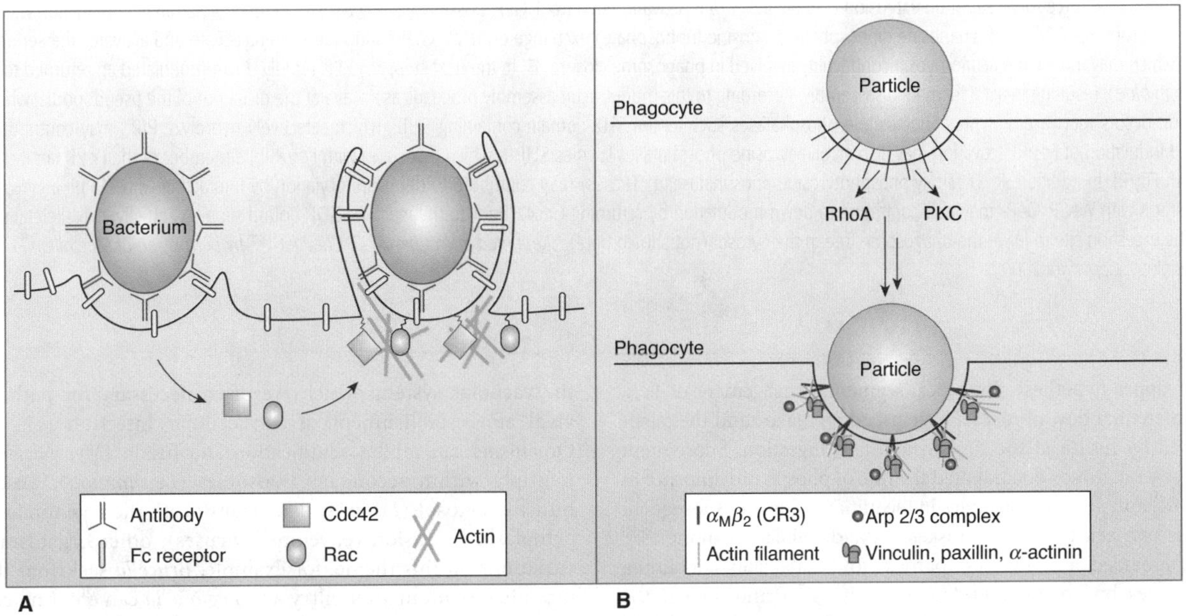

FIGURE 68–8. Phagocytosis. **A.** Fc receptor-mediated phagocytosis. Fc receptors on the surface of macrophages are activated by immunoglobulin-G molecules bound to a bacterium. A signaling cascade that involves Rac, Cdc42, and downstream kinases triggers actin rearrangements, protrusion of the membrane around the bacterium, and its engulfment into a phagosome. *(Reprinted from Conner SD, Schmid SL[110] by permission of Macmillan Publishers Ltd,* Nature. *Copyright 2003.)* **B.** CR3-mediated phagocytosis. Complement receptor type 3 (CR3) binds C3bi molecules on the surface of complement-opsonized particles. Engagement induces activation of protein kinase C and RhoA, which are both required for CR3-mediated phagocytosis. This results in assembly of actin filaments and recruitment of cytoskeletal proteins, including vinculin, paxillin and α-actinin. RhoA-mediated actin assembly may depend on the activation of the nucleating activity of the Arp2/3 complex. *(Reprinted from Chimini G, Chavrier P[67] by permission of Macmillan Publishers Ltd,* Nature Cell Biology. *Copyright 2000.)*

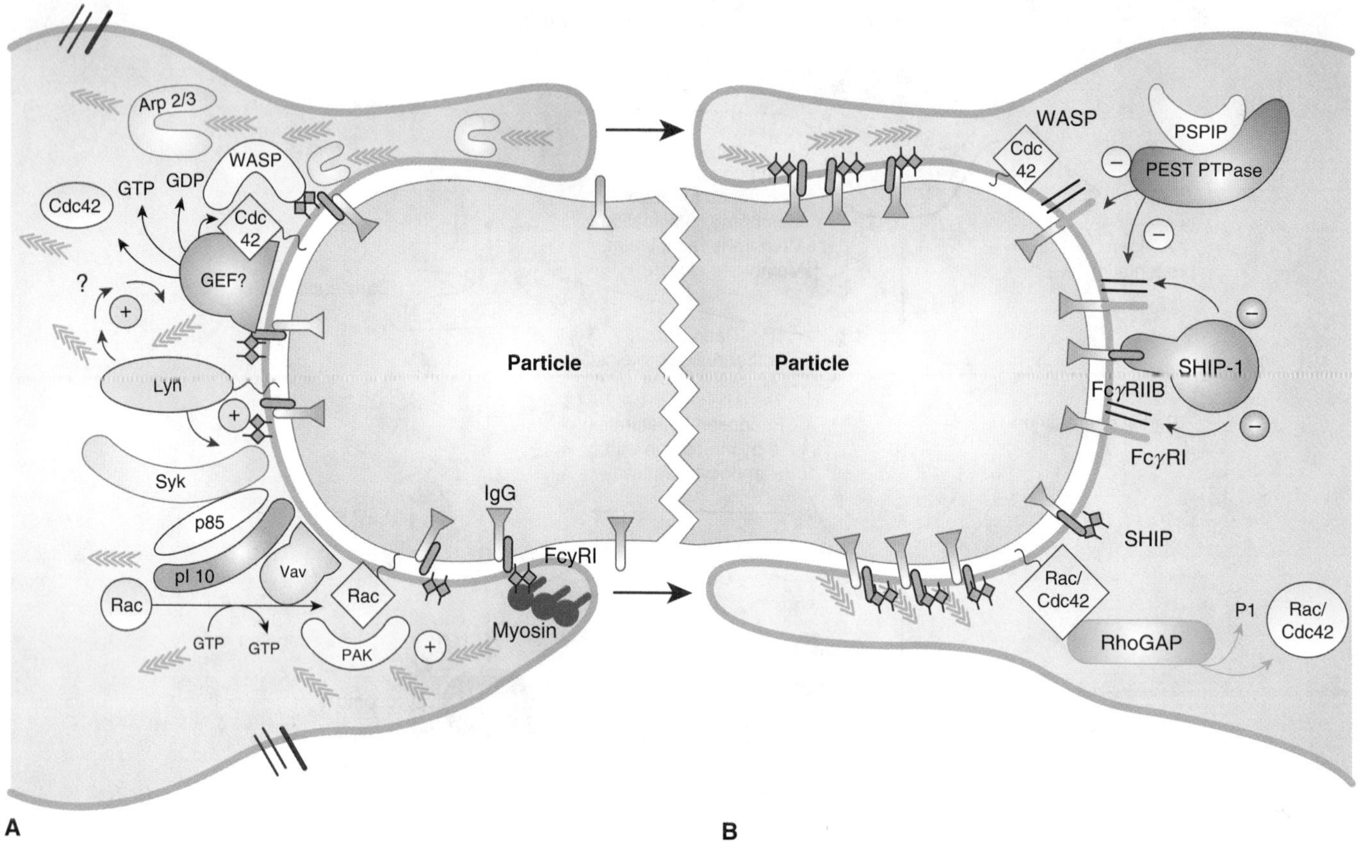

FIGURE 68–9. A model for FcγR-mediated phagocytosis. **A.** Signaling upstream and downstream of Rho guanosine triphosphatases during FcγR-mediated phagocytosis. Immunoglobulin (Ig) G bound to antigen on the particle binds to FcγRI receptors at the surface of the mφ and induces their aggregation (shown in *red*). This activates a Src family tyrosine kinase (probably Lyn). Lyn phosphorylates the receptor γ chain (phosphotyrosine residues in the γ chains are depicted as *red diamonds*) and Syk. Syk is activated and recruited to the phosphotyrosine residues of the γ chain through its two SH2 (Src homology 2) domains. Cdc42 activation by an unknown guanine-nucleotide exchange factor (GEF) allows the recruitment of WASP (Wiskott-Aldrich syndrome protein). In turn, WASP activates the Arp2/3 complex that triggers actin polymerization to generate the protrusive force for pseudopod extension (*red arrowheads*). Activation of a Rac1 GEF, possibly Vav, by tyrosine phosphorylation in conjunction with PI3 kinase products (PIP_3) promotes GDP/GTP (guanosine diphosphate/guanosine triphosphate) exchange on Rac1. GTP-bound Rac1 interacts with and activates the serine/threonine kinase Pak1, which may induce the actinomyosin contractility involved in phagosome closure. **B.** In the next step, FcγRI is rapidly down-modulated an returned to an inactive state (shown in *blue*), resulting in actin filament disassembly. According to this model, actin assembly proceeds as a wave at the distal rim of the pseudopodia, while actin depolymerization occurs rearward. Polyphosphoinositide phosphatases such as the SH2 domain-containing SHIP, which selectively hydrolyze PIP_3, may contribute to down-modulation. Modulation of FcγRI activation may also involve tyrosine phosphatases such as SHP-1, which associates with FcγRIIb, a member of the FcγR family that may be coligated with FcγRI. In addition, PEST family phosphotyrosine phosphatases (PTPases) may contribute to dephosphorylation by interacting with PSPIP, a cytoskeletal protein that interacts with WASP. GAPs may also contribute to down-modulation by returning Cdc42/Rac1 to the inactive, GDP-bound state. Eventually, cytoskeletal proteins are shed from the ingestion site to leave the phagosome free in the cytosol (not shown here). *(Reprinted from Chimini G, Chavrier P*[67] *by permission of Macmillan Publishers Ltd,* Nature Cell Biology. *Copyright 2000.)*

rise to the zipper hypothesis with local segmental engagement of FcR, and circumferential flow of macrophage pseudopodia around the particle, followed by fusion at the tip, closure, and ingestion. Subsequent studies by several groups documented the role of phosphatidylinositol 3-kinase (PI3K) and phosphoinositides in the initial fusion and subsequent associations between the actin cytoskeleton and cellular membranes.[76] Latex has provided a useful test particle to isolate latex-containing phagolysosomes by flotation. Proteomic analyses[77] demonstrated the protein composition of phagosomes and drew attention to functional constituents in the phagolysosomal membrane (Fig. 68–10). It also gave rise to a controversy regarding the contribution of the endoplasmic reticulum to the nascent phagosome.[78]

These observations have provided the basis for numerous investigations regarding the interactions of diverse microorganisms with the vacuolar system, which are often necessary for pathogen survival and establishment of intracellular infection (Fig. 68–11).[6] Organisms can inhibit acidification and fusion (*Mycobacterium*),[25,79] multiply within secondary lysosomes (*Leishmania*),[80] escape free into the cytosol (*Listeria*),[81] or translocate their genomes into the cytoplasm by fusion (enveloped viruses); other organisms induce variations on this theme, for example, *Brucella* seeks out the endoplasmic reticulum after entry and *Legionella* can enter macrophages by inducing a phagosome membrane of unusual composition.[82] Nonpathogenic organisms or pathogens taken up via opsonic receptors or after IFN-γ activation undergo a different fate, with killing and destruction.

The zipper mechanism, with tight apposition of membrane to the particle's surface ligands, does not apply to all forms of ingestion (see

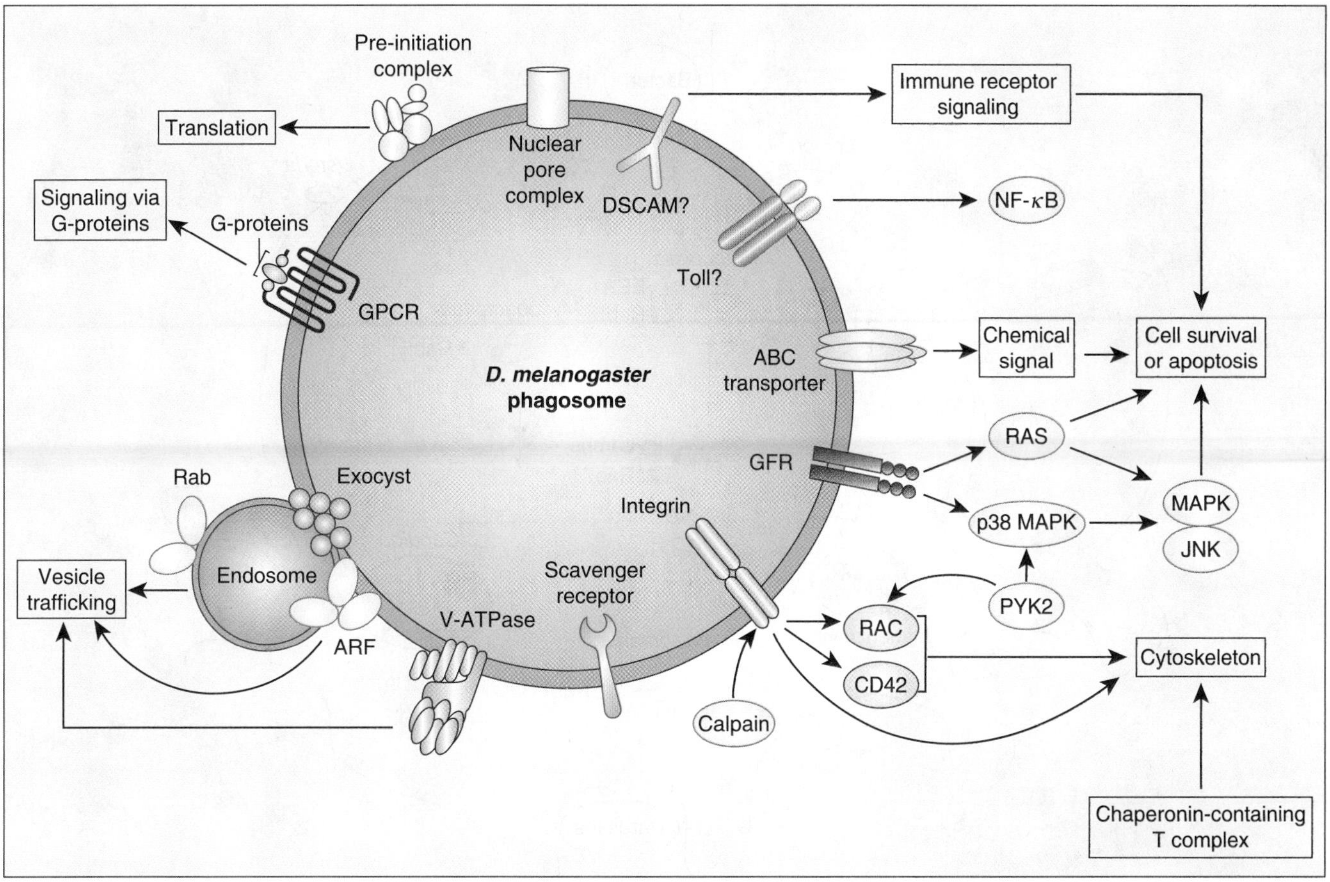

FIGURE 68–10. The phagosome is a multifunctional organelle. Proteomic analysis has identified more than 600 proteins that are associated with the phagosomes of *Drosophila melanogaster*. Bioinformatic analyses of these proteins suggest that numerous protein–protein interactions and macromolecular complexes associate with this organelle. These include the vacuolar-adenosine triphosphatase (V-ATPase), the exocyst, and the chaperonin-containing T complex. In addition, components of multiple signaling pathways are present in association with phagosomes, suggesting this as a point of initiation of signal transduction. These pathways are likely to be downstream of transmembrane proteins found in the phagosome such as G-protein-coupled receptors (GPCRs), scavenger receptors, integrins, the toll receptor, and growth-factor receptors (GFRs). ABC, ATP-binding cassette; ARF, adenosine diphosphate (ADP)-ribosylation factor; DSCAM, Down syndrome cell-adhesion molecule; MAPK, mitogen-activated protein kinase; NF-κB, nuclear factor-κB; PYK2, protein tyrosine kinase 2. *(Reprinted from Stuart LM, Ezekowitz RA[111] by permission of Macmillan Publishers Ltd,* Nature Reviews Immunology. *Copyright 2008.)*

Fig. 68–8). For example, complement opsonized particles seem to sink into the cytoplasm, and other phagosomes can be spacious. A number of key methods of visualization[70] illustrate the dynamic nature of phagocytosis. Figures 68–8 and 68–9 illustrate some of the signaling pathways that control the cytoskeleton.

Macrophages are rich in lysosomal digestive enzymes,[23] activated by a falling pH of ~6.5 within the mature vacuole. Unless captured as peptides by major histocompatibility complex molecules, a feature of antigen processing by DCs, macromolecular substrates can be degraded to their constituent amino acids, sugars, or nucleic acid bases. Early studies by Ehrenreich and Cohn[1] probed the permeability of the lysosomal vacuolar membrane. If the content cannot be fully degraded because of its nature (e.g., sucrose), overload (e.g., lipid), or owing to a genetic deficiency in a catabolic enzyme (lysosomal storage diseases), it accumulates within residual lysosomes, altering macrophage gene expression and secretory output, thus mediating chronic inflammation or metabolic forms of modified inflammation, such as atherosclerosis, foam cell formation and Gaucher disease. Figure 68–12A illustrates the uptake of senescent erythrocytes, the breakdown of heme and storage of Fe^{2+}.[83] Figure 68–12B shows how phagocytosis by DCs can bring about processing and cross-presentation of exogenous antigens.[84] By comparison (Fig. 68–12C), autophagy is the envelopment of damaged intracellular organelles and cytoplasm by cytoplasmic membrane, and sequestration within a digestive vacuole, resembling heterophagy.[82] Its biochemical and cellular basis has become of interest because of its apparent relevance to cancer, infections such as tuberculosis and Legionnaire disease, and inflammatory syndromes such as inflammatory bowel disease (IBD).

Although the phagocytic mechanism has been investigated in depth, we do not understand fully how the process of internalization is controlled. For example, ingestion can be thwarted by attempts to ingest too large a particle or foreign surface, or by close apposition of plasma membrane to noninternalizable immune complexes. This results in redirecting secretory vesicles to the surface, reminiscent of osteoclast adhesion. In other circumstances, as in response to foreign bodies, and especially mycobacteria, and in the presence of the Th2 cytokines interleukin (IL)-4/13, individual macrophages can fuse to form giant cells, with a common cytoplasm and multinucleation. Several fusogenic surface molecules have been identified and DNAX-activating protein

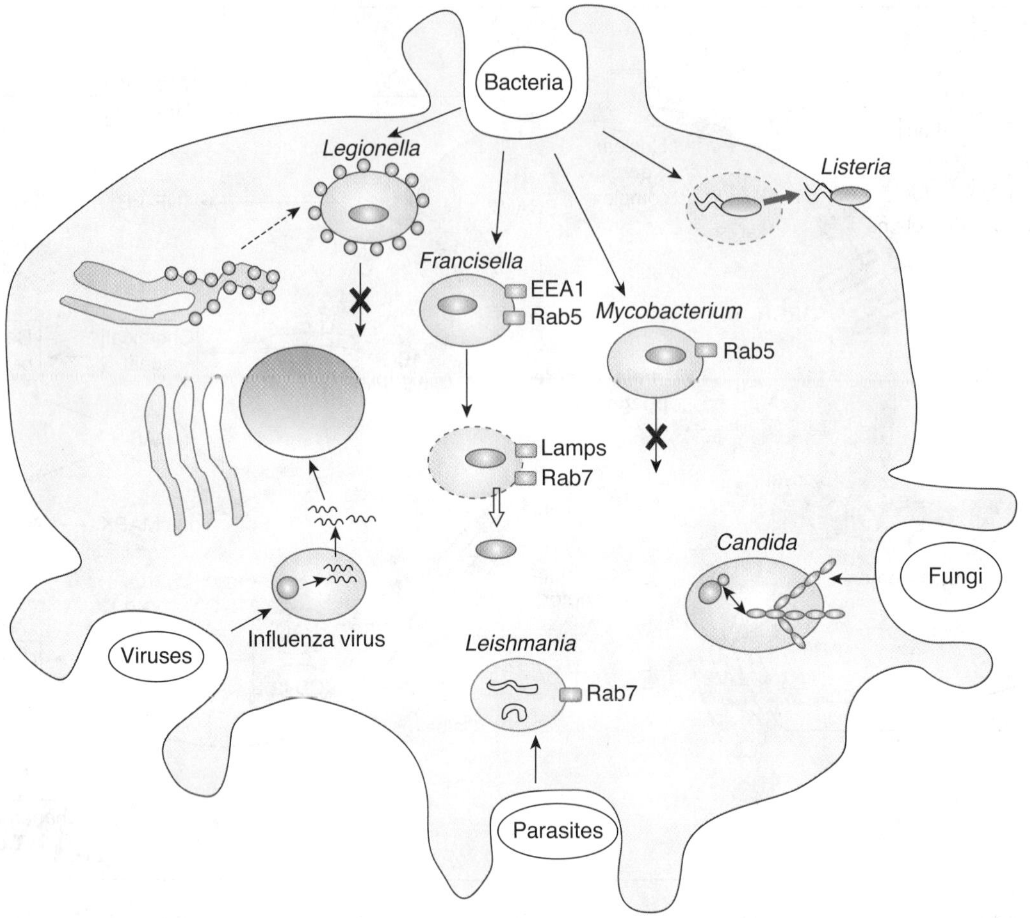

FIGURE 68–11. Selected pathogens evade distinct phagocytic mechanisms. Pathogens have developed several mechanisms to enter and survive inside macrophages. *Legionella pneumophila* resides and multiplies in a vacuole studded with ribosomes as a result of interaction with the rough endoplasmic reticulum. The organism secretes effector molecules via its type IV secretion system into the cell, which inhibit phagosome/lysosome fusion. The *Francisella tularensis* phagosome acquires the early endosome markers EEA1 and Rab5 and then matures into a late endosome defined by the presence of the markers Lamp1, Lamp2, and Rab7. The late endosome does not acidify and the phagosomal membrane is disrupted, releasing the bacteria into the cytosol. The *Mycobacterium tuberculosis* phagosome acquires the early endosome marker Rab5 but excludes the late endosomal Lamps and Rab7. This organism also produces molecules that block fusion with the lysosome and resides and replicates in this early endosome. Acidification of the *Listeria monocytogenes* phagosome is essential for the perforation of the phagosomal membrane and escape of the bacteria into the cytosol. Here they mobilize the actin polymerization machinery to move within the cell and then from cell to cell. *Candida albicans* undergoes a conversion from a unicellular form to a multicellular hyphal form, which allows this fungus to escape the macrophage. The *Leishmania mexicana* phagosome develops into an acidic phagolysosome containing Rab7 where the parasite is able to survive and replicate. Viruses such as the influenza virus are able to inhibit the activation of antiviral mechanisms, such as the activation of interferon regulatory function proteins that induce interferon production upon viral infection, and enter the nucleus. Cytomegalovirus (not shown) incapacitates a range of major histocompatibility complex-antigen presenting pathways.

(DAP) 12 expression and signaling is important in generating a fusogenic differentiation phenotype in macrophages.[85]

CYTOSOLIC RECOGNITION AND SIGNALING

The recognition of the multiprotein inflammasome complex[25] has stimulated intense interest in the recognition by cytosolic proteins of foreign nucleic acid, uric acid-induced injury, and breakdown products of microbial walls, for example, muramyl dipeptide. More complex peptidoglycan structures can also be recognized by surface receptors in *Drosophila*. Several reviews chart the rapid growth in our knowledge of inflammasome function in health and disease.[24,26,86,87] Figure 68–13 illustrates selected nucleotide-binding oligomerization domain (NOD)-like and related receptors (NLRs) with nucleotide oligomerization and other characteristic domains. Mutations in NLR have been implicated in IBD, in periodic familial Mediterranean fever, and in a range of autohyperinflammatory syndromes.[88] Excessive caspase activation and IL-1β release can be countered therapeutically with IL-1 receptor antagonists. Figure 68–14 illustrates the role of inflammasome activation in intracellular infection. Antiviral production of IFN-α and -β involves retinoid-inducible gene (RIG)-I–like helicases, indicating a role for mitochondria in cytosolic sensing.

GENE EXPRESSION, SYNTHESIS, AND SECRETION

The development of microarray technology has had a dramatic impact on the analysis of macrophage gene expression in response to

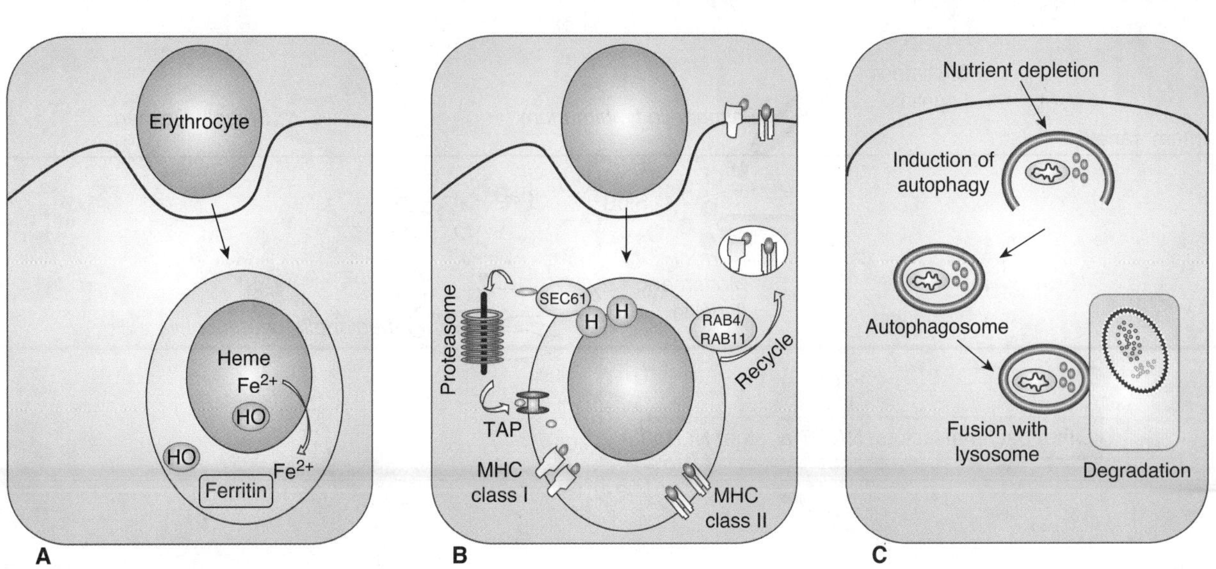

FIGURE 68–12. **A.** Macrophages have an important role in iron metabolism by processing effete erythrocytes, internalized by phagocytosis, and returning iron to the blood (through ferritin) for reuse. Dissociation of iron linked to heme on erythrocytes requires the action of heme oxygenase (HO), an enzyme present in the endoplasmic reticulum (ER). The process allowing the transfer of heme oxygenase from the ER to the phagosome lumen is so far unknown. **B.** Presentation of antigens from intracellular pathogens is mainly carried out by major histocompatibility complex (MHC) class II molecules loaded in phagosomes. Presentation of some pathogen antigens could also involve MHC class I molecules. Current models indicate that antigens generated by hydrolases in the phagosome lumen could use SEC61 for translocation to the cytoplasm. After processing by the proteasome, antigens could be translocated to the phagosome lumen through the transporter for antigen processing (TAP) complex where loading onto MHC class I or MHC class II molecules would occur. Transport to the cell surface from the phagosome lumen could take place by using the existing membrane recycling machinery, involving the small guanosine triphosphatases Rab4 and Rab11. **C.** Autophagy is a conserved membrane traffic pathway that equips eukaryotic cells to capture cytoplasmic components within a double-membrane vacuole, or autophagosome, for delivery to lysosomes. Although best known as a mechanism to survive starvation, autophagy is now recognized as a mechanism to combat infection by a variety of intracellular microbes.

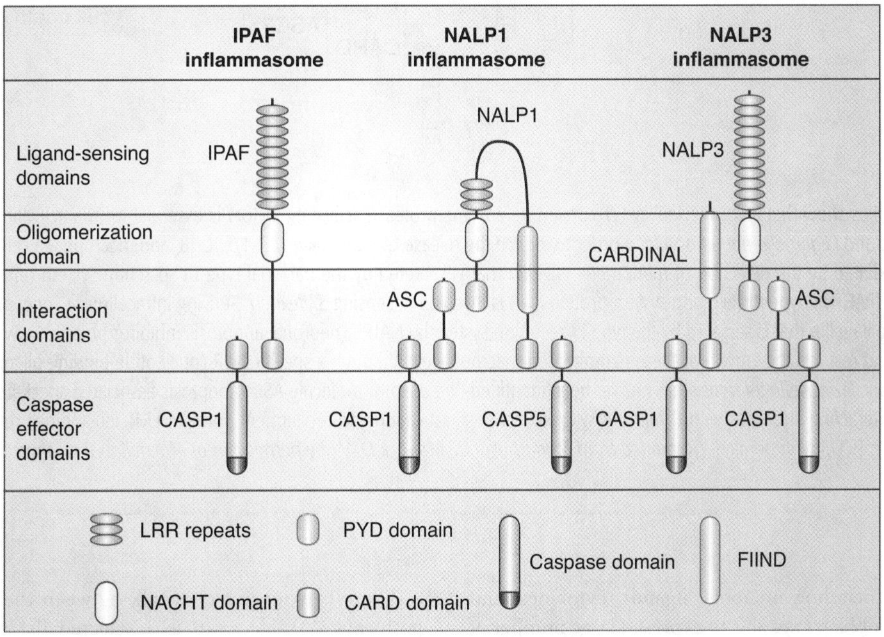

FIGURE 68–13. Nucleotide-binding and oligomerization domain (NOD)–leucine-rich repeat (LRR) and inflammasome structures. NOD-like receptors (NLRs) have three structural domains: The LRR domain at the C-terminus, the NACHT (domain present in NAIP, CIITA HET-E, TP-1) domain, and the N-terminal domain that can be a pyrin domain (PYD), a caspase activation and recruitment domain (CARD), or a baculovirus inhibitor-of-apoptosis protein repeat domain (BIR). The LRR domain is considered as the ligand-sensing motif, thus involved in the interaction with pathogen-associated molecular patterns (PAMPs), in analogy to toll-like receptors (TLRs). The NACHT domain is responsible for the oligomerization and activation of NLRs. The PYD or CARD domain of NLR is the link to downstream adaptors (such as apoptosis-associated speck-like protein containing a CARD [ASC]) or effectors (such as caspase-1). The BIR domain is proposed to act as caspase inhibitor. During NACHT leucine-rich repeat protein (NALP) and NALP1 inflammasome activation, NALP3 or NALP1 interact through PYD–PYD homotypic interactions with ASC, resulting in its activation. Subsequently, the CARD domain of ASC interacts with the CARD domain of caspase-1 and mediates its activation. Of note, NALP1 may also activate directly the caspase-5 through its C-terminal CARD domain. In contrast, NALP3 does not simultaneously activate caspase-5, but NALP3 can recruit a second capsase-1 through the CARD domain of CARD inhibitor of nuclear factor-κB–activating ligand (CARDINAL), a component of the NALP3 inflammasome. Interestingly, interleukin-1β-converting enzyme (ICE)-protease activating factor (IPAF), that can on its own sense PAMPs, possesses a CARD domain at the N-terminal and thus may directly activate caspase-1 without ASC recruitment ("IPAF inflammasome"). *(Reproduced from Sidiropoulos PI, Goulielmos G, Voloudakis GK, et al[86] with permission from BMJ Publishing Group Ltd.)*

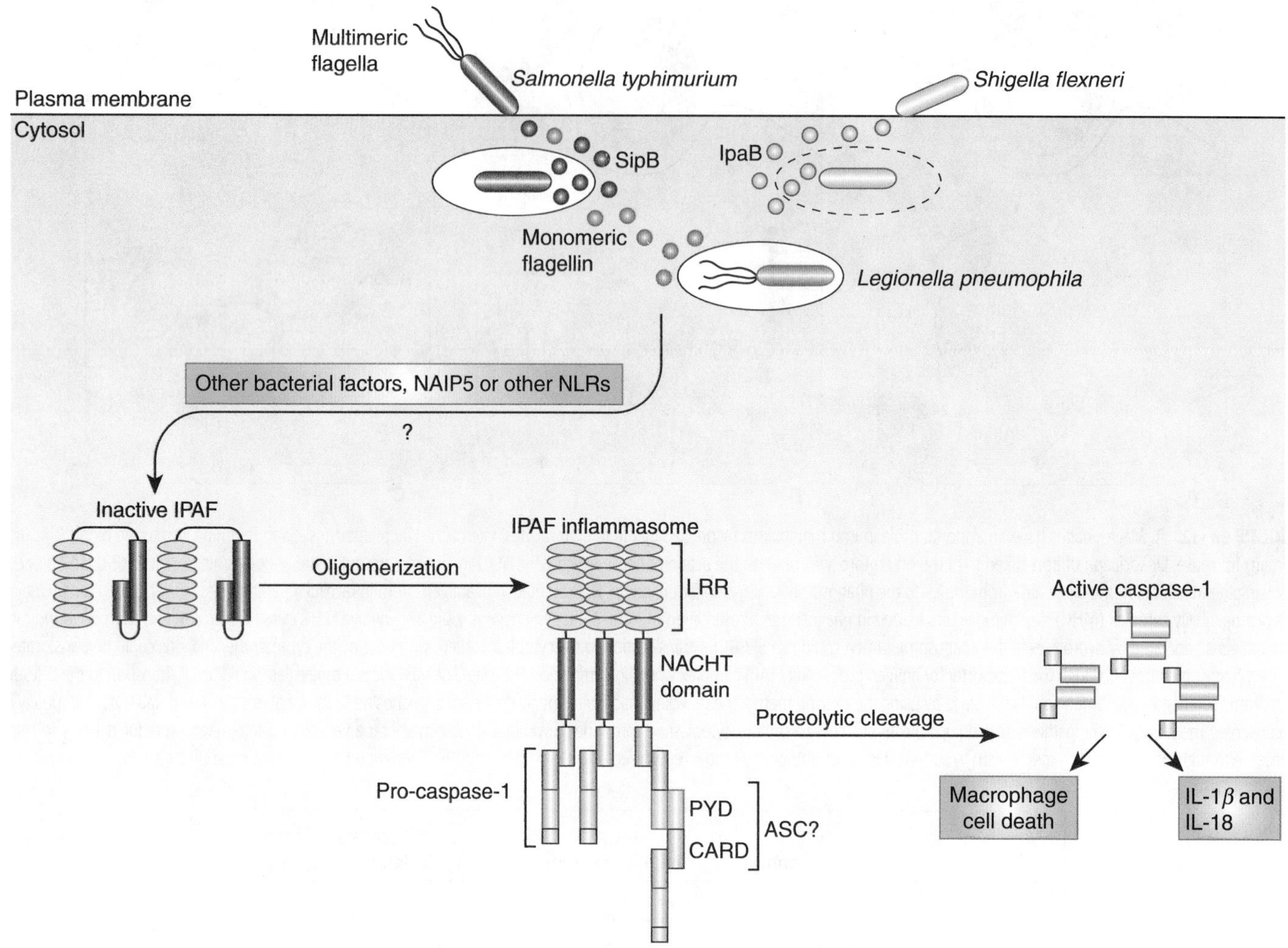

FIGURE 68–14. Knockout studies show that Ipaf (interleukin-1β-converting enzyme-protease activating factor) is essential for the activation of caspase-1 by *Salmonella typhimurium, Shigella flexneri*, and *Legionella pneumophila* in order to induce the release of interleukin (IL)-1β, IL-18, and macrophage cell death. Sensing intracellular *S. typhimurium* seems to be mediated by the detection of monomeric flagellin that is secreted by the bacterial type III secretion system (and is dependent on the protein SipB from *S. typhimurium*) by IPAF. The type III secretion system protein IpaB is involved in sensing *S. flexneri*. Sensing intracellular *L. pneumophila* seems to be mediated by the detection of monomeric flagellin that is secreted by the type IV secretion system by NAIP5 (neuronal apoptosis inhibitor protein 5), which, in conjunction with IPAF, induces caspase-1 activation and restricts the growth of these pathogens in macrophages. Although a specific NLR (nucleotide-binding oligomerization domain-like receptor) protein that detects cytosolic *Francisella tularensis* has not yet been identified, the adaptor molecule ASC (apoptosis-associated speck-like protein containing a CARD) seems to be essential for counteracting infections with *F. tularensis*. CARD, caspase activation and recruitment domain; LRR, leucine-rich repeat; NACHT, domain present in NAIP, CIITA, HET-E, and TP-1; PYD, pyrin domain. *(Reprinted from Mariathasan S, Monack DM[24] by permission of Macmillan Publishers Ltd,* Nature Reviews Immunology. *Copyright 2007.)*

a wide range of stimuli, including microbial ligands, cytokines, and immunomodulators. Macrophages are able to express a large number of genes and are extremely versatile in their responses to environmental cues. It has been possible to discern signatures of particular agonists, for example, IFN-α and -β and IL-4, but many caveats remain in the interpretation of such data. Heterogeneity of cellular origin, differentiation stage, and populations from diverse origins, as well as substantial species differences, make it difficult to compare results within and among experiments. Validation of more quantitative messenger RNA analysis of protein synthesis and modification is difficult, although proteomic analysis is gaining ground. The study of macrophage chromatin organization in relation to gene expression is in its infancy.

There is extensive crosstalk between the secretory and endocytic pathways.[89] Table 68–3 is a selected list of secretory products.[7,90] This includes lysozyme, a major myelomonocytic product that is constitutively expressed *in vitro*, but upregulated in granulomata *in vivo*. The secretion pathway of lysozyme in monocytes and macrophages has not been defined. The well-known pro- and antiinflammatory cytokines are better characterized, both in terms of regulation and the secretion pathway.[90] The response to IL-6 and TNF-α secretion in model systems has shown a more complex pathway than previously recognized.[91–93] In addition to these and other important growth and differentiation factors that regulate angiogenesis, for example, macrophages are able to produce and secrete

TABLE 68–3. Selected Secretion Products of Macrophages

Proteins	Product	Comment
Enzymes	Lysozyme	Bulk product
	Urokinase-type plasminogen activator	Regulated by inflammation
	Collagenase	Regulated by inflammation
	Elastase	Regulated by inflammation
	Metalloproteinases	Also inhibitors
	Complement	All components and regulators
	Arginase	Alternative activation
	Angiotensin-converting enzyme	Induced glucocorticoids, granulomas
	Chitotriosidase	Gaucher disease, lysosomal storage
Inhibitors	Acid hydrolases	All classes (mainly intracellular)
	TIMP	
Chemokines	Many C-C, C-X-C, CX_3C– e.g., MCP, Rantes, IL-8	Initiates acute and chronic recruitment of myeloid and lymphoid cells
Cytokines	IL-1β, TNF-α	Pro- and antiinflammatory
	IL-6, IL-10, IL-12, IL-17, IL-18, IL-23	Also antagonists, e.g., IL-1Ra
	Type I IFN	Autocrine and paracrine amplification
Apolipoproteins	Apolipoprotein E	Local source, marrow origin after adoptive transfer
Growth/differentiation factors	TGF-β	Also other family members (activins), myeloid growth and differentiation
	M-CSF	
	GM-CSF	
	FGF	Fibrosis
	PDGF	Repair
	VEGF	Angiogenesis
Opsonins	Fibronectin, Pentraxin (PTX3)	Also uncharacterized receptor on Mϕ
Soluble receptors	Mannose receptor	Soluble mannose receptor
Cationic peptides	Defensins	Subpopulations and species variation
Lipids	Procoagulant	Initiation clotting
	Arachidonate metabolites:	Pro- and antiinflammatory mediators
	Prostaglandins	
	Leukotrienes	
	Thromboxanes	
	Resolvins	
Metabolites	Reactive oxygen intermediates	
	Reactive nitrogen intermediates	
	Haem breakdown (bile pigments)	
	Iron, B_{12}-binding protein	
	Vitamin D metabolites	

FGF, fibroblast growth factor; GM-CSF, granulocyte-macrophage colony-stimulating factor; IFN, interferon; IL, interleukin; MCP, monocyte chemotactic protein; M-CSF, macrophage colony-stimulating factor; PDGF, platelet-derived growth factor; RANTES, regulated on activation, normal T-cell expressed, presumed secreted; TGF, transforming growth factor; TIMP, tissue inhibitor of metalloproteinase; TNF, tumor necrosis factor; VEGF, vascular endothelial growth factor.

SOURCE: Reproduced with permission from Gordon S.[7]

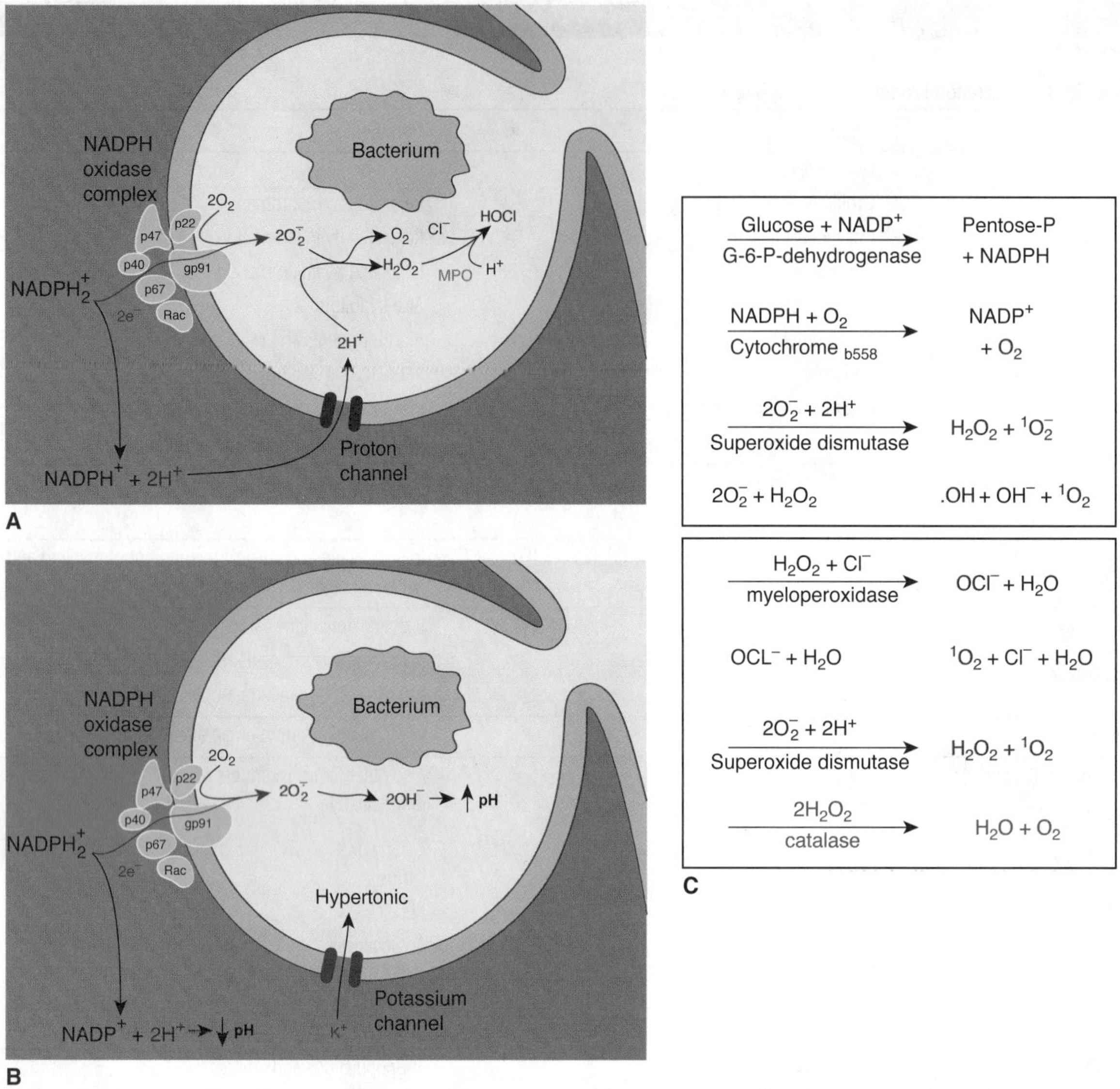

FIGURE 68–15. The respiratory burst in a phagocyte is triggered when a bacterium is phagocytosed. During the phagocytosis of bacteria by macrophages and neutrophils, the phagosome membrane pinches off and the microbe is endocytosed along with a small volume of extracellular fluid. The mechanisms discussed here are based on studies in neutrophils and are still controversial.[112] Electrons are removed from nicotinamide adenine dinucleotide phosphate (NADPH) in the cytoplasm and transferred through the gp91phox component (which includes flavin adenine dinucleotide and two hemes) across the membrane, where they reduce extracellular (or intraphagosomal) O_2 to O_2^-. Protons left behind in the cell are extruded through voltage-gated proton channels (*red*). Some of the reactive oxygen species (ROS) derived from O_2^- are indicated. Spontaneous or superoxide dismutase–catalyzed disproportionation of O_2^- produces hydrogen peroxide (H_2O_2), which may be converted to HOCl (hypochlorous acid, or household bleach) by myeloperoxidase (MPO). **A.** Traditional view of the respiratory burst with charge compensation by proton channels. A perfect match of one proton per electron results in no change in membrane potential, intracellular pH (pHi), or external pH (pHo) and little change in ionic strength. Because proton channels are separate molecules and for the most part operate independently of NADPH oxidase, perfect 1:1 stoichiometry is not obligatory. The large depolarization that occurs during the respiratory burst in intact neutrophils and eosinophils is likely the most important factor that causes proton channels to open, although both pHi and pHo tend to change in a direction that causes proton channels to open. The fact that depolarization occurs demonstrates unequivocally that proton efflux initially lags behind electron efflux. **B.** If any fraction of the total charge compensation were mediated by K+ efflux, pHi would fall, pHo (or phagosomal pH) would increase, and the osmolality of the phagosomal contents would increase. In this model, the elevated pH and osmolality of the phagosomal contents are crucial to activating proteolytic enzymes that actually kill bacteria, as opposed to ROS, which are said to be inert. *(Reproduced with permission from DeCoursey TE.[113])* **C.** Respiratory burst reactions. During phagocytosis glucose is metabolized via the pentose monophosphate shunt and NADPH is formed. Cytochrome B, which was part of the specific granule, combines with the plasma membrane NADPH oxidase and activates it. The activated NADPH oxidase uses oxygen to oxidize the NADPH. The result is the production of superoxide anion. Some of the superoxide anion is converted to H_2O_2 and singlet oxygen by superoxide dismutase. In addition, superoxide anion can react with H_2O_2 resulting in the formation of hydroxyl radical and more singlet oxygen. The result of all of these reactions is the production of the toxic oxygen compounds superoxide anion (O_2^-), H_2O_2, singlet oxygen ($^1O_2$) and hydroxyl radical (OH•). As the azurophilic granules fuse with the phagosome, myeloperoxidase is released into the phagolysosome. Myeloperoxidase utilizes H_2O_2 and halide ions (usually Cl^-) to produce hypochlorite, a highly toxic substance. Some of the hypochlorite can spontaneously break down to yield singlet oxygen. The result of these reactions is the production of toxic hypochlorite (Ocl^-) and singlet oxygen ($^1O_2$).

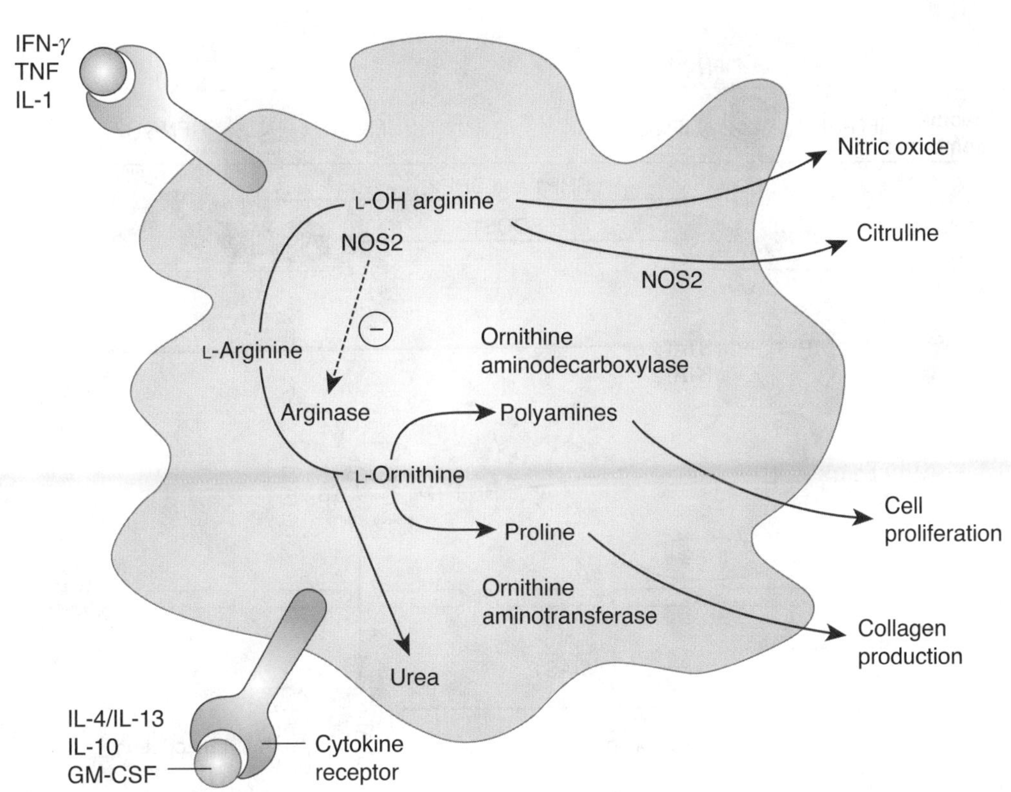

FIGURE 68–16. The role of nitrogen metabolism in mϕ function. Interferon-γ (IFN-γ) enhances the activity of nitric oxide synthase 2 (NOS2) to generate nitric oxide, and inhibits arginase. Interleukin-4 (IL-4) and IL-13 promote arginase-dependent formation of L-ornithine and, ultimately, fibroblast proliferation and collagen production. GM-CSF, granulocyte-macrophage colony-stimulating factor; TNF, tumor necrosis factor. *(Reprinted from Gordon S[114] by permission of Macmillan Publishers Ltd,* Nature Reviews Immunology. *Copyright 2003.)*

enzymes and proenzymes for a range of activities, as well as their inhibitors, for example, proteinases and antiproteinases. Although the amounts of complement proteins produced, for example, are relatively small, they can be significantly concentrated in a local microenvironment. In addition, macrophages can produce a range of antimicrobial peptides and lytic agents, but their most important killing mechanisms depend on oxygen[94,95] and nitrogen metabolites,[80,96] which are illustrated in Figures 68–15 and 68–16. Regulation of the nicotinamide adenine dinucleotide phosphate oxidase and of inducible nitric oxide synthase has been studied extensively in mouse and human, through biochemical and genetic approaches. Apart from their antimicrobial activity, nitrogen metabolites contribute to signaling pathways.[97] IFN-α and -β play an important role in macrophage antiviral activities[98] and perhaps in the cellular response to bacteria.[99] These cytokines also contribute significantly to immune and inflammatory pathways, as well as cancer immunoediting[100] and autoimmunity.[101]

Macrophages may be able to produce IFN-γ, for example, under particular circumstances, but *in vivo* most of the cytokine derives from other sources. IFN-γ has a major impact on macrophage function, including priming of biosynthetic and functional responses associated with cytotoxicity and inflammation in cell-mediated immunity (Fig. 68–17).[102,103] Table 68–4 summarizes the markers and functions associated with various forms of macrophage activation and deactivation, as described in Chap. 69.[104] Intracellular GTPases have been implicated in cell activation by IFN-γ, for example, in resistance to infection in mice,[105] and in relation to IBD. Similarly, the Th2 cytokines IL-4/13 induce characteristic changes in macrophage phenotype, which are associated with an alternative activation pathway. The cellular biology of alternatively activated macrophages is modified extensively (see Fig. 68–16).[106] In the mouse, markers such as arginase, Fizz-1, and Ym1, a chitinase-like protein, are useful markers of alternative activation, but analysis in humans requires development of novel markers. Macrophages also express a range of inhibitory proteins, such as members of the suppressor of cytokine signaling family, that suppress cytokine production, in addition to IL-10[90] and transforming growth factor-β. Lipid metabolites, mainly derived from arachidonate and other lipid precursors, provide another potent source of inflammatory and immunomodulatory products.[21,107] The suppressive functions of monocytes and macrophages in chronic infections and experimental tumors require further study, including the development of new phenotypic markers in mice and humans.

CELLULAR INTERACTIONS

In addition to cytokine and other soluble afferent and efferent responses, macrophages are able to directly interact among themselves, with all other cell types in the body, both viable and injured, as well as with all kinds of microorganisms. Their interactions are

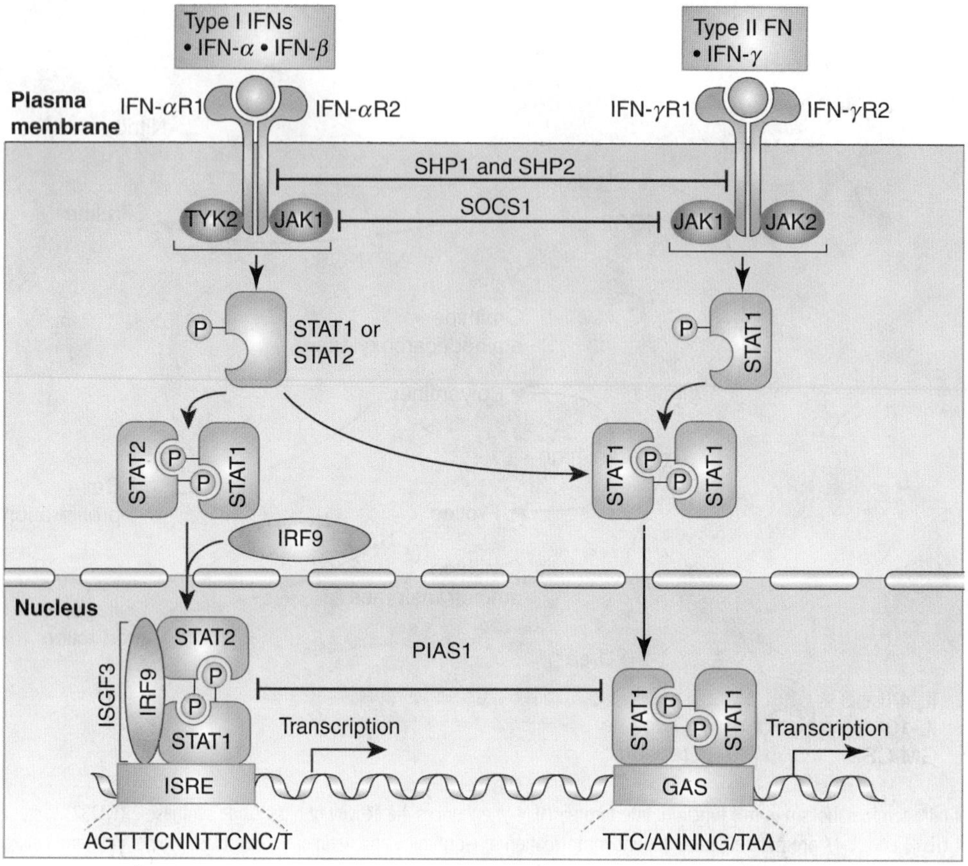

FIGURE 68–17. Signaling pathways induced by type I and type II interferon (IFN). The type I IFNs (IFN-α and IFN-β) bind a receptor that consists of the subunits IFN-αR1 and IFN-αR2, which are constitutively associated with tyrosine kinase 2 (TYK2) and Janus kinase (JAK) 1, respectively. Type-I-IFN-induced JAK–STAT (signal transducer and activator of transcription) signaling is propagated similarly to IFN-γ-induced JAK–STAT signaling (below). Activated TYK2 and JAK1 phosphorylate STAT1 or STAT2. Type I IFN-induced signaling then induces homodimerization of STAT1 and heterodimerization of STAT1 and STAT2. STAT1 and STAT2 associate with the cytosolic transcription factor IFN-regulatory factor 9 (IRF9), forming a trimeric complex known as IFN-stimulated gene factor 3 (ISGF3). On entering the nucleus, ISGF3 binds IFN-stimulated response elements (ISREs). Studies of gene-targeted mice have shown that JAK1, STAT1, STAT2, and IRF9 are required for signaling through the type I IFN receptor. TYK2 is required for optimal type I IFN-induced signaling. IFN-γ signaling: IFN-γ induces reorganization of the IFN-γ receptor (IFN-γR) subunits, IFN-γR1 and IFN-γR2, activating the Janus kinases JAK1 and JAK2, which are constitutively associated with each subunit, respectively. The JAKs phosphorylate a crucial tyrosine residue of IFN-γR1, forming a STAT1-binding site; they then tyrosine phosphorylate receptor-bound STAT1, which homodimerizes through SRC homology 2 (SH2) domain–phosphotyrosine interactions and is fully activated by serine phosphorylation. STAT1 homodimers enter the nucleus and bind promoters at IFN-γ-activated sites (GASs) and induce gene transcription in conjunction with coactivators, such as CBP (cyclic adenosine monophosphate-responsive–element-binding protein [CREB]), p300, and minichromosome maintenance-deficient 5 (MCM5). IFN-γ-mediated signaling is controlled by several mechanisms: by dephosphorylation of IFN-γR1, JAK1, and STAT1 (mediated by SH2 domain-containing protein tyrosine phosphatase 2 [SHP2]); by inhibition of the JAKs (mediated by suppressor of cytokine signaling 1 [SOCS1]); by proteasomal degradation of the JAKs; and by inhibition of STAT1 (mediated by protein inhibitor of activated STAT 1 [PIAS1]). *(Reprinted from Dunn GP, Koebel CM, Schreiber RD[100] by permission of Macmillan Publishers Ltd,* Nature Reviews Immunology. *Copyright 2006.)*

reciprocal and regulated, contributing to homeostasis and to pathogenesis, both acutely and following persistent injury, to chronic inflammation. Storage of poorly degraded materials in lysosomes, for example, results in sustained production of degradation products, whereas massive, acute responses have a profound impact on the systemic circulation, endocrine and nervous systems, and on metabolic pathways. Short-range interactions include giant cell formation during granulomatous inflammation, and also contact-dependent immunoregulation by surface molecules such as CD200/CD200R (see Fig. 68–5) and SIRPα/CD47.[108] Matrix and other surface interactions regulate the induction or suppression of adaptive immune responses, as well as of other functions. The availability of oxygen plays an important role in macrophage interactions with a range of other cells, both normally and in a range of pathologies inducing inflammation, repair, and malignancy (Fig. 68–18).

RELEVANCE TO HEMATOPOIETIC FUNCTIONS AND DISORDERS

In addition to their essential role in host defense (innate and acquired immunity), inflammation, and repair, macrophages contribute

TABLE 68–4. Immunomodulation of Macrophage Phenotype

Stimulus	Category	Markers	Function
Microbial (bacterial)	Innate activation	Induction of MARCO	Enhanced phagocytosis
		Costimulatory molecules	Antigen presentation
		CD200	Inhibition (CD200R)
IFN-γ	Classical activation	Induction MHC II	Cell mediated immunity/delayed type hypersensitivity
		Potentiation innate markers	
		- TNF-α	Proinflammatory
		- iNOS induction	Antimicrobial (NO) signaling
		- NADPH, respiratory burst	Host defense, inflammation
		LGP47 induction	Association with phagosome/intracellular pathogen killing
		Downregulation of MR	Unknown
		Modulation of FcR expression	
		Proteasomal composition	Antigen presentation
IL-4/IL-13	Alternative activation	Enhanced MR	Endocytosis
		Induction arginase	Humoral immunity
		Induction YM1, FIZZ1 (mouse)	Th2-responses, allergy, antiparasitic
		Induction CCL17 (MDC) and CCL22 (TARC)	Immunity, repair/fibrosis
		Fusion, giant cell formation	
	Upregulation	CD23 (FcRε)	
Immune complexes	Modified activation	Selective IL-12 downregulation, IL-10 induction	
IL-10	Deactivation	Downregulation MHC II	
TGF-β	Deactivation	Downregulation of proinflammatory NO and ROI	
Glucocorticoids	Deactivation	CD163 induction, monocyte recruitment downregulated, ACE induction, Stabilin induction	Antiinflammatory Homeostatic clearance of hemoglobin/haptoglobin complexes

IFN, interferon; IL, interleukin; iNOS, inducible nitric oxide synthase; MARCO, macrophage receptor with collagenous structure; MDC, macrophage-derived chemokine; MHC, major histocompatibility complex; MR, mannose receptor; NADPH, nicotinamide adenine dinucleotide phosphate; NO, nitric oxide; ROI, reactive oxygen intermediate; TARC, thymus and activation-regulated chemokine; TGF, transforming growth factor; TNF, tumor necrosis factor.

to hematopoiesis, as well as to the turnover of hematopoietic cells and their products. Macrophages can be induced to take up folate, sense and respond to oxygen levels, and promote vascular growth, regulating the integrity of the hematopoietic microenvironment. However, they also play a central effector role in pathogenesis. Their surface expression and secretion of TNF-α, other proinflammatory cytokines, enzymes, and metabolites contribute to vascular injury and increased permeability of the microvasculature, as well as to local and systemic catabolic effects associated with chronic inflammation. In this regard, anti–TNF-α therapy is of considerable value in selected inflammatory conditions and may be extended to the treatment of cancer.[109] Stromal and other resident macrophage populations provide a niche for acute and persistent infections in marrow and elsewhere, and these macrophages also contribute to trophic support of hematopoietic malignancies, such as multiple myeloma. The macrophage, therefore, provides an important target cell for selective therapeutic intervention, without undue enhancement of vulnerability to infection. Additional molecular targets are needed, based on more detailed analysis of macrophage functions within their native hematopoietic tissue environment. A deeper understanding of macrophage physiologic functions and of their role in a broad range of diseases should lead to the development of fresh insights into the pathogenesis and management of hematologic disorders.

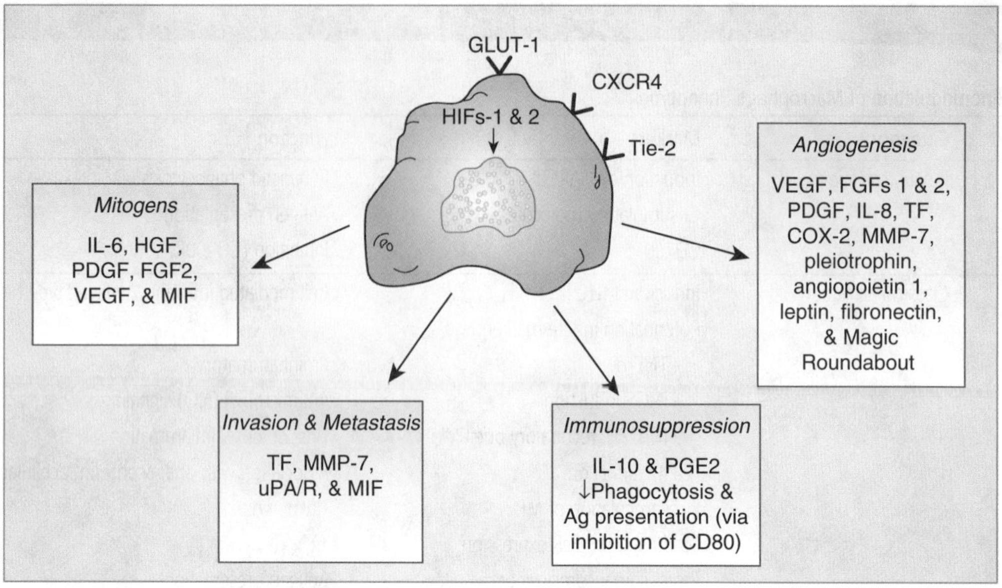

FIGURE 68–18. Hypoxia induces marked changes in the phenotype of macrophages. Macrophages upregulate hypoxia-inducible transcription factor (HIF)-1 and HIF-2 in hypoxia, which translocate to the nucleus to induce the expression of a wide array of target genes. Several important cell-surface receptors are upregulated in hypoxia, including the glucose receptor GLUT-1 (for increased glucose uptake as the cell switches to anaerobic glycolysis to make ATP in the absence of oxygen), the chemokine stromal cell-derived factor-1 (SDF-1) receptor CXCR4, and the angiopoietin receptor Tie-2. Hypoxia also stimulates the expression of a wide array of other pro-tumor cytokines, enzymes, and receptors, grouped here according to their known function in tumors. Downregulation of a factor or tumor-associated macrophage function is indicated by an *arrow*. Ag, antigen; COX, cyclooxygenase; FGF, fibroblast growth factor; HGF, hepatocyte growth factor; MIF, macrophage migration inhibitory factor; MMP, matrix metalloproteinase; PDGF, platelet-derived growth factor; PGE_2, prostaglandin E_2; TF, tissue factor; uPA/R, urokinase-type plasminogen activator receptor; VEGF, vascular endothelial growth factor. *(Reprinted from Lewis CE, Hughes R[115] with permission from BioMed Central. Copyright 2007.)*

REFERENCES

1. Steinman RM, Moberg CL: Zanvil Alexander Cohn 1926–1993. *J Exp Med* 179:1, 1994.
2. Steinman RM, Kaplan G, Witmer MD, Cohn ZA: Identification of a novel cell type in peripheral lymphoid organs of mice. V. Purification of spleen dendritic cells, new surface markers, and maintenance *in vitro*. *J Exp Med* 149:1, 1979.
3. Steinman RM, Witmer MD, Nussenzweig MC, et al: Dendritic cells of the mouse: identification and characterization. *J Invest Dermatol* 75:14, 1980.
4. Taylor PR, Martinez-Pomares L, Stacey M, et al: Macrophage receptors and immune recognition. *Annu Rev Immunol* 23:901, 2005.
5. Gordon S, Taylor PR: Monocyte and macrophage heterogeneity. *Nat Rev Immunol* 5:953, 2005.
6. Russell DG, Gordon S (eds): *Phagocyte-Pathogen Interactions: Macrophages and the Host Response to Infection*. ASM Press, Washington, DC, 2009.
7. Gordon S: Mononuclear phagocytes in rheumatic diseases, in *Kelley's Textbook of Rheumatology*, edited by GS Firestein, RC Budd, ED Harris, IB McInnes, S Ruddy, JS Sergent, p 135–154. WB Saunders, Philadelphia, 2008.
8. Gordon S: Macrophages and the immune response, in *Fundamental Immunology*, 6th ed, edited by W Paul, p 481. Lippincott Williams and Wilkins, Philadelphia, 2008.
9. Williams TJ, Rankin SM: Chemokines and phagocyte trafficking, in *Phagocyte-Pathogen Interactions: Macrophages and the Host Response to Infection*, edited by DG Russell, S Gordon, p 93. ASM Press, Washington, DC, 2009.
10. Ross R: Atherosclerosis—An inflammatory disease. *N Engl J Med* 340:115, 1999.
11. Janeway CA Jr, Medzhitov R: Innate immune recognition. *Annu Rev Immunol* 20:197, 2002.
12. Jiang A, Bloom O, Ono S, et al: Disruption of E-cadherin-mediated adhesion induces a functionally distinct pathway of dendritic cell maturation. *Immunity* 27:610, 2007.
13. Hazenbos WLW, Brown EJ: Integrins on phagocytes, in *Phagocyte-Pathogen Interactions: Macrophages and the Host Response to Infection*, edited by DG Russell, S Gordon, p 137. ASM Press, Washington, DC, 2009.
14. Auffray C, Sieweke MH, Geissmann F: Blood monocytes: Development, heterogeneity, and relationship with dendritic cells. *Annu Rev Immunol* 27:669, 2009.
15. Wheeler A, Ridley AJ: Leukocyte chemotaxis, in *Phagocyte-Pathogen Interactions: Macrophages and the Host Response to Infection*, edited by DG Russell, S Gordon, p 183. ASM Press, Washington, DC, 2009.
16. Lattin JE, Schroder K, Su AI, et al: Expression analysis of G Protein-Coupled Receptors in mouse macrophages. *Immunome Res* 4:5, 2008.
17. Yona S, Lin HH, Siu WO, et al: Adhesion-GPCRs: Emerging roles for novel receptors. *Trends Biochem Sci* 33:491, 2008.
18. Rosen H, Gordon S: The role of the type 3 complement receptor in the induced recruitment of myelomonocytic cells to inflammatory sites in the mouse. *Am J Respir Cell Mol Biol* 3:3, 1990.
19. Fraser I, Hughes D, Gordon S: Divalent cation-independent macrophage adhesion inhibited by monoclonal antibody to murine scavenger receptor. *Nature* 364:343, 1993.
20. Gordon S, Unkeless JC, Cohn ZA: Induction of macrophage plasminogen activator by endotoxin stimulation and phagocytosis: Evidence for a two-stage process. *J Exp Med* 140:995, 1974.
21. Serhan CN, Aliberti J: Novel anti-inflammatory and proresolution lipid mediators in induction and modulation of phagocyte function, in *Phagocyte-Pathogen Interactions: Macrophages and the Host Response to Infection*, edited by DG Russell, S Gordon, p 267. ASM Press, Washington, DC, 2009.
22. Henson PM, Bratton DL: Recognition and removal of apoptotic cells, in *Phagocyte-Pathogen Interactions: Macrophages and the Host Response to Infection*, edited by DG Russell, S Gordon, p 341. ASM Press, Washington, DC, 2009.
23. Delamarre L, Pack M, Chang H, et al: Differential lysosomal proteolysis in antigen-presenting cells determines antigen fate. *Science* 307:1630, 2005.
24. Mariathasan S, Monack DM: Inflammasome adaptors and sensors: Intracellular regulators of infection and inflammation. *Nat Rev Immunol* 7:31, 2007.
25. Martinon F, Burns K, Tschopp J: The inflammasome: A molecular platform triggering activation of inflammatory caspases and processing of proIL-beta. *Mol Cell* 10:417, 2002.
26. Martinon F, Mayor A, Tschopp J: The inflammasomes: Guardians of the body. *Annu Rev Immunol* 27:229, 2009.
27. Deretic V: Autophagy: A fundamental cytoplasmic sanitation process operational in all cell types including macrophages, in *Phagocyte-Pathogen Interactions: Macrophages and the Host Response to Infection*, edited by DG Russell, S Gordon, p 419. ASM Press, Washington, DC, 2009.
28. Rabinovitch M: Professional and non-professional phagocytes: An introduction. *Trends Cell Biol* 5:85, 1995.
29. Plüddemann A, Hoe JC, Makepeace K, et al: The macrophage scavenger receptor a is host-protective in experimental meningococcal septicaemia. *PLoS Pathog* 5:e1000297, 2009.
30. Plüddemann A, Mukhopadhyay S, Gordon S: The interaction of macrophage receptors with bacterial ligands. *Expert Rev Mol Med* 8:1, 2006.
31. Plüddemann A, Neyen C, Gordon S: Macrophage scavenger receptors and host-derived ligands. *Methods* 43:207, 2007.
32. van Kooyk Y, Rabinovich GA: Protein-glycan interactions in the control of innate and adaptive immune responses. *Nat Immunol* 9:593, 2008.
33. Carroll MC: The complement system in regulation of adaptive immunity. *Nat Immunol* 5:981, 2004.

34. Nimmerjahn F, Ravetch JV: Fcgamma receptors as regulators of immune responses. *Nat Rev Immunol* 8:34, 2008.
35. Savill J, Dransfield I, Gregory C, Haslett C: A blast from the past: Clearance of apoptotic cells regulates immune responses. *Nat Rev Immunol* 2:965, 2002.
36. Medzhitov R: Origin and physiological roles of inflammation. *Nature* 454:428, 2008.
37. Areschoug T, Gordon S: Pattern recognition receptors and their role in innate immunity: focus on microbial protein ligands. *Contrib Microbiol* 15:45, 2008.
38. Gazzinelli RT, Fitzgerald K, Golenbock DT: Toll-like receptors, in *Phagocyte-Pathogen Interactions: Macrophages and the Host Response to Infection*, edited by DG Russell, S Gordon, p 107. ASM Press, Washington, DC, 2009.
39. McCoy CE, O'Neill LA: The role of toll-like receptors in macrophages. *Front Biosci* 13:62, 2008.
40. O'Neill LA: The interleukin-1 receptor/toll-like receptor superfamily: 10 years of progress. *Immunol Rev* 226:10, 2008.
41. Davidson DJ, Currie AJ, Bowdish DM, et al: IRAK-4 mutation (Q293X): Rapid detection and characterization of defective post-transcriptional TLR/IL-1R responses in human myeloid and non-myeloid cells. *J Immunol* 177:8202, 2006.
42. Khor CC, Chapman SJ, Vannberg FO, et al: A Mal functional variant is associated with protection against invasive pneumococcal disease, bacteremia, malaria and tuberculosis. *Nat Genet* 39:523, 2007.
43. Park BS, Song DH, Kim HM, et al: The structural basis of lipopolysaccharide recognition by the TLR4-MD-2 complex. *Nature* 458:1191, 2009.
44. Kagan JC, Su T, Horng T, et al: TRAM couples endocytosis of toll-like receptor 4 to the induction of interferon-beta. *Nat Immunol* 9:361, 2008.
45. Trinchieri G, Sher A: Cooperation of toll-like receptor signals in innate immune defence. *Nat Rev Immunol* 7:179, 2007.
46. Blander JM, Medzhitov R: Regulation of phagosome maturation by signals from toll-like receptors. *Science* 304:1014, 2004.
47. Blander JM, Medzhitov R: On regulation of phagosome maturation and antigen presentation. *Nat Immunol* 7:1029, 2006.
48. Beutler BA: TLRs and innate immunity. *Blood* 113:1399, 2009.
49. Awomoyi AA, Rallabhandi P, Pollin TI, et al: Association of TLR4 polymorphisms with symptomatic respiratory syncytial virus infection in high-risk infants and young children. *J Immunol* 179:3171, 2007.
50. Rosas M, Liddiard K, Kimberg M, et al: The induction of inflammation by dectin-1 *in vivo* is dependent on myeloid cell programming and the progression of phagocytosis. *J Immunol* 181:3549, 2008.
51. Taylor PR, Tsoni SV, Willment JA, et al: Dectin-1 is required for beta-glucan recognition and control of fungal infection. *Nat Immunol* 8:31, 2007.
52. Taylor PR, Gordon S, Martinez-Pomares L: The mannose receptor: Linking homeostasis and immunity through sugar recognition. *Trends Immunol* 26:104, 2005.
53. Gazi U, Martinez-Pomares L: Influence of the mannose receptor in host immune responses. *Immunobiology* 2009.
54. McKenzie EJ, Taylor PR, Stillion RJ, et al: Mannose receptor expression and function define a new population of murine dendritic cells. *J Immunol* 178:4975, 2007.
55. Brown GD: Dectin-1: A signalling non-TLR pattern-recognition receptor. *Nat Rev Immunol* 6:33, 2006.
56. Crocker PR, Paulson JC, Varki A: Siglecs and their roles in the immune system. *Nat Rev Immunol* 7:255, 2007.
57. Mukhopadhyay S, Gordon S: The role of scavenger receptors in pathogen recognition and innate immunity. *Immunobiology* 209:39, 2004.
58. Peiser L, Makepeace K, Plüddemann A, et al: Identification of *Neisseria meningitidis* nonlipopolysaccharide ligands for class A macrophage scavenger receptor by using a novel assay. *Infect Immun* 74:5191, 2006.
59. Hoebe K, Georgel P, Rutschmann S, et al: CD36 is a sensor of diacylglycerides. *Nature* 433:523, 2005.
60. Krieger M: Charting the fate of the "good cholesterol": Identification and characterization of the high-density lipoprotein receptor SR-BI. *Annu Rev Biochem* 68:523, 1999.
61. Means TK, Mylonakis E, Tampakakis E, et al: Evolutionarily conserved recognition and innate immunity to fungal pathogens by the scavenger receptors SCARF1 and CD36. *J Exp Med* 206:637, 2009.
62. Mantovani A, Bottazzi B, Doni A, Salvatori G: Phagocytes are a source of the fluid-phase pattern recognition receptor PTX3: Interplay between cellular and humoral innate immunity, in *Phagocyte-Pathogen Interactions: Macrophages and the Host Response to Infection*, edited by DG Russell, S Gordon, p 171. ASM Press, Washington, DC, 2009.
63. Helming L, Winter J, Gordon S: The scavenger receptor CD36 plays a role in cytokine-induced macrophage fusion. *J Cell Sci* 122:453, 2009.
64. Xia W, Hilgenbrink AR, Matteson EL, et al: A functional folate receptor is induced during macrophage activation and can be used to target drugs to activated macrophages. *Blood* 113:438, 2009.
65. Kristiansen M, Graversen JH, Jacobsen C, et al: Identification of the haemoglobin scavenger receptor. *Nature* 409:198, 2001.
66. Allen LA, Aderem A: Mechanisms of phagocytosis. *Curr Opin Immunol* 8:36, 1996.
67. Chimini G, Chavrier P: Function of Rho family proteins in actin dynamics during phagocytosis and engulfment. *Nat Cell Biol* 2: E191, 2000.
68. Fairn GD, Gershenzon E, Grinstein S: Membrane trafficking during phagosome formation and maturation, in *Phagocyte-Pathogen Interactions: Macrophages and the Host Response to Infection*, edited by DG Russell, S Gordon, p 209. ASM Press, Washington, DC, 2009.
69. Mukherjee S, Maxfield FR: Acidification of endosomes and phagosomes, in *Phagocyte-Pathogen Interactions: Macrophages and the Host Response to Infection*, edited by DG Russell, S Gordon, p 225. ASM Press, Washington, DC, 2009.
70. Swanson JA: Signaling for phagocytosis, in *Phagocyte-Pathogen Interactions: Macrophages and the Host Response to Infection*, edited by DG Russell, S Gordon, p 195. ASM Press, Washington, DC, 2009.
71. Greenberg S, Dale BM: Fc receptors and phagocytosis, in *Phagocyte-Pathogen Interactions: Macrophages and the Host Response to Infection*, edited by DG Russell, S Gordon, p 71. ASM Press, Washington, DC, 2009.
72. Kzhyshkowska J, Gordon S (eds): Vesicular trafficking in immune cells, in *Immunobiology* vol 24, pp 493–642. Elsevier GmbH, 2009.
73. Ridley AJ, Hall A: Snails, Swiss, and serum: The solution for Rac 'n' Rho. *Cell* 116:S23, 2004.
74. Bezbradica JS, Medzhitov R: Integration of cytokine and heterologous receptor signaling pathways. *Nat Immunol* 10:333, 2009.
75. Michl J, Pieczonka MM, Unkeless JC, Silverstein SC: Effects of immobilized immune complexes on Fc- and complement-receptor function in resident and thioglycollate-elicited mouse peritoneal macrophages. *J Exp Med* 150:607, 1979.
76. Swanson JA: Shaping cups into phagosomes and macropinosomes. *Nat Rev Mol Cell Biol* 9:639, 2008.
77. Jutras I, Desjardins M: Phagocytosis: At the crossroads of innate and adaptive immunity. *Annu Rev Cell Dev Biol* 21:511, 2005.
78. Touret N, Paroutis P, Terebiznik M, et al: Quantitative and dynamic assessment of the contribution of the ER to phagosome formation. *Cell* 123:157, 2005.
79. Rohde K, Yates RM, Purdy GE, Russell DG: Mycobacterium tuberculosis and the environment within the phagosome. *Immunol Rev* 219:37, 2007.
80. Bogdan C: Mechanisms and consequences of persistence of intracellular pathogens: Leishmaniasis as an example. *Cell Microbiol* 10:1221, 2008.
81. Portnoy DA, Auerbuch V, Glomski IJ: The cell biology of *Listeria* monocytogenes infection: The intersection of bacterial pathogenesis and cell-mediated immunity. *J Cell Biol* 158:409, 2002.
82. Swanson MS: Autophagy: Eating for good health. *J Immunol* 177:4945, 2006.
83. Ganz T: Iron in innate immunity: Starve the invaders. *Curr Opin Immunol* 21:63, 2009.
84. Giodini A, Rahner C, Cresswell P: Receptor-mediated phagocytosis elicits cross-presentation in nonprofessional antigen-presenting cells. *Proc Natl Acad Sci U S A* 106:3324, 2009.
85. Helming L, Tomasello E, Kyriakides TR, et al: Essential role of DAP12 signaling in macrophage programming into a fusion-competent state. *Sci Signal* 1:ra11, 2008.
86. Sidiropoulos PI, Goulielmos G, Voloudakis GK, et al: Inflammasomes and rheumatic diseases: Evolving concepts. *Ann Rheum Dis* 67:1382, 2008.
87. Ye Z, Ting JP: NLR, the nucleotide-binding domain leucine-rich repeat containing gene family. *Curr Opin Immunol* 20:3, 2008.
88. Ryan JG, Kastner DL: Fevers, genes, and innate immunity. *Curr Top Microbiol Immunol* 321:169, 2008.
89. Kzhyshkowska J, Krusell L: Cross-talk between endocytic clearance and secretion in macrophages. *Immunobiology* 241:576, 2009.
90. Kaiser F, O'Garra A: Cytokines and macrophages and dendritic cells: key modulators of immune response, in *Phagocyte-Pathogen Interactions: Macrophages and the Host Response to Infection*, edited by DG Russell, S Gordon, p 281. ASM Press, Washington, DC, 2009.
91. Lieu ZZ, Lock JG, Hammond LA, et al: A *trans*-Golgi network golgin is required for the regulated secretion of TNF in activated macrophages *in vivo*. *Proc Natl Acad Sci U S A* 105:3351, 2008.
92. Shurety W, Merino-Trigo A, Brown D, et al: Localization and post-Golgi trafficking of tumor necrosis factor-alpha in macrophages. *J Interferon Cytokine Res* 20:427, 2000.
93. Stow JL, Ching Low P, Offenhauser C, Sangermani D: Cytokine secretion in macrophages and other cells: Pathways and mediators. *Immunobiology* 214:601, 2009.
94. Kuijpers TW, van den Berg TK, Roos D: Neutrophils forever. . . in *Phagocyte-Pathogen Interactions: Macrophages and the Host Response to Infection*, edited by DG Russell, S Gordon, p 3. ASM Press, Washington, DC, 2009.
95. McPhail LC: SH3-dependent assembly of the phagocyte NADPH oxidase. *J Exp Med* 180:2011, 1994.
96. Bogdan C: Regulation and antimicrobial function of inducible nitric oxide synthase in phagocytes, in *Phagocyte-Pathogen Interactions: Macrophages and the Host Response to Infection*, edited by DG Russell, S Gordon, p 367. ASM Press, Washington, DC, 2009.
97. O'Shea JJ, Murray PJ: Cytokine signaling modules in inflammatory responses. *Immunity* 28:477, 2008.
98. Garcia-Sastre A, Biron CA: Type 1 interferons and the virus-host relationship: A lesson in detente. *Science* 312:879, 2006.
99. Bogdan C, Mattner J, Schleicher U: The role of type I interferons in non-viral infections. *Immunol Rev* 202:33, 2004.
100. Dunn GP, Koebel CM, Schreiber RD: Interferons, immunity and cancer immunoediting. *Nat Rev Immunol* 6:836, 2006.
101. Sharif MN, Tassiulas I, Hu Y, et al: IFN-alpha priming results in a gain of proinflammatory function by IL-10: Implications for systemic lupus erythematosus pathogenesis. *J Immunol* 172:6476, 2004.

102. Herrero C, Hu X, Li WP, et al: Reprogramming of IL-10 activity and signaling by IFN-gamma. *J Immunol* 171:5034, 2003.
103. Vinh DC, Holland SM: Macrophage classical activation, in *Phagocyte-Pathogen Interactions: Macrophages and the Host Response to Infection*, edited by DG Russell, S Gordon, p 301. ASM Press, Washington, DC, 2009.
104. Martinez FO, Helming L, Gordon S: Alternative activation of macrophages: An immunologic functional perspective. *Annu Rev Immunol* 27:451, 2009.
105. Henry SC, Daniell XG, Burroughs AR, et al: Balance of Irgm protein activities determines IFN-gamma-induced host defense. *J Leukoc Biol* 85:877, 2009.
106. Varin A, Gordon S: Alternative activation of macrophages: Immune function and cellular biology. *Immunobiology* 214:630, 2009.
107. Lin DA, Boyce JA: Lysophospholipids as mediators of immunity. *Adv Immunol* 89:141, 2006.
108. Barclay AN, Wright GJ, Brooke G, Brown MH: CD200 and membrane protein interactions in the control of myeloid cells. *Trends Immunol* 23:285, 2002.
109. Balkwill F: Tumour necrosis factor and cancer. *Nat Rev Cancer* 9:361, 2009.
110. Conner SD, Schmid SL: Regulated portals of entry into the cell. *Nature* 422:37, 2003.
111. Stuart LM, Ezekowitz RA: Phagocytosis and comparative innate immunity: Learning on the fly. *Nat Rev Immunol* 8:131, 2008.
112. Cross AR, Segal AW: The NADPH oxidase of professional phagocytes—Prototype of the NOX electron transport chain systems. *Biochim Biophys Acta* 1657:1, 2004.
113. DeCoursey TE: During the respiratory burst, do phagocytes need proton channels or potassium channels, or both? *Sci STKE* 2004:pe21, 2004.
114. Gordon S: Alternative activation of macrophages. *Nat Rev Immunol* 3:23, 2003.
115. Lewis CE, Hughes R: Inflammation and breast cancer. Microenvironmental factors regulating macrophage function in breast tumours: Hypoxia and angiopoietin-2. *Breast Cancer Res* 9:209, 2007.
116. Lattin J, Zidar DA, Schroder K, et al: G-protein-coupled receptor expression, function, and signaling in macrophages. *J Leukoc Biol* 82:16, 2007.

CHAPTER 69

PRODUCTION, DISTRIBUTION, AND FATE OF MONOCYTES AND MACROPHAGES

Siamon Gordon and Annette Plüddemann

SUMMARY

Monocytes and macrophages play an important role in hematology, both as a component of the hematopoietic system and within the stroma and tissue microenvironment where they contribute trophic and clearance functions. They constitute a widely dispersed cellular system throughout the body, interacting with host cells and foreign invaders through their versatile biosynthetic and secretory responses, to maintain physiologic homeostasis. They are specialized migratory or sessile phagocytes, present within the circulation and extravascular tissue compartment, contributing to diverse hematologic diseases, directly and by production of bioactive products. Because of extensive heterogeneity and plasticity, their centrality has not always been recognized by hematologists. The origin, life span, and functions of the monocyte are the focus of this chapter, including their relevance to hematologic health and disease in humans, based on current understanding of their properties. The relationship of monocytes and macrophages to dendritic cells, and monocyte-derived cells with a specialized immunologic role in T-lymphocyte activation, are described. Together, macrophages and dendritic cells are major antigen-presenting cells, contributing to host defense, innate and acquired immunity, and inflammation, as well as noninfectious disease processes, both within and outside the lymphohematopoietic organs.

METHODS OF MACROPHAGE STUDY

The history[1] and nomenclature of the family of macrophages and closely related cells have been reviewed extensively. We refer to the mononuclear phagocyte system (MPS), collectively, and consider macrophage heterogeneity in different tissue compartments in detail. Aspects of their morphology and contribution to clinical conditions are found in Chap. 68. This chapter deals with the basic cellular and molecular properties of monocytes and macrophages in general, as well as more specifically within the hematopoietic system. There are many useful texts and reviews available for further study; a selection is found in the references section of this chapter and Chap. 68.[2–6] A recent set of recorded lectures on relevant topics is available from Henry Stewart Talks.[7]

Our current knowledge is based on long-standing methods of intravital labeling with carbon or carmine; *in situ* phenotyping with gene expression analysis and immunocytochemistry (antigen markers); cell isolation and characterization (fluorescence-activated cell sorting [FACS]); and *in vitro* culture (colony growth in semisolid media, and liquid cultures with or without growth factors and cytokines) of cells obtained from fetal liver, marrow, and spleen. Peritoneal macrophages harvested from unstimulated mice or after injection of inflammatory stimuli such as thioglycollate broth and Biogel polyacrylamide beads have been particularly useful.[8,9] More complex stromal mixed cultures supplemented with dexamethasone yield macrophages with different properties, perhaps closer to an *in vivo* phenotype than conventional culture. Other standard methods have been used to reconstitute irradiated mice with donor marrow, which repopulates the radiosensitive macrophages in tissue. Adoptive transfer of mature macrophages is less satisfactory.[10] Clearance studies with labeled particles have been employed traditionally to probe phagocytic function *in vivo*. Clodronate-loaded liposomes have also proved useful to deplete phagocytic subpopulations *in vivo*.[11]

There has been a resurgence of interest in the *in situ* analysis of macrophages in the intact, living animal. Genetic/ribonucleic acid interference manipulation, more recently with macrophage-specific/restricted promoters, has been used to knock down macrophage genes or messenger RNA, and to mark cells with fluorescent labels such as green fluorescent protein. Of particular value in tracing cell origins and distribution has been the use of fractalkine receptor-transgenics,[12] and myeloid-specific lysozyme-Cre for targeted ablation.[13] Diphtheria-toxin species differences in sensitivity have also proved useful.[14] Random chemical mutagenesis has been spectacularly successful in validating known, and discovering novel gene targets that affect macrophage functions.[15,16] A wider range of experimental models (*Drosophila*, zebra fish) have facilitated interspecies comparisons of macrophage migration and phagocytosis *in vivo*.[17–19] The analysis of microRNA expression[20] and functions is still in its infancy and is likely to generate important insights into gene expression in health and disease. Combined with improved imaging methods (fluorescent, nuclear magnetic resonance imaging-based, 2-photon microscopy), new insights have been obtained regarding the dynamic behavior of macrophages and dendritic cells (DCs) *in vivo*.[21] *In vitro*, there has been progress in harnessing embryonic stem cell differentiation into macrophages and DCs, opening the possibility of introducing mutations into human genes, to complement the naturally occurring material derived from human inborn errors and resultant genetic diseases.[22,23]

However, there are still formidable problems in the interpretation and exploitation of these methods of analysis. Although individual-labeled cells can be followed in accessible tissues or *ex vivo*, the resolution, isolation, and characterization of important embedded macrophage populations are limiting. Methods of isolation from solid organs, for example, brain and even liver and gut, are prone to artifact and macrophages are profoundly affected by removal from their natural tissue environment. Many of the genetic manipulations introduced by transgenesis are leaky and not uniform, not surprising in the light of macrophage heterogeneity. Although the fate of recently recruited cells from blood into tissues can be tracked more easily, the slowly turning over resident populations are less easily accessed, resulting in bias. Above all, it remains difficult to obtain quantitative information about cell markers and functions within the living host.

Abbreviations and acronyms that appear in this chapter include: CR, complement receptor; DC, dendritic cell; DC-SIGN, dendritic cell-specific intercellular adhesion molecule-3–grabbing nonintegrin; EMR, epidermal growth factor module-containing mucin-like hormone receptor; FACS, fluorescence-activated cell sorting; FcR, Fc receptor; GM-CSF, granulocyte-macrophage colony-stimulating factor; IFN-γ, interferon-γ; IL, interleukin; LPS, lipopolysaccharide; MARCO, macrophage receptor with a collagenous structure; M-CSF, macrophage colony-stimulating factor; M-CSFR, macrophage colony-stimulating factor receptor; MR, mannose receptor; Sn, sialoadhesin; SR-A, scavenger receptor A; TGF, transforming growth factor; TLR, toll-like receptor; TNF-α, tumor necrosis factor-α.

Finally, there are obvious difficulties with human experimentation *in vivo*. Induced skin blisters, for example, make it possible to collect fluid and cells from sites of inflammation.[24] However, the low frequency of monocytes compared with neutrophils limits the use of *ex vivo* indium-labeled cells for transfer studies *in vivo*. Nevertheless, clinical syndromes provide a rich resource, the natural history of human disease, providing new information of monocyte and macrophage distribution, fate, and function within the intact organism.

MACROPHAGE DEVELOPMENT

Macrophages and related ameboid phagocytic cells, ancient in the evolution of multicellular organisms, are the main leukocytes responsible for innate immunity and tissue remodeling, as documented by Metchnikoff in his pioneering studies on invertebrates,[25] and confirmed by contemporary studies on *Drosophila melanogaster*.[19] In mammals, much of our knowledge of macrophage ontogeny derives from studies in the mouse. After origins from an aortic mesonephric site, the best understood phases of macrophage development occur during mid fetal development, in the yolk sac, followed by fetal liver, spleen, and marrow, before and after birth.[26] The association of macrophages with definitive erythropoiesis is a striking feature of fetal liver hematopoiesis from approximately day 12 of mouse development; macrophages then, for the first time, become intimately associated with nucleated erythroblasts, reaching a peak of hematopoietic cluster formation at day 14. The role of stromal macrophages in hematopoiesis within the adult is illustrated and discussed further below (see "Growth, Differentiation, and Turnover of Monocytes and Macrophages" below).

The association of macrophages with erythroblasts is mediated by surface adhesion molecules,[27,28] including a poorly characterized divalent cation-dependent receptor and the sialic acid-binding molecule sialoadhesin (Siglec1).[29] The potential trophic functions of stromal macrophages in hematopoietic clusters is poorly understood, as is the considerable role of macrophages in iron and heme metabolism. Macrophages interact with cells in numerous ways; however, during erythropoiesis a special phagocytic process allows for the removal of pyknotic erythroid nuclei during the final stages of erythropoiesis. The mechanism of recognition of membrane-bound erythroid nuclei is not clear, nor its relationship to the uptake of apoptotic cells elsewhere during development. The production of granulocytes from progenitors also involves macrophage–myeloblast clusters and similar adhesion receptors. Once fetal liver hematopoiesis declines before and after birth, the macrophages in the liver adopt the features of resident Kupffer cells. The stromal macrophages associate with developing blood cells within islands of clustered cells, a feature of hematopoiesis throughout life, as observed in animals and in humans.[30] During fetal life, monocytes and macrophages are distributed through the developing vasculature, providing ameboid, phagocytic cells implicated in tissue remodeling, for example, sculpting of digits,[31] and growth of the central nervous system.[32] Blood monocytes seed resident tissue macrophage populations throughout the organism, and these cells proliferate more readily in the fetus than in later life; the adhesion molecules, chemotactic signals, and receptors involved during this constitutive phase of distribution are poorly defined, but it is independent of the β_2-integrin CD11b/CD18, which plays a role in myelomonocytic cell recruitment induced by inflammation in the adult.[33,34] The appearance of macrophages during development has been correlated with fibrous scar formation after injury.[31] In sum, macrophages play a major role during development, both in hematopoiesis and in extravascular tissues, and much remains to be learned regarding their properties in the fetus, not least in humans.

GROWTH, DIFFERENTIATION, AND TURNOVER OF MONOCYTES AND MACROPHAGES

Figure 69–1 gives an overview of differentiation of monocytic cells in the adult.[35] The origins of monocytes from multipotential hematopoietic (progenitors colony-forming units, spleen [CFU-S]) and committed precursors (colony-forming units, culture [CFU-C]) and the role of lineage-restricted growth factors such as macrophage colony-stimulating factor (M-CSF) and granulocyte-macrophage colony-stimulating factor (GM-CSF) have been studied extensively, but new details are still emerging. Monocytes share precursors with other hematopoietic cells and are closely related to granulocytes. Monocytic precursors are the source of adult tissue macrophages, as well as of myeloid DCs and osteoclasts. Their relationship to B lymphocytes and to plasmacytoid DCs is still unclear, as plasmacytoid DCs express a range of myeloid as well as lymphoid markers. There is a considerable body of knowledge about the specific growth factors and their receptors, and growing knowledge of the nature and role of transcription factors involved in monocyte/macrophage differentiation.[36] Figure 69–2 illustrates how the balance of repressive and activating transcription factors, especially PU.1, is thought to regulate the expression and the formation of active chromatin at macrophage colony-stimulating factor receptor (M-CSFR), a prototypic macrophage-specific gene.[37–39] Genetic and cellular abnormalities in growth and differentiation pathways underlie myeloid leukemogenesis, though rarely giving rise to monocytic leukemia.

Growth Factors

M-CSF and GM-CSF are the major growth factors implicated in monocyte and macrophage differentiation. Others such as interleukin (IL)-3 and IL-4 are not specific for this lineage, nor do they result in such marked proliferative expansion. M-CSF promotes survival as well as growth and differentiation of macrophages, acting through a specific receptor (M-CSFR), also known as c-fms, an oncogene that has been extensively used as a lineage marker for FACS analysis (CD115) and transgenesis.[40,41] The biology of M-CSF has been reviewed[42] and its role in macrophage and osteoclast development is illustrated in Figure 69–3. The naturally occurring mouse mutant, op/op, gives rise to M-CSF deficiency and osteopetrosis, with marked or partial deficiency in monocyte and selected tissue macrophage populations; DC numbers are unaffected.[43] Unlike PU.1 deficiency, the op/op mouse is viable, though its reproductive ability is impaired, because M-CSF also plays an important role in the reproductive system. Uterine epithelium is a rich source of M-CSF, inducing monocyte-macrophage recruitment, growth and differentiation, and upregulating scavenger receptor expression, cell adhesion, and endocytosis of modified low-density lipoproteins and other polyanionic ligands. M-CSF is produced in a soluble and proteoglycan-linked form, is present in plasma, and has been implicated in atherosclerosis and tumor-dependent recruitment of monocytes and macrophages. The size of the growth burst induced by M-CSF depends on the differentiation of the target cell, decreasing markedly as the precursors mature into monocytes and macrophages. Adhesion and inflammatory stimuli enhance the response to growth factors and can result in macrophage proliferation at peripheral sites, for example, in granulomata.

GM-CSF has a broader myeloid target profile. It is produced by many cells, including macrophages themselves, especially after inflammatory stimuli such as lipopolysaccharide (LPS), and it enhances production of monocytes and macrophages with a different morphology to that induced by M-CSF. GM-CSF is required for myeloid DC differentiation *in vitro* and has been widely used, alone and in combination with cytokines such as IL-4 or transforming growth factor (TGF)-β, to produce DC from mouse marrow or from human monocytes in cell

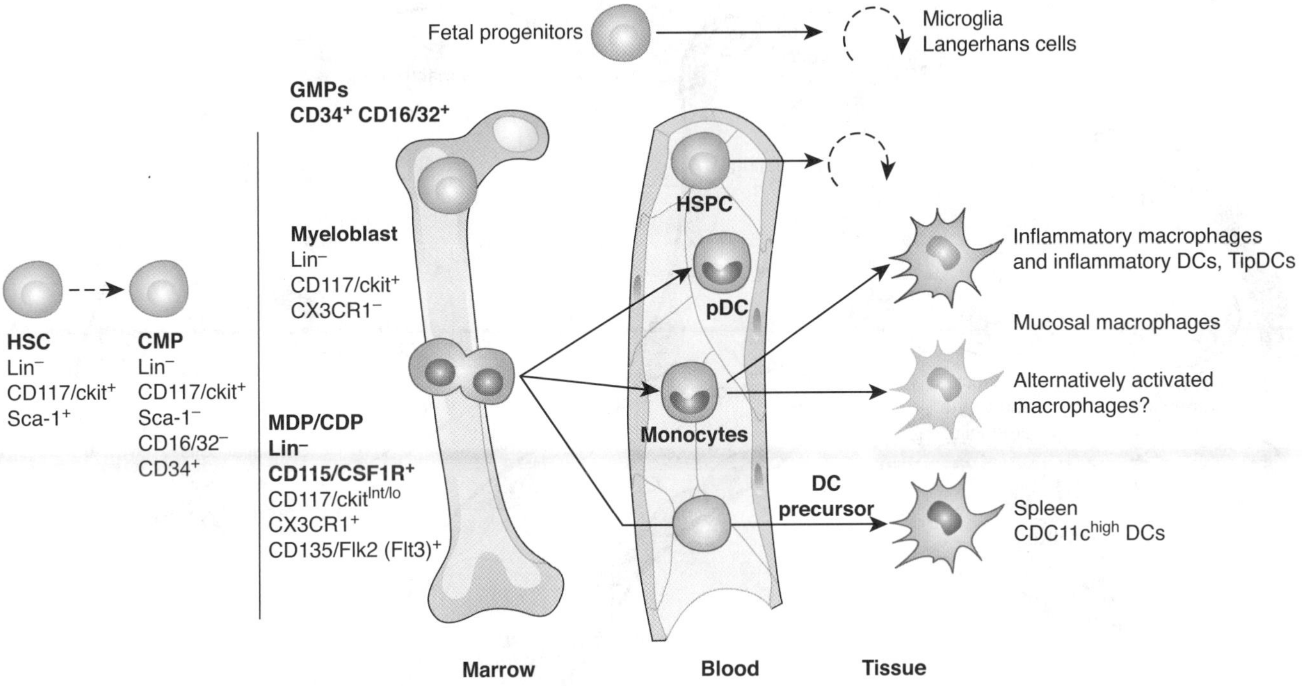

FIGURE 69–1. Differentiation of the macrophage/dendritic cell (DC) progenitor and origin of macrophage and DC subsets. CDP, common dendritic cell precursor; CMP, common myeloid progenitor; GMP, granulocyte/macrophage progenitor; HSC, hematopoietic stem cell; HSPCs, hematopoietic stem and progenitor cells; MDP, macrophage/DC progenitor; pDC, plasmacytoid dendritic cell. For further details see Auffray C, Sieweke MH, Geissmann F.[35] *(Reprinted with permission from Auffray C, Sieweke MH, Geissmann F[35] and the* Annual Review of Immunology, *Volume 27, copyright 2009, by Annual Reviews, www.annualreviews.org.)*

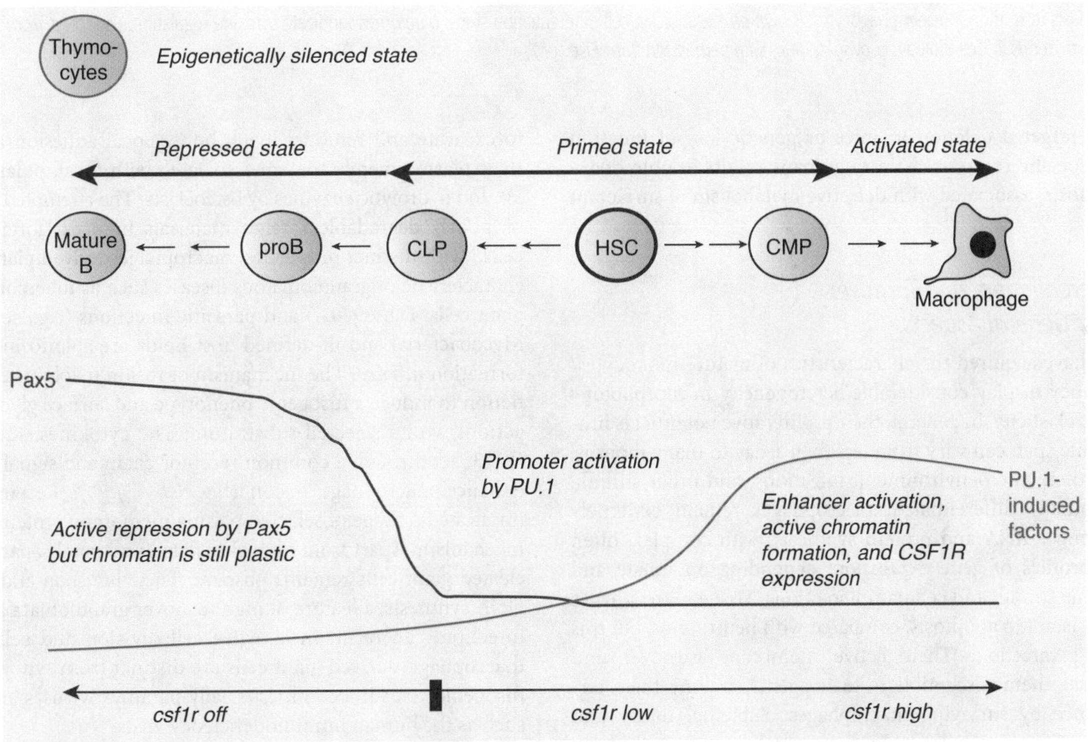

FIGURE 69–2. The balance of repressive and activating transcription factors regulates the expression and the formation of active chromatin at *M-CSFR*. The transcription factor PU.1 and the macrophage colony-stimulating factor (M-CSF) receptor (M-CSFR) are both central to myelopoiesis and macrophage differentiation. *PU.1* is essential for correct myelopoiesis. Expression of both genes is switched on at the onset of hematopoietic development, but their tissue-specific expression is regulated differently. *M-CSFR* is crucial for macrophage development and its expression is dependent on the expression of PU.1. The B-cell–specific transcription factor Pax5 is crucial for the activation of a B-cell–specific gene expression program, as well as for the repression of lineage inappropriate genes. *(Reprinted from Bonifer C, Hoogenkamp M, Krysinska H, Tagoh H,[37] from* Seminars in Immunology, *copyright 2008, with permission of Elsevier.)*

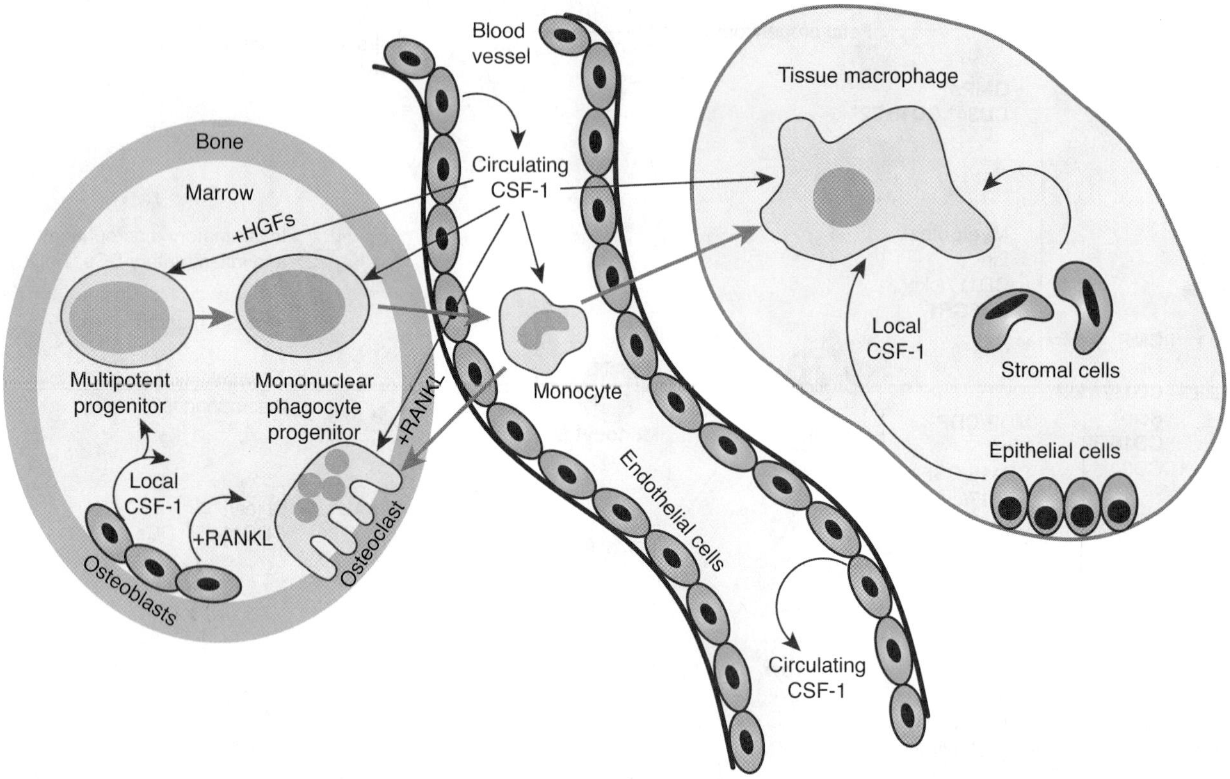

FIGURE 69–3. Regulation of macrophage and osteoclast development by macrophage colony-stimulating factor (M-CSF). Circulating M-CSF, produced by endothelial cells in blood vessels, together with locally produced M-CSF regulates the survival, proliferation, and differentiation of mononuclear phagocytes and osteoclasts. The cytokine synergizes with hematopoietic growth factors (HGFs) to generate mononuclear progenitor cells from multipotent progenitors, and with receptor activator of nuclear factor-κB ligand (RANKL) to generate osteoclasts from mononuclear phagocytes. *Brown arrows* indicate cell differentiation steps; *blue arrows* indicate cytokine regulation. *(Adapted from Pixley FJ, Stanley ER.[42] Reprinted from* Trends in Cell Biology, *copyright 2004, with permission from Elsevier.)*

culture.[44,45] Its targeted deletion in mice or genetic loss of function mutants of its specific receptor chain in humans results in pulmonary alveolar proteinosis, associated with defective metabolism of surfactant in the lung.[46]

Survival, Differentiation, and Turnover of Monocytes: General Aspects

Once the cells have acquired the characteristics of mature monocytes/macrophages, they display considerable heterogeneity in morphology and phenotypic plasticity. In general, their proliferative potential is limited, and their life span can vary from less than 1 day to many months, depending on their microenvironment, infections, and other stimuli. Although terminally differentiated, macrophages remain extremely active in messenger RNA and protein synthesis, with complex, often characteristic profiles of gene expression, depending on innate and acquired immune stimuli and cellular interactions. Tissue macrophages are relatively resistant to apoptosis, compared with neutrophils, but this changes during infection. Their active membrane turnover and endocytosis make them susceptible to toxic agents, making them targets for clearance by surviving macrophages. Sublethal injury and infection can also induce autophagy, increasingly recognized as an important component of inflammatory and infectious diseases.

The remarkable ability of macrophages to undergo homotypic cell–cell fusion results in giant cell formation. This is a feature of osteoclast differentiation, depending on M-CSF and the tumor necrosis factor (TNF) family member receptor activator of nuclear factor-κB (RANK) ligand, which act on monocytic precursors to yield catabolic cells able to excavate and remodel living bone. Local adhesion and ruffling of their plasma membrane are associated with focal, polarized release of H^+ and hydrolytic enzymes by osteoclasts. The attempted uptake of non- or poorly degradable foreign materials induces "foreign body giant cells," with distinct properties; macrophage-derived giant cells are also characteristic of granulomatous diseases such as tuberculosis (Langhans giant cells; Fig. 69–4A) and parasitic infections (e.g., schistosomiasis). Mycobacterial and ill-defined host lipids are able to induce giant-cell formation *in vitro*. The mechanism of fusion involves cellular differentiation to induce a fusogenic phenotype and surface glycoprotein interactions with a selected substratum; Th2 cytokines, such as IL-4 and IL-13, act through a common receptor chain and signaling pathway to enhance macrophage fusion (Fig. 69–4B).[47–50] Recent research has implicated a range of selected plasma membrane proteins in the fusion mechanism. Apart from osteoclasts, the functional capacity of multinucleated giant cells remains obscure. Their life span and stability vary; DNA synthesis, a feature of high turnover granulomata associated with infection, can result in abortive cell division and cell death. These macrophage-derived giant cells are distinct from syncytia induced by fusogenic virus infection, especially paramyxoviruses and retroviruses such as the human immunodeficiency virus.

MONOCYTE HETEROGENEITY

Monocytes are defined as the population of differentiated cells present in the circulation, with classical morphologic features (see Chap. 68), and include the less-defined precursors able to give rise to myeloid DCs and osteoclasts. Because of their ready availability from human blood

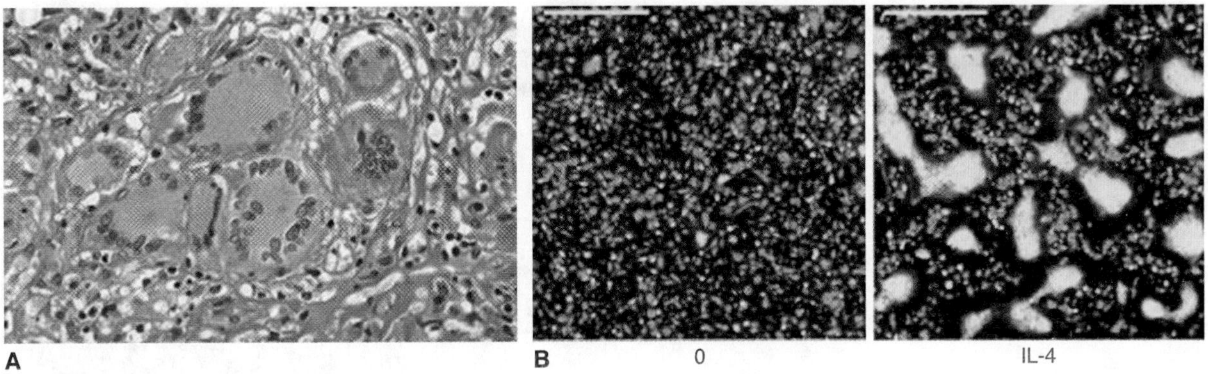

FIGURE 69–4. A. Microscopic image of Langhans giant cells, tuberculosis induced. *(Reproduced with permission from http://granuloma.homestead.com/giant_cell_images.html.)* **B.** Homotypic macrophage fusion induced *in vitro* by the Th2 cytokine, interleukin (IL)-4. Thioglycollate-elicited mouse peritoneal macrophages were labeled separately with green and red fluorescent markers, mixed and cultivated overnight in the presence of IL-4. Cell fusion is indicated by the appearance of yellow macrophage giant cells. For further details see Helming L, Gordon S.[48]

and the sensitive methods now available to analyze their phenotype *ex vivo* (FACS, microarray, immuno-, and cytochemistry), human monocytes have been more amenable to study, whereas in the mouse, analysis of precursor–product relationship and tissue distribution have provided new insights into the fate and heterogeneity of the circulating population. The number of monocytes in the circulation depends on constitutive, steady-state production and delivery from marrow, possibly from marginated pools in spleen, as well as adhesion and diapedesis in response to unknown stimuli and enhanced recruitment in response to peripheral stimuli such as infection and inflammation. M-CSF and glucocorticosteroids affect their level and phenotype, as do metabolic stimuli; Chap. 71 describes clinical conditions that give rise to monocytosis. The biochemical properties and functions of monocytes are described in Chap. 68. They are relatively radioresistant once entering the circulation, where they persist for 12 to 48 hours as motile cells, with an ability to phagocytose particles and to adhere transiently or more stably to arterial as well as microvascular endothelium, thus modulating their phagocytic ability. Depending on interactions with the vessel wall and local differentiation, monocytes are able to crawl along and patrol the intravascular surface utilizing CD11a, a β_2-integrin-dependent property.[35] Monocytes enter tissues to become macrophages or may be able to reverse migrate into the circulatory pool as myeloid DC.[51] Mature macrophages lining the endothelium can also detach and recirculate, for example, filled with lipid stores as foam cells in atherosclerosis, and circulate heavily laden with erythroid breakdown products in malaria.

The precursors of myeloid DC and osteoclasts may represent a subpopulation, whose further differentiation depends on cytokines and local factors in the vessel wall, marrow, and other tissues. *Ex vivo* substantial numbers of monocytes give rise to myeloid DC after treatment with GM-CSF and IL-4.[45] Monocytes that differentiate into macrophages do not recirculate for the most part, but persist for varying times as "resident" tissue cells that turn over locally, especially in lymph nodes. It is not known if the constitutive exit from blood is a stochastic process or whether such precursors are postcoded for particular tissues.

Phenotypic heterogeneity of monocyte populations has become a topic of intense interest to investigators, thanks to the availability of surface antigens/receptors such as CD14, CD16 (human), and Ly6C (mouse), and analysis of chemokine/receptor expression, especially fractalkine receptor (CX_3CR) and CCR2.[52] Figure 69–5 illustrates the subsets and tissue progeny established by the use of genetically manipulated mice and Table 69–1 compares expression of markers to characterize monocyte subsets in mouse and human blood. The relationship of monocyte precursor subsets that give rise to inflammatory tissue macrophages and DCs is better defined than to resident cells, which turn over more slowly. Current studies aim to elucidate the subset origin of other recruited populations, for example, in atherosclerosis, normal CNS, and tumors, and in response to metabolic, traumatic, or degenerative injury. Conceptually, it is still not clear how stable these apparently distinct subsets are or whether they represent part of a continuous phenotypic spectrum, arising by modulation of subpopulations rather than irreversible, true differentiation. Separation and microarray analysis of freshly isolated monocytes will yield further information regarding this question, providing novel markers and diagnostic signatures. Removal from an *in vivo* environment, as well as *in vitro* artifacts, can profoundly alter the phenotype and function of monocytes in such studies. Imaging and *in situ* analysis may enable single-cell direct studies of their fate.

Resident Macrophage Populations in Adult Tissues: General Considerations

It is important to describe first the nature of those macrophages present throughout the body as resident populations, in the absence of overt inflammation, before considering the altered monocyte-derived macrophages recruited to local sites by infectious or sterile inflammatory (e.g., metabolic) stimuli. Although the properties of such elicited macrophages are well established and are described in Chap. 68, the functions of resident macrophages, especially in different organs, are still mysterious and are considered in outline here, with further details in Chap. 68.

The use of differentiation antigens such as F4/80 and cd68 (mouse) and CD68 (human) has made it possible to define resident macrophage populations in mouse tissues,[53] and to compare their anatomic relationships in the two species (Table 69–2). F4/80 (EMR1), a member of a family of epidermal growth factor-7 transmembrane (EGF-TM7) plasma membrane molecules, is broadly present and almost exclusive to macrophages (Fig. 69–6A–C).[54,55] It is related to G-protein–coupled chemokine receptors in structure, but has a large epidermal growth factor domain extracellular extension, thought to be involved in adhesion to extracellular matrix. The human members of this family are more broadly present on myeloid cells; epidermal growth factor module-containing mucin-like hormone receptor 2 (EMR2) is a useful tissue marker for human macrophages, although it is also present in neutrophils and immature DCs (Fig. 69–6A). The F4/80 antigen has been implicated in peripheral tolerance,

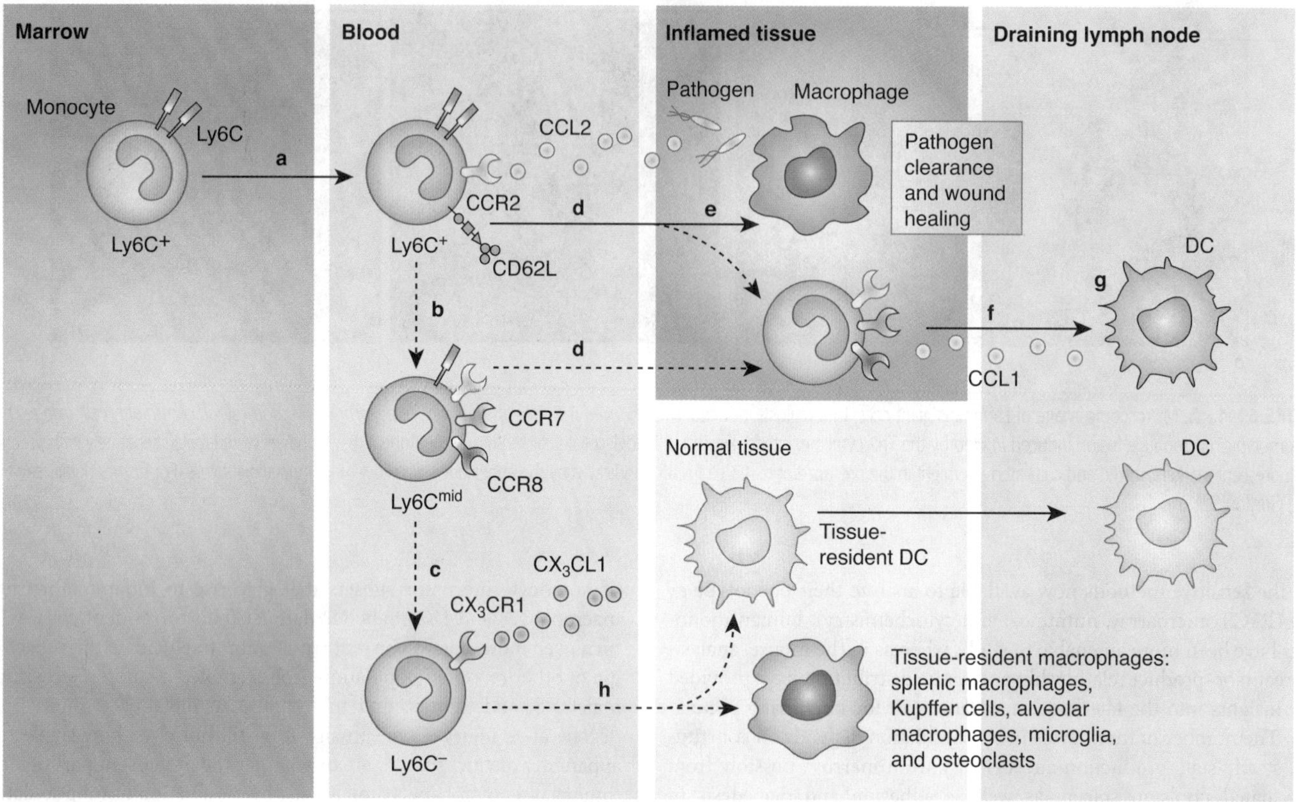

FIGURE 69–5. Heterogeneity of monocytes in blood and the contribution of different subsets to resident and inflammatory macrophages and dendritic cells (DCs) in tissues. For further details see Gordon S, Taylor PR.[52] *(Reproduced with permission from Gordon S, Taylor PR,[52] copyright Wiley-VCH Verlag GmbH & Co. KGaA.)*

by studies in wild-type and F4/80 knockout mice.[56] CD68 is a pan-macrophage endosomal/lysosomal antigen, modulated by phagocytosis and inflammation.[57] Additional macrophage antigen markers useful for immunocytochemical and FACS analysis include Siglec1 (Fig. 69–6D), a sialic acid-binding lectin, the β_2 integrins CD11b/CD18 (Mac1, CR3) and CD11c, present on DCs and selected, especially alveolar, macrophages.[58] Receptor antigen markers include scavenger receptor (SR)-A,[59] a broadly expressed macrophage receptor additionally found on sinusoidal endothelium, whereas MARCO (macrophage receptor with collagenous structure), a related collagenous SR, is more restricted in expression.[60] Additional markers include lectins such as the macrophage mannose/fucose receptor (MR; Fig. 69–6E).[61] CD163, a receptor for hemoglobin–haptoglobin complexes, is induced by glucocorticosteroids and IL-10.[62] Other complement receptors (CRs) and Fc receptors (FcRs) are described in Chap. 68.

The F4/80 antigen is remarkably stable to fixation and is mainly expressed on the plasma membrane, making it possible to define intercellular relationships of mouse macrophages with precision[63] and to reconstruct a putative map of extravascular migration of macrophages in tissue. F4/80+ macrophages can themselves be endothelial in location, or adopt a perivascular distribution. They are found at most interstitial sites and in association with simple or more complex epithelia, which they can cross to be "free" in serosal cavities (peritoneal, pleural, pericardial) and in the pulmonary alveoli. Although relatively "fixed" in tissues ("histiocytes") and more adherent than DCs, macrophages are induced to migrate by inflammatory stimuli, often ending up in draining lymph nodes, their graveyard.

Taken together, the resident macrophages in tissues constitute a major dispersed organ system, responsive to endogenous and exogenous stimuli; they are highly active in uptake of particles and soluble ligands, providing not only sentinels for defense at portals of entry, but also mediating the clearance of damaged or dying cells and modulating the properties of viable neighboring cells. In sum, these cells provide a homeostatic, trophic function that is often overlooked in considering their role in cytotoxicity and antimicrobial host defense. The properties of macrophages in hematolymphoid organs and other tissues, with special relevance to hematologic aspects, are discussed in detail. The constitutive distribution and heterogeneity of DCs are described elsewhere.[64–66]

HEMATOPOIETIC ORGANS

Marrow

It is often overlooked that mature macrophages are important constituents of the hematopoietic stroma,[67] along with fibroblastic mesenchymal cells, osteoblasts, and endothelial cells, contributing to hematopoiesis beyond their own differentiation (Figs. 69–7 to 69–9). Stromal macrophages in hematopoietic island clusters associate with developing erythroid and other granulocytic cells through nonphagocytic, cell–cell adhesion receptors, such as sialoadhesin and a divalent cation-dependent receptor,[28] as described for fetal liver. Care is required in isolating such cells because of their fragile processes and the disruption of clusters. The potential trophic functions provided by stromal macrophages are ill-defined but include surface-expressed and secreted growth factors and cytokines. Stromal macrophages are actively endocytic and clear erythroid nuclei and apoptotic hematopoietic cells as required, rapidly degrading them for possible reutilization of iron and other nutrients. Stromal macrophages also interact with less-differentiated hematopoietic precursors through release of potent secretory products, such as IL-1, and with lymphocytic populations, including plasma cells, through IL-6. They are targets for infectious agents, for example, mycobacteria,

TABLE 69–1. Selected Markers of Different Monocyte Subsets in Mouse and Human Blood

Antigen	Human $CD14^{hi}$ CD16–	Human CD14+ CD16+	Mouse CCR2+ CX_3CR1^{low}	Mouse CCR2– CX_3CR1^{hi}
Chemokine receptors				
CCR1	+	–	ND	ND
CCR2	+	–	+	–
CCR4	+	–	ND	ND
CCR5	–	+	ND	ND
CCR7	+	–	ND	ND
CXCR1	+	–	ND	ND
CXCR2	+	–	ND	ND
CXCR4	+	++	ND	ND
CX_3CR1	+	++	+	++
Other receptors				
CD4	+	+	ND	ND
CD11a	ND	ND	+	++
CD11b	++	++	++	++
CD11c	++	+++	–	+
CD14	+++	+	ND	ND
CD31	+++	+++	++	+
CD32	+++	+	ND	ND
CD33	+++	+	ND	ND
CD43	ND	ND	–	+
CD49b	ND	ND	+	–
CD62L	++	–	+	–
CD86	+	++	ND	ND
CD115	++	++	++	++
CD116	++	++	++	++
F4/80	ND	ND	+	+
Ly6C	ND	ND	+	–
7/4	ND	ND	+	–
MHC class II	+	++	–	–

SOURCE: Adapted from Gordon S, Taylor PR.[52]

TABLE 69–2. Selected Markers of Mononuclear Phagocytes and Related Cells

Cell Type	Antigen Markers	Other Properties
Monocytes/ macrophages	F4/80 (mouse) EMR2 (human) CD68 CR3 (CD11b) Sialoadhesin (Siglec-1) Scavenger receptors (SR-A, MARCO) Mannose receptor M-CSF receptor	Opsonic phagocytosis; lysozyme secretion; abundant acid hydrolases
Myeloid dendritic cells	MHC II Costimulatory molecules CD11c CD8α+/– DEC205 DC-SIGN DC-LAMP	Activation of naïve CD4 T lymphocytes
Plasmacytoid dendritic cells	CD123 B220 Lectin-like receptors (Siglec-H)	Type I interferon production; *in vitro* growth by flt-3 ligand
Osteoclasts	CD68 TRAP Calcitonin receptor $\alpha_v\beta_3$	Vacuolar H^+ ATPase; proteinase K; resorption of living bone

ATPase, adenosine triphosphatase; DC, dendritic cell; DC-LAMP, dendritic cell lysosomal-associated membrane protein; DC-SIGN, dendritic cell-specific intercellular adhesion molecule-3–grabbing nonintegrin; EMR, epidermal growth factor module-containing mucin-like hormone receptor; MARCO, macrophage receptor with collagenous structure; M-CSF, macrophage colony-stimulating factor; MHC, major histocompatibility complex; TRAP, tartrate-resistant acid phosphatase.

NOTE: Marker expression is variable, depending on cell localization, maturation, and activation. Some markers are also present on other myeloid cells, e.g., polymorphonuclear cells, and selected endothelial cells.

Structure and functions of receptor antigens are described in Chap. 68.

lentiviruses, and retroviruses, and serve as reservoirs in many chronic infections, while expressing a reduced killing capacity, as demonstrated for other resident macrophage populations.

It is intriguing that several monocyte and macrophage populations coexist in the marrow compartment; a network of stromal macrophages, clustered in hematopoietic islands, the developing monocytes, as well as osteoclasts and isolated macrophages apposed to bone surfaces.[68] Mature macrophages in human marrow contain prominent inclusions in storage disorders, such as Gaucher disease and hemosiderosis. Hemophagocytosis, a consequence of perforin deficiency in some patients, and seen in genetic syndromes and postviral infection, is a striking manifestation of excessive macrophage cytopathic activity in the marrow.[69,70] Uptake of opsonized platelets by macrophage FcR and CRs in stromal and other resident tissue macrophages are important features of thrombocytopenic syndromes.

Spleen

From the macrophage point of view, the spleen is the most complex organ in the body (Fig. 69–10).[71,72] Our knowledge is based mainly on the mouse and we know there is considerable species variation,[73] as well as constitutive hematopoiesis in mouse spleen. Subpopulations observed in the mouse by marker and genetic knockout experiments include (1) macrophages in the red pulp, white pulp, and in the marginal zone, itself M-CSF dependent,[43] and (2) heterogeneous, more phagocytic "metallophilic" macrophages in the outer marginal zone. Characteristic phenotypic markers are available to identify macrophages in mouse spleen (see Fig. 69–6C–E). The F4/80 antigen and the MR are restricted to mature macrophages in the red pulp, whereas CD68 is a marker for all macrophages, as well as DCs, although the mainly intracellular expression of CD68 is less prominent in DCs. There are several well-characterized markers for mouse metallophilic macrophages, including sialoadhesin (Sn), a poorly characterized protein recognized by the MOMA-1

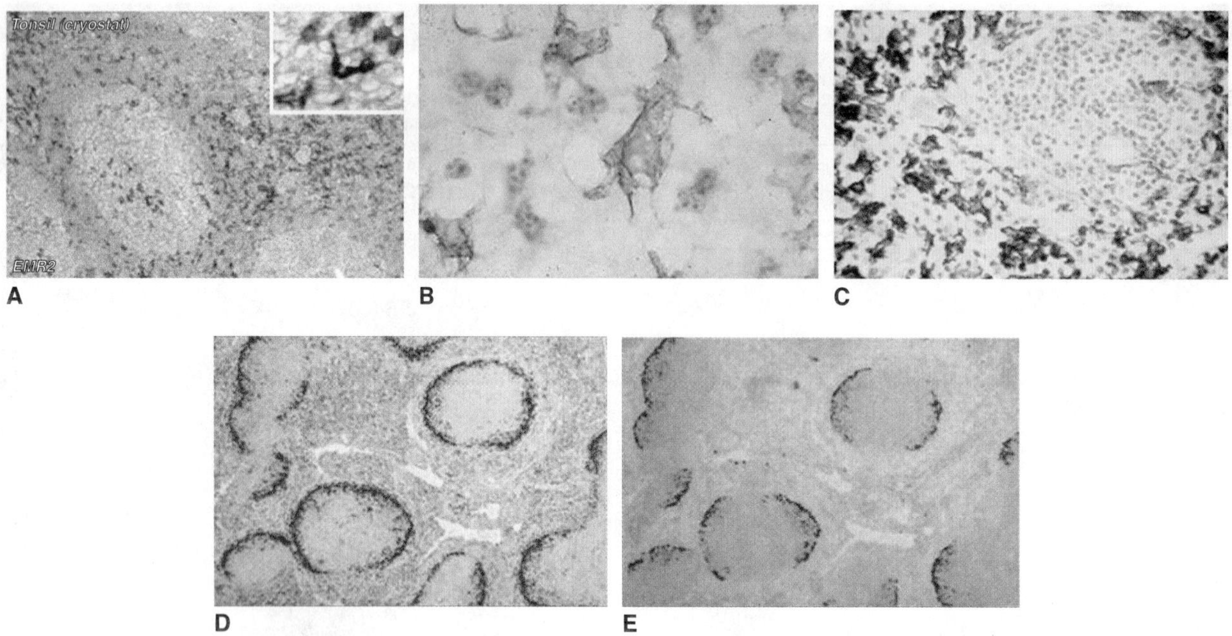

FIGURE 69–6. Immunocytochemical detection of macrophages in human **(A)** and mouse **(B–E)** lymphohematopoietic tissues. **A.** Tonsil. EMR2-positive macrophages are scattered throughout follicles and interfollicular areas. *(Courtesy of T. Marafioti.)* **B.** Liver. Kupffer cells are F4/80+, unlike sinusoidal endothelium and hepatocytes. **C–E.** Spleen. **C.** Red pulp macrophages express F4/80, unlike marginal zone cells. Macrophages in T-cell area are F4/80–, except for periarteriolar processes. **D.** Marginal metallophilic macrophages express sialoadhesin (Siglec1) strongly; red pulp macrophages are weakly positive. **E.** A subset of marginal metallophils binds a chimeric protein probe of the cysteine-rich domain of the MR-human Fc. For details see Taylor PR, Zamze S, Stillion RJ, et al.[86] *(Reproduced from Taylor PR, Zamze S, Stillion RJ, et al[86] with permission of the National Academy of Sciences, USA. Copyright 2004.)*

monoclonal antibody, and ligands for MR cysteine-rich domain-Fc chimeric proteins (see Fig. 69–6E). The splenic marginal zone macrophage population develops postnatally,[74] in parallel with antipolysaccharide responses to encapsulated bacteria. Functions of splenic marginal zone macrophages include clearance of senescent erythrocytes and neutrophils (red pulp), targeting of circulating antigens and pathogens (marginal zone), interferon (IFN) production, induction of secondary adaptive immune responses, regulation of hematopoiesis, and iron storage. Markers for the outer marginal zone macrophages include MARCO and SIGNR1, a mouse homologue of DC-SIGN. The spleen is also a site for storage and rapid deployment of monocytes, which participate in wound healing and play a role regulation of inflammation.[74a]

Lymph Nodes

Lymph node macrophages are also heterogeneous, with distinctive Sialoadhesin subcapsular cells, corresponding to marginal metallophils in their marker expression, and F4/80+ macrophages in germinal follicles and in the hilus. Macrophages in T-lymphocyte–rich areas are F4/80– or dim, as in T-cell areas in spleen, but express CD68. It is thought that antigen enters lymph nodes via afferent lymphatics and two photon experiments have defined the possible transfer of viral and other antigens and immune complexes to B lymphocytes after capture by the subcapsular sinus macrophages.[75] Their contributions to the initiation of adaptive immune responses, compared with DCs, are unclear. Tingible body macrophages arise from the clearance of apoptotic B cells in germinal centers, as in the spleen.

Thymus

The possible role of macrophages in thymic selection and tolerance has been neglected. Thymic macrophages are present in both the cortex and medulla and play a prominent role in the clearance of apoptotic thymocytes. Less appreciated is their presence in clusters with viable thymocytes.[6] Again, CD68 is a striking marker of macrophage populations in the developing thymus or during enhanced phagocytosis of apoptotic thymocytes, for example, after glucocorticosteroid treatment or irradiation.

Peyer Patch

Macrophages lie beneath the dome and mucosal cells, and are present with DCs, in association with lymphoid cells, where they express CD68 and low levels of F4/80.

Nonlymphohematopoietic Organs

In bulk, the gastrointestinal tract represents the largest accumulation of F4/80+ macrophages in the body, extending throughout the upper and lower gut. The small intestine is essentially sterile, and the abundant F4/80+ resident macrophages in the lamina propria express a distinct phenotype, ascribed to TGF-β production by adjacent cells.[67,76–78] The liver contains an abundant population of sinusoidal F4/80+ Kupffer cells, which share some properties (FcR, MR, SR-A) with sinusoidal endothelium, which lacks F4/80. The skin has F4/80+ epidermal Langerhans cells and F4/80+ dermal macrophages, which can migrate to draining lymph nodes and differentiate into antigen-presenting DCs.[79,80] The lung has a distinctive F4/80– or dim alveolar macrophage population, as well as interstitial F4/80+ macrophages. Alveolar macrophages are CD11c+ and express a range of nonopsonic phagocytic receptors (MR, SR-A), as well as FcR, but lack CR3. These cells also contain particle debris, cigarette smoke residue, and abundant lysozyme, because of exposure to irritants and uptake of carbon and dust particles, as well as of mucosal secretions in the airway.

The central nervous system contains an extensive network of F4/80+ CR3+ microglia, derived from monocytes during development, when they remove apoptotic neurons.[32] They differentiate into characteristic membrane-rich arborized forms within the neuropil and persist

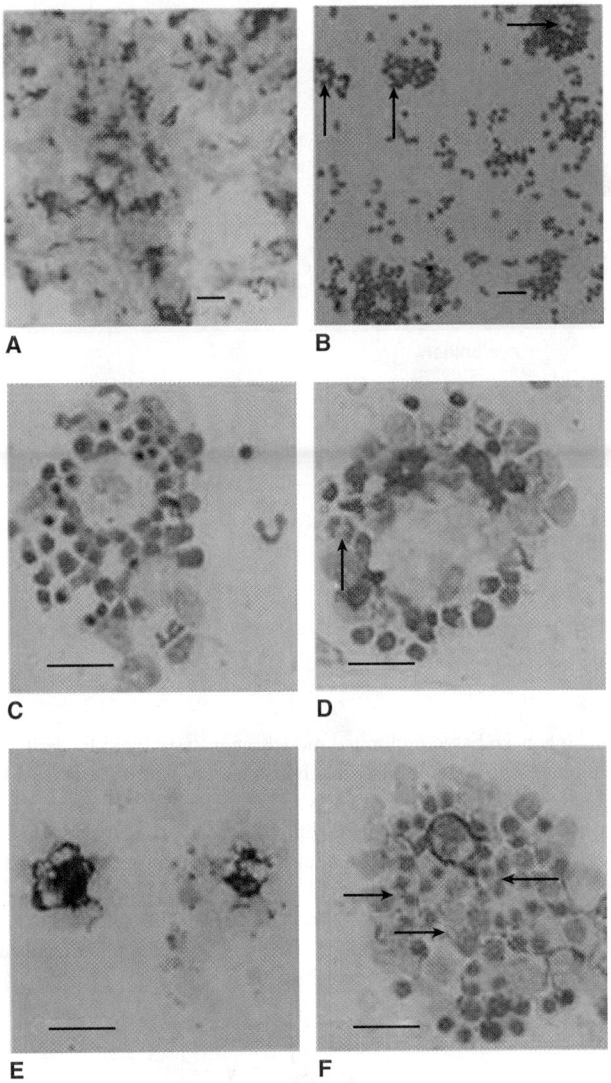

FIGURE 69–7. **A.** Stromal macrophages in human marrow associate with developing hematopoietic cells in islands/clusters. Immunocytochemical staining with antimacrophage monoclonal antibody Y1/82A of marrow section reveals a network of arborizing stromal macrophages uniformly distributed throughout the marrow interstitium (alkaline phosphatase-antialkaline phosphatase [APAAP] stain; hematoxylin counterstain). **B.** Marrow cells depleted of red cells and other single cells are enriched for cell clusters, most of which are erythroid clusters with a central stromal macrophage (*arrows*; Giemsa). **C.** Isolated erythroid cluster with intermediate and late normoblasts surrounding a central stromal macrophage (Giemsa). **D.** Isolated mixed cluster with both myeloid and erythroid cells attached to a central stromal macrophage. A dividing cell (*arrow*) is seen (Giemsa). **E.** Isolated erythroid clusters from a pathologic marrow sample show intense staining for hemosiderin of stromal macrophages with cellular processes extending between attached erythroblasts (Perl acid ferrocyanide reaction; counterstain neutral red). **F.** Immunocytochemical stain with antibody Y1/82A of isolated erythroid cluster. Both the stromal macrophage cell body and processes (*arrows*) between attached erythroblasts are visible (APAAP stain; hematoxylin counterstain). Bar = 50 μm. *(Reproduced from Lee SH, Crocker PR, Westaby S, et al,[87] with permission.)*

throughout adult life. Their function is obscure but may involve homeostasis and catabolism of neurotransmitters. In addition, there are perivascular F4/80+ macrophages (also MR+ SR-A+) and other F4/80+ populations in the meningeal space and choroid plexus. The endocrine, exocrine, reproductive, and urinary tracts all contain macrophage populations at sites of phagocytosis (ovary, testes) and hormonal metabolism (adrenal, thyroid, for example).[76] Further details can be found elsewhere.[6]

RECRUITMENT OF MONOCYTES IN RESPONSE TO INFLAMMATION

The stimuli that give rise to induced recruitment of monocytes, with or without accompanying myeloid and/or lymphoid cells, and the mechanisms involved are better understood than those of constitutive recruitment. Bacterial infections induce enhanced myelomonocytic cell recruitment and follow the stages established for neutrophils, transient arrest, and rolling on the microvascular endothelium, mediated by L-selectin, and initiated by chemotactic stimuli acting via G-protein-coupled chemokine receptors (Fig. 69–11). The β_2 integrins CD11a/CD18 and CD11b/CD18 mediate more stable adhesion. This is followed by diapedesis and interactions with CD31. Receptors implicated in subsequent extravascular migration are less defined but may include the fractalkine receptor, also involved intravascularly, β_1- and β_2-integrin, CD44, and EMR2. The evidence for an important role of L-selectin and β_2 integrins in human phagocyte recruitment to inflammatory stimuli comes from human inborn error syndromes, mouse genetic experiments, and antibody inhibition. The role of the common β_2-integrin chain (CD18) and definition of leukocyte adhesion deficiency syndrome provided a powerful paradigm for further experimental study of CD11/CD18.[81,82] Cellular signaling gives rise to dynamic changes in migration/adhesion and cytoskeletal reorganization outlined further in Chap. 68.

Mononuclear cell recruitment without that of other myeloid cells is a feature of viral infection and modified forms of inflammation observed in metabolic diseases, atherosclerosis, storage disorders, autoimmunity, and tumors. Different chemokine receptors and cell adhesion molecules account, in part, for more selective monocytic recruitment, although some are shared. The phenotypic heterogeneity in monocyte subsets is characterized by quantitative differences in expression of plasma membrane molecules resulting in differential recruitment of subsets in response to different stimuli. Once in the tissues, their subsequent fate also varies markedly, depending on the local environment, where newly recruited monocytes respond to tissue-specific factors. A striking example is that observed in the neurophil, where monocytes can differentiate over a few days into highly arborized, activated microglia, resembling locally reactivated resident microglia.[32] Thus, it becomes progressively more difficult to distinguish newly recruited from initially resident cells through marker analysis. Direct observation by fluorescent imaging *in vivo* may define precursor–product relationships more clearly. Similar issues arise in other organs, for example, lung, liver, gut, and even in skin, where static observations can be misleading. There are also common features of recruited cells irrespective of the local tissue environment, including the expression of CD11b/CD18 and of monocytic adhesion molecules, and metabolic markers, such as the ability to undergo a respiratory burst and an increased proliferative potential and high cell turnover rate. These monocytic markers tend to decline upon further macrophage differentiation, and in the case of myeloperoxidase may not be renewed after degranulation.

HETEROGENEITY OF MACROPHAGE IN TISSUES: IMMUNOMODULATION

Characterization of the macrophages found in tissues has yielded insights into their versatility in response to microbial constituents and cytokines produced by lymphoid, other immune and nonimmune cells.

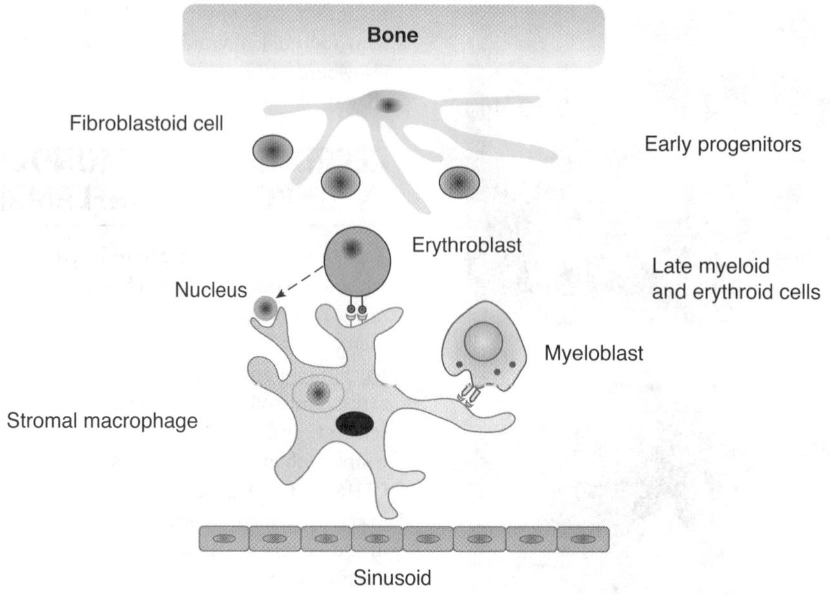

FIGURE 69–8. Stromal macrophages associate with later stages of developing hematopoietic cells in marrow. Developing myeloblasts and erythroblasts adhere selectively to stromal macrophages through nonphagocytic receptors (sialoadhesin and a divalent cation-dependent receptor), whereas erythroid nuclei are avidly ingested.

Adhesion to extracellular matrix, metabolites, vascular, and hormonal changes all influence the macrophage phenotype. This variety of stimuli can selectively activate or deactivate macrophage gene and protein expression, regulating their function. Figure 69–12 illustrates some of the stereotypic signature phenotypes, and Chap. 68 further describes the innate recognition mechanisms and functional responses.

Broadly considered, it is convenient to distinguish several clusters of activation properties; innate, classical, and alternative activation, and deactivation. The definition of activation has a long and confusing history, has mainly been based on limited models of analysis, typically peritoneal macrophages *in vivo* and *in vitro*, and on studies with macrophage-like cell lines. The advent of microarrays and of proteomics and systems biology has generated increasingly detailed information. It makes sense to schematize the interactions of monocytes and macrophages with microorganisms, microbial products, and Th1/Th2 lymphocytes, although this is subject to revision as CD4 T-lymphocyte heterogeneity continues to grow in complexity, with the description of Th17, $FoxP_3$+, and other regulatory T cells. Further details are given in Chap. 68.

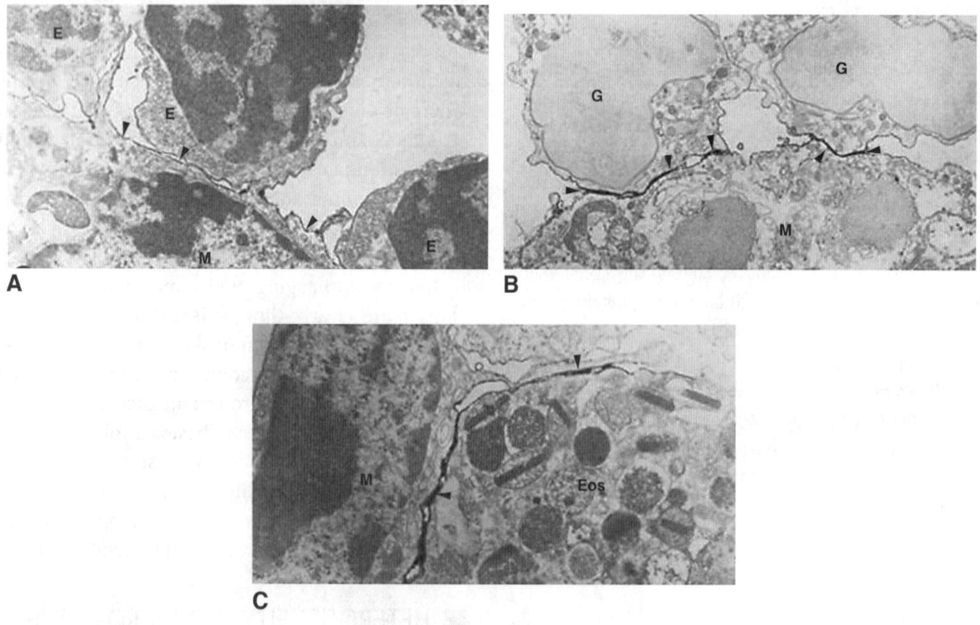

FIGURE 69–9. Sialoadhesin (Siglec-1) (*arrow heads*) is clustered at sites of stromal macrophage adhesion to developing cells (**B**, granulocytes; **C**, eosinophils) but diffusely present in association with erythroblasts (**A**). For details see Crocker PR, Werb Z, Gordon S, Bainton DF.[88] *(This research was originally published in* Blood. *PR, Werb Z, Gordon S, Bainton DF: Ultrastructural localization of a macrophage-restricted sialic acid binding hemagglutinin, SER, in macrophage-hematopoietic cell clusters.* Blood *76:1131–1138, 1990. Copyright the American Society of Hematology.)*

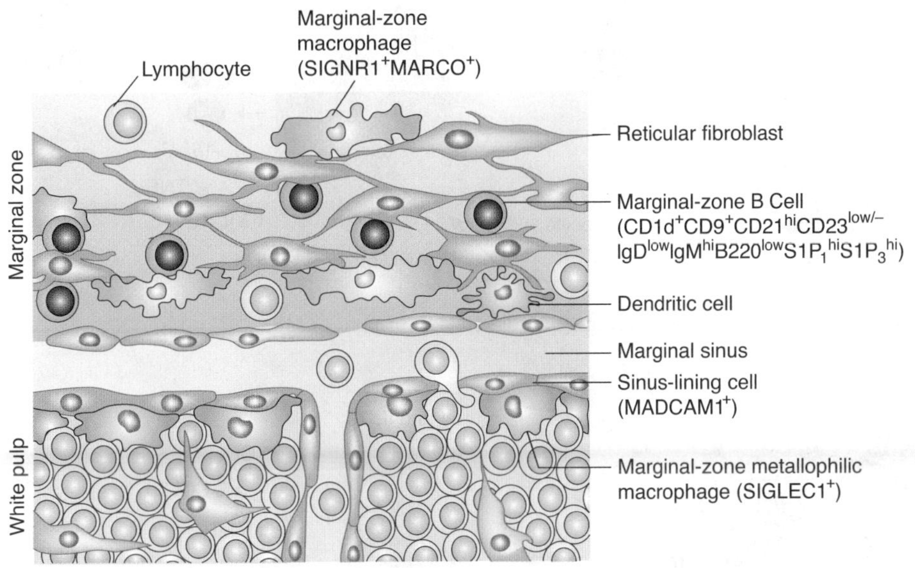

FIGURE 69–10. Microanatomy of the marginal zone of mouse spleen. A framework of reticular fibroblasts forms the basis of the marginal zone and is continuous with the reticular fibroblasts in the red pulp and the sinus-lining cells of the marginal sinus. In this framework, the most distinctive cell type is the marginal-zone macrophage, which expresses both MARCO (macrophage receptor with collagenous structure) and SIGNR1 (a mouse homologue of DC-SIGN [dendritic cell-specific intercellular adhesion molecule-3–grabbing nonintegrin]). Another important cell type in the marginal zone is the marginal zone B cell. In addition to these two resident cells, many lymphocytes and dendritic cells, as well as granulocytes, can also be found in transit, because part of the bloodstream flows through the marginal zone into the red pulp. Lymphocytes and dendritic cells can enter the white pulp from the marginal sinus by passing through a layer of sinus-lining cells that form a barrier between the marginal zone and the white pulp. These sinus-lining cells express mucosal vascular addressin cell-adhesion molecule 1 (MADCAM1). Directly beneath the sinus-lining cells is a ring of sialic-acid-binding immunoglobulin-like lectin 1 (SIGLEC1)+ macrophages, which are known as marginal zone metallophilic macrophages. $S1P_1$, sphingosine 1-phosphate receptor 1; $S1P_3$, sphingosine 1-phosphate receptor 3. *(Reprinted from Mebius RE, Kraal G*[72] *by permission of Macmillan Publishers Ltd,* Nature Reviews Immunology. *Copyright 2005.)*

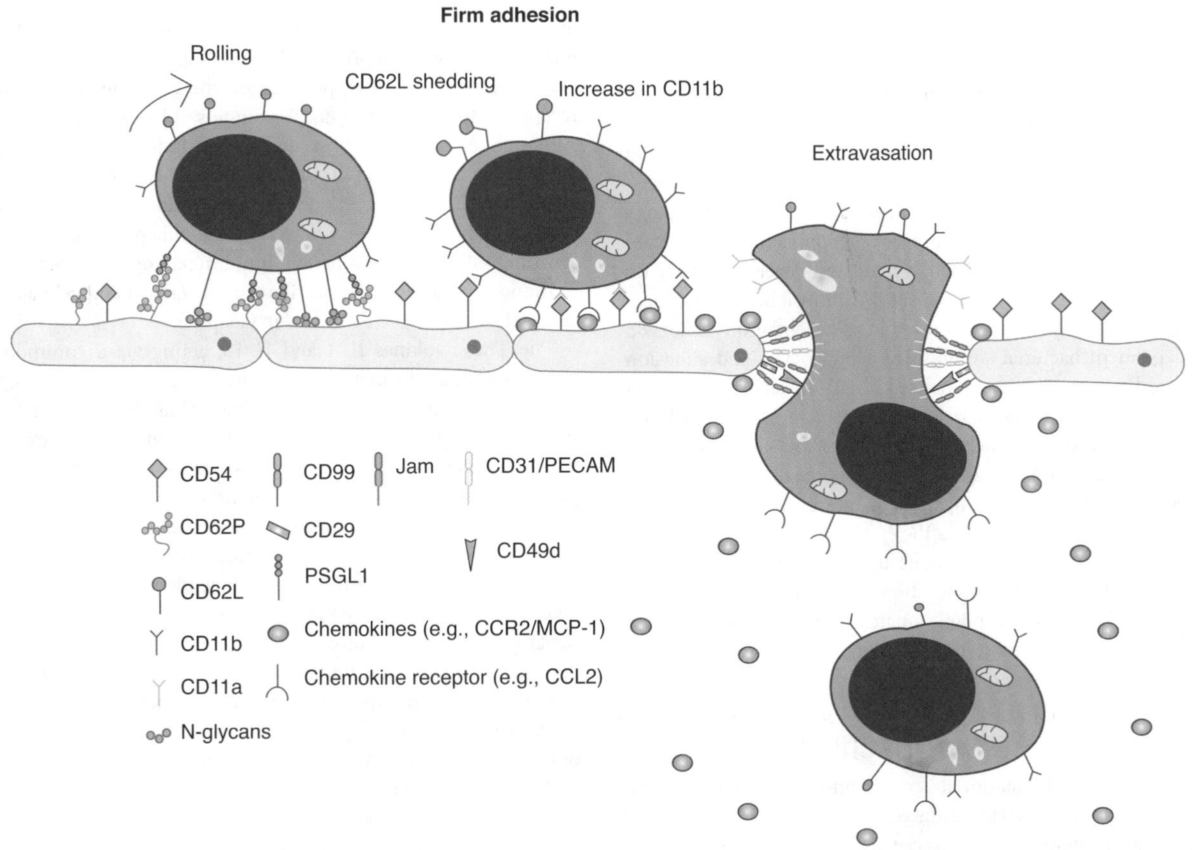

FIGURE 69–11. Recruitment. Stages of monocyte adherence to endothelium and diapedesis, induced by inflammatory stimuli. The model is mainly based on the recruitment of neutrophils, with which it shares many features, although monocyte-specific chemokines, receptors, and adhesion ligands exist, especially in constitutive and noninfectious, metabolic forms of inflammation.

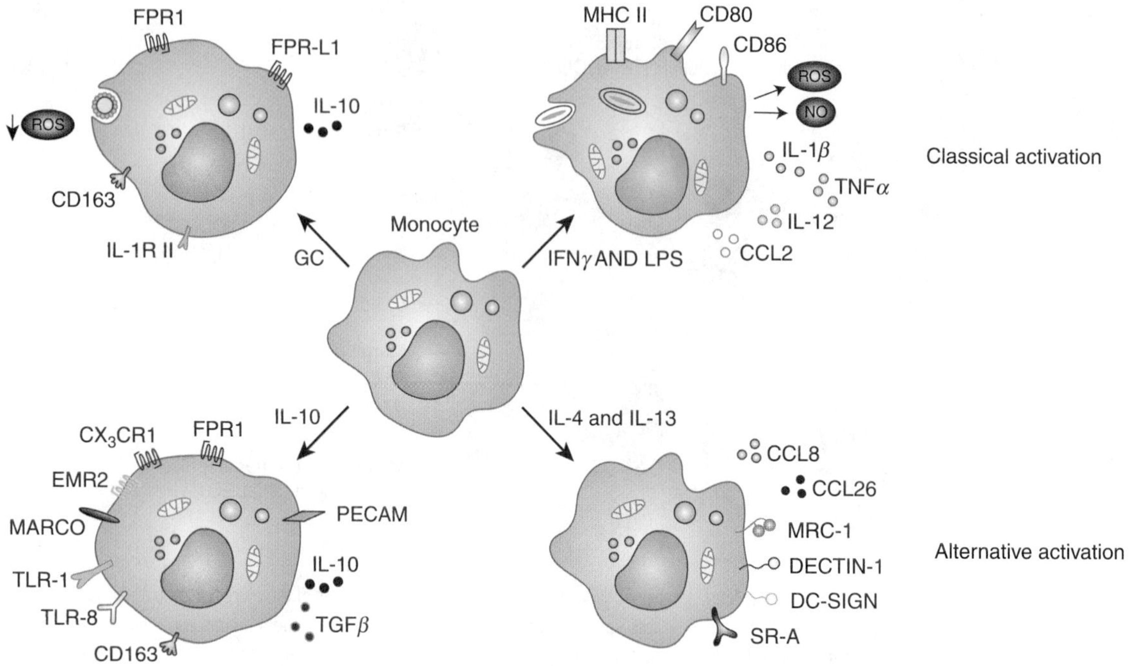

FIGURE 69–12. Immunomodulation of macrophage phenotype by cytokines, microbial constituents, and glucocorticosteroids. CCL, chemokines; CR, complement receptor; DC-SIGN, dendritic cell-specific intercellular adhesion molecule-3–grabbing nonintegrin; EMR, epidermal growth factor module-containing mucin-like hormone receptor; FPR1, formyl-peptide receptor 1; FPRL-1, formyl-peptide receptor-like 1; GC, glucocorticoids; IL, interleukin; INFγ, interferon-γ; LPS, lipopolysaccharide; MARCO, macrophage receptor with a collagenous structure; MRC-1, mannose receptor C-type 1; NO, nitric oxide; PECAM, platelet endothelial cell adhesion molecule-1; ROS, reactive oxygen species; SR-A, scavenger receptor A; TLR, toll-like receptor; TNF-α, tumor necrosis factor-α. Further details on innate modulation of phenotype by microbial products are given in Chap. 68. *(Adapted with permission from Yona S, Gordon S.[54])*

INNATE ACTIVATION

For this discussion innate activation is defined as direct microbial stimulation by intact bacteria or their constituents, such as LPS acting via toll-like receptor (TLR) sensors, in the absence of the major Th1/2 cytokines. For example, ethanol-killed *Neisseria meningitidis*, a potent immunomodulator with adjuvant-like properties, stimulates the expression of two useful markers on macrophages: MARCO and CD200. Expression of MARCO, a class A scavenger receptor, is remarkably specific for macrophages (and DCs) and is regulated developmentally on the outer marginal zone macrophages, but it is inducible on most macrophage populations by TLR and myeloid differentiation factor 88 (MyD88)-dependent bacterial stimuli. It is a phagocytic and adhesion receptor providing an adaptive, enhanced ability to take up *Neisseria* and other bacteria, after innate activation. CD200, an immunoglobulin (Ig) superfamily member, is widely expressed on many cells, but not on resident macrophages, and part of an immunoregulatory receptor pair with CD200 R, is also induced on macrophages by innate stimuli (S. Mukhopadhyay, unpublished observation).

Lectins such as Dectin-1 control innate activation of macrophages by β glucans in fungal walls,[83] in collaboration with TLR pathways, as discussed in Chap. 68. TLR-independent innate activation by viruses, parasites, and other pathogen-associated stimuli requires further study.

CYTOKINE-INDUCED PRIMING AND ACTIVATION: CLASSICAL AND ALTERNATIVE ACTIVATION

IFN-γ, produced mainly by natural killer cells and activated Th1 CD4+ and CD8+ cytotoxic lymphocytes, induces a set of macrophage biosynthetic and effector responses, known as classical activation, because of its well-established role in enhanced macrophage functions in cell-mediated immunity, inflammation, and host defense, particularly against intracellular pathogens. Full activation of effector functions, such as the respiratory burst and generation of oxidative nitrogen metabolites, depends on a two-stage mechanism of priming by the cytokine, via specific IFN-γ receptors, followed by a local stimulus, LPS or other TLR ligands. Although essential for host defense, including against opportunistic pathogens such as found in patients with the acquired immunodeficiency syndrome, classical activation is responsible for tissue injury and its consequences in inflammatory bowel disease, tuberculosis, and rheumatoid arthritis, although additional immunopathogenic agents, such as immune complexes, also contribute. Biochemical and cellular aspects of classical activation are described in Chap. 68.

The Th2 cytokines IL-4 and IL-13, acting via a common receptor chain as well as distinct receptors, induce a characteristic signature of altered gene expression in macrophages known as alternative activation.[84,85] Such primed macrophages can be induced to respond further to local, TLR-dependent phagocytic stimuli to secrete enhanced levels of proinflammatory cytokines, analogous to classically activated macrophages (A. Varin and S. Gordon, unpublished). Alternative activation is associated with allergy and parasitic infection, and has been implicated in humoral immunity, control of Th1-dependent inflammation, and host defense to extracellular pathogens, such as helminths. It can promote repair or, if excessive, fibrosis. Other forms of alternative activation have been described after stimulation of macrophages by immune complexes, acting via FcR. An important caveat is that there are substantial species differences in the marker changes associated with IL-4/13 pretreatment of macrophages from man and mouse, depending on the differentiation and prior activation state of the macrophages (F. Martinez-Estrada, L. Helming, and S. Gordon, unpublished).

IL-10 is a major deactivating cytokine for macrophages, produced by the macrophages themselves, as well as by Th2 lymphocytes and other sources. Acting through its own receptor, it counteracts IFN-γ, and can potentiate IL-4–induced actions. Other antiinflammatory regulators of macrophages activation include glucocorticosteroids and prostaglandin E_2. Although less-well defined, the overall gene and protein expression profiles of macrophages are also markedly influenced by the extracellular matrix, hormones, and other immunomodulators, so that modified forms of inflammation are associated with macrophages present in lipid-rich environments, tumors, and metabolic diseases. Finally, cell–cell interactions, as well as intracellular regulatory networks, profoundly influence the functions of macrophages, and are described in Chap. 68.

It is important to test in man concepts so far mainly derived *in vitro* and from experimental models and genetically manipulated mice. The influence of specific tissue microenvironments on the properties of resident, as well as of recruited macrophages, has hardly begun to be analyzed *in situ*. Imaging and direct observations, with appropriate markers, are far easier to perform in model organisms and need to be validated for humans. Naturally occurring human inborn errors provide a rich source of clinical material for study. The hematopoietic system is particularly valuable in providing access to circulatory monocytes, as well as macrophages in tissues such as marrow, but further progress will depend on awareness of the contributions of macrophages to the full range of their homeostatic and cytopathic functions in health and disease.

REFERENCES

1. Gordon S: The macrophage: Past, present and future. *Eur J Immunol* 37(Suppl 1):S9, 2007.
2. Akira S: Innate recognition: Receptors and signaling [special issue]. *Immunol Rev* 227:1, 2009.
3. Gordon S, Trinchieri G: Innate resistance and inflammation. *Curr Opin Immunol* 21:1, 2009.
4. Russell DG, Gordon S (eds): *Phagocyte-Pathogen interactions: Macrophages and the Host Response to Infection*. ASM Press, Washington, DC, 2009.
5. Van Furth R: *Mononuclear Phagocytes: Biology of Monocytes and Macrophages*. Kluwer Academic, Dordrecht, The Netherlands, 1992.
6. Gordon S: Macrophages and the immune response in *Fundamental Immunology*, 6th ed, edited by W Paul, p 481. Lippincott Williams and Wilkins, Philadelphia, 2008.
7. Talks HS: Innate immunity: Host recognition and response in health and disease. *Henry Stewart Talks* [online seminar]. Available at: www.hstalks.com/main/browse_talks.php?father_id=437&c=252, 2009.
8. Martinez-Pomares L, Gordon S: Murine macrophages: A technical approach. *Methods Mol Biol* 415:255, 2008.
9. Davies JQ, Gordon S: Isolation and culture of murine macrophages. *Methods Mol Biol* 290:91, 2005.
10. Rosen H, Gordon S: Adoptive transfer of fluorescence-labeled cells shows that resident peritoneal macrophages are able to migrate into specialized lymphoid organs and inflammatory sites in the mouse. *Eur J Immunol* 20:1251, 1990.
11. van Rooijen N: Liposomes for targeting of antigens and drugs: Immunoadjuvant activity and liposome-mediated depletion of macrophages. *J Drug Target* 16:529, 2008.
12. Jung S, Aliberti J, Graemmel P, et al: Analysis of fractalkine receptor CX(3)CR1 function by targeted deletion and green fluorescent protein reporter gene insertion. *Mol Cell Biol* 20:4106, 2000.
13. Herbert DR, Holscher C, Mohrs M, et al: Alternative macrophage activation is essential for survival during schistosomiasis and downmodulates T helper 1 responses and immunopathology. *Immunity* 20:623, 2004.
14. Lang RA, Bishop JM: Macrophages are required for cell death and tissue remodeling in the developing mouse eye. *Cell* 74:453, 1993.
15. Beutler B, Casanova JL: New frontiers in immunology. Workshop on the road ahead: Future directions in fundamental and clinical immunology. *EMBO Rep* 6:620, 2005.
16. Georgel P, Du X, Hoebe K, Beutler B: ENU mutagenesis in mice. *Methods Mol Biol* 415:1, 2008.
17. Davis JM, Ramakrishnan L: The zebrafish as a model of host-pathogen interactions, in *Phagocyte-Pathogen Interactions: Macrophages and the Host Response to Infection*, edited by DG Russell, S Gordon, p 523. ASM Press, Washington, DC, 2009.
18. Herbomel P, Levraud JP: Imaging early macrophage differentiation, migration, and behaviors in live zebrafish embryos. *Methods Mol Med* 105:199, 2005.
19. Lemaitre B, Hoffmann J: The host defense of *Drosophila melanogaster*. *Annu Rev Immunol* 25:697, 2007.
20. Frankel LB, Christoffersen NR, Jacobsen A, et al: Programmed cell death 4 (PDCD4) is an important functional target of the microRNA miR-21 in breast cancer cells. *J Biol Chem* 283:1026, 2008.
21. Egen JG, Rothfuchs AG, Feng CG, et al: Macrophage and T cell dynamics during the development and disintegration of mycobacterial granulomas. *Immunity* 28:271, 2008.
22. Fairchild PJ, Nolan KF, Waldmann H: Genetic modification of dendritic cells through the directed differentiation of embryonic stem cells. *Methods Mol Biol* 380:59, 2007.
23. Karlsson KR, Cowley S, Martinez FO, et al: Homogeneous monocytes and macrophages from human embryonic stem cells following coculture-free differentiation in M-CSF and IL-3. *Exp Hematol* 36:1167, 2008.
24. Day RM, Harbord M, Forbes A, Segal AW: Cantharidin blisters: A technique for investigating leukocyte trafficking and cytokine production at sites of inflammation in humans. *J Immunol Methods* 257:213, 2001.
25. Gordon S: Elie Metchnikoff: Father of natural immunity. *Eur J Immunol* 38:3257, 2008.
26. Crocker PR, Morris L, Gordon S: Novel cell surface adhesion receptors involved in interactions between stromal macrophages and haematopoietic cells. *J Cell Sci Suppl* 9:185, 1988.
27. Fabriek BO, Polfliet MM, Vloet RP, et al: The macrophage CD163 surface glycoprotein is an erythroblast adhesion receptor. *Blood* 109:5223, 2007.
28. Morris L, Crocker PR, Gordon S: Murine fetal liver macrophages bind developing erythroblasts by a divalent cation-dependent hemagglutinin. *J Cell Biol* 106:649, 1988.
29. Crocker PR, Gordon S: Mouse macrophage hemagglutinin (sheep erythrocyte receptor) with specificity for sialylated glycoconjugates characterized by a monoclonal antibody. *J Exp Med* 169:1333, 1989.
30. Bessis M, Mize C, Prenant M: Erythropoiesis: Comparison of *in vivo* and *in vitro* amplification. *Blood Cells* 4:155, 1978.
31. Redd MJ, Cooper L, Wood W, et al: Wound healing and inflammation: Embryos reveal the way to perfect repair. *Philos Trans R Soc Lond B Biol Sci* 359:777, 2004.
32. Perry VH, Andersson PB, Gordon S: Macrophages and inflammation in the central nervous system. *Trends Neurosci* 16:268, 1993.
33. Hughes DA, Gordon S: Expression and function of the type 3 complement receptor in tissues of the developing mouse. *J Immunol* 160:4543, 1998.
34. Rosen H, Gordon S: Monoclonal antibody to the murine type 3 complement receptor inhibits adhesion of myelomonocytic cells *in vitro* and inflammatory cell recruitment *in vivo*. *J Exp Med* 166:1685, 1987.
35. Auffray C, Sieweke MH, Geissmann F: Blood monocytes: Development, heterogeneity, and relationship with dendritic cells. *Annu Rev Immunol* 27:669, 2009.
36. Glass CK, Ogawa S: Combinatorial roles of nuclear receptors in inflammation and immunity. *Nat Rev Immunol* 6:44, 2006.
37. Bonifer C, Hoogenkamp M, Krysinska H, Tagoh H: How transcription factors program chromatin—Lessons from studies of the regulation of myeloid-specific genes. *Semin Immunol* 20:257, 2008.
38. Bonifer C, Hume DA: The transcriptional regulation of the colony-stimulating factor 1 receptor (csf1r) gene during hematopoiesis. *Front Biosci* 13:549, 2008.
39. Feng R, Desbordes SC, Xie H, et al: PU.1 and C/EBPalpha/beta convert fibroblasts into macrophage-like cells. *Proc Natl Acad Sci U S A* 105:6057, 2008.
40. Hume DA: Macrophages as APC and the dendritic cell myth. *J Immunol* 181:5829, 2008.
41. Yu W, Chen J, Xiong Y, et al: CSF-1 receptor structure/function in MacCsf1r–/– macrophages: Regulation of proliferation, differentiation, and morphology. *J Leukoc Biol* 84:852, 2008.
42. Pixley FJ, Stanley ER: CSF-1 regulation of the wandering macrophage: Complexity in action. *Trends Cell Biol* 14:628, 2004.
43. Witmer-Pack MD, Hughes DA, Schuler G, et al: Identification of macrophages and dendritic cells in the osteopetrotic (op/op) mouse. *J Cell Sci* 104(Pt 4):1021, 1993.
44. Inaba K, Swiggard WJ, Steinman RM, et al: Isolation of dendritic cells. *Curr Protoc Immunol* Chapter 3:Unit 3.7, 2001.
45. Sallusto F, Lanzavecchia A: Efficient presentation of soluble antigen by cultured human dendritic cells is maintained by granulocyte/macrophage colony-stimulating factor plus interleukin 4 and downregulated by tumor necrosis factor alpha. *J Exp Med* 179:1109, 1994.
46. Dranoff G, Mulligan RC: Activities of granulocyte-macrophage colony-stimulating factor revealed by gene transfer and gene knockout studies. *Stem Cells* 12 (Suppl 1):173, 1994.
47. Helming L, Gordon S: The molecular basis of macrophage fusion. *Immunobiology* 212:785, 2007.
48. Helming L, Gordon S: Macrophage fusion induced by IL-4 alternative activation is a multistage process involving multiple target molecules. *Eur J Immunol* 37:33, 2007.
49. Helming L, Tomasello E, Kyriakides TR, et al: Essential role of DAP12 signaling in macrophage programming into a fusion-competent state. *Sci Signal* 1:Ra11, 2008.
50. Helming L, Winter J, Gordon S: The scavenger receptor CD36 plays a role in cytokine-induced macrophage fusion. *J Cell Sci* 122:453, 2009.
51. Randolph GJ, Beaulieu S, Lebecque S, et al: Differentiation of monocytes into dendritic cells in a model of transendothelial trafficking. *Science* 282:480, 1998.
52. Gordon S, Taylor PR: Monocyte and macrophage heterogeneity. *Nat Rev Immunol* 5:953, 2005.
53. Taylor PR, Martinez-Pomares L, Stacey M, et al: Macrophage receptors and immune recognition. *Annu Rev Immunol* 23:901, 2005.
54. Yona S, Gordon S: Inflammation: Glucocorticoids turn the monocyte switch. *Immunol Cell Biol* 85:81, 2007.
55. Yona S, Lin HH, Siu WO, et al: Adhesion-GPCRs: Emerging roles for novel receptors. *Trends Biochem Sci* 33:491, 2008.
56. Lin HH, Faunce DE, Stacey M, et al: The macrophage F4/80 receptor is required for the induction of antigen-specific efferent regulatory T cells in peripheral tolerance. *J Exp Med* 201:1615, 2005.

57. da Silva RP, Gordon S: Phagocytosis stimulates alternative glycosylation of macrosialin (mouse CD68), a macrophage-specific endosomal protein. *Biochem J* 338(Pt 3):687, 1999.
58. Holt PG, Oliver J, Bilyk N, et al: Downregulation of the antigen presenting cell function(s) of pulmonary dendritic cells in vivo by resident alveolar macrophages. *J Exp Med* 177:397, 1993.
59. Fraser I, Hughes D, Gordon S: Divalent cation-independent macrophage adhesion inhibited by monoclonal antibody to murine scavenger receptor. *Nature* 364:343, 1993.
60. van der Laan LJ, Kangas M, Dopp EA, et al: Macrophage scavenger receptor MARCO: In vitro and in vivo regulation and involvement in the anti-bacterial host defense. *Immunol Lett* 57:203, 1997.
61. Taylor PR, Gordon S, Martinez-Pomares L: The mannose receptor: Linking homeostasis and immunity through sugar recognition. *Trends Immunol* 26:104, 2005.
62. Kristiansen M, Graversen JH, Jacobsen C, et al: Identification of the haemoglobin scavenger receptor. *Nature* 409:198, 2001.
63. Hume DA, Perry VH, Gordon S: Immunohistochemical localization of a macrophage-specific antigen in developing mouse retina: Phagocytosis of dying neurons and differentiation of microglial cells to form a regular array in the plexiform layers. *J Cell Biol* 97:253, 1983.
64. Merad M, Ginhoux F, Collin M: Origin, homeostasis and function of Langerhans cells and other langerin-expressing dendritic cells. *Nat Rev Immunol* 8:935, 2008.
65. Merad M, Manz MG: Dendritic cell homeostasis. *Blood* 113:3418, 2009.
66. Naik SH: Demystifying the development of dendritic cell subtypes, a little. *Immunol Cell Biol* 86:439, 2008.
67. Hume DA, Robinson AP, MacPherson GG, Gordon S: The mononuclear phagocyte system of the mouse defined by immunohistochemical localization of antigen F4/80. Relationship between macrophages, Langerhans cells, reticular cells, and dendritic cells in lymphoid and hematopoietic organs. *J Exp Med* 158:1522, 1983.
68. Hume DA, Loutit JF, Gordon S: The mononuclear phagocyte system of the mouse defined by immunohistochemical localization of antigen F4/80: Macrophages of bone and associated connective tissue. *J Cell Sci* 66:189, 1984.
69. Chu T, Jaffe R: The normal Langerhans cell and the LCH cell. *Br J Cancer Suppl* 23:S4, 1994.
70. Favara BE, Jaffe R, Egeler RM: Macrophage activation and hemophagocytic syndrome in Langerhans cell histiocytosis: Report of 30 cases. *Pediatr Dev Pathol* 5:130, 2002.
71. Martinez-Pomares L, Kosco-Vilbois M, Darley E, et al: Fc chimeric protein containing the cysteine-rich domain of the murine mannose receptor binds to macrophages from splenic marginal zone and lymph node subcapsular sinus and to germinal centers. *J Exp Med* 184:1927, 1996.
72. Mebius RE, Kraal G: Structure and function of the spleen. *Nat Rev Immunol* 5:606, 2005.
73. Martinez-Pomares L, Hanitsch LG, Stillion R, et al: Expression of mannose receptor and ligands for its cysteine-rich domain in venous sinuses of human spleen. *Lab Invest* 85:1238, 2005.
74. Morris L, Crocker PR, Hill M, Gordon S: Developmental regulation of sialoadhesin (sheep erythrocyte receptor), a macrophage-cell interaction molecule expressed in lymphohemopoietic tissues. *Dev Immunol* 2:7, 1992.
74a. Swirski, FK, Nahrendorf M, Etzrodt M, et al: Identification of splenic reservoir monocytes and their deployment to inflammatory sites. *Science* 325:612, 2009.
75. Martinez-Pomares L, Gordon S: Antigen presentation the macrophage way. *Cell* 131:641, 2007.
76. Hume DA, Halpin D, Charlton H, Gordon S: The mononuclear phagocyte system of the mouse defined by immunohistochemical localization of antigen F4/80: Macrophages of endocrine organs. *Proc Natl Acad Sci U S A* 81:4174, 1984.
77. Smythies LE, Maheshwari A, Clements R, et al: Mucosal IL-8 and TGF-beta recruit blood monocytes: Evidence for cross-talk between the lamina propria stroma and myeloid cells. *J Leukoc Biol* 80:492, 2006.
78. Smythies LE, Sellers M, Clements RH, et al: Human intestinal macrophages display profound inflammatory anergy despite avid phagocytic and bacteriocidal activity. *J Clin Invest* 115:66, 2005.
79. Haniffa M, Ginhoux F, Wang XN, et al: Differential rates of replacement of human dermal dendritic cells and macrophages during hematopoietic stem cell transplantation. *J Exp Med* 206:371, 2009.
80. McKenzie EJ, Taylor PR, Stillion RJ, et al: Mannose receptor expression and function define a new population of murine dendritic cells. *J Immunol* 178:4975, 2007.
81. Arnaout MA: Leukocyte adhesion molecules deficiency: Its structural basis, pathophysiology and implications for modulating the inflammatory response. *Immunol Rev* 114:145, 1990.
82. Luo BH, Carman CV, Springer TA: Structural basis of integrin regulation and signaling. *Annu Rev Immunol* 25:619, 2007.
83. Brown GD: Dectin-1: A signalling non-TLR pattern-recognition receptor. *Nat Rev Immunol* 6:33, 2006.
84. Gordon S: Alternative activation of macrophages. *Nat Rev Immunol* 3:23, 2003.
85. Martinez FO, Helming L, Gordon S: Alternative activation of macrophages: An immunologic functional perspective. *Annu Rev Immunol* 27:451, 2009.
86. Taylor PR, Zamze S, Stillion RJ, et al: Development of a specific system for targeting protein to metallophilic macrophages. *Proc Natl Acad Sci U S A* 101:1963, 2004.
87. Lee SH, Crocker PR, Westaby S, et al: Isolation and immunocytochemical characterization of human bone marrow stromal macrophages in hemopoietic clusters. *J Exp Med* 168:1193, 1988.
88. Crocker PR, Werb Z, Gordon S, Bainton DF: Ultrastructural localization of a macrophage-restricted sialic acid binding hemagglutinin, SER, in macrophage-hematopoietic cell clusters. *Blood* 76:1131, 1990.

CHAPTER 70

CLASSIFICATION AND CLINICAL MANIFESTATIONS OF DISORDERS OF MONOCYTES AND MACROPHAGES

Marshall A. Lichtman

SUMMARY

Disorders that exclusively result in abnormalities of monocytes, macrophages, or dendritic cells are uncommon and usually are referred to pathologically as histiocytosis. These disorders can be inherited, such as familial hemophagocytic lymphohistiocytosis; inflammatory, such as infectious hemophagocytic lymphohistiocytic syndrome; or clonal, such as Langerhans cell histiocytosis. They can result from an inherited enzyme insufficiency in macrophages that lead to exaggerated storage of macromolecules, such as in Gaucher disease. Monocytes are critical sources for proinflammatory and inflammatory cytokines and, when inappropriately activated, can result in the lymphohistiocytic hemophagocytic syndrome with fever, intravascular coagulation, and organ pathology. A variety of hematopoietic neoplasms may have a phenotype expressed by a large proportion of monocytes. Idiopathic (clonal) monocytosis is an uncommon myelodysplastic syndrome. Some cases of myelogenous leukemia have progenitor cells that mature preferentially into leukemic monocytes, including acute monoblastic or monocytic leukemia, chronic myelomonocytic leukemia, and juvenile myelomonocytic leukemia. Two acquired diseases, hairy cell leukemia and aplastic anemia, result in a severe depression of blood monocytes (along with other blood cell types). Inherited disorders affecting white cells, such as chronic granulomatous disease and Chédiak-Higashi syndrome, result in impaired monocyte function. Monocyte dysfunction may accompany a variety of severe illnesses, such as in sepsis, trauma, and cancer. Monocytes also contribute to a variety of diseases, such as Crohn disease and rheumatoid arthritis, by virtue of their being a principal source of tumor necrosis factor. Monocytes play a pathogenetic role in other complex, acquired disorders, such as thrombosis and atherogenesis. Table 70–1 categorizes the qualitative and quantitative abnormalities of monocytes, macrophages, and dendritic cells.

CLASSIFICATION

Classification of monocytic disorders is difficult because few abnormalities result solely in a disturbance of monocytes or macrophages.

Abbreviations and acronyms that appear in this chapter include: CD, cluster of differentiation; GM-CSF, granulocyte-macrophage colony-stimulating factor; HLA, human leukocyte antigen; HLA-DR, human leukocyte antigen-D related; IL, interleukin; TNF, tumor necrosis factor.

However, the presence of monocytopenia, monocytosis, histiocytosis, or qualitative disorders of monocytes may be an important diagnostic feature or contribute to the functional abnormality in the patient.

The terms *histiocyte* and *macrophage* are synonymous. The latter term is customary when discussing the biology of the cells of the *mononuclear phagocyte system*, which is the total pool of marrow, blood, and tissue monocytes and macrophages, formerly referred to as the *reticuloendothelial system*. In disease nosology, the terms *histiocyte* and *histiocytosis* continue to be used for diseases that principally involve cells derived from blood monocytes, that is, macrophages and monocyte-derived dendritic cells.

The physician should consider the absolute monocyte count and not the percent of cells that are monocytes when evaluating the differential blood cell count before concluding that there is an inappropriate content of blood monocytes (see Chap. 71).

Table 70–1 lists a classification of monocyte and macrophage disorders of relevance to hematologists.

MONOCYTOPENIA

Table 70–1 contains several important causes of monocytopenia. Two notable examples of disorders accompanied by severe monocytopenia are aplastic anemia and hairy cell leukemia. Pancytopenia is usual in both conditions, but the predisposition to serious infection is heightened by the deficiency in monocyte production. In hairy cell leukemia, the severe monocytopenia represents an important diagnostic clue because of its constancy.

MONOCYTOSIS AND HISTIOCYTOSIS

Table 70–1 contains a comprehensive list of causes of monocytosis. Monocytosis is often the manifestation of an inflammatory or a neoplastic disease. Certain hematopoietic tumors, especially acute monocytic and chronic myelomonocytic leukemia, have as their principal manifestation a predominance of monocytic cells in marrow and blood. Occasionally, chronic monocytosis can precede the onset of acute myelogenous leukemia, representing an uncommon manifestation of the myelodysplastic syndromes. Dendritic cell variants of acute myelogenous leukemia have also been discovered since the advent of immunophenotyping and genotyping of acute leukemias. The precise derivation of these myeloid dendritic cells is uncertain (i.e., granulocytic or monocytic). In some cases of monocytic leukemia, the malignant clone does not appear to include precursors of red cells and platelets. Such cases are not likely to be the result of a mutation of a multipotential hematopoietic cell. This so-called progenitor cell monocytic leukemia and other histiocytic or dendritic cell tumors support the concept that primitive cells, committed to the monocyte-macrophage lineage, can undergo malignant transformation (see Chaps. 85 and 89).

Several uncommon types of histiocytosis are serious systemic diseases that may masquerade as malignant disease. However, in such cases the cytopathologic changes in monocytes or macrophages do not constitute a malignant transformation and are not monoclonal. Familial and sporadic hemophagocytic lymphohistiocytosis, infection-induced hemophagocytic syndromes, and sinus histiocytosis with massive lymphadenopathy are among such disorders (see Chap. 72). Infectious hemophagocytic histiocytosis caused by Epstein-Barr virus may be a hybrid disease because of the association with an underlying monoclonal or oligoclonal proliferation of virus-infected lymphocytes. The striking activation of macrophages and the resulting cytokine elaboration and organ pathology seen in some patients with juvenile rheumatoid arthritis, referred to as the "macrophage-activation

TABLE 70–1. Disorders of Monocytes and Macrophages

I. Monocytopenia
- A. Aplastic anemia[1]
- B. Hairy cell leukemia[2]
- C. Glucocorticoid therapy[3,4]

II. Monocytosis
- A. Benign
  - (1) Reactive monocytosis[5]
  - (2) Exercise-induced[5a]
- B. Clonal monocytosis
  - Indolent
    - (1) Chronic idiopathic monocytosis[6]
    - (2) Oligoblastic myelogenous leukemia (myelodysplasia)[7]
  - Progressive
    - (1) Acute monocytic leukemia[8–10]
    - (2) Dendritic cell leukemia[11–13]
    - (3) Progenitor cell monocytic leukemia[14]
    - (4) Chronic myelomonocytic leukemia[15,16]
    - (5) Juvenile myelomonocytic leukemia[17]

III. Macrophage Deficiency
- A. Osteopetrosis (isolated osteoclast deficiency)[18,19]

IV. Inflammatory Histiocytosis (see Chap. 72)
- A. Primary hemophagocytic lymphohistiocytosis[20–22]
  - (1) Familial
  - (2) Sporadic
- B. Other inherited syndromes with hemophagocytosis lymphohistiocytosis: Chédiak-Higashi, X-linked lymphoproliferative, Gracelli[23]
- C. Infectious hemophagocytic histiocytosis[22,24]
- D. Tumor-associated hemophagocytic histiocytosis[25,26]
- E. Drug-associated hemophagocytic histiocytosis[25,26]
- F. Disease-associated hemophagocytic histiocytosis[23,26,27]
- G. Juvenile rheumatoid arthritis[23]
- H. Sinus histiocytosis with massive lymphadenopathy[28,29]

V. Storage Histiocytosis (see Chap. 73)
- A. Gaucher disease[30]
- B. Niemann-Pick disease[31]
- C. Gangliosidosis[32]
- D. Sea-blue histiocytosis syndrome[33]

VI. Clonal (Neoplastic) Histiocytosis (see Chap. 72)
- A. Langerhans cell histiocytosis[34,35]
  - (1) Localized
  - (2) Systemic
- B. Tumors or sarcomas of histiocytes and dendritic cells[36]
  - (1) Histiocytic sarcoma
  - (2) Langerhans cell sarcoma
  - (3) Interdigitating dendritic cell sarcoma
  - (4) Follicular dendritic cell sarcoma

VII. Monocyte and Macrophage Dysfunction[37–39]
- A. α_1-Proteinase inhibitor deficiency[40,41]
- B. Chédiak-Higashi syndrome[42]
- C. Chronic granulomatous disease[43,44]
- D. Chronic lymphocytic leukemia[45,46]
- E. Disseminated mucocutaneous candidiasis[47,48]
- F. Glucocorticoid therapy[49,50]
- G. Kawasaki disease[51,52]
- H. Malakoplakia[53]
- I. Mycobacteriosis syndrome[54–56]
- J. Leprosy[57]
- K. Posttraumatic[58,59]
- L. Septic shock-induced[60–63]
- M. Critically ill subjects[64]
- N. Solid tumors[65,66]
- O. Tobacco smoking[67,68]
- P. Marijuana smoking or cocaine inhalation[68,69]
- Q. Whipple disease[70,71]
- R. Human interleukin (IL)-10 effects; Epstein-Barr virus IL-10–like gene product (vIL-10)[72,73]

VIII. Atherogenesis[74–78]

IX. Thrombogenesis[78–81]

X. Obesity[82]

syndrome," is closely related to other types of hemophagocytic syndromes (see Chap 72). Pediatric rheumatologists refer to the hemophagocytic syndrome in patients with juvenile rheumatoid arthritis as the "macrophage activation syndrome," but the clinical expression is closely analogous to other acquired hemophagocytic lymphohistiocytic syndromes. In these hemophagocytic syndromes, it is currently thought that the inherited or acquired inability of natural killer cells and cytotoxic T lymphocytes to modulate and, eventually, abrogate the immune response is responsible for the pathologic events of cytokine storm, fever, intravascular coagulation, organ dysfunction, and intense hemophagocytosis. Tumors of histiocytes (or dendritic cells) are rare, but can be classified into several groups with a combination of morphologic and immunophenotypic markers (see Chap. 72).

QUALITATIVE DISORDERS OF MONOCYTES

Inherited abnormalities can result in dysfunctional macrophages (see Table 70–1). In these situations the abnormality is usually shared by other leukocytes, as in chronic granulomatous disease, which results from a defect in oxygen-dependent microbial killing. In Chédiak-Higashi disease, defective macrophages result from an abnormality in their cell-granule membranes (see Chap. 66). An indomethacin-sensitive monocyte-killing defect in children is associated with a predisposition to atypical mycobacterial disease. Also, inherited or enzyme deficiencies in macrophages can result in accumulation of undegraded macromolecules, leading to various types of storage diseases. A classic example is Gaucher disease, a disorder that results from an inherited deficiency of the enzyme glucocerebrosidase, in which tissue damage results from the engorgement of macrophages with the enzyme substrate. Recombinant glucocerebrosidase, which enters macrophage lysosomes by endocytosis, can ameliorate this macrophagic disease (see Chap. 73).

Acquired functional abnormalities of monocytes occur in a variety of diseases and circumstances (see "VII. Monocyte and Macrophage Dysfunction" in Table 70–1). Monocyte dysfunction occurs after severe trauma, sepsis, in other critically ill patients, and in patients with metastatic cancer. Monocyte production of interleukin (IL)-12 or maturation to dendritic cells also can be impaired in cases of severe trauma, critical illness, or metastatic cancer.

Some factors, such as IL-10, impair monocyte functions. A viral IL-10–like molecule encoded by the Epstein-Barr virus *BCRF1* gene also might play a role in the pathogenesis of that virus infection, and may act, in part, by inhibiting monocyte function. Tobacco smoking and marijuana smoking can result in impairment of alveolar macrophage function. In several diseases, including chronic lymphocytic leukemia, Kawasaki disease, Whipple disease, and malakoplakia, specific abnormalities of monocyte function play a significant role in the immune impairment in each disorder.

CLINICAL MANIFESTATIONS OF MONOCYTE DISORDERS

MONOCYTOPENIA OR MONOCYTE DYSFUNCTION

Isolated monocytopenia has not been reported. Theoretically, such a clinical syndrome could occur if there was a mutation in the gene for the synthesis of monocyte-macrophage colony stimulating factor (M-CSF) or its receptor. The manifestations of such a clinical state (amonocytosis) must be inferred. Neutrophils, endothelial cells, and other cell types can substitute in part for some monocyte functions. Monocytes have antibacterial, antiviral, antifungal, and antiparasitic capabilities. They are effective phagocytes that are involved in the ingestion and inactivation of microbes, such as mycobacteria, *Listeria, Brucella,* trypanosomes, and other granuloma-producing organisms. Thus their deficiency or functional abnormality predisposes to such infections. Macrophages can serve as a reservoir for the human immunodeficiency virus and is the principal locus for the virus in the brain and in neural tissue.

Deficiency in a specific subset of macrophages, the osteoclasts, results in *osteopetrosis*, an imbalance in bone metabolism that favors accretion. Osteoclasts normally play a key role in the closely regulated process of bone resorption and accretion, mediating the former process. Monocyte derivatives are, thereby, involved in the development of osteoporosis and other metabolic bone diseases in which the balance tips toward resorption. Bisphosphonates can inhibit osteoclast action by interfering with its function of bone resorption and by inhibiting the mevalonate pathway to geranylgeranyl diphosphate, which prevents the transformation of monocytes to osteoclasts. Thus, the deleterious clinical manifestations of macrophages are being subdued by making the monocyte a target of therapy, in this case the prevention and amelioration of postmenopausal osteoporosis, tumor-induced bone lysis, and Paget disease, as well as of others.

Macrophages and their derivatives, monocyte-derived dendritic cells, process and present antigens and play a role in immune regulation. In complex systems, such as that of antibody production, abnormal macrophages might lead to defects in humoral immunity. Activated monocytes secrete more than 50 chemical mediators or monokines, which, among other things, play a vital role in cellular immunity and inflammation. In effect, they are a critical endocrine (hormone-elaborating) apparatus. The absence of monocytes from the inflammatory response and the failure to elaborate, or the inappropriate elaboration, of monokines such as IL-1, α_1-proteinase inhibitor, prostaglandins, leukotrienes, plasminogen activator, elastase, tumor necrosis factor, IL-6, IL-12, and other cytokines, may cause or contribute to disease manifestations. A deficiency or impairment of monocytes has the potential of influencing several functions and systems, because monocytes are such important sources of inflammatory cytokines (see Chap. 68). Contrariwise, the unregulated activation of monocytes can lead to deleterious cytokine elaboration. Central to this process is tumor necrosis factor (TNF). The monocyte is a major source of TNF, which is a principal proinflammatory cytokine, triggering the elaboration of IL-1, IL-6, and others. Monocyte-derived TNF is also the primary chemical inducer of granuloma formation. The appreciation of its latter roles resulted in therapy to sequester TNF by antibody neutralization or receptor blockade and has resulted in substantial therapeutic effects in adult and juvenile rheumatoid arthritis, psoriasis, psoriatic arthritis, and Crohn disease. The side effects of such therapy confirm the key role of TNF in suppression of intracellular pathogens, such as *Mycobacterium tuberculosis* (potentiation of microbial diseases by TNF sequestrants), and in the role of the monocyte in modulating demyelinization (exacerbation of multiple sclerosis in patients treated with anti-TNF). The therapeutic administration of granulocyte-monocyte colony-stimulating factor also activates monocytes to elaborate cytokines, and this effect is being used to augment cancer vaccine therapy.

Monocytopenia and decreased monocyte entry into inflammatory sites occur after glucocorticoid administration. This may explain why patients treated with glucocorticoids are predisposed to infections in which monocytes play a protective role, such as those resulting from fungal, mycobacterial, and other opportunistic organisms. Dysfunctional monocytes, incapable of killing ingested microorganisms, are present in chronic granulomatous disease (see Chap. 66), as well as in hematopoietic stem cell diseases, such as monocytic variants of acute myelogenous leukemia.

TISSUE EFFECTS OF MONOCYTOSIS

Benign monocytosis is not associated with specific clinical manifestations. All forms of myelogenous leukemia with a predominance of monocytes are associated with a predisposition to troublesome tissue infiltrates, especially in the skin, gingiva, lymph nodes, meninges, and anal canal. The higher the monocyte count and the higher the proportion of leukemic monocytes, the more prevalent is tissue infiltration. In some cases, the tissue infiltration of leukemic monocytes can produce symptoms: lung dysfunction, laryngeal obstruction, and intracranial vessel rupture, as well as others. Release of procoagulants leading to intravascular coagulation also occurs in myelogenous leukemia with a high proportion of monocytes. The hyperleukocytic syndrome can occur in acute monocytic leukemia with markedly elevated white cell counts (see Chaps. 85 and 89).

EFFECTS OF HISTIOCYTOSIS

Hemophagocytic lymphohistiocytosis usually refers to the accumulation of activated macrophages (histiocytes) in tissue sites. The cells become intensely cytophagocytic; ingestion of red cells and occasionally of leukocytes, platelets, erythroblasts in marrow, or cells in other tissue sites is an important feature of these inflammatory histiocytoses (see Chap. 72). Because morphology has been misleading, the diagnosis of histiocytosis requires identification of specific cell markers. A histiocytosis may be inflammatory (polyclonal) or neoplastic (clonal). Because tissue macrophages can take on highly specialized phenotypes and localize in different tissues, histiocytosis is further defined by whether they carry markers of these cell types (e.g., Langerhans cells, interdigitating dendritic cells; see Chap. 72).

THROMBOATHEROGENESIS

The complex interrelationships among monocytes, atherogenesis,[74–78] and coagulation[78–81] are discussed in several other chapters in the text (see Chaps. 117 and 135). Monocytes may play a central role in the pathologic aspects of both processes, as a repository for tissue factor, inflammatory cytokines, and a key element in the inflammatory precursor lesions of atheroma formation.

BLOOD DENDRITIC CELLS

Dendritic cells and macrophages belong to a family of antigen-presenting cells and in the laboratory can be generated from a common precursor. So-called monocyte-derived dendritic cells are easily produced in the culture vessel by the appropriate cytokines. Indeed, the use of granulocyte-macrophage colony-stimulating factor (GM-CSF) as an adjuvant in cancer vaccines may relate in part to the cytokine's ability to activate monocytes and foster conversion to dendritic (antigen-presenting) cells *in vivo* (see Chaps. 24 and 25). Dendritic cells can be defined by phenotype into two principal types—myeloid and lymphoid (plasmacytoid) dendritic cells—of which there are likely subtypes. Monocyte-derived dendritic cells are probably a subset of the myeloid type. There is still uncertainty about the derivation of specific types of dendritic cells *in vivo* (see Chaps. 18 and 19).

Flow cytometry using cluster of differentiation (CD) markers and antidendritic cell surface antibodies have permitted the enumeration of myeloid (human leukocyte antigen-D related [HLA-DR]+, CD11c+, CD123–) and lymphocytic-plasmacytoid (HLA-DR+, CD11c–, CD123+, CD303+) dendritic cells in human blood in normal subjects and subjects with disease.[83,84] The analysis of changes in blood dendritic cell concentrations and distributions (myeloid-to-plasmacytoid ratios) is at an early stage; specific diagnostic correlations may be forthcoming. It is likely, however, that their centrality in the immune response as premier antigen-presenting cells may result in nonspecific alterations in their blood concentration or function in many generalized or localized inflammatory, infectious, and neoplastic diseases. Plasmacytoid dendritic cells may be decreased in numbers with aging, further impairing the immune response of older individuals (see Chap. 8).[85] Dendritic cells are also profoundly decreased in patients with hairy cell leukemia[2] and are dysfunctional in chronic lymphocytic leukemia.[45,46]

REFERENCES

1. Twomey JJ, Douglas CC, Sharkey O Jr: The monocytopenia of aplastic anemia. *Blood* 41:187, 1973.
2. Bourguin-Plonquet A, Rouard H, Roudot-Thoraval F: Severe decrease in peripheral blood dendritic cells in hairy cell leukaemia. *Br J Haematol* 116:595, 2002.
3. Fauci AS, Dale DC: The effect of in vivo hydrocortisone on subpopulations of human lymphocytes. *J Clin Invest* 53:240, 1974.
4. Viegas LR, Hoijman E, Beato M, Pecci A: Mechanisms involved in tissue-specific apoptosis regulated by glucocorticoids. *J Steroid Biochem Mol Biol* 109:273, 2008.
5. Maldonado GE, Hanlon DG: Monocytosis. *Mayo Clin Proc* 40:248, 1965.
5a. Lippi G, Banfi G, Montagnana M, et al: Acute variation of leucocytes counts following a half-marathon run. *Int J Lab Hematol* 2009.
6. Jaworkowsky LI, Solovey DY, Rhausova LY, Udris OY: Monocytosis as a sign of subsequent leukemia in patients with cytopenias (preleukemia). *Folia Haematol Int Mag Klin Morphol Blutforsch* 110:395, 1983.
7. Rigolin GM, Cuneo A, Roberti MG, et al: Myelodysplastic syndrome with monocytic component: hematologic and cytologic characterization. *Haematologica* 82:25, 1997.
8. Haferlach T, Schoch C, Schnittger S, et al: Distinct genetic patterns can be identified in acute monoblastic leukaemia (FAB AML M5a and M5b): A study of 124 patients. *Br J Haematol* 118:426, 2002.
9. Villeneuve P, Kim DT, Xu W, Brandwein J, Chang H: The morphological subcategories of acute monocytic leukemia (M5a and M5b) share similar immunophenotypic and cytogenetic features and clinical outcomes. *Leuk Res* 32:269, 2008.
10. de Fonseca LM, Brunetti IL, Campa A, et al: Assessment of monocytic component in acute myelomonocytic and monocytic/monoblastic leukemias by a chemoluminescence assay. *Hematol J* 4:26, 2003.
11. Ferran M, Gallardo F, Ferrer AM, et al: Acute myeloid dendritic cell leukaemia with specific cutaneous involvement: A diagnostic challenge. *Br J Dermatol* 158:1129, 2008.
12. Santiago-Schwartz F, Coppock DL, Hindenberg AA, Kern J: Identification of a malignant counterpart of the monocytic-dendritic cell progenitor in an acute myeloid leukemia. *Blood* 84:3054, 1994.
13. Srivastava HI, Srivistava A, Srivastava MD: Phenotype, genotype and cytokine production in acute leukemia involving progenitors of dendritic Langerhans' cell. *Leuk Res* 18:499, 1994.
14. Ferraris AM, Broccia G, Meloni T, et al: Clonal origin of cells restricted to monocytic differentiation in acute nonlymphocytic leukemia. *Blood* 64:817, 1984.
15. Beran M: Chronic myelomonocytic leukemia. *Cancer Treat Res* 142:107, 2008.
16. Onida F, Kantarjian HM, Smith TL, et al: Prognostic scoring factors and scoring systems in chronic myelomonocytic leukemia: A retrospective analysis of 213 patients. *Blood* 99:840, 2002.
17. Kratz CP, Niemeyer CM: Juvenile myelomonocytic leukemia. *Hematology* 1:100, 2005.
18. Del Fattore A, Cappariello A, Teti A. Genetics, pathogenesis and complications of osteopetrosis. *Bone* 42:19, 2008.
19. Helfrich MH: Osteoclast diseases. *Microsc Res Tech* 61:514, 2003.
20. Aricò M, Janka G, Fischer A, et al, for the FHL Study Group of the Histiocyte Society: hemophagocytic lymphohistiocytosis. Report of 122 children from the international registry. *Leukemia* 10:197, 1996.
21. Janka GE: Familial and acquired hemophagocytic lymphohistiocytosis. *Eur J Pediatr* 166:95, 2007.
22. Filipovich AH: Hemophagocytic lymphohistiocytosis and related disorders. *Curr Opin Allergy Clin Immunol* 6:410, 2006.
23. Rouphael NG, Talati NJ, Vaughan C, et al: Infections associated with haemophagocytic syndrome. *Lancet Infect Dis* 7:814, 2007.
24. Grom AA: Macrophage activation syndrome and reactive hemophagocytic lymphohistiocytosis: the same entities? *Curr Opin Rheumatol* 15:587, 2003.
25. Larroche C, Mouthon L: Pathogenesis of hemophagocytic syndrome (HPS). *Autoimmun Rev* 3:69, 2004.
26. Janka GE: Hemophagocytic syndromes. *Blood Rev* 21:245, 2007.
27. Imashuku S: Clinical features and treatment strategies of Epstein-Barr virus-associated hemophagocytic lymphohistiocytosis. *Crit Rev Oncol Hematol* 44:259, 2002.
28. Foucar E, Rosai J, Dorfman RF: Sinus histiocytosis with massive lymphadenopathy. *Cancer* 54:1834, 1984.
29. Pauli M, Bergamashi G, Tonon L, et al: Evidence of a polyclonal nature of the cell infiltrate in sinus histiocytosis with massive lymphadenopathy (Rosai-Dorfman disease). *Br J Haematol* 91:415, 1995.
30. Beutler E: Gaucher disease: Multiple lessons from a single gene disorder. *Acta Paediatr Suppl* 95:103, 2006.
31. Schuchman EH: The pathogenesis and treatment of acid sphingomyelinase-deficient Niemann-Pick disease. *J Inherit Metab Dis* 30:654, 2007.
32. Brunetti-Pierri N, Scaglia F: GM(1) gangliosidosis: Review of clinical, molecular, and therapeutic aspects. *Mol Genet Metab* 94:391, 2008.
33. Hirayama Y, Kohada K, Andoh M, et al: Syndrome of the sea-blue histiocyte. *Intern Med* 35:419, 1996.
34. Chang KL, Snyder DS: Langerhans cell histiocytosis. *Cancer Treat Res* 142:383, 2008.
35. Bechan GI, Egeler RM, Arceci RJ: Biology of Langerhans cells and Langerhans cell histiocytosis. *Int Rev Cytol* 254:1, 2006.
36. Jaffe ES, Harris NL, Stein H, Vardiman JW: Tumors of haematopoietic and lymphoid tissues, chapter 10. Histiocytic and dendritic cell neoplasms, in *World Health Organization Classification of Tumors*, pp 273–289. IARC Press, Lyon, 2001.
37. Lopez-Berestein G, Klostergaard J (eds): *Mononuclear Phagocytes in Cell Biology*, pp 1–239. CRC Press, Boca Raton, FL, 1993.
38. Cline MJ: Histiocytes and histiocytosis. *Blood* 84:2840, 1994.
39. Asherson GL, Zembala M: Monocyte abnormalities in disease, in *Human Monocytes*, edited by M Zembala, GL Asherson, pp 395–415. Academic Press, London, 1989.
40. Abboud RT, Vimalanathan S: Pathogenesis of COPD. Part I. The role of protease-antiprotease imbalance in emphysema. *Int J Tuberc Lung Dis* 12:361, 2008.
41. Aldonyte R, Jansson L, Piitulainen E, Janciauskiene S: Circulating monocytes from healthy individuals and COPD patients. *Respir Res* 4:11, 2003.

42. Kaplan J, De Domenico I, Ward DM: Chediak-Higashi syndrome. *Curr Opin Hematol* 15:22, 2008.
43. Davis WC, Huber H, Douglas SD, Fudenberg HH: A defect in circulating mononuclear phagocytes in chronic granulomatous disease of childhood. *J Immunol* 101:1093, 1968.
44. Stasia MJ, Li XJ: Genetics and immunopathology of chronic granulomatous disease. *Semin Immunopathol* 30:209, 2008.
45. Orsini E, Guarini A, Chiaretti S, et al: The circulating dendritic cell compartment in patients with chronic lymphocytic leukemia is severely defective and unable to stimulate an effective T cell response. *Cancer Res* 63:4497, 2003.
46. Mami NB, Mohty M, Aurran-Schleinitz T, et al: Blood dendritic cells in patients with chronic lymphocytic leukaemia. *Immunobiology* 213:493, 2008.
47. Snyderman R, Altman LC, Frankel A, Blaese RM: Defective mononuclear leukocyte chemotaxis. *Ann Intern Med* 78:509, 1973.
48. Komiyama A, Ichikawa M, Kanda H, et al: Defective interleukin 1 production in a familial monocyte disorder with a combined abnormality of mobility and phagocytosis-killing. *Clin Exp Immunol* 73:500, 1988.
49. Bhavsar PK, Sukkar MB, Khorasani N, et al: Glucocorticoid suppression of CX3CL1 (fractalkine) by reduced gene promoter recruitment of NF-kappaB. *FASEB J* 22:1807, 2008.
50. Ehrchen J, Steinmüller L, Barczyk K, et al: Glucocorticoids induce differentiation of a specifically activated, anti-inflammatory subtype of human monocytes. *Blood* 109:1265, 2007.
51. Nomura I, Abe J, Noma S, et al: Adrenomedullin is highly expressed in blood monocytes associated with acute Kawasaki disease: A microarray gene expression study. *Pediatr Res* 57:49, 2005.
52. Matsubara T, Ichiyama T, Furukawa S: Immunological profile of peripheral blood lymphocytes and monocytes/macrophages in Kawasaki disease. *Clin Exp Immunol* 141:381, 2005.
53. Van Crevel R, Curfs J, van der Ven AJ et al: Functional and morphological monocyte abnormalities in a patient with malakoplakia. *Am J Med* 105:74, 1998.
54. Ridgeway D, Wolff LJ, Wall M, Bouzy MS, et al: Indomethacin-sensitive monocyte killing defect in a child with disseminated atypical mycobacterial disease. *J Clin Immunol* 11:357, 1991.
55. Onwubalili JK: Defective monocyte chemotactic responsiveness in patients with active tuberculosis. *Immunol Lett* 16:39, 1987.
56. Welin A, Winberg ME, Abdalla H, et al: Incorporation of *Mycobacterium tuberculosis* lipoarabinomannan into macrophage membrane rafts is a prerequisite for the phagosomal maturation block. *Infect Immun* 76:2882, 2008.
57. Murray RA, Siddiqui MR, Mendillo M, Krahenbuhl J, Kaplan G. *Mycobacterium leprae* inhibits dendritic cell activation and maturation. *J Immunol* 178:338, 2007.
58. Spolarics Z,Siddiqi M, Siege4l JH, et al: Depressed interleukin-12-producing activity by monocytes correlates with adverse clinical course and a shift toward Th2-type lymphocyte pattern in severely injured male trauma patients. *Crit Care Med* 31:1722, 2003.
59. De AK, Laudanski K, Miller-Graziano CL: Failure of monocytes of trauma patients to convert to immature dendritic cells is related to preferential macrophage-colony-stimulating factor-driven macrophage differentiation. *J Immunol* 170:6355, 2003.
60. Venet F, Tissot S, Debard AL, et al: Decreased monocyte human leukocyte antigen-DR expression after severe burn injury: Correlation with severity and secondary septic shock. *Crit Care Med* 35:1910, 2007.
61. Pachot A, Cazalis MA, Venet F, et al: Decreased expression of the fractalkine receptor CX3CR1 on circulating monocytes as new feature of sepsis-induced immunosuppression. *J Immunol* 180:6421, 2008.
62. Tsujimoto H, Ono S, Efron PA, et al: Role of Toll-like receptors in the development of sepsis. *Shock* 29:315, 2008.
63. Albaiceta GM, Pedreira PR, García-Prieto E, Taboada F: Therapeutic implications of immunoparalysis in critically ill patients. *Inflamm Allergy Drug Targets* 6:191, 2007.
64. Sica A, Schioppa T, Mantovani A, Allavena P: Tumour-associated macrophages are a distinct M2 polarised population promoting tumour progression: Potential targets of anti-cancer therapy. *Eur J Cancer* 42:717, 2006.
65. Allavena P, Sica A, Solinas G, et al: The inflammatory micro-environment in tumor progression: The role of tumor-associated macrophages. *Crit Rev Oncol Hematol* 66:1, 2008.
66. Ryder MI, Saghizadeh M, Ding Y, et al: Effects of tobacco smoke on secretion of interleukin 1-beta,tumor necrosis factor-alpha, and transforming growth-beta from peripheral blood mononuclear cells. *Oral Microbiol Immunol* 17:331, 2002.
67. Chen H, Cowan MJ, Hasday JD, et al: Tobacco smoking inhibits expression of proinflammatory cytokines and activation of IL-1R-associated kinase, p38, and NF-kappaB in alveolar macrophages stimulated with TLR2 and TLR4 agonists. *J Immunol* 179:6097, 2007.
68. Shay AH, Choi R, Whittaker K, et al: Impairment of antimicrobial activity and nitric acid production by alveolar macrophages from smokers of marijuana and cocaine. *J Infect Dis* 187:700, 2003.
69. Klein TW, Cabral GA: Cannabinoid-induced immune suppression and modulation of antigen-presenting cells. *J Neuroimmune Pharmacol* 1:50, 2006.
70. Marth T, Neurath M, Cuccherini BA, Strober W: Defects of monocyte interleukin 12 production an humoral immunity in Whipple's disease. *Gastroenterology* 113:442, 1997.
71. Desnues B, Ihrig M, Raoult D, Mege JL: Whipple's disease: A macrophage disease. *Clin Vaccine Immunol* 13:170, 2006.
72. Moore KW, de Waal Maleyt R, Coffman RL, O'Garra A: Interleukin-10 and the interleukin 10 receptor. *Annu Rev Immunol* 19:683, 2001.
73. Dobrovolskaia MA, Vogel SN: Toll receptors, CD14, and macrophage activation and deactivation by LPS. *Microbes Infect* 4:903, 2002.
74. Tousoulis D, Davies G, Stefanadis C, et al: Inflammatory and thrombotic mechanisms in coronary atherosclerosis. *Heart* 89:993, 2003.
75. Oliveira RT, Mamoni RL, Souza JR, et al: Differential expression of cytokines, chemokines and chemokine receptors in patients with coronary artery disease. *Int J Cardiol* 24:17, 2009.
76. Murphy AJ, Woollard KJ, Hoang A, et al: High-density lipoprotein reduces the human monocyte inflammatory response. *Arterioscler Thromb Vasc Biol* 28:2071, 2008.
77. Jawie J: New insights into immunological aspects of atherosclerosis. *Pol Arch Med Wewn* 118:127, 2008.
78. Brambilla M, Camera M, Colnago D, et al: Tissue factor in patients with acute coronary syndromes: Expression in platelets, leukocytes, and platelet-leukocyte aggregates. *Arterioscler Thromb Vasc Biol* 28:947, 2008.
79. Martin J, Collot-Teixeira S, McGregor L, McGregor JL: The dialogue between endothelial cells and monocytes/macrophages in vascular syndromes. *Curr Pharm Des* 13:1751, 2007.
80. Napoleone E, di Santo A, Peri G, et al: The long pentraxin PTX3 up-regulates tissue factor in activated monocytes: Another link between inflammation and clotting activation. *J Leukoc Biol* 76:203, 2004.
81. Key NS: Platelet tissue factor: How did it get there and is it important? *Semin Hematol* 45(Suppl 1):S16, 2008.
82. Weisberg SP, McCann D, Desai M, et al: Obesity is associated with macrophage accumulation in adipose tissue. *J Clin Invest* 112:1796, 2003.
83. Giannelli S, Taddeo A, Presicce P, et al: A six-color flow cytometric assay for the analysis of peripheral blood dendritic cells. *Cytometry B Clin Cytom* 74:349, 2008.
84. Koga Y, Matsuzaki A, Suminoe A, et al: Expression of cytokine-associated genes in dendritic cells (DCs): Comparison between adult peripheral blood- and umbilical cord blood-derived DCs by cDNA microarray. *Immunol Lett* 116:55, 2008.
85. Pérez-Cabezas B, Naranjo-Gómez M, Fernández MA, et al: Reduced numbers of plasmacytoid dendritic cells in aged blood donors. *Exp Gerontol* 42:1033, 2007.

CHAPTER 71
MONOCYTOSIS AND MONOCYTOPENIA

Marshall A. Lichtman

SUMMARY

The blood monocyte is in transit between the marrow and tissues where it transforms (matures) into a macrophage. In tissues, the monocyte develops a phenotype characteristic of the specific tissue of residence (e.g., Kupffer cells of liver, microglia of brain, osteoclasts of bone). Because the monocyte participates in virtually all inflammatory and immune reactions, its concentration may be increased in many such conditions, including autoimmune diseases, gastrointestinal disorders, sarcoidosis, and several viral and bacterial infections. Monocytosis, an increase in the blood absolute monocyte count to more than 800/μL (0.8×10^9/L), may occur in some patients with cancer and several unrelated conditions, such as postsplenectomy states, inflammatory bowel disease, and some chronic infections (e.g., bacterial endocarditis, tuberculosis, and brucellosis). The inconsistency and unpredictability in the blood monocyte concentration among patients with the same disease is a function of its relatively small blood pool size, the damping effect of a large tissue pool, its relatively long life span, the number and complexity of effectors in the relevant cytokine network that can influence the response, and, perhaps, the ability to expand macrophage numbers by local mitosis in tissues. The most striking increase in blood monocyte concentration occurs with hematopoietic malignancies, especially clonal monocytosis (MDS), and monocytic or myelomonocytic leukemia. Depression, myocardial infarction, parturition, thermal injuries, and marathon competition are closely associated with monocytosis. Table 71–1 is a comprehensive list of causes of monocytosis. Monocytopenia is rare as an isolated finding. It is, however, notable in patients with aplastic anemia or hairy cell leukemia as a feature of pancytopenia. Although other cytopenias accompany the monocytopenia, the latter contributes significantly to the predisposition to infection and in hairy cell leukemia is an aid to diagnosis because of its constancy.

The blood monocyte is a cell in transit from marrow to tissues.[1] There are two major populations of blood monocytes: a smaller population represents a less mature stage, has a higher buoyant density, a smaller cell volume, lacks Fc receptors, and has greater tumoricidal activity; the larger population represents a more mature stage, has a lower buoyant density, has a larger cell volume, displays Fc receptors, expresses more peroxidase activity, secretes larger amounts of interleukin (IL)-1, and presents antigen and mediates antibody-dependent cell-mediated cytotoxicity more efficiently. The larger population, which composes approximately 90 percent of blood monocytes, strongly expresses CD14 (lipopolysaccharide receptor) and does not express CD16 (FcγR-III), the CD14++CD16– subset, whereas, 10 percent of blood monocytes have weak expression of CD14 and strong expression of CD16, the CD14+CD16++ subset.[2] The latter subset contains dendritic cell precursors.[3] The two major subsets can each be further stratified based on the expression of CD64 (FcγR-I).[4] (See Chaps. 68 and 69.)

Acronyms and abbreviations that appear in this chapter include: CD, cluster of differentiation; G-CSF, granulocyte colony-stimulating factor; GM-CSF, granulocyte-monocyte colony-stimulating factor; IL, interleukin; LPS, lipopolysaccharide; M-CSF, monocyte/macrophage colony-stimulating factor; MDS, myelodysplastic syndrome.

In tissues the monocyte is capable of transformation, under the influence of local environmental factors, into a macrophage. The monocyte plays an important role in acute and chronic inflammatory reactions, including granulomatous inflammation; immunologic reactions, including those involved in delayed hypersensitivity; tissue repair and reorganization; atheroma and thrombus formation; and the reaction to neoplasia and allografts. Because of the key role of monocytes in a variety of pathophysiologic reactions, a modest elevation in blood monocyte count can occur in many disparate conditions. In addition, in circumstances in which large increases in the number of macrophages are required in tissue sites, the demand may be met by local proliferation of macrophages and not be reflected either in increased transit of monocytes through the blood compartment from marrow to tissue or in an increased concentration of blood monocytes.[5] The evidence for local proliferation of macrophages is suggestive but inconclusive. Occasionally T-cell clones release only macrophage/monocyte colony-stimulating factor (M-CSF) and their conditioned medium stimulates growth only of macrophage colonies, providing a hypothetical model for local control of macrophage proliferation.[6]

NORMAL BLOOD MONOCYTE CONCENTRATION

In the first 2 weeks of life, the average absolute blood monocyte count is approximately 1000/μL (1×10^9/L; see Chap. 6). There is a gradual decline in the normal monocyte count to a mean of 400/μL (0.4×10^9/L) in adulthood, at which time monocytes constitute 1 to 9 percent (mean: 4 percent) of blood leukocytes (see Chap. 2). Monocytosis is present when the absolute count exceeds 800/μL (0.8×10^9/L) in adults. Men tend to have slightly higher monocyte counts than women.[7] Increments in the number of blood monocytes correlate directly with increases in the total blood monocyte pool and the monocyte turnover rate.[8] The blood monocyte count cycles with a periodicity of 5 days.[9] Older persons have a striking decrease in the proportion of CD14++CD16– to CD14+CD16+ monocytes as compared to younger persons.[10]

DISORDERS ASSOCIATED WITH MONOCYTOSIS

Table 71–1 outlines the diseases reported to be associated with monocytosis. In one review, hematologic disorders represented more than 50 percent, collagen vascular diseases approximately 10 percent, and malignant disease approximately 8 percent of cases of monocytosis.[11]

HEMATOLOGIC DISORDERS

Approximately 25 percent of patients with myelodysplastic states have an increase in the absolute monocyte count.[12–17] Occasional patients with a myelodysplastic state may develop an absolute monocyte count as high as 30,000/μL (30×10^9/L). Chronic monocytosis may be the principal feature of a clonal myeloid disease and precede by years the development of acute myelogenous leukemia. Patients with myelodysplasia and monocytosis have a high propensity to evolve into acute or chronic myelomonocytic leukemia. The number of promonocytes and monocytes may be increased in patients with acute myelogenous leukemia of the monocytic[18,19] or myelomonocytic type.[20] Acute myelogenous leukemic cells with a histiocytic (macrophagic) [21] or dendritic cell phenotype have been described.[22–24]

TABLE 71–1. Disorders Associated with Monocytosis

I. Hematologic Disorders
  A. Myeloid neoplasms
    1. Myelodysplastic states (12–17)
    2. Acute monocytic leukemia (18, 19)
    3. Acute myelomonocytic leukemia (20)
    4. Acute monocytic leukemia with histiocytic features (21)
    5. Acute myeloid dendritic cell leukemia (22–24)
    6. Chronic myelomonocytic leukemia (25–27)
    7. Juvenile myelomonocytic leukemia (28)
    8. Chronic myelogenous leukemia (m-*BCR*–positive type) (29, 30)
    9. Polycythemia vera (11)
  B. Chronic neutropenias (31–36)
  C. Drug-induced neutropenia (37–39)
  D. Postagranulocytic recovery (40,41)
  E. Lymphocytic neoplasms
    1. Lymphoma (43)
    2. Hodgkin lymphoma (44, 45)
    3. Myeloma (46, 47)
    4. Macroglobulinemia (48)
    5. T-cell lymphoma (49)
  F. Drug-induced pseudolymphoma (50)
  G. Immune hemolytic anemia (11)
  H. Idiopathic thrombocytopenic purpura (11)
  I. Postsplenectomy state (51, 52)

II. Inflammatory and Immune Disorders
  A. Connective tissue diseases
    1. Rheumatoid arthritis (53)
    2. Systemic lupus erythematosus (54)
    3. Temporal arteritis (11)
    4. Myositis (11)
    5. Polyarteritis nodosa (11)
    6. Sarcoidosis (55, 56)
  B. Infections
    1. Mycobacterial infections (57–60)
    2. Subacute bacterial endocarditis (61–63)
    3. Brucellosis (64)
    4. Dengue hemorrhagic fever (65)
    5. Resolution phase of acute bacterial infections (66)
    6. Syphilis (67, 68)
    7. Cytomegalovirus infection (69)
    8. Varicella-zoster virus (70)

III. Gastrointestinal Disorders
  A. Alcoholic liver disease (71)
  B. Inflammatory bowel disease (72)
  C. Sprue (11)

IV. Nonhematopoietic Malignancies (73–76)

V. Exogenous Cytokine Administration (77–83)

VI. Myocardial Infarction (84–87)

VII. Cardiac Bypass Surgery (88)

VIII. Miscellaneous Conditions
  A. Tetrachloroethane poisoning (89)
  B. Parturition (90, 91)
  C. Glucocorticoid administration (92–94)
  D. Depression (95–97)
  E. Thermal injury (98, 99)
  F. Marathon running (100, 101)
  G. Holoprosencephaly (102)
  H. Kawasaki disease (103)
  I. Wiskott-Aldrich syndrome (104)

Patients with chronic myelomonocytic leukemia have, by definition, an increased proportion of monocytes in the blood. The monocytosis may be striking in some cases.[25–27] Juvenile myelomonocytic leukemia, also, is defined in part by the increased proportion of monocytes in the blood.[28] In some cases of acute monocytic leukemia, the monocytes are immature and have features of monoblasts or promonocytes, but in many cases they are indistinguishable by light microscopy from normal blood monocytes. Some automated instruments are dependent on the α-naphthol acetate esterase reaction to detect the proportion of monocytes in white cell differential counts. These instruments may underestimate leukemic monocytes counts, especially in cases of chronic myelomonocytic leukemia, because the leukemic monocytes have a decreased activity of the enzyme.[25] An uncommon variant of Ph-positive chronic myelogenous leukemia (CML), expressing a p190 BCR-ABL transcript, is associated with a striking monocytosis in approximately 50 percent of cases.[29,30]

Monocytosis occurs in a number of neutropenic states: cyclic neutropenia,[31] chronic granulocytopenia of childhood,[32] familial benign chronic neutropenia,[33] infantile genetic agranulocytosis[34,35] and chronic hypoplastic neutropenia.[36] In human cyclic neutropenia, monocyte oscillation is reciprocal to the neutrophil cycle; the peak monocytosis, which often exceeds 2000/μL (2.0×10^9/L), occurs at the end of the neutropenic period. Monocytes often stay above 500/μL (0.5×10^9/L) throughout the cycle. In the variety of other neutropenias mentioned, monocytopoiesis often is preserved in the face of neutropenia. Transient elevations of the monocyte count have been reported in the acute phases of drug-induced agranulocytosis.[37–39] Monocytosis characteristically appears later in the recovery phase of agranulocytosis and may be a harbinger of recovery.[37,40,41] Some researchers dispute the validity of this observation.[42]

Monocytosis can occur with lymphomas and can increase with exacerbation of disease activity.[43] Monocytosis has been noted in approximately 25 percent of cases of Hodgkin lymphoma, although it does not correlate with prognosis.[43,44] In contrast, one treatise on the disease reports the hematologic values of patients with Hodgkin lymphoma at the time of diagnosis; only 4 of 100 have nominal increases in absolute blood monocyte counts.[45] A statistically significant increase in blood monocyte concentration has been reported in myeloma and has been correlated with the presence of λ light chains containing monoclonal immunoglobulin.[46,47] Rare cases of M-CSF secreting lymphoid tumors have been associated with monocytosis.[48,49] Pseudolymphoma syndrome, induced by drugs such as carbamazepine, phenytoin, phenobarbital, and valproic acid, is associated with monocytosis.[50]

SPLENECTOMY

Monocytosis is a common feature in individuals who have had splenectomy.[51,52]

INFLAMMATORY AND IMMUNE DISORDERS

Connective tissue diseases, including rheumatoid arthritis,[53] systemic lupus erythematosus, temporal arteritis, myositis, and periarteritis nodosa, may be associated with monocytosis, although monocytosis is not common in these diseases.[11] The usual alterations of the white cell count in systemic lupus erythematosus, for example, are neutropenia and lymphopenia, but 10 percent of patients have a mild monocytosis.[54] An elevation of the blood monocyte count occurs in sarcoidosis[55] and is inversely related to a reduction in circulating T lymphocytes.[56]

Infectious diseases are an uncommon cause of monocytosis. Only a few instances of infection were noted in a comprehensive review of causes of monocytosis, including tonsillitis, dental infection, recurrent liver abscesses, candidiasis, and one instance of tuberculous peritonitis.[11] Tuberculosis was once a leading cause of monocytosis, because of the role of monocytes in granuloma (tubercle) formation. Neither the monocyte count nor the ratio of monocytes to lymphocytes correlates with the stage or activity of tuberculosis.[57–59] *Mycobacterium fortuitum* infection, usually in the setting of AIDS, also is associated with monocytosis.[60]

Monocytosis is found in 15 to 20 percent of patients with subacute bacterial endocarditis[61,62] but is not correlated with the presence of blood macrophages, which may be present in this disease.[63]

A number of infections formerly thought to be associated with monocytosis are not, when examined systematically. These include rickettsial diseases, leishmaniasis, typhoid fever, malaria, and disseminated candidiasis. Brucellosis[64] and dengue hemorrhagic fever.[65]

A monocytosis in the resolution phase of acute infections has been noted,[66] and monocytosis appears in neonatal, primary, and secondary syphilis.[67,68] Certain viruses, especially cytomegalovirus and varicella-zoster virus, induce an increase in blood monocytes.[69,70]

GASTROINTESTINAL DISEASES

Sprue, ulcerative colitis, regional enteritis, and alcoholic liver disease are associated with monocytosis.[11,71,72]

NONHEMATOPOIETIC MALIGNANCIES

Sixty percent of patients with nonhematologic malignancy exhibit a monocytosis that is independent of the presence or absence of metastatic disease.[73] An inverse relationship of monocyte count (elevated) and T-lymphocyte concentration (decreased) has also been noted in patients with malignant disease.[74] Reports of hematologic values in metastatic colon cancer and soft-tissue sarcoma have emphasized the frequency of monocytosis in patients with cancer.[75,76] Consequently, if *unexplained* monocytosis persists, malignancy should be considered.

EXOGENOUS CYTOKINE ADMINISTRATION

The administration of granulocyte-macrophage colony-stimulating factor (GM-CSF),[77] interleukin-10,[78] or granulocyte colony-stimulating factor (G-CSF)[79,80] may result in mild increases in blood monocyte counts. Administration of M-CSF [81,82] results in an invariable increase in blood monocytes. Doses of 40 to 120 mcg/kg per day result in the peak increase, which may reach three- to fourfold baseline, in about 8 days. Administration of human macrophage inflammatory protein-1α to patients or normal volunteers is associated with a brief monocytopenia followed by a monocytosis that is proportional to the dose administered.[83]

MYOCARDIAL INFARCTION

Monocytosis occurs after myocardial infarction, reaching a peak on day 3. A correlation exists between serum creatine kinase activity and monocyte count, suggesting a relationship between extent of infarction and monocytosis.[84] After myocardial infarction, persistent monocytosis is correlated also with pump failure.[85–87] Monocytosis is a frequent finding after cardiopulmonary bypass surgery.[88] In the latter circumstance, CD14 (lipopolysaccharide [LPS] receptor) is markedly decreased on the monocyte surface and plasma-soluble CD14 is increased, which changes are compatible with monocyte activation.

MISCELLANEOUS CONDITIONS

Other disorders associated with monocytosis include tetrachloroethane poisoning.[89] Monocytosis is a frequent finding at the time of parturition.[90,91] An increase in blood monocytes occurs in healthy volunteers[92,93] and in patients with myelodysplastic syndrome (MDS)[94] who are given moderately high, therapeutic-level doses of glucocorticoids. Psychiatric depression is associated with a conjoint increase in neutrophils and monocytes.[95–97] The monocytosis in depressive and anxiety disorders is associated with high plasma levels of β endorphins and dysfunctional (hypophagocytic) monocytes.[97] Thermal injury is accompanied by monocytosis.[98,99] Competitive marathon runners have a monocytosis associated with elevated plasma levels of several cytokines, including M-CSF.[100,101] An increase in blood monocytes accompanies several rare syndromes: holoprosencephaly,[102] Kawasaki disease,[103] and Wiskott-Aldrich.[104]

BLOOD MONOCYTE SUBSET COUNTS IN DISEASE

Differential monocyte subset responses (CD14++CD16– vs. CD14+CD16+) without deviation of total monocyte counts outside the normal range have been observed in older subjects and those with sepsis, AIDS, allergic disorders, dermatitides, hemodialysis, and atherosclerosis.[4,10,88,105] These monocytic subset variations usually are not measured in clinical laboratories and probably have little diagnostic importance, as yet.

DISORDERS ASSOCIATED WITH MONOCYTOPENIA

Although monocytopenia may occur in any hematopoietic stem cell disease associated with pancytopenia (e.g., myelogenous leukemia), a decrease in monocytes is notable and constant in aplastic anemia.[106] It is also a constant feature of hairy cell leukemia, in which monocytopenia can be a helpful diagnostic clue and also a contributor to the predisposition to infection, which is an important, morbid feature of the disease.[107] Monocytopenia occurs in a small proportion of patients with chronic lymphocytic leukemia and these patients may have a higher frequency of infections, especially by viruses.[108] Severe thermal injuries also can result in monocytopenia.[109] Cyclic neutropenia is also notable for intermittent periods of monocytopenia.[110] Rare cases of conjoint severe neutropenia and monocytopenia occur.[111] Transient monocytopenia is a feature of hemodialysis, but monocyte counts return to normal within hours after the procedure ends.[105]

In contrast, to reports of monocytosis noted above in "Inflammatory and Immune Disorders," automated blood cell counts in large numbers of subjects find that a decreased absolute monocyte count is frequent in patients with rheumatoid arthritis[112] or systemic lupus erythematosus,[113] and in those with human immunodeficiency virus infection.[114] One has to presume that these contrasting results relate to stage or activity of disease at the time of measurement.

Glucocorticoid hormones produce a monocytopenia, transiently, about 6 hours after administration to human volunteers[115] or to patients.[92,120] Administration of interferon-α and tumor necrosis factor-α may also cause monocytopenia.[117] Monocytopenia may follow radiotherapy.[118]

BLOOD DENDRITIC CELL COUNTS

Blood dendritic cells are composed of two phenotypic subtypes: myeloid-derived (HLA-Dr+CD11c+CD123+) and lymphoid/plasmacytoid-derived (HLA-Dr+CD11c–CD123+). The total blood dendritic cell count can be measured by flow cytometry.[119–121] Dendritic cells make up approximately 0.6 percent of blood cells (range: 0.15 to 1.30 percent) and represent 14×10^6 cells/L (range: 3 to 30×10^6 cells/L). Approximately one-third of these cells are lymphoid-plasmacytoid–derived type and two-thirds are myeloid-derived type.[121–123] Blood dendritic cell counts decrease with aging[124] and increase with surgical stress[123] (and presumably other stressful reactions) in relation to plasma cortisol levels. Fluctuations in blood dendritic cells are often independent of changes in total blood monocyte count.

REFERENCES

1. Turpin JA, Lopez-Bernstein G: Differentiation, maturation, and activation of monocytes and macrophages: Functional activity is controlled by a continuum of activation, in *Mononuclear Phagocytes in Cell Biology*, edited by G Lopez-Berestein, J Klostergaard, p 71. CRC Press, Boca Raton, FL, 1993.
2. Zeigler-Heitbrock HW: Heterogeneity of human blood monocytes: The CD14+ CD16+ subpopulation. *Immunol Today* 17:424, 1996.
3. Thomas R, Lipsky PE: Human peripheral blood dendritic cell subsets. Isolation and characterization of precursor and mature antigen-presenting cells. *J Immunol* 153:4016, 1994.
4. Grage-Griebenow E, Flad H-D, Ernst M: Heterogeneity of peripheral blood monocyte subsets. *J Leukoc Biol* 69:11, 2001.
5. Hume DA, Ross IL, Himes SR, et al: The mononuclear phagocyte system revisited. *J Leukoc Biol* 72:621, 2001.
6. Griffin JD, Meuer SC, Schlossman SF, Reinherz EL: T-cell regulation of myelopoiesis: Analysis at a clonal level. *J Immunol* 133:1863, 1984.
7. Munan L, Kelly A: Age-dependent changes in blood monocyte populations in man. *Clin Exp Immunol* 35:161, 1979.
8. Meuret G, Hoffman G: Monocyte kinetic studies in normal and disease states. *Br J Haematol* 24:275, 1973.
9. Meuret G, Bremer C, Bammert J, Ewen J: Oscillation of blood monocyte counts in healthy individuals. *Cell Tissue Kinet* 7:223, 1974.
10. Sadeghi HM, Schnelle JF, Thoma JK, et al: Phenotypic and functional characteristics of circulating monocytes of elderly persons. *Exp Gerontol* 34:959, 1999.
11. Maldonado JE, Hanlon DG: Monocytosis: A current appraisal. *Mayo Clin Proc* 40:248, 1965.
12. Rigolin GM, Cuneo A, Roberti MG, et al: Myelodysplastic syndromes with monocytic component: Hematologic and cytogenetic characterization. *Haematologia (Budap)* 82:25, 1997.
13. Cunningham I, MacCallum SJ, Nicholls MD, et al: The myelodysplastic syndromes: An analysis of prognostic factors in 226 cases from a single institution. *Br J Haematol* 90:602, 1995.
14. Castaldi G, Rigolin GM: The monocytic component in myelodysplastic syndromes. *Cancer Treat Res* 108:81, 2001.
15. Jaworkowsky LI, Solovey DY, Rhausova LY, Udris OY: Monocytosis as a sign of subsequent leukemia in patients with cytopenias (preleukemia). *Folia Haematol Int Mag Klin Morphol Blutforsch* 110:395, 1983.
16. Ruggiero G, Sica M, Luciano L, et al: A case of myelodysplastic syndrome associated with CD14(+)CD56(+) monocytosis, expansion of NK lymphocytes and defect of HLA-E expression. *Leuk Res* 33:181, 2009.
17. Cunha BA, Hamid N, Krol V, Eisenstein L: Fever of unknown origin due to preleukemia/myelodysplastic syndrome: the diagnostic importance of monocytosis with elevated serum ferritin levels. *Heart Lung* 35:277, 2006.
18. Haferlach T, Schoch C, Schnittger S, et al: Distinct genetic patterns can be identified in acute monoblastic leukaemia (FAB AML M5a and M5b): A study of 124 patients. *Br J Haematol* 118:426, 2002.
19. Villeneuve P, Kim DT, Xu W, Brandwein J, Chang H: The morphological subcategories of acute monocytic leukemia (M5a and M5b) share similar immunophenotypic and cytogenetic features and clinical outcomes. *Leuk Res* 32:269, 2008.
20. Sun X, Zhang W, Ramdas L, et al: Comparative analysis of genes regulated in acute myelomonocytic leukemia with and without inv(16)(p13q22) using microarray techniques, real-time PCR, immunohistochemistry, and flow cytometry immunophenotyping. *Mod Pathol* 20:811, 2007.
21. Laurencet FM, Chapius B, Roux-Lombard P, et al: Malignant histiocytosis in the leukaemic stage: A new entity (M5c-AML) in the FAB classification? *Leukemia* 8:502, 1994.
22. Ferran M, Gallardo F, Ferrer AM, et al: Acute myeloid dendritic cell leukaemia with specific cutaneous involvement: A diagnostic challenge. *Br J Dermatol* 158:1129, 2008.
23. Santiago-Schwartz F, Coppock DL, Hindenberg AA, Kern J: Identification of a malignant counterpart of the monocytic-dendritic cell progenitor in an acute myeloid leukemia. *Blood* 84:3054, 1994.
24. Lichtman MA, Segel GB: Uncommon phenotypes of acute myelogenous leukemia: Basophilic, mast cell, eosinophilic, and myeloid dendritic cell subtypes: A review. *Blood Cells Mol Dis* 35:370, 2005.
25. Frew ME, Donaldson K: Monocyte analysis in chronic myelomonocytic leukaemia. *Br J Biomed Sci* 54:244, 1997.
26. Onida F, Kantarjian HM, Smith TL, et al: Prognostic scoring factors and scoring systems in chronic myelomonocytic leukemia: A retrospective analysis of 213 patients. *Blood* 99:840, 2002.
27. Xu Y, McKenna RW, Karandikar NJ, et al: Flow cytometric analysis of monocytes as a tool for distinguishing chronic myelomonocytic leukemia from reactive monocytosis. *Am J Clin Pathol* 124:799, 2005.
28. Kratz CP, Niemeyer CM: Juvenile myelomonocytic leukemia. *Hematology* 1:100, 2005.
29. Ohsaka A, Shiina S, Kobayashi M, et al: Philadelphia chromosome-positive chronic myeloid leukemia expressing p190(BCR-ABL). *Intern Med* 41:1092, 2002.
30. Hur M, Song HM, Kang SH, et al: Lymphoid predominance and the absence of basophilia and splenomegaly are frequent in m-bcr-positive chronic myelogenous leukemia. *Ann Hematol* 81:219, 2002.
31. Wright D, Dale DC, Fauci AS, Wolff SM: Human cyclic neutropenia: Clinical review and long-term follow-up of patients. *Medicine (Baltimore)* 60:1, 1981.
32. Zuelzer WW, Bajoghli M: Chronic granulocytopenia in childhood. *Blood* 23:359, 1964.
33. Cutting HO, Lang JE: Familial benign chronic neutropenia. *Ann Intern Med* 61:876, 1964.
34. Krill CE, Mauer AM: Congenital agranulocytosis. *J Pediatr* 68:361, 1966.
35. Lang JE, Cutting HO: Infantile genetic agranulocytosis. *Pediatrics* 35:596, 1965.
36. Spaet TH, Dameshek W: Chronic hypoplastic neutropenia. *Am J Med* 13:35, 1952.
37. Robinson RL, Burk MS, Raman S: Fever, delirium, autonomic instability, and monocytosis associated with olanzapine. *J Postgrad Med* 49:96, 2003.
38. Graf M, Tarlov A: Agranulocytosis with monohistiocytosis associated with ampicillin therapy. *Ann Intern Med* 69:91, 1968.
39. Thöne J, Kessler E: Monocytosis subsequent to ziprasidone treatment: A possible side effect. *Prim Care Companion J Clin Psychiatry* 9:465, 2007.
40. Reznikoff P: The etiologic importance of fatigue and the prognostic significance of monocytosis in neutropenia (agranulocytosis). *Am J Clin Pathol* 6:205, 1936.
41. Rosenthal N, Abel HA: The significance of the monocytes in agranulocytosis (leukopenic infectious agranulocytosis). *Am J Clin Pathol* 6:205, 1936.
42. Pretty HM, Gosselin G, Colprian G, Long LA: Agranulocytosis: A report of 30 cases. *Can Med Assoc* J 93:1058, 1965.
43. Rosenberg SA, Diamond HD, Jaslowitz B, Craver LF: Lymphosarcoma: A review of 1269 cases. *Medicine (Baltimore)* 40: 31, 1961.
44. Ultmann JE: Clinical features and diagnosis of Hodgkin's disease. *Cancer* 9:297, 1966.
45. Kaplan HS: *Hodgkin's Disease*, 2nd ed, Table 4.1, pp 127–128. Harvard University Press, Cambridge, MA, 1980.
46. Sewell RL: Lymphocyte abnormalities in myeloma. *Br J Haematol* 36:545, 1977.
47. Blom J, Nielsen H, Larsen SO, et al: A study of certain functional parameters of monocytes from patients with multiple myeloma: Comparison with monocytes from healthy individuals. *Scand J Haematol* 33:425, 1984.
48. Nakajima H, Mori S, Takeuchi T, et al: Monocytosis and high serum macrophage colony-stimulating factor in Waldenström's macroglobulinemia. *Blood* 86:2863, 1995.

49. Tokioka T, Shimamoto Y, Motoyoshi K, Yamaguchi M: Clinical significance of monocytosis and human monocytic colony stimulating factor in patients with adult T-Cell leukaemia/lymphoma. *Haematologia (Budap)* 26:1, 1994.
50. Choi TS, Doh KS, Kim SH, et al: Clinicopathological and genotypic aspects of anti-convulsant-induced pseudolymphoma syndrome. *Br J Dermatol* 148:730, 2003.
51. Durig M, Landmann RMA, Harder F: Lymphocyte subsets in human peripheral blood after splenectomy and autotransplantation of splenic tissue. *J Lab Clin Med* 104:110, 1984.
52. Lanng Nielson J, Romer FK, Ellegaard J: Serum angiotensin-converting enzyme and blood monocytes in splenectomized individuals. *Acta Haematol* 67:132, 1982.
53. Buchan GS, Palmer DG, Gibbins BL: The response of human peripheral blood mononuclear phagocytes to rheumatoid arthritis. *J Leukoc Biol* 37:221, 1985.
54. Budman DR, Steinberg AD: Hematologic aspects of systemic lupus erythematosus. Current concepts. *Ann Intern Med* 86:220, 1977.
55. Goodwin JS, DeHaratius R, Israel H, et al: Suppressor cell function in sarcoidosis. *Ann Intern Med* 90:169, 1979.
56. Daniele RP, Dauber JH, Rossman MD: Immunologic abnormalities in sarcoidosis. *Ann Intern Med* 92:406, 1980.
57. Stobie W, England NJ, McMenemy WH: The interpretation of haemograms in pulmonary tuberculosis. *Am Rev Tuberc* 46:1, 1942.
58. Flinn JW: A study of the differential blood count in 1000 cases of active pulmonary tuberculosis. *Ann Intern Med* 2:622, 1929.
59. Singh KJ, Ahluwalia G, Sharma SK, et al: Significance of haematological reactions in patients with tuberculosis. *J Assoc Physicians India* 49:788, 2001.
60. Smith MB, Schnadig VJ, Boyars MC, Woods GL: Clinical and pathological features of Mycobacterium fortuitum infections: An emerging pathogen in patients with AIDS. Am *J Clin Pathol* 116:225, 2001.
61. Daland GA, Gottlieb L, Wallerstein RO, et al: Hematologic observations in bacterial endocarditis. *J Lab Clin Med* 48:827, 1956.
62. Myhre EB, Braconier JH, Sjögren U: Automated cytochemical differential leukocyte count in patients hospitalized with acute bacterial infections. *Scand J Infect Dis* 17:201, 1985.
63. Hill RW, Bayrd ED: Phagocytic reticuloendothelial cells in subacute bacterial endocarditis with negative cultures. *Ann Intern Med* 52:310, 1960.
64. Tsolia M, Drakonaki S, Messaritaki A et al: Clinical features, complications and treatment outcome of childhood brucellosis in central Greece. *J Infect* 44:257, 2002.
65. Khan E, Siddiqui J, Shakoor S, et al: Dengue outbreak in Karachi, Pakistan, 2006: Experience at a tertiary care center. *Trans R Soc Trop Med Hyg* 101:1114, 2007.
66. Hickling RA: The monocytes in pneumonia: A clinical and hematologic study. *Arch Intern Med* 40:594, 1927.
67. Rosahn PD, Pearce L: The blood cytology in untreated and treated syphilis. *Am J Med Sci* 187:88, 1934.
68. Karyalcin G, Khanijou A, Kim KY, et al: Monocytosis in congenital syphilis. *Am J Dis Child* 131:782, 1977.
69. Klemola E: Cytomegalovirus infection in previously healthy adults. *Ann Intern Med* 79:267, 1973.
70. Tsukahara T, Yogushi A, Horiuchi Y: Significance of monocytosis in varicella herpes zoster. *J Dermatol* 19:94, 1992.
71. McKeever UM, O'Mahoney C, Lawlor E, et al: Monocytosis: A feature of alcoholic liver disease. *Lancet* 2:1492, 1983.
72. Mees AS, Berney J, Jewell DP: Monocytes in inflammatory bowel disease: Absolute monocyte counts. *J Clin Pathol* 33:917, 1980.
73. Barrett O Jr: Monocytosis in malignant disease. *Ann Intern Med* 73:991, 1970.
74. Wood GW, Neff JE, Stephens R: Relationship between monocytosis and T-lymphocyte function in human cancer. *J Natl Cancer Inst* 63:587, 1979.
75. Melichar B, Touskova M, Vesely P: Effect of irinotecan on the phenotype of peripheral blood leukocyte populations in patients with metastatic colorectal cancer. *Hepatogastroenterology* 49:967, 2002.
76. Ruka W, Rutkowski p, Kaminska J, et al: Alterations of routine blood tests in adult patients with soft tissue sarcomas: Relationships to cytokine serum levels and prognostic significance. *Ann Oncol* 12: 1423, 2001.
77. Schmitz LL, McClure JS, Litz CE, et al: Morphologic and quantitative changes in blood and marrow cells following growth factor therapy *Am J Clin Pathol* 101:67, 1994.
78. Chernoff AE, Granowitz EV, Shapiro L, et al: A randomized controlled trial of IL -10 in humans. *J Immunol* 154:5492, 1995.
79. Ranaghan L, Drake M, Humphreys MW, Morris TC: Leukaemoid monocytosis in M4 AML following chemotherapy: G-CSF. *Clin Lab Haematol* 20:49, 1998.
80. Liu CZ, Persad R, Inghirami G, et al: Transient atypical monocytosis mimic acute myelomonocytic leukemia in post-chemotherapy patients receiving G-CSF: Report of two cases. *Clin Lab Haematol* 26:359, 2004.
81. Weiner LM, Li W, Holmes M, et al: Phase I trial of recombinant macrophage colony-stimulating factor and recombinant gamma-interferon: Toxicity, monocytosis, and clinical effects. *Cancer Res* 54:4084, 1994.
82. Minasian LM, Yao TJ, Steffens TA, et al: A phase I study of anti-GD3 ganglioside monoclonal antibody R24 and recombinant human macrophage-colony stimulating factor in patients with metastatic melanoma. *Cancer* 75:2251, 1995.
83. Marshall E, Howell AH, Powles R, et al: Clinical effects of human macrophage inflammatory protein-1 alpha MIP-1 alpha (LD78) administration in humans. *Eur J Cancer* 34:1023, 1998.
84. Meisel SR, Panzner H, Schecter M, et al: Peripheral monocytosis following myocardial infarction. *Cardiology* 90:52, 1998.
85. Maekawa y, Anzai t, Yoshikawa T, et al: Prognostic significance of peripheral monocytosis after reperfusion acute myocardial infarction: Possible role for left ventricular remodeling. *J Am Coll Cardiol* 16:241, 2002.
86. Gibson WJ, Gibson CM: The association of impaired myocardial perfusion and monocytosis with late recovery of left ventricular function following primary percutaneous coronary intervention. *Eur Heart J* 27:2487, 2006.
87. Hong YJ, Jeong MH, Ahn Y, et al: Relationship between peripheral monocytosis and nonrecovery of left ventricular function in patients with left ventricular dysfunction complicated with acute myocardial infarction. *Circ J* 71:1219, 2007.
88. Fingerle-Rowson G, Auers J, Kreuzer E, et al: Down-regulation of surface monocyte lipopolysaccharide-receptor CD14 in patients on cardiopulmonary bypass undergoing aorta-coronary bypass operation. *J Thorac Cardiovasc Surg* 115:1172, 1998.
89. Minot GR, Smith LW: The blood in tetrachloroethane poisoning. *Arch Intern Med* 28:687, 1921.
90. Siegal I, Gleichner N: Peripheral white blood cells alterations in early labor. *Diagn Gynecol Obstet* 3:123, 1981.
91. Buchan GS, Gibbins BL, Griffin JFT: The influence of parturition on peripheral blood mononuclear phagocyte subpopulation in pregnant women. *J Leukoc Biol* 37:231, 1985.
92. Rinehard JJ, Sagone AL, Balcerzak SP, et al: Effects of corticosteroid therapy on human monocyte function. *N Engl J Med* 292:236, 1975.
93. Shoenfeld Y, Gurewich Y, Gallant LA, et al: Prednisone-induced leukocytosis. *Am J Med* 71:773, 1981.
94. Morales M, Wilkes J, Lowder JN: Monocytic leukemoid reaction, glucocorticoid therapy, and myelodysplastic syndrome. *Cleve Clin J Med* 6:571, 1990.
95. Maes M, VanDerPlanken M, Stevens WJ, et al: Leukocytosis, monocytosis and neutrophilia: Hallmarks of severe depression. *J Psychiatr Res* 26:125, 1992.
96. Maes M, Lambrechts J, Suy E, et al: Absolute number and percentage of circulating natural killer, non-MHC-restricted T cytotoxic, and phagocytic cells in unipolar depression. *Neuropsychobiology* 29:157, 1994.
97. Castilla-Cortazar I, Castilla A, Gurpegui M: Opioid peptides and immunodysfunction in a patient with major depression and anxiety disorders. *J Physiol Biochem* 54:203, 1998.
98. Santangelo S, Gamelli RL, Shankar R: Myeloid commitment shifts toward monocytopoiesis after thermal injury and sepsis. *Ann Surg* 233:97, 2001.
99. Lovell R, Madden L, McNaughton LR, Carroll S: Effects of active and passive hyperthermia on heat shock protein 70 (HSP70). *Amino Acids* 34:203, 2008.
100. Kratz A, Lewandrowski KB, Siegel AJ, et al: Effect of marathon running on hematologic and biochemical laboratory parameters, including cardiac markers. *Am J Clin Pathol* 118:856, 2002.
101. Suzuki K, Nakaji S, Yamadi M, et al: Impact of a competitive marathon race on systemic cytokine and neutrophil responses. *Med Sci Sports Exerc* 35:348, 2003.
102. Jubinsky PT, Shanske AL, Pixley FJ, et al: A syndrome of holoprosencephaly, recurrent infections, and monocytosis. *Am J Med Genet A* 140:2742, 2006.
103. Kuo HC, Wang CL, Liang CD, et al: Persistent monocytosis after intravenous immunoglobulin therapy correlated with the development of coronary artery lesions in patients with Kawasaki disease. *J Microbiol Immunol Infect* 40:395, 2007.
104. Watanabe N, Yoshimi A, Kamachi Y, et al: Wiskott-Aldrich syndrome is an important differential diagnosis in male infants with juvenile myelomonocytic leukemia like features. *J Pediatr Hematol Oncol* 29:836, 2007.
105. Nockher WA, Wiemer J, Scherberich JE: Hemodialysis monocytopenia: Differential sequestration kinetics of CD14+CD16+ and CD14++ blood monocyte subsets. *Clin Exp Immunol* 123:49, 2001.
106. Twormey JJ, Douglas CC, Sharkey O Jr: The monocytopenia of aplastic anemia. *Blood* 41:187, 1973.
107. den Ottolander GJ, van der Burgh FJ, Lopes Cardozo P, et al: The Hemalog D automated differential counter in the diagnosis of hairy cell leukemia. *Leuk Res* 7:309, 1983.
108. DeRossi G, Mauro FR, Ialongo P, et al: Monocytopenia and infections in chronic lymphocytic leukemia (CLL). *Eur J Haemat* 46(2):119, 1991.
109. Peterson V, Hensbrough J, Buerk C, et al: Regulation of granulopoiesis following severe thermal injury. *J Trauma* 23:19, 1983.
110. Adams WH, Liu YK: Periodic neutropenia and monocytopenia. *Am J Hematol* 13:73, 1982.
111. Marinone G, Roncoli B, Marinone MG Jr: Pure white cell aplasia. *Semin Hematol* 28:298, 1991.
112. Isenberg DA, Martin P, Hajirousou V, et al: Haematological reassessment of rheumatoid arthritis using an automated method. *Br J Rheumatol* 25:152, 1986.
113. Isenberg DA, Patterson KG, Todd-Pokropek A, et al: Haematological aspects of systemic lupus erythematosus: A reappraisal using automated methods. *Acta Haematol* 67:242, 1982.
114. Treacy M, Lai L, Costello C, et al: Peripheral blood and bone marrow abnormalities in patients with HIV related disease. *Br J Haematol* 65:289, 1987.
115. Steer JH, Vuong Q, Joyce DA: Suppression of human monocyte tumor necrosis factor-alpha release by glucocorticoid therapy: Relationship to systemic monocytopenia and cortisol suppression. *Br J Clin Pharmacol* 43:383, 1997.
116. Fauci AS, Dale DC: Monocytopenia after prednisone. *N Engl J Med* 292:928, 1975.

117. Aulitzky WE, Tilg H, Vogel W, et al: Acute hematologic effects of interferon alpha, interferon gamma, tumor necrosis factor alpha and interleukin 2. *Ann Hematol* 62:25, 1991.
118. Rotman M, Ansley H, Rogow L, et al: Monocytosis: A new observation during radiotherapy. *Int J Radiat Oncol Biol Phys* 2:117, 1977.
119. Fearnley DB, Whyte LF, Carnoutosis SA, et al: The monitoring of human blood dendritic cell numbers. *Blood* 93:728, 1999.
120. Szabolcs P, Park K-D, Reese M, et al: Absolute values of dendritic cell subsets in bone marrow, cord blood, and peripheral blood enumerated by a novel method. *Stem Cells* 21:269, 2003.
121. Giannelli S, Taddeo A, Presicce P, et al: A six-color flow cytometric assay for the analysis of peripheral blood dendritic cells. *Cytometry B Clin Cytom* 74:349, 2008.
122. Koga Y, Matsuzaki A, Suminoe A, et al: Expression of cytokine-associated genes in dendritic cells (DCs): Comparison between adult peripheral blood- and umbilical cord blood-derived DCs by cDNA microarray. *Immunol Lett* 116:55, 2008.
123. Ho CSK, López JA, Vuckovic S, et al: Surgical and physical stress increases circulatory blood dendritic cell counts independently of monocyte counts. *Blood* 98:140, 2001.
124. Pérez-Cabezas B, Naranjo-Gómez M, Fernández MA, et al: Reduced numbers of plasmacytoid dendritic cells in aged blood donors. *Exp Gerontol* 42:1033, 2007.

CHAPTER 72

INFLAMMATORY AND MALIGNANT HISTIOCYTOSIS

Kenneth L. McClain and Carl E. Allen

SUMMARY

Diseases of the histiocyte (macrophage) lineage are divided into four groups based upon the final maturation steps from their myeloid progenitor cells. These disease groups include Langerhans cell histiocytosis (LCH), malignant histiocytoses or dendritic cell sarcomas, juvenile xanthogranuloma/Erdheim-Chester disease, and hemophagocytic lymphohistiocytosis syndromes/Rosai-Dorfman disease. Storage diseases of macrophages are discussed in Chap. 73. The distinction among these diseases is based upon clinical characteristics and histopathologic staining for unique surface markers. LCH may present at birth or in adulthood with skin rash, bone pain, draining ears, oral ulcers, gingivitis, pulmonary dysfunction, chronic diarrhea, diabetes insipidus, and marrow or liver failure. Therapy for LCH in children has been studied in clinical trials of the Histiocyte Society, resulting in improvement in outcome. Treatment for adults is based primarily on case series and extrapolation from the pediatric data. Treatment is still unsatisfactory for patients with LCH who relapse and have chronic abnormalities of endocrine and central nervous system. The diagnostic criteria for the malignant histiocytosis has been clarified by cell-surface marker studies. Treatment options and prognosis vary widely. Erdheim-Chester disease and juvenile xanthogranuloma derive from an abnormality in the same cell, but are treated differently. Erdheim-Chester disease is found almost exclusively in adults and juvenile xanthogranuloma occurs primarily in children. Rosai-Dorfman disease presents with massive cervical lymphadenopathy in most patients, but may also involve other parts of the body. There are several treatment options for Rosai-Dorfman disease, Erdheim-Chester disease, and juvenile xanthogranuloma, but no clinical trials of specific drugs have been published. Patients with a hemophagocytic lymphohistiocytosis syndrome may present in ways suggesting they have infections, hepatitis, meningitis, or autoimmune diseases. Fifty-five percent of patients with hemophagocytic lymphohistiocytosis syndrome can be cured with combined chemotherapy and immunotherapy or by hematopoietic stem cell transplantation.

Abbreviations and acronyms used in this chapter include: ALL, acute lymphoblastic leukemia; ATG, antithymocyte globulin; CD, cluster designation; CT, computed tomography; DAL, Deutsche Arbeitsgemeinschaft für Leukaemieforschung und therapie in Kindersalter; DC, dendritic cell; DI, diabetes insipidus; ECD, Erdheim-Chester disease; HLH, hemophagocytic lymphohistiocytosis; HUMARA, human androgen antigen receptor assay; HX, histiocytosis X; JLCHSG, Japan Langerhans Cell Histiocytosis Study Group; JXG, juvenile xanthogranuloma; IL-1, interleukin 1; LC, Langerhans cell; LCH, Langerhans cell histiocytosis; M-CSF, macrophage colony-stimulating factor; M/M, macrophage/monocyte; MRI, magnetic resonance imaging; NF, neurofibromatosis; PET, positron emission tomography; RDD, Rosai-Dorfman disease; TGF-β, transforming growth factor-beta.

CLASSIFICATION OF THE HISTIOCYTOSES

The description of cells in the monocyte-macrophage system (mononuclear phagocyte system) has been largely clarified (see Chaps. 67, 68, and 69). One historical aberrancy is the term "histiocyte" and the set of diseases termed "the histiocytoses." Histiocyte, a designation assigned in the 19th century to certain tissue cells, is a synonym for the more recent designation "macrophage," and the diseases under discussion are diseases of macrophages or related cells (e.g., monocyte-derived dendritic cells [DCs]; see Chap. 19). For historical reasons, the pathologist and clinician refer to them as histiocytoses, a deeply ingrained term. The distinctions among diseases in this category are determined by (1) clinical findings, (2) histopathology, (3) immunocytology to define the antigens on the surface of the pathologic cells, and (4) cytogenetic or genetic features (Table 72–1).

The histiocytic disorders have been classified based upon whether they are (1) DC related, (2) monocyte-macrophage related, or (3) malignancies of macrophages or DCs (Table 72–2).[1,2]

The DC disorders include Langerhans cell histiocytosis (LCH), derived from the Langerhans cells (LCs) found at the dermal–epidermal junction in the skin, as well as lung, lymph nodes, spleen, and marrow. LCs are the most avid antigen-presenting cells of the immune system.[1] The unique staining of these cells with anti-CD207 (anti-langerin) has provided a specific tool to identify this protein, associated with Birbeck granules, seen in the LC by electron microscopy.[3,3a] Birbeck granules are racket-shaped inclusions in LCs of LCH. Their function has not been resolved but they are likely organelles that either exocytose or endocytose contents. Cells staining with anti-CD207 and/or anti-CD1a are required for the diagnosis of LCH. Other antigens, such as S100 or HLA-DR (human leukocyte antigen-D related) are not specific for LC. Other DC disorders derive from the dermal-interstitial dendrocyte that stains with antibodies to CD68, fascin, and factor XIIIa, and are found in patients with Erdheim-Chester disease (ECD) and juvenile xanthogranuloma (JXG). The DCs in these disorders lack CD1a and CD207. Macrophages and dermal dendrocytes come from a common precursor. These cells develop under the influence of macrophage colony-stimulating factor (M-CSF) to produce a cell that is CD163-positive and shares many of the same epitopes as the dermal dendrocyte.

The monocyte-macrophage disorders include hemophagocytic lymphohistiocytosis (HLH), which is different from the aforementioned diseases, except for the macrophage activation syndrome, which can be seen, also, in LCH. The other macrophage disease is Rosai-Dorfman disease (RDD), also known as sinus histiocytosis with massive lymphadenopathy, which has the telltale histopathologic finding of intact lymphocytes in the cytoplasm of macrophages (emperipolesis), a feature that must be present to diagnose this disorder.

Malignant histiocytosis has evolved as a specific diagnostic entity, after excluding cases of anaplastic large-cell lymphoma and other lymphomas by identifying their unique immunophenotype. There are several subsets of malignant histiocytosis, depending on the dendritic cell of origin. The interdigitating DCs serve as antigen-gathering and antigen-presenting cells (like the LCs) in other organs, except the cornea and brain. When either of these cells contacts an antigen and migrates toward a lymph node, their morphology changes to *veiled or indeterminate cells*. Interdigitating DC reside in the T-cell areas of lymph and splenic tissue. During this stage the cells have the same surface markers as LCs, but lack Birbeck granules, a specialized cytoplasmic inclusion specific to LCs, and complex interdigitating cellular junctions. Follicular DCs are found in the germinal center (B-cell region) of lymph nodes and have the characteristic immunophenotype, CD21+, CD35+, CD1a–, and S100+/–.

TABLE 72–1. Distinctions in Antibodies to Cell-Surface Epitopes and Microscopic Findings among the Histiocytic Diseases

Clinical Findings	Langerhans Cell Histiocytosis	Malignant Histiocytosis	Erdheim-Chester Disease/ Juvenile Xanthogranuloma	Hemophagocytic Lymphohistiocytosis	Rosai-Dorfman Disease
	Langerhans cell	Interdigitating dendritic cell	Dermal dendritic cell	Monocyte-macrophage	Sinus histiocyte
HLH-DR	++	+	–	+	+
CD1a	++	–	–	–	–
CD14	–	–	++	++	++
CD68	+/–	+/–	++	++	++
CD163	–	–	–	++	++
CD 207 (Langerin)	+++	+	–	–	–
Factor XIIIa	–	–	++	–	–
Fascin	–	++	++	+/–	+
Birbeck granules	+	–	–	–	–
Hemophagocytosis	+/–	–	–	+/–	–
Emperipolesis					+

SOURCE: Adapted from Jaffe R[1]; Chikwava K, Jaffe R[3]; and Lau SK.[3a]

TABLE 72–2. Classification of Histiocytic Disorders*

1. Disorders of varying biologic behavior, lacking cytologic atypia
   a. Dendritic-cell related
      - Langerhans cell histiocytosis
      - Juvenile xanthogranuloma
      - Erdheim-Chester disease
   b. Monocyte-macrophage related
      - Hemophagocytic lymphohistiocytosis
        - Familial and/or with identified dysfunctional gene mutation
      - Secondary hemophagocytic syndromes
        - Infection associated
        - Malignancy associated
        - Autoimmune associated
        - Other
      - Sinus histiocytosis with massive lymphadenopathy (Rosai-Dorfman disease)
      - Solitary histiocytoma of macrophage phenotype
2. Malignant disorders
   - Dendritic-cell related
   - Histiocytic sarcoma
   - Monocyte-macrophage related
   - Leukemias: acute monocytic, acute myelomonocytic, and chronic myelomonocytic leukemias

*Histiocytic disorders are broadly characterized as nonmalignant or malignant as defined by neoplastic cytologic changes, specific clonal chromosomal abnormalities, and clinical behavior. Some of the nonmalignant histiocytic disorders can be aggressive and fatal despite having neither of the first two characteristics. Within the first group, "Disorders of varying biologic behavior," it is divided into those derived from dendritic cells versus those from macrophages.

SOURCE: Adapted from Jaffe R[1] and Favara BE, Feller AC, Pauli M, et al.[2]

LANGERHANS CELL HISTIOCYTOSIS

DEFINITION AND HISTORY

In 1868, Paul Langerhans used a colloidal gold stain to identify cells with multiple branching appendages in skin and called them dendritic cells thinking they were part of the nervous system.[4] In 1973, Christian Nezelof and colleagues used electron microscopy to evaluate the biopsies of a disease then known as histiocytosis X.[5] They found pentalaminar granules in the cells that were identical to those of the LCs at the dermal–epidermal border. These cells are now known to be sentinels of the immune system that contact and take up antigen, migrate to lymph nodes, and present the antigen to T cells. The current standard for identifying these cells is staining with an antibody to CD207 (Fig. 72–1), which is the protein, langerin, of the Birbeck granules, the latter seen only by electron microscopy.[3,3a] Anti-CD1a staining of cells is also considered diagnostic of LCH.

LCH results from the proliferation of immunophenotypically and functionally immature, rounded LCs, along with eosinophils, macrophages, lymphocytes, and, sometimes, multinucleated giant cells. The clonal proliferation of LCs is sufficient to consider LCH a neoplasm, but as noted, the lesions contain additional, prominent, nonclonal inflammatory cells.[6] In some ways, the histopathologic reaction is akin to Hodgkin lymphoma in the sense that a relatively small, clonal (neoplastic) population of cells (Reed-Sternberg cells) results, through cytokine activation, in diverse appearances of the lesion, involving reactive cells (e.g., lymphocytes, eosinophils, macrophages). Treatment outcomes for LCH have improved with chemotherapeutic agents with activity against malignant and activated immune cells.

LCH is the preferred term for the disease, replacing histiocytosis-X, eosinophilic granuloma, Abt-Letterer-Siwe disease, Hand-Schüller-Christian disease or diffuse reticuloendotheliosis, now obsolete terms. This change is the result of showing that the pathologic LC is the cell type common to all of these diagnoses.[5,7,8]

EPIDEMIOLOGY

The incidence of LCH is 2 to 10 cases per 1 million children younger than age 15 years.[9] A survey of LCH patients in France revealed an

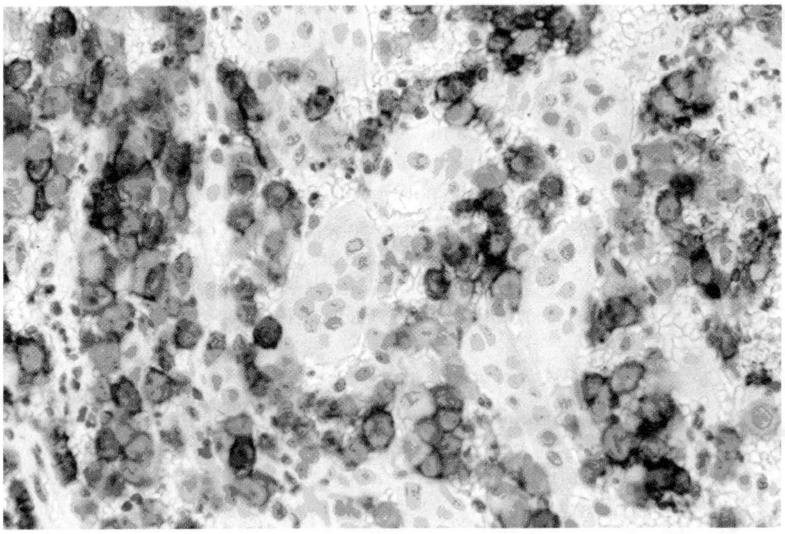

FIGURE 72–1. Biopsy of a bone lesion in a patient with Langerhans cell histiocytosis. Langerhans cells cytoplasm and membrane stain positively for CD207 (immunoperoxidase stain with hematoxylin and eosin [H&E] counterstain).

incidence of 4 to 6 per 1 million in children younger than age 15 years.[10] The male-to-female ratio is close to 1 and the median age of presentation is 30 months, although patients may present with the disease from birth through the ninth decade. Identical and fraternal twins with early onset of LCH have been described. There are occasional reports of affected nontwin siblings and multiple cases in one family.[11] However, strong evidence of a genetic basis in most cases of LCH is lacking. Solvent exposure in parents and perinatal infections has a weak association with LCH, an association that has not reached the level of scientific certainty. There is no increase in cases after viral epidemics.[12] An increased frequency of family members with thyroid disease has been reported.[13]

ETIOLOGY AND PATHOGENESIS

Cells and Cytokines

The etiology of LCH is unknown. Efforts to define a viral cause have not been successful.[14,15] Normally, the activated LC presents antigen to naïve T-lymphocytes. In LCH the LC cell does not stimulate primary T-lymphocyte responses efficiently.[16] Antibody staining for the DC markers, CD80, CD86, and class II antigens, show that in LCH, the abnormal cells are phenotypically similar to immature DC, present antigen poorly, and proliferate at a low rate.[17] Transforming growth factor-β (TGF-β) as well as interleukin (IL)-10 are possibly responsible for preventing LC maturation in LCH.[17] An expansion of regulatory T cells occurs in LCH patients.[18] The population of CD4+ CD25^{high} FoxP3^{high} cells comprise 20 percent of T cells and appear to be in contact with LC in LCH lesions. These T cells are present in higher numbers in the blood of LCH patients than in controls and return to a normal level when patients are in remission.

Chromosome Studies

Studies show clonality in LCH based on polymorphisms of methylation-specific restriction enzyme sites on the X-chromosome regions coding for the human androgen receptor (HUMARA), as well as polymorphism for three other loci.[19,20] Biopsies of lesions with single system or multisystem disease were both found to have a proliferation of LCs from a single clone. In contrast, pulmonary LCH in adults is nonclonal.[21] Cytogenetic abnormalities in LCH rarely have been reported. Three reports on use of comparative genomic hybridization have detailed loss of heterozygosity at loci of possible tumor suppressor genes, but there have been no DNA sequencing studies to confirm these results. A study using array comparative genomic hybridization failed to identify any mutations in CD207 cells.[22–24]

Gene Expression by Microarray Analysis

Laser capture microdissection can be used to purify LCs from frozen biopsy specimens or normal LCs from the skin.[25] The level of cytokine and growth factor gene expression in the control LCs versus those from patient biopsies showed a striking similarity for expression of RNA of the tumor necrosis factor family of genes and several interleukins. Only M-CSF, TGF-β receptor, and IL-1α transcripts were expressed at higher levels in the LCs from LCH patients. A different approach using LCs generated from CD34-positive cells *in vitro*, followed by a serial analysis of a gene expression library was used to identify highly expressed genes in the LCs.[26] Several of the highly expressed genes were then chosen and the expression of RNA in LCH patient biopsy specimens was examined. High expression of *FSCN1, GSN, MMP12, CCL22, CD1a,* and *CD207* was observed.

Plasma Markers

Markedly elevated levels of the FMS-like tyrosine kinase 3 ligand (FLT-3) and M-CSF have been found in the plasma of LCH patients with good correlation of these levels with circulating immature myeloid dendritic cells and the extent of disease. The degree of decrease in these levels correlate with response to treatment.[27] A higher concentration of circulating myeloid dendritic cells in LCH patients was not confirmed in another study.[18] Elevated levels of another regulator of the immune system and bone metabolism, osteoprotegerin, are present in the plasma of patients with active LCH.[28,29] Osteoprotegerin levels reported in this study were highest in patients with multisystem disease and decreased with response to therapy, similar to the findings with *FLT-3* ligand and M-CSF.

CLINICAL FEATURES

LCH usually presents with a skin rash or painful bone lesion. Systemic symptoms of fever, weight loss, diarrhea, edema, dyspnea, polydipsia, and polyuria relate to specific organ involvement.

In LCH, specific organs are considered "high-risk" or "low-risk" when involved at the time of diagnosis. High-risk organs include liver, spleen, lung, and marrow. Low-risk organs include skin, bone, lymph nodes, and pituitary gland. Patients may present with disease in one site or organ (single site or single system) or in multiple sites or organs (multisystem). Treatment decisions for patients are based on whether or not high-risk or low-risk organs are involved and if LCH presents as a single site or as a multisystem disease. Patients can have LCH of the skin, bone, lymph nodes, and pituitary in any combination and still be considered to have low-risk disease.

Single-Site Disease Presentation

In this situation the disease presents with involvement of skin and oral mucosa, bone, lymph nodes, pituitary, or thymus.

Skin Lesions simulating seborrheic dermatitis of the scalp, a manifestation of LCH, may be mistaken for prolonged "cradle cap" in infants. The lesions may be localized to intertriginous areas or diffuse (Fig. 72–2). The most common skin flexures affected are the groin, the perianal area,

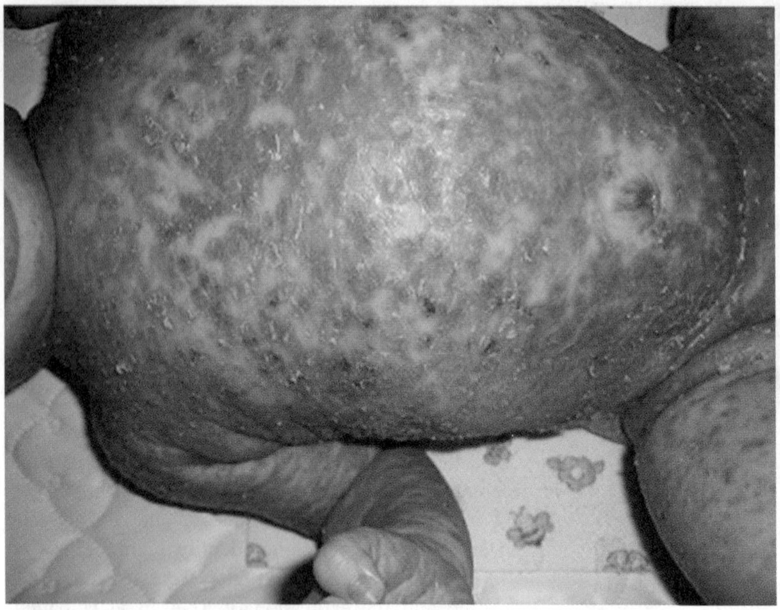

FIGURE 72–2. Langerhans cell histiocytosis. Diffuse skin involvement in an infant. Confluent erythematous rash with scaling lesions.

back of the ears, the neck, the armpits, and in women, the crease below the breasts. Infants may also present with brown to purplish papules over any part of their body (Hashimoto-Pritzker disease).[30] Similar to that of stage IV-S neuroblastoma, this manifestation may be self-limited, as the lesions often disappear during the first year of life with no therapy. However, these patients should be observed closely for systemic disease, which may present after the initial skin lesions.[31,32] In a report of 61 neonatal LCH cases from 1069 patients, nearly 60 percent had multisystem disease and 72 percent had high-risk organ involvement.[33] The overall survival was poorer in neonates with high-risk organ involvement compared to infants and children with the same extent of disease. Response to therapy at 12 weeks was more important than patient age in determining outcome.

Children and Adults Children and adults may develop red papular lesions in the scalp, skin of the groin, abdomen, back, or chest that resemble the diffuse rash of *Candida* infection. Seborrhea-like involvement of the scalp may be mistaken for a severe case of dandruff in older individuals. Ulcerative lesions behind the ears, involving the scalp, skin of the genitalia, or perianal region are often misdiagnosed as bacterial or fungal infections.

Oral Mucosa Presenting symptoms include gingival hypertrophy, ulcers of the soft or hard palate, buccal mucosa, or on the tongue and lips. Lesions of the oral mucosa may precede evidence of LCH elsewhere.[34]

Bone The most frequent site of LCH in children is a lytic lesion of the skull, which may be asymptomatic or painful.[35] LCH can occur in any bone. The most frequently involved skeletal sites are skull, femur, ribs, vertebrae, and humerus. Spine lesions are most often located in the cervical vertebrae and are frequently associated with other bone lesions. Proptosis from a LCH mass in the orbit mimics rhabdomyosarcoma, neuroblastoma, and benign fatty tumors of the eye. Some skull lesions are not only lytic but may have an accompanying mass that impinges on the dura. Lesions of the facial bones or anterior or middle cranial fossae (e.g., temporal, sphenoid, ethmoid, or zygomatic bone) with intracranial tumor extension comprise part of a "CNS-risk" group. These patients have a threefold increased risk for developing diabetes insipidus and an increased risk of other CNS disease (see "Central Nervous System" below).

Lymph Nodes and Thymus The cervical nodes are most frequently involved and may be soft or hard-matted masses with accompanying lymphedema. An enlarged thymus or mediastinal node involvement can mimic lymphoma or an infectious process and may cause asthma-like symptoms. Biopsy of the node or mass with histologic examination and microbial cultures is mandatory for these presentations.

Pituitary Gland The posterior part of the pituitary gland can be affected in LCH patients causing central diabetes insipidus (DI; see "Endocrine System" below). Anterior pituitary involvement often results in failure of growth and sexual maturation.

Multisystem Disease

In multisystem LCH, the disease presents in multiple organs or body systems, including liver and spleen, lung, marrow (high-risk sites) or bones, skin, lymph nodes endocrine system, gastrointestinal system (low-risk sites), and central nervous system (intermediate-risk site depending on extent).

Liver and Spleen These are considered high-risk organs. Hepatic enlargement can be accompanied by dysfunction, leading to hypoalbuminemia with ascites, hyperbilirubinemia, and clotting factor deficiencies. Sonographic, computed tomography (CT), or magnetic resonance imaging (MRI) of the liver will show hypoechoic or low-signal intensity along the portal veins or biliary tracts when the liver is involved.[36] One of the most serious complications of hepatic LCH is cholestasis and sclerosing cholangitis.[37]

The median age of children with hepatic LCH is 23 months and they present with hepatomegaly with or without splenomegaly, elevated alkaline phosphatase, liver transaminases, and -glutamyl transpeptidase. Biopsies do not show LCs and it is thought that cytokines elaborated by lymphocytes damage the bile ducts. Seventy-five percent of children with sclerosing cholangitis will not respond to chemotherapy and all of these patients require liver transplantation.[37] Massive splenomegaly may lead to cytopenias because of hypersplenism and to respiratory compromise. Performing a splenectomy for these patients is not customary, although one may be forced to do this when salvage chemotherapy is not working fast enough. Unfortunately, splenectomy only provides transient relief of cytopenias, as increased liver size and mononuclear phagocyte system activation results in blood cell sequestration and destruction.

Lung The lung is a high-risk organ, but is less frequently involved in children than in adults, in whom smoking is a key etiologic factor.[38] Chest radiographs may show a nonspecific interstitial infiltrate. A high-resolution CT image of the chest is needed to visualize the cystic and nodular pattern of LCH that leads to the destruction of lung tissue. "Spontaneous" pneumothorax can be the first sign of LCH in the lung. These patients may present with tachypnea or dyspnea. Ultimately, widespread fibrosis and destruction of lung tissue leads to severe pulmonary insufficiency. A study reporting outcomes for children with only low-risk organ disease (skin, bone, lymph nodes, or pituitary gland) or pulmonary plus low-risk organs revealed that patients with pulmonary involvement had a 5-year survival of 83 percent, as opposed to 94 percent for those with only low-risk organ involvement.[39] Declining diffusion capacity may also herald the onset of pulmonary hypertension.[40] In young children with diffuse disease, therapy can halt progress of the tissue destruction and normal repair mechanisms may restore some function.

Marrow Most patients with marrow involvement are young children who have diffuse disease in the liver, spleen, lymph nodes, and skin, and significant thrombocytopenia or neutropenia.[41] Others have only mild cytopenias and are found to have marrow involvement with LCH by immunohistochemical or flow cytometric analysis.[42] Patients with LCH who are considered at very high risk sometimes present with hemophagocytosis involving the marrow.[43] The cytokine milieu driving LCH is probably responsible for the epiphenomenon of macrophage activation. These patients may be confusing as to which histiocytic syndrome is primary: HLH or LCH. Evidence of bone involvement or the characteristic LCH skin rash can often point to the diagnosis.

Endocrine System DI is the most frequent endocrine manifestation of LCH. Some patients may present with an apparent "idiopathic" DI before other lesions are identified. Approximately half of these patients will have other lesions diagnostic of LCH within a year of identifying the DI.[44] The 10-year risk of pituitary involvement is 24 percent.[45] This incidence rate of DI did not decrease in chemotherapy-treated patients (see "Central Nervous System" below). However, in another study the incidence of DI decreased from 40 to 20 percent after 6 months of treatment that included vinblastine and prednisone for CNS-risk patients.[46] DI followed initial LCH diagnosis by a mean of 1 year and growth hormone deficiency occurred 5 years later.

Patients with multisystem disease and craniofacial involvement at the time of diagnosis, particularly of the ear, eye, and oral region, carried a significantly increased risk of developing DI during their course (relative risk of 4.6).[47] This risk increased when the disease remained active for a longer period of time or reactivated. The risk for development of DI in this population was 20 percent at 15 years after diagnosis. Additional data showed that 56 percent of DI patients will develop anterior pituitary hormone deficiencies (growth, thyroid, or gonad-stimulating hormones) within 10 years of the onset of DI.[45] DI occurs in 10 percent of patients treated with multiagent chemotherapy and occurs in up to 50 percent of patients treated when less-aggressive management is used.[51,52]

Gastrointestinal System A few patients with diarrhea, hematochezia, perianal fistulas, or malabsorption have been reported.[48,49] Diagnosing gastrointestinal lesions in LCH is difficult because of the patchy involvement. Endoscopic evaluation including multiple biopsies are usually needed.

Central Nervous System **Diabetes Insipidus** DI (considered both an endocrine and a central nervous system manifestation of LCH) can present as an early or late condition. DI caused by damage to the posterior pituitary is the most frequent initial sign (and early manifestation) of LCH in the central nervous system.[50] DI is the presenting symptom in approximately 4 percent of patients subsequently found to have LCH. Between 15 and 20 percent of patients will develop DI sometime before or during the course of the disease. One series reported 2 percent before diagnosis, 4 percent at diagnosis, and 12 percent after the initial diagnosis of LCH. Pituitary biopsies are rarely done and only if the stalk is larger than 6.5 mm or there is a hypothalamic mass. Most often the diagnosis of LCH is established by biopsy of skin, bone, or lymph node of a patient who also has the pituitary abnormalities noted above.

Other Chronic Central Nervous System Disease Manifestations LCH patients may develop mass lesions of the choroid plexus, or gray or white matter.[53] These lesions contain CD1a-positive Langerhans cells as well as CD8+ lymphocytes.[54]

Another chronic CNS problem that occurs in 1 to 4 percent of LCH patients is a neurodegenerative syndrome manifested by dysarthria, ataxia, dysmetria, and sometimes behavior changes.[52] It is called the "LCH central nervous system neurodegenerative syndrome." MRI in these patients shows hyperintensity of the dentate nucleus and white matter of the cerebellum on T2-weighted images or hyperintense lesions of the basal ganglia on T1-weighted images. Atrophy of the cerebellum also may be seen (Fig. 72–3).[53] The radiologic findings may precede the onset of symptoms by many years or can be found coincidently. Among 83 LCH patients who had at least two MRI studies of the brain for evaluation of cranio-facial lesions, diabetes insipidus or other endocrine deficiencies, or neuropsychological symptoms, 57 percent had radiological neurodegenerative changes at a median time of 34 months after diagnosis. Of these patients, one-quarter had clinical neurological deficits develop 3 to 15 years after LCH diagnosis.[55]

LABORATORY FEATURES

A biopsy of an affected organ is necessary to make the diagnosis of LCH by staining of the LC for CD1a or CD207.[1] Patients with high-risk disease may present with anemia and thrombocytopenia, if the marrow is involved.[41,42] An elevated sedimentation rate and thrombocytosis may correlate with active LCH.[56] When the liver is involved hypoalbuminemia, elevated liver enzymes, and elevated bilirubin are present. Intestinal involvement may also cause hypoalbuminemia. Lytic lesions of the bone are found by plain films, CT imaging, MRI, bone scan, or positron emission tomography (PET) scan. PET scans are useful for detecting lesions not found by bone scan or plain films and comparison PET scans are particularly good for providing evidence of healing after 6 to 12 weeks of therapy.[57]

DIFFERENTIAL DIAGNOSIS

The varied cutaneous presentations of LCH may mimic a fungal diaper rash, seborrheic scalp rash or cradle cap, congenital viral infections or

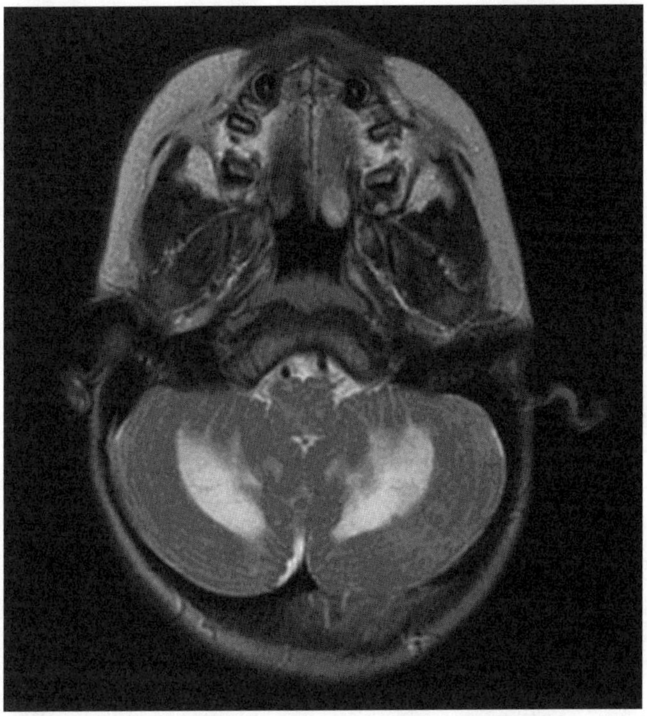

FIGURE 72–3. Radiologic evidence of Langerhans cells histiocytosis and CNS neurodegenerative syndrome. T2-weighted MRI image of the brain of a patient with Langerhans cells histiocytosis showing hyperintense changes of the cerebellar white matter.

neuroblastoma, contact dermatitis, or psoriasis. Women or men with genital lesions may be thought to have a sexually transmitted disease or other infection. Oral lesions mimic other ulcerative lesions, gingival infections, or dental caries. The copious white or green discharge that may come from the ears resemble otitis externa. Lytic bone lesions are often thought to be evidence of a malignancy such as neuroblastoma, rhabdomyosarcoma, or Ewing sarcoma. Collapsed vertebrae from LCH may mimic tuberculosis, trauma, or osteomyelitis. The interstitial infiltrates found in LCH patients with pulmonary involvement may initially look like a viral pneumonia. An enlarged thymus or mediastinal lymph nodes can cause respiratory distress and wheezing similar to asthma. Enlarged lymph nodes from LCH resemble any infiltrative condition such as lymphomas, other histiocytic diseases, infections, or immune-related conditions. Likewise, hepatosplenomegaly of LCH patients could result from the same conditions. Chronic diarrhea in LCH patients may initially be considered to be an infectious or inflammatory bowel disease. Isolated diabetes insipidus with enlargement of the pituitary may suggest a germinoma or hypophysitis. LCH should be strongly considered when symptoms of other more common confounding conditions do not respond to therapy.

Occasionally infiltrates of LC are found in various malignancies and as such represent an attempt of the immune system to respond to that disease.[58–61] Similarly LCH are found in the thymus of patients with myasthenia gravis.[62]

TREATMENT

The optimal treatment of childhood and adults LCH patients is on clinical trials sponsored by the Histiocyte Society (www.histiocytesociety.org/) or a similar international consortium. The NCI Website and the Histiocytosis Association of America (1–856–589–6606) also may be useful resources.

Patients with only skin LCH, some single-bone lesions (non–CNS-risk), and isolated DI have not been included in these trials, but are discussed in this section.

Skin Involvement Only

The approach to this circumstance can be observation, the use of topical glucocorticoids,[32] although topical glucocorticoid creams are rarely effective in the authors' experience, oral methotrexate (20 mg/m^2) weekly for 6 months,[63] or oral thalidomide 50 to 200 mg nightly.[64] Topical application of nitrogen mustard is effective for cutaneous LCH that is resistant to oral therapies, but not for disease involving large areas of skin.[65] Psoralen plus long-wave ultraviolet A radiation (PUVA) has been used as well.[66] The approach is limited by the severity and distribution of the skin involvement.

Single Skull Lesions of the Frontal, Parietal, or Occipital Regions, or Single Lesions of Any Other Bone

In this situation, curettage or curettage plus injection of methylprednisolone may be used.[67]

Skull Lesions in the Mastoid, Temporal, or Orbital Bones (CNS-Risk Lesions)

The purpose of treating these patients is to decrease the risk of developing DI.[68] Six months of vinblastine and prednisone using weekly vinblastine, 6 mg/m^2, for 7 weeks, then every 3 weeks if there is a good response accompanied by daily prednisone, 40 mg/m^2 for 4 weeks then tapered over the next 2 weeks. Thereafter, prednisone is given for 5 days at 40 mg/m^2 every 3 weeks with the vinblastine injections.[69]

A series of patients with orbital or mastoid lesions have received only surgical curettage.[70] None of these patients developed DI. However, in patients who received little or no chemotherapy there was a 20 to 50 percent incidence of DI compared to incidence rates of 10 percent in patients treated for LCH. The weight of evidence supports chemotherapy treatment to prevent DI in patients with the mastoid, temporal, or orbital bones.[52,68]

Multiple Bone Lesions or Combinations of Skin, Lymph Node, or Pituitary Gland Involvement with or without Bone Lesions

Vinblastine and prednisone should be used as outlined for the CNS-risk lesions. A short (<6 months) treatment course with only a single agent (e.g., prednisone) is not sufficient, and the number of relapses is higher than with combination chemotherapy. An 18 percent reactivation rate with a two-drug regimen has been reported versus 50 to 80 percent with only surgery or single-drug treatments.[47,71,72]

Spleen, Liver, Marrow, or Lung (May or May Not Include Skin, Bone, Lymph Node, or Pituitary Gland Involvement)

The standard length of therapy used for LCH in high-risk organs, the spleen, liver, marrow, or lung, is based upon LCH-I, LCH-II, and the DAL-HX 83 studies and varies from 6 months (LCH-I and LCH-II) to 1 year (DAL-HX-83 and LCH-III).[51,69] The LCH-II study was a randomized trial to compare treatment of patients with vinblastine/prednisone/6-mercaptopurine or vinblastine/etoposide/prednisone/6-mercaptopurine.[73] There was no significant difference in the response at 6 weeks, 5-year probability of survival, relapses, and permanent consequences between the two treatment arms. Etoposide has not been used in subsequent Histiocyte Society trials. However, in comparison with historical data, use of etoposide may result in reduced mortality of patients with high-risk organ involvement. Although controversial, this comparison of patients in the LCH-I to LCH-II trials suggested that increased treatment intensity promotes additional early responses and reduced mortality. The DAL treatment regimen used much the same concept, but with more etoposide in the first week of therapy and the addition of methotrexate, 500 mg/m^2, intravenously every 3 weeks, during continuation therapy. Another more intensive regimen (JLSG-96) has been reported that includes cytarabine, vincristine, prednisolone, and methotrexate for good responders or a salvage therapy with daunorubicin, cyclophosphamide, vincristine, and prednisolone for poor responders.[74] Both treatments lasted 7.5 months. Table 72–3 compares the results of the four trials noted above.

TABLE 72–3. Comparison of Treatment Outcomes in High-Risk Patients with Langerhans Cell Histiocytosis

	Protocol Used			
	DAL-HX	LCH-I	LCH-II	JLSG-96
No. patients	63	143	193	59
Median age at diagnosis (years)	0.9	1.5	1	0.9
Therapy duration (months)	12	6	6	7.5
Response (% of patients)	79	53	63*, 71†	76
Reactivation (% of patients with a response)	30	50	47	45
Survival (% at 3 years)	94	93	88	97

DAL, Deutsche Arbeitsgemeinschaft für Leukaemieforschung und therapie in Kindersalter; LCH-I and LCH-II: Histiocyte Society, Langerhans cell histiocytosis treatment protocols I and II; JLCHSG, Japan Langerhans Cell Histiocytosis Study Group.

*Arm A (Velban, prednisone).

†Arm B (Velban, prednisone, etoposide).

Vertebral or Femoral Bone Lesions at Risk for Collapse

Isolated radiation therapy is indicated for patients with single bone lesions of a vertebrae or the femoral neck, which are at risk of collapse.[75,76] When instability of the cervical vertebrae and neurologic symptoms are present, bracing or spinal fusion may be needed.[77] Certain skull lesions, not in the CNS-risk region, could also be considered for radiation therapy.

Central Nervous System

Treatment of mass lesions, including enlargement of the hypothalamic–pituitary axis, parenchymal mass lesions, and leptomeningeal involvement, with cladribine has been effective in thirteen reported cases.[78–80] Doses of cladribine ranged from 5 to 13 mg/m^2 given at varying frequencies.[80]

Treatment of the CNS neurodegenerative syndrome with clinical signs has included the combination of dexamethasone, cladribine, all-*trans* retinoic acid, and intravenous immunoglobulin.[81,82] All-*trans* retinoic acid was given at a dose of 45 mg/m^2 daily for 6 weeks, then 2 weeks a month for 1 year.[82] Intravenous immunoglobulin, 400 mg/m^2, monthly and chemotherapy with oral prednisolone with or without oral or intravenous methotrexate and oral 6-mercaptopurine were given for at least 1 year.[81] MRI findings were stable, but clinical efficacy was difficult to judge as patients were reported to have no progression in their neurologic symptoms. Intravenous cytarabine with or without vincristine was effective in decreasing neurologic symptoms and improving the MRI images in 5 of 8 patients.[82a]

Treatment of Recurrent, Refractory, or Progressive Childhood Langerhans Cell Histiocytosis

Recurrent "Low-Risk" Organ Involvement The optimal therapy for patients with relapsed or recurrent disease has not been determined. Several regimens exist. Patients with recurrent bone disease who reoccur more than 6 months after stopping vinblastine and prednisone can benefit from treatment with a "reinduction" of vinblastine weekly and daily prednisone for 6 weeks. If there is no active disease, or at least very little evidence of active disease, then treatment can be changed to every 3 weeks with the addition of oral methotrexate weekly and mercaptopurine nightly. This protocol concept is currently under discussion in the Histiocyte Society. As mentioned above cladribine is an effective agent for patients with recurrent bone disease.[83,83a] An alternative treatment regimen employs vincristine and cytosine arabinoside.[84]

A phase II trial of thalidomide for LCH patients (10 low-risk patients; 6 high-risk patients) who failed primary and at least one secondary regimen had a complete response in 4 of 10 and a partial responses in 3 of 10 low-risk patients. However, dose-limiting toxicities may limit the overall usefulness of thalidomide.[64]

Recurrent High-Risk Organ Involvement The current Histiocyte Society clinical trial for patients with refractory high-risk organ (liver, spleen, or marrow) involvement is an intensive, acute myelogenous leukemia-like protocol. Prompt change of therapy to this protocol, which includes cladribine and cytosine arabinoside, may provide an improvement in overall survival.[85] This is a very intense regimen and requires that physicians are able to treat infectious and metabolic complications. Responses may be delayed. Stem cell transplantation has been used for patients with multisystem high-risk organ involvement that is refractory to chemotherapy. Reduced-intensity conditioning regimens are curative and associated with less toxicity.[86–88]

A new treatment plan is indicated when a patient with multisystem involvement progresses after 6 weeks of standard treatment, or has not had a partial response by 12 weeks. Data from the DAL studies have shown that these children have only a 10 percent chance of surviving.[69] Results of the LCH-II study revealed that patients treated with vinblastine/prednisone who did not respond well by 6 weeks had a 27 percent chance of survival.[73] Those treated with vinblastine, prednisone, and etoposide who had a poor response at 6 weeks had a 52 percent chance of survival. Cladribine and pentostatin have been used as salvage therapies for LCH.[83a] These drugs were more often effective for patients with bone, skin, or lymph node involvement. Only one-third of patients with LCH of the liver, marrow, spleen, or lung responded. Another study demonstrated that patients with multiple reactivations or high-risk disease could be treated with continuous infusion cladribine for 3 days.[83] Seven of 10 patients on this trial required no more therapy.

Treatment Options No Longer Considered Effective

Treatments for LCH in any location that have been used in the past but are no longer recommended include cyclosporine[89] and interferon-α.[90] Extensive surgery is also not indicated. For lesions of the mandible, extensive surgery may destroy any possibility of secondary tooth development. Surgical resection or radiotherapy of groin or genital lesions is contraindicated as chemotherapy can heal bone or skin lesions.

COURSE AND PROGNOSIS

LCH patients with low-risk disease treated with vinblastine and prednisone have a 99 percent chance of being cured of their disease, but up to 46 percent relapse when treated for only 6 months or with just those two drugs.[51,74,91] Nearly 100 percent of these patients are ultimately cured of LCH despite suffering two to four relapses after initial treatment. Cure required multiple treatments.[91] Table 72–3 summarizes the outcome of high-risk patients. Patients with high-risk disease who do not respond adequately by 6 to 12 weeks of treatment have a 35 percent chance of long-term survival. Most of these patients died of LCH until the advent of a salvage protocol with cladribine and cytosine arabinoside.[85] Although this is a very intensive regimen with extreme cytopenias and risk of infection, it has been successful in a majority of patients or may provide sufficient control of disease to allow the patient to undergo a hematopoietic stem cell transplantation. Reduced-intensity conditioning has led to nearly an 80 percent survival of LCH patients who required this salvage treatment.[88] Although several other treatments for LCH such as pamidronate, cyclosporine, and interferon-α have been reported in the literature, they have not become standard treatments.[92]

Permanent Consequences or Late Effects of Treatment Children with low-risk organ involvement (skin, bones, lymph nodes, or pituitary gland) have a 24 percent chance of developing long-term sequelae.[93] Those with DI are at risk for panhypopituitarism and should be monitored carefully for adequacy of growth and development. In a retrospective review of 141 patients with LCH and DI, 43 percent developed growth hormone deficiency.[94–96] The 5- and 10-year risks of growth hormone deficiency among children with LCH and DI were 35 percent and 54 percent, respectively. There was no increased reactivation of LCH in patients who received replacement growth hormone compared to those who did not.[94]

Patients with multisystem involvement have a 71 percent incidence of long-term problems.[93–96] Hearing loss has been found in 13 percent of children treated for LCH.[96] Neurologic symptoms secondary to vertebral compression of cervical lesions have been reported in LCH patients with spinal lesions. Cognitive defects and MRI abnormalities may develop in some long-term survivors with CNS-risk skull lesions.[97] Some patients have markedly abnormal cerebellar function and behavior abnormalities, while others have subtle deficits in brain stem–evoked potentials and short-term memory.[98]

Orthopedic problems from lesions of the spine, femur, tibia, or humerus may be seen in 20 percent of patients. These problems include vertebral collapse or instability of the spine that may lead to scoliosis, and facial or limb asymmetry.

Diffuse pulmonary disease may result in poor lung function with higher risk for infections and decreased exercise tolerance. These patients should be followed with pulmonary function testing including the diffusing capacity of carbon monoxide and ratio of residual volume to total lung capacity.[40]

Liver disease may lead to later sclerosing cholangitis, which responds to chemotherapy in only 25 percent of cases and liver transplantation usually is indicated.[37]

Dental problems characterized by loss of teeth have been significant for some patients, usually related to overly aggressive dental surgery.[93]

Marrow failure secondary to LCH or from therapy is rare but is associated with a higher risk of malignancy. Patients with LCH have a higher than normal risk of developing secondary cancers.[99] Leukemia (usually acute myelogenous) occurs after treatment as does lymphoblastic lymphoma. Concurrent LCH and a malignancy have been reported in a few patients, and some patients have had their malignancy initially followed by development of LCH. Three patients with T-cell acute lymphoblastic leukemia (T-ALL) and aggressive LCH, for which the two disorders had shared clonal markers have been reported.[100,101] Two cases in which clonality of the same T-cell receptor genotype were found.[100] The authors considered the plasticity of lymphocytes permitting development into Langerhans cells. One patient with LCH after T-ALL had the same T-cell receptor gene rearrangements and activating mutations of the *NOTCH1* gene in the LC and ALL cells.[101]

The concurrence of retinoblastoma, brain tumors, hepatocellular carcinoma, and Ewing sarcoma with LCH has also been reported.[99]

ADULT LANGERHANS CELL HISTIOCYTOSIS

Incidence

It is estimated that one to two adult cases of LCH occur per 1 million population.[102] The true incidence of this disease is impossible to know because large published studies usually are from referral centers and the disorder often is underdiagnosed. A survey from Germany reported that 66 percent of the adult LCH patients were women with an average age of 43.5 years.[103]

Presentation of Adult Langerhans Cell Histiocytosis

Adult LCH patients may have symptoms and signs for many months before a definitive diagnosis is made and treatment instituted. LCH in adults is often similar to that in children, except that isolated adult pulmonary LCH is closely associated with smoking. Presenting symptoms are (in order of decreasing frequency) dyspnea or tachypnea, polydipsia and polyuria, bone pain, lymphadenopathy, weight loss, fever, gingival hypertrophy, ataxia, and memory problems. Among the signs of LCH are skin rash, scalp nodules, soft-tissue swelling near bone lesions, lymphadenopathy, gingival hypertrophy, hepatosplenomegaly. Patients who present with isolated DI should be carefully observed for onset of other symptoms or signs characteristic of LCH. At least 80 percent of patients with DI had involvement of other organ systems: bone (68%), skin (57%), lung (39%), and lymph nodes (18%).[104]

Many patients have a papular rash with brown, red, or crusted areas ranging in size from a pinhead to a dime. In the scalp, the rash is similar to that of seborrhea. Skin in the inguinal region, genitalia, or around the anus may have open ulcers that do not heal after antibacterial or antifungal therapy. In the mouth, swollen gums or ulcers along the cheeks, roof of the mouth, or tongue occur.

The frequency of bone involvement in adults differs from that of children. The frequency in adults versus children, of lesions in the mandible, is 30 versus 7 percent and in the skull is 21 versus 40 percent.[35,103] The frequency of LCH lesions in the vertebrae (13%), pelvis (13%), extremities (17%), and ribs (6%) of adults is similar to that found in children.[102]

Pulmonary LCH is slightly more prevalent in smokers than in nonsmokers and the male-to-female ratio may be near unity depending on the incidence of smoking in the population studied.[38,105] Patients with pulmonary LCH usually present with cough, dyspnea, or chest pain, although nearly 20 percent of adults with lung involvement have no symptoms.[106,107] The presence of chest pain may indicate the presence of a spontaneous pneumothorax. The LCs in adult lung lesions are mature dendritic cells expressing high levels of the accessory molecules CD80 and CD86, unlike LCs found in other lung disorders.[108] In addition, pulmonary LCH in adults is primarily a reactive process, rather than a clonal proliferation as seen in childhood LCH.[108]

The most frequent pulmonary function abnormality finding in patients with pulmonary LCH is a reduced carbon monoxide diffusing capacity in approximately 80 percent of cases.[109,110] A high-resolution CT scan can uncover cysts and nodules, usually in the upper lobes characteristic of LCH. Despite the typical CT findings, a lung biopsy is needed to confirm the diagnosis.[111] The presence of cystic abnormalities on high-resolution CT scans does not predict which patients will have progressive disease.[112]

Adults with pulmonary LCH can have multisystem disease, including bone (18%) and skin (13%) lesions, and DI (5%).

Therapy of Adult LCH

Although adult patients have been treated with vinblastine and prednisone similar to childhood cases, vinblastine often causes significant neurologic toxicity in adults when given weekly for 6 weeks, and glucocorticoids are not tolerated as well by adults as children. A better approach in adults, we believe, is to use either cytarabine or cladribine. Extensive or mutilating surgery to remove teeth or jaw bones is not indicated. Systemic chemotherapy will cause bone lesions to regress and the involved teeth and jaw bones can reform. Thalidomide and oral methotrexate have been effective in adults with skin disease.[63,64]

Results from LCH studies in children show that the rate of recurrent disease is appreciably reduced when patients receive 6 months of treatment with vinblastine and prednisone as opposed to either single-agent treatment or irradiation of multiple bone lesions.[47] Anecdotal reports have described the successful use of the bisphosphonate pamidronate in controlling severe bone pain in patients with multiple osteolytic lesions.[113,114]

Another approach using antiinflammatory agents coupled with trofosfamide, a cyclophosphamide congener, in a specific timed sequence was successful in two patients with disease resistant to standard chemotherapy treatment.[115]

Treatment Options for Adults Under Clinical Evaluation

There are no published clinical trial results for adult LCH patients.

The LCH-A1 trial for adult patients using vinblastine and prednisone with 6-mercaptopurine was opened in 2008. Early toxicity data show severe neuropathy secondary to vinblastine in many patients. For patients who do not respond to this "front-line" therapy, cladribine is effective for adults with skin, bone, lymph node, and probably pulmonary and central nervous system disease.[33,116,117]

Special Considerations on the LCH-A1 Trial for Adult LCH Patients with Lung Disease and Who Smoke Cigarettes Glucocorticoid efficacy for treating adult LCH is controversial because past case-series reports on LCH patients with pulmonary disease did not control for smoking cessation. Most adult patients with LCH have gradual disease progression with continued smoking. The disease may regress or progress with the cessation of smoking.[118] In the LCH-A1 trial, patients are first offered a smoking cessation program and observation. If the smoking cessation program does not work, glucocorticoid treatment is started. Treatment of progressive disease after 6 months of steroids is up to the investigator's choice, but usually includes vinblastine and mercaptopurine or 2-chlorodeoxyadenosine.

Lung transplantation may be necessary for adults with extensive pulmonary destruction from LCH.[119] A multicenter study documented a 54 percent survival at 10 years posttransplantation, with 20 percent of patients having recurrent LCH, which did not impact on survival, but longer followup of these patients is needed.

MALIGNANT HISTIOCYTIC DISEASES

DEFINITION AND HISTORY

The original description of this group of malignant histiocytosis is attributed to Scott and Robb-Smith who, in 1939, reported cases of a rapidly fatal disease with jaundice, lymphadenopathy, anemia, leucopenia, and hepatosplenomegaly that they called *histiocytic medullary reticulosis*.[120] They believed the malignant cell was a histiocyte based upon the accepted morphologic criteria of that time. Advanced immunohistochemical techniques resulted in identifying cells as either lymphocytes or histiocytes. The disease was labeled *giant cell reticulosis* and the cells *reticulum cells* based upon their large size, but revealed little as to the place of these cells in the immune system. Later Rappaport introduced the term *malignant histiocytosis*,[121] as he believed the morphologic characteristics identified the histiocyte as the malignant cell. There has been considerable debate about the identity of malignancies of LC histiocytes as the majority of patients with "histiocytic lymphoma or malignant histiocytosis" reported in the literature had one of the variants of large cell lymphoma.[122,123] By excluding patients with anaplastic large cell lymphomas and other T- or B-lineage large cell lymphomas, the residual number with malignancies of histiocytes becomes very small. Favara and colleagues suggested that such diseases should be considered sarcomas of histiocytic or macrophage-related lineage.[2] Acute myelogenous leukemias with a dominant monocytic phenotype represent the other group of malignant disorders involving monocytic cells. Descriptions of the clinical presentation, biology, and treatment of the monocytic leukemias and large cell lymphomas are presented elsewhere in this book (see Chaps. 89 and 100, respectively).

The markers most specific for histiocytic cells include M-CSF receptor, lysozyme, Ki-M8, S100+ large cells, Ki-M4, cathepsin D and E, CD21−, and CD35−.[2] If a dendritic/histiocytic cell proliferation meets a combination of criteria as "malignant," such as having a clonal cytogenetic abnormality, aneuploid DNA profile, malignant histocytomorphology, monoclonality, and an aggressive clinical course, it is classified as a histiocytic sarcoma.

An international panel of experts carefully reviewed 61 cases of tumors of histiocytes and accessory dendritic cells.[124] Seventeen cases (27%) were classified as histiocytic sarcoma and were CD68+, lysozyme+, CD1a−, S100−/+, CD21−, and CD35−. LC tumors (24 cases, 38%) were CD68+, lysozyme−/+, CD1a+, S100+, and CD21/35−. Interdigitating dendritic cell sarcomas (4 cases, 7%) were CD68+/−, lysozyme−, CD1a−, S100−/+, and CD21/35−. Follicular dendritic cell tumors (13 cases, 21%) were CD68+/−, lysozyme−, CD1a−, S100−/+, and CD21/35+. Four cases were unclassifiable.

EPIDEMIOLOGY

Although malignant dendritic/histiocytic cell tumors affect all age groups, the median age is 33 years.[124] Males are affected more often than females in the subsets, with the most patients having histiocytic sarcomas and LC tumors. One review of more than 2000 lymphoma cases found 8 patients with histiocytic sarcomas (4 of 1000).[125]

CLINICAL FEATURES

Systemic symptoms of fever, headache, malaise, weight loss, dyspnea, and sweating occur in patients with diffuse disease.[124–126] Infiltration of the marrow ultimately is found in approximately 25 percent of the patients.

Dendritic or Langerhans Cell Sarcomas

These patients may have systemic symptoms of fever, pain, or weight loss. They usually present with erythematous nodules or skin rash, but may also have involvement of bone, lymph nodes, lung, liver, or brain.[127,128] A series of histiocytic-dendritic cell sarcomas in patients with follicular lymphomas showed a clonal evolution from the B-cell lymphoma to myeloid-derived sarcomas.[129]

Extranodal Histiocytic Sarcomas

These tumors occur equally in males and females and present at a median age of 55 years.[130] Tumors are found in the soft tissue of extremities, gastrointestinal tract, nasal cavity, and lung, sometimes with involvement of regional lymph nodes. Gastrointestinal masses were usually painful. Extremity tumors often present as painless masses. Patients had symptoms or signs for 1 month to 2 years before diagnosis. Most tumors are stage I or II at the time of diagnosis.

Interdigitating Dendritic Cell Sarcomas

These may occur as extranodal tumors in children and primarily affect lymph nodes in adults.[131] A series of four pediatric cases had involvement of the chest wall, vertebrae, lymph nodes, marrow, and pelvic space.[131] The other 7 pediatric and 26 adult cases published by 2004 reported extranodal presentations in 17. Many of the 17 cases had intestinal or mediastinal tumors. These tumors were very aggressive in a third of cases.[132,133]

Follicular Dendritic Cell Tumors

These malignancies affect males and female equally and present at a median age of 47 years (range: 14–77).[132] Nodal and extranodal sites can be affected. Most frequent nodal presentations are cervical, axillary, and supraclavicular, but mediastinal and mesenteric nodes can also be affected. These tumors are usually slow growing and painless. Although local invasion is common, metastasis to sites other than the lungs is uncommon.

LABORATORY FINDINGS

Patients with diffuse disease may have pancytopenia although leukocytosis occurs in some with as a secondary response. Hemophagocytosis is occasionally seen in the marrow. An elevated lactate dehydrogenase and erythrocyte sedimentation rate may be found.

DIFFERENTIAL DIAGNOSIS

A diagnostic biopsy with full immunophenotype panel should be done for these rare tumors, which have been mistaken for Hodgkin lymphoma, anaplastic large cell lymphoma, or large cell lymphomas of T- and B-cell subtypes. The dendritic cell neoplasms do not express T- or B-lymphocyte markers and do not have rearrangements of immunoglobulin or T-cell receptor genes.[124,132,134] Malignant fibrous histiocytoma, fibrosarcoma leiomyosarcoma, rhabdomyosarcoma, or melanoma may simulate interdigitating dendritic cell sarcoma, as well as inflammatory pseudotumor. Although follicular dendritic cell sarcoma and histiocytic lymphoma may have a similar presentation, the unique immunophenotype-immunohistochemical characteristics of the tumors

TABLE 72–4. Treatment Results: Histiocytic and Dendritic Cell Sarcomas

Study	Number of Patients*	Disease Stage	Chemotherapy	Radiotherapy (R) Surgery (S)	Chemotherapy Responses	Survival
Lauritzen et al[124]	8	I–III	Multiagent		2	6.5 months
Kamel et al[125]	11	I–II	Multiagent		5	0.5–36 months
Pileri et al[123]	9	I/IV	Multiagent	2R, 2S	3	NA
Hornick et al[129]	14	I/II	CHOP	4R, 5S	5/6	21 months–10 years

CHOP, Cytoxan, Adriamycin, vincristine, prednisone; NA, not available.

*Number with sufficient followup information.

helps differentiate them from interdigitating dendritic cell sarcoma. Thymomas, meningiomas, and malignant fibrous histiocytomas can mimic follicular dendritic cell sarcoma they but lack CD21 and CD35.

TREATMENT, COURSE, AND PROGNOSIS

Therapy for dendritic and LC sarcomas has usually been unsuccessful.[129] However, case reports of long-term remissions with thalidomide[135] or MESNA, doxorubicin, ifosfamide, and dacarbazine have been published.[136] In some instances, surgical resection of a localized mass with radiotherapy has been adequate (Table 72–4).

Interdigitating dendritic cell sarcomas have been successfully treated with surgery alone or a combination of surgery and radiotherapy when the tumor is localized.[131] Patients with stage III/IV tumors generally do not respond multidrug chemotherapy, such as cyclophosphamide, doxorubicin, vincristine, and prednisone with or without the addition of actinomycin D.

MALIGNANT FIBROUS HISTIOCYTOMA AND GIANT CELL TUMOR OF THE BONE

Gene profiling experiments have shown that these tumors are not derived from histocytes, but are poorly differentiated fibrosarcomas, myosarcomas, fibromyxosarcomas, or liposarcomas.[137–139] They are treated similarly to osteosarcomas.[140–142]

HEMOPHAGOCYTIC LYMPHOHISTOCYTOSIS

DEFINITION AND HISTORY

Farquhar and Claireux first described this disease in siblings in 1952.[143] Although many case reports using several eponyms ensued, Henter and Elinder provided a logical organization of the diverse clinical presentations.[144] HLH is an aggressive and potentially fatal syndrome that results from inappropriate prolonged activation of lymphocytes and macrophages. The name describes the characteristic (but not diagnostic) pathologic finding of macrophages engulfing all types of blood cells in marrow, lymph nodes, spleen, or liver biopsies (Fig. 72–4). HLH is also known as autosomal recessive familial hemophagocytic lymphohistiocytosis, familial erythrophagocytic lymphohistiocytosis, viral-associated hemophagocytic syndrome, and infection-associated hemophagocytosis. "Primary" HLH has been used to describe young children with HLH with known gene mutations or a family history of HLH. Older children with HLH, or children without identifiable mutations, are sometimes described as having "secondary" or "acquired" HLH with the assumption that the condition is caused by infection or other stimulus and not a result of genetic predisposition. The same mutations may be present in both situations, and there is no rapid and definitive gene-testing strategy to identify the two groups. In general, presentation and outcome are the same for primary and acquired HLH. Thus this distinction is not clinically useful in the acute setting as they both must be diagnosed promptly and treated aggressively.

EPIDEMIOLOGY

The incidence of HLH in Sweden was estimated at 1.2 children per 1 million children per year, or 1 in 50,000 livebirths with equal sex distribution.[144] At the Baylor College of Medicine, HLH was diagnosed in 1 of 3000 inpatient admissions in a 2-year study.[145]

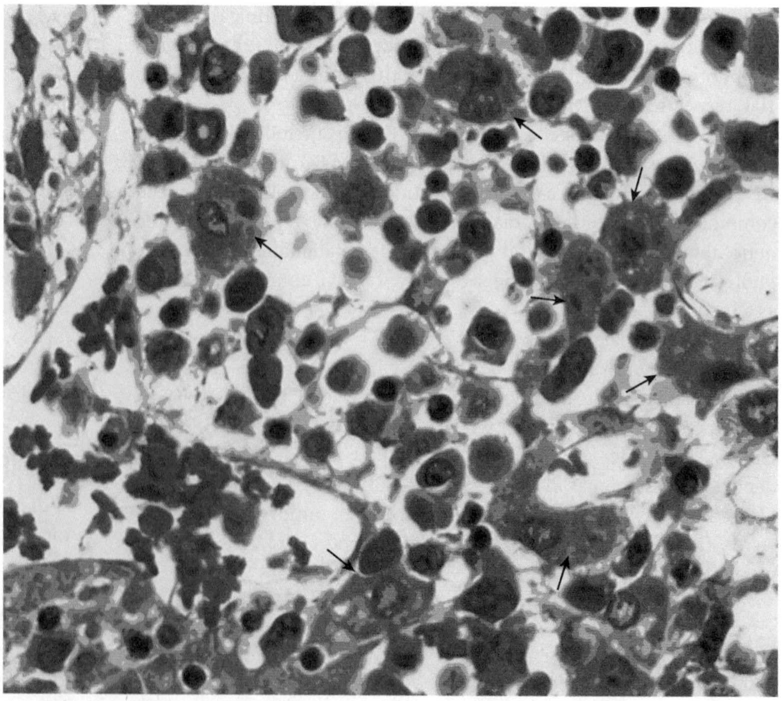

FIGURE 72–4. Hemophagocytosis by macrophages. Marrow aspirate treated with Wright-Giemsa stain illustrating prominent hemophagocytosis of multiple cell types by macrophages (*arrows*) in the marrow of a patient with HLH.

ETIOLOGY AND PATHOGENESIS

Defects in the function of natural killer (NK) cells and cytotoxic T cells have been found in HLH patients. This results in the inappropriate activation of T cells and macrophages, which produce proinflammatory cytokines, including interferon-γ, tumor necrosis factor-α, IL-6, IL-10, IL-12, and soluble IL-2 receptor-α (sCD25).[146,147] Hypercytokinemia generated by activated T cells and macrophages results in multiorgan dysfunction that can rapidly lead to death.

Perforin Expression

Perforin was identified as a candidate HLH gene by gene mapping and was confirmed by poor expression of perforin in NK cells and cytotoxic T lymphocytes of HLH patients.[148] Some HLH characteristics were reproducible in *PRF1* knockout mice.[149] Perforin is secreted from NK cells and cytotoxic T cells upon activation by target cells and introduces pores in the target cell membrane, allowing granzyme to enter and trigger apoptosis.[150]

Other Defects Causing HLH

Mutations in other genes encoding proteins involved in NK and cytotoxic T-cell–mediated killing of target cells have also been discovered in patients with HLH, including *granzyme B*, *MUNC13–4*, and *syntaxin 11*.[151] Mutations in the gene that encodes rab27a (protein that controls secretion of lytic granules) have been identified in patients with Griscelli syndrome.[152]

Immune Deficiencies Associated with HLH

Patients with other immune deficiencies associated with lysosomal trafficking defects (e.g., Chédiak-Higashi syndrome, Hermansky-Pudlak syndrome type II) also have a high frequency of HLH.[151] HLH, often associated with infection by the Epstein-Barr virus, is the commonest fatal complication of X-linked lymphoproliferative disease.[153]

CLINICAL FEATURES

Initial signs and symptoms of HLH mimic more common problems (e.g., fever of unknown origin or sepsis).[154] Confounding diagnoses such as infection, autoimmune disease, hepatitis, multisystem organ failure, encephalitis, and malignancy do not exclude a diagnosis of HLH. Important clues are an acutely ill patient with unexplained fever, rash, or neurologic symptoms. A medical history of immune deficiency should bring HLH to mind. Family history of consanguinity, recurrent spontaneous abortions, or HLH in siblings (or symptoms suggesting undiagnosed HLH) should prompt full evaluation for HLH.

Prominent early clinical signs in one study included fever (91%), hepatomegaly (90%), splenomegaly (84%), neurologic signs (47%), rash (43%), and lymphadenopathy (42%).[155] Another study found 75 percent of patients with HLH to have CNS symptoms that may mimic encephalitis.[156] Patients with HLH develop liver failure with markedly elevated bilirubin, pancytopenia, coagulopathy, renal failure heralded by hyponatremia, and pulmonary failure similar to acute respiratory distress syndrome with interstitial infiltrates on chest radiography.

Diagnostic Criteria

The cumulative experiences from the first prospective international treatment protocol sponsored by the Histiocyte Society, HLH-94, as well as other observations and studies, have led to the Histiocyte Society treatment protocol HLH-2004, which includes diagnostic guidelines (Table 72–5).[156] Mutations in *PRF1* (encodes perforin),[157] *UNC13D* (encodes MUNC13–4),[158] or *syntaxin 11* genes[159] are diagnostic. Gene mutation studies may be helpful in the acute setting if polymerase chain reaction methodology is readily available. In the absence of a known gene mutation, a diagnosis of HLH can be made with at least five of eight criteria (Table 72–5).

TABLE 72–5. Clinical Criteria for Diagnosis of HLH*

HLH diagnosis is established with at least five of the following:
Fever
Splenomegaly
Cytopenias in at least two cell lines:
Hemoglobin <90 g/L
Platelets <100 × 10^9/L
Neutrophils <1 × 10^9/L
Hypertriglyceridemia and/or hypofibrinogenemia:
Fasting triglycerides >3 mmol/L (>265 mg/dL)
Fibrinogen <1.5 g/L
Hemophagocytosis in marrow or spleen or lymph nodes
Low or absent activity of natural killer cells (specialized laboratory test)
Ferritin >500 mcg/L
Soluble cD25 (soluble interleukin-2 receptor) >2400 units/mL

*Five of these eight clinical or laboratory findings are sufficient to make the diagnosis of HLH. It is important to obtain serial measurements of ferritin as well as the complete blood count, coagulation, and liver function tests when evaluating a patient.

Hemophagocytosis is sometimes misunderstood as pathognomonic and necessary for the diagnosis of HLH, but biopsies fail to demonstrate hemophagocytosis in approximately one-third of patients.[160] HLH changes over time such that the cytokine stimulation resulting in hemophagocytosis may be modest early in the disease, or the marrow may progress to become aplastic with few macrophages available to engage in hemophagocytosis. Repeat marrow aspirates and biopsies, as well as lymph node or liver biopsies, may be helpful. Finding hemophagocytosis is highly suggestive of HLH, but is neither necessary nor sufficient to make the diagnosis. HLH. Cerebrospinal fluid should be tested in patients with signs of CNS abnormalities; pleocytosis and hyperproteinemia support HLH with CNS involvement. The clonal proliferation of lymphocytes in lymph nodes may be confused with a lymphomatous infiltrate.[161]

LABORATORY FEATURES

Ferritin

Although no one diagnostic criterion is sufficient to make the diagnosis of HLH, a highly elevated serum ferritin along with four other criteria is strongly indicative. A ferritin concentration of more than 500 mcg/L was included because a survey found that most children with infectious diseases had levels less than that level and those with rheumatologic diagnoses only rarely had higher levels. Ferritin concentrations greater than 500 mcg/L were 100 percent sensitive for HLH in a retrospective review of ferritin concentrations of more than 500 mcg/L over a 2-year period.[145] However, at this level there is considerable overlap with other disorders. Ferritin concentrations more than 10,000 mcg/L were 90 percent sensitive and 96 percent specific for HLH with very minimal overlap with sepsis, infections, and liver failure.

The following tests should be done on a previously healthy patient who presents with persistent fevers, hepatosplenomegaly, and cytopenia of at least two cell lines: serum ferritin, aspartate aminotransferase/alanine aminotransferase, lactate dehydrogenase, bilirubin, coagulation studies, fibrinogen, triglycerides. A marrow biopsy and aspirate is needed as well as a lumbar puncture for spinal fluid examination. NK-cell function, perforin expression of T cells and NK cells, and sCD25 concentrations should be measured if four or more of the HLH diagnostic criteria are met.[162] Following daily serum ferritin levels is useful because rapidly rising ferritin is a strong indicator of HLH. It may be necessary to repeat the marrow biopsy or biopsy an enlarged liver or lymph nodes, if the first marrow biopsy fails to show hemophagocytosis and clinical suspicion of HLH is high. Other conditions should be evaluated and treated as sepsis, viral infection, autoimmune disease, and malignancy do not exclude a concurrent diagnosis of HLH.

DIFFERENTIAL DIAGNOSIS

Patients with fever of unknown origin, moderate infections, sepsis, multiorgan dysfunction, hepatitis, anemia and thrombocytopenia, and autoimmune phenomena such as Kawasaki disease, lupus erythematosus, or rheumatoid arthritis may present with features that overlap the diagnostic criteria for HLH. One must consider HLH if no clear diagnosis is established for the above mentioned entities and the patient is deteriorating. Identification of an underlying immune deficiency such as X-linked lymphoproliferative disease (Chap. 84), Griscelli syndrome (Chap. 65), or Chédiak-Higashi syndrome (Chap. 66) should increase the suspicion of HLH. Epstein-Barr virus, cytomegalovirus, and other herpes virus infections are the most frequent viral infections associated with HLH. A wide variety of bacterial fungal and protozoal infections may also lead to HLH.

THERAPY

Before treatment with immune-modulating therapy fewer than 10 percent of patients with HLH survived.[155] After case reports and case series described patients successfully treated with strategies that included aggressive immune suppression, podophyllotoxin derivatives, or a combination of immune suppression with etoposide, a prospective treatment protocol was developed that included induction therapy with dexamethasone and etoposide, followed by continuous treatment with cyclosporine and pulses of dexamethasone and etoposide.[156,163–165] Patients with CNS symptoms or cerebrospinal fluid lymphocytosis or pleocytosis also received intrathecal methotrexate. Patients with resistant disease, recurrent disease, or familial HLH had hematopoietic stem cell transplant. The overall estimated 3-year survival on the HLH-94 protocol is 55 percent.[165] Some physicians prefer to start treatment with dexamethasone and cyclosporine before adding etoposide. If the patient deteriorates etoposide treatment is necessary.

A second protocol containing minor modifications from the first included starting cyclosporine at the onset of induction therapy, adding glucocorticoids to intrathecal therapy in patients with CNS disease, adding etoposide to conditioning in patients who undergo stem cell transplantation, and considering depletion of T cells in patients who receive stem cells from unrelated donors.[166] This protocol should be used for patients who fit the diagnostic criteria for HLH, with the exception of patients with systemic juvenile rheumatoid arthritis or systemic lupus erythematosus with macrophage activation syndrome (see "Macrophage Activation Syndrome" below). Treatment may be modified for patients with HIV-associated HLH and patients with iatrogenic immune suppression. The protocol outlines specific treatment modifications for marrow toxicity, nephrotoxicity, hepatotoxicity, and neurotoxicity. One must be especially careful of cyclosporine levels greater than 200 ng/mL if a patient is hypertensive or has renal or hepatic failure.[167] In such patients, seizures and encephalopathy, accompanied by the imaging findings of the posterior reversible encephalopathy syndrome (PRES) can occur. Patients may require multiple transfusions of red cells, platelets, and fresh frozen plasma. Prophylaxis against *Pneumocystis carinii* infection with sulfamethoxazole and against fungi with fluconazole is necessary. Newly diagnosed HLH patients should have HLA typing done and a donor search initiated in case allogeneic hematopoietic stem cell transplantation is required for therapy.

Antithymocyte globulin (ATG) has been used as a primary treatment of 38 cases of familial HLH.[168] It was intended that all of these patients undergo stem cell transplantation, which ultimately cured 16 of 19 cases. ATG was ineffective for patients who had been previously treated with etoposide, dexamethasone, and cyclosporine and who had relapsed while on therapy.

Stem cell transplantation is needed for all patients with familial HLH or with gene defects, CNS disease, or who relapse either on or off HLH therapy. Survival ranges from 45 to 60 percent in several series, which included use of matched-related and matched-unrelated donor stem cell transplantation with conventional or reduced-intensity conditioning.[169–171]

Macrophage Activation Syndrome

This syndrome describes patients with symptoms and signs of HLH in the setting of juvenile rheumatoid arthritis or systemic lupus erythematosus.[172] Similar to classic HLH, macrophage activation is characterized by proliferation of macrophages and T cells. Patients present with continuous fever, purpura, hepatosplenomegaly, mental status changes, cytopenias, coagulopathy, and hypofibrinogenemia. Laboratory findings may include defective NK-cell function and low perforin expression, as seen in HLH. Unlike classic HLH, patients with macrophage activation syndrome may be successfully treated with cyclosporine and glucocorticoids without etoposide.[173] Full HLH-2004 therapy is recommended if patients fail to improve after 2 days of glucocorticoid and cyclosporine therapy.

COURSE AND PROGNOSIS

Patients with HLH are often critically ill, functionally immunosuppressed, and receive highly toxic chemotherapy. They should be treated at institutions familiar with the complications of chemotherapy and immune suppression. Splenectomy is recommended only in the case of life-threatening respiratory compromise. Some patients have an initial good response to therapy with etoposide, dexamethasone, and cyclosporine, but then have progressive disease as evidenced by elevation of the serum ferritin, worsening coagulopathy, or need for increased respiratory, blood pressure, or renal support. Despite being profoundly neutropenic, it is important to continue etoposide because it is the only medication that will cause apoptosis of the macrophages. Treatment of active Epstein-Barr virus infection with rituximab[174] or addition of anti-tumor necrosis factor-α agents such as infliximab or etanercept has proven useful.[175–177]

SINUS HISTIOCYTOSIS WITH MASSIVE LYMPHADENOPATHY (ROSAI-DORFMAN DISEASE)

DEFINITION AND HISTORY

Rosai and Dorfman recognized this nonmalignant proliferation of histiocytes as a unique histopathologic entity, which is part of the differential diagnosis of massive lymphadenopathy.[178] Although this disease is self-limited in some patients, others with airway obstruction or orbital or brain tumors may require therapy.[179]

EPIDEMIOLOGY

Rosai-Dorfman disease is found throughout the world as a disease of children and young adults (mean age: 20.6 years). Most of our knowledge about it is the result of analysis of the 423 cases in the registry developed by Drs. Rosai and Dorfman in which there is no gender, ethnic, or socioeconomic predilection. Persons of African and European descent are equally represented; people of Asian descent less so. In cases of digestive system disease, males and persons of African descent were more commonly affected.[180] Intracranial disease is found in patients with a mean age of 37.5 years.[181] There is an apparent increase in rheumatologic disorders and hemolytic anemia among these patients.[182]

ETIOLOGY AND PATHOGENESIS

Although associations with various herpes virus infections have been reported, these most likely represent detection of lymphocytes or macrophages harboring these viruses with no relation to etiology. A possible model for the key histopathologic finding, emperipolesis of lymphocytes by macrophages, has been reported.[183] These authors hypothesized that macrophage-activating cytokines could stimulate the macrophages to ingest lymphocytes. The cells in the lesions of this disorder are polyclonal.[184]

CLINICAL FEATURES

Massive, painless bilateral cervical adenopathy is the presenting finding in 87 percent of patients. Some have fever, night sweats, malaise, and weight loss. A few patients have polyarthralgia, rheumatoid arthritis, glomerulonephritis, asthma, and diabetes mellitus. Painless maculopapular eruptions, sometimes reddish or bluish, or yellow xanthomatous rashes occur in 16 percent of patients. Subcutaneous nodules can be found anywhere in the body. Another 16 percent of patients have nasal cavity and paranasal sinus involvement with obstruction of the airways, epistaxis, septal displacement, and mass lesions infiltrating the sinuses. Ten percent have eyelid or orbital masses with proptosis. Unlike patients with LCH, patients with Rosai-Dorfman disease rarely (10%) have osteolytic bone lesions that have irregular borders but may have sclerotic bone lesions. Bilateral parotid or submandibular gland swelling may also be a sign of Rosai-Dorfman disease. Less than 10 percent of patients have central nervous system, intracranial, epidural, or dural masses, as solitary or multiple lesions leading to headaches, nerve palsies, or syncope. Other organ system involvement in 1 to 3 percent of cases include the kidney, genitourinary tract, lungs, larynx, liver, tonsil, breast, gastrointestinal tract, and heart. Up to 43 percent of patients will have lymphadenopathy, as well as extranodal involvement: skin, soft tissue, upper respiratory tract, bone, eye, or retroorbital tissue.[185]

LABORATORY FEATURES

Patients may have a hemolytic anemia or anemia of chronic disease, elevated erythrocyte sedimentation rate, and polyclonal hyperimmunoglobulinemia. Elevation of liver enzymes and other laboratory abnormalities depend on the organs involved.[186] Hepatic features include capsular and pericapsular fibrosis. The lymph node sinuses are enlarged by a proliferation of histiocytes with large round or oval vesicular nuclei and a prominent nucleolus. Mitoses are rare. The cytoplasm is pale and eosinophilic, although some may have a foamy cytoplasm. The key diagnostic finding is intact lymphocytes in macrophages (lymphophagocytosis, active ingestion, or emperipolesis, the penetration of a smaller cell into larger one). Because the lymphocytes are inside vacuoles, they are not degraded. Accompanying the histiocytes are numerous plasma cells. The pathologic macrophages in this disease infiltrate the sinuses of lymph nodes and are phagocytosing lymphocytes and plasma cells as well as erythrocytes.[179] Although the histiocytes are S100-positive, they are CD1a-negative, unlike the LCs, which are positive for both markers. The macrophages express CD68, CD14, CD15, lysozyme, transferrin receptor, interleukin-2 receptor, and CD163.[179]

DIFFERENTIAL DIAGNOSIS

Any other cause of lymphadenopathy, such as infections, lymphomas, leukemias, Gaucher disease, melanoma, and other malignancies, should be ruled out by a biopsy. The massive cervical lymph nodes are strikingly similar to those of patients with the autoimmune lymphoproliferative syndrome.[187] Inflammatory pseudotumor and Rosai-Dorfman disease have been found in the same patient suggesting a histologic continuum.[188]

Clinicians should be aware that the sinuses of many reactive lymph nodes contain macrophages (histiocytes) and pathologists will report that presence as "sinus histiocytes or sinus histiocytosis." This is not evidence for Rosai-Dorfman disease because in those cases the sinus histiocytes do not have lymphocytes within their cytoplasm.

THERAPY

Many cases are self-limited and do not require therapy. Surgery may be useful for symptomatic treatment of large lymph nodes. Multiorgan involvement or dysfunction, and association with immune dysfunction are poor prognostic indicators and indicate the necessity of treatment.[189] Several therapies have been used including glucocorticoids and chemotherapy with success in some cases. Several case reports have described improvement or cure of patients with the disease with dexamethasone, methotrexate, 6-mercaptopurine, cladribine, or vinorelbine plus methotrexate.[190–193]

COURSE AND PROGNOSIS

Most patients will have a slow but steady decrease in the size of their lymph nodes over months to years. For those patients requiring treatment because of impingement on vital organs responses are variable. Because no clinical trials have been done, treatment has been based on anecdotal reports.

ERDHEIM-CHESTER DISEASE

DEFINITION AND HISTORY

In 1930, two cases of "lipid granulomatosis" were described by William Chester and Jakob Erdheim.[194] Jaffe coined the term *Erdheim-Chester disease*.[195] This histopathologic characteristics of ECD overlap xanthogranuloma and distinctions between the two are made on clinical and radiologic findings. Lipid-laden histocytes with foamy or eosinophilic cytoplasm infiltrate bones and various organs and generate a fibroblastic response that leads to critical organ failure. The histocytes are CD68+, factor XIIIa+ CD1a–, S100–, and lack Birbeck granules. Touton-like giant cells are commonly found.

EPIDEMIOLOGY/ETIOLOGY

This disease primarily affects adults (mean age: 53 years; range: 7–84 years).[196] There is no known etiology. Cells from ECD biopsies have been found to be clonal in three cases and polyclonal in two.[197–199] Elevated levels of osteopontin in ECD tissue have been found at diagnosis and then declined after treatment with prednisolone.[200] It is difficult to judge the exact role of osteopontin in ECD as it has many functions as a noncollagenous extracellular matrix protein that may affect cell adhesion, migration, and other functions. Immunohistochemical staining of ECD tissue show expression of CCL2 (monocyte chemotactic protein 1), CCL4 (macrophage inflammatory protein-1β [MIP1β]), CCL5 (RANTES [regulated on activation, normal T-cell expressed, presumed secreted]), CCL20 (MIP-3α), and CCL19 (MIP-3β), along with their receptors CCR1, CCR2, CCR3, CCR5, CCR6, and CCR7.[201] Elevated expression of an interferon-γ-inducible protein, IL-6, and RANKL (receptor activator of nuclear factor-B ligand) were described. The latter two are important for bone remodeling. Biopsies of 32 of 37 patients with ECD had prominent staining for the platelet-derived growth factor receptor-β.

CLINICAL FEATURES

Many patients have fever, weakness, and weight loss. Symmetric osteosclerosis of long bones with infiltrating and encasing masses around various organs are characteristic of ECD. Patients present with bone pain, especially in the lower extremities. The second most common presenting symptom is DI. Some patients have cerebellar signs and focal neurologic deficits.[202] Bilateral painless exophthalmos may also occur. Fifty percent of patients have extraskeletal disease. It is unusual for lymph nodes, liver, spleen, or axial skeleton to be affected, whereas these areas are frequently affected in LCH and RDD. Retroperitoneal and renal involvement occurs in one-third of ECD patients and causes abdominal pain, dysuria, and hydronephrosis. Pulmonary involvement may present in 20 percent of patients and causes dyspnea. Skin manifestations of ECD include xanthomatous lesions that may begin as reddish-brown papules similar to xanthoma disseminatum. Cardiac dysfunction occurs because of circumferential sheathing of the aorta, and aortic branches, including coronary arteries. There may also be endocardial, myocardial, or pericardial involvement, leading to pericardial effusions with risk of tamponade.[203,204]

LABORATORY FEATURES

There are no specific laboratory findings, but elevated sedimentation rate and alkaline phosphatase have been reported in about one-fifth of cases. Radiographs show bilateral patchy osteosclerosis of the metaphysis and diaphysis of the femur, proximal tibia, and fibula. Lytic lesions are found in approximately one-third of patients. Chest CT imaging findings include diffuse interstitial infiltrates, and pleural and interlobular septal thickening.[204] Perirenal infiltration, extending through the fat of the anterior or posterior pararenal spaces, leading to the classic "hairy kidney" appearance and circumferential sheathing of the aorta, can be seen on an abdominal CT scan in some patients.

DIFFERENTIAL DIAGNOSIS

Although histologically distinct, the clinical features may suggest LCH, RDD, juvenile xanthogranuloma, or xanthoma disseminatum. Some clinical features overlap with sarcoidosis, amyloidosis, Paget disease, Ormond disease (idiopathic retroperitoneal fibrosis), and Whipple disease. The histologic features can be confused with Gaucher disease, Niemann-Pick disease, mucopolysaccharidosis, or malakoplakia.[205]

THERAPY

In a review of 37 patients, glucocorticoids, usually 1 mg/kg per day, decreased exophthalmos or general symptoms in 20 patients.[196] Among these patients, glucocorticoids were effective in six patients, transiently effective in four, and ineffective in eight. Of eight patients treated with a variety of chemotherapy agents and glucocorticoids, four had improvement. Radiation was ineffective for orbital masses but transiently relieved bone pain. Long-term responses occurred with interferon-α in three patients.[206] These patients had marked decrease in their fatigue, improvement of bone films, and in one case, nearly complete resolution of DI. Treatments continued for months or years. Another case with favorable response to interferon-α has been reported.[198] A series of eight cases treated with interferon-α was reported, with four patients failing and four improving after several months of treatment.[207] The same group published a series of six patients treated with imatinib mesylate.[208] Two patients had stable disease and one an initial response before worsening.

COURSE AND PROGNOSIS

Nearly 60 percent of ECD patients die of their disease; 36 percent die within 6 months. The mean survival duration is less than 3 years. Cardiac, pulmonary, or renal failure are the primary causes of death.

JUVENILE XANTHOGRANULOMA

DEFINITION AND HISTORY

JXG is a histiocytic disorder that affects the skin with multiple nodules in the head, neck, and trunk primarily in children, although adults can also be affected.[209] The lesional cells are derived from dermal dendrocytes. Systemic involvement occurs in a few cases. Rudolf Virchow may have been the first to describe a child with "cutaneous xanthomas" in 1871, as noted in a 1954 report of this condition.[210] Other early reports of JXG were published in 1905 by Adamson and in 1912 by McDonagh.[211,212]

EPIDEMIOLOGY

Children with solitary lesions have a median age of onset of 2 years with a male-to-female ratio of 1.5:1. Children with multiple lesions have a median age of onset of 5 months and have a male-to-female ratio of 12:1. No population study of JXG has been reported, so the precise incidence is unknown. However, a review of JXG from the Kiel Pediatric Tumor Registry recorded 129 (0.52%) cases of JXG and 800 (3.25%) cases of LCH among 24,600 children over a 36-year period.[213]

ETIOLOGY AND PATHOGENESIS

There is no known cause of JXG. Patients with JXG and neurofibromatosis types 1 and 2, as well as the triad of the aforementioned diseases with juvenile chronic myelogenous leukemia, have been reported.[214–216] These and other cases have led to discussion of apparent increased risk of leukemia in neurofibromatosis patients with JXG, but there is no rigorous proof for this association.[217,218]

CLINICAL FEATURES

The majority of patients are children younger than 2 years of age who have solitary skin nodules on their head, neck, or trunk.[209,213] The lesion is most often the same color as surrounding skin, but may be erythematous or yellowish. Rarely nodules may be in the subcutaneous fat, deep soft tissue, or skeletal muscle. Organ involvement is very rare but has been reported in the soft tissue, central nervous system, bone, lung, liver, spleen, pancreas, adrenal, intestines, kidneys, lymph nodes, marrow, and heart.[209,213,219] Systemic symptoms and signs occur only if these organ systems are involved.

LABORATORY FEATURES

Immunohistochemical staining of biopsies is necessary to differentiate JXG from other histiocytic lesions. JXG classically stains with a macrophage marker such as CD68 or Ki-M1P, anti-factor XIIIa, vimentin, and often anti-CD4. They are most often negative for S100 and anti-CD1a. There are three characteristic histologic patterns: early JXG, classic JXG, and transitional JXG.[213] Early JXG is characterized by small to intermediate-sized mononuclear histiocytes in a sheet-like infiltrate. The cells in this category have only small quantities of lipid in the cytoplasm and Touton-type giant cells are absent. This type has relatively more mitoses than the others, but there is no cytologic atypia. Classic JXG exhibits abundant vacuolated, foamy histiocytes with Touton giant cells (lipid-laden histiocytes with multiple nuclei with a small amount of centrally oriented cytoplasm).

Transitional JXG has a predominance of spindle-shaped cells resembling benign fibrous histiocytoma with foamy histiocytes and occasional giant cells.[213] Biopsies also contain lymphocytes, eosinophils, and occasionally Charcot-Leyden crystals.

If the marrow is involved patients may have cytopenias. Liver infiltration may cause elevation of liver enzymes, hypoalbuminemia, and an elevated erythrocyte sedimentation rate. Pituitary involvement may lead to DI. Hypercalcemia has been reported.

DIFFERENTIAL DIAGNOSIS

LCH is the disease most often confused with JXG.[213] Others include fibrohistiocytic lesion not otherwise specified, reticulohistiocytoma, hemangioendothelioma, Spitz nevus, malignant fibrous histiocytoma, and rhabdomyosarcoma or other malignancies.

THERAPY

Patients with a single or only a few lesions need no therapy. An excisional biopsy can be used, if desired for cosmetic reasons. For the rare patients who have systemic disease and require treatment a wide variety of chemotherapy and radiotherapy regimens have been reported.[219,220] Inclusion of a vinca alkaloid and glucocorticoid is associated with better overall response rates. A child with CNS JXG who failed to respond to vinblastine was successfully treated with cladribine.[221]

COURSE AND PROGNOSIS

Patients with only skin or soft-tissue involvement all survive and in a majority of cases, the lesions spontaneously disappear over time. Infants with large retroperitoneal masses, liver, marrow, or central nervous system involvement usually survive with chemotherapy treatment. Two of 17 patients with multisystem JXG reported in the literature died despite multiagent chemotherapy.[220]

REFERENCES

1. Jaffe R: The diagnostic histopathology of Langerhans cell histiocytosis, in *Histiocytic Disorders of Children and Adults. Basic Science Clinical Features, and Therapy*, edited by S Weitzman, RM Egeler, p 14. Cambridge University Press, Cambridge, UK, 2005.
2. Favara BE, Feller AC, Pauli M, et al: Contemporary classification of histiocytic disorders. The WHO Committee on Histiocytic/Reticulum Cell Proliferations. Reclassification Working Group of the Histiocyte Society. *Med Pediatr Oncol* 29:157, 1997.
3. Chikwava K, Jaffe R: Langerin (CD207) staining in normal pediatric tissues, reactive lymph nodes, and childhood histiocytic disorders. *Pediatr Dev Pathol* 7:607, 2004.

3a. Lau SK, Chu PG, Weiss LM: Immunohistochemical expression of Langerin in Langerhans cell histiocytosis and non-Langerhans cell histiocytic disorders. *Am J Surg Pathol* 32:615, 2008.

4. Langerhans P: Ueber die nerven der menschlichen Haut. *Virchows Arch A* 325, 1868.
5. Nezelof C, Basset F, Rousseau MF: Histiocytosis X histogenetic arguments for a Langerhans cell origin. *Biomedicine* 18:365, 1973.
6. Laman JD, Leenen PJ, Annels NE, et al: Langerhans-cell histiocytosis "insight into DC biology." *Trends Immunol* 24:190, 2003.
7. Coppes-Zantinga A, Egeler RM: The Langerhans cell histiocytosis X files revealed. *Br J Haematol* 116:3, 2002.
8. Arceci R: Langerhans cell histiocytosis in children and adults: Pathogenesis, clinical manifestations, and treatment. *Hematology Am Soc Hematol Educ Program* 297, 2002.
9. Carstensen H, Ornvold K: The epidemiology of LCH in children in Denmark, 1975–89. *Med Pediatr Oncol* 21:387, 1993.
10. Guyot-Goubin A, Donadieu J, Barkaoui M, et al: Descriptive epidemiology of childhood Langerhans cell histiocytosis in France, 2000–2004. *Pediatr Blood Cancer* 51:71, 2008.
11. Arico M, Nichols K, Whitlock JA, et al: Familial clustering of Langerhans cell histiocytosis. *Br J Haematol* 107:883, 1999.
12. Nicholson HS, Egeler RM, Nesbit ME: The epidemiology of Langerhans cell histiocytosis. *Hematol Oncol Clin North Am* 12:379, 1998.
13. Bhatia S, Nesbit ME Jr, Egeler RM, et al: Epidemiologic study of Langerhans cell histiocytosis in children. *J Pediatr* 130:774, 1997.
14. McClain K, Jin H, Gresik V, Favara B: Langerhans cell histiocytosis: Lack of a viral etiology. *Am J Hematol* 47:16, 1994.
15. Jeziorski E, Senechal B, Molina TJ, et al: Herpes-virus infection in patients with Langerhans cell histiocytosis: A case-controlled sero-epidemiological study, and in situ analysis. *PLoS One* 3:e3262, 2008.
16. Yu RC, Morris JF, Pritchard J, Chu TC: Defective alloantigen-presenting capacity of "Langerhans cell histiocytosis cells." *Arch Dis Child* 67:1370, 1992.
17. Geissmann F, Lepelletier Y, Fraitag S, et al: Differentiation of Langerhans cells in Langerhans cell histiocytosis. *Blood* 97:1241, 2001.
18. Senechal B, Elain G, Jeziorski E, et al: Expansion of regulatory T cells in patients with Langerhans cell histiocytosis. *PLoS Med* 4:e253, 2007.
19. Willman CL, Busque L, Griffith BB, et al: Langerhans'-cell histiocytosis (histiocytosis X)—a clonal proliferative disease. *N Engl J Med* 331:154, 1994.
20. Yu RC, Chu C, Buluwela L, Chu AC: Clonal proliferation of Langerhans cells in Langerhans cell histiocytosis. *Lancet* 343:767, 1994.
21. Yousem SA, Colby TV, Chen YY, et al: Pulmonary Langerhans' cell histiocytosis: Molecular analysis of clonality. *Am J Surg Pathol* 25:630, 2001.
22. Chikwava KR, Hunt JL, Mantha GS, et al: Analysis of loss of heterozygosity in single-system and multisystem Langerhans' cell histiocytosis. *Pediatr Dev Pathol* 10:18, 2007.
23. da Costa CE, Szuhai K, van Eijk R, et al: No genomic aberrations in Langerhans cell histiocytosis as assessed by diverse molecular technologies. *Genes Chromosomes Cancer* 48:239, 2009.
24. Murakami I, Gogusev J, Fournet JC, et al: Detection of molecular cytogenetic aberrations in Langerhans cell histiocytosis of bone. *Hum Pathol* 33:555, 2002.
25. McClain KL, Cai YH, Hicks J, et al: Expression profiling using human tissues in combination with RNA amplification and microarray analysis: Assessment of Langerhans cell histiocytosis. *Amino Acids* 28:279, 2005.
26. Rus R, Kluiver J, Viser L: Gene expression analysis of dendritic/Langerhans cells and Langerhans cell histiocytosis. *J Pathol* 209:474, 2006.
27. Rolland A, Guyon L, Gill M, et al: Increased blood myeloid dendritic cells and dendritic cell-poietins in Langerhans cell histiocytosis. *J Immunol* 174:3067, 2005.
28. Ishii R, Morimoto A, Ikushima S, et al: High serum values of soluble CD154, IL-2 receptor, RANKL and osteoprotegerin in Langerhans cell histiocytosis. *Pediatr Blood Cancer* 47:194, 2006.
29. Rosso DA, Karis J, Braier JL, et al: B. Elevated serum levels of the decoy receptor osteoprotegerin in children with Langerhans cell histiocytosis. *Pediatr Res* 59:281, 2006.
30. Munn S, Chu AC: Langerhans cell histiocytosis of the skin. *Hematol Oncol Clin North Am* 12:269, 1998.
31. Stein SL, Paller AS, Haut PR, Mancini AJ: Langerhans cell histiocytosis presenting in the neonatal period: A retrospective case series. *Arch Pediatr Adolesc Med* 155:778, 2001.
32. Lau L, Krafchik B, Trebo MM, Weitzman S: Cutaneous Langerhans cell histiocytosis in children under one year. *Pediatr Blood Cancer* 46:66, 2006.
33. Minkov M, Prosch H, Steiner M, et al: Langerhans cell histiocytosis in neonates. *Pediatr Blood Cancer* 45:802, 2005.
34. Hicks J, Flaitz CM: Langerhans cell histiocytosis: Current insights in a molecular age with emphasis on clinical oral and maxillofacial pathology practice. *Oral Surg Oral Med Oral Pathol Oral Radiol Endod* 100(2 Suppl):S42, 2005.
35. Slater JM, Swarm OJ: Eosinophilic granuloma of bone. *Med Pediatr Oncol* 8:151, 1980.
36. Wong A, Ortiz-Neira CL, Reslan WA, et al: Liver involvement in Langerhans cell histiocytosis. *Pediatr Radiol* 36:1105, 2006.
37. Braier J, Ciocca M, Latella A, et al: Cholestasis, sclerosing cholangitis, and liver transplantation in Langerhans cell histiocytosis. *Med Pediatr Oncol* 38:178, 2002.
38. Vassallo R, Ryu JH, Colby TV, et al: Pulmonary Langerhans' cell histiocytosis. *N Engl J Med* 342:1969, 2000.
39. Braier J, Latella A, Balancini B, et al: Outcome in children with pulmonary Langerhans cell histiocytosis. *Pediatr Blood Cancer* 43:765, 2004.
40. Bernstrand C, Cederlund K, Henter JI: Pulmonary function testing and pulmonary Langerhans cell histiocytosis. *Pediatr Blood Cancer* 49:323, 2007.
41. McClain K, Ramsay NK, Robison L, et al: Bone marrow involvement in histiocytosis X. *Med Pediatr Oncol* 11:167, 1983.
42. Minkov M, Potschger U, Grois N, et al: Bone marrow assessment in Langerhans cell histiocytosis. *Pediatr Blood Cancer* 49:694, 2007.
43. Favara BE, Jaffe R, Egeler RM: Macrophage activation and hemophagocytic syndrome in Langerhans cell histiocytosis: Report of 30 cases. *Pediatr Dev Pathol* 5:130, 2002.
44. Prosch H, Grois N, Prayer D, et al: Central diabetes insipidus as presenting symptom of Langerhans cell histiocytosis. *Pediatr Blood Cancer* 43:594, 2004.

45. Donadieu J, Rolon MA, Thomas C, et al: Endocrine involvement in pediatric-onset Langerhans' cell histiocytosis: A population-based study. *J Pediatr* 144:344, 2004.
46. Grois N, Potschger U, Prosch H, et al: Risk factors for diabetes insipidus in Langerhans cell histiocytosis. *Pediatr Blood Cancer* 46:228, 2006.
47. Titgemeyer C, Grois N, Minkov M, et al: Pattern and course of single-system disease in Langerhans cell histiocytosis data from the DAL-HX 83- and 90-study. *Med Pediatr Oncol* 37:108, 2001.
48. Hait E, Liang M, Degar B, et al: Gastrointestinal tract involvement in Langerhans cell histiocytosis: Case report and literature review. *Pediatrics* 118:e1593, 2006.
49. Geissmann F, Thomas C, Emile JF, et al: Digestive tract involvement in Langerhans cell histiocytosis. The French Langerhans Cell Histiocytosis Study Group. *J Pediatr* 129:836, 1996.
50. Grois N, Prayer D, Prosch H, et al: Course and clinical impact of magnetic resonance imaging findings in diabetes insipidus associated with Langerhans cell histiocytosis. *Pediatr Blood Cancer* 43:59, 2004.
51. Gadner H, Heitger A, Grois N, et al: Treatment strategy for disseminated Langerhans cell histiocytosis. DAL HX-83 Study Group. *Med Pediatr Oncol* 23:72, 1994.
52. Grois NG, Favara BE, Mostbeck GH, et al: Central nervous system disease in Langerhans cell histiocytosis. *Hematol Oncol Clin North Am* 12:287, 1998.
53. Prayer D, Grois N, Prosch H, et al: MR imaging presentation of intracranial disease associated with Langerhans cell histiocytosis. *AJNR Am J Neuroradiol* 25:880, 2004.
54. Grois N, Prayer D, Prosch H, et al: Neuropathology of CNS disease in Langerhans cell histiocytosis. *Brain* 128:829, 2005.
55. Wnorowski M, Prosch H, Prayer D, et al: Pattern and course of neurodegeneration in Langerhans cell histiocytosis. *J Pediatr* 153:127, 2008.
56. Calming U, Henter JI: Elevated erythrocyte sedimentation rate and thrombocytosis as possible indicators of active disease in Langerhans' cell histiocytosis. *Acta Paediatr* 87:1085, 1998.
57. Phillips M, Allen C, Gerson P, McClain K: Comparison of FDG-PET scans to conventional radiography and bone scans in management of Langerhans cell histiocytosis. *Pediatr Blood Cancer* 52:97, 2009.
58. Burns BF, Colby TV, Dorfman RF: Langerhans' cell granulomatosis (histiocytosis X) associated with malignant lymphomas. *Am J Surg Pathol* 7:529, 1983.
59. Almanaseer IY, Kosova L, Pellettiere EV: Composite lymphoma with immunoblastic features and Langerhans' cell granulomatosis (histiocytosis X). *Am J Clin Pathol* 85:111, 1986.
60. Egeler RM, Neglia JP, Arico M, et al: The relation of Langerhans cell histiocytosis to acute leukemia, lymphomas, and other solid tumors. The LCH-Malignancy Study Group of the Histiocyte Society. *Hematol Oncol Clin North Am* 12:369, 1998.
61. Bonetti F, Knowles DM, Chilosi M, et al: A distinctive cutaneous malignant neoplasm expressing the Langerhans cell phenotype. Synchronous occurrence with B-chronic lymphocytic leukemia. *Cancer* 55:2417, 1985.
62. Bramwell NH, Burns BF: Histiocytosis X of the thymus in association with myasthenia gravis. *Am J Clin Pathol* 86:224, 1986.
63. Steen AE, Steen KH, Bauer R, Bieber T: Successful treatment of cutaneous Langerhans cell histiocytosis with low-dose methotrexate. *Br J Dermatol* 145:137, 2001.
64. McClain K, Kozinetz C: A phase II trial using thalidomide for Langerhans cell histiocytosis. *Pediatr Blood Cancer* 48:44, 2007.
65. Hoeger PH, Nanduri VR, Harper JI, et al: Long term follow up of topical mustine treatment for cutaneous Langerhans cell histiocytosis. *Arch Dis Child* 82:483, 2000.
66. Kwon OS, Cho KH, Song KY: Primary cutaneous Langerhans cell histiocytosis treated with photochemotherapy. *J Dermatol* 24:54, 1997.
67. Nauert C, Zornoza J, Ayala A, et al: Eosinophilic granuloma of bone: Diagnosis and management. *Skeletal Radiol* 10:227, 1983.
68. Grois N, Potschger U, Prosch H, et al: Risk factors for diabetes insipidus in Langerhans cell histiocytosis. *Pediatr Blood Cancer* 46:228, 2006.
69. Gadner H, Grois N, Arico M, et al: A randomized trial of treatment for multisystem Langerhans' cell histiocytosis. *J Pediatr* 138:728, 2001.
70. Woo KI, Harris GJ: Eosinophilic granuloma of the orbit: Understanding the paradox of aggressive destruction responsive to minimal intervention. *Ophthal Plast Reconstr Surg* 19:429, 2003.
71. McCullough C: Eosinophilic granuloma of bone. *Acta Orthop Scand* 51:389, 1980.
72. Raney RB Jr, D'Angio GJ: Langerhans' cell histiocytosis (histiocytosis X): Experience at the Children's Hospital of Philadelphia, 1970–1984. *Med Pediatr Oncol* 17:20, 1989.
73. Gadner H, Grois N, Potschger U, et al: Improved outcome in multisystem Langerhans cell histiocytosis is associated with therapy intensification. *Blood* 111:2556, 2008.
74. Morimoto A, Ikushima S, Kinugawa N, et al: Improved outcome in the treatment of pediatric multifocal Langerhans cell histiocytosis: Results from the Japan Langerhans Cell Histiocytosis Study Group-96 protocol study. *Cancer* 107:613, 2006.
75. Nesbit ME, Kieffer S, D'Angio GJ: Reconstitution of vertebral height in histiocytosis X: A long-term follow-up. *J Bone Joint Surg Am* 51:1360, 1969.
76. Womer RB, Raney RB Jr, D'Angio GJ: Healing rates of treated and untreated bone lesions in histiocytosis X. *Pediatrics* 76:286, 1985.
77. Mammano S, Candiotto S, Balsano M: Cast and brace treatment of eosinophilic granuloma of the spine: Long-term follow-up. *J Pediatr Orthop* 17:821, 1997.
78. Buchler T, Cervinek L, Belohlavek O, et al: Langerhans cell histiocytosis with central nervous system involvement: Follow-up by FDG-PET during treatment with cladribine. *Pediatr Blood Cancer* 44:286, 2005.
79. Watts J, Files B: Langerhans cell histiocytosis: Central nervous system involvement treated successfully with 2-chlorodeoxyadenosine. *Pediatr Hematol Oncol* 18:199, 2001.
80. Dhall G, Finlay JL, Dunkel IJ, et al: Analysis of outcome for patients with mass lesions of the central nervous system due to Langerhans cell histiocytosis treated with 2-chlorodeoxyadenosine. *Pediatr Blood Cancer* 50:72, 2008.
81. Imashuku S, Ishida S, Koike K, et al: Cerebellar ataxia in pediatric patients with Langerhans cell histiocytosis. *J Pediatr Hematol Oncol* 26:735, 2004.
82. Idbaih A, Donadieu J, Barthez MA, et al: Retinoic acid therapy in "degenerative-like" neuro-Langerhans cell histiocytosis: A prospective pilot study. *Pediatr Blood Cancer* 43:55, 2004.
82a. Allen CE, Flores R, Rauch R, et al. Neurodegenerative central nervous system Langerhans cell histiocytosis and coincident hydrocephalus: Treated with vincristine cytosine arabinoside treatment. *Pediatr Blood Cancer* 2009 Nov 11. [Epub ahead of print].
83. Stine KC, Saylors RL, Saccente S, et al: Efficacy of continuous infusion 2-CDA (cladribine) in pediatric patients with Langerhans cell histiocytosis. *Pediatr Blood Cancer* 43:81, 2004.
83a. Weitzman S, Braier J, Donadieu J, et al: 2′-Chlorodeoxyadenosine (2-CdA) as salvage therapy for Langerhans cell histiocytosis (LCH), Results of the LCH-S-98 protocol of the histiocyte society. *Pediatr Blood Cancer* 53:1271, 2009.
84. Egeler RM, de Kraker J, Voute PA: Cytosine-arabinoside, vincristine, and prednisolone in the treatment of children with disseminated Langerhans cell histiocytosis with organ dysfunction: Experience at a single institution. *Med Pediatr Oncol* 21:265, 1993.
85. Bernard F, Thomas C, Bertrand Y, et al: Multi-centre pilot study of 2-chlorodeoxyadenosine and cytosine arabinoside combined chemotherapy in refractory Langerhans cell histiocytosis with haematological dysfunction. *Eur J Cancer* 41:2682, 2005.
86. Akkari V, Donadieu J, Piguet C, et al: Hematopoietic stem cell transplantation in patients with severe Langerhans cell histiocytosis and hematological dysfunction: Experience of the French Langerhans Cell Study Group. *Bone Marrow Transplant* 31:1097, 2003.
87. Nagarajan R, Neglia J, Ramsay N, Baker KS: Successful treatment of refractory Langerhans cell histiocytosis with unrelated cord blood transplantation. *J Pediatr Hematol Oncol* 23:629, 2001.
88. Cooper N, Rao K, Goulden N, et al: The use of reduced-intensity stem cell transplantation in haemophagocytic lymphohistiocytosis and Langerhans cell histiocytosis. *Bone Marrow Transplant* 42 Suppl 2:S47, 2008.
89. Minkov M, Grois N, Broadbent V, et al: Cyclosporine A therapy for multisystem Langerhans cell histiocytosis. *Med Pediatr Oncol* 33:482, 1999.
90. Lukina EA, Kuznetsov VP, Beliaev DL, et al: [The treatment of histiocytosis X (Langerhans-cell histiocytosis) with alpha-interferon preparations]. *Ter Arkh* 65:67, 1993.
91. Minkov M, Steiner M, Potschger U, et al: Reactivations in multisystem Langerhans cell histiocytosis: Data of the international LCH registry. *J Pediatr* 153:700, 705, 2008.
92. Allen CE, McClain KL: Langerhans cell histiocytosis: A review of past, current and future therapies. *Drugs Today (Barc)* 43:627, 2007.
93. Haupt R, Nanduri V, Calevo MG, et al: Permanent consequences in Langerhans cell histiocytosis patients: A pilot study from the Histiocyte Society-Late Effects Study Group. *Pediatr Blood Cancer* 42:438, 2004.
94. Donadieu J, Rolon MA, Pion I, et al: Incidence of growth hormone deficiency in pediatric-onset Langerhans cell histiocytosis: Efficacy and safety of growth hormone treatment. *J Clin Endocrinol Metab* 89:604, 2004.
95. Komp DM: Long-term sequelae of histiocytosis X. *Am J Pediatr Hematol Oncol* 3:163, 1981.
96. Willis B, Ablin A, Weinberg V, et al: Disease course and late sequelae of Langerhans' cell histiocytosis: 25-year experience at the University of California, San Francisco. *J Clin Oncol* 14:2073, 1996.
97. Nanduri VR, Lillywhite L, Chapman C, et al: Cognitive outcome of long-term survivors of multisystem Langerhans cell histiocytosis: A single-institution, cross-sectional study. *J Clin Oncol* 21:2961, 2003.
98. Mittheisz E, Seidl R, Prayer D, et al: Central nervous system-related permanent consequences in patients with Langerhans cell histiocytosis. *Pediatr Blood Cancer* 48:50, 2007.
99. Egeler RM, Neglia JP, Puccetti DM, et al: Association of Langerhans cell histiocytosis with malignant neoplasms. *Cancer* 71:865, 1993.
100. Feldman AL, Berthold F, Arceci RJ, et al: Clonal relationship between precursor T-lymphoblastic leukaemia/lymphoma and Langerhans-cell histiocytosis. *Lancet Oncol* 6:435, 2005.
101. Rodig SJ, Payne EG, Degar BA, et al: Aggressive Langerhans cell histiocytosis following T-ALL: Clonally related neoplasms with persistent expression of constitutively active NOTCH1. *Am J Hematol* 83:116, 2008.
102. Baumgartner I, von Hochstetter A, Baumert B, et al: Langerhans'-cell histiocytosis in adults. *Med Pediatr Oncol* 28:9, 1997.
103. Gotz G, Fichter J: Langerhans' cell histiocytosis in 58 adults. *Eur J Med Res* 9:510, 2004.
104. Kaltsas GA, Powles TB, Evanson J, et al: Hypothalamo-pituitary abnormalities in adult patients with Langerhans cell histiocytosis: Clinical, endocrinological, and radiological features and response to treatment. *J Clin Endocrinol Metab* 85:1370, 2000.
105. Schonfeld N, Frank W, Wenig S, et al: Clinical and radiologic features, lung function and therapeutic results in pulmonary histiocytosis X. *Respiration* 60:38, 1993.
106 Travis WD, Borok Z, Roum JH, et al: Pulmonary Langerhans cell granulomatosis (histiocytosis X). A clinicopathologic study of 48 cases. *Am J Surg Pathol* 17:971, 1993.
107. Tazi A, Moreau J, Bergeron A, et al: Evidence that Langerhans cells in adult pulmonary Langerhans cell histiocytosis are mature dendritic cells: Importance of the cytokine microenvironment. *J Immunol* 163:3511, 1999.

108. Yousem SA, Colby TV, Chen YY, et al: Pulmonary Langerhans' cell histiocytosis: Molecular analysis of clonality. *Am J Surg Pathol* 25:630, 2001.
109. Delobbe A, Durieu J, Duhamel A, Wallaert B: Determinants of survival in pulmonary Langerhans' cell granulomatosis (histiocytosis X). Groupe d'Etude en Pathologie Interstitielle de la Societe de Pathologie Thoracique du Nord. *Eur Respir J* 9:2002, 1996.
110. Crausman RS, Jennings CA, Tuder RM, et al: Pulmonary histiocytosis X: Pulmonary function and exercise pathophysiology. *Am J Respir Crit Care Med* 153:426, 1996.
111. Diette GB, Scatarige JC, Haponik EF, et al: Do high-resolution CT findings of usual interstitial pneumonitis obviate lung biopsy? Views of pulmonologists. *Respiration* 72:134, 2005.
112. Soler P, Bergeron A, Kambouchner M, et al: Is high-resolution computed tomography a reliable tool to predict the histopathological activity of pulmonary Langerhans cell histiocytosis? *Am J Respir Crit Care Med* 162:264, 2000.
113. Farran RP, Zaretski E, Egeler RM: Treatment of Langerhans cell histiocytosis with pamidronate. *J Pediatr Hematol Oncol* 23:54, 2001.
114. Brown RE: Bisphosphonates as antialveolar macrophage therapy in pulmonary Langerhans cell histiocytosis? *Med Pediatr Oncol* 36:641, 2001.
115. Reichle A, Vogt T, Kunz-Schughart L, et al: Anti-inflammatory and angiostatic therapy in chemorefractory multisystem Langerhans' cell histiocytosis of adults. *Br J Haematol* 128:730, 2005.
116. Saven A, Foon KA, Piro LD: 2-Chlorodeoxyadenosine-induced complete remissions in Langerhans-cell histiocytosis. *Ann Intern Med* 121:430, 1994.
117. Pardanani A, Phyliky RL, Li CY, Tefferi A: 2-Chlorodeoxyadenosine therapy for disseminated Langerhans cell histiocytosis. *Mayo Clin Proc* 78:301, 2003.
118. Mogulkoc N, Veral A, Bishop PW, et al: Pulmonary Langerhans' cell histiocytosis: Radiologic resolution following smoking cessation. *Chest* 115:1452, 1999.
119. Dauriat G, Mal H, Thabut G, et al: Lung transplantation for pulmonary Langerhans' cell histiocytosis: A multicenter analysis. *Transplantation* 81:746, 2006.
120. Scott R, Robb-Smith AHT: Histiocytic Medullary Reticulosis. *Lancet* ii:194, 1939.
121. Tumors of the hematopoietic system. *Atlas of Tumor Pathology* Section III, Fascicle 8. By Henry Rappaport, MD, Armed Forces Institute of Pathology, Washington, DC, 1966. pp 49–63.
122. Wilson MS, Weiss LM, Gatter KC, et al: Malignant histiocytosis. A reassessment of cases previously reported in 1975 based on paraffin section immunophenotyping studies. *Cancer* 66:530, 1990.
123. Fonseca R, Tefferi A, Strickler JG: Follicular dendritic cell sarcoma mimicking diffuse large cell lymphoma: A case report. *Am J Hematol* 55:148, 1997.
124. Pileri SA, Grogan TM, Harris NL, et al: Tumours of histiocytes and accessory dendritic cells: An immunohistochemical approach to classification from the International Lymphoma Study Group based on 61 cases. *Histopathology* 41:1, 2002.
125. Lauritzen AF, Delsol G, Hansen NE, et al: Histiocytic sarcomas and monoblastic leukemias. A clinical, histologic, and immunophenotypical study. *Am J Clin Pathol* 102:45, 1994.
126. Kamel OW, Gocke CD, Kell DL, et al: True histiocytic lymphoma: A study of 12 cases based on current definition. *Leuk Lymphoma* 18:81, 1995.
127. Newman B, Hu W, Nigro K, Gilliam AC: Aggressive histiocytic disorders that can involve the skin. *J Am Acad Dermatol* 56:302, 2007.
128. Julg BD, Weidner S, Mayr D: Pulmonary manifestation of a Langerhans cell sarcoma: Case report and review of the literature. *Virchows Arch* 448:369, 2006.
129. Feldman AL, Arber DA, Pittaluga S, et al: Clonally related follicular lymphomas and histiocytic/dendritic cell sarcomas: Evidence for transdifferentiation of the follicular lymphoma clone. *Blood* 111:5433, 2008.
130. Hornick JL, Jaffe ES, Fletcher CD: Extranodal histiocytic sarcoma: Clinicopathologic analysis of 14 cases of a rare epithelioid malignancy. *Am J Surg Pathol* 28:1133, 2004.
131. Pillay K, Solomon R, Daubenton JD, Sinclair-Smith CC: Interdigitating dendritic cell sarcoma: A report of four paediatric cases and review of the literature. *Histopathology* 44:283, 2004.
132. Kairouz S, Hashash J, Kabbara W, et al: Dendritic cell neoplasms: An overview. *Am J Hematol* 82:924, 2007.
133. Porter DW, Gupte GL, Brown RM, et al: Histiocytic sarcoma with interdigitating dendritic cell differentiation. *J Pediatr Hematol Oncol* 26:827, 2004.
134. Soriano AO, Thompson MA, Admirand JH, et al: Follicular dendritic cell sarcoma: A report of 14 cases and a review of the literature. *Am J Hematol* 82:725, 2007.
135. Abidi MH, Tove I, Ibrahim RB, et al: Thalidomide for the treatment of histiocytic sarcoma after hematopoietic stem cell transplant. *Am J Hematol* 82:932, 2007.
136. Uchida K, Kobayashi S, Inukai T, et al: Langerhans cell sarcoma emanating from the upper arm skin: Successful treatment by MAID regimen. *J Orthop Sci* 13:89, 2008.
137. Nakayama R, Nemoto T, Takahashi H, et al: Gene expression analysis of soft tissue sarcomas: Characterization and reclassification of malignant fibrous histiocytoma. *Mod Pathol* 20:749, 2007.
138. Lee Y, John M, Edwards S: Molecular classification of synovial sarcomas, leiomyosarcomas and malignant fibrous histiocytomas by gene expression profiling. *Br J Cancer* 88:510, 2003.
139. Gazziola C, Cordani N, Wasserman B, et al: Malignant fibrous histiocytoma: A proposed cellular origin and identification of its characterizing gene transcripts. *Int J Oncol* 23:343, 2003.
140. Picci P, Bacci G, Ferrari S, Mercuri M: Neoadjuvant chemotherapy in malignant fibrous histiocytoma of bone and in osteosarcoma located in the extremities: Analogies and differences between the two tumors. *Ann Oncol* 8:1107, 1997.
141. Bramwell VH, Steward WP, Nooij M, et al: Neoadjuvant chemotherapy with doxorubicin and cisplatin in malignant fibrous histiocytoma of bone: A European Osteosarcoma Intergroup study. *J Clin Oncol* 17:3260, 1999.
142. Daw NC, Billups CA, Pappo AS, et al: Malignant fibrous histiocytoma and other fibrohistiocytic tumors in pediatric patients: The St. Jude Children's Research Hospital experience. *Cancer* 97:2839, 2003.
143. Farquhar JW, Claireaux AE: Familial haemophagocytic reticulosis. *Arch Dis Child* 27:519, 1952.
144. Henter JI, Elinder G, Soder O, Ost A: Incidence in Sweden and clinical features of familial hemophagocytic lymphohistiocytosis. *Acta Paediatr Scand* 80:428, 1991.
145. Allen CE, Yu X, Kozinetz CA, McClain KL: Highly elevated ferritin levels and the diagnosis of hemophagocytic lymphohistiocytosis. *Pediatr Blood Cancer* 50:1227, 2008.
146. Henter JI, Elinder G, Soder O, et al: Hypercytokinemia in familial hemophagocytic lymphohistiocytosis. *Blood* 78:2918, 1991.
147. Imashuku S, Hibi S, Sako M, et al: Heterogeneity of immune markers in hemophagocytic lymphohistiocytosis: Comparative study of 9 familial and 14 familial inheritance-unproved cases. *J Pediatr Hematol Oncol* 20:207, 1998.
148. Stepp SE, Dufourcq-Lagelouse R, Le DF, et al: Perforin gene defects in familial hemophagocytic lymphohistiocytosis. *Science* 286:1957, 1999.
149. Jordan MB, Hildeman D, Kappler J, Marrack P: An animal model of hemophagocytic lymphohistiocytosis (HLH): CD8+ T cells and interferon gamma are essential for the disorder. *Blood* 104:735, 2004.
150. Stepp SE, Mathew PA, Bennett M, et al: Perforin: More than just an effector molecule. *Immunol Today* 21:254, 2000.
151. Filipovich AH: Hemophagocytic lymphohistiocytosis and related disorders. *Curr Opin Allergy Clin Immunol* 6:410, 2006.
152. Menasche G, Pastural E, Feldmann J, et al: Mutations in RAB27A cause Griscelli syndrome associated with haemophagocytic syndrome. *Nat Genet* 25:173, 2000.
153. Arico M, Imashuku S, Clementi R, et al: Hemophagocytic lymphohistiocytosis due to germ line mutations in SH2D1A, the X-linked lymphoproliferative disease gene. *Blood* 97:1131, 2001.
154. Palazzi DL, McClain KL, Kaplan SL: Hemophagocytic syndrome in children: An important diagnostic consideration in fever of unknown origin. *Clin Infect Dis* 36:306, 2003.
155. Janka GE: Familial hemophagocytic lymphohistiocytosis. *Eur J Pediatr* 140:221, 1983.
156. Horne A, Trottestam H, Aricò M, et al: Frequency and spectrum of central nervous system involvement in 193 children with haemophagocytic lymphohistiocytosis. *Br J Haematol* 140:327, 2008.
157. Molleran Lee S, Villanueva J, Sumegi J, et al: Characterisation of diverse PRF1 mutations leading to decreased natural killer cell activity in North American families with haemophagocytic lymphohistiocytosis. *J Med Genet* 137, 2004.
158. Ueda I, Ishii E, Morimoto A, et al: Correlation between phenotypic heterogeneity and gene mutational characteristics in familial hemophagocytic lymphohistiocytosis (FHL). *Pediatr Blood Cancer* 46:482, 2006.
159. Bryceson YT, Rudd E, Zheng C, et al: Defective cytotoxic lymphocyte degranulation in syntaxin-11 deficient familial hemophagocytic lymphohistiocytosis 4 (FHL4) patients. *Blood* 110:1906, 2007.
160. Gupta A, Weitzman S, Abdelhaleem M: The role of hemophagocytosis in bone marrow aspirates in the diagnosis of hemophagocytic lymphohistiocytosis. *Pediatr Blood Cancer* 50:192, 2008.
161. Nagano M, Kimura N, Ishii E, et al: Clonal expansion of alphabeta-T lymphocytes with inverted Jbeta1 bias in familial hemophagocytic lymphohistiocytosis. *Blood* 94:2374, 1999.
162. Kogawa K, Lee SM, Villanueva J, et al: Perforin expression in cytotoxic lymphocytes from patients with hemophagocytic lymphohistiocytosis and their family members. *Blood* 99:61, 2002.
163. Ambruso DR, Hays T, Zwartjes WJ, et al: Successful treatment of lymphohistiocytic reticulosis with phagocytosis with epipodophyllotoxin VP 16–213. *Cancer* 45:2516, 1980.
164. Fischer A, Virelizier JL, Renzana-Seisdedos F, et al: Treatment of four patients with erythrophagocytic lymphohistiocytosis by a combination of epipodophyllotoxin, steroids, intrathecal methotrexate, and cranial irradiation. *Pediatrics* 76:263, 1985.
165. Henter JI, Samuelsson-Horne A, Arico M, et al: Treatment of hemophagocytic lymphohistiocytosis with HLH-94 immunochemotherapy and bone marrow transplantation. *Blood* 100:2367, 2002.
166. Henter JI, Horne A, Arico M, et al: HLH-2004: Diagnostic and therapeutic guidelines for hemophagocytic lymphohistiocytosis. *Pediatr Blood Cancer* 48:124, 2007.
167. Thompson PA, Allen CE, Horton T, et al: Severe neurologic side effects in patients being treated for hemophagocytic lymphohistiocytosis. *Pediatr Blood Cancer* 52:621, 2009.
168. Mahlaoui N, Ouachee-Chardin M, de Saint BG, et al: Immunotherapy of familial hemophagocytic lymphohistiocytosis with antithymocyte globulins: A single-center retrospective report of 38 patients. *Pediatrics* 120:e622, 2007.
169. Baker KS, Filipovich AH, Gross TG, et al: Unrelated donor hematopoietic cell transplantation for hemophagocytic lymphohistiocytosis. *Bone Marrow Transplant* 42:175, 2008.
170. Baker KS, DeLaat CA, Steinbuch M, et al: Successful correction of hemophagocytic lymphohistiocytosis with related or unrelated bone marrow transplantation. *Blood* 89:3857, 1997.
171. Cooper N, Rao K, Gilmour K, et al: Stem cell transplantation with reduced-intensity conditioning for hemophagocytic lymphohistiocytosis. *Blood* 107:1233, 2006.

172. Villanueva J, Lee S, Giannini EH, et al: Natural killer cell dysfunction is a distinguishing feature of systemic onset juvenile rheumatoid arthritis and macrophage activation syndrome. *Arthritis Res Ther* 7:R30, 2005.
173. Mouy R, Stephan JL, Pillet P, et al: Efficacy of cyclosporine A in the treatment of macrophage activation syndrome in juvenile arthritis: Report of five cases. *J Pediatr* 129:750, 1996.
174. Balamuth NJ, Nichols KE, Paessler M, Teachey DT: Use of rituximab in conjunction with immunosuppressive chemotherapy as a novel therapy for Epstein-Barr virus-associated hemophagocytic lymphohistiocytosis. *J Pediatr Hematol Oncol* 29:569, 2007.
175. Mischler M, Fleming GM, Shanley TP, et al: Epstein-Barr virus-induced hemophagocytic lymphohistiocytosis and X-linked lymphoproliferative disease: A mimicker of sepsis in the pediatric intensive care unit. *Pediatrics* 119:e1212, 2007.
176. Henzan T, Nagafuji K, Tsukamoto H, et al: Success with infliximab in treating refractory hemophagocytic lymphohistiocytosis. *Am J Hematol* 81:59, 2006.
177. Makay B, Yilmaz S, Turkyilmaz Z, et al: Etanercept for therapy-resistant macrophage activation syndrome. *Pediatr Blood Cancer* 50:419, 2008.
178. Rosai J, Dorfman RF: Sinus histiocytosis with massive lymphadenopathy. A newly recognized benign clinicopathological entity. *Arch Pathol* 87:63, 1969.
179. McClain, KL, Natkunam Y, Swerdlow *SH*: Atypical Cellular Disorders: an update. Hematology (Amer Soc Hematol Education Book), p283, 2004. An update.
180. Lauwers GY, Perez-Atayde A, Dorfman RF, Rosai J: The digestive system manifestations of Rosai-Dorfman disease (sinus histiocytosis with massive lymphadenopathy): Review of 11 cases. *Hum Pathol* 31:380, 2000.
181. Deodhare SS, Ang LC, Bilbao JM: Isolated intracranial involvement in Rosai-Dorfman disease: A report of two cases and review of the literature. *Arch Pathol Lab Med* 122:161, 1998.
182. Grabczynska SA, Toh CT, Francis N, et al: Rosai-Dorfman disease complicated by autoimmune haemolytic anaemia: Case report and review of a multisystem disease with cutaneous infiltrates. *Br J Dermatol* 145:323, 2001.
183. Jadus MR, Sekhon S, Barton BE, Wepsic HT: Macrophage colony stimulatory factor-activated bone marrow macrophages suppress lymphocytic responses through phagocytosis: A tentative in vitro model of Rosai-Dorfman disease. *J Leukoc Biol* 57:936, 1995.
184. Paulli M, Bergamaschi G, Tonon L, et al: Evidence for a polyclonal nature of the cell infiltrate in sinus histiocytosis with massive lymphadenopathy (Rosai-Dorfman disease). *Br J Haematol* 91:415, 1995.
185. Foucar E, Rosai J, Dorfman R: Sinus histiocytosis with massive lymphadenopathy (Rosai-Dorfman disease): Review of the entity. *Semin Diagn Pathol* 7:19, 1990.
186. Chow CP, Ho HK, Chan GC, et al: Congenital Rosai-Dorfman disease presenting with anemia, thrombocytopenia, and hepatomegaly. *Pediatr Blood Cancer* 52:415, 2009.
187. Sneller MC, Wang J, Dale JK, et al: Clinical, immunologic, and genetic features of an autoimmune lymphoproliferative syndrome associated with abnormal lymphocyte apoptosis. *Blood* 89:1341, 1997.
188. Govender D, Chetty R: Inflammatory pseudotumour and Rosai-Dorfman disease of soft tissue: A histological continuum? *J Clin Pathol* 50:79, 1997.
189. Pulsoni A, Anghel G, Falcucci P, et al. Treatment of sinus histiocytosis with massive lymphadenopathy (Rosai-Dorfman disease): Report of a case and literature review. *Am J Hematol* 69:67, 2002.
190. Horneff G, Jurgens H, Hort W, et al: Sinus histiocytosis with massive lymphadenopathy (Rosai-Dorfman disease): Response to methotrexate and mercaptopurine. *Med Pediatr Oncol* 27:187, 1996.
191. Stine KC, Westfall C: Sinus histiocytosis with massive lymphadenopathy (SHML) prednisone resistant but dexamethasone sensitive. *Pediatr Blood Cancer* 44:92, 2005.
192. Rodriguez-Galindo C, Helton KJ, Sanchez ND, et al: Extranodal Rosai-Dorfman disease in children. *J Pediatr Hematol Oncol* 26:19, 2004.
193. Perry R, Penk J, Kapoor N, Shah A: Vinorelbine and methotrexate for the treatment of Rosai-Dorfman Disease in children. *Pediatr Blood Cancer* 45:84–85, 2005.
194. Chester W: Uber lipoidgranulomatose [Over lipoid granulomatosis]. *Virchows Arch Pathol Anat Physiol* 279:561, 1930.
195. Jaffe HS: *Metabolic, Degenerative, and Inflammatory Diseases of Bones and Joints*. Lea and Febiger, Philadelphia, 1972.
196. Veyssier-Belot C, Cacoub P, Caparros-Lefebvre D, et al: Erdheim-Chester disease. Clinical and radiologic characteristics of 59 cases. *Medicine (Baltimore)* 75:157, 1996.
197. Al-Quran S, Reith J, Bradley J, Rimsza L: Erdheim-Chester disease: Case report, PCR-based analysis of clonality, and review of literature. *Mod Pathol* 15:666, 2002.
198. Loddenkemper K, Hoyer B, Loddenkemper C, et al: A case of Erdheim-Chester disease initially mistaken for Ormond's disease. *Nat Clin Pract Rheumatol* 4:50, 2008.
199. Chetritt J, Paradis V, Dargere D, et al: Chester-Erdheim disease: A neoplastic disorder. *Hum Pathol* 30:1093, 1999.
200. Taguchi T, Iwasaki Y, Asaba K, et al: Erdheim-Chester disease: Report of a case with PCR-based analysis of the expression of osteopontin and survivin in Xanthogranulomas following glucocorticoid treatment. *Endocr J* 55:217, 2008.
201. Stoppacciaro A, Ferrarini M, Salmaggi C, et al: Immunohistochemical evidence of a cytokine and chemokine network in three patients with Erdheim-Chester disease: Implications for pathogenesis. *Arthritis Rheum* 54:4018, 2006.
202. Caparros-Lefebvre D, Pruvo JP, et al: Neuroradiologic aspects of Chester-Erdheim disease. *AJNR Am J Neuroradiol* 16:735, 1995.
203. Dion E, Graef C, Haroche J, et al: Imaging of thoracoabdominal involvement in Erdheim-Chester disease. *AJR Am J Roentgenol* 183:1253, 2004.
204. Gupta A, Kelly B, McGuigan JE: Erdheim-Chester disease with prominent pericardial involvement: Clinical, radiologic, and histologic findings. *Am J Med Sci* 324:96, 2002.
205. Caputo R, Marzano AV, Passoni E, Berti E: Unusual variants of non-Langerhans cell histiocytoses. *J Am Acad Dermatol* 57:1031, 2007.
206. Braiteh F, Boxrud C, Esmaeli B, Kurzrock R: Successful treatment of Erdheim-Chester disease, a non-Langerhans-cell histiocytosis, with interferon-alpha. *Blood* 106:2992, 2005.
207. Haroche J, Amoura Z, Trad SG, et al: Variability in the efficacy of interferon-alpha in Erdheim-Chester disease by patient and site of involvement: Results in eight patients. *Arthritis Rheum* 54:3330, 2006.
208. Haroche J, Amoura Z, Charlotte F, et al: Imatinib mesylate for platelet-derived growth factor receptor-beta-positive Erdheim-Chester histiocytosis. *Blood* 111:5413, 2008.
209. Dehner LP: Juvenile xanthogranulomas in the first two decades of life: A clinicopathologic study of 174 cases with cutaneous and extracutaneous manifestations. *Am J Surg Pathol* 27:579, 2003.
210. Helwig EB, Hackney VC: Juvenile xanthogranuloma (nevoxanthoendothelioma). *Am J Pathol* 625, 1954.
211. Adamson HG: Society intelligence: The Dermatological Society of London. *Br J Dermatol* 17:222, 1905.
212. McDonagh JER: A contribution to our knowledge of the naevoxantho-endotheliomata. *Br J Dermatol* 24:85, 1912.
213. Janssen D, Harms D: Juvenile xanthogranuloma in childhood and adolescence: A clinicopathologic study of 129 patients from the Kiel pediatric tumor registry. *Am J Surg Pathol* 29:21, 2005.
214. Tan HH, Tay YK: Juvenile xanthogranuloma and neurofibromatosis 1. *Dermatology* 197:43, 1998.
215. Iyengar V, Golumb CA, Schachner L: Neurilemmomatosis, NF2, and juvenile xanthogranuloma. *J Am Acad Dermatol* 5 pt 2:831, 1998.
216. van Leeuwen RL, Berretty PJ, Knots E, Tan-Go I: Triad of juvenile xanthogranuloma, von Recklinghausen's neurofibromatosis and trisomy 21 in a young girl. *Clin Exp Dermatol* 21:248, 1996.
217. Zvulunov A, Barak Y, Metzker A: Juvenile xanthogranuloma, neurofibromatosis, and juvenile chronic myelogenous leukemia. World statistical analysis. *Arch Dermatol* 131:904, 1995.
218. Gutmann DH, Gurney JG, Shannon KM: Juvenile xanthogranuloma, neurofibromatosis 1, and juvenile chronic myeloid leukemia. *Arch Dermatol* 132:1390, 1996.
219. Freyer DR, Kennedy R, Bostrom BC, et al: Juvenile xanthogranuloma: Forms of systemic disease and their clinical implications. *J Pediatr* 129:227, 1996.
220. Stover DG, Alapati S, Regueira O, et al: Treatment of juvenile xanthogranuloma. *Pediatr Blood Cancer* 51:130, 2008.
221. Rajendra B, Duncan A, Parslew R, Pizer BL: Successful treatment of central nervous system juvenile xanthogranulomatosis with cladribine. *Pediatr Blood Cancer* 52:413, 2009.

CHAPTER 73
LIPID STORAGE DISEASES

Ari Zimran and Deborah Elstein

SUMMARY

Gaucher disease and Niemann-Pick disease are the two lipid storage disorders that are most likely to be encountered by the hematologist because both may cause hepatosplenomegaly and cytopenias.

Gaucher disease is the most common autosomal recessive lipid storage disorder. It is most prevalent in Ashkenazi Jews, in whom the disease genotype occurs in approximately 1 in 850 births. Deficiency of the enzyme *β*-glucocerebrosidase results in accumulation of the glycolipid glucocerebroside in the cells of the macrophage-monocyte system. Patients with the common type 1 disease have no primary neuronopathic symptoms, but there is involvement of the central nervous system in type 2 and type 3 diseases. Diagnosis of Gaucher disease depends on demonstration of deficiency of *β*-glucocerebrosidase or identification of mutations in the *β*-glucocerebrosidase gene. Disease manifestations include hepatosplenomegaly, thrombocytopenia, anemia, osteoporosis with pathologic fractures and osteonecrosis, and, less commonly, pulmonary infiltration. Many patients, especially those who are homozygous for the common N370S (1226C→G) mutation, are protected against neurologic involvement, probably because of some residual glucocerebrosidase activity, and may manifest a mild disease that does not require specific therapy. There has been some concern about an increased incidence of malignancies and parkinsonism in patients with type 1 disease. For patients who have more severe signs and symptoms, effective enzyme replacement therapy with imiglucerase is available. The glucocerebroside substrate reduction therapy is also available but may cause adverse events.

Niemann-Pick disease is a heterogeneous group of autosomal recessive disorders. Type A and type B result from deficiency of the enzyme sphingomyelinase, whereas type C results from mutations in the *NPC1* or *NPC2* genes that appear to be involved in cholesterol trafficking, and results in accumulation of cholesterol as well as sphingomyelin. Type A is a severe lethal infantile form of the disease with marked progressive neurologic involvement. Type B is a later-onset form of the disease with no neurologic involvement but with hepatosplenomegaly in many patients. Patients with type C disease manifest neurologic signs and hepatosplenomegaly and may survive into adulthood. The marrow of these patients contains typical foam cells with small droplets in the cytoplasm and sea-blue histiocytes. Miglustat therapy was approved for patients with type C disease in 2008 in Europe.

DEFINITIONS

The glycolipid storage diseases are hereditary disorders in which one or more tissues become engorged with specific lipids, because of deficiencies of specific lysosomal enzymes required for hydrolysis of one of the glycosidic bonds. Figure 73–1 shows the catabolic pathway of glycosphingolipids and lists the diseases that are involved in impaired degradation because of specific enzyme deficiencies. The type of lipid and its tissue distribution have a characteristic pattern in each disorder. This chapter deals mainly with Gaucher disease, in which glucocerebroside is stored. It is the most common lysosomal storage disorder and also the one with the most hematologic features. The second storage disorder with some hematologic features is Niemann-Pick disease, in which the accumulated material is sphingomyelin and/or cholesterol. The remaining lysosomal diseases in which there are no hematologic abnormalities, except for sometimes slight hepatosplenomegaly, are not reviewed in this chapter.

Acronyms and abbreviations that appear in this chapter include: cDNA, complementary DNA; ERT, enzyme replacement therapy; HSGP, horizontal supranuclear gaze palsy; MRI, magnetic resonance imaging; SRT, substrate reduction therapy.

GAUCHER DISEASE

HISTORY

Gaucher disease was first described by Philippe Gaucher in 1882, who thought that the peculiar large cells in the spleen were evidence of a primary neoplasm.[1] The term *Gaucher disease* appeared first in 1905, when the autosomal recessive genetic nature of the disorder was described.[2] In 1934, it was shown that glucocerebroside is the storage material,[3] and in 1965, the primary defect was recognized as the inability of the glucocerebrosidase to degrade glucocerebroside.[4,5] The purification of the enzyme ultimately led to the cloning of the gene in 1985,[6,7] elucidation of its structure, and identification of many mutations that cause the disease.[8] Enzyme replacement therapy (ERT) was introduced in 1991,[9] and glucocerebroside substrate reduction therapy (SRT) was introduced in 2002.

EPIDEMIOLOGY

Gaucher disease is inherited as an autosomal recessive disorder. Although pan ethnic, it is most common among the Ashkenazi Jews, with a carriership prevalence of 1 in 17 and an expected frequency of the disease of 1 in 850 births.[10] Two distinct forms of Gaucher disease are also relatively common in Norrbottnia in northern Sweden,[11] and near the Palestinian town of Jenin, respectively.[12] In the general population, the estimated frequency is in the range of 1:50,000 to 1:100,000.[13]

The high prevalence of more than one Gaucher mutation among Ashkenazi Jews, and the existence of other lysosomal diseases within this ethnic group may reflect in addition to a founder effect, a selective advantage. However, a selective advantage, because of greater resistance to tuberculosis,[14] superior intelligence,[15] or increased fertility[16] have not been proven. Animal studies suggest that the selective advantage may be the higher circulating serum levels of glucocerebroside that have antiinflammatory and beneficial immunomodulary effects.[17]

ETIOLOGY AND PATHOGENESIS

Enzymatic Basis

During normal growth, development, and senescence, parts of or whole cells are continually replaced. Breakdown of complex constituents of cells requires sequential enzymatic degradation. Such degradation occurs largely in secondary lysosomes, organelles formed by the fusion of primary lysosomes with phagocytic vacuoles containing ingested material.

Gaucher disease is the result of a hereditary deficiency in the activity of a lysosomal enzyme required for glycolipid degradation: glucocerebrosidase. The reduced activity of glucocerebrosidase results in accumulation of glucocerebroside (Fig. 73–1) in macrophages wherein storage induces increased size: These are the "Gaucher cells." Inherent in subsequent lysosomal dysfunction is disregulation of metabolites and consequent lack of coordination of cellular metabolism. These changes may explain elaboration of various cytokines and other biomarkers because of chronic storage.

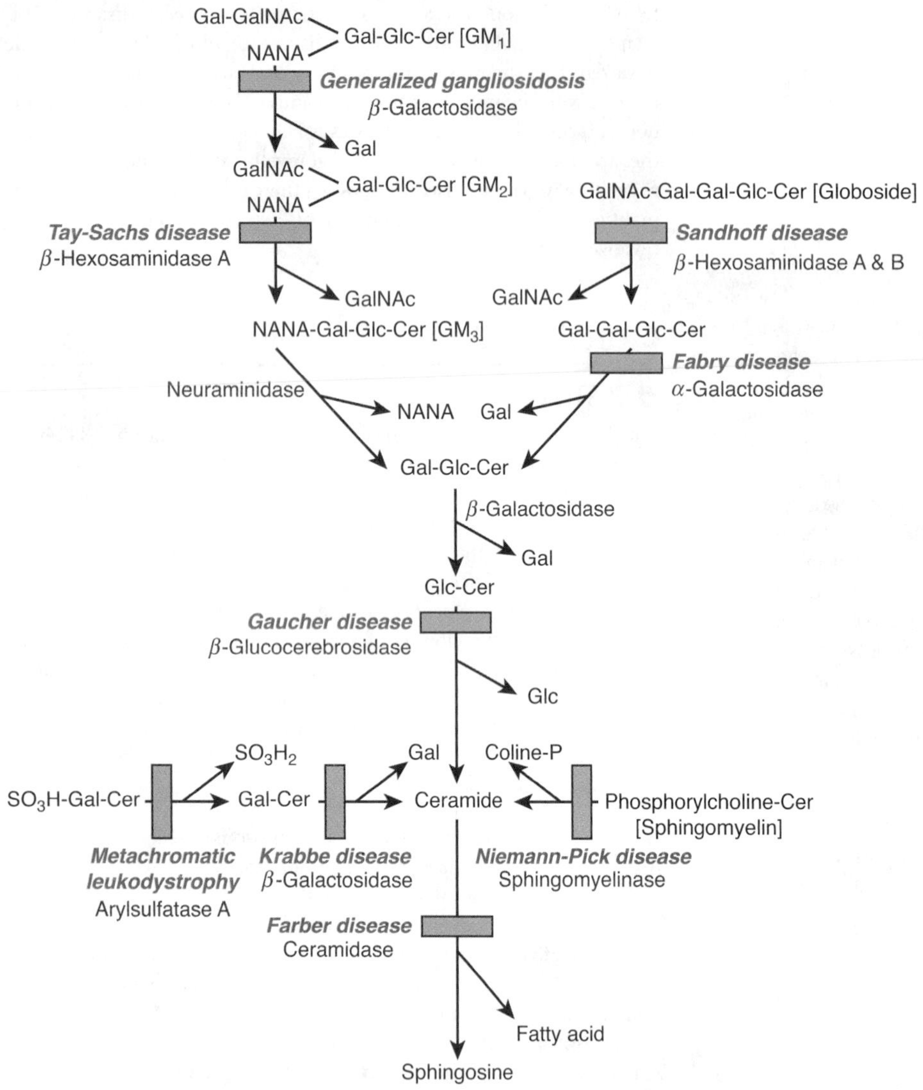

FIGURE 73–1. The catabolic pathways of selected glycosphingolipids involved in some of the glycolipid storage diseases. *Solid squares* depict the blocked pathways caused by specific inherited deficiencies of enzymes, which give rise to the accumulation of the respective substrates. The names of the various diseases are shown above the names of the deficient enzymes. *(Used with permission from* Lichtman's Atlas of Hematology, *www.accessmedicine.com.)*

In rare instances, severe forms of Gaucher disease have been associated with deficiency of saposin C, a heat-stable glucocerebrosidase cofactor.[18,19]

GENETIC BASIS OF GAUCHER DISEASE

The glucocerebrosidase gene is located on chromosome 1q21. A pseudogene, with 96 percent sequence homology, has been identified approximately 16 kb downstream from the functional gene. More than 300 mutations causing Gaucher disease have been described[8]; most are point mutations, missense, nonsense, frameshift, and splice-site mutations, but there are also insertions, deletions, and recombinant alleles. Some mutations result from recombinant events between the functional gene and its pseudogene.[8] An updated list of all published mutations was published in 2008.[20]

Among Ashkenazi Jews, the predominant mutation is at complementary DNA (cDNA) nucleotide 1226, causing an Asn370Ser substitution. This mutation accounts for approximately 75 percent of mutant alleles among Jewish patients and approximately 30 percent of the alleles among non-Jewish patients. Homozygosity for Asn370Ser is displayed by a relatively mild disease and some residual glucocerebrosidase activity that is considered "protective" against the development of neuronopathic features. The second common mutation found almost exclusively among Ashkenazi Jews is 84GG an insertion of a guanine at nucleotide 84 of the cDNA. This mutation creates a null allele that causes a more severe phenotype than the Asn370Ser mutation. Five or six common mutations account for approximately 97 percent of alleles among Jews, but for less than 75 percent of alleles among non-Jews.[8,21–23] Although controversial, premarital/prenatal screening for common mutations has become popular among Ashkenazi Jews.[24,25]

The common mutation observed in Norrbottnians is Leu444Pro, which also accounts for most patients with neuronopathic Gaucher disease and is prevalent in Asians and Arabs. Patients with the unique variant of progressive calcifications of cardiac valves are uniformly homozygous for the mutation at nucleotide 1342 (D409H).[12]

Despite some relationship between specific mutations and the clinical course, genotype–phenotype correlation is usually not good. The elucidation of the three-dimensional structure of the glucocerebrosidase by crystallography[26] has not improved prediction of disease severity based on location of mutations in the native protein.

Several mutations cause glucocerebrosidase misfolding, which may lead to early degradation of the enzyme in the endoplasmic reticulum.[27,28] The investigation of the proteotoxic effect of the misfolded mutant enzyme in the endoplasmic reticulum has led to the development of the new therapeutic modality of pharmacologic chaperones. Such chaperones are targeted to stabilize the mutated glucocerebrosidase and allow its appropriate trafficking from endoplasmic reticulum to Golgi and finally to the lysosome.

CLINICAL FEATURES

Three major types of Gaucher disease are differentiated clinically based on absence (type 1) or presence of neurologic features (types 2 and 3).[29] Table 73–1 summarizes key clinical, genetic, and demographic features. Although it has been suggested that there is a phenotypic continuum,[30,31] it is still useful to think of Gaucher disease as three distinct forms to facilitate genetic counseling and management decisions.

There is great variability in disease severity of all types of Gaucher disease. Type 1 disease may be asymptomatic and be discovered in the course of population surveys of Ashkenazi Jews,[24] or incidentally during evaluation of an unrelated hematologic disorder.

In symptomatic patients, the spleen is typically enlarged.[32] The spleen may be barely palpable or massively enlarged causing positional symptoms, such as early satiety or abdominal discomfort. Pain caused

TABLE 73–1. Features of the Different Types of Gaucher Disease

	Type 1		Type 2		Type 3		
Subtype	**Asymptomatic**	**Symptomatic**	**Neonatal**	**Infantile**	**3a**	**3b**	**3c**
Common genotype	N370S/N370S or two mild mutations	N370S/other or two mild mutations	Two null or recombinant mutations	One null and one severe mutations	None	L444P/L444P	D409H/D409H
Ethnic predilection	Ashkenazi Jews	Ashkenazi Jews	None	None	None	Norbottnians; Asians; Arabs	Palestinian Arabs, Japanese
Common presenting features	None	Hepatosplenomegaly; hypersplenism; bleeding bone pains	Hydrops fetalis; congenital ichthyosis	SNGP; strabismus opisthotonus; trismus	SNGP; myoclonic seizures	SNGP; hepatosplenomegaly growth retardation	SNGP; cardiac valves' calcifications
CNS involvement	Parkinsonism?	None	Lethal	Severe	SNGP; slowly progressive neurologic deterioration	SNGP; gradual cognitive deterioration	SNGP; brachycephalus
Bone involvement	None	Mild to severe (variable)	None	None	Mild	Moderate to severe; kyphosis (gibbus)	Minimal
Lung involvement	None	None to (rarely) severe	Severe	Severe	Mild to moderate	Moderate to severe	Minimal
Life Expectancy	Normal	Normal/near-normal	Neonatal death	Death before 2 years of age	Death during childhood	Death in mid-adulthood	Death in early adulthood

SNGP, supranuclear gaze palsy.

by splenic infarction or subcapsular hematoma is uncommon. Hepatomegaly, like splenomegaly, may cause positional symptoms, and in very severe cases, for example, in those who undergo splenectomy, liver fibrosis and/or cirrhosis with or without portal hypertension occur. In most patients, liver function tests are within normal limits unless there is a hepatic comorbidity such as viral or autoimmune hepatitis.[32]

Epistaxis, easy bruising, hemorrhage after surgical or dental procedures or bleeding during labor are common presenting symptoms. These manifestations usually are related to thrombocytopenia caused by hypersplenism or marrow replacement by Gaucher cells. Platelet dysfunctions and decreased levels of coagulation factors have been described.[33–35]

Fatigue is another common complaint, usually but not invariably related to anemia. Reduced hemoglobin levels are also primarily a result of hypersplenism, but additional causes include iron deficiency, vitamin B_{12} deficiency, and autoimmune hemolysis.[36,37]

An increased tendency to infections is uncommon, but can be present in splenectomized patients or severely affected patients, some of whom have defective neutrophil chemotaxis.[38,39] Bacterial osteomyelitis is most often iatrogenic following surgical intervention at the site of a bone crisis. In children, linear growth retardation is common regardless of disease severity.[40]

Severe pulmonary disease with cyanosis and clubbing occurs in some patients with advanced liver involvement. Infiltration of the lungs by Gaucher cells has been described.[41,42] Mild pulmonary hypertension is present in many patients, and splenectomized patients are particularly at risk for developing severe pulmonary hypertension.[43] Pulmonary function tests may reveal abnormalities, such as reduced diffusion capacity in approximately two-thirds of patients.[44]

Bone involvement can occur in any long bone.[45] Patchy areas of bone demineralization and infarction are seen (Fig. 73–2A), and widening of the distal femur known as "Erlenmeyer flask" deformity is very common (Fig. 73–2B). Bone metabolism markers indicate that bone resorption predominates,[46] but the mechanisms underlying development of bone lesions are poorly understood. Children may have delayed bone age and delayed eruption of the teeth.[47] Bone pain is probably the most troublesome symptom of Gaucher disease. Bone pain may be related to the pathologic processes evident by radiography, magnetic resonance imaging (MRI), and computerized tomography, or have the character of a "crisis" which is a self-limiting, albeit exquisitely painful event, associated with signs of acute local and/or systemic inflammation (Fig. 73–2D). Aseptic necrosis of femoral heads and vertebral collapse are particularly common (Fig. 73–2C,E), and constitute the most devastating complications.[29,48]

Gynecologic and obstetric problems are common, which may explain why females are more likely to be diagnosed. Delayed menarche, and menorrhagia are common, and increased risk of recurrent abortions has been reported.[49] Fertility is unaffected in males and females.

Organs other than the spleen, liver, bones, and lungs may be affected. Brownish masses of Gaucher cells can be found at the corneoscleral limbus of the eye giving rise to pinguecula and pterygium.[50] Uncommon ophthalmic features include uveitis and white preretinal spots.[51]

Renal manifestations are distinctly rare and limited to case reports of independently sorting kidney diseases; nonetheless, many patients seem to have benign urinary hyperfiltration.[52]

Neurologic symptoms constitute the hallmark of types 2 and 3 diseases. Particularly notable and pathognomonic are oculomotor abnormalities. Patients with type 2 disease can develop hypertonia of the neck muscles with extreme arching of the neck (opisthotonus), bulbar signs, limb rigidity, seizures, and sometimes choreoathetoid movements. Patients with type 3a disease exhibit progressive neurologic abnormalities such as myoclonus and dementia.[53] Patients with type 3b disease display aggressive visceral and skeletal involvement, and neurologic manifestations largely limited to horizontal supranuclear gaze palsy (HSGP).[53] Patients with type 3c disease exhibit HSGP, mild visceral involvement, and progressive calcifications of cardiac valves and great arteries[12,54–56]

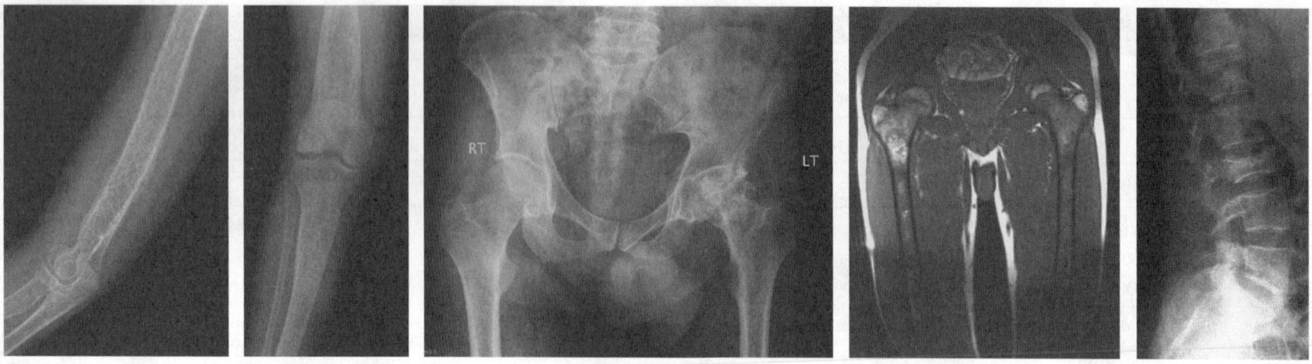

A B C D E

FIGURE 73–2. Gaucher-related skeletal involvement including **(A)** humerus with chevron or herring-bone pattern; **(B)** Erlenmeyer flask deformity of the proximal femur; **(C)** plain radiograph of osteonecrosis of the left hip; **(D)** MRI of pelvis and thighs performed 2 weeks after bone crisis of the right thigh. Bone edema is seen in the upper part of the femur at the level of lesser trochanter. Chronic marrow signal changes are seen in both femurs; **(E)** vertebral collapse. *(Courtesy of Dr. Ehud Lebel, Shaare Zedek Medical Center, Jerusalem, Israel.)*

Several neurologic abnormalities have been observed in patients with type 1 disease, including peripheral neuropathy[57,58] and an increased prevalence of parkinsonism among both patients and heterozygous carriers.[59–62] Carriers of mutations that cause severe disease in homozygotes have a 13.6-fold increased risk for Parkinson disease compared to controls, whereas carriers of the more benign mutations have a 2.2-fold increased risk.[63] A meta-analysis of patients with Parkinson disease has confirmed this strong association between glucocerebrosidase gene mutations and Parkinson disease.[62]

Neoplastic disorders, especially lymphoproliferative diseases, including myeloma, chronic lymphocytic leukemia, lymphoma, Hodgkin lymphoma, and essential monoclonal gammopathy are more prevalent in Gaucher disease than in the general population.[64–66] It was hypothesized that increased levels of interleukin-6 in patients with Gaucher disease link Gaucher disease with lymphoproliferative disorders.[67] A study of non-Jewish European patients revealed an increased incidence of hepatocellular carcinoma and malignant lymphomas.[68]

Local accumulation of Gaucher cells within parenchymatous organs such as liver, spleen, lymph nodes, or marrow, have been shown to develop into pseudotumors or "Gaucheromas" (Fig. 73–3).[69–72]

LABORATORY FEATURES

Blood Count

The complete blood count in patients with Gaucher disease may be normal or may reflect the effects of hypersplenism. A normocytic, normochromic anemia is frequently present, but hemoglobin levels only rarely fall below 8 g/dL. A modest reticulocytosis is often present in anemic patients. The white cell count may be decreased to as low as 1000/ μL, but milder degrees of leukopenia are common. The differential count is normal, yet splenectomized patients tend to show significant lymphocytosis. A defect of leukocyte chemotaxis corrected by enzyme replacement therapy has been reported[38,39]; in some patients this is associated with a tendency to bacterial infections. Thrombocytopenia is typically more prominent than anemia.[32] In an anemic nonsplenectomized patient without thrombocytopenia, there is probably another reason for the low hemoglobin level, which is unrelated to Gaucher disease. Thrombocytopenia may be quite severe, even in an otherwise mildly affected patient. In splenectomized patients, anemia is more likely in the absence of thrombocytopenia; white cell count and platelet counts are usually higher than normal. Severe anisocytosis and

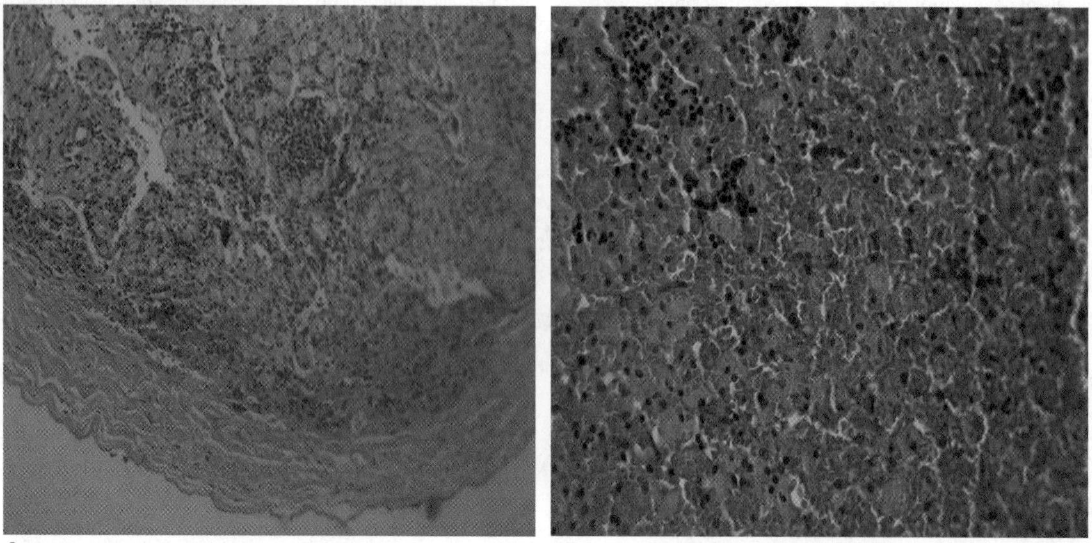

A B

FIGURE 73–3. A. Histologic section of "Gaucheroma" showing hemorrhagic mass with nucleated red blood cells covered by a fibrous capsule. **B.** Histologic section at a higher magnification showing nucleated red blood cells admixed with numerous Gaucher cells. *(Courtesy of Prof. Eliezer Rosenmann, Shaare Zedek Medical Center, Jerusalem, Israel.)*

poikilocytosis also occur in splenectomized patients, with many target cells, some nucleated red cells and Howell-Jolly bodies. During bone crises, leukocytosis, thrombocytosis, and elevated erythrocyte sedimentation are seen. Other markers of inflammation have been noted regardless of disease severity: elevated fibrinogen levels, elevated high-sensitivity C-reactive protein, and increased adhesion and aggregation of red blood cells.[73,74]

Other Hematologic Parameters

Clotting factor abnormalities may be induced by activated macrophages[34] or may be found when there is liver involvement. Factor IX deficiency may be a laboratory artifact related to the effect of accumulated lipid on platelet membranes.[75] Factor XI deficiency is common among Ashkenazi Jewish patients because of its high prevalence in this ethnic group.[76]

Bleeding tendency may also result from defective aggregation or adhesion of platelets,[33] and therefore platelet function should be tested before surgical and dental procedures and labor.[77,78]

Biochemistry and Immunology

A routine chemical test may be entirely normal. In conjunction with more severe disease, splenectomy, and/or comorbidities (hepatitic B and/or C, or autoimmune diseases) abnormal liver function tests may be seen. Because of the increased prevalence of cholelithiasis,[79–80] cholestatic findings may occur. Renal function tests are typically normal.[52]

Many patients present with polyclonal gammopathies. Monoclonal gammopathies are found in 1 to 20 percent of patients, particularly older patients, and are associated with the increased prevalence of myeloma.[66–68] Increased levels of autoantibodies have been reported,[81] and may indicate comorbidity with autoimmune diseases such as Hashimoto thyroiditis, rheumatoid arthritis, or hemolytic anemia.

Biochemical abnormalities have been used as surrogate markers in Gaucher disease. In the past, increased activities of serum acid phosphatase, angiotensin-converting enzyme, serum ferritin, and other hydrolases, such as β-hexosaminidase or β-glucuronidase, were used. Other biomarkers correlate better with the extent of glucocerebroside storage. The most widely used biomarker is chitotriosidase,[82] which is undetectable in healthy subjects (its physiologic role is unknown), but is elevated, often several thousands-fold, in patients with Gaucher disease. Chitotriosidase measurement is useful for monitoring both untreated patients, to assess stability *versus* deterioration, and treated patients, to assess response to therapy. A change in chitotriosidase levels rather than absolute values is used for monitoring. In approximately 6 percent of people, it is undetectable, and for those patients, measurements of CCL18 (chemokine [C-C motif] ligand 18), which is predominantly produced by Gaucher cells, can be used.[83]

Serum iron levels may be low in patients because of iron deficiency related to bleeding or chronic inflammation. Deficiencies of vitamin B_{12} and vitamin D have been described.[84,85]

Gaucher Cells

Gaucher cells, found mainly in the marrow, spleen, and liver (Fig. 73–4), have small, usually eccentrically placed nuclei and cytoplasm with characteristic crinkles or striations. The cytoplasm is stained by the periodic acid-Schiff technique. Electron microscopy features cytoplasm containing spindle- or rod-shaped, membrane-bound inclusion bodies 0.6 to 4 μm in diameter, consisting of numerous small tubules, 130 to 750 Å in diameter, that are composed of twisted multilayers in negatively stained preparations.[86]

DIFFERENTIAL DIAGNOSIS

Diagnosis

The diagnosis of Gaucher disease should be considered in any patient who presents with the clinical features and long-standing splenomegaly, in children with acute or chronic bone pain, splenomegaly, thrombocytopenia, frequent nosebleeds, height retardation, and persons with nontraumatic avascular necrosis of a large joint at any age.

The definitive and gold standard for diagnosis is reduced enzymatic activity of glucocerebrosidase in leukocytes,[87,88] cultured fibroblasts,[64] or amniocytes obtained during prenatal diagnosis. Measurement of glucocerebrosidase is supplemented by mutations analysis. This is important for prognosis particularly in children, and for detection of carriers among affected families. While rapid polymerase chain reaction-based tests are often performed for five or seven common mutations, especially among Ashkenazi Jews as a "first-pass," it is highly recommended to perform whole-gene sequencing to rigorously establish the molecular diagnosis.[8]

Marrow aspiration as a means of diagnosis is only indicated when other hematologic diseases must be ruled out.[89] Gaucher cells are often sparse and thorough examination under low power may be required to find them. Cells indistinguishable by light microscopy from typical Gaucher cells also are seen in patients with chronic myelogenous leukemia, Hodgkin disease, myeloma, and AIDS. The latter patients do not lack the ability to catabolize glucocerebroside, but the great inflow of globoside into phagocytic cells exceeds their capacity to hydrolyze glucocerebroside, forming "pseudo-Gaucher cells."

Prenatal diagnosis can be established by examining cultured amniocytes obtained by amniocentesis for measurement of glucocerebrosidase activity[87] or by examining DNA of amniocytes or chorionic villi DNA for known mutations. Measurement of informative biomarkers may confirm the diagnosis.

Heterozygote Detection

Heterozygotes for Gaucher disease have neither Gaucher cells in their marrow nor stigmata of Gaucher disease. Existence of a carrier state can be demonstrated by reduced glucocerebrosidase activity to approximately 50 percent of normal values. However, regardless of methodology, enzyme activity among heterozygotes overlaps the normal range and hence definitive diagnosis of heterozygous status only can be made by mutation analysis.

THERAPY

Symptomatic Treatment

Symptoms and signs related to massive enlargement of the spleen (e.g., pancytopenia, early satiety, abdominal discomfort, and growth retardation in children) can be resolved by splenectomy. However, because of the efficacy of enzyme therapy, splenectomy should only be a last resort, because it often induces progressive liver and bony complications, and increases the risk of infection with encapsulated organisms. Partial splenectomy has not proved useful.[90]

When bone lesions result in fractures or osteonecrosis (see Fig. 73–2D), orthopedic procedures may be required. Joint replacement is generally uneventful, with good functional outcome and quality of life. The success of arthroplasties is enhanced by adherence to preoperative protocols including assessment of bleeding tendency, prophylactic use of antibiotic therapy, particularly in splenectomized patients, and early postoperative ambulation.[91]

Deficiencies of iron, vitamin B_{12}, or vitamin D should be corrected and calcium supplementation is recommended in patients with

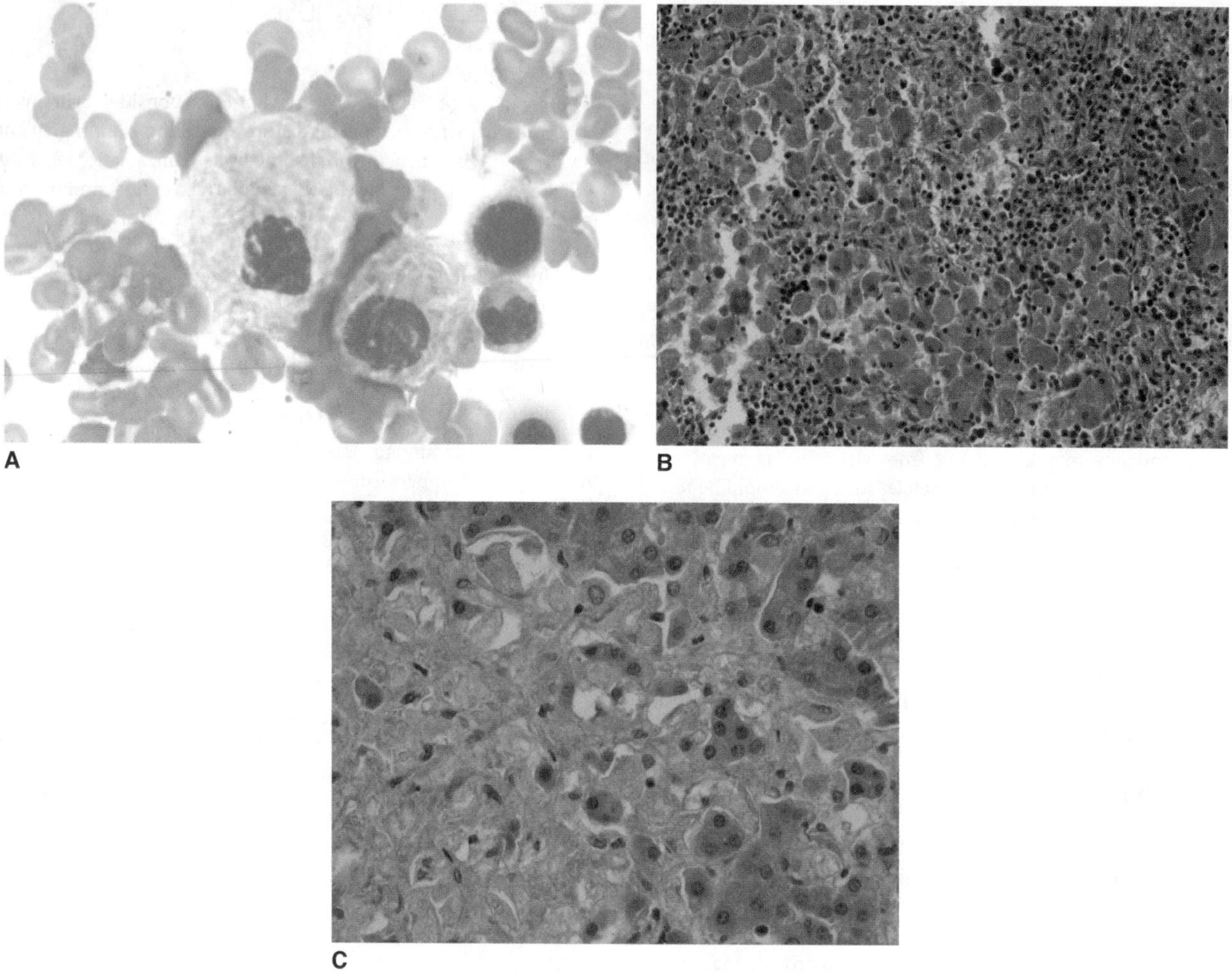

FIGURE 73–4. **A.** "Gaucher cell" from the marrow of a patient with Gaucher disease. **B.** Histomicrograph of a Gaucher spleen with marked infiltration of the red pulp by Gaucher cells. **C.** Liver infiltrated by Gaucher cells (the pale pink cells). *(Marrow picture courtesy of Prof. Chaim Hershko, Shaare Zedek Medical Center, Jerusalem, Israel; spleen and liver pictures courtesy of Prof. Gail Amir, Hadassah Medical Center, Jerusalem, Israel.)*

osteoporosis receiving bisphosphonates.[92] Use of erythropoietin may be required for therapy of anemia because of marrow failure.[93]

Enzyme Replacement Therapy

ERT for Gaucher disease has been attempted intermittently since the middle 1970s but was not successful until sugars were removed from the preparation thereby exposing inner mannose residues. This facilitated targeting of the enzyme to macrophages via mannose receptors.[9] The use of alglucerase (Ceredase),[9] the first mannose-terminated, placental-derived enzyme, was approved in 1991, and the recombinant form, imiglucerase (Cerezyme), was introduced in 1994.[94] In 2009, two enzymatic preparations, one with the perfect native-enzyme sequence and the other, a plant-derived preparation, completed phase 3 clinical trials.[95,96]

The response to enzyme replacement therapy is most gratifying.[9,94,97–100] Decreased spleen and liver volumes and increased hemoglobin levels and platelet counts usually occur within 6 months of therapy with biweekly doses between 15 and 60 U/kg. Platelet counts in patients with massively enlarged spleens may require longer periods to respond, but dramatic improvements continue within the first 2 years of therapy. Thereafter, regardless of dosage, responsiveness of all major disease features and surrogate markers plateau and most patients achieve stabilization even while continuing therapy with the same regimen.

The bone response is slower and less predictable. The best outcome in bones is when therapy is administered prior to onset of irreversible complications, because osteonecrosis and lytic lesions do not respond to enzyme replacement therapy. Various imaging modalities, especially MRI based, are used to document the skeletal status. Quantitative chemical shift imaging is the most sensitive modality to show changes in the marrow, and can demonstrate change in status as with enzyme therapy (Fig. 73–5),[101] but it is a scarce resource.

Enzyme replacement therapy may or may not improve the pulmonary pathologic findings. Because the enzyme used is a large molecule, it does not cross the blood–brain barrier, and hence, it cannot improve neuronopathic features.[102,103] Imiglucerase is safe with few side effects that are usually transient.[104] Hypersensitivity reactions are few (in 6.5% of patients according to the package insert), with rare cases of anaphylaxis. However, most patients who had such reactions can continue therapy with or without administration of glucocorticoids and antihistaminic drugs. Up to 15 percent of treated patients may develop non-neutralizing antibodies within 2 years of treatment. Another side effect is weight gain. Because of the excellent safety profile, many patients receive therapy at home,[105] and many female patients are comfortable continuing with imiglucerase during pregnancy and lactation.[106] The two major disadvantages of imiglucerase are the apparent lifetime dependency on intravenous infusions and its extremely high cost.

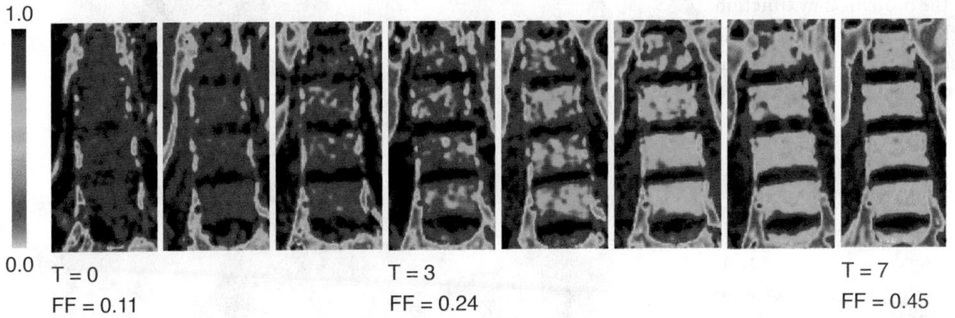

FIGURE 73–5. Color-coded fat fraction measurements using quantitative chemical shift imaging in an adult patient with type 1 Gaucher disease. Annual measurements show increase in fat fraction with specific therapy (mean value in 1994 = 0.11; mean value in 2001 = 0.45). *(Courtesy of Dr. Mario Maas, Academic Medical Center, Amsterdam, The Netherlands.)*

Guidelines and/or expert opinions recommend the use of relatively high doses.[107–110] Yet, it is evident that for most symptomatic patients, there is no justification for doses higher than 30 U/kg per month, and for patients with asymptomatic type 1 disease, enzyme replacement therapy should not be encouraged.[111]

Substrate Reduction Therapy

The amount of glucocerebroside that accumulates in macrophages represents the balance achieved between the rate of synthesis and the rate of degradation. The possibility that decreasing the formation of glucocerebroside from ceramide and glucose might favorably affect the disease was proposed in the 1970s.[112] Among a number of potential inhibitors of glucocerebroside synthase, only miglustat (*N*-butyldeoxynojirimycin, Zavesca) has been licensed for treatment of patients for whom enzyme therapy is not suitable or not a therapeutic option according to the European Medicines Agency and the U.S. Food and Drug Administration definitions, respectively. This circumscribed approval stems from the inferior efficacy of miglustat in comparison with enzyme replacement therapy and a problematic safety profile. Inhibiting glucocerebroside synthesis is referred to as "substrate reduction therapy."[113] Miglustat is effective in reducing hepatosplenomegaly in patients with Gaucher disease when given orally at a starting dose of 100 mg three times daily.[114] Response to miglustat is dose-dependent; lower doses, 50 mg three times daily yield suboptimal improvement without reducing the frequency of side effects.[115] Miglustat has also been studied as maintenance therapy in patients previously treated with imiglucerase.[115] The convenience of oral treatment is undeniable, but there are nontrivial side effects ascribed to miglustat, including peripheral neuropathies, tremor, and memory impairment. A ceramide analogue is currently undergoing clinical trials but unlike miglustat, it cannot cross the blood-brain barrier.

Pharmacologic Chaperones

A new approach to lysosomal storage diseases is "chaperone therapy." This treatment modality is based on *in vitro* experiments showing that some misfolded mutants of glucocerebrosidase are destroyed prior to their export from the endoplasmic reticulum to the lysosome.[116,117] Under these circumstances, a reversible inhibitor was predicted to stabilize the mutant enzyme, enabling its passage to the lysosome without loosing activity. At the time of this writing, two molecules are undergoing clinical testing: isofagomine and ambroxol.

Organ Transplantation

Because the macrophage is a descendant of hematopoietic stem cells, allogeneic marrow transplantation might be expected to cure Gaucher disease.[118] Although some enthusiasm was expressed for this approach, the considerable short-term risk of marrow transplantation markedly limit the number of suitable candidates. The availability of effective enzyme replacement therapy further limits the appropriateness of marrow transplantation. Liver transplantation has been performed in a few patients with severe hepatic failure.

■ COURSE AND PROGNOSIS

Age of onset, severity of clinical manifestations, and degree of progression are partially related to genotype. Patients homozygous for the N370S mutation tend to present with symptoms and signs at an older age with relatively milder manifestations, and usually have a relatively stable disease. By contrast, compound heterozygotes for N370S and a "severe" mutation (N370S/84GG or N370S/L444P) present with the disease during childhood, and if untreated, progress gradually and commonly develop skeletal complications.[91,119–121] Patients homozygous for the L444P mutation develop type 3 disease with neurologic signs and symptoms.

Although the genotype of the patient provides a benchmark for prognosis, there is much variability in patients with the same genotype, including siblings. The availability of ERT has changed the natural course of the disease allowing normal growth and development in most patients, even in those with "severe" genotypes. Nevertheless, some patients still develop skeletal complications despite ERT and there is concern regarding development of associated comorbidities, such as myeloma and parkinsonism.[120]

Prior to the availability of ERT, patients with severe type 1 or type 3, died at an early age because of liver disease, bleeding, or sepsis. With the advent of enzyme therapy, typical causes of death are malignancy, cardiovascular disease, and cerebrovascular disease.[122] In type 2 disease, death usually results from neurologic complications and occurs within the first 4 years of life; there is also a lethal neonatal variant. Total absence of glucocerebrosidase may not be compatible with life. This notion is supported by the absence of homozygous 84GG patients albeit a relative high incidence of 84GG in Ashkenazi Jews.

NIEMANN-PICK DISEASE

■ HISTORY AND CLASSIFICATION

In 1914, Niemann, a Berlin pediatrician, reported the case of an infant who died at age 18 months with a disorder that seemed atypical for Gaucher disease because of its early onset and rapid course.[123] In 1927, Pick identified this as a unique disorder of rapid, progressive neurodegeneration of infants.[124] The first adults identified had massive hepatosplenomegaly but no neurologic involvement. The predominant phospholipid accumulating in this disorder is sphingomyelin. In 1966, a deficiency of sphingomyelinase activity was demonstrated in a patient with Niemann-Pick disease.[125] Niemann-Pick is not a single entity; it comprises a group of disorders in which sphingomyelin storage occurs. Type A and type B disease, the classic forms of the disorder, represent an infantile neuronopathic and a later-onset nonneuronopathic form, respectively.[126] Type C, the most common form of Niemann-Pick disease, is a neuronopathic disorder, usually with an onset in early childhood, that results from an abnormality in cholesterol transport.[127] The sphingomyelinase gene is normal in type C disease, but mutations occur in one of two genes, which have been designated *NPC1* and *NPC2;* the proteins may function in closely related steps of cholesterol transport. The designation type D disease was once applied to a population isolate in Nova Scotia,[128] but because these individuals also had a *NPC1* mutation, this term is no longer used.

EPIDEMIOLOGY

Niemann-Pick type A and type B diseases, also referred to as acid-sphingomyelinase deficiency, are pan-ethnic disorders. There is a relatively high prevalence of type A disease among Ashkenazi Jewish ancestry with a carrier rate of approximately 1:90.[129] Three mutations account for 90 percent of Ashkenazi Jewish patients. Type B is common among individuals from the Mahgreb region and the Arabian peninsula[130] with three and two mutations accounting for 75 percent and 85 percent of Turkish and Arabic patients, respectively. The type C disease is relatively common in a Nova Scotia isolate,[128] in a Hispanic population from the Upper Rio Grande Valley in the United States,[131] and in Western Europe.[132] The prevalence of Niemann-Pick type C disease in European populations is estimated to be 1:120,000 to 150,000.[133]

ETIOLOGY AND PATHOGENESIS

Type A and type B are autosomal recessive diseases caused by loss of function mutations of the gene for sphingomyelinase,[134] which is required for cleaving the bond between ceramide and phosphorylcholine (see Fig. 73–1). Nonsense mutations seem to cause the more severe type A disease, while missense mutations are found in the milder type B disorder.[134] Although sphingomyelinase is believed to be a part of an apoptosis-signaling pathway by generating ceramide from sphingomyelin,[135] no relationship between severity of disease manifestations and this pathway has been established.

Type C disease also is an autosomal recessive disorder and is caused by mutations in either the *NPC1*[136,137] or *NPC2*[137] gene. The function of the proteins encoded by these genes is unknown, but was suggested to be related to intracellular cholesterol transport.[137,138] The *NPC1* gene encodes for a multipass transmembrane protein that localizes to the late endosome. The *NPC2* protein is soluble. The *NPC1* mutations account for more than 95 percent of cases.[138] There are only a few cases of *NPC2* mutations that cause a disease manifested in neonates by severe liver and lung involvement and progressive neurologic involvement leading to death at 4 years of age, and there is a juvenile form in which there seems to be good genotype–phenotype correlation.[139] *NPC1* deficiency is associated with induction of autophagy via the class III-P13K/beclin-1 complex.[140] A naturally occurring murine model of the disease exists.[141]

PATHOLOGY AND CLINICAL MANIFESTATIONS

The most characteristic histopathologic feature of the various forms of Niemann-Pick disease is the presence of foam histiocytes (Fig. 73–6). These cells are found mainly in lymphoid tissues, but they may be present throughout the body. The foam cells contain largely sphingomyelin and cholesterol, the storage of cholesterol being more prominent in type C disease.

Type A Niemann-Pick disease presents in infancy. During the first months of life, affected infants gain weight at a diminished rate, the abdomen enlarges, and development is delayed. The patients usually cannot sit and lose physical capabilities already achieved. They may become blind and deaf. Some infants have a protracted course of jaundice of unknown cause. During the second year of life, the child lies still with nearly flaccid hyporeflexic extremities, the abdomen is enlarged with enormous sizes of the spleen and liver, mild lymphadenopathy, and often a fine xanthomatous rash. Bone lesions may occur.

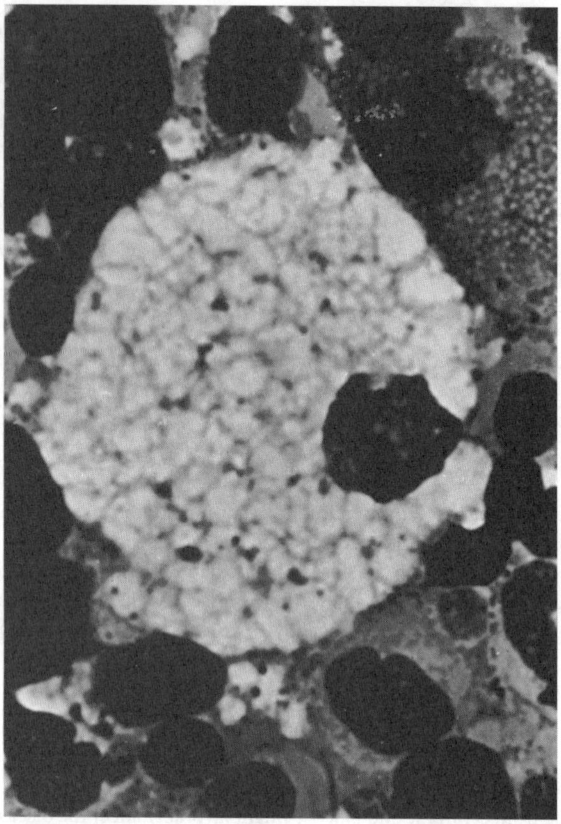

FIGURE 73–6. Typical foam cell from the marrow of a patient with Niemann-Pick disease.

Patients with type B disease usually present in the first decade of life with hepatosplenomegaly, but may not be noted until adult life. Neurologic manifestations are usually absent. Pulmonary infiltrates are common. The absence of a cherry-red spot in the macula and longer life expectancy differentiate type B from type A. Sea-blue histiocytes are sometimes found in the marrow, and a number of patients had been diagnosed as having sea-blue histiocytosis before a deficiency in sphingomyelinase was demonstrated.[142]

Patients with type C disease often have neonatal jaundice, develop normally in early childhood, and then develop dementia, ataxia, dysarthria, dystonia, seizures, and a specific pattern of neurocognitive deficits.[143] Hepatosplenomegaly is commonly observed.[126] This form of the disease can present at any age, even in the seventh decade,[143] but the "classic" description is of juvenile dystonic lipidosis with neonatal icterus and hepatosplenomegaly. In infants and toddlers, hepatosplenomegaly may be the only sign of the disease. In patients with a later-onset, there are variable presentations, but psychiatric signs and symptoms predominate.[143]

LABORATORY FEATURES AND DIFFERENTIAL DIAGNOSIS

Hemoglobin values may be normal, or mild anemia may be present. Approximately 75 percent of the blood lymphocytes contain 1 to 9 vacuoles with a diameter of 2 μm. Electron microscopy reveals that these vacuoles are lipid-filled lysosomes.[144] The marrow contains typical foam cells whose diameter ranges between 20 to 100 μm. Small droplets are scattered throughout the cytoplasm (see Fig. 73–6). The cytoplasm of these cells stains only very faintly with the periodic acid-Schiff reagent. Phase microscopy of unstained preparations clearly reveals droplets in the cytoplasm of Niemann-Pick foam cells that distinguish them from Gaucher cells. The occurrence of sea-blue histiocytes in the spleen and marrow has been documented.[135,141]

Type A and type B Niemann-Pick disease can be distinguished from other disorders by identification of the lipid as sphingomyelin and by demonstration of sphingomyelinase deficiency in leukocytes or cultured fibroblasts.[145,146] Patients with type A disease have acid sphingomyelinase activity levels less than 5 percent of normal in *in vitro* cultures of lymphoblasts or fibroblasts. In type B disease, acid sphingomyelinase activity levels range between 2 and 10 percent of normal levels. Monospecific antibodies against sphingomyelinase are used to differentiate between type A and type B disease. Heterozygotes may be detected by measurement of sphingomyelinase activity of cultured fibroblasts.[146] For patients with type C disease, the presence of foam cells is the only indication of the disease.

Prenatal diagnosis of the 3 types of the disease has been carried out but is difficult in type C disease.[147]

TREATMENT

There is no effective treatment for Niemann-Pick disease. Cholesterol-lowering diets for type C disease have shown no clear benefit. Splenectomy is only rarely required, because death usually occurs from other manifestations of the disease before hypersplenism becomes clinically important. Liver transplantation in type A disease corrects hepatic pathology but has little long-term benefit[148]; similarly, marrow transplantation does not ameliorate the neurologic deterioration in type B disease,[149] nor does it affect the course of type C disease.[150] Somatic cell gene therapy has been attempted in knockout type B mice,[151] and was effective in ameliorating visceral signs but had no effect on neurologic signs.

Substrate reduction therapy was attempted in a patient with Niemann-Pick type C disease.[152] Depletion of glycosphingolipids by miglustat despite having no direct effect on cholesterol metabolism, corrected abnormal lipid trafficking[153] and implied that glycosphingolipid accumulation is a primary pathogenetic event in type C disease.

A clinical trial using miglustat at a dose of 200 mg three times daily in an open-label 12-month trial with extension to 66 months in juvenile and adult patients with Niemann-Pick type C disease and in some children, showed improvement or stabilization.[153]

COURSE AND PROGNOSIS

The prognosis in type A Niemann-Pick disease is very poor; death nearly always occurs before the third year of life. Patients with type B disease may survive into childhood or adult life. Patients with type C disease usually die in the second decade of life, but some patients with mild disease have a normal life span. New hope for adults and children with type C disease emanates from the approval of miglustat by the European Union for the treatment of affected patients (see www.emea.europa.eu/pdfs/human/opinion/Zavesca_33596508en.pdf).

REFERENCES

1. Gaucher PCE: *De L'epithelioma Primitif de la Rate, Hypertrophie Idiopathique del la Rate San Leucemie*. University of Paris, Paris, 1882.
2. Brill N, Mandelbaum F, Libman E: Primary splenomegaly-Gaucher type. Report on one of four cases occurring in a single generation in a family. *Am J Med Sci* 129:491, 1905.
3. Aghion H: *La maladie de Gaucher dans l'enfance* [PhD thesis]. Paris, 1934.
4. Brady RO, Kanfer JN, Shapiro D: Metabolism of glucocerebrosides: II. Evidence of an enzymatic deficiency in Gaucher's disease. *Biochem Biophys Res Commun* 18:221, 1965.
5. Patrick AD: Short communications: A deficiency of glucocerebrosidase in Gaucher's disease. *Biochem J* 97:17C, 1965.
6. Sorge J, West C, Westwood B, Beutler ED: Molecular cloning and nucleotide sequence of human glucocerebrosidase cDNA. *Proc Natl Acad Sci U S A* 82:7289, 1985.
7. Horowitz M, Wilder S, Horowitz Z, et al: The human glucocerebrosidase gene and pseudogene: Structure and evolution. *Genomics* 4:87, 1989.
8. Hruska KS, LaMarca ME, Sidransky E: Gaucher disease: Molecular biology and genotype-phenotype correlations, in *Gaucher Disease*, edited by AH Futerman, A Zimran, p 13. CRC Press, Boca Raton, FL, 2007.
9. Barton NW, Brady RO, Dambrosia JM, et al: Replacement therapy for inherited enzyme deficiency—Macrophage-targeted glucocerebrosidase for Gaucher's disease. *N Engl J Med* 324:1464, 1991.
10. Beutler E, Nguyen NJ, Henneberger MW, et al: Gaucher disease: Gene frequencies in the Ashkenazi Jewish population. *Am J Hum Genet* 52:85, 1993.
11. Svennerholm L, Erikson A, Groth CG, et al: Norrbottnian type of Gaucher disease—Clinical, biochemical and molecular biology aspects: Successful treatment with bone marrow transplantation. *Dev Neurosci* 13:345, 1991.
12. Abrahamov A, Elstein D, Gross-Tsur V, et al: Gaucher's disease variant characterized by progressive calcification of heart valves and unique genotype. *Lancet* 346:1000, 1995.
13. Meikle PJ, Fuller M, Hopwood JJ: Gaucher Disease: Epidemiology and screening policy, in *Gaucher Disease*, edited by AH Futerman, A Zimran, p 321. CRC Press, Boca Raton, FL, 2007.
14. Kannai R, Elstein D, Weiler-Razell D, Zimran A: The selective advantage of Gaucher's disease: TB or not TB? *Isr Med Assoc J* 30:911, 1994.
15. Cochran G, Hardy J, Harpending H: Natural history of Ashkenazi intelligence. *J Biosoc Sci* 38:659, 2006.
16. Sprecher-Levy H, Orr-Urtreger A, Lonai P, Horowitz M: Murine prosaposin: Expression in the reproductive system of a gene implicated in human genetic diseases. *Cell Mol Biol* 39:287, 1993.
17. Zimran A, Ilan Y, Elstein D: Enzyme replacement therapy for mild patients with Gaucher disease. *Am J Hematol* 84:202, 2009.
18. Schnabel D, Schröder M, Sandhoff K: Mutation in the sphingolipid activator protein 2 in a patient with a variant of Gaucher disease. *FEBS Lett* 284:57, 1991.
19. Tylki-Szymaska A, Czartoryska B, Vanier MT, et al: Non-neuronopathic Gaucher disease due to saposin C deficiency. *Clin Genet* 72:538, 2007.
20. Hruska KS, LaMarca ME, Scott CR, Sidransky E: Gaucher disease: Mutations and polymorphism spectrum in the glucocerebrosidase gene (GBA). *Hum Mutat* 29:567, 2008.
21. Beutler E, Gelbart T, Kuhl W, et al: Mutations in Jewish patients with Gaucher disease. *Blood* 79:1662, 1992.
22. Beutler E, Gelbart T: Gaucher disease mutations in non-Jewish patients. *Br J Haematol* 85:401, 1993.
23. Horowitz M, Pasmanik-Chor M, Borochowitz Z, et al: Prevalence of glucocerebrosidase mutations in the Israeli Ashkenazi Jewish population. *Hum Mutat* 12:240, 1998.
24. Zuckerman S, Lahad A, Shmueli A, et al: Carrier screening for Gaucher disease: Lessons for low-penetrance, treatable diseases. *JAMA* 298:1281, 2007.
25. Beutler E: Carrier screening for Gaucher disease: More harm than good? *JAMA* 298:1329, 2007.
26. Dvir H, Harel M, McCarthy AA, et al: X-ray structure of human acid-beta-glucosidase, the defective enzyme in Gaucher disease. *EMBO Rep* 4:704, 2003.
27. Sawkar AR, Adamski-Werner SL, Cheng WC, et al: Gaucher disease-associated glucocerebrosidases show mutation-dependent chemical chaperoning profiles. *Chem Biol* 12:1235, 2005.
28. Ron I, Horowitz M: ER retention and degradation as the molecular basis underlying Gaucher disease heterogeneity. *Hum Mol Genet* 15:2387, 2005.
29. Beutler E, Grabowski G: Gaucher disease, in *The Metabolic and Molecular Bases of Inherited Disease*, edited by CR Scriver, AL Beaudet, WS Sly, D Valle, p 3635. McGraw-Hill, New York, 2001.
30. Sidransky E: Gaucher disease: Complexity in a "simple" disorder. *Mol Genet Metab* 83:6, 2004.
31. Chérin P, Sedel F, Mignot C, Schupbach M, et al: Neurological manifestations of type 1 Gaucher's disease: Is a revision of disease classification needed? *Rev Neurol (Paris)* 162:1076, 2006.
32. Elstein D, Abrahamov A, Hadas-Halpern I, Zimran A: Gaucher's disease. *Lancet* 358:324, 2001.
33. Gillis S, Hyam E, Abrahamov A, et al: Platelet function abnormalities in Gaucher disease patients. *Am J Hematol* 61:103, 1999.
34. Hollak CE, Levi M, Berends F, et al: Coagulation abnormalities in type 1 Gaucher disease are due to low-grade activation and can be partly restored by enzyme supplementation therapy. *Br J Haematol* 96:470, 1997.
35. Aerts JM, Hollak CE: Plasma and metabolic abnormalities in Gaucher's disease. *Baillieres Clin Haematol* 10:691, 1997
36. Zimran A, Altarescu G, Rudensky B, et al: Survey of hematological aspects of Gaucher disease. *Hematology* 10:151, 2005.
37. Hughes D, Cappellini MD, Berger M, et al: Recommendations for the management of the haematological and onco-haematological aspects of Gaucher disease. *Br J Haematol* 138:676, 2007.
38. Aker M, Zimran A, Abrahamov A, et al: Abnormal neutrophil chemotaxis in Gaucher disease. *Br J Haematol* 83:187, 1993.
39. Zimran A, Abrahamov A, Aker M, et al: Correction of neutrophil chemotaxis defect in patients with Gaucher disease by low-dose enzyme replacement therapy. *Am J Hematol* 43:69, 1993.

40. Zevin S, Abrahamov A, Hadas-Halpern I, et al: Adult-type Gaucher disease in children: Genetics, clinical features and enzyme replacement therapy. *Q J Med* 86:565, 1993.
41. Lee RE: The pathology of Gaucher disease, in *Gaucher Disease: A Century of Delineation and Research*, edited by RJ Desnick, S Gatt, GA Grabowski, p 177. Alan R. Liss, New York, 1982.
42. Amir G, Ron N: Pulmonary pathology in Gaucher's disease. *Hum Pathol* 30:666, 1999.
43. Mistry PK, Sirrs S, Chan A, et al: Pulmonary hypertension in type I Gaucher's disease: Genetic and epigenetic determinants of phenotype and response to therapy. *Mol Genet Metab* 77:91, 2002.
44. Kerem E, Elstein D, Abrahamov A, et al: Pulmonary function abnormalities in type I Gaucher disease. *Eur Respir J* 9:340, 1996.
45. Elstein D, Itzchaki M, Mankin HJ: Skeletal involvement in Gaucher's disease. *Baillieres Clin Haematol* 10:793, 1997.
46. Ciana G, Martini C, Leopaldi A, et al: Bone marker alterations in patients with type 1 Gaucher disease. *Calcif Tissue Int* 72:185, 2003.
47. Carter LC, Fischman SL, Mann J, et al: The nature and extent of jaw involvement in Gaucher disease: Observations in a series of 28 patients. *Oral Surg Oral Med Oral Pathol Oral Radiol Endod* 85:233, 1999.
48. Itzchaki M, Lebel E, Dweck A et al: Orthopedic considerations in Gaucher disease since the advent of enzyme replacement therapy. *Acta Orthop Scand* 75:641, 2004.
49. Granovsky-Grisaru S, Aboulafia Y, Diamant YZ, et al: Gynecologic and obstetric aspects of Gaucher's disease: A survey of 53 patients. *Am J Obstet Gynecol* 172:1284, 1995.
50. Petrohelos M, Tricoulis D, Kotsiras I, et al: Ocular manifestations of Gaucher's disease. *Am J Ophthalmol* 80:1006, 1975.
51. Wollstein G, Elstein D, Zimran A: Ocular findings in adult patients with type I Gaucher disease. *Haema, J Hellen Soc Hematol* 6:217, 2003.
52. Becker-Cohen R, Elstein D, Abrahamov A, et al: A comprehensive assessment of renal function in patients with Gaucher disease. *Am J Kidney Dis* 46:837, 2005.
53. Brady RO, Barton NW, Grabowski GA: The role of neurogenetics in Gaucher disease. *Arch Neurol* 50:1212, 1993.
54. Uyama E, Takahashi K, Owada M, et al: Hydrocephalus, corneal opacities, deafness, valvular heart disease, deformed toes and leptomeningeal fibrous thickening in adult siblings: A new syndrome associated with beta-glucocerebrosidase deficiency and a mosaic population of storage cells. *Acta Neurol Scand* 86:407, 1992.
55. Chabas A, Cormand B, Grinberg D, et al: Unusual expression of Gaucher's disease: Cardiovascular calcifications in three sibs homozygous for the D409H mutation. *J Med Genet* 32:740, 1995.
56. Mistry PK: Genotype/phenotype correlations in Gaucher's disease. *Lancet* 346:982, 1995.
57. Pastores GM, Barnett NL, Bathan P, et al: A neurological symptom survey of patients with type I Gaucher disease. *J Inherit Metab Dis* 26:641, 2003.
58. Biegstraaten M, van Schaik IN, Aerts JM, Hollak CE: "Non-neuronopathic" Gaucher disease reconsidered. Prevalence of neurological manifestations in a Dutch cohort of type I Gaucher disease patients and a systematic review of the literature. *J Inherit Metab Dis* 31:337, 2008.
59. Neudorfer O, Giladi N,,Elstein D, et al: Occurrence of Parkinson's syndrome in type I Gaucher disease. *Q J Med* 89:691, 1996.
60. Tayebi N, Callahan M, Madike V, et al: Gaucher disease and parkinsonism: A phenotypic and genotypic characterization. *Mol Genet Metab* 73:313, 2001.
61. Aharon-Peretz J, Rosenbaum H, Gershoni-Baruch R: Mutations in the glucocerebrosidase gene and Parkinson's disease in Ashkenazi Jews. *N Engl J Med* 351:1972, 2004.
62. Sidransky E, Nalls MA, Aasly JO, et al: Multicenter analysis of glucocerebrosidase mutations in Parkinson's disease. *N Engl J Med* 361:1651, 2009.
63. Gan-Or Z, Giladi N, Rozovski U, et al: Genotype-phenotype correlations between GBA mutations and Parkinson disease risk and onset. *Neurology* 70:2277, 2008.
64. Zimran A, Liphshitz I, Barchana M, et al: Incidence of malignancies among patients with type I Gaucher disease from a single referral clinic. *Blood Cells Mol Dis* 34:197, 2005.
65. Rosenbloom BE, Weinreb NJ, Zimran A, et al: Gaucher disease and cancer incidence: A study from the Gaucher registry. *Blood* 105:4569, 2005.
66. de Fost M, Out TA, de Wilde FA, et al: Immunoglobulin and free light chain abnormalities in Gaucher disease type I: Data from an adult cohort of 63 patients and review of the literature. *Ann Hematol* 87:439, 2008.
67. Allen MJ, Myer BJ, Khokher AM, et al: Pro-inflammatory cytokines and the pathogenesis of Gaucher's disease: Increased release of interleukin-6 and interleukin-10. *Q J Med* 90:19, 1997.
68. de Fost M, Vom Dahl S, Weverling GJ, et al: Increased incidence of cancer in adult Gaucher disease in Western Europe. *Blood Cells Mol Dis* 36:53, 2006.
69. Barone R, Pavone V, Nigro F, et al: Extraordinary bone involvement in a Gaucher disease type I patient. *Br J Haematol* 108:838, 2000.
70. Poll, LW: Type I Gaucher disease: Extraosseous extension of skeletal disease. *Skeletal Radiol* 29, 15, 2000.
71. Kaloterakis A, Cholongitas E, Pantelis E, et al: Type I Gaucher disease with severe skeletal destruction, extraosseous extension and monoclonal gammopathy. *Am J Hematol* 77:377, 2004.
72. Burrow TA, Cohen MB, Bokulic R, et al: Gaucher disease: Progressive mesenteric and mediastinal lymphadenopathy despite enzyme therapy. *J Pediatr* 150:202, 2007.
73. Zimran A, Bashkin A, Elstein D, et al: Rheological determinants in patients with Gaucher disease and internal inflammation. *Am J Hematol* 75:190, 2004.
74. Rogowski O, Shapira I, Zimran A, et al: Automated system to detect low-grade underlying inflammatory profile: Gaucher disease as a model. *Blood Cells Mol Dis* 34:26, 2005.
75. Boklan BF, Sawitsky A: Factor IX deficiency in Gaucher disease. An *in vitro* phenomenon. *Arch Intern Med* 136:489, 1976.
76. Berrebi A, Malnick SDH, Vorst EJ, et al: High incidence of Factor XI deficiency in Gaucher's disease. *Am J Hematol* 40:153, 1992.
77. Zimran A, Altarescu G, Rudensky B, et al: Survey of hematological aspects of Gaucher disease. *Hematology* 10:151, 2005.
78. Hughes D, Cappellini MD, Berger M, et al: Recommendations for the management of the haematological and onco-haematological aspects of Gaucher disease. *Br J Haematol* 138:676, 2007.
79. Rosenbaum H, Sidransky E: Cholelithiasis in patients with Gaucher disease. *Blood Cells Mol Dis* 28:21, 2002.
80. Ben Harosh-Katz M, Patlas M, Hadas-Halpern I, et al: Increased prevalence of cholelithiasis in Gaucher disease: Association with splenectomy but not with gilbert syndrome. *J Clin Gastroenterol* 38:586, 2004.
81. Shoenfeld Y, Beresovski A, Zharhary D, et al: Natural autoantibodies in sera of patients with Gaucher's disease. *J Clin Immunol* 15:363, 1995.
82. Hollak CE, van Weely S, van Oers MH, Aerts JM: Marked elevation of plasma chitotriosidase activity. A novel hallmark of Gaucher disease. *J Clin Invest* 93:1288, 1994.
83. Boot RG, Verhoek M, de Fost M: Marked elevation of the chemokine CCL18/PARC in Gaucher disease: A novel surrogate marker for assessing therapeutic intervention. *Blood* 103:33, 2004.
84. Gielchinsky Y, Elstein D, Green R: High prevalence of low serum vitamin B_{12} in a multi-ethnic Israeli population. *Br J Haematol* 115:707, 2001.
85. Mikosch P, Reed M, Stettner H, et al: Patients with Gaucher disease living in England show a high prevalence of vitamin D insufficiency with correlation to osteodensitometry. *Mol Genet Metab* 96:113, 2009.
86. Naito M, Takahashi K, Hojo H: An ultrastructural and experimental study on the development of tubular structures in the lysosomes of Gaucher cells. *Lab Invest* 58:590, 1988.
87. Beutler E, Kuhl W: The diagnosis of the adult type of Gaucher's disease and its carrier state by demonstration of deficiency of beta-glucosidase activity in peripheral blood leukocytes. *J Lab Clin Med* 76:747, 1970.
88. Rudensky B, Paz E, Altarescu G, Raveh D et al: Fluorescent flow cytometric assay: A new diagnostic tool for measuring beta-glucocerebrosidase activity in Gaucher disease. *Blood Cells Mol Dis* 30:97, 2003.
89. Beutler E, Saven A: Misuse of marrow examination in the diagnosis of Gaucher disease. *Blood* 76:646, 1990.
90. Zimran A, Elstein D, Schiffmann R, et al: Outcome of partial splenectomy for type I Gaucher disease. *J Pediatr* 126:596, 1995.
91. Itzchaki M, Lebel E, Dweck A, et al: Orthopedic considerations in Gaucher disease since the advent of enzyme replacement therapy. *Acta Orthop Scand* 75:641, 2004.
92. Wenstrup RJ, Bailey L, Grabowski GA, et al: Gaucher disease: Alendronate disodium improves bone mineral density in adults receiving enzyme therapy. *Blood* 104:1253, 2004.
93. Rodgers GP, Lessin LS: Recombinant erythropoietin improves the anemia associated with Gaucher's disease. *Blood* 73:2228, 1989.
94. Grabowski GA, Barton NW, Pastores G, et al: Enzyme therapy in type 1 Gaucher disease: Comparative efficacy of mannose-terminated glucocerebrosidase from natural and recombinant sources. *Ann Intern Med* 122:33, 1995.
95. Zimran A, Loveday K, Fratazzi C, Elstein D: A pharmacokinetic analysis of a novel enzyme replacement therapy with gene-activated human glucocerebrosidase (GA-GCB) in patients with type 1 Gaucher disease. *Blood Cells Mol Dis* 39:115, 2007.
96. Aviezer D, Brill-Almon E, Shaaltiel Y et al: A plant-derived recombinant human glucocerebrosidase enzyme—A preclinical and phase I investigation. *PLoS ONE* 4e:4792, 2009.
97. Weinreb NJ, Charrow J, Andersson HC, et al: Effectiveness of enzyme replacement therapy in 1028 patients with type 1 Gaucher disease after 2 to 5 years of treatment: A report from the Gaucher Registry. *Am J Med* 113:112, 2002.
98. Brady RO: Enzyme replacement for lysosomal diseases. *Annu Rev Med* 57:283, 2006.
99. Zimran A, Bembi B, Pastores G: Enzyme replacement therapy for type I Gaucher disease, in *Gaucher Disease*, edited by AH Futerman, A Zimran, p 341. CRC Press, Boca Raton, FL, 2007.
100. Grabowski GA, Kacena K, Cole JA, et al: Dose-response relationships for enzyme replacement therapy with imiglucerase/alglucerase in patients with Gaucher disease type 1. *Genet Med* 11:92, 2009.
101. Maas M, Hollak CE, Akkerman EM, et al: Quantification of skeletal involvement in adults with type I Gaucher's disease: Fat fraction measured by Dixon quantitative chemical shift imaging as a valid parameter. *Am J Roentgenol* 179:961, 2002.
102. Altarescu G, Hill S, Wiggs E, et al: The efficacy of enzyme replacement therapy in patients with chronic neuronopathic Gaucher's disease. *J Pediatr* 138:539, 2001.
103. Zimran A, Elstein D: No justification for very high-dose enzyme therapy for patients with type III Gaucher disease. *J Inherit Metab Dis* 30:843, 2007.
104. Starzyk K, Richards S, Yee J, et al: The long-term international safety experience of imiglucerase therapy for Gaucher disease. *Mol Genet Metab* 90:157, 2007.
105. Zimran A, Hollak CEM, Abrahamov A, et al: Home treatment with intravenous enzyme replacement therapy for Gaucher disease: An international collaborative study of 33 patients. *Blood* 82:1107, 1993.
106. Elstein D, Granovsky-Grisaru S, Rabinowitz R et al: Use of enzyme replacement therapy for Gaucher disease during pregnancy. *Am J Obstet Gynecol* 177:1509, 1997.
107. Pastores GM, Weinreb NJ, Aerts H, et al: Therapeutic goals in the treatment of Gaucher disease. *Semin Hematol* 41:4, 2004.

108. Weinreb NJ, Aggio MC, Andersson HC et al: International Collaborative Gaucher Group (ICGG). Gaucher disease type 1: Revised recommendations on evaluations and monitoring for adult patients. *Semin Hematol* 41:15, 2004.
109. Beutler E: Consensus recommendations. *Br J Haematol* 138:673, 2006.
110. Sidransky E, Pastores GM, Mori M: Dosing enzyme replacement therapy for Gaucher disease: Older, but are we wiser? *Genet Med* 11:90, 2009.
111. Zimran A, Ilan Y, Elstein D: Enzyme replacement therapy for mild patients with Gaucher disease. *Am J Hematol* 84:202, 2009.
112. Radin NS: Chemical models and chemotherapy in the sphingolipidoses, in *Current Trends in Sphingolipidoses and Allied Disorders*, edited by BW Volk, L Schneck, p 453. Plenum Press, New York, 1976.
113. Cox T, Lachmann R, Hollak C, et al: Novel oral treatment of Gaucher's disease with *N*-butyldeoxynojirimycin (OGT 918) to decrease substrate biosynthesis. *Lancet* 355:1481, 2000.
114. Heitner R, Elstein D, Aerts J, et al: Low-dose *N*-butyldeoxynojirimycin (OGT 918) for type I Gaucher disease. *Blood Cells Mol Dis* 28:127, 2003.
115. Elstein D, Dweck A, Attias D, et al: Oral maintenance clinical trial with miglustat for type I Gaucher disease: Switch from or combination with intravenous enzyme replacement. *Blood* 110:2296, 2007.
116. Fan JQ: A contradictory treatment for lysosomal storage disorders: Inhibitors enhance mutant enzyme activity. *Trends Pharmacol Sci* 24:355, 2003.
117. Ron I, Horowitz M: ER retention and degradation as the molecular basis underlying Gaucher disease heterogeneity. *Mol Genet Metab* 93:426, 2008.
118. Peters C, Krivit W: Hematopoetic stem cell transplantation, stem cells and gene therapy, in *Gaucher Disease*, edited by AH Futerman, A Zimran, p 423. CRC Press, Boca Raton, FL, 2007.
119. Zimran A, Kay AC, Gelbart T, et al: Gaucher disease: Clinical, laboratory, radiologic and genetic features of 53 patients. *Medicine (Baltimore)* 71:337, 1992.
120. Mistry P, Zimran A: Type I Gaucher disease—Clinical features, in *Gaucher Disease*, edited by AH Futerman, A Zimran, p 155. CRC Press, Boca Raton, FL, 2007.
121. Taddei TH, Kacena KA, Yang M, et al: The underrecognized progressive nature of N370S Gaucher disease and assessment of cancer risk in 403 patients. *Am J Hematol* 84:208, 2009.
122. Weinreb NJ, Deegan P, Kacena KA, et al: Life expectancy in Gaucher disease type 1. *Am J Hematol* 83:896, 2008.
123. Niemann A: Ein unbekanntes Krankheitsbild. *Jahrbuch Kinderheilkunde* 79:1, 1914.
124. Pick L: Uber die lipoidzellige Splenhepatomegalie Typus Niemann-Pick als Stoffwechselerkrankung. *Med Klin* 23:1483, 1927.
125. Brady RO, Kanfer JN, Mock MB, et al: The metabolism of sphingomyelin II. Evidence of an enzymatic deficiency in Niemann-Pick disease. *Proc Natl Acad Sci U S A* 55:366, 1966.
126. Schuchman EH, Desnick RJ: Niemann-Pick disease types A and B: Acid sphingomyelinase deficiencies, in *The Metabolic and Molecular Bases of Inherited Disease*, edited by CR Scriver, AL Beaudet, WS Sly, D Valle, p 2601. McGraw-Hill, New York, 1995.
127. Pentchev PG, Vanier MT, Suzuki K, et al: Niemann-Pick disease type C: A cellular cholesterol lipidosis, in *The Metabolic and Molecular Bases of Inherited Disease*, edited by CR Scriver, AL Beaudet, WS Sly, D Valle, p 2625. McGraw-Hill, New York, 1995.
128. Greer WL, Riddell DC, Murty S, et al: Linkage disequilibrium mapping of the Nova Scotia variant of Niemann-Pick disease. *Clin Genet* 55:248, 1999.
129. Schuchman EH, Miranda SR: Niemann-Pick disease: Mutation update, genotype/phenotype correlations, and prospects for genetic testing. *Genet Test* 1:13,1997.
130. Simonaro CM, Desnick RJ, McGovern MM, et al: The demographics and distribution of type B Niemann-Pick disease: Novel mutations lead to new genotype/phenotype correlations. *Am J Hum Genet* 71:1413, 2002.
131. Wenger DA, Barth G, Githens JH: Nine cases of sphingomyelin lipidosis, a new variant in Spanish-American children. Juvenile variant of Niemann-Pick Disease with foamy and sea-blue histiocytes. *Am J Dis Child* 131:955, 1977.
132. Millat G, Marçais C, Rafi MA, et al: Niemann-Pick C1 disease: The I1061T substitution is a frequent mutant allele in patients of Western European descent and correlates with a classic juvenile phenotype. *Am J Hum Genet* 65:1321, 1999.
133. Patterson MC, Vanier MT, Suzuki K, et al: Niemann-Pick disease type C: A lipid trafficking disorder, in *The Metabolic and Molecular Bases of Inherited Disease*, 8th ed, edited by CR Scriver, AL Beaudet, WS Sly, Valle D, Childs B, Kinzler KW, Vogelstein B, p 3611. McGraw-Hill, New York, 2001.
134. Takahashi T, Suchi M, Desnick RJ, et al: Identification and expression of five mutations in the human acid sphingomyelinase gene causing types A and B Niemann-Pick disease. Molecular evidence for genetic heterogeneity in the neuronopathic and non-neuronopathic forms. *J Biol Chem* 267:12552, 1992.
135. De Maria R, Rippo MR, Schuchman EH, et al: Acidic sphingomyelinase (ASM) is necessary for fas-induced GD3 ganglioside accumulation and efficient apoptosis of lymphoid cells. *J Exp Med* 187:897, 1998.
136. Carstea ED, Morris JA, Coleman KG, et al: Niemann-Pick C1 disease gene: Homology to mediators of cholesterol homeostasis. *Science* 277:228, 1997.
137. Park WD, O'Brien JF, Lundquist PA, et al: Identification of 58 novel mutations in Niemann-Pick disease type C: Correlation with biochemical phenotype and importance of PTC1-like domains in NPC1. *Hum Mutat* 22:313, 2003.
138. Millat G, Chikh K, Naureckiene S, et al: Niemann-Pick disease type C: Spectrum of HE1 mutations and genotype/phenotype correlations in the NPC2 group. *Am J Hum Genet* 69:1013, 2001.
139. Verot L, Chikh K, Freydière E, et al: Niemann-Pick C disease: Functional characterization of three NPC2 mutations and clinical and molecular update on patients with NPC2. *Clin Genet* 71:320, 2007.
140. Pacheco CD, Kunkel R, Lieberman AP: Autophagy in Niemann-Pick C disease is dependent upon Beclin-1 and responsive to lipid trafficking defects. *Hum Mol Genet* 16:1495, 2007.
141. Loftus SK, Morris JA, Carstea ED, et al: Murine model of Niemann-Pick C disease: Mutation in a cholesterol homeostasis gene. *Science* 277:232, 1997.
142. Golde DW, Schneider EL, Bainton EL, et al: Pathogenesis of one variant of sea-blue histiocytosis. *Lab Invest* 33:371, 1975.
143. Patterson MC: A riddle wrapped in a mystery: Understanding Niemann-Pick disease, type C. *Neurologist* 9:301, 2003.
144. Lazarus SS, Vethamany VG, Schneck L, et al: Fine structure and histochemistry of peripheral blood cells in Niemann-Pick disease. *Lab Invest* 17:155, 1967.
145. Brady RO: Sphingomyelin lipidoses: Niemann-Pick disease, in *The Metabolic Basis of Inherited Disease*, edited by JB Stanbury, JB Wyngaarden, DS Fredrickson, JL Goldstein, MS Brown, p 831. McGraw-Hill, New York, 1983.
146. Gal AE, Brady RO, Hibberg SR, et al: A practical chromogenic procedure for the detection of homozygotes and heterozygous carriers of Niemann-Pick disease. *N Engl J Med* 293:632, 1975.
147. Vanier MT. Prenatal diagnosis of Niemann-Pick diseases types A, B and C. *Prenat Diagn* 22:630, 2002.
148. Daloze P, Delvin EE, Glorieux FH, et al: Replacement therapy for inherited enzyme deficiency: Liver orthotopic transplantation in Niemann-Pick disease type A. *Am J Med Genet* 1:229, 1977.
149. Victor S, Coulter JB, Besley GT, et al: Niemann-Pick disease: Sixteen-year follow-up of allogeneic bone marrow transplantation in a type B variant. *J Inherit Metab Dis* 26:775, 2003.
150. Hsu YS, Hwu WL, Huang SF, et al: Niemann-Pick disease type C (a cellular cholesterol lipidosis) treated by bone marrow transplantation. *Bone Marrow Transplant* 24:103, 1999.
151. Miranda SR, Erlich S, Friedrich VL Jr, et al: Hematopoietic stem cell gene therapy leads to marked visceral organ improvements and a delayed onset of neurological abnormalities in the acid sphingomyelinase deficient mouse model of Niemann-Pick disease. *Gene Ther* 7:1768, 2000.
152. Lachmann RH, te Vruchte D, Lloyd-Evans E, et al. Treatment with miglustat reverses the lipid-trafficking defect in Niemann-Pick disease type C. *Neurobiol Dis* 16:654, 2004.
153. Wraith E, Vecchio D, Jacklin E, et al: Disease stability in patients with Niemann-Pick type C treated with miglustat [abstract]. Fifth annual World Symposium, San Diego, CA, 2009.

PART IX

Lymphocytes and Plasma Cells

CHAPTER 74
MORPHOLOGY OF LYMPHOCYTES AND PLASMA CELLS

H. Elizabeth Broome

SUMMARY

Lymphocytes are a heterogeneous collection of cells that can be distinguished from other leukocytes by their characteristic morphology. Blood T and B lymphocytes are indistinguishable by light and electron microscopy. Natural killer cells tend to be larger cells with relatively large granules scattered in their cytoplasm. B cells can mature into plasma cells upon activation by engagement with antigen or with certain B-cell mitogens. There are many lymphocyte subpopulations that can appear similar by morphology but have distinct antigen expression patterns. These subpopulations, as defined by antigen expression, reflect different functional subsets, maturation stages, and activation stages. This chapter describes the light and transmission electron microscopy of lymphocytes and plasma cells and the major surface antigens that are characteristic of each lymphocyte type.

DEFINITION AND HISTORY

Lymphocytes and plasma cells first were described in 1774 and 1875, respectively.[1] Studies during the subsequent 75 years with improved histologic techniques and light microscope optics furthered understanding of the lymphoid organs and the distribution of lymphocytes.[2–6] By mid 20th century, an awareness that the immune system had at least two components, one governing humoral immunity and one governing cellular immunity led to early concepts of different lymphocyte subsets. Also, at the same time came the discovery that the thymus and bursa of Fabricius in birds were the source of what came to be known as T (thymic-derived) and B (bursa-derived) lymphocytes, respectively, and that the marrow was the bursa equivalent in humans (human B cells therefore could represent marrow-derived cells, a happy coincidence). This discovery coupled with descriptions of inherited absence of the thymus leading to loss of cellular immunity but retention of humoral immunity and cases of retention of cellular immunity in children who were deficient in antibody production, eventually led to our current understanding of the division of labor among what originally appeared to be a common lymphocyte pool, morphologically. The later advent of monoclonal antibodies against numerous surface antigens coupled with flow cytometry, *in vitro* functional assays, molecular techniques to distinguish between B cells and T cells, and experiments using inbred strains of mice have brought us to our current state of knowledge of the immune response and its abnormalities.

Acronyms and abbreviations that appear in this chapter include: CD, clusters of differentiation; Ig, immunoglobulin; MHC, major histocompatibility complex; NK, natural killer; TFH, follicular helper T-cells; T_{reg}, T-regulatory cell.

Flow cytometry identifies a multitude of lymphocyte subsets based on antigen expression patterns. These immunophenotypic subsets correlate closely with function as determined by *in vitro* and *in vivo* testing. Three major blood lymphocyte functional subsets have been identified: T lymphocytes, B lymphocytes, and natural killer (NK) cells. The marrow and thymus contain precursor cells that resemble lymphocytes but lack function without differentiation and maturation into various lymphocyte subsets. Plasma cells are terminally differentiated B lymphocytes that produce immunoglobulin and mostly reside in marrow, lymph nodes, and other lymphoid tissues (see Chap. 5).

MICROSCOPY AND HISTOCHEMISTRY OF NORMAL BLOOD LYMPHOCYTES

LIGHT MICROSCOPY

Classic studies of blood and tissues defined lymphocytes as spherical and/or ovoid cells that have diameters from 6 to 15 μm when flattened on glass slides.[3] Some of these studies described two separate broad types of lymphocytes based on size: small lymphocytes with diameters of 6 to 9 μm and large lymphocytes with diameters of 9 to 15 μm. Patients with acute viral illnesses have increased numbers of circulating large, "reactive," lymphocytes. Other illnesses, such as infection with *Bordetella pertussis* and autoimmune disorders, can cause blood to have increased small lymphocytes or lymphocytes with plasma cell-like morphology (see Chap. 80). The mean absolute number of circulating small lymphocytes in normal adults is 2.5×10^9/L (see Chap. 2).[7] Children have higher lymphocyte counts that trend downward until they reach adult levels at about age 8 to 10 years (see Chap. 6).[8]

Most lymphocytes in normal blood are small with an ovoid or kidney-shaped nucleus that stains purple, has densely packed nuclear chromatin, and occupies approximately 90 percent of the cell area (Fig. 74–1A and B) by Romanowsky polychromatic stains (e.g., Giemsa or Wright) of air-dried films. A small rim of cytoplasm stains light blue. Nucleoli rarely are observed in Wright-stained films, but nucleoli in these cells may become visible in certain preparations, such as cytospin slides, or after prolonged storage in anticoagulated blood collection tubes.

A minority of lymphocytes (larger granular lymphocytes [LGLs]) in normal blood have morphology that defines them as large granular lymphocytes.[10] These LGLs are slightly larger than most lymphocytes, having an increased area of light blue or clear cytoplasm. LGL cytoplasm contains a number of coarse pink granules, usually 5 to 15 per cell, and occasional clear vacuoles. In a normal adult, approximately 5 percent but up to 10 to 15 percent of blood lymphocytes are LGLs (see Fig. 74–1E).[10] The LGL cells in blood are composed of NK cells and a subset of CD8+ T lymphocytes, indistinguishable by their morphology.

PHASE-CONTRAST MICROSCOPY

Active movement of lymphocytes is studied by phase-contrast, or interference-contrast, microscopy. Lymphocytes move slowly with a "hand mirror" appearance. Cytoplasmic spreading does not occur. However, during cell movement, a thickening occurs in the cytoplasmic rim, which houses most of the cell's organelles, including the Golgi.

TRANSMISSION ELECTRON MICROSCOPY AND CYTOCHEMISTRY

The blood lymphocyte measures approximately 5 μm in spherical diameter as visualized by transmission electron microscopy.[11] The nucleus has an abundance of electron-dense, condensed heterochromatin, a feature characteristic of nonproliferating cells. The nucleoli are round in section,

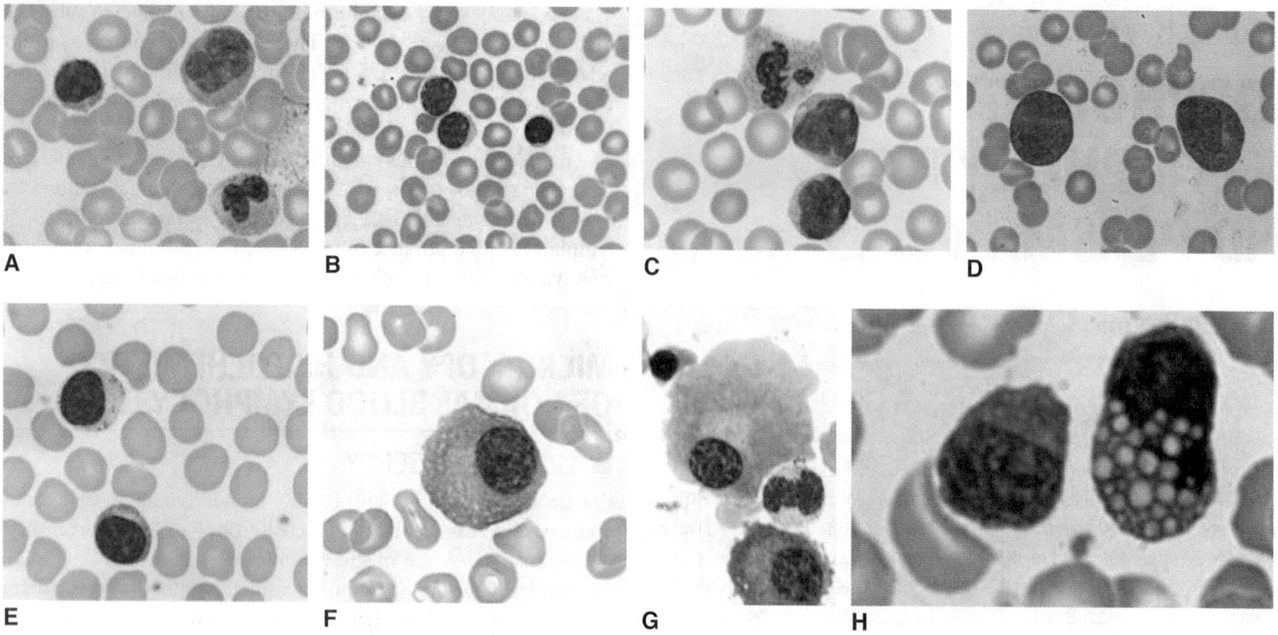

FIGURE 74–1. Wright-Giemsa stained blood films showing **(A)** a normal, small lymphocyte, monocyte, and segmented neutrophil; **(B)** normal small lymphocyte and two medium-sized lymphocytes; **(C)** neutrophil and two lymphocytes with morphologic features characteristic of *Bordetella pertussis* infection (small size, cleaved nuclei, and scant cytoplasm); **(D)** reactive lymphocytes; and **(E)** large granular lymphocyte and small lymphocyte. Wright-Giemsa stained marrow films showing **(F)** normal plasma cell; **(G)** two normal plasma cells, one nucleated red cell, and one neutrophil; and **(H)** two plasma cells with one containing many Russell bodies.

approximately 0.5 to 1.4 μm in diameter. They are composed of three distinct and concentrically arranged structural units: the central region or agranular zone; the middle, fibrillar region; and the granular zone, which contains intranucleolar chromatin. The lymphocyte's nuclear membrane contains nuclear pores and a perinuclear space.

The cytoplasmic organelles of the lymphocytes are characteristic of eukaryotic cells. Some organelles, such as the Golgi zone, are poorly developed. The cytoplasm contains free ribosomes, occasional ribosome clusters, and strands of rough-surfaced endoplasmic reticulum (Fig. 74–2). Centrioles, mitochondria, microtubules (diameter approximately 0.25 μm), and microfilaments (diameter approximately 0.07 μm) are present in the cytoplasm adjacent to the cell membrane. The cytoplasm also contains lysosomes, which are approximately 0.4 μm in diameter, are electron opaque, and contain classic lysosomal enzymes (e.g., acid phosphatase, β-glucuronidase, and acid ribonuclease).[12] The lymphocyte plasma membrane stains with colloidal iron, a marker for membrane sialic acid. Lymphocyte cell membranes and cell coat glycoproteins are shown with other electron-dense markers, including phosphotungstic acid, lanthanum colloid, and ruthenium red.

Most T lymphocytes have a localized "dot" pattern when stained for acid phosphatase, acid and neutral nonspecific esterases, β-glucuronidase, and *N*-acetyl-β-glucosaminidase.[13] LGLs stain for acid hydrolases with a dispersed, granular reaction pattern.[14] B lymphocytes either lack esterase and acid phosphatase or show minimal scattered granular staining.

■ SCANNING ELECTRON MICROSCOPY

Scanning electron microscopy provides three-dimensional information.[15] However, the resolution achieved with scanning electron microscopy, approximately 0.1 μm, is considerably less than that possible with transmission electron microscopy, generally 0.002 to 0.0039 μm. Normal blood lymphocytes, washed and collected on silver membranes and fixed in glutaraldehyde, have a spherical topography with varying numbers of stubby or finger-like microvilli (Fig. 74–3).[16] In contrast, monocytes are much larger, have few microvilli, and display ruffled membranes and ridge-like profiles (see Chap. 67).

Lymphocyte microvilli contain parallel bundles of actin filaments that undergo continuous assembly and disassembly.[17] The function of lymphocyte microvilli probably includes segregating surface receptors involved in extravasation. Two receptors involved in the initial rolling phase of extravasation, L-selectin and $\alpha_4\beta_7$ integrin,[18] localize to microvillar tips. In contrast, the β_2 integrins that mediate stable adhesion and diapedesis localize to nonprotrusive regions of the cell surface. This spatial separation of surface receptors might enable a temporal segregation of adhesive function during extravasation. Lymphocytes expressing chimeric L-selectin constructs that no longer localize to microvilli do not roll on L-selectin ligands, supporting this hypothesis.[19]

MORPHOLOGIC CHANGES ASSOCIATED WITH ACTIVATION

Lymphocyte stimulation is associated with a complex sequence of morphologic and biochemical events. Activation of B and T lymphocytes results in the transformation of the small, resting lymphocyte into proliferating large cells with abundant highly basophilic cytoplasm, irregularly condensed or smudgy chromatin, and round to slightly irregular nuclear outlines (see Fig. 74–1D). Nucleoli may be evident by light microscopy in these cells, but they usually are not prominent. Infection with *B. pertussis* causes an increase in blood lymphocytes with a particular activated morphology characterized by small size, scant cytoplasm, and cleaved nuclei with mature chromatin (see Fig. 74–1C; Chap. 81).

Activated lymphocytes proliferate and mature into effector lymphocytes and memory cells. Effector cells include helper T cells, cytolytic T cells, and plasma cells (see Figs. 74–1F and G, 74–4, and 74–5). *In vitro*, plant lectins, bacterial products, polymeric substances, and enzymes

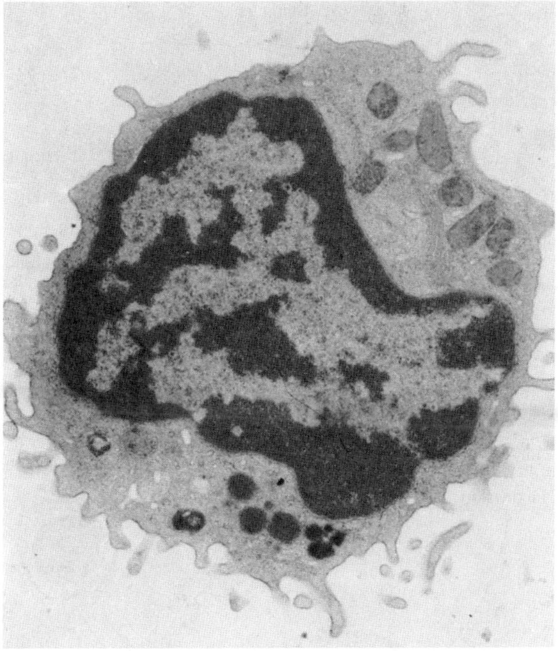

A

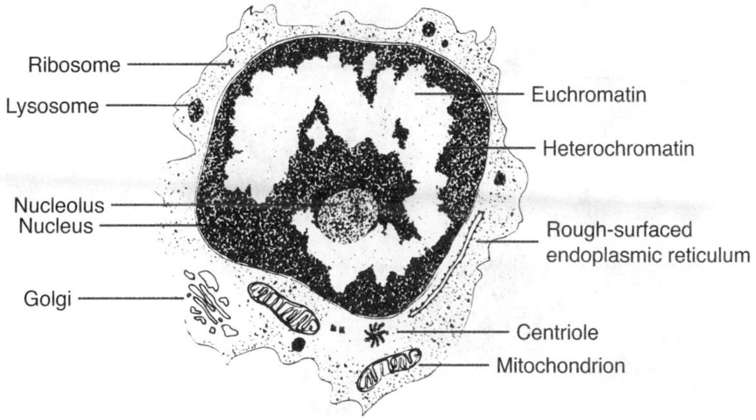

B

FIGURE 74–2. A. Transmission electron micrograph of normal human blood lymphocyte (×12,000). **B.** Diagrammatic representation of normal blood lymphocyte, with organelles labeled.

activate lymphocytes and cause mitosis. Such agents are called *mitogens.* Some mitogens are specific for either B or T lymphocytes, whereas other mitogens stimulate both.[20]

Approximately 4 hours after mitogen stimulation, lymphocytes show increased nucleolar size and an increase in the number and concentration of granules in the granular zone. These changes are followed by an increase in fibrillar zones and increased intranucleolar chromatin. Nucleolar chromatin becomes more electron lucent or dispersed. From 48 to 72 hours following the addition of phytohemagglutinin, the volume of the cytoplasm increases. In addition, the cytoplasm contains an increased number of ribosomal clusters and more rough-surfaced endoplasmic reticulum. The activated cell has increased numbers of lysosomes and a larger Golgi complex with more components.[21] Under some circumstances (e.g., cultures of human lymphocytes stimulated for 7–10 days with pokeweed mitogen), some B cells form well-developed Golgi and plasmacytoid features.[22] Similar plasmacytoid cells are observed in antigen-stimulated lymph nodes, during graft rejection *in vivo*, and in some *in vitro* systems, including the mixed lymphocyte

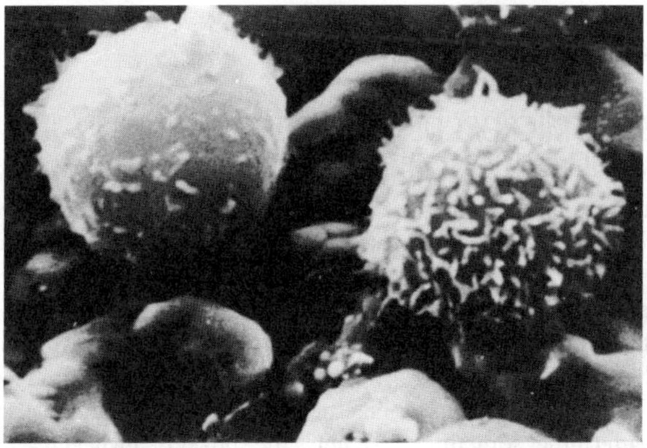

FIGURE 74–3. Scanning electron micrograph of normal blood lymphocytes separated by the Ficoll-Hypaque method. Cells show varying numbers of microvilli (×5000). *(Figs 74–3, 74–5, and 74–6 provided by Dr. Aaron Polliack of the Department of Hematology, Hebrew University Hadassah Medical School, Jerusalem, Israel.)*

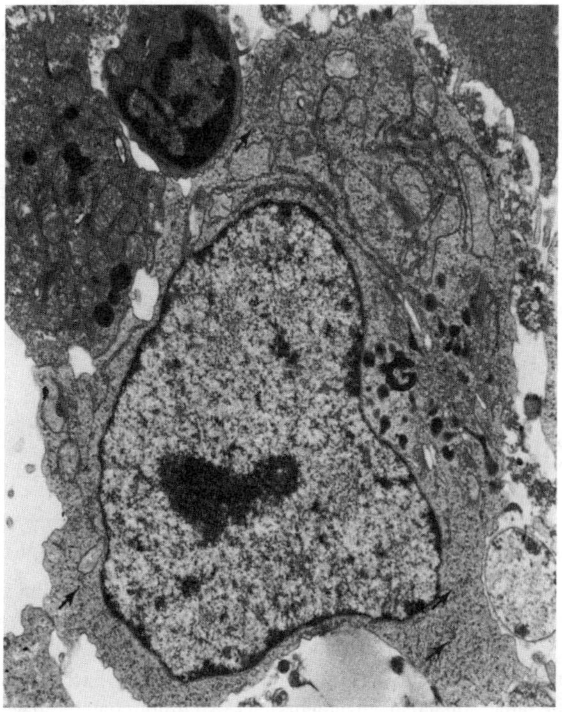

FIGURE 74–4. Transmission electron micrograph of lymphocyte from normal individual incubated with phytohemagglutinin[21] for 3 days. The transformed cell has a large Golgi zone (*G*) and many ribosomal aggregates (*arrows*). The nucleus is euchromatic (×7500).

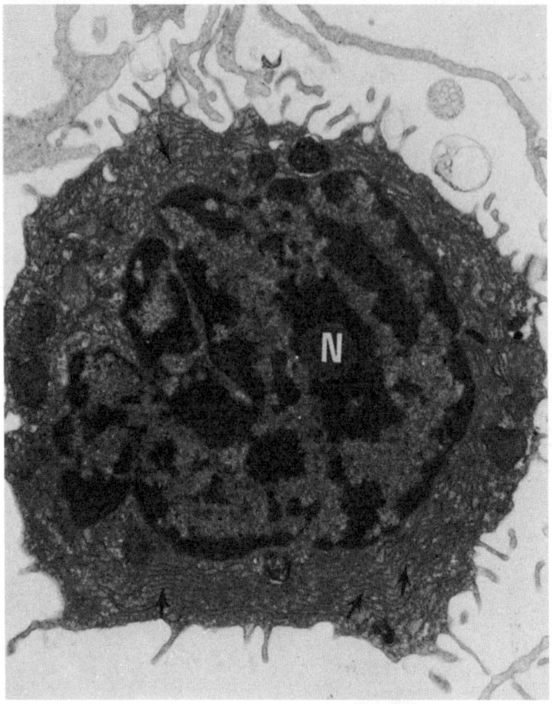

FIGURE 74–5. Transmission electron micrograph of plasmacytoid cell present in culture of lymphocytes from a patient with chronic lymphocytic leukemia incubated with pokeweed mitogen for 7 days. The nucleolus (*N*) and rough-surfaced endoplasmic reticulum (*arrows*) are evident (×9000). *(Reproduced from Cohnen G, Douglas SD, Konig E, Brittinger G: Pokeweed mitogen response of lymphocytes in chronic lymphocytic leukemia: A fine structural study.* Blood *42:591,1973, with permission.)*

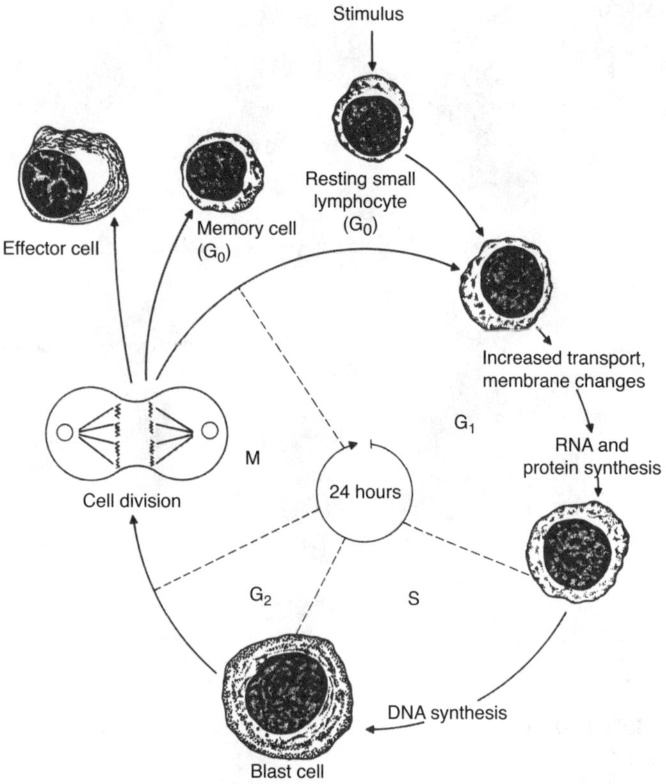

FIGURE 74–6. Diagram of lymphocyte activation displaying the relationship of cell-cycle phases (G_0, G_1, S, and M) with changes in cell metabolism and cell function. A lymphocyte may become an effector cell or a memory cell in G_0 after having traversed the cell cycle. *(Reproduced from Klein J,* Immunology, *p 40. Cambridge, MA, Blackwell, 1990, with permission.)*

culture. In lymph nodes, the stimulated lymphoid cells may be referred to by various pathologists as lymphoblasts, immunoblasts, centroblasts, or large lymphoid cells. Morphologic criteria for these cells overlap.

Following stimulation with antigen or mitogens, the lymphocyte enters the cell cycle. Figure 74–6 summarizes the cell-cycle phases and accompanying genetic or morphologic changes. These parallel genetic and morphologic alterations are necessary correlates of the cell-cycle phases. The fate and function of lymphocytes that traverse the cell cycle can be divided into two pathways. Some lymphocytes undergo several mitotic cycles and then return to the G_0 phase, indistinguishable in morphology from the original nonactivated cells. Some of them then become memory cells, programmed to remember the stimulating antigen and thus respond more rapidly to reexposure to the original antigen. Alternatively, they become terminally differentiated effector lymphocytes, such as plasma cells or cytotoxic T cells.

MICROSCOPY AND HISTOCHEMISTRY OF PLASMA CELLS

■ MORPHOLOGIC STUDIES

Plasma cells derive from small B lymphocytes after activation in the correct environment. The characteristic feature of plasma cells is abundant cytoplasmic and secretory immunoglobulin. A fully mature plasma cell lacks surface immunoglobulin expression. Each plasma cell has the same clonal rearrangement of its VDJ immunoglobulin genes as its predecessor B lymphocyte (see Chap. 77). Several mitotic divisions may occur during cellular differentiation from the resting lymphocyte to the plasmablast to the immature plasma cell. Immature plasma cells can undergo successive waves of mitosis in the medullary cords of lymph nodes in response to antigen.[23] Cell transfer experiments demonstrated that these transformed cells later mature into antibody-producing plasma cells.[24]

Pokeweed mitogen induces B lymphocytes to transform into plasma cells after 7 to 10 days of culture.[25] These plasma cells infrequently contain large electron-dense inclusions (Russell bodies), which may measure 2 to 3 μm in diameter (see Figs. 74–1H and 74–7).[26] Russell bodies, cytoplasmic immunoglobulin (Ig) in the endoplasmic reticulum, sometimes are dissolved during the staining procedure. They usually occur in pathologic states but may be found in plasma cells from normal lymph nodes or marrow.

■ LIGHT MICROSCOPY, HISTOCHEMISTRY, AND ELECTRON MICROSCOPY

The mature plasma cell has a characteristic basophilic cytoplasm and an eccentric nucleus when treated with a polychrome stain. The nuclear polarity is attributable to a large paranuclear zone, which corresponds to the Golgi apparatus. The typical mature plasma cell spread on a slide usually is round or oval and has a diameter of 9 to 20 μm, with a mean cell diameter of 14 μm and a mean nuclear diameter of 8.5 μm (see Fig. 74–1F and G).[27] The nuclear heterochromatin is coarse and distributed in a pattern that sometimes resembles the spokes of a wheel (cartwheel nucleus) on paraffin sections. Normal plasma cells may occasionally have two or more nuclei. Cytochemical features of plasma cells include positive staining for β-glucuronidase and mitochondrial enzyme markers. They do not stain for peroxidase or nonspecific esterase.[28]

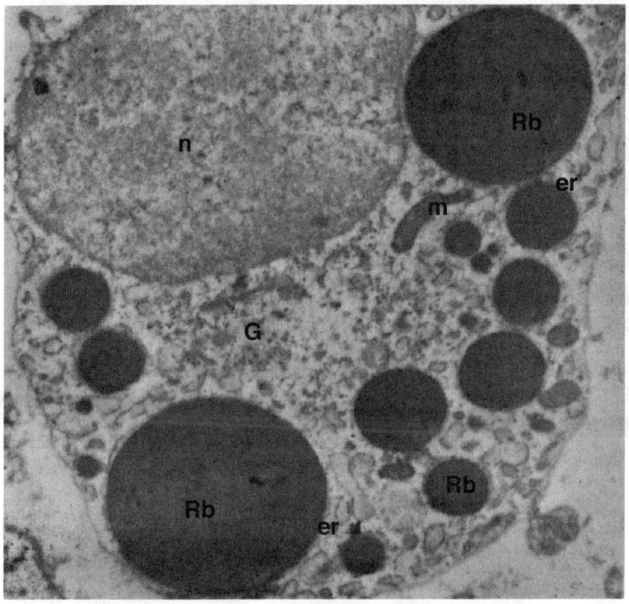

FIGURE 74–7. Intracytoplasmic electron-dense bodies (Russell bodies [*Rbs*]) in plasma cell from the marrow of a patient with myeloma (×12,600, reduced). The large Golgi apparatus (*G*) is in the paranuclear zone. The Rbs vary in size and are surrounded by single membranes of rough-surfaced endoplasmic reticulum (*er*). A mitochondrion (*m*) is adjacent to the Golgi. The nucleus (*n*) is slightly indented by a Rb. *(From Welsh RA: Electron microscopic localization of Russell bodies in the human plasma cell.* Blood *16:1307, 1960.)*

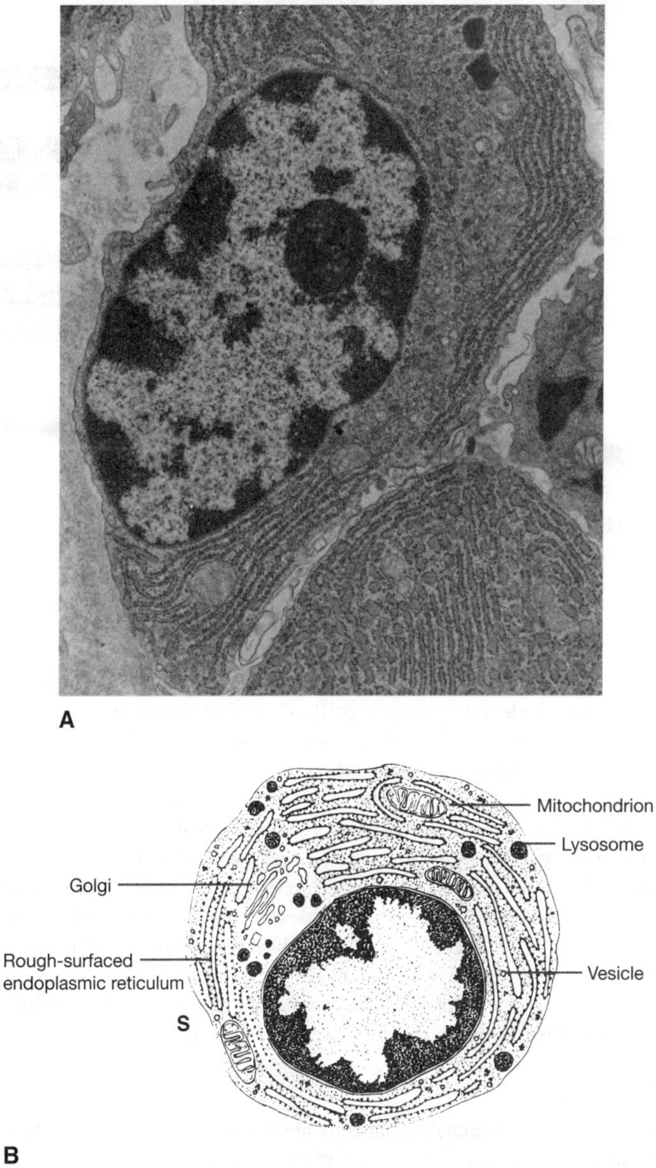

FIGURE 74–8. A. Transmission electron micrograph of mature plasma cells in normal human lymph node (×9000). **B.** Diagrammatic representation of normal plasma cell with organelles labeled.

Plasma cells in patients with certain diseases may have different histochemical properties. Plasma cell size and morphology may be altered substantially in myeloma and macroglobulinemia (see Chap. 109). Plasma cells with two or three nuclei are more frequent in marrows from patients with plasma cell dyscrasias. Periodic acid-Schiff stains may reveal cytoplasmic or nuclear inclusions in clonal plasma cells.[29] Under some circumstances, amyloid inclusions in plasma cells have been detected by electron microscopy.[30] In hemochromatosis and hemosiderosis, plasma cells may contain hemosiderin when examined by electron microscopy.[31]

The plasma cell is packed with a rough-surfaced endoplasmic reticulum having numerous attached ribosomes as seen by electron microscopy. A large, circumscribed Golgi zone forms a paranuclear halo when observed by light microscopy. The nucleus has dense areas of heterochromatin. The Golgi zone contains lamellae, vesicles, vacuoles, and a number of granules. Mitochondria are located between the strands of endoplasmic reticulum (Fig. 74–8).[32]

ANTIGENS OF HUMAN LYMPHOCYTES

B-LYMPHOCYTE ANTIGENS

Figure 74–9 summarizes the expression of antigens on cells of the B-lymphocyte lineage, including committed progenitor B cells and pre-B cells. Chapter 75 discusses these cells and the maturation stages they represent. Figure 74–9 also lists antigens that are expressed or increased upon B-cell activation. Chapter 15 (see Table 15–1) discusses the physiology, structure, and distribution of each of the cluster of differentiation (CD) antigens listed in Figure 74–9.

Of the B-cell–associated antigens that are commonly used, only a few are restricted to cells of the B lineage (see Chap. 15). Of these antigens, only CD20, CD22, and Pax 5 are not found on other cell types. Pax 5, a transcription factor, is a "master regulator" of B-cell development[33,34] that is expressed from the precursor stage through all B-cell maturation until it is lost at the plasma cell stage. Demonstration of monoclonal surface Ig allows diagnosis of clonal, neoplastic B cells. CD20 is the target of rituximab, a monoclonal antibody commonly used for treatment of B-cell neoplasms. CD19 is restricted mostly to B cells, but may be expressed weakly by follicular dendritic cells. CD19 is expressed by B cells at all stages of maturation, including the committed B-cell progenitor and most normal plasma cells. As such, it is the best-defined pan–B-cell surface antigen.

In addition to the CD antigens and Igs, B cells express the three major histocompatibility complex (MHC) class II antigens: DR, DP, DQ. These antigens are heterodimers of heavy chains and light chains that are encoded by genes within the D complex of the human leukocyte antigen (HLA) complex (see Chap. 138). MHC class I antigens are expressed on all nucleated cells.

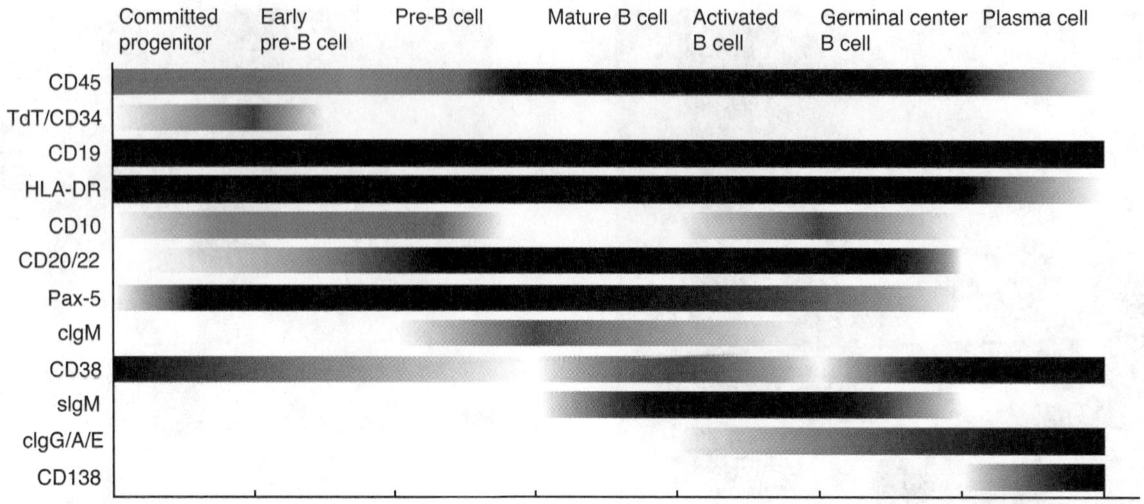

FIGURE 74–9. Clinically useful antigens expressed during B-lymphocyte maturation. The intensity of the antigen expression at each stage of B-lymphocyte maturation is depicted by gradient density of bars on the graph. c, cytoplasmic; s, surface.

B-1 B Cells and CD5+ B Cells

B-1 B cells have distinctive activation requirements and high levels of CD44 and interleukin-5 receptor α (IL-5Rα). They proliferate more rapidly than other B cells to stimuli such as IgM crosslinking, possibly because of having constitutively activated nuclear signal transducer and activator of transcription 3 (STAT3).[35] Many, but not all, B-1 cells express CD5, a 67-kDa transmembrane glycoprotein that is more brightly expressed by T cells (see Chap. 15). These cells are designated CD5 B cells.[36] B-1 B cells do not express other T-cell markers but do express all other pan–B-cell surface antigens. Various agents modulate B-cell expression of CD5.[37] B-1 B cells are found in umbilical cord blood,[38] adult blood, the pleura and peritoneum, and all major secondary lymphoid organs; they are rare in the marrow.[39] These cells apparently are enriched for cells that spontaneously produce polyreactive autoantibodies.[40–42]

Plasma Cells

Many B-cell differentiation antigens are not expressed by the mature plasma cell, including CD20, Pax-5, surface Ig and HLA class II antigens (see Fig. 74–9). Of the cells of the B lineage, plasma cells are distinctive in that they express CD138 and bright CD38.[43] Clonal plasma cell neoplasms usually have antigen expression distinct from normal plasma cells including aberrant expression of CD20, CD28, CD56, and CD117. Clonal plasma cells usually aberrantly lack expression of CD19 and CD27.[44]

■ T-LYMPHOCYTE AND NK CELL ANTIGENS

Figure 74–10 and Table 74–1 summarize the expression of antigens on cells of the T-lymphocyte and NK lineages. All lymphocyte progenitors originate in the marrow, but T lymphocytes have their own special organ for maturation—the thymus (see Chap. 5). Chap. 75 discusses these cells and the maturation stages they represent.

Thymocyte

The thymus promotes the development of antigen-specific T lymphocytes and eliminates self-reactive T lymphocytes. There are three general stages of thymocyte maturation: double negative, double positive, and single positive. These stages have corresponding anatomic localization within the thymus with the least-mature double-negative cells located in the subcapsular area and the most-mature single-positive cells located in the medulla (see Chap. 5). The most immature T lymphocytes in the thymus populate the subcapsular areas and express CD2, CD5, and CD7, antigens present on T lymphocytes of all stages. Capsular, "double-negative" thymocytes also express CD1a, cytoplasmic CD3, and terminal deoxynucleotidyl transferase. The majority of thymocytes are at the "double-positive" stage within the cortical area. These are the cells undergoing positive selection. Once the thymocytes achieve their "education" without dying, they mature to the single-positive stage in the medulla. These varying stages of immature T-cell maturation in the thymus have corresponding cells phenotypes in T-lymphoblastic leukemia/lymphoma.

Mature T Lymphocytes

Small, mature T lymphocytes are the most common lymphocytes in blood. T lymphocytes recognize antigen in the context of the MHC through binding with the T-cell receptor. Signaling from the T-cell

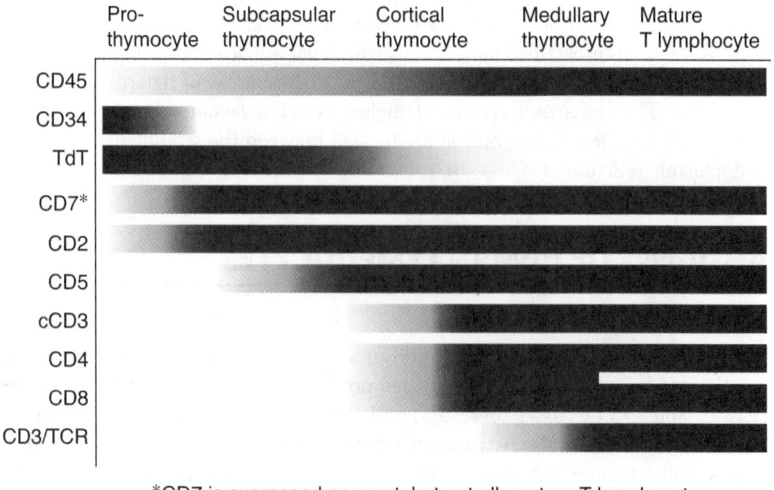

*CD7 is expressed on most, but not all, mature T lymphocytes.

FIGURE 74–10. Clinically useful antigens expressed during T-lymphocyte maturation. The intensity of the antigen expression at each stage of T-lymphocyte maturation is depicted by gradient density of bars on the graph.

TABLE 74–1. Mature Natural Killer and T-Lymphocyte Subsets

NK or T-Cell Subset	Antigens
CD4+ helper T cells	CD2, CD3, CD4, CD5, CD7, and TCR α/β
	Subsets express CD10,[49] CD25,[53] CD57,[54] and Foxp3[55]
CD8+ cytolytic T cells	CD2, CD3, CD5, CD7, CD8, and TCR α/β
	Subsets express CD16,[56] CD56, CD57, cytolytic enzymes[57]
NK cells	CD2, CD7, killer cell immunoglobulin-like receptors (KIRs) (multiple)
	Negative for CD3, TCR (α/β or γ/δ)
	Subsets express either CD16 partial, CD56 bright or CD16 bright, CD56 moderate[58]
	Cytolytic enzymes
γ/δ T cells	CD2, CD3, CD7, TCR γ/δ
	Usually negative for CD4
	Subsets express CD5, CD8, and cytolytic enzymes

TCR, T-cell receptor.

receptor involves many membrane proteins, including CD3, a three-subunit complex expressed by early thymocytes and mature T cells.[45] It is tightly linked to the T-cell antigen receptor (see Chap. 78). Most T lymphocytes have the α/β T-cell receptor on their surface, but a few percent of blood lymphocytes have the γ/δ T-cell receptor.

CD4 and CD8 Lymphocyte Subsets

Mature T cells express either CD4 or CD8 but not both. CD4, a member of the Ig supergene family, is a single-chain transmembrane glycoprotein.[46] CD8 is a 34-kDa dimeric transmembrane glycoprotein.[47] Most T cells express the α and β subunits of CD8. CD4 and CD8 act as coreceptors during T-cell activation by antigen. CD4 recognizes MHC II and CD8 recognizes MHC I (see Chap. 78). CD4 also is a coreceptor for the human immunodeficiency virus[9] (see Chap. 83), as are CCR5 (chemokine receptor 5) and CXCR4 (chemokine-related receptor). The majority of CD8 cells are cytolytic when appropriately activated.

Subsets of CD4+ T cells have helper function for activation and maturation of cytolytic cells or B cells. Other CD4 subsets have regulatory activity including the T-regulatory (T_{reg}) cells that induce immune tolerance and follicular T-helper cells that promote B-cell maturation and differentiation in germinal centers. T_{reg} and follicular T helper cells have unique phenotypes. T_{reg} cells express CD25, the IL-2 receptor α chain, and Foxp3, a transcription factor. Follicular helper T-TFH cells express CD10 and CD57. Malignant counterparts to both subsets occur. Adult T-cell leukemia/lymphoma expresses both CD25 and Foxp3 and is associated with marked immunosuppression.[48] Angioimmunoblastic T-cell lymphoma has characteristic clonal T cells that express CD10 and CD57 just like TFH cells, and this lymphoma is associated with polyclonal hypergammaglobulinemia and the expansion and proliferation of both B cells and CD21+ follicular dendritic cells.[49]

Natural Killer Cells

The NK cell is defined as an effector cell that is not MHC restricted and has the capacity for spontaneous cytotoxicity toward various target cells (see Chap. 79). Most NK cells have LGL morphology (see Fig. 74–1E).[50] However, not all NK cells have LGL morphology, and not all LGL cells are NK cells. Many are cytolytic T lymphocytes. Cytolytic T lymphocytes and NK cells share many granule contents that can be detected by immunohistochemistry or flow cytometry. These include TIA-1, an RNA binding protein, and several granzymes, which are granule enzymes with serine protease activity.

Despite their relative morphologic homogeneity, NK cells comprise several subpopulations with distinct phenotypes. Human NK cells characteristically express CD16 (FcγRIII) and CD56 but not T-cell receptors (α/β or γ/δ), CD3, or CD4.[51] CD8 is found on approximately 30 to 50 percent of NK cells. CD8 on NK cells is dim by flow cytometry and is of the β-homodimer form. CD16 (FcγRIII) is a low-affinity receptor that binds to IgG, which is bound specifically to antigens present on cells targeted for destruction in antibody-dependent cell-mediated cytotoxicity. CD16 is expressed on all NK cells, neutrophils, and tissue macrophages. CD56 is the neural cell adhesion molecule and is seen on most NK cells, albeit at low density.[52] This 200-kDa protein is expressed at higher levels following activation.

REFERENCES

1. Hewson W, Johnson J: No.72, Pauls Church Yard London, 1774, in *Lymphatics, Lymph, and Lymphomyeloid Complex*, edited by JF Yoffey, FC Courtice, p 3. Harvard University Press, Cambridge, MA, 1970.
2. Everett NB, Caffrey RW, Rieke WO: Recirculation of lymphocytes. *Ann N Y Acad Sci* 113:887, 1964.
3. Ford WI, Gowans JL: The traffic of lymphocytes. *Semin Hematol* 6:67, 1969.
4. Nossal GJ, Makela O: Elaboration of antibodies by single cells. *Annu Rev Microbiol* 16:53, 1962.
5. Miller RG: Physical separation of lymphocytes and lymphocyte structure and function, in *Immunology Series*, edited by JJ Marchalonis, p 205. Marcel Dekker, New York, 1977.
6. Ackerman GA: Structual studies of the lymphocyte and lymphocyte development, in *Regulation of Hematopoiesis*, edited by AS Gordon, p 1297. Appleton Century Crofts, New York, 1970.
7. Bain BJ: *Blood Cells, A Practical Guide*. Blackwell Science, London, 1995.
8. Cranendonk E, van Gennip AH, Abeling NG, et al: Reference values for automated cytochemical differential count of leukocytes in children 0–16 years old: Comparison with manually obtained counts from Wright-stained smears. *J Clin Chem Clin Biochem* 23:663, 1985.
9. Dalgleish AG, Beverley PC, Clapham PR, et al: The CD4 (T4) antigen is an essential component of the receptor for the AIDS retrovirus. *Nature* 312:763, 1984.
10. Timonen T, Ortaldo JR, Herberman RB: Characteristics of human large granular lymphocytes and relationship to natural killer and K cells. *J Exp Med* 153:569, 1981.
11. Tanaka T, Goodman JR: *Electron Microscopy of Human Blood Cells*. Harper & Row, New York, 1972.
12. Brittinger G, Hirschhorn R, Douglas SD, Weissmann G: Studies on lysosomes. XI. Characterization of a hydrolase-rich fraction from human lymphocytes. *J Cell Biol* 37:394, 1968.
13. Basso G, Cocito MG, Semenzato G, et al: Cytochemical study of thymocytes and T lymphocytes. *Br J Haematol* 44:577, 1980.
14. Landay A, Clement LT, Grossi CE: Phenotypically and functionally distinct subpopulations of human lymphocytes with T cell markers also exhibit different cytochemical patterns of staining for lysosomal enzymes. *Blood* 63:1067, 1984.
15. Hayes TL: Scanning electron microscope techniques in biology, in *Advanced Techniques in Biological Electron Microscopy*, edited by JK Koehler, p 153. Springer, New York, 1973.
16. Polliack A, Lampen N, Clarkson BD, et al: Identification of human B and T lymphocytes by scanning electron microscopy. *J Exp Med* 138:607, 1973.
17. Majstoravich S, Zhang J, Nicholson-Dykstra S, et al: Lymphocyte microvilli are dynamic, actin-dependent structures that do not require Wiskott-Aldrich syndrome protein (WASP) for their morphology. *Blood* 104:1396, 2004.
18. Berlin C, Bargatze RF, Campbell JJ, et al: Alpha 4 integrins mediate lymphocyte attachment and rolling under physiologic flow. *Cell* 80:413, 1995.
19. von Andrian UH, Hasslen SR, Nelson RD, et al: A central role for microvillous receptor presentation in leukocyte adhesion under flow. *Cell* 82:989, 1995.
20. Handwerger BS, Douglas SD: The cell biology of blastogenesis, in *Handbook of Inflammation*, edited by G Weissman, p 609. Elsevier, North Holland, 1980.
21. Douglas SD, Cohnen G, Brittinger G: Ultrastructural comparison between phytomitogen transformed normal and chronic lymphocytic leukemia lymphocytes. *J Ultrastruct Res* 44:11, 1973.
22. Douglas SD, Fudenberg HH: *In vitro* development of plasma cells from lymphocytes following pokeweed mitogen stimulation: A fine structural study. *Exp Cell Res* 54:277, 1969.

23. Sainte-Marie G: Study on Plasmocytopoiesis. I. Description of plasmocytes and of their mitoses in the mediastinal lymph nodes of ten-week-old rats. *Am J Anat* 114:207, 1964.
24. Sainte-Marie G, Coons AH: Studies on antibody production X. Mode of formation of plasmocytes in cell transfer experiments. *J Exp Med* 119:743, 1964.
25. Parkhouse RME, Janossy G, Greaves MF: Selective stimulation of IgM synthesis in mouse B lymphocytes by pokeweed mitogen. *Nat New Biol* 235:21, 1972.
26. Welsh RA: Electron microscopic localization of Russell bodies in the human plasma cell. *Blood* 16:1307, 1960.
27. Sacchetti C: Plasma cells of the bone marrow in normal and pathological states; quantitative, cytometric and auxological research. *Haematologica* 35:13, 1951.
28. Suzuki A, Shibata A, Onodera S, et al: Histochemical study on plasma cells. *Tohoku J Exp Med* 97:1, 1969.
29. Quaglino D, Torelli U, Sauli S, Mauri C: Cytochemical and autoradiographic investigations on normal and myelomatous plasma cells. *Acta Haematol* 38:79, 1967.
30. Franklin EC, Zucker-Franklin D: Current concepts of amyloid. *Adv Immunol* 15:249, 1972.
31. Lerner RG, Parker JW: Dysglobulinemia and iron in plasma cells. Ferrokinetics and electron microscopy. *Arch Intern Med* 121:284, 1968.
32. Bessis MC: Ultrastructure of lymphoid and plasma cells in relation to globulin and antibody formation. *Lab Invest* 10:1040, 1961.
33. Adams B, Dorfler P, Aguzzi A, et al: Pax-5 encodes the transcription factor BSAP and is expressed in B lymphocytes, the developing CNS, and adult testis. *Genes Dev* 6:1589, 1992.
34. Urbanek P, Wang ZQ, Fetka I, et al: Complete block of early B cell differentiation and altered patterning of the posterior midbrain in mice lacking Pax5/BSAP. *Cell* 79:901, 1994.
35. Karras JG, Wang Z, Huo L, et al: Signal transducer and activator of transcription-3 (STAT3) is constitutively activated in normal, self-renewing B-1 cells but only inducibly expressed in conventional B lymphocytes. *J Exp Med* 185:1035, 1997.
36. Kipps TJ: The CD5 B cell. *Adv Immunol* 47:117, 1989.
37. Defrance T, Vanbervliet B, Durand I, Banchereau J: Human interleukin 4 down-regulates the surface expression of CD5 on normal and leukemic B cells. *Eur J Immunol* 19:293, 1989.
38. Durandy A, Thuillier L, Forveille M, Fischer A: Phenotypic and functional characteristics of human newborns' B lymphocytes. *J Immunol* 144:60, 1990.
39. Caligaris-Cappio F, Gobbi M, Bofill M, Janossy G: Infrequent normal B lymphocytes express features of B-chronic lymphocytic leukemia. *J Exp Med* 155:623, 1982.
40. Casali P, Prabhakar BS, Notkins AL: Characterization of multireactive autoantibodies and identification of Leu-1+ B lymphocytes as cells making antibodies binding multiple self and exogenous molecules. *Int Rev Immunol* 3:17, 1988.
41. Hayakawa K, Hardy RR, Honda M, et al: Ly-1 B cells: Functionally distinct lymphocytes that secrete IgM autoantibodies. *Proc Natl Acad Sci U S A* 81:2494, 1984.
42. Sthoeger ZM, Wakai M, Tse DB, et al: Production of autoantibodies by CD5-expressing B lymphocytes from patients with chronic lymphocytic leukemia. *J Exp Med* 169:255, 1989.
43. Anderson KC, Park EK, Bates MP, et al: Antigens on human plasma cells identified by monoclonal antibodies. *J Immunol* 130:1132, 1983.
44. Rawstron AC, Orfao A, Beksac M, et al: Report of the European Myeloma Network on multiparametric flow cytometry in multiple myeloma and related disorders. *Haematologica* 93:431, 2008.
45. Keegan AD, Paul WE: Multichain immune recognition receptors: Similarities in structure and signaling pathways. *Immunol Today* 13:63, 1992.
46. Maddon PJ, Littman DR, Godfrey M, et al: The isolation and nucleotide sequence of a cDNA encoding the T cell surface protein T4: A new member of the immunoglobulin gene family. *Cell* 42:93, 1985.
47. Snow PM, Terhorst C: The T8 antigen is a multimeric complex of two distinct subunits on human thymocytes but consists of homomultimeric forms on peripheral blood T lymphocytes. *J Biol Chem* 258:14675, 1983.
48. Roncador G, Garcia JF, Maestre L, et al: FOXP3, a selective marker for a subset of adult T-cell leukaemia/lymphoma. *Leukemia* 19:2247, 2005.
49. Grogg KL, Attygalle AD, Macon WR, et al: Expression of CXCL13, a chemokine highly upregulated in germinal center T-helper cells, distinguishes angioimmunoblastic T-cell lymphoma from peripheral T-cell lymphoma, unspecified. *Mod Pathol* 19:1101, 2006.
50. Timonen T, Saksela E: Isolation of human NK cells by density gradient centrifugation. *J Immunol Methods* 36:285, 1980.
51. Hercend T, Griffin JD, Bensussan A, et al: Generation of monoclonal antibodies to a human natural killer clone. Characterization of two natural killer-associated antigens, NKH1A and NKH2, expressed on subsets of large granular lymphocytes. *J Clin Invest* 75:932, 1985.
52. Lanier LL, Le AM, Phillips JH, et al: Subpopulations of human natural killer cells defined by expression of the Leu-7 (HNK-1) and Leu-11 (NK-15) antigens. *J Immunol* 131:1789, 1983.
53. Sakaguchi S, Sajaguchi N, Asano M, et al: Immunologic self-tolerance maintained by activated T cells expressing IL-2 receptor alpha-chains (CD25). Breakdown of a single mechanism of self-tolerance causes various autoimmune diseases. *J Immunol* 131:1789, 1983.
54. Maeda T, Yamada H, Nagamine R, et al: Involvement of CD4+, CD57+, T cells in the disease activity of rheumatoid arthritis. *Arthritis Rheum* 46:379, 2002.
55. Fontenot JD, Gavin MA, Rudensky AY: Foxp3 programs the development and function of CD4+CD25+ regulatory T cells. *Nat Immunol* 4:330, 2003.
56. Bjorkstrom NK, Gonzalez VD, Malmberg KJ, et al: Elevated numbers of Fc gamma RIIIA+ (CD16+) effector CD8 T cells with NK cell-like function in chronic hepatitis C virus infection. *J Immunol* 181:4219, 2008.
57. Chattopadhyay PK, Betts MR, Price DA, et al: The cytolytic enzymes granzyme A, granzyme B, and perforin: Expression patterns, cell distribution, and their relationship to cell maturity and bright CD57 expression. *J Leukoc Biol* 85:88, 2009.
58. Cooper MA, Fehniger TA, Caliguri MA: The biology of human natural killer-cell subsets. *Trends Immunol* 22:633, 2001.

CHAPTER 75

COMPOSITION AND BIOCHEMISTRY OF LYMPHOCYTES AND PLASMA CELLS

Thomas J. Kipps

SUMMARY

Mature lymphocytes can be divided into several functional types and subtypes. The major classes of lymphocytes are the T cells, B cells, and natural killer (NK) cells. T lymphocytes are derived from the thymus (see Chaps. 5 and 76) and are responsible for cell-mediated cytotoxic reactions and for delayed hypersensitivity responses (see Chap. 78). They also produce the cytokines that regulate immune responses and provide helper activity for B cells. B lymphocytes can concentrate and present antigens to T cells and are the precursors of immunoglobulin-secreting plasma cells (see Chap. 77). NK cells account for innate immunity against infectious agents and transformed cells that have altered expression of transplantation antigens (see Chap. 79). This chapter describes methods for isolating lymphocytes and discusses their physical and biochemical properties.

ISOLATION OF LYMPHOCYTES

LYMPHOCYTE DENSITY

Lymphocytes can be isolated from the blood using density gradient centrifugation. Most commonly, this is performed using a step gradient composed of a mixture of the carbohydrate polymer Ficoll and the dense iodine-containing compound sodium metrizoate.[1] This technique takes advantage of the low density of lymphocytes (1.07 g/mL) relative to that of erythrocytes (1.09–1.10 g/mL), granulocytes (1.08–1.09 g/mL), or monocytes (1.08 g/mL).

A Ficoll solution adjusted to a density of 1.077 g/mL is ideal for isolating human lymphocytes. Whole blood is layered onto a cushion of Ficoll-sodium metrizoate prior to centrifugation at 400g for 30 minutes. The denser red blood cells and granulocytes will sediment to the bottom of the tube, and the monocytes will enter into the Ficoll cushion. The lymphocytes can be collected from the interface formed between the Ficoll–sodium metrizoate cushion and the plasma above, which contains the lighter-density platelets (1.04–1.06 g/mL). This layer contains lymphocytes and some monocytes, which can be removed by plating the cells in culture flasks and harvesting the lymphocytes that are not adherent to plastic.

Acronyms and abbreviations that appear in this chapter include: ADAM, a disintegrin and a metalloprotease; ATP, adenosine 5′-triphosphate; Btk, Bruton tyrosine kinase; DHEA, dehydroepiandrosterone; DNA-PK, DNA-dependent protein kinase; DSBR, double-strand break repair; lck, leukocyte tyrosine kinase; NK, natural killer; RAG, recombination-activating gene; S1P, sphingosine 1-phosphate; TdT, terminal deoxynucleotidyl transferase; ZAP-70, zeta-associated protein of 70 kDa.

LYMPHOCYTE SURFACE ANTIGENS

Lymphocyte subsets generally cannot be distinguished from one another by morphology. Most resting lymphocytes appear as small round cells with a dense nucleus and little cytoplasm (see Chap. 74). However, this homogeneous appearance is deceptive, as these cells comprise many functionally distinct subpopulations.

These subsets can be distinguished through the differential expression of cell-surface proteins, each of which can be recognized by a specific monoclonal antibody (see Chap. 15). Coupled with the biochemical analyses of the surface molecules that are recognized by these each of these antibodies, many lymphocyte surface antigens have been defined.

Typically, it is necessary to monitor for coexpression of two or more cell-surface proteins to define a functional subset of lymphocytes. The same cell-surface protein is often expressed by more than one cell subset. For example, both helper and cytotoxic T cells express CD3, the proteins associated with the T-cell receptor for antigen (see Chap. 78). Expression of both CD3 and CD4 helps to distinguish mature helper T cells from cytotoxic T cells that express CD3 and CD8, and from other cells, such as dendritic cells, that express CD4 but lack expression of CD3 (see Chap. 78). Another subset of T cells that regulates the activation of other T cells and is necessary to maintain peripheral tolerance to self-antigens (sometimes referred to "T_{reg} cells") is defined by the coexpression of CD3, CD4, CD25; the low affinity receptor for interleukin-2; and the transcription factor forkhead box P3 (FoxP3).[2] For these and other types of lymphocytes, it is the expression of a characteristic constellation of surface and cytoplasmic molecules, rather than the expression of any one particular marker, that generally helps to distinguish one subset of lymphocytes from another (see Chap. 15).

Fluorescent probes also can be used to identify antigen-specific-lymphocytes.[3] Each clone of B lymphocytes expresses immunoglobulin capable of binding a particular antigen (see Chap. 77). The frequencies of B cells specific for one antigen are estimated to range from 1 in 100,000 to 1,000,000 cells or less. Populations of lymphocytes enriched for B cells binding to a specific antigen can be stained using antigen coupled to probes, allowing for the detection and isolation of antigen-specific B cells using flow cytometry.[4] Alternatively, flow-based techniques can be used to monitor for antigen-specific B cells that are activated by contact with antigen.[5] T lymphocytes, however, generally recognize antigen in the form of peptides nestled into molecules of the major histocompatibility complex (see Chap. 78). Thus identification and isolation of antigen-specific T cells require more complex probes using multimeric complexes comprised of specific peptide antigen complexed with the relevant major histocompatibility complex molecule.[3]

Flow Cytometry

The flow cytometer is a highly effective tool for defining these lymphocyte subsets. This instrument is based on the principle of fluorescence, or the emission of light resulting from the release of energy gained through the absorption of light at a different wavelength. Monoclonal antibodies specific for desired cell-surface proteins can each be coupled to a fluorescent dye, called a fluorochrome, that will fluoresce with a defined spectrum of light when excited by light at a certain wavelength.[6] The flow cytometer can detect cells labeled with such fluorochrome-conjugated antibodies as they pass in a liquid stream through a beam of laser light of defined wavelength. As each cell passes through the laser beam, the laser light is scattered and excites any dye molecules bound to the cell, causing it to fluoresce. Sensitive photomultiplier tubes can detect the scattered light and the fluorescence emissions, respectively, providing information on each cell's granularity and extent to which it bound a given fluorescence dye. This is the most common means used for distinguishing the lymphocyte subsets from one another.

The flow cytometer also can be used to isolate lymphocytes that express selected surface antigens. This requires a fluorescence-activated cell sorter. With this instrument, the fluorescence signals of cells passing through the laser light are passed back to a computer. This, in turn, triggers an electric charge that passes from the nozzle through the liquid stream at the precise time the stream is breaking up into droplets containing the desired cell.[7] Such droplets have a positive or negative charge, allowing for their deflection from the main stream of droplets as they pass between plates of opposite charge. In this way, two different subsets of cells can be isolated from each other and from the unsorted cells in nondeflected droplets.

In addition, the flow cytometer can be used to monitor for lymphocyte cell division[8] and/or to identify lymphocyte subsets that produce specific cytokines[3] or that express specific intracellular proteins or enzymes.[9] Using monoclonal antibodies specific for particular phosphoproteins, flow cytometry also can be used to monitor the biochemical events that occur within lymphocytes that are stimulated with antigen or by crosslinking one or more surface receptor molecules.[10,11] The advent of these new technologies should allow for better understanding how different lymphocyte subpopulation respond to various microenvironmental signals that occur during the immune response to antigen (see Chap. 78).

Other Separation Techniques

An effective way of isolating lymphocyte subpopulations is to expose them to paramagnetic beads coated with a monoclonal antibody specific for a surface molecule that is differentially expressed by the desired versus undesired cell subpopulation.[12,13] The tube of cells then is placed in a strong magnetic field, thereby attracting the cells that are attached to the beads. The cells attached to the beads are retained, allowing for decanting of the cells that lack the specific surface molecule. The decanted cells lacking the surface molecule are designated as being isolated via negative selection. Bead-bound cells can be harvested and released from the magnetic beads by adding an antibody that reacts with the antibody attached to the magnetic beads, thereby displacing the cells that are bound to the magnetic-bound antibody. The released cells are said to have been isolated via positive selection.

Lymphocyte subsets also can be isolated by binding the cells to plates that are coated with antibodies to a selected surface antigen or with selected surface proteins,[14] a technique known as panning. Alternatively, cells binding a specific complement-fixing antibody can be lysed with complement,[15] leaving behind those cells that lack expression of the targeted surface antigen. All these techniques can be used to enrich for a selected cell subset or to deplete an undesired subset, prior to sorting using the fluorescence-activated cell sorter.

COMPOSITION OF LYMPHOCYTES

Unfortunately, few studies of the composition and biochemistry of lymphocytes have used purified lymphocyte subpopulations. Because mature helper T cells are the predominant blood lymphocyte of normal adults, many reported biochemical parameters are most relevant to this subpopulation.

■ ION AND WATER CONTENT

The resting blood lymphocyte has a mean cell volume of 200 μm^3 and contains 71 ± 1.2 percent by weight of water.[16] The total lymphocyte cation content is 35 femtomole per cell, of which 22 to 28 femtomole per cell is potassium, and 7.9 ± 3.2 femtomole per cell is sodium.[17] Lymphocyte membranes have both voltage-gated and calcium-activated potassium channels that regulate cell volume. Pharmacologic inhibition of these channels blocks T-cell activation. The calcium content of resting lymphocytes has been estimated at 580 to 800 pmol/10^6 cells.[18] Cytosolic free calcium concentrations are relatively low in resting lymphocytes (approximately 0.1 μM) but increase severalfold after activation.[19]

■ LYMPHOCYTE MEMBRANE

The lymphocyte plasma membrane is composed of equal parts of weight of protein and glycosphingolipids and 6 percent by weight of carbohydrate.[20] The molar ratio of cholesterol to phospholipid is approximately 0.5.[21,22] Phosphatidylcholine is the predominant phospholipid in the lymphocyte plasma membrane, but phosphatidylethanolamine, phosphatidylinositol, phosphatidylserine, and sphingomyelin are also present. Approximately half the membrane fatty acids are saturated. The membrane proteins are usually glycosylated.

The glycosphingolipids and protein receptors of lymphocytes often are organized in glycolipoprotein microdomains termed *lipid rafts*.[23,24] Such lipid rafts sequester various protein receptors, coreceptors, and accessory molecules that together are involved in lymphocyte cell signaling, cytoskeletal reorganization, and/or membrane trafficking.[25] As such, the surface molecules on lymphocytes are not randomly distributed.

Extracellular Membrane-Associated Enzymes (Ectoenzymes)

Exposed on the exterior surface of lymphocytes are several enzymes called ectoenzymes (Table 75–1). Generally, the number of surface enzyme molecules is low compared with that of other surface molecules, such as those involved in lymphocyte adhesion (see Chap. 15). This probably reflects the fact that these molecules are catalytic and have a higher functional specific activity than do molecules involved in adhesion events, where multiple interactions over large surface areas are required. As such, it is possible that many more enzymes are present than the ones currently recognized because they are expressed at levels that are not detectable by conventional methods using monoclonal antibodies and flow cytometry.

Some of the surface enzymes are involved in nucleotide metabolism (see Table 75–1). For example, CD73 is an ecto-5′-nucleotidase that catalyzes the 5′ dephosphorylation of purine and pyrimidine ribo- and deoxyribonucleoside monophosphates to nucleosides that can be taken up by transport systems.[26] This ecto-5′-nucleotidase is attached to the plasma membrane by a glycerol phosphatidylinositol anchor (see Chap. 15). In addition, lymphocytes express CD26,[27] which is a membrane protein that can associate with adenosine deaminase, the levels of which are increased after activation.[28] The shedding of adenosine deaminase by stimulated cells may explain why plasma levels of this enzyme are increased in early HIV infection and in other diseases associated with immune activation.[29]

The ectoenzymes of nucleotide metabolism may regulate lymphocyte and granulocyte function at sites of inflammation. Activated T lymphocytes can release adenosine 5′-triphosphate (ATP), which, in turn, can bind to specific plasma membrane ATP receptors.[30] In addition, CD38 can catalyze the transient formation of cyclic adenosine 5′-diphosphate-ribose, a new second-messenger molecule directly involved in the control of calcium homeostasis by means of receptor-mediated release of calcium from ryanodine-sensitive intracellular stores.[31] The consequent increase in calcium mobilization and phospholipid breakdown can provoke activation or death, depending on the target cell. Subsequently, the dephosphorylation of ATP generates adenosine, which can interact with A2 receptors on the plasma membranes of neutrophils, monocytes, and lymphocytes.[32] The engagement of A2 receptors elevates adenosine 3′,5′-cyclic phosphate levels, counteracting the effects of ATP on cell activation. The deamination of adenosine permits the cycle to begin anew.

TABLE 75–1. Ectoenzymes Expressed by Lymphocytes

Surface Molecule	Enzymatic Activity	Function	Reference
CD10	Neutral endopeptidase, EC 3.4.24.11	Metalloproteinase that may also play a role in the metabolic stability of glucagon-like peptide-1	33
CD13	Aminopeptidase N, EC 3.4.11.2	Aminopeptidase involved in trimming peptides bound to major histocompatibility complex class II molecules and cleaving macrophage inflammatory protein (MIP)-1 chemokine to alter target cell specificity. Also served as Rc for coronavirus	102
CD26	Dipeptidylpeptidase IV, EC 3.4.14.5	Serine peptidase that may be involved in T cell signaling and T cell activation	34
CD38	ADP-ribosyl cyclase, EC 3.4.14.5	Ectoenzyme with NAD glycohydrolase, ADP ribosyl cyclase, and cyclic ADP ribose hydrolase activities	31
CD39	Ecto (Ca2+, Mg2+)-apyrase (ecto-ATPase)	Ectoenzyme with ADPase and ATPase activities that plays a role in regulating platelet aggregation	103
CD73	Ecto-5′-nucleotidase	Ecto-5′-nucleotidase that may play a role in T-cell signaling	26
CD143	Peptidyl-dipeptide hydrolase (angiotensin-converting enzyme)	Peptidyl-dipeptide hydrolase that is involved in the metabolism of vasoactive peptides angiotensin II and bradykinin	104
CD156a	ADAM8 metalloprotease	Matrix metalloprotease that may play a role in leukocyte extravasation	35
CD156b	ADAM17 metalloprotease	Metalloprotease that cleaves membrane-bound tumor necrosis factor and transforming growth factor-α to release the soluble cytokine	36
CD157	ADP ribosyl cyclase and cyclic ADP ribose hydrolase	ADP ribosyl cyclase and cyclic ADP ribose hydrolase that may play a role in lymphocyte development. Like CD38, this enzyme also is involved in the metabolism of NAD	105
CD224	γ-Glutamyl transpeptidase, EC2.3.2.2	γ-Glutamyl transpeptidase role in γ-glutamyl cycle involving the degradation and neosynthesis of glutathione	106

ADAM, a disintegrin and a metalloprotease; ADP, adenosine 5′-diphosphate; ADPase, adenosine 5′-diphosphatase; ATPase, adenosine 5′-triphosphate; NAD, nicotinamide adenine dinucleotide.

The ectodomains of several other surface antigens can possess proteolytic activity. For example, CD10 (or CALLA) also has neutral endopeptidase activity,[33] and CD26 has dipeptidyl peptidase IV activity.[34] These enzymes may play a role in modulating the binding of lymphocytes to other cells and to the extracellular matrix. In addition, inhibition of the catalytic activity of CD26 can provoke many cellular effects, including induction of tyrosine phosphorylation and p38 mitogen-activated protein kinase activation, as well as suppression of DNA synthesis and reduced production of various cytokines. As such, these ectoenzymes could play an important role in lymphocyte activation.

Some membrane-bound proteases have a disintegrin and a metalloprotease domain, termed ADAM (a disintegrin and a metalloprotease).[35] One such member of this family of proteins is the tumor necrosis factor-α converting enzyme, otherwise known as ADAM17 (CD156b).[36] These enzymes cleave other surface molecules, such as tumor necrosis factor, thereby releasing the soluble active cytokine. In addition, they may play an important role in modifying the activity of cytokines or other cell-surface molecules that are present in the vicinity of the plasma membrane.

Intracellular Membrane-Associated Enzymes

Transmembrane proteins that have cytoplasmic regions with kinase or phosphatase activities are common in biology although relatively few of these are restricted to lymphocytes. Nevertheless, many cytoplasmic domains of transmembrane proteins interact directly with enzymes that are restricted or preferentially expressed by lymphocytes or lymphocyte subsets (see Chaps. 76 and 77). B lymphocytes, for example, selectively express Bruton tyrosine kinase (Btk), a tyrosine kinase that plays a critical role in signal transduction via surface immunoglobulin receptors.[37] Moreover, mutations that disrupt the function of such kinases can impair B-cell development, leading to dysregulated B-cell function or immune deficiency.[38] On the other hand, T-cell development and function rely heavily on cytoplasmic receptor-associated tyrosine kinases, such as the zeta-associated protein of 70 kDa (ZAP-70), leukocyte tyrosine kinase (lck), or fyn. ZAP-70 interacts with the ζ-chain (CD247) of the T-cell receptor for antigen,[39] whereas the latter enzymes, lck and fyn, are Src family tyrosine kinases that interact with cytoplasmic domains of various accessory molecules, including CD2, CD4, CD8, CD44, CD50, and/or CD137.[40] Through such interactions, these receptor protein tyrosine kinases play important roles in signal transduction following immune recognition and/or cognate intercellular immune interactions.

In addition, lymphocytes possess an important class of intracellular molecules, known collectively as adapter proteins, that have no intrinsic enzymatic activity.[41] These adaptor proteins can serve as a scaffolding for the assembly of kinases and other signaling molecules following antigen-receptor ligation. One important adaptor protein expressed in B lymphocytes is B-cell linker protein (BLNK; see Chap. 77).[42] On the other hand, T cells use a distinct adaptor protein called linker for activation of T cells (LAT).[43] These molecules couple proximal biochemical events initiated by surface-receptor ligation with more distal signaling pathways by recruiting other cytosolic proteins (see Chaps. 77 and 78).

CYTOPLASMIC STRUCTURES

■ CYTOMATRIX

Beneath the lymphocyte's plasma membrane is a fully developed cytomatrix with several different structural and mechanical proteins, including tubulin, actin, myosin, tropomyosin, α-actinin, filamin, and a spectrin-like molecule, which are important in the formation of the immunologic synapse that forms during cognate intercellular interactions.[44] These are arranged into typical microfilaments, microtubules, and intermediate filaments. Lymphocyte activation by antigens or mitogens can lead to changes in the interaction of membrane components with the cytoskeleton, allowing for antigen processing, immunoglobulin secretion, or cell-mediated cytotoxic reactions.[45]

■ ORGANELLES

In large part the composition and metabolism of long-lived blood T lymphocytes reflect their resting state. The T cells have a high nuclear-to-cytoplasmic ratio, few ribosomes or mitochondria, and scant endoplasmic reticulum. Glycogen stores are meager. The DNA content of the resting small lymphocyte, 8 pg per cell, is the same amount in other diploid cells. In contrast, the RNA content averages 2.5 pg per cell, yielding an RNA-to-DNA ratio of approximately 0.32.[46] This value is less than in most other human cells, as a result of the small amount of ribosomal RNA in most lymphocytes.

In contrast to most lymphocytes, however, plasma cells have a high RNA-to-DNA ratio. These cells are the end products of B-cell differentiation and are committed to the synthesis, assembly, and secretion of immunoglobulin. Accordingly, these cells have a well-developed rough endoplasmic reticulum and Golgi apparatus, but lack many of the surface receptors found on most lymphocytes. Mature plasma cells are probably terminally differentiated and have a low rate of DNA synthesis and abundant RNA, reflecting the plasma cell's high-level synthesis of immunoglobulin protein.

Lysosomes

The few lysosomes in blood lymphocytes contain several different acid hydrolases including acid phosphatase, β-glucuronidase, β-galactosidase, β-hexosaminidase, α-arabinosidase, α-galactosidase, α-mannosidase, α-glucosidase, and β-glucosidase.[47–49] Acid hydrolase activities are generally higher in T cells than in non-T lymphocytes. Lysosomal acid esterase, assayed histochemically with α-naphthyl acetate as substrate, has a characteristic punctate appearance in mature T lymphocytes.[50] Secretory lysosomes are specialized organelles that combine catabolic functions of conventional lysosomes with the capacity to be secreted upon induction.[51] An example of such secretory lysosomes are the specialized cytoplasmic granules of T cells and natural killer (NK) cells that are responsible for the cytotoxic effector function of these cells.

Cytoplasmic Granules

In contrast to other lymphocytes, cytotoxic T lymphocytes and NK cells possess abundant cytoplasmic granules. These contain a pore-forming proteolytic enzyme, termed perforin, and a series of serine proteinases with specific proapoptotic activity, called granzymes.[52] To protect against possible autolysis by granule contents, cytotoxic lymphocytes possess serine-proteinase inhibitors, termed *serpins*.[53] As an additional safeguard, the granzymes of resting lymphocytes are stored as inactive proenzymes.

Cytotoxic lymphocytes rely primarily on the perforin/granzyme system to kill their targets.[54] Upon contact with its target cell, the cytotoxic lymphocyte converts the granzymes into active forms by a lysosomal cysteine protease called dipeptidyl peptidase I.[55] Then perforin introduces a pore in the membrane, allowing the activated granzymes and other granule contents to pass into the cytoplasm and then the nucleus of the cell targeted for destruction.[52] *In vitro* studies indicate that granzyme nuclear import is independent of ATP, cannot be inhibited by nonhydrolyzable guanosine triphosphate analogues, and involves binding within the nucleus, unlike conventional signal-dependent nuclear protein import. The perforin-dependent nuclear entry of granzymes precedes the nuclear events of apoptosis, such as DNA fragmentation and breakdown of the nuclear envelope (see Chap. 12).

LYMPHOCYTE METABOLISM

■ FATTY ACID AND LIPID SYNTHESIS

Normal lymphocytes synthesize phospholipids from acetate. The cells contain phospholipases A_1, A_2, C, and D, and the enzymes of the inositol phosphate metabolic cycle.[56,57]

In contrast to monocytes, small lymphocytes probably do not synthesize prostaglandins or leukotrienes; however, small lymphocytes may contain prostaglandin receptors. Prostaglandins synthesized by macrophages inhibit lymphocyte function and may be partially responsible for the impaired immunity associated with chronic inflammatory states, such as in Hodgkin lymphoma or systemic fungal infections.[58] Certain natural fatty acid precursors of prostaglandins, such as γ-linoleic acid, suppress immune function, and may be useful for the treatment of autoimmune disorders.[59] However, some prostaglandins may facilitate immunoglobulin class switching and synthesis of selected cytokines or cytokine receptors.[60]

■ CARBOHYDRATE METABOLISM

Quiescent blood lymphocytes have few or no insulin receptors, although these appear following activation. The rate of glucose metabolism is limited by the rate of entry of glucose into the cells by facilitated diffusion. Lymphocytes contain all the enzymes of the glycolytic pathway and the tricarboxylic acid cycle. Although resting lymphocytes consume only small amounts of oxygen *in vitro*, their mitochondria have typically coupled electron transport chains.

The resting lymphocyte requires energy to maintain its ionic milieu, to replace degraded proteins and lipids, and for active locomotion.[61] The recirculation of long-lived lymphocytes through the vascular space to the interstitial tissues and back from the lymphatic drainage system requires directed cell movement and utilizes considerable amounts of ATP. Lymphocytes treated with nonlethal concentrations of drugs that specifically inhibit mitochondrial respiration, but not with agents that inhibit glycolysis, recirculate sluggishly. This suggests that the energy for lymphocyte locomotion is derived largely from oxidative phosphorylation.

The enzymes of the pentose-phosphate pathway account for only a small fraction of energy production in resting lymphocytes.[62] As in other cell types, the pathway provides lymphocytes with phosphorylated ribose derivatives necessary for purine and pyrimidine synthesis and with a source of reducing energy in the form of nicotinamide adenine dinucleotide phosphate.

■ PROTEIN SYNTHESIS AND AMINO ACID METABOLISM

Human blood lymphocytes actively incorporate radioactive amino acids into protein. The protein synthesis is necessary for survival, and inhibition with cycloheximide or puromycin leads to the rapid death of lymphocytes.

The metabolic pathways for the synthesis of two normally nonessential amino acids, L-cysteine and L-asparagine, are inadequate in thymic lymphocytes, and probably in blood T cells.[63] A similar L-asparagine requirement among NK-cell and T-cell leukemias is responsible for the L-asparaginase sensitivity of these neoplasms.[64]

NUCLEIC ACID SYNTHESIS AND REPAIR

Nucleotide Metabolism

The enzymes for the early pathways of *de novo* purine and pyrimidine synthesis have very low activity in blood lymphocytes, consistent with the small nucleotide requirements of these nondividing cells. The lymphocytes also have minimal ribonucleotide reductase activity and a concomitantly low rate of deoxyribonucleotide synthesis. In contrast, enzymes for purine and pyrimidine intraconversion are easily detectable, with the exception of xanthine oxidase and guanase, which are absent in lymphocytes. The lymphocytes have the capacity to utilize preformed purines and pyrimidines in the plasma, when these are available. However, patients with genetic deficiencies of the purine salvage enzymes hypoxanthine-guanine phosphoribosyltransferase (the Lesch-Nyhan syndrome) and adenine phosphoribosyltransferase have normal numbers of lymphocytes and adequate immune function. Hence, the purine salvage pathways are not absolutely necessary for lymphocyte survival.

Genetic deficiencies in two enzymes of purine metabolism, adenosine deaminase and purine nucleoside phosphorylase, are associated with a specific impairment of the development and function of the lymphoid system.[65] The primary function of these enzymes is the catabolism of the potentially toxic nucleosides deoxyadenosine and deoxyguanosine. In adenosine deaminase- and purine nucleoside phosphorylase-deficient patients, phosphorylated derivatives of deoxyadenosine and deoxyguanosine may accumulate in lymphocytes. When compared with other cell types, the lymphocytes have high levels of deoxycytidine kinase, for which the purine deoxyribonucleosides are alternative substrates, and low levels of cytoplasmic deoxynucleotidase.

DNA Repair

In addition to several double-strand break repair (DSBR) enzymes that are found in other cell types, T and B lymphocytes express lymphoid-specific enzymes that are required for the rearrangement of the immunoglobulin (Ig) and T-cell receptor (TCR) genes (see Chaps. 77 and 78). In particular, two proteins, encoded by recombination-activating gene 1 (*RAG-1*) and recombination-activating gene 2 (*RAG-2*), form a tetrameric complex that plays a critical role in Ig and TCR gene rearrangement.[66] The Rag-1 protein acts on the DNA sequence in a manner similar to that of a restriction endonuclease, but only when complexed with the Rag-2 protein (see Chaps. 77 and 78). The Rag-1 protein makes a nick on one DNA strand located between a heptamer recognition sequence and the coding segments of the Ig or TCR that are brought together for recombination. This releases a 3′OH end that attacks the other strand to form a covalent hairpin, thereby completing a double-strand DNA break.[67] The Rag-2 protein, on the other hand, apparently helps bind the Rag-1/Rag-2 tetramer to other proteins, including proteins that "open" receptor gene loci at specific stages of lymphocyte development. The Rag-1/Rag-2 tetramer also holds together the gene segments that are acted upon by Rag-1 and that eventually are joined together to form the rearranged gene encoding the mature Ig or TCR gene (see Chaps. 77 and 78). Mice made genetically deficient in either of these enzymes underscore the importance of these genes in lymphocyte development. Such animals fail to produce Ig or TCR proteins and thus lack mature B and T lymphocytes.

Other enzymes are involved in the process of nonhomologous end joining that mediates DSBR during the process of Ig or TCR gene rearrangement. Ku70 and Ku80 are two DNA end-binding proteins that bind to double-strand DNA breaks and recruit the catalytic subunit of DNA-dependent protein kinase (DNA-PK), which is a double-stranded DNA repair enzyme that phosphorylates and activates another endonuclease called Artemis.[68,69] Artemis opens up the hairpins formed by the activity of Rag-1,[70] allowing the double-strand breaks to be repaired by DNA ligase IV,[71] which functions together with the human protein X-ray repair complementing defective repair in Chinese hamster cells 4 (XRCC4).[72] Mice with the severe combined immunodeficiency (SCID) were found to have a deficiency in DNA-PK,[73] which precluded their capacity to repair the DNA strand breaks formed during the process of Ig or TCR gene rearrangement. Consequently, these animals fail to develop mature T or B cells. Similarly, inactivating mutations in Artemis also can impair the capacity to rearrange Ig and TCR genes, resulting also in impaired T- and B-cell development and SCID.[68] Partial deficiency in Artemis or *RAG-1* or *-2* can lead to a leaky severe combined immune deficiency syndrome, called Omenn syndrome, characterized by enlarged lymphoid tissue and thymus and recurrent viral or fungal pneumonias, chronic diarrhea, and failure to thrive.[74]

Another lymphoid-specific enzyme is terminal deoxynucleotidyl transferase (TdT). TdT acts downstream of the Rag proteins, adding nontemplated nucleotides to the junctions between the gene segments prior to completion of DSBR.[75] TdT acts principally on the gene segments that encode the antigen-binding sites of the Ig or TCR. The activity of this enzyme increases the diversity of Ig or TCR that can be generated, thereby enhancing our repertoire of receptors for antigens (see Chaps. 77 and 78). Similarly, the enzyme activation-induced cytidine deaminase plays a critical role in Ig class switch recombination and Ig somatic mutation.[76] The latter process introduces changes in the amino acid sequence encoding the antigen-binding portion of the Ig molecule and thereby plays an important role in enhancing the diversity of the Ig repertoire for antigens (see Chap. 77).[77]

HORMONES AND VITAMINS

Lymphocytes have receptors for several biologically active peptides, including adrenocorticotropic hormone, corticotrophin-releasing hormone, calcitonin, calcitonin–gene-related peptide, melatonin, endorphins, enkephalins, vasopressin, oxytoxin, thyrotropin, the tachykinins, bombesin, prolactin, growth hormone, prolactin, somatostatin, vasoactive intestinal peptide, sphingosine 1-phosphate (S1P), and chemokines.[78–84] The various neuropeptides can deliver both positive and negative activation signals to lymphocytes,[81] helping to mediate communication between the central nervous system and the immune system. Chemokines are responsible for lymphocyte trafficking to and through lymphoid tissues, helping to organize lymphoid tissues into functional compartments of interacting cells.[82–85] On the other hand, lymphocyte receptors for S1P are involved in orchestrating the egress of T cells and B cells from lymphoid organs.[83]

Lymphocyte activation and proliferation require enhanced cell metabolism, leading to an increased requirement for cofactors required for DNA and protein synthesis. For example, proliferating lymphocytes generally increase biotin uptake presumably to provide adequate coenzyme for biotin-dependent carboxylases.[86] Also, the receptor density for peptide hormones on lymphocytes generally increases markedly following activation of the cells. Furthermore, vitamins A and D are implicated in modulating a broad range of immune functions, such as lymphocyte activation and proliferation, helper T-cell differentiation, tissue-specific lymphocyte trafficking, production of specific antibody isotypes, and regulation of the immune response.[87,88]

Glucocorticoids are also potent immunosuppressive agents. This effect appears partially as a result of their capacity to regulate the expression and function of annexin A_1 (also known as lipocortin I)[89] and to inhibit TCR signaling and release of cytokines, such as interleukin-2.[90,91] At physiologic concentrations, glucocorticoids can direct and enhance immune function by interacting with the high-affinity glucocorticoid receptors of mature lymphocytes.[92] At pharmacologic concentrations, glucocorticoids have a unique lympholytic effect that is not dependent upon cell division. Exposure of lymphocytes to high concentrations of glucocorticoids causes endonuclease activation and DNA fragmentation.[90,93] Among normal lymphocyte subsets, immature T cells in the thymus are most sensitive.

Lymphocytes presumably also have receptors for androgens and estrogens. Androgens can modulate cytokine production and immune function[94,95] and indirectly act to accelerate thymocyte apoptosis.[96] Medical castration reduces the percentage of regulatory CD4+ CD25+ T cells and decreases mitogen-induced expression of interferon-γ by CD8+ T cells.[97] Estrogen, on the other hand, can affect mature CD4 T-cell production of proinflammatory cytokines.[98] The incidence of many autoimmune diseases is higher in females than in males. Androgen therapy may benefit some women with systemic lupus erythematosus, but frequently causes unacceptable masculinizing side effects.

The natural adrenal glucocorticoid dehydroepiandrosterone (DHEA) stimulates lymphocyte function in aged rodents, in part by reversing age-associated decreases in the receptor for activated C kinase.[99] Plasma levels of DHEA decline with age.[100] Whether DHEA supplementation can enhance immune responses in aged humans is still not known.[101]

REFERENCES

1. Bøyum A: Isolation of mononuclear cells and granulocytes from human blood. Isolation of mononuclear cells by one centrifugation, and of granulocytes by combining centrifugation and sedimentation at 1 g. *Scand J Clin Lab Invest Suppl* 97:77, 1968.
2. Sakaguchi S, Yamaguchi T, Nomura T, Ono M: Regulatory T cells and immune tolerance. *Cell* 133:775, 2008.
3. Thiel A, Scheffold A, Radbruch A: Antigen-specific cytometry—New tools arrived! *Clin Immunol* 111:155, 2004.
4. Kodituwakku AP, Jessup C, Zola H, Roberton DM: Isolation of antigen-specific B cells. *Immunol Cell Biol* 81:163, 2003.
5. Kinoshita K, Ozawa T, Tajiri K, et al: Identification of antigen-specific B cells by concurrent monitoring of intracellular Ca(2+) mobilization and antigen binding with microwell array chip system equipped with a CCD imager. *Cytometry A* 75:682, 2009.
6. Wood B: 9-color and 10-color flow cytometry in the clinical laboratory. *Arch Pathol Lab Med* 130:680, 2006.
7. Orfao A, Ruiz-Arguelles A: General concepts about cell sorting techniques. *Clin Biochem* 29:5, 1996.
8. Lyons AB: Analysing cell division *in vivo* and *in vitro* using flow cytometric measurement of CFSE dye dilution. *J Immunol Methods* 243:147, 2000.
9. Francis C, Connelly MC: Rapid single-step method for flow cytometric detection of surface and intracellular antigens using whole blood. *Cytometry* 25:58, 1996.
10. Krutzik PO, Irish JM, Nolan GP, Perez OD: Analysis of protein phosphorylation and cellular signaling events by flow cytometry: Techniques and clinical applications. *Clin Immunol* 110:206, 2004.
11. Krutzik PO, Crane JM, Clutter MR, Nolan GP: High-content single-cell drug screening with phosphospecific flow cytometry. *Nat Chem Biol* 4:132, 2008.
12. Thiel A, Scheffold A, Radbruch A: Immunomagnetic cell sorting—Pushing the limits. *Immunotechnology* 4:89, 1998.
13. Thornton AM: Fractionation of T and B cells using magnetic beads. *Curr Protoc Immunol* Chapter 3:Unit 3.5A, 2003.
14. Sekine K, Revzin A, Tompkins RG, Toner M: Panning of multiple subsets of leukocytes on antibody-decorated poly(ethylene) glycol-coated glass slides. *J Immunol Methods* 313:96, 2006.
15. Kanof ME: Purification of T cell subpopulations. *Curr Protoc Immunol* Chapter 7:Unit 7.3, 2001.
16. Segel GB, Cokelet GR, Lichtman MA: The measurement of lymphocyte volume: Importance of reference particle deformability and counting solution tonicity. *Blood* 57:894, 1981.
17. Segel GB, Simon W, Lichtman MA: Regulation of sodium and potassium transport in phytohemagglutinin-stimulated human blood lymphocytes. *J Clin Invest* 64:834, 1979.
18. Lichtman AH, Segel GB, Lichtman MA: An ultrasensitive method for the measurement of human leukocyte calcium: Lymphocytes. *Clin Chim Acta* 97:107, 1979.
19. Komada H, Nakabayashi H, Nakano H, et al: Measurement of the cytosolic free calcium ion concentration of individual lymphocytes by microfluorometry using quin 2 or fura-2. *Cell Struct Funct* 14:141, 1989.
20. Crumpton MJ, Snary D: Preparation and properties of lymphocyte plasma membrane. *Contemp Top Mol Immunol* 3:27, 1974.
21. Goppelt M, Eichhorn R, Krebs G, Resch K: Lipid composition of functional domains of the lymphocyte plasma membrane. *Biochim Biophys Acta* 854:184, 1986.
22. Johnson SM, Robinson R: The composition and fluidity of normal and leukaemic or lymphomatous lymphocyte plasma membranes in mouse and man. *Biochim Biophys Acta* 558:282, 1979.
23. Jury EC, Flores-Borja F, Kabouridis PS: Lipid rafts in T cell signalling and disease. *Semin Cell Dev Biol* 18:608, 2007.
24. Gupta N, DeFranco AL: Lipid rafts and B cell signaling. *Semin Cell Dev Biol* 18:616, 2007.
25. Landry A, Xavier R: Isolation and analysis of lipid rafts in cell-cell interactions. *Methods Mol Biol* 341:251, 2006.
26. Colgan SP, Eltzschig HK, Eckle T, Thompson LF: Physiological roles for ecto-5′-nucleotidase (CD73). *Purinergic Signal* 2:351, 2006.
27. Havre PA, Abe M, Urasaki Y, et al: The role of CD26/dipeptidyl peptidase IV in cancer. *Front Biosci* 13:1634, 2008.
28. Kameoka J, Tanaka T, Nojima Y, et al: Direct association of adenosine deaminase with a T cell activation antigen, CD26. *Science* 261:466, 1993.
29. Ohtsuki T, Tsuda H, Morimoto C: Good or evil: CD26 and HIV infection. *J Dermatol Sci* 22:152, 2000.
30. Swennen EL, Coolen EJ, Arts IC, et al: Time-dependent effects of ATP and its degradation products on inflammatory markers in human blood *ex vivo*. *Immunobiology* 213:389, 2008.
31. Partida-Sanchez S, Rivero-Nava L, Shi G, Lund FE: CD38: An ecto-enzyme at the crossroads of innate and adaptive immune responses. *Adv Exp Med Biol* 590:171, 2007.
32. Kumar V, Sharma A: Adenosine: An endogenous modulator of innate immune system with therapeutic potential. *Eur J Pharmacol* 616:7, 2009.
33. Plamboeck A, Holst JJ, Carr RD, Deacon CF: Neutral endopeptidase 24.11 and dipeptidyl peptidase IV are both involved in regulating the metabolic stability of glucagon-like peptide-1 *in vivo*. *Adv Exp Med Biol* 524:303, 2003.
34. Ohnuma K, Takahashi N, Yamochi T, et al: Role of CD26/dipeptidyl peptidase IV in human T cell activation and function. *Front Biosci* 13:2299, 2008.
35. Yamamoto S, Higuchi Y, Yoshiyama K, et al: ADAM family proteins in the immune system. *Immunol Today* 20:278, 1999.
36. Black RA: Tumor necrosis factor-alpha converting enzyme. *Int J Biochem Cell Biol* 34:1, 2002.
37. Lindvall JM, Blomberg KE, Valiaho J, et al: Bruton's tyrosine kinase: Cell biology, sequence conservation, mutation spectrum, siRNA modifications, and expression profiling. *Immunol Rev* 203:200, 2005.
38. Kurosaki T, Hikida M: Tyrosine kinases and their substrates in B lymphocytes. *Immunol Rev* 228:132, 2009.
39. Au-Yeung BB, Deindl S, Hsu LY, et al: The structure, regulation, and function of ZAP-70. *Immunol Rev* 228:41, 2009.
40. Salmond RJ, Filby A, Qureshi I, et al: T-cell receptor proximal signaling via the Src-family kinases, Lck and Fyn, influences T-cell activation, differentiation, and tolerance. *Immunol Rev* 228:9, 2009.
41. Leo A, Schraven B: Adapters in lymphocyte signalling. *Curr Opin Immunol* 13:307, 2001.
42. Tsukada S, Baba Y, Watanabe D: Btk and BLNK in B cell development. *Adv Immunol* 77:123, 2001.
43. Aguado E, Martinez-Florensa M, Aparicio P: Activation of T lymphocytes and the role of the adapter LAT. *Transpl Immunol* 17:23, 2006.
44. Rey M, Sanchez-Madrid F, Valenzuela-Fernandez A: The role of actomyosin and the microtubular network in both the immunological synapse and T cell activation. *Front Biosci* 12:437, 2007.
45. Miletic AV, Swat M, Fujikawa K, Swat W: Cytoskeletal remodeling in lymphocyte activation. *Curr Opin Immunol* 15:261, 2003.
46. Glen AC: Measurement of DNA and RNA in human peripheral blood lymphocytes. *Clin Chem* 13:299, 1967.
47. Beaumelle BD, Gibson A, Hopkins CR: Isolation and preliminary characterization of the major membrane boundaries of the endocytic pathway in lymphocytes. *J Cell Biol* 111:1811, 1990.
48. Casey TM, Meade JL, Hewitt EW: Organelle proteomics: Identification of the exocytic machinery associated with the natural killer cell secretory lysosome. *Mol Cell Proteomics* 6:767, 2007.
49. Qu P, Du H, Wilkes DS, Yan C: Critical roles of lysosomal acid lipase in T cell development and function. *Am J Pathol* 174:944, 2009.
50. Kulenkampff J, Janossy G, Greaves MF: Acid esterase in human lymphoid cells and leukaemic blasts: A marker for T lymphocytes. *Br J Haematol* 36:231, 1977.
51. Lettau M, Schmidt H, Kabelitz D, Janssen O: Secretory lysosomes and their cargo in T and NK cells. *Immunol Lett* 108:10, 2007.
52. Chavez-Galan L, Arenas-Del Angel MC, Zenteno E, et al: Cell death mechanisms induced by cytotoxic lymphocytes. *Cell Mol Immunol* 6:15, 2009.
53. Bots M, Medema JP: Serpins in T cell immunity. *J Leukoc Biol* 84:1238, 2008.
54. Trapani JA, Smyth MJ: Functional significance of the perforin/granzyme cell death pathway. *Nat Rev Immunol* 2:735, 2002.
55. Pham CT, Ley TJ: Dipeptidyl peptidase I is required for the processing and activation of granzymes A and B *in vivo*. *Proc Natl Acad Sci U S A* 96:8627, 1999.
56. Bonvini E, DeBell KE, Veri MC, et al: On the mechanism coupling phospholipase Cgamma1 to the B- and T-cell antigen receptors. *Adv Enzyme Regul* 43:245, 2003.
57. Wakelam MJ, Harnett MM: Phospholipase A2 (EC 3.1.1.4) and D (EC 3.1.4.4) signalling in lymphocytes. *Proc Nutr Soc* 57:551, 1998.
58. Brassard P, Larbi A, Grenier A, et al: Modulation of T-cell signalling by non-esterified fatty acids. *Prostaglandins Leukot Essent Fatty Acids* 77:337, 2007.

59. Calder PC, Yaqoob P, Thies F, et al: Fatty acids and lymphocyte functions. *Br J Nutr* 87 Suppl 1:S31, 2002.
60. Fedyk ER, Harris SG, Padilla J, Phipps RP: Prostaglandin receptors of the EP2 and EP4 subtypes regulate B lymphocyte activation and differentiation to IgE-secreting cells. *Adv Exp Med Biol* 433:153, 1997.
61. Freitas AA, Bognacki J: The role of locomotion in lymphocyte migration. *Immunology* 36:247, 1979.
62. Hedeskov CJ: Early effects of phytohaemagglutinin on glucose metabolism of normal human lymphocytes. *Biochem J* 110:373, 1968.
63. Kamatani N, Carson DA: Differential cyst(e)ine requirements in human T and B lymphoblastoid cell lines. *Int Arch Allergy Appl Immunol* 68:84, 1982.
64. Ando M, Sugimoto K, Kitoh T, et al: Selective apoptosis of natural killer-cell tumours by L-asparaginase. *Br J Haematol* 130:860, 2005.
65. Carson DA, Carrera CJ: Immunodeficiency secondary to adenosine deaminase deficiency and purine nucleoside phosphorylation deficiency. *Semin Hematol* 27:260, 1990.
66. Jones JM, Simkus C: The roles of the RAG1 and RAG2 "non core" regions in V(D)J recombination and lymphocyte development. *Arch Immunol Ther Exp (Warsz)* 57:105, 2009.
67. Schatz DG, Spanopoulou E: Biochemistry of V(D)J recombination. *Curr Top Microbiol Immunol* 290:49, 2005.
68. Le Deist F, Poinsignon C, Moshous D, et al: Artemis sheds new light on V(D)J recombination. *Immunol Rev* 200:142, 2004.
69. Meek K, Gupta S, Ramsden DA, Lees-Miller SP: The DNA-dependent protein kinase: The director at the end. *Immunol Rev* 200:132, 2004.
70. Jolly CJ, Cook AJ, Manis JP: Fixing DNA breaks during class switch recombination. *J Exp Med* 205:509, 2008.
71. Han L, Yu K: Altered kinetics of nonhomologous end joining and class switch recombination in ligase IV—Deficient B cells. *J Exp Med* 205:2745, 2008.
72. Yan CT, Boboila C, Souza EK, et al: IgH class switching and translocations use a robust non-classical end-joining pathway. *Nature* 449:478, 2007.
73. Taccioli GE, Amatucci AG, Beamish HJ, et al: Targeted disruption of the catalytic subunit of the DNA-PK gene in mice confers severe combined immunodeficiency and radiosensitivity. *Immunity* 9:355, 1998.
74. Villa A, Notarangelo LD, Roifman CM: Omenn syndrome: Inflammation in leaky severe combined immunodeficiency. *J Allergy Clin Immunol* 122:1082, 2008.
75. Benedict CL, Gilfillan S, Thai TH, Kearney JF: Terminal deoxynucleotidyl transferase and repertoire development. *Immunol Rev* 175:150, 2000.
76. Chaudhuri J, Basu U, Zarrin A, et al: Evolution of the immunoglobulin heavy chain class switch recombination mechanism. *Adv Immunol* 94:157, 2007.
77. Teng G, Papavasiliou FN: Immunoglobulin somatic hypermutation. *Annu Rev Genet* 41:107, 2007.
78. Cyster JG: Chemokines, sphingosine-1-phosphate, and cell migration in secondary lymphoid organs. *Annu Rev Immunol* 23:127, 2005.
79. Carreno PC, Sacedon R, Jimenez E, et al: Prolactin affects both survival and differentiation of T-cell progenitors. *J Neuroimmunol* 160:135, 2005.
80. Franco R, Pacheco R, Lluis C, et al: The emergence of neurotransmitters as immune modulators. *Trends Immunol* 28:400, 2007.
81. Levite M: Neurotransmitters activate T-cells and elicit crucial functions via neurotransmitter receptors. *Curr Opin Pharmacol* 8:460, 2008.
82. Acosta-Rodriguez EV, Merino MC, Montes CL, et al: Cytokines and chemokines shaping the B-cell compartment. *Cytokine Growth Factor Rev* 18:73, 2007.
83. Bono MR, Elgueta R, Sauma D, et al: The essential role of chemokines in the selective regulation of lymphocyte homing. *Cytokine Growth Factor Rev* 18:33, 2007.
84. Viola A, Molon B, Contento RL: Chemokines: Coded messages for T-cell missions. *Front Biosci* 13:6341, 2008.
85. Allen CD, Okada T, Cyster JG: Germinal-center organization and cellular dynamics. *Immunity* 27:190, 2007.
86. Zempleni J, Mock DM: Utilization of biotin in proliferating human lymphocytes. *J Nutr* 130:335S, 2000.
87. Moro JR, Iwata M, and von Andriano UH: Vitamin effects on the immune system: Vitamins A and D take centre stage. *Nat Rev Immunol* 8:685, 2008.
88. Ross AC, Chen Q, Ma Y: Augmentation of antibody responses by retinoic acid and costimulatory molecules. *Semin Immunol* 21:42, 2009.
89. Perretti M, D'Acquisto F: Annexin A1 and glucocorticoids as effectors of the resolution of inflammation. *Nat Rev Immunol* 9:62, 2009.
90. Herold MJ, McPherson KG, Reichardt HM: Glucocorticoids in T cell apoptosis and function. *Cell Mol Life Sci* 63:60, 2006.
91. Lowenberg M, Stahn C, Hommes DW, Buttgereit F: Novel insights into mechanisms of glucocorticoid action and the development of new glucocorticoid receptor ligands. *Steroids* 73:1025, 2008.
92. Liberman AC, Druker J, Garcia FA, et al: Intracellular molecular signaling. Basis for specificity to glucocorticoid anti-inflammatory actions. *Ann N Y Acad Sci* 1153:6, 2009.
93. Thompson EB: Stepping stones in the path of glucocorticoid-driven apoptosis of lymphoid cells. *Acta Biochim Biophys Sin (Shanghai)* 40:595, 2008.
94. Liva SM, Voskuhl RR: Testosterone acts directly on CD4+ T lymphocytes to increase IL-10 production. *J Immunol* 167:2060, 2001.
95. Wunderlich F, Benten WP, Lieberherr M, et al: Testosterone signaling in T cells and macrophages. *Steroids* 67:535, 2002.
96. Dulos GJ, Bagchus WM: Androgens indirectly accelerate thymocyte apoptosis. *Int Immunopharmacol* 1:321, 2001.
97. Page ST, Plymate SR, Bremner WJ, et al: Effect of medical castration on CD4+ CD25+ T cells, CD8+ T cell IFN-gamma expression, and NK cells: A physiological role for testosterone and/or its metabolites. *Am J Physiol Endocrinol Metab* 290:E856, 2006.
98. Pernis AB: Estrogen and CD4+ T cells. *Curr Opin Rheumatol* 19:414, 2007.
99. Corsini E, Lucchi L, Meroni M, et al: *In vivo* dehydroepiandrosterone restores age-associated defects in the protein kinase C signal transduction pathway and related functional responses. *J Immunol* 168:1753, 2002.
100. Sitzmann BD, Urbanski HF, Ottinger MA: Aging in male primates: Reproductive decline, effects of calorie restriction and future research potential. *Age (Dordr)* 30:157, 2008.
101. Genazzani AD, Lanzoni C, Genazzani AR: Might DHEA be considered a beneficial replacement therapy in the elderly? *Drugs Aging* 24:173, 2007.
102. Tani K, Ogushi F, Huang L, et al: CD13/aminopeptidase N, a novel chemoattractant for T lymphocytes in pulmonary sarcoidosis. *Am J Respir Crit Care Med* 161:1636, 2000.
103. Schulte am Esch J 2nd, Sevigny J, Kaczmarek E, et al: Structural elements and limited proteolysis of CD39 influence ATP diphosphohydrolase activity. *Biochemistry* 38:2248, 1999.
104. Bauvois B: Transmembrane proteases in cell growth and invasion: New contributors to angiogenesis? *Oncogene* 23:317, 2004.
105. Ortolan E, Vacca P, Capobianco A, et al: CD157, the Janus of CD38 but with a unique personality. *Cell Biochem Funct* 20:309, 2002.
106. Stark AA, Porat N, Volohonsky G, et al: The role of gamma-glutamyl transpeptidase in the biosynthesis of glutathione. *Biofactors* 17:139, 2003.

CHAPTER 76
LYMPHOPOIESIS

Gay M. Crooks

SUMMARY

Lymphopoiesis refers to the process by which the cellular components of the immune system (i.e., T cells, B cells, and natural killer cells, and certain dendritic cells) are produced during hematopoietic differentiation. This process begins with the hematopoietic stem cell and continues through progenitor stages down a series of mostly diverging lineage pathways, ultimately resulting in the remarkable diversity and flexibility of the immune system. Although the more terminal events in lymphocyte differentiation and function have been defined in detail (see Chaps. 77, 78, and 79), the earliest events during which hematopoietic stem cells undergo lymphoid lineage commitment are less-well understood and still somewhat controversial. Although the conceptual framework for the questions of lymphoid commitment has been established largely on studies in murine species, experimental systems now exist to better understand how such events are controlled in humans. This chapter summarizes what is known about the ontogeny of lymphoid development and the control of lymphoid differentiation and discusses some of the persisting controversies in the field.

LYMPHOPOIESIS DURING PRENATAL DEVELOPMENT

Blood is formed from a succession of sites during embryonic and fetal development, beginning outside the embryo in the yolk sac. Soon afterward, hematopoiesis begins in the embryo proper, initially in the paraaortic splanchnopleure (PAS), and aorto-gonad-mesonephros (AGM) regions, then the fetal liver, spleen, and finally the fetal marrow (see Chap. 6). With each change of anatomical site the range of hematopoiesis becomes progressively more complex and similar to that of the adult (Fig. 76–1).

When assigning hematopoietic function to each developmental stage, it is important to distinguish the lineage "potential" of stem and progenitor cells that arise from certain areas (i.e., the ability to generate specific lineages *in vitro* from immature cells removed from a region) from the spontaneous physiologic production of lineages in each region. The onset of lymphopoiesis during embryogenesis lags behind development of the myeloid and erythroid lineages. Although myeloid, erythroid, and natural killer (NK) cells can be produced from all extraembryonic and embryonic sites, B and T lymphocytes can only be generated from so-called definitive hematopoietic stem cells (HSCs) in the embryo proper.[1]

MURINE HEMATOPOIETIC DEVELOPMENT

Most of the studies exploring embryonic and fetal hematopoiesis have been performed using mouse models. Although the timing of each developmental stage has been carefully mapped, it has long been a source of controversy as to whether hematopoiesis in the embryo is initiated from colonizing precursors from the extraembryonic yolk sac, or whether the embryonic sites of hematopoiesis arise independently from the yolk sac.[2–6] This debate has implications for understanding the lineages generated at different sites of hematopoiesis and thus for tracing the ancestry of the lymphoid cells that are produced in the mammalian embryo. One reason for the difficulty in assigning the exact organ in which lineages are generated, is that each site of hematopoiesis is active during overlapping periods (see Fig. 76–1). In addition, once circulation has been established, it is difficult to rule out the possibility that stem cells and progenitors found in one location did not migrate from another.

The first wave of hematopoiesis in the mouse begins in the extraembryonic tissue of the yolk sac by 7.5 days of gestation (E7.5), before circulation is established.[7,8] This initial stage of so-called primitive hematopoiesis produces mostly erythrocytes and macrophages, and lymphocytes are not detectable at this time.[8] Definitive HSCs that are capable of generating all lymphohematopoietic lineages first appear in the PAS/AGM region at E8.5 to E9.[3,8] High-level, multilineage reconstituting activity typical of definitive HSC can be found in the murine AGM region by E10.5. However, although AGM cells can produce all lineages, including T and B lymphocytes, in culture, lymphocytes do not spontaneously develop in the fetus until hematopoiesis has begun in the fetal liver. Rag-1 expression, one of the earliest lymphoid-specific events, can be found in the E11 murine fetal liver.[8] T-cell differentiation begins with the colonization of the thymus, around E11 of murine gestation,[9,10] and is generated from stem or progenitor cells that migrate to the thymus from the AGM, fetal liver, and later still, the fetal marrow.

HUMAN HEMATOPOIETIC DEVELOPMENT

Hematopoietic cells have been identified in the human yolk sac as early as day 18 of embryonic life, at which time, like the mouse, they are almost exclusively comprised of erythrocytes and to a lesser extent monocytes and macrophages (see Fig. 76–1).[11] Although no lymphocytes are seen in the yolk sac, yolk sac progenitors do have NK cell potential; that is, it is possible to generate NK cells from progenitors removed from the yolk sac and cultured in certain conditions.[11,12] The same yolk sac progenitors, however, do not possess the capacity for B- or T-cell potential, even when placed in culture conditions that permit lymphoid differentiation from definitive HSC.[12]

As in the mouse, definitive hematopoiesis develops first in the AGM region developed from the splanchnopleure, that is, the AGM is the site where CD34+ cells with the capacity for full lymphoid and myeloid differentiation are first found in the human embryo.[12,13] The AGM develops at day 27 of gestation in the human, when human HSCs are generated as clusters of two or three cells arising from the endothelium specifically on the ventral surface of the preumbilical region of the aorta. These cells are clonogenic and highly proliferative, rapidly increasing to several thousand in number and spreading further along the aorta. However, hematopoiesis exists only transiently in the AGM, disappearing entirely by day 40.[11] Although lymphoid cells can be produced in culture from cells extracted from the AGM[11,12] the HSC of the AGM do not produce mature cells *in situ*; instead their role is to migrate and colonize the fetal liver, producing the next wave of hematopoiesis.

Although blood cells are first detectable in the human fetal liver as early as day 23, they exist at this time only as erythroid and myeloid cells associated with hepatic sinusoids. These erythroid cells consist of megaloblasts expressing embryonic hemoglobins (globin chains ζ and ε), and no CD34+ cells are seen in the fetal liver during this early phase. It is likely that this first stage of fetal liver hematopoiesis is secondary to colonization of more mature cells from the yolk sac. By day 30, CD34+ cells appear in the fetal liver[14] and by day 32, these cells are able to

Acronyms and abbreviations that appear in this chapter include: B, bone marrow derived; BCR, B-cell receptor; CLP, common lymphoid progenitor; E, days of gestation; EBF, early B-cell factor; HSC, hematopoietic stem cell; Ig, immunoglobulin; IL, interleukin; LMPP, lymphoid-multipotential primed progenitor; LSK, lin^{neg}sca-1+c-kit+; NK, natural killer; SCID, severe combined immunodeficiency.

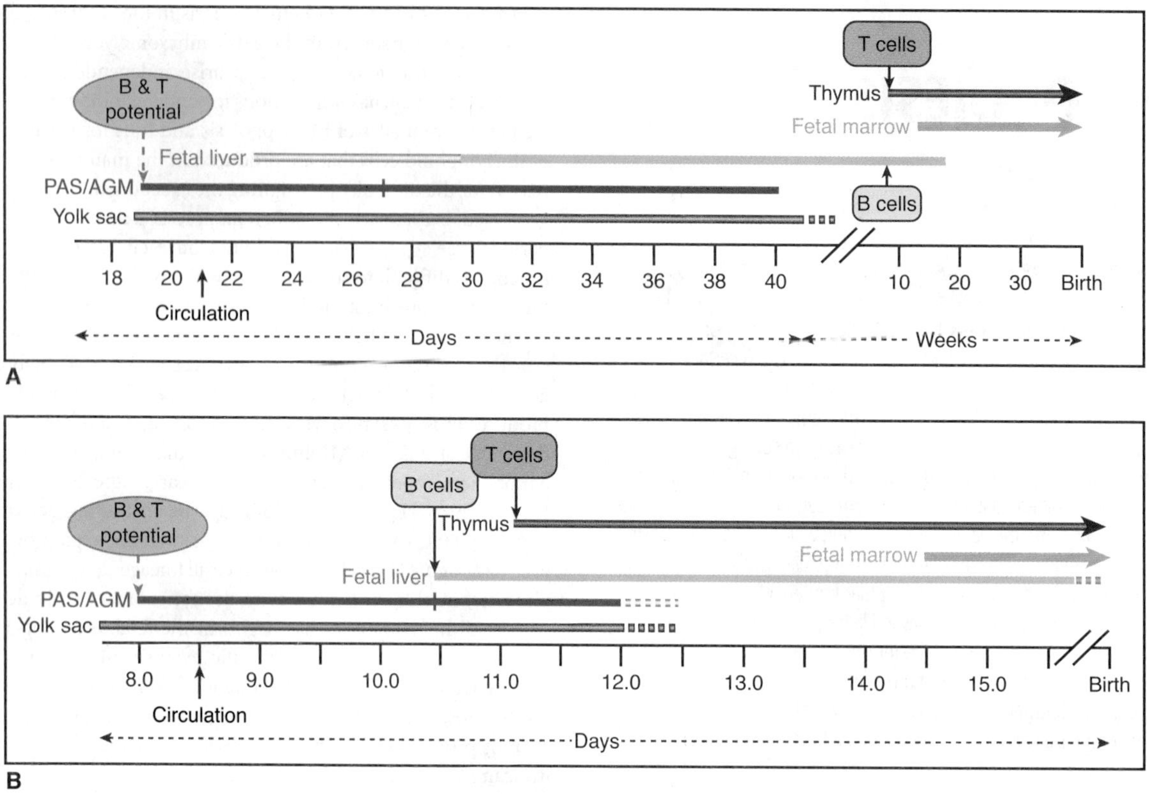

FIGURE 76–1. Timing of lymphohematopoiesis during prenatal development. Shown is the timeline for activity in each site of hematopoiesis in the embryo and fetus of **(A)** human and **(B)** mouse. *Solid lines* show tissues in which long-term reconstituting, multilineage definitive hematopoietic stem cells (HSCs) are present. *Open lines* show sites where only more differentiated hematopoietic cells are present (i.e., HSCs are absent), e.g., myeloid and erythroid cells in yolk sac, thymocytes in thymus. "B- and T-cell potential" (in ovals) refers to the presence of progenitor cells in the paraaortic splanchnopleure (PAS) that can generate T- and B-lymphoid cells when cultured *in vitro*. B and T cells are first detected *in vivo* in fetal liver and thymus, respectively, at times shown in *rectangles*. Not shown here are other sites of hematopoiesis such as omentum, placenta, and spleen, in which exact onset of human lymphoid potential is less clear. AGM, aorto-gonad-mesonephros.

maintain long-term hematopoiesis *in vitro*.[14] Erythroid cells in the fetal liver at this later stage of definitive hematopoiesis consist of enucleated macrocytes producing fetal hemoglobin (globin chains α and γ). It is most likely that the definitive hematopoiesis in the fetal liver is derived from colonizing HSCs that have migrated from the AGM. In normal development, as with the yolk sac and AGM, hematopoiesis in the fetal liver is transient, disappearing by 20 weeks of gestation.[1]

The final wave of hematopoietic development takes place in the fetal marrow, starting around 11 weeks of gestation. The initial cells seen in the marrow are CD15+ myeloid cells and glycophorin A+ erythroid cells, and hematopoiesis is again associated with the endothelium, taking place in the medullary sinusoids before osteoblast formation.[15] Eventually, CD34+ cells are found in the fetal marrow and behave functionally as true HSC, generating B, T, NK, and myeloid and erythroid lineages.[1] HSC have found their final niche, and lifelong, self-renewing lymphohematopoiesis resides permanently in the marrow thereafter.

THYMIC DEVELOPMENT

The human thymic microenvironment begins to develop at approximately 4 weeks' gestation and then undergoes three developmental phases.[16] The first phase occurs between 4 and 8 weeks' gestation, with the appearance of thymic epithelium arising as a product of the third and fourth pharyngeal pouches[17] and the expansion of thymic epithelial cells. The second phase occurs between 9 and 15 weeks' gestation and is characterized by the development of subcapsular, cortical, and medullary regions.[16] Thymic colonization by fetal liver-derived progenitors and lymphocyte production begins at approximately week 9.[17] The ability of thymocytes to respond to the mitogen phytohemagglutinin is detectable as early as 10 weeks' gestation,[18] and alloreactive, phenotypically mature T cells can be found by 13 to 16 weeks' gestation.[19]

The third phase occurs from 16 weeks' gestation until age 1 to 2 years and is characterized by robust intrathymic T-cell maturation (see Chaps. 5 and 77).

An exhaustive study of 136 human postnatal thymuses ranging from neonatal life to more than 90 years old, found that essentially all postnatal thymic growth (based on weight and volume) occurs during the first postnatal year, mostly in the first few months of life.[20] From the age of 12 months, the human thymus undergoes steady involution, with a reduction of thymocytes and thymic epithelium, particularly the medulla, and a corresponding increase in fatty infiltration of the perivascular space.[20]

Whereas mice lose approximately 90 percent of the wet weight of the thymus during life, the increasing fatty infiltration in the perivascular space in the aging human thymus maintains the total size of the thymus in healthy people into late life.[20] Radiologic studies using computed tomography (CT) scans have confirmed that total thymic size remains stable in humans throughout life although parenchymal tissue atrophies dramatically (~95%; see Chap. 8, Fig. 8–1).[21]

B-CELL DEVELOPMENT

The hallmark characteristic of a mature B cell circulating in blood or residing in secondary lymphoid tissue is the expression of cell surface immunoglobulin (Ig). The cell surface Ig consists of μ, δ, γ, α, or ε

heavy chains disulfide-linked to κ or λ light chains (see Chap. 77). The cell surface Ig and the associated signaling molecules Igα (CD79a) and Igβ (CD79b) are referred to as the *B-cell receptor* (BCR). Progenitor (pro-) B cells are defined by the absence of both cytoplasmic μ heavy chains and cell surface BCR. Precursor (pre-) B cells are defined by the presence of cytoplasmic μ heavy chains in the absence of cell surface BCR. This minimal definition of pro-B, pre-B, and B cells forms the basis of the current detailed model of human B-cell development.[22] B-cell development can be divided into two stages: an antigen-independent stage that occurs primarily in fetal liver and fetal and adult marrow, and an antigen-dependent stage that occurs primarily in secondary lymphoid tissue, such as spleen and lymph node.

The first B cells detectable in the human fetus are found in the fetal liver[17] at approximately 8 weeks' gestation, with the appearance of cytoplasmic IgM+ pre-B cells; by 10 to 12 weeks, surface IgM+ B cells are seen in the fetal liver[23] and fetal omentum.[24] B-cell and IgM production move to the fetal marrow and spleen by 17 weeks of gestation (see Chaps. 5, 6, and 77).[25,26] From the end of the second trimester throughout adult life, marrow is the exclusive site of B-cell development.[27] The frequency of early B-lineage cells as a percentage of the total nucleated lymphohematopoietic cell pool is higher in fetal than in adult marrow. However, the ratio between pro-B, pre-B, and immature B cells and the mitotic activity within these fractions is relatively constant.[28]

In murine B-cell development, two functionally and immunophenotypically distinct types of B cells, B-1 and B-2, have been described.[23] Most B cells in adult mice are B-2 cells, which form part of the adaptive immune system by their ability to interact with T cells and undergo immunoglobulin heavy chain class switching. The B-1 cells make up approximately 5 percent of adult murine lymphocytes, but demonstrate a far less diverse immunoglobulin repertoire than the B-2 cells, responding to carbohydrate antigens and other T-cell–independent immunogens and forming part of the innate immune system. Murine B-1 cells are marked by their expression of CD11b, and are found in multiple sites, including the spleen, intestine, and the pleural and peritoneal cavities.[29,30] The B-1 cells can be further divided into B-1a cells (which secrete immunoglobulins spontaneously) and B-1b cells (in which immunoglobulin production is induced) based on the expression of the marker CD5. At present, there is no clear evidence that humans have similar subpopulations of B-1 and B-2 cells during development.[23]

NATURAL KILLER CELL DEVELOPMENT

Functional NK cells can be detected in the human fetal liver as early as 9 to 10 weeks of gestation,[18] but NK cell differentiation can be induced *in vitro* from progenitors derived at all stages of hematopoietic development, even those from the yolk sac.[1,11,12] Thus, the onset of NK potential is not equivalent to the full lymphoid potential of definitive hematopoiesis, as NK potential can be assigned to a range of progenitor types that exist at different stages, including primitive hematopoiesis. NK cell production can be considered as providing an essential defense mechanism for the developing mammalian embryo prior to development of more complex pathways of adaptive immunity.

DENDRITIC CELL DEVELOPMENT

Dendritic-like cells which express Class II major histocompatibility antigens are produced at all stages of embryonic and fetal hematopoiesis, being first detected in the human yolk sac and mesenchyme as early as 4 to 8 weeks, before development of the fetal marrow or thymus.[31] Dendritic cells are detectable at each site of hematopoiesis as soon as they become active, in the human fetal thymus at 11 to 14 weeks, marrow at 14 to 17 weeks, spleen 16 weeks, and tonsils at 23 weeks.[31,32] Dendritic cells and macrophages are closely related and phenotypically similar (see Chap. 19), both expressing major histocompatibility complex class II. Thus, clear discrimination of these two cell types can be difficult, particularly as many studies that provided information on human dendritic cell development were conducted before all the molecular and antibody tools for analysis of dendritic cells were available.

DIFFERENTIATION PATHWAYS FOR LYMPHOCYTE PRODUCTION

The conceptual framework for how the lymphocyte lineages are generated from HSCs has been developed largely from studies using genetically engineered mice and murine transplant models. Although necessary and useful as a starting point, caution should be exercised in translating the results of the murine studies to human lymphopoiesis, or in assuming for any species, that only one pathway to lymphopoiesis exists at all stages of ontogeny.[33,34] Additionally, the conclusions about lineage relationships of isolated populations are influenced by limitations inherent in any of the *in vitro* or *in vivo* assays employed to examine differentiation potential.[35]

For several decades, our understanding of hematopoiesis has been built on a hierarchical schema in which all the pathways of differentiation lead away from a pluripotent HSC, and progress through discrete progenitor stages that mark each branch-point of lineage commitment (see Chap. 16). In the classical paradigm, the earliest differentiation "decision" made by an HSC is to enter one of two pathways, marked by either a common lymphoid progenitor (CLP) or a common myeloid progenitor (CMP), which has full myeloid and erythromegakaryocytic differentiation potential (Fig. 76–2).[36] With each successive stage of differentiation, lineage-specific cell surface markers and transcription factors are upregulated. Consequently, the CLP is defined as a single cell that can give rise to all lymphoid lineages (B, T, and NK), but cannot generate myeloid, erythroid, or megakaryocytic lineages. The concept of progenitor populations marking two mutually exclusive differentiation pathways, one limited to myeloid and erythromegakaryocytic potential and the second defining lymphoid commitment, was held long before cells that satisfied the criteria of CLP were identified.[37–39] In contrast, the existence of single clonogenic cells with myeloid, erythroid, and megakaryocyte lineages was shown more than three decades ago through the use of *in vitro* clonal assays to demonstrate so-called colony-forming unit-granulocyte erythromyeloid megakaryocyte,[40] and later confirmed using markers to prospectively isolate such cells in mice[41] and humans.[42] The lymphocyte lineages were assumed to be closely related because of a number of associations, for example, common anatomical sites of T and B lymphopoiesis (spleen, lymph nodes; see Chap. 5), similar molecular mechanisms that regulate T-cell receptor and B-cell immunoglobulin rearrangements (see Chaps. 77 and 78), and severe B- and T-lymphoid defects that result from single genetic mutations in mice (see Chap. 82).[43]

Development of flow cytometry (synonym: fluorescence-activated cell sorting [FACS]) made possible the isolation of rare hematopoietic cell populations and the subsequent interrogation of lineage potential using *in vitro* cultures and *in vivo* reconstitution studies (see Chaps. 15 and 16). Primitive multilymphoid progenitors with little or no clonogenic myeloid or erythroid potential have now been isolated from human tissue using flow cytometry with combinations of various cell surface markers.[44–47] However, it seems likely that lineage relationships are less-strictly organized than once believed. Studies in mice show that the erythroid and megakaryocytic lineages can branch off at an earlier point in hematopoiesis, and that lymphoid (i.e., T, B, and NK) and myeloid (or at least monocytic) lineages can arise from the same pathway through a so-called lymphoid-myeloid primed progenitor (LMPP).[48] It

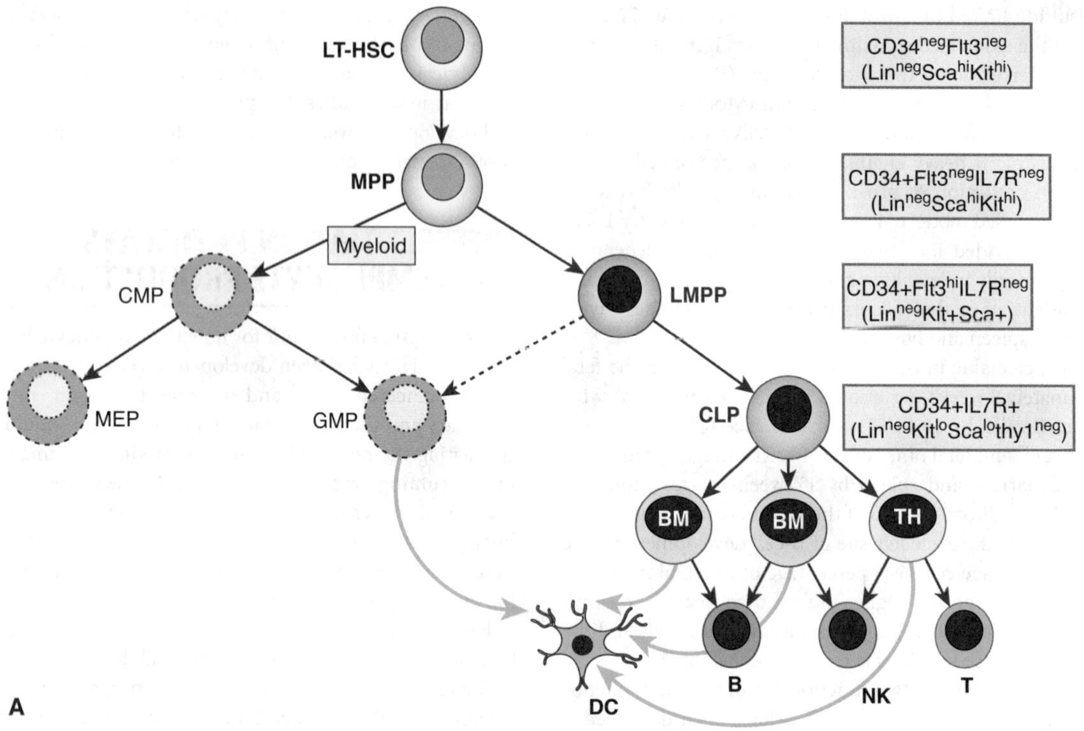

FIGURE 76–2. Postnatal pathways of lymphopoiesis in mice and humans. The key immunophenotype used to isolate each population is shown in boxes on the right. In parentheses under the main immunophenotypes are other markers also associated with each population. Myeloid progenitors are shown in *broken red lines*. The figure also shows that, in both mice and humans, dendritic cells can be produced from all prospectively identified lymphoid progenitors as well as myeloid progenitors. **A.** Murine lymphoid progenitor pathways. Populations with multilineage potential include long-term hematopoietic stem cells (LT-HSCs) and multipotential progenitors (MPPs). Lymphoid commitment begins at the lymphoid-primed multipotential progenitors (LMPPs), which have full lymphoid (T-, B-, and NK cell developmental potential) and limited myeloid (mostly monocyte) potential. With the common lymphoid progenitor (CLP), all myeloid potential is lost and full lymphoid potential remains. BM, bone marrow; CMP, common myeloid progenitor; DC, dendritic cell; GMP, granulocyte-macrophage progenitor; MEP, megakaryocyte-erythroid progenitor; NK, natural killer cell; TH, thymus. (Continued)

remains unclear which of these alternative lineage differentiation pathways are most physiologically significant during steady-state hematopoiesis, but it is likely that more than one pathway can exist simultaneously and alternative pathways may predominate during different stages of ontogeny and from different sites of hematopoiesis.

MURINE LYMPHOID PROGENITORS

In 1997, investigators working with murine marrow cells, isolated progenitors that possessed no myeloid or erythromegakaryocytic potential, but when transplanted into irradiated recipients could rapidly restore T-, B-, and NK cell lineages.[45] Clonal *in vitro* and *in vivo* studies showed that all lymphoid lineages were derived from a single common progenitor, thus proving the existence of the long-assumed CLP and supporting the classical model of lymphopoiesis. This study isolated cells based in part on expression of interleukin (IL)-7 receptor alpha (IL-7Rα).[45] The IL-7Rα+ CLP do not express hematopoietic markers associated with fully differentiated lineages (they are called "lineage negative" or "lin^{neg}" cells). As an indication that they are more differentiated than multilineage HSCs, expression of certain HSC-related cell surface markers (Sca-1, Thy-1, c-kit) is downregulated.[45] Thus the full immunophenotype assigned to the murine CLP is Lin^{neg} IL-7R+Thy-1^{neg} Sca-1^{lo} c-kit^{lo}. This contrasts the murine CLP immunophenotype with that of the murine HSC, which is found within the Lin^{neg} IL-7R^{neg} Thy-1^{lo} Sca-1^{hi} c-kit^{hi} population.[45]

Work with murine marrow has prompted a reexamination of when the lymphoid lineage pathways diverge from those of the myeloid and erythroid lineages (see Fig. 76–2). A population from murine marrow cells, defined largely by expression of the receptor FLT3, has been shown to possess full lymphoid and some myeloid potential, but not erythroid or megakaryocytic potential.[48,49] These lin^{neg}sca-1+c-kit+CD34+FLT3^{hi} (synonym: LSK CD34+FLT3^{hi}) cells are primed for lymphoid commitment in that they have downregulated genes involved in erythromegakaryocytic differentiation and upregulated lymphoid-associated genes.[50] Although they are able to generate monocytes and granulocytes *in vitro*, their differentiation potential is nonetheless skewed heavily to lymphoid cells; after transplantation into irradiated recipients, LSK CD34+FLT3^{hi} cells rapidly reconstitute B and T lymphopoiesis. However, unlike the multipotent LSK CD34+FLT3^{neg} cells, reconstitution of myeloid lineages *in vivo* from LSK CD34+FLT3^{hi} is very limited; LSK CD34+FLT3^{hi} do not reconstitute granulocytes after transplantation, producing only monocytes *in vivo*.[48] They have thus been termed LMPPs.[48,50]

One confusing factor in defining lineage potential is the ability of both myeloid and lymphoid progenitor populations to differentiate into dendritic cells, and the presence of an intermediate "monocyte" stage during differentiation of progenitors into dendritic cells (see Chap. 19).[51–54] As the monocyte and macrophage precursors of dendritic cells express many cell surface markers common to the myeloid lineage, irrespective of the lineage of origin, it can be misleading to assign "myeloid" potential purely on the basis of the ability to generate monocytes. Myeloid and lymphoid progenitors that express FLT3 can generate dendritic cells, and production of dendritic cells depends on FLT3 ligand.[51] Nonetheless, the ability of the FLT3+ LMPPs identified in murine marrow to generate granulocytes, albeit only *in vitro*, suggests that this progenitor population retains some myeloid potential.

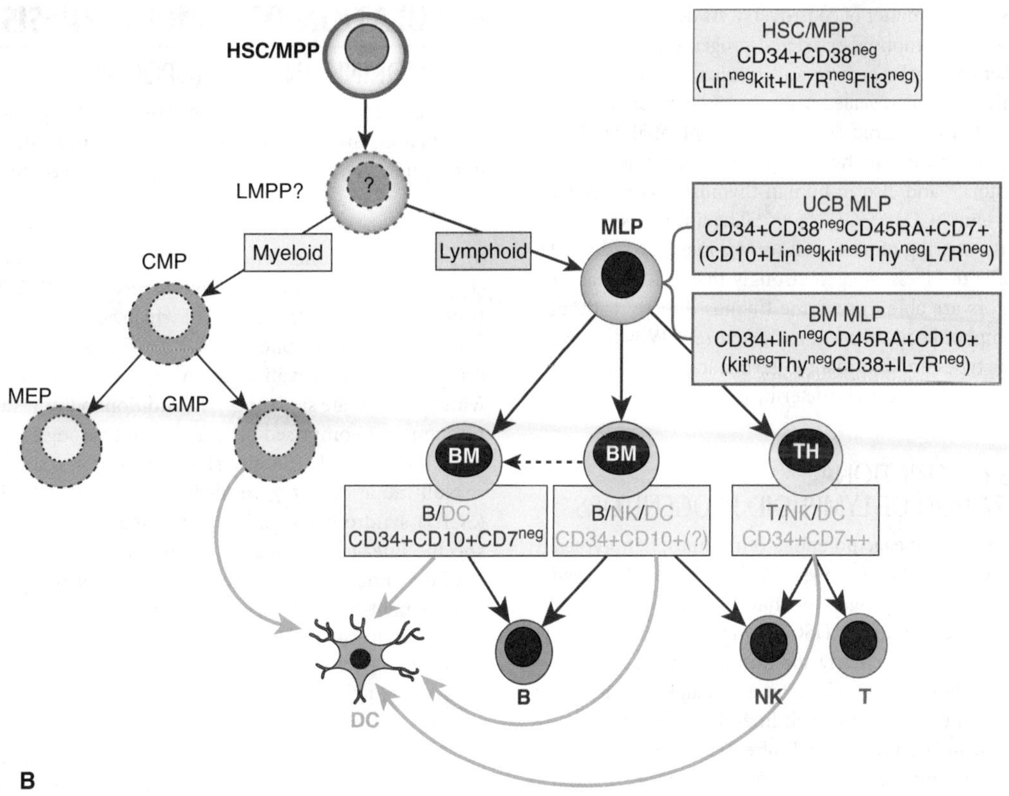

FIGURE 76–2. *(Continued)* Postnatal pathways of lymphopoiesis in mice and humans. The key immunophenotype used to isolate each population is shown in boxes on the right. In parentheses under the main immunophenotypes are other markers also associated with each population. Myeloid progenitors are shown in *broken red lines*. The figure also shows that, in both mice and humans, dendritic cells can be produced from all prospectively identified lymphoid progenitors as well as myeloid progenitors. **B.** Human lymphoid progenitor pathways. The term *multilymphoid progenitor* (MLP) is used rather than CLP, as assay systems have not yet been able to definitively prove full T-, B-, and NK cell potential from a single human progenitor. Clonal analysis, however, has demonstrated single progenitor cells with B-cell and dendritic cell potential, and B-, NK, and dendritic cell potential from human cord blood and human marrow. The exact phenotype of the B, NK, and dendritic progenitor cell is not yet known although such potential can be found within the CD34+CD10+ population. The relationship between B and dendritic progenitor and B, NK, and dendritic progenitor is not yet proven, and therefore is shown as a *dotted line*. Clonal analysis has also shown single progenitors with T-, NK, and dendritic cell potential in human thymus. Not shown is an even more primitive CD34+lin^{neg}CD7^{neg} thymic progenitor that has lymphoid and myeloerythroid potential, and which probably represents an MPP that seeds the human thymus. The human equivalent to the murine LMPP has not been identified. BM, bone marrow; CMP, common myeloid progenitor; DC, dendritic cell; GMP, granulocyte-macrophage progenitor; MEP, megakaryocyte-erythroid progenitor; NK, natural killer cell; TH, thymus.

HUMAN LYMPHOID PROGENITORS

The CD34 cell surface marker is expressed on human HSCs and on a variety of different types of hematopoietic progenitors, including those restricted to lymphoid development (see Chaps. 15 and 16).[55,56] CD34 has been combined with additional cell surface markers to identify human multilymphoid progenitors, for example, CD10,[44,57] CD7,[46,47,58,59] and CD45RA.[44,58] Similar to the mouse CLP, in addition to the upregulation of expression of the aforementioned markers, lymphoid commitment is accompanied by downregulation of certain HSC cell surface markers, such as c-kit and thy-1.[33]

As in murine studies, no one marker used in isolation is able to define a human lymphoid progenitor.[56] For example, although the expression of CD7 can be used to define a subset of CD34+CD38^{neg} cells in cord blood that are multilymphoid progenitors without myeloid or erythroid potential,[46,47] CD34+CD38+CD7+ cells from cord blood have full lineage (lymphoid, myeloid, and erythroid) potential. When comparing the progenitor populations identified in human studies with those described from murine experiments it is important to recognize that species differences exist between cell surface markers.[33] For example, IL-7Rα expression is used to define murine CLP,[45] but CD34+CD38^{neg}CD7+ multilymphoid progenitors in human cord blood do not express IL-7Rα[46] and CD34+CD38+IL-7Rα+ cells in human cord blood have both myeloid and lymphoid potential. A different ontogeny and source of hematopoietic cells will also introduce unexpected variations of progenitor immunophenotype and function.[33] Whereas most murine studies have been conducted with adult murine marrow, most human studies have been performed with umbilical cord blood, a more logistically available source containing progenitors that are significantly more proliferative than marrow.[60] Again using the example of the CD34+CD38^{neg}CD7+ multilymphoid progenitor, although this immunophenotype can be used to identify multilymphoid progenitors in cord blood,[46] the same markers cannot be used in human marrow because CD34+CD38^{neg} marrow cells do not express CD7. No human equivalent of the murine LMPP has yet been described, but dendritic potential has been found in all the primitive lymphoid-restricted human progenitors reported.[44,46,58,61] In fact, the antigen CD33 usually thought of as a myeloid marker, was expressed on dendritic cells from the CD34+lin^{neg}CD45RA+CD10+ marrow CLP.[44]

THYMIC PROGENITORS

It was long assumed that lymphoid commitment in the marrow precedes thymic seeding and T-cell development. However, despite the clear existence of lymphoid-committed progenitors within the marrow, the dominant cell type that migrates from the marrow and seeds the thymus to initiate thymopoiesis is still a matter of controversy. As described above, a variety of marrow-derived lymphoid-restricted progenitors and LMPPs are each able to generate T cells *in vitro* and *in vivo*. However, careful examination of the thymus has revealed primitive progenitors that have not only lymphoid, but also myeloid and erythroid potential. Such rare cells have been identified in murine thymus where they are referred to as early thymic progenitors[62] and also in human thymus where they have the phenotype CD34+lin^{neg}CD1a^{neg}CD7^{neg}.[63,64] The lineage potential of such cells as well as the sharing of many cell surface markers and similar gene expression profile to HSCs, suggest strongly that HSCs or at least multipotent progenitors are able to seed the thymus directly without a preceding stage of lymphoid commitment in the marrow. Which of these alternative progenitor types are dominant in terms of their contribution to steady-state thymopoiesis is yet to be determined.[65]

CHALLENGES IN FUNCTIONAL CHARACTERIZATION OF LYMPHOID PROGENITORS

The accurate assignment of lineage potential to immunophenotypically defined progenitors requires clonal analysis. Although clonal assays for myelo-erythro-megakaryocytic progenitors have existed for more than 30 years,[40] the ability to differentiate HSCs along lymphoid pathways has been relatively recent, particularly for human studies.[35] *In vitro* assays for human lymphoid potential became available when it was observed that selected murine stromal cell lines were capable of supporting B-cell, NK cell, and dendritic cell differentiation from primitive human HSCs.[66–68] T-cell differentiation systems are more complex, requiring an *in vitro* model that recapitulates the unique environment of the thymus. Originally this was only possible using the fetal thymic organ culture method, a system in which large numbers of human progenitors are seeded into whole thymus in so-called hanging drop cultures.[69] A more efficient *in vitro* system for studying murine and human T-cell differentiation has been developed using a murine stromal monolayer that expresses the notch ligand delta-like ligand 1 ("OP9-DL1 stroma").[70] However, none of the *in vitro* T-cell culture systems simultaneously support B-cell development, making proof of full T- and B-lymphoid potential at a clonal level technically problematic. *In vivo* transplantation of a single murine HSC can prove multilineage potential at a clonal level, but this also is technically difficult, especially when studying progenitor populations that are not self-renewing. *In vivo* studies with human cells are particularly challenging as they rely on xenogeneic transplant models with low engraftment efficiency.[33,35]

As mentioned above, one potential source of confusion in studies trying to identify the progenitor stages involved in lymphopoiesis, has been the assignment of myeloid potential to any progenitor that can generate monocytes, a cell type that is defined by a nonspecific morphology and expression of cell surface antigens such as CD33, CD11b, and CD14 (see Chap. 67). Monocytes can be generated by clonogenic myeloerythroid (i.e., CMPs) and granulocyte-monocyte progenitors. These monocytes can then differentiate further into macrophages or dendritic cells.[53,54,71] However, dendritic cells are also readily generated from lymphoid-restricted progenitors including CLPs,[44,46,51,53,58,59] B-lymphoid progenitors,[61] and thymic T/NK progenitors[51,53,72,73] (see Chap. 19). Thus, it may be more relevant to reassign monocytes, like dendritic cells, to a promiscuous differentiation pathway common to both myeloid and lymphoid origins. The infidelity of dendritic differentiation and the unreliability of the markers in assigning lineage origin to dendritic cells is well described.[53,74,75] Although it was once thought that cell surface markers could identify dendritic cells of lymphoid versus myeloid origin, it has been realized in both murine and human studies that these markers are more related to the conditions used in dendritic cell culture than in the lineage of their precursors.[51,53,54,74,75]

REGULATION OF LYMPHOPOIESIS

CYTOKINES IN LYMPHOPOIESIS

The many cytokine pathways that regulate lymphoid development, differentiation, and function are too numerous and complex for a full description here. However, the cytokine receptors of the common gamma (γ_c) chain family should be mentioned particularly because of their biologic importance in lymphopoiesis and their clinical relevance in primary immune deficiency disease. The γ_c subunit is a signaling component of six different cytokine receptors, IL-2,[76] IL-4,[77,78] IL-7,[79,80] IL-9,[81] IL-15,[82] and IL-21,[83] all of which act on different stages and pathways involved in lymphopoiesis.[43,84,85] All six γ_c-dependent receptors are unique in their activation of JAK3, a molecule that directly interacts with γ_c to mediate signaling.[86] In addition to the γ_c subunit, each of these receptors are comprised of an α subunit through which specific ligands bind; IL-2R and IL-15R also share a common β subunit.[43]

Null mutations of γ_c result in severe combined immune deficiency (SCID) syndromes in mice and humans. However differences in the specific lineages affected reveal important species differences in cytokine dependency.[43] The most important of these differences is in the requirement for IL-7 signaling in human and murine B-cell development. Adult murine B-cell development has an absolute requirement for IL-7 to IL-7 receptor interaction and subsequent downstream signaling involving the γ_c subunit of the IL-7 receptor and the JAK3 tyrosine kinase.[87] In contrast, IL-7 is not essential for human B-cell development. X-linked SCID patients with mutations in the γ_c cytokine-receptor subunit exhibit profound thymic hypoplasia and an absence of NK cells but normal or elevated numbers of B cells.[43] SCID patients with mutations in *JAK3*[88,89] or the IL-7 receptor[90] also have normal numbers of blood B cells. Although B-cell numbers are normal, B-cell function in patients with γ_c-deficient SCID is not normal and patients are hypoglobulinemic, presumably partly as a result of the role of IL-4 in B-cell function and the absence of T-cell interactions in antibody production. These collective results indicate IL-7 is not essential for at least the numerically normal development of human B cells.

NK cells are absent in patients with γ_c-deficient and JAK3-deficient SCID, but are normal in IL-7Rα deficiency.[56,90,91] NK cells are also absent in mice deficient in IL-15,[92] IL-15Rα,[93] or IL-2Rβ (a subunit shared by IL-2R and IL-15R),[94] demonstrating the essential role of IL-15, but not IL-7, in NK cell development. Although no null mutations for IL-15 or its receptor have been described in humans, a familial NK cell deficiency has been described in humans in which the response to IL-15 and IL-2 appears to be subnormal.[95]

The production of both B and NK cells in patients with IL-7Rα deficiency, shows that in humans IL-7 is not required for the earliest stages of lymphoid commitment or growth of common lymphoid progenitors. This point is further supported with the finding that multilymphoid CD34+CD38^{neg}CD7+ progenitors in human cord blood do not express IL-7Rα.[46] In contrast to B cells and NK cells, however, T-cell development is absolutely dependent on IL-7 in both mice and humans.[84] In both species, mutations of any portion of the IL-7 signaling pathway, that is, γ_c, IL-7Rα, or JAK3, completely prevents T-cell development.[43] IL-2, in contrast, although an important cytokine in proliferation and function of mature T cells, is not essential for thymopoiesis; mutations in IL-2,[96] IL-2Rα, or IL2Rβ[97] result in functional T-cell defects, but T cells are not absent.

TRANSCRIPTIONAL REGULATION IN LYMPHOPOIESIS

The hierarchical differentiation pathways that lead irreversibly to the diverse array of functionally specialized mature lymphocytes are regulated by groups of genes expressed and repressed in a complex, precisely orchestrated sequence. As with cytokine regulation, our understanding of which transcriptional factors control each stage of differentiation has been developed using a combination of gene expression analyses in isolated progenitors and precursors, and an examination of the functional consequences of genetic mutations in mice and humans. The review in this chapter focuses on genes that regulate the earliest commitment decisions in the production of lymphoid progenitors; regulation of later differentiation stages in each lineage is discussed in Chaps. 77, 78, and 79, respectively.

The complex interplay between groups of genes involved in hematopoietic differentiation has been likened to a multidimensional network whose "regulatory space" is formed by a dynamic balance between certain transcriptional regulators.[98] Expression analysis of multiple genes in defined progenitor populations demonstrates levels of promiscuity at early stages of hematopoiesis, that preclude assignment of any unique gene expression pattern to each stage.[98–100] As differentiation proceeds, a more specific "genetic fingerprint" for each lineage develops.

REGULATION OF EARLY LYMPHOID COMMITMENT

Ikaros

Although no single gene has been identified as a lymphoid-specific master regulator, several transcription factors have been shown to be essential for the early stages of lymphopoiesis. The gene Ikaros, which encodes a family of DNA-binding zinc finger proteins, was identified in murine knockout studies as essential for all fetal lymphopoiesis.[101,102] However, in the postnatal setting, the role of Ikaros is more complex and less specific. Adult Ikaros^{null} mice completely lack B cells, and although T cells are produced, their differentiation is abnormal.[103] A murine study has suggested that Ikaros is not required for the initial lymphomyeloid versus myeloerythroid commitment decision, and that not only lymphoid differentiation, but also certain fate choices in the myeloerythroid pathway are affected by Ikaros.[104] As the expression of two key lymphoid cytokine receptors, FLT3 and IL-7Rα, is dependent on Ikaros, and as these markers are used to isolate murine LMPP and CLP, respectively, it is still not completely clear at which exact lymphoid progenitor stage Ikaros exerts its effects.[104] In addition to lymphoid progenitors, Ikaros isoforms are also expressed in HSCs, and myeloid lineages in mice[104–108] and humans.[108,109] Although Ikaros may act as a typical transcription factor in some settings, Ikaros also affects gene expression through its role in chromatin formation.[110]

PU.1

The transcription factor PU.1 is essential for normal B- and T-lymphocyte development, but its effects are highly dose dependent. At high levels of PU.1, key myeloid regulatory genes are upregulated and macrophage differentiation is induced preferentially over lymphoid differentiation.[111] Low-level expression of PU.1, however, is essential for lymphopoiesis.[112,113] Mice in which PU.1 is completely absent lack B cells and have abnormal fetal thymopoiesis. However, studies with mice in which PU.1 is deleted specifically in B cells show that PU.1 is not essential for B-cell differentiation beyond the pre-B stage.[114] It is likely that the critical role for PU.1 in murine lymphopoiesis lies in its upregulation of expression of the receptor for IL-7, which as mentioned above, is a key cytokine in both B and T lymphopoiesis in mice.[112]

E2A

E2A encodes two basic helix-loop-helix proteins, E12 and E47, through differential splicing.[115] Murine studies suggest that E2A is necessary for lymphoid priming of multipotent progenitors and that the E2A proteins prime expression of a number of lymphoid-associated genes.[116] There is a dose-dependent requirement for E2A expression in the development of LMPP and CLP.[116] Both B- and T-lineage commitment are severely reduced in the absence of E2A, but Ikaros and PU.1 expression are normal.[116–118] E2A affects B lymphopoiesis in part through upregulation of early B-cell factor (EBF)[119] and T lymphopoiesis through upregulation of expression and function of the key T-cell specification factor notch 1.[120]

REGULATION OF B CELL COMMITMENT

The transcription factors Ikaros, PU.1 E2A, EBF, and Pax5 are essential for normal B-cell differentiation. Mice that have functional deletions in any one of these genes have severely abnormal B-cell development; however, of these genes, only EBF and Pax5 are B-cell specific within the hematopoietic system.

Pax5

Pax5 is expressed specifically in B-lineage–committed progenitors and is required for normal expression of the B-lineage genes CD19 and CD79a.[113] Pax5–/– mice are blocked at the pro-B cell stage, but express most early B-cell–related genes.[121] PU.1, E2A, and EBF function earlier than Pax5 in B lymphopoiesis. Forced expression of Pax5 does not rescue the B-cell defect seen in EBF–/– mice or PU.1–/– mice.[113]

EBF

EBF encodes a helix-loop-helix zinc finger protein that induces B lymphoid in preference to myeloid development, in part by antagonizing the expression of genes encoding alternative lineages such as C/EBPα, Id2, and PU.1,[122] and, in part, by inducing Pax5 expression.[113] EBF and E2A function cooperatively in early B lymphopoiesis.[116] EBF–/– lymphoid progenitor populations from mice lack the ability to generate B cells but retain the ability to generate T, NK, and myeloid cells.[122] Overexpression of EBF in multipotential (lympho-myeloid) progenitors promotes B-cell production at the expense of myeloid differentiation.[122] Pax5 overexpression cannot rescue the B-cell defect in EBF–/– mice,[113] demonstrating the critical, Pax5-independent role of EBF in early B-cell fate decisions.

REGULATION OF T CELL COMMITMENT

GATA-3

GATA-3 is a key transcriptional factor for T-cell development, and is essential at various stages of differentiation. However, in addition to T cells, GATA-3 is also expressed in uncommitted HSCs, CLPs, and even in nonhematopoietic cells, and its effects are complex and highly dose dependent.[123,124]

Notch

Upon arrival into the thymus, multipotent progenitors from the marrow become rapidly committed to the T- and NK-cell pathways. The most important environmental cue for T-cell commitment is delivered by the thymic epithelium in the form of the notch ligands, delta-like ligand 1 (DLL1) and delta-like ligand 4 (DLL4).[123] Binding of one of these ligands to the notch 1 receptor expressed on the surface of thymocyte precursors causes activation of intracellular notch and a series of transcriptional programs turn on to switch lineage fate toward the T lineage at the expense of B-cell development.[123] In mice, notch is absolutely required for T-cell differentiation and proliferation, including β selection.[125] However, although notch signaling is necessary for murine thymopoiesis it is not sufficient for activation of the full complement of T-cell genes.[126] The ability of hematopoietic progenitors to respond to notch signaling and commit to T-lineage fate depends on a balance between positive and negative regulators. Combinations of at least four other transcription factors are required to initiate T-cell development, PU.1, Ikaros, Runx family factors, and E2A.[116,123] In addition, leukemia-lymphoma related factor must be downregulated to allow notch signaling to induce T-cell fate decisions.[127] Notch signaling also plays important roles at later stages of thymocyte differentiation.[123]

The effects of notch signaling have been extensively studied in mice, but the exact stages and processes regulated by notch appear to differ between mice and humans. For example, using *in vitro* studies of human T-cell development, it appears that while notch is essential for early thymocyte proliferation, it is not required for β selection or T-cell receptor $\alpha\beta$ differentiation.[128,129] As with so much of the information described in this chapter, the most important challenge that lies ahead is to translate the detailed mechanistic framework developed from murine studies into careful investigations of human lymphopoiesis.

REFERENCES

1. Tavian M, Peault B: Embryonic development of the human hematopoietic system. *Int J Dev Biol* 49:243, 2005.
2. Ueno H, Weissman IL: Stem cells: Blood lines from embryo to adult. *Nature* 446:996, 2007.
3. Medvinsky A, Dzierzak E: Definitive hematopoiesis is autonomously initiated by the AGM region. *Cell* 86:897, 1996.
4. Yoder MC, Hiatt K, Mukherjee P: *In vivo* repopulating hematopoietic stem cells are present in the murine yolk sac at day 9.0 postcoitus. *Proc Natl Acad Sci U S A* 94:6776, 1997.
5. Yoder MC, Hiatt K, Dutt P, et al: Characterization of definitive lymphohematopoietic stem cells in the day 9 murine yolk sac. *Immunity* 7:335, 1997.
6. Yoder MC, Hiatt K: Engraftment of embryonic hematopoietic cells in conditioned newborn recipients. *Blood* 89:2176, 1997.
7. Palis J, Yoder MC: Yolk-sac hematopoiesis: The first blood cells of mouse and man. *Exp Hematol* 29:927, 2001.
8. Yokota T: Tracing the first waves of lymphopoiesis in mice. *Development* 133:2041, 2006.
9. Auerbach R: Experimental analysis of the origin of cell types in the development of the mouse thymus. *Dev Biol* 3:336, 1961.
10. Owen JJ, Ritter MA: Tissue interaction in the development of thymus lymphocytes. *J Exp Med* 129:431, 1969.
11. Oberlin E, Tavian M, Blazsek I, Péault B: Blood-forming potential of vascular endothelium in the human embryo. *Development* 129:4147, 2002.
12. Tavian M, Robin C, Coulombel L, Péault B: The human embryo, but not its yolk sac, generates lympho-myeloid stem cells: Mapping multipotent hematopoietic cell fate in intraembryonic mesoderm. *Immunity* 15:487, 2001.
13. Tavian M, Coulombel L, Luton D, et al: Aorta-associated CD34+ hematopoietic cells in the early human embryo. *Blood* 87:67, 1996.
14. Tavian M, Hallais MF, Peault B: Emergence of intraembryonic hematopoietic precursors in the pre-liver human embryo. *Development* 126:793, 1999.
15. Charbord P, Tavian M, Humeau L, Péault B: Early ontogeny of the human marrow from long bones: An immunohistochemical study of hematopoiesis and its microenvironment. *Blood* 87:4109, 1996.
16. Haynes BF: The human thymic microenvironment. *Adv Immunol* 36:87, 1984.
17. Hayward AR: Development of lymphocyte responses and interactions in the human fetus and newborn. *Immunol Rev* 57:39, 1981.
18. Toivanen P, Uksila J, Leino A: Development of mitogen responding T cells and natural killer cells in the human fetus. *Immunol Rev* 57:89, 1981.
19. Renda MC, Fecarotta E, Dieli F, et al: Evidence of alloreactive T lymphocytes in fetal liver: Implications for fetal hematopoietic stem cell transplantation. *Bone Marrow Transplant* 25:135, 2000.
20. Steinmann GG: Changes in the human thymus during aging. *Curr Top Pathol* 75:43, 1986.
21. Moore AV, Korobkin M, Olanow W, et al: Age-related changes in the thymus gland: CT-pathologic correlation. *AJR Am J Roentgenol* 141:241, 1983.
22. LeBien TW: Fates of human B-cell precursors. *Blood* 96:9, 2000.
23. Dorshkind K, Montecino-Rodriguez E: Fetal B-cell lymphopoiesis and the emergence of B-1-cell potential. *Nat Rev Immunol* 7:213, 2007.
24. Solvason N, Kearney JF: The human fetal omentum: A site of B cell generation. *J Exp Med* 175:397, 1992.
25. Hofman FM, Danilovs J, Husmann L, Taylor CR: Ontogeny of B cell markers in the human fetal liver. *J Immunol* 133:1197, 1984.
26. Gathings WE, Lawton AR, Cooper MD: Immunofluorescent studies of the development of pre-B cells, B lymphocytes and immunoglobulin isotype diversity in humans. *Eur J Immunol* 7:804, 1977.
27. Nunez C, Nishimoto N, Gartland GL, et al: B cells are generated throughout life in humans. *J Immunol* 156:866, 1996.
28. Rossi MI, Yokota T, Medina KL, et al: B lymphopoiesis is active throughout human life, but there are developmental age-related changes. *Blood* 101:576, 2003.
29. Kroese FG, Ammerlaan WA, Deenen GJ: Location and function of B-cell lineages. *Ann N Y Acad Sci* 651:44, 1992.
30. Kantor AB, Herzenberg LA: Origin of murine B cell lineages. *Annu Rev Immunol* 11:501, 1993.
31. Janossy G, Bofill M, Poulter LW, et al: Separate ontogeny of two macrophage-like accessory cell populations in the human fetus. *J Immunol* 136:4354, 1986.
32. Hofman FM, Danilovs JA, Taylor CR: HLA-DR (Ia)-positive dendritic-like cells in human fetal nonlymphoid tissues. *Transplantation* 37:590, 1984.
33. Payne KJ, Crooks GM: Immune-cell lineage commitment: Translation from mice to humans. *Immunity* 26:674, 2007.
34. Kincade PW, Owen JJ, Igarashi H, et al: Nature or nurture? Steady-state lymphocyte formation in adults does not recapitulate ontogeny. *Immunol Rev* 187:116, 2002.
35. Payne KJ, Crooks GM: Human hematopoietic lineage commitment. *Immunol Rev* 187:48, 2002.
36. Reya T, Morrison SJ, Clarke MF, Weissman IL: Stem cells, cancer, and cancer stem cells. *Nature* 414:105, 2001.
37. Hakoda M, Hirai Y, Shimba H, et al: Cloning of phenotypically different human lymphocytes originating from a single stem cell. *J Exp Med* 169:1265, 1989.
38. Gore SD, Kastan MB, Civin CI: Normal human bone marrow precursors that express terminal deoxynucleotidyl transferase include T-cell precursors and possible lymphoid stem cells. *Blood* 77:1681, 1991.
39. Terstappen LW, Huang S, Picker LJ: Flow cytometric assessment of human T-cell differentiation in thymus and bone marrow. *Blood* 79:666, 1992.
40. Johnson GR, Metcalf D: Pure and mixed erythroid colony formation in vitro stimulated by spleen conditioned medium with no detectable erythropoietin. *Proc Natl Acad Sci U S A* 74:3879, 1977.
41. Akashi K, Traver D, Miyamoto T, Weissman IL: A clonogenic common myeloid progenitor that gives rise to all myeloid lineages. *Nature* 404:193, 2000.
42. Manz MG, Miyamoto T, Akashi K, Weissman IL: Prospective isolation of human clonogenic common myeloid progenitors. *Proc Natl Acad Sci U S A* 99:11872, 2002.
43. Leonard WJ: Cytokines and immunodeficiency diseases. *Nat Rev Immunol* 1:200, 2001.
44. Galy A, Travis M, Cen D, Chen B: Human T, B, natural killer, and dendritic cells arise from a common bone marrow progenitor cell subset. *Immunity* 3:459, 1995.
45. Kondo M, Weissman IL, Akashi K: Identification of clonogenic common lymphoid progenitors in mouse bone marrow. *Cell* 91:661, 1997.
46. Hao QL, Zhu J, Price MA, et al: Identification of a novel, human multilymphoid progenitor in cord blood. *Blood* 97:3683, 2001.
47. Hoebeke I, De Smedt M, Stolz F, et al: T-, B- and NK-lymphoid, but not myeloid cells arise from human CD34(+)CD38(−)CD7(+) common lymphoid progenitors expressing lymphoid-specific genes. *Leukemia* 21:311, 2007.
48. Adolfsson J, Månsson R, Buza-Vidas N, et al: Identification of Flt3+ lympho-myeloid stem cells lacking erythro-megakaryocytic potential a revised road map for adult blood lineage commitment. *Cell* 121:295, 2005.
49. Yang L, Bryder D, Adolfsson J, et al: Identification of Lin(−)Sca1(+)kit(+)CD34(+)Flt3-short-term hematopoietic stem cells capable of rapidly reconstituting and rescuing myeloablated transplant recipients. *Blood* 105:2717, 2005.
50. Luc S, Buza-Vidas N, Jacobsen SE: Biological and molecular evidence for existence of lymphoid-primed multipotent progenitors. *Ann N Y Acad Sci* 1106:89, 2007.
51. Wu L, Liu YJ: Development of dendritic-cell lineages. *Immunity* 26:741, 2007.
52. Wu L, Vandenabeele S, Georgopoulos K: Derivation of dendritic cells from myeloid and lymphoid precursors. *Int Rev Immunol* 20:117, 2001.
53. Manz MG, Traver D, Miyamoto T, et al: Dendritic cell potentials of early lymphoid and myeloid progenitors. *Blood* 97:3333, 2001.
54. Chapuis F, Rosenzwajg M, Yagello M, et al: Differentiation of human dendritic cells from monocytes *in vitro*. *Eur J Immunol* 27:431, 1997.
55. Civin CI, Gore SD: Antigenic analysis of hematopoiesis: A review. *J Hematother* 2:137, 1993.
56. Blom B, Spits H: Development of human lymphoid cells. *Annu Rev Immunol* 24:287, 2006.
57. Six EM, Bonhomme D, Monteiro M, et al: A human postnatal lymphoid progenitor capable of circulating and seeding the thymus. *J Exp Med* 204:3085, 2007.
58. Canque B, Camus S, Dalloul A, et al: Characterization of dendritic cell differentiation pathways from cord blood CD34(+)CD7(+)CD45RA(+) hematopoietic progenitor cells. *Blood* 96:3748, 2000.
59. Storms RW, Goodell MA, Fisher A, et al: Hoechst dye efflux reveals a novel CD7(+)CD34(−) lymphoid progenitor in human umbilical cord blood. *Blood* 96:2125, 2000.
60. Hao QL, Shah AJ, Thiemann FT, et al: A functional comparison of CD34+ CD38− cells in cord blood and bone marrow. *Blood* 86:3745, 1995.
61. Bjorck P, Kincade PW: CD19+ pro-B cells can give rise to dendritic cells *in vitro*. *J Immunol* 161:5795, 1998.
62. Allman D, Sambandam A, Kim S, et al: Thymopoiesis independent of common lymphoid progenitors. *Nat Immunol* 4:168, 2003.
63. Hao QL, George AA, Zhu J, et al: Human intrathymic lineage commitment is marked by differential CD7 expression: Identification of CD7− lympho-myeloid thymic progenitors. *Blood* 111:1318, 2008.
64. Weerkamp F, Baert MR, Brugman MH, et al: Human thymus contains multipotent progenitors with T/B lymphoid, myeloid, and erythroid lineage potential. *Blood* 107:3131, 2006.

65. Bhandoola A, Sambandam A, Allman D, et al: Early T lineage progenitors: New insights, but old questions remain. *J Immunol* 171:5653, 2003.
66. Rawlings DJ, Quan S, Hao QL, et al: Differentiation of human CD34+CD38– cord blood stem cells into B cell progenitors *in vitro*. *Exp Hematol* 25:66, 1997.
67. Berardi AC, Meffre E, Pflumio F, et al: Individual CD34+CD38lowCD19–CD10– progenitor cells from human cord blood generate B lymphocytes and granulocytes. *Blood* 89:3554, 1997.
68. Miller JS, McCullar V, Punzel M, et al: Single adult human CD34(+)/Lin–/CD38(–) progenitors give rise to natural killer cells, B-lineage cells, dendritic cells, and myeloid cells. *Blood* 93:96, 1999.
69. Plum J, De Smedt M, Verhasselt B, et al: Human T lymphopoiesis. *In vitro* and *in vivo* study models. *Ann N Y Acad Sci* 917:724, 2000.
70. Awong G, Herer E, Surh CD, et al: Characterization *in vitro* and engraftment potential *in vivo* of human progenitor T cells generated from hematopoietic stem cells. *Blood* 114:972, 2009.
71. Schreurs MW, Eggert AA, de Boer AJ, et al: Generation and functional characterization of mouse monocyte-derived dendritic cells. *Eur J Immunol* 29:2835, 1999.
72. Wu L, Li CL, Shortman K: Thymic dendritic cell precursors: Relationship to the T lymphocyte lineage and phenotype of the dendritic cell progeny. *J Exp Med* 184:903, 1996.
73. Ardavin C, Wu L, Li CL, Shortman K: Thymic dendritic cells and T cells develop simultaneously in the thymus from a common precursor population. *Nature* 362:761, 1993.
74. Ishikawa F, Niiro H, Iino T, et al: The developmental program of human dendritic cells is operated independently of conventional myeloid and lymphoid pathways. *Blood* 110: 3591, 2007.
75. Traver D, Akashi K, Manz M, et al: Development of CD8alpha-positive dendritic cells from a common myeloid progenitor. *Science* 290:2152, 2000.
76. Noguchi M, Yi H, Rosenblatt HM, et al: Interleukin-2 receptor gamma chain mutation results in X-linked severe combined immunodeficiency in humans. *Cell* 73:147, 1993.
77. Kondo M, Takeshita T, Ishii N, et al: Sharing of the interleukin-2 (IL-2) receptor gamma chain between receptors for IL-2 and IL-4. *Science* 262:1874, 1993.
78. Russell SM, Keegan AD, Harada N, et al: Interleukin-2 receptor gamma chain: A functional component of the interleukin-4 receptor. *Science* 262:1880, 1993.
79. Noguchi M, Nakamura Y, Russell SM, et al: Interleukin-2 receptor gamma chain: A functional component of the interleukin-7 receptor. *Science* 262:1877, 1993.
80. Kondo M, Takeshita T, Higuchi M, et al: Functional participation of the IL-2 receptor gamma chain in IL-7 receptor complexes. *Science* 263:1453, 1994.
81. Kimura Y, Takeshita T, Kondo M, et al: Sharing of the IL-2 receptor gamma chain with the functional IL-9 receptor complex. *Int Immunol* 7:115, 1995.
82. Giri JG, Ahdieh M, Eisenman J, et al: Utilization of the beta and gamma chains of the IL-2 receptor by the novel cytokine IL-15. *EMBO J* 13:2822, 1994.
83. Asao H, Okuyama C, Kumaki S, et al: Cutting edge: The common gamma-chain is an indispensable subunit of the IL-21 receptor complex. *J Immunol* 167:1, 2001.
84. Kang J, Der SD: Cytokine functions in the formative stages of a lymphocyte's life. *Curr Opin Immunol* 16:180, 2004.
85. Di Santo JP, Kuhn R, Muller W: Common cytokine receptor gamma chain (gamma c)-dependent cytokines: Understanding in vivo functions by gene targeting. *Immunol Rev* 148:19, 1995.
86. Russell SM, Johnston JA, Noguchi M, et al: Interaction of IL-2R beta and gamma c chains with Jak1 and Jak3: Implications for XSCID and XCID. *Science* 266:1042, 1994.
87. Candeias S, Muegge K, Durum SK: IL-7 receptor and VDJ recombination: Trophic versus mechanistic actions. *Immunity* 6:501, 1997.
88. Macchi P, Villa A, Giliani S, et al: Mutations of Jak-3 gene in patients with autosomal severe combined immune deficiency (SCID). *Nature* 377:65, 1995.
89. Russell SM, Tayebi N, Nakajima H, et al: Mutation of Jak3 in a patient with SCID: Essential role of Jak3 in lymphoid development. *Science* 270:797, 1995.
90. Puel A, Ziegler SF, Buckley RH, Leonard WJ: Defective IL7R expression in T(–)B(+)NK(+) severe combined immunodeficiency. *Nat Genet* 20:394, 1998.
91. Giliani S, Mori L, de Saint Basile G, et al: Interleukin-7 receptor alpha (IL-7Ralpha) deficiency: Cellular and molecular bases. Analysis of clinical, immunological, and molecular features in 16 novel patients. *Immunol Rev* 203:110, 2005.
92. Kennedy MK, Glaccum M, Brown SN, et al: Reversible defects in natural killer and memory CD8 T cell lineages in interleukin 15-deficient mice. *J Exp Med* 191:771, 2000.
93. Lodolce JP, Boone DL, Chai S, et al: IL-15 receptor maintains lymphoid homeostasis by supporting lymphocyte homing and proliferation. *Immunity* 9:669, 1998.
94. Suzuki H, Kündig TM, Furlonger C, et al: Deregulated T cell activation and autoimmunity in mice lacking interleukin-2 receptor beta. *Science* 268:1472, 1995.
95. Eidenschenk C, Jouanguy E, Alcaïs A, et al: Familial NK cell deficiency associated with impaired IL-2- and IL-15-dependent survival of lymphocytes. *J Immunol* 177:8835, 2006.
96. Weinberg K, Parkman R: Severe combined immunodeficiency due to a specific defect in the production of interleukin-2. *N Engl J Med* 322:1718, 1990.
97. Gilmour KC, Fujii H, Cranston T, et al: Defective expression of the interleukin-2/interleukin-15 receptor beta subunit leads to a natural killer cell-deficient form of severe combined immunodeficiency. *Blood* 98:877, 2001.
98. Warren LA, Rothenberg EV: Regulatory coding of lymphoid lineage choice by hematopoietic transcription factors. *Curr Opin Immunol* 15:166, 2003.
99. Akashi K, He X, Chen J, et al: Transcriptional accessibility for genes of multiple tissues and hematopoietic lineages is hierarchically controlled during early hematopoiesis. *Blood* 101:383, 2003.
100. Miyamoto T, Iwasaki H, Reizis B, et al: Myeloid or lymphoid promiscuity as a critical step in hematopoietic lineage commitment. *Dev Cell* 3:137, 2002.
101. Georgopoulos K, Bigby M, Wang JH, et al: The Ikaros gene is required for the development of all lymphoid lineages. *Cell* 79:143, 1994.
102. Wang JH, Nichogiannopoulou A, Wu L, et al: Selective defects in the development of the fetal and adult lymphoid system in mice with an Ikaros null mutation. *Immunity* 5:537, 1996.
103. Georgopoulos K, Winandy S, Avitahl N: The role of the Ikaros gene in lymphocyte development and homeostasis. *Annu Rev Immunol* 15:155, 1997.
104. Yoshida T, Ng SY, Zuniga-Pflucker JC, Georgopoulos K: Early hematopoietic lineage restrictions directed by Ikaros. *Nat Immunol* 7:382, 2006.
105. Nichogiannopoulou A, Trevisan M, Neben S, et al: Defects in hemopoietic stem cell activity in Ikaros mutant mice. *J Exp Med* 190:1201, 1999.
106. Wu L, Nichogiannopoulou A, Shortman K, Georgopoulos K: Cell-autonomous defects in dendritic cell populations of Ikaros mutant mice point to a developmental relationship with the lymphoid lineage. *Immunity* 7:483, 1997.
107. Klug CA, Morrison SJ, Masek M, et al: Hematopoietic stem cells and lymphoid progenitors express different Ikaros isoforms, and Ikaros is localized to heterochromatin in immature lymphocytes. *Proc Natl Acad Sci U S A* 95:657, 1998.
108. Payne KJ, Huang G, Sahakian E, et al: Ikaros isoform x is selectively expressed in myeloid differentiation. *J Immunol* 170:3091, 2003.
109. Payne KJ, Nicolas JH, Zhu JY, et al: Cutting edge: Predominant expression of a novel Ikaros isoform in normal human hemopoiesis. *J Immunol* 167:1867, 2001.
110. Cobb BS, Smale ST: Ikaros-family proteins: In search of molecular functions during lymphocyte development. *Curr Top Microbiol Immunol* 290:29, 2005.
111. DeKoter RP, Walsh JC, Singh H: PU.1 regulates both cytokine-dependent proliferation and differentiation of granulocyte/macrophage progenitors. *EMBO J* 17:4456, 1998.
112. DeKoter RP, Lee HJ, Singh H: PU.1 regulates expression of the interleukin-7 receptor in lymphoid progenitors. *Immunity* 16:297, 2002.
113. Medina KL, Ponqubala JM, Reddy KL, et al: Assembling a gene regulatory network for specification of the B cell fate. *Dev Cell* 7:607, 2004.
114. Polli M, Dakic A, Light A, et al: The development of functional B lymphocytes in conditional PU.1 knock-out mice. *Blood* 106:2083, 2005.
115. Murre C: Helix-loop-helix proteins and lymphocyte development. *Nat Immunol* 6:1079, 2005.
116. Dias S, Månsson R, Gurbuxani S, et al: E2A proteins promote development of lymphoid-primed multipotent progenitors. *Immunity* 29:217, 2008.
117. Bain G, Engel I, Robanus Maandag EC, et al: E2A deficiency leads to abnormalities in alphabeta T-cell development and to rapid development of T-cell lymphomas. *Mol Cell Biol* 17: 4782, 1997.
118. Bain G, Robanus Maandag EC, te Riele HP, et al: Both E12 and E47 allow commitment to the B cell lineage. *Immunity* 6:145, 1997.
119. Kee BL, Murre C: Induction of early B cell factor (EBF) and multiple B lineage genes by the basic helix-loop-helix transcription factor E12. *J Exp Med* 188:699, 1998.
120. Ikawa T, Kawamoto H, Goldrath AW, Murre C: E proteins and Notch signaling cooperate to promote T cell lineage specification and commitment. *J Exp Med* 203:1329, 2006.
121. Nutt SL, Heavey B, Rolink AG, Busslinger M: Commitment to the B-lymphoid lineage depends on the transcription factor Pax5. *Nature* 401:556, 1999.
122. Pongubala JM, Northrup DL, Lancki DW, et al: Transcription factor EBF restricts alternative lineage options and promotes B cell fate commitment independently of Pax5. *Nat Immunol* 9:203, 2008.
123. Rothenberg EV, Moore JE, Yui MA: Launching the T-cell-lineage developmental programme. *Nat Rev Immunol* 8:9, 2008.
124. Taghon T, Yui MA, Rothenberg EV: Mast cell lineage diversion of T lineage precursors by the essential T cell transcription factor GATA-3. *Nat Immunol* 8:845, 2007.
125. Maillard I, Tu L, Sambandam A, et al: The requirement for Notch signaling at the beta-selection checkpoint *in vivo* is absolute and independent of the pre-T cell receptor. *J Exp Med* 203:2239, 2006.
126. Taghon TN, David ES, Zúñiga-Pflücker JC, Rothenberg EV: Delayed, asynchronous, and reversible T-lineage specification induced by Notch/Delta signaling. *Genes Dev* 19:965, 2005.
127. Maeda T, Merghoub T, Hobbs RM, et al: Regulation of B versus T lymphoid lineage fate decision by the proto-oncogene LRF. *Science* 316:860, 2007.
128. Taghon T, Van de Walle I, De Smet G, et al: Notch signaling is required for proliferation but not for differentiation at a well-defined beta-selection checkpoint during human T-cell development. *Blood* 113:3254, 2009.
129. Van de Walle I, De Smet G, De Smedt M, et al: An early decrease in Notch activation is required for human TCR-alphabeta lineage differentiation at the expense of TCR-gammadelta T cells. *Blood* 113:2988, 2009.

CHAPTER 77

FUNCTIONS OF B LYMPHOCYTES AND PLASMA CELLS IN IMMUNOGLOBULIN PRODUCTION

Thomas J. Kipps

SUMMARY

Much of our immune defense against invading organisms is predicated upon the tremendous diversity of immunoglobulin molecules. Immunoglobulins are glycoproteins produced by B lymphocytes and plasma cells. These molecules can be considered receptors because the primary function of the immunoglobulin molecule is to bind antigen. A single person can synthesize 10 to 100 million different immunoglobulin molecules, each having a distinct antigen-binding specificity. The great diversity in this so-called humoral immune system allows us to generate antibodies specific for a variety of substances, including synthetic molecules not naturally present in our environment. Despite the diversity in the specificities of antibody molecules, the binding of antibody to antigen initiates a limited series of biologically important effector functions, such as complement activation and/or adherence of the immune complex to receptors on leukocytes. The eventual outcome is the clearance and degradation of the foreign substance. This chapter describes the structure of immunoglobulins and outlines the mechanisms by which B cells produce molecules of such tremendous diversity with defined effector functions.

Acronyms and abbreviations that appear in this chapter include: ADCC, antibody-dependent cellular cytotoxicity; AID, activation-induced deaminase; BACH2, basic leucine zipper transcription factor 2; BCL-6, B-cell chronic lymphocytic leukemia/lymphoma 6; BiP, immunoglobulin-binding protein; Blimp-1, B-lymphocyte-induced maturation protein-1; BLNK, B-cell linker protein; Btk, Bruton tyrosine kinase; C, constant; CDR, complementarity determining region; CRI, cross-reactive idiotype; CSR, class switch recombination; D, diversity; DLBCL, diffuse large B-cell lymphoma; DNA-PK, DNA protein kinase; E2F1, E2F transcription factor 1; EBF1, early B-cell factor 1; FR, framework region; H, heavy; HMG, high-mobility group protein; Ig, immunoglobulin; IL, interleukin; IRF4, interferon regulatory factor 4; ITAM, immunoreceptor tyrosine-based activation motif; κ, immunoglobulin kappa light chain; Kde, kappa-deleting element; λ, immunoglobulin lambda light chain; L, light; MITF, microphthalmia-associated transcription factor; mRNA, messenger RNA; MYBL1 and 2, v-myb myeloblastosis viral oncogene homolog 1 and 2; NHEJ, nonhomologous DNA end-joining; PAX5, paired box gene 5; PLC, phospholipase C; P-nucleotide, palindromic nucleotide; POU2AF1, Pou domain, class 2, associating factor 1; POU2F2, Pou domain, class 2, factor 2; PRDM1, positive regulatory domain 1-binding factor-1; *RAG*, recombination-activating gene; RSS, recombination signal sequences; SCID, severe combined immunodeficiency; SHP-1, Src homology 2 domain-containing protein tyrosine phosphatase-1; TCFE2A, transcription factor E2a; UNG, uracil-DNA glycosylase; V, variable-region gene; VDJ, exon created by a rearranged immunoglobulin heavy-chain variable-region gene, diversity gene segment, and joining gene segment; XBA1, X-box binding protein-1.

IMMUNOGLOBULIN STRUCTURE AND FUNCTION

BASIC STRUCTURE

All naturally occurring immunoglobulin molecules are composed of one or several basic units consisting of two identical heavy (H) chains and two identical light (L) chains (Fig. 77–1). The four polypeptides are held in a symmetrical, Y-shaped structure by disulfide bonds and noncovalent interactions. The internal disulfide bonds of the heavy and light chains cause the polypeptides to fold into compact globe-shaped regions called domains, each containing approximately 110 to 120 amino acid residues.[1] Each domain forms a common fold of a type of protein structure known as beta-pleated sheets and is stabilized by a conserved disulfide bond (Fig. 77–1). The light chains have two domains; the heavy chains have four or five domains. The amino-terminal domains of the heavy and light chains are designated the variable (V) regions because their primary structure varies markedly among different immunoglobulin molecules.[2] The carboxy-terminal domains are referred to as constant (C) regions because their primary structure is the same among immunoglobulins of the same class or subclass. The amino acids in the light- and heavy-chain variable regions interact to form an antigen-binding site. Each four-chain immunoglobulin basic unit has two identical binding sites. The constant-region domains of the heavy and light chains provide stability for the immunoglobulin molecule. The heavy-chain constant regions also mediate the specific effector functions of the different immunoglobulin classes (Table 77–1).

LIGHT CHAINS

Immunoglobulin light chains have an approximate Mr of 23,000. They are divided into two types, κ and λ, based upon multiple amino acid sequence differences in the single constant-region domain.[2] The λ chains are divided further into subclasses. The proportion of κ-to-λ chains in adult human plasma is approximately 2:1. The immunoglobulin light-chain constant region has no known effector function. Its main purpose may be to allow for proper assembly and release of an intact immunoglobulin molecule. Soon after synthesis, the antibody light-chain constant region associates with the nascent immunoglobulin heavy chain (see Fig. 77–1), releasing the latter from the immunoglobulin-binding protein (BiP). BiP is a heat shock protein that, in the absence of antibody light chain, binds the first constant-region domain of the newly synthesized heavy chain, thereby retaining the heavy-chain polypeptide in the cell's endoplasmic reticulum.[3]

HEAVY CHAINS

Immunoglobulin heavy chains have an Mr of 50,000 to 70,000, depending upon the number and length of the constant-region domains. The five major isotypes of heavy chains—γ, α, μ, δ, and ε—determine the five corresponding classes of immunoglobulin (Ig): IgG, IgA, IgM, IgD, and IgE. The individual immunoglobulin molecules of each isotype may contain either κ or λ light chains, but not both. Tables 77–1 and 77–2 summarize the distinct physical and functional properties of the human immunoglobulin classes.

IgG

Approximately 80 percent of the immunoglobulins in adult plasma are IgG. The IgG molecule is composed of the basic 150-kDa immunoglobulin four-chain structure plus approximately 3 percent carbohydrate. Near the junction of the two arms of the Y-shaped immunoglobulin molecule, the two heavy chains interact to form a flexible "hinge" region

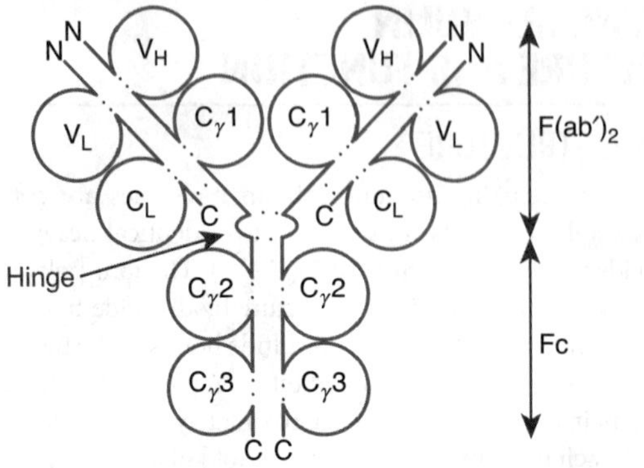

FIGURE 77–1. Model of an immunoglobulin (Ig) G molecule. The light-chain domains V_L and C_L and the heavy-chain domains V_H, $C_\gamma 1$(or $C_H 1$), $C_\gamma 2$ (or $C_H 2$), and $C_\gamma 3$ (or $C_H 3$) are labeled inside the respective immunoglobulin domain. Dotted red colored lines indicate intrachain and interchain disulfide bonds. The amino-terminus (N) and carboxyl-terminus (C) of each polypeptide are indicated. The hinge region also is indicated. Digestion by pepsin cleaves the molecule at the carboxyl side of the hinge region, which generates Fc and $F(ab')_2$ fragments, as indicated on the *right*. The $F(ab')_2$ fragment is bivalent, as it is held together by the disulfide bridges in the hinge region. On the other hand, digestion of the molecule by papain degrades the Fc portion and generates monovalent Fab fragments, as the cleavage site for papain is on the amino-terminal side of the disulfide bridges of the hinge region.

(see Fig. 77–1). Exposed between constant-region globular domains, the hinge region is attacked readily by the proteolytic enzyme papain or pepsin. Figure 77–1 shows the cleavage sites. Digestion of IgG with papain yields three fragments. The single Fc piece contains the carboxy-terminal region of both heavy chains. The two identical F(ab) pieces contain the entire light chain and the amino-terminal portion of the heavy chain. IgG molecules effectively penetrate extravascular spaces and readily cross the placental barrier to provide passive immunity to the newborn.

IgG is the predominant antibody produced during the secondary immune response to antigen. The average half-life of circulating IgG molecules is approximately 21 days, although the exact value varies among the IgG subclasses (Table 77–3). Within the IgG class are four major subclasses, designated IgG_1, IgG_2, IgG_3, and IgG_4. Each subclass has a distinct heavy-chain constant region and mediates different effector functions (Table 77–3).[4] Whereas IgG_1 and IgG_3 proteins activate complement via the classic pathway, IgG_2 molecules fix complement poorly and IgG_4 proteins not at all. IgG_3 myeloma protein may aggregate spontaneously to produce a hyperviscosity syndrome. The most abundant subclass is IgG_1, which constitutes 65 percent of the total IgG in plasma.

For antigens found on pathogens, the bound IgG can: (1) tag the pathogen for ingestion and destruction by phagocytes, a process called *opsonization*; (2) activate complement; and/or (3) direct antibody-dependent cell mediated cytotoxicity (ADCC). Either aggregated IgG or antigen–antibody complexes may bind to specific receptors for the Fc fragment, designated FcRI (CD64), FcRII (CD32), and FcRIII (CD16). Of the IgG subclasses, IgG_1 binds best to FcRI (CD64) and FcRII (CD32), with affinities (dissociation constant [Kd]) of 10 nanomolars and 50 micromolars, respectively (see Table 77–3). IgG_1 and IgG_3 bind equally well to FcRIII (CD16), with a Kd of 2 micromolars (see Table 77–3). This is the Fc receptor expressed by natural killer (NK) cells (or K cells), which mediate ADCC. Proteins of the IgG_4 or IgG_2 subclass bind poorly to FcRI (CD64) or FcRII (CD32), and bind not at all to FcRIII (CD16) (see Table 77–3). IgG_1 is the most proficient subclass at directing ADCC. For this reason, most of the therapeutic monoclonal antibodies are of the IgG_1 subclass, which can be modified further to enhance their capacity to direct ADCC.[5]

IgA

IgA composes only approximately 13 percent of plasma immunoglobulins (see Table 77–1), even though the production of IgA exceeds that of any other immunoglobulin isotype, accounting for 60 to 70 percent of antibodies produced each day.[6] The relatively low amount in plasma is due to the high amount of IgA secreted into the gastrointestinal tract. It is estimated that a normal 70-kg adult secretes approximately 2 g of IgA per day.[6] IgA also circulates in the plasma as a monomer, dimer, or higher polymer containing approximately 8 percent carbohydrate. Within the IgA class are two major subclasses, designated IgA_1 and IgA_2. The most abundant subclass is IgA_1, which constitutes approximately 85 percent of the total IgA in plasma. The half-life of circulating IgA of either subclass is approximately 6 days.

TABLE 77–1. Physical Properties of Human Immunoglobulins

	IgG	IgA	IgM	IgD	IgE
Heavy-chain class	γ	α	μ	δ	ε
Heavy chain subclass	$\gamma 1, \gamma 2, \gamma 3, \gamma 4$	$\alpha 1, \alpha 2$	–	–	–
No. of heavy-chain domains	4	4	5	4	5
Secretory form	Monomer	Monomer, dimer	Pentamer	Monomer	Monomer
Molecular mass (Da)	150,000	160,000 (monomer) 400,000 (secretory)	900,000	184,000	188,000
Antigen-binding valency	2	2 (monomer) 4 (secretory)	10	2	2
Serum concentration (mg/mL)	8–16	1.4–4.0	0.5–2.0	0–0.4	17–450 ng/mL
Percent of total immunoglobulin	80	13	6	1	0.002
Electrophoretic mobility	γ	Fast γ to β	Slow γ	Fast γ	Fast γ
Percent carbohydrate	3	8	12	13	12

TABLE 77–2. Biologic Properties of Human Immunoglobulins

	IgG	IgA	IgM	IgD	IgE
Percent of body pool in intravascular space	45	42	76	75	51
Percent of intravascular pool catabolized per day	6.7	25	18	37	89
Normal synthetic rate (mg/kg per day)	33	24	6.7	0.4	0.02
Serum half-life (days)	21	5.8	10	2.8	2.3
Placental transfer	Yes	No	No	No	No
Cytophilic for mast cells and basophils	No	No	No	No	Yes
Binding to macrophages and other phagocytes	Yes	No	No	No	Yes
Reactivity with staphylococcal protein A	Yes	No	No	No	No
Antibody-dependent cell-mediated cytotoxicity	Yes	No	No	No	No
Complement fixation					
Classic pathway	Yes	No	Yes	No	No
Alternative pathway	No	Yes	No	No	No

The primary role for IgA is in mucosal immunity.[7] Plasma cells in the lamina propria secrete IgA as a dimmer that is held together by a J (joining) chain. The secreted IgA can bind to a *poly-Ig receptor*, which is an integral membrane glycoprotein expressed on the basal membrane of mucosal cells. Following the binding of IgA, the mucosal epithelial cells mediate endocytosis and transport of the IgA–poly-Ig receptor complex in vesicles that are exported to the epithelial luminal surface. Here the poly-Ig receptor is proteolytically cleaved, releasing the extracellular domain, which remains complexed with the secreted IgA as a 70-kDa *secretory protein* that can protect the secreted IgA molecule from proteolytic digestion by enzymes in the intestinal lumen. This modified form of IgA, comprised of an IgA dimer bound to the J chain and secretory protein, is the principal antibody in saliva, tears, colostrum, and the fluids of the gastrointestinal, respiratory, and urinary tracts.[6–8]

IgA can direct various effector functions by cells that bear specific Fc receptors for IgA (FcαR). FcαRI is the principal myeloid IgA receptor and is responsible for directing various IgA-mediated effector responses, such as respiratory burst, degranulation, and phagocytosis by granulocytes, monocytes, or macrophages. Another IgA receptor specific for the secretory protein can elicit powerful effector responses from eosinophils.[9] On the other hand, IgA antibodies do not cross the placenta, fix complement via the classic pathway, or bind efficiently to cell surfaces. Their main function may be to prevent foreign substances from adhering to mucosal surfaces and entering the blood.

Defective glycosylation of IgA_1 can lead to the most common form glomerulonephritis, namely *Berger disease* or *IgA nephropathy*. This is an autoimmune disorder in which neoepitopes caused by defective galactosylation of *O*-linked glycans in the hinge region of human IgA_1 are recognized by antiglycan IgG or IgA_1 antibodies.[10] Some of the resultant immune complexes in the circulation escape normal clearance mechanisms, deposit in the renal mesangium, and induce glomerular injury.[11] Another nephritis associated with glomerular IgA deposits is *Henoch-Schönlein purpura*, a condition that most commonly presents with a characteristic pruritic skin rash, arthritis, and abdominal pain in children or young adults (see Chap. 123).

TABLE 77–3. Characteristics of Major IgG Subclasses

	IgG_1	IgG_2	IgG_3	IgG_4
Heavy-chain subclass	$\gamma 1$	$\gamma 2$	$\gamma 3$	$\gamma 4$
Serum concentration (mg/mL)	9	3	1	0.5
Percent of total IgG	67	22	7	4
Serum half-life (days)	21	20	7	21
Complement fixation				
Classic pathway	++	+/−	+++	−
Alternative pathway	−	−	−	−
FcRI (CD64) binding	++++	+/−	++	+
FcRII (CD32) binding	+++	+/−	+	+
FcRIII (CD16) binding	+	−	+	−
Antibody-dependent cell-mediated cytotoxicity	+	−	+	−
Heterologous skin sensitization	+	−	+	+

IgM

In a normal adult, approximately 6 percent of the total plasma immunoglobulins belong to the IgM class (see Tables 77–1 and 77–2). IgM molecules classically are termed macroglobulins because of their large molecular weight. Circulating IgM molecules contain 12 percent carbohydrate and are formed through the linkage of five identical immunoglobulin units by disulfide bonds and by a J chain (Fig. 77–2).[12] IgM represents the predominant immunoglobulin class formed during a primary immune response. IgM macroglobulins do not penetrate easily into extravascular spaces or readily cross the placenta. Compared to monomeric IgG antibodies, pentavalent IgM antibodies fix complement more efficiently. A single IgM molecule on the surface of a red blood cell can initiate complement-mediated hemolysis. IgM is catabolized rapidly, with a plasma half-life of only 6 days. The monomeric form of IgM, with only two heavy and two light chains, is the major immunoglobulin expressed on the B-cell surface (Fig. 77–3).

IgD

IgD is a trace serum protein that composes less than 1 percent of plasma immunoglobulins. IgD is expressed on most peripheral B cells, as is IgM. The molecule has the basic four-chain constant region and contains 11 percent carbohydrate (see Tables 77–1 and 77–2). IgD antibodies are sensitive to proteolytic degradation. They do not penetrate extravascular spaces efficiently, cross the placental barrier, or fix complement via the classic pathway. Rather, IgD functions primarily as a B cell membrane receptor for antigen that facilitates recruitment of B cells into specific antigen-driven responses.[13]

IgE

Although four human IgE isoforms can be produced by alternative splicing of the epsilon primary transcript,[14] each isoform appears to have similar function. IgE has been called reaginic antibody to denote its association with immediate hypersensitivity. It normally constitutes only 0.004 percent of total plasma immunoglobulin (see Tables 77–1 and 77–2). In patients with parasitic infestation and in some children with atopic diseases, plasma IgE levels may rise to 5 to 20 times normal. The IgE molecule consists of a four-chain basic unit plus 12 percent carbohydrate. Monomeric IgE binds via the Fc region to high-affinity

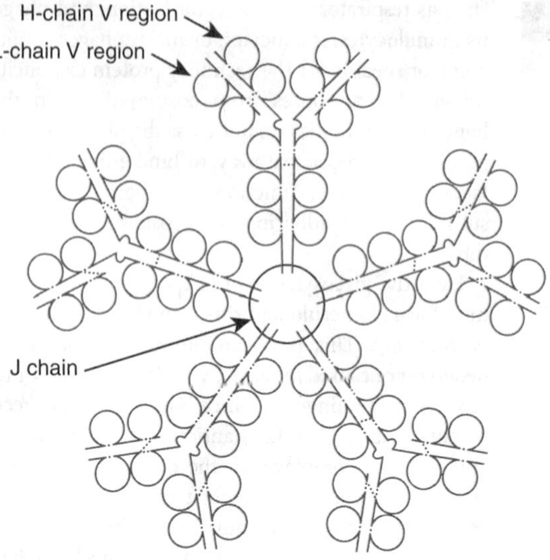

FIGURE 77–2. Schematic model of an IgM pentamer. IgM has 10 binding sites for antigen, each composed of a heavy-chain variable region (H-chain V region) and a light-chain variable region (L-chain V region). Five bivalent IgM molecules are held together by the single joining (J) chain. Broken red colored lines indicate intrachain and interchain disulfide bonds.

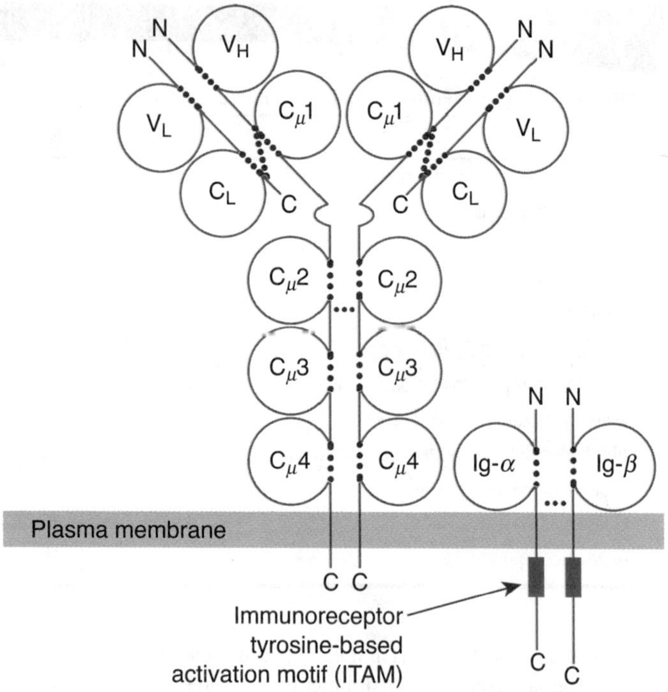

FIGURE 77–3. Schematic model of membrane IgM and its associated accessory proteins Ig-α (CD79a) and Ig-β (CD79b). The light-chain domains V_L and C_L and the heavy-chain domains V_H, $C_\mu1$ (or C_H1), $C_\mu2$ (or C_H2), $C_\mu3$ (or C_H3), and $C\mu4$ (or C_H4) are labeled inside the respective immunoglobulin domain. Each of the cytoplasmic domains of Ig-α (CD79a) and Ig-β (CD79b) has an immunoreceptor tyrosine-based activation motif (ITAM) depicted by a green rectangle. These ITAMs play a critical role in the signaling events that are initiated by ligation of surface immunoglobulin by antigen. Dotted red colored lines indicate intrachain and interchain disulfide bonds.

receptors on the surface membranes of basophils and mast cells. When bound to tissue mast cells, IgE has a much longer half-life than in plasma, in which its half-life is only approximately 2 days (see Table 77–2). Crosslinking of cell-bound IgE antibody by antigen induces the release of vasoactive amines, lipid-derived inflammatory mediators, proteases, proteoglycans, and cytokines, such as tumor necrosis factor-α (cachectin), interferon-γ, granulocyte-macrophage colony-stimulating factor, and interleukins (IL)-1, IL-3, IL-4, IL-5, and IL-6. These substances act on adjacent cells and may regulate the metabolism of the connective tissue extracellular matrix. These lipid mediators and biogenic amines may produce the rapid components of immediate hypersensitivity, such as vascular leakage, vasodilation, and bronchoconstriction. The released cytokines, on the other hand, are responsible for the late phase of the immediate hypersensitivity response. The physiologic function of this response is not clear. Instead, the immediate hypersensitivity response may represent a pathologic systemic exaggeration of a local physiologic process that ordinarily contributes to the inflammatory response to invading organisms.

SURFACE IMMUNOGLOBULIN

Any one of the immunoglobulin isotypes may serve as a B-cell membrane receptor for antigen.[15] However, most B cells express surface IgM with or without IgD. Each immunoglobulin is expressed on the surface membrane as a monomer complexed noncovalently with disulfide-linked heterodimeric glycoproteins that, together with surface immunoglobulin, form the B-cell antigen–receptor complex (see Fig. 77–3). For surface IgM, each heterodimer is composed of CD79a, an IgM α chain of 33 kDa, complexed with CD79b, an Ig β chain of 37 kDa (see Chap. 15). CD79a interacts with the transmembrane domain and C_H4 domain of the immunoglobulin molecule, which mediates B-cell receptor clustering and signaling in response to antigen (see Fig. 77–3).[16] The CD79a chain is a product of the human mb-1 gene (designated *CD79a*) located at 19q13.2, whereas CD79b is the product of *CD79b* located on a different chromosome at 17q23 (see Chap. 15). B cells that lack expression of CD79a or CD79b cannot express surface immunoglobulin. CD79a/CD79b are necessary, not only for transport of the assembled immunoglobulin to the cell surface but also for signal transduction following surface immunoglobulin-receptor crosslinking by antigen. Patients with inherited defects in CD79a have an immune deficiency that is indistinguishable from that of classic X-linked agammaglobulinemia (see Chap. 82).[17] The cytoplasmic tails of CD79a and CD79b each contain immunoreceptor tyrosine-based activation motifs (ITAMs). Such motifs are found in the cytoplasmic domains of several immune system signaling molecules, including those of the T-cell receptor complex (see Chap. 78).

B cells can become activated following ligation of their surface immunoglobulin receptors by antigen, which typically is presented on the surface of dendritic cells or macrophages.[18–21] This can cause microclustering of the immunoglobulin receptor complex into the *immunologic synapse*, which accumulates src family tyrosine kinases (e.g., Lyn, Blk, and Fyn), which can phosphorylate tyrosine residues in the ITAMs of CD79a and CD79b. In turn, the phosphorylated ITAM binds cytoplasmic signaling molecules, the most important of which is $p72^{Syk}$, a 72-kDa tyrosine kinase. Following its recruitment to the activated immunoglobulin receptor complex, $p72^{Syk}$ itself becomes activated through phosphorylation, allowing it to phosphorylate the cytosolic adapter protein BLNK (B-cell linker protein, also known as SLP-65, BASH, or BCA).[22] BLNK serves as a docking site for a number of important signaling molecules, including Bruton tyrosine kinase (Btk), Vav-1, Vav-2, and phospholipase C gamma (PLCγ).[23] Dual phosphorylation and activation of PLCγ by Btk and $p72^{syk}$ allows PLCγ to effect hydrolysis of the polyphosphoinositides into inositol 1,4,5-trisphosphate and diacylglycerol, which, in turn, increase intracellular Ca^{2+} and activate protein kinase C and Ras, respectively. The importance of these activation events in B-cell signaling and development is underscored by patients with inherited defects in Btk, who lack B-cell development and have X-linked agammaglobulinemia (see Chap. 82).[24]

To mitigate the problem of accidental initiation of signal transduction, the signaling cascade is subject to negative controls. The quantity and quality of immunoglobulin receptor signaling are modulated by several transmembrane proteins that are associated with the immunoglobulin-CD79a/CD79b receptor complex. These associated proteins can be either costimulatory (e.g., CD19) or inhibitory (e.g., CD22 and CD72; see Chap. 15).[25,26] In contrast to CD79a and CD79b, CD22 and CD72 have cytoplasmic domains with immunoreceptor tyrosine-based inhibitory motifs. When immunoreceptor tyrosine-based inhibitory motifs are phosphorylated by activated Lyn kinase, the domains recruit Src homology 2 (SH2) domain-containing protein tyrosine phosphatase 1 (SHP-1), otherwise known as protein tyrosine phosphatase 1c.[27,28] Bound SHP-1 can remove the phosphate group from the phosphorylated (and thereby activated) tyrosine kinases, returning these kinases to their inactive state so that they no longer trigger B-cell activation. The importance of SHP-1 in limiting B cell activation is demonstrated by mutant mice that lack this phosphatase.[29] The B lymphocytes of such animals are stimulated by much lower concentrations of antigen than the B lymphocytes of normal mice. Because of this situation, these mice have excessive B-cell proliferation, autoimmune disease, and early mortality.

GENETICS OF IMMUNOGLOBULINS

IMMUNOGLOBULIN GENE COMPLEXES

Immunoglobulin genes are inherited in three unlinked gene complexes: one for the heavy-chain classes, one for κ light chains, and one for λ light chains. The immunoglobulin heavy-chain gene complex is located at band q32 of the long arm of chromosome 14. This complex is composed of 39 functional heavy-chain variable-region (V_H) genes, more than 120 nonfunctional V_H pseudogenes, 25 functional diversity (D) segments, 6 functional J_H minigenes, and exons encoding the constant regions for each of the immunoglobulin heavy-chain isotypes (Fig. 77–4).[30] The κ light-chain gene complex is contained within band p12 on the short arm of chromosome 2. This gene complex consists of approximately 40 functional κ light-chain variable-region genes (V_κ genes), more than 30 nonfunctional V_κ pseudogenes, 5 J_κ segments, 1 constant-region exon, and 1 kappa-deleting element (Kde) (Fig. 77–5).[31] Many of the V_κ genes in the so-called p region most proximal to the J_κ segments are in the opposite orientation of the J_κ segments, thus requiring that the V_κ exons in the proximal region undergo inversion during immunoglobulin gene rearrangement (Fig. 77–5). The λ light-chain gene complex is located at band q11.2 on the long arm of chromosome 22, 6 megabases from the centromere.[32] This gene complex consists of approximately 41 functional λ light-chain variable-region genes (V_λ genes), more than 30 V_λ pseudogenes, 4 functional λ constant-region genes ($C_\lambda 1$, $C_\lambda 2$, $C_\lambda 3$, $C_\lambda 7$), and 3 λ constant-region pseudogenes ($C_\lambda 4$, $C_\lambda 5$, $C_\lambda 6$), each associated with 1 J_λ segment (Fig. 77–5).[33] The constant-region elements of the heavy-chain gene complex are proximal to variable-region segments on chromosome 14, whereas the constant-region segments of the two light chains are in the opposite orientation, telomeric to the variable-region genes.

Each germ-line V gene, D element, and J segment is flanked by recognition sequences that are necessary to direct site-specific recombination (Fig. 77–6). Such sequences consist of a highly conserved palindromic heptamer (5′-CACAGTG-3′) a nonconserved spacer of 12 or 23 bp, and a conserved nonamer (5′ACAAAAACC-3′)[34] Joining usually occurs only between segments flanked by recognition sequences with unequal spacers.[35,36] Each recognition sequence consists of a dyad symmetric heptamer, an A/T-rich nonamer, and a spacer region of conserved length, either 12 bp or 23 bp ± 1 bp. This sequence is referred to as the 12/23 joining rule. The consensus sequences for the heptamer (CACAGTG) and nonamers (ACAAAAACC) are optimal for rearrangement, but considerable deviation from the consensus sequence is observed and tolerated. Each spacer varies in sequence, but its length is conserved and corresponds to one or two turns of the DNA double helix. Each spacer brings the heptamer and nonamer sequences to one side of the DNA helix, where they are bound by the Rag-1/Rag-2 protein complex that catalyzes recombination (Fig. 77–6). Similar recognition sequences flank the elements that rearrange to form the T-cell antigen receptor (see Chap. 78). Because all segments of a particular type (e.g., V_κ gene segments) are flanked by one type of signal sequence and all the segments to which they should be joined (e.g., J_κ segments) are flanked by the opposite type of signal sequence, the 12/23 rule ensures that the joining is restricted to events that could be biologically productive. Such heptamer-spacer-nonamer sequences, often called recombination signal sequences (RSS), are targets of lymphocyte-specific enzymes encoded by recombination activating gene *RAG1* and *RAG2*.[35]

IMMUNOGLOBULIN GENE REARRANGEMENT AND EXPRESSION DURING B-CELL DEVELOPMENT

IMMUNOGLOBULIN GENE REARRANGEMENT

During B-cell ontogeny, the first immunoglobulin gene rearrangements generally occur within the heavy-chain gene complex (Fig. 77–7A). One or more D segments may rearrange and become juxtaposed with a single J_H element, generating a DJ_H complex that then may rearrange with one of the 39 functional V_H genes. Subsequently, gene rearrangements occur in the light-chain loci (Fig. 77–7B). One of the 40 functional V_κ genes can rearrange with any one of five J_κ segments. Should these gene rearrangements fail to generate a functional $V_\kappa J_\kappa$ exon, the Kde may rearrange to a site in or immediately downstream of the $V_\kappa J_\kappa$ exon, thus deleting the kappa light-chain constant-region exon. Subsequent to κ light-chain gene rearrangement, one of the 41 functional V_λ exons can rearrange with any one of the four functional $J_\lambda C_\lambda$ exons to generate a gene that can encode a λ light chain (Fig. 77–7C).[33]

Somatic V-region gene recombination involves introduction of double-strand DNA breaks at RSS, juxtaposition of the broken ends, and then religation through a process called *nonhomologous DNA end-joining* (NHEJ). The most common mode of recombination involves the looping out and deletion of the DNA intervening between two gene segments on the same chromosome. The ends of the heptamer sequences are joined precisely in a head-to-head configuration to form a signal joint in a circular piece of DNA that then is lost from the genome when the cell divides. However, when the RSS are oriented in the same direction along the chromosome, the segments undergo recombination via inversion, in which case the intervening DNA is retained.

The first cleavage step requires a specialized heterodimeric endonuclease complex comprised of Rag-1 and Rag-2 (see Chap. 75 and Fig. 77–6). Rag-1 and Rag-2 are encoded by adjacent genes located on the short arm of chromosome 11 (11p13-p12). They were identified based on their ability to enable fibroblasts to catalyze V(D)J recombination of nonrearranged immunoglobulin genes that were cointroduced via gene transfer. Rag-1 has sequence similarities to bacterial topoisomerases that catalyze the breakage and rejoining of DNA. Rag-1 and Rag-2 normally are coexpressed only in developing lymphocytes that are undergoing receptor gene rearrangement. Mice with either *RAG* gene knocked out cannot undergo immunoglobulin or T-cell receptor gene rearrangements and consequently fail to produce mature B or T lymphocytes.[37]

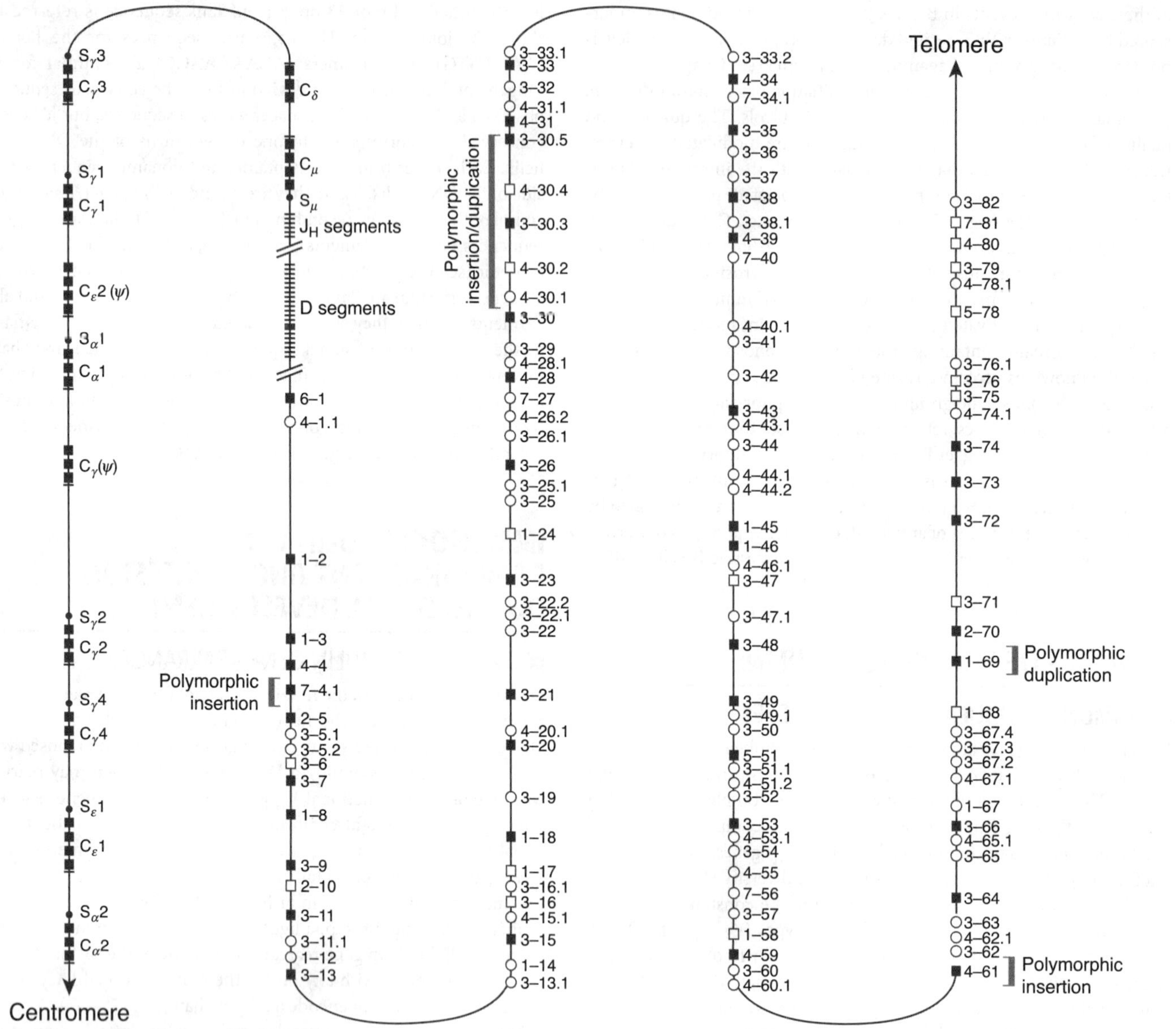

FIGURE 77–4. Human heavy-chain immunoglobulin gene complex on chromosome 14q32. The heavy-chain exons encoding the constant regions are represented by *boxes*, and the associated intronic switch regions (S) are each depicted as a *line*. These exons are labeled to the right of these symbols. A *Ψ* symbol next to the heavy-chain isotype designation indicates the gene is a pseudogene. J_H segments and D segments are indicated by lines. Each V_H gene locus is labeled on the right of each symbol. By convention, the loci encoding each of the various V_H genes are assigned a number corresponding to the V_H gene subgroup, followed by a hyphen and then the rank order distance from the heavy-chain D segments. Identified polymorphic insertions and/or duplications are indicated with brackets. *Blue squares* represent V_H gene loci that are known to be functional. *Open circles* represent V_H pseudogenes. *Open boxes* depict V_H exons that appear to be functional but rarely are found to encode a functional heavy-chain gene rearrangement and, in fact, may be pseudogenes. *Arrows* at the end of the line containing the symbols indicate the direction to the centromere or the telomere.

Mutations that impair, but do not completely abolish, the function of Rag-1 or Rag-2 in humans result in a form of combined immune deficiency called Omenn syndrome.[38]

The Rag-1/Rag-2 endonuclease complex recognizes either the 12-mer–spaced or 23-mer–spaced RSS and then introduces double-stranded DNA breaks (see Fig. 77–6). After introducing these breaks, the Rag-1/Rag-2 complex remains bound to the DNA (see Chap. 75).[39] Mutations that affect the ability of the Rag proteins to bind and maintain the broken ends in a stable post-cleavage complex can lead to misrepair of the double-strand breaks, thereby enhancing the risk for oncogenic chromosomal aberrations.[40,41] Several proteins are involved in the processing and juxtaposition of these double-strand breaks, including high-mobility group protein-1 (HMG1) and high-mobility group protein 2 (HMG2). HMG1 and HMG2 are widely expressed, abundant nuclear proteins that bind and bend DNA without sequence specificity, thereby playing an important role in the assembly of nucleoprotein complexes involved in DNA repair and transcription.[42] HMG1 may facilitate the bending of the DNA to allow the components of one double-stranded-break-Rag complex to bind and cleave the DNA at a different RSS, thus bringing together two disparate RSS in accordance with the 12/23 joining rule.[43]

The double-stranded-break RAG complex also binds several other proteins, including Artemis, DNA-dependent protein kinase (DNA-PK), Ku70, Ku80, the human protein *X-ray repair complementing defective repair in Chinese hamster cells 4* (XRCC4), and DNA ligase IV (Lig4) (see Chap. 75 and Fig. 77–6). DNA-PK is a serine-threonine protein

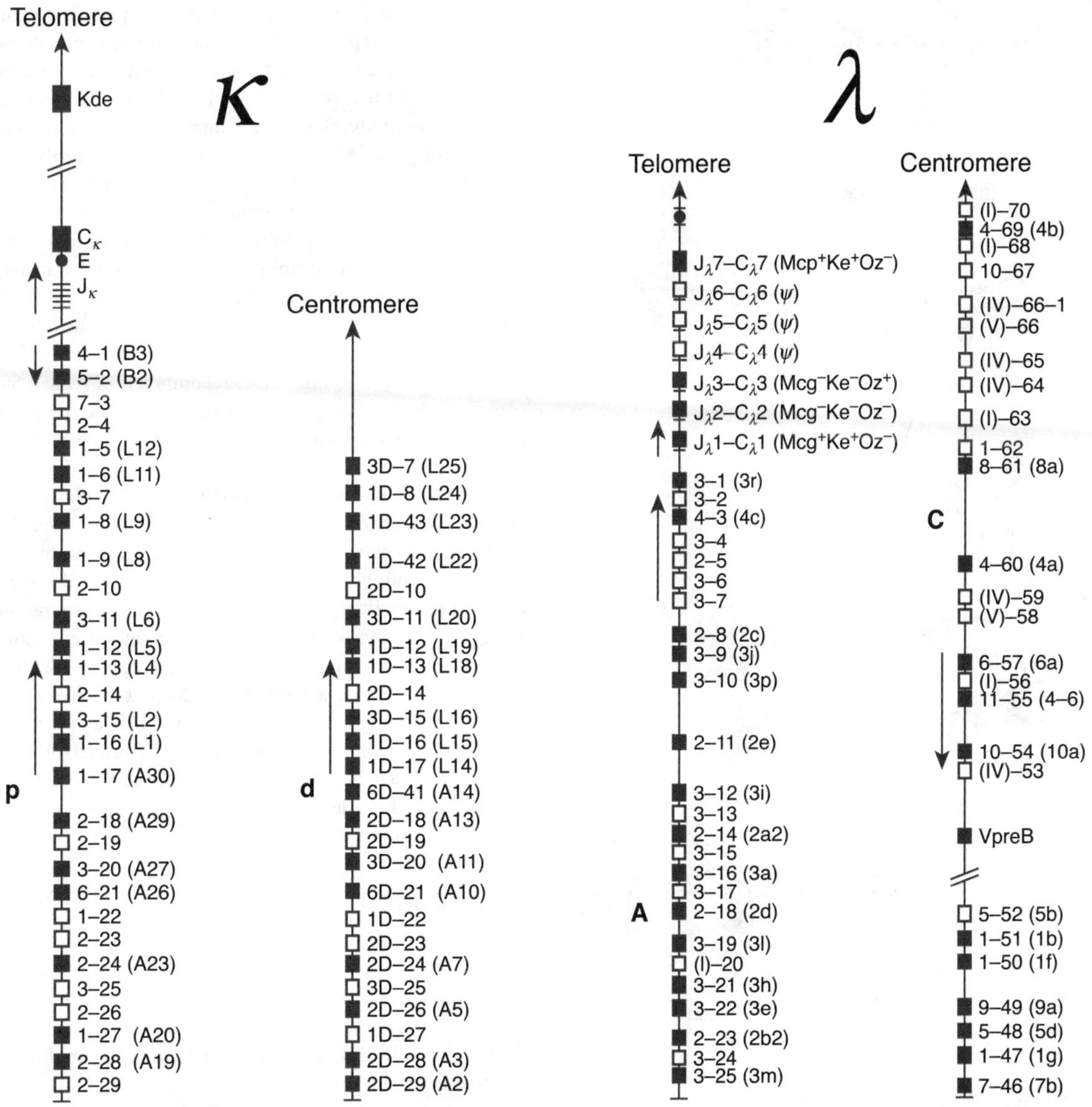

FIGURE 77–5. Immunoglobulin light-chain gene complexes. (*Left*) κ Light-chain gene complex on chromosome 2p11–12. *Blue boxes* represent the kappa-deleting element (Kde) or the C_κ constant-region exon as indicated to the right of each box. The κ light-chain enhancer (E) is positioned between the C_κ constant-region exon and the J_κ segments. J_κ segments are indicated by *lines*. The V_κ genes are clustered in two regions centromeric to the J_κ and C_κ exons, each region spanning approximately 500 kb. Approximately 800 kb separate the two regions. The region proximal to J_κ and C_κ, designated p, contains 40 V_κ genes. The distal region, designated d, contains 36 gene segments. V_κ genes that can encode functional κ light chains are represented by *blue boxes* and are labeled to the right of each symbol. Thirty of the 76 V_κ genes are pseudogenes (*open boxes*). The d region apparently arose through duplication of a large portion of the p region. Consequently, 33 pairs of V_κ genes share 95 to 100 percent nucleic acid sequence homology, accounting for 66 of the 76 V_κ genes in the κ light-chain complex. V_κ genes can be grouped further into four clusters: A, B, L, and O. Three of the clusters (A, L, O) are duplicated and found in both the J_κ-proximal p region and the J_κ-distal d region. The B cluster, containing V_κ genes, B2 and B3, is found only in the J_κ-proximal p region. Each V_κ gene can be assigned to one of three main subgroups (I–III) and several smaller subgroups (IV–VII) based on nucleotide sequence homology. The largest subgroup is $V_\kappa 1$, with 21 functional genes, depicted as *blue boxes*. The next largest subgroups are $V_\kappa 2$, with 11 functional genes, and $V_\kappa 3$, with seven functional genes. The $V_\kappa 6$ subgroup has three functional genes, and the $V_\kappa 4$ and $V_\kappa 5$ subgroups each have one functional gene. The $V_\kappa 7$ subgroup consists of one of the nonfunctional pseudogenes, which are depicted as *open squares*. *Red arrows* indicate the transcriptional orientation of the V genes in the complex. *Arrows* at the end of the line connecting the symbols indicate the direction to the centromere or the telomere. (*Right*) λ Light-chain gene complex on chromosome 22q11.2. *Blue boxes* represent functional genes; *open boxes* represent pseudogenes. The $J_\lambda C_\lambda$ exon pairs are labeled to the right of each symbol. *Blue boxes* also indicate the 39 functional V_λ genes centromeric to the λ constant regions. These V_λ genes are arranged into 10 subgroups, each composed of V_λ genes sharing greater than 75 percent nucleotide sequence homology. The first number in the labels to the right of each V_λ gene is the number of the subgroup, followed by a hyphen and then the relative rank order of the V gene from the constant-region exons. Note that the V_λ genes have been mapped into three clusters within 860 kb of the J_λ and C_λ genes, which are separated from one another in the figure by *double lines*. The cluster most proximal to the $J_\lambda C_\lambda$ exons, designated A, is composed of 18 functional V_λ genes mostly belonging to the $V_\lambda 2$ and $V_\lambda 3$ gene subgroups. The next cluster, B, contains 15 functional V_λ genes of the $V_\lambda 1$, $V_\lambda 5$, $V_\lambda 7$, and $V_\lambda 9$ gene subgroups. The third cluster, C, contains six functional V_λ genes of the $V_\lambda 4$, $V_\lambda 6$, $V_\lambda 8$, $V_\lambda 10$, and $V_\lambda 11$ gene subgroups and the exon encoding VpreB. Some individuals have an insertion of a functional V_λ gene, 5–39 (5a), marked as polymorphic insertion. *Red arrows* indicate the transcriptional orientation of the V genes in the complex.

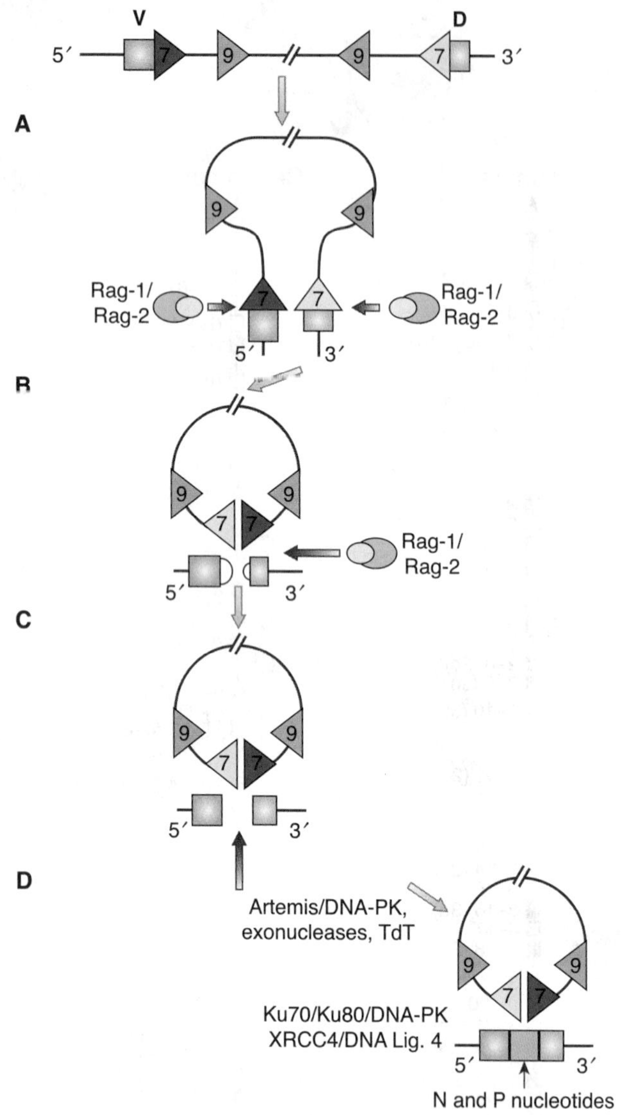

FIGURE 77–6. Schematic depicting the process of VDJ recombination. The Rag-1/Rag-2 complex mediates **(A)** synapsis and **(B)** cleavage of the DNA at the boundaries of the heptamer/coding segments. **(C)** The Artemis/DNA-PK (DNA protein kinase) endonuclease opens the hairpin and **(D)** the broken ends are then repaired by the proteins that mediate nonhomologous end-joining, namely the complex of Ku70, Ku80, DNA-PK, XRCC4, and Lig4.

kinase that is activated by DNA double-stranded breaks and is essential for the normal repair of DNA breaks induced by ionizing radiation, chemical agents, and during VDJ (exon created by a rearranged immunoglobulin heavy-chain variable-region gene, diversity gene segment, and joining gene segment) recombination.[44] Mice deficient in DNA-PK can make only trivial amounts of immunoglobulin or T-cell receptors and are called severe combined immunodeficiency (SCID) mice.[45] Mice deficient in Artemis have a "leaky" SCID phenotype and develop some T and B cells in later life.[46] Ku-deficient mice also are deficient in T and B cells but have a small stature and other nonimmunologic defects, suggesting that these proteins also play important roles in normal development.[47] Defects resulting from mutation in Ku, XRCC4, Lig4, Artemis, or DNA-PK predispose to lymphomagenesis in mice.[48,49]

The process of recombination allows for generation of "junctional diversity" in the sequence of the rearranged gene segments. DNA ends generated by the Rag-1/Rag-2 endonuclease cleavage reaction each is fused by the NHEJ pathway involving the proteins mentioned in the preceding paragraph. The hairpinned termini of gene segments that give rise to the coding joint each is subsequently cleaved at random sites by an exonuclease. Cleavage of a hairpin away from its apex generates an overhanging flap that, if incorporated into the joint, results in addition of palindromic (P) nucleotides that contribute to junctional diversity (see Fig. 77–6). The opened hairpin ends can be modified further by nucleases that can remove a self-complementary overhang or cut further into the original coding sequence. In addition, a lymphocyte-specific enzyme, terminal deoxynucleotidyl transferase, can add non–template-encoded (N) nucleotides (see Fig. 77–6). Finally, additional junctional diversity comes from the nucleolytic activities that remove potential coding end nucleotides prior to the final ligation of the DNA breaks into one intact recombination joint.[50] Such processes contribute to immunoglobulin diversity and are the principal mechanism responsible for somatic diversification of the T-cell repertoire (see Chap. 78).

Under normal conditions, a B-lymphocyte or plasma cell synthesizes only one species of light chain and heavy chain, even though the cell has two different sets of immunoglobulin gene complexes that initially undergo seemingly independent immunoglobulin gene rearrangements. The specificity of the humoral immune response depends upon antigenic selection of unique clones of B cells, each clone expressing a homogeneous set of immunoglobulin receptors. Such restriction is achieved by limiting a given B cell to functional rearrangement and expression of only a single heavy-chain allele and a single light-chain allele. This phenomenon is called *allelic exclusion*. Although occasional neoplastic B-cell populations lack allelic exclusion and express both immunoglobulin alleles, allelic exclusion generally is observed with most B-cell tumors.[51]

SURROGATE λ LIGHT CHAINS

Precursor B cells that only have rearranged D and J_H elements are referred to as progenitor B cells or "pro-B cells." The term *pre-B cells* is reserved for precursor B cells that have completed immunoglobulin heavy-chain gene rearrangement and have a functional VDJ complex. Both pro-B cells and pre-B cells have immunoglobulin light-chain loci in germ-line configuration.

Despite this situation, pre-B cells express some immunoglobulin μ chains in association with "surrogate" λ light chains. One of these proteins, called λ_5, has similarity with known C_λ light-chain domains. Another protein is called *VpreB* because it resembles a V domain but bears an extra N-terminal protein sequence. Both proteins are encoded by genes located on chromosome 22. The λ_5 gene is situated within a λ-like locus that is telomeric to the true λ light-chain locus. The VpreB gene is located within the cluster of immunoglobulin V_λ genes (see Fig. 77–5), defined by breakpoints of chromosomal translocations found in a few leukemias and lymphomas. Together, VpreB and λ_5 pair with the μ heavy chains. Subsequent covalent linkages via an S-S bond between the λ_5 and the first C_H1 domain of the μH chain allow VpreB and λ_5 μ heavy chains to form a primitive immunoglobulin receptor that, with CD79a and CD79b, may be expressed on the surface membrane of the developing pre-B cell. Monoclonal antibodies that recognize λ_5 or VpreB specifically bind to pre-B cells and can react with B lineage acute lymphocytic leukemias.[52]

The pre-B cell receptor complex is expressed only transiently, as production of λ_5 ceases as soon as it is formed. Nevertheless, this protein plays an important role in normal B-cell development. In normal mice, the appearance of the pre-B cell receptor coincides with inactivation of the Rag-2 protein by phosphorylation and degradation of Rag-1 and Rag-2 messenger RNA (mRNA), suggesting that this receptor plays a

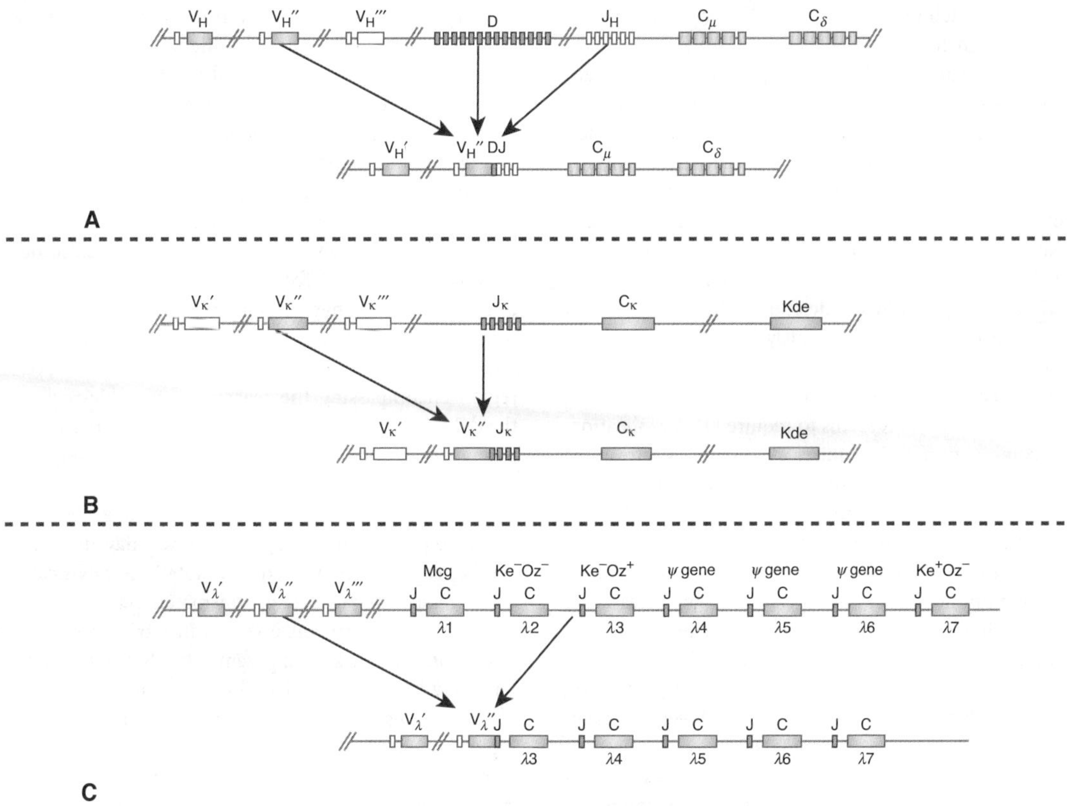

FIGURE 77–7. Immunoglobulin gene complexes and rearrangement. *Diagonal gold double lines* indicate a large DNA distance between the flanking genes depicted as *rectangular boxes* (not drawn to scale). The upper diagrams in **(A)**, **(B)**, and **(C)** show the germ-line DNA configuration of the immunoglobulin heavy-chain genes, κ light-chain genes, and λ light-chain genes, respectively. Exemplary immunoglobulin heavy-chain variable-region genes (V_H', V_H'', V_H'''), immunoglobulin κ light-chain genes (V_κ', V_κ'', V_κ'''), and immunoglobulin λ light-chain variable-region genes (V_λ', V_λ'', V_λ''') are depicted on the left side of each immunoglobulin gene complex. D denotes the diversity gene segments of the antibody heavy-chain locus. J_H, J_κ, and J_λ indicate the joining gene segments of the antibody heavy chain, κ light chain, and λ light chain, respectively. C_μ and C_δ denote the constant-region exons of the μ and δ heavy chains, respectively. Below each is a possible immunoglobulin gene rearrangement composed of a VDJ for the antibody heavy chain or a $V_\kappa J_\kappa$ or $V_\lambda J_\lambda$ for the κ or λ light-chain gene, respectively. Below the representative λ constant-region loci in **(C)** are listed the names of the λ nonallelic genetic markers Mcg, Ke–Oz–, Ke–Oz+, and Ke+Oz– on $C_\lambda 1$, $C_\lambda 2$, $C_\lambda 3$, and $C_\lambda 7$, respectively. As indicated, $C_\lambda 4$, $C_\lambda 5$, and $C_\lambda 6$ are pseudogenes (ψ gene) that do not encode protein.

role in suppressing further immunoglobulin gene rearrangement. However, expression of the pre-B cell receptor on the surface membrane is associated with cell activation and proliferation, leading to generation of small, resting pre-B daughter cells that again express Rag-1 and Rag-2. This situation leads to subsequent light-chain gene rearrangement. As such, expression of the pre–B-cell receptor appears to signal that a complete μ heavy-chain gene has been formed, that further rearrangements at this locus should be suppressed, and that development to the next stage can proceed. Therefore, the surrogate light chains play a critical role in normal B-cell development. This observation is underscored by studies on transgenic mice that lack functional λ_5 genes. In these mice, B-cell development in the marrow is blocked at the pre–B-cell stage, thereby markedly reducing the numbers of functional mature B lymphocytes in the blood and lymphoid tissues.[53] Similarly, humans who have inactivating mutations in the λ_5 genes on both alleles of chromosome 22 have agammaglobulinemia and markedly reduced numbers of B cells.[54]

■ HEAVY-CHAIN CLASS SWITCHING

During differentiation, a single B lymphocyte can synthesize heavy chains with different constant regions coupled to the same variable region through process called *class switch recombination*, which shares features of VDJ recombination.[55] As pre-B cells develop into mature B cells, intact IgM monomers are inserted into the plasma membrane, followed by IgD molecules with the same antigen-binding specificity. The IgM and IgD constant-region genes are closely linked in embryonic DNA (see Fig. 77–4) and may be transcribed together. The differential splicing of the transcript allows simultaneous synthesis of the two immunoglobulin heavy chains from a single species of mRNA. As such, the expression of IgD that occurs during B cell maturation only rarely involves deletion of C_μ.

The switch from IgM to IgG, IgA, or IgE requires active transcription of the downstream constant-region exons encoding the future immunoglobulin isotype. This process requires prior interaction of B lymphocytes with antigen or mitogen and ligation of CD40 via the ligand for CD40 (CD154) expressed by activated T cells. Patients with inherited defects in CD40 or CD154 have an immune deficiency (hyper-IgM syndrome type I) characterized by normal to high serum levels of IgM with extremely low serum levels of other immunoglobulin isotypes (see Chap. 82).[56] Interleukins provided by antigen-reactive T lymphocytes strongly influence (1) which B cells differentiate into IgM-secreting plasma cells and (2) which B cells switch to synthesizing the heavy chain of another immunoglobulin isotype, such as IgG and IgA. Isotype switching to IgA occurs most efficiently in mucosal lymphoid tissue, particularly in Peyer patches and mesenteric lymph nodes (see Chap. 5).[57] Also, class-switched IgA plasmablasts have a propensity to migrate to the lamina propria of the intestine and to other mucosal sites.[58]

Immunoglobulin class switch recombination (CSR) occurs in or near the switch region located in the intron between the rearranged VDJ_H sequence and the μ gene and any one of similar regions located upstream of the C genes encoding each of the other heavy-chain isotypes, with the exception of the δ gene (see Fig. 77–4). The μ switch region, designated S_μ, consists of approximately 150 repeats of the sequence $(GAGCT)_n$ (GGGGGT), where n is generally 3 but can be as many as 7. The sequences of the other switch regions (S_λ, S_δ, S_ε) are similar in that they also contain repeats of the GAGCT and GGGGGT sequences. The switch in heavy-chain classes results from DNA recombination between S_μ, and S_λ, S_δ, or S_ε, accompanied by the deletion of intervening DNA segments and the apposition of the previously rearranged variable-region gene next to the new constant-region gene.

In contrast to VDJ recombination, which mostly occurs in the G_0 and/or G_1 stage of the cell cycle, CSR seems to require DNA replication. Also, unlike VDJ recombination, CSR requires expression of activation-induced deaminase (AID), an enzyme expressed in activated B cells that also is required for somatic hypermutation.[59] Patients with inherited defects in AID have an immune deficiency (hyper-IgM syndrome type II) characterized by relatively high serum levels of IgM and negligible serum levels of other immunoglobulin isotypes.[60] AID is expressed in germinal centers of peripheral lymphoid organs, the site where CSR occurs in B cells activated in response to antigen. AID most likely deaminates the closely positioned cytosines (dC) in the S-region DNA, converting the dC to uracils (dU), which in turn are removed by uracil-DNA glycosylase (UNG). The importance of UNG is underscored by patients who have inherited defects in this enzyme, resulting in an autosomal recessive form of the hyper-IgM immunodeficiency syndrome similar to that of patients with inherited defects in AID (see Chap. 82).[61] The abasic sites generated by UNG are cleaved by AP endonuclease, resulting in closely positioned staggered nicks in the DNA that may result in double-stranded DNA breaks.[62] The end processing, repair, and joining mechanisms for these DNA breaks apparently involve mechanisms and proteins similar to those involved in NHEJ used for VDJ recombination. Because the CSR occurs in the intron between the variable-region exon and the exon encoding the first constant-region domain, this process does not generate mutations in the regions encoding the variable or constant regions of the newly generated immunoglobulin heavy chain.

MECHANISMS FOR GENERATING ANTIBODY DIVERSITY

Several mechanisms contribute to the generation of diversity among immunoglobulin polypeptide variable regions. The mechanisms are (1) the presence in the germ-line DNA of multiple different V, J, and D gene segments; (2) the random joining of these DNA segments to produce a complete variable-region exon; (3) junctional diversity; (4) the coming together of the heavy- and light-chain polypeptides to produce a complete immunoglobulin monomer capable of binding antigen; and (5) somatic mutations within the rearranged DNA segments themselves. The latter occurs through a process called somatic hypermutation.

Somatic hypermutation is not active in all B cells and cannot be triggered merely by mitogen-induced B-cell activation. However, during discrete stages of B-cell differentiation, expressed immunoglobulin V genes may incur new mutations at rates as high as 10^{-3} base substitutions per base pair per generation over several cell divisions, particularly during the secondary humoral immune response to antigen. Hypermutations begin on the 5′ end of rearranged V genes downstream of the transcription initiation site and continue through the V gene and into the 3′ flanking region before tapering off. As such, the mutations are clustered in the region spanning from 300 bp 5′ of the rearranged variable-region exon to approximately 1 kb 3′ of the rearranged minigene J segment. A high frequency of mutations are clustered around "hotspots" defined by the primary DNA sequence. The sequence RGYW (R = purine, A or G; Y = pyrimidine, C or T; W = A/T) and its complement, for example, is a hotspot for mutation that is conserved among species.[63]

The process of somatic hypermutation requires the activity of AID through a process that has some similarly with CSR.[64] In addition to having the hyper-IgM immunodeficiency syndrome type II, patients who have inherited defects in AID have B cells that lack the capacity to undergo somatic hypermutation (see Chap. 82).[60,65] As with CSR, somatic hypermutation requires active transcription of the genes undergoing mutation. AID most likely deaminates the cytosines (dC) in the region encompassing the rearranged variable-region gene, converting the dC to uracils (dU), which are converted to T after DNA replication, giving rise to C/G to T/A transitions. Alternatively, the dU are removed by UNG, resulting in abasic sites that subsequently are cleaved by AP endonuclease. This process generates staggered nick cleavage of the DNA. Repair of these staggered nicks may involve low-fidelity DNA synthesis, giving rise to frequent mutations. DNA cleaving enzymes and DNA repair enzymes (e.g., mismatch repair enzymes, base-excision repair enzymes, proteins involved in NHEJ) form a complex called the *mutasome*, which also apparently binds the target DNA to reduce its tendency to incur complete double-stranded DNA breaks. As a consequence of this process, mostly transitional mutations are introduced at high frequency in the expressed immunoglobulin V genes and in other transcriptionally active genes with "hotspots" that can serve as a substrate for AID, UNG, and the mutasome.[63] Subsequent selection of the B cell and its daughter cells that express mutated V genes encoding an immunoglobulin variable region with improved fitness for binding antigen allows for "affinity maturation" of the antibodies expressed during the immune response to antigen, which typically is retained on follicular dendritic cells.[66] Such selection enhances the frequency of nonconservative base substitutions in the DNA sequences encoding the complementarity-determining region (CDR) that serves as the contact site for antigen binding.[64]

IMMUNOGLOBULIN VARIABLE-REGION STRUCTURE

IMMUNOGLOBULIN VARIABLE-REGION SUBGROUPS

Despite the large number of different immunoglobulin variable regions that can be generated through the mechanisms, each antibody polypeptide can be assigned to one of a relatively small number of variable-region subgroups.[2] Comparisons of the amino acid sequences of a large number of different monoclonal immunoglobulin proteins reveal four segments of limited amino acid sequence diversity between different antibody heavy- or light-chain variable regions. These segments are designated the immunoglobulin variable-region frameworks (FRs; see Fig. 77–7). Each immunoglobulin polypeptide can be assigned to one of a relatively small number of variable-region subgroups based upon the primary structure of its first three frameworks. Moreover, each subgroup has characteristic framework sequences that distinguish it from other variable-region subgroups.

Satisfying expectations that immunoglobulin subgroups defined families of highly related antibody V genes, variable-region amino acid subgroup homologies extend to the nucleic acid sequence level.[67–69] Cloned immunoglobulin V genes whose deduced amino acid sequences belong to a given subgroup generally share greater than 80 percent nucleic acid sequence homology. The human heavy-chain variable regions can be grouped into seven subgroups, whereas κ or λ light chains can be divided into 6 or 11 subgroups, respectively.

Crystallographic data of immunoglobulin variable regions indicate that amino acids within the first and third FRs of either the light or heavy chain form β bonds on the external surface of the molecule. These regions form relatively compact structures on the external solvent-accessible face of the antibody molecule that are not adjacent to the classic antibody-combining site for antigen. Accordingly, amino acid differences noted between the different variable-region subgroups are amenable to recognition by antisubgroup antibodies.[70]

IMMUNOGLOBULIN IDIOTYPES

Antisubgroup antibodies must be distinguished from antiidiotypic antibodies. Positioned between the FRs are three segments of extreme hypervariability in both light- and heavy-chain sequences.[2] The third hypervariable region is generated through the recombinatorial process that joins the antibody light-chain V gene with the J segment of the light chain or the V_H gene with the somatically generated DJ_H segment of the antibody heavy chain. The diversity in first and second hypervariable regions in part reflects germ-line DNA-encoded differences between disparate antibody V genes, a diversity often noted even between V genes of the same subgroup.[2,30] During an immune response, somatic hypermutation subsequent to V gene rearrangement also may play an important role in increasing the amino acid sequence diversity noted within these regions. These hypervariable regions on both chains fold together to form the antigen combining site.[1,42] Hence, each of these regions of hypervariability is designated a CDR (see Fig. 77–7).

During secondary immune responses, extensive amino acid substitutions may occur in the CDRs. In contrast, amino acid replacement mutations occur much less frequently in the FRs than would be anticipated if the nucleic acid substitutions were occurring randomly. As a consequence, the subgroup determinants that characterize an entire variable-region subgroup may be relatively resilient to somatic hypermutation. On the other hand, the CDRs may form determinants of unique specificity that contribute to the epitopes recognized by antiidiotypic antibodies.

Despite the tremendous potential for diversity in Ig V gene expression and genetic polymorphism, antibodies produced by B-cell malignancies or normal B cells of unrelated persons may share common idiotypic determinants.[71] These common idiotypes, designated cross-reactive idiotypes (CRIs), were defined initially on IgM autoantibodies, such as rheumatoid factors. However, CRIs may be found on antibodies that do not have anti-self-reactivity. Molecular studies have demonstrated several of these CRIs represent serologic markers for expression of conserved immunoglobulin variable-region genes with little or no somatic mutation.

IMMUNOGLOBULIN ALLOTYPES

HEAVY-CHAIN ALLOTYPES

Human immunoglobulins have inherited differences in structure, termed allotypes. These genetic markers usually are detected with agglutinating sera from individuals naturally immunized through transfusion or pregnancy. These antibodies recognize minor amino acid sequence variations in the constant regions of γ, α, and κ chains.[72,73] No definite allotypic differences have been detected on μ or δ chains. On ε chains, a monoclonal antibody to IgE defined an allotype that was common to persons of all races except for a few individuals of Asian or Melanesian background.

The α-chain allotypes, designated Am allotypes, are on the heavy chains of the IgA_2 subclass.[73] The γ-chain allotypes are on the heavy chains of the IgG_1, IgG_2, and IgG_3 subclasses and are designated G_1m, G_2m, and G_3m, respectively. More than 24 Gm allotypic markers have been identified serologically. All the heavy-chain constant-region genes reside on chromosome 14. Therefore, different combinations of heavy-chain allotype markers are inherited as haplotypic units, in an autosomal codominant manner. The frequency of the various allelic markers differs among ethnic groups.[74]

Particular immunoglobulin allotypes have been associated with susceptibility or resistance to infectious diseases or the relative immune response to particular vaccines.[75,76] This could reflect linkage disequilibrium between particular polymorphic immunoglobulin variable region genes and constant region genes encoding particular immunoglobulin allotypes. Also, patients treated with humanized IgG_1 monoclonal antibodies may develop antiallotypic antibodies against Gm_1 determinants found on the constant region of the therapeutic antibody.[77]

LIGHT-CHAIN ALLOTYPES

The κ light-chain allotypes are designated Km allotypes (formerly called inv). At least three major Km allotypes exist, designated Km(1),1 Km(1,2), and Km(3), which may be recognized serologically or via molecular techniques.[75] Patients with B-cell malignancies who are treated with allogeneic hematopoietic stem cell transplantation have been noted to have better survival outcomes when there is disparity in the κ light-chain allotypes between donor and recipient, presumably because of an enhanced capacity to mount a graft-versus-leukemia effect.[78]

Seven J_λ-C_λ gene segments are telomeric to the upstream V_λ genes, but only four such segments are functional, namely $J_\lambda1$-$C_\lambda1$, $J_\lambda2$-$C_\lambda2$, $J_\lambda3$-$C_\lambda3$, and $J_\lambda7$-$C_\lambda7$ (see Fig. 77–5). These segments respectively encode the four identified isotypes of λ light chains, termed $Mcg^+Ke^+Oz^-$, $Mcg^-Ke^-Oz^-$, $Mcg^-Ke^-Oz^+$, and $Mcp^+Ke^+Oz^-$, which were defined based on their reactivity with the Oz, Kern, Mcg, and Mcp antisera raised against λ Bence Jones proteins.[79] These isotypes reflect minor nonallelic amino acid differences in the λ light-chain constant regions.[80] A fifth type of λ light-chain, termed $Mcg^-Ke^+Oz^-$ is highly homologous to $Mcg^-Ke^-Oz^-$ and actually results from a polymorphic gene amplification in a functional polymorphic $C_\lambda2$ segment.[80]

IMMUNOGLOBULIN SYNTHESIS AND SECRETION

IMMUNOGLOBULIN SYNTHESIS

The total IgG content of the adult human body is approximately 75 g, of which 2.2 g is synthesized each day. Most immunoglobulin is produced by mature plasma cells, which have abundant rough endoplasmic reticulum, a well-developed Golgi apparatus, and high-level transcription of the immunoglobulin genes. The final mRNAs for immunoglobulin light and heavy chains are derived by the processing of large nuclear RNA transcripts. In plasma cells, the rearranged and spliced mRNA molecules for the heavy-and light-chain polypeptides are translated on separate ribosomal complexes.

The folding and assembly of intact immunoglobulin molecules occur in the endoplasmic reticulum (ER), which contains a large set of redox catalysts and chaperones that guide the folding of nascent proteins.[81] First, an amino-terminal leader peptide approximately 18 to 30 residues long is cleaved prior to the release of the completed light and heavy chains in the cisternae of the ER. In that location, the heavy-chain immunoglobulin polypeptides interact via their C_H1 domains with BiP, a heat-shock chaperone protein that allows for proper folding of the heavy-chain polypeptide and prevents its transport into the Golgi. The nascent immunoglobulin light chain can displace BiP and then spontaneously combine with the heavy chain to form immunoglobulin half molecules that are stabilized by disulfide bonds.[82] The process also requires the redox conditions generated by redox catalysts within ER, a requirement that has handicapped efforts to produce immunoglobulin in prokaryotic cell-free expression systems.[83] The joining of two identical half molecules by disulfide bonds yields a basic four-chain immunoglobulin unit, which then is allowed to transport to the Golgi for glycosylation.

Glycosyltransferase enzymes add a defined sequence of sugars to the assembled immunoglobulin unit to form branched-chain oligosaccharides composed of *N*-acetyl-glucosamine, mannose, galactose, fructose, and sialic acid. The oligosaccharides are attached covalently to the immunoglobulin heavy chain at several sites. The carbohydrate facilitates the transport of the antibody molecule across the plasma membrane and into the extracellular space and increases the solubility of the secreted protein.[84] Specific types of glycosylation also may improve the clinical activity of therapeutic monoclonal antibodies.[85]

Five monomeric units of IgM combine to form a pentameric macroglobulin linked by disulfide bonds and a single J-chain polypeptide. Usually polymerization immediately precedes or occurs simultaneously with IgM secretion. Similarly, IgA molecules form dimers and polymers linked by the J chain just prior to secretion from the plasma cell.

REGULATION OF IMMUNOGLOBULIN SYNTHESIS

GENERATION OF PLASMA CELLS

A normal adult has some preexisting B lymphocytes that can produce immunoglobulin that can bind almost any foreign antigen. Such B cells can be recruited to the immune response against the antigen. In the presence of accessory T-follicular helper cells (T_{FH}; see Chap. 78), an antigen-binding clone of B lymphocytes may transform into antibody-secreting plasma cells.[86]

Transcription factors regulate this differentiation of B cells into antibody-secreting plasma cells. An important factor in plasma cell differentiation is the *B-lymphocyte-induced maturation protein-1* (Blimp-1),[87] which also is called the *positive regulatory domain 1-binding factor-1* (PRDM1) because it initially was identified by its ability to bind to the positive regulatory domain I of the human interferon-β promoter.[88] Blimp-1 is a zinc finger-containing transcription factor encoded by *PRDM1* on human chromosome 6q21 that represses expression of genes encoding transcription factors that inhibit plasma-cell differentiation (e.g., *MYC*, B-cell CLL/lymphoma 6 [*BCL-6*], paired box gene 5 [*PAX5*], microphthalmia-associated transcription factor [*MITF*], and basic leucine zipper transcription factor 2 [*BACH2*]).[87] On the other hand, Blimp-1 directly or indirectly induces expression of other transcription factors that control genes encoding other transcription factors or proteins responsible for plasma-cell differentiation and/or immunoglobulin secretion (e.g., X-box binding protein-1 [*XBP1*], E2F transcription factor 1 [*E2F1*], *v*-myb myeloblastosis viral oncogene homolog 1 and 2 [*MYBL1/MYBL2*], early B-cell factor 1 [*EBF1*], Pou domain, class 2, factor 2, or associating factor 1 [*POU2F2/POU2AF1*], and transcription factor E2a [*TCFE2A*]). This capacity of Blimp-1 to repress and to activate expression of a variety of different transcription factors accounts for its capacity to orchestrate the dramatic changes in B-cell morphology and function associated with plasma-cell differentiation and high-level secretion of immunoglobulin protein. Mice made to have a conditional deletion of *PRDM1* encoding Blimp-1 in the B lineage demonstrate the critical requirement of Blimp-1 in plasma cell development.[89] Although such mice have normal numbers of B cells and develop germinal centers in response to T-dependent antigens, they fail to generate plasma cells or to secrete normal levels of immunoglobulin in response to either T-independent or T-dependent antigens. Furthermore, other studies found that expression of Blimp-1 is required for the maintenance of long-lived plasma cells in the marrow and the long-term expression of antigen-specific immunoglobulin in the plasma.[90]

Some diffuse large B-cell lymphomas (DLBCL) have deletions or inactivating mutations in *PRDM1*, suggesting that this gene also might act as a tumor suppressor.[91] However, *PRDM1* mutations are not found in other lymphoid or myeloid leukemias, and myeloma cells and some DLBCL express abundant levels of Blimp-1, making it appear unlikely that Blimp-1 suppresses tumor development *per se*.[92] Moreover, the DLBCL cases that expressed Blimp-1 lacked detectable plasmacytic features and actually displayed more aggressive behavior.[93] As such, B-cell expression of Blimp-1 appears necessary but not sufficient for plasma-cell differentiation.

The expression of Blimp-1 in B cells is regulated primarily at the level of *PRDM1* transcription, which requires activation by the transcription factor *interferon regulatory factor 4* (IRF4).[87] Transgenic mice that have B cells a conditional deletion of *IRF4* fail to generate immunoglobulin-secreting plasma cells.[94] Substances that activate toll-like receptor 4 (TLR4) or toll-like receptor 9 (TLR9), such as lipopolysaccharide or CpG oligonucleotides, respectively, also can activate expression of Blimp-1.[87,95] Mice lacking such toll-like receptors cannot mount effective antibody responses,[96] except under certain conditions.[97] Several cytokines, including IL-2, IL-5, IL-6, IL-10, and IL-21, also can induce expression of Blimp-1 when applied in the proper context. Indeed, such cytokines can have positive or negative effects on B-cell differentiation and/or survival depending upon the presence or absence of other signals. IL-21, for example, can induce expression of Blimp-1 and plasma cell differentiation primarily in memory B cells or B cells that previously had been activated via ligation of its B-cell receptor, namely surface immunoglobulin, when in the context of receiving T-cell helper signals, such as that caused by ligation of CD40.[98,99] On the other hand, IL-21 can induce apoptosis of B cells that are activated via ligation of its surface immunoglobulin receptor in the absence of such T-cell helper signals.[99]

MEMORY B CELLS

Following a T-cell dependent immune response to antigen, B cells that express high-affinity immunoglobulin for antigen also can differentiate into memory B cells.[100] Memory B cells differ from plasma cells in morphology and function. In contrast to plasma cells, memory B cells do not secrete immunoglobulin, but rather express surface immunoglobulin that can bind antigen and can be induced to differentiate rapidly into immunoglobulin secreting plasma cells rapidly after secondary challenge with antigen.

Human memory B cells can be distinguished by their expression of CD27 and CD148 (see Chap. 15).[101] Memory B cells also have increased expression of immune costimulatory molecules CD80 and CD86,[102] particularly following immune activation, which enhances their capacity induce immune coactivation of T-helper cells (see Chap. 78). In addition, memory B cells have high-level expression of antiapoptotic genes *BCL2* and *BCL-XL*,[103] which help enhance their long-term survival. Finally, memory B cells lack expression of *BCL-6*, which actually can repress memory B-cell development.[104] Because *BCL-6* also can repress expression of *PRDM1*, the lack of *BCL-6* expression makes memory B cells particularly amenable to stimulation by factors that induce expression of Blimp-1,[94] thereby enhancing the capacity of memory B cells that express antigen-binding immunoglobulin to undergo rapid differentiation into plasma cells during the secondary immune response to antigen.[105]

REFERENCES

1. Perkins SJ, Ashton AW, Boehm MK, Chamberlain D: Molecular structures from low angle X-ray and neutron scattering studies. *Int J Biol Macromol* 22:1, 1998.
2. Kabat EA, National Institutes of Health, and Columbia University: *Sequences of Proteins of Immunological Interest*. US Dept of Health and Human Services, Public Health Service, National Institutes of Health, Bethesda, MD, 1991.
3. Lee YK, Brewer JW, Hellman R, Hendershot LM: BiP and immunoglobulin light chain cooperate to control the folding of heavy chain and ensure the fidelity of immunoglobulin assembly. *Mol Biol Cell* 10:2209, 1999.
4. Jefferis R, Lund J, Goodall M: Recognition sites on human IgG for Fc gamma receptors: The role of glycosylation. *Immunol Lett* 44:111, 1995.
5. Niwa R, Natsume A, Uehara A, et al: IgG subclass-independent improvement of antibody-dependent cellular cytotoxicity by fucose removal from Asn297-linked oligosaccharides. *J Immunol Methods* 306:151, 2005.
6. Macpherson AJ, McCoy KD, Johansen FE, Brandtzaeg P: The immune geography of IgA induction and function. *Mucosal Immunol* 1:11, 2008.
7. Cerutti A, Rescigno M: The biology of intestinal immunoglobulin A responses. *Immunity* 28:740, 2008.
8. Brandtzaeg P: Do salivary antibodies reliably reflect both mucosal and systemic immunity? *Ann N Y Acad Sci* 1098:288, 2007.
9. Wines BD, Hogarth PM: IgA receptors in health and disease. *Tissue Antigens* 68:103, 2006.
10. Novak J, Julian BA, Tomana M, Mestecky J: IgA glycosylation and IgA immune complexes in the pathogenesis of IgA nephropathy. *Semin Nephrol* 28:78, 2008.
11. Sanders JT, Wyatt RJ: IgA nephropathy and Henoch-Schönlein purpura nephritis. *Curr Opin Pediatr* 20:163, 2008.
12. Niles MJ, Matsuuchi L, Koshland ME: Polymer IgM assembly and secretion in lymphoid and nonlymphoid cell lines: Evidence that J chain is required for pentamer IgM synthesis. *Proc Natl Acad Sci U S A* 92:2884, 1995.
13. Preud'homme JL, Petit I, Barra A, et al: Structural and functional properties of membrane and secreted IgD. *Mol Immunol* 37:871, 2000.
14. Lyczak JB, Zhang K, Saxon A, Morrison SL: Expression of novel secreted isoforms of human immunoglobulin E proteins. *J Biol Chem* 271:3428, 1996.
15. Brezski RJ, Monroe JG: B-cell receptor. *Adv Exp Med Biol* 640:12, 2008.
16. Tolar P, Hanna J, Krueger PD, Pierce SK: The constant region of the membrane immunoglobulin mediates B cell-receptor clustering and signaling in response to membrane antigens. *Immunity* 30:44, 2009.
17. Wang Y, Kanegane H, Sanal O, et al: Novel Igalpha (CD79a) gene mutation in a Turkish patient with B cell-deficient agammaglobulinemia. *Am J Med Genet* 108:333, 2002.
18. Carrasco YR, Batista FD: B cell recognition of membrane-bound antigen: An exquisite way of sensing ligands. *Curr Opin Immunol* 18:286, 2006.
19. Qi H, Egen JG, Huang AY, Germain RN: Extrafollicular activation of lymph node B cells by antigen-bearing dendritic cells. *Science* 312:1672, 2006.
20. Phan TG, Grigorova I, Okada T, Cyster JG: Subcapsular encounter and complement-dependent transport of immune complexes by lymph node B cells. *Nat Immunol* 8:992, 2007.
21. Junt T, Moseman EA, Iannacone M, et al: Subcapsular sinus macrophages in lymph nodes clear lymph-borne viruses and present them to antiviral B cells. *Nature* 450:110, 2007.
22. Wu JN, Koretzky GA: The SLP-76 family of adapter proteins. *Semin Immunol* 16:379, 2004.
23. Weber M, Treanor B, Depoil D, et al: Phospholipase C-gamma2 and Vav cooperate within signaling microclusters to propagate B cell spreading in response to membrane-bound antigen. *J Exp Med* 205:853, 2008.
24. Fruman DA, Satterthwaite AB, Witte ON: Xid-like phenotypes: A B cell signalosome takes shape. *Immunity* 13:1, 2000.
25. Batista FD, Arana E, Barral P, et al: The role of integrins and coreceptors in refining thresholds for B-cell responses. *Immunol Rev* 218:197, 2007.
26. Depoil D, Weber M, Treanor B, et al: Early events of B cell activation by antigen. *Sci Signal* 2:pt1, 2009.
27. Baba T, Fusaki N, Aoyama A, et al: Dual regulation of BCR-mediated growth inhibition signaling by CD72. *Eur J Immunol* 35:1634, 2005.
28. Zhu C, Sato M, Yanagisawa T, et al: Novel binding site for Src homology 2-containing protein-tyrosine phosphatase-1 in CD22 activated by B lymphocyte stimulation with antigen. *J Biol Chem* 283:1653, 2008.
29. Shultz LD, Rajan TV, Greiner DL: Severe defects in immunity and hematopoiesis caused by SHP-1 protein-tyrosine-phosphatase deficiency. *Trends Biotechnol* 15:302, 1997.
30. Matsuda F, Ishii K, Bourvagnet P, et al: The complete nucleotide sequence of the human immunoglobulin heavy chain variable region locus. *J Exp Med* 188:2151, 1998.
31. Kawasaki K, Minoshima S, Nakato E, et al: Evolutionary dynamics of the human immunoglobulin kappa locus and the germline repertoire of the Vkappa genes. *Eur J Immunol* 31:1017, 2001.
32. Dunham I, Shimizu N, Roe BA, et al: The DNA sequence of human chromosome 22. *Nature* 402:489, 1999.
33. Pallares N, Frippiat JP, Giudicelli V, Lefranc MP: The human immunoglobulin lambda variable (IGLV) genes and joining (IGLJ) segments. *Exp Clin Immunogenet* 15:8, 1998.
34. Bassing CH, Alt FW, Hughes MM, et al: Recombination signal sequences restrict chromosomal V(D)J recombination beyond the 12/23 rule. *Nature* 405:583, 2000.
35. Gellert M: Recent advances in understanding V(D)J recombination. *Adv Immunol* 64:39, 1997.
36. Steen SB, Gomelsky L, Speidel SL, Roth DB: Initiation of V(D)J recombination in vivo: Role of recombination signal sequences in formation of single and paired double-strand breaks. *EMBO J* 16:2656, 1997.
37. Shinkai Y, Rathbun G, Lam KP, et al: RAG-2-deficient mice lack mature lymphocytes owing to inability to initiate V(D)J rearrangement. *Cell* 68:855, 1992.
38. Villa A, Notarangelo LD, Roifman CM: Omenn syndrome: Inflammation in leaky severe combined immunodeficiency. *J Allergy Clin Immunol* 122:1082, 2008.
39. Jones JM, Simkus C: The roles of the RAG1 and RAG2 "non-core" regions in V(D)J recombination and lymphocyte development. *Arch Immunol Ther Exp (Warsz)* 57:105, 2009.
40. Huye LE, Purugganan MM, Jiang MM, Roth DB: Mutational analysis of all conserved basic amino acids in RAG-1 reveals catalytic, step arrest, and joining-deficient mutants in the V(D)J recombinase. *Mol Cell Biol* 22:3460, 2002.
41. Tsai CL, Drejer AH, Schatz DG: Evidence of a critical architectural function for the RAG proteins in end processing, protection, and joining in V(D)J recombination. *Genes Dev* 16:1934, 2002.
42. Thomas JO, Travers AA: HMG1 and 2, and related "architectural" DNA-binding proteins. *Trends Biochem Sci* 26:167, 2001.
43. Schatz DG, Spanopoulou E: Biochemistry of V(D)J recombination. *Curr Top Microbiol Immunol* 290:49, 2005.
44. Meek K, Gupta S, Ramsden DA, Lees-Miller SP: The DNA-dependent protein kinase: The director at the end. *Immunol Rev* 200:132, 2004.
45. Khanna KK, Jackson SP: DNA double-strand breaks: Signaling, repair and the cancer connection. *Nat Genet* 27:247, 2001.
46. Le Deist F, Poinsignon C, Moshous D, et al: Artemis sheds new light on V(D)J recombination. *Immunol Rev* 200:142, 2004.
47. Gu Y, Sekiguchi J, Gao Y, et al: Defective embryonic neurogenesis in Ku-deficient but not DNA-dependent protein kinase catalytic subunit-deficient mice. *Proc Natl Acad Sci U S A* 97:2668, 2000.
48. Surucu B, Bozulic L, Hynx D, et al: *In vivo* analysis of protein kinase B (PKB)/Akt regulation in DNA-PKcs-null mice reveals a role for PKB/Akt in DNA damage response and tumorigenesis. *J Biol Chem* 283:30025, 2008.
49. Roth DB: Amplifying mechanisms of lymphomagenesis. *Mol Cell* 10:1, 2002.
50. Grawunder U, West RB, Lieber MR: Antigen receptor gene rearrangement. *Curr Opin Immunol* 10:172, 1998.
51. Rassenti LZ, Kipps TJ: Lack of allelic exclusion in B cell chronic lymphocytic leukemia. *J Exp Med* 185:1435, 1997.
52. Tsuganezawa K, Kiyokawa N, Matsuo Y, et al: Flow cytometric diagnosis of the cell lineage and developmental stage of acute lymphoblastic leukemia by novel monoclonal antibodies specific to human pre-B-cell receptor. *Blood* 92:4317, 1998.
53. Corcos D, Dunda O, Butor C, et al: Pre-B-cell development in the absence of lambda 5 in transgenic mice expressing a heavy-chain disease protein. *Curr Biol* 5:1140, 1995.
54. Minegishi Y, Coustan-Smith E, Wang YH, et al: Mutations in the human lambda5/14.1 gene result in B cell deficiency and agammaglobulinemia. *J Exp Med* 187:71, 1998.
55. Stavnezer J, Guikema JE, Schrader CE: Mechanism and regulation of class switch recombination. *Annu Rev Immunol* 26:261, 2008.
56. Ferrari S, Plebani A: Cross-talk between CD40 and CD40L: Lessons from primary immune deficiencies. *Curr Opin Allergy Clin Immunol* 2:489, 2002.
57. Cerutti A: The regulation of IgA class switching. *Nat Rev Immunol* 8:421, 2008.
58. Mora JR, von Andrian UH: Differentiation and homing of IgA-secreting cells. *Mucosal Immunol* 1:96, 2008.
59. Dudley DD, Chaudhuri J, Bassing CH, Alt FW: Mechanism and control of V(D)J recombination versus class switch recombination: Similarities and differences. *Adv Immunol* 86:43, 2005.
60. Revy P, Muto T, Levy Y, et al: Activation-induced cytidine deaminase (AID) deficiency causes the autosomal recessive form of the Hyper-IgM syndrome (HIGM2). *Cell* 102:565, 2000.
61. Imai K, Slupphaug G, Lee WI, et al: Human uracil-DNA glycosylase deficiency associated with profoundly impaired immunoglobulin class-switch recombination. *Nat Immunol* 4:1023, 2003.
62. Chen X, Kinoshita K, Honjo T: Variable deletion and duplication at recombination junction ends: Implication for staggered double-strand cleavage in class-switch recombination. *Proc Natl Acad Sci U S A* 98:13860, 2001.
63. Storb U, Shen HM, Michael N, Kim N: Somatic hypermutation of immunoglobulin and non-immunoglobulin genes. *Philos Trans R Soc Lond B Biol Sci* 356:13, 2001.
64. Di Noia JM, Neuberger MS: Molecular mechanisms of antibody somatic hypermutation. *Annu Rev Biochem* 76:1, 2007.
65. Muramatsu M, Kinoshita K, Fagarasan S, et al: Class switch recombination and hypermutation require activation-induced cytidine deaminase (AID), a potential RNA editing enzyme. *Cell* 102:553, 2000.
66. Allen CD, Cyster JG: Follicular dendritic cell networks of primary follicles and germinal centers: Phenotype and function. *Semin Immunol* 20:14, 2008.
67. Cook GP, Tomlinson IM: The human immunoglobulin VH repertoire. *Immunol Today* 16:237, 1995.
68. Kipps TJ: Human B cell biology. *Int Rev Immunol* 15:243, 1997.
69. Frippiat JP, Williams SC, Tomlinson IM, et al: Organization of the human immunoglobulin lambda light-chain locus on chromosome 22q11.2. *Hum Mol Genet* 4:983, 1995.

70. Jefferis R: Nomenclature of V-region markers. *Immunol Today* 16:207, 1995.
71. Kipps TJ, Carson DA: Autoantibodies in chronic lymphocytic leukemia and related systemic autoimmune diseases. *Blood* 81:2475, 1993.
72. Williams RC Jr, Malone CC, Solomon A: Conformational dependency of human IgG heavy chain-associated Gm allotypes. *Mol Immunol* 30:341, 1993.
73. Schanfield MS, van Loghem E: Human immunoglobulin allotypes, in *Handbook of Experimental Immunology*, edited by LA Herzenberg, C Blackwell, LA Herzenberg, DM Weir, p 1. Blackwell Scientific, Oxford, 1986.
74. Schanfield MS, Ferrell RE, Hossaini AA, et al: Immunoglobulin allotypes in Southwest Asia: Populations at the crossroads. *Am J Hum Biol* 20:671, 2008.
75. Pandey JP: Immunoglobulin GM and KM allotypes and vaccine immunity. *Vaccine* 19:613, 2000.
76. Muratori P, Sutherland SE, Muratori L, et al: Immunoglobulin GM and KM allotypes and prevalence of anti-LKM1 autoantibodies in patients with hepatitis C virus infection. *J Virol* 80:5097, 2006.
77. Magdelaine-Beuzelin C, Vermeire S, Goodall M, et al: IgG1 heavy chain-coding gene polymorphism (G1m allotypes) and development of antibodies-to-infliximab. *Pharmacogenet Genomics* 19:383, 2009.
78. Etto TL, Stewart LA, Muirhead J, et al: Kappa immunoglobulin light chain polymorphisms and survival after allogeneic transplantation for B-cell malignancies: A potential graft-vs-leukaemia target. *Tissue Antigens* 69:56, 2007.
79. Niewold TA, Murphy CL, Weiss DT, Solomon A: Characterization of a light chain product of the human JC lambda 7 gene complex. *J Immunol* 157:4474, 1996.
80. van der Burg M, Barendregt BH, van Gastel-Mol EJ, et al: Unraveling of the polymorphic C lambda 2-C lambda 3 amplification and the Ke+Oz– polymorphism in the human Ig lambda locus. *J Immunol* 169:271, 2002.
81. Shimizu Y, Hendershot LM: Organization of the functions and components of the endoplasmic reticulum. *Adv Exp Med Biol* 594:37, 2007.
82. Reddy PS, Corley RB: The contribution of ER quality control to the biologic functions of secretory IgM. *Immunol Today* 20:582, 1999.
83. Frey S, Haslbeck M, Hainzl O, Buchner J: Synthesis and characterization of a functional intact IgG in a prokaryotic cell-free expression system. *Biol Chem* 389:37, 2008.
84. Rudd PM, Elliott T, Cresswell P, et al: Glycosylation and the immune system. *Science* 291:2370, 2001.
85. Jefferis R: Glycosylation as a strategy to improve antibody-based therapeutics. *Nat Rev Drug Discov* 8:226, 2009.
86. Johnston RJ, Poholek AC, Ditoro D, et al: Bcl6 and Blimp-1 are reciprocal and antagonistic regulators of T follicular helper cell differentiation. *Science* 325:1006, 2009.
87. Martins G, Calame K: Regulation and functions of Blimp-1 in T and B lymphocytes. *Annu Rev Immunol* 26:133, 2008.
88. Keller AD, Maniatis T: Identification and characterization of a novel repressor of beta-interferon gene expression. *Genes Dev* 5:868, 1991.
89. Shapiro-Shelef M, Lin KI, McHeyzer-Williams LJ, et al: Blimp-1 is required for the formation of immunoglobulin secreting plasma cells and pre-plasma memory B cells. *Immunity* 19:607, 2003.
90. Shapiro-Shelef M, Lin KI, Savitsky D, et al: Blimp-1 is required for maintenance of long-lived plasma cells in the bone marrow. *J Exp Med* 202:1471, 2005.
91. Tam W, Gomez M, Chadburn A, et al: Mutational analysis of PRDM1 indicates a tumor-suppressor role in diffuse large B-cell lymphomas. *Blood* 107:4090, 2006.
92. Garcia JF, Roncador G, Garcia JF, et al: PRDM1/BLIMP-1 expression in multiple B- and T-cell lymphoma. *Haematologica* 91:467, 2006.
93. Pasqualucci L, Compagno M, Houldsworth J, et al: Inactivation of the PRDM1/BLIMP1 gene in diffuse large B cell lymphoma. *J Exp Med* 203:311, 2006.
94. Klein U, Casola S, Cattoretti G, et al: Transcription factor IRF4 controls plasma cell differentiation and class-switch recombination. *Nat Immunol* 7:773, 2006.
95. Lin KI, Kao YY, Kuo HK, et al: Reishi polysaccharides induce immunoglobulin production through the TLR4/TLR2-mediated induction of transcription factor Blimp-1. *J Biol Chem* 281:24111, 2006.
96. Pasare C, Medzhitov R: Control of B-cell responses by toll-like receptors. *Nature* 438:364, 2005.
97. Nemazee D, Gavin A, Hoebe K, Beutler B: Immunology: Toll-like receptors and antibody responses. *Nature* 441:E4; discussion E4, 2006.
98. Ettinger R, Sims GP, Fairhurst AM, et al: IL-21 induces differentiation of human naive and memory B cells into antibody-secreting plasma cells. *J Immunol* 175:7867, 2005.
99. Konforte D, Simard N, Paige CJ: IL-21: An executor of B cell fate. *J Immunol* 182:1781, 2009.
100. Tarlinton D: B-cell memory: Are subsets necessary? *Nat Rev Immunol* 6:785, 2006.
101. Tangye SG, Liu YJ, Aversa G, et al: Identification of functional human splenic memory B cells by expression of CD148 and CD27. *J Exp Med* 188:1691, 1998.
102. Liu YJ, Barthelemy C, de Bouteiller O, et al: Memory B cells from human tonsils colonize mucosal epithelium and directly present antigen to T cells by rapid up-regulation of B7-1 and B7-2. *Immunity* 2:239, 1995.
103. Klein U, Tu Y, Stolovitzky GA, et al: Transcriptional analysis of the B cell germinal center reaction. *Proc Natl Acad Sci U S A* 100:2639, 2003.
104. Kuo TC, Shaffer AL, Haddad J Jr, et al: Repression of BCL-6 is required for the formation of human memory B cells *in vitro*. *J Exp Med* 204:819, 2007.
105. Good KL, Avery DT, Tangye SG: Resting human memory B cells are intrinsically programmed for enhanced survival and responsiveness to diverse stimuli compared to naive B cells. *J Immunol* 182:890, 2009.

CHAPTER 78

FUNCTIONS OF T LYMPHOCYTES: T-CELL RECEPTORS FOR ANTIGEN

Thomas J. Kipps

SUMMARY

All T cells express a receptor for antigen that is formed by two polymorphic polypeptides that invariably are associated with a collection of invariant proteins called CD3γ, CD3δ, CD3ε, and CD247. These invariant proteins are necessary for the surface expression and signaling by the T-cell receptor. The two polypeptides that form the T-cell receptor on most T cells are termed α and β; whereas a small subset of T cells have receptors formed by different polypeptides termed γ and δ. The polypeptides of the T-cell receptor have a diversity that is comparable to that estimated for immunoglobulin molecules. However, unlike immunoglobulins, the T-cell receptors recognize small fragments of antigen, usually peptides, which are nestled in defined peptide-binding groves of major histocompatibility complex molecules that are present on the plasma membrane of another cell. As such, T-cell immune recognition generally requires cognate intercellular interactions between a T cell and another cell, the antigen-presenting cell. The response of the T cell to antigen depends upon the intensity of the signal generated by ligation of the T-cell receptor. In addition, this signal is modified by the simultaneous ligation of other T-cell receptors for accessory molecules on the plasma membrane of the antigen-presenting cell. Because of this, the outcome of T-cell antigen recognition can range from immune activation and T-cell proliferation to specific T-cell tolerance and/or programmed cell death.

T-LYMPHOCYTE ANTIGEN RECEPTORS

■ T-CELL RECEPTOR HETERODIMERS

The receptor proteins of the T-cell antigen receptor are structurally related to immunoglobulin molecules.[1] The receptor for antigen on most T cells is formed by two polypeptides, termed α and β, that are linked to each other via disulfide bonds and associated with a collection of invariant proteins called invariant CD3 proteins (see Chap. 15). Following the rule of allelic exclusion, the T-cell receptor is clonally distributed, each T cell expressing a single α chain and a single β chain. Each chain has a hydrophobic leader sequence of 18 to 29 amino acids and an amino-terminal domain of 102 to 119 amino acids termed *the variable region*. This designation reflects the variation in the primary structure of these domains among different T-cell receptor polypeptides. Each chain has a carboxyl-terminal region segment of 87 to 113 amino acids, which is termed *the constant region* because this region is invariant among chains of the same class. Owing to their role as surface-membrane receptors, each chain also has a small connecting peptide, a transmembrane region of 20 to 24 amino acids, and a small cytoplasmic region of 5 to 12 residues at the carboxyl terminus anchoring the polypeptide in the cell membrane.

Like the immunoglobulin domains, the variable and constant regions each contain cysteine residues at positions consistent with the presence of a centrally located disulfide loop of 63 to 69 amino acids. Sequence comparisons indicate that several amino acids that are highly conserved in immunoglobulins, including those involved in domain–domain interactions, also are conserved in the T-cell receptor chains. The T-cell receptor chains fold into tertiary structures that are very similar to that of the light and heavy chains of the immunoglobulin molecule. The structural similarities of the T-cell receptor justifiably place the genes encoding these receptor proteins in the so-called immunoglobulin supergene family.

Acronyms and abbreviations that appear in this chapter include: AP-1, activation protein-1 (AP-1); APC, antigen-presenting cell; CTLA-4, cytotoxic T-lymphocyte antigen 4; ERK, extracellular receptor-activated kinase; FoxP3, forkhead box P3; ICAMs, intercellular adhesion molecules; IFN-γ, interferon gamma; IL, interleukin; IPEX syndrome, immune dysregulation, polyendocrinopathy, enteropathy, X-linked syndrome; ITAMs, immunoreceptor tyrosine-based activation motifs; ITIMs, immunoreceptor tyrosine-based inhibitory motifs; iT_{reg}, induced regulatory T cell; JNK, c-Jun N-terminal kinase; LAT, linker of activation of T cells; LFA, lymphocyte-function-associated; MAP, mitogen-activated protein; MHC, major histocompatibility complex; NFAT, nuclear factor of activated T cells; nT_{reg}, natural regulatory T cell; PKC, protein kinase C; PLC-γ1, phospholipase C-1 gamma; RORγt, retinoic acid-related orphan receptor γ thymus isoform; SAP, stress-activated kinase; SH2 domain, Src homology 2 domain; SH3 domain, Src homology 3 domain; STAT, signal transducer and activator of transcription; Tfh cell, follicular helper T cell; TGF-β, transforming growth factor beta; Th17, CD4+ T-cell subset that produces cytokines of the interleukin-17 family; T_{reg}, CD4+CD25+ regulatory T cells; V-like, variable-region-like; VLA, very-late activation; ZAP-70, zeta-associated protein of 70 kDa.

αβ Heterodimers

More than 90 percent of mature T cells express an $\alpha\beta$ heterodimer, making this the major class of T-cell receptor. Without glycan side chains, each α or β polypeptide has a respective size of only 27 kDa or 32 kDa. However, within minutes after being translated into protein, both chains are glycosylated and assembled into a heterodimer composed of a single acidic α glycoprotein of 39 to 46 kDa linked to a more basic 40- to 44-kDa β-glycoprotein via a disulfide bond between the constant regions of the two chains (Fig. 78–1).

γδ Heterodimers

Less than 10 percent of blood T cells and thymocytes exclusively express a different T-cell receptor heterodimer composed of two glycoproteins designated γ and δ.[2] The development of $\gamma\delta$-expressing T cells appears distinct from that of $\alpha\beta$-expressing T cells.[3] In fact, T cells bearing $\gamma\delta$ receptors apparently constitute a distinct cell lineage that can undergo relative expansion in response to infection with certain organisms, such as *Listeria monocytogenes*.[4,5] In secondary lymphoid tissues (see Chap. 5), only approximately 1 to 5 percent of the CD3-positive T cells express $\gamma\delta$ receptors. However, in epithelial tissues most T cells express $\gamma\delta$ receptors, especially in the epidermis and small intestine of the mouse.

The amino acid sequence of the γ chain is more like that of the T-cell receptor β chain, whereas the amino acid sequence of the δ chain is more like that of the α chain. Like the $\alpha\beta$ heterodimer and immunoglobulins, the $\gamma\delta$ heterodimer is clonally distributed. Like the homologous $\alpha\beta$ heterodimer, the $\gamma\delta$ heterodimer also is associated with the CD3 complex and appears capable of stimulating T-cell activation when bound to specific ligand. Together these two chains have structural and size characteristics similar to those of the $\alpha\beta$ heterodimer. However, the tertiary structure of variable regions of $\gamma\delta$ T-cell receptors has a closer resemblance to immunoglobulin variable regions than to the variable regions of $\alpha\beta$ T-cell receptors.

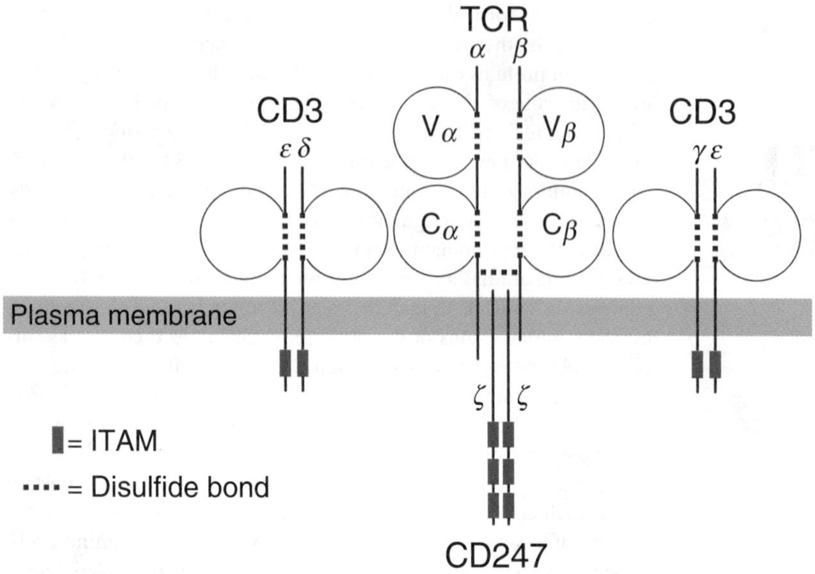

FIGURE 78–1. Schematic of the $\alpha\beta$ T-cell receptor (TCR) complex. The two chains of the $\alpha\beta$ TCR are depicted under the heading TCR and labeled α or β, respectively. The variable (V) domain and constant (C) domains of each chain are depicted within the loop representing the immunoglobulin-like domain of each chain. The heterodimers comprised of CD3ε and CD3δ or CD3γ and CD3ε are, respectively, depicted to the *left* and *right* of the two chains of the $\alpha\beta$ TCR, each under the heading CD3 and labeled ε and δ or γ and ε, respectively. The ζ chain (CD247) homodimer is depicted between the two chains of $\alpha\beta$ TCR. The *dotted lines* represent intrachain or interchain disulfide bridges, as indicated in the legend in the *lower left-hand* corner. The plasma membrane spanned by each of these chains is indicated. The boxes indicate the immunoreceptor tyrosine-based activation motifs (ITAMs) in the cytoplasmic domains of the CD3 polypeptides and the ζ chain.

GENETICS OF T-CELL RECEPTOR HETERODIMERS

Similar to the immunoglobulin genes, each chain of the T-cell receptors is encoded by discrete genetic elements that rearrange during development (Fig. 78–2; see Chap. 77). Evaluation for T-cell receptor gene rearrangements can distinguish between patients who have clonal T-cell lymphoproliferative diseases from those who have nonneoplastic polyclonal T-cell expansion.[6] Molecular analysis for clonal T-cell receptor gene rearrangements can be used to detect minimal residual disease in patients treated for clonal T-cell disorders.[7]

Located at band q35 on the long arm of chromosome 7, the β-chain complex has two closely linked genes, each capable of encoding the β-chain constant region. Each constant region gene is associated with a cluster of functional J_β-gene segments and a single D_β segment. The functional gene encoding the variable region of the β chain is constructed from the rearrangement of any of about 50 variable region gene segments to either one of the two D_β regions and one of 13 J_β regions. The α-chain complex is located at band q11.2 on the long arm of chromosome 14 and thus is linked to the immunoglobulin heavy-chain complex. The α-chain gene complex consists of one constant region gene and at least 50 different variable region gene segments. The functional gene encoding the α-chain variable region is derived from the juxtaposition of any one of the variable region gene segments with one of the many J_α segments through rearrangement that generally involves the deletion of the intervening DNA.

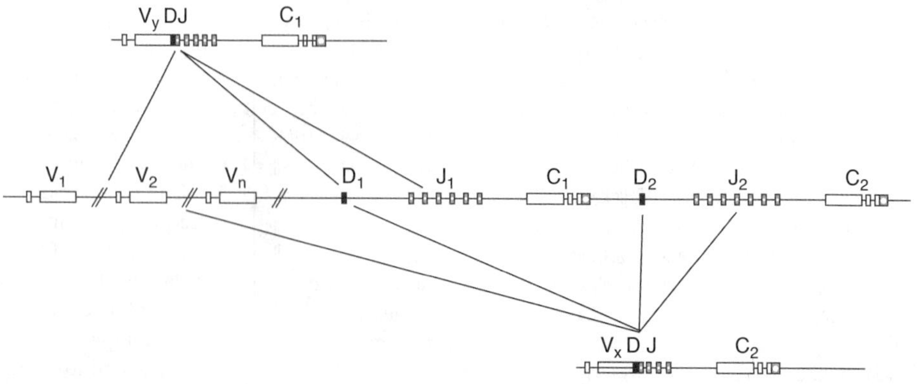

FIGURE 78–2. Schematic of possible rearrangements of the T-cell receptor (TCR)-β-chain genes. The TCR-β-chain genes in the germ-line DNA configuration are depicted in the *middle*. Possible recombination of either the first constant region (C_1, *above*) or the second constant region (C_2, *below*) with the variable region (V), diversity (D), or joining (J) segments are indicated by the *lines*.

The organization of the γ and δ genes is similar to that of the α and β genes except for some significant differences. First, the gene complex encoding the δ genes is located entirely within the α-chain gene complex between the V_α and J_α gene segments. Consequently, any rearrangement of the α-chain genes inactivates the genes encoding the δ chain. Second, there are fewer V gene segments in the γ and δ gene complexes than at either the T-cell receptor α or β gene loci. The γ-gene complex on band p15 on the short arm of chromosome 7, for example, has only about 12 V_γ gene segments, two virtually identical J_γ segments, and two constant region gene segments. Moreover, there are only about four V_δ gene segments, three D_δ gene segments, three J_δ gene segments, and a single constant region gene in the δ gene complex. Consequently, most of the variability in the γ and δ chains is found in the junctional region formed during the process of $\gamma\delta$ T-cell receptor gene rearrangement. The amino acids encoded by this region form the center of the T-cell receptor-binding site.

ANTIGENS RECOGNIZED BY T-CELL RECEPTOR HETERODIMERS

Although highly similar in structure, there are important differences in the ways that T-cell receptors and immunoglobulins recognize antigen. Whereas immunoglobulins can bind antigens directly, T-cell receptors generally recognize peptide antigens that are bound to a molecule of the major histocompatibility complex (MHC) on the surface of another cell.[8]

There are two basic classes of MHC molecules. Class I MHC molecules bind peptides that generally are derived from proteins synthesized and degraded in the cytoplasm of the cell. The human histocompatibility antigens HLA-A, -B, or -C are class I molecules. Class II MHC molecules, such as the HLA-D antigens DP, DQ, and DR, generally bind peptides that are derived from exogenous proteins that are degraded in the intracellular vesicles. Peptides that bind to MHC class I molecules are usually 8 to 10 amino acids long. The binding of such peptides is stabilized by contacts between atoms in the free amino and carboxyl termini of the peptide and the peptide-binding groove of all MHC class I molecules. Peptides that bind to MHC class II molecules, on the other hand, generally are 13 amino acids long or longer. This is because MHC class II molecules do not bind the two ends of the peptide such as the MHC class I molecules.

Nevertheless, for either class I or class II molecules, there exists a discrete binding site for the peptide that lies in a cleft between two α helices of the MHC molecule. Steric factors, hydrogen bonding, and hydrophobic interactions between the peptide and the particular MHC molecule serve to tether the peptide within this cleft, thus generating a tertiary structure that is formed by amino acid residues of both the MHC and the peptide antigen. It is this tertiary structure that is recognized by the T-cell receptor for antigen.

There are several genes for each class of MHC molecule, and each of these is highly polymorphic with many different alleles (see Chap. 138). The particular combination of MHC alleles found on an individual chromosome is known as an MHC haplotype. Both maternal and paternal MHC haplotypes are expressed concomitantly. Polymorphism in the MHC molecules primarily is found in the amino acids lining the clefts that cradle the peptide antigen, allowing the MHC molecules encoded by each allele to bind a distinctive array of different peptides. Structural studies show that the T-cell receptor can recognize both the bound peptide and the amino acid residues that surround the peptide-binding pocket of self or allogeneic MHC molecules.[9,10]

Each MHC allele encodes a MHC molecule that can bind a restricted set of peptides with a discrete sequence motif. Moreover, different alleles of the same MHC molecule will bind peptides with different sequence motifs. This polymorphism combined with biallelic expression of MHC genes and the degeneracy of MHC molecules on any given MHC haplotype ensure that a wide variety of different peptides can be presented to the T cell for immune recognition. Because T cells actually interact with a tertiary structure that is largely dictated by a particular MHC molecule, T cells manifest MHC-restricted antigen recognition.

Some T cells, however, do not recognize peptides bound to a given MHC molecule. Such T cells recognize nonpeptide antigens that are presented by MHC class I-like molecules encoded by genes that map outside the MHC region. One such family of molecules is called CD1, the first defined cluster of differentiation antigen (see Chap. 15). CD1 molecules can present nonpeptide lipid antigens to T cells.[11,12] For example, in cells infected with mycobacteria, the CD1 molecules are able to bind and present the mycobacterial membrane components such as lipoarabinomannan or mycolic acid. T cells that recognize these complexes play an important role in the immune response to Mycobacterium tuberculosis.

Structural studies show that $\gamma\delta$ T-cell receptors assume a different tertiary structure than $\alpha\beta$ T-cell receptors.[2] As such, the T cells that express $\gamma\delta$ receptors (the so-called $\gamma\delta$ T-cells) apparently do not recognize peptides bound to classic MHC class I molecules.[13] Some $\gamma\delta$ T cells recognize products of certain MHC class IB genes, or variants of the standard MHC class I genes that have little polymorphism (see Chap. 138). Other $\gamma\delta$ receptors apparently recognize antigen directly like immunoglobulin molecules. Finally, $\gamma\delta$ T cells also can recognize determinants presented by CD1 molecules.[14] Because increased numbers of $\gamma\delta$ T cells have been found in a variety of infectious and autoimmune diseases, it is speculated that $\gamma\delta$ T-cells play an immunoregulatory role that is complementary to the function of T cells bearing the more conventional $\alpha\beta$ T-cell receptor.[15]

GENERATION OF T-CELL RECEPTOR DIVERSITY

Diversity of the T-cell receptor for antigen is achieved by several mechanisms, some of which are the same as those that generate diversity among immunoglobulin molecules (see Chap. 77). The joining of different V, D, and J elements to produce a complete V gene, the presence of uncorrected errors made during the recombination of these genetic elements, and the combinatorial diversity afforded by the random pairing of two chains encoded by separated gene complexes all function to enhance the diversity of the T-cell antigen receptor repertoire.[16] An important difference between T cells and B cells in how they may enhance receptor diversity, however, is that B cells are capable of somatic hypermutation (see Chap. 77). This process requires expression of activation-induced deaminase along with other enzymes that are expressed primarily by B cells within the germinal center of secondary lymphoid tissue during the immune response to antigen (see Chaps. 5 and 77).

That T-cell receptor genes do not undergo somatic mutation probably relates to the central role that T cells have in directing host immune defenses. During differentiation, immature precursors to $\alpha\beta$-expressing T cells pass through the thymus, where they are "educated" to distinguish self from nonself vis-à-vis the cell-surface proteins of the major histocompatibility complex (see Chaps. 5 and 76). Because the ligand for the $\alpha\beta$ T-cell receptor is "processed" antigen presented by the proteins, close interaction with the molecules of the MHC might be lost if the variable region genes of the T-cell receptor were allowed to diverge significantly from the inherited germ-line repertoire. Furthermore, somatic mutation of expressed T-cell receptor variable region genes may lead to constitutive T-cell activation to processed self-antigen presented by self-MHC molecules. Such a scenario could lead to a breakdown in tolerance to self-antigens and autoimmunity.

THE INVARIANT CHAINS OF THE T-CELL RECEPTOR COMPLEX

COMPOSITION OF THE T-CELL RECEPTOR COMPLEX

Closely associated with and required for the surface expression of the two polypeptides of the T-cell receptor is the CD3 complex of polypeptides and CD247, known as the zeta-chain (ζ chain) of the T-cell receptor.[17] Unlike the T-cell receptor heterodimers, these polypeptides are invariant and are found on all T cells that express $\alpha{:}\beta$ or $\gamma{:}\delta$ heterodimers. The CD3 polypeptides are designated CD3γ, CD3δ, CD3ε. The CD3ε chain couples with either the CD3γ or the CD3δ chain to generate heterodimers that each form a tight association with the $\alpha{:}\beta$ (or $\gamma{:}\delta$) receptor heterodimer on the T-cell surface (see Fig. 78–1). Each CD3 polypeptide has a negatively charged amino acid in the central portion of the hydrophobic transmembrane region that stabilizes the CD3 complex with the two chains of the T-cell receptor. The ζ chain (CD247), on the other hand, forms a disulfide-like homodimer that primarily associates with the two T-cell receptor chains and only weakly associates with the CD3 complex. As such, it cannot be co-immunoprecipitated readily with antibodies to the CD3 polypeptides. Very little of the ζ chain is present on the T-cell surface (see Fig. 78–1).

MOLECULAR FEATURES OF THE T-CELL RECEPTOR COMPLEX

The genes encoding CD3γ, CD3δ, or CD3ε chains are clustered in band q23 on the long arm of chromosome 11. CD3γ has a 16-kDa polypeptide backbone that is heavily glycosylated to assume a final molecular mass of 25 to 28 kDa. CD3δ and CD3ε are each 20 kDa in molecular mass. The CD3δ is a glycoprotein consisting of 30 percent carbohydrate. In contrast, CD3ε is not glycosylated. CD3δ and CD3γ are highly homologous at both the protein and nucleic acid sequence level. The nucleic acid sequence of each predicts CD3δ and CD3γ to have typical signal peptides, respective hydrophilic extracellular domains of 79 to 89 amino acids, hydrophobic transmembrane regions of 27 amino acids, and hydrophilic intracellular domains of 44 to 55 amino acids. CD3ε is similar, with a 22-residue signal peptide, an extracellular domain of 104 amino acids, a transmembrane domain, and a comparatively long intracellular domain of 81 amino acids. Each CD3 polypeptide has one immunoglobulin-like domain in its extracellular domain that is defined by an intrachain disulfide bond (see Fig. 78–1), indicating that these polypeptides are members of the immunoglobulin superfamily. However, unlike the $\alpha\beta$ or $\gamma\delta$ chains of the T-cell receptor, there is no variability in the extracellular domains of the CD3 proteins, indicating that these molecules do not contribute to the specificity of antigen recognition.

The ζ chain has no sequence or structural homology to the other three CD3 chains. It is a nonglycosylated protein of 16-kDa molecular mass that is encoded by a gene found on chromosome 1. The ζ chain has only a very short extracellular domain of 6 to 9 amino acids, a transmembrane domain of 21 amino acids, and a long intracellular domain of 113 amino acids.

The cytoplasmic domains of all the CD3 polypeptides and the ζ chain each contain sequences termed immunoreceptor tyrosine-based activation motifs (ITAMs). Each ITAM contains two copies of the sequence tyrosine-X-X-leucine separated by six to eight amino acid residues, in which X represents an unspecified amino acid. The cytoplasmic domains of each CD3 polypeptide contain one ITAM, whereas each ζ chain contains three ITAMs (see Fig. 78–1). These sequences allow the CD3 proteins to associate with cytosolic protein tyrosine kinases following T-cell receptor ligation, thus transducing a signal to the interior of the T cell. The cytoplasmic domains of CD3ε and CD3ζ are particularly important in this regard.

SIGNAL TRANSDUCTION VIA THE T-CELL RECEPTOR COMPLEX

The CD3 polypeptides and the ζ chain are responsible for signal transduction from the T-cell receptor heterodimer to intracellular proteins.[18] Upon binding to specific ligand, the T-cell receptor $\alpha\beta$ (or $\gamma\delta$) heterodimer undergoes steric changes that result in the phosphorylation of the ITAMs of the ζ chain and each of the CD3 polypeptides (see Fig. 78–1). When the tyrosine residues in the ITAMs become phosphorylated they can act as docking sites for adapter proteins or tyrosine kinases, such as the zeta-associated protein of 70 kDa (ZAP-70), which possesses a pair of Src homology 2 (SH2) domain and an Src homology 3 (SH3) domain. Following ligation of the T-cell receptor, there is recruitment and activation of a Src family protein tyrosine kinase (e.g., Lck), which, in turn, differentially phosphorylate the ITAMs of the accessory molecules in the T-cell receptor complex.[19] ZAP-70 is recruited to the phosphorylated ITAMs of the ζ chain via its SH2 and SH3 domains, and subsequently becomes activated.[20] Activated ZAP-70 can recruit and phosphorylate a membrane-anchored adapter protein called linker of activation of T cells (LAT).[21] Activated LAT, in turn, can recruit several other adapter proteins, including the SH2-binding leukocyte phosphoprotein of 76-kDa (SLP-76) and Grb2 to the site of T-cell receptor clustering.[22] Grb2 in turn can recruit a RAS guanosine triphosphate (GTP)/guanosine diphosphate (GDP) exchange factor termed *SOS* (because of its structural homology to the *Drosophila* protein called "son of sevenless"), which catalyzes GTP for GDP exchange on RAS. This generates a GTP-bound form of RAS that functions as an allosteric activator of successive mitogen-activated protein (MAP) kinases,[23] culminating in the activation of the extracellular receptor-activated kinase 1 and 2 (ERK1/2). Activated ERK phosphorylates Elk, which, in turn, stimulates transcription of Fos, a component of the activation protein-1 (AP-1) factor that is a necessary component of the transcription-factor complex required for expression of interleukin (IL)-2 and other critical T-cell proteins.

In parallel with the activation of ERK, the adapter proteins that are phosphorylated and recruited to the T-cell receptor complex also recruit and activate another GTP/GDP exchange protein, Vav, which in turn acts on a 21-kDa guanine nucleotide-binding protein, Rac. The newly generated GTP-bound form of Rac activates another MAP kinase, called p38, and initiates a parallel enzymatic cascade, resulting in the activation of yet another MAP kinase called c-Jun N-terminal kinase (JNK), otherwise known as stress-activated kinase (SAP). Activated JNK phosphorylates c-Jun, the second component of the AP-1 transcription factor required for IL-2 transcription. The GTP-bound form of Rac also induces cytoskeletal reorganization, thereby facilitating the clustering of the T-cell receptor complex, accessory molecules, and other accessory proteins at the site(s) of contact between the T cell and the antigen-presenting cell.

The activated adapter proteins that are recruited to the T-cell receptor complex also can induce calcium signaling and activation of protein kinase C (PKC) and the phosphoinositide-3 kinase.[24] Upon its phosphorylation by ZAP-70, the recruited LAT molecule can directly bind phospholipase C γ_1 (PLC-γ_1), which, in turn, is activated through phosphorylation by activated ZAP-70. Activated PLC-γ_1 mediates hydrolysis of a plasma membrane phospholipid phosphatidylinositol 4,5-biphosphosphate, generating inositol 1,4,5-triphosphate and diacylglycerol, which respectively induce a rapid increase in cytosolic free calcium and activation of the θ isoform of PKC. Cytosolic free calcium binds to calmodulin, a ubiquitous calcium-dependent regulatory protein. The calcium–calmodulin complex activates the cytoplasmic phosphatase calcineurin, which in turn catalyzes the removal of an inhibitory phosphate group on the nuclear factor of activated T cells (NFAT) that retains NFAT proteins in the cytoplasm. Removal of the phosphates from NFAT1 and NFAT2 by activated calcineurin allows these transcription factors to translocate into the nucleus, where they enhance transcription of a several activation-induced genes, including those encoding IL-2, IL-4, and tumor necrosis factor. The importance of this pathway in T-cell activation is underscored by the strong immunosuppressive activity of the drugs cyclosporine and FK-506, which, respectively, can bind cyclophilin and FK-506 binding protein to form complexes that inhibit the phosphatase activity of calcineurin.

CD4 AND CD8

STRUCTURE OF CD4 AND CD8

CD4 and CD8 are glycoproteins that share structural features with other receptor molecules of the immunoglobulin superfamily. CD8 is expressed as a heterodimer of CD8α and CD8β or as a CD8α/CD8α homodimer. Each chain contains a single immunoglobulin-like domain linked to the membrane by a segment of polypeptide chain that could have an extended conformation. These chains are encoded by genes that are linked closely to the immunoglobulin κ light-chain locus at band p12, on the short arm of chromosome 2. The protein sequence of the amino-terminal domains of each CD8 chain shares greater than 28 percent homology with κ light-chain variable regions. As such, these domains are called the variable-region-like (V-like) domains. Following this V-like domain, the CD8 molecule has a short region rich in prolines, threonines, and serines that resembles the immunoglobulin hinge region. This region also contains sites for *O*-linked glycosylation. A hydrophobic transmembrane region anchors this hinge-like region. The CD8 molecule has a 25-amino-acid cytoplasmic tail consisting of highly basic residues. Two cysteines within the V-like domain form a disulfide bridge that stabilizes the immunoglobulin-like fold. An additional cysteine residue is located each within the V-like domain, the hinge region, the transmembrane segment, and cytoplasmic domain. These cysteines form intermolecular disulfide bridges between two CD8 molecules;

thereby stabilizing the CD8α/CD8β heterodimers or CD8α/CD8α homodimers that are expressed on the T-cell surface. The cell-surface CD8 heterodimer shares structural geometry with the heterodimers formed by the pairing of light chain and heavy chains immunoglobulin.

CD4, on the other hand, is expressed as a monomer on the surface of a subset of peripheral T cells, mononuclear phagocytes and some blood-derived dendritic cells. It is a 55-kDa monomeric glycoprotein that is encoded by a gene that maps to the short arm of chromosome 12. It consists of 5 external domains, a stretch of hydrophobic transmembrane residues, and a highly basic cytoplasmic tail of 38 residues. Similar to CD8, the amino-terminal domain of CD4 also has extensive homology to immunoglobulin light-chain variable regions. However, following this immunoglobulin-like domain is a domain of 270 amino acids that bears little resemblance to other proteins of the immunoglobulin superfamily.

The cytoplasmic regions of CD4 and CD8 are conserved among vertebrates, suggesting that these regions are essential for the function of these molecules. The cytoplasmic region of CD4 contains five serines and threonines, one or more of which is phosphorylated by protein kinase C upon activation of T cells by phorbol esters or exposure to antigen. Subsequent to phosphorylation, the CD4 glycoprotein is internalized concomitant with T-cell activation. Similarly, the CD8 protein also possesses a highly charged and conserved cytoplasmic domain that may be involved in transmembrane signal transduction. In this light, CD4 and CD8 actually may be integral components of the functional T-cell receptor complex required to trigger T-cell activation and/or function upon exposure to specific antigen.

FUNCTION OF CD4 AND CD8

CD4 and CD8 facilitate T-cell antigen recognition by interacting with the glycoproteins of the MHC.[25] Moreover, during antigen recognition, CD4 and CD8 molecules associate on the plasma membrane with components of the T-cell receptor for antigens. For these reasons, these molecules are considered coreceptors of the T-cell receptor for antigen.

The CD8 molecules bind to the nonpolymorphic α_3 domain of the HLA class I molecule (HLA A, B, or C),[26] whereas the CD4 molecule binds to the nonpolymorphic β_2 domain of HLA class II molecules (HLA-D region-encoded molecules: DP, DQ, and DR).[27] CD8 or CD4 enhance by more than 100-fold the adhesion between the T cell's CD3/T-cell receptor complex and the MHC glycoproteins expressed by an antigen-presenting cell (APC) or target cell. These molecules apparently focus MHC molecules of the APC or target cell onto the T-cell surface, allowing for specific recognition of "processed" antigen that is cradled within the MHC glycoproteins. Because CD4 and CD8 differ in their MHC-binding specificities, T cells expressing CD4 or CD8 generally recognize antigens presented by class II or class I MHC glycoproteins, respectively.[28] This selectivity is underscored by studies on knockout mice that lack expression of either of these accessory molecules. Mice lacking CD4 or CD8 fail to develop class II-restricted or class I-restricted T cells, respectively, indicating that these coreceptors play essential roles in the maturation of T cells in the thymus. A similar defect is observed in patients with the bare lymphocyte syndrome who have a congenital immune deficiency caused by genetic defects in their capacity to make MHC class II molecules.[29] Although such patients have normal numbers of B cells and T cells, they have markedly reduced numbers of CD4+ T cells, thus accounting in part for their profound immune deficiency.

In addition to serving as coreceptors, CD4 or CD8 molecules also enhance antigen responsiveness by transducing a signal either directly or in concert with CD3/T-cell receptor complex.[30] Such signal transducing functions are mediated through their interaction with the SRC family tyrosine kinase called *Lck*. Lck is noncovalently associated with the cytoplasmic tails of CD4 and/or CD8. When a T cell recognizes a peptide antigen presented by an appropriate MHC antigen, the interaction of CD4 or CD8 with the MHC molecule brings Lck close to the T-cell receptor complex. Lck then phosphorylates the tyrosine residues in the ITAMs of CD3 polypeptides and the ζ chain, thereby initiating the receptor signaling required for T-cell activation.

Finally, CD4 also is a coreceptor molecule for the human immunodeficiency virus (HIV).[31,32] Binding of CD4 along with the chemokine receptor CCR5 facilitates entry of the virus into those T cells that are stimulated specifically in an antigen-driven immune response. Monoclonal antibodies specific for the CD4 glycoprotein can block infection by HIV. Moreover, genetically engineered soluble CD4 can compete with cell-surface CD4 for HIV binding. Finally, disease progression in patients infected with HIV correlates with depletion of blood T cells that express CD4 (see Chap. 83).

T-CELL SUBSETS

PRECURSOR THYMOCYTES

CD4 and CD8 are expressed by nearly all T-cell precursors. Only a fraction of thymocytes express neither CD4 nor CD8. These cells are thought to be the marrow-derived precursors to the vast majority of thymocytes that express both CD4 and CD8. More mature thymocytes and all peripheral T cells express either CD4 or CD8, but not both (see Chap. 76).

HELPER AND SUPPRESSOR (CYTOLYTIC) T CELLS

The mutually exclusive expression of CD4 or CD8 defines two major blood T-cell subsets. Blood T cells that express CD8 had been designated suppressor T cells. These cells normally constitute 25 to 35 percent of the peripheral T-cell population. CD8 T cells, perhaps more appropriately, should be designated cytolytic T lymphocytes, in that a main function of these cells is to lyse target cells that bear surface antigens for which they are specific. Blood T cells that solely express the CD4 surface antigen are designated helper T cells. These cells normally comprise approximately 65 percent of the blood T cells. Generally, helper T cells produce lymphokines upon activation by foreign antigens presented by MHC molecules expressed on the surface of APCs.

CD4+ T-CELL SUBSETS

Th1 and Th2 Cells

Mature CD4+ T cells may be divided into at least two subsets, Th1 and Th2, each able to elaborate a distinctive profile of cytokines upon activation.[33] Th1 cells are the major helper T-cell source of interferon-γ (IFN-γ), and are the major T cells involved in activating macrophages, eliciting delayed-type hypersensitivity responses, and clearing intracellular pathogens. Th2 cells, on the other hand, are the major helper-T cell source of IL-4 and are important for the generation of immunoglobulin (Ig) E, the production of eosinophils, and the immune defense against infections by parasites.

These CD4+ T-cell subsets are distinguished most effectively by the cytokines that they produce and not by the surface antigens or cytokine receptors that they express. In addition to IFN-γ, Th1 cells also produce lymphotoxin β and IL-2, whereas Th2 cells produce IL-5, IL-13, and IL-25, in addition to IL-4. Nevertheless, human Th1 cells preferentially express CD26, membrane IFN-γ, the chemokine receptors CCR5 (CD195) and CXCR3 (CD183), and the receptor for IL-12 (IL-12R or CD212).[34] Moreover, Th1 cells may express higher levels of the lymphocyte activation gene 3 (LAG-3 or CD223), a ligand for MHC class II antigens that is structurally related to CD4.[35] Th2 cells, on the other hand, preferentially express CD62L, the α chain of the IL-4 receptor (IL-4Rα), the α chain of the IL-33 receptor (IL-33Rα), CD30, and the chemokine receptors CCR3 (CD193), CCR4 (CD194), CCR8 (CDw198), and, to some extent, CXCR4 (CD184).[34,36,37] Distinctive expression levels of these cytokine and chemokine receptors, along with distinctive binding activities for various endothelial selectins, most likely account for the differences in the response to cytokines and tissue-specific migration of these helper T-cell subsets.[38] (See Table 15–1, Chap. 15.)

The cytokines produced by each subset also stimulate differentiation of additional T cells of the same subset. For example, the IFN-γ and IL-12 elaborated by Th1 cells promote further Th1 differentiation and inhibit the proliferation of Th2 cells. In naïve CD4+ T cells, the Th1 cytokine IFN-γ induces or activates the signal transducer and activator of transcription (STAT) 4, STAT1, and the T-box transcription factor T-bet, transcription factors that play critical roles in Th1 cell differentiation (Fig. 78–3).[39–41] On the other hand, IL-4, the archetypical Th2 cytokine, respectively activates or enhances the expression STAT6, STAT5, and GATA3, transcription factors that play important roles in Th2 cell development (Fig. 78–3).[42,43] Another Th2 cytokine, IL-10, inhibits Th1 cell activation, thereby limiting the production of Th1-type cytokines. Because of these self-amplifying and mutually excluding feedback loops, an immune response becomes increasingly polarized once it develops along a Th1 or Th2 pathway, particularly upon protracted stimulation by chronic infection or prolonged exposure to environmental antigens.

Each of these two T-cell subsets has a discrete function.[44] Each can act on monocyte-derived dendritic cells to express a different array of chemokines,[45] thereby influencing the character of the immune response to antigen. The principle functions of Th1 cells are to activate macrophages to kill microorganisms and to induce B cells to make subclasses of IgG antibodies that are very effective at opsonizing extracellular pathogens for uptake by phagocytic cells. In addition, Th1 cells are the major helper T cells involved in delayed-type hypersensitivity. The cytokines elaborated by Th1 cells stimulate macrophage Fc receptor expression, phagocytosis, and antigen presentation, enhancing the capacity of macrophages to kill intracellular pathogens. Th2 cells, on the other hand, initiate the antibody response to antigen by activating naïve antigen-specific B cells to produce IgM antibodies and subsequently stimulate the production of switched immunoglobulin isotypes, including IgA, IgE, and neutralizing and/or weakly opsonizing subtypes of IgG (see Chap. 77). In addition to stimulating the production of IgE antibodies, the cytokines made by Th2 cells induce differentiation of mast cells and eosinophils. Although these effects may contribute to development of allergy,[46,47] these responses are protective in helminth infections.[48,49] Studies demonstrate that eosinophilia and elevated IgE that accompany infection with *Schistosoma mansoni*, for example, are caused by the induction of Th2-type cells in the immune response to parasite ova.[50,51] In addition, because they express the B-cell stimulatory/growth factor IL-4, Th2 cells appear better suited than Th1 cells to induce B-cell responses to antigen.

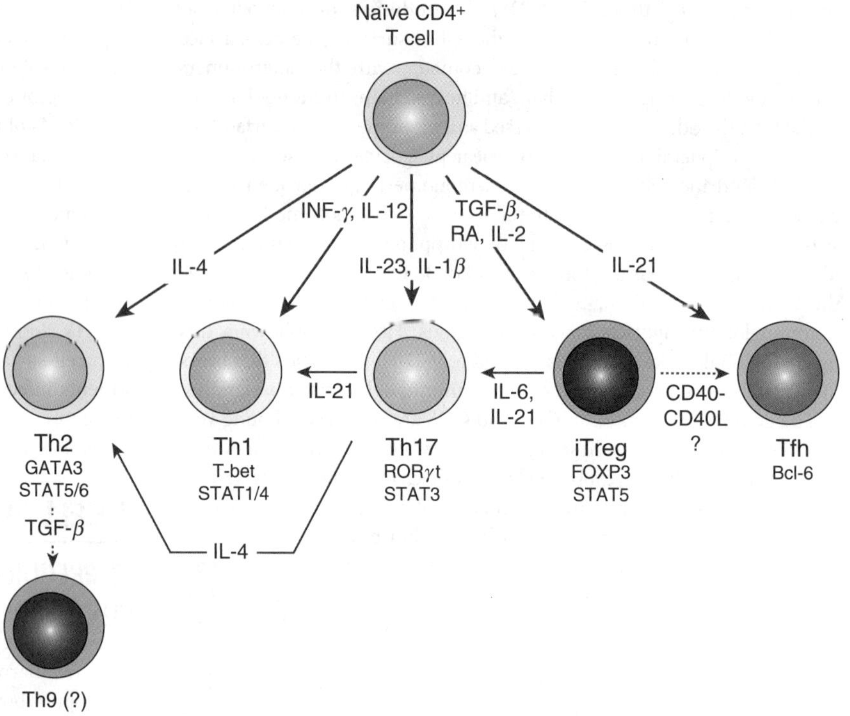

FIGURE 78–3. Differentiation of CD4+ T-cell subsets. During the course of the immune response, a naïve CD4+ T cell (*top of figure*) can differentiate into any one of several distinctive CD4+ T cells, as indicated beneath each differentiated cell type. Beneath the name of each T-cell subset is listed the transcription factor (if known) that is critical for the differentiation and maintenance of the subset. IL-4 is critical for development of Th2 cells (*green*), which triggers activation and/or induction of STAT5, STAT6, and GATA3, transcription factors that are important in Th2 differentiation. On the other hand, interferon-γ and IL-12 pattern the development of Th1 cells (*light red*) through the activation and/or induction of transcription factors STAT1, STAT4, and T-bet. Interleukin (IL)-23 along with IL-1β or transforming growth factor beta (TGF-β) can induce blood CD4+ T cells to express the transcription factors STAT3 and RORγt (retinoic acid-related orphan receptor γ thymus isoform), which programs differentiation into Th17 cells (*light yellow*),[74] whereas TGF-β, retinoic acid (RA), and IL-2 induces these cells to express the transcription factors FoxP3 and STAT5, which are required for differentiation of these cells into iT_{reg} (induced regulatory T cell) cells (*red*).[126] Finally, IL-21 favors differentiation of naïve CD4 T cells into follicular helper T cells (Tfh [*gold*]). There is some plasticity in these differentiated T-cell subsets.[127] IL-6 in combination may induce iT_{reg} cells to differentiate into Th17 cells, whereas B cells stimulated via CD40-CD40-ligand (CD40L or CD154) may induce their differentiation into Tfh cells, as indicated by the *dashed horizontal arrows*. Similarly, IL-21 may induce Th17 cells to differentiate into Th1 cells, whereas IL-4 may induce their differentiation into Th2 cells. Th9 cells (*dark blue*) constitute a putative CD4+ T-cell subset characterized by its ability to secrete IL-9. These cells apparently differentiate from Th2 cells in the context of TGF-β.

Extracellular antigens tend to stimulate the generation of Th2 cells, whereas pathogens that accumulate in large numbers inside macrophage vesicles tend to stimulate differentiation of Th1 cells.[52] CD4+ T cells secrete minute amounts of IL-4 during their initial activation. If the antigen is present at high concentrations and does not trigger inflammation and attendant production of IL-12, then the local concentration of IL-4 increases over time, inducing differentiation of Th2 cells. Because of this, Th2 cells typically develop in response to helminth infections or noninflammatory environmental allergens.[53] On the other hand, pathogens that induce inflammation and/or engage toll-like receptors on accessory cells and macrophages can promote production of IFN-γ and IL-12, thereby stimulating development of the immune response down the Th1 pathway.[41] Immune responses restricted to that of Th1 cells, for example, are observed in patients with leprosy who have developed cellular immunity to *Mycobacterium leprae*, or in patients with arthritis triggered by infection with either *Borrelia burgdorferi* (Lyme disease) or *Yersinia enterocolitica*.[54]

CD4+CD25+ Regulatory T Cells

There is another CD4+ T-cell subset that serves to suppress immune responses rather than to provide the helper activity that typically is associated with CD4+ T cells. These cells express CD3, CD4, and CD25 (the low-affinity receptor for IL-2; see Chap. 15), and play an important role in the maintenance of specific immune tolerance.[55,56] These cells generally are referred to as T_{reg} cells, which is an abbreviation of the term *CD4+ CD25+ regulatory T cells*.[57] T_{regs} also constitutively express the cytotoxic T-lymphocyte antigen 4 (CTLA-4 or CD152), an inhibitory receptor for immune costimulatory molecules CD80 and CD86 that ordinarily is expressed on other types of T cells only after immune activation (see section on T-cell accessory molecules).[56] Finally, T_{regs} express the transcription factor *forkhead box P3* (FoxP3), which stabilizes the phenotype and suppressive function of these T cells by altering a wide spectrum of T_{reg}-specific genes.[58,59] Patients with the *immune dysregulation, polyendocrinopathy, enteropathy, X-linked syndrome* (IPEX syndrome), are found to have inactivating mutations in the gene encoding FoxP3, which maps to the long arm of the X chromosome at Xp11.23[60] (see Chap. 82), resulting in the inability to generate T_{reg} cells. These patients typically have autoimmune skin conditions, such as bullous pemphigoid or alopecia universalis, and autoimmune endocrinopathies similar to those seen in patients with the *autoimmune polyendocrine candidiasis ectodermal dystrophy syndrome* (APECED syndrome), which is associated with genetic defects in the autoimmune regulator (*AIRE*) gene responsible for the generation of T-cell tolerance in the thymus (see Chaps. 5 and 82). The IPEX syndrome demonstrates the importance of T_{regs} cells in maintaining tolerance to self-antigens and in preventing runaway immune responses to environmental antigens that might evolve into cross-reactive autoimmunity.[61,62]

T_{reg} cells can specifically suppress immune responses via several different mechanisms.[56] Upon activation T_{regs} can (1) produce anti-inflammatory cytokines (e.g., IL-10, TGF-β, or IL-35),[63] (2) reduce the availability of interleukin-2 (IL-2), (3) kill other immune effector cells, (4) modulate the activation state and/or function of antigen presenting cells and other immune effector cells,[55] and/or (5) release suppressor factors, such as galectin-1 (a β-galactoside-binding protein that can bind and inhibit the function of many glycoproteins, including CD7, CD43, and CD45; see Chap. 15[64]) and fibrinogen-like protein 2 (FGL2; a member of the fibrinogen family that can stimulate an inhibitory IgG Fc receptor, FcγRIIB, on dendritic cells.[65] These suppressor functions require activation of the T-cell receptors expressed by the T_{reg} cells, allowing their suppressor to be directed against specific target antigens. However, once activated these cells can mediate "bystander" suppression of other immune effector cells, including other types of CD4+ T cells and CD8+ T cells.

T_{reg} cells can be further subdivided into two subtypes, "natural T_{reg}" (nT_{reg}) and "induced T_{reg}" (iT_{reg}).[66] The nT_{reg} cells (sometimes referred to as "thymic T_{reg}" [tT_{reg}]), differentiate from CD4+CD8- T cells that have undergone positive and negative selection to self-antigens presented in the thymus (see Chap. 5).[67] These cells are thought to play a role maintaining tolerance to self-antigens. The iT_{reg} cells, on the other hand, differentiate in mesenteric lymph nodes during induction of oral tolerance[68] or at the sites of chronic inflammation,[69] neoplastic tumors,[70] or nonrejected allografts.[71] As such, iT_{regs} are thought to play an important role in the development of tolerance to environmental antigens, such as those of certain foods or commensal microbes, or to "altered" self-antigens of inflamed tissues or neoplastic cells. Although nT_{reg} cells have subtle features that can distinguish them from iT_{reg} cells,[66] the generation of either type requires the induced and maintained expression of FoxP3 and STAT5,[72] which can result from stimulation of the T-cell receptor of CD4+ T cells in the proper context along with the cytokines transforming growth factor (TGF)-β and IL-2 and/or retinoic acid (Fig. 78–3).[73]

Th17 T Cells

Naïve CD4+ T cells also can differentiate into another type of T-helper cell that plays an important role in the immune responses to certain extracellular pathogens and fungi.[74] These cells produce IL-17 (sometimes referred to as IL-17A) and a closely related cytokine, IL-17F, which can form biologically active homodimers or heterodimers. Because of this, these T cells are called Th17 cells.[74] Principle cytokines involved in the differentiation of naïve blood CD4+ T cells into Th17 cells are IL-23 and IL-1β[75] (Fig. 78–3), although other cytokines apparently are involved in the differentiation of naïve cord blood CD4+ T cells into Th17 cells (e.g., IL-21, TGF-β, and/or IL-23).[74] Prostaglandins, most notably prostaglandin E_2, can synergize with IL-23 and IL-1β to drive differentiation of CD4+ T cells into Th17 cells.[76] These cytokines and factors can induce activation and/or expression of transcription factors that are distinct from those used by Th1 or Th2 cells, including the retinoic acid-related orphan receptor γ (RORγt) and STAT3[77,78] (Fig. 78–3), which in turn can induce expression of IL-17 and IL-17F,[79,80] the hallmark feature of Th17 cells. Th17 also express high levels of the IL-23R, CCR6, CXCR4, CD161, and multiple CD49 integrins, but not CCR2, CCR5, or CCR7.[81,82] In contrast to Th1 or Th2 cells, Th17 cells do not elaborate IFN-γ or IL-4, both of which can inhibit expression of IL-17.[83]

Th17 cells play a role in inflammation and the defense against intestinal bacteria, extracellular pathogens, and fungal infections. Th17 cells are abundant in the intestinal lamina propria, where they are induced and stimulated by commensal bacteria, allowing these cells to play a role in the maintenance of epithelial integrity and clearance of extracellular pathogens. Th17 cells are the principle producers of IL-17 in response to specific immune stimulation. IL-17 is a proinflammatory cytokine that has pleiotropic effects on multiple target cells, resulting in enhanced antigen presentation, antibody production, macrophage activation, cellular extravasation, and neutrophil migration.[84] In addition to IL-17 and IL-17F, Th17 cells elaborate other proinflammatory factors, including chemokines (e.g., CXCL8 (IL-8) and CCL20), cytokines (e.g., IL-6, tumor necrosis factor-α, IL-21, and IL-22), growth factors (e.g., granulocyte colony-stimulating factor and granulocyte-macrophage colony-stimulating factor), acute phase proteins (e.g., C-reactive protein), and antimicrobial peptides and mucins.[72,85] The importance of Th17 cells in the defense against certain microorganisms is reflected in the rare primary immunodeficiency disorder called *autosomal dominant hyper-IgE syndrome*, which results from inactivating mutation(s) in the gene encoding STAT3 that is required for the differentiation of Th17 cells (see Chap. 82).[72] Such patients lack Th17 cells and have an increased susceptibility to infection with the various species of *Staphylococcus* or *Candida*.[86,87] Furthermore, loss of intestinal commensal bacteria that are essential for the induction of Th17 cells through the use of antibiotics can cause depletion in intestinal Th17 cells. Loss of gut-associated Th17 cells might account in part for the increased incidence of gastrointestinal infections with *Candida albicans* or *Clostridium difficile* observed in patients subjected to long-term, broad-spectrum antibiotic therapy.[88]

Because of their capacity to enhance inflammation in an antigen-specific manner, Th17 cells also have been implicated in the development and/or propagation of autoimmune disease. Th17 cells initially were identified as the T-cell subset required for pathogenesis of certain animal models of autoimmune disease, such as experimental autoimmune encephalomyelitis or collagen-induced arthritis.[89] Subsequent studies demonstrated that Th17 cells can play similar roles in human inflammatory diseases, such as Crohn disease or psoriasis.[81,90] Consistent with the major role that IL-23 plays in the development of Th17 cells,[75] polymorphisms in the gene encoding the IL-23 receptor influence the susceptibility to such autoimmune disorders.[91,92]

Tfh Cells

Follicular helper T cells (Tfh cells) constitute another subset of CD4+ T cells that regulates the development of antigen-specific B-cell immunity in the germinal center of secondary lymphoid follicles.[93] Tfh cells express the CXCR5 chemokine receptor, allowing these cells to home to the CXCL13-rich, B-cell zones of lymphoid follicles, where they engage antigen-specific B cells in cognate intercellular interactions. Such interactions play a critical role in B-cell differentiation into plasma cells or memory B cells in response to antigenic stimulation. In addition, Tfh cells express CD154, ICOS (for "inducible costimulator" because of its expression on activated T cells), and SAP, which allows these cells to form stable contacts with antigen-primed B cells, and can elaborate cytokines such as IL-4, IFN-γ, IL-10, and/or IL-21, which help to modify the differentiation fate of B lymphocytes (see Chap. 77). Development of Tfh cells apparently requires stimulation in the context of IL-21 and the transcription factor BCL-6 (Fig. 78–3).[94]

■ MEMORY T CELLS

Following a successful immune response to antigen, antigen-specific T lymphocytes may differentiate into memory T cells.[94,95] These cells may have less stringent requirements for activation and an enhanced capacity for lymphokine production upon rechallenge with the same antigen.[96] Alternatively, these cells may develop an impaired responsiveness to antigen when stimulated in the absence of certain costimulatory factors, thus rendering these cells "anergic."[97] In any case, naïve and memory CD4+ or CD8+ T lymphocytes apparently differ in surface phenotypes, response to recall antigens, rate of cycling, and migration.[98] These subsets may be distinguished using antibodies specific for isoforms of CD45.[99,100]

CD45, also known as leukocyte common antigen or T200, consists of a family of membrane glycoproteins, ranging from 180 to 220 kDa, that are expressed on all leukocytes. Each member is the product of a single complex gene on chromosome 1 that contains 34 exons. Exons 3 through 7 may be spliced differently at the RNA transcript level to generate several distinct messenger RNA and protein products. The deduced amino acid sequences of these protein products have extracellular domains ranging from 391 to 552 amino acids, a transmembrane region, and a highly conserved cytoplasmic domain of 705 amino acids. This large cytoplasmic domain contains an intrinsic tyrosine phosphatase activity that is important in the regulation of various activation pathways involving tyrosine kinase activity, such as those involved in signal transduction via the T-cell receptor for antigen.[101]

Differential glycosylation of the CD45 peptide backbone contributes further to the heterogeneity of the members of this family of proteins. Different isoforms of CD45 have distinct patterns of expression during lymphocyte ontogeny and activation. Monoclonal antibodies have been developed that recognize individual members of this family that are expressed on physiologically distinct lymphocyte subsets (see Chap. 15). Isoforms of CD45 that are expressed on such distinct subsets of cells are designated as CD45R.

Naïve CD4+ T cells express a form of CD45R, called CD45RA, whereas memory CD4+ T cells and CD8+ T cells express another isoform of CD45R, designated CD45RO. These isoforms can be recognized by monoclonal antibodies 2H4 and UCHL1, respectively.[102] Evaluation for the expression level of another isoform of CD45, designated CD45RB, also can be useful for distinguishing memory T cells. Within the CD4+ memory T-cell population, for example, there is an increase of helper activity associated with the shift from a $CD45RB^{bright}$ to a $CD45RB^{dim}$ phenotype.[103] In addition, relative to naïve T cells, memory T cells also express lower levels of L-selectin (CD62L) and higher levels of CD29 and CD44[104] (see Chap. 15). It is still uncertain whether the differentiation of CD4+ T cells with the "naïve" phenotype (i.e., $CD4+CD45RA+CD29^{low}CD44^{low}$) to cells having the "memory" phenotype (i.e., $CD4+CD45RO+CD29^{high}CD44^{high}$) is irreversible,[102] and whether these phenotypic changes are valid for all Th1- and Th2-type CD4+ T cells.[105]

Memory T cells also express higher levels of certain adhesion molecules, such as integrins and CD44, which facilitate homing and migration to sites of inflammation or secondary lymphoid tissues. Some memory T cells migrate preferentially to lymph nodes, where they can be activated rapidly in response to re-exposure to antigen. Other memory T cells circulate in the blood or reside in mucosal or dermal tissue, from where they can be recruited to distant or to local sites of inflammation, respectively.

T CELL ACCESSORY MOLECULES

■ IMMUNE MODULATORY MOLECULES

CD28

CD28 is a 44-kDa disulfide-linked homodimer that is expressed on most resting T cells and plasma cells (see Chap. 15). Mature thymocytes have higher levels of CD28 than the immature cells. Among peripheral T cells, more than 90 percent of CD4+ T cells and approximately 50 percent of CD8 T cells express CD28. In general, activation of T cells induces enhanced expression of CD28, but ligation of CD28 leads to its transient downregulation.[106]

CD28 is another member of the immunoglobulin superfamily that is an important receptor for CD80 and CD86. It binds to both CD80 and CD86 using a highly conserved motif (MYPPPY) in a loop that resembles the third complementarity-determining region of immunoglobulin molecules. CD28 binds to CD80 with relatively low affinity (Kd = 4 μM) and dissociates very rapidly ($K_{off} = 1.6\ s^{-1}$).[107] Its binding to CD86 may be even weaker.[108]

CD28 is one of the major costimulatory molecules that are important in T-cell activation.[109,110] CD28 may enhance signaling by the T-cell receptor complex by stabilizing and prolonging the synapse between T cells and antigen-presenting cells. More importantly, ligation of CD28 by CD80 or CD86 or by anti-CD28 antibodies activates distinct signaling pathways that function together with the signals induced by ligation of the T-cell receptor to allow for T-cell activation and proliferation.[111] Following coligation of CD28, the Src kinases Lck and Fyn may phosphorylate a tyrosine within an ITAM found in the cytoplasmic domain of CD28, allowing the latter to bind and to activate phosphatidylinositide 3-kinase via its SH2 domains.[24] CD28 signaling also facilitates GTP/GDP exchange on Ras, resulting in activation of the MAP kinase pathway, activation of Akt kinase, and activation of the adapter protein Vav, and the associated Rac pathway. These signals enhance the transcription of IL-2 and the stability of IL-2 transcripts, thereby stimulating T-cell proliferation.[112] Although mice lacking CD28 can mount effective T-cell responses, they are defective in T-cell-dependent antibody responses, suggesting that CD28 is necessary for T-cell ↔ B-cell interactions and the proficient generation of antibody responses to antigen.

The requirement for the same cell to present both the specific antigen and the costimulatory signal plays an important role in preventing destructive autoimmune responses to self-tissues.[113] The initiation of T-cell responses requires simultaneous ligation of the T-cell receptor and CD28. This restricts the initiation of T-cell responses to antigen-presenting cells that express both the peptide antigen in the context of self-MHC molecules and the ligands for CD28, namely CD80 and CD86. This is important, as not all self-reactive T cells undergo deletion in the thymus because not all self-peptides are presented in the thymus (see Chap. 5). This is especially true for specialized tissues that express proteins that are never expressed in the thymus. If simultaneous ligation of the T-cell receptor and CD28 was not required, then T cells that recognize the self-peptide expressed by the MHC of such specialized tissues could become activated, leading to autoimmune rejection of the specialized tissue. Instead, ligation of the T-cell receptor in the absence of CD28-ligation leads to a state of anergy, in which the T cell expressing that receptor becomes refractory to activation.[114] Anergic T cells are unable to produce IL-2 following ligation of their antigen receptors. This prevents these T cells from proliferating and differentiating into effector cells when they encounter antigen. This is an important basis for development of peripheral tolerance for self-antigens that are not expressed in the thymus (see Chaps. 5 and 76).

CTLA-4 (CD152)

CTLA-4 (CD152) is another receptor for CD80 and CD86. It is a 50-kDa disulfide-linked homodimer that shares 31 percent identity with CD28. The gene encoding this receptor is closely linked with that encoding CD28 on the long arm of chromosome 2 at 2q33-q34. However, in contrast to the constitutive expression of CD28, T cells other than T_{regs} express CD152 only upon activation. Expression of CD152 peaks at approximately 24 hours after activation and then subsides by 72 hours but is always approximately 30- to 50-fold lower than that of CD28. Ligation of CD28 is particularly effective in inducing CD152.

CD152 binds to both CD80 and CD86 using the same highly conserved motif (MYPPPY) used by CD28, which, like CD28, is also in a loop that resembles the third complementarity-determining region of immunoglobulin molecules. However, CD152 binds to CD80 and CD86 approximately 20 times more avidly than CD28, with a Kd of 0.4 and 2.2 μM, respectively.[107,108]

In contrast to CD28, ligation of CD152 transmits a negative signal to T-cell activation.[111] Instead of an ITAM in its cytoplasmic domain, CD152 possesses an "immunoreceptor tyrosine inhibitory motif" (ITIM). Ligation of CD152 induces tyrosine phosphorylation of the ITIM, which, in turn, recruits the tyrosine phosphatase SHP-2 that can deactivate the phosphorylated ITAMs of the ζ chains (CD247) of the T-cell receptor complex. Mice made genetically deficient in CD152 develop a fatal disorder that is characterized by massive lymphocyte proliferation, indicating that CD152 serves as an important brake on unregulated T-cell activation.[56] Moreover, anti-CD152 monoclonal antibodies that block the interaction of CD152 with CD80 and CD86 can enhance T-cell responses *in vitro* and *in vivo*, prompting their evaluation as immune-enhancing agents in vaccine studies or clinical trials in active immune therapy.

Other Members of the CD28 Receptor Family

Homology-based cloning strategies have identified other proteins that are structurally related to CD28/CTLA-4 or its ligand CD80. These proteins are considered to be members of the CD28 or CD80 (B7) families, respectively. All of these proteins are members of the larger immunoglobulin superfamily. Two other members of the CD28 family are ICOS (CD278) and PDCD1 (CD279) (for "programmed cell death-1" because this molecule initially was thought to regulate programmed cell death of T cells).[115] Whereas CD278 is found primarily on activated T cells, CD279 can be found on activated T cells, B cells, and some myeloid cells. CD278 and CD279, respectively, bind to the ICOS-ligand (ICOS-L or CD275) and the PD-ligands, PD-L1 (CD274) or PD-L2 (CD273). CD275, CD274, and CD273 belong to the CD80 (B7) family of surface molecules and are found or can be induced on B cells, antigen presenting cells, and other tissues. Whereas CD278 primarily functions as a costimulatory molecule for cells bearing CD275,[116] CD279 plays a negative regulatory role on activated T cells.[117,118] Like CD152, CD279 possesses an ITIM motif in its cytoplasmic tail that, upon phosphorylation, can recruit the tyrosine phosphatase SHP-2. In this regard, CD279 may play a role similar to that of CD152, helping to brake cellular activation when expressed in the context of cells expressing CD273 or CD274 (see Chapter 15).[119]

T-CELL ADHESION MOLECULES

DEFINITION

Besides the CD3/T-cell receptor molecules and CD4 or CD8, several other surface proteins are required for efficient T-cell antigen recognition.[120] Some of these surface proteins may be termed adhesion molecules, in that they facilitate the adhesion of the T cell to its appropriate antigen-presenting cell or target cell (Fig. 78–4).[121] By facilitating cell adhesion, these accessory molecules permit the T-cell antigen receptor complex to interact better with the MHC glycoproteins of the other cell, allowing for efficient T-cell antigen recognition and activation. Because each member of this group of accessory molecules has distinctive affinities for the surface molecules expressed by the APC or target cell, differential expression of the accessory molecules may pattern differences in the antigenic specificities and/or cell types with which a given T cell best may interact. As such, the differential expression of these accessory molecules by peripheral T cells may define physiologically distinct T-cell subsets.

LYMPHOCYTE FUNCTION-ASSOCIATED GLYCOPROTEINS

The lymphocyte function-associated (LFA) molecules are an important family of glycoproteins that facilitate efficient cell–cell adhesion.[122,123] The molecules were first identified with monoclonal antibodies that could block T-cell function, such as cytotoxic T-cell–mediated killing of target cells. From these early experiments three major surface molecules were identified and designated LFA-1, LFA-2 (CD2), and LFA-3 (CD58). Following international convention, LFA-2 will be referred to as CD2 and LFA-3 as CD58.

LFA-1 belongs to a family of three related glycoproteins: LFA-1, MAC-1 (CD11b/CD18), and gp150,95 (CD11c/CD18). These proteins also are called "integrins" because they are hypothesized to coordinate the binding of cells to other cell types and to extracellular proteins. Each protein consists of a distinct α subunit noncovalently associated with the common β_2 subunit glycoprotein of 95 kDa, designated as CD18. Because they share a common β_2 subunit, these molecules also are referred to as the β_2 integrins. The α subunit of LFA-1, designated CD11a, is a 180-kDa glycoprotein (see Chap. 15). Coupled together with the common β_2 subunit, this 180-kDa molecule is expressed on more than one-third of all marrow cells, all T cells, B cells, and natural killer cells. The α subunit of MAC-1 is a glycoprotein of 170 kDa, designated CD11b. MAC-1 is expressed on natural killer cells, monocytes, macrophages, granulocytes, and small subpopulations of T and B cells. The α subunit of p150,95, designated CD11c, is a 150-kDa glycoprotein that is not expressed by T lymphocytes.

The LFA-1 family of glycoproteins is comprised of important adhesion molecules.[122] The shared β_2 subunit (CD18) has extensive sequence homology to the β_3 subunit (CD61) of the platelet adhesion receptor glycoprotein IIb/IIIa (CD41/CD61) and the β_1 subunit (CD29) of a family of related adhesion proteins, termed very-late-activation (VLA) antigens. Many of these receptors function in cell–cell interactions and recognize their ligands at sites that contain the amino acid sequence Arg-Gly-Asp. In addition, the α subunit provides some selectivity. LFA-1, because of its α subunit, binds best to cell surface ligands called intercellular adhesion molecules (ICAMs), namely ICAM-1 (CD54), ICAM-2 (CD102), and ICAM-3 (CD50) (see Chap. 15). CD54 and CD102 are expressed on endothelial cells as well as antigen-presenting cells. The binding of LFA-1 on lymphocytes to these molecules allows lymphocytes to migrate through blood vessel walls. CD50 is expressed only on leukocytes, including T cells, and is thought to play an important role in the adhesion of T cells with LFA-1 expressed on antigen-presenting cells (see Fig. 78–4).

The LFA glycoproteins are required for proper T-cell function and host immunity. Monoclonal antibodies specific for LFA-1 may inhibit T-cell–directed cytolysis of target cells. Furthermore, a few CD8+ or CD4+ cytolytic T-cell clones express MAC-1 (CD11b/CD18). Antibodies to CD11b may inhibit conjugate formation between these T-cell clones and their specific target cells and thus block cytotoxic T-lymphocyte–mediated killing. Finally, patients with an inherited deficiency in the ability to produce the common β_2 subunit (CD18) suffer from recurrent life-threatening bacterial and fungal infections and rarely survive beyond childhood.

The LFA molecules are important for initial T-cell interactions with antigen-presenting cells. LFA-1, CD2, and CD50 on the T cell interact with CD54, CD102, LFA-1, and CD58 on the antigen-presenting cell (see Fig. 78–4). This provides time for the T cell to sample large numbers of MHC molecules on the plasma membrane of the antigen-presenting cell for the presence of specific peptide antigen. When a naïve T cell recognizes its specific peptide in the context of the MHC, signaling through the T-cell receptor induces a conformational change in LFA-1 that greatly increases its affinity for CD54 and CD102. This stabilizes the association between the antigen-specific T cell and the antigen-presenting cell. This association can last for several days during which time the naïve T cell proliferates, forming daughter cells that also adhere to the antigen-presenting cell and that differentiate into armed effector T cells.

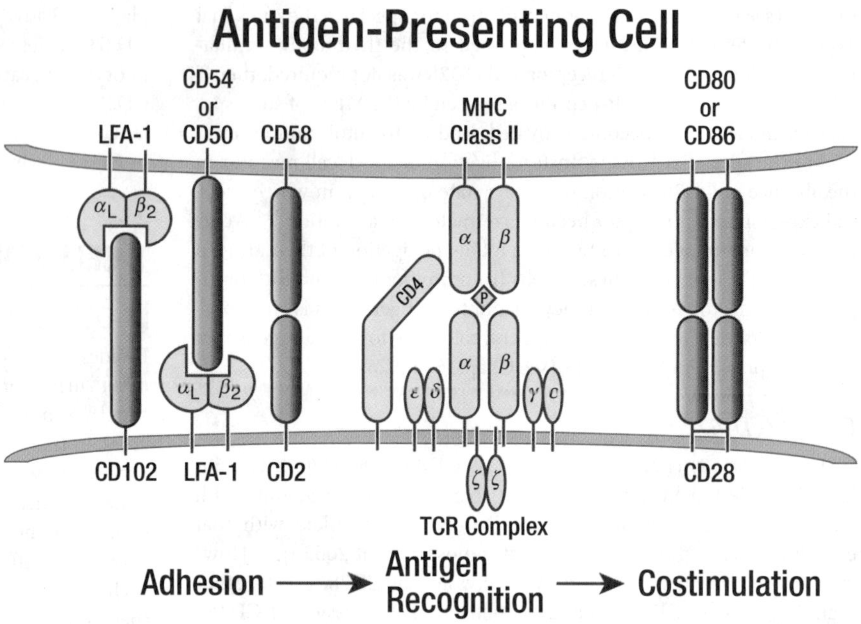

FIGURE 78–4. Schematic of a T-cell interactions with an antigen-presenting cell. The *thick green lines* depict the plasma membranes of the interacting cells. The molecules of the antigen-presenting cell, namely lymphocyte function-associated antigen (LFA)-1, intercellular adhesion molecule (ICAM)-1 or ICAM-3, LFA-3, major histocompatibility complex (MHC) class II, and CD80 or CD86, are displayed on *top*, while the T-cell antigens, ICAM-2, LFA-1, CD2, CD4, the T-cell receptor (TCR) complex, and CD28, are shown on the *bottom* of the diagram. *Thin lines* connecting the stick figures indicate disulfide bridges. The TCR complex consists of the $\alpha\beta$ heterodimer that is noncovalently coupled with the δ, ε, γ, and ζ chains of CD3, as indicated. This complex can recognize peptide antigen (designated by the *diamond labeled P*) that is cradled by the α and β chains of the MHC class II molecule of the antigen-presenting cell. The avidity of this interaction is enhanced by CD4 on the T-cell surface that interacts with nonpolymorphic determinants on the MHC class II molecule. The interaction steps between the T cell and the antigen-presenting cell are listed at the *bottom* of the figure. T-cell molecules ICAM-2 (CD102), LFA-1 (CD11a/CD18), and CD2 bind to LFA-1, ICAM-1 (CD54) or ICAM-3 (CD50), and LFA-3 (CD58), respectively, that are present on the surface of the antigen-presenting cell. These molecules provide for better adhesion between the T cell and the antigen-presenting cell (adhesion), allowing for time for the TCR complex to find the MHC molecule bearing a specific peptide antigen (antigen recognition). Should the antigen-presenting cell express CD80 or CD86, then simultaneous ligation of CD28 will occur (costimulation), leading to activation of the reactive T cell.

VERY-LATE-ACTIVATION ANTIGENS

The VLA molecules are β_1 integrins in that each share a common β_1 unit (CD29) that is paired with any one of six different α chains (α_1 to α_6), designated CD49a-f (see Chap. 15). CD49a, CD49b, CD49c, CD49d, CD49e, and CD49f form molecules called VLA-1, VLA-2, VLA-3, VLA-4, VLA-5, or VLA-6, respectively, when paired with CD29. These molecules are called VLA for "very-late antigens" because the first identified VLA molecules, namely VLA-1 and VLA-2, initially were found on T cells only weeks after repetitive stimulation *in vitro*. However, some of these VLA molecules, most notably VLA-4, are also expressed constitutively by some T cells and are rapidly induced on others. VLA-4 plays an important role in facilitating the attachment of cells that bear this molecule to the endothelium through its binding to vascular cell adhesion molecule-1 (VCAM-1), designated CD106 (see Chap. 15). CD106 can be upregulated by various proinflammatory cytokines. Upregulation of CD106 allows VLA-4 to play an important role in facilitating the homing of T cells to endothelium at sites of inflammation.

CD2

CD2 is a glycoprotein of approximately 50 kDa found on all T lymphocytes, large granular lymphocytes, and thymocytes.[124] CD2 facilitates cell–cell adhesion by binding to CD58, a 55- to 70-kDa surface glycoprotein that is expressed on erythrocytes and leukocytes as well as on endothelial, epithelial, and connective tissue cells in most organ studies (see Fig. 78–4; see Chap. 15). Monoclonal antibodies that bind CD2 may inhibit a variety of T-lymphocyte functions, including antigen-specific T-lymphocyte proliferative responses to lectins, alloantigens, and soluble antigens. Anti-CD2 inhibits cytotoxic T-lymphocyte–mediated cell killing by binding to the T cell rather than to the target, which generally does not express CD2. On the other hand, antibodies directed against CD58 inhibit cytotoxic T-lymphocyte–mediated cell killing by binding to CD58 on the target cell, thus blocking interaction of CD2 with CD58. T cells can be activated by certain monoclonal antibodies to CD2, apparently independent of the CD3/T-cell receptor complex.[125] Thus, aside from being a receptor for CD58, CD2 also plays a role in transmembrane signal transduction leading to T-cell activation in response to antigen.

REFERENCES

1. Garcia KC, Teyton L, Wilson IA: Structural basis of T cell recognition. *Annu Rev Immunol* 17:369, 1999.
2. O'Brien RL, Roark CL, Jin N, et al: Gammadelta T-cell receptors: Functional correlations. *Immunol Rev* 215:77, 2007.
3. Xiong N, Raulet DH: Development and selection of gammadelta T cells. *Immunol Rev* 215:15, 2007.
4. Chien YH, Konigshofer Y: Antigen recognition by gammadelta T cells. *Immunol Rev* 215:46, 2007.
5. Hayes SM, Love PE: A retrospective on the requirements for gammadelta T-cell development. *Immunol Rev* 215:8, 2007.
6. Rockman SP: Determination of clonality in patients who present with diagnostic dilemmas: A laboratory experience and review of the literature. *Leukemia* 11:852, 1997.
7. Dibenedetto SP, Lo Nigro L, Di Cataldo A, Schilirò G: Detection of minimal residual disease: Methods and relationship to outcome in T-lineage acute lymphoblastic leukemia. *Leuk Lymphoma* 32:65, 1998.
8. Housset D, Malissen B: What do TCR-pMHC crystal structures teach us about MHC restriction and alloreactivity? *Trends Immunol* 24:429, 2003.
9. Marchalonis JJ, Jensen I, Schluter SF: Structural, antigenic and evolutionary analyses of immunoglobulins and T cell receptors. *J Mol Recognit* 15:260, 2002.
10. Whitelegg A, Barber LD: The structural basis of T-cell allorecognition. *Tissue Antigens* 63:101, 2004.
11. Barral DC, Brenner MB: CD1 antigen presentation: How it works. *Nat Rev Immunol* 7:929, 2007.
12. Cohen NR, Garg S, Brenner MB: Antigen presentation by CD1 lipids, T cells, and NKT cells in microbial immunity. *Adv Immunol* 102:1, 2009.
13. Thedrez A, Sabourin C, Gertner J, et al: Self/non-self discrimination by human gammadelta T cells: Simple solutions for a complex issue? *Immunol Rev* 215:123, 2007.
14. Cui Y, Cui L, He W: Unraveling the mystery of gammadelta T cell recognizing lipid A. *Cell Mol Immunol* 2:359, 2005.
15. Nanno M, Shiohara T, Yamamoto H, et al: Gammadelta T cells: Firefighters or fire boosters in the front lines of inflammatory responses. *Immunol Rev* 215:103, 2007.
16. Theofilopoulos AN, Baccalà R, González-Quintial R, et al: T-cell repertoires in health and disease. *Ann N Y Acad Sci* 756:53, 1995.
17. Call ME, Wucherpfennig KW: Molecular mechanisms for the assembly of the T cell receptor-CD3 complex. *Mol Immunol* 40:1295, 2004.
18. Peterson EJ, Koretzky GA: Signal transduction in T lymphocytes. *Clin Exp Rheumatol* 17:107, 1999.
19. Guirado M, de Aos I, Orta T, et al: Phosphorylation of the N-terminal and C-terminal CD3-epsilon-ITAM tyrosines is differentially regulated in T cells. *Biochem Biophys Res Commun* 291:574, 2002.
20. Qian D, Weiss A: T cell antigen receptor signal transduction. *Curr Opin Cell Biol* 9:205, 1997.
21. Sommers CL, Samelson LE, Love PE: LAT: A T lymphocyte adapter protein that couples the antigen receptor to downstream signaling pathways. *Bioessays* 26:61, 2004.
22. Saito T, Yamasaki S: Negative feedback of T cell activation through inhibitory adapters and costimulatory receptors. *Immunol Rev* 192:143, 2003.
23. Gudkov AV, Zelnick CR, Kazarov AR, et al: Isolation of genetic suppressor elements, inducing resistance to topoisomerase II-interactive cytotoxic drugs, from human topoisomerase II cDNA. *Proc Natl Acad Sci U S A* 90:3231, 1993.
24. Kane LP, Weiss A: The PI-3 kinase/Akt pathway and T cell activation: Pleiotropic pathways downstream of PIP3. *Immunol Rev* 192:7, 2003.
25. Zamoyska R: CD4 and CD8: Modulators of T-cell receptor recognition of antigen and of immune responses? *Curr Opin Immunol* 10:82, 1998.
26. Gao GF, Jakobsen BK: Molecular interactions of coreceptor CD8 and MHC class I: The molecular basis for functional coordination with the T-cell receptor. *Immunol Today* 21:630, 2000.
27. Reinherz EL, Tan K, Tang L, et al: The crystal structure of a T cell receptor in complex with peptide and MHC class II. *Science* 286:1913, 1999.
28. Janeway CAJ: The co-receptor function of CD4. *Semin Immunol* 3:153, 1991.
29. Reith W, Mach B: The bare lymphocyte syndrome and the regulation of MHC expression. *Annu Rev Immunol* 19:331, 2001.
30. Miceli MC, Parnes JR: Role of CD4 and CD8 in T cell activation and differentiation. *Adv Immunol* 53:59, 1993.
31. Virelizier JL: Blocking HIV co-receptors by chemokines. *Dev Biol Stand* 97:105, 1999.
32. Berger EA, Murphy PM, Farber JM: Chemokine receptors as HIV-1 coreceptors: Roles in viral entry, tropism, and disease. *Annu Rev Immunol* 17:657, 1999.
33. Abbas AK, Murphy KM, Sher A: Functional diversity of helper T lymphocytes. *Nature* 383:787, 1996.
34. Annunziato F, Galli G, Cosmi L, et al: Molecules associated with human Th1 or Th2 cells. *Eur Cytokine Netw* 9:12, 1998.
35. Huard B, Mastrangeli R, Prigent P, et al: Characterization of the major histocompatibility complex class II binding site on LAG-3 protein. *Proc Natl Acad Sci U S A* 94:5744, 1997.
36. Zingoni A, Soto H, Hedrick JA, et al: The chemokine receptor CCR8 is preferentially expressed in Th2 but not Th1 cells. *J Immunol* 161:547, 1998.
37. Kim CH, Broxmeyer HE: Chemokines: Signal lamps for trafficking of T and B cells for development and effector function. *J Leukoc Biol* 65:6, 1999.
38. O'Garra A, McEvoy LM, Zlotnik A: T-cell subsets: Chemokine receptors guide the way. *Curr Biol* 8:R646–649, 1998.
39. Fields PE, Kim ST, Flavell RA: Cutting edge: Changes in histone acetylation at the IL-4 and IFN-gamma loci accompany Th1/Th2 differentiation. *J Immunol* 169:647, 2002.
40. Nishikomori R, Usui T, Wu CY, et al: Activated STAT4 has an essential role in Th1 differentiation and proliferation that is independent of its role in the maintenance of IL-12R beta 2 chain expression and signaling. *J Immunol* 169:4388, 2002.
41. O'Garra A, Robinson D: Development and function of T helper 1 cells. *Adv Immunol* 83:133, 2004.
42. Rao A, Avni O: Molecular aspects of T-cell differentiation. *Br Med Bull* 56:969, 2000.
43. Zhou M, Ouyang W: The function role of GATA-3 in Th1 and Th2 differentiation. *Immunol Res* 28:25, 2003.
44. Lucey DR: Evolution of the type-1 (Th1)-type-2 (Th2) cytokine paradigm. *Infect Dis Clin North Am* 13:1, v, 1999.
45. Lebre MC, Burwell T, Vieira PL, et al: Differential expression of inflammatory chemokines by Th1- and Th2-cell promoting dendritic cells: A role for different mature dendritic cell populations in attracting appropriate effector cells to peripheral sites of inflammation. *Immunol Cell Biol* 83:525, 2005.
46. Del Prete G: Human Th1 and Th2 lymphocytes: Their role in the pathophysiology of atopy. *Allergy* 47:450, 1992.
47. van Reijsen FC, Bruijnzeel-Koomen CA, Kalthoff FS, et al: Skin-derived aeroallergen-specific T-cell clones of Th2 phenotype in patients with atopic dermatitis. *J Allergy Clin Immunol* 90:184, 1992.
48. Sher A, Coffman RL: Regulation of immunity to parasites by T cells and T cell-derived cytokines. *Annu Rev Immunol* 10:385, 1992.
49. King CL, Nutman TB: Biological role of helper T-cell subsets in helminth infections. *Chem Immunol* 54:136, 1992.
50. Vella AT, Pearce EJ: CD4+ Th2 response induced by Schistosoma mansoni eggs develops rapidly, through an early, transient, Th0-like stage. *J Immunol* 148:2283, 1992.
51. Contigli C, Silva-Teixeira DN, Del Prete G, et al: Phenotype and cytokine profile of Schistosoma mansoni specific T cell lines and clones derived from schistosomiasis patients with distinct clinical forms. *Clin Immunol* 91:338, 1999.
52. Constant SL, Bottomly K: Induction of Th1 and Th2 CD4+ T cell responses: The alternative approaches. *Annu Rev Immunol* 15:297, 1997.
53. Stetson DB, Voehringer D, Grogan JL, et al: Th2 cells: Orchestrating barrier immunity. *Adv Immunol* 83:163, 2004.
54. Lahesmaa R, Yssel H, Batsford S, et al: *Yersinia enterocolitica* activates a T helper type 1-like T cell subset in reactive arthritis. *J Immunol* 148:3079, 1992.
55. Shevach EM: Mechanisms of foxp3+ T regulatory cell-mediated suppression. *Immunity* 30:636, 2009.
56. Bour-Jordan H, Bluestone JA: Regulating the regulators: Costimulatory signals control the homeostasis and function of regulatory T cells. *Immunol Rev* 229:41, 2009.
57. Walker LS: CD4+ CD25+ Treg: Divide and rule? *Immunology* 111:129, 2004.
58. Gavin MA, Rasmussen JP, Fontenot JD, et al: Foxp3-dependent programme of regulatory T-cell differentiation. *Nature* 445:771, 2007.
59. Zheng Y, Josefowicz SZ, Kas A, et al: Genome-wide analysis of Foxp3 target genes in developing and mature regulatory T cells. *Nature* 445:936, 2007.
60. Ochs HD, Gambineri E, Torgerson TR: IPEX, FOXP3 and regulatory T-cells: A model for autoimmunity. *Immunol Res* 38:112, 2007.
61. Curotto de Lafaille MA, Lafaille JJ: CD4(+) regulatory T cells in autoimmunity and allergy. *Curr Opin Immunol* 14:771, 2002.
62. Stassen M, Schmitt E, Jonuleit H: Human CD(4+)CD(25+) regulatory T cells and infectious tolerance. *Transplantation* 77:S23–25, 2004.
63. Collison LW, Workman CJ, Kuo TT, et al: The inhibitory cytokine IL-35 contributes to regulatory T-cell function. *Nature* 450:566, 2007.
64. Garin MI, Chu CC, Golshayan D, et al: Galectin-1: A key effector of regulation mediated by CD4+CD25+ T cells. *Blood* 109:2058, 2007.
65. Shevach EM, Stephens GL: The GITR-GITRL interaction: Co-stimulation or contrasuppression of regulatory activity? *Nat Rev Immunol* 6:613, 2006.
66. Curotto de Lafaille MA, Lafaille JJ: Natural and adaptive foxp3+ regulatory T cells: More of the same or a division of labor? *Immunity* 30:626, 2009.
67. Mathis D, Benoist C: Aire. *Annu Rev Immunol* 27:287, 2009.
68. Coombes JL, Siddiqui KR, Arancibia-Carcamo CV, et al: A functionally specialized population of mucosal CD103+ DCs induces Foxp3+ regulatory T cells via a TGF-beta and retinoic acid-dependent mechanism. *J Exp Med* 204:1757, 2007.
69. Curotto de Lafaille MA, Kutchukhidze N, Shen S, et al: Adaptive Foxp3+ regulatory T cell-dependent and -independent control of allergic inflammation. *Immunity* 29:114, 2008.
70. Liu VC, Wong LY, Jang T, et al: Tumor evasion of the immune system by converting CD4+CD25- T cells into CD4+CD25+ T regulatory cells: Role of tumor-derived TGF-beta. *J Immunol* 178:2883, 2007.
71. Cobbold SP, Castejon R, Adams E, et al: Induction of foxP3+ regulatory T cells in the periphery of T cell receptor transgenic mice tolerized to transplants. *J Immunol* 172:6003, 2004.
72. Ochs HD, Oukka M, Torgerson TR: TH17 cells and regulatory T cells in primary immunodeficiency diseases. *J Allergy Clin Immunol* 123:977; quiz 984, 2009.
73. Liu Y, Zhang P, Li J, et al: A critical function for TGF-beta signaling in the development of natural CD4+CD25+Foxp3+ regulatory T cells. *Nat Immunol* 9:632, 2008.
74. Korn T, Bettelli E, Oukka M, Kuchroo VK: IL-17 and Th17 Cells. *Annu Rev Immunol* 27:485, 2009.

75. McGeachy MJ, Chen Y, Tato CM, et al: The interleukin 23 receptor is essential for the terminal differentiation of interleukin 17-producing effector T helper cells *in vivo*. *Nat Immunol* 10:314, 2009.
76. Boniface K, Bak-Jensen KS, Li Y, et al: Prostaglandin E2 regulates Th17 cell differentiation and function through cyclic AMP and EP2/EP4 receptor signaling. *J Exp Med* 206:535, 2009.
77. Ivanov, II, McKenzie BS, Zhou L, et al: The orphan nuclear receptor RORgammat directs the differentiation program of proinflammatory IL-17+ T helper cells. *Cell* 126:1121, 2006.
78. Laurence A, O'Shea JJ: T(H)-17 differentiation: Of mice and men. *Nat Immunol* 8:903, 2007.
79. Bettelli E, Carrier Y, Gao W, et al: Reciprocal developmental pathways for the generation of pathogenic effector TH17 and regulatory T cells. *Nature* 441:235, 2006.
80. Mangan PR, Harrington LE, O'Quinn DB, et al: Transforming growth factor-beta induces development of the T(H)17 lineage. *Nature* 441:231, 2006.
81. Annunziato F, Cosmi L, Santarlasci V, et al: Phenotypic and functional features of human Th17 cells. *J Exp Med* 204:1849, 2007
82. Kryczek I, Banerjee M, Cheng P, et al: Phenotype, distribution, generation, and functional and clinical relevance of Th17 cells in the human tumor environments. *Blood* 114:1141, 2009.
83. Harrington LE, Hatton RD, Mangan PR, et al: Interleukin 17-producing CD4+ effector T cells develop via a lineage distinct from the T helper type 1 and 2 lineages. *Nat Immunol* 6:1123, 2005.
84. Iwakura Y, Nakae S, Saijo S, Ishigame H: The roles of IL-17A in inflammatory immune responses and host defense against pathogens. *Immunol Rev* 226:57, 2008.
85. Gaffen SL: An overview of IL-17 function and signaling. *Cytokine* 43:402, 2008.
86. Milner JD, Brenchley JM, Laurence A, et al: Impaired T(H)17 cell differentiation in subjects with autosomal dominant hyper-IgE syndrome. *Nature* 452:773, 2008.
87. Ma CS, Chew GY, Simpson N, et al: Deficiency of Th17 cells in hyper IgE syndrome due to mutations in STAT3. *J Exp Med* 205:1551, 2008.
88. DuPont HL, Garey K, Caeiro JP, Jiang ZD: New advances in Clostridium difficile infection: Changing epidemiology, diagnosis, treatment and control. *Curr Opin Infect Dis* 21:500, 2008.
89. Langrish CL, Chen Y, Blumenschein WM, et al: IL-23 drives a pathogenic T cell population that induces autoimmune inflammation. *J Exp Med* 201:233, 2005.
90. Wilson NJ, Boniface K, Chan JR, et al: Development, cytokine profile and function of human interleukin 17-producing helper T cells. *Nat Immunol* 8:950, 2007.
91. Duerr RH, Taylor KD, Brant SR, et al: A genome-wide association study identifies IL23R as an inflammatory bowel disease gene. *Science* 314:1461, 2006.
92. Smith RL, Warren RB, Griffiths CE, Worthington J: Genetic susceptibility to psoriasis: An emerging picture. *Genome Med* 1:72, 2009.
93. Fazilleau N, Mark L, McHeyzer-Williams LJ, McHeyzer-Williams MG: Follicular helper T cells: Lineage and location. *Immunity* 30:324, 2009.
94. Sallusto F, Lanzavecchia A: Heterogeneity of CD4(+) memory T cells: Functional modules for tailored immunity. *Eur J Immunol* 39:2076, 2009.
95. Tanchot C, Rocha B: The organization of mature T-cell pools. *Immunol Today* 19:575, 1998.
96. Carter LL, Zhang X, Dubey C, et al: Regulation of T cell subsets from naive to memory. *J Immunother* 21:181, 1998.
97. Jenkins MK, Miller RA: Memory and anergy: Challenges to traditional models of T lymphocyte differentiation. *FASEB J* 6:2428, 1992.
98. McHeyzer-Williams MG, Altman JD, Davis MM: Enumeration and characterization of memory cells in the TH compartment. *Immunol Rev* 150:5, 1996.
99. Plebanski M, Saunders M, Burtles SS, et al: Primary and secondary human in vitro T-cell responses to soluble antigens are mediated by subsets bearing different CD45 isoforms. *Immunology* 75:86, 1992.
100. Mason D: Subsets of CD4+ T cells defined by their expression of different isoforms of the leucocyte-common antigen, CD45. *Biochem Soc Trans* 20:188, 1992.
101. Koretzky GA: Role of the CD45 tyrosine phosphatase in signal transduction in the immune system. *FASEB J* 7:420, 1993.
102. Beverley P: Immunological memory in T cells. *Curr Opin Immunol* 3:355, 1991.
103. Tortorella C, Schulze-Koops H, Thomas R, et al: Expression of CD45RB and CD27 identifies subsets of CD4+ memory T cells with different capacities to induce B cell differentiation. *J Immunol* 155:149, 1995.
104. Sprent J, Tough DF, Sun S: Factors controlling the turnover of T memory cells. *Immunol Rev* 156:79, 1997.
105. Lee WT, Vitetta ES: Changes in expression of CD45R during the development of Th1 and Th2 cell lines. *Eur J Immunol* 22:1455, 1992.
106. Lenschow DJ, Walunas TL, Bluestone JA: CD28/B7 system of T cell costimulation. *Annu Rev Immunol* 14:233, 1996.
107. van der Merwe PA, Bodian DL, Daenke S, et al: CD80 (B7–1) binds both CD28 and CTLA-4 with a low affinity and very fast kinetics. *J Exp Med* 185:393, 1997.
108. Greene JL, Leytze GM, Emswiler J, et al: Covalent dimerization of CD28/CTLA-4 and oligomerization of CD80/CD86 regulate T cell costimulatory interactions. *J Biol Chem* 271:26762, 1996.
109. Yokosuka T, Saito T: Dynamic regulation of T-cell costimulation through TCR-CD28 microclusters. *Immunol Rev* 229:27, 2009.
110. Sharpe AH: Mechanisms of costimulation. *Immunol Rev* 229:5, 2009.
111. Rudd CE, Taylor A, Schneider H: CD28 and CTLA-4 coreceptor expression and signal transduction. *Immunol Rev* 229:12, 2009.
112. Powell JD, Ragheb JA, Kitagawa-Sakakida S, Schwartz RH: Molecular regulation of interleukin-2 expression by CD28 co-stimulation and anergy. *Immunol Rev* 165:287, 1998.
113. Malvey EN, Telander DG, Vanasek TL, Mueller DL: The role of clonal anergy in the avoidance of autoimmunity: Inactivation of autocrine growth without loss of effector function. *Immunol Rev* 165:301, 1998.
114. Appleman LJ, Boussiotis VA: T cell anergy and costimulation. *Immunol Rev* 192:161, 2003.
115. Dong C, Nurieva RI, Prasad DV: Immune regulation by novel costimulatory molecules. *Immunol Res* 28:39, 2003.
116. Yong PF, Salzer U, Grimbacher B: The role of costimulation in antibody deficiencies: ICOS and common variable immunodeficiency. *Immunol Rev* 229:101, 2009.
117. Riley JL: PD-1 signaling in primary T cells. *Immunol Rev* 229:114, 2009.
118. Kaufmann DE, Walker BD: PD-1 and CTLA-4 inhibitory cosignaling pathways in HIV infection and the potential for therapeutic intervention. *J Immunol* 182:5891, 2009.
119. Keir ME, Butte MJ, Freeman GJ, Sharpe AH: PD-1 and its ligands in tolerance and immunity. *Annu Rev Immunol* 26:677, 2008.
120. van Seventer GA, Semnani RT, Palmer EM, et al: Integrins and T helper cell activation [see comments]. *Transplant Proc* 30:4270, 1998.
121. Wang J, Springer TA: Structural specializations of immunoglobulin superfamily members for adhesion to integrins and viruses. *Immunol Rev* 163:197, 1998.
122. Springer TA: Traffic signals for lymphocyte recirculation and leukocyte emigration: The multistep paradigm. *Cell* 76:301, 1994.
123. de Fougerolles A, Springer TA: Ideas crystallized on immunoglobulin superfamily-integrin interactions. *Chem Biol* 2:639, 1995.
124. Davis SJ, Ikemizu S, Wild MK, van der Merwe PA: CD2 and the nature of protein interactions mediating cell-cell recognition. *Immunol Rev* 163:217, 1998.
125. Holter W, Schwarz M, Cerwenka A, Knapp W: The role of CD2 as a regulator of human T-cell cytokine production. *Immunol Rev* 153:107, 1996.
126. Campbell DJ, Ziegler SF: FOXP3 modifies the phenotypic and functional properties of regulatory T cells. *Nat Rev Immunol* 7:305, 2007.
127. Zhou L, Chong MM, Littman DR: Plasticity of CD4+ T cell lineage differentiation. *Immunity* 30:646, 2009.

CHAPTER 79

FUNCTIONS OF NATURAL KILLER CELLS

Giorgio Trinchieri and Lewis L. Lanier

SUMMARY

Natural killer (NK) cells, with a predominant morphology of large granular lymphocytes, represent a third lineage of lymphoid cells with constitutive ability to mediate cytotoxicity of pathologic target cells and secrete cytokines. NK cells participate in the innate resistance to intracellular pathogens and malignancies and have a modulatory effect on adaptive immunity and hematopoiesis. NK cell activity is regulated by the opposite effects of activating and inhibitory receptors. Malignant expansions of NK cells, either acute or chronic, are rare but represent well-identified clinical entities.

IDENTIFICATION AND DEFINITION OF NATURAL KILLER CELLS

DEFINITION

Natural killer (NK) cells originally were identified in the blood and other lymphoid organs of humans and experimental animals as cells capable of killing a variety of cell types, including tumor-derived cell lines, virus-infected cells, and, in some instances, normal cells in the absence of previous deliberate or known sensitization.[1,2] NK cells are defined as cytotoxic cells with the predominant morphology of large granular lymphocytes (LGLs) that (1) neither productively rearrange any of the genes encoding the T-cell antigen receptor (TCR) chains nor express on their surface the CD3 antigen complex or any TCR chain; (2) express on the majority of cells the CD16 (FcγRIIIA), CD335 (NKp46), and CD56 (NCAM) antigens in humans (see Chap. 15, Table 15–1), the NK1.1 (NKR-P1C), NKp46 (Ly94), and DX5 (VLA-2/CD49d) antigens in the mouse, and the NKR-P1 antigen in the rat; (3) mediate cytolytic reactions even in the absence of major histocompatibility complex (MHC) class I or class II antigen expression on the target cells. Target cell recognition by NK cells is clearly distinct from cytotoxic T lymphocytes (CTLs), which recognize specific antigenic peptides in association with MHC class I molecules. Cytotoxicity mediated by NK cells often is defined as non-MHC requiring, distinguishing it from the MHC-restricted cytotoxicity mediated by CTL. Nonetheless, the presence of MHC class I on target cells can affect NK cell recognition, in some cases inhibiting an NK cell response against cells expressing MHC class I. Certain T lymphocytes that express either an $\alpha\beta$ or a $\gamma\delta$ TCR may exhibit, particularly upon activation, TCR-independent cytolytic activity that resembles that of NK cells. Among the T lymphocytes displaying NK-like cytotoxicity or non–MHC-requiring cytotoxicity, NK T cells are a subset of cytotoxic T cells expressing in the mouse NK1.1 and with a restricted $\alpha\beta$ TCR diversity. The majority of NK T cells recognize glycolipids presented by CD1d, a nonclassical MHC molecule, and upon stimulation rapidly produce large amounts of interferon (IFN)-γ, granulocyte-macrophage colony stimulating factor (GM-CSF), interleukin (IL)-4, and IL-13.[3]

Acronyms and abbreviations that appear in this chapter include: CTL, cytotoxic T lymphocyte; GM-CSF, granulocyte-macrophage colony-stimulating factor; HLA, human leukocyte antigen; IFN, interferon; Ig, immunoglobulin; IL, interleukin; ITAM, immunoreceptor tyrosine-based activation motif; ITIM, immunoreceptor tyrosine-based inhibitory motif; KIR, killer cell immunoglobulin-like receptor; LCMV, lymphocytic choriomeningitis virus; LGL, large granular lymphocyte; M-CSF, macrophage colony-stimulating factor; MHC, major histocompatibility complex; NK, natural killer; NKG2, killer cell lectin-like receptor family; R, receptor; Syk, spleen tyrosine kinase; TCR, T-cell antigen receptor; TNF, tumor necrosis factor; YIMN, tyrosine-containing motif.

MORPHOLOGY

Human LGLs are medium- to large-size lymphocytes with round or indented nuclei, condensed chromatin, and usually prominent nucleoli (see Chap 96, Fig. 96–1). The cytoplasm is abundant and contains a variety of organelles. Circular membrane-bound granules (primary lysosomes), which are characteristic of these cells, range in diameter from 50 to 800 nm and contain an electron-dense core (internum) surrounded by a layer of lesser opacity (externum). In addition to lysosomal enzymes, the granules contain phospholipids, proteoglycans, and proteins important for cytotoxic lymphocyte function, such as serine esterases (granzymes) and pore-forming proteins (perforin).[4] Although many NK cells have the morphology typical of LGLs, a significant proportion of NK cells are indistinguishable from other lymphocytes and may even be agranular.[5]

ORIGIN AND TISSUE DISTRIBUTION

NK cells originate in the marrow from the common lymphoid progenitor cell that gives rise to T, B, and NK cells, and some dendritic cells.[6] Most are relatively short-lived, with calculated life spans ranging from a few days to a few weeks,[7] although studies in mice demonstrate that some NK cells may persist for months after exposure to viral challenge.[8] The cytokine IL-15 bound to IL-15Rα on accessory cells and its receptor chains CD122 (IL-2Rβ) and CD132 (common γ chain) on NK cell precursors play a particularly important role in the differentiation and expansion of NK cells.[9,10] NK cell differentiation does not require the presence of the thymus, although NK cell progenitors can be demonstrated in the thymus, particularly during fetal development. Also a new pathway of NK cell differentiation in the thymus from an NK precursor expressing the CD127 (IL-7Rα) antigen has been described.[6] Recent evidence suggests that secondary lymphoid tissues may also be a site of NK cell development in humans.[9] The increased number of NK cells and altered anatomical distribution in response to infection or other stimuli are primarily the result of increased NK cell production in the marrow and possibly proliferation of immature or mature peripheral NK cells.[11,12]

Mature NK cells are present in blood, where they represent approximately 5 to 15 percent of lymphocytes (but with large individual variations).[13] Most blood NK cells express low amounts of CD56 and high amounts of CD16, have high cytotoxic activity, and are able to produce cytokines. A few NK cells, however, express high amounts of CD56, lack CD16, and have low cytotoxic activity.[9] NK cells are present in the red pulp of the spleen and are found at a very low frequency in other lymphoid organs.[2] NK cells have been detected in lymph nodes.[14] These NK cells display an antigenic phenotype distinct from most NK cells in blood and resemble the CD56 high subset.[14] In the marrow, mature NK cells represent less than 1 percent of the cells, indicating that a pool of preformed NK cells is not sequestered in the marrow. Small numbers of NK cells can be identified in the liver (pit cells), lung, and intestinal mucosa.[15,16] Upon activation, for example, in response to interferon or viral or bacterial infections, NK cells may accumulate in organs in which they normally are rare, particularly the liver, marrow, and lymph nodes where they may produce large amounts of pro-inflammatory and immunomodulatory cytokines.[12] Cells with characteristics of activated CD56^{bright} CD16− NK cells (decidual granulocytes) with low cytotoxic activity and ability to produce cytokines, chemokines, and proangiogenic factors represent the predominant cell type present in the human early pregnancy decidua.[17] The physiologic significance of these cells in the decidua is not clear, but they have tissue remodeling capacity and play a role in facilitating embryonic implantation, allowing placenta and embryo growth, monitoring mucosal integrity throughout the menstrual cycle, controlling trophoblast invasion during pregnancy, and modulating the maternal immune response against embryo antigens.[17]

MECHANISMS OF NK CELL FUNCTIONS

CELL-MEDIATED CYTOTOXICITY

Cytotoxicity mediated by NK cells depends on binding to the target cells, followed by activation of the lytic mechanism, which usually involves secretion of the granules, including molecules with lytic ability, such as the pore-forming protein perforin and granzymes.[4] In some cases, cytotoxicity also is mediated through the interaction of surface molecules, for example, the interaction of Fas ligand, membrane tumor necrosis factor alpha (TNF), or TNF-related apoptosis-inducing ligand (TRAIL or CD253) on NK cells with their death-inducing receptors on target cells. Lysis of the target cells results from alteration of membrane permeability and induction of apoptosis.[4]

The initial interaction between an NK cell and a potential target requires cell-to-cell contact, which often involves CD11a/CD18 (LFA-1) on the NK cell interacting with an intercellular adhesion molecule (ICAM; CD54, CD102, CD50, CD242, and/or ICAM-5) on the target cell. Several surface molecules on NK cells have been identified that, when stimulated, activate the cytotoxic mechanism and induce cytokine secretion (Fig. 79–1).[18] One of these molecules is the low-affinity receptor for the Fc fragment of immunoglobulin (Ig) G (FcγIIIA or CD16), which is expressed on most human NK cells in association with the signal-transducing CD247 (CD3ζ) or FcεRIγ chains. When CD16 is crosslinked by IgG antibodies bound to a target cell surface, it triggers antibody-dependent cell-mediated cytotoxicity.[19] CD16 is not required, in the absence of antibodies, for NK cell-mediated cytotoxicity.[18] In the case of "natural killing," this process can be accomplished using several different receptors, depending upon the presence of a relevant ligand on the potential target cell. CD314 (NKG2D), a receptor expressed on all NK cells, has been implicated in NK cell recognition of transformed and virus-infected cells.[20] This receptor recognizes a family of MHC class I-related glycoproteins (including MICA, MICB, ULBP1, ULBP2, ULBP3, ULBP4, and RAET1E-1), which are absent or expressed at only low levels on healthy cells but are induced or upregulated upon cell transformation or viral infection.[21]

Some tumors secrete soluble forms of these CD314 (NKG2D) ligands, which serve as a decoy to avoid NK cell attack.[22] Certain viruses, such as cytomegalovirus, have devised strategies to prevent the expression of CD314 (NKG2D) ligands in the infected cells,[23] presumably to escape NK cell-mediated immunity. NK cells express many other activating receptors that have been implicated in their recognition of tumors, including CD226 (DNAM-1)[24] and the "natural cytotoxicity" receptors CD337 (NKp30), CD336 (NKp44), and CD335 (NKp46).[25] Ligands for these "natural cytotoxicity" receptors have not been identified.

Based on the observation that NK cells preferentially kill certain tumor cells lacking expression of MHC class I molecules, NK cells may detect and eliminate autologous cells lacking MHC class I.[26] NK cells may be regulated by positive signals initiated by activating receptors and negative signals transmitted by interactions between inhibitory receptors for MHC class I on the NK cells and autologous MHC class I molecules on potential target cells. A mechanism for immune surveillance against cells that lose expression of MHC class I would be advantageous because, in the absence of class I, these abnormal cells would escape elimination by CTL. Numerous viruses inhibit the synthesis or transport of MHC class I proteins, presumably to avoid detection by CTLs.[27] In addition, frequent loss of MHC class I expression on tumor cells has been documented.[28] However, NK cells are capable of killing cells expressing MHC class I if they received sufficiently strong activation signals.

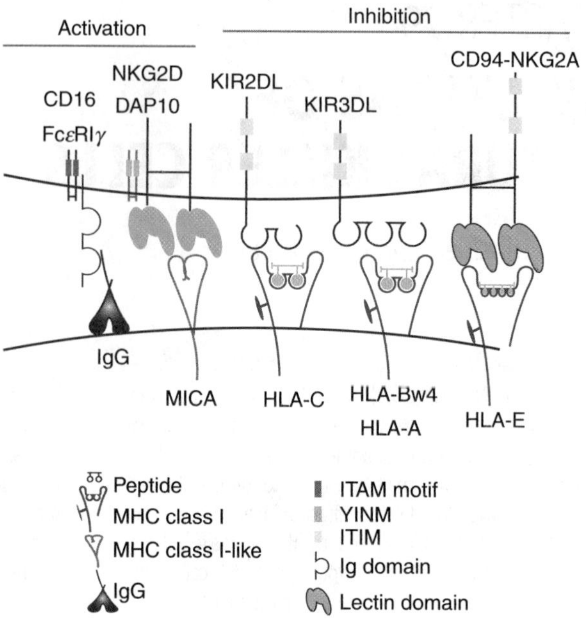

FIGURE 79–1. Schematic of selected inhibitory and activating NK cell receptors regulating NK cell responses.

Two families of NK cell receptors for MHC class I have been identified in humans. The killer cell immunoglobulin-like receptors (KIRs; CD158) are encoded by approximately 15 genes present on human chromosome 19q13.4 (see Chap. 15, Table 15–1).[29] *KIR* genes are polymorphic and appear to be evolving rapidly and diversifying by gene duplication and conversion events. Certain KIRs (CD158) bind human leukocyte antigen (HLA)-C ligands, whereas other KIRs recognize certain alleles of HLA-B or HLA-A. Another class of NK cell receptors for MHC class I are heterodimeric glycoproteins composed of a CD94 subunit that is disulfide bonded to a killer cell lectin-like receptor family (CD159a) molecule.[29] The genes encoding CD94 (*KLRD1*) and CD159a (*KLRC1*; NKG2A) are on human chromosome 12p12-p13 and are members of the C-type lectin superfamily. The CD94–CD159a (NKG2A) receptor binds to a nonclassical MHC class I molecule, HLA-E, which is unusual because the peptides present in the HLA-E binding groove are leader segments derived from HLA-A, HLA-B, HLA-C, or HLA-G proteins.[30] When synthesis of HLA-A, HLA-B, HLA-C, or HLA-G is disrupted, possibly by viral infection or transformation of the host cell, HLA-E cannot be transported to the cell surface for presentation to the CD94–CD159a (NKG2A) receptor.

The various KIR (CD158) and CD94–CD159a (NKG2A) receptors are expressed on overlapping subsets within the NK cell population and on certain memory T cells, usually CD8+ T cells, although a minor subset of CD4+ T cells also express KIR (CD158). The observation that F1 mice reject marrow grafts from their parents can be explained by the existence of NK cell subpopulations in the F1 recipient that lack appropriate inhibitory NK cell receptors for the grafted parental cells.[31] The inhibitory KIR (CD158) molecules and the CD94–D159a (NKG2A) receptor have an immunoreceptor tyrosine-based inhibitory motif (ITIM) sequence in their cytoplasmic domains, which binds to the cytoplasmic tyrosine phosphatase nonreceptor type 6 (SHP-1), resulting in inhibition of NK cell cytotoxicity and cytokine secretion.[29] Therefore, the functional behavior of NK and T cells expressing KIR (CD158) or CD94–CD159a (NKG2A) is regulated by the balance of positive signals transmitted by a variety of activating receptors and negative signals (resulting in phosphatase recruitment) provided by the inhibitory MHC class I receptors. Although the expression of NK cell inhibitory receptors is variegated and polymorphic, most NK cells express at least one inhibitory receptor recognizing self-MHC and thus are not self reactive. This is accomplished at least in part by the requirement of interaction of an inhibitory receptor with its ligands during NK cell development for full functional maturation and possibly expansion (NK cell "licensing").[32] The small subset of NK cells in an individual that lack inhibitory receptors for self-MHC class I appear anergic, thereby preventing autoimmunity.

Certain receptors of the KIR (CD158) and CD94–CD159a (NKG2A) families do not possess ITIM sequences and activate, rather than suppress, NK and T-cell responses (see Chap. 15).[29] These receptors noncovalently associate with the homodimeric adapter protein DAP12.[33] Like the CD247 (CD3ζ) and the FcεRI-γ subunits, DAP12 contains an immunoreceptor tyrosine-based activation motif (ITAM) in the cytoplasmic domain. Upon receptor ligation, DAP12 becomes tyrosine phosphorylated, recruits the ZAP70 and Syk (spleen tyrosine kinase) cytoplasmic tyrosine kinases, and induces cellular activation.[33] The physiologic role of activating NK cell receptors for MHC class I has not been determined, but these receptors may have consequences in allogeneic marrow transplantation. In mice, one activating receptor in the Ly49 family (the functional counterpart of KIR [CD158] in humans) recognizes the m157 viral glycoprotein encoded by cytomegalovirus and protects the mice from this pathogen.[34,35] This finding suggests that certain activating KIRs (CD158) in humans may also recognize pathogens.

Although resting blood NK cells are cytotoxic, their activity can be greatly enhanced by both *in vivo* and *in vitro* exposure to cytokines such as IFN-α/β, IL-2, IL-12, IL-15, and IL-18.[36–38] Resting NK cells constitutively express intermediate-affinity IL-2 receptors, and IL-2 induces the progression of most NK cells into the cell cycle.[39]

■ PRODUCTION OF CYTOKINES

Many of the physiologic functions of NK cells are mediated at least partly by their ability to secrete cytokines. NK cells are powerful producers of IFN-γ and GM-CSF. They also can produce TNF-α, macrophage colony-stimulating factor (M-CSF), IL-3, IL-5, IL-8, IL-10, IL-13, and other cytokines and chemokines. Stimulation by cytokines, such as IL-2, IL-12, IL-18, TNF-α, and IL-1,[2,37,40,41] and triggering by activating receptors, such as CD16 interacting with immune complexes, are among the stimuli that, acting individually or often in synergistic combination, induce NK cells to produce cytokines.[2,42,43]

PHYSIOLOGIC ROLES OF NK CELLS

■ INNATE MICROBIAL RESISTANCE

Because of their ability to respond to external stimuli without previous sensitization, NK cells can respond rapidly to the presence of infectious microorganisms or, in some cases, neoplastic cells. Together with phagocytic cells, NK cells are effectors of the innate or natural resistance, which represents the first line of defense against infection (Fig. 79–2).

The ability of NK cells to participate in the resistance against infection by certain viruses is well documented in experimental animals and is strongly suggested by the recurrent viral infections in the few patients described to have a selective deficiency of NK cells.[44] NK cells selectively kill virus-infected cells by a mechanism that is at least partly dependent on the production of IFN-α, a potent stimulator of NK cell activity.[45,46] *In vivo* viral infection and IFN production usually are accompanied by rapid activation of, and increase in the number of, NK cells, both systemically and localized in the infected area.[12] The NK response to virus infection usually peaks 2 to 3 days postinfection and is followed by an antigen-specific T-helper cell and CTL response, which peaks 7 to 9 days postinfection.[12] The early NK response induces a significant reduction in the titer of certain viruses, including mouse cytomegalovirus.[47,48] NK cells from certain resistant mouse strains specifically recognize the m157 protein of mouse cytomegalovirus through the DAP12-linked activating receptor Ly49H and respond by killing the virus-infected cells and secreting IFN-γ.[35,48,49] Other viruses, such as lymphocytic choriomeningitis virus (LCMV), are resistant to the antiviral effects of NK

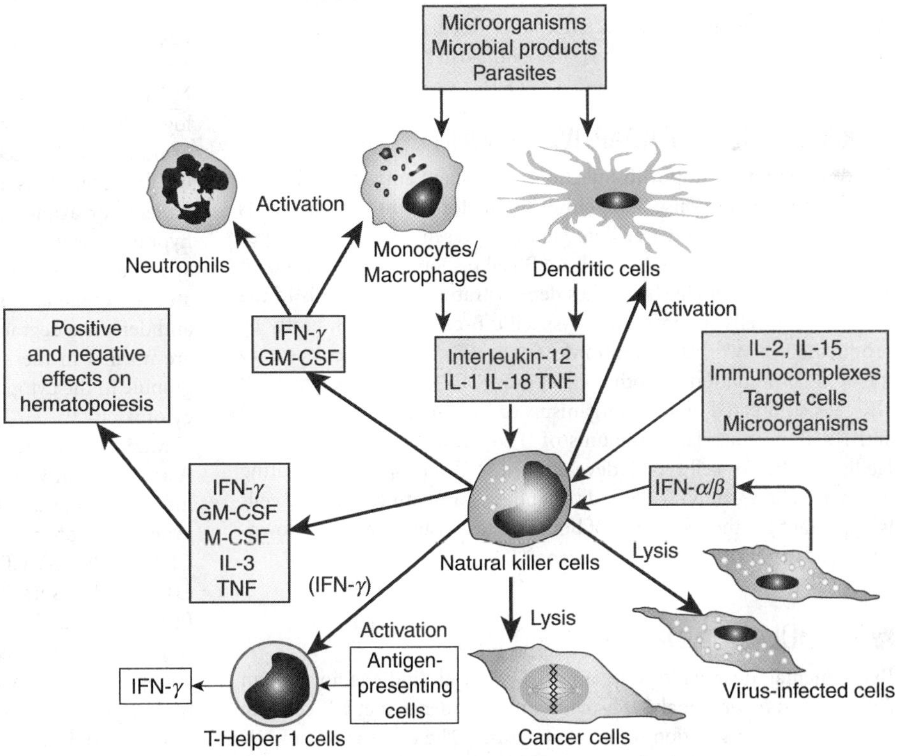

FIGURE 79–2. Schematic of some of the functions and regulatory pathways of NK cells as effector cells of natural resistance. In addition to mediating cytotoxicity, NK cells exert their physiologic roles by releasing several cytokines that affect the functions of other cell types, including hematopoietic progenitor cells. Natural killer cell activity also is regulated by cytokines. Cytokines IFN-α/β, IL-2, IL-15, and IL-12 enhance NK cell-mediated cytotoxicity. IL-2, IL-12, IL-15, IL-18, TNF, and IL-1 induce NK cell lymphokine production. IL-2 and IL-12 induce NK cell proliferation. *Blue arrows* indicate conditions that activate NK cells whereas the *red arrows* indicate innate, proinflammatory, and immunoregulatory functions of NK cells.

cells. NK cell activation induced by the resistant viruses may have pathogenic effects.[47] Although innate resistance, unlike adaptive immunity, is not characterized by immunologic memory, studies demonstrate that Ly49H+ NK cells remained increased in number and activation state for several months after expansion in response to murine cytomegalovirus infection and were able to rapidly respond to a subsequent infection, thus mimicking immunologic memory.[8] Similarly hapten-specific memory was demonstrated in a subset of Ly49C/I+ liver NK cells that could mediate contact hypersensitivity responses.[50]

NK cells enhance the response of phagocytic cells to microorganisms, especially intracellular bacteria and parasites, by producing high levels of the phagocyte-activating cytokines IFN-γ and GM-CSF in response to the microorganisms themselves or to factors, such as IL-12 and TNF-α, produced by infected phagocytic cells.[51,52]

The observation that NK cells kill *in vitro*-transformed or tumor-derived cell lines has been used to support the theory that, in immune surveillance, NK cells, rather than T cells, can recognize and kill newly arising malignant tumor cells.[53,54] In experimental animals, it has been clearly shown that NK cells can destroy tumor cells *in vivo* and are particularly effective in eliminating circulating tumor cells and prevent metastasis, with some evidence also suggesting an effective role of NK cells in resistance to spontaneously arising tumors.[55] An activating receptor expressed by NK cells (NKG2D;CD314) recognizes ligands that are upregulated on tumor cells and virally infected cells but are not expressed well by normal cells[56] and may contribute to immune surveillance against cancer.[57] NK-mediated rejection of tumor cells then may facilitate tumor-antigen presentation to T cells and induce an antigen-specific antitumor immune response.[58,59] NK cell cytotoxic activity often is decreased in human cancer patients. Several studies have suggested that increased NK cell activity tends to correlate with increased survival times and longer intervals before metastasis.[60]

REGULATION OF ADAPTIVE IMMUNITY

NK cells, by interacting with infectious agents and antigens early during the immune response, have either stimulatory or inhibitory effects on the function of B and T cells and antigen-presenting cells.[2] Evidence for an enhancing effect of NK cells on B-cell responses has been shown both *in vitro* and *in vivo* by studies demonstrating that NK cells in the absence of T cells support antigen-specific B-cell responses, partly by producing IFN-γ.[61,62] In certain infections, NK cells may be necessary for optimal induction of both a CD4+ and CD8+ T-cell response.[63,64] NK cells stimulated by microorganisms or by cytokines, such as IL-12 and IL-18, produce large amounts of IFN-γ and other cytokines that facilitate T-helper cell type 1 development.[65] The reciprocal activating interaction between NK cells and the antigen-presenting dendritic cells is important for the regulation of both innate resistance and the downstream adaptive response to pathogens.[66,67]

MODULATION OF HEMATOPOIESIS

Experimental observations in animals, clinical findings in human patients, and *in vitro* analyses provide strong evidence that NK cells are involved in the regulation of hematopoiesis.[68] The effector role of NK cells in rejection of parental marrow graft in irradiated F1 mice[69] and in suppressing erythropoiesis and phagocytopoiesis in mice infected with LCMV[70] demonstrated that *in vivo*-activated NK cells can affect both allogeneic and syngeneic hematopoietic progenitor cells. Because of the ability of NK cells to kill malignant hematopoietic cells, NK cells have been postulated to play an important role in the graft-versus-leukemia reaction in allogeneic marrow transplantation, but only a modest, if any, role in graft-versus-host disease.[71] In haploidentical or mismatched hematopoietic transplantation, the presence on donor NK cells of KIR not recognizing inhibiting ligands on host hematopoietic and malignant cells results in protection from leukemia relapse.[72] A reduced incidence of graft-versus-host disease also was observed and thought to result from the elimination of recipient antigen-presenting cells by donor NK cells.[72]

In vivo depletion of NK cells produces differential effects on various cell lineages. NK cell depletion in normal mice increases phagocytopoiesis and decreases erythropoiesis and megakaryopoiesis.[73,74] Consistent with these results, depletion of NK cells in mice receiving myelosuppressive irradiation results in faster recovery of phagocytopoiesis and slower recovery of megakaryopoiesis and erythropoiesis.[75] Clinical evidence for a role of NK cells in the regulation of human hematopoiesis is provided by the demonstration that NK cells are the effector cells mediating suppression of hematopoiesis in some cases of acquired aplastic anemia in both acute and chronic monoclonal NK lymphocytosis and possibly in other clinical conditions.[68] *In vitro* studies show that NK cells have a prevalent inhibitory effect on colony formation from hematopoietic progenitor cells.[76,77] However, NK cells enhance formation of megakaryocytic colonies and, in some experimental conditions, of erythroid and granulocyte-macrophage colonies.[78,79] The effect of NK cells is mostly mediated by secretion of humoral factors.[72] NK cells, constitutively or upon activation, produce several lymphokines, some with mostly inhibitory effects on hematopoiesis, such as TNF and IFN-γ, and some with mostly positive effects, such as GM-CSF, M-CSF, and IL-3.[40,78]

PATHOLOGIC ALTERATIONS IN NK CELL NUMBER AND FUNCTIONS

NK cell function and NK cell numbers often are decreased in pathologic conditions, including cancer and AIDS.[2,80] The reduced activity or number of NK cells may contribute to disease pathology by decreasing the innate resistance against tumor growth and metastasis in cancer patients or against opportunistic infections in AIDS patients. A NK hyporesponsiveness is observed in patients with Chédiak-Higashi syndrome[81] (see Chap. 66), a rare autosomal recessive disease associated with cellular dysfunction, including fusion of cytoplasmic granules and defective degranulation of neutrophil lysosomes. NK cell numbers are normal in these patients, but the NK cells present a single, large granule in the cytoplasm and have a severely reduced ability to mediate cytotoxicity.[81]

Malignant acute expansion of NK cells is rare; more frequent in Asians than in whites, and often is associated with Epstein-Barr virus infection.[82] Extranodal NK cell lymphomas occur in both the nasopharyngeal region and in nonnasal areas as a NK cell (CD2+, CD3−, CD56+, CD16−, CD57−) leukemia or lymphoma that mostly affects extranodal tissues.[83] It affects predominantly men typically in their fifth decade and usually has an extremely aggressive clinical course. Aggressive NK cells leukemia is a catastrophic disease that affects young adults and is characterized by the systemic presence of neoplastic NK cells in blood and marrow.[83] The blastic NK cell lymphomas, characterized by CD4+CD56+ cells with dermal tropism, are now recognized to represent an expansion of plasmacytoid dendritic cells rather than NK cells.[83] A chronic monoclonal proliferative disorder of LGLs with a clinical course that is often relatively indolent is more commonly observed (see Chap. 96).[84] Most patients have lymphocytic infiltration of the marrow. Severe neutropenia and anemia often are observed. Associated diseases, most commonly rheumatoid arthritis, hepatitis, or cancer, are present in up to half of patients.[84] Although cells from all these patients are characterized by an LGL morphology, in approximately two-thirds of the cases they represent a monoclonal expansion of CD8+ T cells, and in only less than one-third of cases they have the typical phenotype and genotype of CD3–, CD56+, CD57+, and, in some patients, CD16+ NK cells.[84]

REFERENCES

1. Takasugi M, Mickey MR, Terasaki PI: Reactivity of lymphocytes from normal persons on cultured tumor cells. *Cancer Res* 33:2898, 1973.
2. Trinchieri G: Biology of natural killer cells. *Adv Immunol* 47:187, 1989.
3. Tupin E, Kinjo Y, Kronenberg M: The unique role of natural killer T cells in the response to microorganisms. *Nat Rev Microbiol* 5:405, 2007.
4. Young JDE, Cohn ZA: Cellular and humoral mechanisms of cytotoxicity: Structural and functional analogies. *Adv Immunol* 41:269, 1987.
5. Ortaldo JR, Winkler-Pickett R, Kopp W, et al: Relationship of large and small CD3– CD56+ lymphocytes mediating NK-associated activities. *J Leukoc Biol* 52:287, 1992.
6. Di Santo JP, Vosshenrich CA: Bone marrow versus thymic pathways of natural killer cell development. *Immunol Rev* 214:35, 2006.
7. Miller SC: Production and renewal of murine killer cells in the spleen and bone marrow. *J Immunol* 129:2282, 1982.
8. Sun JC, Beilke JN, Lanier LL: Adaptive immune features of natural killer cells. *Nature* 457:557, 2009.
9. Freud AG, Caligiuri MA: Human natural killer cell development. *Immunol Rev* 214:56, 2006.
10. Liu CC, Perussia B, Young JD: The emerging role of IL-15 in NK-cell development. *Immunol Today* 21:113, 2000.
11. Lian RH, Kumar V: Murine natural killer cell progenitors and their requirements for development. *Semin Immunol* 14:453, 2002.
12. Biron CA, Nguyen KB, Pien CG, et al: Natural killer cells in antiviral defense: Function and regulation by innate cytokines. *Annu Rev Immunol* 17:189, 1999.
13. Perussia B, Acuto O, Terhorst C, et al: Human natural killer cells analyzed by B73.1, a monoclonal antibody blocking FcR functions. II. Studies of B73.1 antibody-antigen interaction on the lymphocyte membrane. *J Immunol* 130:2142, 1983.
14. Fehniger TA, Cooper MA, Nuovo GJ, et al: CD56bright natural killer cells are present in human lymph nodes and are activated by T cell-derived IL-2: A potential new link between adaptive and innate immunity. *Blood* 101:3052, 2003.
15. Bouwens L, Wisse E: Pit cells in the liver. *Liver* 12:3, 1992.
16. Weissler JC, Nicod LP, et al: Natural killer cell function in human lung is compartmentalized. *Am Rev Respir Dis* 135:941, 1987.
17. Kitaya K: Accumulation of uterine CD16(–) natural killer (NK) cells: Friends, foes, or Jekyll-and-Hyde relationship for the conceptus? *Immunol Invest* 37:467, 2008.
18. Lanier LL: On guard—Activating NK cell receptors. *Nat Immunol* 2:23, 2001.
19. Sulica A, Morel P, Metes D, et al: Ig-binding receptors on human NK cells as effector and regulatory surface molecules. *Int Rev Immunol* 20:371, 2001.
20. Bauer S, Groh V, Wu J, et al: Activation of NK cells and T cells by NKG2D, a receptor for stress-inducible MICA. *Science* 285:727, 1999.
21. Cerwenka A, Lanier LL: NKG2D ligands: Unconventional MHC class I-like molecules exploited by viruses and cancer. *Tissue Antigens* 61:335, 2003.
22. Groh V, Wu J, Yee C, Spies T: Tumour-derived soluble MIC ligands impair expression of NKG2D and T-cell activation. *Nature* 419:734, 2002.
23. Cosman D, Mullberg J, Sutherland CL, et al: ULBPs, novel MHC class I-related molecules, bind to CMV glycoprotein UL16 and stimulate NK cytotoxicity through the NKG2D receptor. *Immunity* 14:123, 2001.
24. Shibuya A, Campbell D, Hannum C, et al: DNAM-1, a novel adhesion molecule involved in the cytolytic function of T lymphocytes. *Immunity* 4:573, 1996.
25. Moretta A, Bottino C, Vitale M, et al: Activating receptors and coreceptors involved in human natural killer cell-mediated cytolysis. *Annu Rev Immunol* 19:197, 2001.
26. Karre K, Ljunggren HG, Piontek G, Kiessling R: Selective rejection of H-2-deficient lymphoma variants suggests alternative immune defence strategy. *Nature* 319:675, 1986.
27. Ploegh HL: Viral strategies of immune evasion. *Science* 280:248, 1998.
28. Garcia-Lora A, Algarra I, Garrido F: MHC class I antigens, immune surveillance, and tumor immune escape. *J Cell Physiol* 195:346, 2003.
29. Long EO: Regulation of immune responses through inhibitory receptors. *Annu Rev Immunol* 17:875, 1999.
30. Braud VM, Allan DS, O'Callaghan CA, et al: HLA-E binds to natural killer cell receptors CD94/NKG2A, B and C. *Nature* 391:795, 1998.
31. Yu YY, George T, Dorfman JR, et al: The role of Ly49A and 5E6(Ly49C) molecules in hybrid resistance mediated by murine natural killer cells against normal T cell blasts. *Immunity* 4:67, 1996.
32. Kim S, Poursine-Laurent J, Truscott SM, et al: Licensing of natural killer cells by host major histocompatibility complex class I molecules. *Nature* 436:709, 2005.
33. Lanier LL, Corliss BC, Wu J, et al: Immunoreceptor DAP12 bearing a tyrosine-based activation motif is involved in activating NK cells. *Nature* 391:703, 1998.
34. Brown MG, Dokun AO, Heusel JW, et al: Vital involvement of a natural killer cell activation receptor in resistance to viral infection. *Science* 292:934, 2001.
35. Arase H, Mocarski ES, Campbell AE, et al: Direct recognition of cytomegalovirus by activating and inhibitory NK cell receptors. *Science* 296:1323, 2002.
36. Trinchieri G, Santoli D: Antiviral activity induced by culturing lymphocytes with tumor-derived or virus-transformed cells. Enhancement of human natural killer cell activity by interferon and antagonistic inhibition of susceptibility of target cells to lysis. *J Exp Med* 147:1314, 1978.
37. Trinchieri G, Matsumoto-Kobayashi M, Clark SC, et al: Response of resting human peripheral blood natural killer cells to interleukin-2. *J Exp Med* 160:1147, 1984.
38. Kobayashi M, Fitz L, Ryan M, et al: Identification and purification of Natural Killer cell stimulatory factor (NKSF), a cytokine with multiple biologic effects on human lymphocytes. *J Exp Med* 170:827, 1989.
39. London L, Perussia B, Trinchieri G: Induction of proliferation in vitro of resting human natural killer cells: IL-2 induces into cell cycle most peripheral blood NK cells, but only a minor subset of low density T cells. *J Immunol* 137:3845, 1986.
40. Cuturi MC, Anegon I, Sherman F, et al: Production of hematopoietic colony-stimulating factors by human natural killer cells. *J Exp Med* 169:569, 1989.
41. Peritt D, Robertson S, Gri G, et al: Differentiation of human NK cells into NK1 and NK2 subsets. *J Immunol* 161:5821, 1998.
42. Anegon I, Cuturi MC, Trinchieri G, Perussia B: Interaction of Fcg receptor (CD16) with ligands induces transcription of IL-2 receptor (CD25) and lymphokine genes and expression of their products in human natural killer cells. *J Exp Med* 167:452, 1988.
43. Chan SH, Perussia B, Gupta JW, et al: Induction of interferon gamma production by natural killer cell stimulatory factor: Characterization of the responder cells and synergy with other inducers. *J Exp Med* 173:869, 1991.
44. Biron CA, Byron KS, Sullivan JL: Severe herpesvirus infections in an adolescent without natural killer cells. *N Engl J Med* 320:1731, 1989.
45. Santoli D, Trinchieri G, Koproswki H: Cell-mediated cytotoxicity in humans against virus-infected target cells. II. Interferon induction and activation of natural killer cells. *J Immunol* 121:532, 1978.
46. Bandyopadhyay S, Perussia B, Trinchieri G, et al: Requirement for HLA-DR positive accessory cells in natural killing of cytomegalovirus-infected fibroblasts. *J Exp Med* 164:180, 1986.
47. Welsh RM: Regulation of virus infections by natural killer cells. A review. *Nat Immun Cell Growth Regul* 5:169, 1986.
48. Arase H, Lanier LL: Virus-driven evolution of natural killer cell receptors. *Microbes Infect* 4:1505, 2002.
49. Smith HR, Heusel JW, Mehta IK, et al: Recognition of a virus-encoded ligand by a natural killer cell activation receptor. *Proc Natl Acad Sci U S A* 99:8826, 2002.
50. O'Leary JG, Goodarzi M, Drayton DL, von Andrian UH: T cell- and B cell-independent adaptive immunity mediated by natural killer cells. *Nat Immunol* 7:507, 2006.
51. Bancroft GJ, Schreiber RD, Bosma GC, et al: A T cell-independent mechanism of macrophage activation by interferon-gamma. *J Immunol* 139:1104, 1987.
52. Gazzinelli RT, Hieny S, Wynn TA, et al: Interleukin 12 is required for the T-lymphocyte-independent induction of interferon gamma by an intracellular parasite and induces resistance in T-cell-deficient hosts [see comments]. *Proc Natl Acad Sci U S A* 90:6115, 1993.
53. Bloom ET: Density gradient fractionation of effector cells in human natural cell-mediated cytotoxicity. *Cell Immunol* 61:231, 1981.
54. Bloom BR: Natural killers to rescue immune surveillance? *Nature* 300:214, 1982.
55. Smyth MJ, Hayakawa Y, Takeda K, Yagita H: New aspects of natural-killer-cell surveillance and therapy of cancer. *Nat Rev Cancer* 2:850, 2002.
56. Diefenbach A, Raulet DH: The innate immune response to tumors and its role in the induction of T-cell immunity. *Immunol Rev* 188:9, 2002.
57. Guerra N, Tan YX, Joncker NT, et al: NKG2D-deficient mice are defective in tumor surveillance in models of spontaneous malignancy. *Immunity* 28:571, 2008.
58. Kelly JM, Darcy PK, Markby JL, et al: Induction of tumor-specific T cell memory by NK cell-mediated tumor rejection. *Nat Immunol* 3:83, 2002.
59. Mocikat R, Braumuller H, Gumy A, et al: Natural killer cells activated by MHC class I (low) targets prime dendritic cells to induce protective CD8 T cell responses. *Immunity* 19:561, 2003.
60. Brittenden J, Heys SD, Ross J, Eremin O: Natural killer cells and cancer. *Cancer* 77:1226, 1996.
61. Mond JJ, Brunswick M: A role for IFN-gamma and NK cells in immune response to T cell-regulated antigens types 1 and 2. *Immunol Rev* 99:105, 1987.
62. Yuan D, Wilder J, Dang T, et al: Activation of B lymphocytes by NK cells. *Int Immunol* 4:1373, 1992.
63. Goldszmid RS, Bafica A, Jankovic D, et al: TAP-1 indirectly regulates CD4+ T cell priming in *Toxoplasma gondii* infection by controlling NK cell IFN-gamma production. *J Exp Med* 204:2591, 2007.
64. Scharton TM, Scott P: Natural killer cells are a source of interferon gamma that drives differentiation of CD4+ T cell subsets and induces early resistance to Leishmania major of mice. *J Exp Med* 178:567, 1993.
65. Trinchieri G: Interleukin-12 and the regulation of innate resistance and adaptive immunity. *Nat Rev Immunol* 3:133, 2003.
66. Gerosa F, Gobbi A, Zorzi P, et al: The reciprocal interaction of NK cells with plasmacytoid or myeloid dendritic cells profoundly affects innate resistance functions. *J Immunol* 174:727, 2005.
67. Moretta A: Natural killer cells and dendritic cells: Rendezvous in abused tissues. *Nat Rev Immunol* 2:957, 2002.
68. Trinchieri G: Natural killer cells in hematopoiesis, in *The Natural Immune System: Natural Killer Cells*, edited by CE Lewis, p 41. Oxford University Press, Oxford, UK, 1992.

69. Cudkowicz G, Hochman PS: Do natural killer cells engage in regulated reaction against self to ensure homeostasis? *Immunol Rev* 44:13, 1979.
70. Randrup-Thomsen A, Pisa P, Bro-Jørgensen K, Kiessling R: Mechanisms of lymphocytic choriomeningitis virus-induced hemopoietic dysfunction. *J Virol* 59:428, 1986.
71. Jiang YZ, Barrett AJ, Goldman JM, Mavroudis DA: Association of natural killer cell immune recovery with a graft-versus-leukemia effect independent of graft-versus-host disease following allogeneic bone marrow transplantation. *Ann Hematol* 74:1, 1997.
72. Velardi A, Ruggeri L, Alessandro, Moretta, Moretta L: NK cells: A lesson from mismatched hematopoietic transplantation. *Trends Immunol* 23:438, 2002.
73. Hansson M, Petersson M, Koo GC, et al: *In vivo* function of natural killer cells as regulators of myeloid precursor cells in the spleen. *Eur J Immunol* 18:485, 1988.
74. Pantel K, Nakeff A: Differential effect of natural killer cells on modulating CFU-Meg and BFU-E proliferation *in situ*. *Exp Hematol* 17:1017, 1989.
75. Pantel K, Boertman J, Nakeff A: Inhibition of hematopoietic recovery from radiation-induced myelosuppression by natural killer cells. *Radiat Res* 122:168, 1990.
76. Hansson M, Beran M, Andersson B, Kiessling R: Inhibition of *in vitro* granulopoiesis by autologous and allogeneic human NK cells. *J Immunol* 129:126, 1982.
77. Degliantoni G, Murphy M, Kobayashi M, et al: Natural killer (NK) cell-derived hematopoietic colony-inhibiting activity and NK cytotoxic factor. Relationship with tumor necrosis factor and synergism with immune interferon. *J Exp Med* 162:1512, 1985.
78. Murphy WJ, Keller JR, Harrision CL, et al: Interleukin-2-activated natural killer cells can support hematopoiesis *in vitro* and promote marrow engraftment *in vivo*. *Blood* 80:670, 1992.
79. Gewirtz AM, Xu WY, Mangan KF: Role of natural killer cells, in comparison with T lymphocytes and monocytes, in the regulation of normal human megakaryocytopoiesis in vitro. *J Immunol* 139:2915, 1987.
80. Chehimi J, Starr SE, Frank I, et al: Natural killer (NK) cell stimulatory factor increases the cytotoxic activity of NK cells from both healthy donors and human immunodeficiency virus-infected patients. *J Exp Med* 175:789, 1992.
81. Haliotis T, Roder J, Klein M, et al: Chédiak-Higashi gene in humans. I. Impairment of natural-killer function. *J Exp Med* 151:1039, 1980.
82. Kanavaros P, Lescs MC, Briere J, et al: Nasal T-cell lymphoma: A clinicopathologic entity associated with peculiar phenotype and with Epstein-Barr virus. *Blood* 81:2688, 1993.
83. Liang X, Graham DK: Natural killer cell neoplasms. *Cancer* 112:1425, 2008.
84. Reynolds CW, Foon KA: T gamma-lymphoproliferative disease and related disorders in humans and experimental animals: A review of the clinical, cellular and functional characteristics. *Blood* 64:1146, 1984.

CHAPTER 80

CLASSIFICATION AND CLINICAL MANIFESTATIONS OF LYMPHOCYTE AND PLASMA CELL DISORDERS

Thomas J. Kipps

SUMMARY

This chapter outlines the major categories of lymphocyte and plasma cell disorders. The disorders can be sorted into three main groups. The first is composed of diseases caused by defects intrinsic to lymphoid cells. The second is caused by disorders that result from factors extrinsic to lymphoid cells. The third is composed of disorders caused by neoplastic or preneoplastic lymphoid cells and is outlined in Chap. 92 using the World Health Organization classification of tumors of lymphoid tissues. The clinical manifestations of diseases in any one of the three groups may be difficult to distinguish, but this grouping can provide a framework with which to proceed in evaluating patients with known or suspected lymphocyte disorders. This chapter introduces the framework and presents a roadmap to other chapters in this book that discuss each of the disorders in greater detail.

CLASSIFICATION

Lymphocyte and plasma cell disorders can be classified into three major groups. The first group is composed of lymphocyte disorders caused by intrinsic defects in lymphoid cells that result in functional abnormalities of marrow-derived (B) lymphocytes, thymic-derived (T) lymphocytes, both (impaired humoral and cellular immunity), or natural killer (NK) cells (Table 80–1). These disorders primarily result from inborn errors in lymphocyte metabolism (see Chaps. 75, 76, 77, and 82) and/or receptor–ligand expression (see Chaps. 14 and 82). Table 80–1 groups these disorders together as "primary disorders." The second group consists of disorders caused by factors extrinsic to lymphocytes resulting in immune dysfunction. These conditions most commonly result from infection with viruses or other cellular pathogens (see Chaps. 81, 83, and 84), but they also may be caused by drugs or systemic disease of nonlymphoid cells. Table 80–1 lists these disorders as "acquired disorders." The third group of diseases is composed of preneoplastic and neoplastic lymphocyte disorders (see Chap. 92).

Acronyms and abbreviations that appear in this chapter include: AIRE gene, autoimmune regulator gene; APECED syndrome, autoimmune polyglandular, candidiasis, and ectodermal dystrophy syndrome; Ig, immunoglobulin; IPEX syndrome, immune dysregulation, polyendocrinopathy, enteropathy, X-linked syndrome; NK, natural killer; Th, T helper; T_{regs}, CD4+ regulatory T cells; WHIM syndrome, warts, hypogammaglobulinemia, infections, myelokathexis syndrome.

Different categories of lymphocyte and plasma cell disorders may be difficult to distinguish clinically for several reasons. Lymphocyte disorders can have many clinical manifestations that are not restricted to cells of the immune system. Also, disparate disorders can have similar clinical manifestations, and any one disorder can be associated with a diverse array of clinical pathologies.

In some cases, however, the classification of lymphocyte disorders is influenced by the manifestations of the disease. For example, autoimmune hemolytic disease (see Chap. 53) and autoimmune thrombocytopenia (see Chap. 119) are caused by inappropriate secretion of autoantibodies by B lymphocytes. The blood cell that is coated with autoantibody presumably is normal, yet we classify the disease that can result from hemolytic autoantibodies as an acquired hemolytic anemia because that aspect of the disease is more visible and better understood than is the inappropriate synthesis of antierythrocyte antibody by the disturbed lymphocyte population(s). These disorders are not considered here.

Many diseases, especially infection (e.g., tuberculous adenitis), inflammatory states (e.g., rheumatoid arthritis), autoimmune disease (e.g., systemic lupus erythematosus), and metastatic carcinoma can involve lymph nodes or the spleen as a secondary alteration. These disorders also may be associated with abnormal production of antibodies, such as those resulting in the lupus anticoagulant (see Chap. 132). These disorders also are not considered here because the primary disease is not generally considered a lymphocyte disorder per se.

CLINICAL MANIFESTATIONS

B LYMPHOCYTE DISORDERS

Immunoglobulin Deficiency

The clinical manifestations of B-lymphocyte disorders include the consequences of B-lymphocyte deficiency, dysfunction, or malignant transformation. The manifestations may consist of a specific deficiency of one of the Ig isotypes or of several or all normal immunoglobulin (Ig) molecules (panhypogammaglobulinemia; see Chap. 77). Inability to synthesize or secrete antibodies impairs the clearance of pathogens because of the inability to opsonize microorganisms for phagocytosis, resulting in immune deficiency (see Chap. 82).

Abnormal Immunoglobulin Production

Excess production of Ig by a clone of B cells can result in essential monoclonal gammopathy (see Chap. 108). This situation could result from a primary defect in the B-cell clone or expansion of a clone in response to chronic antigen stimulation. Essential monoclonal gammopathy can a harbinger for development of B-cell neoplastic disease, such as plasma cell myeloma (see Chap. 109) or Waldenström macroglobulinemia (see Chap. 111). Production of abnormal Ig molecules or Ig fragments can be seen in association with chronic infection, leading to development of Ig heavy-chain disease (see Chap. 112). Deposition of Ig or Ig fragments can contribute to amyloid formation (see Chap. 110). Reactivity of the Ig with self-antigen(s), such as those found on the red cell membrane (see Chap. 53), can result in systemic autoimmune disease.

T LYMPHOCYTE DISORDERS

Impaired Immunoregulation

The clinical manifestations of deficiencies or excesses of T lymphocytes depend on the subset of T lymphocytes involved. For example, delayed

TABLE 80–1. Classification of Disorders of Lymphocytes and Plasma Cells

I. Primary disorders
- A. B-lymphocyte deficiency or dysfunction (see Chap. 82)[5]
  - 1. Agammaglobulinemia
    - a. Acquired agammaglobulinemia[6]
    - b. Associated with plasma cell myeloma or chronic lymphocytic leukemia (see Chaps. 94 and 109)[7]
    - c. Associated with celiac disease[8]
    - d. X-linked agammaglobulinemia of Bruton[9]
  - 2. Selective agammaglobulinemia (see Chap. 82)
    - a. IgM deficiency
      - 1. Bloom syndrome[10]
      - 2. Isolated[11]
      - 3. Wiskott-Aldrich syndrome[12]
    - b. Selective IgG deficiency (see Chap. 82)
    - c. IgA deficiency[13]
      - 1. Isolated asymptomatic
      - 2. Steatorrheic[14]
    - d. IgA and IgM deficiency[15]
  - 3. Hyper-IgA[16,17]
  - 4. Hyper-IgD[16,18,19]
  - 5. Hyper-IgE (see Chap. 82)[20]
  - 6. Hyper-IgE associated with HIV infection[21]
  - 7. Hyper-IgM immunodeficiency (see Chap. 82)
  - 8. X-linked lymphoproliferative disease[22,23]
- B. T-lymphocyte deficiency or dysfunction (see Chap. 82)[24]
  - 1. Cartilage-hair hypoplasia (see Chap. 82)[25,26]
  - 2. Lymphocyte function antigen-1 deficiency[27]
  - 3. Thymic aplasia (DiGeorge syndrome)[28]
  - 4. Thymic dysplasia (Nezelof syndrome)[29]
  - 5. Thymic hypoplasia[30]
  - 6. Wiskott-Aldrich syndrome (see Chaps. 82 and 121)[31]
  - 7. ZAP-70 deficiency (see Chap. 82)[32,33]
  - 8. Purine nucleoside phosphorylase deficiency (see Chap. 82)
  - 9. Interleukin-7 receptor deficiency (see Chap. 82)
  - 10. Major histocompatibility complex class I deficiency (see Chap. 82)
  - 11. Coronin-1A deficiency (see Chap. 82)
  - 12. IPEX syndrome caused by mutations in FoxP3 that cause a deficiency of CD4+ regulatory T cells (T_{regs}) (see Chaps. 78 and 82)
  - 13. APECED syndrome caused by mutations in the autoimmune regulator gene (AIRE) gene (see Chaps. 5, 78, and 82)
  - 14. Autoimmune lymphoproliferative syndrome (see Chap. 82)
  - 15. Calcium entry channel deficiency caused by mutations in *ORAI1* or *STIM1* (see Chap. 82)[34]
- C. Combined T- and B-cell deficiency or dysfunction (see Chap. 82)
  - 1. Ataxia-telangiectasia[35]
  - 2. Combined immunodeficiency syndrome (see Chap. 82)
    - a. Adenosine deaminase deficiency[36,37]
    - b. Thymic alymphoplasia[38]
  - 3. Major histocompatibility complex class II deficiency–bare lymphocyte syndrome (see Chap. 82)[39,40]
  - 4. IgG and IgA deficiency and impaired cellular immunity (type I dysgammaglobulinemia)[41]
  - 5. Immunodeficiency with thymoma[42]
  - 6. Pyridoxine deficiency[43]
  - 7. Reticular agenesis (congenital aleukocytosis)[44]
  - 8. Omenn syndrome (see Chap. 82)[45,46]
  - 9. WHIM syndrome resulting from mutation in the CXCR4 gene (see Chap. 82)
  - 10. Nijmegen breakage syndrome (see Chap. 82)
- D. Natural killer cells (see Chaps. 79 and 96)
  - 1. Chronic natural killer cell lymphocytosis[1,47–51]

II. Acquired disorders
- A. Acquired immunodeficiency syndrome (see Chap. 83)
- B. Reactive lymphocytosis or plasmacytosis (see Chap. 81)[52]
  - 1. *Bordetella pertussis* lymphocytosis (see Chap. 81)[53]
  - 2. Cytomegalovirus mononucleosis (see Chap. 84)[54]
  - 3. Drug-induced lymphocytosis[55]
  - 4. Epstein-Barr virus mononucleosis (see Chap. 84)
  - 5. Inflammatory (secondary) plasmacytosis of marrow
  - 6. Large granular lymphocytosis (see Chap. 96)[56,57]
  - 7. Other viral mononucleosis (see Chap. 84)[52,58]
  - 8. Polyclonal lymphocytosis (see Chap. 81)[59,60]
  - 9. Serum sickness[61,62]
  - 10. T-cell lymphocytosis associated with thymoma (see Chap. 81)
  - 11. *Toxoplasma gondii* mononucleosis (see Chap. 84)
  - 12. Viral infectious lymphocytosis (see Chap. 81)
- C. T-lymphocyte dysfunction or depletion associated with systemic disease
  - 1. B-cell chronic lymphocytic leukemia (see Chap. 94)
  - 2. Hodgkin lymphoma (see Chap. 99)
  - 3. Leprosy[63,64]
  - 4. Lupus erythematosus[65]
  - 5. Sjögren syndrome[66]
  - 6. Sarcoidosis[67,68]

hypersensitivity normally is mediated by CD4+ helper T cells (Th cells) and, more specifically, Th1-type cells (see Chap. 78). A deficit or functional disturbance in these T cells can impair the cellular immune response to mycobacteria, listeria, brucella, fungi, or other intracellular organisms associated with formation of immune granulomas. Th2-type CD4+ helper T cells, on the other hand, appear better suited to induce B-cell responses to antigen and direct the immune response against parasitic infestations (see Chap. 78). Deficiency or defects in CD4+ regulator T cells (T_{regs}) can result in autoimmune disease, whereas depletion or deficiency of Th17 cells can result in impaired resistance to opportunistic infection (see Chap 78). Depletion of CD4+ T cells in patients infected with human immunodeficiency virus accounts in large part for the acquired immune deficiency that develops in patients infected with the virus (see Chap. 83).

T lymphocytes within a marrow allograft are responsible for initiation of the graft-versus-host reaction (see Chap. 21). The acute form of the reaction can lead to severe dermatitis, gastroenteritis, and hepatitis. The chronic syndrome simulates a collage of connective tissue diseases, such as scleroderma, xerophthalmia, xerostomia, and pulmonary insufficiency. Eosinophilia, hypergammaglobulinemia, development of autoantibodies, and plasmacytosis can occur. Infection with classic or opportunistic pathogens is a common complication of both acute and chronic graft-versus-host disease. A similar qualitative reaction, albeit more limited, is seen in mononucleosis resulting from Epstein-Barr virus infection (see Chap. 84).

NATURAL KILLER CELL DISORDERS

Chronic Natural Killer Cell Lymphocytosis

Chronic natural killer (NK) cell lymphocytosis is a rare proliferative disorder that can be distinguished from NK cell leukemia and lymphoma by its indolent nature.[1] Patients typically have neutropenia, anemia, vasculitic syndromes, fever of unknown origin, constitutional symptoms, and autoimmune disorders, including rheumatoid arthritis, Sjögren syndrome, and/or polymyalgia rheumatica, and often have cutaneous lesions.[2] Studies seeking to define this condition as a clonal disorder using X-linked gene analysis have not yielded consistent findings (see Chap. 79).

The association of such conditions with chronic expansions in the numbers of NK cells implicates the NK cell as playing a role in autoimmunity. Consistent with this notion are animal studies implicating a deficiency of NK cells and/or NK-like T cells as a contributing factor in the pathogenesis of type 1 diabetes.[3] Moreover, NK cells play a role in regulating stem cell engraftment and in graft-versus-host disease following allogeneic hematopoietic stem cell transplantation.[4]

REFERENCES

1. Morice WG, Leibson PJ, Tefferi A: Natural killer cells and the syndrome of chronic natural killer cell lymphocytosis. *Leuk Lymphoma* 41:277, 2001.
2. Fujita Y, Fujii T, Takeda N, et al: Successful treatment of primary Sjögren's syndrome with chronic natural killer lymphocytosis by high-dose prednisolone and indomethacin farnesil. *Intern Med* 46:251, 2007.
3. Rodacki M, Milech A, de Oliveira JE: NK cells and type 1 diabetes. *Clin Dev Immunol* 13:101, 2006.
4. Moretta A, Locatelli F, Moretta L: Human NK cells: From HLA class I-specific killer Ig-like receptors to the therapy of acute leukemias. *Immunol Rev* 224:58, 2008.
5. Conley ME, Dobbs AK, Farmer DM, et al: Primary B cell immunodeficiencies: Comparisons and contrasts. *Annu Rev Immunol* 27:199, 2009.
6. Ballow M: Primary immunodeficiency disorders: Antibody deficiency. *J Allergy Clin Immunol* 109:581, 2002.
7. Kyrtsonis MC, Mouzaki A, Maniatis A: Mechanisms of polyclonal hypogammaglobulinaemia in multiple myeloma (MM). *Med Oncol* 16:73, 1999.
8. Halfdanarson TR, Litzow MR, Murray JA: Hematologic manifestations of celiac disease. *Blood* 109:412, 2007.
9. Schiff C, Lemmers B, Deville A, et al: Autosomal primary immunodeficiencies affecting human bone marrow B-cell differentiation. *Immunol Rev* 178:91, 2000.
10. Amor-Gueret M: Bloom syndrome, genomic instability and cancer: The SOS-like hypothesis. *Cancer Lett* 236:1, 2006.
11. Callard RE, Smith SH, Matthews DJ: Regulation of human B cell growth and differentiation: Lessons from the primary immunodeficiencies. *Chem Immunol* 67:114, 1997.
12. Notarangelo LD, Notarangelo LD, Ochs HD: WASP and the phenotypic range associated with deficiency. *Curr Opin Allergy Clin Immunol* 5:485, 2005.
13. Latiff AH, Kerr MA: The clinical significance of immunoglobulin A deficiency. *Ann Clin Biochem* 44:131, 2007.
14. Ojuawo A, St Louis D, Lindley KJ, Milla PJ: Non-infective colitis in infancy: Evidence in favour of minor immunodeficiency in its pathogenesis. *Arch Dis Child* 76:345, 1997.
15. Schroeder HW Jr, Schroeder HW 3rd, Sheikh SM: The complex genetics of common variable immunodeficiency. *J Investig Med* 52:90, 2004.
16. Klasen IS, Goertz JH, van de Wiel GA, et al: Hyper-immunoglobulin A in the hyperimmunoglobulinemia D syndrome. *Clin Diagn Lab Immunol* 8:58, 2001.
17. Bermejo JF, Carbone J, Rodriguez JJ, et al: Macroamylasaemia, IgA hypergammaglobulinaemia and autoimmunity in a patient with Down syndrome and coeliac disease. *Scand J Gastroenterol* 38:445, 2003.
18. Yoshimura K, Wakiguchi H: Hyperimmunoglobulinemia D syndrome successfully treated with a corticosteroid. *Pediatr Int* 44:326, 2002.
19. Simon A, Mariman EC, van der Meer JW, Drenth JP: A founder effect in the hyperimmunoglobulinemia D and periodic fever syndrome. *Am J Med* 114:148, 2003.
20. Paulson ML, Freeman AF, Holland SM: Hyper IgE syndrome: An update on clinical aspects and the role of signal transducer and activator of transcription 3. *Curr Opin Allergy Clin Immunol* 8:527, 2008.
21. Burastero SE, Paolucci C, Breda D, et al: Immunological basis for IgE hyper-production in enfuvirtide-treated HIV-positive patients. *J Clin Immunol* 26:168, 2006.
22. Engel P, Eck MJ, Terhorst C: The SAP and SLAM families in immune responses and X-linked lymphoproliferative disease. *Nat Rev Immunol* 3:813, 2003.
23. Gilmour KC, Gaspar HB: Pathogenesis and diagnosis of X-linked lymphoproliferative disease. *Expert Rev Mol Diagn* 3:549, 2003.
24. Elder ME: T-cell immunodeficiencies. *Pediatr Clin North Am* 47:1253, 2000.
25. Notarangelo LD, Roifman CM, Giliani S: Cartilage-hair hypoplasia: Molecular basis and heterogeneity of the immunological phenotype. *Curr Opin Allergy Clin Immunol* 8:534, 2008.
26. Maida Y, Yasukawa M, Furuuchi M, et al: An RNA-dependent RNA polymerase formed by TERT and the RMRP RNA. *Nature* 461:230-5, 2009.
27. Smith A, Stanley P, Jones K, et al: The role of the integrin LFA-1 in T-lymphocyte migration. *Immunol Rev* 218:135, 2007.
28. McLean-Tooke A, Spickett GP, Gennery AR: Immunodeficiency and autoimmunity in 22q11.2 deletion syndrome. *Scand J Immunol* 66:1, 2007.
29. Nezelof C: Thymic pathology in primary and secondary immunodeficiencies. *Histopathology* 21:499, 1992.
30. Sullivan KE, McDonald-McGinn D, Zackai EH: CD4(+) CD25(+) T-cell production in healthy humans and in patients with thymic hypoplasia. *Clin Diagn Lab Immunol* 9:1129, 2002.
31. Bosticardo M, Marangoni F, Aiuti A, et al: Recent advances in understanding the pathophysiology of Wiskott-Aldrich syndrome. *Blood* 113:6288, 2009.
32. Grunebaum E, Sharfe N, Roifman CM: Human T cell immunodeficiency: When signal transduction goes wrong. *Immunol Res* 35:117, 2006.
33. Picard C, Dogniaux S, Chemin K, et al: Hypomorphic mutation of ZAP70 in human results in a late onset immunodeficiency and no autoimmunity. *Eur J Immunol* 39:1966, 2009.
34. Feske S, Gwack Y, Prakriya M, et al: A mutation in Orai1 causes immune deficiency by abrogating CRAC channel function. *Nature* 441:179, 2006.
35. Nowak-Wegrzyn A, Crawford TO, Winkelstein JA, et al: Immunodeficiency and infections in ataxia-telangiectasia. *J Pediatr* 144:505, 2004.
36. Cassani B, Mirolo M, Cattaneo F, et al: Altered intracellular and extracellular signaling leads to impaired T-cell functions in ADA-SCID patients. *Blood* 111:4209, 2008.
37. Aiuti A, Cattaneo F, Galimberti S, et al: Gene therapy for immunodeficiency due to adenosine deaminase deficiency. *N Engl J Med* 360:447, 2009.
38. Buckley RH: Immunodeficiency diseases. *JAMA* 268:2797, 1992.
39. Reith W, Mach B: The bare lymphocyte syndrome and the regulation of MHC expression. *Annu Rev Immunol* 19:331, 2001.
40. Nekrep N, Fontes JD, Geyer M, Peterlin BM: When the lymphocyte loses its clothes. *Immunity* 18:453, 2003.
41. Sutor G, Fabel H: Sarcoidosis and common variable immunodeficiency. A case of a malignant course of sarcoidosis in conjunction with severe impairment of the cellular and humoral immune system. *Respiration* 67:204, 2000.
42. Agarwal S, and Cunningham-Rundles C: Thymoma and immunodeficiency (Good syndrome): A report of 2 unusual cases and review of the literature. *Ann Allergy Asthma Immunol* 98:185, 2007.
43. Trakatellis A, Dimitriadou A, Trakatelli M: Pyridoxine deficiency: New approaches in immunosuppression and chemotherapy. *Postgrad Med J* 73:617, 1997.
44. Small TN, Wall DA, Kurtzberg J, et al: Association of reticular dysgenesis (thymic alymphoplasia and congenital aleukocytosis) with bilateral sensorineural deafness. *J Pediatr* 135:387, 1999.
45. Marrella V, Poliani PL, Sobacchi C, et al: Of Omenn and mice. *Trends Immunol* 29:133, 2008.
46. Poliani PL, Facchetti F, Ravanini M, et al: Early defects in human T-cell development severely affect distribution and maturation of thymic stromal cells: Possible implications for the pathophysiology of Omenn syndrome. *Blood* 114:105, 2009.
47. Vanness ER, Davis MD, Tefferi A: Cutaneous findings associated with chronic natural killer cell lymphocytosis. *Int J Dermatol* 41:852, 2002.
48. Tefferi A, Greipp PR, Leibson PJ, Thibodeau SN: Demonstration of clonality, by X-linked DNA analysis, in chronic natural killer cell lymphocytosis and successful therapy with oral cyclophosphamide. *Leukemia* 6:477, 1992.

49. Nash R, McSweeney P, Zambello R, et al: Clonal studies of CD3- lymphoproliferative disease of granular lymphocytes. *Blood* 81:2363, 1993.
50. Kukreja A, Maclaren NK: NKT cells and type-1 diabetes and the "hygiene hypothesis" to explain the rising incidence rates. *Diabetes Technol Ther* 4:323, 2002.
51. Lowdell MW: Natural killer cells in haematopoietic stem cell transplantation. *Transfus Med* 13:399, 2003.
52. Brown KA: Nonmalignant disorders of lymphocytes. *Clin Lab Sci* 10:329, 1997.
53. Agarwal RK, Sun SH, Su SB, et al: Pertussis toxin alters the innate and the adaptive immune responses in a pertussis-dependent model of autoimmunity. *J Neuroimmunol* 129:133, 2002.
54. Rodriguez-Caballero A, Garcia-Montero AC, Barcena P, et al: Expanded cells in monoclonal TCR-alphabeta+/CD4+/NKa+/CD8-/+dim T-LGL lymphocytosis recognize hCMV antigens. *Blood* 112:4609, 2008.
55. Kano Y, Shiohara T: The variable clinical picture of drug-induced hypersensitivity syndrome/drug rash with eosinophilia and systemic symptoms in relation to the eliciting drug. *Immunol Allergy Clin North Am* 29:481, 2009.
56. O'Malley DP: T-cell large granular leukemia and related proliferations. *Am J Clin Pathol* 127:850, 2007.
57. Sokol L, Loughran TP Jr: Large granular lymphocyte leukemia. *Oncologist* 11:263, 2006.
58. Greenberg MS: Herpesvirus infections. *Dent Clin North Am* 40:359, 1996.
59. Lawrie CH, Shilling R, Troussard X, et al: Expression profiling of persistent polyclonal B-cell lymphocytosis suggests constitutive expression of the AP-1 transcription complex and downregulation of Fas-apoptotic and TGFbeta signalling pathways. *Leukemia* 23:581, 2009.
60. Cornet E, Lesesve JF, Mossafa H, et al: Long-term follow-up of 111 patients with persistent polyclonal B-cell lymphocytosis with binucleated lymphocytes. *Leukemia* 23:419, 2009.
61. Erffmeyer JE: Serum sickness. *Ann Allergy* 56:105, 1986.
62. Virella G: Immune complex diseases. *Immunol Ser* 50:395, 1990.
63. Chattree V, Khanna N, Rao DN: Alterations in T cell signal transduction by M. leprae antigens is associated with downregulation of second messengers PKC, calcium, calcineurin, MAPK and various transcription factors in leprosy patients. *Mol Immunol* 44:2066, 2007.
64. Im JS, Kang TJ, Lee SB, et al: Alteration of the relative levels of iNKT cell subsets is associated with chronic mycobacterial infections. *Clin Immunol* 127:214, 2008.
65. Wenzel J, Gerdsen R, Uerlich M, et al: Lymphocytopenia in lupus erythematosus: Close in vivo association to autoantibodies targeting nuclear antigens. *Br J Dermatol* 150:994, 2004.
66. Mandl T, Bredberg A, Jacobsson LT, et al: CD4+ T-lymphocytopenia—A frequent finding in anti-SSA antibody seropositive patients with primary Sjögren's syndrome. *J Rheumatol* 31:726, 2004.
67. Morell F, Levy G, Orriols R, et al: Delayed cutaneous hypersensitivity tests and lymphopenia as activity markers in sarcoidosis. *Chest* 121:1239, 2002.
68. Gentil B, Cottin V, Girard P, Cordier JF: Ambivalence of CD4 lymphocytopenia in sarcoidosis. *Sarcoidosis Vasc Diffuse Lung Dis* 20:74, 2003.

CHAPTER 81

LYMPHOCYTOSIS AND LYMPHOCYTOPENIA

Thomas J. Kipps

SUMMARY

Lymphocytosis is defined as an absolute lymphocyte count exceeding 4×10^9/L (4000/μL), whereas *lymphocytopenia* is defined as a total lymphocyte count less than 1.0×10^9/L (1000/μL). The causes of each are many and varied. Lymphocytosis can be categorized as either polyclonal or monoclonal. *Monoclonal lymphocytosis* generally reflects an underlying lymphoproliferative disease in which the numbers of lymphocytes are increased because of an intrinsic defect in the expanded lymphocyte population, whereas *polyclonal lymphocytosis* most commonly is secondary to stimulation or reaction to factors extrinsic to lymphocytes, generally infections and/or inflammation. Lymphocytopenia, on the other hand, typically reflects depletion of T cells, the most abundant lymphocyte subtype in the blood. The most common cause of such T-cell depletion is viral infection, such as infection with the human immunodeficiency virus, although other causes exist. This chapter outlines the conditions associated with abnormalities in the numbers of circulating lymphocytes in the blood. It also serves as a useful road map to other chapters in the book that describe in detail those conditions that commonly are associated with abnormalities in the absolute numbers of circulating lymphocytes.

LYMPHOCYTOSIS

DEFINITION

Lymphocytosis is defined as an absolute lymphocyte count exceeding 4×10^9/L (4000/μL), although somewhat higher threshold values (e.g., >5.0×10^9/L [>5000/μL]) are sometimes used. The normal absolute lymphocyte count is significantly higher in childhood. Chapter 2 describes the methods for determining the absolute lymphocyte count and the normal range for such counts in older children and adults (see Chap. 2, Tables 2–1 and 2–2). Chapter 6, Tables 6–3 and 6–4, provides the lymphocyte counts and lymphocyte subset counts in newborns and infants.

The blood film of patients with lymphocytosis should be evaluated for a predominance of reactive lymphocytes associated with infectious mononucleosis (see Chap. 84), large granular lymphocytes associated with large granular lymphocytic leukemia (see Chap. 96), smudge cells associated with chronic lymphocytic leukemia (CLL; see Chap. 94), or blasts of acute lymphocytic leukemia (see Chap. 93). Chapter 74 provides a description of normal lymphocyte morphology.

Characterization of cell surface markers is valuable in distinguishing primary lymphocytosis (leukemic) from secondary lymphocytosis (reactive). New improvements in flow cytometric techniques and reagents have allowed clinical laboratories to perform flow cytometric immunophenotyping to distinguish benign from neoplastic lymphoproliferative disease (see Chap. 15). Analysis for immunoglobulin or T-cell receptor gene rearrangement also may provide evidence for monoclonal B-cell or T-cell proliferation, respectively.[1]

Acronyms and abbreviations that appear in this chapter include: CLL, chronic lymphocytic leukemia; EBV, Epstein-Barr virus; HIV, human immunodeficiency virus; Ig, immunoglobulin; NK, natural killer; PPBL, persistent polyclonal B-cell lymphocytosis.

PRIMARY LYMPHOCYTOSIS

Primary lymphocytosis defines conditions associated with an increase in the absolute number of lymphocytes secondary to an intrinsic defect in the expanded lymphocyte population (Table 81–1). These conditions also are referred to as *lymphoproliferative disorders* and most commonly are secondary to the neoplastic accumulation of monoclonal B cells, T cells, natural killer (NK) cells, or less fully differentiated cells of the lymphoid lineage. Table 81–1 lists the chapters describing each of these conditions.

Although patients with lymphocytosis secondary to lymphoproliferative disease generally maintain abnormal lymphocyte counts that may rise over time, this finding is not invariable. Patients with large granular lymphocytic leukemia (see Chap. 96) may have only transient lymphocytosis that is induced by stress or exercise.[2]

Monoclonal B-Cell Lymphocytosis

The advent of multiparameter flow cytometric and molecular diagnostic techniques has identified a syndrome in patients who have expanded populations of monoclonal B cells without other associated clinical signs or symptoms.[3] High-sensitivity flow cytometric techniques, developed to monitor disease in patients with CLL undergoing treatment, have allowed for identification of monoclonal or oligoclonal B-cell populations in more than 5 to 12 percent of healthy individuals who are older than age 60 years, independent of whether they have lymphocytosis.[3,4]

Termed *monoclonal B-cell lymphocytosis*,[5] this condition may portend development of CLL, especially in individuals with CLL-immunophenotype monoclonal B-cell lymphocytosis. Such persons have monoclonal blood B cells with immunophenotypic features of CLL cells (see Chap. 94), but at numbers that are less than the 5000/μL, required to satisfy diagnostic criteria for CLL.[6] CLL requiring treatment develops in patients who have lymphocytosis caused by CLL-phenotype monoclonal B-cell lymphocytosis at the rate of approximately 1.1 percent per year.[3] For such patients, the B-cell count and the absolute lymphocyte count have roughly equivalent value for predicting treatment-free survival as continuous variables, but as binary factors, the absolute B-cell count is the better predictor of treatment-free and overall survival.[7]

Persistent Polyclonal Lymphocytosis of B Lymphocytes

Persistent polyclonal B-cell lymphocytosis (PPBL) is defined as a chronic, moderate increase in absolute lymphocyte counts (>4×10^9/L) without evidence for infection or other conditions that can increase the lymphocyte count. In perhaps the most common manifestation of PPBL, the patients have an accumulation of polyclonal B cells that have an unusual binucleated appearance on the blood film.[8,9] These lymphocytes typically have low-to-negligible expression of CD5 or CD23 found in patients with chronic lymphocytic leukemia[10] and are polyclonal with respect to light-chain expression and immunoglobulin heavy-chain gene rearrangements (Fig. 81–1).[11]

The B cells in PPBL commonly express relatively high levels of immunoglobulin (Ig)D and CD27,[12] a phenotype shared with that of memory B cells (see Chap. 77). Consistent with this phenotype, the immunoglobulin variable-region genes used by the B cells in PPBL most commonly have evidence of somatic mutations, implying that the

TABLE 81–1. Causes of Lymphocytosis

I. Primary lymphocytosis
A. Lymphocytic malignancies
1. Acute lymphocytic leukemia (Chap. 93)
2. Chronic lymphocytic leukemia and related disorders (Chap. 94)
3. Prolymphocytic leukemia (Chap. 94)
4. Hairy cell leukemia[151] (Chap. 95)
5. Adult T-cell leukemia (Chaps. 94 and 106)
6. Leukemic phase of B-cell lymphomas[152] (Chap. 97)
7. Large granular lymphocytic leukemia[153] (Chap. 96)
a. Natural killer (NK) cell leukemia[154] (Chap. 106)
b. CD8+ T-cell large granular lymphocytic leukemia[155–157]
c. CD4+ T-cell large granular lymphocytic leukemia[47,158]
d. γ/δ T-cell large granular lymphocytic leukemia[159]
B. Monoclonal B-cell lymphocytosis[5] (Chap. 94)
C. Persistent polyclonal B cell lymphocytosis[34,160]
II. Reactive lymphocytosis
A. Mononucleosis syndromes (Chap. 84)
1. Epstein-Barr virus[36]
2. Cytomegalovirus[161]
3. Human immunodeficiency virus[162] (Chap. 83)
4. Herpes simplex virus type II
5. Rubella virus[163]
6. *Toxoplasma gondii*[164]
7. Adenovirus
8. Infectious hepatitis virus[165]
9. Dengue fever virus[166–168]
10. Human herpes virus type 6 (HHV-6)[169]
11. Human herpes virus type 8 (HHV-8)[170]
12. Varicella zoster virus[171]
B. *Bordetella pertussis*[172]
C. NK cell lymphocytosis[50,154]
D. Stress lymphocytosis (acute)[66,71]
1. Cardiovascular collapse[65]
a. Acute cardiac failure
b. Myocardial infarction
2. Staphylococcal toxic shock syndrome[173]
3. Drug-induced[70,79,174]
4. Major surgery
5. Sickle cell crisis[175]
6. Status epilepticus
7. Trauma[64,65]
E. Hypersensitivity reactions
1. Insect bite[75–77]
2. Drugs[80,81,83,87,176]
F. Persistent lymphocytosis (subacute or chronic)
1. Cancer[91]
2. Cigarette smoking[20,31,177]
3. Hyposplenism[94]
4. Chronic infection
a. Leishmaniasis[178]
b. Leprosy[179]
c. Strongyloidiasis[54,55,180]
5. Thymoma[90,181]

expanded B cells have undergone germinal center maturation in an immune response(s) to antigen(s).[13,14] Analyses of the immunoglobulin variable-region genes expressed by memory-type B cells of patients with PPBL failed to reveal evidence of positive antigenic selection, suggesting that inappropriate clearance of B cells expressing low-affinity immunoglobulin receptors plays a role in this disorder.[13,15]

The cause(s) of PPBL is unknown. Gender and genotype may be important in the pathogenesis, as the patients most commonly are young to middle-age women who often are HLA-DR7 positive.[8] In addition, there are shared cases of PPBL among identical twins[16] and in families.[17] Moreover, evaluation of first-degree relatives of individuals with PPBL may identify new patients who have all the criteria for diagnosis of PPBL or have slight increases in serum IgM,[18] suggesting a possible hereditary or genetic contribution to the pathogenesis.[19]

Patients with PPBL can have features resembling those of patients with various monoclonal B-cell malignancies. Patients may have mild splenomegaly and raised serum IgM levels, which appears more common among cigarette smokers[20] and persons with the HLA-DR7 haplotype.[8] In some cases, there is modest infiltration of the marrow by polyclonal B cells that can be mistaken for neoplastic disease.[21] Histologic examination of marrow and secondary lymphoid tissues from patients with progressive splenomegaly can reveal features resembling marginal zone B-cell lymphoma (see Chap. 103).[22] In possibly another manifestation of this syndrome, first identified in Japan as hairy B-cell lymphoproliferative disorder,[23] the patients can present with anemia, thrombocytopenia, and splenomegaly and have an excess of polyclonal B lymphocytes that appear similar in morphology and immune phenotype to the neoplastic B cells in hairy cell leukemia (see Chap. 95).[24]

Although the lymphocytosis of PPBL generally is not progressive, most patients have small numbers of blood B cells with chromosomal abnormalities. These abnormalities can include an additional isochromosome +i(3q) and premature chromosome condensation,[9,25–27] and/or the t(14;18) translocation involving the *BCL-2* and immunoglobulin heavy-chain loci that typically is found in the neoplastic B cells of patients with follicular lymphoma (see Chap. 101).[11,17,28,29] In another study of 43 patients with PPBL, two-thirds of patients had lymphocytes with independent chromosomal abnormalities, such as del(6q), +der,[8] +8, or other polyploidy karyotypic abnormalities.[30] In any one patient, these chromosomal abnormalities are restricted to B lymphocytes independent of their expression of immunoglobulin or light chains.[9] For PPBL associated with smoking, these cytogenetic abnormalities apparently persist after the discontinuation of tobacco use.[8] The finding of such chromosome

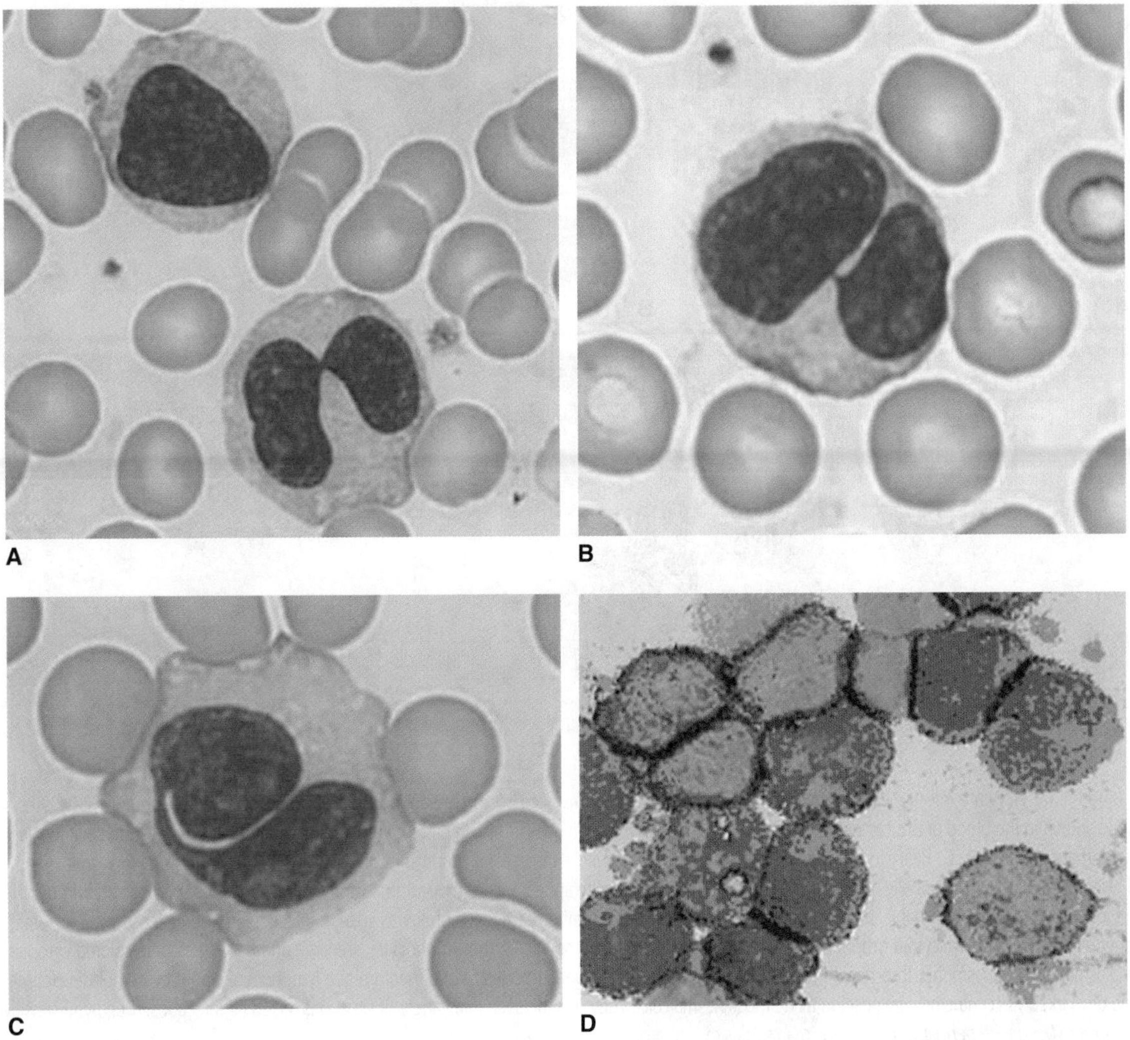

FIGURE 81–1. Persistent polyclonal lymphocytosis of B lymphocytes. Blood film. **A–C.** Examples of the nuclear abnormality of lymphocytes in this disorder. The lymphocyte nucleus may be bilobed or segmented although not fully bilobed. Some are monolobed. **D.** Light chain analysis. Immunoenzymatic method. Cytocentrifuge cell preparation. Anti-kappa immunoglobulin light chain tagged with peroxidase and anti-lambda light chain tagged with alkaline phosphatase. Note polyclonal reactivity of lymphocytes; some cells with surface kappa light chains (*brownish*) and some with surface lambda light chains (*reddish*). Molecular studies did not show immunoglobulin gene rearrangement. *(Used with permission from* Lichtman's Atlas of Hematology, *www.accessmedicine.com. These Atlas images were generously provided by Dr. Xavier Troussard, Laboratoire d'Hématologie CHU Côte de Nacre, Caen, France.)*

abnormalities is consistent with the notion that PPBL represents a preneoplastic state. Occasional reports of clonal immunoglobulin rearrangements in this disorder suggest that polyclonal expansion in some cases may be followed by the emergence of one predominant clone.[8,21,31] Moreover, a small proportion of patients with PPBL ultimately develop monoclonal B-cell lymphoma or B-cell leukemia.[32–34]

■ SECONDARY (REACTIVE) LYMPHOCYTOSIS

Secondary lymphocytosis defines conditions associated with an increase in the absolute number of lymphocytes secondary to a physiologic or pathophysiologic response to infection, toxins, cytokines, or unknown factors.[35]

Infectious Mononucleosis

The most common reactive lymphocytosis is infectious mononucleosis (see Table 81–1). In cases of mononucleosis secondary to infection with Epstein-Barr virus (EBV), the atypical lymphocytes commonly consist of polyclonal populations of CD8+ T cells, γ/δ T cells, and CD16+CD56+ NK cells that are stimulated in response to EBV-infected B cells (see Chap. 84, Fig. 84–1).[36] Typically, no changes in the absolute CD4+ T-cell and CD19+ B-cell counts are observed.

Acute Infection Lymphocytosis

Acute infection lymphocytosis is a disorder that occurs in children usually between the ages of 2 and 10 years. It is characterized by an increase in blood lymphocytes, often to 20 to 30 × 10^9/L (20,000–30,000/μL)[37] and occasionally to as high as 100 × 10^9/L (100,000/μL), which might be mistaken for acute leukemia.[38] The lymphocytes may have some variation in size but they are similar in features to normal blood lymphocytes (Fig. 81–2). Patients usually are asymptomatic but may have fever, abdominal pain, or diarrhea. Lymph node enlargement and splenomegaly do not occur, and the patient's serum usually is negative for heterophile antibodies found in patients with infectious mononucleosis caused by EBV. In this regard, the disease resembles infectious mononucleosis

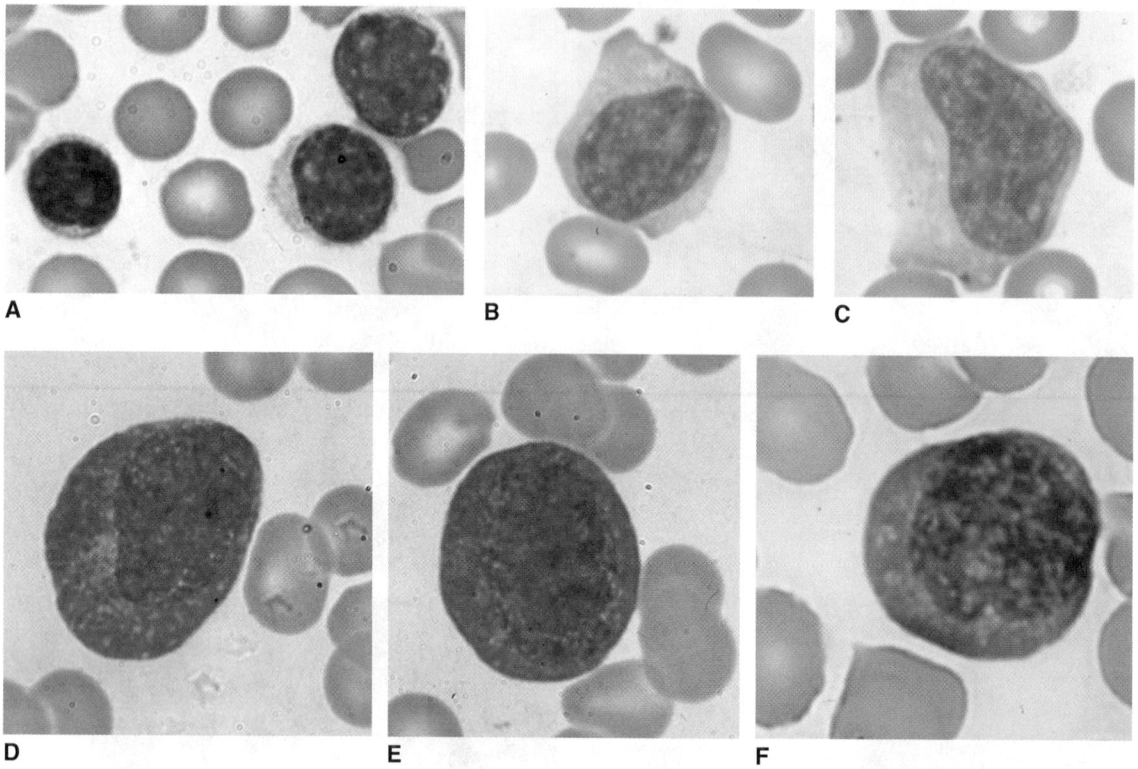

FIGURE 81–2. Blood films. **A.** Acute infectious lymphocytosis. The lymphocytosis in this disorder of childhood is composed of normal appearing lymphocytes, which may vary somewhat in size as shown in the blood of this case. Note typical small lymphocyte with dense chromatin pattern and scant rim of cytoplasm and somewhat two larger lymphocytes with less dense chromatin pattern. **B, C.** Reactive lymphocytes. Large lymphocytes with an increased proportion of cytoplasm with basophilic cytoplasmic edges, often engaging neighboring red cells. Nucleoli may occasionally be evident. This variation in lymphocyte appearance can occur in a variety of disorders that provoke an immunologic response, including viral illnesses. They are indistinguishable in appearance by light microscopy from the reactive lymphocytes seen in infectious mononucleosis, viral hepatitis, or other conditions such as Dengue fever. **D–F.** Plasmacytoid lymphocytes. In this type of reactive lymphocytosis, the lymphocytes are large and have deep blue-colored cytoplasm, approaching the coloration of plasma cell cytoplasm, but they retain the nuclear appearance, cell shape, and cell size of a medium-size lymphocyte, and they do not develop a prominent paranuclear clear zone or markedly eccentric nuclear position as do most plasma cells. They may be seen in a variety of situations including infections, drug hypersensitivity, and serum-sickness-type reactions. *(Used with permission from* Lichtman's Atlas of Hematology, *www.accessmedicine.com.)*

caused by viruses other than EBV, such as cytomegalovirus (see Chap. 84).[39,40] Clinical symptoms last for a few days, but the lymphocytosis may persist for several weeks. Eosinophilia may be present.[41] Examination of marrow from a few patients has shown minimal increases in lymphocytes, but marked infiltration with lymphocytes also has been observed. In some cases, the lymphocytosis has been found in association with acute infection by coxsackievirus B2.[42]

Bordetella Pertussis

A marked increase in the number of lymphocytes occurs in patients infected with the Gram-negative bacterium *Bordetella pertussis*. Absolute lymphocyte counts range from 8 to 70 × 10^9/L (8000–70,000/μL), with a mean of approximately 30 × 10^9/L (30,000/μL), involving all lymphocyte subsets.[43] A notable proportion of lymphocytes have clefted nuclei, characteristic of the cells in cases of pertussis (see Chap. 74, Fig. 74–1C).

Lymphocytosis primarily results from failure of lymphocytes to leave the blood because of *pertussis toxin*, which is released by the bacteria.[44] Pertussis toxin is an adenosine diphosphate ribosylase that modifies Gi proteins in mammalian lymphocytes. This inhibits the capacity of lymphocytes to traffic from blood into lymphoid tissues, primarily through inhibition of chemokine receptors. Pertussis toxin also may stimulate egress of maturing T cells from the thymus[45] and may bind to neuraminic acid residues of T-cell surface glycoproteins to induce T-cell activation.[46]

Large Granular Lymphocytosis

Large granular lymphocytosis can result from expansions of NK cells, CD8+ T cells, or, more rarely, CD4+ T cells.[47–49] In the most common form, the lymphocytosis is secondary to CD3– CD16+ CD56+ NK cells and is termed *NK lymphocytosis*, in which NK cell counts typically approximate 4 × 10^9/L (4000/μL), but can sometimes exceed 15 × 10^9/L (15,000/μL).[50] The blood lymphocytes of patients with T-cell large granular lymphocytosis should be evaluated for clonal rearrangements in the T-cell receptor genes (see Chap. 78),[51] which would be indicative of T-cell large granular lymphocytic leukemia (see Chap. 96, Fig. 96–1).

Expansion of NK cells or T cells may represent an exaggerated response to systemic infection and/or immune deregulation. T-cell large granular lymphocytosis may be secondary to an exaggerated cellular immune response to infection with human cytomegalovirus.[48,52,53] Also, there are reports describing an association between NK lymphocytosis and strongyloidiasis.[54,55] A high incidence of NK lymphocytosis has been reported associated with the use of the kinase inhibitor, dasatinib, for treatment of Philadelphia-chromosome-positive leukemia.[56]

Patients with NK lymphocytosis frequently have recurrent cutaneous lesions, such as livedoid vasculopathy, urticarial vasculitis, or complex recurrent aphthous stomatitis.[57,58] Other reports noted an association between NK lymphocytosis and various cytopenias, including severe aplastic anemia.[50,59] Large granular lymphocytosis also may be associated with rheumatoid arthritis. Occurring in less than 0.6 percent of patients with rheumatoid arthritis, large granular lymphocytic lymphocytosis almost invariably is associated with neutropenia in the absence of splenomegaly and thus may represent a subset disorder of patients with Felty syndrome.[60,61] Patients with autoimmune pure red cell aplasia or immune thrombocytopenia also may have large granular lymphocytosis secondary to expanded numbers of polyclonal T cells[62] or NK cells.[50,59,63]

Stress Lymphocytosis

Trauma, surgery, acute cardiac failure, septic shock, myocardial infarction, sickle cell crisis, or status epilepticus may be associated with an elevated lymphocyte count, often greater than 5×10^9/L (5000/μL),[64–68] which may revert to normal or below-normal levels within hours.[69] The increased lymphocyte count appears promptly after the event and appears secondary to lymphocyte redistribution affecting all major lymphocyte subsets.[70,71] A transient lymphocytosis can be induced by the adrenaline released and/or administered in response to the medical episode.[72–74] Characteristically, two phases are recognized after catecholamine administration: a quick (<30 minutes) mobilization of lymphocytes, followed by an increase in granulocyte numbers with decreasing lymphocyte numbers.[73]

Hypersensitivity Reactions

Delayed hypersensitivity reactions to insect bites, especially mosquitos, may be associated with a large granular lymphocytic lymphocytosis and adenopathy.[75–78] Idiosyncratic drug reactions also may be associated with subacute lymphocytosis, typically developing 2 to 8 weeks after initiating administration of the responsible drug.[79–86] An infectious mononucleosis-like syndrome can be induced in some patients by salazosulfapyridine[87] or sulfasalazine (see Fig. 81–2).[81]

Persistent Lymphocytosis

Patients may have subacute or chronic lymphocytosis, termed *persistent lymphocytosis*, in association with a variety of clinical conditions (see Table 81–1).

Cancer Patients with lymphocytosis may have underlying neoplastic disease. Most notably, patients with malignant thymoma may have a polyclonal T-cell lymphocytosis thought to be secondary to the aberrant release of thymic hormones by the neoplastic thymic epithelium.[88–90] A reactive lymphocytosis or plasmacytosis may be detected in patients with acute myeloid leukemia[91,92] or systemic mastocytosis.[93] Patients with solid tumors also may develop lymphocytosis following cancer chemotherapy.[75]

Postsplenectomy Lymphocytosis Patients may develop polyclonal lymphocytosis following splenectomy.[57,94,95] An absolute lymphocyte count ranging from 4.0 to 8.7×10^9/L often is noted 4 to 242 (median 70) months after splenectomy and can persist for prolonged periods (e.g., >50 months).

Chronic Infections A reactive lymphocytosis commonly is associated with many viral and certain bacterial infections, which, if protracted, can result in subacute or chronic lymphocytosis (see Table 81–1).[35]

LYMPHOCYTOPENIA

DEFINITION

Chapter 2 presents the methods for determining the absolute lymphocyte count and the normal range for such counts. *Lymphocytopenia* is defined as a total lymphocyte count less than 1.0×10^9/L (1000/μL), but some consider the lower limit of normal to be 1.5×10^9/L (1500/μL). Because approximately 80 percent of normal adult blood lymphocytes are T lymphocytes and nearly two-thirds of blood T lymphocytes are CD4+ (helper) T lymphocytes, most patients with lymphocytopenia have reductions in the absolute numbers of T lymphocytes, particularly CD4+ T lymphocytes. The average absolute number of T lymphocytes in normal adult blood is 1.9×10^9/L (1900/μL), ranging from 1.0 to 2.3×10^9/L (1000–2300/μL).[96] The average absolute number of CD4+ T lymphocytes is 1.1×10^9/L (1100/μL), ranging from 7.2 to 14×10^8/L (720–1400/μL). The average absolute number of cells of the other major T-cell subgroup, CD8+ T lymphocytes, is 6.5×10^8/L (650/μL), ranging from 3.8 to 9.7×10^8/L (380–970/μL).

Table 81–2 summarizes the conditions associated with lymphocytopenia. The mechanism of lymphocytopenia is not established for many of these disorders, and several possible mechanisms exist. Further discussion of lymphocytes and of the diseases associated with lymphocytopenia are presented in the cited reports (Table 81–2).

The relative incidence of each of these conditions varies, depending upon the patient population. In one New Zealand survey of patients who had significant lymphocytopenia (<0.6×10^9/L), the patients fell into several categories with some overlap.[97] In order of decreasing frequency, the factors associated with lymphocytopenia were bacterial or fungal sepsis (250 patients), major surgery (228 patients), definite (153 patients) or suspected (53 patients) glucocorticoid therapy, malignancy (180 patients), cytotoxic therapy and/or radiotherapy (90 patients), recent trauma or hemorrhage (86 patients), renal allograft (38 patients), marrow allograft (35 patients), "viral infections" other than human immunodeficiency virus (HIV; 26 patients), or infection with HIV (13 patients). Only one patient was suspected of having idiopathic CD4+ T lymphocytopenia.

INHERITED CAUSES

Patients with inherited immunodeficiency diseases may have associated lymphocytopenia (see Table 81–2 and see Chap. 82, Table 82–2). Inherited immunodeficiency disorders may have a quantitative or qualitative stem cell abnormality, resulting in ineffective lymphopoiesis (see references cited in Table 81–2). Moreover, mutations in the genes that are critical for T-cell development can results in severe combined immunodeficiency and lymphocytopenia as a consequence of the inability to generate mature T cells (see Chap. 78).[98] Other immune deficiencies, such as the Wiskott-Aldrich syndrome, have associated lymphopenia because of premature destruction of T cells secondary to a defect in the lymphocyte cytoskeleton.[99] Studies have reported that certain ethnic groups have lower CD4+ T-cell counts in the absence of other identified factors, for example, Ethiopians[100] and Chukotka natives.[101]

ACQUIRED LYMPHOCYTOPENIA

Acquired lymphocytopenia defines syndromes associated with depletion of blood lymphocytes that are not secondary to inherited disease.

Infectious Diseases

The most common infectious disease associated with lymphopenia is the acquired immunodeficiency syndrome (see Chap. 83). The lymphocytopenia results in part from destruction and/or clearance of CD4+ T cells infected with HIV-1 or HIV-2.[96,102,103]

Other viral and bacterial diseases may be associated with lymphocytopenia (see Table 81–2). Patients presenting with active tuberculosis often have lymphocytopenia that usually resolves 2 weeks after initiating appropriate antimicrobial therapy[104–106] and/or recombinant

TABLE 81–2. Causes of Lymphocytopenia

I. Inherited causes
- A. Congenital immunodeficiency diseases[182] (Chap. 82)
  1. Severe combined immunodeficiency disease[98]
     a. Aplasia of lymphopoietic stem cells
     b. Adenosine deaminase deficiency[183]
     c. Absence of histocompatibility antigens[184]
     d. Absence of CD4+ helper cells[185]
     e. Thymic alymphoplasia with aleukocytosis (reticular dysgenesis)[186]
     f. Mutations in genes required for T-cell development[98]
  2. Common variable immune deficiency[187,188]
  3. Ataxia-telangiectasia[189]
  4. Wiskott-Aldrich syndrome[190]
  5. Immunodeficiency with short-limbed dwarfism (cartilage-hair hypoplasia)[191]
  6. Immunodeficiency with thymoma[192]
  7. Purine nucleoside phosphorylase deficiency[193]
  8. Immunodeficiency with venoocclusive disease of the liver[194]
- B. Lymphopenia resulting from genetic polymorphism[100,101]

II. Acquired causes
- A. Aplastic anemia[195] (Chap. 34)
- B. Infectious diseases
  1. Viral diseases
     a. Acquired immunodeficiency syndrome[196] (Chap. 83)
     b. Severe acute respiratory syndrome[1,97,109,110,198–201]
     c. West Nile encephalitis[202–204]
     d. Hepatitis[96]
     e. Influenza[205,206]
     f. Herpes simplex virus[207]
     g. Herpes virus type 6 (HHV-6)[208,209]
     h. Herpes virus type 8 (HHV-8)[210,211]
     i. Measles virus[111,112]
     j. Other[212]
  2. Bacterial diseases
     a. Tuberculosis[104–106,213]
     b. Typhoid fever[214]
     c. Pneumonia[215]
     d. Rickettsiosis[216]
     e. Ehrlichiosis[217]
     f. Sepsis[218,219]
  3. Parasitic diseases
     a. Acute phase of malaria infection[220–222]
- C. Iatrogenic
  1. Immunosuppressive agents[223,224]
     a. Antilymphocyte globulin therapy[225]
     b. Alemtuzumab (CAMPATH 1-H)[226]
     c. Glucocorticoids[227]
  2. High-dose psoralen plus ultraviolet A treatment[113]
  3. Stevens-Johnson syndrome[228]
  4. Chemotherapy[229]
  5. Platelet or stem cell apheresis procedures[119,120]
  6. Radiation[230]
  7. Major surgery[231,232]
  8. Extracorporeal bypass circulation[233,234]
  9. Renal or marrow transplant[235]
  10. Thoracic duct drainage[118]
  11. Hemodialysis[236]
  12. Pheresis for donor lymphocyte infusion[237]
- D. Systemic disease associated
  1. Autoimmune diseases[121]
     a. Arthritis[238]
     b. Systemic lupus erythematosus[123,124,239,240]
     c. Sjögren syndrome[241]
     d. Myasthenia gravis[242]
     e. Systemic vasculitis[240]
     f. Behçet-like syndrome[243]
     g. Dermatomyositis[244]
     h. Wegener granulomatosis[245]
  2. Hodgkin lymphoma[246] (Chap. 99)
  3. Carcinoma[246]
  4. Idiopathic myelofibrosis[247]
  5. Protein-losing enteropathy[248,249]
  6. Renal failure[250]
  7. Sarcoidosis[251–254]
  8. Thermal injury[125]
  9. Severe acute pancreatitis[255]
  10. Strenuous exercise[256,257]
  11. Silicosis[258]
  12. Celiac disease[259]
- E. Nutritional and dietary
  1. Ethanol abuse[128]
  2. Zinc deficiency[126,127]

III. Idiopathic
- A. Idiopathic CD4+ T lymphocytopenia[132,135,142,149,150]

interleukin-2.[107] Patients with severe acute respiratory syndrome resulting from infection with coronavirus typically have lymphocytopenia that resolves following recovery.[108–110] Several other common viral diseases, such as measles,[111,112] typically are associated with transient lymphocytopenia during the acute phases of infection, which in turn is thought to contribute to a disease course-related immunodeficiency that can predispose patients to infection with opportunistic infectious agents (see Table 81–2).

Iatrogenic

Radiotherapy, cytotoxic chemotherapy, glucocorticoids, or administration of antilymphocyte globulin or alemtuzumab (CAMPATH-1H) each can lead to lymphocytopenia by destroying circulating lymphocytes (see Table 81–2). Long-term treatment of psoriasis with psoralen and ultraviolet A irradiation may result in T-lymphocyte lymphopenia, possibly through destruction of cells circulating through the cutaneous vasculature.[113] The mechanism by which glucocorticoids cause lymphocytopenia is not clear, but may be secondary to a glucocorticoid-induced redistribution of lymphocytes[114,115] in addition to induced cell destruction.[115,116] Redistribution also may be responsible for the lymphocytopenia occurring after surgery.[117] In thoracic duct drainage, the lymphocytes are lost from the body.[118] Platelet or stem cell apheresis similarly lowers the lymphocyte count because of inadvertent removal of lymphocytes with the platelets.[119,120]

Systematic Disease Associated with Lymphocytopenia

Patients with systemic autoimmune disease can have lymphocytopenia, secondary to either the underlying disease or therapy.[121,122] Patients who present with systemic lupus erythematosus may have autoantibody-mediated lymphocytopenia prior to therapy.[123,124] Similarly, patients with primary Sjögren syndrome sometimes have lymphocytopenia even prior to therapy.[122] In conditions such as protein-losing enteropathy, lymphocytes may be lost from the body. Severe thermal injury may result in profound T-cell lymphopenia secondary to redistribution of blood T cells to the tissues.[125]

Nutritional or Dietary

Zinc is essential for normal T-cell development and function.[126,127] Zinc therapy corrects the lymphocytopenia of zinc deficiency, and lymphocytic function is restored. Excessive intake of ethanol and/or chronic ethanol use may result in impaired lymphocyte proliferative responses and lymphopenia, which may resolve with abstinence from alcohol.[128] Concerns over whether the soy isoflavones found in soy protein can factor in the development of lymphocytopenia appear unjustified.[129]

IDIOPATHIC CD4+ T LYMPHOCYTOPENIA

The advent of immunophenotyping and HIV serologic testing has identified a syndrome of isolated CD4+ T-cell depletion in the absence of evidence for retroviral infection.[130,131] The syndrome, termed *idiopathic CD4+ T lymphocytopenia* by the Centers for Disease Control and Prevention in 1993, is defined by a CD4+ T-lymphocyte count less than 3×10^8/L (300/μL) on two separate occasions in patients without serologic or virologic evidence of HIV-1 or HIV-2 infection.[132] Unlike HIV infection, the decrease in the CD4 cell counts of patients with idiopathic CD4+ T-lymphocytopenia is generally slow.[131] It is important to exclude congenital immunodeficiency diseases, such as common variable immunodeficiency, which may lead to altered CD4+ T-cell counts that are recognized in later life (see Chap. 82).[96,133] The pathogenesis of this disorder is not known, although one study found that the CD4+ T cells from patients with this abnormality were unusually sensitive to programmed cell death induced by T-cell receptor crosslinking.[134]

Although some patients with idiopathic CD4+ T lymphocytopenia do not have any clinical manifestations,[135,136] more than half of all reported cases had prior opportunistic infections indicative of a cellular immunodeficiency (e.g., recurrent herpes zoster, pulmonary *Mycobacterium avium*, *Pneumocystis carinii* pneumonia, toxoplasmosis, or cryptococcal infections).[131,137–145] The World Health Organization classifies such patients as having idiopathic CD4+ T-lymphocytopenia and severe unexplained HIV-seronegative immune suppression.[96]

The exact proportion of patients with this disorder is unknown because patients who are not affected clinically by the isolated CD4+ T-cell depletion may not come to medical attention. There are several reports of this abnormality in aged individuals, suggesting that the incidence is increased in the aged population.[146–148] CD4+ T-lymphocytopenic patients with this condition differ from those infected with HIV in that they generally have stable CD4+ counts over time and may manifest reductions in other lymphocyte subgroups.[149,150] Also, patients with this abnormality may have a complete or partial spontaneous reversal in the CD4+ T lymphocytopenia.[149]

REFERENCES

1. Rockman SP: Determination of clonality in patients who present with diagnostic dilemmas: A laboratory experience and review of the literature. *Leukemia* 11:852, 1997.
2. de Pasquale A, Ginaldi L, di Leonardo G, et al: Exercise-induced variations of lymphocytosis in the lymphoproliferative disease of large granular lymphocytes [letter]. *Br J Haematol* 82:178, 1992.
3. Rawstron AC, Bennett FL, O'Connor SJ, et al: Monoclonal B-cell lymphocytosis and chronic lymphocytic leukemia. *N Engl J Med* 359:575, 2008.
4. Nieto WG, Almeida J, Romero A, et al: Increased frequency (12%) of circulating chronic lymphocytic leukemia-like B-cell clones in healthy subjects using a highly sensitive multicolor flow cytometry approach. *Blood* 114:33, 2009.
5. Marti G, Abbasi F, Raveche E, et al: Overview of monoclonal B-cell lymphocytosis. *Br J Haematol* 139:701, 2007.
6. Hallek M, Cheson BD, Catovsky D, et al: Guidelines for the diagnosis and treatment of chronic lymphocytic leukemia: A report from the International Workshop on Chronic Lymphocytic Leukemia updating the National Cancer Institute-Working Group 1996 guidelines. *Blood* 111:5446, 2008.
7. Shanafelt TD, Kay NE, Jenkins G, et al: B-cell count and survival: Differentiating chronic lymphocytic leukemia from monoclonal B-cell lymphocytosis based on clinical outcome. *Blood* 113:4188, 2009.
8. Troussard X, Flandrin G: Chronic B-cell lymphocytosis with binucleated lymphocytes (LWBL): A review of 38 cases. *Leuk Lymphoma* 20:275, 1996.
9. Mossafa H, Malaure H, Maynadie M, et al: Persistent polyclonal B lymphocytosis with binucleated lymphocytes: A study of 25 cases. Groupe Français d'Hématologie Cellulaire. *Br J Haematol* 104:486, 1999.
10. Schmidt-Hieber M, Burmeister T, Weimann A, et al: Combined automated cell and flow cytometric analysis enables recognition of persistent polyclonal B-cell lymphocytosis (PPBL), a study of 25 patients. *Ann Hematol* 87:829, 2008.
11. Delage R, Roy J, Jacques L, et al: Multiple bcl-2/Ig gene rearrangements in persistent polyclonal B-cell lymphocytosis. *Br J Haematol* 97:589, 1997.
12. Himmelmann A, Gautschi O, Nawrath M, et al: Persistent polyclonal B-cell lymphocytosis is an expansion of functional IgD(+)CD27(+) memory B cells. *Br J Haematol* 114:400, 2001.
13. Loembe MM, Neron S, Delage R, Darveau A: Analysis of expressed V(H) genes in persistent polyclonal B cell lymphocytosis reveals absence of selection in CD27+IgM+IgD+ memory B cells. *Eur J Immunol* 32:3678, 2002.
14. Salcedo I, Campos-Caro A, Sampalo A, et al: Persistent polyclonal B lymphocytosis: An expansion of cells showing IgVH gene mutations and phenotypic features of normal lymphocytes from the CD27+ marginal zone B-cell compartment. *Br J Haematol* 116:662, 2002.
15. Roussel M, Roue G, Sola B, et al: Dysfunction of the Fas apoptotic signaling pathway in persistent polyclonal B-cell lymphocytosis. *Haematologica* 88:239, 2003.
16. Carr R, Fishlock K, Matutes E: Persistent polyclonal B-cell lymphocytosis in identical twins. *Br J Haematol* 96:272, 1997.
17. Himmelmann A, Ruegg R, Fehr J: Familial persistent polyclonal B-cell lymphocytosis. *Leuk Lymphoma* 41:157, 2001.
18. Delage R, Jacques L, Massinga-Loembe M, et al: Persistent polyclonal B-cell lymphocytosis: Further evidence for a genetic disorder associated with B-cell abnormalities. *Br J Haematol* 114:666, 2001.
19. Wolowiec D, Nowak J, Majewski M, et al: High incidence of ancestral HLA haplotype 8.1 and monoclonal incomplete DH-JH immunoglobulin heavy chain gene rearrangement in persistent polyclonal B-cell lymphocytosis. *Ann Hematol* 87:597, 2008.
20. Delannoy A, Djian D, Wallef G, et al: Cigarette smoking and chronic polyclonal B-cell lymphocytosis. *Nouv Rev Fr Hematol* 35:141, 1993.
21. Feugier P, De March AK, Lesesve JF, et al: Intravascular bone marrow accumulation in persistent polyclonal lymphocytosis: A misleading feature for B-cell neoplasm. *Mod Pathol* 17:1087, 2004.
22. Del Giudice I, Pileri SA, Rossi M, et al: Histopathological and molecular features of persistent polyclonal B-cell lymphocytosis (PPBL) with progressive splenomegaly. *Br J Haematol* 144:726, 2009.
23. Machii T, Yamaguchi M, Inoue R, et al: Polyclonal B-cell lymphocytosis with features resembling hairy cell leukemia-Japanese variant [see comments]. *Blood* 89:2008, 1997.

24. Okamoto A, Inaba T, and Fujita N: The role of interleukin-6 in a patient with polyclonal hairy B-cell lymphoproliferative disorder: A case report. *Lab Hematol* 13:124, 2007.
25. Callet-Bauchu E, Renard N, Gazzo S, et al: Distribution of the cytogenetic abnormality +i(3)(q10) in persistent polyclonal B-cell lymphocytosis: A FICTION study in three cases. *Br J Haematol* 99:531, 1997.
26. Espinet B, Florensa L, Sole F, et al: Isochromosome +i(3)(q10) in a new case of persistent polyclonal B-cell lymphocytosis (PPBL). *Eur J Haematol* 64:344, 2000.
27. Samson T, Mossafa H, Lusina D, et al: Dicentric chromosome 3 associated with binucleated lymphocytes in atypical B-cell chronic lymphoproliferative disorder. *Leuk Lymphoma* 43:1749, 2002.
28. Granados E, Llamas P, Pinilla I, et al: Persistent polyclonal B lymphocytosis with multiple bcl-2/IgH rearrangements: A benign disorder. *Haematologica* 83:369, 1998.
29. Lancry L, Roulland S, Roue G, et al: No BCL-2 protein over expression but BCL-2/IgH rearrangements in B cells of patients with persistent polyclonal B-cell lymphocytosis. *Hematol J* 2:228, 2001.
30. Mossafa H, Tapia S, Flandrin G, Troussard X: Chromosomal instability and ATR amplification gene in patients with persistent and polyclonal B-cell lymphocytosis (PPBL). *Leuk Lymphoma* 45:1401, 2004.
31. Chan MA, Benedict SH, Carstairs KC, et al: Expansion of B lymphocytes with an unusual immunoglobulin rearrangement associated with atypical lymphocytosis and cigarette smoking. *Am J Respir Cell Mol Biol* 2:549, 1990.
32. Bassan R, Spinelli O, Rambaldi A, Barbui T: The course of monoclonal 'villous' lymphocytosis over 15 years of follow-up: Progression to SLVL or spontaneous clinical but not molecular remission. *Leukemia* 17:2243, 2003.
33. Radossi P, Dazzi F, De Franchis G, et al: Myasthenic syndrome and oligoclonal lymphocytosis: Evolution into chronic lymphocytic leukemia. *Ann Hematol* 76:45, 1998.
34. Cornet E, Lesesve JF, Mossafa H, et al: Long-term follow-up of 111 patients with persistent polyclonal B-cell lymphocytosis with binucleated lymphocytes. *Leukemia* 23:419, 2009.
35. Brown KA: Nonmalignant disorders of lymphocytes. *Clin Lab Sci* 10:329, 1997.
36. Hudnall SD, Patel J, Schwab H, and Martinez J: Comparative immunophenotypic features of EBV-positive and EBV-negative atypical lymphocytosis. *Cytometry B Clin Cytom* 55:22, 2003.
37. Horwitz MS, and Moore GT: Acute infectious lymphocytosis: An etiologic and epidemilogic study of an outbreak. *N Engl J Med* 279:399, 1968.
38. Yetgin S, Kuskonmaz B, Aytac S, Tavil B: An unusual case of reactive lymphocytosis mimicking acute leukemia. *Pediatr Hematol Oncol* 24:129, 2007.
39. Kunno A, Abe M, Yamada M, Murakami K: Clinical and histological features of cytomegalovirus hepatitis in previously healthy adults. *Liver* 17:129, 1997.
40. Labalette M, Salez F, Pruvot FR, et al: CD8 lymphocytosis in primary cytomegalovirus (CMV) infection of allograft recipients: Expansion of an uncommon CD8+ CD57− subset and its progressive replacement by CD8+ CD57+ T cells. *Clin Exp Immunol* 95:465, 1994.
41. Roumier AS, Grardel N, Lai JL, et al: Hypereosinophilia with abnormal T cells, trisomy 7 and elevated TARC serum level. *Haematologica* 88:ECR24, 2003.
42. Arnez M, Cizman M, Jazbec J, Kotnik A: Acute infectious lymphocytosis caused by coxsackievirus B2. *Pediatr Infect Dis J* 15:1127, 1996.
43. Hodge G, Hodge S, Markus C, et al: A marked decrease in L-selectin expression by leucocytes in infants with Bordetella pertussis infection: Leucocytosis explained? *Respirology* 8:157, 2003.
44. Verschueren H, Dewit J, Van der Wegen A, et al: The lymphocytosis promoting action of pertussis toxin can be mimicked *in vitro*. Holotoxin but not the B subunit inhibits invasion of human T lymphoma cells through fibroblast monolayers. *J Immunol Methods* 144:231, 1991.
45. Suzuki G, Sawa H, Kobayashi Y, et al: Pertussis toxin-sensitive signal controls the trafficking of thymocytes across the corticomedullary junction in the thymus. *J Immunol* 162:5981, 1999.
46. Witvliet MH, Vogel ML, Wiertz EJ, Poolman JT: Interaction of pertussis toxin with human T lymphocytes. *Infect Immun* 60:5085, 1992.
47. Lima M, Almeida J, Dos Anjos Teixeira M, et al: TCRalphabeta+/CD4+ large granular lymphocytosis: A new clonal T-cell lymphoproliferative disorder. *Am J Pathol* 163:763, 2003.
48. van Steensel MA, van Gelder M, van Marion AM, et al: T-cell large granular lymphocytic leukaemia with an uncommon clinical and immunological phenotype. *Acta Derm Venereol* 89:172, 2009.
49. Moura J, Rodrigues J, Santos AH, et al: Chemokine receptor repertoire reflects mature T-cell lymphoproliferative disorder clinical presentation. *Blood Cells Mol Dis* 42:57, 2009.
50. Rabbani G, Phyliky R, Tefferi A: A long-term study of patients with chronic natural killer cell lymphocytosis. *Br J Haematol* 106:960, 1999.
51. O'Malley DP: T-cell large granular leukemia and related proliferations. *Am J Clin Pathol* 127:850, 2007.
52. Rossi D, Franceschetti S, Capello D, et al: Transient monoclonal expansion of CD8+/CD57+ T-cell large granular lymphocytes after primary cytomegalovirus infection. *Am J Hematol* 82:1103, 2007.
53. Crompton L, Khan N, Khanna R, et al: CD4+ T cells specific for glycoprotein B from cytomegalovirus exhibit extreme conservation of T-cell receptor usage between different individuals. *Blood* 111:2053, 2008.
54. del Giudice P: Strongyloidiasis and natural killer cell lymphocytosis. *Br J Dermatol* 142:1066, 2000.
55. Myers B, Speight EL, Huissoon AP, Davies JM: Natural killer-cell lymphocytosis and strongyloides infection. *Clin Lab Haematol* 22:237, 2000.
56. Kim DH, Kamel-Reid S, Chang H, et al: Natural killer or natural killer/T cell lineage large granular lymphocytosis associated with dasatinib therapy for Philadelphia chromosome positive leukemia. *Haematologica* 94:135, 2009.
57. Granjo E, Lima M, Fraga M, et al: Abnormal NK cell lymphocytosis detected after splenectomy: Association with repeated infections, relapsing neutropenia, and persistent polyclonal B-cell proliferation. *Int J Hematol* 75:484, 2002.
58. Vanness ER, Davis MD, Tefferi A: Cutaneous findings associated with chronic natural killer cell lymphocytosis. *Int J Dermatol* 41:852, 2002.
59. Kaito K, Otsubo H, Ogasawara Y, et al: Severe aplastic anemia associated with chronic natural killer cell lymphocytosis. *Int J Hematol* 72:463, 2000.
60. Agarwal V, Sachdev A, Lehl S, Basu S: Unusual haematological alterations in rheumatoid arthritis. *J Postgrad Med* 50:60, 2004.
61. Prochorec-Sobieszek M, Rymkiewicz G, Makuch-Lasica H, et al: Characteristics of T-cell large granular lymphocyte proliferations associated with neutropenia and inflammatory arthropathy. *Arthritis Res Ther* 10:R55, 2008.
62. Grossi A, Nozzoli C, Gheri R, et al: Pure red cell aplasia in autoimmune polyglandular syndrome with T lymphocytosis [letter]. *Haematologica* 83:1043, 1998.
63. Garcia-Suarez J, Prieto A, Reyes E, et al: Persistent lymphocytosis of natural killer cells in autoimmune thrombocytopenic purpura (ATP) patients after splenectomy [see comments]. *Br J Haematol* 89:653, 1995.
64. Pinkerton PH, McLellan BA, Quantz MC, Robinson JB: Acute lymphocytosis after trauma—early recognition of the high-risk patient? *J Trauma* 29:749, 1989.
65. Teggatz JR, Parkin J, Peterson L: Transient atypical lymphocytosis in patients with emergency medical conditions. *Arch Pathol Lab Med* 111:712, 1987.
66. Bosch JA, Berntson GG, Cacioppo JT, et al: Acute stress evokes selective mobilization of T cells that differ in chemokine receptor expression: A potential pathway linking immunologic reactivity to cardiovascular disease. *Brain Behav Immun* 17:251, 2003.
67. Mignini F, Traini E, Tomassoni D, et al: Leucocyte subset redistribution in a human model of physical stress. *Clin Exp Hypertens* 30:720, 2008.
68. Anane LH, Edwards KM, Burns VE, et al: Mobilization of gammadelta T lymphocytes in response to psychological stress, exercise, and beta-agonist infusion. *Brain Behav Immun* 23:823, 2009.
69. Thommasen HV, Boyko WJ, Montaner JS, et al: Absolute lymphocytosis associated with nonsurgical trauma. *Am J Clin Pathol* 86:480, 1986.
70. Toft P, Tonnesen E, Svendsen P, et al: The redistribution of lymphocytes during adrenaline infusion. An *in vivo* study with radiolabelled cells. *APMIS* 100:593, 1992.
71. Karandikar NJ, Hotchkiss EC, McKenna RW, Kroft SH: Transient stress lymphocytosis: An immunophenotypic characterization of the most common cause of newly identified adult lymphocytosis in a tertiary hospital. *Am J Clin Pathol* 117:819, 2002.
72. Tonnesen E, Hohndorf K, Lerbjerg G, et al: Immunological and hormonal responses to lung surgery during one-lung ventilation. *Eur J Anaesthesiol* 10:189, 1993.
73. Benschop RJ, Rodriguez-Feuerhahn M, Schedlowski M: Catecholamine-induced leukocytosis: Early observations, current research, and future directions. *Brain Behav Immun* 10:77, 1996.
74. Bergmann M, Sautner T: Immunomodulatory effects of vasoactive catecholamines. *Wien Klin Wochenschr* 114:752, 2002.
75. Chung JS, Shin HJ, Lee EY, Cho GJ: Hypersensitivity to mosquito bites associated with natural killer cell-derived large granular lymphocyte lymphocytosis: A case report in Korea. *Korean J Intern Med* 18:50, 2003.
76. Satoh M, Oyama N, Akiba H, et al: Hypersensitivity to mosquito bites with natural-killer cell lymphocytosis: The possible implication of Epstein-Barr virus reactivation. *Eur J Dermatol* 12:381, 2002.
77. Asada H, Miyagawa S, Sumikawa Y, et al: CD4+ T-lymphocyte-induced Epstein-Barr virus reactivation in a patient with severe hypersensitivity to mosquito bites and Epstein-Barr virus-infected NK cell lymphocytosis. *Arch Dermatol* 139:1601, 2003.
78. Konuma T, Uchimaru K, Sekine R, et al: Atypical hypersensitivity to mosquito bites without natural killer cell proliferative disease in an adult patient. *Int J Hematol* 82:441, 2005.
79. Enomoto M, Ochi M, Teramae K, et al: Codeine phosphate-induced hypersensitivity syndrome. *Ann Pharmacother* 38:799, 2004.
80. Sakai C, Takagi T, Oguro M, et al: Erythroderma and marked atypical lymphocytosis mimicking cutaneous T-cell lymphoma probably caused by phenobarbital. *Intern Med* 32:182, 1993.
81. Halmos B, Anastopoulos HT, Schnipper LE, Ballesteros E: Extreme lymphoplasmacytosis and hepatic failure associated with sulfasalazine hypersensitivity reaction and a concurrent EBV infection—case report and review of the literature. *Ann Hematol* 83:242, 2004.
82. Choi TS, Doh KS, Kim SH, et al: Clinicopathological and genotypic aspects of anticonvulsant-induced pseudolymphoma syndrome. *Br J Dermatol* 148:730, 2003.
83. Leslie KS, Gaffney K, Ross CN, et al: A near fatal case of the dapsone hypersensitivity syndrome in a patient with urticarial vasculitis. *Clin Exp Dermatol* 28:496, 2003.
84. Karande S, Gogtay NJ, Kanchan S, Kshirsagar NA: Anticonvulsant hypersensitivity syndrome to lamotrigine confirmed by lymphocyte stimulation *in vitro*. *Indian J Med Sci* 60:59, 2006.
85. Tsuruta D, Someda Y, Sowa J, et al: Drug hypersensitivity syndrome caused by minocycline. *J Cutan Med Surg* 10:131, 2006.
86. Kano Y, Shiohara T: The variable clinical picture of drug-induced hypersensitivity syndrome/drug rash with eosinophilia and systemic symptoms in relation to the eliciting drug. *Immunol Allergy Clin North Am* 29:481, 2009.

87. Ohtani T, Hiroi A, Sakurane M, Furukawa F: Slow acetylator genotypes as a possible risk factor for infectious mononucleosis-like syndrome induced by salazosulfapyridine. *Br J Dermatol* 148:1035, 2003.
88. Medeiros LJ, Bhagat SK, Naylor P, et al: Malignant thymoma associated with T-cell lymphocytosis. A case report with immunophenotypic and gene rearrangement analysis. *Arch Pathol Lab Med* 117:279, 1993.
89. Cranney A, Markman S, Lach B, Karsh J: Polymyositis in a patient with thymoma and T cell lymphocytosis. *J Rheumatol* 24:1413, 1997.
90. Morales M, Trujillo M, del Carmen Maeso M, Piris MA: Thymoma and progressive T-cell lymphocytosis. *Ann Oncol* 18:603, 2007.
91. Rosenthal NS, Farhi DC: Reactive plasmacytosis and lymphocytosis in acute myeloid leukemia. *Hematol Pathol* 8:43, 1994.
92. Janik-Moszant A, Barc-Czarnecka M, van der Burg M, et al: Concomitant EBV-related B-cell proliferation and juvenile myelomonocytic leukemia in a 2-year-old child. *Leuk Res* 32:181, 2008.
93. Horny HP, Lange K, Sotlar K, Valent P: Increase of bone marrow lymphocytes in systemic mastocytosis: Reactive lymphocytosis or malignant lymphoma? Immunohistochemical and molecular findings on routinely processed bone marrow biopsy specimens. *J Clin Pathol* 56:575, 2003.
94. Juneja S, Januszewicz E, Wolf M, Cooper I: Post-splenectomy lymphocytosis. *Clin Lab Haematol* 17:335, 1995.
95. Domingo P, Fuster M, Muñiz-Diaz E, et al: Spurious post-splenectomy CD4 and CD8 lymphocytosis in HIV-infected patients [letter]. *AIDS* 10:106, 1996.
96. Laurence J: T-cell subsets in health, infectious disease, and idiopathic CD4+ T lymphocytopenia. *Ann Intern Med* 119:55, 1993.
97. Castelino DJ, McNair P, Kay TW: Lymphocytopenia in a hospital population—What does it signify? [see comments]. *Aust N Z J Med*27:170, 1997.
98. Kalman L, Lindegren ML, Kobrynski L, et al: Mutations in genes required for T-cell development: IL7R, CD45, IL2RG, JAK3, RAG1, RAG2, ARTEMIS, and ADA and severe combined immunodeficiency: HuGE review. *Genet Med* 6:16, 2004.
99. Molina IJ, Kenney DM, Rosen FS, Remold-O'Donnell E: T cell lines characterize events in the pathogenesis of the Wiskott-Aldrich syndrome. *J Exp Med* 176:867, 1992.
100. Wolday D, Tsegaye A, Messele T: Low absolute CD4 counts in Ethiopians. *Ethiop Med J* 40 Suppl 1:11, 2002.
101. Gyrgolkay LA, Nikitin YP: Leukogram and white blood cells count in native people of Chukotka. *Int J Circumpolar Health* 60:534, 2001.
102. Phillips AN: CD4 lymphocyte depletion prior to the development of AIDS [editorial; comment]. *AIDS* 6:735, 1992.
103. Daniel V, Melk A, Süsal C, et al: CD4 depletion in HIV-infected haemophilia patients is associated with rapid clearance of immune complex-coated CD4+ lymphocytes. *Clin Exp Immunol* 115:477, 1999.
104. Pilheu JA, De Salvo MC, Gonzalez J, et al: CD4+ T-lymphocytopenia in severe pulmonary tuberculosis without evidence of human immunodeficiency virus infection [see comments]. *Int J Tuberc Lung Dis* 1:422, 1997.
105. Singh KJ, Ahluwalia G, Sharma SK, et al: Significance of haematological manifestations in patients with tuberculosis. *J Assoc Physicians India* 49:788, 790–784, 2001.
106. Olaniyi JA, Aken'Ova YA: Haematological profile of patients with pulmonary tuberculosis in Ibadan, Nigeria. *Afr J Med Med Sci* 32:239, 2003.
107. Trojan T, Collins R, and Khan DA: Safety and efficacy of treatment using interleukin-2 in a patient with idiopathic CD4(+) lymphopenia and *Mycobacterium avium-intracellulare. Clin Exp Immunol* 156:440, 2009.
108. Lin PY, Chiu CH, Wang YH, et al: *Bordetella pertussis* infection in northern Taiwan, 1997–2001. *J Microbiol Immunol Infect* 37:288, 2004.
109. Peiris JS, Lai ST, Poon LL, et al: Coronavirus as a possible cause of severe acute respiratory syndrome. *Lancet* 361:1319, 2003.
110. Yang M, Li CK, Li K, et al: Hematological findings in SARS patients and possible mechanisms (review). *Int J Mol Med* 14:311, 2004.
111. Okada H, Kobune F, Sato TA, et al: Extensive lymphopenia due to apoptosis of uninfected lymphocytes in acute measles patients. *Arch Virol* 145:905, 2000.
112. Am J: Influenza A (H5N1) in Hong Kong: An overview. *Vaccine* 20:S77, 2002.
113. Borroni G, Zaccone C, Vignati G, et al: Lymphopenia and decrease in the total number of circulating CD3+ and CD4+ T cells during "long-term" PUVA treatment for psoriasis. *Dermatologica* 183:10, 1991.
114. Bloemena E, Weinreich S, Schellekens PT: The influence of prednisolone on the recirculation of peripheral blood lymphocytes in vivo. *Clin Exp Immunol* 80:460, 1990.
115. Bloemena E, Koopmans RP, Weinreich S, et al: Pharmacodynamic modeling of lymphocytopenia and whole blood lymphocyte cultures in prednisolone-treated individuals. *Clin Immunol Immunopathol* 57:374, 1990.
116. Braat MC, Oosterhuis B, Koopmans RP, et al: Kinetic-dynamic modeling of lymphocytopenia induced by the combined action of dexamethasone and hydrocortisone in humans, after inhalation and intravenous administration of dexamethasone. *J Pharmacol Exp Ther* 262:509, 1992.
117. Hauser GJ, Chan MM, Casey WF, et al: Immune dysfunction in children after corrective surgery for congenital heart disease [see comments]. *Crit Care Med* 19:874, 1991.
118. Ueo T, Tanaka S, Tominaga Y, et al: The effect of thoracic duct drainage on lymphocyte dynamics and clinical symptoms in patients with rheumatoid arthritis. *Arthritis Rheum* 22:1405, 1979.
119. Prior CR, Coghlan PJ, Hall JM, Jacobs P: In vitro study of immunologic changes in long-term cytapheresis donors. *J Clin Apheresis* 6:69, 1991.
120. Novotny J, Kadar J, Hertenstein B, et al: Sustained decrease of peripheral lymphocytes after allogeneic blood stem cell aphereses. *Br J Haematol* 100:695, 1998.
121. Martin-Suarez I, D'Cruz D, Mansoor M, et al: Immunosuppressive treatment in severe connective tissue diseases: Effects of low dose intravenous cyclophosphamide. *Ann Rheum Dis* 56:481, 1997.
122. Mandl T, Bredberg A, Jacobsson LT, et al: CD4+ T-lymphocytopenia—A frequent finding in anti-SSA antibody seropositive patients with primary Sjögren's syndrome. *J Rheumatol* 31:726, 2004.
123. Wenzel J, Gerdsen R, Uerlich M, et al: Lymphocytopenia in lupus erythematosus: Close *in vivo* association to autoantibodies targeting nuclear antigens. *Br J Dermatol* 150:994, 2004.
124. Ng WL, Chu CM, Wu AK, et al: Lymphopenia at presentation is associated with increased risk of infections in patients with systemic lupus erythematosus. *QJM* 99:37, 2006.
125. Maldonado MD, Venturoli A, Franco A, Nunez-Roldan A: Specific changes in peripheral blood lymphocyte phenotype from burn patients. Probable origin of the thermal injury-related lymphocytopenia. *Burns* 17:188, 1991.
126. Taylor CG, Giesbrecht JA: Dietary zinc deficiency and expression of T lymphocyte signal transduction proteins. *Can J Physiol Pharmacol* 78:823, 2000.
127. Fraker PJ, King LE: Reprogramming of the immune system during zinc deficiency. *Annu Rev Nutr* 24:277, 2004.
128. Kapasi AA, Patel G, Goenka A, et al: Ethanol promotes T cell apoptosis through the mitochondrial pathway. *Immunology* 108:313, 2003.
129. Soung do Y, Patade A, Khalil DA, et al: Soy protein supplementation does not cause lymphocytopenia in postmenopausal women. *Nutr J* 5:12, 2006.
130. Walker UA, Warnatz K: Idiopathic CD4 lymphocytopenia. *Curr Opin Rheumatol* 18:389, 2006.
131. Zonios DI, Falloon J, Bennett JE, et al: Idiopathic CD4+ lymphocytopenia: Natural history and prognostic factors. *Blood* 112:287, 2008.
132. Smith DK, Neal JJ, Holmberg SD: Unexplained opportunistic infections and CD4+ T-lymphocytopenia without HIV infection. An investigation of cases in the United States. The Centers for Disease Control Idiopathic CD4+ T-lymphocytopenia Task Force [see comments]. *N Engl J Med* 328:373, 1993.
133. al-Attas RA, Rahi AH, Ahmed el FE: Common variable immunodeficiency with CD4+ T lymphocytopenia and overproduction of soluble IL-2 receptor associated with Turner's syndrome and dorsal kyphoscoliosis. *J Clin Pathol* 50:876, 1997.
134. Laurence J, Mitra D, Steiner M, et al: Apoptotic depletion of CD4+ T cells in idiopathic CD4+ T lymphocytopenia. *J Clin Invest* 97:672, 1996.
135. Spira TJ, Jones BM, Nicholson JK, et al: Idiopathic CD4+ T-lymphocytopenia—An analysis of five patients with unexplained opportunistic infections [see comments]. *N Engl J Med* 328:386, 1993.
136. Cascio G, Massobrio AM, Cascio B, Anania A: Undefined CD4 lymphocytopenia without clinical complications. A report of two cases. *Panminerva Med* 40:69, 1998.
137. Sinicco A, Maiello A, Raiteri R, et al: Pneumocystis carinii in a patient with pulmonary sarcoidosis and idiopathic CD4+ T lymphocytopenia. *Thorax* 51:446; discussion 448, 1996.
138. Kumlin U, Elmqvist LG, Granlund M, et al: CD4 lymphopenia in a patient with cryptococcal osteomyelitis. *Scand J Infect Dis* 29:205, 1997.
139. Zanelli G, Sansoni A, Ricciardi B, et al: Muscular-skeletal cryptococcosis in a patient with idiopathic CD4+ lymphopenia. *Mycopathologia* 149:137, 2001.
140. Cheung MC, Rachlis AR, Shumak SL: A cryptic cause of cryptococcal meningitis. *CMAJ* 168:451, 2003.
141. Plonquet A, Bassez G, Authier FJ, et al: Toxoplasmic myositis as a presenting manifestation of idiopathic CD4 lymphocytopenia. *Muscle Nerve* 27:761, 2003.
142. Netea MG, Brouwer AE, Hoogendoorn EH, et al: Two patients with cryptococcal meningitis and idiopathic CD4 lymphopenia: Defective cytokine production and reversal by recombinant interferon- gamma therapy. *Clin Infect Dis* 39:e83, 2004.
143. Yuanjie Z, Julin G, Fubing C, Jianghan C: Recurrent pulmonary cryptococcosis in a patient with idiopathic CD4 lymphocytopenia. *Med Mycol* 46:729, 2008.
144. Warnatz K: Review: Cryptococcosis in HIV-negative immunodeficiency. *Clin Adv Hematol Oncol* 6:448, 2008.
145. Luo L, Li T: Idiopathic CD4 lymphocytopenia and opportunistic infection—an update. *FEMS Immunol Med Microbiol* 54:283, 2008.
146. Matsuyama W, Mizoguchi A, Hamasaki T, et al: Idiopathic CD4+ T-lymphocytopenia in chronic obstructive pulmonary disease [letter]. *Intern Med* 38:71, 1999.
147. Belmin J, Ortega MN, Bruhat A, et al: CD4 lymphopenia in elderly patients [letter; comment] [see comments]. *Lancet* 347:911; discussion 912, 1996.
148. McBride M: CD4 lymphopenia in elderly patients [letter; comment]. *Lancet* 347:911; discussion 912, 1996.
149. Ho DD, Cao Y, Zhu T, et al: Idiopathic CD4+ T-lymphocytopenia—Immunodeficiency without evidence of HIV infection [see comments]. *N Engl J Med* 328:380, 1993.
150. Duncan RA, von Reyn CF, Alliegro GM, et al: Idiopathic CD4+ T-lymphocytopenia—Four patients with opportunistic infections and no evidence of HIV infection [see comments]. *N Engl J Med* 328:393, 1993.
151. Adley BP, Sun X, Shaw JM, Variakojis D: Hairy cell leukemia with marked lymphocytosis. *Arch Pathol Lab Med* 127:253, 2003.
152. Nelson BP, Variakojis D, Peterson LC: Leukemic phase of B-cell lymphomas mimicking chronic lymphocytic leukemia and variants at presentation. *Mod Pathol* 15:1111, 2002.

153. Lamy T, Loughran TP Jr: Clinical features of large granular lymphocyte leukemia. *Semin Hematol* 40:185, 2003.
154. Oshimi K: Leukemia and lymphoma of natural killer lineage cells. *Int J Hematol* 78:18, 2003.
155. Granjo E, Lima M, Correia T, et al: Cd8(+)/V beta 5.1(+) large granular lymphocyte leukemia associated with autoimmune cytopenias, rheumatoid arthritis and vascular mammary skin lesions: Successful response to 2-deoxycoformycin. *Hematol Oncol* 20:87, 2002.
156. Krishna MT, Hodges E, Lavender FL, et al: CD3+CD4–CD8+NK– large granular lymphocytosis with neutropenia and evidence for clonality and T-cell receptor gene rearrangement: Two pediatric cases. *J Pediatr Hematol Oncol* 24:495, 2002.
157. Narumi H, Kojima K, Matsuo Y, et al: T-cell large granular lymphocytic leukemia occurring after autologous peripheral blood stem cell transplantation. *Bone Marrow Transplant* 33:99, 2004.
158. Schleinitz N, Brunet C, Pascal V, et al: A CD4+ V(beta)13.6+ CD56+ large granular lymphocyte expansion with decreased expression of CD95 and an indolent clinical course. *Haematologica* 87:ECR35, 2002.
159. Vartholomatos G, Alymara V, Dova L, et al: T-cell receptor gammadelta-large granular lymphocytic leukemia associated with an aberrant phenotype and TCR-Vbeta20 clonality. *Haematologica* 89:ECR16, 2004.
160. Lawrie CH, Shilling R, Troussard X, et al: Expression profiling of persistent polyclonal B-cell lymphocytosis suggests constitutive expression of the AP-1 transcription complex and downregulation of Fas-apoptotic and TGFbeta signalling pathways. *Leukemia* 23:581, 2009.
161. Rodriguez-Caballero A, Garcia-Montero AC, Barcena P, et al: Expanded cells in monoclonal TCR-alphabeta+/CD4+/NKa+/CD8-/+dim T-LGL lymphocytosis recognize hCMV antigens. *Blood* 112:4609, 2008.
162. Basu D, Williams FM, Ahn CW, Reveille JD: Changing spectrum of the diffuse infiltrative lymphocytosis syndrome. *Arthritis Rheum* 55:466, 2006.
163. Amor B, Dougados M, Carlioz R, Menkes CJ: [Lymphocytic arthritis. 54 cases, of which 25 appear to be idiopathic]. *Rev Rhum Mal Osteoartic* 50:507, 1983.
164. Brown KA: Nonmalignant disorders of lymphocytes. *Clin Lab Sci* 10:329, 1997.
165. Carmack S, Taddei T, Robert ME, et al: Increased T-cell sinusoidal lymphocytosis in liver biopsies in patients with chronic hepatitis C and mixed cryoglobulinemia. *Am J Gastroenterol* 103:705, 2008.
166. Gawoski JM, Ooi WW: Dengue fever mimicking plasma cell leukemia. *Arch Pathol Lab Med* 127:1026, 2003.
167. Wiwanitkit V: Bleeding and other presentations in Thai patients with dengue infection. *Clin Appl Thromb Hemost* 10:397, 2004.
168. Liu CC, Huang KJ, Lin YS, et al: Transient CD4/CD8 ratio inversion and aberrant immune activation during dengue virus infection. *J Med Virol* 68:241, 2002.
169. Tsaparas YF, Brigden ML, Mathias R, et al: Proportion positive for Epstein-Barr virus, cytomegalovirus, human herpesvirus 6, Toxoplasma, and human immunodeficiency virus types 1 and 2 in heterophile-negative patients with an absolute lymphocytosis or an instrument-generated atypical lymphocyte flag. *Arch Pathol Lab Med* 124:1324, 2000.
170. Bernit E, Veit V, Zandotti C, et al: Chronic lymphadenopathies and human herpes virus type 8. *Scand J Infect Dis* 34:625, 2002.
171. Buyukavci M, Tan H, Keskin Z: Profound lymphocytosis preceding chickenpox. *Pediatr Infect Dis J* 23:693, 2004.
172. Heininger U, Klich K, Stehr K, Cherry JD: Clinical findings in Bordetella pertussis infections: Results of a prospective multicenter surveillance study. *Pediatrics* 100:E10, 1997.
173. Carulli G, Lagomarsini G, Azzara A, et al: Expansion of TcRalphabeta+CD3+CD4-CD8- (CD4/CD8 double-negative) T lymphocytes in a case of staphylococcal toxic shock syndrome. *Acta Haematol* 111:163, 2004.
174. Tiberghien P, Racadot E, Deschaseaux ML, et al: Interleukin-2-induced increase of a monoclonal B-cell lymphocytosis. A novel *in vivo* interleukin-2 effect? *Cancer* 69:2583, 1992.
175. Groom DA, Kunkel LA, Brynes RK, et al: Transient stress lymphocytosis during crisis of sickle cell anemia and emergency trauma and medical conditions. An immunophenotyping study [see comments]. *Arch Pathol Lab Med* 114:570, 1990.
176. Higa K, Hirata K, Dan K: Mexiletine-induced severe skin eruption, fever, eosinophilia, atypical lymphocytosis, and liver dysfunction. *Pain* 73:97, 1997.
177. Tollerud DJ, Brown LM, Blattner WA, et al: T cell subsets in healthy black smokers and nonsmokers. Evidence for ethnic group as an important response modifier. *Am Rev Respir Dis* 144:612, 1991.
178. Sever-Prebilic M, Prebilic I, Seili-Bekafigo I, et al: A case of visceral leishmaniasis in the Northern Adriatic region. *Coll Antropol* 26:545, 2002.
179. Halim NK, Ogbeide E: Haematological alterations in leprosy patients treated with dapsone. *East Afr Med J* 79:100, 2002.
180. Speight EL, Myers B, Davies JM: Stronglyoidiasis, angio-oedema and natural killer cell lymphocytosis. *Br J Dermatol* 140:1179, 1999.
181. Chen HK, Huang WT, Eng HL, et al: Ossifying thymoma clinically presenting with peripheral T-cell lymphocytosis. *Ann Thorac Surg* 88:e5–7, 2009.
182. Buckley RH: Primary cellular immunodeficiencies. *J Allergy Clin Immunol* 109:747, 2002.
183. Hartel C, Strunk T, Bucsky P, Schultz C: Failure to thrive in a 14-month-old boy with lymphopenia and eosinophilia. *Klin Padiatr* 216:24, 2004.
184. Touraine JL, Betuel H, Souillet G, Jeune M: Combined immunodeficiency disease associated with absence of cell-surface HLA-A and -B antigens. *J Pediatr* 93:47, 1978.
185. Freier S, Kerem E, Dranitzki Z, et al: Hereditary CD4+ T lymphocytopenia. *Arch Dis Child* 78:371, 1998.
186. Roper M, Parmley RT, Crist WM, et al: Severe congenital leukopenia (reticular dysgenesis). Immunologic and morphologic characterizations of leukocytes. *Am J Dis Child* 139:832, 1985.
187. Di Renzo M, Zhou Z, George I, et al: Enhanced apoptosis of T cells in common variable immunodeficiency (CVID): Role of defective CD28 co-stimulation. *Clin Exp Immunol* 120:503, 2000.
188. Sawabe T, Horiuchi T, Nakamura M, et al: Defect of lck in a patient with common variable immunodeficiency. *Int J Mol Med* 7:609, 2001.
189. Staples ER, McDermott EM, Reiman A, et al: Immunodeficiency in ataxia telangiectasia is correlated strongly with the presence of two null mutations in the ataxia telangiectasia mutated gene. *Clin Exp Immunol* 153:214, 2008.
190. Ochs HD: The Wiskott-Aldrich syndrome. *Semin Hematol* 35:332, 1998.
191. Kavadas FD, Giliani S, Gu Y, et al: Variability of clinical and laboratory features among patients with ribonuclease mitochondrial RNA processing endoribonuclease gene mutations. *J Allergy Clin Immunol* 122:1178, 2008.
192. Montella L, Masci AM, Merkabaoui G, et al: B-cell lymphopenia and hypogammaglobulinemia in thymoma patients. *Ann Hematol* 82:343, 2003.
193. Myers LA, Hershfield MS, Neale WT, et al: Purine nucleoside phosphorylase deficiency (PNP-def) presenting with lymphopenia and developmental delay: Successful correction with umbilical cord blood transplantation. *J Pediatr* 145:710, 2004.
194. Etzioni A, Benderly A, Rosenthal E, et al: Defective humoral and cellular immune functions associated with veno-occlusive disease of the liver. *J Pediatr* 110:549, 1987.
195. Zeng W, Maciejewski JP, Chen G, et al: Selective reduction of natural killer T cells in the bone marrow of aplastic anaemia. *Br J Haematol* 119:803, 2002.
196. Douek DC, Picker LJ, and Koup RA: T cell dynamics in HIV-1 infection. *Annu Rev Immunol* 21:265, 2003.
197. Lawlor E, Murray M, O'Briain DS, et al: Persistent polyclonal B lymphocytosis with Epstein-Barr virus antibodies and subsequent malignant pulmonary blastoma [see comments]. *J Clin Pathol* 44:341, 1991.
198. Panesar NS: Lymphopenia in SARS. *Lancet* 361:1985, 2003.
199. Wang JT, Chang SC: Severe acute respiratory syndrome. *Curr Opin Infect Dis* 17:143, 2004.
200. Wang JT, Sheng WH, Fang CT, et al: Clinical manifestations, laboratory findings, and treatment outcomes of SARS patients. *Emerg Infect Dis* 10:818, 2004.
201. Hui DS, Chan MC, Wu AK, Ng PC: Severe acute respiratory syndrome (SARS): Epidemiology and clinical features. *Postgrad Med J* 80:373, 2004.
202. Cunha BA, Minnaganti V, Johnson DH, Klein NC: Profound and prolonged lymphocytopenia with West Nile encephalitis. *Clin Infect Dis* 31:1116, 2000.
203. Huhn GD, Sejvar JJ, Montgomery SP, Dworkin MS: West Nile virus in the United States: An update on an emerging infectious disease. *Am Fam Physician* 68:653, 2003.
204. Cunha BA: Profound and prolonged lymphocytopenia with West Nile encephalitis. *Clin Infect Dis* 31:1116, 2004.
205. Servet-Delprat C, Vidalain PO, Valentin H, Rabourdin-Combe C: Measles virus and dendritic cell functions: How specific response cohabits with immunosuppression. *Curr Top Microbiol Immunol* 276:103, 2003.
206. Vuorinen T, Peri P, Vainionpaa R: Measles virus induces apoptosis in uninfected bystander T cells and leads to granzyme B and caspase activation in peripheral blood mononuclear cell cultures. *Eur J Clin Invest* 33:434, 2003.
207. Wollenberg A, Zoch C, Wetzel S, et al: Predisposing factors and clinical features of eczema herpeticum: A retrospective analysis of 100 cases. *J Am Acad Dermatol* 49:198, 2003.
208. Wang FZ, Linde A, Dahl H, Ljungman P: Human herpesvirus 6 infection inhibits specific lymphocyte proliferation responses and is related to lymphocytopenia after allogeneic stem cell transplantation. *Bone Marrow Transplant* 24:1201, 1999.
209. Yoshikawa T, Ihira M, Asano Y, et al: Fatal adult case of severe lymphocytopenia associated with reactivation of human herpesvirus 6. *J Med Virol* 66:82, 2002.
210. García-Silva J, Almagro M, Peña C, et al: CD4+ T-lymphocytopenia, Kaposi's sarcoma, HHV-8 infection, severe seborrheic dermatitis, and onychomycosis in a homosexual man without HIV infection [letter]. *Int J Dermatol* 38:231, 1999.
211. Mazzucchelli I, Vezzoli M, Ottini E, et al: A complex immunodeficiency. Idiopathic CD4+ T-lymphocytopenia and hypogammaglobulinemia associated with HHV8 infection, Kaposi's sarcoma and gastric cancer [letter]. *Haematologica* 84:378, 1999.
212. Kim SK, Welsh RM: Comprehensive early and lasting loss of memory CD8 T cells and functional memory during acute and persistent viral infections. *J Immunol* 172:3139, 2004.
213. Mert A, Bilir M, Tabak F, et al: Miliary tuberculosis: Clinical manifestations, diagnosis and outcome in 38 adults. *Respirology* 6:217, 2001.
214. Abdool Gaffar MS, Seedat YK, Coovadia YM, Khan Q: The white cell count in typhoid fever. *Trop Geogr Med* 44:23, 1992.
215. Kemp K, Bruunsgaard H, Skinhoj P, Klarlund Pedersen B: Pneumococcal infections in humans are associated with increased apoptosis and trafficking of type 1 cytokine-producing T cells. *Infect Immun* 70:5019, 2002.
216. Jensenius M, Fournier PE, Hellum KB, et al: Sequential changes in hematologic and biochemical parameters in African tick bite fever. *Clin Microbiol Infect* 9:678, 2003.
217. Bakken JS, Aguero-Rosenfeld ME, Tilden RL, et al: Serial measurements of hematologic counts during the active phase of human granulocytic ehrlichiosis. *Clin Infect Dis* 32:862, 2001.

218. Le Tulzo Y, Pangault C, Gacouin A, et al: Early circulating lymphocyte apoptosis in human septic shock is associated with poor outcome. *Shock* 18:487, 2002.
219. Hotchkiss RS, Tinsley KW, Swanson PE, et al: Sepsis-induced apoptosis causes progressive profound depletion of B and CD4+ T lymphocytes in humans. *J Immunol* 166:6952, 2001.
220. Aubouy A, Deloron P, Migot-Nabias F: Plasma and in vitro levels of cytokines during and after a *Plasmodium falciparum* malaria attack in Gabon. *Acta Trop* 83:195, 2002.
221. Kern P, Dietrich M, Hemmer C, Wellinghausen N: Increased levels of soluble Fas ligand in serum in *Plasmodium falciparum* malaria. *Infect Immun* 68:3061, 2000.
222. Lee HK, Lim J, Kim M, et al: Immunological alterations associated with *Plasmodium vivax* malaria in South Korea. *Ann Trop Med Parasitol* 95:31, 2001.
223. Hutchinson P, Chadban SJ, Atkins RC, Holdsworth SR: Laboratory assessment of immune function in renal transplant patients. *Nephrol Dial Transplant* 18:983, 2003.
224. Bohler T, Waiser J, Schutz M, et al: FTY720 mediates apoptosis-independent lymphopenia in human renal allograft recipients: Different effects on CD62L+ and CCR5+ T lymphocytes. *Transplantation* 77:1424, 2004.
225. Schatz DA, Riley WJ, Silverstein JH, Barrett DJ: Long-term immunoregulatory effects of therapy with corticosteroids and anti-thymocyte globulin. *Immunopharmacol Immunotoxicol* 11:269, 1989.
226. Dearden C: Alemtuzumab in peripheral T-cell malignancies. *Cancer Biother Radiopharm* 19:391, 2004.
227. Buysmann S, van Diepen FN, Yong SL, et al: Mechanism of lymphocytopenia following administration of corticosteroids. *Transplant Proc* 27:871, 1995.
228. Wang L, Hong KC, Lin FC, Yang KD: Mycoplasma pneumoniae-associated Stevens-Johnson syndrome exhibits lymphopenia and redistribution of CD4+ T cells. *J Formos Med Assoc* 102:55, 2003.
229. Tolaney SM, Najita J, Winer EP, Burstein HJ: Lymphopenia associated with adjuvant anthracycline/ taxane regimens. *Clin Breast Cancer* 8:352, 2008.
230. Standish LJ, Torkelson C, Hamill FA, et al: Immune defects in breast cancer patients after radiotherapy. *J Soc Integr Oncol* 6:110, 2008.
231. Bolla G, Tuzzato G: Immunologic postoperative competence after laparoscopy versus laparotomy. *Surg Endosc* 17:1247, 2003.
232. Leung KL, Tsang KS, Ng MH, et al: Lymphocyte subsets and natural killer cell cytotoxicity after laparoscopically assisted resection of rectosigmoid carcinoma. *Surg Endosc* 17:1305, 2003.
233. Tayama E, hayashida N, Oda T: Recovery from lymphocytopenia following extracorporeal circulation: Simple indicator to assess surgical stress. *Artif Organs* 23:736, 1999.
234. Shi SS, Shi CC, Zhao ZY, et al: Effect of open heart surgery with cardiopulmonary bypass on peripheral blood lymphocyte apoptosis in children. *Pediatr Cardiol* 30:153, 2009.
235. Guichard G, Rebibou JM, Ducloux D, et al: Lymphocyte subsets in renal transplant recipients with *de novo* genitourinary malignancies. *Urol Int* 80:257, 2008.
236. Bhaskaran M, Ranjan R, Shah H, et al: Lymphopenia in dialysis patients: A preliminary study indicating a possible role of apoptosis. *Clin Nephrol* 57:221, 2002.
237. Nicolini FE, Wattel E, Michallet AS, et al: Long-term persistent lymphopenia in hematopoietic stem cell donors after donation for donor lymphocyte infusion. *Exp Hematol* 32:1033, 2004.
238. Wagner U, Kaltenhauser S, Pierer M, et al: B lymphocytopenia in rheumatoid arthritis is associated with the DRB1 shared epitope and increased acute phase response. *Arthritis Res* 4:R1, 2002.
239. Silva LM, Garcia AB, Donadi EA: Increased lymphocyte death by neglect-apoptosis is associated with lymphopenia and autoantibodies in lupus patients presenting with neuropsychiatric manifestations. *J Neurol* 249:1048, 2002.
240. Yu HH, Wang LC, Lee JH, et al: Lymphopenia is associated with neuropsychiatric manifestations and disease activity in paediatric systemic lupus erythematosus patients. *Rheumatology (Oxford)* 46:1492, 2007.
241. Wladis EJ, Kapila R, Chu DS: Idiopathic CD4+ lymphocytopenia and Sjögren syndrome. *Arch Ophthalmol* 123:1012, 2005.
242. Gerli R, Paganelli R, Cossarizza A, et al: Long-term immunologic effects of thymectomy in patients with myasthenia gravis. *J Allergy Clin Immunol* 103:865, 1999.
243. Venzor J, Hua Q, Bressler RB, et al: Behçet's-like syndrome associated with idiopathic CD4+ T-lymphocytopenia, opportunistic infections, and a large population of TCR alpha beta+ CD4– CD8- T cells. *Am J Med Sci* 313:236, 1997.
244. Viguier M, Fouere S, de la Salmoniere P, et al: Peripheral blood lymphocyte subset counts in patients with dermatomyositis: Clinical correlations and changes following therapy. *Medicine (Baltimore)* 82:82, 2003.
245. Izzedine H, Cacoub P, Launay-Vacher V, et al: Lymphopenia in Wegener's granulomatosis. A new clinical activity index? *Nephron* 92:466, 2002.
246. Ray-Coquard I, Cropet C, Van Glabbeke M, et al: Lymphopenia as a prognostic factor for overall survival in advanced carcinomas, sarcomas, and lymphomas. *Cancer Res* 69:5383, 2009.
247. Cervantes F, Hernandez-Boluda JC, Villamor N, et al: Assessment of peripheral blood lymphocyte subsets in idiopathic myelofibrosis. *Eur J Haematol* 65:104, 2000.
248. Garty BZ: Deficiency of CD4+ lymphocytes due to intestinal loss after Fontan procedure. *Eur J Pediatr* 160:58, 2001.
249. Chakrabarti S, Keeton BR, Salmon AP, Vettukattil JJ: Acquired combined immunodeficiency associated with protein losing enteropathy complicating Fontan operation. *Heart* 89:1130, 2003.
250. Meier P, Dayer E, Blanc E, Wauters JP: Early T cell activation correlates with expression of apoptosis markers in patients with end-stage renal disease. *J Am Soc Nephrol* 13:204, 2002.
251. Gupta D, Rao VM, Aggarwal AN, et al: Haematological abnormalities in patients of sarcoidosis. *Indian J Chest Dis Allied Sci* 44:233, 2002.
252. Morell F, Levy G, Orriols R, et al: Delayed cutaneous hypersensitivity tests and lymphopenia as activity markers in sarcoidosis. *Chest* 121:1239, 2002.
253. Gentil B, Cottin V, Girard P, Cordier JF: Ambivalence of CD4 lymphocytopenia in sarcoidosis. *Sarcoidosis Vasc Diffuse Lung Dis* 20:74, 2003.
254. Yanardag H, Pamuk GE, Karayel T, Demirci S: Bone marrow involvement in sarcoidosis: An analysis of 50 bone marrow samples. *Haematologia (Budap)* 32:419, 2002.
255. Takeyama Y, Takas K, Ueda T, et al: Peripheral lymphocyte reduction in severe acute pancreatitis is caused by apoptotic cell death. *J Gastrointest Surg* 4:379, 2000.
256. Mooren FC, Bloming D, Lechtermann A, et al: Lymphocyte apoptosis after exhaustive and moderate exercise. *J Appl Physiol* 93:147, 2002.
257. Steensberg A, Morrow J, Toft AD, et al: Prolonged exercise, lymphocyte apoptosis and F2-isoprostanes. *Eur J Appl Physiol* 87:38, 2002.
258. Subra JF, Renier G, Reboul P, et al: Lymphopenia in occupational pulmonary silicosis with or without autoimmune disease. *Clin Exp Immunol* 126:540, 2001.
259. Di Sabatino A, D'Alo S, Millimaggi D, et al: Apoptosis and peripheral blood lymphocyte depletion in coeliac disease. *Immunology* 103:435, 2001.

CHAPTER 82
IMMUNODEFICIENCY DISEASES

Hans D. Ochs and Luigi D. Notarangelo

SUMMARY

Primary immune deficiency diseases (PIDDs) are characterized by increased susceptibility to infections, often associated with autoimmunity and inflammation and an increased risk of malignancies because of impaired immune homeostasis and surveillance. Depending on the nature of the immune defect, the clinical presentation of PIDD may vary and may include recurrence of upper and lower respiratory tract infections, invasive bacterial infections, purulent lymphadenitis, skin or deep abscesses, infections sustained by poorly virulent or opportunistic pathogens (*Pneumocystis jiroveci*, cytomegalovirus, environmental mycobacteria, *Cryptosporidium*, *Giardia lamblia*), persistent or recurrent candidiasis, autoimmunity, increased susceptibility to malignancies, and association with typical signs of specific immunodeficiency syndromes.

With the exception of immunoglobulin (Ig) A deficiency, PIDDs are generally rare, with a prevalence of approximately 1:10,000 to 1:50,000. However, prompt recognition of PIDD is of importance, because diagnostic delay is associated with increased risk of death and of irreversible complications. Most forms of PIDD follow mendelian inheritance; however, some, for example, common variable immunodeficiency (CVID), have a multifactorial origin. In most cases, PIDDs present in childhood, but late presentations may occur or even predominate in some forms, such as CVID.

The diagnostic approach to PIDD is based on a detailed family and clinical history, physical examination and appropriate laboratory tests. Lymphopenia is characteristic of severe combined immune deficiency. Abnormalities of the neutrophil count can be observed in patients with disorders of neutrophil production (e.g., congenital neutropenia) or function (e.g., chronic granulomatous disease), respectively. Evaluation of serum immunoglobulin levels and of antibody responses to immunization antigens is important for patients with a history of recurrent infections. The clinical presentation and the results of these preliminary evaluations may prompt additional laboratory testing. For instance, patients with a profound hypogammaglobulinemia and a history of recurrent infections should be tested for the presence of circulating B lymphocytes (CD19+ or CD20+ cells), which are absent or markedly reduced in X-linked agammaglobulinemia. On the other hand, early presentation with severe and/or opportunistic infections, especially if associated with lymphopenia, should prompt enumeration of lymphocyte subsets. A severe reduction of circulating CD3+ T cells is typically observed in severe combined immune deficiency, and may be associated with defects of B and/or natural killer cells. Deep bacterial infections, or infections sustained by *Aspergillus*, require evaluation of neutrophil count and function, to identify patients with congenital neutropenia and chronic granulomatous disease, respectively. Invasive recurrent infections sustained by *Neisseria* species are an indication for assessing complement levels and function. On the other hand, complement component deficiencies may also lead to systemic lupus erythematosus-like features or to autoimmune disorders. Laboratory results should be compared to age-matched control values, as white blood cell counts, lymphocyte subsets, complement components and immunoglobulin levels, and antibody production (especially to polysaccharide antigens) undergo significant changes and progressive maturation in the first years of life. It is important to rule out secondary forms of immunodeficiency, such as human immunodeficiency virus infection, protein loss, immunodeficiency secondary to use of immunosuppressive drugs, as well as anatomical and/or functional problems (e.g., asplenia) that may lead to increased susceptibility to infections.

Recognition of PIDDs is essential to start optimal therapies at an early age. These include immunoglobulin substitution for patients with antibody deficiency; allogeneic hematopoietic stem cell transplantation for patients with severe combined immune deficiency; and in some cases, gene therapy or enzyme replacement therapy may be considered. Antimicrobial prophylaxis and aggressive treatment of infections is necessary in most cases of PIDD. Some patients with significant immune dysregulation may benefit from immunosuppressive therapy.

This chapter focuses on defects that primarily affect T and B lymphocytes, the complement system, and innate immunity. The chapter discusses specific immunodeficiency syndromes, reviews etiology and pathogenesis, clinical and laboratory features, treatment, and prognosis. Chaps. 65 and 66 discuss in detail disorders of neutrophil number and function.

Acronyms and abbreviations used in this chapter include: AD, autosomal dominant; ADA, adenosine deaminase; AD-HIES, autosomal dominant hyperimmunoglobulin E syndrome; AIRE, autoimmune regulator; AK, adenylate kinase; AK2 adenylate kinase 2; ALPS, autoimmune lymphoproliferative syndrome; APECED, autoimmune polyendocrinopathy, candidiasis, and ectodermal dystrophy; AT, ataxia-telangiectasia; ATLD, ataxia-telangiectasia–like disorder; ATM, ataxia-telangiectasia mutated; BS, Bloom syndrome; BTK, Bruton tyrosine kinase; CD40L, CD40 ligand; CID, combined immune deficiency; CMV, cytomegalovirus; CSR, class switch recombination; CTL, cytotoxic T lymphocyte; CVID, common variable immunodeficiency; D, diversity; FHL, familial hemophagocytic lymphohistiocytosis; G-CSF, granulocyte colony-stimulating-factor; HIES, hyperimmunoglobulin E syndrome; HSE, herpes simplex virus encephalitis; IL, interleukin; IL-7R, IL-7 receptor; IPEX, immune dysregulation, polyendocrinopathy, enteropathy, X-linked; IRAK, IL-1 receptor-associated kinase; J, joining; JAK3, Janus-associated tyrosine kinase 3; LIG4, DNA ligase IV; NBS, Nijmegen breakage syndrome; NEMO, nuclear factor-κB essential modulator; NK, natural killer; PNP, purine nucleoside phosphorylase; RMRP, ribonuclease mitochondrial RNA processing; SAP, signaling lymphocyte activation molecule-associated protein; SCID, severe combined immune deficiency; SHM, somatic hypermutation; TLR, toll-like receptor; UNG, uracil N-glycosylase; V, variable; WAS, Wiskott-Aldrich syndrome; WASP, Wiskott-Aldrich syndrome protein; WHIM, warts, hypogammaglobulinemia, infections, myelokathexis; XHIGM, X-linked hyperimmunoglobulin M; XLA, X-linked agammaglobulinemia; XLP1 and XLP2, X-linked lymphoproliferative syndrome types 1 and 2; XLT, X-linked thrombocytopenia; ZAP-70, zeta-associated protein of 70 kDa.

PREDOMINANT ANTIBODY DEFICIENCIES

X-LINKED AND AUTOSOMAL RECESSIVE AGAMMAGLOBULINEMIA

Definition and Genetic Features

X-linked agammaglobulinemia (XLA) is the prototypic antibody deficiency characterized by profound hypogammaglobulinemia caused by a maturation defect in B-cell development.[1,2] XLA, described in 1953, is one of the first primary immunodeficiencies in which the underlying defect, a mutation of the Bruton tyrosine kinase (BTK) was identified. Autosomal recessive agammaglobulinemia, a variant form of agammaglobulinemia, has been reported in patients with a clinical phenotype resembling XLA including very low B-cell numbers and severe bacterial infections but normal BTK.[2] Several responsible gene mutations have been identified, including those involving the B-cell receptor complex μ heavy chain (IGHM), the surrogate light chain component $\lambda 5$ (IGLL1), the signal transducer complex of the pre-B cell receptors immunoglobulin (Ig) α (CD79a), Igβ (CD79b), and mutations in the B-cell adaptor molecule BLINK.

Clinical Features

Because IgG is actively transported across the placenta, infants born with XLA have normal levels of IgG at birth and are frequently asymptomatic for the first few months of life. Following metabolism of the maternal antibodies, affected boys begin to develop recurrent infections usually between 4 and 12 months of age. In a review of 96 XLA patients, 20 percent experienced initial clinical systems after their first birthday and approximately 10 percent after 18 months of age.[3] In an Italian study of 73 patients with mutation-verified XLA, the mean age of onset of symptoms was 2 years.[4] The presenting symptoms vary greatly and may be mild or severe (Table 82–1). Otitis media and chronic sinusitis, pneumonia, pyoderma, and diarrhea are frequent clinical presentations. Serious complications include septicemia, meningitis, septic arthritis, and osteomyelitis. In young children with XLA, acute infections are often associated with neutropenia. Pyogenic bacteria, such as *Haemophilus influenzae, Streptococcus pneumoniae,* and *Staphylococcus aureus* are the most common pathogens observed in XLA. Opportunistic infections such as *Pneumocystis jiroveci*, are rarely observed. Infections with *Ureaplasma urealyticum* have been reported in XLA patients with mycoplasma arthritis.[5] Although resistance to viral infections is generally intact, XLA patients are unusually susceptible to enteroviruses such as echovirus, coxsackievirus, and poliovirus. Poliomyelitis after live attenuated (Sabin) poliovirus vaccine, especially if given at a time when maternal antibodies had disappeared, is associated with high morbidity and mortality.[3] Before the introduction of intravenous immunoglobulin (IVIg), XLA patients frequently developed chronic, disseminated echo- and coxsackievirus infections presenting as meningoencephalitis, dermatomyositis/fasciitis, and hepatitis.[6] Gastroenteritis caused by *Giardia lamblia, Campylobacter* species, or rotavirus is not uncommon and may be associated with malabsorption. Chronic intestinal inflammation resembling Crohn disease may develop in children and adults with XLA. Interestingly, an increased incidence of rectosigmoid cancer with high mortality has been reported.[7]

TABLE 82–1. Principal Clinical Features of Primary Immunodeficiency Disorders

Neutrophils Numerical or Functional Defects	Complement Deficiencies	Antibody Deficiencies	Combined Immune Deficiencies
Severe bacterial and fungal infections Skin or deep bacterial and fungal abscesses Infections sustained by unusual bacteria and fungi	Recurrent or severe infections sustained by encapsulated pathogens Recurrent *Neisseria meningitidis* infections Autoimmune manifestations (systemic lupus erythematosus-like) Atypical hemolytic-uremic syndrome Recurrent angioedema (C1-INH deficiency)	Recurrent infections after 4 to 6 months of age Intestinal *Giardia lamblia* infection Enterovirus meningoencephalitis	Early onset respiratory and gut infections Opportunistic infections Growth failure Persistent candidiasis Erythroderma

Laboratory Features

Most patients have markedly reduced levels of all classes of immunoglobulins; circulating B cells are less than 1 percent of total lymphocytes and tonsils are absent. Because of the maturation arrest at the pre–B-cell stage, very few B cells undergo differentiation into plasma cells. As a result lymph nodes, lymphoid follicles, germinal centers, and intestinal mucosal biopsies lack plasma cells. As expected, specific antibodies to microorganisms or vaccines are markedly reduced or undetectable (see Table 82–2).

BTK, a cytoplasmic protein tyrosine kinase known to interact with other cytoplasmic proteins, plays an important role in the pre–B-cell expansion and the survival of mature B cells by facilitating signaling through the B-cell antigen receptor. BTK is present in all hematopoietic cells except T cells, natural killer (NK) cells, and plasma cells. The presence of BTK in normal monocytes and platelets allows assessment of BTK in most XLA patients with low or absent BTK levels using flow cytometry, and to identify carrier females.[8] Sequence analysis of the *BTK* gene confirms the diagnosis and allows prenatal diagnosis.

Treatment

Intravenous or subcutaneous IgG infusions at a dose of 400 to 600 mg/kg every 4 weeks are highly effective in preventing chronic infections in agammaglobulinemic patients. Prophylactic antibiotics are indicated in those with chronic lung disease. Adequate IVIg replacement has markedly reduced the incidence of enteroviral infections, but other complications, such as Crohn-like disease, are difficult to prevent, and progressive neurodegeneration has been observed in a small number of XLA patients without identification of an infectious agent.[9]

■ HYPERIMMUNOGLOBULIN M SYNDROMES

Definition and Genetic Abnormalities

Hyper-IgM syndromes are characterized by recurrent infections associated with low serum levels of IgG, IgA, and IgE, but normal or increased levels of IgM. They are the direct result of mutations affecting genes involved in B-cell activation, class switch recombination (CSR), and somatic hypermutation (SHM). Mutations in the genes encoding CD40 ligand (CD40L) or CD40 interfere with the triggering of events that lead to CSR and SHM. Mutations in the B-cell intrinsic enzymes, activation-induced cytosine deaminase (AID) and uracil N-glycosylase (UNG), directly affect CSR and SHM. Mutations in the *NEMO* gene (nuclear factor [NF]-κB essential modulator), a protein crucial for NF-κB activation, cause clinical features of anhydrotic ectodermal dysplasia with associated immune deficiency in males and incontinentia pigmenta in females.[10] A novel B-cell–intrinsic CSR deficiency was associated with mutations in the gene encoding the PMS2 component of the mismatch repair machinery.[11]

X-Linked Hyper-IgM as a Result of CD40L Deficiency

Clinical Features In addition to recurrent bacterial infections, affected infants with X-linked hyperimmunoglobulin M (XHIGM) often present with interstitial pneumonia caused by *Pneumocystis jiroveci*; approximately 50 percent of affected males will develop neutropenia.[12] Patients with XHIGM are at high risk of developing chronic *Cryptosporidium* infections complicated by ascending cholangiolitis and chronic liver disease. Progressive neurodegeneration in XHIGM patients similar to those with XLA has been reported.[9] Abortive germinal center

TABLE 82–2. Common Primary Immunodeficiencies: Laboratory and Clinical Features*

	Lymphocytes			Cellular Immunity	Humoral Immunity: Serum Immunoglobulins				Humoral Immunity: Antibody Responses	Common Infections
	B	T	NK		M	G	A	E		
Predominantly antibody deficiency										
X-linked agammaglobulinemia (BTK)	–	+	+	+	↓	↓	↓	↓	–	Bacteria, *Giardia lamblia*
Autosomal recessive agammaglobulinemia λ5, Igα, Igβ, or BLNK deficiency	–	+	+	+	↓	↓	↓	↓	–	Bacteria
Hypogammaglobulinemia (AR) ICOS, CD19, CD21, BAFF-R	–	+		+	↓	↓	↓	↓	–	Bacteria
Transient hypogammaglobulinemia of infancy	+	+	+	+	N/↓	N/↓	N/↓	N/↓	+/–	Bacteria
Selective IgA deficiency	+	+	+	+	N	N	↓	N	+/–	Bacteria, *G. lamblia*
Common variable immune deficiency	+	+	+	+	N/↓		↓		–	Bacteria, *G. lamblia*
IgG subclass deficiencies	+	+	+	+	N	N/↓	N/↓	N	+/–	Bacteria
Hyper-IgM syndrome										
Activation-induced cytidine deaminase deficiency	+	+	+	+	N/↑	↓	↓	↓	+/–	Bacteria
Uracil-DNA glycosylase deficiency	+	+	+	+	N/↑	↓	↓	↓	+/–	Bacteria
X-linked CD40 ligand deficiency	+	+	+	+	N/↑	↓	N/↓	↓	+/–	Bacteria, viruses, fungi
CD40 deficiency	+	+	+	+	N/↑	↓	N/↓	↓	+/–	Bacteria, viruses, fungi
X-linked IKK-γ (NEMO) deficiency	+	+	+	+	N/↑	↓	↓	↓	+/–	Bacteria, viruses, fungi
Severe combined immunodeficiency (SCID)										
Interleukin receptor γ-chain deficiency (X-linked SCID)	+	–	–	–	N	↓	↓	↓	–	Bacteria, viruses, fungi
Janus-associated kinase 3 (JAK3) deficiency	+	–	–	–	N	↓	↓	↓	–	Bacteria, viruses, fungi
Interleukin-7 receptor α-chain deficiency	+	–	–	–	N	↓	↓	↓	–	Bacteria, viruses, fungi
Zap-70 tyrosine kinase deficiency	+	+/–	+	–	N	N/↓	N/↓	N/↓	+/–	Bacteria, viruses, fungi
Adenosine deaminase (ADA) deficiency	–	–	–	–	↓	↓	↓	↓	–	Bacteria, viruses, fungi
Purine nucleotide phosphorylase (PNP) deficiency	+	–	+	–	N	↓	↓	↓	+/–	Bacteria, viruses, fungi
Recombinase activating gene (RAG 1/2) deficiency	–	–	+	–	↓	↓	↓	↓	–	Bacteria, viruses, fungi
Artemis deficiency	–	–	+	–	↓	↓	↓	↓	–	Bacteria, viruses, fungi
Reticular dysgenesis (AK2 deficiency)	–	–	–	–	↓	↓	↓	↓	–	Bacteria, viruses, fungi
Primary T-cell deficiency										
Congenital thymic aplasia (DiGeorge syndrome)	+	–	+	–	N	N	N	N	+/–	Bacteria, viruses, fungi
Major histocompatibility complex (MHC) class II deficiency	+	+/–	+	+	N	↓	↓	↓	+/–	Bacteria, viruses, fungi
Transport-associated protein (TAP)-1 or TAP-2 deficiency (MHC class I deficiency)	+	+/–	+	–	N	N	N	N	+	Bacteria, viruses, fungi
Th1 deficiency										
Interferon-γ and interferon-γ receptor deficiency	+	+	+	+	N	N	N	N	+	Mycobacteria, *Salmonella*
Interleukin-12 and interleukin-12 receptor deficiency	+	+	+	+	N	N	N	N	+	Mycobacteria, *Salmonella*
Other well-defined immunodeficiency syndromes										
Ataxia-telangiectasia	+	+	+	+	N/↑	N/↓	N/↓	↓	+/–	Bacteria
Wiskott-Aldrich syndrome	+	+/–	+	+/–	↓	N	↑	↑	+/–	Bacteria

*Natural killer lymphocytes (NK), T cells (T), B cells (B).

Normal levels (+), reduced or absent levels (–); normal (N), elevated (↑), or reduced (↓) serum immunoglobulins.

formation and severe depletion of follicular dendritic cells of lymph nodes occurs. Affected patients are at risk to develop neoplasms, most often lymphomas, but also tumors of the biliary and gastrointestinal tract,[13] which are rarely observed in other primary immunodeficiencies.

Laboratory Features Circulating lymphocyte subsets are present in normal numbers but B cells are predominantly naïve and few are of the switched memory B-cell subtype (IgD– CD27+).[14] Lymphocyte proliferation in response to mitogens is normal, but responses to specific antigens are often reduced.[15] XHIGM is caused by mutations in CD40L, a surface protein expressed by activated CD4+ lymphocytes. CD40L interacts with the CD40 membrane protein constitutively expressed by B cells, macrophages, and dendritic cells. The interaction of CD40L/CD40 sets in motion a signaling event that results in the expression of AID and UNG, and induces CSR and SHM. Mutations in CD40L are distributed throughout the gene and may result in nonfunctional or absent protein.[12] Several patients with mild cases of XHIGM not treated with IVIg have developed chronic pure red cell aplasia as a result of persistent parvovirus B19 infection.[16]

Treatment Prophylactic treatment with trimethoprim-sulfamethoxazole is indicated during infancy and childhood to prevent *P. jiroveci* pneumonia. Intravenous or subcutaneous immunoglobulin at doses similar to patients with XLA is used to prevent chronic infections, including parvovirus B19. Exposure to *Cryptosporidium* should be prevented by avoiding the use of potentially contaminated water. Because of the high incidence of serious complications and the unfavorable long-term outcome,[17] allogeneic stem cell transplantation should be considered if an optimal donor can be identified. Severe and persistent neutropenia may require treatment with granulocyte colony-stimulating factor (G-CSF), at least on a temporary basis.

Autosomal Recessive Hyper-IgM with CD40 Mutations

A few unrelated families with autosomal recessive hyperimmunoglobulin M caused by mutations of CD40 have been reported. Affected members have similar clinical and laboratory findings as those with CD40L mutations. Treatment and prognosis of CD40 deficiency is similar to XHIGM.

Autosomal Recessive Hyper-IgM Syndrome Caused by an Intrinsic B-Cell Defect

Definition AID is expressed only in B cells undergoing CSR or SHM and is thought to affect DNA editing.[18] Because of milder symptoms, the diagnosis of AID deficiency is often established later in life.

Clinical Features AID-deficient patients present with recurrent bacterial infections, mostly affecting the upper and lower respiratory tract. In contrast to patients with XHIGM, AID-deficient individuals have an excellent long-term prognosis, especially if given IVIg prophylaxis. Most affected individuals present with striking lymphoid hyperplasia involving tonsils and lymph nodes as a result of marked follicular hyperplasia. The number of circulating T- and B-cell subsets are normal, including normal proportion of memory B cells; however, all CD27+ memory B cells fail to isotype switch and express IgM and IgD. Mutations of *AID* affect the entire gene and include missense, nonsense mutations, and small deletions.

UNG is expressed in proliferating cells, including B cells undergoing CSR. Following AID-induced deamination of cytosine into uracil residues on single-stranded DNA, UNG deglycosylates and removes uracil residues, thus leading to a single-stranded DNA break. The repair of the DNA nick leads to successful CSR and SHM. Because AID and UNG are functionally closely linked, lack of UNG results in a clinical phenotype similar to AID deficiency. The three UNG deficient patients reported to date have a history of frequent bacterial infections, lymphadenopathy, and an excellent response to IVIg therapy.[18]

X-Linked Anhydrotic Ectodermal Dysplasia with Immunodeficiency Caused by Mutations of NEMO

Definition Anhydrotic (or hypohidrotic) ectodermal dysplasia is a rare syndrome with partial or complete absence of sweat glands, sparse hair growth, and abnormal dentition. A subset of these patients has an X-linked mode of inheritance and immunodeficiency characterized by low-serum IgG levels, variably elevated IgM levels, and decreased antibody responses. This syndrome results from mutations in the IKBKG gene encoding NEMO, a key subunit of IκB-kinase that regulates NF-κB dimerization and nuclear transfer.[19] Most affected boys have a hypomorphic NEMO mutation that allows some function, and present with bacterial (*Streptococcus pneumoniae*, *S. aureus*) and often atypical mycobacterial infections. Loss-of-function mutations cause the X-linked dominant condition of incontinentia pigmenti in females and are embryonically lethal in males.

Clinical Features A review of 72 individuals with NEMO mutations has demonstrated a wide spectrum of clinical phenotypes.[20] Thirty-two different mutations of NEMO were identified, with 70 percent being associated with ectodermal dysplasia, 86 percent with serious pyogenic infections, 39 percent with mycobacterial infections, 19 percent with serious viral infections, and 21 percent with inflammatory bowel disease. One-third of this cohort of NEMO patients died prematurely (mean age: 6.4 years).

Treatment Treatment with IVIg is useful but does not prevent the occurrence of serious complications. Symptomatic treatment depends on those complications

COMMON VARIABLE IMMUNODEFICIENCY AND SELECTIVE IgA DEFICIENCY

Definition

Common variable immunodeficiency (CVID) is a clinically and molecularly heterogeneous disorder, presenting at any age, but most often during adulthood. CVID is characterized by recurrent bacterial infections, hypogammaglobulinemia, and impaired antibody responses. Together with selective IgA deficiency, CVID is the most common primary immune deficiency, with an incidence of 1 in 10,000 individuals. Familial inheritance is observed in approximately 20 percent of cases and CVID and IgA deficiency may be present in the same families. In rare instances, patients with selective IgA deficiency may progress to CVID. Attempts have been made to associate CVID with genes on chromosome 6; however, no specific genes within this region have been identified. A small proportion of patients with CVID have been molecularly defined as having mutations in several genes involved directly or indirectly with B-cell differentiation, including *ICOS*, *TACI*, *BAFF*-receptor, CD19, and CD21.[21] In addition, patients with mutations in BTK, CD40L, and SH2D1A have been mistakenly diagnosed as CVID.

Clinical Features and Treatment of Common Variable Immunodeficiency

The majority of CVID patients present with recurring sinopulmonary infections, most often bacterial pneumonia.[21] If the diagnosis is delayed or if treatment is inadequate, bronchiectasis and chronic lung disease may develop. Gastrointestinal complaints are frequent and may be caused by chronic *Giardia lamblia* or *Campylobacter* infections, resembling chronic inflammatory bowel disease. Lymphoid hyperplasia of the small bowel is a frequent finding. Autoimmune disorders are common and may resemble rheumatoid arthritis, dermatomyositis, or scleroderma. In addition, CVID patients may develop autoimmune hemolytic anemia, autoimmune thrombocytopenia purpura, autoimmune neutropenia, pernicious anemia, and chronic active hepatitis. Lymphadenopathy and splenomegaly are common, the result of follicular hyperplasia. Caseating granulomas of the lung, spleen, liver, skin, and other tissues may develop at any age, and a condition resembling sarcoidosis has been described. The cause of this devastating granuloma formation is unknown. A high incidence of lymphoma and gastrointestinal malignancies have been reported in older CVID patients,[22] with a 438-fold increase in the risk of lymphomas in affected women during the fifth and sixth decades.[23] Despite normal numbers of blood B lymphocytes and the presence of lymphoid cortical follicles, CVID patients have hypogammaglobulinemia that may be as profound as in XLA. Antibody responses to recall and to neoantigens are diminished and some CVID patients have decreased numbers of memory B cells, especially of switched memory B cells. A subset of CVID patients have a substantial T-cell deficiency characterized by decreased expression of CD40L by activated CD4+ T cells (without a mutation of CD40L) and by reversed CD4:CD8 ratio. Treatment with IVIg substitution and prophylactic antibiotics is beneficial but often insufficient to prevent serious complications. Allogeneic hematopoietic stem cell marrow transplantation is generally not recommended, except in patients with lymphoid malignancies. There is a rare association between immune deficiency and thymoma, which is estimated to be present in 4 percent of patients with hypogammaglobulinemia.[24]

Clinical Features and Treatment of Selective IgA Deficiency

The incidence of selective IgA deficiency, defined as IgA less than 5 to 10 mg/dL, differs greatly between ethnic groups, being highest in Scandinavia (1 in 396 in a Finnish study) and lowest in Asian populations (1 in 23,000 in Japan).[21] Because secretory IgA is considered to be most important in protecting mucus surfaces, it is surprising that most IgA-deficient patients remain healthy. Other defense systems, for example, noncirculatory IgM or neutrophils, may compensate for this deficiency. Symptomatic individuals are not only IgA deficient, but have deficient antibody responses to certain antigens. IgA deficiency may be associated with IgG_2 and IgG_3 deficiency and poor responses to polysaccharide antigens.[21,25] Selective IgA deficiency, if associated with symptoms, often leads to recurrent sinopulmonary infections and atopic symptoms including allergic conjunctivitis, rhinitis, and eczema. Food allergy may be more common in IgA-deficient patients and asthma associated with IgA deficiency appears to be more refractory to therapy. Gastrointestinal tract disorders include chronic giardiasis, malabsorption, celiac disease, primary biliary cirrhosis, pernicious anemia, and nodular lymphoid hyperplasia. A number of autoimmune diseases are associated with selective IgA deficiency, including rheumatoid arthritis, systemic lupus erythematous, thyroiditis, myasthenia gravis, and ulcerative colitis.

A significant proportion of IgA-deficient individuals have anti-IgA antibodies in their serum and may react to blood products containing IgA, including IVIg preparations with low IgA content. However, patients with selective IgA deficiency who make normal IgG antibody do not need IVIg therapy.

The fundamental defect in selective IgA deficiency is the failure of IgA-bearing B lymphocytes to mature into IgA-secreting plasma cells. There is no specific treatment that would correct this problem. Intermittent or continuous prophylactic antibiotics may be helpful in patients with recurrent respiratory tract infections, who develop chronic symptoms of lung disease. On the other hand, if IgA deficiency is associated with poor antibody responses to selected antigens, for example, to polysaccharides, an attempt with IVIg substitution should be made.

SEVERE COMBINED IMMUNODEFICIENCIES

DEFINITION AND HISTORY

The first description of severe combined immunodeficiencies (SCID) dates back to 1950, when Glanzmann and Riniker described infants who died with overwhelming infections, intractable diarrhea, thrush, and profound lymphophenia.[26] The SCID phenotype represents a heterogeneous group of genetic disorders that are characterized by a severe impairment of T-lymphocyte development and function (Fig. 82–1).[27–29] Depending on whether the development of B and/or NK lymphocytes is also affected, SCID can be classified into four distinct immunologic phenotypes: (1) T–B+NK– SCID (the most common variant); (2) T–B+NK+ SCID; (3) T–B–NK+ SCID; or, (4) T–B–NK– SCID. The term "combined immune deficiency" (CID) is used to define disorders with residual development and/or function of T lymphocytes. Unless treated by allogeneic hematopoietic stem cell transplantation or, in selected cases, by gene therapy or enzyme replacement therapy, SCID is inevitably fatal.

MOLECULAR DEFECTS AND PATHOGENESIS OF SCID

SCIDs are mendelian disorders, and their overall prevalence is estimated to be 1:50,000 births. In Western countries, the most common form of SCID is inherited as an X-linked trait; however, a variety of autosomal recessive forms are also known. SCID can be grouped in

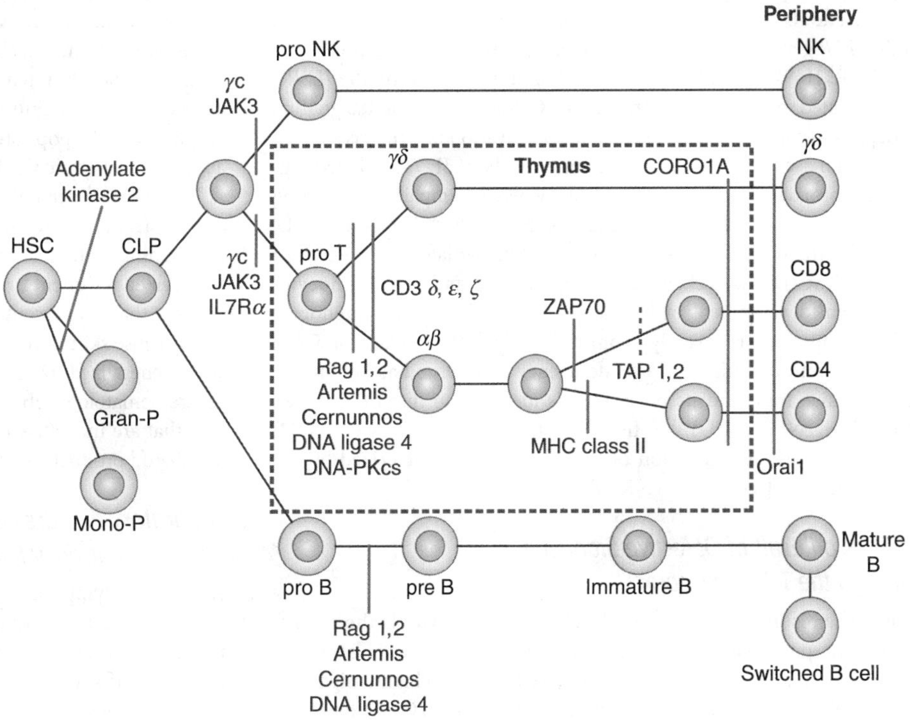

FIGURE 82–1. Disruption of the normal T-cell development by mutations of genes known to cause a severe combined immunodeficiency disease phenotype.

different categories that illustrate the various pathogenetic mechanisms involved in T-cell development.

SCID as a Result of Increased Apoptosis of Lymphocyte Precursors

Adenosine Deaminase Deficiency Approximately 5 to 10 percent of infants with SCID have a deficiency of adenosine deaminase (ADA), the enzyme that converts adenosine and deoxyadenosine into inosine and deoxyinosine, respectively.[30] In the absence of ADA, high intracellular levels of adenosine, deoxyadenosine, and their toxic phosphorylated metabolites cause apoptosis of lymphoid precursors, and hence result in the virtual absence of T lymphocytes, that is usually associated with marked reduction of B and NK lymphocytes (T–B–NK–SCID).[31,32] ADA-SCID is inherited as an autosomal recessive trait, and its clinical manifestations extend beyond the immune system, reflecting the fact that ADA is a general housekeeping enzyme.

Purine Nucleoside Phosphorylase Deficiency Purine nucleoside phosphorylase (PNP) is another enzyme of the purine salvage pathway. PNP catalyzes the phosphorylation of inosine, guanosine, and deoxyguanosine.[30] In the absence of PNP, high intracellular levels of deoxyguanosine triphosphatase cause lymphoid and neuronal toxicity. Immature thymocytes are particularly susceptible to PNP deficiency.[33] Accordingly, the immunologic phenotype of PNP deficiency is characterized by decreased T-cell counts, whereas B and NK lymphocytes are often unaffected.[34] PNP deficiency accounts for 1 to 2 percent of all forms of SCID, and is inherited as an autosomal recessive trait.

Adenylate Kinase 2 Deficiency Another rare variant of autosomal recessive SCID, reticular dysgenesis, is characterized by extreme lymphopenia, absence of neutrophils, and sensorineural deafness.[35] The disease is caused by mutations of adenylate kinase 2 that result in apoptosis of myeloid precursors of neutrophils, and of lymphoid progenitor cells.[36,37]

SCID as a Result of Defects of Cytokine-Mediated Signaling

Thymic T-cell progenitors depend on interleukin (IL)-7 for cell proliferation. The IL-7 receptor (IL-7R) is composed of an α chain (encoded by the *IL7R* gene) and a common γ chain (γc), that is shared also by IL-2R, IL-4R, IL-9R, IL-15R, and IL-21R,[38] and is encoded by the *IL2RG* gene, located on the X chromosome. Cytokine-mediated signaling through γc—containing receptors involves activation of Janus-associated tyrosine kinase 3 (JAK3).[39] In humans, defects of IL-7–mediated signaling abrogate T-cell development, whereas impaired signaling through IL-15R affects development of NK cells.[38] X-linked SCID, caused by *IL2RG* mutations,[40] represents approximately 40 percent of all cases of SCID, and is characterized by lack of T and NK lymphocytes but normal development of B cells (T–B+NK– SCID). B-lymphocyte function, however, is severely compromised by both the lack of T-cell help and nonfunctional γc. JAK3 deficiency is inherited as an autosomal recessive trait, and its phenotype is identical to that of X-linked SCID (T–B+NK– SCID).[41,42] In contrast, autosomal recessive IL-7R deficiency caused by mutation of the α chain is characterized by the selective lack of T cells (T–B+NK+ SCID).[43]

SCID as a Result of Defective Signaling Through the T-Cell Receptor

One of the distinctive features of developing thymocytes is the expression of the pre–T-cell receptor (TCR), that is composed of a pre-Tα chain, a TCRβ chain, and the CD3 γ, δ, ε, and ζ chains. Signaling through the pre-TCR permits rearrangement of the TCRα chain and expression of a mature TCR$\alpha\beta$. Alternatively, thymocytes may express the $\gamma\delta$ chains of the TCR. Rearrangement of the TCR loci is accomplished by means of the V(D)J recombination, whereby the lymphoid specific RAG1 and RAG2 proteins mediate DNA cleavage at the variable (V), diversity (D), and joining (J) elements of the TCR loci. The DNA double-strand break of the coding ends is initially sealed as a hairpin, that is resolved by Artemis (encoded by the *DCLRE1C* gene). Eventually, joining of coding (and signal) elements is mediated by a series of proteins, that include the Ku70/80 heterodimer, XRCC4, DNA ligase IV (LIG4), DNA-protein kinase catalytic subunit, and Cernunnos/XLF. Defects in V(D)J recombination affect both T- and B-cell development and hence cause T–B–NK+ SCID, because this process is also essential to mediate rearrangement of the immunoglobulin genes, a key step in B-cell development. RAG1 or RAG2 deficiencies account for 3 to 20 percent of all SCID cases in different series.[27,44] Artemis (*DCLRE1C*),[45] DNA-protein kinase catalytic subunit,[46] LIG4,[47,48] and Cernunnos/XLF[49] deficiencies are less frequent and their cellular and clinical phenotype extends beyond impaired T and B cells development, because enzymes that mediate DNA double-strand break repair are ubiquitously expressed, and their deficiency results in increased cellular radiosensitivity.[45–49] The phenotype of LIG4 deficiency can be extremely variable, from T–B–NK+ SCID to mild or no immunodeficiency whereas Cernunnos/XLF deficiency is characterized by significant T-cell lymphopenia and progressive decrease in the number of B cells.

Defects of the CD3 δ, ε, or ζ chains affect signaling through the pre-TCR and the TCR and hence cause autosomal recessive T–B+NK+ SCID.[50–52] In contrast, CD3γ deficiency is associated with mild T-cell lymphopenia and a variable clinical phenotype.[53,54]

Mutations of CD45, a pan-leukocyte tyrosine phosphatase that has been implicated in signaling through the TCR and the B-cell receptor, have been reported in few patients with T–B+NK+ SCID.[55,56]

Clinical Features of Severe Combined Immunodeficiency Syndromes

Despite genetic heterogeneity, SCID is characterized by a consistent clinical phenotype. Interstitial pneumonia, often sustained by *P. jiroveci*, cytomegalovirus (CMV), adenovirus, parainfluenza 3 virus, respiratory syncytial virus, chronic diarrhea, failure to thrive, and persistent candidiasis are common features. Typically, infections develop in the first months of life. Skin manifestations (maculopapular rash, erythroderma, alopecia) are also common, especially in infants with maternal T-cell engraftment. Hypoplastic lymphoid tissue (tonsils, lymph nodes), and absence of a thymic shadow on chest radiography are characteristic.[57,58]

Because of the inability to control replication of live microorganisms, administration of live-attenuated vaccines often leads to severe, life-threatening complications in infants with SCID.[59–61]

T-cell engraftment from maternal transplacentally derived cells occurs in more than 50 percent of infants with SCID. Most often asymptomatic, it may cause skin rash or, less frequently, typical graft-versus-host disease with generalized rash, liver disease, profuse diarrhea, jaundice, and severe hematologic abnormalities (thrombocytopenia, anemia, leukopenia) that are indicative of marrow damage.[62,63] Transfusion of unirradiated blood products often leads to fatal graft-versus-host disease.

Laboratory Features of Severe Combined Immunodeficiency Syndromes

An absolute lymphocyte count less than 2000/μL should prompt immediate investigation for SCID, regardless of the severity of clinical symptoms.[27] However, a normal absolute lymphocyte count does not rule out SCID, if suggestive clinical features are present. Typically, infants with SCID have markedly reduced or absent circulating T cells, hence circulating CD3+ cells should be determined in infants suspected of having SCID, and values should be compared to healthy age-matched controls.[64] Lymphocytes fail to proliferate *in vitro* to mitogens and specific antigens.[27,57]

Normal absolute lymphocyte counts in SCID may reflect maternal T-cell engraftment, hypomorphic mutations, or somatic reversions that allow for some autologous T-cell development.[65,66] Maternal T-cell engraftment and "leaky" SCID with residual development of autologous T cells are characterized by the expression of the CD45R0 memory/activation antigen on the surface of circulating T lymphocytes (whereas most T cells in normal infants have a naïve CD45RA+ phenotype) and failure to respond *in vitro* to mitogens.

T-cell receptor excision circles, consisting of circularized signal joints, are a byproduct of V(D)J recombination and are exported to the blood by recent thymic emigrants. Levels of T-cell receptor excision circles in circulating lymphocytes are particularly high in newborns and infants, and progressively decline with age. Because T-cell receptor excision circles cannot be detected in infants with SCID, assessment of T-cell receptor excision circle levels by polymerase chain reaction has been proposed for newborn screening for SCID[67]; two pilot studies of this approach have started in the United States.

Although the number of circulating B lymphocytes can vary, depending on the nature of the genetic defect, serum immunoglobulin levels are low in infants with SCID. Normal serum IgG levels early in life reflect transplacental passage of maternal immunoglobulins. Antibody response to immunization antigens is abolished. PNP deficiency represents an exception, as in this disease humoral immunity is often spared.

Eosinophilia and elevated IgE levels are common in SCID. Anemia, thrombocytopenia, and neutropenia, caused by infections or marrow damage, may also be present. Autoimmune hemolytic anemia is frequent in PNP deficiency.[34] Marrow abnormalities (dysplasia or aplasia) can be observed in ADA,[68] PNP,[69] Cernunnos/XLF,[70,71] and LIG4[72] deficiencies.

The diagnosis of ADA and PNP deficiency is facilitated by the demonstration of increased levels of deoxyadenosine triphosphate and deoxyguanosine triphosphate, respectively, in red blood cells.

Differential diagnosis of SCID includes secondary forms of immunodeficiencies, especially HIV infection, congenital rubella, and CMV infections, severe malnutrition, marrow failure syndromes,[73] and defects of vitamin B_{12} and folate metabolism.[74,75]

Therapy, Course, and Prognosis of Severe Combined Immunodeficiency Syndromes

SCID is a medical emergency and is inevitably fatal if untreated. Confirmation of diagnosis by appropriate laboratory assays, referral to a tertiary care center, and aggressive treatment of infections should be immediately initiated in infants with possible SCID. High-dose intravenous sulfamethoxazole/trimethoprim (20 mg/kg) is effective in treating *P. jiroveci* pneumonia. CMV or adenoviral infections should be treated with ganciclovir or cidofovir, respectively. Infants who have received bacillus Calmette-Guerin vaccination at birth should receive isoniazid and rifampicin, regardless of the presence of overt signs of mycobacteriosis. Administration of intravenous immunoglobulins and antimicrobial prophylaxis are necessary to reduce the risk of infections. Parenteral nutrition may be necessary, especially if chronic diarrhea and failure to thrive are present.

Survival, however, is ultimately dependent on immune reconstitution. Allogeneic stem cell transplantation was first performed in 1968 in an infant with X-linked SCID,[76] and is the treatment of choice. Survival following stem cell transplantation from an human leukocyte antigen (HLA)-identical sibling is currently as high as 90 percent.[27,77,78] T-cell–depleted transplantation from haploidentical donors results in excellent results if the transplantation is performed in the neonatal period[79] or in the first 3.5 months of life,[27] but survival is only 50 to 65 percent if performed at a later age.[77] Haploidentical transplantation is more successful in B+ SCID than in B– SCID,[77] but is problematic in patients with the Artemis gene mutation or ADA deficiency, or with reticular dysgenesis. Although graft rejection should in theory be impossible in patients with SCID (making the use of pretransplantation chemotherapy unnecessary), full and durable immune reconstitution is more easily achieved following pretransplantation nonmyeloablative conditioning, which favors engraftment of donor stem cells. Promising results have been achieved with stem cell transplantation from matched-unrelated donors and unrelated cord blood.[78,80]

Failure to achieve sufficient T- and B-cell reconstitution is associated with prolonged morbidity after transplantation, but most patients with SCID enjoy good quality of life after transplantion,[81] except for those with ADA or PNP deficiency and SCID with increased cellular radiosensitivity, who often develop neurologic deterioration and developmental problems even after transplantation.[82–84]

Enzyme replacement therapy offers rapid normalization of the toxic metabolites in ADA deficiency in those who do not have a matched donor, and may result in immune reconstitution and significant clinical improvement in patients with ADA deficiency,[85] although T-cell counts often remain low.[86]

A proof of principle that gene therapy may cure SCID has been achieved in X-linked SCID[87,88]; however, some of the patients have developed leukemia because of insertional mutagenesis.[89,90] In contrast, efficacy of gene therapy without adverse events has been reported in ADA deficiency.[91]

OTHER COMBINED IMMUNODEFICIENCIES

In some cases, significant impairment of T-cell immunity is associated with residual development and function of T lymphocytes. These conditions are also known as CID to distinguish them from SCID, in which T-cell development and function are abrogated. The clinical features of CID overlap with SCID, but also include autoimmunity and/or inflammatory manifestations reflecting unbalanced immune homeostasis. CID is caused by two main mechanisms: (1) hypomorphic mutations in SCID-causing genes that allow for some T-cell development; and (2) genetic defects that affect late stages in T-cell development or peripheral T-cell function.

■ OMENN SYNDROME

Definition

Originally described in 1965, Omenn syndrome is characterized by severe infections, associated with early onset diffuse rash or generalized erythroderma, alopecia, eosinophilia, lymphadenopathy, hepatosplenomegaly, hypoproteinemia with edema, and oligoclonal expansion of anergic, activated autologous T lymphocytes that infiltrate and damage target tissues.[92,93]

Genetic Abnormalities

Various gene defects can cause this syndrome. Hypomorphic mutations in the *RAG1* and *RAG2* genes are most common,[94] but mutations of *DCLRE1C* (Artemis),[95] *IL7R*,[96] *LIG4*,[97] *RMRP*,[98] *IL2RG*,[99] *ADA*,[100] and *ZAP70*[101] have been also reported. All these defects severely restrict, but do not completely abrogate, T-cell development.

Pathophysiology

Defects of immunologic tolerance have been implied in the pathophysiology of Omenn syndrome. Thymic expression of AIRE (autoimmune regulator), a transcription factor involved in presentation of self-antigens and negative selection of autoreactive thymocytes, is reduced.[102] Impaired generation of natural regulatory T cells, and homeostatic proliferation of T lymphocytes in a lymphopenic environment, may also play a critical role in the pathophysiology of the disease.[103]

Laboratory Features

Laboratory investigations show that leukocytosis with eosinophilia is common, immunoglobulin levels are low, but serum IgE is often elevated. The number of circulating T lymphocytes may vary, but they have a characteristic activated/memory (CD45R0+) phenotype. T cells have a restricted repertoire, and the distribution of CD4 and CD8 subsets is generally skewed. There is also a skewing to a Th2 profile, with increased production of IL-4 and IL-5. The *in vitro* lymphocyte response to antigens is abrogated; responses to mitogens are variable, but in general are reduced.[104] The number of circulating B and NK lymphocytes may vary, depending on the nature of the underlying genetic defect. Absence of invariant natural killer T cells has been reported in RAG-deficient Omenn syndrome.[105]

Differential Diagnosis

Differential diagnosis includes maternal T-cell engraftment in patients with SCID, complete atypical DiGeorge syndrome, and CHARGE syndrome.[106,107] CHARGE is an acronym derived from coloboma of the eye, heart defects, atresia of the nasal choanae, retardation of growth and development, genital and urinary abnormalities, and ear abnormalities and deafness. Those features are no longer used in making a diagnosis of this complex disorder. The syndrome is considered if a nonrandom pattern of congenital anomalies occurs together more frequently than one would expect on the basis of chance. Very few children with CHARGE will have all of its known features. Most cases have a mutation of the *CHD7* gene on chromosome 8. Male infants with NEMO deficiency can also present with severe skin manifestations resembling Omenn syndrome.

Treatment

In preparation for allogeneic hematopoietic stem cell transplantation, the only curative treatment available,[81] patients require aggressive nutritional support, correction of hypoproteinemia, and treatment or prevention of infections with antibiotics, antifungals, and immunoglobulin replacement therapy. Immune suppression with glucocorticoids or cyclosporine A is beneficial in controlling T-cell–mediated tissue damage.

ZAP-70 DEFICIENCY

Definition

The zeta-associated protein of 70 kDa (ZAP-70) is recruited to phosphorylated CD3ζ chains following TCR ligation, and participates in intracellular signaling. Mutations of ZAP-70 result in a rare form of SCID, with inability to support positive selection of CD8+ lymphocytes in the thymus, whereas development of CD4+ T cells is unaffected.[101,108,109]

Clinical and Laboratory Features

Patients present with clinical features of SCID, with early onset and severe infections. However, lymph nodes are palpable, and a thymic shadow can be visualized by chest radiography. Although the number of circulating CD8+ T cells is severely reduced in patients with ZAP-70 deficiency, the absolute lymphocyte count is normal or can even be elevated. The *in vitro* response to mitogens is markedly reduced, indicating that CD4+ lymphocytes are functionally defective. Profound hypogammaglobulinemia has been demonstrated in some patients, but normal antibody responses to immunization antigens have been recorded in others.

Differential Diagnosis

Differential diagnosis includes major histocompatibility complex (MHC) class I deficiency and CD8α deficiency, two conditions characterized by a severe reduction of CD8+ lymphocytes. Patients with CD8α deficiency have an unusual population of CD3+ TCR $\alpha\beta$+ CD4− CD8− cells that have a normal proliferative responses and usually survive to adulthood, although a late death from infections has been reported.[110,111]

Treatment

The only curative treatment of ZAP-70 deficiency is allogeneic hematopoietic stem cell transplantation.

MHC CLASS I DEFICIENCY

Definition

MHC class I deficiency is characterized by reduced expression of MHC class I molecules at the cell surface. The disease is inherited as an autosomal recessive trait, and may be caused by defects in the *TAP1*,[112] *TAP2*,[113] or Tapasin[114] genes. These defects interfere with intracellular transport of peptide antigens and their loading onto MHC class I molecules, and cell surface expression of the complex.

Clinical and Laboratory Features

The clinical presentation of MHC class I deficiency includes recurrent respiratory infections in childhood, and chronic inflammatory lung disease and skin lesions, mimicking Wegener granulomatosis in patients with transporter associated with antigen-processing (TAP) 1 and TAP2 deficiencies.[115,116] Chronic lung disease is a prominent cause of death. Glomerulonephritis and herpes zoster infections have been reported in the only patient described to date with Tapasin deficiency.[114]

The number of circulating CD8+ T cells is reduced, because positive selection of CD8+ lymphocytes in the thymus depends on the recognition of MHC class I molecules. Although the proportion of TCR$\gamma\delta$+ T cells is increased, *in vitro* T-cell function is normal, which facilitates differential diagnosis with ZAP-70 deficiency in patients who have significantly reduced CD8+ cells. The NK cytolytic activity is usually significantly reduced. Serum immunoglobulin levels are variable.

Treatment

Prophylactic measures, similar to those used in cystic fibrosis, may be beneficial. Treatment of the granulomatous lesions is based on use of topical antiseptics; immunosuppressive drugs may worsen symptoms and should be avoided.

MHC CLASS II DEFICIENCY

Definition

MHC class II deficiency is defined by the lack of MHC class II expression and autosomal recessive inheritance. There is a higher prevalence in populations of North African origin. MHC class II deficiency is caused by mutations of transcription factors that control MHC class II antigen expression by binding to the proximal promotors of the MHC class II gene. Four different gene defects are known and include mutations of the *CIITA*, *RFXANK*, *RFX5*, and *RFXAP* genes.[117]

Clinical and Laboratory Features

Typically, patients present early in life with increased susceptibility to bacterial, viral, and opportunistic infections. Severe lung infections, chronic diarrhea, and sclerosing cholangitis, often secondary to *Cryptosporidium* or CMV infection, are frequently observed. Less-severe presentations and survival into adulthood have been reported.[118,119]

The number of circulating CD4+ T cells is markedly reduced, reflecting an impairment of positive selection in the thymus. Delayed-type hypersensitivity responses are absent, but *in vitro* proliferative responses to mitogens are preserved. Hypogammaglobulinemia is common and poor antibody response to immunization antigens is consistently observed.[118] The diagnosis is based on demonstrating lack of MHC class II expression on monocytes, B lymphocytes and *in vitro* activated T cells. In most patients, expression of MHC class I molecules at the cell surface is also reduced. Differential diagnoses include HIV infection and idiopathic CD4 lymphopenia; however, in these conditions expression of MHC class II molecules is preserved.

Treatment and Course

MHC class II deficiency has a severe prognosis. If untreated, most patients die in infancy or childhood. Respiratory infections are the predominant cause of death. Liver failure is observed in patients who develop sclerosing cholangitis. Nutritional support is often needed and antibiotic prophylaxis and immunoglobulin replacement therapy are required, with marginal impact on long-term prognosis. In some cases, correction of the disease has been achieved by allogeneic hematopoietic stem cell transplantation, but the overall results of this procedure are unsatisfactory, even with an HLA-identical sibling donor.[77] Graft-versus-host disease is common after transplantation, especially in patients with preexisting viral infections.[120]

■ CORONIN-1A DEFICIENCY

Coronin 1A, an actin regulator that is predominantly expressed in hematopoietic cells, plays a key role in regulating egress of thymocytes and trafficking of naïve T lymphocytes to secondary lymphoid organs. Mutations affecting both alleles of the *CORO1A* gene have been reported in a patient with CID who presented at 13 months of age with severe vaccine-related varicella and recurrent respiratory tract infections. The immunologic phenotype includes T-cell lymphopenia with normal numbers of B and NK cells. *In vitro* proliferative responses to mitogens were slightly decreased. Immunoglobulin serum levels were low, but detectable, and antibody responses to antigens were absent. The disease can be treated by allogeneic hematopoietic stem cell transplantation.[121]

■ SIGNAL TRANSDUCERS AND ACTIVATOR OF TRANSCRIPTION 5b DEFICIENCY

Signal transduction and transcription protein, STAT5b, is activated in response to hormones (such as growth hormone) and cytokines (including IL-2) and promotes the transcription of both immune and nonimmune genes. STAT5b deficiency is a rare autosomal recessive disease, characterized by the association of growth hormone insensitivity and a variable degree of immune deficiency.[122,123] Patients have normal length at birth, but then develop short stature. Levels of growth hormone are normal to elevated, but insulin growth factor levels are very low. Patients fail to respond to growth hormone replacement therapy. When present, immune deficiency is manifested by pulmonary infections, including *P. jiroveci* pneumonia, lung fibrosis, and increased susceptibility to severe viral diseases (hemorrhagic varicella, herpes zoster, herpetic keratitis). Autoimmune manifestations also have been reported. Prompt treatment of infections is required to prevent bronchiectasis. Glucocorticoids may be beneficial if there is evidence of lung fibrosis.

■ Ca^{2+} ENTRY CHANNEL DEFICIENCY

Calcium mobilization is a key event in the activation process of lymphocytes and nonimmune cells. Two molecules, ORAI1 and STIM1, mediate the function of Ca^{2+} entry channels. ORAI1 is a ubiquitously expressed protein that constitutes the pore-forming subunits of the Ca^{2+} release-activated channels located in the cell membrane. STIM1 senses the Ca^{2+} concentration in the endoplasmic reticulum and activates Ca^{2+} release-activated channels. Mutations of both the *ORAI1* and *STIM1* genes in humans result in an autosomal recessive immunodeficiency, the clinical manifestations of which resemble SCID with the additional features of nonprogressive myopathy, ectodermal dysplasia, hepatosplenomegaly, hemolytic anemia, and thrombocytopenia.[124,125] Although T-cell development is unaffected, *in vitro* proliferation of circulating T cells to mitogens and to a combination of phorbol ester and ionomycin is drastically reduced, and the Ca^{2+} influx following T-cell activation is absent. In spite of hypergammaglobulinemia, specific antibody responses are typically absent. Allogeneic hematopoietic stem cell transplantation has been used in some patients to correct the defect.[125]

DEFECTIVE THYMIC DEVELOPMENT

■ DIGEORGE SYNDROME (22q 11.2 DELETION SYNDROME)

Definition

The DiGeorge syndrome is a developmental disorder caused by abnormal cephalic neural crest cell migration and differentiation in the third and fourth pharyngeal arches during early embryonic development.[126] The aortic arch anomalies have been created in transgenic mice with haploinsufficiency because of a deletion affecting the murine chromosome 16 that is homologous to human chromosome 22q11.2 which contains the Tpx1 gene known to encode a transcription factor with a T-box DNA binding domain. TBX1 mutations were observed in a few patients with classic features of DiGeorge syndrome, but also in patients with less classic manifestations.[127] However, a significant fraction (10–45%) of patients with DiGeorge syndrome do not have a chromosome 22q11.2 deletion and some 2 percent have small deletions in chromosome 10p.

Clinical and Laboratory Features

The clinical phenotype of DiGeorge syndrome varies considerably. The complete DiGeorge syndrome phenotype consists of the triad congenital cardiac defects, hypocalcemia as a result of parathyroid insufficiency, and immune deficiency as a consequence of aplasia or hypoplasia of the thymus.[126] Most patients have a mild to moderate immune deficiency involving T-cell maturation and function with often T-cell numbers of less than 1500/μL during the first few months of life. A small number of DiGeorge patients lack T cells completely and resemble SCID patients. A few patients with severe T-cell deficiency may present with an atypical phenotype characterized by a pronounced erythematous rash and lymphadenopathy; autoaggressive oligoclonal T cells may be present, similar to patients with Omenn syndrome.[128] As in other cellular immunodeficiencies, patients with DiGeorge syndrome have a high incidence of autoimmune diseases such as rheumatoid arthritis and thyroiditis, and those with profound T-cell deficiency may develop B-cell lymphomas. Cardiac defects occur in 50 to 80 percent of patients with 22q11.2 deletion and hypocalcemia is observed in 50 to 60 percent. A third of DiGeorge syndrome patients have velopharyngeal incompetence, leading to feeding difficulties and speech delay; 10 percent have a cleft palate. As young adults, many develop social, behavioral, and psychiatric problems. Infants suspected of having DiGeorge syndrome should be evaluated for 22q11.2 deletion by the fluorescence *in situ* hybridization assay. DiGeorge syndrome may also occur in the absence of a 22q11.2 deletion.

Treatment

Cardiovascular anomalies require prompt attention and hypocalcemia appropriate medical treatment. Depending on the extent of the immune deficiency, patients may require antibiotic prophylaxis, IVIg therapy, and if T-cell function is absent, immune reconstitution. Transplantation of T-cell–depleted thymic fragments obtained from unrelated donors undergoing partial thymectomy have restored T-cell immunity.[129] Patients with complete lack of thymic function receiving allogeneic hematopoietic stem cells from a matched donor have been successfully reconstituted with a normal immune system that has persisted for up to 20 years.[130]

CONGENITAL ALOPECIA AND ABSENCE OF THYMUS

A homozygous nonsense mutation of the transcription factor FOXN1 resulting in the absence of the thymus has been found in two sisters with a SCID phenotype, congenital alopecia, nail dystrophy, and a severe neural tube defect.[131] FOXN1 is associated with the mouse nude/scid phenotype.

PRIMARY IMMUNODEFICIENCY DISORDERS PRESENTING AS AUTOIMMUNE DISEASES

The concept of a link between immune dysregulation and autoimmunity has been strengthened by the discovery of distinct single gene defects resulting in unusual susceptibility to autoimmune diseases. Three syndromes in this category are (1) immune dysregulation, polyendocrinopathy, enteropathy, and X-linked (IPEX), (2) autoimmune polyendocrinopathy, candidiasis, and ectodermal dystrophy (APECED), and (3) the autoimmune lymphoproliferative syndrome (ALPS).

IPEX SYNDROME

Clinical Findings

The most prominent IPEX symptoms include early onset diarrhea secondary to autoimmune enteropathy, multiple endocrinopathies including insulin-dependent type 1 diabetes mellitus, thyroiditis, and, rarely, adrenal insufficiency. Autoimmune hemolytic anemia, thrombocytopenia, and neutropenia are common complications. Eczema is the most frequent pathology of the skin, but erythematous and psoriasiform dermatitis and alopecia universalis have been reported. Lymphadenopathy and hepatosplenomegaly are less common.[132] There is loss of small bowel villi, and lymphocytic infiltrates in the intestinal mucosa, the pancreas, thyroid, lung, and liver. Immunologic abnormalities include elevated serum IgA and IgE concentrations and the absence of CD4+CD25+ FOXP3+ regulatory T cells.

IPEX is caused by mutations in the *FOXP3* gene located in the centromeric region of the X chromosome.[133] The transcription factor FOXP3 acts as a transcriptional repressor of the IL-2, IL-4, and Interferon (IFN)-γ promoters by interfering with the cytokine regulator, NFAT (nuclear factor of activated T cells).[134]

Treatment

Immunosuppressive drugs such as cyclosporine A, tacrolimus, sirolimus, and glucocorticoids provide temporary remission. Allogeneic hematopoietic stem cell transplantation can cure this disease.[135]

An IPEX-like phenotype has been associated with mutations in CD25, resulting in a complete lack of the IL-2 receptor α chain (CD25). In addition to the characteristic autoimmune manifestations of IPEX, both patients with CD25 deficiency suffered from opportunistic infections, as expected from defective IL-2R signaling.[136,137] Because of these SCID-like features, one patient was successfully transplanted with hematopoietic stem cells from a matched sibling.[136]

AUTOIMMUNE POLYENDOCRINOPATHY, CANDIDIASIS, AND ECTODERMAL DYSTROPHY SYNDROME

APECED is a rare autosomal recessive disorder, also known as autoimmune polyglandular syndrome (APS) type I. The incidence is high in certain isolated populations, for example, Finns, Iranian Jews, and Sardinians. Most patients with APECED present with chronic mucocutaneous candidiasis and endocrinopathies predominantly involving the parathyroid and adrenal glands, less frequently the thyroid and the pancreas. The syndrome is often associated with ectodermal manifestations such as dystrophic dental enamel and fingernails.[138] APECED results from mutations in the *AIRE* gene. AIRE expression is limited to medullary thymic epithelial cells which express MHC class II and the costimulatory molecule CD80. These cells are endowed with the remarkable ability to "promiscuously" express a wide variety of tissue-restricted antigens derived from nearly all organs in the body.[139] Expression of these organ specific proteins allows for the negative selection of autoreactive T cells or the generation of immunoregulatory FOXP3+ T cells in the thymus. A lack of AIRE function causes decreased expression of tissue restricted antigens in the thymus, resulting in the escape of autoreactive T-cell clones into the periphery.[140]

AUTOIMMUNE LYMPHOPROLIFERATIVE SYNDROME (ALPS)

Definition, Clinical Features, and Pathogenesis

ALPS is caused by defective apoptosis of lymphocytes, resulting in nonmalignant lymphadenopathy, hepatosplenomegaly, and autoimmune disorders, which most commonly include Coombs-positive autoimmune hemolytic anemia, thrombocytopenia, and neutropenia. The incidence of lymphoma is estimated to be 9 percent in the National Institutes of Health cohort of 79 probands[141] and consist of both Hodgkin and non-Hodgkin lymphoma. Both lymph nodes and spleen show pronounced hyperplasia and contain a T-cell population of which a large proportion consists of TCRα/β+ CD4–CD8– cells. This phenomenon is also observed in blood lymphocytes from ALPS patients in which the proportion of double-negative T cells is typically between 5 and 20 percent (range: 1–68%).[141] Many of these cells express MHC class II and secrete high levels of IL-4, IL-5, and IL-10.

The Fas-mediated apoptosis pathway is important for the downregulation of antigen induced immune responses and the elimination of autoreactive lymphocytes. ALPS patients have mutations in genes required for "programmed cell death." The most common defect involves the gene encoding T-cell surface molecule Fas, also known as CD95 or TNFRSF6 (ALPS type Ia). In some patients, somatic mutations of Fas have been identified in double-negative T cells (ALPS type 1m). A few families have been identified with mutations affecting the Fas ligand (CD95L; TNFSF6 responsible for ALPS type Ib). Approximately 3 percent of ALPS patients have mutations of caspase 10 or caspase 8 (ALPS type II). Ten to 20 percent of patients with the ALPS phenotype do not have mutations of Fas, FasL, or caspases and are classified as ALPS type III. Because three Fas molecules form a trimeric complex to interact with a FasL trimer, most families with ALPS have autosomal dominant inheritance with variable penetrance (mutations in caspase 8 and 10 are autosomal recessive).

Treatment

Immunosuppressive therapy has been used with variable success to treat autoimmune symptoms. Splenectomy is recommended only in patients with excessively large spleens or splenic rupture and afterwards require lifetime antibiotic prophylaxis. The long-term prognosis is poor.

OTHER WELL-DEFINED IMMUNODEFICIENCY SYNDROMES

WISKOTT-ALDRICH SYNDROME

Definition

The Wiskott-Aldrich syndrome (WAS) is a rare X-linked disorder characterized by thrombocytopenia, small platelets, eczema, recurrent infections, immunodeficiency, and a high incidence of autoimmune diseases and malignancies (see Chap. 121). A classic WAS phenotype is generally associated with null-mutations of the gene that encode the WAS protein (WASP). WASP is the key regulator of actin polymerization in hematopoietic cells and has well-defined domains that are involved in cytoplasmic signaling, cell locomotion, and immunologic synapse formation. A milder phenotype, X-linked thrombocytopenia (XLT), is often associated with mutations that result in expression of mutated protein. XLT patients have either no or very mild eczema and few problems, if any, with infections, autoimmunity, and malignancy.[142] Amino acid substitutions within the guanosine triphosphatase-binding domain of WASP interfere with the intramolecular autoinhibitory mechanism, resulting in gain of function impaired actin polymerization, causing X-linked neutropenia.[143]

Clinical and Laboratory Features

By definition, WAS and XLT patients have congenital thrombocytopenia in the range of 20,000 to 60,000/μL and microplatelets, but normal numbers of megakaryocytes. Hemorrhagic problems may be mild, consisting of bruises and petechiae, or serious, including gastrointestinal and central nervous system hemorrhages. Patients with classic WAS acquire bacterial, fungal, and viral infections.

Treatment Patients may require antibiotic prophylaxis and IVIg replacement therapy. Immunosuppressive therapy may be needed if autoimmune symptoms occur. Because of the poor long-term outcome, early allogeneic hematopoietic stem cell transplantation is the treatment of choice. The outcome is excellent if a matched-related or matched-unrelated donor can be identified, or if a partially matched cord blood unit is available.[144] Haploidentical transplantation is not recommended. Splenectomy ameliorates the bleeding tendency by increasing the number of blood platelets. However, splenectomy substantially increases the risk of septicemia, sometimes in spite of antibiotic prophylaxis, and often results in fatal bacterial infections. Patients with XLT have an excellent prognosis, but may develop complications including serious bleeding, autoimmune diseases, and malignancies. Therefore, allogeneic stem cell transplantation for XLT may be considered if an appropriate donor is available. Because complete myeloid and lymphoid engraftment is required to correct all aspects of WAS/XLT, standard-conditioning using myeloablative protocols (busulfan, cyclophosphamide, with or without antithymocyte globulin) is required. A followup study of WAS patients who received transplantations in Europe reports a strong association of autoimmunity with mixed chimerism, clearly demonstrating that reduced intensity conditioning is not sufficient.[145]

THE HYPERIMMUNOGLOBULIN E SYNDROMES

Autosomal Dominant Hyper IgE Syndrome

Hyperimmunoglobulin E syndrome (HIES) is a rare autosomal dominant (AD) or sporadic multisystem immunodeficiency characterized by eczema, *S. aureus*-induced skin abscesses, recurrent pneumonia with abscess and pneumatocele formation, *Candida* infections, and skeletal and connective tissue abnormalities.[146] In 1966, two girls suffering from eczema, recurrent respiratory tract infections, and "cold" staphylococcus skin abscesses were described as having Job syndrome because of the phenotypic similarity to the biblical figure Job, who had been "smitten with sore boils from the soles of his feet unto his crown."[147] Subsequently, patients with similar clinical findings were reported to have very high serum IgE concentrations[148] and additional characteristic abnormalities were recognized, including distinct facial features, often described as "coarse," hyperextensive joints, pathologic bone fractures, scoliosis, craniosynostosis, and retained primary teeth.[149,150] Serum IgE levels of greater than 2000 IU/mL have been used as arbitrary diagnostic values, but often are greater than 10,000 IU/mL. Other abnormal laboratory tests include eosinophilia, abnormal antibody responses to neoantigens, chemotactic defects of neutrophils, and reduced lymphocyte proliferation to specific antigens.

Most patients with HIES are noted to arise sporadically from unaffected, healthy parents. With the advent of improved antibiotic therapy, patients survived into adulthood and had affected children, suggesting autosomal dominant inheritance.[149] This observation was validated by the finding that heterozygous mutations of the gene encoding the transcription factor STAT3 are the cause of AD-HIES. All STAT3 mutations identified to date in patients with AD-HIES are either amino acid substitutions or in-frame deletions strongly supporting the concept that coexpression of wild-type and mutant STAT3 protein is required to cause the syndrome. The notable lack of nonsense or frameshift mutations strengthens the notion that AD-HIES is a result of a dominant-negative effect.[151–153] The molecular analysis of a large cohort of patients (n = 38) with "classic" HIES and a score of greater than 40 points using the National Institutes of Health clinical scoring system, identified STAT3 mutations in all but one individual. The mutations clustered in three domains of the STAT3 protein known to have distinct functional characteristics, the DNA-binding, and the SH2 and the transactivation domains. This finding suggests that more than one molecular mechanism causes the AD-HIES phenotype. This notion is supported by the observation that mutations in the SH2 domain, but not those in the DNA-binding domain affect tyrosine phosphorylation of STAT3, whereas mutations in the DNA-binding domain interfere with nuclear import and DNA-binding.[153] Because STAT3 plays a key role in the development of IL-17 producing Th17 cells, AD-HIES patients have a marked decrease in circulating Th17 cells.[154] Given that IL-17 plays an important role in host defense against extracellular bacteria and fungi and upregulates production of β defensins and S100 proteins by neutrophils,[155] the absence of Th17 cells may directly affect susceptibility to *S. aureus* and *Candida albicans*.

Treatment To prevent progressive lung destruction, prophylactic antibiotic therapy to decrease the frequency of *S. aureus* infections are important. Antifungal therapy is indicated to prevent recurrent *Candida* infections. A surgical approach to treating chronic lung disease should be avoided, if possible. Allogeneic hematopoietic stem cell transplantation has been performed in a few patients without clear benefit.[156,157]

Autosomal Recessive Hyper IgE Syndromes

In 2004, a cohort of patients from consanguineous families were reported to have markedly elevated serum IgE levels, recurrent bacterial, fungal, and viral infections including herpes simplex, therapy-resistant molluscum contagiosum, and recurrent varicella zoster. Decreased lymphocyte proliferation suggested a significant T-cell defect. In contrast to HIES due to STAT3 mutations, AR-HIES patients frequently present with neurologic complications but do not develop skeletal abnormalities nor postpneumonia pneumatoceles. Most, if not all, have mutations in the DOCK8 gene.[157a] A single adult patient with eczema; moderately elevated serum IgE; a history of bacterial, fungal, and viral infections including molluscum contagiosum; and a mild T-cell deficiency was found to have a mutation in TYK2, a receptor-associated cytoplasmatic tyrosine kinase which plays an important role in multiple cytokine signaling in T cells.[157b]

IMMUNOOSSEOUS DYSPLASIAS

Cartilage Hair Hypoplasia

Cartilage hair hypoplasia is an autosomal recessive condition characterized by short-limbed dwarfism and light-colored hypoplastic hair.[158] Patients may also present with marrow cell dysplasia, increased susceptibility to malignancies, Hirschsprung disease, defects of spermatogenesis, and a variable degree of immunodeficiency (SCID, Omenn syndrome, partial T-cell deficiency) or may have normal immune function.[159] The rare disorder is more common in certain populations, such as the Amish and the Finns, and is caused by mutations of the gene encoding for untranslated RNA component of the ribonuclease mitochondrial RNA processing (*RMRP*) complex, that is involved in cleavage of ribosomal RNA, processing of mitochondrial RNA, and cell-cycle control.[160] Decreased number of T lymphocytes, reduced number of CD8+ cells, and impaired *in vitro* proliferative responses to mitogens have been reported.[161] Impairment of cellular immunity may cause increased susceptibility to severe varicella or other viral diseases, and administration of live-attenuated viral vaccines should be avoided. Defects of humoral immunity are less frequent, and may contribute to recurrent infections. Autoimmune manifestations (hemolytic anemia, neutropenia, and thrombocytopenia) may also occur. Similar to what has been observed in other disorders of ribosomal biogenesis (Diamond-Blackfan anemia, Shwachman-Diamond syndrome), disturbances of hematopoiesis, such as anemia, leukopenia, thrombocytopenia, and marrow dysplasia, are frequent manifestations of cartilage hair hypoplasia. Allogeneic hematopoietic stem cell transplantation has been successfully used to correct those forms of cartilage hair hypoplasia presenting with a SCID or Omenn syndrome phenotype.[161,162]

Schimke Syndrome

Schimke syndrome is an autosomal recessive condition characterized by dwarfism with short neck and trunk because of spondyloepiphyseal dysplasia, progressive renal impairment evolving to renal failure, facial dysmorphisms, lentigines, immunodeficiency (ranging from T-cell lymphopenia to SCID), and increased occurrence of marrow failure and of early onset arteriosclerosis associated with cerebral infarcts.[163] Microcephaly and cognitive, motor, or social abnormalities have been reported in a significant proportion of the patients.[164] The disease is caused by mutations of the *SMARCAL1* gene, that encodes for a chromatin remodeling protein.[165] Recurrent infections of bacterial, viral, and fungal origin, and opportunistic infections (*P. jiroveci* pneumonia) are seen in half of the patients. Severe presentations lead to death in the first decade of life, and development of renal failure is common among those who survive. A combined hematopoietic stem cell and renal transplantation has been used to correct immune deficiency and renal problems.[163]

WHIM Syndrome

Warts, hypogammaglobulinemia, infections, and myelokathexis (WHIM) syndrome[166] is an autosomal dominant disorder, caused by heterozygous mutations in the *CXCR4* gene that encodes for the receptor for the CXCL12 chemokine, involved in leukocyte trafficking.[167] The term *myelokathexis* indicates retention of mature neutrophils in the marrow. WHIM mutations result in truncation or structural abnormalities in the intracytoplasmic tail of CXCR4, that interfere with ligand-induced internalization and ultimately cause increased cellular responsiveness to CXCL12.[168]

Patients with WHIM syndrome may present with early onset recurrent bacterial infections, but the clinical phenotype may vary greatly.[169] Warts, caused by human papillomavirus, tend to develop in the second decade of life. Severe neutropenia contrasts with accumulation of mature neutrophils in the marrow. Spontaneous apoptosis of neutrophils has been reported.[170] Lymphopenia including low B-cell numbers is a frequent finding. Hypogammaglobulinemia of variable degree can be observed, and immunizations result in short-lived antibody responses. Epstein-Barr virus (EBV)-positive B-cell lymphoma can occur.

Immunoglobulin replacement therapy and antibiotic prophylaxis may reduce the incidence of infections. Recombinant G-CSF can be used to increase the absolute neutrophil count. Warts are resistant to local therapy and need to be monitored for neoplastic transformation.

CHROMOSOMAL INSTABILITY SYNDROMES ASSOCIATED WITH IMMUNODEFICIENCY

Chromosomal instability syndromes have in common increased spontaneous or induced DNA breaks, susceptibility to infections secondary to immune deficiency, and an increased risk of malignancies. Disease-specific abnormalities involving growth and development, the central nervous system, and the skin provide useful diagnostic clues. The classic chromosomal instability syndromes include ataxia-telangiectasia (AT), Nijmegen breakage syndrome (NBS), Bloom syndrome (BS), and ataxia-telangiectasia–like disorder (ATLD). The genes responsible for these syndromes protect human genome integrity by contributing to the complex task of double-strand break repair. Together with the proteins associated with Fanconi anemia, the gene products of the chromosomal instability syndromes form or regulate a large protein complex which is active in the surveillance and maintenance of genomic integrity.[171] The triad of immunodeficiency, neoplasia, and infertility is the direct consequence of defective double-strand break repair, and involves nonhomologous end-joining or homologous rejoining. Because nonhomologous end-joining is crucial for the generation of T-cell receptor diversity and polyclonal immunoglobulins, any interruption of this process will predictably result in defective adaptive immunity. Tumor development and infertility may be a direct consequence of defective DNA repair during miotic recombination of lymphocytes, other somatic cells, or germ cells, respectively.

ATAXIA-TELANGIECTASIA

AT is a multisystem disorder, characterized by immunodeficiency, progressive neurologic impairment, and ocular and cutaneous telangiectasia.

The immune deficiency in AT is highly variable, involving both cellular and humoral immunity. Respiratory infections are common and often result in chronic lung disease. Opportunistic infections are rare. The majority of AT patients have low or absent IgA and IgE, often combined with IgG_2 and IgG_4 deficiency.[172] Specific antibody responses may be depressed or normal. The number of circulating lymphocytes is often reduced, and proliferation in response to mitogens is variably depressed. Spontaneous cytogenetic abnormalities include chromosomal breaks, translocations, rearrangements, and inversions; these defects increase following *in vitro* exposure to radiation. The thymus is often small, showing marked paucity of thymocytes and absence of Hassall corpuscles. The most consistent laboratory abnormality, an elevation of serum α-fetoprotein, is diagnostic in adults and children older than age 8 months as it is not observed in the other chromosomal instability syndromes.

Cancer is the second most common cause of death, after infections. Most malignancies are non-Hodgkin lymphomas (40%), leukemias (25%), and solid tumors (25%); 10 percent are Hodgkin lymphoma. In contrast to other immune deficiency syndromes with increased incidence of malignancies, the leukemias and lymphomas observed in AT are predominantly of T-cell origin. The solid tumors in AT patients include adenocarcinoma, dysgerminoma, gonadoblastoma, and medulloblastoma.

Cerebellar ataxia is the earliest clinical manifestation of AT and becomes evident when a child begins to walk at the end of the first year of life. The ataxic gait persists, and most patients never develop normal speech. Eventually, involuntary movements become a major handicap and the child may require a wheelchair by the end of the first decade of life. Cortical cerebellar degeneration involves primarily Purkinje and granular cells; progressive changes to the central nervous system also occur.

A variety of other features have been reported. Growth retardation is present in 30 percent of the patients. Female hypogonadism is common and associated with hypoplasia of the ovaries. Hypogonadism is also observed in male AT patients.

The AT gene (*AT mutated [ATM]*) encodes a large transcript that predicts a protein of 3056 amino acids.[173] ATM is a predominantly nuclear protein with a strong serine-threonine kinase activity. Its major function is to rapidly respond to the induction of double-stranded breaks in DNA. The activation of ATM leads to phosphorylation of an extensive array of target proteins, each of which plays a key role in a unique damage response pathway. Specifically, ATM is involved in cell-cycle checkpoint control and delays the passage of cells through the various phases of the cell cycle, allowing time for DNA damage repair. Additionally, ATM is functionally linked to telomere maintenance, a process crucial to aging and cancer.[174] The more than 400 unique mutations of ATM described to date are distributed throughout the gene with a majority predicted to cause premature termination resulting in unstable truncated proteins.

ATAXIA-TELANGIECTASIA–LIKE DISORDER

An AT-like disorder(ATLD) that has many features of AT[175] is the result of mutations in the hMre11 protein which is part of the DNA-repair complex (Mre11/Rad50/Nbs1).[176] Affected patients have progressive ataxia, but show less-severe neurodegeneration and may be ambulatory until their early twenties. They do not develop telangiectasia and α-fetoprotein levels are normal. However, similar to AT, ATLD patients have increased spontaneous chromosomal abnormalities in blood lymphocytes and show increased radiation sensitivity.

NIJMEGEN BREAKAGE SYNDROME

NBS is characterized by short stature, microcephaly, a bird-like face, immunodeficiency, chromosomal instability, increased radiosensitivity, and a high percentage of malignancies.[177] Although NBS shares many characteristics with AT and ATLD, it can be distinguished from these disorders by an absence of neurodegeneration, impressive microcephaly with mild to moderate mental retardation, and absence of telangiectasia.

Most NBS patients develop respiratory tract infections, including recurrent pneumonia that may result in bronchiectasis and premature death from respiratory failure. Both humoral and cellular immunity are defective and include hypogammaglobulinemia, except for normal or elevated IgM, abnormal antibody responses to protein and polysaccharide antigens, suggesting a defect in class switch recombination, reduced numbers of T lymphocytes, and abnormal lymphoproliferation to mitogens and specific antigens.[171]

NBS lymphocytes show the typical features of chromosomal instability syndromes characterized by increased chromatid and chromosome breaks, rearrangement/translocations of chromosome 7 and 14, telomere fusions, radio-resistant DNA synthesis, and hypersensitivity to ionizing radiation and radiomimetic agents.

The extensive immunodeficiency and the chromosomal instability explain the high incidence of lymphoid malignancies, including non-Hodgkin lymphoma (both of B- and T-cell origin), lymphoblastic leukemia/lymphoma, and less frequently Hodgkin lymphoma and acute myeloblastic leukemia. Solid tumors are less frequent and include medulloblastoma and rhabdomyosarcoma. Because of hypersensitivity to radiation and radiomimetic/alkylating agents, tumor therapy is limited. However, several patients have been successfully treated with allogeneic hematopoietic stem cell transplantation. Prophylactic therapy with antibiotics and IVIg is indicated in patients with recurrent infections.

BLOOM SYNDROME

BS is characterized by short stature, hypersensitivity to sunlight, increased susceptibility to infections, and a predisposition to early development of a variety of cancers.[171] Susceptibility to bacterial infections, affecting mainly the upper and lower respiratory tract, is associated with hypogammaglobulinemia and variable T-cell deficiency. Most affected patients have decreased fertility and some may develop early onset type II diabetes mellitus. By age 25 years, approximately half of the patients with BS will have developed one or more malignancies. Leukemia and non-Hodgkin lymphoma predominate during the first two decades; later, carcinoma affecting the colon, skin, and breast are common. The diagnosis of BS can be confirmed by demonstrating excessive numbers of sister-chromatid exchanges, increased chromatid gaps and breaks, and the presence of quadriradial configuration composed of two homologous chromosomes. The causative gene, BLM, encodes a 1417-amino-acid protein with homology to the RecQ family of helicases. This family of helicases include the WRN protein, which is mutated in Werner syndrome. BLM is a member of a group of proteins that associate with BRCA1 to form a large complex that colocalizes to large nuclear foci if cells are treated with agents that interfere with DNA synthesis. As part of this complex, BLM plays a role in sensing DNA damage and contributes to the maintenance and genomic integrity during the process of DNA replication and repair. More than 60 unique mutations in the BLM gene have been identified. The most common mutation is a 6bp deletion/7bp insertion in exon 10 causing BS in Ashkenazi Jews.

Patients with chromosomal instability may benefit from antibiotic prophylaxis and IVIg therapy, if immune deficiency is documented. Because of increased radiation sensitivity, exposure to any form of irradiation should be restricted.

CYTOTOXICITY DISORDERS

Defense against viruses is primarily dependent on cell-mediated cytotoxicity. Cytotoxic T lymphocytes (CTLs) and NK cells are capable of killing virus-infected target cells using pore-forming perforin and cytolytic granzymes A and B. Different genetic defects can affect various steps in the formation, intracellular transport, and delivery of cytolytic granules,[178,179] and result in different defects of cell-mediated cytotoxicity, that include various forms of familial hemophagocytic lymphohistiocytosis (FHL), Chédiak-Higashi syndrome, Griscelli syndrome type II, and Hermansky-Pudlak syndrome type II. Overall, these disorders are characterized by increased susceptibility to severe viral infections that in some cases is associated with defects of hair and skin pigmentation, and neurological problems. Dysregulation in CTL and NK homeostasis, with increased production of inflammatory cytokines and accumulation of activated lymphocytes, characterizes the two genetic variants of X-linked lymphoproliferative syndrome (XLP1 and XLP2).

FAMILIAL HEMOPHAGOCYTIC LYMPHOHISTIOCYTOSIS

FHL includes a group of genetically heterogeneous conditions that are characterized by the uncontrolled proliferation of activated lymphocytes and histiocytes that secrete large amounts of proinflammatory cytokines. This results in life-threatening manifestations, characterized by fever, hepatosplenomegaly, marrow infiltration and pancytopenia, and severe neurologic manifestations (see Chap. 72).

There are at least four different forms of FHL, three of which have been defined at the molecular level. FHL2 is caused by mutations of the *PRF1* gene, which encodes perforin.[180] FHL3 is caused by mutations in *UNC13D*, also known as MUNC 13–4,[181] whereas FHL4 is caused by defects of the *STX11* gene, that encodes syntaxin 11.[182] Each of these defects interferes with a specific step of the cytolytic machinery, and ultimately causes inefficient pathogen clearance, uncontrolled activation of CTLs, and release of IFN-$\gamma$and other inflammatory cytokines, resulting in recruitment and activation of macrophages, and inhibition of hematopoiesis.

Clinical and Laboratory Features

In approximately 85 percent of the cases, FHL becomes clinically evident within the first year of life,[183] but late presentations may occur in patients with hypomorphic mutations.[184–186] High fever, severe hepatosplenomegaly, lymphadenopathy, hemorrhagic manifestations as a result of thrombocytopenia, and edema are common. Neurologic symptoms, including seizures and decreased level of consciousness, may lead to long-term disability.[187]

The FHL diagnostic guidelines were updated in 2007.[188] Anemia and thrombocytopenia are early symptoms followed by increased serum levels of triglycerides, bilirubin, liver enzymes, ferritin, and coagulation abnormalities. Hemophagocytosis can be observed in the marrow, lymph nodes, and cerebrospinal fluid, which often shows abundant mononuclear cells and increased proteins, even in the absence of overt neurologic symptoms. Immunologic findings include persistently impaired cytolytic activity of NK cells and elevated levels of inflammatory cytokines (IFN-γ, IL-1, IL-6, tumor necrosis factor-γ) in the blood. Monitoring circulating soluble CD25 (IL-2Rα) is also useful as a measure of increased cellular activation.

Flow-cytometry enables analysis of perforin expression except for hypomorphic mutations, and may thus facilitate diagnosis of FHL2. The diagnosis of FHL forms that are characterized by reduced NK cell degranulation (such as *UNC13D* and *STX11* defects) may be facilitated by the analysis of membrane expression of the lysosomal marker CD107a.[189]

Treatment and Prognosis

Without treatment, FHL is usually rapidly fatal. Treatment of active disease includes antimicrobials, etoposide, immune suppression (antithymocyte globulin), cyclosporine A, and dexamethasone.[188,190] However, a permanent cure for FHL can be only provided by allogeneic hematopoietic stem cell transplantation. A higher success rate is obtained when HLA-matched related or unrelated donors are used; partial chimerism is enough to achieve disease control.[191]

X-LINKED LYMPHOPROLIFERATIVE DISEASE

Definition and History

In 1975, Purtilo described a family in which multiple males in multiple generations presented with fulminant infectious mononucleosis, lymphoma, or hypogammaglobulinemia after primary EBV infection.[192] X-linked lymphoproliferative disease type 1 (XLP1) is caused by mutations in the *SH2D1A* gene[193,194] that encodes an adaptor protein (SLAM [signaling lymphocyte activation molecule]-associated protein [SAP]) involved in T- and NK cell signaling.[195] Thus, defects of SAP drastically affect both T- and NK-mediated cytotoxicity.[196–198] SAP, also, plays an important role in germinal center formation and antibody production by modulating development and function of follicular helper T cells.[199] Finally, SAP is required for the development of invariant NKT cells, which are immunoregulatory cells that are involved in the responses to pathogens and cancer cells.[200] In the absence of SAP, EBV and other virus infections result in dysregulated immune responses, because of persistent antigenic stimulation that leads to hyperactive cytotoxic T lymphocytes and macrophages, with increased production of IFN-γ.

However, not all males with XLP-features have mutations in *SH2D1A* and mutations in another X-chromosome-associated gene (*XIAP*; X-linked inhibitor of apoptosis, also known as *BIRC4*) have been identified,[201] resulting in XLP2. Similar to XLP1, patients with XLP2 lack NKT cells. Based on the role played by XIAP/BIRC4 in inhibiting caspase-3, caspase-7, and caspase-9, lymphocytes from XLP2 patients display increased susceptibility to apoptosis upon *in vitro* activation, but the precise pathophysiology is not well understood.

Clinical and Laboratory Features

Most often XLP1 and XLP2 become clinically manifest following EBV infection in childhood, although later presentations are possible. Fulminant infectious mononucleosis has been observed in 50 to 60 percent of cases, and EBV-related lymphoma in 30 percent of the cases. Most lymphomas are of B-cell origin, and about half are of the Burkitt type. Persistent dysgammaglobulinemia, with low IgG and low to increased levels of IgM, is common among survivors. Other clinical manifestations of XLP include vasculitis, marrow aplasia secondary to hemophagocytic lymphohistiocytosis, and lymphoid granulomatosis.

Although less frequently encountered, other viral infections (CMV, other herpesviruses) may unmask the clinical phenotype of XLP.[202]

Fulminant infectious mononucleosis is marked by a rapid increase of liver enzymes, followed by impaired coagulation, hepatic encephalopathy, and signs of hemophagocytic lymphohistiocytosis, associated with a high EBV viral load in the blood and other tissues. B-cell lymphomas carry monoclonal immunoglobulin gene rearrangements. Patients who develop dysgammaglobulinemia show impaired antibody responses. Antibody levels to the EBV nuclear antigen usually remain undetectable, even in patients who survive the acute EBV infection. In contrast, antibodies to the EBV viral capsid antigen can be low to elevated. During clinical manifestations of XLP, the proportion of CD8+ T cells carrying activation markers is increased and the number of memory (CD27+), and specifically switched memory (CD27+IgD–) B cells are reduced. NK cell cytotoxicity is usually normal, when measured in a conventional K562 killing assay. However, NK cytolytic activity is markedly reduced in XLP1, when costimulation through CD244 is provided.[196] Flow cytometry can be used to detect a lack of SAP protein expression in circulating T and NK lymphocytes in patients with XLP1.[203]

Treatment and Prognosis

If untreated, approximately 70 percent of XLP patients die within 10 years of onset. The mortality rate is particularly high (96%) in patients who present with fulminant infectious mononucleosis.[204] Allogeneic stem cell transplantation is the treatment of choice, yielding the best results when the transplant is performed early in life, prior to EBV infection. However, transplantation using reduced-intensity conditioning may permit correction of the disease in EBV-positive patients with severe organ toxicity.[205] The use of anti-CD20 monoclonal antibody can reduce viral load and improve the clinical status, and antitumor necrosis factor-α therapy or etoposide may be beneficial in patients with active EBV infection and severe systemic inflammatory response.[206–208] Administration of immunoglobulins may reduce the risk of infections in XLP patients with hypogammaglobulinemia, but does not prevent or attenuate the symptoms of primary EBV infection.

■ CHÉDIAK-HIGASHI SYNDROME

Definition and Clinical Features

Chédiak-Higashi syndrome is an autosomal recessive disorder characterized by immune dysregulation with impaired cellular cytotoxicity, partial oculocutaneous albinism, platelet functional abnormalities, and neurologic involvement (see Chaps. 66 and 121).[209] The disease is caused by mutations in the *lysosomal trafficking regulator* (*LYST*) gene.[210] LYST plays an important role in sorting of lysosomal proteins, and in docking and fusion of lysosomal vesicles.[178]

Patients are susceptible to recurrent pyogenic and viral infections. Bruises are common and reflect deficiency of the platelet specific granules responsible for secondary aggregation. Both bacterial and viral infections may trigger the life-threatening "accelerated phase" of the disease, characterized by high fever, hepatosplenomegaly, coagulation abnormalities, increase of liver enzymes and bilirubin (with possible jaundice), edema, and neurologic symptoms, with seizures, ataxia, cranial nerve palsies, and peripheral neuropathy.[209]

Abnormally large granules in lymphocytes, neutrophils, platelets, melanocytes, and neurons represent a morphologic hallmark of the disease. Light microscopy examination of hair reveals large and evenly distributed granules of melanin. Reduced NK cytotoxic activity, and prolonged bleeding time are typical findings.

Treatment

Treatment requires control of infections, and immunosuppressive intervention during the accelerated phase. Allogeneic hematopoietic stem cell transplantation, best performed during remission, is the only permanent cure of the immunohematologic problems.[211] However, hematopoietic stem cell transplantation does not seem to prevent progressive neurologic involvement.[212]

■ GRISCELLI SYNDROME TYPE 2

Griscelli syndrome type 2 (GS2) is an autosomal recessive syndrome characterized by immunodeficiency and hypopigmentation, and a variable degree of neurologic involvement. The presence of immune deficiency distinguishes GS2 from GS1 (marked by the association of partial albinism and neurologic involvement) and GS3 (with isolated hypopigmentation). GS2 is caused by mutations of the *RAB27A* gene,[213] which encodes for a guanosine triphosphatase involved in intracellular transport of granules.

GS2 patients are highly susceptible to recurrent pyogenic infections and to episodes of "accelerated phase" of the disease, with high fever, hepatosplenomegaly, neutropenia, and thrombocytopenia. Prominent hypopigmentation is a result of large clumps of melanin in the hair shafts. NK cytotoxicity is defective and impaired CD107 expression at the cell membrane is observed upon *in vitro* coculture of NK lymphocytes with target cells. Treatment is based on hematopoietic stem cell transplantation early in life.

■ HERMANSKY-PUDLAK TYPE 2

This autosomal recessive disease is characterized by oculocutaneous albinism, bleeding tendency, recurrent infections, and moderate to severe neutropenia (see Chap. 121).[214] Bone anomalies (with dysplastic acetabulae), facial dysmorphisms and development of pulmonary fibrosis are also part of the clinical phenotype. Hermansky-Pudlak type 2 is caused by mutations of the *AP3B1* gene that encode for the β_1 subunit of the AP-3 endosomal protein, which is required for sorting of lysosomal membrane proteins to the granules.[215] Missorting of tyrosinase in melanocytes accounts for oculocutaneous albinism. Reduced platelet dense granules and impaired platelet degranulation are responsible for increased susceptibility to bleeding. Absence of AP-3 leads to low intracellular content of neutrophil elastase in myeloid progenitors causing neutropenia. CTL and NK cell cytolytic activity is defective[216] and progression to acute episodes of hemophagocytic lymphohistiocytosis has been occasionally observed.[217] Control of infections is important in the management of these patients. G-CSF may improve the chronic neutropenia.

IMMUNODEFICIENCIES WITH SELECTIVE SUSCEPTIBILITY TO PATHOGENS

Although classical forms of primary immune deficiency disease are characterized by susceptibility to a broad range of pathogens, several disorders have been identified with selective susceptibility to certain microorganisms. Some of these diseases (e.g., mendelian susceptibility to herpes simplex encephalitis or to pyogenic infections, especially *S. pneumoniae*) are a result of defects of innate immunity, in particular toll-like receptor (TLR) signaling. Others (mendelian susceptibility to mycobacterial disease) involve defects of the IL-12/IFN-γ axis at the interface of innate and adaptive immunity. Susceptibility to recurrent meningitis caused by *Neisseria meningitidis* is discussed under "Genetically Determined Deficiencies of the Complement System".

■ IMMUNODEFICIENCIES WITH IMPAIRED SIGNALING THROUGH TOLL-LIKE RECEPTORS

TLRs are transmembrane proteins expressed on a variety of cell types that recognize pathogen-associated molecular patterns, such as lipopolysaccharide derived from Gram-negative bacteria, lipopeptide, double-stranded RNA that is generated during viral replication, viral single-stranded RNA, viral cytosine phosphate guanine DNA moieties and flagellin. Most TLRs are expressed at the cell surface, however TLRs 7, 8, and 9 are expressed on the membrane of endosomal vesicles.

Binding of pathogen-associated molecular patterns to TLRs induces characteristic intracellular signalling. The classical pathway of TLR activation involves the adaptor molecules MyD88 (myeloid differentiation factor 88) and toll-interleukin 1 receptor domain-containing adaptor protein, and the intracellular kinases IL-1 receptor-associated kinase (IRAK)-4 and IRAK-1, ultimately resulting in the nuclear transfer of NF-κB and the production of inflammatory cytokines (IL-1, IL-6, tumor necrosis factor-α, IL-12). TLRs 3, 7, 8, and 9 activate an alternative pathway that involves other adaptor molecules, such as toll-interleukin 1 receptor domain-containing adaptor-inducing IFN-β (TRIF), TRIF-related adaptor molecule, and the UNC-93B protein, and ultimately results in the induction of type 1 interferons (IFN-α/β). Deficiencies of IRAK-4, MyD88, TLR3, and UNC-93B have been identified in humans, and are associated with two distinct phenotypes.

TLR-Signaling Defects with Increased Susceptibility to Herpes Simplex Virus Encephalitis

Two unrelated patients with *herpes simplex virus encephalitis* (HSE) from consanguineous families were found to carry homozygous mutations in the *UNC-93B1* gene.[218] Blood mononuclear cells from these patients failed to produce IFN-α, -β, and -γ in response to TLR3, TLR7, TLR8, and TLR9 agonists.

Heterozygous, dominant-negative mutations of *TLR3* have also been identified in patients with recurrent HSE.[219] Because TLR3 recognizes double-stranded RNA and is normally expressed in CNS resident cells, *TLR3* mutations impair the response of these cells to actively replicating herpes simplex virus-1. Because cellular responsiveness to type 1 IFN is intact in both UNC-93B– and in TLR3-deficient patients, the use of IFN-α along with acyclovir should be considered to treat HSE in these patients.[219]

HSE may also be a result of null mutations of STAT1, a transcription factor that is activated upon interaction of type 1 IFN with their receptors, and is critical for the induction of IFN-responsive genes. Because STAT1 is also involved in the response to IFN-γ, patients with null *STAT1* mutations are also at risk for mycobacterial disease.[220]

TLR-Signaling Defects with Increased Susceptibility to Pyogenic Infections

IRAK-4 and MyD88 deficiencies are characterized by recurrent and invasive pyogenic bacterial infections, particularly from *S. pneumoniae* and *S. aureus*.[221,222] These infections are common especially during the first years of life (when lethality rate can be as high as 50%), but their frequency tends to decline with age.[223] Fever and systemic inflammatory responses are absent or unusually modest, reflecting poor induction of inflammatory cytokines and reduced response through the IL-1R. Failure to sustain antibody responses to T-cell–dependent and T-cell–independent antigens has been reported in patients with IRAK-4 deficiency.[224] Diagnosis can be suspected based on the infection history associated with poor inflammatory responses. Defective shedding of CD62L from the surface of granulocytes upon addition of TLR agonists can be used as a flow cytometry-based screening assay.[225]

Use of antimicrobic prophylaxis is important to prevent invasive pyogenic infections, especially in childhood. Substitution therapy with immunoglobulins may be beneficial in patients with impaired antibody responses.

Defects Involving Other Pattern-Recognition Signaling Pathways with Increased Susceptibility to Fungal Infections

Chronic mucocutaneous candidiasis is a common complication affecting patients with APECED due to mutation in the transcription factor AIRE[138] and those with autosomal dominant HIES due to mutations in the transcription factor STAT3.[146] Genetic evaluation of a large consanguineous family in which four members had recurrent mucocutaneous candidiasis and two additional members had died of invasive candidiasis of the brain.[225A] Homozygosity mapping identified a region within chromosome 9 that encompassed CARD9 encoding the caspase recruitment domain-containing protein 9. Affected members of this family had a homozygous point mutation in CARD9, resulting in a premature termination codon. CARD9 is recruited by Dectin-1, a transmembrane pattern-recognition receptor that senses the beta-glucan component of fungal cell walls, and together with other cytoplasmatic proteins, forms an intracellular signaling complex that leads to the nuclear import of NFkB and the induction of key cytokines including IL-1, IL-6, IL-23, and the generation of IL-17 cells, which are required to control antifungal immune responses.

MENDELIAN SUSCEPTIBILITY TO MYCOBACTERIAL DISEASE

The IL-12/IFN-γ axis is essential for controlling mycobacterial infections. Following phagocytosis of mycobacteria, macrophages secrete IL-12, a heterodimer composed of IL-12p40 and IL-12p70. IL-12 binds to the heterodimeric IL-12R (composed of IL12Rβ_1 and IL-12Rβ_2 chains) expressed by Th1 and NK cells. This results in activation of the JAK-STAT4 pathway and ultimately in the production of IFN-γ, which binds to its receptor (comprising IFN-γR1 and IFN-γR2 chains) on the surface of macrophages, triggering a signalling cascade that involves the transcription factor STAT1 and induction of IFN-γ-responsive genes that are essential to contain the infection and kill the mycobacteria. A variety of defects along this pathway have been shown to account for mendelian susceptibility to mycobacterial disease in humans.[60,226] The basis for increased susceptibility to mycobacterial disease in patients with NEMO deficiency was discussed above in the section "X-Linked Anhydrotic Ectodermal Dysplasia with Immunodeficiency."

IL-12p40 Deficiency

Autosomal recessive IL-12p40 deficiency is the only genetically-determined cytokine deficiency known in humans. Affected patients are at increased risk of severe infections due to bacillus Calmette-Guerin and environmental mycobacteria, but *Salmonella*, *Nocardia,* and *Mycobacterium tuberculosis* infections have also been reported.[227] The clinical course is variable, but approximately 40 percent of the IL-12p40-deficient patients have died prematurely of infections. Treatment with antibiotics and IFN-γ is indicated.

IL-12Rβ_1 Deficiency

Autosomal recessive IL-12Rβ_1 deficiency is characterized by infections with mycobacteria of low virulence and *Salmonella* species. However, infections with *M. tuberculosis* have also been reported.[228] Unlike salmonellosis, mycobacterial infections tend not to recur and the overall prognosis is good. In most cases, IL-12Rβ_1 expression on the cell surface is absent, and *in vitro* IFN-γ production in response to IL-12 is abrogated. Treatment with appropriate antibiotics and IFN-γ is effective.

IFN-γR1 and IFN-γR2 Deficiencies

The genetic and biochemical pathophysiology of IFN-γR1 and IFN-γR2 deficiencies are remarkably complex. Autosomal recessive forms are most often associated with mutations that abrogate cell surface expression of IFN-γR1 or result in the expression of receptors that do not bind IFN-γ. Partial autosomal recessive deficiency is the result of hypomorphic mutations, with residual IFN-γ binding and signaling. Dominant partial forms reflect the presence of heterozygous mutations in the cytoplasmic tail of IFN-γR1, allowing the expression of mutant molecules on the cell surface (often in increased density due to defective receptor shedding) which are unable to mediate signal transduction.[229]

The severity of the clinical features reflects the nature of the biochemical defect.[230] Patients with complete deficiency develop severe infections with environmental mycobacteria infections early in life, with lack of granuloma formation.[230] Osteomyelitis caused by bacillus Calmette-Guerin or by environmental mycobacteria has been reported in several patients with dominant partial IFN-γR1 deficiency.

Treatment of partial deficiency should be based on careful identification and typing of the mycobacterial strains and appropriate antimicrobial therapy; addition of IFN-γ may be useful. Recessive forms are resistant to medical treatment. Although allogeneic hematopoietic stem cell transplantation has been attempted,[231] a high rate of graft failure has been observed as a consequence of the inhibitory effect of high levels of circulating IFN-γ.[232]

STAT1 Deficiency

Complete STAT1 deficiency causes increased susceptibility to mycobacterial disease with a severe clinical course.[220] Correction of the defect can be achieved with hematopoietic stem cell transplantation (Notarangelo, unpublished).

Dominant partial STAT1 deficiency is caused by a heterozygous mutation that allows formation of the IFN-α/β-dependent ISGF3 transcription factor, but abrogates expression of the γ-activating factor, composed of STAT1 homodimers. Affected individuals have either a mild clinical course, characterized by selective susceptibility to mycobacterial infections, or are asymptomatic.[233]

GENETICALLY DETERMINED DEFICIENCIES OF THE COMPLEMENT SYSTEM

The complement (C) system consists of the classical and alternative pathways and the membrane attack complex, and is composed of a series of plasma proteins that play an important role in host defense, inflammation, clearance of immune complexes and apoptotic cells, and induction of a normal humoral immune response (see Chap. 17).[234] Mutations in the classical pathway (C1q, C1r/C1s, C4, C2, and C3) result in pyogenic infections and autoimmune diseases. Mutations affecting the alternative pathway (factors B, D, H, properidin) result in meningococcal and pneumococcal sepsis. Mutations in the terminal components (C5–C9) are associated with an increased susceptibility to *Neisseria* species, especially meningococcal sepsis and meningitis. C1 inhibitor deficiency, an autosomal dominant disorder, is the cause of hereditary angioedema. The other complement-component deficiencies have an autosomal recessive mode of inheritance with the exception of properidin deficiency, which is X-linked.

The most important screening tests for complement deficiencies are those utilizing the assessment of the hemolytic function of both the classic and alternative pathways, CH50 and AH50, respectively. If both tests are normal, a complement deficiency is unlikely. If CH50 is absent and AH50 normal, a defect of C1, C4, or C2 is likely. Normal CH50 but absent AH50 suggests a defect of properdin or factor D. If both tests are abnormal, the defect most likely affects C3 to C8. Deficiency of C9 results usually in a CH50 value that is approximately half of normal. To pinpoint the specific complement component deficiency, immunochemical tests using component specific antibodies or functional assays using *in vitro* reconstitution of the hemolytic function are recommended. Treatment of complement-component deficiencies depends on the defect and may include frequent immunizations using the appropriate vaccines, antibiotic prophylaxis, and workup for sepsis if the clinical symptoms suggest bacterial infections. Autoimmune disorders are treated symptomatically, using the same immunosuppressive agents and antiinflammatory medications as those used in the general population. Management of angioedema has been revolutionized by the recent release in the United States of C1 esterase inhibitor concentrate, which is most effective for the treatment of acute attacks.

REFERENCES

1. Winkelstein JA, Marino MC, Lederman HM, et al: X-linked agammaglobulinemia: Report on a United States registry of 201 patients. *Medicine (Baltimore)* 85:93, 2006.
2. Conley ME, Dobbs AK, Farmer DM, et al: Primary B cell immunodeficiencies: Comparisons and contrasts. *Annu Rev Immunol* 27:199, 2009.
3. Lederman HM, Winkelstein JA: X-linked agammaglobulinemia: An analysis of 96 patients. *Medicine (Baltimore)* 64:145, 1985.
4. Plebani A, Soresina A, Rondelli R, et al: Clinical, immunological, and molecular analysis in a large cohort of patients with X-linked agammaglobulinemia: An Italian multicenter study. *Clin Immunol* 104:221, 2002.
5. Franz A, Webster AD, Furr PM, Taylor-Robinson D: Mycoplasmal arthritis in patients with primary immunoglobulin deficiency: Clinical features and outcome in 18 patients. *Br J Rheumatol* 36:661, 1997.
6. McKinney RE Jr, Katz SL, Wilfert CM: Chronic enteroviral meningoencephalitis in agammaglobulinemic patients. *Rev Infect Dis* 9:334, 1987.
7. van der Meer JW, Weening RS, Schellekens PT, et al: Colorectal cancer in patients with X-linked agammaglobulinaemia. *Lancet* 341:1439, 1993.
8. Futatani T, Watanabe C, Baba Y, et al: Bruton's tyrosine kinase is present in normal platelets and its absence identifies patients with X-linked agammaglobulinaemia and carrier females. *Br J Haematol* 114:141, 2001.
9. Ziegner UH, Kobayashi RH, Cunningham-Rundles C, et al: Progressive neurodegeneration in patients with primary immunodeficiency disease on IVIG treatment. *Clin Immunol* 102:19, 2002.
10. Jain A, Ma CA, Liu S, et al: Specific missense mutations in NEMO result in hyper-IgM syndrome with hypohydrotic ectodermal dysplasia. *Nat Immunol* 2:223, 2001.
11. Peron S, Metin A, Gardes P, et al: Human PMS2 deficiency is associated with impaired immunoglobulin class switch recombination. *J Exp Med* 205:2465, 2008.
12. Geha RS PA, Notarangelo LD: CD40 CD40 ligand and the hyper-IgM syndrome, in *Primary Immunodeficiency Diseases, A Molecular and Genetic Approach,* 2nd ed, edited by HD Ochs, CIE Smith, JM Puck, p 251. Oxford University Press, New York, 2007.
13. Hayward AR, Levy J, Facchetti F, et al: Cholangiopathy and tumors of the pancreas, liver, and biliary tree in boys with X-linked immunodeficiency with hyper-IgM. *J Immunol* 158:977, 1997.
14. Agematsu K, Nagumo H, Shinozaki K, et al: Absence of IgD-CD27(+) memory B cell population in X-linked hyper-IgM syndrome. *J Clin Invest* 102:853, 1998.
15. Ameratunga R, Lederman HM, Sullivan KE, et al: Defective antigen-induced lymphocyte proliferation in the X-linked hyper-IgM syndrome. *J Pediatr* 131:147, 1997.
16. Seyama K, Kobayashi R, Hasle H, et al: Parvovirus B19-induced anemia as the presenting manifestation of X-linked hyper-IgM syndrome. *J Infect Dis* 178:318, 1998.
17. Levy J, Espanol-Boren T, Thomas C, et al: Clinical spectrum of X-linked hyper-IgM syndrome. *J Pediatr* 131:47, 1997.
18. Durandy A, Revy RP, Fischer A: Autosomal hyper-IgM syndromes caused by an intrinsic B cell defect, in *Primary Immunodeficiency Diseases, A Molecular and Genetic Approach,* 2nd ed, edited by HD Ochs, CIE Smith, JM Puck, p 269. Oxford University Press, New York, 2007.
19. Abinun M, Kaitila KI, Casanova J-L: Immunodeficiencies with associated manifestations of skin, hair, teeth, and skeleton, in *Primary Immunodeficiency Diseases, A Molecular and Genetic Approach,* 2nd ed, edited by HD Ochs, CIE Smith, JM Puck, p 513. Oxford University Press, New York, 2007.
20. Hanson EP, Monaco-Shawver L, Solt LA, et al: Hypomorphic nuclear factor-kappaB essential modulator mutation database and reconstitution system identifies phenotypic and immunologic diversity. *J Allergy Clin Immunol* 122:1169, 2008.
21. Hammarström L, Smith CIE: Genetic approach to common variable immunodeficiency and IgA deficiency, in *Primary Immunodeficiency Diseases, A Molecular and Genetic Approach,* 2nd ed, edited by HD Ochs, CIE Smith, JM Puck, p 313. Oxford University Press, New York, 2007.
22. Cunningham-Rundles C, Siegal FP, Cunningham-Rundles S, Lieberman P: Incidence of cancer in 98 patients with common varied immunodeficiency. *J Clin Immunol* 7:294, 1987.
23. Cunningham-Rundles C, Cooper DL, Duffy TP, Strauchen J: Lymphomas of mucosal-associated lymphoid tissue in common variable immunodeficiency. *Am J Hematol* 69:171, 2002.
24. Van der Hilst JC, Smits BW, van der Meer JW: Hypogammaglobulinaemia: Cumulative experience in 49 patients in a tertiary care institution. *Neth J Med* 60:140, 2002.
25. Oxelius VA, Laurell AB, Lindquist B, et al: IgG subclasses in selective IgA deficiency: Importance of IgG_2-IgA deficiency. *N Engl J Med* 304:1476, 1981.
26. Glanzman E RP: Essentielle lymphocytophtise. Ein neues Krankheitsbild aus der Sauglingspathologie. *Ann Paediatr* 175:1, 1950.
27. Buckley RH: Molecular defects in human severe combined immunodeficiency and approaches to immune reconstitution. *Annu Rev Immunol* 22:625, 2004.
28. Fischer A, Le Deist F, Hacein-Bey-Abina S, et al: Severe combined immunodeficiency. A model disease for molecular immunology and therapy. *Immunol Rev* 203:98, 2005.
29. Notarangelo LD, Fischer A, Geha RS, et al: Primary Immunodeficiencies: 2009 update (International Union of Immunological Societies Expert Committee on Primary Immunodeficiencies). *J Allergy Clin Immunol* 124:1161, 2009.
30. Nyhan WL: Disorders of purine and pyrimidine metabolism. *Mol Genet Metab* 86:25, 2005.
31. Malacarne F, Benicchi T, Notarangelo LD, et al: Reduced thymic output, increased spontaneous apoptosis and oligoclonal B cells in polyethylene glycol-adenosine deaminase-treated patients. *Eur J Immunol* 35:3376, 2005.
32. Cassani B, Mirolo M, Cattaneo F, et al: Altered intracellular and extracellular signaling leads to impaired T-cell functions in ADA-SCID patients. *Blood* 111:4209, 2008.

33. Arpaia E, Benveniste P, Di Cristofano A, et al: Mitochondrial basis for immune deficiency. Evidence from purine nucleoside phosphorylase-deficient mice. *J Exp Med* 191:2197, 2000.
34. Cohen A GE, Arpaia E, Roifman CM: Immunodeficiency caused by purine nucleoside phosphorylase deficiency. *Immunol Allergy Clin North Am* 20:143, 2000.
35. Small TN, Wall DA, Kurtzberg J, et al: Association of reticular dysgenesis (thymic alymphoplasia and congenital aleukocytosis) with bilateral sensorineural deafness. *J Pediatr* 135:387, 1999.
36. Pannicke U, Honig M, Hess I, et al: Reticular dysgenesis (aleukocytosis) is caused by mutations in the gene encoding mitochondrial adenylate kinase 2. *Nat Genet* 41:101, 2009.
37. Lagresle-Peyrou C, Six EM, Picard C, et al: Human adenylate kinase 2 deficiency causes a profound hematopoietic defect associated with sensorineural deafness. *Nat Genet* 41:106, 2009.
38. Kovanen PE, Leonard WJ: Cytokines and immunodeficiency diseases: Critical roles of the gamma(c)-dependent cytokines interleukins 2, 4, 7, 9, 15 and 21 and their signaling pathways. *Immunol Rev* 202:67, 2004.
39. Johnston JA, Bacon CM, Finbloom DS, et al: Tyrosine phosphorylation and activation of STAT5 STAT3 and Janus kinases by interleukins 2 and 15. *Proc Natl Acad Sci U S A* 92:8705, 1995.
40. Noguchi M, Yi H, Rosenblatt HM, et al: Interleukin-2 receptor gamma chain mutation results in X-linked severe combined immunodeficiency in humans. *Cell* 73:147, 1993.
41. Macchi P, Villa A, Giliani S, et al: Mutations of Jak-3 gene in patients with autosomal severe combined immune deficiency (SCID). *Nature* 377:65, 1995.
42. Russell SM, Tayebi N, Nakajima H, et al: Mutation of Jak3 in a patient with SCID: Essential role of Jak3 in lymphoid development. *Science* 270:797, 1995.
43. Puel A, Ziegler SF, Buckley RH, Leonard WJ: Defective IL7R expression in T(−) B(+)NK(+) severe combined immunodeficiency. *Nat Genet* 20:394, 1998.
44. Neven B, Leroy S, Decaluwe H, et al: Long-term outcome after hematopoietic stem cell transplantation of a single-center cohort of 90 patients with severe combined immunodeficiency. *Blood* 113:4114, 2009.
45. Moshous D, Callebaut I, de Chasseval R, et al: Artemis, a novel DNA double-strand break repair/V(D)J recombination protein, is mutated in human severe combined immune deficiency. *Cell* 105:177, 2001.
46. van der Burg M, Ijspeert H, Verkaik NS, et al: A DNA-PKcs mutation in a radiosensitive T-B- SCID patient inhibits Artemis activation and nonhomologous end-joining. *J Clin Invest* 119:91, 2009.
47. Buck D, Moshous D, de Chasseval R, et al: Severe combined immunodeficiency and microcephaly in siblings with hypomorphic mutations in DNA ligase IV. *Eur J Immunol* 36:224, 2006.
48. van der Burg M, van Veelen LR, Verkaik NS, et al: A new type of radiosensitive T–B–NK+ severe combined immunodeficiency caused by a LIG4 mutation. *J Clin Invest* 116:137, 2006.
49. Ahnesorg P, Smith P, Jackson SP: XLF interacts with the XRCC4-DNA ligase IV complex to promote DNA nonhomologous end-joining. *Cell* 124:301, 2006.
50. Dadi HK, Simon AJ, Roifman CM: Effect of CD3delta deficiency on maturation of alpha/beta and gamma/delta T-cell lineages in severe combined immunodeficiency. *N Engl J Med* 349:1821, 2003.
51. de Saint Basile G, Geissmann F, Flori E, et al: Severe combined immunodeficiency caused by deficiency in either the delta or the epsilon subunit of CD3. *J Clin Invest* 114:1512, 2004.
52. Rieux-Laucat F, Hivroz C, Lim A, et al: Inherited and somatic CD3zeta mutations in a patient with T-cell deficiency. *N Engl J Med* 354:1913, 2006.
53. Arnaiz-Villena A, Timon M, Corell A, et al: Brief report: Primary immunodeficiency caused by mutations in the gene encoding the CD3-gamma subunit of the T-lymphocyte receptor. *N Engl J Med* 327:529, 1992.
54. Recio MJ, Moreno-Pelayo MA, Kilic SS, et al: Differential biological role of CD3 chains revealed by human immunodeficiencies. *J Immunol* 178:2556, 2007.
55. Kung C, Pingel JT, Heikinheimo M, et al: Mutations in the tyrosine phosphatase CD45 gene in a child with severe combined immunodeficiency disease. *Nat Med* 6:343, 2000.
56. Tchilian EZ, Wallace DL, Wells RS, et al: A deletion in the gene encoding the CD45 antigen in a patient with SCID. *J Immunol* 166:1308, 2001.
57. Stephan JL, Vlekova V, Le Deist F, et al: Severe combined immunodeficiency: A retrospective single-center study of clinical presentation and outcome in 117 patients. *J Pediatr* 123:564, 1993.
58. Buckley RH, Schiff RI, Schiff SE, et al: Human severe combined immunodeficiency: Genetic, phenotypic, and functional diversity in one hundred eight infants. *J Pediatr* 130:378, 1997.
59. Jean-Philippe P, Freedman A, Chang MW, et al: Severe varicella caused by varicella-vaccine strain in a child with significant T-cell dysfunction. *Pediatrics* 120:e1345, 2007.
60. Casanova JL, Jouanguy E, Lamhamedi S, et al: Immunological conditions of children with BCG disseminated infection. *Lancet* 346:581, 1995.
61. Yeganeh M, Heidarzade M, Pourpak Z, et al: Severe combined immunodeficiency: A cohort of 40 patients. *Pediatr Allergy Immunol* 19:303, 2008.
62. Muller SM, Ege M, Pottharst A, et al: Transplacentally acquired maternal T lymphocytes in severe combined immunodeficiency: A study of 121 patients. *Blood* 98:1847, 2001.
63. Palmer K, Green TD, Roberts JL, et al: Unusual clinical and immunologic manifestations of transplacentally acquired maternal T cells in severe combined immunodeficiency. *J Allergy Clin Immunol* 120:423, 2007.
64. Shearer WT, Rosenblatt HM, Gelman RS, et al: Lymphocyte subsets in healthy children from birth through 18 years of age: The Pediatric AIDS Clinical Trials Group P1009 study. *J Allergy Clin Immunol* 112:973, 2003.
65. Hirschhorn R, Yang DR, Israni A, et al: Somatic mosaicism for a newly identified splice-site mutation in a patient with adenosine deaminase-deficient immunodeficiency and spontaneous clinical recovery. *Am J Hum Genet* 55:59, 1994.
66. Speckmann C, Pannicke U, Wiech E, et al: Clinical and immunologic consequences of a somatic reversion in a patient with X-linked severe combined immunodeficiency. *Blood* 112:4090, 2008.
67. Puck JM: Population-based newborn screening for severe combined immunodeficiency: Steps toward implementation. *J Allergy Clin Immunol* 120:760, 2007.
68. Engel BC, Podsakoff GM, Ireland JL, et al: Prolonged pancytopenia in a gene therapy patient with ADA-deficient SCID and trisomy 8 mosaicism: A case report. *Blood* 109:503, 2007.
69. Dror Y, Grunebaum E, Hitzler J, et al: Purine nucleoside phosphorylase deficiency associated with a dysplastic marrow morphology. *Pediatr Res* 55:472, 2004.
70. Buck D, Malivert L, de Chasseval R, et al: Cernunnos, a novel nonhomologous end join ing factor, is mutated in human immunodeficiency with microcephaly. *Cell* 124:287, 2006.
71. Faraci M, Lanino E, Micalizzi C, et al: Unrelated hematopoietic stem cell transplantation for Cernunnos-XLF deficiency. *Pediatr Transplant* 3:785, 2009.
72. Gruhn B, Seidel J, Zintl F, et al: Successful bone marrow transplantation in a patient with DNA ligase IV deficiency and bone marrow failure. *Orphanet J Rare Dis* 2:5, 2007.
73. Cossu F, Vulliamy TJ, Marrone A, et al: A novel DKC1 mutation, severe combined immunodeficiency (T+B-NK- SCID) and bone marrow transplantation in an infant with Hoyeraal-Hreidarsson syndrome. *Br J Haematol* 119(3):765, 2002.
74. Hitzig WH, Kenny AB: The role of vitamin B12 and its transport globulins in the production of antibodies. *Clin Exp Immunol* 20:105, 1975.
75. Wong SN, Low LC, Lau YL, et al: Immunodeficiency in methylmalonic acidaemia. *J Paediatr Child Health* 28:180, 1992.
76. Gatti RA, Meuwissen HJ, Allen HD, et al: Immunological reconstitution of sex-linked lymphopenic immunological deficiency. *Lancet* 2:1366, 1968.
77. Antoine C, Muller S, Cant A, et al: Long-term survival and transplantation of haemopoietic stem cells for immunodeficiencies: Report of the European experience 1968–99. *Lancet* 361:553, 2003.
78. Grunebaum E, Mazzolari E, Porta F, et al: Bone marrow transplantation for severe combined immune deficiency. *JAMA* 295:508, 2006.
79. Myers LA, Patel DD, Puck JM, Buckley RH: Hematopoietic stem cell transplantation for severe combined immunodeficiency in the neonatal period leads to superior thymic output and improved survival. *Blood* 99:872, 2002.
80. Gennery AR, Cant AJ: Cord blood stem cell transplantation in primary immune deficiencies. *Curr Opin Allergy Clin Immunol* 7:528, 2007.
81. Mazzolari E, de Martiis D, Forino C, et al: Single-center analysis of long-term outcome after hematopoietic cell transplantation in children with congenital severe T cell immunodeficiency. *Immunol Res* 44:4, 2009.
82. Honig M, Albert MH, Schulz A, et al: Patients with adenosine deaminase deficiency surviving after hematopoietic stem cell transplantation are at high risk of CNS complications. *Blood* 109:3595, 2007.
83. Baguette C, Vermylen C, Brichard B, et al: Persistent developmental delay despite successful bone marrow transplantation for purine nucleoside phosphorylase deficiency. *J Pediatr Hematol Oncol* 24:69, 2002.
84. Titman P, Pink E, Skucek E, et al: Cognitive and behavioral abnormalities in children after hematopoietic stem cell transplantation for severe congenital immunodeficiencies. *Blood* 112:3907, 2008.
85. Booth C, Hershfield M, Notarangelo L, et al: Management options for adenosine deaminase deficiency; proceedings of the EBMT satellite workshop (Hamburg, March 2006). *Clin Immunol* 123:139, 2007.
86. Chan B, Wara D, Bastian J, et al: Long-term efficacy of enzyme replacement therapy for adenosine deaminase (ADA)-deficient severe combined immunodeficiency (SCID). *Clin Immunol* 117:133, 2005.
87. Hacein-Bey-Abina S, Le Deist F, Carlier F, et al: Sustained correction of X-linked severe combined immunodeficiency by *ex vivo* gene therapy. *N Engl J Med* 346:1185, 2002.
88. Gaspar HB, Parsley KL, Howe S, et al: Gene therapy of X-linked severe combined immunodeficiency by use of a pseudotyped gammaretroviral vector. *Lancet* 364:2181, 2004.
89. Hacein-Bey-Abina S, Garrigue A, Wang GP, et al: Insertional oncogenesis in 4 patients after retrovirus-mediated gene therapy of SCID-X1. *J Clin Invest* 118:3132, 2008.
90. Howe SJ, Mansour MR, Schwarzwaelder K, et al: Insertional mutagenesis combined with acquired somatic mutations causes leukemogenesis following gene therapy of SCID-X1 patients. *J Clin Invest* 118:3143, 2008.
91. Aiuti A, Slavin S, Aker M, Ficara F, et al: Correction of ADA-SCID by stem cell gene therapy combined with nonmyeloablative conditioning. *Science* 296:2410, 2002.
92. Omenn GS: Familial reticuloendotheliosis with eosinophilia. *N Engl J Med* 273:427, 1965.
93. Signorini S, Imberti L, Pirovano S, et al: Intrathymic restriction and peripheral expansion of the T-cell repertoire in Omenn syndrome. *Blood* 94:3468, 1999.
94. Villa A, Santagata S, Bozzi F, et al: Partial V(D)J recombination activity leads to Omenn syndrome. *Cell* 93:885, 1998.

95. Ege M, Ma Y, Manfras B, et al: Omenn syndrome due to ARTEMIS mutations. *Blood* 105:4179, 2005.
96. Giliani S, Bonfim C, de Saint Basile G, et al: Omenn syndrome in an infant with IL7RA gene mutation. *J Pediatr* 148:272, 2006.
97. Grunebaum E, Bates A, Roifman CM: Omenn syndrome is associated with mutations in DNA ligase IV. *J Allergy Clin Immunol* 122:1219, 2008.
98. Roifman CM, Gu Y, Cohen A: Mutations in the RNA component of RNase mitochondrial RNA processing might cause Omenn syndrome. *J Allergy Clin Immunol* 117:897, 2006.
99. Wada T, Yasui M, Toma T, et al: Detection of T lymphocytes with a second-site mutation in skin lesions of atypical X-linked severe combined immunodeficiency mimicking Omenn syndrome. *Blood* 112:1872, 2008.
100. Roifman CM, Zhang J, Atkinson A, et al: Adenosine deaminase deficiency can present with features of Omenn syndrome. *J Allergy Clin Immunol* 121:1056, 2008.
101. Turul T, Tezcan I, Artac H, et al: Clinical heterogeneity can hamper the diagnosis of patients with ZAP70 deficiency. *Eur J Pediatr* 168:87, 2009.
102. Cavadini P, Vermi W, Facchetti F, et al: AIRE deficiency in thymus of 2 patients with Omenn syndrome. *J Clin Invest* 115:728, 2005.
103. Villa A, Marrella V, Rucci F, Notarangelo LD: Genetically determined lymphopenia and autoimmune manifestations. *Curr Opin Immunol* 20:318, 2008.
104. Villa A, Notarangelo LD, Roifman CM: Omenn syndrome: Inflammation in leaky severe combined immunodeficiency. *J Allergy Clin Immunol* 122:1082, 2008.
105. Matangkasombut P, Pichavant M, Saez DE, et al: Lack of iNKT cells in patients with combined immune deficiency due to hypomorphic RAG mutations. *Blood* 111:271, 2008.
106. Markert ML, Alexieff MJ, Li J, et al: Complete DiGeorge syndrome: Development of rash, lymphadenopathy, and oligoclonal T cells in 5 cases. *J Allergy Clin Immunol* 113:734, 2004.
107. Gennery AR, Slatter MA, Rice J, et al: Mutations in CHD7 in patients with CHARGE syndrome cause T-B + natural killer cell + severe combined immune deficiency and may cause Omenn-like syndrome. *Clin Exp Immunol* 153:75, 2008.
108. Chan AC, Kadlecek TA, Elder ME, et al: ZAP-70 deficiency in an autosomal recessive form of severe combined immunodeficiency. *Science* 264:1599, 1994.
109. Elder ME, Lin D, Clever J, et al: Human severe combined immunodeficiency due to a defect in ZAP-70 a T cell tyrosine kinase. *Science* 264:1596, 1994.
110. de la Calle-Martin O, Hernandez M, Ordi J, et al: Familial CD8 deficiency due to a mutation in the CD8 alpha gene. *J Clin Invest* 108:117, 2001.
111. Mancebo E, Moreno-Pelayo MA, Mencia A, et al: Gly111Ser mutation in CD8A gene causing CD8 immunodeficiency is found in Spanish Gypsies. *Mol Immunol* 45:479, 2008.
112. de la Salle H, Zimmer J, Fricker D, et al: HLA class I deficiencies due to mutations in subunit 1 of the peptide transporter TAP1. *J Clin Invest* 103:R9, 1999.
113. de la Salle H, Hanau D, Fricker D, et al: Homozygous human TAP peptide transporter mutation in HLA class I deficiency. *Science* 265:237, 1994.
114. Yabe T, Kawamura S, Sato M, et al: A subject with a novel type I bare lymphocyte syndrome has tapasin deficiency due to deletion of 4 exons by Alu-mediated recombination. *Blood* 100:1496, 2002.
115. Gadola SD, Moins-Teisserenc HT, Trowsdale J, et al: TAP deficiency syndrome. *Clin Exp Immunol* 121:173, 2000.
116. Zimmer J, Andres E, Donato L, et al: Clinical and immunological aspects of HLA class I deficiency. *QJM* 98:719, 2005.
117. Reith W, Lisowska-Grospierre B, Fischer A: Molecular basis of major histocompatibility complex class II deficiency, in *Primary Immunodeficiency Diseases, A Molecular and Genetic Approach*, 2nd ed., edited by HD Ochs, CIE Smith, J Puck, p 227. Oxford University Press, New York, 2007.
118. Klein C, Lisowska-Grospierre B, LeDeist F, et al: Major histocompatibility complex class II deficiency: Clinical manifestations, immunologic features, and outcome. *J Pediatr* 123:921, 1993.
119. Saleem MA, Arkwright PD, Davies EG, et al: Clinical course of patients with major histocompatibility complex class II deficiency. *Arch Dis Child* 83:356, 2000.
120. Renella R, Picard C, Neven B, et al: Human leucocyte antigen-identical haematopoietic stem cell transplantation in major histocompatibility complex class II immunodeficiency: Reduced survival correlates with an increased incidence of acute graft-versus-host disease and pre-existing viral infections. *Br J Haematol* 134:510, 2006.
121. Shiow LR, Roadcap DW, Paris K, et al: The actin regulator coronin 1A is mutant in a thymic egress-deficient mouse strain and in a patient with severe combined immunodeficiency. *Nat Immunol* 9:1307, 2008.
122. Kofoed EM, Hwa V, Little B, et al: Growth hormone insensitivity associated with a STAT5b mutation. *N Engl J Med* 349:1139, 2003.
123. Bernasconi A, Marino R, Ribas A, et al: Characterization of immunodeficiency in a patient with growth hormone insensitivity secondary to a novel STAT5b gene mutation. *Pediatrics* 118:e1584, 2006.
124. Feske S, Gwack Y, Prakriya M, et al: A mutation in Orai1 causes immune deficiency by abrogating CRAC channel function. *Nature* 441:179, 2006.
125. Picard C, McCarl CA, Papolos A, et al: STIM1 mutation associated with a syndrome of immunodeficiency and autoimmunity. *N Engl J Med* 360:1971, 2009.
126. Driscoll DA, Sullivan KA: DiGeorge syndrome: A chromosome 22q11.2 deletion syndrome, in *Primary Immunodeficiency Diseases, A Molecular and Genetic Approach,* 2nd ed, edited by HD Ochs, CIE Smith, JM Puck, p 485. Oxford University Press, New York, 2007.
127. Yagi H, Furutani Y, Hamada H, et al: Role of TBX1 in human del22q11.2 syndrome. *Lancet* 362:1366, 2003.
128. Markert ML, Devlin BH, Alexieff MJ, et al: Review of 54 patients with complete DiGeorge anomaly enrolled in protocols for thymus transplantation: Outcome of 44 consecutive transplants. *Blood* 109:4539, 2007.
129. Markert ML, Devlin BH, Chinn IK, et al: Factors affecting success of thymus transplantation for complete DiGeorge anomaly. *Am J Transplant* 8:1729, 2008.
130. Land MH, Garcia-Lloret MI, Borzy MS, et al: Long-term results of bone marrow transplantation in complete DiGeorge syndrome. *J Allergy Clin Immunol* 120:908, 2007.
131. Pignata C, Fiore M, Guzzetta V, et al: Congenital alopecia and nail dystrophy associated with severe functional T-cell immunodeficiency in two sibs. *Am J Med Genet* 65:167, 1996.
132. Moraes-Vasconcelos D, Costa-Carvalho BT, Torgerson TR, Ochs HD: Primary immune deficiency disorders presenting as autoimmune diseases: IPEX and APECED. *J Clin Immunol* 28 Suppl 1:S11, 2008.
133. Bennett CL, Christie J, Ramsdell F, et al: The immune dysregulation, polyendocrinopathy, enteropathy, X-linked syndrome (IPEX) is caused by mutations of FOXP3. *Nat Genet* 27:20, 2001.
134. Torgerson TR, Genin A, Chen C, et al: FOXP3 inhibits activation-induced NFAT2 expression in T cells thereby limiting effector cytokine expression. *J Immunol* 183:907, 2009.
135. Rao A, Kamani N, Filipovich A, et al: Successful bone marrow transplantation for IPEX syndrome after reduced-intensity conditioning. *Blood* 109:383, 2007.
136. Roifman CM: Human IL-2 receptor alpha chain deficiency. *Pediatr Res* 48:6, 2000.
137. Caudy AA, Reddy ST, Chatila T, et al: CD25 deficiency causes an immune dysregulation, polyendocrinopathy, enteropathy, X-linked-like syndrome, and defective IL-10 expression from CD4 lymphocytes. *J Allergy Clin Immunol* 119:482, 2007.
138. Ahonen P, Myllarniemi S, Sipila I, Perheentupa J: Clinical variation of autoimmune polyendocrinopathy-candidiasis-ectodermal dystrophy (APECED) in a series of 68 patients. *N Engl J Med* 322:1829, 1990.
139. Anderson MS, Venanzi ES, Klein L, et al: Projection of an immunological self shadow within the thymus by the AIRE protein. *Science* 298:1395, 2002.
140. Kont V, Laan M, Kisand K, et al: Modulation of AIRE regulates the expression of tissue-restricted antigens. *Mol Immunol* 45:25, 2008.
141. Puck JM, Rieux-Laucat F, Le Diest F, Straus SE: Autoimmune lymphoproliferative syndrome, in *Primary Immunodeficiency Diseases, A Molecular and Genetic Approach*, 2nd ed, edited by HD Ochs, CIE Smith, JM Puck, p 326. Oxford University Press, New York, 2007.
142. Ochs HD, Rosen F: Wiskott-Aldrich syndrome, in *Primary Immunodeficiency Diseases, A Molecular and Genetic Approach*, 2nd ed, edited by HD Ochs, CIE Smith, JM Puck, p 454. Oxford University Press, New York, 2007.
143. Ancliff PJ, Blundell MP, Cory GO, et al: Two novel activating mutations in the Wiskott-Aldrich syndrome protein result in congenital neutropenia. *Blood* 108:2182, 2006.
144. Notarangelo LD, Miao CH, Ochs HD: Wiskott-Aldrich syndrome. *Curr Opin Hematol* 15:30, 2008.
145. Ozsahin H, Cavazzana-Calvo M, Notarangelo LD, et al: Long-term outcome following hematopoietic stem-cell transplantation in Wiskott-Aldrich syndrome: Collaborative study of the European Society for Immunodeficiencies and European Group for Blood and Marrow Transplantation. *Blood* 111:439, 2008.
146. Grimbacher B, Holland SM, Gallin JI, et al: Hyper-IgE syndrome with recurrent infections—An autosomal dominant multisystem disorder. *N Engl J Med* 340:692, 1999.
147. Davis SD, Schaller J, Wedgwood RJ: Job's syndrome. Recurrent, "cold," staphylococcal abscesses. *Lancet* 1:1013, 1996.
148. Buckley RH, Wray BB, Belmaker EZ: Extreme hyperimmunoglobulinemia E and undue susceptibility to infection. *Pediatrics* 49:59, 1972.
149. Grimbacher B, Schaffer AA, Holland SM, et al: Genetic linkage of hyper-IgE syndrome to chromosome 4. *Am J Hum Genet* 65:735, 1999.
150. Borges WG, Hensley T, Carey JC, et al: The face of Job. *J Pediatr* 133:303, 1998.
151. Renner ED, Torgerson TR, Rylaarsdam S, et al: STAT3 mutation in the original patient with Job's syndrome. *N Engl J Med* 357:1667, 2007.
152. Holland SM, DeLeo FR, Elloumi HZ, et al: STAT3 mutations in the hyper-IgE syndrome. *N Engl J Med* 357:1608, 2007.
153. Minegishi Y, Saito M, Tsuchiya S, et al: Dominant-negative mutations in the DNA-binding domain of STAT3 cause hyper-IgE syndrome. *Nature* 448:1058, 2007.
154. Renner ED, Rylaarsdam S, Anover-Sombke S, et al: Novel signal transducer and activator of transcription 3, (STAT3) mutations, reduced T(H)17 cell numbers, and variably defective STAT3 phosphorylation in hyper-IgE syndrome. *J Allergy Clin Immunol* 122:181, 2008.
155. Huang W, Na L, Fidel PL, Schwarzenberger P: Requirement of interleukin-17A for systemic anti-*Candida albicans* host defense in mice. *J Infect Dis* 190:624, 2004.
156. Gennery AR, Flood TJ, Abinun M, Cant AJ: Bone marrow transplantation does not correct the hyper IgE syndrome. *Bone Marrow Transplant* 25:1303, 2000.
157. Nester TA, Wagnon AH, Reilly WF, et al: Effects of allogeneic peripheral stem cell transplantation in a patient with job syndrome of hyperimmunoglobulinemia E and recurrent infections. *Am J Med* 105:162, 1998.
157a. Zhang Q, Davis JC, Lamborn IT, et al: Combined immunodeficiency associated with DOCK8 mutations. *N Engl J Med*, 2009 [Epub ahead of print].
157b. Minegishi Y, Saito M, Morio T, et al: Human tyrosine kinase 2 deficiency reveals its requisite roles in multiple cytokine signals involved in innate and acquired immunity. *Immunity* 25:745, 2006.

158. McKusick VA, Eldridge R, Hostetler JA, et al: Dwarfism in the Amish. II. Cartilage-hair hypoplasia. *Bull Johns Hopkins Hosp* 116:285, 1965.
159. Notarangelo LD, Roifman CM, Giliani S: Cartilage-hair hypoplasia: Molecular basis and heterogeneity of the immunological phenotype. *Curr Opin Allergy Clin Immunol* 8:534, 2008.
160. Ridanpaa M, van Eenennaam H, Pelin K, et al: Mutations in the RNA component of RNase MRP cause a pleiotropic human disease, cartilage-hair hypoplasia. *Cell* 104:195, 2001.
161. Kavadas FD, Giliani S, Gu Y, et al: Variability of clinical and laboratory features among patients with ribonuclease mitochondrial RNA processing endoribonuclease gene mutations. *J Allergy Clin Immunol* 122:1178, 2008.
162. Guggenheim R, Somech R, Grunebaum E, et al: Bone marrow transplantation for cartilage-hair-hypoplasia. *Bone Marrow Transplant* 38:751, 2006.
163. Boerkoel CF, O'Neill S, Andre JL, et al: Manifestations and treatment of Schimke immuno-osseous dysplasia: 14 new cases and a review of the literature. *Eur J Pediatr* 159:1, 2000.
164. Deguchi K, Clewing JM, Elizondo LI, et al: Neurologic phenotype of Schimke immuno-osseous dysplasia and neurodevelopmental expression of SMARCAL1. *J Neuropathol Exp Neurol* 67:565, 2008.
165. Boerkoel CF, Takashima H, John J, et al: Mutant chromatin remodeling protein SMARCAL1 causes Schimke immuno-osseous dysplasia. *Nat Genet* 30:215, 2002.
166. Gorlin RJ, Gelb B, Diaz GA, et al: WHIM syndrome, an autosomal dominant disorder: Clinical, hematological, and molecular studies. *Am J Med Genet* 91:368, 2000.
167. Hernandez PA, Gorlin RJ, Lukens JN, et al: Mutations in the chemokine receptor gene CXCR4 are associated with WHIM syndrome, a combined immunodeficiency disease. *Nat Genet* 34:70, 2003.
168. Gulino AV, Moratto D, Sozzani S, et al: Altered leukocyte response to CXCL12 in patients with warts hypogammaglobulinemia, infections, myelokathexis (WHIM) syndrome. *Blood* 104:444, 2004.
169. Tassone L, Notarangelo LD, Bonomi V, et al: Clinical and genetic diagnosis of warts, hypogammaglobulinemia, infections, and myelokathexis syndrome in 10 patients. *J Allergy Clin Immunol* 123:1170, 2009.
170. Sanmun D, Garwicz D, Smith CI, et al: Stromal-derived factor-1 abolishes constitutive apoptosis of WHIM syndrome neutrophils harbouring a truncating CXCR4 mutation. *Br J Haematol* 134:640, 2006.
171. Wegner R-D, German JJ, Chrzanowska KH, et al: Chromosomal instability syndromes other than ataxia-telangiectasia, in *Primary Immunodeficiency Diseases, A Molecular and Genetic Approach*, 2nd ed, edited by HD Ochs, CIE Smith, JM Puck, p 427. Oxford University Press, New York, 2007.
172. Nowak-Wegrzyn A, Crawford TO, Winkelstein JA, et al: Immunodeficiency and infections in ataxia-telangiectasia. *J Pediatr* 144:505, 2004.
173. Savitsky K, Bar-Shira A, Gilad S, et al: A single ataxia telangiectasia gene with a product similar to PI-3 kinase. *Science* 268:1749, 1995.
174. Pandita TK: The role of ATM in telomere structure and function. *Radiat Res* 156(5 Pt 2):642, 2001.
175. Klein C, Wenning GK, Quinn NP, Marsden CD: Ataxia without telangiectasia masquerading as benign hereditary chorea. *Mov Disord* 11:217, 1996.
176. Stewart GS, Maser RS, Stankovic T, et al: The DNA double-strand break repair gene hMRE11 is mutated in individuals with an ataxia-telangiectasia-like disorder. *Cell* 99:577, 1999.
177. Weemaes CM, Smeets DF, van der Burgt CJ: Nijmegen Breakage syndrome: A progress report. *Int J Radiat Biol* 66(6 Suppl):S185, 1994.
178. Huizing M, Helip-Wooley A, Westbroek W, et al: Disorders of lysosome-related organelle biogenesis: Clinical and molecular genetics. *Annu Rev Genomics Hum Genet* 9:359, 2008.
179. Filipovich AH: Hemophagocytic lymphohistiocytosis and other hemophagocytic disorders. *Immunol Allergy Clin North Am* 28:293, 2008.
180. Stepp SE, Dufourcq-Lagelouse R, Le Deist F, et al: Perforin gene defects in familial hemophagocytic lymphohistiocytosis. *Science* 286:1957, 1999.
181. Feldmann J, Callebaut I, Raposo G, et al: Munc13–4 is essential for cytolytic granules fusion and is mutated in a form of familial hemophagocytic lymphohistiocytosis (FHL3). *Cell* 115:461, 2003.
182. zur Stadt U, Schmidt S, Kasper B, et al: Linkage of familial hemophagocytic lymphohistiocytosis (FHL) type-4 to chromosome 6q24 and identification of mutations in syntaxin 11. *Hum Mol Genet* 14:827, 2005.
183. Janka GE: Hemophagocytic syndromes. *Blood Rev* 21:245, 2007.
184. Ueda I, Kurokawa Y, Koike K, et al: Late-onset cases of familial hemophagocytic lymphohistiocytosis with missense perforin gene mutations. *Am J Hematol* 82:427, 2007.
185. Trizzino A, zur Stadt U, Ueda I, et al: Genotype-phenotype study of familial haemophagocytic lymphohistiocytosis due to perforin mutations. *J Med Genet* 45:15, 2008.
186. Rudd E, Bryceson YT, Zheng C, et al: Spectrum, and clinical and functional implications of UNC13D mutations in familial haemophagocytic lymphohistiocytosis. *J Med Genet* 45:134, 2008.
187. Horne A, Trottestam H, Arico M, et al: Frequency and spectrum of central nervous system involvement in 193 children with haemophagocytic lymphohistiocytosis. *Br J Haematol* 140:327, 2008.
188. Henter JI, Horne A, Arico M, et al: HLH-2004: Diagnostic and therapeutic guidelines for hemophagocytic lymphohistiocytosis. *Pediatr Blood Cancer* 48:124, 2007.
189. Marcenaro S, Gallo F, Martini S, et al: Analysis of natural killer-cell function in familial hemophagocytic lymphohistiocytosis (FHL): Defective CD107a surface expression heralds Munc13–4 defect and discriminates between genetic subtypes of the disease. *Blood* 108:2316, 2006.
190. Mahlaoui N, Ouachee-Chardin M, de Saint Basile G, et al: Immunotherapy of familial hemophagocytic lymphohistiocytosis with antithymocyte globulins: A single-center retrospective report of 38 patients. *Pediatrics* 120:e622, 2007.
191. Ouachee-Chardin M, Elie C, de Saint Basile G, et al: Hematopoietic stem cell transplantation in hemophagocytic lymphohistiocytosis: A single-center report of 48 patients. *Pediatrics* 117:e743, 2006.
192. Purtilo DT, Constantian HM, DeGirolami E: Letter: Epsilon-aminocaproic acid in haematuria. *Lancet* 1:755, 1975.
193. Coffey AJ, Brooksbank RA, Brandau O, et al: Host response to EBV infection in X-linked lymphoproliferative disease results from mutations in an SH2-domain encoding gene. *Nat Genet* 20:129, 1998.
194. Sayos J, Wu C, Morra M, et al: The X-linked lymphoproliferative-disease gene product SAP regulates signals induced through the co-receptor SLAM. *Nature* 395:462, 1998.
195. Calpe S, Wang N, Romero X, et al: The SLAM and SAP gene families control innate and adaptive immune responses. *Adv Immunol* 97:177, 2008.
196. Parolini S, Bottino C, Falco M, et al: X-linked lymphoproliferative disease. 2B4 molecules displaying inhibitory rather than activating function are responsible for the inability of natural killer cells to kill Epstein-Barr virus-infected cells. *J Exp Med* 192:337, 2000.
197. Bottino C, Falco M, Parolini S, et al: NTB-A [correction of GNTB-A], a novel SH2D1A-associated surface molecule contributing to the inability of natural killer cells to kill Epstein-Barr virus-infected B cells in X-linked lymphoproliferative disease. *J Exp Med* 194:235, 2001.
198. Dupre L, Andolfi G, Tangye SG, et al: SAP controls the cytolytic activity of CD8+ T cells against EBV-infected cells. *Blood* 105:4383, 2005.
199. Qi H, Cannons JL, Klauschen F, et al: SAP-controlled T-B cell interactions underlie germinal centre formation. *Nature* 455:764, 2008.
200. Pasquier B, Yin L, Fondaneche MC, et al: Defective NKT cell development in mice and humans lacking the adapter SAP, the X-linked lymphoproliferative syndrome gene product. *J Exp Med* 201:695, 2005.
201. Rigaud S, Fondaneche MC, Lambert N, et al: XIAP deficiency in humans causes an X-linked lymphoproliferative syndrome. *Nature* 444:110, 2006.
202. Sumegi J, Huang D, Lanyi A, et al: Correlation of mutations of the SH2D1A gene and Epstein-Barr virus infection with clinical phenotype and outcome in X-linked lymphoproliferative disease. *Blood* 96:3118, 2000.
203. Tabata Y, Villanueva J, Lee SM, et al: Rapid detection of intracellular SH2D1A protein in cytotoxic lymphocytes from patients with X-linked lymphoproliferative disease and their family members. *Blood* 105:3066, 2005.
204. Seemayer TA, Gross TG, Egeler RM, et al: X-linked lymphoproliferative disease: Twenty-five years after the discovery. *Pediatr Res* 38:471, 1994.
205. Lankester AC, Visser LF, Hartwig NG, et al: Allogeneic stem cell transplantation in X-linked lymphoproliferative disease: Two cases in one family and review of the literature. *Bone Marrow Transplant* 36:99, 2005.
206. Milone MC, Tsai DE, Hodinka RL, et al: Treatment of primary Epstein-Barr virus infection in patients with X-linked lymphoproliferative disease using B-cell-directed therapy. *Blood* 105:994, 2005.
207. Mischler M, Fleming GM, Shanley TP, et al: Epstein-Barr virus-induced hemophagocytic lymphohistiocytosis and X-linked lymphoproliferative disease: A mimicker of sepsis in the pediatric intensive care unit. *Pediatrics* 119(5):e1212, 2007.
208. Migliorati R, Castaldo A, Russo S, et al: Treatment of EBV-induced lymphoproliferative disorder with epipodophyllotoxin VP16–213. *Acta Paediatr* 83:1322, 1994.
209. Kaplan J, De Domenico I, Ward DM: Chédiak-Higashi syndrome. *Curr Opin Hematol* 15:22, 2008.
210. Nagle DL, Karim MA, Woolf EA, et al: Identification and mutation analysis of the complete gene for Chédiak-Higashi syndrome. *Nat Genet* 14:307, 1996.
211. Eapen M, DeLaat CA, Baker KS, et al: Hematopoietic cell transplantation for Chédiak-Higashi syndrome. *Bone Marrow Transplant* 39:411, 2007.
212. Tardieu M, Lacroix C, Neven B, et al: Progressive neurologic dysfunctions 20 years after allogeneic bone marrow transplantation for Chédiak-Higashi syndrome. *Blood* 106:40, 2005.
213. Menasche G, Pastural E, Feldmann J, et al: Mutations in RAB27A cause Griscelli syndrome associated with haemophagocytic syndrome. *Nat Genet* 25:173, 2000.
214. Badolato R, Parolini S: Novel insights from adaptor protein 3 complex deficiency. *J Allergy Clin Immunol* 120:735, 2007.
215. Dell'Angelica EC, Shotelersuk V, Aguilar RC, et al: Altered trafficking of lysosomal proteins in Hermansky-Pudlak syndrome due to mutations in the beta 3A subunit of the AP-3 adaptor. *Mol Cell* 3:11, 1999.
216. Fontana S, Parolini S, Vermi W, et al: Innate immunity defects in Hermansky-Pudlak type 2 syndrome. *Blood* 107:4857, 2006.
217. Enders A, Zieger B, Schwarz K, et al: Lethal hemophagocytic lymphohistiocytosis in Hermansky-Pudlak syndrome type II. *Blood* 108:81, 2006.
218. Casrouge A, Zhang SY, Eidenschenk C, et al: Herpes simplex virus encephalitis in human UNC-93B deficiency. *Science* 314:308, 2006.
219. Zhang SY, Jouanguy E, Ugolini S, et al: TLR3 deficiency in patients with herpes simplex encephalitis. *Science* 317:1522, 2007.
220. Dupuis S, Jouanguy E, Al-Hajjar S, Fieschi C, et al: Impaired response to interferon-alpha/beta and lethal viral disease in human STAT1 deficiency. *Nat Genet* 33:388, 2003.
221. Picard C, Puel A, Bonnet M, et al: Pyogenic bacterial infections in humans with IRAK-4 deficiency. *Science* 299:2076, 2003.

222. von Bernuth H, Picard C, Jin Z, et al: Pyogenic bacterial infections in humans with MyD88 deficiency. *Science* 321:691, 2008.
223. Ku CL, von Bernuth H, Picard C, et al: Selective predisposition to bacterial infections in IRAK-4-deficient children: IRAK-4-dependent TLRs are otherwise redundant in protective immunity. *J Exp Med* 204:2407, 2007.
224. Day N, Tangsinmankong N, Ochs H, et al: Interleukin receptor-associated kinase (IRAK-4) deficiency associated with bacterial infections and failure to sustain antibody responses. *J Pediatr* 144:524, 2004.
225. von Bernuth H, Ku CL, Rodriguez-Gallego C, et al: A fast procedure for the detection of defects in Toll-like receptor signaling. *Pediatrics* 118:2498, 2006.
225a. Glocker E-O, Hennings A, Mohammad N, et al: A homozygous CARD9 mutation in a family with susceptibility to fungal infections. *N Engl J Med* 361:1727, 2009.
226. Al-Muhsen S, Casanova JL: The genetic heterogeneity of mendelian susceptibility to mycobacterial diseases. *J Allergy Clin Immunol* 122:1043, 2008.
227. Altare F, Lammas D, Revy P, et al: Inherited interleukin 12 deficiency in a child with bacille Calmette-Guerin and Salmonella enteritidis disseminated infection. *J Clin Invest* 102:2035, 1998.
228. Altare F, Durandy A, Lammas D, et al: Impairment of mycobacterial immunity in human interleukin-12 receptor deficiency. *Science* 280:1432, 1998.
229. Jouanguy E, Lamhamedi-Cherradi S, Lammas D, et al: A human IFNGR1 small deletion hotspot associated with dominant susceptibility to mycobacterial infection. *Nat Genet* 21:370, 1999.
230. Dorman SE, Picard C, Lammas D, et al: Clinical features of dominant and recessive interferon gamma receptor 1 deficiencies. *Lancet* 364:2113, 2004.
231. Roesler J, Horwitz ME, Picard C, et al: Hematopoietic stem cell transplantation for complete IFN-gamma receptor 1 deficiency: A multi-institutional survey. *J Pediatr* 145:806, 2004.
232. Rottman M, Soudais C, Vogt G, et al: IFN-gamma mediates the rejection of haematopoietic stem cells in IFN-gammaR1-deficient hosts. *PLoS Med* 5:e26, 2008.
233. Dupuis S, Dargemont C, Fieschi C, et al: Impairment of mycobacterial but not viral immunity by a germline human STAT1 mutation. *Science* 293:300, 2001.
234. Sullivan KE, Winkelstein JA: Genetically determined deficiencies of the complement system, in *Primary Immunodeficiency Diseases, A Molecular and Genetic Approach*, 2nd ed, edited by HD Ochs, CIE Smith, JM Puck, p 589. Oxford University Press, New York, 2007.

CHAPTER 83
HEMATOLOGIC MANIFESTATIONS OF ACQUIRED IMMUNODEFICIENCY SYNDROME

Erin Gourley Reid

SUMMARY

Persons infected with the human immunodeficiency virus (HIV) are living longer in the era of highly active antiretroviral therapy (HAART) as a result of significant advances in both the understanding of the immunopathogenesis and the clinical management of the acquired immunodeficiency syndrome (AIDS). HIV may affect virtually any organ system, including abnormalities of the marrow and blood. The hematologic abnormalities associated with HIV are numerous and often profound, but many of these abnormalities may be prevented, ameliorated, or corrected by the use of HAART. The manifestations of disease include the direct effects of HIV on hematopoietic tissue, immune dysregulation, complications of secondary infections, and medications, and associated malignancies. Widespread use of HAART has been associated with a marked decrease in new AIDS-defining illnesses and in mortality from AIDS. Malignancies associated with HIV include lymphoma, Kaposi sarcoma, and cervical cancer. The pathogenesis of these neoplastic disorders has been elucidated in large part, by the effects of new treatment strategies attempting to address the various steps involved in the development of these tumors.

DEFINITION AND HISTORY

The definition of acquired immunodeficiency syndrome (AIDS) initially was based exclusively upon clinical symptoms and signs.[1] As knowledge of the viral etiopathogenesis evolved, the case definition of AIDS underwent multiple revisions by the Centers for Disease Control and Prevention (CDC). Inclusion of specific clinical illnesses in a patient with serologic evidence of infection with the human immunodeficiency virus (HIV) was classified as "clinical AIDS," whereas an HIV-infected patient with a blood CD4+ lymphocyte count of less than 200 CD4+ cells/μL or 14 percent of total lymphocytes was considered to have "immunological AIDS."[2–4] The World Health Organization (WHO) adopted alternative case-definition systems for diagnosis of AIDS in resource-poor countries where serologic and immunologic testing is not readily available (Table 83–1).[5,6]

The United Nations estimated that 30 to 35 million people worldwide were living with HIV in 2007.[5] The majority were infected by heterosexual contact, but homosexual contact and injection drug use were the predominant modes of transmission in the United States and Western Europe. Vertical transmission from infected mother to child is now decreasing in developed countries, although such transmission continues to increase in resource-poor regions of the world.

Acronyms and abbreviations that appear in this chapter include: ABVD, Adriamycin, bleomycin, vinblastine, dacarbazine; AIDS, acquired immunodeficiency syndrome; ANC, absolute neutrophil count; AZT, zidovudine; BEACOPP, bleomycin, etoposide, doxorubicin, cyclophosphamide, vincristine, procarbazine, prednisone; CDC, Centers for Disease Control and Prevention; CI, confidence interval; CNS, central nervous system; EBV, Epstein-Barr virus; ELISA, enzyme-linked immunosorbent assay; G-CSF, granulocyte colony-stimulating factor; GM-CSF, granulocyte-macrophage colony-stimulating factor; GP, glycoprotein; HAART, highly active antiretroviral therapy; HHV, human herpesvirus; HIV, human immunodeficiency virus; HL, Hodgkin lymphoma; IFN, interferon; Ig, immunoglobulin; IL, interleukin; ITP, immune thrombocytopenic purpura; IV, intravenous; IVIg, intravenous γ-globulin; KS, Kaposi sarcoma; LASA, linear analogue scale; m-BACOD, methotrexate, bleomycin, Adriamycin (doxorubicin), cyclophosphamide, Oncovin (vincristine) dexamethasone; NCI, National Cancer Institute; NK, natural killer; OR, odds ratio; PCR, polymerase chain reaction; PET, positron emission tomography; PHAT, primary HIV-associated thrombocytopenia; QOL, quality of life; SIR, standardized incidence ratio; TNF, tumor necrosis factor; WHO, World Health Organization; WIHS, Women's Interagency HIV Study.

ETIOLOGY AND PATHOGENESIS

HUMAN IMMUNODEFICIENCY VIRUS 1

HIV-1 is a member of the primate Lentivirinae subfamily of retroviruses,[6,7] RNA viruses that induce a chronic cellular infection by converting their RNA genome into a DNA provirus that is integrated into the genome of the infected cell. Infection by these lentiviruses is characterized by long periods of clinical latency followed by a gradual onset of disease-related symptoms.[8–10]

Transmission of Human Immunodeficiency Virus

HIV can be transmitted by sexual contact with an infected partner, parenteral drug use with a blood-contaminated needle, exposure to infected blood or blood products, and perinatal exposure from an infected mother to her infant.

General Mechanisms of Sexual Transmission HIV-1 has been isolated from the semen of HIV-infected men[11] and from cell-free seminal fluid.[12] It can be detected during the first 2 to 4 weeks after primary infection.[13] Factors associated with increased viral burden in semen include more advanced symptomatic HIV disease, higher levels of HIV RNA in blood, CD4 cell counts less than 200/μL, and presence of seminal fluid leukocytosis. HIV infection has been reported after exposure to infected semen during artificial insemination.[14]

HIV has been recovered from cervical and vaginal secretions of HIV-infected women.[15,16] HIV-infected endothelial cells and macrophages have been detected in cervical biopsies.[17] Factors that influence the levels of HIV-1 in female genital tract secretions include the stage of HIV disease, menstruation status, hormonal parameters, concomitant vaginal infection, age, HIV-1 RNA level in plasma, and antiviral therapy.[18] Female-to-female transmission of HIV has been reported[19,20] but appears to be relatively unusual.

HIV transmission may be facilitated by the presence of other sexually transmitted diseases, both with and without ulceration[21]; HIV has been isolated directly from genital ulcers.[22] Prevention or treatment of sexually transmitted disease has been associated with decreased HIV-1 transmission.[23]

Transmission Through Parenteral Drug Use Sharing needles and syringes is an important mode of transmission among parenteral drug users.[24] Use of cocaine, methamphetamine, or other such nonparenteral drugs also is associated with an increased risk for HIV infection,[25] through their association with engagement in sexual risk-taking behaviors.

TABLE 83–1. Definition of AIDS in the United States

Clinical AIDS-defining conditions in persons infected with human immunodeficiency syndrome
Opportunistic infections
Lymphomas (non-Hodgkin)
Kaposi sarcoma
Cervical cancer
Wasting syndrome
AIDS dementia syndrome
Recurrent bacteria pneumonia (≥2 episodes/years)
Mycobacterium infections
Immunologic AIDS
CD4+ cell counts <200/μL
CD4+ percent of lymphocytes <14%

Transmission Through Infected Blood Products The risk of infection with HIV after receiving 1 U of infected blood is approximately 90 percent.[26] Transfusion of blood products derived from multiple units of pooled blood can transmit HIV. This effect accounts for the initially high prevalence of HIV infection among patients with hemophilia who received coagulation factor replacement derived from many units of blood. Screening of all donated blood, beginning in March 1985, and the subsequent routine heat or solvent detergent treatment of clotting factor concentrates have resulted in a marked decrease in new transfusion-associated HIV infections. Guidelines for proper inactivation of HIV in clotting factor concentrates have been developed.[27,28] Currently, the risk of acquiring HIV through receipt of 1 U of blood that tests negative for antibodies to HIV-1 is approximately 1 in 493,000.[29]

Mother-to-Child Transmission The risk of transmission of HIV from mother to infant differs in various parts of the world, ranging from approximately 15 percent in Europe to 15 to 30 percent in the United States and 40 to 50 percent in Africa.[30–32] HIV-1 may be transmitted *in utero*,[33,34] intrapartum,[35,36] or postpartum through ingestion of HIV-1 infected mother's milk.[37,38] Several factors predict an increased risk of perinatal transmission. In terms of the mother, more advanced HIV disease,[39,40] higher HIV-1 viral load in the plasma,[41,42] cigarette smoking,[43] and active injected-drug use[44] all are associated with increased risk of transmission. In terms of the details of delivery, premature rupture of the amniotic membranes (>4 hours),[45,46] presence of chorioamnionitis,[44] and vaginal delivery, as opposed to elective cesarean section,[47,48] each is associated with increased rates of transmission. In terms of the infant, breast-feeding, prematurity, and low gestational age are risk factors.[45–49] The CDC has made formal recommendations regarding the optimal care for HIV-1 infected pregnant women.[50] These recommendations differ for resource-rich and resource-poor settings. In the United States, use of antiretroviral agents in pregnancy and delivery, with subsequent administration to the infant for the first 6 weeks of life, has resulted in a dramatically reduced rate of transmission, from approximately 25 to 8 percent with zidovudine alone and even lower with use of highly active antiretroviral therapy (HAART).[51] With the further use of elective cesarean section and avoidance of breast-feeding, transmission rates have dropped to approximately 2 percent.[47] The efficacy of shorter courses of zidovudine or nevirapine (a nonnucleoside reverse transcriptase inhibitor) have been demonstrated and may be more practically feasible in resource-poor regions of the world.[52,53] The long-term toxicities of *in utero* exposure to antiretroviral agents are unknown. Nonetheless, their use during pregnancy resulted in a 43 percent decrease in the number of children with perinatally acquired HIV infection in the United States when comparing data from 1992 and 1996.[54]

PATHOGENESIS OF HUMAN IMMUNODEFICIENCY VIRUS INFECTION

HIV infection results in aberrant immune regulation and immunodeficiency. The numerous *in vitro* and *in vivo* defects in cellular immune response observed with HIV infection include decreased lymphocyte proliferative response to soluble antigens *in vitro*,[55] decreased helper response in immunoglobulin (Ig) synthesis,[56] impaired delayed hypersensitivity,[1,2] decreased interferon (IFN)-γ production,[57] and decreased T-cell–mediated cytotoxicity of virally infected cells.[58]

Depletion of CD4+ T cells

Infection with HIV-1 results in a progressive loss of CD4+ T lymphocytes, resulting from the direct cytopathic effect of HIV on these cells. Formation of syncytial multinucleated giant cells by a mechanism involving fusion of infected cells expressing viral gp120 with noninfected CD4+ T lymphocytes is another mechanism of CD4 depletion.[59] The propensity of certain viral strains to form syncytia appears to be associated with an aggressive clinical course.[58,59] Experimental data suggest that an HIV-1 phenotypic switch from a macrophage-tropic (nonsyncytial) to a T-lymphocyte–tropic (syncytial) virus may be the central event in acceleration of HIV-induced immunodepletion.[60]

The host immunologic response against HIV-infected lymphocytes may contribute to the progressive loss of CD4+ lymphocytes by antibody-mediated and cytotoxic T-cell–mediated mechanisms.[61,62] Noninfected lymphocytes may become "innocent bystander" targets for immunologic destruction by binding free gp120 to their surface CD4 protein.

Defective production of immunostimulatory cytokines, such as interleukin (IL)-2,[63–65] or exaggerated expression of inhibitors of T-lymphocyte proliferation, such as transforming growth factor-β,[66] can contribute to the progressive decline in CD4+ lymphocytes. High-level replication and budding of virus, resulting in membrane injury, has also been proposed as a mechanism for lymphocyte cytotoxicity.

Combination antiretroviral therapy has resulted in marked suppression of viral replication, with resulting reductions of blood and tissue viral reservoirs.[67,68] Efficient viral suppression has resulted in significant and prolonged immunologic reconstitution characterized by increased CD4+ lymphocyte numbers, reduced opportunistic infections, and prolonged survival.[69,70] However, significant deficits in the immunologic repertoire persist, and complete immunologic reconstitution has not yet been attained.[71,72]

Defects in B-Cell Immunity

A number of defects in humoral immunity are associated with HIV infection. Pronounced polyclonal activation of B lymphocytes is common, resulting in polyclonal hypergammaglobulinemia.[73,74] Spontaneous proliferation of B cells is observed in patients with advanced HIV infection.[75] In contrast, antigen-specific B-cell proliferation and antibody production are decreased in patients with AIDS.[76] This finding may result from the loss of helper T-lymphocyte activity.

The aberrant B-lymphocyte regulation in HIV infection is associated with a pronounced increase in autoimmune phenomena and an increased risk of B-cell lymphomas.[74] In addition to an increased frequency of positive antiglobulin test results, antibodies against neutrophils,[78,79] lymphocytes,[80] and platelets[81–83] have developed.

Defects in Immune Accessory Cells and Natural Killer Cells

Monocytes, macrophages, and follicular dendritic cells of the lymph nodes express CD4 antigen and can be infected by HIV.[84,85] Monocytes and macrophages are resistant to HIV-induced cytotoxicity and serve as a chronic reservoir of HIV expression.[84] Although functional abnormalities in the chemotaxis of HIV-infected monocytes have been reported,[86] most studies have failed to demonstrate consistent defects.[87,88] The follicular dendritic cells appear to play an important role in HIV clearance in early asymptomatic HIV disease. However, a progressive depletion of these cells is observed over time, resulting in increasing plasma viremia. The loss of follicular dendritic cells results in defective antigen processing in patients with advanced HIV disease.

Natural killer (NK) cell activity is decreased in the blood of HIV-infected individuals.[88,89] In combination with helper T-lymphocyte depletion, decreased NK cell activity results in defective clearance of virally infected cells. Although the number of NK cells is normal,[88,89] the defect results from a deficiency in the signals for NK cell activation. The addition of exogenous IL-2 can improve NK lymphocyte function.[90]

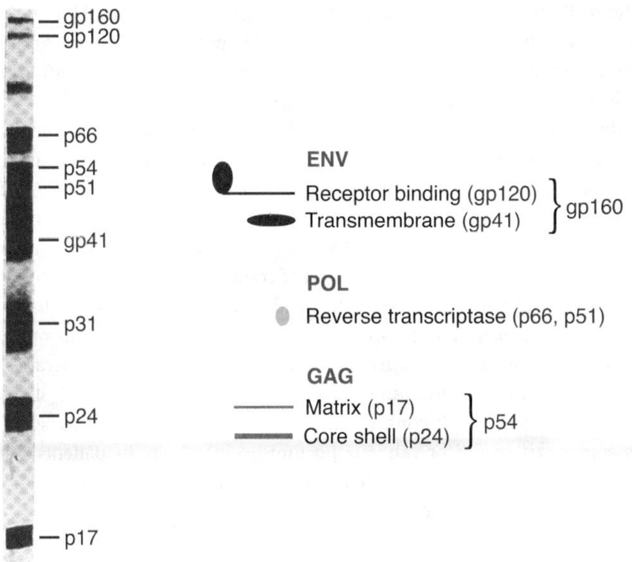

FIGURE 83–1. Western blot analysis of antibodies against human immunodeficiency virus proteins from the serum of a patient with acquired immunodeficiency syndrome.

DIAGNOSIS OF HUMAN IMMUNODEFICIENCY VIRUS INFECTION

The primary diagnostic screening tool for HIV infection is detection of antibody via the enzyme-linked immunosorbent assay (ELISA). However, because a positive ELISA result may not be specific for HIV-1 infection, all positive ELISA screening test results should be verified by immunoblotting of HIV-1 antigens (Fig. 83–1).

By ELISA and immunoblot techniques, the median time from initial infection to first detection of HIV antibody is estimated to be approximately 2 to 4 weeks. Ninety-five percent of patients are expected to seroconvert within 5.8 months (Fig. 83–2).[91] HIV infection for longer than 6 months without detectable antibody is extremely uncommon.[92–94]

The presence of the p24 antigen or HIV RNA in serum or plasma may precede seroconversion by several weeks.[95] This initial rise in p24 antigen correlates with the burst of viremia that occurs shortly after primary HIV infection.[96] Despite these observations, p24 antigen screening of donated units of blood appears to provide no benefit over conventional ELISA and immunoblot techniques.[97]

Testing by polymerase chain reaction (PCR) may detect the presence of HIV within days or 1 week of initial infection. However, PCR is not used as a screening tool because false-positive results have been detected in as many as 9 percent of individuals.

COURSE AND PROGNOSIS

Untreated HIV infection results in a progressive process characterized by gradual depletion of immune function and eventual development of rather nonspecific symptoms, followed by specific infections and/or neoplastic disease. Without effective antiretroviral therapy, patients who develop AIDS generally experience relentless deterioration in physical health and ultimately die of one or more complications secondary to acquired immunodeficiency, organ dysfunction, and/or malignancy associated with HIV infection. However, many persons with AIDS who are compliant with HAART will experience at least a partial restoration of immune function and general health.

Use of monitoring by assessment of the quantity of HIV-1 RNA in the plasma has allowed a more rational basis upon which to predict the course of disease in individual patients. In a study performed through the Multicenter AIDS Cohort, a longitudinal cohort study of HIV disease in homosexual and bisexual men, the earliest, baseline level of HIV RNA in plasma was found to correlate significantly with prognosis over time.[98] In a subsequent study, use of both viral load and concentration of blood CD4+ cells was found to more accurately predict the prognosis of HIV-infected men.[99] Current guidelines from the United

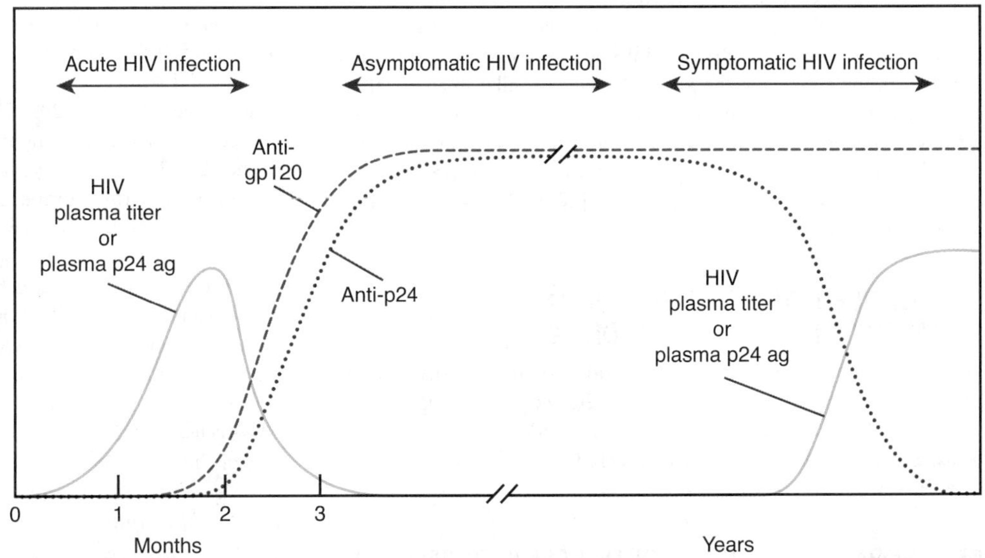

FIGURE 83–2. Virologic, serologic, and clinical course of human immunodeficiency virus (HIV) infection. Antibodies against HIV can first be detected between 2 and 5 months after infection. ag, Antigen.

States Public Health Service propose institution of HAART in all patients with symptomatic HIV or AIDS, pregnant women, and in asymptomatic HIV-infected individuals when the CD4+ cell count falls below 350 CD4+ cells/μL (0.35×10^9/L).[100]

In addition to the use of viral load monitoring, the development of potent antiretroviral agents has led to a remarkable improvement in the natural history of HIV infection.[70,100] The use of combinations of HAART was found to be associated with a 73 percent decrease in the incidence of new opportunistic infections and a 49 percent decrease in death resulting from AIDS when data from 1994 were compared to data from 1997 to 1998.[70] Remarkable decreases in the incidence of cytomegalovirus disease, atypical *Mycobacterium intracellulare* infection, and other serious opportunistic infections have occurred as a consequence of HAART therapy,[103] and improvement in immune function has been documented.[104] It may now be possible to discontinue the routine use of prophylaxis against *Pneumocystis carinii* or other opportunistic infections in patients who have been successfully treated with HAART.[105] These remarkable improvements in disease outcome have been maintained over time.[106]

ACUTE RETROVIRAL SYNDROME

An acute clinical illness often is associated with initial HIV infection, occurring in approximately 50 to 90 percent of individuals.[96,107,108] This syndrome begins approximately 1 to 3 weeks (range: 5 days to 3 months) after primary infection and usually lasts for 1 to 2 weeks. Prominent symptoms include significant fatigue and malaise; fever, which may be as high as 40°C; headache; photophobia; myalgia; and a morbilliform rash, seen in approximately 40 to 50 percent of patients. Generalized lymphadenopathy may occur toward the end of the acute illness. The symptoms are similar to those of other viral illnesses, such as infectious mononucleosis (see Chap. 84). Most symptoms of this acute retroviral syndrome subside within several weeks. However, headache may persist as an intermittent complaint, as may generalized lymphadenopathy, termed *persistent generalized lymphadenopathy*, which occurs in approximately 75 percent of patients.[96,108]

EARLY ASYMPTOMATIC HUMAN IMMUNODEFICIENCY VIRUS DISEASE

After resolution of the acute retroviral syndrome, the patient usually returns to a state of well being. During this period, the patient harbors HIV in blood and in genital secretions and may transmit the virus to others. This phase of asymptomatic infection persists for approximately 1 decade in the absence of therapy and appears similar in all racial and ethnic groups, all geographic areas, both genders, and all risk groups for HIV infection.[109–112] Certain genetic polymorphisms have been described in the chemokine receptor genes that serve as coreceptors for HIV (e.g., $\Delta 32$ deletion of CCR4), which predict for better prognosis and longer periods of AIDS-free survival.[113]

ADVANCED SYMPTOMATIC HUMAN IMMUNODEFICIENCY VIRUS DISEASE

With time, more significant manifestations of disease occur if left untreated, with more extensive fatigue, fevers, weight loss, night sweats, and eventual development of opportunistic infections, neurologic symptoms, and/or neoplasms that are considered AIDS-defining conditions (see Table 83–1).

LABORATORY FEATURES OF DISEASE PROGRESSION

With progression from the initial acute infection to the subsequent asymptomatic period, various laboratory measurements can be used to predict development of more advanced disease.[98,99,114] Quantitation of plasma HIV RNA (viral load) and CD4+ lymphocyte count are the most useful parameters. CD4+ lymphocyte count falls during the acute retroviral infection and then stabilizes during early asymptomatic infection and may appear relatively normal. The CD4+ count then decreases by approximately 40 to 80 μL per year in the absence of antiretroviral medications,[115] although there is significant variability among patients.[116]

An initial measurement of plasma viral load by reverse transcriptase PCR or branched-DNA methods provides important prognostic information that can be useful in determining when to start antiretroviral medications.[98,99] Serial assessment of plasma HIV viral load also allows for rapid assessment of efficacy of antiretroviral medications. Changes in viral load usually precede significant alterations in CD4+ lymphocyte counts.[69,99]

Several nonspecific markers of disease progression have been defined, including β_2-microglobulin[117] and neopterin,[118] each of which has an independent predictive value in estimating the probability of progression to AIDS. However, each of these surrogate markers has been largely replaced by the more specific molecular assays to quantify plasma HIV viral load.

HEMATOLOGIC ABNORMALITIES

ANEMIA IN HUMAN IMMUNODEFICIENCY VIRUS INFECTION

Incidence of Anemia

Anemia is common in HIV-infected individuals, occurring in approximately 10 to 20 percent at initial presentation and diagnosed in approximately 70 to 80 percent of patients over the course of disease.[119–121] In an attempt to ascertain the precise incidence of anemia in the setting of HIV infection, data derived from the case records of 32,867 HIV-infected persons followed from 1990 through 1996 were evaluated.[121] This cohort, termed the *Multistate Adult and Adolescent Spectrum of HIV Disease Surveillance Project*, consists of individuals who receive HIV care in hospitals and HIV clinics in nine U.S. cities. Using a hemoglobin level of less than 10 g/dL to define anemia, the 1-year incidence of anemia was 37 percent among patients with clinical AIDS; 12 percent among patients with immunologic AIDS, as defined by a count of less than 200 CD4+cells/μL; and 3 percent among HIV-infected individuals with neither clinical nor immunologic AIDS. Using a hemoglobin cutoff value of 12 g/dL as the criterion for anemia in a large group of participants from the Women's Interagency HIV Study (WIHS), a higher prevalence of anemia was found in HIV-infected women compared to HIV-uninfected controls.[122] Thus, 37 percent of the 2056 HIV infected women were anemic at baseline, compared to 17 percent of the 569 HIV negative controls ($p < 0.001$). In the HAART era, an observational cohort study of 6725 HIV-infected patients from across Europe also found a high prevalence of anemia.[123] Thus, 58.2 percent had mild anemia, defined as hemoglobin level of 8 to 14 g/dL in males or 8 to 12 g/dL in females; whereas 1.4 percent had severe anemia, defined as a hemoglobin level of less than 8 g/dL.[123] These data confirm the high incidence of anemia among HIV-infected patients in both the pre-HAART and HAART eras. Furthermore, the frequency and severity of anemia in HIV-infected patients appear to correlate with HIV-related factors, such as counts of less than 200 CD4+cells/μL (0.2×10^9/L), higher plasma HIV-1 RNA levels, and a history of clinical AIDS-defining condition.[122,123]

Causes of Anemia

Numerous causes for anemia exist in HIV-infected patients (Table 83–2).

Anemia Resulting from Decreased Production of Red Blood Cells A decrease in red blood cell production may result from factors suppressing the

TABLE 83–2. Mechanisms and Causes of Anemia in Human Immunodeficiency Virus Infection

Mechanism of Anemia	Cause of Anemia
Decreased red cell production	Neoplasm infiltrating the marrow
	Lymphoma
	Kaposi sarcoma
	Other
	Infection
	Atypical *Mycobacterium* (*Mycobacterium avium intracellulare* or *Mycobacterium avium* complex)
	Mycobacterium tuberculosis
	Cytomegalovirus
	Parvovirus B19
	Fungal infection
	Medications
	HIV infection
	Abnormal growth of burst-forming unit–erythroid
	Anemia of chronic disease
	Blunted erythropoietin production and response
	Iron-deficiency anemia secondary to chronic blood loss
Ineffective production	Folic acid deficiency
	Vitamin B_{12} deficiency
Increased red cell destruction	Coombs-positive hemolytic anemia
	Hemophagocytic syndrome
	Thrombotic thrombocytopenic purpura
	Disseminated intravascular coagulation
	Medications and recreational drugs
	Sulfonamides, dapsone
	Oxidant drugs in glucose-6-phosphate dehydrogenase deficiency
	Nitrite "poppers"

CD34+ colony-forming unit–granulocyte-erythroid-macrophage, such as inflammatory cytokines or the virus itself.[119,120] In addition, blunted production of erythropoietin has been documented in anemic HIV-infected patients, similar to the suppression observed in other states of chronic infection or inflammation.[124] Infiltration of the marrow by tumor, such as lymphoma,[125] or infection, such as *Mycobacterium avium* complex, may lead to the decreased production of red cells. *M. avium* complex may also be associated with cytokine-induced marrow suppression. Involvement of the gastrointestinal tract by various infections or tumors may lead to chronic blood loss, with eventual iron-deficiency anemia. Another prominent cause of hypoproliferative anemia in patients with HIV infection is the common use of multiple medications, many of which may cause suppression of erythropoiesis. Zidovudine (AZT), the first licensed antiretroviral agent, is uniformly associated with macrocytosis (mean cell volume >100 fL), which can be used as an objective indication that the patient has been compliant with this medication.[126] Of note, transfusion-dependent anemia (hemoglobin <8.5 g/dL) has been reported in approximately 30 percent of patients with full-blown AIDS who were receiving zidovudine at doses of 600 mg/day. However, the incidence of severe anemia is only 1 percent when the same dose of zidovudine is used in patients with asymptomatic HIV disease.[127]

Infection of the marrow by parvovirus B19 is another cause of hypoproliferative anemia in HIV-infected patients, resulting in specific infection of the pronormoblast.[128,129] Thus, although marrow failure affecting all three lines has been described in association with parvovirus B19 infection, a pure red cell aplasia is the usual consequence. Parvovirus infection usually is acquired during childhood, leading to "fifth disease," one of the common childhood exanthems. Exposure to the virus leads to an antibody response, with subsequent resistance to further infection. Approximately 85 percent of adults have serologic evidence of prior parvovirus infection. However, the seroprevalence of such antibodies among HIV-infected patients is only 64 percent. These individuals may have an ineffective immune response against newly acquired infection, or they may have lost prior seropositivity. The diagnosis of parvovirus B19 can be made on marrow examination, revealing giant pronormoblasts with clumped basophilic chromatin and clear cytoplasmic vacuoles (see Chap. 35, Fig. 35–1). Diagnosis can be confirmed by *in situ* hybridization using sequence-specific DNA probes for parvovirus B19. Therapy for parvovirus-induced red cell aplasia consists of infusions of intravenous (IV) gamma-immunoglobulin (IVIg) that contain antibodies from plasma donors, most of whom have been exposed to parvovirus. Relapse of parvovirus B19-induced red cell aplasia may occur, necessitating retreatment in these individuals.[128,129]

Anemia Resulting from Increased Red Cell Destruction Increased red cell destruction may be seen in HIV-infected patients with glucose-6-phosphate dehydrogenase deficiency if exposed to oxidant drugs and in HIV-infected patients with disseminated intravascular coagulation or thrombotic thrombocytopenic purpura.[130] Presence of fragmented red cells and thrombocytopenia on blood film is seen in the latter two conditions (see Chaps. 130 and 133). Heinz bodies are seen in association with glucose-6-phosphate dehydrogenase deficiency using the supravital stain (see Chap. 29, Fig. 29–12). Hemophagocytic syndrome has been described in association with HIV infection.[131,132] An additional cause of red cell destruction in HIV-infected patients is the development of autoantibodies, with resultant positive direct antiglobulin (Coombs) test and shortened red cell survival (see Chap. 53). Of interest, a positive direct antiglobulin test has been reported in 18 to 77 percent of HIV-infected patients, although the incidence of clinically significant hemolysis is low.[133] When present, anti-i antibody and antibody against auto-U antigens have been described, occurring in 64 percent and 32 percent of HIV-infected patients, respectively.[133–135] A high incidence of positive direct antiglobulin test results has been detected in patients with other hypergammaglobulinemic states, indicating that a positive test results in HIV may be secondary to the polyclonal hypergammaglobulinemia known to occur in the setting of HIV infection.[136]

Anemia Resulting from Ineffective Production of Red Cells (Vitamin B_{12} and/or Folic Acid Deficiency) Folic acid is absorbed in the jejunum and is responsible for one carbon transfer required in the synthesis of DNA. A deficiency of folic acid leads to a megaloblastic anemia, with large ovalocytes in the blood, hypersegmented neutrophils, and a decrease in all three lines, with resultant anemia, neutropenia, and thrombocytopenia (see Chap. 41, Figs. 41–12 and 41–13). Because tissue stores of folate are relatively small, a deficiency of folate in the diet lasting as few as 2 to 4 months may lead to anemia. Thus, HIV-infected patients who are ill and not eating properly and those with underlying disease of the jejunum may be unable to absorb sufficient folic acid. The classic changes of megaloblastic anemia are detected upon examination of the marrow, whereas serum and red cell folate levels are low.

Ineffective production of red cells, with pancytopenia in the blood, elevated indirect bilirubin level, and low reticulocyte count may be seen in vitamin B_{12} deficiency (see Chap. 41). Absorption of vitamin B_{12} requires initial production of intrinsic factor by parietal cells in the stomach, with subsequent absorption of the complex of B_{12} and intrinsic factor within the ileum. Thus, malabsorption of vitamin B_{12} can occur in various disorders of the stomach, by production of antibodies to the H^+-K^+ ATP pump or to intrinsic factor (pernicious anemia), or by various disorders of the small bowel and ileum (infection or Crohn disease). Although vitamin B_{12} deficiency based on diet alone is highly unlikely, patients with HIV infection appear to be prone to vitamin B_{12} malabsorption, presumably because of the myriad of infections and other disorders that may occur in the small intestine. Negative vitamin B_{12} balance has been documented in approximately one-third of patients with AIDS, the majority demonstrating defective absorption of the vitamin.[137] Diagnosis of vitamin B_{12} deficiency can be made by documenting low serum vitamin B_{12} levels. The earliest indication of negative vitamin B_{12} balance is the finding of low vitamin B_{12} levels in blood in patients taking transcobalamin II.[138] Monthly administration of parenteral vitamin B_{12} corrects the deficiency and the resultant pancytopenia. Because vitamin B_{12} deficiency may cause neurologic dysfunction (subacute combined degeneration of the cord), with motor, sensory, and higher cortical dysfunction, the possibility of vitamin B_{12} deficiency should be considered in HIV-infected patients with these neurologic symptoms and signs.

Consequences of Anemia in Human Immunodeficiency Virus Infection

Decreased Survival Several large cohort studies have shown that anemia is an independent risk factor for shorter survival in HIV-infected patients.[139–142] In the Multistate Adult and Adolescent Spectrum of HIV Disease Surveillance Project, anemia, defined as a hemoglobin level less than 10 g/dL or a physician's diagnosis of anemia, was found to be associated with an increased risk of death regardless of CD4+ cell count in this cohort.[139] However, the greatest risk of death was noted in patients with baseline counts greater than 200 CD4+ cells/μL (0.2×10^9/L), with a relative risk of death 150 percent higher than for individuals in the same CD4+ cell count strata without anemia (relative risk [RR]: 2.3; $p < 0.001$). In comparison, the risk of death was increased by approximately 60 percent for anemic patients with baseline counts of less than 200 CD4+ cells/μL (0.2×10^9/L). Recovery from anemia was shown to be independently associated with improved survival. Thus, among anemic patients with baseline counts less than 50 CD4+ cells/μL (0.05×10^9/L), those who remained anemic (hemoglobin level <10 g/dL) had a 160 percent higher risk of death than patients who recovered from anemia following treatment. In another series of 2348 HIV-infected patients from Baltimore, Maryland, development of any grade of anemia was found to be independently associated with decreased survival, with the risk of death approximately threefold increased in those with a hemoglobin level of 7 to 8 g/dL and fourfold increased in those with a hemoglobin level less than 6.5 g/dL.[140] Use of erythropoietin was associated with a decreased risk of death, as was use of antiretroviral therapy. Similarly, an additional study of 6725 European HIV-infected patients demonstrated that hemoglobin level at baseline, CD4+ count, and viral load were independent prognostic factors for survival.[106] For each 1 g/dL decrease in hemoglobin level, the relative hazard of death was 1.39 (95% confidence interval [CI] 1.34–1.43; $p < 0.0001$). A large multicenter prospective study of 2056 HIV-infected women (WIHS) confirmed the independent association between anemia and decreased survival.[142] Further work is required to elucidate the precise mechanisms underlying this strong prognostic association. It is conceivable that anemia may simply serve as a surrogate marker for more advanced systemic illness.

Disease Progression Anemia has been shown to be independently associated with more rapid clinical progression of HIV infection. In one large European study aimed at identifying predictive factors for disease progression among HIV-infected patients receiving HAART, the most recent measured hemoglobin level, CD4+ cell count, HIV-1 viral load, and a history of clinical AIDS before initiation of HAART all were independently related to the risk of disease progression.[143] Thus, with mild anemia (hemoglobin 8–14 g/dL for men and 8–12 g/dL for women) the relative hazard of disease progression or death was 2.2 (95% CI 1.6–2.9; $p < 0.0001$), whereas for severe anemia (hemoglobin <8 g/dL) the relative hazard was 7.1 (95% CI 2.5–20.1; $p = 0.0002$).

Quality-of-Life Parameters Anemia has been associated with decreases in quality of life (QOL), as measured by the linear analogue self-assessment (LASA) scale and other such instruments.[144,145]

Prevention or Correction of Anemia with Highly Active Antiretroviral Therapy

HAART can correct or improve the anemia of HIV infection. In a study of 6725 HIV-infected patients from across Europe,[141] use of HAART was statistically associated with improvement in hemoglobin levels. In addition, prolonged HAART use was associated with a greater likelihood of correcting anemia. Thus, 65.5 percent of the cohort was anemic before the use of HAART, 53 percent were anemic after 6 months of HAART, and 46 percent were anemic after 12 months of HAART. In a study of 905 HIV-infected patients from Baltimore, Maryland, use of HAART was associated with an increase in hemoglobin levels after 1-year followup.[146] Among the patients with a baseline hemoglobin level less than 14 g/dL, 21 percent of patients receiving HAART recovered from anemia (hemoglobin >14 g/dL) compared to only 8 percent of patients not receiving HAART ($p = 0.0006$).[146] In multivariate analysis, use of HAART was strongly associated with freedom from anemia, after adjusting for CD4+ cell count, HIV-1 RNA level, sex, race, history of injection drug use, and use of various therapies for anemia. The WIHS study concluded that use of HAART for as few as 6 months was independently associated with a higher likelihood of resolution of anemia, and longer use was associated with more profound improvements.[142] The use of HAART for at least 12 months was associated significantly with a reduced risk of developing anemia.[142] However, patients with CD4+ counts under 200 cells/μL and 100 cells/μL were less likely to have improvement in anemia in both the WIHS study and a longitudinal study of 2493 HIV infected persons in Seattle from 1996 to 2002, respectively.[142,101]

The mechanisms whereby HAART may protect against development of anemia or correct preexisting anemia are not yet fully understood. Nonetheless, because HIV infection directly contributes to the development of anemia, it is conceivable that HAART may protect against or correct anemia simply by decreasing the level of HIV-1 viral burden and/or by overcoming the factors responsible for the anemia of chronic disease. The use of HAART is associated with an increase in hematopoietic progenitor cell growth,[147] whereas ritonavir, a protease inhibitor, directly stimulates progenitor cell growth and inhibits apoptosis of hematopoietic progenitors *in vitro*.[148]

Use of Erythropoietin in Human Immunodeficiency Virus Infected Patients with Anemia Low erythropoietin levels and blunted response to erythropoietin are extremely common in the setting of HIV infection.[141,149,150] The mechanism of this decreased production of erythropoietin likely is a posttranscriptional defect, as levels of messenger RNA for erythropoietin are normal although erythropoietin protein levels are decreased. In addition, development of autoantibodies to erythropoietin has been described in HIV-infected patients.[151] Multiple studies confirm the beneficial effect of erythropoietin in HIV-infected patients with anemia, in whom marrow function is suppressed as a result of HIV or other chronic infectious or inflammatory diseases.[140,152–154] Erythropoietin also is effective in treating anemia resulting from zidovudine or other medications, including cancer chemotherapy, which suppress the marrow.[154]

The baseline level of endogenous serum erythropoietin can predict which patients will respond to therapeutic use of erythropoietin. Thus, patients with a baseline endogenous erythropoietin level of 500 IU/L or less are expected to respond to erythropoietin therapy, whereas those with endogenous levels greater than 500 IU/L are not. Erythropoietin 100 to 200 U/kg body weight is administered subcutaneously three times per week until improvement of the hemoglobin concentration and then approximately once every week or every other week to maintain a hemoglobin concentration of approximately 11 to 12 g/dL. Clinical trials have demonstrated the equivalent efficacy of 40,000 U of erythropoietin given weekly compared with the original thrice-weekly schedule in anemic HIV-infected patients.[145]

Correction of anemia is associated with improvement in QOL measures after erythropoietin use,[144,145,155] with the mean LASA QOL score increasing by 41 percent and the Medical Outcomes Study-HIV overall QOL score increasing by as much as 37 percent in one study.[144]

Toxicity of erythropoietin is uncommon, consisting primarily of local pain at the site of injection, influenza-like syndrome, headache, hypertension, and rash. Adverse cardiovascular effects have been reported if the target hemoglobin levels are greater than 12 g/dL. Development of pure red cell aplasia has been described in HIV-negative patients receiving the Eprex product (erythropoietin alfa) from Europe, although this complication is uncommon and has not been reported in the patients with HIV.[156]

NEUTROPENIA

Etiology of Neutropenia and Decreased Granulocyte Function in Human Immunodeficiency Virus

Neutropenia is reported in approximately 10 percent of patients with early, asymptomatic HIV infection and in more than 50 percent of individuals with more advanced HIV-related immunodeficiency.[119,120,154] As with other blood cytopenias in the setting of HIV infection, multiple etiologies may be present, either singly or in combination.[158] Decreased colony growth of the progenitor cell colony-forming unit–granulocyte-macrophage[159] may lead to decreased production of both granulocytes and monocytes. Soluble inhibitory substances produced by HIV-infected cells can suppress neutrophil production *in vitro*, suggesting that autoimmunity plays a part in the development of neutropenia in HIV infection.[160] However, other studies show that the presence of neutrophil-bound Ig correlates best with stage of disease rather than with neutropenia per se.[161] Decreased serum levels of granulocyte colony-stimulating factor (G-CSF) have been described in HIV-seropositive subjects with afebrile neutropenia (<1000 neutrophils/μL), indicating that a relative deficiency of this specific hematopoietic growth factor also may contribute to persistent neutropenia.[162] The other causes of neutropenia in HIV infection include the presence of opportunistic infections, malignancies, and HIV-related myelodysplasia affecting marrow function.[163] Myelosuppression and neutropenia may result from any one of several medications that are commonly prescribed for HIV-infected patients.

Aside from absolute neutropenia, patients with HIV infection also may experience decreased function of granulocytes and monocytes. Abnormal Fc processing by macrophages has been described. Decreased opsonization and intracellular killing of bacterial or fungal organisms by granulocytes also have been noted.[164]

Risk Factors for Infection in Neutropenic Patients with Human Immunodeficiency Virus

Multiple studies show that in patients with cancer who receive chemotherapy, the risk of bacterial infection rises when the absolute neutrophil count (ANC) falls below 1000 cells/μL and increases further when the ANC falls below 500 cells/μL.[165] Several studies have confirmed the same relationship in patients with HIV infection. Thus, the risk of bacterial infection increased 2.3-fold for HIV-infected individuals with ANC less than 1000 cells/μL and rose by 7.9-fold in those with ANC levels less than 500 cells/μL.[166] Lower ANCs have been associated with increased risk of hospitalization for serious infection, as shown in a review of 2047 HIV-positive patients.[167] On multivariate analysis, the severity and duration of neutropenia were found to be a significant predictor of the incidence of hospitalization for serious bacterial infections.[167]

In a study of 62 HIV-infected patients with ANCs of 1000 cells/μL or less, 24 percent developed infectious complications, most commonly within 24 hours after onset of neutropenia.[168] On multivariate analysis, the three factors independently associated with infectious complications were presence of a central venous catheter, neutropenia in the previous 3 months, and a lower nadir of granulocyte count (250 cells/μL in those with infections vs. 622 cells/μL in those without infections). Among patients with medication-associated neutropenia, the most common cause was zidovudine, followed by trimethoprim-sulfamethoxazole and ganciclovir. Neutropenia was less likely to be associated with infection in these patients than in individuals who were neutropenic because of cancer chemotherapy.[168]

Another study, however, has suggested that the risk of serious infectious complications in neutropenic HIV-infected patients is low.[169] In this prospective study of neutropenia (defined as ANC ≤1000 cells/μL) in 87 consecutive HIV-infected patients, all except three episodes of neutropenia were associated with known myelosuppressive medications. The majority of patients had received cotrimoxazole (62%), lamivudine (56%), and/or zidovudine (40%).[169] The mean ANC of these individuals was 660 cells/μL (range: 100–900 cells/μL), and the median duration of neutropenia was 13 days. However, severe neutropenia was uncommon; only three patients had ANC nadirs less than 200 cells/μL. Serious neutropenia-related sepsis in this setting was uncommon, with culture-proven infection occurring in only 8 percent of patients and presumed infection in another 8 percent. No patient died of infection. As expected, patients with infections had significantly lower ANC nadirs (mean: 460 vs. 710 cells/μL) and significantly lower CD4 cell counts (mean: 64 vs. 126 cells/μL) but did not have a longer duration of neutropenia than patients who did not develop infection.

Impact of Effective Antiretroviral Therapy on Neutropenia

The use of HAART can be associated with improvement of leukopenia and neutropenia in treated patients. Use of HAART and higher CD4+ counts was associated with reduced risk and resolution of neutropenia in the WIHS cohort.[157] A prospective trial that included 66 HIV-infected patients treated with HAART found significant increases in total leukocyte counts and absolute granulocyte counts after 6 months of HAART.[148] A direct stimulatory effect of protease inhibitors on human hematopoiesis has been demonstrated.[170] These data indicate that mild to moderate levels of neutropenia may be managed by use of HAART alone.

Use of Granulocyte-Macrophage Colony-Stimulating Factor in Neutropenic Patients with Human Immunodeficiency Virus Infection

When administered subcutaneously to HIV-infected patients with neutropenia, granulocyte-macrophage colony-stimulating factor (GM-CSF) results in dose-dependent increases in granulocytes, monocytes, and eosinophils.[171,172] Therapy with GM-CSF may improve neutrophil function by enhancing phagocytosis, degranulation, leukotriene B_4 synthesis, release of arachidonic acid, superoxide anion generation, and antibody-dependent cellular cytotoxicity.[173–175] Although there were initial concerns that GM-CSF may increase HIV replication,[176] *in vitro* studies indicated that GM-CSF inhibits HIV-1 replication in monocytes and macrophages.[177]

Granulocyte-Macrophage Colony Stimulating Factor In one study comparing 123 HIV-positive leukopenic patients (defined as a white blood cell count $<3 \times 10^9$/L) treated with subcutaneous GM-CSF with 121 nontreated leukopenic HIV-positive controls, administration of GM-CSF for 12 weeks significantly increased the total leukocyte count of treated patients.[176] In patients receiving GM-CSF, the total leukocyte count increased by 22 percent at week 1 and by 65 percent at week 12 over baseline values ($p < 0.001$), whereas the circulating monocyte levels increased by twofold to threefold at week 12 ($p < 0.001$). In contrast, the total leukocyte count decreased by 24 percent below baseline values at week 12 ($p < 0.001$) in the control group. Of importance, no statistically significant change occurred in HIV p24 antigen levels in patients treated with GM-CSF, even among those who were not receiving antiretroviral therapy.[176–178]

The safety and efficacy of GM-CSF in HIV-infected patients receiving antiretroviral therapy has also been confirmed in another randomized placebo-controlled trial involving a group of 105 HIV-infected patients.[179] GM-CSF 125 mcg/m^2 was given twice weekly for 6 months. Patients randomized to antiretroviral therapy plus GM-CSF achieved a greater reduction in plasma viral load, were more likely to achieve HIV-1 RNA levels below the limit of detection, and demonstrated a lower frequency of zidovudine resistance mutations than those who received antiretroviral agents plus placebo. Side effects of GM-CSF include primarily an influenza-like syndrome, with fever, bone pain, myalgia, fatigue, malaise, and headache.

Granulocyte Colony-Stimulating Factor G-CSF is effective at preventing severe neutropenia and reducing the incidence of bacterial infections and the number of days of hospitalization in neutropenic HIV-infected patients.[180] A study that randomized 258 such patients with counts less than 200 CD4+ cells/μL and moderate neutropenia (defined as ANC 750–1000 cells/μL) to receive G-CSF (1 mcg/kg per day or 300 mcg three times per week) versus no treatment for 24 weeks.[180] Patients in the control group who developed severe neutropenia (ANC <500 cells/μL) were re-randomized to receive G-CSF according to one of the two treatment groups. Treatment with G-CSF was effective at preventing the development of severe neutropenia and reducing the incidence of bacterial infections, independent of CD4+ count, number of prior opportunistic infections, and baseline use of zidovudine. Thus, in an intention-to-treat analysis, the incidence of severe neutropenia was 1.7 percent in the treated group versus 22 percent in the control group, whereas the incidence of bacterial infections was 31 percent lower in the treated group (2.93 vs. 4.25/1000 patient-days). Furthermore, patients treated with G-CSF had 54 percent fewer severe bacterial infections and 45 percent fewer hospital days for bacterial infections. There was no difference between the groups in terms of toxicity or HIV RNA levels in plasma. The most frequently reported adverse events were fever, diarrhea, fatigue, nausea, headache, anemia, abdominal pain, vomiting, and myalgia. Thus, administration of G-CSF when patients are mildly neutropenic appears to be superior to waiting for patients to become severely neutropenic. However, use of HAART may be equally efficacious in resolving mild to moderate neutropenia.

The early recommendations for dosing of G-CSF included use of 5 mcg/kg per day given subcutaneously. Evidence suggests, however, that much lower doses of G-CSF may be effective in HIV-infected persons. Thus, an initial dose of 1 mcg/kg per day often is initiated and used until the neutrophil count rises to acceptable levels (>1000 cells/μL). This is followed by a titration of dosing, often requiring therapy only once or twice per week, as necessary to maintain the desired response.

Thus, use of G-CSF or GM-CSF to improve neutropenia in HIV-infected patients is both safe and effective. Although patient survival has not increased as a consequence of G-CSF or GM-CSF,[181] these drugs allow safer administration of other medications and potentially reduce both the incidence of bacterial infections and number of hospital days.[172,180,181]

THROMBOCYTOPENIA

Thrombocytopenia is relatively common during the course of HIV infection, occurring in approximately 40 percent of patients and serving as the first symptom or sign of infection in approximately 10 percent.[182,183] Evaluation of the 1-year incidence of thrombocytopenia (<50,000 cells/μL) in a group of 30,214 HIV-infected patients as part of the retrospective Adult and Adolescent Spectrum of Disease Project[183] found the incidence of thrombocytopenia over 1 year was 8.7 percent in patients with clinical AIDS, 3.1 percent in patients with immunologic AIDS (<200 CD4+ cells/μL), and 1.7 percent in patients with neither clinical nor immunologic AIDS. Development of thrombocytopenia was associated with (1) history of clinical or immunologic AIDS, (2) injection drug use, (3) history of anemia or lymphoma, and (4) being an American of African descent. After controlling for multiple factors (AIDS, CD4 count, anemia, neutropenia, antiviral therapy, receipt of prophylaxis against *P. carinii*), thrombocytopenia was significantly associated with shorter survival (risk ratio 1.7; 95% CI 1.6–1.8).[183]

The WIHS data found thrombocytopenia was a significant predictor of both all-cause and AIDS-related mortality among women infected with HIV. HIV-infected women with a platelet count less than 50,000/μL had a fivefold increased risk of death from any cause compared to women with normal platelet counts (hazard ratio [HR] = 5.10; 95% CI 2.71–9.58) and an approximate threefold increased risk of death from AIDS (HR = 3.36; 95% CI 1.44–7.83).[184]

In addition to thrombocytopenia related to the HIV virus, persons with HIV infection have a high risk of secondary thrombocytopenia because of increased risk of other infections, malignancies, hypersplenism as a result of coexisting hepatitis or cirrhosis, and treatment with infection prophylaxis regimens that often include myelosuppressive medications.

Mechanisms of Thrombocytopenia in Human Immunodeficiency Virus-Related Thrombocytopenia

Primary HIV-Associated Thrombocytopenia What has previously been described as HIV-associated immune thrombocytopenic purpura (ITP) is increasingly characterized as "primary HIV-associated thrombocytopenia (PHAT)" to highlight differences from *de novo* ITP. PHAT is the most common cause of thrombocytopenia in persons with HIV. In contrast to *de novo* ITP, PHAT is associated with a higher rate of splenomegaly, typically less-severe thrombocytopenia, and a 20 percent spontaneous remission rate.[77] The etiology of the thrombocytopenia is multifactorial including both increased platelet destruction and decreased platelet production.[80]

Increased Platelet Destruction As in *de novo* ITP, patients with PHAT also have increased platelet destruction via phagocytosis by macrophages in the spleen.[185] In PHAT, however, several mechanisms for development of platelet-associated antibody have been described, often occurring simultaneously in a given patient. Presence of platelet-specific antibodies, against both glycoprotein (GP) IIb and GPIIIa, have been detected in patients with PHAT, indicating a mechanism similar to that described in *de novo* ITP. However, in HIV patients, antibodies against platelet GPIIb-IIIa have been demonstrated to be cross-reactive with HIV GP160/120.[187] Thus, molecular mimicry between HIV GP160/120 and platelet GPIIb-IIIa may be operative in the immune destruction of platelets in some cases of PHAT. Autoantibodies against a specific peptide sequence of GPIIIa (49–66) have been recovered from patient plasma in the form of immune complexes consisting of autoantibody and platelet fragments. These antibodies are unique in that they cause complement-independent platelet fragmentation through activation of oxidases generating reactive oxygen species.[194]

A further mechanism of antibody-induced destruction of platelets arises from the absorption of immune complexes against HIV onto the platelet Fc receptor, thus providing a "free" Fc portion for subsequent macrophage binding and phagocytosis.[186]

Decreased Platelet Production Kinetic studies of platelet production and destruction have been performed in patients with PHAT, with results compared to a group of normal control subjects and to a group of patients with *de novo* ITP.[185] Mean platelet survival was significantly decreased in patients with PHAT, occurring to the same extent in patients receiving zidovudine and in those who were untreated. Mean platelet survival also was significantly decreased in HIV-infected patients with normal platelet counts. In addition to increased destruction of platelets, mean platelet production was significantly decreased in patients with untreated PHAT, although those patients receiving zidovudine demonstrated a subsequent increase in platelet production, occurring even in zidovudine-treated HIV-infected individuals without thrombocytopenia. Thus, patients with PHAT, while experiencing a moderate increase in platelet destruction, also face a significant decrease in platelet production, which occurs even in HIV-infected individuals with normal platelet counts.[185]

Infection of Megakaryocytes by Human Immunodeficiency Virus The cause of reduced production of platelets in the setting of HIV infection may be direct infection of the megakaryocyte by HIV. Human megakaryocytes bear a CD4+ receptor capable of binding HIV-1,[188] and HIV-1 can be internalized by human megakaryocytes.[189] The HIV-1 coreceptor CXCR4 is present on megakaryocytic progenitors, megakaryocytes, and platelets.[190] Using *in situ* hybridization techniques and a ^{35}S HIV riboprobe (antisense to an HIV *ENV* sequence), HIV transcripts have been detected in megakaryocytes of 5 of 10 patients with PHAT, indicating the megakaryocyte had been infected by HIV in these cases.[191] Expression of viral RNA was also detected in all 10 patients using *in situ* hybridization techniques. Specific ultrastructural damage in the HIV-infected megakaryocytes has been noted, consisting of blebbing and vacuolization of the surface membrane.[192] Documentation of significant increases in platelet production after receipt of zidovudine[193] is consistent with the hypothesis that a major mechanism of this disorder is the direct infection of the megakaryocyte by HIV.

Therapy for Primary Human Immunodeficiency Virus-Associated Thrombocytopenia

As with ITP, the diagnosis of PHAT is clinical and requires the exclusion of secondary causes of thrombocytopenia and discontinuation of potentially myelosuppressive medications and herbal preparations. Treatment considerations are similar to ITP in that several factors need to be considered prior to initiation of treatment including comorbidities influencing the risk of bleeding and the degree of thrombocytopenia.

Zidovudine The Swiss Group for HIV Studies was the first to demonstrate the efficacy of zidovudine therapy in patients with PHAT.[193] Ten seropositive patients, with platelet counts ranging from 20,000 to 100,000/μL, received zidovudine 2 g/day for 2 weeks, followed by 1 g/day for 6 weeks. This treatment was followed by 8 weeks of placebo. All 10 patients experienced an increase in platelet counts while receiving zidovudine, with a mean increase of 54,600/μL (range: 53,200–107,800/μL). In contrast, no patient experienced an increase in platelet count while receiving placebo. The time to onset of response was approximately 8 days, with full response achieved by day 30. These results were subsequently confirmed by other studies.[195,196]

The appropriate dose of zidovudine for treatment of PHAT was studied by comparing a dose of 500 mg/day in 35 patients with 1000 mg/day in another group of 36 individuals.[197] The majority of patients in both groups were injection drug users, with similar mean platelet counts (~ 23,000/μL) and mean lymphocyte counts (~ 400 CD4+ cells/μL). A response rate of 57 percent was achieved in the low-dose group, with 11 percent experiencing complete response. In contrast, a response rate of 72 percent was achieved in those receiving zidovudine 1000 mg/day, with complete response in 39 percent. At month 6, a significant difference remained between the groups, with a mean platelet count of 56,000/μL in the low-dose group versus 98,200/μL in those receiving high-dose zidovudine. It is apparent from this study that high-dose zidovudine is advantageous in patients with PHAT.[197]

Highly Active Antiretroviral Therapy in Primary HIV-Associated Thrombocytopenia HAART is effective for treatment of PHAT. In a report of 37 patients with PHAT, effective use of HAART was associated with a significantly increased platelet count after 3 months, independent of baseline platelet count or concomitant use of zidovudine.[198] Similarly, in a retrospective study involving 15 patients with PHAT treated with HAART, 11 (73%) had an increase in platelet count to values of 50,000/μL or greater, and 8 (53%) had an increase in platelet count to values of 100,000/μL or greater after 6 months of HAART therapy.[199] Consistent with these findings, data from the WIHS demonstrated a strong association between use of HAART and resolution of thrombocytopenia (defined as a platelet count >150,000/μL).[184] Thus, compared to thrombocytopenic women not receiving antiretroviral therapy, women taking a non–AZT-containing HAART regimen were nearly two times more likely to improve their thrombocytopenia (odds ratio [OR], 1.84; 95% CI 1.31–2.59; $p < 0.001$), whereas women taking an AZT-containing HAART regimen were even more likely to resolve their thrombocytopenia (OR 2.85; 95% CI 1.96–4.15; $p < 0.0001$).[184] Thus, HAART is an important treatment modality in patients with PHAT and should be the initial treatment of choice in these patients. Effective use of HAART probably significantly decreases HIV viral load and, in so doing, ameliorates many of the effects of HIV on megakaryocytes, platelet production, and destruction.

Interferon-α A prospective, randomized, double-blind, placebo-controlled trial of IFN-α 3,000,000 U given subcutaneously three times per week was conducted in 15 patients with PHAT.[200] A platelet response was documented in 66 percent, with a mean increase of 60,000/μL. The average time to response was 3 weeks. When IFN therapy was discontinued, platelet counts returned to baseline values within 3 months, indicating the necessity to maintain IFN-α therapy over time. IFN-α was found to prolong platelet survival, whereas no significant increase in platelet production was noted.[201]

High-Dose Intravenous Gammaglobulin IVIg 1000 to 2000 mg/kg has been used effectively in pediatric and adult patients with *de novo* ITP, resulting in a significant rise in platelet counts within 24 to 72 hours in the majority of individuals.[202] Twenty-two patients with PHAT were treated with IVIg 1 to 2 g/kg during a 2- to 5-day period, depending upon the platelet response.[203] The average platelet count prior to therapy was 22,000/μL and rose to a mean of 182,000/μL (range: 10,000–404,000/μL) within 2 to 5 days. Only two patients did not respond, whereas 77 percent experienced an increase to greater than 100,000/μL, and 86 percent had an increase to greater than 50,000/μL. However, when IVIg was discontinued, only 25 percent of patients maintained the increased platelet count, whereas the remainder required repeat infusions approximately every 21 days. The major problem with IVIg appears to be its significant cost. For this reason, IVIg often is reserved for use in patients who are acutely bleeding or require an immediate increase in platelet count, for example, prior to an invasive procedure.

Anti-Rh Immunoglobulin Use of anti-Rh immunoglobulin in nonsplenectomized Rh-positive patients with PHAT is another potential mode of therapy.[204] Requirements for effective therapy with anti-Rh (D) include presence of Rh+ red cells in the patient, a baseline hemoglobin level adequate to permit a 1- to 2-g decrease as a result of hemolysis, and presence of a spleen, the site at which red cells preferentially are phagocytized. Fourteen patients with PHAT were treated with 25 mg/kg IV over 30 minutes on 2 consecutive days.[205] Nine of 11 (83%) Rh-positive patients responded with a platelet count greater than 50,000/μL, with response first noted at a median of 4 days (range: 3 to 12 days), and median response duration of 13 days (range: 0–37 days). Maintenance therapy of 13 to 25 mg/kg intravenously was administered every 2 to 4 weeks, resulting in a long-term response (>6 months) in 70 percent of patients. Subclinical hemolysis occurred in all patients, with a decrease in hemoglobin of 0.4 to 2.2 g. These results were confirmed, and use of intramuscular anti-D immunoglobulin was examined for maintenance treatment after successful induction therapy by the intravenous route.[204] Patients self-administered anti-Rh immunoglobulin intramuscularly at a dosage of 6 to 13 mg/kg per week. After induction, 83 percent of patients had achieved a platelet count greater than 50,000/μL, a response that was maintained in 85 percent of patients over time. Thus it is apparent that anti-Rh immunoglobulin can be used safely and effectively in patients with PHAT, providing an alternative that in some institutions may be half the cost of high-dose IVIg.[204,205]

Splenectomy Splenectomy has been used effectively in *de novo* ITP refractory to glucocorticoids. At the onset of the AIDS epidemic, several anecdotal case reports described a rapid progression of AIDS postsplenectomy, and the procedure was largely abandoned. Long-term experience with splenectomy in a cohort of 185 patients with PHAT has been reported.[206] Splenectomy eventually was performed in 68 such patients, at an average of 13 months from initial diagnosis of PHAT. The mean platelet count presplenectomy was 18,000/μL and rose to 223,000/μL postoperatively. A response was seen in 92 percent of patients, with complete response (platelet count >100,000/μL) in 85 percent. Maintenance of the elevated platelet count for longer than 6 months was documented in 82 percent. No difference was found when the survival or rate of progression to AIDS in the 68 splenectomized patients was compared with the rate in the 117 patients who did not undergo the procedure, indicating that splenectomy was not associated with more rapid progression of HIV disease. Another study reached similar conclusions.[207] However, 5.8 percent of patients who underwent splenectomy in one series experienced fulminant infection, consisting of *Streptococcus pneumoniae* meningitis in two and *Haemophilus influenzae* sepsis in one.[206] Thus patients should undergo prophylactic vaccination prior to splenectomy and such surgery may be safer in HIV-infected patients who can still achieve an appropriate antibody response to vaccination against *S. pneumoniae* or *H. influenzae*.

Glucocorticoids Glucocorticoids remain the initial therapy of choice in patients with *de novo* ITP and at a dosage of 1 mg/kg per day are associated with an 80 to 90 percent response rate. Similar results were documented in patients with HIV-related disease. However, the immunosuppressive effects of high-dose glucocorticoids have made such therapy suboptimal in HIV-infected patients. Furthermore, the potential development of fulminant Kaposi sarcoma (KS) in dually HIV-infected and human herpes virus (HHV)-8–infected patients after use of glucocorticoids has further dampened enthusiasm for this therapeutic modality.

■ THROMBOTIC DISEASE

Venous Thrombosis

There may be an increased incidence of venous thromboembolic disease in persons with HIV infection.[208–215] In the Multistate Adult and Adolescent Spectrum of HIV Disease Surveillance Project sponsored by the CDC, the incidence of thrombosis among 42,935 HIV-infected individuals was 2.6 per 1000 person-years.[212] The incidence was lower for individuals with immunologic AIDS (1.8 per 1000 person-years) or asymptomatic HIV infection (1.3 per 1000 person-years) than for persons with clinical AIDS (6.2 per 1000 person-years). Factors significantly associated with the risk of thrombosis included age 45 years or older, cytomegalovirus retinitis or other infection, other AIDS-defining opportunistic infections, hospitalization, use of megestrol acetate, and use of indinavir.[212] Use of other antiretroviral agents, sex, race, and a history of injection drug use were not associated with an increased risk for thrombosis.

However, in another study that directly compared the risk of venous thromboembolism in HIV-infected patients and HIV-negative controls, no statistically significant difference in the rate of thrombotic disease was reported between the groups as a whole (HIV-infected patients 2.8% vs. HIV-negative controls 1.8%).[214] However, in patients younger than age 50 years, the frequencies were significantly different (HIV-infected patients 3.31% vs. HIV-negative controls 0.53%, $p < 0.0001$).

In an attempt to determine the incidence of venous thrombosis in HIV-infected patients compared to individuals without HIV infection and to determine whether the introduction of combination antiretroviral therapy altered the rates of thrombotic disease, a retrospective review was conducted of the medical charts of 37,535 HIV-infected veterans and 37,535 age-, race-, and site-matched controls.[215] Compared to HIV-negative controls, HIV infection was associated with a 39 percent increased incidence of thromboembolism in the pre-HAART era (standardized incidence ratio [SIR] 1.39; 95% CI 1.26–1.52) and a 33 percent increased incidence in the post-1996 era (SIR 1.33; 95% CI 1.24–1.43). This increased risk of thrombosis was independent of a diagnosis of malignancy, HIV-related opportunistic infection, or use of central venous catheters. Furthermore, thrombosis was significantly associated with increased mortality in all groups. Thus, venous thrombotic disease is increased in the setting of HIV infection, independent of many of the more commonly known risk factors.

HIV infection is known to result in increased levels of proinflammatory cytokines, such as tumor necrosis factor (TNF)-α, IL-1, and IL-6, which can contribute to the development of a procoagulant state by increased levels of factor VIII and decreased levels of protein S.[216–218] These same cytokines downregulate the expression of several proteins necessary for fibrinolysis.[219] Several studies suggest that progressive HIV infection may be associated with the development of such a hypercoagulable state. Thus, one study comparing 94 HIV-infected women and 50 HIV-negative controls documented a clear relationship between progressive stages of HIV disease, progressive increases in factor VIII activity, and progressively decreasing levels of protein S. Other studies report abnormalities of coagulation proteins in HIV-infected patients, such as acquired deficiencies in protein S,[221–226] protein C,[226,227] and heparin cofactor II,[228] and higher titers of anticardiolipin antibodies.[229] Thus, although the mechanisms leading to thromboembolism in HIV are not completely elucidated, the progressive proinflammatory milieu of HIV infection may be important.

Thrombotic Thrombocytopenic Purpura

Thrombotic thrombocytopenic purpura is associated with advanced HIV disease. The Collaborations in HIV Outcomes Research/United States (CHORUS) cohort, which included 6022 persons with HIV infection in the HAART era, found a 0.3 percent incidence of thrombotic microangiopathy. Factors associated with thrombotic thrombocytopenic purpura included higher HIV viral loads, lower CD4+ counts, and increased incidence of AIDS diagnoses, as well as infections with *M. avium* complex and hepatitis C. The incidence is decreasing in the HAART era.[220]

HUMAN IMMUNODEFICIENCY VIRUS-ASSOCIATED MALIGNANCIES

More than 40 percent of all HIV-infected patients eventually are diagnosed with cancer.[230] In the HAART era, malignancies account for 20 percent of deaths in persons with HIV-infection.[231] Furthermore, the spectrum of neoplastic disease appears to be wider than initially thought.[230] Three cancers currently considered AIDS-defining in HIV-infected persons are (1) KS, associated with the epidemic from the onset in 1981; (2) intermediate- or high-grade B-cell lymphoma, added to the case definition for AIDS in 1985; and (3) cervical carcinoma, which became an AIDS-defining illness on January 1, 1993. Although not considered an AIDS-defining condition, data from cohort studies have consistently shown an increased risk of Hodgkin lymphoma (HL) among patients infected with HIV.

■ ACQUIRED IMMUNODEFICIENCY SYNDROME–RELATED LYMPHOMA

Epidemiology

Patients with AIDS have a risk of developing lymphoma that is nearly 100 times greater than that of the general population.[232–234] The incidence of lymphoma increases with prolonged survival in HIV and may approach 20 percent for patients with prolonged, far-advanced immunodeficiency.[235,236] In one study that linked AIDS and cancer registries in selected areas in the United States, the relative risk of developing lymphoma within 3 years of an AIDS diagnosis was increased by 165-fold compared to people without AIDS.[237] The same study also demonstrated that the increase in risk ranged from 652-fold for high-grade diffuse immunoblastic tumors to 261-fold for Burkitt lymphomas, 113-fold for intermediate-grade lymphomas, and 14-fold for low-grade lymphomas.

As a percentage of first AIDS-defining illness, lymphomas have increased since the widespread use of HAART.[238–241] In one prospective observational multicenter study of more than 7300 patients from Europe, the proportion of AIDS-defining illness attributable to AIDS-related lymphoma rose from less than 4 percent in 1994 to almost 16 percent in 1998.[239] A similar trend has been observed in the United States and Australia.[210,241]

Although use of HAART has led to a major and dramatic decline in the incidence of KS, results from studies evaluating the impact of HAART on the incidence of lymphoma have been inconsistent. The Swiss HIV Cohort study and the Multicenter AIDS Cohort Study (MACS) found no decline in the incidence rates of lymphoma between the pre-HAART and HAART eras,[242,243] but the International Collaboration on HIV and Cancer and the EuroSIDA studies documented a significant decline of lymphoma in the HAART era.[244,245] However, these studies have primarily examined the influence of HAART by dividing the study population into two different time intervals, without considering the actual effects of HAART on individual patients.

Data from a French study suggest that the incidence of lymphoma will decline when HAART is effective in a population. Using data from the French Hospital Database on HIV, the incidence of systemic AIDS-related lymphoma decreased from 86.0 per 10,000 person-years during the pre-HAART era (defined as 1993 to 1994) to 42.9 per 10,000 person-years during the HAART era (defined as 1997 to 1998).[246] In both the pre-HAART and HAART periods, patients with lower CD4+ cell counts were more likely to develop lymphoma. Nonetheless, within strata of patients with similar CD4+ cell counts, the French study showed no change in the incidence of AIDS-related lymphoma between the two periods.[246] Although the risk of lymphoma did not change between the periods among patients with similar CD4+ cell counts, the proportion of patients with low counts (<200 CD4+ cells/μL [0.2×10^9/L]) decreased from 49.5 to 24.5 percent between the pre-HAART and HAART periods, thus decreasing the overall proportion of individuals at risk for AIDS-related lymphoma in the second period. The observed decrease in the incidence of lymphoma in the French study resulted from the overall decrease in the proportion of patients with low CD4+ counts. Taken together, these data indicate that the incidence of AIDS-related lymphoma in a population depends on the effectiveness of HAART in improving the immune status of that population. If access to HAART is not uniformly available or if HAART is ineffective in increasing CD4+ cell counts or decreasing HIV RNA levels, the incidence of lymphoma in that population will not decline.

Etiology and Pathogenesis

The mechanisms underlying the development of lymphoma in the setting of HIV are not fully understood. One factor may be immune suppression itself, which is associated with an increased incidence of lymphoma in certain congenital immunodeficiency diseases,[247] autoimmune disorders,[248] or in patients chronically using immunosuppressive drugs, as in the setting of organ transplantation.[249,250] The lymphomas that develop in these settings are similar to the AIDS lymphomas in terms of the pathologic types, the high frequency of extranodal disease at presentation, and the relatively poor prognosis.

Infection by HIV is associated with a myriad of immunologic aberrations (Fig. 83–3). These abnormalities include functional and quantitative defects of CD4+ T cells[66,73,251] and chronic antigenic stimulation of B lymphocytes by antigens, mitogens, or viruses, including Epstein-Barr virus (EBV)[252] and HIV itself.[75,253] Ongoing B-cell expansion and activation result in the development of reactive B cell hyperplasia in lymphoid tissues (persistent generalized lymphadenopathy)[73,65,88,251] and polyclonal hypergammaglobulinemia in the serum.[74] Lymphomas may develop after acquisition of genetic errors occurring during the course of polyclonal B-cell proliferation in the setting of underlying immunodeficiency. This finding has been observed in a primate model, in which high-grade B-cell lymphoma develops between 5 and 15 months after infection with the simian immune deficiency virus, coincident with development of severe immunodeficiency.[254]

Cytokine Networks Dysregulated expression of cytokines and cell surface receptors may contribute to the chronic B-cell proliferation that characterizes HIV disease. B-cell proliferation and maturation may be induced by several cytokines, including IL-4, IL-6, IL-10, and TNF-α.[255] B cells from HIV-infected patients with hypergammaglobulinemia constitutively express TNF-α and IL-6.[256] High levels of IL-6 gene expression have been noted in myeloma, chronic lymphocytic leukemia, and both HIV-positive and HIV-negative cases of immunoblastic and large-cell lymphoma, independent of EBV status.[259] Although not unique to AIDS-related lymphoma, IL-6 may play a role in the pathogenesis of diverse types of B-cell neoplasia. Moreover, elevated serum IL-6 levels can be detected in the sera of patients with symptomatic HIV infection who later develop large cell lymphoma.[236]

IL-10 may play a role in the development of AIDS-related lymphoma. Constitutive expression of IL-10 has been shown in EBV-positive B-cell lines derived from patients with AIDS-related Burkitt lymphoma,[260] and

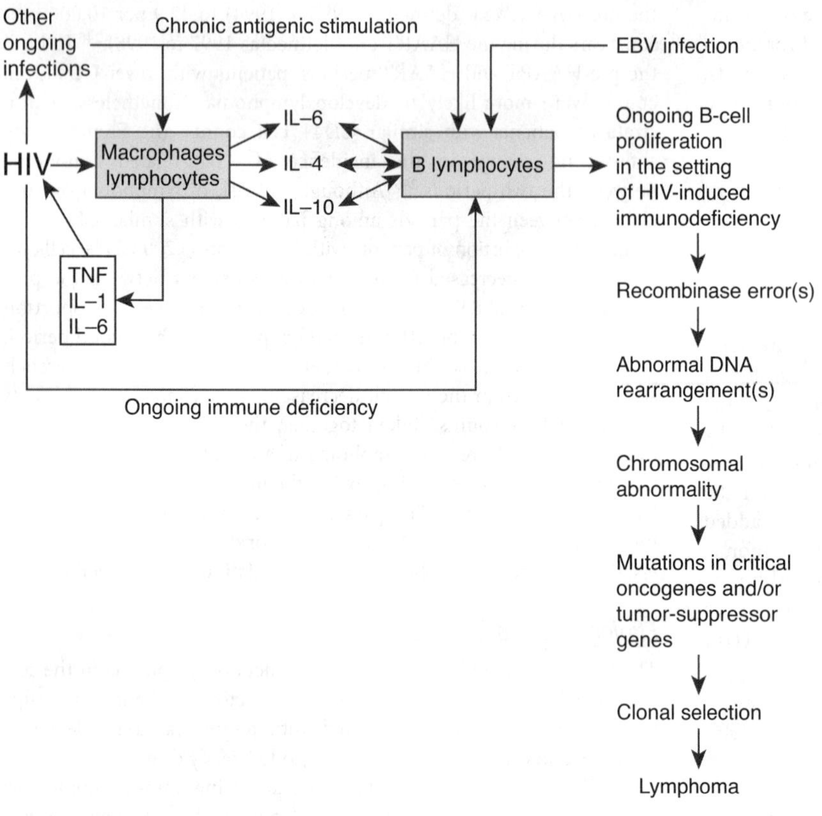

FIGURE 83–3. Schematic representation of the possible sequence of events resulting in the development of lymphoma in human immunodeficiency virus (HIV) disease. EBV, Epstein-Barr virus; IL, interleukin; TNF, tumor necrosis factor. *(Reproduced and modified with permission from Martin JN, Ganem DE, Osmond DH, et al.[379])*

IL-10 has been shown to function as an autocrine growth factor in B-cell lines.[261] Soluble CD44, involved in inflammation, tumor cell growth, and metastasis, was found to be increased before the development of HIV-related lymphoma in a longitudinal cohort study.[257] HIV may induce aberrant expression of these cytokines and cell surface receptors, thus stimulating pathologic B-cell proliferation and differentiation and allowing for neoplastic transformation.

Epstein-Barr Virus EBV is implicated in the pathogenesis of at least a subset of AIDS-related lymphoma, perhaps related to the impaired immunosurveillance against EBV-infected cells.[252] EBV DNA has been found in the affected lymph nodes of 35 percent of HIV-infected patients with reactive lymphadenopathy.[263] These individuals were shown to have an increased incidence of lymphoma over time.[263]

Patients with large cell or immunoblastic lymphoma primary to the brain uniformly have latent EBV infections.[264] EBV-associated latent small nuclear RNAs can be detected in essentially all such patients and the EBV latent membrane protein in 45 percent.[264] Latent membrane protein has transforming and oncogenic properties.[265]

Approximately 50 percent of systemic AIDS-related lymphoma cases have detectable EBV DNA within tumor nuclei.[266,267] Immunoblastic lymphomas and, to a lesser extent, diffuse large B-cell lymphomas are most commonly EBV positive.[268] Evidence for clonal EBV infection has been demonstrated in all cases examined, indicating that EBV integration occurred before clonal B-cell expansion.[269] Loss of EBV-specific CD4 and CD8 T cells was significantly more prominent in HIV-positive individuals who went on to develop an EBV-positive lymphoma than in those who progressed to non-EBV-related AIDS diagnoses and slow progressors.[258] These findings suggest, but do not prove, that EBV plays a role in the etiopathogenesis of these lymphomas.

Abnormal DNA Rearrangements During AIDS-related B-cell stimulation induced by HIV, EBV, and/or or other antigens, genetic "errors" in immunoglobulin gene rearrangement, and/or expression may occur, leading to chromosomal translocations involving the immunoglobulin heavy- or light-chain genes. Thus, specific chromosomal translocations have been described in AIDS-related Burkitt lymphoma, including t(8;14), t(8;22), and t(8;2).[270–272]

c-myc Translocations involving chromosome 8 can result in dysregulation of the *MYC* oncogene. Dependent upon the specific breakpoint position on chromosome 8 and the locus on chromosome 14, 2, or 22, different mechanisms for *MYC* dysregulation may apply, as described in the distinct forms of Burkitt lymphoma and in distinct geographic regions of the world.[273,274] However, dysregulation of this gene is not seen in all cases of AIDS-related lymphoma. Activation was detected in 100 percent of small noncleaved lymphomas in one series,[269] but such activation was found in only a minority of large cell or immunoblastic lymphomas.[275] Moreover, the specific mechanisms leading to *MYC* dysregulation are diverse.[269,276,277] Thus, HIV-1 infection of immortalized B-cell lines in itself can result in upregulation of *MYC* transcripts,[278] whereas HIV may also affect cellular *MYC* gene expression directly.[277] Whatever the mechanism, dysregulation may contribute to transformation of human B cells *in vitro* and may cause B-cell lymphoma in transgenic animals carrying *Ig-MYC* chimeric constructs.[279,280]

BCL-6 Dysregulation and Other Genetic Abnormalities In AIDS-related, diffuse, large B-cell lymphoma, the primary molecular alteration involves mutations of *BCL-6*.[281,282] Although gross rearrangements or chromosomal translocations involving *BCL-6* usually are absent, mutations in the 5′ regions of the gene are detectable in as many as 60 percent of cases.[281–283] These mutations are markers of germinal center derivation of B cells, indicating that diffuse large B-cell lymphomas in AIDS are related to germinal center B cells.[284]

Aside from these genetic abnormalities, other molecular aberrations have been noted, including p53 mutations or deletions, which may occur in as many as 60 percent of AIDS-related small noncleaved lymphomas.[275,285] In addition, mutations of *RAS* have been described in some cases of AIDS-related Burkitt lymphoma.[275]

Diverse molecular mechanisms are responsible for the various types of AIDS-related lymphoma.[284] Small noncleaved lymphomas are most often associated with *MYC* aberrations, mutations in p53, and occasionally *RAS*. Diffuse large B-cell lymphomas are associated with mutations in the *BCL-6* gene, whereas immunoblastic and large cell lymphomas appear to be driven primarily by EBV.

Pathology

Eighty to 90 percent of lymphomas associated with AIDS are intermediate- or high-grade B-cell tumors,[285–289] including immunoblastic or large B-cell types and small noncleaved or Burkitt lymphomas, which is in sharp contrast to non–HIV-infected patients, in whom high-grade lymphomas are expected in only 10 to 15 percent of cases.[290] In an effort to standardize the nomenclature, the WHO has classified AIDS-related lymphoma into three groups: (1) those occurring specifically in HIV-infected patients, (2) those also occurring in other immunodeficiency states, and (3) those that also arise in immunocompetent

TABLE 83–3. Categories of HIV-Associated Lymphomas: World Health Organization Classification

Lymphomas also occurring in immunocompetent patients
Burkitt lymphoma
Classic
With plasmacytoid differentiation
Atypical
Diffuse large B-cell lymphoma
Centroblastic
Immunoblastic
Extranodal marginal zone B cell lymphoma of mucosa-associated lymphoid tissue (MALT) lymphoma (rare)
Peripheral T-cell lymphoma (rare)
Classic Hodgkin lymphoma
Lymphomas occurring more specifically in patients who are HIV positive
Primary effusion lymphoma
Plasmablastic lymphoma of the oral cavity
Lymphomas occurring in other immunodeficiency states
Polymorphic B-cell lymphoma

patients (Table 83–3).[291] The two most common histologic subtypes of lymphoma in HIV-infected patients are Burkitt lymphoma and diffuse large B-cell lymphoma.

Burkitt Lymphoma In patients with HIV-related Burkitt lymphoma, histology may resemble classic Burkitt lymphoma as seen in the general population or, more commonly, may demonstrate atypical features.[292–295] Histologically, classic Burkitt lymphoma is characterized by sheets of intermediate-size lymphoid cells with regular round or oval nuclear outlines or slight nuclear irregularities. A "starry sky" appearance resulting from the presence of tangible body macrophages is characteristically found (see Chap. 98, Fig. 98–28 and Chap. 104, Fig 104–1). The neoplastic cells have an extremely high mitotic rate, with a Ki67 score approaching 100 percent. In atypical Burkitt lymphoma, the cells are more varied in size and shape and show greater nuclear pleomorphism.[295] In some cases, the cells have a plasmacytoid appearance, characterized by medium-size cells with abundant cytoplasm and eccentric nuclei. This type of Burkitt lymphoma is termed *Burkitt lymphoma with plasmacytoid differentiation* in the WHO classification, an entity unique to patients with HIV.[296]

Diffuse Large B-Cell Lymphoma In the WHO classification, AIDS-related diffuse large B-cell lymphomas are divided into centroblastic and immunoblastic subtypes. The centroblastic subtype has features of large cell lymphomas similar to those seen in the general population without HIV (see Chap. 100). The immunoblastic subtype (approximately 20% of cases) is more typical of HIV infection. It is characterized by large cells, each containing a single prominent nucleolus and plasmacytoid features in the cytoplasm. Compared to the centroblastic subtype, the immunoblastic subtype more frequently involves extranodal sites, particularly the central nervous system (CNS), and is more commonly associated with EBV infection, with EBV-encoded LMP antigen found in 90 percent compared to 30 percent in the centroblastic variant.[268,297,298] Furthermore, amplification of *BCL-6* is associated with the centroblastic but usually not the immunoblastic subtype, whereas CD138/syndecan-1, normally expressed by B cells in late stages of B-cell differentiation, is more commonly expressed in the immunoblastic subtype. These phenotypic differences suggest that the two variants of diffuse large B-cell lymphoma have differing histogenesis, with the centroblastic subtype arising from germinal centers and the immunoblastic variant arising from postgerminal center lymphocytes.

Primary Effusion Lymphoma Primary effusion lymphoma and plasmablastic lymphoma of the oral cavity occur more specifically in patients with HIV infection. Primary effusion lymphoma is uncommon, representing only a small fraction of all AIDS-related lymphomas, and is caused by HHV-8.[299–301] Morphologically, primary effusion lymphoma is characterized by large neoplastic cells with cytologic features that range between immunoblastic, plasmablastic, and anaplastic large cells.[301] The malignant cell usually lacks B-cell markers on its surface but is B lymphoid in origin, as Ig gene rearrangement is consistently present. In addition to HHV-8, the tumor cells often harbor EBV.[301] Plasmablastic lymphoma of the oral cavity, another uncommon entity, is characterized by rapidly growing large lymphoid cells with marked plasma cell differentiation.[302,303] Phenotypically, these lymphomas usually do not express conventional B-cell markers such as CD20 but stain strongly with plasma cell markers CD138/syndecan-1 and VS38c.[302,303] They are positive for EBV-associated latent small nuclear RNAs by *in situ* hybridization, variably positive for EBV LMP-1, and negative for EBV nuclear antigen 2 (EBNA2); HHV-8 is typically negative.[304] However, plasmablastic lymphoma of the oral cavity remains a rare and poorly understood entity and the mechanisms responsible for its pathogenesis remain to be elucidated.

T-Cell Lymphoma Patients with AIDS are at an increased risk for developing T-cell lymphomas. One study reported a 15-fold increased risk for developing T-cell lymphoma 2 years after a diagnosis of AIDS.[235] The prevalence of T-cell lymphomas among patients with AIDS-related lymphoma is approximately 3 percent.[235,305] A wide spectrum of T-cell malignancies in the setting of HIV infection has been reported.[306–308] However, the majority of cases consist of peripheral T-cell lymphomas, occurring in 45 percent, or anaplastic large cell lymphomas, occurring in 27 percent of a small series.[305] Morphologically, they resemble peripheral T-cell lymphomas seen in the general population (see Chap. 98, Figs. 98–30 and 98–31).

Low-Grade B-Cell Lymphoma Occasionally HIV-infected patients with low-grade B-cell lymphomas have been reported,[285,289,309] as have relatively young individuals with myeloma or solitary plasmacytoma.[310] The natural history of low-grade lymphoma appears similar in the presence or absence of underlying HIV infection.[309,311]

Clinical Features

B symptoms, such as fever, night sweats, and weight loss, are present at diagnosis in 80 to 90 percent of patients with AIDS-related lymphoma,[312,313] and 61 to 90 percent have far-advanced disease presenting in extranodal sites.[285–289,310,313] This finding is in contrast to non–AIDS-related lymphoma, in which approximately 40 percent of individuals present with extranodal lymphomatous disease.[314]

Virtually any anatomic site may be involved.[312] The more common sites of initial extranodal disease include the CNS (17–42%), gastrointestinal tract (4–28%), marrow (21–33%), and liver (9–26%).[285–289,312]

Staging evaluation should include computed tomographic scanning of the chest, abdomen, and pelvis; a gallium-67 scan[315] or positron emission tomography (PET) scan; marrow aspirate and biopsy; and other studies as clinically indicated. Lumbar puncture should routinely be performed, because approximately 20 percent of patients have leptomeningeal lymphoma, even in the absence of specific symptoms or signs.[316] Intrathecal methotrexate or cytosine arabinoside is often given to prevent isolated CNS relapse.[316]

Primary Central Nervous System Lymphoma Approximately 75 percent of patients with primary CNS lymphoma have far-advanced HIV disease, with median CD4+ cell counts less than 50/μL, and a prior history of AIDS.[231,313,317–319] Initial symptoms and signs may be variable, with seizures, headache, and/or focal neurologic dysfunction noted in most patients. However, subtle changes in behavior may be the only presenting complaint.[317]

Radiographic scanning reveals relatively large mass lesions (2–4 cm), which tend to be few in number (one to three lesions). Ring enhancement may be seen.[318,319] There is no specific radiographic picture. PET scanning may be useful in differentiating cerebral lymphoma from toxoplasmosis.[320] In addition, thallium-201 single-photon emission computerized tomography scanning may be useful, with a median T1 uptake index greater than 1.5 and a lesion size greater than 2.5 cm serving as independent predictors of primary CNS lymphoma.[321]

Pathologically, almost all such lymphomas are of diffuse large B-cell or immunoblastic subtypes and are uniformly associated with EBV infection within malignant cells.[322] Thus, detection of EBV DNA (Epstein-Barr nuclear antigen) in cerebrospinal fluid by polymerase chain reaction may be used as a diagnostic criterion for primary central nervous lymphoma. One study reported a sensitivity of 80 percent and a specificity of 100 percent.[323]

Optimal therapy for primary CNS lymphoma remains to be defined. Use of cranial radiation is associated with a complete remission rate of only 50 percent and median survival of only 2 or 3 months. Although median survival times have not been prolonged with radiation, approximately 75 percent of patients experience an improvement in QOL.[306] Use of HAART is associated with significantly prolonged survival of these patients.[324] A small pilot trial conducted by the National Cancer Institute AIDS Malignancy Consortium demonstrated activity of an antiviral strategy employing high-dose ganciclovir, zidovudine, and IL-2. One of 4 subjects had a complete remission; the trial was closed early because of slow accrual.[335] Intravenous methotrexate also demonstrated activity in a pilot trial where complete remission was found in 7 of 15 subjects.[336]

T-Cell Lymphomas Systemic B symptoms, consisting of fever, drenching night sweats, and/or unexplained weight loss, are extremely common in patients with T-cell lymphomas; one study reported such symptoms occurred in 82 percent of patients.[305] Like B-cell lymphomas in the setting of HIV, T-cell lymphomas also present with advanced lymphomatous disease, with stage IV disease confirmed in up to 90 percent.[305] Compared to HIV-infected patients with aggressive B-cell lymphomas, patients with T-cell lymphomas more likely present with cutaneous and marrow involvement.[305]

Primary Effusion Lymphoma Primary effusion lymphoma has been reported in both HIV-positive and HIV-negative patients but appears to be more common in the former. Of note, primary effusion lymphoma was diagnosed in an HIV-negative cardiac transplant recipient whose original explanted heart was retrospectively found to be infected by HHV-8.[325] Patients present with effusions in the pleura, pericardium, or peritoneal cavity. Most patients do not have mass lesions, although such masses have been reported, most commonly in the gastrointestinal tract. Optimal therapy is unknown. Outcome with polychemotherapy has generally been poor, with median survival of approximately 2 months.[326] Immune reconstitution with HAART likely plays an important role in the control of this condition. Several studies reported complete remissions in patients treated with HAART alone.[327–329] Palliative measures include draining effusions and therapeutic radiation to affected areas.

Prognostic Factors in Acquired Immunodeficiency Syndrome–Related Lymphoma

The age-adjusted international prognostic index (IPI) established for immunocompetent patients with intermediate grade lymphoma is also predictive of outcome in AIDS patients with lymphoma.[313] A prognostic index designed specifically for HIV-associated lymphoma found the IPI risk group and CD4+ cell count as the only two predictors of death. According to the four risk strata generated, 1-year survival rates were 82, 47, 20, and 15 percent. Although it had not been previously shown to be an important prognostic factor, one retrospective study evaluating prognostic factors in 363 patients with systemic AIDS-related lymphoma treated with standard chemotherapy, such as cyclophosphamide, doxorubicin (Adriamycin), vincristine (Oncovin), and prednisone (CHOP) or methotrexate, bleomycin, Adriamycin (doxorubicin), cyclophosphamide, Oncovin (vincristine) dexamethasone (m-BACOD), in the HAART era found that a histology of Burkitt lymphoma was an independent poor prognostic factor for survival.[331]

Gene expression profiling and immunophenotyping have segregated immunocompetent diffuse large B-cell lymphoma into differentiation categories that are prognostically significant: germinal center B-like type and postgerminal center or activated B-cell type. When immunohistochemical expression patterns were studied in AIDS lymphomas, it was similarly prognostic. Using Cox regression analysis for disease-free survival, low IPI and postgerminal center differentiation were identified as independent prognostic factors for disease-free survival, with postgerminal center differentiation associated with a 35-fold relative hazard compared with germinal center-type histology.[332]

Patients with systemic lymphoma with leptomeningeal involvement have decreased survival.[333]

Treatment

Standard versus Low-Dose Chemotherapy At the outset of the AIDS epidemic, very dose-intensive regimens were used in patients with AIDS-related lymphoma, but these were associated with low complete remission rates (20–33%) and high rates of serious infectious complications, leading to death in 28 to 78 percent of patients.[318,319,334,335] These observations led to the design and implementation of a low-dose modification of the m-BACOD regimen.[316] In an attempt to clarify the value of low-dose therapy, the AIDS Clinical Trials Group in the United States compared standard-dose m-BACOD and GM-CSF support with reduced-dose m-BACOD without GM-CSF in 198 HIV-infected patients with aggressive lymphomas.[336] No differences were found in either response rate (standard dose 52% vs. reduced dose 41%) or median survival (standard dose 6.8 months vs. reduced dose 7.7 months). However, reduced dose m-BACOD was associated with a statistically significant lower toxicity. Thus, in the pre-HAART era, this trial indicated that low-dose m-BACOD was preferable to standard-dose therapy in patients with AIDS lymphoma.[336]

Since these early efforts, a significant advance in the management of patients with AIDS-related lymphoma has been made, with survival of many of these patients now comparable to that of patients without HIV infection.[333,337] Apart from the contribution of HAART, this improvement in prognosis can be attributed to new initiatives in treatment, such as the use of infusion regimens and the feasibility of high-dose therapy with blood stem cell rescue for relapsed or refractory disease, and better supportive care. However, several controversial issues, such as the optimal timing of HAART with combination chemotherapy and the role of rituximab, remain.

Infusional Dose-Adjusted EPOCH Regimen Investigators at the National Cancer Institute (NCI) reported on the dose-adjusted EPOCH (etoposide, prednisone, vincristine, cyclophosphamide, doxorubicin) regimen (Table 83–4), used in 39 patients with newly diagnosed AIDS-related lymphoma. The EPOCH regimen consists of a 96-hour continuous infusion of etoposide, vincristine, and doxorubicin, and a bolus of cyclophosphamide, which was dose adjusted based on the patient's

TABLE 83–4. Dose-Adjusted EPOCH in Acquired Immunodeficiency Syndrome–Related Lymphoma

Agent	Dose	Day
Etoposide	50 mg/m²/day	1–4
Oncovin	0.4 mg/m²/day	1–4
Doxorubicin	10 mg/m²/day	1–4
Prednisolone	60 mg/m²/day	1–5
Cytoxan		
CD4+ cells <100/μL	187 mg/m²	5
CD4+ cells >100/μL	375 mg/m²	

SOURCE: Reproduced with permission from Little RF, Pittaluga S, Grant N, et al.[333]

CD4+ cell count and neutrophil count at the nadir.[333] Oral prednisone also was given. HAART was omitted during the administration of chemotherapy to prevent potential drug interactions but was restarted immediately upon completion of chemotherapy. The overall complete remission rate was 74 percent. Among patients with CD4+ cell counts greater than 100 cells/μL, the complete remission rate was 87 percent, and the overall survival was 87 percent at 56 months. However, patients with CD4+ cell counts less than 100 cells/μL continued to do poorly, with a complete remission rate of 56 percent and an overall survival of only 16 percent at 56 months.

Role of Rituximab The role of rituximab in patients with AIDS-related lymphoma has been investigated. In a randomized phase III trial conducted by the AIDS Malignancy Consortium of the National Cancer Institute (NCI), standard-dose CHOP was compared to CHOP with rituximab (R-CHOP).[341] Although complete remission was higher in the 99 patients who received R-CHOP (58%) compared to the 50 patients who received CHOP alone (47%), this difference did not reach statistical significance. With a median followup of 137 weeks, the progression-free survival (R-CHOP 45 weeks vs. CHOP 38 weeks) and overall survival (R-CHOP 139 weeks vs. CHOP 110 weeks) were not statistically different. This study documented a statistically increased risk of infectious deaths in the R-CHOP arm. Overall, 15 of the 16 infectious deaths occurred in the group receiving R-CHOP. This study notably included a maintenance period of rituximab after completion of the 6 cycles of R-CHOP. Six of the 14 infectious deaths occurred in this maintenance or postmaintenance period, which raises the question of whether these deaths would have occurred without maintenance rituximab. Nine of the 15 patients who died had a CD4+ cell count less than 50 cells/μL (0.05×10^9/L), suggesting that the higher infectious death rate observed was related to the severely immunodeficient state of these individuals. In this regard, a CD4+ cell count less than 50 cells/μL (0.05×10^9/L) has been associated with an increased risk of neutropenia, neutropenic infections, and death in patients with HIV infection without lymphoma.[342]

Investigators in Europe have investigated the role of rituximab in patients with AIDS-related lymphoma.[343] The pooled results of three phase II trials evaluating rituximab in combination with 96-hour continuous infusion of cyclophosphamide, doxorubicin, and etoposide (R-CDE) in 74 patients with AIDS-related lymphoma has been reported.[343] All patients received G-CSF as prophylaxis, and most patients (76%) received concurrent HAART.[343] The overall response rate was 75 percent, with complete remission in 52 patients (70%) and partial remission in 4 (5%). With a median followup of 23 months, the estimated 2-year overall survival and disease-free survival rates were 64 percent (95% CI 52–76%) and 89 percent (95% CI 81–97%), respectively. These results were superior to the complete remission rate of 45 percent and 2-year overall survival rate of 38 percent reported in a multicenter trial of infusional CDE without rituximab in 55 patients with AIDS-related lymphoma conducted by the Eastern Cooperative Oncology Group.

Compared to the infection rates in patients receiving infusional CDE in the Eastern Cooperative Oncology Group study,[343] infusional R-CDE was associated with a higher incidence of grades 3 to 4 infection (31% vs. 20%) and lethal infection (2% vs. 0%), although no differences in the proportions of patients with grades 3 to 4 neutropenia (78% vs. 90%) were apparent. Thus, consistent with the AIDS Malignancy Consortium data on R-CHOP,[342] the study also suggested that rituximab increased the risk for severe and life-threatening infection when used in combination with chemotherapy in patients with AIDS, particularly in those who are severely immunocompromised.[343] However, the addition of rituximab to infusional CDE was associated with an improvement in complete remission rate and overall survival despite the higher rates of infectious complications.[343]

The AIDS Malignancy Consortium performed a multicenter prospective randomized trial comparing dose-adjusted EPOCH with either concurrent or sequential rituximab in 106 patients with AIDS non-Hodgkin lymphoma.[344] The complete remission rate was 69 percent (90% CI 56–79%) in the concurrent arm, where 69 percent of subjects had an IPI of 2 to 3. No increase in toxicity was seen compared with the sequential arm of this study where not all subjects received rituximab and the complete remission rate was 53 percent (90% CI 41–64%). These studies compare favorably against the historical comparison of CHOP and R-CHOP from both response and toxicity profiles.[341]

A particular survival advantage in patients with CD4+ cell counts of less than 100/μL was reported by adding rituximab to EPOCH. R-EPOCH (rituximab on days 1 and 5) was given to 21 subjects with AIDS-related lymphoma.[345] Subjects with CD4+ cell counts less than 100/μL fared similarly after EPOCH with or without rituximab whereas, subjects with CD4 cell counts less than 100/μL had survival of 57 percent with R-EPOCH versus 16 percent with EPOCH alone. R-EPOCH results were achieved with 50 percent fewer cycles than EPOCH alone. Although increased neutropenia, including late onset neutropenia, occurred with R-EPOCH, these were managed without subject deaths.

These data suggest a role for rituximab in improving response rates in CD20+ AIDS-related lymphoma but with a concern for increased infectious complications, including death, particularly with advanced immunosuppression and/or without the use of HAART. However, subjects with the most advanced immunosuppression may have the most to gain in terms of additional response benefit from addition of rituximab to chemotherapy. The addition of aggressive neutropenic and antibiotic prophylaxis to rituximab-containing regimens appears to improve the infectious complication rates.

Optimal Timing of Highly Active Antiretroviral Therapy Consistent with the NCI data on dose-adjusted EPOCH, a prospective study evaluating the safety and efficacy of liposomal doxorubicin, cyclophosphamide, vincristine, and prednisone in 24 patients with AIDS-related lymphoma found no statistically significant relationship between virologic response to HAART and antitumor response to chemotherapy.[337] Nonetheless, in this study, concurrent use of HAART during administration of chemotherapy was generally well tolerated, and treatment-related toxicities were comparable to those previously reported with low-dose or standard-dose m-BACOD. In another study investigating the pharmacokinetic interactions resulting from simultaneous combination chemotherapy (low-dose or standard-dose CHOP) and HAART for patients with AIDS-related lymphoma, no clinically significant interactions were documented, although the clearance of cyclophosphamide was 1.5-fold reduced compared to historical controls.[338] Thus, delaying HAART until completion of chemotherapy is reasonable but does not appear to be obligatory. Furthermore, including HAART therapy with chemotherapy in patients with counts less than 100 CD4+ cells/μL (0.1×10^9/L) clearly seems important given the poor survival rates in this group when HAART is not employed.

Although the optimal timing of HAART during chemotherapy remains controversial, use of HAART is associated with improved survival in patients with AIDS-related lymphoma.[339,340] Thus, in a multicenter cohort study from Germany involving 203 patients, response to HAART therapy, defined as an increase in CD4+ cell count to 100 cells/μL (0.1×10^9/L) or greater and/or at least one viral load less than 500 copies/mL during the first 2 years following diagnosis of lymphoma, were each independently associated with prolonged survival.[339] Among patients with both a response to HAART and complete tumor remission, 83 percent were still alive at 39 months. Complete remission to chemotherapy without a HAART response in terms of HIV resulted in significantly decreased survival compared to HAART responders. Similarly, a retrospective study from Italy also reported that a good virologic response to HAART therapy was associated with a prolongation in survival.[340] In contrast to the NCI data on dose-adjusted EPOCH, the Italian study showed that virologic response to HAART was the only factor correlated with response to chemotherapy; but the study was retrospective and examined only a small number of patients.

Taken together, these data suggest that use of HAART, concurrently or sequentially with combination chemotherapy, improves survival in patients with AIDS-related lymphoma. Although attainment of virologic control does not appear to be mandatory for achievement of complete response to chemotherapy, institution of HAART prior to chemotherapy, while completing lymphoma-staging studies, should be considered, particularly in subjects with low CD4+ cell counts.

Role of Central Nervous System Prophylaxis The incidence of CNS involvement at presentation in patients with systemic AIDS-related lymphoma has ranged from 10 to 20 percent.[333] Although CNS chemoprophylaxis is generally recommended for patients with Burkitt lymphoma or in those with marrow, paraspinal, paranasal, epidural, testicular, or widespread systemic involvement, the higher rates of neural disease warrant consideration of prophylactic intrathecal chemotherapy in all patients with AIDS-related lymphoma. Of importance, in the NCI trial of dose-adjusted EPOCH, CNS prophylaxis was not uniformly given.[333] However, relapse in the CNS occurred rather quickly in two patients, resulting in a change in the protocol to mandate such prophylaxis.[333]

Management of Relapsed or Refractory Acquired Immunodeficiency Syndrome–Related Lymphoma In the pre-HAART era, patients with relapsed or refractory lymphoma had little possibility of cure with standard-dose salvage regimens. Complete response rates with salvage chemotherapy ranged from 10 to 30 percent, with median survival ranging from 2 to 7 months. One study of 21 such patients treated with etoposide, mitoxantrone, and prednimustine (VMP) reported a complete response rate of 26 percent and an overall median survival of only 2 months.[346] Similarly, in another study involving 40 patients with resistant or recurrent AIDS-related lymphoma, infusional CDE was associated with a low complete remission rate of 10 percent and overall median survival of only 4 months.[347] Slightly more encouraging results were reported in another retrospective study evaluating the use of the etoposide, methylprednisolone, cytosine arabinoside, cisplatin (ESHAP) regimen as treatment in patients with relapsed or refractory AIDS-related lymphoma.[348] Among the 13 treated patients, 4 patients (31%) achieved complete remission and 3 patients (23%) attained partial remission, with a median survival of 7.1 months. One of these patients remained well more than 5 years after completion of ESHAP after having failed three prior regimens.[348]

With the advent of HAART and improvement in supportive care, HIV-infected patients with relapsed or refractory lymphoma now can be effectively retreated with high-dose chemotherapy and peripheral stem cell transplantation. In one reported series of 20 patients with relapsed or refractory patients with AIDS-related lymphoma, 17 (85%) remained alive and in complete remission a median of 31.8 months after transplantation.[349] Both the ability to collect adequate CD34+ cells and the time required for white cell engraftment were comparable to that in non–HIV-infected individuals. Encouraging results have been reported by other investigators.[350] These studies suggest that chemotherapy followed by high-dose therapy with blood progenitor stem cell transplantation is a useful option for selected patients with relapsed or refractory AIDS-related lymphoma.

Hodgkin Lymphoma in the Setting of Human Immunodeficiency Virus Infection

Epidemiology of Human Immunodeficiency Virus–Related Hodgkin Lymphoma HL is the most common non–AIDS-defining cancer in HIV-infected patients, accounting for approximately 4 percent of all malignancies in this population.[351] Large epidemiologic studies show that HIV-infected individuals have an increased risk of developing HL—up to 13-fold of that expected in the general population.[351] The incidence of HL is increasing in the HAART era, with a peak incidence in persons with CD4+ cell counts between 225 and 249/μL.[351] HIV-related HL is distinguished from non–HIV-related HL by a higher proportion of mixed cellularity as the histologic subtype, higher EBV association, and higher proportion of patients with advanced stage and extranodal disease at presentation (see Chap. 99).[351–353]

Immunosuppression and Human Immunodeficiency Virus-Related Hodgkin Lymphoma The relationship between immunosuppression and HIV-related HL risk is complex. Earlier studies reported a wide range of CD4+ cell counts in patients with HIV-related HL, ranging from a median of 113 CD4+ cells/μL in a group of 21 patients treated prospectively as part of the AIDS Clinical Trials Group[359] to 306 CD4+cells/μL in a comparable study from France.[360] The precise level of immune dysfunction in patients with HIV-related HL from these earlier studies was uncertain. HIV-related HL seems to be associated with more profound immunodeficiency. A statistically increased risk of HIV-related HL is present in the period after initial diagnosis of AIDS compared to the period immediately prior to diagnosis of AIDS.[361] Also, using linked population-based AIDS and cancer registry data from diverse areas in the United States, a fourfold increase in the relative risk of HL has been observed in the period immediately prior to development of AIDS (RR = 9.8) compared to the period 60 to 25 months before development of AIDS (RR = 2.6).[362] Similarly, in studies conducted in Australia, no case of HL was observed in the period 5 years prior to diagnosis of AIDS compared to 10 cases in the period within 6 months following an AIDS diagnosis (SIR = 59.1) and one case in the period 6 months to 2 years after diagnosis of AIDS (SIR = 7.34).[363]

Paradoxically, the highest risk of HIV-related HL is found in persons with counts between 225 and 250 CD4+ cells/μL, which is above the level required to establish an immunologic AIDS diagnosis. The risks decline with CD4+ cell counts both above and below that range with the lowest risks seen with counts less than 75 CD4+ cells/μL.[351] This may be a result of the nature of the malignant clone, the Reed-Sternberg cell, which typically induces a Th2 lymphoid response that forms CD4+-rich lymphocyte rosettes around Reed-Sternberg clones.[367] These rosettes are thought to prevent an immune response against the clones along with Reed-Sternberg secretion of immunosuppressive IL-10 and transforming growth factor-β. The Th2 CD4+ cells likely support Reed-Sternberg cell development further through CD40L/CD40 signaling and IL-4.[368]

Pathology In Europe and the United States, nodular sclerosis is the most common subtype of *de novo* HL, described in 52 to 62 percent of patients.[364] Lymphocyte-predominant disease accounts for 8 to 21 percent, whereas mixed cellularity HL is seen in 24 percent and lymphocyte depletion subtype in 3 to 6 percent of patients.[364] In contrast, HIV-related HL is characterized by the preponderance of more aggressive histologic subtypes, with mixed cellularity HL and lymphocyte depletion HL diagnosed in 41 to 100 percent of patients.[360,364–366] These patterns may be changing in the HAART era where an increasing proportion of nodular sclerosing subtypes are reported, albeit still less than in *de novo* HL.[353] Another distinguishing feature of HIV-related HL is its close association with EBV, which can be detected within the nuclei of Reed-Sternberg cells in almost all cases.[297,353, 370] In contrast, EBV is associated with only one-third of *de novo* HL cases[371] and one-half of *de novo* cases of mixed cellularity.[372]

Clinical Features Systemic B symptoms such as fever, drenching night sweats, and/or weight loss occur in 70 to 100 percent of patients with HIV-related HL compared to 30 to 60 percent of patients with *de novo* HL.[355,360,364–366] Furthermore, compared to patients with *de novo* HL, those with HIV-related HL are more likely to present with advanced stages of disease.[357,360,368] Marrow involvement is present in 50 percent of patients with underlying HIV infection, often presenting with pancytopenia and systemic B symptoms.[373]

Staging evaluation should include a thorough history; physical examination; standard laboratory tests; computed tomographic scans of the chest, abdomen, and pelvis; gallium or PET scans; and bilateral marrow biopsies. Because determining the precise etiology of constitutional symptoms such as fever and night sweats often is difficult, microbiologic tests to exclude *M. aviumintracellulare*, cytomegalovirus disease, and other opportunistic infections should be performed, as clinically indicated.

Therapy In the pre-HAART era, treatment of HIV-related HL with chemotherapy was associated with poor treatment outcomes. Treatment-related toxicities, especially hematologic, were substantial, even when hematopoietic growth factors were used. The AIDS Clinical Trials Group conducted a nonrandomized, prospective, multiinstitutional clinical trial in 21 HIV-infected patients with HL using the standard Adriamycin (doxorubicin), bleomycin, vinblastine, dacarbazine (ABVD) regimen with G-CSF.[359] No antiretroviral therapy was used. Despite routine use of G-CSF, nine opportunistic infections occurred in six patients during the study or shortly thereafter. Results were poor, with complete remission attained in only 43 percent of treated patients and a median survival of only 1.5 years.

Similarly, in another prospective study from Italy, a disappointing overall survival rate of 32 percent at 36 months in 35 HIV-infected patients with HL treated with a regimen consisting of epirubicin, bleomycin, vinblastine, and prednisolone (EBVP) with concomitant antiretroviral therapy and G-CSF support was reported.[374]

With the availability of HAART, better treatment outcomes with combination chemotherapy have been reported. In a retrospective analysis of 104 patients with HL, HAART was employed with chemotherapy (primarily ABVD) in 83 subjects resulting in a complete remission in 91 percent of patients. Median time to progression was not reached at median follow up of 3 years. Multivariate analysis demonstrated that achieving a complete remission was independently associated with use of HAART, baseline CD4+ cell count of greater than 100/μL and having received therapy appropriate to stage of disease.[369]

A phase II study of the Stanford V regimen in 59 patients with HIV-related HL had an overall response rate of 89 percent and a complete response rate of 81 percent, with an estimated 3-year overall survival and disease-free survival of 51 percent and 68 percent, respectively.[375] The regimen consisted of mechlorethamine (6 mg/m^2 on day 1), doxorubicin (25 mg/m^2 on days 1 and 15), vinblastine (6 mg/m^2 on 1 and 15), vincristine (2 mg/m^2 IV on days 8 and 22), bleomycin (5 U/m^2 on days 8 and 22), etoposide (60 mg/m^2 on days 15 and 16), and prednisone (40 mg/m^2 orally, every other day). This regimen was given every 28 days for a total of three cycles. Involved-field radiation was planned for all patients who achieved partial remission or who had initial bulky mediastinal disease. Fifty-two (88%) of the 59 patients received HAART concomitantly with the Stanford V regimen.

In another retrospective study evaluating the impact of HAART on patients with HIV-related HL, an improvement in complete response rate from 64.5 percent in the pre-HAART to 74.5 percent in the HAART period was observed, with an improvement in the estimated 2-year survival probability from 45 percent to 62 percent, respectively.[376] Although the median survival of patients treated in the pre-HAART era was only 19 months, the median survival of patients treated in the post-HAART era had not been reached after a median followup of 20 months. Improvements in response rate and survival were achieved without significant change in the chemotherapy regimens used between the two periods. Furthermore, the response to HAART therapy, defined as an increase of at least 100 CD4+ cells/μL (0.1×10^9/L) and/or at least one viral load less than 500 copies/mL during the first 2 years following diagnosis of HIV-related HL, was associated with prolonged survival.[377]

The German Hodgkin's Study Group reported results of a small phase II study evaluating the efficacy and safety of six cycles of a regimen consisting of bleomycin, etoposide, doxorubicin, cyclophosphamide, vincristine, procarbazine, and prednisone (BEACOPP) at standard doses in 12 patients with HIV-related HL.[378] The median age of the patients treated in this study was 33 years, and 92 percent had advanced stage disease. Eight of the 12 treated patients received the intended six cycles of BEACOPP. Overall, toxicity with BEACOPP was notable for grade 3 or 4 neutropenia occurring in 75 percent, and two deaths caused by opportunistic infections during the treatment period. Efficacy results from this study were impressive; all 12 patients attained complete remission of disease, although 2 died of infection. With a median followup of 49 months, nine patients remained alive and in continuous complete remission. Although the results of this trial are encouraging, further confirmation is required, especially considering the apparent toxicity encountered.

Although improved outcomes have been reported in the HAART era, results still are inferior compared to those in HIV-negative patients with HL, among whom even those with stage IV disease have a cure rate of approximately 70 percent. Nonetheless, at the current time, it is reasonable to treat patients with HIV-related HL using standard regimens such as ABVD or the Stanford V regimen.

Multicentric Castleman Disease in the Setting of Human Immunodeficiency Virus Infection

Multicentric Castleman disease (MCD) is a diffuse lymphoproliferative disorder associated with HIV that is often progressive and potentially fatal. MCD is characterized histologically by angiofollicular hyperplasia and plasma cell infiltration.[380] It manifests itself as a systemic syndrome with elevated IL-6 and C-reactive protein that may flare for several days to weeks, resolving spontaneously at times.[381] Clinical features include lymphadenopathy, splenomegaly, fevers, weight loss, hypotension, pancytopenia, hypoalbuminemia, and oligo- or monoclonal gammopathy.[380–383] In the setting of HIV, persons with MCD are at increased risk of both KS and lymphoma.[380,382] In one series of 60 HIV-infected subjects with MCD, the 2-year probability of developing lymphoma was 24 percent.[382] Neither HIV viral load nor CD4+ cell count has been predictive of the risk of developing MCD, MCD flares, or MCD-related lymphoma. MCD can lead to death via complications of associated malignancies or directly as a consequence of systemic effects resulting in respiratory, renal, or other organ failure.[380]

In the setting of HIV-related infection, MCD is universally associated with HHV-8.[380] It is distinguished from other HHV-8–associated neoplasms, including KS and primary effusion lymphoma, by high levels of HHV-8 lytic gene products including ORF5, ORF59, ORF65, and K8.[384] High levels of HHV-8 viremia are seen in MCD; the degree of viremia within a patient typically correlates directly with clinical severity of the exacerbation.[381]

Optimal treatment of HIV-associated MCD remains unclear. There are few data regarding the effects of HAART on MCD. Both clinical improvements and exacerbations after initiating HAART have been described.[380] Case reports have described activity of antiviral agents (ganciclovir), immunomodulatory agents (glucocorticoids, interferon-α), cytoreductive chemotherapy with agents active in lymphomas, and the monoclonal antibody, rituximab. Except for rituximab, remissions obtained with each of the interventions did not persist significantly beyond the duration of the treatment period.[380] Although rituximab resulted in MCD remissions in 3 of 5 HIV-infected patients, 1 of which lasted longer than 14 months, 2 of the 4 patients with coexisting KS experienced exacerbation of KS with ritiuximab.[383]

REFERENCES

1. Centers for Disease Control: Case definition of acquired immunodeficiency syndrome. *MMWR Morb Mortal Wkly Rep* 30:250, 1981.
2. Centers for Disease Control: Revision of the case definition of acquired immunodeficiency syndrome for national reporting. *MMWR Morb Mortal Wkly Rep* 34:373, 1985.
3. Centers for Disease Control: Revision of the CDC surveillance case definition for acquired immunodeficiency syndrome. *MMWR Morb Mortal Wkly Rep* 36(1S):1, 1987.
4. Centers for Disease Control: New case definition of HIV/AIDS. *MMWR Morb Mortal Wkly Rep* 41:RR17, 1992.
5. Joint United Nations Programme on HIV/AIDS (UNAIDS): *Report on the Global HIV/AIDS Epidemic 2008*. UNAIDS, Geneva, 2008.
6. Varmus H: Retroviruses. *Science* 240:1427, 1988.
7. Sharp PM, Robertson F, Gao F, Hahn B: Origins and diversity of human immunodeficiency viruses. *AIDS* 8(Suppl 1):S27, 1994.
8. Gonda MA, Wong-Staal F, Gallo RC, et al: Sequence homology and morphologic similarity of HTLV-III and visna virus, a pathogenic lentivirus. *Science* 227:173, 1985.
9. Daniel MD, Letvin NL, King NW, et al: Isolation of T-cell tropic HTLVIII-like retrovirus from macaques. *Science* 228:1201, 1985.
10. Overbaugh J, Donahue PR, Quackenbush SL, et al: Molecular cloning of a feline leukemia virus that induces fatal immunodeficiency disease in cats. *Science* 239:906, 1988.
11. Ho DD, Schooley RT, Rota TR, et al: HTLV-III in the semen and blood of a healthy homosexual man. *Science* 226:451, 1984.
12. Levy JA: Human immunodeficiency viruses and the pathogenesis of AIDS. *JAMA* 261:2997, 1989.
13. Tindall B, Evans L, Cunningham P, et al: Identification of HIV-1 in semen following primary HIV-1 infection. *AIDS* 6:949, 1992.
14. Chiasson MA, Stoneburner RI, Joseph SC: Human immunodeficiency virus transmission through artificial insemination. *J Acquir Immune Defic Syndr* 3:69, 1990.
15. Vogt MW, Witt DJ, Craven DE, et al: Isolation of HTLV-III/LAV from cervical secretions of women at risk for AIDS. *Lancet* 1:525, 1986.
16. Wofsy C, Cohen J, Hauer I, et al: Isolation of AIDS associated retrovirus from genital secretions of women with antibodies to the virus. *Lancet* 1:527, 1986.
17. Pomerants RJ, de la Monte SM, Donegan SP, et al: Human immunodeficiency virus (HIV) infection of the uterine cervix. *Ann Intern Med* 108:321, 1988.
18. Anderson DA, Voeller B: AIDS and contraception, in *Clinical Perspective in Obstetrics and Gynecology*, edited by F Haseltine, D Shoupe, p 192. Springer-Verlag, New York, 1993.
19. Marmor M, Weiss LR, Lyden M, et al: Possible female to female transmission of human immunodeficiency virus. *Ann Intern Med* 105:969, 1986.
20. Monzon OT, Capellan JM: Female to female transmission of HIV. *Lancet* 2:40, 1987.
21. Stamm WE, Handsfield HH, Rompalo AM, et al: The association between genital ulcer disease and acquisition of HIV infection in homosexual men. *JAMA* 260:1429, 1988.
22. Kreiss JK, Coombs R, Plummer F, et al: Isolation of human immunodeficiency virus from genital ulcers in Nairobi prostitutes. *J Infect Dis* 160:380, 1989.
23. Grosskurth H, Mosha F, Todd J, et al: Impact of improved treatment of sexually transmitted diseases on HIV infection in rural Tanzania: Randomized controlled trial. *Lancet* 356:530, 1995.
24. Sasse H, Salmaso S, Conti S: Risk behaviors for HIV-1 infection in Italian drug users: Report from a multicenter study. First Drug User Multicenter Study Group. *J Acquir Immune Defic Syndr* 2:486, 1989.
25. Chaisson RE, Bacchetti P, Osmond D, et al: Cocaine use and HIV infection in intravenous drug users in San Francisco. *JAMA* 261:561, 1989.
26. Donegan E, Stuart M, Niland JC, et al: Infection with human immunodeficiency virus type 1 (HIV-1) among recipients of antibody-positive blood donations. *Ann Intern Med* 113:733, 1990.
27. Centers for Disease Control: Safety of therapeutic products used for hemophilia patients. *MMWR Morb Mortal Wkly Rep* 37:441, 1988.
28. Pierce GF, Lusher JM, Brownstein AP, et al: The use of purified clotting factor concentrates in hemophilia: Influence of viral safety, cost and supply on therapy. *JAMA* 261:3434, 1989.
29. Schreiber GB, Busch MP, Kleinman SH, Korelitz JJ: The risk of transfusion transmitted viral infections. *N Engl J Med* 334:1685, 1996.
30. Goedert JJ, Mendez H, Drummond JE, et al: Mother to infant transmission of human immunodeficiency virus type 1: Association with prematurity or low anti-gp 120. *Lancet* 2:1351, 1989.
31. Hira SK, Kamanga J, Bhat GJ, et al: Perinatal transmission of HIV-1 in Zambia. *BMJ* 299:1250, 1989.
32. European Collaborative Study: Risk factors for mother-to-child transmission of HIV-1. *Lancet* 339:1007, 1992.
33. Courgnaud V, Laure F, Brossard A, et al: Frequent and early *in utero* HIV-1 infection. *AIDS Res Hum Retroviruses* 7:337, 1991.
34. Rouzioux C, Costagliola D, Burgard M, et al: Timing of mother-to-child HIV-1 transmission depends on maternal status: The HIV infection in newborns French Collaborative Study Group. *AIDS* 7(Suppl 2):S49, 1993.
35. Burgard M, Mayaux MJ, Blanche S, et al: The use of viral culture and p24 antigen testing to HIV infection in neonates: The HIV infection in newborns French Collaborative Study Group. *N Engl J Med* 327:1192, 1992.
36. Ehrns A, Lindgren S, Dictor M, et al: HIV in pregnant women and their offspring: Evidence for late transmission. *Lancet* 337:203, 1991.
37. van de Perre P, Simonon A, Msellati P, et al: Postnatal transmission of human immunodeficiency virus type 1 from mother to infant: A prospective cohort study in Kigali, Rwanda. *N Engl J Med* 325:593, 1991.
38. Dunn DT, Newell ML, Ades AE, Peckham CS: Risk of human immunodeficiency virus type 1 transmission through breast-feeding. *Lancet* 340:585, 1992.
39. European Collaborative Study: Risk factors for mother-to-child transmission of HIV-1. *Lancet* 339:1007, 1992.
40. Mayzux M-J, Blanche S, Rouzioux C, et al: Maternal factors associated with perinatal HIV-1 transmission: The French cohort study, seven years of follow-up observation. *J Acquir Immune Defic Syndr* 8:188, 1995.
41. Fang G, Burger H, Grimson R, et al: Maternal plasma human immunodeficiency virus type 1 RNA level: A determinant and projected threshold for mother-to-child transmission. *Proc Natl Acad Sci U S A* 92:12100, 1995.
42. Weiser B, Nachman S, Tropper P, et al: Quantitation of human immunodeficiency virus type 1 during pregnancy: Relationship of viral titer to mother-to-child transmission and stability of viral load. *Proc Natl Acad Sci U S A* 91:8031, 1994.
43. Burns DN, Landesman S, Muenz LR, et al: Cigarette smoking, premature rupture of membranes, and vertical transmission of HIV-1 among women with low CD4 levels. *J Acquir Immune Defic Syndr* 7:718, 1994.
44. Nair P, Alger L, Hines S, et al: Maternal and neonatal characteristics associated with HIV infection in infants of seropositive women. *J Acquir Immune Defic Syndr* 6:298, 1993.
45. Landesman SH, Kalish LA, Burns DN, et al: Obstetrical factors and the transmission of human immunodeficiency virus type 1 from mother to child. *N Engl J Med* 334:1617, 1996.
46. Simonds RJ, Steketee R, Nesheim S, et al: Impact of zidovudine use on risk and risk factors for perinatal transmission of HIV. *AIDS* 12:301, 1998.
47. The International Perinatal HIV Group: The mode of delivery and the risk of vertical transmission of human immunodeficiency virus type 1: A meta-analysis of 15 prospective cohort studies. *N Engl J Med* 340:977, 1999.
48. European Collaborative Study: Caesarean section and the risk of vertical transmission of HIV-1 infection. *Lancet* 343:1464, 1994.
49. Stratton P, Tuomala RE, Abboud R, et al: Obstetric and newborn outcomes in a cohort of HIV-infected pregnant women: A report of the Women and Infants Transmission Study. *J Acquir Immune Defic Syndr Hum Retrovirol* 20:179, 1999.
50. Centers for Disease Control and Prevention: Public Health Service Task Force recommendations for the use of antiretroviral drugs in pregnant women infected with HIV-1 for maternal health and for reducing perinatal HIV-1 transmission in the United States. *MMWR Morb Mortal Wkly Rep* 47:1, 1998.
51. Connor EM, Sperling RS, Gelver R, et al: Reduction of maternal-infant transmission of human immunodeficiency virus type 1 with zidovudine treatment. *N Engl J Med* 331:1173, 1994.
52. Shaffer N, Chauchoowong R, Mock PA, et al: Short-course zidovudine for perinatal HIV-1 transmission in Bangkok, Thailand: A randomized controlled trial. *Lancet* 353:773, 1999.
53. Jackson B, Fleming TR: Executive Summary, HIVNET 012. Available at: www.niaid.nih.gov/newsroom/simple/exec.htm. Last accessed July 14, 1999.
54. Centers for Disease Control and Prevention: Update: Perinatally acquired HIV/AIDS—United States 1997. *MMWR Morb Mortal Wkly Rep* 46:1086, 1997.

55. Pahwa SG, Quilop MTJ, Lane M, et al: Defective B-lymphocyte function in homosexual men in relation to the acquired immunodeficiency syndrome. *Ann Intern Med* 101:757, 1984.
56. Murry HW, Rubin BY, Masur H, Roberts RB: Impaired production of lymphokines and immune (gamma) interferon in the acquired immunodeficiency syndrome. *N Engl J Med* 310:883, 1984.
57. Rook AH, Masur H, Lane HC, et al: Interleukin-2 enhances the depressed natural killer and cytomegalovirus-specific cytotoxic activities of lymphocytes from patients with the acquired immunodeficiency syndrome. *J Clin Invest* 72:398, 1983.
58. Tersmette M, de Goede REY, Al BJM, et al: Differential syncytium-inducing capacity of human immunodeficiency virus isolates: Frequent detection of syncytium-inducing isolates in patients with acquired immunodeficiency syndrome (AIDS) and AIDS-related complex. *J Virol* 62:2026, 1988.
59. Pantaleo G, Graziosi C, Demarest JF, et al: HIV infection is active and progressive in lymphoid tissue during the clinically latent stage of disease. *Nature* 362:355, 1993.
60. Glushakova S, Grivel J-C, Fitzgerald W, et al: Evidence for the HIV-1 phenotype switch as a causal factor in acquired immunodeficiency. *Nat Med* 4:346, 1998.
61. Walker BD, Chakrabarti S, Moss B, et al: HIV-specific cytotoxic T lymphocytes in seropositive individuals. *Nature* 328:345, 1987.
62. Tsuchiya S, Imaizumi M, Minegishi M, et al: Lack of interleukin-2 production in a patient with OKT4+ T-cell deficiency. *N Engl J Med* 308:1294, 1983.
63. Ebert EC, Stoll DB, Cassens BJ, et al: Diminished interleukin production and receptor generation characterize the acquired immunodeficiency syndrome. *Clin Immunol Immunopathol* 37:283, 1985.
64. Prince HE, Kermani-Arab V, Fahey J: Depressed interleukin-2 receptor expression in acquired immune deficiency and lymphadenopathy syndromes. *J Immunol* 133:1313, 1984.
65. Kekow J, Wachsman W, Gross WL, et al: Transforming growth factor-beta and suppression of humoral immune responses in HIV infection. *J Clin Invest* 87:1010, 1991.
66. Ammann AJ, Abrams D, Conant M, et al: Acquired immune dysfunction in homosexual men: Immunologic profiles. *Clin Immunol Immunopathol* 27:315, 1983.
67. Wong JK, Gunthard HF, Havir DV, et al: Reduction of HIV-1 in blood and lymph nodes following potent antiretroviral therapy of HIV-1 infection. *Proc Natl Acad Sci U S A* 94:2574, 1997.
68. Cavert W, Notermans DW, Staskus K, et al: Kinetics of response in lymphoid tissues to antiretroviral therapy of HIV-1 infection. *Science* 276:960, 1997.
69. Hammer SM, Squires KE, Hughes MD, et al: A controlled trial of two nucleoside analogues plus indinavir in persons with human immunodeficiency virus infection and CD4 cell counts of 200 per cubic millimeter or less. *N Engl J Med* 337:725, 1997.
70. Palella FJ Jr, Delaney KM, Moorman AC, et al: Declining morbidity and mortality among patients with advanced human immunodeficiency virus infection. *N Engl J Med* 338:853, 1998.
71. Connors M, Kovacs JA, Krevat S, et al: HIV infection induces changes in CD4+ T-cell phenotype and depletions within the CD4+ T-cell repertoire that are not immediately restored by antiviral or immune-based therapies. *Nat Med* 3:533, 1997.
72. Gorochov G, Neumann AU, Kereveur A, et al: Perturbation of CD4+ and CD8+ T-cell repertoire during progression to AIDS and regulation of the CD4+ repertoire during antiviral therapy. *Nat Med* 4:215, 1998.
73. Chess Q, Daniels J, North E, et al: Serum immunoglobulin elevations in the acquired immunodeficiency syndrome (AIDS): IgG, IgA, IgM, and IgD. *Diagn Immunol* 2:148, 1984.
74. Lane HC, Masur H, Edgar LC, et al: Abnormalities of B-cell activation and immunoregulation in patients with the acquired immunodeficiency syndrome. *N Engl J Med* 309:453, 1983.
75. Pahwa S, Pahwa R, Saxinger C, et al: Influence of the human T-lymphotropic virus/lymphadenopathy–associated virus on functions of human lymphocytes: Evidence for immunosuppressive effects and polyclonal B-cell activation by banded viral preparations. *Proc Natl Acad Sci U S A* 82:8198, 1985.
76. Kopelman RG, Zolla-Pazner S: Association of human immunodeficiency virus infection and autoimmune phenomena. *Am J Med* 84:82, 1988.
77. Walsh C, Kirgel R, Lennette E, Karpatkin S: Prognosis, response to therapy and prevalence of antibody to the retrovirus associated with the acquired immunodeficiency syndrome. *Ann Intern Med* 103:542, 1985.
78. van der Lelie J, Lange JMA, Vos JJE, et al: Autoimmunity against blood cells in human immunodeficiency virus infection. *Br J Haematol* 67:755, 1987.
79. Stricker RB, McHugh TM, Moody D, et al: An AIDS-related cytotoxic autoantibody reacts with a specific antigen on stimulated CD4+ cells. *Nature* 327:170, 1987.
80. Rossi G, Goria R, Stellini R, et al: Prevalence, clinical, and laboratory features of thrombocytopenia in HIV-infected individuals. *AIDS Res Hum Retroviruses* 6:261, 1990.
81. Murphy MF, Metcalfe P, Waters AH, et al: Incidence and mechanism of neutropenia and thrombocytopenia in patients with human immunodeficiency virus infection. *Br J Haematol* 66:337, 1987.
82. Ballem PJ, Belzberg A, Devine DV, et al: Kinetic studies of the mechanism of thrombocytopenia in patients with human immunodeficiency virus infection. *N Engl J Med* 327:1179, 1992.
83. Gartner S, Markovits P, Markovitz DM, et al: The role of mononuclear phagocytes in HTLV-III/LAV infection. *Science* 233:215, 1986.
84. Armstrong GA, Horne R: Follicular dendritic cells and virus-like particles in AIDS-related lymphadenopathy. *Lancet* 2:370, 1984.
85. Poli G, Bottazzi B, Acero R, et al: Monocyte function in intravenous drug abusers with lymphadenopathy syndrome and in patients with the acquired immunodeficiency syndrome: Selective impairment of chemotaxis. *Clin Exp Immunol* 62:136, 1985.
86. Murray HW, Gellene RA, Libby DM, et al: Activation of tissue macrophages from AIDS patients: *In vitro* response of alveolar macrophages to lymphokines and interferon-gamma. *J Immunol* 135:1501, 1985.
87. Kleinerman ES, Ceccorulli LM, Zwelling LA, et al: Activation of monocyte-mediated tumoricidal activity in patients with acquired immunodeficiency syndrome. *J Clin Oncol* 3:1005, 1985.
88. Creemers PC, Stark DF, Boyko WJ: Evaluation of natural killer cell activity in patients with persistent generalized lymphadenopathy and acquired immunodeficiency syndrome. *J Clin Lab Immunol* 14:114, 1984.
89. Klatzman M, Lederman MM: Defective postbinding lysis underlies the impaired natural killer activity in factor VIII–treated human T lymphotropic virus type III seropositive hemophiliacs. *J Clin Invest* 45:406, 1986.
90. Reddy MM, Chinoy P, Grieco MH: Differential effects of interferon alpha and interleukin-2 on natural killer cell activity in patients with the acquired immune deficiency syndrome. *J Biol Response Mod* 3:379, 1984.
91. Horsburgh CR Jr, Ou CY, Jason J, et al: Duration of human immunodeficiency virus infection before detection of antibody. *Lancet* 2:637, 1989.
92. Imagawa DT, Lee MH, Wolinsky SM, et al: HIV-1 infection in homosexual men who remain seronegative for prolonged periods. *N Engl J Med* 320:1458, 1989.
93. Brettler DB, Somasundaran M, Forsberg AF, et al: Silent human immunodeficiency virus type 1 infection: A rare occurrence in a high-risk heterosexual population. *Blood* 80:2396, 1992.
94. Read S, Cassol S, Coates R, et al: Detection of incident HIV infection by PCR compared to serology. *J Acquir Immune Defic Syndr* 5:1075, 1992.
95. Goudsmit J, Lange JM, Krone WJ, et al: Pathogenesis of HIV and its implications for serodiagnosis and monitoring of antiviral therapy. *J Virol Methods* 17:19, 1987.
96. Tindall B, Cooper DA, Donovan B, et al: Primary human immunodeficiency virus infection: Clinical and serologic aspects. *Infect Dis Clin North Am* 2:329, 1988.
97. Alter HJ, Epstein JS, Swensen SG, et al: Prevalence of human immunodeficiency virus type 1 p24 antigen in U.S. blood donors: An assessment of the efficacy of testing in donor screening. *N Engl J Med* 323:1312, 1990.
98. Mellors JW, Rinaldo CR Jr, Gupta P, et al: Prognosis in HIV-1 infection predicted by the quantity of virus in plasma. *Science* 272:1167, 1996.
99. Mellors JW, Munoz A, Giorgi J, et al: Plasma viral load and CD4+ lymphocytes as prognostic markers of HIV-1 infection. *Ann Intern Med* 126:946, 1997.
100. Department of Health and Human Services: *Guidelines for the Use of Antiretroviral Agents of HIV-1-Infected Adults and Adolescents*. Available at: www.aidsinfo.nih.gov. Last accessed August 15, 2009.
101. Buskin SE, Sullivan PS: Anemia and its treatment and outcomes in persons infected with human immunodeficiency virus. *Transfusion* 44:826, 2004.
102. Centers for Disease Control and Prevention: Guidelines for the use of antiretroviral agents in HIV-infected adults and adolescents. *MMWR Morb Mortal Wkly Rep* 48:1-22, 1999.
103. Tural C, Romeu J, Sirera G, et al: Long lasting remission of cytomegalovirus retinitis without maintenance therapy in human immunodeficiency virus infected patients. *J Infect Dis* 177:1080, 1998.
104. Li TS, Tubiana R, Katlama C, et al: Long-lasting recovery in CD4 T cell function and viral load reduction after highly active antiretroviral therapy in advanced HIV-1 disease. *Lancet* 351:1682, 1998.
105. Furrer H, Egger M, Opravil M, et al: Discontinuation of primary prophylaxis against *Pneumocystis carinii* pneumonia in HIV-1 infected adults treated with combination antiretroviral therapy. *N Engl J Med* 340:1301, 1999.
106. Mocroft A, Ledergerber B, Katlama C, et al: Decline in the AIDS and death rates in the EuroSIDA study: An observational study. *Lancet* 362:22, 2003.
107. Cooper DA, Maclean P, Finlayson R, et al: Acute AIDS retrovirus infection. *Lancet* 1:537, 1985.
108. Fox R, Eldred LJ, Fuchs EJ, et al: Clinical manifestations of acute infection with human immunodeficiency virus in a cohort of gay men. *AIDS* 1:35, 1987.
109. Lemp GF, Payne SF, Rutherford GW, et al: Projections of AIDS morbidity and mortality in San Francisco. *JAMA* 263:1497, 1990.
110. Moss AR, Bacchetti P: Editorial review: Natural history of HIV infection. *AIDS* 3:55, 1989.
111. Schoenbaum EE, Hartel D, Friedland G: HIV infection and intravenous drug use. *Curr Opin Infect Dis* 3:80, 1990.
112. Volberding P: Clinical spectrum of HIV disease, in *AIDS: Etiology, Diagnosis, Treatment and Prevention*, 3rd ed, edited by VT DeVita Jr, S Hellman, SA Rosenberg, p 123. Lippincott, Philadelphia, 1992.
113. Samson M, Libert F, Doranz BJ: Resistance to HIV-1 infection in Caucasian individuals bearing mutant alleles of the CCR-5 chemokine receptor gene. *Nature* 382:722, 1996.
114. Phillips AN: Studies of prognostic markers in HIV infection: Implications for pathogenesis. *AIDS* 6:1391, 1992.
115. Munoz A, Carey V, Saah AJ, et al: Predictors of decline in CD4 lymphocytes in a cohort of homosexual men infected with human immunodeficiency virus. *J Acquir Immune Defic Syndr* 1:396, 1988.
116. Malone JL, Simms TE, Gray GC, et al: Sources of variability in repeated T-helper lymphocyte counts from human immunodeficiency virus type 1 infected patients:

Total lymphocyte count fluctuations and diurnal cycle are important. *J Acquir Immune Defic Syndr* 3:144, 1990.
117. Anderson RE, Lang W, Shiboski S, et al: Use of beta 2 microglobulin level and CD4 lymphocyte count to predict development of acquired immunodeficiency syndrome in persons with human immunodeficiency virus infection. *Arch Intern Med* 150:73, 1990.
118. Melmed RN, Taylor JMG, Detels R, et al: Serum neopterin changes in HIV infected subjects: Indicator of significant pathology, CD4 T cell changes, and the development of AIDS. *J Acquir Immune Defic Syndr* 2:70, 1989.
119. Mitsuyasu R: Clinical uses of hematopoietic growth hormones in HIV-related illnesses. *AIDS Clin Rev* 189, 1993-1994.
120. Zon LI, Arkin C, Groopman JE: Hematologic manifestations of the human immunodeficiency virus (HIV). *Semin Hematol* 25:208, 1988.
121. Sullivan PS, Hanson DL, Chu SY, et al: Epidemiology of anemia in human immunodeficiency virus infected persons: Results from the Multistate Adult and Adolescent Spectrum of HIV Disease Surveillance Project. *Blood* 91:301, 1998.
122. Levine AM, Berhane K, Masri-Lavine L: Prevalençe and correlates of anemia in a large cohort of HIV-infected women: Women's Interagency HIV Study. *J Acquir Immune Defic Syndr* 26:28, 2001.
123. Mocroft A, Kirk O, Barton SE, et al: Anaemia is an independent predictive marker for clinical prognosis in HIV infected patients from across Europe. *AIDS* 13:943, 1999.
124. Spivak JL, Barnes DC, Fuchs E, Quinn TC: Serum immunoreactive erythropoietin in HIV infected patients. *JAMA* 261:310, 1989.
125. Seneviratne LS, Tulpule A, Mummaneni M, et al: Clinical, immunological, and pathologic correlates of bone marrow involvement in 253 patients with AIDS-related lymphoma. *Blood* 92:244A, 1998.
126. Walker RE, Parker RI, Kovacs JA, et al: Anemia and erythropoiesis in patients with the acquired immunodeficiency syndrome (AIDS) and Kaposi sarcoma treated with zidovudine. *Ann Intern Med* 108:372, 1988.
127. Richman DD, Fischl MA, Grieco MH, et al: The toxicity of azidothymidine (AZT) in the treatment of patients with AIDS and AIDS-related complex: A double-blind, placebo-controlled trial. *N Engl J Med* 317:192, 1987.
128. Anderson LJ: Human parvoviruses. *J Infect Dis* 161:603, 1990.
129. Frickhofen N, Abkowitz JL, Safford M, et al: Persistent B19 parvovirus infection in patients infected with human immunodeficiency virus type 1 (HIV-1): A treatable cause of anemia in AIDS. *Ann Intern Med* 113:926, 1990.
130. Rarick MU, Espina B, Mocharnuk R, et al: Thrombotic thrombocytopenic purpura in patients with human immunodeficiency virus infection: A report of three cases and review of the literature. *Am J Hematol* 40:103, 1992.
131. Sasadeusz J, Buchanan M, Speed B: Reactive haemophagocytic syndrome in human immunodeficiency virus infection. *J Infect* 20:65, 1990.
132. Sproat LO, Pantanowitz L, Lu CM, et al: Human immunodeficiency virus-associated hemophagocytosis with iron-deficiency anemia and massive splenomegaly. *Clin Infect Dis* 37:170, 2003.
133. Telen MJ, Roberts KB, Bartlett JA: HIV associated autoimmune hemolytic anemia: Report of a case and review of the literature. *AIDS* 3:933, 1990.
134. McGinniss MH, Macher AM, Rook AH, Alter HJ: Red cell autoantibodies in patients with acquired immune deficiency syndrome. *Transfusion* 26:405, 1986.
135. Gupta S, Licorish K: The Coombs' test and the acquired immunodeficiency syndrome. *Ann Intern Med* 100:462, 1984.
136. Toy PTCY, Reid ME, Burns M: Positive direct antiglobulin test associated with hyperglobulinemia in AIDS. *Am J Hematol* 19:145, 1985.
137. Harriman GR, Smith PD, Horne MK, et al: Vitamin B_{12} malabsorption in patients with acquired immunodeficiency syndrome. *Arch Intern Med* 149:2039, 1989.
138. Herbert V, Fong W, Gulle V, Stopler T: Low holotranscobalamin II is the earliest serum marker for subnormal vitamin B_{12} (cobalamin) absorption in patients with AIDS. *Am J Hematol* 34:132, 1990.
139. Sullivan PS, Hanson DL, Chu SY, et al: Epidemiology of anemia in human immunodeficiency virus infected persons: Results from the Multistate Adult and Adolescent Spectrum of HIV Disease Surveillance Project. *Blood* 91:301, 1998.
140. Moore RD, Keruly JC, Chaisson RE: Anemia and survival in HIV infection. *J Acquir Immune Defic Syndr* 19:29, 1998.
141. Mocroft A, Kirk O, Barton SE, et al: Anaemia is an independent predictive marker for clinical prognosis in HIV infected patients from across Europe. *AIDS* 13:943, 1999.
142. Berhane K, Karim R, Cohen MH: Impact of highly active antiretroviral therapy on anemia and relationship between anemia and survival in a large cohort of HIV-infected women: Women's Interagency HIV Study. *J Acquir Immune Defic Syndr* 37:1245, 2004.
143. Lundgren JD, Mocroft A, Gatell JM, et al: A clinically prognostic scoring system for patients receiving highly active antiretroviral therapy: Results from the EuroSIDA Study. *J Infect Dis* 185:178, 2002.
144. Saag MS, Bowers P, Leitz GJ, et al: Once-weekly epoetin alfa improves quality of life and increases hemoglobin in anemic HIV+ patients. *AIDS Res Hum Retroviruses* 20:1037, 2004.
145. Grossman HA, Goon B, Bowers P, et al: Once-weekly epoetin alfa dosing is as effective as three times-weekly dosing in increasing hemoglobin levels and is associated with improved quality of life in anemic HIV-infected patients. *J Acquir Immune Defic Syndr* 34:368, 2003.
146. Moore RD, Forney D: Anemia in HIV-infected patients receiving highly active antiretroviral therapy. *J Acquir Immune Defic Syndr* 29:54, 2002.
147. Isgro A, Mezzaroma I, Aiuti A, et al: Recovery of hematopoietic activity in bone marrow from human immunodeficiency virus type 1 infected patients during highly active antiretroviral therapy. *AIDS Res Hum Retroviruses* 16:1471, 2000.
148. Huang SS, Barbour JD, Deeks SG, et al: Reversal of human immunodeficiency virus type 1 associated hematosuppression by effective anti-retroviral therapy. *Clin Infect Dis* 30:504, 2000.
149. Spivak JL, Barnes DC, Fuchs E, et al: Serum immunoreactive erythropoietin in HIV-infected patients. *JAMA* 261:3104, 1989.
150. Moore RD: Human immunodeficiency virus infection, anemia, and survival. *Clin Infect Dis* 29:44, 1999.
151. Sipsas NV, Kokori SI, Ionnidis JPA, et al: Circulating autoantibodies to erythropoietin are associated with human immunodeficiency virus type 1 related anemia. *J Infect Dis* 180:2044, 1999.
152. Henry DH, Beall GN, Benson CA, et al: Recombinant human erythropoietin in the treatment of anemia associated with human immunodeficiency virus (HIV) infection and zidovudine therapy: Overview of four clinical trials. *Ann Intern Med* 117:739, 1992.
153. Demetri G, Wade J, Cella D, et al: Epoetin alfa improves quality of life in cancer patients receiving cytotoxic treatment independent of disease response: Prospective clinical trial results. *Blood* 90:175a, 1997.
154. Miles SA: The use of hematopoietic growth factors in HIV infection and AIDS-related malignancies. *Cancer Invest* 9:229, 1991.
155. Abrams DI, Steinhart C, Frascino R: Epoetin alfa therapy for anemia in HIV infected patients: Impact on quality of life. *Int J STD AIDS* 11:659, 2000.
156. Bennett CL, Luminari S, Nissenson AR, et al: Pure red-cell aplasia and epoetin therapy. *N Engl J Med* 351:1403, 2004.
157. Levine AM, Karim R, MackW et al: Neutropenia in human immunodeficiency virus infection: Data from the women's interagency HIV study. *Arch Intern Med* 116:405, 2006.
158. Murphy M, Metcalfe P, Waters A: Incidence and mechanism of neutropenia and thrombocytopenia in patients with human immunodeficiency virus infection. *Br J Haematol* 66:337, 1987.
159. Bagnara GP, Zauli G, Giovannini M, et al: Early loss of circulating hemopoietic progenitors in HIV-1 infected subjects. *Exp Hematol* 18:426, 1990.
160. Leiderman I, Greenberg M, Adelsberg B, et al: A glycoprotein inhibitor of in vitro granulopoiesis associated with AIDS. *Blood* 70:1267, 1987.
161. Klaassen RJ, Mulder JW, Vlekke AB, et al: Autoantibodies against peripheral blood cells appear early in HIV infection and their prevalence increases with disease progression. *Clin Exp Immunol* 81:11, 1990.
162. Mauss S, Steinmetz HT, Willers R, et al: Induction of granulocyte colony-stimulating factor by acute febrile infection but not by neutropenia in HIV seropositive individuals. *J Acquir Immune Defic Syndr* 14:430, 1997.
163. Karcher DS, Frost AR: The bone marrow in human immunodeficiency virus (HIV)-related disease. Morphology and clinical correlation. *Am J Clin Pathol* 95:63, 1991.
164. Elis M, Gupta S, Galant S, et al: Impaired neutrophil function in patients with AIDS or AIDS-related complex: A comprehensive evaluation. *J Infect Dis* 158:1268, 1988.
165. Bodey GP, Buckley M, Sathe US, et al: Qualitative relationships between circulating leukocytes and infection in patients with acute leukemia. *Ann Intern Med* 64:328, 1966.
166. Moore RD, Keruly J, Chaisson RE, et al: Neutropenia and bacterial infection in acquired immunodeficiency syndrome. *Arch Intern Med* 155:1965, 1995.
167. Jacobson MA, Cohen PT, Liu RC, et al: Risk of hospitalization for serious bacterial infection associated with neutropenia severity in patients with HIV [abstract 231]. 11th International Conference on AIDS, Vancouver, Canada, 1996.
168. Meynard J-L, Guiguet M, Arsac S, et al: Frequency and risk factors of infectious complications in neutropenic patients infected with HIV. *AIDS* 11:995, 1997.
169. Moore DAJ, Benepal T, Portsmouth S, et al: Etiology and natural history of neutropenia in human immunodeficiency virus disease: A prospective study. *Clin Infect Dis* 32:469, 2001.
170. Sloand EM, Maciejewski J, Kumar P, et al: Protease inhibitors stimulate hematopoiesis and decrease apoptosis and ICE expression in CD34+ cells. *Blood* 96:2735, 2000.
171. Groopman JE, Feder D: Hematopoietic growth factors in AIDS. *Semin Oncol* 19:408, 1992.
172. Groopman JE, Mitsuyasu RT, DeLeo MJ, et al: Effect of recombinant human granulocyte-macrophage colony stimulating factor on myelopoiesis in the acquired immunodeficiency syndrome. *N Engl J Med* 317:593, 1987.
173. Lieschke GJ, Burgess AW: Granulocyte colony-stimulating factor and granulocyte-macrophage colony-stimulating factor (1). *N Engl J Med* 327:28, 1992.
174. Lieschke GJ, Burgess AW: Granulocyte colony-stimulating factor and granulocyte-macrophage colony-stimulating factor (2). *N Engl J Med* 327:99, 1992.
175. Avalos BR, Parker JM, Ware DA, et al: Dissociation of the Jak kinase pathway from G-CSF receptor signaling in neutrophils. *Exp Hematol* 25:160, 1997.
176. Kaplan LD, Kahn JO, Crowe S, et al: Clinical and virologic effects of recombinant human granulocyte-macrophage colony-stimulating factor in patients receiving chemotherapy for human immunodeficiency virus-associated non-Hodgkin's lymphoma: Results of a randomized trial. *J Clin Oncol* 9:929, 1991.
177. Kedzierska K, Maerz A, Warby T, et al: Granulocyte-macrophage colony-stimulating factor inhibits HIV-1 replication in monocyte-derived macrophages. *AIDS* 14:1739, 2000.
178. Barbaro G, Di Lorenzo G, Grisorio B, et al: Effect of recombinant human granulocyte-macrophage colony-stimulating factor on HIV-related leukopenia: A randomized, controlled clinical study. *AIDS* 11:1453, 1997.

179. Brites C, Gilbert MJ, Pedral-Sampaio D, et al: A randomized, placebo-controlled trial of granulocyte-macrophage colony-stimulating factor and nucleoside analogue therapy in AIDS. *J Infect Dis* 182:1531, 2000.
180. Kuritzkes DR, Parenti D, Ward DJ, et al: Filgrastim prevents severe neutropenia and reduces infective morbidity in patients with advanced HIV infection: Results of a randomized, multicenter, controlled trial. GCSF 930101 Study Group *AIDS* 12:65, 1998.
181. Keiser P, Higgs E, Scanton J: Neutropenia is associated with bacteremia in patients with HIV. *Am J Med Sci* 312:118, 1996.
182. Pechere M, Samii K, Hirschel B: HIV related thrombocytopenia. *N Engl J Med* 328:1785, 1993.
183. Sullivan PS, Hanson DL, Chu SY, et al: Surveillance for thrombocytopenia in persons infected with HIV: Results from the multistate Adult and Adolescent Spectrum of Disease Project. *J Acquir Immune Defic Syndr* 14:374, 1997.
184. Pearce CL, Wendy JM, Levine AM, et al: *Thrombocytopenia Is a Strong Predictor of All-Cause and AIDS-Specific Mortality in Women with HIV: The Women's Interagency HIV Study*. 46th Annual Meeting of the American Society of Hematology, San Diego, California, 2004.
185. Ballem PJ, Belzberg A, Devine DV, et al: Kinetic studies of the mechanism of thrombocytopenia in patients with human immunodeficiency virus infection. *N Engl J Med* 327:1779, 1992.
186. Walsh CM, Nardi MA, Karpatkin S: On the mechanism of thrombocytopenic purpura in sexually active homosexual men. *N Engl J Med* 311:635, 1984.
187. Bettaieb A, Fromont P, Louache F, et al: Presence of cross-reactive antibody between human immunodeficiency virus (HIV) and platelet glycoproteins in HIV related immune thrombocytopenic purpura. *Blood* 80:162, 1992.
188. Kouri Y, Borkowsky W, Nardi M, et al: Human megakaryocytes have a CD4+ molecule capable of binding human immunodeficiency virus-1. *Blood* 81:2664, 1993.
189. Zucker-Franklin D, Seremetis S, Heng ZY: Internalization of human immunodeficiency virus type I and other retroviruses by megakaryocytes and platelets. *Blood* 75:1920, 1990.
190. Wang J-F, Liu Z-Y, Groopman JE: The alpha-chemokine receptor CXCR4 is expressed on the megakaryocytic lineage from progenitor to platelets, and modulates migration and adhesion. *Blood* 92:756, 1998.
191. Zucker-Franklin D, Cao Y: Megakaryocytes of human immunodeficiency virus-infected individuals express viral RNA. *Proc Natl Acad Sci U S A* 86:5595, 1989.
192. Zucker-Franklin D, Termin CS, Cooper MC: Structural changes in the megakaryocytes of patients infected with the human immunodeficiency virus (HIV-1). *Am J Pathol* 134:1295, 1989.
193. Swiss Group for Clinical Studies on AIDS: Zidovudine for the treatment of thrombocytopenia associated with HIV: A prospective study. *Ann Intern Med* 109:718, 1988.
194. Nardi M, Feinmark SJ, Hu L, et al: Complement-independent Ab-induced peroxide lysis of platelets requires 12-lipoxygenase and a platelet NADPH oxidase pathway. *J Clin Invest* 113:973, 2004.
195. Oksenhendler E, Bierling P, Farcet JP, et al: Response to therapy in 37 patients with HIV related thrombocytopenic purpura. *Br J Haematol* 66:49, 1987.
196. Oksenhendler E, Bierling P, Ferchal F, et al: Zidovudine for thrombocytopenic purpura related to human immunodeficiency virus (HIV) infection. *Ann Intern Med* 110:365, 1989.
197. Landonio G, Cinque P, Nosari A, et al: Comparison of two dose regimens of zidovudine in an open, randomized, multicenter study for severe HIV related thrombocytopenia. *AIDS* 7:209, 1993.
198. Caso JAA, Mingo CS, Tena JG: Effect of highly active antiretroviral therapy on thrombocytopenia in patients with HIV infection. *N Engl J Med* 16:1239, 1999.
199. Carbonara S, Fiorentino G, Serio G, et al: Response of severe HIV-associated thrombocytopenia to highly active antiretroviral therapy including protease inhibitors. *J Infect* 42:251, 2001.
200. Marroni M, Gresele P, Landonio G, et al: Interferon-a is effective in the treatment of HIV-1 related, severe, zidovudine-resistant thrombocytopenia: A prospective, placebo-controlled, double-blind trial. *Ann Intern Med* 121:423, 1994.
201. Vianelli N, Catani L, Gugliotta L, et al: Recombinant alpha-interferon 2b in the treatment of HIV related thrombocytopenia. *AIDS* 7:823, 1993.
202. Imbach P, D'Apuzzo V, Hirt A, et al: High dose intravenous gammaglobulin for idiopathic thrombocytopenic purpura in childhood. *Lancet* 1:1228, 1981.
203. Bussel JB, Saimi JS: Isolated thrombocytopenia in patients infected with HIV: Treatment with intravenous gammaglobulin. *Am J Hematol* 28:79, 1998.
204. Gringeri A, Cattaneo M, Santagostino E, Mannucci PM: Intramuscular anti-D immunoglobulins for home treatment of chronic immune thrombocytopenic purpura. *Br J Haematol* 80:337, 1992.
205. Oksenhendler E, Bierling P, Brossard Y, et al: Anti-Rh immunoglobulin therapy for human immunodeficiency virus-related immune thrombocytopenic purpura. *Blood* 71:1499, 1988.
206. Oksenhendler E, Bierling P, Chevret S, et al: Splenectomy is safe and effective in human immunodeficiency virus related immune thrombocytopenia. *Blood* 82:29, 1993.
207. Kemeny MM, Cooke V, Melester TS, et al: Splenectomy in patients with AIDS and AIDS-related complex. *AIDS* 7:1063, 1993.
208. Becker DM, Saunders TJ, Wispelwey B, Schain DC: Case report: Venous thromboembolism in AIDS. *Am J Med Sci* 303:395, 1992.
209. Roberts SP, Haefs TMP: Central retinal vein occlusion in a middle aged adult with HIV infection. *Optom Vis Sci* 210:108, 1992.
210. Tanimowo M: Deep vein thrombosis as a manifestation of acquired immunodeficiency syndrome? A case report. *Cent Afr J Med* 42:327, 1996.
211. Narayanan TS, Narawane NM, Phadke AY, et al: Multiple abdominal venous thrombosis in HIV seropositive patient. *Indian J Gastroenterol* 17:105, 1998.
212. Sullivan PS, Dworkin MS, Jones JL, et al: Epidemiology of thrombosis in HIV-infected individuals. *AIDS* 14:321, 2000.
213. Jacobson MC, Dezube BJ, Aboulafia DM: Thrombotic complications in patients infected with HIV in the era of highly active antiretroviral therapy: A case series. *Clin Infect Dis* 39:1214, 2004.
214. Copur AS, Smith PR, Gomez V, et al: HIV infection is a risk factor for venous thromboembolism. *AIDS Patient Care STDS* 16:205, 2002.
215. Fultz SL, McGinnis KA, Skanderson M, et al: Association of venous thromboembolism with human immunodeficiency virus and mortality in veterans. *Am J Med* 116:420, 2004.
216. Birx DL, Redfield RR, Tencer K, et al: Induction of interleukin 6 during human immunodeficiency virus infection. *Blood* 76:2303, 1990.
217. Emilie D, Peuchmaur M, Maillot MC, et al: Production of interleukins in HIV-1 replicating lymph nodes. *J Clin Invest* 86:148, 1990.
218. Hack EC: Tissue factor pathway of coagulation in sepsis. *Crit Care Med* 28 (Suppl):25S, 2000.
219. Nawroth PP, Handley DA, Esmon CT, Stern DM: Interleukin 1 induces endothelial cell pro-coagulant while suppressing cell-surface anti coagulant activity. *Proc Natl Acad Sci U S A* 83:3460, 1986.
220. Becker S, Fusco G, Fusco J, et al: HIV-associated thrombotic microangiopathy in the era of highly active antiretroviral therapy; an observational study. *Clin Infect Dis* 39:S5:S267:2004.
221. Iranzo A, Domingo P, Cadafalch J, Sambeat MA: Intracranial venous and dural sinus thrombosis due to protein S deficiency in a patient with AIDS. *J Neurol Neurosurg Psychiatry* 64:688, 1998.
222. Bissuel F, Berruyer M, Causse X, et al: Acquired Protein S deficiency: Correlation with advanced disease in HIV 1 infected patients. *J Acquir Immune Defic Syndr* 5:484, 1992.
223. Pulik M, Lebret-Lerolle D: Acquired protein S deficiency in HIV infections. *Ann Med Interne (Paris)* 143:57, 1992.
224. Stahl CP, Wideman CS, Spira TJ, et al: Protein S deficiency in men with long term human immunodeficiency virus infection. *Blood* 81:1801, 1993.
225. Sorice M, Griggi T, Acieri P, et al: Protein S and HIV infection. The role of anticardiolipin and anti-protein S antibodies. *Thromb Res* 73:165, 1992.
226. Erbe M, Rickerts V, Bauersachs RM, et al: Acquired protein C and protein S deficiency in HIV-infected patients. *Clin Appl Thromb Hemost* 9:325, 2003.
227. Feffer SE, Fox FL, Orsen MM, et al: Thrombotic tendencies and correlation with clinical status in patients infected with HIV. *South Med J* 88:1126, 1995.
228. Toulon P, Lamine M, Ledjev I, et al: Heparin cofactor II deficiency in patients infected with the human immunodeficiency virus. *Thromb Haemost* 70:730, 1993.
229. Bloom EJ, Abrams DI, Rodgers G, et al: Lupus anticoagulant in the Acquired Immunodeficiency Syndrome. *JAMA* 256:491, 1986.
230. Peters BS, Beck EJ, Coleman DG, et al: Changing disease patterns in patients with AIDS in a referral center in the United Kingdom: The changing face of AIDS. *BMJ* 302:203, 1991.
231. Krentz HB, Kliewer G, Gill MJ: Changing mortality rates and casues of death for HIV-infected individuals living in Southern Alberta, Canada from 1984 to 2003. *HIV Med* 6:99, 2005.
232. Gail MH, Pluda JM, Rabkin CS, et al: Projections of the incidence of non-Hodgkin's lymphoma related to acquired immunodeficiency syndrome. *J Natl Cancer Inst* 83:695, 1991.
233. Rabkin CS, Biggar RJ, Horm JW: Increasing incidence of cancers associated with the human immunodeficiency virus epidemic. *Int J Cancer* 47:692, 1991.
234. Beral V, Peterman T, Berkelman R, Jaffe H: AIDS-associated non-Hodgkin lymphoma. *Lancet* 337:805, 1991.
235. Biggar RJ, Rabkin CS: The epidemiology of acquired immunodeficiency syndrome-related lymphomas. *Curr Opin Oncol* 4:883, 1992.
236. Pluda JM, Vanzon D, Tosato G, et al: Factors which predict for the development of non-Hodgkin's lymphoma in patients with HIV infection receiving antiretroviral therapy. *Blood* 78:285a, 1991.
237. Cote TR, Biggar RJ, Rosenberg PS, et al: Non-Hodgkin's lymphoma among people with AIDS: Incidence, presentation, and public health burden. AIDS/Cancer Study Group. *Int J Cancer* 73:645, 1997.
238. Franceschi S, Dal Maso L, La Vecchia C: Advances in the epidemiology of HIV-associated non-Hodgkin's lymphoma and other lymphoid neoplasms. *Int J Cancer* 83:481, 1999.
239. Mocroft A, Katlama C, Johnson AM, et al: AIDS across Europe 1994–98: The EuroSIDA study. *Lancet* 356:291, 2000.
240. Rabkin CS, Testa MA, Huang J, et al: Kaposi's sarcoma and non-Hodgkin's lymphoma incidence trends in AIDS Clinical Trial Group study participants. *J Acquir Immune Defic Syndr* 21(Suppl 1):S31, 1999.
241. Dore GJ, Li Y, McDonald A, et al: Impact of highly active antiretroviral therapy on individual AIDS-defining illness incidence and survival in Australia. *J Acquir Immune Defic Syndr* 4:388, 2002.
242. Ledergerber B, Telenti A, Egger M, et al: Risk of HIV-related Kaposi's sarcoma and non-Hodgkin's lymphoma with potent antiretroviral therapy: Prospective cohort study. *BMJ* 319:23, 1999.

243. Jacobson LP: Impact of highly effective anti-retroviral therapy on the incidence of malignancies among HIV infected individuals [abstract S5]. *J Acquir Immune Defic Syndr* 17:A39, 1998.
244. International Collaboration on HIV and Cancer: Highly active antiretroviral therapy and incidence of cancer in human immunodeficiency virus-infected adults. *J Natl Cancer Inst* 92:1823, 2000.
245. Kirk O, Pedersen C, Cozzi-Lepri A, et al: Non-Hodgkin lymphoma in HIV-infected patients in the era of highly active antiretroviral therapy. *Blood* 98:3406, 2001.
246. Besson C, Goubar A, Gabarre J, et al: Changes in AIDS-related lymphoma since the era of highly active antiretroviral therapy. *Blood* 98:2339, 2001.
247. Purtilo DT: Opportunistic non-Hodgkin's lymphoma in X-linked recessive immunodeficiency and lymphoproliferative syndromes. *Semin Oncol* 4:335, 1977.
248. Levine AM, Taylor CR, Schneider DR, et al: Immunoblastic sarcoma of T cell versus B cell origin: I. Clinical features. *Blood* 58:52, 1981.
249. Penn I: Tumors of the immunocompromised patient. *Annu Rev Med* 39:63, 1988.
250. Swinnen LJ, Costanzo-Nordin MR, Fisher SG, et al: Increased incidence of lymphoproliferative disorder after immunosuppression with the monoclonal antibody OKT3 in cardiac transplant recipients. *N Engl J Med* 323:1723, 1990.
251. Pantaleo G, Graziosi C, Fauci AS: Mechanisms of disease: The immunopathogenesis of human immunodeficiency virus infection. *N Engl J Med* 328:327, 1993.
252. Birx DI, Redfield RR, Tosato G: Defective regulation of Epstein-Barr virus infection in patients with acquired immunodeficiency syndrome (AIDS) or AIDS-related disorders. *N Engl J Med* 314:874, 1986.
253. Shear GM, Salahuddin SZ, Markham PD, et al: Prospective study of cytotoxic T lymphocyte responses to influenza virus and antibodies to human T lymphotropic virus-III in homosexual men: Selective loss of influenza-specific human leukocyte antigen-restricted cytotoxic lymphocyte response to human T lymphotropic virus-III positive individuals with symptoms of acquired immunodeficiency syndrome. *J Clin Invest* 76:1699, 1985.
254. Feichtinger H, Rutkonen P, Parravicini C, et al: Malignant lymphomas in *Cynomolgus* monkeys infected with simian immunodeficiency virus. *Am J Pathol* 137:1311, 1990.
255. Jelinek DF, Lipsky PE: Enhancement of human B cell proliferation and differentiation by tumor necrosis factor-alpha and interleukin 1. *J Immunol* 139:2970, 1987.
256. Fauci A, Schnittman SM, Poli G, et al: Immunopathogenetic mechanisms in human immunodeficiency virus (HIV) infection. *Ann Intern Med* 114:678, 1991.
257. Breen EC, Epeldegui M, Boscardin WJ, et al: Elevated levels of soluble CD44 precede the development of AIDS-associated non-Hodgkin's B-cell lymphoma. *AIDS* 19:1711, 2005.
258. Piriou E, van Dort NM, Nanlohy NM, et al: Loss of EBNA1-specific memory CD4 and CD8 T cells in HIV-infected patients progressing to AIDS-related non-Hodgkin lymphoma. *Blood* 106:3166, 2005.
259. Emillie D, Coumbaras J, Raphael M, et al: IL-6 production in high grade B lymphomas: Correlation with presence of malignant immunoblasts in AIDS and in HIV-seronegative patients. *Blood* 80:498, 1992.
260. Benjamin D, Knobloch TJ, Abrams J, Dayton MA: Human B cell IL-10: B cell lines derived from patients with AIDS and Burkitt's lymphoma constitutively secrete large quantities of IL-10.*Blood* 78:384a, 1991.
261. Masood R, Bond M, Scadden D, et al: Interleukin-10: An autocrine B cell growth for human B-cell lymphomas and their progenitors. *Blood* 80:115a, 1992.
262. Poli G, Fauci AS: The effect of cytokines and pharmacologic agents on chronic HIV infection. *AIDS Res Hum Retroviruses* 8:191, 1992.
263. Shibata D, Weiss LM, Nathwani BN, et al: Epstein-Barr virus in benign lymph node biopsies from individuals infected with the human immunodeficiency virus is associated with concurrent or subsequent development of non-Hodgkin's lymphoma. *Blood* 77:1527, 1991.
264. MacMahon EME, Glass JD, Hayward SD, et al: Epstein-Barr virus in AIDS-related primary central nervous system lymphoma. *Lancet* 338:969, 1991.
265. Wang D, Liebowitz D, Kieff E: An EBV membrane protein expressed in immortalized lymphocytes transforms established rodent cells. *Cell* 43:831, 1985.
266. Subar M, Neri A, Inghirami G, et al: Frequent c-myc oncogene activation and infrequent presence of Epstein-Barr virus genome in AIDS-associated lymphoma. *Blood* 72:667, 1988.
267. Shibata D, Weiss LM, Hernandez AM, et al: Epstein-Barr virus–associated non-Hodgkin's lymphoma in patients infected with the human immunodeficiency virus. *Blood* 81:2102, 1993.
268. Hamilton-Dutoit SJ, Raphael M, Audouin M, et al: In situ demonstration of Epstein-Barr virus small RNAs (EBER 1) in AIDS related lymphomas: Correlation with tumor morphology and primary site. *Blood* 82:619, 1993.
269. Neri A, Barriga F, Inghirami G, et al: Epstein-Barr virus infection precedes clonal expansion in Burkitt's and acquired immunodeficiency associated lymphoma. *Blood* 77:1092, 1991.
270. Chaganti RSK, Jhanwar SC, Koziner B, et al: Specific translocations characterize Burkitt's-like lymphoma of homosexual men with the acquired immunodeficiency syndrome. *Blood* 61:1269, 1983.
271. Peterson JM, Tubbs RR, Savage RA, et al: Small noncleaved B cell Burkitt-like lymphoma with chromosome t(8;14) translocation and Epstein-Barr virus nuclear associated antigen in a homosexual man with acquired immunodeficiency syndrome. *Am J Med* 78:141, 1985.
272. Rechavi G, Ben-Bassat M, Berkowicz U, et al: Molecular analysis of Burkitt's leukemia in two hemophilic brothers with AIDS. *Blood* 70:1713, 1987.
273. Pelicci PG, Knowles DM, McGrath IT, Dalla-Favera R: Chromosomal breakpoints and structural alterations of the c-myc locus differ in endemic and sporadic forms of Burkitt lymphoma. *Proc Natl Acad Sci U S A* 83:2984, 1986.
274. Shiramizu B, Barriga F, Neequaye J, et al: Patterns of chromosomal breakpoint locations in Burkitt's lymphoma: Relevance to geography and Epstein-Barr virus association. *Blood* 77:1516, 1991.
275. Ballerini P, Gaidano G, Gong JZ, et al: Molecular pathogenesis of HIV-associated lymphomas. *AIDS Res Hum Retroviruses* 8:731, 1992.
276. Pelicci PG, Knowles DM II, Arlin ZA, et al: Multiple monoclonal B cell expansions and c-myc oncogene rearrangements in acquired immune deficiency syndrome-related lymphoproliferative disorders: Implications for lymphomagenesis. *J Exp Med* 164:2049, 1986.
277. Pauza CD, Galindo J, Richman DD: Human immunodeficiency virus infection of monoblastoid cells: Cellular differentiation determines the pattern of virus replication. *J Virol* 62:3558, 1988.
278. Laurence J, Astrin SM: Human immunodeficiency virus induction of malignant transformation in human B lymphocytes. *Proc Natl Acad Sci U S A* 88:7635, 1991.
279. Lombardi L, Newcomb EW, Dalla-Favera R: Pathogenesis of Burkitt lymphoma: Expression of an activated c-myc oncogene causes the tumorigenic conversion of EBV infected human B lymphoblasts. *Cell* 46:161, 1987.
280. Adams JM, Harris AW, Pinkert CA, et al: The c-myc oncogene driven by immunoglobulin enhancers induces lymphoid malignancy in transgenic mice. *Nature* 318:553, 1985.
281. Gaidano G, Lo Coco F, Ye BH, et al: Rearrangements of the BCL-6 gene in AIDS associated non-Hodgkin's lymphoma: Association with diffuse large cell subtype. *Blood* 84:397, 1994.
282. Gaidano G, Carbone A, Pastore C, et al: Frequent mutations of the 5′ noncoding region of the BCL-6 gene in acquired immunodeficiency syndrome-related non-Hodgkin's lymphomas. *Blood* 89:3755, 1997.
283. Gaidano G, Dalla-Favera R: Biologic aspects of human immunodeficiency virus-related lymphoma. *Curr Opin Oncol* 4:900, 1992.
284. Gaidano G, Carbone A, Dalla-Favera R: Pathogenesis of AIDS-related lymphomas: Molecular and histogenetic heterogeneity. *Am J Pathol* 152:623, 1998.
285. Ziegler JL, Beckstead JA, Volberding PA, et al: Non-Hodgkin's lymphoma in 90 homosexual men: Relation to generalized lymphadenopathy and the acquired immunodeficiency syndrome. *N Engl J Med* 311:565, 1984.
286. Kaplan LD, Abrams DI, Feigal E, et al: AIDS-associated non-Hodgkin's lymphoma in San Francisco. *JAMA* 261:719, 1989.
287. Knowles DM, Chamulak GA, Subar M, et al: Lymphoid neoplasia associated with the acquired immunodeficiency syndrome (AIDS): The New York University experience with 105 cases during 1981 through 1986. *Ann Intern Med* 108:744, 1988.
288. Lowenthal DA, Straus DJ, Campbell SW, et al: AIDS-related lymphoid neoplasia: The Memorial Hospital experience. *Cancer* 61:2325, 1988.
289. Ioachim HL, Dorsett B, Cronin W, et al: Acquired immunodeficiency syndrome associated lymphomas: Clinical, pathological, immunologic, and viral characteristics of 111 cases. *Hum Pathol* 22:659, 1991.
290. Lukes RJ, Parker JW, Taylor CR, et al: Immunologic approach to non-Hodgkin's lymphomas and related leukemias: Analysis of the results of multiparameter studies of 425 cases. *Semin Hematol* 15:322, 1978.
291. Jaffe ES, Harris NL, Stein H, Vardinan JW: *World Health Organization Classification of Tumors. Pathology & Genetics. Tumours of Haematopoietic and Lymphoma Tissues*, p 260. IARC Press, Lyon, France, 2001.
292. Bellas C, Santon A, Manzanal A, et al: Pathological, immunological, and molecular features of Hodgkin's disease associated with HIV infection. Comparison with ordinary Hodgkin's disease. *Am J Surg Pathol* 12:1520, 1996
293. Raphael M, Gentilhomme O, Tulliez M, et al: Histopathologic features of high-grade non-Hodgkin's lymphomas in acquired immunodeficiency syndrome. The French Study Group of Pathology for Human Immunodeficiency Virus-Associated Tumors. *Arch Pathol Lab Med* 115:15, 1991.
294. Carbone A, Gloghini A, Gaidano G, et al: AIDS-related Burkitt's lymphoma. Morphologic and immunophenotypic study of biopsy specimens. *Am J Clin Pathol* 103:561, 1995.
295. Delecluse HJ, Raphael M, Magaud JP, et al: Variable morphology of human immunodeficiency virus-associated lymphomas with c-myc rearrangements. The French Study Group of Pathology for Human Immunodeficiency Virus-Associated Tumors I. *Blood* 82:552, 1993.
296. Davi F, Delecluse HJ, Guiet P, et al: Burkitt-like lymphomas in AIDS patients: Characterization within a series of 103 human immunodeficiency virus-associated non-Hodgkin's lymphomas. Burkitt's Lymphoma Study Group. *J Clin Oncol* 12:3788, 1998.
297. Ambinder RF: Epstein-Barr virus associated lymphoproliferations in the AIDS setting. *Eur J Cancer* 10:1209, 2001.
298. Carbone A, Gaidano G, Gloghini, et al: BCL-6 protein expression in AIDS-related non-Hodgkin's lymphomas: Inverse relationship with Epstein-Barr virus-encoded latent membrane protein-1 expression. *Am J Pathol* 1:155, 1997.
299. Nador RG, Cesarman E, Chadburn A, et al: Primary effusion lymphomas: A distinct clinicopathologic entity associated with the Kaposi's sarcoma-associated herpes virus. *Blood* 88:645, 1996.
300. Chang Y, Cesarman E, Pessin MS, et al: Identification of herpesviruslike DNA sequences in AIDS associated Kaposi's sarcoma. *Science* 266:1865, 1994.
301. Cesarman E, Chang Y, Moore PS, et al: Kaposi's sarcoma associated herpesvirus like DNA sequences in AIDS-related body cavity based lymphomas. *N Engl J Med* 332:1186, 1995.

302. Flaitz CM, Nichols CM, Walling DM, et al: Plasmablastic lymphoma: An HIV-associated entity with primary oral manifestations. *Oral Oncol* 38:96, 2002.
303. Delecluse HJ, Anagnostopoulos I, Dallenbach F, et al: Plasmablastic lymphomas of the oral cavity: A new entity associated with the human immunodeficiency virus infection. *Blood* 89:1413, 1997.
304. Gaidano G, Cerri M, Capello D, et al: Molecular histogenesis of plasmablastic lymphoma of the oral cavity. *Br J Haematol* 119:622, 2002.
305. Arzoo KK, Bu X, Espina BM, et al: T-Cell lymphoma in HIV-infected patients. *J Acquir Immune Defic Syndr* 36:1020, 2004.
306. Jhala DN, Medeiros LJ, Lopez-Terrada D, et al: Neutrophil-rich anaplastic large cell lymphoma of T-cell lineage. A report of two cases arising in HIV-positive patients. *Am J Clin Pathol* 114:478, 2000.
307. Gonzalez-Clemente JM, Ribera JM, Campo E, et al: Ki-1+ anaplastic large-cell lymphoma of T-cell origin in an HIV-infected patient. *AIDS* 5:751 1991.
308. Arber DA, Chang KL, Weiss LM: Peripheral T-cell lymphoma with Touton like tumor giant cells associated with HIV infection: Report of two cases. *Am J Surg Pathol* 23:519, 1999.
309. Levine AM, Burkes RL, Walker M, et al: Development of B cell lymphoma in two monogamous homosexual men. *Arch Intern Med* 145:479, 1985.
310. Dezube BJ, Aboulafia DM, Pantanowitz L: Plasma cell disorders in HIV-infected patients: From benign gammopathy to multiple myeloma. *AIDS Read* 14:372, 2004.
311. Horning SJ, Rosenberg SA: The natural history of initially untreated low grade non-Hodgkin's lymphomas. *N Engl J Med* 311:1471, 1984.
312. Levine AM: Acquired immunodeficiency syndrome-related lymphoma [review]. *Blood* 80:8, 1992.
313. Lim ST, Karim R, Tulpule A, et al: Prognostic factors in HIV-related diffuse large-cell lymphoma: Before versus after highly active antiretroviral therapy. *J Clin Oncol* 23:8477, 2005.
314. Jones SE, Fuks Z, Bellm M, et al: Non-Hodgkin's lymphoma: IV. Clinicopathologic correlation of 405 cases. *Cancer* 31:806, 1973.
315. Podzamczer D, Ricat I, Bolao F, et al: Gallium-67 scan for distinguishing follicular hyperplasia from other AIDS associated diseases in lymph nodes. *AIDS* 4:683, 1990.
316. Levine AM, Wernz JC, Kaplan L, et al: Low dose chemotherapy with central nervous system prophylaxis and azidothymidine maintenance in AIDS-related lymphoma: A prospective multi-institutional trial. *JAMA* 266:84, 1991.
317. Gill PS, Levine AM, Meyer PR, et al: Primary central nervous system lymphoma in homosexual men: Clinical, immunologic, and pathologic features. *Am J Med* 78:742, 1985.
318. Gill PS, Graham RA, Boswell W, et al: A comparison of imaging, clinical, and pathologic aspects of space occupying lesions within the brain in patients with acquired immunodeficiency syndrome. *Am J Physiol Imaging* 1:134, 1986.
319. Ciricillo SF, Rosenblum ML: Use of CT and MR imaging to distinguish intracranial lesions and to define the need for biopsy in AIDS patients. *J Neurosurg* 73:720, 1990.
320. Hoffman JM, Waskin HA, Schifter T, et al: PDG-PET in differentiating lymphoma from nonmalignant central nervous system lesions in patients with AIDS. *J Nucl Med* 34:567, 1993.
321. Alcaide FG, Lomena F, Cruceta A, et al: Predictive value of thallium-201 SPECT in the diagnosis of primary central nervous system lymphoma in AIDS patients [abstract 22291]. 12th World AIDS Conference, Geneva, Switzerland, 1998.
322. MacMahon EME, Glass JD, Hayward SDC, et al: Epstein-Barr virus in AIDS related primary central nervous system lymphoma. *Lancet* 338:969, 1991.
323. Cingolani A, De Luca A, Larocca LM, et al: Minimally invasive diagnosis of acquired immunodeficiency syndrome-related primary central nervous system lymphoma. *J Natl Cancer Inst* 5:364, 1998.
324. Ribera JM, Navarro JT, Oriol A, et al: Prognostic impact of highly active antiretroviral therapy in HIV-related Hodgkin's disease. *AIDS* 27:1973, 2002.
325. Jones D, Ballestas ME, Kaye KM, et al: Primary effusion lymphoma and Kaposi's sarcoma in a cardiac transplant recipient. *N Engl J Med* 339:444, 1998.
326. Simonelli C, Spina M, Cinelli R, et al: Clinical features and outcome of primary effusion lymphoma in HIV-infected patients: A single-institution study. *J Clin Oncol* 21:3948, 2003.
327. Oksenhendler E, Clauvel JP, Jouveshomme S, et al: Complete remission of a primary effusion lymphoma with antiretroviral therapy. *Am J Hematol* 57:266, 1998.
328. Hocqueloux L, Agbalika F, Oksenhendler E: Long-term remission of an AIDS-related primary effusion lymphoma with antiviral therapy. *AIDS* 15:280, 2001.
329. Spina M, Gaidano G, Carbone A: Highly active antiretroviral therapy in human herpesvirus-8-related body-cavity-based lymphoma. *AIDS* 12:955, 1998.
330. Bower M, Gazzard B, Mandalia S, et al: A prognostic index for systemic AIDS-related non-Hodgkin lymphoma treated in the era of highly active antiretroviral therapy. *Ann Intern Med* 143:265, 2005.
331. Lim ST, Espina B, Tulpule A, et al: AIDS related small non-cleaved (Burkitt or atypical burkitt) lymphoma versus diffuse large cell lymphoma in the pre- and post-HAART eras: Significant differences in survival. 46th Annual Meeting of the American Society of Hematology, San Diego, California, December 6, 2004.
332. Hoffmann C, Tiemann M, Schrader C, et al: AIDS-related B-cell lymphoma (ARL): Correlation of prognosis with differentiation profiles assessed by immunophenotyping. *Blood* 106:1762, 2005.
333. Little RF, Pittaluga S, Grant N, et al: Highly effective treatment of acquired immunodeficiency syndrome-related lymphoma with dose-adjusted EPOCH: Impact of antiretroviral therapy suspension and tumor biology. *Blood* 101:4653, 2003.
334. Dugan M, Subar M, Odajnyk C, et al: Intensive multiagent chemotherapy for AIDS related diffuse large cell lymphoma. *Blood* 68:124a, 1986.
335. Odajnyk C, Subar M, Dugan M, et al: Clinical features and correlates with immunopathology and molecular biology of a large group of patients with AIDS associated small non-cleaved lymphoma (SNCL). *Blood* 68:1331a, 1986.
336. Kaplan LD, Straus DH, Testa MA, et al: Low dose compared with standard dose m-BACOD chemotherapy for non-Hodgkin's lymphoma associated with human immunodeficiency virus infection. *N Engl J Med* 336:1641, 1997.
337. Levine AM, Tulpule A, Espina B, et al: Liposome-encapsulated doxorubicin in combination with standard agents (cyclophosphamide, vincristine, prednisone) in patients with newly diagnosed AIDS-related non-Hodgkin's lymphoma: Results of therapy and correlates of response. *J Clin Oncol* 22:2662, 2004.
338. Ratner L, Lee J, Tang S, et al: Chemotherapy for human immunodeficiency virus-associated non-Hodgkin's lymphoma in combination with highly active antiretroviral therapy. *J Clin Oncol* 19:2171, 2001.
339. Hoffmann C, Wolf E, Fatkenheuer G, et al: Response to highly active antiretroviral therapy strongly predicts outcome in patients with AIDS-related lymphoma *AIDS* 10:1521, 2003.
340. Antinori A, Cingolani A, Alba L, et al: Better response to chemotherapy and prolonged survival in AIDS-related lymphomas responding to highly active antiretroviral therapy. *AIDS* 15:1483, 2001.
341. Kaplan LD, Lee JY, Ambinder RF, et al: Rituximab does not improve clinical outcome in a randomized phase 3 trial of CHOP with or without rituximab in patients with HIV-associated non-Hodgkin lymphoma: AIDS-Malignancies Consortium Trial 010. *Blood* 106:1538, 2005.
342. Vlahov D, Graham N, Hoover D: Prognostic indicators for AIDS and infectious disease death in HIV-infected injection drug users: Plasma viral load and CD4+ cell count. *JAMA* 279:35,1998.
343. Spina M, Jaeger U, Sparano JA, et al: Rituximab plus infusional cyclophosphamide, doxorubicin, and etoposide in HIV-associated non-Hodgkin lymphoma: Pooled results from 3 phase 2 trials. *Blood* 105:1891, 2005.
344. Levine AM, Lee J, Kaplan L, et al: Efficacy and toxicity of concurrent rituximab plus infusional EPOCH in HIV associated lymphoma: AIDS Malignancy Consortium Trial 034 [abstract 8527]. *Proceedings of American Society of Clinical Oncology (ASCO)* 26:460S, 2008.
345. Dunleavy, K, et al: The case for rituximab in AIDS-related lymphoma. *Blood* 107:3014, 2006.
346. Tirelli U, Errante D, Spina M, et al: Second-line chemotherapy in human immunodeficiency virus-related non-Hodgkin's lymphoma: Evidence of activity of a combination of etoposide, mitoxantrone, and prednimustine in relapsed patients. *Cancer* 77:2127, 1996.
347. Spina M, Vaccher E, Juzbasic S, et al: Human immunodeficiency virus-related non-Hodgkin lymphoma: Activity of infusional cyclophosphamide, doxorubicin, and etoposide as second-line chemotherapy in 40 patients. *Cancer* 92:200, 2001.
348. Bi J, Espina BM, Tulpule A, et al: High-dose cytosine-arabinoside and cisplatin regimens as salvage therapy for refractory or relapsed AIDS-related non-Hodgkin's lymphoma. *J Acquir Immune Defic Syndr* 28:416,2001.
349. Krishnan A, Molina A, Zaia J, et al: Durable remissions with autologous stem cell transplantation for high risk HIV-associated lymphomas. *Blood* 105:874, 2004.
350. Re A, Cattaneo C, Michieli M, et al: High-dose therapy and autologous peripheral-blood stem-cell transplantation as salvage treatment for HIV-associated lymphoma in patients receiving highly active antiretroviral therapy. *J Clin Oncol* 23:4423, 2003.
351. Biggar RJ, Jaffe ES, Goedert JJ, et al: Hodgkin lymphoma and immunodeficiency in persons with HIV/AIDS. *Blood* 108:3786, 2006.
352. Engels EA, Pfeiffer RM, Goedert JJ, et al: Trends in cancer risk among people with AIDS in the United States 1980–2002. *AIDS* 20:1645, 2006.
353. Glaser SL, Clarke CA, Gulley ML, et al: Population-based patterns of human immunodeficiency virus-related Hodgkin lymphoma in the Greater San Francisco Bay Area, 1988–1998. *Cancer* 98:300, 2003.
354. Spina M, Vaccher E, Nasti G, Tirelli U: Human immunodeficiency virus-associated Hodgkin's disease. *Semin Oncol* 27:480, 2000.
355. Ames ED, Conjalka MS, Goldberg AF, et al: Hodgkin's disease and AIDS. Twenty-three new cases and a review of the literature. *Hematol Oncol Clin North Am* 5:343, 1991.
356. Re A, Casari S, Cattaneo C, et al: Hodgkin disease developing in patients infected by human immunodeficiency virus results in clinical features and a prognosis similar to those in patients with human immunodeficiency virus-related non-Hodgkin lymphoma. *Cancer* 92:2739, 2001.
357. Bellas C, Santon A, Manzanal A, et al: Pathological, immunological, and molecular features of Hodgkin's disease associated with HIV infection. Comparison with ordinary Hodgkin's disease. *Am J Surg Pathol* 20:1520, 1996.
358. Cooley TP: Non-AIDS-defining cancer in HIV-infected people. *Hematol Oncol Clin North Am* 17:889, 2003.
359. Levine AM, Li P, Cheung T, et al: Chemotherapy consisting of doxorubicin, bleomycin, vinblastine, and dacarbazine with granulocyte-colony-stimulating factor in HIV-infected patients with newly diagnosed Hodgkin's disease: A prospective, multi-institutional AIDS clinical trials group study (ACTG 149). *J Acquir Immune Defic Syndr* 24:444, 2000.
360. Andrieu JM, Roithmann S, Tourani JM, et al: Hodgkin's disease during HIV1 infection: The French registry experience. French Registry of HIV-associated tumors. *Ann Oncol* 4:635, 1993.
361. Goedert JJ, Cote TR, Virgo P, et al: Spectrum of AIDS-associated malignant disorders. *Lancet* 351:1833, 1998.

362. Frisch M, Biggar RJ, Engels EA, et al: Association of cancer with AIDS-related immunosuppression in adults. *JAMA* 285:1736, 2001.
363. Grulich AE, Li Y, McDonald A, et al: Rates of non-AIDS-defining cancers in people with HIV infection before and after AIDS diagnosis. *AIDS* 16:1155, 2002.
364. Rubio R: Hodgkin's disease associated with human immunodeficiency virus infection. A clinical study of 46 cases. Cooperative Study Group of Malignancies Associated with HIV Infection of Madrid. *Cancer* 73:2400, 1994.
365. Monfardini S, Tirelli U, Vaccher E, et al: Hodgkin's disease in 63 intravenous drug users infected with human immunodeficiency virus. Gruppo Italiano Cooperativo AIDS & Tumori (GICAT). *Ann Oncol* 2(Suppl 2):201, 1991.
366. Tirelli U, Errante D, Vaccher E, et al: Hodgkin's disease in 92 patients with HIV infection: The Italian experience. GICAT (Italian Cooperative Group on AIDS & Tumors). *Ann Oncol* 3(Suppl 4):69, 1992.
367. Ohshima K, Tutiya T, Yamaguchi T, et al: Infiltration of Th1 and Th2 lymphocytes around Hodgkin and Reed-Sternberg (H&RS) cells in Hodgkin disease: Relation with expression of CXC and CC chemokines on H&RS cells. *Int J Cancer* 98:567, 2002.
368. Skinnider BF, Mak TW: The role of cytokines in classical Hodgkin lymphoma. *Blood* 99:4283, 2002.
369. Berenguer J, Miralles P, Ribera JM, et al: Characteristics and outcome of AIDS-related Hodgkin lymphoma before and after the introduction of highly active antiretroviral therapy. *J Acquir Immune Defic Syndr* 47:422, 2008.
370. Dolcetti R, Boiocchi M, Gloghini A, et al: Pathogenetic and histogenetic features of HIV-associated Hodgkin's disease. *Eur J Cancer* 37:1276, 2001.
371. Glaser SL, Lin RJ, Stewart SL, et al: Epstein-Barr virus-associated Hodgkin's disease: Epidemiologic characteristics in international data. *Int J Cancer* 70:375, 1997.
372. Herbst H, Steinbrecher E, Niedobitek G, et al: Distribution and phenotype of Epstein-Barr virus-harboring cells in Hodgkin's disease. *Blood* 80:484, 1992.
373. Levine AM: Hodgkin's disease in the setting of human immunodeficiency virus infection. *J Natl Cancer Inst Monogr* 23:37, 1998.
374. Errante D, Gabarre J, Ridolfo AL, et al: Hodgkin's disease in 35 patients with HIV infection: An experience with epirubicin, bleomycin, vinblastine and prednisone chemotherapy in combination with antiretroviral therapy and primary use of G-CSF. *Ann Oncol* 10:189, 1999.
375. Spina M, Gabarre J, Rossi G, et al: Stanford V regimen and concomitant HAART in 59 patients with Hodgkin disease and HIV infection. *Blood* 100:1984, 2002.
376. Gerard L, Galicier L, Boulanger E, et al: Improved survival in HIV-related Hodgkin's lymphoma since the introduction of highly active anti-retroviral therapy. *AIDS* 17:81, 2003.
377. Hoffmann C, Chow KU, Wolf E, et al: Strong impact of highly active antiretroviral therapy on survival in patients with human immunodeficiency virus-associated Hodgkin's disease. *Br J Haematol* 125:455, 2004.
378. Hartmann P, Rehwald U, Salzberger B, et al: BEACOPP therapeutic regimen for patients with Hodgkin's disease and HIV infection. *Ann Oncol* 14:1562, 2003.
379. Martin JN, Ganem DE, Osmond DH, et al: Sexual transmission and the natural history of human herpesvirus 8 infection. *N Engl J Med* 338:948, 1998.
380. Casper C: The aetiology and management of Castleman disease at 50 years: Translating pathophysiology to patient care. *Br J Haematol* 129:3, 2005.
381. Oksenhendler E, Carcelain G, Aoki Y, et al: High levels of human herpesvirus 8 viral load, human interleukin-6, interleukin-10, and C reactive protein correlate with exacerbation of multicentric Castleman disease in HIV-infected patients. *Blood* 96:2069, 2000.
382. Oksenhendler E, Boulanger E, Galicier L, et al: High incidence of Kaposi sarcoma-associated herpesvirus-related non-Hodgkin lymphoma in patients with HIV infection and multicentric Castleman disease. *Blood* 99:2331, 2002.
383. Marcelin A, Aaron L, Mateus C, et al: Rituximab therapy for HIV-associated Castleman disease. *Blood* 102:2786, 2003.
384. Abe Y, Matsubara D, Gatanaga H,et al: Distinct expression of Kaposi's sarcoma-associated herpesvirus-encoded proteins in Kaposi's sarcoma and multicentric Castleman's disease. *Pathol Int* 56:617, 2006.
385. Aboulafia DM, Ratner L, Miles SA, et al. Antiviral and immunomodulatory treatment for an AIDS-related primary central nervous system lymphoma: AIDS Malignancies Consortium Pilot Study 019. *Clin Lymphoma Myeloma* 6:399, 2006.
386. Jacomet C, Girard P, Lebrette M, et al: Intravenous methotrexate fro primary central nervous system non-Hodgkin's lymphoma in AIDS. *AIDS* 11:1725, 1997.

CHAPTER 84

MONONUCLEOSIS SYNDROMES

Robert F. Betts

SUMMARY

The defining clinical features of a mononucleosis syndrome are fever and reactive lymphocytes in the blood. The two most common causes of mononucleosis are Epstein-Barr virus (EBV) and cytomegalovirus (CMV) infection. The clinical manifestations of EBV and CMV mononucleosis depend on a vigorous host response to the viral infection. Patients who become infected without a host response develop antibodies to the virus but no or minimal clinical manifestations. Several clinical similarities exist between EBV and CMV mononucleosis. Both infections have a febrile prodrome before the mononucleosis phase develops. Both infections can induce fever, an enlarged spleen, and an erythematous skin rash–the mononucleosis phase. The disease is self-limited in the vast majority of patients, although resolution may take several weeks, especially in older individuals. In both viral infections, lymphocytes represent greater than 50 percent of blood cells, and at least 10 percent are reactive lymphocytes. Differences in clinical and laboratory findings are observed. Severe pharyngitis and tender lymph node enlargement, often in several lymph node groups, occur in infection with EBV and perhaps with some unknown agents, but not to the same degree in infections with CMV. The majority of cases of EBV mononucleosis occur in teenagers and young adults, whereas CMV-induced disease occurs most commonly in adults in their thirties to sixties. A much larger percentage of adults have unrecognized primary infection with CMV than with EBV. EBV results in the development of heterophile antibodies, active against sheep and horse red cells among others, but this development does not occur in CMV. The pathway leading to lymphocytosis and reactive lymphocytes differs between the two agents. The B cell is infected in EBV infection, which eventually may lead to hematologic malignancy, whereas the macrophage is infected in CMV. This may explain its important role posttransplantation. In both infections, the T lymphocyte is the reactive cell. Other agents, such as *Toxoplasma gondii*, human immune deficiency virus type 1, and several other viruses, can cause a mononucleosis-like syndrome with reactive lymphocytes in the blood.

DEFINITION AND HISTORY

The first clinical description of a syndrome resembling infectious mononucleosis was published in 1885 when Pfeiffer[1] described a disorder termed *Drüsenfieber* (glandular fever). In 1920, Sprunt and Evans[2] introduced the term *infectious mononucleosis* for an acute, self-limited syndrome of mononuclear leukocytosis in febrile patients. In 1932, Paul and Bunnell[3] showed that the sera from patients with infectious mononucleosis agglutinated red cells from sheep and horses, a reaction that was termed the *heterophile antibody test*. Paul had become interested in heterophile antibodies that were phylogenetically unrelated to the antigen with which they reacted, the so-called Forssmann antigen. For this reason, he was studying human sera that reacted with sheep red cells. He inadvertently found that the highest titer came from an individual recovering from infectious mononucleosis. Davidson showed that the heterophil antibody of infectious mononucleosis after absorption by guinea pig kidney cells, no longer reacted with sheep or horse cells. Guinea pig kidney absorption of serum made this test very specific for Epstein-Barr virus (EBV) infection.[4] In 1964, Epstein, Ashong, and Barr reported the isolation of a virus from the cells of a patient with African Burkitt lymphoma. The virus later was named after two of the investigators. The etiologic role of EBV in infectious mononucleosis was discovered serendipitously in the laboratory of Gertrude and Werner Henle.[5] A technician in their laboratory whose serum had been negative for EBV antibodies was restudied (as a control) after she recovered from infectious mononucleosis. Her serum was found to contain antibodies to EBV. The association later was confirmed by large seroepidemiologic studies in college students.[6–9]

Acronyms and abbreviations that appear in this chapter include: CMV, cytomegalovirus; EA, early antigen; EBNA, Epstein-Barr nuclear antigen; EBV, Epstein-Barr virus; HIV, human immunodeficiency virus; NK, natural killer; PCR, polymerase chain reaction; PTLD, posttransplantation lymphoproliferative disease; VCA, virus capsid antigen.

Much of the clinical nature and the incubation period of mononucleosis was documented by Hoagland,[10] in studies of cadets at West Point. His work led to mononucleosis being dubbed the "kissing disease," after he established that oral transmission was the principal route of viral transmission. He also noted that cadets developed the disease approximately 6 weeks after they returned from their vacation.[11]

Although EBV is the most common cause of infectious mononucleosis, other agents produce a febrile syndrome with a blood lymphocytosis that mimics some aspects of EBV mononucleosis.

ETIOLOGY AND PATHOGENESIS

The infectious mononucleosis syndrome is caused most commonly by one of two members of the herpes virus family: EBV or cytomegalovirus (CMV). Occasionally, the human immunodeficiency virus-1 (HIV) and, less commonly, the parasite *Toxoplasma gondii* produce a febrile illness with lymphocytosis. Other viral agents produce the blood picture of mononucleosis, but only infrequently (Table 84–1). After the early phase of fever, which lasts for 3 to 7 days, laboratory abnormalities include a blood lymphocyte proportion greater than 50 percent, often with greater than 10 percent reactive lymphocytes. Liver function test abnormalities that occur with cholestasis predominate over hepatocellular changes resulting in elevations in alkaline phosphatase and proportionately lower elevations in transaminases. Bilirubin elevation is uncommon in EBV infection in the young but occurs in the older patient, and is of similar frequency to that of CMV in the older age group. Severe jaundice is rare. Table 84–2 lists other complications of EBV and CMV mononucleosis.

FEATURES OF MONONUCEOSIS CAUSED BY EACH ETIOLOGIC AGENT

Distinct epidemiologic, clinical, and cytopathologic differences exist between EBV and CMV mononucleosis. However, those who develop CMV mononucleosis at a very young age (1–5 years) usually have pharyngitis and lymphadenopathy[12] at a similar frequency to those who develop EBV as young adults, as shown in Table 84–3. EBV occurs most commonly in the age group from 15 to 25 years, whereas CMV is more common in older individuals, often those older than age 50 years. The greatest clinical differences between EBV and CMV are manifest when comparing those whose disease occurs between ages 12 and 25 years. In the few older individuals in whom EBV occurs, EBV and

TABLE 84–1. Etiologic Agents Associated with Mononucleosis Syndrome

Epstein-Barr virus	Hepatitis A
Cytomegalovirus	Adenovirus
Human immunodeficiency virus	*Toxoplasma gondii*
Human herpes virus-6	*Bartonella henselae*
Metapneumovirus	*Brucella abortus*
Rubella	

CMV more closely resemble one another in their clinical manifestations. Finally, the target cell for infection in EBV is the B lymphocyte, whereas it is the macrophage in CMV. In both, the "mononucleosis" cell is the reactive T lymphocyte. CMV infection of the macrophage leads to its role in disease following transplant, especially in posttransplantation pneumonia. Table 84–3 compares the clinical manifestations of EBV infection with CMV infection in a young and old population. These are also detailed in the description that follows.

TABLE 84–3. Signs and Symptoms of Epstein-Barr Virus and Cytomegalovirus Mononucleosis: Effect of Age (Percent of Patients)

Signs and Symptoms	EBV (Age 14–35 Years*)	EBV (Age 40–72 Years†)	CMV (Age 30–70 Years‡)
Fever	95	94	85
Pharyngitis	95	46	15
Lymphadenopathy	98	49	24
Splenomegaly	65	33	3
Hepatomegaly	23	42	N/A
Jaundice	8	27	24

*Data from Hoagland RJ.[10]

†Data from Axelrod P and Finestone AJ;[30] Hurwitz CA, Henle W, Henle G, et al;[31] and Schmader KE, van der Horst CM, and Klotman ME.[32]

‡Data from Wreghitt TG, Teare O, Sule O, et al.[109]

EPSTEIN-BARR VIRUS MONONUCLEOSIS

VIROLOGY AND PATHOGENESIS

EBV is a DNA virus of the Gammaherpesvirinae subfamily. The virus is estimated to infect 90 percent of the world's population. Initially, EBV intercalates itself into the B cell and thereafter establishes lifelong residence in its host. It infects primarily the long-lived memory B cells and not naïve B cells.[13,14] Early after infection, the virus is continuously shed into oral secretions. Varying severity of disease ensues. The virus then usually undergoes latency, but it may be reactivated periodically.[15]

There is increasing evidence that host genetic factors are important in predicting the severity and duration of disease following primary EBV infection. Interferon-γ plus 874T/A and the interleukin-10–592C/A polymorphisms, acting together, are prominent genetic factors.[16] Persons with interferon-γ plus 874TT allele (high interferon producers) have a striking increase in frequency of high fever, fatigue, and myalgias (more severe illness) than do those with interferon-γ plus 874A allele and the interleukin-10-592 polymorphism. Other factors in host response, such as cytokine polymorphisms, also might influence the response to the infection.[17,18] Also, when EBV mononucleosis occurs between the ages of 12 and 25 years, some individuals with primary infection do not have a vigorous cellular response. Thus, if seronegative subjects are followed prospectively, when they develop immunoglobulin (Ig)M antibody to EBV as the method of diagnosis, they are less likely to have fever, pharyngitis, lymphocytosis, and elevated liver enzymes than patients of other age groups.[19]

In those who develop the classical syndrome, within a few days to 1 week after onset of EBV infection, T lymphocytes recognize viral replicative antigens on the infected B cell as foreign, and an exuberant polyclonal cytotoxic T-cell response ensues. CD8+ T cells are estimated to be approximately 50 percent of the population of cells proliferating per day, which translates into a population doubling time of 1.5 days, a rate that is approximately two orders of magnitude greater than normal.[20] The surface marker signaling lymphocyte activation molecule (SLAM)-associated protein (SAP) on T lymphocytes engenders cell activation in response to a signal from CD244 and CD150 (SLAM) on the T-cell surface.[21] In the healthy individual, the process and the signs and symptoms of the infection subside over days to weeks.

TABLE 84–2. Complications of Epstein-Barr Virus and Cytomegalovirus Mononucleosis

	EBV	CMV
Hemolytic anemia	++	+
Thrombocytopenia	+	+
Aplastic anemia	+	–
Splenic rupture	+	–
Jaundice (>age 25 years)	++	++
Guillain-Barré syndrome	+	++
Encephalitis*	++	+/–
Pneumonitis*	+/–	+
Myocarditis*	+	–
B-cell lymphoma	+	–
Agammaglobulinemia	+	–

++, Common; +, less common; +/–, uncommon; –, not observed; CMV cytomegalovirus; EBV, Epstein Barr virus.

*Can occur without the mononucleosis syndrome.

EPIDEMIOLOGY

Close contact is required for transmission. There is an apparent seasonal disease pattern with a peak incidence during summer months.[19] Epidemics rarely occur and perinatal infection and transmission from breast milk are very uncommon.[22] Frequent reactivation of EBV in the previously infected subject provides the opportunity for transmission at all ages. In the developing world and in the lowest socioeconomic strata of the developed world, nearly everyone is subclinically infected by age 5 years and mononucleosis is rarely clinically apparent. In the upper socioeconomic strata of the developed world, persons avoid infection in infancy; instead they become exposed to the virus between the ages of 12 and 25 years by contact with a latently infected asymptomatic individual. Characteristically, primary infection occurs in an individual a few months after he or she develops a relationship with an individual who has latent infection.[15] Individuals who are raised in more protected environments or in single-child families may reach an age of 30 years or older before they are infected. If both individuals in a relationship are seronegative, years may pass before they become infected, usually from their children. Individuals who are seropositive usually do not develop clinical disease upon reexposure, although a second infection with a different strain may occur.[23–25]

CLINICAL MANIFESTATIONS

Clinical manifestations vary by age.[12,26–32] When young children acquire infection with EBV, they develop a typical childhood illness of respiratory tract infection (43%), otitis media (29%), pharyngitis (21%), gastroenteritis (7%), or typical mononucleosis (<10%). Rashes and eyelid or periorbital swelling occur more frequently in younger children. In the classical presentation, in the age group 12 to 25 years, the earliest manifestations of disease—fever and lassitude—develop 30 to 45 days after patients become infected. Initial symptoms of pharyngitis, tonsillar enlargement, sometimes massive, and fever result from infection and proliferation of the B lymphocytes that are found in the Waldeyer ring. Infection occurs via virus attachment to the cell-surface CD21 glycoprotein, a 140-kDa complement receptor type 2. Infection induces polyclonal proliferation of infected B cells in the nodes of the pharynx. From the nodes of the pharynx, virus-infected cells make their way into the circulating lymphocyte pool.[33,34] Subsequent massive T-lymphocyte response to the neoantigens on infected B lymphocytes is evident by the lymphocytosis with reactive blood T lymphocytes and other disease manifestations, such as lymphadenopathy, hepatic inflammation, and splenomegaly.[35] Liver function abnormalities occur, although hyperbilirubinemia is very uncommon. The liver is not an organ rich in lymphocytes but CD4+ and CD8+ lymphocytes are trapped in the liver and their release of cytokines contributes to the hepatic inflammation. Hepatocytes are not damaged directly by EBV.[36] The frequency of each clinical finding of the typical syndrome in newly infected patients is variable (see Table 84–3).[11,19]

Group A streptococcus infection occurs occasionally in concert with an EBV primary infection. Several studies show that this concurrence is uncommon (3–4% of cases). Although treatment of the streptococcus eradicates the organism, the severe pharyngitis changes little, and the disease follows its usual course. Thus, treatment should be administered only if the test result for β-streptococcus is positive. If a penicillin-type antibiotic is used, a rash almost always develops[37,38] and the patient is erroneously diagnosed as "penicillin allergic." The patient should be re-evaluated after the mononucleosis resolves to determine if the patient has a true allergy to penicillin-type drugs.

The disease abates with the occurrence of a T-cell-mediated counter-response to the virus-induced polyclonal B-cell proliferation. During this time, dramatic clinical improvement can occur within 24 to 48 hours. Subsequently, EBV remains in the patient's B cells throughout life, but expresses only Epstein-Barr nuclear antigen-1 (EBNA-1), which does not elicit a T-cell response because of a glycine-alanine repeat that inhibits its processing.[39]

Most individuals become infected by age 25 years. However, if the individual has escaped infection until middle age or late adulthood, primary infection is much less likely to be accompanied by lymphadenopathy and pharyngitis (see Table 84–3).[30–32] Fever is present in almost all older patients. Abdominal pain, hepatomegaly, and liver function abnormalities occur in substantial proportions of patients, frequently leading to an initial clinical impression of hepatitis or an intraabdominal process, such as cholecystitis. Older adults have less-significant lymphocytosis and fewer reactive lymphocytes in the blood. Splenomegaly is less evident and the illness tends to be more protracted.

LABORATORY FINDINGS

Antibody Responses

A heterophile antibody response occurs in approximately 85 percent of cases by week 3 of illness. The rapid slide test for heterophil antibody may be falsely negative in approximately 6 percent of patients,[40] especially in young children.[26] The infection of the B cell elicits a polyclonal response. Among the clones expanded are those preprogrammed to make specific antibody, including antibodies against other infectious agents, such as, *Brucella, Chlamydia, Borrelia burgdorferi*, the yellow fever virus, and others. If the patient's disease is approached as a fever of unknown origin, the serologic results can be misleading. A variety of other antibodies also are produced nonspecifically because of polyclonal B cell activation. These antibodies include antiplatelet, antired cell (anti-i cold agglutinin), and antinuclear antibodies.

At the time clinical disease is evident, IgM and IgG antibodies to Epstein-Barr virus capsid antigen (VCA) are detectable. Later, antibody to early antigen (EA) develops. A small proportion of individuals will have antibody to EBNA-1 on presentation, but usually this appears during recovery. For patients suspected of having infectious mononucleosis but who do not have a positive heterophile antibody test result, a positive reaction for IgG and IgM antibodies to EBV and usually a negative antibody reaction to EBNA-1[41] are diagnostic of acute infection. A real-time polymerase chain reaction (PCR) is sometimes useful.[42]

Reactive Lymphocytosis

Expansion of cytotoxic T lymphocytes produces lymphocytosis. Reactive lymphocytes are larger than lymphocytes normally found in the blood (Fig. 84–1). They may have a vacuolated cytoplasm, lobulated, and eccentrically placed nucleus, and a cell membrane that often is indented by neighboring erythrocytes. A more darkly staining peripheral cytoplasm "skirting" occurs. Reactive lymphocytes are a hematologic hallmark of infectious mononucleosis, but they are not always found[19] and are not pathognomonic. They also are found in CMV infection, roseola (caused by human herpes virus-6), viral hepatitis, toxoplasmosis, rubella, mumps, and drug reactions.

Sheets of lymphocytes are noted on a stained slide preparation of tonsillar exudate. If β-streptococcal infection accompanies the EBV infection, segmented neutrophils are seen. The immunophenotype of lymphocytes in mononucleosis syndromes assessed by multiparametric flow cytometry has confirmed that lymphocytosis results from CD8+ T cells. CD4+ cells and B cells are not increased. In EBV mononucleosis, the notable populations increased are CD8+CD57– and CD3+$\gamma\delta$+ T cells.[43]

Other Blood Test Abnormalities

Liver function abnormalities are common, predominantly elevated serum alkaline phosphatase and γ-aminotransferase activity with no or only slight elevation of bilirubin in most patients. Studies in Israel found a higher frequency of hyperbilirubinemia (15%), a lower incidence of leukocytosis (46%), and elevated liver enzymes (58%) than previously reported, but the differences may be geographical or genetic. Lymphadenopathy and reactive lymphocytes were each noted in approximately 90 percent of the 590 young adults studied.[19]

COURSE AND PROGNOSIS

Complications of EBV Mononucleosis

Hematologic Virtually all subjects with acute mononucleosis develop a mildly decreased platelet count (see Table 84–2). More severe hematologic complications occur infrequently, but include severe immune thrombocytopenia with petechiae, immune hemolytic anemia, immune-mediated

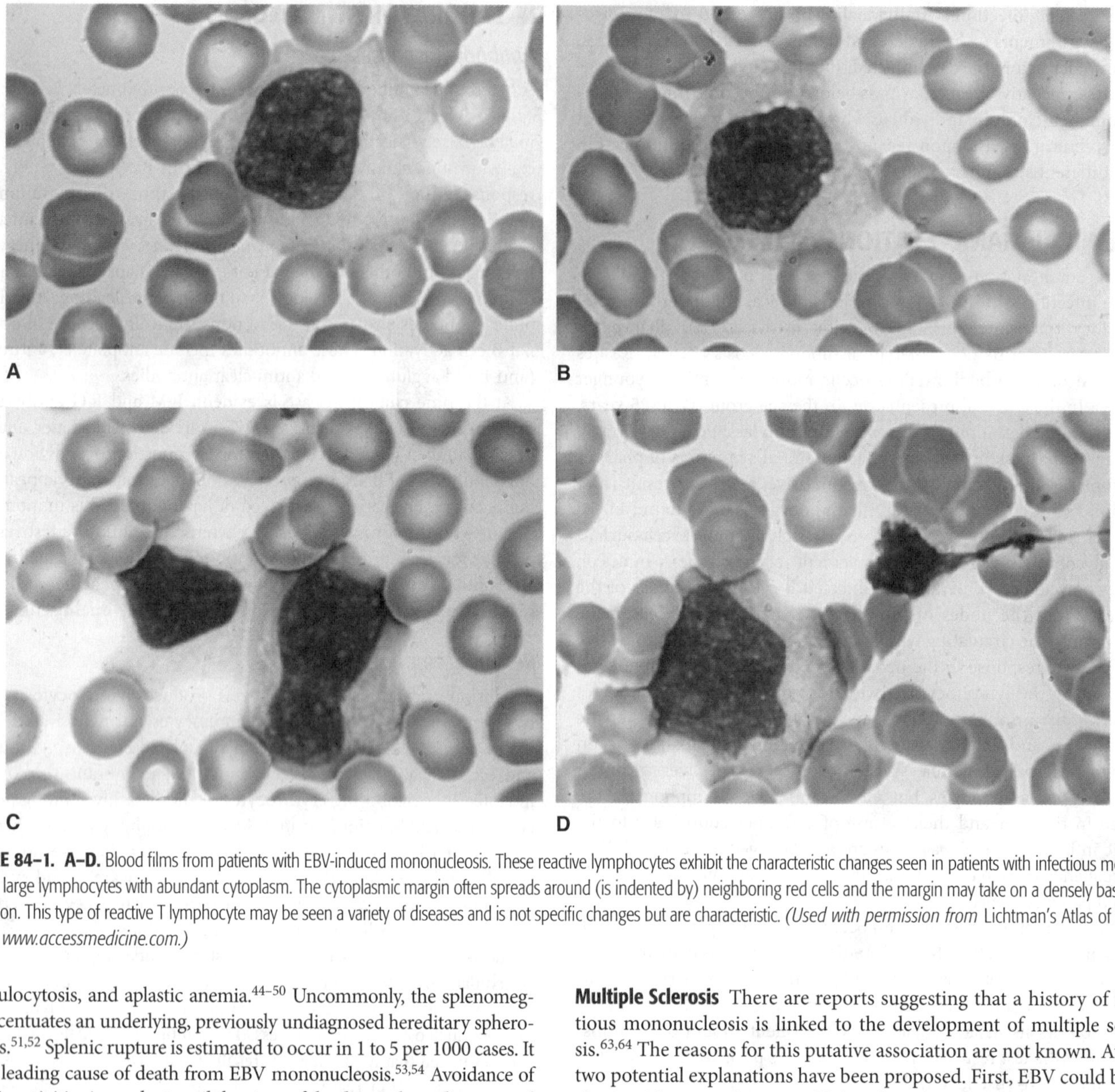

FIGURE 84–1. A–D. Blood films from patients with EBV-induced mononucleosis. These reactive lymphocytes exhibit the characteristic changes seen in patients with infectious mononucleosis: large lymphocytes with abundant cytoplasm. The cytoplasmic margin often spreads around (is indented by) neighboring red cells and the margin may take on a densely basophilic coloration. This type of reactive T lymphocyte may be seen a variety of diseases and is not specific changes but are characteristic. *(Used with permission from* Lichtman's Atlas of Hematology, *www.accessmedicine.com.)*

agranulocytosis, and aplastic anemia.[44–50] Uncommonly, the splenomegaly accentuates an underlying, previously undiagnosed hereditary spherocytosis.[51,52] Splenic rupture is estimated to occur in 1 to 5 per 1000 cases. It is the leading cause of death from EBV mononucleosis.[53,54] Avoidance of athletic activities is prudent until the signs of the disease have disappeared and the spleen has returned to normal size.[54]

Neurologic Neurologic complications include acute encephalitis, acute disseminated encephalomyelitis (*Alice in Wonderland* syndrome), acute cerebellar ataxia, viral meningitis, Guillain-Barré syndrome, transverse myelitis, and cranial nerve palsies.[49,50,55–57] There is evidence that antibodies to gangliosides play a role in the pathogenesis of Guillain-Barré syndrome.[58,59] Neurologic complications can occur in the absence of clinical mononucleosis. Diagnosis of EBV-induced disease requires studies of EBV-specific antibodies (see "Antibody Responses" above) and PCR for EBV on cerebrospinal fluid.[55] Neurologic disease can be associated with primary infection, reactivated infection, or chronic EBV infection.[55] Table 84–2 lists other complications.

Chronic Fatigue Most subjects with EBV mononucleosis recover completely fairly promptly. However, there are a few who remain fatigued for a very long period of time. The source of the fatigue is not certain but there is indirect evidence that it may be midbrain dysfunction. Furthermore, there were genetic associations found in those who have had prolonged fatigue.[60,61] There is also suggestive evidence that treatment of this small subset with antiviral agents leads to improvement.[62]

Multiple Sclerosis There are reports suggesting that a history of infectious mononucleosis is linked to the development of multiple sclerosis.[63,64] The reasons for this putative association are not known. At least two potential explanations have been proposed. First, EBV could be etiologic. Alternatively, it could be that those who have the genetic makeup that predisposes to a more severe mononucleosis following primary EBV infection have a similar vigorous response to CNS tissue.

Systemic Lupus Erythematosus and Rheumatoid Arthritis There are epidemiologic links between previous infection with EBV and development of systemic lupus erythematosus (SLE). Virtually everyone with lupus erythematosus has had previous infection with Epstein-Barr virus.[65] Because of the high incidence of EBV infection the link may be fortuitous. Alternatively, a history of infection with EBV might be involved with induction of autoimmunity.[66,67] There also has been suggested a relationship between increased EBV load in rheumatoid arthritis leading to an expansion of CD8+ cells and its consequences.[68]

Chronic Progressive EBV Infection, T or NK Lymphoproliferation, Lymphoma, and Hemophagocytic Syndrome Chronic EBV infection is a rare outcome of primary EBV infection.[69,70] In chronic EBV infection, fever, marrow hypoplasia, interstitial pneumonia, hepatosplenomegaly, persistent hepatitis often to the point of hepatic failure, lymphadenitis, and uveitis are frequent clinical manifestations. The syndrome may persist for months or years and has a relatively high fatality rate.[68] The EBV-related antibodies, including IgG to VCA, may be greater than 1:5120 and anti-EA greater than 1:640, accompanied by a low to undetectable EBNA-1 titer. A persistently high EBV load in circulating lymphocytes is measured by PCR for EBV DNA. The more severe form of the syndrome may evolve into an NK or T-cell lymphoproliferative disease[71–72] that ranges from chronic to fulminant.[72] EBV-induced hemophagocytic syndrome can be another concomitant feature of chronic active EBV infection. The latter disease is a severe multiorgan, inflammatory disease provoked by massive inflammatory cytokine elaboration and, in some cases, clonal lymphocyte expansion induced by EBV infection (discussed in Chap. 72).[73–75]

OTHER EBV-ASSOCIATED DISEASE PROCESSES

Neoplastic Potential of the Virus

EBV was the first human tumor virus identified, isolated from the cultured cells of a patient with African Burkitt lymphoma.[76] EBV can confer unlimited growth potential on infected B lymphocytes in culture.[77] EBV has since been associated with tumors other than Burkitt lymphoma, including approximately one-third of patients with Hodgkin lymphoma[78–81]; lymphoma in immunodeficient individuals, including the immunodeficiency state posttransplantation[82–84]; X chromosome-linked lymphoproliferative disease[85,86]; T-cell and NK-cell lymphomas that follow chronic EBV infection[87,88]; nasopharyngeal carcinoma in patients in the Far East[89,90]; leiomyomas and leiomyosarcomas in persons infected with HIV or immunodeficient posttransplantation[91,92]; and a small fraction of cases of gastric carcinoma[93] (Table 84–4). In the three principal lymphomas—Burkitt, Hodgkin, and posttransplantation—the cell that mutates to produce the clonal disease is a germinal-center B cell[94] with a circular viral genome in the tumor cells and the expression of EBV-encoded latent genes.[95]

EBV is detectable in the neoplastic B cells (Reed-Sternberg cells) of approximately 35 percent of patients with Hodgkin lymphoma.[78] The precise etiologic role of EBV in this subset of patients with Hodgkin lymphoma is uncertain.[81]

In the case of posttransplantation lymphoproliferative disease (PTLD), the most characteristic clinical pattern involves an EBV-seronegative person receiving an organ from an EBV-seropositive donor.[82] EBV is latent in the B lymphocytes of the transplanted marrow or solid organ. Immunosuppression allows reactivation of the virus. If the recipient is not immune there is no T-cell response and the B cells proliferate unchecked, sometimes eventuating in PTLD. Occasionally PTLD occurs in a subject known to be EBV seropositive pretransplantation, usually longer than 1 year posttransplantation.[82,83] In a recipient who was seronegative at the time of transplantation, disease usually becomes manifest within the first year after transplantation and often in the first few months. In its initial stages, the disease may respond to lowering the immunosuppressive medications. The abnormally proliferating cell almost always is a B cell and the process at an early stage may be monoclonal. Although antiviral prophylaxis seems to reduce the incidence of PTLD,[84] antiviral therapy is ineffective once the disease develops. Primary therapy is a reduction in immunosuppressive medications and use of anti-CD20 therapy with rituximab.

In young males with an X-linked lymphoproliferative syndrome, primary EBV infection leads to unabated B-cell proliferation and evolution into a frank B-cell lymphoma, the so-called Duncan syndrome.[85,86] These young males do not develop a T-cell response and hence do not develop mononucleosis. Although control of this effect of EBV infection by treatment with antiviral agents and/or chemotherapy has been attempted, the Duncan syndrome usually is fatal.

Oral hairy leukoplakia, a characteristic white lingual lesion with hairy projections seen in patients with HIV infection, results from EBV infection of the lingual epithelium.[96]

TABLE 84–4. Special Problems with Epstein-Barr Virus or Cytomegalovirus Infection

Epstein-Barr Virus	Cytomegalovirus
Rare congenital infection[133,134]	Congenital infection[104]
Chronic progressive mononucleosis[68–70]	Posttransplantation primary infection[107,112]
Hemophagocytic syndrome[73–75]	
X-linked B-cell lymphoma[85–86]	Graft-versus-host disease association[116]
Posttransplantation lymphoproliferative disease[82,83]	Transfusion-related infection[106]
T- or NK-cell lymphoproliferative disease[86–88]	*Aspergillus* and/or *Pneumocystis* infection[117,118]
African Burkitt lymphoma[76]	
Approximately 20% of Burkitt lymphoma in the United States[86]	
Approximately 35% of Hodgkin lymphoma[78–81,86]	
Nasopharyngeal carcinoma[89,90]	
Approximately 5% of gastric carcinoma[93]	
Leiomyoma and leiomyosarcoma in HIV or immunosuppressed patients[91,92]	
Oral hairy leukoplakia[96]	

FUTURE THERAPEUTIC APPROACHES TO EBV INFECTION AND NEOPLASIA

Because of the severe consequences of EBV infection, several approaches to preventing or treating these disorders are under way, such as development of an EBV vaccine,[97,98] adoptive transfer of activated cytotoxic T cells,[99] and the development of peptides that inhibit viral replication.[97]

CYTOMEGALOVIRUS MONONUCLEOSIS

HISTORY

The early description of CMV-related disease was that of an uncommon congenital syndrome with thrombocytopenia and petechiae and abnormal liver function tests.[101] Subsequently, primary CMV infection was recognized in previously healthy young children with abnormal liver function, hepatosplenomegaly, lymphocytosis, and thrombocytopenia.[102] Later, primary CMV infection was linked to a febrile mononucleosis syndrome.[103]

EPIDEMIOLOGY

In the developing world, CMV, like EBV, infects the majority of individuals at an early age for three reasons. Teenage mothers carrying CMV in their cervix transmit it to their newborn children and transmission also occurs through breast milk. Transmission from contact with infected young children also plays a role. As the individual ages, infection with CMV is acquired by several routes. Sexual transmission occurs because male semen has one of the highest concentrations of virus among the body fluids. It explains why nearly all homosexual males, but only 15 to 20 percent of heterosexual males, are infected by age 20 years and why increase in the incidence of primary infection occurs at a younger age in women then in men. This genital infection has no symptoms. If congenital infection occurs severe fetal abnormalities can occur (see below).[104]

In developed societies, transmission of infection also occurs when children congregate in settings such as daycare centers. For unexplained reasons, college-age individuals, except for homosexual males, are relatively resistant to primary CMV infection. In classic studies of students at Yale and at West Point[8,105] seroconversion reflecting CMV primary infection was rare, whereas annual seroconversion to EBV was high. Because of that difference there are a large number of susceptible subjects age 20 years and older in the developed world. Thus, primary CMV infection, unlike EBV, begins in the twenties and continues into the eighth decade. At least one of the reasons that primary infection occurs in the older population is that children in daycare centers acquire primary CMV infection from their playmates. They bring the virus home and then transmit it to parents or grandparents, thus accounting for primary CMV infection in adults. If the mother is pregnant, primary infection can lead to congenital CMV, which may be severe.[101] In grandparents, primary infection can lead to CMV mononucleosis, although the latter is uncommon. CMV can also be transmitted by blood transfusion or by a donated organ.[106–108]

CLINICAL MANIFESTATIONS

CMV has a broad spectrum of clinical manifestations.[109] The basic clinical disease is fever, often as high as 40°C (104°F), with a palpable spleen and laboratory abnormalities. Tables 84–2 and 84–3 list additional complications and clinical findings of CMV infection, respectively. Because no classic manifestation, such as severe exudative pharyngitis occurs, the disease often is not considered in the differential diagnosis. Fever, weight loss, and associated malaise and myalgia are common. As in EBV infection, administration of a penicillin can result in development of a rash that is not a reflection of future sensitivity to the drugs. Because the disease occurs in the older population, including those older than age 50 years, the causes of fever of unknown origin often are pursued in an expensive evaluation prior to the diagnosis.[110] The development of antinuclear factor and thrombocytopenia (Table 84–5) often results in an evaluation for a collagen-vascular disease or, because of the splenomegaly, for lymphoma. Similar studies as have been carried out in EBV suggest that host factors play a role in manifestation of CMV disease after infection.[111,112]

TABLE 84–5. Laboratory Findings in Mononucleosis

	EBV	CMV
Heterophile antibody	+++	–
Lymphocytosis	+++	++
Reactive lymphocytes	+++	++
Abnormal liver function	++	++
Antinuclear factor	+	+
Cold agglutinins	+	+
Cryoglobulins	+	+
Decreased platelets	++	+

+++, Characteristic; ++, common; +, occurs.

LABORATORY FINDINGS

Neutrophilia with band neutrophils in the blood can occur early in the infection. Lymphocytosis that develops later is indistinguishable from that of EBV. In the case of CMV, the macrophage[110] is the target cell infected and the lymphocyte responds to infection of that cell. Hence exudative pharyngitis, polyclonal antibody, and heterophile antibody response do not occur, but specific anti-CMV antibodies do develop. Because the incubation period ranges between 30 and 40 days, IgM and IgG antibodies to CMV usually are positive at presentation. The PCR of a blood sample for CMV usually is positive, and CMV can be isolated from urine or saliva specimens. Liver function changes mimic those of the older group of EBV primary infection (see Tables 84–2 and 84–3). Bilirubin elevation and jaundice may occur in up to 25 percent of patients.[109]

COMPLICATIONS

Hemolytic anemia and thrombocytopenia occur in primary CMV infection and are other factors that may lead the clinician initially to consider a diagnosis of lymphoma. The most prominent neurologic complications are Guillain-Barré syndrome and, less commonly, transverse myelitis and aseptic meningitis (see Table 84–2). The antibody that develops to CMV-infected cells cross-reacts with GM2 antigen, which may explain the development of the Guillain-Barré syndrome in some patients. This antibody can be adsorbed from the plasma of patients with Guillain-Barré syndrome by CMV-infected, but not uninfected, fibroblasts.[59,113]

The macrophage is the cell infected with CMV.[114] A T-cell response to the macrophage neoantigen leads to reactive lymphocytosis. Because of the mechanism provoking T-cell response, evolution to unrestrained B-cell replication, lymphoma, and PTLD do not occur.

THE COMPROMISED HOST AND CMV

Primary CMV infection is a major problem in solid-organ transplantation. There are two explanations for this phenomenon. First, CMV infects all the major organs during primary infection. It then evolves to a latent state, presumably in the parenchymal cells. The highest risk for symptomatic infection occurs when a CMV-seronegative recipient receives an organ from a seropositive donor.[107,108] CMV latent in tissue macrophages can reactivate as a result of immunosuppression. Two phenomena may result. The first occurs when a seronegative recipient gets a solid organ donation from a person who is seropositive. The classic situation involves a parent donating a kidney to a seronegative child.[115] Infection may lead to organ-specific rejection and CMV-induced bowel disease in recipients. Superinfection for the seropositive recipient is less of a problem. Seronegative solid-organ recipients from a CMV-seropositive donor who receive ganciclovir prophylaxis for the first 3 months posttransplantation often present several months after discontinuing prophylaxis with late CMV disease, manifesting as severe diarrhea and cytomegalic inclusion cells in their colon. In addition, the pretransplantation seropositive patient who is treated posttransplantation with immunoregulatory agents such as antithymocyte globulin (ATG) may develop severe CMV disease as a result. It is common practice to provide ganciclovir with the ATG. The other phenomenon is an alteration of the surface antigen of tissue macrophages in transplanted organs. When CMV is reactivated the tissue it is in may behave like a "foreign tissue" to which the host responds, resulting in rejection or disease in that organ. The pulmonary macrophage is an example. Seronegative recipients of a lung transplant are the only solid organ recipients who frequently develop CMV pneumonia. This reaction is thought to be the result of reactivated CMV making the pulmonary macrophage a target for the recipient's immune response with consequent cytokine release and lung disease.[116–118]

In allogeneic stem cell transplantation, the situation is somewhat reversed. A higher risk occurs if the donor is negative and the recipient of the transplant was previously infected with CMV. The donor cells undergo primary infection. The recipient reactivates their CMV, which replicates in pulmonary macrophages. The previously uninfected donor T cells may recognize neoantigens on the infected macrophages and respond to the neoantigens. Thus, pneumonitis develops in concert with graft-versus-host disease. Once pneumonia becomes manifest, both immunoglobulin and ganciclovir are required to control this process.[116] IgG 400 mg/kg administered once per week for 4 weeks and ganciclovir 5 mg/kg every 12 hours for 2 weeks then once per day for 2 weeks is one of several approaches to therapy, depending on circumstances. However, antiviral therapy alone when given at the first sign of CMV in the blood detected by PCR prevents the development of pneumonia. For slightly different reasons, lung transplant recipients are at higher risk for CMV pneumonitis. The donor's CMV reactivates in the pulmonary macrophage and the recipient's immune cells in turn react against infected macrophages, releasing cytokines eventuating in pneumonitis.

In all of the above settings, CMV can produce a syndrome of fever, leukopenia, and inflammatory gastrointestinal disease. Clinically significant CMV infection often is followed by other opportunistic infections, such as *Pneumocystis carinii* or *Aspergillus* spp. (see Table 84–4).[117,118] Two approaches have been taken to prevent CMV-induced disease in the early posttransplantation period. One is treatment with ganciclovir for 90 days from the time of transplantation. The other method is monitoring for evidence of CMV infection either by measuring circulating CMV antigen or CMV DNA using quantitative PCR. Therapy with ganciclovir is initiated when evidence for infection is detected. No trial comparing these two approaches has been conducted, but use of the latter approach leads to treatment of far fewer subjects and a shorter course of therapy among the treated patients.

Other compromised populations where CMV plays a role is in the rapidity of progression of CD4 lymphocyte depletion in the HIV infected subject and in the otherwise normal host in the intensive care unit setting.

PRIMARY HIV INFECTION

At the time of development of primary infection with HIV, an acute syndrome develops.[119–123] The frequency with which the HIV mononucleosis syndrome develops is uncertain, but for this discussion the difference in features is more important (Table 84–6). Fever is sudden in onset, followed by sore throat, lymphadenopathy, tonsillar hypertrophy, painful oral ulcerations, conjunctivitis, and rash. Nausea, vomiting, and diarrhea also occur. Leukopenia, thrombocytopenia, a relative increase in band neutrophils, and a small proportion of reactive lymphocytes usually can be identified on the blood film. Although absolute lymphocytosis is uncommon, the syndrome is referred to as *HIV mononucleosis*. Uncommonly, patients may also develop a heterophile antibody. Among a group of 563 heterophile antibody-positive patient samples retrospectively tested for HIV-1 RNA and p24 antigen, approximately 1 percent had evidence of primary HIV-1 infection.[121] In another study, none of 132 cases was positive.[122] The acute retroviral syndrome must be recognized for both the patient's health and the public health. In this situation, before an anti-HIV antibody response develops, HIV load in the blood should be measured by PCR to make a diagnosis of HIV infection. Usually, viral load is very high (greater than 50,000 viral particles per milliliter of blood). Early treatment may reduce the incidence of HIV-1 complications (see Chap. 83). Acute

TABLE 84–6. Clinical Findings in Primary HIV Infection

Finding	Frequency (%)
Fever	79
Pharyngitis	48
Oral ulcers	29
Lymphadenopathy	44
Splenomegaly	5
Hepatomegaly	<1
Reactive lymphocytes	Uncommon

HIV-1 infection may be particularly contagious. Physician intervention may prevent further transmission.

OTHER AGENTS LINKED TO THE MONONUCLEOSIS SYNDROME

Human herpes virus-6 occasionally has been associated with a mononucleosis-type picture as has metapneumovirus (see Table 84–1).[124–125] Hepatitis A and rubella virus infection have produced the typical lymphocytic changes. Pharyngitis is not a prominent feature in patients infected with *T. gondii*. Lymphocytosis is mild, and liver functions are normal even when the liver is enlarged. Usually toxoplasmosis presents as posterior cervical lymphadenopathy. In the United States, exposure to oocysts from cat feces is the primary route of infection. In overseas countries, ingestion of partially cooked meat, especially from sheep, is a route of infection. The IgM immunofluorescent antibody test for *T. gondii* is useful in diagnosing the disease.

Catscratch disease, *Corynebacterium diphtheriae* pharyngitis, infection with brucellosis, and lymphoma can be mistaken for mononucleosis. Other as yet unidentified agents probably produce the classic syndrome because laboratory studies do not implicate one of the several agents in a small percentage of mononucleosis cases.

DIFFERENTIAL DIAGNOSIS

At a very young age, EBV and CMV mimic one another presenting as one of the many febrile illnesses in young children.[12] The difference here, compared to other viral illness, is that these children develop abnormal liver function tests. The importance of establishing a diagnosis rests in the ability then to prevent transmission to a pregnant mother who might not be immune. By so doing, a severe congenital CMV infection may be avoided.[104] That possibility is much more likely for CMV as only 20 percent of young women have been infected before they reach reproductive age. In the older, teenage child, both EBV and CMV may cause the mononucleosis-like illness, but the former is far more common. The presence of exudative pharyngitis plays a critical role in the differential diagnosis. In the individual who is sexually active between the ages of 15 and 25 years and who has a febrile illness with lymphadenopathy, evidence for infection with EBV and HIV should be sought, but CMV remains a possibility.[103] Simultaneous infection with HIV and EBV, although not common, may occur. Mononucleosis-like changes in blood lymphocytes occur in HIV but are uncommon. Exudative pharyngitis suggests infection by EBV rather than by HIV, whereas intraoral ulcers suggest infection with HIV. Rarely, heterophile antibodies occur in conjunction with primary HIV.[121,122]

β-Hemolytic streptococcus, adenovirus, or *Arcanobacterium haemolyticum* also can produce exudative pharyngitis.

In adults in their thirties or forties, mononucleosis more likely results from infection with CMV than EBV simply because the vast majority of individuals in this age group have already been infected by EBV. Absence of exudative pharyngitis points to CMV although some with primary EBV may lack this finding; however, HIV must be considered in this age group. Patients infected with either CMV or HIV can present with blood neutrophilia with an increased proportion of band neutrophils. Rash or aseptic meningitis is more common in patients infected with HIV than CMV. In the middle-aged patient, primary CMV infection is by far the most important possibility, although the unusual individual who has escaped infection with EBV earlier in life can present with clinical manifestations similar to patients with primary CMV infection at that age.[30–32]

THERAPY AND COURSE

For the majority of patients with primary CMV or EBV infection, treatment is supportive. Salicylates or other analgesics are appropriate for control of fever, headache, and sore throat. Splenic rupture can occur in the first few weeks after diagnosis. Thus, contact sports should be avoided until the spleen has returned to normal size. The vast majority of subjects improve and have resolution of most symptoms. Almost half of patients recovering from EBV mononucleosis still feel fatigued at 60 days and a small percent at 6 months. Severe fatigue can persist after CMV mononucleosis also.

Antiviral or glucocorticoid therapy may be considered in special settings for treatment of EBV mononucleosis. The nucleoside analogue acyclovir blocks EBV replication through inhibition of viral DNA polymerase and can prevent viral shedding from the oropharynx.[126,127] However, acyclovir has little, if any, effect on the course of mononucleosis, presumably because the disease at that point results from the immunopathologic process and not virus proliferation. Antiviral therapy may be useful in chronic aggressive EBV infection and in EBV infection posttransplantation. Glucocorticoids have been used for management of specific complications. Their specific benefit is difficult to determine because glucocorticoids often are started only late in the clinical course, when immunologic reaction to infection is leading to improvement and the response is credited to the treatment. One carefully controlled trial showed little benefit from glucocorticoids, and the treated group did less well at 30 days than the placebo group.[128] Nevertheless, treatment with glucocorticoid is indicated when the tonsils are touching in the midline and airway obstruction is imminent. For impending airway obstruction in patients with EBV, prednisone 40 to 60 mg/day can be given for 7 to 10 days, then rapidly tapered once a clinical response is achieved. Urgent tonsillectomy and adenoidectomy may be required.[129] The same regimen is used for severe immune hemolytic anemia (see Chap. 53), severe symptomatic immune thrombocytopenia (see Chap. 119),[130–132] neurologic complications, pancreatitis, and myocarditis.

The same dose of glucocorticoid has been used for the hematologic or neurologic complications of CMV mononucleosis. Ganciclovir, 5 mg/kg per day, given intravenously for 14 days for severe CMV mononucleosis occasionally has resulted in excellent responses. However, ganciclovir is seldom used because of the potential long-term risk to spermatogenesis (aspermia) or potentially on female fertility. Antiretroviral therapy has been suggested for severe HIV primary disease. However, when the disease appears to be self-limited, many therapists do not begin therapy. Therapy that already was started is stopped after a few weeks.

Acyclovir use for other manifestations of EBV infection not resulting from host response but from a high titer of EBV replication, such as the oral hairy leukoplakia of AIDS, rapidly resolves the lingual lesions.[131] However, treatment with acyclovir does not appear to be effective for the carrier state.[132]

MONONUCLEOSIS IN PREGNANCY

EBV and CMV Infection

When EBV mononucleosis occurs during pregnancy, severe congenital abnormalities similar to those described in primary CMV infection during pregnancy can occur (see Table 84–4).[133,134] Microcephaly, mental retardation, cataracts, hepatosplenomegaly, and fetal loss or postnatal death have been described. For CMV, immunity does not necessarily protect against congenital infection. Two percent of livebirths in all societies are infected at the time of birth as manifested by viruria, but most of the newborns are asymptomatic at birth. Some go on to develop unilateral or bilateral hearing loss. The fact that high titers of CMV are found in semen and that infection and conception may occur simultaneously may explain the failure of protection. If primary CMV infection occurs during gestation, severe abnormalities similar to those produced by EBV noted above may occur.[104] Antiviral therapy with famciclovir or valacyclovir has been used for EBV primary infection during pregnancy, but the number of patients treated is too small to draw conclusions. Ganciclovir for primary CMV infection is being studied. It is, however, well documented that cervical- or breast-milk-acquired infection does not lead to symptomatic disease or hearing loss.

HIV Infection

Primary infection with HIV during pregnancy is seldom recognized because HIV antibody is absent early in infection and the antibody screening process is performed at the first prenatal visit. If suspicion of primary infection is raised during pregnancy, then viral load should be measured. If positive, antiretroviral therapy for the mother to prevent HIV transmission to the fetus or newborn is indicated.[135]

Toxoplasma Infection

T. gondii producing primary infection during pregnancy can lead to congenital abnormalities. Although no controlled trials are available, treatment of the mother with pyrimethamine plus sulfonamides or spiramycin may eradicate parasites from the infant and the placenta.[136–137]

REFERENCES

1. Pfeiffer E: Drüsenfieber. *Jahrbuch für Kinderheilkunde* 23:257, 1885.
2. Sprunt TP, Evans FA: Mononucleosis in reaction to acute infections ("infectious mononucleosis"). *Johns Hopkins Bull* 31:410, 1920.
3. Paul JR, Bunnell WW: The presence of heterophile antibodies in infectious mononucleosis. *Am J Med Sci* 183:91, 1932.
4. Davidson I, Walker PH: The nature of the heterophile antibodies in infectious mononucleosis. *Am J Clin Pathol* 5:455, 1935.
5. Henle G, Henle W, Diehl V: Relation of Burkitt's tumor associated herpes type virus to infectious mononucleosis. *Proc Natl Acad Sci U S A* 59:94, 1968.
6. Niederman JC, McCollum RW, Henle G, et al: Infectious mononucleosis: Clinical manifestations in relation to EB virus antibodies. *JAMA* 203:205, 1968.
7. Evans AS, Niederman JC, McCollum RW: Seroepidemiologic studies of infectious mononucleosis with EB virus. *N Engl J Med* 279:1121, 1968.
8. Sawyer RN, Evans AS, Niederman JC, et al: Prospective studies of a group of Yale University freshman: I. Occurrence of infectious mononucleosis. *J Infect Dis* 123:263 1971.
9. University Health Physicians, PHLS Laboratories: A joint investigation of infectious mononucleosis and it relationship to EB virus antibody. *Br Med J* 4:643 1971.

10. Hoagland RJ: The clinical manifestations of infectious mononucleosis: A report of 200 cases. *Am J Med Sci* 240:55, 1960.
11. Hoagland RJ: The incubation period of infectious mononucleosis. *Am J Public Health* 54:1699, 1964.
12. Lajo A, Borque C, Del Castillo F, Martin-Ancel A: Mononucleosis caused by Epstein-Barr virus and cytomegalovirus in children: A comparative study of 124 cases. *Pediatr Infect Dis J* 13(1):56, 1994.
13. Macsween KF, Crawford DH: Epstein-Barr virus-recent advances. *Lancet Infect Dis* 3:131, 2003.
14. Hochberg D, Souza T, Catalina M, et al: Acute infection with Epstein-Barr virus targets and overwhelms peripheral memory B-cell compartment with resting, latently infected cells. *J Virol* 78:5194, 2004.
15. Yao QY, Rickinson AB, Epstein MA: A re-examination of the Epstein-Barr virus carrier state in healthy seropositive individuals. *Int J Cancer* 35:35, 1985.
16. McAuley KA, Higgins CD, Macsween KF, et al: HLA class I polymorphisms are associated with development of infectious mononucleosis upon primary EBV infection. *J Clin Invest* 117(10):3042, 2007.
17. Vollmer-Conner U, Piraino B, Cameron B, et al: Cytokine polymorphisms have a synergistic effect on the acute sickness response to infection. *Clin Infect Dis* 47:1418, 2008.
18. Scherrenburg J, Piriou ER, Nantohy NM, Baarle D: Detailed analysis of Epstein-Barr virus specific CD4+ and CD8+ T cell response during infectious mononucleosis. *Clin Exp Immunol* 153(2):231, 2008.
19. Grotto I, Mimouni D, Huerta M, et al: Clinical and laboratory presentation of EBV positive infectious mononucleosis in young adults. *Epidemiol Infect* 131:683, 2003.
20. Macallan DC, Wallace DL, Irvine AJ, et al: Rapid turnover of T cells in acute infectious mononucleosis. *Eur J Immunol* 33:2655, 2003.
21. Williams H, Macsween K, McAulay K, et al: Analysis of immune activation and clinical events in acute infectious mononucleosis. *J Infect Dis* 190:63, 2004.
22. KusuHara K, Takabayashi A, Ueda k, et al: Breast milk is not a significant source of early Epstein-Barr virus or human herpes 6 infection in infants: A sero-epidemiologic study in 2 endemic areas of human T-cell lymphotropic virus type 1 in Japan. *Microbiol Immunol* 41(4):309, 1997.
23. Sixbey JW, Shirley P, Chesney PJ, et al: Detection of a second widespread strain of Epstein-Barr virus. *Lancet* 2:76, 1989.
24. Yao QY, Croom-Carter DSG, Tierney RJ, et al: Epidemiology of infection with Epstein-Barr virus types 1 and 2: Lessons from the study of a T cell immunocompromised hemophiliac cohort. *J Virol* 72:4352, 1998.
25. Pichler R, Berg J, Hengstschlager A, et al: Recurrent infectious mononucleosis caused by Epstein-Barr virus with persistent splenomegaly. *Mil Med* 166:733, 2001.
26. Sumaya CV, Ench Y: Epstein-Barr virus infectious mononucleosis in children: I. Clinical and general laboratory findings. *Pediatrics* 75:1003, 1985.
27. Sumaya CV, Ench Y: Epstein-Barr virus infectious mononucleosis in children: II. Heterophil antibody and viral specific responses. *Pediatrics* 75:1011, 1985.
28. Fleisher G, Henle W, Henle G, et al: Primary infection with Epstein-Barr virus in infants in the United States: Clinical and serologic observations. *J Infect Dis* 139:553 1979.
29. Hickey SM, Strasburger VC: What every pediatrician should know about infectious mononucleosis in adolescents. *Pediatr Clin North Am* 44:1541, 1997.
30. Axelrod P, Finestone AJ: Infectious mononucleosis in older adults. *Am Fam Physician* 42:1599, 1990.
31. Hurwitz CA, Henle W, Henle G, et al: Infectious mononucleosis in patients aged 40 to 72 years: Report of 27 cases, including 3 without heterophile-antibody responses. *Medicine (Baltimore)* 62:256, 1983.
32. Schmader KE, van der Horst CM, Klotman ME: Epstein-Barr virus and the elderly host. *Rev Infect Dis* 11:64, 1989.
33. Karajannis MA, Hummel M, Anagnostopoulos I, Stein H: Strict lymphotropism of Epstein-Barr virus during acute infectious mononucleosis in non-immunocompromised individuals. *Blood* 89:2856, 1997.
34. Yefenof E, Bakacs T, Einhorn L, et al: Epstein-Barr virus (EBV) receptors, complement receptors and EBV infectibility of different lymphocyte fractions of human peripheral blood: I. Complement receptor distribution and complement binding by separated lymphocyte subpopulations. *Cell Immunol* 35:34, 1978.
35. Thorley-Lawson DA: Immunological responses to Epstein-Barr virus infection and the pathogenesis of EBV-induced disease. *Biochim Biophys Acta* 948:263, 1988.
36. Drebber U, Kasper HU, Krupacz J, et al: The role of Epstein-Barr virus in acute and chronic hepatitis. *J Hepatol* 44:879, 2006.
37. Renn CN, Straff W, Dorfmuller A, et al: Amoxicillin-induced exanthema in young adults with infectious mononucleosis: Demonstration of drug-specific lymphocyte reactivity. *Br J Dermatol* 147:1166, 2002.
38. Haverkos HW, Amsel Z, Drotman DP: Adverse virus-drug interactions. *Rev Infect Dis* 13:697, 1991.
39. Levitskaya J, Coram M, Levitsky V, et al: Inhibition of antigen processing by the internal repeat region of the Epstein-Barr virus nuclear antigen-1 *Nature* 375:685, 1995.
40. Linderholm M, Boman J, Juto P, Linde A: Comparative evaluation of nine kits for rapid diagnosis of infectious mononucleosis and Epstein-Barr virus-specific serology. *J Clin Microbiol* 32:259, 1994.
41. Rea TD, Ashley TL, Russo JE, Buchwald DS: A systematic study of Epstein-Barr virus serologic assays following acute infection. *Am J Clin Pathol* 117:156, 2002.
42. Pitetti RD, Laus S, Wadowsky RM: Clinical evaluation of a quantitative realtime polymerase chain reaction assay for diagnosis of primary Epstein-Barr virus infection in children. *Pediatr Infect Dis J* 22:736, 2003.
43. Hudnall SD, Patel JU, Schwab H, Martinez J: Comparative immunophenotypic features of EBV-positive and EBV-negative atypical lymphocytosis. *Cytometry* 55B:22, 2003.
44. Matsukawa Y, Okano M, Ishikawa N, Imasi S: Severe thrombocytopenic purpura associated with primary Epstein-Barr virus infection. *J Infect* 29:107, 1994.
45. Whitelaw F, Brook MG, Kennedy N, Weir WR: Haemolytic anemia complicating Epstein-Barr virus infection. *Br J Clin Pract* 49:212, 1995.
46. Lazarus KH, Baehner RL: Aplastic anemia complicating infectious mononucleosis: A case report and review of the literature. *Pediatrics* 67:907, 1981.
47. Auvin S, Dalle JH, Ganga-Zandzou PS, Ythier H: Is agranulocytosis following infectious mononucleosis caused by autoimmunity? *Pediatr Hematol Oncol* 20:611, 2003.
48. Tanaka M, Kamijo T, Koike T, et al: Specific autoantibodies to platelet glycoprotein in Epstein-Barr virus-associated immune thrombocytopenia. *Int J Hematol* 78:168, 2003.
49. Evans AS: Infectious mononucleosis and related syndromes. *Am J Med Sci* 276:325, 1978.
50. Jones JF: A perspective on Epstein-Barr virus diseases. *Adv Pediatr* 36:307, 1989.
51. Bhaskaran J, Harkness DR: Hereditary spherocytosis unmasked by infectious mononucleosis with autoimmune hemolytic anemia. *J Fla Med Assoc* 67:483, 1980.
52. Taylor JJ: Haemolysis in infectious mononucleosis: Inapparent congenital spherocytosis. *Br Med J* 4:525, 1973.
53. Asgari MM, Begos DG: Spontaneous splenic rupture in infectious mononucleosis: A review. *Yale J Biol Med* 70:175, 1997.
54. Kinderknecht JJ: Infectious mononucleosis and the spleen. *Curr Sports Med Rep* 1:116, 2002.
55. Fujimoto H, Asaoka K, Imaaizumi T, et al: Epstein-Barr virus infections of the central nervous system. *Intern Med* 42:33, 2003.
56. Connelly KP, DeWitt LD: Neurologic complications of infectious mononucleosis. *Pediatr Neurol* 10:181, 1994.
57. Jacobs BC, Rothbarth PH, van der Meché FG, et al: The spectrum of antecedent infections in Guillain-Barré syndrome. *Neurology* 51:1110, 1998.
58. Hughes RA, Hadden RD, Gregson NA, Smith KJ: Pathogenesis of Guillain-Barré syndrome. *J Neuroimmunol* 100:74, 1999.
59. Ang CW, Jacobs BC, Laman JD: The Guillain-Barré syndrome: a true case of molecular mimicry. *Trends Immunol* 25:61, 2004.
60. Cameron B, Galbraith S, Zhang Y, et al: Gene expression correlates of post fatigue syndrome after infectious mononucleosis *J Infect Dis* 196:56, 2007.
61. Lerner AM, Benqaj SM, Deeter RG, Fitzgerald JT: Valacyclovir treatment in Epstein-Barr virus subset chronic fatigue syndrome—36 month follow up. *In Vivo* 21(5):707, 2007.
62. White PD: What causes prolonged fatigue after infectious mononucleosis—And does it tell us anything about chronic fatigue syndrome? *J Infect Dis* 196:4, 2007.
63. Thacker EL, Mirzaei F, Ascherio A: Infectious mononucleosis and risk for multiple sclerosis: A meta-analysis. *Ann Neurol* 59(3):499, 2006.
64. Zaadstra BM, Chorus AM, van Buuren S, et al: Selective association of multiple sclerosis with infectious mononucleosis. *Mult Scler* 14(3):307, 2008.
65. James JA, Neas BR Moser KL, et al: Systemic lupus in adults is associated with previous Epstein-Barr virus exposure. *Arthritis Rheum* 44(5):1122, 2001.
66. Harley JB, Harley IT, Guthridge JM, James JA: The curiously suspicious: a role of Epstein-Barr virus in lupus. *Lupus* 15(11):768, 2006.
67. Lunemann JD, Frey O, Eidner T, et al: Increased frequency of EBV-specific effector memory CD8+ T cells correlates with higher viral load in rheumatoid arthritis. *J Immunol* 181(2):991, 2008.
68. Kimura H, Morishima T, Kanegane H, et al: Prognostic factors for chronic active Epstein-Barr virus infection. *J Infect Dis* 187:527, 2003.
69. Buchwald DS, Rea TD, Katon WJ, et al: Acute infectious mononucleosis: Characteristics of patients who report failure to recover. *Am J Med* 109:531, 2000.
70. Okano M: Overview and problematic standpoints of severe chronic active Epstein-Barr virus infection syndrome. *Crit Rev Oncol Hematol* 44:273, 2002.
71. Ohga S, Monura A, Takada H, Hara T: Immunological aspects of Epstein-Barr virus infection. *Crit Rev Oncol Hematol* 44:203, 2002.
72. Suzuki K, Ohshima K, Karube K, et al: Clinicopathological states of Epstein-Barr virus-associated T/NK cell proliferative disorders (severe chronic active EBV infection) of children and young adults. *Int J Oncol* 24:1165, 2004.
73. Chen CJ, Huang YC, Jaing TH, et al: Hemophagocytic syndrome: A review of 18 pediatric cases. *J Microbiol Immunol Infect* 37:157, 2004.
74. Imashuku S, Kuriyama K, Sakai R, et al: Treatment of Epstein-Barr virus-associated hemophagocytic lymphohistiocytosis (EBV-HLH) in young adults: A report from HLH study center. *Med Pediatr Oncol* 41:103, 2003.
75. Imashuku S, Teramura T, Tauchi H, et al: Longitudinal follow-up of patients with Epstein-Barr virus-associated hemophagocytic lymphohistiocytosis. *Haematologica* 89:183, 2004.
76. Pagano JS: Epstein-Barr virus: The first human tumor virus and its role in cancer. *Proc Assoc Am Physicians* 111:573, 1999.
77. Endo R, Kikuta H, Ebihara T, et al: Possible involvement in oncogenesis of a single base mutation in internal ribosome entry site of Epstein-Barr nuclear antigen 1 mRNA. *J Med Virol* 72:630, 2004.

78. Flavell KJ, Murray PG: Hodgkin disease and Epstein-Barr virus. *Mol Pathol* 53:262, 2000.
79. Hjalgrim H, Askling J, Rostgaard K, et al: Characteristics of Hodgkin's lymphoma after infectious mononucleosis. *N Engl J Med* 349:1324, 2003.
80. Jarrett RF: Risk factors for Hodgkin lymphoma by EBV status and significance of detection of EBV genomes in serum of patients with EBV-associated Hodgkin's lymphoma. *Leuk Lymphoma* 44(Suppl 3):S27, 2003.
81. Jarrett RF, Stark GL, White J, et al: Impact of tumor Epstein-Barr virus status on presenting features and outcome in age-defined subgroups of patients with classic Hodgkin lymphoma: A population-based study. *Blood* 106(7):2444, 2005.
82. Zangwill SD, Hsu DT, Kichuk MR, et al: Incidence and outcome of Epstein-Barr virus infection and lymphoproliferative disease in pediatric heart transplant recipients. *J Heart Lung Transplant* 17:1161, 1998.
83. Gao SZ, Chapparro SV, Perlroth M, et al: Post-transplant lymphoproliferative disease in heart and heart-lung transplant recipients: 30-year experience at Stanford University. *J Heart Lung Transplant* 22:505, 2003.
84. Malouf MA, Chajed PN, Hopkins P, et al: Anti-viral prophylaxis reduces the incidence of lymphoproliferative disease in lung transplant recipients. *J Heart Lung Transplant* 21:547, 2002.
85. MacGinnitie AJ, Geha R: X-linked lymphoproliferative disease: Genetic lesions and clinical consequences. *Curr Allergy Asthma Rep* 2:361, 2002.
86. Cohen JI: Benign and malignant Epstein-Barr virus-associated B-cell lymphoproliferative diseases. *Semin Hematol* 40:116, 2003.
87. Yachie A, Kanegane H, Kasahara Y: Epstein-Barr virus associated T-/natural killer cell lymphoproliferative diseases. *Semin Hematol* 40:124, 2003.
88. Kawa K, Okamura T, Yasui M, et al: Allogeneic hematopoietic stem cell transplantation for Epstein-Barr virus-associated T/NK-cell lymphoproliferative disease. *Crit Rev Oncol Hematol* 44:251, 2002.
89. Cheng WM, Chan KH, Chen HL, et al: Assessing the risk of nasopharyngeal cancer on the basis of EBV antibody spectrum. *Int J Cancer* 97:489, 2002.
90. Moss DJ, Khanna R, Bharadwaj M: Will a vaccine to nasopharyngeal carcinoma retain orphan status? *Dev Biol* 110:67, 2002.
91. McClain K, Leach CT, Jenson HB, et al: Association of Epstein-Barr virus with leiomyosarcomas in young people with AIDS. *N Engl J Med* 332:12, 1995.
92. Lee ES, Locker J, Nalesnik M, et al: The association of Epstein-Barr virus with smooth muscle tumors occurring after organ transplantation. *N Engl J Med* 332:19, 1995.
93. Oda K, Koda K, Takiguchi N, et al: Detection of Epstein-Barr virus in gastric carcinoma cells and surrounding lymphocytes. *Gastric Cancer* 6:173, 2003.
94. Kuppers R: B cells under influence: Transformation of B cells by Epstein-Barr virus. *Nat Rev Immunol* 3:801, 2003.
95. Murry PG, Young LS: Epstein-Barr virus infection: Basis of malignancy and potential for therapy. *Expert Rev Mol Med* 15:2001, 2001.
96. Greenspan JS, Greenspan D, Lennette ET: Replication of Epstein-Barr virus within epithelial cells of hairy oral leukoplakia an AIDS associated lesion. *N Engl J Med* 332:19, 1986.
97. Bharadwaj M, Moss DJ: Epstein-Barr virus vaccine: A cytotoxic T-cell-based approach. *Expert Rev Vaccines* 1:467, 2002.
98. Sokal EM, Hoppenbrouwers K, Vandermeulen C, et al: Recombinant gp350 vaccine for infectious mononucleosis: A phase 2, randomized, double-blind, placebo controlled trial to evaluate the safety, immunogenicity, and efficacy of Epstein-Barr virus vaccine in healthy young adults. *J Infect Dis* 196(12):1749, 2007.
99. Davis JE, Moss DJ: Treatment options for post-transplant lymphoproliferative disorders and other Epstein-Barr virus associated malignancies. *Tissue Antigens* 63:285, 2004.
100. Farrell CJ, Lee JM, Shin EC, et al: Inhibition of Epstein-Barr virus-induced growth proliferation by nuclear antigen EBNA-2 peptide. *Proc Natl Acad Sci U S A* 101:4625, 2004.
101. Weller TH, Hanshaw JB: Virologic and clinical observations in cytomegalic inclusion disease. *N Engl J Med* 266:1233, 1962.
102. Hanshaw JB, Betts RF, Simon G, Boynton RC: Acquired cytomegalovirus infection. *N Engl J Med* 272:602, 1965.
103. Klemola E, Von Essen R, Henle G, et al: Infectious mononucleosis like disease with negative heterophile agglutination test. Clinical features in relation to Epstein-Barr virus and cytomegalovirus antibodies. *J Infect Dis* 121:608, 1970.
104. Stagno S, Pass RF, Dworsky ME, et al: Congenital cytomegalovirus infection: The relative importance of primary or recurrent maternal infection. *N Engl J Med* 306:945, 1982.
105. Hallee TJ, Evans AS, Niederman JC, et al: Infectious mononucleosis at the United States Military Academy. A prospective study of a single class over 4 years. *Yale J Biol Med* 47:182, 1974.
106. Yeager AS: Transfusion-acquired cytomegalovirus infection in newborn infants. *Am J Dis Child* 128:478, 1974.
107. Betts RF, Freeman RB, Douglas RG Jr, et al: Transmission of cytomegalovirus with renal allograft. *Kidney Int* 8:385, 1975.
108. Ho M, Suwansirkul S, Dowling JN, et al. The transplanted kidney as a source of cytomegalovirus infection. *N Engl J Med* 293:1109, 1975.
109. Wreghitt TG, Teare O, Sule O, et al: Cytomegalovirus infection in immunocompetent patients. *Clin Infect Dis* 37:1603, 2003.
110. Rodriguez-Bano J, Muniain MA, Borobio MV, et al: Cytomegalovirus mononucleosis as a cause of prolonged fever and prominent weight loss in immunocompetent adults. *Clin Microbiol Infect* 10:468, 2004.
111. Alberola J, Tarnarit A, Iguai R, et al: Early neutralizing and glycoprotein B (gB) specific antibody responses to human cytomegalovirus (HCMV) in immunocompetent individuals with distinct clinical presentations of primary HCMV infection. *J Clin Virol* 16(2):113, 2000.
112. Scalzo AA, Corbett AJ, Rawlinson WD, et al: The interplay between host and viral factors in shaping the outcome of cytomegalovirus infection. *Immunol Cell Biol* 85(1):46, 2007.
113. Smith MS, Bentz GL, Alexander JS, Yurochko AD: Human cytomegalovirus induces monocyte differentiation and migration as a strategy for dissemination and persistence. *J Virol* 78:4444, 2004.
114. Ang CW, Jacobs BC, Brandenburg AH, et al: Cross-reactive antibodies against GM2 and CMV-infected fibroblasts in Guillain-Barré syndrome. *Neurology* 54:1453, 200.
115. Betts RF, Freeman RB, Douglas RG Jr, Talley TE: Clinical manifestations of renal allograft derived primary cytomegalovirus infection. *Am J Dis Child* 131:759, 1977.
116. Meyers JD, Spencer HC Jr, Watts JC, et al: Cytomegalovirus pneumonia after human marrow transplantation. *Ann Intern Med* 82:181, 1975.
117. Schooley RT, Hirsch MS, Colvin RB, et al: Association of Herpesvirus infections with T-lymphocyte subset alterations, glomerulopathy, and opportunistic infections after renal transplantation. *N Engl J Med* 308:307, 1983.
118. George MJ, Snydman DR, Werner BG, et al: The independent role of cytomegalovirus for invasive fungal disease in orthotopic liver transplant recipients: The Boston Center for Liver Transplantation CMV IgG-Study Group: Cytogam, MedImmune Inc., Gaithersburg, Md. *Am J Med* 103:106, 1997.
119. Tindall B, Cooper DA, Donovan B, Penny R: Primary human immunodeficiency infection. Clinical and serologic aspects. *Infect Dis Clin North Am* 2:329, 1988.
120. Vanhems P, Allard R, Cooper DA, et al: Acute human immunodeficiency virus type 1 disease as a mononucleosis-like illness: Is the diagnosis too restrictive? *Clin Infect Dis* 24:965, 1997.
121. Rosenberg ES, Caliendo AM, Walker BD: Acute HIV among patients tested for mononucleosis [letter]. *N Engl J Med* 340:969, 1999.
122. Walensky RP, Rosenberg ES, Ferraro MJ, et al: Investigation of primary human immunodeficiency virus infection in patients who test positive for heterophile antibody. *Clin Infect Dis* 33:570, 2001.
123. Dalmau J, Puertas MC, Azuara M, et al: Contribution of Immunologic and virological factors to the extremely severe primary HIV type 1 infection. *Clin Infect Dis* 48:229, 2009.
124. Steeper TA, Horwitz CA, Ablashi DV, et al: The spectrum of clinical and laboratory findings resulting from human herpesvirus-6 (HHV-6) in patients with mononucleosis-like illness not resulting from Epstein-Barr virus or cytomegalovirus. *Am J Clin Pathol* 93:776, 1990.
125. Li IW, To Kk, Tang BS, et al: Human metapneumovirus infection in a human immunocompetent adult presenting as mononucleosis-like illness. *J Infect* 56(5):389, 2008.
126. Andersson J, Britton S, Ernberg I, et al: Effect of acyclovir on infectious mononucleosis: A double-blinded, placebo-controlled study. *J Infect Dis* 153:283, 1986.
127. Torre D, Tambini R: Acyclovir for treatment of infectious mononucleosis: A meta-analysis. *Scand J Infect Dis* 31:543, 1999.
128. Collins M, Fleisher G, Kreisberg J, Fager S: Role of steroids in the treatment of infectious mononucleosis in the ambulatory college student. *J Am Coll Health* 33:101, 1984.
129. Chan SC, Dawes PJ: The management of severe infectious mononucleosis tonsillitis and upper airway obstruction. *J Laryngol Otol* 115:973; 2001.
130. Peter J, Ray GG: Infectious mononucleosis. *Pediatr Rev* 19:276, 1998.
131. Walling DM, Flaitz CM, Nichols CM, et al: Persistent productive Epstein-Barr virus replication in normal epithelial cells *in vivo*. *J Infect Dis* 184:1499, 2001.
132. Yao QY, Ogan P, Rowe M, et al: Epstein-Barr virus-infected B cells persist in the circulation of acyclovir-treated virus carriers. *Int J Cancer* 43:67, 1989.
133. Goldberg GN, Fulginiti VA, Ray CG, et al: *In utero* Epstein-Barr virus (infectious mononucleosis) infection. *JAMA* 246:1579, 1981.
134. Avgil M, Ornoy A: Herpes simplex virus and Epstein-Barr virus infections in pregnancy: Consequences of neonatal or intrauterine infection. *Reprod Toxicol* 21(4):436, 2006.
135. Connor EM, Sperling RS, Gelber R, et al: Reduction of maternal-infant transmission of human immunodeficiency virus type 1 with zidovudine treatment. Pediatrics AIDS Clinical Trials Group Protocol 076 Study Group. *N Engl J Med* 331:1173, 1994.
136. Cengir SD, Ortac F, Soylemez F: Treatment and results of chronic toxoplasmosis. Analysis of 33 cases. *Gynecol Obstet Invest* 33:105, 1992.
137. Stray-Pedersen B: Treatment of toxoplasmosis in the pregnant mother and newborn child. *Scand J Infect Dis* 84:23, 1992.

PART X

Neoplastic Myeloid Diseases

CHAPTER 85

CLASSIFICATION AND CLINICAL MANIFESTATIONS OF THE CLONAL MYELOID DISORDERS

Marshall A. Lichtman

SUMMARY

The clonal myeloid disorders result from acquired mutations within a multipotential marrow cell or very early progenitor cell. The chromosomal alteration resulting in the primary mutation sometimes is evident when cytogenetic analysis is performed. Translocations, inversions, and deletions of chromosomes can result in (1) the expression of fusion genes that encode fusion proteins that are oncogenic or (2) the overexpression or underexpression of genes that encode molecules critical to the control of cell growth, programmed cell death, or other regulatory pathways. Duplication of chromosomes, such as trisomy, also results in deregulated cellular behavior. Gene and miRNA (microribonucleic acid) expression profiling has also identified potentially leukemogenic gene mutations in cases without a cytogenetic abnormality. The different mutations may result in phenotypes that range from mild impairment of the steady-state levels of blood cells, insignificant functional impairment of cells, and little consequence on longevity to severe cytopenias and death in days, if the disorder is untreated. The somatically mutated (neoplastic) multipotential cell from which the clonal expansion of hematopoietic cells derives retains the ability, with various degrees of imperfection, to differentiate and mature into each blood cell lineage. The particular syndrome may have altered blood cell concentrations, structure, and function, and minimal to severe effects on a particular blood cell lineage. The effect on any one lineage occurs in an unpredictable way, even in subjects within the same category of disease. The resulting phenotypes are, therefore, innumerable and varied. In polycythemia vera or thrombocythemia, maturation of progenitors results in cells nearly normal in appearance and function, but their level in the blood is excessive. Moreover, overlapping features are common, such as thrombocytosis as a feature of polycythemia vera, essential thrombocythemia, primary myelofibrosis, or chronic myelogenous leukemia. The clonal anemias may be accompanied by insignificant or very severe neutropenia or thrombocytopenia or sometimes thrombocytosis. These findings reflect the unpredictable expression of the mutant multipotential cell's differentiation capabilities for which the genetic explanations are largely unknown. Tight relationships between the cytogenetic alteration and the phenotype occur in only a few circumstances, and even these are imperfect, for example, translocation (t) (9;22)(q34;q11)(*BCR-ABL*;p210) with chronic myelogenous leukemia and t(15;17)(q22;q21) (*PML-RARα*) with acute promyelocytic leukemia. However, most patients can be grouped into the classic diagnostic designations listed in Table 85–1. An important feature of the clonal myeloid diseases is the potentially reversible suppression of normal (polyclonal) stem cells by the clonally expanded cells. This coexistence and competition forms the basis for the remission-relapse pattern seen in acute myelogenous leukemia after intensive chemotherapy and for the reappearance of polyclonal, normal hematopoiesis in many patients with chronic myelogenous leukemia after tyrosine kinase inhibitor therapy.

Acronyms and abbreviations that appear in this chapter include: ALL, acute lymphocytic leukemia; AML, acute myelogenous leukemia; CD, cluster of differentiation; CML, chronic myelogenous leukemia; FGFR, fibroblast growth factor receptor; FLT-3, FMS-like tyrosine kinase 3; G-banding, Giemsa banding; GPI, glycosylphosphatidylinisotol; JAK2, Janus kinase 2; miRNA, microribonucleic acid; ^{32}P, phosphorus-32; PDGFR, platelet-derived growth factor receptor; PNH, paroxysmal nocturnal hemoglobinuria; P_{O2}, pressure of oxygen; t, translocation; WHO, World Health Organization.

A wide array of clonal (neoplastic) syndromes or diseases can result from a somatic mutation in a multipotential hematopoietic progenitor cell (Table 85–1). This mutated cell behaves like a stem cell, self-replicating and feeding cells into the various hematopoietic lineages. Strong circumstantial evidence has existed for a myelogenous leukemia stem cell for approximately 60 years. This concept has been buttressed by experimental verification of such cells by transplantation of human leukemia cells into immunodeficient mice[1,2] and by techniques to isolate and characterize their phenotype.[3] Although most attention has been given to the leukemic stem cell in acute myelogenous leukemia (AML) and chronic myelogenous leukemia (CML), it is very likely that a similar cell underlies (initiates and sustains) each of the clonal myeloid diseases.

The clonal myeloid diseases can be grouped, somewhat arbitrarily, by their degree of malignancy, using the classic terminology of experimental carcinogenesis, which considers the degree of loss of differentiation and maturation potential and the rate of progression of the disease. The term *deviation* relates to the relationship to normal cellular differentiation and maturation potential and the regulation of cell population homeostasis (birth and death rates). This terminology has been used to array the diagnostic categories of clonal hematopoietic diseases into a framework related to their pathogenesis for the reader.

MINIMAL-DEVIATION CLONAL MYELOID DISORDERS

The neoplasms in this category in Table 85–1 retain a higher degree of differentiation and maturation capability and permit median life spans measured in decades without treatment or with minimally toxic treatment approaches.[4] Use of the term *minimal deviation* should not be construed as indicating these conditions do not have morbidity, shorten life, and have other consequences to the patient. The term is used relative to AML, in which differentiation and maturation and regulation of cell proliferation and cell death are profoundly disturbed, and in which expected life span is measured in days to weeks, if untreated.

PRECURSOR APOPTOSIS PROMINENT

The clonal (refractory) anemias and bi- and tricytopenias are characteristic of this category. Cytopenias resulting from exaggerated apoptosis of marrow late precursors (referred to as ineffective hematopoiesis) are a principal feature of this subgroup of clonal hematopoietic multipotential cell diseases. A common additional characteristic is striking dysmorphogenesis of blood cells.[5] These cytologic abnormalities, characteristic of the clonal anemias, bicytopenias, or pancytopenias, include changes in the size (macrocytosis and microcytosis), shape (poikilocytosis), and nuclear or organelle structure (hypogranulation or hypergranulation, nuclear hypolobulation) of blood cells and their precursors (see Chap. 88).

TABLE 85–1. Neoplastic (Clonal) Myeloid Disorders

I. Minimal-deviation neoplasms (no leukemic blast cells are evident in marrow)
- A. Underproduction of mature cells is prominent
  1. Clonal (refractory) sideroblastic anemia[a] (Chap. 88)
  2. Clonal (refractory) nonsideroblastic anemia[a] (Chap. 88)
  3. Clonal bi- or tricytopenia[a] (Chap. 88)
  4. Paroxysmal nocturnal hemoglobinuria (Chap. 40)
- B. Overproduction of mature cells is prominent
  1. Polycythemia vera[b] (Chap. 86)
  2. Primary thrombocythemia[b] (Chap. 87)

II. Moderate-deviation neoplasms (small proportions of leukemic blast cells usually present in marrow)
- A. Chronic myelogenous leukemia (Chap. 90)
  1. Ph chromosome-positive, *BCR* rearrangement positive (~90%)
  2. Ph chromosome-negative, *BCR* rearrangement positive (~6%)
  3. Ph chromosome-negative, *BCR* rearrangement negative (~4%)
- B. Primary myelofibrosis[b] (chronic megakaryocytic leukemia) (Chap. 91)
- C. Chronic eosinophilic leukemia (Chaps. 62 and 90)
  1. *PDGFR* rearrangement-positive
  2. *FGFR1* rearrangement-positive
- D. Chronic neutrophilic leukemia (Chap. 90)
- E. Chronic basophilic leukemia (Chap. 90)
- F. Systemic mastocytosis (chronic mast cell leukemia) (Chap. 63)
  1. KIT^{D816V} mutation-positive (~90 %)
  2. KIT^{V560G} mutation-positive (rare)

III. Moderately severe deviation neoplasms (moderate concentration of leukemic blast cells present in marrow)
- A. Oligoblastic myelogenous leukemia (refractory anemia with excess blasts)[a] (Chap. 88)
- B. Subacute myelomonocytic leukemia (Chap. 90)
  1. *PDGFR* rearrangement positive (rare)
- C. Juvenile myelomonocytic leukemia (Chap. 90)

IV. Severe deviation neoplasms (leukemic blast or early progenitor cells frequent in the marrow and blood)
- A. Phenotypic variants of acute myelogenous leukemia (Chap. 89)
  1. Myeloblastic (granuloblastic)
  2. Myelomonocytic (granulomonoblastic)
  3. Promyelocytic
  4. Erythroid
  5. Monocytic
  6. Megakaryocytic
  7. Eosinophilic[c]
  8. Basophilic[d]
  9. Mastocytic[e]
  10. Histiocytic or Dendritic[f]
- B. High-frequency genotypic variants of acute myelogenous leukemia [t(8;21), Inv16 or t(16;16), t(15;17), or (11q23)][g]
- C. Myeloid sarcoma
- D. Acute biphenotypic (myeloid and lymphoid markers) leukemia[h]
- E. Acute leukemia with lymphoid markers evolving from a prior clonal myeloid disease

[a]The World Health Organization includes these four disorders under the rubric of the "Myelodysplastic Syndromes," the classification of which is discussed in Chap. 88.

[b]The World Health Organization includes these three disorders under the rubric of the "Myeloproliferative Syndromes," the classification of which is discussed in Chaps. 86, 87, and 90.

[c]Acute eosinophilic leukemia is rare. Most cases are subacute or chronic and formerly were included in the category of the hypereosinophilic syndrome (see Chaps. 62, 89, and 90).

[d]Rare cases of acute basophilic leukemia are Ph-negative and are variants of acute myelogenous leukemia. Most cases have the Ph chromosome and evolve from chronic myelogenous leukemia (see Chaps. 63, 89, and 90).

[e]See Chap. 63.

[f]See Chap. 72.

[g]The World Health Organization has designated these subtypes as separate entities even though they also have phenotypes listed under phenotypic variants.[1]

[h]Approximately 10 percent of cases of acute myeloblastic leukemia may be biphenotypic (myeloid and lymphoid markers on individual cells) when studied with antimyeloid and antilymphoid monoclonal antibodies (see Chap. 89).

Abnormal maturation of blood cells leads to morphologic, biochemical, and functional alterations of the cells. Ineffective erythropoiesis, the intramedullary, apoptotic death of late erythroblasts before they reach full maturation, is a common feature. Ineffective granulopoiesis and thrombopoiesis also can occur, resulting in neutropenia and thrombocytopenia, despite a cellular marrow.

There is no clinical distinction in the presenting manifestation or the course of clonal anemia with less than 15 or greater than 15 percent pathologic sideroblasts in the marrow. Therefore, this distinction, nonsideroblastic vis-à-vis sideroblastic clonal (refractory) anemia, has no nosologic or clinical utility, yet the World Health Organization (WHO) has retained it.[6] Indeed, the clonal anemias nearly invariably have pathologic sideroblasts in the marrow, and, thus, are virtually all sideroblastic, in fact. Leukemic blast cells are not evident in these syndromes. If marrow blasts are elevated above the normal upper limit of 2 percent, the disorder should be considered oligoblastic myelogenous leukemia (synonym: *refractory anemia with excess blasts*; see below, "Moderately Severe Deviation Disorders"). The WHO has defined "acute myelogenous leukemia" as having ≥20 percent leukemic blast cells in marrow; whereas, a marrow with fewer blasts (5 to 20 percent) is referred to as refractory anemia with excess blasts (e.g., myelodysplasia). The use of 5 percent blasts as a threshold is an anachronism that dates back approximately 50 years to a time when supportive care was inadequate (no platelets for transfusion, limited antibiotics, etc.). At that time, the risk of "overtreating" children with acute lymphocytic leukemia (ALL) was so great and the presence of atypical lymphoid cells in the marrow after treatment so common, that an arbitrary threshold of 5 percent blasts was used to avoid an unnecessarily long period of posttreatment-induced aplasia. It is too high a threshold at the time of diagnosis. In no other cancer is the diagnosis defined by the proportion of cancer cells in histologic or cytologic examinations, thus using ≥20 percent blasts as the basis for diagnosis of leukemia versus myelodysplasia represents an aberration in cancer diagnosis.[7] Because the differential cell count in a marrow aspirate (or biopsy) is variable and represents a small sample of marrow, such distinctions also are made arbitrary by problems of sampling at the time of diagnosis.

The term *hematopoietic dysplasia*, later simplified to *myelodysplasia*, has become ensconced as the category into which clonal anemia, clonal multicytopenia, and refractory anemia with excess blasts (oligoblastic myelogenous leukemia) have been grouped. In strict pathologic terms, a dysplasia is a polyclonal, and thus nonmalignant, change in the cells of a tissue. These myeloid syndromes are clonal, often have aneuploid or pseudodiploid cells in the clone, and can be associated with significant morbidity and premature death; thus, they are neoplasias not dysplasias. They demonstrate clonal instability, and each has a propensity to evolve into polyblastic AML that far exceeds that of the general population. The term *dysplasia* was instituted in the early 1970s at a time when prominent dysmorphogenesis and cytopenias were thought to be the singular abnormalities and arguments existed as to whether these syndromes represented a preneoplastic (polyclonal) or neoplastic (clonal) condition.[8] They have long been established as the latter, but the terminology has not been rectified.

■ OVERPRODUCTION OF CELLS PROMINENT

Polycythemia vera (see Chap. 86) and essential thrombocythemia (see Chap. 87) are clonal myeloid disorders. They are so named because of the overaccumulation of red cells, and often neutrophils, and platelets in polycythemia, and of platelets, and to a lesser extent neutrophils, in thrombocythemia.[9] Each cell lineage is affected in each disorder, reflecting a multipotential hematopoietic cell origin, but the magnitude of the effects on each lineage differs. The decrease in red cell production in essential thrombocythemia usually is mild. Polycythemia vera and essential thrombocythemia do not show morphologic evidence of leukemic hematopoiesis; the proportion of blast cells in the marrow is not increased above normal, and blast cells are not present in the blood. Hematopoietic differentiation and maturation are maintained. These disorders do not have a specific cytogenetic abnormality, but approximately 95 percent of cases of polycythemia and approximately 40 percent of cases of essential thrombocythemia have an acquired mutation in the Janus kinase 2 (*JAK2*) gene.[9] The survival of cohorts of patients with these diseases is only slightly less than expected for age- and gender-matched unaffected persons.[4,10,11] Two exceptions are the uncommon onset of polycythemia vera in childhood in which there is a shortened life span,[12] and adults with the homozygous *JAK2* V61F mutation who have a more aggressive form of the disease (Chap 86).

■ MODERATE-DEVIATION CLONAL MYELOID DISORDERS

CML (see Chap. 90) and primary myelofibrosis (see Chap. 91) classically share the features of overproduction of granulocytes and platelets and impaired production of red cells. In contrast to the minimally deviated clonal myeloid neoplasms, CML and primary myelofibrosis have a small proportion of leukemic blast cells in marrow and often blood. The most constant feature in primary myelofibrosis is the abundance of dysmorphic megakaryocytes and the resultant predisposition to marrow reticulin and collagen fibrosis, extramedullary fibrohematopoietic tumors, splenomegaly, and teardrop-shaped red cells (dacryocytes) in every oil immersion field on the blood film. The megakaryocytic abnormalities are so dominant and consistent in this disorder that it could be called chronic megakaryocytic leukemia.[13] The cells in this disorder have no specific cytogenetic change, but approximately 40 to 50 percent of cases carry a mutation in the *JAK2* gene (see Chaps. 87 and 91). CML, in contrast, has a rearrangement of the *BCR* gene on chromosome 22. The shortening of the long arm of chromosome 22 gives it the designation of the Philadelphia chromosome, now called the Ph chromosome. It can be identified by Giemsa (G)-banding cytogenetic study in approximately 90 percent of patients with CML. This mutation is caused by and reflected in translocation t(9;22)(q34;q11)(*BCR-ABL*). The *BCR-ABL* fusion in CML cells can be found in virtually all cases studied by fluorescence in situ hybridization. An unrelenting increase in the white cell (granulocyte) count, splenomegaly, and a progressive course are common features. Blast cells are very slightly increased in marrow and often blood in most patients with these two disorders. CML has a very high (nearly universal) propensity to transform to acute leukemia. Primary myelofibrosis terminates in acute leukemia in approximately 15 percent of patients. Median life span in these disorders is measured in years but is significantly decreased compared to age- and gender-matched unaffected cohorts. Therapy is required in all cases of CML and in some but not all cases of primary myelofibrosis at the time of diagnosis. Both diseases can be cured by stem cell transplantation. Median life span is projected to be increased by decades in CML with the use of tyrosine kinase inhibitors (see Chap. 90).[14]

Chronic eosinophilic leukemia, chronic neutrophilic leukemia, chronic basophilic leukemia, and systemic mastocytosis are included in this category. Chronic basophilic leukemia is a rare disease, thus far only reported by the Mayo Clinic.[15] Chronic neutrophilic leukemia is uncommon but well described and defined (see Chap. 90). Chronic eosinophilic leukemia represents cases previously called hypereosinophilic syndrome with evidence of clonal hematopoiesis involving eosinopoiesis. Some cases are associated with a rearrangement of the platelet-derived growth factor receptor-β (*PDGFR*-β) gene and these are called out in Table 85–1 because they are specifically responsive to the tyrosine kinase inhibitor, imatinib mesylate (see Chaps. 62 and 90). Chronic clonal eosinophilia may also be associated with a *PDGFR*-α gene rearrangement, but histopathologic examination may be consistent also with systemic mastocytosis. This rearrangement is usually the result of a *FIP1L1-PDGFR*-α fusion gene. Identification of this fusion gene in cases of eosinophilia-mastocytosis is important because of the sensitivity of those gene products to imatinib mesylate. A clonal myeloid syndrome that includes eosinophilia and a translocation between 8p11, at the site of the tyrosine kinase domain of the fibroblast growth factor receptor-1 (*FGFR1*) gene, and several different partner chromosomes, is not responsive to imatinib mesylate. Systemic mastocytosis may have several types of *KIT* gene mutation; KIT^{V560G} is sensitive to imatinib mesylate and KIT^{D816V} is insensitive to imatinib but may be responsive to second-generation tyrosine kinase inhibitors. *PDGFR*-α mutations also may be present in the cells of patients with systemic mastocytosis and be responsive to imatinib mesylate.[16]

■ MODERATELY SEVERE DEVIATION CLONAL MYELOID DISORDERS

These disorders fall into a group that progresses less rapidly than acute leukemia and more rapidly than chronic leukemia.[17,18] They have a predisposition to develop with a granulocytic and monocytic phenotype, either morphologically or cytochemically. These diseases include oligoblastic myelogenous leukemia (refractory anemia with excess blasts), subacute myelomonocytic leukemia, and juvenile myelomonocytic leukemia. Occasional patients have an atypical or unclassifiable syndrome. The latter designation is used for uncommon cases that do not fall into a classical or easily classifiable designation and usually are seen in patients older than age 70 years.

The subacute syndromes produce more morbidity than do the chronic syndromes, and patients have a shorter life expectancy. These are leukemic states that have low or moderate concentrations of leukemic blast cells in marrow and often blood, anemia, often thrombocytopenia, and usually prominent monocytic maturation of cells (see Chap. 88). The oligoblastic myelogenous leukemias compose approximately 50 percent of the cases that have been grouped under the title *myelodysplastic syndromes.* In all other malignancies, the presence of tumor cells determines the diagnosis, such as carcinoma of the colon or the uterine cervix, whether in situ, invasive, or metastatic. Use of the percentage of tumor (leukemic blast) cells as a threshold for the diagnosis of leukemia versus "dysplasia" is not consistent with usual practice; hence, the preference for oligoblastic myelogenous leukemia rather than myelodysplasia for patients with increased blast cells (leukemia) and dysmorphic cell maturation. Moreover, chronic myelogenous "leukemia," chronic neutrophilic "leukemia," subacute myelomonocytic "leukemia," acute promyelocytic "leukemia," and other subtypes of AML invariably have fewer than 20 percent blasts in the marrow. Thus, the criteria used in the WHO classification system for clonal myeloid diseases have internal inconsistencies that can be dealt with by experts but are confusing to the uninitiated.

SEVERE-DEVIATION CLONAL MYELOID DISORDERS

Morphologic, histochemical, immunologic, and cytogenetic characteristics of cells in the blood and marrow provide the major basis for the diagnosis and classification of AML and its subtypes (see Chaps. 11 and 89). Correlation among observers and between the morphologic method of classification and the monoclonal antibody reactivity-dependent classification of AML is imperfect.[19–21] The approach that uses morphology, immunocytochemistry, and immunophenotype is the most inclusive because virtually all cases can be placed into a morphologic subtype. Because immunophenotyping is a standard procedure in most laboratories, the results are readily available. Classification by cytogenetics is more limited because many cases have different infrequent abnormalities, making this approach complex. Approximately 900 unique cytogenetic abnormalities have been reported in cells of patients with AML, including unbalanced structural abnormalities, such as loss of part or all of chromosome 5 or 7, numerical abnormalities, such as an additional chromosome 8 (trisomy 8), or balanced structural abnormalities, such as translocation between chromosomes 8 and 21, 15 and 17, or between chromosome 11 and many other chromosome partners, or any one of numerous other abnormalities involving other chromosomes (genes).[22] Despite this heterogeneity, knowing the cytogenetic alterations is useful for estimating the probability of entering a sustained remission (risk category). For example, AML patients whose cells contain t(8;21), t(16;16) or Inv16 (approximately 20 percent of cases) are more likely to enter a prolonged remission. The cytogenetic findings may influence the drugs used for remission-induction therapy. Notably, patients with t(15;17) AML (approximately 7 percent of all AML cases), uniquely require use of all-*trans*-retinoic acid and arsenic trioxide to result in the best long-term outcome, and in many cases, a cure. Thus, combined light microscopy of blood and marrow, immunocytochemistry, and immunophenotyping to designate the phenotypic subtype, supplemented by cytogenetics or molecular diagnostic methods, currently is the best approach to categorization of the AML subtype. The polymerase chain reaction may be particularly useful for determining subclinical (minimal) residual disease and monitoring therapy in cases in which an appropriate genetic marker is available, such as the t(8;21) or t(15;17) (see Chaps. 89 and 90).

Gene expression profiling using chips containing tens, hundreds, or thousands of relevant genes can be used to further genotype and subclassify AML into prognostic groups.[23] One would predict, based on cytogenetics, a large and diverse group of gene expression profiles for cases of AML. This tool is currently most useful in analyzing cases with prior stratification by some relevant variable. For example, a study of patients with AML who have normal karyotypes by standard cytogenetic methods (e.g., G-banding) has identified two groups by hierarchical gene clustering with significantly different survival after current therapy.[24] Patients with AML whose cells contain a FMS-like tyrosine kinase 3 (FLT-3) internal tandem duplication also can be stratified into more discriminating prognostic groups using hierarchical gene cluster analysis.[25] Gene expression profiling also can identify groups of patients with AML who have previously covert gene abnormalities, such as a mutation in the nucleophosmin 1 gene that encodes a protein that shuttles between the nucleus and cytoplasm. Gene expression studies in AML are important because they (1) identify genes that cooperate or interact to result in a fully malignant phenotype, (2) provide potential new targets for therapy, and (3) help identify patients who might benefit from early stem cell transplantation. At this time, these methods and their interpretation are complex and not available in many clinical laboratories. Moreover, they require interpretation based on the time during the course of the disease that gene analyses are performed; gene expression profiles can differ over time as clonal evolution or selection occurs. Also, studies are best focused on the most primitive multipotential cells in the clone to avoid secondary changes in the mass of derivative leukemic cells.

Another molecular technique applied to understanding the molecular pathology of AML and to defining prognostic groups is the leukemic cell microribonucleic acid (miRNA) signature.[26,27] miRNAs are small (19–25 nucleotides), noncoding RNAs that regulate translation of protein by messenger RNA. miRNA signatures can be analyzed by polymerase chain reaction technology of RNA samples from leukemic cells and compared to normal or compared among different categories of AML cases. For example, miRNA analysis can distinguish among cytogenetically normal cases of AML as to their expression of different genes that influence prognosis, such as the nucleophosmin 1 gene (*NPM1*) and the CCAAT/enhancer binding protein α gene (*CEPBA*).

Specific miRNAs may regulate lineage differentiation of stem cells, indicating critical roles for these molecules in the regulation of hematopoiesis and in leukemogenesis.[28]

In general, at this time, these techniques are principally research tools because therapists do not have significantly different drug regimens to permit special treatment of poor prognosis groups identified prospectively.

TRANSITIONS AMONG CLONAL MYELOID DISEASES

Patients with minimal, moderate, and moderately severe deviation clonal myeloid disorders have an increased likelihood of progressing to florid (polyblastic) AML, with a frequency ranging from approximately less than 1 percent of patients with paroxysmal nocturnal hemoglobinuria, to 10 percent of patients with clonal sideroblastic anemia, and to 35 percent of patients with clonal bi- or tricytopenia. Approximately 15 percent of patients with polycythemia vera evolve to a syndrome indistinguishable from primary myelofibrosis.[29] AML develops as a terminal event in approximately 1 percent of patients with polycythemia vera not treated with phosphorus-32 (^{32}P) or an alkylating agent and in a larger proportion of patients who are treated with cytotoxic agents.[30] Occasional cases of apparent essential thrombocythemia or rare cases of primary myelofibrosis can evolve into polycythemia vera. Apparent

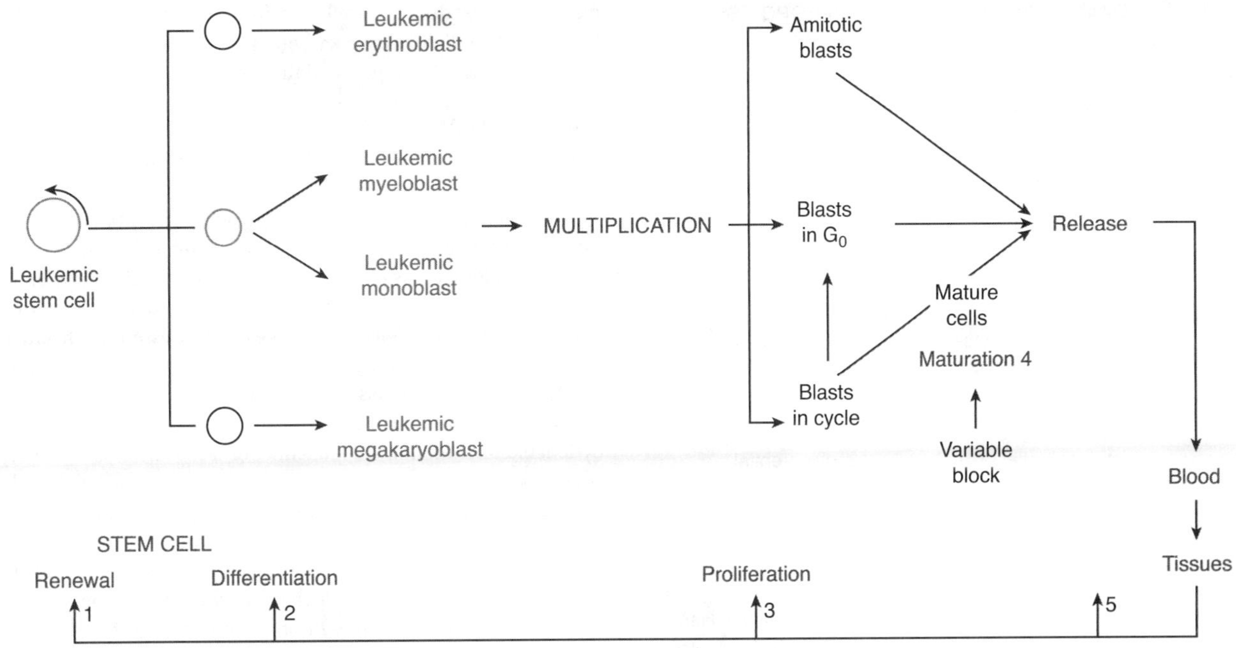

FIGURE 85–1. Hematopoiesis in acute myelogenous leukemia. The malignant process evolves from a single mutant multipotential cell. This cell is represented at either level 1 or level 2 in Figure 85–2. This cell is capable of multivariate commitment to leukemic erythroid, granulocytic, and megakaryocytic progenitors. In most cases, granulocytic commitment predominates, and myeloblasts and monoblasts or their immediate derivatives are the dominant cell types. Leukemic blast cells accumulate in the marrow. The leukemic blast cells may become amitotic (sterile) and undergo programmed cell death, may stop dividing for prolonged periods (blasts in G_0) but have the potential to reenter the mitotic cycle, or may divide and undergo varying degrees of maturation. Maturation may lead to mature cells, such as red cells, segmented neutrophils, monocytes, or platelets. A severe block in maturation is characteristic of AML, whereas a high proportion of leukemic blast cells mature into terminally differentiated cells in patients with CML. The disturbance in commitment and maturation in myelogenous leukemia is quantitative, thus many patterns are possible. At least five major steps in hematopoiesis are regulated: (1) stem cell self-renewal, (2) differentiation into hematopoietic cell lineages (e.g., red cells, granulocytes, platelets), (3) proliferation (cell multiplication) and maturation of progenitor and precursor cells, (4) maturation of progenitor and precursor cells, and (5) release of mature cells into the blood. These control points are defective in myelogenous leukemia. Premature or delayed apoptosis of cells may be another key abnormality contributing to premature death or cell accumulation.

essential thrombocythemia with cells containing the *BCR-ABL* fusion gene may progress to CML or acute blast crisis of CML.

A very small percentage of patients with essential thrombocythemia and approximately 15 percent of patients with primary myelofibrosis progress to overt AML. The rate of conversion to AML in polycythemia and thrombocythemia is increased by prior radiotherapy or chemotherapy, depending on the dose, duration, and type of drug. Virtually all patients with CML have the potential to progress to acute leukemia of any subtype, including lymphoid phenotypes, although in some cases the patient enters an accelerated phase that behaves like oligoblastic leukemia before it progresses to acute leukemia. The accelerated phase of CML is associated with inadequate response to therapy, progressive anemia, bone pain, enlarging spleen, thrombocytopenia, among other changes (see Chap. 90). The progression from chronic to accelerated phase of CML, however, has been delayed in the majority of patients by the application of tyrosine kinase inhibitor therapy during the chronic phase of the disease. Determining the frequency of evolution to AML in those patients with CML who enter a complete cytogenetic or major or complete molecular remission with tyrosine kinase inhibitors must await observations over the next several decades.

PATHOGENESIS OF CLONAL MYELOID DISEASES

In AML, a sequence of mutations in a single multipotential cell results in a clone that is severely defective and contains precursor cells that are unable to mature.[31,32] Proliferation of primitive progenitors is excessive when considered in absolute terms, that is, the total number of blast cells proliferating. AML is a clinical disease with many forms of morphologic expression. This variation of phenotype is consistent with the large number of genetic lesions identified and the behavior of the leukemic multipotential cell, which is capable of differentiation into all the blood cell lineages (Fig. 85–1). Hence, the asymmetrical and uncoordinated maturation of leukemic progenitor cells may allow one or another cell type to predominate.[33] These different morphologic or cytogenetic variants of AML are each rapidly progressive, however, if not treated successfully (see Chap. 89).

Important epiphenomena are related to certain morphologic types of AML, such as tissue infiltration, including into the central nervous system (monocytic leukemia), disseminated intravascular coagulation, fibrinolysis, and hemorrhage (promyelocytic leukemia), hepatosplenomegaly (eosinophilic leukemia), mediator-release syndromes (basophilic or mast cell leukemia), and intense marrow fibrosis (megakaryocytic leukemia) (see Chap. 89).

In CML, injury to a single cell results in a clone in which there is an enormous expansion of progenitors for granulocytic and, often, megakaryocytic cells. Erythropoiesis is effective but decreased. Unlike AML, maturation of progenitor cells in CML is nearly normal; hence, the predominant leukemic cells in the blood are amitotic, mature, or partially matured cells, such as myelocytes and segmented neutrophils, erythrocytes, and platelets. This process of multilineage differentiation and maturation to cells with virtually normal function accounts for the relative infrequency of severe hemorrhage or recurrent infection in the chronic phase of CML.

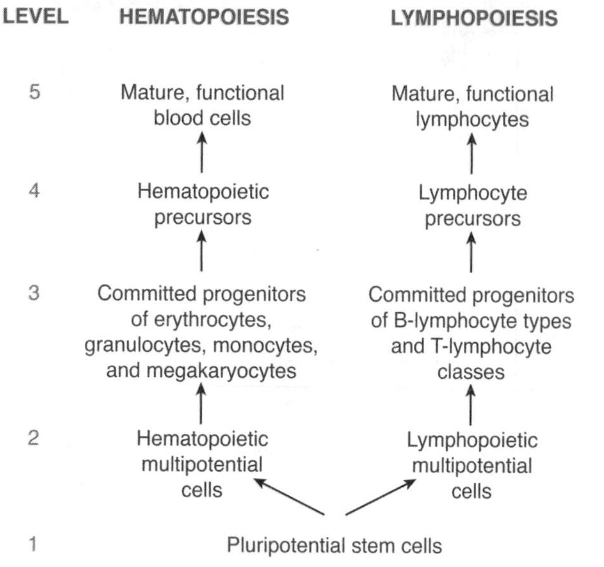

FIGURE 85–2. Differentiation and maturation of hematopoietic stem cells. The functioning stem cell pool is thought to be at *level 1*, the pluripotential cells. In healthy humans, two multipotential progenitor cell pools may be operative (*level 2*). The multipotential progenitors differentiate further to unipotential progenitors, which are sensitive to specific cytokines (*level 3*). The committed progenitor cells are referred to as colony-forming units or colony-forming cells because they form colonies of cells in semisolid medium in the presence of the appropriate growth factors. These growth factors are capable of inducing proliferation and maturation of the committed progenitor cells so that they achieve *level 4*, at which the first morphologically identifiable precursors have developed, such as myeloblasts and proerythroblasts, and, ultimately, *level 5*, the mature, functional blood cells.

Because hematopoiesis is generated by a leukemic stem cell, erythropoiesis, thrombopoiesis, and granulopoiesis are leukemic in most patients with AML, CML, and other clonal myeloid diseases. Thus, qualitative abnormalities of structure and function and clonal cytogenetic abnormalities are present in erythroblasts, megakaryocytes, and granulocyte precursors in most cases of AML (see Chap. 89) and in all cases of CML (see Chap. 90).

PHENOTYPE OF MYELOID CLONAL DISEASES AS A RESULT OF THE MATRIX OF DIFFERENTIATION AND MATURATION

The phenotype of clonal myeloid diseases is a reflection of a neoplastic stem cell's capability to differentiate into abnormal committed progenitor cells and the ability of progenitor cells to mature into identifiable cells of the erythroid, granulocytic (neutrophilic, basophilic, mastocytic, eosinophilic), monocytic, dendritic, and megakaryocytic lineages (Fig. 85–3).[31,34,35]

Under normal circumstances, differentiation represents the changes from a multipotential cell to multiple unipotential lineage progenitors. Maturation represents the physical and chemical changes from a unipotential progenitor through a sequence of precursors to the fully mature and functional blood cell, including progression from a burst-forming unit–erythroid to proerythroblast to erythrocyte; from a colony-forming unit–granulocyte to myeloblast to segmented neutrophil; from a colony-forming unit–eosinophil to a segmented eosinophil; from a colony-forming unit–basophil to a mature basophil; from a colony-forming unit–mast cell to a mature mast cell; from a colony-forming unit–monocyte-macrophage to promonocyte to monocyte to macrophage or dendritic cell; and from a colony-forming unit–megakaryocyte to a diploid megakaryoblast to the polyploid megakaryocyte. A matrix, which is composed of the options of commitment to different lineages and the progressive stages of maturation at which partial or complete arrest can occur, results in the potential for a wide array of morphologic syndromes by which a leukemic stem cell can dominate hematopoiesis (see Fig. 85–2).

In the clonal myeloid diseases in which differentiation and maturation capability are retained, one of the cell lines, for example, erythrocytes, granulocytes, or platelets, tends to accumulate in the blood more prominently and results in a phenotypic expression of the disease that determines the nosology (e.g., platelets and essential thrombocythemia). In AML, the phenotypic expression may be predominantly myeloblastic (granuloblastic), erythroid, monocytic, megakaryocytic, or combinations thereof. Certain patterns are favored. In AML, myelocytic leukemia, monocytic leukemia, or a mosaic of the two cell types (myelomonocytic leukemia) are more common than erythroid, megakaryocytic, or eosinophilic leukemia. However, AML usually has a disturbance in all cell lines. In myeloblastic or myelomonocytic leukemia, overt, qualitative abnormalities of erythroblasts and megakaryocytes may occur. The prevalence of the abnormalities in the latter two lineages may not be great enough or evident enough for the observer to designate a case as erythroid or megakaryocytic leukemia. In the latter two cases, identification of markers unique for erythroid (e.g., cluster of differentiation [CD] 71) or megakaryocytic cells (e.g., CD41, CD42, or CD61), rather than reliance solely on light microscopy, has increased the frequency of identification of these variants.

The continuum of maturation can be completely or partially blocked at various levels, leading to morphologic variants such as acute myeloblastic, acute promyelocytic, acute myelogenous leukemia with maturation, and CML.

PLURIPOTENTIAL STEM CELL POOL AS SITE OF THE LESION

Evidence points to a lesion in the multipotential hematopoietic cell pool in most of the clonal myeloid diseases, explaining the involvement of erythropoiesis, granulopoiesis, and thrombopoiesis. In CML patients, the mutation is in the pluripotential stem cell; in other syndromes, evidence for involvement of B and T lymphocytes is variable. B lymphocytes are derived from the clone in most cases. The evidence for T lymphocyte involvement is less compelling. Evidence that affected T lymphocytes undergo apoptosis before entering the blood in patients with CML may explain the absence of clonal markers in T lymphocytes in some cases of CML and other clonal myeloid disorders.[36]

Thus, the mutation of the cell may be at level 1, between levels 1 and 2, or at level 2 in Figure 85–2 in different clonal myeloid diseases and in different patients.

PROGENITOR CELL LEUKEMIA

Analysis of cases of AML in girls and women who were heterozygous for isotypes A and B of the enzyme glucose-6-phosphate dehydrogenase indicated that the AML clone in the girls was restricted to the granulocyte–monocyte pathway, whereas monoclonality was expressed in all cell lines in the women. These findings are in keeping with all prior CML and AML studies using enzymes or chromosome markers.[37,38] These findings support the possibility that a leukemic transformation in some (young) patients can occur in progenitor cells (e.g., colony-forming unit—granulocyte-monocyte; level 3 in Fig. 85–2) and result in a true acute "granulocytic" leukemia. If progenitor cell myelog-

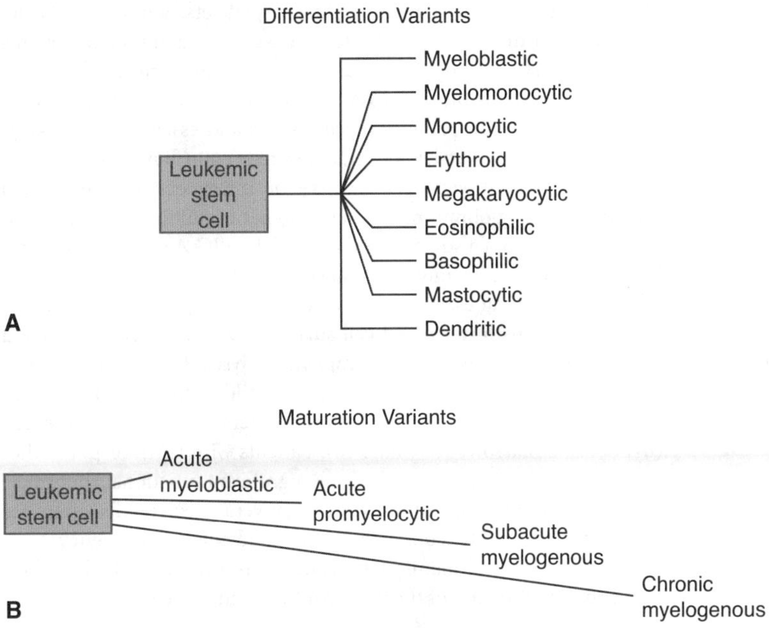

FIGURE 85–3. Phenotypic subtypes of acute myelogenous leukemia. Acute myelogenous leukemia has variable morphologic expression and a variable degree of maturation of leukemic cells into recognizable precursors of each blood cell type. This phenotypic variation results because the leukemic lesion resides in a multipotential cell normally capable of all the commitment decisions. **A.** Morphologic variants of AML can be considered differentiation variants in which the cells derived from one of the options of commitment accumulate prominently (e.g., leukemic erythroblasts, leukemic monocytes, leukemic megakaryocytes). In promyelocytic leukemia and in some cases of acute leukemia in younger individuals, the somatic mutation may arise in a more differentiated progenitor. **B.** Acute myeloblastic leukemia, promyelocytic leukemia, subacute myelogenous leukemia, and chronic myelogenous leukemia can be considered maturation variants in which blocks at different levels of maturation are present or do not exist.

enous leukemia is common in younger patients, this pattern could explain their better response to treatment. In a subset of patients with acute monocytic leukemia,[39] t(8;21) AML,[40] and t(15;17) AML,[41] the leukemia derives from the neoplastic transformation of a progenitor cell. The acute transformation of CML also appears to occur in a granulocyte-monocyte progenitor (see Chap. 90).

QUANTITATIVENESS OF CLONAL MYELOID DISEASES

The lesions of the primitive hematopoietic multipotential cell compartment are qualitative in the sense that a distinct alteration from normal is seen in the function of that cell pool. The alteration reflects a change in the genome of one primitive hematopoietic cell.[11] This qualitative change, however, is such that the mutant multipotential cell can express all or some of the normal differentiation and maturation options. This expression can mimic the differentiation (commitment) and maturation expected of normal hematopoietic cells, as occurs in CML, essential thrombocythemia, and polycythemia vera. Most cases tend to conform to readily recognized patterns, but the opportunity for a large number of variations on the most common themes is possible. Thus, some mixed and "in-between" syndromes occur in which features of ineffective hematopoiesis and myeloproliferation of different cell lineages are present. For example, extreme thrombocytosis, usually confined to primary thrombocythemia, may accompany CML, primary myelofibrosis, or clonal bicytopenia. Erythrocytosis may rarely accompany CML. Atypical myeloproliferative syndromes or other clonal myeloid diseases may have mixtures of anemia, granulocytopenia, and thrombocytosis or of anemia, granulocytosis, and thrombocytopenia rather than pancytopenia. Qualitative abnormalities of red cell, granulocyte, or platelet structure or function may be more or less prominent in a given patient. For example, qualitative abnormalities of erythroblast development may result in acquired α-thalassemia (acquired hemoglobin H disease), especially in patients with primary myelofibrosis or occasionally other clonal myeloid diseases. In AML, unusual patterns of phenotypic expression occur frequently. For example, prominent leukemic erythroblasts and monocytes or eosinophils and monocytes may be seen in patients. So much opportunity for variation in disease expression exists among patients with AML that observation of patients in whom the phenotype of their leukemic cells is identical to the phenotype of other patients is unusual. Choice of treatment is little affected by these variations. Decisions about whether to treat and which drugs to use are greatly influenced by whether a patient has a chronic, subacute, or acute clonal myeloid disease; by the rate of progression of the disease; by the extent of the leukemic blast cell infiltrate; by the cytogenetic findings; and by the severity of the cytopenias. The diagnostician and therapist usually can identify variants as a clonal myeloid disorder and can manage the disorder as dictated by their manifestations regardless of their precise subclassification.

INTERPLAY OF CLONAL AND POLYCLONAL HEMATOPOIESIS

Although potentially curative chemotherapy of myelogenous leukemia was introduced in the mid-20th century to kill "the last leukemic cell," two important factors were not explicitly appreciated. The first was whether residual normal stem cells coexisted in marrow to restore polyclonal (normal) hematopoiesis if ablation of the leukemia was accomplished. The second was whether, given the estimates of 1 trillion leukemic cells in a patient, the therapist had to eliminate all the leukemic cells to achieve a cure. A corollary of the latter was whether the disease was the result of a leukemic stem cell and, if it was, were the replicates of the leukemic cell the only cells that mattered, ultimately, in the eradication process. We know that remissions result from sufficient suppression of the leukemic population by intensive chemotherapy to permit restitution of polyclonal hematopoiesis by normal stem cells (Fig. 85–4).[42] Why monoclonal leukemic hematopoiesis is so difficult to subdue, even temporarily, with intensive chemotherapy (pretyrosine kinase therapy) in the chronic myeloid neoplasms (e.g., CML) compared to the acute myeloid neoplasms (AML) is unclear. Prolonged remission (>3 years) may occur in some cases of AML with late relapse occurring from the same clone, suggesting a new symbiotic relationship occurs after intensive therapy that suppresses the growth potential of leukemic cells. However, this phenomenon is more evident in lymphoid than myeloid neoplasms.

CLINICAL MANIFESTATIONS

■ DEFICIENCY, EXCESS, OR DYSFUNCTION OF BLOOD CELLS

Alterations in blood cell concentration are the primary manifestations of clonal hematopoietic disorders. The clinical manifestations of deficiencies

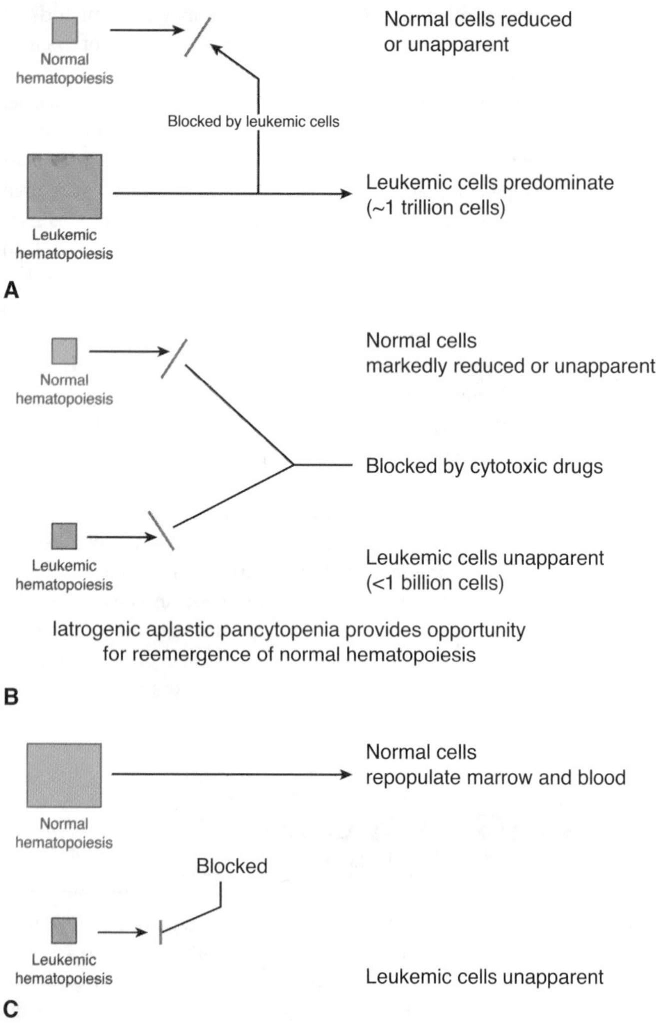

FIGURE 85–4. Remission–relapse pattern of acute myelogenous leukemia. **A.** Acute myelogenous leukemia at diagnosis or in relapse. Monoclonal leukemic hematopoiesis predominates. Normal polyclonal stem cell function is suppressed. **B.** Following effective cytotoxic treatment leukemic cells are unapparent in marrow and blood. Severe pancytopenia exists as a result of cytotoxic therapy. The reduction in leukemic cells can release inhibition of normal polyclonal stem cell function. **C.** If reconstitution of normal hematopoiesis ensues, a remission is established and blood cells return to near normal as a result of the recovery of polyclonal hematopoiesis. This relapse–remission pattern has not been seen in the subacute and chronic myeloid leukemias because it has not been possible to minimize the leukemic cell population with cytotoxic therapy to a point at which polyclonal hematopoiesis is restored. The only exception is the effect of BCR-ABL inhibitor therapy in which suppression of BCR-ABL–positive cells in CML can be achieved with return of polyclonal hematopoiesis. Uncommon examples of tyrosine kinase inhibitor responses in myeloid neoplasms with *PDGFR* or certain *KIT* mutations may also show this pattern. In a proportion of cases, BCR-ABL transcripts (minimal residual disease) can be detectable along with normal, polyclonal hematopoiesis. *(Reproduced from MA Lichtman,[42] with permission of Alpha Med Press.)*

or excesses of individual blood cell types are described in the chapters on clinical manifestations of disorders of erythrocytes (Chap. 33), granulocytes (Chap. 64), monocytes (Chap. 70), and platelets (Chap. 118).

Several clonal hematopoietic diseases frequently manifest as qualitative abnormalities of blood cells. Abnormal red cell shapes, red cell or granulocyte enzyme deficiencies, abnormal neutrophil granules, bizarre nuclear configurations, disorders of neutrophil chemotaxis, phagocytosis or microbial killing, giant platelets, abnormal platelet granules, and disturbed platelet function can occur in some patients with oligoblastic myelogenous leukemia and primary myelofibrosis. In oligoblastic myelogenous leukemia, the effects of severe cytopenia usually dominate. In primary myelofibrosis and essential thrombocythemia, functional platelet abnormalities may contribute to the hemorrhagic diathesis, especially if surgery or injury occurs. Paroxysmal nocturnal hemoglobinuria is a hematopoietic multipotential cell disease resulting from a somatic mutation of the *PIG-A* gene on the active X chromosome. The mutation causes a highly specific alteration in blood cell membranes, a deficiency in the glycosylphosphatidylinisotol (GPI) anchor, with decreased cell surface CD59, rendering the blood cells exquisitely sensitive to complement lysis. In its classic form, chronic hemolytic anemia is coupled with mild decreases in neutrophil and platelet counts but depressions in hematopoiesis often occur (hypoplastic marrow; see Chap. 40). Patients with CML or polycythemia vera usually do not have clinically significant functional abnormalities of cells, although in polycythemia vera, neutrophils often are activated with heightened metabolic rates and enhanced phagocytosis.

Secondary clinical manifestations occur as a result of the proliferation and accumulation of the malignant (leukemic) cells.

EFFECTS OF LEUKEMIC BLAST CELLS

Extramedullary Tumors

Myeloid (granulocytic) sarcomas (also called *chloromas* or *myeloblastomas*) are discrete tumors of leukemic cells that form in skin and soft tissues, breast, periosteum and bone, lymph nodes, mediastinum, lung, pleura, gastrointestinal tract, gonads, urinary tract, uterus, central nervous system, and virtually any other site (see Chap. 89).[43–45] They can develop in patients with AML or the accelerated phase of CML and, occasionally, may be the first manifestation of AML, preceding the onset in marrow and blood by months or years. Myeloid sarcomas can be mistaken for large cell lymphomas because of the similarity of the histopathology in biopsy specimens from soft tissues. In the past, approximately 50 percent of cases that occur in the absence of blood and marrow involvement initially were misdiagnosed, usually as lymphoma.[43] The presence of eosinophils or other granulocytes may arouse suspicion of a myeloid sarcoma; however, immunohistochemistry should be used on such lesions to identify myeloperoxidase, lysozyme, CD117, CD61, CD68/KP1, and other relevant CD markers of myeloid cells. One of four histopathologic patterns usually is evident by immunocytochemistry: myeloblastic, monoblastic, myelomonoblastic, or megakaryoblastic.

More diffuse collections of leukemic promonocytes or monoblasts can invade the skin, gingiva, anal canal, lymph nodes, central nervous system, or other tissues of patients with AML of the monocytic subtype and may form tumors in those locations. Leukemic monocytes tend to mature to the point at which they develop many of the cytoplasmic and membrane features required for motility and tissue entry.[46–48] Moreover, leukemic monocytes proliferate and survive in tissues for long periods. Consequently, this AML phenotype has a higher frequency of overt infiltrative tissue lesions than do other forms of AML.

Extramedullary tumors may usher in the accelerated phase of CML. These tumors may be composed of myeloblasts or lymphoblasts, although in each case the Ph chromosome or the *BCR-ABL* fusion is present in the cells, indicating the extramedullary Ph-positive lymphoblastomas are the tissue variant of the predisposition of CML to transform into a terminal deoxynucleotidyl transferase-positive lymphoblastic leukemia in approximately 30 percent of patients who enter blast crisis (see Chap. 90).

Release of Procoagulants and Fibrinolytic Activators

Microvascular thrombosis is a feature of AML of promyelocytic type, although thrombosis can occur in other forms of acute leukemia, especially in cases with elevated white cell counts or monocytic phenotypes.[49,50] The leukemic promyelocytes liberate tissue factor and other procoagulants, giving rise to disseminated intravascular coagulation, and annexin II, which augments conversion of plasminogen to plasmin and contributes to the activation of fibrinolysis (see Chaps. 89, 130, and 136). Each mechanism contributes to hypofibrinogenemia and hemorrhage. Thrombin generation may mediate the microvascular thrombotic aspect of this process, which can occur in acute promyelocytic, acute monocytic, or acute myelomonocytic leukemia, either before or after cytotoxic treatment.[51,52] The increased fibrinolytic activity further complicates coagulopathy in patients with promyelocytic leukemia.

Large-vessel arterial thrombosis is very rare as a presenting feature or complication of leukemia but has occurred in the setting of hyperleukocytosis and as a presenting feature of acute promyelocytic leukemia.[53,54]

The plasma levels of protein C antigen, functional protein C, free protein S, and antithrombin are decreased in some patients with AML. Although these changes are particularly notable in acute promyelocytic leukemia, they occur occasionally in other morphologic variants of AML. The changes are not related to liver disease or white cell count.[55,56]

Hyperleukocytic Syndromes

A proportion of patients with AML (5 to 15 percent) and CML (10 to 20 percent) manifest extraordinarily high blood leukocyte counts.[57–61] These patients present special problems because of the effects of blast cells in the microcirculation of the lung, brain, eye, ear, and penis, and the metabolic effects that result when massive numbers of leukemic cells in blood, marrow, and tissues are simultaneously killed by cytotoxic drugs. Cell concentrations greater than 100,000/μL (100×10^9/L) in AML and greater than 300,000/μL (300×10^9/L) in CML usually are required to produce such problems. In CML, the manifestations of hyperleukocytosis are usually reversed by cytoreduction and may not portend a poor outcome with antityrosine kinase therapy. In AML, intracerebral hemorrhage and the impairment of pulmonary function are the most serious manifestations in predicting early death.[60,61] A respiratory distress syndrome attributed to pulmonary leukostasis occurs in some patients with acute promyelocytic leukemia after all-*trans*-retinoic acid therapy.[62] The syndrome is usually, but not always, associated with prominent neutrophilia.

The viscosity of blood is related to the total cytocrit and usually is not increased in hyperleukocytic leukemias because the reduced hematocrit compensates for increased leukocrit. This compensatory change is invariably present in AML. In CML there is a very close negative correlation of hematocrit with leukocrit, preventing an increase in bulk viscosity.[57] Occasional patients with hyperleukocytic CML who are transfused initially with red cells may have a blood viscosity increased above normal.

Pathologic studies of patients who have died with hyperleukocytosis have identified leuko-occlusion, and vascular invasion in small vessels of the lung, brain, or other sites. Because viscosity in the microcirculation is a function of the plasma viscosity and the deformability of individual cells in capillaries, leukocytes should transiently raise the viscosity in such small channels. Flow in microvascular channels decreases if poorly deformable blast cells enter capillary channels.[63] With high leukocyte counts, chronically reduced flow may reduce oxygen transport to tissues because the probability of leukocytes being in microchannels should increase as a function of white cell count. Moreover, trapped leukemic cells have an oxygen consumption rate that contributes to deleterious effects in the microcirculation. Leukocyte aggregation, leukocyte microthrombi, release of toxic products from leukocytes, endothelial cell damage, and microvascular invasion can contribute to vascular injury and flow impedance. Adhesive interactions between leukemic blast cells and endothelium may also be involved but have not been defined.

TABLE 85–2. Clinical Features of the Hyperleukocytic Syndrome

I.	Pulmonary circulation
	A. Tachypnea, dyspnea, cyanosis
	B. Alveolar–capillary block
	C. Pulmonary infiltrates
	D. Postchemotherapy respiratory dysfunction
II.	Predisposition to tumor lysis syndrome
III.	Central nervous system circulation
	A. Dizziness, slurred speech, delirium, stupor
	B. Intracranial (cerebral) hemorrhage
IV.	Special sensory organ circulation
	A. Visual blurring
	B. Papilledema
	C. Diplopia
	D. Tinnitus, impaired hearing
	E. Retinal vein distention, retinal hemorrhages
V.	Penile circulation
	A. Priapism
VI.	Spurious laboratory results
	A. Decreased blood partial pressure of oxygen (P_{O2}); increased serum potassium
	B. Decreased plasma glucose; increased mean corpuscular volume, red cell count, hemoglobin, and hematocrit

High leukemic blast cell counts in AML and CML may be associated with pulmonary, central nervous system, special sensory, or penile circulatory impairment (Table 85–2). Sudden death can occur in patients with hyperleukocytic acute leukemia as a result of intracranial hemorrhage.[60,61] Hyperleukocytosis can be treated initially with hydration, leukapheresis, and/or cytotoxic therapy, usually hydroxyurea (see Chaps. 89 and 90). In patients with CML, leukapheresis reverses the hyperleukocytic syndrome and can reduce the extent of cytolysis-induced hyperuricemia, hyperkalemia, and hyperphosphatemia by reducing tumor cell mass before cytotoxic therapy. Hydroxyurea may follow as, or soon after, the tumor cell burden is decreased. Unfortunately, the specific effect of leukapheresis, hydroxyurea therapy, or cranial irradiation in patients with hyperleukocytic AML on duration of survival appears to be negligible.[59–61]

THROMBOCYTHEMIC SYNDROMES: HEMORRHAGE AND THROMBOPHILIA

Hemorrhagic or thrombotic episodes can develop during the course of essential thrombocythemia or thrombocythemia associated with other clonal myeloid diseases.[62–64] Arterial vascular insufficiency and venous thrombosis are the major vascular manifestations of thrombocythemia. Peripheral vascular insufficiency with gangrene and cerebral vascular thrombi can occur. Thrombosis of superficial or deep veins of the extremities occurs frequently.[65] Mesenteric, hepatic, portal, splenic, or penile venous thrombosis can develop. Hemorrhage is an occasional manifestation of thrombocythemia and can occur concomitantly with thrombotic episodes. Gastrointestinal hemorrhage and cutaneous hemorrhage, the latter especially after trauma, happen most frequently, but bleeding from other sites also can occur (see Chap. 87).

Procoagulant factors, such as the content of platelet tissue factor and blood platelet neutrophil aggregates, are higher in patients with essential thrombocythemia than normal subjects and are higher among patients with the V617F JAK2 mutation than patients with wild-type gene structure.[65,66]

Thrombotic complications occur in approximately 40 percent of patients with polycythemia vera.[65,67] Erythrocytosis and thrombocytosis may interact and cause hypercoagulability, especially in the abdominal venous circulation. A syndrome of splanchnic venous thrombosis associated with endogenous erythroid colony growth, the latter characteristic of polycythemia vera, but without blood cell count changes indicative of a myeloproliferative disease, has accounted for a high proportion of patients with apparent idiopathic hepatic or portal vein thrombosis.[68,69] These cases may have blood cells with the Janus kinase 2 (JAK2) gene mutation without a clinically apparent myeloproliferative phenotype.[70]

Nearly half of patients with paroxysmal nocturnal hemoglobinuria have thrombosis, especially in the venous system. Thrombosis of the veins of the abdomen, liver, and other organs, characteristic complications of paroxysmal nocturnal hemoglobinuria, may result from a complex thrombophilic state related to nitric oxide depletion, formation of prothrombotic platelet microvesicles, the dysfunction of tissue factor pathway inhibitor, and other factors.[71,72] Thrombosis is more common in paroxysmal nocturnal hemoglobinuria (PNH) patients with the classical hemolytic syndrome than in those with the PNH-aplastic anemia hybrid (see Chap. 40).

■ SYSTEMIC SYMPTOMS

Fever, weight loss, and malaise occur as early manifestations of AML. At the time of diagnosis, low-grade fever is present in nearly 50 percent of patients.[73] Although minor infections may be present, severe systemic infections are relatively uncommon at the time of AML diagnosis.[74] However, fever during cytotoxic therapy, when neutrophil counts are extremely low, nearly always is a sign of infection. Fever also may be a manifestation of the acute leukemic transformation of CML and can occur in patients with oligoblastic myelogenous leukemia (refractory anemia with excess blasts).

Weight loss occurs in nearly 20 percent of patients with AML.[74] Loss of well-being and intolerance to exertion may be disproportionate to the extent of anemia and may not be corrected by red cell transfusions. The pathogenesis of these effects is unknown.

■ METABOLIC SIGNS

Hyperuricemia and hyperuricosuria are common manifestations of AML and CML. Acute gouty arthritis and hyperuricosuric nephropathy are less common. If therapy is instituted without a reduction in plasma uric acid and without adequate hydration, saturation of the urine with uric acid can lead to precipitation of urate (gravel) and obstructive uropathy. If the uropathy is severe, urine flow can be obliterated, and renal failure ensues. Hyponatremia can occur in AML, and in some cases results from inappropriate antidiuretic hormone secretion. Hyponatremia also can result from an osmotic diuresis of urea, creatinine, urate, and other substances released from blast cells and wasting muscles. Hypernatremia is rare but may be seen in cases with central diabetes insipidus. Hypokalemia is commonly seen in AML[74–76] and is thought to be caused by injury to the kidney by increased plasma and urine lysozyme and subsequent kaliuresis. Hypokalemia is related to excessive urinary potassium loss, but the correlation with lysozymuria is imperfect. Other mechanisms probably are responsible in most cases, including osmotic diuresis and tubular dysfunction. Kaliuretic antibiotics, often administered to patients with AML, may accentuate the hypokalemia. Hyperkalemia is very unusual, but may be seen with tumor lysis syndrome. Hypercalcemia occurs in occasional patients with AML. Several causes have been proposed, including bone resorption as a result of leukemic infiltration. This explanation is in keeping with the normal serum inorganic phosphate in most patients. Occasional patients with hypercalcemia, and hypophosphatemia can have ectopic parathyroid hormone secretion by leukemic blast cells. Hypophosphatemia also can occur because of rapid utilization of plasma inorganic phosphate in some cases of myelogenous leukemia with a high blood blast cell count and a high fraction of proliferative cells. Hyperphosphatemia is uncommon, except as a reflection of the tumor lysis syndrome. Approximately 10 percent of persons with AML show varying degrees of tumor lysis syndrome in the week after onset of therapy, reflected in at least doubling of baseline creatinine, and increases in serum phosphate (>1.6 mmol/L [>5 mg/dL]), uric acid (>416 mmol/L [>7mg/dL]), or potassium (>5 mmol/L [>5 mEq/L]).[77] Hypomagnesemia is common as a result of low intake coupled with gastrointestinal loss and a shift of magnesium to the intracellular compartment.

Acid–base disturbances occur in approximately 25 percent of patients, the majority having respiratory or metabolic alkalosis.[76] The latter may be secondary to volume depletion, upper gastrointestinal fluid loss, and hypokalemia. Lactic acidosis also has been observed in association with AML, although the mechanism is obscure. True hypoxia can result from the hyperleukocytic syndrome as a consequence of pulmonary vascular leukostasis (see also "Factitious Laboratory Results" below)

Increased serum concentrations of lipoprotein (a) and decreased concentrations of both low-density and high-density lipoproteins have been observed in a high proportion of patients with AML.[78] The increased level of lipoprotein (a), which returns to normal after successful treatment, correlates with the presence of leukemic blast cells. Serum prolactin also is increased in some patients with AML.[79] Leukemic blast cells may be an ectopic source of this hormone.[79]

Colony-stimulating factor-1 is elevated in a variety of lymphoid and hemopoietic malignancies, including AML and CML.[80] The malignant cells have been proposed as the source of excess cytokine.

■ FACTITIOUS LABORATORY RESULTS

Elevations of serum potassium levels have resulted from the release of potassium from platelets or, less often, leukocytes in patients with myeloproliferative diseases and extreme elevations in those blood cell concentrations. If blood is collected in a tube that contains an anticoagulant and the plasma is removed after high-speed centrifugation, the potassium concentration is normal. Glucose can be falsely decreased, especially because autoanalyzer techniques call for omission of glycolytic inhibitors such as sodium fluoride in collection tubes. Blood with high leukocyte counts, if it stands prior to separation of the plasma, may have a significant amount of glucose metabolism by leukocytes. Factitious hypoglycemia also can occur as a result of red cell utilization of glucose, especially in polycythemic patients. True hypoglycemia has been observed rarely in patients with leukemia. Arterial blood oxygen content also can be lowered spuriously as a result of in vitro utilization by large numbers of leukocytes, while the anticoagulated blood awaits measurement.

■ SPECIFIC ORGAN INVOLVEMENT

Clonal myeloid diseases lead to disturbances principally in marrow, blood, and spleen. Although clusters of cells may be found in all organs, major infiltrates and organ dysfunction are unusual. In AML and the acute blastic phase of CML, clinically significant infiltration of the larynx, central nervous system, heart, lungs, bone, joints, gastrointestinal tract, genitourinary tract, skin, or virtually any other organ can occur.

Splenomegaly

In AML, palpable splenomegaly is present in approximately one-third of cases but usually is slight in extent. In the chronic myeloproliferative diseases, palpable splenomegaly is present in a high proportion of cases (polycythemia vera ~80 percent, CML ~90 percent, primary myelofibrosis ~100 percent). In essential thrombocythemia, splenic enlargement is present in approximately 60 percent of patients. A predisposition to silent splenic vascular thrombi, infarction, and subsequent splenic atrophy, analogous to that occurring in sickle cell anemia, is postulated as the cause of the lower frequency of splenic enlargement in essential thrombocythemia. Early satiety, left-upper-quadrant discomfort, splenic infarctions with painful perisplenitis, diaphragmatic pleuritis, and shoulder pain may occur in patients with splenomegaly, especially in the acute phase of CML and in primary myelofibrosis. In primary myelofibrosis, the spleen can become enormous, occupying the left hemiabdomen. Blood flow through the splenic vein can be so great as to lead to portal hypertension and gastroesophageal varices. Usually, reduced hepatic venous compliance also is present (see Chap. 91). Bleeding and, occasionally, encephalopathy can result from portal–systemic venous shunts.

Marrow Necrosis

Extensive marrow necrosis, an uncommon event, can occur in any clonal myeloid disease, especially AML, and less often, primary myelofibrosis, CML, essential thrombocythemia, and polycythemia vera. Bone pain and fever are the most common initial findings. Anemia and thrombocytopenia are very common, as are nucleated red cells and myelocytes in the blood (leukoerythroblastic reaction).[81,82] Marrow aspiration does not result in a useful sample but biopsy early in the process usually shows hypocellularity with loss of marrow cell structural definition (blurred staining of residual cells), evidence of cell necrosis, gelatinous transformation of marrow, and, often, an amorphous eosinophilic material throughout. The mechanism is thought to be microvascular dysfunction. Restitution of marrow and repopulation of hematopoietic tissue often may follow. The prognosis is a function of the underlying disease.

REFERENCES

1. Dick JE, Lapidot T: Biology of normal and acute myeloid leukemia stem cells. *Int J Hematol* 82:389, 2005.
2. Jordan CT: Searching for leukemia stem cells—Not yet the end of the road. *Cancer Cell* 10:253, 2006.
3. Jordan CT, Guzman ML, Noble M: Cancer stem cells. *N Engl J Med* 355:1253, 2006.
4. Rozman CGM, Feliu E, Rubio D, et al: Life expectancy of patients with chronic non-leukemic myeloproliferative disorders. *Cancer* 67:2658, 1991.
5. Germing U, Gattermann N, Aivado M, et al: Two types of acquired idiopathic sideroblastic anaemia (AISA): A time-tested distinction. *Br J Haematol* 108:724, 2000.
6. Jaffe ES, Harris NL, Stein H, Vardiman JW: *World Health Organization Classification of Tumours: Pathology and Genetics of Tumours of Haematopoietic and Lymphoid Tissues*. IARC Press, Lyon, 2001.
7. Lichtman MA: Myelodysplasia or myeloneoplasia: Thoughts on the nosology of clonal myeloid diseases. *Blood Cells Mol Dis* 26:572, 2000.
8. Bessis M, Bernard J: Hematopoietic dysplasias (preleukemic states) *Blood Cells* 2:5, 1976.
9. Spivak JL, Silver RT: The revised World Health Organization diagnostic criteria for polycythemia vera, essential thrombocytosis, and primary myelofibrosis: An alternative proposal. *Blood* 112:231, 2008.
10. Kiladjian JJ, Gardin C, Renoux M, et al: Long-term outcomes of polycythemia vera patients treated with pipobroman as initial therapy. *Hematol J* 4:198, 2003.
11. Tefferi A, Fonesca R, Pereira DL, Hoagland HC: A long-term retrospective study of young women with essential thrombocythemia. *Mayo Clin Proc* 76:22, 2001.
12. Passamonti F, Malabarba L, Orlandi E, et al: Polycythemia in young patients: A study on the long-term risk of thrombosis, myelofibrosis and leukemia. *Haematologica* 88:13, 2003.
13. Lichtman MA: Is it chronic idiopathic myelofibrosis, myelofibrosis with myeloid metaplasia, chronic megakaryocytic-granulocytic myelosis, or chronic megakaryocytic leukemia? Further thoughts on the nosology of the clonal myeloid disorders. *Leukemia* 19:1139, 2005.
14. Simon W, Segel GB, Lichtman MA: Early allogeneic stem cell transplantation for chronic myelogenous leukemia in the imatinib era: A preliminary assessment. *Blood Cells Mol Dis* 37:116, 2006.
15. Tefferi A, Elliott MA, Pardanani A: Atypical myeloproliferative disorders: Diagnosis and management. *Mayo Clin Proc* 81:553, 2006.
16. Tefferi A, Vardiman JW: Classification and diagnosis of myeloproliferative neoplasms: the 2008 World Health Organization criteria and point-of-care diagnostic algorithms. *Leukemia* 22:14, 2008.
17. Breccia M, Cannella L, Frustaci A, et al: Chronic myelomonocytic leukemia with antecedent refractory anemia with excess blasts: further evidence for the arbitrary nature of current classification systems. *Leuk Lymphoma* 49:1292, 2008.
18. Breccia M, Latagliata R, Cannella L, et al: Analysis of prognostic factors in patients with refractory anemia with excess of blasts (RAEB) reclassified according to WHO proposal. *Leuk Res* 33:391, 2009.
19. Barnard DR, Kalousek DK, Wiersma SR, et al: Morphologic, immunologic, and cytogenetic classification of acute myeloid leukemia and myelodysplastic syndrome in childhood. *Leukemia* 10:5,1996.
20. Bene MC, Castoldi G, Knapp W, et al: Proposals for the immunological classification of acute leukemias. *Leukemia* 9:1783, 1995.
21. Jennings CD, Foon KA: Recent advances in flow cytometry: Application to the diagnosis of hematologic malignancy. *Blood* 90:2863, 1997.
22. http://cgap.nci.nih.gov/Chromosomes/Mitelman (accessed August 2008).
23. Oyan AM, Bø TH, Jonassen I, et al: Global gene expression in classification, pathogenetic understanding and identification of therapeutic targets in acute myeloid leukemia. *Curr Pharm Biotechnol* 8:344, 2007.
24. Valk PJM, Verhaak RGW, Beijen A, et al: Prognostically useful gene expression profiles in acute myeloid leukemia. *N Engl J Med* 350:1617, 2004.
25. Bullinger L, Döhner K, Kranz R, et al: An FLT3 gene-expression signature predicts clinical outcome in normal karyotype AML. *Blood* 111:4490, 2008.
26. Jongen-Lavrencic M, Sun SM, Dijkstra MK, et al: MicroRNA expression profiling in relation to the genetic heterogeneity of acute myeloid leukemia. *Blood* 111:5078, 2008.
27. Garzon R, Croce CM: MicroRNAs in normal and malignant hematopoiesis. *Curr Opin Hematol* 15:352 2008.
28. Mills K I. Gene expression profiling for the diagnosis and prognosis of acute myeloid leukemia. *Front Biosci* 13:4605, 2008.
29. Andrieux J, Demory JL, Caulier MT, et al: Karyotype abnormalities in myelofibrosis following polycythemia vera. *Cancer Genet Cytogenet* 140:118, 2003.
30. Finazzi G, Caruso V, Marchioli R, et al: Acute leukemia in polycythemia vera: An analysis of 1638 patients enrolled in a prospective observational study. *Blood* 105:2664, 2005.
31. Lichtman MA: The stem cell in the pathogenesis and treatment of myelogenous leukemia: A perspective. *Leukemia* 15:1489, 2001.
32. Gilliland DG: Molecular genetics of human leukemias: New insights into therapy. *Semin Hematol* 39:6, 2002.
33. Lichtman MA, Segel GB: Uncommon phenotypes of acute myelogenous leukemia: Basophilic, mast cell, eosinophilic, and myeloid dendritic cell subtypes: A review. *Blood Cells Mol Dis* 35:370, 2005.
34. Ploemacher RE: Characterization and biology of normal human haematopoietic stem cells. *Haematologica* 84:4(EHA-4), 1999.
35. Bonnet D, Dick J: Human acute myeloid leukemia is organized as a hierarchy that originates from a primitive hematopoietic cell. *Nat Med* 3:730, 1997.
36. Takahashi N, Maura I, Saitoh K, Miura AB: Lineage involvement of stem cells bearing the Philadelphia chromosome in chronic myeloid leukemia in the chronic phase as shown by combination of fluorescence-activated cell sorting and fluorescence in situ hybridization. *Blood* 92:4758, 1998.
37. Fialkow PJ, Singer JW, Adamson JW, et al: Acute nonlymphocytic leukemia: Expression in cells restricted to granulocytic and monocytic differentiation. *N Engl J Med* 301:1, 1979.
38. Fialkow PJ, Singer JW, Adamson JW, et al: Acute nonlymphocytic leukemia: Heterogeneity of stem cell origin. *Blood* 57:1068, 1981.
39. Ferraris AM, Broccia G, Meloni T, et al: Clonal origin of cells restricted to monocytic differentiation in acute nonlymphocytic leukemia. *Blood* 64:817, 1984.
40. Van Lom K, Hagenmaijer A, Vandekerckhove F, et al: Clonality analysis of hematopoietic cell lineages in acute myeloid leukemia and trans-location (8;21): Only myeloid cells are part of the malignant clone. *Leukemia* 11:202, 1997.
41. Grimwade D, Enver T: Acute promyelocytic leukemia: Where does it stem from? *Leukemia* 18:375, 2004.
42. Lichtman MA: Interrupting the inhibition of normal hematopoiesis in myelogenous leukemia: A hypothetical approach to therapy. *Stem Cells* 18(5):304, 2000.
43. Menasce LP, Banerjee SS, Becket E, Harris M: Extramedullary myeloid tumor (granulocytic sarcoma) is often misdiagnosed. A study of 26 cases. *Histopathology* 34:391, 1999.

44. Pileri SA, Ascani S, Cox MC, et al: Myeloid sarcoma: clinico-pathologic, phenotypic and cytogenetic analysis of 92 adult patients. *Leukemia* 21:340, 2007.
45. Tsimberidou AM, Kantarjian HM, Wen S, et al: Myeloid sarcoma is associated with superior event-free survival and overall survival compared with acute myeloid leukemia. *Cancer* 113:1370, 2008 .
46. Lichtman MA, Weed RI: Peripheral cytoplasmic characteristics of leukemia cells in monocytic leukemia: Relationship to clinical manifestations. *Blood* 40:52, 1972.
47. Peterson L, Dekner LP, Brunning RD: Extramedullary masses as presenting features of acute monoblastic leukemia. *Am J Clin Pathol* 75:140, 1981.
48. Tobelem G, Jacquillat C, Chastang C, et al: Acute monoblastic leukemia: A clinical and biologic study of 74 cases. *Blood* 55:71, 1980.
49. Weltermann A, Pabinger I, Geissler K, et al: Hypofibrinogenemia in non-M3 acute myeloid leukemia. Incidence, clinical and laboratory characteristics and prognosis. *Leukemia* 12:1182, 1998.
50. Uchiumi H, Matsushima T, Yamane A, et al: Prevalence and clinical characteristics of acute myeloid leukemia associated with disseminated intravascular coagulation. *Int J Hematol* 86:137, 2007.
51. Falanga A, Rickles FR: Pathogenesis and management of the bleeding diathesis in acute promyelocytic leukaemia. *Best Pract Res Clin Haematol* 16:463, 2003.
52. Tallman MS, Abutalib SA, Altman JK: The double hazard of thrombophilia and bleeding in acute promyelocytic leukemia. *Semin Thromb Hemost* 33:330, 2007.
53. Kalk E, Goede A, Rose P: Acute arterial thrombosis in acute promyelocytic leukaemia. *Clin Lab Haematol* 25:267, 2003.
54. Reisch N, Roehnisch T, Sadeghi M, et al: AML M1 presenting with recurrent acute large arterial vessel thromboembolism. *Leuk Res* 31:869, 2007.
55. Troy K, Essex D, Rand J, et al: Protein C and S levels in acute leukemia. *Am J Hematol* 37:159, 1991.
56. Dixit A, Kannan M, Mahapatra M, et al: Roles of protein C, protein S, and antithrombin III in acute leukemia. *Am J Hematol* 81:171, 2006.
57. Lichtman MA, Heal J, Rowe JM: Hyperleukocytic leukaemia: Rheological and clinical features and management. *Baillieres Clin Haematol* 1:725, 1987.
58. Rowe JM, Lichtman MA: Hyperleukocytosis and leukostasis: common features of childhood chronic myelogenous leukemia. *Blood* 63:1230, 1984.
59. Porcu P, Cripe LD, Ng EW, et al: Hyperleukocytic leukemias and leukostasis: A review of pathophysiology, clinical presentation and management. *Leuk Lymphoma* 39:1, 2000.
60. Marbello L, Ricci F, Nosari AM: Outcome of hyperleukocytic adult acute myeloid leukaemia: A single-center retrospective study and review of literature. *Leuk Res* 32:1221, 2008.
61. Chang MC, Chen TY, Tang JL, et al: Leukapheresis and cranial irradiation in patients with hyperleukocytic acute myeloid leukemia: No impact on early mortality and intracranial hemorrhage. *Am J Hematol* 82:976, 2007.
62. Patatanian E, Thompson DF: Retinoic acid syndrome: A review. *J Clin Pharm Ther* 33:331, 2008.
63. Östergren J, Fagrell B, Björkholm M: Hyperleukocytic effects on skin capillary circulation in patients with leukaemia. *J Intern Med* 231:19, 1992.
64. Cortelazzo S, Vicero P, Finazzi G, et al: Incidence and risk factors for thrombotic complications in a historical cohort of 100 patients with thrombocythemia. *J Clin Oncol* 8:556, 1990.
65. Falanga A, Barbui T, Rickles FR: Hypercoagulability and tissue factor gene upregulation in hematologic malignancies. *Semin Thromb Hemost* 34:204, 2008.
66. Dahabreh IJ, Zoi K, Giannouli S, et al: Is JAK2 V617F mutation more than a diagnostic index? A meta-analysis of clinical outcomes in essential thrombocythemia. *Leuk Res* 33:67, 2009.
67. Landolfi R: Bleeding and thrombosis in myeloproliferative disorders. *Curr Opin Hematol* 5:327, 1998.
68. Anger B, Haugh U, Seidler R, Heimpel H: Polycythemia vera: A clinical study of 141 patients. *Blut* 59:493, 1989.
69. Teofili L, De Stefano V, Leone G, et al: Hematologic causes of venous thrombosis in young people: High incidence of myeloproliferative disorder as underlying disease in patients with splanchnic venous thrombosis. *Thromb Haemost* 67:297, 1992.
70. Colaizzo D, Amitrano L, Tiscia GL, et al: Occurrence of the JAK2 V617F mutation in the Budd-Chiari syndrome. *Blood Coagul Fibrinolysis* 19:459, 2008.
71. Peffault de Latour R, Mary JY, Salanoubat C, et al: Paroxysmal nocturnal hemoglobinuria: natural history of disease subcategories. *Blood* 112:3099, 2008.
72. Brodsky RA: Advances in the diagnosis and therapy of paroxysmal nocturnal hemoglobinuria. *Blood Rev* 22:65, 2008.
73. Burke PJ, Braine HG, Rathbun HK, Owens AH Jr: The clinical significance of fever in acute myelocytic leukemia. *Johns Hopkins Med J* 139:1, 1976.
74. Burns CP, Armitage JO, Frey AL, et al: Analysis of the presenting features of adult acute leukemia. *Cancer* 47:2460, 1981.
75. Mir MA, Delamore JW: Metabolic disorders in acute myeloid leukaemia. *Br J Haematol* 40:79, 1978.
76. Filippatos TD, Milionis HJ, Elisaf MS: Alterations in electrolyte equilibrium in patients with acute leukemia. *Eur J Haematol* 75:449, 2005.
77. Mato AR, Riccio BE, Qin L, et al: A predictive model for the detection of tumor lysis syndrome during AML induction therapy. *Leuk Lymphoma* 47:877, 2006.
78. Niendorf A, Stang A, Beisiegel U, et al: Elevated lipoprotein (a) levels in patients with acute myeloblastic leukaemia decrease after successful chemotherapeutic treatment. *Clin Investig* 70:683, 1990.
79. Hatfill SJ, Kirby R, Hanley M, et al: Hyperprolactinemia in acute myeloid leukemia and indication of ectopic expression of human prolactin in blast cells of a patient of subtype M4. *Leuk Res* 14:57, 1990.
80. Janowska-Wieczarek A, Belch AR, Jacobs A, et al: Increased circulating colony-stimulating factor-1 in patients with preleukemia, leukemia and lymphoid malignancies. *Blood* 77:1796, 1991.
81. Janssens AM, Offner FC, Van Hove WZ: Bone marrow necrosis. *Cancer* 88:1769, 2000.
82. Paydas S, Ergin M, Baslamisli F, et al: Bone marrow necrosis: clinicopathologic analysis of 20 cases and review of the literature. *Am J Hematol* 70:300, 2002.

CHAPTER 86
POLYCYTHEMIA VERA

Josef T. Prchal and Jaroslav F. Prchal

SUMMARY

Polycythemia vera is a disorder in the group of chronic myeloproliferative disorders (MPDs), also refered to as myeloproliferative neoplasms, that includes essential thrombocythemia (ET), primary myelofibrosis (PMF), and chronic myelogenous leukemia (CML). Polycythemia vera is an acquired clonal primary polycythemic disorder. Primary polycythemias result from abnormal intrinsic properties of erythroid progenitors that proliferate independently or excessively in response to extrinsic regulators; low serum erythropoietin is their hallmark. The most common primary polycythemia is polycythemia vera. Polycythemia vera arises from mutations in a multipotential hematopoietic stem cell, which results in an excess production of functionally normal erythrocytes, a variable overproduction of granulocytes and monocytes, and of platelets. It is usually accompanied by splenomegaly. Most patients with polycythemia vera have a somatic mutations of the Janus-type tyrosine kinase-2 gene (*JAK2*) that is detectable in blood myeloid cells. This mutation, *JAK2* V617F, results in constitutive hyperactivity of JAK2 stemming from the loss-of-function of its negative regulatory domain. *JAK2* V617F is present in virtually all cases of polycythemia vera; however, ET, MF, and, much less commonly, other hematologic neoplastic disorders are also associated with this mutation, albeit at lower frequency. As with other clonal hematologic disorders, polycythemia vera can undergo a clonal evolution to PMF (typically *JAK2* V617-positive) and acute leukemia (often *JAK2* V617-negative). In virtually all PV *JAK2* V617F-positive patients at least some progenitors exist that became homozygous for the *JAK2* V617F mutation by uniparenteral disomy acquired by mitotic recombination and the majority of these account for the erythropoietin-independent erythroid colonies detected *in vitro* by clonogenic burst-forming unit–erythroid assay (BFU-E). The *JAK2* V617F mutation is not a cause of clonal proliferation of these disorders but is preceded by other germ-line and somatic mutation(s) that remain to be identified. Arterial and venous thromboses are the major causes of morbidity and mortality of polycythemia vera. A small proportion of patients develop secondary myelofibrosis (*spent phase*) and/or an invariably fatal acute leukemic transformation. Myelosuppressive therapy has been an effective mode of therapy, with drugs such as hydroxyurea, busulfan, and radioactive phosphorus useful in controlling proliferation of all blood cell lineages. Myelosuppressive therapy decreases the incidence of thrombotic complications but these drugs have variable leukemogenic potential. Newer, better-tolerated preparations of interferon such as pegylated interferon-α may lead to complete hematologic remission and restoration of polyclonal hematopoiesis. Targeted therapy with JAK2 kinase inhibitors is currently being evaluated for effects on splenomegaly and splenomegaly-associated symptoms, hypercoagulability, and control of the polycythemia vera clone.

Acronyms and abbreviations used in this chapter include: *bcl-x,* an antiapoptotic protein; BFU-E, burst-forming unit–erythroid; EEC, endogenous erythroid colonies; EPO, erythropoietin; ET, essential thrombocytosis; c-MPL, thrombopoietin receptor; JAK2, Janus-type tyrosine kinase 2; MPDs, myeloproliferative disorders; PFCP, primary familial and congenital polycythemia; PMF, primary myelofibrosis; PV, polycythemia vera; PRV-1, a receptor named polycythemia rubra vera 1.

DEFINITION AND HISTORY

The term *polycythemia,* denoting an increased amount of blood, has traditionally been applied to those conditions in which the mass of erythrocytes is increased. In polycythemia vera (PV), an increase in the erythroid mass is frequently accompanied by an increase in neutrophils and in platelets. Chapter 56 and Table 33–2 present a classification of the polycythemias.

PV, the sole clonal form of primary polycythemia, was first described in 1892 by Vaquez.[1] In 1903, Osler reviewed four cases of his own and an additional five cases from the literature. He wrote, "The condition is characterized by chronic cyanosis, polycythemia, and moderate enlargement of the spleen. The chief symptoms have been weakness, prostration, constipation, headache, and vertigo."[2] The increased proliferation of granulocyte precursors and megakaryocytes was first described by Türk in 1904.[3]

EPIDEMIOLOGY

Mayo Clinic data indicate that 2.8 per 100,000 men and 1.3 per 100,000 women[4] have PV, estimates that are similar to those from epidemiologic data in Sweden[5]; other studies and estimates indicate a higher incidence among Ashkenazi Jews.[6,7] The true incidence may be higher, as many cases are asymptomatic, and thus not diagnosed. JAK2 V617F mutation testing can uncover hidden cases of PV among subjects with thrombosis or concomitant iron deficiency.

Although most patients with PV do not endorse a history of polycythemia in the family, familial incidence of the disorder is known to occur[8–10] and is very likely underreported. In the familial cases, an inherited predisposition, perhaps in the form of a germ-line mutation, presumably facilitates the acquired somatic mutation(s) necessary for disease onset.[9,11]

ETIOLOGY AND PATHOGENESIS

PV arises from the neoplastic transformation of a single normal hematopoietic multipotential cell, which provides both a selective growth and survival advantage that results in the cells produced in the clone suppressing and replacing normal polyclonal hematopoiesis. The clonal origin of PV has been demonstrated in women heterozygous for a polymorphic X-chromosome marker, glucose-6-phosphate dehydrogenase,[12] as well as by more modern clonality assays (see Chap. 9).[13] In each case, all hematopoietic cell lineages[9,12,16] express either only one isoform of the enzyme or the X-chromosome polymorphic allele encoded by the maternal or paternal X chromosome, whereas nonhematopoietic cells are a mosaic of both enzyme types.

In vitro marrow- or blood-derived erythroid colonies of PV patients arise from both burst-forming unit–erythroid (BFU-E) precursors with normal erythropoietin sensitivity along with BFU-E that grow in the absence of erythropoietin and form so-called endogenous erythroid colonies (EEC),[14,15] the latter a characteristic of PV. However, most of the BFU-E progenitors with normal erythropoietin sensitivity are also part of the PV clone.[16] The fibroblasts that accumulate in the marrow of patients with PV as the disease progresses are not a part of the abnormal clone. Rather, they seem to be a response to the proliferating marrow cells, perhaps to the platelet-derived fibroblast growth factor elaborated by megakaryocytes (see Chap. 91).

Other abnormalities that have been described include (1) decreased levels of the platelet thrombopoietin receptor,[17] (2) deregulation of BCL-x, an inhibitor of apoptosis,[18] (3) increased expression of protein tyrosine phosphatase activity by red cell precursors,[19] (4) increased messenger RNA (mRNA) levels of the PRV-1 ("a receptor named polycythemia rubra vera 1") gene in granulocytes,[20] and (5) acquired loss-of-heterozygosity of chromosome 9p as a result of uniparental disomy.[11] This last observation led to the discovery of the Janus-type tyrosine kinase 2 (*JAK2*) V617F mutation located on chromosome 9p,[11,21] which has improved our understanding of disease pathogenesis, improved the specificity of diagnosis and has led to an explosion of research in myeloproliferative disorders (see "*JAK2 V617F* Mutation" below).

There are no specific karyotypic markers occurring with high frequency in PV. Fewer than 25 percent of patients have karyotypic abnormalities at diagnosis,[22–26] but the incidence rises with the increasing duration of the disease,[23,27] suggesting that karyotypic abnormalities represent secondary genetic events.[28]

JAK2 V617F MUTATION

JAK2 is present in virtually all hematopoietic cells and is essential for proliferative intracellular signaling in response to a variety of hematopoietic growth factors (see Chaps. 33 and 56). The *V617F* mutation was first identified in PV in 2004[21] and was then reported by several other laboratories.[29–31] The *V617F* mutation is identified in virtually all patients with PV and in more than 50 percent of patients with essential thrombocytosis (ET) and myelofibrosis; rarely is it found in a minority of patients with other myeloproliferative disorders.[32,33] In PV (unlike in ET), it is often in its homozygous form, at least in some of the progenitors.[24,34] In some of the rare PV patients who are *JAK2 V617F*-negative, other *JAK2* mutations have been identified in exon 12.[35]

Studies of families of MPD patients, in which several different MPDs occur in a single pedigree,[9,36] indicate that *JAK2* mutations may not be solely responsible for the disease phenotype, and may not even represent the disease-initiating event. A number of compelling lines of evidence support this conclusion. First, in familial PV, there is no clear linkage between the disease and chromosome 9p, the genetic site of *JAK2*, suggesting an independent germ-line predisposition to PV.[11] Second, in familial PV, affected members can be either *JAK2 V617F*-negative or -positive.[37] Third, the acquisition of the *JAK2 V617F* mutation is a late genetic event in PV.[38] Fourth, in sporadic PV, only a proportion of clonal PV cells are *JAK2 V617F*-positive.[34] Fifth, although the BFU-Es responsible for EEC, a hallmark of PV, are mostly *JAK2 V617F*-homozygous, some are heterozygous and some have a wild sequence at the *JAK2* locus.[34] And sixth, the acute leukemic transformation of any *JAK2*-positive MPDs is frequently negative for the *JAK2 V617F* mutation.[32,39] These diverse observations strongly suggest that the somatic mutation of *JAK2* gene is not the initiating or sole pathogenic process in PV.

A genomic chromosome 9p functional variant might also be relevant to the pathogenesis of the *JAK2 V617F* mutation. The genotypes of PV, ET, and PMF have a specific constitutional JAK2 haplotype associated with *JAK2 V617F* somatic mutation.[40,41] This haplotype is not associated with increased *JAK2* transcription or with augmented erythroid proliferation when measured in *in vitro* erythroid cultures.[40] The acquisition of the *V617F* mutation of *JAK2* is a late genetic event in patients with myeloproliferative disorders.[38,41] This finding was determined by examining the genomic composition in individual erythroid colonies. An independent occurrence of the *JAK2 V617F* mutation present on different haplotypes was found, although a specific constitutional inherited *JAK2* haplotype (*GGCC*) associated with the *JAK2 V617F* somatic mutation was also found in most *JAK2 V617F*-positive individuals and colonies.[41] This *GGCC* haplotype of *JAK2* also confers susceptibility to *JAK2* exon 12 mutation-positive PV.[42] These studies suggest that pre-JAK2 hypermutability events exist and that germ-line genetics play an important role in the early pathogenesis of MPDs.

In addition to the important role of *JAK2 V617F* and other *JAK2* mutations in the etiology of PV and other MPDs, mutations in other genes may be important to the full genesis of these disorders. *TET2* is a homologue of the gene originally discovered at the chromosome 10-11 translocation (TET) site in a subset of patients with acute leukemia. *TET2* mutations and deletions in this gene were found in marrow cells from a significant proportion of patients with PV and other MPDs,[43] and it was established that *TET2* loss-of-function mutations originate in pluripotential hematopoietic stem cells but seem to favor myeloid rather than lymphoid proliferation, and that in many patients both alleles were affected. However, studies in familial PV demonstrated that *TET2* mutations cannot be disease initiating, as the mutations differ among affected relatives and in some instances the *TET2* mutations followed, rather than preceded, the appearance of the *JAK2 V617F* mutation.[44]

CLINICAL FEATURES

SIGNS AND SYMPTOMS

PV usually has an insidious onset, most commonly during the sixth decade of life, although the onset may occur from childhood to old age.[45] Presenting symptoms and signs include headache, plethora, pruritus, thrombosis, and gastrointestinal bleeding, but many patients are diagnosed because elevated hemoglobin and blood cell counts are found on a periodic medical examination. Others cases may be uncovered during investigation for blood loss, iron-deficiency anemia, or thrombosis. Symptoms are reported by at least 30 percent of patients with polycythemia at the time of diagnosis; the most common in decreasing order of frequency are headache, weakness, pruritus, dizziness, and sweating.[45]

PV generally occurs in an older population and, thus, many of the vascular abnormalities (e.g., coronary artery disease) have a high prevalence related to the changes of aging. The prevalence of these events, however, is increased when complicated by PV.

Thrombosis and Hemorrhage

Thrombotic episodes are the most common and the most important complications of PV, occurring in about one-third of the patients.[46] From one half to three-quarters of these events are arterial[47]; ischemic strokes and transient ischemic attacks account for the majority of arterial complications. In some studies, it has been stated that over a period of 10 years, 40 to 60 percent of patients develop at least one thrombotic event, the annual incidence being approximately equal throughout this period.[48] However, in prospective studies, thrombosis was most common just prior to and in the first few years after diagnosis.[49,50] The most common serious complication is a cerebrovascular accident, which accounts for about one-third of the thrombotic events, followed in frequency by myocardial infarction, deep vein thrombosis, and pulmonary embolism.[48]

Bleeding and bruising is a common complication of PV, occurring in approximately one-quarter of the patients in some series.[46] Although such episodes are usually minor, such as gingival bleeding, nose bleeding, or easy bruising, serious gastrointestinal and other hemorrhagic complications with a fatal outcome also can occur.[28,47,51]

Hepatic Vein Thrombosis (Budd-Chiari Syndrome) Budd-Chiari syndrome is a catastrophic and often fatal complication of PV; it occurred in 10 percent of 140 patients in one series,[52] but was less common in a European collaborative study.[47] Budd-Chiari syndrome is caused by thrombosis of hepatic venous outflow leading to ischemia from reduced perfusion through hepatic arterioles and necrosis of hepatocytes. Budd-Chiari syndrome may present as ascites with or without right upper quadrant abdominal pain, hepatosplenomegaly, and jaundice.

The Budd-Chiari syndrome may be the first clinical manifestation of PV preceding the elevated blood counts; endogenous erythroid colony formation and the *JAK2 V617* mutation have been described in many of these patients before clinical evidence of polycythemia occurred. PV is the most frequent underlying disease associated with Budd-Chiari syndrome. In some series it accounts for the majority of this serious condition, frequently requiring a liver transplant for treatment.[53–55] The association of Budd-Chiari syndrome and PV is so strong that many experts advocate screening for PV in all patients who present with hepatic vein thrombosis.

Cutaneous Findings

Pruritus occurs in approximately 40 percent of patients.[56] It is usually aggravated by bathing or showering and may be so severe as to markedly compromise the quality of life of the patient. Its cause is unclear, and it has been attributed to increased numbers of mast cells in the skin[57] and to elevated histamine levels,[58] although these associations were not found in other studies.[59]

Several patients have developed the dermatologic disorder acute febrile neutrophilic dermatosis (Sweet syndrome).[60,61]

Erythromelalgia Erythromelalgia is a syndrome of warmth of the extremities, painful, reddened digits, a burning sensation, and erythema of the fingers and hands (Fig. 86–1) and feet that is associated with thrombocytosis and, characteristically, responds rapidly to low-dose aspirin therapy. In severe cases, it results in ischemic necrosis of the digits and may lead to their amputation. This syndrome occurs in less than 5 percent of PV patients.[47,51] It is not specific to PV or other myeloproliferative disorders, and in one series of 168 patients with erythromelalgia, less than 10 percent had PV.[62] It is frequently associated with essential thrombocythemia, and a role for transient microvascular occlusion by platelet aggregates has been proposed (Chap. 123).[63,64]

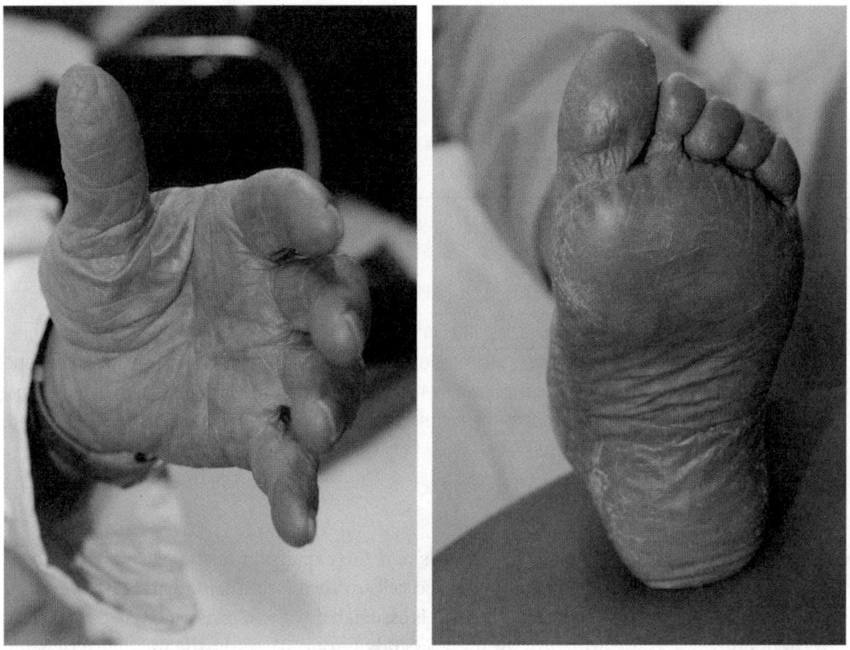

FIGURE 86–1. A recently diagnosed 82-year-old man with a JAK2 V617F positive myeloproliferative disorder and elevated platelets and hematocrit complaining of a burning sensation of hand and fingers. **A.** Erythromelalgia of his hands and finger. **B.** Erythromelalgia of his foot and toes.

Gastrointestinal Findings

The occurrence of Budd-Chiari syndrome is noted above (see "Hepatic Vein Thrombosis [Budd-Chiari Syndrome]"). Portal hypertension, varices, and abdominal pain are not uncommon,[65] and are often caused by unrecognized splenic or hepatic vein thromboses. The incidence of peptic ulcer is four to five times as great as in the general population.[66] Gastrointestinal bleeding may be the first presenting symptom of PV, with iron deficiency caused by gastrointestinal blood loss frequently masking the erythrocytosis of PV.

Cardiovascular Findings

Cardiovascular symptoms and complications include angina, myocardial infarction, and congestive heart failure, related to a predisposition to thrombosis in the coronary circulation.[28,47,49]

Pulmonary Hypertension

Pulmonary hypertension occurs in a higher than expected frequency in patients with PV. The suggested etiologies include smooth muscle hyperplasia induced by the release of platelet-derived growth factor from activated platelets, obstruction of pulmonary circulation by megakaryocytes, extramedullary hematopoiesis, and unrecognized recurrent thrombotic events[67,68]; however, none of these etiologies is clearly established.

Neurologic Findings

Neurologic symptoms such as dizziness are very common.[28,47,49,51,69] Spinal cord compression secondary to extramedullary hematopoiesis is documented.[70]

Other Organ Systems Findings

The increased nucleic acid turnover that results from the excessive proliferation of marrow cells often leads to an increase in blood uric acid concentration; gout can be exacerbated in some patients.[28]

SPECIAL CONSIDERATIONS

Surgery

More than 75 percent of patients with uncontrolled PV develop complications during or after major surgery because both bleeding and thrombosis are common.[71] Thus, it is often advised to bring the blood volume to normal before surgical interventions, which lowers the frequency of intraoperative and postoperative complications.

Pregnancy

Chapter 7 discusses the complications of PV in pregnancy.

THE SPENT PHASE OF POLYCYTHEMIA VERA

The spent phase of PV, also known as postpolycythemia myelofibrosis or secondary myelofibrosis, is a frequent and often terminal complication of the disease.[47,50,72] It is characterized by a combination of anemia not due to iron deficiency, recent and often progressive increase of splenic size (Fig. 86–2), and marrow fibrosis (see Chap. 91). The phase may be first

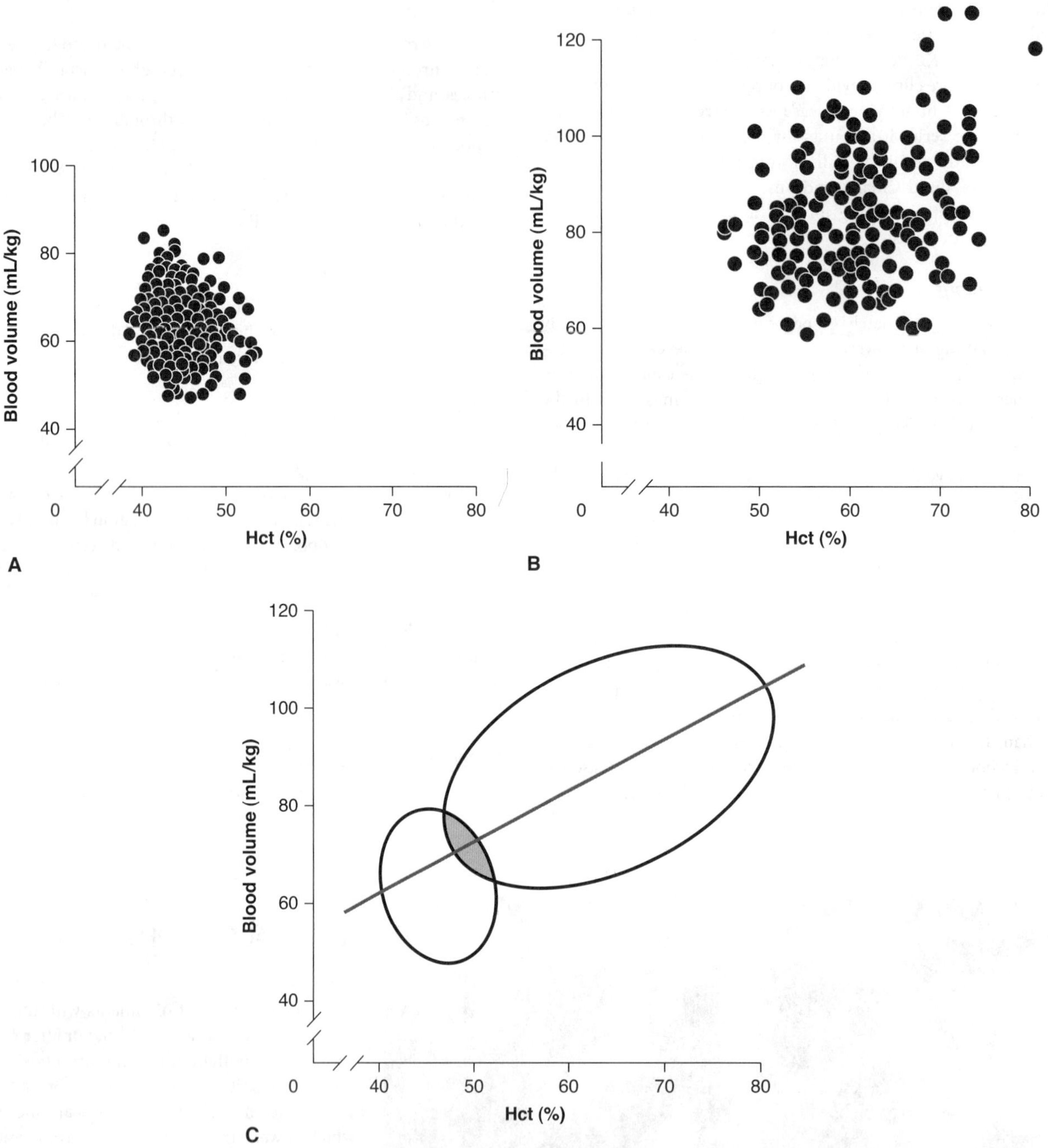

FIGURE 86–2. The correlation of blood volume (mL/kg) and venous blood hematocrit (Hct) in 306 normal males, 140 normal females, and 157 patients with PV when measured by labeling of erythrocytes with ^{32}P or ^{51}Cr, as recommended by the International Committee on Standardization in Haematology. **A.** Blood volume versus Hct in normal males and females. **B.** Blood volume versus Hct in patients with polycythemia vera. **C.** Comparison of the two populations shown in *A* and *B*. The *leftward oval* includes most of the normal subjects, and the *overlapping rightward oval* includes most of the polycythemia patients. The *diagonal line* is the regression line calculated for both groups when combined. *(Data compiled from references 198-201.)*

evident by a decrease in the frequency of phlebotomy needed to control the red cell mass. The other frequently associated features are thrombocytosis or thrombocytopenia, granulocytosis often with immature myeloid cells, or granulocytopenia. The affected individuals are frequently symptomatic from anemia, bleeding, and splenic enlargement with early satiety, splenic infarcts. Most patients become transfusion or erythropoietin therapy dependent.[28,47,49,51,72] The anemia that characterizes the spent phase of PV is usually multifactorial in origin. Splenomegaly results in the pooling of red cells and the expansion of the plasma volume, as well as in shortening of red cell survival (see Chaps. 5 and 55). Development of the "spent phase" is associated with an increased risk of leukemic transformation. In the PV Study Group-01 study, the incidence of acute leukemia was 24 percent in those with myelofibrosis compared to 7 percent in patients without myelofibrosis,[50] although the relatively high incidence of leukemia in this older study is likely related to the widespread use of alkylating agents and ^{32}P in most of these patients.

LEUKEMIC AND MYELODYSPLASTIC TRANSFORMATION OF POLYCYTHEMIA VERA

Patients with PV have an increased risk of developing leukemia. This contrasts with other nonclonal polycythemic disorders wherein progression to leukemia is not part of the disease process. Acute leukemia, usually myelogenous, is a nearly invariably fatal complication of PV. The European multicenter observational study of 1638 patients reported a 6.3 percent relative risk of developing leukemia by 10 years after the diagnosis of PV.[47] In the PV Study Group-01 randomized trial, the incidence of acute leukemia at 18 years of followup was 1.5 percent on the phlebotomy-only treatment arm, 10 percent on the ^{32}P treatment arm, and 13 percent on the chlorambucil treatment arm.[51] The measurable increase in acute leukemia incidence with ^{32}P therapy does not occur until after 5 millicuries have been administered.

Acute leukemia as the terminal PV event may arise from either the *JAK2 V617F*-positive clone or, more frequently, from a hematopoietic cell that does not carry the *JAK2* mutation.[32,36,39]

LABORATORY FEATURES

JAK2 V617F AND EXON 12 MUTATIONS

JAK2 G1849T Creating V617F

Mutations within the *JAK2* gene cause a deregulation of the hematopoietic process, which is expressed in a wide spectrum of disorders involving the expansion of erythrocytes, granulocytes, or leukocytes. The primary lesion associated with these disorders was discovered in exon 14 and is a single nucleotide change *JAK2 G1849T* creating *V617F*. The detection of the *JAK2 V617F* mutation provides a qualitative diagnostic marker for the identification of Philadelphia-chromosome-negative subgroup of myeloproliferative disorders and their differentiation from congenital and acquired reactive hematopoietic disorders. In general, PMF patients have the highest, PV patients an intermediate, and ET patients the lowest *JAK2 V617F* allelic burden. In virtually all PV *JAK2 V617F*-positive patients at least some progenitors exist that became homozygous for *JAK2 V617F* mutation by uniparenteral disomy acquired by mitotic recombination. Allele-specific polymerase chain reaction (PCR) is widely used for single nucleotide polymorphism (SNP) genotyping, and the technique is based on amplification of DNA by an allele-specific primer matching the polymorphism at the 3′ position. This approach is directly applicable to analysis of *JAK2* V617F because the mutation (*G1849T*) is analogous to a SNP. In theory, the allele-specific primer containing the mismatched nucleoside at the 3′ end should not be extended by Taq DNA polymerase. However, this DNA polymerase can extend mismatched allele-specific primers, generating false-positive results and decreasing sensitivity of mutation detection. To improve the specificity, sensitivity, and reliability, an *allele-specific quantitative PCR* method for quantitating the *JAK2 V617F* allele burden, two modifications into the basic technique were incorporated: (1) inclusion of a second mismatch at the −1 positions; (2) substitution of a modified locked nucleic acid (LNA) at the −2 position.[34] A study comparing 11 different techniques was undertaken and carried out in 16 laboratories using various equipment.[73] Although 5 of the 11 techniques were similarly reliable for the quantification of *JAK2 V617F* loads ≥1 percent of total *JAK2*, the *allele-specific quantitative PCR* technique could detect 0.2% *JAK2 V617F*.

The majority of laboratories analyze the *JAK2 V617F* allele burden from (clonal) granulocytes; the nonquantitative analyses use total leukocytes, whole blood, or marrow for screening. A proportion of *JAK2 V617F*-negative assays are positive using sensitive quantitative analyses.[73] Plasma has been used for detection of the *JAK2 V617F* DNA and mRNA mutation and zygosity state.[74,75] Detection of *JAK2 V617F* DNA and mRNA in plasma is, however, the result of the lysis of granulocytes during storage, compounded by decreased viability of the *JAK2 V617F*-bearing cells and is a storage artifact[76]; as such it should not be used in clinical practice to detect, quantify *JAK2 V617F*, or address zygosity.

JAK2 Exon 12 Mutations

Although the most common *JAK2* mutation is a single SNP in exon 14, many MPD cases negative for the exon 14 mutation *JAK2 V617F* carry one of a number of mutations in the 3′ terminus of exon 12. These mutations occur within codons 537 to 544 and consist of single and multiple base substitutions and small deletions. Ten different mutations comprising base substitutions have been identified thus far with small base deletions and sequence duplication through this region.[77–81] These mutations have been observed primarily in patients with isolated erythrocytosis. In addition to the varied types of mutations observed in this region, the proportion of mutation within a sample may be small and therefore difficult to detect in a high background of a normal sequence.

PCR amplification in the presence of a short blocking oligonucleotide homologous to exon 12 (codons 537–544) of the wild-type *JAK2* gene. The oligonucleotide is designed to specifically suppress PCR amplification of the wild-type *JAK2* exon 12 sequence. In contrast, *JAK2* exon 12 mutations located between *JAK2* codons 537 and 544 disrupt proper binding of the blocking oligonucleotide during PCR amplification, resulting in a product of approximately 225 base pairs. Each assay includes control DNA from mutation-positive and wild-type–negative samples; all samples are tested in paired reactions with and without blocking oligonucleotide. When a PCR product is formed solely in the presence of a blocking oligonucleotide, the sample is suspected of harboring a mutation and is sent for confirmatory sequencing. An alternative approach has been to use one of the modifications of the high-resolution melting analysis.[77]

A *V617F*-negative patient may have PV and require a search for other *JAK2* mutations, or they may have another type of polycythemia (see Chap. 56).

V617-positive patients may have another MPD and require additional studies (see Chaps. 87, 91).

MARROW FINDINGS

The marrow is characteristically hypercellular with an increase in erythroid and granulocytic precursor cells and megakaryocytes. Whereas marrow morphology is part of a World Health Organization (WHO) diagnostic criteria of PV,[82] the morphologic features have not yet been validated and may be subject to inter- and intraobserver variations. Unpublished data suggest that the marrow in PV patients with exon 12 mutations is morphologically normal.[83] Marrow morphology in the related myeloproliferative disorder ET was unreliable as a criterion for diagnosis.[84] Absent or decreased iron stores are seen in the marrow of most PV patients. There are no characteristic cytogenetic findings, but occasional clonal chromosomal changes, none of which is very specific for PV, are observed in a minority of patients (see Chap. 11).

BLOOD FINDINGS

Erythrocytes

The hemoglobin concentration, erythrocyte count, and hematocrit are usually increased and the mean cell volume is usually low-normal or low in untreated patients; in patients who have undergone phlebotomy or who have had gastrointestinal bleeding episodes, the erythrocyte count may be increased disproportionately to the increase in the hemoglobin and hematocrit, resulting in marked hypochromia and microcytosis. The plasma iron in such patients is decreased, the iron-binding capacity increased, and plasma ferritin levels are low. The red cell mass is usually increased in proportion to the hemoglobin concentration (see Fig. 86–2). However, because of the expanded plasma volume, the hemoglobin may be normal.[85] In some series, the hemoglobin was falsely lower compared to the red cell mass without any apparent reason.[86,87] Aniso- and poikilocytosis and teardrop cells herald the onset of the spent phase.

Red Cell Mass Determination

The polycythemia vera study group employed the direct determination of the red cell mass as the *sine qua non* of the diagnosis of PV in patients entered into their studies.[48] Some believe that even in the routine clinical setting, this procedure should be performed on all patients to establish this diagnosis.[48,88] Unfortunately, the determination of the red cell mass is expensive, requires the use of radioactive isotopes in patients, and, when performed by the inexperienced, is often inaccurate.[89] It is not useful in distinguishing PV from secondary polycythemia, the differentiation that is usually needed, because it is increased in both disorders. The principal value of a red cell mass determination might then be to distinguish apparent or spurious polycythemia from PV and secondary polycythemia, since the elevated red blood cell mass was masked by simultaneous elevation of plasma volume.[86,87] It may be useful in distinguishing some cases of "hidden PV" from cases of essential thrombocythemia.[85] Ideally, the red cell volume and plasma volume should be measured separately. The availability of the *JAK2* assay has made the blood cell mass determination only very rarely important.

The effect of the elevated red cell mass on blood viscosity is discussed under "Treatment" below.

Leukocytes

An absolute neutrophilia occurs in about two-thirds of the patients.[45] Occasional myelocytes and metamyelocytes are present in the blood, and considerable degrees of immaturity are present in patients with long-standing, advanced disease. Again, these abnormalities herald the onset of the spent phase (see Chap. 91). Basophilia occurs in approximately two-thirds of patients with uncontrolled disease.[28,51,90] In PV, the proportion of activated neutrophils is increased[91] and it is possible that neutrophils may be an important factor in PV-associated thrombosis.

The leukocyte alkaline phosphatase level is elevated in approximately 70 percent of patients with PV,[45] but this assay has now become largely obsolete.[45]

Platelets

The platelet count is increased in approximately 50 percent of patients at the time of diagnosis, and in approximately 10 percent if it is greater than $1000 \times 10^9/L$.[45] In contrast to normal individuals in whom phlebotomy results in an increase in the platelet count, platelet levels may not be affected by phlebotomy in patients with PV.[92] There are no consistent abnormalities of thrombopoietin levels.[93] A significant proportion of PV patients first present with isolated thrombocytosis without an elevated hemoglobin and are sometimes misdiagnosed as having essential thrombocythemia.[94]

Qualitative abnormalities of the platelets have been described. *In vitro* spontaneous platelet aggregation is accelerated. On the other hand, patients with PV, ET, and other MPDs have a nearly pathognomonic defect in the primary wave of platelet aggregation induced by epinephrine.[95] In contrast, there is increased platelet thromboxane A_2 generation[96] and increased excretion of thromboxane metabolites,[97] even though the response to thromboxane A_2 may be subnormal.[98] Platelet factor-4 levels are elevated[99] and platelet survival is normal[100] or shortened.[92,99] Fibrinogen binding after stimulation with a platelet activating factor is diminished[101] and there is reduced expression of the thrombopoietin receptor.[17] However, none of these so far described changes is specific for PV. Platelet counts over 1 to 1.5 millions are associated with progressive decrease of von Willebrand factor and increase risk of bleeding but not thrombosis.[102]

In a prospective study, the PI^{A2} polymorphism of the platelet glycoprotein (GP) IIIa was associated with an increased risk of arterial thrombosis in PV patients.[103] However, polymorphisms of GPIb and GPIa, or the presence of the prothrombin G20210A mutation or factor V Leiden mutation, did not correlate with thrombohemorrhagic events.[103]

Plasma

Serum lysozyme levels are slightly increased in some patients,[104] and because of the increased leukocyte turnover and increased B12 binding protein, the levels of vitamin B_{12} are usually increased.[105] Hyperuricemia, a consequence of hyperproliferative myelopoiesis, is frequently encountered.[28]

DIFFERENTIAL DIAGNOSIS

Also refer to Chap. 33, Table 33–2, and Chap. 56, Figure 56–6.

The diagnostic task has been greatly facilitated by the discovery of the *JAK2 V617F* mutation that is present in 95% or more of all PV patients.

When a patient presents with polycythemia, the initial step should be a repeat of the blood counts as the hemoglobin concentration may reflect a transient decrease of plasma volume (spurious polycythemia). If the hemoglobin concentration is persistently elevated, hypoxia should be considered as a possible cause. An arterial oxygen saturation level (SaO_2) of <92% suggests cardiac or pulmonary etiologies. However, in PV, the partial pressure of oxygen of the arterial blood (PaO_2) is often slightly decreased,[106] complicating the differential diagnosis.

When hypoxia is ruled out, determining whether the increased hemoglobin is acquired or congenital and whether there are other family members involved is essential. The following tests should be employed, depending on availability and other specific circumstances to aid with the diagnosis of PV: (1) The *JAK2 V617F* mutation assay (see *JAK2 V617F* AND EXON 12 MUTATIONS) (2) Complete blood counts. In the 5 percent of PV patients without the *JAK2 V617F* mutation, the most important diagnostic features of PV are erythrocytosis, leukocytosis (especially basophilia or eosinophilia), thrombocytosis, and splenomegaly. Frequently, only two or three of these features are found at presentation and, if sufficiently pronounced, suffice to establish (at least preliminary) diagnosis. In some patients, only one of these features is found initially, most commonly erythrocytosis, but occasionally only thrombocytosis[94] and, less often, leukocytosis or splenomegaly. Such patients represent more difficult diagnostic challenges. A subset of patients with erythrocytosis do not develop the other features of PV, even after they have been followed for many years.[107,108] Such patients have been designated as manifesting pure erythrocytosis or idiopathic erythrocytosis.[109] Some of these PV patients will have exon 12 *JAK2* mutations.[78,81] In JAK2 V617F negative patients: (3) Serum erythropoietin (EPO) level is usually low (see Fig. 56–6). In a small proportion of PV patients the EPO level may be normal. Such cases are often found in the presence of Budd-Chiari syndrome, iron deficiency, or postphlebotomy. (4) If the EPO level is normal or elevated, the P_{50} level (partial pressure of oxygen in the blood at which 50% of the hemoglobin is saturated with oxygen) should be measured (see Chaps. 48, 49 and 56). Polycythemic disorders resulting from high-affinity hemoglobin mutants (see Chap. 48) or low 2,3-bisphosphoglycerate (2,3-BPG) concentrations (see Chap. 46) are diagnosed with a decreased P_{50} from a Hemox-Analyzer, an instrument that records blood oxygen equilibrium curves. If a Hemox-Analyzer is not available, the P_{50} value can be calculated from freshly obtained venous blood gasses using a formula that can be calculated in Excel computer software.[110] (5) Red cell and plasma volume studies (see Red Cell Mass Determination) to rule out spurious polycythemia (see Chaps. 33 and 56) caused by chronic contraction of plasma volume (Gaisbock syndrome) and unsuspected polycythemia in the face of normal hemoglobin. (6) If there is no evidence of congenital and familial history (see Chap. 56), search for *exon 12 JAK2* mutations.

Distinguishing between PV and other polycythemic disorders may, at times, be challenging. Although the diagnosis of PV may be straightforward if patients have the classic criteria as defined by the most recent WHO criteria,[82] (Table 86–1) patients often present with an incomplete phenotype. Some of the clinical and laboratory features that can be helpful for differential diagnosis are summarized in Table 33–2 and in Fig. 56–6. The current WHO diagnostic criteria, presented in Table 86–1,[82] represent an improvement over the previous ones, although they do not necessarily discriminate between individual MPDs[111] and they are yet to be validated by clinical studies. Children with PV are especially unlikely to fit the most recent WHO criteria.[112]

ERYTHROID COLONY CULTURES

In vitro assays of erythroid progenitor cells permit the study of their responsiveness to erythropoietin. In PV, erythroid BFU-E progenitors grow in serum containing cultures without added erythropoietin[14] and the colonies are referred to as EECs. Detection of EECs in cultures of blood or marrow or blood may be the most specific test for PV.[13,14,113,114] In one study, all patients with PV but none with secondary or other causes of polycythemia formed EECs *in vitro*.[115] However, rare EECs may, at times, be observed in primary and familial polycythemia (PFCP) and in Chuvash polycythemia, but unlike the EEC of PV, these are abrogated by pretreatment with erythropoietin and erythropoietin receptor-blocking antibodies.[116,117]

In experienced hands, the EEC assay is a specific and sensitive means for detecting PV and may be useful in diagnosing patients with unusual presentations of PV, such as Budd-Chiari syndrome,[53,55,118,119] isolated thrombocytosis, or in *V617F*-negative patients. In the era of *JAK2 V617F*, this test, which has not been standardized and is expensive and laborious, is useful primarily in a research setting where it remains the gold standard for the diagnosis of PV.

Studies of red cell progenitors suggest that patients who have been diagnosed as having pure erythrocytosis can be divided into two groups of about equal size, those with erythropoietin-independent BFU-E and those without such precursors.[107,115] It is possible that EEC negative pure erythrocytosis is a distinct entity, but those with EEC should be considered to have PV.

TABLE 86–1. World Health Organization Criteria for the Diagnosis of Polycythemia Vera, 2008

	Major Criteria	Minor Criteria
A1	Hgb >18.5 g/dL (men) >16.5 g/dL (women) or Hgb >17 g/dL (men), or >15 g/dL (women) if associated with a sustained increase of ≥2 g/dL from baseline that cannot be attributed to correction of iron deficiency	Marrow trilineage myeloproliferation
A2	Presence of *JAK2 V617F* or similar mutation	Subnormal serum EPO level
		EEC growth

EEC, endogenous erythroid colony; EPO, erythropoietin; Hgb, hemoglobin.

Both major and 1 minor or first major and 2 minor.

ERYTHROPOIETIN LEVELS

Because PV is distinguished by the fact that erythroid cells proliferate even in the absence of normal levels of erythropoietin, one would expect that at high hematocrit levels the production of EPO would be reduced and the serum EPO levels would consequently be low. Several studies have indeed documented serum EPO levels below the normal reference range in patients with PV.[120-122] In contrast to normal individuals, the serum EPO levels remain low even after phlebotomy.[120] Patients with secondary polycythemia usually have normal to elevated erythropoietin levels, although considerable overlap exists in the range of erythropoietin levels between patients with PV and those with secondary polycythemia.[121,123] Although an elevated EPO level generally excludes the diagnosis of polycythemia vera, a low EPO level is not pathognomonic of PV. Patients with PFCP also have as low EPO levels.[124] Some PV patients with exon 12 JAK2 mutations were noted to have normal serum EPO levels.[35]

CLONALITY IN FEMALE SUBJECTS USING ASSAYS EMPLOYING X-CHROMOSOME–BASED POLYMORPHISM ASSAYS

PV results from an acquired mutation in a pluripotential hematopoietic cell. Clonality studies based on the phenomenon of X-chromosome inactivation[125] show that red cells, granulocytes, platelets, monocytes, and B lymphocytes are all part of the neoplastic clone.[12,13,126] The majority of T lymphocytes and natural killer cells are polyclonal, but a small proportion of these cells are also derived from the PV clone.[11] This is presumed to be a result of the detection of the presence of long-lived normal T cells that preceded the development of the clone. Unfortunately, the applicability of X-chromosome inactivation for the differential diagnosis of PV is hampered by the many methodologic and conceptual differences that have drawn conflicting conclusions. Some of discrepancies are a result of two different approaches comparable[127] that are used to distinguish the active from the inactive X-chromosome; one using X-chromosome differential methylation,[128] typically using the polymorphic CAG repeat in the human androgen-receptor gene,[129] versus the more biologically sound but more technically demanding transcriptional analysis of the active X-chromosome[130,131] (see Chap. 9). Furthermore, the wide range of skewing of the X-chromosome allelic usage that is normally present[132] is often misinterpreted as monoclonality, and the potentially clonal myeloid cells are not compared to the polyclonal control cells of the same origin.[13] In approximately 100 female PV patients, the reticulocytes, platelets, and granulocytes were always clonal with the exception of a few patients who converted to polyclonal hematopoiesis after therapy with interferon-α.[13]

OTHER PROPOSED TESTS OF PROPOSED DIAGNOSTIC UTILITY

Assay for MPL

Thrombopoietin, the primary regulator of platelet production, is produced in the liver and its levels are regulated, in large part, by binding to its receptor, c-MPL. Levels of c-MPL on platelets and megakaryocytes are decreased in patients with PV.[17] The major limitations of an assay of c-MPL levels in the diagnosis of PV are its difficulty and nonspecificity.[11]

Assay for bcl-x

Increased expression of *bcl-x*, an antiapoptotic gene, occurs in PV erythroid progenitors[18] but this is not specific for PV.

Assay for Polycythemia Rubra Vera-1

Increased mRNA levels of a receptor termed *polycythemia rubra vera-1* (PRV-1) have been reported in PV granulocytes but not their progenitors.[20] The exact function of PRV-1 in normal hematopoiesis is unclear and likely plays no significant role in PV pathophysiology because there are no differences in the amount of this protein between normal and PV progenitors. Approximately 80 to 100 percent of PV patients have increased granulocyte PRV-1 mRNA.

TABLE 86–2. Definition of Clinical and Hematologic Response in Polycythemia Vera

Complete Response:

1. Hematocrit <45% without phlebotomy *and*
2. Platelet count ≤400 × 10^9/L *and*
3. White blood cell count ≤10 × 10^9/L, *and*
4. Normal spleen size on imaging, *and*
5. No disease-related symptoms

Partial Response:

The patients who do not fulfill the criteria for complete response, hematocrit <45% without phlebotomy, or response in three or more of the other criteria.

TREATMENT

An increased incidence of vascular complications and a progression to myelofibrosis or acute leukemia/myelodysplasia are the major causes of morbidity and mortality. In a large randomized PV trial, previous thrombosis, age, phlebotomy, and rate of phlebotomies contributed to the increased risk of thrombosis.[49] The age of the patient (>60 years) and previous thrombotic events are now universally acknowledged major risk factors for new major vascular complications in PV.[133] Thus, PV patients are staged to low risk and high risk, with previous thrombotic events, including transient ischemic attacks and age greater than 60 years, defining the high-risk category. The assigned risk factor has a major impact on therapeutic decisions; high-risk patients are treated with cytoreductive drugs. Other stratifications of risk include a formulation of an intermediate-risk category that includes PV patients with other cardiovascular factors, such as hypertension.[134] Other risk factors also play a role in the pathogenesis of thrombosis, including the presence of leukocytosis[135,136] and the *JAK2 V617F* mutational allele burden,[137,138] but have not yet been incorporated into therapeutic decision making. Bleeding is more frequent in patients with platelet counts in excess of 1500 × 10^9/L and this is thought to be a result of an acquired von Willebrand disease. An increased platelet count does not increase the risk of thrombosis.[102]

There is a need for prospective clinical studies with stratification of patients according to their baseline leukocyte counts and mutant JAK2 allele burden. A number of criteria of response essential for prospective studies have been formulated (Table 86–2).[139] However, until such evidence is available, the decision on how to manage patients with high leukocyte levels and/or high *JAK2 V617F* mutational burden should continue to follow conventional criteria.

The mainstay of therapy of PV remains nonspecific myelosuppression, which many practitioners supplement by phlebotomies. Additional measures are medications to prevent thrombotic events (aspirin) and to relieve symptoms. Promising therapies are pegylated interferon preparations, which are better tolerated, and JAK2 inhibitors, which are being evaluated mainly in the post-PV–myelofibrotic stage.

It is useful to consider treatments in the plethoric and the spent phases separately.

THE PLETHORIC PHASE

The treatment of patients in the plethoric phase of the disease is aimed at ameliorating symptoms and decreasing the risk of thrombosis or bleeding by reducing the blood counts. This is best accomplished by the use of myelosuppressive drugs and, in some patients, by combination therapy consisting of myelosuppression, phlebotomies, and platelet-reducing agents, or, alternatively, by using interferon-α therapy. Table 86–3 summarizes the advantages and disadvantages of various forms of therapy.

Myelosuppression

Myelosuppression decreases blood counts, decreases the risk of vascular events, and ameliorates symptoms, thus increasing an overall sense of well-being. Although there is also a clinical impression that it increases patients' long-term survival, there are no long-term clinical studies to document this.

TABLE 86–3. Treatment of Polycythemia Vera

Treatment	Advantages	Disadvantages
Phlebotomy	Low risk. Simple to perform.	Does not control thrombocytosis or leukocytosis.
Hydroxyurea	Controls leukocytosis and thrombocytosis. Low leukemogenic risk.	Continuous therapy required.
Busulfan	Easy to administer. Prolonged remissions. Risk of leukemogenesis probably not high.	Overdose produces prolonged marrow suppression. Risks of leukemogenesis, long-term pulmonary and cutaneous toxicity.
^{32}P	Patient compliance not required. Prolonged control of thrombocytosis and leukocytosis.	Expensive and relatively inconvenient. Moderate leukemogenic risk.
Chlorambucil	Easy to administer. Good control of thrombocytosis and leukocytosis.	High risk of leukemogenesis.
Interferon	Low leukemogenic potential. Effect on pruritus.	Inconvenient, costly, frequent side effects.
Anagrelide	Selective effect on platelets.	Selective effect on platelets.

Hydroxyurea Hydroxyurea is the most common myelosuppressive agent used in the treatment of PV. Hydroxyurea is effective therapy for controlling the erythrocyte, leukocyte, and platelet count and it decreases the risk of thrombosis during the first few years of therapy when compared to an historical cohort treated with phlebotomy alone.[50] Its suppressive effect is of short duration; consequently, continuous rather than intermittent therapy is required. Because it is short acting, it is relatively safe to use, as the blood counts rise within a few days of decreasing the dose or of stopping the drug. Moreover, because it is not an alkylating agent, it has less potential for causing acute leukemic transformation than other myelosuppressive agents. Although some studies suggest that hydroxyurea presents a higher risk of acute leukemic transformation, the observations did not reach statistical significance. An analysis of 1638 PV patients enrolled in a prospective observational study did not find an increased incidence of leukemic or myelodysplastic transformation (hazard ratio: 0.86; 95% confidence interval 0.26-2.88; P = 0.8021).[143] In one study, the incidence of acute leukemia was slightly, but not significantly, higher than that in patients treated with phlebotomy alone,[140] a trend that remains controversial because many, if not all, patients treated with hydroxyurea who developed leukemia had also received an alkylating agent at some time in their disease course. Experience in the use of hydroxyurea in the treatment of ET has indicated a marked reduction of thrombosis to approximately 30 percent of the untreated patient.[141] Limited evidence indicates that hydroxyurea treatment in adults with sickle cell disease is not associated with leukemia.[142] Unfortunately, despite its safety and effectiveness, a number of patients administered hydroxyurea discontinue the drug because of adverse effects (skin ulcers or gastrointestinal intolerance).

Busulfan Busulfan is a useful second-line agent in patients whose disease is difficult to control or who have adverse reactions to hydroxyurea. The administration of busulfan is a convenient and effective means for the treatment of PV. Marrow suppression produced by this drug is long-lasting and, as a consequence, it can be given intermittently at a dose of 2 to 6 mg daily for a period not exceeding several weeks; the counts continue to fall for several weeks after drug administration is discontinued and may then remain within normal range for many months or even years. In one large study, the median first remission duration of busulfan-treated patients was 4 years.[144] This prolonged depression of marrow activity that is brought about by busulfan is its major advantage in the treatment of PV, but it also poses a hazard of long-term pancytopenia. The incidence of transformation to acute leukemia in patients treated intermittently with busulfan is relatively low. Of 145 patients followed from 2 to 11 years, 3 developed acute leukemia.[144] Exposure to busulfan had an independent role in producing an excess risk for progression to acute leukemia in the multicenter study of more than 1600 PV patients.[143]

Radioactive Phosphorus ^{32}P therapy was one of the first effective modes of treatment used. Extensive investigations of the long-term outcome of treatment with ^{32}P have been documented.[48,145] Good control of the disease usually can be achieved with initial doses of 2 to 4 mCi. It is rarely used at present, but it may be the treatment of choice for older patients and patients who may be difficult to follow on chemotherapy.[146,147]

Phlebotomy

Often, the initial treatment for patients with uncomplicated PV is phlebotomy.[28,148] The rationale for phlebotomy of patients with PV is based on a widely quoted study that suggested that the risk of thrombosis in PV was proportional to the elevation in hematocrit.[149] The underlying mechanisms causing thrombosis in PV are not fully understood, but the hematocrit is unlikely to be the only risk factor. The lack of a significant risk of thrombosis in large studies of patients with polycythemia caused by chronic exposure to high altitude or by Eisenmenger syndrome[150] and other cyanotic heart diseases[151] argue against hematocrit as the only factor causing thrombosis. For example, when 100 cyanotic patients with congenital heart disease were observed for a total of 748 patient-years, no patient with polycythemia developed cerebral arterial thrombosis.[152] Studies of transgenic mouse with extreme polycythemia caused by constitutive overexpression of erythropoietin did not have an increase in thrombotic complications.[153] Additionally, the increased risk of strokes in Chuvash polycythemia is not statistically different in those affected patients whose hematocrit is controlled by phlebotomies. Furthermore, the European Collaboration on Low-Dose Aspirin in the Polycythemia Vera study, which included 1638 patients from 12 participating countries and 94 centers, has not found differences in thrombotic complications in the range of hematocrits between 40 and 50 percent.

When phlebotomy is instituted, the hemoglobin may be reduced to normal or near-normal values by the removal of 450 mL of blood at intervals of 2 to 4 days for average-size patients, with removal of smaller amounts being from patients who weigh less than 50 kg. Patients with impaired cardiovascular function are better treated with smaller phlebotomies at more frequent intervals.

Phlebotomy is an effective way in which to lower or normalize the elevated blood viscosity of patients with PV. Phlebotomy may result in improvement of symptoms such as headaches or a feeling of "increased pressure" in some patients. It neither reduces the leukocyte nor platelet count, nor does it affect symptoms such as pruritus or gout. Iron deficiency and a resulting microcytosis are the usual consequences of repeated phlebotomies. The iron-deficient state may help to control the hemoglobin concentration in the long run but it increases the sense of fatigue. It may increase the platelet count in some patients. Viscosity of the blood is a function of the hematocrit, and is independent of the number of red cells[154]; deformability of iron-deficient erythrocytes is virtually normal.[155]

A randomized study[156] comparing phlebotomy alone with treatment with ^{32}P or with chlorambucil indicated that the life span of patients treated only with phlebotomy was better than that of patients treated with chlorambucil and no worse than of those given ^{32}P. However, patients undergoing phlebotomy suffered more thrombotic episodes than patients treated with myelosuppressive therapy, although the risk seemed limited to the first 3 years of therapy. This documented increased risk of phlebotomy is balanced by a lower incidence of acute leukemia late in the patient's course. Surprisingly, there was no correlation between the level of the platelet count and the development of thrombotic complications. Many patients can be well controlled by phlebotomy alone during much or all of their disease course; the role of myelosuppressive therapy in the treatment of PV has sometimes been questioned.[157] Patients younger than age 50 years who have no prior history of thrombosis might be treated with phlebotomy alone,[158] but no rigorous data are available to support this recommendation.

Anagrelide

Among 113 patients with PV who had thrombocytosis, the administration of anagrelide produced a platelet response in 85 cases (75%).[159] The starting dose was 0.5 or 1.0 mg given four times daily, and a response was noted in most patients within a week. The average dose required to control the platelet count was 2.4 mg per day. Adverse events included headache, palpitations, diarrhea, and fluid retention and were occasionally sufficiently severe to require discontinuation of the treatment.[160] The United Kingdom randomized trial indicated superior results for hydroxyurea compared to anagrelide for the control of elevated platelet count, myelofibrosis, and hemorrhagic complications in essential thrombocythemia.[24]

Symptomatic Therapy for Pruritus

Many of the symptoms of polycythemia are controlled either with myelosuppressive therapy or by phlebotomy. Pruritus is sometimes an exception. It tends to be more severe when the disease is active and becomes milder or disappears when control is achieved by myelosuppression. Evidence indicates that the mutant JAK2 can stimulate an agonist of pruritus in basophils[161] and the *JAK2 V617F* allelic burden correlates with thromboses on multivariate analysis.[162] The same analysis suggested a negative correlation between arterial thrombosis and pruritus.[162] Nonetheless, in some patients pruritus becomes a nearly intolerable annoyance. Because bathing or showering usually intensifies the itching, often the best advice that can be offered is to bathe less frequently. Photochemotherapy with psoralens and ultraviolet light is helpful.[163] Antihistamines are often given but are usually not very effective. Aspirin[164] and cyproheptadine[90] may be useful. Interferon-α has been helpful in some patients.[165–167] The use of JAK2 inhibitors can decrease pruritus in patients with post-PV PMF.[168,169]

Aspirin

An aspirin and dipyridamole have been used to prevent thromboembolic events in PV. The early trials using 300 mg of aspirin daily showed an increase in the incidence of bleeding without a measurable impact on the incidence of thrombotic episodes.[170] The administration of low-dose aspirin has been suggested in patients who have a vascular occlusion.[171] A pilot-controlled trial showed that low-dose aspirin was well tolerated by PV patients and is sufficient to fully inhibit synthesis of the platelet aggregating compound thromboxane, but not the endothelial cell protectant prostacyclin.[172] The European Collaboration on Low-Dose Aspirin in Polycythemia Vera study showed that daily low-dose aspirin decreases arterial and venous thromboses, albeit to a small extent.[47] Because most of the thrombotic complications were not prevented, this study suggests that only a minor fraction of thromboses are attributable to platelets and raises a question regarding the mechanism of thrombosis in PV. The studies showed a correlation between the neutrophil count and the incidence of thrombosis. Multivariate analysis of a study of hydroxyurea in sickle cell disease revealed a benefit to decreasing blood neutrophil levels in prevention of sickle cell vascular events.[173] The possibility that cytoreductive agents affect platelets and/or endothelial cells is being explored.

Interferon

Since the pioneering work of interferon-α in PV,[174] many other studies documenting the efficacy of interferons in PV have been reported.[175] Although these studies have many design similarities, they do not lend themselves to accurate meta-analysis as various formulations of interferon (α_{2a}, α_{2b}, human leukocyte interferon, peg-α_{2a}, peg-α_{2b}) were used and because heterogeneous criteria were employed to measure response. For example, in studies of PV, complete response was defined in some cases as control of hematocrit with freedom from phlebotomy, whereas in other studies it was defined as normalization of platelet count, disappearance of splenomegaly, and resolution of disease-related symptoms such as pruritus. Furthermore, in the small number of patients studied thus far, administration of interferon-α has led to the *JAK2 V617F* mutation becoming undetectable[175,176] and clonal hematopoiesis converting to a polyclonal state.[13] In addition to its capacity to induce hematologic responses and to ameliorate disease-related symptoms, studies show molecular responses in a subset of patients treated with pegylated interferon-α (Pegasys). Using *JAK2 V617F* as a molecular marker, a French group[175] studied 40 patients with PV treated with Pegasys and reported that of 37 evaluable patients, 94 percent had a complete hematologic response. Approximately 25 percent of patients with PV and ET treated with interferon discontinue treatment, half within the first year. The hematologic toxicities include anemia, thrombocytopenia, and neutropenia. Other potential untoward effects of interferon include depression, mood changes, skin toxicity, hair loss, nausea, diarrhea, weight loss, liver function abnormalities, and cardiac and neurologic toxicity. Immunologic abnormalities in the form of autoimmune processes (e.g., hypothyroidism, autoimmune hemolytic anemia, polyarthritis, glomerulonephritis, connective tissue diseases, and asymptomatic antinuclear antibodies) may occur as a consequence of interferon therapy.[177] Conceivably, the development of interferon-induced autoimmune processes reflects the immunomodulatory activity of the drug through which at least part of its antitumor activity is mediated. Using serologic analysis of tumor antigens through screening an expression complementary DNA library, tumor antigens that elicit immune responses in chronic myelogenous leukemia[178] and PV patients who achieved remission after treatment with interferon were identified.[179–181] Interferon is the drug of choice in pregnant patients with PV (see Chap. 7).

JAK2 Inhibitors

Currently available JAK2 inhibitors target the catalytic site of the enzyme and are therefore active against wild-type JAK2 and *JAK2 V617F*; some also inhibit other JAKs, including JAK3.[182] In addition to technical obstacles, certain pathobiologic characteristics of the *JAK2 V617F*-positive myeloproliferative disorders suggest that targeting *JAK2 V617F* is a suboptimal therapeutic strategy; data from several laboratories indicate that the mutant enzyme is not the disease-initiating step in Philadelphia-chromosome-negative MPDs[34,183] and that these disease processes are characterized by clonal heterogeneity that is a consequence of genetic instability.[184] Indeed, initial studies in humans suggest that currently available inhibitors of JAK2 have modest clinical activity and little, if any, effect on the mutant allele burden.[169,185] The clinical studies of the inhibitors have been largely confined to *JAK2 V617F*-positive PMF. Five JAK2 inhibitors are already in clinical testing (INCB018424, TG101348, CEP-701, AZD1480, and XL019). Overall, these JAK2 inhibitors have reduced myelofibrosis symptoms. The Incyte compound INCB018424 has completed phase II studies and has reduced spleen size and splenomegaly-associated symptoms, as well as general symptomatology such as night sweats, itching, and fatigue; however, the clinical, hematologic, and molecular responses have not matched that of imatinib mesylate use in chronic myelogenous leukemia and do not induce a complete or substantial remission of the disease.[168,186]

Epigenetic Modulation

There is growing evidence of abnormal epigenetic gene regulation as a mechanism potentially contributing to the pathogenesis and the phenotypic diversity of myeloproliferative disorders, especially PMF or post-PV myelofibrosis.[187] The clinical trials with epigenetic drug modifiers are in progress. The use of these agents holds considerable promise.[187]

Summary of Therapeutic Approach

The current general approach to treatment of patients not participating in clinical trials is:

1. Myelosuppression with hydroxyurea daily, both as initial therapy (1500 mg qd) and long-term treatment (500–2000 mg QD), aiming to maintain neutrophil counts at low-normal levels. Interferon may be given instead of hydroxyurea. In addition, some patients will require the use of phlebotomies and/or anagrelide to maintain the hemoglobin and platelet levels in normal ranges.
2. Aspirin at a dose of 80–100 mg QD is given to all patients without histories of major bleeding or gastric intolerance.
3. Allopurinol and medication to control pruritus may be added if required.

4. Judicious phlebotomies with isovolemic replacement in patients with hematocrits greater than 55 percent and in patients who report immediate improvement of symptoms after phlebotomy. The symptoms that may be related to hyperviscosity are headaches, difficulty concentrating, and fatigue.

THE SPENT PHASE

Ultimately, sometimes after only a few years and usually after 15 or more years, erythrocytosis of PV patients gradually abates, phlebotomy requirements decrease and cease, and anemia develops. During this "spent" phase of the disease, marrow fibrosis becomes more marked and the spleen becomes greatly enlarged (Fig. 86–3A). Instead of phlebotomies, transfusions or erythropoietin may be required.[188] The platelet count may remain high or may decline, even to thrombocytopenic levels. Marked leukocytosis may occur with the appearance of immature granulocytes in the blood. At this point, the disease mimics closely primary myelofibrosis (Chap. 91) and the condition is termed *post-PV myelofibrosis*. Treatment of this phase of the disease is difficult and requires the judicious use of a combination of therapeutic approaches, depending on the circumstances of each individual patient. Hydroxyurea given together with erythropoiesis-stimulating agents is often helpful and splenectomy should be considered in selected patients. Allogeneic stem cell transplantation should be considered in younger patients; nonmyeloablative allogenic marrow transplantation has been successful in clinical trials of patients up to 65 years of age.[188]

Splenectomy

Splenectomy may be warranted (see Fig. 86–3B), particularly in patients with severe fatigue, with cytopenias, and in those where a greatly enlarged spleen produces physical discomfort.[189] However, a large Mayo Clinic series reported significant mortality and morbidity of splenectomy at this stage of the disease.[190]

Hematopoietic Stem Cell Transplantation

A few younger patients have undergone successful allogeneic stem cell transplantation.[191] Nonmyeloablative stem cell transplantation, a procedure that may be performed in otherwise healthy people even in the sixth decade of life (see Chap. 21), shows promise[192] and is, at present, the only curative approach to this disease stage.[188]

COURSE AND PROGNOSIS

Thrombotic complications discussed in the preceding sections are the dominant cause of morbidity and mortality in patients with PV. In addition and in contrast to other polycythemic disorders, PV has an increased risk of evolution to acute leukemia. Although several clinical stages of PV are recognized (plethoric or proliferative phase, stable phase, spent phase or postpolycythemic myelofibrosis phase, and acute leukemia), it is not clear that these stages represent a sequential progression of the disease.

The Polycythemia Vera Study Group[48] found that the median survival from the beginning of treatment was 13.9 years for those treated by phlebotomy alone, 11.8 years for ^{32}P-treated patients, and 8.9 years for chlorambucil-treated patients. Thrombosis was the most common cause of death, accounting for 31 percent of the fatalities. Nineteen percent of the patients died of acute leukemia, 15 percent from other neoplasms, and approximately 5 percent each from hemorrhage or the development of the spent phase. Similarly, a large French study revealed a median survival of 13.5 years of PV patients initially treated with ^{32}P, only slightly less that the 15.2 years of age-matched controls.[193] Others suggested that PV is a disease that is compatible with normal or near-normal life for many years.[194,195] However, most studies agree that there is excess mortality attributable to thrombotic complications and acute leukemia transformation as a direct consequence of PV.[47] Acute leukemia occurs even in patients who have been treated only by phlebotomy, although its incidence is increased by the various forms of cytotoxic therapy that have been employed. While acute

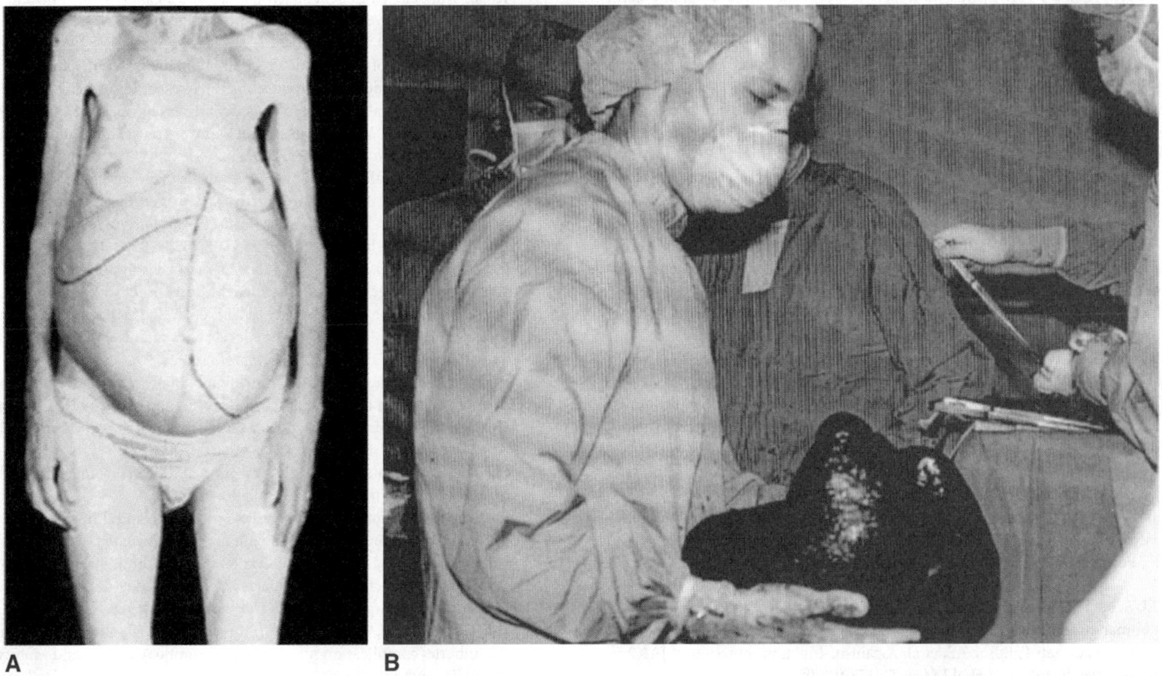

FIGURE 86–3. Patient with spent phase of PV with a massive increase of splenic size **(A)** and surgically removed spleen **(B)**. *(Courtesy of Steven Fruchtman, MD, Allos Therapeutics, Princeton, NJ.)*

myelogenous leukemia is most common, acute lymphoid leukemia[196] and chronic neutrophilic leukemia[197] have occurred as well.

REFERENCES

1. Vaquez MH: Sur une forme spéciale de cyanose s'accompagnant d'hyperglobulie excessive et persistante. *CR Soc Biol* 44:384, 1892.
2. Osler W: Chronic cyanosis, with polycythemia and enlarged spleen: A new clinical entity. *Am J Med Sci* 126:187, 1903.
3. Türk W: Beitrage zur Kenntnis des Symptomenbildes Polycythamie mit Milztumor und Zyanose. *Wien Klin Wochenschr* 17:153, 1904.
4. Ania BJ, Suman VJ, Sobell JL, et al: Trends in the incidence of polycythemia vera among Olmsted County, Minnesota residents, 1935–1989. *Am J Hematol* 47:89, 1994.
5. Kutti J, Ridell B: Epidemiology of the myeloproliferative disorders: Essential thrombocythaemia, polycythaemia vera and idiopathic myelofibrosis. *Pathol Biol (Paris)* 49:164, 2001.
6. Chaiter Y, Brenner B, Aghai E, et al: High incidence of myeloproliferative disorders in Ashkenazi Jews in northern Israel. *Leuk Lymphoma* 7:251, 1992.
7. Modan B, Kallner H, Zemer D, et al: A note on the increased risk of polycythemia vera in Jews. *Blood* 37:172, 1971.
8. Bellanne-Chantelot C, Chaumarel I, Labopin M, et al: Genetic and clinical implications of the Val617Phe JAK2 mutation in 72 families with myeloproliferative disorders. *Blood* 108:346, 2006.
9. Kralovics R, Stockton DW, Prchal JT: Clonal hematopoiesis in familial polycythemia vera suggests the involvement of multiple mutational events in the early pathogenesis of the disease. *Blood* 102:3793, 2003.
10. Landgren O, Goldin LR, Kristinsson SY, et al: Increased risks of polycythemia vera, essential thrombocythemia, and myelofibrosis among 24,577 first-degree relatives of 11,039 patients with myeloproliferative neoplasms in Sweden. *Blood* 112:2199, 2008.
11. Kralovics R, Guan Y, Prchal JT: Acquired uniparental disomy of chromosome 9p is a frequent stem cell defect in polycythemia vera. *Exp Hematol* 30:229, 2002.
12. Adamson JW, Fialkow PJ, Murphy S, et al: Polycythemia vera: Stem-cell and probable clonal origin of the disease. *N Engl J Med* 295:913, 1976.
13. Liu E, Jelinek J, Pastore YD, et al: Discrimination of polycythemias and thrombocytoses by novel, simple, accurate clonality assays and comparison with PRV-1 expression and BFU-E response to erythropoietin. *Blood* 101:3294, 2003.
14. Prchal JF, Axelrad AA: Letter: Bone-marrow responses in polycythemia vera. *N Engl J Med* 290:1382, 1974.
15. Eaves CJ, Eaves AC: Erythropoietin (Ep) dose-response curves for three classes of erythroid progenitors in normal human marrow and in patients with polycythemia vera. *Blood* 52:1196, 1978.
16. Prchal JF, Adamson JW, Murphy S, et al: Polycythemia vera. The *in vitro* response of normal and abnormal stem cell lines to erythropoietin. *J Clin Invest* 61:1044, 1978.
17. Moliterno AR, Hankins WD, Spivak JL: Impaired expression of the thrombopoietin receptor by platelets from patients with polycythemia vera. *N Engl J Med* 338:572, 1998.
18. Silva M, Richard C, Benito A, et al: Expression of Bcl-x in erythroid precursors from patients with polycythemia vera. *N Engl J Med* 338:564, 1998.
19. Sui X, Krantz SB, Zhao Z: Identification of increased protein tyrosine phosphatase activity in polycythemia vera erythroid progenitor cells. *Blood* 90:651, 1997.
20. Klippel S, Strunck E, Busse CE, et al: Biochemical characterization of PRV-1, a novel hematopoietic cell surface receptor, which is overexpressed in polycythemia rubra vera. *Blood* 100:2441, 2002.
21. James C, Ugo V, Le Couedic JP, et al: A unique clonal JAK2 mutation leading to constitutive signalling causes polycythaemia vera. *Nature* 434:1144, 2005.
22. Bench AJ, Nacheva EP, Champion KM, et al: Molecular genetics and cytogenetics of myeloproliferative disorders. *Baillieres Clin Haematol* 11:819, 1998.
23. Diez-Martin JL, Graham DL, Petitt RM, et al: Chromosome studies in 104 patients with polycythemia vera. *Mayo Clin Proc* 66:287, 1991.
24. Green A, Campbell P, Buck G, et al: The Medical Research Council PT1 Trial in Essential Thrombocythemia. *Blood* 104(suppl 1):5a, 2004.
25. Najfeld V, Montella L, Scalise A, et al: Exploring polycythaemia vera with fluorescence in situ hybridization: Additional cryptic 9p is the most frequent abnormality detected. *Br J Haematol* 119:558, 2002.
26. Wurster-Hill D, Whang-Peng J, McIntyre OR, et al: Cytogenetic studies in polycythemia vera. *Semin Hematol* 13:13, 1976.
27. Swolin B, Weinfeld A, Westin J: A prospective long-term cytogenetic study in polycythemia vera in relation to treatment and clinical course. *Blood* 72:386, 1988.
28. Spivak JL: Polycythemia vera: Myths, mechanisms, and management. *Blood* 100:4272, 2002.
29. Baxter EJ, Scott LM, Campbell PJ, et al: Acquired mutation of the tyrosine kinase JAK2 in human myeloproliferative disorders. *Lancet* 365:1054, 2005.
30. Kralovics R, Passamonti F, Buser AS, et al: A gain-of-function mutation of JAK2 in myeloproliferative disorders. *N Engl J Med* 352:1779, 2005.
31. Levine RL, Wadleigh M, Cools J, et al: Activating mutation in the tyrosine kinase JAK2 in polycythemia vera, essential thrombocythemia, and myeloid metaplasia with myelofibrosis. *Cancer Cell* 7:387, 2005.
32. Jelinek J, Oki Y, Gharibyan V, et al: JAK2 mutation 1849G>T is rare in acute leukemias but can be found in CMML, Philadelphia chromosome-negative CML, and megakaryocytic leukemia. *Blood* 106:3370, 2005.
33. Jones AV, Kreil S, Zoi K, et al: Widespread occurrence of the JAK2 V617F mutation in chronic myeloproliferative disorders. *Blood* 106:2162, 2005.
34. Nussenzveig RH, Swierczek SI, Jelinek J, et al: Polycythemia vera is not initiated by JAK2V617F mutation. *Exp Hematol* 35:32, 2007.
35. Scott LM, Tong W, Levine RL, et al: JAK2 exon 12 mutations in polycythemia vera and idiopathic erythrocytosis. *N Engl J Med* 356:459, 2007.
36. Skoda R, Prchal JT: Lessons from familial myeloproliferative disorders. *Semin Hematol* 42:266, 2005.
37. Cario H, Schwarz K, Herter JM, et al: Clinical and molecular characterisation of a prospectively collected cohort of children and adolescents with polycythemia vera. *Br J Haematol* 142:622, 2008.
38. Kralovics R, Teo SS, Buser AS, et al: Altered gene expression in myeloproliferative disorders correlates with activation of signaling by the V617F mutation of Jak2. *Blood* 106:3374, 2005.
39. Theocharides A, Boissinot M, Girodon F, et al: Leukemic blasts in transformed JAK2-V617F-positive myeloproliferative disorders are frequently negative for the JAK2-V617F mutation. *Blood* 110:375, 2007.
40. Jones AV, Chase A, Silver RT, et al: JAK2 haplotype is a major risk factor for the development of myeloproliferative neoplasms. *Nat Genet* 41:446, 2009.
41. Olcaydu D, Harutyunyan A, Jager R, et al: A common JAK2 haplotype confers susceptibility to myeloproliferative neoplasms. *Nat Genet* 41:450, 2009.
42. Olcaydu D, Skoda RC, Looser R, et al: The "GGCC" haplotype of JAK2 confers susceptibility to JAK2 exon 12 mutation-positive polycythemia vera. Leukemia 23:1924, 2009
43. Delhommeau F, Dupont S, Della Valle V, et al: Mutation in TET2 in myeloid cancers. *N Engl J Med* 360:2289, 2009.
44. Saint-Martin C, Leroy G, Delhommeau F, et al: Analysis of the ten-eleven translocation 2 (TET2) gene in familial myeloproliferative neoplasms. *Blood* 114:1628, 2009.
45. Berlin NI: Diagnosis and classification of the polycythemias. *Semin Hematol* 12:339, 1975.
46. Wehmeier A, Daum I, Jamin H, et al: Incidence and clinical risk factors for bleeding and thrombotic complications in myeloproliferative disorders. A retrospective analysis of 260 patients. *Ann Hematol* 63:101, 1991.
47. Landolfi R, Marchioli R, Kutti J, et al: Efficacy and safety of low-dose aspirin in polycythemia vera. *N Engl J Med* 350:114, 2004.
48. Berk PD, Goldberg JD, Donovan PB, et al: Therapeutic recommendations in polycythemia vera based on Polycythemia Vera Study Group protocols. *Semin Hematol* 23:132, 1986.
49. Polycythemia vera: The natural history of 1213 patients followed for 20 years. Gruppo Italiano Studio Policitemia. *Ann Intern Med* 123:656, 1995.
50. Berk P, Wasserman L, Fruchtman S: Treatment of polycythemia vera. A summary of clinical trials conducted by the Polycythemia Study Group in *Polycythemia Vera and the Myeloproliferative Disorders,* edited by L Wasserman, P Berk, N Berlin, p 166. WB Saunders, Philadelphia, 1995.
51. Spivak JL, Barosi G, Tognoni G, et al: Chronic myeloproliferative disorders. *Hematology Am Soc Hematol Educ Program* 200, 2003.
52. Anger BR, Seifried E, Scheppach J, et al: Budd-Chiari syndrome and thrombosis of other abdominal vessels in the chronic myeloproliferative diseases. *Klin Wochenschr* 67:818, 1989.
53. De Stefano V, Teofili L, Leone G, et al: Spontaneous erythroid colony formation as the clue to an underlying myeloproliferative disorder in patients with Budd-Chiari syndrome or portal vein thrombosis. *Semin Thromb Hemost* 23:411, 1997.
54. Srinivasan P, Rela M, Prachalias A, et al: Liver transplantation for Budd-Chiari syndrome. *Transplantation* 73:973, 2002.
55. Valla D, Casadevall N, Lacombe C, et al: Primary myeloproliferative disorder and hepatic vein thrombosis. A prospective study of erythroid colony formation in vitro in 20 patients with Budd-Chiari syndrome. *Ann Intern Med* 103:329, 1985.
56. Murphy S: Polycythemia vera. *Dis Mon* 38:153, 1992.
57. Jackson N, Burt D, Crocker J, et al: Skin mast cells in polycythaemia vera: Relationship to the pathogenesis and treatment of pruritus. *Br J Dermatol* 116:21, 1987.
58. Steinman HK, Kobza-Black A, Lotti TM, et al: Polycythaemia rubra vera and water-induced pruritus: Blood histamine levels and cutaneous fibrinolytic activity before and after water challenge. *Br J Dermatol* 116:329, 1987.
59. Buchanan JG, Ameratunga RV, Hawkins RC: Polycythemia vera and water-induced pruritus: Evidence against mast cell involvement. *Pathology* 26:43, 1994.
60. Cox NH, Leggat H: Sweet's syndrome associated with polycythemia rubra vera. *J Am Acad Dermatol* 23:1171, 1990.
61. Furukawa T, Takahashi M, Shimada H, et al: Polycythaemia vera with Sweet's syndrome. *Clin Lab Haematol* 11:67, 1989.
62. Davis MD, O'Fallon WM, Rogers RS 3rd, et al: Natural history of erythromelalgia: Presentation and outcome in 168 patients. *Arch Dermatol* 136:330, 2000.
63. van Genderen PJ, Lucas IS, van Strik R, et al: Erythromelalgia in essential thrombocythemia is characterized by platelet activation and endothelial cell damage but not by thrombin generation. *Thromb Haemost* 76:333, 1996.
64. van Genderen PJ, Michiels JJ: Erythromelalgia: A pathognomonic microvascular thrombotic complication in essential thrombocythemia and polycythemia vera. *Semin Thromb Hemost* 23:357, 1997.
65. Wanless IR, Peterson P, Das A, et al: Hepatic vascular disease and portal hypertension in polycythemia vera and agnogenic myeloid metaplasia: A clinicopathological study of 145 patients examined at autopsy. *Hepatology* 12:1166, 1990.

66. Tinney WS, Hall BE, Giffin HZ: Polycythemia vera and peptic ulcer. *Mayo Clin Proc* 18:24, 1943.
67. Dingli D, Utz JP, Krowka MJ, et al: Unexplained pulmonary hypertension in chronic myeloproliferative disorders. *Chest* 120:801, 2001.
68. Garcia-Manero G, Schuster SJ, Patrick H, et al: Pulmonary hypertension in patients with myelofibrosis secondary to myeloproliferative diseases. *Am J Hematol* 60:130, 1999.
69. Newton LK: Neurologic complications of polycythemia and their impact on therapy. *Oncology (Williston Park)* 4:59, 1990.
70. Jackson A, Burton IE: Retroperitoneal mass and spinal cord compression due to extramedullary haemopoiesis in polycythaemia rubra vera. *Br J Radiol* 62:944, 1989.
71. Wasserman LR, Gilbert HS: Surgical bleeding in polycythemia vera. *Ann N Y Acad Sci* 115:122, 1964.
72. Gilbert HS: Modern treatment strategies in polycythemia vera. *Semin Hematol* 40:26, 2003.
73. Lippert E, Girodon F, Hammond E, et al: Concordance of assays designed for the quantification of JAK2V617F: A multicenter study. *Haematologica* 94:38, 2009.
74. Ma W, Kantarjian H, Verstovsek S, et al: Hemizygous/homozygous and heterozygous JAK2 mutation detected in plasma of patients with myeloproliferative diseases: Correlation with clinical behaviour. *Br J Haematol* 134:341, 2006.
75. Ma W, Kantarjian H, Zhang X, et al: Higher detection rate of JAK2 mutation using plasma. *Blood* 111:3906, 2008.
76. Salama ME, Swierczek SI, Hickman K, et al: Plasma quantitation of JAK2 mutation is not suitable as a clinical test: An artifact of storage. *Blood* 114:223, 2009.
77. Jones AV, Cross NC, White HE, et al: Rapid identification of JAK2 exon 12 mutations using high resolution melting analysis. *Haematologica* 93:1560, 2008.
78. Percy MJ, Scott LM, Erber WN, et al: The frequency of JAK2 exon 12 mutations in idiopathic erythrocytosis patients with low serum erythropoietin levels. *Haematologica* 92:1607, 2007.
79. Pietra D, Li S, Brisci A, et al: Somatic mutations of JAK2 exon 12 in patients with JAK2 (V617F)-negative myeloproliferative disorders. *Blood* 111:1686, 2008.
80. Rapado I, Grande S, Albizua E, et al: High resolution melting analysis for JAK2 Exon 14 and Exon 12 mutations: A diagnostic tool for myeloproliferative neoplasms. *J Mol Diagn* 11:155, 2009.
81. Schnittger S, Bacher U, Haferlach C, et al: Detection of JAK2 exon 12 mutations in 15 patients with JAK2V617F negative polycythemia vera. *Haematologica* 94:414, 2009.
82. Tefferi A, Thiele J, Vardiman JW: The 2008 World Health Organization classification system for myeloproliferative neoplasms: Order out of chaos. *Cancer* 115:3842, 2009.
83. McMullin MF. Personal communication and presentation at the European Society of Haematology Meeting to Josef T. Prchal, MD. Berlin, 2009.
84. Wilkins BS, Erber WN, Bareford D, et al: Bone marrow pathology in essential thrombocythemia: Interobserver reliability and utility for identifying disease subtypes. *Blood* 111:60, 2008.
85. Spivak JL, Silver RT: The revised World Health Organization diagnostic criteria for polycythemia vera, essential thrombocytosis, and primary myelofibrosis: An alternative proposal. *Blood* 112:231, 2008.
86. Cassinat B, Laguillier C, Gardin C, et al: Classification of myeloproliferative disorders in the JAK2 era: Is there a role for red cell mass? *Leukemia* 22:452, 2008.
87. Johansson PL, Safai-Kutti S, Kutti J: An elevated venous haemoglobin concentration cannot be used as a surrogate marker for absolute erythrocytosis: A study of patients with polycythaemia vera and apparent polycythaemia. *Br J Haematol* 129:701, 2005.
88. Spivak JL: Diagnosis of the myeloproliferative disorders: Resolving phenotypic mimicry. *Semin Hematol* 40:1, 2003.
89. Beutler E: Polycythemia. *Med Grand Rounds* 3:142, 1984.
90. Gilbert HS, Warner RR, Wasserman LR: A study of histamine in myeloproliferative disease. *Blood* 28:795, 1966.
91. Falanga A, Marchetti M, Evangelista V, et al: Polymorphonuclear leukocyte activation and hemostasis in patients with essential thrombocythemia and polycythemia vera. *Blood* 96:4261, 2000.
92. Kutti J, Weinfeld A: Platelet survival in active polycythaemia vera with reference to the haematocrit level. An experimental study before and after phlebotomy. *Scand J Haematol* 8:405, 1971.
93. Cerutti A, Custodi P, Duranti M, et al: Thrombopoietin levels in patients with primary and reactive thrombocytosis. *Br J Haematol* 99:281, 1997.
94. Shih LY, Lee CT: Identification of masked polycythemia vera from patients with idiopathic marked thrombocytosis by endogenous erythroid colony assay. *Blood* 83:744, 1994.
95. Yamamoto K, Sekiguchi E, Takatani O: Abnormalities of epinephrine-induced platelet aggregation and adenine nucleotides in myeloproliferative disorders. *Thromb Haemost* 52:292, 1984.
96. Mehta P, Mehta J, Ross M, et al: Decreased platelet aggregation but increased thromboxane A2 generation in polycythemia vera. *Arch Intern Med* 145:1225, 1985.
97. Landolfi R, Ciabattoni G, Patrignani P, et al: Increased thromboxane biosynthesis in patients with polycythemia vera: Evidence for aspirin-suppressible platelet activation in vivo. *Blood* 80:1965, 1992.
98. Ushikubi F, Ishibashi T, Narumiya S, et al: Analysis of the defective signal transduction mechanism through the platelet thromboxane A2 receptor in a patient with polycythemia vera. *Thromb Haemost* 67:144, 1992.
99. Berild D, Hasselbalch H, Knudsen JB: Platelet survival, platelet factor-4 and bleeding time in myeloproliferative disorders. *Scand J Clin Lab Invest* 47:497, 1987.
100. Harker LA, Finch CA: Thrombokinetics in man. *J Clin Invest* 48:963, 1969.
101. Le Blanc K, Lindahl T, Rosendahl K, et al: Impaired platelet binding of fibrinogen due to a lower number of GPIIB/IIIA receptors in polycythemia vera. *Thromb Res* 91:287, 1998.
102. Landolfi R, Cipriani MC, Novarese L: Thrombosis and bleeding in polycythemia vera and essential thrombocythemia: Pathogenetic mechanisms and prevention. *Best Pract Res Clin Haematol* 19:617, 2006.
103. Afshar-Kharghan V, Lopez JA, Gray LA, et al: Hemostatic gene polymorphisms and the prevalence of thrombotic complications in polycythemia vera and essential thrombocythemia. *Blood Coagul Fibrinolysis* 15:21, 2004.
104. Binder RA, Gilbert HS: Muramidase in polycythemia vera. *Blood* 36:228, 1970.
105. Gilbert HS, Krauss S, Pasternack B, et al: Serum vitamin B12 content and unsaturated vitamin B12-binding capacity in myeloproliferative disease. Value in differential diagnosis and as indicators of disease activity. *Ann Intern Med* 71:719, 1969.
106. Lertzman M, Frome BM, Israels LG, et al: Hypoxia in polycythemia vera. *Ann Intern Med* 60:409, 1964.
107. Clement S, Eberlin A, Najean Y, et al: Two different *in vitro* growth patterns for erythroid precursors in 18 patients with pure erythrocytosis. *Scand J Haematol* 29:319, 1982.
108. Najean Y, Triebel F, Dresch C: Pure erythrocytosis: Reappraisal of a study of 51 cases. *Am J Hematol* 10:129, 1981.
109. Pearson TC, Wetherley-Mein G: The course and complications of idiopathic erythrocytosis. *Clin Lab Haematol* 1:189, 1979.
110. Agarwal N, Mojica-Henshaw MP, Simmons ED, et al: Familial polycythemia caused by a novel mutation in the beta globin gene: Essential role of P50 in evaluation of familial polycythemia. *Int J Med Sci* 4:232, 2007.
111. Samuelson SJ, Parker CJ, Prchal JT: Revised criteria for the myeloproliferative disorders: Too much too soon? *Blood* 111:1741; author reply 1742, 2008.
112. Teofili L, Giona F, Martini M, et al: The revised WHO diagnostic criteria for Ph-negative myeloproliferative diseases are not appropriate for the diagnostic screening of childhood polycythemia vera and essential thrombocythemia. *Blood* 110:3384, 2007.
113. Kralovics R, Buser AS, Teo SS, et al: Comparison of molecular markers in a cohort of patients with chronic myeloproliferative disorders. *Blood* 102:1869, 2003.
114. Weinberg RS: *In vitro* erythropoiesis in polycythemia vera and other myeloproliferative disorders. *Semin Hematol* 34:64, 1997.
115. Shih LY, Lee CT, See LC, et al: *In vitro* culture growth of erythroid progenitors and serum erythropoietin assay in the differential diagnosis of polycythaemia. *Eur J Clin Invest* 28:569, 1998.
116. Fisher MJ, Prchal JF, Prchal JT, et al: Anti-erythropoietin (EPO) receptor monoclonal antibodies distinguish EPO-dependent and EPO-independent erythroid progenitors in polycythemia vera. *Blood* 84:1982, 1994.
117. Kralovics R, Sokol L, Prchal JT: Absence of polycythemia in a child with a unique erythropoietin receptor mutation in a family with autosomal dominant primary polycythemia. *J Clin Invest* 102:124, 1998.
118. Acharya J, Westwood NB, Sawyer BM, et al: Identification of latent myeloproliferative disease in patients with Budd-Chiari syndrome using X-chromosome inactivation patterns and *in vitro* erythroid colony formation. *Eur J Haematol* 55:315, 1995.
119. Pagliuca A, Mufti GJ, Janossa-Tahernia M, et al: *In vitro* colony culture and chromosomal studies in hepatic and portal vein thrombosis—Possible evidence of an occult myeloproliferative state. *Q J Med* 76:981, 1990.
120. Birgegard G, Wide L: Serum erythropoietin in the diagnosis of polycythaemia and after phlebotomy treatment. *Br J Haematol* 81:603, 1992.
121. Messinezy M, Westwood NB, El-Hemaidi I, et al: Serum erythropoietin values in erythrocytoses and in primary thrombocythaemia. *Br J Haematol* 117:47, 2002.
122. Mossuz P, Girodon F, Donnard M, et al: Diagnostic value of serum erythropoietin level in patients with absolute erythrocytosis. *Haematologica* 89:1194, 2004.
123. Remacha AF, Montserrat I, Santamaria A, et al: Serum erythropoietin in the diagnosis of polycythemia vera. A follow-up study. *Haematologica* 82:406, 1997.
124. Prchal JT: Classification and molecular biology of polycythemias (erythrocytoses) and thrombocytosis. *Hematol Oncol Clin North Am* 17:1151, 2003.
125. Beutler E, Yeh M, Fairbanks VF: The normal human female as a mosaic of X-chromosome activity: Studies using the gene for C-6-PD-deficiency as a marker. *Proc Natl Acad Sci U S A* 48:9, 1962.
126. Prchal JT: Pathogenetic mechanisms of polycythemia vera and congenital polycythemic disorders. *Semin Hematol* 38:10, 2001.
127. Swierczek SI, Agarwal N, Nussenzveig RH, et al: Hematopoiesis is not clonal in healthy elderly women. *Blood* 112:3186, 2008.
128. Vogelstein B, Fearon ER, Hamilton SR, et al: Use of restriction fragment length polymorphisms to determine the clonal origin of human tumors. *Science* 227:642, 1985.
129. Allen RC, Zoghbi HY, Moseley AB, et al: Methylation of HpaII and HhaI sites near the polymorphic CAG repeat in the human androgen-receptor gene correlates with X chromosome inactivation. *Am J Hum Genet* 51:1229, 1992.
130. Curnutte JT, Hopkins PJ, Kuhl W, et al: Studying X inactivation. *Lancet* 339:749, 1992.
131. Prchal JT, Guan YL, Prchal JF, et al: Transcriptional analysis of the active X-chromosome in normal and clonal hematopoiesis. *Blood* 81:269, 1993.
132. Prchal JT, Prchal JF, Belickova M, et al: Clonal stability of blood cell lineages indicated by X-chromosomal transcriptional polymorphism. *J Exp Med* 183:561, 1996.
133. Marchioli R, Finazzi G, Landolfi R, et al: Vascular and neoplastic risk in a large cohort of patients with polycythemia vera. *J Clin Oncol* 23:2224, 2005.
134. Finazzi G, Barbui T: Evidence and expertise in the management of polycythemia vera and essential thrombocythemia. *Leukemia* 22:1494, 2008.

135. Barbui T, Carobbio A, Rambaldi A, et al: Perspectives on thrombosis in essential thrombocythemia and polycythemia vera: Is leukocytosis a causative factor? *Blood* 114:759, 2009.
136. Caramazza D, Caracciolo C, Barone R, et al: Correlation between leukocytosis and thrombosis in Philadelphia-negative chronic myeloproliferative neoplasms. *Ann Hematol* 88:967, 2009.
137. Carobbio A, Finazzi G, Antonioli E, et al: JAK2V617F allele burden and thrombosis: A direct comparison in essential thrombocythemia and polycythemia vera. *Exp Hematol* 37:1016, 2009.
138. Vannucchi AM, Antonioli E, Guglielmelli P, et al: Clinical correlates of JAK2V617F presence or allele burden in myeloproliferative neoplasms: A critical reappraisal. *Leukemia* 22:1299, 2008.
139. Barosi G, Birgegard G, Finazzi G, et al: Response criteria for essential thrombocythemia and polycythemia vera: Result of a European LeukemiaNet consensus conference. *Blood* 113:4829, 2009.
140. Kaplan ME, Mack K, Goldberg JD, et al: Long-term management of polycythemia vera with hydroxyurea: A progress report. *Semin Hematol* 23:167, 1986.
141. Cortelazzo S, Finazzi G, Ruggeri M, et al: Hydroxyurea for patients with essential thrombocythemia and a high risk of thrombosis. *N Engl J Med* 332:1132, 1995.
142. Lanzkron S, Strouse JJ, Wilson R, et al: Systematic review: Hydroxyurea for the treatment of adults with sickle cell disease. *Ann Intern Med* 148:939, 2008.
143. Finazzi G, Caruso V, Marchioli R, et al: Acute leukemia in polycythemia vera: An analysis of 1638 patients enrolled in a prospective observational study. *Blood* 105:2664, 2005.
144. Treatment of polycythaemia vera by radiophosphorus or busulphan: A randomized trial. "Leukemia and Hematosarcoma" Cooperative Group, European Organization for Research on Treatment of Cancer (E.O.R.T.C.). *Br J Cancer* 44:75, 1981.
145. Randi ML, Fabris F, Varotto L, et al: Haematological complications in polycythaemia vera and thrombocythaemia patients treated with radiophosphorus (32P). *Folia Haematol Int Mag Klin Morphol Blutforsch* 117:461, 1990.
146. Balan KK, Critchley M: Outcome of 259 patients with primary proliferative polycythaemia (PPP) and idiopathic thrombocythaemia (IT) treated in a regional nuclear medicine department with phosphorus-32—A 15 year review. *Br J Radiol* 70:1169, 1997.
147. Roberts BE, Smith AH: Use of radioactive phosphorus in haematology. *Blood Rev* 11:146, 1997.
148. Tefferi A: Polycythemia vera: A comprehensive review and clinical recommendations. *Mayo Clin Proc* 78:174, 2003.
149. Pearson TC, Wetherley-Mein G: Vascular occlusive episodes and venous haematocrit in primary proliferative polycythaemia. *Lancet* 2:1219, 1978.
150. Vongpatanasin W, Brickner ME, Hillis LD, et al: The Eisenmenger syndrome in adults. *Ann Intern Med* 128:745, 1998.
151. Thorne SA: Management of polycythaemia in adults with cyanotic congenital heart disease. *Heart* 79:315, 1998.
152. Perloff JK, Marelli AJ, Miner PD: Risk of stroke in adults with cyanotic congenital heart disease. *Circulation* 87:1954, 1993.
153. Shibata J, Hasegawa J, Siemens HJ, et al: Hemostasis and coagulation at a hematocrit level of 0.85: Functional consequences of erythrocytosis. *Blood* 101:4416, 2003.
154. Van de Pette JE, Guthrie DL, Pearson TC: Whole blood viscosity in polycythaemia: The effect of iron deficiency at a range of haemoglobin and packed cell volumes. *Br J Haematol* 63:369, 1986.
155. Reinhart WH: The influence of iron deficiency on erythrocyte deformability. *Br J Haematol* 80:550, 1992.
156. Berlin NI, Wasserman LR: Polycythemia vera: A retrospective and reprise. *J Lab Clin Med* 130:365, 1997.
157. Nand S, Messmore H, Fisher SG, et al: Leukemic transformation in polycythemia vera: Analysis of risk factors. *Am J Hematol* 34:32, 1990.
158. Hocking WG, Golde DW: Polycythemia: Evaluation and management. *Blood Rev* 3:59, 1989.
159. Petitt RM, Silverstein MN, Petrone ME: Anagrelide for control of thrombocythemia in polycythemia and other myeloproliferative disorders. *Semin Hematol* 34:51, 1997.
160. Storen EC, Tefferi A: Long-term use of anagrelide in young patients with essential thrombocythemia. *Blood* 97:863, 2001.
161. Pieri L, Bogani C, Guglielmelli P, et al: The JAK2V617 mutation induces constitutive activation and agonist hypersensitivity in basophils of polycythemia vera. *Haematologica* Jul 16. [Epub ahead of print] 2009.
162. Gangat N, Strand JJ, Lasho TL, et al: Pruritus in polycythemia vera is associated with a lower risk of arterial thrombosis. *Am J Hematol* 83:451, 2008.
163. Swerlick RA: Photochemotherapy treatment of pruritus associated with polycythemia vera. *J Am Acad Dermatol* 13:675, 1985.
164. Bircher AJ: Water-induced itching. *Dermatologica* 181:83, 1990.
165. de Wolf JT, Hendriks DW, Egger RC, et al: Alpha-interferon for intractable pruritus in polycythaemia vera. *Lancet* 337:241, 1991.
166. Foa P, Massaro P, Caldiera S, et al: Long-term therapeutic efficacy and toxicity of recombinant interferon-alpha 2a in polycythaemia vera. *Eur J Haematol* 60:273, 1998.
167. Ozturk A, Gunay A, Uskent N: Therapeutic efficacy of recombinant interferon-alpha in polycythaemia vera. *Acta Haematol* 99:89, 1998.
168. Mesa RA, Tefferi A: Emerging drugs for the therapy of primary and post essential thrombocythemia, post polycythemia vera myelofibrosis. *Expert Opin Emerg Drugs* 14:471, 2009.
169. Verstovsek S. KH, Pardanani AD, et al: Characterization of JAK2 V617F allele burden in advanced myelofibrosis (MF) patients: No change in V617F:WT JAK2 ratio in patients with high allele burdens despite profound clinical improvement following treatment with the JAK inhibitor, INCB018424. In: *ASH Annual Meeting*. San Francisco, 2008.
170. Tartaglia AP, Goldberg JD, Berk PD, et al: Adverse effects of antiaggregating platelet therapy in the treatment of polycythemia vera. *Semin Hematol* 23:172, 1986.
171. Willoughby S, Pearson TC: The use of aspirin in polycythaemia vera and primary thrombocythaemia. *Blood Rev* 12:12, 1998.
172. Landolfi R, Marchioli R: European Collaboration on Low-dose Aspirin in Polycythemia Vera (ECLAP): A randomized trial. *Semin Thromb Hemost* 23:473, 1997.
173. Buchanan GR, DeBaun MR, Quinn CT, et al: Sickle cell disease. *Hematology Am Soc Hematol Educ Program* 35, 2004.
174. Silver RT: Recombinant interferon-alpha for treatment of polycythaemia vera. *Lancet* 2:403, 1988.
175. Kiladjian JJ, Cassinat B, Chevret S, et al: Pegylated interferon-alfa-2a induces complete hematologic and molecular responses with low toxicity in polycythemia vera. *Blood* 112:3065, 2008.
176. Kiladjian JJ, Cassinat B, Turlure P, et al: High molecular response rate of polycythemia vera patients treated with pegylated interferon alpha-2a. *Blood* 108:2037, 2006.
177. Steegmann JL, Requena MJ, Martin-Regueira P, et al: High incidence of autoimmune alterations in chronic myeloid leukemia patients treated with interferon-alpha. *Am J Hematol* 72:170, 2003.
178. Yang XF, Wu CJ, McLaughlin S, et al: CML66, a broadly immunogenic tumor antigen, elicits a humoral immune response associated with remission of chronic myelogenous leukemia. *Proc Natl Acad Sci U S A* 98:7492, 2001.
179. Xiong Z, Liu E, Yan Y, et al: An unconventional antigen translated by a novel internal ribosome entry site elicits antitumor humoral immune reactions. *J Immunol* 177:4907, 2006.
180. Xiong Z, Liu E, Yan Y, et al: A novel unconventional antigen MPD5 elicits anti-tumor humoral immune responses in a subset of patients with polycythemia vera. *Int J Immunopathol Pharmacol* 20:373, 2007.
181. Xiong Z, Yan Y, Liu E, et al: Novel tumor antigens elicit anti-tumor humoral immune reactions in a subset of patients with polycythemia vera. *Clin Immunol* 122:279, 2007.
182. Pardanani A: JAK2 inhibitor therapy in myeloproliferative disorders: Rationale, preclinical studies and ongoing clinical trials. *Leukemia* 22:23, 2008.
183. Kralovics R, Teo SS, Li S, et al: Acquisition of the V617F mutation of JAK2 is a late genetic event in a subset of patients with myeloproliferative disorders. *Blood* 108:1377, 2006.
184. Plo I, Nakatake M, Malivert L, et al: JAK2 stimulates homologous recombination and genetic instability: Potential implication in the heterogeneity of myeloproliferative disorders. *Blood* 112:1402, 2008.
185. Mesa RA, Tefferi A. Emerging drugs for the therapy of primary and postessential thrombocythemia, post polycythemia vera myelofibrosis. *Expert Opin Emerg Drugs* 14:471, 2009.
186. Garber K: JAK2 inhibitors: Not the next imatinib but researchers see other possibilities. *J Natl Cancer Inst* 101:980, 2009.
187. Vannucchi AM, Guglielmelli P, Rambaldi A, et al: Epigenetic therapy in myeloproliferative neoplasms: Evidence and perspectives. *J Cell Mol Med* 3:1437, 2009.
188. Hoffman R, Prchal JT, Samuelson S, et al: Philadelphia chromosome-negative myeloproliferative disorders: Biology and treatment. *Biol Blood Marrow Transplant* 13:64, 2007.
189. Rosenthal DS: Clinical aspects of chronic myeloproliferative diseases. *Am J Med Sci* 304:109, 1992.
190. Tefferi A, Mesa RA, Nagorney DM, et al: Splenectomy in myelofibrosis with myeloid metaplasia: A single-institution experience with 223 patients. *Blood* 95:2226, 2000.
191. Anderson JE, Sale G, Appelbaum FR, et al: Allogeneic marrow transplantation for primary myelofibrosis and myelofibrosis secondary to polycythaemia vera or essential thrombocytosis. *Br J Haematol* 98:1010, 1997.
192. Devine SM, Hoffman R, Verma A, et al: Allogeneic blood cell transplantation following reduced-intensity conditioning is effective therapy for older patients with myelofibrosis with myeloid metaplasia. *Blood* 99:2255, 2002.
193. Silver RT: Interferon alfa: Effects of long-term treatment for polycythemia vera. *Semin Hematol* 34:40, 1997.
194. Passamonti F, Malabarba L, Orlandi E, et al: Polycythemia vera in young patients: A study on the long-term risk of thrombosis, myelofibrosis and leukemia. *Haematologica* 88:13, 2003.
195. Rozman C, Giralt M, Feliu E, et al: Life expectancy of patients with chronic nonleukemic myeloproliferative disorders. *Cancer* 67:2658, 1991.
196. Camos M, Cervantes F, Montoto S, et al: Acute lymphoid leukemia following polycythemia vera. *Leuk Lymphoma* 32:395, 1999.
197. Higuchi T, Oba R, Endo M, et al: Transition of polycythemia vera to chronic neutrophilic leukemia. *Leuk Lymphoma* 33:203, 1999.
198. Berlin NI, Lawrence JH, Gartland J: Blood volume in polycythemia as determined by P32 labeled red blood cells. *Am J Med* 9:747, 1950.
199. Fairbanks VF, Klee GG, Wiseman GA, et al: Measurement of blood volume and red cell mass: Re-examination of 51Cr and 125I methods. *Blood Cells Mol Dis* 22:169, 1996.
200. Huber H, Lewis SM, Szur L: [The indications for determination of blood volume and the circulating erythrocyte volume in polycythemia vera and polyglobulia]. *Acta Haematol* 34:116, 1965.
201. Najean Y, Dresch C, Rain J, et al: Radioisotope investigations for the diagnosis and follow-up of polycythemic patients, in *Polycythemia Vera and the Myeloproliferative Disorders*, edited by LR Wasserman, PD Berk, NI Berlin, p 361. WB Saunders, Philadelphia, 1995.

CHAPTER 87

ESSENTIAL THROMBOCYTHEMIA

Philip A. Beer and Anthony R. Green

SUMMARY

Essential thrombocythemia is a clonal stem cell disorder characterized by an overproduction of platelets and associated with mutations in *JAK2* or *MPL*. Complications include thrombosis (predominantly arterial), hemorrhage, and progression to myelofibrosis or acute myeloid leukemia. Diagnosis requires exclusion of reactive thrombocytosis and other myeloid malignancies associated with a raised platelet count. Therapy is aimed at reducing thrombotic complications and includes modification of known cardiovascular risk factors and antiplatelet therapy for the majority of patients. Those at high risk of thrombosis are also considered for cytoreductive therapy with agents such as hydroxyurea, anagrelide, or interferon-α. Although survival in the first decade following diagnosis appears similar to controls, mortality rates increase thereafter as a consequence of disease complications.

DEFINITION AND HISTORY

Essential thrombocythemia (ET), one of the myeloproliferative neoplasms, is a clonal hematopoietic stem cell disorder characterized by an isolated thrombocytosis and associated with thrombotic and hemorrhagic complications. First recognized as a specific disease entity in 1934,[1] ET shares clinical and pathologic similarities with other myeloproliferative neoplasms, particularly polycythemia vera (PV) and primary myelofibrosis (PMF).

EPIDEMIOLOGY

The annual incidence of ET is in the order of 1 to 2.5 per 100,000 population and appears slightly more common in females.[2,3] Patients may present at any age, although ET is largely a disorder of later life with a peak incidence between the ages of 50 and 70 years. Presentation in childhood is rare but well recognized.

ETIOLOGY AND PATHOGENESIS

Little is known about the precise etiology of this disorder, although environmental factors such as exposure to radiation have been implicated in the genesis of other myeloproliferative neoplasms.[4] Both registry data and kindred studies suggest a familial tendency to develop myeloproliferative neoplasms, including ET.[5–7] This predisposition appears to be explained in part by inheritance of a specific haplotype that contains the *JAK2* gene.[8–10]

Although shown to be a clonal disorder in 1981,[11] little was known about the molecular pathogenesis of ET until 2005, when an acquired mutation in the *JAK2* gene (*JAK2* V617F) was identified in approximately 50 percent of patients with ET or PMF and the majority of those with PV.[12–15] JAK2, one of the JAK family of cytoplasmic tyrosine kinases, is essential for signaling by the erythropoietin and thrombopoietin receptors,[16,17] and also contributes to signaling by the granulocyte colony-stimulating factor, granulocyte-macrophage colony-stimulating factor,[18] and interferon- receptors.[19] Studies of the erythropoietin receptor have demonstrated that erythropoietin binding leads to a conformation change in the JAK2-receptor complex,[20] with consequent activation of JAK2 kinase activity and recruitment of downstream signaling pathways.[16] The *JAK2* V617F mutation alters a highly conserved residue within the autoinhibitory pseudokinase (JH2) domain of the protein. Current evidence suggests that alteration of this autoinhibitory domain leads to increased basal kinase activity, resulting in activation of the JAK2-receptor complex in the absence of cognate ligand binding.[21] The central role of JAK2 in erythropoiesis is highlighted by a *JAK2* knock-out mouse, which dies in mid-gestation as a result of severe anemia.[19]

The *JAK2* V617F mutation arises in a hematopoietic stem cell with B-cell, T-cell, natural killer cell, and myeloid lineage potential.[22] The cellular consequences of mutant *JAK2* expression include increased proliferation,[23] cytokine hypersensitivity,[24] cytokine-independent differentiation,[13,25] and inhibition of apoptosis.[26,27] In human disease, mutant *JAK2* appears to act at multiple levels, leading to an erythroid lineage bias in stem cells[28] and resulting in a cellular expansion at the later stages of erythroid differentiation.[24] The association of the *JAK2* V617F mutation with three apparently distinct clinical phenotypes (ET, PV, and PMF) is discussed below.

Despite evidence indicating a central role for *JAK2* mutations in myeloproliferative neoplasm pathogenesis, several observations suggest that a mutation in *JAK2* may not be the disease-initiating event. A familial tendency to develop a myeloproliferative neoplasm[5–7] has led to speculation that *JAK2* mutations are insufficient alone to cause a clinical phenotype, with additional genetic events being inherited in familial cases or acquired in sporadic disease. In female myeloproliferative neoplasm patients, granulocyte clonality measured by X chromosome inactivation pattern or quantitation of a cytogenetic abnormality was found to be in excess of clonality measured by mutant allele burden in a proportion of cases.[29,30] Furthermore, patients with a *JAK2* V617F-positive myeloproliferative neoplasm may develop *JAK2* wild-type leukemia[31,32] or produce erythroid colonies in the absence of erythropoietin that are negative for the *JAK2* mutation.[33,34] Although these studies may be interpreted as evidence for clonal hematopoiesis preceding acquisition of a *JAK2* mutation, alternative explanations exist in some patients, such as the presence of two independent clonal expansions.[35] However, it has been reported that a minority of myeloproliferative neoplasm patients harbor *TET2* mutations, which may precede acquisition of a *JAK2* mutation.[36] This finding indicates that *JAK2* mutations are not the disease-initiating event in some patients, but the frequency of this phenomenon is not yet clear.

Acquired mutations in *MPL*, the thrombopoietin receptor, are found in an additional 4 percent of ET patients.[37,38] These mutations alter residues in the transmembrane (*MPL* S505N) or juxtamembrane regions (*MPL* W515) and lead to constitutive activation of the receptor complex.[39,40] Rarely, ET patients harbor more than one mutation, for example, both *JAK2* V617F and *MPL* W515L.[35]

Acronyms and abbreviations that appear in this chapter include: AML, acute myeloid leukemia; CML, chronic myeloid leukemia; ET, essential thrombocythemia; JAK2, Janus family of tyrosine kinases type 2; PMF, primary myelofibrosis; PV, polycythemia vera; RARS-t, refractory anemia with ringed sideroblasts and thrombocytosis.

CLINICAL FEATURES

SYMPTOMS AND SIGNS

ET is often diagnosed following the incidental finding of a high platelet count, although a proportion of patients present with thrombotic or hemorrhage complications. A detailed clinical history and physical examination is necessary to exclude causes for a reactive thrombocytosis. Approximately 10 percent of ET patients have a mild degree of palpable splenomegaly at diagnosis,[41] although significant splenic enlargement should raise the possibility of another myeloproliferative neoplasm such as PMF or chronic myeloid leukemia (CML).

THROMBOSIS

Thrombotic complications are the major source of morbidity and mortality in ET, with a prospective study indicating a cumulative incidence of 24 percent over 27 months for untreated high-risk patients.[42] The strongest predictive factors for thrombotic complications are age older than 60 years or a history of previous thrombosis.[43–45] Other reported risk factors include predisposition to cardiovascular disease,[44,46,47] leukocytosis at diagnosis,[48,49] and increased marrow fibrosis at diagnosis.[50] Arterial thrombosis predominates, affecting the central nervous system (stroke, transient ischemic attack) and cardiovascular system (myocardial infarction, unstable angina, peripheral arterial occlusion).[41,42] Erythromelalgia, a distinct clinicopathologic syndrome caused by occlusion of small blood vessels, is manifest by discomfort and burning sensations in the fingers or toes, sometimes accompanied by mottling or discoloration of the skin.[51] Venous events mainly comprise deep vein thrombosis and pulmonary embolism. Involvement of unusual sites such as hepatic, portal, or mesenteric veins also occurs and may precede the onset of clinically overt ET (Fig. 87–1A). In one series, half of all patients presenting with hepatic vein thrombosis and a normal blood count tested positive for the *JAK2* V617F mutation, and a quarter of these subsequently developed a clinically overt myeloproliferative neoplasm, most commonly ET.[52]

HEMORRHAGE

Serious bleeding is less common than thrombosis and mainly affects the nasal and buccal mucosa and the gastrointestinal tract, although central nervous system hemorrhage may occur.[41,42] ET patients often demonstrate prolongation of the bleeding time and various abnormalities of *in vitro* coagulation studies, including abnormal platelet aggregation or loss of large von Willebrand factor multimers[53]; however, the relationship of these findings to episodes of clinical bleeding is unclear.[54,55] In a prospective study, rates of major hemorrhage appeared higher in patients with increased marrow fibrosis at diagnosis.[50] Small studies suggest an increased bleeding risk in patients with very high platelet counts and in those receiving antiplatelet therapy, although the data are contradictory and prospective studies are lacking.[47,55–58]

MYELOFIBROTIC TRANSFORMATION

Evolution to myelofibrosis is seen in a proportion of ET patients, although the reported prevalence varies widely, reflecting differences in study design, therapeutic intervention, and diagnostic criteria for post-ET myelofibrosis. Retrospective studies suggest that disease duration is a major predictor of progressive disease, with rates of myelofibrosis in the first decade after diagnosis of 3 to 10 percent rising to 6 to 30 percent in the second decade.[45,48,59] The presence of marrow fibrosis at diagnosis also appears to presage progression to myelofibrosis,[50] although the predictive value of other histologic features of early-stage PMF such as megakaryocyte dysplasia remains controversial.[60] Mutations in *JAK2*[61,62] or *MPL*[37,38] appear to lack prognostic significance with respect to myelofibrotic transformation. A prospective study of high-risk ET patients indicated increased progression to myelofibrosis with anagrelide therapy, with a 5-year cumulative incidence of 7 percent for anagrelide-treated versus 2 percent for hydroxyurea-treated patients.[41] The clinical consequences of post-ET myelofibrosis are similar to *de novo* myelofibrosis, and the conditions are managed in the same way.

LEUKEMIC TRANSFORMATION

Progression to acute myeloid leukemia (AML) occurs in a small minority of patients, with retrospective studies suggesting a prevalence of 1 to 2.5 percent in the first decade after diagnosis, 5 to 8 percent in the second decade, and continuing to rise thereafter.[45,48,63] Therapeutic heterogeneity in theses studies, however, renders their findings difficult to interpret. Studies in PV demonstrated a significantly increased risk of AML in patients receiving genotoxic agents such as radioactive phosphorus or alkylating drugs,[64–66] with ET studies showing an increased incidence of AML in those receiving sequential therapy with alkylating drugs and hydroxyurea.[67,68] The potential leukemogenicity of single agent therapy with hydroxyurea or pipobroman remains controversial (see "Choice of Cytoreductive Agent" below). However, transformation to leukemia has been reported in the absence of prior cytoreductive therapy,[32,69–71] indicating that AML is part of the natural history of this disorder. Of note, patients with *JAK2* V617F-positive ET may develop AML that is negative for the *JAK2* mutation.[31,32]

Therapy of post-ET AML is often limited by the older age of the affected patients, in whom palliative treatment may be the most appropriate strategy. Overall the prognosis of secondary AML is poor (see Chap. 89). Younger patients who do achieve remission with AML induction therapy may be considered for marrow transplantation.

LABORATORY FEATURES

An unexplained and persistently raised platelet count generally warrants further investigation. Establishing a diagnosis of ET requires exclusion of both reactive conditions and other myeloproliferative or myelodysplastic disorders that may present with an isolated thrombocytosis (Tables 87–1 and 87–2).

HEMATOLOGIC AND BIOCHEMICAL PARAMETERS

The blood count in ET shows an elevated platelet count usually with normal hemoglobin and white cell levels, although a mild neutrophilia may be present. The degree of thrombocytosis varies markedly between patients. Examination of the blood film often reveals large platelets that may stain poorly, and is useful in excluding features of PMF such as tear-drop cells (dacryocytes) or circulating progenitor cells. Blood tests should be performed to exclude iron deficiency and look for evidence of inflammation (e.g., by measuring C-reactive protein or erythrocyte sedimentation rate). Levels of thrombopoietin are normal or slightly elevated in ET and have no diagnostic utility.[72] ET patients may show a spurious increase in serum potassium level as a consequence of *in vitro* activation of platelets and leukocytes; this phenomenon can be circumvented by using a plasma sample for biochemical analysis. Growth of cytokine independent erythroid and/or megakaryocyte colonies is observed in approximately one-half of ET patients,[61,73] although limited availability and lack of standardization reduces the diagnostic utility of this test.

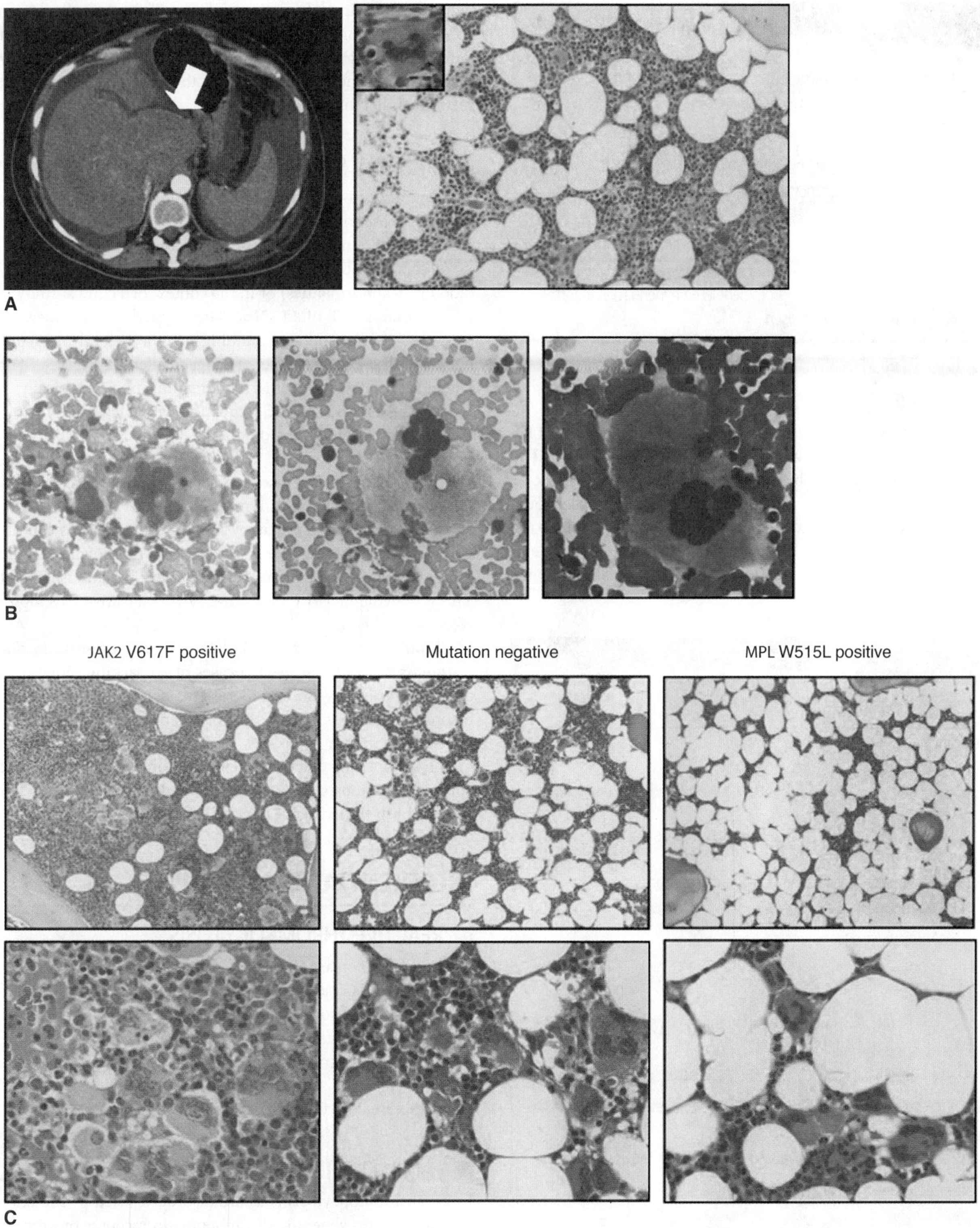

FIGURE 87–1. Morphologic features of essential thrombocythemia. **A.** Contrast enhanced abdominal computed tomographic scan showing features of established hepatic vein thrombosis in a 53-year-old female, including hypertrophy of the caudate lobe (*arrow*) with atrophy of the remaining liver and surrounding ascites; the spleen is of normal size. Hematoxylin-and-eosin stained marrow trephine biopsy showing normal cellularity and increased megakaryocytes with occasional hyperlobulated forms (*inset*). Although the patient was *JAK2* V617F-positive, other investigations performed at this time, including blood count, red cell mass, and cytogenetic analysis, were normal. **B.** Marrow aspirate from a *JAK2* V617F-positive ET patient showing large, hyperlobulated megakaryocytes (slide stained with Wright-Giemsa). **C.** Low- and high-power views of hematoxylin-and-eosin stained marrow trephine biopsies obtained at diagnosis of ET from a *JAK2* V617F-positive 73-year-old female showing increased cellularity and clusters of large, hyperlobulated megakaryocytes; a 69-year-old male without a *JAK2* V617F or *MPL* exon 10 mutation showing normal cellularity and large, hyperlobulated megakaryocytes; and an *MPL* W515L-positive 71-year-old female showing reduced cellularity with occasional loose clusters of hyperlobulated megakaryocytes.

TABLE 87–1. Proposed Diagnostic Criteria for Essential Thrombocythemia

Diagnosis requires A1 to A3 or A1 + A3 to A5	
A1	Sustained platelet count >450 × 10^9/L
A2	Presence of an acquired pathogenic mutation (e.g., in *JAK2* or *MPL*)
A3	No other myeloid malignancy, especially PV, PMF, CML, or myelodysplastic syndrome
A4	No reactive cause for thrombocytosis and normal iron stores
A5	Marrow studies showing increased megakaryocytes displaying a spectrum of morphology with prominent large hyperlobulated forms; reticulin is generally not increased

■ MOLECULAR TESTING

The *JAK2* V617F mutation is present in approximately 50 percent of ET patients and testing is recommended in all suspected cases. The method used should be of suitable sensitivity, such as allele-specific or real-time polymerase chain reaction, given that the mutant allele burden is low in a proportion of patients.[13] Mutations in *MPL* exon 10 are present in a further 4 percent of patients, with five different alleles reported to date (*MPL* S505N and *MPL* W515L/K/A/R). Strategies for detection may include testing only for the most common mutation (*MPL* W515L) or using a technology such as melting curve analysis to detect all mutations within exon 10. In the absence of marrow cytogenetic analysis, molecular testing for the *BCR-ABL1* fusion gene is also recommended to exclude CML.

TABLE 87–2. Causes of Thrombocytosis

Clonal thrombocytosis
Essential thrombocythemia
Polycythemia vera
Primary myelofibrosis
Chronic myeloid leukemia
Refractory anemia with ringed sideroblasts and thrombocytosis
5q-minus syndrome
Reactive (secondary) thrombocytosis
Transient thrombocytosis
Acute blood loss
Recovery from thrombocytopenia (rebound thrombocytosis)
Acute infection or inflammation
Response to exercise
Response to drugs (vincristine, epinephrine, all-*trans*-retinoic acid)
Sustained thrombocytosis
Iron deficiency
Splenectomy or congenital absence of spleen
Malignancy
Chronic infection or inflammation
Hemolytic anemia
Familial thrombocytosis
Spurious thrombocytosis
Cryoglobulinemia
Cytoplasmic fragmentation in acute leukemia
Red cell fragmentation
Bacteremia

■ MARROW STUDIES

Marrow aspiration and trephine biopsy is particularly recommended in suspected cases of ET that are negative for mutations in *JAK2* and *MPL*. Marrow studies may also be useful in cases showing atypical clinical or laboratory features (e.g., palpable splenomegaly, unexplained anemia, blood film abnormalities) or in the context of a clinical study. The marrow aspirate in ET often shows large hyperlobulated megakaryocytes (see Fig. 87–1B), and iron staining may be helpful in excluding iron deficiency or the presence of ringed sideroblasts (see "Differential Diagnosis" below). The marrow trephine biopsy typically shows an increase in megakaryocyte frequency with megakaryocyte clustering and nuclear hyperlobulation in the absence of significant reticulin fibrosis (see Fig. 87–1C). Cellularity is usually normal or slightly increased, but occasional cases may show a hypocellular marrow, for example a proportion of those with mutations in *MPL* (see Fig. 87–1C).[37,61] It has been suggested that marrow trephine appearances can distinguish ET from the early stages of PMF,[74] but the reproducibility and clinical utility of this distinction is unclear[60] (see "Relationship of Essential Thrombocythemia to Other *JAK2* V617F-Positive Myeloproliferative Neoplasms" below).

Chromosomal analysis, by G-banding or fluorescent *in situ* hybridization, is helpful in suspected cases of ET lacking mutations in *JAK2* and *MPL*, primarily to exclude lesions associated with other myeloid disorders such as t(9:22) (CML) or deletions of chromosome 5q ("5q-minus syndrome"; see Chap. 90). Other karyotypic abnormalities, mainly comprising deletions of chromosomes 20q or 13q or additional copies of chromosomes 8 or 9, are found in 5 percent of ET patients[75] and establish the existence of clonal hematopoiesis.

DIFFERENTIAL DIAGNOSIS

■ REACTIVE THROMBOCYTOSIS

A secondary increase in platelet count, mediated by cytokines such as interleukin-6, is associated with a number of infectious, inflammatory and malignant disorders (see Table 87–2; Chap. 120). In reports of unselected patients attending various hospital departments, an increased platelet count was as a result of reactive causes in more than 80 percent of cases, with the degree of thrombocytosis not predictive of a clonal versus reactive etiology.[76,77]

■ FAMILIAL THROMBOCYTOSIS

Familial thrombocytosis is a rare disorder caused by mutations in the thrombopoietin gene, the thrombopoietin receptor or other unknown genes. Mutations in the 5′-untranslated region of the thrombopoietin gene are associated with increased translation of thrombopoietin and consequent thrombocytosis.[78] These mutations are dominantly inherited and have not been seen in sporadic disease.[79] A mutation in the thrombopoietin receptor (*MPL* S505N) has been reported in Japanese and Italian kindreds.[80,81] This mutation is also dominantly inherited and results in ligand-independent activation of the receptor.[40] Of interest, the same mutation may be acquired in patients with a sporadic myeloproliferative neoplasm.[37] Although complicated by occasional thrombotic or bleeding episodes, the clinical phenotype of familial thrombocytosis appears to be mild.[82] The genetic cause underlying the majority of familial cases remains to be elucidated.

■ OTHER MYELOID MALIGNANCIES

Other myeloid malignancies that may present with thrombocytosis and an otherwise normal blood count include PV, PMF, CML or myeloproliferative-myelodysplastic syndromes. PV is often associated with thrombocytosis, and may present with a normal hemoglobin level in the presence of iron depletion. Marrow studies will confirm the absence of storage iron and usually show an increase in granulocytic activity and an increased proportion of small megakaryocytes compared to ET. PMF may present with an isolated thrombocytosis, but palpable splenomegaly, circulating tear-drop red cells and progenitor cells and marrow fibrosis are usually present (see Chap. 91).

Occasional patients with CML present with an isolated thrombocytosis. Such cases are predominantly females with absent or minimal splenomegaly and a normal or marginally elevated white cell count, often without basophilia or circulating myeloid progenitors.[83] Marrow studies, however, are usually informative, showing small hypolobulated megakaryocytes typical of CML, and not the large hyperlobulated forms observed in ET. Given the significant impact of tyrosine kinase inhibitors on the prognosis of CML, it is important that this unusual presentation is not overlooked. It is therefore recommended that suspected cases of ET that are negative for a known pathogenic lesion (e.g., a mutation in *MPL* or *JAK2*) undergo either marrow aspiration, trephine biopsy and cytogenetic analysis or molecular analysis of blood for the *BCR-ABL1* fusion.

Thrombocytosis, usually in association with anemia, may be seen in the myelodysplastic disorder associated with an isolated deletion of chromosome 5q ("5q-minus syndrome"). Although often increased in number, megakaryocytes are generally small and hypolobulated,[74] in contrast to the large hyperlobulated forms typical of ET. A raised platelet count is also a feature of refractory anemia with ringed sideroblasts and thrombocytosis (RARS-t). Approximately half of such patients harbor a *JAK2* V617F mutation, or, rarely, a mutation in *MPL*, and may experience thrombotic complications.[84] At present it is not clear whether RARS-t is best considered as a variant of ET or as a separate myelodysplastic/myeloproliferative disorder.

■ RELATIONSHIP OF ESSENTIAL THROMBOCYTHEMIA TO OTHER *JAK2* V617F-POSITIVE MYELOPROLIFERATIVE NEOPLASMS

Relationship of Essential Thrombocythemia to Polycythemia Vera

The same *JAK2* V617F mutation is present in the vast majority of patients with PV and in approximately half of those with ET, raising questions as to how a single mutation is commonly associated with apparently distinct clinical phenotypes. Compared to V617F-negative ET, patients with V617F-positive ET were found to have multiple features resembling PV, including higher hemoglobin levels and white cell counts, lower erythropoietin levels (Fig. 87–2A), increased marrow erythroid and granulocytic activity, and higher rates of venous thrombosis.[61] These findings suggest that ET and PV may form part of a phenotypic continuum, with *JAK2* V617F-positive ET representing a *forme fruste* of PV. According to this concept, the precise phenotype manifested following acquisition of a *JAK2* mutation will depend on additional constitutional and/or acquired modifiers (Fig. 87–2B). A role for genetic background in the modulation of disease phenotype is evidenced by mouse models of disease, where expression of *JAK2* V617F *in vivo* produces variable phenotypic manifestations, depending on the genetic strain of the recipient animal.[85] At the molecular level, the majority of PV patients harbor a clone that is homozygous for the *JAK2* V617F mutation, whereas such clones are rare in ET,[86] suggesting that the ratio of mutant to wild-type *JAK2* may be important in the determination of disease phenotype. Support for this hypothesis again comes from animal models, wherein mice with a low mutant-to-wild-type *JAK2* ratio developed thrombocytosis whereas a high mutant-to-wild-type ratio was associated with erythrocytosis.[87,88] Also consistent with this notion is the observation that mutations of *JAK2* exon 12, which are associated with stronger activation of JAK2 and downstream pathways compared to *JAK2* V617F, are seen in patients with PV but not in those with ET.[89] Furthermore, activation of STAT5 in human CD34-positive cells favors erythroid differentiation, whereas reduced levels favor a megakaryocyte fate.[90] Taken together, these findings suggest that the level of JAK2-STAT5 signaling may modulate the disease phenotype, with homozygosity for the *JAK2* V617F mutation leading to stronger JAK2-STAT5 activation and a predominantly erythroid proliferation.

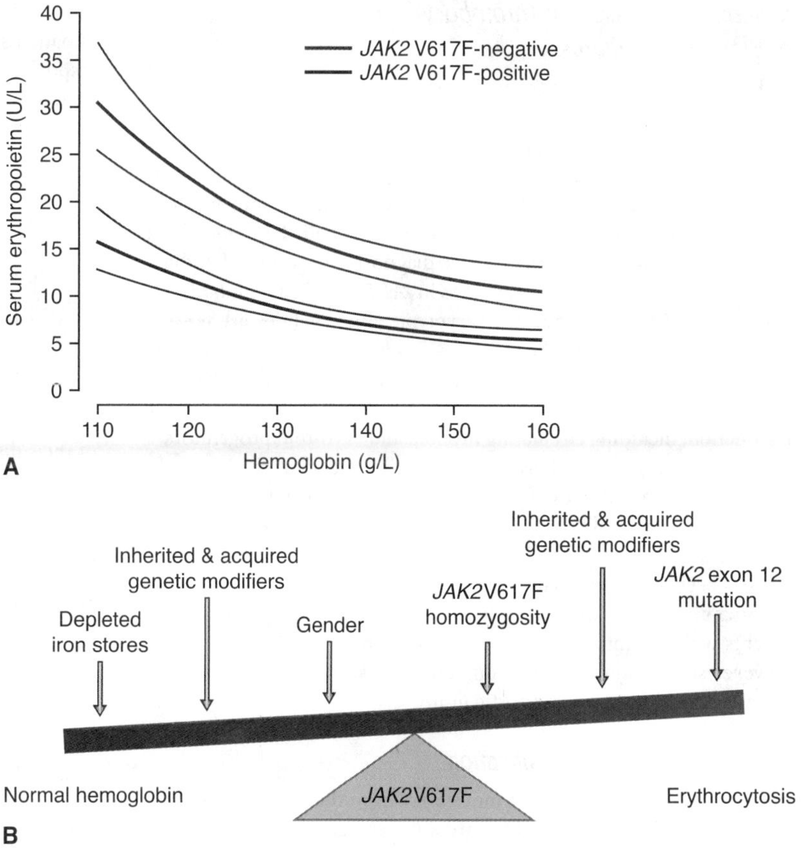

FIGURE 87–2. Relationship of *JAK2* V617F-positive essential thrombocythemia to polycythemia vera. **A.** Estimated mean population serum erythropoietin levels plotted against hemoglobin concentration with simultaneously fitted 95 percent confidence intervals for the mean curves in patients with V617F-positive and V617F-negative ET.[61] **B.** Representation of the relationship of *JAK2* V617F-positive ET to PV, highlighting the interplay of host factors and the acquired *JAK2* V617F mutation.[61]

Relationship of Essential Thrombocythemia to Primary Myelofibrosis

PMF is characterized by marrow fibrosis, extramedullary hematopoiesis, and marrow failure (see Chap. 91). Although traditionally considered as a distinct clinical syndrome, it has been suggested that PMF may represent presentation with accelerated phase disease.[91] In support of this hypothesis, PMF is clinically indistinguishable from myelofibrotic transformation of ET or PV, and patients with PMF may have thrombocytosis for many years prior to diagnosis, suggestive of undiagnosed ET. The prevalence of mutations in *JAK2* or *MPL* is similar in ET compared to PMF[13,37]; however, karyotypic abnormalities are present in up to 50 percent of PMF patients[92,93] compared to only 5 percent in ET,[75] suggesting a greater degree of genetic instability within the PMF clone. Moreover PMF is associated with features of increasing stem cell dysfunction, including circulating myeloid and erythroid progenitors,[94] increased levels of lactate dehydrogenase indicative of ineffective erythropoiesis,[95] increased rates of progression to acute leukemia, and shortened overall survival,[96,97] features that are all consistent with the presence of advanced phase disease.

It has been suggested that marrow histology may be of use in distinguishing biologically distinct subtypes of ET, and that a proportion of patients with thrombocytosis may represent an early stage of PMF.[74,98] However such distinctions are difficult to make in everyday practice, and may lack clinical or prognostic utility.[60]

Toward a Molecular Classification

Recent insights are catalyzing a move away from the traditional definitions of ET, PV, and PMF and toward a molecular classification of the myeloproliferative neoplasms (Fig. 87–3).[91] *JAK2* V617F-positive ET shares multiple laboratory and clinical features with PV. By contrast, *JAK2* V617F-negative ET is biologically distinct, both in presenting features and clinical outcome,[61] and is also heterogeneous, with 10 percent of patients harboring mutations in *MPL*[37,38] and the molecular lesion(s) responsible for the remainder currently unknown. The relationship between PMF and the other myeloproliferative neoplasms is also becoming more blurred. It is likely that in patients with ET or PV, a gradual and variable accumulation of reticulin fibrosis is an inherent part of the disease process. Support for this notion comes from histologic studies in myeloproliferative neoplasm patients[99,100] and mouse models in which the development of postpolycythemic myelofibrosis is common.[85] The rate at which fibrosis develops may be influenced by inherited genetic modifiers (as evidenced by differences in the development of fibrosis among different strains of mice expressing *JAK2* V617F[85]), environmental factors, and acquired genetic or epigenetic changes.[101] In a proportion of patients with chronic phase ET or PV the accumulation of genetic or epigenetic changes results in an acceleration of their disease, which may present as leukocytosis, cytopenia, or overt myelofibrotic transformation, the latter defined as marrow fibrosis associated with anemia, splenomegaly, and the presence of progenitor cells in the blood. According to this concept, at least some patients labeled as primary myelofibrosis may in fact represent individuals presenting in accelerated phase of a preexisting myeloproliferative neoplasm. This model is consistent with the fact that the clinical and laboratory features of PMF are indistinguishable from those of post-ET/PV myelofibrosis and also predicts that the initiating or early genetic lesions responsible for ET will be found in a similar proportion of patients with PMF, as is the case for both *JAK2* V617F and *MPL* mutations.

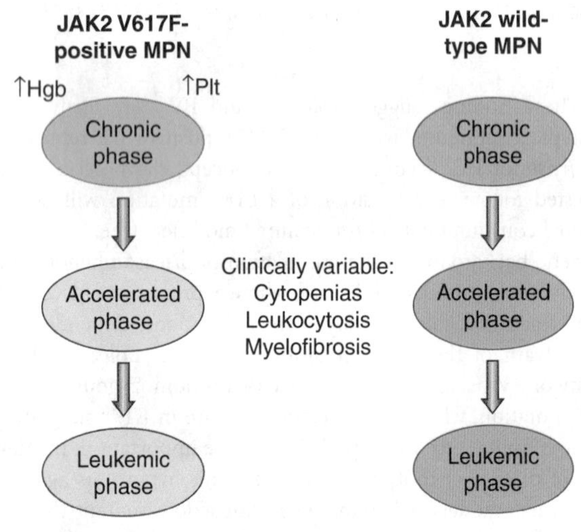

FIGURE 87–3. Toward a molecular classification model to explain the relationship of essential thrombocythemia, polycythemia vera, and primary myelofibrosis. *JAK2* V617F-positive polycythemia and thrombocythemia form part of a phenotypic continuum, whereas *JAK2* V617F-negative ET is both biologically distinct and heterogeneous, including 10 percent of patients with *MPL* mutations and 90 percent in whom the molecular cause is currently unknown. Accelerated phase disease may follow *JAK2* V617F-positive or -negative disease, is clinically variable, and may include marrow fibrosis, leukocytosis, cytopenias, and splenomegaly. A minority of patients undergo disease evolution to acute myeloid leukemia. This model suggests that patients currently labeled as having primary myelofibrosis may in fact be presenting in accelerated phase of a preexisting myeloproliferative neoplasm. Hgb, hemoglobin; Plt, platelet count.

THERAPY

MODIFICATION OF CARDIOVASCULAR RISK FACTORS

Established risk factors for cardiovascular disease, such as hypertension, diabetes, smoking, hypercholesterolemia, and obesity, should be identified and treated accordingly. The broad efficacy of the cholesterol-lowering statin drugs in the prevention of atherosclerotic disease has raised the possibility that such agents may be useful in ET, although this has yet to be tested in a prospective study.

ANTIPLATELET THERAPY

A large randomized trial in polycythemia vera demonstrated a reduction in thrombotic events in those taking low-dose aspirin (100 mg daily) without a concomitant increase in the risk of hemorrhage.[102] Although retrospective studies suggest a similar protective effect in ET,[51,58] prospective trials have not been performed. Based on current evidence, aspirin is recommended for all ET patients unless contraindicated. Although there are few data concerning the use of newer antiplatelet agents such as clopidogrel in ET, their proven track record in preventing complications of atherosclerotic disease suggests they may be appropriate for patients unable to tolerate aspirin.

CYTOREDUCTIVE THERAPY

Indications to Treat

A prospective randomized trial demonstrated a clear role for cytoreductive therapy with hydroxyurea in reducing thrombotic events in high-risk ET patients (age >60 years or history of prior thrombosis), approximately 70 percent of whom were also receiving antiplatelet agents.[42] Although retrospective studies suggest that thrombotic complications in those younger than 60 years of age without additional risk factors may be no higher than controls,[46,56,103] prospective data

TABLE 87–3. Risk Stratification for Patients with Essential Thrombocythemia

	No High-Risk Features	
High Risk	Low Risk	Intermediate Risk
Age >60 years	Age <40 years	Age 40–60 years
Prior thrombosis		
Platelets >1500 × 10⁹/L		

are lacking. Patients with ET are currently stratified on the basis of their risk of thrombotic complications (Table 87–3), with cytoreductive therapy likely to benefit high-risk patients. Patients without high-risk features can be divided into low risk (age less than 40 years) and intermediate risk (age 40–60 years). Cytoreductive therapy is unlikely to offer a significant protective effect for those with low-risk disease, in whom the *a priori* risk of thrombosis is small. There is currently little evidence available to guide treatment decisions in the intermediate risk group. The ongoing PT-1 trials (http://www.ctsu.ox.ac.uk/projects/leuk/pt1/), comprising a randomized trial of hydroxyurea and aspirin versus aspirin alone for intermediate-risk patients and an observational study of low-risk patients treated with aspirin alone, will provide prospective data to help clarify therapeutic decisions for these patients. Once cytoreductive therapy is instituted, most physicians advise dose adjustment to maintain the platelet count within the normal range.

Choice of Cytoreductive Agent (Table 87–4)

Hydroxyurea, a ribonucleotide reductase inhibitor also known as hydroxycarbamide, is widely regarded as first-line therapy for patients requiring treatment, and is the only cytoreductive agent proven to reduce thrombotic events in a randomized controlled trial.[42] Major complications of this drug include reversible myelosuppression and ulceration of the buccal mucosa or lower leg. Although hydroxyurea appears nonleukemogenic when used to treat sickle cell disease,[104] controversy remains about potential leukemogenicity in the myeloproliferative neoplasms.[105] Some studies have suggested an increased risk of acute leukemia in hydroxyurea-treated ET patients,[106–108] but others have failed to observe this association.[67–69] Problems with these studies include small patient numbers, inclusion of patients who have received multiple cytotoxic agents, lack of proper controls, retrospective data collection, and relatively short followup. Of note, analysis of blood cells from sickle cell and myeloproliferative neoplasm patients receiving hydroxyurea showed equivalent rates of DNA mutations to normal controls, suggesting that the mutagenic potential of hydroxyurea is low.[109] At present it is not clear whether hydroxyurea used as a single agent is associated with an increased risk of acute leukemia; however, any increased risk is likely to be small and should be balanced against the reduction in thrombotic complications.

Anagrelide, a quinazoline derivative, reduces the platelet count by inhibition of megakaryocyte differentiation.[110] Although the white cell count is unaffected, anemia is common and often progressive.[50] Up to one-third of patients cannot tolerate anagrelide because of side effects, many of which result from its vasodilatory and positive inotropic actions, including palpitations and arrhythmias, fluid retention, heart failure, and headaches.[41,111] Use of this drug requires particular caution in elderly patients and in those with preexisting cardiac disease. Although anagrelide is not cytotoxic, and therefore unlikely to be leukemogenic, the PT-1 randomized trial demonstrated that anagrelide plus aspirin was inferior to hydroxyurea plus aspirin in high-risk ET patients (Fig. 87–4). In this study, anagrelide treated patients experienced reduced event-free survival ($p = 0.03$) with higher rates of arterial thrombosis ($p = 0.004$), major hemorrhage ($p = 0.008$), and progression to myelofibrosis ($p = 0.01$), despite equivalent control of the platelet count, although rates of venous thrombosis were decreased ($p = 0.006$).[41] In contrast to hydroxyurea, anagrelide therapy was also associated with an increase in marrow reticulin over time.[50] Comparison of patients in the PT-1 (comparison of hydroxyurea vs. anagrelide) and Italian (comparison of hydroxyurea vs. no cytoreductive therapy) prospective studies suggests that anagrelide does provide partial protection from thrombosis[112] and thus may be suitable as second-line therapy for patients in whom hydroxyurea therapy is inadequate or not tolerated. It has been suggested that the results of the ANAHYDRET trial (comparing hydroxyurea to anagrelide) show that anagrelide is not inferior to hydroxyurea in the treatment of ET.[113] However, the number of patients enrolled, duration of followup, and primary endpoints recorded were relatively small (Table 87–5), and as such this trial was not powered to see the differences observed in the PT-1 study.

Recombinant interferon-α is effective at controlling the platelet count in ET, although there is little direct evidence of efficacy in prevention of thrombosis.[114] Treatment is often associated with significant side effects, including flulike symptoms and psychiatric disturbance that may mandate cessation of therapy. As this agent is free from leukemogenic or teratogenic effects, interferon-α is often used for younger patients or during conception and pregnancy. The adverse side-effect profile, however, means that it is generally avoided in older patients. Pegylated interferon-α, for which less-frequent administration is required, may be more convenient, but studies in CML suggest that toxicity is similar to the native compound.[115]

Radioactive phosphorus and alkylating agents such as busulphan are effective at controlling the platelet count, but are associated with an increased risk of progression to acute leukemia, particularly when used sequentially with hydroxyurea,[64,108] and thus should be avoided in younger patients. Both radioactive phosphorus and busulphan can be given intermittently with long intervals between doses and may be useful in treating older patients who are unable to attend the clinic on a regular basis. Pipobroman, a piperazine derivative, is effective at reducing the platelet count in ET, although there is little direct evidence for efficacy in thrombosis prevention.[116] Despite structural similarities to other alkylating agents, pipobroman does not appear to be associated with high rates of leukemic transformation,[63,116] but nonetheless should be avoided in the treatment of younger patients.

TABLE 87–4. Choice of Cytoreductive Agent in Essential Thrombocythemia

Age Group	First Line	Second Line
<40 years old	Interferon-α	Hydroxyurea
		Anagrelide
40–75 years	Hydroxyurea	Interferon-α
		Anagrelide
>75 years	Hydroxyurea	Anagrelide
		Pipobroman
		Busulphan
		Radioactive phosphorus

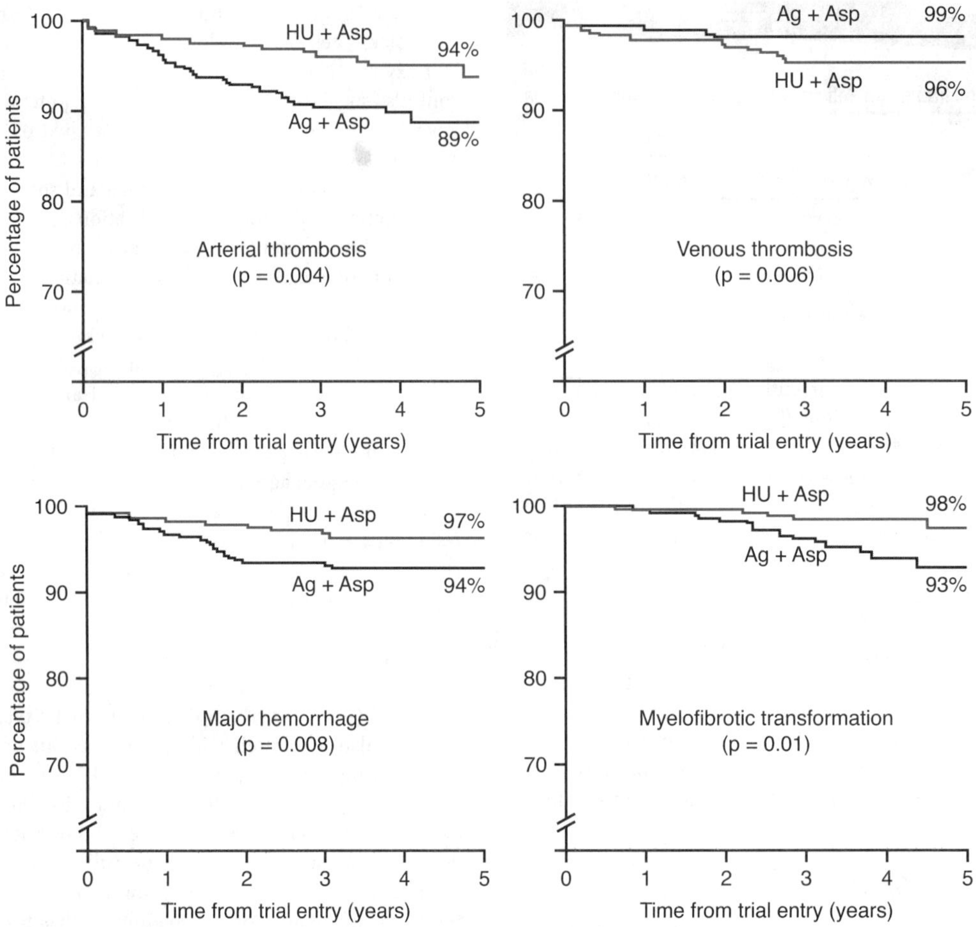

FIGURE 87–4. Hydroxyurea versus anagrelide in the treatment of essential thrombocythemia. Kaplan-Meier estimates of survival free from arterial thrombosis, venous thrombosis, major hemorrhage, and myelofibrotic transformation in high-risk ET patients treated with hydroxyurea (*HU*) plus aspirin (*Asp*) versus anagrelide (*Ag*) plus aspirin.[41]

TABLE 87–5. ANAHYDRET and PT-1 Randomized Controlled Trials of Anagrelide versus Hydroxyurea for the Treatment of Essential Thrombocythemia

	ANAHYDRET Trial[113]	PT-1 Trial[41]
Diagnosis	WHO criteria (2001)	PVSG criteria
	Central review of histology*	Diagnosis by treating physician
Patients	High risk	High risk
	Treatment naïve	Treated or untreated
Median age: AN/HU	58/56	61/62
Patient number: AN/HU	122/136	405/404
Followup	539 patient-years	2,653 patient-years
Total events:		
Arterial thrombosis	10	54
Venous thrombosis	7	17
Hemorrhage	6	30
Transformation to MF	0	21

AN, anagrelide; HU, hydroxyurea; MF, myelofibrosis; WHO, World Health Organization.
*82.2% of patients met WHO 2001 diagnostic criteria for ET.

SPECIAL CONSIDERATIONS

Conception and Pregnancy

First trimester fetal loss complicates up to 50 percent of pregnancies in ET patients, with other complications such as intrauterine growth retardation, still birth, and preeclampsia also occurring more frequently.[117–120] Such complications occur irrespective of the platelet count prior to conception,[117–120] but may be more prominent in those with *JAK2* V617F-positive disease.[120] Whether the use of aspirin or cytoreductive agents can improve pregnancy outcome is uncertain, with studies reporting contradictory results.[117–121] However, a large meta-analysis of preeclampsia patients without ET suggested that aspirin use in pregnancy is safe for both mother and fetus,[122] and it therefore seems reasonable to consider its use for all pregnant ET patients. Although hydroxyurea has been used during pregnancy, usually without adverse effects for mother or fetus, it is teratogenic in various nonhuman mammals[123] and should be avoided if possible. Anagrelide can cross the placenta with unknown effects on fetal development and should also be avoided. Interferon-α is nonteratogenic and is the agent of choice for patients with high-risk disease should cytoreductive therapy be required during pregnancy. Although studies in ET patients are lacking, thromboprophylaxis appears safe in pregnancy (e.g., with low doses of low-molecular-weight heparin),[124] and may be considered for patients with a history of thrombosis or pregnancy loss; in those with prior thrombosis, treatment should be continued for 6 weeks postpartum. Ideally, pregnant ET patients should be managed in a center where regular fetal monitoring can be performed and that has good communication between the obstetric, hematology, and anesthetic departments. Pregnancy does not appear to affect the natural history of the disease,[118] although the platelet count often falls during gestation. In animal studies, hydroxyurea is associated with reduced spermatogenesis and genetic damage to spermatogonia.[123] Consequently, male patients requiring cytoreductive treatment should consider interferon-α therapy prior to attempted conception.

Surgery

Although thrombotic and bleeding complications appear increased in ET patients undergoing surgical procedures, it is not clear whether these risks can be ameliorated by specific therapeutic interventions.[125] In general, antiplatelet agents should be stopped 7 to 10 days prior to major surgery or surgery to critical sites, and recommenced as soon as the surgeon is confident of secure hemostasis. Postoperative thromboprophylaxis should be administered according to local protocols. For patients receiving cytoreductive therapy, control of blood counts should be optimized preoperatively and interruptions in therapy kept to a minimum. For patients not receiving treatment, temporary cytoreductive therapy may be considered on a case-by-case basis, taking into account the individual's thrombotic risk profile, the degree of thrombocytosis, and the nature of the surgery.

Splenectomy in ET patients generally results in an increase in the platelet count and also in increased thrombotic and hemorrhagic complications. Consequently, normalization of the platelet count is advisable for all ET patients prior to elective splenectomy. Thromboprophylaxis and daily monitoring of blood counts is recommended during the postoperative period.

TABLE 87–6. Risk Factors for Complications in Essential Thrombocythemia

Thrombosis	Hemorrhage	Myelofibrotic Transformation	Acute Myeloid Leukemia
Age >60 years	Marrow fibrosis†	Disease duration	Disease duration
Prior thrombosis		Anagrelide therapy§	Genotoxic therapy
Cardiovascular risk*		Marrow fibrosis†	Use of >1 cytoreductive agent
Leukocytosis†			
Marrow fibrosis†			
JAK2 V617F mutation‡			

*Diabetes, hypertension, hypercholesterolemia, or tobacco use.

†At diagnosis.

‡Venous thrombosis and total thrombotic events.

§Compared to hydroxyurea.

COURSE AND PROGNOSIS

There is a lack of good quality prospective data concerning long-term survival in ET. From retrospective studies, mortality rates are similar to population controls in the first decade after diagnosis,[48,68] but appear to increase thereafter.[48] This excess mortality results from disease complications such as thrombosis and transformation to myelofibrosis or AML. However, management paradigms have changed significantly over the last 20 years, and so the relevance of these data for current patients is unclear.

A number of predictive factors for thrombotic complications have been identified (Table 87–6), the best established of which are age older than 60 years or a history of previous thrombosis.[43–45] Risk factors associated with atherosclerotic disease in general, such as diabetes, hypertension, hypercholesterolemia, and tobacco use, also predict for thrombosis in ET patients[44,46,47] and should be managed accordingly. It is unclear, however, if patients with cardiovascular risk factors but no features of high-risk ET (age older than 60 years or history of thrombosis) will benefit from cytoreductive therapy. Leukocyte count at diagnosis has been reported as an independent predictor of thrombotic events,[48,49] but prospective data are lacking. It remains to be seen if this risk can be modulated by therapeutic reduction in the white cell count. Patients with *JAK2* V617F-positive ET are reported to exhibit higher rates of venous thrombosis[61] and higher overall rates of thrombosis[126] compared to those without the mutation, although a direct association between *JAK2* V617F-positive ET and arterial events is not well established.[126] Increased marrow fibrosis at diagnosis also predicts for subsequent thrombotic complications.[50] At the present time, age older than 60 years or history of previous thrombosis are generally considered to mandate cytoreductive therapy in ET patients. The role of other risk factors in altering management decisions is currently unclear. Although the degree of thrombocytosis is not a reliable indicator of thrombotic risk,[44,45,56,127] many physicians consider cytoreductive therapy in patients with a very high platelet count (e.g., greater than 1500×10^9/L).

In contrast to thrombotic complications, there are few identifiable factors that predict for progression to myelofibrosis or acute leukemia. The incidence of both complications increases progressively with disease duration.[45,48,59,63] Choice of therapy also plays a role, with anagrelide increasing the risk of myelofibrotic transformation compared to hydroxyurea[41] and genotoxic agents increasing the risk of leukemia, especially when used sequentially with hydroxyurea.[67,68] Marrow fibrosis at diagnosis was associated with an increased risk of subsequent myelofibrosis in a prospective study,[50] but other markers have failed to show a consistent association with either myelofibrotic or leukemic transformation.

REFERENCES

1. Epstein E, Goedel A: Haemorrhagische thrombocythamie bei vascularer schrumpfmilz. *Virchow's Archiv Abteilung* 293:233, 1934.
2. McNally RJ, Rowland D, Roman E, Cartwright RA: Age and sex distributions of hematological malignancies in the U.K. *Hematol Oncol* 15:173, 1997.
3. Mesa RA, Silverstein MN, Jacobsen SJ, et al: Population-based incidence and survival figures in essential thrombocythemia and agnogenic myeloid metaplasia: An Olmsted County Study, 1976–1995. *Am J Hematol* 61:10, 1999.
4. Anderson RE, Hoshino T, Yamamoto T: Myelofibrosis with myeloid metaplasia in survivors of the atomic bomb in Hiroshima. *Ann Intern Med* 60:1, 1964.
5. Kralovics R, Stockton DW, Prchal JT: Clonal hematopoiesis in familial polycythemia vera suggests the involvement of multiple mutational events in the early pathogenesis of the disease. *Blood* 102:3793, 2003.
6. Landgren O, Goldin LR, Kristinsson SY, et al: Increased risks of polycythemia vera, essential thrombocythemia, and myelofibrosis among 24,577 first-degree relatives of 11,039 patients with myeloproliferative neoplasms in Sweden. *Blood* 112:2199, 2008.
7. Bellanne-Chantelot C, Chaumarel I, Labopin M, et al: Genetic and clinical implications of the Val617Phe JAK2 mutation in 72 families with myeloproliferative disorders. *Blood* 108:346, 2006.
8. Kilpivaara O, Mukherjee S, Schram AM, et al: A germline JAK2 SNP is associated with predisposition to the development of JAK2(V617F)-positive myeloproliferative neoplasms. *Nat Genet* 41:455, 2009.
9. Jones AV, Chase A, Silver RT, et al: JAK2 haplotype is a major risk factor for the development of myeloproliferative neoplasms. *Nat Genet* 41:446, 2009.

10. Olcaydu D, Harutyunyan A, Jager R, et al: A common JAK2 haplotype confers susceptibility to myeloproliferative neoplasms. *Nat Genet* 41:450, 2009.
11. Fialkow PJ, Faguet GB, Jacobson RJ, et al: Evidence that essential thrombocythemia is a clonal disorder with origin in a multipotent stem cell. *Blood* 58:916, 1981.
12. James C, Ugo V, Le Couedic JP, et al: A unique clonal JAK2 mutation leading to constitutive signalling causes polycythaemia vera. *Nature* 434:1144, 2005.
13. Baxter EJ, Scott LM, Campbell PJ, et al: Acquired mutation of the tyrosine kinase JAK2 in human myeloproliferative disorders. *Lancet* 365:1054, 2005.
14. Levine RL, Wadleigh M, Cools J, et al: Activating mutation in the tyrosine kinase JAK2 in polycythemia vera, essential thrombocythemia, and myeloid metaplasia with myelofibrosis. *Cancer Cell* 7:387, 2005.
15. Kralovics R, Passamonti F, Buser AS, et al: A gain-of-function mutation of JAK2 in myeloproliferative disorders. *N Engl J Med* 352:1779, 2005.
16. Witthuhn BA, Quelle FW, Silvennoinen O, et al: JAK2 associates with the erythropoietin receptor and is tyrosine phosphorylated and activated following stimulation with erythropoietin. *Cell* 74:227, 1993.
17. Drachman JG, Millett KM, Kaushansky K: Thrombopoietin signal transduction requires functional JAK2, not TYK2. *J Biol Chem* 274:13480, 1999.
18. Sandberg EM, Wallace TA, Godeny MD, et al: Jak2 tyrosine kinase: A true jak of all trades? *Cell Biochem Biophys* 41:207, 2004.
19. Parganas E, Wang D, Stravopodis D, et al: Jak2 is essential for signaling through a variety of cytokine receptors. *Cell* 93:385, 1998.
20. Remy I, Wilson IA, Michnick SW: Erythropoietin receptor activation by a ligand-induced conformation change. *Science* 283:990, 1999.
21. Levine RL, Pardanani A, Tefferi A, Gilliland DG: Role of JAK2 in the pathogenesis and therapy of myeloproliferative disorders. *Nat Rev Cancer* 7:673, 2007.
22. Delhommeau F, Dupont S, Tonetti C, et al: Evidence that the JAK2 G1849T (V617F) mutation occurs in a lymphomyeloid progenitor in polycythemia vera and idiopathic myelofibrosis. *Blood* 109:71, 2007.
23. Walz C, Crowley BJ, Hudon HE, et al: Activated Jak2 with the V617F Point Mutation Promotes G1/S Phase Transition. *J Biol Chem* 281:18177, 2006.
24. Dupont S, Masse A, James C, et al: The JAK2 V617F mutation triggers erythropoietin hypersensitivity and terminal erythroid amplification in primary cells from patients with polycythemia vera. *Blood* 110:1013, 2007.
25. Garcon L, Rivat C, James C, et al: Constitutive activation of STAT5 and Bcl-xL overexpression can induce endogenous erythroid colony formation in human primary cells. *Blood* 108:1551, 2006.
26. Zeuner A, Pedini F, Signore M, et al: Increased death receptor resistance and FLIPshort expression in polycythemia vera erythroid precursor cells. *Blood* 107:3495, 2006.
27. Zhao R, Follows GA, Beer PA, et al: Inhibition of the Bcl-xL deamidation pathway in myeloproliferative disorders. *N Engl J Med* 359:2778, 2008.
28. Jamieson CHM, Gotlib J, Durocher JA, et al: The JAK2 V617F mutation occurs in hematopoietic stem cells in polycythemia vera and predisposes toward erythroid differentiation. *Proc Natl Acad Sci U S A* 103:6224, 2006.
29. Kralovics R, Teo SS, Li S, et al: Acquisition of the V617F mutation of JAK2 is a late genetic event in a subset of patients with myeloproliferative disorders. *Blood* 108:1377, 2006.
30. Levine RL, Belisle C, Wadleigh M, et al: X-inactivation-based clonality analysis and quantitative JAK2V617F assessment reveal a strong association between clonality and JAK2V617F in PV but not ET/MMM, and identifies a subset of JAK2V617F-negative ET and MMM patients with clonal hematopoiesis. *Blood* 107:4139, 2006.
31. Campbell PJ, Baxter EJ, Beer PA, et al: Mutation of JAK2 in the myeloproliferative disorders: Timing, clonality studies, cytogenetic associations, and role in leukemic transformation. *Blood* 108:3548, 2006.
32. Theocharides A, Boissinot M, Girodon F, et al: Leukemic blasts in transformed JAK2-V617F-positive myeloproliferative disorders are frequently negative for the JAK2-V617F mutation. *Blood* 110:375, 2007.
33. Nussenzveig RH, Swierczek SI, Jelinek J, et al: Polycythemia vera is not initiated by JAK2V617F mutation. *Exp Hematol* 35:32, 2007.
34. Li S, Kralovics R, De Libero G, et al: Clonal heterogeneity in polycythemia vera patients with JAK2 exon12 and JAK2-V617F mutations. *Blood* 111:3863, 2008.
35. Beer PA, Jones AV, Bench AJ, et al: Clonal diversity in the myeloproliferative neoplasms: Independent origins of genetically distinct clones. *Br J Haematol* 144:904, 2009.
36. Delhommeau F, Dupont S, James C, et al: TET2 Is a Novel Tumor Suppressor Gene Inactivated in Myeloproliferative Neoplasms: Identification of a Pre-JAK2 V617F Event. *N Engl J Med* 360:2289, 2009.
37. Beer PA, Campbell PJ, Scott LM, et al: MPL mutations in myeloproliferative disorders: Analysis of the PT-1 cohort. *Blood* 112:141, 2008.
38. Vannucchi AM, Antonioli E, Guglielmelli P, et al: Characteristics and clinical correlates of MPL 515W>L/K mutation in essential thrombocythemia. *Blood* 112:844, 2008.
39. Staerk J, Lacout C, Sato T, et al: An amphipathic motif at the transmembrane-cytoplasmic junction prevents autonomous activation of the thrombopoietin receptor. *Blood* 107:1864, 2006.
40. Ding J, Komatsu H, Iida S, et al: The Asn505 mutation of c-MPL gene, which causes familial essential thrombocythemia, induces autonomous homodimerization of the c-Mpl protein due to strong amino acid polarity. *Blood* May 29. [Epub ahead of print] 2009.
41. Harrison CN, Campbell PJ, Buck G, et al: Hydroxyurea compared with anagrelide in high-risk essential thrombocythemia. *N Engl J Med* 353:33, 2005.
42. Cortelazzo S, Finazzi G, Ruggeri M, et al: Hydroxyurea for patients with essential thrombocythemia and a high risk of thrombosis. *N Engl J Med* 332:1132, 1995.
43. Cortelazzo S, Viero P, Finazzi G, et al: Incidence and risk factors for thrombotic complications in a historical cohort of 100 patients with essential thrombocythemia. *J Clin Oncol* 8:556, 1990.
44. Besses C, Cervantes F, Pereira A, et al: Major vascular complications in essential thrombocythemia: A study of the predictive factors in a series of 148 patients. *Leukemia* 13:150, 1999.
45. Passamonti F, Rumi E, Arcaini L, et al: Prognostic factors for thrombosis, myelofibrosis, and leukemia in essential thrombocythemia: A study of 605 patients. *Haematologica* 93:1645, 2008.
46. Alvarez-Larran A, Cervantes F, Bellosillo B, et al: Essential thrombocythemia in young individuals: Frequency and risk factors for vascular events and evolution to myelofibrosis in 126 patients. *Leukemia* 21:1218, 2007.
47. Radaelli F, Colombi M, Calori R, et al: Analysis of risk factors predicting thrombotic and/or haemorrhagic complications in 306 patients with essential thrombocythemia. *Hematol Oncol* 25:115, 2007.
48. Wolanskyj AP, Schwager SM, McClure RF, Larson DR, Tefferi A: Essential thrombocythemia beyond the first decade: Life expectancy, long-term complication rates, and prognostic factors. *Mayo Clin Proc* 81:159, 2006.
49. Carobbio A, Finazzi G, Antonioli E, et al: Thrombocytosis and leukocytosis interaction in vascular complications of essential thrombocythemia. *Blood* 112:3135, 2008.
50. Campbell PJ, Bareford D, Erber WN, et al: Reticulin accumulation in essential thrombocythemia: Prognostic significance and relationship to therapy. *J Clin Oncol* 27:2991, 2009.
51. Michiels JJ, van Genderen PJ, Lindemans J, van Vliet HH: Erythromelalgic, thrombotic and hemorrhagic manifestations in 50 cases of thrombocythemia. *Leuk Lymphoma* 22 Suppl 1:47, 1996.
52. Patel RK, Lea NC, Heneghan MA, et al: Prevalence of the activating JAK2 tyrosine kinase mutation V617F in the Budd-Chiari syndrome. *Gastroenterology* 130:2031, 2006.
53. Elliott MA, Tefferi A: Thrombosis and haemorrhage in polycythaemia vera and essential thrombocythaemia. *Br J Haematol* 128:275, 2005.
54. Schafer AI: Bleeding and thrombosis in the myeloproliferative disorders. *Blood* 64:1, 1984.
55. Fenaux P, Simon M, Caulier MT, et al: Clinical course of essential thrombocythemia in 147 cases. *Cancer* 66:549, 1990.
56. Tefferi A, Fonseca R, Pereira DL, Hoagland HC: A long-term retrospective study of young women with essential thrombocythemia. *Mayo Clin Proc* 76:22, 2001.
57. Tartaglia AP, Goldberg JD, Berk PD, Wasserman LR: Adverse effects of antiaggregating platelet therapy in the treatment of polycythemia vera. *Semin Hematol* 23:172, 1986.
58. Jensen MK, de Nully Brown P, Nielsen OJ, Hasselbalch HC: Incidence, clinical features and outcome of essential thrombocythaemia in a well defined geographical area. *Eur J Haematol* 65:132, 2000.
59. Cervantes F, Alvarez-Larran A, Talarn C, et al: Myelofibrosis with myeloid metaplasia following essential thrombocythaemia: Actuarial probability, presenting characteristics and evolution in a series of 195 patients. *Br J Haematol* 118:786, 2002.
60. Wilkins BS, Erber WN, Bareford D, et al: Bone marrow pathology in essential thrombocythemia: Interobserver reliability and utility for identifying disease subtypes. *Blood* 111:60, 2008.
61. Campbell PJ, Scott LM, Buck G, et al: Definition of subtypes of essential thrombocythaemia and relation to polycythaemia vera based on JAK2 V617F mutation status: A prospective study. *Lancet* 366:1945, 2005.
62. Vannucchi AM, Antonioli E, Guglielmelli P, et al: Clinical correlates of JAK2V617F presence or allele burden in myeloproliferative neoplasms: A critical reappraisal. *Leukemia* 22:1299, 2008.
63. Kiladjian JJ, Rain JD, Bernard JF, et al: Long-term incidence of hematological evolution in three French prospective studies of hydroxyurea and pipobroman in polycythemia vera and essential thrombocythemia. *Semin Thromb Hemost* 32:417, 2006.
64. Finazzi G, Caruso V, Marchioli R, et al: Acute leukemia in polycythemia vera: An analysis of 1638 patients enrolled in a prospective observational study. *Blood* 105:2664, 2005.
65. Modan B, Lilienfeld AM: Polycythemia vera and leukemia—The role of radiation treatment. A study of 1222 patients. *Medicine (Baltimore)* 44:305, 1965.
66. Berk PD, Goldberg JD, Silverstein MN, et al: Increased incidence of acute leukemia in polycythemia vera associated with chlorambucil therapy. *N Engl J Med* 304:441, 1981.
67. Finazzi G, Ruggeri M, Rodeghiero F, Barbui T: Second malignancies in patients with essential thrombocythaemia treated with busulphan and hydroxyurea: Long-term follow-up of a randomized clinical trial. *Br J Haematol* 110:577, 2000.
68. Passamonti F, Rumi E, Pungolino E, et al: Life expectancy and prognostic factors for survival in patients with polycythemia vera and essential thrombocythemia. *Am J Med* 117:755, 2004.
69. Gangat N, Wolanskyj AP, McClure RF, et al: Risk stratification for survival and leukemic transformation in essential thrombocythemia: A single institutional study of 605 patients. *Leukemia* 21:270, 2007.
70. Andersson PO, Ridell B, Wadenvik H, Kutti J: Leukemic transformation of essential thrombocythemia without previous cytoreductive treatment. *Ann Hematol* 79:40, 2000.

71. Gugliotta L, Marchioli R, Fiacchini M: Epidemiological, diagnostic, therapeutic and prognostic aspects of essential thrombocythemia in a retrospective study of the GIMMC group in two thousand patients [abstract]. *Blood* 90(Suppl 1):172, 1997.
72. Panteli KE, Hatzimichael EC, Bouranta PK, et al: Serum interleukin (IL)-1, IL-2, sIL-2Ra, IL-6 and thrombopoietin levels in patients with chronic myeloproliferative diseases. *Br J Haematol* 130:709, 2005.
73. Florensa L, Besses C, Woessner S, et al: Endogenous megakaryocyte and erythroid colony formation from blood in essential thrombocythaemia. *Leukemia* 9:271, 1995.
74. Swerdlow SH, Campo E, Harris NL, et al: *WHO classification of Tumours of Haematopoietic and Lymphoid Tissues.* IARC Press, Lyon, 2008.
75. Bench AJ, Nacheva EP, Champion KM, Green AR: Molecular genetics and cytogenetics of myeloproliferative disorders. *Baillieres Clin Haematol* 11:819, 1998.
76. Griesshammer M, Bangerter M, Sauer T, et al: Aetiology and clinical significance of thrombocytosis: Analysis of 732 patients with an elevated platelet count. *J Intern Med* 245:295, 1999.
77. Buss DH, Cashell AW, O'Connor ML, et al: Occurrence, etiology, and clinical significance of extreme thrombocytosis: A study of 280 cases. *Am J Med* 96:247, 1994.
78. Wiestner A, Schlemper RJ, van der Maas AP, Skoda RC: An activating splice donor mutation in the thrombopoietin gene causes hereditary thrombocythaemia. *Nat Genet* 18:49, 1998.
79. Harrison CN, Gale RE, Wiestner AC, et al: The activating splice mutation in intron 3 of the thrombopoietin gene is not found in patients with non-familial essential thrombocythaemia. *Br J Haematol* 102:1341, 1998.
80. Ding J, Komatsu H, Wakita A, et al: Familial essential thrombocythemia associated with a dominant-positive activating mutation of the c-MPL gene, which encodes for the receptor for thrombopoietin. *Blood* 103:4198, 2004.
81. Teofili L, Giona F, Martini M, et al: Markers of myeloproliferative diseases in childhood polycythemia vera and essential thrombocythemia. *J Clin Oncol* 25:1048, 2007.
82. Skoda R: The genetic basis of myeloproliferative disorders. *Hematology* 2007:1, 2007.
83. Michiels JJ, Berneman Z, Schroyens W, et al: Philadelphia (Ph) chromosome-positive thrombocythemia without features of chronic myeloid leukemia in peripheral blood: Natural history and diagnostic differentiation from Ph-negative essential thrombocythemia. *Ann Hematol* 83:504, 2004.
84. Schmitt-Graeff AH, Teo SS, Olschewski M, et al: JAK2V617F mutation status identifies subtypes of refractory anemia with ringed sideroblasts associated with marked thrombocytosis. *Haematologica* 93:34, 2008.
85. Wernig G, Mercher T, Okabe R, et al: Expression of Jak2V617F causes a polycythemia vera-like disease with associated myelofibrosis in a murine bone marrow transplant model. *Blood* 107:4274, 2006.
86. Scott LM, Scott MA, Campbell PJ, Green AR: Progenitors homozygous for the V617F mutation occur in most patients with polycythemia vera, but not essential thrombocythemia. *Blood* 108:2435, 2006.
87. Tiedt R, Hao-Shen H, Sobas MA, et al: Ratio of mutant JAK2-V617F to wild-type Jak2 determines the MPD phenotypes in transgenic mice. *Blood* 111:3931, 2008.
88. Shide K, Shimoda HK, Kumano T, et al: Development of ET, primary myelofibrosis and PV in mice expressing JAK2 V617F. *Leukemia* 22:87, 2008.
89. Scott LM, Tong W, Levine RL, et al: JAK2 exon 12 mutations in polycythemia vera and idiopathic erythrocytosis. *N Engl J Med* 356:459, 2007.
90. Olthof SG, Fatrai S, Drayer AL, et al: Downregulation of signal transducer and activator of transcription 5 (STAT5) in CD34+ cells promotes megakaryocytic development, whereas activation of STAT5 drives erythropoiesis. *Stem Cells* 26:1732, 2008.
91. Campbell PJ, Green AR: The myeloproliferative disorders. *N Engl J Med* 355:2452, 2006.
92. Mertens F, Johansson B, Heim S, et al: Karyotypic patterns in chronic myeloproliferative disorders: Report on 74 cases and review of the literature. *Leukemia* 5:214, 1991.
93. Tefferi A, Mesa RA, Schroeder G, et al: Cytogenetic findings and their clinical relevance in myelofibrosis with myeloid metaplasia. *Br J Haematol* 113:763, 2001.
94. Oppliger Leibundgut E, Horn MP, Brunold C, et al: Hematopoietic and endothelial progenitor cell trafficking in patients with myeloproliferative diseases. *Haematologica* 91:1465, 2006.
95. Cervantes F, Pereira A, Esteve J, et al: Identification of "short-lived" and "long-lived" patients at presentation of idiopathic myelofibrosis. *Br J Haematol* 97:635, 1997.
96. Dupriez B, Morel P, Demory JL, et al: Prognostic factors in agnogenic myeloid metaplasia: A report on 195 cases with a new scoring system. *Blood* 88:1013, 1996.
97. Barosi G, Ambrosetti A, Centra A, et al: Splenectomy and risk of blast transformation in myelofibrosis with myeloid metaplasia. Italian Cooperative Study Group on Myeloid with Myeloid Metaplasia. *Blood* 91:3630, 1998.
98. Thiele J, Kvasnicka HM, Zankovich R, Diehl V: Relevance of bone marrow features in the differential diagnosis between essential thrombocythemia and early stage idiopathic myelofibrosis. *Haematologica* 85:1126, 2000.
99. Roberts BE, Miles DW, Woods CG: Polycythaemia vera and myelosclerosis: A bone marrow study. *Br J Haematol* 16:75, 1969.
100. Burston J, Pinniger JL: The reticulin content of bone marrow in haematological disorders. *Br J Haematol* 9:172, 1963.
101. Jost E, do O N, Dahl E, et al: Epigenetic alterations complement mutation of JAK2 tyrosine kinase in patients with BCR/ABL-negative myeloproliferative disorders. *Leukemia* 21:505, 2007.
102. Landolfi R, Marchioli R, Kutti J, et al: Efficacy and safety of low-dose aspirin in polycythemia vera. *N Engl J Med* 350:114, 2004.
103. Ruggeri M, Finazzi G, Tosetto A, et al: No treatment for low-risk thrombocythaemia: Results from a prospective study. *Br J Haematol* 103:772, 1998.
104. Lanzkron S, Strouse JJ, Wilson R, et al: Systematic review: Hydroxyurea for the treatment of adults with sickle cell disease. *Ann Intern Med* 148:939, 2008.
105. Spivak JL: Polycythemia vera: Myths, mechanisms, and management. *Blood* 100:4272, 2002.
106. Weinfeld A, Swolin B, Westin J: Acute leukaemia after hydroxyurea therapy in polycythaemia vera and allied disorders: Prospective study of efficacy and leukaemogenicity with therapeutic implications. *Eur J Haematol* 52:134, 1994.
107. Sterkers Y, Preudhomme C, Lai JL, et al: Acute myeloid leukemia and myelodysplastic syndromes following essential thrombocythemia treated with hydroxyurea: High proportion of cases with 17p deletion. *Blood* 91:616, 1998.
108. Nielsen I, Hasselbalch HC: Acute leukemia and myelodysplasia in patients with a Philadelphia chromosome negative chronic myeloproliferative disorder treated with hydroxyurea alone or with hydroxyurea after busulphan. *Am J Hematol* 74:26, 2003.
109. Hanft VN, Fruchtman SR, Pickens CV, et al: Acquired DNA mutations associated with in vivo hydroxyurea exposure. *Blood* 95:3589, 2000.
110. Solberg LA Jr, Tefferi A, Oles KJ, et al: The effects of anagrelide on human megakaryocytopoiesis. *Br J Haematol* 99:174, 1997.
111. Storen EC, Tefferi A: Long-term use of anagrelide in young patients with essential thrombocythemia. *Blood* 97:863, 2001.
112. Campbell PJ, Green AR: Management of polycythemia vera and essential thrombocythemia. *Hematology* 2005:201, 2005.
113. Gisslinger H, Gotic M, Holowiecki J, et al: Final results of the ANAHYDRET study: Non-inferiority of anagrelide compared to hydroxyurea in newly diagnosed WHO-essential thrombocythemia patients. *ASH Annu Meet Abstr* 112:661, 2008.
114. Kiladjian JJ, Chomienne C, Fenaux P: Interferon-alpha therapy in BCR-ABL-negative myeloproliferative neoplasms. *Leukemia* 22:1990, 2008.
115. Michallet M, Maloisel F, Delain M, et al: Pegylated recombinant interferon alpha-2b vs recombinant interferon alpha-2b for the initial treatment of chronic-phase chronic myelogenous leukemia: A phase III study. *Leukemia* 18:309, 2004.
116. Passamonti F, Rumi E, Malabarba L, et al: Long-term follow-up of young patients with essential thrombocythemia treated with pipobroman. *Ann Hematol* 83:495, 2004.
117. Niittyvuopio R, Juvonen E, Kaaja R, et al: Pregnancy in essential thrombocythaemia: Experience with 40 pregnancies. *Eur J Haematol* 73:431, 2004.
118. Beressi AH, Tefferi A, Silverstein MN, et al: Outcome analysis of 34 pregnancies in women with essential thrombocythemia. *Arch Intern Med* 155:1217, 1995.
119. Wright CA, Tefferi A: A single institutional experience with 43 pregnancies in essential thrombocythemia. *Eur J Haematol* 66:152, 2001.
120. Passamonti F, Randi ML, Rumi E, et al: Increased risk of pregnancy complications in patients with essential thrombocythemia carrying the JAK2 (617V>F) mutation. *Blood* 110:485, 2007.
121. Griesshammer M, Bergmann L, Pearson T: Fertility, pregnancy and the management of myeloproliferative disorders. *Baillieres Clin Haematol* 11:859, 1998.
122. Askie LM, Duley L, Henderson-Smart DJ, Stewart LA: Antiplatelet agents for prevention of pre-eclampsia: A meta-analysis of individual patient data. *Lancet* 369:1791, 2007.
123. Liebelt EL, Balk SJ, Faber W, et al: NTP-CERHR expert panel report on the reproductive and developmental toxicity of hydroxyurea. *Birth Defects Res B Dev Reprod Toxicol* 80:259, 2007.
124. Patel JP, Hunt BJ: Where do we go now with low molecular weight heparin use in obstetric care? *J Thromb Haemost* 6:1461, 2008.
125. Ruggeri M, Rodeghiero F, Tosetto A, et al: Postsurgery outcomes in patients with polycythemia vera and essential thrombocythemia: A retrospective survey. *Blood* 111:666, 2008.
126. Finazzi G, Rambaldi A, Guerini V, et al: Risk of thrombosis in patients with essential thrombocythemia and polycythemia vera according to JAK2 V617F mutation status. *Haematologica* 92:135, 2007.
127. Carobbio A, Antonioli E, Guglielmelli P, et al: Leukocytosis and risk stratification assessment in essential thrombocythemia. *J Clin Oncol* 26:2732, 2008.

CHAPTER 88

MYELODYSPLASTIC SYNDROMES (CLONAL CYTOPENIAS AND OLIGOBLASTIC MYELOGENOUS LEUKEMIA)

Jane L. Liesveld and Marshall A. Lichtman

SUMMARY

In contrast to florid (polyblastic) acute myelogenous leukemia (AML), the myelodysplastic syndrome (MDS) encompasses a group of neoplastic (clonal) myeloid disorders that range from nonprogressive to more slowly progressive than AML. The disorders may appear uncommonly in childhood or young adulthood, especially after cytotoxic therapy for another cancer, but the incidence increases exponentially after age 40 years. The disorders also may develop as a result of inherited syndromes that predispose to MDS or AML, such as Fanconi anemia. Most cases occur between the ages of 50 and 90 years. Cases usually occur *de novo*, but a proportion result from hematopoietic cell injury during treatment of lymphomas or solid tumors with cytotoxic therapy. The disorders range from clonally derived (refractory) anemias to oligoblastic myelogenous leukemia (refractory anemia with excess blasts). The diseases share a propensity to the development of (1) cytopenias, as a result of exaggerated apoptosis of late-stage marrow precursor cells, and (2) multilineage dysmorphogenesis of blood cells. Red cells often have readily discernible poikilocytosis, anisocytosis, anisochromia, and basophilic stippling. The marrow usually contains increased erythroid precursors with dysmorphic features, including nuclear distortions and scanty, poorly hemoglobinized cytoplasm or macroerythroblasts. Ringed sideroblasts are a frequent feature. Neutrophils have anomalies, including bilobed or hypersegmented nuclei and hypogranulated cytoplasm, in association with increased marrow granulocyte precursors. Giant and microcytic platelets, sometimes with abnormal or absent granulation, in the blood are associated with megakaryocytic hyperplasia and atypical lobulation of the nucleus and decreased marrow megakaryocyte size. In the nonprogressive syndromes, anemia may be accompanied by mild variations in other cell counts, usually decreases in neutrophil and platelet levels, and blast cells are not increased in the marrow (<2%). Clonal cytogenetic abnormalities occur in approximately 50 percent of patients. Chromosomes 5, 7, and 8 are most frequently involved. The classic 5q− syndrome is categorized within the myelodysplastic disorders. The syndrome primarily affects older women, and features anemia and hypercellular and dysmorphic erythropoiesis with lobulated erythroblast nuclei and hypolobulated micromegakaryocyte nuclei, but usually normal or elevated platelet counts. It is the most indolent form of the myelodysplastic syndromes with the lowest propensity to evolve into AML. In the more progressive syndromes, leukemic blast cells are increased, cytopenias are more severe, and the disease has high morbidity and mortality from infection and bleeding. Each of the syndromes has a propensity to evolve into polyblastic AML, ranging from approximately 10 to 15 percent in the clonal (refractory) anemia to approximately 40 percent of patients with trilineage cytopenias and increased marrow blast cells. Mortality from infection is a risk in patients with severe neutropenia. Various scoring systems have been developed to help predict outcome and the timing of various treatments. In the most indolent forms, therapy may not be required. Erythropoietin plus granulocyte colony-stimulating factor may improve the anemia or decrease transfusion requirements, if clonal anemia is the principal feature. Cyclosporine or antithymocyte globulin may transiently improve the anemia in patients with clonal anemia, hypoplastic marrows, and low blast counts. Therapy with cytotoxic drugs, red cell or platelet transfusions, and antibiotics may palliate the progressive syndrome (oligoblastic myelogenous leukemia). Lenalidomide and inhibitors of DNA methylation, such as 5-azacytidine or decitabine, have been useful in some patients. Allogeneic stem cell transplantation may be curative in younger patients, and nonmyeloablative stem cell transplantation is being explored in older patients.

Acronyms and abbreviations that appear in this chapter include: ALIP, abnormal localized immature precursors; ALL, acute lymphocytic leukemia; AML, acute myelogenous leukemia; ATG, antithymocyte globulin; ATRA, all-*trans*-retinoic acid; CFU-GM, colony forming unit–granulocyte-monocyte; CI, confidence interval; FISH, fluorescence *in situ* hybridization; G-CSF, granulocyte colony-stimulating factor; GM-CSF, granulocyte-macrophage colony-stimulating factor; IL, interleukin; IPSS, International Prognosis Scoring System; M-CSF, monocyte colony-stimulating factor; MDS, myelodysplastic syndromes; RAEB, refractory anemia with excess blasts; TNF, tumor necrosis factor; WHO, World Health Organization.

DEFINITION

Myelodysplasia is a term used to encompass a spectrum of clonal (neoplastic) myeloid disorders marked by ineffective hematopoiesis (exaggerated marrow cell apoptosis), cytopenias, qualitative disorders of blood cells and their precursors, clonal chromosomal abnormalities, and a variable predilection to undergo clonal evolution to florid acute myelogenous leukemia (AML).[1] The disorders range from relatively indolent clonally derived anemias, with a relatively lower frequency of progression to AML, to more troublesome clonal multilineage cytopenias or to oligoblastic myelogenous leukemias that often progress to overt AML. The somatic mutations leading to these disorders arise in a multipotential hematopoietic cell. *Dysplasia* is a term that classically implies a polyclonal and, therefore, nonneoplastic process. The choice of the term *myelodysplasia* to denote clonal (neoplastic) disorders was unfortunate because the term does not assist students and patients in understanding the relationship of myelodysplasia to other clonal multipotential progenitor stem cell disorders. In addition, diseases such as primary myelofibrosis or paroxysmal nocturnal hemoglobinuria can have the features of "myelodysplasia" but are excluded in its classification. Moreover, drawing diagnostic distinctions among 5, 10, and 20 percent leukemic blast cells is inconsistent with the biologic behavior of cancer and medicine's classification of cancer.[1] Also, separation of clonal anemias into two categories based on whether the anemia has greater than or less than 15 percent pathologic sideroblasts is arbitrary and is not based on the pathobiology of the two variants. The term *myelodysplasia* and its subsidiary syndromes, for example, refractory anemia, are, however, widely used and deeply ensconced in the medical lexicon.[2]

The term *clonal cytopenias* refers to (1) neoplasms arising in a multipotential hematopoietic marrow cell that result in diseases with no discernible leukemic blast cells in the marrow or blood (e.g., refractory anemias or refractory multicytopenias) and (2) *oligoblastic myelogenous leukemia* (refractory anemia with excess blasts [RAEB] in which an increased proportion of (leukemic) blast cells is present in the marrow but in which, untreated, the course is smoldering or subacute compared to AML.[3]

The boundary between clonal anemia and oligoblastic myelogenous leukemia may be indistinct because of the insensitivity of the marrow examination; however, continued observation clarifies the situation. If leukemic myeloblasts are evident in marrow, the diagnosis of oligoblastic myelogenous leukemia can be made, maintaining the principle that the histopathologic diagnosis depends on the presence or absence of tumor cells and not the rate of progression or severity of the manifestations of the malignancy. The proportion of marrow myeloblasts is not increased in reactive states, for example, granulocytic hyperplasia as a result of infection, noninfectious inflammation, solid tumors, and drug-induced granulocytosis (e.g., glucocorticoids, lithium). The proportion of blasts usually is less than the normal value of 1.0 ± 0.4 SD percent. A finding of greater than 2.0 percent myeloblasts in a normal marrow is rare in healthy older children and adults. Higher proportions, for example, greater than 2 percent, are confined to cases of oligoblastic myelogenous leukemia. Some patients treated with granulocytic growth factors may have a slight transient increase in blast cells.

Clonal proliferation of multipotential hemopoietic cells in this group of disorders is accompanied by variable effects on all blood cell lineages and usually is associated with pathologically enhanced apoptosis of marrow precursor cells such that leukopenia and thrombocytopenia of varying severity often accompany the anemia. Qualitative abnormalities of cell shape, organelle structure, biochemical pathways, and function can occur in each lineage. The range of clinical expression is broad. Thus, clonal cytopenias can occur with isolated anemia and a nearly normal-appearing marrow, or with severe pancytopenia, profoundly hypercellular marrow, and alterations in blood cell shape, size, and function. The more profound the disorder, the more likely the finding of oligoblastic leukemia on marrow examination.

HISTORY

At the beginning of the 20th century, reports of highly morbid cytopenic disorders that were refractory to treatment began to appear in the medical literature.[4] In 1942, Chevallier and colleagues[5] discussed formally the "odo-leukemias." They chose the Greek word *odo*, meaning threshold, to highlight disorders on the threshold of leukemia. Chevallier proposed *leucoses* as the generic term for the leukemias so that marked variations in white cell counts and other highly variable presenting features would not engender inappropriate terminology. His proposal was sage but neglected.

In 1949, Hamilton-Paterson[6] used the term *preleukemic anemia* to describe patients with refractory anemia antecedent to AML development. In 1953, Block and coworkers[7] expanded the concept to include cytopenias of all lineages and described cases that closely fit with our current concepts of a clonal myeloid hemopathy prior to evolution to overt AML. By mid-20th century, the relationship of acquired idiopathic cytopenias to the subsequent onset of AML had become broadly appreciated.[8–15] Terms such as *herald state of leukemia, refractory anemia, sideroachrestic anemia, idiopathic refractory sideroblastic anemia, pancytopenia with hyperplastic marrow*, and others were coined to describe the various manifestations of the hematopoietic derangement that preceded the onset of florid AML. In the late 1960s numerous reports discussing "refractory anemia," "refractory sideroblastic anemia," and "preleukemia" appeared that described cases we now consider "myelodysplastic" syndromes. In 1970, the designation "les anémies réfractaires avec excès de myeloblasts" was proposed,[3] and in 1976 a preliminary classification of these syndromes was discussed by Dreyfus in which refractory anemia with an excess of myeloblasts was amplified, parenthetically, as smoldering acute leukemia.[13] The synonym, *oligoblastic leukemia*, had been used also to describe those cases with low proportions of leukemic myeloblasts and relatively protracted courses.[16,17]

In 1976, at a conference held in Paris, Marcel Bessis and Jean Bernard used the term *hematopoietic dysplasia*, later shortened to *myelodysplasia*, for the group of disorders having a more indolent course than AML.[18] The concept that neoplasia is a tissue abnormality defined by its origin in the mutation(s) within a single cell (monoclonality) and that dysplasia is a polyclonal tissue change, not neoplasia, was ignored and took a back seat to the participants' primary interest in the dysmorphia of cells that characterized most of these syndromes, hence the application of the term *dysplasia*, which has become entrenched.

CLASSIFICATION

The World Health Organization (WHO) classification designates six categories in the spectrum of the myelodysplastic syndromes (MDSs): (1) refractory cytopenia with unilineage dysplasia, (2) refractory anemia with ringed sideroblasts, (3) refractory cytopenia with multilineage dysplasia, (4) refractory anemia with excess blasts (type 1 with less than 10 percent blasts in the marrow and type 2 with 10 to 19 percent blasts in the marrow), (5) myelodysplastic syndrome, unclassified, and (6) isolated 5q− abnormality (Table 88–1).[19] MDSs include entities that have marrow blast percentages ranging from a mean of less than 2 percent in refractory anemia to a mean of approximately 10 percent and upper limit of 19 percent in RAEB.[20] The distinction between refractory anemia in which less than 15 percent of nucleated red cells in marrow are ringed sideroblasts and refractory anemia with ringed sideroblasts in which greater than 15 percent of nucleated red cells are ringed sideroblasts uses the same arbitrary boundary as does classifying a patient as having RAEB if less than 20 percent of nucleated marrow cells are blasts or as having AML if greater than 19 percent of nucleated marrow cells

TABLE 88–1. Classification of the Myelodysplastic Syndromes (Clonal Cytopenias and Oligoblastic Leukemia)

1. Clonal (refractory) anemia (with pathologic sideroblasts).*
2. Clonal bicytopenia or tricytopenia (overt multilineage dysmorphic cytopenias).
3. Oligoblastic myelogenous leukemia (refractory anemia with excess myeloblasts).
4. Apparent clonal myeloid disease that does not fit in any category shown above (e.g., chronic clonal monocytosis; isolated thrombocytopenia or isolated neutropenia, only if clonal)[19,20] Clonal isolated neutropenia or thrombocytopenia are rare occurrences as initial manifestations of a clonal myeloid disease and their inclusion by the WHO is arguable. Nonclonal diseases should not be in this category.
5. Classical 5q− syndrome.

*The WHO classification distinguishes refractory "nonsideroblastic" from sideroblastic anemia based on whether the case has ≥15% or <15% pathologic sideroblasts in marrow erythroid cells. No basis exists for distinguishing the anemia based on proportion of pathologic sideroblasts because most patients with clonal anemia have pathologic sideroblasts, and the manifestations and course of the disease are virtually identical in patients with a high or low prevalence of pathologic sideroblasts. Given the relatively crude nature of quantification of pathologic sideroblasts and the biologic illegitimacy of such distinctions in any case, it is unjustified to consider them two different diagnostic categories. Indeed, recent survival studies have collapsed the two groups into one category.[275]

NOTE: Other acute and chronic clonal myeloid diseases are categorized in Table 85–1.

are myeloblasts. This approach to categorization is unfortunate because in no other neoplasm is the designation of the cancer, in this case myelogenous leukemia, which all such patients have, called by another name when a greater or fewer number of tumor cells are present.

Several laboratories that explored the use of flow cytometry in the classification of these heterogenous disorders have found it to be of limited value or largely confirmatory of the findings on blood film and marrow examination.[20,21]

Clonal (refractory) cytopenia or oligoblastic myelogenous leukemia arising *de novo* in children is very infrequent. These syndromes may occur somewhat more frequently after radiation or chemotherapeutic treatment of children with other cancers. Although some pediatric oncologists have included juvenile myelomonocytic leukemia and chronic myelomonocytic leukemia in children among the myelodysplastic syndromes, they stand alone and are discussed in Chap. 90 with the chronic myelogenous leukemias.

EPIDEMIOLOGY

INCIDENCE BY AGE, SEX, AND OCCUPATION

Disease onset before age 50 years is uncommon except in cases preceded by irradiation or chemotherapy given for another malignancy.[22–25] MDS, as defined by the WHO classification, occurs in children ages 5 months to 15 years at a rate of approximately 1 per 1 million children per year. In contrast to adults, most pediatric cases are oligoblastic myelogenous leukemia (RAEB); clonal sideroblastic anemia is rare.[26–29] A proportion of childhood cases evolve from inherited predisposing diseases, such as Down syndrome and Fanconi anemia. The annual incidence of MDS increases logarithmically after age 40 years from about 2 per 1 million persons to more than 40 per 100,000 persons in septuagenarians (see Fig. 88–1).[24] In the United States, the annual incidence is approximately equivalent to that of annual new cases of AML.[30] Reporting of clonal anemia and other low-risk MDSs is inadequate and, thus, population age-adjusted incidence estimates of MDS (~3/100,000 population) are underestimates.[31] Males are affected approximately 1.5 times as often as females. Case-control studies of possible occupational or environmental associations have provided many possible candidates as contributors to MDS, but none other than benzene (exposure of ≥40 parts per million [ppm]-years) has reached a level of scientific validity.[32,33]

ETIOLOGY AND PATHOGENESIS

ETIOLOGY

Not unexpectedly, the etiologic factors that increase the incidence of MDS are similar to the factors affecting the incidence of AML. Exposure to prolonged, high levels of benzene,[34,35] chemotherapeutic agents, particularly alkylating agents and topoisomerase inhibitors,[36–43] and radiation[44,45] increase the risk of these clonal hemopathies. These agents may cause DNA damage, impair DNA repair enzymes, and induce loss of chromosome integrity. Most cases of secondary or posttreatment MDS occur in patients treated for a lymphoma or a solid tumor. Increasing reports of MDS as a complication of treatment of myeloid diseases, such as acute

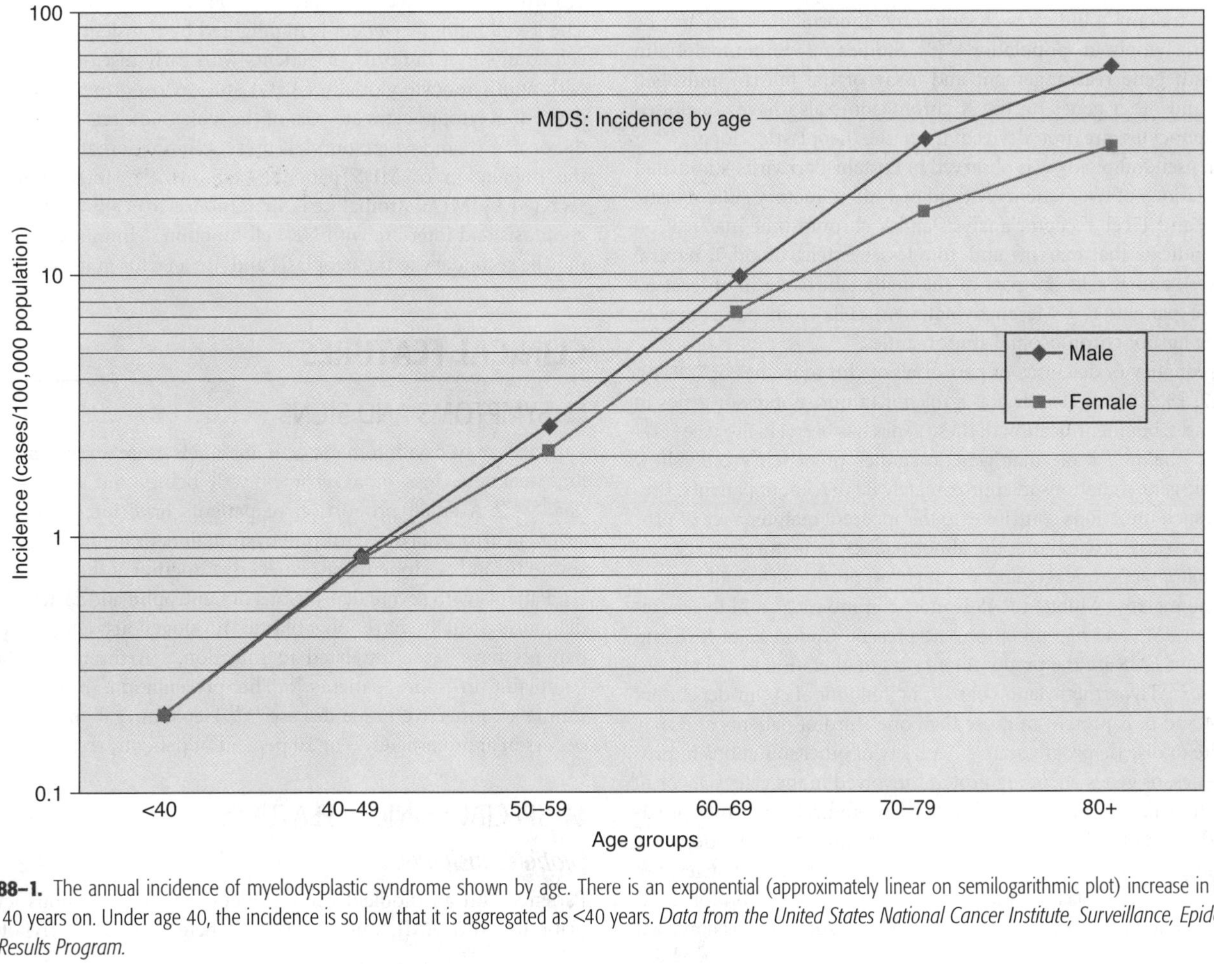

FIGURE 88–1. The annual incidence of myelodysplastic syndrome shown by age. There is an exponential (approximately linear on semilogarithmic plot) increase in incidence from age 40 years on. Under age 40, the incidence is so low that it is aggregated as <40 years. *Data from the United States National Cancer Institute, Surveillance, Epidemiology, and End-Results Program.*

promyelocytic leukemia, reflect a second clonal myeloid disease from another primitive hematopoietic cell injured during therapy.[43] The increased life span of patients with acute promyelocytic leukemia after effective therapy may make this event more common.

Inherited diseases, such as Fanconi anemia, known to predispose to AML development occasionally evolve instead into a clonal myeloid hemopathy.[46] In addition, as is the case in all hematologic malignancies,[47] familial myelodysplasia occurs rarely as a result of as-yet undefined germ-line susceptibility genes.[48–50]

Acquired copper deficiency, especially after gastric bypass surgery, intestinal surgery, parenteral nutrition, and sometimes without an evident cause may result in a reversible low-risk MDS picture with anemia, neutropenia, sometimes thrombocytopenia, and marrow dysplasia, including ringed sideroblasts. Neurologic changes mimicking subacute combined degeneration may also occur.[51,52]

PATHOGENESIS

These disorders arise from the clonal expansion of a multipotential hematopoietic cell. The clonal origin is supported by studies of women who were heterozygotes for glucose-6-phosphate dehydrogenase isoenzymes A and B and who had such a syndrome. The hematopoietic progenitors,[53,54] and in some cases B lymphocytes,[55] of such patients had only one isoenzyme present, supporting the concept of clonal expansion of a neoplastic marrow cell. Clonal studies using X-linked restriction fragment length polymorphisms with probes for hypoxanthine phosphoribosyl transferase or phosphoglycerate kinase also supported the origin of these disorders from a single multipotential stem cell.[56–58]

Fluorescence *in situ* hybridization (FISH) of interphase blood cell populations with probes for chromosome 7 or 8 in patients with monosomy 7 or trisomy 8 indicates chromosome abnormalities may not be present in lymphoid populations.[58,59] Studies of immunoglobulin heavy-chain gene rearrangement and assay of the human androgen receptor and other genes on the X chromosome also have concluded that lymphocytes are not derived from the neoplastic clone.[57,60–62] However, pseudodiploidy was observed in Epstein-Barr virus-stimulated cell populations of two patients with idiopathic refractory sideroblastic anemia[63]; and T-cell receptor analysis and X chromosome inactivation analysis indicate that marrow and, to a lesser extent, blood T, natural killer (NK), and B cells are part of the malignant clone in at least 50 percent of patients.[64,65] Mesenchymal stem cells from patients with MDS may harbor chromosomal abnormalities.[66]

The frequency of deletions of part or all of chromosomes 5, 7, 9, 11, 12, 13, 17, 18, 20, and 21 indicates a role for tumor suppressor genes in disease onset, but identification of these genes has been elusive (see "5q– Syndrome" below). Molecular genetic studies of patient's cells show identifiable gene mutations in approximately 60 percent of patients. Presumably, such mutations contribute to the apparent maintenance of proliferation of early progenitors, the abnormalities in maturation seen in each hematopoietic lineage, and the high proportional loss of mature cells in the marrow. Mutated *RAS* is most common,[67–71] and lower frequencies of *FMS* and *p53* mutations are present. Codon 12 of *RAS* and codon 969 of *FMS* are the predominant sites of alteration in the respective genes.[72,73] Hypermethylation of p15, an inhibitor of cyclin-dependent kinases 4 and 6, is present in more than one-third of patients and may contribute to disease progression.[74] A variety of other mutations in protooncogenes, or genes encoding proteins involved in the cell cycle, or of transcription factors have been described sporadically.[72,73] Interpretation of these molecular studies is difficult because the mutations are present in patients with advanced disease and may be late changes, not seminal in the neoplastic transformation. Overexpression of DLK (delta-like) and GATA-1 and GATA-2 have been suggested as a marker for MDS in the former case and as contributing to the maturation abnormalities in the case of the latter two genes.[75,76] The role of mutations in mitochondrial DNA in the cells of older persons and in the hematopoietic cells of patients with MDS and AML has not been integrated into the pathogenesis of the disease.[77]

The major specific pathophysiologic mechanism in MDS is ineffective hematopoiesis, that is, defective maturation and death of marrow precursor cells.[78–80] The specific characteristics of ineffective erythropoiesis and granulopoiesis include a decreased proportion of cells in the DNA synthesis phase of the mitotic cycle and a marked increase in the fraction of late precursor cells undergoing apoptosis.[81] Increased levels of apoptotic mediators are present in cells, including tumor necrosis factor (TNF)-α, FAS antigen (CD95), and calcium-dependent nuclease activity.[82–84] Stepwise degradation of DNA, which is characteristic of apoptosis, is evident in late precursors.[82–84] The apoptosis of erythroid precursors may involve BCL-2 related proteins in the endoplasmic reticulum upstream of the mitochondria, and downstream of FAS. Erythropoietin may protect against FAS-induced apoptosis.[85] The proliferation of progenitor and early precursor cells usually is normal or enhanced, resulting in a hypercellular marrow, but failure to accumulate adequate numbers of mature cells has been observed. Mild shortening of cell life span also contributes to the cytopenias.

Immune dysregulation involving B and T lymphocytes in MDS has been described. CD40 expression on monocytes is increased, as is CD40L on T lymphocytes, and has been postulated as being a contributing factor to hematopoietic failure in some patients with less-advanced disease.[86] Heightened apoptosis of marrow B lymphocytes is a feature of the disease.[87] Depletion of autologous T lymphocytes in cultures of the marrow of patients with early MDS (clonal anemia) results in improved growth of marrow cells, apparently from residual normal stem cells.[88] The T-cell inhibitory effect is highlighted by transient improvement in cell counts in a minority of patients with early disease after treatment with antithymocyte globulin (ATG) and cyclosporine.[89] However, evidence that lymphocytes are part of the leukemic clone has been contradictory,[60,89,90] and when found, is present in no more than 50 percent of the population of MDS patients examined.[64,65] Interleukin (IL)-32, secreted by MDS stromal cells in response to TNF-α may modulate apoptosis and interfere with NK cell function.[91] Immune dysregulation may be secondary to the neoplasia and not a factor in its origin.[92]

CLINICAL FEATURES

SYMPTOMS AND SIGNS

Patients can be asymptomatic or, if anemia is more severe, can have pallor, weakness, loss of a sense of well being, and exertional dyspnea.[14,93,94] A small proportion of patients have infections related to severe neutropenia or neutrophil dysfunction, or hemorrhage related to severe thrombocytopenia or platelet dysfunction at the time of diagnosis. Patients with severe depressions of neutrophil and platelet counts at diagnosis usually have oligoblastic myelogenous leukemia. Rarely, patients have fever unrelated to infection.[95] Arthralgia is the initial complaint in some patients.[84] The presentation, infrequently, can mimic a connective tissue disease.[96,97] Hepatomegaly or splenomegaly occurs in approximately 5 or 10 percent of patients, respectively.

SPECIAL CLINICAL FEATURES

Diabetes Insipidus

Patients with an indolent phase (oligoblastic myelogenous leukemia) prior to overt AML may develop diabetes insipidus. Hypothalamic involvement can lead to polyuria, polydipsia, and decreased libido. Hypothalamic-posterior hypophysis insufficiency in clonal myeloid states is associated with monosomy 7 in hematopoietic cells.[98,99] Hypodipsia can occur with extensive hypothalamic involvement. The syndrome lacks the signs of thirst, polyuria, and polydipsia because signals transmitted by the thirst center to the cerebral cortex are blocked.[99]

Neutrophilic Dermatosis

Acute neutrophilic dermatosis (Sweet disease) is an acute febrile illness characterized by erythematous patches on the arms, face, and legs that progress to painful brown plaques. The plaques may ulcerate and produce large necrotizing skin lesions. The histopathology of the skin is that of a dense dermal neutrophilic infiltrate.[100,101] The syndrome, which occurs principally in middle-aged women, lasts for 6 to 10 weeks, often is associated with blood neutrophilia, and may recur. At least 10 percent of patients with Sweet disease develop AML or another clonal myeloid disease. Occasional cases have been associated with monocytosis or cytogenic abnormalities in marrow cells prior to AML onset. Granulocyte colony-stimulating factor (G-CSF) and all *trans*-retinoic acid (ATRA) administration has been followed by Sweet disease in some cases.[101] Other dermatopathic conditions also have been associated with clonal myeloid diseases.[102]

Inflammatory Syndromes

Immune or inflammatory syndromes may be seen in as many as 10 percent of patients. A symptom complex that mimics systemic lupus erythematosus; fever, pleurisy, symmetric arthritis, plasma antinuclear antibody, and pancytopenia with a hyperplastic marrow) may precede AML.[96] Several patients with signs of systemic lupus erythematosus and the lupus erythematosus cell phenomenon were reported in a review of the clonal myeloid syndromes.[96,103] Behçet disease, glomerulonephritis, seronegative arthritis, systemic vasculitis, polychondritis, polyneuropathy, panniculitis, and inflammatory bowel disease also have been associated with clonal myeloid disorders.[96,97,104–109]

Other Cancers

The incidence of other cancers may be higher in subjects with myelodysplastic diseases.[110–112]

LABORATORY FEATURES

■ BLOOD

Red Cells

Anemia is present in greater than 85 percent of patients.[14,93,94] In approximately 4 percent of patients, the anemia results from erythroid aplasia.[113] Mean cell volume often is increased. Red cell shape abnormalities include oval, elliptical, teardrop, spherical, and fragmented cells. Red cell findings occur in a spectrum. Some patients have only slight anisocytosis. Elliptical red cells sometimes dominate. Basophilic stippling of red cells occurs (Fig. 88–2). Nucleated red cells are seen in the blood film in approximately 10 percent of cases. Reticulocyte counts usually are low for the degree of anemia. Other abnormalities of red cells occur, such as an increased proportion of hemoglobin F[114] and decreased red cell enzyme activities, especially acquired pyruvate kinase deficiency.[115] Hemolysis has occurred in some patients with the latter deficiency. Enhanced sensitivity of membranes to complement[116] and modification of red cell blood group antigens may be observed.[117] Acquired hemoglobin H disease, a rare superimposition, results in red cell morphology similar to thalassemia (microcytosis, anisocytosis, basophilic stippling, poikilocytosis with target cells, fragmented cells, and tear-drop cells). Intracellular precipitates of β-chain tetramers (identified by crystal violet stain) reflect an acquired decrease in the rate of α-chain synthesis in erythroblasts.[118–120] The decrease in α-globin–chain synthesis is profound, involves each of the four α-chain loci, and results from a transcription abnormality. No gross alterations in genes (e.g., insertions, deletions) are seen in these cases.[118] Acquired hemoglobin H disease in this setting has been dubbed the α-thalassemia–myelodysplastic syndrome and is the consequence of acquired mutations in ATRX, the gene associated with the X-linked alpha-thalassemia/mental retardation (ATR-X) syndrome.[120]

Granulocytes and Monocytes

Neutropenia is present in approximately 50 percent of patients at the time of diagnosis.[121] The proportion of monocytes often is increased, and monocytosis per se can be the dominant manifestation of the hematopoietic abnormality for months or years.[122–124] Morphologic abnormalities of neutrophils can occur, sometimes resulting in the acquired Pelger-Huët anomaly (see Fig. 88–2E). In this condition, neutrophils have very condensed chromatin and unilobed or bilobed nuclei that often have a pince-nez shape. The neutrophils may be in the process of apoptosis.[125] Ring-shaped nuclei also can occur in neutrophils (see Fig. 88–2F).[126] Neutrophil alkaline phosphatase activity is decreased in some patients.[14] Expression of normal surface antigens on neutrophils and monocytes is decreased, and abnormal surface antigen expression occurs in some cases.[127] Defective primary granules of abnormal size and shape with decreased myeloperoxidase content can be present.[128] Specific neutrophil granules can be decreased in number, producing hypogranular cells.[129] Neutrophil granule membranes frequently are deficient in glycoprotein.[130] Chemotactic, phagocytic, and bactericidal capability may be impaired.[131–133] Formylleucyl-methionyl-phenylamine receptor signaling and actin polymerization can be abnormal.[134,135] Muramidase (lysozyme) activity in blood and urine may be increased, reflecting granulocytic hyperplasia, heightened monocytopoiesis, and monocyte turnover.

Platelets

Approximately 25 to 50 percent of patients have mild to moderate thrombocytopenia at the time of diagnosis.[14,121] Mild thrombocytosis also can occur.[14,121] Platelets may be abnormally large, have poor granulation, or have large, fused central granules (see Fig. 88–2H).[136,137] Abnormal platelet function can contribute to a prolonged bleeding time, easy bruising, or exaggerated bleeding. Decreased platelet aggregation in response to collagen or epinephrine is a frequent functional abnormality.[138]

Lymphocytes

Patients with clonal hemopathies may have immunologic deficiencies, such as a decrease in natural killer cells in the blood but no decrease in large granular lymphocytes,[139–142] a decrease in helper T lymphocytes,[140] and a decrease in Epstein-Barr virus receptors on B lymphocytes.[140–143] Antibody-dependent cellular cytotoxicity is normal.[140] Thymidine incorporation after mitogenic stimulation[144,145] and colony growth of T lymphocytes are decreased.[140] Lymphocytes may have an increased sensitivity to irradiation.[144] The defects in lymphoid cells could reflect the level of the somatic mutation in a primitive multipotential cell in different cases. Intrinsic, rather than secondary, alterations in lymphocytes are determined by whether no lymphocytes are generated from the clone, B cells are part of the clone, or B and T cells are part of the clone.[63] Clonally derived, CD8+CD57+CD244+CD28−CD62L− T lymphocytes are present in marrow and to a lesser extent in blood in approximately 50 percent of patients, independent of type of

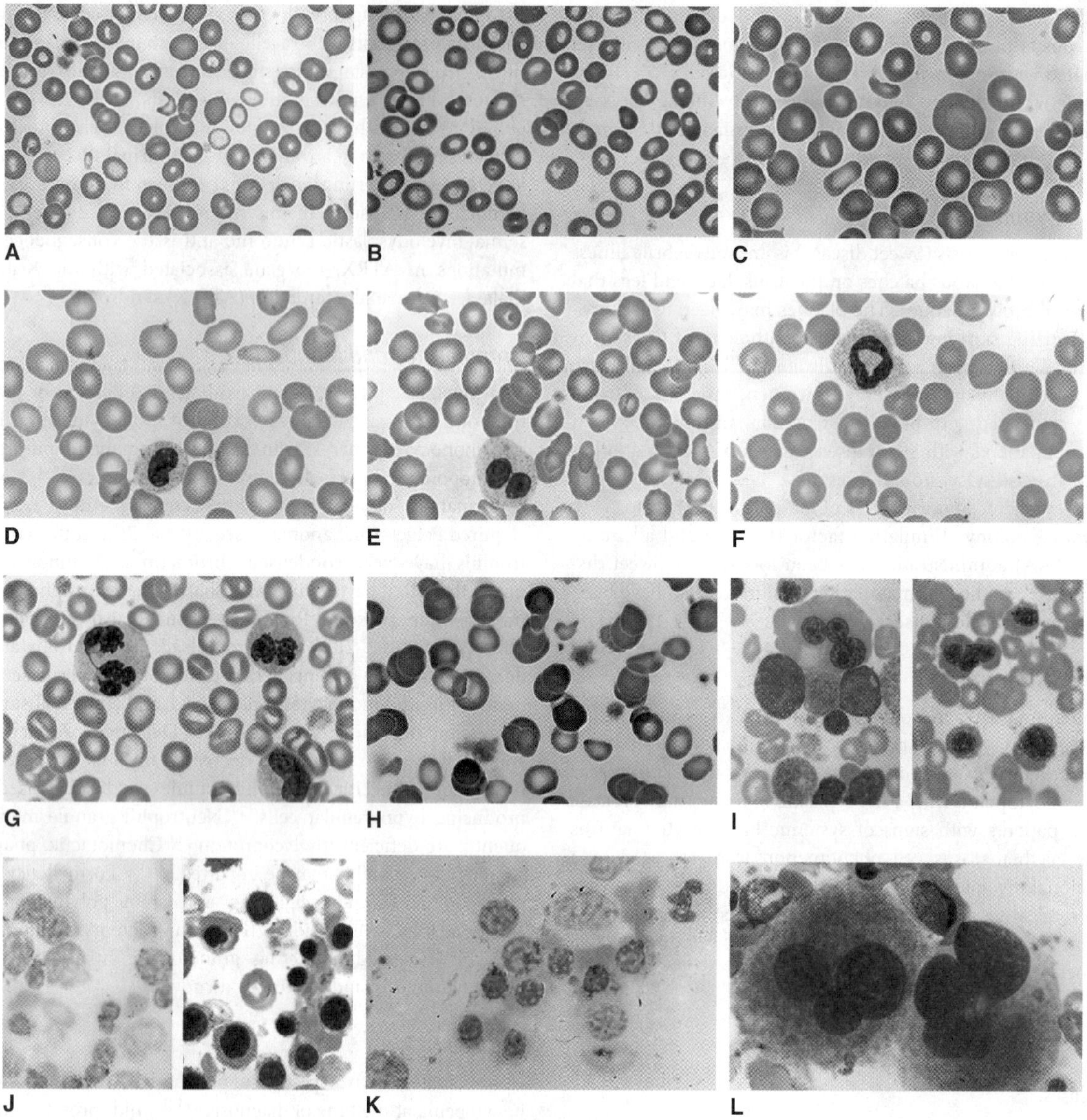

FIGURE 88–2. Blood and marrow films from patients with clonal cytopenias (MDS). **A.** Blood film. Anisocytosis. Poikilocytosis with occasional fragmented cells. Marked anisochromia with marked hypochromia, mild hypochromia and normochromic cells. **B.** Blood film. Marked anisocytosis. Mild anisochromia. Poikilocytes with occasional fragmented cells and oval and elliptical cells. Two polychromatophilic macrocytes. **C.** Blood film. Striking anisocytosis with giant macrocytes and microcytes. Poikilocytes with tiny red cell fragment and elliptocyte. **D.** Blood film. Mild anisocytosis. Ovalocytes and elliptocytes. Dacryocyte. Hyposegmented neutrophil with poor granulation. **E.** Blood film. Marked anisocytosis (macrocytes and microcytes). Ovalocytes and elliptocytes. Acquired Pelger-Hüet nuclear anomaly (classic pince-nez shape) in neutrophil. **F.** Blood film. Mild anisocytosis. Abnormal neutrophil with ring nucleus. **G.** Blood film. Anisochromia. Stomatocytes. Abnormal neutrophil nuclei with hyperlobulation and hyperchromatic staining. Note abnormal elongated nuclear bridge in neutrophil on left. **H.** Blood film. Atypical platelets. Two macrothrombocytes with excess cytoplasm and atypical central granules. Anisocytosis (conspicuous microcytes). Anisochromia (conspicuous hypochromic cells). Poikilocytosis with occasional fragmented red cells. **I.** Marrow film. Wright stain. Trilobed megakaryocyte. Wright stain. Macroerythroblasts. **J.** Marrow films. Prussian blue stain. Ringed sideroblasts. Wright stain. Erythroid hyperplasia with macroerythroblasts. **K.** Marrow film. Prussian blue stain. Ringed sideroblasts. **L.** Marrow film. Wright stain. Trilobed megakaryocytes. *(Used with permission from* Lichtman's Atlas of Hematology, *www.accessmedicine.com.)*

myelodysplastic syndrome, age, and sex of the patient,[64,65] as are NK and B cells (see "Pathogenesis" above).[65]

PLASMA ABNORMALITIES

Serum iron, transferrin, and ferritin levels may be elevated as a result of anemia and the shift of erythron iron to plasma and storage compartments. Lactic dehydrogenase and uric acid concentrations can be increased as a result of ineffective hematopoiesis and a high death fraction of maturing marrow precursors. Monoclonal gammopathy, polyclonal hypergammaglobulinemia, and hypogammaglobulinemia each occur with increased frequency.[146,147] The frequency of autoantibodies was increased in one report[133] but not in another.[146] β_2-Microglobulin serum levels are increased in proportion to the prognostic category of the disease.[148]

MARROW

Magnetic Resonance Imaging

Although rarely used clinically, magnetic resonance imaging scans of human femoral marrow correlate with disease severity. Approximately 85 percent of patients with refractory anemia have images consistent with fatty marrow, whereas approximately 85 percent of patients with oligoblastic leukemia have images showing marrow fat replaced by abnormal hematopoietic tissue.[149]

Cellularity

Marrow cellularity usually is normal or increased.[14,150,151] Cellularity is decreased in approximately 15 percent of cases[151] and may simulate hypoplastic or aplastic anemia.[152] However, islands of dysmorphic cells, especially atypical megakaryocytes, usually are present (see Fig. 88–2L). An increased proportion of blast cells in this setting suggests hypoplastic myelogenous leukemia (see Chap. 89).

Erythropoiesis

Erythroid hyperplasia is frequent. Very large or small erythroblasts, nuclear fragmentation, stippled erythroblasts, and poor hemoglobinization may be seen.[14,150,151] Proerythroblasts may be present in excess, and the marrow may lack normal clusters or islets of erythroblasts. Erythroblasts may resemble megaloblasts that have nuclear-cytoplasmic maturation asynchrony, nuclear fragmentation, or cytoplasmic nuclear remnants. The asynchrony is manifest morphologically by nuclear immaturity with prominent euchromatin in cells with more advanced cytoplasmic maturation. This pattern is referred to as *megaloblastoid erythropoiesis* (see Fig. 88–2I). Erythroid aplasia seen in occasional cases results in a hypocellular marrow.[113]

Pathologic sideroblasts may be identified when the marrow is stained with Prussian blue stain (see Fig. 88–2J and 2K). The sideroblasts include erythroblasts with an increased number and size of siderosomes (cytoplasmic ferritin-containing vacuoles), referred to as *intermediate sideroblasts*, or erythroblasts with mitochondrial iron aggregates that take the form of a partial or complete circumnuclear ring of iron globules, referred to as *ringed sideroblasts*. Macrophage iron often is increased. Ringed sideroblasts are uncommon or present only in very low proportions in clonal myeloid disorders other than refractory anemia.

Granulopoiesis

Granulocytic hyperplasia is frequent.[14,121,150,151] Marrow monocytes may be increased in number. Abnormalities of granulocytes include hypogranulation, a monocytoid appearance of neutrophilic granulocytes, and the acquired Pelger-Huët nuclear abnormality of neutrophils.[125,153] Progranulocytes and myelocytes may be increased. The proportion of blast cells is not increased in clonal hemopathies that are categorized as refractory anemia (i.e., <2%); a blast percentage of greater than 2 percent can be considered oligoblastic leukemia. Marrow biopsy may show abnormal localized immature precursors (ALIP),[154,155] which are clusters of immature myeloid, CD34+ cells[156] located centrally rather than subjacent to the endosteum. These clusters of atypical cells are present in almost all cases of oligoblastic leukemia where blast cells compose 3 percent or more of nucleated marrow cells (RAEB) and in approximately one-third of patients with refractory anemia, suggesting these patients have a disorder closely approaching oligoblastic leukemia. Patients with this abnormality are more prone to develop overt AML. Vascular endothelial growth factor and its receptor are expressed on cells forming ALIP clusters and has been proposed as providing an autocrine loop to promote leukemia progenitor cell formation.[157] The number of plasma cells may be slightly increased. Marrow basophilia or eosinophilia occurs in approximately 1 in 7 patients and is associated with a higher probability of evolution to AML.[158]

Thrombopoiesis

Megakaryocytes are present in normal or increased numbers.[14,150,151] Micromegakaryocytes (dwarf megakaryocytes) may occur.[150,159,160] Megakaryocytes with unilobed or bilobed nuclei may be increased, and hypersegmented and hyposegmented megakaryocytes may be present (see Fig. 88–2L). Clusters of megakaryocytes may be seen. Megakaryocytes may be distributed laterally from their usual parasinusoidal location.[161]

Fibrosis and Angiogenesis

An increase in reticulin and collagen fibers of varying degree is common (approximately 15% of cases), especially in oligoblastic myelogenous leukemia.[156] When fibrosis is prominent, the disorder can resemble primary myelofibrosis, although, in contrast to the latter, splenomegaly usually is not marked. Because primary myelofibrosis is an oligoblastic leukemia with striking dysmorphogenesis of cells, some confusion in classification with other fibrotic clonal myeloid disorders may occur.[162] Marrow fibrosis is correlated with higher blast counts and poor-risk cytogenetics.[156] Some physicians have proposed a category of myelofibrotic myelodysplasia, but all clonal myeloid diseases, including AML, chronic myelogenous leukemia, and chronic myelomonocytic leukemia may have within their spectrum of expression occasional cases with intense myelofibrosis. Like numerous other epiphenomena that occur in the expression of hematopoietic stem cell diseases, extending the general classifications is not warranted.

Increased angiogenesis is a feature of MDS. Microvessel density increases with more advanced stages of the disease.[163] Mast cell frequency and mast cell tryptase activity are highly correlated with microvessel density.[164] Circulating endothelial cells are also increased in concentration in patients with MDS and their concentration is correlated with marrow neoangiogenesis (microvessel density).[165]

Cell Culture

Clonal growth of marrow progenitors in soft agar or other viscous culture systems usually is abnormal in patients with clonal hemopathies.[166] Most reports indicate growth of multipotential (colony-forming unit–granulocyte-erythrocyte-monocyte-megakaryocyte) and erythroid progenitors (burst forming unit–erythroid, colony forming unit–erythroid) in the blood or marrow is markedly decreased in subjects with clonal myeloid disorders.[166–169] Biochemical abnormalities of erythroid precursors also have been found. Colony-forming units for granulocytes and monocytes (CFU-GM) are decreased.[166,167] Very small colonies or clusters with impaired maturation often dominate the cultures. Abnormally small and infrequent CFU-GM may be found when blood neutrophil and monocyte counts are nearly normal. Occasionally, overabundant growth is present. Usually, cell culture results become more abnormal as the blood cell abnormalities in the patient worsen.

In overt AML, CFU-GM colony growth usually is absent. Some studies indicate very abnormal growth of progenitors in culture (decreased colonies or predominance of small clusters) is a poor prognostic sign and may be a harbinger of overt leukemia.[170,171] Growth occurring in clonal myeloid hemopathies (and AML) usually remains dependent on growth factors such as erythropoietin and granulocyte-macrophage colony-stimulating factor (GM-CSF).[172] Colony growth in children with the monosomy 7 syndrome may occur without added growth factors, supporting the view of autocrine and paracrine stimulation of progenitor cells.[173–176] Colony-forming unit–blast cell progenitors may be increased in patients with oligoblastic leukemia.[169] The long-term marrow initiating cell is decreased in some patients,[175,176] and the ability of marrow stromal layers to support *in vitro* hematopoiesis can be impaired.[177]

Circulating monocyte colony-stimulating factor (M-CSF) is increased in some patients with MDS, AML, and other hematologic malignancies.[178] IL-1α and GM-CSF levels have been undetectable in most patients. IL-6, G-CSF, and erythropoietin concentrations have been variable. TNF has been inversely related to hematocrit.[179] Stem cell factor, a multilineage hematopoietin, has been decreased in some patients.[180] The FLT-3 ligand, another multilineage growth factor, is increased in patients with indolent clonal hemopathies but not oligoblastic leukemia.[181] The inverse relationship between platelet count and thrombopoietin levels is maintained in clonal anemia but not oligoblastic leukemia.[182]

Cytogenetics

An altered number or form of chromosomes occur in approximately 50 percent of patients with clonal hemopathies, depending on the severity of the syndrome.[183–185] The chromosome abnormalities are nonrandom and often involve chromosomes that are abnormal in patients with AML, although certain chromosomal rearrangements seen in AML, such as t(15;17), t(8;21), and inv16, only are seen rarely (see Chap. 11).[186–188]

Chromosomal abnormalities involving virtually every chromosome have been noted in marrow cells, and approximately 60 percent of chromosomal abnormalities are very uncommon, occurring in less than 2 percent of patients in large series.[168–170] The most common abnormalities are 5q−, -7/7q−, +8, −18/18q−,and 20q−. Losses of part or all of chromosomes 5 and 7 and complex chromosome aberrations are particularly common in the oligoblastic myelogenous leukemias associated with prior treatment with cytotoxic drugs, radiation, or a high exposure to benzene.[32,42,185,189] In this circumstance, the deletion in 5q is at band 5q31.1, in distinction to the classic 5q− syndrome (see "5q− Syndrome" below) in which the deletions occur at band q32–33.3. The Philadelphia (Ph) chromosome t(9;22) and a variety of other chromosome abnormalities not characteristically seen in MDS have been described on rare occasion.[190]

Categories of cytogenetic abnormalities correlated with median survival have been determined. The more favorable risk category (survival longer than 3 years) includes a normal karyotype and isolated deletions of 5q32–33.3, 20q, or loss of the Y chromosome. Loss of the Y chromosome is an age-dependent variable, usually evident in a proportion of cell metaphases in older men. Only an absence of the Y chromosome in all metaphases is indicative of a clonal myeloid disorder.[191] The poor-risk category (median survival less than 1 year) includes −5q31.1, −7 or 7q−, and complex chromosomal abnormalities (three or more abnormalities). The intermediate-risk group (median survival about 2 years) includes deletions of 17p, 11q translocations, trisomy 9 or 19, and 3q abnormalities, among other alterations. In treatment-induced MDS, complex cytogenetic abnormalities are very common, whereas in *de novo* MDS such abnormalities occur in approximately 15 percent of cases.[42,190]

The proportion of cases with chromosome abnormalities differs depending on the severity of clinical manifestations. Chromosome abnormalities are more frequent in patients with oligoblastic myelogenous leukemia (RAEB) than in patients with clonal (refractory) anemia. In general, prevalence of chromosome abnormalities and the likelihood of progression to overt AML are a function of the number of cell lines involved, the severity of the cytopenias, and the proportion of blast cells present.

Allelotype analysis of chromosomes of patients with MDS using microsatellite markers mapped to most of the arms of autosomes have found loss of heterozygosity on chromosomes 5q, 7q, 17p, and 20q, in keeping with the most prevalent chromosome abnormalities in MDS patients. Loss of heterozygosity on three other segments, 1p, 1q, and 18q, also were identified. These segments are presumed to contain tumor suppressor genes that may play a role in the initiation of this neoplasm.[192]

Gene expression studies using primitive multipotential cells (CD34+) from patients with MDS and confirmed by real-time polymerase chain reaction studies have identified 11 selected genes by hierarchical clustering that differ from the CD34+ cells of normal persons.[193] In addition, distinctions in gene expression were identified that distinguished high-risk (more blast cells) from low-risk MDS patients. In low-risk patients three genes (retinoic acid-induced gene; radiation-inducible, immediate early response gene; stress-induced phosphoprotein 1 gene) were downregulated. Apparently, MDS patients accumulate gene defects that interfere with hematopoietic regulation.

MDS Stem Cells MDS stem and progenitor cells do not engraft well in nonobese diabetic-severe combined immunodeficiency (NOD-SCID) mice.[194] CD34+ cells circulate in MDS and may increase in number before AML transformation.[195] In CD34+ CD38− cells in 5q− MDS, few distinct differences were found between MDS and normal stem cells.[196] BMI1 was upregulated, and CEBPA was downregulated.

SPECIFIC MYELODYSPLASTIC SYNDROMES

These syndromes highlight the variability in expression of the MDS (see Table 88–1). Most patients have one of the syndromes described below.

■ 5Q− SYNDROME

Van Den Berge and colleagues are credited with the description of this syndrome in 1974.[197] Patients with the 5q− syndrome have clonal anemia and dysmorphic cells in the marrow containing, as the sole cytogenetic abnormality, a deletion in the long arm of chromosome 5 (5q).[198–200] The anemia, observed most frequently in older women, is associated with marked dyserythropoiesis, erythroid multinuclearity, and hypolobulated and frequently small ("dwarf") megakaryocytes (Fig. 88–3). Neutropenia and thrombocytopenia are highly uncommon. The syndrome occurs infrequently in children.

The somatic mutation in this syndrome resides in a very primitive multipotential cell, which has been defined as a myeloid progenitor in

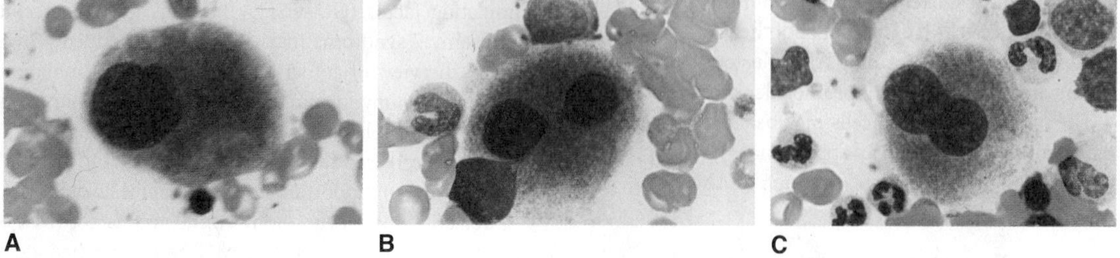

FIGURE 88–3. Composite from marrow films of patient with the 5q− syndrome. Characteristic hypolobulated megakaryocytes. **A.** Monolobed megakaryocyte. **B.** Bilobed megakaryocyte. Lobes connected by a nuclear bridge. **C.** Bilobed megakaryocyte. *(Used with permission from* Lichtman's Atlas of Hematology, *www.accessmedicine.com.)*

some studies[201,202] and as a lymphohematopoietic progenitor in other studies.[203,204] Patients with this disorder have a risk of developing AML (approximately 10%) that is similar to the risk of patients with clonal anemia and marrow cells without 5q−. Patients in whom 5q− is a single abnormality by FISH and whose blood and marrow correspond to the morphologic criteria for the 5q− syndrome have a median survival of approximately 7 years.[205] Patients who appear to have a solitary 5q− by standard cytogenetics but who have other abnormalities when studied by FISH have a median survival of less than 3 years. With the application of FISH, complex abnormalities involving 5q− are unlikely to represent the classic syndrome with its very favorable prognosis. The less-morbid course of the classic 5q− syndrome is associated with a lower degree of pathologic apoptosis.[206]

Deletion of 5q− may be a feature of other clonal cytopenias, oligoblastic myelogenous leukemia, or AML. In these situations, two of the classic features of the 5q− syndrome often are absent: macrocytic red cells and normal or elevated platelet count. Blast cells are evident in the oligoblastic leukemias, and basophilia and eosinophilia have been found in more than half of patients.[207] The 5q− cytogenetic finding still confers a somewhat better prognosis in these atypical situations if the marrow blast percentage is less than 10. In some cases, the 5q deletion may be a translocation or insertion as judged by FISH. Cells in cases of T- or B-cell acute lymphoblastic leukemia also have contained a 5q− abnormality.[200]

Extensive studies of the deleted region of the long arm of chromosome 5 have demonstrated a common deleted region and the spectrum of genes that reside in that region and may be involved in the initiation of this clonal syndrome. In the 5q− syndrome, the deletion is at q13-q31, whereas in other MDS with a 5q−, the region involved is 5q22 to q33.[208] The studies of the deleted regions of chromosome 5q− in cases with the syndrome have resulted in discrepant findings regarding (1) the size of the common deleted region, (2) the proximal and distal breakpoints on the long arm of chromosome 5 involved, (3) the candidate genes that might represent the tumor suppressor genes lost on 5q−, and, more specifically, (4) the gene or genes required to transform a multipotential hematopoietic cell into the cell that sustains the clone, causing the 5q− syndrome.[209] Using short hairpin RNA functional screens of normal CD34+ cells, the inhibition of RPS14 simulates a syndrome akin to that of 5q− with decreased erythropoiesis and increased megakaryocytopoiesis.[210] The loss of this gene, part of the ribosomal protein complex, could lead to dysregulation of messenger RNA translation and disturb hematopoiesis and result in oncogenesis.[211] An RNA processing defect has been observed in CD34+ cells from patients with the 5q− syndrome.[212] Other genes, such as *EGR1*, *CTNNA1* (α-catenin), and *NPM1* have been examined for a role in the pathogenesis of the 5q− syndrome.[213] Mutations have not been found on the normal homologous region of chromosome 5, and an epigenetic change such as hypermethylation of the allelic gene likely accounts for the loss of tumor suppressor activity. Alternatively, haploinsufficiency may induce the dysregulation of ribosomal protein apparently associated with this syndrome.

Therapy

Lenalidomide, a thalidomide analogue, induces improvement in approximately 85 percent of patients with the classical 5q− syndrome.[214–216] One approach is to administer 10 mg/day until improvement or toxicity requiring cessation. The improvement ranges from complete remission with disappearance of abnormal cytogenetics and normalization of blood counts to improvement in blood hemoglobin and loss of transfusion requirement to a maintenance of the low hemoglobin at a level sufficient to markedly decrease the frequency of transfusion. Some patients derive no benefit. The response may occur as soon as 1 week, but on average in about 5 weeks, and may take as long as 7 weeks to occur. In many cases, these patients had been unresponsive to prior erythropoietin treatment. Neutropenia and thrombocytopenia can be adverse effects of lenalidomide. The results are less favorable if additional cytogenetic abnormalities accompany the 5q− change.

MONOSOMY 7–ASSOCIATED SYNDROMES

Monosomy 7 is the second most frequent cytogenetic abnormality in the marrow cells of patients with myelodysplasia. It often occurs in marrow cells of subjects exposed to chemicals or radiation and is associated with a poor prognosis and rapid transformation to AML.[217–221] A critical region carrying the gene responsible for the neoplastic transformation may reside within bands 7q35–36.[222,223] Monosomy 7 syndromes are difficult to classify. The syndromes usually are not associated with special clinical features in adults, but in children they are characterized by an atypical myeloproliferative disorder or myelomonocytic leukemia with abnormal expression of the neurofibromatosis (*NF1*) and Wilms tumor (*WT1*) genes, unusual susceptibility to infection, and a rapid termination in acute leukemia.[217,220] Chapter 90 discusses juvenile chronic myelomonocytic leukemia. Monosomy 7 also occurs in a familial form and in the leukemic evolution of Down syndrome and Fanconi anemia.[223–226] A variant of the monosomy 7 syndrome, translocation 1;7, also is seen in adults and children and may be preceded by exposure to cytotoxic treatment.[117,227] The *ERBB* gene, which encodes a shortened form of the epidermal growth factor receptor, is amplified in this syndrome.[228] Patients with aplastic anemia have a predisposition to evolving into a clonal myeloid disease with a monosomy 7 cytogenetic abnormality (see Chap. 34).[229,230]

CLONAL (REFRACTORY) SIDEROBLASTIC ANEMIA

History

The term *refractory anemia* has been used for nearly a century to define erythropoietic insufficiencies that cannot be assigned to a specific vitamin or mineral deficiency and, thus, are unresponsive to the known hematinics.[1] At the time, the knowledge base was insufficient to determine the disorder was a neoplasm behaving in a relatively benign fashion. One sage observer likened the disorder to an adenoma in relationship to a carcinoma.[1] In 1956, Bjorkman[231] defined a subset of refractory anemias by the presence of ringed sideroblasts in the marrow. The intramitochondrial location of the iron in the ringed sideroblasts was described 1 year later.[232] Because the finding of ringed sideroblasts was a constant feature of marrow stained with Prussian blue in this situation, the designation *refractory anemia with ringed sideroblasts* was coined.

Pathogenesis

The disorder is a clonal multipotential hemopoietic stem cell defect in which ineffective erythropoiesis with normal or slightly shortened red cell survival and only slight impairment of the maturation of other cell lineages occur. Plasma iron turnover is increased, but incorporation of radioactive iron into heme and its delivery to blood as newly synthesized hemoglobin are depressed. These early ferrokinetic studies presaged the evidence that erythroid precursors were subject to aberrant maturation and pathologic apoptosis.[78,79] Low levels of the iron transporter gene, *ABCB7*, have been found in clonal sideroblastic anemia, and this gene is also associated with X-linked sideroblastic anemia with ataxia.[233] The genes somatically mutated to initiate this disorder have not been identified, but the frequency of deleted chromosome arms suggests a tumor suppressor gene on the affected chromosome is involved.[185]

Clinical Features

The disease is very uncommon in individuals younger than age 50 years,[24,26,234] except in patients in whom the disease occurs as a result of radiotherapy or chemotherapy of a malignant tumor. The rare concurrence of familial sideroblastic anemia has been reported.[235] Males and females are affected almost equally. The signs and symptoms are those of anemia: pallor, easy fatigue, weakness, dyspnea, and palpitations on exertion.[232,234] In most patients the anemia is detected as a result of blood cell analysis for other medical reasons. The liver may be slightly enlarged. The spleen is slightly increased in size in approximately 5 percent of patients. Splenic and hepatic enlargement do not necessarily occur together, and more than slight enlargement is unusual.

Laboratory Features

Most patients have mild to severe macrocytic anemia.[232,234] The blood film often contains a population of hypochromic cells (dimorphic red cell changes) and, hence, a widened red cell distribution width.[232,234–236] Red cell anisocytosis, basophilic stippling, and slight poikilocytosis may be present. The total white cell count and platelet count usually are normal, but mild abnormalities may be seen, including a decreased white cell count and an increased or decreased platelet count. Occasionally, the white cell count or platelet count is increased markedly, or nucleated red cells are present in the blood film. The reticulocyte percentage usually is between 0.5 and 2.0. Hemoglobin F concentration may be increased slightly. The disease may express a subtle phenotype: either mild macrocytic anemia in older patients with few other features of clonal anemia,[237,238] or in patients with clonal cytogenetic abnormalities with cytopenia but no unequivocal morphologic evidence of clonal dysmorphic hematopoiesis.[239]

Marrow cellularity usually is increased as a result of erythroid hyperplasia. Evidence of dyserythropoiesis in the form of vacuolated, small, large, or binucleate erythroblasts may be present. Prussian blue stain of the marrow invariably shows pathologic sideroblasts. The latter may have Prussian blue-positive cytoplasmic granules in a partial or complete circumnuclear pattern (ringed sideroblasts) in 15 or more percent of cells or an increased number (more than five) of Prussian blue-positive granules in their cytoplasm. If the disease progresses to oligoblastic leukemia, sideroblasts may become less prominent.[240] Granulopoiesis and thrombopoiesis are not altered significantly in two-thirds of patients.[236,241] In the other third of patients, dysgranulopoiesis (hypogranulation, acquired Pelger-Huët anomaly, hypersegmented nuclei, granule abnormalities) or dysmegakaryocytopoiesis (micromegakaryocytes, large lobulated cells) may be present. Marrow iron stores often are increased.

Cytogenetic abnormalities in marrow cells of patients with acquired refractory sideroblastic anemia provide evidence for the clonal character of the disease. Approximately half of the reported patients with sideroblastic anemia in whom cytogenetic studies have been performed have a chromosomal abnormality.[235] Involvement of chromosomes 8, 11, and 20 has been notable.[184,242,243] The Philadelphia chromosome has been reported.[244] Involvement of chromosome 3 has been associated with thrombocytosis.[245] The absence of the Y chromosome, only in the pathologic sideroblasts in one report (45;X/46;XY mosaic), substantiates the dimorphic nature of the erythroid lineage involvement and parallels the hypochromic and normochromic red cell populations.[246] Involvement of the X chromosome (a breakpoint at Xq13) of female patients with sideroblastic anemia[247] is noteworthy because a type of hereditary sideroblastic anemia is X chromosome linked (see Chap. 58).

Serum iron levels and saturation of transferrin are increased. Serum ferritin concentration is increased, reflecting an increase in body iron stores. Bilirubin-proteinate levels (indirect-reacting fraction) may be increased as a result of ineffective erythropoiesis and intramedullary hemolysis.

Special Clinical Feature: Thrombocytosis

A proportion of patients with clonal sideroblastic anemia have thrombocytosis, generally considered a platelet count greater than 450×10^9/L (450,000/μL). This syndrome is referred to as refractory anemia with ringed sideroblasts with thrombocytosis (RARS-T) in the WHO classification. A proportion (approximately 40%) of these patients have a mutation in the *JAK2* (Janus kinase 2) gene. The presence of the *JAK2* mutation confers a better prognosis on these patients.[248–250]

Differential Diagnosis

The principal considerations are the anemias with an inadequate reticulocyte response in which erythrocytes are hypochromic. Iron-deficiency anemia in contradistinction to sideroblastic anemia is associated with low serum iron levels, saturation of transferrin of less than 16 percent, low serum ferritin concentration, elevated serum transferrin receptors, and absent marrow sideroblasts and macrophage iron. The anemia of chronic disease can simulate some features of clonal anemia, although the low serum iron in the former and the presence of an overt chronic inflammatory disease, such as rheumatoid arthritis, are important distinctions. β-Thalassemia minor is characterized by normal to elevated serum iron and ferritin, low mean red cell volume, elevated hemoglobin A_2 concentration, and evidence of the disease in a parent, siblings, or offspring. α-Thalassemia trait is common among Americans of African descent. It can be distinguished from MDS by several features. It is microcytic, and often the red cell count is normal or elevated in relationship to the hemoglobin concentration. Target cells are more prominent than in MDS. Similar red cell changes may be present in a parent, sibling, or child supporting its hereditary nature. Molecular techniques are available to detect the α loci deletions in the usual $-\alpha/-\alpha,^{-3.7\text{ kb del}}$ type. Confusion may be engendered because the individual also may have a "low" white cell count based on laboratory normal values not corrected for the lower white cell counts in persons of African descent. Copper deficiency following gastric bypass surgery can also simulate myelodysplasia.[51,52] Detection of secondary forms of sideroblastic anemia requires evaluation for exposure to lead or other agents or diseases listed in Chap. 58, as do the hereditary sideroblastic anemias.

Therapy

Some patients do not require treatment because the moderate decrease in hemoglobin concentration is tolerated without limitation of usual activities.

Folic Acid, Pyridoxal, and Danazol Occasional patients who have low serum and red cell folate concentrations may have partial improvement in blood hemoglobin concentration after administration of folic acid (1 mg/day orally). Rare patients benefit temporarily from pharmacologic doses of pyridoxine (200 mg/day orally for at least 3 months) or danazol.[251] A therapeutic trial with folic acid and pyridoxine is worthwhile if the anemia is symptomatic, even though only a small percentage of patients are responsive. The attenuated androgen danazol has increased the platelet count and decreased the frequency of platelet transfusions in patients with all categories of MDS.[252] Danazol also has been combined with retinoic acid and low-dose prednisone.[253]

Transfusion of Red Cells If anemia is severe or symptoms of heart failure or coronary insufficiency are present, periodic transfusion of red cells is required.

Iron Chelation Iron overload is an important therapeutic consideration in transfusion-dependent patients who have a life expectancy measured in years. Cardiac, liver, and other organ dysfunction secondary to iron-overload from transfusion can result. Circumstantial evidence indicates that iron-overload may shorten survival in chronically transfused patients with clonal anemia. Guidelines for initiation of iron chelating agents are not definitive; if a patient has received 20 or more transfusions, has a ferritin level greater than 1000 mcg/L, and has a prognosis for at least 1-year survival, administration of an iron chelating agent should be strongly considered.[254–257] Deferasirox, an available oral iron chelator that can be administered once per day (20 mg/kg), has been approved by the FDA for use in transfusion-dependent patients.[258] The most common adverse events associated with deferasirox treatment include nausea, vomiting, abdominal pain, constipation or diarrhea, and skin rash. Elevated serum creatinine and, less frequently, elevated liver enzymes may develop. Thus, renal and hepatic function should be evaluated prior to use. Visual and auditory dysfunction has been reported. Careful monitoring of the drug is important since its toxicity profile in older patients is still being assessed.

Erythropoietin and G-CSF Recombinant human erythropoietin generally is not useful unless the pretreatment serum erythropoietin level is low for the blood hemoglobin concentration (less than 500 U/L) and the transfusion requirement is less than 2 U per month, an infrequent finding in these patients. In eligible patients, the combination of G-CSF with erythropoietin increases the response rate.[259–262] Response rates in various studies range widely. On average approximately 40 percent of eligible patients get some benefit from therapy. Duration of response is also variable but averages about 2 years. Improvement in quality of life has been variable among studies. Darbepoetin (long-acting erythropoietin) is probably equally effective as erythropoietin. Serum iron should be maintained at a normal level by oral or intravenous supplementation, if needed, to ensure an optimal erythropoietic response from erythropoietin administration.

Demethylating Agents Azacitidine, 75 mg/m^2 per day, subcutaneously (or intravenously), for 7 days every 28 days, can be useful in the patient with significant anemia and a transfusion requirement, unresponsive to erythropoietin and G-CSF. Approximately 40 percent of patients have a complete or partial response with improvement in hemoglobin level and either a cessation of transfusion requirements or a significant decrease in transfusion frequency. Patients who respond to the drug have an increase in survival and a longer period before progression to AML or death.[263–266] These differences are proportionally great (approximately 80%) but are measured only in months. Decreased blood counts are a common initial response and, thus, transfusion requirements may increase temporarily in the first weeks of treatment, even in good responders. The response to the drug may be evident by the end of two treatment cycles, but it may require four or five cycles to obtain a response, and maximal responses may not occur for eight or nine cycles. Thus, the drug should be continued until disease progression or a serious adverse response requires cessation and until improvement is maximized. Nausea and vomiting may be adverse events but they can be treated with antiemetics and usually do not require stopping therapy. If patient tolerance is good, the dose can be increased to 100 mg/m^2, if a response is not evident by the second or third cycle. Phase 1 trials are under way to examine the efficacy of an oral preparation of 5-azacytadine. Early results have been promising with decreased side effects. Decitabine has also been approved as a demethylating agent in this situation (see "Therapy for Patients with High-Intermediate (INT-2) Prognostic Scores: Demethylating Agent and Histone Deacetylation Inhibitor Therapy" below).

Course and Prognosis

In many patients, the disorder lasts for years without progression of the anemia or symptoms and without need for specific therapy. A small proportion of patients may have progressive marrow failure, severe cytopenias, and morbidity from infections or hemorrhage. Iron overload is a function of increased absorption related to chronic anemia and, more importantly, repeated red cell transfusions over prolonged periods. Improvement of the anemia and the adverse effects of iron overload in parenchymal tissues can result from iron-chelation therapy.[254–258,267]

Over a 10- to 15-year period, approximately 10 percent of patients with clonal (sideroblastic) anemia develop AML.[268–272] Progression to leukemia is correlated with the degree of abnormal hematopoiesis and trilineage abnormalities.[205,240] Transformation to acute lymphocytic leukemia (ALL) also has occurred.[273] In one series of 37 patients, 25 had abnormalities confined to the erythroid series, transfusion dependence occurred in 26, and iron overload was common. Five patients progressed to marrow failure and five to AML. Median survival was 72 months.[274] Survival in other series has ranged from 85 to more than 100 months.[205,274,275] The presence of thrombocytosis (and the *JAK2* gene mutation) may confer a better prognosis.[248] Survival is better in patients without significant abnormalities in lineages other than the erythroid series and with favorable cytogenetic findings.[274,275] This latter prognostic indicator also applies to clonal nonsideroblastic anemias and oligoblastic leukemia.[275]

■ CLONAL (REFRACTORY) NONSIDEROBLASTIC ANEMIA

This clonal disorder, another arbitrary misnomer, closely mimics clonal sideroblastic anemia. No significant difference is observed in any of comparative variables (age, gender, blood cell counts, marrow findings), except that the frequency of ringed sideroblasts is by definition less than 15 percent, but, almost invariably, present. The requirement for sideroblasts to have at least five Prussian blue-staining circumnuclear aggregates further complicates determining the incidence of clonal sideroblastic anemia.[278] If one assumes the presence of any percentage of ringed sideroblasts in marrow is abnormal and is consistent with "sideroblastic anemia" as a descriptive term, virtually all patients with clonal anemia without overt multilineage findings and an increase in myeloblasts in marrow have clonal sideroblastic anemia. The presence of pathologic sideroblasts is a useful indication of the presence of dysmorphic erythropoiesis, regardless of their prevalence. The anemia is mild to moderate, with a tendency to macrocytosis. Leukopenia and thrombocytopenia, if present, usually are mild.[275,279] Hyposegmented and hypersegmented neutrophils, giant platelets, and red cell shape, size, and hemoglobinization abnormalities may be present. The marrow usually is cellular, and the precursors may show morphologic evidence of dysmorphic erythropoiesis. Because anemia predominates and other cytopenias are slight, the course and management are similar to those of clonal sideroblastic anemia. Patients with low erythropoietin levels may have a significant increase in hemoglobin concentration with weekly injections of the hormone. The proportion of patients transforming into AML and the median survival of patients are similar to patients with clonal sideroblastic anemia.[275] Cytopenias and blood and marrow dysmorphic changes can become more severe, and the course and management in that instance are similar to clonal multilineal cytopenias.

In a study of MDS in which 382 patients were categorized as clonal anemia (with higher or lower proportions of recognizable sideroblasts), 94 percent of patients were in the low or low-intermediate risk category of the International Prognostic Scoring System (IPSS). In each case (higher or lower proportions of sideroblasts), approximately 50 percent of patients were at low risk of progression, and approximately 50 percent were low-intermediate risk. The median survival of patients with clonal anemia who were categorized as low risk was 9 years, and for patients categorized as low-intermediate risk, median survival was 5 years. Because of equivalent numbers in each group, the overall median survival for patients with clonal anemia of either type was approximately 7 years. In a study of 374 patients, the patients with clonal anemia with either high or low proportions of sideroblasts had a median survival of 9 years (108 months) (Table 88–2).[275]

Treatment

Therapy in this situation follows the guidelines described in "Clonal (Refractory) Sideroblastic Anemia" above.

TABLE 88–2. Distribution of Five Principal Categories of MDS among 374 Patients

MDS Subtype	% of Patients	% Marrow Blasts Median (Range)	Median Survival (Months)
Clonal anemia with low (<15%)[1] or high (≥15%)[2] proportion of pathologic sideroblasts	30	3 (0–4)	108
Clonal multicytopenias[3]	25	4 (0–4)	49
Oligoblastic myelogenous leukemia[4]	35	11 (5–19)	24
5q– syndrome[5]	7.5	4 (2–4)	Not statistically different from clonal anemia; DNS
Unclassifiable[6]	2.5	3 (2–4)	DNS

DNS, data not shown.

WHO classification: [1]refractory anemia; [2]refractory sideroblastic anemia; [3]refractory anemia with multicytopenia; [4]refractory anemia with excess blasts types 1 and 2; [5]5q– syndrome; [6]unclassifiable category. Among the oligoblastic myelogenous leukemia patients, the survival was better the lower the diagnostic marrow blast count.

SOURCE: Data derived from Malcovati L, Porta MG, Pascutto C, et al.[275]

CLONAL MULTILINEAL CYTOPENIAS

At least two-thirds of patients with clonal cytopenia present with some degree of neutropenia and/or thrombocytopenia in addition to anemia. There is considerable variability in the pattern with a range of white cell counts from leucopenia to mild leukocytosis and platelet counts from thrombocytopenia to thrombocytosis.[275] Patients with clonal multilineal cytopenias (refractory cytopenia with multilineal dysplasia) represent a subset of myelodysplastic disorders that has greater morbidity and significantly decreased life expectancy than the clonal anemias. If the cytopenias are not functionally significant, some patients can be observed for very long periods without specific therapy. The increased risk of infection or hemorrhage if severe neutropenia, neutrophil qualitative abnormalities, severe thrombocytopenia, and platelet qualitative abnormalities are present in patients augurs morbidity and decreased survival.

Clinical Findings

Patients present with anemia, neutropenia, and thrombocytopenia; anemia and neutropenia; or anemia and thrombocytopenia. The blood and marrow features are as described in "Laboratory Features" above and lead to the diagnosis, especially in the patient who is older than age 50 years.[14,15,280–282] The patient usually seeks medical attention for symptoms of anemia: fatigue, dyspnea, and palpitations on exertion, headache, or dizziness. Exaggerated bleeding associated with thrombocytopenia may be present. Mild hepatomegaly and/or splenomegaly occasionally may be present.

Dysmorphic blood and marrow cell changes are common. Marrow myeloblasts range from 0 to 4 percent and usually are absent from the blood. Cytogenetic abnormalities may be present as described in "Cytogenetics" above. If monocytosis is greater than 1000×10^6/L, the disorder can merge with chronic myelomonocytic leukemia (see Chap. 90).

Differential Diagnosis

Mild to moderate bicytopenia (anemia and neutropenia) and sometimes tricytopenia with dysmorphic blood and marrow findings and hypercellular marrow occur in patients with the acquired immune deficiency syndrome,[283,284] but are not associated with progression to acute leukemia. Pancytopenia with hyperplastic marrow is associated with nonhemopoietic cancers (paraneoplastic syndrome).[285] Megaloblastic anemia can be simulated and distinguished by the normal concentration of serum or red cell folate and serum vitamin B_{12}. In the small proportion of patients with a hypocellular marrow, aplastic anemia or paroxysmal nocturnal hemoglobinuria should be considered (see "Relationship Among Aplastic Anemia, Paroxysmal Nocturnal Hemoglobinuria, and Clonal Myeloid Diseases" in Chap. 34). Dysmorphic cells are not a feature of aplastic anemia. Paroxysmal nocturnal hemoglobinemia may have markedly dysmorphic red cells, but they have a marked deficiency of CD55 and CD59 on red blood cells as measured by flow cytometry.

Treatment

In patients with pancytopenia and cellular but dysmorphic marrow, cytopenias that are not troublesome should not be treated.

Anemia The treatment for the anemia in this syndrome is similar to that described above in "Clonal (Refractory) Sideroblastic Anemia: Therapy." Transfusion of blood components when necessary is the mainstay of treatment. Erythropoietin plus G-CSF administration may increase hemoglobin concentration and eliminate or decrease transfusion requirements. The response is best in patients with low erythropoietin levels for the degree of anemia (<500 U/L) and requiring less than 2 U of red cells per month. Regular transfusion of red cells may be used for patients who do not adapt to moderate anemia or in whom medical conditions, such as angina pectoris, require a higher packed red cell volume. Cytokines (erythropoietin and G-CSF) have not been shown to increase survival and can produce troubling side effects, such as local skin reactions, fever, bone pain, and a capillary leak syndrome.[261,262] They also can lead to increased immature granulocytes, including blast cells, in the marrow and blood.[286] The target hemoglobin for erythropoietin plus G-CSF therapy is usually about 10 g/dL.

Iron-chelation therapy should be considered for patients who require chronic transfusion therapy (see "Clonal (Refractory) Sideroblastic Anemia: Therapy" above).

Thrombocytopenia Thrombocytopenia and infections are more troublesome in this category of disease. Thrombocytopenia may not be so severe as to require treatment. If thrombocytopenic bleeding occurs, platelet transfusions should be used. Antifibrinolytic agents such as epsilon-aminocaproic acid may be a useful adjunct to platelet transfusion to minimize thrombocytopenic bleeding. Platelet-stimulating agents may be useful (see "Therapy for Patients with High-Intermediate (INT-2) Prognostic Scores: Management of Thrombocytopenia" below).

Neutropenia and Fever Asymptomatic neutropenia should not be treated, but fever should be evaluated promptly and suspected infection treated with broad-spectrum bactericidal antibiotics until the results of cultures are known. In appropriate situations, oral antibiotics can be used in patients treated at home.[287,288]

Hypocellular Marrow In uncommon cases with hypoplastic marrows (usually less than 30 percent marrow cellularity), cyclosporine and rabbit ATG have been used,[289,290] analogous to the responsiveness of the hypoplasia of many cases of aplastic anemia to such approaches (see "Therapy for Patients with Low and Low-Intermediate (INT-1) Prognostic Scores: Immunotherapy" below). The response rate to cyclosporine and ATG is approximately 25 percent in this category of disease. A variety of chemotherapeutic agents have been used, especially when the disease evolves to oligoblastic or frank AML (see "Oligoblastic Myelogenous Leukemia: Treatment" below).

Demethylating Agents 5-Azacytidine or decitabine may be useful in these patients.[263–266] The initial response, however, may be further suppression of blood counts, which can be very troublesome, especially if an improvement does not follow soon. Older patients also may not tolerate these drugs and a decreased dose may be required, initially. The combination of valproic acid and decitabine is under study for this type of high-intermediate risk disease (see "Therapy for Patients with High–Intermediate (INT-2) Prognostic Scores: Demethylating Agent and Histone Deacetylation Inhibitor Therapy" below).

AML-Type Therapy If patients' cytopenias are very severe and morbidity high, consideration can be given to either AML induction therapy (see Chap. 89) or allogeneic hematopoietic stem cell transplantation (see "Therapy for Patients with High-Intermediate (INT-2) or High-Risk Prognostic Scores: Hematopoietic Stem Cell Transplantation" below).

Course and Prognosis

Morbidity is high in patients with multicytopenias. Lassitude, severe, symptomatic anemia, severe infections, and exaggerated bleeding may occur. Mortality from infection or hemorrhage occurs in approximately 25 percent of patients. AML develops in approximately 50 percent of patients. The likelihood of transformation to overt AML is greater if the patient has severe cytopenias, more overt qualitative disorders of cells, abnormal localized immature myeloid precursors (increased CD34+ cells) in marrow, complex chromosome abnormalities, and abnormalities of marrow cell colony growth in culture (excessive growth or decreased growth).[277,291–293] Median survival of patients with clonal hemopathy and multicytopenias is approximately 30 to 50 months.[275,292,293]

OLIGOBLASTIC MYELOGENOUS LEUKEMIA (REFRACTORY ANEMIA WITH EXCESS BLASTS)

Definition and History

In 1963, the term *smoldering acute leukemia* was introduced to highlight a subset of patients, usually those older than age 50 years, who had a low proportion of leukemic blast cells in marrow (3–20%) and blood (0–7%) and who survived for months or years without specific therapy for leukemia.[294–296] The terms "smoldering," "pauciblastic," "low-infiltrate," and "oligoblastic" myelogenous leukemia for this type of process are synonyms. Oligoblastic myelogenous leukemia is called *refractory anemia with excess myeloblasts* in various classification schemes.[2,3] This is a peculiar turn of phrase as these are not excess normal myeloblasts but malignant myeloblasts, which if present in the marrow examination imply an overt malignancy (leukemia not an anemia). When the blast count increases to greater than 19 percent, a diagnosis of AML is made. Chronic myelomonocytic leukemia, another type of oligoblastic subacute leukemia, previously included under the rubric myelodysplasia, is better linked to the subacute and chronic myelogenous leukemias discussed in Chap. 90.

Clinical Findings

Oligoblastic leukemia composes approximately 30 to 50 percent of all cases of myelodysplasia, if one uses a definition of ≥4 percent marrow blasts as a requirement. Most patients are older than age 50 years. Males are affected more often than females by approximately 1.5:1. Reticulocytopenic anemia, granulocytopenia, and/or thrombocytopenia are usually present. Qualitative abnormalities of blood cells usually are overt (see "Laboratory Features" above). Myeloblasts constitute from 5 to 19 percent of nucleated marrow cells by definition, but marrow blasts greater than 2 percent are almost never seen in normal marrows, and a lower threshold would increase the proportion of patients with oligoblastic myelogenous leukemia markedly. Auer rods may be present in blast cells. Dysmorphic changes that occur in abnormal marrow precursor cells are described in "Laboratory Features" above. This syndrome evolves into overt AML in approximately 50 percent of cases. Median survival of patients with oligoblastic leukemia is approximately 12 to 24 months, although occasional long-term survival has been reported.[275,297]

Treatment

Treatment of oligoblastic myelogenous leukemia should be individualized. In some cases, no active treatment is required. Periodic evaluation is essential to detect deterioration in well-being or blood cell counts. Most patients require treatment in weeks to months. The response to cytotoxic therapy is poor, and symptomatic therapy with component transfusion and antibiotics, as required, is the preferable management if that approach can sustain a reasonable functional status. If the disease progresses such that cytopenias lead to infection, hemorrhage, or anemia and require inordinate amounts of transfusions or if the disease progresses to AML and the patient is fit, intensive cytotoxic therapy for AML may be warranted (see Chap. 89). If the patient has a poor performance status or has comorbid medical conditions that would lower the tolerance for intensive cytotoxic therapy, attenuation of doses should be considered. Cytarabine combined with anthracycline antibiotics, etoposide, or topotecan has produced remissions in approximately half of a group of selected patients.[298–304] Recovery may be slow, and remissions tend to be short, however. Patients with a poor performance status or of advanced age, or who choose not to be treated with combined-agent chemotherapy, can be treated with either low-dose cytarabine or 5-azacytidine or decitabine.[264–267] Other agents that have been used include etoposide, hydroxyurea, retinoids, butyrates, and other therapies coupled with transfusion therapy for palliation of the disease. Although some patients have improved, these approaches have been of limited benefit. Patients younger than age 50 years of age with a histocompatible donor should be considered for allogeneic hematopoietic stem cell transplantation.[307] Older patients may be considered for nonmyeloablative allogeneic transplantation. Some patients in remission can be considered for intensive therapy and autologous stem cell rescue (see "Hematopoietic Stem Cell Transplantation" below).[308]

Course and Prognosis

The median survival in published series of patients with oligoblastic leukemia varies from 6 to 36 months, with survival of individual patients ranging from 1 to 160 months. In a very large single series that included refractory anemia, median survival was 15 months.[272] Approximately half of the patients died of infection associated with severe neutropenia or dysfunctional neutrophils and monocytes, and approximately 25 percent died of bleeding complications resulting from thrombocytopenia. Approximately 30 percent of cases evolved into AML. Length of survival of patients with oligoblastic leukemia after diagnosis is inversely correlated with a higher risk category of the cytogenetic abnormality, a higher proportion of blast cells in the marrow, the presence of N-*RAS* mutations, greater severity of the neutropenia and thrombocytopenia, and higher serum level of β_2-microglobulin.[148,275,309–315]

A rare case of spontaneous disappearance of oligoblastic leukemia has been documented.[316]

THERAPY-RELATED MYELODYSPLASTIC SYNDROMES

Therapy-related myelodysplastic syndromes are increasing in frequency as the utilization of intensive chemotherapy and radiation increases in other solid tumors and lymphoma.[36–43] These cases have a poor prognosis and are not included in the International Prognostic Scoring System (IPSS). Cellular abnormalities of chromosomes 5, 7, and 8 are common in these cases.[317] MDS following breast cancer is associated with older age, presence of other cancers, and multiple first-degree relatives with cancer.[318] As compared to patients with myeloma or germ cell tumors, patients with lymphoma undergoing autologous stem cell transplantation have a higher incidence of treatment-related MDS. In this group, pretransplantation therapy, total-body irradiation, and other transplantation-related factors play a role, as do inherited polymorphisms in genes governing drug metabolism and DNA repair.[319] Therapy-related MDS has been reported after high-dose melphalan for myeloma treatment, but the risk is relatively low.[320] Accelerated telomere shortening precedes development of therapy-related myelodysplasia after autologous transplantation for lymphoma.[321] Treatment-related MDS is managed as are *de novo* cases of MDS, but are very refractory to treatment. Allogeneic hematopoietic stem cell transplantation can result in long-term disease-free survival, but most patients with therapy-related MDS are not candidates because of advanced age, comorbidities, or the inability to control the primary cancer.[322]

TREATMENT OF MYELODYSPLASTIC SYNDROME BASED ON PROGNOSTIC SCORE

Therapeutic decisions in MDS patients can be based on the category of disease, such as 5q– syndrome or clonal anemia. These approaches are outlined after each category of specific syndrome. Because the syndromes are a continuum and have irregular manifestations, an IPSS was devised to assign patients at the time of diagnosis to a category that estimates the likelihood of early progression, the average time by which patients with those characteristics will evolve to AML, and incorporates information beyond the MDS subtype.[277,279,309] Multivariate analysis combines the impact of (1) percentage of marrow blasts, (2) three cytogenetic subgroups (favorable, unfavorable, intermediate), and (3) number of cytopenias (Table 88–3). In large numbers of patients, the following frequency distribution of patients has been observed: low-risk group (i.e., longest time to evolve to AML) in 15 to 30 percent of patients; intermediate-1 risk group in 30 to 40 percent of patients; intermediate-2 risk group in 20 to 25 percent of patients; and high-risk group in 5 to 10 percent of patients.[277,279,323]

Using the IPSS to classify patients, survival is worse as risk category increases in four defined groups from low-risk to high-risk (Table 88–4), and this effect is influenced by age at diagnosis within the same prognostic category (Table 88–5).

The prognostic score should not be the sole guide to treatment because many patients deviate from the average expectation of disease behavior. Unexpected progression may necessitate changes in treatment approach and in the case of patients who are candidates for allogeneic hematopoietic stem cell transplantation; their course may require rec-

TABLE 88–3. International Prognostic Scoring System for Myelodysplastic Syndromes[277]

Prognostic Variable	Score Value			
	0	0.5	1.0	1.5
Marrow Blast (%)	<5	5–10		11–20
Karyotype	Good	Intermediate	Poor	
Cytopenias	0, 1	2, 3		

Risk groups: Low, 0; INT-1, 0.5–1.0; INT-2, 1.5–2.0; High, ≥2.5.

Karyotype: Good score, -Y, del(5q); poor score, complex abnormalities and chromosome 7 abnormalities; intermediate score, other abnormalities. See "Marrow: Cytogenetics" above for further details.

TABLE 88–4. Survival of Patients with Clonal Cytopenias and Oligoblastic Myelogenous Leukemia Based on the International Prognostic Scoring System

IPSS Score at Diagnosis	No. of Patients	2-Year Survival	5-Year Survival	10-Year Survival	15-Year Survival
Low	267	85%	55%	28%	20%
Intermediate-1	314	70%	35%	17%	12%
Intermediate-2	179	30%	8%	0	–
High	56	5%	0	–	–

IPSS, International Prognostic Scoring System.

These data were extrapolated from curves in Figure 6 of reference 277. Data are expressed as percent of all patients in that risk category surviving at the time interval shown.

TABLE 88–5. Survival of Patients with Clonal Cytopenias and Oligoblastic Myelogenous Leukemia Based on the International Prognostic Scoring System Stratified by Age

IPSS Score and Age	2-Year Survival	5-Year Survival	10-Year Survival	15-Year Survival
Low ≤60 years	95%	80%	65%	30%
Low >60 years	80%	45%	18%	18%
Intermediate-1 ≤60 years	85%	50%	37%	18%
Intermediate-1 >60 years	62%	30%	12%	ND
Intermediate-2 ≤60 years	50%	15%	ND	–
Intermediate-2 >60 years	25%	5%	0	–
High ≤60 years	0	–	–	–
High >60 years	7%	0		

IPSS, International Prognostic Scoring System; ND, no data.

These data were extrapolated from curves in Figure 7 of reference 277. Data are expressed as percent of all patients in that risk category surviving at the time interval shown.

ommending the procedure. Furthermore, several refinements to the original IPSS score have been proposed to incorporate factors such as ALIP and CD34 expression,[324] duration of MDS and prior therapy,[325] and lactate dehydrogenase.[326,327] Also, other time-dependent prognostic scoring systems have been proposed, including the WHO Prognositc scoring System.[328] Although these systems have benefit in defining populations and allowing comparisons between defined groups, they are often of little aid in making treatment decisions in individual patients and in understanding the biology of MDS.[329]

Treatments based on the IPSS can be considered (1) supportive care, (2) low-intensity therapy, or (3) high-intensity treatment.[330–332] Treatment response is judged based on the MDS subtype and IPSS score of the patient and the presence of treatment-induced (secondary) MDS.[333]

THERAPY FOR PATIENTS WITH LOW AND LOW-INTERMEDIATE (INT-1) PROGNOSTIC SCORES

Supportive care consists of improving quality of life with specific treatment of cytopenias or their complications and providing psychosocial support, while monitoring the patient's clinical status at intervals.[334,335]

Management of Anemia

Red Cell Transfusion Red cell transfusions should be administered for symptomatic anemia. Often patients will tolerate hemoglobin levels as low as 8 g/dL, but the level at which symptoms develop varies from patient to patient. Higher thresholds have been suggested to prevent cardiac consequences of prolonged anemia.[336]

Erythropoiesis-Stimulating Agents Red cell transfusion dependency may have a negative impact on clinical outcomes in MDS probably related to more severe marrow failure in those cases, increased iron overload, and possibly correlation with increased risk of transformation to AML.[337] Some studies found that neither the serum ferritin nor the number of red blood cell transfusions impacted survival in clonal sideroblastic anemia.[338] Recombinant erythropoietin can be used to treat anemia in patients who are transfusion-dependent, if the serum erythropoietin level is low for the hemoglobin level. Responses are best with low erythropoietin levels, normal blast counts, lower IPSS scores,[339] normal cytogenetics,[340] and in patients who do not require transfusion.[341] Hemolysis, or iron, vitamin B_{12}, or folate deficiency should be ruled out as a cause of anemia before erythropoietin therapy is started. Iron stores should be kept replete during erythropoietin therapy. Erythropoietin 150 to 300 U/kg per day or single weekly doses of 40,000 U are effective.[340] Darbepoetin alpha in various schedules of administration has also been found effective in increasing hemoglobin levels and in enhancing quality of life.[343,344] The probability of a response increases with duration of therapy; for example, optimal at 26 weeks compared to 12 weeks.[345] Meta-analysis has confirmed erythropoietic response rates are similar for those treated either with epoetin alfa or with the longer-acting darbepoetin alfa.[346] Unlike the case in patients with solid tumors or renal failure, there is no evidence that erythropoietic agents increase thromboembolic disease or accelerate progress to leukemia, but followup in these studies has been short.[347] G-CSF combined with erythropoietin may produce a response more frequently.[348,349] This combination does not appear to affect the risk of leukemic transformation and may have a positive impact on survival in those with low transfusion needs.[350] This approach is not recommended for those with intermediate-2 risk or high-risk IPSS scores.[351] There is evidence that marrow erythroid cells of MDS patients who respond to erythropoietin have a different gene expression pattern than do those of nonresponders.[352]

Iron-Chelation Therapy Chelation may be necessary to prevent iron overload in patients receiving frequent transfusions. Numerous consensus guidelines have been published regarding the treatment of iron overload in myelodysplastic syndromes.[353–355] These emphasize that there is no prospectively validated threshold for (1) the number of units of transfused blood or (2) the level of serum ferritin that should trigger iron chelation.[355] Several of these guidelines use a serum ferritin >1000 mcg/L as a threshold for starting iron-chelation therapy. They also take into account the patient's candidacy for allogeneic stem cell transplantation, life expectancy, and evidence of iron-related organ damage.[355] Both deferoxamine given subcutaneously or intravenously and deferasirox given orally are available for chelation therapy in MDS patients.[356] Cardiac magnetic resonance imaging may provide more reliable means of assessing myocardial iron overload than does measurement of serum ferritin.[357]

Low-Dose Cytarabine Low-dose cytarabine 5 to 20 mg/m^2 per day by subcutaneous injection every 12 hours for up to 8 to 16 weeks or by continuous intravenous infusion has been used in lieu of intensive chemotherapy.[358,359] Although this approach led to remission in approximately 20 percent of patients with oligoblastic leukemia, the median duration of remission is approximately 10 months, and survival has not been prolonged compared with supportive care alone. Moreover, low-dose cytosine arabinoside usually is cytotoxic, inducing marrow hypoplasia and worsening cytopenias. Although occasional reports of remission following low-dose cytarabine have been consistent with an effect on leukemia cell maturation, most patients experience suppression of the malignant cell clone, leading to marrow repopulation with polyclonal hemopoiesis.[304,309,330] This treatment approach is now utilized less often since the advent of other FDA-approved agents for MDS, but may still have a role in some patients, especially when combined with G-CSF.[360]

Immunotherapy Cyclosporine and Antithymocyte Globulin In some patients with MDS, T-lymphocyte–mediated inhibition of hematopoiesis occurs and contributes to cytopenias. The cytopenias can be ameliorated by treatment with immunosuppressive agents.[361] In patients who recovered effective hematopoiesis after treatment, the $V\beta$ (T-cell receptor-β) spectra-type representative of clonal or oligoclonal T-cell populations reverted to normal patterns.[361] A nonclonal X-chromosome inactivation pattern in the marrow, as assessed by the human androgen receptor gene assay and the phosphoglycerated kinase-1 assay, was associated with a response to ATG. This finding was attributed to incomplete clonal expansion, with ATG improving normal hematopoiesis by relieving the immunologic pressure on the remaining normal progenitors.[362] Others have postulated that responses may result from suppression of interferon-γ secretion by CD4+ T cells.[363] Some series have reported response rates to ATG of 15 to 60 percent[364–366] and longer survival times in patients who respond. Human leukocyte antigen (HLA)-DR15 (DR2) is overrepresented in MDS and predicts a response to immunosuppressive therapy.[367] In one series of 60 patients treated with ATG and cyclosporine, 60 percent had hematologic improvement, and more responders had good karyotype or DRB1 1501.[368] Most of the patients in this series had refractory anemia and an IPSS score of intermediate-1. Most, but not all, responses have occurred in patients with hypocellular marrows.[369,370] In a series of 129 patients who were treated with immunosuppressive therapy at a single institution, 30 percent had either a complete or partial response, and younger age and intermediate or low IPSS score favored survival.[371] Other groups have reported lack of response to ATG and prednisone. One study was stopped early because of lack of efficacy and development of adverse reactions.[372] Other studies also have reported lack of efficacy of single-agent cyclosporine.[373]

Other Treatment Options in Low- or Intermediate-1–Risk Patients For those patients not likely to respond to supportive care measures alone or for those who are not likely to respond to immune suppressive therapies, azacytidine, decitabine, or lenalidomide can be used. In those not responding to these approved agents, in appropriate patients, allogeneic stem cell transplantation or other investigational options can be considered (see Hematopoietic Stem Cell Transplantation).

THERAPY FOR PATIENTS WITH HIGH-INTERMEDIATE (INT-2) PROGNOSTIC SCORES

Demethylating Agent and Histone Deacetylation Inhibitor Therapy

Oligoblastic and secondary myelogenous leukemias have a high prevalence of tumor suppressor gene hypermethylation.[374] 5-Azacytidine is a pyrimidine analogue that inhibits DNA methyltransferase, reduces cytosine methylation, and induces maturation of some leukemic cell lines. It also is an antiproliferative drug. Administration of the drug and its congener decitabine has resulted in improvement of some patients with oligoblastic leukemia.[267,375] 5-Azacytidine at a dose of 75 mg/m^2 once per day given subcutaneously for 7 consecutive days each month provided significantly more frequent benefit to two-thirds of patients than did supportive care. Quality of life was enhanced, and disease progression was delayed.[267,275,376] Complete responses were seen in approximately 15 percent of 5-azacytidine–treated patients, and up to 36 percent had hematologic improvement.[375] Ninety percent of responses were seen by cycle 6. In another series,[377] subclasses of MDS did not predict for response to 5-azacytidine. A decrease in the white blood count during the initial cycle correlated with a higher response rate. 5-Azacytidine was approved by the FDA in 2004 for treatment of all subtypes of myelodysplastic syndrome. Treatment with this agent can usually be accomplished on an outpatient basis,[378] and intravenous[379] and oral formulations have been examined.[380] Other schedules of administration to accommodate outpatient therapy have been reported to have benefit but have not been directly compared to the 75 mg/m^2 daily dose for 7 days every 4 weeks.[381]

5-Aza-2′-deoxycytidine (decitabine) is also FDA approved for all MDS risk categories. Seventeen percent of patients in one series had a major cytogenetic response on an intention-to-treat basis after a median of three courses. The median duration of cytogenetic response was 7.5 months in all IPSS groups.[382] Patients who responded had improved survival compared with patients in whom the cytogenetically abnormal clone persisted.[383,384] A 5-day intravenous schedule was found to be optimal in one series, which examined several schedules of administration[385]; examination of optimal doses and schedules continues.[386] Decitabine probably works partly through demethylation, as it has resulted in demethylation of a hypermethylated *p15/INK4B* gene in patients.[383] Demethylation was associated with clinical responses.[384] Oligodeoxynucleotide antisense approaches to DNA methyltransferase-1 inhibition are also being explored in MDS.[387]

Inhibitors of histone deacetylation may have activity in MDS and are under investigation. Numerous agents are being studied and include depsipeptide, butyrate derivatives, suberoylanilide hydroxamic acid, and valproic acid.[388] Phase I trials have been completed in MDS with LBH589, a cinnamic hydroxamic acid analogue[389] and with MGCD0103.[390] There is interest in combining histone deacetylation inhibitors with DNA methyltransferase inhibitors.[391]

Management of Thrombocytopenia

Thrombocytopenia is common in MDS and has a higher prevalence in higher-risk IPSS categories.[392] Furthermore, many therapies used in MDS may exacerbate thrombocytopenia. Platelet transfusions may be required if the platelet count falls below 10×10^9 cells/L or in support of chemotherapeutic-induced thrombocytopenia. Antifibrinolytic agents such as aminocaproic acid can be used in patients who have bleeding despite platelet transfusion or to decrease the need of platelet transfusions.[393] Low-dose IL-11 is being studied as a means of increasing the platelet count in patients with symptomatic thrombocytopenia as are thrombopoietin-receptor agonists. AMG-531 (Romiplostim) and Eltrombopag may increase platelet counts in a subset of MDS patients[394–396] and are under investigation for this purpose.

Neutropenia, Fever, and Infections

Granulocyte-Stimulating Factors Randomized, double-blind studies have not shown that any cytokine prolongs survival or reduces morbidity in oligoblastic leukemia. GM-CSF and G-CSF[397–399] increase neutrophil counts and functions in some patients. G-CSF receptor expression may be low in some patients with MDS and prevents a good response to endogenous or administered G-CSF.[400] Complete remissions have been reported in hypoplastic AML/MDS with G-CSF alone.[401] Granulocyte transfusions are rarely used in MDS.[402] Rare serious complications, such as splenic rupture, have been reported with use of G-CSF.[403] Cytokines do not delay progression to acute leukemia; however, they increase the percentage of blasts in the blood in a proportion of patients, an event that is not always reversible with cessation of cytokine.[397,398] In one review, 22 of 83 reported cases of myelodysplasia treated with G-CSF or GM-CSF had an increase in marrow blast percentage, and AML evolved in 12 of 69 patients. An increased percentage of abnormal macrophages has been reported.[404] Use of these agents without chemotherapy in oligoblastic leukemias carries a risk of promoting expansion of leukemic blast cells.[405] Combinations of growth factors alone or coupled with maturing agents have not significantly improved response or survival rates.[406,407]

Antibiotics Febrile events are common in higher-risk syndromes because of the frequency of moderately severe neutropenia and functional disorders of neutrophils and monocytes. Also, chemotherapy is more likely to be used in these situations, inducing severe neutropenia. Careful cultures and use of broad-spectrum antibiotics until and if a specific organism are found is important (see Chap. 20).

THERAPY FOR PATIENTS WITH HIGH-INTERMEDIATE (INT-2) OR HIGH-RISK PROGNOSTIC SCORES

Demethylating Agent Therapy

Patients in higher-risk IPSS categories can be treated with demethylating agents if they are not suitable candidates for allogeneic hematopoietic stem cell transplantation. In one study of higher-risk MDS patients where 5-azacytidine was compared to conventional care regimens that included supportive care, low-dose cytarabine treatment, or intensive induction chemotherapy, 5-azacytidine increased survival as compared to standard care regimens.[408] With the exception of allogeneic hematopoietic stem cell transplantation, however, all of these treatments are palliative.[409]

Acute Myelogenous Leukemia Chemotherapy

Chemotherapeutic regimens containing standard doses of cytarabine, an anthracycline antibiotic, and/or etoposide (see Chap. 89) result in remission in fewer than 20 percent of patients with high-risk MDS. Moreover, a proportion of patients become worse with intensive chemotherapy. The advanced age and the high frequency of cardiac, renal, immunologic, and other organ system impairment in most patients with oligoblastic leukemia are largely responsible for the poor outcome. Patients who are younger than age 60 years have higher remission rates of up to 50 percent[410] and can be considered for intensive therapy. Patients older than age 60 years have a median survival of only 9.5 months with this approach and the survival is reduced to 4 months in those with unfavorable karyotypes, indicating a lack of benefit in this group.[411] In addition to the standard combination of anthracycline and cytarabine, other regimens, such as liposomal daunorubicin and topotecan with or without thalidomide, did not result in clinical benefit in patients with AML or high-risk MDS.[412] The so-called FLAG-Ida regimen (fludarabine, cytarabine, idarubicin, and G-CSF) resulted in 53 percent complete remissions and 11 percent improvement in 45 patients with high-risk myeloid malignancies, 13 of whom had MDS.[413] Gemtuzumab ozogamicin (Mylotarg), which is approved for treatment of relapsed AML in elderly patients, has not been useful for treatment of MDS.[414,415]

Hematopoietic Stem Cell Transplantation

Allogeneic Stem Cell Transplantation This approach has been used to treat various MDS in patients ranging in age from 1 month to older than 70 years.[416–418] It remains the only treatment with curative potential for MDS. Conditioning regimens have consisted of cyclophosphamide plus irradiation or busulfan plus cyclophosphamide. Most patients have received transplants from histocompatible sibling donors, although some experience with partially mismatched, related, and unrelated donors has been reported. A good representation of the results of this traditional approach using marrow stem cells is a study of 93 patients (age range: 1 month to older than 60 years; median age: 30 years).[419] The most favorable results were seen in patients younger than age 40 years with shorter duration of disease and with less than 5 percent blast cells in the marrow at the time of transplant. These patients may have a disease-free survival of 60 percent at 4 years and an overall disease-free survival estimated at 40 percent. Older patients had higher peritransplantation mortality and relapse rates. Actuarial relapse probability at 4 years was 30 percent for the entire group and 50 percent for patients with greater than 5 percent marrow blasts. Cytogenetic abnormalities did not predict outcome in this study, but adverse cytogenetics were an important prognostic factor in other studies. With targeted busulfan therapy, stem cell transplantation can be successfully performed in patients as old as 66 years of age.[420,421] Numerous factors such as disease stage, patient age, comorbidities, prior therapies, type of donor, and source of stem cells need to be weighed when recommending stem cell transplantation to MDS patients.

An International Bone Marrow Transplant Registry report of 452 patients with MDS who received allogeneic transplantation found that young age and platelet counts greater then 100×10^9/L prior to transplantation were associated with lower transplantation mortality, higher disease-free survival, and overall survival. Patients with higher percentage of blasts and high IPSS scores had higher relapse rates.[422] Blood or marrow stem cell sources can be utilized. One report showed superior results with mobilized blood versus marrow stem cells.[423]

The National Marrow Donor Program transplantation experience in MDS included 510 patients. Median age was 38 years, and the probability of disease-free survival at 2 years was 29 percent (confidence interval [CI] 25–33%). The 2-year incidence of treatment-related mortality was 54 percent, which was the major barrier to success in this patient population.[424] Unrelated cord blood transplantation for adult and pediatric patients with MDS has been successfully performed,[425] but results with unrelated marrow donors are inferior to the results of matched sibling transplants. It is anticipated that these results will improve in the era of high-resolution HLA matching between donor and recipient.[426]

Stem cell transplantation for MDS should be performed before the disease progresses to AML.[427] When T-cell depletion is used to prevent graft-versus-host disease, the best outcomes occur in those who are transplanted while in remission.[428] Poor cytogenetics may impact risk of relapse but not nonrelapse mortality.[429] In one retrospective series, blast percentage less than 5 percent at time of transplantation was the best predictor of improved disease-free survival, and myeloablative conditioning was associated with lower relapse risk but could not overcome increased disease burden.[430] Patients with secondary MDS have comparable outcomes after stem cell transplantation as those with *de novo* MDS when high-risk cytogenetics are considered.[431,432] Pretransplantation neutropenia is also associated with inferior outcomes as a result of infection-related mortality.[433] Prior therapy with demethylating agents does not appear to increase the toxicity of transplantation and whether it will improve outcomes by decreasing disease burden remains to be studied systematically.[434] The morbidity and mortality of various transplantation approaches remain high, and some patients are not candidates for ablative transplantation because of age or comorbid conditions.[435]

Reduced-intensity conditioning with allogeneic hematopoietic stem cell transplantation from HLA-identical family members or unrelated donors has been examined for MDS treatment.[436] In one series of 16 patients (median age: 54 years) receiving a conditioning regimen of fludarabine and cyclophosphamide, no day 100 transplantation-related mortality was observed, and the 2-year actuarial event-free survival was 56 percent (CI 30–68%). Other fludarabine-containing conditioning regimens have been reported.[437,438] One series compared reduced intensity to standard transplantation in MDS patients and noted similar 2-year overall and disease-free survival with different patterns of toxicity.[439] In some series, patients older than 70 years of age have undergone transplantation[440]; the future role this will play in therapy of older MDS patients is under investigation.[441] For those patients who relapse after reduced-intensity stem cell transplantation, salvage therapy with donor lymphocyte infusions, second transplantations, or chemotherapy may be feasible.[442,443]

Autologous Stem Cell Infusion Patients with oligoblastic leukemia have been infused with their own stem cells after intensive chemotherapy.[444] The approach may be limited by contamination of the stem cell product with a repopulating leukemic cell and the absence of a graft-versus-leukemia effect. The absence of a graft-versus-host reaction makes the approach more applicable to the age group usually affected. In selected patients, peritransplantation mortality with intensive therapy and stem cell rescue has been approximately 10 percent, and approximately 50 percent of selected patients had extended survivals.[445] The more advanced the disease at the time of treatment, the worse the outcome. With the increasing use of reduced-intensity allogeneic transplantation, autologous stem cell transplantation has been used less often. Interestingly, when autologous transplantations for AML are performed in patients with antecedent myelodysplasia, no impact on stem cell mobilization or hematopoietic recovery has been noted.[446]

■ OTHER THERAPIES IN USE OR UNDER STUDY IN MDS

Other Single-Agent Cytotoxic Drugs

Hydroxyurea and low-dose etoposide are useful in controlling leukemic cell proliferation but usually produce only partial responses and do not influence survival duration.[331] Occasional patients have achieved remissions with etoposide (50 mg as a 2-hour infusion, two to seven times weekly for 4 weeks; or 100 mg/day orally for 3 days and then 50 mg twice weekly).[447] Low-dose melphalan,[448] gemcitabine,[449] CPT-11, a DNA topoisomerase I inhibitor,[450] troxacitabine, an enantiomer of cytarabine,[451] and weekly doses of oral idarubicin[452] have each resulted in responses in some patients. Clofarabine, a purine nucleoside analogue, has activity in MDS.[453] Oral topotecan has only modest activity in MDS.[454] ABT-751, a microtubule inhibitor, is being studied in MDS.[455]

Antiangiogenesis Agents

Thalidomide has shown effectiveness in MDS therapy.[456] Patients receiving 100 to 400 mg/day for 12 or more weeks had no cytogenetic or complete responses, but 16 patients had hematologic improvement.[457] In another series of 34 patients in whom 400 mg/day was the median dose tolerated, 6 patients had progressive disease, 4 patients had stable disease, and 11 patients had partial remissions (5 major responses and 6 minor responses), accounting for a 56 percent response rate. Hematologic improvement was not noted until after a median of 2 months.[458] Cytogenetic responses have been seen in cases of monosomy 7, the 5q– syndrome, and with complex karyotypic abnormalities. Although thalidomide has antiangiogenesis activity, it also decreases vascular endothelial growth factor and basic fibroblast growth factor levels.[459] The drug may have a particular role in patients with marrow fibrosis.[460] Thromboembolic events have occurred in patients receiving thalidomide in combination with darbepoietin-α.[461]

The thalidomide derivative lenalidomide (Revlimid) lowers levels of proangiogenic cytokines, inhibits attachment of stromal cells, promotes cell-cycle arrest and apoptosis, and affects function of natural killer and cytotoxic T lymphocytes. In patients who have chromosome 5q deletion, lenalidomide has been found to reduce transfusion requirements and reverses cytogenetic abnormalities.[462] In patients without deletion 5q, reduction in transfusion requirements occur in approximately 43 percent with some patients becoming independent of transfusions. This trial included only low- or Int-1-risk MDS,[463] whereas 5q– patients who have high-risk MDS can show responses. Additional cytogenetic abnormalities limit the responses.[464] Unlike the case with thalidomide, dose reduction for myelosuppression often was required, and myelosuppression appears to be lenalidomide's primary toxicity.[465] In those patients with 5q deletion, cytopenias during therapy may be indicative of a response.[466]

Anti-Tumor Necrosis Factor Therapy

The soluble TNF receptor fusion protein etanercept (p75 TNFR:Fc) has produced mixed results in MDS. In one pilot series, moderate improvement in cytopenias was noted,[467] whereas in another trial, no responses were noted in 10 patients.[468] In another pilot study of 3 months duration, one patient became transfusion independent temporarily, but overall efficacy was low.[469] The chimeric anti–TNF-α monoclonal antibody infliximab resulted in two sustained erythroid responses (one major and one minor), and a decreased percentage of apoptotic cells in the marrow.[470] It is anticipated that therapies such as TNF inhibitors, which inhibit apoptosis, might be useful in low-grade MDS, whereas in high-grade MDS, therapies that promote apoptosis might be more effective.[471]

Agents That Alter Oxidation State

Amifostine has had minimal activity in MDS.[472] TLK199, a glutathione analogue inhibitor of glutathione S-transferase has resulted in hematologic improvement in early phase studies[473] and is still undergoing evaluation.

Retinoids, Vitamin D Derivatives, Arsenic Trioxide, and Other Potentially Maturation-Enhancing Agents

Glucocorticoids, vitamin A analogues (retinoids), vitamin D analogues (dihydroxyvitamin D_3), pyrimidine analogues (cytarabine), hexamethylene bisacetamide, and interferon are among other agents that can induce *in vitro* maturation of mouse and human leukemic cells.[474–476] Use of *cis*-retinoic acid, 20 to 100 mg/m^2, isotretinoin, 25 mg/m^2, or ATRA, 45 mg/ m^2, orally given daily for up to 3 months, has produced only slight, transient (few weeks) improvement in a very small proportion of patients with oligoblastic leukemia.[477,478]

A combination of low-dose cytarabine, retinoic acid, and 1,25-dihydroxyvitamin D_3 in 44 patients with oligoblastic leukemias produced 50 percent response rates, with longer survival in responders than in nonresponders.[479] Hexamethylene bisacetamide given intravenously at a dosage of 20 to 24 g/m^2 per day for 10 days, followed by an 18- to 75-day observation period, resulted in increased neutrophil counts and reduced marrow blasts in 4 of 16 patients with oligoblastic leukemia.[480] In another study, no responses were observed.[475] Sodium phenylbutyrate is an agent that has shown some activity against oligoblastic leukemia and is in clinical trials.[481]

Arsenic trioxide, used as a single agent, results in responses in approximately 20 percent of cases.[482] Low-risk MDS patients are most likely to show benefit.[483] Whether the drug affects cell maturation, apoptosis, or proliferation in this disease remains to be determined.[484–486]

Tyrosine Kinase and Other Cell-Signaling Inhibitors

Imatinib mesylate, the tyrosine kinase inhibitor of ABL, KIT, and platelet-derived growth factor receptor, has not resulted in clinical responses in patients with MDS.[487,488] Inhibitors of RAF protein kinase such as sorafenib,[489] and inhibitors of farnesyltransferase such as lonafarnib,[490] tipifarnib,[491,492] and BMS-214662,[493] have been examined in MDS. Statins that inhibit geranylgeranylation are being studied for treatment of AML and MDS.[494] Agents such as bortezomib, which indirectly target nuclear factor-κB, are being examined in MDS,[495–497] as are agents which target mTOR (mammalian target of rapamycin).[498] Progenitors involved in MDS rarely express FLT-3 mutations,[499] so FLT-3 inhibitors are not thought to be useful in the treatment of MDS.

UNCOMMON ACQUIRED SYNDROMES WITH INCREASED RISK OF ACUTE MYELOGENOUS LEUKEMIA

AMEGAKARYOCYTIC THROMBOCYTOPENIA

Amegakaryocytic thrombocytopenia may be congenital, associated with *MPL* gene mutations, or acquired,[500,501] and are both very uncommon preleukemic syndromes (<1%), although bona fide cases have transformed into AML months or years after diagnosis.[502,503] Among 1220 cases of MDS, 11 cases of isolated thrombocytopenia were associated with clonal chromosome abnormalities, usually involving chromosome 3, 5, 8, or 20. Antiplatelet antibodies were not present, and glucocorticoids were ineffective. Five of the 11 patients progressed to acute myelogenous leukemia (Table 88–6; see Chap. 119).[502]

ISOLATED NEUTROPENIA

Acquired, isolated, chronic neutropenic states are very rare antecedents of AML. Congenital neutropenia can evolve into AML.[504] The latter evolution is associated with mutations in the G-CSF-receptor (*CSF3R*) gene (see Chap. 65). Evolution of Shwachman-Diamond syndrome (neutropenia and exocrine pancreatic insufficiency) into oligoblastic or overt acute leukemia has been documented.[505] The related disorder, Pearson

TABLE 88–6. Hypocellular Marrow Syndromes That May Precede Onset of Acute Myelogenous Leukemia

Amegakaryocytic thrombocytopenia (Chap. 110)
Chronic hypoplastic neutropenia (Chap. 65)
Apparent aplastic anemia with evidence of clonal hematopoiesis (Chap. 34)
Paroxysmal nocturnal hemoglobinuria–aplastic anemia syndrome (Chaps. 34 and 40)

syndrome (sideroblastic anemia, neutropenia, and exocrine pancreatic insufficiency), is a preleukemia disorder in children (see Chap. 34).[506]

CHRONIC MONOCYTOSIS

In a small proportion of patients, unexplained persistent monocytosis may be the most striking blood cell abnormality for months or years before development of acute leukemia.[122–124]

APLASTIC ANEMIA, PAROXYSMAL NOCTURNAL HEMOGLOBINURIA, AND EOSINOPHILIC FASCIITIS

AML or MDS occurs in a proportion of patients with acquired aplastic anemia.[507,508] Since the advent of immunotherapy, the propensity to myelodysplasia and leukemia has increased, partly because of the greater longevity of patients and the often incomplete restitution of hematopoiesis. Patients who initially responded to immunosuppressive therapy have later developed MDS (see Chap. 34 for a discussion of the interrelationship among aplastic anemia, MDS, and paroxysmal nocturnal hemoglobinuria).[509]

Paroxysmal nocturnal hemoglobinuria is a clonal stem cell disease that often is associated with marrow hypoplasia (see Chap. 40). AML may ensue in approximately 0.5 percent of patients. It is a clonally derived syndrome with a low incidence of leukemic transformation relative to other clonal myeloid diseases. All chronic clonal hemopoietic stem cell disorders (e.g., polycythemia vera, essential thrombocythemia, idiopathic myelofibrosis, chronic myelogenous leukemia) have a propensity to undergo clonal evolution to AML (see Chap. 85). Patients with indolent myeloid clonal disorders may have a paroxysmal nocturnal hemoglobinuria-like defect of their blood cell membranes.

Eosinophilic fasciitis mimics the cutaneous manifestations of scleroderma. Symmetrical swelling and induration of arms and legs, sparing the hands and feet, are common.[510,511] Eosinophilia and hypergammaglobulinemia are frequent. Immune cytopenias, aplastic anemia, myelodysplasia, AML, and lymphoma have been associated with the disease.[512] An immune mechanism has been postulated for all the disease manifestations. The risk of developing AML is greatly increased compared with healthy individuals.[510–512] Marrow transplantation has been used to treat the aplastic anemia.[513]

PRODROMAL SYNDROMES ANTEDATING LYMPHOCYTIC LEUKEMIA

The indolent clonal disorders usually imply conditions that are an antecedent of myelogenous leukemia. A significant proportion of cases of AML are preceded by MDS. Even in *de novo* AML many cases have protracted periods of symptoms and signs before onset. ALL usually begins explosively, and symptoms rarely are present for more than a few weeks prior to diagnosis (see Chap. 93). Intermediate syndromes (e.g., smoldering or oligoblastic lymphocytic leukemia or prodromal anemias) are rare, but the latter have been reported, occasionally in children,[514] but especially in adults who develop ALL.[515–521]

Apparent aplastic anemia[522–526] or erythroid hypoplasia[527] has been described as an antecedent to ALL in approximately 2 percent of childhood cases and much less commonly in adult cases. The aplasia is promptly improved by glucocorticoids, and ALL ensues soon, usually within 1 to 8 months. The brief interval between remission of aplastic anemia and onset of leukemia suggests the leukemia, although inapparent on marrow biopsy, in some way initiates the aplasia.[522,528] Remission of aplasia followed shortly by ALL has occurred in the absence of glucocorticoid or other specific therapy in several cases. The aplastic marrow prodrome of ALL may be distinguishable by its very high prevalence in females (approximately 90%), high prevalence of fibrosis on marrow biopsy (approximately 90%), frequent marrow lymphocytosis (approximately 60%), and spontaneous, temporary recovery (>90%).[529]

INDOLENT CLONAL MYELOID DISORDERS OR OLIGOBLASTIC (MYELOGENOUS) LEUKEMIA PRECEDING OR EMERGING IN LYMPHOID MALIGNANCIES OTHER THAN ACUTE LYMPHOCYTIC LEUKEMIA

Sideroblastic anemia sometimes associated with qualitative disorders of other blood cell lines (such as thrombopathy) has developed in patients who had, or later developed, a lymphoproliferative disease, such as hairy cell leukemia, lymphocytic lymphoma, myeloma, chronic lymphocytic leukemia, or Hodgkin lymphoma.[530–538] The sideroblastic anemia in these cases was not preceded by cytotoxic therapy. Similar associations have been reported in patients who received chemotherapy or radiotherapy for a lymphoproliferative disease or a solid tumor and who later developed a preleukemic syndrome presumed to result from the prior treatment. Other types of myelodysplasia can occur concurrent with B- or T-lymphocyte–derived tumors.[530–539]

REFERENCES

1. Lichtman MA: Myelodysplasia or myeloneoplasia: Thoughts on the nosology of the clonal myeloid disorders. *Blood Cells Mol Dis* 26:572, 2000.
2. Brunning RD, Porwit A, Orazi A, et al: Myelodysplastic syndromes, in *WHO Classification of Tumors; Tumors of Haematopoietic and Lymphoid Tissues,* edited by SH Swerdlow, E Campo, NL Harris, ES Jaffe, SA Pileri, H Stein, J Thiele, JW Vardiman, p 87. IARC Press, Lyon, 2008.
3. Dreyfus B, Rochant H, Sultan C, et al: Les anémies réfractaires avec excès de myeloblastes dans la moelle. Etude de onze observations. *Presse Med* 78:359, 1970.
4. Layton DM, Mufti GJ: Myelodysplastic syndromes: Their history, evolution, and relation to acute myeloid leukemia. *Blut* 53:423, 1986.
5. Chevallier P: Sur la terminologie des leucoses et des affection frontières. Les odoleucoses. *Sang* 15:587, 1942–43.
6. Hamilton-Paterson JL: Preleukaemic anemia. *Acta Haematol* 2:309, 1949.
7. Block M, Jacobson LO, Bethard WJ: Preleukemic acute human leukemia. *JAMA* 152:1018, 1953.
8. Vilter RW, Jarrold T, Will JJ, et al: Refractory anemia with hyperplastic bone marrow. *Blood* 15:1, 1960.
9. Schiller M, Rachmilewitz EA, Izak G: Pancytopenia with hypercellular hemopoietic tissue. *Isr J Med Sci* 5:69, 1969.
10. Saarni MI, Linman JW: Preleukemia. *Am J Med* 55:38, 1973.
11. Linman JW, Saarni MI: The preleukemic syndrome. *Semin Hematol* 11:93, 1974.
12. Pierre RV: Preleukemic states. *Semin Hematol* 11:73, 1974.
13. Dreyfus B: Preleukemic states. I. Definition and classification. II. Refractory anemia with an excess of myeloblasts in the bone marrow (smoldering acute leukemia) *Blood Cells* 2:33, 1976.
14. Linman JW, Bagby GC Jr: The preleukemic syndrome: Clinical and laboratory features, natural course and management. *Blood Cells* 2:11, 1976.
15. Linman JW, Bagby GC Jr: The preleukemic syndrome (hemopoietic dysplasia). *Cancer* 42:854, 1978.
16. Izrael V, Jacquillat C, Chastang C, et al: New data about oligoblastic leukemias. Apropos of an analysis of 120 cases. *Nouv Presse Med* 4:947, 1975.
17. Bernard J, Izrael V, Jacquillat C: Oligoblastic leukemias. *Nouv Presse Med* 4:943, 1975.
18. Bessis M, Bernard J: Hematopoietic dysplasias. *Blood Cells* 2:5, 1976.
19. *WHO Classification of Tumors of Hematopoietic and Lymphoid Tissues, 4th ed.,* edited by SH Swerdlow, E Campo, NL Harris, ES Jaffe, SA Pileri, H Stein, J Thiele, JW Vardiman. WHO Press, Lyons, 2008.
20. Maynadie M, Picard F, Husson B, et al: Immunophenotypic clustering of myelodysplastic syndromes. *Blood* 100:2349, 2002.
21. Stetler-Stevenson M, Arthur DC, Jabbour N, et al: Diagnostic utility of flow cytometric immunophenotyping in myelodysplastic syndrome. *Blood* 98:979, 2001.
22. Groupe Francais de Morphologie Hématologique: French registry of acute leukemia and myelodysplastic syndromes. *Cancer* 60:1385, 1987.
23. Aul C, Gatterman N, Schneider W: Age-related incidence and other epidemiologic aspects of myelodysplastic syndrome. *Br J Haematol* 82:358, 1992.

24. McNally RJO, Rowland D, Roman E, Cartwright RA: Age and sex distributions of hematological malignancies in the U.K. *Hematol Oncol* 15:173, 1997.
25. Luna-Fineman S, Shannon KM, Atwater SK, et al: Myelodysplastic and myeloproliferative disorders of childhood: A study of 167 patients. *Blood* 93:459, 1999.
26. Novitzky N, Prindull G, for the European Society of Paediatric Haematology and Immunology: Myelodysplastic syndromes in children. *Am J Hematol* 63:212, 2000.
27. Hasle H, Niemeyer CM, Chessells JM, et al: A pediatric approach to the WHO classification of myelodysplastic and myeloproliferative diseases. *Leukemia* 17:277, 2003.
28. Sasaki H, Manabe A, Kojima S, et al: Myelodysplastic syndrome in childhood. *Leukemia* 15:713, 2001.
29. Kardos G, Baumann I, Passmore SJ, et al: Refractory anemia in childhood: A retrospective analysis of 67 patients with particular reference to monosomy 7. *Blood* 102:1997, 2003.
30. Ma X, Does M, Raza A, Mayne ST: Myelodysplastic syndromes: Incidence and survival in the United States. *Cancer* 109:1536, 2007.
31. Rollison DE, Howlader N, Smith MT, et al: Epidemiology of myelodysplastic syndromes and chronic myeloproliferative disorders in the United States, 2001–2004, using data from the NAACCR and SEER programs. *Blood* 112:45, 2008.
32. West RR, Stafford DA, White DT, et al: Cytogenetic abnormalities in the myelodysplastic syndromes and occupational or environmental exposure. *Blood* 95:2093, 2000.
33. Nisse C, Haguenoer JM, Grandbastien B, et al: Occupational and environmental risk factors of the myelodysplastic syndromes in the North of France. *Br J Haematol* 112:927, 2001.
34. Yin SN, Hayes RB, Linet MS, et al: A cohort study of cancer among benzene-exposed workers in China: Overall results. *Am J Ind Med* 29:227, 1996.
35. Snyder R: Benzene and leukemia. *Crit Rev Toxicol* 32:155, 2002.
36. Park DJ, Koeffler HP: Therapy-related myelodysplastic syndromes. *Semin Hematol* 33:256, 1996.
37. Rigolin GM, Cuneo A, Roberti MG, et al: Exposure to myelotoxic agents and myelodysplasia: Case-control study and correlation with clinicobiological findings. *Br J Haematol* 103:189, 1998.
38. Sterkers Y, Preudhomme C, Lai JL, et al: Acute myeloid leukemia and myelodysplastic syndromes following essential thrombocythemia treated with hydroxyurea: High proportion of cases with 17p deletion. *Blood* 91:616, 1998.
39. Van Den Neste E, Louviaux I, Michaux JL, et al: Myelodysplastic syndrome with monosomy 5 and/or 7 following therapy with 2-chloro-2′-deoxyadenosine. *Br J Haematol* 105:268, 1999.
40. Krishnan A, Bhatia S, Slovak ML, et al: Predictors of therapy-related leukemia and myelodysplasia following autologous transplantation for lymphoma. *Blood* 95:1588, 2000.
41. Abruzzese E, Radford JE, Miller JS, et al: Detection of abnormal pretransplant clones in progenitor cells of patients who developed myelodysplasia after autologous transplantation. *Blood* 94:1814, 2000.
42. Smith SH, Le Beau MM, Huo D, et al: Clinical-cytogenetic associations in 306 patients with therapy-related myelodysplasia and myeloid leukemia: The University of Chicago series. *Blood* 102:43, 2003.
43. Lobe I, Rigal-Huguet F, Vekhoff A, et al: Myelodysplastic syndrome after acute promyelocytic leukemia: The European APL group experience. *Leukemia* 17:1600, 2003.
44. Nakanishi M, Tanaka K, Shintani T, et al: Chromosomal instability in acute myelocytic leukemia and myelodysplastic syndrome patients among atomic bomb survivors. *J Radiat Res (Tokyo)* 40:159, 1999.
45. Finch SC: Myelodysplasia and radiation. *Radiat Res* 161:603, 2004.
46. Alter BP: Cancer in Fanconi's anemia 1923–2001. *Cancer* 97:425, 2003.
47. Segel GB, Lichtman MA: Familial (inherited) leukemia, lymphoma, and myeloma. *Blood Cells Mol Dis* 32:2004.
48. Horwitz M, Sabath DE, Smithson WA, Radich J: A family inheriting different subtypes of acute myelogenous leukemia. *Am J Hematol* 52:295, 1996.
49. Pradhan A, Mijovic A, Mills K, et al: Differentially expressed genes in adult familial myelodysplastic syndromes. *Leukemia* 18:449, 2004.
50. Kumar T, Mandla SG, Greer WL: Familial myelodysplastic syndrome with early age onset. *Am J Hematol* 64:53, 2000.
51. Griffith DP, Liff DA, Ziegler TR, et al: Acquired copper deficiency: A potentially serious and preventable complication following gastric bypass surgery. *Obesity (Silver Spring)* 17:827, 2009.
52. Fong T, Vij R, Vijayan A, et al: Copper deficiency: An important consideration in the differential diagnosis of myelodysplastic syndrome. *Haematologica* 92:1429, 2007.
53. Abkowitz JL, Fialkow PJ, Niebrugge DJ, et al: Pancytopenia as a clonal disorder of a multipotent hemopoietic stem cell. *J Clin Invest* 73:258, 1984.
54. Rasking WH, Tirumali N, Jacobson R, et al: Evidence for a multistep pathogenesis of a myelodysplastic syndrome. *Blood* 63:1318, 1984.
55. Mongkonsritragoon W, Letendre L, Li CY: Multiple lymphoid nodules in bone marrow have the same clonality as underlying myelodysplastic syndrome recognized with fluorescent in situ hybridization technique. *Am J Hematol* 59:252, 1998.
56. Janssen JWG, Buschle M, Layton M, et al: Clonal analysis of myelodysplastic syndromes: Evidence of multipotent stem cell origin. *Blood* 73:248, 1989.
57. Boultwood J, Weainscot JS: Clonality in the myelodysplastic syndromes. *Int J Hematol* 73:411, 2001.
58. Gerritsen WR, Donohue J, Bauman J, et al: Clonal analysis of myelodysplastic syndrome: Monosomy 7 is expressed in the myeloid lineage but not in the lymphoid lineage as detected by fluorescent in situ hybridization. *Blood* 80:217, 1992.
59. Anastasi J, Fang J, LeBeau MM, et al: Cytogenetic clonality in myelodysplastic syndromes studied with fluorescence *in situ* hybridization: Lineage, response to growth factor therapy, and clone expansion. *Blood* 81:1580, 1993.
60. Culligan DJ, Cachia P, Whittaker A, et al: Clonal lymphocytes are detectable in only some cases of MDS. *Br J Haematol* 81:346, 1992.
61. Abrahamson G, Boultwod J, Madden J, et al: Clonality of cell population in refractory anaemia using combined approach of gene loss and X-linked restricting fragment length polymorphism–methylation analysis. *Br J Haematol* 79:550, 1991.
62. Delforge M, Demuynck H, Verhoef G, et al: Patients with high risk myelodysplastic syndrome can have polyclonal or clonal haemopoiesis in complete haematological remission. *Br J Haematol* 102:486, 1998.
63. Lawrence HJ, Broudy VC, Magenis RE, et al: Cytogenetic evidence for involvement of B-lymphocytes in acquired idiopathic sideroblastic anemia. *Blood* 70:1003, 1982.
64. Meers S, Vandenberghe P, Boogaerts M, et al: The clinical significance of activated lymphocytes in patients with myelodysplastic syndromes: A single centre study of 131 patients. *Leuk Res* 32:1026, 2008.
65. Epling-Burnette PK, Painter JS, Rollison DE, et al: Prevalence and clinical association of clonal T-cell expansions in myelodysplastic syndrome. *Leukemia* 21:659, 2007.
66. Flores-Figueroa E, Montesinos JJ, Flores-Guzm·n P, et al: Functional analysis of myelodysplastic syndromes-derived mesenchymal stem cells. *Leuk Res* 32:1407, 2008.
67. Nakagawa T, Saitoh S, Imoto S, et al: Multiple point mutation of N-ras and K-ras oncogenes in myelodysplastic syndrome and acute myelogenous leukemia. *Oncology* 49:114, 1992.
68. VanKamp H, DePijper C, Verlaan-de Vries M, et al: Longitudinal analysis of point mutations of the N-ras protooncogene in patients with myelodysplasia using archival blood smears. *Blood* 79:1266, 1992.
69. Paquette RL, Landau EM, Pierre RV, et al: N-ras mutations are associated with poor prognosis and increased risk of leukemia in myelodysplastic syndrome. *Blood* 82:590, 1993.
70. Bartram CR: Molecular genetic aspects of myelodysplastic syndromes. *Semin Hematol* 33:139, 1996.
71. Parker J, Mufti GJ: Ras and myelodysplasia: Lessons from the last decade. *Semin Hematol* 33:206, 1996.
72. Padua RA, Guinn BA, Al-Sabah AI, et al: RAS, FMS and p53 mutations and poor clinical outcome in myelodysplasias: A 10-year follow-up. *Leukemia* 12:887, 1998.
73. Plata E, Viniou N, Abazis D, et al: Cytogenetic analysis and RAS mutations in primary myelodysplastic syndromes. *Cancer Genet Cytogenet* 111:124, 1999.
74. Quesnel B, Guillerm G, Vereecque R, et al: Methylation of the p15 (INK4b) gene in myelodysplastic syndromes is frequent and acquired during disease progression. *Blood* 91:2985, 1998.
75. Miyazato A, Ueno S, Ohmine K, et al: Identification of myelodysplastic syndrome-specific genes by DNA microarray analysis with purified hematopoietic stem cell fraction. *Blood* 98:422, 2001.
76. Fadilah SAW, Cheong SK, Roslan H, et al: *GATA-1* and *GATA-2* gene expression is related to the severity of dysplasia in myelodysplastic syndrome. *Leukemia* 16:1563, 2002.
77. Wulfert M, Küpper AC, Tapprich C, et al: Analysis of mitochondrial DNA in 104 patients with myelodysplastic syndromes. *Exp Hematol* 36:577, 2008.
78. Greenberg PL: Apoptosis and its role in the myelodysplastic syndromes: Implications for disease natural history and treatment. *Leuk Res* 22:1123, 1998.
79. Van de Loosdrecht AA, Vellenga E: Myelodysplasia and apoptosis. *Med Oncol* 17:16, 2000.
80. Huh YO, Jilani I, Estey E, et al: More cell death in refractory anemia with excess blasts in transformation than in acute myeloid leukemia. *Leukemia* 16:2249, 2002.
81. Raza A, Alvi S, Broady-Robinson L, et al: Cell cycle kinetic studies in 68 patients with myelodysplastic syndromes following intravenous iodo- and/or bromodeoxyuridine. *Exp Hematol* 25:530, 1997.
82. Gersuk GM, Beckham C, Loken MR, et al: A role for tumour necrosis factor-alpha, Fas and Fas-ligand in marrow failure associated with myelodysplastic syndrome. *Br J Haematol* 103:176, 1998.
83. Mundle SD, Ali A, Cartlidge JD, et al: Evidence for involvement of tumor necrosis factor-alpha in apoptotic death of bone marrow cells in myelodysplastic syndromes. *Am J Hematol* 60:36, 1999.
84. Parker JE, Fishlock KL, Mijovic A, et al: "Low-risk" myelodysplastic syndrome is associated with excessive apoptosis and an increased ratio of pro- versus anti-apoptotic bcl-2-related proteins. *Br J Haematol* 103:1075, 1998.
85. Gyan E, Frisan E, Beyne-Rauzy O, et al: Spontaneous and Fas-induced apoptosis of low-grade MDS erythroid precursors involves the endoplasmic reticulum. *Leukemia* 22:1864, 2008.
86. Meers S, Kasran A, Boon L, et al: Monocytes are activated in patients with myelodysplastic syndromes and can contribute to bone marrow failure through CD40-CD40L interactions with T helper cells. *Leukemia* 21:2411, 2007.
87. Amin HM, Jilani I, Estey EH, et al: Increased apoptosis in bone marrow B lymphocytes but not T lymphocytes in myelodysplastic syndrome. *Blood* 102:1866, 2003.
88. Baumann I, Scheid C, Koref MS, et al: Autologous lymphocytes inhibit hemopoiesis in long-term culture in patients with myelodysplastic syndrome. *Exp Hematol* 30:1045, 2002.
89. Moldrem J, Jiang Y, Stetler-Stevenson M, et al: Haematologic response of patients with myelodysplastic syndrome to antithymocyte globulin is associated with a loss of lymphocyte-mediated inhibition of CFU-GM and alterations in T cell receptor Vβ profiles. *Br J Haematol* 102:1314, 1998.

90. Epperson D, Nakamura R, Saunthararajah Y, et al: Oligoclonal T cell expansion in myelodysplastic syndrome: Evidence for an autoimmune process. *Leuk Res* 25:1075, 2001.
91. Marcondes AM, Mhyre AJ, Stirewalt DL, et al: Dysregulation of IL-32 in myelodysplastic syndrome and chronic myelomonocytic leukemia modulates apoptosis and impairs NK function. *Proc Natl Acad Sci U S A* 105:2865, 2008.
92. Rosenfeld C, List A: A hypothesis for the pathogenesis of myelodysplastic syndromes: Implications for new therapies. *Leukemia* 14:2, 2000.
93. Bagby GC: The preleukemic syndrome (hematopoietic dysplasia). *Blood Rev* 2:194, 1988.
94. Noel P, Solberg LA Jr: Myelodysplastic syndromes: Pathogenesis, diagnosis and treatment. *Crit Rev Oncol Hematol* 12:193, 1992.
95. Ahmad YH, Kiehl R, Papac RJ: Myelodysplasia. The clinical spectrum of 51 patients. *Cancer* 76:869, 1995.
96. Hebbar M, Hebbar-Savean K, Fenaux P: Systemic diseases in myelodysplastic syndromes. *Rev Med Interne* 16:897, 1995.
97. Saif MW, Hopkins JL, Gore SD: Autoimmune phenomena in patients with myelodysplastic syndromes and chronic myelomonocytic leukemia. *Leuk Lymphoma* 43:2409, 2002.
98. de la Chapelle A, Lahtinen R: Monosomy 7 predisposes to diabetes insipidus in leukaemia and myelodysplastic syndrome. *Eur J Haematol* 39:404, 1987.
99. Nakamura F, Kishimoto Y, Handa T, et al: Diabetes insipidus manifesting hypodipsic hypernatremia and dehydration. *Am J Hematol* 75:213, 2004.
100. Soppi E, Nousiainen T, Seppa A, et al: Acute febrile neutrophilic dermatosis (Sweet's syndrome) in association with myelodysplastic syndromes: A report of three cases and a review of the literature. *Br J Haematol* 73:43, 1989.
101. Arbetter KR, Hubbard KW, Markovic SN, et al: Case of granulocyte colony-stimulating factor-induced Sweet's syndrome. *Am J Hematol* 61:126, 1999.
102. Avi I, Rosenbaum H, Levy Y, Rowe J: Myelodysplastic syndrome and associated skin lesions: A review of the literature. *Leuk Res* 23:323, 1999.
103. Weber RFA, Geraedts JPM, Kerkhofs H, Leeksma CHW: The preleukemic syndrome. *Acta Med Scand* 207:391, 1980.
104. Ohno E, Ohtsuka E, Watanabe K, et al: Behçet's disease associated with myelodysplastic syndromes. A case report and a review of the literature. *Cancer* 79:262, 1997.
105. Komatsuda A, Miura I, Ohtani H, et al: Crescentic glomerulonephritis accompanied by myeloperoxidase-antineutrophil cytoplasmic antibodies in a patient having myelodysplastic syndrome with trisomy 7. *Am J Kidney Dis* 31:336, 1998.
106. Saitoh T, Murakami H, Uchiumi H, et al: Myelodysplastic syndromes with nephrotic syndrome. *Am J Hematol* 60:200, 1999.
107. Harewood GC, Loftus EV Jr, Tefferi A, et al: Concurrent inflammatory bowel disease and myelodysplastic syndromes. *Inflamm Bowel Dis* 5:98, 1999.
108. Lesprit P, Piette AM, Baumelou E, et al: Panniculitis and myelodysplasia: Report of 2 cases. *Eur J Med* 2:500, 1993.
109. Saif MW, Hopkins JL, Gore SD: Autoimmune phenomena in patients with myelodysplastic syndromes and chronic myelomonocytic leukemia. *Leuk Lymphoma* 43:2083, 2002.
110. Clark RE, Payne HE, Jacobs A: Primary myelodysplastic syndrome and cancer. *Br Med J* 294:937, 1987.
111. Sans-Sabrafen J, Buxó-Costa J, Woessner S, et al: Myelodysplastic syndromes and malignant solid tumors. *Am J Hematol* 41:1, 1992.
112. Florensa L, Vallespi T, Woessner S, et al: Incidence and characteristics of lymphoid malignancies in untreated myelodysplastic syndromes. *Leuk Lymphoma* 23:609, 1996.
113. Park S, Merlat A, Guesnu M, et al: Pure red cell aplasia associated with myelodysplastic syndromes. *Leukemia* 14:1709, 2000.
114. Choi JW, Kim Y, Fujino M, Ito M: Significance of fetal hemoglobin-containing erythroblasts (F blasts) and the F blast/F cell ratio in myelodysplastic syndromes. *Leukemia* 19:1478, 2002.
115. Kornberg A, Goldfarb A: Preleukemia manifested by hemolytic anemia with pyruvate-kinase deficiency. *Arch Intern Med* 146:785, 1986.
116. Harris JW, Koscick R, Lazarus HM, et al: Leukemia arising out of paroxysmal nocturnal hemoglobinuria. *Leuk Lymphoma* 32:401, 1999.
117. Lopez M, Bonnet-Gajdos M, Reviron M, et al: Acute leukemia augured before clinical signs by blood group antigen abnormalities and low levels of A and H blood group transferase activities in erythrocytes. *Br J Haematol* 63:535, 1986.
118. Anagnou NP, Ley TJ, Chesbro B, et al: Acquired α-thalassemia in pre-leukemia is due to decreased expression of all four α-globin genes. *Proc Natl Acad Sci U S A* 80:6051, 1983.
119. Helder J, Deisseroth A: S1 nuclease analysis of α-globin gene expression in preleukemic patients with acquired hemoglobin H disease after transfer to mouse erythroleukemia cells. *Proc Natl Acad Sci U S A* 84:2387, 1987.
120. Steensma DP, Higgs DR, Fisher CA, Gibbons RJ: Acquired somatic *ATRX* mutations in myelodysplastic syndrome associated with α-thalassemia (ATMDS) convey a more severe hematological phenotype than germline *ATRX* mutations. *Blood* 103:2019, 2004.
121. Group Française de Morphologie Hématologique: French registry of acute leukemia and myelodysplastic syndromes. *Cancer* 60:1385, 1987.
122. Jaworkowsky LI, Solovey DY, Rhausova LY, Udris OY: Monocytosis as a sign of subsequent leukemia in patients with cytopenias (preleukemia). *Folia Haematol (Frankf)* 110:395, 1983.
123. Friedland ML, Ward H, Wittels EG, Arlin ZA: A monocytic leukemoid reaction: A manifestation of preleukemia. *R I Med J* 68:173, 1985.
124. Economopoulos T, Stathakis N, Maragoyannis Z, et al: Myelodysplastic syndrome. Clinical significance of monocyte concentration, degree of blastic infiltration and ring sideroblasts. *Acta Haematol* 65:97, 1981.
125. Shetty VT, Mundle SD, Raza A: Pseudo Pelger-Huët anomaly in myelodysplastic syndrome: Hyposegmented or apoptotic neutrophil? *Blood* 98:1273, 2001.
126. Langenhuijsen MM: Neutrophils with ring-shaped nuclei in myeloproliferative disease. *Br J Haematol* 58:227, 1984.
127. Clark RE, Smith SA, Jacobs A: Myeloid surface antigen abnormalities in myelodysplasia: Relation to prognosis and modification by 13-*cis* retinoic acid. *J Clin Pathol* 40:652, 1987.
128. Cech P, Markert M, Perrin LH: Partial myeloperoxidase deficiency in preleukemia. *Blut* 47:21, 1983.
129. Schofield KP, Stone PCW, Kelsey P, et al: Quantitative cytochemistry of blood neutrophils in myelodysplastic syndromes and chronic granulocytic leukaemia. *Cell Biochem Funct* 1:92, 1983.
130. Elghetany MT, Peterson B, MacCallum J, et al: Deficiency of neutrophilic granule membrane glycoproteins in the myelodysplastic syndromes: A common deficiency in 216 patients studied by the Cancer and Leukemia Group B. *Leuk Res* 21:801, 1997.
131. Ruutu P: Granulocyte function in myelodysplastic syndromes. *Scand J Haematol* 36(Suppl 45):66, 1986.
132. Prodan M, Tulissi P, Perticarari S, et al: Flow cytometric assay for the evaluation of phagocytosis and oxidative burst of polymorphonuclear leukocytes and monocytes in myelodysplastic disorders. *Haematologica* 80:212, 1995.
133. Piva E, De Toni S, Caenazzo A, et al: Neutrophil NADPH oxidase activity in chronic myeloproliferative and myelodysplastic diseases by microscopic and photometric assays. *Acta Haematol* 94:16, 1995.
134. Carulli G, Sbrana S, Minnucci S, et al: Actin polymerization in neutrophils from patients affected by myelodysplastic syndromes—A flow cytometric study. *Leuk Res* 21:513, 1997.
135. Nakaseko C, Asai T, Wakita H, et al: Signaling defect in FMLP-induced neutrophil respiratory burst in myelodysplastic syndromes. *Br J Haematol* 95:482, 1996.
136. Pamphilon DH, Aparicio SR, Roberts BE, et al: The myelodysplastic syndromes—A study of haemostatic function and platelet ultrastructure. *Scand J Haematol* 33:486, 1984.
137. Payne CM, Glasser L: An ultrastructural morphometric analysis of platelet grant and fusion granules. *Blood* 67:299, 1986.
138. Rasi V, Lintula R: Platelet-function in the myelodysplastic syndromes. *Scand J Haematol* 36(Suppl 45):71, 1986.
139. Hamblin TJ: Immunological abnormalities in myelodysplastic syndromes. *Semin Hematol* 33:150, 1996.
140. Anderson RW, Volsky DJ, Greenberg B, et al: Lymphocyte abnormalities in preleukemia: I. Decreased NK activity, anomalous immunoregulatory cell subsets and deficient EBV receptors. *Leuk Res* 7:389, 1983.
141. Kerndrup G, Meyer K, Ellegaard J, Hokland P: Natural killer (NK)-cell activity and antibody-dependent cellular cytotoxicity (ADCC) in primary preleukemic syndrome. *Leuk Res* 8:239, 1984.
142. Takagi S, Kitagawa S, Takeda A, et al: Natural killer–interferon system in patients with preleukaemic states. *Br J Haematol* 58:71, 1984.
143. Volsky DJ, Anderson RW: Deficiency in Epstein-Barr virus receptors on B lymphocytes of preleukemia patients. *Cancer Res* 43:3923, 1983.
144. Knox SJ, Greenberg BR, Anderson RW, Rosenblatt LS: Studies of T lymphocytes in preleukemic disorders and acute nonlymphocytic leukemia: In vitro radiosensitivity, mitogenic responsiveness, colony formation, and enumeration of lymphocytic subpopulations. *Blood* 61:449, 1983.
145. Baumann MA, Milson TJ, Patrick CW, et al: Immunoregulatory abnormalities in myelodysplastic disorders. *Am J Hematol* 22:17, 1986.
146. Economopoulos T, Economidou J, Giannopoulos G, et al: Immune abnormalities in myelodysplastic syndromes. *J Clin Pathol* 38:908, 1985.
147. Mufti GJ, Figes A, Hamblin TJ, et al: Immunological abnormalities in myelodysplastic syndromes. *Br J Haematol* 63:143, 1986.
148. Gatto S, Ball G, Onida F, et al: Contribution of β-2 microglobulin levels to the prognostic stratification of survival in patients with myelodysplastic syndrome (MDS). *Blood* 102:1622, 2003.
149. Takagi S, Tanaka O, Miura Y: Magnetic resonance imaging of femoral marrow in patients with myelodysplastic syndromes or leukemia. *Blood* 86:316, 1995.
150. Delacretaz F, Schmidt PM, Piguet D, et al: Histopathology and myelodysplastic syndromes: The FAB classification (proposals) applied to bone marrow biopsy. *Am J Clin Pathol* 87:180, 1987.
151. Yue G, Hao S, Fadare O, et al: Hypocellularity in myelodysplastic syndrome is an independent factor which predicts a favorable outcome. *Leuk Res* 32:553, 2008.
152. Fohlmeister I, Fischer R, Modder B, et al: Aplastic anemia and hypocellular myelodysplastic syndrome. *J Clin Pathol* 38:1218, 1985.
153. Kuriyama K, Tomonaga M, Matsuo T, et al: Diagnostic significance of pseudo Pelger Huët anomalies and micro-megakaryocytes in myelodysplastic syndrome. *Br J Haematol* 63:665, 1986.
154. Tricot G, DeWolf-Peeters C, Vlietinck R, Verwilghen RL: Bone marrow histology in myelodysplastic syndromes. II. Prognostic value of ALIP in MDS. *Br J Haematol* 58:217, 1984.
155. Mangi MH, Mufti GJ: Primary myelodysplastic syndromes: Diagnostic and prognostic significance of immunohistochemical assessment of bone marrow biopsies. *Blood* 79:198, 1992.
156. Della Porta MG, Malcovati L, Boveri E, et al: Clinical relevance of bone marrow fibrosis and cd34-positive cell clusters in primary myelodysplastic syndromes. *J Clin Oncol* 27:754, 2009.

157. Bellamy WT, Richter L, Sirjani D, et al: Vascular endothelial cell growth factor (VEGF) is an autocrine promoter of abnormal localized immature precursors (ALIP) and leukemia progenitor formation in myelodysplastic syndromes. *Blood* 97:1427, 2001.
158. Matsushima T, Handa H, Yokohama A, et al: Prevalence and clinical characteristics of myelodysplastic syndrome with bone marrow eosinophilia or basophilia. *Blood* 101:3386, 2003.
159. Smith WB, Ablin A, Goodman JR, Brecher J: Atypical megakaryocytes in the preleukemic phase of AML. *Blood* 42:535, 1973.
160. Queisser W, Queisser U, Ansmann M, et al: Megakaryocyte polyploidization in acute leukemia and preleukemia. *Br J Haematol* 28:261, 1974.
161. Bartl R, Frisch B, Baumgart R: Morphologic classification of the myelodysplastic syndromes (MDS): Combined utilization of bone marrow aspirates and trephine biopsies. *Leuk Res* 16:15, 1992.
162. Maschek H, Georgii A, Kaloutsi V, et al: Myelofibrosis in primary myelodysplastic syndromes: A retrospective study of 352 patients. *Eur J Haematol* 148:208, 1992.
163. Moehler TM, Ho AD, Goldschmidt H, Barlogie B: Angiogenesis in hematological malignancies. *Crit Rev Oncol Hematol* 45:227, 2003.
164. Ribatti D, Polimeno G, Vacca A, et al: Correlation of bone marrow angiogenesis and mast cells with tryptase activity in myelodysplastic syndromes. *Leukemia* 16:1680, 2002.
165. Della Porta MG, Malcovati L, Rigolin GM, et al: Immunophenotypic, cytogenetic and functional characterization of circulating endothelial cells in myelodysplastic syndromes. *Leukemia* 22:530, 2008.
166. Greenberg PL: Biologic and clinical implications of marrow culture studies in the myelodysplastic syndromes. *Semin Hematol* 33:163, 1996.
167. Chui DHK, Clarke BJ: Abnormal erythroid progenitor cells in human preleukemia. *Blood* 60:362, 1982.
168. Senn JS, Messner HA, Pinkerton PH, et al: Peripheral blood blast cell progenitors in human preleukemia. *Blood* 59:106, 1982.
169. Juvonen E, Partanen S, Knuutila S, Ruutu T: Megakaryocyte colony formation by bone marrow progenitors in myelodysplastic syndrome. *Br J Haematol* 63:331, 1986.
170. Lidbeck J: In vitro colony and cluster growth haemopoietic dysplasia (the preleukaemic syndrome): I. Clinical correlations. *Scand J Haematol* 24:412, 1980.
171. Raymakers R, DeWitte T, Joziasse J, et al: *In vitro* growth pattern and differentiation predict for progression of myelodysplastic syndromes to acute nonlymphocytic leukemia. *Br J Haematol* 78:35, 1991.
172. Konwalinka G, Peschel C, Schmalzl F, et al: CFU-GM assay, cytochemical and electron microscopic studies in agar in patients with preleukemia syndrome and aplastic anemia. *Int J Cell Cloning* 3:367, 1985.
173. Cambier N, Baruchel A, Schlageter MH, et al: Chronic myelomonocytic leukemia: From biology to therapy. *Hematol Cell Ther* 39:41, 1997.
174. Aul C, Gatterman N, Schneider W: Comparison of in vitro growth characteristics of blast cell progenitors (CFU-BL) in patients with myelodysplastic syndromes and acute myeloid leukemia. *Blood* 80:625, 1992.
175. Flores-Figueroa E, Gutierrez-Espindola G, Guerrero-Rivera S, et al: Hematopoietic progenitor cells from patients with myelodysplastic syndromes: *In vitro* colony growth and long-term proliferation. *Leuk Res* 23:385, 1999.
176. Sato T, Kim S, Selleri C, et al: Measurement of secondary colony formation after 5 weeks in long-term cultures in patients with myelodysplastic syndrome. *Leukemia* 12:1187, 1998.
177. Aizawa S, Nakano M, Iwase O, et al: Bone marrow stroma from refractory anemia of myelodysplastic syndrome is defective in its ability to support normal CD34-positive cell proliferation and differentiation in vitro. *Leuk Res* 23:239, 1999.
178. Janowska-Wieczorek A, Bilch AR, Jacobs A: Increased circulating colony-stimulating factor-1 in patients with preleukemia, leukemia, and lymphoid malignancies. *Blood* 77:1796, 1991.
179. Verhoef GEG, DeSchouder P, Ceuppens JL: Measurement of serum cytokine levels in patients with myelodysplastic syndromes. *Leukemia* 6:1268, 1992.
180. Bowen D, Yancik S, Bennett L, et al: Serum stem cell factor concentration in patients with myelodysplastic syndromes. *Br J Haematol* 85:63, 1993.
181. Zwierzina H, Anderson JE, Rollinger-Holzinger I, et al: Endogenous FLT-3 ligand serum levels are associated with disease stage in patients with myelodysplastic syndromes. *Leukemia* 13:553, 1999.
182. Tamura H, Ogata K, Luo S, et al: Plasma thrombopoietin (TPO) levels and expression of TPO receptor on platelets in patients with myelodysplastic syndromes. *Br J Haematol* 103:778, 1998.
183. Mecucci C, La Starza R: Cytogenetics of myelodysplastic syndromes. *Forum (Genova)* 9:4, 1999.
184. Haase D: Cytogenetic features in myelodysplastic syndromes. *Ann Hematol* 87:515, 2008.
185. Solé F, Luño E, Sanzo C, et al: Identification of novel cytogenetic markers with prognostic significance in a series of 968 patients with primary myelodysplastic syndromes. *Haematologica* 90:1168, 2005.
186. Estey E, Trujillo JM, Cork A, et al: AML-associated cytogenetic abnormalities inv ((16), del (16), t(8;21)) in patients with myelodysplastic syndromes. *Hematol Pathol* 6:43, 1992.
187. Block AW, Carroll AJ, Hagemeijer A, et al: Rare recurring balanced chromosome abnormalities in therapy-related myelodysplastic syndromes and acute leukemia. *Genes Chromosomes Cancer* 33:401, 2002.
188. Rossi G, Pelizzari AM, Bellotti D, et al: Cytogenetic analogy between myelodysplastic syndrome and acute myeloid leukemia of elderly patients. *Leukemia* 14:636, 2000.
189. Zhang L, Rothman N, Wang Y, et al: Increased aneusomy and long arm deletion of chromosomes 5 and 7 in the lymphocytes of Chinese workers exposed to benzene. *Carcinogenesis* 19:1955, 1998.
190. Olney HJ, Le Beau MM: The cytogenetics and molecular biology of myelodysplastic syndromes, in *The Myelodysplastic Syndromes*, edited by JM Bennett, p 89. Marcel Dekker, New York, 2002.
191. Wong AK, Fang B, Zhang L, et al: Loss of the Y chromosome: An age-related or clonal phenomenon in acute myelogenous leukemia/myelodysplastic syndrome? *Arch Pathol Lab Med* 132:1329, 2008.
192. Xie D, Hofmann W-K, Mori N, et al: Allelotype analysis of the myelodysplastic syndrome. *Leukemia* 14:805, 2000.
193. Hoffman W-K, De Vos S, Komor M, et al: Characterization of gene expression of CD34+ cells from normal and myelodysplastic bone marrow. *Blood* 100:3553, 2002.
194. Bernasconi P: Molecular pathways in myelodysplastic syndromes and acute myeloid leukemia: Relationships and distinctions: A review. *Br J Haematol* 142:695, 2008.
195. Cesana C, Klersy C, Brando B, et al: Prognostic value of circulating CD34+ cells in myelodysplastic syndromes. *Leuk Res* 32:1715, 2008.
196. Nilsson L, EdÈn P, Olsson E, et al: The molecular signature of MDS stem cells supports a stem-cell origin of 5q myelodysplastic syndromes. *Blood* 110:3005, 2007.
197. Van den Berghe H, Cassiman JJ, David G, et al: Distinct haematological disorder with deletion of long arm of no. 5 chromosome. *Nature* 251:437, 1974.
198. Boultwood J, Lewis S, Wainscoat JS, et al: The 5q− syndrome. *Blood* 84:3253, 1994.
199. Washington LT, Doherty D, Glassman A, et al: Myeloid disorders with deletion 5q as the sole karyotypic abnormality: The clinical spectrum and pathological spectrum. *Leuk Lymphoma* 43:761, 2002.
200. Van den Berghe H, Michaux L: 5q-, twenty-five years later: A synopsis. *Cancer Genet Cytogenet* 94:1, 1997.
201. Bigoni R, Cuneo A, Milani R, et al: Multilineage involvement in the 5q− syndrome: A fluorescent *in situ* hybridization study on bone marrow smears. *Haematologica* 86:375, 2001.
202. Anderson K, Arvidsson I, Jacobsson B, Hast R: Fluorescence in situ hybridization for the study of cell lineage involvement in myelodysplastic syndromes with chromosome 5 anomalies. *Cancer Genet Cytogenet* 136:101, 2002.
203. Jaju RJ, Jones M, Boultwood J, et al: Combined immunophenotyping and FISH identifies the involvement of B-C cells in 5q− syndrome. *Genes Chromosomes Cancer* 29:276, 2000.
204. Nilsson L, Astrand-Grundastrom I, Arvidsson I, et al: Isolation and characterization of hematopoietic progenitor/stem cells in 5q-deleted myelodysplastic syndromes: Evidence for involvement at the hematopoietic stem cell level. *Blood* 96:2012, 2000.
205. Cermak J, Michalova K, Brezinova J, Zemanova Z: A prognostic impact of separation of refractory cytopenia with multilineage dysplasia and 5q− syndrome from refractory anemia in primary myelodysplastic syndrome. *Leuk Res* 27:221, 2003.
206. Giagounidis AAN, Germing U, Haase S, et al: Clinical, morphological, cytogenetics, and prognostic features of patients with myelodysplastic syndrome and del(5q) including band q31. *Leukemia* 18:113, 2004.
207. Washington LT, Dherty D, Glassman A, et al: Myeloid disorders with deletion of 5q as sole karyotypic abnormality: The clinical and pathological spectrum. *Leuk Lymphoma* 43:761, 2002.
208. Pedersen B: Anatomy of the 5q− deletion: Different sex ratios and deleted 5q bands in MDS and AML. *Leukemia* 10:1883, 1996.
209. Mohamedali A, Mufti GJ: Van-den Berghe's 5q− syndrome in 2008. *Br J Haematol* 144:157, 2009.
210. Ebert BL, Pretz J, Bosco J, et al: Identification of RPS14 as a 5q− syndrome gene by RNA interference screen. *Nature* 451:335, 2008.
211. Mauro VP, Edelman GM: The ribosome filter redux. *Cell Cycle* 6:2246, 2007.
212. Pellagatti A, Hellström-Lindberg E, Giagounidis A, et al: Haploinsufficiency of RPS14 in 5q− syndrome is associated with deregulation of ribosomal- and translation-related genes. *Br J Haematol* 142:57, 2008.
213. Joslin JM, Fernald AA, Tennant TR, et al: Haploinsufficiency of EGR1, a candidate gene in the del(5q), leads to the development of myeloid disorders. *Blood* 110:719, 2007.
214. Kelaidi C, Eclache V, Fenaux P: The role of lenalidomide in the management of myelodysplasia with del 5q. *Br J Haematol* 140:267, 2008.
215. Melchert M, Kale V, List A: The role of lenalidomide in the treatment of patients with chromosome 5q deletion and other myelodysplastic syndromes. *Curr Opin Hematol* 14:123, 2007.
216. Mohr B, Oelschlaegel U, Thiede C, et al; The response to lenalidomide of myelodysplastic syndrome patients with deletion del(5q) can be sequentially monitored in CD34+ progenitor cells. *Haematologica* 94:430, 2009.
217. Bernstein R, Philip P, Ueshima Y: Fourth international workshop on chromosomes in leukemia 1982. Abnormalities of chromosome 7 resulting in monosomy 7 or in deletion of the long arm (7q−): Review of translocations, breakpoints, and associated abnormalities. *Cancer Genet Cytogenet* 11:300, 1984.
218. Michiels JJ, Mallios-Zorbala H, Prins MEF, et al: Simple monosomy 7 and myelodysplastic syndrome in thirteen patients without previous cytostatic treatment. *Br J Haematol* 64:425, 1986.
219. Pasquali F, Bernasconi P, Cosalone R, et al: Pathogenetic significance of "pure" monosomy 7 in myeloproliferative disorders. Analysis of 14 cases. *Hum Genet* 62:40, 1982.
220. Kardos G, Baumann I, Passmore SJ, et al: Refractory anemia in childhood: A retrospective analysis of 67 patients with particular reference to monosomy 7. *Blood* 102:1997, 2003.

221. Brozek I, Babinska M, Kardas I, et al: Cytogenetic analysis and clinical significance of chromosome 7 aberrations in acute leukemia. *J Appl Genet* 44:401, 2003.
222. Dohner K, Brown J, Hehmann U, et al: Molecular cytogenetic characterization of a critical region in bands 7q35-q36 commonly deleted in malignant myeloid disorders. *Blood* 92:4031, 1998.
223. Sessarego M, Fugazza G, Gobbi M, et al: Complex structural involvement of chromosome 7 in primary myelodysplastic syndromes determined by fluorescence in situ hybridization. *Cancer Genet Cytogenet* 106:110, 1998.
224. Hayashi Y, Egushi M, Sugita K, et al: Cytogenetic findings and clinical features in acute leukemia and transient myeloproliferation disorder in Down's syndrome. *Blood* 72:15, 1988.
225. Berger R, LeConiat M, Schaison G: Chromosome abnormalities in bone marrow of Fanconi anemia patients. *Cancer Genet Cytogenet* 65:47, 1993.
226. Minelli A, Maserati E, Giudici G, et al: Familial partial monosomy 7 and myelodysplasia: Different parental origin of monosomy 7 suggests action of a mutator gene. *Cancer Genet Cytogenet* 124:147, 2001.
227. Smadja N, Krulik M, DeGramont A, et al: Translocation 1;7 in preleukemic states. *Cancer Genet Cytogenet* 18:189, 1985.
228. Woloschak GF, Dewald GW, Gahn RS, et al: Amplification of RNA and DNA specific for erb B in unbalanced 1;7 chromosomal translocation associated with myelodysplastic syndrome. *J Cell Biochem* 32:23, 1986.
229. Ueda H, Tashiro S, Kojima S, et al: Instability of chromosome 7 in colony forming cells of patients with aplastic anemia. *Int J Hematol* 70:13, 1999.
230. Kaito K, Kobayashi M, Katayama T, et al: Long-term administration of G-CSF for aplastic anemia is closely related too the early evolution of monosomy 7 MDS in adults. *Br J Haematol* 103:297, 1998.
231. Bjorkman SE: Chronic refractory anemia with sideroblastic bone marrow. A study of four cases. *Blood* 11:250, 1956.
232. Kushner JP, Lee GR, Wintrobe MM, et al: Idiopathic refractory sideroblastic anemia. *Medicine (Baltimore)* 50:139, 1971.
233. Boultwood J, Pellagatti A, Nikpour M, et al: The role of the iron transporter ABCB7 in refractory anemia with ring sideroblasts. *PLoS ONE* 3:e1970, 2008.
234. Chang KL, O'Donnell MR, Slovak ML, et al: Primary myelodysplasia occurring in adults under 50 years old: A clinicopathologic study of 52 patients. *Leukemia* 16:623, 2002.
235. Kardos G, Veerman AJ, De Waal FC, et al: Familial sideroblastic anemia with emergence of monosomy 5 and myelodysplastic syndrome. *Med Pediatr Oncol* 26:54, 1996.
236. Garand R, Gardars J, Bizet M, et al: Heterogeneity of acquired idiopathic sideroblastic anemia (AISA). *Leuk Res* 16:463, 1992.
237. Bowen DT, Jacobs A: Primary acquired sideroblastic erythropoiesis in non-anaemic and minimally anaemic subjects. *J Clin Pathol* 42:56, 1989.
238. Antilla P, Thalainen J, Salo A, et al: Idiopathic macrocytic anaemia in the aged: Molecular and cytogenetic findings. *Br J Haematol* 90:797, 1995.
239. Steensma DP, Dewald GW, Hodnfield JM, et al: Clonal cytogenetic abnormalities in bone marrow specimens without clear morphologic evidence of dysplasia: A form fruste of myelodysplasia? *Leuk Res* 27:235, 2003.
240. Yoshida Y, Oguma S, Tohyama K, et al: Diagnostic and biological significance of sideroblastic erythropoiesis in the myelodysplastic syndromes. *Int J Hematol* 67:137, 1998.
241. Beris PH, Graf J, Miescher PA: Primary acquired sideroblastic and primary acquired refractory anemia. *Semin Hematol* 20:101, 1983.
242. Mecucci C, Van Orshoven A, Vermaelen K, et al: 11q– chromosome is associated with abnormal iron stores in myelodysplastic syndromes. *Cancer Genet Cytogenet* 27:39, 1987.
243. Parlier V, Van Melle G, Beris PH, et al: Hematological, clinical, and cytogenetic analysis in 109 in patients with primary myelodysplastic syndrome. *Cancer Genet Cytogenet* 78:219, 1994.
244. Berrebi A, Bruck R, Shtalrid M, Chemke J: Philadelphia chromosome in idiopathic acquired sideroblastic anemia. *Acta Haematol* 72:343, 1984.
245. Carroll AJ, Poon M-C, Robinson NC, Christ WM: Sideroblastic anemia associated with thrombocytosis and a chromosome 3 abnormality. *Cancer Genet Cytogenet* 22:183, 1986.
246. Bennett DD, Stanley WS, Johnson CB: Combined phenotypic and genotypic analysis of ringed sideroblasts in acquired idiopathic sideroblastic anemia. *Acta Haematol* 73:235, 1985.
247. DeWald GW, Brecher M, Travis LB, Stupea PJ: Twenty-six patients with hematologic disorders and X-chromosome abnormalities. *Cancer Genet Cytogenet* 42:173, 1989.
248. Remacha AF, Nomdedéu JF, Puget G, et al: Occurrence of the JAK2 V617F mutation in the WHO provisional entity: Myelodysplastic/myeloproliferative disease, unclassifiable-refractory anemia with ringed sideroblasts associated with marked thrombocytosis. *Haematologica* 91:719, 2006.
249. Szpurka H, Tiu R, Murugesan G, et al: Refractory anemia with ringed sideroblasts associated with marked thrombocytosis (RARS-T), another myeloproliferative condition characterized by JAK2 V617F mutation. *Blood* 108:2173, 2006.
250. Schmitt-Graeff AH, Teo SS, Olschewski M, et al: JAK2V617F mutation status identifies subtypes of refractory anemia with ringed sideroblasts associated with marked thrombocytosis. *Haematologica* 93:34, 2008.
251. Chabannori G, Molina L, Pegouri-Bandelier B, et al: A review of 76 patients with myelodysplastic syndromes treated with danazol. *Cancer* 73:3073, 1994.
252. Chan G, DiVenuti G, Miller K: Danazol for the treatment of thrombocytopenia in patients with myelodysplastic syndrome. *Am J Hematol* 71:166, 2002.
253. Sadek I, Zayed E, Hayne O, Fernandez L: Prolonged complete remission of myelodysplastic syndrome treated with danazol, retinoic acid and low-dose prednisone. *Am J Hematol* 64:306, 2000.
254. Dreyfus F: The deleterious effects of iron overload in patients with myelodysplastic syndromes. *Blood Rev* 22(Suppl 2):S29, 2008.
255. Steensma DP: Myelodysplasia paranoia: Iron as the new radon. *Leuk Res* 33:1158, 2009.
256. Messa E, Cilloni D, Messa F, et al: Deferasirox treatment improved the hemoglobin level and decreased transfusion requirements in four patients with the myelodysplastic syndrome and primary myelofibrosis. *Acta Haematol* 120:70, 2008.
257. Bennett JM: MDS Foundation's Working Group on Transfusional Iron Overload. Consensus statement on iron overload in myelodysplastic syndromes. *Am J Hematol* 83:858, 2008.
258. Yang LP, Keam SJ, Keating GM: Deferasirox: A review of its use in the management of transfusional chronic iron overload. *Drugs* 67:2211, 2007.
259. Hellström-Lindberg E, Gulbrandsen N, Lindberg G, et al: A validated decision model for treating the anaemia of myelodysplastic syndromes with erythropoietin + granulocyte colony-stimulating factor: Significant effects on quality of life. *Br J Haematol* 120:1037, 2003.
260. Casadevall N, Durieux P, Dubois S, et al: Health, economic, and quality-of-life effects of erythropoietin and granulocyte colony-stimulating factor for the treatment of myelodysplastic syndromes: A randomized, controlled trial. *Blood* 104:321, 2004.
261. Balleari E, Rossi E, Clavio M, et al: Erythropoietin plus granulocyte colony-stimulating factor is better than erythropoietin alone to treat anemia in low-risk myelodysplastic syndromes: Results from a randomized single-centre study. *Ann Hematol* 85:174, 2006.
262. Jädersten M, Malcovati L, Dybedal I, et al: Erythropoietin and granulocyte-colony stimulating factor treatment associated with improved survival in myelodysplastic syndrome. *J Clin Oncol* 26:3607, 2008.
263. Silverman LR, McKenzie DR, Peterson BL, et al: Further analysis of trials with azacitidine in patients with myelodysplastic syndrome: Studies 8421, 8921, and 9221 by the Cancer and Leukemia Group B. *J Clin Oncol* 24:3895, 2006.
264. Müller-Thomas C, Schuster T, Peschel C, Götze KS: A limited number of 5-azacitidine cycles can be effective treatment in MDS. *Ann Hematol* 88:213, 2009.
265. Kaminskas E, Farrell A, Abraham S, et al: Approval summary: Azacitidine for treatment of myelodysplastic syndrome subtypes. *Clin Cancer Res* 11:3604, 2005.
266. Gore SD, Hermes-DeSantis ER: Future directions in myelodysplastic syndrome: Newer agents and the role of combination approaches. *Cancer Control* 15(Suppl):40, 2008.
267. Kornblith AB, Herndon JE II, Silverman EP, et al: Impact of azacytidine on the quality of life of patients with myelodysplastic syndrome treated in a randomized phase III trial. *J Clin Oncol* 15:2441, 2002.
268. Cazzola M, Barosi G, Gobbi PG, et al: Natural history of idiopathic refractory sideroblastic anemia. *Blood* 71:305, 1988.
269. Lewy RI, Kansu E, Gabuzda T: Leukemia in patients with acquired idiopathic sideroblastic anemia. *Am J Hematol* 6:323, 1979.
270. Cheng DS, Kushner JP, Wintrobe MM: Idiopathic refractory sideroblastic anemia. Incidence and risk factors for leukemic transformation. *Cancer* 44:724, 1979.
271. Hast R, Reizenstein P: Sideroblastic anemia and development of leukemia. *Blut* 42:203, 1981.
272. Streeter RR, Presant CA, Reinhard E: Prognostic significance of thrombocytosis in idiopathic sideroblastic anemia. *Blood* 50:427, 1977.
273. Barton JC, Conrad ME, Parmley R: Acute lymphoblastic leukemia in idiopathic refractory sideroblastic anemia. *Am J Hematol* 9:109, 1980.
274. Cazzola M, Barosi G, Gobbi PG: Natural history of idiopathic refractory sideroblastic anemia. *Blood* 71:305, 1988.
275. Malcovati L, Porta MG, Pascutto C, et al: Prognostic factors and life expectancy in myelodysplastic syndromes classified according to WHO criteria: A basis for clinical decision making. *J Clin Oncol* 23:7594, 2005.
276. Gattermann N, Aul C, Schneider W: Two types of acquired idiopathic sideroblastic anemia (AISA). *Br J Haematol* 74:45, 1990.
277. Greenberg P, Cox C, LeBeau MM, et al: International scoring system for evaluating prognosis in myelodysplastic syndromes. *Blood* 89:2079, 1997.
278. Mufti GJ, Bennett JM, Goasguen J, et al: Diagnosis and classification of myelodysplastic syndrome: International Working Group on Morphology of myelodysplastic syndrome (IWGM-MDS) consensus proposals for the definition and enumeration of myeloblasts and ring sideroblasts. *Haematologica* 93:1712, 2008.
279. Maes B, Meeus P, Michaux L, et al: Application of the International Prognostic Scoring System for myelodysplastic syndromes. *Ann Oncol* 10:825, 1999.
280. Rosati S, Mick R, Xu F, et al: Refractory cytopenia with multilineage dysplasia: Further characterization of an "unclassifiable" myelodysplastic syndrome. *Leukemia* 10:20, 1996.
281. Matsuda A, Jinnai I, Yagasaki F, et al: Refractory anemia with severe dysplasia: Clinical significance of morphological features in refractory anemia. *Leukemia* 12:482, 1998.
282. Vallespi T, Imbert M, Meccuci C, et al: Diagnosis, classification, and cytogenetics of myelodysplastic syndromes. *Haematologia (Budap)* 83:258, 1998.
283. Zon LI, Arkin C, Groopman JE: Haematologic manifestations of the human immune deficiency virus (HIV). *Br J Haematol* 66:251, 1987.
284. Thiele J, Zirbas TK, Bertsch HP, et al: AIDS-related bone marrow lesions—Myelodysplastic features or predominant inflammatory-reactive changes (HIV-myelopa-

thy)? A comparative morphometric study by immunohistochemistry with special emphasis on apoptosis and PCNA-labeling. *Anal Cell Pathol* 11:141, 1996.
285. Haznedar R: Pancytopenia with hypercellular bone marrow as a possible paraneoplastic syndrome. *Am J Hematol* 19:205, 1985.
286. Meyerson HJ, Farhi DC, Rosenthal NS: Transient increase in blasts mimicking acute leukemia and progressing myelodysplasia in patients receiving growth factor [comments]. *Am J Clin Pathol* 109:675, 1998.
287. Freifeld A, Marchigiani D, Walsh T, et al: A double-blind comparison of empirical oral and intravenous antibiotic therapy for low-risk febrile patients with neutropenia during cancer chemotherapy. *N Engl J Med* 341:305, 1999.
288. Malik IA, Moid I, Aziz Z, et al: A randomized comparison of fluconazole with amphotericin B as empiric anti-fungal agents in cancer patients with prolonged fever and neutropenia. *Am J Med* 105:478, 1998.
289. Jonasova A, Neuwirtova R, Cermak J, et al: Cyclosporin A therapy in hypoplastic MDS patients and certain refractory anaemias without hypoplastic bone marrow. *Br J Haematol* 100:304, 1998.
290. Molldrem JJ, Jiang YZ, Stetler-Stevenson M, et al: Haematological response of patients with myelodysplastic syndrome to antithymocyte globulin is associated with a loss of lymphocyte-mediated inhibition of CFU-GM and alterations in T-cell receptor V-beta profiles. *Br J Haematol* 102:1314, 1998.
291. Coiffier B, Adeleine P, Viala JJ, et al: Dysmyelopoietic syndromes: A search for prognostic factors in 193 patients. *Cancer* 52:83, 1983.
292. Garcia S, Sanz MA, Amigo V, et al: Prognostic factors in chronic myelodysplastic syndromes: A multivariate analysis in 107 cases. *Am J Hematol* 27:163, 1988.
293. Dunkley SM, Manoharan A, Kwan YL: Myelodysplastic syndromes: Prognostic significance of multilineage dysplasia in patients with refractory anemia or refractory anemia with ringed sideroblasts. *Blood* 99:3870, 2002.
294. Joseph AS, Cinkotal KI, Hunt L, Geary CG: Natural history of smoldering leukemia. *Br J Cancer* 46:160, 1982.
295. Greenberg PL: The smoldering myeloid leukemic states: Clinical and biological features. *Blood* 61:1035, 1983.
296. Maddox A-M, Keating MJ, Smith TL, et al: Prognostic factors for survival of 194 patients with low infiltrate leukemia. *Leuk Res* 10:995, 1986.
297. Foucar K, Langdon RM II, Armitage JO, et al: Myelodysplastic syndromes. A clinical and pathologic analysis of 109 cases. *Cancer* 56:553, 1985.
298. Hiddemann W, Jahns-Streubel G, Verbeek W, et al: Intensive therapy for high-risk myelodysplastic syndromes and the biological significance of karyotype abnormalities. *Leuk Res* 22(Suppl 1):S23, 1998.
299. Invernizzi R, Pecci A, Rossi G, et al: Idarubicin and cytosine arabinoside in the induction and maintenance therapy of high-risk myelodysplastic syndromes. *Haematologica* 82:660, 1997.
300. Kuriya S, Murai K, Miyairi Y, et al: A combination chemotherapy with low doses of cytarabine and etoposide for high risk myelodysplastic syndromes and their leukemic stage. A pilot study. *Cancer* 78:422, 1996.
301. Estey EH: Incorporating new modalities into guidelines. Topotecan for myelodysplastic syndromes. *Oncology* 12:81, 1998.
302. Estey EH, Thall PF, Pierce S, et al: Randomized phase II study of fludarabine + cytosine arabinoside + idarubicin +/– all-*trans* retinoic acid +/- granulocyte colony-stimulating factor in poor prognosis newly diagnosed acute myeloid leukemia and myelodysplastic syndrome. *Blood* 93:2478, 1999.
303. Sanz GF, Sanz MA: Progress in intensive chemotherapy for high-risk myelodysplastic syndromes. *Forum (Genova)* 9:63, 1999.
304. Cheson BD: Standard and low-dose chemotherapy for the treatment of myelodysplastic syndromes. *Leuk Res* 22(Suppl 1):S17, 1998.
305. Gassmann W, Schmitz N, Loffler H, De Witte T: Intensive chemotherapy and bone marrow transplantation for myelodysplastic syndromes. *Semin Hematol* 33:196, 1996.
306. Appelbaum FR, Anderson J: Allogeneic bone marrow transplantation for myelodysplastic syndrome: Outcomes analysis according to IPSS score. *Leukemia* 12(Suppl 1):S25, 1998.
307. Runde V, De Witte T, Arnold R, et al: Bone marrow transplantation from HLA-identical siblings as first-line treatment in patients with myelodysplastic syndromes: Early transplantation is associated with improved outcome. Chronic Leukemia Working Party of the European Group for Blood and Marrow Transplantation. *Bone Marrow Transplant* 21:255, 1998.
308. Wattel E, Solary E, Leleu X, et al: A prospective study of autologous bone marrow or peripheral blood stem cell transplantation after intensive chemotherapy in myelodysplastic syndromes. Groupe Francais des Myelodysplasies. Group Ouest-Est d'etude des Leucemies aigues myeloides. *Leukemia* 13:524, 1999.
309. Sanz GF, Sanz MA, Vallespi T, et al: Two regression models and a scoring system for predicting survival and planning treatment in myelodysplastic syndromes: A multivariate analysis of prognostic factors in 370 patients. *Blood* 74:395, 1989.
310. Ganser A, Hoelzer D: Clinical course of myelodysplastic syndromes. *Hematol Oncol Clin North Am* 6:607, 1992.
311. White AD, Culligan DJ, Hoy TG, Jacobs A: Extended cytogenetic follow-up of patients with myelodysplastic syndrome (MDS). *Br J Haematol* 81:499, 1992.
312. Mufti GJ: A guide to risk assessment in the primary myelodysplastic syndrome. *Hematol Oncol Clin North Am* 6:587, 1992.
313. Pfeilstocker M, Reisner R, Nosslinger T, et al: Cross validation of prognostic scores in myelodysplastic syndromes on 386 patients from a single institution confirms importance of cytogenetics. *Br J Haematol* 106:455, 1999.
314. Greenberg PL, Sanz GF, Sanz MA: Prognostic scoring systems for risk assessment in myelodysplastic syndromes. *Forum (Genova)* 9:17, 1999.
315. Muller-Berndorff H, Haas PS, Kunzmann R, et al: Comparison of five prognostic scoring systems, the French-American-British (FAB) and World Health Organization (WHO) classifications in patients with myelodysplastic syndromes: Results of a single-center analysis. *Ann Hematol* 85:502, 2006.
316. Brown ER, Heerma NA, Tricot G: Spontaneous remission in myelodysplastic syndrome. *Cancer Genet Cytogenet* 46:125, 1990.
317. Karp JE, Sarkodee-Adoo CB: Therapy-related acute leukemia. *Clin Lab Med* 20:71, 2000.
318. Padmanabhan A, Baker JA, Zirpoli G, et al: Acute myeloid leukemia and myelodysplastic syndrome following breast cancer: Increased frequency of other cancers and of cancers in multiple family members. *Leuk Res* 32:1820, 2008.
319. Hake CR, Graubert TA, Fenske TS: Does autologous transplantation directly increase the risk of secondary leukemia in lymphoma patients? *Bone Marrow Transplant* 39:59, 207.
320. Barlogie B, Tricot G, Haessler J, et al: Cytogenetically defined myelodysplasia after melphalan-based autotransplantation for multiple myeloma linked to poor hematopoietic stem-cell mobilization: The Arkansas experience in more than 3,000 patients treated since 1989. *Blood* 111:94, 2008.
321. Chakraborty S, Sun CL, Francisco L, et al: Accelerated telomere shortening precedes development of therapy-related myelodysplasia or acute myelogenous leukemia after autologous transplantation for lymphoma. *J Clin Oncol* 27:791, 2009.
322. Fukumoto JS, Greenberg PL: Management of patients with higher risk myelodysplastic syndromes. *Crit Rev Oncol Hematol* 56:179, 2005.
323. Estey E, Keating M, Pierce S, et al: Application of the International Scoring System for myelodysplasia to M.D. Anderson patients. *Blood* 90:2843, 1997.
324. Verburgh E, Achten R, Maes B, et al: Additional prognostic value of bone marrow histology in patients subclassified according to the International Prognostic Scoring System for myelodysplastic syndromes. *J Clin Oncol* 21:273, 2003.
325. Kantarjian H, O'Brien S, Ravandi F, et al: Proposal for a new risk model in myelodysplastic syndrome that accounts for events not considered in the original International Prognostic Scoring System. *Cancer* 113:1351, 2008.
326. Germing U, Hildebrandt B, Pfeilstöcker M, et al: Refinement of the international prognostic scoring system (IPSS) by including LDH as an additional prognostic variable to improve risk assessment in patients with primary myelodysplastic syndromes (MDS). *Leukemia* 19:2223, 2005.
327. Wimazal F, Sperr WR, Kundi M, et al: Prognostic significance of serial determinations of lactate dehydrogenase (LDH) in the follow-up of patients with myelodysplastic syndromes. *Ann Oncol* 19:970, 2008.
328. Malcovati L, Germing U, Kuendgen A, et al: Time-dependent prognostic scoring system for predicting survival and leukemic evolution in myelodysplastic syndromes. *J Clin Oncol* 25:3503, 2007.
329. Schiffer CA: World Health Organization and international prognostic scoring system: The limitations of current classification systems in assessing prognosis and determining appropriate therapy in myelodysplastic syndromes. *Semin Hematol* 45:3, 2008.
330. National Comprehensive Cancer Network: Myelodysplastic syndromes. *J Natl Compr Canc Netw* 1:456, 2003.
331. Alessandrino EP, Amadori S, Bardsi G, et al: Evidence and consensus-based practice guidelines for the therapy of primary myelodysplastic syndromes: A statement from the Italian Society of Hematology. *Haematologica* 87:1286, 2002.
332. Bowen D, Culligan D, Jowitt S, et al: Guidelines for diagnosis and therapy of the myelodysplastic syndromes. *Br J Haematol* 120:187, 2003.
333. Cheson BD, Bennett JM, Kantarjian H, et al: Report of an international working group to standardize response criteria for myelodysplastic syndromes. *Blood* 96:3671, 2000.
334. Erba HP: Recent progress in the treatment of myelodysplastic syndrome in adult patients. *Curr Opin Oncol* 15:1, 2003.
335. Jansen AJ, Essink-Bot ML, Beckers EA, et al: Quality of life measurement in patients with transfusion-dependent myelodysplastic syndromes. *Br J Haematol* 1 21:270, 2003.
336. Oliva EN, Dimitrov BD, Benedetto F, et al: Hemoglobin level threshold for cardiac remodeling and quality of life in myelodysplastic syndrome. *Leuk Res* 29:1217, 2005.
337. Cazzola M, Della Porta MG, Malcovati L: Clinical relevance of anemia and transfusion iron overload in myelodysplastic syndromes. *Hematology Am Soc Hematol Educ Program* 2008:166, 2008.
338. Chee CE, Steensma DP, Wu W, et al: Neither serum ferritin nor the number of red blood cell transfusions affect overall survival in refractory anemia with ringed sideroblasts. *Am J Hematol* 83:611, 2008.
339. Park S, Grabar S, Kelaidi C, et al: Predictive factors of response and survival in myelodysplastic syndrome treated with erythropoietin and G-CSF: The GFM experience. *Blood* 111:574, 2008.
340. Rigolin GM, Porta MD, Bigoni R, et al: RHuEpo administration in patients with low-risk myelodysplastic syndromes: Evaluation of erythroid precursors' response by fluorescence in situ hybridization on May-Grünwald-Giemsa-stained bone marrow samples. *Br J Haematol* 119:652, 2002.
341. Wallvik J, Stenke L, Bernell P, et al: Serum erythropoietin (EPO) levels correlate with survival and independently predict response to EPO treatment in patients with myelodysplastic syndromes. *Eur J Haematol* 68:180, 2002.
342. Musto P, Falcone A, Sanpaolo G, et al: Efficacy of a single, weekly dose of recombinant erythropoietin in myelodysplastic syndromes. *Br J Haematol* 122:269, 2003.

343. Gabrilove J, Paquette R, Lyons RM, et al: Phase 2, single-arm trial to evaluate the effectiveness of darbepoetin alfa for correcting anaemia in patients with myelodysplastic syndromes. *Br J Haematol* 142:379, 2008.
344. Stasi R, Abruzzese E, Lanzetta G, et al: Darbepoetin alfa for the treatment of anemic patients with low- and intermediate-1–risk myelodysplastic syndromes. *Ann Oncol* 16:1921, 2005.
345. Terpos E, Mougiou A, Kouraklis A, et al: Prolonged administration of erythropoietin increases erythroid response rate in myelodysplastic syndromes: A phase II trail in 281 patients. *Br J Haematol* 118:174, 2002.
346. Moyo V, Lefebvre P, Duh MS, et al: Erythropoiesis-stimulating agents in the treatment of anemia in myelodysplastic syndromes: A meta-analysis. *Ann Hematol* 87:527, 2008.
347. Nordstrom BL, Luo W, Fraeman K, et al: Use of erythropoiesis-stimulating agents among chemotherapy patients with hemoglobin exceeding 12 grams per deciliter. *J Manag Care Pharm* 14:858, 2008.
348. Thompson JA, Gillilland DG, Prchal JT, et al: Effect of recombinant human erythropoietin combined with granulocyte/macrophage colony-stimulating factor in the treatment of patients with myelodysplastic syndrome. *Blood* 95:1175, 2000.
349. Stein RS: The role of erythropoietin in the anemia of myelodysplastic syndrome. *Clin Lymphoma* 1:S36, 2003.
350. Mundle S, Lebebvre P, Vekeman F, et al: An assessment of erythroid response to epoetin alpha as a single agent versus in combination with granulocyte-or granulocyte-macrophage-colony-stimulating factor in myelodysplastic syndromes using a meta-analysis approach. *Cancer* 115:706, 2009.
351. Jädersten M, Montgomery SM, Dybedal I, et al: Long-term outcome of treatment of anemia in MDS with erythropoietin and G-CSF. *Blood* 106:803, 2005.
352. Cortelezzi A, Colombo G, Pellegrini C, et al: Bone marrow glycophorin-positive erythroid cells of myelodysplastic patients responding to high-dose rHuEPO therapy have a different gene expression pattern from those of nonresponders. *Am J Hematol* 83:531, 2008.
353. Jabbour E, Garcia-Manero G, Taher A, Kantarjian HM: Managing iron overload in patients with myelodysplastic syndromes with oral deferasirox therapy. *Oncologist* 14:489, 2009.
354. Gattermann N: Guidelines on iron chelation therapy in patients with myelodysplastic syndromes and transfusional iron overload. *Leuk Res* 31 Suppl 3:S10, 2007.
355. Wells RA, Leber B, Buckstein R, et al: Iron overload in myelodysplastic syndromes: A Canadian consensus guideline. *Leuk Res* 32:1338, 2008.
356. Wimazal F, Nösslinger T, Baumgartner C, et al: Deferasirox induces regression of iron overload in patients with myelodysplastic syndromes. *Eur J Clin Invest* 39:406, 2009.
357. Di Tucci AA, Matta G, Deplano S, et al: Myocardial iron overload assessment by T2* magnetic resonance imaging in adult transfusion dependent patients with acquired anemias. *Haematologica* 93:1385, 2008.
358. Hellström-Lindberg E, Robért K-H, Gahrton G, et al: A predictive model for the clinical response to low dose ARA-C: A study of 102 patients with myelodysplastic syndromes and acute leukemia. *Br J Haematol* 81:503, 1992.
359. Ganser A, Seipelt G, Eder M, et al: Treatment of myelodysplastic syndromes with cytokines and cytotoxic drugs. *Semin Oncol* 19:95, 1992.
360. Visani G, Malagola M, Piccaluga PP, Isidori A: Low dose Ara-C for myelodysplastic syndromes: Is it still a current therapy? *Leuk Lymphoma* 45:1531, 2004.
361. Kochenderfer JH, Kobayashi S, Wieder ED, et al: Loss of T-lymphocyte clonal dominance in patients with myelodysplastic syndrome responsive to immunosuppression. *Blood* 100:3639, 2002.
362. Aivado M, Rong A, Stadler M: Favourable response to antithymocyte or antilymphocyte globulin in low-risk myelodysplastic syndrome patients with a "non-clonal" pattern of X-chromosome inactivation in bone marrow cells. *Eur J Haematol* 68:210, 2002.
363. Selleri C, Maciejewski JP, Catalano L: Effects of cyclosporine on hematopoietic and immune functions in patients with hypoplastic myelodysplasia: *In vitro* and *in vivo* studies. *Cancer* 95:1911, 2002.
364. Yazji S, Giles FJ, Tsimberidou A-M, et al: Antithymocyte globulin (ATG)-based therapy in patients with myelodysplastic syndromes. *Leukemia* 17:2101, 2003.
365. Molldrem JJ, Leufer E, Bahceci E, et al: Antithymocyte globulin for treatment of the bone marrow failure associated with myelodysplastic syndromes. *Ann Intern Med* 137:156, 2002.
366. Killick SB, Mufti G, Cavenagh JD, et al: A pilot study of antithymocyte globulin (ATG) in the treatment of patients with "low-risk" myelodysplasia. *Br J Haematol* 120:679, 2003.
367. Sauntharajah Y, Nakamura R, Nam JM, et al: HLA-DR15 (DR2) is over represented in myelodysplastic syndrome and aplastic anemia and predicts a response to immunosuppression in myelodysplastic syndrome. *Blood* 100:1570, 2002.
368. Sauntharajah Y, Nakamura R, Wesley R, et al: A simple method to predict response to immunosuppressive therapy in patients with myelodysplastic syndrome. *Blood* 102:3025, 2003.
369. Shimamoto T, Iguchi T, Ando K, et al: Successful treatment with cyclosporin A for myelodysplastic syndrome with erythroid hypoplasia associated with T-cell receptor gene rearrangements. *Br J Haematol* 114:358, 2001.
370. Lim ZY, Killick S, Germing U, et al: Low IPSS score and bone marrow hypocellularity in MDS patients predict hematological responses to antithymocyte globulin. *Leukemia* 21:1436, 2007.
371. Sloand EM, Wu CO, Greenberg P, et al: Factors affecting response and survival in patients with myelodysplasia treated with immunosuppressive therapy. *J Clin Oncol* 26:2505, 2008.
372. Steensma DP, Dispenzieri A, Moore B, et al: Antithymocyte globulin has limited efficacy and substantial toxicity in unselected anemic patients with myelodysplastic syndrome. *Blood* 101:2156, 2003.
373. Atoyebi W, Bywater L, Rawlings L, et al: Treatment of myelodysplasia with oral cyclosporin. *Clin Lab Haematol* 24:211, 2002.
374. Leone G, Teofili L, Voso MT: DNA methylation and demethylating drugs in myelodysplastic syndromes and secondary leukemias. *Haematologica* 87:1324, 2002.
375. Garcia-Manero G: Demethylating agents in myeloid malignancies. *Curr Opin Oncol* 6:506, 2008.
376. Stone R, Sekeres M, Garcia-Manero G, et al: Recent advances in low-and intermediate-1-risk myelodysplastic syndrome: Developing a consensus for optimal therapy. *Clin Adv Hematol Oncol* 6:1, 2008.
377. Gryn J, Zeigler ZR, Shadduck RK, et al: Treatment of myelodysplastic syndromes with 5-azacytidine. *Leuk Res* 26:893, 2002.
378. Sudan N, Rossetti JM, Shadduck RK, et al: Treatment of acute myelogenous leukemia with outpatient azacitidine. *Cancer* 107:1839, 2006.
379. Gore SD: Intravenous azacitidine for MDS. *Clin Adv Hematol Oncol* 5:234, 2007.
380. Garcia-Manero G, Stoltz ML, Ward MR, et al: A pilot pharmacokinetic study of oral azacitidine. *Leukemia* 22:1680, 2008.
381. Lyons RM, Cosgriff TM, Modi SS, et al: Hematologic response to three alternative dosing schedules of azacitidine in patients with myelodysplastic syndromes. *J Clin Oncol* 27:1850, 2009.
382. Lubbert M, Wijermans P, Kunzmann R, et al: Cytogenetic responses in high-risk myelodysplastic syndrome following low-dose treatment with the DNA methylation inhibitor 5-aza-2′-deoxycytidine. *Br J Haematol* 114:349, 2001.
383. Daskalakis M, Nguyen TT, Nguyen C, et al: Demethylation of a hyper-methylated P15/INK4B gene in patients with myelodysplastic syndrome by 5-Aza-2′-deoxycytidine (decitabine) treatment. *Blood* 100:2957, 2002.
384. Sigalotti L, Altomonte M, Colizzi F, et al: Correspondence: 5-Aza-2′-deoxycytidine (decitabine) treatment of hematopoietic malignancies: A multimechanism therapeutic approach? *Blood* 101:4644, 2003.
385. Kantarjian H, Oki Y, Garcia-Manero G, et al: Results of a randomized study of 3 schedules of low-dose decitabine in higher-risk myelodysplastic syndrome and chronic myelomonocytic leukemia. *Blood* 109:52, 2007.
386. Jabbour E, Issa JP, Garcia-Manero G, Kantarjian H: Evolution of decitabine development: Accomplishments, ongoing investigations, and future strategies. *Cancer* 112:2341, 2008.
387. Klisovic RB, Stock W, Cataland S, et al: A phase I biological study of MG98, an oligodeoxynucleotide antisense to DNA methyltransferase 1, in patients with high-risk myelodysplasia and acute myeloid leukemia. *Clin Cancer Res* 14:2444, 2008.
388. Oki Y, Issa JP: Review: Recent clinical trials in epigenetic therapy. *Rev Recent Clin Trials* 1:169, 2006.
389. Giles F, Fischer T, Cortes J, et al: A phase I study of intravenous LBH589, a novel cinnamic hydroxamic acid analogue histone deacetylase inhibitor, in patients with refractory hematologic malignancies. *Clin Cancer Res* 12:4628, 2006.
390. Garcia-Manero G, Assouline S, Cortes J, et al: Phase 1 study of the oral isotype specific histone deacetylase inhibitor MGCD0103 in leukemia. *Blood* 112:981, 2008.
391. Griffiths EA, Gore SD: DNA methyltransferase and histone deacetylase inhibitors in the treatment of myelodysplastic syndromes. *Semin Hematol* 45:23, 2008.
392. Kantarjian H, Giles F, List A, et al: The incidence and impact of thrombocytopenia in myelodysplastic syndromes. *Cancer* 109:1705, 2007.
393. Zeigler ZR: Effects of epsilon aminocaproic acid on primary hemostasis. *Haemostasis* 21:313, 1991.
394. Hellström-Lindberg E, Malcovati L: Supportive care and use of hematopoietic growth factors in myelodysplastic syndromes. *Semin Hematol* 45:14, 2008.
395. Montero AJ, Estrov Z, Freireich EJ, et al: Phase II study of low-dose interleukin-11 in patients with myelodysplastic syndrome. *Leuk Lymphoma* 47:2049, 2006.
396. Tiu RV, Sekeres MA: The role of AMG-531 in the treatment of thrombocytopenia in idiopathic thrombocytopenic purpura and myelodysplastic syndromes. *Expert Opin Biol Ther* 8:1021, 2008.
397. Vadhan-Raj S, Keating M, LeMaistre A, et al: Effects of recombinant human granulocyte-macrophage colony-stimulating factor in patients with myelodysplastic syndromes. *N Engl J Med* 317:1545, 1987.
398. Thompson JA, Gilliland DG, Prchal JT, et al: Effect of recombinant human erythropoietin combined with granulocyte/macrophage colony-stimulating factor in the treatment of patients with myelodysplastic syndrome. *Blood* 95:1175, 2000.
399. Chuncharunee S, Intragumtornchai T, Chaimongkol B, et al: Treatment of myelodysplastic syndrome with low-dose human granulocyte colony-stimulating factor: A multicenter study. *Int J Hematol* 74:144, 2001.
400. Sultana TA, Harada H, Ito K, et al: Expression and functional analysis of granulocyte colony-stimulating factor receptors on CD34++ cells in patients with myelodysplastic syndrome (MDS) and MDS-acute myeloid leukaemia. *Br J Haematol* 212:63, 2003.
401. Nimubona S, Grulois I, Bernard M, et al: Complete remission in hypoplastic acute myeloid leukemia induced by G-CSF without chemotherapy: Report on three cases. *Leukemia* 16:1871, 2002.
402. Cesaro S, Chinello P, De Silvestro G, et al: Granulocyte transfusions from G-CSF-stimulated donors for the treatment of severe infections in neutropenic pediatric patients with onco-hematological diseases. *Support Care Cancer* 11:101, 2003.
403. O'Malley DP, Whalen M, Banks PM: Spontaneous splenic rupture with fatal outcome following G-CSF administration for myelodysplastic syndrome. *Am J Hematol* 73:294, 2003.

404. Verhoef G, VandDenBerghe HV, Boogaerts M: Cytogenetic effects on cells derived from patients with myelodysplastic syndromes during treatment with hemopoietic growth factors. *Leukemia* 6:766, 1992.
405. Tohyama K, Ohmori S, Michishita M: Effects of recombinant G-CSF and GM-CSF on in vitro differentiation of the blast cells of RAEB and RAEB-T. *Eur J Haematol* 42:348, 1989.
406. Ferrero D, Bruno B, Pregno P, et al: Combined differentiating therapy for myelodysplastic syndromes: A phase II study. *Leuk Res* 20:867, 1996.
407. Hofmann WK, Ganser A, Seipelt G, et al: Treatment of patients with low-risk myelodysplastic syndromes using a combination of all-trans retinoic acid, interferon alpha, and granulocyte colony-stimulating factor. *Ann Hematol* 78:125, 1999.
408. Fenaux P, Mufti GJ, Hellstrom-Lindberg E, et al: Efficacy of azacitidine compared with that of conventional care regimens in the treatment of higher-risk myelodysplastic syndromes: A randomised, open-label, phase III study. *Lancet Oncol* 10:223, 2009.
409. Nachtkamp K, Kündgen A, Strupp C, et al: Impact on survival of different treatments for myelodysplastic syndromes (MDS). *Leuk Res* 33:1024, 2009.
410. Beran M: Intensive chemotherapy for patients with high-risk myelodysplastic syndrome. *Int J Hematol* 72:139, 2000.
411. Knipp S, Hildebrand B, Kündgen A, et al: Intensive chemotherapy is not recommended for patients aged >60 years who have myelodysplastic syndromes or acute myeloid leukemia with high-risk karyotypes. *Cancer* 110:345, 2007.
412. Cortes J, Kantarjian H, Albitar M, et al: A randomized trial of liposomal daunorubicin and cytarabine versus liposomal daunorubicin and topotecan with or without thalidomide as initial therapy for patients with poor prognosis acute myelogenous leukemia or myelodysplastic syndrome. *Cancer* 97:1234, 2003.
413. De la Rubia J, Regadera A, Martin G, et al: FLAG-IDA regimen (fludarabine, cytarabine, idarubicin and G-CSF) in the treatment of patients with high-risk myeloid malignancies. *Leuk Res* 26:725, 2002.
414. Voutsadakis IA: Gemtuzumab ozogamicin (CMA-676, Mylotarg) for the treatment of CD33+ acute myeloid leukemia. *Anticancer Drugs* 13:685, 2002.
415. Cohen AD, Luger SM, Sickles C, et al: Gemtuzumab ozogamicin (Mylotarg) monotherapy for relapsed AML after hematopoietic stem cell transplantation: Efficacy and incidence of hepatic veno-occlusive disease. *Bone Marrow Transplant* 30:23, 2002.
416. Marcondes M, Deeg HJ: Hematopoietic cell transplantation for patients with myelodysplastic syndromes (MDS): When, how and for whom? *Best Pract Res Clin Haematol* 21:67, 2008.
417. Oliansky DM, Antin JH, Bennett JM, et al: The role of cytotoxic therapy with hematopoietic stem cell transplantation in the therapy of myelodysplastic syndromes: An evidence-based review. *Biol Blood Marrow Transplant* 15:137, 2009.
418. Luger S, Sacks N: Bone marrow transplantation for myelodysplastic syndrome—Who? When? and Which? *Bone Marrow Transplant* 30:199, 2002.
419. Anderson JE, Appelbaum FR, Schoch G, et al: Allogeneic marrow transplantation for myelodysplastic syndrome with advanced disease morphology: A phase II study of busulfan, cyclophosphamide, and total-body irradiation and analysis of prognostic factors. *J Clin Oncol* 14:220, 1996.
420. Deeg HJ, Shulman HM, Anderson JE, et al: Allogeneic and syngeneic marrow transplantation for myelodysplastic syndrome in patients 55 to 66 years of age. *Blood* 95:1188, 2000.
421. Deeg HJ, Storer B, Slattery JT, et al: Conditioning with targeted busulfan and cyclophosphamide for hemopoeitic stem cell transplantation related and unrelated donors in patients with myelodysplastic syndrome. *Blood* 100:1201, 2002.
422. Sierra J, Perez WS, Rozman C, et al: Bone marrow transplantation from HLA-identical siblings as treatment for myelodysplasia. *Blood* 100:1997, 2002.
423. Guardiola P, Runder V, Bacigalupo A, et al: Retrospective comparison of bone marrow and granulocyte colony-stimulating factor-mobilized peripheral blood progenitor cells for allogeneic stem cell transplantation using HLA identical sibling donors in myelodysplastic syndromes. *Blood* 99:4370, 2002.
424. Castro-Malaspina H, Harris RE, Gajewski J, et al: Unrelated donor marrow transplantation for myelodysplastic syndromes: Outcome analysis in 510 transplants facilitated by the National Marrow Donor Program. *Blood* 99:1943, 2002.
425. Ooi J, Iseki T, Nagayama H, et al: Unrelated cord blood transplantation for adult patients with myelodysplastic syndrome-related secondary acute myeloid leukaemia. *Br J Haematol* 114:834, 2001.
426. Maury S, Balère-Appert ML, Chir Z, et al: Unrelated stem cell transplantation for severe acquired aplastic anemia: Improved outcome in the era of high-resolution HLA matching between donor and recipient. *Haematologica* 92:589, 2007.
427. Cutler CS, Lee SJ, Greenberg P, et al: A decision analysis of allogeneic bone marrow transplantation for the myelodysplastic syndromes: Delayed transplantation for low-risk myelodysplasia is associated with improved outcome. *Blood* 104:579, 2004.
428. Castro-Malaspina H, Jabubowski AA, Papadopoulos EB, et al: Transplantation in remission improves the disease-free survival of patients with advanced myelodysplastic syndromes treated with myeloablative T cell-depleted stem cell transplants from HLA-identical siblings. *Biol Blood Marrow Transplant* 14:458, 2008.
429. Armand P, Kim HT, DeAngelo DJ, et al: Impact of cytogenetics on outcome of de novo and therapy-related AML and MDS after allogeneic transplantation. *Biol Blood Marrow Transplant* 13:655, 2007.
430. Warlick ED, Cioc A, Defor T, et al: Allogeneic stem cell transplantation for adults with myelodysplastic syndromes: Importance of pretransplant disease burden. *Biol Blood Marrow Transplant* 15:30, 2009.
431. Chang C, Storer BE, Scott BL, et al: Hematopoietic cell transplantation in patients with myelodysplastic syndrome or acute myeloid leukemia arising from myelodysplastic syndrome: Similar outcomes in patients with *de novo* disease and disease following prior therapy or antecedent hematologic disorders. *Blood* 110:1379, 2007.
432. Kröger N, Brand R, van Biezen A, et al: Risk factors for therapy-related myelodysplastic syndrome and acute myeloid leukemia treated with allogeneic stem cell transplantation. *Haematologica* 94:542, 2009.
433. Scott BL, Park JY, Deeg HJ, et al: Pretransplant neutropenia is associated with poor-risk cytogenetic features and increased infection-related mortality in patients with myelodysplastic syndromes. *Biol Blood Marrow Transplant* 14:799, 2008.
434. De Padua Silva L, de Lima M, Kantarjian H, et al: Feasibility of allo-SCT after hypomethylating therapy with decitabine for myelodysplastic syndrome. *Bone Marrow Transplant* 43:839, 2009.
435. Luger S, Sacks N: Bone marrow transplantation for myelodysplastic syndrome—Who? When? and Which? *Bone Marrow Transplant* 30:199, 2002.
436. Taussig Dc, Davies AJ, Cavenagh JD: Durable remissions of myelodysplastic syndrome and acute myeloid leukemia after reduced-intensity allografting. *J Clin Oncol* 21:3060, 2003.
437. Mielcarek M, Storb R: Non-myeloablative hematopoietic cell transplantation as immunotherapy for hematologic malignancies. *Cancer Treat Rev* 29:283, 2003.
438. Kroger N, Schetelig J, Zabelina T, et al: A fludarabine-based dose-reduced conditioning regimen followed by allogeneic stem cell transplantation from related or unrelated donors in patients with myelodysplastic syndrome. *Bone Marrow Transplant* 28:643, 2001.
439. Parker JE, Shafi T, Pagliuca A, et al: Allogeneic stem cell transplantation in the myelodysplastic syndromes: Interim results of outcomes following reduced-intense conditioning compared with standard preparative regimens. *Br J Haematol* 119:144, 2002.
440. Gupta V, Daly A, Lipton JH, et al: Nonmyeloablative stem cell transplantation for myelodysplastic syndrome or acute myeloid leukemia in patients 60 years or older. *Biol Blood Marrow Transplant* 11:764, 2005.
441. Finke J, Nagler A: Viewpoint: What is the role of allogeneic haematopoietic cell transplantation in the era of reduced-intensity conditioning—is there still an upper age limit? A focus on myeloid neoplasia. *Leukemia* 21:1357, 2007.
442. Pollyea DA, Artz AS, Stock W, et al: Outcomes of patients with AML and MDS who relapse or progress after reduced intensity allogeneic hematopoietic cell transplantation. *Bone Marrow Transplant* 40:1027, 2007.
443. Campregher PV, Gooley T, Scott BL, et al: Results of donor lymphocyte infusions for relapsed myelodysplastic syndrome after hematopoietic cell transplantation. *Bone Marrow Transplant* 40:965, 2007.
444. Testoni N, Lemoli RM, Martinelli G, et al: Autologous peripheral blood stem cell transplantation in acute myeloblastic leukaemia and myelodysplastic syndrome patients: Evaluation of tumour cell contamination of leukaphereses by cytogenetic and molecular methods. *Bone Marrow Transplant* 22:1065, 1998.
445. Wattel E, Solary E, Leleu X, et al: A prospective study of autologous bone marrow or peripheral blood stem cell transplantation after intensive chemotherapy in myelodysplastic syndromes. Groupe Francais des Myelodysplasies. Group Ouest-Est d'etude des Leucemies aigues myeloides. *Leukemia* 13:524, 1999.
446. Viola A, Falco C, D'Elia R, et al: An antecedent diagnosis of refractory anemia with excess blasts has no influence on mobilization of peripheral blood stem cells and hematopoietic recovery after autologous stem cell transplantation in acute myeloid leukemia. *Eur J Haematol* 78:41, 2007.
447. Ogata K, Yamada T, Ito T, et al: Low-dose etoposide: A potential therapy for myelodysplastic syndromes. *Br J Haematol* 82:354, 1992.
448. Robak T, Szmigielska-Kaplon A, Urbanska-Rys H, et al: Efficacy and toxicity of low-dose melphalan in myelodysplastic syndromes and acute myeloid leukemia with multilineage dysplasia. *Neoplasma* 50:172, 2003.
449. Mario AD, Pagano L, Mele L, et al: Use of gemcitabine (GEM) in advanced myelodysplastic syndromes. *Ann Oncol* 12:1494, 2001.
450. Ribrag V, Suzan F, Ravoet C, et al: Phase II trial of CPT-11 in myelodysplastic syndromes with excess of marrow blasts. *Leukemia* 17:319, 2003.
451. Giles FJ, Faderl S, Thomas DA, et al: Randomizing phase I/II study of troxacitabine combined with cytarabine, idarubicin, or topotecan in patients with refractory myeloid leukemias. *J Clin Oncol* 21:1050, 2003.
452. Bouabdallah R, Lefrere F, Rose C, et al: A phase II trial of induction and consolidation therapy of acute myeloid leukemia with weekly oral idarubicin alone in poor risk elderly patients. *Leukemia* 13:1491, 1999.
453. Kantarjian HM, Jeha S, Gandhi V, et al: Clofarabine: Past, present, and future. *Leuk Lymphoma* 48:1922, 2007.
454. Grinblatt DL, Yu D, Hars V, et al: Treatment of myelodysplastic syndrome with 2 schedules and doses of oral topotecan: A randomized phase 2 trial by the Cancer and Leukemia Group B (CALGB19803). *Cancer* 115:84, 2009.
455. Yee KW, Hagey A, Verstovsek S, et al: Phase 1 study of ABT-751, a novel microtubule inhibitor, in patients with refractory hematologic malignancies. *Clin Cancer Res* 11:6615, 2005.
456. Tamburini J, Elie C, Park S, et al: Effectiveness and tolerance of low to very low dose thalidomide in low-risk myelodysplastic syndromes. *Leuk Res* 33:547, 2009.
457. Raza A, Meyer P, Dutt D, et al: Thalidomide produces transfusion independence in long-standing refractory anemias of patients with myelodysplastic syndromes. *Blood* 98:958, 2001.
458. Strupp C, Germing U, Aivado M, et al: Thalidomide for the treatment of patients with myelodysplastic syndromes. *Leukemia* 16:1, 2002.

459. Bertolini F, Mingrone W, Alietti A, et al: Thalidomide in multiple myeloma, myelodysplastic syndromes and histiocytosis. Analysis of clinical results and of surrogate angiogenesis markers. *Ann Oncol* 12:1333, 2001.
460. Tsirigotis P, Venetis E, Rontogianni D, et al: Thalidomide in the treatment of myelodysplastic syndrome with fibrosis. *Leuk Res* 26:965, 2002.
461. Steurer M, Sudmeier I, Stauder R, Gastl G: Thromboembolic events in patients with myelodysplastic syndrome receiving thalidomide in combination with darbepoetin-alpha. *Br J Haematol* 121:101, 2003.
462. List A, Dewald G, Bennett J, et al: Lenalidomide in the myelodysplastic syndrome with chromosome 5q deletion. *N Engl J Med* 355:1456, 2006.
463. Raza A, Reeves JA, Feldman EJ, et al: Phase 2 study of lenalidomide in transfusion-dependent, low-risk, and intermediate-1 risk myelodysplastic syndromes with karyotypes other than deletion 5q. *Blood* 111:86, 2008.
464. Adès L, Boehrer S, Prebet T, et al: Efficacy and safety of lenalidomide in intermediate-2 or high-risk myelodysplastic syndromes with 5q deletion: Results of a phase 2 study. *Blood* 113:3947, 2009.
465. List AF, Kurtin S, Glinsmann-Gibson B, et al: Efficacy and safety of CC 5013 for treatment of anemia in patients with myelodysplastic syndromes (MDS). *Blood* 102:184a, 2003.
466. Sekeres MA, Maciejewski JP, Giagounidis AA, et al: Relationship of treatment-related cytopenias and response to lenalidomide in patients with lower-risk myelodysplastic syndromes. *J Clin Oncol* 26:5943, 2008.
467. Deeg HJ, Gotlib J, Beckham C, et al: Soluble TNF receptor fusion protein (etanercept) for the treatment of myelodysplastic syndrome: A pilot study. *Leukemia* 16:162, 2002.
468. Rosenfeld C, Bedell C: Pilot study of recombinant human soluble tumor necrosis factor receptor (TNFR:Fc) in patients with low risk myelodysplasia syndrome. *Leuk Res* 26:721, 2002.
469. Maciejewski JP, Risitano Am, Sloand EM, et al: A pilot study of the recombinant soluble human tumour necrosis factor receptor (p75)-Fc fusion protein in patients with myelodysplastic syndrome. *Br J Haematol* 117:119, 2002.
470. Stasi R, Amadori S: Infliximab chimaeric anti-tumour necrosis factor alpha monoclonal antibody treatment for patients with myelodysplastic syndromes. *Br J Haematol* 116:334, 2002.
471. Stone RM: Are new agents really making a difference in MDS? *Best Pract Res Clin Haematol* 21:639, 2008.
472. Invernizzi R, Pecci A, Travaglino E, et al: Clinical and biological effects of treatment with amifostine in myelodysplastic syndromes. *Br J Haematol* 118:246, 2002.
473. Callander N, Ochoa-Bayona JF, Piro L, et al: Hematologic improvement following treatment with TLK199 (Telintra™), a novel glutathione analog inhibitor of GST P1–1, in myelodysplastic syndrome (MDS): Interim results of a dose-ranging phase 2a study. *Blood* 104:4001, 2004.
474. Nagler A, Rikilis I, Tatarsky I, Fabian I: Effect of 1,25-dihydroxyvitamin D_3 and 13-*cis*-retinoic acid on *in vitro* hematopoiesis in the myelodysplastic syndromes. *J Lab Clin Med* 110:237, 1987.
475. Rowinsky EK, Conley BA, Jones RJ, et al: Hexamethylene bisacetamide in myelodysplastic syndrome: Effect of five-day exposure to maximal therapeutic concentrations. *Leukemia* 6:526, 1992.
476. List AF: Hematopoietic stimulation by amifostine and sodium phenylbutyrate: What is the potential in MDS? *Leuk Res* 22(Suppl 1):S7, 1998.
477. Hast R, Lauren SAL, Reizenstein P: Absent clinical effects of retinoic acid and isotretinoin treatment on the myelodysplastic syndrome. *Hematol Oncol* 7:297, 1989.
478. Ohno R, Naoe T, Hirano M, et al: Treatment of myelodysplastic syndromes with all-trans retinoic acid. *Blood* 81:1152, 1993.
479. DeRosa L, Montuoro A, DeLaurenzi A: Therapy of "high risk" myelodysplastic syndromes with an association of low-dose ara-c, retinoic acid and 1,25-dihydroxyvitamin D_3. *Biomed Pharmacother* 46:211, 1992.
480. Andreeff M, Stone R, Michaeli J, et al: Hexamethylene bisacetamide in myelodysplastic syndrome and acute myelogenous leukemia: A phase II clinical trial with a differentiation-inducing agent. *Blood* 80:2604, 1992.
481. Gore SD, Weng LJ, Zhai S, et al: Impact of the putative differentiating agent sodium phenylbutyrate on myelodysplastic syndromes and acute myeloid leukemia. *Clin Cancer Res* 7:2330, 2001.
482. Sekeres MA: New data with arsenic trioxide in leukemias and myelodysplastic syndromes. *Clin Lymphoma Myeloma* 8 Suppl 1:S7, 2007.
483. Schiller GJ, Slack J, Hainsworth JD, et al: Phase II multicenter study of arsenic trioxide in patients with myelodysplastic syndromes. *J Clin Oncol* 24:2456, 2006.
484. Miller WH Jr: Molecular targets of arsenic trioxide in malignant cells. *Oncologist* 7(Suppl 1):14, 2002.
485. Slack JL, Waxman S, Tricot G, et al: Advances in the management of acute promyelocytic leukemia and other hematologic malignancies with arsenic trioxide. *Oncologist* 7(Suppl 1):1, 2002.
486. List A, Beran M, DiPersio J, Slack J, et al: Opportunities for Trisenox® (arsenic trioxide in the treatment of myelodysplastic syndromes. *Leukemia* 17:1499, 2003.
487. Cortes J, Giles F, O'Brien S, et al: Results of imatinib mesylate therapy in patients with refractory or recurrent acute myeloid leukemia, high-risk myelodysplastic syndrome, and myeloproliferative disorders. *Cancer* 97:2760, 2003.
488. Drummond MW, Lush CJ, Vickers MA, et al: Imatinib mesylate-induced molecular remission of Philadelphia chromosome-positive myelodysplastic syndrome. *Leukemia* 17:463, 2003.
489. Crump M: Inhibition of raf kinase in the treatment of acute myeloid leukemia. *Curr Pharm Des* 8:2243, 2002.
490. Feldman EJ, Cortes J, DeAngelo DJ, et al: On the use of lonafarnib in myelodysplastic syndrome and chronic myelomonocytic leukemia. *Leukemia* 22:1707, 2008.
491. Kurzrock R, Albitar M, Cortes JE, et al: Phase II study of R115777, a farnesyl transferase inhibitor, in myelodysplastic syndrome. *J Clin Oncol* 22:1287, 2004.
492. Fenaux P, Raza A, Mufti GJ, et al: A multicenter phase 2 study of the farnesyltransferase inhibitor tipifarnib in intermediate- to high-risk myelodysplastic syndrome. *Blood* 109:4158, 2007.
493. Cortes J, Faderl S, Estey E, et al: Phase I study of BMS-214662, a farnesyl transferase inhibitor in patients with acute leukemias and high-risk myelodysplastic syndromes. *J Clin Oncol* 23:2805, 2005.
494. Xia Z, Tan MM, Wong WW, et al: Blocking protein geranylgeranylation is essential for lovastatin-induced apoptosis of human acute myeloid leukemia cells. *Leukemia* 15:1398, 2001.
495. Armand JP, Burnett AK, Drach J, et al: The emerging role of targeted therapy for hematologic malignancies: Update on bortezomib and tipifarnib. *Oncologist* 12:281, 2007.
496. Terpos E, Verrou E, Banti A, et al: Bortezomib is an effective agent for MDS/MPD syndrome with 5q– anomaly and thrombocytosis. *Leuk Res* 31:559, 2007.
497. Cilloni D, Martinelli G, Messa F, et al: Nuclear factor κB as a target for new drug development in myeloid malignancies. *Haematologica* 92:1224, 2007.
498. Rizzieri DA, Feldman E, Dipersio JF, et al: A phase 2 clinical trial of deforolimus (AP23573, MK-8669), a novel mammalian target of rapamycin inhibitor, in patients with relapsed or refractory hematologic malignancies. *Clin Cancer Res* 14:2756, 2008.
499. Sawyers CL: Finding the next Gleevec: FLT3 targeted kinase inhibitor therapy for acute myeloid leukemia. *Cancer Cell* 1:413, 2002.
500. Maserati E, Panarello C, Morerio C, et al: Clonal chromosome anomalies and propensity to myeloid malignancies in congenital amegakaryocytic thrombocytopenia. *Haematologica* 93:1271, 2008.
501. Niparuck P, Atichartakarn V, Chuncharunee S: Successful treatment of acquired amegakaryocytic thrombocytopenic purpura refractory to corticosteroids and intravenous immunoglobulin with antithymocyte globulin and cyclosporin. *Int J Hematol* 88:223, 2008.
502. Minke DM, Colon-Otero G, Cockerill KJ, et al: Refractory thrombocytopenia: A myelodysplastic syndrome that may mimic immune thrombocytopenic purpura. *Am J Clin Pathol* 98:502, 1992.
503. Hoffman R: Acquired pure amegakaryocytic thrombocytopenia purpura. *Semin Hematol* 28:303, 1991.
504. Zeidler C, Germeshausen M, Klein C, Welte K: Clinical implications of ELA2-, HAX1-, and G-CSF-receptor (CSF3R) mutations in severe congenital neutropenia. *Br J Haematol* 2008.
505. Dror Y: Shwachman-Diamond syndrome: Implications for understanding the molecular basis of leukaemia. *Expert Rev Mol Med* 10:e38, 2008.
506. Finsterer J: Hematological manifestations of primary mitochondrial disorders. *Acta Haematol* 118:88, 2007.
507. Orlandi E, Alessandrino EP, Caldera D, Bernasconi C: Adult leukemia after aplastic anemia: Report of 8 cases. *Acta Haematol* 79:174, 1988.
508. DePlanque MM, Bacigalupo A, Wüsch A, et al: Long-term follow up of severe aplastic anemia patients treated with antithymocyte globulin. *Br J Haematol* 73:121, 1989.
509. Dunn DE, Tanawattanacharoen P, Boccuni P, et al: Paroxysmal nocturnal hemoglobinuria cells in patients with bone marrow failure syndromes. *Ann Intern Med* 131:401, 1999.
510. Bischoff L, Derk CT: Eosinophilic fasciitis: Demographics, disease pattern and response to treatment: Report of 12 cases and review of the literature. *Int J Dermatol* 47:29, 2008.
511. Lakhanpal S, Ginsburg WW, Michet CJ, et al: Eosinophilic fasciitis: Clinical spectrum and therapeutic response in 52 cases. *Semin Arthritis Rheum* 17:221, 1988.
512. Naschitz JE, Boss JH, Misselevich I, et al: The fasciitis-panniculitis syndromes. Clinical and pathologic features. *Medicine (Baltimore)* 75:6, 1996.
513. Kim SW, Rice L, Champlin R, Udden MM: Aplastic anemia in eosinophilic fasciitis: Response to immunotherapy and marrow transplantation. *Haematologia (Budap)* 28:131, 1997.
514. Goel R, Kumar R, Bakhshi S:Transformation of childhood MDS-refractory anemia to acute lymphoblastic leukemia. *J Pediatr Hematol Oncol* 29:725, 2007.
515. Disperati P, Ichim CV, Tkachuk D, et al: Progression of myelodysplasia to acute lymphoblastic leukaemia: Implications for disease biology. *Leuk Res* 30:233, 2006.
516. Brusamolino E, Isernia P, Alessandrino EP, et al: Terminal deoxynucleotidyl transferase–positive acute leukemias evolving from a myelodysplastic syndrome. *Am J Hematol* 20:187, 1985.
517. Berneman ZN, Van Bockstaele D, DeMeyer P, et al: A myelodysplastic syndrome preceding acute lymphoblastic leukaemia. *Br J Haematol* 60:353, 1985.
518. Ascensao JL, Kay NE, Wright JJ, et al: Lymphoblastic transformation of myelodysplastic syndrome. *Am J Hematol* 22:431, 1986.
519. Bonati A, Delia D, Starcich R: Progression of a myelodysplastic syndrome to pre-B-acute lymphoblastic leukaemia with unusual phenotype. *Br J Haematol* 64:487, 1986.
520. Dayton MA, VanBesien K, Tricot G, et al: Preleukemic state preceding adult acute lymphoblastic leukemia. *Am J Med* 89:657, 1990.
521. Escudier SM, Albitar M, Robertson LE, et al: Acute lymphoblastic leukemia following preleukemic syndromes in adults. *Leukemia* 10:473, 1996.
522. Saarinen UM, Wegelius R: Preleukemic syndrome in children. Report of four cases and review of literature. *Am J Pediatr Hematol Oncol* 6:137, 1984.

523. Breatnach F, Chessells JM, Greaves MF: The aplastic presentation of childhood leukemia: A feature of common ALL. *Br J Haematol* 49:387, 1981.
524. Klingemann H-G, Storb R, Sanders J, et al: Acute lymphoblastic leukaemia after bone marrow transplantation for aplastic anaemia. *Br J Haematol* 63:47, 1986.
525. Nakamori Y, Takahashi M, Moriyama Y, et al: The aplastic presentation of adult acute lymphoblastic leukaemia. *Br J Haematol* 62:782, 1986.
526. Homans AC, Cohen JL, Barker BE, Marzur EM: Aplastic presentation of acute lymphoblastic leukemia: Evidence for cellular inhibition of normal hematopoietic progenitors. *Am J Pediatr Hematol Oncol* 11:456, 1989.
527. DeAlarcon P, Miller M, Stuart MJ: Erythroid hypoplasia: An unusual presentation of childhood leukemia. *Am J Dis Child* 132:763, 1978.
528. Horsley SW, Colman S, McKinley M, et al: Genetic lesions in a preleukemic aplasia phase in a child with acute lymphoblastic leukemia. *Genes Chromosomes Cancer* 47:333, 2008.
529. Reid MM, Summerfield GP: Distinction between aleukaemic prodrome of childhood acute lymphoblastic leukaemia and aplastic anemia. *J Clin Pathol* 45:697, 1992.
530. MacSween JM, Langley GR: Light-chain disease and sideroblastic anemia–preleukemic chronic granulocytic leukemia. *Can Med Assoc J* 106:995, 1972.
531. Trachida L, Palutke M, Poylik MD, Prasad AS: Primary acquired sideroblastic anemia preceding monoclonal gammopathy and malignant lymphoma. *Am J Med* 55:559, 1973.
532. Papayannis AG, Stathakis NE, Kyrkou K, et al: Primary acquired sideroblastic anemia associated with chronic lymphocytic leukemia. *Br J Haematol* 28:125, 1974.
533. Berkowitz LR, Ross DW, Orringe EP: Hairy cell leukemia with acquired dyserythropoiesis. *JAMA* 140:554, 1980.
534. Catovsky D, Shaw MT, Hoffbrand AV, Dacie JV: Sideroblastic anemia and its association with leukemia and myelomatosis. A report of five cases. *Br J Haematol* 20:385, 1971.
535. Dahlke MA, Nowell PC: Chromosomal abnormalities and dyserythropoiesis in the preleukaemic phase of multiple myeloma. *Br J Haematol* 31:111, 1975.
536. Meckenstock G, Bonatsch CH, Heyll A, et al: T-cell receptor α/δ expressing acute leukemia emerging from sideroblastic anemia: Morphologic, immunological, and cytogenetic features. *Leuk Res* 16:379, 1992.
537. Khaleeli M, Keane WM, Lee GR: Sideroblastic anemia in multiple myeloma. A preleukemic change. *Blood* 41:17, 1973.
538. Greenberg BR, Miller C, Cardoff RD, et al: Concurrent development of preleukaemic lymphoproliferative and plasma cell disorders. *Br J Haematol* 53:125, 1983.
539. Copplestone JA, Mufti GJ, Hamblin TJ, Oscier DG: Immunological abnormalities in myelodysplastic syndromes. *Br J Haematol* 63:149, 1986.

CHAPTER 89
ACUTE MYELOGENOUS LEUKEMIA

Jane L. Liesveld and Marshall A. Lichtman

SUMMARY

Acute myelogenous leukemia (AML) is the result of a sequence of somatic mutations in a multipotential primitive hematopoietic cell or, in some cases, a more differentiated progenitor cell. Exposure to radiation, chronic exposure to high doses of benzene, and chronic, heavy inhalation of tobacco smoke increase the incidence of the disease. A small but increasing proportion of cases develop after a patient with lymphoma or a nonhematologic cancer is exposed to intensive chemotherapy, especially with alkylating agents or topoisomerase II inhibitors. The mutant hematopoietic cell gains a growth and/or survival advantage in relationship to the normal pool of stem cells. As the progeny of this mutant, now leukemic, multipotential cell proliferates to form approximately 11 billion or more cells, normal hematopoiesis is inhibited, and normal red cell, neutrophil, and platelet blood levels fall. The resultant anemia leads to weakness, exertional limitations, and pallor; the thrombocytopenia to spontaneous hemorrhage, usually in the skin; and the neutropenia and monocytopenia to poor wound healing and minor infections. Severe infection usually does not occur at diagnosis but will if the disease progresses because of lack of treatment or if chemotherapy intensifies the decrease of blood neutrophil and monocyte levels. The diagnosis is made by measurement of blood cell counts and examination of blood and marrow cells and is based on identification of leukemic blast cells in the marrow and blood. The diagnosis of AML specifically is confirmed by identification of myeloperoxidase activity in blast cells or by identifying characteristic cluster of differentiation (CD) antigens on the blast cells (e.g., CD13, CD33). The leukemic stem cell is capable of imperfect differentiation and maturation. The clone may contain cells that have the morphologic or immunophenotypic features of erythroblasts, megakaryocytes, monocytes, eosinophils, or, rarely, basophils or mast cells, in addition to myeloblasts or promyelocytes. When one cell line is sufficiently dominant, the leukemia may be referred to as acute erythroid, acute megakaryocytic, acute monocytic, and so on. Certain cytogenetic alterations are more frequent and include t(8;21), t(15;17), inversion 16, trisomy 8, and deletions of all or part of chromosome 5 or 7. A translocation involving chromosome 17 at the site of the retinoic acid receptor alpha (RAR-α) gene is uniquely associated with acute promyelocytic leukemia. AML usually is treated with cytarabine and an anthracycline antibiotic, although other drugs may be added or substituted in poor-prognosis, refractory, or relapsed patients. The exception to this approach is the treatment of acute promyelocytic leukemia with all-*trans*-retinoic acid, arsenic trioxide, and an anthracycline antibiotic. High-dose chemotherapy and either autologous stem cell infusion or allogeneic stem cell transplantation may be used in an effort to treat relapse or patients at high risk to relapse after chemotherapy treatment. The probability of remission ranges from approximately 80 percent in children to less than 25 percent in octogenarians. The probability for cure decreases from approximately 50 percent in children to virtually zero in octogenarians.

Acronyms and abbreviations that appear in this chapter include: AIDS, acquired immunodeficiency syndrome; ALL, acute lymphocytic leukemia; AML, acute myelogenous leukemia; APL, acute promyelocytic leukemia; As_2O_3, arsenic trioxide; ATRA, all-*trans*-retinoic acid; CD, cluster of differentiation; CEBPA, CCAAT-enhancer binding protein A; CML, chronic myelogenous leukemia; CNS, central nervous system; FAB, French-American-British classification; FISH, fluorescence *in situ* hybridization; G-CSF, granulocyte colony-stimulating factor; GM-CSF, granulocyte-monocyte colony-stimulating factor; GVHD, graft-versus-host disease; HIV, human immunodeficiency virus; HLA, human leukocyte antigen; Ig, immunoglobulin; MDR, multidrug resistance; MDS, myelodysplastic syndrome; PAS, periodic acid-Schiff; PCR, polymerase chain reaction; PDGF, platelet-derived growth factor; P-gp, permeability glycoprotein; RT, reverse transcriptase; TdT, terminal deoxynucleotidyl transferase; TMD, transient myeloproliferative disease; TNF, tumor necrosis factor; VEGF, vascular endothelial growth factor; VEGFR, vascular endothelial growth factor receptor; WHO, World Health Organization.

DEFINITION AND HISTORY

Acute myelogenous leukemia (AML) is a clonal, malignant disease of hematopoietic tissues that is characterized by (1) accumulation of abnormal (leukemic) blast cells, principally in the marrow, and (2) impaired production of normal blood cells. Thus, the leukemic cell infiltration in marrow is accompanied, nearly invariably, by anemia and thrombocytopenia. The absolute neutrophil count may be low or normal, depending on the total white cell count.

The first well-documented case of acute leukemia is attributed to Friedreich,[1] but Ebstein[2] was the first to use the term *acute leukämie* in 1889. This work led to the general appreciation of the clinical distinctions between AML and chronic myelogenous leukemia (CML).[3] In 1878, Neumann,[4] who proposed that marrow was the site of blood cell production, first suggested that leukemia originated in the marrow and used the term *myelogene* (myelogenous) leukemia. The availability of polychromatic stains, as a result of the work of Ehrlich,[5] the description of the myeloblast and myelocyte by Naegeli,[6] and the earliest appreciation of the common origin of red cells and leukocytes by Hirschfield[7] laid the foundation for our current understanding of the disease.

Although Theodor Boveri proposed a critical role for chromosomal abnormalities in the development of cancer in 1914, a series of technical developments in the 1950s was needed to permit informed examination of the chromosomes of cancer cells. Thereafter, the discovery that a G group chromosome consistently had a foreshortened long arm in the cells of patients with CML (Philadelphia chromosome) supported the concept that chromosome abnormalities may be specifically linked to a cancer phenotype. This finding was followed by the introduction of banding of chromosomes, which enhanced the specific identification of individual chromosomes and the point at which they break in the formation of a translocation, inversion, or deletion. This technologic advance unleashed the power of cancer cytogenetics and initiated an era of leukemia study based not solely on the appearance of cells under the microscope (phenotype) but also by their chromosomal or genetic abnormality (genotype).[8] The completion of the major phase of the human genome project further enhanced the specificity of the identification of gene alterations.[9] These advances permitted (1) more precise understanding of the molecular pathology of specific leukemia subtypes, (2) improvement of diagnostic and prognostic methods for the study of AML, and (3) identification of molecular targets for therapy.

The introduction to the clinic by Holland, Ellison, and colleagues[10] of arabinosyl cytosine (cytarabine) in the late 1960s as the first potent drug for treatment of AML, followed by their introduction of the combination of 7 days of cytosine arabinoside and 3 days of daunomycin in the early 1970s (the "7 and 3 regimen")[11] opened the era of effective therapy for AML. This drug combination or its congeners remains the mainstay of treatment nearly four decades later. The description of allogeneic marrow (stem cell) transplantation as a curative therapy for AML by Thomas and colleagues[12] in 1977 ushered in the era of hematopoietic stem cell transplantation as a modality to cure eligible patients with AML.

ETIOLOGY AND PATHOGENESIS

ENVIRONMENTAL FACTORS

Table 89–1 lists the major conditions that predispose to development of AML. Only four environmental factors are established causal agents: tobacco smoking, high-dose radiation exposure,[13,14] chronic benzene exposure,[14–18] and chemotherapeutic (DNA-damaging) agents.[19–25] Most patients have not been exposed to an antecedent causative factor. Exposure to high-linear energy transfer radiation from α-emitting radioisotopes such as thorium dioxide increases the risk of AML.[26] Case-control studies have sometimes found a relationship between AML and organic solvents, petroleum products, radon exposure, pesticides, and herbicides, but these data have been inconsistent, have shown no association in several studies, and have not reached a level comparable to the strong association that exists for benzene, high-dose external irradiation, and certain chemotherapeutic agents.[27] The increased incidence of AML related to benzene exposure has not been seen in studies of industrial sites in which stringent regulations regarding benzene exposure have been implemented.[14] There is a significant association between tobacco smoking and AML with a relative risk of about 1.5 to 2.0.[28–30]

EVOLUTION FROM A CHRONIC CLONAL HEMOPATHY

AML may develop from the progression of other clonal disorders of a multipotential hematopoietic cell, including CML, polycythemia vera, primary myelofibrosis, essential thrombocythemia, and clonal sideroblastic anemia or oligoblastic myelogenous leukemia (MDS; see Table 89–1). Clonal progression can occur spontaneously, although with a different probability of occurrence in each chronic disorder (see Chap. 85). The frequency of clonal progression to AML is enhanced by radiation or chemotherapy in patients with polycythemia vera (see Chap. 86) or essential thrombocythemia (see Chap. 87).[23,31]

PREDISPOSING DISEASES

Patients who develop AML may have an antecedent predisposing nonmyeloid disease, such as aplastic anemia (polyclonal T-cell disorder), myeloma (monoclonal B-cell disorder),[32,33] or, rarely, AIDS (HIV-induced polyclonal T-cell disorder).[34] An association between immune thyroid diseases and familial polyendocrine disorder and AML has been reported.[35,36] A number of inherited conditions carry an increased risk of AML (see Table 89–1).[37–79] In the inherited syndromes, at least several pathogenetic types of gene alterations are represented: (1) DNA repair defects, e.g., Fanconi anemia; (2) susceptibility genes favoring a second mutation, e.g., familial platelet syndrome; (3) tumor-suppressor defects, e.g., dyskeratosis congenita; and (4) unknown mechanisms, e.g., ataxia-pancytopenia (see Chap. 34 and reference 46 for further details of each pathogenetic process).

MOLECULAR PATHOGENESIS

AML results from a series of somatic mutations in either a hematopoietic multipotential cell or, occasionally, a more differentiated, lineage-restricted progenitor cell.[78] Some cases of monocytic leukemia, promyelocytic

TABLE 89–1. Conditions Pedisposing to Development of Acute Myelogenous Leukemia

Environmental factors
Radiation[13,14,25]
Benzene[14–18]
Alkylating agents, topoisomerase II inhibitors, and other cytotoxic drugs[14,19–25]
Tobacco smoke[27,28]
Acquired diseases
Clonal myeloid diseases
Chronic myelogenous leukemia (Chap. 90)
Primary myelofibrosis (Chap. 91)
Essential thrombocythemia (Chap. 87)
Polycythemia vera (Chap. 86)
Clonal cytopenias (Chap. 88)
Paroxysmal nocturnal hemoglobinuria (Chap. 40)
Other hematopoietic disorders
Aplastic anemia (Chap. 34)
Eosinophilic fasciitis (Chap. 88)
Myeloma[32,33]
Other disorders
Human immunodeficiency virus infection[34]
Thyroid disorders[35]
Polyendocrine disorders[36]
Inherited or Congenital Conditions
Sibling with AML[37–39]
Amegakaryocytic thrombocytopenia, congenital[40,41]
Ataxia-pancytopenia[42,43]
Bloom syndrome[44,45]
Congenital agranulocytosis (Kostmann syndrome)[46–49]
Chronic thrombocytopenia with chromosome 21q 22.12 microdeletion[50]
Diamond-Blackfan syndrome[51,52]
Down syndrome[53,54]
Dubowitz syndrome[55]
Dyskeratosis congenita[56,57]
Familial (pure, nonsyndromic) AML[58]
Familial platelet disorder[59,60]
Fanconi anemia[61,62]
Naxos syndrome[63]
Neurofibromatosis 1[64,65]
Noonan syndrome[66,67]
Poland syndrome[68]
Rothmund-Thomson syndrome[69,70]
Seckel syndrome[71]
Shwachman syndrome[72–74]
Werner syndrome (progeria)[75–77]
Wolf-Hirschhorn syndrome[78]
WT syndrome[79]

leukemia, and AML in younger individuals more likely arise in a progenitor cell with lineage restrictions (progenitor cell leukemia).[80–84] Other morphologic phenotypes and older patients likely have disease that originates in a primitive multipotential cell.[78] In the latter case, all blood cell lineages can be derived from the leukemic stem cell because it retains the ability for some degree of differentiation and maturation (see Chap. 85).

The AML stem cell has been defined by its immunophenotype, CD123+CD45dimCD34+CD38–. These stem cells can be isolated from cases of AML at presentation or at relapse. In remission, the AML stem cell can be found using a panel of antigens—CLL-1, CD5, CD7, CD19, CD56—to identify leukemic stem cells bearing CD45dim,CD34+Cd38–.[85] Attempts to find agents that selectively target AML stem cells are under way.[86]

Somatic mutation results from a chromosomal translocation in the majority of patients.[87] The translocation results in rearrangement of a critical region of a protooncogene. Fusion of portions of two genes usually does not prevent the processes of transcription and translation; thus, the fusion gene encodes a fusion protein that, because of its abnormal structure, disrupts a normal cell pathway and predisposes to a malignant transformation of the cell. The mutant protein product often is a transcription factor or an element in the transcription pathway that disrupts the regulatory sequences controlling growth rate or survival of blood cell progenitors and their differentiation and maturation.[87–89] Examples of genes often mutated are core binding factor, retinoic acid receptor-α (*RAR-α*), *HOX* family, *MLL*, and others. Core binding factor (*CBF*) has two subunits: *CBF-β* and *RUNX1* (formerly*AML1*). Approximately 10 percent of AML cases have translocations involving one or the other of these latter two genes, although the percentage varies depending on the patient's age at onset. In patients younger than age 50 years, the frequency is approximately 20 percent. In patients older than age 50 years, the frequency is approximately 6 percent. Core binding factor activates genes involved in myeloid and lymphoid differentiation and maturation. These primary mutations are not sufficient to cause AML. Additional activating mutations, for example, in hematopoietic tyrosine kinases *FLT3* and *KIT* or in N-*RAS* and K-*RAS*, are required to induce a proliferative advantage in the affected primitive cell.[85] Other protooncogene mutations occur in leukemic cells involving *FES, FOS, GATA-1, JUN B, MPL, MYC,* p53, *PU.1, RB, WT1, WNT, NPM1, CEPBA,* and other genes.[90–101] Their interaction with loss-of-function mutations in hematopoietic transcription factors probably causes the acute leukemia phenotype characterized by a disorder of proliferation, programmed cell death, differentiation, and maturation.[89,100] A minimum of two classes of genes has been proposed: class I gene mutations, for example, *RUNX1*, which lead to a proliferation and survival advantage to the cells in the clone, and class II gene mutations, for example, core binding factor, which interacts with the class I mutation, conferring severely disturbed differentiation and maturation patterns on the mutated cell and fostering the evolution of a classic AML phenotype.[89] Because the mutant stem or early progenitor cell can proliferate and retains the capability to differentiate, a wide variety of phenotypes can emerge from a leukemic transformation.

FLT3 encodes a tyrosine kinase receptor in normal myeloid and lymphoid progenitors. Internal tandem duplications of *FLT3* on chromosome 13 occurs in approximately one-fourth to one-third of adult AML cases but occurs more frequently in cases of AML with normal cytogenetic patterns, monocytic phenotype, and *PML-RAR-α* or *DEK-CAN* translocations.[102] The *FLT3*-internal tandem duplication *(ITD)* mutation confers a poor prognosis if the ratio of mutant to wild-type expression is high.[103,104] Hypermethylation of the death-associated protein kinase has been observed in approximately 25 percent of AML cases and is twice as prevalent in cases of AML following cytotoxic therapy.

Deletions of all or part of a chromosome (e.g., chromosome 5, 7, or 9) or additional chromosomes (such as trisomy 4, 8, or 13) are common cytogenetic abnormalities (see Chap. 11), although the specific causative oncogenes or tumor suppressor genes in these latter circumstances have not been defined. Deletions in chromosomes 5 and 7 and complex cytogenetic abnormalities are increased in frequency in older patients and cases of AML following cytotoxic therapy compared to *de novo* cases.[105] Because the genes residing on the undeleted homologous segment of chromosome 5 are not mutated, an epigenetic lesion, such as hypermethylation of a gene allelic to one on the deleted segment on chromosome 5, may result in the leukemogenic event.

In acute promyelocytic leukemia, *PML-RAR-α* fusion protein represses retinoic acid-inducible genes, which prevent appropriate maturation of promyelocytes. The induced disruption, which involves corepressor–histone deacetylase complexes, results in the leukemic phenotype (see "Acute Promyelocytic Leukemia" below).[106,107]

DEREGULATED SIGNALING PATHWAYS

The mutations in AML result in deregulation of any of several signal transduction pathways, which disrupt pathways that ensure the normal behavior of (1) differentiation and maturation, (2) proliferation, and (3) survival signals in hematopoietic cells. The pathways involved are myriad but several represent the majority of cases. These include the (1) PI3K-AKT, (2) RAS-RAF-MEK-ERK, and (3) STAT3 signaling sequences.[108] The expectation is that a relative small number of downstream signaling pathways mediate the leukemogenic effect of gene mutations, making the potential targets for therapy less diffuse than suggested by the number of gene mutations involved in AML.

MODE OF INHERITANCE

In most cases, little evidence is seen for a strong influence of inherited factors. The identical twin of a child with acute leukemia has a heightened risk of developing the disease. However, the risk appears to be related to intraplacental metastasis and thus falls to the risk of a nonidentical sibling after the first few years of life.[109,110] The risk of AML in a nonidentical sibling in the United States is elevated, perhaps twofold to threefold, compared to the risk of AML in unrelated American children of European descent younger than age 15 years.[109,111] Clusters of AML cases in families have been documented, but their frequency is low.[58] Clusters of AML in unrelated persons in a community are uncommon and, when investigated, usually prove to be a chance occurrence.

EPIDEMIOLOGY

AML is the predominant form of leukemia during the neonatal period but represents a small proportion of cases during childhood and adolescence. Approximately 15,000 new cases of AML occur annually, representing approximately 35 percent of the annual new cases of leukemia in the United States. Approximately 9000 patients with AML in the United States die each year as a result of the disease. The incidence rate of AML is approximately 1.5 per 100,000 in infants younger than 1 year of age, decreases to approximately 0.4 per 100,000 children ages 5 to 9 years, increases gradually to approximately 1.0 persons per 100,000 until age 25 years, and thereafter increases exponentially until the rate reaches approximately 25 per 100,000 persons in octogenarians (Fig. 89–1). The exception to this exponential age-related increase in incidence is acute promyelocytic leukemia (APL), which does not change greatly in incidence with age.[112]

AML accounts for 15 to 20 percent of the acute leukemias in children and 80 percent of the acute leukemias in adults. It is slightly more common in males. Little difference in incidence is seen between individuals of African or European descent at any age. A somewhat lower incidence is

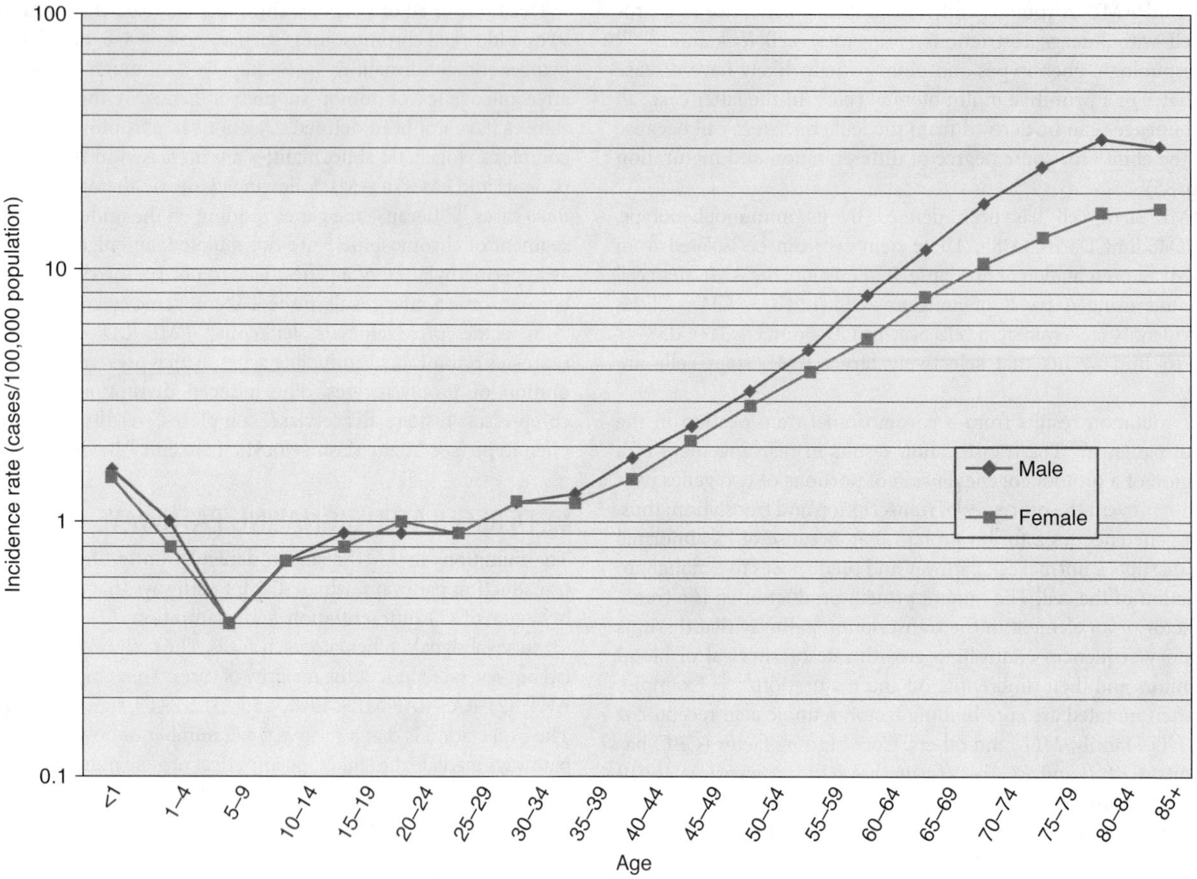

FIGURE 89–1. The annual incidence of acute myelogenous leukemia as a function of age. There is a relatively small increase to about 1.5 cases per 100,000 population in the first year of life year representing congenital, neonatal, and infant AML. The incidence falls to a nadir of 0.4 new cases per 100,000 population over the first 10 years of life and then rises again to 1 case per 100,000 in the second decade of life. From about 25 years of age, the incidence increases exponentially (log-linear) to about 20 cases per 100,000 population in octogenarians.

seen in persons of Asian descent. An increase in the frequency of AML is seen in Jews, especially those of Eastern European descent. The acute promyelocytic variant of AML is somewhat more common in Latinos.[113,114]

CLASSIFICATION

Variants of AML can be identified by morphologic features of blood films using polychromatic stains and histochemical reactions,[115] monoclonal antibodies against surface markers,[115–120] or by the presence of specific chromosome translocations.[121] The epitopes on the progenitor cells of several phenotypic variants overlap, and several monoclonal antibodies are required to make specific distinctions among cell types (Table 89–2; see also "Morphologic Variants of Acute Myelogenous Leukemia" and Table 89–4 below). Correlation between morphologic and immunologic phenotyping of AML is poor. However, poor correlation is expected because the former method is more subjective, given to observer variation, and is based on qualitative factors, whereas the latter method, which characterizes surface molecular features, is more accurate and reproducible. The correlation is improved only somewhat if morphology and histochemistry are coupled.[122] Gene expression profiling is early in its use as a classification technique for AML but may prove to be more specific and informative than current methods.[123,124] The outcome will depend on the simplification and automation of such techniques, and the availability of drugs that make such distinctions in the prognostic category of practical utility. Chapter 85 contains the classification of morphologic variants of AML (see Table 85–1 and Fig. 85–2). The need to consider functional markers for drug resistance, such as *MDR* expression, has been proposed to separate more-responsive from less-responsive AML. However, a cogent argument has been made that, for practical purposes, a classification that initially considers morphologic phenotype and immunophenotype is advisable. Cytogenetics, molecular genetics, gene expression

TABLE 89–2. Immunologic Phenotypes of AML

Phenotype	Usually Positive
Myeloblastic	CD11b, CD13, CD15, CD33, CD117, HLA-DR
Myelomonocytic	CD11b, CD13, CD14, CD15, CD32, CD33, HLA-DR
Erythroid	Glycophorin, spectrin, ABH antigens, carbonic anhydrase I, HLA-DR
Promyelocytic	CD13, CD33
Monocytic	CD11b, 11c, CD13, CD14, CD33, CD65, HLA-DR
Megakaryoblastic	CD34, CD41, CD42, CD61, anti-von Willebrand factor
Basophilic	CD11b, CD13, CD33, CD123, CD203c
Mast cell	CD13, CD33, CD117

NOTE: Chapter 14 provides the definition of the antigen that represents a cluster of differentiation (CD).

profiling, *MDR* expression, and other considerations can, and should, be layered on as available and useful in influencing therapy.[125]

CLINICAL FEATURES

SIGNS AND SYMPTOMS

General

Signs and symptoms that signal the onset of AML include pallor, fatigue, weakness, palpitations, and dyspnea on exertion. The signs and symptoms reflect the development of anemia; however, weakness, loss of sense of well-being, and fatigue on exertion can be disproportionate to the severity of anemia.[126–130]

Easy bruising, petechiae, epistaxis, gingival bleeding, conjunctival hemorrhages, and prolonged bleeding from skin injuries reflect thrombocytopenia and are frequent early manifestations of the disease. Very infrequently, gastrointestinal, genitourinary, bronchopulmonary, or central nervous system (CNS) bleeding occurs at the onset of disease.

Pustules or other minor pyogenic infections of the skin and of minor cuts or wounds are most common. Major infections, such as sinusitis, pneumonia, pyelonephritis, and meningitis, are uncommon presenting features of the disease, partly because absolute neutrophil counts less than 500/μL (0.5×10^9/L) are uncommon until chemotherapy starts. With intensification of neutropenia and monocytopenia after chemotherapy, major bacterial, fungal, or viral infections become more frequent. Anorexia and weight loss are frequent findings. Fever is present in many patients at the time of diagnosis.[129,131–133] Palpable splenomegaly or hepatomegaly occurs in approximately one-third of patients.[126,127,130] Lymphadenopathy is extremely uncommon,[130,134,135] except in the monocytic variant of AML.[136]

Specific Organ System Involvement

Leukemic blast cells circulate and enter most tissues in small numbers. Occasionally, biopsy or autopsy uncovers marked aggregates or infiltrates of leukemic cells. Collections of such cells may cause functional disturbances. Extramedullary involvement is most common in monocytic or myelomonocytic leukemia.[137,138]

Skin involvement may be of three types: nonspecific lesions, leukemia cutis, or granulocytic (myeloid) sarcoma of skin and subcutis.[139–142] Nonspecific lesions include macules, papules, vesicles, pyoderma gangrenosum, vasculitis,[143–145] neutrophilic dermatitis (Sweet syndrome),[146] cutis vertices gyrata,[147] and erythema multiforme or nodosum.[140,141] Skin involvement preceding marrow and blood involvement or relapse occurs but is rare.[148–151]

Sensory organ involvement is very unusual, but retinal, choroidal, iridial, and optic nerve infiltration can occur.[152] Otitis externa and interna, inner ear hemorrhage, and mastoid tumors with seventh nerve involvement may be presenting signs.[153–155]

The *gastrointestinal tract* may be involved at any point, but functional disturbances are unusual.[156,157] The mouth, colon, and anal canal are sites of involvement that most commonly lead to symptoms. Oral manifestations may prompt the patient to visit the dentist. Gingival or periodontal infiltration and dental abscesses may lead to an extraction, followed by prolonged bleeding of an infected tooth socket.[158] Ileotyphlitis (enterocolitis), a necrotizing inflammatory lesion involving the terminal ileum, cecum, and ascending colon, can be a presenting syndrome or occur during treatment.[159–162] Fever, abdominal pain, bloody diarrhea, or ileus may be present and occasionally mimic appendicitis. Intestinal perforation, an inflammatory mass, and associated infection with enteric gram-negative bacilli or clostridial species often are associated with a fatal outcome. Isolated involvement of the gastrointestinal tract is rare.[163,164] Proctitis, especially common in the monocytic variant of AML, can be a presenting sign or a vexing problem during periods of severe granulocytopenia and diarrhea.[156]

The *respiratory tract* can be involved by infiltrates or tumors, leading to laryngeal obstruction, parenchymal infiltrates, alveolar septal infiltration, or pleural seeding. Each of these events can result in severe symptoms and radiologic findings.[165–169]

Cardiac involvement is frequent but rarely causes symptoms. Symptomatic pericardial infiltrates, transmural ventricular infiltrates with hemorrhage, and endocardial foci with associated intracavitary thrombi can occasionally cause heart failure, arrhythmia, and death.[170] Infiltration of the conducting system or valve leaflets or myocardial infarction has occurred.[171]

The *urogenital system* can be affected. The kidneys are infiltrated with leukemic cells in a high proportion of cases, but functional abnormalities are rare. Hemorrhage in the pelvis or collecting system is frequent.[172,173] Cases of vulvar, bladder neck, prostatic, and testicular involvement have been described.[174–176]

Osteoarticular symptoms may occur. Bone pain, joint pain, and bone necrosis can occur, and, rarely, arthritis with effusion is present.[177] Crystal-induced arthritis of either calcium pyrophosphate dihydrate (pseudogout) or monosodium urate (gout) may be responsible for the synovitis in some cases.[178]

Central or peripheral *nervous system* involvement by infiltration of leukemic cells is very uncommon, although meningeal involvement is an important consideration in the treatment of the monocytic type of AML.[179,180] An association of CNS involvement and diabetes insipidus in AML with monosomy 7[181] and inversion of chromosome 16[182,183] has been reported.

Myeloid (Granulocytic) Sarcoma

Myeloid sarcoma (also known as granulocytic sarcoma, chloroma, myeloblastoma, monocytoma) is a tumor composed of myeloblasts, monoblasts, or megakaryocyes.[184–189] The tumors may occur as extramedullary masses without evidence of leukemia in blood or marrow, so-called nonleukemic myeloid sarcomas, or in association with AML. When the tumors appear as isolated lesions, they initially may be misdiagnosed as extranodal lymphoma because they look like lymphoid cells on biopsy.[186] They may be found in virtually any location, including the skin; orbit; paranasal sinuses; bone; chest wall; breast; heart; gastrointestinal, respiratory, or genitourinary tract; central or peripheral nervous system; or lymph nodes and spleen. The tumors originally were called *chloromas* because of the green color imparted by the high concentration of the enzyme myeloperoxidase present in myelogenous leukemic cells. Biopsy specimens are positive for chloracetate esterase, lysozyme, myeloperoxidase, and cluster of differentiation (CD) markers of myeloid cells. When myeloid sarcomas are the initial manifestation of AML, the appearance of the disease in the blood and marrow may follow weeks or months later. Abnormalities in chromosome 8 are the most frequent cytogenetic disturbance in nonleukemic sarcomas.[187] Systemic chemotherapy, rather than local therapy, should be used for treatment, although the long-term outcome in such cases usually is poor.[189–191] Patients having AML with t(8;21) have a propensity to develop extramedullary leukemia,[192–195] and such patients with myeloid sarcomas have a poorer outcome after treatment.[192,194]

LABORATORY FEATURES

BLOOD CELL FINDINGS

Anemia is a constant feature.[126–130] Red cell life span may be mildly shortened, but the principal cause of anemia is inadequate production of red cells. The reticulocyte count usually is between 0.5 and 2.0 percent. Occasionally patients have rapid destruction of autologous and transfused red cells as a result of an unknown mechanism (milieu hemolysis). The presence of red cell autoantibodies (positive Coombs test) is very uncommon and may be nonspecific (anti-C_3), perhaps related to circulating immune complexes. Red cell morphology is mildly abnormal, with exaggerated variation in cell size and occasional poikilocytes. Nucleated red cells or stippled erythrocytes may be present. Less often, extreme abnormalities of red cell size, shape, and hemoglobin content occur (AML with trilineage dysmorphia), but these changes are seen more often in oligoblastic myelogenous leukemia (see Chap. 88).

Thrombocytopenia is nearly always present at the time of diagnosis. The mechanism of thrombocytopenia is a combination of inadequate production and decreased survival of platelets. More than half of patients have a platelet count less than 50,000/μL (50×10^9/L) at the time of diagnosis.[196] Giant platelets and poorly granulated platelets with functional abnormalities can occur.[197] Defects in platelet aggregation and 5-hydroxytryptamine release are frequent.[197]

The total leukocyte count is less than 5000/μL (5×10^9/L) in approximately half of patients at the time of diagnosis.[126–130] The absolute neutrophil count is less than 1000/μL (1×10^9/L) in more than half of cases at diagnosis.[126–130] Patients with very elevated total leukocyte counts have a low proportion of mature neutrophils but may have a normal absolute neutrophil count. Hypersegmented, hyposegmented, and hypogranular mature neutrophils may be present. Cytochemical abnormalities of blood neutrophils include low or absent myeloperoxidase or low alkaline phosphatase activity.[198] Defects in phagocytosis or microbial killing are common.[199]

Myeloblasts almost always are present in the blood but may be infrequent in severely leukopenic patients. Diligent search may uncover the myeloblasts, or examination of a white cell concentrate (buffy coat) may permit their identification. Classic leukemic blast cells are agranular, but mixtures of immature cells, including agranular and slightly granular cells ranging up to overt progranulocytes, can occur. Auer rods are elliptical cytoplasmic inclusions approximately 1.5 μm long and 0.5 μm wide that derive from azurophilic granules (see Fig. 89–2B). The inclusions are present in the blast cells of approximately 15 percent of cases. When present, the inclusions are found in only a small percentage of blast cells when examined with polychrome stains.[115,200] An exception is APL, in which a high proportion of cells have Auer rods and some have multiple (bundles) of rods. This finding can be dramatic if peroxidase stain is used to highlight the Auer rods.

MARROW FINDINGS

Morphology

The marrow always contains leukemic blast cells. From 3 to 95 percent of marrow cells are blasts at the time of diagnosis or relapse. The World Health Organization (WHO) has invoked an arbitrary breakpoint of 20 percent of marrow nucleated cells being blast cells to distinguish polyblastic AML (≥20% blasts) from oligoblastic myelogenous leukemia (<20% blasts).[126–130,200] The latter situation is referred to as refractory anemia with excess blasts, a myelodysplastic syndrome (see Chap. 88). The WHO choice of ≥20 percent blasts is an arbitrary, inconsistent, and confusing standard. Acute monocytic leukemia, acute promyelocytic leukemia, acute erythroid leukemia, and other variants often have less than 20 percent blast cells at the time of diagnosis. Moreover, relapse of AML can be identified at any increase in blast count >1 percent. Myeloblasts are distinguished from lymphoblasts by any of three pathognomonic features: reactivity with specific histochemical stains; Auer rods in the cells; or reactivity with a panel of monoclonal antibodies against epitopes present on myeloblasts (e.g., CD13, CD33, CD117). Leukemic myeloblasts give positive histochemical reactions for peroxidase, Sudan black B, or naphthyl AS-D-chloroacetate esterase stains. Auer rods can be found in the marrow blast cells in approximately one-sixth of cases. Blast cells may express granulocytic (CD15, CD65) or monocytic (CD11b, CD11c, CD14, CD64) surface antigens. They typically do not express either lymphoid surface markers or membrane or cytoplasmic immunoglobulin. No immunoglobulin gene rearrangement or T-lymphocyte receptor gene rearrangement is evident with molecular probes (see "Hybrid and Mixed Leukemias" below). In a proportion of otherwise typical cases of AML, the cells may contain terminal deoxynucleotidyl transferase (TdT).[201,202] Variations in marrow findings are discussed further below in "Morphologic Variants of Acute Myelogenous Leukemia." Normal erythropoiesis, megakaryocytopoiesis, and granulopoiesis are decreased or absent in the marrow aspirate. The biopsy may contain residual islands of erythroblasts or megakaryocytes. Dysmorphic changes in hematopoietic cells, including very small or large erythroblasts with nuclear fragmentation or binucleation or delayed nuclear condensation; small or monolobed megakaryocytes; or hypogranulated, bilobed, or monolobed neutrophils, may occur in 30 to 50 percent of patients with *de novo* AML.[203] Marrow reticulin fibrosis is common but usually is slight to moderate except in cases of megakaryoblastic leukemia, in which intense fibrosis is the rule.[204] Increased blood vessel density (angiogenesis) is present in the marrow of patients with AML compared to normal subjects.[205,206] Various angiogenic factors, including vascular endothelial growth factor (VEGF), basic fibroblast growth factor, angiogenin, and angiopoietin-1, are increased. VEGF detected histochemically in human marrow is closely correlated with the prevalence of leukemic myeloblasts in the various AML subtypes.[207] AML cytogenetic variants may result in marrow basophilia (usually t(6;9))[208] or marrow eosinophilia (usually inv16 or t(16;16)).[209]

Marrow Cell Culture

Progenitor cells for granulocytes, monocytes and macrophages, or both granulocytes and macrophages form colonies when normal marrow cells are grown in a viscous medium with a source of growth factors. Marrow cells from patients with AML have heterogeneous growth patterns. The marrow of approximately 85 percent of patients does not have colony-forming cells, but the marrow of 60 percent of patients has cells capable of forming small clusters (4–40 cells) *in vitro*. Approximately 15 percent of patients retain colony-forming cells, but often in reduced numbers and with abnormal maturation patterns.[210,211] Restoration of colony-forming cells in the marrow of treated patients often precedes morphologic evidence of remission.[212] The correlation of pretreatment marrow colonial growth pattern *in vitro* with the outcome of intensive chemotherapy is insufficiently strong to use growth pattern as a prognostic variable.[213]

Cytogenetic and Genic Features

An abnormal number (aneuploidy) or structure (pseudodiploidy) of chromosomes or both are evident in approximately 60 percent of cases.[214–217] The most prevalent abnormalities are trisomy 8, monosomy 7, monosomy 21, trisomy 21, and loss of an X or Y chromosome. However, any chromosome can be rearranged, added, or lost. In cases of AML following chemotherapy or radiotherapy, loss of part or all of chromosome 5 is a common feature,[218–220] as are the cytogenetic findings noted above for AML, occurring *de novo*. Table 89–3 lists the most frequent abnormalities and translocations seen in AML (see Chap. 11). The translocations 8;21 and 15;17 and inversion 16 confer a more favorable outcome on average. Deletion of all or part of chromosomes 5 and 7 or the presence of complex changes confers an unfavorable prognosis. Other findings (e.g., normal karyotype, +8, 11q23) generally confer an intermediate prognosis (see Chap. 11 for further details).[214–216]

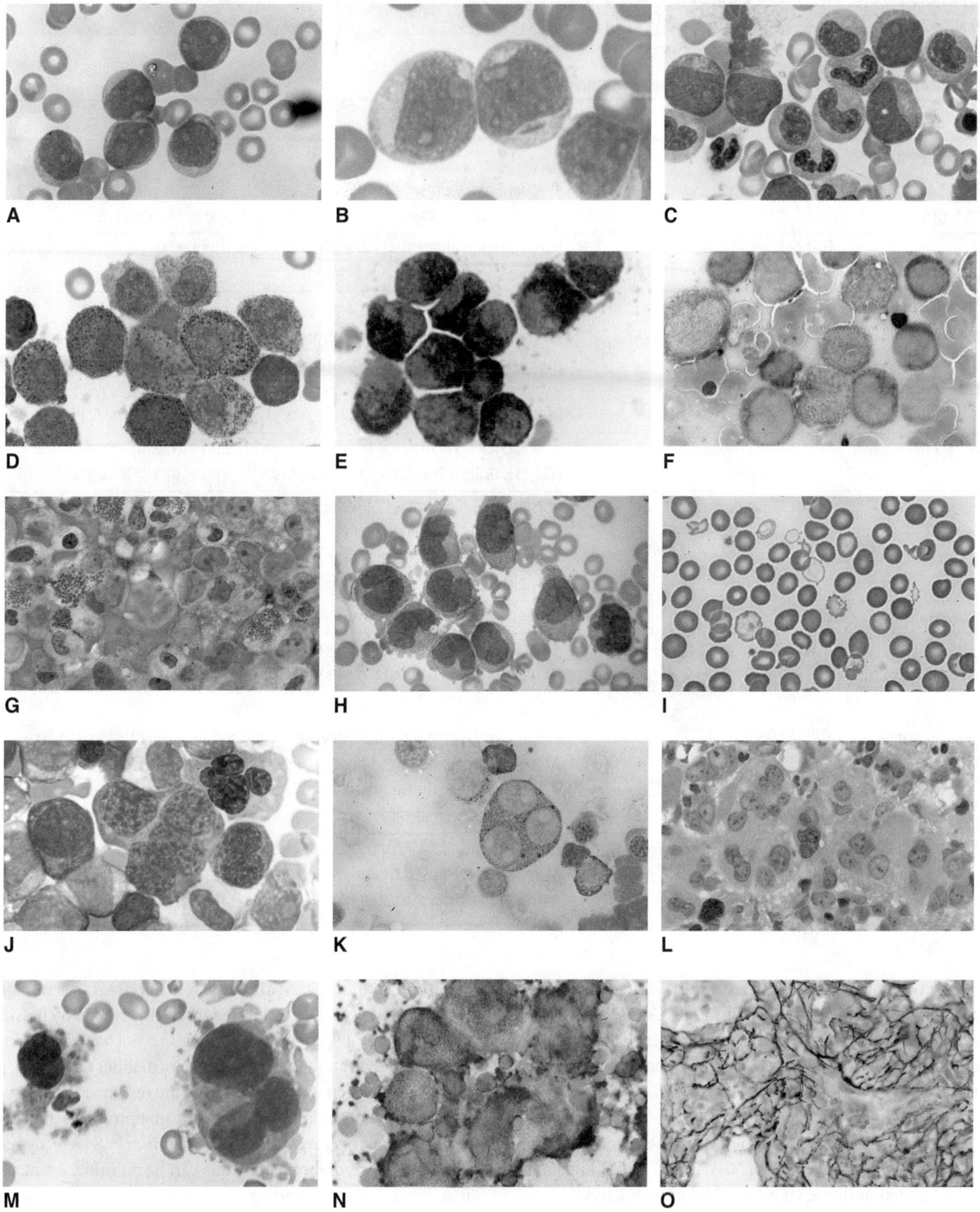

FIGURE 89–2. Blood and marrow images of major subtypes of acute myelogenous leukemia. **A.** Blood film of AML without maturation (acute myeloblastic leukemia). Five myeloblasts are evident. High nuclear-to-cytoplasmic ratio. Agranular cells. Nucleoli in each cell. **B.** Blood film. AML without maturation (acute myeloblastic leukemia). Three myeloblasts, one containing an Auer rod. **C.** Marrow film. AML with maturation. Three leukemic myeloblasts admixed with myelocytes, bands, and segmented neutrophils. **D.** Blood film. Acute promyelocytic leukemia. Majority of cells are heavily granulated leukemic promyelocytes. **E.** Blood film. Acute promyelocytic leukemia. Myeloperoxidase stain. Intensely positive. Numerous stained (black) granules in cytoplasm of leukemic progranulocytes. **F.** Blood film. Acute myelomonocytic leukemia. Double esterase stain. Leukemic monocytic cells stained dark blue and leukemic neutrophil precursors stained reddish-brown. **G.** Marrow film. AML with inv16. Note high proportion of eosinophils in field. Note myeloblasts with very large nucleoli at upper right. Also, intermediate leukemic granulocytic forms. **H.** Blood film. Acute monocytic leukemia. Leukemic cells have characteristics of monocytes with agranular gray cytoplasm and reniform or folded nuclei with characteristic chromatin staining. This case had hyperleukocytosis as evident by leukemic monocyte frequency in blood film. **I.** Blood film. Acute erythroid leukemia. Note population of extremely hypochromic cells with scattered bizarre-shaped poikilocytes admixed with normal-appearing red cells. **J.** Marrow film. Acute erythroid leukemia. Giant erythroblasts with multilobulated nuclei. **K.** Marrow film. Acute erythroid leukemia. Note giant trinucleate erythroblast and other leukemic erythroblasts with periodic acid-Schiff–positive cytoplasmic staining (reddish granules). **L.** Marrow section. Acute megakaryoblastic leukemia. Marrow replaced with atypical two- and three-lobed leukemic megakaryocytes with bold nucleoli. **M.** Marrow film. Acute megakaryoblastic leukemia. Marrow replaced with atypical megakaryocytes and megakaryoblasts with cytoplasmic disorganization, fragmentation, and budding. **N.** Marrow film. Acute megakaryoblastic leukemia. Marrow replaced with atypical megakaryocytes and megakaryoblasts staining for platelet glycoprotein IIIA (reddish-brown). Platelets in background also stained. **O.** Marrow section. Acute megakaryoblastic leukemia. Argentophilic (silver) stain shows marked increase in collagen, type III fibrils (marrow reticulin fibrosis), characteristic of this AML subtype. *(Images reproduced from* Lichtman's Atlas of Hematology, *www.accessmedicine.com, with permission.)*

TABLE 89–3. Clinical Correlates of Frequent Cytogenetic Abnormalities Observed in AML

Chromosome Abnormality	Genes Affected	Clinical Correlation
Loss or Gain of Chromosome		
Deletions of part or all of chromosome 5 or 7	Not defined	Frequent in patients with AML occurring *de novo* and in patients with history of chemical, drug, or radiation exposure and/or previous hematologic disease.[214,215,218,219]
Trisomy 8	Not defined	Very common abnormality in acute myeloblastic leukemia. Poor prognosis, often a secondary change.[215,222]
Translocation		
t(8;21) (q22;q22)	*RUNX1(AML1)–RUNX1T1(ETO)*	Present in ~8% of patients <50 years old and in 3% of patients >50 years old with AML.[220] Approximately 75% of cases have additional cytogenetic abnormalities, including loss of Y in males or X in females. Secondary cooperative mutations of *KRAS, NRAS, KIT* common. Present in ~40% of myelomonocytic phenotype. Higher frequency of myeloid sarcomas.[192–195]
t(15;17) (q31; q22)	*PML-RAR-α*	Represents ~6% of cases of AML.[220] Translocation involving chromosome 17, t(15;17), (t11;17), or t(5;17) is present in most cases of promyelocytic leukemia.[106,107,223,224]
t(9;11); (p22; q23)	*MLL(especially MLLT3)*	Present in ~7% of cases of AML.[225–229] Associated with monocytic leukemia.[226–227] 11q23 translocations in 60% of infants with AML and carries poor prognosis. Rearranges *MLL* gene.[225–229] Many translocation partners for 11q23 translocation.[228–231] *MLL1,MLL4,MLL10* may also result in AML phenotype.
t(9;22) (q34; q22)	*BCR–ABL*	Present in ~2% of patients with AML[232,233]
t(1;22)(p13;q13)	*RBMIS-MKL1*	<1% of cases of AML. Admixture of myeloblasts, megakaryoblasts, micromegakaryocytes with cytoplasmic blebbing, dysmorphic megakaryocytes. Reticulin fibrosis common.[234]
Inversion		
Inv (16) (p13.1;q22) or t(16;16) (p13.1;q22)	*CBF-βMYH11*	Present in ~8% of patients <50 years of age and in ~3% of patients >50 years of age with AML[220]; often acute myelomonocytic phenotype; associated with increased marrow eosinophils; predisposition to cervical lymphadenopathy,[235] better response to therapy.[236–239] Predisposed to myeloid sarcoma.
Inv(3)(q21q26.2)	*RPN1-EVI1*	~1% of cases of AML. Approximately 85% of cases with normal or increased platelet count. Marrow has increased dysmorphic, hypolobulated megakaryocytes. Hepatosplenomegaly more frequent than usual in AML.[240]

Approximately 50 percent of cases of AML contain cells that are cytogenetically normal. When five genes—*NPM1*, *FLT3*, *CEPBA*, *MLL*, and *NRAS*—were examined in 872 adults who were younger than 60 years of age with a normal karyotype, approximately 85 percent had a mutation in at least one of these genes. Mutations in *NPM1* or *CEPBA* were associated with more favorable outcomes, analogous to the category of favorable cytogenetics noted above. Mutations in *FLT3* resulting from an internal tandem duplication (ITD) or wild-type expression of *NPM1* and *CEPBA* in patients' cells without a *FLT3* mutation (triple wild-type) had poor outcomes.[101]

The microarray expression signature in patients with AML younger than age 60 years who have cytogenetically normal cells but high-risk molecular features, especially *FLT3-ITD* and/or wild-type *NMP1* expression, is correlated with outcome of therapy. MicroRNAs regulate gene expression and the downregulation of the microRNA-181 family predicts a poor outcome. The microRNAs studied also revealed several important gene families that appear to be involved in the pathogenesis of AML, including genes involved in innate immunity (e.g., toll-like receptors and interleukin-1B expression and regulation).[221] (See Chaps. 10 and 85 for further discussion of gene array profiling and microRNA analysis.)

PLASMA CHEMICAL FINDINGS

Prior to treatment, mild to moderate increases in serum uric acid and lactic dehydrogenase levels are frequent. Both levels are higher in myelomonocytic and monocytic AML than in other AML phenotypes.[129,130] Occasional patients have very elevated uric acid levels, which usually occur after chemotherapy if proper precautions are not taken (e.g., hypouricosemic agents and hydration therapy).[241] Abnormalities of sodium, potassium, calcium, or hydrogen ion concentration are infrequent and usually mild.[242,243] Severe hyponatremia associated with inappropriate antidiuretic hormone secretion has occurred at presentation.[242,243] Severe hypernatremia as a consequence of diabetes insipidus can be an initial event.[244] Hypokalemia is a more frequent finding at presentation and is related to kaliuresis, although the reason for the proximal renal tubular dysfunction is unclear.[242,243,245] The hypokalemia can be severe and often is worsened by the effects of treatment, especially use of kaliuretic antibiotics.[245] Factitious elevations in serum potassium levels have been reported in patients with hyperleukocytosis as a result of leakage from white cells *in vitro*.[246,247] Factitious hypoglycemia and spurious hypoxia from the effects of high blast cell counts in blood can occur.[244,248]

Hypercalcemia can occur. The pathogenesis probably is multifactorial,[249] but cases with increased ectopic parathormone-like activity in the plasma have been described.[250] Severe lactic acidosis prior to treatment has been reported.[242,251,252] Hypophosphatemia as a result of phosphate uptake by leukemic cells can occur.[253] Ectopic adrenocorticotropic hormone secretion,[254] circulating immune complexes,[255] and abnormal concentrations of coagulation factors or their inhibitors[256] may be present.

Although prothrombin and partial thromboplastin times usually are normal or near normal, abnormal concentrations of coagulation factors are frequent. Elevations of platelet factor 4 and thromboxane B_2 occur often.[257] Decreases in α_2-antiplasmin, protein C, and antithrombin III levels occur often[257] and may be associated with venous thrombosis.[258] Acute promyelocytic and acute monocytic leukemia are associated with hypofibrinogenemia and other indicators of activation of coagulation or fibrinolysis (see "Morphologic Variants of Acute Myelogenous Leukemia" below).[259]

The levels of the shed form of L-selectin[260] and anticardiolipin antibodies[261] in plasma frequently are elevated as are the levels of soluble VEGF receptor-1 (VEGFR-1) and VEGFR-2. The ratio of soluble VEGFR-1 to VEGF correlates with greater leukemic blast cell burden and with less favorable outcome.[262]

SPECIAL CLINICAL FEATURES

Hyperleukocytosis

Leukocyte count is an independent prognostic factor in the outcome of AML treatment.[263] Approximately 5 percent of patients with AML develop signs or symptoms attributable to a markedly elevated blood blast cell count, usually greater than 100×10^9/L (see Chap. 85).[264] The circulations of the CNS, lungs, and penis are most sensitive to the effects of leukostasis. Intracerebral hemorrhage from vascular occlusion, invasion, and disruption, sometimes complicated by thrombocytopenia and vascular insufficiency are the most virulent manifestations of the syndrome.[265–269] Dizziness, stupor, dyspnea, and priapism may occur.[246–251] Diabetes insipidus is another association.[270,271] Other severe organ involvement may occur infrequently, also. A high early mortality in patients with AML correlates with hyperleukocytosis greater than 100×10^9/L.[267–269,272,273] Chemotherapy in hyperleukocytic patients may lead to a pulmonary leukostatic syndrome, presumably from the effects of rigid, effete blast cells, or the discharge of large amounts of cell contents and resultant cell aggregation or other effects.[274–276] Larger-vessel vascular occlusion as a result of white thrombi or masses of leukemic cells is rare.[277–281] The upregulation of endothelial cell intercellular adhesion molecule-1 and of leukemic blast cell lymphocyte function-associated antigen-1 may mediate the vessel wall interaction contributing to leukostasis.[282]

Hypoplastic Leukemia

Approximately 10 percent of patients with AML present with a syndrome that includes pancytopenia, often with inapparent blood blast cells, and absence of hepatic, splenic, or lymph nodal enlargement.[283–285] If one corrects for the decrease in marrow cellularity with age, hypoplastic AML occurs in approximately 2 percent of cases.[286] Approximately 75 percent of these patients are men older than 50 years of age. Marrow biopsy is hypocellular, which is the unusual feature of the syndrome, but leukemic blast cells are evident and present in a proportion of 10 to 90 percent of marrow cells. Response to intensive chemotherapeutic treatment, often with low-dose cytarabine because of the patients' very advanced age, has been relatively good, and 3-year survival rates are approximately the same as the rates of other age-matched patients.[287]

Oligoblastic (Subacute, Smoldering) Leukemia

In approximately 10 percent of cases, usually in patients older than 50 years of age, myelogenous leukemia is manifested by anemia and often thrombocytopenia. The leukocyte count may be low, normal, or increased, and a small proportion of blast cells are present in the blood (0–15%) and marrow (3–20%). Such cases have been referred to as *oligoblastic myelogenous leukemia, subacute,* or *smoldering leukemia,*[288–290] or classified as a myelodysplastic syndrome, particularly refractory anemia with excess blasts. The clinical course of the untreated disease can be protracted. The disease has a high morbidity and mortality from infection and hemorrhage and can evolve into overt (polyblastic) AML. The smoldering or oligoblastic leukemias historically have been grouped with the clonal cytopenias as part of the myelodysplastic syndromes (refractory anemia with excess blasts); thus, the diagnosis and treatment of these variants are discussed in Chap. 88. Biologically and clinically, the disorders in this subset of the myelodysplastic syndrome with blast cell proportions in the marrow above normal are leukemias, not dysplasias, but they have a slower rate of progression than polyblastic myelogenous leukemia. Dysmorphogenesis of red cells, neutrophils, and platelets is more frequent and more striking than in the average case of polyblastic AML (see Chap. 88), but such dysmorphogenesis also occurs in polyblastic leukemia, so-called AML with trilineage dysmorphia.[203]

Ph-Chromosome–Positive Acute Myelogenous Leukemia

Approximately 2 percent of patients with acute myelogenous leukemias have the Ph (Philadelphia) chromosome t(9;22)(q34;q11) in a significant proportion (10–100%) of leukemic blast cells.[291–293] The blast cells have surface antigens, such as CD13 and CD33, characteristic of myeloid leukemias.[294,295] One interpretation of the concurrence of AML with t(9;22) is that it represents CML presenting in myeloid blast crisis.[296–298] The arguments in favor of this proposal are as follows: (1) Blast crisis may occur within days after diagnosis of Ph-chromosome–positive CML. (2) Cases can present with additional cytogenetic changes comparable to CML in blast crisis.[296,298] (3) Marked hepatosplenomegaly, uncharacteristic of AML, may be present.[297,298] (4) Platelet counts may be normal, and basophils can be increased.[296,298] (5) A long prodromal period of weakness and weight loss may occur, and some features of CML, such as granulocytosis, can appear after treatment with chemotherapy.[299] (6) Ph-chromosome–positive AML has a very poor prognosis, as in myeloid blast crisis of CML. (7) The breakpoint on chromosome 22 in the M-bcr may be typical of CML, and the product of the fusion *BCR-ABL* gene is a p210 tyrosine kinase identical to that in classic CML.[295,297–303] (8) Occasional cases express p210 and p190 tyrosine kinases, now known to be features of CML.[303] (9) Some patients enter a remission by converting to a phenotype analogous to chronic phase CML. An alternative view has been promulgated because (1) cases of Ph-chromosome–positive AML can be a mosaic (normal and abnormal karyotypes),[295] (2) the Ph chromosome may appear later in the course of the disease,[304] (3) additional chromosomal abnormalities often are different from those seen in the myeloblastic crisis of CML,[295,305,306] and (4) in some cases, the *BCR-ABL* gene is not encoding a p210 but a p190 mutant tyrosine kinase,[292,300,302,303,307] the former being most characteristic of CML. Moreover, Ph-chromosome–positive AML has developed following Ph-chromosome–negative oligoblastic leukemia.[292,308,309] Many cases of Ph-chromosome–positive acute leukemia are myeloid-lymphoid hybrids.[299,303,305,310] Thus, Ph-chromosome–positive AML comes in two varieties: one with a break in M-BCR of chromosome 22 with a p210 product, which could be considered analogous to acute blast crisis of CML, and one with a molecular pathology resulting in the oncogene product being a p190 protein (m-BCR) that could be considered a *de novo* case.

Marrow Necrosis

Necrosis of the marrow is an uncommon event and can be seen in a wide variety of malignant and nonmalignant clinical disorders, but about two-thirds of cases are associated with lymphoid or myeloid malignancies and about one-quarter of cases occur in patients with AML.[311] Bone pain (~80% of patients) and fever (~70% of patients) are the two most common symptoms or signs. Anemia and thrombocytopenia, if not already present, results. White cell counts may be low or high. The blood may contain nucleated red cells and myeloid immaturity (~50% of cases). Lactic dehydrogenase and alkaline phosphatase are elevated in about half the cases. Marrow aspirate is often watery and serosanguineous. An amorphous extracellular eosinophilic background with disintegrating cells that have lost their staining characteristics with indistinct margins and varying degrees of pyknosis and karyorrhexis is characteristic. Rare cases have been described in which the marrow contained Charcot-Leyden crystals without an increase in eosinophils or basophils.[312] Boney spicules may also show evidence of necrosis. Destruction of spicule architecture with loss of osteocytes, osteoblasts, and osteocytes may be seen. It is important not to identify these changes as artifact. Usually more than 50 percent of the biopsy is involved. Careful search may identify the underlying hematological disorder in small islands of intact cells. Technetium-99m sulfur colloid scans show little or no uptake. Magnetic resonance imaging (MRI) may not be diagnostic but can show the extent of the necrosis by changes in signal intensity signifying an increase in water content in relation to fat. Both scanning and MRI can point to areas of intact marrow that may be used to make a diagnosis of the underlying disease, if it is unknown. The pathophysiology is uncertain but is thought to be related to marrow vascular injury and or thrombosis secondary to inflammatory or immune factors and cytokines. The prognosis of marrow necrosis is largely related to the underlying disease. Repair of marrow can occur, if the patient enters remission.

NEONATAL MYELOPROLIFERATION AND LEUKEMIA

Four myeloproliferative syndromes related to AML have been identified in the neonate: transient myeloproliferative disorder, transient leukemia, congenital leukemia, and neonatal leukemia. Transient myeloproliferative disorder and transient leukemia are considered to represent the same phenomenon.

Transient myeloproliferative disease (TMD) can be present at birth or occur shortly thereafter in approximately 10 percent of infants with Down syndrome.[313–319] The leukocyte count is markedly elevated, blast cells are present in the blood and marrow, and anemia and thrombocytopenia may be present, but the latter are not constant findings. The liver and spleen may be enlarged. Results of cytogenetic studies and marrow cell culture studies are normal, except for trisomy 21, which is characteristic of Down syndrome. The blast cells usually have the immunophenotype of megakaryocytes. In contrast to congenital leukemia, the elevated white cell and blast cell counts disappear in most patients (~80%) over a period of weeks to months. In approximately 20 percent of patients, severe and potentially lethal complications of hydrops fetalis, hepatic fibrosis, or cardiorespiratory failure may occur.

In some cases, an additional cytogenetic abnormality is present, which disappears after regression of the myeloproliferative syndrome, suggesting a reversible clonal disorder (transient leukemia) that is replaced by normal hematopoiesis. The presence of a trisomy of chromosome 21 is essential for the disease as judged by three observations: the trisomy occurs in (1) the TMD clone of patients with constitutional trisomy 21, (2) the TMD clone in patients with Down syndrome with a cell mosaic pattern of trisomy 21, and (3) in the TMD clone of phenotypically normal infants without a constitutional trisomy 21, but with TMD. In the last case, trisomy 21 disappears with resolution of the myeloproliferation.[320] Candidate oncogenes on chromosome 21 responsible for the phenomenon include *FPDMM, RUNX1* (*CBF-β*), and *IFNAR*, among others.[320] *GATA-1* mutations have been found in nearly all patients with TMD and in acute megakaryocytic leukemia in Down patients.[321] The TMD syndrome may disappear, only to be followed shortly thereafter by acute leukemia, predominantly AML, but occasionally acute lymphocytic leukemia (ALL).

One hypothesis for TMD is that the disorder originates in a primitive cell of fetal hepatic hematopoiesis. The cell involutes and is replaced with marrow stem cells. Approximately 25 percent of newborns with Down syndrome and transient leukemia develop acute megakaryocytic leukemia in the first 4 years of life.[322–324]

Very low dose cytarabine has been suggested for those patients with severe hepatic fibrosis, very high white cell counts, or hydrops fetalis.[320] TMD cells in these infants are very sensitive to cytarabine.[325,326]

Children with Down syndrome have a 150-fold risk of AML and about a 40-fold risk of ALL by age five years. A slightly increased risk of acute leukemia persists into older age. Myelogenous leukemia in patients with Down syndrome often has a megakaryoblastic or erythroid phenotype and may have an interstitial deletion of chromosome 21.[315,316,327–330] The response rate of infants with Down syndrome and AML to chemotherapy is very high over prolonged followup and better than the response of patients without Down syndrome.[322,326,331,332] The response to adjusted-dose anthracycline antibiotic and cytarabine in Down syndrome children with AML is approximately 90 percent and the event-free 5-year survival is approximately 80 percent.[329] ALL may occur, and the response to therapy is similar to the response of patients without Down syndrome of the same age. Most solid tumors occur less frequently in Down syndrome patients.[325]

Congenital or neonatal leukemia, a rare syndrome, occurs less than one-tenth as frequently in infants without Down syndrome than in newborns with Down syndrome.[327,328] Leukocytosis, blood and marrow blast cells, hepatosplenomegaly, thrombocytopenia, purpura, anemia, and skin infiltrates are usual. The disease has been diagnosed prenatally. Cytogenetic abnormalities can occur and mark the leukemic clone.[328,333,334] Monocytic leukemia and t(4;11) are the most common phenotype and karyotype.[334–336] A case of vertical (transplacental) transmission of acute monocytic leukemia from mother to son has been reported.[337]

Infants who are normal at birth but develop AML in the first few weeks of life (neonatal leukemia) often display pallor, inadequate food intake, insufficient weight gain, diarrhea, and lethargy. The presence of a cytogenetic abnormality on band q23 of chromosome 11 is a very poor prognostic sign. Most infants with congenital or neonatal leukemia do not survive for more than a few weeks or months. Because treatment has been largely ineffective, observation to ascertain if TMD or a transient leukemia is present has been recommended if the clinical picture is unclear.[338]

HYBRID AND MIXED LEUKEMIAS

Hybrid Leukemias

Although coincidental myeloid and lymphoid clonal diseases have been reported for more than 50 years, the availability of techniques to identify surface antigens with monoclonal antibodies, immunoglobulin gene, and T-lymphocyte receptor gene rearrangements with molecular methods, and chromosome translocations by chromosome banding cytogenetic techniques has led to the appreciation of several types of hybrid acute leukemia.[339–347]

In bilineal (interlineal) acute leukemias, a proportion of cells (>10%) have lymphoid and myeloid markers; *interlineal* here refers to lymphopoietic and myeloid gene expression. Bilineal (biphenotypic) leukemias are heterogeneous. Some patients have cells with both lymphoid and myeloid markers (chimeric), whereas other patients have cells with either lymphoid or myeloid markers but evidence that all the cells are part of the same malignant clone (mosaic). The bilineal leukemias may be synchronous (lymphoid and myeloid cells are present simultaneously) or asynchronous (in which lymphoid cells are succeeded by myeloid cells or vice versa), but evidence exists for their origin from the same clone.

Cases of biphenotypic leukemia that are morphologically or cytochemically indicative of myelogenous leukemia have been referred to as LY+AML; the cases that are more indicative of lymphocytic leukemia are referred to as MY+ALL. As a group, interlineal hybrid leukemias treated with current regimens respond to therapy at approximately the same rate as AML cases without lymphoid markers.[339] Some observers suggest altering drug regimens, depending on the balance between lymphoid and myeloid biochemical (drug-response) patterns.[348]

Acute leukemias may be intralineal hybrids in that the blast cells have markers for two or more myeloid lineages (e.g., erythroid, granulocytic, and megakaryocytic) or, in the case of lymphocytic leukemias, both immunoglobulin gene rearrangement (B-lymphocyte type) and T-cell receptor gene rearrangement (T-lymphocyte type).

Myeloid–Natural Killer Cell Hybrids and t(8;13) Myeloid–Lymphoid Leukemias

Although most hybrid leukemias share myeloid and either B- or T-lymphocyte markers, two notable syndromes are associated with hybrid leukemias: (1) the myeloid leukemia and natural killer cell hybrid (CD56+, CD7+, CD13+, CD33+)[349–355] and (2) the lymphoma, eosinophilia, and t(8;13) myeloid leukemia hybrid.[356,357] Signs of lymphoma, such as mediastinal or other lymphadenopathy and extranodal lymphoid tumor, are mixed with findings compatible with AML in both syndromes. The morphology of the myeloid–natural killer cell leukemia often simulates APL, with hypergranular cytoplasm present but abnormality of chromosome 17 absent. The hybrids can appear *de novo* or after relapse of a lymphoma, T-cell leukemia, or blast crisis of CML. The hybrid leukemias usually have a poor prognosis. Myeloid antigens may not be evident at diagnosis in the natural killer cell hybrid but appear later in the course.[358] Hematopoietic stem cell transplantation should be considered in an eligible patient.[359]

Hybrid leukemias may result from either lineage infidelity caused by genetic misprogramming[349] or promiscuous gene expression, which occurs transiently in the differentiation of normal pluripotential hematopoietic stem cells. In the case of promiscuity, persistence of the transient normal event is thought to be present because of the block in differentiation that occurs.[343,344] Genetic misprogramming (infidelity) could result from rearrangements of the DNA sequences that control the transcription of genes designating differentiation antigens.[360]

Mixed Leukemias

In these cases, lymphoid and myeloid cells are present simultaneously but are derived from separate clones, or sequential myeloid and lymphoid leukemia are present but the two lineages are derived from separate clones.

■ MEDIASTINAL GERM CELL TUMORS AND ACUTE MYELOGENOUS LEUKEMIA

An unusual but significant concordance has been reported between nonseminomatous mediastinal germ cell tumors and AML, especially the megakaryoblastic variant.[361–366] Mediastinal tumors are rare variants of germ cell tumors. The latter ordinarily occur as testicular teratomas and seminomas in men or as ovarian teratomas in women. They are thought to be derived from yolk sac cells that failed to migrate.[364,365] AML is a hematopoietic stem cell tumor derived from a cell type that is present in the yolk sac. Cytogenetic studies are compatible with a clonal relationship (identity) of mediastinal germ cells and myelogenous leukemia cells.[362,363] Apparently, hematopoietic lineage genes are predisposed to expression in extragonadal (mediastinal) germ cell tumors. Use of etoposide, platinum, and related cytotoxic drugs for treatment of mediastinal germ cell tumors may induce secondary AML in a predisposed cell population.[367]

■ GASTROINTESTINAL TUMORS AND ACUTE MYELOGENOUS LEUKEMIA

A study of 1892 patients with KIT-positive mesenchymal tumors of the gastrointestinal tract (gastrointestinal stromal tumors or GISTs) found a significant subsequent incidence of AML (9 patients). The standardized incidence ratio was about 3.0 (confidence interval: 1.1–5.8). The patients had not received prior chemotherapy or radiotherapy and the median duration of GIST before onset of AML was 6 years.[368]

MORPHOLOGIC VARIANTS OF ACUTE MYELOGENOUS LEUKEMIA

Morphologic variants of AML (Table 89–4) may occur *de novo* or may be the manifestation of clonal evolution from essential thrombocythemia, idiopathic myelofibrosis, CML, or other chronic clonal myeloid disorders. For example, every phenotypic variant of AML can occur as the blast crisis of CML (see Chap. 90).

■ ACUTE MYELOBLASTIC LEUKEMIA

The designation *acute myeloblastic leukemia* came into existence in the second decade of the 20th century,[4] following the specific description of the myeloblast.[6] Approximately 25 percent of AML cases have the features of acute myeloblastic leukemia, a variant in which the leukemic myeloblast is the predominant cell in the marrow. Acute myeloblastic leukemia has been divided into two forms, designated *M0* and *M1* in the French-American-British (FAB) classification which converts the descriptive term for a leukemic phenotype into a number. In either type, little evidence of maturation of myeloblasts exists, and the marrow is replaced by a monotonous population of blasts. In acute myeloblastic leukemia (M0), the patient's age distribution, presenting white cell count, and cytogenetic abnormalities are not distinctive. The blasts are nonreactive when stained for myeloperoxidase activity, and Auer rods are not seen. The blasts react with antibodies to myeloperoxidase and antibodies to CD13, CD33, and CD34. Human leukocyte antigen (HLA)-DR is positive in most patients. Occasional cases require *in situ* hybridization to identify the myeloperoxidase gene[369] or genomic profiling for early myeloid-associated genes.[370] Abnormal and unfavorable karyotypes (e.g., 5q–,7q–) and higher expression of the multidrug resistance glycoprotein (p170) are more frequent. This phenotypic variant has a poor prognosis.[371–374] In the other type of myeloblastic leukemia, designated *M1*, myeloblasts are present in the blood and compose more than 70 percent of marrow cells. Less than 15 percent of marrow cells are promyelocytes and myelocytes. Auer rods may be present in occasional blasts, but azurophilic granules are not evident in the blasts by light microscopy. At least 3 percent, but usually a much higher percentage, of the blast cells have a positive reaction when stained for peroxidase or with Sudan black or react with monoclonal antibodies specific to myeloblasts, such as CD33. This morphologic subtype is denoted as M1 in the FAB classification. The WHO has divided acute myeloblastic leukemia into three types, designated AML without differentiation, AML without maturation, and AML with maturation. The category without differentiation seems inappropriate as immunophenotypic markers, and often myeloperoxidase assays, unequivocally place it into the acute myeloblastic category, and hence differentiation into myeloblastic leukemia is evident as "differentiation" in the WHO classification implies markers of myeloid or lymphoid lineages. There is no

TABLE 89–4. Morphologic Variants of AML

Variant	Cytologic Features	Special Clinical Features	Special Laboratory Features
Acute myeloblastic leukemia (M0,M1,M2)	1. Myeloblasts range from 20 to 90% of marrow cells. Cytoplasm occasionally contains Auer bodies. Nucleus shows fine reticular pattern and distinct nucleolus (1 or 2 usually). 2. Blast cells are sudanophilic. They are positive for myeloperoxidase and chloroacetate esterase, negative for nonspecific esterase, and negative or diffusely positive for PAS (no clumps or blocks). 3. Electron microscopy shows cytoplasmic primary granules.	1. Most common in adults, and most frequent variety in infants. 2. Three morphologic-cytochemical types (M0, M1, M2)	1. Chromosomes +8, −5, −7, del(11q) and complex abnormalities common. *RUNX1(AML1)* and *FLT3* mutations occur in approximately 20–25% of cases. 2. M0 type blast cells positive with antibody to myeloperoxidase and anti-CD34 and CD13 or CD33 coexpression. *AML1* mutations in ~25%. 3. M1 expresses CD13 and CD33. Positive for myeloperoxidase by cytochemistry. 4. M2 AML with maturation often associated with t(8;21) karyotype. 5. M2 AML with t(6;9)(p23;q34), an uncommon variant, is associated with marrow basophilia, a high blast count, a high frequency of *FLT3*-ITD, and a poor outcome.
Acute promyelocytic leukemia (M3, M3v)	1. Leukemic cells resemble promyelocytes. They have large atypical primary granules and a kidney-shaped nucleus. Branched or adherent Auer rods are common. 2. Peroxidase stain intensely positive. 3. A variant has microgranules (M3v), otherwise the same course and prognosis.	1. Usually in adults. 2. Hypofibrinogenemia and hemorrhage common. 3. Leukemic cells mature in response to all-*trans*-retinoic acid.	1. Cell contains t(15;17) or other translocation involving chromosome 17 (*RAR-α* gene). 2. Cells are HLA-DR negative.
Acute myelomonocytic leukemia (M4, M4Eo)	1. Both myeloblastic and monoblastic leukemic cells in blood and marrow. 2. Peroxidase-, Sudan-, chloroacetate esterase-, and nonspecific esterase-positive cells. 3. M4Eo variant has marrow eosinophilia.	1. Similar to myeloblastic leukemia but with more frequent extramedullary disease. 2. Mildly elevated serum and urine lysozyme.	1. Leukemic cells in eosinophilic variant (M4Eo) usually have inversion or translocation of chromosome 16.
Acute monocytic leukemia (M5)	1. Leukemia cells are large; nuclear cytoplasmic ratio lower than myeloblast. Cytoplasm contains fine granules. Auer rods are rare. Nucleus is convoluted and cell simulates promonocytes (M5a) or may simulate monoblasts (M5b) and contain large nucleoli. 2. Nonspecific esterase-positive inhibited by NaF; Sudan-, peroxidase-, and chloroacetate esterase-negative. PAS occurs in granules, blocks.	1. Seen in children or young adults. 2. Gum, CNS, lymph node, and extramedullary infiltrations are common. 3. DIC occurs. 4. Plasma and urine lysozyme elevated. 5. Hyperleukocytosis common.	1. t(4;11) common in infants. 2. Rearrangement of q11;q23 very frequent.
Acute erythroid leukemia (M6)	1. Abnormal erythroblasts are in abundance initially in marrow and often in blood. Later the morphologic findings may be indistinguishable from those of AML.	1. Pancytopenia common at diagnosis.	1. Cells reactive with antihemoglobin antibody. Erythroblasts usually are strongly PAS and CD71-positive, express ABH blood group antigens, and react with antihemoglobin antibody. 2. Cells reactive with anti–Rc-84 (antihuman erythroleukemia cell-line antigen).

(*continued*)

TABLE 89–4. Morphologic Variants of AML (Continued)

Variant	Cytologic Features	Special Clinical Features	Special Laboratory Features
Acute megakaryocytic leukemia (M7)	1. Small blasts with pale agranular cytoplasm and cytoplasmic blebs. May mimic lymphoblasts of medium to larger size. 2. Leukemic cells with megakaryocytic morphology may coexist with megakaryoblasts.	1. Usually presents with pancytopenia. 2. Markedly elevated serum lactic dehydrogenase levels. 3. Marrow aspirates are usually "dry taps" because of the invariable presence of myelofibrosis. 4. Common phenotype in the AML of Down syndrome.	1. Antigens of von Willebrand factor, and glycoprotein Ib (CD42), IIb/IIIa (CD41), IIIa (CD61) on blast cells. 2. Platelet peroxidase positive.
Acute eosinophilic leukemia	1. Mixture of blasts and cells with dysmorphic eosinophilic granules (smaller and less refractile).	1. Hepatomegaly, splenomegaly, lymphadenopathy may be prominent. 2. Absence of neurologic, respiratory, or cardiac signs or symptoms characteristic of chronic eosinophilic leukemia (clonal hypereosinophilic syndrome).	1. Cyanide-resistant peroxidase stains eosinophilic granules. TEM shows eosinophilic granules to be smaller and missing central crystalloid. 2. Biopsy may show Charcot-Leyden crystals in skin, marrow, or other sites of eosinophil accumulation.
Acute basophilic leukemia	Mixture of blast cells and cells with basophilic granules in blood and marrow.	1. Often has hepatomegaly and or splenomegaly; symptoms often present. 2. Rash with urticaria, headaches, prominent gastrointestinal symptoms.	1. CD9-, CD11b-, CD25-, CD123-positive cells are usually present. 2. Toluidine blue-positive cells. 3. Hyperhistaminemia and hyperhistaminuria. 4. Cells negative for tryptase but positive for histidine decarboxylase.
Acute mast cell leukemia	1. Mast cells in blood and marrow. Most contain granules but some are agranular and may simulate monocytes.	1. Fever, headache, flushing of face and trunk, pruritus may be present. 2. Abdominal pain, peptic ulcer, bone pain, diarrhea more common than other AML subtypes. 3. Hepatomegaly, splenomegaly common. 4. Hemorrhagic diathesis may be evident.	1. CD13, CD33, CD68, CD117 often positive. 2. Cells positive for tryptase staining and serum tryptase elevated. 3. Hyperhistaminemia and hyperhistaminuria.

DIC, disseminated intravascular coagulation; NaF, sodium fluoride; PAS, periodic acid-Schiff; TEM, transmission electron microscopy.

NOTE: Parentheses indicate French-American-British (FAB) designation M0 through M7.

evidence of a clinical distinction in response to therapy or in prognosis within these rarified designations.

In many cases of myeloblastic leukemia, more prominent granulocytic maturation is evident (FAB type *M2* or WHO designation AML with maturation). This variant is present in approximately 15 percent of AML cases; thus, approximately 45 percent of cases of AML are myeloblastic leukemia with or without maturation. Blasts usually constitute at least 20 percent of the marrow cells. Auer rods may be present in blast cells. Promyelocytes, myelocytes, and segmented neutrophils, the latter often with the acquired Pelger-Hüet anomaly, may constitute 20 to 60 percent of marrow granulocytes. The anomaly is reflected in bilobed or monolobed neutrophils. Histochemical and surface markers of blast cells are typical of myeloblastic leukemia, and monocytic markers are absent or infrequent. Monocytes represent less than 10 percent of cells. A translocation between chromosomes 8 and 21 t(8;21)(q22; q22), often concomitant with loss of the Y chromosome in men or loss of an X chromosome in women, is associated with the phenotype and occurs in younger patients (average age approximately 30 years).[375–377] Patients whose cells contain t(8;21) are more prone to develop myeloid sarcoma.[192,195]

ACUTE MYELOMONOCYTIC LEUKEMIA

The ability of AML to express cells of the monocytic and granulocytic lineages was first highlighted in the early 1900s by Naegeli. Later, Downey proposed the eponym *Naegeli type* for myelomonocytic leukemia.[378] Approximately 15 percent of patients with AML present with this variant, and they are more likely to have extramedullary infiltrates in gingiva, skin, or CNS than patients with acute myeloblastic leukemia (see "Myeloid [Granulocytic] Sarcoma" above).[379] A mixture of myeloblasts and monoblasts is found in the blood and marrow. More than 30 percent of marrow cells are a mixed population of myeloblasts, which react with peroxidase or chloracetate esterase, and monoblasts or promonocytes, which react with fluoride-inhibitable nonspecific esterase (Fig. 89–2F). More than 20 percent of cells are monoblasts or promonocytes in blood and marrow. In some cases, individual cells react with monocytic and granulocytic histochemical stains.[380] Serum and urinary lysozyme levels are increased in most cases. This variant of AML is referred to as *M4* in the FAB classification and as acute myelomonocytic leukemia in the WHO classification. Translocations involving chromosome 3 have been associated with this phenotype.[381]

The proportion of marrow eosinophils[382] or basophils[383] may be increased. A particular variant of myelomonocytic leukemia has increased numbers of marrow eosinophils (10–50%), Auer rods in blast cells, and inversion or rearrangement of chromosome 16 (see Fig. 89–2G).[236–239] The eosinophils are abnormally large, and the eosinophilic myelocytes contain large basophilic granules. Macrophages with ingested Charcot-Leyden crystals may be present. This phenotypic variant of AML has been designated *M4Eo* in the FAB classification. Although this variant has an increased risk of CNS involvement, it carries a more favorable prognosis than the average case of AML. Fluorescence *in situ* hybridization (FISH) is a more accurate method for detection of cryptic 16q22 gene rearrangements and is useful in conjunction with conventional cytogenetics for patients with M4Eo AML. AML with t(6;9)(p23;q34) is an uncommon variant, occurring in approximately 1 percent of cases, and may express itself as acute myelomonocytic or acute myeloblastic leukemia. Anemia, thrombocytopenia, a variable white cell count, and prevalent myeloblasts are frequent. The myeloblasts often contain Auer rods. Marrow basophilia is present in about half the cases.[208,384] The variant occurs at a younger age, has a poor prognosis, and has a tendency to trilineage dysmorphia and ringed sideroblasts.[385]

ACUTE ERYTHROID LEUKEMIA

Prominence of erythroid cell proliferation in AML cases was noted by Copelli[386] and DiGuglielmo[387] in the early 20th century. Moeschlin[388] used the term *erythroleukemia*. Dameshek[389] suggested the name *DiGuglielmo syndrome* and dissected the disorder into three phases depending on the decreasing prevalence of dysmorphic erythroblasts and the reciprocal increasing prevalence of myeloblasts. Erythroid leukemia makes up approximately 5 percent of AML cases and is referred to as *M6* in the FAB classification.[390] Familial erythroleukemia has been described.[391,392] Erythroid leukemia is arbitrarily divided into three degrees of severity: (1) *erythroleukemia* in which more than 50 percent of the marrow cells are dysmorphic; (2) erythroblasts admixed with myeloblasts, the latter composing approximately 20 percent of non-erythroid cells or approximately 5 to 10 percent of total marrow cells; and (3) a form in which dysmorphic erythroblasts dominate the marrow, *pure erythroid leukemia*, in which more than 80 percent of marrow cells are dysmorphic erythroblasts with a trivial granulocytic proportion of cells and very few if any myeloblasts. This last form of the disease may start in as a milder variant, formerly called *erythremic myelosis*, in which granulopoiesis, and thrombopoiesis may be only mildly abnormal. This phase, dominated morphologically by bizarre dysmorphia of erythroblasts, can be protracted but eventually evolves into a dimorphic phase in which myeloblasts are more prominent, severe neutropenia and thrombocytopenia develop, and the patient progresses to erythroleukemia. The disease may evolve further into polyblastic AML.[393–396] In the erythremic myelosis variant, erythropoiesis is ineffective. However, some normal regulation may remain because hypertransfusion decreases both erythropoietin levels and the amount of abnormal erythropoiesis.[397] Spontaneous growth of leukemic erythroid clonogenic cells is a feature of the disease.[398] Periodic acid-Schiff (PAS)-positive erythroblasts are evident in almost all cases.[393,396]

The erythroid leukemias are characterized by a striking population of dysmorphic erythroblasts in marrow and red cells in blood (see Fig. 89–2I, 2J, and 2K). Anemia and thrombocytopenia are present in nearly all cases. Some patients may have elevated total leukocyte counts. The red cells show marked anisocytosis, poikilocytosis, anisochromia, and basophilic stippling. Nucleated red cells are present in the blood. The marrow erythroblasts are extremely abnormal, with giant multinucleate forms, nuclear budding, and nuclear fragmentation. Cytogenetic abnormalities are present in approximately two-thirds of patients. The frequency of erythroid leukemia is increased if methods for detecting erythroid differentiation more sensitive than light microscopy are used. These cell features include glycophorin A, spectrin, carbonic anhydrase I, ABH blood group antigens, and other antigens that occur on early erythroid progenitors.[399–401] Antihemoglobin antibody and antihuman erythroleukemic cell line antibody often are positive.[394]

Erythremic myelosis can have an indolent course and may be managed for a time without intensive chemotherapy. Treatment is warranted in patients with erythroleukemia and acute erythroid leukemia, and the results are approximately the same as with other phenotypes in patients of similar age.[396] The more predominant the erythroid component and the lower the proportion of myeloblasts, the better the response to therapy.[399]

ACUTE PROMYELOCYTIC LEUKEMIA

The association of an exaggerated hemorrhagic syndrome with certain leukemias was described by French hematologists in 1949.[402] In 1957, Hillstad[403] bestowed the appellation *promyelocytic leukemia* upon this morphologic-clinical subtype of AML. This variant, which is called *M3* in the FAB classification and acute promyelocytic leukemia in the WHO classification, occurs at any age and constitutes approximately 10 percent of AML cases.[223,224,404,405] This subtype of AML occurs with greater than expected frequency among Latinos from Europe and South and Central America[113,114] and among patients with an increased body mass index.[406] Unlike all other major variants of AML, which increase in incidence logarithmically with age, the incidence of APL is constant over the human life span.[112] Hemorrhagic manifestations are prominent including hemoptysis, hematuria, vaginal bleeding, melena, hematemesis, and pulmonary and intracranial bleeding, as well as the more typical skin and mucous membrane bleeding. In severely leukopenic patients, blasts may not be evident in the blood. Moderately severe thrombocytopenia $<50 \times 10^9$/L is present in most cases. The marrow contains few agranular blast cells and some blast-like cells with scant granules. The dominant cells are promyelocytes, which comprise 30 to 90 percent of marrow cells (see Fig. 89–2D and 2E). Auer rods and cells with multiple Auer rods (1–10%) are present in nearly every case. Promyelocytes with multiple Auer rods have been referred to as *faggot cells*. Leukemic promyelocytes stain intensely with myeloperoxidase and Sudan black and express CD 9, CD13, and CD33, but not CD34 or HLA-DR.[223,224,404,405]

A variant type of promyelocytic leukemia is referred to as *microgranular* (*M3v* in the FAB nomenclature).[407–410] Microgranular cases represent approximately 20 percent of patients with promyelocytic leukemia. The leukemic cells may mimic promonocytes with convoluted or lobulated nuclei. Auer rods may be present but are less evident. The majority of the leukemic cells contain azurophilic granules that are so small they are not visible by light microscopy, but the peroxidase stain usually is strongly positive. Typical hypergranulated promyelocytes usually are present on careful inspection. The total white cell count often is highly elevated, and severe coagulopathy is prominent in microgranular cases.[408] Rarely, the cells contain eosinophilic or basophilic granules, but t(15;17) is present, and the response to all-*trans*-retinoic acid (ATRA) persists,[411–413] although the basophilic variant can be virulent.[414]

A translocation between chromosome 17 and another chromosome is present in almost all cases of APL and in the acute promyelocytic transformation of CML; it is not found in other AML variants. The t(15;17) is the most frequent (>95%), but variant translocations between chromosome 5 or 11 and 17, isochromosome 17, and other less common variants have been described.[106,223,404,415,416] In some cases, cytogenetic analysis is inadequate, and Southern blot analysis is required to identify the rearrangement of the *RAR-α* gene. A functional distinction is that t(15;17), *PML-RAR-α* fusion, and t(5:17), *NPM-RAR-α* fusion, confer retinoid therapy responsiveness, whereas t(11;17), *PLZF-RAR-α* fusion, usually is retinoid resistant. In cells with t(11;17), Auer rods are absent and CD56 expression usually is present, offering some clinical variables to provoke special molecular investigations.[417] The retinoid resistance may not always be present.[418]

The breakpoint on chromosome 17 is within the gene for the RAR-α, and the breakpoint on chromosome 15 is within the locus of a gene originally referred to as *MYL* and renamed *PML*.[223,419] The gene encodes a unique transcription factor. The translocation results in two new chimeric or fusion genes: *RAR-α-PML*, which is actively transcribed in APL, and *PML-RAR-α*, which also is transcribed and may account for the aberrancy in hematopoiesis. The *PML-RAR-α* gene has two isoforms that produce a short- and a long-type fusion messenger RNA (mRNA), respectively.[420] Patients with the short isoform may have a worse outcome than those with the longer form. Polymerase chain reaction (PCR) for the mRNA of the fusion gene can be used to identify residual cells during remission and may predict relapse. The *PML-RAR-α* transgene can reproduce the disease in mice,[421] although in some models a superimposed *FLT3* mutation is required to express the disease.[107] *FLT3* mutations are frequently found in human disease, especially in the hypogranular variant.[106]

A propensity to hemorrhage is a striking feature of this subtype. The prothrombin and partial thromboplastin times are prolonged, and the plasma fibrinogen level is decreased in most cases. The disturbance in coagulation first was thought to principally result from intravascular coagulation initiated by procoagulant released from the granules of the leukemic promyelocytes. Elevated thrombin–antithrombin complexes, prothrombin fragment 1+2, and fibrinopeptide A plasma levels support that supposition. Increased levels of fibrinogen–fibrin degradation products, D-dimer, and evidence of plasminogen activation indicate fibrinolysis.[422–424] Furthermore, decreased levels of plasminogen, increased expression of annexin II on the leukemic cells,[425] and reports of responses to tranexamic acid support a role for fibrinolysis in the bleeding in APL.[426] Release of nonspecific proteases may further contribute to fibrinogenolysis. Thus, the coagulopathy is now considered tripartite.[427]

Although APL responded to chemotherapy regimens for AML, especially those containing an anthracycline antibiotic such as daunomycin or rubidazone,[428] the cytologic pattern of response in the marrow often was paradoxical.[429–432] Persistence of leukemic promyelocytes preceded remission in the absence of further therapy, whereas induction of marrow cell hypoplasia was classically considered a requirement for remission in patients with AML. Generally, if leukemic blast cells persist after therapy for AML, relapse ensues unless hypoplasia is induced by more cytotoxic therapy. The unusual pattern of response in APL was put into context by reports of successful treatment with isomers of retinoic acid, an agent that leads to maturation of leukemic promyelocytes *in vitro*.[432] In 1988, the success of ATRA in remission induction was reported[433,434] and confirmed.[223,224] Relapse occurs invariably, however, so chemotherapy regimens also are required. Use of ATRA has decreased the risk of early hemorrhagic complications and death and has enhanced the long-term response to chemotherapy. Despite the improvement in therapy, approximately 10 percent of patients die during remission induction, most of hemorrhage, often into the brain. The prolonged remissions of patients with promyelocytic leukemia has been marred in approximately 1 to 5 percent of cases by the later appearance of oligoblastic leukemia with deletions of all or part of chromosome 5 or 7 and no evidence of involvement of chromosome 17, compatible with a myelogenous leukemia secondary to therapy.[435,436] The approach to therapy and is discussed in the "Therapy" section below.

ACUTE MONOCYTIC LEUKEMIA

Monocytic leukemia was first reported by Reschad and Schilling-Torgau[437] in 1913. Approximately 8 percent of patients with AML present with monocytic leukemia, which is referred to as *M5* in the FAB classification. Patients with monocytic leukemia have a higher prevalence (50%) of extramedullary tumors in the skin, gingiva, eyes, larynx, lung, rectum and anal canal, bladder, lymph nodes, meninges, CNS, and other sites than do other phenotypes (<5%). Hepatomegaly and splenomegaly are more frequent in monocytic leukemia.[136,438–440]

The proportion of monocytic cells is usually greater than 75 percent. The total leukocyte count is higher in a larger proportion of patients, and hyperleukocytosis occurs more frequently (approximately 35%) than in other variants.[441–443] The marrow and blood cells may be largely monoblasts (acute monoblastic leukemia) or more mature-appearing promonocytes and monocytes (acute monocytic leukemia) (see Fig. 89–2H). When the blood contains more mature-appearing monocytic cells, the marrow contains a lower proportion of blast cells, approximately 15 to 50 percent. When the blood monocytes are largely blast cells, the marrow contains approximately 50 to 90 percent blasts. In nearly all cases, 10 to 90 percent of monocytic cells react for nonspecific esterase stains, α-naphthyl acetate esterase, and naphthol AS-D-chloroacetate esterase; in a cytochemical or chemoluminescence assay; or with monoclonal antibodies against monocyte surface antigens, especially CD14. Immunoreactivity of cells for lysozyme is characteristic. Serum and urine lysozyme levels are elevated in most patients. Serum lactic dehydrogenase and β_2-microglobulin concentrations are increased in greater than 80 percent of patients.[444] Plasminogen activator inhibitor-2 is present in the plasma and the cells of a high proportion of patients.[445] Auer rods are absent when monoblasts dominate but are present frequently in cases where promonocytes and monocytes are prevalent in blood and marrow. Leukemic monocytes have Fc receptors and can ingest and kill microorganisms in some cases.[446,447]

There is an association between translocations involving chromosome 11, especially region 11q23, and monocytic leukemia.[225–227] In particular, t(9;11) is found in leukemic monocytes.[228,229,440,441] In t(9;11) the β_1-interferon gene is translocated to chromosome 11, and the protooncogene *ETS*-1 is translocated to chromosome 9 adjacent to the α-interferon gene. The latter juxtaposition may be important in the pathogenesis of monocytic leukemia.[448]

The expression of *FOS* is closely correlated with monocytic maturation of cells in myelomonocytic and monocytic leukemia and in normal monocytopoiesis.[449,450] Absence or markedly decreased expression of the retinoblastoma gene growth suppressor product (p105) is present in approximately half of patients with monocytic leukemia. Patients express a more dramatic phenotype.[451] A variant of acute monocytic leukemia in which the leukemic cells have monocytoid features and are positive for early and late monocytic lineage antigens and for TdT activity often occurs after prior radiotherapy or chemotherapy and is relatively resistant to treatment.[452] A syndrome of acute monoblastic leukemia with t(8;16), resulting in *MOZ-CBP* fusion gene, is characterized by mildly granular promonocytes (simulating hypogranular promyelocytes), intense phagocytosis of red cells, erythroblasts, and sometimes neutrophils and platelets in blood and marrow, simulating macrophagic hemophagocytic syndrome, intravascular coagulation or primary fibrinolysis, and a high frequency of extramedullary disease.[453]

The management of monocytic leukemia is complicated by a greater incidence of CNS or meningeal disease either at the time of diagnosis or as a form of relapse during remission. Thus, examination of cerebrospinal fluid should be performed even in the absence of symptoms when remission has been achieved.[137,440,441] Most therapists recommend prophylactic intrathecal therapy with methotrexate or cytosine arabinoside for patients who enter remission after having presented with hyperleukocytic acute monocytic leukemia because of the risk of subclinical meningeal involvement.

Rare cases of dendritic cell or Langerhans cell phenotype have been described (see Chap. 72).[454,455] Uncommon cases of histiocytic sarcoma are the tissue or extramedullary variant of monocytic leukemia (see Chap. 72).[456,457] The outcome of treatment, once thought to be less favorable than with other forms of AML, is comparable to the outcome of other subtypes.[458]

■ ACUTE MEGAKARYOBLASTIC LEUKEMIA

In 1963, Szur and Lewis[459] reported patients with pancytopenia, low percentages of blast cells, and intense myelofibrosis but an absence of teardrop red cells, splenomegaly, leukocytosis, and thrombocytosis, the usual features of primary myelofibrosis. They designated the syndrome *malignant myelosclerosis*.[459] Reports of similar cases ensued, with some investigators referring to the syndrome as *acute myelofibrosis*.[460] The development of methods to phenotype megakaryoblasts indicated the cases were variants of AML rather than of primary myelofibrosis and have been designated *acute megakaryocytic* or *acute megakaryoblastic leukemia*.[326,461,462] This leukemia is referred to as *M7* in the FAB classification. The prevalence of this phenotype is approximately 5 percent of all AML cases if appropriate cell markers are used in the diagnosis, and is at least twice that frequency in childhood AML.[463,464] The syndrome is an especially prevalent variant of AML that develops in patients with Down syndrome[332,465] or in patients with mediastinal germ cell tumors and coincident AML.[361–365]

Leukemic megakaryoblasts and promegakaryocytes can be difficult to identify by light microscopy using polychrome staining. However, with experience, heightened suspicion can be engendered by blasts in the blood with abundant budding cytoplasm or blasts having a lymphoid appearance, especially if the marrow cannot be aspirated because of intense myelofibrosis, which is evident on the marrow biopsy. Initially high-resolution histochemistry for platelet peroxidase and identification of the demarcation membrane system using transmission electron microscopy were required for diagnosis. Now antibodies to von Willebrand factor or to platelet glycoprotein Ib (CD42), IIb/IIIa (CD41), or IIIa (CD61) can be used to identify very primitive megakaryocytic cells.[461,462] A small proportion of megakaryoblasts may be present in other cases of AML, but in megakaryocytic leukemia they are the prominent or the dominant leukemic cells (see Fig. 89–2L through 2O). Moreover, the other key features of the syndrome usually are present, especially severe myelofibrosis.[463]

Patients usually present with pallor, weakness, excessive bleeding and anemia, and leukopenia. Lymphadenopathy or hepatosplenomegaly is uncommon at the time of diagnosis. High leukocyte and blood blast cell counts may be present initially or may develop later. The platelet count may be normal or elevated in many patients at the time of presentation. Abnormal platelets or megakaryocytic cytoplasmic fragments may be found in the blood. Marrow aspiration often is unsuccessful ("dry tap") because of extensive marrow fibrosis in most cases, although not all. The marrow biopsy contains small blast cells, large blast cells, or a combination of both. The former have a high nuclear-to-cytoplasmic ratio, have dense chromatin with distinct nucleoli, and resemble lymphoblasts. Cases have been mistaken for ALL. The larger blasts may have some features of maturing megakaryocytes with agranular cytoplasm with cytoplasmic protrusions, clusters of platelet-like structures, or shedding of cytoplasmic blebs. The blast cells are peroxidase negative and tend to aggregate. Confirmation of their megakaryoblastic maturation requires immunocytologic studies for the presence of von Willebrand factor and the immunoreactivity to CD41, CD42, or CD61. The more mature megakaryocytes, which often coexist in the marrow, stain with PAS reagent, contain sodium fluoride-inhibitable nonspecific esterase, and fail to react for α-naphthylbutyrate esterase or myeloperoxidase. The thrombopoietin receptor gene (*MPL*) is expressed in megakaryocytes and exhibits the gain of function point mutation W515K/L in approximately 25 percent of cases of acute megakaryoblastic leukemia.[466]

The serum lactic acid dehydrogenase level frequently is strikingly increased and has an isomorphic pattern unlike that seen with other acute leukemias. Complex chromosome aberrations are common.[467] An association of megakaryoblastic leukemia in infants with t(1;22)(p13;q13) has been reported.[467–470] Abnormalities of chromosome 3 have been linked to clonal hemopathies expressing a prominent megakaryocytic phenotype.[471,472] Progression of primary myelofibrosis or essential thrombocythemia to AML may have the phenotype of acute megakaryocytic leukemia. Paradoxically, in children with Down syndrome the disease can be treated with modified doses of chemotherapy, with a very high remission rate and long-term event-free survival.[473,474] The result is thought to be related to the exquisite sensitivity of the leukemic cells to drug-induced apoptosis,[475] whereas the long-term remission rate as a result of chemotherapy in children without Down syndrome or in adults are not as good.[476,477]

■ ACUTE EOSINOPHILIC LEUKEMIA

Acute eosinophilic leukemia is rare. Increased eosinophils in the marrow but not in the blood is a variant of acute myelomonocytic leukemia and inversion 16 or other abnormalities of chromosome 16 but is not considered an acute eosinophilic leukemia.[236–239] First described in 1912,[478] acute eosinophilic leukemia is a distinct entity that can arise *de novo* as AML, with 50 to 80 percent of eosinophilic cells in the blood and marrow.[479–482] Anemia, thrombocytopenia, and blast cells in blood and marrow are present. There is apparent eosinophilic differentiation in striking proportions. The eosinophilic cells are dysmorphic and the cytoplasm hypogranulated with smaller than normal eosinophilic granules. The granules stain less intensely and are less refractile with polychrome stains. These findings are the result of the loss of the central crystalloid in the eosinophilic granules that can be identified with electron microscopic analysis. Biopsy of skin, marrow, or other sites of eosinophil accumulation often shows Charcot-Leyden crystals. A specific histochemical reaction, cyanide-resistant peroxidase, permits identification of leukemic cells with eosinophilic differentiation and diagnosis of acute eosinoblastic leukemia in some cases of AML with fewer identifiable eosinophils in blood or marrow.[483] Eosinophilia, not part of the malignant clone, may be a feature of occasional patients with AML, an uncommon reactive phenomenon. In many cases, idiopathic eosinophilia (hypereosinophilic syndrome) is a monoclonal disorder representing a spectrum of more indolent chronic or subacute eosinophilic leukemia to more progressive acute leukemia (see Chaps. 62 and 90).[484] Acute eosinophilic leukemia may develop in patients having the chronic form of a hypereosinophilic syndrome. Overexpression of Wilms tumor gene expression has been proposed as a means of distinguishing acute eosinophilic leukemia from a polyclonal, reactive eosinophilia.[485]

Patients with acute eosinophilic leukemia do not usually develop bronchospastic signs, neurologic signs, and heart failure from endomyocardial fibrosis as is seen in chronic eosinophilic leukemia, probably because those tissue changes are the result of release of toxins in the granule crystalloid, absent in most eosinophils in acute eosinophilic leukemia and because of the shorter duration of survival in acute eosinophilic leukemia. Hepatomegaly, splenomegaly, and lymphadenopathy are more common than in other variants of AML. The treatment approach is similar to other types of AML. A combination of cytarabine and an anthracycline antibiotic is an appropriate choice for treatment. Response to treatment is approximately the same as in other types of AML.[483]

ACUTE BASOPHILIC AND MAST CELL LEUKEMIA

First described in 1906,[486] basophilic differentiation as a feature of AML is an uncommon event, occurring in about 1 in 100 cases of AML.[482] Most cases of acute basophilic leukemia evolve from the chronic phase of CML,[487] but *de novo* acute basophilic leukemia, in which the cells do not contain the Philadelphia chromosome, does occur.[482,488–493] The cells stain with toluidine blue, and the basophilic granules can be most striking in myelocytes. In some cases of acute myelomonocytic leukemia associated with t(6;9)(p23;q34), basophils may be increased in the marrow but not in the blood. Because CML with t(9;22)(q34;q11) has the same breakpoint (q34) on chromosome 9 as AML with t(6;9) and both diseases are strongly associated with marrow basophilia, a gene(s) at the breakpoint on chromosome 9 may influence basophilopoiesis.[384]

Anemia, thrombocytopenia, and blast cells in the blood are present at the time of diagnosis. The blood leukocyte count usually is elevated, and proportions of the cells are basophils. The marrow is cellular with a high proportion of blasts and early and late basophilic myelocytes. Special staining with toluidine blue or Astra blue often is necessary to distinguish basophilic from neutrophilic promyelocytes and myelocytes. Immunophenotyping may show myeloid markers (CD33, CD13) that are not specific. Presence of CD9, CD25, or both is characteristic of basophilic differentiation. Cells may have granules with ultrastructural features of basophils and mast cells.[491] Electron microscopy can be useful in identifying basophilic granules in cases where no granules are evident by light microscopy and the phenotype simulates M0.[491] Basophilic leukemia can be confused with promyelocytic leukemia if the basophilic early myelocytes are mistaken for promyelocytes.[494] On the contrary, promyelocytic leukemia may have basophilic maturation and can be mistaken for basophilic leukemia. However, if the cells contain t(15;17), the disease should respond to ATRA and an anthracycline antibiotic.[408,411,412] Prolonged clotting time, intravascular coagulation, and hemorrhage are uncommon presenting features in patients with basophilic leukemia, but are common in patients with promyelocytic leukemia. Coagulopathy can occur after chemotherapy. Cluster headaches, skin rashes, often with an urticarial component, and gastrointestinal symptoms may be present. Elevated blood and urine histamine and urinary methylhistamine levels are characteristic features. Rare cases of a chronic course in *BCR-ABL*–negative basophilic leukemia preceding the onset of rapid progression have occurred.[495] Treatment for acute (Ph-negative) basophilic leukemia is similar to that for other variants of AML.

Mast cell leukemia is a rare manifestation of systemic mast cell disease (see Chap. 63).[482,496] It can be related to a mutation of the *KIT* gene.[440] The leukemic mast cells are CD117 positive, naphthol AS-D-chloracetate esterase positive, tryptase positive, myeloperoxidase negative, and CD25 negative.[498] Plasma tryptase is elevated. In some cases, electron microscopy of the granule-containing cells, which demonstrates the characteristic scroll-like granules of mast cells, may aid in distinguishing basophils from mast cells (see Chap. 63). Extensive, apparently reactive, mast cell tissue infiltrations may be provoked by cytokines during the course of AML.[499,500]

The key laboratory distinctions between acute basophilic leukemia and acute mast cell leukemia are that the cells in the former are naphthol AS-D-chloracetate esterase negative, CD11b positive, CD117 negative or weakly positive, CD123 positive, have no increase in cell or plasma tryptase, and have basophilic-like granules on electron microscopy; whereas, the cells in mast cell leukemia are naphthol AS-D-chloracetate esterase positive, CD11b negative, CD117 positive, CD123 negative, have an increase in cell and plasma tryptase, and have mast cell-like granules on electron microscopy.[482]

HISTIOCYTIC AND ACUTE MYELOID DENDRITIC CELL LEUKEMIA

Chapter 72 discusses histiocytic and myeloid dendritic cell leukemia.

DIFFERENTIAL DIAGNOSIS

Acute leukemia in infants with Down syndrome should be differentiated from TMD (see "Neonatal Myeloproliferation and Leukemia" above). In adults, the term *pseudoleukemia* has been applied to circumstances that mimic the marrow appearance of promyelocytic leukemia. Recovery from drug-induced or *Pseudomonas aeruginosa*–induced agranulocytosis is characterized by a striking cohort of promyelocytes in the marrow, which upon inspection of the marrow aspirate or biopsy mimics promyelocytic leukemia.[501–503]

In pseudoleukemia, the platelet count may be normal; the degree of leukopenia often is more profound ($<1.0 \times 10^9$/L) than usually seen in AML[444,445]; promyelocytes contain a prominent paranuclear clear (Golgi) zone not covered with granules; and promyelocytes do not have Auer rods.[503–505] Similar reactions have been reported after granulocyte colony-stimulating factor (G-CSF) administration.[506] In patients suspected of having pseudoleukemia, observation for a few days usually clarifies the significance of the marrow appearance, because progressive maturation to segmented neutrophils normalizes the marrow and leads to an increased blood neutrophil count.

In patients with hypoplastic marrows, careful examination of specimens is required to distinguish among aplastic anemia, hypoplastic acute leukemia,[283–285] and hypoplastic oligoblastic leukemia.[507] Leukemic blast cells are evident in the marrow in hypoplastic leukemia, and islands of dysmorphic cells, especially megakaryocytes, are present in hypoplastic oligoblastic leukemia.

Leukemoid reactions and nonleukemic pancytopenias can be distinguished from AML by the absence of leukemic blast cells in the blood or marrow.[508] In older children and adults, myeloblasts usually do not constitute more than 2 percent of marrow cells except in patients with leukemia, and the proportion of blast cells usually decreases in the marrow with neutrophilic leukemoid reactions.

THERAPY

OVERVIEW OF TREATMENT PLAN

The usual treatment of AML includes an initial program termed the *induction* phase. Induction may involve the simultaneous use of multiple agents or a planned sequence of therapy called *timed sequential treatment*. Once a remission is obtained, further treatment is indicated to preserve the remission state. Remission is defined as elimination of the leukemic cell population in marrow as judged by microscopy and flow cytometry and the restitution of normal or virtually normal white cell, hemoglobin, and platelet concentrations in the blood. The postinduction treatment can consist of cytotoxic chemotherapy, hematopoietic stem cell transplantation, or low-dose maintenance chemotherapy, depending upon patient performance status and risk factors. If relapse occurs, treatment options may include different chemotherapy regimens, allogeneic hematopoietic stem cell transplantation, or other investigational regimens.

DECISION TO TREAT

Most patients with AML should be advised to undergo treatment promptly after diagnosis. Patients younger than 60 years of age have a poorer outcome as the time from diagnosis to treatment lengthens.[509] Although remission rates are lower in older patients, a significant proportion enter remission. Occasionally, very elderly patients refuse treatment or are so ill from unrelated illnesses that treatment may be unreasonable. Age per se is not a contraindication to treatment, and septuagenarians and octogenarians who are fit can enter remissions. Treatment can be tailored to the decreased tolerance of older patients, some of whom have a smoldering course (see "Treatment of Older Patients" below). Associated problems, such as hemorrhagic manifestations, severe anemia, or infections, should be treated in parallel.

PREPARATION OF THE PATIENT

Orientation of the patient and the family should provide them with an understanding of the disease, the treatment planned, and the adverse effects of treatment, as well as information about long-term prognosis to the extent this can be provided while awaiting cytogenetic and molecular markers. Socioeconomic status and distance from the treatment center have minimal effects on survival in AML,[510] but impaired Karnofsky performance status and instrumental activities of daily living score do impact outcomes.[511]

Pretreatment laboratory examination should include blood cell counts, cytochemistry analysis and immunophenotyping of leukemic cells from blood or marrow, marrow examination including cytogenetic and molecular analyses to include *FLT-3* ITD, *NPM-1*, and *KIT* mutation status, if available, blood chemistry studies, chest radiography, electrocardiogram, and determination of partial thromboplastin time, prothrombin time, and fibrinogen level. More extensive evaluation of coagulation factors should be made if (1) clotting times are abnormal, (2) bleeding is exaggerated for the level of the platelet count, or (3) acute promyelocytic or monocytic leukemia is the phenotype. Early HLA typing is useful so that compatible platelet products can be provided if alloimmunization (see Chap. 141) occurs and for patients who will become marrow transplantation candidates (see Chap. 21). *Herpes simplex* virus and cytomegalovirus serotyping may be helpful, especially if transplantation is a consideration. HIV and hepatitis serology is indicated in patients with appropriate risk factors, and patients should have a baseline cardiac scan to determine ejection fraction prior to administration of an anthracycline antibiotic.

A tunneled central venous catheter should be placed. This access to the circulation facilitates administration of chemotherapy, blood components, antibiotics, and other intravenous fluids and medications. It also permits sampling blood for analysis without patient discomfort or concern about venous access. Meticulous skin care at the catheter exit site is required to minimize tunnel infections. Central venous catheters have become a major source of infection during neutropenia, especially with Gram-positive organisms.[512]

Therapy for hyperuricemia is required if (1) the pretreatment uric acid level is greater than 7 mg/dL (0.4 mmol/L), (2) the marrow is packed with blast cells, or (3) the blood blast cell count is moderately or markedly elevated. Allopurinol 300 mg/day orally should be given. Allopurinol can cause allergic dermatitis and should not be used if the uric acid level is less than 7 mg/dL and the total white cell count is less than approximately 20,000/μL (20×10^9/L), as long as hydration is adequate and urine flow is high (>150 mL/h). The dermatitis may appear when antibiotics are instituted. This concurrence may confound the decision to continue antibiotics. Thus, allopurinol should be discontinued after the risk of acute hyperuricosuria or tumor lysis has passed (usually 4 to 7 days). Recombinant urate oxidase (rasburicase) can be used to prevent urate-induced nephropathy. This preparation, although costly, can reduce plasma urate levels by approximately 80 percent within 4 hours of the first drug dose. It is well tolerated, and the recommended dose of rasburicase is 0.2 mg/kg daily for 5 to 7 days, although shorter courses are usually effective.[513]

Attention to decreasing pathogen exposure by assiduous hand washing and meticulous care of catheter and intravenous sites is important, especially when the total neutrophil count is less than 500/μL (0.5×10^9/L). Care of the patient in *a single room* is advisable to provide privacy during periods of intensive care and to help decrease the risk of exogenously acquired infection until the neutrophil count recovers.

REMISSION-INDUCTION THERAPY

Principles

The cytotoxic therapy of AML rests on two tenets: (1) two competing populations of cells are present in marrow—a normal polyclonal and a leukemic monoclonal population; and (2) profound suppression of the leukemic cells to the point they are inapparent in the marrow aspirate and biopsy is required to permit restoration of polyclonal hematopoiesis.[514,515] Although these two principles hold in most cases, two deviations from these guidelines are (1) the predisposition of patients with APL to enter remission despite cellular posttherapy marrow[516] and (2) the occasional presence of monoclonal hematopoiesis in some cases of AML during remission (see "Results of Treatment" below). AML is a heterogeneous disease, and subgroups with different prognosis can be identified. In the future, incorporation of knowledge about the biology of the particular AML subtype may be utilized for adapted therapies, but at present, all subtypes of AML classified by cytogenetics or molecular changes with the exception of acute promyelocytic leukemia are approached similarly.[517]

The goal of induction therapy in AML is achievement of complete remission (<2% blasts in the marrow), a neutrophil count greater than 1000/μL, and a platelet count greater than 100,000/μL. An International Working Group for Diagnosis, Standardization of Response Criteria, Treatment Outcomes, and Reporting Standards has redefined outcomes in an effort to standardize reporting and comparison of data.[518] Other treatment guidelines have been published.[519,520] Most adults enter remission with standard induction therapy, but for patients with high-risk disease, consideration can be given to an experimental approach. How durable a complete remission will be attained in an individual patient often is difficult to predict at diagnosis. Gene expression profiling can separate some patients into prognostic groups that may indicate patients with a high risk of not responding to standard approaches.[123,124]

Cytotoxic Regimens

Anthracycline Antibiotic or Anthraquinone and Cytarabine Current standard induction treatment for AML involves drug regimens with two or more agents that include an anthracycline antibiotic or an anthraquinone and cytarabine [521, 522] Remission rates in the studies cited range from approximately 55 to 90 percent in adult subjects, depending on the composition of the population treated (Table 89–5). The two most important variables are the age of the patients and the proportion of patients with therapy-induced leukemia or an antecedent clonal myeloid disease. In the studies listed in Table 89–5, the median age of the

TABLE 89–5. Remission Induction for AML: Examples of Cytosine Arabinoside and Anthracycline Antibiotic Combinations

Cytarabine	Anthracycline Antibiotic ± Another Agent	No. of Patients	Age Range in Years (Median)	Complete Remissions (%)	Year of Report	Reference
100 mg/m², days 1-7	DNR 45 mg/m², days 1-3	330	17–60 (47)	57	2009	525
100 mg/m², days 1-7	DNR 90 mg/m², days 1-3	327	18–60 (48)	71	2009	525
200 mg/m², days 1–7	DNR 60 mg/m², days 1–3	200	16–60 (45)	72	2004	537
200 mg/m², days 1–7	DNR 60 mg/m², days 1–3 Cladribine 5 mg/m², days 1–5	200	16–60 (45)	69	2004	537
200 mg/m² twice per day for 10 days (some in this report received FLAG-Ida vs. H-DAT)	DNR 50 mg/m², days 1, 3, 5 Thioguanine 100 mg/m² twice per day, days 10–20 Gemtuzumab ozogamicin 3 mg/m², day 1	64	18–59 (46.5)	91	2003	535
3 g/m² every 12 h for 8 doses	60 mg/m² DNR daily for 2 days	122	Adults	80	2000	529
100 mg/m² daily for 7 days (2 courses always given)	IDA 12 mg/m² daily for 3 days	153	NR	63	2000	522
500 mg/m² by continuous infusion, days 1–3, 8–10	Mitoxantrone 12 mg/m² for 3 days Etoposide 200 mg/m² IV, days 8–10	133	15–70 (43)	60	1996	532
100 mg/m² daily for 7 days	DNR 45 mg/m² for 3 days	113	NR (55)	59	1992	521
100 mg/m² daily for 7 days	IDA 13 mg/m² for 3 days	101	NR (56)	70	1992	521

DNR, daunorubicin; FLAG, fludarabine, cytarabine, and granulocyte colony-stimulating factor; H-DAT, hydroxydaunorubicin, cytarabine, and thioguanine; IDA, idarubicin; NR, not reported.

NOTE: The reader is advised to consult the original reports for details of induction and ancillary therapy and consolidation or continuation therapy, which may vary from protocol to protocol.

patient populations was much younger (~50 years) than the median age of the population of AML patients at large (~70 years); thus the results cannot be generalized (see "Treatment of Older Patients" below). A combination of anthracycline and cytarabine has been the standard induction therapy since 1973.[11] A now classic standard induction regimen is cytarabine 100 mg/m² daily by continuous infusion on days 1 through 7 and daunorubicin at 45 to 60 mg/m² on days 1 through 3, the so-called 7-and-3 regimen. Dose or schedule modulation of the anthracycline or cytarabine, addition of other agents such as etoposide, in various schedules of administration, represent attempts to improve upon results obtained with "7-and-3" therapy.

Choice of Anthracycline Development of drug resistance is reduced with idarubicin relative to other anthracyclines. Idarubicin does not induce P-glycoprotein expression, but daunorubicin, doxorubicin, and epirubicin do.[523] Idarubicin 12 mg/m² gives better complete remission rates in younger adults than does daunorubicin 45 mg/m², each given for 3 days. Amsacrine, aclarubicin, and mitoxantrone give improved results over standard-dose daunorubicin. In older adults, mitoxantrone may reduce cardiotoxicity, but this is controversial.[524] In two randomized studies, high dose daunorubicin (90 mg per square meter) for 3 days resulted in superior complete remission rates as compared to 45 mg per square meter for 3 days when combined with cytarabine.[525,526] Dexrazoxane may be given during induction to reduce the risk of cardiotoxicity in patients at higher than usual risk because of a history of coronary artery disease or congestive heart failure.[527]

High-Dose Versus Standard-Dose Cytarabine High-dose cytarabine does not increase complete remission rates and increases toxicity compared to conventional doses, especially in older patients (for doses of these regimens, see "Intensive Consolidation Therapy" below). Patients receiving high-dose cytarabine have more leukopenia, thrombocytopenia, gastrointestinal distress, and eye toxicity. Disease-free survival and overall survival may be better than that achieved with standard therapy, leading some investigators to suggest use of high-dose therapy for induction in patients younger than age 50 years, but this approach is not a standard one, and these studies do not take into account the role of high-dose cytarabine in postremission therapy.[528] Complete remission rates of greater than 60 percent have been noted with high-dose cytarabine in patients with poor-risk cytogenetics.[529,530]

Timed Sequential Therapy and Other Drugs Timed sequential therapy, which uses agents in a scheduled sequence rather than concurrently, may prolong remission duration.[531–533] Timed sequential chemotherapy combining mitoxantrone on days 1 to 3, etoposide on days 8 to 10, and cytarabine on days 1 to 3 and 8 to 10 resulted in a complete remission in 60 percent of patients, but treatment-related death in 9 percent of patients. Median disease-free survival was 9 months.[531]

Adding ATRA,[534] gemtuzumab ozogamicin,[535] fludarabine,[536] cladribine[537] or topotecan[538] to induction regimens has not improved results significantly. There are preliminary reports suggesting that the addition of gemtuzumab ozogamicin to standard induction chemotherapy may increase disease-free survival in patients with low- and standard-risk cytogenetic abnormalities,[539] and inhibitors of FLT-3 ITD are now being examined in this setting, as well in those patients who express the mutation, but no data are available regarding utility of this approach.[540] Thus, the practice guideline for AML, other than promyelocytic leukemia, recommends standard-dose cytarabine plus an anthracycline antibiotic as treatment.[520]

Hematopoietic Cytokines to Enhance Chemotherapy G-CSF and granulocyte-monocyte colony-stimulating factor (GM-CSF), when used in untreated leukemia, can increase the percentage of leukemic cells in the DNA synthetic phase, resulting in blast population expansion during short-term administration. This process could render the cells more sensitive to simultaneous chemotherapy, but clinical benefit from growth-factor priming has not been observed[541,542] despite an increased ratio of intracellular cytosine arabinoside triphosphate to deoxycytidine-5′-triphosphate and enhanced cytarabine incorporation into the DNA of AML blasts.[542] Remission rates or overall survival did not differ among adult patients who received cytarabine plus idarubicin or cytarabine plus amsacrine with or without G-CSF given concurrently, but relapse rates decreased in patients who received G-CSF.[543] GM-CSF priming in a younger patient group treated with timed-sequential therapy increased complete remission rates but did not impact overall survival.[544] Thus, these growth factors are not generally considered useful as enhancers of chemotherapy. However, complete remissions have occurred in hypoplastic AML after G-CSF treatment without chemotherapy.[545]

Duration of Induction Therapy Patients who have persistent leukemia after the first course of induction chemotherapy generally are given a second course of the same drugs. The patient's long-term outcome is worse if two courses of treatment are required even if a complete remission is achieved. Approximately 40 percent of patients with persistent AML after one course of induction therapy have a complete remission after a second course,[546] and disease-free survival at 5 years is approximately 10 percent. In some European centers, two courses of induction chemotherapy are given routinely, but impact on remission rates or overall survival is uncertain.[547] The longer the time to remission after the first induction therapy, the shorter the duration of disease-free survival.[548] High-risk cytogenetic abnormalities, antecedent hematologic disorders, and other poor prognostic factors can be used to assign nonresponders to an experimental chemotherapy regimen designed to treat refractory disease, rather than repeating induction therapy. In one study, overall response to reinduction was 53 percent. Those patients with poor risk cytogenetics and those with marrow blast percentage ≥60 percent following the 7-and-3 regimen induction treatment were found to have a low probability of achieving a complete remission with reinduction.[549] Mortality during induction therapy is correlated with age[550] and, perhaps, leukocyte count.[551] The effect of polymorphisms of detoxification genes and DNA repair enzymes, such as the glutathione-S-transferase gene on the response to antileukemic therapies is under study.[552,553]

Special Considerations during Induction Therapy

Hyperleukocytosis Patients with blast counts greater than 100,000/μL (100×10^9/L) require prompt treatment to prevent the most serious complications of hyperleukocytosis: intracranial hemorrhage or pulmonary insufficiency. Hydration should be administered promptly to maintain urine flow greater than 100 mL/hour per m^2. Cytoreduction therapy can be initiated with hydroxyurea 1.5 to 2.5 g orally every 6 hours (total dose 6 to 10 g/day) for approximately 36 hours. Appropriate remission-induction therapy should be initiated as soon as possible after the leukocyte count has been decreased significantly. Simultaneous leukapheresis can decrease blast cell concentration by approximately 30 percent within several hours,[264,554,555] without contributing to uric acid or cellular phosphate release. Leukapheresis may improve acute disturbances resulting from the vascular effects of blast cells, but the procedure may not alter the long-term outcome with current therapeutic programs[272,273,554] Inhaled nitric oxide reportedly improves hypoxemia related to hyperleukocytosis.[555]

Antibiotic Therapy Pancytopenia is worsened or induced shortly after treatment is instituted. Absolute neutrophil counts less than 100/μL (0.1×10^9/L) are expected and are a sign of effective drug action. The patient usually becomes febrile (>38°C), often with associated rigors. Cultures of urine, blood, nasopharynx, and, if available, sputum should be obtained. Because the inflammatory response is blunted by severe neutropenia and monocytopenia, evidence of exudates on physical examination or imaging studies may be minimal or absent. Antibiotics should be started immediately after cultures are obtained.[556] Chapter 22 describes antibiotic usage in the setting of intensive chemotherapy. Infections remain a major cause of therapy-associated morbidity and mortality.[557,558] Gram-positive bacterial isolates now outnumber Gram-negative organisms.[558] Cultures are often negative but if fever and other signs are present, antibiotic therapy should be continued.

Some centers use prophylactic antibacterial, antifungal, and/or antiviral antibiotics, whereas other centers do not. Antifungal prophylaxis can consist of low-dose amphotericin, fluconazole, itraconazole, posaconazole, or voriconazole.[559,560] Acyclovir, valacyclovir, or famciclovir prophylaxis during remission-induction therapy of patients with AML does not affect the duration of fever or the need for antibiotics. The incidence of bacteremia is not reduced, but acute oral infections are less severe.[561] The caspofungins and azoles are available for treatment of established fungal infections.[562] Some centers use outpatient supportive therapy immediately after induction therapy in adult AML. One approach is use of cotrimoxazole, itraconazole, or fluconazole administered orally until the granulocyte count is greater than 1000/μL, and every-other-day platelet transfusions until the platelet count is greater than 20,000/μL.[563]

Hematopoietic Growth Factors to Treat Cytopenias Cytokine therapy as an adjunctive treatment for AML remains controversial.[564] Although GM-CSF and G-CSF accelerate neutrophil recovery, neither GM-CSF nor G-CSF reproducibly decreases major morbidity or mortality. However, one study has shown decreased mortality from fungal infections in older patients.[565] Use of cytokines during periods of cytopenia following induction therapy is safe, and nearly all trials have shown a modestly reduced duration of severe neutropenia with a variable effect on the incidence of severe infections, antibiotic usage, and duration of hospital stays. Although no increase in relapse has been noted when growth factors are started after completion of chemotherapy, no consistent enhancement of remission, event-free survival, or overall survival has been noted.[566] Therefore, the cost-effectiveness of growth factor usage is doubtful.

Component Transfusion Therapy Red cell transfusions should be used to keep the hemoglobin level greater than 8.0 g/dL, or higher in special cases (e.g., symptomatic coronary artery disease; see Chap. 140). Platelet transfusions should be used for hemorrhagic manifestations related to thrombocytopenia and prophylactically if necessary to maintain the platelet count between 5000/μL (5×10^9/L) and 10,000/μL (10×10^9/L).[567] Patients without coagulation abnormalities, anticoagulant use, sepsis, or other complications usually can maintain hemostasis with platelet counts of 5000 to 10,000/μL ($5–10 \times 10^9$/L). Initially, random donor platelets can be used, although single-donor platelets or HLA-matched platelets may be preferable products and should be tried if random-donor platelets do not raise the platelet count significantly. Family members may be effective donors, if allogeneic transplantation is not being considered (see Chap. 141). There are data that fever should result in increasing the platelet count used as a transfusion threshold, and there is some suggestion that higher hemoglobin values protect against bleeding related to thrombocytopenia.[568]

All red cell and platelet products should be depleted of leukocytes, and all products, including granulocytes for transfusions, should be irradiated to prevent transfusion-associated graft-versus-host disease (GVHD) in this immunosuppressed population (see Chap. 141).

Granulocyte transfusion should not be used prophylactically for neutropenia but can be used in patients with high fever, rigors, and bacteremia unresponsive to antibiotics, with blood fungal infections, or with septic shock. G-CSF administration to a volunteer donor increases neutrophil yield fourfold and results in posttransfusion blood neutrophil increments for more than 24 hours after transfusion.[569] GM-CSF administration may be warranted for treatment of major fungal infections (see Chap. 22).

Jehovah's Witnesses and others who refuse blood product support can survive tailored chemotherapy.[570] In general, phlebotomy is minimized, and antifibrinolytics, hematinics, and growth factors are used to support such patients during severe cytopenias.

Therapy for Hypofibrinogenemic Hemorrhage Patients with evidence of intravascular coagulation (see Chap. 130) or exaggerated primary fibrinolysis (see Chap. 136) should be considered for platelet and fresh-frozen plasma administration before antileukemic therapy is started. If the findings are equivocal, patients should be monitored closely with measurements of fibrinogen levels, fibrin(ogen) degradation products, D dimer assay, and coagulation times. Intravascular coagulation or primary fibrinolysis may occur in patients with APL and acute monocytic leukemia, but also may occur in occasional patients with other AML subtypes.

Management of Central Nervous System Disease CNS disease occurs in approximately 1 in 50 cases at presentation.[571] Prophylactic therapy usually is not indicated, but examination of the spinal fluid after remission should be considered in (1) monocytic subtypes,[441] (2) cases with extramedullary disease, (3) cases with inversion 16[183] and t(8;21)[192,195] cytogenetics, (4) CD7- and CD56-positive (neural-cell adhesion molecule) immunophenotypes,[572] and (5) patients who present with very high blood blast cell counts. In these situations, the risk of meningeal leukemia or a brain myeloid sarcoma is heightened, but prophylactic intrathecal chemotherapy is not recommended if high dose cytarabine is used for consolidation. Treatment of meningeal leukemia can include high-dose intravenous cytarabine (which penetrates the blood–brain barrier), intrathecal methotrexate, intrathecal cytarabine, cranial radiation, or chemotherapy and radiation in combination.[571] Systemic relapse commonly follows relapse in the meninges, and concurrent systemic treatment usually is indicated. Long-term success is unusual unless allogeneic hematopoietic stem cell transplantation is possible. Unless the patient has neurologic symptoms, lumbar puncture generally is deferred until blood blast cells have cleared. No consensus exists on a trigger for platelet transfusion in adults with AML undergoing lumbar puncture, but a platelet count less than 20,000/μL (20×10^9/L) has been proposed as such a trigger.[573]

Management of Nonleukemic Myeloid Sarcoma Some patients present with myeloid (granulocytic) sarcomas without evidence of leukemia in the blood or marrow (see "Myeloid [Granulocytic] Sarcoma" above). Myeloid sarcoma may be the presenting finding in approximately 2 percent of patients with AML. Such patients should receive intensive AML induction therapy.[191] Intensive therapy results in a longer nonleukemic period than patients who have undergone surgical resection or resection followed by local irradiation.[179] Median relapse-free survival is about 12 months after AML-type chemotherapy.[191] Patients with trisomy 8 have poorer survival rates.[189]

POSTREMISSION THERAPY

Cytotoxic Therapy

General Considerations Postremission therapy is intended to prolong remission duration and overall survival, but no consensus exists regarding the best approach. Postremission chemotherapy that does not produce profound prolonged cytopenias, closely simulating intensive induction therapy, has produced on average only slight prolongation of remission or life. Regimens that fall between these intensities have been used, with equivocal results. Intensive consolidation therapy after remission results in a somewhat longer remission duration and, more significantly, a subset of patients who have a remission of more than 3 years. The issue of postremission therapy and its impact is complicated by the large proportion of patients with AML who are older than 60 years of age and have limited tolerance for intensive therapy in the later decades of life. In addition, a very small pool of leukemic stem cells may sustain the process, and elimination of these cells may require approaches other than intensive chemotherapy, especially in adults.

Several randomized trials have studied whether AML patients in first remission should receive consolidation chemotherapy alone, autologous transplantation, or allogeneic marrow transplantation, without reaching a consensus. Allogeneic transplantation was compared to autologous transplantation using unpurged marrow and two courses of intensive chemotherapy in 623 patients who had a complete remission after induction chemotherapy.[574] Disease-free survival was 53 percent at 4 years for those receiving allogeneic transplantation, 48 percent for those receiving autologous transplantation, and 30 percent for patients receiving intensive chemotherapy. Overall survival after complete remission was similar in all three groups because patients who relapsed after chemotherapy could be rescued with stem cell transplantation. No significant difference in the 4-year disease-free survival between allogeneic stem cell transplantation (42%) and other types of intensive postremission therapy (40%) has been found.[575] In another study, only patients younger than 15 to 35 years of age with poor-risk cytogenetics had improved disease-free survival if they had a sibling donor and underwent allogeneic transplantation (43.5% vs. 18.5% at 4 years).[576] Thus, in several studies, the early mortality after allogeneic transplantation and the chemotherapy-induced remissions in patients who relapse following autologous transplantation or chemotherapy have led to comparable overall survival rates. However, leukemia-free survival was greater after allogeneic transplantation.[577] When quality of life was measured for patients in complete remission for 1 to 7 years, those treated with chemotherapy had the highest quality of life whereas those who underwent allogeneic stem cell transplantation had the lowest.[578]

The decision to utilize autologous or allogeneic stem cell transplantation or high-dose cytarabine alone for consolidation is individualized based on the patient's age and other prognostic factors, such as high-risk cytogenetic findings and antecedent hematologic disease. Patients with good-risk cytogenetics should receive up to four cycles of high-dose cytarabine. Patients with poor-risk cytogenetics should be considered for allogeneic or autologous stem cell transplantation after one or two cycles of high-dose cytarabine. A meta analysis has shown that compared with non-allogeneic therapies, allogeneic hematopoietic stem cell transplant has superior relapse-free survival and overall survival for cases of AML classified intermediate and poor-risk but not for cases considered good-risk AML in first remission.[579]

Intensive Consolidation Therapy For patients who do not receive high-dose chemotherapy with autologous or allogeneic transplantation in first remission, consolidation chemotherapy regimens containing high-dose cytarabine provide better results than intermediate-dose cytarabine,[580,581] but these regimens are not universally accepted.[582] Patients who have ablative allogeneic hematopoietic stem cell transplantation do not require four cycles of high-dose cytarabine.[583] *RAS* mutations have been associated with benefit from high-dose cytarabine therapy.[584] Patients with t(8;21) also have particularly favorable responses to repetitive cycles of high-dose cytarabine. In patients who received three or more cycles, a relapse rate of 19 percent was reported.[585]

Other regimens, such as those containing gemtuzumab ozogamicin and fludarabine, have been used in postremission therapy, but whether they provide benefit over use of high-dose cytarabine has not been studied.[586] Long-term disease-free survival at 5 years generally is approximately 30 percent when two to four cytarabine-containing regimens are administered.[587,588] Most centers use four cycles of therapy. A cycle is 3 g/m^2 twice daily on days 1, 3, and 5, providing six doses per cycle, with cycle durations dependent on normal blood count recovery. The optimal number of cycles for this therapy is not known.[589] High-dose cytarabine can be administered at a dose of 3 g/m^2 in a 1- to 3-hour intravenous infusion every 12 hours for up to 6 days (12 doses), but this schedule is almost never used because of its toxicity. High-dose cytarabine frequently causes conjunctivitis and photophobia, and glucocorticoid eye drops are usually used every 6 hours until 24 hours after the last dose of the drug.[590] Cerebellar function abnormalities also may occur, and these require cessation of drug administration. A 1-hour duration infusion of high-dose or reduced-dose (e.g., 2 g/m^2) cytarabine may decrease the likelihood of severe cerebellar toxicity.[590] Older patients and patients with renal insufficiency require dose attenuation (i.e., to 1–2 g/m^2).[591]

Additional Maintenance Therapy Various forms of less-intensive maintenance chemotherapy have been attempted after completion of intensive consolidation chemotherapy. Many of the regimens consist of monthly chemotherapy, for example, low-dose 6-thioguanine or cytarabine. Although improved disease-free survival was noted in some studies, no improvement in overall survival has been demonstrated in most studies.[592] Some groups are examining the role of demethylating agents (e.g., 5-azacytidine) as maintenance therapy.

Autologous Stem Cell Infusion after Ablative Chemotherapy or Chemoradiotherapy for Consolidation

Removal and cryopreservation of postremission marrow or collection of mobilized blood stem cells from patients with AML and reinfusion of these products following intensive chemotherapy and/or radiotherapy is a form of postremission therapy (see Chap. 21).[593] Autologous marrow or blood stem cell rescue can be used in patients with AML who achieve a remission, do not have a compatible stem cell donor, and are as old as 70 years.

Various preparative regimens for autologous transplantation in AML have been utilized,[594] such as busulfan-cyclophosphamide, busulfan-etoposide-cytarabine, high-dose cytarabine-mitoxantrone plus total-body irradiation, melphalan plus total-body irradiation, and cyclophosphamide plus total-body irradiation. A disease-free survival rate of approximately 40 percent at 3 years is average after such regimens in the age-range treated.[595,596] Long-term disease-free survival can occur in patients who undergo this treatment for AML in second remission.[597] Patients older than age 50 years have inferior outcomes, but no strict upper-age limit for this procedure has been determined.[598] Administration of two or more courses of consolidation chemotherapy prior to harvest and transplant is associated with decreased relapse rates and improved disease-free survival. A marrow nucleated cell dose greater than 2×10^8/kg improves disease-free survival.[599] Chemotherapy agents such as 4-hydroperoxycyclophosphamide have been utilized for purging residual leukemic cells,[600,601] and antisense agents reportedly diminish leukemic cell contamination.[602] Use of marrow grafts purged of residual leukemia cells has not significantly improved the results obtained with unpurged marrow in many studies, suggesting that low proportions of leukemic stem cells may not transplant easily or that they do not survive the freeze–thaw cycle to which autologous marrow is subjected as well as do normal stem cells.[603] In addition, residual leukemia in the patient may contribute to relapse. For these reasons, marrow purging is rarely utilized in AML autografting (see Chap. 21). In long-term cultures from patients newly diagnosed with AML, normal progenitors can be detected, and their numbers are increased by *in vitro* culture with cytokines.[604] In oligoblastic leukemia (myelodysplasia), secondary AML, and therapy-related AML, leukapheresis products obtained after chemotherapy and growth factor treatment contain normal progenitors,[605] indicating mobilized stem cells may be relatively free of leukemic counterparts even in the absence of *ex vivo* purging.[606] Early mortality may be decreased using blood stem cells because they engraft more rapidly, but relapse rates may be higher.[607] The Center for International Bone Marrow Transplantation reported that in 2007 the majority of autologous stem cell transplantations in AML used blood stem cell collections. Mobilized stem cells can be collected after high-dose cytarabine plus G-CSF or after G-CSF alone.[608] There is a plateau in the survival curve after autologous stem cell transplantation at about 2.2 years,[609] and there is evidence that autologous transplantations improve disease-free survival but not overall survival.[610] The total number of CD34+ cells infused influences early engraftment, but durable engraftment is associated more closely with the CD34+/CD38– subset in the graft.[611] Myeloablative chemotherapy followed by autologous stem cell rescue may overcome the adverse prognosis associated with FLT3 mutations.[612]

Chemoradiotherapy Plus Allogeneic Stem Cell Transplantation for Consolidation Therapy

General Considerations Utilization of allogeneic hematopoietic stem cell transplantation for AML is increasing in Europe and the United States.[613] No strict upper-age limit for transplantation exists,[614] but many centers use age 60 or 65 years for transplants following ablation of hematopoiesis and 70 years for transplants not preceded by ablation of hematopoiesis (nonmyeloablative transplants). Decisions to proceed to allogeneic transplantation should be individualized, and feasibility depends on (1) the availability of a suitable donor, (2) the recipient's age and health status, and (3) whether AML is in remission.

For ablative transplantations, the patient is prepared with a regimen that includes total-body irradiation and/or high-dose chemotherapy, after which the donor stem cells are infused by vein. Patients given allogeneic blood stem cells have more rapid hematopoietic reconstitution than patients given marrow stem cells.[615] Chapter 21 describes the indications, procedure, and preparative regimens for stem cell transplantation. For standard-risk leukemia, blood and marrow appear to be equivalent sources for allografting.[616] Engraftment is faster, but chronic GVHD may be more frequent when blood stem cells are used, and longer followup is needed to determine the ultimate effects of blood versus marrow allografts when the donor is a matched sibling.[617] G-CSF–primed donor-marrow stem cells may result in less GVHD compared with G-CSF–mobilized blood stem cells.[618] In general, no single preparative regimen is superior for patients with AML in first remission.[619] In one study, cyclophosphamide and total-body irradiation lowered relapse risk, but overall results were comparable to conditioning with chemotherapy alone.[620] Postremission consolidation with cytarabine before allogeneic transplantation for AML in first remission does not improve outcome compared with immediate transplant after successful induction.[621] It is unclear that this result will also hold in the setting of reduced-intensity transplants or for transplants performed beyond first remission.[622]

Related Donors When matched-sibling transplantation is performed for AML in first remission, approximately half of patients have a disease-free survival of 4 years. Small series using T-cell depletion have reported 4-year disease-free survival of 65 percent.[623] Leukemia relapses occur in approximately 20 percent of patients who receive an allogeneic transplant.[618] Patients who are alive with good performance status 3 years after transplantation have excellent prospects of long-term survival.[623] In the posttransplantation period, approximately one-third of patients die of severe GVHD, opportunistic infection, or interstitial pneumonitis. Marrow transplantation therapy is superior to chemotherapy in that the proportion of subjects who have leukemia relapse is lower, but whether marrow transplantation provides an advantage in overall survival at 3 years is uncertain.[624] The outlook for long-term survival is improved if (1) the AML is in remission prior to transplantation, (2) grade III to IV acute GVHD does not occur, and (3) chronic GVHD is low grade.[625,626] For patients with unfavorable cytogenetics, an allogeneic sibling transplantation in first remission is often recommended.[627] Patients with FLT3/ITD-positive AML may also benefit from stem cell transplantation in first remission.[628] When AML patients in first remission were compared on a donor versus no donor basis, and more than 80 percent of patients with a donor went on to transplantation, patients with a donor had a significantly better disease-free survival, although treatment-related mortality was higher.[629] For patients with intermediate-risk cytogenetics, where the decision is made to delay transplantation until first relapse, physicians should identify a source of a hematopoietic stem cell graft and ensure that careful monitoring of the patient occurs so that transplantation can be instituted as quickly as possible.[630]

In an attempt to decrease the relapse rate after stem cell transplantation for advanced acute leukemia, ^{131}I-labeled anti-CD45 antibody to deliver radiation to leukemic cells, followed by a standard transplant preparative regimen, has been used. Nine of 13 patients with AML were disease free 8 to 41 months after transplantation. With this regimen, more radiation can be delivered to hematopoietic tissues compared with liver, lung, or kidney, which may improve the efficacy of the transplantation.[631]

Unrelated Donors Approximately 70 percent of all patients with AML are older than 50 years of age, and the current mean family size in the United States is slightly more than two children per family. Thus, only approximately 10 to 15 percent of subjects with AML are within the age range and have a sibling donor for marrow transplantation. The ability to extend the proportion of patients who can be transplanted has led to histocompatible, unrelated donors or HLA type-mismatched sibling or parent (haploidentical) donor transplants.[632] Molecular matching of class I and II HLA alleles adds to the clinical success of unrelated donor transplantations but makes finding a donor more difficult.[633] Treatment of high-risk acute leukemia with T-cell–depleted stem cells from related donors with one mismatched HLA haplotype with standard conditioning regimens has been successful, with an acceptable incidence of GVHD. However, infectious complications were high.[634] HLA-matched or HLA-mismatched cord blood stem cells can be used in adults with acute leukemia but generally not for patients in first remission.[635,636] In adults, the numbers of stem cells available in a single cord product may not result in engraftment, which has led to the use of two-cord blood units for grafting (see Chap. 21).[637]

Nonmyeloablative Transplantation Patients who, based upon comorbidities or performance status, are deemed too old or too ill to undergo a myeloablative stem cell transplantation may be offered a reduced-intensity transplantation procedure, provided a suitable donor is available. This type of transplantation relies upon the graft versus leukemia effect as primary therapy.[638] Use of this approach, specific to AML and a variety of hematologic malignancies, has been described.[639,640] These regimens have moderate hematologic and nonhematologic toxicity, and often can be performed on an outpatient basis. Engraftment and establishment of complete donor chimerism are successful in most patients. GVHD rates have been variable, and the ultimate risk of acute and chronic GVHD with these regimens is unclear. A variety of low-intensity regimens have been proposed.[641] In AML in first remission, the 1-year progression-free survival is approximately 55 percent.[642,643] The role of this approach in the treatment of AML remains to be defined, and comparative trials with longer followup are needed. Nonmyeloablative conditioning with unrelated donors has been used successfully.[644,645] Although randomized trials of ablative versus reduced-dose-intensity conditioning regimens for transplantation of AML patients in first remission have not been done, there is evidence that reduced-dose intensity is an inferior option for disease control, but that disadvantage is offset by the decreased treatment-related mortality.[646] In one retrospective study, stratified outcomes based on comorbidity and disease status did not differ significantly between reduced-dose and full-dose conditioning of patients, with the exception of lessened nonrelapse mortality in the high-risk group.[647] In a multivariate analysis, active disease at transplant and development of grades II to IV GVHD after transplantation had a negative impact on survival in reduced-dose-intensity transplantations.[648] Reduced-dose-intensity transplantations are feasible in elderly patients, but donor availability and coexisting medical problems often limit its use.[649]

Use of Transplantation in Relapsed Patients Some form of allograft usually is recommended for patients in early first relapse or second remission, because long-term survival with chemotherapy alone is improbable, whereas histocompatible sibling transplants have a 25 percent survival rate. For patients who lack a sibling donor, matched-unrelated donor transplants can be effective, but treatment-related mortality is high, suggesting that patients with unfavorable cytogenetics should undergo a matched-unrelated donor transplant in first complete remission, if an acceptable donor can be found.[650] However, when transplantation was compared to chemotherapy for AML in second remission, the 3-year probability of event-free survival was 17 percent with chemotherapy and 16 percent with transplant. Patients younger than 30 years of age who were in remission for at least 1 year fared best.[651] Development of chronic GVHD, an unrelated donor, a young age of donor, and blast cell count <30 percent at transplant were found in another series to be favorable predictors of survival for transplants performed in leukemia relapse.[652] Patients with extramedullary sites of leukemia are more likely to relapse after allogeneic marrow transplantation.[653]

Patients with AML who relapse after allogeneic stem cell transplantation can have a long-term remission if they undergo retransplantation.[654] The mechanism of benefit of stem cell transplantation was thought to result from high-dose ablative chemoradiotherapy followed by marrow "rescue." The increased relapse rate of AML in patients transplanted with marrow from identical twins, compared to nonidentical siblings, or transplanted with T-lymphocyte–depleted marrow has indicated an immunologic effect of donor lymphocytes may determine the results of transplantation. This immunologic response, referred to as *graft-versus-leukemia effect*, may play a role in preventing leukemia relapses.[655]

Donor Leukocyte Infusion In an attempt to enhance graft-versus-leukemia effects, adoptive immunotherapy with donor mononuclear cell infusions is sometimes used to treat relapse of leukemia after allografting.[656,657] These infusions have been successful in only a minority of patients with AML, but given the high mortality associated with alternative procedures such as second transplantations, the infusions are a reasonable approach for patients who relapse after allogeneic transplantation.[658] GVHD and marrow aplasia are the major complications of this form of treatment.[659] The graft-versus-leukemia reaction is thought to be directed against minor histocompatibility antigens on the cell surface of hematopoietic cells, but reactions against leukemia-specific antigens are possible. Relapses after donor leukocyte infusions for recurring acute leukemia have a higher probability of being extramedullary.[660] Donor lymphocyte infusions are most effective in early relapses and in the absence of extensive of chronic GVHD.[661] Some patients also enter a new remission upon withdrawal of immune suppression. Patients who enter remission by donor lymphocyte infusion or cessation of immune suppressive agents have a better survival than those who entered remission with chemotherapy alone or after a second transplant.[662] Unrelated-donor leukocyte infusions can be used to treat relapsed leukemia after unrelated donor stem cell transplantation.[663] Approximately 40 percent of AML patients enter remission with this treatment. G-CSF has been used as an alternative to donor leukocyte infusions after AML relapse posttransplant.[664] Donor blood stem cells can be combined with chemotherapy for early relapse of AML after allogeneic stem cell transplantation.[665] Strategies with donor leukocyte infusions are anticipated to become more effective once the effector cells are identified and the tumor target antigens better understood.[666]

Adjunct Therapy with Interleukin-2 and Vaccines Interleukin-2 has been used to modulate natural killer cell and T-cell activity after both autologous and allogeneic transplantation. The efficacy of this approach has not yet been determined.[667] Minor histocompatibility antigens restricted to hematopoietic cells are an ideal target for antileukemic immune responses. Modification of leukemic cells to express costimulatory molecules identical to professional antigen-presenting cells to generate cytotoxic T lymphocyte responses against myeloid leukemia cells may be possible.[668] Dendritic cells derived *in vitro* from AML cells also can be used to stimulate leukemia-specific cytolytic activity in autologous or allogeneic lymphocytes.[669]

Recurrent Leukemia in Donor Cells or New Leukemia in Recipient Cells Recurrence of AML in donor cells has been reported in patients who received stem cell transplants from healthy siblings. These recurrences in donor cells occurred in approximately 1 in 18 relapsed patients who received marrow from a donor of the opposite sex.[670] A similar frequency of relapsed AML is observed in recipient cells but with a different clonal cytogenetic abnormality, suggesting a "new" leukemia.[670] The frequencies are dependent on the sensitivity and specificity of cytogenetic techniques, which have been challenged. AML developing in a stem cell recipient but of donor cell origin long after transplantation has been documented in rare cases.[671]

TREATMENT OF RELAPSED OR REFRACTORY PATIENTS

Chemotherapy

Patients who relapse after remission-induction and postinduction therapy have a decreased probability of entering a subsequent remission, and the duration of any remission that occurs is usually shorter. In patients who relapse more than 1 year after the first remission, the original remission-induction regimen can be readministered or a combination salvage chemotherapy regimen can be administered.

Refractory leukemia is defined as leukemia that does not respond to initial induction chemotherapy with cytarabine and an anthracycline antibiotic or anthraquinone. Patients with refractory disease are more likely to have disease with adverse cytogenetic findings, a history of antecedent clonal myeloid disease, adverse immunophenotypic features, and expression of multidrug resistance (MDR).[672]

Relapsed leukemia is leukemia that recurs following a remission. The duration of remission greatly affects the patient's prognosis and response to additional treatment. The wide range of response rates may not only reflect the regimen used but may also reflect variability in patient selection, age, and other prognostic factors.[672,673]

Chemotherapy regimens can be divided into cytarabine-based, noncytarabine-based, and timed sequential therapy with growth factors and cytotoxic drugs. Table 89–6 lists the response rates; the duration of response usually is measured in months. The duration of response is difficult to define because many patients go on to other therapies, including stem cell transplantation.

Results from second remission-induction therapy are better in younger patients and in those with longer first remissions, longer durations since last chemotherapy, and better general health. The probability of a second remission is approximately 50 percent in younger subjects (ages 15–60 years) and approximately 25 percent in older patients (ages 60–80 years), but the duration of remission nearly always is much shorter than the first remission. An eventual fatal outcome is nearly certain unless allogeneic hematopoietic stem cell transplantation can be performed. Rare patients may have a third (or more) relapse followed by a remission when treated with cytotoxic drugs, but each remission is shorter than the preceding one and usually is measured in weeks. For those who have favorable or normal karyotype, long second remission, and no previous stem cell transplantation, intensive chemotherapy can be useful.[674] In one study, approximately 17 percent of 124 patients had a second remission duration at least 2 months longer than the first remission.[675] In patients in relapse treated with the sequential high-dose cytosine arabinoside and mitoxantrone (S-HAM) regimen, the duration of the first remission was the only factor associated with a successful outcome, and unfavorable karyotype was the only factor related to duration of survival.[676] Patients who relapse less than 1 year from remission should be treated with investigational agents, whereas patients who relapse more than 1 year later may benefit from standard reinduction therapy.[677] No standard chemotherapy regimen provides durable remission of AML patients who relapse (see Table 89–6),[678–685] and all such patients should be considered for clinical trials if available.

Allogeneic Hematopoietic Stem Cell Transplantation

Allogeneic stem cell transplantation may be the only means to induce a sustained remission in patients with AML who do not enter remission with cytotoxic drug therapy or who relapse after a first remission. Approximately 25 percent of patients with refractory or relapsed AML have a sustained remission of at least 3 years.[686] Transplant-related mortality at 3 years is approximately 50 percent. Relapse rates are higher after sibling than matched-unrelated transplantation.[687,688] If a histocompatible donor is available and the patient is younger than age 50 years, stem cell transplantation can be as successful if it is performed when the patient is in early relapse compared with in second remission.[689]

Relapse after Stem Cell Transplantation For patients who relapse after allogeneic stem cell transplantation, the prognosis is extremely poor and available chemotherapy, donor leukocyte infusions, or second transplants do not result in consistent durable remissions.[690] For patients who relapse after reduced-dose-intensity allogeneic transplantations, median overall survival after relapse was found to be 6 months, and no advantage was found for donor leukocyte infusions or second transplantations as compared with chemotherapy.[691] Patients who relapse after autologous stem cell transplantation can sometimes be salvaged with reduced-dose-intensity allogeneic transplantations or with full-dose-intensity allogeneic transplantations with high treatment-related mortality rates even in younger patients.

OTHER TREATMENT MODALITIES

Chemotherapy

Several newer chemotherapeutic agents are being examined for treatment of AML. Troxacitabine, an isomer of cytarabine, has entered into phase I and II trials in AML and has been combined with cytarabine, idarubicin, or topotecan.[692,693] Temozolomide[694] and clofarabine,[695] a nucleoside analogue, induced responses in refractory or relapsed acute leukemias,[696] High-dose hydroxyurea can result in remission in 42 percent of patients with poor-risk leukemias when given at a dosage of 100 mg/kg per day until marrow aplasia occurs or for a maximum of 30 days.[697] Cloretazine is a new sulfonylhydrazine alkylating agent with activity in relapsed AML and in elderly patients with untreated AML. It has also been studied in combination with cytarabine.[698,699]

Epigenetic Modulation

Methylation of DNA at critical sites can cause transcriptional inactivation of genes or chromosomal instability. In AML, aberrant methylation,

TABLE 89–6. Examples of Chemotherapy Used for Relapsed or Refractory Patients

Regimen	No. of Patients	% of Patients Entering a Complete Remission (Median Duration)	Year	Reference
Gemtuzumab ozogamicin 6 mg/m^2 IV, days 1 and 13 Idarubicin 12 mg/m^2, days 2–4 Cytarabine 1.5 g/m^2, days 2–5	15	21 (27 weeks)	2003	679
Mitoxantrone 12 mg/m^2, days 1–3 Cytarabine 500 mg/m^2, days 1–3 Followed (at count recovery) by Etoposide 200 mg/m^2, days 1–3 Cytarabine 500 mg/m^2, days 1–3	66	36 (5 months)	2003	680
Cladribine 5 mg/m^2, days 1–5 Cytarabine 2 g/m^2, days 1–5 2 h after 2-CdA G-CSF 10 mcg/kg/day, days 1–5	58	50 (29% disease-free at 1 year)	2003	681
Fludarabine 30 mg/m^2, days 1–5 Cytarabine 2 g/m^2, days 1–5 Idarubicin 10/m^2 days 1–3 G-CSF 5 mcg/kg per day, day +6 until neutrophil recovery	46	52 (13 months)	2003	682
Gemtuzumab ozogamicin 9 mg/m^2, days 1 and 15	43	9	2002	683
Mitoxantrone 4 mg/m^2, days 1–3 Etoposide 40 mg/m^2, days 1–3 Cytarabine 1 g/m^2, days 1–3, ± PSC-833	37	32	1999	684
Fludarabine 30 mg/m^2, days 1–5 Cytarabine 2 g/m^2, days 1–5± Idarubicin 12 mg/m^2, days 1–3 G-CSF 400 mcg/m^2 daily until complete remission	85	66	1995	685

DNR, daunorubicin; FLAG, fludarabine, cytarabine, and granulocyte colony-stimulating factor; H-DAT, hydroxydauorubicin, cytarabine, and thioguanine; IDA, idarubicin; NR, not reported.

NOTE: The reader is advised to consult the original reference for details of chemotherapy regimen administration.

especially preferential methylation of chromosome 11, has been described.[700] Epigenetic gene silencing caused by DNA methylation is a target for demethylating agents such as 5-azacytidine or decitabine, and silencing mediated by histone deacetylation is a target for histone deacetylases.[701] Decitabine, a potent hypomethylating agent, can cause maturation and growth arrest of AML cells.[702–704] 5-Azacytidine also has activity in AML, and it is being studied in an oral formulation.[705] These demethylating agents, singly or in combination, have resulted in response rates of 25 to 60 percent.[706] Histone deacetylase inhibitors can restore retinoic acid-dependent transcriptional activation and maturation in AML blasts.[707] Depsipeptide can promote histone acetylation and gene transcription in RUNX1/ETO-positive leukemic cells.[708] Depsipeptide (romidepsin),[709] LBH589,[710] vorinostat (suberoylanilide hydroxamic acid [SAHA]),[711] and MGCD0103[712] have each been studied in early phase trials in leukemia. Combination therapy of demethylating agents with other targeted therapies is being explored,[713] and combination therapy with demethylating agents and histone deacetylase inhibitors have been reported.[714]

Growth Factors and Receptor Targets

A ricin fusion toxin attached to human GM-CSF[715] and a diphtheria toxin attached to GM-CSF to form a fusion protein are toxic to AML cells.[716] GM-CSF can alter the cellular metabolism of cytarabine and fludarabine in AML patients.[717] A diphtheria toxin—interleukin (IL)-3 fusion protein is cytotoxic for blasts that express high-affinity interleukin-3 receptor (CD123),[718] and progenitor cells from patients with CD87+ urokinase receptor are sensitive to a diphtheria toxin–urokinase fusion protein.[719]A phase I study has been completed with the diphtheria toxin–IL-3 fusion protein with some responses noted.[720]

Antibodies to CD33

The CD33 antigen is expressed on approximately 90 percent of AML blasts and is a target for antibody-mediated destruction. Gemtuzumab ozogamicin is a recombinant humanized anti-CD33 monoclonal immunoglobulin (Ig) G_4 antibody conjugated to the cytotoxin calicheamicin.[721] The conjugated antibody is rapidly internalized and causes subsequent apoptosis.[722] Gemtuzumab ozogamicin administered to AML patients with CD33+ blast cells in untreated first relapse at a dose of 9 mg/m^2 twice, 14 days apart, produced complete remission in 16 percent of patients and complete remission with incomplete platelet recovery in an another 14 percent of patients.[723] It has been approved by the U.S. Food and Drug Administration for use in patients older than age 65 years.[724] This agent produces myelosuppression and is associated with an infusional syndrome that can be minimized with glucocorticoids.[725] It does not cause alopecia or mucositis. Hyperbilirubinemia and transaminase elevations can occur. Although it results in similar survival rates as standard chemotherapy reinduction, its use was associated with fewer days of hospitalization.[726] In patients who relapsed between 3 to 11 months, gemtuzumab ozogamicin resulted in higher remission rates compared to regimens containing high-dose cytarabine in different trials. However, in patients who had prolonged first remissions of greater than 19 months, cytarabine resulted in superior remission rates.[727] Prior gemtuzumab ozogamicin exposure may increase the risk of venoocclusive disease in patients who later undergo myeloablative allogeneic stem cell transplant procedures.[728] Cytotoxic activity of gemtuzumab ozogamicin correlates with expression of syk.[729] Studies are examining its role in induction coupled with standard chemotherapy, in postremission therapy, and in the treatment of acute promyelocytic leukemia.[730,731]

Therapies Targeted to Signal Transduction Mediators

Tyrosine Kinase Inhibitors: *FLT3* Inhibitors Constitutively activating FLT3 receptor mutations have been found in approximately 30 percent of patients with AML. Several small-molecule *FLT3* tyrosine kinase inhibitors have been formulated, including PKC412 (midostaurin),[732] CT83518,[733] CEP-701 (lestaurtinib),[734] SU5416,[735] and MLN518.[736] These agents inhibit *FLT3-ITD* phosphorylation, induce cell apoptosis *in vitro*, and have efficacy in mouse models of human leukemia. Targeted inhibition of *FLT3* can overcome blockade of myeloid differentiation.[737] These agents are in phase I and II trials, in which they have induced a decline in blood blast cells, but rarely result in complete remissions.[738,739] Sorafenib, a multikinase inhibitor, has also been reported to have activity against *FLT3-ITD*–positive blast cells *in vitro* and *in vivo*.[740] Trials are now under way to examine inhibitors such as midostaurin (PKC412) in combination with cytostatic drugs for AML.[741]

KIT Tyrosine Kinase Inhibitors: Imatinib Mesylate Activation of the KIT tyrosine kinase by somatic mutation has been documented in a small minority of AML cases. Paracrine or autocrine activation of *KIT* may occur in AML cells.[742] In culture systems, KIT ligand (stem cell factor)-independent, KIT phosphorylation usually is not detected, suggesting that imatinib mesylate would have only limited activity.[743] Imatinib mesylate also inhibits the activity of the platelet-derived growth factor receptor and mutant tyrosine kinase (BCR-ABL). Imatinib mesylate has induced a complete remission of refractory secondary AML,[744] but this is a very uncommon result of its use.[745]

Nuclear Factor-Kappa B Inhibitors AML initiating or stem cells have activated nuclear factor-κB (NF-κB) unlike normal hematopoietic stem cells.[746] Proteasome inhibitors such as bortezomib inhibit NF-κB and have been examined in AML. They have been found to increase sensitivity to chemotherapy agents in *NPM1*-mutated AML.[747] Bortezomib is also being combined with chemotherapy agents in AML patients.[748]

Other Signal Transduction and Tyrosine Kinase Inhibitors Numerous inhibitors of activated tyrosine kinases have been examined for AML therapy.[749,750] These include mammalian target of rapamycin (mTOR) inhibitors,[751,752] phosphoinositol 3 kinase inhibitors,[753,754] AKT inhibitors such as perifosine,[755] small-molecule mitogen-activated protein kinase (MEK) kinase inhibitors,[756] Aurora kinase inhibitors,[757] and heat shock protein inhibitors.[758] None of these agents have had impact on AML survival as single agents, but using a combination of agents that target multiple pathways or using multitargeted tyrosine kinase inhibitors may hold promise for incremental improvements in AML therapy.[759] There is some indication that extramedullary disease may increase in incidence in cases treated with signal transduction agents alone.[760]

Other Inhibitors of Signal Transduction and Apoptosis Pathways Many malignancies overexpress antiapoptotic proteins, such as BCL-2 and BCL-x_L.[761] Antisense agents to BCL-2 mRNA in combination with chemotherapy are being tested in patients with AML.[762] The 18-merphosphorothioate BCL-2 antisense molecule G3139 (Genasense) has been combined with fludarabine, arabinosyl cytosine, and G-CSF (FLAG) therapy. It downregulates its target BCL-2.[762] Small-molecule BCL-2 homology domain-3 (BH3) mimetics such as ABT-737[763] and GX15–070 (obatoclax)[764] inhibit BCL-2. CDDO-Me, a triterpenoid, studied *in vitro* induces apoptosis and differentiation in AML cells through activation of caspase-8 and caspase-3 and induction of mitochondrial cytochrome *c* release.[765] It can facilitate the maturation of cells by ATRA; downregulate the FAS-associated death domain-like IL-1β-converting enzyme (FLICE) like inhibitory protein (FLIP), an antagonist of caspase-8; and result in tumor necrosis factor (TNF)-related apoptosis-inducing ligand (TRAIL)-induced apoptosis via a TNF-family death pathway.[766] TRAIL itself may have a therapeutic role in AML.[767] The cyclin-dependent kinase inhibitor flavopiridol potentiates apoptosis in AML cells,[768] and it has entered trials of timed sequential therapy in AML.[769]

Prenylation Inhibitors: Farnesyltransferase Inhibitors Mutation or activation of *RAS* occurs in the cells of approximately 15 percent of AML patients. Because posttranslational processing by farnesyltransferase is necessary for RAS translocation to the cell membrane, inhibitors of this enzyme are postulated to inhibit RAS activity.[770] Several farnesyltransferase inhibitors are being studied as inhibitors of AML cell growth (BMS-214662, L-778,123, R-115777 [Tipifarnib], and SCH66336 [Lonafarnib]).[771–774] In a phase I trial of R-115777 in adults with refractory and relapsed AML, clinical responses occurred in 10 of 34 evaluable patients, including 2 complete remissions.[774] It is anticipated that these agents will need to be combined with standard cytotoxic agents for maximum effectiveness[775] as their effectiveness as single agents has been minimal in untreated AML/MDS patients.[776] There is some evidence that these agents could be of benefit in maintenance phases of therapy.[777]

Geranylgeranyltransferase-1 Inhibitors Because many proteins subject to farnesylation also undergo geranylgeranylation, geranylgeranyltransferase-1 inhibitors may have activity in AML and may explain resistance to farnesyltransferase inhibitor monotherapy in patients with AML.[778] Several of these inhibitors are being screened. The statins inhibit geranylation, and cases of responses of AML to lovastatin have been reported.[779] Simvastatin adds to the effect of cytarabine's inhibition of AML cell lines.[780] Other studies suggest that the statins may mediate antileukemic effects independent of RAS/RHO prenylation through blockade of cholesterol responses to cellular injury.[781]

Maturation Therapies Several analogues of vitamin D inhibit AML cells by inducing inhibition of cyclin-dependent kinases.[782] In general, AML cells have not responded to retinoids. Single-strand conformational polymorphism analysis and DNA sequencing of leukemic cells from AML, other than APL, have not found mutations of RAR-α.[783] Nevertheless, combinations of retinoids, growth factors, and chemotherapeutic agents are being examined for therapeutic potential in AML.[784] Leukemias with 11q, –5, and –7 chromosome abnormalities have high telomerase activity, which can be inhibited by maturation-inducing agents.[785] In one study, addition of ATRA to chemotherapy did not improve patient outcome but did result in a 25 percent increase in apoptosis in AML marrow cells *in vitro*.[786] ATRA has induced a complete remission in a patient with acute myelomonocytic leukemia.[787,788] Arsenic trioxide (As_2O_3) induces apoptosis and cytotoxic effects in blasts from patients with AML other than APL, and it is not influenced by permeability glycoprotein (P-gp) expression.[789,790]

Antiangiogenesis Agents and Agents That Inhibit Microenvironmental Interactions

Targeting the increased vascular density of marrow noted in AML or cytokines secreted by marrow endothelium has been examined as means to inhibit AML cell growth. Amifostine,[791] thalidomide,[790] sunitinib,[791] and other agents that target VEGF and IL-8,[792] as well as of the angiopoietin signaling pathway,[793] are potential antiangiogenic agents in the treatment of AML. Lenalidomide, which also has antiangiogenic properties, is used to treat deletion 5q− AML.[794] Antagonists of the chemokine receptor CXCR4, which plays a role in retention of hematopoietic cells in marrow, have been proposed as therapeutic agents to overcome stromal-mediated resistance and to enhance chemotherapy-induced cell death.[795,796]

Modulation of Drug Resistance

Numerous mechanisms of drug resistance occur in AML,[797] and several attempts to overcome this resistance have been instituted. P-gp, MDR protein-1 (MRP-1), and breast cancer resistance protein (BCRP) expression all have been found in AML.[798] P-gp expression is correlated with decreased rates and shorter duration of remission.[799] Homozygous *MDR-1* gene expression, which encodes P-gp, is associated with shorter relapse-free intervals and poor survival rates and does not vary between diagnosis and relapse in paired samples.[800] PSC-833 has been used to modulate P-gp and has been combined with daunorubicin[801] and with mitoxantrone, etoposide, and cytarabine.[802] PSC-833 reduces the clearance of etoposide and mitoxantrone. Idarubicin does not appear to be as affected by P-gp expression.[803] In a phase II study of PSC-833 in previously untreated older patients with AML, considerable early toxicity was noted with the addition of PSC-833 to daunorubicin, etoposide, and cytarabine.[804] Use of PSC-833 necessitates a two-thirds reduction in mitoxantrone and etoposide doses.[805] In a randomized study, addition of cyclosporine A to infusional daunorubicin reduced drug resistance, prolonged remission duration, and improved overall survival. Whether this response resulted entirely from drug efflux modulation or from other immune modulatory effects of cyclosporine was not determined.[806]

Other Immunotherapy and Antisense DNA Approaches

Culture of AML blasts upregulates costimulatory molecules, and the role of dendritic cells in antileukemia therapy is being examined.[807–809] Other approaches to generating autologous T-cell antileukemic activity include vaccination with AML-specific peptides, immunization with AML blasts exhibiting dendritic cell phenotype and function,[810,811] and pulsing normal dendritic cells with AML-specific peptide sequences.[812] Natural killer cells may mediate antileukemia effects.[813] Low doses of interleukin-2 have been used in the maintenance phase of AML, and some patients have remained on this regimen for 10 or more years without significant side effects.[814] However, low dose interleukin-2 does not improve outcomes when used as maintenance treatment in older AML patients.[815] Wilms tumor gene *WT1* is expressed on AML blasts, and a *WT1* vaccine may elicit cytotoxic T-cell responses against this protein.[816] Other proteins against which such humoral responses have been elicited include minor HLA antigens and proteinase-3.[817] Small interfering RNA (siRNA) targeting of transcription factors,[818] and GTI-2040, an antisense to ribonucleotide reductase have been utilized in AML therapy.[819] In addition to CD33, CD45, CD66, and CD38 have been examined as targets for immunotherapy of AML.[820,821]

■ SPECIAL THERAPEUTIC CONSIDERATIONS

Acute Promyelocytic Leukemia

Induction Treatment ATRA has become a standard component of induction therapy for APL. Used alone, ATRA can induce a short-term remission in at least 80 percent of patients.[822] However, ATRA should be combined with an anthracycline such as idarubicin during induction treatment for most benefit and to prevent drug resistance.[823] Idarubicin by itself can induce remission in approximately 75 percent of patients.[824] A typical induction regimen for APL is ATRA 45 mg/m^2 daily in divided doses with idarubicin at standard induction doses (e.g., 12 mg/m^2 on days 1 to 3).[825,826] Although cytarabine has been largely abandoned as part of induction, some studies have shown a high degree of efficacy of high-dose cytarabine combined with ATRA.[827] There is evidence that in patients who present with a white cell count of 10,000/μL (10×10^9/L) or greater, the complete remission rate and overall survival may be superior when cytarabine is added to induction or consolidation regimens.[828] Older patients generally tolerate a combination of ATRA and an anthracycline.[829] Combinations that include gemtuzumab ozogamicin are being examined for their effectiveness in APL induction therapy.[830] The combination of ATRA and As_2O_3 results in more rapid remissions and lower PML-RAR-α transcript levels than either agent alone.[831] Despite the high remission rates and frequency of long-term event-free survival achieved in this disease, controversies remain regarding therapy because of the 5 to 10 percent early death rate, as a result of fatal intracranial hemorrhages.[832]

All-*Trans*-Retinoic Acid: Dose and Mechanism of Action ATRA, an analogue of vitamin A, has been used to initiate the therapy of APL since 1987 in the United States. ATRA induces complete remissions in approximately 80 percent of previously untreated patients.[833] *In vitro*, ATRA is 10 times more potent in inducing maturation of leukemic promyelocytes to neutrophils than 13-*cis*-retinoic acid, the other naturally occurring isomer.[834] ATRA induces maturation of the leukemic cells and their apoptosis results in the reappearance of normal polyclonal hematopoiesis and a remission in most cases.[835] ATRA may induce synthesis of a protein that selectively degrades PML-RAR-α. ATRA can overcome the recruitment of histone deacetylase activity by the *PML-RAR-α* fusion gene through interference with a nuclear corepressor.[836] Signal transducer and activator of transcription factor STAT-1 is induced and activated by ATRA. Promyelocytic leukemia cells with PML-RAR-α break-fusion sites in *PML* exon 6 have decreased *in vitro* responsiveness to ATRA.[837] The t(11;17) variant of APL in which the promyelocytic leukemia zinc finger *(PLZF)* gene is fused to *RAR-α* does not respond to ATRA.[838] Other nonpromyelocytic leukemia subtypes of AML have not responded to ATRA therapy. ATRA is beneficial in APL during the induction and maintenance phases of disease,[839] and improved outcome with ATRA is reflected in the 5-year survival rates of 75 to 80 percent.[840] Additional cytogenetic changes do not influence treatment outcomes with ATRA plus an anthracycline.[841] ATRA induction therapy can result in favorable results without blood product support.[842]

Toxic Effects ATRA therapy is associated with dryness of the skin and lips, occasionally leading to mild exfoliation, nausea, headache, arthralgia, and bone pain. The white cell count may rise dramatically in the first week or two of therapy. Serum glutamic-pyruvate transaminase and triglyceride concentrations often increase. Leukemic promyelocytes disappear from the blood in 2 to 4 weeks, and a normal marrow aspirate may be obtained in 4 to 10 weeks. Anemia improves gradually. The majority of patients become PML-RAR-α–negative by PCR after the second consolidation therapy in conjunction with ATRA.[843] ATRA has been used successfully to treat promyelocytic leukemia diagnosed during pregnancy.[844] ATRA has been used from week 3 of gestation, but may result in fetal malformations when it is used during the first trimester.[845]

A rapid increase in the total blood leukocyte count to as high as 80,000/μL (80×10^9/L) in the first several weeks of therapy, referred to as the *retinoic acid syndrome*, is a potential cause of early death during therapy.[846,847] The median time of onset is 11 days, but the syndrome has occurred up to 47 days after therapy starts.[847] Two approaches to treatment of this phenomenon have been suggested: early use of cytotoxic chemotherapy[848,849] and glucocorticoid administration.[850,851] The syndrome consists of fever, weight gain, dependent edema, pleural or pericardial effusion, and bouts of hypotension. Respiratory distress is the key feature. In fatal cases, pulmonary interstitial infiltration with maturing granulocytes is prominent. Once respiratory distress is evident, the patient should receive dexamethasone 10 mg intravenously every 12 hours for several days. Because the syndrome may occur at relatively low total white cell counts and its onset is unpredictable, high-dose glucocorticoid therapy should be instituted if respiratory symptoms develop even in the absence of pulmonary infiltrates or an elevated white cell count.[846,849] ATRA can be continued or resumed with glucocorticoids or with concurrent cytotoxic chemotherapy, but the syndrome may recur.[846] This syndrome is not observed during maintenance therapy.

Treatment of Coagulopathy Reducing the risk of early death from hemorrhage as a result of the coagulopathy accompanying APL requires use of fresh-frozen plasma, platelet replacement, and fibrinogen replacement.[422,423,852] Targeted levels for platelet counts are usually 30,000/L or higher and for fibrinogen levels, 1.5 g/L or higher, but these levels are often difficult to achieve in patients with active hemorrhage.[853] Heparin treatment was utilized during induction chemotherapy to prevent onset of disseminated intravascular coagulopathy during treatment in the past, but rarely is used now.[854] ATRA may have some corrective effect on coagulation disorders in promyelocytic leukemia.[855] However, a reduction of 5 to 10 percent of fatal hemorrhages has not been significant with ATRA utilized early during treatment. Paradoxically, hypercoagulable clotting tendency may occur in patients during the first months of ATRA therapy.[835]

Chemotherapy Induction of remission with ATRA is followed by relapse in weeks to months unless intensive chemotherapy is used concomitantly.[856] At relapse, cells show high levels of a cytosolic retinoic-acid-binding protein not detected prior to ATRA therapy.[836] The mechanism of retinoid resistance in leukemic cells may involve cytochrome P450 and P-gp because of induction of various enzymes that may alter ATRA metabolism.[857] ATRA, whether administered as part of induction therapy or as maintenance therapy, confers a disease-free survival advantage. More than 70 percent of patients receiving ATRA at any point were in continuous remission at 2.5 years versus less than 20 percent of patients who never received ATRA.[840] The acquired *in vivo* resistance that occurs rapidly to ATRA as a single agent requires consolidation of ATRA-induced complete remission with intensive chemotherapy using an anthracycline antibiotic. Customary treatment today involves simultaneous administration of ATRA and an anthracycline. Some therapists have returned to combining an anthracycline antibiotic with cytarabine in an effort to decrease CNS relapse, especially in patients younger than 60 years with white counts greater than 10,000/μL at presentation.[858] Maintenance therapy with ATRA alone or with the combination of ATRA, mercaptopurine, or methotrexate has been recommended.[826] This additional therapy has not been examined in a randomized trial of ATRA dosing and scheduling, but ATRA usually is given in an interrupted fashion. Intensified maintenance therapy may have a negative impact on those patients who have become negative for the PML-RAR-α fusion transcript after induction plus consolidation therapy.[859] Some have proposed that elderly patients can be treated with ATRA and arsenic trioxide without chemotherapy and with addition of gemtuzumab ozogamicin in the event of an elevated white counts at the time of diagnosis.[860]

Arsenic Trioxide As_2O_3 can be useful for patients who relapse.[861,862] As_2O_3 can trigger apoptosis of promyelocytic leukemia cells at high concentrations and maturation at low concentrations. The presence of PML-RAR-α is important for the response.[777] Apoptosis may occur through induction of activation of caspase-1 and caspase-3 after changes in the mitochondrial membrane potential with increase in H_2O_2.[863,864] It also may function through NF-κB inhibition.[865] Death-associated protein 5 also contributes to As_2O_3-induced apoptosis in promyelocytic leukemia.[866] As_2O_3 given at 0.06 to 0.12 mg/kg body weight per day until leukemic cells were eliminated from the marrow induced remission within 12 to 89 days in 11 of 12 patients.[867] Suppression of hematopoiesis did not occur. Rash, light-headedness, fatigue, and musculoskeletal pain were the main side effects. As_2O_3 can be combined with idarubicin in relapsed patients; it also has been used with ATRA.[868,869] A retinoic acid-like syndrome (see "All-*Trans*-Retinoic Acid: Dose and Mechanism of Action" above) has been described in patients with APL treated with As_2O_3.[870] Torsade de pointes, an uncommon variant of ventricular tachycardia in which the underlying etiology and management are different from those of the usual variety of ventricular tachycardia, has been described with As_2O_3 use,[871] and monitoring of electrocardiographic QTc intervals during therapy is recommended.[872]

Other Treatments for Relapsed Acute Promyelocytic Leukemia Conventional chemotherapy can be effective after relapse. Patients younger than age 60 years should be considered for allogeneic or autologous hematopoietic stem cell transplantation after they have achieved a second remission or for allogeneic transplantation if a second remission cannot be induced.[873] Other treatments for patients in relapse include the combination of ATRA, As_2O_3, and gemtuzumab ozogamicin, which have resulted in durable remissions.[874] Transplantation generally is not recommended for patients with APL in first remission given the prolonged remissions after standard treatments. Allogeneic stem cell transplant is best used in advanced APL, especially in patients with persistent disease by PCR.[875] The outcome of autologous stem cell transplantation in second complete remission is excellent if the stem cells used are negative for PML-RAR-α.[845] A direct comparison of autologous transplantation, allogeneic transplantation, and arsenic or ATRA with standard chemotherapy has not been studied in patients with APL in a second remission after relapse.[876] Many cases of extramedullary relapse in APL have been reported.[877] Many of the relapses occur in patients who received ATRA and who initially were diagnosed with hyperleukocytosis,[878] and many of the patients are in marrow remission. Relapses occurring more than 5 years after diagnosis have been reported, some at extramedullary sites such as in the mastoid bone.[879] Early detection of relapse is important as those with molecular relapse before hematologic relapse has occurred fare best.[880] Patients should be monitored with PCR every 3 months for 2 years after remission induction.

Myelodysplastic syndrome can occur in patients in remission with APL, usually 24 months or more after diagnosis. The complication results from a second (drug-induced) clonal disease in long-term responders.[881–883] Cases of therapy-related APL have been described.[884] Patients with APL who are FLT3-ITD positive generally have worse overall outcomes than do those persons who present with elevated white cell counts and older age.[885]

SECONDARY ACUTE MYELOGENOUS LEUKEMIA

Secondary leukemias arise after a myelodysplastic syndrome or after treatment of another malignancy with cytotoxic chemotherapy or radiation. Secondary AML responds more poorly to chemotherapy and stem cell transplantation than does *de novo* AML. Secondary AML accounts for approximately 15 percent of all AML cases, although this percentage is increasing.[886,887] The leukemogenic risk of treatment regimens depends on the agents used. Future development of agents with lower risk of inducing AML is important.[888]

Effect of Topoisomerase II Inhibitors

Exposure to topoisomerase II inhibitors (e.g., etoposide, mitoxantrone, amsacrine) can lead to AML with *MLL* gene rearrangements on chromosome 11q32.[889] Inversion 16 is an uncommon aberration in secondary AML and, like balanced translocations of chromosome bands 11q32, 21q22, and t(15;17), is associated with prior chemotherapy with topoisomerase II inhibitors when seen in the setting of treatment-induced leukemias. The site of breakpoints within the *MYH*11 gene involved in inversion 16 may vary between therapy-induced AML and AML occurring *de novo*.[890] The latency period for development of AML after topoisomerase II inhibitors is approximately 2 years. No relationship with higher cumulative dose has been identified. Studies of single nucleotide polymorphisms to ascertain genetic predisposition are ongoing.[891] Polymorphisms in detoxification genes and in genes involved in DNA repair pathways might be involved.[892] Even the use of low-dose or oral etoposide can be associated with development of secondary AML.

Effect of Alkylating Agents and Cisplatin

Alkylating agents cause secondary AML, often preceded by myelodysplasia. The mean latency period after onset of treatment is approximately 6 years. Deletions of all or part of chromosome 5 or 7 are the most common cytogenetic changes. The risk is related to cumulative alkylating agent dose. Germ-line aberrancies of NFI and p53 may increase the risk of AML. Cisplatin used for treatment of ovarian cancer also increases the risk of secondary leukemia.[893]

Other Cytotoxic Agents

Other drugs that may increase the risk of secondary leukemias include low-dose weekly methotrexate for rheumatoid arthritis,[894] etanercept therapy,[895] temozolamide,[896] growth hormone administration,[897] and G-CSF given to patients with congenital, but not idiopathic or cyclic, neutropenia.[898] In the latter case, a cause-and-effect relationship between MDS/AML and G-CSF therapy was not established. Improved survival duration with G-CSF may allow expression of an underlying leukemic predisposition.

Other Settings for Secondary Leukemia

Patients with APL in remission may develop a new oligoblastic leukemia, presumably secondary to therapy.[899] Series of children with treatment-related myelodysplasia or AML have the same latency period as do adults treated with alkylating agents or topoisomerase II inhibitors for AML.[900] Breast cancer patients receiving doxorubicin and cyclophosphamide regimens of such intensity that they required G-CSF support had increased rates of posttherapy AML. Breast and prostate radiotherapy are associated with an increased risk of AML.[901,902] In patients with non-Hodgkin lymphoma, up to 10 percent of patients treated with either conventional chemotherapy or high-dose therapy may develop secondary AML within 10 years.[903] Secondary leukemia is seen after autologous marrow or blood stem cell transplants involving high-dose chemotherapy and/or radiotherapy. In a study of 83 patients after autografting, 12 had nonclonal cytogenetic abnormalities and 10 had clonal abnormalities, 5 of whom developed secondary AML. Onset occurred 12 to 48 months after autografting. The relative contribution of the underlying disease and conditioning therapy is uncertain.[904] Clonality analysis utilizing an X chromosome gene, based on methylation of the human androgen receptor locus in cell samples in patients with lymphoma, found a clonal marrow cell population 6 months after autologous transplantation at a time when no morphologic or clinical evidence of AML was present. AML appeared later in some patients.[905] More than 10 percent of patients with non-Hodgkin lymphoma who underwent stem cell rescue after total body irradiation and cyclophosphamide developed AML at a median followup of 6 years.[906] Using a triple FISH assay to detect loss of chromosomal material from 5q31, 7q22, or 13q14, abnormal cells were detected before high-dose therapy was given to non-Hodgkin lymphoma patients.[907] Thus, some patients are at increased risk for developing secondary AML based on pretreatment chromosome studies.

Treatment of Secondary Leukemia

Secondary leukemia generally is treated similarly to *de novo* leukemia. However, given the lower response rates and remission durations of secondary leukemia, patients can be treated in clinical trials examining new therapies or treated initially with chemotherapy regimens used for refractory disease.[908] Some patients may benefit from early hematopoietic stem cell transplantation.[909] Autologous transplant can be successful if stem cells are harvested prior to the secondary AML.[910] In those who have low blood blast counts, allogeneic stem cell transplantation as initial therapy may be superior to induction chemotherapy followed by transplantation, but this remains an area of controversy.[911] Although patients may have a response rate to standard induction chemotherapy of approximately 50 percent, most soon relapse, and long-term survival is approximately 10 percent.[912] Secondary AML more often has unfavorable cytogenetic features compared to *de novo* leukemia.[913]

TREATMENT OF Ph-CHROMOSOME–POSITIVE AML

This cytogenetic variant of acute leukemia is characterized by extraordinary drug resistance. Imatinib mesylate in doses of 600 to 800 mg/day may produce a hematologic remission in a small proportion of patients with Ph-chromosome–positive AML, based on the response in patients with CML who go on to a myeloid blast crisis. No formal studies of the response to imatinib mesylate of *de novo* Ph-chromosome–positive AML have been performed. In myeloid blast crisis of CML, the uncommon full hematologic response (blood and marrow) usually is short lived, measured in weeks or a few months. This outcome also seems to be the case when therapy with other drugs (e.g., cytarabine, etoposide, anthracycline antibiotics) is included. Occasional cases in which chemotherapy has induced remission in Ph-chromosome–positive AML and imatinib mesylate has appeared to help induce and sustain the remission have been reported.[914] Thus, in Ph-chromosome–positive AML, a matched-related or matched-unrelated donor stem cell transplant should be considered if the patient is younger than age 50 years. This approach may have the highest probability of a long-term remission.

TREATMENT OF OLDER PATIENTS

Biologic Features

Approximately 65 percent of patients with AML are older than age 60 years at the time of diagnosis.[915] The disease in this patient age group is less responsive to therapy, and this age group has a higher proportion of patients who have oligoblastic myelogenous leukemia (MDS); an antecedent clonal myeloid disease; prior chemotherapy for cancer of the breast, ovary, or another site; and comorbid conditions that decrease the tolerance to intensive chemotherapy programs.[916–919] The AML cells of elderly patients often have more CD34 expression, suggesting origin from a more primitive multipotential (? stem) cell. This finding is thought to contribute to longer duration of postchemotherapy aplasia and to the increased risk of induction deaths in this age group.[920] Patients older than age 60 years also have a high frequency of unfavorable cytogenetic findings (32%) and higher *MDR1* expression (71%) and functional drug efflux (58%).[921]

Chemotherapy

The therapist and patient determine whether a standard regimen, a standard regimen with dose reductions, or a special regimen is used.[922]

Decisions based on chronologic age should be supplanted by measurements of cognitive, neurologic, and physical fitness used by geriatricians to evaluate the wisdom of considering intensive treatment.[923] In patients older than age 60 years who are fit and otherwise are considered good candidates, standard two-drug therapy can be used: cytarabine and an anthracycline antibiotic, and on some occasions the addition of a third drug, etoposide. Remission rates of approximately 35 percent can be achieved. Based on case studies, those who are able to receive induction chemotherapy may have a median survival slightly better than those who receive supportive care alone,[924] but there are no randomized trials that address this issue.[925] Chemotherapy has been combined with growth factor support to accelerate neutrophil recovery in older patients.[926] In a study in which patients older than 55 years were randomized to receive either placebo or G-CSF after induction therapy, no reduction in the duration of hospitalization, survival prolongation, or costs of supportive care was noted.[927] In previously untreated elderly patients with AML, mitoxantrone induction therapy produces a slightly higher remission rate than does daunorubicin but had no significant effect on remission duration and survival.[928] Oral idarubicin alone has been used with success.[929]

Attenuated standard regimens can be used in older patients. An example of an attenuated regimen is cytarabine 100 mg/m^2 subcutaneously every 12 hours for 10 doses on days 1 through 5 and daunorubicin 30 mg/m^2 intravenously on days 1 through 3 of treatment. One induction regimen is not superior to another in older patients. Outcomes achieved with cytarabine and daunorubicin are comparable to results with mitoxantrone and etoposide.[930] Other regimens for older patients include lower total doses of idarubicin, etoposide, and cytarabine (DIVA regimen)[931] and a combination of continuous infusion low-dose cytarabine with etoposide and G-CSF.[932] Addition of PSC833 to mitoxantrone and etoposide was well tolerated, but a reduction in chemotherapy dose was required to avoid undue toxicity.[933] Temozolomide has been used in this age group,[934] and clofarabine is also being tested in patients age 60 years and older.[935] Several investigational therapies, including 5-azacytidine, decitabine, cloretazine, and depsipeptide, are also being studied.

Autologous Stem Cell Infusion or Nonmyeloablative Allogeneic Transplantation

Autologous stem cell transplantation has been used in fit patients older than age 60 years.[936] The incidence of relapse is lower when marrow stem cells are used compared to blood stem cells. Some patients older than age 60 years may be eligible for reduced-dose intensity allogeneic stem cell transplantation from related or unrelated donors, but more data regarding outcomes are needed.[937]

Postremission Therapy in Older Patients

No consensus exists regarding the best regimen or the number of treatment cycles for postremission therapy in older adults. Regardless of the consolidation regimen, the duration of the leukemia-free survival is longer with high-dose cytarabine and autologous stem cell transplantation, just as it is in younger patients,[933] but fewer older patients can tolerate this degree of therapeutic intensity. High-dose cytarabine can be used in older adults with AML, but usually at a reduced dose.[938] Older patients treated with attenuated high-dose cytarabine at 750 mg/m^2 intravenously for 12 doses and then consolidated with 4 to 6 doses had an approximately 50 percent remission rate with a median duration of remission of 326 days.[939] Fifty-one percent of 110 patients older than 60 years of age had a 9-month median remission duration when consolidated with high-dose cytarabine.[940] Older patients are at higher risk for relapse despite successfully completing intensive consolidation therapy, regardless of whether other adverse prognostic features are present. Cytarabine as maintenance therapy may prolong disease-free survival but does not improve overall survival.[941] In one randomized study, those receiving consolidation therapy had more hospitalizations and more transfusion requirements.[942]

Patients older than 80 years of age do not tolerate treatments well. Remission rates are approximately 30 percent, but the median survival of treated patients is approximately 1 month. Less than 10 percent of patients survive for 1 year.[943]

Unlike the case in younger patients, the treatment outcomes for older patients have not improved over the last two decades.[944] Treatment options in older patients include (1) no treatment, (2) supportive care, (3) palliative low-dose chemotherapy, (4) attenuated induction chemotherapy, or (5) high-dose chemotherapy regimens. Investigative agents should also be given strong consideration in this population.[945] Comorbidities are independent predictors of complete remission and should be taken into account during decision making,[946] as should performance status.[947] Some argue that the approximately 15 percent rate of death in those older than 60 years of age in the first month after standard induction chemotherapy is unacceptable given the less than 1 year median survival expected.[948] Lower-dose regimens can also be toxic and can lead to severe cytopenias. Use of colony-stimulating factor permits more older patients to tolerate full-dose induction therapy. The Medical Research Council of the United Kingdom observed remission rates of 80 percent in children, 70 percent in adults younger than 50 years of age, 68 percent in adults 50 to 59 years old, 53 percent in adults 60 to 69 years old, 39 percent in adults 70 to 75 years old, and 22 percent in adults older than 75 years of age.[949] In one study of patients older than 60 years of age, the 2-, 5-, and 10-year survivals were 22, 11, and 8 percent, respectively.[950,951] The older patients who remain free of leukemia beyond 1 year have a reasonable quality of life.[952,953] The National Cancer Institute 5-year relative survival rates for patients with AML are 5 percent for adults ages 65 to 74 years and 2 percent for adults ages 75 years and older.[954]

TREATMENT OF PREGNANT PATIENTS

Leukemia (AML, ALL, CML) is the second most common malignancy of women in the childbearing age group and is expected to occur in approximately 1 in 75,000 to 100,000 pregnancies.[955,956] No systematic studies of the (1) effects of leukemia on pregnancy or delivery, (2) effects of the leukemia or its treatment on the fetus, or (3) postnatal development of the offspring exposed to maternal chemotherapy *in utero* have been performed. Folic acid inhibitors, purine, pyrimidine, or retinoid analogues given during the first trimester of pregnancy increase the probability of major congenital malformations. In a French study of 37 patients with acute leukemia during pregnancy, 34 patients achieved remission, and disease-free survival appeared equivalent to that of patients who were not treated during pregnancy.[957]

If the pregnancy is not terminated, leukapheresis might be useful in the first trimester, when chemotherapy poses a high risk to the embryo. Intensive chemotherapy given to women in the second and third trimesters of pregnancy does not present an inordinate risk to fetal or neonatal development,[958,959] although an increased frequency of premature delivery, higher perinatal mortality, and lower birth-weight for gestational age are observed, especially if the fetus is exposed to chemotherapy.

Cytarabine is highly teratogenic in animal models and malformations have been described in women who were treated in the first trimester of pregnancy. Doxorubicin is the preferred anthracycline antibiotic to treat pregnant women as it has lower transplacental transfer. Doxorubicin is considered relatively safe when used in pregnant women.[960] Newborn infants may be transiently cytopenic if the mother receives chemotherapy near the time of delivery. Development of the newborn usually is normal after intensive chemotherapy for AML during pregnancy, if therapy is started after the first trimester.[955,958,959] Vaginal delivery should be used whenever possible. Pregnant women with AML who enter remission have little difficulty with childbirth or postparturition. The remission rates of AML are approximately the rates expected for the age group, and long-term remissions can occur with current therapy. Leukemic infiltrates can be found on the maternal side of the placenta, but usually not in the villi. One case of maternal-to-fetal transmission of AML has been documented.[961] Transmission of AML from one identical twin to another through a shared placental circulation accounts for the dual occurrence in twins in the first several years of life.[109] There are reports of the use of ATRA for APL treatment during pregnancy, but use during the first trimester is discouraged, and data are sparse.[845,962,963]

TREATMENT OF CHILDREN

AML represents approximately 15 percent of the acute leukemias in children (younger than 20 years of age) or approximately 600 children per year in the United States. APL is treated as in adults, with ATRA and an anthracycline antibiotic. In other phenotypes of AML, intensive treatment—including initial therapy with cytarabine and daunomycin or doxorubicin and a third drug such as mitoxantrone or 6-thioguanine, followed by intensive multidrug consolidation therapy including additional agents such as etoposide, and intrathecal cytarabine—has resulted in remission in approximately 80 percent of children and 5-year relapse-free remissions in approximately 50 percent of treated children.[964–967] Most of the children in long-term remission are considered cured.

Monocytic leukemia and hyperleukocytic (>100,000/μL [>100 × 10^9/L]) myelogenous leukemia are unfavorable phenotypes. In children, *FLT3-ITD* mutations are approximately half as common (15%) as in adults (30%), but are a very poor prognostic indicator.[968] Therapy can be adjusted for children based on the presence of poor prognostic variables, which include age younger than 2 years or older than 10 years; abnormalities of chromosome 3, 5, or 7, complex karyotypes, *FLT3* mutations, elevated white cell count (>50,000/μL [50 × 10^9/L]), male gender; and, perhaps, most importantly, because it reflects the effect of all factors, the presence of greater than 15 percent blast cells in the marrow examined 14 days after onset of treatment.[966–970] The presence of residual blast cells detected by flow cytometry after induction therapy is a very poor prognostic finding.[971] The duration of first remission predicts the subsequent remission rate and long-term survival in children with relapse.

Translocations 8;21, 15;17, or inv16 are good prognostic markers. Loss of a sex chromosome in the t(8;21) group is especially favorable. Monosomy 7 and abnormalities of chromosomes 3 or 5 are poor prognostic features.[972]

In the United Kingdom Medical Research Council Trial 12, completed in 2002, using daunorubicin, mitoxantrone cytarabine, etoposide, and asparaginase in different combinations, approximately 90 percent of children with AML had a remission, 60 percent of children had a 5-year disease-free survival, and most were considered cured.[972] Approximately 4 percent of children are drug resistant with this program and approximately 4 percent die during induction and intensification therapy. Studies are under way to examine the effects of using fludarabine in the regimen (Medical Research Council 15 Trial).

Autologous stem cell transplantation has not improved outcome compared to current intensive chemotherapy treatment regimens.[973] Allogeneic stem cell transplantation from a histocompatible sibling should be considered in children in first remission with a donor and poor prognostic indicators or in children who relapse.[973] Children younger than age 2 years previously had a very poor prognosis. They tend to present with myelomonocytic or monocytic leukemia with high blast counts and CNS involvement. The t(9;11) abnormality has a more favorable prognosis. Intensive multidrug regimens have resulted in 3-year survivals approaching 70 percent of all infants treated. Thus, most infants can be successfully treated with intensive chemotherapy or allogeneic stem cell transplantation.[974,975] Cord blood may be a suitable graft option for children with AML who lack an acceptably matched unrelated marrow donor.[976]

Growth failure, neurocognitive abnormalities, endocrine deficiencies, and cardiac abnormalities are found in children treated at a young age.[977] The occurrence of a second malignancy in cured children is approximately 10-fold greater than expected in a matched population by age.[978] Indefinite followup of children in remission or believed to be cured is important to assess developmental and intellectual progress and to evaluate long-term adverse events.

NONHEMATOPOIETIC ADVERSE EFFECTS OF TREATMENT

Skin Rashes

More than 50 percent of patients with AML develop skin lesions during remission-induction or remission-consolidation therapy. The rash may be on the trunk and extremities. The rash usually is maculopapular initially but can become hemorrhagic in patients who have thrombocytopenia. Allopurinol, trimethoprim-sulfamethoxazole, and other β-lactam antibiotics are commonly implicated causes. Use of multiple drugs enhances the probability of skin reactivity of patients.[979] Cytostatic therapy coupled with the effects of leukemia predisposes patients to an increased frequency of allergic dermatitis.

Cardiac Toxicity

Alterations in cardiac function, especially left ventricular and intraventricular septal diastolic wall motion abnormalities, occur frequently in patients after they are exposed to the anthracycline antibiotics, daunorubicin, or doxorubicin.[980] The risk of serious cardiac effects is correlated with increasing dose of anthracycline antibiotic, increasing patient age, and presence of underlying heart disease. Adverse effects include electrocardiographic changes, such as prolonged QT interval, myocarditis, pericarditis, myocardial infarction, and congestive heart failure. The incidence of congestive heart failure is dose related and ranges from approximately 5 percent at doses of 550 mg/m^2 to greater than 30 percent at doses of 600 mg/m^2. Chapter 20 discusses the toxicity further. The frequency and long-term sequelae increase as anthracycline dose increases. However, even lower doses of these agents exert negative effects on cardiac myocytes. Measurement of heart wall behavior, valvular competence, and ejection fraction by ultrasonography can assist in assessing the risk of proceeding with anthracycline treatment in patients with or without pretreatment heart disease.[981,982] In younger patients, transient abnormalities, although frequent, often improve after therapy is completed. Increased long-term remissions in children and younger adults have led to an increase in serious ventricular and valvular disturbances years after therapy in some patients. Periodic evaluation of cardiac status by ultrasonography should be undertaken in long-term survivors.[982] Cardiomyopathy and heart failure can occur 10 to 15 years after therapy. Two approaches that may ameliorate the cardiomyopathic effect of anthracycline antibiotics are the use of these agents in liposome encapsulated preparations[983] and the use of dexrazoxane. Either approach may reduce the cardiotoxicity of anthracycline antibiotics.[984]

Hepatitis

Hepatitis may occur in multiply transfused patients and usually is mild, but persistent hepatitis can develop, although hepatitis viruses A and B infection are not increased above the expected incidence in the general population.[985] Persistent elevation in serum transaminases occurring after initiation of chemotherapy in patients with AML usually results from blood transfusion-transmitted hepatitis. Hepatitis caused by type A virus is nearly nonexistent early in the course of AML. Cases of type B hepatitis can occur infrequently in patients who are carriers of the B virus and in whom chemotherapy and transient immunosuppression reactivate the virus.[986,987] These rare cases of fibrosing cholestatic hepatitis can be fulminant. Screening blood products for hepatitis virus C has markedly decreased the risk of hepatitis C.[988] Reactivation of carriers of the C virus after chemotherapy is unusual.[989]

Systemic Candidiasis Syndrome

Although microbial sepsis is a common complication of AML treatment, chronic systemic candidiasis syndrome has become of special concern.[990] Protracted posttherapy neutropenia, severe mucositis, colonization with *Candida*, and use of high-dose cytarabine are frequent antecedents of the syndrome.[991] The syndrome is manifested by fever, abdominal pain, and hepatomegaly. Increased serum alkaline phosphatase activity often is noted. Blood cultures are often negative. Abdominal ultrasonography, computed tomography, and magnetic resonance imaging show characteristic hepatic lesions: circular areas of decreased attenuation of liver and often spleen, kidney, lung, or paraspinal muscles by imaging.[992] Ultrasonography reveals multiple hypoechogenic areas with a bull's-eye appearance. Laparoscopic-guided liver biopsy reveals yellow nodules on the liver surface, which on microscopic examination are large granulomas with *Candida* and pseudohyphae. Cure of this infection is possible with long-term (2–10 months) amphotericin B, supplemented with fluconazole or itraconazole.[993] Hepatosplenic candidiasis is seen less frequently when azoles are used for fungal prophylaxis.

Neutropenic Typhlitis

Necrotizing inflammation of the cecum with secondary infection can occur in patients with acute leukemia on intensive chemotherapy.[162] Right lower abdominal pain and fever can simulate appendicitis. The diagnosis can be confirmed by sonography or computerized tomographic scanning in which a characteristic mucosal thickening and polypoid appearance are evident.[994,995] Management includes bowel rest, nasogastric suction, parenteral nutrition, and antibiotics. Restoration of the neutrophil count after chemotherapy is an important feature of resolution. In the absence of resolution, right hemicolectomy should be considered but is a last resort in neutropenic patients, usually imposed if hemodynamic stability is lost.[162]

Thrombotic Thrombocytopenic Purpura

This syndrome has been reported in patients with solid tumors treated with cisplatin, bleomycin, vinca alkaloids, or mitomycin C. It also has been reported in patients in remission of AML during consolidation chemotherapy.[996] Patients with AML undergoing allogeneic stem cell transplantation also may develop posttransplantation thrombotic thrombocytopenic purpura, which rarely responds to plasmapheresis (see Chap. 133).

Fertility and Gonadal Function

Patients treated for AML, especially patients undergoing conditioning for allogeneic stem cell transplantation, have decreased gonadal function.[997–999] Men may develop oligospermia. Women may develop ovarian dysfunction and very high gonadotropin levels. Men recover gonadal function more often and sooner than do women. Recovery of ovarian function in women is partly dependent on a younger age at the time of treatment. Women in remission following treatment for AML with allogeneic transplantation can become pregnant and deliver healthy infants[1000,1001]; however, this preservation of fertility is not invariable.[1002] Histologic studies of the testes show marked suppression of spermatogenesis as a function of duration of treatment for AML and not of the specific agents used or the patient's age. Residual spermatogenesis in intensively treated patients enables recovery of reproductive function in males.[1003] Males receiving intensive daunorubicin, cytosine arabinoside, or 6-thioguanine treatment for AML have conceived children during therapy.[1004] Banking of sperm should be offered, and experimental cryopreservation of ova can be attempted prior to institution of cytotoxic therapy, but often neither is logistically possible or successful in patients with AML who are acutely ill at presentation and require urgent chemotherapy.[997] Banking of sperm or ova should be considered before myeloablative conditioning regimens for transplantation are administered.

COURSE AND PROGNOSIS

RESULTS OF TREATMENT

Remission rates have improved dramatically, but remission, 5-year survival, and cure rates are most dependent on the patient's age when AML occurs.[1005,1006] Initial remission rates now approach 90 percent in children, 70 percent in young adults, 60 percent in middle-aged subjects, and 40 percent in older patients. Within age groups, remission is related to other variables such as cytogenetic risk category and expression of *MDR* genes in leukemic cells, but these variables also are correlated with age at onset. For example, the more favorable cytogenetic patterns t(8;21), t(15;17), inv16, or t(16;16) are present in approximately 30 percent of patients between 10 and 39 years old, 15 percent of patients between 40 and 59 years old, and 5 percent of patients 60 to 90 years old (Table 89–7).[1006] Other factors, such as AML evolving from a prior clonal myeloid disease or developing as a result of cytotoxic treatment for another cancer or immune disorder, can decrease the expected remission and survival rates for the age group. Age-related comorbid conditions may limit the appropriateness or tolerance of intensive therapy, decreasing the opportunity for remission. The expected increase in the proportion of old and old-old individuals in the population may decrease remission rates and their duration unless counteracting

TABLE 89–7. Frequency of Cytogenetic Findings with a More Favorable Prognosis by Age Group

Age (Years)	No. of Cases Studied	t(8;21) (No. of Cases)	t(15;17) (No. of Cases)	Inv16/t(16;16) (No. of Cases)	Total (No. of Cases)	Favorable Karyotypes (% of All Cases)
10–39	307	27	38	33	98	32
40–59	584	36	28	28	92	16
60–69	579	18	24	21	63	11
70–79	381	5	7	5	17	4.5
>80	45	1	2	0	3	6.6
Total	1896	87	99	87	273	22

SOURCE: These observations were made in Germany by Claudia Schock and colleagues and kindly provided to the authors. (See also Schoch C, Kern W, Krawitz P, et al: Dependence of age-specific incidence of acute myeloid leukemia on karyotype. *Blood* 98:3500, 2001.

improvements in treatment approaches are developed. In one study of 1069 consecutive AML patients in first complete remission treated between 1991 and 2003, the yearly risk of treatment failure was 69.1 in the first year, 37.7 in the second year, 17 in the third year, 7.6 in the fourth year, and 6.6 in the fifth year. The effects of cytogenetics remained constant during the first 3 years, but the effect of age increased with time. The probability of relapse-free survival at 6 years was 84 percent for those in remission at 3 years, but for the group older than 60 years old, it was only 56 percent, suggesting that different variables contribute differently over time to overall outcomes.[1007]

CLONAL REMISSIONS

A small proportion of patients who enter remission have apparently normal hematopoiesis supported by a single clone rather than the expected polyclonal hematopoiesis. Evidence points to this clone being a preleukemic cell rather than a normal stem cell.[1008–1011] This finding is in keeping with previous hypotheses about the possible patterns of remission and relapse in AML[1012–1015] and has implications for minimal residual disease detection.

TABLE 89–8. Acute Myelogenous Leukemia: Five-Year Relative Survival Rates (1996–2004)

Age (Years)	Acute Myelogenous Leukemia*
<45	50.0
45–54	28.5
55–64	17.9
65–74	7.4
>75	1.8
<65	35.8
>65	4.5

*Rates expressed as number of cases per 100.

SOURCE: Data from SEER Cancer Statistics. Table XIII-13. National Cancer Institute, Washington, DC. Available at: http://seer.cancer.gov/csr/1975_2005/results_merged/sect_13_leukemia.pdf

SPONTANEOUS REMISSIONS

Spontaneous disappearance of AML has been reported for more than 100 years; however, most cases reported before 1960 had poor documentation of the diagnosis. Bona fide cases of AML patients who entered complete remission, usually after or concurrent with an infection, occur but are very rare.[1015–1018] The occurrence of spontaneous remission with infection is consistent with the observation that the antibody response to *Pseudomonas* vaccine[1019] correlates with improved probability of chemotherapy-induced remission. Spontaneous remissions often are short lived but have lasted up to 3 years in adults and more than 9 years in children.[1020] A particularly notable case of remission for more than 60 years has been documented following "treatment" prior to the introduction of chemotherapeutic drugs. The regimen included arsenic.[1021]

LONG-TERM SURVIVAL

Prior to the introduction of chemotherapy for AML 55 years ago, the median survival of patients was approximately 6 weeks,[1022] the 1-year survival was approximately 3 percent, and longer survival occurred in less than 1 percent of patients. Five-year relative survival rates of patients in the United States from 1999 to 2004, based on the Surveillance, Epidemiology, and End Results Program of the National Cancer Institute, are approximately 50 percent for patients younger than age 45 years, 29 percent for patients 45 to 54 years old, 18 percent for patients 55 to 64 years old, 7.0 percent for patients 65 to 74 years old, and 2.0 percent for patients older than age 75 years at the time of diagnosis (Table 89–8).[954] Considering that the median age at disease onset is approximately 70 years and that 75 percent of patients are older than 45 years, the overall median survival is approximately 12 months. A study of the cost of care of older AML patients using Medicare data found that in adults older than age 65 years who were diagnosed between 1991 and 1996, the median survival was 2 months and the 2-year survival was 6 percent.[1023] Very similar results were found in a study of nearly 10,000 patients in Sweden.[1024] Better survival has been reported for younger patients who have received allogeneic stem cell transplantation in first remission, but the confidence limits for remission duration and survival are overlapping for drug-treated and drug- and transplantation-treated groups, and the proportion of AML patients receiving transplantation is very small.[1005,1025–1028]

Relapse (or a new leukemic event) in long-term survivors occurring as late as 8 years after remission has been reported in adults[1020,1021] and after more than 16 years in children.[1020,1021] Relapse in long-term survivors nearly always occurs in the marrow in adults and usually in the marrow in children, with occasional childhood cases of CNS or gonadal relapses occurring initially, followed by relapse in the marrow.[1026] Studies of long-term survivors of AML have shown that most can return to work and that, at a median followup of 9 years, no increased risk of secondary invasive cancer or secondary AML had occurred.[1027,1028] An exception to this finding is the occasional report of myelodysplasia or presumably secondary AML in long-term survivors of APL. Health-related quality of life in long-term survivors appears to recover completely as related to physical, psychological, and emotional well-being, but continued sexual dysfunction has been reported.[1029] The quality of life at the time of diagnosis and during the course of therapy usually is poor.[1029,1030]

FEATURES INFLUENCING OUTCOME OF THERAPY IN ACUTE MYELOGENOUS LEUKEMIA

Numerous features are related to outcome of AML treatment. Older age and less-favorable cytogenetic risk group are the two most compelling determinants of a poor outcome. Even with multivariate analysis, dissecting which other features are themselves important or are associations that segregate with another prognostic factor is difficult (Table 89–9).

Determining useful prognostic variables in patients with AML is imprecise because negative prognostic factors may be eliminated by better treatment protocols. Moreover, several prognostic factors are significant only when AML is stratified by age or by morphologic phenotype. Conflicting findings are common among studies. In addition, although a prognostic variable may be correlated significantly with a favorable outcome, the lack of a very strong statistical correlation with the outcome of treatment makes the variable's presence or absence of little prognostic value in an individual patient. If a stem cell donor is available, unfavorable prognostic factors could influence the therapist to use allogeneic stem cell transplantation as a means of remission maintenance in patients entering remission. The impact of prognostic factors may change in patients treated with allogeneic stem cell transplantation compared with conventional cytotoxic treatment.[1113,1114]

DETECTION OF MINIMAL RESIDUAL DISEASE

General Considerations

The tumor cell burden in acute leukemia at presentation is approximately 1 trillion (10^{12}) cells. Apparent marrow aplasia followed by

TABLE 89–9. Prognostic Factors in Acute Myelogenous Leukemia

Better prognosis than average of all patients
Early blast clearance during remission induction therapy[1031,1032]
Leukemic cells contain t(8;21), t(15;17), inv(16) t(16;16), trisomy 21[214,216,1033]
CEBPA mutations in cytogenetically normal AML[1034]
Absence of exaggerated dysmyelopoiesis[1035]
Residual normal metaphases admixed with clonal cytogenetic abnormalities[1036]
High telomerase activity levels[1037]
Low levels of TdT expression by flow cytometry (<5%)[1038]
High BAX expression[1039] and high BAX/BCL-2 ratios[1040]
High expression of integrin CD11b[1041]
Absence of VLA-4 expression on AML blast cells[1042]
High levels of soluble VCAM-1 binding to AML blast cells[1043]
High levels of caspase-3[1044]
Mutant CEBPA expression[1045]
NPM1 gene expression in adults or children (usually present in cytogenetically normal cases)[1046]
Higher neutrophil and higher platelet counts at time of complete remission[1047]
<5% blasts on day 14 marrow predicts for complete remission but not for overall survival[1048]
Poorer prognosis than average of all patients
Older age: Age at the time of diagnosis has the greatest impact on the probability of remission and on duration of survival. Children in the first 15 years of life, exclusive of the neonatal period, have the highest rate of remission and longest relapse-free remission; patients older than age 60 years have only half the chance of a young adult to enter remission and less likelihood of a long relapse-free remission.[1006] There is a gradient of poor response to treatment through adulthood, with the largest decrease after the sixth decade of life.[94]
Unfavorable karyotypes: The cytogenetic pattern of leukemic blast cells influences outcome, but the relationship is complex.[214–216] The presence of 5−, 7−, 5q−, 7q−, or of exaggerated hyperdiploidy (>47 chromosomes), trisomy 8, t(6;9), trisomy 11, and multiple chromosomal abnormalities in leukemic cells are poor prognostic signs.
Multidrug resistance phenotype: Leukemic cells expressing P-glycoprotein, a unidirectional drug efflux pump, encoded by the *MDR1*.[1049] Expression of this gene product can result in decreased accumulation of anthracyclines, amsacrine, mitoxantrone, and etoposide. Expression of P-glycoprotein does not influence outcome of treatment, but if rhodamine-123 efflux also is increased, relapse is more common.[1050–1053] Frequently observed in AML cells after relapse. Associated with CD34 expression and chromosome 7 abnormalities.[1052] Alternative non-*MDR1*–mediated drug efflux mechanisms are important also.[1053–1056] *MDR1* expression is low in favorable prognosis subtypes of AML.[1057]
Presence of mutated KIT with t(8;21): Associated with higher relapse risk and poorer overall survival.[1058]
Prior clonal hemopathy: Chemotherapy or radiotherapy remission rates are one-third to one-half that of *de novo* AML in the same age group. Remission duration is shorter with remissions >3 years very uncommon.[1059–1060] AML developing from the clonal hemopathy may relapse as a smoldering leukemia. It then reverts to AML but can be treated with remissions lasting several years.[1061–1065]
Higher white cell count: Count >30,000/μL (30 × 10^9/L) or a blast cell count >15,000/μL (>15 × 10^9/L).[1066–1068]
Very low platelet count (<30,000/μL [<30 × 10^9/L])[1067]
High serum lactic dehydrogenase[1069]
High stem cell mobilizing capacity during complete remission predicts for relapse risk[1070]
Another medical disorder: extreme obesity, diabetes mellitus, chronic renal disease
Low serum albumin or prealbumin
Need for intubation or ventilator support during induction therapy[1071]
Autonomous clonal growth of leukemic blast cells[1072]
High BCL-2 expression[1073]
High MCL-1 expression: Elevated at the time of leukemic relapse. Suggests prognostic importance or that chemotherapeutic regimen selects for leukemia cells with elevated levels of apoptosis inhibitors.[1074]
Low expression of retinoblastoma gene[1075]
High levels of WAF/Cip1 protein: This is a regulator at the G1 checkpoint of cell cycle.[1076]
High CD34 expression: High CD34 antigen expression often in AML subtypes M0, M1, and M4.[1077] Remission rate of 61% vs. to 88% in AML not expressing CD34. Correlation is stronger between high-intensity expression of CD34 and lower remission rate.[1077–1078] CD34 expression in APL.[1079]
GATA-1 expression[1080]
Neural cell adhesion molecule (CD56) expression[1081]
Elevated soluble L-selectin: Seen especially in extramedullary disease.[082]
Higher expression of interleukin-1β gene[1083]
Low *FMS* expression[1083]
Expression of the thrombopoietin receptor (c-*MPL*) mRNA[1084]
FLT3 mutations[103,104,472,1085]
Increased angiogenesis/vascular endothelial growth factor levels[1086]
High β_2-microglobulin levels in adults younger than 60 years old[1087]
MN1 (meningioma 1) gene overexpression in AML patients with normal cytogenetics[1088]
Young adults with the genotype WT1(mutation)/FLT3-ITD(positive) have a lower complete remission rate and an inferior relapse-free and overall survival compared to those with the genotype WT1(mutation)/FLT3-ITD(negative).[1089]
WT1 gene mutations in patients with AML and a normal karyotype[1167,1168]
Patients with AML with a large number of AML stem cells
Elevated expression of IL-3Rα[1090]
MLL tandem duplications[1091] and 11p23/MLL abnormalities[1092]
CD56 expression in APL.[1093] High incidence of CNS involvement, especially with CD7 expression.[1094] Also contributes to poorer outcomes in t(8;21) cases.[1095]
P15 methylation[1096]
Microsatellite instability[1097] (may not be independent of age and t-AML).
AC133 expression (shorter remissions and disease-free survival)[1098]
Constitutive activity of signal transducer and activator of transcription 3 protein (shorter disease-free survival)[1099]
BAALC gene expression[1100]
High S-phase activity in cells surviving after 7 days of induction[1101]
High EVI1 expression[1102,1103]
Overexpression of CXCR4 [1104]
Increased marrow angiogenesis as measured by magnetic resonance imaging[1165]
The presence of the CTLA4 CT60 A/G genotype adult patients with AML[1166]
Factors with no or uncertain prognostic findings
Complex karyotype or secondary aberrations in patients with t(8;21), inv(16) t(16;16), or t(9;11)[1105]
Myeloid antigens: CD11b expression may be predictive of shorter survival.[1106]
Detection of the WT1 (Wilms tumor) transcript[1107]
FLT3-ITD or Asp835 mutations in APL[1108]
Levels of initiator caspase[1109]
Persistent thrombocytopenia after remission induction[1110]
Lung resistance protein: Functional test is needed to assess activity.[1111] Expression may predict poor outcome in *de novo* AML.[1055,1112]

restitution of normal hematopoiesis can occur with at least a three-log reduction in leukemic cell numbers, which represents a residual tumor cell burden of approximately 1 billion cells. Intensification therapy is intended to decrease further the residual cell numbers. With the advent of specific monoclonal antibodies for leukemic cell antigens and FISH coupled with flow cytometry and DNA amplification by PCR, residual leukemic cell populations at or below the level of one billion cells, which are undetectable by light microscopy of stained marrow films, can be quantified.[1115] When real-time PCR is used to quantify PML-RAR-α, RUNX1/ETO, or CBF-β/MYH11, risk for treatment failure can be determined by the levels of the fusion gene at diagnosis and after the first 3 to 4 months of therapy.[1116] Sampling remains an important problem because marrow aspiration contains approximately 1/10,000 of the marrow cell population, and variation among sites of aspiration is well documented. In addition, the markers of the leukemic cell used for detection can change during the course of the disease. For example, persistence of circulating cells containing t(8;21) in patients with AML in long-term remission has been established using PCR.[1117]

There are many other pitfalls when interpreting these studies, including timing of sampling in relationship to therapy, sensitivity of the PCR reaction for target genes, interlaboratory standardization, selection of patients, and retrospective or prospective design of the study.[1118] Detection of minimal residual disease in the postallogeneic stem cell transplantation setting is also potentially important, and sensitive chimerism assays have been developed using PCR-based technology to detect short tandem repeat polymorphisms. Whether these will have impact on treatment of posttransplantation relapses is still unclear.[1119,1120]

Marrow examinations are not needed in the majority of AML patients in first complete remission.[1121] Because of increased myeloid precursors in regenerating marrow, detection of residual disease may be difficult early after a given therapeutic modality.[1122] Cytogenetic followup usually is not helpful. Emergence of a karyotypically unrelated clone of AML cells, especially containing chromosome 7, can occur. Studies using multiparameter flow cytometry to identify leukemic cells by aberrant antigen expression have a high positive predictive value with regard to the incidence of relapse.[1123] Detection of residual disease in AML patients using double immunologic marker analysis for terminal deoxynucleotidyl transferase and myeloid CD antigens can be useful because these two markers are expressed on leukemic cells in the majority of AML patients. These findings are rare in normal marrow cells.[1124,1125] In other cases, aberrant combinations of surface antigens[1124,1126] or increased expression of various surface antigens such as CD34 are seen.[1127] Immunophenotype may change at relapse and has implications for minimal disease detection.[1128] Five-color staining has been reported to improve the percentage of AML cases in which a leukemia-associated aberrant immunophenotype is identified.[1129] Various markers, such as CLL-1 (C-type lectin-like molecule-1) and other lineage markers and marker-combinations, have been found aberrantly expressed on leukemic CD34+CD38−, cells allowing residual disease detection at the stem cell level.[1130] Other methods for detecting minimal residual disease include magnetic resonance imaging; fluorescence DNA in FISH[1131,1132]; reverse transcriptase (RT)-PCR to detect amplification of abnormal fusion genes such as t(15;17), t(8;21), inversion 16, and 11q23; and DNA PCR for mutations in the *RAS* coding regions.[1115] Quantitative assessment of WT1 expression[1133] or presence of *FLT3* mutation[1134] can also be evaluated for MDR monitoring. Real-time quantitative PCR can be used to quantitate MDR more precisely than other methods, but this test requires standardized criteria and is not widely available clinically.[1135]

Multiparameter flow cytometry is applicable to most AML cases, whereas real-time quantitative PCR is applicable in just above half the cases when *NPM1* and *FLT3* mutations are examined in addition to fusion genes.[1136] Gene profiling of CD34+CD38− cells, a fraction that contains both normal and leukemic stem cells, might be important in minimal residual disease measurement, but 34 percent of genes modulated in AML stem cells are shared with normal stem cells.[1137]

Detecting Inversion 16

Minimal residual disease in acute myelomonocytic leukemia with inversion 16 can be detected by nested PCR with allele-specific amplifications (*CBF-β* on 16q and *MYH11* on 16p).[1138,1139] This fusion transcript occurs not only in the majority of cases of acute myelomonocytic leukemia with marrow eosinophilia (M4Eo), but also in 10 percent of acute myelomonocytic leukemia M4 without eosinophilic abnormalities, a much higher incidence than suggested by the sporadic reports of chromosome 16 abnormalities in AML. Additional screening by either RT-PCR or FISH should be performed in patients with acute myelomonocytic leukemia, regardless of morphologic features, to evaluate the prognostic usefulness of this fusion transcript in minimal disease detection.[1140] Following completion of chemotherapy (induction and consolidation), patients who had a CBF-β/MYH11 fusion transcript copy number greater than 10 had a shorter remission duration and higher risk for relapse than did patients with a copy number less than 10.[1139] Evidence indicates transcript ratios of samples may have utility in establishing thresholds for curability and for relapse risk in standard clinical complete remission states in the future.[1141]

Detecting t(8;21)

Translocation 8;21 is one of the most common translocations in AML, especially in younger patients (see Table 89–7). This translocation fuses the *RUNX1* gene on chromosome 21p to ETO on chromosome 8p to produce the fusion gene.[1142,1143] The fusion has been detected in the majority of patients in remission. One study found its persistence in all patients with t(8;21) after chemotherapy or autologous marrow transplantation.[1144–1146] Using PCR measurement, *RUNX1/ETO* was found in patients in complete remission for 12 to 150 months but not in patients who received allogeneic hematopoietic stem cell transplantation. The *PGK* allele, used as a tracking marker, was identical to that detected in the leukemic blasts from the time of initial diagnosis, confirming the persistence and reappearance of leukemic cells from the same clone.[1146] This marker may persist after allogeneic stem cell transplantation but is compatible with continued remission.[1147] Quantitation of the amount of the fusion transcript during remission may be more predictive of cure or relapse than a simple qualitative assessment.[1148,1149] Real-time quantitative RT-PCR can be used for this purpose.[1021] Quantitative RT-PCR can predict relapse up to 4 months before clinical onset.[1150] In a study of 45 t(8;21) positive AML cases, the quality of molecular response after induction, as well as after consolidation therapies, was correlated with relapse, event-free survival, and overall survival.[1151] Serial RT-PCR quantification of cases with residual t(8;21) indicates at least 0.1 fg of *RUNX1/ETO* competitor dose is present before cytogenetic relapse occurs.[1152] Both ETO and *RUNX1* are expressed in normal CD34+ progenitors.[1153] Blood can be used as an alternative to marrow for quantitating RUNX1/ETO transcripts.[1154]

Detecting t(15;17)

Unlike AML with the fusion transcript t(8;21), in APL the t(15;17) fusion transcript usually disappears after intensive therapy.[1155] At least 1 in 100,000 cells with the *PML-RAR-α* transcript can be detected by RT-PCR.[1155] FISH also can be used.[1156] Molecular monitoring has shown treatment capable of achieving a molecular remission (negative RT-PCR).[1157] Nested PCR can be used to determine the need for additional treatment at the end of consolidation, to determine the advisability of autologous stem cell transplantation in second remission, and to predict relapse after transplantation.[1158] Real-time quantitative RT-PCR may improve the predictive value of MDR assessment and aid in laboratory standardization.[1159]

Detecting NPM-1 and FLT-3 Mutations

In AML patients who have normal cytogenetics, mutational status of *NPM1, FLT3, CEPBA, MLL,* and *RAS* may have implications for treatment outcomes and prognosis.[101] Whether detection of these mutations in a state of minimal residual disease will have implications for relapse and therapy remains undetermined. There is evidence in *NPM1*—mutated cases, relapse was always accompanied by an increase of mutant gene copy numbers, and it has been concluded that quantitative PCR monitoring may have prognostic impact in such patients.[1160]

The technology to detect minimal residual disease has increased in sensitivity and availability. Detection of minimal residual disease to determine a patient's treatment or prognosis remains an evolving area of investigation. The role that proteomic[1161,1162] and microRNA profiles[1163,1164] will play in minimal residual disease detection is currently under study.

REFERENCES

1. Friedreich N: Ein neuer Fall von Leukämie. *Arch Pathol* 12:37, 1857.
2. Ebstein W: Ueber die acute Leukämie und Pseudoleukämie. *Dtsch Arch Klin Med* 44:343, 1889.
3. Fraenkel A: Ueber acute Leukämie. *Dtsch Med Wochenschr* 21:639, 1895.
4. Neumann E: Ueber myelogene leukäemie. *Berl Klin Wochenschr* 15:69, 1878.
5. Ehrlich P: *Farbenanolytische Untersuchungen zur Histologie und Klinik des Blutes.* Hirschwald, Berlin, 1891.
6. Naegeli O: Ueber rothes Knochenmark und Myeloblasten. *Dtsch Med Wochenschr* 26:287, 1900.
7. Hirschfield H: Zur Kenntnis der Histogenese der granulirten Knochenmarkzellen. *Arch Pathol* 153:335, 1898.
8. Hsu TC: *Human and Mammalian Cytogenetics: An Historical Perspective.* Springer-Verlag, New York, 1979.
9. Subramanian G, Adams MD, Venter JC, Broder S: Implications of the human genome for understanding human biology and medicine. *JAMA* 286:2296, 2001.
10. Ellison RR, Holland JF, Weil M, et al: Arabinosyl cytosine: A useful agent in the treatment of acute leukemia in adults. *Blood* 33:507, 1968.
11. Yates JW, Wallace HJ, Ellison RR, Holland JF: Cytosine arabinoside and daunorubicin therapy in acute non-lymphocytic leukemia. *Cancer Chemother Rep* 52:485, 1973.
12. Thomas ED, Buckner CD, Banaji M, et al: One hundred patients with acute leukemia treated by chemotherapy, total body irradiation, and allogeneic bone marrow transplantation. *Blood* 49:511, 1977.
13. Preston DL, Kusumi S, Tomonaga M, et al: Cancer incidence in atomic bomb survivors. Part III. Leukemia, lymphoma and multiple myeloma, 1950–1987. *Radiat Res* 137(2 Suppl):S68, 1994.
14. Lichtman MA: Is there an entity of chemically induced BCR-ABL-positive chronic myelogenous leukemia? *Oncologist* 13:645, 2008.
15. Schnatter AR, Rosamilia K, Wojcik NC: Review of the literature on benzene exposure and leukemia subtypes. *Chem Biol Interact* 153–154:9, 2005.
16. Schattner AR, Nicholich MJ, Bird MG: Determination of leukemogenic benzene exposure concentrations. *Risk Anal* 16:833, 1996.
17. Pyatt D: Benzene and hematopoietic malignancies. *Clin Occup Environ Med* 4:529–55, 2004.
18. Yin S-N, Hayes RB, Linet MS, et al: A cohort study of cancer among benzene-exposed workers in China: Overall results. *Am J Ind Med* 29:227, 1996.
19. Rund D, Ben-Yehuda D: Therapy-related leukemia and myelodysplasia: Evolving concepts of pathogenesis and treatment. *Hematology* 9:179, 2004.
20. Larson RA, Le Beau MM: Therapy-related myeloid leukaemia: A model for leukemogenesis in humans. *Chem Biol Interact* 153–154:187, 2005.
21. Pui CH, Relling MV, Behn FG, et al: L-Asparaginases may potentiate the leukemogenic effect of the epipodophyllotoxins. *Leukemia* 9:1680, 1995.
22. Travis LB, Holowty EF, Bergfeldt K, et al: Risk of leukemia after platinum-based chemotherapy for ovarian cancer. *N Engl J Med* 340:351, 1999.
23. Finazzi G, Harrison C: Essential thrombocythemia. *Semin Hematol* 42:230, 2005.
24. Van Leeuwen FE: Risk of acute myelogenous leukemia and myelodysplasia following cancer treatment. *Baillieres Clin Haematol* 9:57, 1996.
25. Yeasmin S, Nakayama K, Ishibashi M, et al: Therapy-related myelodysplasia and acute myeloid leukemia following paclitaxel- and carboplatin-based chemotherapy in an ovarian cancer patient: A case report and literature review. *Int J Gynecol Cancer* 18:1371, 2008.
26. Visfeldt J, Anderson M: Pathoanatomical aspects of malignant haematological disorders among Danish patients exposed to thorium dioxide. *APMIS* 103:29, 1995.
27. Rodella S, Ciccone G, Rege-Cambrin G, et al: Cytogenetics and occupational exposures in acute nonlymphocytic leukemia and myelodysplastic syndrome. *Scand J Work Environ Health* 19:369, 1993.
28. Brownson RC, Novotny TE, Perry MC: Cigarette smoking and adult leukemia: A meta-analysis. *Arch Intern Med* 153:469, 1993.
29. Lichtman MA: Cigarette smoking, cytogenetic abnormalities, and acute myelogenous leukemia. *Leukemia* 21:1137, 2007.
30. Stewart SL, Cardinez CJ, Richardson LC, et al: Surveillance for cancers associated with tobacco use—United States, 1999–2004. *MMWR Surveill Summ* 57:1, 2008.
31. Swolin B, Rödjer S, Westin J: Therapy-related patterns of cytogenetic abnormalities in acute myeloid leukemia and myelodysplastic syndrome post polycythemia vera: Single center experience and review of literature. *Ann Hematol* 87:467, 2008.
32. Wiernik P: Leukemias and plasma cell myeloma. *Cancer Chemother Biol Response Modif* 17:390, 1997.
33. Luca DC, Almanaseer IY: Simultaneous presentation of multiple myeloma and acute monocytic leukemia. *Arch Pathol Lab Med* 127:1506, 2003.
34. Pulik M, Genet P, Jary L, et al: Acute myeloid leukemias, multiple myelomas, and chronic leukemias in the setting of HIV infection. *AIDS Patient Care STDS* 12:913, 1998.
35. Moskowitz C, Dutcher JP, Wiernik PH: Association of thyroid disease with acute leukemia. *Am J Hematol* 39:102, 1992.
36. Willems E, Valdes-Socin H, Betea D, et al: Association of acute leukemia and autoimmune polyendocrine syndrome in two kindreds. *Leukemia* 17:1912, 2003.
37. Lichtenstein P, Holm NV, Verkasalo PK, et al: Environmental and hereditable factors in causation of cancer—Analyses of cohorts of twins from Sweden, Denmark, and Finland. *N Engl J Med* 343:78, 2000.
38. Risch N: The genetic epidemiology of cancer. Interpreting family and twin studies and their implications for molecular genetic approaches. *Cancer Epidemiol Biomarkers Prev* 10:733, 2001.
39. Hemminki K, Vaittinen P, Dong C, Easton D: Sibling risks in cancer: Clues to recessive or X-linked genes? *Br J Cancer* 84:388, 2001.
40. Germeshausen M, Ballmaier M, Welte K: Implications of mutations in hematopoietic growth factor receptor genes in congenital cytopenias. *Ann N Y Acad Sci* 938:305, 2001.
41. Tonelli R, Scardovi AL, Pession A, et al: Compound heterozygosity for two different amino-acid substitution mutations in the thrombopoietin receptor (c-mpl gene) in congenital amegakaryocytic thrombocytopenia (CAMT). *Hum Genet* 107:225, 2000.
42. Li FP, Hecht F, Kaiser-McCaw B, et al: Ataxia-pancytopenia: Syndrome of cerebellar ataxia, hypoplastic anemia, monosomy 7, and acute myelogenous leukemia. *Cancer Genet Cytogenet* 4:189, 1981.
43. Gonzales-del Angel A, Cervera M, Gomez L, et al: Ataxia-pancytopenia syndrome. *Am J Med Genet* 90:252, 2000.
44. German J: Bloom's syndrome: Incidence, age of onset, and types of leukemia in the Bloom's syndrome registry, in *Genetics in Hematologic Disorders*, edited by CS Bartsocas, D Loukopoulos, p 241. Hemisphere, Washington, 1992.
45. Poppe B, Van Limbergen H, Van Roy N, et al: Chromosomal aberrations in Bloom syndrome patients with myeloid malignancies. *Cancer Genet Cytogenet* 128:39, 2001.
46. Freedman MH, Alter BP: Risk of myelodysplastic syndrome and acute myeloid leukemia in congenital neutropenia. *Semin Hematol* 39:128, 2002.
47. Aprikyan AA, Kutyavin T, Stein S, et al: Cellular and molecular abnormalities in severe congenital neutropenia predisposing to leukemia. *Exp Hematol* 31:372, 2003.
48. Rosenberg PS, Alter BP, Link DC, et al: Neutrophil elastase mutations and risk of leukaemia in severe congenital neutropenia. *Br J Haematol* 140:210, 2008.
49. Link DC, Kunter G, Kasai Y, et al: Distinct patterns of mutations occurring in *de novo* AML versus AML arising in the setting of severe congenital neutropenia. *Blood* 110:1648, 2007.
50. Shinawi M, Erez A, Shardy DL, et al: Syndromic thrombocytopenia and predisposition to acute myelogenous leukemia caused by constitutional microdeletions on chromosome 21q. *Blood* 112:1042, 2008.
51. Janov AJ, Leong T, Nathan DG, Guinan EC: Diamond-Blackfan anemia: Natural history and sequelae of treatment. *Medicine (Baltimore)* 75:77, 1996.
52. Vlachos A, Klein G, Lipton J: The Blackfan-Diamond anemia registry: Tool for investigating the epidemiology and biology of Diamond-Blackfan anemia. *Pediatr Hematol Oncol* 23:377, 2001.
53. Forestier E, Izraeli S, Beverloo B, et al: Cytogenetic features of acute lymphoblastic and myeloid leukemias in pediatric patients with Down syndrome: An iBFM-SG study. *Blood* 111:1575, 2008.
54. Puumala SE, Ross JA, Olshan AF, et al: Reproductive history, infertility treatment, and the risk of acute leukemia in children with down syndrome: A report from the Children's Oncology Group. *Cancer* 110:2067, 2007.
55. Andrade-Machado R, Machado-Rojas A, de la Torre-Santos ME: Dubowitz syndrome, polymyositis, and aleucemic myeloblastic leukemia. A new association. *Rev Neurol* 35:500, 2001.

56. Savage SA, Alter BP: The role of telomere biology in bone marrow failure and other disorders. *Mech Ageing Dev* 129:35, 2008.
57. Röth A, Baerlocher GM: Dyskeratosis congenita. *Br J Haematol* 141:412, 2008.
58. Segel GB, Lichtman MA: Familial (inherited) leukemia, lymphoma, and myeloma. *Blood Cells Mol Dis* 32:246, 2004.
59. Owen CJ, Toze CL, Koochin A, et al: Five new pedigrees with inherited RUNX1 mutations causing familial platelet disorder with propensity to myeloid malignancy (FPD/AML). *Blood* 112:4639, 2008.
60. Minelli A, Maserati E, Rossi G, et al: Familial platelet disorder with propensity to acute myelogenous leukemia: Genetic heterogeneity and progression to leukemia via acquisition of clonal chromosome anomalies. *Genes Chromosomes Cancer* 40:165, 2004.
61. Rosenberg PS, Greene MH, Alter BP: Cancer incidence in persons with Fanconi anemia. *Blood* 101:822, 2003.
62. Rosenberg PS, Alter BP, Ebell W: Cancer risks in Fanconi anemia: Findings from the German Fanconi Anemia Registry. *Haematologica* 93:511, 2008.
63. Polychronopoulou S, Tsatsopoulou A, Papadhimitriou SI, et al: Myelodysplasia and Naxos disease: A novel pathogenetic association? *Leukemia* 16:2335, 2002.
64. Kratz CP, Antonietti L, Shannon KM, et al: Acute myeloid leukemia associated with t(8;21) or trisomy 8 in children with neurofibromatosis type 1. *Pediatr Hematol Oncol* 25:343, 2003.
65. Lurgaespada DA, Brannan CI, Shaughnessy JD, et al: The neurofibromatosis type 1 (NF1) tumor suppressor gene and myeloid leukemia. *Curr Top Microbiol Immunol* 211:233, 1996.
66. Bader-Meunier B, Tchernia G, Miélot F, et al: Occurrence of myeloproliferative disorder in patients with Noonan syndrome. *J Pediatr* 130:885, 1997.
67. Bentires-Alj M, Paez JG, David FS, et al: Activating mutations of the Noonan syndrome-associated SHP2/PTPN11 gene in human solid tumors and adult acute myelogenous leukemia. *Cancer Res* 64:8816,2004.
68. Fokin AA, Robicsek F: Poland's syndrome revisited. *Ann Thorac Surg* 74:2218, 2002.
69. Pianigiani E, DeAloe G, Andreassi A, et al: Rothmund-Thomson syndrome (Thomson type) and myelodysplasia. *Pediatr Dermatol* 18:422, 2001.
70. Duker NJ: Chromosome breakage syndromes and cancer. *Am J Med Genet* 115:125, 2002.
71. Hayani A, Suarez CR, Molnar Z, et al: Acute myeloid leukemia in a patient with Seckel syndrome. *J Med Genet* 31:148, 1994.
72. Boocock GR, Morrison JA, Popovic M, et al: Mutations in SBDS are associated with Shwachman-Diamond syndrome. *Nat Genet* 33:97, 2003.
73. Rujkijyanont P, Beyene J, Wei K, et al: Leukaemia-related gene expression in bone marrow cells from patients with the preleukaemic disorder Shwachman-Diamond syndrome. *Br J Haematol* 137:537, 2007.
74. Mitsui T, Kawakami T, Sendo D, et al: Successful unrelated donor bone marrow transplantation for Shwachman-Diamond syndrome with leukemia. *Int J Hematol* 79:189, 2004.
75. Yamada T, Tsurumi H, Murakami N, et al: Werner's syndrome developing acute megakaryoblastic leukemia with der(1;7). *Rinsho Ketsueki* 38:28, 1997.
76. Tao LC, Stecker E, Gardner HA: Werner's syndrome and acute myeloid leukemia. *CMAJ* 105:951, 1971.
77. Muftuoglu M, Oshima J, von Kobbe C, et al: The clinical characteristics of Werner syndrome: Molecular and biochemical diagnosis. *Hum Genet* 124:369, 2008.
78. Sharathkumar A, Kirby M, Freedman M, et al: Malignant hematological disorders in children with Wolf-Hirschhorn syndrome. *Am J Med Genet* 119A:194, 2003.
79. Gonzalez CH, Durkin-Stamm MV, Geimer NF, et al: The WT syndrome—A "new" autosomal dominant pleiotropic trait of radial/ulnar hypoplasia with high risk of bone marrow failure and/or leukemia. *Birth Defects Orig Artic Ser* 13:31, 1977.
80. Fialkow PH, Singer JW, Adamson JW, et al: Acute nonlymphocytic leukemia. Heterogeneity of stem cell origin. *Blood* 57:1068, 1991.
81. Ferraris AM, Broccia G, Meloni T, et al: Clonal origin of cells restricted to monocytic differentiation in acute nonlymphocytic leukemia. *Blood* 64:817, 1984.
82. Greaves MF: Stem cell origins of leukaemia and curability. *Br J Cancer* 67:413, 1993.
83. Turhan AG, Lemoire FB, Debert C, et al: Highly purified primitive hematopoietic stem cells are PML-RARA negative and generate nonclonal progenitors in acute promyelocytic leukemia. *Blood* 85:2154, 1995.
84. Van Lom K, Hagenmeijer A, Vandekerckhove F, et al: Clonality analysis of hematopoietic cell lineages in acute myeloid leukemia and translocation (8;21): Only myeloid cells are part of malignant clone. *Leukemia* 11:202, 1997.
85. van Rhenen A, van Dongen GA, et al: The novel AML stem cell associated antigen CLL-1 aids in discrimination between normal and leukemic stem cells. *Blood* 110:2659, 2007.
86. Guzman ML, Rossi RM, Karnischky L, et al: The sesquiterpene lactone parthenolide induces apoptosis of human acute myelogenous leukemia stem and progenitor cells. *Blood* 105:4163, 2005.
87. Look AT: Oncogene transcription factors in human acute leukemias. *Science* 278:1059, 1997.
88. Pabst T, Mueller BU: Transcriptional dysregulation during myeloid transformation in AML. *Oncogene* 26:6829, 2007.
89. Kelly LM, Gilliland DG: Genetics of myeloid leukemias. *Annu Rev Genomics Hum Genet* 3:179, 2002.
90. Adams JM, Cosy S: Oncogene cooperation in leukaemogenesis. *Cancer Surv* 15:119, 1992.
91. Bashey A, Gill R, Levi S, et al: Mutational activation of the N-ras oncogene assessed in primary clonogenic culture of acute myeloid leukemia (AML): Implications for the role of N-ras mutation in AML pathogenesis. *Blood* 79:981, 1992.
92. Preisler HD, Kinniburgh AJ, Wei-Dong G, Khan S: Expression of the protooncogenes *c-myc, c-fos*, and *c-fms* in acute myelocytic leukemia at diagnosis and in remission. *Cancer Res* 47:874, 1987.
93. Buesco-Ramos DE, Yang Y, De Leon E: The human MDM-2 oncogene is overexposed in leukemia. *Blood* 82:2617, 1993.
94. Mori N, Hidai H, Yokota J, et al: Mutations of the p53 gene in myelodysplastic syndrome and overt leukaemia. *Leuk Res* 19:869, 1995.
95. Wiede R, Parviz B, Pflüger K-H, et al: The role of decreased retinoblastoma protein expression in acute myelomonocytic and monoblastic leukemias. *Leuk Lymphoma* 17:135, 1995.
96. Ridge SA, Worwood M, Oscier D, et al: FMS mutations in myelodysplastic, leukemic and normal subjects. *Proc Natl Acad Sci U S A* 87:1377, 1990.
97. Menssen HD, Renki HJ, Rodeck U, et al: Presence of Wilm's tumor gene (wt1) transcripts and the WT1 nuclear protein on the majority of human acute leukemias. *Leukemia* 9:1060, 1995.
98. Wellman CL, Whittaker MH: The molecular biology of acute myeloid leukemia. *Clin Lab Med* 10:769, 1990.
99. Vigon I, Dreyfus F, Melle J, et al: Expression of the c-mpl protooncogene in human hematologic malignancies. *Blood* 82:877, 1993.
100. Mills K: Gene expression profiling for the diagnosis and prognosis of acute myeloid leukaemia. *Front Biosci* 13:4605, 2008.
101. Schlenk RF, Döhner K, Krauter J, et al: Mutations and treatment outcome in cytogenetically normal acute myeloid leukemia. *N Engl J Med* 358:1909, 2008.
102. Renneville A, Roumier C, Biggio V, et al: Cooperating gene mutations in acute myeloid leukemia: A review of the literature. *Leukemia* 22:915, 2008.
103. Libura M, Asnafi V, Delabesse E, et al: *FLT3* and *MLL* intragenic abnormalities in AML reflect a common category of genotoxic stress. *Blood* 1902:2198, 2003.
104. Small D: Targeting FLT3 for the treatment of leukemia. *Semin Hematol* 45(3 Suppl 2):S17, 2008.
105. Mauritzson N, Albin M, Rylander L, et al: Pooled analysis of clinical and cytogenetic features in treatment-related and de novo adult acute myeloid leukemia and myelodysplastic syndromes based on consecutive series of 761 patients analyzed 1976–1993 and on 5098 unselected cases reported in the literature 1974–2001. *Leukemia* 16:2366, 2002.
106. Grimwade D, Enver T: Acute promyelocytic leukemia: Where does it stem from? *Leukemia* 18:375, 2004.
107. Zeisig BB, Kwok C, Zelent A, et al: Recruitment of RXR by homotetrameric RARalpha fusion proteins is essential for Transformation. *Cancer Cell* 12:36, 2007.
108. Scholl C, Gilliland DG, Fröhling S: Deregulation of signaling pathways in acute myeloid leukemia. *Semin Oncol* 35:336, 2008.
109. Greaves MF, Maia AT, Wiemels JL, Ford AM: Leukemia in twins: Lessons in natural history. *Blood* 102:2321, 2003.
110. Wiemels JL, Xiao Z, Buffler PA, et al: *In utero* origin of t(8;21) AML1-ETO translocation in childhood acute leukemia. *Blood* 99:3801, 2002.
111. Groves FD, Linet MS, Devesa SS: Epidemiology of leukemia, in *Leukemia*, 6th ed, edited by ES Henderson, TA Lister, MF Greaves, p 145. WB Saunders, New York, 1986.
112. Vickers M, Jackson G, Taylor P: The incidence of acute promyelocytic leukemia appears constant over most of a human life span, implying only one rate limiting mutation. *Leukemia* 14:727, 2000.
113. Douer D, Santillana S, Ramezani L, et al: Acute promyelocytic leukaemia in patients originating in Latin America is associated with an increased frequency of the bcr1 subtype of the PML/RARalpha fusion gene. *Br J Haematol* 122:563, 2003.
114. Otero JC, Santillana S, Fereyros G: High frequency of acute promyelocytic leukemia among Latinos with acute myeloid leukemias. *Blood* 88:377, 1996.
115. Stanley M, McKenna RW, Ellinger G, Brunning RD: Classification of 358 cases of acute myeloid leukemia by FAB criteria: Analysis of clinical and morphologic features, in *Chronic and Acute Leukemias in Adults*, edited by CD Bloomfield, p 147. Martinus Nijhoff, Boston, 1985.
116. Scott CS, Den Ottolander GJ, Swirsky D, et al: Recommended procedures for the classification of acute leukaemias. *Leuk Lymphoma* 11:37, 1993.
117. Jennings CD, Foon KA: Recent advances in flow cytometry: Application to the diagnosis of hematologic malignancy. *Blood* 90:2863, 1997.
118. Cassanovas RD, Campos L, Mugneret F, et al: Immunophenotypic patterns and cytogenetic anomalies in acute non-lymphoblastic leukemia subtypes: A prospective study of 432 patients. *Leukemia* 12:34, 1998.
119. Del Vecchio L, Di Noto R, Lo Pardo C, et al: Immunological classification of acute leukemias: Comments on the EGIL proposals. *Leukemia* 10:1832, 1996.
120. Paietta E: Classification of acute leukemias: Proposals for the immunological classification of acute leukemias. *Leukemia* 9:2147, 1995.
121. De Greef GE, Hagemeiger A: Molecular and cytogenetic abnormalities in acute myeloid leukemia and myelodysplastic syndromes. *Baillieres Clin Haematol* 9:1, 1996.
122. Kheiri SA, MacKerrell T, Bonagura VR, et al: Flow cytometry with or without cytochemistry for the diagnosis of acute leukemias? *Cytometry* 34:82, 1998.
123. Valik PJM, Verhaak RGW, Beijin A, et al: Prognostically useful gene expression profiles in acute myeloid leukemia. *N Engl J Med* 350:1617 2004.

124. Bullinger L, Dohner K, Bair E, et al: Use of gene-expression profiling to identify prognostic subclasses in adult acute myeloid leukemia. *N Engl J Med* 350:1605, 2004.
125. Head DR: Revised classification of acute myeloid leukemia. *Leukemia* 10:1826, 1996.
126. Boggs DR, Wintrobe MM, Cartwright GE: The acute leukemias. Analysis of 322 cases and review of the literature. *Medicine (Baltimore)* 41:163, 1962.
127. Roath S, Israëls MCG, Wilkinson JF: The acute leukemias: A study of 580 patients. *Q J Med* 33:256, 1964.
128. Choi S-I, Simone JV: Acute non-lymphocytic leukemia in 171 children. *Med Pediatr Oncol* 2:119, 1976.
129. Chessels JM, O'Calloghan U, Hardisty RM: Acute myeloid leukaemia in childhood: Clinical features and prognosis. *Br J Haematol* 63:555, 1986.
130. Burns CP, Armitage JO, Frey AL, et al: Analysis of presenting features of adult leukemia. *Cancer* 47:2460, 1981.
131. Goodall PT, Vosti KL: Fever in acute myelogenous leukemia. *Arch Intern Med* 135:1197, 1975.
132. Burke PJ, Braine HG, Rothbun HK, Owens AH: The clinical significance and management of fever in acute myelocytic leukemia. *Johns Hopkins Med J* 139:1, 1976.
133. Chang JC: How to differentiate neoplastic fever from infectious fever in patients with cancer. Usefulness of the naproxen test. *Heart Lung* 16:122, 1987.
134. Gollard RP, Robbins BA, Piro L, Saven A: Acute myelogenous leukemia presenting with bulky lymphadenopathy. *Acta Haematol* 95:129, 1996.
135. Davey DD, Fourcar K, Burns CP, Goekin JA: Acute myelocytic leukemia manifested by prominent generalized lymphadenopathy. *Am J Hematol* 21:89, 1986.
136. Tobelem G, Jacquillat C, Chastang C, et al: Acute monoblastic leukemia: A clinical and biologic study of 74 cases. *Blood* 55:71, 1980.
137. Sipp N, Radaszkiemicz T, Meijer CJLM, et al: Specific skin manifestations in acute leukemia with monocytic differentiation. *Cancer* 71:124, 1993.
138. Hejmadi RK,Thompson D, Shah F, Naresh KN: Cutaneous presentation of aleukemic monoblastic leukemia cutis—A case report and review of literature with focus on immunohistochemistry. *J Cutan Pathol* 35:46, 2008.
139. Cibull TL, Thomas AB, O'Malley DP, Billings SD: Myeloid leukemia cutis: A histologic and immunohistochemical review. *J Cutan Pathol* 35:180, 2008.
140. Kaiserling E, Horny H-P, Geerts M-L, Schmid U: Skin involvement in myelogenous leukemia. Morphologic and immunophenotypic heterogeneity of skin infiltrates. *Mod Pathol* 7:771, 1994.
141. Longacre TA, Smoller BR: Leukemia cutis: Analysis of 50 biopsy-proven cases with an emphasis on occurrences in myelodysplastic syndromes. *Am J Clin Pathol* 100:276, 1993.
142. Cho-Vega JH, Medeiros LJ, Prieto VG, Vega F: Leukemia cutis. *Am J Clin Pathol* 129:130, 2008.
143. Bourantas K, Malamou-Mitsi V, Christou L, et al: Cutaneous vasculitis as the initial manifestation in acute myelomonocytic leukemia. *Ann Intern Med* 121:942, 1994.
144. Sheps M, Shapero H, Ramsay C: Bullous pyoderma gangrenosum and acute leukemia. *Arch Dermatol* 114:1842, 1978.
145. Lewis SJ, Poh-Fitzpatrick MB, Walther RR: A typical pyoderma gangrenosum with leukemia. *JAMA* 239:935, 1978.
146. Cohen PR: Sweet's syndrome—A comprehensive review of an acute febrile neutrophilic dermatosis. *Orphanet J Rare Dis* 26(2):34, 2007.
147. Cheson BD, Christensen RM: Cutis verticis gyrata: Unusual chloromatous disease in acute myelogenous leukemia. *Am J Hematol* 8:415, 1980.
148. Stern M, Halter J, Buser A, et al: Leukemia cutis preceding systemic relapse of acute myeloid leukemia. *Int J Hematol* 87:108, 2008.
149. Markowski TR, Martin DB, Kao GF, et al: Leukemia cutis: A presenting sign in acute promyelocytic leukemia. *Arch Dermatol* 143:1220, 2007.
150. Long JC, Mihm MC: Multiple granulocytic tumors of the skin: Report of six cases of myelogenous leukemia with initial manifestations in the skin. *Cancer* 39:2004, 1977.
151. Rallis E, Stavropoulou E, Michalakeas I, et al: Monoblastic sarcoma cutis preceding acute monoblastic leukemia. *Am J Hematol* 2008 .
152. Kincaid MC, Green WR: Ocular and orbital involvement in leukemia. *Surv Ophthalmol* 27:211, 1983.
153. Paparella MM, Berlinger NT, Oda M: Otological manifestations of leukemia. *Laryngoscope* 83:1510, 1973.
154. Bertrand Y, Lefrère J-J, L'Evergren G, et al: Acute myeloblastic leukemia presenting as apparent acute otitis media. *Am J Hematol* 27:136, 1988.
155. Shiknecht HF, Igarashi M, Chasin WD: Inner ear hemorrhage in leukemia. *Laryngoscope* 75:662, 1965.
156. Dewar GJ, Lim C-NH, Michalyshyn B, Akabutu J: Gastrointestinal complications in patients with acute and chronic leukemia. *Can J Surg* 24:67, 1981.
157. Hunter TB, Bjelland JC: Gastrointestinal complications of leukemia and its treatment. *AJR Am J Roentgenol* 142:513, 1984.
158. Duffy JH, Driscoll EJ: Oral manifestations of leukemia. *Oral Surg Oral Med Oral Pathol* 11:484, 1958.
159. Ahsan N, Schen-Chih, JS, John DD: Acute ileotyphlitis as presenting manifestation of acute myelogenous leukemia. *Am J Clin Pathol* 89:407, 1988.
160. Rodgers B, Seibert JJ: Unusual combination of an appendicolith in a leukemic patient with typhlitis-ultrasound diagnosis. *J Clin Ultrasound* 18:141, 1990.
161. Abramson SJ, Berdon WE, Baker DH: Childhood typhlitis: Its increasing association with acute myelogenous leukemia. *Radiology* 146:61, 1983.
162. Bagnoli P, Castagna L, Cozzaglio L, et al: Neutropenic enterocolitis: Is there a right timing for surgery? Assessment of a clinical case. *Tumori* 93:608, 2007.
163. Roy J, Vercellotti G, Fenderson M, et al: Isolated relapse of acute myelogenous leukemia presenting as a gastric ulcer. *Am J Hematol* 37:270, 1991.
164. Thompson BC, Feczko PJ, Mezwa DG: Dysphagia caused by acute leukemia infiltration of the esophagus. *AJR Am J Roentgenol* 155:654, 1990.
165. Ti M, Villafuerte R, Chase PH, Dosik H: Acute leukemia presenting as laryngeal obstruction. *Cancer* 34:427, 1974.
166. Bodey GP, Powell RD, Hersh EM, et al: Pulmonary complications of acute leukemia. *Cancer* 19:781, 1966.
167. Maile CW, Moore AV, Ulreich S, Putnam CE: Chest radiographic pathologic correlation in adult leukemia patients. *Invest Radiol* 18:495, 1983.
168. Armstrong P, Dyer R, Alford BA, O'Hara M: Leukemic pulmonary infiltrates. Rapid development mimicking pulmonary edema. *AJR Am J Roentgenol* 135:373, 1980.
169. Wu KK, Burns CP: Leukemic pleural infiltrates during bone marrow remission of acute myelocytic leukemia. *Cancer* 33:1179, 1974.
170. Roberts WC, Bodey GP, Wertlake PT: The heart in acute leukemia. A study of 420 autopsy cases. *Am J Cardiol* 21:388, 1968.
171. Lisker SA, Finkelstein D, Brody JI, Beizer LH: Myocardial infarction in acute leukemia. *Arch Intern Med* 119:332, 1967.
172. Norris NH, Weiner J: The renal lesions in leukemia. *Am J Med Sci* 241:512, 1961.
173. Uno Y: Histopathological study of leukemic cell infiltration in the kidney. *Med J Osaka Univ* 18:185, 1967.
174. Russo A, Basquez E, Russo G, Schilvio G: Testicular relapse in acute myelogenous leukemia after 3 1/2 years of complete remission. *Acta Haematol* 65:131, 1981.
175. Quien ET, Wallach B, Sandhaus L, et al: Primary extramedullary leukemia of the prostate. *Am J Hematol* 53:267, 1996.
176. Vanden Broecke R, Van Droogenbroek J, Dhont M: Vulvovaginal manifestations of acute myeloblastic leukemia. *Obstet Gynecol* 88:735, 1996.
177. Marsh WL, Byland DJ, Heath VC, Anderson MJ: Osteoarticular and pulmonary manifestations of acute leukemia. *Cancer* 57:385, 1986.
178. Weinberger A, Schumacher R, Schimmer BM, et al: Arthritis in acute leukemia. *Arch Intern Med* 141:1183, 1981.
179. Pavlovsky S, Eppinger-Helft M, Murill FS: Factors that influence the appearance of central nervous system leukemia. *Blood* 42:935, 1973.
180. Meyer RJ, Ferreira PP, Cuttner J, et al: Central nervous system involvement at presentation in acute granulocytic leukemia. *Am J Med* 68:691, 1980.
181. Castagnola C, Morra E, Bernasconi P, et al: Acute myeloid leukemia and diabetes insipidus: Results in five patients. *Acta Haematol* 93:1, 1995.
182. Holmes R, Keating MJ, Cork A, et al: A unique pattern of central nervous system leukemia in acute myelomonocytic leukemia associated with inv (16) (p13;q32). *Blood* 65:1071, 1985.
183. Glass JP, VanTassel P, Keating MJ, et al: Central nervous system complications of a newly recognized subtype of leukemia: AMML with a pencentric inversion of chromosome 16. *Neurology* 38:639, 1987.
184. Neiman RS, Barcos M, Berard C, et al: Granulocytic sarcoma: A clinicopathologic study of 61 biopsied cases. *Cancer* 48:426, 1981.
185. Byrd JC, Edenfield WJ, Shields DJ, Dawson NA: Extramedullary myeloid cell tumors in acute nonlymphocytic leukemia. A clinical review. *J Clin Oncol* 13:1800, 1995.
186. Menasce LP, Banerjee SS, Becket E, Harris M: Extramedullary myeloid tumor (granulocytic sarcoma) is often misdiagnosed. A study of 26 cases. *Histopathology* 34:391, 1999.
187. Audouin J, Comperat E, Le Tourneau A, et al: Myeloid sarcoma: Clinical and morphologic criteria useful for diagnosis. *Int J Surg Pathol* 11:271, 2003.
188. Hernandez JA, Navarro JT, Rozman M, et al: Primary myeloid sarcoma of the gynecologic tract: A report of two cases progressing to acute leukemia. *Leuk Lymphoma* 43:2151, 2002.
189. Tsimberidou AM, Kantarjian HM, Estey E, et al: Outcome in patients with nonleukemic granulocytic sarcoma treated with chemotherapy with or without radiotherapy. *Leukemia* 17:1100, 2003.
190. Yamauchi K, Yasuda M: Comparison of nonleukenic granulocytic sarcoma. *Cancer* 94:1739, 2002.
191. Tsimberidou AM, Kantarjian HM, Wen S, et al: Myeloid sarcoma is associated with superior event-free survival and overall survival compared with acute myeloid leukemia. *Cancer* 113:1370, 2008.
192. Byrd JC, Weiss RB, Arthur DC, et al: Extramedullary leukemia adversely affects hematologic complete remission rate and overall survival in patients with t(8;21) (q22;q22): Results from Cancer and Leukemia Group B 8461. *J Clin Oncol* 15:466, 1997.
193. Andrieu V, Radford-Weill I, Troussand X, et al: Molecular detection of t(8;21)/AML1-ETO in AML M1/M2: Correlation with cytogenetics, morphology and immunophenotype. *Br J Haematol* 92:855, 1996.
194. Rege K, Swansbury GJ, Atra AA, et al: Disease features in acute myeloid leukemia with t(8;21)(q22;q22). Influence of age, secondary karyotypic abnormalities, CD19 status, and extramedullary leukemia. *Leuk Lymphoma* 40:67, 2000.
195. Nguyen S, Leblanc T, Fenaux P, et al: A white blood cell index as the main prognostic factor in t(8;21) acute myeloid leukemia (AML): A survey of 161 cases from the French AML intergroup. *Blood* 99:3517, 2002.
196. Rowe JM: Clinical and laboratory features of the myeloid and lymphoid leukemias. *Am J Med Technol* 49:103, 1983.

197. Woodcock BE, Cooper PC, Brown PR, et al: The platelet defect in acute myeloid leukemia. *J Clin Pathol* 37:1339, 1984.
198. Hofmann WK, Stauch M, Höffken K: Impaired granulocytic function in patients with acute leukaemia: Only partial normalization after successful remission-inducing treatment. *J Clin Res Clin Oncol* 124:113, 1998.
199. Suda T, Onai T, Maekawa T: Studies on abnormal polymorphonuclear neutrophils in acute myelogenous leukemia. *Am J Hematol* 15:45, 1983.
200. Glick AD, Paniker K, Flexner JM, et al: Acute leukemia of adults: Ultrastructural, cytochemical, and histological observations in 100 cases. *Am J Pathol* 73:459, 1980.
201. San Miguel JF, Conzalez M, Canizo MC, et al: TdT activity in acute myeloid leukemias defined by monoclonal antibodies. *Am J Hematol* 23:9, 1986.
202. Kaplan SS, Penchansky L, Krause JR, et al: Simultaneous evaluation of terminal deoxynucleotidyl transferase and myeloperoxidase in acute leukemias using an immunocytochemical method. *Am J Clin Pathol* 87:732, 1987.
203. Kahl C, Florschü tz A, Müller G, et al: Prognostic significance of dysplastic features of hematopoiesis in patients with de novo acute myelogenous leukemia. *Ann Hematol* 75:91, 1997.
204. Manoharan A, Horsley R, Pitney WR: The reticulin content of bone marrow in acute leukemia in adults. *Br J Haematol* 43:185, 1979.
205. Moehler TM, Ho AD, Goldschmidt H, Barlogie B: Angiogenesis in hematologic malignancies. *Crit Rev Oncol Hematol* 45:227, 2003.
206. Albitar M: Angiogenesis in acute myeloid leukemia and myelodysplastic syndrome. *Acta Haematol* 106:170, 2001.
207. Ghannadan M, Wimazal F, Simonitsch I, et al: Immunohistochemical detection of VEGF in the bone marrow of patients with acute myeloid leukemia. Correlation between VEGF expression and the FAB category. *Am J Clin Pathol* 119:663, 2003.
208. Chi Y, Lindgren V, Quigley S, Gaitonde S: Acute myelogenous leukemia with t(6;9)(p23;q34) and marrow basophilia: An overview. *Arch Pathol Lab Med* 132:1835, 2008.
209. Seiter K: Diagnosis and management of core-binding factor leukemias. *Curr Hematol Rep* 2:78, 2003.
210. Moore MAS, Spitzer G, Williams N, et al: Agar culture studies in 127 cases of untreated acute leukemia: The prognostic value of reclassification of leukemia according to in vitro growth characteristics. *Blood* 44:1, 1974.
211. Knudtzon S: *In vitro* culture of leukaemic cells from 81 patients with acute leukemia. *Scand J Haematol* 18:377, 1977.
212. Spitzer G, Dicke KA, McCredre KB, Barlogie B: The early detection of remission in acute myelogenous leukaemia by *in vitro* cultures. *Br J Haematol* 35:411, 1977.
213. Goldberg J, Tice D, Nelson DA, Gottliev AJ: Predictive value of *in vitro* colony and cluster formation in acute nonlymphocytic leukemia. *Am J Med Sci* 277:81, 1979.
214. Mrózek K, Heinonen K, De la Chapelle A, Bloomfield C: Clinical significance of cytogenetics in acute myeloid leukemia. *Semin Oncol* 24:17, 1997.
215. Schoch C, Haferlach T, Haase D, et al: Patients with *de novo* acute myeloid leukaemia and complex karyotype aberrations show a poor prognosis despite intensive treatment: A study of 90 patients. *Br J Haematol* 112:118, 2001.
216. Weltermann A, Fonatsch C, Haas OA, et al: Impact of cytogenetics on the prognosis of adults with *de novo* AML in first relapse. *Leukemia* 18:293, 2004.
217. Martinez-Climent JA, Lane NJ, Rubin CM, et al: Clinical and prognostic significance of chromosomal abnormalities in childhood acute myeloid leukemia de novo. *Leukemia* 9:95, 1995.
218. Pedersen-Bjergaard J, Philip P: Chromosome characteristics of therapy-related acute nonlymphocytic leukemia and preleukemia: Possible implications for pathogenesis of the disease. *Leuk Res* 11:315, 1987.
219. Zaccarea A, Alimena G, Baccarani M, et al: Cytogenetic analyses in 89 patients with secondary hematologic disorders: Results of a cooperative study. *Cancer Genet Cytogenet* 26:65, 1987.
220. Schoch C, Kern W, Krawitz P, et al: Dependence of age-specific incidence of acute myeloid leukemia on karyotype. *Blood* 98:3500, 2002.
221. Marcucci G, Radmacher MD, Maharry K, et al: MicroRNA expression in cytogenetically normal acute myeloid leukemia. *N Engl J Med* 358:1919, 2008.
222. Byrd JC, Lawrence D, Arthur DC, et al: Patients with isolated trisomy 8 in acute myeloid leukemia are not cured with cytarabine-based chemotherapy: Results from Cancer and Leukemia Group B 8461. *Clin Cancer Res* 4:1235, 1998.
223. Melnick A, Licht J: Deconstructing a disease, RARalpha, its fusion partners, and their roles in the pathogenesis of acute promyelocytic leukemia. *Blood* 93:3167, 1999.
224. LoCoco F, Diverio D, Falini B, et al: Genetic diagnosis and molecular monitoring in the management of acute promyelocytic leukemia. *Blood* 94:12, 1999.
225. Mrózek K, Heinonen K, Lawrence D, et al: Adult patients with *de novo* acute myeloid leukemia and t(9;11) (p22;q23) have a superior outcome to patients with other translocations involving band 11q23: A Cancer and Leukemia Group B study. *Blood* 90:4532, 1997.
226. Poirel H, Rack K, Dalbesse E, et al: Incidence and characterization of MLL gene (11q23) rearrangements in acute myeloid leukemia M1 and M5. *Blood* 87:2496, 1996.
227. Schoch C, Schnittger S, Klaus M, et al: AML with 11q23/MLL abnormalities as defined by the WHO classification: Incidence, partner chromosomes, FAB subtype, age distribution, and prognostic impact in an unselected series of 1897 cytogenetically analyzed AML cases. *Blood* 102:2395, 2003.
228. Swansbury GJ, Slater R, Bain BJ, et al: Hematologic malignancies with t(9;11) (p21–22; q23)—A laboratory and clinical study of 125 cases. *Leukemia* 12:792, 1998.
229. Huret JL, Dessen P, Bernheim A, et al: An atlas on chromosomes in hematological malignancies. Example 11q23 and MLL. *Leukemia* 15:987, 2001.
230. Scholl C, Breitinger H, Schlenk RF, et al: Development of a real-time RT-PCR assay for the quantification of the most frequent MLL/AF9 fusion types resulting from translocation t(9;11)(p22;q23) in acute myeloid leukemia. *Genes Chromosomes Cancer* 38:274, 2003.
231. Meyer C, Schneider B, Jakob S, et al: The MLL recombinome of acute leukemias. *Leukemia* 20:777, 2006.
232. Soupir CP, Vergilio JA, Dal Cin P, et al: Philadelphia chromosome-positive acute myeloid leukemia: A rare aggressive leukemia with clinicopathologic features distinct from chronic myeloid leukemia in myeloid blast crisis, *Am J Clin Pathol* 127:642, 2007.
233. Tien H-F, Wang C-W, Chuang S-M, et al: Characterization of Philadelphia-chromosome-positive acute leukemia by clinical, cytochemical, and gene analysis. *Leukemia* 6:907, 1992.
234. Duchayne E, Fenneteau O, Pages MP, et al: Acute megakaryoblastic leukaemia: A national clinical and biological study of 53 adult and childhood cases by the Groupe Français d'Hématologie Cellulaire (GFHC). *Leuk Lymphoma* 44:49, 2003.
235. Billstrom R, Ahlgren T, Bekassy AN, et al: Acute myeloid leukemia with inv(16)(p13q22): Involvement of cervical lymph nodes and tonsils is common and may be a negative prognostic sign. *Am J Hematol* 71:15, 2002.
236. Speck NA, Gilliland DG: Core-binding factors in haematopoiesis and leukaemia. *Nat Rev Cancer* 2:502, 2002.
237. Delauney J, Ve3y N, Leblanc T, et al: Prognosis of Inv 16/t(16;16) acute myeloid leukemia (AML): A survey of 110 cases from the French AML Intergroup. *Blood* 102:462, 2003.
238. Poirel H, Radford-Weiss I, Rack K, et al: Detection of the chromosome 16 CBFβ-MYH11 fusion transcript in myelomonocytic leukemias. *Blood* 85:1313, 1995.
239. Haferlach T, Winkemann M, Löffler H, et al: The abnormal eosinophils are part of the leukemic cell population in acute myelomonocytic leukemia with abnormal eosinophils (AML M4 Eo) and carry pericentric inversion 16: A combination of May-Grünwald-Giemsa a staining and fluorescence *in situ* hybridization. *Blood* 87:2459, 1996.
240. Secker-Walker LM, Mehta A, Bain B: Abnormalities of 3q21 and 3q26 in myeloid malignancy: A United Kingdom Cancer Cytogenetic Group study. *Br J Haematol* 91:490, 1995.
241. Kjellstrand CM, Campbell DC, Von Hartitzsch B, Buselmeier TJ: Hyperuricemic acute renal failure. *Arch Intern Med* 133:349, 1974.
242. O'Regan S, Carson S, Chesney RW, Drummond KN: Electrolyte and acid–base disturbances in the management of leukemia. *Blood* 49:345, 1977.
243. Mir MA, Delamore IW: Metabolic disorders in acute myeloid leukaemia. *Br J Haematol* 40:79, 1978.
244. Bergman GE, Baluarte HJ, Naiman JL: Diabetes insipidus as a presenting manifestation of acute myelogenous leukemia. *J Pediatr* 88:355, 1976.
245. Mir MA, Brabin B, Tang OT, et al: Hypokalemia in acute myeloid leukaemia. *Ann Intern Med* 82:54, 1975.
246. Salomon J: Spurious hypoglycemia and hyperkalemia in myelomonocytic leukemia. *Am J Med Sci* 267:359, 1974.
247. Bellevue R, Disik H, Speigel G, Gussoff BD: Pseudohyperkalemia and extreme leukocytosis. *J Lab Clin Med* 85:660, 1975.
248. Fox MJ, Brody JS, Weintraub LR, et al: Leukocyte larceny: A cause of spurious hypoxia. *Am J Med* 67:742, 1979.
249. Palva IP, Salokannel SJ: Hypercalcemia in acute leukemia. *Blut* 24:209, 1972.
250. Zidar BL, Shadduck RK, Winkelstein A, et al: Acute myeloblastic leukemia and hypercalcemia. *N Engl J Med* 295:692, 1976.
251. Roth GJ, Poite D: Chronic lactic acidosis and acute leukemia. *Arch Intern Med* 125:317, 1970.
252. Wainer RA, Wiernik PH, Thompson WL: Metabolic and therapeutic studies of a patient with acute leukemia and severe lactic acidosis of prolonged duration. *Am J Med* 55:255, 1973.
253. Zamkoff KW, Kirshner JJ: Marked hypophosphatemia associated with acute myelomonocytic leukemia. *Arch Intern Med* 140:1523, 1980.
254. Pflüger K-H, Gramse M, Gropp C, Havemann K: Ectopic ACTH production with autoantibody formation in a patient with acute myeloblastic leukemia. *N Engl J Med* 305:1632, 1981.
255. Carpenter NA, Fiere DM, Schuh D, et al: Circulating immune complexes and the prognosis of acute myeloid leukemia. *N Engl J Med* 307:1174, 1982.
256. Bratt G, Bromback M, Paul C, et al: Factors and inhibitors of blood coagulation and fibrinolysis in acute nonlymphoblastic leukaemia. *Scand J Haematol* 34:332, 1985.
257. Reddy VB, Kowal-Vern A, Hoppensteadt DA, et al: Global and molecular hemostatic markers in acute myeloid leukemia. *Am J Clin Pathol* 94:397, 1990.
258. Tsumita Y, Matsushima T, Uchiumi H, et al: Acute myeloid leukemia accompanied by multiple thrombophlebitis. *Intern Med* 36:595, 1997.
259. Weltermann A, Pabinger I, Geiseler K, et al: Hypofibrinogenemia in non-M3 acute myeloid leukemia. Incidence, clinical and laboratory characteristics and prognosis. *Leukemia* 12:1182, 1998.
260. Spertini O, Callegari P, Cordey A-S, et al: High levels of the shed form of L-selectin are present in patients with acute leukemia and inhibit blast cell adhesion to activated endothelium. *Blood* 84:1249, 1994.
261. Lossos IS, Bogomolski-Yahalom V, Matzner Y: Anticardiolipin antibodies in acute myeloid leukemia: Prevalence and significance. *Am J Hematol* 57:139, 1998.

262. Wierzbowska A, Robak T, Wrzesien-Kus A, et al: Circulating VEGF and its soluble receptors sVEGFR-1 and sVEGFR-2 in patients with acute leukemia. *Eur Cytokine Netw* 14:149, 2003.
263. Greenwood MJ, Seftel MD, Richardson C, et al: Leukocyte count as a predictor of death during remission induction in acute myeloid leukemia. *Leuk Lymphoma* 47:1245, 2006.
264. Lichtman MA, Heal J, Rowe JM: Hyperleukocytic leukaemia: Rheological and clinical features and management. *Baillieres Clin Haematol* 1:725, 1987.
265. Nowacki P, Zdziarska B, Fryze C, Urasinski I: Co-existence of thrombocytopenia and hyperleukocytosis ("critical period") as a risk factor of haemorrhage into the central nervous system in patients with acute leukaemias. *Haematologia (Budap)* 31:347, 2002.
266. Wurthner JU, Kohler G, Behringer D, et al: Leukostasis followed by hemorrhage complicating the initiation of chemotherapy in patients with acute myeloid leukemia and hyperleukocytosis: A clinicopathologic report of four cases. *Cancer* 85:368, 1999.
267. Ventura GJ, Hester JP, Smith TL, Keating MJ: Acute myeloblastic leukemia with hyperleukocytosis: Risk factors for early mortality in induction. *Am J Hematol* 27:34, 1988.
268. Dutcher J, Schiffer CA, Wiernik PH: Hyperleukocytosis in adult acute nonlymphocytic leukemia: Impact on remission rate, duration, and survival. *J Clin Oncol* 5:1364, 1987.
269. VanBuchem MA, Te Velde J, Willemze R, Spaander PJ: Leucostasis, an underestimated cause of death in leukaemia. *Blut* 56:39, 1988.
270. Dilek I, Uysal A, Demirer T, et al: Acute myeloblastic leukemia associated with hyperleukocytosis and diabetes insipidus. *Leuk Lymphoma* 30:657, 1998.
271. Lavabre-Bertrand T, Bourquard P, Chiesa J, et al: Diabetes insipidus revealing acute myelogenous leukaemia with a high platelet count, monosomy 7 and abnormalities of chromosome 3: A new entity? *Eur J Haematol* 66:66, 2001.
272. Inaba H, Fan Y, Pounds S, et al: Clinical and biologic features and treatment outcome of children with newly diagnosed acute myeloid leukemia and hyperleukocytosis. *Cancer* 113:522, 2008.
273. Bug G, Anargyrou K, Tonn T, et al: Impact of leukapheresis on early death rate in adult acute myeloid leukemia presenting with hyperleukocytosis. *Transfusion* 47:1843, 2007.
274. Nagler A, Brenner B, Zuckerman E, et al: Acute respiratory failure in hyperleukocytic acute myeloid leukemia. *Am J Hematol* 27:65, 1988.
275. Von Eyben FE, Siddiqui MZ, Spanosi G: High-voltage irradiation and hydroxyurea for pulmonary leukostasis in acute myelomonocytic leukemia. *Acta Haematol* 77:180, 1987.
276. Azoulay E, Fieux F, Moreau D, et al: Acute monocytic leukemia presenting as respiratory failure. *Am J Respir Crit Care Med* 167:1329, 2003.
277. Koote AMM, Thompson J, Bruijn JA: Acute myelocytic leukemia with acute aortic occlusion as presenting symptoms. *Acta Haematol* 75:120, 1986.
278. Foss R, Haddad M, Zaizov R, et al: Recurrent peripheral arterial occlusion by leukemic cells sedimentation in acute promyelocytic leukemia. *J Pediatr Surg* 27:665, 1992.
279. Mataix R, Gómez-Casares MT, Campo C, et al: Acute leg ischaemia as a presentation of hyperleukocytosis syndrome in acute myeloid leukaemia. *Am J Hematol* 51:250, 1996.
280. Murray JC, Dorfman SR, Brandt ML, Dreyer ZE: Renal venous thrombosis complicating acute myeloid leukemia in the hyperleukocytosis. *J Pediatr Hematol Oncol* 18:327, 1996.
281. Cohen Y, Amir G, Da'as N, et al: Acute myocardial infarction as the presenting symptom of acute myeloblastic leukemia with extreme hyperleukocytosis. *Am J Hematol* 71:47, 2002.
282. Zhang W, Zhang X, Fan X, et al: Effect of ICAM-1 and LFA-1 in hyperleukocytic acute myeloid leukaemia. *Clin Lab Haematol* 28:177, 2006.
283. Berdeaux DH, Glosser L, Serokmann R: Hypoplastic acute leukemia. Review of 70 cases with multivariate regression analysis. *Hematol Oncol* 4:291, 1986.
284. Tuzuner N, Cox C, Rowe JM, Bennett JM: Hypocellular acute leukemia. *Hematol Pathol* 9:195, 1995.
285. Nagai K, Kohno T, Chen Y-X, et al: Diagnostic criteria for hypocellular acute leukemia. *Leuk Res* 7:563, 1996.
286. Bennett JM, Orazi A: Diagnostic criteria to distinguish hypocellular acute myeloid leukemia from hypocellular myelodysplastic syndromes and aplastic anemia: Recommendations for a standardized approach. *Haematologica* 94:264, 2009.
287. Iwakiri R, Ohta M, Mikoshiba M, et al: Prognosis of elderly patients with acute myelogenous leukemia: Analysis of 126 AML cases. *Int J Hematol* 75:45, 2002.
288. Barlogie B, Johnston DA, Keating M, et al: Evolution of oligoleukemia. *Cancer* 53:2115, 1984.
289. Maddox A-M, Keating MJ, Smith TL, et al: Prognostic factors for survival of 194 patients with low infiltrate leukemia. *Leuk Res* 10:995, 1986.
290. Niissler V, Sauer H, Pelka-Fleischer R, et al: Clinical, biochemical and cytokinetic parameters for distinguishing smouldering and rapidly proliferating variants of acute leukaemia. *Eur J Haematol* 45:19, 1990.
291. Paietta E, Racevskis J, Bennett JM, et al: Biologic heterogeneity in Philadelphia chromosome-positive acute leukemia with myeloid morphology. *Leukemia* 12:1881, 1998.
292. Keung YK, Beaty M, Powell BL, et al: Philadelphia chromosome positive myelodysplastic syndrome and acute myeloid leukemia—Retrospective study and review of literature. *Leuk Res* 28:579, 2004.
293. Saikevych IA, Kerrigan DP, McConnell TS, et al: Multiparameter analysis of acute mixed lineage leukemia: Correlation of a B/myeloid immunophenotype and immunoglobulin and T-cell receptor gene rearrangements with the presence of the Philadelphia chromosome translocation in acute leukemias with myeloid morphology. *Leukemia* 5:373, 1991.
294. Neuman MP, deSolas I, Parkin JL, et al: Monoclonal antibody study of Philadelphia chromosome-positive blastic leukemias using the alkaline phosphatase anti-alkaline phosphatase (APAAP) technique. *Am J Clin Pathol* 85:564, 1986.
295. Cuneo A, Ferrant A, Michaux JL, et al: Philadelphia chromosome-positive acute myeloid leukemia: Cytoimmunologic and cytogenetic features. *Haematologica* 81:423, 1996.
296. Bornstein RS, Nesbit M, Kennedy BJ: Chronic myelogenous leukemia presenting in blast crisis. *Cancer* 30:939, 1972.
297. Peterson LC, Bloomfield CD, Brunning RD: Blast crisis as an initial or terminal manifestation of chronic myeloid leukemia. *Am J Med* 60:209, 1976.
298. Worm A-M, Pedersen-Bjergaard J: Chronic myelocytic leukemia presenting in blast transformation. *Scand J Haematol* 18:288, 1977.
299. Kantarjian HM, Talpaz M, Chingra K, et al: Significance of the p210 versus p190 molecular abnormalities in adults with Philadelphia chromosome-positive acute leukemia. *Blood* 78:2411, 1991.
300. Chen SJ, Flandrin G, Daniel M-T, et al: Philadelphia-positive acute leukemia: Lineage promiscuity and inconsistently rearranged breakpoint cluster region. *Leukemia* 2:261, 1988.
301. Price CM, Rasool F, Shirji MKK, et al: Rearrangement of the breakpoint cluster region and expression of p210 BCR-ABL in a "masked" Philadelphia chromosome-positive acute myeloid leukemia. *Blood* 72:1829, 1988.
302. Westbrook CA, Hooberman AL, Spino C, et al: Clinical significance of the BCR-ABL fusion gene in adult acute lymphoblastic leukemia: A Cancer and Leukemia Group B study. *Blood* 80:2983, 1992.
303. Lim LC, Heng KK, Vellupillai M, et al: Molecular and phenotypic spectrum of de novo Philadelphia positive acute leukemia. *Int J Mol Med* 4:665, 1999.
304. Vandenberghe E, Martiat P, Baens M, et al: Megakaryoblastic leukemia with an N-ras mutation and late acquisition of a Philadelphia chromosome. *Leukemia* 5:683, 1991.
305. Helenglass G, Testa JR, Schiffer CA: Philadelphia chromosome-positive acute leukemia. *Am J Hematol* 25:311, 1987.
306. Mecucci C, Noens L, Aventin A, et al: Philadelphia-positive acute myelomonocytic leukemia with inversion of chromosome 16 and eosinobasophils. *Am J Hematol* 27:69, 1988.
307. Kurzrock R, Shtalrid M, Talpaz M, et al: Expression of c-abl in Philadelphia-positive acute myelogenous leukemia. *Blood* 70:1584, 1987.
308. Smadja N, Krulik M, DeGramont A, et al: Acquisition of Philadelphia chromosome concomitant with transformation of a refractory anemia into acute leukemia. *Cancer* 55:1477, 1985.
309. Primo D, Tabernero MD, Rasillo A, et al: Patterns of BCR/ABL gene rearrangements by interphase fluorescence in situ hybridization (FISH) in BCR/ABL+ leukemia: Incidence and underlying genetic abnormalities. *Leukemia* 17:1124, 2003.
310. LoCoco F, Basso G, DiCello PF, et al: Molecular characterization of Ph^1+ hybrid acute leukemia. *Leuk Res* 13:1061, 1989.
311. Janssens AM, Offner FC, Van Hove WZ: Bone marrow necrosis. *Cancer* 88:1769, 2000.
312. Vermeersch P, Zachee P, Brusselmans C: Acute myeloid leukemia with bone marrow necrosis and Charcot Leyden crystals. *Am J Hematol* 82:1029, 2007.
313. Yumura-Yagi K, Hara J, Talva A, Kawa-Ha K: Phenotypic characteristics of acute megakaryocytic leukemia and transient myelopoiesis. *Leuk Lymphoma* 13:393, 1994.
314. Bhatt S, Schreck R, Graham JM, et al: Transient leukemia with trisomy 21. *Am J Med Genet* 58:310, 1995.
315. Litz CE, Davies S, Brunning RD, et al: Acute leukemia and the transient myeloproliferative disorder associated with Down syndrome: Morphologic immunophenotypic and cytogenetic manifestations. *Leukemia* 9:1432, 1999.
316. Ito E, Kasai M, Hayashi Y, et al: Expression of erythroid-specific genes in acute megakaryoblastic leukaemia and transient myeloproliferative disorder in Down syndrome. *Br J Haematol* 90:607, 1995.
317. Kurukashi H, Junichi H, Keiko Y, et al: Monoclonal nature of transient abnormal myelopoiesis in Down's syndrome. *Blood* 77:1161, 1991.
318. Apollonsky N, Shende A, Ouansafi I, et al: Transient myeloproliferative disorder in neonates with and without Down syndrome: A tale of 2 syndromes. *J Pediatr Hematol Oncol* 30:860, 2008.
319. Muramatsu H, Kato K, Watanabe N, et al: Risk factors for early death in neonates with Down syndrome and transient leukaemia. *Br J Haematol* 142:610, 2008.
320. Gamis AS, Hilden J: Transient myeloproliferative disorder. *J Pediatr Hematol Oncol* 241:2, 2002.
321. Gurbuxani S, Vyas P, Crispino JD: Recent insights into the mechanism of myeloid leukemogenesis in Down syndrome. *Blood* 103:399, 2004.
322. Zipursky A, Poon A, Doyle J: Leukemia in Down syndrome: A review. *Pediatr Hematol Oncol* 9:139, 1992.
323. Creutzig U, Ritter J, Vormoor J, et al: Myelodysplasia and acute myelogenous leukemia in Down's syndrome. *Leukemia* 10:1677, 1996.
324. Avet-Loiseau H, Mechinaud F, Harousseau J-L: Clonal hematologic disorders in Down syndrome. *J Pediatr Hematol Oncol* 17:19, 1995.
325. Taub J, Huang X, Ge Y, et al: Cystathionine-beta-synthase cDNA transfection alters sensitivity and metabolism of 1-beta-D-arabinofuranosylcytosine in CCRF-CEM leukemic cells *in vitro* and *in vivo*: A model of leukemia in Down syndrome. *Cancer Res* 60:6421, 2000.
326. Lange BJ, Kobrinsky N, Barnard DR, et al: Distinctive demography, biology, and outcome of acute myeloid leukemia and myelodysplastic syndrome in children with Down syndrome: Children's Cancer Group Studies 2861 and 2891. *Blood* 91:608, 1998.

327. McCoy JP Jr, Overton WR: Immunophenotyping of congenital leukemia. *Cytometry* 22:85, 1995.
328. Kempski HM, Chessells JM, Reeves BR: Deletions of chromosome 21 restricted to the leukemia cells of children with Down syndrome and leukemia. *Leukemia* 11:1973, 1997.
329. Hama A, Yagasaki H, Takahashi Y, et al: Acute megakaryoblastic leukaemia (AMKL) in children: A comparison of AMKL with and without Down syndrome. *Br J Haematol* 140:552, 2008.
330. Hasle H, Abrahamsson J, Arola M, et al: Myeloid leukemia in children 4 years or older with Down syndrome often lacks GATA1 mutation and cytogenetics and risk of relapse are more akin to sporadic AML. *Leukemia* 22:1428, 2008.
331. Ravindranath Y, Abella E, Kruscher JP, et al: Acute myeloid leukemia (AML) in Down's syndrome is highly responsive to chemotherapy: Experience on Pediatric Oncology Group AML Study 8498. *Blood* 80:2210, 1992.
332. Pui C-H, Kane JR, Crist WM: Biology and treatment of infant leukemias. *Leukemia* 9:762, 1995.
333. Lampert F, Harbott J, Ritterbach J: Cytogenetic findings in acute leukaemias of infants. *Br J Cancer* 66(suppl XVII):S20, 1992.
334. Nagasaka M, Maeda S, Maeda H, et al: Four cases of t(4;11) acute leukemia and its myelomonocytic nature in infants. *Blood* 61:1174, 1983.
335. Hunger SP, Cleary ML: What significance should we attribute to the detection of MLL fusion transcripts? *Blood* 92:709, 1998.
336. Bresters D, Reus AC, Veerman AJ, et al: Congenital leukaemia: The Dutch experience and review of the literature. *Br J Haematol* 7:513, 2002.
337. Osada S, Horibe K, Oiwa K, et al: A case of infantile acute monocytic leukemia caused by vertical transmission of the mother's leukemic cells. *Cancer* 65:1146, 1990.
338. Lampkin BC, Peipon JJ, Price JK, et al: Spontaneous remission of presumed congenital acute nonlymphoblastic leukemia (ANLL) in a karyotypically normal neonate. *Am J Pediatr Hematol Oncol* 7:346, 1985.
339. Lauria F, Raspadori D, Ventura MA, et al: The presence of lymphoid-associated antigens in adult acute myeloid leukemia is devoid of prognostic relevance. *Stem Cells* 13:428, 1995.
340. Carbonell F, Swansbury J, Min T, et al: Cytogenetic findings in acute biphenotypic leukaemia. *Leukemia* 10:1283, 1996.
341. Gagnon GA, Childs CC, LeMaistre A, et al: Molecular heterogeneity in acute leukemia lineage switch. *Blood* 74:2088, 1989.
342. Greaves MF, Chan LC: Mixed lineage leukemia: The implication for hemopoietic differentiation [letter]. *Blood* 68:598, 1986.
343. Greaves MF, Chan LC, Furley AJW, et al: Lineage promiscuity in hemopoietic differentiation and leukemia. *Blood* 67:1, 1986.
344. Schmidt CA, Przybylski GK: What can we learn from leukemia as for the process of lineage commitment in hematopoiesis? *Int Rev Immunol* 20:107, 2001.
345. Neame PB, Soamboonsrup P, Browman G, et al: Simultaneous or sequential expression of lymphoid and myeloid phenotypes in acute leukemia. *Blood* 65:142, 1985.
346. Scott CS, Vulliamy T, Catovsky D, et al: DNA genotypic conservation during phenotypic switch from T-cell acute lymphoblastic leukaemia to acute myeloblastic leukaemia. *Leuk Lymphoma* 1:21, 1989.
347. Jensen AW, Hokland M, Jorgensen H, et al: Solitary expression of CD 7 among T-cell antigens in acute myeloid leukemia. *Blood* 78:1291, 1991.
348. Ferra F, DelVecchio L: Clinical relevance of acute mixed-lineage leukemia. *Blood* 79:2799, 1992.
349. Miwa H, Nakase K, Kita K: Biological characteristics of CD7(+) acute leukemia. *Leuk Lymphoma* 21:239, 1996.
350. Suzuki R, Yamamoto K, Seto M, et al: CD7+ and CD56+ myeloid/ natural killer cell precursor acute leukemia: A distinct hematolymphoid disease entity. *Blood* 90:2417, 1997.
351. Scott AA, Head DR, Kropecky KJ, et al: HLA-DR–, CD33+, CD56+, CD16– myeloid/natural killer cell acute leukemia. *Blood* 84:244, 1994.
352. Paietta E, Gallagher RE, Wiernik PH: Myeloid/natural killer cell acute leukemia. *Blood* 84:2824, 1994.
353. Lee PS, Lin CN, Liu C, et al: Acute leukemia with myeloid, B-, and natural killer cell differentiation. *Arch Pathol Lab Med* 127:E93, 2003.
354. Handa H, Motohashi S, Isozumi K, et al: CD7+ and CD56+ myeloid/ natural killer cell precursor acute leukemia treated with idarubicin and cytosine arabinoside. *Acta Haematol* 108:47, 2002.
355. Oshimi K: Progress in understanding and managing natural killer-cell malignancies. *Br J Haematol* 139:532, 2007.
356. Inhorn RC, Aster JC, Roach SA, et al: A syndrome of lymphoblastic lymphoma, eosinophilia, and myeloid hyperplasia malignancy associated with t(8;13) (p11;q11): Description of a distinctive clinical entity. *Blood* 85:1881, 1995.
357. Still IH, Chernova O, Hurd D, et al: Molecular characterization of the t(8;13) (p11;q12) translocation associated with an atypical myeloproliferative disorder: Evidence for three discrete loci involved in myeloid leukemias on 8 p11. *Blood* 90:3136, 1997.
358. Ogura K, Kimura F, Kobayashi S, et al: Myeloid/NK cell precursor acute leukemia lost both CD13 and CD33 at first diagnosis. *Leuk Res* 30:761, 2006.
359. Suzuki R, Suzumiya J, Nakamura S, et al: NK-cell Tumor Study Group. Hematopoietic stem cell transplantation for natural killer-cell lineage neoplasms. *Bone Marrow Transplant* 37:425, 2006.
360. Mirro J, Kitchingman GR, Williams DL, Murphy SB: Mixed lineage leukemia: The implication for hemopoietic differentiation [letter]. *Blood* 68:597, 1986.
361. Ladanyi M, Samaniego F, Reuter VE, et al: Cytogenetic and immunohistochemical evidence for the germ cell origin of a subset of acute leukemias associated with mediastinal germ cell tumors. *J Natl Cancer Inst* 82:221, 1990.
362. DeMent, CR, Roth BJ, Heerema N, et al: Hematologic neoplasia associated with primary mediastinal germ-cell tumors. *Hum Pathol* 21:699, 1990.
363. Nichols CR, Roth BJ, Heerema N, et al: Hematologic neoplasia associated with primary mediastinal germ-cell tumors. *N Engl J Med* 322:1425, 1990.
364. Kiffer JD, Sandeman TF: Primary malignant mediastinal germ cell tumors: A study of eleven cases and a review of the literature. *Int J Radiat Oncol Biol Phys* 17:835, 1990.
365. Nichols CR: Mediastinal germ cell tumors: Clinical features and biologic correlates. *Chest* 99:472, 1991.
366. Brahmanday GR, Gheorghe G, Jaiyesimi IA, et al: Primary mediastinal germ cell tumor evolving into an extramedullary acute megakaryoblastic leukemia causing cord compression. *J Clin Oncol* 26:4686, 2008.
367. Kollmannsberger C, Beyer J, Droz JP, et al: Secondary leukemia following high cumulative doses of etoposide in patients treated for advanced germ cell tumors. *J Clin Oncol* 16:3386, 1998.
368. Miettinen M, Kraszewska E, Sobin LH, Lasota J: A nonrandom association between gastrointestinal stromal tumors and myeloid leukemia. *Cancer* 112:645, 2008.
369. Miyazato H, Sono H, Nasiki Y, et al: Detection of myeloperoxidase gene expression by in situ hybridization in a case of granulocytic sarcoma associated with AML-M0. *Leukemia* 14:1797, 2001.
370. Testa U, Torelli GF, Riccioni R, et al: Human acute stem cell leukemia with multilineage differentiation potential via cascade activation of growth factor receptors. *Blood* 99:4534, 2002.
371. Cuneo A, Ferrant A, Michaux JL, et al: Cytogenetic profile of minimally differentiated (FAB M0) acute myeloid leukemia: Correlation with clinicobiologic findings. *Blood* 85:3688, 1995.
372. Venditti A, Del Poeta G, Buccisano F, et al: Minimally differentiated acute myeloid leukemia (AML M0): Comparison of 25 cases with other French-American-British subtypes. *Blood* 89:621, 1997.
373. Villamor N, Zarco M-A, Rozman M, et al: Acute myeloblastic leukemia with minimal myeloid differentiation: Phenotypical and ultrastructural characteristics. *Leukemia* 12:1071, 1998.
374. Roumier C, Eclache V, Imbert M, et al: M0 AML, clinical and biologic features of the disease, including *AML1* gene mutations. *Blood* 101:1277, 2003.
375. Maruyami F, Stass SA, Estey EH, et al: Detection of AML1/ETO fusion transcript as a tool for diagnosing t(8;21) positive acute myelogenous leukemia. *Leukemia* 8:40, 1994.
376. Schoch C, Haase D, Haferlach T, et al: Fifty-one patients with acute myeloid leukemia and translocation t(8;21) (q22; q22): An additional deletion in 9q is an adverse prognostic factor. *Leukemia* 10:1288, 1996.
377. Wang J, Wang M, Liu JM: Transformation properties of the ETO gene, fusion partner in t(8;21) leukemias. *Cancer Res* 57:2951, 1997.
378. Watkins CH, Hall BE: Monocytic leukemia of the Naegeli and Schilling types. *Am J Clin Pathol* 10:387, 1940.
379. Huhn D, Twardzik L: Acute myelomonocytic leukemia and the French-American-British classification. *Acta Haematol* 69:36, 1983.
380. Scott CS, Morgan M, Limbert HJ, et al: Cytochemical, immunological and ANAE-isoenzyme studies in acute myelomonocytic leukaemia: A study of 39 cases. *Scand J Haematol* 35:284, 1985.
381. Bloomfield CD, Garson OM, Knuutila S, De la Chapelle A: T(1;3)(p36; q21) in acute nonlymphocytic leukemia: A new cytogenetic-clinicopathologic association. *Blood* 66:1409, 1985.
382. Creictzig U, Niederbiermann G, Kitter J, et al: Prognostic significance of eosinophilia in acute myelomonocytic leukemia in relation to induction treatment. *Haematol Blood Transfus* 33:226, 1990.
383. Hoyle CF, Sherrington PD, Fischer P, Hayhoc FGT: Basophils in acute leukemia. *J Clin Pathol* 42:785, 1989.
384. Pearson MG, Vardiman JW, LeBeau MM, et al: Increased numbers of marrow basophils may be associated with t(6;9) in ANLL. *Am J Hematol* 18:393, 1985.
385. Alsabeh R, Byrnes RK, Slovak ML, Arber DA: Acute myeloid leukemia with t(6;9) (p23;q34): Association with myelodysplasia, basophilia, and initial CD34 negative phenotype. *Am J Clin Pathol* 107:430, 1997.
386. Copelli M: Di una emopatia sistemizzata rappresentata da una iperplasia eritroblastica (eritromatosis). *Path Riv Quindicin* 4:460, 1912.
387. DiGuglielmo G: Richerche di hematologia: I. Una casa di eritroleucemia. *Folia Med* 13:386, 1917.
388. Moeschlin S: Erythroblastosen, erythroleukemien und erythroblastamien. *Folia Haematol (Frankf)* 64:262, 1940.
389. Dameshek W: The Di Guglielmo syndrome. *Blood* 13:192, 1940.
390. Fouillard L, Labopin M, Gorin N-C, et al: Hematopoietic stem cell transplantation for *de novo* erythroleukemia: A study of the European Group for Blood and Marrow Transplantation (EBMT). *Blood* 100:3135, 2002.
391. Novick Y, Marino P, Makower DF, Wiernik PH: Familial erythroleukemia: A distinct clinical and genetic type of familial leukemia. *Leuk Lymphoma* 80:395, 1998.
392. Lee EJ, Schiffer CA, Misawa S, Testa JR: Clinical and cytogenetic features of familial erythroleukaemia. *Br J Haematol* 65:313, 1987.

393. Cuneo A, VanOrshoven A, Michaux JL, et al: Morphologic, immunologic and cytogenetic studies in erythroleukemia: Evidence for multilineage involvement and identification of two distinct cytogenetic clinicopathologic types. *Br J Haematol* 75:346, 1990.
394. Goldberg SL, Noel P, Klumpp TR, Dewald GW: The erythroid leukemias. *Am J Clin Oncol* 21:42, 1998.
395. Olopade OI, Thangavelu M, Larson RA, et al: Clinical, morphologic, and cytogenetic characteristics of 26 patients with acute erythroblastic leukemia. *Blood* 80:2873, 1992.
396. Davey FR, Abraham N Jr, Bronetto VL, et al: Morphologic characteristics of erythroleukemia (Acute myeloid leukemia; FAB-M6): A CALGB study. *Am J Hematol* 49:29, 1995.
397. Adamson JW, Finch CA: Erythropoietin and the regulation of erythropoiesis in di Guglielmo's syndrome. *Blood* 36:590, 1970.
398. Mitjavila MT, Villeval JL, Cramer P, et al: Effects of granulocyte-macrophage colony-stimulating factor and erythropoietin on leukemic erythroid colony formation in human early erythroblastic leukemias. *Blood* 70:965, 1987.
399. Mazzella FM, Kowel-Vern A, Shrit MA, et al: Acute erythroleukemia evaluation of 48 cases with reference to classification, cell proliferation, cytogenetics, and prognosis. *Am J Clin Pathol* 110:590, 1998.
400. Breton-Gorius J: Phenotypes of blasts in acute erythroblastic and megakaryoblastic leukemia—A review. *Keio J Med* 36:23, 1987.
401. Peterson BA, Levine EG: Uncommon subtypes of acute nonlymphocytic leukemia: Clinical features and management of FAB M5, M6 and M7. *Semin Oncol* 14:425, 1987.
402. Croizat P, Favre-Gilly J: Les aspects du syndrome hémorrhagiue des leucémies. *Sang* 20:417, 1949.
403. Hillstad LK: Acute promyelocytic leukemia. *Acta Med Scand* 159:189, 1957.
404. LoCoco F, Nervi C, Avvisati G, Mandelli F: Acute promyelocytic leukemia: A curable disease. *Leukemia* 12:1866, 1998.
405. Avvisati G, Lo Coco F, Mandelli F: Acute promyelocytic leukemia: Clinical and morphological features and prognostic factors. *Semin Hematol* 38:4, 2001.
406. Estey E, Thall P, Kantarjian H, et al: Association between increased body mass index and a diagnosis of acute promyelocytic leukemia in patients with acute myeloid leukemia. *Leukemia* 11:1661, 1997.
407. Golomb HM, Rowley JD, Vardiman J, et al: "Microgranular" acute promyelocytic leukemia: A distinct clinical, ultrastructural, and cyto-genetic entity. *Blood* 55:253, 1980.
408. McKenna RW, Parkin J, Bloomfield C, et al: Acute promyelocytic leukaemia: A study of 39 cases with identification of a hyperbasophilic microgranular variant. *Br J Haematol* 50:201, 1982.
409. Rovelli A, Biondi A, Rajnoldi AC, et al: Microgranular variant of acute promyelocytic leukemia in children. *J Clin Oncol* 10:1413, 1992.
410. Castoldi GL, Liso V, Speechia G, Thomasi P: Acute promyelocytic leukemia: Morphological aspects. *Leukemia* 8(Suppl 2):S27, 1994.
411. Umeda M, Nojima Z, Yamaguchi R, et al: Two cases of acute promyelocytic leukemia with marked basophilia—A variant type of APL with the capability of differentiating into basophils. *Rinsho Ketsueki* 28:2004, 1987.
412. Gotoh H, Murakani S, Oku N, et al: Translocation t(15;17) and t(9;14) (q34;q22) in a case of acute promyelocytic leukemia with increased number of basophils. *Cancer Genet Cytogenet* 36:103, 1988.
413. Yu R-Q, Huang W, Chen S-J, et al: A case of acute eosinophilic granulocytic leukemia with PML-RAR alpha fusion gene expression and response to all-*trans*-retinoic acid. *Leukemia* 11:609, 1997.
414. Invernizzi R, Iannone AM, Bernuzzi S, et al: Acute promyelocytic leukemia toluidine blue subtype. *Leuk Lymphoma* 18(Suppl 1):57, 1995.
415. Rowley JD, Golomb HM, Dogherty C: 15/17 translocation, a consistent chromosomal change in acute promyelocytic leukaemia. *Lancet* 1:549, 1977.
416. Lavau C, Dejean A: The t(15;17) translocation in acute promyelocytic leukemia. *Leukemia* 8:1615, 1994.
417. Sainty D, Liso V, Cantu-Rajnoldi A, et al: A new morphologic classification system for acute promyelocytic leukemia distinguishes cases with underlying PLZF/RARA gene rearrangements. *Blood* 96:1287, 2000.
418. Petti MC, Fazi F, Gentile M, et al: Complete remission through blast differentiation in PLZF/RARα-positive acute promyelocytic leukemia: *In vitro* and *in vivo* studies. *Blood* 100:1065, 2002.
419. DeThé H, Chomienne C, Lanotte M, et al: The t(15;17) translocation of acute promyelocytic leukaemia fuses the retinoic acid receptor α-gene to a novel transcribed locus. *Nature* 347:558, 1990.
420. Huang W, Sun G-L, Li X-S, et al: Acute promyelocytic leukemia: Clinical relevance of two major PML-RARα isoforms and detection of minimal residual disease by retrotranscriptase/polymerase chain reaction to predict relapse. *Blood* 82:1264, 1993.
421. Rego EM, Pandolfi PP: Analysis of molecular genetics of acute promyelocytic leukemia in mouse models. *Semin Hematol* 38:54, 2001.
422. Dombret H, Scrobohaci ML, Ghorra P, et al: Coagulation disorder associated with acute promyelocytic leukemia: Correct effect of all-*trans* retinoic acid. *Leukemia* 7:2, 1993.
423. Tallman MS, Kwaan HC: Reassessing the hemostatic disorder associated with acute promyelocytic leukemia. *Blood* 79:543, 1992.
424. Barbui T, Finazzi G, Falanga A: The impact of all-*trans* retinoic acid on the coagulopathy of acute promyelocytic leukemia. *Blood* 91:3093, 1998.
425. Menell JS, Cesarman GM, Jacovina AT, et al: Annexin II and bleeding in acute promyelocytic leukemia. *N Engl J Med* 340:994, 1999.
426. Avvisati G, Ten Cate JW, Büller H, Mandelli F: Tranexamic acid for control of haemorrhage in patients with acute promyelocyte leukaemia. *Lancet* ii:122, 1989.
427. Tallman MS, Abutalib SA, Altman JK: The double hazard of thrombophilia and bleeding in acute promyelocytic leukemia. *Semin Thromb Hemost* 33:330, 2007.
428. Fenaux P, Tertian G, Castaigne S, et al: A randomized trial of amsacrine and rubidazone on 39 patients with acute promyelocytic leukemia. *J Clin Oncol* 9:1556, 1991.
429. Craddock CG, Crandall BF, Como R: Restoration of effective hemopoiesis preceding suppression of leukemia clone in myeloblastic leukemia. *Am J Med* 59:737, 1975.
430. Amato R, Kantarjian H, Walter R, Keating M: Rebound peripheral blastosis with subsequent remission during induction in a patient with acute promyelocytic leukemia. *Cancer* 61:650, 1988.
431. Stone RM, Maguire M, Goldberg MA, et al: Complete remission in acute promyelocytic leukemia despite persistence of abnormal marrow promyelocytes during induction therapy: Experience in 34 patients. *Blood* 71:690, 1988.
432. Breitman TR, Collins SJ, Keene BR: Terminal differentiation of human promyelocytic leukemic cells in primary culture in response to retinoic acid. *Blood* 57:1000, 1981.
433. Huang ME, Ye YC, Chen SR, et al: Use of all-*trans* retinoic acid in the treatment of acute promyelocytic leukemia. *Blood* 72:567, 1988.
434. Wu X, Wang X, Qen X, et al: Four years experience with treatment of all-*trans* retinoic acid in acute promyelocytic leukemia. *Am J Hematol* 43:183, 1993.
435. Lobe I, Regal-Huguet FR, Vekhoff A, et al: Myelodysplastic syndrome after acute promyelocytic leukemia: The European APLK group experience. *Leukemia* 17:1600, 2003.
436. Garcia-Manero G, Kantarjian HM, Kornblau S, Estey E: Therapy-related myelodysplastic syndrome or acute myelogenous leukemia in patients with acute promyelocytic leukemia. *Leukemia* 17:1888, 2002.
437. Reschad H, Schilling-Torgau V: Ueber eine neue Leukämie durch echte Uebergangsformen (Splenozyten-leukämie) und ihre Bedeutung für die Selbstständigkeit dieser Zellen. *Munch Med Wochenschr* 60:1981, 1913.
438. Straus DJ, Mertelsmann R, Koziner B, et al: The acute monocytic leukemias. *Medicine (Baltimore)* 59:409, 1980.
439. Janvier M, Tobelem G, Daniel MT, et al: Acute monoblastic leukaemia. Clinical, biological data and survival in 45 cases. *Scand J Haematol* 32:385, 1984.
440. Finaux P, Vanhaesbroucke C, Estienne MH, et al: Acute monocytic leukaemia in adults: Treatment and prognosis in 99 cases. *Br J Haematol* 75:41, 1990.
441. Fung H, Shepard JD, Naiman SC, et al: Acute monocytic leukemia: A single institution experience. *Leuk Lymphoma* 19:259, 1995.
442. Cuttner J, Conjalka MS, Reilly M, et al: Association of monocyte leukemia in patients with extreme leukocytosis. *Am J Med* 69:555, 1980.
443. Jourdan E, Dombret H, Glaisner S, et al: Unexpected high incidence of intracranial subdural haematoma during intensive chemotherapy for acute myeloid leukaemia with a monoblastic component. *Br J Haematol* 89:527, 1995.
444. Scott CS, Stark AN, Limbert HJ, et al: Diagnostic and prognostic factors in acute monocytic leukemia: An analysis of 51 cases. *Br J Haematol* 69:247, 1988.
445. Scherrer A, Kruithof EKO, Grob J-P: Plasminogen activator inhibitor-2 in patients with monocytic leukemia. *Leukemia* 5:479, 1991.
446. Van Furth R, Van Zwet TL: Cytochemical, functional, and proliferative characteristics of promonocytes and monocytes from patients with monocytic leukemia. *Blood* 62:298, 1983.
447. Van Furth R, Leijh PCJ, Van Zwet TL, Van den Barselaar MT: Phagocytic and intracellular killing by peripheral blood monocytes of patients with monocytic leukemia. *Blood* 59:1234, 1982.
448. Diaz MO, LeBeau MM, Pitha P, Rowley JD: Interferon and *c-est-1* genes in the translocation (9;11)(p22;q23) in human acute monocytic leukemia. *Science* 231:265, 1986.
449. Mavilo F, Testa U, Sposi NM, et al: Selective expression of *fos* protooncogene in human acute myelomonocytic and monocytic leukemias: A molecular marker of terminal differentiation. *Blood* 69:160, 1987.
450. Pinto A, Colletta G, DeVecchio L, et al: *C-fos* oncogene expression in human hemopoietic malignancies is restricted to acute leukemias with monocytic phenotype and to subsets of B cell leukemias. *Blood* 70:1450, 1987.
451. Weide R, Parviz B, Pflüger K-H, Haveman K: Altered expression of the human retinoblastoma gene in monocytic leukaemias. *Br J Haematol* 83:428, 1993.
452. Cuttner J, Seremetis S, Najfield V, et al: TdT-positive acute leukemia with monocytoid characteristics: Clinical, cytochemical, cytogenetic, and immunologic findings. *Blood* 64:237, 1984.
453. Sun T, Wu E: Acute monoblastic leukemia with t(8;16): A distinct clinicopathologic entity. *Am J Hematol* 66:207, 2001.
454. Santiago-Schwarz F, Coppock DL, Hindenburg A, Kern J: Identification of a malignant counterpart of the monocytic-dendritic cell progenitor in acute myeloid leukemia. *Blood* 84:3054, 1994.
455. Pileri SA, Grogan TM, Harris NL, et al: Tumors of histiocytes and accessory dendritic cells: An immunohistochemical approach to classification from the International Lymphoma Study Group based on 61 cases. *Histopathology* 41:1, 2002.
456. Elghetany MT: True histiocytic lymphoma: Is it an entity? *Leukemia* 11:762, 1997.
457. Esteve J, Rozman M, Campo E, et al: Leukemia after true histiocytic lymphoma: Another type of acute monocytic leukemia with histiocytic differentiation (AML-M5c). *Leukemia* 9:1389, 1995.
458. Tallman MS, Kim HT, Paietta E, et al: Acute monocytic leukemia (French-American-British classification M5) does not have a worse prognosis than other subtypes of acute myeloid leukemia: Report from the Eastern Cooperative Group. *J Clin Oncol* 22:1276, 2004.
459. Lewis SM, Szur L: Malignant myelosclerosis. *Br Med J* 2:472, 1963.
460. Bergsman KL, VanSlyck EJ: Acute myelofibrosis. *Ann Intern Med* 74:232, 1971.

461. Huang MJ, Li CY, Nichols WL, et al: Acute leukemia with megakaryocytic differentiation. A study of twelve cases identified immunocytochemically. *Blood* 64:427, 1984.
462. Gassman W, Löffler H: Acute megakaryoblastic leukemia. *Leuk Lymphoma* 18:69, 1995.
463. Cripe LD, Hromas R: Malignant disorders of megakaryocytes. *Semin Hematol* 35:200, 1998.
464. Paredes-Aguilera R, Romero-Guzman L, Lopez-Santiago N, Trejo RA: Biological, clinical, and hematological features of acute megakaryoblastic leukemia in children. *Am J Hematol* 73:71, 2003.
465. Zipursky A, Brown E, Christensen H, et al: Leukemia and/or myeloproliferative syndrome in neonates with Down syndrome. *Semin Perinatol* 21:97, 1997.
466. Hussein K, Bock O, Theophile K, et al: MPL(W515L) mutation in acute megakaryoblastic leukaemia. *Leukemia* 23:852, 2009.
467. Dastugue N, Lafage-Pochitaloff M, Pages MP, et al: Cytogenetic profile of childhood and adult megakaryoblastic leukemia (M7): A study of the Groupe Francais de Cytogenetique Hematologique (GFCH). *Blood* 100:618, 2002.
468. Carroll A, Civin C, Schneider N, et al: The t(1;22)(p13;q13) is non-random and restricted to infants with acute megakaryoblastic leukemia: A pediatric oncology group study. *Blood* 78:748, 1991.
469. Duchayne F, Fenneteau O, Pages MP, et al: Acute megakaryoblastic leukaemia: A national clinical and biological study of adult and childhood cases by the Group Francais d'Hematologie Cellulaire (GFHC). *Leuk Lymphoma* 44:49, 2003.
470. Bernstein J, Dastugue N, Haas OA, et al: Nineteen cases of the t(1;22)(p13;q13) acute megakaryoblastic leukaemia of infants/children and a review of 39 cases: Report from a t(1;22) study group. *Leukemia* 14:216, 2000.
471. Cuneo A, Mecucci C, Kerim S, et al: Multipotent stem cell involvement in megakaryoblastic leukemia: Cytologic and cytogenetic evidence in 15 patients. *Blood* 74:1781, 1989.
472. Dhyashiki K, Ohyashiki JH, Hojo H, et al: Cytogenetic findings in adult acute leukemia in myeloproliferative disorders with an involvement of megakaryocytic lineage. *Cancer* 65:940, 1990.
473. Kojima S, Sako M, Kato K, et al: An effective chemotherapeutic regimen for acute myeloid leukemia and myelodysplastic syndrome in children with Down's syndrome. *Leukemia* 14:786, 2000.
474. Athale UH, Razzouk BI, Raimondi SC, et al: Biology and outcome of childhood acute megakaryoblastic leukemia: A single institution's experience. *Blood* 97:3727, 2001.
475. Yamada S, Hongo T, Okada S, et al: Distinctive multidrug sensitivity and outcome of acute erythroblastic and megakaryoblastic leukemia in children with Down syndrome. *Int J Hematol* 74:428, 2001.
476. Tallman MS, Neuberg D, Bennett JM, et al: Acute megakaryocytic leukemia: The Eastern Cooperative Group experience. *Blood* 96:2405, 2000.
477. Pagano L, Pulsoni A, Vignetti M, et al: Acute megakaryoblastic leukemia: Experience of GIMEMA trial. *Leukemia* 16:1622, 2002.
478. Stillman RG: A case of myeloid leukemia with predominance of eosinophilic cells. *Med Rec* 81:594, 1912.
479. Harrington DS, Peterson C, Ness M, et al: Acute myelogenous leukemia with eosinophilic differentiation. *Am J Clin Pathol* 90:464, 1988.
480. Kueck BD, Smith RE, Parkin J, et al: Eosinophilic leukemia: A myeloproliferative disorder distinct from the hypereosinophilic syndrome. *Hematol Pathol* 5:195, 1991.
481. Sanada I, Asou N, Kajima S, et al: Acute myelogenous leukemia (FABM1) associated with t(5;16) and eosinophilia. *Cancer Genet Cytogenet* 43:139, 1989.
482. Lichtman MA, Segel GB: Uncommon phenotypes of acute myelogenous leukemia: Basophilic, mast cell, eosinophilic, and myeloid dendritic cell subtypes: A review. *Blood Cells Mol Dis* 35:370, 2005.
483. Gabbas AG, Li CF: Acute non-lymphocytic leukemia with eosinophilic differentiation. *Am J Hematol* 21:29, 1986.
484. Brito-Babapulle F: Clonal eosinophilic disorders and the hypereosinophilic syndrome. *Blood Rev* 11:129, 1997.
485. Menssen HD, Renkl H-J, Rieder H, et al: Distinction of eosinophilic leukaemia from idiopathic hypereosinophilic syndrome by analysis of Wilms tumor gene expression. *Br J Haematol* 101:325, 1998.
486. Joachim G: Über mastzellenleukämien. *Dtsch Arch Klin Med* 87:437, 1906.
487. Goh KO, Anderson FW: Cytogenetic studies in basophilic chronic myelocytic leukemia. *Arch Pathol Lab Med* 193:288, 1979.
488. Shvidel L, Shaft D, Stark B, et al: Acute basophilic leukaemia: Eight unsuspected new cases diagnosed by electron microscopy. *Br J Haematol* 120:774, 2003.
489. Yokohama A, Tsukamoto N, Hatsumi N, et al: Acute basophilic leukemia lacking basophil-specific antigens: The importance of cytokine receptor expression in differential diagnosis. *Int J Hematol* 75:309, 2002.
490. Kubota M, Akiyama Y, Tabata Y, et al: Acute nonlymphocytic leukemia with basophilic differentiation and t(9;11)(p22;q23) in a child. *Am J Hematol* 31:133, 1989.
491. Mezger J, Permanetter W, Gerhartz H, et al: Philadelphia chromosome-negative acute hematopoietic malignancy: Ultrastructural, cytochemical, and immunocytochemical evidence of mast cell and basophil differentiation. *Leuk Res* 14:169, 1990.
492. Duchayne E, Demur C, Rubie H, et al: Diagnosis of acute basophilic leukemia. *Leuk Lymphoma* 32:269, 1999.
493. Petersen LC, Parkin JL, Arthur DC, Brunning RD: Acute basophilic leukemia. A clinical, morphologic, and cytogenetic study of eight cases. *Am J Clin Pathol* 96:160, 1991.
494. Kubonishi I, Fijishita M, Niiya K, et al: Basophilic differentiation in acute promyelocytic leukaemia. *Nippon Ketsueki Gakkai Zasshi* 48:1390, 1985.
495. Pardanani AD, Morice WG, Hoyer JD, Tefferi A: Chronic basophilic leukemia: A distinct clinico-pathologic entity. *Eur J Haematol* 71:18, 2003.
496. Travis WD, Li C-Y, Hoaglan HC, et al: Mast cell leukemia. Report of a case and review of the literature. *Mayo Clin Proc* 61:957, 1986.
497. Beghini A, Cairoli R, Morra E, Larizza L: In vivo differentiation of mast cells from acute myeloid leukemia blasts carrying a novel activating ligand-independent c-Kit mutation. *Blood Cells Mol Dis* 24:262, 1998.
498. Sperr WR, Horny HP, Lechner K, Valent P: Clinical and biological diversity of leukemias occurring in patients with mastocytosis. *Leuk Lymphoma* 37:473, 2000.
499. Fukuda T, Kakihara T, Kamishima T, et al: Leukemic cell membrane from acute myelogenous leukemias with massive mast cell infiltration has a mast cell differentiation activity under culture condition containing interleukin 3. *Leuk Res* 18:749, 1994.
500. Valent P, Sperr WR, Samorapoompichit P, et al: Myelomastocytic overlap syndromes: Biology, criteria, and relationship to mastocytosis. *Leuk Res* 25:595, 2001.
501. Levine PH, Weintraub LR: Pseudoleukemia during recovery from dapsone-induced agranulocytosis. *Ann Intern Med* 68:1060, 1968.
502. Sanal SM, Campbell EW, Bowdler AJ, Brat PJ: Pseudoleukemia. *Postgrad Med* 65:143, 1979.
503. Dreskin SC, Iberti TJ, Watson-Williams EJ: Pseudoleukemia due to infection. *J Med* 14:147, 1983.
504. Lanham GR, Dahl GV, Billings FT, Stass SA: *Pseudomonas aeruginosa* infection with marrow suppression simulating acute promyelocytic leukemia. *Am J Clin Pathol* 80:404, 1983.
505. Orchard PJ, Moffet HL, Hafez R, Sondel PM: Pseudomonas sepsis simulating acute promyelocytic leukemia. *Pediatr Infect Dis J* 7:66, 1988.
506. Reykdal S, Sham R, Phatak P, Kouides P: Pseudoleukemia following the use of G-CSF. *Am J Hematol* 49:258, 1995.
507. Innes DJ, Hess CE, Bertholf MF, Wade P: Promyelocyte morphology: Differentiation of acute promyelocytic leukemia from benign myeloid proliferations. *Am J Clin Pathol* 88:725, 1987.
508. Ahmed MA: Promyelocytic leukaemoid reaction: An atypical presentation of mycobacterial infection. *Acta Haematol* 85:143, 1991.
509. Sekeres MA, Elson P, Kalaycio ME: Time from diagnosis to treatment initiation predicts survival in younger, but not older, acute myeloid leukemia patients. *Blood* 113:28, 2009.
510. Rodriguez CP, Baz R, Jawde RA, et al: Impact of socioeconomic status and distance from treatment center on survival in patients receiving remission induction therapy for newly diagnosed acute myeloid leukemia. *Leuk Res* 32:413, 2008.
511. Wedding U, Röhrig B, Klippstein A, et al: Impairment in functional status and survival in patients with acute myeloid leukaemia. *J Cancer Res Clin Oncol* 132:665, 2006.
512. Karthaus M, Doellmann T, Klimasch T, et al: Central venous catheter infections in patients with acute leukemia. *Chemotherapy* 48:154, 2002.
513. Hummel M, Duchheidt D, Reiter S, et al: Successful treatment of hyperuricemia with low doses of recombinant urate oxidase in four patients with hematologic malignancy and tumor lysis syndrome. *Leukemia* 17:2542, 2003.
514. LoCoco F, Pelicci PG, D'Adamo F, et al: Polyclonal hematopoietic reconstitution in leukemia patients in remission after suppression of specific gene rearrangements. *Blood* 82:606, 1993.
515. Lichtman MA: The stem cell in the pathogenesis and treatment of myelogenous leukemia. *Leukemia* 15:1489, 2001.
516. Sanz MA, Jarque I, Martin G, et al: Acute promyelocytic leukemia. *Cancer* 6:7, 1988.
517. Hiddemann W, Spiekermann K, Buske C, et al: Towards a pathogenesis-oriented therapy of acute myeloid leukemia. *Crit Rev Oncol Hematol* 56:235, 2005.
518. Cheson BD, Bennett JM, Kopecky KJ, et al: Revised recommendations of the International Working Group for Diagnosis, Standards for Therapeutic Trials in Acute Myeloid Leukemia. *J Clin Oncol* 21:4642, 2003.
519. Fey M, Dreyling M: ESMO Guidelines Working Group: Acute myeloblastic leukemia in adult patients: ESMO clinical recommendations for diagnosis, treatment and follow-up. *Ann Oncol* 19 Suppl 2:ii58, 2008.
520. National Comprehensive Cancer Network (NCCN) Clinical Practice Guidelines in Oncology. Acute Myeloid Leukemia V.I.2009 http://www.nccn.org/professionals/physician_gls/f_guidelines.asp (last accessed June 2009).
521. Wiernik PH, Banks PLC, Case DC Jr, et al: Cytarabine plus idarubicin or daunorubicin as induction and consolidation therapy for previously untreated adult patients with acute myeloid leukemia. *Blood* 79:313, 1992.
522. Flasshove M, Meusers P, Schutte J, et al: Long-term survival after induction therapy with idarubicin and cytosine arabinoside for *de novo* acute myeloid leukemia. *Ann Hematol* 79:533, 2000.
523. Hargrave RM, Davey MW, Davey RA, Kidman AD: Development of drug resistance in reduced idarubicin relative to other anthracyclines. *Anticancer Drugs* 6:432, 1995.
524. Feldman EJ: High-dose mitoxantrone in acute leukaemia: New York Medical College experience. *Eur J Cancer Care (Engl)* 6:27, 1997.
525. Fernandez HF, Sun Z, Yao X, et al: Anthracycline dose intensification in acute myeloid leukemia. *N Engl J Med* 361:1249, 2009.
526. Lowenberg B, Ossenkoppele GJ, van Putten W, et al: High-dose daunorubicin in older patients with acute myeloid leukema. *N Engl J Med* 361:1235, 2009.
527. Woodlock TJ, Lifton R, DiSalle M: Coincident acute myelogenous leukemia and ischemic heart disease: Use of the cardioprotectant dexrazoxane during induction chemotherapy. *Am J Hematol* 59:246, 1998.
528. Kern W, Estey EH: High-dose cytosine arabinoside in the treatment of acute myeloid leukemia: Review of three randomized trials. *Cancer* 107:116, 2006.

529. Stein AS, O'Donnell MR, Slovak ML, et al: High-dose cytosine arabinoside and daunorubicin induction therapy for adult patients with *de novo* non M3 acute myelogenous leukemia: Impact of cytogenetics on achieving a complete remission. *Leukemia* 14:1191, 2000.
530. Mehta J, Powles R, Treleaven J, et al: The impact of karyotype on remission rates in adult patients with de novo acute myeloid leukemia receiving high-dose cytarabine-based induction chemotherapy. *Leuk Lymphoma* 34:553, 1999.
531. Archimbaud E, Thomas X, Leblond V, et al: Timed sequential chemotherapy for previously treated patients with acute myeloid leukemia: Long-term follow-up of the etoposide, mitoxantrone, and cytarabine-86 trial. *J Clin Oncol* 13:11, 1995.
532. Archimbaud E, Leblond V, Fenaux P, et al: Timed sequential chemotherapy for advanced acute myeloid leukemia. *Hematol Cell Ther* 38:161, 1996.
533. Thomas X, Dombret H: Timed-sequential chemotherapy as induction and/or consolidation regimen for younger adults with acute myelogenous leukemia. *Hematology* 12:15, 2007.
534. Bolanos-Meade J, Karp JE, Guo C, et al: Timed sequential therapy of acute myelogenous leukemia in adults: A phase II study of retinoids in combination with the sequential administration of cytosine arabinoside, idarubicin and etoposide. *Leuk Res* 27:313, 2003.
535. Kell WJ, Burnett AK, Chopra R, et al: A feasibility study of simultaneous administration of gemtuzumab ozogamicin with intensive chemotherapy in induction and consolidation in younger patients with acute myeloid leukemia. *Blood* 102:4277, 2003.
536. Borthakur G, Kantarjian H, Wang X, et al: Treatment of core-binding-factor in acute myelogenous leukemia with fludarabine, cytarabine, and granulocyte colony-stimulating factor results in improved event-free survival. *Cancer* 113:3181, 2008.
537. Holowiecki J, Grosicki S, Robak T, et al: Addition of cladribine to daunomycin and cytarabine increases remission rate after a single course of induction treatment in acute myeloid leukemia. Multicenter phase III study. *Leukemia* 18:989, 2004.
538. Estey EH, Thall PF, Cortes JE, et al: Comparison of idarubicin + ara-C, and topotecan + ara-C-, and topotecan + ara-C-based regimens in treatment of newly diagnosed acute myeloid leukemia, refractory anemia with excess blasts in transformation, or refractory anemia with excess blasts. *Blood* 98:3575, 2001.
539. Giles F: Gemtuzumab ozogamicin: A component of induction therapy in AML? *Leuk Res* 29:1, 2005.
540. Tallman M: Existing and emerging therapeutic options for the treatment of acute myeloid leukemia. *Clin Adv Hematol Oncol* 6:3, 2008.
541. Rowe JM, Neuberg D, Friedenberg W, et al: A phase 3 study of three induction regimens and of priming with GM-CSF in older adults with acute myeloid leukemia: A trial by the Eastern Cooperative Oncology Group. *Blood* 103:479, 2004.
542. Ganser A, Heil G: Use of hematopoietic growth factors in the treatment of acute myelogenous leukemia. *Curr Opin Hematol* 4:191, 1997.
543. Lowenberg B, Van Putten W, Theobald M, et al: Effect of priming with granulocyte colony-stimulating factor on the outcome of chemo-therapy for acute myeloid leukemia. *N Engl J Med* 348:743, 2003.
544. Thomas X, Raffoux E, Botton S, et al: Effect of priming with granulocyte-macrophage colony-stimulating factor in younger adults with newly diagnosed acute myeloid leukemia: A trial by the Acute Leukemia French Association (ALFA) Group. *Leukemia* 21:453, 2007.
545. Nimubona S, Grulois I, Bernard M, et al: Complete remission in hypoplastic acute myeloid leukemia induced by G-CSF without chemo-therapy: Report on three cases. *Leukemia* 16:1872, 2002.
546. Schlenk RF, Benner A, Hartmann F, et al: Risk-adapted postremission therapy in acute myeloid leukemia: Results of the German multicenter AML HD93 treatment trial. *Leuk Res* 17:1521, 2003.
547. Anderlini P, Ghaddar HM, Smith TL, et al: Factors predicting complete remission and subsequent disease-free survival after a second course of induction therapy in patients with acute myelogenous leukemia resistant to the first. *Leukemia* 10:964, 1996.
548. Estey EH, Shen Yu, Thall PF: Effect of time to complete remission on subsequent survival and disease-free survival time in AML, RAEB-t, and RAEB. *Blood* 95:72, 2000.
549. Brandwein JM, Gupta V, Schuh AC, et al: Predictors of response to reinduction chemotherapy for patients with acute myeloid leukemia who do not achieve complete remission with frontline induction chemotherapy. *Am J Hematol* 83:54, 2008.
550. Tsimberidou AM, Estey E: Induction mortality risk in adult acute myeloid leukemia. *Leuk Lymphoma* 47:1199, 2006.
551. Greenwood MJ, Seftel MD, Richardson C, et al: Leukocyte count as a predictor of death during remission induction in acute myeloid leukemia. *Leuk Lymphoma* 47:1245, 2006.
552. Voso MT, Hohaus S, Guidi F, et al: Prognostic role of glutathione S-transferase polymorphisms in acute myeloid leukemia. *Leukemia* 22:1685, 2008.
553. Voso MT, Fabiani E, D'Alo' F, et al: Increased risk of acute myeloid leukaemia due to polymorphisms in detoxification and DNA repair enzymes. *Ann Oncol* 18:1523, 2007.
554. Blum W, Porcu P: Therapeutic apheresis in hyperleukocytosis and hyperviscosity syndrome. *Semin Thromb Hemost* 33:350, 2007.
555. Schmidt JE, Tamburro RF, Sillos EM, et al: Pathophysiology-directed therapy for acute hypoxemic respiratory failure in acute myeloid leukemia with hyperleukocytosis. *J Pediatr Hematol Oncol* 25:569, 2003.
556. Hughes WT, Armstrong D, Bodey GP, et al: 1997 guidelines for the use of antimicrobial agents in neutropenic patients with unexplained fever. Infectious Diseases Society of America. *Clin Infect Dis* 25:551, 1997.
557. Lehrenbecher T, Varig D, Kaiser J, et al: Infectious complications in pediatric acute myeloid leukemia: Analysis of the prospective multi-institutional clinical trial AML-BFM 93. *Leukemia* 18:72, 2004.
558. Jagarlamidi R, Kumar L, Kochupillai V, et al: Infections in acute leukemia: An analysis of 240 febrile episodes. *Med Oncol* 17:111, 2000.
559. Uzun O, Anaissie EJ: Antifungal prophylaxis in patients with hematologic malignancies: A reappraisal. *Blood* 86:2063, 1995.
560. Glasmacher A, Molitor E, Hahn C, et al: Antifungal prophylaxis with itraconazole in neutropenic patients with acute leukaemia. *Leukemia* 12:1338, 1998.
561. Bergmann OJ, Mogensen SC, Ellermann-Eriksen S, Ellegaard J: Acyclovir prophylaxis and fever during remission-induction therapy of patients with acute myeloid leukemia: A randomized, double-blind, placebo-controlled trial. *J Clin Oncol* 15:2269, 1997.
562. Marr KA: New approaches to invasive fungal infections. *Curr Opin Hematol* 10:445, 2003.
563. Ruiz-Arguelles GJ, Apreza-Molina MG, Aleman-Hoey DD, et al: Out-patient supportive therapy after induction to remission therapy in adult acute myelogenous leukaemia (AML) is feasible: A multicentre study. *Eur J Haematol* 54:18, 1995.
564. Ravandi F: Role of cytokines in the treatment of acute leukemias: A review. *Leukemia* 20:563, 2006.
565. Rowe J, Anderson JW, Mazza JJ, et al: A randomized placebo-controlled phase III study of granulocyte-macrophage colony-stimulating factor in adult patients (>55 to 70 years of age) with acute myelogenous leukemia: A study of the Eastern Cooperative Oncology Group (E1490). *Blood* 86:457, 1995.
566. Hoelzer D, Seipelt G: Granulocyte colony-stimulating factor and granulocyte-macrophage colony-stimulating factor in the treatment of myeloid leukemia. *Curr Opin Hematol* 2:196, 1995.
567. Beutler E: Platelet transfusions: The 20,000/microL trigger. *Blood* 81:1441, 1993.
568. Webert K, Cook RJ, Sigouin CS, et al: The risk of bleeding in thrombocytopenic patients with acute myeloid leukemia. *Haematologica* 91:1530, 2006.
569. Schiffer CA: Granulocyte transfusion therapy. *Curr Opin Hematol* 6:3, 1999.
570. Cullis JO, Duncombe AS, Dudley JM, et al: Acute leukaemia in Jehovah's Witnesses. *Br J Haematol* 100:664, 1998.
571. Castagnola C, Nozza A, Corso A, Bernasconi C: The value of combination therapy in adult acute myeloid leukemia with central nervous system involvement. *Haematologia (Budap)* 82:577, 1997.
572. Hatano Y, Miura I, Horiuchi T, et al: Cerebellar myeloblastoma formation in CD7-positive, neural cell adhesion molecule (CD56)-positive acute myelogenous leukemia (M1). *Ann Hematol* 75:125, 1997.
573. Vavricka SR, Walter RB, Irani S, et al: Safety of lumbar puncture for adults with acute leukemia and restrictive prophylactic platelet trans-fusion. *Ann Hematol* 82:570, 2003.
574. Zittoun RA, Madelli F, Willemze R, et al: Autologous or allogeneic bone marrow transplantation compared with intensive chemotherapy in acute myelogenous leukemia. European Organization for Research and Treatment of Cancer (EORTC) and the Gruppo Italiano Malattie Ematologiche Maligne dell-Adulto (GIMEMA) Leukemia Cooperative Groups. *N Engl J Med* 332:217, 1995.
575. Harousseau JL, Cahn JY, Pignon B, et al: Comparison of autologous bone marrow transplantation and intensive chemotherapy as postremission therapy in adult acute myeloid leukemia. The Group Ouest Est Leucemies Aigues Myeloblastiques (GOELAM). *Blood* 90:2978, 1997.
576. Suciu S, Mandelli F, De Witte T, et al: Allogeneic compared with autologous stem cell transplantation in the treatment of patients younger than 46 years with acute myeloid leukemia (AML) in first complete remission (CR1): An intention-to-treat analysis of the EORTC/GIMEMAAML-10 trial. *Blood* 102:1232, 2003.
577. Bassara N, Schulze A, Wedding U, et al: Early related or unrelated haematopoietic cell transplantation results in higher overall survival and leukaemia-free survival compared with conventional chemotherapy in high-risk acute myeloid leukaemia patients in first complete remission. *Leukemia* 23:635, 2009.
578. Messerer D, Engel J, Hasford J, et al: Impact of different post-remission strategies on quality of life in patients with acute myeloid leukemia. *Haematologica* 93:826, 2008.
579. Koreth J, Schlenk R, Kopecky KJ, et al: Allogeneic stem cell transplantation for acute myeloid leukemia in first complete remission: systematic review and meta-analysis of prospective clinical trials. *JAMA* 301:2349, 2009.
580. Shpilberg O, Haddad N, Sofer O, et al: Postremission therapy with two different dose regimens of cytarabine in adults with acute myelogenous leukemia. *Leuk Res* 19:893, 1995.
581. Heil G, Mitrou PS, Hoeizer D, et al: High-dose cytosine arabinoside and daunorubicin postremission therapy in adults with *de novo* acute myeloid leukemia. Long-term follow-up of a prospective multicenter trial. *Ann Hematol* 71:219, 1995.
582. Rowe JM: Uncertainties in the standard care of acute myelogenous leukemia. *Leukemia* 15:677, 2001.
583. Cahn JY, Labopin M, Sierra J, et al: No impact of high-dose cytarabine on the outcome of patients transplanted for acute myeloblastic leukemia in first remission. Acute Leukemia Working Party of the European Group for Blood and Marrow Transplantation (EBMT). *Br J Haematol* 110:308, 2000.
584. Neubauer A, Maharry K, Mrózek K, et al: Patients with acute myeloid leukemia and RAS mutations benefit most from postremission high-dose cytarabine: A Cancer and Leukemia Group B study. *J Clin Oncol* 26:4603, 2008.
585. Byrd JC, Dodge RK, Carroll A, et al: Patients with t(8;21) (q22) and acute myeloid leukemia have superior failure-free and overall survival when repetitive cycles of high-dose cytarabine are administered. *J Clin Oncol* 17:3767, 1999.

586. Tsimberidou AM, Estey E, Cortes JE, et al: Mylotarg, fludarabine, cytarabine (ara-C), and cyclosporine (MFAC) regimen as post-remission therapy in acute myelogenous leukemia. *Cancer Chemother Pharmacol* 52:449, 2003.
587. Schiller G: Dose-intensive treatment of acute myelogenous leukemia: Improved survival [letter, comment]. *J Clin Oncol* 13:1828, 1995.
588. Mayer RJ, Davis RB, Schiffer CA, et al: Intensive postremission chemotherapy in adults with acute myeloid leukemia. Cancer and Leukemia Group B. *N Engl J Med* 331:896, 1994.
589. Elonen E, Almqvist A, Hanninen A, et al: Comparison between four and eight cycles of intensive chemotherapy in adult acute myeloid leukemia: A randomized trial of the Finnish Leukemia Group. *Leukemia* 12:1041, 1998.
590. Graves T, Hooks MA: Drug-induced toxicities associated with high-dose cytosine arabinoside infusions. *Pharmacotherapy* 9:23, 1989.
591. Smith GA, Damon LE, Rugo HS, et al: High-dose cytarabine dose modification reduces the incidence of neurotoxicity in patients with renal insufficiency. *J Clin Oncol* 15:833, 1997.
592. Hewlett J, Kopecky KJ, Head D, et al: A prospective evaluation of the roles of allogeneic marrow transplantation and low-dose monthly maintenance chemotherapy in the treatment of adult acute myelogenous leukemia (AML): A Southwest Oncology Group study. *Leukemia* 9:562, 1995.
593. Breems DA, Löwenberg B: Autologous stem cell transplantation in the treatment of adults with acute myeloid leukaemia. *Br J Haematol* 130:825, 2005.
594. Gorin NC: Autologous stem cell transplantation in acute myelocytic leukemia. *Blood* 92:1073, 1998.
595. Schiller G, Lee M, Miller T, et al: Transplantation of autologous peripheral blood progenitor cells procured after high-dose cytarabine-based consolidation chemotherapy for adults with acute myelogenous leukemia in first remission. *Leukemia* 11:1533, 1997.
596. Gondo H, Harada M, Miyamoto T, et al: Autologous peripheral blood stem cell transplantation for acute myelogenous leukemia. *Bone Marrow Transplant* 20:821, 1997.
597. Meloni G, Vignetti M, Avvisati G, et al: BAVC regimen and autograft for acute myelogenous leukemia in second complete remission. *Bone Marrow Transplant* 18:693, 1996.
598. Kusnierz-Glaz CR, Schlegel PG, Wong RM, et al: Influence of age on the outcome of 500 autologous bone marrow transplant procedures for hematologic malignancies. *J Clin Oncol* 15:18, 1997.
599. Mehta J, Powles R, Singhal S, et al: Autologous bone marrow transplantation for acute myeloid leukemia in first remission: Identification of modifiable prognostic factors. *Bone Marrow Transplant* 16:499, 1995.
600. Miller CB, Rowlings PA, Zhang MJ, et al: The effect of graft purging with 4-hydroperoxycyclophosphamie in autologous bone marrow transplantation or acute myelogenous leukemia. *Exp Hematol* 29:1336, 2001.
601. Abdallah A, Egerer G, Weberf-Nordt RM, et al: Long-term outcome in acute myelogenous leukemia autografted with mafosfamide-purged marrow in a single institution: Adverse events and incidence of secondary myelodysplasia. *Bone Marrow Transplant* 30:15, 2002.
602. Bishop MR, Jackson JD, Tarantolo SR, et al: Ex vivo treatment of bone marrow with phosphorothioate oligonucleotide OL(l) p53 for autologous transplantation in acute myelogenous leukemia and myelodysplastic syndrome. *J Hematother* 6:441, 1997.
603. To LB, Haylock DN, Thorp D, et al: The optimization of collection of peripheral blood stem cells for autotransplantation in acute myeloid leukaemia. *Bone Marrow Transplant* 4:41, 1989.
604. Hogge DE, Ailles LE, Gerhard B: Cytokine responsiveness of primitive progenitors in acute myelogenous leukemia. *Leukemia* 11:2220, 1997.
605. Carella AM, Dejana A, Lerma E, et al: In vivo mobilization of karyotypically normal peripheral blood progenitor cells in high-risk MDS, secondary or therapy-related acute myelogenous leukaemia. *Br J Haematol* 95:127, 1996.
606. Mehta J, Powles R, Horton C, et al: Factors affecting engraftment and hematopoietic recovery after unpurged autografting in acute leukemia. *Bone Marrow Transplant* 18:319, 1996.
607. Gorin N-C, Labopin M, Blaiise D, et al: Higher incidence of relapse with peripheral blood rather than marrow as a source of stem cells in adults with acute myelocytic leukemia autografted during the first remission. *J Clin Oncol* 27:3987, 2009.
608. Voog E, Le QH, Philip I, et al: Autologous transplantation in acute myeloid leukemia: Peripheral blood stem cell harvest after mobilization in steady state by granulocyte colony-stimulating factor alone. *Ann Hematol* 80:584, 2001.
609. Ganguly S, Singh J, Divine CL, et al: Is there a plateau in the survival curve after autologous transplantation in patients with intermediate and high-risk acute myeloid leukemia? A 20-year single institution experience. *Leuk Res* 31:1253, 2007.
610. Chauncey TR: Autologous bone marrow transplantation improves disease free survival but not overall survival in people with acute myeloid leukaemia. *Cancer Treat Rev* 30:483, 2004.
611. Specchia G, Pastore D, Mestice A, et al: Early and long-term engraftment after autologous peripheral stem cell transplantation in acute myeloid leukemia patients. *Acta Haematol* 116:229, 2006.
612. Palmieri S, Ferrara F, Leoni F, et al: Myeloablative chemotherapy followed by autologous stem cell infusion may overcome the adverse prognostic impact of FLT3 (foetal liver tyrosine kinase 3) mutations in patients with acute myeloid leukaemia and normal karyotype. *Hematol Oncol* 25:1, 2007.
613. Gratwohl S, Bslfomero H, Honisberger B, et al: Current trends in hematopoietic stem cell transplantation in Europe. *Blood* 100:2374, 2002.
614. Popplewell LL, Forman SJ: Is there an upper age limit for bone marrow transplantation? *Bone Marrow Transplant* 29:277, 2002.
615. Lemoli RM, Bandini G, Leopardi G, et al: Allogeneic peripheral blood stem cell transplantation in patients with early-phase hematologic malignancy: A retrospective comparison of short-term outcome with bone marrow transplantation. *Haematologica* 83:48, 1998.
616. Gorin NC, Labopin M, Rocha V, et al: Marrow versus peripheral blood for geno-identical allogeneic stem cell transplantation in acute myelocytic leukemia: Influence of dose and stem cell source shows better outcome with rich marrow. *Blood* 102:3043, 2003.
617. Champlin RE, Schmitz N, Horowitz MM, et al: Blood stem cells compared with bone marrow as a source of hematopoietic cells for allogeneic transplantation. IBMTR Histocompatibility and Stem Cell Sources Working Committee and the European Group for Blood and Marrow Transplantation (EBMT). *Blood* 95:3702, 2000.
618. Morton J, Hutchins C, Durrant S: Granulocyte-colony-stimulating factor (G-CSF)-primed allogeneic bone marrow: Significantly less graft-versus-host disease and comparable engraftment to G-CSF-mobilized peripheral blood stem cells. *Blood* 98:3186, 2001.
619. Applebaum FR: Is there a best transplant conditioning regimen for acute myeloid leukemia? *Leukemia* 14:497, 2000.
620. Litzow MR, Perez WS, Klein JP, et al: Comparison of outcome following allogeneic bone marrow transplantation with cyclophosphamide-total body irradiation versus busulphan-cyclophosphamide conditioning regimens for acute myelogenous leukaemia in first remission. *Br J Haematol* 119:1115, 2002.
621. Tallman MS, Rowlings PA, Milone G, et al: Effect of postremission chemotherapy before human leukocyte antigen-identical sibling transplantation for acute myelogenous leukemia in first complete remission. *Blood* 96:1254, 2000.
622. Rowe JM: Is there a role for consolidation therapy pre-transplantation? *Best Pract Res Clin Haematol* 19:301, 2006.
623. Mehta J, Powles R, Treleaven J, et al: Long-term follow-up of patients undergoing allogeneic bone marrow transplantation for acute myeloid leukemia in first complete remission after cyclophosphamide-total body irradiation and cyclosporine. *Bone Marrow Transplant* 18:741, 1996.
624. Messner HA: Long-term outcome of allogeneic transplants in acute myeloid leukemia. *Leukemia* 16:751, 2002.
625. Robin M, Guardiola P, Dombret H, et al: Allogeneic bone marrow transplantation for acute myeloblastic leukaemic in remission: Risk factors for long-term morbidity and mortality. *Bone Marrow Transplant* 31:877, 2003.
626. Greinex HT, Nachbaur D, Krieger O, et al: Factors affecting long-term outcome after allogeneic haematopoietic stem cell transplantation for acute myelogenous leukaemia: A retrospective study of 172 adult patients reported to the Austrian Stem Cell Transplant Registry. *Br J Haematol* 117:914, 2002.
627. Mathews V, DiPersio JF: Stem cell transplantation in acute myelogenous leukemia in first remission: What are the options? *Curr Hematol Rep* 3:235, 2004.
628. Bornhäuser M, Illmer T, Schaich M, et al: Improved outcome after stem-cell transplantation in FLT3/ITD-positive AML. *Blood* 109:2264, 2007.
629. Cornelissen JJ, van Putten WL, Verdonck LF, et al: Results of a HOVON/SAKK donor versus no-donor analysis of myeloablative HLA-identical sibling stem cell transplantation in first remission acute myeloid leukemia in young and middle-aged adults: Benefits for whom? *Blood* 109:3658, 2007.
630. Appelbaum FR, Pearce SF: Hematopoietic cell transplantation in first complete remission versus early relapse. *Best Pract Res Clin Haematol* 19:333, 2006.
631. Matthews DC, Appelbaum FR, Eary JF, et al: Development of a marrow transplant regimen for acute leukemia using targeted hematopoietic irradiation delivered by ^{131}I-labeled anti-CD45 antibody, combined with cyclophosphamide and total body irradiation. *Blood* 85:1122, 1995.
632. Zuckerman T, Rowe JM: Alternative donor transplantation in acute myeloid leukemia: Which source and when? *Curr Opin Hematol* 14:152, 2007.
633. Sasazuki T, Juji T, Morishima Y, et al: Effect of matching of class I HLA alleles on clinical outcome after transplantation of hematopoietic stem cells from an unrelated donor. Japan Marrow Donor Program. *N Engl J Med* 339:1177, 1998.
634. Aversa F, Tabilio A, Velardi A, et al: Treatment of high-risk acute leukemia with T-cell-depleted stem cells from related donors with one fully mismatched HLA haplotype. *N Engl J Med* 339:1186, 1998.
635. Ooi J, Iseki T, Takahashi S, et al: Unrelated cord blood transplantation for adult patients with de novo acute myeloid leukemia. *Blood* 103:489, 2004.
636. Michel G, Rocha V, Chevret S, et al: Unrelated cord blood transplantation for childhood acute myeloid leukemia: A Eurocord Group Analysis. *Blood* 102:4290, 2003.
637. Haspel RL, Ballen KK: Double cord blood transplants: Filling a niche? *Stem Cell Rev* 2:81, 2006.
638. Storb R: Mixed allogeneic chimerism and graft-versus-leukemia effects in acute myeloid leukemia. *Leukemia* 16:753, 2002.
639. Lekakis L, de Lima M: Reduced-intensity conditioning and allogeneic hematopoietic stem cell transplantation for acute myeloid leukemia. *Expert Rev Anticancer Ther* 8:785, 2008.
640. Blaise D, Vey N, Faucher C, Mohty M: Current status of reduced-intensity-conditioning allogeneic stem cell transplantation for acute myeloid leukemia. *Haematologica* 92:533, 2007.
641. Schlenk RF, Hartmann F, Hensel M, et al: Less intense conditioning with fludarabine, cyclophosphamide, idarubicin and etoposide (FCIE) followed by allogeneic unselected peripheral blood stem cell transplantation in elderly patients with leukemia. *Leukemia* 16:581, 2002.
642. Massenkeil G, Nagy M, Lawang M, et al: Reduced intensity conditioning and prophylactic DLI can cure patients with high-risk acute leukaemia if complete donor chimerism can be achieved. *Bone Marrow Transplant* 31:339, 2003.

643. Giralt S, Anagnastopoulos A, Shahjahanan M, Champlin R: Nonablative stem cell transplantation for older patients with acute leukemias and myelodysplastic syndromes. *Semin Hematol* 39:57, 2002.
644. Maris MB, Niederwieser D, Sandmaier BM, et al: HLA-matched unrelated donor hematopoietic cell transplantation after nonmyeloablative conditioning for patients with hematologic malignancies. *Blood* 102:2021, 2003.
645. Chakraverly R, Peggs K, Chopra R, et al: Limiting transplantation-related mortality following unrelated donor stem cell transplantation by using a nonmyeloablative conditioning regimen. *Blood* 99:1071, 2002.
646. Alyea EP, Kim HT, Ho V, et al: Impact of conditioning regimen intensity on outcome of allogeneic hematopoietic cell transplantation for advanced acute myelogenous leukemia and myelodysplastic syndrome. *Biol Blood Marrow Transplant* 12:1047, 2006.
647. Sorror ML, Sandmaier BM, Storer BE, et al: Comorbidity and disease status based risk stratification of outcomes among patients with acute myeloid leukemia or myelodysplasia receiving allogeneic hematopoietic cell transplantation. *J Clin Oncol* 25:4246, 2007.
648. Oran B, Giralt S, Saliba R, et al: Allogeneic hematopoietic stem cell transplantation for the treatment of high-risk acute myelogenous leukemia and myelodysplastic syndrome using reduced-intensity conditioning with fludarabine and melphalan. *Biol Blood Marrow Transplant* 13:454, 2007.
649. Estey E, de Lima M, Tibes R, et al: Prospective feasibility analysis of reduced-intensity conditioning (RIC) regimens for hematopoietic stem cell transplantation (HSCT) in elderly patients with acute myeloid leukemia (AML) and high-risk myelodysplastic syndrome (MDS). *Blood* 109:1395, 2007.
650. Tallman MS, Dewald GW, Gandham S, et al: Impact of cytogenetics on outcome of matched unrelated donor hematopoietic stem cell transplantation for acute myeloid leukemia in first or second complete remission. *Blood* 110:409, 2007.
651. Gale RP, Horowitz MM, Rees JK, et al: Chemotherapy versus transplants for acute myelogenous leukemia in second remission. *Leukemia* 10:13, 1996.
652. Bacigalupo A, Lamparelli T, Gualandi F, et al: Allogeneic hemopoietic stem cell transplants for patients with relapsed acute leukemia: Long-term outcome. *Bone Marrow Transplant* 39:341, 2007.
653. Michel G, Boulad F, Small TN, et al: Risk of extramedullary relapse following allogeneic bone marrow transplantation for acute myelogenous leukemia with leukemia cutis. *Bone Marrow Transplant* 20:107, 1997.
654. Blau IW, Basara N, Bischoff M, et al: Second allogeneic hematopoietic stem cell transplantation as treatment for leukemia relapsing following a first transplant. *Bone Marrow Transplant* 25:41, 2000.
655. Shlomchik WD, Emerson SG: The immunobiology of T cell therapies for leukemias. *Acta Haematol* 96:189, 1996.
656. Porter DL, Roth MS, Lee SJ, et al: Adoptive immunotherapy with donor mononuclear cell infusions to treat relapse of acute leukemia or myelodysplasia after allogeneic bone marrow transplantation. *Bone Marrow Transplant* 18:975, 1996.
657. Porter DL: Donor leukocyte infusions in acute myelogenous leukemia. *Leukemia* 17:1035, 2003.
658. Greinix NT: DLI or second transplant. *Ann Hematol* 81:S34, 2002.
659. Van Rhee F, Kolb HJ: Donor leukocyte transfusions for leukemic relapse. *Curr Opin Hematol* 2:423, 1995.
660. Berthou C, Leglise MC, Herry A, et al: Extramedullary relapse after favorable molecular response to donor leukocyte infusions for recurring acute leukemia. *Leukemia* 12:1676, 1998.
661. Carlens S, Remberger M, Aschan J, Ringden O: The role of disease stage in the response to donor lymphocyte infusions as treatment for leukemic relapse. *Biol Blood Marrow Transplant* 7:31, 2001.
662. Keil F, Prinz E, Kalhs P, et al: Treatment of leukemic relapse after allogeneic stem cell transplantation with cytotoreductive chemotherapy and/or second transplants. *Leukemia* 15:355, 2001.
663. Porter DL, Collins RH, Hardy C, et al: Treatment of relapsed leukemia after unrelated donor marrow transplantation with unrelated donor leukocyte infusions. *Blood* 95:1214, 2000.
664. Bishop MR, Tarantolo SR, Pavletic ZS, et al: Filgrastim as an alternative to donor leukocyte infusion for relapse after allogeneic stem-cell transplantation *J Clin Oncol* 18:2269, 2000.
665. Trenschel R, Bernier M, Stryckmans P, et al: Complete remission following donor PBSC after low-dose cytarabine chemotherapy for early relapse of acute myelogenous leukemia after allogeneic stem cell transplantation. *Bone Marrow Transplant* 19:381, 1997.
666. Porter DL, Antin JH: Donor leukocyte infusions in myeloid malignancies: New strategies. *Best Pract Res Clin Haematol* 19:737, 2006.
667. Goodman M, Cabral L, Cassileth P: Interleukin-2 and leukemia. *Leukemia* 12:1671, 1998.
668. Falkenburg JH, Smit WM, Willemze R: Cytotoxic T-lymphocyte (CTL) responses against acute or chronic myeloid leukemia. *Immunol Rev* 157:223, 1997.
669. Choudhury A, Toubert A, Sutaria S, et al: Human leukemia-derived dendritic cells: Ex vivo development of specific antileukemic cytotoxicity. *Crit Rev Immunol* 18:121, 1998.
670. Murata M, Ishikawa Y, Ohashi H, et al: Donor cell leukemia after allogeneic peripheral blood stem cell transplantation: A case report and literature review. *Int J Hematol* 88:111, 2008.
671. Reichard KK, Zhang QY, Sanchez L, et al: Acute myeloid leukemia of donor origin after allogeneic bone marrow transplantation for precursor T-cell acute lymphoblastic leukemia: Case report and review of the literature. *Am J Hematol* 81:178, 2006.
672. Estey E: Treatment of refractory AML. *Leukemia* 10:932, 1996.
673. Estey E, Kornblau S, Pierce S, et al: A stratification system for evaluating and selecting therapies in patients with relapsed or primary refractory acute myelogenous leukemia. *Blood* 88:756, 1996.
674. Stolser B, Knobl P, Fonatsch C, et al: Prognosis of patients with second relapse of acute myeloid leukemia. *Leukemia* 14:2059, 2000.
675. Lee S, Tallman MS, Oken MM, et al: Duration of second complete remission compared with first complete remission in patients with acute myeloid leukemia. *Leukemia* 14:1345, 2000.
676. Kern W, Schoch C, Haferlach T, et al: Multivariate analysis of prognostic factors in patients with refractory and relapsed acute myeloid leukemia undergoing sequential high-dose cytosine arabinoside and mitoxantrone (S-HAM) salvage therapy: Relevance of cytogenetic abnormalities. *Leukemia* 14:226, 2000.
677. Estey EH: Treatment of relapsed and refractory acute myelogenous leukemia. *Leukemia* 14:476, 2000.
678. Leopold LH, Willemze R: The treatment of acute myeloid leukemia in first relapse: A comprehensive review of the literature. *Leuk Lymphoma* 43:1715, 2002.
679. Alvarado Y, Tsimberidou A, Kantarjian H, et al: Pilot study of Mylotarg, idarubicin and cytarabine combination regimen in patients with primary resistant or relapsed acute myeloid leukemia. *Cancer Chemother Pharmacol* 51:87, 2003.
680. Revesz D, Chelghoum Y, Le QH, et al: Salvage by timed sequential chemotherapy in primary resistant acute myeloid leukemia: Analysis of prognostic factors. *Ann Hematol* 82:684, 2003.
681. Wrzesien-Kus A, Robak T, Lech-Maranda E, et al: A multicenter, open, non-comparative, phase II study of the combination of cladribine (2-chlorodeoxyadenosine), cytarabine, and G-CSF as induction therapy in refractory acute myeloid leukemia: A report of the Polish Adult Leukemia Group (PALG). *Eur J Haematol* 71:155, 2003.
682. Pastore D, Specchia G, Carluccio P, et al: FLAG-IDA in the treatment of refractory/relapsed acute myeloid leukemia: Single-center experience. *Ann Hematol* 82:231, 2003.
683. Roboz GJ, Knovich MA, Bayer RL, et al: Efficacy and safety of gemtuzumab ozogamicin in patients with poor-prognosis acute myeloid leukemia. *Leuk Lymphoma* 43:1951, 2002.
684. Advani R, Saba HI, Tallman MS, et al: Treatment of refractory and relapsed acute myelogenous leukemia with combination chemotherapy plus the multidrug resistance modulator PSC 833 (Valspodar). *Blood* 93:787, 1999.
685. Estey EH, Kantarjian HM, O'Brien S, et al: High remission rate, short remission duration in patients with refractory anemia with excess blasts (RAEB) in transformation (RAEB-t) given acute myelogenous leukemia (AML)-type chemotherapy in combination with granulocyte-CSF (G-CSF). *Cytokines Mol Ther* 1:21, 1995.
686. Greinix HT, Keil F, Brugger SA, et al: Long-term leukemia-free survival after allogeneic marrow transplantation in patients with acute myelogenous leukemia. *Ann Hematol* 72:53, 1996.
687. Appelbaum FR: Hematopoietic cell transplantation beyond first remission. *Leukemia* 16:157, 2002.
688. Singhal S, Powles R, Henslee-Downey PJ, et al: Allogeneic transplantation from HLA-matched sibling or partially HLA-missmatched related donors for primary refractory acute leukemia. *Bone Marrow Transplant* 29:291, 2002.
689. Biggs JC, Horowitz MM, Gale RP, et al: Bone marrow transplants may cure patients with acute leukemia never achieving remission with chemotherapy. *Blood* 80:1090, 1992.
690. Arellano ML, Langston A, Winton E, et al: Treatment of relapsed acute leukemia after allogeneic transplantation: A single center experience. *Biol Blood Marrow Transplant* 13:116, 2007.
691. Pollyea DA, Artz AS, Stock W, et al: Outcomes of patients with AML and MDS who relapse or progress after reduced intensity allogeneic hematopoietic cell transplantation. *Bone Marrow Transplant* 40:1027, 2007.
692. Giles FJ, Faderl S, Thomas DA, et al: Randomized phase I/II study of troxacitabine combined with cytarabine, idarubicin, or topotecan in patients with refractory myeloid leukemias. *J Clin Oncol* 21:1050, 2003.
693. Roboz GJ, Giles FJ, Ritchie EK, et al: Phase I/II study of continuous-infusion troxacitabine in refractory acute myeloid leukemia. *J Clin Oncol* 25:10, 2007.
694. Seiter K, Liu D, Loughran T, et al: Phase I study of temozolomide in relapsed/refractory acute leukemia. *J Clin Oncol* 20:3249, 2002.
695. Kantarjian H, Gandhi V, Cortes J, et al: Phase 2 clinical and pharmacologic study of clofarabine in patients with refractory or relapsed acute leukemia. *Blood* 102:2379, 2003.
696. Kantarjian HM, Jeha S, Gandhi V, et al: Clofarabine: Past, present, and future. *Leuk Lymphoma* 48:1922, 2007.
697. Petti MC, Tafuri A, Latagliata R, et al: High-dose hydroxyurea in the treatment of poor-risk myeloid leukemia. *Ann Hematol* 82:476, 2003.
698. Vey N, Giles F: Cloretazine for the treatment of acute myeloid leukemia. *Expert Rev Anticancer Ther* 6:321, 2006.
699. Penketh PG, Baumann RP, Ishiguro K, et al: Lethality to leukemia cell lines of DNA interstrand cross-links generated by Cloretazine derived alkylating species. *Leuk Res* 32:1546, 2008.
700. Rush LJ, Dai Z, Smiraglia DJ, et al: Novel methylation targets in *de novo* acute myeloid leukemia with prevalence of chromosome 11 loci. *Blood* 97:3226, 2001.
701. Blum W, Marcucci G: Targeting epigenetic changes in acute myeloid leukemia. *Clin Adv Hematol Oncol* 3:855, 2005.
702. Lübbert M, Minden M: Decitabine in acute myeloid leukemia. *Semin Hematol* 42(Suppl 2):S38, 2005.

703. Kihslinger JE, Godley LA: The use of hypomethylating agents in the treatment of hematologic malignancies. *Leuk Lymphoma* 48:1676, 2007.
704. Plimack ER, Kantarjian HM, Issa JP, et al: Decitabine and its role in the treatment of hematopoietic malignancies. *Leuk Lymphoma* 48:1472, 2007.
705. Garcia-Manero G, Stoltz ML, Ward MR, et al: A pilot pharmacokinetic study of oral azacitidine. *Leukemia* 22:1680, 2008.
706. Kantarjian HM, O'Brien SM, Estey E, et al: Decitabine studies in chronic and acute myelogenous leukemia. *Leukemia* 11(Suppl 1):S35, 1997.
707. Ferrara EF, Fazi F, Bianchini A, et al: Histone deacetylase-targeted treatment restores retinoic acid signaling and differentiation in acute myeloid leukemia. *Cancer Res* 61:2, 2001.
708. Klisovic MI, Maghraby EA, Parthun MR, et al: Depsipeptide (FR 901228) promotes histone acetylation, gene transcription, apoptosis and its activity is enhanced by DNA methyltransferase inhibitors in AML1/ETO-positive leukemic cells. *Leukemia* 17:350, 2003.
709. Klimek VM, Fircanis S, Maslak P, et al: Tolerability, pharmacodynamics, and pharmacokinetics studies of depsipeptide (romidepsin) in patients with acute myelogenous leukemia or advanced myelodysplastic syndromes. *Clin Cancer Res* 14:826, 2008.
710. Giles F, Fischer T, Cortes J, et al: A phase I study of intravenous LBH589, a novel cinnamic hydroxamic acid analogue histone deacetylase inhibitor, in patients with refractory hematologic malignancies. *Clin Cancer Res* 12:4628, 2006.
711. Garcia-Manero G, Yang H, Bueso-Ramos C, et al: Phase 1 study of the histone deacetylase inhibitor vorinostat (suberoylanilide hydroxamic acid [SAHA]) in patients with advanced leukemias and myelodysplastic syndromes. *Blood* 111:1060, 2008.
712. Garcia-Manero G, Assouline S, Cortes J, et al: Phase 1 study of the oral isotype specific histone deacetylase inhibitor MGCD0103 in leukemia. *Blood* 112:981, 2008.
713. Gore SD: Combination therapy with DNA methyltransferase inhibitors in hematologic malignancies. *Nat Clin Pract Oncol* 2 Suppl 1:S30, 2005.
714. Blum W, Klisovic RB, Hackanson B, et al: Phase I study of decitabine alone or in combination with valproic acid in acute myeloid leukemia. *J Clin Oncol* 25:3884, 2007.
715. Burbage C, Tagge EP, Harris B, et al: Ricin fusion toxin targeted to the human granulocyte-macrophage colony stimulating factor receptor is selectively toxic to acute myeloid leukemia cells. *Leuk Res* 21:681, 1997.
716. Hogge DE, Willman CL, Kreitman RJ, et al: Malignant progenitors from patients with acute myelogenous leukemia are sensitive to a diphtheria toxin-granulocyte-macrophage colony-stimulating factor fusion protein. *Blood* 92:589, 1998.
717. Lanza F, Rigolin GM, Castagnari B, et al: Potential clinical pplications of rhGM-CSF in acute myeloid leukemia based on its biologic activity and receptor interaction. *Haematologica* 82:239, 1997.
718. Du X, Ho M, Pastan I, et al: New immunotoxins targeting CD123, a stem cell antigen on acute myeloid leukemia cells. *J Immunother* 30:607, 2007.
719. Frankel AE, Beran M, Hogge DE, et al: Malignant progenitors from patients with CD87+ acute myelogenous leukemia are sensitive to a diphtheria toxin-urokinase fusion protein. *Exp Hematol* 30:1316, 2002.
720. Frankel A, Liu JS, Rizzieri D, Hogge D: Phase I clinical study of diphtheria toxin-interleukin 3 fusion protein in patients with acute myeloid leukemia and myelodysplasia. *Leuk Lymphoma* 49:543, 2008.
721. Larson RA: Current use and future development of gemtuzumab ozogamicin. *Semin Hematol* 38:24, 2001.
722. Van DerVelden VH, Te Marvelde JG, Hoogeveen PG, et al: Targeting of the CD33-calicheamicin immunoconjugate Mylotarg (CMA-676) in acute myeloid leukemia: *In vivo* and *in vitro* saturation and internalization by leukemic and normal myeloid cells. *Blood* 97:3197, 2001.
723. Larson RA, Boogaerts M, Estey E, et al: Antibody-targeted chemotherapy of older patients with acute myeloid leukemia in first relapse using Mylotarg (gemtuzumab ozogamicin). *Leukemia* 16:1627, 2002.
724. Bross PF, Beitz J, Chen G, et al: Approval summary: Gemtuzumab ozogamicin in relapsed acute myeloid leukemia. *Clin Cancer Res* 8:300, 2002.
725. Giles FJ, Cortes JE, Halliburton TA, et al: Intravenous corticosteroids to reduce gemtuzumab ozogamicin infusion reactions. *Ann Pharmacother* 37:1182, 2003.
726. Lang K, Menzin J, Earle CC, Mallick R: Outcomes in patients treated with gemtuzumab ozogamicin for relapsed acute myelogenous leukemia. *Am J Health Syst Pharm* 59:941, 2002.
727. Leopold LH, Berger MS, Cheng S-C, et al: Comparative efficacy and safety of Gemtuzumab ozogamicin monotherapy and high-dose cytarabine combination therapy in patients with acute myeloid leukemia in first relapse. *Clin Adv Hematol Oncol* 1:220, 2003.
728. Wadleigh M, Richardson PG, Zahrieh D, et al: Prior gemtuzumab ozogamicin exposure significantly increases the risk of veno-occlusive disease in patients who undergo myeloablative allogeneic stem cell transplantation. *Blood* 102:1578, 2003.
729. Balaian L, Ball ED: Cytotoxic activity of gemtuzumab ozogamicin (Mylotarg) in acute myeloid leukemia correlates with the expression of protein kinase Syk. *Leukemia* 20:2093, 2006.
730. Stasi R, Evangelista ML, Buccisano F, et al: Gemtuzumab ozogamicin in the treatment of acute myeloid leukemia. *Cancer Treat Rev* 34:49, 2008.
731. Tsimberidou AM, Giles FJ, Estey E, et al: The role of gemtuzumab ozogamicin in acute leukaemia therapy. *Br J Haematol* 132:398, 2006.
732. Weisberg E, Boulton C, Kelly LM, et al: Inhibition of mutant FLT3 receptors in leukemia cells by the small molecule tyrosine kinase inhibitor PKC412. *Cancer Cell* 1:433, 2002.
733. Kelly LM, Yu JC, Boulton CL, et al: CT53518, a novel selective FLT3 antagonist for the treatment of acute myelogenous leukemia (AML). *Cancer Cell* 1:421, 2002.
734. Levis M, Allebach J, Tse KF, et al: A FLT3-targeted tyrosine kinase inhibitor is cytotoxic to leukemia cells *in vitro* and *in vivo*. *Blood* 99:3885, 2002.
735. Spiekermann K, Dirschinger RJ, Schwab R, et al: The protein tyrosine kinase inhibitor SU5614 inhibits FLT3 and induces growth arrest and apoptosis in AML-derived cell lines expressing a constitutively activated FLT3. *Blood* 101:1494, 2003.
736. DeAngelo DJ, Stone RM, Heaney ML, et al: Phase 1 clinical results with tandutinib (MLN518), a novel FLT3 antagonist, in patients with acute myelogenous leukemia or high-risk myelodysplastic syndrome: Safety, pharmacokinetics, and pharmacodynamics. *Blood* 108:3674, 2006.
737. Tickenbrock L, Müller-Tidow C, Berdel WE, Serve H: Emerging Flt3 kinase inhibitors in the treatment of leukaemia. *Expert Opin Emerg Drugs* 11:153, 2006.
738. Stone RM, De Angelo DJ, Klimek V, et al: Patients with acute myeloid leukemia and an activating mutation in FLT3 respond to a small molecule FLT3 tyrosine kinase inhibitor. *Blood* 105:54, 2005.
739. Knapper S, Burnett AK, Littlewood T, et al: A phase 2 trial of the FLT3 inhibitor lestaurtinib (CEP701) as first-line treatment for older patients with acute myeloid leukemia not considered fit for intensive chemotherapy. *Blood* 108:3262, 2006.
740. Safaian NN, Czibere A, Bruns I, et al: Sorafenib (Nexavar) induces molecular remission and regression of extramedullary disease in a patient with FLT3-ITD+ acute myeloid leukemia. *Leuk Res* 33:348, 2009.
741. Möllgård L, Deneberg S, Nahi H, et al: The FLT3 inhibitor PKC412 in combination with cytostatic drugs *in vitro* in acute myeloid leukemia. *Cancer Chemother Pharmacol* 62:439, 2008.
742. Heinrich MC, Blanke CD, Druker BJ, Corless CL: Inhibition of KIT tyrosine kinase activity: A novel molecular approach to the treatment of KIT-positive malignancies. *J Clin Oncol* 20:1692, 2002.
743. Scappini B, Onida F, Kantarjian HM, et al: Effects of signal transduction inhibitor 571 in acute myelogenous leukemia cells. *Clin Cancer Res* 7:3884, 2001.
744. Kindler T, Breitenbuecher F, Marx A, et al: Sustained complete hematologic remission after administration of the tyrosine kinase inhibitor imatinib mesylate in a patient with refractory, secondary AML. *Blood* 101:2960, 2003.
745. Kindler T, Breitenbuecher F, Marx A, et al: Efficacy and safety of imatinib in adult patients with C-kit-positive acute myeloid leukemia. *Blood* 103:3644, 2004.
746. Guzman ML, Jordan CT: Considerations for targeting malignant stem cells in leukemia. *Cancer Control* 11:97, 2004.
747. Cilloni D, Messa F, Rosso V, et al: Increase sensitivity to chemotherapeutical agents and cytoplasmatic interaction between NPM leukemic mutant and NF-kappaB in AML carrying NPM1 mutations. *Leukemia* 22:1234, 2008.
748. Minderman H, Zhou Y, O'Loughlin KL, Baer MR: Bortezomib activity and *in vitro* interactions with anthracyclines and cytarabine in acute myeloid leukemia cells are independent of multidrug resistance mechanisms and p53 status. *Cancer Chemother Pharmacol* 60:245, 2007.
749. Stone RM: Novel therapeutic agents in acute myeloid leukemia. *Exp Hematol* 35(Suppl 1):163, 2007.
750. Chalandon Y, Schwaller J: Targeting mutated protein tyrosine kinases and their signaling pathways in hematologic malignancies. *Haematologica* 90:949, 2005.
751. Tamburini J, Chapuis N, Bardet V, et al: Mammalian target of rapamycin (mTOR) inhibition activates phosphatidylinositol 3-kinase/Akt by up-regulating insulin-like growth factor-1 receptor signaling in acute myeloid leukemia: Rationale for therapeutic inhibition of both pathways. *Blood* 111:379, 2008.
752. Wei G, Twomey D, Lamb J, et al: Gene expression-based chemical genomics identifies rapamycin as a modulator of MCL1 and glucocorticoid resistance. *Cancer Cell* 10:331, 2006.
753. Kojima K, Shimanuki M, Shikami M, et al: The dual PI3 kinase/mTOR inhibitor PI-103 prevents p53 induction by Mdm2 inhibition but enhances p53-mediated mitochondrial apoptosis in p53 wild-type AML. *Leukemia* 22:1728, 2008.
754. Martelli AM, Nyåkern M, Tabellini G, et al: Phosphoinositide 3-kinase/Akt signaling pathway and its therapeutical implications for human acute myeloid leukemia. *Leukemia* 20:911, 2006.
755. Papa V, Tazzari PL, Chiarini F, et al: Proapoptotic activity and chemosensitizing effect of the novel Akt inhibitor perifosine in acute myelogenous leukemia cells. *Leukemia* 22:147, 2008.
756. Milella M, Kornblau SM, Estrov Z, et al: Therapeutic targeting of the MEK/MAPK signal transduction module in acute myeloid leukemia. *J Clin Invest* 108:851, 2001.
757. Ikezoe T, Yang J, Nishioka C, et al: A novel treatment strategy targeting Aurora kinases in acute Myelogenous leukemia. *Mol Cancer Ther* 6:1851, 2007.
758. Thomas X, Campos L, Le QH, Guyotat D: Heat shock proteins and acute leukemias. *Hematology* 10:225, 2005.
759. Hu S, Niu H, Minkin P, et al: Comparison of antitumor effects of multitargeted tyrosine kinase inhibitors in acute myelogenous leukemia. *Mol Cancer Ther* 7:1110, 2008.
760. Raanani P, Shpilberg O, Ben-Bassat I, et al: Extramedullary disease and targeted therapies for hematological malignancies—Is the association real? *Ann Oncol* 18:7, 2007.
761. Shangary S, Johnson DE: Recent advances in the development of anticancer agents targeting cell death inhibitors in the Bcl-2 protein family. *Leukemia* 17:1470, 2003.
762. Marucci G, Byrd JC, Dai G, et al: Phase 1 and pharmacodynamic studies of G3139, a Bcl-2 antisense oligonucleotide, in combination with chemotherapy in refractory or relapsed acute leukemia. *Blood* 101:425, 2003.

763. Konopleva M, Contractor R, Tsao T, et al: Mechanisms of apoptosis sensitivity and resistance to the BH3 mimetic ABT-737 in acute myeloid leukemia. *Cancer Cell* 10:375, 2006.
764. Konopleva M, Watt J, Contractor R, et al: Mechanisms of antileukemic activity of the novel Bcl-2 homology domain-3 mimetic GX15–070 (obatoclax). *Cancer Res* 68:3413, 2008.
765. Konopleva M, Tsao T, Ruvolo P, et al: Novel triterpenoid CDDO-Me is a potent inducer of apoptosis and differentiation in acute myelogenous leukemia. *Blood* 99:326, 2002.
766. Suh WS, Kim YS, Schimmer AD, et al: Synthetic triterpenoids activate a pathway for apoptosis in AML cells involving downregulation of FLIP and sensitization of TRAIL. *Leukemia* 17:2122, 2003.
767. Kaufmann SH, Steensma DP: On the TRAIL of a new therapy for leukemia. *Leukemia* 19:2195, 2005.
768. Rosato RR, Almenara JA, Cartree L, et al: The cyclin-dependent kinase inhibitor flavopiridol disrupts sodium butyrate-induced p21WAF1/CIP1 expression and maturation while reciprocally potentiating apoptosis in human leukemia cells. *Mol Cancer Ther* 1:253, 2002.
769. Karp JE, Ross DD, Yang W, et al: Timed sequential therapy of acute leukemia with flavopiridol: In vitro model for a phase I clinical trial. *Clin Cancer Res* 9:307, 2003.
770. Le DT, Shannon KM: Ras processing as a therapeutic target in hematologic malignancies. *Curr Opin Hematol* 9:308, 2002.
771. Morgan MA, Ganser A, Reuter CWM: Therapeutic efficacy of prenylation inhibitors in the treatment of myeloid leukemia. *Leukemia* 17:1482, 2003.
772. Kurzrock R, Cortes J, Kantarjian H: Clinical development of farnesyltransferase inhibitors in leukemias and myelodysplastic syndrome. *Semin Hematol* 39:20, 2002.
773. Brunner TB, Hahn SM, Gupta AK, et al: Farnesyltransferase inhibitors: An overview of the results of preclinical and clinical investigations. *Cancer Res* 63:5656, 2003.
774. Karp JE, Lancet JE, Kaufmann SH, et al: Clinical and biologic activity of the farnesyltransferase inhibitor R115777 in adults with refractory and relapsed acute leukemias: A phase 1 clinical-laboratory correlative trial. *Blood* 97:3361, 2001.
775. Martinelli G, Iacobucci I, Paolini S, Ottaviani E: Farnesyltransferase inhibition in hematologic malignancies: The clinical experience with tipifarnib. *Clin Adv Hematol Oncol* 6:303, 2008.
776. Harousseau JL, Lancet JE, Reiffers J, et al: A phase 2 study of the oral farnesyltransferase inhibitor tipifarnib in patients with refractory or relapsed acute myeloid leukemia. *Blood* 109:5151, 2007.
777. Karp JE, Smith BD, Gojo I, et al: Phase II trial of tipifarnib as maintenance therapy in first complete remission in adults with acute myelogenous leukemia and poor-risk features. *Clin Cancer Res* 14:3077, 2008.
778. Morgan MA, Wegner J, Aydilek E, et al: Synergistic cytotoxic effects in myeloid leukemia cells upon cotreatment with farnesyltransferase and geranylgeranyl transferase-1 inhibitors. *Leukemia* 17:1508, 2003.
779. Minden MD, Dimitroulakos J, Nohynek D, Penn LZ: Lovastatin induced control of blast cell growth in an elderly patient with acute myeloblastic leukemia. *Leuk Lymphoma* 40:659, 2001.
780. Lishner M, Bar-Sef A, Elis A, Fabian I: Effect of simvastatin alone and in combination with cytosine arabinoside on the proliferation of myeloid leukemia cell lines. *J Investig Med* 49:319, 2001.
781. Li HY, Appelbaum FR, Willman CL, et al: Cholesterol-modulating agents kill acute myeloid leukemia cells and sensitize them to therapeutics by blocking adaptive cholesterol responses. *Blood* 101:3628, 2003.
782. Munker R, Kobayashi T, Eistner E, et al: A new series of vitamin D analogs is highly active for clonal inhibition, differentiation, and induction of WAF1 in myeloid leukemia. *Blood* 88:2201, 1996.
783. Morosetti R, Grignani F, Liberatore C, et al: Infrequent alterations of the RAR alpha gene in acute myelogenous leukemias, retinoic acid-resistant acute promyelocytic leukemias, myelodysplastic syndromes, and cell lines. *Blood* 87:4399, 1996.
784. Usuki K, Kitazume K, Endo M, et al: Combination therapy with granulocyte colony-stimulating factor, all-*trans* retinoic acid, and low-dose cytotoxic drugs for acute myelogenous leukemia. *Intern Med* 34:1186, 1995.
785. Zhang W, Piatyszek MA, Kobayashi T, et al: Telomerase activity in human acute myelogenous leukemia: Inhibition of telomerase activity by differentiation-inducing agents. *Clin Cancer Res* 2:799, 1996.
786. Seiter K, Feldman EJ, Dorota Halicka H, et al: Clinical and laboratory evaluation of all-trans retinoic acid modulation of chemotherapy in patients with acute myelogenous leukaemia. *Br J Haematol* 108:40, 2000.
787. Chen Z, Wang Y, Wang W, et al: All-trans retinoic acid as a single agent induces complete remission in a patient with acute leukemia of M2a subtype. *Chin Med J* 115:58, 2002.
788. Lehman S, Bengtzen S, Paul A, et al: Effects of arsenic trioxide (As_2O_3) on leukemic cells from patients with non-M3 acute myelogenous leukemia: Studies of cytotoxicity, apoptosis and the pattern of resistance. *Eur J Haematol* 66:357, 2001.
789. Ozturk A, Orhan B, Turken O, et al: Acute myeloblastic leukemia achieving complete remission with amifostine alone. *Leuk Lymphoma* 43:451, 2002.
790. Steins MB, Padro T, Bieker R, et al: Efficacy and safety of thalidomide in patients with acute myeloid leukemia. *Blood* 99:834, 2002.
791. Cabebe E, Wakelee H: Sunitinib, et al: A newly approved small-molecule inhibitor of angiogenesis. *Drugs Today (Barc)* 42:387, 2006.
792. Hatfield KJ, Olsnes AM, Gjertsen BT, Bruserud Ø: Antiangiogenic therapy in acute myelogenous leukemia: Targeting of vascular endothelial growth factor and interleukin 8 as possible antileukemic strategies. *Curr Cancer Drug Targets* 5:229, 2005.
793. Kitagawa M: The angiopoietin signaling pathway as a promising target for the treatment of acute myeloid leukemia. *Haematologica* 91:1155B, 2006.
794. Lancet JE, List AF, Moscinski LC, et al: Treatment of deletion 5q acute myeloid leukemia with lenalidomide. *Leukemia* 21:586, 2007.
795. Burger JA, Bürkle A: The CXCR4 chemokine receptor in acute and chronic leukaemia: A marrow homing receptor and potential therapeutic target. *Br J Haematol* 137:288, 2007.
796. Zeng Z, Samudio IJ, Munsell M, et al: Inhibition of CXCR4 with the novel RCP168 peptide overcomes stroma-mediated chemoresistance in chronic and acute leukemias. *Mol Cancer Ther* 5:3113, 2006.
797. Andreeff M, Konopleva M: Mechanisms of drug resistance in AML. *Cancer Treat Res* 112:237, 2002.
798. Van der Kolk DM, De Vries EG, Muller M, Vellenga E: The role of drug efflux pumps in acute myeloid leukemia. *Leuk Lymphoma* 43:685, 2002.
799. Tothova E, Elbertova A, Fricova M, et al: P-glycoprotein expression in adult acute myeloid leukemia: Correlation with induction treatment outcome. *Neoplasma* 48:393, 2001.
800. Van den Heuvel-Eibrink MM, Wiemer EAC, DeBoevere MJ, et al: MDR1 gene-related clonal selection and P-glycoprotein function and expression in relapsed or refractory acute myeloid leukemia. *Blood* 97:3605, 2001.
801. Sonneveld P, Burnett A, Vossebeld P, et al: Dose-finding study of valspodar (PSC 833) with daunorubicin and cytarabine to reverse multidrug resistance in elderly patients with previously untreated acute myeloid leukemia. *Hematol J* 1:411, 2000.
802. Visani G, Milligan D, Leoni F, et al: Combined action of PSC 833 (Valspodar), a novel MDR reversing agent, with mitoxantrone, etoposide and cytarabine in poor-prognosis acute myeloid leukemia. *Leukemia* 15:764, 2001.
803. Tsimberidou AM, Paterakis G, Androutsos G, et al: Evaluation of the clinical relevance of the expression and function of P-glycoprotein, multidrug resistance protein and lung resistance protein in patients with primary acute myelogenous leukemia. *Leuk Res* 26:143, 2002.
804. Baer MR, George SL, Dodge RK, et al: Phase 3 study of the multidrug resistance modulator PSC-833 in previously untreated patients 60 years of age or older with acute myeloid leukemia: Cancer and Leukemia Group B Study 9720. *Blood* 100:1224, 2002.
805. Kornblau SM, Estry E, Madden T, et al: Phase I study of mitoxantrone plus etopside with multidrug blockade by SDZ PSC-833 in relapsed or refractory acute myelogenous leukemia. *J Clin Oncol* 15:1796, 1997.
806. List AF, Kopecky KJ, Willman CL, et al: Benefit of cyclosporine modulation of drug resistance in patients with poor-risk acute myeloid leukemia: A Southwest Oncology Group study. *Blood* 98:3212, 2001.
807. Claxton D, Choudhury A: Potential for therapy with AML-derived dendritic cells. *Leukemia* 15:668, 2001.
808. Rosenblatt J, Avigan D: Can leukemia-derived dendritic cells generate antileukemia immunity? *Expert Rev Vaccines* 5:467, 2006.
809. Panoskaltsis N: Dendritic cells in MDS and AML—Cause, effect or solution to the immune pathogenesis of disease? *Leukemia* 19:354, 2005.
810. Woiciechowsky A, Regn S, Kolb H-J, Roskrow M: Leukemic dendritic cells generated in the presence of FLT3 ligand have the capacity to stimulate an autologous leukemia-specfic cytotoxic T cell response from patients with acute myeloid leukemia. *Leukemia* 15:246, 2001.
811. Stripecke R, Levine AM, Pullarkat V, Cardoso AA: Immunotherapy with acute leukemia cells modified into antigen-presenting cells: *Ex vivo* culture and gene transfer methods. *Leukemia* 16:1974, 2002.
812. Galea-Lauri J, Darling D, Mufti G, et al: Eliciting cytotoxic T lymphocytes against acute myeloid leukemia-derived antigens: Evaluation of dendritic cell-leukemia cell hybrids and other antigen-loading strategies for dendritic cell-based vaccination. *Cancer Immunol Immunother* 51:299, 2002.
813. Cooper MA, Caligiuri MA: Immunologic manipulation in AML: From bench to bedside. *Leukemia* 16:736, 2002.
814. Meloni G, Trisolini SM, Capria S, et al: How long can we give interleukin-2? Clinical and immunological evaluation of AML patients after 10 or more years of IL2 administration. *Leukemia* 16:2016, 2002.
815. Baer MR, George SL, Caligiuri MA, et al: Low-dose interleukin-2 immunotherapy does not improve outcome of patients age 60 years and older with acute myeloid leukemia in first complete remission: Cancer and Leukemia Group B Study 9720. *J Clin Oncol* 26:4934, 2008.
816. Elisseeva OA, Oka Y, Tsuboi A, et al: Humoral immune responses against Wilms tumor gene WT1 product in patients with hematopoietic malignancies. *Blood* 99:3272, 2002.
817. Molldrem J: Immune therapy of AML. *Cytotherapy* 4:437, 2002.
818. Choo A, Palladinetti P, Holmes T, et al: SiRNA targeting the IRF2 transcription factor inhibits leukaemic cell growth. *Int J Oncol* 33:175, 2008.
819. Klisovic RB, Blum W, Wei X, et al: Phase I study of GTI-2040, an antisense to ribonucleotide reductase, in combination with high-dose cytarabine in patients with acute myeloid leukemia. *Clin Cancer Res* 14:3889, 2008.
820. Stevenson GT: CD38 as a therapeutic target. *Mol Med* 12:345, 2006.
821. Abutalib SA, Tallman MS: Monoclonal antibodies for the treatment of acute myeloid leukemia. *Curr Pharm Biotechnol* 7:343, 2006.
822. Sanz MA, Martin G, Gonzalez M, et al: Risk-adapted treatment of acute promyelocytic leukemia with all-trans-retinoic acid and anthracycline monochemotherapy: A multicenter study by the PETHEMA. *Blood* 103:1237, 2004.
823. Avvisati G, Petti MC, Lo-Coco F, et al: Induction therapy with idarubicin alone significantly influences event-free survival duration in patients with newly diagnosed

hypergranular acute promyelocytic leukemia: Final results of the GIMEMA randomized study LAP 0389 with 7 years of minimal follow-up. *Blood* 100:3141, 2002.
824. Sanz MA, Tallman MS, Lo-Coco F, et al: Practice points, consensus, and controversial issues in the management of patients with newly diagnosed acute promyelocytic leukemia. *Oncologist* 10:806, 2005.
825. Sanz MA, Lo Coco F: Standard practice and controversial issues in front-line therapy of acute promyelocytic leukemia. *Haematologica* 90:840, 2005.
826. Sanz MA, Grimwade D, Tallman MS, et al: Management of acute promyelocytic leukemia: Recommendations from an expert panel on behalf of the European LeukemiaNet. *Blood* 113:1875, 2009.
827. Lengfelder E, Reichert A, Schoch C, et al: Double induction strategy including high dose cytarbine in combination with all-trans retinoic acid: Effects in patients with newly diagnosed acute promyelocytic leukemia. German AML Cooperative Group. *Leukemia* 14:1362, 2000.
828. Adès L, Sanz MA, Chevret S, et al: Treatment of newly diagnosed acute promyelocytic leukemia (APL): A comparison of French-Belgian-Swiss and PETHEMA results. *Blood* 111:1078, 2008.
829. Mandelli F, Latagliata R, Avvisati G, et al: Treatment of elderly patients (> or = 60 years) with newly diagnosed acute promyelocytic leukemia. Results of the Italian multicenter group GIMEMA with ATRA and idarubicin (AIDA) protocols. *Leukemia* 17:1085, 2003.
830. Estey EH, Giles FJ, Beran M, et al: Experience with gemtuzumab ozogamycin ("mylotarg") and all-trans retinoic acid in untreated acute promyelocytic leukemia. *Blood* 99:4222, 2002.
831. Shen Z-X, Shi Z-Z, Fang J, et al: All-*trans* retinoic acid/As_2O_3 combination yields a high quality remission and survival in newly diagnosed acute promyelocytic leukemia. *Proc Natl Acad Sci U S A* 10:1073, 2004.
832. Tallman MS, Rowe JM: Long-term follow-up and potential for cure in acute promyelocytic leukaemia. *Best Pract Res Clin Haematol* 16:535, 2003.
833. Tallman MS, Andersen JW, Schiffer CA, et al: All-*trans*-retinoic acid in acute promyelocytic leukemia. *N Engl J Med* 337:1021, 1997.
834. Chomienne C, Ballerini P, Balitrans N, et al: All-*trans* retinoic acid in acute promyelocytic leukemia: II. *In vitro* studies: Structure–function relationship. *Blood* 76:1710, 1990.
835. Degos L: Is acute promyelocytic leukemia a curable disease? Treatment strategy for a long-term survival. *Leukemia* 8:911, 1994.
836. Degos L, Dombret H, Chomienne C, et al: All-*trans*-retinoic acid as a differentiating agent in the treatment of acute promyelocytic leukemia. *Blood* 85:2643, 1995.
837. Gallagher RE, Li YP, Rao S, et al: Characterization of acute promyelocytic leukemia cases with PML-RAR alpha break/fusion sites in PML exon 6: Identification of a subgroup with decreased in vitro responsiveness to all-*trans* retinoic acid. *Blood* 86:1540, 1995.
838. Licht JD, Chomienne C, Goy A, et al: Clinical and molecular characterization of a rare syndrome of acute promyelocytic leukemia associated with translocation (11;17). *Blood* 85:1083, 1995.
839. Jansen JH, De Ridder MC, Geertsma WM, et al: Complete remission of t(11;17) positive acute promyelocytic leukemia induced by all-*trans* retinoic acid and granulocyte colony-stimulating factor. *Blood* 94:39, 1999.
840. Tallman MS, Andersen JW, Schiffer CA, et al: All-trans retinoic acid in acute promyelocytic leukemia: Long-term outcome and prognostic factor analysis from the North American Intergroup protocol. *Blood* 100:4298, 2002.
841. Hernandez JM, Martin G, Gutierrez MC, et al: Additional cytogenetic changes do not influence the outcome of patients with newly diagnosed acute promyelocytic leukemia treated with an ATRA plus anthracyclin based protocol. A report of the Spanish group PETHEMA. *Haematologica* 86:807, 2001.
842. Kennedy GA, Marlton P, Cobcroft R, Gill D: Molecular remission without blood product support using all-trans retinoic acid (ATRA) induction and combined arsenic trioxide/ATRA consolidation in a Jehovah's Witness with *de novo* acute promyelocytic leukemia. *Br J Haematol* 111:1103, 2000.
843. Martinelli G, Ottaviani E, Testoni N, et al: Disappearance of PML/RAR alpha acute promyelocytic leukemia associated transcript during consolidation chemotherapy. *Haematologica* 83:985, 1998.
844. Fadilah SA, Hatta AZ, Keng CS, et al: Successful treatment of acute promyelocytic leukemia in pregnancy with all-trans retinoic acid. *Leukemia* 15:1665, 2001.
845. Carridice D, Austin N, Bayston K, Ganly PS: Successful treatment of acute promyelocytic leukaemia during pregnancy. *Clin Lab Haematol* 24:307, 2002.
846. Tallman MS, Andersen JW, Schiffer CA, et al: Clinical description of 44 patients with acute promyelocytic leukemia who developed the retinoic acid syndrome. *Blood* 95:90, 2000.
847. Larsen RS, Tallman MS: Retinoic acid syndrome: Manifestations, pathogenesis, and treatment. *Best Pract Res Clin Haematol* 16:453, 2003.
848. Frankel SR, Eardley A, Lauwers G, et al: The "retinoic acid syndrome" in acute promyelocytic leukemia. *Ann Intern Med* 117:292, 1992.
849. De Botton S, Dombret H, Sanz M, et al: Incidence, clinical features, and outcome of all *trans*-retinoic acid syndrome in 413 cases of newly diagnosed acute promyelocytic leukemia. The European APL Group. *Blood* 92:2712, 1998.
850. Azlin ZA, Ahmed T: Cure in acute promyelocytic leukemia—Now more readily achievable with less toxic therapy. *Blood* 79:2492, 1992.
851. Tallman MS: Retinoic acid syndrome: A problem of the past? *Leukemia* 16:160, 2002
852. Falanga A, Barbui T: Coagulopathy of acute promyelocytic leukemia. *Acta Haematol* 106:43, 2001.
853. Yanada M, Matsushita T, Asou N, et al: Severe hemorrhagic complications during remission induction therapy for acute promyelocytic leukemia: Incidence, risk factors, and influence on outcome. *Eur J Haematol* 78:213, 2007.
854. Goldberg MA, Ginsburg D, Mayer RJ, et al: Is heparin administration necessary during induction chemotherapy for patients with acute promyelocytic leukemia? *Blood* 69:187, 1987.
855. Visani G, Gugliotta L, Tosi P, et al: All-trans retinoic acid significantly reduces the incidence of early hemorrhagic death during induction therapy of acute promyelocytic leukemia. *Eur J Haematol* 64:139, 2000.
856. Petti MC, Avvisati G, Amadori S, et al: Acute promyelocytic leukaemia: Clinical aspects and results of treatment in 62 patients. *Haematologica* 72:151, 1987.
857. Kizaki M, Ueno H, Yamazoe Y, et al: Mechanisms of retinoid resistance in leukemic cells: Possible role of cytochrome P450 and P-glycoprotein. *Blood* 87:725, 1996.
858. Adès L, Chevret S, Raffoux E, et al: Is cytarabine useful in the treatment of acute promyelocytic leukemia? Results of a randomized trial from the European Acute Promyelocytic Leukemia Group. *J Clin Oncol* 24:5703, 2006
859. Asou N, Kishimoto Y, Kiyoi H, et al: A randomized study with or without intensified maintenance chemotherapy in patients with acute promyelocytic leukemia who have become negative for PML-RARalpha transcript after consolidation therapy: The Japan Adult Leukemia Study Group (JALSG) APL97 study. *Blood* 110:59, 2007.
860. Tsimberidou AM, Kantarjian H, Keating MJ, Estey E: Optimizing treatment for elderly patients with acute promyelocytic leukemia: Is it time to replace chemotherapy with all-*trans* retinoic acid and arsenic trioxide? *Leuk Lymphoma* 47:2282, 2006.
861. Dombret H, Fenaux P, Soignet SL, Tallman MS: Established practice in the treatment of patients with acute promyelocytic leukemia and the introduction of arsenic trioxide as a novel therapy. *Semin Hematol* 39:8, 2002.
862. Sanz MA, Fenaux P, Lo Coco F, et al: Arsenic trioxide in the treatment of acute promyelocytic leukemia. A review of current evidence. *Haematologica* 90:1231, 2005.
863. Chen GQ, Shi XG, Tang W, et al: Use of arsenic trioxide (As_2O_3) in the treatment of acute promyelocytic leukemia (APL): 1. As_2O_3 exerts dose-dependent dual effects on APL cells. *Blood* 89:3345, 1997.
864. Jing Y, Dai J, Chalmers-Redman RME, et al: Arsenic trioxide selectively induces acute promyelocytic leukemia cell apoptosis via a hydrogen peroxide-dependent pathway. *Blood* 94:2102, 1999.
865. Mathas S, Lietz A, Janz M, et al: Inhibition of NF-kappaB essentially contributes to arsenic-induced apoptosis. *Blood* 102:1028, 2003.
866. Ozpolat B, Akar U, Zorrilla-Calancha I, et al: Death-associated protein 5 (DAP5/p97/NAT1) contributes to retinoic acid-induced granulocytic differentiation and arsenic trioxide-induced apoptosis in acute promyelocytic leukemia. *Apoptosis* 13:915, 2008.
867. Soignet SL, Maslak P, Wang ZG, et al: Complete remission after treatment of acute promyelocytic leukemia with arsenic trioxide. *N Engl J Med* 339:1341, 1998.
868. Kwong YL, Au WY, Chim CS, et al: Arsenic trioxide- and idarubicin-induced remissions in relapsed acute promyelocytic leukaemia: Clinicopathological and molecular features of a pilot study. *Am J Hematol* 66:274, 2001.
869. Raffoux E, Rousselot P, Poupon J, et al: Combined treatment with arsenic trioxide and all-trans-retinoic acid in patients with relapsed acute promyelocytic leukemia. *J Clin Oncol* 21:2326, 2003.
870. Comacho LH, Soignet SL, Chanel S, et al: Leukocytosis and the retinoic acid syndrome in patients with acute promyelocytic leukemia treated with arsenic trioxide. *J Clin Oncol* 18:2620, 2000.
871. Unnikrishnan D, Dutcher JP, Varshneya N, et al: Torsades de pointes in 3 patients with leukemia treated with arsenic trioxide. *Blood* 97:1514, 2001.
872. Zhou J, Meng R, Li X, et al: The effect of arsenic trioxide on QT interval prolongation during APL therapy. *Chin Med J* 116:1764, 2003.
873. Estey EH: Treatment options for relapsed acute promyelocytic leukaemia. *Best Pract Res Clin Haematol* 16:521, 2003.
874. Aribi A, Kantarjian HM, Estey EH, et al: Combination therapy with arsenic trioxide, all-trans retinoic acid, and gemtuzumab ozogamicin in recurrent acute promyelocytic leukemia. *Cancer* 109:1355, 2007.
875. Lo-Coco F, Romano A, Mengarelli A, et al: Allogeneic stem cell transplantation for advanced acute promyelocytic leukemia: Results in patients treated in second molecular remission or with molecularly persistent disease. *Leukemia* 17:1930, 2003.
876. Nabhan C, Mehta J, Tallman MS: The role of bone marrow transplantation in acute promyelocytic leukemia. *Bone Marrow Transplant* 28:219, 2001.
877. Colvic N, Bogdanovic A, Miljic P, et al: Central nervous system relapse in acute promyelocytic leukemia. *Am J Hematol* 71:60–2002.
878. Sanz MA, Larrea L, Sanz G, et al: Cutaneous promyelocytic sarcoma at sites of vascular access and marrow aspiration. A characteristic localization of chloromas in acute promyelocytic leukemia? *Haematologica* 85:758, 2000.
879. Latagliata R, Carmosino I, Breccia M, et al: Late relapses in acute promyelocytic leukaemia. *Acta Haematol* 117:106, 2007.
880. Esteve J, Escoda L, Martín G, et al: Outcome of patients with acute promyelocytic leukemia failing to front-line treatment with all-*trans* retinoic acid and anthracycline-based chemotherapy (PETHEMA protocols LPA96 and LPA99): Benefit of an early intervention. *Leukemia* 21:446, 2007.
881. Latagliata R, Petti MC, Fenu S, et al: Therapy-related myelodysplastic syndrome-acute myelogenous leukemia in patients treated for acute promyelocytic leukemia: An emerging problem. *Blood* 99:822, 2002.
882. Lobe I, Rigal-Huguet F, Vekhoff A, et al: Myelodysplastic syndrome after acute promyelocytic leukemia: The European APL group. *Leukemia* 17:1600, 2003.

883. Garcia-Manero G, Kantarjian HM, Kornblau S, Estey E: Therapy-related myelodysplastic syndrome or acute myelogenous leukemia in patients with acute promyelocytic leukemia (APL). *Leukemia* 16:1888, 2002.
884. Jantunen E, Heinonen K, Mahlamäki E, et al: Secondary acute promyelocytic leukemia: An increasingly common entity. *Leuk Lymphoma* 48:190, 2007.
885. Yoo SJ, Park CJ, Jang S, et al: Inferior prognostic outcome in acute promyelocytic leukemia with alterations of FLT3 gene. *Leuk Lymphoma* 47:1788, 2006.
886. Smith MA, McCaffrey RP, Karp JE: The secondary leukemias: Challenges and research directions. *J Natl Cancer Inst* 88:407, 1996.
887. Smith MA, Rubinstein L, Anderson JR, et al: Secondary leukemia or myelodysplastic syndrome after treatment with epipodophyllotoxins. *J Clin Oncol* 17:569, 1999.
888. Ng A, Taylor GM, Eden OB: Treatment-related leukaemia: A clinical and scientific challenge. *Cancer Treat Rev* 26:377, 2000.
889. Super HJ, McCabe NR, Thirman MJ, et al: Rearrangements of the MLL gene in therapy-related acute myeloid leukemia in patients previously treated with agents targeting DNA-topoisomerase 11. *Blood* 82:3705, 1993.
890. Dissing M, Le Beau MM, Pedersen-Bjergaard J: Inversion of chromosome 16 and uncommon rearrangements of the CBFB and MYHl1 genes in therapy-related acute myeloid leukemia: Rare events related to DNA-topoisomerase II inhibitors? *J Clin Oncol* 16:1890, 1998.
891. Gondek LP, Tiu R, O'Keefe CL, et al: Chromosomal lesions and uniparental disomy detected by SNP arrays in MDS, MDS/MPD, and MDS-derived AML. *Blood* 111:1534, 2008.
892. Seedhouse C, Russell N: Advances in the understanding of susceptibility to treatment-related acute myeloid leukaemia. *Br J Haematol* 137:513, 2007.
893. Pogliani EM, Pioltelli P, Russini F, et al: Acute leukemia following cisplatin for ovarian cancer [letter]. *Haematologica* 72:184, 1987.
894. Kolte B, Baer AN, Sait SN, et al: Acute myeloid leukemia in the setting of low dose weekly methotrexate therapy for rheumatoid arthritis. *Leuk Lymphoma* 42:371, 2001.
895. Bakland G, Nossent H: Acute myelogenous leukemia following etanercept therapy. *Rheumatology (Oxford)* 42:900, 2003.
896. Noronha V, Berliner N, Ballen KK, et al: Treatment-related myelodysplasia/AML in a patient with a history of breast cancer and an oligodendroglioma treated with temozolomide: Case study and review of the literature. *Neuro Oncol* 8:280, 2006.
897. Aktan M, Tanakol R, Nalcaci M, Dincol G: Leukemia in a patient treated with growth hormone. *Endocr J* 47:471, 2000.
898. Freedman MH, Bonilla MA, Fier C, et al: Myelodysplasia syndrome and acute myeloid leukemia in patients with congenital neutropenia receiving G-CSF therapy. *Blood* 96:429, 2000.
899. Andersen MK, Pedersen-Bjergaard J: Therapy-related MDS and AML in acute promyelocytic leukemia. *Blood* 100:1928, 2002.
900. Barnard DR, Lange B, Alonzo TA, et al: Acute myeloid leukemia and myelodysplastic syndrome in children treated for cancer: Comparison with primary presentation. *Blood* 100:427, 2002.
901. Smith RE, Bryant J, DeCillis A, et al: Acute myeloid leukemia and myelodysplastic syndrome after doxorubicin-cyclophosphamide adjuvant therapy for operable breast cancer: The National Surgical Adjuvant Breast and Bowel Project Experience. *J Clin Oncol* 21:1195, 2003.
902. Gershkevitsh E, Rosenberg I, Dearnaley DP, Trott KR: Bone marrow doses and leukemia risk in radiotherapy of prostate cancer. *Radiother Oncol* 53:189, 1999.
903. Armitage JO, Carbone PP, Connors JM, et al: Treatment-related myelodysplasia and acute leukemia in non-Hodgkin's lymphoma. *J Clin Oncol* 21:897, 2003.
904. Lambertenghi Deliliers G, Annaloro C, Pozzoli E, et al: Cytogenetic and myelodysplastic alterations after autologous hemopoietic stem cell transplantation. *Leuk Res* 23:291, 1999.
905. Legare RD, Gribben JG, Maragh M, et al: Prediction of therapy-related acute myelogenous leukemia (AML) and myelodysplastic syndrome (MDS) after autologous bone marrow transplant (ABMT) for lymphoma. *Am J Hematol* 56:45, 1997.
906. Micallef IN, Lillington DM, Apostolidis J, et al: Therapy-related myelodysplasia and secondary acute myelogenous leukemia after high-dose therapy with autologous hematopoietic progenitor-cell support for lymphoid malignancies. *J Clin Oncol* 18:847, 2000.
907. Lillington DM, Micallef IN, Carpenter E, et al: Detection of chromosome abnormalities pre-high-dose treatment in patients developing therapy-related myelodysplasia and secondary acute myelogenous leukemia after treatment for non-Hodgkin's lymphoma. *J Clin Oncol* 19:2472, 2001.
908. Estey EH: Treatment of acute myelogenous leukemia and myelodys-plastic syndromes. *Semin Hematol* 32:132, 1995.
909. Witherspoon RP, Deeg HJ, Storer B, et al: Hematopoietic stem-cell transplantation for treatment-related leukemia or myelodysplasia. *J Clin Oncol* 19:2134, 2001.
910. Costa LJ, Rodriguez V, Porrata LF, et al: Autologous HSC transplant in t-MDS/AML using cells harvested prior to the development of the secondary malignancy. *Bone Marrow Transplant* 42:497, 2008.
911. Anderson JE, Gooley TA, Schoch G, et al: Stem cell transplantation for secondary acute myeloid leukemia: Evaluation of transplantation as initial therapy or following induction chemotherapy. *Blood* 89:2578, 1997.
912. Rowe JM: Therapy of secondary leukemia. *Leukemia* 16:748, 2002.
913. Rosenfield C, Kantarjian H: Is myelodysplastic related acute myelogenous leukemia a distinct entity from *de novo* acute myelogenous leukemia? Potential for targeted therapies. *Leuk Lymphoma* 41:493, 2001.
914. Viniou NA, Vassilakopoulos TP, Giakoumi X, et al: Ida-FLAG plus imatinib mesylate-induced remission with chemoresistant Ph1+ acute myeloid leukemia. *Eur J Haematol* 72:58, 2004.
915. Brincker H: Estimate of overall treatment results in acute nonlymphocytic leukemia based on age-specific rates of incidence and complete remission. *Cancer Treat Rep* 69:5, 1985.
916. Büchner T, Berdel WE, Haferlach C, et al: Age-related risk profile and chemotherapy dose response in acute myeloid leukemia: A study by the German Acute Myeloid Leukemia Cooperative Group. *J Clin Oncol* 27:61, 2009.
917. Kuendgen A, Germing U: Emerging treatment strategies for acute myeloid leukemia (AML) in the elderly. *Cancer Treat Rev* 35:97, 2009.
918. Dombret H, Raffoux E, Gardin C: Acute myeloid leukemia in the elderly. *Semin Oncol* 35:430, 2008.
919. Ferrara F, Pinto A: Acute myeloid leukemia in the elderly: Current therapeutic results and perspectives for clinical research. *Rev Recent Clin Trials* 2:33, 2007.
920. Pinto A, Zulian GB, Archimbaud E: Acute myelogenous leukaemia. *Crit Rev Oncol Hematol* 27:161, 1998.
921. Leith CP, Kopecky KJ, Godwin J, et al: Acute myeloid leukemia in the elderly: Assessment of multidrug resistance (MDR1) and cytogenetics distinguishes biologic subgroups with remarkably distinct responses to standard chemotherapy. A Southwest Oncology Group study. *Blood* 89:3323, 1997.
922. Ballester O, Moscinski LC, Morris D, Balducci L: Acute myelogenous leukemia in the elderly. *J Am Geriatr Soc* 40:277, 1992.
923. Balducci L: Geriatric oncology. *Crit Rev Oncol Hematol* 46:211, 2003.
924. Baz R, Rodriguez C, Fu AZ, et al: Impact of remission induction chemotherapy on survival in older adults with acute myeloid leukemia. *Cancer* 110:1752, 2007.
925. Deschler B, de Witte T, Mertelsmann R, Lübbert M: Treatment decision-making for older patients with high-risk myelodysplastic syndrome or acute myeloid leukemia: Problems and approaches. *Haematologica* 91:1513, 2006.
926. Kalaycio M, Pohlman B, Elson P, et al: Chemotherapy for acute myelogenous leukemia in the elderly with cytarabine, mitoxanthrone, and granulocyte-macrophage colony-stimulating factor. *Am J Clin Oncol* 24:58, 2001.
927. Bennett CL, Hynes D, Godwin J, et al: Economic analysis of granulocyte colony stimulating factor as adjunct therapy for older patients with acute myelogenous leukemia (AML): Estimates from a Southwest Oncology Group clinical trial. *Cancer Invest* 19:603, 2001.
928. Lowenberg B, Suciu S, Archimbaud E, et al: Mitoxantrone versus daunorubicin in induction-consolidation chemotherapy—The value of low-dose cytarabine for maintenance of remission, and an assessment of prognostic factors in acute myeloid leukemia in the elderly: Final report. European Organization for the Research and Treatment of Cancer and the Dutch-Belgian Hemato-Oncology Cooperative Hovon Group. *J Clin Oncol* 16:872, 1998.
929. Harousseau JF, Rigal-Huguet F, Hurteloup P, et al: Treatment of acute myeloid leukemia in elderly patients with oral idarubicin as a single agent. *Eur J Haematol* 42:182, 1989.
930. Anderson JE, Kopecky KJ, Willman CL, et al: Outcome after induction chemotherapy for older patients with acute myeloid leukemia is not improved with mitoxantrone and etoposide compared to cytarabine and daunorubicin: A Southwest Oncology Group study. *Blood* 100:3869, 2002.
931. Hartman F, Jacobs G, Gotto H, et al: Cytosine arabinoside, idarubicin and divided dose etoposide for the treatment of acute myeloid leukemia in elderly patients. *Leuk Lymphoma* 42:347, 2001.
932. Kanemura N, Tsurumi H, Kasahara S, et al: Continuous drip infusion of low dose cytarabine and etoposide with granulocyte colony-stimulating factor for elderly patients with acute myeloid leukaemia ineligible for intensive chemotherapy. *Hematol Oncol* 26:33, 2008.
933. Chauncey TR, Rankin C, Anderson JE, et al: A phase I study of induction chemotherapy for older patients with newly diagnosed acute myeloid leukemia (AML) using mitoxantrone, etoposide, and the MDR modulator PSC 833: A Southwest Oncology Group study 9617. *Leuk Res* 24:567, 2000.
934. Brandwein JM, Yang L, Schimmer AD, et al: A phase II study of temozolomide therapy for poor-risk patients aged > or = 60 years with acute myeloid leukemia: Low levels of MGMT predict for response. *Leukemia* 21:821, 2007.
935. Faderl S, Ravandi F, Huang X, et al: A randomized study of clofarabine versus clofarabine plus low-dose cytarabine as front-line therapy for patients aged 60 years and older with acute myeloid leukemia and high-risk myelodysplastic syndrome. *Blood* 112:1638, 2008.
936. Schiller GJ: Postremission therapy of acute myeloid leukemia in older adults. *Leukemia* 10(Suppl 1):S18, 1996.
937. Kiss TL, Sabry W, Lazarus HM, Lipton JH: Blood and marrow transplantation in elderly acute myeloid leukaemia patients—Older certainly is not better. *Bone Marrow Transplant* 40:405, 2007.
938. Herzig RH: High-dose ara-C in older adults with acute leukemia. *Leukemia* 10(Suppl 1):S10, 1996.
939. Letendre L, Noel P, Litzow MR, et al: Treatment of acute myelogenous leukemia in the older patient with attenuated high-dose ara-C. *Am J Clin Oncol* 21:142, 1998.
940. Schiller G, Lee M: Long-term outcome of high-dose cytarabine-based consolidation chemotherapy for older patients with acute myelogenous leukemia. *Leuk Lymphoma* 25:111, 1997.
941. Lowenberg B: Post-remission treatment of acute myelogenous leukemia. *N Engl J Med* 332:260, 1995.

942. Gardin C, Turlure P, Fagot T, et al: Postremission treatment of elderly patients with acute myeloid leukemia in first complete remission after intensive induction chemotherapy: Results of the multicenter randomized Acute Leukemia French Association (ALFA) 9803 trial. *Blood* 109:5129, 2007.
943. DeLima M, Ghaddar H, Pierce S, Estey E: Treatment of newly-diagnosed acute myelogenous leukaemia in patients aged 80 years and above. *Br J Haematol* 93:89, 1996.
944. Burnett AK, Mohite U: Treatment of older patients with acute myeloid leukemia—new agents. *Semin Hematol* 43:96, 2006.
945. Estey EH: Older adults: Should the paradigm shift from standard therapy? *Best Pract Res Clin Haematol* 21:61, 2008.
946. Etienne A, Esterni B, Charbonnier A, et al: Comorbidity is an independent predictor of complete remission in elderly patients receiving induction chemotherapy for acute myeloid leukemia. *Cancer* 109:1376, 2007.
947. Gupta V, Xu W, Keng C, et al: The outcome of intensive induction therapy in patients > or = 70 years with acute myeloid leukemia. *Leukemia* 21:1321, 2007.
948. Estey EH: General approach to, and perspectives on clinical research in, older patients with newly diagnosed acute myeloid leukemia. *Semin Hematol* 43:89, 2006
949. Johnson PR, Yin JA: Prognostic factors in elderly patients with acute myeloid leukaemia. *Leuk Lymphoma* 16:51, 1994.
950. Oberg G, Killander A, Bjoreman M, et al: Long-term follow-up of patients > or = 60 yr old with acute myeloid leukaemia. *Eur J Haematol* 68:376, 2002.
951. Stone RM: The difficult problem of acute myeloid leukemia in the older adult. *CA Cancer J Clin* 52:363, 2002.
952. Alibhai SM, Leach M, Kermalli H, et al: The impact of acute myeloid leukemia and its treatment on quality of life and functional status in older adults. *Crit Rev Oncol Hematol* 64:19, 2007.
953. Büchner T, Berdel WE, Wörmann B, et al: Treatment of older patients with AML. *Crit Rev Oncol Hematol* 56:247, 2005.
954. http://seer.concer.gov/csr/1975_2005/results+mreger/sect_13_leukemia.pdf
955. Renosos EE, Shepard FA, Messner HA, et al: Acute leukemia during pregnancy: The Toronto Leukemia Study Group Experience with long-term follow-up of children exposed in utero to chemotherapeutic agents. *J Clin Oncol* 5:1098, 1987.
956. Caligiuri MA, Mayer RJ: Pregnancy and leukemia. *Semin Oncol* 16:388, 1989.
957. Chelghoum Y, Vey N, Raffoux E, et al: Acute leukemia during pregnancy: A report on 37 patients and a review of the literature. *Cancer* 104:110, 2005.
958. Aviles A, Neri N: Hematological malignancies and pregnancy: A final report of 84 children who received chemotherapy in utero. *Clin Lymphoma* 2:173, 2001.
959. Greenlund LJ, Letendre L, Tefferi A: Acute leukemia during pregnancy: A single institutional experience with 17 cases. *Leuk Lymphoma* 41:571, 2001.
960. Shapira T, Pereg D, Lishner M: How I treat acute and chronic leukemia in pregnancy. *Blood Rev* 22:247, 2008.
961. Osada S, Horibe K, Oiwa K, et al: A case of infantile acute monocytic leukemia caused by vertical transmission of the mother's leukemic cells. *Cancer* 65:1146, 1990.
962. Lipovsky MM, Biesma DH, Christiaens GC, Petersen EJ: Successful treatment of acute promyelocytic leukaemia with all-*trans* retinoic acid during late pregnancy. *Br J Haematol* 94:669, 1996.
963. Valappil S, Kurkar M, Howell R, et al: Outcome of pregnancy in women treated with all-trans retinoic acid; a case report and review of literature. *Hematology* 12:415, 2007.
964. Gregory J, Arceci R: Acute myeloid leukemia in children: A review of risk factors and recent trials. *Cancer Invest* 20:1027, 2002.
965. Clark JJ, Smith FO, Arceci RJ: Update in childhood myeloid leukemia: Recent developments in the molecular basis of disease and novel therapies. *Curr Opin Hematol* 10:31, 2002.
966. Arceci RJ: Progress and controversies in the treatment of pediatric acute myelogenous leukemia. *Curr Opin Hematol* 9:353, 2002.
967. Webb DKH, Harrison G, Stevens RF, et al: Relationships between age at diagnosis, clinical featuures, and outome of therapy in children in the Medical Research Council AML 10 and 12 trials for acute myeloid leukemia. *Blood* 98:1714, 2001.
968. Zwaan CM, Meshinchi S, Radich JP, et al: FLT3 internal tandem duplication in 234 children with acute myeloid leukemia: Prognostic significance and relation to cellular drug resistance. *Blood* 102:2387, 2002.
969. Wheatley K, Burnett AK, Goldstone AH, et al: A simple robust, validated and highly predictive index for the determination of risk-directed therapy in acute myeloid leukaemia derived from the MRC AML 10 trial. *Br J Haematol* 107:69, 1999.
970. Wells RJ, Arthur DC, Srivastava A, et al: Prognostic variables in newly diagnosed children and adolescents with acute myeloid leukemia. *Leukemia* 16:601, 2002.
971. Sievers EL, Lange BJ, Alonzo TA, et al: Immunophenotypic evidence of leukemia after induction therapy predicts relapse: Results from a prospective Children's Cancer Group study of 252 patients with acute myeloid leukemia. *Blood* 101:3398, 2003.
972. Hann IM, Webb DK, Gibson BE, Harrison CJ: MRC trials in childhood acute myeloid leukaemia. *Ann Hematol* 83 Suppl 1:S108, 2004.
973. Woods WG, Neudorf S, Gold S, et al: A comparison of allogeneic bone marrow transplantaion, autologous bone marrow transplantation, and aggressive chemotherapy in children with acute myeloid leukemia in remission: A report from the Children's Cancer Group. *Blood* 97:56, 2001.
974. Kawasaki H, Isoyama K, Eguchi M, et al: Superior outcome of infant acute myeloid leukemia with intensive chemotherapy: Results of the Japan Infant Leukemia Study Group. *Blood* 98:3589, 2001.
975. Chessels JM, Harrison CJ, Kempski H, et al: Clinical features, cytogenetics, and outcome in acute lymphoblastic and myeloid leukemia of infancy: Report from the MRC Childhood Leukemia working party. *Leukemia* 16:776, 2002.
976. Rocha V, Cornish J, Sievers EL, et al: Comparison of outcomes of unrelated bone marrow and umbilical cord blood transplants in children with acute leukemia. *Blood* 97:2962, 2001.
977. Leung W, Hudson MM, Strickland DK, et al: Late effects of treatment in survivors of childhood acute myeloid leukemia. *J Clin Oncol* 18:3273, 2000.
978. Leung W, Ribiero RC, Hudson MM, et al: Second malignancy after treatment of childhood acute myeloid leukemia. *Leukemia* 15:41, 2001.
979. Verhagen C, Stalpers LJA, DePauw BE, Haanen C: Drug-induced skin reactions in patients with acute non-lymphocytic leukaemia. *Eur J Haematol* 38:225, 1987.
980. Kapusta L, Groot-Loonen J, Thijssen JM, et al: Regional cardiac wall motion abnormalities during and shortly after anthracyclines therapy. *Med Pediatr Oncol* 41:426, 2003.
981. Benvenuto GM, Ometto R, Fontanelli A, et al: Chemotherapy-related cardiotoxicity: New diagnostic and preventive strategies. *Ital Heart J* 4:655, 2003.
982. Dietz B, Van der Hem KG: Late-onset cardiotoxicity of chemotherapy and radiotherapy. *Neth J Med* 61:228, 2003.
983. Theodoulou M, Hudis C: Cardiac profiles of liposomal anthracyclines: Greater cardiac safety versus conventional doxorubicin? *Cancer* 100:2052, 2004.
984. Swain SM, Vici P: The current and future role of dexrazoxane as a cardioprotectant in anthracycline treatment: Expert panel review. *J Cancer Res Clin Oncol* 130:1, 2004.
985. Anderson LA, Pfeiffer R, Warren JL, et al: Hematopoietic malignancies associated with viral and alcoholic hepatitis. *Cancer Epidemiol Biomarkers Prev* 17:3069, 2008.
986. Kojima H, Abei M, Takei N, et al: Fatal reactivation of hepatitis B virus following cytotoxic chemotherapy for acute myelogenous leukemia: Fibrosing cholestatic hepatitis. *Eur J Haematol* 69:101, 2002.
987. Ishiga K, Kawatani T, Suou T, et al: Fulminant hepatitis type B after chemotherapy in a serologically negative hepatitis B virus carrier with acute myelogenous leukemia. *Int J Hematol* 73:115, 2001.
988. Bianco E, Marcucci F, Mele A, et al: Italian Multi-Center case-control study. Prevalence of hepatitis C virus infection in lymphoproliferative diseases other than B-cell non-Hodgkin's lymphoma, and in myeloproliferative diseases: An Italian Multi-Center case-control study. *Haematologica* 89:70, 2004.
989. Zuckerman E, Zuckerman T, Douer D, et al: Liver dysfunction in patients infected with hepatitis C virus undergoing chemotherapy for hematologic malignancies. *Cancer* 15:1224, 1998.
990. Roozrokh HC, Stahlfeld KR: Disseminated hepatic candidiasis. *J Am Coll Surg* 194:231, 2002.
991. Sallah S, Wan JY, Nguyen NP, et al: Analysis of factors related to the occurrence of chronic disseminated candidiasis in patients with acute leukemia in a non-bone marrow transplant setting: A follow-up study. *Cancer* 15:1349, 2001.
992. Colovic M, Lazarevic V, Colovic R, et al: Hepatosplenic candidiasis after neutropenic phase of acute leukaemia. *Med Oncol* 16:139, 1999.
993. Sallah S, Semelka R, Kelekis N, et al: Diagnosis and monitoring response to treatment of hepatosplenic candidiasis in patients with acute leukemia using magnetic resonance imaging. *Acta Haematol* 100:77, 1998.
994. Teefey SA, Montana MA, Goldfogel GA, Shuman WP: Sonographic diagnosis of neutropenic typhlitis. *AJR Am J Roentgenol* 149:731.
995. Keidan RD, Fanning J, Gatenby RA, Weese JL: Recurrent typhlitis. A disease resulting from aggressive chemotherapy. *Dis Colon Rectum* 32:206, 1989.
996. Byrnes JJ, Baqueriro H, Gonzalez M, Henseley GT: Thrombotic thrombocytopenic purpura subsequent to acute myelogenous leukemia chemotherapy. *Am J Hematol* 21:299, 1986.
997. Blumenfeld Z, Avivi I, Ritter M, Rowe JM: Preservation of fertility and ovarian function and minimizing chemotherapy-induced gonadotoxicity in young women. *J Soc Gynecol Investig* 6:229, 1999.
998. Lopez Andreu JA, Fernandez PJ, et al: Persistent altered spermatogenesis in long-term childhood cancer survivors. *Pediatr Hematol Oncol* 17:21, 2000.
999. Relander T, Cavallin-Stahl E, Garwicz S, et al: Gonadal and sexual function in men treated for childhood cancer. *Med Pediatr Oncol* 35:52, 2000.
1000. Hinterberger-Fischer M, Kier P, Kalhs P, et al: Fertility, pregnancies and offsing complications after bone marrow transplantation. *Bone Marrow Transplant* 7:5, 1991.
1001. Giri N, Vowels MR, Barr AL, Mameghan H: Successful pregnancy after total body irradiation and bone marrow transplantation for acute leukaemia. *Bone Marrow Transplant* 10:93, 1992.
1002. Lemez P, Urbánek V: Chemotherapy for acute myeloid leukemias with cytosine arabinoside, daunorubicin, etoposide, and mitoxantrone may cause permanent oligoasthenozoospermia or amenorrhea in middle-aged patients. *Neoplasma* 52:398, 2005.
1003. Maguire LC, Dick FR, Sherman BM: The effects of anti-leukemic therapy on gonadal histology in adult males. *Cancer* 48:1967, 1981.
1004. Matthews JH, Wood JK: Male fertility during chemotherapy for acute leukemia. *N Engl J Med* 303:1235, 1980.
1005. Wahlin A, Markevarn B, Gololeva I, et al: Improved outcome in adult acute myeloid leukemia is almost entirely restricted to young patients and associated stem cell transplantation. *Eur J Haematol* 68:54, 2002.
1006. Lichtman MA, Rowe JM: The relationship of patient age to the pathobiology of the clonal myeloid disease. *Semin Oncol* 31:185, 2004.

1007. Yanada M, Garcia-Manero G, Borthakur G, et al: Potential cure of acute myeloid leukemia : Analysis of 1069 consecutive patients in first complete remission. *Cancer* 110:2756, 2007.
1008. Fialkow PJ, Singer JW, Roskind WH, et al: Clonal development, stem cell differentiation and the nature of clinical remissions in acute nonlymphocytic leukemia: Studies of patients heterozygous for glucose-6-phosphate dehydrogenase. *N Engl J Med* 317:468, 1987.
1009. Bartram CR, Ludwig W-D, Hiddemann W, et al: Acute myeloid leukemia: Analysis of *ras* gene mutations and clonality defined by polymorphic X-linked loci. *Leukemia* 3:247, 1989.
1010. Fialkow PJ, Janssen JWG, Bartram CR: Clonal remissions in acute nonlymphocytic leukemia: Evidence for a multistep pathogenesis of the malignancy. *Blood* 77:1415, 1991.
1011. Busque L, Gilliland DG: Clonal evolution in acute myeloid leukemia. *Blood* 82:337, 1993.
1012. Gale RE, Wheadon H, Goldstone AH, et al: Frequency of clonal remission in acute myeloid leukaemia. *Lancet* 341:138, 1993.
1013. Killman S-A: Acute leukemia: Development, remission/relapse pattern, relationship between normal and leukaemic haemopoiesis, and the "sleeper-to-feeder" stem cell hypothesis. *Baillieres Clin Haematol* 4:577, 1991.
1014. Kudoh S, Asou H, Kyo T, et al: Emergence of karyotypically unrelated clone in remission of de novo acute myeloblastic leukaemias. *Br J Haematol* 89:531, 1995.
1015. Jinnai 1, Nagai K, Yoshida S, et al: Incidence and characteristics of clonal hematopoiesis in remission of acute myeloid leukemia in relation to morphological dysplasia. *Leukemia* 9:1756, 1995.
1016. Robert EE: Spontaneous complete remission in acute promyelocytic leukemia. *N Y State J Med* 86:662, 1985.
1017. Takue Y, Culbert SJ, Van Eys J, et al: Spontaneous cure of end-stage acute nonlymphocytic leukemia complicated with chloroma (granulocytic sarcoma). *Cancer* 58:1101, 1986.
1018. Jehn UW, Mempel MA: Spontaneous remission of acute myeloid leukemia. *Blut* 52:165, 1986.
1019. Passe S, Miké V, Mertelsmann R, et al: Acute nonlymphoblastic leukemia: Prognostic factors in adults with long-term follow-up. *Cancer* 50:1462, 1982.
1020. Evansen SA, Stavem P: Long-term survival in acute leukemia. *Acta Med Scand* 219:79, 1986.
1021. Grunwald HW: The cure of acute myeloblastic leukemia in adults. *JAMA* 247:1698, 1982.
1022. MacMahon B, Forman D: Variations in the duration of survival of patients with acute leukemia. *Blood* 12:683, 1957.
1023. Menzin J, Lang K, Earle C, et al: The outcomes and costs of acute myeloid leukemia among the elderly. *Arch Intern Med* 162:1597, 2002.
1024. Derolf AR, Kristinsson SY, Andersson TM, et al: Improved patient survival for acute myeloid leukemia: A population-based study of 9,729 patients diagnosed in Sweden 1973–2005. *Blood* 113:3666, 2009.
1025. Burnett AK: Transplantation in first remission of acute myeloid leukemia. *N Engl J Med* 339:1698, 1998.
1026. Burnett AK, Goldstone AH, Stevens RM, et al: Randomised comparison of addition of autologous bone-marrow transplantation to intensive chemotherapy for acute myeloid leukaemia in first remission: Results of MRC AML 10 trial. U.K. Medical Research Council Adult and Children's Leukaemia Working Parties. *Lancet* 351:700, 1998.
1027. Clift RA, Buckner CD: Marrow transplantation for acute myeloid leukemia. *Cancer Invest* 16:53, 1998.
1028. Gale RP, Butturini A: Transplants for acute myelogenous leukemia. *Cancer Invest* 16:66, 1998.
1029. Redaelli A, Stephens JM, Brandt S, et al: Short- and long-term effects of acute myeloid leukemia on patient health-related quality of life. *Cancer Treat Rev* 30:103, 2004.
1030. Hsu C, Wang JD, Hwang JS, et al: Survival-weighted health profile for long-term survivors of acute myelogenous leukemia. *Qual Life Res* 12:519, 2003.
1031. Kern W, Haferlach T, Schoch C, et al: Early blast clearance by remission induction therapy is a major independent prognostic factor for both achievement of complete remission and long-term outcome in acute myeloid leukemia: Data from the German AML Cooperative Group (AMLCG) 1992 Trial. *Blood* 101:64, 2003.
1032. Elliott MA, Litzow MR, Letendre LL, et al: Early peripheral blood blast clearance during induction chemotherapy for acute myeloid leukemia predicts superior relapse-free survival. *Blood* 110:4172, 2007.
1033. Cortes JE, Kantarjian H, O'Brien S, et al: Clinical and prognostic significance of trisomy 21 in adult patients with acute myelogenous leukemia and myelodysplastic syndromes. *Leukemia* 9:115, 1995.
1034. Marcucci G, Maharry K, Radmacher MD, et al: Prognostic significance of, and gene and microRNA expression signatures associated with, CEBPA mutations in cytogenetically normal acute myeloid leukemia with high-risk molecular features: A Cancer and Leukemia Group B Study. *J Clin Oncol* 26:5078, 2008.
1035. Buchner T, Heinecke A: The role of prognostic factors in acute myeloid leukemia. *Leukemia* 10(Suppl 1):S28, 1996.
1036. Ghaddar HM, Pierce S, Reed P, Estey EH: Prognostic value of residual normal metaphases in acute myelogenous leukemia patients presenting with abnormal karyotype. *Leukemia* 9:779, 1995.
1037. Seol JG, Kim ES, Park WH, et al: Telomerase activity in acute myelogenous leukaemia: Clinical and biological implications. *Br J Haematol* 100:156, 1998.
1038. Huh Y, Smith TL, Collins P, et al: Terminal deoxynucleotidyl transferase expression in acute myelogenous leukemia and myelodysplasia as determined by flow cytometry. *Leuk Lymphoma* 37:319, 2000.
1039. Del Poeta G, Venditti A, Del Principe MI, et al: Amount of spontaneous apoptosis detected by Bax/Bcl-2 ratio predicts outcome in acute myeloid leukemia (AML). *Blood* 101:2125, 2003.
1040. Ong YL, McMullin MF, Bailie KE, et al: High bax expression is a good prognostic indicator in acute myeloid leukaemia. *Br J Haematol* 111:182, 2000.
1041. Amirghofran Z, Zakerinia M, Shamseddin A: Significant association between expression of the CD11b surface molecule and favorable outcome for patients with acute myeloblastic leukemia. *Int J Hematol* 73:502, 2001.
1042. Matsunaga T, Takemoto N, Sato T, et al: Interaction between leukemic-cell VLA-4 and stromal fibronectin is a decisive factor for minimal residual disease of acute myelogenous leukemia. *Nat Med* 9:1158, 2003.
1043. Becker PS, Kopecky KJ, Wilks AN, et al: Very late antigen-4 (VLA-4) function of myeloblasts correlates with improved overall survival for patients with acute myeloid leukemia. *Blood* 113:866, 2009.
1044. Estrov Z, Thall PF, Talpaz M, et al: Caspase 2 and caspase 3 protein levels as predictors of survival in acute myelogenous leukemia. *Blood* 92:3090, 1998.
1045. Frehling S, Schlenk RF, Stolze I, et al: CEBPA mutation in younger adults with acute myeloid leukemia and normal cytogenetics: Prognostic relevance and analysis of cooperating mutations. *J Clin Oncol* 22:624, 2004.
1046. Hollink IH, Zwaan CM, Zimmermann M, et al: Favorable prognostic impact of NPM1 gene mutations in childhood acute myeloid leukemia, with emphasis on cytogenetically normal AML. *Leukemia* 23:262, 2009.
1047. Yanada M, Borthakur G, Garcia-Manero G, et al: Blood counts at time of complete remission provide additional independent prognostic information in acute myeloid leukemia. *Leuk Res* 32:1505, 2008.
1048. Hussein K, Jahagirdar B, Gupta P, et al: Day 14 bone marrow biopsy in predicting complete remission and survival in acute myeloid leukemia. *Am J Hematol* 83:446, 2008.
1049. Paietta E: Classical multidrug resistance in acute myeloid leukaemia. *Med Oncol* 14:53, 1997.
1050. Ino T, Miyazaki H, Isogai M, et al: Expression of P-glycoprotein in de novo acute myelogenous leukemia at initial diagnosis: Results of molecular and functional assays and correlation with treatment outcome. *Leukemia* 8:1492, 1994.
1051. Hart SM, Ganeshaguru K, Hoffbrand AV: Expression of the multidrug resistance-associated protein (MRP) in acute leukaemia. *Leukemia* 8:2163, 1994.
1052. Guerci A, Merlin JL, Missoum N, et al: Predictive value for treatment outcome in acute myeloid leukemia of cellular daunorubicin accumulation and P-glycoprotein expression simultaneously determined by flow cytometry. *Blood* 85:2147, 1995.
1053. Leith CP, Chen IM, Kopecky KJ, et al: Correlation of multidrug resistance (MDR1) protein expression with functional dye/drug efflux in acute myeloid leukemia by multiparameter flow cytometry: Identification of discordant MDR/efflux+ and MDR1+/efflux- cases. *Blood* 86:2329, 1995.
1054. Kohler T, Eller J, Leiblein S, et al: Mechanisms responsible for therapy resistance of acute myelogenous leukemia (AML). *Int J Clin Pharmacol Ther* 36:97, 1998.
1055. Filipits M, Stranzl T, Pohl G, et al: Drug resistance factors in acute myeloid leukemia: A comparative analysis. *Leukemia* 14:68, 2000.
1056. Massaad-Massade L, Ribrag V, Marie JP, et al: Glutathione system, topoisomerase II level and multidrug resistance phenotype in acute myelogenous leukemia before treatment and at relapse. *Anticancer Res* 17:4647, 1997.
1057. Drach D, Zhao S, Drach J, Andreeff M: Low incidence of MDR1 expression in acute promyelocytic leukaemia. *Br J Haematol* 90:369, 1995.
1058. Paschka P, Marcucci G, Ruppert AS, et al: Adverse prognostic significance of KIT mutations in adult acute myeloid leukemia with inv(16) and t(8;21): A Cancer and Leukemia Group B Study. *J Clin Oncol* 24:3904, 2006.
1059. Hoyle CF, DeBastos M, Wheatley K, et al: AML associated with previous cytotoxic therapy, MDS or myeloproliferative disorders: Results from the MRC's 9th AML trial. *Br J Haematol* 72:45, 1989.
1060. DeWitte T, Muus P, DePauw B, Haanen C: Intensive antileukemic treatment of patients younger than 65 years with myelodysplastic syndromes and secondary acute myelogenous leukemia. *Cancer* 66:831, 1990.
1061. Brito-Babapulle F, Catovsky D, Galton DAG: Clinical and laboratory features of de novo acute myeloid leukaemia with trilineage myelodysplasia. *Br J Haematol* 66:445, 1987.
1062. Brito-Babapulle F, Catovsky D, Galton DAG: Myelodysplastic relapse of *de novo* acute myeloid leukaemia with trilineage myelodysplasia. *Br J Haematol* 68:411, 1988.
1063. Rosenthal NS, Farhi DC: Dysmegakaryopoiesis resembling acute megakaryoblastic leukemia in treated acute myeloid leukemia. *Am J Clin Pathol* 95:556, 1991.
1064. Layton DM, Ireland RM, Mufti GJ, Bellingham AJ: Myelodysplastic relapse of *de novo* AML: A heterogenous entity. *Leuk Res* 11:1055, 1987.
1065. Jowitt SN, Yin JAL, Saunders MJ: Relapsed myelodysplastic clone differs from acute onset clone as shown by X-linked DNA polymorphism patterns in a patient with acute myeloid leukemia. *Blood* 82:613, 1993.
1066. O'Brien S, Kantarjian HM, Keating M, et al: Association of granulocytosis with poor prognosis in patients with acute myelogenous leukemia and translocation of chromosomes 8 and 21. *J Clin Oncol* 7:1081, 1989.
1067. Krykowski E, Polkowska-Kulesza E, Robak T, et al: Analysis of prognostic factors in acute leukemias in adults. *Haematol Blood Transfus* 30:369, 1987.

1068. Greenwood MJ, Seftel MD, Richardson C, et al: Leukocyte count as a predictor of death during remission induction in acute myeloid leukemia. *Leuk Lymphoma* 47:1245, 2006.
1069. Bernard P, Reiffers J, LaComb F, et al: A stage classification for prognosis in adult acute myelogenous leukaemia based upon patient's age, bone marrow karyotype, and clinical features. *Scand J Haematol* 32:429, 1984.
1070. Keating S, Suciu S, De Witte T, et al: The stem cell mobilizing capacity of patients with acute myeloid leukemia in complete remission correlates with relapse risk: Results of the EORTC-GIMEMA AML-10 trial. *Leukemia* 17:60, 2003.
1071. Tremblay LN, Hyland RH, Schouten BD, Hanly PJ: Survival of acute myelogenous leukemia patients requiring intubation/ventilatory support. *Clin Invest Med* 18:19, 1995.
1072. Hunter AE, Rogers SY, Roberts IAG, et al: Autonomous growth of blast cells is associated with reduced survival in acute myeloblastic leukemia. *Blood* 82:399, 1993.
1073. Campos L, Rouault JP, Sabido O, et al: High expression of bcl-2 protein in acute myeloid leukemia cells is associated with poor response to chemotherapy. *Blood* 81:3091, 1993.
1074. Kaufmann SH, Karp JE, Svingen PA, et al: Elevated expression of the apoptotic regulator Mcl-1 at the time of leukemic relapse. *Blood* 91:991, 1998.
1075. Zhang W, Xu HJ, Kornblau SM, et al: Growth-factor stimulation reveals two mechanisms of retinoblastoma gene inactivation in human myelogenous leukemia cells. *Leuk Lymphoma* 16:191, 1995.
1076. Zhang W, Kornblau SM, Kobayashi T, et al: High levels of constitutive WAFl/Cipl protein are associated with chemoresistance in acute myelogenous leukemia. *Clin Cancer Res* 1:1051, 1995.
1077. Raspadori D, Lauria F, Ventura MA, et al: Incidence and prognostic relevance of CD34 expression in acute myeloblastic leukemia: Analysis of 141 cases. *Leuk Res* 21:603, 1997.
1078. Dalal Bi, Wu V, Barnett MJ, et al: Induction failure in de novo acute myelogenous leukemia is associated with expression of high levels of CD34 antigen by the leukemic blasts. *Leuk Lymphoma* 26:299, 1997.
1079. Lee JJ, Cho D, Chung IJ, et al: CD34 expression is associated with poor clinical outcome in patients with acute promyelocytic leukemia. *Am J Hematol* 73:149, 2003.
1080. Shimamoto T, Ohyashiki K, Ohyashiki JH, et al: The expression pattern of erythrocyte/megakaryocyte-related transcription factors GATA-1 and the stem cell leukemia gene correlates with hematopoietic differentiation and is associated with outcome of acute myeloid leukemia. *Blood* 86:3173, 1995.
1081. Baer MR, Stewart CC, Lawrence D, et al: Expression of the neural cell adhesion molecule CD56 is associated with short remission duration and survival in acute myeloid leukemia with t(8;21)(q22;q22). *Blood* 90:1643, 1997.
1082. Extermann M, Bacchi M, Monai N, et al: Relationship between cleaved L-selectin levels and the outcome of acute myeloid leukemia. *Blood* 92:3115, 1998.
1083. Raza A, Preisler HD, Li YQ, et al: Biologic characteristics of newly diagnosed poor prognosis acute myelogenous leukemia. *Am J Hematol* 42:359, 1993.
1084. Wetzler M, Baer MR, Bernstein SH, et al: Expression of c-mpl MRNA, the receptor for thrombopoietin, in acute myeloid leukemia blasts identifies a group of patients with poor response to intensive chemotherapy. *J Clin Oncol* 15:2262, 1997.
1085. Small D: Targeting FLT3 for the treatment of leukemia. *Semin Hematol* 45(3 Suppl 2):S17, 2008.
1086. Kim DH, Lee NY, Lee MH, et al: Vascular endothelial growth factor (VEGF) gene (VEGFA) polymorphism can predictthe prognosis in acute myeloid leukaemia patients. *Br J Haematol* 140:71, 2008.
1087. Tsimberidou AM, Kantarjian HM, Wen S, et al: The prognostic significance of serum beta2 microglobulin levels in acute myeloid leukemia and prognostic scores predicting survival: Analysis of 1,180 patients. *Clin Cancer Res* 14:721, 2008.
1088. Heuser M, Beutel G, Krauter J, et al: High meningioma 1 (MN1) expression as a predictor for poor outcome in acute myeloid leukemia with normal cytogenetics. *Blood* 108:3898, 2006.
1089. Gaidzik VI, Schlenk RF, Moschny S, et al: Prognostic impact of WT1 mutations in cytogenetically normal acute myeloid leukemia (AML): A study of the German-Austrian AML Study Group (AMLSG). *Blood* 113:4505, 2009.
1090. Testa U, Riccioni R, Militi S, et al: Elevated expression of IL-3Ralpha in acute myelogenous leukemia is associated with enhanced blast proliferation, increased cellularity, and poor prognosis. *Blood* 100:2980, 2002.
1091. Schnittger S, Kinkelin U, Schoch C, et al: Screening for MLL tandem duplication in 387 unselected patients with AML identify a prognostically unfavorable subset of AML. *Leukemia* 14:796, 2000.
1092. Schoch C, Schnittger S, Klaus M, et al: AML with 11q23/MLL abnormalities as defined by the WHO classification: Incidence, partner chromosomes, FAB subtype, age distribution, and prognostic impact in an unselected series of 1897 cytogenetically analyzed AML cases. *Blood* 102:2395, 2003.
1093. Di Bono E, Sartori R, Zambello R, et al: Prognostic significance of CD56 antigen expresssion in acute myeloid leukemia. *Haematologica* 87:250, 2002.
1094. Kahl C, Florschutz A, Jentsch-Ullrich K, et al: Primary intracranial manifestation of CD7/CD56-positive acute myelogenous leukemia. *Onkologie* 23:580, 2000.
1095. Yang DH, Lee JJ, Mun YC, et al: Predictable prognostic factor of CD56 expression in patients with acute myeloid leukemia with t(8:21) after high dose cytarabine or allogeneic hematopoietic stem cell transplantation. *Am J Hematol* 82:1, 2007.
1096. Chim CS, Liang R, Tam CY, Kwong YL: Methylation of p15 and p16 genes in acute promyelocytic leukemia: Potential diagnostic and prognostic significance. *J Clin Oncol* 19:2033, 2001.
1097. Das-Gupta EP, Seedhouse CH, Russell NH: Microsatellite instability occurs in defined subsets of patients with acute myeloblastic leukaemia. *Br J Haematol* 114:307, 2001.
1098. Lee ST, Jang JH, Min YH, et al: AC133 antigen as a prognostic factor in acute leukemia. *Leuk Res* 25:757, 2001.
1099. Benekle M, Xia Z, Donohue KA, et al: Constitutive activity of signal transducer and activator of transcription 3 protein in acute myeloid leukemia blasts is associated with short disease-free survival. *Blood* 99:252, 2002.
1110. Baldus CD, Tanner SM, Ruppert AS, et al: *BAALC* expression predicts clinical outcome of de novo acyte myeloid leukemia patients with normal cytogenetics. *Blood* 102:1613, 2003.
1101. Smith MA, Luxton RW, Pallister CJ, Smith JG: A novel predictive model of outcome in de novo AML based on S-phase activity and proliferative response of blast cells to haemopoietic growth factors. *Leuk Res* 26:345, 2002.
1102. Van Doorn-Khosrovani, Erpelinck C, Van Putten WLJ, et al: High *EVI1* expression predicts poor survival in acute myeloid leukemia *Blood* 101:837, 2003.
1103. Lugthart S, van Drunen E, van Norden Y, et al: High EVI1 levels predict adverse outcome in acute myeloid leukemia: Prevalence of EVI1 overexpression and chromosome 3q26 abnormalities underestimated. *Blood* 111:4329, 2008.
1104. Konoplev S, Rassidakis GZ, Estey E, et al: Overexpression of CXCR4 predicts adverse overall and event-free survival in patients with unmutated FLT3 acute myeloid leukemia with normal karyotype. *Cancer* 109:1152, 2007.
1105. Byrd JC, Mrozek K, Dodge RK, et al: Pretreatment cytogenetic abnormalities are predictive of induction success, cumulative incidence of relapse, and overall survival in adult patients with de novo acute myeloid leukemia: Results from Cancer and Leukemia Group B (CALGB 8461). *Blood* 100:4325, 2002.
1106. Bradstock K, Matthews J, Benson E, et al: Prognostic value of immunophenotyping in acute myeloid leukemia. Australian Leukaemia Study Group. *Blood* 84:1220, 1994.
1107. Gaiger A, Schmid D, Heinze G, et al: Detection of the WT1 transcript by RT-PCR in complete remission has no prognostic relevance in de novo acute myeloid leukemia. *Leukemia* 12:1886, 1998.
1108. Shih LY, Kuo MC, Liang DC, et al: Internal tandem duplication and Asp835 mutations of the FMS-like tyrosine kinase 3 (FLT3) gene in acute promyelocytic leukemia. *Cancer* 98:1206, 2003.
1109. Svingen PA, Karp JE, Krajewski S, et al: Evaluation of Apaf-1 and procaspases-2, -3, -7, -8, and -9 as potential prognostic markers in acute leukemia. *Blood* 96:3922, 2000.
1110. Heckman KD, Weiner GJ, Burns CP: Persistent thrombocytopenia during remission in acute leukemia does not preclude long-term disease-free survival. *Am J Hematol* 71:236, 2002.
1111. Legrand O, Simonin G, Zittoun R, Marie JP: Lung resistance protein (LRP) gene expression in adult acute myeloid leukemia: A critical evaluation by three techniques. *Leukemia* 12:1367, 1998.
1112. Filipits M, Pohl G, Stranzl T, et al: Expression of the lung resistance protein predicts poor outcome in *de novo* acute myeloid leukemia. *Blood* 91:1508, 1998.
1113. Gale RP, Horowitz MM, Weiner RS, et al: Impact of cytogenetic abnormalities on outcome of bone marrow transplants in acute myelogenous leukemia in first remission. *Bone Marrow Transplant* 16:203, 1995.
1114. Zapatero A, Martin de Vidales C, Pinar B, et al: Prognostic factors affecting leukemia relapse after allogeneic BMT conditioned with cyclophosphamide and fractionated TBI. *Bone Marrow Transplant* 18:591, 1996.
1115. Sievers EL, Loken MR: Detection of minimal residual disease in acute myelogenous leukemia. *J Pediatr Hematol Oncol* 17:123, 1995.
1116. Schnittger S, Weisser M, Schoch C, et al: New score predicting for prognosis in PML-RARA+, AML1-ETO+, or CBFBMYH11+ acute myeloid leukemia based on quantification of fusion transcripts. *Blood* 102:2746, 2003.
1117. Nucifora G, Larson RA, Rowley JD: Persistence of the 8;21 translocation in patients with acute myeloid leukemia type M2 in long-term remission. *Blood* 82:712, 1993.
1118. Cazzaniga G, Gaipa G, Rossi V, Biondi A: Monitoring of minimal residual disease in leukemia, advantages and pitfalls. *Ann Med* 38:512, 2006.
1119. Bacher U, Zander AR, Haferlach T, et al: Minimal residual disease diagnostics in myeloid malignancies in the post transplant period. *Bone Marrow Transplant* 42:145, 2008.
1120. Huisman C, de Weger RA, de Vries L, et al: Chimerism analysis within 6 months of allogeneic stem cell transplantation predicts relapse in acute myeloid leukemia. *Bone Marrow Transplant* 39:285, 2007.
1121. Estey E, Pierce S: Routine bone marrow exam during first remission of acute myeloid leukemia. *Blood* 87:3899, 1996.
1122. Zeleznikova T, Stevulova L, Kovarikova A, Babusikova O: Increased myeloid precursors in regenerating bone marrow; implications for detection of minimal residual disease in acute myeloid leukemia. *Neoplasma* 54:471, 2007.
1123. Campana D, Coustan-Smith E: Detection of minimal residual disease in acute leukemia by flow cytometry. *Cytometry* 38:139, 1999.
1124. Adriaansen HJ, Jacobs BC, Kappers-Klunne MC, et al: Detection of residual disease in AML patients by use of double immunological marker analysis for terminal deoxynucleotidyl transferase and myeloid markers. *Leukemia* 7:472, 1993.
1125. Reading CL, Estey EH, Huh YO, et al: Expression of unusual immunophenotype combinations in acute myelogenous leukemia. *Blood* 81:3083, 1993.
1126. Kita K, Miwa H, Nakase K, et al: Clinical importance of CD7 expression in acute myelocytic leukemia. The Japan Cooperative Group of Leukemia/Lymphoma. *Blood* 81:2399, 1993.
1127. Porwit-MacDonald A, Janossy G, Ivory K, et al: Leukemia-associated changes identified by quantitative flow cytometry: IV. CD34 overexpression in acute myelogenous leukemia M2 with t(8;21). *Blood* 87:1162, 1996.

1128. Baer MR, Stewart CC, Dodge RK, et al: High frequency of immunophenotype changes in acute myeloid leukemia at relapse: Implications for residual disease detection (Cancer and Leukemia Group B Study 8361). *Blood* 97:3574, 2001.
1129. Voskova D, Schnittger S, Schoch C, et al: Use of five-color staining improves the sensitivity of multiparameter flow cytomeric assessment of minimal residual disease in patients with acute myeloid leukemia. *Leuk Lymphoma* 48:80, 2007.
1130. van Rhenen A, Moshaver B, Kelder A, et al: Aberrant marker expression patterns on the CD34+CD38– stem cell compartment in acute myeloid leukemia allows to distinguish the malignant from the normal stem cell compartment both at diagnosis and in remission. *Leukemia* 21:1700, 2007.
1131. Arkesteijn GJ, Erpelinck SL, Martens AC, et al: The use of FISH with chromosome specific repetitive DNA probes for the follow-up of leukemia patients. Correlations and discrepancies with bone marrow cytology. *Cancer Genet Cytogenet* 88:69;1996.
1132. Engel H, Drach J, Keyhani A, et al: Quantitation of minimal residual disease in acute myelogenous leukemia and myelodysplastic syndromes in complete remission by molecular cytogenetics of prognitor cells. *Leukemia* 13:568, 1999.
1133. Cilloni D, Gottardi E, De Micheli D, et al: Quantitative assessment of WT1 expression by real time quantitative PCR may be a useful tool for monitoring minimal residual disease in acute leukemia patients. *Leukemia* 16:2115, 2002.
1134. Elmaagacli AH: Molecular methods used for detection of minimal residual disease following hematopoietic stem cell transplantation in myeloid disorders. *Methods Mol Med* 134:161, 2007.
1135. Van der Velden VHJ, Hochhaus A, Gazzaniga G, et al: Detection of minimal residual disease in hematologic malignancies by real-time quantitative PCR: Principles, approaches, and laboratory aspects. *Leukemia* 17:1013, 2003.
1136. Kern W, Haferlach C, Haferlach T, Schnittger S: Monitoring of minimal residual disease in acute myeloid leukemia. *Cancer* 112:4, 2008.
1137. Gal H, Amariglio N, Trakhtenbrot L, et al: Gene expression profiles of AML derived stem cells; similarity to hematopoietic stem cells. *Leukemia* 20:2147, 2006.
1138. Laczika K, Novak M, Hilgarth B, et al: Competitive CBFbeta/MYH11 reverse-transcriptase polymerase chain reaction for quantitative assessment of minimal residual disease during postremission therapy in acute myeloid leukemia with inversion(16): A pilot study. *J Clin Oncol* 16:1519, 1998.
1139. Marucci G, Caligiuri MA, Dohner H, et al: Quantification of CBFbeta/MYH11 fusion transcript by real time RT-PCR in patients with INV(16) acute myeloid leukemia. *Leukemia* 15:1072, 2001.
1140. Poirel H, Radford-Weiss 1, Rack K, et al: Detection of the chromosome 16 CBF beta-MYH11 fusion transcript in myelomonocytic leukemias. *Blood* 85:1313, 1995.
1141. Buonamici S, Ottaviani E, Testoni N, et al: Real-time quantitation of minimal residual disease in inv(16)-positive acute myeloid leukemia may indicate risk for clinical relapse and may identify patients in a curable state. *Blood* 99:443, 2002.
1142. Nucifora G, Birn DJ, Erickson P, et al: Detection of DNA rearrangements in the AML1 and ETO loci and of an AML 1/ETO fusion mRNA in patients with t(8;21) acute myeloid leukemia. *Blood* 81:1573, 1993.
1143. Maseki N, Miyoshi H, Shimuzu K, et al: The 8;21 chromosome trans-location in acute myeloid leukemia is always detectable by molecular analysis using AML 1. *Blood* 81:1573, 1993.
1144. Kusec R, Laczika K, Knobl P, et al: AML1/ETO fusion mRNA can be detected in remission blood samples of all patients with t(8;21) acute myeloid leukemia after chemotherapy or autologous bone marrow transplantation. *Leukemia* 8:735, 1994.
1145. Marcucci G, Livak KJ, Bi W, et al: Detection of minimal residual disease in patients with AML1/ETO-associated acute myeloid leukemia using a novel quantitative reverse transcription polymerase chain reaction assay. *Leukemia* 12:1482, 1998.
1146. Miyamoto T, Nagafuji K, Akashi K, et al: Persistence of multipotent progenitors expressing AML1/ETO transcripts in long-term remission patients with t(8;21) acute myelogenous leukemia. *Blood* 87:4789, 1996.
1147. Jurlander J, Caligiuri MA, Ruutu T, et al: Persistence of the AML1/ETO fusion transcript in patients treated with allogeneic bone marrow transplantation for t(8;21) leukemia. *Blood* 88:2183, 1996.
1148. Miyamoto T, Nagafuji K, Harada M, et al: Quantitative analysis of AML1/ETO transcripts in peripheral blood stem cell harvests from patients with t(8;21) acute myelogenous leukaemia. *Br J Haematol* 91:132, 1995.
1149. Miyamoto T, Nagafuji K, Harada M, Niho Y: Significance of quantitative analysis of AML1/ETO transcripts in peripheral blood stem cells from t(8;21) acute myelogenous leukemia. *Leuk Lymphoma* 25:69, 1997.
1150. Tobal K, Liu Yin JA: Molecular monitoring of minimal residual disease in acute myeloblastic leukemia with t(8;21) by RT-PCR. *Leuk Lymphoma* 31:115, 1998.
1151. Weisser M, Haferlach C, Hiddemann W, Schnittger S: The quality of molecular response to chemotherapy is predictive for the outcome of AML1-ETO-positive AML and is independent of pretreatment risk factors. *Leukemia* 21:1177, 2007.
1152. Muto A, Mori S, Matsushita H, et al: Serial quantification of minimal residual disease of t(8;21) acute myelogenous leukaemia with RT-competitive PCR assay. *Br J Haematol* 95:85, 1996.
1153. Erickson PF, Dessev G, Lasher RS, et al: ETO and AML1 phospho-proteins are expressed in CD34+ hematopoietic progenitors: Implications for t(8;21) leukemogenesis and monitoring residual disease. *Blood* 88:1813, 1996.
1154. Tobal K, Newton J, Macheta M, et al: Molecular quantitation of minimal residual disease in acute myeloid leukemia with t(8;21) can identify patients in durable remission and predict clinical relapse. *Blood* 95:815, 2000.
1155. Takatsuki H, Umemura T, Sadamura S, et al: Detection of minimal residual disease by reverse transcriptase polymerase chain reaction for the PML/RAR alpha fusion MRNA: A study in patients with acute promyelocytic leukemia following peripheral stem cell transplantation. *Leukemia* 9:889, 1995.
1156. Zhao L, Chang KS, Estey EH, et al: Detection of residual leukemic cells in patients with acute promyelocytic leukemia by the fluorescence *in situ* hybridization method: Potential for predicting relapse. *Blood* 85:495, 1995.
1157. Grimwade D, Lo Coco F: Acute promyelocytic leukemia: A model for the role of molecular diagnosis and residual disease monitoring in a directing treatment approach in acute myeloid leukemia. *Leukemia* 16:1959, 2002.
1158. Lo Coco F, Breccia M, Diverio D: The importance of molecular monitoring in acute promyelocytic leukaemia. *Best Pract Res Clin Haematol* 16:503, 2003.
1159. Tobal K, Moore H, Macheta M, Liu Yin JA: Monitoring minimal residual diease and predicting relapse in APL by quantitating *PML-RAR* α transcripts with a sensitive competitive RT-PCR method. *Leukemia* 15:1060, 2001.
1160. Chou WC, Tang JL, Wu SJ, et al: Clinical implications of minimal residual disease monitoring by quantitative polymerase chain reaction in acute myeloid leukemia patients bearing nucleophosmin (NPM1) mutations. *Leukemia* 21:998, 2007.
1161. Sjøholt G, Anensen N, Wergeland L, et al: Proteomics in acute myelogenous leukaemia (AML): Methodological strategies and identification of protein targets for novel antileukaemic therapy. *Curr Drug Targets* 6:631, 2005.
1162. Czibere A, Grall F, Aivado M: Perspectives of proteomics in acute myeloid leukemia. *Expert Rev Anticancer Ther* 6:1663, 2006.
1163. Wang XS, Zhang JW: The microRNAs involved in human myeloid differentiation and myelogenous/myeloblastic leukemia. *J Cell Mol Med* 12:1445, 2008.
1164. Garzon R, Volinia S, Liu CG, et al: MicroRNA signatures associated with cytogenetics and prognosis in acute myeloid leukemia. *Blood* 111:3183, 2008.
1165. Shih TT, Hou HA, Liu CY, et al: Bone marrow angiogenesis magnetic resonance imaging in patients with acute myeloid leukemia: Peak enhancement ratio is an independent predictor for overall survival. *Blood* 113:3161, 2009.
1166. Pérez-García A, Brunet S, Berlanga JJ, et al: CTLA-4 genotype and relapse incidence in patients with acute myeloid leukemia in first complete remission after induction chemotherapy. *Leukemia* 23:486, 2009.
1167. Virappane P, Gale R, Hills R, et al: Mutation of the Wilms' tumor 1 gene is a poor prognostic factor associated with chemotherapy resistance in normal karyotype acute myeloid leukemia: The United Kingdom Medical Research Council Adult Leukaemia Working Party. *J Clin Oncol* 26:5429, 2008.
1168. Paschka P, Marcucci G, Ruppert AS, et al: Wilms' tumor 1 gene mutations independently predict poor outcome in adults with cytogenetically normal acute myeloid leukemia: A cancer and leukemia group B study. *J Clin Oncol* 26:4595, 2008.

CHAPTER 90

CHRONIC MYELOGENOUS LEUKEMIA AND RELATED DISORDERS

Jane L. Liesveld and Marshall A. Lichtman

SUMMARY

The chronic myelogenous leukemias (CMLs) include *BCR* rearrangement-positive CML, chronic myelomonocytic leukemia, juvenile myelomonocytic leukemia, chronic neutrophilic leukemia, chronic eosinophilic leukemia, chronic basophilic leukemia, and possibly chronic monocytic leukemia. The term *chronic*, in contrast to *acute*, once had prognostic implications. However, although the terms remain useful for nosology, they no longer reflect an invariable difference in prognosis. For example, acute myelogenous leukemia in children and young adults has higher remission and cure rates than juvenile or chronic myelomonocytic leukemia in children or adults, respectively. *BCR* rearrangement-positive CML presents with anemia, exaggerated granulocytosis, a large proportion of myelocytes and mature neutrophils, absolute basophilia, normal or elevated platelet counts, and, frequently, splenomegaly. The marrow is hypercellular, and marrow cells contain the Philadelphia (Ph) chromosome in approximately 90 percent of cases by cytogenetic analysis. A rearrangement of the *BCR* gene on chromosome 22 is present in approximately 96 percent of cases by molecular diagnostic analysis. The disease usually responds to imatinib mesylate, a specific tyrosine kinase inhibitor, and median survival has been extended significantly. Allogeneic stem cell transplantation can cure the disease, especially if the transplantation is applied early in the chronic phase. The effect of stem cell transplantation is related in part to a robust graft-versus-leukemia effect, engendered by donor T lymphocytes. The chronic phase usually is followed by an accelerated phase that often terminates in acute leukemia (blast crisis), at which point therapy with imatinib mesylate and other agents may induce a remission in a proportion of patients, but median survival is measured in months. Blast crisis results in a myelogenous leukemic phenotype in 75 percent of cases and a lymphoblastic leukemic phenotype in approximately 25 percent of cases. Ph-chromosome–positive acute myeloblastic leukemia (AML) may appear *de novo* in approximately 1 percent of cases of AML, and Ph-chromosome–positive acute lymphocytic leukemia (ALL) may occur *de novo* in approximately 20 percent of cases of adult ALL and approximately 5 percent of childhood ALL cases. In Ph-chromosome–positive ALL, the translocation between chromosomes 9 and 22 results in the fusion gene encoding a mutant tyrosine kinase oncoprotein that may be identical in size to that in classic CML (210 kDa) in approximately one-third of cases. A smaller mutant tyrosine kinase (190 kDa) is encoded in approximately two-thirds of cases. In children, the cells in approximately 90 percent of cases contain a 190-kDa mutant tyrosine kinase. These acute leukemias may reflect (1) the presentation of CML in acute blastic transformation without a preceding chronic phase or (2) *de novo* cases resulting from a *BCR-ABL* mutation occurring in a different hematopoietic cell from the event in CML or with as yet unidentified modifying gene alterations. Chronic myelomonocytic leukemia has variable presenting features. Anemia may be accompanied by mildly or moderately elevated leukocyte counts; an elevated total monocyte count; a low, normal, or elevated platelet count; and sometimes splenomegaly. Although cytogenetic abnormalities may be present, there is no specific genetic marker of the disease. In a very small proportion of cases, a translocation involving the platelet-derived growth factor receptor-beta (PDGFR-β) gene is associated with eosinophilia and is responsive to imatinib mesylate. Juvenile myelomonocytic leukemia occurs in infancy or very early childhood. Anemia, thrombocytopenia, and leukocytosis with monocytosis are usual. The disease is refractory to treatment and, even with current maximal therapy and stem cell rescue, cures are uncommon. Chronic neutrophilic leukemia presents with mild anemia and exaggerated neutrophilia, with very few immature cells in the blood. Splenomegaly is common. The disease usually occurs after age 60 years and is refractory to current treatment approaches. Chronic and juvenile myelomonocytic leukemia and chronic neutrophilic leukemia have a propensity to evolve into acute myelogenous leukemia. Prior to that evolution, morbidity and mortality are related to infection, hemorrhage, and complicating medical conditions. Chronic eosinophilic leukemia represents the major subset of the hypereosinophilic syndrome. It is a clonal disorder with a striking absolute eosinophilia, often neurologic and cardiac manifestations secondary to toxic effects of eosinophil granules, and sometimes a translocation involving the platelet-derived growth factor receptor-alpha (PDGFR-α) gene that encodes a mutant tyrosine kinase, imparting sensitivity to imatinib mesylate.

Acronyms and abbreviations that appear in this chapter include: AGP, α_1-acid glycoprotein; ALL, acute lymphocytic leukemia; BCR, breakpoint cluster region; CCyR, complete cytogenetic remission; CFU-GM, colony-forming unit–granulocyte-monocyte; CHR, complete hematologic response; CLL, chronic lymphocytic leukemia; CML, chronic myelogenous leukemia; CMML, chronic myelomonocytic leukemia; DLI, donor lymphocyte infusion; FISH, fluorescence *in situ* hybridization; G-CSF, granulocyte colony-stimulating factor; GM-CSF, granulocyte-monocyte colony-stimulating factor; GRB2, growth factor receptor-bound protein-2; GTP, guanosine triphosphate; GTPase, guanosine triphosphatase; GVHD, graft-versus-host disease; HLA, human leukocyte antigen; HPRT, hypoxanthine phosphoribosyltransferase; HR, hematologic response; hsp, heat shock protein; HUMARA, human androgen receptor assay; IFN, interferon; IL, interleukin; JAK, Janus-associated kinase; LTC-IC, long-term culture-initiating cell; MCP, monocyte chemotactic protein; MCyR, major cytogenetic response; mCyR, minor cytogenetic response; MDS, myelodysplastic syndrome; MIP, macrophage inflammatory protein; MMR, major molecular response; mRNA, messenger RNA; NF-κB, nuclear factor-κB; *NF1*, neurofibromatosis tumor suppressor gene; NK, natural killer; NOD, nonobese diabetic; PCR, polymerase chain reaction; PDGF, platelet-derived growth factor; PDGFR, platelet-derived growth factor receptor; PHR, partial hematologic response; Ph, Philadelphia chromosome; PI3K, phosphatidylinositol 3′-kinase; Rb, retinoblastoma; RT-PCR, reverse transcriptase polymerase chain reaction; SCID, severe combined immunodeficiency; STAT, signal transducer and activator of transcription; TBI, total-body irradiation; TdT, terminal deoxynucleotidyl transferase; TGF, transforming growth factor; VEGF, vascular endothelial growth factor; WT, Wilms tumor.

DEFINITION AND HISTORY

Chronic myelogenous leukemia (CML) is a pluripotential stem cell disease characterized by anemia, extreme blood granulocytosis and granulocytic immaturity, basophilia, often thrombocytosis, and splenomegaly. The hematopoietic cells contain a reciprocal translocation between chromosomes 9 and 22 in more than 95 percent of patients, which leads to an overtly foreshortened long arm of one of the chromosome pair 22 (i.e., 22, 22q–) referred to as the *Philadelphia (Ph) chromosome*. A rearrangement of the breakpoint cluster gene on the long arm of chromosome 22 defines this form of CML and is present even in the 10 percent of patients without an overt 22q abnormality by Giemsa banding. The natural history of the disease is to undergo clonal evolution into an accelerated phase and/or a rapidly progressive phase resembling acute leukemia, which is refractory to therapy.

In 1845, Bennett[1] in Scotland and Virchow[2] in Germany described patients with splenic enlargement, severe anemia, and enormous concentrations of leukocytes in their blood at autopsy. Bennett initially favored an extreme pyemia as the explanation, but Virchow argued against suppuration as a cause. Additional cases were reported by Craige[3] and others, and in 1847 Virchow[4] introduced the designation *weisses Blut* and *leukämie* (leukemia). In 1878, Neumann[5] proposed that the marrow not only was the site of normal blood cell production, but also was the site from which leukemia originated and used the term *myelogene* (myelogenous) leukemia. Subsequent observations amplified the clinical and laboratory features of the disease, but few fundamental insights were gained until the discovery by Nowell and Hungerford,[6] who reported in 1960 that two patients with the disease had an apparent loss of the long arm of chromosome 21 or 22, an abnormality that was quickly confirmed[7–9] and designated the Philadelphia chromosome.[7] This observation led to a new approach to diagnosis, a marker to study the pathogenesis of the disease, and a focus for future studies of the molecular pathology of the disease. The availability of banding techniques to define the fine structure of chromosomes[10,11] led to the discovery by Rowley[12] that the apparent lost chromosomal material on chromosome 22 was part of a reciprocal translocation between chromosomes 9 and 22. The discovery that the cellular oncogene *ABL* on chromosome number 9 and a segment of chromosome 22, the breakpoint cluster region (BCR), fuse as a result of the translocation provided a basis for the study of the molecular cause of the disease.[13,14] The appreciation that the fusion gene encoded a constitutively active tyrosine kinase (*BCR-ABL*) that was capable of inducing the disease in mice established the fusion gene product as the proximate cause of the malignant transformation. The search for, identification of, and clinical development of a small molecule inhibitor of the mutant tyrosine kinase has provided a specific agent, imatinib mesylate, with which to inhibit the molecule that incites the disease.[15] Several more potent congeners have also been synthesized (see "Etiology and Pathogenesis" below). Thomas and colleagues established that allogeneic hematopoietic stem cell transplantation could cure the disease.[16]

EPIDEMIOLOGY

CML accounts for approximately 15 percent of all cases of leukemia, or approximately 5000 new cases per year in the United States. The age-adjusted incidence rate in the United States is approximately 2.0 per 100,000 persons for men and approximately 1.1 per 100,000 persons for women. The incidence around the world varies by a factor of approximately twofold. The lowest incidence is in Sweden and China (approximately 0.7 per 100,000 persons), and the highest incidence is in Switzerland and the United States (approximately 1.5 per 100,000 persons).[17] The age-specific incidence rate for CML in the United States increases logarithmically with age, from approximately 0.2 per 100,000 persons younger than 20 years to a rate of approximately 10.0 per 100,000 octogenarians per year (Fig. 90–1). Although CML occurs in children and adolescents, less than 10 percent of all cases occur in subjects between 1 and 20 years old. CML represents approximately 3 percent of all childhood leukemias. Multiple occurrences of CML in families are rare. There is no concordance of the disease between identical twins. Analytical epidemiologic evidence for a familial predisposition in CML was not found in a Swedish database.[18]

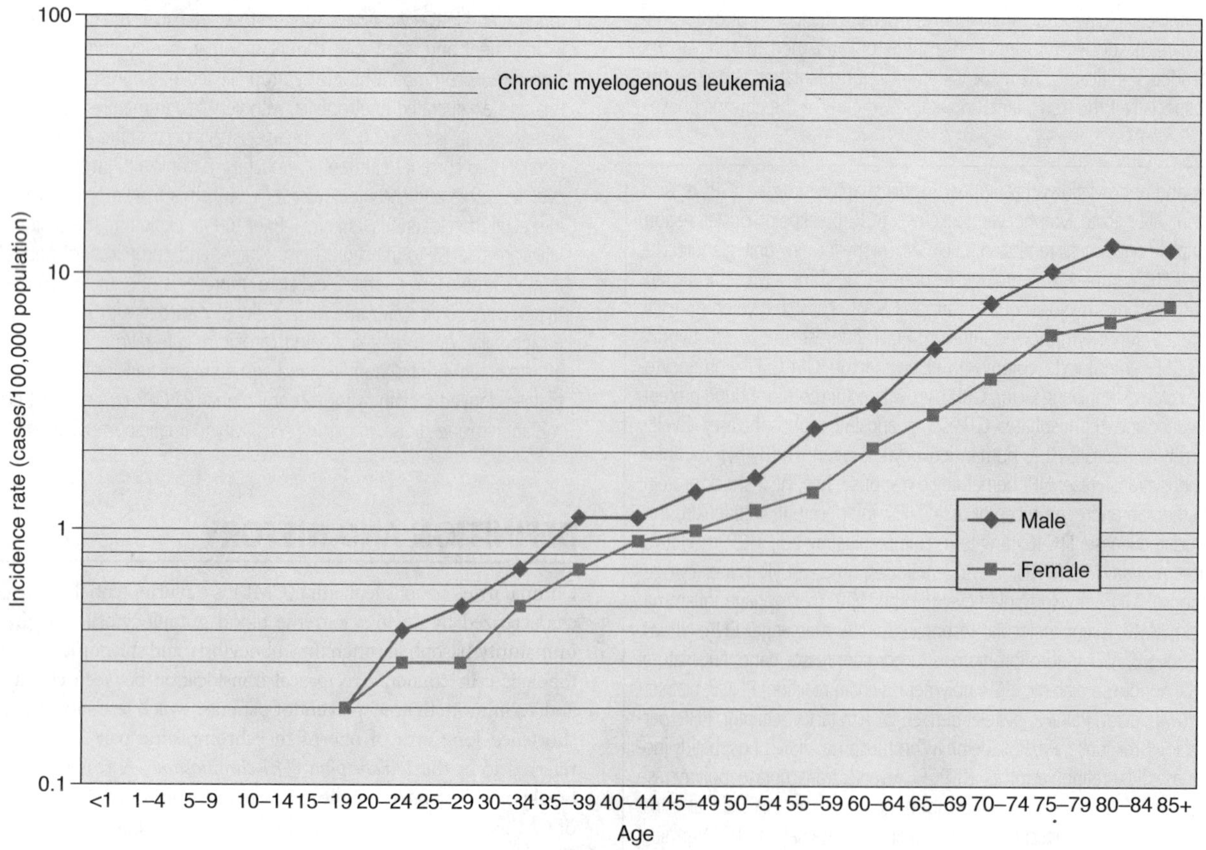

FIGURE 90–1. Incidence of chronic myelogenous leukemia by age. Note the exponential increase in incidence with age from about teenagers to octogenarians. Rare cases occur in younger children but too few to generate an incidence rate.

ETIOLOGY AND PATHOGENESIS

ENVIRONMENTAL LEUKEMOGENS

Exposure to very high doses of ionizing radiation can increase the occurrence of CML above the expected frequency in comparable populations. Three major populations—the Japanese exposed to the radiation released by the atomic bomb detonations at Nagasaki and Hiroshima,[19] British patients with ankylosing spondylitis treated with spine irradiation,[20,21] and women with uterine cervical carcinoma who received radiation therapy[22]—had a frequency of CML (as well as acute leukemia) significantly above the frequency expected in comparable unexposed groups. The median latent period was approximately 4 years in irradiated spondylitics, among whom approximately 20 percent of the leukemia cases were CML; 9 years in the uterine cervical cancer patients, of whom approximately 30 percent had CML; and 11 years in the Japanese survivors of the atomic bombs, of whom approximately 30 percent of the leukemia patients had CML.[23] Chemical leukemogens, such as benzene and alkylating agents, are not causative agents of CML, although they are well established to produce a dose-dependent increase in acute myelogenous leukemia.[24]

ORIGIN FROM A HEMATOPOIETIC STEM CELL CLONE

CML results from the malignant transformation of a single multipotential hematopoietic cell. The disease is acquired (somatic mutation), given that the identical twin of patients with CML and the offspring of mothers with the disease neither carry the Ph chromosome nor develop the disease.[25] The origin of CML from a single multipotential hematopoietic cell is supported by the following lines of evidence:

1. Involvement of erythropoiesis, neutrophilopoiesis, eosinophilopoiesis, basophilopoiesis, monocytopoiesis, and thrombopoiesis in chronic phase CML[26]
2. Presence of the Ph chromosome (22q−) in erythroblasts; neutrophilic, eosinophilic, and basophilic granulocytes; macrophages; and megakaryocytes[27]
3. Presence of a single glucose-6-phosphate dehydrogenase isoenzyme in red cells, neutrophils, eosinophils, basophils, monocytes, and platelets, but not in fibroblasts or other somatic cells in women with CML who are heterozygotes for isoenzymes A and B[28–30]
4. Presence of the Ph translocation only on a structurally anomalous chromosome 9 or 22 of each chromosome pair in every cell analyzed in occasional patients with a structurally dissimilar 9 or 22 chromosome within the pair[31–33]
5. Presence of the Ph chromosome in one but not the other cell lineage of patients who are a mosaic for sex chromosomes, as in Turner syndrome (45X/46XX)[34] and Klinefelter syndrome (46XY/47XXY)[35]
6. Molecular studies showing variation in the breakpoint of chromosome 22 among different patients with CML but precisely the same breakpoint among cells within a single patient with CML[36,37]
7. Combined DNA hybridization-methylation analysis of women who have restriction fragment length polymorphisms at the X-linked locus for hypoxanthine phosphoribosyltransferase (HPRT), which enables distinction of the two alleles of the HPRT gene in heterozygous females, coupled with methylation-sensitive restriction-enzyme cleavage patterns, which permits delineation of whether cells contain either the maternally derived or the paternally derived copy of the gene[38]

The foregoing observations place the parent cell of the clone at least at the level of the hematopoietic stem cell.

THE CHRONIC MYELOGENOUS LEUKEMIA STEM CELL

Acquisition of the *BCR-ABL* fusion gene as a result of the t(9;22)(q34;q11.2) in a single multipotential hematopoietic cell results in the CML stem cell, necessary for the initiation and maintenance of the chronic phase of CML.[39,40] The phenotype of the CML stem cell is not fully defined but they are among the CD34+CD33− fraction of CML cells. A large proportion of CML stem cells are in the G_0 phase of the cell cycle and are resistant to therapy with *BCR-ABL* inhibitors. These cells represent a pool for the regrowth of the tumor, if suppressive therapy is interrupted. The acquisition of genetic and epigenetic events in a derivative *BCR-ABL*–positive cell can result in evolution to accelerated phase and blastic transformation[41] (see "Accelerated Phase and Blast Crisis of CML" below).

PLURIPOTENTIAL VERSUS HEMATOPOIETIC STEM CELL LESION

Some patients in chronic phase CML have lymphocytes that are derived from the primordial malignant cell. Evidence for this finding includes the following: A single isoenzyme for glucose-6-phosphate dehydrogenase has been found in some T and B lymphocytes in women with CML who are heterozygous for isoenzymes A and B;[42] blood cells from patients with CML induced to proliferate with Epstein-Barr virus (presumptive B lymphocytes) are of the same glucose-6-phosphate dehydrogenase isoenzyme type, have cytoplasmic immunoglobulin heavy and light chains, and contain the Ph chromosome;[43] blood lymphocytes stimulated with B lymphocyte mitogens contain the Ph chromosome;[44,45] purified B lymphocytes from the blood in chronic phase CML contain an abnormal, elongated phosphoprotein coded for by the chimeric gene resulting from the t(9;22);[46] and fluorescence *in situ* hybridization (FISH) has detected the *BCR-ABL* fusion gene in approximately 25 percent of B lymphocytes in some, but not all, patients in chronic phase.[47,48] These findings suggest that B lymphocytes are derived from the malignant clone, placing the lesion closer to, if not in, the pluripotential stem cell.[42–46] Almost all studies find that the B lymphocyte pool is a mosaic, containing both Ph-chromosome– and *BCR-ABL*–positive cells and Ph-chromosome– or *BCR-ABL*–negative cells. Results of studies examining the derivation of T lymphocytes from the malignant clone are more ambiguous but indicate that T lymphocytes are derived from the malignant clone in some, but not most, patients.[42,44,49–58] Natural killer (NK) cells isolated from patients with chronic phase CML do not contain the *BCR-ABL* fusion gene.[59] It is possible that myelopoiesis is invariably clonal and lymphopoiesis is an unpredictable mosaic derived largely from normal residual stem cells. This conclusion is supported by the finding that progenitors of T, B, and NK lymphocytes contain the Ph chromosome and *BCR-ABL*, but most B-cell and all T-cell progenitors derived from the leukemic clone undergo apoptosis, leaving unaffected cells in the blood.[60–63]

The cell in which the mutation occurs may be even more primitive in that some endothelial cells generated *in vitro* express the *BCR-ABL* fusion gene, as do some cells in the patient's vascular endothelium.[64]

ETIOLOGIC ROLE OF THE Ph CHROMOSOME

Early studies indicated that the Ph chromosome may appear after the initial leukemogenic event.[65–68] Patients with CML have developed the Ph chromosome during the course of the disease, have experienced periods of the disease when the Ph chromosome disappeared,[69] or have had Ph-chromosome–positive and Ph-chromosome–negative cells concurrently.[70–74]

Nearly all, if not all, patients with CML have an abnormality of chromosome 22 at a molecular level (*BCR* rearrangement). Thus, earlier studies indicating an absence of a Ph chromosome were not a valid measure of the normality of chromosome 22. The molecular abnormality in CML involving the *ABL* gene on chromosome 9 and the *BCR* gene on chromosome 22 has been established as being the proximate cause of the chronic phase of the disease (see "Molecular Pathology" below).

COEXISTENCE OF NORMAL STEM CELLS

Most, if not all, patients with CML have hematopoietic stem cells that, after treatment[75–77] or culture *in vitro*,[78–80] use of special cell isolation techniques,[81,82] or use of cell transfer to nonobese diabetic (NOD)/severe combined immunodeficiency (SCID) mice[83] do not have the Ph chromosome[84,85] or the *BCR-ABL* fusion gene.[86–90] The switch to Ph-chromosome–negative cells *in vitro* is associated with a loss of monoclonal glucose-6-phosphate dehydrogenase isoenzyme patterns, indicating the persistence and reemergence of normal polyclonal hematopoiesis rather than reversion to a Ph-chromosome–negative clone.[91] In confirmation, *BCR-ABL*+, CD34+, human leukocyte antigen (HLA)-DR– cells isolated from women with early phase CML are polyclonal using the human androgen receptor assay (HUMARA) to assess X chromosome inactivation patterns.[92] Very primitive hematopoietic cells, the long-term culture-initiating cells (LTC-ICs), are present in Ph-chromosome–negative cytapheresis samples collected during early recovery after chemotherapy for CML.[93] These LTC-ICs are most commonly present when samples are collected within 3 months of diagnosis.[94] Variable levels of *BCR-ABL*–negative progenitors are found in the CD34+DR– population, but low levels are found in the CD34+CD38– population.[90,95] Preprogenitors for the CD34+DR– cells are predominantly *BCR-ABL*–negative in both marrow and blood at diagnosis.[96] However, some cells with surface marker characteristics of very primitive normal hematopoietic cells do express the *BCR-ABL* gene.[97] Both normal and leukemic SCID-repopulating cells coexist in the marrow and blood from CML patients in chronic phase, whereas only leukemic SCID-repopulating cells are detected in blast crisis.[98,99]

PROGENITOR CELL CHARACTERISTICS

Progenitor Cell Dysfunction

The leukemic transformation resulting from the *BCR-ABL* fusion oncogene is maintained by a relatively small number of BCR-ABL stem cells that favor differentiation over self-renewal.[100] This predisposition to differentiation and progenitor cell expansion is mediated by an autocrine interleukin (IL)-3–granulocyte colony-stimulating factor (G-CSF) loop.[100] The earliest progenitors have the capacity to undergo marked expansion of erythroid, granulocytic, and megakaryocytic cell populations, and have a decreased sensitivity to regulation.[100–102] This expansion is especially dramatic in the more mature progenitor cell compartment.[100,103] The proliferative capacity of individual granulocytic progenitors is decreased compared to normal cells. Thus, the progenitor cell population in marrow and blood expands proportionately more than the increase in granulopoiesis.[104,105] Moreover, the progenitors have buoyant density that is lighter than that of their normal counterparts but similar to that of hepatic fetal granulopoietic progenitors, suggesting an oncofetal pattern.[104] The marked expansion of the total blood granulocyte pool results from a total expansion of granulopoiesis,[103,106] with a minor contribution from prolonged intravascular circulation time.[107] BCR-ABL reduces growth factor dependence of progenitor cells.

Erythroid progenitors are expanded, erythroid precursor maturation is blocked at the basophilic erythroblast stage, and the extent of erythropoiesis is inversely proportional to the total white cell count.[108]

Progenitor Cell Characterization

Phenotypic differences of stem and progenitor cells in CML patients compared to normal subjects have been identified.[109] For example, a greater proportion of the circulating leukemic colony-forming unit–granulocyte-monocytes (CFU-GMs) express high levels of the adhesion receptor CD44[110] and low levels of L-selectin[111] in contrast to normal cells. Leukemic CD34+ cells overexpress the P glycoprotein that determines the multidrug resistance phenotype.[112]

BCR-ABL–positive progenitors survive less well in long-term culture than do their normal counterparts. Leukemic CFU-GM colonies, unlike normal colonies, decrease in long-term cultures that are deficient in KIT ligand,[113] whereas their proliferation is favored in the presence of KIT ligand.[114] Macrophage inflammatory protein (MIP)-1α does not inhibit growth factor-mediated proliferation of CD34+ cells from CML patients, as it does CD34+ cells from normal subjects, even though the MIP-1α receptor is expressed.[115] Another chemokine, monocyte chemotactic protein (MCP)-1, unlike MIP-1α, is an endogenous chemokine that cooperates with transforming growth factor beta (TGF-β) to inhibit the cycling of primitive normal, but not CML, progenitors in long-term human marrow cultures.[116] Leukemic progenitors are less sensitive than normal progenitors to the antiproliferative effects of TGF-β.[117]

EFFECTS OF *BCR-ABL* ON CELL ADHESION

Primitive progenitors and blast colony-forming cells from patients with CML have decreased adherence to marrow stromal cells.[118,119] This defect is normalized if stromal cells are treated with interferon (IFN)-α.[119,120] As a result, *BCR-ABL*–negative progenitors are enriched in the adherent fraction of circulating CD34+ cells in chronic phase CML patients. The most primitive *BCR-ABL*–positive cells in the blood of patients with CML differ from their normal counterparts. They are increased in frequency and are activated, such that signals that block cell mitosis are bypassed.[121]

Ph-chromosome–positive colony-forming cells adhere less to fibronectin (and to marrow stroma) than do their normal counterparts. Adhesion is fostered as a result of restoration of cooperation between activated β_1 integrins and the altered epitopes of CD44.[122–124] CML granulocytes have reduced and altered binding to P-selectin because of modification in the CD15 antigens.[125] *BCR-ABL*–induced defects in integrin function may underlie the abnormal circulation and proliferation of progenitors[126,127] because growth signaling can occur through the fibronectin receptor.[128] IFN-α restores normal integrin-mediated inhibition of hematopoietic progenitor proliferation by the marrow microenvironment.[129] There are conflicting data regarding the effects of tyrosine kinase inhibitor effects on adhesion of CML cells to stroma.[130,131]

BCR-ABL–encoded fusion protein $p210^{BCR-ABL}$ binds to actin, and several cytoskeletal proteins are thereby phosphorylated. The $p210^{BCR-ABL}$ interacts with actin filaments through an actin-binding domain. *BCR-ABL* transfection is associated with increased spontaneous motility, membrane ruffling, formation of long actin extensions (filopodia), and accelerated rate of protrusion and retraction of pseudopodia on fibronectin-coated surfaces. IFN-α treatment slowly converts the abnormal motility phenotype of *BCR-ABL*–transformed cells toward normal.[132] Integrins regulate the c-*ABL*–encoded tyrosine kinase activity and its cytoplasmic nuclear transport.[133] The $p210^{BCR-ABL}$ abrogates the anchorage requirement but not the growth factor requirement for proliferation.[134]

In normal cells exposed to IL-3, paxillin tyrosine residues are phosphorylated. In cells transformed by $p210^{BCR-ABL}$, the tyrosines of paxillin, vinculin, $p125^{FAK}$, talin, and tensin are constitutively phosphorylated. Pseudopodia enriched in focal adhesion proteins[134,135] are present in cells expressing $p210^{BCR-ABL}$.

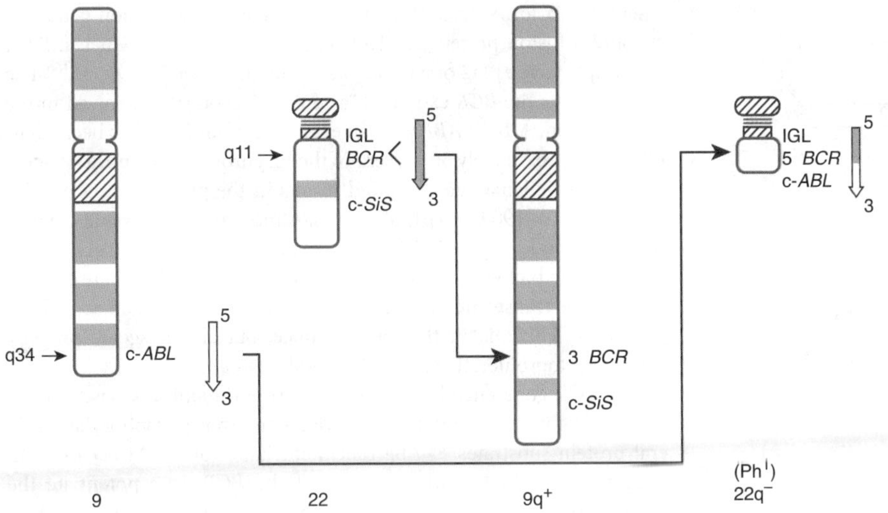

FIGURE 90–2. Schematic of normal chromosome 9 showing the *ABL* gene between band q34 and qter of chromosome 22, which has the *BCR* and *SIS* genes between band q11 and qter. The t(9;22) is shown on the *right*. The *ABL* from chromosome 9 is transposed to the chromosome 22 M-*bcr* sequences, and the terminal portion of chromosome 22 is transposed to the long arm of chromosome 9. The 22q– is the Ph chromosome. bcr, breakpoint cluster region; c-SiS, cellular homologue of the viral simian sarcoma virus-transforming gene; IGL, gene for immunoglobulin light chains. *(From De Klein A: Oncogene activation by chromosomal rearrangement in chronic myelocytic leukemia.* Mutat Res *186:161, 1987, with permission.)*

The sum of evidence suggests that defects in adhesion (contact and anchoring) of CML primitive cells remove them from their controlling signals normally received from microenvironmental cells via cytokine messages. These signals retain the balance among cell survival, cell death, cell proliferation, and cell differentiation. Inappropriate phosphorylation of cytoskeletal proteins, possibly independent of tyrosine kinase, is thought to be the key factor in disturbed integrin function of CML cells.

MOLECULAR PATHOLOGY

Ph Chromosome

The genic disturbance became evident with the knowledge that CML was derived from a primitive cell containing a 22q– abnormality.[6,11] The abnormal chromosome contained only 60 percent of the DNA in other G-group chromosomes.[136] Cytogenetic analysis indicated the G-group chromosome involved was different from the extra G-group chromosome in Down syndrome, which had been assigned number 21. Thus, the former was assigned number 22—even though it proved to be slightly longer than the chromosome involved in Down syndrome.[11,137] The Paris Conference on Nomenclature decided not to undo the concept that Down syndrome is trisomy 21 and assigned the Ph chromosome and its normal counterpart, 22.[138] Using quinacrine (Q) and Giemsa (G) banding, Rowley[12] reported in 1973 that the material missing from chromosome 22 was not lost (deleted) from the cell, but was translocated to the distal portion of the long arm of chromosome 9. The amount of material translocated to chromosome 9 was approximately equivalent to that lost from 22, and the translocation was predicted to be balanced.[12] Moreover, the breaks were localized to band 34 on the long arm of 9 and band 11 on the long arm of 22. Therefore, the classic Ph chromosome is t(9;22)(q34;q11), abbreviated t(Ph) (Fig. 90–2). The Ph chromosome can develop on either the maternal or the paternal member of the pair.[139]

Mutation of ABL and BCR Genes

Mutations of the *ABL* gene on chromosome 9 and of the *BCR* gene on chromosome 22 are central to the development of CML (Fig. 90–3).[140–142]

In 1982, the human cellular homologue *ABL* of the transforming sequence of the Abelson murine leukemia virus was localized to human chromosome 9.[143] In 1983, *ABL* was shown to be on the segment of chromosome 9 that is translocated to chromosome 22[144] by demonstrating reaction to hybridization probes for *ABL* only in somatic cell hybrids of human CML cells containing 22q– but not those containing 9q+. v-*abl* is the viral oncogenic homologue of the normal cellular *ABL* gene. This gene (v-*abl*) can induce malignant transformation of cells in culture and can induce leukemia in susceptible mice.[145]

The *ABL* gene is rearranged and amplified in cell lines from patients with CML.[146] Cell lines and fresh isolates of CML cells contain an

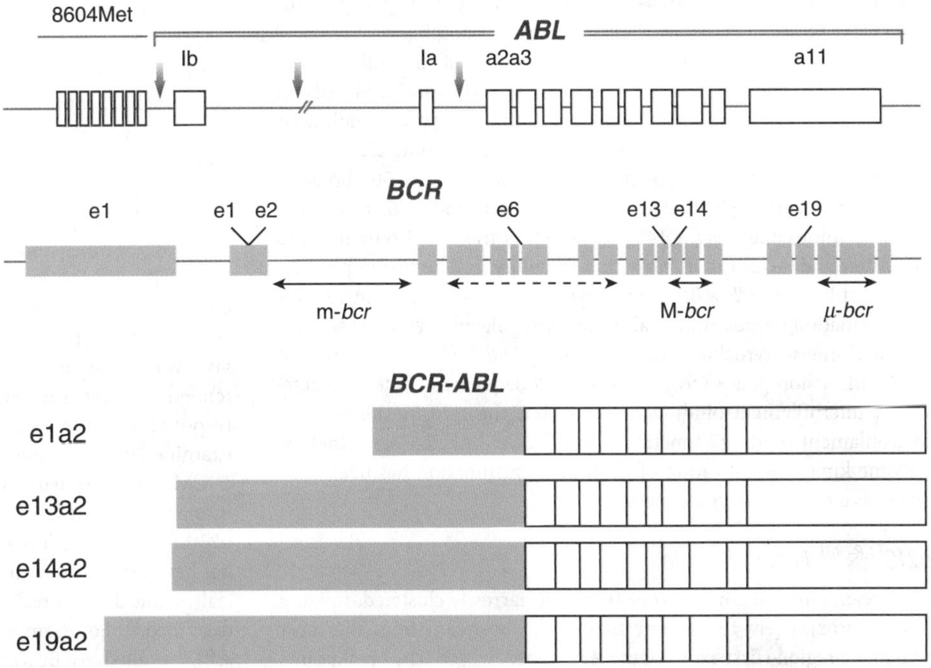

FIGURE 90–3. Schematic of the normal *ABL* and *BCR* genes and of the *BCR-ABL* fusion transcripts. In the *upper panel* of the diagram, the possible breakpoint positions in *ABL* are marked by *vertical arrows*. Note the position immediately upstream of the *ABL* locus of the *8604Met* gene. The *BCR* gene contains 25 exons, including first (e1) and second (e2) exons. The positions of the three breakpoint cluster regions, m-*bcr*, M-*bcr*, and *μ-bcr*, are shown. The *lower panel* of the figure shows the structure of the *BCR-ABL* messenger RNA fusion transcripts. Breakpoints in *μ-bcr* result in *BCR-ABL* transcripts with an e19a2 junction. The associated number designates the exon (location) at which the break occurs in each gene. *(From Verschraegen CF, Kantarjian HM, Hirsch-Ginsberg C, et al,[179] with permission.)*

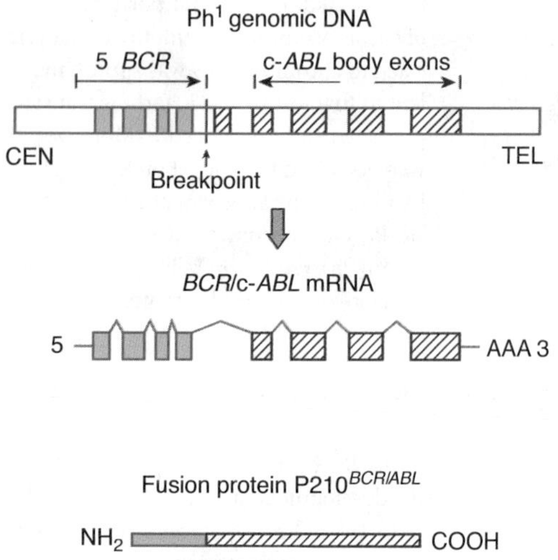

FIGURE 90–4. Molecular effects of the Ph chromosome translocation t(9;22)(q34;q11). The *upper panel* shows the physically joined 5′ *BCR* and the 3′ *ABL* regions on chromosome 22. The exons are *solid* (from chromosome 22, *BCR*) and *hatched* (from chromosome 9, *ABL*). The *middle panel* depicts transcription of chimeric messenger RNA. The *lower panel* shows the translated fusion protein with the amino-terminus derived from the *BCR* of chromosome 22 and the carboxy-terminus from the *ABL* of chromosome 9. *(From De Klein A: Oncogene activation by chromosomal rearrangement in chronic myelocytic leukemia.* Mutat Res *186:161, 1987, with permission.)*

abnormal, elongated 8-kb RNA transcript,[147–150] which is transcribed from the new chimeric gene produced by the fusion of the 5′ portion of the *BCR* gene left on chromosome 22 with the 3′ portion of the *ABL* gene translocated from chromosome 9[144] (Fig. 90–4). The fusion messenger RNA (mRNA) leads to the translation of a unique tyrosine phosphoprotein kinase of 210 kDa ($p210^{BCR-ABL}$), which can phosphorylate tyrosine residues on cellular proteins similar to the action of the v-*abl* protein product.[151–155] The anomalous tyrosine kinase is difficult to identify in chronic phase cells because of inhibitors in granulocytes;[155] molecular variants reflect variations in the breakpoint on chromosome 22.[156]

The *ABL* locus contains at least two alleles, one having a 500-bp deletion.[157] In normal cells, the *ABL* protooncogene codes for a tyrosine kinase of molecular weight 145,000, which is translated only in trace quantities and lacks any *in vitro* kinase activity.[152] The fusion product expressed by the *BCR-ABL* gene is hypothesized to lead to malignant transformation because of the abnormally regulated enzymatic activity of the chimeric tyrosine protein kinase.[153,154,158,159] Construction of *BCR-ABL* fusion genes indicated that *BCR* sequences could also activate a microfilament-binding function, but the tyrosine kinase and microfilament-binding functions were not linked. Nevertheless, tyrosine kinase modification of actin filament function has been proposed as a step in leukemogenesis.[160]

$p210^{BCR-ABL}$ Fusion Protein

The breakpoints on chromosome 9 are not narrowly clustered, ranging from approximately 15 to more than 40 kb upstream from the most proximate region (first exon) of the *ABL* gene.[143,144,161] The breakpoints on chromosome 22 occur over a very short, approximately 5 to 6 kb, stretch of DNA referred to as the breakpoint cluster region (M-*bcr*),[162,163] which is part of a much longer breakpoint cluster region gene, *BCR*[164,165] (see Fig. 90–4). Three main breakpoint cluster regions have been characterized on chromosome 22: major (M-*bcr*), minor (m-*bcr*), and micro (μ-*bcr*). The three different breakpoints result in a p210, p190, and p230 fusion protein, respectively (see Fig. 90–3). The overwhelming majority of CML patients have a *BCR-ABL* fusion gene that encodes a fusion protein of 210 kDa ($p210^{BCR-ABL}$), for which mRNA transcripts have e14a2 or a e13a2 fusion junction (see Fig. 90–3).[166] The "e" represents the *BCR* exon and "a" the *ABL* exon sites involved in the translocation. A *BCR-ABL* with an e1a2 type of junction has been identified in approximately 50 percent of the Ph chromosome–positive acute lymphoblastic leukemia cases and results in the production of a *BCR-ABL* protein of 190 kDa ($p190^{BCR-ABL}$). Almost all CML cases at diagnosis that encode a $p210^{BCR-ABL}$ also express *BCR-ABL* transcripts for p190.[167] The biologic or clinical significance of these dual transcripts is not known. Transgenic mice expressing $p210^{BCR-ABL}$ develop acute lymphoblastic leukemia in the founder mice, but all transgenic progeny have a myeloproliferative disorder resembling CML.[168]

The *BCR* gene encodes a 160-kDa serine-threonine kinase, which, when it oligomerizes, autophosphorylates and transphosphorylates several protein substrates.[169] Aberrant methylation of the M-*bcr* in CML occurs.[166] The first exon sequences of the *BCR* gene potentiate the tyrosine kinase of *ABL* when they fuse as a result of the translocation.[170] The central portion of *BCR* has homology to *DBL*, a gene involved in the control of cell division after the S phase of the cell cycle. The C-terminus of *BCR* has a guanosine triphosphatase (GTPase)-activating protein for $p21^{rac}$, a member of the *RAS* family of guanosine triphosphate (GTP)-binding proteins.[171] A reciprocal hybrid gene *ABL-BCR* is formed on chromosome 9q+ when *BCR-ABL* fuses on chromosome 22. The *ABL-BCR* fusion gene actively transcribes in most patients with CML.[172]

Variations in breakpoints involving smaller stretches of chromosome 9 and rearrangements outside the M-*bcr* of chromosome 22 can occur.[37] In a few cases of CML with no evident elongation of chromosome 9, molecular probes have shown that *ABL* still is translocated to chromosome 22.[173] In occasional patients with Ph-chromosome–positive CML, the break in chromosome 22 is outside the M-*bcr*, and transcription of a fusion RNA of the usual type fails or a fusion RNA is transcribed that does not hybridize with the classic M-*bcr* complementary DNA (cDNA) probe.[174]

In cases in which the Ph chromosome is not found, *BCR-ABL* still may be located on chromosome 9 (a masked Ph chromosome).[175] The *BCR* gene can recombine with genomically distinct sites on band 11q13 in complex translocations in a region rich in Alu repeat elements.[176] ETV6/ABL fusion genes have also been found in *BCR-ABL*–negative CML.[177]

The *BCR* breakpoint site has been examined as a factor in disease prognosis. Some studies have shown no correlation between CML chronicity and breakpoint site, although thrombocytosis may be more common with 3′ breakpoint sites and basophilia with 5′ breakpoint sites.[178] No difference in response to IFN-α therapy was noted, and survival was not significantly different, although patients with 3′ deletions tended to have shorter survival.[179] Others have observed a better response to IFN-α in patients with a 3′ rearrangement, which is being examined with imatinib mesylate therapy.[180]

CML patients with m-*bcr* breakpoints develop a blast crisis with monocytosis and an absence of splenomegaly and basophilia.[181] The p230 (e19a2 RNA junction) encoded by μ-*bcr* is rarely expressed but has been associated with neutrophilic CML or thrombocytosis (see "Special Clinical Features" below). Other rare breakpoints have been described.[182] For example, a case with a 12-bp insert between BCR1 and ABL1 resulted in a *BCR-ABL*–negative (false-negative), Ph-chromosome–positive CML with thrombocythemia.[183] Another novel *BCR-ABL* fusion gene (e6a2) in a patient with Ph-chromosome–negative CML encoded an oncoprotein of 185 kDa.[184] Typical CML also has been associated with an e19a2 junction *BCR-ABL* transcript.[185]

Experimental support for the hypothesis that $p210^{BCR-ABL}$ tyrosine phosphoprotein kinase is transforming is provided by a retroviral gene transfer system that permits expression of the protein. Mouse marrow cells transfected with *BCR-ABL* develop clonal outgrowths of immature cells expressing the p210$^{BCR-ABL}$ tyrosine kinase. Some clones progress to a malignant phenotype, can be transplanted, and can induce tumors in syngeneic mice.[186] Similar studies suggest that the p210$^{BCR-ABL}$ can transform 3T3 murine fibroblasts if the *gag* gene sequence from a helper virus cooperates.[187] The *BCR-ABL* gene from a retroviral vector has been expressed in an IL-3–dependent cell line. Clones derived from the infected line transform over months to IL-3 independency, are capable of increased proliferation, and develop chromosomal abnormalities.[188]

A series of mouse models in which the *BCR-ABL* was used to induce leukemogenesis have been described.[189–197] Lethally irradiated mice have been reconstituted with marrow enriched for cycling stem cells infected with a *BCR-ABL*–bearing retrovirus. Fatal diseases with abnormal accumulations of macrophagic, erythroid, mast, and lymphoid cells develop.[188] Classic CML did not occur, and complete transformation was not documented. The cell lines from spleen and marrow from mice with a *BCR-ABL* retrovirus infection were predominantly mast cells; however, in some cases these cell lines spontaneously switched to either erythroid and megakaryocytic, erythroid, or granulocytic lineages displaying maturation. They were transplantable (transformed) and contained the same proviral inserts as the original mast cell line.[198] Murine marrow also has been infected with a retrovirus encoding p210$^{BCR-ABL}$ and transplanted into irradiated syngeneic recipients.[189] Although several types of hematologic malignancies developed, a syndrome mimicking human CML also occurred. Mice transgenic for a p190$^{BCR-ABL}$ develop an acute lymphocytic leukemia (ALL) lymphoma syndrome[190] that resembles human Ph-chromosome–positive ALL. When a p210$^{BCR-ABL}$ transcript is introduced into a mouse germ line (one-cell fertilized eggs), the p210 founder and progeny transgenic animals developed leukemia of B or T lymphoid or of myeloid origin after a relatively long latency period. In contrast, p190 transgenic mice exclusively developed leukemia of B-cell origin, with a relatively short period of latency. This finding was believed to be consistent with the apparent indolent nature of human CML during the chronic phase.[191] When transgenic mice express p210$^{BCR-ABL}$, the transgenes develop ALL, whereas the progeny develop a myeloproliferative disorder.[192]

Mouse models remain important for exploring the pathogenesis of the acute and chronic BCR-ABL–mediated leukemias *in vivo* and in examining the potential effects of new drugs targeted at BCR-ABL.[199]

BCR-ABL IN HEALTHY SUBJECTS

BCR-ABL fusion genes can be found in the leukocytes of some normal individuals using a two-step reverse transcriptase polymerase chain reaction assay. Thus, although *BCR-ABL* may be expressed relatively frequently at very low levels in hematopoietic cells, only infrequently do the cells acquire the additional changes necessary to produce leukemia. This may be a dosage effect.[200]

BCR-ABL AND SIGNAL TRANSDUCTION

The tyrosine phosphoprotein kinase activity of p210$^{BCR-ABL}$ has been causally linked to the development of Ph-chromosome–positive leukemia in man.[201–212] p210$^{BCR-ABL}$ is, unlike the ABL protein that is located principally in the nucleus, located in the cytoplasm making it accessible to a large number of interactions, especially components of signal transduction pathways.[205,206,213] It binds and/or phosphorylates more than 20 cellular proteins in its role as an oncoprotein.[206] A subunit of phosphatidylinositol 3′-kinase (PI3K) associates with p210$^{BCR-ABL}$; this interaction is required for the proliferation of *BCR-ABL*–dependent cell lines and primary CML cells. Wortmannin, a nonspecific inhibitor of the p110 subunit of the kinase, inhibits growth of these cells.[207]

The pathways and interactions invoked by BCR-ABL acting on mitogen-activated protein kinases are multiple and complex.[214,215]

An RAF-encoded serine-threonine kinase activity is regulated by p210$^{BCR-ABL}$. Downregulation of RAF expression inhibits both *BCR-ABL*–dependent growth of CML cells and growth factor–dependent proliferation of normal hematopoietic progenitors.[208]

The efficiency of cell transformation by *BCR-ABL* is affected by an adaptor protein that can relate tyrosine kinase signals to RAS. This involves growth factor receptor-bound protein-2 (GRB2). p210$^{BCR-ABL}$ also activates multiple alternative pathways of RAS.[209] PI3K is constitutively activated by BCR-ABL, generates inositol lipids, and is dysregulated by the downregulation by BCR-ABL of polyinositol phosphate tumor suppressors, such as PTEN and SHIP1.[213] Figure 90–5 demonstrates interaction of p210$^{BCR-ABL}$ with various mediators of signal transduction.

Reactive oxygen species are increased in BCR-ABL–transformed cells and may act as a second messenger to modulate enzymes regulated by the redox equilibrium. An increase in these reactive oxygen products is

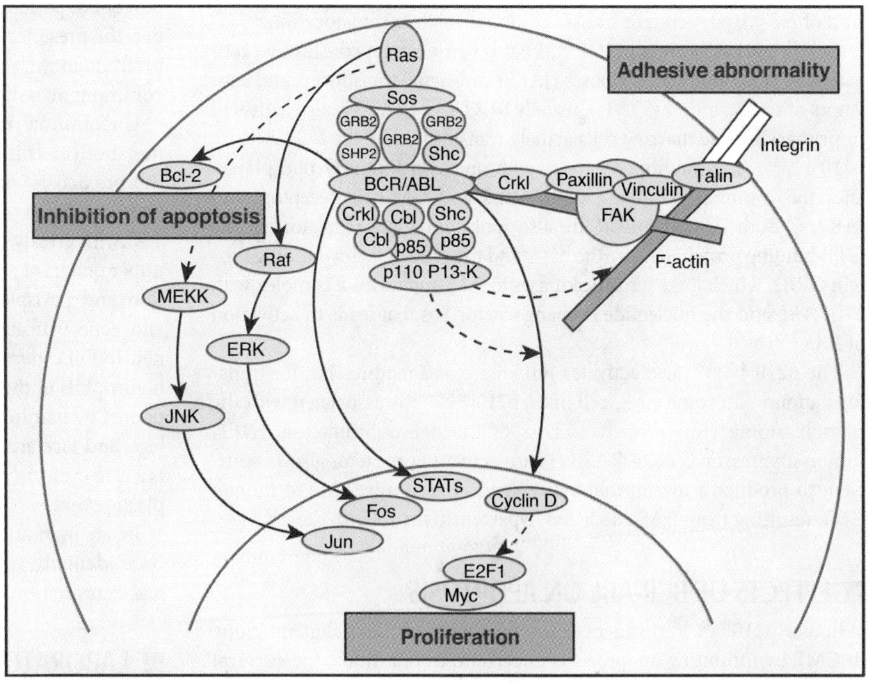

FIGURE 90–5. Major intracellular signaling events associated with *BCR/ABL*. Constitutive activation of ABL protein tyrosine kinase (PTK) induces phosphorylation of the tyrosine moiety of various substrates, including autophosphorylation of *BCR/ABL* and complex formation of *BCR/ABL* with adaptor proteins. This process subsequently activates multiple intracellular signaling pathways, including *RAS* activation and phosphatidylinositol 3′-kinase (PI3-K) activation pathways. *BCR/ABL* also activates the c-MYC pathway, which involves *ABL*-SH2 domain. *BCR/ABL* inhibits apoptosis, possibly in part through upregulation of Bcl-2, and alters cellular adhesive properties, possibly by interacting with focal adhesion proteins and the actin cytomatrix. *Broken lines* indicate hypothetical pathways. ERK, extracellular signal-regulated kinase; FAK, focal adhesion kinase; JNK, Jun N-terminal kinase; MEKK, MEK kinase; Sos, Son-of-sevenless; STAT, signal transducer and activator of transcription. *(From Gotoh A, Broxmeyer HE: The function of BCR/ABL and related proto-oncogenes.* Curr Opin Hematol *4:3, 1997, with permission.)*

postulated to play a role in the acquisition of additional mutations as a result of production of reactive oxygen species through the chronic phase, contributing to the progression to accelerated phase.[213,216]

The adaptor molecule CRKL is a major *in vivo* substrate for $p210^{BCR-ABL}$, and it acts to relate $p210^{BCR-ABL}$ to downstream effectors. CRKL is a linker protein that has homology to the v-*crk* oncogene product. Antibodies to CRKL can immunoprecipitate paxillin. Paxillin is a focal adhesion protein[210] that is phosphorylated by $p210^{BCR-ABL}$. The $p210^{BCR-ABL}$ may be physically linked to paxillin by CRKL. CRKL binds to CBL, an oncogene product that induces B cell and myeloid leukemias in mice.[211] The Src homology 3 domains of CRKL do not bind to CBL, but they do bind *BCR-ABL*. Therefore, CRKL mediates the oncogenic signal of *BCR-ABL* to CBL. The $p120^{CBL}$ and the adaptor proteins CRKL and c-CRK also link c-abl, $p190^{BCR-ABL}$, and $p210^{BCR-ABL}$ to the PI3K pathway.[212] The $p120^{CBL}$ also coprecipitates with the p85 subunit of PI3K, CRKL, and c-CRK. The $p210^{BCR-ABL}$ may, therefore, induce the formation of multimeric complexes of signaling proteins.[217] These complexes contain paxillin and talin and may explain some of the adhesive defects of CML cells.[218]

Hef2 also binds to CRKL in leukemic tissues of $p190^{BCR-ABL}$ transgenic mice. Hef2 is involved in the integrin signaling pathway[219] and encodes a protein that accelerates GTP hydrolysis of RAS-encoded proteins and neurofibromin. The latter negatively regulates granulocyte-monocyte colony-stimulating factor (GM-CSF) signaling through RAS in hematopoietic cells.[220] $P62^{DOK}$, a constitutively tyrosine-phosphorylated, $p120^{RAS}$ GAP-associated protein, which is rapidly tyrosine phosphorylated upon activation of the *c-kit* receptor,[221] is also associated with ABL.[222]

Nuclear factor (NF)-κB activation is also required for $p210^{BCR-ABL}$-mediated transformation.[223] Expression of $p210^{BCR-ABL}$ leads to activation of NF-κB–dependent transcription via nuclear translocation.[224]

Cell lines that express $p210^{BCR-ABL}$ also demonstrate constitutive activation of Janus-associated kinases (JAKs) and signal transducers and activators of transcription (STATs), usually STAT5.[225] STAT5 is also activated in primary mouse marrow cells acutely transformed by the *BCR-ABL*[226]; $p210^{BCR-ABL}$ coimmunoprecipitates with and constitutively phosphorylates the common β subunit of the IL-3 and GM-CSF receptors and JAK2.[227] Both *ABL* and *BCR* are also multifunctional regulators of the GTP-binding protein family Rho[228,229] and the growth factor-binding protein GRB2, which links tyrosine kinases to RAS and forms a complex with *BCR-ABL* and the nucleotide exchange factor Sos that leads to activation of *RAS*.[230]

The $p210^{BCR-ABL}$ also activates Jun kinase and requires Jun for transformation.[231] In some CML cell lines, $p210^{BCR-ABL}$ is associated with the retinoblastoma (Rb) protein.[232] Loss of the neurofibromatosis (*NF1*) tumor-suppressor gene, a RAS GTPase-activating protein, also is sufficient to produce a myeloproliferative syndrome in mice akin to human CML resulting from RAS-mediated hypersensitivity to GM-CSF.[233]

EFFECTS OF BCR-ABL ON APOPTOSIS

Whether $p210^{BCR-ABL}$ influences the expansion of the malignant clone in CML by inhibiting apoptosis is uncertain. In one study, the survival of normal and CML progenitors was the same after *in vitro* incubation in serum-deprived conditions and after treatment with X-irradiation or glucocorticoids.[234] $p210^{BCR-ABL}$ inhibits apoptosis by delaying the G_2/M transition of the cell cycle after DNA damage.[235] The $p210^{BCR-ABL}$ also may exert an antiapoptotic effect in factor-dependent hematopoietic cells.[236,237]

$p210^{BCR-ABL}$ does not prevent apoptotic death induced by human NK or lymphokine-activated killer cells directed against CML or normal cells.[238] In accelerated and blast phases, apoptosis rates were lower in CML neutrophils. G-CSF and GM-CSF considerably decreased the rate of apoptosis in CML neutrophils.[239]

TELOMERE LENGTH

Patients with CML present with a somewhat shortened mean telomere length in granulocytic cells but not blood T lymphocytes at diagnosis, but considerable overlap exists in the distribution of telomere length with healthy individuals.[240–242] The rate of shortening of telomere length during the chronic phase is correlated with a more rapid onset of accelerated phase.[240,242] Telomerase reverse transcriptase (TERT) is the catalytic subunit, expression of which is closely correlated with telomerase activity. In CML CD34+ cells containing BCR-ABL, the expression of TERT is significantly lower than in normal CD34+ cells, consistent with accelerated shortening of telomeres in CML cells.[243] A further significant decrease in telomere length occurs in the accelerated phase of CML. Telomerase activity is increased in the accelerated phase.[244] When therapy permits restoration of Ph-negative cells in the blood, these cells have telomere length comparable to that in matched healthy controls.[245]

CLINICAL FEATURES

SIGNS AND SYMPTOMS

In the 70 percent of patients who are symptomatic at diagnosis, the most frequent complaints include easy fatigability, loss of sense of well-being, decreased tolerance to exertion, anorexia, abdominal discomfort, early satiety (related to splenic enlargement), weight loss, and excessive sweating.[246–248] The symptoms are vague, nonspecific, and gradual in onset (weeks to months). A physical examination may detect pallor and splenomegaly. The latter was present in approximately 90 percent of patients at diagnosis, but with medical care being sought earlier, the presence of splenomegaly at the time of diagnosis is decreasing in frequency.[247] Sternal tenderness, especially the lower portion, is common; occasionally, patients notice it themselves.

Uncommon presenting symptoms include those of dramatic hypermetabolism (night sweats, heat intolerance, weight loss) simulating thyrotoxicosis; acute gouty arthritis, presumably related in part to hyperuricemia; priapism, tinnitus, or stupor from the leukostasis associated with greatly exaggerated blood leukocyte count elevations[249–251]; left upper quadrant and left shoulder pain as a consequence of splenic infarction and perisplenitis; vasopressin-responsive diabetes insipidus[252,253]; and acne urticata associated with hyperhistaminemia.[254] Acute febrile neutrophilic dermatosis (Sweet syndrome), a perivascular infiltrate of neutrophils in the dermis, can occur. In the latter situation, fever accompanied by painful maculonodular violaceous lesions on the trunk, arms, legs, and face are characteristic.[255,256] Spontaneous rupture of the spleen is a rare event.[257,258] Digital necrosis has been reported as a rare paraneoplastic event.[259,260]

In an increasing proportion of patients, the disease is discovered, coincidentally, when blood cell counts are measured at a periodic medical examination.

LABORATORY FINDINGS

Blood

The presumptive diagnosis of CML can be made from the results of the blood cell counts and examination of the blood film.[26,246,247] The blood hemoglobin concentration is decreased in most patients at the time of diagnosis. Red cells usually are only slightly altered, with an increase in variation from small to large size and only occasional misshapen (elliptical or irregular) erythrocytes. Small numbers of nucleated red cells are commonly present. The reticulocyte count is normal or slightly elevated, but clinically significant hemolysis is rare.[246,261,262] Rare cases of mild erythrocytosis[263,264] or erythroid aplasia[265,266] have been documented.

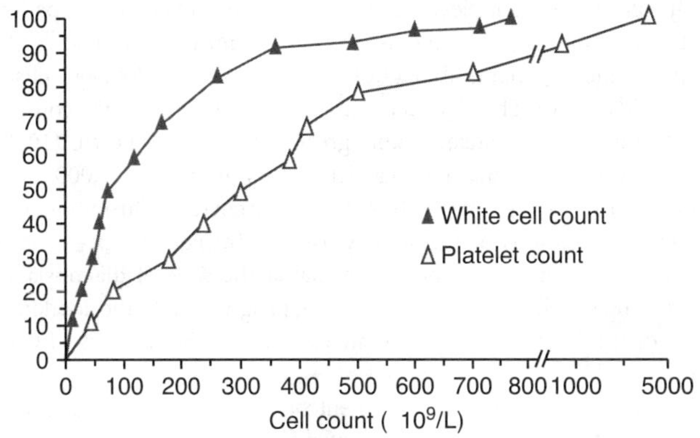

FIGURE 90–6. Total white cell count and platelet count of 90 patients with CML at the time of diagnosis. The cumulative percent of patients is on the *ordinate*, and the cell count is on the *abscissa*. Fifty percent of patients had a white cell count greater than 100×10^9/L and a platelet count greater than approximately 300×10^9/L at the time of diagnosis.

The total leukocyte count is always elevated at the time of diagnosis and is nearly always greater than 25,000/μL (25×10^9/L); at least half the patients have total white counts greater than 100,000/μL (100×10^9/L) (Fig. 90–6).[26,246,247] The total leukocyte count rises progressively in untreated patients. Rare patients may have dramatic cyclic variations in white cell counts as much as an order of magnitude with cycle intervals of approximately 60 days.[267,268] Granulocytes at all stages of development are present in the blood and are generally normal in appearance (Fig. 90–7). The mean blast cell prevalence is approximately 3 percent but can range from 0 to 10 percent; progranulocyte prevalence is approximately 4 percent; myelocytes, metamyelocytes, and bands account for approximately 40 percent; and segmented neutrophils account for approximately 35 percent of total leukocytes (Table 90–1). Often, there is a "myelocyte bulge" in which the differential count shows an exaggerated proportion of myelocytes compared to the proportion observed in normal persons. Hypersegmented neutrophils are commonly present.

Neutrophil alkaline phosphatase activity is low or absent in more than 90 percent of patients with CML.[269–271] The mRNA for alkaline phosphatase is undetectable in neutrophils of patients with CML.[272] The activity increases toward or to normal in the presence of intense inflammation or infection and when the total leukocytic count is decreased to or near normal with treatment.[271,273] CML neutrophils regain alkaline phosphatase activity after infusion into leukopenic recipients, suggesting the effect of regulators or factors extrinsic to the neutrophils.[274] *In vitro*, a monocyte-derived soluble mediator is capable of inducing increased alkaline phosphatase activity in neutrophils from CML patients.[275] Neutrophil alkaline phosphate is decreased sporadically in a variety of disorders and conditions,[276] but is decreased markedly

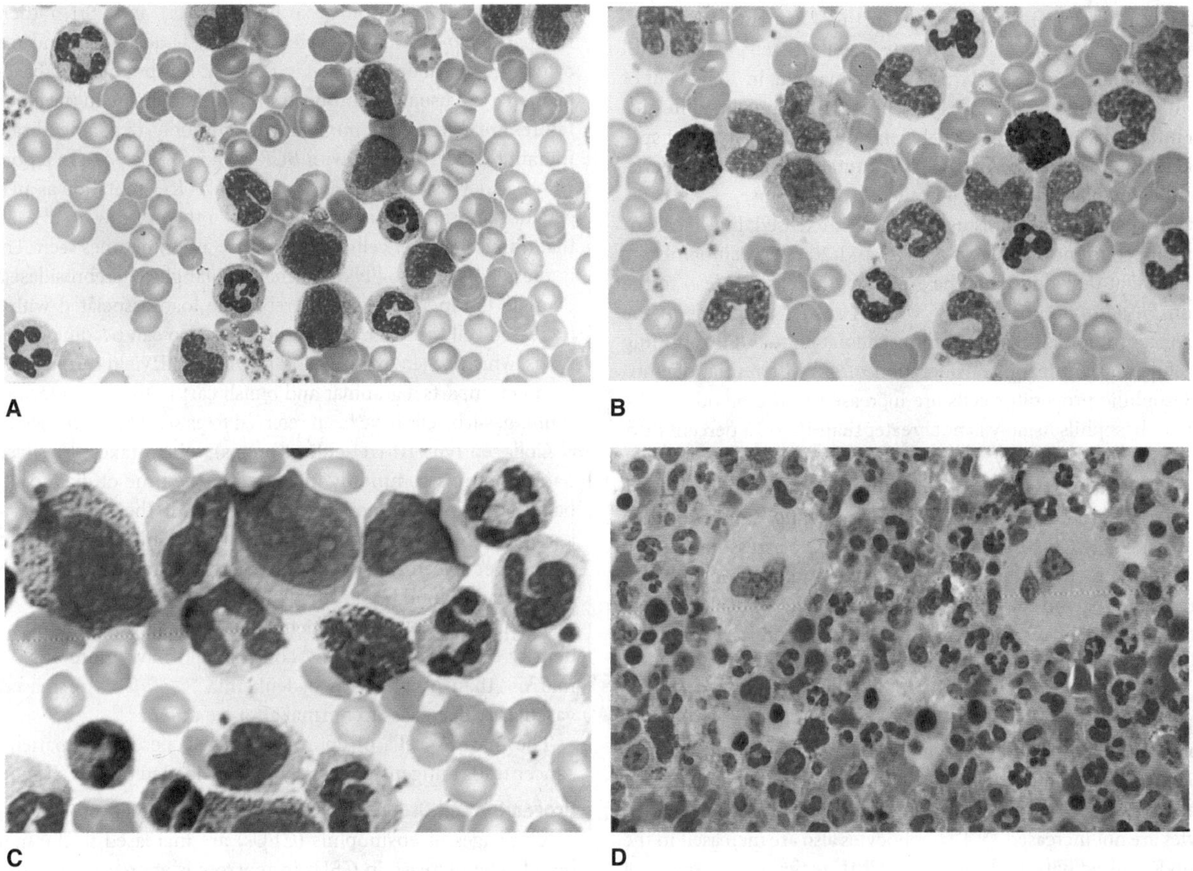

FIGURE 90–7. Blood and marrow cells characteristic of chronic myelogenous leukemia. **A.** Blood film. Elevated leukocyte count. Elevated platelet count (aggregates). Characteristic array of immature (myelocytes, metamyelocytes, band forms) and mature neutrophils. **B.** Blood film. Elevated leukocyte count. Characteristic array of immature (myelocytes, metamyelocytes, band forms) and mature neutrophils. Two basophils in the field. Absolute basophilia is a constant finding in CML. **C.** Blood film. Elevated leukocyte count. Characteristic array of immature (promyelocytes, myelocytes, metamyelocytes, band forms) and mature neutrophils. Basophil in the field. Two myeloblasts in upper center. Note multiple nucleoli (abnormal) and agranular cytoplasm. **D.** Marrow section. Hypercellular. Replacement of fatty tissue (normally approximately 60% of marrow volume in adults of this patient's age) with hematopoietic cells. Intense granulopoiesis and evident megakaryocytopoiesis. Decreased erythropoiesis. *(Reproduced from* Lichtman's Atlas of Hematology, *www.accessmedicine.com, with permission.)*

TABLE 90–1. White Blood Cell Differential Count at the Time of Diagnosis in 90 Cases of Ph-Chromosome–Positive Chronic Myelogenous Leukemia

	Percent of Total Leukocytes (Mean Values)
Myeloblasts	3
Promyelocytes	4
Myelocytes	12
Metamyelocytes	7
Band forms	14
Segmented forms	38
Basophils	3
Eosinophils	2
Nucleated red cells	0.5
Monocytes	8
Lymphocytes	8

NOTE: In these 90 patients, the mean hematocrit was 31 mL/dL, mean total white cell count was 160 × 10^9/L, and mean platelet count was 442 × 10^9/L at the time of diagnosis.

SOURCE: Hematology Unit, University of Rochester Medical Center.

and consistently in paroxysmal nocturnal hemoglobinuria,[276] in hypophosphatasia,[277] in approximately one-fourth of patients with idiopathic myelofibrosis, and in patients using androgens. Neutrophil alkaline phosphatase is increased in polycythemia vera, in 25 percent of patients with idiopathic myelofibrosis, in pregnant women, and in subjects with inflammatory disorders or infections. With the advent of specific markers, BCR-ABL in CML and JAK2 mutations in polycythemia, leukocyte alkaline phosphatase is of limited diagnostic use.

The proportion of eosinophils usually is not increased, but the absolute eosinophil count nearly always is increased. Rarely, eosinophils are so prominent that they dominate the granulocytic cells and lead to the designation *Ph-positive eosinophilic CML*. An absolute increase in the basophil concentration is present in almost all patients, and this finding can be useful in preliminary consideration of the differential diagnosis.[26,278] Basophilic progenitor cells are increased in the blood.[279] The proportion of basophils usually is not greater than 10 to 15 percent during the chronic phase but may, in rare patients, represent 30 to 80 percent of the total leukocyte count during chronic phase and lead to the designation of Ph-chromosome–positive basophilic CML.[280] Flow cytometry using anti-CD203c provides very accurate assessment of the basophil frequency. Basophils may be hypogranulated or have an immature phenotype and may be left uncounted in an optical differential count. Anti-CD203c recognizes these cells as basophils.[281] Granules of basophils in patients with CML, unlike normal basophils, contain mast cell α-tryptase.[281,282] Granulocytes containing both eosinophilic and basophilic granules (mixed granulation) are commonly present.[283]

The total absolute lymphocyte count is increased (mean: approximately 15 × 10^9/L) in patients with CML at the time of diagnosis[284] as a result of the balanced increase in T-helper and T-suppressor cells.[285] B lymphocytes are not increased.[288] T lymphocytes also are increased in the spleen.[286] NK cell activity is defective in CML patients as a result of decreased maturation of these cells *in vivo*[287,288] and a decrease in the absolute number of circulating NK cells in patients with CML. The latter change can perhaps be related to increased apoptosis.[289] The CD56 bright subset of NK cells is particularly decreased. These cells are reduced more as CML progresses, and they respond less to stimuli that recruit clonogenic NK cells compared to NK cells from normal subjects.[290]

The platelet count is elevated in approximately 50 percent of patients at the time of diagnosis and is normal in most of the rest.[291] The median value in patients at diagnosis is approximately 400,000 cells/μL (400 × 10^9 cells/L). The platelet count may increase during the course of the chronic phase. Platelet counts greater than 1,000,000/μL (1000 × 10^9/L) are not unusual, and platelet counts as high as 5,000,000 to 7,000,000/μL (5000–7000 × 10^9/L) have occurred. Thrombohemorrhagic complications of thrombocytosis are infrequent. Occasionally, the platelet count may be below normal at the time of diagnosis, but this finding usually signals an impending progression to the accelerated phase of the disease (see "Accelerated Phase and Blast Crisis of CML" below).

Functional abnormalities of neutrophils (adhesion, emigration, phagocytosis) are mild; are compensated for by high neutrophil concentrations; and do not predispose patients in chronic phase to infections by either the usual or opportunistic organisms.[292–294] Platelet dysfunction can occur but is not associated with spontaneous or exaggerated bleeding. A decrease in the second wave of epinephrine-induced platelet aggregation is the most common abnormality and is associated with a deficiency of adenine nucleotides in the storage pool.[295,296]

Marrow

Morphology The marrow is markedly hypercellular, and hematopoietic tissue takes up 75 to 90 percent of the marrow volume, with fat markedly reduced (see Fig. 90–7).[297,298] Granulopoiesis is dominant, with a granulocytic-to-erythroid ratio between 10:1 and 30:1, rather than the normal 2:1 to 4:1. Erythropoiesis usually is decreased, and megakaryocytes are normal or increased in number. Eosinophils and basophils may be increased, usually in proportion to their increase in the blood. Mitotic figures are increased in number. Uncommonly a juxtamembrane domain mutant of *KIT* coincides with *BCR-ABL* in CML.[299] Rare reports of marrow mastocytosis have been explained by a *KIT* mutation as an additional genetic abnormality or by dual clones in the marrow.[300,301] Macrophages that mimic Gaucher cells in appearance are sometimes seen. This finding is a result of the inability of normal cellular glucocerebrosidase activity to degrade the increased glucocerebroside load associated with markedly increased cell turnover.[302] Macrophages also can become engorged with lipids, which, when oxidized and polymerized, yield ceroid pigment. This pigment imparts a granular and bluish cast to the cells after polychrome staining; such cells have been referred to as *sea-blue histiocytes*.[302]

Collagen type III (reticulin fibrosis), which takes the silver impregnation stain, is commonly increased at the time of diagnosis in nearly half the patients,[303] and is correlated with the proportion of megakaryocytes in the marrow.[304,305] Increased fibrosis also is correlated with larger spleen size, more severe anemia, and a higher proportion of marrow and blood blast cells.

The marrows of CML patients have a mean doubling of microvessel density compared to healthy controls and have more angiogenesis in marrow than other forms of leukemia.[306–308] This increased marrow vascularity decreases to normal after treatment.[309]

The marrow cells of approximately 50 percent of patients express cancer testis antigens, especially those encoded by *HAGE* genes.[310]

Progenitor Cell Growth Cells that form colonies of neutrophils and macrophages or eosinophils (CFUs) are increased in the marrow and blood. The increase in CFUs in marrow is approximately 20-fold normal and in blood approximately 500-fold normal. The CFUs are of lighter buoyant density than those in normal marrow.[95] More primitive progenitors that can initiate long-term cultures of hematopoiesis also are markedly increased.[311] Spontaneous blood-derived granulocyte-macrophage colony growth is common, although CFUs also respond to growth factor stimulation.[105]

Cytogenetics The marrow and nucleated blood cells of more than 90 percent of patients with clinical and laboratory signs that fall within the criteria for the diagnosis of CML contain the Ph chromosome (22q−) as measured by G-banding, and virtually all patients have the t(9;22)(q34;q11)(*BCR-ABL*) by fluorescence in situ hybridization. The Ph chromosome is present in all blood cell lineages (erythroblasts, granulocytes, monocytes, megakaryocytes, T- and B-cell progenitors) but is not present in the majority of blood B lymphocytes or in most T lymphocytes.[49,51] Approximately 70 percent of patients in the chronic phase have the classic Ph chromosome in their cells.[312] The remaining 20 percent also have a missing Y chromosome [t(Ph),−Y]; an additional C-group chromosome, usually number 8 [t(Ph),+8]; an additional chromosome 22q− but without the 9q+ [t(Ph), 22q−]; or t(Ph) plus either another stable translocation or another minor clone.[75] These variations have not been shown to affect the duration of the chronic phase. Deletion of the Y chromosome occurs in approximately 10 percent of healthy men older than 60 years.[313,314]

Variant Ph chromosome translocations occur in approximately 5 percent of subjects with CML and involve complex rearrangements (three chromosomes), and every chromosome except the Y chromosome can be involved.[315–319] The Ph chromosome, that is, 22q−, is present, but the gross exchange of chromosomal material involves a chromosome other than 9 (simple variant) or involves exchange of material among chromosomes 9 and 22 and a third or more chromosomes (complex variant; see Fig. 90–8). High-resolution techniques have indicated that 9q34-qter is transposed to 22q11 in simple and in complex translocations.[320,321] Thus, the fusion of 9q34 with 22q11 seems to occur in the cells of most patients with CML.[323] Complex translocations involving chromosome 3 have been notable.[322–324] In rare cases, a reciprocal translocation with a chromosome other than 9 to chromosome 22 is larger than usual, and the posttranslocation shortening of the long arms of 22 is not apparent. This circumstance has been referred to as a *masked Ph chromosome* or *masked translocation* because the 22q− is not evident by microscopic examination,[325,326] although t(9;22) may occur as judged by banding techniques or molecular probes.[327]

Approximately 10 percent of patients have a deletion of the derivative 9 chromosome adjacent to the chromosome breakpoint. Although this deletion is thought to be an important factor in resistance to drug effects with IFN therapy, it does not appear to be significant with the use of imatinib.[214]

Molecular Probes In a small proportion of patients with a clinical disease analogous to CML, cytogenetic studies do not disclose a classic, variant, or masked Ph chromosome. In these cases, use of a panel of restriction enzymes and Southern blot analyses with a molecular probe for the breakpoint cluster region on chromosome 22 nearly always detects rearrangement of fragments. This finding has led to the conclusion that almost all cases of CML have an abnormality of the long arm of chromosome number 22 (*BCR* rearrangement).[328–332] Ph-chromosome–negative CML cells with *BCR* rearrangement can express $p210^{BCR-ABL}$, and such patients have a clinical course similar to Ph-chromosome–positive CML.[328,333–336]

The ability to identify the molecular consequences of the t(9;22), that is, *BCR* rearrangement, mRNA transcripts of the mutant fusion gene, and $p210^{BCR-ABL}$, has resulted in diagnostic tests supplementary to cytogenetic analysis.[332] These tests include Southern blot analysis of *BCR* rearrangement,[334–338] polymerase chain reaction (PCR) amplification of the abnormal mRNA,[339] and a less complex variation on the latter, a hybridization protection assay.[340]

PCR can achieve a sensitivity of one positive cell in approximately 500,000 to 1 million cells. This extreme sensitivity requires special care in analysis and the inclusion of negative controls.[341–344] Immunodiagnosis of CML by identification of $p210^{BCR-ABL}$ also is possible. This tumor-specific protein for CML is unique, based on the amino acids at the junction between the *ABL* and *BCR* sequences. Oligopeptides corresponding to the junctional amino acids have been synthesized and used as antigens[345–348] to develop specific antibodies to $p210^{BCR-ABL}$.

A multicolor FISH method to detect the *BCR-ABL* fusion in patients with CML is a rapid and sensitive alternative to Southern blot and PCR-dependent methods.[349] For diagnostic purposes, FISH is simple, accurate, and sensitive, and can detect the various molecular fusions (e.g., e13a2, e14a2, e1a2).[350–354] Interphase FISH is faster and more sensitive than cytogenetics in identifying the Ph chromosome. If the concentration of CML cells is very low, interphase FISH may not detect *BCR-ABL*, so it has limited use for detecting minimal residual disease.[355] Hypermetaphase FISH allows analysis of up to 500 metaphases per sample in 1 day. Several factors influence the false-positive and false-negative rates of FISH identification of *BCR-ABL*, including definition of a fusion signal, nuclear size, and the genomic position of the ABL breakpoint.[356] Double BCR-ABL fusion signals (double-fusion [D]-FISH) have been proposed as being more accurate than the fusion signal used in dual color (single-fusion) S-FISH, because in the latter case a small percentage of the normal BCR and ABL signals overlap.[357]

The frequency of cytogenetic analysis can be reduced if patients are monitored by molecular methods such as quantitative Southern blotting, FISH, quantitative Western blotting, or competitive reverse transcriptase (RT)-PCR. Molecular analyses

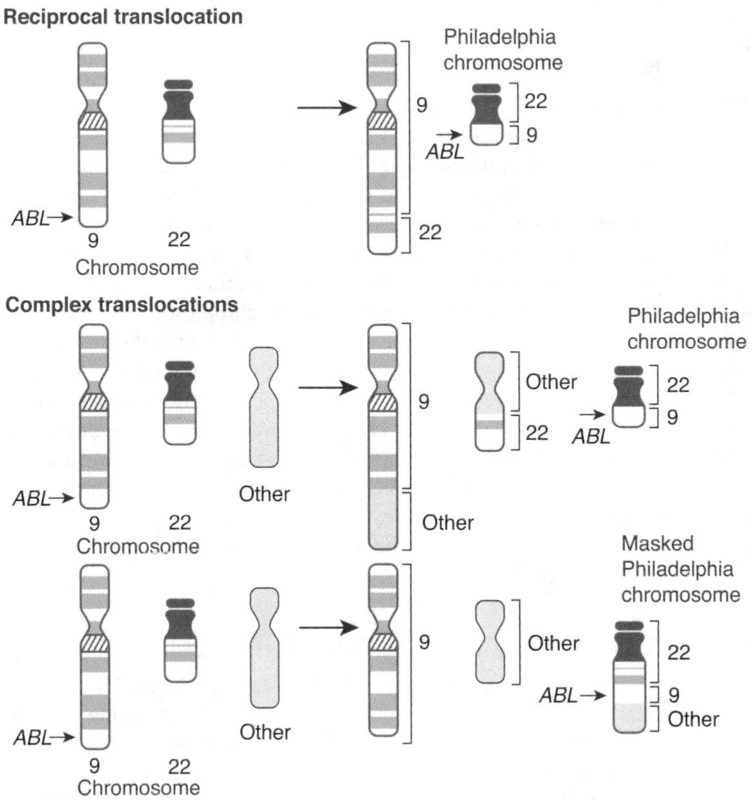

FIGURE 90–8. Translocations involved in chronic myelogenous leukemia. The positions of the *ABL* gene in each of the chromosomes before and after the translocation are noted. The origin of the chromosomal segments in each of the translocated chromosomes is indicated by a *bracket* on the side of the chromosome. *(From Rosson D, Reddy EP: Activation of the abl oncogene and its involvement in chromosomal translocations in human leukemia.* Mutat Res *195:231, 1988, with permission.)*

can be performed on blood samples and therefore are much easier to use than cytogenetic analysis of marrow cell metaphases. Quantitative RT-PCR is the method of choice for monitoring patients for residual disease or reappearance of disease after marrow transplantation and for following response to tyrosine kinase inhibitors once routine cytogenetics and FISH are negative for the Philadelphia chromosome. Competitive PCR can detect reappearance of or increasing levels of RNA *BCR-ABL* transcripts prior to clinical relapse in patients after transplantation.[358–360]

Chemical Abnormalities

Uric Acid An increased production of uric acid with hyperuricemia and hyperuricosuria occurs in untreated CML.[361] Uric acid excretion often is two to three times normal in patients with CML. If aggressive therapy leads to rapid cell lysis, excretion of the additional purine load may produce urinary tract blockage from uric acid precipitates. Formation of urinary urate stones is common in patients with CML, and some patients with latent gout may develop acute gouty arthritis or uric acid nephropathy.[362] The likelihood of complications from urate overproduction is greatly increased by starvation, acidosis, renal disease, or diuretic drug therapy.

Serum Vitamin B_{12}-Binding Proteins and Vitamin B_{12} Neutrophils contain vitamin B_{12}-binding proteins, including transcobalamin I and III (synonym: R-type B_{12}-binding protein or cobalophilin).[363–366] Patients with myeloproliferative diseases have an increased serum level of B_{12}-binding capacity, and the source of the protein is principally mature neutrophilic granulocytes.[363,364] The increase in transcobalamin level and the resultant increase in vitamin B_{12} concentration are particularly notable in CML, although any increase in the number of neutrophilic granulocytes, as in leukemoid reactions, can be accompanied by an increase in serum B_{12}-binding protein levels and vitamin B_{12} concentration.[366] The serum B_{12} level in CML patients is increased on average to more than 10 times normal.[367] The increase is proportional to the total leukocyte count in untreated patients and falls toward normal levels with treatment, although increased B_{12} levels commonly persist even after the white cell count is lowered to near normal with therapy.

Pernicious anemia and CML may rarely coexist. In this situation, the tissues are vitamin B_{12} deficient, but the serum vitamin B_{12} level may be normal because of the elevated level of transcobalamin I, a binder with a very high affinity for vitamin B_{12}.[367]

Whole Blood Histamine Mean histamine levels are markedly increased in patients in chronic phase (median: ~5000 ng/mL) compared to healthy individuals (median: ~50 ng/mL); and, this elevation is correlated with the blood basophil count.[368] Cases of exaggerated basophilia and disabling pruritus, urticaria, and gastric hyperacidity have occurred, associated with enormous increases (several hundred-fold) of blood histamine concentration.[369,370]

Serum Lactic Dehydrogenase, Potassium, Calcium, and Cholesterol The level of serum lactic acid dehydrogenase (LDH) is elevated in CML.[371] Pseudohyperkalemia resulting from the release of potassium from white cells during clotting[372] and spurious hypoxemia or pseudohypoglycemia from *in vitro* utilization of oxygen or glucose by granulocytes can occur. Hypercalcemia[373] or hypokalemia[374] has occurred during the chronic phase of the disease, but such complications are very rare until the disorder transforms to acute leukemia. Elevated serum and urinary lysozyme levels are features of leukemia with greater monocytic components and are not features of CML.[375] Serum cholesterol is decreased in patients with CML.[376,377]

Serum Angiogenic Factors Angiogenin, endoglin (CD105), vascular endothelial growth factor (VEGF), β-fibroblast growth factor, and hepatocyte growth factor are increased strikingly in the serum of CML patients.[307,308,378,379]

SPECIAL CLINICAL FEATURES

■ *BCR-ABL*–POSITIVE THROMBOCYTHEMIA

Either of two syndromes—thrombocythemia with the Ph chromosome and *BCR-ABL* rearrangement or thrombocythemia without a Ph chromosome but with the *BCR-ABL* rearrangement—may precede the overt signs of CML or its accelerated phase.[380–386] In general, the disease closely mimics classic thrombocythemia initially: marked platelet elevation, extreme megakaryocytic hyperplasia, normal or mildly elevated white cell count, no or very slight myeloid immaturity in the blood, and minimal anemia. Minor bleeding, such as epistaxis, erythromelalgia, or signs of thrombosis, such as cerebral or limb ischemia, are occasionally present.[387] In some cases the absolute basophil count is mildly elevated. Using immunostaining, Ph-positive thrombocythemia is proposed to be distinctive from Ph-negative thrombocythemia by small megakaryocytes in the former and by large clusters of megakaryocytes in the latter.[387] However, this distinction was not found in other studies,[388] has to be validated, and is difficult to use as a discriminator. In two studies, approximately 5 percent of patients with apparent essential thrombocythemia had a Ph chromosome.[382,389] In another study, 2 of 121 patients with essential thrombocythemia had *BCR-ABL* transcripts, and 1 of these patients also had a Ph chromosome in the marrow cells,[390] whereas in a different study, 4 of 32 patients with thrombocythemia had low levels of *BCR-ABL* transcripts in blood cells.[391] Approximately 1 in 20 patients with CML present with the features of essential thrombocythemia.[383,384] Evolution to blast crisis may occur.[381,392,393] Thus, the frequency of Ph-chromosome–negative, *BCR-ABL*–positive thrombocythemia ranges from approximately 1.6 to 13 percent of patients, which may reflect in part the range of sensitivity of the detection method.[389–391,394,395]

■ NEUTROPHILIC CML

A rare variant of *BCR-ABL*–positive CML has been described in which the elevated white cell count is composed principally of mature neutrophils.[396,397] The white cell count is lower on average (30,000–50,000/μL) at the time of diagnosis than is the case with classic CML (median, 100,000–150,000/μL). Moreover, patients with neutrophilic CML usually do not have basophilia, notable myeloid immaturity in the blood, prominent splenomegaly, or low leukocyte alkaline phosphatase scores. The cells of these patients have the Ph chromosome but have an unusual *BCR-ABL* fusion gene in that the breakpoint in the *BCR* gene is between exons 19 and 20. This breakpoint location results in fusion of most of the *BCR* gene with *ABL* (e19a2 type *BCR-ABL*), which leads to a larger fusion protein (230 kDa) compared to the fusion protein in classic CML (210 kDa; see Fig. 90–3). This correlation between genotype and phenotype has not been observed in all cases.[398] This variant usually has an indolent course, which may be the result of very low levels of mRNA for p230 and the undetectable or barely detectable p230 protein in cells.[399]

■ MINOR-BCR BREAKPOINT–POSITIVE CML

A small proportion of patients with BCR-ABL–positive CML have the breakpoint on the *BCR* gene in the first intron (m-*bcr*), resulting in a 190-kDa fusion protein instead of the classic 210-kDa protein observed in most patients with CML (see Fig. 90–3). The m-*bcr* molecular lesion is similar to that observed in approximately 60 percent of patients with *BCR* rearrangement-positive ALL. In patients with m-*bcr* CML, monocytes are more prominent, the white cell count is lower on average, and basophilia and splenomegaly are less prominent than in disease with classic *BCR* breakpoint (M-*bcr*). The few reported cases had a short interval before either myeloid or lymphoid blast transformation developed.[400,401]

HYPERLEUKOCYTOSIS

Approximately 15 percent of patients present with symptoms or signs referable to leukostasis as a result of the intravascular flow-impeding effects of white cell counts greater than 300,000/μL (300×10^9/L).[249] Hyperleukocytosis is more prevalent in children with Ph-chromosome–positive CML.[250] The effects of total leukocyte counts from 300,000 to 800,000/μL ($300–800 \times 10^9$/L) include impaired circulation of the lung, central nervous system, special sensory organs, and penis, resulting in some combination of tachypnea, dyspnea, cyanosis, dizziness, slurred speech, delirium, stupor, visual blurring, diplopia, retinal vein distention, retinal hemorrhages, papilledema, tinnitus, impaired hearing, and priapism.[251] In asymptomatic patients with hyperleukocytosis, initial treatment with hydration and hydroxyurea usually can be used to decrease the white cell count. Hydroxyurea treatment should be designed to accomplish a gradual decrease in white cell count over a few days so as to avoid the tumor lysis syndrome. If signs of hyperleukocytosis are present, hydration, leukapheresis, and hydroxyurea can be used simultaneously; hydroxyurea dose should be selected to avoid exaggerated tumor lysis.

CONCURRENCE OF LYMPHOID MALIGNANCIES

CML has an association with lymphoproliferation that can take four principal forms. (1) Patients may develop CML years after irradiation treatment of non-Hodgkin or Hodgkin lymphoma. (2) Approximately one-third of CML patients enter the accelerated phase of the disease by evolution and dedifferentiation of the CML clone into one that supports lymphoblastic proliferation (acute lymphoblastic transformation). (3) Patients may have concurrent lymphoproliferative or plasmacytic malignancies and CML. Lymphoma or lymphoblastic leukemia,[402–408] essential monoclonal gammopathy,[409,410] myeloma,[411–413] and Waldenström macroglobulinemia[414] have occurred in association with CML. Several cases of CML emergence in patients with established chronic lymphocytic leukemia (CLL) have been reported.[415–417] A few patients have presented with simultaneous occurrence of the two diseases.[418,419] A single case of lymphocytic leukemoid reaction simulating CLL that regressed as CML emerged has been reported.[420] In some cases, the CLL lymphocytes did not contain the Ph chromosome, whereas the CML cells did, suggesting the presence of two independent clonal disorders.[415,416,421,422] In other cases, the Ph chromosome was present in the myeloid and lymphoid cells, indicating a common origin.[419] (4) Patients may present with Ph-chromosome–positive acute lymphoblastic leukemia and, following chemotherapy-induced remission, develop the features of typical CML.[420]

DIFFERENTIAL DIAGNOSIS

DISEASES MIMICKING CML

The diagnosis of CML is made based on the characteristic granulocytosis, white cell differential count, increased absolute basophil count, and splenomegaly coupled with the presence of the Ph chromosome or its variants (90% of patients) or a *BCR* rearrangement on chromosome 22 (>95% of patients).

Patients with other chronic hematopoietic stem cell diseases, such as polycythemia vera, essential thrombocythemia, or primary myelofibrosis, only occasionally have closely overlapping features. For example, the total white cell count is greater than 30×10^9/L in more than 90 percent of patients with CML and increases inexorably over weeks or months of observation, whereas the total white cell count is less than 30×10^9/L in more than 90 percent of patients with the three other classic chronic clonal myeloid diseases and usually does not change significantly over months to years. Polycythemia vera is associated with increased red cell mass and hemoglobin concentration and displays clinical signs of plethora; CML does not have these features. Patients with primary myelofibrosis invariably have marked teardrop poikilocytes and other severe red cell shape, size, and chromicity changes, as well as prominent nucleated red cells in the blood; CML rarely has these features. Patients with essential thrombocythemia have a platelet count greater than 450,000/μL (450×10^9/L) and usually only mild neutrophilia (<20,000/μL); the slight neutrophilia distinguishes it from the proportion (~25%) of CML patients with platelet counts greater than 450,000/μL (450×10^9/L), who at the time of diagnosis have white cell counts above 25,000/μL. In addition, patients with the clinical features of polycythemia vera or primary myelofibrosis do not have the Ph chromosome or *BCR* rearrangement in their blood and marrow cells, except in extremely rare cases. A very small proportion of patients with apparent essential thrombocythemia have BCR-ABL transcripts in their marrow and blood cells, and occasionally a Ph chromosome and may represent an atypical initial phase of CML (see "*BCR-ABL*–Positive Thrombocythemia" above). The presence of a mutation in the JAK2 gene in approximately 95 percent of patients with polycythemia vera and in approximately 40 to 50 percent of patients with primary myelofibrosis or essential thrombocythemia by current assay techniques is a very useful distinguishing feature when present. More sensitive assays for JAK2 may make this marker even more useful in discrimination of these myeloproliferative diseases from CML.[423]

Increased awareness of the features of related disorders, such as chronic myelomonocytic leukemia (CMML) and chronic neutrophilic leukemia, and an appreciation that older patients are prone to atypical clonal myeloid diseases, have minimized the inappropriate diagnosis of Ph-chromosome–negative CML, which should be avoided unless the clinical features are characteristic of classic CML and a masked Ph chromosome or *BCR* rearrangement is not found.

Reactive leukocytosis can occur with absolute neutrophil counts of 30,000 to 100,000/μL ($30–100 \times 10^9$/L). Usually these leukemoid reactions occur in the setting of an overt inflammatory disease (e.g., pancreatitis), cancer (e.g., lung), or infection (e.g., pneumococcal pneumonia). If the incitant is not apparent, the absence of granulocytic immaturity, basophilia, splenomegaly, and decreased neutrophil alkaline phosphatase activity argue against CML. The absence of a cytogenetic or molecular abnormality in chromosome 22 virtually eliminates classic CML as a consideration.

The precise diagnosis of CML is helpful in estimating the patient's prognosis, determining the potential response to tyrosine kinase inhibitors, and assessing the timing of special therapies, such as allogeneic hematopoietic stem cell transplantation.

PH-CHROMOSOME–POSITIVE CLONAL MYELOID DISEASES AND APLASTIC ANEMIA

The Ph chromosome has been found rarely in patients with apparent polycythemia vera,[27,424] polycythemia vera that later evolves into Ph-chromosome–positive CML,[425–427] idiopathic myelofibrosis,[428,429] and myelodysplastic syndrome (MDS).[430,431] Molecular studies to determine the presence of the *BCR-ABL* were not performed in cases reported before 1985. Primary (essential) thrombocythemia with a Ph chromosome and/or *BCR-ABL* rearrangement in blood cells was discussed earlier (see "Special Clinical Features" above). Rare cases of aplastic anemia have presented with *BCR-ABL*–positive cells or have evolved into BCR-ABL CML.[432,433] The frequency of this association is uncertain because of the inability to have sufficient cells for a cytogenetic analysis during the period of aplasia and the unavailability in past years of FISH or PCR to test for the *BCR-ABL* gene in patients with this clinical presentation.

THERAPY

HYPERURICEMIA

Hyperuricemia and hyperuricosuria are frequent features of CML at diagnosis or in relapse.[434] The need for treatment of hyperuricemia is a function of the elevated pretreatment serum uric acid concentration, blood white cell concentration, spleen size, and dose of chemotherapy planned. If these variables suggest a high risk for a significant amount of cell lysis, allopurinol 300 mg/day orally and adequate hydration to maintain a good urine flow should be instituted prior to therapy. Allopurinol is associated with a high frequency of allergic skin reactions and should be discontinued after the blood leukocyte count and spleen size have decreased and the risk of exaggerated cell lysis has passed. If hyperuricemia is extreme, usually over 9 mg/dL, alkalinization of urine can be achieved with sodium bicarbonate, and rasburicase can be administered.[435] Rasburicase is a recombinant urate oxidase that converts uric acid to allantoin. Rasburicase, unlike allopurinol, reduces the uric acid pool very rapidly, does not result in the accumulation of xanthine or hypoxanthine, and does not require alkalinization of urine facilitating phosphate excretion.[436] Although the manufacturer recommends a dose every day for 5 days, several reports have indicated that one injection will produce a rapid and sustained decrease in serum uric acid, significantly decreasing the cost of therapy.[437] Another alternative is to use allopurinol for a few days after one injection of rasburicase. A dose of 0.2 mg/kg of ideal body weight of rasburicase intravenously has been used.[438]

INITIAL CYTOREDUCTION THERAPY

Imatinib mesylate (imatinib) is now used as initial therapy in almost all patients with CML presenting in the chronic phase. In cases where the white cell count is markedly elevated, hydroxyurea can be used prior to or in conjunction with imatinib. If rapid cytoreduction is required because of signs of the hyperleukocytic syndrome, leukapheresis and hydroxyurea often are combined.

Leukapheresis

Leukapheresis can control CML only temporarily. For this reason, it is rarely used in chronic phase CML and is useful in only two types of patients: the hyperleukocytic patient in whom rapid cytoreduction can reverse symptoms and signs of leukostasis (e.g., stupor, hypoxia, tinnitus, papilledema, priapism),[249–251] and in the pregnant patient with CML who can be controlled by leukapheresis treatment without other therapy either during the early months of pregnancy when therapy poses a higher risk to the fetus or, in some cases, throughout the pregnancy.[439,440] Because of the large body burden of leukocytes in marrow, blood, and spleen, and the high proliferative rate in CML, leukocyte reduction by apheresis is less efficient than in other types of leukemias.[249,251] Leukapheresis reduces the burden of tumor cells subject to chemotherapeutically induced cytolysis and thus the production and the excretion of uric acid. In hyperleukocytic nonpregnant patients, leukapheresis is best used in conjunction with hydroxyurea to ensure rapid and optimal reduction in white cell count.

Hydroxyurea

Hydroxyurea 1 to 6 g/day orally, depending on the height of the white cell count, can be used to initiate elective therapy.[441] Urgent treatment of extraordinary total white cell counts may require higher doses. The dose of hydroxyurea should be decreased as the total white cell count decreases and usually is given at 1 to 2 g/day when the total white cell count reaches 20,000/μL (20×10^9/L). The drug should be temporarily discontinued if the white cell count drops below 5000/μL (5×10^9/L). If hydroxyurea is being used in combination with imatinib, the hydroxyurea usually is tapered and discontinued once a hematologic response to imatinib is observed.

Anagrelide

Anagrelide can be used for platelet reduction in patients who present with elevated platelet counts. This agent acts directly to decrease megakaryocyte mass, and it can lead to a precipitous fall in platelet counts. In occasional patients who still have significant thrombocythemia after imatinib is initiated, the combination of imatinib and anagrelide is associated with a normalization of platelet counts.[442]

TYROSINE KINASE INHIBITOR THERAPY

Imatinib Mesylate Patients with newly diagnosed chronic phase CML should be started on imatinib, 400 mg/day by mouth. Imatinib is easier to use, induces a higher frequency of hematologic remission, a higher frequency of complete cytogenetic remission, and greater suppression of the CML clone (molecular remission) than therapy with interferon (INF)-α. The goal of imatinib therapy is to decrease the cells bearing the t(9;22) translocation (leukemic cells) to the lowest levels possible, under which conditions normal (polyclonal) hematopoiesis is restored. The efficacy of imatinib is judged by measuring the three benchmarks: hematologic response, cytogenetic response, and molecular response (Table 90–2).[443,444] These are used to determine its maximal effect. The time to achieve a maximal effect is variable and can range from months to years. Thus, as long as a patient is having a continued reduction in the size of the leukemic clone as judged by cytogenetic or PCR measurements, the drug is continued at 400 mg/day. If the patient stops responding before a complete cytogenetic remission or complete molecular remission is achieved, the dose can be increased to 600 mg/day or to 800 mg/day (400 mg every 12 hours), if tolerated. About two-thirds of patients who do not have a significant hematologic response or who relapse while receiving imatinib at a dose of 400 mg/day achieve a complete or partial hematologic response with higher doses, but few cytogenetic responses occur.[445] Some patients without a cytogenetic response can enter a partial or complete cytogenetic response with higher doses of imatinib. Unfortunately, the responses to higher doses of imatinib in patients lacking a hematologic or cytogenetic response at 400 mg/day usually are transient.[446,447]

TABLE 90–2. Criteria for Extent of Imatinib Treatment Response

Hematologic response	White cell count <10×10^9/L, platelet count <450×10^9/L, no immature myeloid cells in the blood, and disappearance of all signs and symptoms related to leukemia (including palpable splenomegaly) lasting for at least 4 weeks.
Major cytogenetic response	Less than 35% of cells containing the Ph chromosome by cytogenetic analysis of marrow cells.
Complete cytogenetic response	No cells containing the Ph chromosome by cytogenetic analysis of marrow cells.
Major molecular response	Blood cell BCR-ABL/ABL ratio <0.05% (3-log reduction in PCR signal from mean pretreatment baseline value).
Complete molecular response	Blood cell BCR-ABL levels undetectable (usually by nested RT-PCR method).

Patients with newly diagnosed chronic phase CML treated with imatinib, 800 mg/day, administered in two 400 mg doses every 12 hours had a frequency of 90 percent complete cytogenetic responses and 96 percent had at least a major cytogenetic response. At a median of 15 months, no patients had progressed and 63 percent showed blood BCR-ABL/ABL percentage ratios of less than 0.05 percent. Twenty-eight percent of patients had undetectable BCR-ABL blood levels.[448] Despite these reports the current starting dose is customarily 400 mg/day, balancing both effectiveness and tolerability in newly diagnosed patients. Moreover, the more rapid response with higher doses of imatinib may not translate into a better long-term survival.

Doses of imatinib lower than 400 mg/day result in fewer complete cytogenetic responses and a shorter duration of complete cytogenetic response. Patients who are older and who have lower body weight may only tolerate a lower dose but they are less likely to achieve a complete cytogenetic response.[449] If however, a patient is on a lower dose (e.g., 300 mg/day) for a special reason (body size or tolerance level) and achieves a complete hematologic and cytogenetic response within 12 months of onset of therapy, acceptable outcomes without excess toxicity may result.[450]

After 5 years of experience with imatinib, the proportion of patients achieving a complete molecular response continues to increase. Imatinib has been shown to be safe and well tolerated in the majority of patients during this period of observation.[451] Some patients have been studied for up to 7 years; the proportion with an undetectable BCR-ABL level in blood cells increased from 7 percent at 36 months to 52 percent at 84 months. During this time a major molecular response was lost in approximately 25 percent of patients with a detectable blood cell BCR-ABL signal. No patients with an undetectable blood cell BCR-ABL signal lost their major molecular response status after a median followup of 33 months.[452]

At 5 years, of the patients treated, the cumulative incidence of complete cytogenetic response was reached in more than 75 percent and of major molecular response was reached in more than 50 percent. The estimated overall survival and progression-free survival was approximately 80 percent of patients treated with imatinib at 400 mg/day for that period. By 5 years, 25 percent had discontinued imatinib treatment because of an unsatisfactory response or toxicity. The 5-year probability of remaining in major cytogenetic response while still receiving imatinib was approximately 60 percent. Achieving a complete cytogenetic response correlated with progression-free survival, but achieving a major molecular response conferred no further survival benefit.[453]

Use of Imatinib in Patients with Variant Chromosomal Translocations or Breakpoints Patients with variant Ph chromosome translocations have a similar prognosis to that of patients with classic Ph chromosome translocations who are treated with imatinib.[454] (See Fig. 90–3 for a diagram of breakpoints.) Patients with the e13a2 (formerly designated b2a2) $p210^{BCR\text{-}ABL}$ translocation respond well to imatinib, with similar rates of complete cytogenetic remission.[455] The e13a2 transcript may be more sensitive to imatinib than the e14a2 (formerly designated b3a2) transcript.[456] In a patient with both e1a2 and e14a2 fusion transcripts, only the p210 e14a2 transcript disappeared, whereas the e1a2 transcript persisted during progression to blast phase. No mutation in the kinase domain of ABL was found.[457] This finding indicates that different clones in an individual patient may have a different sensitivity to imatinib.

Response to Imatinib in Children and Older Patients More than 80 percent of children with chronic phase CML who are treated with imatinib, 260 to 570 mg/m^2, enter a complete cytogenetic remission. Weight gain is the most common side effect of imatinib.[458] In patients who were older than age 60 years, similar cytogenetic response rates and survival rates were noted as in younger patients in the late chronic phase who were treated concurrently, suggesting that age is not usually a factor in response.[459,460]

Side Effects and Special Treatment Considerations Imatinib is relatively well tolerated. Most adverse effects are manageable and seldom require permanent cessation of therapy. Reduction to subtherapeutic doses is not recommended; it is better to interrupt therapy for a time.[461]

Myelosuppression is common in CML patients, especially at treatment onset when the CML clone accounts for most of blood cells. Dose reduction to less than 300 mg/day is not advisable for myelosuppression. The drug should be stopped until blood counts recover. G-CSF and GM-CSF can prevent or treat neutropenia.[462,463] Platelet transfusion may be used for severe thrombocytopenia. Patients with imatinib-induced chronic cytopenias have inferior responses.[464] Myelosuppression is an independent adverse factor for achieving cytogenetic responses with imatinib.[465] Severe irreversible marrow aplasia after imatinib exposure has been reported.[466]

The main side effects noted with imatinib include fatigue, edema, nausea, diarrhea, muscle cramps, and rash.[467] Elevated hepatic transaminases can occur. Mild transaminase elevations often respond to glucocorticoid use.[468] Hepatotoxicity is uncommon, occurring in approximately 3 percent of patients, usually within 6 months of onset of imatinib use. Acute liver failure has been described.[469] The severe periorbital edema occasionally observed is postulated to be an effect on platelet-derived growth factor receptor (PDGFR) and KIT expressed by dermal dendrocytes. Surgical decompression of severe edema rarely has been required.[470] Although no effects on spermatogenesis have been reported, women of child-bearing age are at risk of teratogenic effects on a fetus.[470]

Uncommon side effects include splenic rupture,[471] cerebral edema and visual disturbances resulting from retinal edema,[472] varicella-zoster infection,[473] gynecomastia,[474] immune-mediated hemolytic anemia,[475] severe muscle edema,[476] severe fluid retention,[477] interstitial lung disease,[478,479] and panniculitis.[480] Hypophosphatemia[481] and altered bone and mineral metabolism have occurred.[482,483]

Cutaneous reactions with imatinib therapy occur in approximately 15 percent of patients.[484] Except for severe reactions (approximately 5% of patients), such as Stevens-Johnson syndrome, exfoliative dermatitis, and erythema multiforme, cutaneous reactions rarely require permanent discontinuation of therapy. With milder reactions, concomitant glucocorticoid therapy or brief discontinuation of imatinib with gradual reintroduction at a lower dose and then a gradual increase in dose can be accomplished.[485,486] With very mild cases, concurrent treatment with antihistamine or other symptomatic therapy may be successful. Oral desensitization regimens have been described that allow some patients to continue imatinib therapy.[487] Sweet syndrome with CML cell infiltration has been reported at the time of molecular remission.[488] Pityriasis rosea,[489] palmoplantar hyperkeratosis,[490] and oral and cutaneous lichenoid reactions,[491] have also been described. Hair repigmentation[492] and hypopigmentation of the skin,[493] probably related to the inhibition of the KIT receptor tyrosine kinase by imatinib, have been reported. Imatinib has been proposed as a therapy for vitiligo.[494]

Other Effects of Imatinib Imatinib has been found to cause regression of marrow fibrosis.[495] One study found that the extent of marrow fibrosis in CML is not a prognostic factor with imatinib therapy,[496] whereas another study observed that although imatinib reverses marrow fibrosis in patients with CML, it does not change the unfavorable prognosis associated with fibrosis.[497]

Imatinib reverses exaggerated VEGF secretion in patients with CML,[498] and it may reverse exaggerated marrow angiogenesis.[499] It can reduce marrow cellularity and normalize morphologic features regardless of cytogenetic response.

Pharmacokinetic Considerations during Imatinib Therapy Mean plasma trough concentration of imatinib and its metabolite CGP74588 obtained at about 1 month (presumptive steady state) was 979 ± 530 ng/mL. The rate of complete cytogenetic response and major molecular response was higher within the highest quartiles of imatinib trough levels.[500] Some therapists suggest that imatinib plasma levels be checked in cases of suboptimal response in order to adjust the dose.[501] Comedications and population covariates such as body weight and white cell count had no or minimal effect on imatinib clearance.[502] Patients with CML on hemodialysis have been successfully treated with imatinib.[503] Therapy interruptions and nonadherence with oral imatinib usage are common, and patient education and close monitoring are important to ensure compliance.[504]

No significant clinical responses to imatinib have been noted in patients with acute myelogenous leukemia (AML), MDS, Ph-chromosome–negative CML, or CMML without *PDGFR* or *KIT* mutations.[505]

Defining a Response to Imatinib Table 90–2 contains definitions of hematologic, cytogenetic, and molecular responses. The median BCR-ABL levels for imatinib-treated patients can continue to decrease over at least 5 years. Table 90–3 lists the approximate milestones expected of patients treated with 400 mg/day of imatinib.[444] There is variation in an individual patient's time of maximal response. Consequently, if a patient has not met those precise milestones but shows a continued decrease in the proportion of Ph-chromosome–positive cells on cytogenetic examination of marrow, or if in a complete cytogenetic remission, a continued decrease in the level of the PCR signal for the BCR-ABL, imatinib should be continued. Loss of response is defined as loss of a complete hematologic or complete cytogenetic response, an increase of 30 or more percent in the number of Ph-chromosome–positive metaphases examined at 3-month intervals, development of new cytogenetic abnormalities, or an increase in the BCR-ABL/ABL ratio of one log or more on serial RT-PCR testing or into the range associated with metaphase positivity. Because of variability in PCR testing, these changes should be confirmed within 1 month. Patients who have 100 percent Ph-chromosome–positive cells after 6 months of therapy have a minimal chance of later achieving a major or complete cytogenetic response and may be offered allogeneic stem cell transplantation, if applicable.[444,506]

Stopping Imatinib Therapy Discontinuation of imatinib in 12 patients who had undetectable disease for at least 2 years resulted in 6 patients having a molecular relapse within 1 to 5 months (imatinib was reintroduced with a response) and 6 others remaining in molecular complete remission for a median of 18 months.[507] There are numerous anecdotes of patients relapsing when imatinib was stopped. In patients with intolerable side effects on imatinib, the dose may be reduced in some cases without the loss of a complete molecular response.[508] In occasional patients in whom imatinib is stopped, a cytogenetic response of up to 15 months has persisted.[509–512] Because early, quiescent Ph-chromosome–positive cells (CD34+Lin–) are insensitive to imatinib *in vitro*,[513] at present it is advisable to maintain treatment indefinitely until the criteria for cessation, if any, can be established in clinical trials.

Use of Imatinib in Pregnancy Imatinib is possibly teratogenic. Normal newborns have been delivered by patients who conceived and ingested imatinib during early pregnancy.[514–517] In 125 women exposed to imatinib during pregnancy, 50 percent delivered normal infants, and 25 percent underwent elective terminations, three of the latter following the identification of fetal abnormalities. Twelve other infants had abnormalities.[518] The majority of patients who discontinue imatinib during pregnancy lose their complete hematologic remission and their cytogenetic responses.[519] One fetal fatality during pregnancy as a result of a meningocele has been reported. Males treated with imatinib have fathered healthy infants.[520] Current recommendations are to practice contraception during imatinib treatment or if pregnant at the onset of the disease, to consider IFN treatment until delivery.[517,521] Imatinib does appear in breast milk.[522]

Secondary Chromosomal Changes with Imatinib Mesylate Clonal abnormalities in cells lacking a detectable Ph chromosome or *BCR-ABL* rearrangements have been detected in patients undergoing imatinib therapy who previously were treated with IFN-α.[523,524] These cytogenetic changes were noted in 7 patients at a median of 13 months of imatinib therapy, and trisomy 8 was the most frequent abnormality. All of these patients had major cytogenetic responses to imatinib.[523] In some patients, clonal evolution may be related to imatinib resistance.[525] Clonal abnormalities may be present in up to 10 percent of patients taking imatinib.[526] Some of these cases may be associated with an MDS, especially in those patients with previous exposure to cytarabine and idarubicin. The antiproliferative effect of imatinib allows restoration of a polyclonal hematopoiesis in complete cytogenetic remission, which might favor the manifestation of a Ph-chromosome–negative disorder.[527] Some investigators have found that, with the possible exception of +8, +Ph, and i(17), additional chromosomal abnormalities at diagnosis are not associated with an inferior outcome.[528,529] In contrast, another group found that development of trisomy 8 in patients taking imatinib, while associated with pancytopenia, did not result in signs of disease progression. In a series of 34 CML patients who developed Ph-chromosome–negative clones while taking imatinib, the most common abnormalities were trisomy 8 and monosomy 7. In 11 of these patients, no archival evidence of these clones was present before imatinib therapy was initiated, and none of the patients developed myelodysplasia.[530] In patients treated at diagnosis with imatinib, 9 percent developed chromosomal abnormalities in Ph-negative metaphases. These appeared at a median of 18 months, and the most common abnormalities were –Y and +8. Most were temporary and had disappeared within 5 months. Only one patient with –7 progressed to AML.[531] Cytogenetic clonal evolution may not be an important impediment to achieving a major or complete cytogenetic response with imatinib, but it is an independent poor prognostic factor for survival of patients in chronic and accelerated phases of CML.[532] Imatinib therapy may overcome the poor prognostic significance of derivative chromosome 9 in CML.[533]

Development of Imatinib Mesylate Resistance The development of resistance to imatinib is not surprising.[534–538] Its specificity and "snug fit" into

TABLE 90–3. Guidelines for Response to Imatinab Mesylate[443,444]

Time of Observation (months)	Disease Response		
	Unsatisfactory	Suboptimal Response	Optimal Response
3	No HR	PHR	CHR
6	No mCyR	mCyR	MCyR
12	No MCyR	MCyR	CCyR
18	No CCyR	CCyR	MMR

CHR, complete hematologic response; CCyR, complete cytogenetic response; HR, hematologic response; mCyR, minor cytogenetic response; MCyR, major cytogenetic response; MMR, major molecular response; PHR, partial hematologic response.

NOTE: Response is defined in Table 90–2. These data are applicable to therapy with imatinib, 400 mg/day, as initial therapy in chronic phase. Unsatisfactory or suboptimal implies need to consider change in treatment approach, as appropriate for that patient. Usually this change is an increase in the dose of imatinib, a shift to a second-generation tyrosine kinase inhibitor, or allogeneic stem cell transplantation, if eligible. These guidelines are approximate in that a patient showing continued response to imatinib can be continued on that therapy until a response plateau has been reached, at which time the response can be evaluated using the benchmarks noted. See text for further details.

the ABL-kinase pocket provide the ideal circumstance for resistance.[539] Some cases demonstrate primary resistance to imatinib, and gene profiling has demonstrated differential expression of about 46 genes in responders compared to nonresponders.[540] Even in patients with complete cytogenetic response, malignant progenitors at the LTC-IC stage persist. Chronic phase CML stem cells are resistant to imatinib and are genetically unstable.[541] These cells have a high level of BCR-ABL transcription, and they are thought to express transporter proteins that result in abnormal imatinib flux.[542] Mathematical models suggest that imatinib rapidly eliminates differentiated leukemic progenitors, but does not deplete leukemic stem cells. Such models predict the probability of developing resistant mutations and can estimate the time that resistance will emerge.[543] Intermittent administration of G-CSF exposure may promote elimination of CML CD34+ cells.[544,545] Imatinib upregulates CXCR4 expression, and thus might promote survival of quiescent CML stem cells by enhancing their interaction with marrow stroma.[546]

Several potential mechanisms of resistance include *BCR-ABL* amplification in the presence of imatinib,[547–549] P-glycoprotein–mediated drug efflux,[550,551] altered drug metabolism,[538] acquisition of BCR-ABL–independent signaling characteristics,[549] and point mutations in the ABL kinase domain that alter imatinib binding. There is evidence that each of these mechanisms of resistance may have clinical relevance.

Expression of the OCT-1 cellular transporter, which mediates drug influx, is thought to be important for imatinib but not dasatinib effectiveness.[553,554] Many CML patients who have a suboptimal response to imatinib have low OCT-1 activity but this can be overcome with higher doses of imatinib or use of dasatinib.[554,554] CML CD34+ cells overexpress the drug transporter ABCG2, but imatinib mesylate is not a substrate for this protein.[555]

Amplified gene expression and increased BCR-ABL protein expression are often reported in resistant patients. Duplication of the Ph-chromosome and isodicentric chromosomes are a possible mechanism of resistance to imatinib.[556,557]

Mutations in the ABL kinase domain may predate imatinib treatment,[558] and several BCR-ABL kinase domain mutants associated with imatinib resistance remain sensitive to the drug, suggesting a need for characterization before a resistant phenotype can be attributed to the given mutation.[559] The mutant clone does not always have a proliferative advantage.[560] Some of these mutations may lie outside the kinase domain, and more than 40 such mutations have been described. Screening early phase CML patients for mutations before the start of imatinib therapy is not cost-effective because of their low incidence, but in patients with evidence of an increase in CML cells while on imatinib, mutation searches are indicated.[561] BCR-ABL kinase domain point mutations are rare in those who have had good cytogenetic responses to imatinib, and when detected in that setting, their presence does not always predict relapse.[562] Mutations in the ABL portion of the *BCR-ABL* oncogene are present in approximately 40 percent of patients who do not achieve a hematologic or cytogenetic response to imatinib. ABL mutations were found in those patients with both primary and acquired resistance. Amino acid substitutions in seven residues accounted for 85 percent of all mutations associated with resistance.[563] The mutations most associated with resistance are Thr315ILe, Gly250Glu, Glu255Lys, and Thr253His substitutions. Few of the described mutations directly affect imatinib binding.[537,564] Mutations in the ABL–ATP phosphate-binding loop (P-loop) are most closely associated with a poor prognosis,[565] and these P-loop mutations predict for disease progression. Overall survival is worse for P-loop and for T315I mutations but not significantly different for other mutations.[566]

Second-generation BCR-ABL inhibitors (see "Dasatinib and Nilotinib" below) are able to overcome imatinib-resistant mutants, with the exception of the T315I mutations. This mutation results in steric hindrance which precludes access of some inhibitors to the ATP-binding pocket of the ABL kinase domain.[567] Based on the crystal structure, the kinase domain of ABL T315I can be predicted by Aurora kinase inhibitors. The inhibitor binds in an active conformation of the kinase domain in the ATP-binding pocket.[568] In a series of 27 patients with T315I mutation, survival was dependent on stage of disease, with many of the chronic phase patients described as having an indolent course.[569] Agents such as IFN-α and homoharringtonine have been proposed as salvage therapy for those with the T315I mutation.[570]

In some cases of resistance associated with imatinib, other signal pathways independent of BCR-ABL may become important in cell proliferation.[571] These include heat shock protein 70,[572] survivin,[573] LYN kinase,[574] SRC,[575] and GRB2.[576]

Dose escalation, combination therapy, and treatment interruption have been proposed as means to overcome drug resistance.[577] Combination therapy from the outset[578] also has been proposed to prevent development of resistance. Treatment interruption to stop clonal selection of resistant cells has been proposed.[575] Gene expression profiles may be useful to predict the clinical effectiveness of imatinib for CML treatment, thereby allowing individualized therapy from the outset.[578] In patients with relapse or resistance, alternative approaches include increasing the dose of imatinib or switching to dasatinib or nilotinib.[579]

Dasatinib and Nilotinib Dasatinib and nilotinib, two second-generation tyrosine kinase inhibitors, are used in cases of imatinib resistance or intolerance. Trials are underway to ascertain whether use of these agents at time of diagnosis will improve response rates and obviate later resistance.

Dasatinib is 325-fold more potent than imatinib and responses occur among all ABL mutant genotypes with the exception of T315I.[580] As a dual inhibitor of SRC and ABL kinases, dasatinib is able to bind to BCR-ABL with less stringent conformational requirements.[581] Dasatinib,100 mg/day, is administered in chronic phase CML.[582,583] The major cytogenetic response rate is approximately 50 percent, and molecular responses occur as well.[584] In patients resistant to imatinib, dasatinib, 140 mg/day (70 mg q12h), resulted in a higher proportion of major cytogenetic responses, complete cytogenetic responses, and major molecular responses than did 800 mg/day (400 mg q12h) of imatinib. Treatment failure was decreased and progression-free survival was improved with dasatinib.[585] Unlike imatinib, dasatinib penetrates the blood–brain barrier.[586]

The major adverse event with dasatinib use is cytopenia. In addition to hematologic toxicity, fluid retention, diarrhea, and skin rash also can occur. Dasatinib may be more effective in the presence of F359I ABL mutation as compared with imatinib and nilotinib.[587] Unlike the case with imatinib, dasatinib cellular uptake is not affected by OCT-1 activity, which is a substrate of the efflux proteins, ABCB1 and ABCG2.[588] Resistance to dasatinib is often found with point mutations at residue 315 or 317.[589]

Nilotinib is an orally bioavailable, ATP-competitive inhibitor of BCR-ABL. It is FDA approved for patients in chronic phase CML resistant or who are intolerant to imatinib. It is approximately 30 times more potent than imatinib.[590] Like imatinib, it does not induce apoptosis in CD34+ CML cells.[591] A dose of 400 mg every 12 hours induced approximately 40 percent of patients who were resistant to or intolerant of imatinib into a major cytogenetic response, and approximately 30 percent into a complete cytogenetic response, with all resistance-inducing ABL mutations except T315I.

Adverse effects included neutropenia and minimal other side effects such as hyperbilirubinemia and hypophosphatemia.[592] Nilotinib can cause electrocardiographic QT interval prolongation, so caution is required with concurrent medications that can prolong the QT interval.[593] There is preclinical data to show that despite binding at the same site in the same target kinase, use of imatinib and nilotinib in combination may have additive or synergistic effects as BCR-ABL inhibitors.[594]

Combined Therapy Agents that have been proposed for use in combination to improve response rates or to overcome resistance to imatinib have included IFN-α, cytarabine, daunorubicin, homoharringtonine, multiagent chemotherapy, arsenic trioxide, and decitabine, with some supporting *in vitro* data.[595–600] Combining imatinib with chemotherapeutic agents is more myelosuppressive, and final effects on response rates and survival have yet to be determined.[601] Trials examining combinations of imatinib and either dasatinib or nilotinib are underway.[602]

Other Combinations Proposed to Overcome Imatinib Resistance Several inhibitors of other signal transduction mediators involved in the downstream effects of BCR-ABL have been proposed for use in imatinib-resistant CML. These inhibitors include the JAK2 inhibitor AG490,[603] SRC kinase inhibitors, mTOR (mammalian target of rapamycin) inhibitors, such as rapamycin,[604] the proteasome inhibitor bortezomib,[605,606] histone deacetylators,[607,608] PI3K or MEK (mitogen-activated kinase) inhibitors, such as wortmannin and LY294002,[609] and inhibitors of prenylation of RAS-related proteins downstream of BCR-ABL. These agents include the bisphosphonate zolendronate[610] and farnesyltransferase inhibitors.[611,612] The farnesyltransferase inhibitors SCH66336 and R115777 have shown some activity in CML.[613–616] Imatinib resistance often is associated with restored activation of the BCR-ABL signal transduction pathway, suggesting that BCR-ABL remains a valid target to overcome resistance in these cases.[617] BCR-ABL point mutations isolated from patients with imatinib-resistant CML remain sensitive to inhibitors of the BCR-ABL chaperone heat shock protein (hsp) 90, such as geldanamycin.[618] Many of these agents have not yet entered clinical trials. Some are being used in conjunction with imatinib in resistant cases.

Disease Prognosis and Monitoring during Imatinib Therapy Treatment failure should lead to alterations in therapeutic strategy.[619] For patients treated initially with imatinib, BCR-ABL expression in cytogenetic responders and nonresponders was similar. BCR-ABL expression became significantly different 3 months after treatment and became increasingly different between responders and nonresponders with continued therapy at 6, 9, and 12 months.[620]

One mode of monitoring patients undergoing imatinib therapy is to measure blood counts at least once per month and to obtain marrow samples every 6 months until a complete cytogenetic remission is obtained.[621] Thereafter, marrow samples are obtained yearly to monitor for other clonal abnormalities. Quantitative RT-PCR is performed every 3 months on blood or marrow. A one log increase in the level of BCR-ABL reactivity, confirmed on a repeat sample at least 1 month later, suggests a loss of response to treatment. In patients who do not have a complete hematologic response at 3 months, or a major cytogenetic response after 6 to 12 months, other therapeutic options are considered.[622] The molecular response after 2 to 3 months of therapy is a strong predictor of clinical and cytogenetic response.[623] Sequencing the BCR-ABL kinase domain can reveal emergence of resistant clones and is useful if there is an insufficient initial response to imatinib (see Table 90–3) or any sign of loss of response, such as relapse to Ph-positive status, a 1-log increase in BCR/ABL transcript ratio, or loss of a major molecular response (MMR).[444] In patients receiving second-generation tyrosine kinase inhibitors, those who have no cytogenetic response at 3 to 6 months should be considered for allogeneic transplantation or switched to an alternative therapy in a clinical trial. After 12 months, those with a major cytogenetic response had a significant survival advantage over those with lesser responses.[624]

Summary of Imatinib Effects Imatinib was first used experimentally for CML treatment in June 1998. Although it has completely altered the treatment approach to CML, its use has raised several questions. Studies require long-term followup of survival, but the degree of cytogenetic response, and degree of molecular response can be used as surrogate endpoints.[625,626] The durability of cytogenetic and molecular responses in the face of persistent minimal residual disease during imatinib therapy require further followup of larger numbers of patients, especially because more than 95 percent of cases have molecular evidence of disease at 2 years.[626]

The success of imatinib therapy has diminished the use of allogeneic stem cell transplantation in chronic phase CML.[627] Imatinib trials show a 95 percent progression-free survival at 24 months, but patients usually have evidence of ongoing molecular disease. Because stem cell transplantation is associated with high toxicity and mortality rates, deciding when and for whom to use this modality while responses to imatinib are ongoing can be difficult. For patients who lose or never achieve an imatinib-induced major cytogenic response and for whom an acceptable donor is available, allogeneic stem cell transplantation should be considered.[628] Another therapeutic issue that has arisen is whether to use dasatinib or nilotinib before allogeneic stem cell transplantation in those in whom imatinib response has been absent or suboptimal.[629] Some therapists would first increase the dose of imatinib, and if unsuccessful try dasatinib or nilotinib, and only if those steps were unsuccessful consider allogeneic transplantation.

Interferon-α

Prior to the approval of imatinib mesylate for upfront therapy in CML, INF-α was often used as initial therapy. A complete cytogenetic response with IFN-α was uncommon (13%), but 10-year survival rates in responders were approximately 70 percent.[630] Cytogenetic responses to IFN-α were stable and durable.[631] Approximately 50 percent of complete responders become long-term survivors. Common toxicities of INF-α use include fatigue, low-grade fever, weight loss, liver function test abnormalities, hematologic changes, and neuropsychiatric symptoms. Most studies have shown no benefit of high-dose IFN-α compared with low-dose IFN-α for chronic phase CML (5 million units/m^2 per day vs. 3 million units/m^2 five times per week).[632] Low-dose IFN-α minimizes toxicity and cost. Pegylated IFN-α, which has a longer half-life, can be administered as a once-per-week injection at 6 mcg/kg per week.[633] Dose-limiting toxicities are neurotoxicity, thrombocytopenia, fatigue, and liver dysfunction. In later studies, 4.5 mcg/kg per week was proposed as the optimal dose because of the toxicity at higher doses. A single weekly dose of 450 mcg pegylated IFN-α has also compared favorably to the standard IFN-α dose in terms of toxicity and response rates.[634] Pegylated IFN-α plus low-dose cytosine arabinoside administered weekly is effective but has significant toxicity in patients with CML.[635]

Overall survival is improved in imatinib-treated patients compared with patients treated with IFN-α or IFN-α plus cytarabine.[636] Nevertheless, among all patients who attained a major or complete cytogenetic response at 12 months, the survival rate was comparable in either case. IFN-α has also been proposed as an immune stimulant to consolidate imatinib remissions because additive effects have been noted.[637,638] Conversely, those treated initially with INF-α who achieve a complete cytogenetic response have an improved molecular response with imatinib.[639,640] Some patients intolerant to a tyrosine kinase inhibitor may be treated successfully with INF-α.

Use of Other Chemotherapeutic Agents in Chronic Phase

Hydroxyurea The major side effect of hydroxyurea is an extension of its pharmacologic effect, that is, reversible suppression of hematopoiesis, often with megaloblastic erythropoiesis. The median survival of patients with CML treated with hydroxyurea alone is approximately 5 years. Studies with high-dose hydroxyurea indicate that marrow metaphase cells in some patients lose the Ph chromosome either partially or completely after such therapy.[641] The drug may be very useful in patients of advanced age, in patients with comorbid conditions, and in patients in whom imatinib and IFN cannot be tolerated or are ineffective. Hydroxyurea often is used for initial cytoreduction. Chronic use of hydroxyurea is associated with leg ulcers.[642]

Cytarabine IFN-α_{2b} combined with cytarabine (20 mg/m^2 per day for 10 days per month) in the chronic phase was associated with a greater proportion of major cytogenetic response at 12 months after randomization and with greater survival prolongation than was IFN alone.[643] Toxicities with these drug combinations were greater, and this combination has been replaced by tyrosine kinase inhibitor therapy.

Busulfan Once the mainstay of treatment for the chronic phase, busulfan usage now is rare.[644] It is used primarily as part of the preparative regimen for allografting or autografting. It may be used occasionally in older patients who do not tolerate tyrosine kinase inhibitors.

Homoharringtonine Homoharringtonine, a plant alkaloid, can induce responses, including cytogenetic responses, in patients in the late chronic phase.[645]

Other Cytotoxic Agents Intensive multidrug regimens have been used in an attempt to eradicate the Ph-chromosome–positive clone and have lead to prolongation of remission or cure of the disease. This approach has not significantly increased survival.[646]

Other Potential Therapeutic Agents in CML The farnesyltransferase inhibitors lonafarnib and tipifarnib have been combined with imatinib and have activity after imatinib failure.[647,648] The hypomethylation agent decitabine has activity in imatinib refractory CML.[649] Berbamine, a natural small molecular compound, has *in vitro* activity against primary CML cells.[650] Adaphostin, a tyrphostin, inhibits CML cell growth, including those cell populations resistant to imatinib by inducing oxidative stress.[651] INNO-406, a dual BCR-ABL/LYN inhibitor, suppresses the growth of CML cells in the central nervous system where imatinib has limited penetration.[652] This agent also enhances autophagy in CML cells.[653] Agents that disrupt autophagy when combined with histone deacetylase inhibitors such as suberoylanilide hydroxamic acid (SAHA) are able to overcome imatinib resistance in preclinical models.[654] The SRC-ABL inhibitor, SKI-606 (bosutinib), is able to overcome most resistance-mediating ABL mutations, except T315I, and it has entered clinical trials.[655] Several third-generation inhibitors are being developed for inhibition of the T315I mutation.[656] MicroRNA technology may eventually play a role in CML treatment,[657] and synthetic BCR-ABL siRNA (small interfering ribonucleic acid) has been used in a patient with resistant CML, postallografting with inhibition of BCR-ABL noted.[658]

Ribozymes targeting BCR-ABL mRNA have been used as CML treatment,[659,660] and these approaches probably will have the most utility for *in vitro* purging of CML marrow cells before autotransplantation.[661,662]

IMMUNOTHERAPY

Several antigens have been proposed as targets of immune therapy for CML. These antigens include BCR-ABL itself, PR1, Wilms tumor protein-1 (WT1), minor histocompatibility antigens, CML-66, CML-28, and survivin.[663,664] Other targets are VEGF and hsp90.[665] A BCR-ABL fusion peptide, used as a vaccine, can elicit a specific T-cell immune response.[666,667] CML-derived dendritic cells can process and present endogenous BCR-ABL fusion proteins to CD4+ T lymphocytes in an HLA class II-restricted antigen presentation.[668] NM23-H2, an HLA-A32 restricted tumor associated antigen aberrantly expressed in tumors such as CML, can generate reactive T cells after transplantation.[669] Immunization with GM-CSF–producing tumor vaccines to enhance a vaccine antitumor effect is being studied in CML.[670] Numerous peptides from the BCR-ABL fusion region have been identified as vaccine candidates.[671] Peptides from the e14a2 BCR-ABL junction have been examined in vaccine trials, elicit T-cell responses, and demonstrate molecular responses of a delayed nature in those who have had a major cytogenetic response to imatinib. Randomized trials with these vaccines have not yet been reported.[672]

RADIOTHERAPY

Splenic irradiation may be useful occasionally in subjects who have entered the accelerated or advanced chronic phase and are troubled with extreme splenomegaly with splenic pain, perisplenitis, and encroachment of the spleen on the gastrointestinal tract.[673] Splenic irradiation may palliate symptoms for a short time.[674]

Radiotherapy may be useful for extramedullary tumors, which may occur occasionally in bone or soft tissue during the late chronic or accelerated phase.

SPLENECTOMY

Splenectomy does not prolong the chronic phase of CML, delay the onset of the accelerated phase, enhance sensitivity to standard or intensive chemotherapy, or prolong survival of patients.[675] In carefully selected patients with symptomatic thrombocytopenia unresponsive to therapy, mechanical discomfort, hypercatabolic symptoms, and portal hypertension, splenectomy may be useful. Postoperative morbidity from infection, thrombosis, or hemorrhage has been high, with mortality rates up to 10 percent reported.[676] Splenectomy performed before allografting has not been found to influence the severity of graft-versus-host disease (GVHD) or survival after allogeneic stem cell transplantation.[677] Splenectomy may reverse poor graft function after allogeneic transplantation, but hyposplenism may trigger or worsen chronic extensive GVHD, leading to increased morbidity and mortality.[678]

TREATMENT OF CHRONIC PHASE CML DURING PREGNANCY

Treatment of chronic phase CML during pregnancy is sometimes needed to prevent placental insufficiency from hyperleukocytosis. Imatinib use during pregnancy has the risk of a teratogenic effect.[514–517] IFN can be used during pregnancy with minimum risk of teratogenicity. Eight patients treated with IFN from the first trimester have been described, and each of these pregnancies resulted in normal infants, except for one with mild neonatal thrombocytopenia. All infants had normal growth.[680] Hydroxyurea may be useful during the second and third trimester but should be avoided in the first trimester.[517,679] Leukapheresis in the first trimester (or longer) also can be used to avoid fetal drug exposure early in pregnancy (see "Leukapheresis" above). It is important to use imatinib after delivery to achieve the best outcome. Further observation may show it to be safe later in pregnancy. Although controversial, stopping and later restarting imatinib may not result in as favorable an outcome of therapy. [517]

HIGH-DOSE CHEMOTHERAPY WITH AUTOLOGOUS STEM CELL INFUSION

Since the availability of imatinib, autografting in CML is rarely used.[681] Ph-chromosome–negative stem cells are present in most patients with CML at the time of diagnosis. Techniques that use these cells to reconstitute hematopoiesis after high-dose therapy have been developed.[682] Ph-chromosome–negative progenitors can be mobilized with G-CSF and collected from the blood of patients who have responded to prior treatment with IFN or imatinib.[683] Such cells also can be collected after recovery from chemotherapy regimens, such as after idarubicin and cytarabine, followed by G-CSF stimulation.[682] G-CSF was used for at least 4 days while imatinib treatment was continued for stem cell mobilization in 58 patients with a complete cytogenetic response. The cells were collected in two cytapheresis procedures in 74 percent of patients, and the cells of 84 percent of those cytapheresis products were negative for the Ph chromosome.[684]

In another series, stem cells were mobilized in 32 patients in complete cytogenetic remission after imatinib, with uninterrupted imatinib therapy in 50 percent of patients and with imatinib temporarily withheld in approximately 50 percent. Blood levels of BCR-ABL were not changed by the use of G-CSF.[685] In yet another series, 13 of 15 patients were successfully mobilized with G-CSF while receiving imatinib, and 28 percent of stem cell harvests were negative for BCR-ABL mRNA. No change in blood BCR-ABL transcript level was noted after stem cell mobilization as assessed by RT-PCR.[686] No series of patients autografted with cells mobilized while they were receiving imatinib have been reported.[687] Autografting might find a role in cases of imatinib resistance,[688] or to reduce the level of residual disease in cases without a molecular response.[689] Imatinib can be effective and safe in chronic phase CML patients who have previously undergone autografting,[690] although increased hematologic toxicity occurs.

ALLOGENEIC STEM CELL TRANSPLANTATION

Until imatinib became available in 2000, allogeneic transplantation was used in most new patients with CML who were younger than 65 years of age and who had a suitable donor. The advent of imatinib treatment and the projected survival of patients with a complete cytogenetic remission has changed the indications for transplantation in CML.[691,692] There has been a marked reduction in number of transplants performed for CML worldwide and a decline in the proportion performed in first chronic phase.[693,694] Although no randomized trials of imatinib versus transplantation have been or are likely to be conducted, there is circumstantial evidence that survival is superior for populations of patients treated with drugs who have a complete cytogenetic remission as compared to transplantation.[695] Allografting continues to play a prominent role in the treatment of patients with suboptimal imatinib responses, who are refractory or intolerant to tyrosine kinase inhibitors, and remains the optimal therapy in those who progress to accelerated phase or blast crisis.

Patients in the chronic phase of CML who are younger than 65 years and who have an identical twin,[696] or a histocompatible sibling,[697,698] or who are younger than 55 years with access to a histocompatible unrelated donor,[699] can be transplanted after intensive therapy, usually with cyclophosphamide and fractionated total-body irradiation (TBI) or a combination of busulfan and cyclophosphamide. Busulfan can be administered as an intravenous preparation and as a single daily dose.[700] When targeted steady-state busulfan levels are utilized, a 3-year survival rate of 86 percent and a disease-free survival rate of 78 percent with no age effect is achieved.[701] With nonmyeloablative or "reduced-intensity" conditioning regimens, older patients and those with comorbidities can undergo successful allografting.

Myeloablative Allogeneic Transplants

Stem cell transplantation from HLA-compatible siblings results in engraftment and an actual or projected long-term survival in 45 to 70 percent of recipients.[702–704] In patients older than age 50 years, survival rates are slightly less at 5 years. The risk of CML relapse is approximately 20 percent, with a plateau of relapse at 5 to 7 years. Transplanted T lymphocytes, especially if activated by a (mild) GVHD, may be an important factor in preventing leukemic relapse. This phenomenon, referred to as *graft-versus-leukemia reaction*, is thought to suppress the leukemic process through T-cell–mediated cytotoxicity.[697] The relative benefit of marrow compared to mobilized blood stem cells as the source of the allograft has not been established.[705,706] Mobilized blood stem cells engraft more rapidly but may be associated with more chronic GVHD. The majority of survivors have no evidence of residual leukemia.[707]

For younger patients who do not have a histocompatible sibling, an unrelated donor or a mismatched family member as a source of stem cells is feasible. The toxicity of this procedure is greater than that of an HLA-identical sibling donor transplant. Five-year disease-free survival is approximately 40 percent.[708] Younger patients with cytomegalovirus-seronegative donors who are matched at the HLA-DRB1 allele by molecular methods fare better.[709] When class I HLA genes are typed with molecular methods, an improvement in matching and better outcomes using unrelated donors are expected. When matched-unrelated donor and sibling donor transplants were compared, unrelated donor transplants had increased risk of graft failure and acute GVHD, but only a slightly poorer survival and disease-free survival. For patients who survived to 1 year, only a slightly inferior disease-free survival was observed.[710] The rate of extensive chronic GVHD is up to 60 percent with unrelated donor transplants, but 63 percent disease-free survival in younger CML chronic phase patients has been reported. Cord blood stem cell transplantation from an unrelated donor has also been used in adults with CML.[711]

Pretransplantation imatinib is not associated with increased transplant-related morbidity or decreased survival, but those who are transplanted with suboptimal response to imatinib or loss of response to imatinib do poorer, probably related to a higher disease burden at the time of transplantation and more aggressive disease.[712,713] Second-generation tyrosine kinase inhibitors do not increase transplant-related toxicity.[714] Disease status after allografting can be monitored with cytogenetic studies, PCR, or FISH analysis. A positive PCR assay 3 months after allogeneic transplantation has not been found to correlate with an increased risk of relapse compared with PCR-negative patients. A positive assay at 6 months and beyond is associated with subsequent relapse. In one series, 42 percent of patients with a positive PCR assay at 6 to 12 months relapsed versus 3 percent with a negative assay.[715] Paradoxically, patients who remain *BCR-ABL* positive more than 36 months after transplantation have little propensity for relapse.[715] Serial quantitative RT-PCR analysis of blood specimens has been proposed to distinguish patients destined to relapse.[716] Patients who remain in remission have undetectable, low, or falling BCR-ABL levels on sequential analysis. After 6 to 9 months, these levels are undetectable in most cases. Recognition of relapse at the molecular level may allow for early therapeutic intervention.

Killer immunoglobulin-like receptors (KIRs) are expressed by NK cells and subpopulations of T cells. NK clones from a single individual can vary substantially in the type of KIR molecules they express. The ligands for several of the inhibitory KIR have been shown to be subsets of HLA class I molecules. Missing KIR ligands in recipients lead to less relapse and increased GVHD based on NK alloreactivity.[717] KIR ligand mismatch has also been found to be an important prognostic factor in achieving molecular responses after transplantation for CML.[718] Increased frequency of Treg cells characterized as CD4+, CD25-high are associated with higher rates of relapse after allografting in CML.[719]

Nonmyeloablative Allogeneic Transplants

Nonablative regimens have been developed in an attempt to expand the indication for allogeneic transplantation to older patients. These regimens rely on immunosuppressive therapy to allow engraftment of cells that potentially will generate a graft-versus-leukemia effect. These procedures in general are associated with acceptable degrees of engraftment, less mortality, similar rates of GVHD, and possible durable effects on persistent or recurrent disease.[720] Approximately 60 percent of patients, mostly in initial chronic phase (median age: 50 years) and transplanted with reduced-intensity conditioning regimens, had a 3-year survival and about one-third had a 3-year progression-free survival.[721] Patients no longer in first chronic phase do not fare as well.[722] Conditioning regimens include fludarabine and busulfan,[723,724] low-dose TBI and fludarabine, and low-dose TBI and cyclophosphamide, but no prospective randomized trials comparing regimens or comparing ablative and nonmyeloablative transplant approaches have been conducted.[723,725,726] In one case, imatinib given concurrently with nonmyeloablative stem cell transplantation did not compromise engraftment and resulted in a cytogenetic remission in a patient with CML in blast crisis.[727]

USE OF TYROSINE KINASE INHIBITORS AFTER STEM CELL TRANSPLANT

In patients treated with stem cell transplantation before the wide availability of imatinib, complete cytogenetic remissions with imatinib treatment can occur if treated at relapse after allografting and after donor lymphocyte infusion (DLI) fails to give a response. Such remissions may include a molecular response.[728] Complete responses after imatinib therapy have been noted in accelerated or blast phase CML persisting after stem cell transplantation.[729] In another series, 45 percent of relapsed patients had a complete cytogenetic response of up to 28 months and without significant GVHD.[730] In a series of 28 adults with relapse after allogeneic stem cell transplantation who then received imatinib, the response rate was 74 percent, and the complete cytogenetic remission rate was 35 percent. Five patients had recurrence of GVHD, and 13 had previous DLI infusions.[728] In one series, imatinib was able to generate complete molecular remissions in 26 percent of chronic phase patients after allografting, with full donor chimerism usually observed.[731] Prophylactic administration of imatinib after transplantation has been used for patients at high risk of relapse.[732] Posttransplantation imatinib may also postpone the requirement for donor leukocyte infusions with its attendant risks of GVHD and marrow aplasia.[733] Some have found that donor leukocyte infusions are superior to imatinib therapy in preventing relapse and increasing leukemia-free survival.[734] Today, virtually all patients receive imatinib initially and receive transplantation only if refractory to or relapse after imatinib and a second-generation tyrosine kinase inhibitor.

IMMUNOTHERAPY: ADOPTIVE CELL THERAPY FOR POSTTRANSPLANTATION RELAPSE

Substantial evidence indicates that the effectiveness of allografting in CML does not result solely from the eradication of the leukemic clone with high-dose chemoradiotherapy conditioning regimens, but also from adoptive immunotherapy provided by lymphocytes in the allograft, the graft-versus-leukemia effect (see "Myeloablative Allogeneic Transplants" above).[735] This phenomenon has been recreated to produce a therapeutic response by infusing the lymphocytes from the stem cell donor after a relapse following allogeneic stem cell transplantation.[736,737] The overall response rate to DLI is approximately 75 percent. The response rate is higher when this approach is used early after detecting a relapse by PCR,[738] compared to use after a hematologic or cytogenetic relapse. Patients with a short interval between transplantation and DLI have a higher probability of response than patients with longer intervals. Responses are the same with related versus unrelated donors.[739] Some patients show a very rapid decline of BCR-ABL transcript levels (<6 months after DLI), whereas other patients demonstrate PCR negativity only over a longer period.[740] The responses to DLI can be durable.[741] Molecular responses can occur in up to two-thirds of patients.[742]

The main toxicities of DLI have been the induction of GVHD and myelosuppression. Chronic GVHD can occur in up to 60 percent of cases.[743] Attempts to diminish these toxicities have included use of CD8-depleted DLIs and infusion of smaller numbers of T cells.[744,745] Lower initial cell dose is associated with less myelosuppression, the same response rate, better survival, and less DLI-related mortality, leading to suggestions that the initial dose should not exceed 0.2×10^8 mononuclear cells/kg.[746] The initial doses should be lower when matched unrelated donors are used. Donor lymphocytes can also be transfected with vectors containing the herpes simplex virus genome in a replication defective form. If GVHD occurs, the lymphocytes can be eradicated with systemic ganciclovir treatment. The ultimate utility of such currently experimental approaches is still unmeasured.[747] IFN after DLI may improve responses,[748,749] and imatinib may synergize with DLI to foster rapid molecular responses after relapse.[750] Methods for administering more specific immune effector cells have been sought, but these approaches are not in widespread clinical use.[751]

COURSE AND PROGNOSIS

Several large studies of treatment during the 1970s and early 1980s reported similar survival rates of patients with CML who were treated with standard chemotherapy, that is, busulfan or hydroxyurea, during the chronic phase.[752–760] Median survival ranged from 39 to 47 months, the 5-year survival rate was approximately 25 to 35 percent of patients, and the 8-year survival rate was 8 to 17 percent of patients. A large randomized study comparing hydroxyurea to busulfan showed a significant prolongation of chronic phase with hydroxyurea[644] and a further prolongation with IFN therapy. Only a small fraction of patients remained in the chronic phase from 10 to 25 years.[761–768] The Surveillance, Epidemiology, and End Results Program of the National Cancer Institute gathers national statistics based on cancer registries in the United States. Table 90–4 lists the 5-year survival rates from these observations. Because these data are a mixture of the pre- and postimatinib therapy periods, they underestimate the 5-year life expectancy of patients with CML who are given imatinib treatment.

At the time of diagnosis, the variables most closely associated with duration of chronic phase and thus survival are percent blasts in the blood, liver and spleen size, and total basophil plus eosinophil count. Using these variables in large numbers of patients, the population segregates into three risk groups: better risk, with a median survival of approximately 5.0 years; intermediate risk, with a median survival of 3.5 years; and poor risk, with a median survival of 2.5 years.[769–771] In the

TABLE 90–4. Chronic Myelogenous Leukemia: 5-Year Relative Survival Rates (1996–2004)

Age (years)	Percent of Patients
<45	77.2
45–54	76.5
55–64	62.3
65–74	38.7
>75	23.9

NOTE: These most recent data underestimate the effects of imatinib mesylate treatment between 2005 and the current date.

SOURCE: Data from Surveillance, Epidemiology, End Results Cancer Statistics, 5-Year Survival Rates, Table 13-15, All Races and Sexes. National Cancer Institute, Washington, DC. Available at www.seer.cancer.gov.

better-risk group, 40 percent are alive at 7 years; in the poor-risk group, 10 percent or fewer are alive at 7 years. These figures are based on patients who were treated principally with busulfan. Treatment of chronic phase by hydroxyurea and then by IFN extended the median survival by approximately 18 months with the former, and by approximately 36 months with the latter drug in patients treated with these agents. Generalizations to all patients with CML based on these studies are not possible because many patients, especially those older than age 65 years, could not tolerate optimal doses of IFN. Thus, the results are for the select group of patients who remained on treatment with these agents. The median survival also has been dramatically improved by imatinib treatment. One projection indicated the median survival for all patients so treated will exceed 15 years.[772] It is as yet uncertain how long patients on imatinib can remain in remission on average.[691,773] In a 5-year followup of patients receiving imatinib for newly diagnosed CML, complete cytogenetic responses were seen in approximately 70 percent by 12 months and in nearly 90 percent by 60 months. In a major study, an estimated overall survival at 84 months of followup was 86 percent.[774] Resistance rates decline with each passing year, and adverse effects have not emerged over time.[775] Those who require 1 year or more of imatinib therapy to attain a complete cytogenetic remission have comparable rates of molecular response, progression-free, and overall survival to those who achieve cytogenetic remission sooner.[776] In patients with failure to respond or intolerance to imatinib the estimated 3-year survival rate was approximately 70 percent for patients in chronic phase. Survival in chronic phase was better when subsequent therapy was nilotinib or dasatinib as compared to allogeneic hematopoietic stem cell transplantation or to others agents. This result was at a median followup of 2 years.[777] Older patients have lower response rates when treated in late chronic phase, but if they attain a complete cytogenetic response, no difference was found in the level of molecular response.[776]

Studies linking the precise (3′) location of the breakpoint in the *BCR* gene with shortened duration of chronic phase[778] have not been confirmed.[779] Prior to the introduction of imatinib therapy, most patients died as a result of conversion from the chronic to the accelerated phase of the disease or blast crisis.[780] It is too soon to determine the cause of death in patients treated with inhibitors of the BCR-ABL kinase. Very rare spontaneous cytogenetic, but not molecular, remissions of CML have been reported,[781,782] but the disease may reappear in that case.[783]

Several other ancillary factors are associated with poor prognosis in CML, including marrow angiogenesis and marrow fibrosis[784]; telomere length shortening[785]; cellular VEGF expression[786]; large deletions at the t(9;22) breakpoint[787]; derivative chromosome 9 deletions[788,789]; increased marrow fiber content and reduction of medullary erythropoiesis[790]; higher CD7 expression by CD34-positive cells[791]; absence of cadherin 13 expression[792]; and persistence of malignant hematopoietic progenitors in CML in complete cytogenetic remission after imatinib.[793] Deletion of the 5′ abl region on der(9), present in approximately 9 percent of patients with CML, occurs at the time of formation of the t(9;22) translocation and may be associated with a slightly worse prognosis.[794] The prognosis may not be worse with imatinib therapy. The type of BCR breakpoint (5′ or 3′) does not affect the course of chronic phase CML.[779,795] CML that occurs after treatment of other cancers appears to have comparable clinical and survival characteristics as *de novo* CML.[796] Histamine levels during treatment with imatinib have been found to be of prognostic importance.[797]

Several prognostic scales have been proposed in CML, including the Sokal and Hasford systems for patients at the time of diagnosis and the European Bone Marrow Transplantation Consortium Risk Score for patients undergoing allogeneic stem cell transplantation,[798] in which performance status is added to the five original variables (age, spleen size, blast cell count, basophil and eosinophil count, and platelet count [Hasford score]), which has been validated with good discrimination for survival.[799] The Sokal score based on age, spleen size, platelet count, and percent myeloblasts was developed much earlier during the busulfan era of treatment and was less accurate in patients treated with IFN. A simple prognostic scale that includes donor type, stage of disease at time of transplantation, age of recipient, sex of donor and recipient, and interval between diagnosis and transplantation has been proposed to predict outcome of allogeneic stem cell transplantation.[800] These prognostic scales require revalidation given the dramatic impact of conversion to universal imatinib therapy. There is evidence that a patient with chronic phase CML and a favorable Sokal Score at the time of diagnosis has a higher proportion of hematologic and cytogenetic responses than other patients.[801] Low neutrophil count and poor cytogenetic response at 3 months of imatinib therapy may predict a poor overall outcome,[802] but this observation requires validation.[803] Cytogenetic response as a surrogate marker for survival appears to be useful in patients undergoing imatinib therapy.[804]

DETECTION OF MINIMAL RESIDUAL DISEASE

Detection of minimal residual disease by molecular probes makes possible the identification of approximately 1 cell in 1,000,000 that is derived from the CML clone.[805] Techniques used to monitor residual disease have been reviewed.[806–808] PCR permits observation of regression or persistence of subclinical disease following therapy and of progression of subclinical disease prior to the disease becoming overt, and it is therefore critical for monitoring responses to CML treatment.[809,810] The stable persistence of subclinical disease does not invariably predict early relapse.[811,812]

The risk of misinterpreting negative results of RT-PCR is increased when very small numbers of transcripts are present.[806] The dilution threshold for reproducible amplification is 250,000 cells. $mRNA^{BCR-ABL}$ can also be detected in single progenitor colonies after culture.[813] A good correlation has been found between the proportion of Ph-chromosome–positive metaphase cells and levels of $mRNA^{BCR-ABL}$.[814–816] Efforts are underway to standardize the technique for measuring and reporting real-time RT-PCR,[817] and serial measurements are required for treatment decisions based on rises in transcript numbers.[818] Some studies show that marrow values tend to be higher than blood in real-time RT-PCR assays, but both follow a similar trend during treatment.[819] Interchanging these may lead to misinterpretation of disease status.[819] In patients on imatinib, who have major molecular responses, confirmed by real-time quantitative PCR, no marrow cell cytogenetic abnormalities were found, indicating that patients with major molecular responses do not require regular marrow examinations for cytogenetics.

Through utilization of quantitative PCR, an increase of $mRNA^{BCR-ABL}$ expression has been found to precede disease progression. This increase was detected up to 16 months before laboratory or clinical parameters showed phenotypic transformation of the malignant clone.[820] The technique of detecting minimal residual disease is highly sensitive and is subject to false-positive reactions. Nested, competitive RT-PCR is more sensitive than RT-PCR, but RT-PCR, when normalized for the total ABL transcripts, can be used to monitor CML patients during therapy.[821] Patients who achieve a major molecular remission (expressed as a 3-log reduction from median baseline value) at the time of achieving a complete cytogenetic response have been found to have longer cytogenetic remissions than those without this magnitude of molecular response.[822] The achievement of a 2-log molecular response at the time of a complete cytogenetic response or a 3-log response anytime thereafter is an independent prognostic marker of progression-free survival.[823] Other studies, however, show that patients who achieve complete cytogenetic response do not derive additional benefit from a complete molecular response.[824]

Interphase FISH may have a false-positive rate of 5 to 10 percent.[825,826] FISH is not standardized, but a large number of cells can be rapidly analyzed (100–500). With D-FISH probes, which flank the breakpoints of the *BCR* and *ABL* genes, the false-positive rate is only approximately 0.2 percent.[825] Fixation, specimen preparation, and hybridization conditions may account for differing false-positive ranges and scoring criteria.[827] In CML patients treated with imatinib, FISH for *BCR-ABL* on interphase blood neutrophils, but not unselected white cells, correlates with marrow cytogenetics.[828] FISH and RT-PCR can be useful complementary techniques,[829] but FISH is generally not suitable for monitoring minimal residual disease.[830]

For patients who are undergoing allogeneic stem cell transplantation, the kinetics of minimal residual disease in either standard or nonmyeloablative transplants differ. BCR-ABL/ABL ratios were 0.2 percent with reduced-intensity transplants versus 0.01 percent in transplantation patients with traditional conditioning regimens in the first 3 months. By 12 months, however, 20 percent of patients who received standard transplants and 50 percent of patients who received reduced-intensity transplants had reached a level less than 0.01 percent, supporting the concept of different kinetics of disease eradication between the two transplantation modalities.[831] Patients who relapse after allografting have reappearance and/or rising levels of BCR-ABL transcripts.[832] Use of quantitative RT-PCR early (3–5 months) after stem cell transplantation can project long-term outcomes.[833] When RT-PCR was negative, the 3-year risk of relapse was 16.7 percent; when RT-PCR was positive at a ratio of less than 0.02 percent, the relapse rate was 42.9 percent; and when RT-PCR was positive at a level greater than 0.02 percent, the relapse rate was 86.5 percent. Another group found that detection of blood BCR-ABL at 18 or more months after transplantation was associated with a highly significant risk of relapse and that patients who had a positive test result but failed to relapse generally had only one positive test result at a low copy number.[834] Performance of qualitative PCR at regular intervals after allogeneic transplant (every 2–4 months in the first year and every 6 months thereafter) is appropriate. If the PCR results are persistently positive or become positive, quantitative PCR should be performed at monthly or shorter intervals. Molecular relapse is defined as a 10-fold increase of PCR positivity without any signs of cytogenetic relapse.[835] Detection of increasing recipient chimerism by FISH for the male chromosome in sex-mismatched donor–recipient pairs or variable number of tandem repeats after allogeneic transplantation or after DLI infusion also is usually associated with a relapse.[836,837]

Imatinib therapy is associated with a rapid decrease in BCR-ABL transcript levels. Nested PCR transcript levels parallel cytogenetic response, and imatinib is superior to IFN or cytarabine in terms of the speed and degree of molecular responses, but residual disease is rarely eliminated.[838] When quantitative RT-PCR is utilized for patients undergoing imatinib therapy, almost all patients have evidence of residual disease.[839,840] Disadvantages of quantitative RT-PCR in monitoring imatinib response include lack of standardization, inability to detect clonal evolution, and current lack of widespread availability.[825] The use of random pentadecamer primers may improve detection of BCR-ABL transcripts in CML,[841] and flow cytometric assays of phosphotyrosine levels may be valuable for serial evaluation of disease response.[842] Table 90–5 outlines suggested monitoring for chronic phase patients undergoing imatinib therapy.

TABLE 90–5. Guidelines for Monitoring of Patients in Chronic Phase Who Are Undergoing Imatinib Mesylate Therapy

1. At diagnosis, before starting therapy, obtain Giemsa-banding cytogenetics and measure BCR-ABL transcript numbers by quantitative PCR using marrow cells. If marrow cannot be obtained, use FISH on a blood specimen to confirm the diagnosis.
2. At 3, 6, 9, and 12 months after initiating therapy, perform FISH for t(9;22) on blood cells and quantitative PCR for BCR-ABL transcripts.
3. At 6 months obtain marrow cytogenetics for cells with Ph chromosome. Repeat every 6 months until complete cytogenic response. If there is a CCyR at 6 months, this does not need to be done at 12 months.
4. Once CCyR is obtained, monitor quantitative PCR on blood cells every 3 months. Continue yearly marrow examination of marrow cytogenetics to identify clonal evolution, if indicated.
5. These guidelines presume continued response to imatinib until complete cytogenetic response achieved. If this does not occur see text for approach.

CCyR, complete cytogenetic response; FISH, fluorescence *in situ* hybridization.

SOURCE: Adapted in part from: www.nccn.org/professionals/physicians_gls/PDF/cml.pdf.

ACCELERATED PHASE AND BLAST CRISIS OF CML

DEFINITION

In all patients with chronic phase CML, the disease has the potential to evolve into a more aggressive, more symptomatic, and troublesome phase, which is poorly responsive to the therapy that formerly controlled the chronic phase. The failure of therapy to restore or maintain near-normal red cell and white cell counts, increased spleen size, increased numbers of marrow blasts and blood basophils, loss of the sense of well-being, and appearance of extramedullary tumors are the most consistent clinical hallmarks of the metamorphosis of the chronic to the accelerated phase of CML. The most objective findings are a blood blast percentage greater than 10, a platelet count less than 100,000/μL (100×10^9/L), blood basophils greater than 20 percent, and new clonal cytogenetic abnormalities accompanying the Philadelphia chromosome.[843]

The terminology used has included *accelerated phase, acute phase, acute transformation*, or, in its most dramatic expression, *blast crisis*, but the metamorphosis, which can be acute, that is, myeloblastic or lymphoblastic crisis, often is more gradual and manifested by severe dysmorphic hematopoiesis, refractory splenomegaly, and extramedullary tumor masses, hence the preference for *transformation* or *accelerated phase* to describe this transition from a controllable to a poorly controlled malignancy. Blast crisis is the most severe manifestation of the accelerated phase and can occur abruptly or after a period of worsening disease. Blast crisis is in effect the evolution to overt acute leukemia.

PATHOGENESIS

Effect of Tyrosine Kinase Inhibitors in Rate of Progression

The advent of tyrosine kinase inhibitor therapy for CML has resulted in a marked increase in the duration of a subclinical chronic phase, with normal blood counts and spleen size, often with the loss of identifiable Ph chromosome-bearing cells in blood and marrow, and sometimes with the loss of laboratory evidence of the *BCR-ABL* oncogene as judged by PCR. This therapeutic advance has greatly delayed the evolution to accelerated phase and blast crisis, but the risk for such a conversion exists since under experimental conditions CML stem cells do not undergo apoptosis when exposed to BCR-ABL tyrosine kinase inhibitors and BCR-ABL-positive cells return in virtually all patients if tyrosine kinase therapy is interrupted.

Blast Crisis Stem Cells

The onset of accelerated phase is thought to occur in a BCR-ABL-bearing granulocyte-monocyte progenitor. Experimental[844,845] and theoretical[846] evidence supports this concept. This locale for clonal evolution also could explain the reversion to chronic phase in some patients in whom the suppression of the advanced phase of the disease is achieved. Thus, during chronic phase there is the interplay between polyclonal normal hematopoietic stem cells and CML stem cells (see Chap. 85, Fig. 85–4) and in the acute phase a third stem cell pool (second cancer stem cell pool) is added that initiates and sustains accelerated phase and blast crisis.

Molecular and Genetic Alterations

The transformation of chronic phase CML to accelerated phase and then blast crisis or directly to blast crisis is thought to be the result of seven or more molecular processes: (1) maturation arrest, (2) failure of genome surveillance, (3) failure of adequate DNA repair, (4) development of a mutator phenotype, (5) telomere shortening, (6) loss of tumor-suppressor function, and (7) unknown factors.[847,848]

Progression of chronic phase to accelerated phase is marked by an increase in *BCR-ABL* expression.[849,850] Superimposed on the increased transcription of $mRNA^{BCR-ABL}$ are additional cytogenetic abnormalities that are added to the persistent Ph chromosome in approximately 50 to 65 percent of patients.[843,850–853] In lymphoid blast crisis, in which the blast cells have a lymphocytic phenotype, acquisition of p16/*ARF* mutations occurs in approximately 50 percent of cases, and *RB* gene mutations occurs in approximately 20 percent of cases. In myeloid blast crisis, in which blast cells have a myeloid phenotype, approximately 25 percent of cases have cells containing a p53 mutation.[854] The possible role of loss of p53 function in fostering transformation of a human chronic phase CML clone has been demonstrated in transgenic mice in which p53 function was abrogated.[855] p51/p63 is a member of the p53 gene family that is not mutated in chronic phase but is mutated in approximately 8 percent of patients in blast crisis.[856]

Progression of the clone to a more malignant clone is reflected in a more disordered growth and maturation pattern of progenitor cells in culture, ultimately mimicking the growth failure of acute leukemia,[851] and in increased morphologic and functional abnormalities of blood cells,[857,858] eventuating in a block in maturation and replacement of blood and marrow by blast cells.

Approximately 65 percent of patients have cytogenetic abnormalities in addition to the Ph chromosome. A double Ph chromosome, trisomy 8, and isochromosome 17p are the secondary changes most commonly seen.[854,859] Because the frequency of trisomy 8 was greater after treatment with busulfan compared to hydroxyurea, the frequency of secondary chromosomal changes may be quite different after imatinib mesylate therapy.[854] Clonal instability has also been found in cases of lymphoid blast crisis. Clones distinct from those identified later may be detected before overt lymphoid transformation. Identification of these abortive clones suggests clonal instability before the onset of transformation, which might have prognostic value.[860] FISH has been used to determine which cells have secondary cytogenetic abnormalities, and these cells often are not the blast cells. This finding suggests that some chromosomal abnormalities merely denote genomic instability.[861] The abnormal mRNA and protein product $p210^{BCR-ABL}$ are present in the marrow and blood cells of patients who have transformed to acute leukemia.[862–864]

Although the breakpoint site on M-*bcr* was thought to be correlated with the time of the onset of the accelerated phase,[865] subsequent studies have not indicated a correlation between length of chronic phase and the specific site of the *BCR-ABL* fusion.[866] Rare cases have displayed deletion of the *BCR-ABL* fusion gene, loss of transcription of the message, and loss of expression of the p210 tyrosine kinase after transformation, the latter finding indicating the abnormal protein kinase may not always play a unique role in sustaining the acute state.[867] In contrast, the frequent response, albeit temporary, to imatinib suggests that the *mutant BCR-ABL* product usually plays a role at this stage of the disease.

Numerous molecular changes identified in the cells of patients with acute transformation that might contribute to the increased malignant behavior of the CML clone, include activation of the *N-RAS* gene,[868,869] rearrangement of the p53 gene,[869–872] hypermethylation of the calcitonin gene,[873] and methylation of the *ABL1* gene.[874] One report described p53 mutations in 17 percent of blast crisis patients. An association between the failure of CML cells to express the retinoblastoma 1 gene product and acute blast crisis with a megakaryoblastic phenotype has been reported.[875] Homozygous deletions of the p16 tumor-suppressor gene are associated with lymphoid transformation of CML,[876] but such deletions are not seen in the chronic phase and in myeloid blast crisis. p16 is also known as the *cyclin-dependent kinase 4 inhibitor gene* and is located on chromosome 9p21.[877,878] This gene inhibits the kinase CDK-4, which regulates a cell-cycle checkpoint prior to commitment to DNA synthesis. The *WT* gene on chromosome 11p13 encodes a zinc finger motif-containing transcription factor found in CML patients only after progression to blast crisis.[879] Overexpression of the *EVI*-1 gene has also been found in CML blast crisis.[880,881] Microsatellite instability has not been found to be involved with progression to blast crisis.[882] *BCL-2, c-MYC*, and various other genes have also been implicated in the evolution of CML.[883–886]

Approximately 50 genes have been identified that could play a role in the progression to accelerated phase or blast crisis,[847] including genes identified by expression profiling that are dysregulated in accelerated phase compared to chronic phase.[887,888] These include the WNT-β-catenin and JunB pathways.

■ CLINICAL FEATURES

Signs and Symptoms

The features that might signal the conversion of the chronic to the accelerated phase include unexplained fever, bone pain, weakness, night sweats, weight loss, loss of sense of well-being, arthralgia, and left upper quadrant pain related to splenic enlargement or infarcts. These features may occur weeks in advance of laboratory evidence of the accelerated phase. Localized or diffuse lymphadenopathy or enlarging masses in extralymphatic and extramedullary sites containing *BCR-ABL*–positive myeloblasts or lymphoblasts may develop. A poor response of blood cell counts and splenic enlargement despite previously effective therapy may be evident.[843,854,889–891] Symptoms caused by histamine excess in basophilic crisis can be present.[892]

Several of these changes may occur in series or in parallel. The time of onset of transformation and the appearance of a blastic crisis and its clinical expression are unpredictable.

■ LABORATORY FEATURES

Blood Findings[854,889–891]

Anemia may worsen and be associated with increasing poikilocytosis, anisocytosis, and anisochromia. The number of nucleated red cells in the blood may increase. These red cell changes may be accentuated further if advancing marrow fibrosis is a feature of the disease.

The total leukocyte count may fall without treatment. The proportion of blasts increases to greater than 10 percent in blood and marrow in the accelerated phase and when blast crisis ensues represents 20 to 90 percent of the cells. The morphology of the blast cells may be lymphoid or myeloid. Myelocytes decrease in number. Hyposegmented neutrophils (Pelger-Huët cells) and other dysmorphic changes may become evident. Basophils increase and often represent 20 to 80 percent of the total blood leukocytes. A decrease of the platelet count to less than 100,000/μL ($<100 \times 10^9$/L) develops. Giant platelets, micromegakaryocytes, and megakaryocyte fragments may enter the blood. Decreased progenitor cell growth in culture is present, akin to that in acute leukemia.

Marrow Findings[854,889–891]

The marrow findings are widely variable. Marked dysmorphic changes in one, two, or three of the major cell lineages; an increase in blast count to greater than 10 percent; marrow morphology simulating subacute myelomonocytic leukemia; or, in the extreme, florid blastic transformation with blast counts greater than 30 percent can occur. Reticulin fibers may increase in prominence, and occasionally severe reticulin and collagen fibrosis develop. Additional clonal cytogenetic abnormalities develop in as many as half the patients in accelerated phase (see "Cytogenetic Studies" below).

EXTRAMEDULLARY BLAST CRISIS

A variety of symptoms or signs may occur as a result of the specific effects of new extramedullary blastic tumors, referred to as *extramedullary blast crisis*.[893–896] Extramedullary blast crisis is the first manifestation of accelerated phase in approximately 10 percent of patients with CML. Lymph nodes,[894,895] serosal surfaces,[897,898] skin and soft tissue,[893–896] breast,[896,899] gastrointestinal or genitourinary tract,[894,896] bone,[894,896,900–903] and central nervous system[894,904–906] are among the principal areas involved. Isolated or diffuse lymphadenopathy may occur. Bone involvement may lead to severe pain, tenderness, and pathologic fracture, and may be evident on imaging of the involved area. Central nervous system involvement usually is meningeal and may be preceded by headache, vomiting, stupor, cranial nerve palsies, and papilledema and is associated with an increase in cells, protein, and the presence of blasts in the spinal fluid.[896,904–906]

Appropriate histochemical and immunologic tests are required to determine if the extramedullary disease is composed of phenotypic myeloblasts or lymphoblasts. Because the tumor cells may have features of lymphoma cells, the terms *myeloid* or *granulocytic sarcoma, chloroma,* and *myeloblastoma* can be misnomers, and the term *extramedullary blast crisis* is used for this circumstance in CML.[905,907–909] The lymphoblasts, like the myeloblasts, are Ph chromosome-positive. A combination of morphology, histochemistry (e.g., peroxidase, lysozyme), terminal deoxynucleotidyl transferase assay, and monoclonal antibodies specific for lymphoid or myeloid cells can be used to classify the extramedullary blast cells. Older reports (1930s–1960s) of concurrent lymphoma and CML probably were, in many cases, examples of extramedullary lymphoblast crisis in lymph nodes or other sites.

MARROW BLAST CRISIS

Approximately half of patients with CML enter the accelerated phase by developing acute leukemia. The onset of blast crisis can develop from days[910–912] to decades after diagnosis of CML. The signs and symptoms may include fever, hemorrhage, bone pain, and lymphadenopathy.[848,910–912] The morphology of the acute leukemia usually is myeloblastic or myelomonocytic.[848,913] A substantial proportion of myeloid leukemia in this setting may not have myeloperoxidase demonstrable by cytochemistry.[914] The proportion of cases classified as erythroblastic leukemia is approximately 10 percent, based on morphologic features,[915] but may be as high as 20 percent if expression of glycophorin-A is used as the determinant.[916] Occasional cases have megakaryoblastic transformation.[875,917] These cases may be difficult to identify by light microscopy because the megakaryoblasts may be mistaken for lymphoid cells or undifferentiated blasts. Myelofibrosis is a feature of this variant. Antiplatelet glycoprotein antibodies and other monoclonal antiplatelet antibodies now are available as reagents to identify megakaryoblasts without the need for ultrastructural studies.[917] Promyelocytic[918–920] and eosinophilic[921] blast crises also can occur. Basophilic leukemia is a known variant of CML.[922] Patients with promyelocytic crisis often have t(15;17) in addition to the Ph chromosome, and some have presented with disseminated intravascular coagulation.[923]

CML may transform into acute lymphoblastic leukemia in approximately 30 percent of CML patients in blastic crisis.[843,924–928] The lymphoid cells generally express terminal deoxynucleotidyl transferase (TdT)[924,925] and are of the B cell lineage,[928–930] as judged by antiimmunoglobulin staining. TdT is a DNA polymerase that adds deoxynucleoside monophosphates from triphosphate substrates to single-stranded DNA by end addition, differing in the latter respect from replicative polymerases.[931] The enzyme is present in normal immature thymocytes and in the blast cells of nearly all patients with acute lymphoblastic leukemia. Rare patients have blasts with a T-lymphocyte phenotype.[907,908,932,934] Some cases are biphenotypic; the blasts have both lymphoid and myeloid markers.[913,935–937] Some cases may have myeloperoxidase activity in blast cells and express CD33 or CD13. Myeloid to lymphoid clonal succession following autologous transplantation in the second chronic phase has been described.[938] Patients with lymphoid blast crisis seldom have an intermediate accelerated phase, have less splenomegaly and basophilia, and usually have a higher degree of marrow blast infiltration. With non-tyrosine-kinase-inhibitor therapy, remission rate and survival were somewhat longer in cases of lymphoid than in myeloid blast crisis.[939]

CYTOGENETIC STUDIES

Most large studies have shown seven recurrent changes in patients' cells prior to, or during, the accelerated phase: trisomy 8 (33% of cases), additional 22q– (30% of cases), isochromosome 17 (20% of cases), trisomy 19 (12% of cases), loss of Y chromosome (8% of males), trisomy 21 (7% of cases), and monosomy 7 (5% of cases).[940–943] In addition, a large number of other chromosome abnormalities have been described.[944–948] In one study, 46 (63%) of 73 blast crisis patients had secondary cytogenetic abnormalities. These abnormalities were more common in myeloid blast crisis and were associated with shorter remission.[860] The changes may be features of myeloid blast crisis compared to lymphoid crisis.[941,946] Some abnormalities, such as inv16, are associated with early transformation to AML.[942,946,949] A significant proportion (50%) of patients in the accelerated phase or blast crisis have no additional cytogenetic abnormalities beyond t(9;22)(q34;q11) after banding and multicolor FISH analysis.[948] In cases where the blastic transformation is in extramedullary sites, such as lymph nodes or spleen, the additional cytogenetic abnormalities may be in the cells at those sites but not in cells in the blood or marrow.[950]

TREATMENT

Optimal treatment is allogeneic stem cell transplantation if the patient is eligible because of the patient's age and donor availability. The role of stem cell transplantation is also evolving as tyrosine kinase inhibitor use in these phases of diseases becomes better defined.

Tyrosine Kinase Inhibitors in Accelerated and Blast Crisis

The initial dose of imatinib in accelerated phase is 600 mg/day.[951] Imatinib, dasatinib, and nilotinib have been utilized as bridging therapies to permit allogeneic stem cell transplantation in accelerated phase.[952] Dasatinib and nilotinib can achieve a better molecular response, and thus the role for and timing of transplantation in accelerated phase CML is being redefined. Combination therapies are being explored in the accelerated phase of disease, including dasatinib plus imatinib.[953] Imatinib can be combined with mitoxantrone plus etoposide or cytarabine for patients in myeloid blast crisis.[954] Imatinib has produced complete hematologic remissions in approximately 20 percent of patients.[955,956] However, complete cytogenetic responses are uncommon. Central nervous system and other extramedullary blast crisis can occur during imatinib therapy for accelerated phase disease,[957,958] and all types of blast crisis, including promyelocytic blast crisis,[959] can occur during imatinib therapy. Compared to historical controls in which various combinations of chemotherapy were utilized, imatinib used alone results in comparable outcomes (6-month median survival of patients in blast crisis).[960] Although dasatinib therapy can result in complete cytogenetic responses in 29 percent of blast crisis CML, and nilotinib can result in complete cytogenetic response in 27 percent of myeloid blast crisis and in 43 percent of lymphoid blast crisis, these responses are rarely durable, so in a patient of appropriate age with an acceptable donor, transplantation options should be considered with the second-line tyrosine kinase inhibitors utilized as a bridge to transplantation therapy.[961,962]

Chemotherapy

The treatment approach is predicated on the phenotype of the blast cells in CML patients with blast crisis and is rarely used in accelerated phase. In patients with myeloid phenotypes, the approach has been similar to that used for acute myelogenous leukemia: combinations of an anthracycline antibiotic, such as idarubicin or daunorubicin, with high-dose cytosine arabinoside and sometimes etoposide.[963] Because this approach produces few remissions that are of short duration (median survival approximately 6 months), a variety of other drug combinations incorporating 5-azacytidine, busulfan, cladribine, fludarabine, clofarabine, high-dose cytosine, arabinoside, decitabine, etoposide, farnesyl transferase inhibitors, hydroxyurea, methotrexate, mitoxantrone, plicamycin, tiazofurin, or troxacitabine have been used, but with no significant improvement in outcome.[960]

In patients with lymphoid phenotypes, vincristine sulfate 1.4 mg/m^2 (not to exceed 2 mg/dose) given intravenously once per week and prednisone 60 mg/m^2 per day given orally are the mainstay of treatment. A minimum of two cycles of treatment (2 weeks) should be given to judge responsivity. Approximately one-third of patients with lymphoid blast transformation reenter the chronic phase after such treatment. However, because only about one-third of patients have lymphoid blasts, this number represents a remission rate of only approximately 10 percent of patients who enter blast crisis using this approach. Some relapsed patients become TdT-negative (myeloblastic relapse). However, even if relapsed patients remain TdT-positive, they are not likely to respond to a second treatment. Some therapists argue for a more intensive induction regimen for patients with lymphoblastic crisis, akin to regimens for *de novo* adult ALL or high-risk childhood ALL, and report somewhat better results: higher remission rates and longer remissions. The benefit of such an intensive approach has been small because remission durations have been modest. TdT-positive, CD10 (CALLA)-positive lymphoblasts may be the lymphoblast phenotype most responsive to vincristine and prednisone.[927] mTOR inhibitors may be useful in lymphoid blast crisis.[964]

Allogeneic Stem Cell Transplantation

Stem cell transplantation from an identical twin or sibling has been used in some patients after entry into the blastic phase. Occasional patients have had long-term survival. The 3-year survival rate is approximately 15 to 20 percent,[965–967] unlike transplantation in the chronic phase, in which the 3-year survival rate is 50 to 60 percent. However, for patients who present in blast crisis, who develop blast crisis in the first year of the chronic phase, or who delay transplantation for other reasons, transplantation remains the best hope for long-term survival if a histocompatible donor is available.[904,905] Relapse of accelerated phase after allogeneic stem cell transplantation has responded to infusion of donor cytotoxic T lymphocytes.[968] The utilization of agents such as imatinib before allogeneic stem cell transplantation for patients in advanced phases of disease may favorably improve transplantation outcomes, especially when major cytogenetic response occurs before transplantation.[969]

Autologous Stem Cell Transplantation

Autografting in the accelerated phase or blast crisis, either with stem cells collected during chronic phase or with mobilized Ph-chromosome–negative progenitor cells collected upon cell rebound after intensive chemotherapy, has resulted in apparent prolonged remission in some patients, but this procedure is rarely used in advanced disease because of the high rate of relapse.[970] Whether Ph-chromosome–negative cells collected during imatinib therapy have the same potential is unknown.

Splenectomy

Splenectomy may be performed for palliation of painful splenic infarctions or hemorrhage. However, the complication rates are high, and the procedure performed in this setting should be avoided if possible.[971]

■ COURSE AND PROGNOSIS

The accelerated phase of CML generally is very poorly responsive or refractory to treatment and is a morbid state that can be fatal in weeks to months in all but a few patients who undergo a successful stem cell transplant from a histocompatible donor. Patients with myeloid blast crisis have a median survival of approximately 6 months, whereas patients with lymphoid blast crisis have a median survival of approximately 12 months.[960–972] In the earliest study of imatinib mesylate in blast crisis, patients with myeloblastic crisis had a slightly longer median survival (about 5 months) than patients with lymphoid blast crisis plus Ph-chromosome–positive ALL (3 months). The results are poor in either case. The median survival after evidence of clonal evolution in patients in the chronic phase is approximately 15 months. A worse survival was seen with abnormalities of chromosome 17, other superimposed translocations, or a high percentage of abnormal metaphases.[973] Severe cytopenias from repeated courses of cytotoxic therapy contribute to infections, hemorrhage, and organ dysfunction, especially liver and kidney dysfunction. Opportunistic infections with herpes viruses, cytomegalovirus, or fungi often supervene. The addition of imatinib mesylate therapy has made only a small difference in long-term outcome, although formal studies of combinations of chemotherapy and imatinib mesylate at a higher dose (600 mg/day) have not been completed, and the results of trials with second-generation tyrosine kinase inhibitors are anticipated.

RELATED CLONAL MYELOID DISEASES WITHOUT THE BCR REARRANGEMENT (Table 90–6)

■ CHRONIC MYELOMONOCYTIC LEUKEMIA

This leukemia is part of the spectrum of clonal myeloid diseases that may have findings that simulate CML. In the past, when rigorous criteria for the diagnosis of CML were not applied, CMML was among a heterogenous group of related diseases that sometimes were referred to as *Ph-chromosome–negative CML*. These diseases share the feature of originating in the clonal expansion of a primitive multipotential hematopoietic cell.[974]

TABLE 90–6. Types of Chronic Myelogenous Leukemia

Type of Chronic Myelogenous Leukemia	Molecular Genetics	Major Clinical Features	Further Details
BCR rearrangement-positive chronic myelogenous leukemia	>95% p210$^{BCR\text{-}ABL}$; <5% p190 or p230	Splenomegaly in 80% of cases; WBC >25,000/μL; blood blasts <5%; Ph chromosome in 90% of cases; *BCR* gene rearrangement in 100% of cases	Page 1338
Chronic myelomonocytic leukemia	Various cytogenetic abnormalities	Anemia, monocytosis >1000/μL; blood blasts <10%; increased plasma and urine lysozyme; *BCR* rearrangement absent; rare cases with *PDGFR-β* mutation respond to imatinib	Page 1356
Chronic eosinophilic leukemia	Various cytogenetic abnormalities	Blood eosinophil count >1500/μL; cardiac and neurologic manifestations common; a proportion of cases have *PDGFR-α* mutations and are responsive to imatinib mesylate	Page 1358
Chronic basophilic leukemia	Various cytogenetic abnormalities	Only 5 cases reported; hemoglobin 6–13 g/dL; basophilia of 3.4–41 × 10^9/μL; 2 of 5 cases with splenomegaly; very cellular marrow (>90%) in each case with mild increase in type III collagen, and megakaryocytic dysmorphia; increase in marrow mast cells in 3 of 5 cases	Page 1359
Chronic monocytic leukemia	Various cytogenetic changes	Proportion of monocytes elevated; very rare form of leukemia	Page 1359
Juvenile myelomonocytic leukemia	Various cytogenetic changes	Infants and children <4 years; eczematoid or maculopapular rash; anemia and thrombocytopenia; increased Hgb F in 70% of cases; neurofibromatosis in 10% of cases; abnormality of chromosome 7 (e.g., del 7, del 7q, etc.) in approximately 20% of patients; *BCR* rearrangement absent	Page 1360
Chronic neutrophilic leukemia	Various cytogenetic changes	Segmented neutrophilia >20,000/μL; splenomegaly >90% of cases; no blood blasts; platelets >100,000/μL; 75% of cases have normal cytogenetics; *BCR* rearrangement absent	Page 1361
BCR rearrangement-negative chronic myelogenous leukemia	Various cytogenetic changes	Clinical findings indistinguishable from *BCR* rearrangement-positive CML; Ph chromosome and *BCR-ABL* fusion gene absent	Page 1362

Epidemiology

Most patients with CMML are older than age 50 years, and approximately 75 percent of patients are older than age 60 years at the time of diagnosis. The median age at diagnosis is approximately 70 years. Occasional cases have been reported in older children and younger adults. Men are affected somewhat more frequently than women (approximately 1.4:1).[975,976]

Clinical Findings

Signs and Symptoms The onset usually is insidious, and weakness, infection, or exaggerated bleeding may bring patients to medical attention.[975,976] Hepatomegaly and splenomegaly occur in approximately 50 percent of patients. Leukemia cutis occurs in a small proportion of patients and usually has a monocytic phenotype: CD45, CD68, and lysozyme positive by immunostaining.[977] Immune manifestations, such as vasculitis, pyoderma gangrenosum, immune cytopenias, and connective tissue diseases, may occur in coincidence with CMML.[978]

Blood and Marrow Findings The disease is characterized by anemia and blood monocytosis greater than 1000/μL (1 × 10^9/L).[979] The white cell count may be slightly decreased, normal, or moderately elevated. Occasional patients may have hyperleukocytosis with total white cell counts of 250,000 to 300,000/μL (250–300 × 10^9/L) associated with respiratory insufficiency resulting from pulmonary leukostasis.[980] Immature granulocytes may be present in the blood. Blood myeloblasts may be absent or, when present, do not exceed 10 percent of total white cells. Most patients have thrombocytopenia, but normal or elevated platelet counts may occur. Eosinophilia may be so prominent in occasional cases that the designation *chronic eosinophilic leukemia* may be appropriate.[975,976,981]

The marrow is hypercellular as a result of granulomonocytic hyperplasia; the dominant cells are early myelocytes. The proportion of progranulocytes is increased. Promonocytes also are increased in number. Distinction between poorly granulated myelocytes and promonocytes with primary granules can be difficult. Macronormoblasts and hypersegmented or hyposegmented, often bilobed (acquired Pelger-Huët anomaly), neutrophils are frequent. Despite thrombocytopenia, megakaryocytes usually are present in the marrow. Microvessel density is increased in the marrow, and myelomonocytic cells contain cytoplasmic mRNA for VEGF and membrane VEGF receptors.[981,982] *In vitro* colony studies suggest that autocrine stimulation of cell growth by VEGF may occur. "Spontaneous" cluster/colony growth of granulocyte-monocyte colony-forming cells occurs *in vitro*. The spontaneous growth may result from autocrine or paracrine production of GM-CSF, based on anti–GM-CSF inhibition of colony growth.[984]

Cytogenetic Findings Patients with CMML have an approximately 35 percent frequency of chromosomal abnormalities. Monosomy 7 and trisomy 8 are the most prevalent findings. Approximately 35 percent of patients have point mutations of the *K-RAS* or *N-RAS* gene. The *RAS* gene also may be involved in the transforming events. Abnormal methylation of p15^{INK4B} is a common finding in CMML.[985] Translocation between the gene *PDGFR-β* on chromosome 5(q33) and four partner genes—*TEL* at 12(p13), *HIP-1* at 7(q11.2), *H4* at 10(q22), and Rabaptin-5 at 17(p13)—occur in a very small proportion of patients (approximately 3–4%).[975,986–989] This mutation juxtaposes the gene encoding the PDGFR-*β* with a partner gene, which results in the encoding of a mutant tyrosine kinase that is constitutively activated and sensitive to inhibition by imatinib mesylate[990] (see "Treatment" below). The cases with *PDGFR-β* translocations are more likely to be accompanied by eosinophilia than are cases with other cytogenetic abnormalities.

Serum and Urine Findings Plasma and urine lysozyme concentrations nearly always are elevated. Plasma levels of VEGF, hepatocyte growth factor, and tumor necrosis factor alpha are elevated. Serum B_{12}, β_2-microglobulin, and LDH levels often are elevated.[975,976]

Treatment

Treatment of most patients with CMML has been unsatisfactory, and remissions of any duration are uncommon. The age and performance status of the patient are considered in determining the intensity of treatment. Cytarabine, either standard or low-dose, etoposide, hydroxyurea, and other approaches used for the oligoblastic myelogenous leukemias have been attempted, but with little success (see Chap. 88). Decitabine and 5-azacytidine have been useful in a small proportion of patients.[975,976] Unfortunately, although a particular approach may confer significant benefit in a small proportion of cases, determining which patients will respond is not possible, except by trial and error. An exception is the patient with a translocation involving PDGFR-β, which itself occurs in only a small percentage of patients. In the case of PDGFR-β fusion genes with several of the partner genes, imatinib mesylate 400 mg/day has resulted in normal blood counts, cytogenetic remissions, and, occasionally, molecular remission.[985–987,991,992] These fortunate patients probably will benefit from this treatment, as evidenced by prolonged remissions and survival, compared to other drug options, but the number of patients and duration of followup do not permit quantitative estimates at this point. Allogeneic stem cell transplantation is an option for the small proportion of younger patients with an appropriate matched-related or unrelated donor.[993]

Course and Prognosis

Median survival in CMML is approximately 12 months, with a range from approximately 1 to more than 60 months. Approximately 20 percent of patients progress to frank AML. Arbitrary stratification of CMML into types 1 and 2 based on the height of the blast count has been proposed, but distinguishing patients by whether they have 8 or 12 percent blasts on a marrow examination is useless for patient care. It is well established that blast percentage usually is a significant correlate with outcome in any patient with a clonal myeloid disease, and this factor among several others should guide therapy. Clusters of prognostic variables have been used to stratify patients into risk groups for survival duration. In general, the severity of the anemia and the height of the blast percentage are the most important. Other variables that may confer a shorter life expectancy are height of the absolute lymphocyte count, high spontaneous rates of myelomonocytic colony growth, higher total leukocyte counts, higher LDH level, and larger spleen size.[994–996] Unfortunately, at this time, unless the patient is a candidate for imatinib therapy or stem cell transplantation, long-term salutary therapeutic effects are uncommon.

■ CHRONIC EOSINOPHILIC LEUKEMIA

History and Definition

The recognition of eosinophilic lineage prominence in myelogenous leukemia dates to a case published in 1912.[997] In 1968, the term *hypereosinophilic syndrome* was introduced to encompass a group of disorders with (1) prolonged exaggerated eosinophilia without an apparent cause, (2) frequent cardiac and neurologic tissue damage, (3) a poor or transient response to therapy, and (4) a progressive course and a high fatality rate. Shortly thereafter, Benvenisti and Ultmann[998] presented five cases of eosinophilic leukemia and reviewed the literature regarding that phenotypic designation. In 1975, Chusid and colleagues[999] described 14 cases of hypereosinophilic syndrome, highlighted the frequency of secondary cardiac and neurologic disorders, and suggested the existence of a continuum of manifestations. Because some cases had clonal cytogenetic abnormalities and hematologic findings compatible with a clonal myeloid disease, the presence of eosinophilic leukemia was suspected in this apparently heterogeneous group of patients.

The relationship of blood eosinophilia to clonal myeloid diseases is complex because the former can be reactive or represent acute eosinophilic leukemia, chronic eosinophilic leukemia, or eosinophilia associated with a different category of disease, such as BCR-ABL–positive CML, idiopathic myelofibrosis, oligoblastic leukemia (MDS), or mastocytosis.[1000] Chronic eosinophilic leukemia is a BCR-ABL–negative, clonal myeloid disease with a striking eosinophilia in the blood and marrow, often with clonal cytogenetic abnormalities that have features including, when present, cytogenetic findings that usually distinguish chronic eosinophilic leukemia from other clonal myeloid diseases that may have an associated eosinophilia, such as CMML. The phenotype of the eosinophilic variant of CMML overlaps somewhat with that of chronic eosinophilic leukemia. However, the fusion gene associated with CMML involves the *PDGFR-β* (see "Chronic Myelomonocytic Leukemia" above), whereas in chronic eosinophilic leukemia the cytogenetic findings are different and in some cases involve *PDGFR-α*. This definition of chronic eosinophilic leukemia recognizes that, at the margins, classification may be arbitrary. Studies in cases with the *FIP1L1-PDGFR-α* translocation were consistent with multilineage involvement, consistent with an origin in a pluripotential lymphohematopoietic cell.[1001] Another report found multilineage involvement but with a presumptive lesion in a multipotential, not pluripotential, hematopoietic cell.[1002]

Signs and Symptoms

Fever, cough, weakness, easy fatigability, dyspnea, abdominal pain, maculopapular rash, cardiac symptoms and signs of heart failure, and a variety of neurologic manifestations ranging from peripheral neuropathy to cerebral encephalomalacia may occur, ranging from mild to severe in expression. Splenomegaly often is evident.

Laboratory Findings

Eosinophilia is a constant finding (see Chap. 62, Fig. 62–3). Anemia usually but not always is present at the time of presentation. The leukocyte count may be high-normal or more often elevated. Platelet counts often are normal or mildly decreased. The marrow shows myelocytic and eosinophilic hyperplasia and occasionally Charcot-Leyden crystals. Mast cells may be increased. Megakaryocytes usually are present but may appear dysmorphic. Reticulin fibrosis is common. Immunophenotyping and PCR does not show evidence of either a clonal T-cell population or T-cell-receptor rearrangement. Pulmonary function studies may provide evidence of fibrotic (restrictive) lung disease. Echocardiography may detect mural thrombi, thickening (fibrosis) of the ventricular wall, valvular dysfunction from papillary muscle, and chordae fibrosis. Magnetic resonance imaging can detect subendocardial fibrosis, thickening of ventricles, and markedly reduced ventricular lumen volume. Serum immunoglobulin (Ig) E, vitamin B_{12}, and tryptase levels usually are elevated. Skin biopsy of lesions uncovers intense eosinophilic infiltrates. Neural or brain biopsy may disclose eosinophilic infiltrates, often perivascular, with microthrombi, axonal degeneration, and gliosis.

Cytogenetic Findings A wide array of cytogenetic findings have been reported in cases of chronic eosinophilic leukemia.[1003] Notable translocations include a high frequency of translocations involving chromosome 5, t(1;5), t(2;5), t(5;12), t(6;11), 8p11, trisomy 8, and numerous others infrequently. Chromosome 5 often is translocated at the site of the *PDGFR-β* gene, and the phenotype usually is more compatible with CMML with eosinophilia. Chromosome 5 from band q31-35 contains several genes relevant to eosinophilopoiesis, including those encoding IL-5, IL-3, GM-CSF, and PDGFR-β. A cryptic interstitial deletion on chromosome 4(q12;q12) results in the fusion gene *FIL1L1-PDGFR-α* and in a phenotype of chronic eosinophilic leukemia, which is of particular note because, like the *PDGFR-β* mutations in CMML with eosinophilia, of a near-universal response to treatment with imatinib mesylate.[1003–1005]

Serum Tryptase Level Elevation Versus Normal Levels

The elevation of serum tryptase level (>11.5 ng/mL) has been used to distinguish a subset of patients who (1) are male, (2) have marrows that are intensely hypercellular with a higher proportion of immature eosinophils and with dysmorphic mast cells with a CD117–CD25+CD2– genotype and phenotype (distinguishing these cells from classic mastocytosis, which are CD117+CD25+CD2+), (3) have dramatically higher serum B_{12} and IgE levels, (4) are more prone to restrictive pulmonary disease and endomyocardial fibrosis, (5) have the *FIP1L1-PDGFR-α* fusion gene, and (6) are responsive to imatinib mesylate.[941] Patients with normal serum tryptase levels are more prone to obstructive pulmonary restrictive disease, eosinophilic dermatitis, and gastrointestinal complaints.

Differential Diagnosis

Eosinophilia can occur for many reasons (see Chap. 62). The first step is to identify signs that may point to a clonal myeloid disease. These signs include anemia, thrombocytopenia, splenomegaly, immature eosinophils in the marrow examination, evidence of dysmorphic cells in blood or marrow, for example, atypical megakaryocytes or dysmorphic mast cells, cardiac or pulmonary manifestations, which may occur secondary to chronic eosinophilic leukemia, and markedly elevated serum tryptase or vitamin B_{12} level. The former signs, especially in the aggregate, are highly suggestive, but the presence of a cytogenetic abnormality in myeloid cells is diagnostic of a clonal myeloid disease (leukemia). If the latter is not evident, PCR and/or flow cytometry to search for a clonal T lymphocyte abnormality should be performed. Whether the eosinophilic leukemia is typical or represents an eosinophilia with idiopathic myelofibrosis, CMML, or MDS is less important than if it has a mutation that is imatinib mesylate sensitive (e.g., *PDGFR* mutation).

Therapy

Patients (nearly always men) whose cells display a *FIP1L1–PDGFR-α* have a very high probability of responding to imatinib mesylate at a dose of 100 to 400 mg/day.[1004–1008] The tyrosine kinase activity of this fusion protein is two orders of magnitude more sensitive to imatinib than that of BCR-ABL. However, because not all patients taking 400 mg/day achieve a molecular remission, and that goal may be more likely to result in long-term remission, initial therapy remains at 400 mg/day and PCR monitoring is appropriate. Dose adjustment upward if molecular remission is not achieved can be considered. Unlike the case in CML, patients with chronic eosinophilic leukemia with significant side effects when taking imatinib mesylate, 400 mg/day, have a reasonable probability of having a good response at lower doses.[1008] Responses to dasatinib and nilotinib have also been reported.[1009]

In patients with eosinophilic leukemia without an imatinib mesylate-sensitive mutation or in patients who become resistant to imatinib mesylate and unresponsive to second-generation tyrosine kinase inhibitor (e.g., dasatinib) and who are progressing, ablative or nonablative allogeneic stem cell transplantation can be considered if they are in an acceptable age range and have access to a matched-related or matched-unrelated donor.[1010,1011]

In imatinib mesylate-insensitive patients without the option of transplantation, empirical treatment with glucocorticoids, hydroxyurea, or anti-IL5[1012,1013] to decrease eosinophil counts and mute the progress of eosinophil-mediated cutaneous, cardiac, pulmonary, and neurologic tissue damage should be considered. These approaches may relieve symptoms for a time, but are temporizing if therapy with drugs that might be effective in inhibiting clonal expansion or evolution is not effective (e.g., cytarabine, anthracycline antibiotic, etoposide).

Course and Prognosis

If chronic eosinophilic leukemia is not imatinib sensitive, the long-term outlook is one of probable progressive cardiac and neurologic disability. Transformation to acute eosinophilic or myelogenous leukemia can occur. Allogeneic stem cell transplantation is potentially curative. In imatinib-sensitive cases, hematologic normalization, reversal of marrow fibrosis and mastocytosis, resolution of skin lesions, normalization of spleen size, and restoration of well-being occurs in the great preponderance of cases. Cardiac, neurologic, and pulmonary changes usually cannot be reversed but should be stabilized. The long-term outlook with imatinib mesylate therapy is uncertain. However, imatinib likely will decisively and dramatically improve survival compared to other prior therapy and should greatly improve the prognosis of patients with a molecular target for the drug.

■ CHRONIC BASOPHILIC LEUKEMIA

This type of clinical disorder, in which the patient has marrow and blood basophilia and other findings compatible with a clonal myeloid disease without evidence of the *BCR-ABL* translocation, is rare. Two reports of such a syndrome occurring in five patients have been published.[1014,1015] The marrow was intensely hypercellular in the three major lineages. Dysmorphic megakaryocytes were evident. Basophilia in marrow and blood was striking, although eosinophilia also was evident in two patients and increased mast cells in three patients. The clinical effects of basophilic mediator release were evident in two patients. One patient evolved to AML; another recovered after allogeneic transplantation. The cases had similar findings, leading to the suggestion they represented Ph-negative chronic basophilic leukemia. In one case, a *PRKG2-PDGFR-β* fusion gene was evident and the patient responded to imatinib mesylate.

■ CHRONIC MONOCYTIC LEUKEMIA

History

In 1937, Osgood[1016] reviewed his experience with monocytic leukemia and included a case that probably represented the rare disorder chronic monocytic leukemia. In 1981, approximately 28 bona fide cases had been reported, 5 cases were added, and the characteristics were reviewed.[1017]

Clinical Findings

Patients range in age from 30 to 80 years. Males are affected more frequently than females. Fever, fatigue, and left upper quadrant pain are the most common complaints. Splenomegaly and hepatomegaly are nearly constant findings.[1017–1019]

Laboratory Findings

Anemia is mild. Anisocytosis and poikilocytosis usually are present. The leukocyte count usually is normal or low but can be elevated in a minority of patients. The percentage of monocytes is increased, but the absolute monocyte count often is normal, ranging from 300 to 1500/μL ($0.3–1.5 \times 10^9$/L), or mildly elevated. Occasional patients have more striking monocyte counts. The platelet count may be normal or decreased. Rare nucleated red cells may be present in the blood. The monocytes in the blood contain α-naphthol acetate esterase, tartrate-sensitive acid phosphatase, fluoride-sensitive naphthol AS-D acetate esterase, and peroxidase as judged by histochemical tests. The marrow is cellular, often without an increase in monocytes. The Ph chromosome is absent. The leukemic cells are similar to mature monocytes with abundant cytoplasm. Erythrophagocytosis or thrombocytophagocytosis by monocytes may be seen.

The disease often is not recognized because the total white cell count, monocyte count, and number of marrow monocytes may not be elevated until the spleen is removed, usually for diagnostic purposes.[1017] Following splenectomy, a gradual leukocytosis of 3000 to 100,000/μL ($3–100 \times 10^9$/L) may develop.[1017] The absolute monocyte count increases dramatically, often from less than 1000/μL (1×10^9/L) to as high as 75,000/μL (75×10^9/L). The marrow may contain more than 50 percent mature monocytes following splenectomy.

The spleen is enlarged (300–2500 g). The red pulp is infiltrated with mononuclear cells, often obliterating sinus lumens. Erythrophagocytosis by the mononuclear cells frequently is evident. Liver biopsy may show a mononuclear infiltrate in the sinusoids. Although clinical lymph node enlargement is rare, lymph node biopsies show striking infiltration by leukemic monocytes.

Course, Prognosis, and Treatment

Median survival is approximately 25 months. Patients often die of septicemia[1017–1019] or acute monocytic leukemia.[1020,1021] Therapy has not been studied systematically, but neither intensive combination chemotherapy nor glucocorticoids have changed the course of the disease.

The World Health Organization Committee on the Lymphohematopoietic Tumors does not describe a disease called chronic monocytic leukemia and recent reports of cases are very rare. A few well-documented cases of chronic monocytosis, presumably clonal, evolving into myelogenous leukemia could also satisfy this designation (see Chap. 88).

JUVENILE MYELOMONOCYTIC LEUKEMIA

Epidemiology

Ph-chromosome–positive, adult-type CML occurring in children younger than age 15 years composes approximately 3 percent of childhood leukemias and approximately 10 percent of all cases of CML.[1022] Although CML occurs in children of all ages, it is rare in children younger than age 5 years. With the exception of a propensity to present with higher total leukocyte counts and with leukostatic signs or symptoms, CML in children has the typical manifestations and course of the disorder seen in adults.

A disorder different from adult-type CML, designated *juvenile myelomonocytic leukemia* (juvenile CML), represents approximately 1.5 percent of childhood leukemias. It occurs most often in infants and children younger than age 4 years and is similar in some respects to adult subacute or chronic myelomonocytic leukemia because the two diseases share a prominent monocytic component in the leukemic cell population.[1023–1026]

Pathogenesis

This disorder is a clonal myeloid disease that originates in an early hematopoietic multipotential cell. Evidence indicates this cell may be pluripotential (myeloid-lymphoid) in some cases and myeloid in others.[1027–1030] *RAS* mutations in hematopoietic cells are present in approximately 20 percent of patients.[1031] Approximately 1 in 10 patients with juvenile myelomonocytic leukemia have mutations of *NF1* and manifest type 1 neurofibromatosis. This frequency is approximately 400 times the expected occurrence in a comparable pediatric population.[1032–1034] The linkage between neurofibromin, the protein encoded by the *NF1* gene, guanosine triphosphatase activity proteins, and the activation state of *RAS*-encoded proteins has led to a postulated sequence of events that may be triggered by the extraordinarily heightened sensitivity of the colony-forming cells in the marrow and blood of infants with the disease to the proliferative effects of GM-CSF. The latter initiates signal transduction from the cell membrane to the nucleus via *RAS* protein activation.[1035,1036] Mutations in the *PTPN11* gene have been found in approximately one-third of children with juvenile CML, and the mutations in *NF1, RAS*, and *PTPN11* usually do not coincide.[1035,1036] However, they each may act through a common pathway. *PTPN11* encodes SHP-2, a nonreceptor tyrosine kinase, which is an upstream regulator of RAS; thus, all three mutations can contribute to deregulation of RAS signaling. As an aside, children with Noonan syndrome, which is characterized by short stature, dysmorphic facies, skeletal abnormalities, and cardiac defects, have a germ-cell mutation of *PTPN1*. These children may have a transient disorder that closely mimics juvenile myelomonocytic leukemia.[1036]

Clinical Findings

Symptoms and Signs Infants present with failure to thrive, and children present with malaise, fever, persistent infections, and exaggerated skin, oral, or nasal bleeding. Hepatomegaly can occur. Splenomegaly, sometimes massive, is present in almost all cases. Lymphadenopathy is frequent.[1023–1026] More than half of the patients have eczematoid or maculopapular skin lesions[1037] and xanthomatous lesions, and multiple *café-au-lait* spots (neurofibromatosis type 1) may occur.[1024] The xanthomas may be the earliest signs of neurofibromatosis.[1024,1025] Noonan syndrome (dysmorphic facies, short stature, heart disease, mental retardation, cryptorchidism, webbed neck, chest deformities, and bleeding diathesis) may coexist.[1025]

Laboratory Findings Anemia, thrombocytopenia, and mild to moderate leukocytosis are common. The leukocyte count usually is greater than 10,000/μL (10×10^9/L) with a median leukocyte count at diagnosis of about 35,000/μL (35×10^9/L). The blood has an increased monocyte concentration of 1000 to 100,000/μL ($1–100 \times 10^9$/L), immature granulocytes including a small percentage of blast cells, and nucleated red cells. Fetal hemoglobin concentration is increased in approximately two-thirds of the patients. The marrow aspirate is hypercellular as a result of granulocytic hyperplasia; the number of erythroblasts and megakaryocytes usually are decreased. Monocytic cells are increased but may not be as striking as in the blood. Leukemic blast cells are present in modest proportions (<20%).

Cell culture of blood and marrow shows a striking preponderance of monocytic progenitors, even in the absence of overt monocytosis in the marrow.[1038,1039] Granulocyte-monocyte colony-forming cells show a marked tendency to spontaneous growth if adherent (monocytic) cells are not depleted from culture.[1039] The effect is mediated by a release of large quantities of GM-CSF by monocytes in culture.[1040]

Although clonal chromosome abnormalities have been found in some cases,[1041] the cytogenetic abnormalities have no consistent pattern, and more than half of the patients have normal karyotypes. The *BCR-ABL* fusion gene is not present.[1041–1043] The phenotype of monosomy 7 syndrome overlaps with juvenile myelomonocytic leukemia, and an abnormality of chromosome 7 (del 7, del 7q, others) is present in approximately one-fifth of patients.[1023]

Course, Prognosis, and Treatment

The median survival of patients with juvenile CML has been less than 2 years.[1023,1024] Younger children (younger than 2 years) are more likely to have a protracted course.[955] The disease has been refractory to most chemotherapy. In a study of 9 patients, 4 of whom were treated with a 5- or 6-drug intensive regimen, remissions were 11 to more than 27 months, compared with untreated or lightly treated patients, 4 of whom died within 7 months.[1044] Even in the treated patients, complete suppression of the disease did not occur, and treatment protocols to induce and sustain remissions were lacking.[1039] A program of cytosine arabinoside, etoposide, vincristine, and isotretinoin resulted in a highly favorable response in five children treated. Three patients relapsed and were treated with cytarabine by infusion and subcutaneously and with etoposide. All patients were alive, and the range of survival at the time of publication was 8 to 89 months, with a median survival of 27 months. The resistance of these cells to currently available therapy is gruesomely highlighted by the sense of success in prolonging the life of infants and young children by a few years. Intensive therapy can control disease, but curative chemotherapy has been elusive.[1045] The inclusion of isotretinoin was based on a prior report of responsiveness to the drug used alone; however, this observation has not been confirmed.[1046] The GM-CSF antagonist E21R, inhibitors of *RAF-1* gene expression, blockers of RAS protein farnesylation, and angiogenesis inhibitors are among other drug approaches to the disease being studied.[1026,1047]

Allogeneic stem cell transplantation is an important approach to therapy and may provide the best chance of long-term survival in selected children.[1048,1049] Hence, a rapid search for a matched-unrelated donor is important in patients without matched sibling donors. Transplantation from a histocompatible sibling or matched-unrelated donor resulted in an event-free survival at 4 years of 54 percent in one study of 27 patients that used a variety of conditioning regimens. A cytogenetic abnormality, such as monosomy 7, was a dismal prognostic finding in that study, and children transplanted before age 1 year had better results than did older children.[1048] DLI has placed a posttransplantation patient in relapse into remission,[1050] but in general this procedure is ineffective in patients who relapse after transplantation.

A minority of patients have a smoldering course for 2 to 4 years. Thereafter, the disease usually rapidly progresses, and patients die of infection or hemorrhage. Occasional patients have a very long survival (>10 years) despite persistence of abnormal blood counts and splenomegaly, independent of the type or intensity of therapy. Some children convert to a full-blown acute myelogenous leukemia with a rapidly fatal outcome. Cases of juvenile myelomonocytic leukemia may be associated with transformation to acute lymphoblastic leukemia.[1051]

■ CHRONIC NEUTROPHILIC LEUKEMIA

History, Pathogenesis, and Epidemiology

In 1920, Tuohey[1052] described the first recorded case of an unusual sustained neutrophilia with splenomegaly without fever, inflammation, cancer, or other cause of a leukemoid reaction. Use of X-chromosome-linked polymorphic genes in blood cells and FISH of chromosome abnormalities have been indicative of a clonal myeloid disorder.[1053–1055] Some cases may arise in the hematopoietic multipotential cell, others in a neutrophil progenitor cell (see Chap. 85).[1053–1057] Evidence points to defective apoptotic signals accounting, in part, for the striking accumulation of segmented neutrophils in the blood.[1058] The median age at onset is approximately age 65 years. Younger patients may be affected.[1059] As in most clonal myeloid diseases, men are affected more frequently than are women.

Clinical Features

Symptoms and Signs Patients may complain of weakness, anorexia, weight loss, abdominal pain, and easy bruising. Symptoms and signs of gouty arthritis occur in approximately one-third of cases. The spleen is enlarged in almost all cases, and the liver frequently is enlarged. Lymphadenopathy is very infrequent.[1057] A hemorrhagic tendency is present in some patients.

Laboratory Findings Although some patients have a normal hemoglobin concentration at the time of presentation, most have mild to moderate anemia on presentation. The reticulocyte count usually is between 0.5 and 3.0 percent. The platelet count rarely is less than 125,000/μL (125×10^9/L) and usually is normal. Coagulation times are normal. The total leukocyte count usually is between 25,000 and 75,000/μL (25 and 75×10^9/L) in most cases, and only rarely is less than 20,000/μL (20×10^9/L) or exceeds 100,000/μL (100×10^9/L). Neutrophils compose 85 to 95 percent of the white cells. Although segmented cells usually dominate, occasional cases have a high proportion of band forms. Very infrequently, metamyelocytes, myelocytes, and nucleated red cells may be present in patients. Basophil and eosinophil counts are not increased. Blasts nearly always are absent from the blood. Neutrophil alkaline phosphatase activity is increased in almost all cases.

The marrow invariably shows granulocytic hyperplasia with myeloid-to-erythroid (M:E) ratios as high as 10:1. Myeloblasts are not overtly increased in number (0.5–3.0%). Megakaryocytes are either normal or slightly increased in number and have normal distribution and morphology. Erythropoiesis usually is mildly decreased. Unlike CML, reticulin fibrosis is unusual. A few cases with dysmorphic features in the marrow (acquired Pelger-Hüet anomaly, erythroid, dysplasia, micromegakaryocytes) have been reported. By definition, the Ph chromosome, *BCR* gene rearrangements, and *BCR-ABL* transcripts are absent.[1059–1062] Most patients have normal karyotypes, but approximately 25 percent of patients have nonrandom abnormalities of chromosomes.[1062] Deletions of chromosome 20q and trisomy 21 or 9 are the most common abnormalities. Serum vitamin B_{12}-binding protein and vitamin B_{12} levels both are markedly increased above normal. Serum uric acid concentration is increased, and serum lactic dehydrogenase activity may be increased.

Almost every case examined postmortem had liver and splenic enlargement. Portal hepatic and splenic red pulp infiltrates of neutrophils or islands of extramedullary hematopoiesis with immature myeloid cells and megakaryocytes are characteristic.

Differential Diagnosis

Most leukemoid reactions are associated with an obvious underlying cause, such as pancreatitis, carcinoma, connective tissue disease, smoker's neutrophilia, and chronic bacterial or fungal infection. The leukocyte alkaline phosphatase level usually is markedly elevated in chronic neutrophilic leukemia and markedly decreased in CML. More to the point, molecular studies identifying *BCR* gene rearrangement or the presence of *BCR-ABL* transcripts should distinguish chronic neutrophilic leukemia (*BCR-ABL*–negative) from neutrophilic CML (*BCR-ABL*–positive; see "Special Clinical Features" above). In the latter case, more than half of the patients have thrombocytosis and megakaryocytic hyperplasia, which are uncharacteristic of chronic neutrophilic leukemia.

Treatment

No systematic studies of treatment have been reported. Although hydroxyurea, IFN-α, or cytarabine may decrease the white count and spleen size, long-term benefit is unusual.[1059–1062] Intensive therapy has led to early posttreatment deaths. Allogeneic stem cell transplantation in eligible patients may be curative.[1063]

Course and Prognosis

The disease is fatal, with a median survival of approximately 2.5 years and a range of 0.5 to 6 years.[1059–1062] A case of spontaneous remission has been reported. The prognosis is considerably worse than the prognosis for CML despite the prevalence of mature neutrophils and the paucity of blasts. Causes of death have included (1) intracranial hemorrhage, sometimes in the presence of adequate platelet counts and coagulation times, suggesting a vascular infiltrative process; (2) severe infection; (3) transformation to acute myelogenous leukemia; and (4) the toxic effects of intensive therapy. The disease usually afflicts older subjects, and cardiac, pulmonary, and vascular diseases contribute to a fatal outcome.

A remarkable frequency of concordant essential monoclonal gammopathy or myeloma has been described.[1055,1064–1072] In two cases, the extreme neutrophilia proved to be a polyclonal response to a plasma cell disorder.[1055,1073] Chronic neutrophilic leukemia has evolved from polycythemia vera or oligoblastic leukemia,[1074–1078] supporting its relationship to the clonal hemopathies.[1055,1079,1080]

BCR REARRANGEMENT-NEGATIVE CHRONIC MYELOGENOUS LEUKEMIA

A very small proportion of patients (~4%) with clinical manifestations within the limits usually applied to the diagnosis of CML have neither a Ph chromosome (classic, variant, or masked) nor evidence of rearrangement of *BCR* on chromosome 22. This circumstance represents *BCR*-negative CML. The literature describing Ph-chromosome–negative CML prior to 1987 is difficult to evaluate because many cases were not studied carefully for masked or variant translocations and for the *BCR* gene rearrangement. Ph-chromosome–negative CML is a clonal disease[974] that has the propensity for lymphoid and myeloid transformation.[1081,1082] Although most cases of *BCR* rearrangement-negative CML are closer in manifestations to CMML,[996,974,1083–1086] some cases are indistinguishable from classic CML but without the *BCR-ABL* after exhaustive molecular diagnostic evaluation.[1087–1091] In a report of 76 such patients, the median age was 66 years (range: 24–88), splenomegaly was present in 50 percent of cases, the median white cell count was 38,000 cells/μL (38 × 109 cells/L; range: 11–296), and the median hemoglobin was 11 g/dL (range: 7 to 16), with classical morphologic features in blood and marrow.[1091] As the disease progressed, patients developed severe cytopenias.[1088] Median survival was 24 months and only 7 percent survived for more than 5 years. Myeloid blast crisis occurred in one-third of those followed until their death. Occasional patients had extended complete remissions with INF-γ therapy.[1090] Hydroxyurea can be useful as palliative therapy.

Some patients have transposition of *ABL* to chromosome 22 but not the classic translocation. In such cases, including TEL-ABL translocations, transient responses to imatinib mesylate have been observed.[1092]

Uncommon cases of coexisting BCR– and BCR+ clones have been described, and the basis for such cases is in dispute.[1093] One proposed explanation is that this case is an example of "field carcinogenesis" in which multiple clones coexist.[1093] An alternative explanation is that these cases represent the dual progeny of a single unstable clone.[1094] The long-term survival of patients with CML may permit the emergence of a drug-induced or spontaneous second malignancy, and in the former it may be notably associated with imatinib (see above "Secondary Chromosomal Changes with Imatinib Mesylate" under "Tyrosine Kinase Inhibitors").[1095–1097]

REFERENCES

1. Bennett JH: Case of hypertrophy of the spleen and liver, in which death took place from suppuration of the blood. *Edinburgh Med Surg J* 64:313, 1845.
2. Virchow R: Weisses blut. *Froieps Notizen* 36:151, 1845.
3. Craige D: Case of disease of the spleen in which death took place in consequence of the presence of purulent matter in the blood. *Edinburgh Med Surg J* 64:400, 1845.
4. Virchow R: *Die Leukaemie in Gesammelte Abhandlungen zur Wissen-Schaftlichen Medizin*. Meidinger, Frankfort, 1865.
5. Neumann E: Ueber myelogene leukämie. *Berl Klin Wochenschr* 15:69, 1878.
6. Nowell PC, Hungerford DA: A minute chromosome in human chronic granulocytic leukemia. *J Natl Cancer Inst* 25:85, 1960.
7. Baike AG, Court Brown WM, Buckton KE, et al: A possible specific chromosome abnormality in human chronic myeloid leukemia. *Nature* 188:1165, 1960.
8. Nowell PC, Hungerford DA: Chromosome studies in human leukemia: II. Chronic granulocytic leukemia. *J Natl Cancer Inst* 27:1013, 1961.
9. Tough IM, Court Brown WM, Buckton KE, et al: Cytogenetic studies in chronic leukemia and acute leukemia associated with mongolism. *Lancet* 1:411, 1961.
10. Caspersson T, Zech L, Johansson C, Modest EJ: Identification of human chromosomes by DNA binding fluorescent agents. *Chromosoma* 30:215, 1970.
11. Caspersson T, Gahrton G, Lindsten J, Zech L: Identification of the Philadelphia chromosome as a number 22 by quinacrine mustard fluorescence analysis. *Exp Cell Res* 63:238, 1970.
12. Rowley JD: A new consistent abnormality in chronic myelogenous leukemia identified by quinacrine fluorescence and Giemsa staining. *Nature* 243:290, 1973.
13. de Klein A, Van Kessel AG, Grosveld G, et al: A cellular oncogene is translocated to the Philadelphia chromosome in chronic myelocytic leukemia. *Nature* 300:765, 1982.
14. Bartram CR, de Klein A, Hagemeijer A, et al: Translocation of c-abl oncogene correlates with the presence of a Philadelphia chromosome in chronic myelocytic leukemia. *Nature* 306:277, 1983.
15. Drucker BJ, Tamura S, Buchdunger E, et al: Effects of a selective inhibitor of the ABL tyrosine kinase in the growth of BCR-ABL positive cells. *Nat Med* 2:561, 1996.
16. Thomas ED, Clift RA, Fefer A, et al: Marrow transplantation for the treatment of chronic myelogenous leukemia. *Ann Intern Med* 104:155, 1986.
17. Redaelli A, Bell C, Casagrande J, et al: Clinical and epidemiologic burden of chronic myelogenous leukemia. *Expert Rev Anticancer Ther* 4:85, 2004.
18. Hemminki K, Jiang Y: Familial myeloid leukemias from the Swedish Family-Cancer database. *Leuk Res* 26:611, 2002.
19. Ichimaru M, Ichimaru T, Belsky JL: Incidence of leukemia in atomic bomb survivors belonging to a fixed cohort in Hiroshima and Nagasaki 1950–1971. *J Radiat Res (Tokyo)* 19:262, 1978.
20. Court Brown WM, Doll R: Adult leukemia: Trends in mortality in relation to etiology. *Br Med J* 1:1063, 1959.
21. Court Brown WM, Doll R: Adult leukemia. *Br Med J* 1:1753, 1960.
22. Boice JD Jr, Day NE, Anderson A, et al: Second cancers following radiation treatment for cervical cancer. *J Natl Cancer Inst* 74:955, 1985.
23. Maloney WC: Radiation leukemia revisited. *Blood* 70:905, 1987.
24. Lichtman MA: Is there an entity of chemically induced BCR-ABL-positive chronic myelogenous leukemia? *Oncologist* 13:645, 2008.
25. Whang-Peng J, Knutsen T: Chromosomal abnormalities, in *Chronic Granulocytic Leukaemia*, edited by MT Shaw, p 49. Praeger, East Sussex, UK, 1982.
26. Spiers ASD, Bain BJ, Turner JE: The peripheral blood in chronic granulocytic leukemia: A study of 50 untreated Philadelphia positive cases. *Scand J Haematol* 18:25, 1977.
27. Sandberg AA: The leukemias: The Philadelphia chromosome, in *The Chromosomes in Human Cancer and Leukemia*, 2nd ed, p 183. Elsevier, New York, 1990.
28. Fialkow PJ, Garther SM, Yoshida A: Clonal origin of chronic myelocytic leukemia in men. *Proc Natl Acad Sci U S A* 58:1468, 1967.
29. Fialkow PJ, Jacobsen RJ, Papayannopoulou T: Chronic myelocytic leukemia: Clonal origin in a stem cell common to granulocyte, erythrocyte, platelet, and monocyte/macrophage. *Am J Med* 63:125, 1977.
30. Koeffler HP, Levine AM, Sparkes LM, Sparkes RS: Chronic myelocytic leukemia: Eosinophils involved in the malignant clone. *Blood* 55:1063, 1980.
31. Hayata I, Kakati S, Sandberg AA: On the monoclonal origin of chronic myelocytic leukemia. *Proc Jpn Acad* 30:351, 1974.
32. Lawler SD, O'Malley F, Lobb DS: Chromosome banding studies in Philadelphia chromosome positive myeloid leukemia. *Scand J Haematol* 17:17, 1976.
33. Harrison CJ, Chang J, Johnson D, et al: Chromosomal evidence of a common stem cell in acute lymphoblastic leukemia and chronic granulocytic leukemia. *Cancer Genet Cytogenet* 13:331, 1984.
34. Chaganti RSK, Bailey RB, Jhanwar SC, et al: Chronic myelogenous leukemia in the monosomic cell line of a fertile Turner syndrome mosaic (45, X/46, XX). *Cancer Genet Cytogenet* 5:215, 1982.
35. Fitzgerald PH, Pickering AF, Eiby JR: Clonal origin of the Philadelphia chromosome and chronic leukemia. *Br J Haematol* 21:473, 1971.
36. Groffen J, Stephenson JR, Heisterkamp N, et al: Philadelphia chromosomal breakpoints are clustered within a limited region, bcr, on chromosome 22. *Cell* 36:93, 1984.
37. Leibowitz D, Schaefer-Rego K, Popenoe DW, et al: Variable breakpoints on the Philadelphia chromosome in chronic myelogenous leukemia. *Blood* 66:243, 1985.
38. Yoffe G, Chinault AG, Talpaz M, et al: Clonal nature of Philadelphia chromosome positive and negative chronic myelogenous leukemia by DNA hybridization analysis. *Exp Hematol* 15:725, 1987.
39. Kavalerchik E, Goff D, Jamieson CH: Chronic myeloid leukemia stem cells. *J Clin Oncol* 26:2911, 2008.
40. Savona M, Talpaz M: Getting to the stem of chronic myeloid leukaemia. *Nat Rev Cancer* 8:341, 2008.
41. Radich JP, Dai H, Mao M, et al: Gene expression changes associated with progression and response in chronic myeloid leukemia. *Proc Natl Acad Sci U S A* 103:2794, 2006.
42. Fialkow PJ, Denman AM, Jacobsen RJ, Lowenthal MN: Chronic myelocytic leukemia. Origin of some lymphocytes from leukemic stem cells. *J Clin Invest* 62:815, 1978.
43. Martin PJ, Najfeld V, Hansen JA, et al: Involvement of the B-lymphoid system in chronic myelogenous leukaemia. *Nature* 287:49, 1980.
44. Boggs DR: Hematopoietic stem cell theory in relation to possible lymphoblastic conversion in chronic myeloid leukemia. *Blood* 44:449, 1974.

45. Bernheim A, Berger R, Preud'homme JL, et al: Philadelphia chromosome positive blood B lymphocytes in chronic myelocytic leukemia. *Leuk Res* 5:331, 1981.
46. Collins S, Coleman H, Groudine M: Expression of bcr and bcr-abl fusion transcripts in normal and leukemic cells. *Mol Cell Biol* 7:2870, 1987.
47. Al-Amin A, Lennartz K, Runde V, et al: Frequency of clonal B lymphocytes in chronic myelogenous leukemia evaluated by fluorescence in situ hybridization. *Cancer Genet Cytogenet* 104:45, 1998.
48. Torlakovic E, Litz CE, McClure JS, Brunning RD: Direct detection of the Philadelphia chromosome in CD20-positive lymphocytes in chronic myelogenous leukemia by tri-color immunophenotyping/FISH. *Leukemia* 8:1940, 1994.
49. Kearney L, Orchard KH, Hibbin JA, Goldman JM: T-cell cytogenetics in chronic granulocytic leukaemia. *Lancet* 1:858, 1981.
50. Nogueira-Costa R, Spitzer G, Cock A, Trijillo JM: E rosette-positive agar colonies containing the Philadelphia chromosome in chronic myeloid leukemia. *Scand J Haematol* 34:184, 1985.
51. Bartram CR, Raghavachar A, Anger B, et al: T lymphocytes lack rearrangement of the bcr gene in Philadelphia chromosome-positive chronic myelogenous leukemia. *Blood* 69:1682, 1985.
52. Fauser AA, Kanz L, Bross KJ, et al: T cells and probably B cells arise from the malignant clone in chronic myelogenous leukemia. *J Clin Invest* 75:1080, 1985.
53. Nitta M, Kato Y, Strife A, et al: Incidence of the B and T lymphocyte lineages in chronic myelogenous leukemia. *Blood* 66:1053, 1985.
54. Ariad S, Dajee D, Willem P, Bezwoda WR: Lack of involvement of T-lymphocytes in the leukaemic population during prolonged chronic phase of Philadelphia chromosome positive chronic myeloid leukaemia. *Leuk Lymphoma* 10:217, 1993.
55. Tsukamoto N, Karasawa M, Maehara T, et al: The majority of T lymphocytes are polyclonal during the chronic phase of chronic myelogenous leukemia. *Ann Hematol* 72:61, 1996.
56. Garicochea B, Chase A, Lazaridou A, Goldman JM: T lymphocytes in chronic myelogenous leukaemia (CML). *Leukemia* 8:1197, 1994.
57. Jonas D, Lubbert M, Kawasaki ES, et al: Clonal analysis of bcr-abl rearrangement in T lymphocytes from patients in the chronic myelogenous leukemia. *Blood* 79:1017, 1992.
58. Haferlach T, Winkemann M, Nickening C, et al: Which components are involved in Philadelphia-chromosome-positive chronic leukemia? *Br J Haematol* 97:99, 1997.
59. Verfaillie C, Miller W, Kay N, McClave P: Adherent lymphokine-activated killer cells in chronic myelogenous leukemia: A benign cell population with potent cytotoxic activity. *Blood* 74:793, 1989.
60. Takahashi N, Miura I, Saitoh K, Miura AB: Lineage involvement of stem cells bearing the Philadelphia chromosome in chronic myeloid leukemia in the chronic phase as shown by a combination of fluorescence-activated cell sorting and fluorescence in situ hybridization. *Blood* 92:4758, 1998.
61. Muñoz L, Bellido M, Sierra J, Nomdedéu JF: Flow cytometric detection of B cell abnormal maturation in chronic myeloid leukemia. *Leukemia* 14:339, 2000.
62. Miura A: Progress in laboratory medicine in chronic myeloid leukemia. *Rinsho Byori* 46:1226, 1998.
63. Muñoz L, Bellido M, Sierra J, Nomdedéu JF: Flow cytometric detection of B cell abnormal maturation in chronic myeloid leukemia. *Leukemia* 14:339, 1999.
64. Gunsilius E, Duba H-C, Petzer AL, et al: Evidence from a leukaemia model for maintenance of vascular endothelium by bone-marrow-derived endothelial cells. *Lancet* 355:1688, 2000.
65. Fialkow PJ, Martin PJ, Najfeld V, et al: Evidence for a multistep pathogenesis of chronic myelogenous leukemia. *Blood* 58:158, 1981.
66. Lisker R, Casas L, Mutchinick O, et al: Late-appearing Philadelphia chromosome in two patients with chronic myelogenous leukemia. *Blood* 56:812, 1980.
67. Kamada N, Uchino H: Chronologic sequence in appearance of clinical and laboratory findings characteristic of chronic myelogenous leukemia. *Blood* 51:843, 1978.
68. Smadja N, Krulik M, DeGramont A, et al: Acquisition of a Philadelphia chromosome concomitant with transformation of a refractory anemia into an acute leukemia. *Cancer* 55:1477, 1985.
69. Fegan C, Morgan G, Whittaker JA: Spontaneous remission in a patient with chronic myeloid leukaemia. *Br J Haematol* 72:594, 1989.
70. Brandt L, Mitelman F, Panani A, Lenner HC: Extremely long duration of chronic myeloid leukaemia with Ph^1 negative and Ph^1 positive bone marrow cells. *Scand J Haematol* 16:321, 1976.
71. Hagemeijer A, Smith EME, Lowenberg B, Abels J: Chronic myeloid leukemia with permanent disappearance of the Ph^1 chromosome and development of new clonal subpopulations. *Blood* 53:1, 1979.
72. Singer JN, Arlin ZA, Najfeld V, et al: Restoration of nonclonal hematopoiesis in chronic myelogenous leukemia (CML) following a chemotherapy induced loss of the Ph^1 chromosome. *Blood* 56:356, 1980.
73. Sokal JE: Significance of Ph^1-negative marrow cells in Ph^1 positive chronic granulocytic leukemia. *Blood* 56:1072, 1980.
74. Smadja N, Krulik M, Audebert AA, et al: Spontaneous regression of cytogenetic and haematologic anomalies in Ph^1-positive chronic myelogenous leukaemia. *Br J Haematol* 63:257, 1986.
75. Goldman JM, Kearney L, Pittman S, et al: Hemopoietic stem cell grafting for chronic granulocytic leukemia. *Exp Hematol* 10:76, 1982.
76. Reiffers J, Vezon G, David B, et al: Philadelphia negative cells in a patient treated with autografting for Ph^1 positive chronic granulocytic leukaemia in transformation. *Br J Haematol* 55:382, 1983.
77. Reiffers J, Broustet A, Goldman JM: Philadelphia chromosome-negative progenitors in chronic granulocytic leukemia. *N Engl J Med* 309:1460, 1983.
78. Coulombel L, Kalousek DK, Eaves CJ, et al: Long-term marrow culture reveals chromosomally normal hemopoietic progenitor cells in patients with Philadelphia chromosome-positive chronic myelogenous leukemia. *N Engl J Med* 308:1493, 1983.
79. Degliantoni G, Mangori L, Rizzoli V: *In vitro* restoration of polyclonal hematopoiesis in a chronic myelogenous leukemia after *in vitro* treatment with 4-hydroperoxycyclophosphamide. *Blood* 65:753, 1985.
80. Barnett MJ, Eaves CJ, Phillips GL, et al: Successful autografting in chronic myeloid leukemia after maintenance of marrow in culture. *Bone Marrow Transplant* 4:345, 1989.
81. Verfaillie CM, Miller WJ, Boylan K, McGlave PB: Selection of benign primitive hematopoietic progenitors in chronic myelogenous leukemia on the basis of HLA-DR antigen expression. *Blood* 79:1003, 1992.
82. Leemhuis T, Leibowitz D, Cox G, et al: Identification of BCR/ABL-negative primitive hematopoietic progenitor cells within chronic myeloid leukemia marrow. *Blood* 81:801, 1993.
83. Wang JCY, Lapidot T, Cashman JD, et al: High level engraftment of NOD/SCID mice by primitive normal and leukemic hemopoietic cells from patients with chronic myeloid leukemia in chronic phase. *Blood* 91:2406, 1998.
84. Dunbar CE, Stewart FM: Separating the wheat from the chaff: Selection of benign hematopoietic cells in chronic myeloid leukemia. *Blood* 79:1107, 1992.
85. Strife A, Clarkson B: Biology of chronic myelogenous leukemia: Is discordant maturation the primary defect? *Semin Hematol* 25:1, 1988.
86. Heinzinger M, Waller CF, Rosentiel A, et al: Quality of IL-3 and GCSF-mobilized peripheral blood stem cells in patients with early chronic phase CML. *Leukemia* 12:333, 1998.
87. Verfaillie CM, Bhatia R, Miller W, et al: BCR/ABL-negative primitive progenitors suitable for transplantation can be selected from the marrow of most early-chronic phase but not accelerated-phase chronic myelogenous leukemia patients. *Blood* 87:4770, 1996.
88. Grand FH, Marley SB, Chase A, et al: BCR/ABL-negative progenitors are enriched in the adherent fraction of CD34+ cells circulating in the blood of chronic phase chronic myeloid leukemia patients. *Leukemia* 11:1486, 1997.
89. Carella AM, Podesta M, Frassoni R, et al: Collection of "normal" blood repopulating cells during early hemopoietic recovery after intensive conventional chemotherapy in chronic myelogenous leukemia. *Bone Marrow Transplant* 12:267, 1993.
90. Guyootat D, Wahabi K, Viallet A, et al: Selection of BCR/ABL-negative stem cells from marrow or blood of patients with chronic myeloid leukemia. *Leukemia* 13:991, 1999.
91. Hogge DE, Coulumbel L, Kalousek D, et al: Nonclonal hemopoietic progenitors in a G6PD heterozygote with chronic myelogenous leukemia revealed after long-term marrow culture. *Am J Hematol* 24:389, 1987.
92. Deforge M, Boogaerts MA, McGlave PB, Verfaillie CM: BCR/ABL-CD34+HLA-DR– progenitor cells in early phase, but not in more advanced phases, of chronic myelogenous leukemia are polyclonal. *Blood* 93:284, 1999.
93. Van den Berg D, Wessman M, Murray L, et al: Leukemic burden in subpopulations of CD34+ cells isolated from the mobilized peripheral blood of alpha-interferon-resistant or -intolerant patients with chronic myeloid leukemia. *Blood* 87:4348, 1996.
94. Podesta M, Piaggio G, Frassoni F, et al: Very primitive hemopoietic cells (LTC-IC) are present in Philadelphia negative cytaphereses collected during early recovery after chemotherapy for chronic myeloid leukemia (CML). *Bone Marrow Transplant* 16:549, 1995.
95. Kirk JA, Reems JA, Roecklein BA, et al: Benign marrow progenitors are enriched in the CD34+/HLA-DRlo population but not in the CD34+/CD38lo population in chronic myeloid leukemia: An analysis using interphase fluorescence in situ hybridization. *Blood* 86:737, 1995.
96. Lewis ID, Haylock DN, Moore S, et al: Peripheral blood is a source of BCR-ABL–negative pre-progenitors in early chronic phase chronic myeloid leukemia. *Leukemia* 11:581, 1997.
97. Maguer-Satta V, Petzer AL, Eaves AC, Eaves CJ: BCR-ABL expression in different subpopulations of functionally characterized Ph+ CD34+ cells from patients with chronic myeloid leukemia. *Blood* 88:1796, 1996.
98. Sirard C, Lapidot T, Vormoor J, et al: Normal and leukemia SCID-repopulating cells (SRC) coexist in the bone marrow and peripheral blood from CML patients in chronic phase, whereas leukemic SRC are detected in blast crisis. *Blood* 87:1539, 1996.
99. Dazzi F, Capelli D, Hasserjian R, et al: The kinetics and extent of engraftment of chronic myelogenous leukemia cells in nonobese diabetic/severe combined immunodeficiency mice reflect the phase of the donor's disease: An *in vivo* model for chronic myelogenous leukemia biology. *Blood* 92:1390, 1998.
100. Holyoake TL, Jiang X, Drummond MW, et al: Elucidating critical mechanisms of deregulated stem cell turnover in the chronic phase of chronic myelogenous leukemia. *Leukemia* 16:549, 2002.
101. Eaves C, Cashman J, Eaves A: Defective regulation of leukemic hematopoiesis in chronic myeloid leukemia. *Leuk Res* 22:1085, 1998.
102. Clarkson BD, Strife A, Wisniewski D, et al: New understanding of the pathogenesis of CML: A prototype of early neoplasia. *Leukemia* 11:1404, 1997.
103. Bedi A, Zehnbauer BA, Collector MI, et al: BCR-ABL gene rearrangement and expression of primitive hematopoietic progenitors in chronic myeloid leukemia. *Blood* 81:2898, 1993.
104. Moore MA: *In vitro* culture studies in chronic granulocytic leukaemia. *Clin Haematol* 6:97, 1977.

105. Siitonen T, Zheng A, Savolainen E-R, Koistinen P: Spontaneous granulocyte-macrophage colony growth by peripheral blood mononuclear cells in myeloproliferative disorders. *Leuk Res* 20:187, 1996.
106. Eaves CJ, Eaves AC: Cell culture studies in CML. *Baillieres Clin Haematol* 1:931, 1987.
107. Galbraith PR, Abu-Zahra HT: Granulopoiesis in chronic granulocytic leukemia. *Br J Haematol* 22:135, 1972.
108. Sjögren U, Brandt L: Composition and mitotic activity of the erythropoietic part of the bone marrow in chronic myeloid leukaemia. *Scand J Haematol* 12:18, 1974.
109. Verfaillie CM: Stem cells in chronic myelogenous leukemia. *Hematol Oncol Clin North Am* 11:1079, 1997.
110. Ghaffari S, Dougherty GJ, Lansdorp PM, et al: Differentiation-associated changes in CD44 isoform expression during normal hematopoiesis and their alteration in chronic myeloid leukemia. *Blood* 86:2976, 1995.
111. Kawaishi K, Kimura A, Katch O, et al: Decreased L-selectin expression in CD34-positive cells from patients with chronic myelocytic leukaemia. *Br J Haematol* 93:367, 1996.
112. Turkina AG, Baryshnikov AY, Sedyakhina NP, et al: Studies of P-glycoprotein in chronic myelogenous leukaemia patients: Expression, activity and correlations with CD34 antigen. *Br J Haematol* 92:88, 1996.
113. Agarwal R, Doren S, Hicks B, Dunbar CE: Long-term culture of chronic myelogenous leukemia marrow cells on stem cell factor-deficient stroma favors benign progenitors. *Blood* 85:1306, 1995.
114. Moore S, Haylock DN, Levesque J-P, et al: Stem cell factor as a single agent induces selective proliferation of the Philadelphia chromosome positive fraction of chronic myeloid leukemia CD34+ cells. *Blood* 92:2461, 1998.
115. Chasty RC, Lucas GS, Owen-Lynch PJ, et al: Macrophage inflammatory protein-1 alpha receptors are present on cells enriched for CD34 expression from patients with chronic myeloid leukemia. *Blood* 86:4270, 1995.
116. Cashman JD, Eaves CJ, Sarris AH, Eaves AC: MCP-1, not MIP-1α, is the endogenous chemokine that cooperates with TGF-β to inhibit the cycling of primitive normal but not leukemic (CML) progenitors in long-term human marrow cultures. *Blood* 92:2338, 1998.
117. Murohashi I, Endho K, Nishida S, et al: Differential effects of TGF-beta 1 on normal and leukemic human hematopoietic cell proliferation. *Exp Hematol* 23:970, 1995.
118. Gordon MY, Dowding C, Riley G, et al: Altered adhesive interactions with marrow stroma of haematopoietic progenitor cells in chronic myeloid leukaemia. *Nature* 328:342, 1987.
119. Dowding C, Guo A-P, Osterholz J, et al: Interferon-α overrides the deficient adhesion of chronic myeloid leukemia primitive progenitor cells to bone marrow stromal cells. *Blood* 78:499, 1991.
120. Bhatia R, Wayner EA, McGlave PB, Verfaillie CM: Interferon-α restores normal adhesion of chronic myelogenous leukemia hematopoietic progenitors to bone marrow stroma by correcting impaired β1 integrin receptor function. *J Clin Invest* 94:384, 1994.
121. Verfaillie CM: Stem cells in chronic myelogenous leukemia. *Hematol Oncol Clin North Am* 11:1079, 1997.
122. Bhatia R, Munthe HA, Verfaillie CM: Tyrphostin AG957, a tyrosine kinase inhibitor with anti-BCR/ABL tyrosine activity restores β_1 integrin-mediated adhesion and inhibiting signaling in chronic myelogenous leukemia hematopoietic progenitors. *Leukemia* 12:1708, 1998.
123. Lundell BI, McCarthy JB, Kovach NL, Verfaillie CM: Activation of beta 1 integrins on CML progenitors reveals cooperation between beta1 integrins and CD44 in the regulation of adhesion and proliferation. *Leukemia* 11:822, 1997.
124. Ghaffari S, Dougherty GJ, Eaves AC, Eaves CJ: Altered patterns of CD44 epitope expression in human chronic and acute myeloid leukemia. *Leukemia* 10:1773, 1996.
125. Vijayan KV, Advani SH, Zingde SM: Chronic myeloid leukemic granulocytes exhibit reduced and altered binding to P-selectin; modification in the CD15 antigens and sialylation. *Leuk Res* 21:59, 1997.
126. Deininger MW, Vieira S, Mendiola R, et al: BCR-ABL tyrosine kinase activity regulates the expression of multiple genes implicated in the pathogenesis of chronic myeloid leukemia. *Cancer Res* 60:2049, 2000.
127. Verfaillie CM, Hurley R, Lundell BI, et al: Integrin-mediated regulation of hematopoiesis: Do BCR/ABL-induced defects in integrin function underlie the abnormal circulation and proliferation of CML progenitors? *Acta Haematol* 29:40, 1997.
128. Symington BE: Growth signalling through the alpha 5 beta 1 fibronectin receptor. *Biochem Biophys Res Commun* 208:126, 1995.
129. Bhatia R, McCarthy JB, Verfaillie CM: Interferon-alpha restores normal beta 1 integrin-mediated inhibition of hematopoietic progenitor proliferation by the marrow microenvironment in chronic myelogenous leukemia. *Blood* 87:3883, 1996.
130. Wertheim JA, Forsythe K, Druker BJ, et al: BCR-ABL-induced adhesion defects are tyrosine kinase-independent. *Blood* 99:4122, 2002.
131. Fruehauf S, Topaly J, Schad M, Paschka P, et al: Imatinib restores expression of CD62L in BCR-ABL-positive cells. *J Leukoc Biol* 73:600, 2003.
132. Salgia R, Li JL, Ewaniuk DS, et al: BCR/ABL induces multiple abnormalities of cytoskeletal function. *J Clin Invest* 100:46, 1997.
133. Lewis JM, Baskaran R, Taagepera S, et al: Integrin regulation of c-ABL tyrosine kinase activity and cytoplasmic-nuclear transport. *Proc Natl Acad Sci U S A* 93:15174, 1996.
134. Renshaw MW, McWhirter JR, Wang JY: The human leukemia onco-gene bcr-abl abrogates the anchorage requirement but not the growth factor requirement for proliferation. *Mol Cell Biol* 15:1286, 1995.
135. Salgia R, Brunkhorst B, Pisick E, et al: Increased tyrosine phosphorylation of focal adhesion proteins in myeloid cell lines expressing p210BCR/ABL. *Oncogene* 11:1149, 1995.
136. Rudkin GT, Hungerford DA, Nowell PC: DNA content of chromosome Ph[1] and chromosome 21 in human chronic granulocytic leukemia. *Science* 144:1229, 1964.
137. O'Riordan ML, Robinson JA, Buckton KE, Evans HJ: Distinguishing between the chromosome involved in Down's syndrome (trisomy 21) and chronic myeloid leukaemia (Ph[1]) by fluorescence. *Nature* 230:167, 1971.
138. Lawler SD: The cytogenetics of chronic granulocytic leukemia. *Clin Haematol* 6:55, 1977.
139. Melo JV, Yan XH, Diamond J, Goldman JM: Balanced parental contribution to the ABL component of the BCR-ABL gene in chronic myeloid leukemia. *Leukemia* 9:734, 1995.
140. Chissoe SL, Bodenteich A, Wang YF, et al: Sequence and analysis of the human ABL gene, the BCR gene, and regions involved in the Philadelphia chromosomal translocation. *Genomics* 27:67, 1995.
141. Melo JV, Deininger MW: Biology of chronic myelogenous leukemia-signaling pathways of initiation and transformation. *Hematol Oncol Clin North Am* 18:545, 2004.
142. Daley GQ, Beu Neriah Y: Implicating the bcr/abl gene in the pathogenesis of Philadelphia chromosome-positive human leukemia. *Adv Cancer Res* 57:151, 1991.
143. Heisterkamp N, Groffen J, Stephenson JR, et al: Chromosomal localization of human cellular homologues of two viral oncogenes. *Nature* 299:747, 1982.
144. Heisterkamp N, Stephenson JR, Groffen J, et al: Localization of the c-abl oncogene adjacent to a translocation breakpoint in chronic myelocytic leukemia. *Nature* 306:239, 1983.
145. Konopka JB, Witte ON: Activation of the abl oncogene in murine and human leukemias. *Biochim Biophys Acta* 823:1, 1985.
146. Collins SJ, Groudine MT: Rearrangements and amplification of c-abl sequences in the human chronic myelogenous leukemia cell line K562. *Proc Natl Acad Sci U S A* 80:4813, 1983.
147. Canaani E, Gale RP, Steiner-Seltz D, et al: Altered transcription of an oncogene in chronic myelocytic leukemia. *Lancet* 1:593, 1984.
148. Gale RP, Canaani E: An 8 kilobase abl RNA transcript in chronic myelogenous leukemia. *Proc Natl Acad Sci U S A* 81:5648, 1984.
149. Collins SJ, Kubonishi I, Miyoshi I, Groudine MT: Altered transcription of the c-abl oncogene in K562 and other chronic myelogenous leukemia cells. *Science* 225:72, 1984.
150. Leibowitz D, Cubbon RM, Bank A: Increased expression of a novel c-abl related RNA in K562 cells. *Blood* 65:526, 1985.
151. Konopka JB, Watanabe SM, Witte ON: An alteration of the human c-abl protein in K562 leukemia cells unmasks associated tyrosine kinase activity. *Cell* 37:1035, 1984.
152. Konopka JB, Watanabe SM, Singer JW, et al: Cell lines and clinical isolates derived from Ph1-positive chronic myelogenous leukemia patients express c-abl proteins with a common structural alteration. *Proc Natl Acad Sci U S A* 82:1810, 1985.
153. Stam K, Heisterkamp N, Grosveld G, et al: Evidence of a new chimeric bcr/c-abl mRNA in patients with chronic myelocytic leukemia and the Philadelphia chromosome. *N Engl J Med* 313:1429, 1985.
154. Ben-Neriah Y, Daley GQ, Mes-Masson A-M, et al: The chronic myelogenous leukemia-specific P210 protein is the product of the bcr/abl hybrid gene. *Science* 233:212, 1985.
155. Maxwell SA, Kurzrock R, Parson SJ, et al: Analysis of P210bcr/abl tyrosine protein kinase activity in various subtypes of Philadelphia chromosome-positive cells from chronic myelogenous leukemia patients. *Cancer Res* 47:1731, 1987.
156. Kurzrock R, Kloetzer WS, Talpaz M, et al: Identification of molecular variants of $P210^{BCR-ABL}$ in chronic myelogenous leukemia. *Blood* 70:233, 1987.
157. Xu DQ, Galibert F: Restriction fragment length polymorphism caused by a deletion within the human c-abl gene (ABL). *Proc Natl Acad Sci U S A* 83:3447, 1986.
158. Popenoe DW, Schaefer-Rego K, Mears JC, et al: Frequent and extensive deletion during the 9,22 translocation in CML. *Blood* 68:1123, 1986.
159. Shtivelman E, Gale RP, Dreazen O, et al: Bcr-abl RNA in patients with chronic granulocytic leukemia. *Blood* 69:971, 1987.
160. McWhirter JR, Wang JJ: Activation of tyrosine kinase and microfilament-binding functions of *c-abl* by *bcr* sequences in *bcr/abl* fusion proteins. *Mol Cell Biol* 11:1553, 1991.
161. Bernards A, Rubin CM, Westbrook CA, et al: The first intron in the human c-abl gene is at least 200 kilobases long and is the target for translocations in chronic myelogenous leukemia. *Mol Cell Biol* 7:3231, 1987.
162. Eisenberg A, Silver R, Soper L, et al: The location of breakpoints within the breakpoint cluster region (bcr) of chromosome 22 in chronic myeloid leukemia. *Leukemia* 2:642, 1988.
163. Collins SJ: Breakpoints on chromosomes 9 and 22 in Philadelphia chromosome-positive chronic myelogenous leukemia. *J Clin Invest* 78:1392, 1986.
164. Heisterkamp N, Stam K, Groffen J, et al: Structural organization of the bcr gene and its role in the Ph[1] translocation. *Nature* 315:758, 1985.
165. Gao L-M, Goldman J: Long-range mapping of the normal BCR gene. *Leukemia* 5:555, 1991.
166. Melo JV: BCR-ABL gene variants. *Baillieres Clin Haematol* 10:203, 1997.
167. Saglio G, Pane F, Gottardi E, et al: Consistent amounts of acute leukemia-associated P190BCR/ABL transcripts are expressed by chronic myelogenous leukemia patients at diagnosis. *Blood* 87:1075, 1996.
168. Honda H, Oda H, Suzuki T, et al: Development of acute lymphoblastic leukemia and myeloproliferative disorder in transgenic mice expressing p210bcr/abl: A novel transgenic model for human Ph1-positive leukemias. *Blood* 91:2067, 1998.
169. Maru Y, Witte ON: The BCR gene encodes a novel serine/threonine kinase activity within a single exon. *Cell* 67:459, 1991.

170. Muller AJ, Young JC, Pendergast A-M, et al: BCR first exon sequences specifically activate the BCR/ABL tyrosine kinase oncogene of Philadelphia chromosome-positive human leukemia. *Mol Cell Biol* 11:1785, 1991.
171. Diekmann D, Brill S, Garrett MD, et al: BCR encodes a GTPase-activating protein for $p21^{rac}$. *Nature* 351:400, 1991.
172. Melo JV, Gordon DE, Goldman JM: The ABL-BCR fusion gene is expressed in chronic myeloid leukemia. *Blood* 81:158, 1993.
173. Bartram CR, de Klein A, Hagemeijer A, et al: Translocation of the human c-abl oncogene correlates with the presence of a Philadelphia chromosome in chronic myelocytic leukaemia. *Nature* 306:277, 1983.
174. Selleri L, Narni F, Emilia G, et al: Philadelphia-positive chronic myeloid leukemia with a chromosome 22 breakpoint outside the breakpoint cluster region. *Blood* 70:1659, 1987.
175. Mohamed AN, Koppitch F, Varterasian M, et al: BCR/ABL fusion located on chromosome 9 in chronic myeloid leukemia with a masked Ph chromosome. *Genes Chromosomes Cancer* 13:133, 1995.
176. Morris C, Jeffs A, Smith T, et al: BCR gene recombines with genomically distinct sites on band 11Q13 in complex BCR-ABL translocations of chronic myeloid leukemia. *Oncogene* 12:677, 1996.
177. Andreasson P, Johansson B, Carlsson M, et al: BCR/ABL-negative chronic myeloid leukemia with ETV6/ABL fusion. *Genes Chromosomes Cancer* 20:299, 1997.
178. Rozman C, Urbano-Ispizua A, Cervantes F, et al: Analysis of the clinical relevance of the breakpoint location within M-BCR and the type of chimeric mRNA in chronic myelogenous leukemia. *Leukemia* 9:1104, 1995.
179. Verschraegen CF, Kantarjian HM, Hirsch-Ginsberg C, et al: The breakpoint cluster region site in patients with Philadelphia chromosome-positive chronic myelogenous leukemia. Clinical, laboratory, and prognostic correlations. *Cancer* 76:992, 1995.
180. Zaccaria A, Martinelli G, Testoni N, et al: Does the type of BCR/ABL junction predict the survival of patients with Ph1-positive chronic myeloid leukemia? *Leuk Lymphoma* 16:231, 1995.
181. Ohno T, Hada S, Sugiyama T, et al: Chronic myeloid leukemia with minor bcr breakpoint developed hybrid type of blast crisis. *Am J Hematol* 57:320, 1998.
182. Melo JV: The diversity of BCR-ABL fusion proteins and their relationship to leukemia phenotype. *Blood* 88:2375, 1996.
183. Rubinstein R, Purves LR: A novel BCR-ABL rearrangement in a Philadelphia chromosome-positive chronic myelogenous leukaemia variant with thrombocythaemia. *Leukemia* 12:230, 1998.
184. Hochhaus A, Reither A, Skladny H, et al: A novel BCR-ABL fusion gene (e6a2) in a patient with Philadelphia chromosome-negative chronic myelogenous leukemia. *Blood* 88:2236, 1996.
185. Briz M, Vilches C, Cabrera R, et al: Typical chronic myelogenous leukemia with e19a2 junction BCR/ABL transcript. *Blood* 90:5024, 1997.
186. McLaughlin J, Chianese E, Witte ON: In vitro transformation of immature hemopoietic cells by P210 bcr/abl oncogene product of the Philadelphia chromosome. *Proc Natl Acad Sci U S A* 84:6558, 1987.
187. Daley GQ, McLaughlin J, Witte ON, Baltimore D: The CML-specific P210 bcr/abl protein, unlike v-abl, does not transform NIH/3T3 fibroblasts. *Science* 237:532, 1987.
188. Elefanty AG, Hariharan IK, Cory S: *Bcr-abl*, the hallmark of chronic myeloid leukaemia in man, induces multiple haemopoietic neoplasms in mice. *EMBO J* 9:1069, 1990.
189. Daley GQ, VanEtten RA, Baltimore D: Induction of chronic myelogenous leukemia in mice by the $p210^{bcr/abl}$ gene of the Philadelphia chromosome. *Science* 247:824, 1990.
190. Voncken JW, Morris C, Pattengale P, et al: Clonal development and karyotype evolution during leukemogenesis of BCR/ABL transgenic mice. *Blood* 79:1029, 1992.
191. Gishizky ML, Johnson-White J, Witte O: Efficient transplantation of BCR-ABL-induced chronic myelogenous leukemia-like syndrome in mice. *Proc Natl Acad Sci U S A* 90:3755, 1993.
192. Daley GQ: Animal models of BCR/ABL-induced leukemias. *Leuk Lymphoma* 11:57, 1993.
193. Voncken JW, Kaartinen V, Pattengale PK, et al: BCR/ABL P210 and P190 cause distinct leukemia in transgenic mice. *Blood* 86:4603, 1995.
194. Honda H, Oda H, Suzuki T, et al: Development of acute lymphoblastic leukemia and myeloproliferative disorder in transgenic mice expressing p210bcr/abl: A novel transgenic model for human Ph 1-positive leukemias. *Blood* 91:2067, 1998.
195. Pear WS, Miller JP, Xu L, et al: Efficient and rapid induction of a chronic myelogenous leukemia-like myeloproliferative disease in mice receiving P210 bcr/abl-transduced bone marrow. *Blood* 92:3780, 1998.
196. Honda M, Ohno S, Takahashi T, et al: Establishment, characterization, and chromosomal analysis of new leukemic cell lines derived from MT/p210/bcr/abl transgenic mice. *Exp Hematol* 26:188, 1998.
197. Zhang X, Ren R: Bcr-Abl efficiency induces in a myeloproliferative disease and production of excess interleukin-3 and granulocyte-macrophage colony-stimulating factor in mice: A novel model for chronic myelogenous leukemia. *Blood* 92:3829, 1998.
198. Elefanty AG, Corsy S: *Bcr-abl*-induced cell lines can switch from mast cell to erythroid or myeloid differentiation in vitro. *Blood* 79:1271, 1992.
199. Van Etten RA: Pathogenesis and treatment of Ph+ leukemia: Recent insights from mouse models. *Curr Opin Hematol* 8:224, 2001.
200. Bose S, Deininger M, Goora-Tybor J, et al: The presence of typical and atypical BCR-ABL fusion genes in leukocytes of normal individuals: Biological significance and implications for the assessment of minimal residual disease. *Blood* 92:3362, 1998.
201. Hirai HS, Tanaka M, Azuma Y, et al: Transforming genes in human leukemia cells. *Blood* 66:1371, 1985.
202. Clarkson BD, Strife A, Wisniewski D, et al: New understanding of the pathogenesis of CML: A prototype of early neoplasia. *Leukemia* 11:1404, 1997.
203. Verfaillie CM: Chronic myelogenous leukemia: From pathogenesis to therapy. *J Hematother* 8:3, 1999.
204. Pasternak G, Hochhaus A, Schultheis B, Hehlmann R: Chronic myelogenous leukemia: Molecular and cellular aspects. *J Cancer Res Clin Oncol* 124:643, 1998.
205. Gotoh A, Broxmeyer HE: The function of BCR/ABL and related protooncogenes. *Curr Opin Hematol* 4:3, 1997.
206. Sattler M, Salgia R: Activation of hematopoietic growth factor signal transduction pathways by the human oncogene BCR/ABL. *Cytokine Growth Factor Rev* 8:63, 1997.
207. Skorski T, Kanakaraj P, Nieborowska-Skorska M, et al: Phosphatidylinositol-3 kinase activity is regulated by BCR/ABL and is required for the growth of Philadelphia chromosome-positive cells. *Blood* 86:726, 1995.
208. Skorski T, Nieborowska-Skorska M, Szczylik C, et al: C-RAF-1 serine/threonine kinase is required in BCR/ABL-dependent and normal hematopoiesis. *Cancer Res* 55:2275, 1995.
209. Goga A, McLaughlin J, Afar DE, et al: Alternative signals to RAS for hematopoietic transformation by the BCR-ABL oncogene. *Cell* 82:981, 1995.
210. Salgia R, Uemura N, Okuda K, et al: CRKL links p210BCR/ABL with paxillin in chronic myelogenous leukemia cells. *J Biol Chem* 270:29145, 1995.
211. De Jong R, ten Hoeve J, Heisterkamp N, Groffen J: Crkl is complexed with tyrosine-phosphorylated Cbl in Ph-positive leukemia. *J Biol Chem* 270:21468, 1995.
212. Salgia R, Pisick E, Sattler M, et al: P130CAS forms a signalling complex with the adapter protein CRKL in hematopoietic cells transformed by the BCR/ABL oncogene. *J Biol Chem* 271:25198, 1996.
213. Sattler M, Griffin JD: Molecular mechanisms of transformation by the *BCR-ABL* oncogene. *Semin Hematol* 40:4, 2003.
214. Melo JV, Deininger MW: Biology of chronic myelogenous-signaling pathways of initiation and transformation. *Hematol Oncol Clin North Am* 18:545, 2004.
215. Wong S, Witte ON: The BCR-ABL story: Bench to bedside and back. *Annu Rev Immunol* 22:247, 2004.
216. Sattler M, Verma S, Shrinkhande G, et al: The BCR/ABL tyrosine kinase induces production of reactive species in hematopoietic cells. *J Biol Chem* 275:24273, 2000.
217. Sattler M, Salgia R, Okuda K, et al: The proto-oncogene product $p120^{CBL}$ and the adaptor proteins CRKL and c-CR link c-ABL, p190BCR/ABL and p210BCR/ABL to the phosphatidylinositol-3; kinase pathway. *Oncogene* 12:832, 1996.
218. Salgia R, Sattler M, Pisick E, et al: P210BCR/ABL induces formation of complexes containing focal adhesion proteins and the protooncogene product p120c-CBL. *Exp Hematol* 24:310, 1996.
219. De Jong R, van Wijk A, Haataja L, et al: BCR/ABL-induced leukemogenesis causes phosphorylation of Hef2 and its association with Crkl. *J Biol Chem* 272:32649, 1997.
220. Bollag G, Clapp DW, Shih S, et al: Loss of NF1 results in activation of the Ras signaling pathway and leads to aberrant growth in haematopoietic cells. *Nat Genet* 12:144, 1996.
221. Carpino N, Wisniewski D, Strife A, et al: P62dok: A constitutively tyrosine-phosphorylated, GAP-associated protein in chronic myelogenous leukemia progenitor cells. *Cell* 88:197, 1997.
222. Yamanashi Y, Baltimore D: Identification of the Abl- and ras GAP-associated 62 kDa protein as a docking protein, Dok. *Cell* 88:205, 1997.
223. Reuther JY, Reuther GW, Cortez D, et al: A requirement for NFkappaB activation in BCR/ABL-mediated transformation. *Genes Dev* 1:12:968, 1998.
224. LaMontagne KR, Flint AJ, Franza BR, et al: Protein tyrosine phosphatase 1B antagonizes signalling by oncoprotein tyrosine kinase p210 bcr/abl in vivo. *Mol Cell Biol* 18:2965, 1998.
225. Chai SK, Nichols GL, Rothman P: Constitutive activation of JAKs and STATs in BCR-abl-expressing cell lines and peripheral blood cells derived from leukemic patients. *J Immunol* 159:4720, 1997.
226. Shuai K, Halpern J, ten Hoeve J, et al: Constitutive activation of STAT5 by the BCR-ABL oncogene in chronic myelogenous leukemia. *Oncogene* 13:247, 1996.
227. Wilson-Rawls J, Xie S, Liu J, et al: P210 Bcr-Abl interacts with the interleukin 3 receptor beta (c) subunit and constitutively induces its tyrosine phosphorylation. *Cancer Res* 56:3426, 1996.
228. Chuang TH, Xu X, Kaartinen V, et al: Abl and Bcr are multifunctional regulators of the Rho GTP-binding protein family. *Proc Natl Acad Sci U S A* 92:10282, 1995.
229. Afar DE, Witte O: Characterization of breakpoint cluster region kinase and SH2-binding activities. *Methods Enzymol* 256:125, 1995.
230. Gishizky ML, Cortez D, Pendergast AM: Mutant forms of growth factor-binding protein-2 reverse BCR-ABL-induced transformation. *Proc Natl Acad Sci U S A* 92:10889, 1995.
231. Raitano AB, Halpern JR, Hambuch TM, Sawyers CL: The Bcr-Abl leukemia oncogene activates Jun kinase and requires Jun for transformation. *Proc Natl Acad Sci U S A* 92:11746, 1995.
232. Miyamura T, Nishimura J, Yufu Y, Nawata H: Interaction of BCRABL with the retinoblastoma protein in Philadelphia chromosome-positive cell lines. *Int J Hematol* 67:115, 1997.
233. Largaespada DA, Brannan CI, Jenkins NA, Copeland NG: NF1 deficiency causes Ras-mediated granulocyte/macrophage colony stimulating factor hypersensitivity and chronic myeloid leukaemia. *Nat Genet* 12:137, 1996.

234. Amos TA, Lewis JL, Grand FH, et al: Apoptosis in chronic myeloid leukaemia: Normal responses by progenitor cells to growth factor deprivation, X-irradiation and glucocorticoids. *Br J Haematol* 91:387, 1995.
235. Bedi A, Barber JP, Bedi GC, et al: BCR-ABL-mediated inhibition of apoptosis with delay of G2/M transition after DNA damage: A mechanism of resistance to multiple anticancer agents. *Blood* 86:1148, 1995.
236. Amarante-Mendes GP, Naekyung KC, Liu L, et al: Bcr-Abl exerts its antiapoptotic effect against diverse apoptotic stimuli through blockage of mitochondrial release of cytochrome C and activation of caspase-3. *Blood* 92:1700, 1998.
237. Maguer-Satta V, Burl S, Liu L, et al: BCR-ABL accelerates C2-ceramide-induced apoptosis. *Oncogene* 16:237, 1998.
238. Pierson BA, Miller JS: CD56+bright and CD56+dim natural killer cells in patients with chronic myelogenous leukemia progressively decrease in number, respond less to stimuli that recruit clonogenic natural killer cells, and exhibit decreased proliferation on a per cell basis. *Blood* 88:2279, 1996.
239. Gissinger H, Kurzrock R, Wetzler M, et al: Apoptosis in chronic myelogenous leukemia: Studies of stage-specific differences. *Leuk Lymphoma* 25:121, 1997.
240. Boultwood J, Peniket A, Watkins F, et al: Telomere length shortening in chronic myelogenous leukemia is associated with reduced time to accelerated phase. *Blood* 96:358, 2000.
241. Terasaki Y, Okamura H, Ohtake S, Nakao S: Accelerated telomere length shortening in granulocytes: A diagnostic marker for myeloproliferative diseases. *Exp Hematol* 30:1399, 2002.
242. Drummond MW, Lennard A, Brummendorf TH, Holyoake TL: Telomere shortening correlates with prognostic score at diagnosis and proceeds rapidly during progression of chronic myeloid leukemia. *Leuk Lymphoma* 45:1775, 2004.
243. Campbell LJ, Fidler C, Eagleton H, et al: HTERT, the catalytic component of telomerase, is downregulated in the haematopoietic stem cells of patients with chronic myeloid leukaemia. *Leukemia* 20:671, 2006.
244. Ohyashiki K, Ohyashiki JH, Iwama H, et al: Telomerase activity and cytogenetic changes in chronic myeloid leukemia with disease progression. *Leukemia* 11:190, 1997.
245. Brümmendorf TH, Ersöz I, Hartmann U, et al: Telomere length in peripheral blood granulocytes reflects response to treatment with imatinib in patients with chronic myeloid leukemia. *Blood* 101:375, 2003.
246. Thompson RB, Stainsby D: The clinical and haematological features of chronic granulocytic leukaemia in the chronic phase, in *Chronic Granulocytic Leukaemia*, edited by MT Shaw, p 137. Praeger, East Sussex, UK, 1982.
247. Cortes JE, Talpaz M, Kantarkian H: Chronic myelogenous leukemia: A review. *Am J Med* 100:555, 1996.
248. Goldman JM: Chronic myeloid leukemia. *Curr Opin Hematol* 4:277, 1997.
249. Lichtman MA, Rowe JM: Hyperleukocytic leukemias: Rheological, clinical and therapeutic considerations. *Blood* 60:279, 1982.
250. Rowe JM, Lichtman MA: Hyperleukocytosis and leukostasis: Common features of childhood chronic myelogenous leukemia. *Blood* 63:1230, 1984.
251. Lichtman MA, Heal J, Rowe JM: Hyperleukocytic leukaemia. *Baillieres Clin Haematol* 1:725, 1987.
252. Ungaro PC, Gonzalez JJ, Werk EE, MacKay JC: Chronic myelogenous leukemia presenting clinically as diabetes insipidus. *N C Med J* 45:640, 1984.
253. Juan D, Hsu S-D, Hunter J: Case report of vasopressin-responsive diabetes insipidus associated with chronic myelogenous leukemia. *Cancer* 56:1468, 1985.
254. Brydon J, Lucky PA, Duffy T: Acne urticaria associated with chronic myelogenous leukemia. *Cancer* 56:2083, 1985.
255. Cohen PR, Talpaz M, Kurzrock R: Malignancy-associated Sweet's syndrome: A review of the world's literature. *J Clin Oncol* 6:1887, 1988.
256. López JLB, Fonseca E, Mauso F: Sweet's syndrome during the chronic phase of chronic myeloid leukemia. *Acta Haematol* 84:207, 1990.
257. Nestok BR, Goldstein JD, Lipkovic P: Splenic rupture as a cause of sudden death in undiagnosed chronic myelogenous leukemia. *Am J Forensic Med Pathol* 9:241, 1988.
258. Giagounidis AAN, Burk M, Meckenstock G, et al: Pathological rupture of the spleen in hematologic malignancies. *Ann Hematol* 73:297, 1996.
259. Hild DH, Myers TJ: Hyperviscosity in chronic granulocytic leukemia. *Cancer* 46:1418, 1980.
260. D'Hondt L, Guillaume TH, Hemblit Y, Symann M: Digital necrosis associated with chronic myeloid leukemia. *Acta Clin Belg* 52:49, 1997.
261. Arbaje YM, Betran G: Chronic myelogenous leukemia complicated by autoimmune hemolytic anemia. *Am J Med* 88:197, 1990.
262. Steegman JL, Pinilla I, Requena MJ, et al: The direct antiglobulin test is frequently positive in chronic myeloid leukemia patients treated with interferon-α. *Transfusion* 37:446, 1997.
263. Hoppin EC, Lewis JP: Polycythemia rubra vera progressing to Ph^1-positive chronic myelogenous leukemia. *Ann Intern Med* 83:820, 1975.
264. Shenkenberg TD, Waddell CC, Rice L: Erythrocytosis and marked leukocytosis in overlapping myeloproliferative diseases. *South Med J* 75:868, 1982.
265. Haas O, Hinterberger W, Morz R: Pure red cell aplasia as possible early manifestation of chronic myeloid leukemia. *Am J Hematol* 27:20, 1986.
266. Mijovic A, Rolovic Z, Novak A, et al: Chronic myeloid leukemia associated with pure red cell aplasia and terminating in promyelocytic transformation. *Am J Hematol* 31:128, 1989.
267. Inbal A, Aktein E, Barak I, Meytes D: Cyclic leukocytosis and long survival in chronic myeloid leukemia. *Acta Haematol* 69:353, 1983.
268. Umemura T, Hirata J, Kaneko S, et al: Periodic appearance of erythropoietin-independent erythropoiesis in chronic myelogenous leukemia with cyclic oscillation. *Acta Haematol* 76:230, 1986.
269. Mitus WJ, Kiossoglou KA: Leukocyte alkaline phosphatase in myeloproliferative syndrome. *Ann N Y Acad Sci* 155:976, 1968.
270. DePalma L, Delgado P, Werner M: Diagnostic discrimination and cost-effective assay strategy for leukocyte alkaline phosphate. *Clin Chim Acta* 6:83, 1996.
271. Pedersen F: Functional and biochemical phenotype in relation to cellular age of differentiated neutrophils in chronic myeloid leukemia. *Br J Haematol* 51:339, 1982.
272. Rambaldi A, Terao M, Bettoni S, et al: Differences in the expression of alkaline phosphatase in mRNA in chronic myelogenous leukemia and paroxysmal nocturnal hemoglobinuria polymorphonuclear leukocytes. *Blood* 73:1113, 1989.
273. Perillie PE: Studies of the changes in leukocyte alkaline phosphatase following pyrogen stimulation in chronic granulocytic leukemia. *Blood* 29:401, 1967.
274. Rustin GJS, Goldman JM, McCarthy D, et al: An extracellular factor controls neutrophil alkaline phosphatase in chronic granulocytic leukemia. *Br J Haematol* 45:381, 1980.
275. Matsuo T: In vitro modulation of alkaline phosphatase activity in neutrophils from patients with chronic myelogenous leukemia by monocyte-derived activity. *Blood* 67:492, 1986.
276. Tanaka KR, Valentine WN, Fredricks RE: Diseases or clinical conditions associated with low leukocyte alkaline phosphatase. *N Engl J Med* 262:912, 1960.
277. Stinson RA, McPhee J, Lewanczk R, Dinwoodie A: Neutrophil alkaline phosphatase in hypophosphatasia. *N Engl J Med* 312:1642, 1985.
278. Kamada N, Uchino H: Chronologic sequence in appearance of clinical and laboratory findings characteristic of chronic myelocytic leukemia. *Blood* 51:843, 1978.
279. Denberg JA, Wilson WEC, Goodacre R, Brenenstock J: Chronic myeloid leukemia—Evidence for basophil differentiation and histamine synthesis from cultured peripheral blood cells. *Br J Haematol* 45:13, 1980.
280. Goh K-O, Anderson FW: Cytogenetic studies in basophilic chronic myelocytic leukemia. *Arch Pathol Lab Med* 103:288, 1979.
281. Valent P, Agis H, Sperr W, et al: Diagnostic and prognostic value of new biochemical and immunohistochemical parameters in chronic myeloid leukemia. *Leuk Lymphoma* 49:635, 2008.
282. Samorapoompichit P, Kiener HP, Schernthaner G-H, et al: Detection of tryptase in cytoplasmic granules of basophils in patients with chronic myeloid leukemia and other myeloid neoplasms. *Blood* 98:2580, 2001.
283. Weil SC, Hrisinko MA: A hybrid eosinophilic-basophilic granulocyte in chronic granulocytic leukemia. *Am J Clin Pathol* 87:66, 1987.
284. Velardi A, Rambotti P, Cernetti C, et al: Monoclonal antibody defined T-cell phenotypes and phytohemagglutinin reactivity of E-rosette forming circulating lymphocytes from untreated chronic myelocyte leukemia patients. *Cancer* 53:913, 1984.
285. Dowding C, Th'ng KH, Goldman JM, Galton DAG: Increased T-lymphocyte numbers in chronic granulocytic leukemia before treatment. *Exp Hematol* 12:811, 1984.
286. Kaur J, Catovsky D, Spiers ASD, Galton DAG: Increase of T-lymphocytes in the spleen in chronic granulocytic leukaemia. *Lancet* 1:834, 1974.
287. Fujimiya Y, Bakke A, Chang WC, et al: Natural killer-cell immunodeficiency in patients with chronic myelogenous leukemia. *Int J Cancer* 37:639, 1986.
288. Fujimiya Y, Chang WC, Bakke A, et al: Natural killer cell immunodeficiency in patients with chronic myelogenous leukemia. *Cancer Immunol Immunother* 24:213, 1987.
289. Mellqvist U-H, Hansson M, Brune M, et al: Natural killer cell dysfunction and apoptosis induced by chronic myelogenous leukemia cells: Role of reactive oxygen species and regulation by histamine. *Blood* 96:1961, 2000.
290. Pierson BA, Miller JS: The role of autologous natural killer cells in chronic myelogenous leukemia. *Leukemia* 11:1404, 1997.
291. Mason JE, DeVita VT, Canellos GP: Thrombocytosis in chronic granulocytic leukemia: Incidence and clinical significance. *Blood* 44:483, 1974.
292. Pederson B: Kinetics and cell function, in *Chronic Granulocytic Leukaemia*, edited by MT Shaw, p 93. Praeger, East Sussex, UK, 1982.
293. Radhika V, Thennarasu S, Naik NR, et al: Granulocytes from chronic myeloid leukemia (CML) patients show differential response to different chemoattractants. *Am J Hematol* 52:155, 1996.
294. Kasimir-Bauer S, Ottinger H, Brittinger G, König W: Philadelphia chromosome-positive chronic myelogenous leukemia: Functional defects in circulating mature neutrophils of untreated and interferon-α-treated patients. *Exp Hematol* 22:426, 1994.
295. Adams T, Schultz L, Goldberg L: Platelet function abnormalities in the myeloproliferative disorders. *Scand J Haematol* 13:215, 1974.
296. Gerrard JM, Stoddard SF, Shapiro RS, et al: Platelet storage pool deficiency and prostaglandin synthesis in chronic granulocytic leukaemia. *Br J Haematol* 40:597, 1978.
297. Knox WF, Bhavani M, Davson J, Geary CG: Histological classification of chronic granulocytic leukemia. *Clin Lab Haematol* 6:171, 1984.
298. Lorand-Metze I, Vassalo J, Souza CA: Histological and cytological heterogeneity of bone marrow in Philadelphia-positive chronic myelogenous leukaemia at diagnosis. *Br J Haematol* 67:45, 1987.
299. Inokuchi K, Yamaguchi H, Tarusawa M, et al: Abnormality of c-kit oncoprotein in certain patients with chronic myelogenous leukaemia—Potential clinical significance. *Leukemia* 16:170, 2002.
300. Cairoli R, Grillo G, Beghini A, et al: Chronic myelogenous leukemia with acquired c-kit activating mutation and transient bone marrow mastocytosis. *Hematol J* 5:273, 2004.
301. Agis H, Sotlar K, Valent P, Horny HP: Ph-Chromosome-positive chronic myeloid leukemia with associated bone marrow mastocytosis. *Leuk Res* 29:1227, 2005.

302. Kelsey PR, Geary CG: Sea-blue histiocytes and Gaucher's cells in bone marrow of patients with chronic myeloid leukaemia. *J Clin Pathol* 41:960, 1988.
303. Dezmezian R, Kantarjian HM, Keating MJ, et al: The relevance of reticulin stain-measured fibrosis at diagnosis in chronic myelogenous leukemia. *Cancer* 59:1739, 1987.
304. Ghosh K, Varma N, Varma S, Dash S: Cellular composition and reticulin fibrosis in chronic myeloid leukaemia. *Indian J Cancer* 25:128, 1988.
305. Buhr T, Choritz H, Georgü A: The impact of megakaryocyte proliferation for the evolution of myelofibrosis. *Virchows Arch* 420:473, 1992.
306. Korkolopoulou P, Viniou N, Kavantzas N, et al: Clinicopathologic correlations of bone marrow angiogenesis in chronic myeloid leukemia: A morphometric study. *Leukemia* 17:89, 2003.
307. Aguayo A, Kantarjian H, Manshouri T, et al: Angiogenesis in acute and chronic leukemias and myelodysplastic syndromes. *Blood* 96:2240, 2000.
308. Zhelyazkova AG, Tonchev AB, Kolova P, et al: Prognostic significance of hepatocyte growth factor and microvessel bone marrow density in patients with chronic myeloid leukaemia. *Scand J Clin Lab Invest* 18:1, 2008.
309. Rumpel M, Friedrich T, Deininger MWN: Imatinib normalizes bone marrow vascularity in patients with chronic myeloid leukemia in first chronic phase. *Blood* 101:4641, 2003.
310. Adams SP, Sahota SS, Mijovic A, et al: Frequent expression of HAGE in presentation chronic myeloid leukemias. *Leukemia* 16:2238, 2002.
311. Udomsakdi C, Eaves CJ, Lansdorp PM, Eaves AC: Phenotypic heterogeneity of primitive leukemic hematopoietic cells in patients with chronic myeloid leukemia. *Blood* 80:2522, 1992.
312. Huret JL: Complex translocations, simple variant translocation and Ph-negative cases in chronic myelogenous leukaemia. *Hum Genet* 85:565, 1990.
313. Sakurai M, Sandberg AA: The chromosomes and causation of human cancer and leukemia: XVIII. The missing Y in acute myeloblastic leukemia (AML) and Ph[1]-positive chronic myelocytic leukemia. *Cancer* 38:762, 1976.
314. Berger R, Bernheim A: Y chromosome loss in leukemias. *Cancer Genet Cytogenet* 1:1, 1979.
315. Ishihara T, Sasaki M, Oshimura M, et al: A summary of cytogenetic studies on 534 cases of chronic myelogenous leukemia in Japan. *Cancer Genet Cytogenet* 9:81, 1983.
316. Mitelman F: Catalogue of chromosomal aberrations in cancer. *Cytogenet Cell Genet* 36:9, 1983.
317. Heim S, Billstrom R, Kristoffersson U, et al: Variant Ph translocations in chronic myeloid leukemia. *Cancer Genet Cytogenet* 18:215, 1985.
318. Bartram CR, Anger B, Carbonell F, Kleihauer E: Involvement of chromosome 9 in variant Ph[1] translocation. *Leuk Res* 9:1133, 1985.
319. Morris CM, Rosman I, Archer SA, et al: A cytogenetic and molecular analysis of five variant Philadelphia translocations in chronic myeloid leukemia. *Cancer Genet Cytogenet* 35:179, 1988.
320. Teyssier JR, Bartram CR, DeVille J, et al: C-abl oncogene and chromosome 22 "bcr" juxtaposition in chronic myelogenous leukemia. *N Engl J Med* 312:1393, 1985.
321. Hagemeijer A, Bartram CR, Smith EME, et al: Is the chromosomal region 9q34 always involved in variants of the Ph[1] translocation? *Cancer Genet Cytogenet* 13:1, 1984.
322. DeBraikeleer M, Chiu H-K, Fiser J, Gardner HA: A further case of Philadelphia chromosome-positive chronic myeloid leukemia with t(3;9;22). *Cancer Genet Cytogenet* 35:279, 1988.
323. Latoge-Pochitaloff-Huvalé M, Sainty D, Adriaansen HJ, et al: Translocation (3;21) in Philadelphia positive chronic myeloid leukemia. *Leukemia* 3:554, 1989.
324. Thompson PW, Whittaker JA: Translocation 3;21 in Philadelphia chromosome positive chronic myeloid leukemia at diagnosis. *Cancer* 39:143, 1989.
325. Engel E, McGee BJ, Flexner JM, et al: Philadelphia chromosome (Ph[1]) translocation in an apparently Ph[1] negative, minus G22, case of chronic myeloid leukemia. *N Engl J Med* 291:154, 1974.
326. Verma RS, Dosik H: "Masked" Ph[1] chromosome in chronic myelogenous leukaemia (CML). *Blut* 50:129, 1985.
327. Hagemeijer A, de Klein A, Godde-Salz E, et al: Translocation of c-abl to "masked" Ph in chronic myeloid leukemia. *Cancer Genet Cytogenet* 18:95, 1985.
328. Melo JV: The diversity of BCR-ABL fusion proteins and their relationship to leukemic phenotype. *Blood* 88:2375, 1996.
329. O'Brien S, Thall PR, Siciliano MJ: Cytogenetics of chronic myeloid leukemia. *Baillieres Clin Haematol* 10:259, 1997.
330. Bartram CR, Carbonell F: Bcr rearrangement in Ph-negative CML. *Cancer Genet Cytogenet* 21:183, 1986.
331. Bartram CR: Rearrangement of bcr and c-abl sequences in Ph-positive acute leukemias and Ph-negative CML—An update. *Curr Stud Hematol Blood Transfus* 31:160, 1987.
332. Ganesan TS, Rassool F, Guo A-P, et al: Rearrangement of the bcr gene in Philadelphia-chromosome negative chronic myeloid leukemia. *Curr Stud Hematol Blood Transfus* 31:153, 1987.
333. Wiedemann LM, Karhi K, Chan LC: Similar molecular alterations occur in related leukemias with and without the Philadelphia chromosome. *Curr Stud Hematol Blood Transfus* 31:149, 1987.
334. Benn P, Loper L, Eisenberg A, et al: Utility of molecular genetic analysis of bcr rearrangement in the diagnosis of chronic myeloid leukemia. *Cancer Genet Cytogenet* 29:1, 1987.
335. Epner DE, Koeffler AP: Molecular genetic advances in chronic myelogenous leukemia. *Ann Intern Med* 113:3, 1990.
336. Dubé I, Dixon J, Beckett T, et al: Location of breakpoints within the major breakpoint cluster region (bcr) in 33 patients with *bcr* rearrangement-positive chronic myeloid leukemia with complex or absent Philadelphia chromosomes. *Genes Chromosomes Cancer* 1:106, 1989.
337. Morris C, Heisterkamp N, Kennedy MA, et al: Ph-negative chronic myeloid leukemia: Molecular analysis of ABL insertion into M-BCR on chromosome 22. *Blood* 76:1812, 1990.
338. Blennerhassett GT, Furth ME, Anderson A, et al: Clinical evaluation of DNA probe assay for the Philadelphia (Ph[1]) translocation in chronic myelogenous leukemia. *Leukemia* 2:648, 1988.
339. Lange W, Snyder DS, Castro R, et al: Detection by enzymatic amplification of bcr-abl mRNA in peripheral blood and bone marrow cells of patients with chronic myelogenous leukemia. *Blood* 73:1735, 1989.
340. Dhingra K, Talpaz M, Riggs MC, et al: Hybridization protection assay: A rapid, sensitive, and specific method for detection of Philadelphia chromosome-positive leukemias. *Blood* 77:238, 1991.
341. Stock W, Westbrook CA, Peterson B, et al: Value of molcular monitoring during the treatment of chronic myeloid leukemia: A Cancer and Leukemia Group B study. *J Clin Oncol* 15:26, 1997.
342. Frenoy N, Chabli A, Sol D, et al: Application of a new protocol for nested PCR to the detection of minimal residual bcr/abl transcripts. *Leukemia* 8:1411, 1994.
343. Melo JV, Yan XH, Diamond J, et al: Reverse transcription/polymerase chain reaction (RT/PCR) amplification of very small numbers of transcripts: The risk in misinterpreting negative results. *Leukemia* 10:1217, 1996.
344. Lin F, Chase A, Bunget J, et al: Correlation between the proportion of Philadelphia chromosome-positive metaphase cells and levels of BCRABL mRNA in chronic myeloid leukaemia. *Genes Chromosomes Cancer* 13:110, 1995.
345. VanDenderen J, Hermans A, Meeuwsen T, et al: Antibody recognition of the tumor-specific bcr-abl joining region in chronic myeloid leukemia. *J Exp Med* 169:87, 1989.
346. Hagemeyer A, vanderPlas DC, Solkarman D, et al: The Philadelphia translocation in CML and ALL: Recent investigations, new detection methods. *Nouv Rev Fr Hematol* 32:83, 1990.
347. Maxwell SA, Kurzrock R, Parsons SJ, et al: Analysis of p210 bcr-abl tyrosine protein kinase activity in various subtypes of Philadelphia chromosome-positive cells from chronic myelogenous leukemia patients. *Cancer Res* 47:1731, 1987.
348. Guo JQ, Lian JY, Xian YM, et al: BCR-ABL protein expression in peripheral blood cells of chronic myelogenous leukemia patients undergoing therapy. *Blood* 83:3629, 1994.
349. Dewald GW, Schad CR, Christensen ER, et al: The application of in situ fluorescent hybridization to detect M bcr/abl fusion in variant Ph chromosomes in CML and ALL. *Cancer Genet Cytogenet* 71:7, 1993.
350. Cox MC, Maffei L, Buffolino S, et al: A comparative analysis of FISH, RT-PCR, and cytogenetics for the diagnosis of bcr-abl-positive leukemias. *Am J Clin Pathol* 109:24, 1998.
351. Sinclair PB, Green AR, Grace C, Nacheva EP: Improved sensitivity of BCR-ABL detection: A triple-probe three-color fluorescence in situ hybridization system. *Blood* 90:1395, 1997.
352. Acar H, Stewart J, Boyd E, Connor MJ: Identification of variant translocations in chronic myeloid leukemia by fluorescence in situ hybridization. *Cancer Genet Cytogenet* 93:115, 1997.
353. Schoch C, Schnittger S, Bursch S, et al: Comparison of chromosome banding analysis, interphase- and hypermetaphase-FISH, qualitative and quantitative PCR for diagnosis and for follow-up in chronic myeloid leukemia: A study of 350 cases. *Leukemia* 16:53, 2002.
354. Yanagi M, Shinjo K, Takeshita A, et al: Simple and reliably sensitive diagnosis and monitoring of Philadelphia chromosome-positive cells in chronic myeloid leukemia by interphase fluorescence in situ hybridization of peripheral blood cells. *Leukemia* 13:542, 1999.
355. Werner M, Ewig M, Nasarek A, et al: Value of fluorescence in situ hybridization for detecting the bcr/abl gene fusion in interphase cells of routine bone marrow specimens. *Diagn Mol Pathol* 6:282, 1997.
356. Chase A, Grand F, Zhang JG, et al: Factors influencing the false positive and negative rates of BCR-ABL fluorescence in situ hybridization. *Genes Chromosomes Cancer* 18:246, 1997.
357. Pelz AF, Kroning H, Franke A, Wieacker P: High reliability and sensitivity of the BCR/ABL1 D-FISH test for the detection of BCR/ABL rearrangements. *Ann Hematol* 81:147, 2002.
358. Hochhaus A, Reiter A, Skladny H, et al: Molecular monitoring of residual disease in chronic myelogenous leukemia patients after therapy. *Recent Results Cancer Res* 144:36, 1998.
359. Wells SJ, Phillips CN, Winton EF, Farhi DC: Reverse transcriptase polymerase chain reaction for bcr-abl fusion in chronic myelogenous leukemia. *Am J Clin Pathol* 105:756, 1996.
360. Cox MC, Maffei L, Buffolino S, et al: A comparative analysis of FISH, RT-PCR, and cytogenetics for the diagnosis of bcr-abl-positive leukemias. *Am J Clin Pathol* 109:24, 1998.
361. Krackoff IH: Studies of uric acid biosynthesis in the chronic leukemias. *Arthritis Rheum* 8:772, 1965.
362. Vogler WR, Bain JA, Huguley CM Jr, et al: Metabolic and therapeutic effects of allopurinol in patients with leukemia and gout. *Am J Med* 40:548, 1966.
363. Zittoun J, Marquet J, Zittoun R: The intracellular content of the three cobalamins at various stages of normal and leukaemic myeloid cell development. *Br J Haematol* 31:299, 1975.
364. Zittoun J, Zittoun R, Marquet J, Sultan C: The three transcobalamins in myeloproliferative disorders and acute leukemia. *Br J Haematol* 31:287, 1975.

365. Rosner F, Schreiber ZA: Serum vitamin B_{12} and vitamin B_{12} binding capacity in chronic myelogenous leukemia and other disorders. *Am J Med Sci* 263:473, 1972.
366. Sternman U-H: Intrinsic factor and the B_{12} binding proteins. *Clin Haematol* 5:473, 1976.
367. Corcino JJ, Zalusky R, Greenberg M, Herbert V: Coexistence of pernicious anaemia and chronic myeloid leukaemia: An experiment of nature involving vitamin B_{12} metabolism. *Br J Haematol* 20:511, 1971.
368. Agis H, Sperr WR, Herndlhofer S, et al: Clinical and prognostic significance of histamine monitoring in patients with CML during treatment with imatinib (STI571). *Ann Oncol* 18:1834, 2007.
369. Youman JD, Taddeini L, Cooper T: Histamine excess symptoms in basophilic chronic granulocytic leukemia. *Arch Intern Med* 131:560, 1973.
370. Rosenthal S, Schwartz JH, Canellos GP: Basophilic chronic granulocytic leukemia with hyperhistaminemia. *Br J Haematol* 36:367, 1977.
371. Gomez GA, Sokal JE, Walsh D: Prognostic features at diagnosis of chronic myelocytic leukemia. *Cancer* 47:2470, 1981.
372. Bellevue R, Dosik H, Spergel G, Gussoff BD: Pseudohyperkalemia and extreme leukocytosis. *J Lab Clin Med* 85:660, 1975.
373. Ballard HS, Marcus AJ: Hypercalcemia in chronic myelogenous leukemia. *N Engl J Med* 282:663, 1970.
374. Evans JJ, Bozdech MJ: Hypokalemia in nonblastic chronic myelogenous leukemia. *Arch Intern Med* 141:786, 1981.
375. Perillie PE, Finch SC: Muramidase studies in Philadelphia-chromosome-positive and chromosome-negative chronic granulocytic leukemia. *N Engl J Med* 283:456, 1970.
376. Gilbert HS, Ginsberg H: Hypocholesterolemia as a manifestation of disease activity in chronic myeloid leukemia. *Cancer* 51:1428, 1983.
377. Muller CP, Wagner AN, Maucher C, Steinke B: Hypocholesterolemia, an unfavorable feature of prognostic value in chronic myeloid leukemia. *Eur J Haematol* 43:235, 1989.
378. Musolino C, Alonci A, Bellomo G, et al: Levels of soluble angiogenin in chronic myeloid malignancies. *Eur J Haematol* 72:416, 2004.
379. Calabro L, Fonsatti E, Bellomo G, et al: Differential levels of soluble endoglin (CD105) in myeloid malignancies. *J Cell Physiol* 194:171, 2003.
380. Morris CM, Fitzgerald PH, Hollings PE, et al: Essential thrombocythemia and the Philadelphia chromosome. *Br J Haematol* 70:13, 1988.
381. Stoll DB, Peterson P, Exten R, et al: Clinical presentation and natural history of patients with essential thrombocythemia and the Philadelphia chromosome. *Am J Hematol* 27:77, 1988.
382. Sessarego M, Defferrari R, Dejana AM, et al: Cytogenetic analysis in essential thrombocythemia at diagnosis and at transformation. *Cancer Genet Cytogenet* 43:57, 1989.
383. Pajor L, Kereskai L, Zsdral K, et al: Philadelphia chromosome and/or bcr-abl mRNA-positive primary thrombocytosis: Morphometric evidence for the transition from essential thrombocythemia to chronic myeloid leukaemia type myeloproliferation. *Histopathology* 42:53, 2003.
384. Blickstein D, Aviram A, Luboshitz J, et al: BCR-ABL transcripts in bone marrow aspirates of Philadelphia-negative essential thrombocythemia patients: Clinical presentation. *Blood* 90:2768, 1997.
385. Cervantes F, Colomer D, Vives-Corrons JL, et al: Chronic myeloid leukemia of thrombocythemic onset: A CML subtype with distinct hematological and molecular features. *Leukemia* 10:1241, 1996.
386. Martiat P, Ifrah N, Rassool F, et al: Molecular analysis of Philadelphia positive essential thrombocythemia. *Leukemia* 3:563, 1989.
387. Michiels JJ, Berneman Z, Schroyens W, et al: Philadelphia (Ph) chromosome–positive thrombocythemia without features of chronic myeloid leukemia in peripheral blood; natural history and diagnostic differentiation from Ph-negative essential thrombocythemia. *Ann Hematol* 83:504, 2004.
388. Blickstein D, Aviram A, Luboshitz J, et al: BCR-ABC transcripts in bone marrow aspirates of Philadelphia-negative essential thrombocythemia patients: Clinical presentation. *Blood* 90:2768, 1997.
389. Pajor L, Kereskai L, Zsdral K, et al: Philadelphia chromosome and/or bcr-abl mRNA positive primary thrombocytosis: Morphometric evidence for the transition from essential thrombocythaemia to chronic myeloid leukaemia type of myeloproliferation. *Histopathology* 42:53, 2003.
390. Damaj G, delabesse E, Le Bihan C, et al: Typical essential thrombocythaemia does not express bcr-abelson fusion transcript. *Br J Haematol* 116:812, 2002.
391. Hsu H-C, Tan L-Y, Au L-C, et al: Detection of bcr-abl gene expression at a low level in blood cells of some patients with essential thrombocythemia. *J Lab Clin Med* 143:125, 2004.
392. Paietta E, Rosen N, Roberts M, et al: Philadelphia chromosome positive essential thrombocythemia evolving into lymphoid blast crisis. *Cancer Genet Cytogenet* 25:227, 1987.
393. Michiels JJ, Prins ME, Hagermeijer A, et al: Philadelphia chromosome-positive thrombocythemia and megakaryoblast leukemia. *Am J Clin Pathol* 88:645, 1987.
394. Kwong YL, Chiu EK, Liang RH, et al: Essential thrombocythemia with BCR/ABL rearrangement. *Cancer Genet Cytogenet* 89:74, 1996.
395. Marasca R, Luppi M, Zucchini P, et al: Might essential thrombocythemia carry Ph anomaly? *Blood* 91:3084, 1998.
396. Sanadi I, Yamamoto S, Ogata M, et al: Detection of the Philadelphia chromosome in chronic neutrophilic leukemia. *Jpn J Clin Oncol* 15:553, 1985.
397. Christopoulus C, Kottoris K, Mikraki V, Anevlavis E: Presence of bcr/abl rearrangement in a patient with chronic neutrophilic leukaemia. *J Clin Pathol* 49:1013, 1996.
398. Pane F, Frigeri F, Sindina M, et al: Neutrophilic-chronic myeloid leukemia: A distinct disease with a specific molecular marker (BCR/ABL with C3/A2 junction). *Blood* 88:2410, 1996.
399. Verstovsek S, Lin H, Kantarjian H, et al: Neutrophilic-chronic myeloid leukemia: Low levels of p 230 BCR/ABL mRNA and undetectable BCR/ABL protein may predict an indolent course. *Cancer* 94:2416, 2002.
400. Ohsaka A, Shiina S, Kobayashi M, et al: Philadelphia chromosome-positive chronic myeloid leukemia expressing p190(BCR-ABL). *Intern Med* 41:1183, 2002.
401. Barnes DJ, Melo JV: Cytogenetic and molecular genetic aspects of chronic myeloid leukaemia. *Acta Haematol* 108:180, 2002.
402. Knowles DM: Thymoma and chronic myelogenous leukemia. *Cancer* 38:414, 1976.
403. Vannier JP, Bizet M, Bastard C, et al: Simultaneous occurrence of a T-cell lymphoma and a chronic myelogenous leukemia with an unusual karyotype. *Leuk Res* 8:647, 1984.
404. Djulbegovi B, Hadley T, Yen F: Occurrence of high-grade T-cell lymphoma in a patient with Philadelphia chromosome-negative chronic myelogenous leukemia with breakpoint cluster region rearrangement. *Am J Hematol* 36:63, 1991.
405. Tittley P, Trempe JM, van der Jagt R, et al: Occurrence of T-cell lymphoma in a patient with Philadelphia chromosome-positive chronic myelogenous leukemia with rearrangements of BCR and TCR-β genes in the lymph nodes. *Am J Hematol* 42:229, 1993.
406. Hornstein P, Nordenson I, Wahlin A: Philadelphia chromosome negative acute lymphoblastic leukemia preceding Philadelphia positive chronic myelogenous leukemia. *Cancer Genet Cytogenet* 39:147, 1989.
407. Ichinohasama R, Miura I, Takahashi N, et al: Ph-negative non-Hodgkin's lymphoma occurring in chronic phase of Ph-positive chronic myelogenous leukemia is defined as a genetically different neoplasm from extramedullary localized blast crisis: Report of two cases and review of the literature. *Leukemia* 14:169, 2000.
408. Rodler E, Welborn J, Hatcher S, et al: Blastic mantle cell lymphoma developing concurrently in a patient with chronic myelogenous leukemia and a review of the literature. *Am J Hematol* 75:231, 2004.
409. Naparstek Y, Zlotnick A, Polliack A: Coexistent chronic myeloid leukemia and IgA monoclonal gammopathy: Report of a case and review of the literature. *Am J Med Sci* 292:111, 1980.
410. Shoenfeld Y, Berliner S, Ayalone A, et al: Monoclonal gammopathy in patients with chronic and acute myeloid leukemia. *Cancer* 54:280, 1984.
411. Tanaka M, Kimura R, Matsutani A, et al: Coexistence of chronic myelogenous leukemia and multiple myeloma. *Acta Haematol* 99:221, 1998.
412. Schwartzmeier JD, Shehata M, Ackermann J, et al: Simultaneous occurrence of chronic myeloid leukemia and multiple myeloma: Evaluation by FISH analysis and in vitro expansion of bone marrow cells. *Leukemia* 17:1426, 2003.
413. Nitta M, Tsuboi K, Yamashita S, et al: Multiple myeloma preceding development of chronic myelogenous leukemia. *Int J Hematol* 69:170, 1999.
414. Vitali C, Bombardieri S, Spremolla G: Chronic myeloid leukemia in Waldenström's macroglobulinemia. *Arch Intern Med* 141:1349, 1981.
415. Whang-Peng J, Gralnick HR, Johnson RE, et al: Chronic granulocytic leukemia (CGL) during the course of chronic lymphocytic leukemia (CLL): Correlation of blood, marrow, and spleen morphology and cytogenetics. *Blood* 43:333, 1974.
416. Schrieber ZA, Axelrod MR, Abebe LS: Coexistence of chronic myelogenous leukemia and chronic lymphocytic leukemia. *Cancer* 54:697, 1984.
417. Specchia G, Buquicchio C, Albano F, et al: Non-treatment-related chronic myeloid leukemia as a second malignancy. *Leuk Res* 28:115, 2004.
418. Esteve J, Cervantes F, Rives S, et al: Simultaneous occurrence of B-cell chronic lymphocytic leukemia and chronic myeloid leukemia with further evolution to lymphoid blast status. *Haematologica* 82:596, 1997.
419. Leoni F, Ferrini PR, Castoldi GL, et al: Simultaneous occurrence of chronic granulocytic leukemia and chronic lymphoid leukemia. *Haematologica* 72:253, 1987.
420. Faguet GB, Little T, Agee JF, Garver FA: Chronic lymphatic leukemia evolving into chronic myelocytic leukemia. *Cancer* 52:1647, 1983.
421. Crescenzi B, Sacchi S, Marasca R, et al: Distinct genomic events in the myeloid and lymphoid lineages in simultaneous presentation of chronic myeloid leukemia and B-chronic lymphocytic leukemia. *Leukemia* 16:955, 2002.
422. Mansat-De Mas V, Regal-Huguet F, Cassar G, et al: Chronic myeloid leukemia associated with B-cell chronic lymphocytic leukemia: Evidence of two separate clones as shown by combined cell-sorting and fluorescence *in situ* hybridization. *Leuk Lymphoma* 44:867, 2003.
423. Lucia E, Martino B, Mammi C, et al: The incidence of JAK2 V617F mutation in bcr/abl-negative chronic myeloproliferative disorders: Assessment by two different detection methods. *Leuk Lymphoma* 18:1, 2008.
424. Jantunen E, Nousiainen T: Ph-positive chronic myelogenous leukemia evolving after polycythemia vera. *Am J Hematol* 37:212, 1991.
425. Hoppen EC, Lewis JP: Polycythemia rubra vera progressing to Ph-positive chronic myelogenous leukemia. *Ann Intern Med* 83:820, 1975.
426. Haq AU: Transformation of polycythemia vera to Ph-positive chronic myelogenous leukemia. *Am J Hematol* 356:110, 1990.
427. Roth AD, Oral A, Przepiorka D, et al: Chronic myelogenous leukemia and acute lymphoblastic leukemia occurring in the course of polycythemia vera. *Am J Hematol* 43:123, 1993.
428. Foviester RH, Louro JM: Philadelphia chromosome abnormality in angiogenic myeloid metaplasia. *Ann Intern Med* 64:622, 1966.
429. Nowell PC, Kant JA, Finan JB, et al: Marrow fibrosis associated with a Philadelphia chromosome. *Cancer Genet Cytogenet* 59:89, 1992.

430. Roth DG, Richman CM, Rowley JD: Chronic myelodysplastic syndrome (preleukemia) with the Philadelphia chromosome. *Blood* 56:262, 1980.
431. Berrebi A, Bruck R, Shtalrid M, Chemke J: Philadelphia chromosome in idiopathic acquired sideroblastic anemia. *Acta Haematol* 72:343, 1984.
432. Suzan F, Terré C, Garcia I, et al: Three cases of typical aplastic anaemia associated with a Philadelphia chromosome. *Br J Haematol* 112:385, 2001.
433. Sica S, Chiusolo P, Zollino M, et al: The association of severe aplastic anaemia with the Philadelphia chromosome and the bcr/abl transcript. *Br J Haematol* 114:961, 2001.
434. Hande K: Hyperuricemia, uric acid nephropathy and the tumor lysis syndrome, in *Renal Complications of Neoplasia*, edited by TD McKinney, p 134. Praeger, New York, 1986.
435. Navolanic PM, Pui CH, Larson RA, et al: Elitek^{TM}-rasburicase: An effective means to prevent and treat hyperuricemia associated with tumor lysis syndrome, a Meeting Report, Dallas, TX, January, 2002. *Leukemia* 17:499, 2003.
436. Jeha S, Pui CH: Recombinant urate oxidase (rasburicase) in the prophylaxis and treatment of tumor lysis syndrome. *Contrib Nephrol* 147:69, 2005.
437. Liu CY, Sims-McCallum RP, Schiffer CA: A single dose of rasburicase is sufficient for the treatment of hyperuricemia in patients receiving chemotherapy. *Leuk Res* 29:463, 2005.
438. Arnold TM, Reuter JP, Delman BS, Shanholtz CB: Use of single-dose rasburicase in an obese female. *Ann Pharmacother* 38:1428, 2004.
439. Bazatbashi MS, Smith MR, Karanes C, et al: Successful management of Ph chromosome chronic myelogenous leukemia with leukapheresis during pregnancy. *Am J Hematol* 38:235, 1991.
440. Strobl FJ, Voelkerding KY, Smith EP: Management of chronic myeloid leukemia during pregnancy with leukapheresis. *J Clin Apher* 14:42, 1999.
441. Kennedy BJ: The evolution of hydroxyurea therapy in chronic myelogenous leukemia. *Semin Oncol* 19(Suppl 9):21, 1992.
442. Tsimberidou AM, Colburn DE, Welch MA, et al: Anagrelide and imatinib mesylate combination therapy in patients with chronic myeloproliferative disorders. *Cancer Chemother Pharmacol* 52:229, 2003.
443. Baccarani M, Saglio G, Goldman J, et al: Evolving concepts in the management of chronic myeloid leukemia. Recommendations from an expert panel of behalf of the European LeukemiaNet. *Blood* 108:1809, 2006.
444. *NCCN Practice Guidelines in Oncology*. v.3.2008. Available at: www.nccn.org/professionsals/physician_gls/.
445. Kantarjian HM, Talpaz M, O'Brien S, et al: Dose escalation of imatinib mesylate can overcome resistance to standard-dose therapy in patients with chronic myelogenous leukemia. *Blood* 101:473, 2003.
446. Marin D, Goldman JM, Olavarria E, Apperley JF: Transient benefit only from increasing the imatinib dose in CML patients who do not achieve complete cytogenetic remissions on conventional doses. *Blood* 102:2702, 2003.
447. Zonder JA, Pemberton P, Brandt H, et al: The effect of dose increase of imatinib mesylate in patients with chronic or accelerated phase chronic myelogenous leukemia with inadequate hematologic or cytogenetic response to initial treatment. *Clin Cancer Res* 9:2092, 2003.
448. Kantarjian H, Talpaz M, O'Brien S, et al: High-dose imatinib mesylate therapy in newly diagnosed Philadelphia chromosome-positive chronic phase chronic myeloid leukemia. *Blood* 103:2873, 2004.
449. Kanda Y, Okamoto S, Tauchi T, et al: Multicenter prospective trial evaluating the tolerability of imatinib for Japanese patients with chronic myelogenous leukemia in the chronic phase: Does body weight matter? *Am J Hematol* 83:835, 2008.
450. Kobayashi S, Kimura F, Kobayashi A, et al: Efficacy of low-dose imatinib in chronic-phase chronic myelogenous leukemia patients. *Ann Hematol* 88:311, 2009.
451. Atallah E, Cortes J: Optimal initial therapy for patients with newly diagnosed chronic myeloid leukemia in chronic phase. *Curr Opin Hematol* 14:138, 2007.
452. Branford S, Seymour JF, Grigg A, et al: BCR-ABL messenger RNA levels continue to decline in patients with chronic phase chronic myeloid leukemia treated with imatinib for more than 5 years and approximately half of all first-line treated patients have stable undetectable BCR-ABL using strict sensitivity criteria. *Clin Cancer Res* 13:7080, 2007.
453. de Lavallade H, Apperley JF, Khorashad JS, et al: Imatinib for newly diagnosed patients with chronic myeloid leukemia: Incidence of sustained responses in an intention-to-treat analysis. *J Clin Oncol* 26:3358, 2008.
454. El-Zimaity MM, Kantarjian H, Talpaz M, et al: Results of imatinib mesylate therapy in chronic myelogenous leukaemia with variant Philadelphia chromosome. *Br J Haematol* 125:187, 2004.
455. Synder DS, McMahon R, Cohen SR, Slovak ML: Chronic myeloid leukemia with an e13a3 BCR-ABL fusion: Benign course responsive to imatinib with an RT-PCR advisory. *Am J Hematol* 75:92, 2004.
456. de Lemos JA, de Oliveira CM, Scerni AC, et al: Differential molecular response of the transcripts B2A2 and B3A2 to imatinib mesylate in chronic myeloid leukemia. *Genet Mol Res* 4:803, 2005.
457. Agirre X, Román-Gómez J, Vázquez I, et al: Coexistence of different clonal populations harboring the b3a2 (p210) and e1a2 (p190) BCR-ABL1 fusion transcripts in chronic myelogenous leukemia resistant to imatinib. *Cancer Genet Cytogenet* 160:22, 2005.
458. Champagne MA, Capdeville R, Krailo M, et al: Imatinib mesylate (STI571) for treatment of children with Philadelphia chromosome-positive leukemia: Results from a Children's Oncology Group phase I study. *Blood* 104:2655, 2004.
459. Cortes J, Talpaz M, O'Brien S, et al: Effects of age on prognosis with imatinib mesylate therapy for patients with Philadelphia chromosome-positive chronic myelogenous leukemia. *Cancer* 98:1105, 2003.
460. Latagliata R, Breccia M, Carmosino I, et al: Elderly patients with Ph+ chronic myelogenous leukemia (CML): Results of imatinib mesylate treatment. *Leuk Res* 29:287, 2005.
461. Guilhot F: Indications for imatinib mesylate therapy and clinical management. *Oncologist* 9:271, 2004.
462. Marin D, Marktel S, Foot N, et al: Granulocyte colony-stimulating factor reverses cytopenia and may permit cytogenetic responses in patients with chronic myeloid leukemia treated with imatinib mesylate. *Haematologica* 88:227, 2003.
463. Quintas-Cardama A, Kantarjian H, O'Brien S, et al: Granulocyte-colony-stimulating factor (filgrastim) may overcome imatinib-induced neutropenia in patients with chronic-phase chronic myelogenous leukemia. *Cancer* 100:2592, 2004.
464. van Deventer HW, Hall MD, Orlowski RZ, et al: Clinical course of thrombocytopenia in patients treated with imatinib mesylate for accelerated phase chronic myelogenous leukemia. *Am J Hematol* 71:184, 2002.
465. Sneed TB, Kantarjian HM, Talpaz M, et al: The significance of myelosuppression during therapy with imatinib mesylate in patients with chronic myelogenous leukemia in chronic phase. *Cancer* 100:116, 2004.
466. Lokeshwar N, Kumar L, Kumari M: Severe bone marrow aplasia following imatinib mesylate in a patient with chronic myelogenous leukemia. *Leuk Lymphoma* 46:781, 2005.
467. Hensley ML, Ford JM: Imatinib treatment: Specific issues related to safety, fertility, and pregnancy. *Semin Hematol* 40:21, 2003.
468. Ferrero D, Pogliani EM, Rege-Cambrin G, et al: Corticosteroids can reverse severe imatinib-induced hepatotoxicity. *Haematologica* 91(6 Suppl):ECR27, 2006.
469. Cross TJ, Bagot C, Portmann B, et al: Imatinib mesylate as a cause of acute liver failure. *Am J Hematol* 83:189, 2006.
470. Esmaeli B, Prieto VG, Butler CE, et al: Severe periorbital edema secondary to STI571 (Gleevec). *Cancer* 95:881, 2002.
471. Elliott MA, Mesa RA, Tefferi A: Adverse events after imatinib mesylate therapy. *N Engl J Med* 346:712, 2002.
472. Kusumi E, Arakawa A, Kami M, et al: Visual disturbance due to retinal edema as a complication of imatinib. *Leukemia* 18:1138, 2004.
473. Mattiuzzi GN, Cortes JE, Talpaz M, et al: Development of Varicella-Zoster virus infection in patients with chronic myelogenous leukemia treated with imatinib mesylate. *Clin Cancer Res* 9:976, 2003.
474. Gambacorti-Passerini C, Tornaghi L, Cavagnini F, et al: Gynaecomastia in men with chronic myeloid leukaemia after imatinib. *Lancet* 361:1954, 2003.
475. Novaretti MCZ, Fonseca GHH, Conchon M, et al: First case of immune-mediated haemolytic anaemia associated with imatinib mesylate. *Eur J Haematol* 71:455, 2003.
476. Kyathari S, Chao K, Liu D, Seiter K: Severe imatinib-associated muscle edema in patients with chronic Myelogenous leukemia and marked leukocytosis. *Leuk Lymphoma* 49:1002, 2008.
477. Ostro D, Lipton J: Unusual fluid retention with imatinib therapy for chronic myeloid leukemia. *Leuk Lymphoma* 48:195, 2007.
478. Ohnishi K, Sakai F, Kudoh S, Ohno R: Twenty-seven cases of drug-induced interstitial lung disease associated with imatinib mesylate. *Leukemia* 20:1162, 2006.
479. Rajda J, Phatak PD: Reversible drug-induced interstitial pneumonitis following imatinib mesylate therapy. *Am J Hematol* 79:80, 2005.
480. Assouline S, Laneuville P, Gambacorti-Passerini C: Panniculitis during dasatinib therapy for imatinib-resistant chronic myelogenous leukemia. *N Engl J Med* 354:2623, 2006.
481. Osorio S, Noblejas AG, Durán A, Steegmann JL: Imatinib mesylate induces hypophosphatemia in patients with chronic myeloid leukemia in late chronic phase, and this effect is associated with response. *Am J Hematol* 82:394, 2007.
482. Fitter S, Dewar AL, Kostakis P, et al: Long-term imatinib therapy promotes bone formation in CML patients. *Blood* 111:2538, 2008.
483. Berman E, Nicolaides M, Maki RG, et al: Altered bone and mineral metabolism in patients receiving imatinib mesylate. *N Engl J Med* 354:2006, 2006.
484. Sanchez-Gonzalez B, Pascual-Ramirez JC, Fernandez-Abellian P, et al: Severe skin reaction to imatinib in a case of Philadelphia-positive acute lymphoblastic leukemia. *Blood* 101:2446, 2003.
485. Drummond A, Micallef-Eynaud P, Douglas WS, et al: A spectrum of skin reactions caused by the tyrosine kinase inhibitor imatinib mesylate (STI 571, Glivec). *Br J Haematol* 120:911, 2003.
486. Rule SAJ, O'Brien SG, Crossman LC: Managing cutaneous reactions to imatinib therapy. *Blood* 100:3434, 2002.
487. Nelson RP Jr, Cornetta K, Ward KE:, et al Desensitization to imatinib in patients with leukemia. *Ann Allergy Asthma Immunol* 97:216, 2006.
488. Liu D, Seiter K, Mathews T, et al: Sweet's syndrome with CML cell infiltration of the skin in a patient with chronic-phase CML while taking imatinib mesylate. *Leuk Res* 28SI:S61, 2004.
489. Brazzelli V, Prestinari F, Roveda E, et al: Pityriasis rosea-like eruption during treatment with imatinib mesylate: Description of 3 cases. *J Am Acad Dermatol* 53(Suppl 1):S240, 2005.
490. Deguchi N, Kawamura T, Shimizu A, et al: Imatinib mesylate causes palmoplantar hyperkeratosis and nail dystrophy in three patients with chronic myeloid leukaemia. *Br J Dermatol* 154:1216, 2006.
491. Pascual JC, Matarredona J, Miralles J, et al: Oral and cutaneous lichenoid reaction secondary to imatinib: Report of two cases. *Int J Dermatol* 45:1471, 2006.

492. Etienne G, Cony-Makhoul P, Mahon FX: Imatinib mesylate and gray hair. *N Engl J Med* 346:645, 2002.
493. Tjao AS, Kantarjian H, Cortes J, et al: Imatinib mesylate causes hypopigmentation in the skin. *Cancer* 98:2483, 2003.
494. Legros L, Cassuto JP, Ortonne JP: Imatinib mesilate (Glivec): A systemic depigmenting agent for extensive vitiligo? *Br J Dermatol* 153:691, 2005.
495. Beham-Schmid C, Apfelbeck U, Sill H, et al: Treatment of chronic myelogenous leukemia with the tyrosine kinase inhibitor STI571 results in marked regression of bone marrow fibrosis. *Blood* 99:381, 2002.
496. Kantarjian HM, Bueso-Ramos CE, Talpaz M, et al: The degree of bone marrow fibrosis in chronic myelogenous leukemia is not a prognostic factor with imatinib mesylate therapy. *Leuk Lymphoma* 46:993, 2005.
497. Buesche G, Ganser A, Schlegelberger B, et al: Marrow fibrosis and its relevance during imatinib treatment of chronic myeloid leukemia. *Leukemia* 21:2420, 2007.
498. Ebos JM, Tran J, Master Z, et al: Imatinib mesylate (STI-571) reduces the Bcr-Abl-mediated vascular endothelial growth factor secretion in chronic myelogenous leukemia. *Mol Cancer Res* 1:89, 2002.
499. Kvasnicka HM, Thiele J, Staib P, et al: Reversal of bone marrow angiogenesis in chronic myeloid leukemia following imatinib mesylate (STI571) therapy. *Blood* 103:3549, 2004.
500. Larson RA, Druker BJ, Guilhot F, et al: Imatinib pharmacokinetics and its correlation with response and safety in chronic-phase chronic myeloid leukemia: A subanalysis of the IRIS study. *Blood* 111:4022, 2008.
501. Picard S, Titier K, Etienne G, et al: Trough imatinib plasma levels are associated with both cytogenetic and molecular responses to standard-dose imatinib in chronic myeloid leukemia. *Blood* 109:3496, 2007.
502. Schmidli H, Peng B, Riviere GJ, et al: Population pharmacokinetics of imatinib mesylate in patients with chronic-phase chronic myeloid leukaemia: Results of a phase III study. *Br J Clin Pharmacol* 60:35, 2005.
503. Ozdemir E, Koc Y, Kansu E: Successful treatment of chronic myeloid leukemia with imatinib mesylate in a patient with chronic renal failure on hemodialysis. *Am J Hematol* 81:474, 2006.
504. Darkow T, Henk HJ, Thomas SK, et al: Treatment interruptions and non-adherence with imatinib and associated healthcare costs: A retrospective analysis among managed care patients with chronic myelogenous leukaemia. *Pharmacoeconomics* 25:481, 2007.
505. Cortes J, Giles F, O'Brien S, et al: Results of imatinib mesylate therapy in patients with refractory or recurrent acute myeloid leukemia, high-risk myelodysplastic syndrome, and myeloproliferative disorders. *Cancer* 97:2760, 2003.
506. Kantarjian H, Talpaz M, O'Brien S, et al: Prediction of initial cytogenetic response for subsequent major and complete cytogenetic response to imatinib mesylate therapy in patients with Philadelphia chromosome-positive chronic myelogenous leukemia. *Cancer* 98:1776, 2003.
507. Rousselot P, Huguet F, Rea D, et al: Imatinib mesylate discontinuation in patients with chronic myelogenous leukemia in complete molecular remission for more than 2 years. *Blood* 109:58, 2007.
508. Carella AM, Lerma E: Durable responses in chronic myeloid leukemia patients maintained with lower doses of imatinib mesylate after achieving molecular remission. *Ann Hematol* 86:749, 2007.
509. Ghanima W, Kahrs J, Dahl TG 3rd, Tjonnfjord GE: Sustained cytogenetic response after discontinuation of imatinib mesylate in a patient with chronic myeloid leukaemia. *Eur J Haematol* 72:441, 2004.
510. Cortes J, O'Brien S, Kantarjian H: Discontinuation of imatinib therapy after achieving a molecular response. *Blood* 104:2204, 2004.
511. Okabe S, Tauchi T, Ishii Y, et al: Sustained complete cytogenetic remission in a patient with chronic myeloid leukemia after discontinuation of imatinib mesylate therapy. *Int J Hematol* 85:173, 2007.
512. Merante S, Orlandi E, Bernasconi P, et al: Outcome of four patients with chronic myeloid leukemia after imatinib mesylate discontinuation. *Haematologica* 90:979, 2005.
513. Graham SM, Jorgensen HG, Allan E, et al: Primitive, quiescent, Philadelphia-positive stem cells from patients with chronic myeloid leukemia are insensitive to STI571 in vitro. *Blood* 99:319, 2002.
514. Meera V, Jijina F, Shrikande M, et al: Twin pregnancy in a patient of chronic myeloid leukemia on imatinib therapy. *Leuk Res* 32:1620, 2008.
515. Skoumalova I, Vondrakova J, Rohon P, et al: Successful childbirth in a patient with chronic myelogenous leukemia treated with imatinib mesylate during early pregnancy. *Biomed Pap Med Fac Univ Palacky Olomouc Czech Repub* 152:121, 2008.
516. Ali R, Ozkalemka F, Ozçelik T, et al: Pregnancy under treatment of imatinib and successful labor in a patient with chronic myelogenous leukemia (CML). Outcome of discontinuation of imatinib therapy after achieving a molecular remission. *Leuk Res* 29:971, 2005.
517. Shapira T, Pereg D, Lishner M: How I treat acute and chronic leukemia in pregnancy. *Blood Rev* 22:247, 2008.
518. Pye SM, Cortes J, Ault P, Hatfield A, et al: The effects of imatinib on pregnancy outcome. *Blood* 111:5505, 2008.
519. Ault P, Kantarjian H, O'Brien S, et al: Pregnancy among patients with chronic myeloid leukemia treated with imatinib. *J Clin Oncol* 24:1204, 2006.
520. Ramasamy K, Hayden J, Lim Z, et al: Successful pregnancies involving men with chronic myeloid leukaemia on imatinib therapy. *Br J Haematol* 137:374, 2007.
521. Breccia M, Cannella L, Montefusco E, et al: Male patients with chronic myeloid leukemia treated with imatinib involved in healthy pregnancies: Report of five cases. *Leuk Res* 32:519, 2008.
522. Gambacorti-Passerini CB, Tornaghi L, Marangon E, et al: Imatinib concentrations in human milk. *Blood* 109:1790, 2007.
523. O'Dwyer ME, Gatter KM, Loriaux M, et al: Demonstration of Philadelphia chromosome negative abnormal clones in patients with chronic myelogenous leukemia during major cytogenetic responses induced by imatinib mesylate. *Leukemia* 17:481, 2003.
524. Guilbert-Douet N, Morel F, LeBris M-J, et al: Clonal chromosomal abnormalities in the Philadelphia chromosome negative cells of chronic myeloid leukemia patients treated with imatinib. *Leukemia* 18:1140, 2004.
525. Deininger MWN: Cytogenetic studies in patients on imatinib. *Semin Hematol* 40:50, 2003.
526. Bumm T, Muller C, Al-Ali K, et al: Emergence of clonal cytogenetic abnormalities in Ph-cells in some CML patients in cytogenetic remission to imatinib but restoration of polyclonal hematopoiesis in the majority. *Blood* 101:1941, 2003.
527. Goldberg SL, Medan RA, Rowley SD, et al: Myelodysplastic subclones in chronic myeloid leukemia: Implications for imatinib mesylate therapy. *Blood* 101:781, 2003.
528. Farag SS, Ruppert AS, Mrozek K, et al: Prognostic significance of additional cytogenetic abnormalities in newly diagnosed patients with Philadelphia chromosome-positive chronic myelogenous leukemia treated with interferon-α: A Cancer and Leukemia Group B study. *Int J Oncol* 25:143, 2004.
529. Andersen MK, Pedersen-Bjergaard J, Kjeldsen I, et al: Clonal Ph-negative hematopoiesis in CML after therapy with imatinib mesylate is frequently characterized by trisomy 8. *Leukemia* 16:1390, 2002.
530. Terre C, Eclache V, Rousselot P, et al: Report of 34 patients with clonal chromosomal abnormalities in Philadelphia-negative cells during imatinib treatment of Philadelphia-positive chronic myeloid leukemia. *Leukemia* 18:1340, 2004.
531. Jabbour E, Kantarjian HM, Abruzzo LV, et al: Chromosomal abnormalities in Philadelphia chromosome negative metaphases appearing during imatinib mesylate therapy in patients with newly diagnosed chronic myeloid leukemia in chronic phase. *Blood* 110:2991, 2007.
532. Cortes JE, Talpaz M, Giles F, et al: Prognostic significance of cytogenetic clonal evolution in patients with chronic myelogenous leukemia on imatinib mesylate therapy. *Blood* 101:3794, 2003.
533. Chee YL, Vickers MA, Stevenson D, et al: Fatal myelodysplastic syndrome developing during therapy with imatinib mesylate and characterised by the emergence of complex Philadelphia negative clones. *Leukemia* 17:634, 2003.
534. Nimmanapalli R, O'Bryan E, Huang M, et al: Molecular characterization and sensitivity of STI-571 (imatinib mesylate, Gleevec)-resistant, Bcr-Abl-positive, human acute leukemia cells to SRC kinase inhibitor PD180970 and 17-allylamino-17-demethoxygeldanamycin. *Cancer Res* 62:5761, 2002.
535. Paterson SC, Smith KD, Holyoake TL, Jorgensen HG: Is there a cloud in the silver lining for imatinib? *Br J Cancer* 88:983, 2003.
536. Hochhaus A, La Rosse P: Imatinib therapy in chronic myelogenous leukemia: Strategies to avoid and overcome resistance. *Leukemia* 18:1320, 2004.
537. Cowan-Jacob SW, Guez V, Fendrich G, et al: Imatinib (STI571) resistance in chronic myelogenous leukemia: Molecular basis of the underlying mechanism and potential strategies for treatment. *Mini Rev Med Chem* 4:285, 2004.
538. Weisberg E, Griffin JD: Resistance to imatinib (Glivec): Update on clinical mechanisms. *Drug Resist Updat* 6:231, 2003.
539. Melo JV: Resistance to imatinib mesylate in CML: All BCR-ABL mutations "are created equal but some are more equal than others." *Blood* 101:4231, 2003.
540. Villuendas R, Steegmann JL, Pollán M, et al: Identification of genes involved in imatinib resistance in CML: A gene-expression profiling approach. *Leukemia* 20:1047, 2006.
541. Jiang X, Zhao Y, Forrest D, et al: Stem cell biomarkers in chronic myeloid leukemia. *Dis Markers* 24:201, 2008.
542. Barnes DJ, Melo JV: Primitive, quiescent and difficult to kill: The role of non-proliferating stem cells in chronic myeloid leukemia. *Cell Cycle* 5:2862, 2006.
543. Michor F, Hughes TP, Iwasa Y, et al: Dynamics of chronic myeloid leukaemia. *Nature* 435:1267, 2005.
544. Jørgensen HG, Copland M, Allan EK, et al: Intermittent exposure of primitive quiescent chronic myeloid leukemia cells to granulocyte-colony stimulating factor in vitro promotes their elimination by imatinib mesylate. *Clin Cancer Res* 12:626, 2006.
545. Holtz M, Forman SJ, Bhatia R: Growth factor stimulation reduces residual quiescent chronic myelogenous leukemia progenitors remaining after imatinib treatment. *Cancer Res* 67:1113, 2007.
546. Jin L, Tabe Y, Konoplev S, et al: CXCR4 up-regulation by imatinib induces chronic myelogenous leukemia (CML) cell migration to bone marrow stroma and promotes survival of quiescent CML cells. *Mol Cancer Ther* 7:48, 2008.
547. le Coutre P, Tassi E, Varella-Garcia M, et al: Induction of resistance to the Abelson inhibitor STI571 in human leukemic cells through gene amplification. *Blood* 95:1758, 2000.
548. Campbell LJ, Patsouris C, Rayeroux KC, et al: BCR/ABL amplification in chronic myelocytic leukemia blast crisis following imatinib mesylate administration. *Cancer Genet Cytogenet* 139:30, 2002.
549. Donato NJ, Wu JY, Stapley J, et al: BCR-ABL independence and LYN kinase overexpression in chronic myelogenous leukemia cells selected for resistance to STI571. *Blood* 101:690, 2003.
550. Illmer T, Schaich M, Platzbecker U, et al: P-glycoprotein-mediated drug efflux is a resistance mechanism of chronic myelogenous leukemia cells to treatment with imatinib mesylate. *Leukemia* 18:401, 2004.

551. Mahon FX, Belloc F, Lagarde V, et al: MDR1 gene overexpression confers resistance to imatinib mesylate in leukemia cell line models. *Blood* 101:2368, 2003.
552. Gambacorti-Passerini C, Barni R, le Coutre P, et al: Role of alpha$_1$ acid glycoprotein in the in vivo resistance of human BCR-ABL(+) leukemic cells to the abl inhibitor STI571. *J Natl Cancer Inst* 92:1641, 2000.
553. White DL, Saunders VA, Dang P, et al: OCT-1-mediated influx is a key determinant of the intracellular uptake of imatinib but not nilotinib (AMN107): Reduced OCT-1 activity is the cause of low in vitro sensitivity to imatinib. *Blood* 108:697, 2006.
554. Hiwase DK, Saunders V, Hewett D, et al: Dasatinib cellular uptake and efflux in chronic myeloid leukemia cells: Therapeutic implications. *Clin Cancer Res* 14:3881, 2008.
555. Jordanides NE, Jorgensen HG, Holyoake TL, et al: Functional ABCG2 is overexpressed on primary CML CD34+ cells and is inhibited by imatinib mesylate. *Blood* 108:1370, 2006.
556. Ossard-Receveur A, Bernheim A, Clausse B, et al: Duplication of the Ph-chromosome as a possible mechanism of resistance to imatinib mesylate in patients with chronic myelogenous leukemia. *Cancer Genet Cytogenet* 163:189, 2005.
557. Szych CM, Liesveld JL, Iqbal MA, et al: Isodicentric Philadelphia chromosomes in imatinib mesylate (Gleevec)-resistant patients. *Cancer Genet Cytogenet* 174:132, 2007.
558. Roche-Lestienne C, Preudhomme C: Mutations in the ABL kinase domain pre-exist the onset of imatinib treatment. *Semin Hematol* 21:80, 2003.
559. Corbin AS, LaRosee P, Stoffregen EP, et al: Several Bcr-Abl kinase domain mutants associated with imatinib mesylate resistance remain sensitive to imatinib. *Blood* 101:4611, 2003.
560. Khorashad JS, Anand M, Marin D, et al: The presence of a BCR-ABL mutant allele in CML does not always explain clinical resistance to imatinib. *Leukemia* 20:658, 2006.
561. Wei Y, Hardling M, Olsson B, et al: Not all imatinib resistance in CML are BCR-ABL kinase domain mutations. *Ann Hematol* 85:841, 2006.
562. Soverini S, Colarossi S, Gnani A, et al: Contribution of ABL kinase domain mutations to imatinib resistance in different subsets of Philadelphia-positive patients: By the GIMEMA Working Party on Chronic Myeloid Leukemia. *Clin Cancer Res* 12:7374, 2006.
563. Sherbenou DW, Wong MJ, Humayun A, et al: Mutations of the BCR-ABL-kinase domain occur in a minority of patients with stable complete cytogenetic response to imatinib. *Leukemia* 21:489, 2007.
564. Miething C, Mugler C, Grundler R, et al: Phosphorylation of tyrosine 393 in the kinase domain of Bcr-Abl influences the sensitivity towards imatinib in vivo. *Leukemia* 17:1695, 2003.
565. Branford S, Rudzki Z, Walsh S, et al: Detection of BRC-ABL mutations in patients with CML treated with imatinib is virtually always accompanied by clinical resistance, and mutations in the ATP phosphate-binding loop (P-loop) are associated with a poor prognosis. *Blood* 102:276, 2003.
566. Nicolini FE, Corm S, Lê QH, et al: Mutation status and clinical outcome of 89 imatinib mesylate-resistant chronic myelogenous leukemia patients: A retrospective analysis from the French intergroup of CML (Fi(phi)-LMC GROUP). *Leukemia* 20:1061, 2006.
567. Quintás-Cardama A, Cortes J: Therapeutic options against BCR-ABL1 T315I-positive chronic myelogenous leukemia. *Clin Cancer Res* 14:4392, 2008.
568. Modugno M, Casale E, Soncini C, et al: Crystal structure of the T315I Abl mutant in complex with the aurora kinases inhibitor PHA-739358. *Cancer Res* 67:7987, 2007.
569. Jabbour E, Kantarjian H, Jones D, et al: Characteristics and outcomes of patients with chronic myeloid leukemia and T315I mutation following failure of imatinib mesylate therapy. *Blood* 112:53, 2008.
570. de Lavallade H, Khorashad JS, Davis HP, et al: Interferon-alpha or homoharringtonine as salvage treatment for chronic myeloid leukemia patients who acquire the T315I BCR-ABL mutation. *Blood* 110:2779, 2007.
571. Jilani I, Kantarjian H, Gorre M, et al: Phosphorylation levels of BCR-ABL, CrkL, AKT and STAT5 in imatinib-resistant chronic myeloid leukemia cells implicate alternative pathway usage as a survival strategy. *Leuk Res* 32:643, 2008.
572. Pocaly M, Lagarde V, Etienne G, et al: Overexpression of the heat-shock protein 70 is associated to imatinib resistance in chronic myeloid leukemia. *Leukemia* 21:93, 2007.
573. Carter BZ, Mak DH, Schober WD, et al: Regulation of survivin expression through Bcr-Abl/MAPK cascade: Targeting survivin overcomes imatinib resistance and increases imatinib sensitivity in imatinib-responsive CML cells. *Blood* 107:1555, 2006.
574. Wu J, Meng F, Kong LY, et al: Association between imatinib-resistant BCR-ABL mutation-negative leukemia and persistent activation of LYN kinase. *J Natl Cancer Inst* 100:926, 2008.
575. Hochhaus A, Erben P, Ernst T, Mueller MC: Resistance to targeted therapy in chronic myelogenous leukemia. *Semin Hematol* 44:S15, 2007.
576. Feller SM, Tuchscherer G, Voss J: Hihg affinity molecular disruption of GRB2 protein complexes as a therapeutic strategy for chronic myelogenous leukemia. *Leuk Lymphoma* 44:411, 2003.
577. Hochhaus A: Cytogenetic and molecular mechanisms of resistance to imatinib. *Semin Hematol* 40:69, 2003.
578. Ohno R, Nakamura Y: Prediction of response to imatinib by cDNA microarray analysis. *Semin Hematol* 40:42, 2003.
579. Cortes J, Kantarjian H: Beyond dose escalation: Clinical options for relapse or resistance in chronic myelogenous leukemia. *J Natl Compr Canc Netw* 6 Suppl 2:S22, 2008.
580. Talpaz M, Shah NP, Kantarjian H, et al: Dasatinib in imatinib-resistant Philadelphia chromosome-positive leukemias. *N Engl J Med* 354:2531, 2006.
581. Martinelli G, Soverini S, Rosti G, Baccarani M: Dual tyrosine kinase inhibitors in chronic myeloid leukemia. *Leukemia* 19:1872, 2005.
582. Wong SF: Dasatinib dosing strategies in Philadelphia chromosome-positive leukemia. *J Oncol Pharm Pract* 15:17, 2009.
583. Shah NP, Kantarjian HM, Kim DW, et al: Intermittent target inhibition with dasatinib 100 mg once daily preserves efficacy and improves tolerability in imatinib-resistant and -intolerant chronic-phase chronic myeloid leukemia. *J Clin Oncol* 26:3204, 2008.
584. Hochhaus A, Kantarjian HM, Baccarani M, et al: Dasatinib induces notable hematologic and cytogenetic responses in chronic-phase chronic myeloid leukemia after failure of imatinib therapy. *Blood* 109:2303, 2007.
585. Kantarjian H, Pasquini R, Hamerschlak N, et al: Dasatinib or high-dose imatinib for chronic-phase chronic myeloid leukemia after failure of first-line imatinib: A randomized phase 2 trial. *Blood* 109:5143, 2007.
586. Porkka K, Koskenvesa P, Lundán T, et al: Dasatinib crosses the blood-brain barrier and is an efficient therapy for central nervous system Philadelphia chromosome-positive leukemia. *Blood* 112:1005, 2008.
587. Baraska M, Lewandowski K, Gniot M, et al: Dasatinib treatment can overcome imatinib and nilotinib resistance in CML patient carrying F359I mutation of BCR-ABL oncogene. *J Appl Genet* 49:201, 2008.
588. Hiwase DK, Saunders V, Hewett D, et al: Dasatinib cellular uptake and efflux in chronic myeloid leukemia cells: Therapeutic implications. *Clin Cancer Res* 14:3881, 2008.
589. Soverini S, Colarossi S, Gnani A, et al: Resistance to dasatinib in Philadelphia-positive leukemia patients and the presence or the selection of mutations at residues 315 and 317 in the BCR-ABL kinase domain. *Haematologica* 92:401, 2007.
590. Golemovic M, Verstovsek S, Giles F, et al: AMN107, a novel amino pyrimidine inhibitor of Bcr-Abl, has *in vitro* activity against imatinib-resistant chronic myeloid leukemia. *Clin Cancer Res* 11:4941, 2005.
591. Jørgensen HG, Allan EK, Jordanides NE, et al: Nilotinib exerts equipotent antiproliferative effects to imatinib and does not induce apoptosis in CD34+ CML cells. *Blood* 109:4016, 2007.
592. Kantarjian HM, Giles F, Gattermann N, et al: Nilotinib (formerly AMN107), a highly selective BCR-ABL tyrosine kinase inhibitor, is effective in patients with Philadelphia chromosome-positive chronic myelogenous leukemia in chronic phase following imatinib resistance and intolerance. *Blood* 110:3540, 2007.
593. Hazarika M, Jiang X, Liu Q, et al: Tasigna for chronic and accelerated phase Philadelphia chromosome-positive chronic myelogenous leukemia resistant to or intolerant of imatinib. *Clin Cancer Res* 14:5325, 2008.
594. Weisberg E, Catley L, Wright RD, et al: Beneficial effects of combining nilotinib and imatinib in preclinical models of BCR-ABL+ leukemias. *Blood* 109:2112, 2007.
595. Tipping AJ, Mahon FX, Zafirides G, et al: Drug responses of imatinib mesylate-resistant cells: Synergism of imatinib with other chemotherapeutic drugs. *Leukemia* 16:2349, 2002.
596. Tipping AJ, Melo JV: Imatinib mesylate in combination with other hemotherapeutic drugs: *In vitro* studies. *Semin Hematol* 40:83, 2003.
597. Kantarjian HM, Talpaz M, Smith TL, et al: Homoharringtonine and low-dose cytarabine in the management of late chronic-phase chronic myelogenous leukemia. *J Clin Oncol* 18:3513, 2000.
598. O'Dwyer ME, La Rosee P, Nimmanapalli R, et al: Recent advances in Philadelphia chromosome-positive malignancies: The potential role of arsenic trioxide. *Semin Hematol* 39:18, 2002.
599. Kantarjian HM, O'Brien S, Corteo J, et al: Results of decitabine (5-aza-2′-deoxycytidine) therapy in 130 patients with chronic myelogenous leukemia. *Cancer* 98:522, 2003.
600. Issa JP, Garcia-Manero G, Giles FJ, et al: Phase 1 study of low-dose prolonged exposure schedules of the hypomethylating agent 5-aza-2′-deoxycytidine (decitabine) in hematopoietic malignancies. *Blood* 103:1635, 2004.
601. Chand M, Thakuri M, Keung YK: Imatinib mesylate associated with delayed hematopoietic recovery after concomitant chemotherapy. *Leukemia* 18:886, 2004.
602. O'Hare T, Walters DK, Stoffregen EP, et al: Combined Abl inhibitor therapy for minimizing drug resistance in chronic myelogenous leukemia. Src/Abl inhibitors are compatible with imatinib. *Clin Cancer Res* 11:6987, 2005.
603. Sun X, Layton JE, Elefanty A, Lieschke GJ: Comparison of effects of the tyrosine kinase inhibitors AG957, AG490, and STI571 on BCRABL-expressing cells, demonstrating synergy between AG490 and STI571. *Blood* 97:2008, 2001.
604. Mohi MG, Boulton C, Gu TL, et al: Combination of rapamycin and protein tyrosine kinase (PTK) inhibitors for the treatment of leukemias caused by oncogenic PTKs. *Proc Natl Acad Sci U S A* 101:3130, 2004.
605. Gatto S, Scappini B, Pham L, et al: The proteasome inhibitor PS-341 inhibits growth and induces apoptosis in Bcr/Abl-positive cell lines sensitive and resistant to imatinib mesylate. *Haematologica* 88:853, 2003.
606. Dai Y, Rahmani M, Pei XY, et al: Bortezomib and flavopiridol interact synergistically to induce apoptosis in chronic myeloid leukemia cells resistant to imatinib mesylate through both Bcr/Abl-dependent and -independent mechanisms. *Blood* 104:509, 2004.
607. Yu C, Rahmani M, Conrad D, et al: The proteasome inhibitor bortezomib interacts synergistically with histone deacetylase inhibitors to induce apoptosis in Bcr/Abl+ cells sensitive and resistant to STI571. *Blood* 102:3765, 2003.
608. Fiskus W, Pranpat M, Bali P, et al: Combined effects of novel tyrosine kinase inhibitor AMN107 and histone deacetylase inhibitor LBH589 against Bcr-Abl-expressing human leukemia cells. *Blood* 108:645, 2006.
609. Chu S, Holtz M, Gupta M, Bhatia R: BCR/ABL kinase inhibition by imatinib mesylate enhances MAP kinase activity in chronic myelogenous leukemia CD34+ cells. *Blood* 103:3167, 2004.

610. Kuroda J, Kimura S, Segawa H, et al: The third-generation bisphosphonate zoledronate synergistically augments the anti-Ph+ leukemia activity of imatinib mesylate. *Blood* 102:2229, 2003.
611. Keating A: Chronic myeloid leukemia: Current therapies and the potential role of farnesyltransferase inhibitors. *Semin Hematol* 39:11, 2002.
612. Daley GQ: Towards combination target-directed chemotherapy for chronic myeloid leukemia: Role of farnesyl transferase inhibitors. *Semin Hematol* 40:11, 2003.
613. Nakajima A, Tauchi T, Sumi M, et al: Efficacy of SCH66336, a farnesyl transferase inhibitor, in conjunction with imatinib against BCRABL-positive cells. *Mol Cancer Ther* 2:219, 2003.
614. Hoover RR, Mahon FX, Melo JV, Daley GQ: Overcoming STI571 resistance with the farnesyl transferase inhibitor SCH66336. *Blood* 100:1068, 2002.
615. Druker BJ: Overcoming resistance to imatinib by combining targeted agents. *Mol Cancer Ther* 2:225, 2003.
616. Cortes J, Albitar M, Thomas D, et al: Efficacy of the farnesyl transferase inhibitor R115777 in chronic myeloid leukemia and other hematologic malignancies. *Blood* 101:1692, 2003.
617. Sawyers CL, Hochhaus A, Feldman E, et al: Imatinib induces hematologic and cytogenetic responses in patients with chronic myelogenous leukemia in myeloid blast crisis: Results of a phase II study. *Blood* 99:3530, 2002.
618. Gorre ME, Ellwood-Yen K, Chiosis G, et al: BCR-ABL point mutants isolated from patients with imatinib mesylate-resistant chronic myeloid leukemia remain sensitive to inhibitors of the BCR-ABL chaperone heat shock protein 90. *Blood* 100:3041, 2002.
619. Deininger M: Resistance and relapse with imatinib in CML: Causes and consequences. *J Natl Compr Canc Netw* 6 Suppl 2:S11, 2008.
620. Wu CJ, Neuberg D, Chillemi A, et al: Quantitative monitoring of BCR/ABL transcript during STI-571 therapy. *Leuk Lymphoma* 43:2281, 2002.
621. Druker BJ: Imatinib as a paradigm of targeted therapies. *J Clin Oncol* 21:239, 2003.
622. Druker BJ: STI571 (Gleevec) as a paradigm for cancer therapy. *Trends Mol Med* 8:S14, 2002.
623. Merx K, Muller MC, Kreil S, et al: Early reduction of BCR-ABL mRNA transcript levels predicts cytogenetic response in chronic phase CML patients treated with imatinib after failure of interferon alpha. *Leukemia* 16:1579, 2002.
624. Tam CS, Kantarjian H, Garcia-Manero G, et al: Failure to achieve a major cytogenetic response by 12 months defines inadequate response in patients receiving nilotinib or dasatinib as second or subsequent line therapy for chronic myeloid leukemia. *Blood* 112:516, 2008.
625. Carella AM: Questioning the aim of CML therapy in the era of Imatinib? *Leukemia* 17:1199, 2003.
626. DeAngelo DJ, Ritz J: Imatinib therapy for patients with chronic myelogenous leukemia: Are patients living longer? *Clin Cancer Res* 10:1, 2004.
627. Goldman JM, Marin D, Olavarria E, Apperley JF: Clinical decisions for chronic myeloid leukemia in the imatinib era. *Semin Hematol* 40:98, 2003.
628. Goldman JM: Chronic myeloid leukemia—Still a few questions. *Exp Hematol* 32:2, 2004.
629. Goldman JM: How I treat chronic myeloid leukemia in the imatinib era. *Blood* 110:2828, 2007.
630. Bonifazi F, Bandini G, Rondelli D, et al: Reduced incidence of GVHD without increase in relapse with low-dose rabbit ATG in the preparative regimen for unrelated bone marrow transplants in CML. *Bone Marrow Transplant* 32:237, 2003.
631. Baccarani M, Russo D, Rosti G, Martinelli G: Interferon-alpha for chronic myeloid leukemia. *Semin Hematol* 40:22, 2003.
632. Kluin-Nelemans HC, Buck G, Le Cessie S, et al: Randomized comparison of low-dose versus high-dose interferon-alfa in chronic myeloid leukemia: Prospective collaboration of 3 joint trials by the MRC and HOVON groups. *Blood* 103:4408, 2004.
633. Michallet M, Maloisel F, Delain M, et al: Pegylated recombinant interferon alpha-2b vs recombinant interferon alpha-2b for the initial treatment of chronic-phase chronic myelogenous leukemia: A phase III study. *Leukemia* 18:309, 2004.
634. Lipton JH, Khoroshko N, Golenkov A, et al: Phase II, randomized, multicenter, comparative study of peginterferon-alpha-2a (40 kD) (Pegasys) versus interferon alpha-2a (Roferon-A) in patients with treatment-naïve, chronic-phase chronic myelogenous leukemia. *Leuk Lymphoma* 48:497, 2007.
635. Garcia-Manero G, Talpaz M, Giles FJ, et al: Treatment of Philadelphia chromosome-positive chronic myelogenous leukemia with weekly polyethylene glycol formulation of interferon-alpha-2b and low-dose cytosine arabinoside. *Cancer* 97:3010, 2003.
636. Roy L, Guilhot J, Krahnke T, et al: Survival advantage from imatinib compared with the combination interferon-alpha plus cytarabine in chronic-phase chronic myelogenous leukemia: Historical comparison between two phase 3 trials. *Blood* 108:1478, 2006.
637. Talpaz M: Interferon-alfa-based treatment of chronic myeloid leukemia and implications of signal transduction inhibition. *Semin Hematol* 38:22, 2001.
638. Kujawski LA, Talpaz M: The role of interferon-alpha in the treatment of chronic myeloid leukemia. *Cytokine Growth Factor Rev* 18:459, 2007.
639. Alimena G, Breccia M, Luciano L, et al: Imatinib mesylate therapy in chronic myeloid leukemia patients in stable complete cytogenic response after interferon-alpha results in a very high complete molecular response rate. *Leuk Res* 32:255, 2008.
640. Branford S, Hughes T, Milner A, et al: Efficacy and safety of imatinib in patients with chronic myeloid leukemia and complete or near-complete cytogenetic response to interferon-alpha. *Cancer* 110:801, 2007.
641. Kolitz JE, Kempin SF, Schluger A, et al: A phase II trial of high-dose hydroxyurea in chronic myelogenous leukemia. *Semin Oncol* 19:27, 1992.
642. Abhyankar D, Shende C, Saikia T, Advani SH: Hydroxyurea induced leg ulcers. *J Assoc Physicians India* 48:926, 2000.
643. Guilhot F, Chastang C, Michallet M, et al: Interferon alfa-2b combined with cytarabine versus interferon alone in chronic myelogenous leukemia. *N Engl J Med* 337:223, 1997.
644. Hehlmann R, Heimpel H, Hasford J, et al: Randomized comparison of busulfan and hydroxyurea in chronic myelogenous leukemia: Prolongation of survival by hydroxyurea. *Blood* 82:398, 1993.
645. O'Brien S, Kantarjian H, Keating M, et al: Homoharringtonine therapy induces responses in patients with chronic myelogenous leukemia in late chronic phase. *Blood* 86:3322, 1995.
646. Clarkson B: Chronic myelogenous leukemia: Is aggressive treatment indicated? *J Clin Oncol* 3:135, 1985.
647. Cortes J, Jabbour E, Daley GQ, et al: Phase 1 study of lonafarnib (SCH 66336) and imatinib mesylate in patients with chronic myeloid leukemia who have failed prior single-agent therapy with imatinib. *Cancer* 110:1295, 2007.
648. Cortes J, Quintás-Cardama A, Garcia-Manero G, et al: Phase 1 study of tipifarnib in combination with imatinib for patients with chronic myelogenous leukemia in chronic phase after imatinib failure. *Cancer* 110:2000, 2007.
649. Issa JP, Gharibyan V, Cortes J, et al: Phase II study of low-dose decitabine in patients with chronic Myelogenous leukemia resistant to imatinib mesylate. *J Clin Oncol* 23:3948, 2005.
650. Xu R, Dong Q, Yu Y, et al: Berbamine: A novel inhibitor of bcr/abl fusion gene with potent anti-leukemia activity. *Leuk Res* 30:17, 2006.
651. Chandra J, Tracy J, Loegering D, et al: Adaphostin-induced oxidative stress overcomes BCR/ABL mutation-dependent and -independent imatinib resistance. *Blood* 107:2501, 2006.
652. Yokota A, Kimura S, Masuda S, et al: INNO-406, a novel BCR-ABL/Lyn dual tyrosine kinase inhibitor, suppresses the growth of Ph+ leukemia cells in the central nervous system, and cyclosporine A augments its in vivo activity. *Blood* 109:306, 2007.
653. Kamitsuji Y, Kuroda J, Kimura S, et al: The Bcr-Abl kinase inhibitor INNO-406 induces autophagy and different modes of cell death execution in Bcr-Abl-positive leukemias. *Cell Death Differ* 15:1712, 2008.
654. Carew JS, Nawrocki ST, Kahue CN, et al: Targeting autophagy augments the anticancer activity of the histone deacetylase inhibitor SAHA to overcome Bcr-Abl-mediated drug resistance. *Blood* 110:313, 2007.
655. Puttini M, Coluccia AM, Boschelli F, et al: In vitro and in vivo activity of SKI-606, a novel Src-Abl inhibitor, against imatinib-resistant Bcr-Abl+ neoplastic cells. *Cancer Res* 66:11314, 2006.
656. Noronha G, Cao J, Chow CP, et al: Inhibitors of ABL and the ABL-T315I mutation. *Curr Top Med Chem* 8:905, 2008.
657. Barbarotto E, Calin GA: Potential therapeutic applications of miRNA-based technology in hematological malignancies. *Curr Pharm Des* 14:2040, 2008.
658. Koldehoff M, Steckel NK, Beelen DW, Elmaagacli AH: Therapeutic application of small interfering RNA directed against bcr-abl transcripts to a patient with imatinib-resistant chronic myeloid leukaemia. *Clin Exp Med* 7:47, 2007.
659. James HA: The potential application of ribozymes for the treatment of hematological disorders. *J Leukoc Biol* 66:361, 1999.
660. Mendoza-Maldonado R, Zentilin L, Fanin R, Giacca M: Purging of chronic myelogenous leukemia cells by retrovirally expressed anti-bcrabl ribozymes with specific cellular compartmentalization. *Cancer Gene Ther* 9:71, 2002.
661. Cotter FE: Antisense oligonucleotides for haematological malignancies. *Haematologica* 84:19, 1999.
662. Verfaillie CM, McIvor S, Zhao RCH: Gene therapy for chronic myelogenous leukemia. *Mol Med Today* 5:359, 1999.
663. Clark RE, Dodi A, Hill SC, et al: Direct evidence that leukemic cells present HLA-associated immunogenic peptides derived from the BCRABL b3a2 fusion protein. *Blood* 98:2887, 2001.
664. Schwartz J, Pinilla-Ibarz J, Yuan RR, Scheinberg DA: Novel targeted and immunotherapeutic strategies in chronic myeloid leukemia. *Semin Hematol* 40:87, 2003.
665. Nossner E, Gastpar R, Milani V, et al: Tumor-derived heat shock protein 90 peptide complexes are cross-presented by human dendritic cells. *J Immunol* 169:5424, 2002.
666. Pinilla-Ibarz J, Cathcart K, Korontsvit T, et al: Vaccination of patients with chronic myelogenous leukemia with bcr-abl oncogene breakpoint fusion peptides generates specific immune responses. *Blood* 95:1781, 2000.
667. Maslak PG, Dao T, Gomez M, et al: A pilot vaccination trial of synthetic analog peptides derived from the BCR-ABL breakpoints in CML patients with minimal disease. *Leukemia* 22:1613, 2008.
668. Yasukawa M, Ohminami H, Kojima K, et al: HLA class II-restricted antigen presentation of endogenous bcr-abl fusion protein by chronic myelogenous leukemia-derived dendritic cells to CD4+ T lymphocytes. *Blood* 98:1498, 2001.
669. Tschiedel S, Gentilini C, Lange T, et al: Identification of NM23-H2 as a tumour-associated antigen in chronic myeloid leukaemia. *Leukemia* 22:1542, 2008.
670. Borrello I, Sotomayor EM, Rattis F-M, et al: Sustaining the graft-versus-tumor effect through posttransplant immunization with granulocyte-macrophage colony-stimulating factor (GM-CSF)-producing tumor vaccines. *Blood* 95:3011, 2000.
671. Kessler JH, Bres-Vloemans SA, van Veelen PA, et al: BCR-ABL fusion regions as a source of multiple leukemia-specific CD8+ T-cell epitopes. *Leukemia* 20:1738, 2006.
672. Rojas JM, Knight K, Wang L, Clark RE: Clinical evaluation of BCR-ABL peptide immunisation in chronic myeloid leukaemia: Results of the EPIC study. *Leukemia* 21:2287, 2007.

673. Wagner H, McKeough PG, Desforges J, Madoc-Jones H: Splenic irradiation in the treatment of patients with chronic myelogenous leukemia or myelofibrosis and myeloid metaplasia. *Cancer* 58:1204, 1986.
674. McFarland JT, Kuzma C, Millard FE, Johnstone PA: Palliative irradiation of the spleen. *Am J Clin Oncol* 26:178, 2003.
675. The Italian Cooperative Study Group on Chronic Myeloid Leukemia: Results of a prospective randomized trial of early splenectomy in chronic myeloid leukemia. *Cancer* 54:333, 1984.
676. Mesa RA, Elliott MA, Tefferi A: Splenectomy in chronic myeloid leukemia and myelofibrosis with myeloid metaplasia. *Blood Rev* 14:121, 2000.
677. Kalhs P, Schwarzinger I, Anderson G, et al: A retrospective analysis of the long-term effect of splenectomy on late infections, graft-versus-host disease, relapse, and survival after allogeneic marrow transplantation for chronic myelogenous leukemia. *Blood* 86:2028, 1995.
678. Rodrigues CA, Fermino FA, Vasconcelos Y, De Oliveira JS: Refractory chronic GVHD emerging after splenectomy in a marrow transplant recipient with accelerated phase CML. *Bone Marrow Transplant* 32:333, 2003.
679. Fadilah SA, Ahmad-Zailani R, Soon-Keng C, Norlaila M: Successful treatment of chronic myeloid leukemia during pregnancy with hydroxyurea. *Leukemia* 16:1202, 2002.
680. Mubarek AA, Kakil IR, Al-Homsi U, et al: Normal outcome of pregnancy in chronic myeloid leukemia treated with interferon-alpha in 1st trimester: Report of 3 cases and review of the literature. *Am J Hematol* 69:115, 2002.
681. CML Autograft Trials Collaboration: Autologous stem cell transplantation in chronic myeloid leukaemia: A meta-analysis of six randomized trials. *Cancer Treat Rev* 33:39, 2007.
682. Goldman J: Autologous stem-cell transplantation for chronic myelogenous leukemia. *Semin Hematol* 30:53, 1993.
683. Talpaz M, Kantarjian H, Liang J, et al: Percentage of Philadelphia chromosome (Ph)-negative and Ph-positive cells found after autologous transplantation for chronic myelogenous leukemia depends on percentage of diploid cells induced by conventional dose chemotherapy before collection of autologous cells. *Blood* 85:3257, 1995.
684. Drummond MW, Marin D, Clark RE, et al: Mobilization of Ph chromosome-negative peripheral blood stem cells in chronic myeloid leukaemia patients with imatinib mesylate-induced complete cytogenetic remission. *Br J Haematol* 123:479, 2003.
685. Hui CH, Goh KY, White D, et al: Successful peripheral blood stem cell mobilisation with filgrastim in patients with chronic myeloid leukaemia achieving complete cytogenetic response with imatinib, without increasing disease burden as measured by quantitative real-time PCR. *Leukemia* 17:821, 2003.
686. Kreuzer KA, Kluhs C, Baskaynak G, et al: Filgastrim-induced stem cell mobilization in chronic myeloid leukaemia patients during imatinib therapy: Safety, feasibility and evidence for an efficient in vivo purging. *Br J Haematol* 124:195, 2004.
687. Gordon MK, Sher D, Karrison T, et al: Successful autologous stem cell collection in patients with chronic myeloid leukemia in complete cytogenetic response, with quantitative measurement of BCR-ABL expression in blood, marrow, and apheresis products. *Leuk Lymphoma* 49:531, 2008.
688. Olavarria E: Autologous stem cell transplantation in chronic myeloid leukemia. *Semin Hematol* 44:252, 2007.
689. Perseghin P, Gambacorti-Passerini C, Tornaghi L, et al: Peripheral blood progenitor cell collection in chronic myeloid leukemia patients with complete cytogenetic response after treatment with imatinib mesylate. *Transfusion* 45:1214, 2005.
690. Cervantes F, Hernandez-Boluda JC, Odriozola J, et al: Imatinib mesylate (STI571) treatment in patients with chronic-phase chronic myelogenous leukaemia previously submitted to autologous stem cell transplantation. *Br J Haematol* 120:500, 2003.
691. Simon W, Segel GB, Lichtman MA: Early allogeneic stem cell transplantation for chronic myelogenous leukemia in the imatinib era: A preliminary assessment. *Blood Cells Mol Dis* 37:116, 2006.
692. Goldman J: Allogeneic stem cell transplantation for chronic myeloid leukemia—Status in 2007. *Bone Marrow Transplant* 42:S11, 2008.
693. Giralt SA, Arora M, Goldman JM, et al: Chronic Leukemia Working Committee, Center for International Blood and Marrow Transplant Research. Impact of imatinib therapy on the use of allogeneic haematopoietic progenitor cell transplantation for the treatment of chronic myeloid leukaemia. *Br J Haematol* 137:461, 2007.
694. Maziarz RT: Who with chronic myelogenous leukemia to transplant in the era of tyrosine kinase inhibitors? *Curr Opin Hematol* 15:127, 2008.
695. Hehlmann R, Berger U, Pfirrmann M, et al: Drug treatment is superior to allografting as first-line therapy in chronic myeloid leukemia. *Blood* 109:4686, 2007.
696. Thomas ED, Clift RA, Fefer A, et al: Marrow transplantation for the treatment of chronic myelogenous leukemia. *Ann Intern Med* 104:155, 1986.
697. Apperley JF: Hematopoietic stem cell transplantation in chronic myeloid leukemia. *Curr Opin Hematol* 5:445, 1998.
698. Cooperative Study Group on Chromosomes in Transplanted Patients: Cytogenetic follow-up of 100 patients submitted to bone marrow transplantation for Philadelphia chromosome-positive chronic myeloid leukemia. *Eur J Haematol* 40:50, 1988.
699. McGlave P, Bartoch G, Anasetti C, et al: Unrelated donor marrow transplantation therapy for chronic myelogenous leukemia. *Blood* 81:543, 1993.
700. Fernandez HF, Tran HT, Albrecht F, et al: Evaluation of safety and pharmacokinetics of administering intravenous busulfan in a twice-daily or daily schedule to patients with advanced hematologic malignant disease undergoing stem cell transplantation. *Biol Blood Marrow Transplant* 8:486, 2002.
701. Radich JP, Gooley T, Bensinger W, et al: HLA-matched related hematopoietic cell transplantation for chronic-phase CML using a targeted busulfan and cyclophosphamide preparative regimen. *Blood* 102:31, 2003.
702. Goldman J: Implications of imatinib mesylate for hematopoietic stem cell transplantation. *Semin Hematol* 38:28, 2001.
703. Barrett J: Allogeneic stem cell transplantation for chronic myeloid leukemia. *Semin Hematol* 40:59, 2003.
704. Messner HA, Curtis JE, Lipton JL, et al: Three decades of allogeneic bone marrow transplants at the Princess Margaret Hospital. *Clin Transplant* 289, 1999.
705. Byrne JL, Stainer C, Hyde H, et al: Low incidence of acute graft-versus-host disease and recurrent leukaemia in patients undergoing allogeneic haemopoietic stem cell transplantation from sibling donors with methotrexate and dose-monitored cyclosporin A prophylaxis. *Bone Marrow Transplant* 22:541, 1988.
706. Goldman J, Apperley J, Kanfer E, et al: Imatinib or transplant for chronic myeloid leukemia? *Lancet* 362:172, 2003.
707. Van Rhee F, Szydlo RM, Hermans J, et al: Long-term results after allogeneic bone marrow transplantation for chronic myelogenous leukemia in chronic phase: A report from the Chronic Leukemia Working Party of the European Groups for Blood and Marrow Transplantation. *Bone Marrow Transplant* 20:553, 1997.
708. Szydlo R, Goldman JM, Klein JP, et al: Results of allogeneic bone marrow transplants using donors other than HLA-identical siblings. *J Clin Oncol* 15:1767, 1997.
709. Petersdorf EW, Longton GM, Anasetti C, et al: The significance of HLA-DRBI matching on clinical outcome after HLA-A band DR identical unrelated donor transplantation. *Blood* 86:1606, 1995.
710. Weisdorf DJ, Anasetti C, Antin JH, et al: Allogeneic bone marrow transplantation for chronic myelogenous leukemia: Comparative analysis of unrelated versus matched sibling donor transplantation. *Blood* 99:1971, 2002.
711. Laporte JP, Gorin NC, Rubinstein P, et al: Cord-blood transplantation from an unrelated donor in an adult with chronic myelogenous leukemia. *N Engl J Med* 335:167, 1997.
712. Oehler VG, Gooley T, Snyder DS, et al: The effects of imatinib mesylate treatment before allogeneic transplantation for chronic myeloid leukemia. *Blood* 109:1782, 2007.
713. Weisser M, Schmid C, Schoch C, et al: Resistance to pretransplant imatinib therapy may adversely affect the outcome of allogeneic stem cell transplantation in CML. *Bone Marrow Transplant* 36:1017, 2005.
714. Jabbour E, Cortes J, Kantarjian H, et al: Novel tyrosine kinase inhibitor therapy before allogeneic stem cell transplantation in patients with chronic myeloid leukemia: No evidence for increased transplant-related toxicity. *Cancer* 110:340, 2007.
715. Radich JP, Gehly G, Gooley T, et al: Polymerase chain reaction detection of the BCR-ABL fusion transcript after allogeneic marrow transplantation for chronic myeloid leukemia: Results and implications in 346 patients. *Blood* 85:2632, 1995.
716. Goldman JM: Therapeutic strategies for chronic myeloid leukemia in chronic (stable) phase. *Semin Hematol* 40:10, 2003.
717. Miller JS, Cooley S, Parham P, et al: Missing KIR ligands are associated with less relapse and increased graft-versus-host disease (GVHD) following unrelated donor allogeneic HCT. *Blood* 109:5058, 2007.
718. Elmaagacli AH, Ottinger H, Koldehoff M, et al: Reduced risk for molecular disease in patients with chronic myeloid leukemia after transplantation from a KIR-mismatched donor. *Transplantation* 79:1741, 2005.
719. Nadal E, Garin M, Kaeda J, et al: Increased frequencies of CD4(+)CD25(high) T(regs) correlate with disease relapse after allogeneic stem cell transplantation for chronic myeloid leukemia. *Leukemia* 21:472, 2007.
720. Crawley C, Szydlo R, Lalancette M, et al: Outcomes of reduced-intensity transplantation for chronic myeloid leukemia: An analysis of prognostic factors from the Chronic Leukemia Working Party of the EBMT. *Blood* 106:2969, 2005.
721. Kebriaei P, Detry MA, Giralt S: Long-term follow-up of allogeneic hematopoietic stem-cell transplantation with reduced-intensity conditioning for patients with chronic myeloid leukemia. *Blood* 110:3456, 2007.
722. Uzunel M, Mattsson J, Brune M, et al: Kinetics of minimal residual disease and chimerism in patients with chronic myeloid leukemia after nonmyeloablative conditioning and allogeneic stem cell transplantation. *Blood* 101:469, 2003.
723. Or R, Shapira MY, Resnick I, et al: Nonmyeloablative allogeneic stem cell transplantation for the treatment of chronic myeloid leukemia in first chronic phase. *Blood* 101:441, 2003.
724. Bornhauser M, Kiehl M, Siegert W, et al: Dose-reduced conditioning for allografting in 44 patients with chronic myeloid leukaemia: A retrospective analysis. *Br J Haematol* 115:119, 2001.
725. Das M, Saikia TK, Advani SH, et al: Use of a reduced-intensity conditioning regimen for allogeneic transplantation in patients with chronic myeloid leukemia. *Bone Marrow Transplant* 32:125, 2003.
726. Feinstein L, Storb R: Reducing transplant toxicity. *Curr Opin Hematol* 8:342, 2001.
727. Koh LP, Hwang WY, Chuah CT, et al: Imatinib mesylate (STI-571) given concurrently with nonmyeloablative stem cell transplantation did not compromise engraftment and resulted in cytogenetic remission in a patient with chronic myeloid leukemia in blast crisis. *Bone Marrow Transplant* 31:305, 2003.
728. McCann SR: Molecular response to imatinib mesylate following relapse after allogeneic SCT for CML. *Blood* 101:1200, 2003.
729. Vandenberghe P, Boeckx N, Ronsyn E, et al: Imatinib mesylate induces durable complete remission of advanced CML persisting after allogeneic bone marrow transplantation. *Leukemia* 17:458, 2003.

730. Ullmann AJ, Hess G, Kolbe K, et al: Current results on the use of imatinib mesylate in patients with relapsed Philadelphia chromosome positive leukemia after allogeneic or syngeneic hematopoietic stem cell transplantation. *Keio J Med* 52:182, 2003.
731. Olavarria E, Craddock C, Dazzi F, et al: Imatinib mesylate (STI571) in the treatment of relapse of chronic myeloid leukemia after allogeneic stem cell transplantation. *Blood* 99:3861, 2002.
732. Carpenter PA, Snyder DS, Flowers ME, et al: Prophylactic administration of imatinib after hematopoietic cell transplantation for high-risk Philadelphia chromosome-positive leukemia. *Blood* 109:2791, 2007.
733. Olavarria E, Siddique S, Griffiths MJ, et al: Posttransplantation imatinib as a strategy to postpone the requirement for immunotherapy in patients undergoing reduced-intensity allografts for chronic myeloid leukemia. *Blood* 110:4614, 2007.
734. Weisser M, Tischer J, Schnittger S, et al: A comparison of donor lymphocyte infusions or imatinib mesylate for patients with chronic myelogenous leukemia who have relapsed after allogeneic stem cell transplantation. *Haematologica* 91:663, 2006.
735. Sullivan KM: Marrow transplantation for disorders of hematopoiesis. *Leukemia* 7:1098, 1993.
736. Kolb HJ, Mittermuller J, Clemm CH, et al: Donor leukocyte transfusions for treatment of recurrent chronic myelogenous leukemia in marrow transplant patients. *Blood* 76:2462, 1990.
737. Dazzi F, Szydlo RM, Goldman JM: Donor lymphocyte infusion for relapse of chronic myeloid leukemia after allogeneic stem cell transplant: Where we now stand. *Exp Hematol* 27:1477, 1999.
738. Van Rhee F, Lin F, Cullis JO, et al: Relapse of chronic myeloid leukemia after allogeneic bone marrow transplant: The case of giving donor leukocyte transfusions before the onset of hematologic relapse. *Blood* 83:3377, 1994.
739. Leis J, Porter DL: Unrelated donor leukocyte infusions to treat relapse after unrelated donor bone marrow transplantation. *Leuk Lymphoma* 43:9, 2002.
740. Dazzi F, Goldman J: Donor lymphocyte infusions. *Curr Opin Hematol* 6:394, 1999.
741. Dazzi F, Szydlo RM, Cross NCP, et al: Durability of responses following donor lymphocyte infusions for patients who relapse after allogeneic stem cell transplantation for chronic myeloid leukemia. *Blood* 96:2712, 2000.
742. Dazzi F: Monitoring of minimal residual disease after allografting: A requirement to guide DLI treatment. *Ann Hematol* 81:S29, 2002.
743. Porter D, Levine JE: Graft-versus-host disease and graft-versus-leukemia after donor leukocyte infusion. *Semin Hematol* 43:53, 2006.
744. Makinnon S: Donor leukocyte infusions. *Baillieres Clin Haematol* 10:357, 1997.
745. Giralt S, Hester J, Huh T, et al: CD8-depleted donor lymphocyte infusion as treatment for relapsed chronic myelogenous leukemia after allogeneic bone marrow transplantation. *Blood* 86:4337, 1995.
746. Guglielma C, Arcese W, Dazzi F, et al: Donor lymphocyte infusion for relapsed chronic myelogenous leukemia: Prognostic relevance of the initial cell dose. *Blood* 100:397, 2002.
747. Verzeletti S, Bonini C, Marktel S, et al: Herpes simplex virus thymidine kinase gene transfer for controlled graft-versus-host disease and graft-versus-leukemia: Clinical follow-up and improved new vectors. *Hum Gene Ther* 9:2243, 1998.
748. Maravcova J, Nadvornikova S, Zmekova V, et al: Molecular monitoring of responses to DLI and DLI + IFN treatment of post-SCT relapse in patients with CML. *Leuk Res* 27:719, 2003.
749. Vela-Ojeda J, Garcia-Ruiz Esparza MA, Reyes-Maldonado E, et al: Donor lymphocyte infusions for relapse of chronic myeloid leukemia after allogeneic stem cell transplantation: Prognostic significance of the dose of CD3+ and CD4+ lymphocytes. *Ann Hematol* 83:295, 2004.
750. Savani BN, Montero A, Kurlander R, et al: Imatinib synergizes with donor lymphocyte infusions to achieve rapid molecular remission of CML relapsing after allogeneic stem cell transplantation. *Bone Marrow Transplant* 36:1009, 2005.
751. Porter DL, Antin JH: Donor leukocyte infusions in myeloid malignancies: New strategies. *Best Pract Res Clin Haematol* 19:737, 2006.
752. Kardinal CG, Bateman JR, Weiner J: Chronic myeloid leukemia. Review of 356 cases. *Arch Intern Med* 136:305, 1976.
753. Tura S, Baccarini M, Corbelli G: Staging of chronic myeloid leukemia. *Br J Haematol* 47:105, 1981.
754. Gomez GA, Sokal JE, Walsh D: Prognostic features at diagnosis of chronic myelogenous leukemia. *Cancer* 47:2470, 1981.
755. Cervantes F, Rozman C: A multivariate analysis of prognostic factors in chronic myeloid leukemia. *Blood* 60:1298, 1982.
756. Sokal JE, Cox EB, Baccarani M, et al: Prognostic discrimination in "good-risk" chronic granulocytic leukemia. *Blood* 63:789, 1984.
757. Sokal JE, Baccarini M, Tura S, et al: Prognostic discrimination among younger patients with chronic granulocytic leukemia: Relevance to bone marrow transplantation. *Blood* 66:1352, 1985.
758. Kantarjian HM, Keating MJ, Walters RS, et al: Clinical and prognostic features of Philadelphia chromosome-negative chronic myelogenous leukemia. *Cancer* 58:2023, 1986.
759. Sokal JE, Baccarini M, Russo D, Tura S: Staging and prognosis in chronic myelogenous leukemia. *Semin Hematol* 25:49, 1988.
760. Kantarjian HM, Keating MK, Smith TL, et al: Proposal for a single synthesis prognostic staging system in chronic myelogenous leukemia. *Am J Med* 88:1, 1990.
761. Dreazen I, Berman M, Gaoe RP: Molecular abnormalities of *bcr* and *c-abl* in chronic myelogenous leukemia associated with a long chronic phase. *Blood* 71:797, 1988.
762. Nowell PC, Jackson L, Weiss A, Kurzrock P: Historical communication: Philadelphia positive chronic myelogenous leukemia followed for 27 years. *Cancer Genet Cytogenet* 34:57, 1988.
763. Selleir L, Emilia G, Temperani P, et al: Philadelphia-positive chronic myelogenous leukemia with typical *bcr/abl* molecular features and atypical, prolonged survival. *Leukemia* 3:538, 1989.
764. Birnie GD, MacKenzie ED, Goyns MH, Pollock A: Sequestration of Philadelphia chromosome-positive cells in the bone marrow of a chronic myeloid leukemia patient in very prolonged remission. *Leukemia* 4:452, 1990.
765. Lamy TH, Dauriac C, Le Prise PY: Long-term survival in chronic granulocytic leukemia. *Br J Haematol* 73:279, 1989.
766. Johansson B, Martens F, Fioretos T, et al: Remarkably long survival of a patient with Ph1-positive chronic myeloid leukemia and 5/bcr rearrangement. *Leukemia* 4:448, 1990.
767. Singer CRJ, McDonald GA, Douglas AS: Twenty-five year survival of chronic granulocytic leukemia with spontaneous karyotype conversion. *Br J Haematol* 57:309, 1984.
768. Wodzinski MA, Potter AM, Lawence ACK: Prolonged survival in chronic granulocytic leukemia associated with loss of the Philadelphia chromosome. *Br J Haematol* 71:296, 1989.
769. Kantarjian HM, Smith TL, McCredie KB, et al: Chronic myelogenous leukemia: A multivariate analysis of the associations of patient characteristics and therapy with survival. *Blood* 66:1326, 1985.
770. Kantarjian HM, Talpaz M: Treatment of chronic myelogenous leukemia. *Hematology* 14:105, 1991.
771. Baccarini M, Russo D, Zuffa E, et al: The prognosis of chronic myeloid leukemia. *Bone Marrow Transplant* 1:126, 1989.
772. Hasford J, Pfirrmann M, Hockhaus A: How long will chronic myeloid leukemia patients treated with imatinib live? *Leukemia* 19:497, 2005.
773. Hasford J, Pfirrmann M, Hochhaus A: How long will chronic myeloid leukemia patients treated with imatinib mesylate live? *Leukemia*. 19:497, 2005.
774. O'Brien SG, Guilhot F, Goldman JM, et al: International randomized study of interferon versus STI571 (IRIS) 7-year follow-up: Sustained survival, low rate of transformation, and increased rate of major molecular response (MMR) in patients (pts) with newly diagnosed chronic myeloid leukemia in chronic phase (CML-CP) treated with imatinib (IM). *Blood* 112:76, 2008.
775. Druker BJ, Guilhot F, O'Brien SG, et al: Five-year follow-up of patients receiving imatinib for chronic myeloid leukemia. *N Engl J Med* 355:2408, 2006.
776. Rosti G, Iacobucci I, Bassi S, et al: Impact of age on the outcome of patients with chronic myeloid leukemia in late chronic phase: Results of a phase II study of the GIMEMA CML Working Party. *Haematologica* 92:101, 2007.
777. Kantarjian H, O'Brien S, Talpaz M, et al: Outcome of patients with Philadelphia chromosome-positive chronic Myelogenous leukemia post-imatinib mesylate failure. *Cancer* 109:1556, 2007.
778. Grossman A, Silver RT, Arlin Z, et al: Fine mapping of chromosome 22 breakpoints within the breakpoint cluster region (bcr) implies a role for bcr exon 3 in determining disease duration in chronic myeloid leukemia. *Am J Hum Genet* 45:729, 1989.
779. Morris SW, Daniel L, Ahmed CMI, et al: Relationship of bcr breakpoint to chronic phase duration, survival, and blast crisis lineage in chronic myelogenous leukemia patients presenting in early chronic phase. *Blood* 75:2035, 1990.
780. Giralt S, Kantarjian H, Talpaz M: The natural history of chronic myelogenous leukemia in the interferon era. *Semin Hematol* 32:152, 1995.
781. Smadja N, Krulik M, Audebert AA, et al: Spontaneous regression of cytogenetic and hematologic anomalies in Ph1-positive chronic myelogenous leukemia. *Br J Haematol* 63:257, 1986.
782. Musashi M, Abe S, Yamada T, et al: Spontaneous remission in a patient with chronic myelogenous leukemia. *N Engl J Med* 336:337, 1997.
783. Provan AB, Smith AG: Re-emergence of Philadelphia chromosome positive clone on a patient with previous spontaneous remission of chronic myeloid leukemia. *Leukemia* 9:1600, 1995.
784. Korkolopoulou P, Viniou N, Kavantzas N, et al: Clinicopathologic correlations of bone marrow angiogenesis in chronic myeloid leukemia: A morphometric study. *Leukemia* 17L:89, 2003.
785. Boultwood J, Peniket A, Watkins F, et al: Telomere length shortening in chronic myelogenous leukemia is associated with reduced time to accelerated phase. *Blood* 96:358, 2000.
786. Verstovsek S, Kantarjian H, Manshouri T, et al: Prognostic significance of cellular vascular endothelial growth factor expression in chronic phase chronic myeloid leukemia. *Blood* 99:2265, 2002.
787. Sinclair PB, Nacheva EP, Leversha M, et al: Large deletions at the t(9;22) breakpoint are common and may identify a poor-prognosis subgroup of patients with chronic myeloid leukemia. *Blood* 95:738, 2000.
788. Huntly BJP, Reid AG, Bench AJ, et al: Deletions of the derivative chromosome 9 occur at the time of the Philadelphia translocation and provide a powerful and independent prognostic indicator in chronic myeloid leukemia. *Blood* 98:1732, 2001.
789. Cohen N, Rozenfeld-Granot G, Hardan I, et al: Subgroup of patients with Philadelphia-positive chronic myelogenous leukemia characterized by a deletion of 9q proximal to ABL gene: Expression profiling, resistance to interferon therapy, and poor prognosis. *Cancer Genet Cytogenet* 128:114, 2001.
790. Kvasnicka HM, Thiele J, Schmitt-Graeff A, et al: Prognostic impact of bone marrow erythropoietic precursor cells and myelofibrosis at diagnosis of Ph^{1+} chronic

myelogenous leukaemia—A multicentre study on 495 patients. *Br J Haematol* 112:727, 2001.
791. Normann AP, Egeland T, Madshus IH, et al: CD7 expression by CD34+ cells in CML patients, of prognostic significance? *Eur J Haematol* 71:266, 2003.
792. Roman-Gomez J, Castillejo JA, Jimenez A, et al: Cadherin-13, a mediator of calcium-dependent cell-cell adhesion, is silenced by methylation in chronic myeloid leukemia and correlates with pretreatment risk profile and cytogenetic response to interferon alfa. *J Clin Oncol* 21:1472, 2003.
793. Bhatia R, Holtz M, Niu N, et al: Persistence of malignant hematopoietic progenitors in chronic myelogenous leukemia patients in complete cytogenetic remission following imatinib mesylate treatment. *Blood* 101:4701, 2003.
794. Morel F, Ka C, Le Bris MJ, et al: Deletion of the 5′ ABL region in Philadelphia chromosome positive chronic myeloid leukemia: Frequency, origin and prognosis. *Leuk Lymphoma* 44:1333, 2003.
795. Prejzner W: Relationship of the BCR gene breakpoint and the type of BCR/ABL transcript to clinical course, prognostic indexes and survival in patients with chronic myeloid leukemia. *Med Sci Monit* 8:193, 2002.
796. Bauduer F, Ducout L, Dastugue N, Marolleau JP: Chronic myeloid leukemia as a secondary neoplasm after anti-cancer radiotherapy: A report of three cases and a brief review of the literature. *Leuk Lymphoma* 43:1057, 2002.
797. Agis H, Sperr WR, Herndlhofer S, et al: Clinical and prognostic significance of histamine monitoring in patients with CML during treatment with imatinib (STI571). *Ann Oncol* 18:1834, 2007.
798. Passweg JR, Walker I, Sobocinski KA, et al: Validation and extension of the EBMT Risk Score for patients with chronic myeloid leukaemia (CML) receiving allogeneic haematopoietic stem cell transplants. *Br J Haematol* 125:613, 2004.
799. Hasford J, Pfirrmann M, Hehlmann R, et al: Prognosis and prognostic factors for patients with chronic myeloid leukemia: Nontransplant therapy. *Semin Hematol* 40:4, 2003.
800. Qazilbash MH, Devetten MP, Abraham J, et al: Utility of a prognostic scoring system for allogeneic stem cell transplantation in patients with chronic myeloid leukemia. *Acta Haematol* 109:119, 2003.
801. Usman M, Syed NN, Kakepoto GN, et al: Chronic phase chronic myeloid leukemia: Response of imatinib mesylate and significance of Sokal score, age and disease duration in predicting the hematological and cytogenetic response. *J Assoc Physicians India* 55:103, 2007.
802. Marin D, Marktel S, Bua M, et al: Prognostic factors for patients with chronic myeloid leukemia in chronic phase treated with imatinib mesylate after failure of interferon alfa. *Leukemia* 17:1448, 2003.
803. Kantarjian HM, O'Brien S, Cortes JE, et al: Complete cytogenetic and molecular responses to interferon-alpha-based therapy for chronic myelogenous leukemia are associated with excellent long-term prognosis. *Cancer* 97:1033, 2003.
804. Rosti G, Martinelli G, Bassi S, et al: Molecular response to imatinib in late chronic-phase chronic myeloid leukemia. *Blood* 103:2284, 2004.
805. Yee K, Anglin P, Keating A: Molecular approaches to the detection and monitoring of chronic myeloid leukemia: Theory and practice. *Blood Rev* 13:105, 1999.
806. Kaeda J, Chase A, Goldman JM: Cytogenetic and molecular monitoring of residual disease in chronic myeloid leukaemia. *Acta Haematol* 107:64, 2002.
807. Hughes T, Branford S: Molecular monitoring of chronic myeloid leukemia. *Semin Hematol* 40:62, 2003.
808. Kantarjian H, Schiffer C, Jones D, Cortes J: Monitoring the response and course of chronic myeloid leukemia in the modern era of BCR-ABL tyrosine kinase inhibitors: Practical advice on the use and interpretation of monitoring methods. *Blood* 111(4):1774, 2008.
809. Lowenberg B: Minimal residual disease in chronic myeloid leukemia. *N Engl J Med* 349:1399, 2003.
810. Gabert J: Detection of recurrent translocations using real time PCR; assessment of the technique for diagnosis and detection of minimal residual disease. *Haematologica* 84:107, 1999.
811. Negrin RS, Blume KG: The use of polymerase chain reaction for the detection of minimal residual malignant disease. *Blood* 78:255, 1991.
812. Lee M-S, Kantarjian H, Talpaz M, et al: Detection of minimal residual disease by polymerase chain reaction in Philadelphia chromosome-positive chronic myelogenous leukemia following interferon therapy. *Blood* 79:1920, 1992.
813. Schulze E, Krahl R, Thalmeier K, Helbig W: Detection of bcr-abl mRNA in single progenitor colonies from patients with chronic myeloid leukemia by PCR: Comparison with cytogenetics and PCR from uncultured cells. *Exp Hematol* 23:1649, 1995.
814. Lin F, Chase A, Bungey J, et al: Correlation between the proportion of Philadelphia chromosome-positive metaphase cells and levels of BCR-ABL mRNA in chronic myeloid leukaemia. *Genes Chromosomes Cancer* 13:110, 1995.
815. Thompson JD, Brodsky I, Yunis JJ: Molecular quantification of residual disease in chronic myelogenous leukemia after bone marrow transplantation. *Blood* 79:1629, 1992.
816. Lin F, Chase A, Bungey J, et al: Correlation between the proportion of Philadelphia chromosome-positive metaphase cells and levels of BCR-ABL mRNA in chronic myeloid leukaemia. *Genes Chromosomes Cancer* 18:110, 1995.
817. Branford S, Fletcher L, Cross NC, et al: Desirable performance characteristics for BCR-ABL measurement on an international reporting scale to allow consistent interpretation of individual patient response and comparison of response rates between clinical trials. *Blood* 112:3330, 2008.
818. Sahay T, Schiffer CA: Monitoring minimal residual disease in patients with chronic myeloid leukemia after treatment with tyrosine kinase inhibitors. *Curr Opin Hematol* 15:134, 2008.
819. Stock W, Yu D, Karrison T, et al: Quantitative real-time RT-PCR monitoring of BCR-ABL in chronic Myelogenous leukemia shows lack of agreement in blood and bone marrow samples. *Int J Oncol* 28:1099, 2006.
820. Gaiger A, Henn T, Horth E, et al: Increase of bcr-abl chimeric mRNA expression in tumor cells of patients with chronic myeloid leukemia precedes disease progression. *Blood* 86:2371, 1995.
821. Guo JQ, Lin H, Kantarjian H, et al: Comparison of competitive-nested PCR and real-time PCR in detecting BCR-ABL fusion transcripts in chronic myeloid leukemia patients. *Leukemia* 16:2447, 2002.
822. Iacobucci I, Saglio G, Rosti G, et al: Achieving a major molecular response at the time of a complete cytogenetic response (CCgR) predicts a better duration of CCgR in imatinib-treated chronic myeloid leukemia patients. *Clin Cancer Res* 12:3037, 2006.
823. Press RD, Love Z, Tronnes AA, et al: BCR-ABL mRNA levels at and after the time of a complete cytogenetic response (CCR) predict the duration of CCR in imatinib mesylate-treated patients with CML. *Blood* 107:4250, 2006.
824. Jabbour E, Cortes JE, Kantarjian HM: Molecular monitoring in chronic myeloid leukemia: Response to tyrosine kinase inhibitors and prognostic implications. *Cancer* 112:2112, 2008.
825. O'Dwyer ME: How to monitor patients with chronic myelogenous leukemia. *JNCCN* 1:513, 2003.
826. Landstrom AP, Tefferi A: Fluorescent in situ hybridization in the diagnosis, prognosis, and treatment monitoring of chronic myeloid leukemia. *Leuk Lymphoma* 47:397, 2006.
827. Cohen N, Novikov I, Hardan I, et al: Standardization criteria for the detection of BCR/ABL fusion in interphase nuclei of chronic myelogenous leukemia patients by fluorescence in situ hybridization. *Cancer Genet Cytogenet* 123:102, 2000.
828. Rheinhold U, Hennig E, Leiblein S, et al: FISH for BCR-ABL on interphases of peripheral blood neutrophils but not of unselected white cells correlates with bone marrow cytogenetics in CML patients treated with imatinib. *Leukemia* 17:1925, 2003.
829. Kim YJ, Kim DW, Lee S, et al: Comprehensive comparison of FISH, RT-PCR, and RQ-PCR for monitoring the BCR-ABL gene after hematopoietic stem cell transplantation in CML. *Eur J Haematol* 68:272, 2002.
830. Bao F, Munker R, Lowery C, et al: Comparison of FISH and quantitative RT-PCR for the diagnosis and follow-up of BCR-ABL-positive leukemias. *Mol Diagn Ther* 11:239, 2007.
831. Uzunel M, Mattsson J, Brune M, et al: Kinetics of minimal residual disease and chimerism in patients with chronic myeloid leukemia after nonmyeloablative conditioning and allogeneic stem cell transplantation. *Blood* 101:469, 2003.
832. Hochhaus A, Weisser A, LaRosee P, et al: Detection and quantification of residual disease in chronic myelogenous leukemia. *Leukemia* 14:998, 2000.
833. Olavarria E, Kanfer E, Szydlo R, et al: Early detection of *BCR-ABL* transcripts by quantitative reverse transcriptase-polymerase chain reaction predicts outcome after allogeneic stem cell transplantation for chronic myeloid leukemia. *Blood* 97:1560, 2001.
834. Radich JP, Gooley T, Bryant E, et al: The significance of *bcr-abl* molecular detection in chronic myeloid leukemia patients "late" 18 months or more after transplantation. *Blood* 98:1701, 2001.
835. Lion T: Minimal residual disease. *Curr Opin Hematol* 6:406, 1999.
836. Thiele J, Wickenhauser C, Kvasnicka HM, et al: Mixed chimerism of bone marow CD34+ progenitor cells (genotyping, bcr/abl analysis) after allogeneic transplantation for chronic myelogenous leukemia. *Transplantation* 74:982, 2002.
837. Serrano J, Roman J, Sanchez J, et al: Molecular analysis of lineage specific chimerism and minimal residual disease by RT-PCR of p210 (BCR-ABL) and p190 (BCR-ABL) after allogeneic bone marrow transplantation for chronic myeloid leukemia: Increasing mixed myeloid chimerism and p190 (BCR-ABL) detection precede cytogenetic relapse. *Blood* 15:2659, 2000.
838. Muller MC, Gattermann N, Lahaye T, et al: Dynamics of BCR-ABL mRNA expression in first-line therapy of chronic myelogenous leukemia patients with imatinib or interferon alpha/ara-C. *Leukemia* 17:2392, 2003.
839. Hochhaus A: Minimal residual disease in chronic myeloid leukaemia patients. *Best Pract Res Clin Haematol* 15:159, 2002.
840. Lin F, Drummond M, O'Brien S, et al: Molecular monitoring in chronic myeloid leukemia patients who achieve complete cytogenetic remission on imatinib. *Blood* 102:1143, 2003.
841. Ross DM, Watkins DB, Hughes TP, Branford S: Reverse transcription with random pentadecamer primers improves the detection limit of a quantitative PCR assay for BCR-ABL transcripts in chronic myeloid leukemia: Implications for defining sensitivity in minimal residual disease. *Clin Chem* 54:1568, 2008.
842. Sun X, Li J, Chen J, et al: Flow cytometric assay of phosphotyrosine levels in Bcr-Abl-positive chronic myelogenous leukemias: A potential prognostic marker. *Ann Hematol* 88:29, 2009.
843. Giles FJ, Cortes JE, Kantarjian HM, O'Brien S: Accelerated and blastic phase of chronic myelogenous leukemia. *Hematol Oncol Clin North Am* 18:753, 2004.
844. Jamieson CH, Ailles LE, Dylla SJ, et al: Granulocyte-macrophage progenitors as candidate leukemic stem cells in blast-crisis CML. *N Engl J Med* 351:657, 2004.
845. Michor F: Chronic myeloid leukemia blast crisis arises from progenitors. *Stem Cells* 25:1114, 2007.

846. Wodarz D: Stem cell regulation and the development of blast crisis in chronic myeloid leukemia: Implications for the outcome of Imatinib treatment and discontinuation. *Med Hypotheses* 70:128, 2008.
847. Melo JV, Barnes DJ: Chronic myeloid leukaemia as a model of disease evolution in human cancer. *Nat Rev Cancer* 7:441, 2007.
848. Brazma D, Grace C, Howard J, et al: Genomic profile of chronic myelogenous leukemia: Imbalances associated with disease progression. *Genes Chromosomes Cancer* 46:1039, 2007.
849. Gaiger A, Henn T, Horth E, et al: Increase of bcr/abl chimeric mRNA expression in tumor cells of patients with chronic myeloid leukemia precedes disease progression. *Blood* 86:2371, 1995.
850. Elmaaglacli AH, Beelen DW, Opalka B, et al: The amount of BCR/ABL fusion transcripts detected by real-time quantitative polymerase chain reaction method in patients with Philadelphia chromosome positive chronic myeloid leukemia disease stages correlates with the disease stages. *Ann Hematol* 79:424, 2000.
851. Lowenberg B, Hagemeijer A, Swart K, Abels J: Serial follow-up of patients with chronic myeloid leukemia (CML) with combined cytogenetic and colony culture methods. *Exp Hematol* 10:123, 1982.
852. Haas OA, Schwarzmeier JD, Nachera E, et al: Investigations on karyotype evolution in patients with chronic myeloid leukemia (CML). *Blut* 48:33, 1984.
853. Swolin B, Weinfeld A, Westin J, et al: Karyotypic evolution in Ph-positive chronic myeloid leukemia in relation to management and disease progression. *Cancer Genet Cytogenet* 18:65, 1985.
854. Cortes J, O'Dwyer ME: Clonal evolution in chronic myelogenous leukemia. *Hematol Oncol Clin North Am* 18:671, 2004.
855. Honda H, Ushijima K, Oda H, et al: Acquired loss of p53 induces blast transformation in p210bcr/abl-expressing hematopoietic cells: A transgenic study for blast crisis in human CML. *Blood* 95:1144, 2000.
856. Yamaguchi H, Inokuchi K, Sakuma Y, Dan K: Mutation of p51/p63 gene is associated with blast crisis in chronic myelogenous leukemia. *Leukemia* 15:1729, 2001.
857. Coiffier B, Byron PA, Flere D, et al: Chronic granulocytic leukemia: Early detection of metamorphosis with "in vitro" culture of granulocytic progenitors. *Biomedicine* 33:96, 1980.
858. Todd MB, Waldron JA, Jennings TA, et al: Loss of myeloid differentiation antigens precedes blastic transformation in chronic myelogenous leukemia. *Blood* 70:122, 1987.
859. Grinesshammer M, Heinze B, Bangerter M, et al: Karyotype abnormalities and their clinical significance in blast crisis of chronic myeloid leukemia. *J Mol Med* 75:8836, 1997.
860. Spencer A, Vulliamy T, Kaeda J, et al: Clonal instability preceding lymphoid blastic transformation of chronic myeloid leukemia. *Leukemia* 11:195, 1997.
861. Anastasi J, Feng J, LeBeau MM, et al: The relationship between secondary chromosomal abnormalities and blast transformation in chronic myelogenous leukemia. *Leukemia* 9:628, 1995.
862. Bartram CR, de Klein A, Hagemeijer A, et al: Additional C-abl/bcr rearrangements in a CML patient exhibiting two Ph[1] chromosomes during blast crisis. *Leuk Res* 10:221, 1986.
863. Collins SJ, Grudine MT: Chronic myelogenous leukemia: Amplification of a rearranged c-abl oncogene in both chronic phase and blast crisis. *Blood* 69:893, 1987.
864. Mughal TI, Goldman JM: Chronic myeloid leukemia: Why does it evolve from chronic phase to blast transformation? *Front Biosci* 11:198, 2006.
865. Schaefer-Rego K, Dudik H, Popenoe D, et al: CML patients in blast crisis have breakpoints localized to a specific region of the bcr. *Blood* 70:448, 1987.
866. Mills KI, Benn P, Birnie GD: Does the breakpoint within the major breakpoint region (M-bcr) influence the duration of the chronic phase in chronic myeloid leukemia? An analytical comparison of current literature. *Blood* 78:1155, 1991.
867. Bartram CR, Janssen JWG, Becher R, et al: Persistence of chronic myelocytic leukemia despite deletion of rearranged bcr/c-abl sequences in blast crisis. *J Exp Med* 164:1389, 1986.
868. Okabe M, Matsushima S: Philadelphia chromosome-positive leukemia: Molecular analysis of *bcr* and *abl* genes and transforming genes. *Nippon Ketsueki Gakkai Zasshi* 51:1471, 1988.
869. Ahuja H, Bar-Eli M, Arlin Z, et al: The spectrum of molecular alterations in the evolution of chronic myelocytic leukemia. *J Clin Invest* 87:2042, 1991.
870. Kelman Z, Prokocimer M, Peller S, et al: Rearrangements in the p53 gene in Philadelphia chromosome positive chronic myelogenous leukemia. *Blood* 74:2318, 1989.
871. Mashal R, Shtalrid M, Talpaz M, et al: Rearrangement and expression of p53 in the chronic phase and blast crisis of chronic myelocytic leukemia. *Blood* 75:180, 1990.
872. Guinn BA, Mello KI: P53 mutations, methylation and genomic instability in the progression of chronic myeloid leukemia. *Leuk Lymphoma* 26:241, 1997.
873. Malinen T, Palotie A, Pakkala S, et al: Acceleration of chronic myeloid leukemia correlates with calcitonin gene methylation. *Blood* 77:2435, 1991.
874. Asimakopoolos FA, Shteper PJ, Krichevsky S, et al: *ABL1* methylation is a distinct molecular event associated with clonal evolution of chronic myeloid leukemia. *Blood* 94:2452, 1999.
875. Towatari M, Adachi K, Kato H, Saito H: Absence of the human retinoblastoma gene product in the megakaryoblastic crisis of chronic myelogenous leukemia. *Blood* 78:2178, 1991.
876. Sill H, Goldman JM, Cross NC: Homozygous deletions of the p16 tumor-suppressor gene are associated with lymphoid transformation of chronic myeloid leukemia. *Blood* 85:2013, 1995.
877. Hernandez-Boluda J-C, Cervantes F, Colomer D, et al: Genomic p16 abnormalities in the progression of chronic myeloid leukemia into blast crisis. *Exp Hematol* 31:204, 2003.
878. Serra A, Gottardi E, Della Ragione F, et al: Involvement at the cyclin-dependent kinase-4 inhibitor (CDKN2) gene in the pathogenesis of lymphoid blast crisis of chronic myelogenous leukaemia. *Br J Haematol* 91:625, 1995.
879. Menssen HD, Renki JMJ, Rodeck U, et al: Presence of Wilms' tumor gene (wt1) transcripts and the WT1 nuclear protein in the majority of human acute leukemias. *Leukemia* 9:1060, 1995.
880. Mitarri K, Ogawa S, Tanaka T, et al: Generation of the AML1-EVI-1 fusion gene in the t(3;21) (q26;q22) causes blastic crisis in chronic myelocytic leukemia. *EMBO J* 13:504, 1994.
881. Carapeti M, Goldman JM, Cross NC: Overexpression of EV-l in blast crisis of chronic myeloid leukemia. *Leukemia* 10:1561, 1996.
882. Mori N, Takeuchi S, Tasaka T, et al: Absence of microsatellite instability during the progression of chronic myelocytic leukemia. *Leukemia* 11:151, 1997.
883. Handa H, Hegde UP, Kuteninikov VM, et al: Bcl-2 and c-myc expressions, cell cycle kinetics and apoptosis during the progression of chronic myelogenous leukemia from diagnosis to blastic phase. *Leuk Res* 21:479, 1997.
884. Daheron L, Salmeron S, Patri S, et al: Identification of several genes differentially expressed during progression of chronic myelogenous leukemia. *Leukemia* 12:326, 1998.
885. Foti A, Ahuja HG, Allen SL, et al: Correlation between molecular and clinical events in the evolution of chronic myelocytic leukemia to blast crisis. *Blood* 77:2441, 1991.
886. Mori N, Morosetti R, Loe S, et al: Allelotype analysis in the evolution of chronic myelocytic leukemia. *Blood* 90:2010, 1997.
887. Radich JP, Dai H, Mao M, et al: Gene expression changes associated with progression and response in chronic myeloid leukemia. *Proc Natl Acad Sci U S A* 103:2794, 2006.
888. Yong AS, Szydlo RM, Goldman JM, et al: Molecular profiling of CD34+ cells identifies low expression of CD7, along with high expression of proteinase 3 or elastase, as predictors of longer survival in patients with CML. *Blood* 107:205, 2006.
889. Spiers ASD: Metamorphosis of chronic granulocytic leukemia: Diagnosis, classification and management. *Br J Haematol* 49:1, 1979.
890. Grignani F: Chronic myelogenous leukemia. *Crit Rev Oncol Hematol* 4:31, 1985.
891. Matsuo T, Tomonaga M, Kuriyama K, et al: Prognostic significance of the morphological dysplastic changes in chronic myelogenous leukemia. *Leuk Res* 10:331, 1986.
892. Ishii N, Murakami H, Matsushima T, et al: Histamine excess symptoms in basophilic crisis of chronic myelogenous leukemia. *J Med* 26:235, 1995.
893. Specchia G, Palumbo G, Pastore D, et al: Extramedullary blast crisis in chronic myeloid leukemia. *Leuk Res* 20:905, 1996.
894. Inveradi D, Lazzarino M, Morra E, et al: Extramedullary disease in Ph-positive chronic myelogenous leukemia: Frequency, clinical features, prognostic significance. *Haematologica* 75:146, 1990.
895. Jacknow J, Fizzera G, Gajl-Peczalska K, et al: Extramedullary presentation of the blast crisis of chronic myelogenous leukemia. *Br J Haematol* 61:225, 1985.
896. Terjanian T, Kantarjian H, Keating M, et al: Clinical and prognostic features of patients with Philadelphia chromosome-positive chronic myelogenous leukemia and extramedullary disease. *Cancer* 59:297, 1987.
897. Miksanek T, Reyes CV, Semkuo Z, Molnar ZJ: Granulocytic sarcoma of the peritoneum. *CA Cancer J Clin* 33:40, 1983.
898. Jones TI: Pleural blast crisis in chronic myelogenous leukemia. *Am J Hematol* 44:75, 1993.
899. Pascoe HR: Tumors composed of immature granulocytes occurring in the breast in chronic granulocytic leukemia. *Cancer* 25:697, 1970.
900. Chabner BA, Haskell CM, Canellos GP: Destructive bone lesions in chronic granulocytic leukemia. *Medicine (Baltimore)* 48:401, 1969.
901. Licht A, Many N, Rachmilewitz EA: Myelofibrosis, osteolytic bone lesions and hypercalcemia in chronic myeloid leukemia. *Acta Haematol* 49:182, 1973.
902. Lee CH, Morris TCM: Bone marrow necrosis and extramedullary myeloid tumor necrosis in aggressive chronic myeloid leukemia. *Pathology* 11:551, 1979.
903. Asarro S, Sato N, Ueshima Y, et al: Localized blastoma preceding blastic transformation in Ph[1]-positive chronic myelogenous leukemia. *Scand J Haematol* 25:251, 1980.
904. Ohyashiki K, Ito H: Characterization of extramedullary tumors in a case of Ph-positive chronic myelogenous leukemia. *Cancer Genet Cytogenet* 15:119, 1985.
905. Sun T, Susin M, Koduru P, et al: Extramedullary blast crisis in chronic myelogenous leukemia. *Cancer* 68:605, 1991.
906. Saikia TK, Dhabhar B, Iyer RS, et al: High incidence of meningeal leukemia in lymphoid blast crisis of chronic myelogenous leukemia. *Am J Hematol* 43:10, 1993.
907. Falini B, Tabilio A, Pelicci PG, et al: T-cell receptor B-chain gene rearrangement in a case of Ph[1]-positive chronic myeloid leukaemia blast crisis. *Br J Haematol* 62:776, 1986.
908. Giannone L, Whitlock JA, Kinney MC, et al: Use of the BCR probe to demonstrate extramedullary recurrence of CML with a T cell lymphoid phenotype following bone marrow transplantation. *Bone Marrow Transplant* 3:631, 1988.
909. Ohyashiki J, Ohyashiki K, Shimizu H, et al: Testicular tumor as the first manifestation of B-lymphoid blastic crisis in a case of Ph-positive chronic myelogenous leukemia. *Am J Hematol* 29:164, 1988.
910. Rosenthal S, Canellos GP, DeVita VT, Gralnick HR: Characteristics of blast crisis in chronic granulocytic leukemia. *Blood* 49:705, 1977.
911. Barton JC, Conrad ME: Current status of blastic transformation in chronic myelogenous leukemia. *Am J Hematol* 4:281, 1978.

912. Peterson LC, Bloomfield CD, Brunning RD: Blast crisis as an initial or terminal manifestation of chronic myeloid leukemia. *Am J Med* 60:209, 1976.
913. Bettelheim P, Lutz D, Majdic O, et al: Cell lineage heterogeneity in blast crisis of chronic myeloid leukaemia. *Br J Haematol* 59:395, 1985.
914. Nair C, Chopra M, Shinde S, et al: Immunophenotype and ultrastructural studies in blast crisis of chronic myeloid leukemia. *Leuk Lymphoma* 19:309, 1995.
915. Rosenthal S, Canellos GP, Gralnick HR: Erythroblastic transformation of chronic granulocytic leukemia. *Am J Med* 63:116, 1977.
916. Ekblom M, Borgstrom G, von Willebrand E, et al: Erythroid blast crisis in chronic myelogenous leukemia. *Blood* 62:591, 1983.
917. Lingg G, Schmalzl F, Breton-Gorius J, et al: Megakaryoblastic micro-megakaryocytic crisis in chronic myeloid leukemia. *Blut* 51:275, 1985.
918. Castaigne S, Berger R, Jolly V, et al: Promyelocytic blast crisis of chronic myelocytic leukemia with both t(9;22) and t(15;17) in M3 cells. *Cancer* 54:2409, 1984.
919. Berger R, Bernheim A, Daniel MT, Flandrin G: T(15;17) in a promyelocytic form of chronic myeloid leukemia blastic crisis. *Cancer Genet Cytogenet* 8:149, 1983.
920. Misawa S, Lee E, Schiffer CA, et al: Association of translocation (15;17) with malignant proliferation of promyelocytes in acute leukemia and chronic myelogenous leukemia in blast crisis. *Blood* 67:270, 1986.
921. Marinone G, Rossi G, Verzura P: Eosinophilic blast crisis in a case of chronic myeloid leukaemia. *Br J Haematol* 55:251, 1983.
922. Goh K-O, Anderson FW: Cytogenetic studies in basophilic chronic myelocytic leukemia. *Arch Pathol Lab Med* 103:288, 1979.
923. Rosenthal NS, Knapp D, Farhi DC: Promyelocytic blast crisis of chronic myelogenous leukemia. A rare subtype associated with disseminated intravascular coagulation. *Am J Clin Pathol* 103:185, 1995.
924. Lemes A, Gomez Casares MT, de la Iglesia S, et al: P190 BCR-ABL rearrangement in chronic myeloid leukemia and acute lymphoblastic leukemia. *Cancer Genet Cytogenet* 113:100, 1999.
925. Bertazzoni U, Brusamolino E, Isernia P, et al: Diagnostic significance of terminal transferase and adenosine deaminase in acute and chronic myeloid leukemia. *Blood* 60:685, 1982.
926. Schuh AC, Sutherland DR, Horsfall W, et al: Chronic myeloid leukemia arising in a progenitor common to T cells and myeloid cells. *Leukemia* 4:631, 1990.
927. Uike N, Takeichi N, Kimura N, et al: Dual arrangement of immunoglobulin and T-cell receptor genes in blast crisis of CML. *Eur J Haematol* 42:460, 1989.
928. Greaves MF, Verbi W, Reeves, BR, et al: "Pre-B" phenotypes in blast crisis of Ph[1] positive CML: Evidence for a pluripotential stem cell "target." *Leuk Res* 3:181, 1979.
929. Bakhshi A, Minowada J, Arnold A, et al: Lymphoid blast crisis of chronic myelogenous leukemia represents stages in the development of B-cell precursors. *N Engl J Med* 309:826, 1983.
930. Griffin JD, Todd RF, Ritz J, et al: Differentiation patterns in the blastic phase of chronic myeloid leukemia. *Blood* 61:85, 1983.
931. Bollum FJ: Terminal deoxynucleotidyl transferase, in *The Enzymes*, edited by RD Boyer, p 145. Academic, New York, 1974.
932. Dorfman DM, Longtine JA, Fox EA, et al: T-cell blast crisis in chronic myelogenous leukemia. *Am J Clin Pathol* 107:168, 1997.
933. Allouche M, Bourinbaiar A, Georgoulias V, et al: T-cell lineage involvement in lymphoid blast crisis of chronic myeloid leukemia. *Blood* 66:1155, 1985.
934. Gramatzki M, Bartram CR, Muller D, et al: Early T-cell differentiated chronic myeloid leukemia blast crisis with rearrangement of the breakpoint cluster region but not of the T-cell receptor beta chain genes. *Blood* 69:1082, 1987.
935. Dastugue N, Kuhlein E, Duchayne E, et al: T(14:14)(q11;q32) in biphenotypic blastic phase of chronic myeloid leukemia. *Blood* 68:949, 1986.
936. Kuriyama K, Tomonaga M, Yao E, et al: Dual expression of lymphoid/basophil markers on single blast cells transformed from chronic myeloid leukemia. *Leuk Res* 10:1015, 1986.
937. Yasukawa M, Iwamasa K, Kawamura S, et al: Phenotypic and genotypic analysis of chronic myelogenous leukaemia with T lymphoblastic and megakaryoblastic mixed crisis. *Br J Haematol* 66:331, 1987.
938. Spencer A, Vulliamy T, Chase A, et al: Myeloid to lymphoid clonal suppression following autologous transplantation in second chronic phase of chronic myeloid leukemia. *Leukemia* 9:2138, 1995.
939. Cervantes F, Villamor N, Esteve J, et al: "Lymphoid" blast crisis of chronic myeloid leukaemia is associated with distinct clinicohaematological features. *Br J Haematol* 100:123, 1998.
940. Stoll C, Oberline F: Non-random clonal evolution in 45 cases of chronic myeloid leukemia. *Leuk Res* 46:61, 1980.
941. Sandberg AA: The cytogenetics of chronic myelocytic leukemia (CML): Chronic phase and blastic crisis. *Cancer Genet Cytogenet* 1:217, 1980.
942. Myint H, Ross FM, Hall JL, et al: Early transformation to acute myeloblastic leukaemia with the acquisition of inv(16) in Ph positive chronic granulocytic leukaemia. *Leuk Res* 21:473, 1997.
943. Johansson B, Fioretos T, Mitelman F: Cytogenetic and molecular genetic evolution of chronic myeloid leukemia. *Acta Haematol* 107:76, 2002.
944. Sandberg AA: Chronic myelocytic leukemia, in *The Chromosomes in Human Cancer and Leukemia*, 2nd ed, p 465. Elsevier North Holland, New York, 1990.
945. Mitani K, Miyazono K, Urabe A, Takaku F: Karyotypic changes during the course of blastic crisis of chronic myelogenous leukemia. *Cancer Genet Cytogenet* 39:299, 1989.
946. Diez-Martin JL, DeWald GW, Pierre RV, et al: Possible cytogenetic distinction between lymphoid and myeloid blast crisis in chronic granulocytic leukemia. *Am J Hematol* 27:194, 1988.
947. Feinstein E, Cimino G, Gale RP, Canaani E: Initiation and progression of chronic myelogenous leukemia. *Leukemia* 6(Suppl 1):37, 1992.
948. Brizard F, Cividin M, Villalva C, et al: Comparison of M-FISH and conventional cytogenetic analysis in accelerated and acute phases of CML. *Leuk Res* 28:345, 2004.
949. Heim S, Christensen EB, Fioretos T, et al: Acute myelomonocytic leukemia with inv(16) (p13q22) complicating Philadelphia chromosome positive chronic myeloid leukemia. *Cancer Genet Cytogenet* 59:35, 1992.
950. Hogge DE, Misawa S, Testa JR, et al: Unusual karyotypic changes and B-cell involvement in a case of lymph node blast crisis of chronic myelogenous leukemia. *Blood* 64:123, 1984.
951. Kantarjian H, Talpaz M, O'Brien S, et al: Survival benefit with imatinib mesylate therapy in patients with accelerated-phase chronic myelogenous leukemia—Comparison with historic experience. *Cancer* 103:2099, 2005.
952. Shah NP: Advanced CML: Therapeutic options for patients in accelerated and blast phases. *J Natl Compr Canc Netw*. 6:S31, 2008.
953. Oki Y, Kantarjian HM, Gharibyan V, et al: Phase II study of low-dose decitabine in combination with imatinib mesylate in patients with accelerated or myeloid blastic phase of chronic Myelogenous leukemia. *Cancer* 109:899, 2007.
954. Fruehauf S, Topaly J, Buss EC, et al: Imatinib combined with mitoxantrone/etoposide and cytarabine is an effective induction therapy for patients with chronic myeloid leukemia in myeloid blast crisis. *Cancer* 109:1543, 2007.
955. Cortes J, Kantarjian H: Advanced-phase chronic myeloid leukemia. *Semin Hematol* 40:79, 2003.
956. Druker BJ, Sawyers CL, Kantarjian H, et al: Activity of a specific inhibitor of the BCR-ABL tyrosine kinase in the blast crisis of chronic myeloid leukemia and acute lymphoblastic leukemia with the Philadelphia chromosome. *N Engl J Med* 344:1038, 2001.
957. Altintas A, Cil T, Kilinc I, et al: Central nervous system blastic crisis in chronic myeloid leukemia on imatinib mesylate therapy: A case report. *J Neurooncol* 84:103, 2007.
958. Simpson E, O'Brien SG, Reilly JT: Extramedullary blast crises in CML patients in complete hematological remission treated with imatinib mesylate. *Clin Lab Haematol* 28:215, 2006.
959. Gozzetti A, Bocchia M, Calabrese S, et al: Promyelocytic blast crisis of chronic myelogenous leukemia during imatinib treatment. *Acta Haematol* 117:236, 2007.
960. Kantarjian HM, Cortes J, O'Brien S, et al: Imatinib mesylate (STI571) therapy for Philadelphia chromosome–positive chronic myelogenous leukemia in blast phase. *Blood* 99:3547, 2002.
961. Giles FJ, Larson RA, Kantarjian HM, et al: Nilotinib in patients with Philadelphia chromosome-positive chronic myelogenous leukemia in blast crisis (CML-BC) who are resistant or intolerant to imatinib. *J Clin Oncol* 26:376, 2008.
962. Cortes J, Rousselot P, Kin DW, et al: Dasatinib induces complete hematologic and cytogenetic responses in patients with imatinib-resistant or intolerant chronic myeloid leukemia in blast crisis. *Blood* 109:3207, 2007.
963. Barone S, Baer MR, Sait SNJ, et al: High-dose cytosine arabinoside and idarubicin treatment of chronic myeloid leukemia in myeloid blast crisis. *Am J Hematol* 67:119, 2001.
964. Hirase C, Maeda Y, Takai S, Kanamaru A: Hypersensitivity of Ph-positive lymphoid cell lines to rapamycin: Possible clinical application of mTOR inhibitor. *Leuk Res* 33:450, 2009.
965. Champlain R, Ho W, Arenson E, Gale RP: Allogeneic bone marrow transplantation for chronic myelogenous leukemia in chronic or accelerated phase. *Blood* 60:1038, 1982.
966. McGlave PB, Kim TH, Hard DD, et al: Successful allogeneic bone-marrow transplantation for patients in the accelerated phase of chronic granulocytic leukaemia. *Lancet* 2:625, 1982.
967. Martin PJ, Clift RA, Fisher LD, et al: HLA-identical marrow transplantation during accelerated-phase chronic myelogenous leukemia: Analysis of survival and remission duration. *Blood* 77:1978, 1988.
968. Falkenberg JHF, Wafelman AR, Joosten P, et al: Complete remission of accelerated phase chronic myeloid leukemia by treatment with leukemia-reactive cytotoxic T lymphocytes. *Blood* 94:1201, 1999.
969. Weisser M, Schleuning M, Haferlach C, et al: Allogeneic stem-cell transplantation provides excellent results in advanced stage chronic myeloid leukemia with major cytogenetic response to pre-transplant imatinib therapy. *Leuk Lymphoma* 48:295, 2007.
970. Carella AM, Gaozza E, Raffo MR, et al: Therapy of acute phase chronic myelogenous leukemia with intensive chemotherapy, blood cell autotransplant and cyclosporin A. *Leukemia* 5:517, 1991.
971. Bouvet M, Babiera GV, Termuhlen PM, et al: Splenectomy in the accelerated or blastic phase of chronic myelogenous leukemia: A single-institution 25-year experience. *Surgery* 122:20, 1997.
972. Wadhwa J, Szydio RM, Apperley J, et al: Factors affecting duration of survival after onset of blastic transformation of chronic myeloid leukemia. *Blood* 99:2304, 2002.
973. Majiis A, Smith TL, Talpaz M, et al: Signficance of cytogenetic clonal evolution in chronic myelogenous leukemia. *J Clin Oncol* 14:196, 1996.
974. Fialkow PJ, Jacobsen RJ, Singer JW, et al: Philadelphia chromosome (Ph[1])-negative chronic myelogenous leukemia (CML): A clonal disease with origin in a multipotent stem cell. *Blood* 56:70, 1980.

975. Cortes J: CMML: A biologically distinct disease. *Curr Hematol Rep* 2:202, 2003.
976. Onida F, Beran M: Chronic myelomonocytic leukemia: Myeloproliferative variant. *Curr Hematol Rep* 3:218, 2004.
977. McCollum A, Bigelow CL, Elkins SL, et al: Unusual skin lesions in chronic myelomonocytic leukemia. *South Med J* 96:681, 2003.
978. Saif MW, Hopkins JL, Gore SD: Autoimmune phenomena in patients with myelodysplastic syndromes and chronic myelomonocytic leukemia. *Leuk Lymphoma* 43:2083, 2002.
979. Cambier N, Baruchel A, Schlageter MH, et al: Chronic myelomonocytic leukemia: From biology to therapy. *Hematol Cell Ther* 39:41, 1997.
980. Stemmler J, Wittman GW, Hacker U, Heinemann V: Leukapheresis in chronic myelomonocytic leukemia with leukostasis syndrome: Elevated serum lactate levels as an early sign of microcirculation failure. *Leuk Lymphoma* 43:1427, 2002.
981. Bain BJ: Hypereosinophilia. *Curr Opin Hematol* 7:21, 2000.
982. Aguayo A, Kantarjian H, Manshouri T, et al: Angiogenesis in acute and chronic leukemias and myelodysplastic syndromes. *Blood* 96:2240, 2000.
983. Bellemy WI, Richter L, Sirjani D, et al: Vascular endothelial cell growth factor in autocrine promoter of abnormal localized precursors and leukemia progenitor formation in myelodysplastic syndromes. *Blood* 97:1427, 2001.
984. Ramshaw HS, Bardy PG, Lee MA, Lopez AQF: Chronic myelomonocytic leukemia requires granulocytic-macrophage colony-stimulating factor for growth in vitro and in vivo. *Exp Hematol* 30:1124, 2002.
985. Tessema M, Länger F, Dingemann J, et al: Aberrant methylation and impaired expression of the p14INK4B cell cycle regulatory gene in chronic myelomonocytic leukemia (CMML). *Leukemia* 17:910, 2003.
986. Magnusson MK, Meade KE, Nakamura R, et al: Activity of STI571 in chronic myelomonocytic leukemia with a platelet-derived growth factor B receptor fusion oncogene. *Blood* 100:1088, 2002.
987. Apperley JF, Gardembas M, Melo JV, et al: Response to imatinib mesylate in patients with chronic myeloproliferative diseases with rearrangements of the platelet-derived growth factor receptor beta. *N Engl J Med* 347:481, 2002.
988. Wessels JW, Fibbe WE, van der Keur D, et al: T(5;12)(q31;p12): A clinical entity with features of both myeloid leukemia and chronic myelomonocytic leukemia. *Cancer Genet Cytogenet* 65:7, 1993.
989. Golub TR, Barker GF, Love HM, Gilliland DG: Fusion of PDGF receptor β to a novel *ets*-like gen, *tel*, in chronic myelomonocytic leukemia with t(5;12) chromosomal translocation. *Cell* 77:307, 1994.
990. Cross NCP, Reiter A: Tyrosine kinase genes in chronic myeloproliferative diseases. *Leukemia* 16:1207, 2002.
991. Gunby RH, Cazzaniga G, Tassi E, et al: Sensitivity to imatinib but low frequency of the TEL/PDGFRβ fusion protein in chronic myelomonocytic leukemia. *Haematologica* 88:408, 2003.
992. Pitini V, Arrigo C, Teti D, et al: Response to STI571 in chronic myelomonocytic leukemia with platelet derived growth factor beta receptor involvement: A new case report. *Haematologica* 88:ECR18, 2003.
993. Kröger N, Zabelina T, Guardiola P, et al: Allogeneic stem cell transplantation of adult chronic myelomonocytic leukemia. *Br J Haematol* 118:67, 2002.
994. Onida F, Kantarjian HM, Smith TL, et al: Prognostic factors and scoring systems in chronic myelomonocytic leukemia: A prospective analysis of 213 patients. *Blood* 99:840, 2002.
995. Germing U, Strupp C, Alvado M, Gattermann N: New prognostic parameters for chronic myelomonocytic leukemia? *Blood* 100:731, 2002.
996. Sagaster V, Ohler L, Berer A, et al: High spontaneous colony growth in chronic myelomonocytic leukemia correlates with increased disease activity and is a novel prognostic factor for predicting short survival. *Ann Hematol* 83:9, 2004.
997. Stillman RG: A case of myeloid leukemia with predominance of eosinophil cells. *Med Rec* 81:594, 1912.
998. Benvenisti DS, Ultmann JE: Eosinophilic leukemia. *Ann Intern Med* 71:731, 1969.
999. Chusid MJ, Dale D, West BG, Wolff SM: The hypereosinophilic syndrome: Analysis of fourteen cases with a review of the literature. *Medicine (Baltimore)* 54:1, 1975.
1000. Brito-Babapulle F: The eosinophilias: Including the idiopathic hypereosinophilic syndrome. *Br J Haematol* 121:203, 2003.
1001. Robyn J, Lemery S, McCoy JP, et al: Multilineage involvement of the fusion gene in patients with FIP1L1/PDGFRA-positive hypereosinophilic syndrome. *Br J Haematol* 132:286, 2006.
1002. Crescenzi B, Chase A, Starza RL, et al: FIP1L1-PDGFRA in chronic eosinophilic leukemia and BCR-ABL1 in chronic myeloid leukemia affect different leukemic cells. *Leukemia* 21:397, 2007.
1003. Bain BJ: Cytogenetic and molecular genetic aspects of eosinophilic leukemia. *Br J Haematol* 122:173, 2003.
1004. Gotlib J, Cools J, Malone JM III, et al: The FIP1L1-PDGFRA fusion tyrosine kinase in hypereosinophilic syndrome and chronic eosinophilic leukemia: Implications for diagnosis, classification, and management. *Blood* 103:2879, 2004.
1005. Vandenberghe P, Wlodarska I, Michaux L, et al: Clinical and molecular features of *FIP1L1-PDFGRA* (+) chronic eosinophilic leukemia. *Leukemia* 18:734, 2004.
1006. Klion AD, Noel P, Akin C, et al: Elevated serum tryptase levels identify a subset of patients with a myeloproliferative variant of idiopathic hypereosinophilic syndrome associated with tissue fibrosis, poor prognosis, and imatinib responsiveness. *Blood* 101:4660, 2003.
1007. Florian S, Esterbauer H, Binder T, et al: Systemic mastocytosis (SM) associated with chronic eosinophilic leukemia (SM-CEL): Detection of FIP1L1/PDGFRalpha, classification by WHO criteria, and response to therapy with imatinib. *Leuk Res* 30:1201, 2006.
1008. Klion AD, Robyn J, Maric I, et al: Relapse following discontinuation of imatinib mesylate therapy for FIP1L1/PDGFRA-positive chronic eosinophilic leukemia: Implications for optimal dosing. *Blood* 110:3552, 2007.
1009. Verstovsek S, Tefferi A, Cortes J, et al: Phase II study of dasatinib in Philadelphia chromosome-negative acute and chronic myeloid disease, including systemic mastocytosis. *Clin Cancer Res* 14:3906, 2008.
1010. Esteva-Lorenzo FJ, Meehan KR, Spitzer TR, Mazumder A: Allogeneic bone marrow transplantation in a patient with hypereosinophilic syndrome. *Am J Hematol* 51:164, 1996.
1011. Juvonen E, Volin L, Koponen A, Ruutu T: Allogeneic blood stem cell transplantation following non-myeloablative conditioning for hypereosinophilic syndrome. *Bone Marrow Transplant* 29:457, 2002.
1012. Plotz S-G, Simon H-U, Darsow U, et al: Use of anti-interleukin-5 antibody in the hypereosinophilic syndrome with eosinophilic dermatitis. *N Engl J Med* 349:2334, 2003.
1013. Klion AD, Law MA, Noel P, et al: Safety and efficacy of the monoclonal anti-interleukin-5 antibody SCHJ55700 in the treatment of patients with hypereosinophilic syndrome. *Blood* 103:2939, 2004.
1014. Ardanani AD, Morice WG, Hoyer JD, Tefferi A: Chronic basophilic leukemia: A distinct clinical entity. *Eur J Haematol* 71:18, 2003.
1015. Lahortiga I, Akin C, Cools J, et al: Activity of imatinib in systemic mastocytosis with chronic basophilic leukemia and a PRKG2-PDGFRB fusion. *Haematologica* 93:49, 2008.
1016. Osgood EE: Monocytic leukemia. Report of six cases and review of one hundred and twenty-seven cases. *Arch Intern Med* 59:931, 1937.
1017. Bearman RM, Kjeldsberg CR, Pangalis GA, et al: Chronic monocytic leukemia in adults. *Cancer* 48:2239, 1981.
1018. Beattie JW, Seal RME, Crowther KV: Chronic monocytic leukemia. *Q J Med* 20:131, 1951.
1019. Sinn CW, Dick FW: Monocytic leukemia. *Am J Med* 20:588, 1956.
1020. Rodgers GM, Carrera CJ, Ries CA, Bainton DF: Blastic transformation of a well differentiated monocytic leukemia. Changes in cytochemical and cell surface markers. *Leuk Res* 6:613, 1982.
1021. Wahlin A, Nordenson I, Roos G: Chronic monocytic leukemia terminating in blastic transformation. *Blut* 53:405, 1986.
1022. Castro-Malaspina H, Schaison G, Brier J, et al: Philadelphia chromosome positive chronic myelocytic leukemia in children: Survival and prognostic factors. *Cancer* 51:721, 1983.
1023. Arico M, Biondi A, Pui C-H: Juvenile myelomonocytic leukemia. *Blood* 90:479, 1997.
1024. Neimeyer CM, Arico M, Basso A, et al: Chronic myelomonocytic leukemia in childhood. *Blood* 89:3535, 1997.
1025. Emanuel PD: Juvenile myelomonocytic leukemia and chronic myelomonocytic leukemia. *Leukemia* 22:1335, 2008.
1026. Niemeyer CM, Kratz C: Juvenile myelomonocytic leukemia. *Curr Oncol Rep* 5:510, 2003.
1027. Busque L, Gilliland DG, Prchal JT, et al: Clonality in juvenile chronic myelogenous leukemia. *Blood* 85:21, 1995.
1028. Cooper LJN, Shannon KM, Loken MR, et al: Evidence that juvenile chronic myelomonocytic leukemia can arise from a pluripotential stem cell. *Blood* 96:2310, 2000.
1029. Emanuel PD: RAS pathway mutations in juvenile myelomonocytic leukemia. *Acta Haematol* 119:207, 2008.
1030. Guilbert-Douet N, Morel F, Le Bris M-J, et al: Somatic *PTPN11* mutation with a heterogeneous clonal origin in children with juvenile myelomonocytic leukemia. *Leukemia* 18:1142, 2004.
1031. Miyauchi J, Asada M, Sasaki M, et al: Mutations of the N-*ras* gene in juvenile chronic myelogenous leukemia. *Blood* 83:2248, 1994.
1032. Bader JL, Miller RW: Neurofibromatosis and childhood leukemia. *J Pediatr* 92:925, 1978.
1033. Brodeur GM: The NF1 gene in myelopoiesis and childhood myelodysplastic syndrome. *N Engl J Med* 330:637, 1994.
1034. Shannon KM: Loss of normal NF1 allele from the bone marrow of children with type 1 neurofibromatosis and malignant myeloid disorders. *N Engl J Med* 330:597, 1994.
1035. Bollag G: Loss of NF1 results in activation of RAS signaling pathway and leads to aberrant growth in haematopoietic cells. *Nat Genet* 12:137, 1996.
1036. Tartaglia M, Niemeyer CM, Fragale A, et al: Somatic mutations in PTPN11 in juvenile myelomonocytic leukemia, myelodysplastic syndrome and acute myeloid leukemia. *Nat Genet* 34:148, 2003.
1037. Owen G, Lewis IJ, Morgan M, et al: Prognostic factors in juvenile chronic granulocytic leukaemia. *Br J CancerSuppl* 18:S68, 1992.
1038. Estrov Z, Grunberger T, Chan HSL, Freedman MH: Juvenile chronic myelogenous leukemia. Characterization of the disease using cell cultures. *Blood* 67:1382, 1986.
1039. Estrov Z, Dube ID, Chan HSL, Freedman MH: Residual juvenile chronic myelogenous leukemia cells detected in peripheral blood during clinical remission. *Blood* 70:1466, 1987.
1040. Emanuel PD, Bates LJ, Zhu S-W, et al: The role of monocyte-derived hemopoietic growth factors in the regulation of myeloproliferation in juvenile chronic myelogenous leukemia. *Exp Hematol* 19:1017, 1991.
1041. Morerio C, Acquila M, Rosanda C, et al: HCMOGT-1 is a novel fusion partner to *PDGFRB* in juvenile myelomonocytic leukemia with t(5;17)(q33;p11.2). *Cancer Res* 64:2649, 2004.

1042. Inoue S, Ravindranath Y, Thompson RI, et al: Cytogenetics of juvenile type chronic granulocytic leukemia. *Cancer* 39:2017, 1977.
1043. Brodeur GM, Dow LW, Williams DL: Cytogenetic features of juvenile chronic myelogenous leukemia. *Blood* 53:812, 1979.
1044. Chan HSL, Estrov Z, Weitzman SS, Freedman MH: The value of intensive combination chemotherapy for juvenile chronic myelogenous leukemia. *J Clin Oncol* 5:1960, 1987.
1045. Kang HJ, Shin HY, Choi HS, Ahn HS: Novel regimen for the treatment of juvenile myelomonocytic leukemia (JMML). *Leuk Res* 28:167, 2004.
1046. Pui CH, Arico M: Isotretinoin for juvenile chronic myelogenous leukemia. *N Engl J Med* 332:1520, 1995.
1047. Bernard F, Thomas C, Emile JF, et al: Transient hematologic and clinical effects of E21R in a child with end-stage juvenile myelomonocytic leukemia. *Blood* 99:2615, 2002.
1048. Locatelli F, Niemeyer C, Angelucci E, et al: Allogeneic bone marrow transplantation for chronic myelomonocytic leukemia in childhood. *J Clin Oncol* 15:556, 1997.
1049. Manabe A, Okamura J, Yumura-Yagi K, et al: Allogeneic hematopoietic stem cell transplantation for 27 children with juvenile myelomonocytic leukemia diagnosed based on the criteria of the International JMML Working Group. *Leukemia* 16:645, 2002.
1050. Worth A, Rao K, Webb D, et al: Successful treatment of juvenile myelomonocytic leukemia relapsing after stem cell transplantation using donor lymphocyte infusion. *Blood* 101:1713, 2003.
1051. Scrideli CA, Baruffi MR, Rogatto SR, et al: B lineage acute lymphoblastic leukemia transformation in a child with juvenile myelomonocytic leukemia, type 1 neurofibromatosis and monosomy of chromosome 7. Possible implications in the leukemogenesis. *Leuk Res* 27:371, 2003.
1052. Tuohey EL: A case of splenomegaly with polymorphonuclear neutrophil hyperleukocytosis. *Am J Med Sci* 160:18, 1920.
1053. Froberg MK, Brunning RD, Dorion P, et al: Demonstration of clonality in neutrophils using FISH in a case of chronic neutrophilic leukemia. *Leukemia* 12:623, 1998.
1054. Böhm J, Schaefer HE: Chronic neutrophilic leukemia:14 new cases of an uncommon myeloproliferative disorder. *J Clin Pathol* 55:862, 2002.
1055. Standen GR, Steers FJ, Jones L: Clonality in chronic neutrophilic leukemia associated with myeloma: Analysis using the X-linked probe M27β. *J Clin Pathol* 46:297, 1993.
1056. Bohm J, Kock S, Schaefer HE, Fisch P: Evidence of clonality in chronic neutrophilic leukaemia. *J Clin Pathol* 56:292, 2003.
1057. Yanagisawa K, Ohminami H, Sato M, et al: Neoplastic involvement of granulocytic lineage, not granulocytic-monocytic, monocytic, or erythrocytic lineage, in a patient with chronic neutrophilic leukemia. *Am J Hematol* 57:221, 1998.
1058. Hasegawa T, Suzuki K, Sakamoto C, et al: Expression of the inhibitor of apoptosis (IAP) family members in human neutrophils: Up-regulation of cIAP2 in chronic neutrophilic leukemia. *Blood* 101:1164, 2003.
1059. Hasle H, Olesen G, Kerndrup G, et al: Chronic neutrophilic leukaemia in adolescence and young adulthood. *Br J Haematol* 94:628, 1996.
1060. Elliott MA, Dewald GW, Tefferi A, Hanson CA: Chronic neutrophilic leukemia (CNL): A clinical and pathological entity. *Leukemia* 15:35, 2001.
1061. Reilly JT: Chronic neutrophilic leukaemia: A distinct clinical entity? *Br J Haematol* 116:10, 2002.
1062. Elliott MA: Chronic neutrophilic leukemia. *Curr Hematol Rep* 3:210, 2004.
1063. Piliotis E, Kutas G, Lipton JH: Allogeneic bone marrow transplantation in the management of chronic neutrophilic leukemia. *Leuk Lymphoma* 43:2051, 2002.
1064. Ito T, Kojima H, Otani K, et al: Chronic neutrophilic leukemia associated with monoclonal gammopathy of undetermined significance. *Acta Haematol* 95:140, 1996.
1065. Vorobiof DA, Benjamin A, Kaplan H, Dvilansky A: Chronic granulocytic leukemia, neutrophilic type with paraproteinemia (IgA type K). *Acta Haematol* 60:316, 1978.
1066. Carcassonne Y, Gastaut JA, Sebahoun G, Gratecos N: Découverte simultanée chez un même malade d'un myélome, d'une leucémie granuleuse (à polynucléaires neutrophils) et d'une maladie de Paget. *Nouv Rev Fr Hematol* 18:240, 1977.
1067. Franchi F, Seminara P, Gruinchi G: Chronic neutrophilic leukemia and myeloma. Report on long survival. *Tumori* 70:105, 1984.
1068. Lewis MJ, Oelbaum MH, Coleman M, Allen S: An association between chronic neutrophilic leukaemia and multiple myeloma with a study of cobalamin-binding proteins. *Br J Haematol* 63:173, 1986.
1069. Rovira M, Cervantes F, Namdedeu B, Rozman C: Chronic neutrophilic leukaemia preceding for seven years the development of multiple myeloma. *Acta Haematol* 3:94, 1990.
1070. Standen GR, Jasani B, Wagstaff M, Wardrop CAJ: Chronic neutrophilic leukemia and multiple myeloma. *Cancer* 66:162, 1990.
1071. Nagai M, Oda S, Iwamoto M, et al: Granulocyte-colony stimulating factor concentrates in a patient with plasma cell dyscrasia and clinical features of chronic neutrophilic leukaemia. *J Clin Pathol* 49:858, 1996.
1072. Dinçol G, Nalçaci M, Dogan O, et al: Coexistence of chronic neutrophilic leukemia with multiple myeloma. *Leuk Lymphoma* 43:649, 2002.
1073. Masini L, Salvarani C, Macchioni P, et al: Chronic neutrophilic leukemia (CNL) with karyotype abnormalities associated with plasma cell dyscrasia. *Haematologica* 77:277, 1992.
1074. Pascucci M, Dorion P, Makary A, Froberg MK: Chronic neutrophilic leukemia evolving from the myelodysplastic syndrome. *Acta Haematol* 98:163, 1997.
1075. Takamatsu Y, Kondo S, Inoue M, Tamura K: Chronic neutrophilic leukemia with dysplastic features mimicking myelodysplastic syndrome. *Int J Hematol* 63:65, 1996.
1076. Higuchi T, Oba R, Endo M, et al: Transition of polycythemia vera to chronic neutrophilic leukemia. *Leuk Lymphoma* 33:203, 1999.
1077. Billio A, Venturi R, Morello E, et al: Chronic neutrophilic leukemia evolving from polycythemia vera with multiple chromosome rearrangements: A case report. *Haematologica* 86:1225, 2001.
1078. Foa P, Iurlo A, Saglio G, et al: Chronic neutrophilic leukemia associated with polycythemia vera. *Br J Haematol* 78:286, 1991.
1079. Higuchi T, Oba R, Endo M, et al: Transition of polycythemia vera to chronic neutrophilic leukemia. *Leuk Lymphoma* 33:203, 1999.
1080. Iurlo A, Foa P, Mailo AT, et al: Polycythemia vera terminating in chronic neutrophilic leukemia. *Am J Hematol* 35:139, 1990.
1081. Soda H, Kuriyama K, Tomonaga M, et al: Lymphoid crisis with T-cell phenotypes in a patient with Philadelphia chromosome negative chronic myeloid leukemia. *Br J Haematol* 59:671, 1985.
1082. Kessler JF, Grogan TM, Greenberg BR: Philadelphia-chromosome-negative chronic myelogenous leukemia with lymphoid stem cell blastic transformation. *Am J Hematol* 18:201, 1985.
1083. Dobrovic A, Morley AA, Seshadri R, Januszewicz EH: Molecular diagnosis of Philadelphia negative CML using the polymerase chain reaction and DNA analysis: Clinical features and course of M-bcr negative and M-bcr positive CML. *Leukemia* 5:187, 1990.
1084. Martiat P, Michaux JL, Rodhain J, et al: Philadelphia-negative (Ph–) chronic myeloid leukemia (CML): Comparison with Ph+ CML and chronic myelomonocytic leukemia. *Blood* 78:205, 1991.
1085. VanderPlas DC, Grosveld G, Hagemeijer A: Review of clinical, cytogenetic, and molecular aspects of Ph-negative CML. *Cancer Genet Cytogenet* 52:143, 1991.
1086. Galton DA: Haematological differences between chronic granulocytic leukemia, atypical chronic myeloid leukaemia and chronic myelomonocytic leukaemia. *Leuk Lymphoma* 7:343, 1992.
1087. Kato Y, Sawada H, Tashima M et al: Heterogeneous features of Ph-negative CML—Possible existence of Ph-negative, bcr-rearrangement-negative CML. *Acta Haematol* 52:1004, 1989.
1088. Selleri L, Emilia G, Luppi M, et al: Chronic myelogenous leukemia with typical clinical and morphological features can be Philadelphia chromosome negative and "bcr negative". *Hematol Pathol* 4:67, 1990.
1089. Costello R, Sainty D, LaFage-Pochitaloff M, Gabert J: Clinical and biological aspects of Philadelphia-negative/BCR-negative chronic myeloid leukemia. *Leuk Lymphoma* 25:225, 1997.
1090. Kurzrock R, Bueso-Ramos CE, Kantarjian H, et al: BCR rearrangement-negative chronic myelogenous leukemia revisited. *J Clin Oncol* 19:2915, 2001.
1091. Onida F, Ball G, Kantarjian HM, et al: Characteristics and outcome of patients with Philadelphia chromosome negative, bcr/abl negative chronic myelogenous leukemia. *Cancer* 95:1673, 2002.
1092. O'Brien SG, Viera SA, Connors S, et al: Transient response to imatinib mesylate (STI571) in a patient with ETV6-ABL t(9;12) translocation. *Blood* 99:3465, 2002.
1093. Mauro MJ, Loriaux M, Deininger MW: Ph-positive and -negative myeloproliferative syndromes may coexist. *Leukemia* 18:1305, 2004.
1094. Raskind WH, Ferraris AM, Najfeld V, et al: Further evidence for the existence of a clonal Ph-negative stage in some cases of Ph-positive chronic myelocytic leukemia. *Leukemia* 18:1305, 2004.
1095. Chee YL, Vickers MA, Stevenson D, et al: Fatal myelodysplastic syndrome developing during therapy with imatinib mesylate and characterized by the emergence of complex Philadelphia negative clones. *Leukemia* 17:634, 2003.
1096. Meeus P, Demuynck H, Martiat P, et al: Sustained clonal karyotype abnormalities in the Philadelphia chromosome negative cells of CML patients successfully treated with imatinib. *Leukemia* 17:465, 2003.
1097. Bumm T, Muller C, Al Ali HK, et al: Emergence of clonal cytogenetic abnormalities in Ph-cells in some CML patients in cytogenetic remission to imatinib but restoration of polyclonal hematopoiesis in the majority. *Blood* 101:1941, 2001.

CHAPTER 91
PRIMARY MYELOFIBROSIS

Marshall A. Lichtman and Ayalew Tefferi

SUMMARY

Primary myelofibrosis is one of several disorders in the spectrum of clonal myeloid diseases, malignant diseases that originate in the clonal expansion of a single neoplastic hematopoietic multipotential cell. Approximately 50 percent of cases have a mutation in the Janus kinase 2 (*JAK2*) gene. It is characterized, classically, by anemia, mild neutrophilia, thrombocytosis, and splenomegaly. Occasional cases may present with bi- or tricytopenias (~10%). Immature myeloid and erythroid precursors, teardrop-shaped erythrocytes, and large platelets are constant features of the blood film. The marrow contains an increased number of pathologic megakaryocytes and increased reticulin fibers and, often later, collagen fibrosis. This reactive, polyclonal fibroplasia is the result of cytokines (e.g., transforming growth factor [TGF]-β) released locally by the numerous abnormal megakaryocytes. The disease may be complicated by portal hypertension as a result of a very large splenic blood flow and loss of compliance of hepatic vessels and by fibrohematopoietic tumors that can develop in any tissue and lead to symptoms by compression of vital structures. Treatment may include hydroxyurea for thrombocytosis and massive splenomegaly, androgens, erythropoietin, or red cell transfusions for severe anemia, local irradiation of fibrohematopoietic tumors or of the spleen, and splenectomy. Trials of newly developed JAK2 inhibitors show beneficial effects but require further study. Portosystemic shunt surgery may be required for gastroesophageal variceal bleeding. In younger patients, allogeneic hematopoietic stem cell transplantation can be curative and nonmyeloablative transplantation has been successful, at least up to age 65 years, and may become the approach of choice at any age. The disease may remain indolent for years or may progress rapidly by further deterioration in hematopoiesis, by massive splenic enlargement and its sequelae, or by transformation to acute myelogenous leukemia. Overall median survival is approximately 5 years.

DEFINITION AND HISTORY

Primary myelofibrosis is a chronic clonal myeloid disorder characterized by (1) anemia; (2) splenomegaly; (3) immature granulocytes, increased CD34+ cells, erythroblasts, and teardrop-shaped red cells in the blood; (4) marrow fibrosis; and (5) osteosclerosis. The disorder originally was described by Heuck[1] in 1879 under the title "Two Cases of Leukemia and Peculiar Blood and Bone Marrow Findings." In his monograph, Silverstein traced the history of the concepts set forth during the first half of the 20th century to explain the pathogenesis of this disease, including its origin in the marrow, the appearance of extramedullary hematopoiesis, and the relationship of fibrosis to hematopoietic changes.[2] More than 20 designations for the disease have been proposed or used, and different designations were preferred in different countries.[3] *Primary myelofibrosis* has been designated the most recent "official" name of the disease by a working group on nomenclature.[3] This compromise selection is debatable as the fibrosis is secondary, not primary, and the choice omits focusing on the central pathologic change: a clonal myeloid disease with singular neoplastic megakaryocytopoiesis.[4] The discovery that the mutated Janus kinase 2 (*JAK2*) gene plays a role in the causation and behavior of myeloproliferative diseases[5] and that approximately 50 percent of cases have a mutation of the *JAK2* gene[6] has led to better understanding of the pathogenesis of the disease and its relationship to other myeloproliferative diseases. The *JAK2* mutation also represents an important new target for therapy.

Acronyms and abbreviations that appear in this chapter include: AML, acute myelogenous leukemia; bFGF, basic fibroblast growth factor; CD, cluster of differentiation; CML, chronic myelogenous leukemia; FISH, fluorescence *in situ* hybridization; G-6-PD, glucose-6-phosphate dehydrogenase; G-CSF, granulocyte colony-stimulating factor; IL, interleukin; MRI, magnetic resonance imaging; PDGF, platelet-derived growth factor; TGF, transforming growth factor; TNF-R, tumor necrosis factor-receptor.

EPIDEMIOLOGY

INCIDENCE

Age and Sex

Primary myelofibrosis characteristically occurs after age 50 years.[2,7–15] The median age at diagnosis is approximately 65 to 70 years,[7,11–13,16] but the disease can occur from the neonatal period to the ninth decade of life.[2,11,13,17–19] In infants, the disorder can mimic the classic disease or show certain features but not others, such as absence of hepatosplenomegaly.[18] Familial infantile myelofibrosis mimics the adult disease and in some cases is transmitted by autosomal recessive inheritance.[20–22] The occurrence of primary myelofibrosis in children usually is in the first 3 years of life.[19,23,24] In young children, girls are afflicted with the disease twice as frequently as boys.[18] In young and middle-aged adults, the disease is similar to that in older subjects, although the proportion of indolent cases may be higher.[17,19,25] In adults, the disease occurs with about equal frequency in men and women.[7,11–15] Like virtually all clonal myeloid diseases,[26] primary myelofibrosis can cluster in families, suggesting transmission of an unidentified predisposition gene.[27–29] A large Swedish study found a significant relative risk (five- to sevenfold) for a familial occurrence of another myeloproliferative disease neoplasm, although not specifically primary myelofibrosis. The latter finding may relate to the small number of cases of primary myelofibrosis in that study.[16] The incidence of the disease is approximately 0.5 cases per 100,000 population per year in northern European countries.[30–33] A survey in Olmstead County, MN, reported an incidence of 1.5 case per 100,000 population per year and a median age of onset of 67 years. This median age is in keeping with several reports based on other studies (see above in this section).[34]

ETIOLOGY AND PATHOGENESIS

EXOGENOUS FACTORS

Exposure to benzene[35–37] or very-high-dose ionizing radiation[38] preceded the development of primary myelofibrosis in a very small proportion of patients with the disease. The former inciting agent, in exposures greater than 40 ppm-years, is associated with an increased relative risk of acute myelogenous leukemia (AML). Radiation is a well-established environmental cause of AML and chronic myelogenous leukemia (CML; see Chaps. 89 and 90).

IMMUNE MECHANISMS

Reports of myelofibrosis in patients with lupus erythematosus, have suggested the possibility of immunologic-mediated hyperplasia of marrow connective tissue[2] (see "Immune and Inflammatory Manifestations" on page 1385). These forms of myelofibrosis are different from the monoclonal multipotential hematopoietic stem cell disease, which is the principal subject considered in this chapter.

■ CLONAL HEMOPATHY, ANIMAL MODELS, AND ACTIVATING MUTATIONS

The disease arises from the neoplastic transformation of a single hematopoietic multipotential cell, a conclusion derived from the presence of clonal cytogenetic abnormalities in patients with an identifiable chromosomal abnormality and in studies in women with primary myelofibrosis who also were heterozygous for isotypes A and B of glucose-6-phosphate dehydrogenase (G-6-PD).[39,40] Although the nonhematopoietic tissues of these patients expressed both isotypes, each patient had blood cells with only one G-6-PD isotype. The findings strongly imply the blood cells of each patient arose from only one transformed stem cell. Furthermore, chromosome studies of colonies of hematopoietic progenitor cells in primary myelofibrosis established that the same clonal cytogenetic abnormality is present in erythroblasts, neutrophils, macrophages, basophils, and megakaryocytes.[41] These studies were confirmed by (1) examining X-linked restriction fragment length polymorphisms in women with primary myelofibrosis with heterozygosity for X chromosome-linked genes[42,43] and (2) verifying the presence of a mutation of codon 12 of the N-*ras* gene in five blood cell lineages of a patient with the disease.[44,45] Lymphocyte derivation from the clone has been noted using mutation in codon 12 of the *RAS* gene as the marker.[44] Using fluorescence *in situ* hybridization (FISH) analysis, T and B lymphocytes were found to be derived from clonal expansion of a multipotential hematopoietic cell in 3 of 4 patients with primary myelofibrosis with a 13q− or 20q− clonal cytogenetic abnormality.[46] Primary myelofibrosis can be distinguished from secondary myelofibrosis in women by clonality studies.[47] The advent of the *JAK2* V617F mutation has permitted this marker to be used in assessing clonality. Mutated *JAK2*-containing cells were identified in all blood lineages and in the common lymphomyeloid cell.[48]

The neoplastic hematopoietic stem cells in primary myelofibrosis containing the *JAK2* V617F mutation behave differently from the same cell population in polycythemia vera when studied in nonobese diabetic severe combined immunodeficient mice. Although studied in a nonhuman environment, the findings provide some explanation for the presence of *JAK2* V617F mutations in three phenotypically different myeloproliferative diseases: polycythemia vera, essential thrombocythemia, and clonal myelofibrosis.[49]

Animal models followed the derivation of the murine myeloproliferative leukemia virus, carrying the oncogene v-*mpl*, which in mice produced a syndrome having features of a mixed idiopathic myelofibrotic–polycythemic disorder (see Chap. 113).[50] The availability of v-*mpl* led to the isolation of the thrombopoietin receptor and its ligand thrombopoietin.[51] Later models of myelofibrosis and osteosclerosis, mimicking some of the important features of human primary myelofibrosis, were induced in mice by retroviral-mediated overexpression of thrombopoietin.[52,53] The concomitant high levels of fibroblastic factors (transforming growth factor [TGF]-β_1 and platelet-derived growth factor [PDGF]) resulted in intense fibrosis.[54] In this model, increased osteoprotegerin was thought to be the principal cause of osteosclerosis.[55] The disease was cured by murine hematopoietic stem cell transplantation.[52]

A syndrome in mice that results from the *GATA-1* (low) mutation also leads to a phenotype that closely simulates human myelofibrosis. The mice gradually develop anemia, teardrop poikilocytes, myeloid immaturity, marrow fibrosis, extramedullary hematopoiesis, and overexpression of profibrotic cytokines in marrow.[56] GATA-1 is a transcription factor required for normal megakaryocyte development. GATA-1 deficiency in mice leads to increased megakaryocytic proliferation, followed by myelofibrosis and osteosclerosis, as a result of exaggerated elaboration of fibroblast-inducing and osteoblast-stimulating factors.[57,58]

The discovery in 2005 that a somatic mutation in *JAK2* was associated with the three major myeloproliferative diseases—polycythemia vera, essential thrombocythemia, and primary myelofibrosis—has rapidly led to a fuller understanding of the pathogenesis of these diseases.[44,59] A dominant, gain-of-function mutation in the gene *JAK2* residing on the short arm of chromosome 9, which encodes the JAK2 tyrosine kinase, is present in approximately 50 percent of patients with primary myelofibrosis, in approximately 95 percent of patients with polycythemia vera (see Chap. 86), and in approximately 40 percent of patients with essential thrombocythemia (see Chap. 87), but is absent in healthy individuals.[60,61] In confirmation, the expression of the mutated human *JAK2* gene transferred into mice can induce a myeloproliferative disease with features characteristic of the human disorders.[62–64] Homozygosity results from allelic duplication as a result of uniparental disomy of chromosome 9p, not loss of the normal allele corresponding to the mutation.[65]

It is not yet precisely known how *JAK2 V617F*, the most prevalent mutation, links the three diseases and what modifiers explain the dramatically different phenotype and expected survival of the patients with polycythemia and primary myelofibrosis. At least four other modifying factors have been proposed to account for the different phenotypes and the apparent absence of the mutation in a high proportion of patients with primary myelofibrosis: (1) gene dosage, (2) germ line modifiers, (3) predisposition alleles, and (4) additional somatic mutations.[59,61,66] An example of each influence follows. There is an increasing *JAK2* V617F allele burden from essential thrombocythemia, to polycythemia vera, to primary myelofibrosis.[67] For example, the *JAK2* V617F allele burden may be a key determinant of the degree of myeloproliferation and myeloid metaplasia reflected by significantly higher levels of white blood cell counts, CD34+ cell counts, lower platelet counts, and a higher frequency of splenomegaly in homozygous polycythemia vera patients compared to their heterozygous counterparts. These findings are consistent with *JAK2* V617F-positive chronic myeloproliferative disorders as a biologic continuum with phenotypic presentation in part influenced by *JAK2* V617F mutational load.[67] Also, single nucleotide polymorphisms may influence the phenotype that results from the *JAK2* mutation. Myeloproliferative neoplasm predisposition alleles could provide a selective advantage for the development of mutations in the *JAK2* signaling pathway. As yet unidentified, pre-*JAK2* alleles, which arise in cells prior to *JAK2* mutation, may contribute to the phenotype displayed.[61]

A mutation in the thrombopoietin receptor gene, *MPL*, has been found in some mutant *JAK2*-negative patients with primary myelofibrosis. The finding of an activating *JAK2* (~50% of patients) or *MPL* (~10% of patients) mutation, which employs JAK2 for signaling, reinforces the critical role of unregulated activation of the JAK-STAT (signal transducer and activator of transcription) signaling pathway in the pathogenesis of primary myelofibrosis.[68–70]

Isolated genetic findings in individual patients have included (13q14) deletions, mutation or overexpression of the retinoblastoma gene,[71,72] *NF1* (17q11) deletions,[73] *RAS* mutations in approximately 1 in 20 patients studied, and occasional patients with mutations in *KIT*.[71] Mutational analysis of the class III receptor tyrosine kinase genes *KIT*, *FMS*, and *FLT3* in 40 to 60 patients with idiopathic myelofibrosis found only 2 mutation in *FMS*.[71] Uniparental disomy has been found on chromosomes 9p (site of *JAK2*) and 1p.[72]

HMGA2, a gene on chromosome 12, normally is not expressed in humans and is implicated in mesenchymal tumors. *HMGA2* was expressed in 12 of 12 patients with idiopathic myelofibrosis studied, implying that, if confirmed, expression of this gene in myeloid cells may play a role in the disease.[73]

CENTRALITY OF CD34+ CELL EGRESS AND NEOPLASTIC MEGAKARYOCYTOPOIESIS

Increased neoplastic megakaryopoiesis is the most prominent alteration in this clonal disease and is responsible for most of its major manifestations. Constitutive mobilization and circulation of CD34+ cells are a prominent feature of the clonal expansion. This phenomenon is the result of epigenetic methylation of the CXCR4 promotor, a resultant decrease in CXCR4 messenger ribonucleic acid (mRNA), decreased expression of CXCR4 on CD34+ cells, and their resultant enhanced migration into the blood in primary myelofibrosis patients.[74]

Circulating CD34+ cells in patients with primary myelofibrosis generate about 24-fold the number of megakaryocytes in culture than do CD34+ cells from normal subjects, express increased levels of BCL-XL, and have delayed apoptosis.[75,76] Media conditioned with CD61-positive cells (presumptive megakaryocytes) elaborated greater quantities of growth factors and proteases, including TGF-β and metalloprotease-9, than did CD61-positive cells generated from normal CD34+ cells.

Circulating CD34+ cells in patients with primary myelofibrosis also had a higher expression of eight genes (CD9, GAS2, DLK1, CDH1, WT1, NFE2, HMGA2, and CXCR4) than did normal CD34+ cells. These genes or subsets of them are likely related to disease pathogenesis and were shown to be related to specific manifestations in patients (e.g., CD9 and DLK1 with platelet count, WT1 with severity score).[77]

ENHANCED ANGIOGENESIS

Microvessel density and marrow blood flow are increased in patients with myelofibrosis. These changes may be related to an increase in circulating endothelial cell progenitors.[78]

DYSFUNCTION OF HEMATOPOIESIS

Neoplastic myeloproliferation usually is the dominant marrow abnormality in the granulocytic and megakaryocytic lineages resulting in intensely cellular marrows and mild to moderate blood granulocytosis and thrombocytosis. Ineffective or hypoplastic hematopoiesis, resulting from exaggerated apoptosis of very early precursors, can be present initially or emerge later as the dominant pathogenetic process, leading to granulocytopenia and/or thrombocytopenia. Anemia is a frequent finding and results from a combination of decreased erythropoiesis, shortened red cell survival, and the effects of splenomegaly on the distribution of red cells in the circulation. Hemolysis can be a prominent factor in some cases. Megakaryocytosis and intense dysmorphogenesis of megakaryocytes are constant features of the disease. Even in intensely fibrotic marrows with severe decreases in erythroid and granulocytic precursors, clusters of megakaryocytes are easily found interspersed between collagen bundles. The term "megakaryocytic myelosis," one of the many synonymous terms for the disease, catches the constancy of this finding. The dominance of megakaryopoiesis may relate to the average fivefold overexpression of *FKBP51* in megakaryocytes in primary myelofibrosis and the marked predisposition of CD34+ cells to differentiate into megakaryocytes (see "Centrality of CD34+ Cell Egress and Neoplastic Megakaryocytopoiesis" above). *FKBP51* increases resistance to apoptosis, possibly by an effect through the calcineurin pathway.[79] The disease has all the hallmarks of chronic megakaryocytic leukemia.[7] Although elevated levels of thrombopoietin (and interleukin [IL]-6 and IL-11) are found in the serum of patients with primary myelofibrosis, their etiologic role in the human disease is unresolved.[80] A marked increase in the thrombopoietin receptor MPL is observed on the platelets and megakaryocytes of a proportion of patients with primary myelofibrosis.[81] Expression of the polycythemia rubra vera gene *PRV-1*, also is increased on neutrophils in some patients with the disease.[82,83] The latter group may include patients whose disease is evolving from polycythemia vera to myelofibrosis. In contrast, congenital overexpression of thrombopoietin produces a syndrome that resembles essential thrombocythemia. Despite the animal models of thrombopoietin-induced myeloproliferation and osteomyelofibrosis and the apparent abnormality of MPL receptor sites on human megakaryocytes, autonomous megakaryocyte growth, characteristic of human primary myelofibrosis marrow in culture, has not been associated with either an autocrine effect of MPL ligand (thrombopoietin) or of a mutation in *MPL*.

FIBROPLASIA

Four of the five major types of collagen[84] are present in normal marrow: type I in bone, type III in blood vessels, and types IV and V in basement membranes. The fine reticulin fibers that appear after silver impregnation of marrow are principally type III collagen. They do not stain with trichrome dyes. The thicker collagen fibers are principally type I collagen and stain with trichrome dyes, but do not impregnate with silver. The amount of the very fine fibrous network barely perceptible in normal marrow that is stained by silver impregnation techniques[85] increases in the marrow of patients with primary myelofibrosis (Table 91–1).[86] The fibrous network contains collagen and occasionally progresses to include thick collagen bands that are evident with trichrome stains. Collagen types I, III, IV, and V are increased in myelofibrosis, but type III collagen is increased uniformly and preferentially.[87–90] The latter occurrence accounts for the increased plasma concentration of procollagen III amino-terminal peptide, a component of collagen type III, which is

TABLE 91–1. Fibroplasia in Idiopathic Myelofibrosis

I. Marrow Stroma
   A. *Increased amount of*
      1. Total collagen (hydroxyproline)[87,91]
      2. Type I collagen[87–89,93]
      3. Type III collagen[87–89,93]
      4. Type III procollagen[88–91,93,94]
      5. Type IV collagen[88,95,96]
      6. Matrix metalloproteinase-14[97]
      7. Bone morphogenetic protein[98]
      8. Laminin[88,95,99]
      9. Fibronectin[100,101]
      10. Tenascin[102]
      11. Vitronectin[103]
      12. Microenvironment TGF-β,[104] bFGF,[104] and substance P[105]
   B. *Decreased amount of*
      1. Collagenase[97]
II. Plasma
   A. *Increased concentration of*
      1. Prolylhydroxylase[106]
      2. C-terminal peptide of procollagen type I[90]
      3. N-terminal peptide of procollagen type III[89,91,107,108]
      4. Type IV collagen[89,99]
      5. Laminin[89,99]
      6. Fibronectin[101]
      7. Hyaluronan[109]

cleaved during collagen biosynthesis.[86,91,92] Serum prolyl-hydroxylase and marrow and plasma fibronectin also increase in patients with idiopathic myelofibrosis or myelofibrosis from other causes.[88,89]

Marrow fibrosis in primary myelofibrosis is most closely correlated with increased dysmorphic megakaryocytes in the marrow. Even densely fibrotic marrow with little residual granulopoiesis or erythropoiesis usually has numerous megakaryocytes scattered throughout the fibrotic areas.[86,92,110] The increased pathologic emperipolesis (the entry of neutrophils and other marrow cells into the canalicular system of megakaryocytes) of neutrophils in megakaryocytes, evident in human primary myelofibrosis and in mouse models, suggests this may be an additional mechanism of α-granule injury and release of TGF-β and PDGF.[111] Animal models also indicate that marrow monocytes and macrophages may play a subsidiary role in the induction of fibrosis.[111–113] Secretion of PDGF, basic fibroblast growth factor (bFGF), and TGF-β from monocytes that are part of the clone have the potential to act as myeloproliferative growth factors and profibrotic cytokines.[104]

The increased content of marrow collagen types I and III results from release of fibroblast growth factors, which include PDGF,[114,115] epidermal growth factor,[116] endothelial cell growth factor,[116] TGF-β,[103,117,118] and bFGF,[109,119] each of which is present in megakaryocyte α granules. Other factors, such as tumor necrosis factor alpha, IL-1α, and IL-1β, which can be released from marrow cells, also can stimulate fibroblasts.[120,121] Platelet factor 4, also derived from megakaryocytes, inhibits collagenase and could contribute to collagen accumulation,[110] although studies showing a poor correlation between plasma platelet factor 4 concentration and marrow fibrosis have dampened enthusiasm for the role of this factor.[122] Substance P, a peptide that acts as a neurotransmitter and a modulator of immune and hematopoietic functions, is increased in the fibrotic marrow and colocalizes with fibronectin. It is angiogenic and is a fibroblast mitogen.[104] Its precise role in the complex interactions among fibroblasts, cytokines, and matrix protein deposition is not clear. The high urinary excretion of platelet-derived calmodulin, a putative fibroblast growth factor, in patients with myelofibrosis has added this compound to the array of factors that may contribute to the fibroplasia.[120] The plasma level of matrix metalloprotein III is decreased and the level of tissue inhibitor of metalloproteinase is increased in patients with idiopathic myelofibrosis.[123] The expression of matrix metalloproteinase-14 in marrow increases by nearly two orders of magnitude as fibroplasia progresses during the course of the disease; and, megakaryocytes and endothelial cells are the major sources of this protein.[97] Neutrophil collagenase (matrix metalloproteinase-8) content is decreased early in the disease.[97] Bone morphogenetic proteins (BMPs) also have been implicated as a contributory factor in fibroplasia. BMP1, 6, and 7, and BMP-receptor 2 are increased in marrow in myelofibrosis as a result of release from megakaryocytes and stromal cells. These proteins are activators of latent TGF-β_1 and processors of collagen precursors. In addition, TGF-β_1 induces release of BMP6.[98]

This complex combination of alterations contributes to matrix deposition. The pathogenetic role of released growth factors in fibroplasia is not completely understood. Generalizations from *in vitro* experiments or correlation between two variables provide only a limited perspective. For example, TGF-β can stimulate or inhibit fibroblast growth, depending on the repertoire of other growth factors in the environment.[117,118]

Fibroplasia is associated with an increase in the number and size of marrow sinuses,[101] the number of endothelial cells,[125] an increase in vascular volume in the marrow,[103] and an increase in blood flow through the marrow.[95,126,127] These processes are responsible for the increase in marrow collagen types IV and V and laminin synthesized by endothelial cells in the marrow of patients.[116]

The fibroblastic proliferation in marrow is not an intrinsic part of the abnormal clonal expansion of hematopoiesis.[128] In cases of primary myelofibrosis in which G-6-PD isoenzyme studies or chromosome karyotyping establish monoclonal growth of hematopoietic cells, marrow fibroblasts contain both G-6-PD isoenzymes and do not share the clonal chromosome abnormality.[129] The findings strongly imply that the fibroblasts differentiate from a primordial cell different from the neoplastic hematopoietic stem cell in primary myelofibrosis and that fibroblast proliferation and enhanced collagen synthesis are secondary results of abnormal hematopoiesis.

EXTRAMEDULLARY HEMATOPOIESIS

Extramedullary hemopoiesis is consistently present in liver and spleen, where it contributes to organ enlargement.[7–9] Escape of progenitor cells from marrow and their lodgment in other organs contributes to extramedullary blood cell formation. Reversion of the liver and spleen to their fetal hematopoietic functions (metaplasia) is not a major factor in extramedullary hematopoiesis, and quantitatively significant, effective hematopoiesis does not occur outside of the marrow (see "Fibrohematopoietic Extramedullary Tumors" below).

CLINICAL FEATURES

PRESENTING SYMPTOMS

About one-fourth of patients are asymptomatic at the time of diagnosis; the disease is detected by medical examination for an unrelated reason. In symptomatic patients, fatigue, weakness, shortness of breath, pruritus, and palpitations are nonspecific but frequent complaints.[8–12] Weight loss is common, but anorexia is less so and night sweats occur infrequently. A dragging sensation in the left upper abdomen caused by an enlarged spleen or early satiety from encroachment of the spleen on the stomach may occur. Severe left upper quadrant or left shoulder pain can occur from splenic infarction and perisplenitis. Patients may report unexpected bleeding. Occasionally, bone pain is prominent, especially in the lower extremities. Fever, weight loss, night sweats, and bone pain are more frequent later in the course of the disease.

PRESENTING SIGNS

Hepatomegaly is detectable in two-thirds of patients, and splenomegaly is present on palpation or imaging studies in almost all patients at the time of diagnosis.[7–11] The spleen is mildly enlarged in one-fourth, moderately enlarged in half, and massively enlarged in approximately one-fourth of patients. Muscle wasting, peripheral edema, and purpura are present infrequently. Bone tenderness may be present. The latter signs may develop in a larger proportion of patients over the course of the disease.

Neutrophilic dermatosis, a syndrome that closely mimics the raised and tender plaques of Sweet syndrome, may occur.[130–132] It can be the presenting or a significant complicating feature, and can progress to bullae or pyoderma gangrenosum.[130,133] The dermatopathology of neutrophilic dermatosis is different from leukemia cutis and is unrelated to infection or vasculitis. The predominant histologic lesion is an intense polymorphonuclear neutrophilic infiltrate.

Skin infiltrates related to hematopoietic cells (leukemia cutis) are uncommon.[134] These cutaneous lesions may have myeloid cells with giant cells carrying CD61 markers characteristic of megakaryocytes.[135,136] Skin lesions representing cutaneous fibrohematopoietic tumors may occur.

SPECIAL CLINICAL FEATURES

Prefibrotic Primary Myelofibrosis

The presenting findings of the clonal myeloid diseases are changing because of more and earlier access to healthcare in industrialized

TABLE 91–2. Diagnostic Findings in Idiopathic Myelofibrosis

Prefibrotic stage
Anemia may be absent or mild
Leukocytosis may be absent or slight
Thrombocythemia very frequent
BCR-ABL fusion gene absent
Presence of *JAK2* mutation indicative of diagnosis of myeloproliferative disease
Cellular marrow with mild increase in granulopoiesis; increased megakaryocytes, clusters of very dysmorphic megakaryocytes and megakaryocytic nuclei; no to very slight increase in reticular fibers on silver stain
Palpable splenomegaly infrequent
Absent or slight anisopoikilocytosis including teardrop red cells
Fully developed stage
Marrow reticulin fibrosis plus or minus collagen fibrosis
BCR-ABL fusion gene absent
JAK2 mutation in approximately 50% of patients
Splenomegaly
Anisopoikilocytosis with teardrop red cells in every oil immersion field
Immature myeloid cells in blood
Increased CD34-positive cells in blood
Erythroblasts in blood
Marrow usually hypercellular but invariably has increased megakaryocytes, clusters of highly dysmorphic megakaryocytes, and megakaryocyte bare nuclei regardless of overall marrow cellularity

countries (Table 91–2). A subset of patients, perhaps as many as 25 percent, with primary myelofibrosis present without overt reticulin fibrosis in the marrow.[137,138] Blood hemoglobin may be normal and white cell count mildly elevated. The classic findings of frequent teardrop red cells, myelocytes, and nucleated red cells in the blood film and palpable splenomegaly often are absent. Thrombocytosis is a nearly constant finding. Essential thrombocythemia is closely simulated, but observation eventually shows evolution to primary myelofibrosis. The most important distinction with essential thrombocythemia is the nature of the megakaryocytic expansion.[139] In primary myelofibrosis, bizarre changes are evident with wide variation in megakaryocyte size from very-small- to giant-size cells. Nuclear lobulation is abnormal, with bulky multilobulation, hypolobulation, and free megakaryocyte nuclei in the marrow spaces. In essential thrombocythemia, megakaryocytes are increased but they do not display the dysmorphia observed in myelofibrosis. The prefibrotic disease usually evolves into fully developed myelofibrosis over a period of years. Although blinded studies have raised questions about the ability to identify a prefibrotic stage, the presence of JAK2 617F mutations does lend support to such a concept.

Fibrohematopoietic Extramedullary Tumors

The appearance of symptoms or signs leading to (1) identification of a mass on imaging regardless of location, (2) appearance of signs or symptoms of an effusion in the thorax or abdomen, (3) unexpected neurologic signs, or (4) another finding that appears unexpected in a patient with primary myelofibrosis should be considered a fibrohematopoietic tumor(s) until proven otherwise. Foci of hematopoiesis may become clinically apparent as fibrohematopoietic tumors in the adrenal glands,[140,141] renal parenchyma,[142–144] and lymph nodes.[145–147] Tumors composed of hematopoietic tissue, sometimes with intense fibrosis, can develop in the bowel,[148–151] breast,[152–154] liver,[155,156] lungs,[157–159] mediastinum,[160] pleura and mesentery,[157,159,161] skin,[162,163] synovium,[164] thymus,[157] thyroid,[165] thorax,[166] prostate,[167] spleen,[168] or urinary tract.[166,169–172]

Extramedullary hematopoiesis in the intracranial or intraspinal epidural space can lead to serious neurologic complications, including subdural hemorrhage,[173] delirium,[173,174] increased intracranial pressure,[175] orbital apex syndrome,[176] papilledema,[177] cerebral tumor,[178] coma,[179] motor and sensory impairment,[180,181] spinal cord compression,[182,183] and limb paralysis.[183,184] Intraspinal myelography,[181–193] computed axial tomography,[173,175,179–185] positron emission tomography after ^{57}Fe infusion,[171] and magnetic resonance imaging[186,187] each has been used to define the location and nature of the masses.

Hematopoietic foci on serosal surfaces can produce effusions, sometimes massive, in the thorax,[166,188] abdomen,[160,161,189,190] and pericardial space.[191–194] The effusion fluid often contains megakaryocytes, immature granulocytes, and occasionally erythroblasts.[195–197] Splenectomy is sometimes followed by extramedullary hematopoietic tumors in soft tissues,[198] in body cavities, or on serosal surfaces,[197] perhaps as a result of an increase in circulating hematopoietic progenitors[199] and loss of the filtration function of the spleen. In rare cases, extramedullary soft tissue megakaryoblastic tumors simulate the myeloid sarcomas of other types of myelogenous leukemia.[200,201]

Portal Hypertension and Varices and Pulmonary Arterial Hypertension

In patients with primary myelofibrosis, there can be a massive increase in splenoportal blood flow and a decrease in hepatic vascular compliance or the presence of hepatic vein thrombosis, either of which can result in severe portal hypertension, ascites, esophageal and gastric varices, intraluminal gastrointestinal bleeding, and hepatic encephalopathy.[202–204] The hepatic venous pressure gradient, normally less than 6 torr, is markedly elevated.[205]

Perisinusoidal fibrosis,[206–208] collagen bundles in the spaces of Disse,[207] perisinusoidal fibroplasia,[206–209] and foci of hematopoietic cells[207,210] each appears to contribute to the decreased sinusoidal compliance. Portal vein thrombosis is a complication of primary myelofibrosis and occasionally precedes disease onset.[211]

Rarely, portal hypertension is accompanied by pulmonary hypertension and may result from pulmonary fibrosis[159] or hydrodynamic factors.[212] Pulmonary arterial hypertension, also, may be the principal problem.[213,214] Although as many as one-third of patients with primary myelofibrosis have an elevated systolic pulmonary artery pressures (>35 torr), the fraction that is symptomatic is very small. Elevated vascular endothelial growth factor (VEGF) levels, elevated circulating endothelial cells, and elevated marrow microvessel density in patients suggest that proangiogenic factors may contribute to the hypertension.[215] Contrariwise, secondary myelofibrosis with polyclonal hematopoiesis and normal blood CD34 cell concentrations frequently occurs in patients with primary pulmonary hypertension.[216]

Immune and Inflammatory Manifestations

Abnormalities of humoral immune mechanisms have been observed in up to half of patients with primary myelofibrosis.[217–222] The array of immune products and events reported includes anti–red cell antibodies,[221,223–225] antiplatelet antibodies,[226,227] antinuclear antibodies,[217,218,222] elevated plasma-soluble IL-2 receptor,[228] anti-Gal (galactosidic determinants) antibodies,[229] anti–γ-globulins,[217,219,222] antiphospholipid antibodies,[222,230] antitissue or organ-specific antibodies,[219,221] and circulating immune complexes,[222,231–233] as well as complement activation,[222,234] immune complex deposition,[219] interstitial immunoglobulin deposition,[219] increased numbers of marrow plasmacytoid lymphocytes,[219,231] and development of amyloidosis.[232–235]

Inflammatory cytokines including IL-1β, IL-6, IL-8, TNF-α, TNF-RII, and C-reactive protein also are markedly elevated and play a role in the constitutional symptoms seen in patients with progressive disease.[236]

Occasional reports of nonclonal secondary myelofibrosis associated with lupus erythematosus,[237–242] vasculitis,[243] polyarteritis nodosa,[222,243] ulcerative colitis,[244] scleroderma,[245] biliary cirrhosis,[225,247] Sjögren syndrome,[248] and acute reversible myelofibrosis responsive to glucocorticoids,[249] although fundamentally different processes from primary myelofibrosis, have raised the possibility that immune mechanisms play a role in the development of marrow fibrosis in some circumstances.

Bone Changes

A large proportion of patients have osteosclerosis at diagnosis or develop osteosclerosis during the course of the disease,[10–14,250–253] as reflected by increased bone density on imaging studies and histomorphometric analysis of a bone biopsy (Table 91–3).[251–256] The proximal femur and humerus, pelvis, vertebrae, ribs, and skull may be involved. Magnetic resonance imaging (MRI) can uncover evidence of new bone formation and periosteal thickening. Lumbar spine dual-energy x-ray absorption studies and quantitative computed tomography provide evidence for increased bone formation, bone thickening, and higher proportions of cancellous and of woven bone.[256,257] Osteolytic lesions are rare[258] and may reflect a myeloid sarcoma.[259] Periostitis, although infrequent, can lead to debilitating bone pain.[260]

Thrombosis

The risk of arterial and venous thrombosis is elevated in patients with primary myelofibrosis, although not to the degree seen in polycythemia vera or essential thrombocythemia.[261] Approximately 10 percent of patients with myelofibrosis will develop a significant thrombotic event during the first 4 years of the disease. The two principal risk factors are an elevated platelet count and a cardiovascular risk factor, such as hypertension, hypercholesterolemia, or smoking. Multiple thrombotic episodes may occur and the thrombotic event may occur at or just before diagnosis.

TABLE 91–3. Serum, Urine, and Bone Changes Reflecting Osteosclerosis[243,244]

- Increased serum alkaline phosphatase
- Increased serum bone GLA-protein
- Increased serum carboxytelopeptidase
- Increased urinary deoxypyridinoline
- Increased bone density by dual-energy x-ray absorption
- Increased bone density by quantitative computed tomography
- Histomorphometry
  - Increased percentage of cancellous bone volume to tissue volume
  - Increased bone formation and resorption (high turnover)
  - Increased trabecular plate thickness
  - Increased percentage of woven bone volume
  - Increased percentage of fibrous area
  - No evidence of mineralization defect

LABORATORY FEATURES

BLOOD CELL COUNTS AND MORPHOLOGY

The range of values for blood cell counts at the time of diagnosis is very broad. Normocytic–normochromic anemia is present in most, but not all, patients (see Table 91–2).[7–15,262–265] Mean hemoglobin concentration in a series of patients at diagnosis is approximately 9.0 to 12.0 g/dL (range: 4–20 g/dL).[7–15,264,265] Anisocytosis and poikilocytosis are a constant finding. In all cases, teardrop-shaped red cells (dacryocytes) are present in sufficient number to be found in every oil immersion field (Fig. 91–1). Nucleated red cells are present in the blood film of most patients and average 2 percent of nucleated cells (range: 0–30%). The percentage of reticulocytes is mildly increased but may vary widely in a given case. Anemia may be worsened by expansion of plasma volume and a higher than normal proportion of the red cell volume in an enlarged spleen. Ineffective erythropoiesis can result in a decrease in red cell mass.[262] Erythroid hypoplasia is present in many patients.[266,267] In some patients, hemolysis may be prominent, and polychromatophilia and very elevated reticulocyte counts can occur.[263,264] The antiglobulin (Coombs) test usually is negative, but red cell autoantibodies can develop and lead to immune-mediated hemolysis,[222,223,268] which rarely has been the presenting finding of the disease.[224] Occasional patients have a positive acid hemolysis and sucrose hemolysis test, reflecting a concurrent clone of cells consistent with paroxysmal nocturnal hemoglobinuria.[269] Acquired hemoglobin H disease, coincident with typical white cells and platelet changes of myelofibrosis, can occur[270] and results in hemolysis, hypochromic–microcytic red cells, marked poikilocytosis, and hemoglobin H inclusions that stain with brilliant cresyl blue. Red cell aplasia, in association with myelofibrosis, has been observed.[265,271]

The total white cell count usually is mildly elevated as a result of granulocytosis.[7–15] The mean total blood white cell count was 10,000 to 14,000/μL (10 to 14 × 10^9/L) in four large studies. The range of white cell counts was 400 to 237,000/μL (0.4 to 237 × 10^9/L) at the time of diagnosis.[7–14,263,264] Myelocytes and promyelocytes are present in small proportions in most patients, and a low proportion of blast cells (0.5–2%) may be found in the blood film. The blood blast cells range from 0 to 20 percent at the time of diagnosis. In patients with blast counts at the high end, which is unusual at presentation, the disease has converged with AML. Hypersegmentation, hyposegmentation (acquired Pelger-Huët anomaly), and abnormal granulation of neutrophils may be present.[7–15] Neutrophil alkaline phosphatase scores may be elevated (25% of patients) or decreased (25% of patients).[272] The percentage of basophils may be slightly increased.[264] Neutropenia is present in approximately 20 percent of patients at the time of diagnosis.[7–15]

The mean platelet count in patient series range from 175,000 to 580,000/μL (175 to 580 × 10^9/L) at the time of diagnosis. Individual platelet counts can range from 15,000 to 3,215,000/μL (15.0 to 3215 × 10^9/L).[7–15,263,264] The platelet count is elevated in approximately 40 percent of patients.[264] Mild to moderate thrombocytopenia is present in approximately one-third of patients at the time of diagnosis. Giant platelets and abnormal platelet granulation are characteristic features of the disease.

Approximately 10 percent of patients present with pancytopenia because of severe impairment of hematopoiesis affecting each cell lineage, coupled with sequestration in a massively enlarged spleen. Pancytopenia usually is associated with intense marrow fibrosis.

Increased concentrations of multipotential,[273,274] granulocytic,[275,276] monocytic,[276] erythroid,[277] and megakaryocytic[278] progenitor cells are present in the blood of patients, as measured by clonogenic assays in semisolid cultures. The frequency of hematopoietic progenitor cells in the blood is correlated with the extent of marrow reticular fiber density.[278]

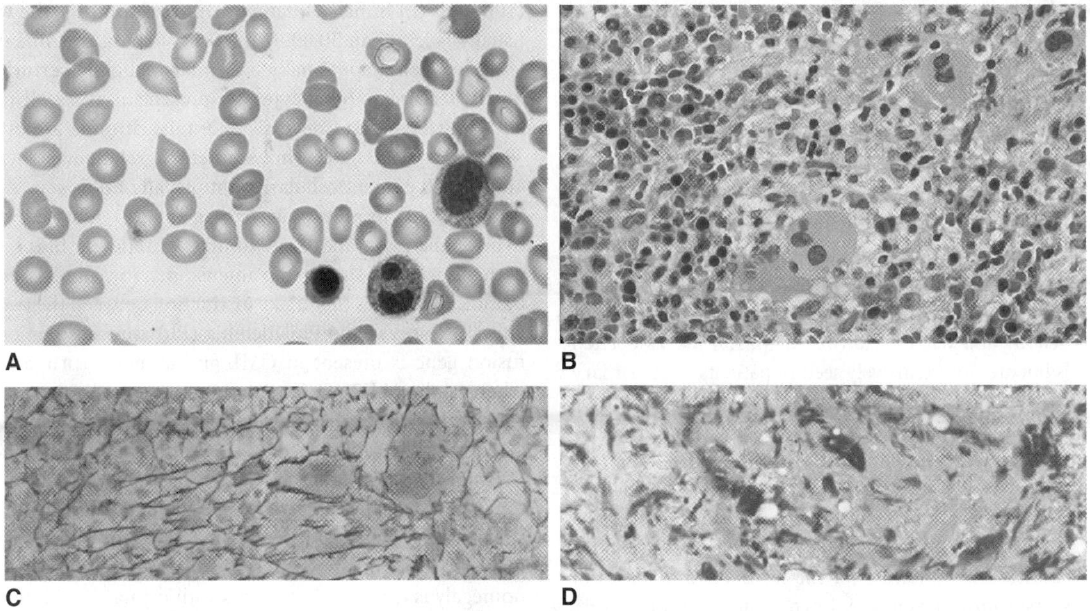

FIGURE 91–1. Blood film and marrow sections from patients with primary myelofibrosis. **A.** Blood film. Characteristic teardrop poikilocytes, a nucleated red cell, and a segmented neutrophil with a dysmorphic nucleus are evident. **B.** Marrow section. Low power. Hypercellular marrow with increased number of hypolobular megakaryocytes. **C.** Marrow section. Silver impregnation stain. Marked increase in argentophilic fibers representing collagen type III (reticulin). **D.** Marrow section. Collagen fibrosis with extensive replacement of marrow with swirls of collagen fibers. *(Used with permission from* Lichtman's Atlas of Hematology, *www.accessmedicine.com.)*

Megakaryocytes also are present in the systemic venous blood.[279] An increase in blood CD34+ cells is very characteristic of primary myelofibrosis, and the concentration of these cells lends weight to the diagnosis. The height of the CD34+ cell count is correlated with the extent of disease and disease progression. Greater than 15 × 10^6/L blood CD34+ cells is virtually diagnostic of primary myelofibrosis, and patients with greater than 300 × 10^6/L CD34+ cells have more rapid progression of disease than patients with fewer CD34+ cells.[274]

Endothelial progenitor cells (CD+CD133+ and VEGFR2-positive cells) are significantly higher in the blood of primary myelofibrosis patients than of normal subjects.[78]

Mild lymphocytopenia resulting from decreased CD3+, CD4+, CD8+, and CD3–/CD56+ T cells is the rule.[280]

FUNCTIONAL ABNORMALITIES OF BLOOD CELLS

The neutrophils of some patients have impaired phagocytosis, oxygen consumption, nitroblue tetrazolium reduction, and hydrogen peroxide generation, and decreased myeloperoxidase[281,282] and glutathione reductase activities.[282] CD34+ cells have impaired *in vitro* differentiation to natural killer cells, which appear to be related to a dysregulation in control of IL-15.[283]

Bleeding time can be prolonged out of proportion to the platelet count.[284,285] Platelet abnormalities include impaired aggregation in response to epinephrine, depletion of dense granule adenosine diphosphate content,[286] decreased platelet lipoxygenase pathway activity,[287] and others.[288,289] The correlation of bleeding or thrombosis with platelet functional abnormalities is weak.[288,289] The lupus anticoagulant has been present, rarely.[230]

MARROW EXAMINATION

Morphology

In the fibrotic phase, marrow aspiration often is unsuccessful because of the fibrosis.[7–15,86,87] The marrow biopsy specimen usually is cellular and shows granulocytic and megakaryocytic hyperplasia (see Fig. 91–1).[7–15,273,274] Erythroid cells may be decreased, normal, or increased in number. Silver stain usually shows an increase in reticular fibers, and in half of patients a striking increase in reticular fibers is seen.[274] Hematoxylin and eosin stains of the biopsy specimen may show mild collagen fibrosis; occasionally the fibrosis is extreme (see Fig. 91–1). Collagen fibrosis may be more evident using a Gomori trichrome stain with which collagen characteristically stains green. In intensely fibrotic marrows, cellularity may be markedly decreased but megakaryocytes usually remain evident.[274] Giant megakaryocytes and micromegakaryocytes, abnormal nuclear lobulation, and naked megakaryocyte nuclei are present.[7–15,290] Thrombopoietin receptors are decreased on megakaryocytes and platelets.[81] Granulocytes may show hyperlobulation and hypolobulation of the nucleus, acquired Pelger-Huët anomaly, nuclear blebs, and nuclear–cytoplasmic maturation asynchrony.[291] Clusters of blasts and CD34-positive cells are often present. Dilated marrow sinusoids are common. Intrasinusoidal, immature hematopoietic cells, and megakaryocytes are present.[86] As a reflection of the high blood flow to marrow-bearing bone and the widened sinusoidal system, microvessel density is significantly increased in approximately 70 percent of patients.[291] Histomorphometric analysis of marrow biopsies permit detection of osteosclerosis,[251,253,254] but imaging is more readily available (see below).

The marrow in the prefibrotic stage usually has no or slight reticular fibrosis. The marrow is cellular and there is often an increase proportion of late neutrophil precursors (myelocytes, metamyelocytes, bands). Myeloblasts and CD34-positive cells are inconspicuous. Erythropoiesis may be slightly decreased. Increased and abnormal megakaroyocytopoiesis is the hallmark of this phase. Clusters of megakaryocytes are present. Megakaryocytes are large and admixed with small megakaryocytes. Nuclei are often ballooned and have scalloped margins. Bare megakaryocyte nuclei are present. Megakaryocyte involvement is facilitated by staining the marrow with a megakaryocyte marker such as CD61.

Cytogenetic Findings

Chromosome abnormalities of hematopoietic cells are evident in approximately 40 to 60 percent of patients at the time of diagnosis.[293–298] The most frequent findings are partial trisomy 1q, interstitial deletion of a segment of the long arm of chromosome 13, del(13)(q12-22), which bears the retinoblastoma gene,[55,294–296,299] del 20q, and trisomy 8.[300] Involvement of chromosome 5, 6, 7, 9, 13, 20, or 21 occurs with heightened frequency.[300] The 5q– abnormality is more prevalent in primary myelofibrosis that any chronic myeloproliferative disorder. Abnormality of chromosome 12 resulting from several translocations or deletion or inversion occurs in approximately 3 percent of patients.[301] The del(13) and der(6)t(1;6)(q21-23;p21.3) are associated with myelofibrosis but are not exclusively seen in patients with primary myelofibrosis.[302] Aneuploidy as a result of monosomy or trisomy is common. Pseudodiploidy, manifested by partial deletions and translocations, occurs. Patients with the clinical features of typical primary myelofibrosis very, very rarely have the Ph chromosome in their marrow cells.[303] With increasing knowledge of the chromosomes commonly affected, interphase FISH of blood cells is used to look for prevalent abnormalities, compensating for the technical difficulties of harvesting cell suspensions, given the intense marrow fibrosis.[296] Clonal chromosomal abnormalities found in hematopoietic cells have not been observed in marrow fibroblasts.[129]

Magnetic Resonance Imaging

Marrow fibrosis alters the hyperintensity of T1-weighted images that normally results from marrow fat. As cellularity and fibrosis progress, hypointensity of T1-weighted and T2-weighted images develops. MRI does not distinguish between primary myelofibrosis and secondary causes of fibrosis,[251,304,305] but the clinical distinctions usually are very evident from the results of prior physical, blood, and marrow examinations. Patchy or diffuse osteosclerosis is a common finding, as are "sandwich vertebrae," so called because of marked radiodensity of superior and inferior margins of the vertebral body. MRI can identify the uncommon periosteal reactions that usually occur in the distal femur, proximal tibia, or ankle. The reactions represent expansion of marrow cellularity into normally inactive regions of long bones or extramedullary space-occupying lesions of fibrohematopoietic tissue.[252] The findings of sodium fluoride (^{18}F) positron emission tomography can be virtually specific for osteosclerosis of primary myelofibrosis.[306]

■ PLASMA AND URINE CHEMICAL CHANGES

Serum levels of uric acid, lactic dehydrogenase, bilirubin, alkaline phosphatase, and high-density lipoprotein frequently are elevated.[7–15] Serum levels of albumin and cholesterol frequently are decreased.[307] Hypocalcemia[308] or hypercalcemia[309] may occur. Plasma levels of thrombopoietin and IL-6 are elevated but do not correlate with either platelet or megakaryocyte mass.[310,311] Elevated thrombopoietin is not explained by increased marrow hematopoietic or stromal cell production.[312] Serum-soluble IL-2 receptor[313] and serum vascular endothelial growth factor[314] levels are increased. Urinary excretion of calmodulin is approximately three times normal.[120] The serum contains evidence of increased collagen (see Table 91–1) and bone (see Table 91–2) synthesis.

DIFFERENTIAL DIAGNOSIS

CML (see Chap. 90) should be considered in the differential diagnosis of primary myelofibrosis. In CML, the white cell count is greater than 30,000/μL (30 × 10^9/L) in almost all patients and greater than 100,000/μL (100 × 10^9/L) in half of patients. In myelofibrosis, the white cell count usually is less than 30,000/μL (30 × 10^9/L) at the time of diagnosis. In CML, red cell shape usually is normal or slightly perturbed. In myelofibrosis, teardrop poikilocytes are present in every oil immersion field and exaggerated anisocytosis and anisochromia are often prominent. The marrow in CML shows intense granulocytic hyperplasia, with almost 100 percent cellularity and usually no or very slight fibrosis.[315] In myelofibrosis, the marrow has mildly increased cellularity or is hypocellular, with moderate to marked reticulin fibrosis. Occasionally, patients with CML develop intense marrow fibrosis and dysmorphic blood cell changes that make distinction between the two diseases difficult.[301] However, the Philadelphia (Ph) chromosome or the *BCR-ABL* fusion gene is present in CML and absent in primary myelofibrosis; whereas, the *JAK2V617F* mutation is present in approximately 50 percent of cases of primary myelofibrosis and absent in CML. Most cases are readily separable based on the aforementioned distinctions.

Patients with primary myelofibrosis may have pancytopenia or bicytopenia and in that respect mimic patients with oligoblastic leukemia (myelodysplasia [MDS]; see Chap. 88). Contrariwise, patients with oligoblastic leukemia may rarely have intense fibrosis.[316] Prominent splenomegaly is expected in patients with primary myelofibrosis but not in patients with oligoblastic leukemia, which helps to distinguish the former from the latter patients. The absence of a high frequency of teardrop-shaped red cells, nucleated red cells, and striking anisopoikilocytosis in the blood film mitigates against primary myelofibrosis.

Because some patients with primary myelofibrosis have platelet counts greater than 450,000/μL (450 × 10^9/L), the diagnosis of primary thrombocythemia may be considered. The anisopoikilocytosis, nucleated red cells, and myeloid immaturity in the blood film characteristic of myelofibrosis are not present in patients with thrombocythemia. Marrow fibrosis usually is insignificant in thrombocythemia, and splenic enlargement often is absent or slight. For these reasons, a clear distinction usually exists between the two disorders.[264,317] The prefibrotic phase of primary myelofibrosis may mimic essential thrombocythemia, but the more prominent splenomegaly and the more disordered megakaryopoiesis in primary myelofibrosis can be used to distinguish the two entities, as does careful observation of disease evolution.[318]

Hairy cell leukemia (see Chap. 95), when associated with shape abnormalities of red cells, pancytopenia, splenomegaly, and fibrotic marrow, can closely mimic primary myelofibrosis.[316,319] Usually, careful scrutiny of the blood and marrow by microscopy, histochemistry, and cell immunophenotype shows evidence of the abnormal mononuclear (hairy) cells characteristic of the disease.

Hepatic disease can be associated with cytopenias and splenomegaly, although the specific blood and marrow findings usually make the distinction with primary myelofibrosis obvious. In a review of 170 cases of splenomegaly in a county hospital, hepatic disease was the second most common cause of massive splenomegaly after primary myelofibrosis.[320]

Primary autoimmune myelofibrosis is characterized by intense marrow fibrosis and an increase in marrow polyclonal T and B lymphocytes.[321,322] Serologic or clinical evidence of lupus erythematosus or other connective tissue diseases is absent, giving primary autoimmune myelofibrosis a definitive diagnostic niche. Cytopenias that occur may be immune mediated (e.g., immune hemolytic disease), and the blood cell findings (anisopoikilocytosis, nucleated red cells, myeloid immaturity) characteristic of primary myelofibrosis usually are absent. The marrow may be cellular with increased megakaryocytes, but strikingly dysmorphic megakaryocytopoiesis is absent. Splenomegaly, a nearly constant feature of primary myelofibrosis, usually is absent. Polyclonal hyperglobulinemia may be present.

Patients with sporadic idiopathic or familial pulmonary hypertension have significant marrow fibrosis. They can be distinguished from patients with primary myelofibrosis with pulmonary hypertension by the latter's high-circulating CD34+ cell count, the presence of clonal platelets and granulocytes, a high frequency of dacryocytes in the blood film, and a *JAK2* V617F mutation.[323]

Metastatic carcinoma, especially derived from carcinoma of breast or prostate[324–329] or disseminated mycobacterial infection,[330,331] can induce reactive marrow fibrosis and occasionally simulate primary myelofibrosis. Demonstration of metastatic carcinoma cells or mycobacteria in the marrow indicates the etiology. Other disorders reported with secondary myelofibrosis include mastocytosis,[332–335] angioimmunoblastic lymphadenopathy,[336] angiosarcoma,[337] lymphoma,[338–340] multiple myeloma,[341–343] renal osteodystrophy,[344] hypertrophic osteoarthropathy,[345] gray platelet syndrome,[346] systemic lupus erythematosus,[239–242] polyarteritis nodosa,[245] hypereosinophilic syndrome,[347,348] kala azar,[349] primary thrombocytopenic purpura,[350] thrombotic thrombocytopenic purpura,[351] tretinoin administration,[352] neuroblastoma,[353] giant lymph node hyperplasia,[354] vitamin D-deficiency rickets,[355–358] Langerhans cell histiocytosis,[359] acute promyelocytic leukemia,[360,361] and malignant histiocytosis.[362] Correction or amelioration of the primary disorder can lead to disappearance of the marrow fibrosis.

Lymphoma,[363,364] chronic lymphocytic leukemia,[365,366] hairy cell leukemia,[319,367] systemic mastocytosis,[368] macroglobulinemia,[369] amyloidosis,[232,233] myeloma,[370,371] malignant teratoma,[372] and essential monoclonal gammopathy[373] can coincide with primary myelofibrosis.

TRANSITIONS TO AND FROM MYELOFIBROSIS AMONG CLONAL HEMOPATHIES

All clonal hematopoietic diseases (AML, CML, oligoblastic myelogenous leukemia [MDS], lymphomas) may have increased marrow reticulin fibers but only infrequently have collagen fibrosis.[374] Acute megakaryoblastic leukemia is accompanied by intense marrow fibrosis (see Chap. 89). Approximately 15 percent of patients with polycythemia vera, whether treated by phlebotomy, alkylating agents, or ^{32}P, develop a clinical state indistinguishable from primary myelofibrosis during 20 years of observation (see Chap. 86).[375–377] Essential thrombocythemia may evolve into a myelofibrotic stage, estimated to occur in approximately 7 percent of cases (see Chap. 87). This estimate is complicated by the question of whether some cases of essential thrombocythemia actually are very early (prefibrotic) primary myelofibrosis.[319] Sideroblastic anemia has progressed to primary myelofibrosis.[378] Rarely, primary myelofibrosis reverts to polycythemia vera, with disappearance of marrow fibrosis.[379,380] Even more rarely, primary myelofibrosis, carrying the *JAK2* mutation, has undergone clonal evolution to BCR-ABL-positive CML or vice-versa.[381,382]

THERAPY

DECISION TO TREAT

A significant proportion (~25%) of asymptomatic patients remain stable for years and do not require specific treatment. Symptomatic anemia, thrombocytopenia, and splenomegaly are the principal initial reasons for therapy. A hemoglobin less than 10 g/dL,[11,13,19] a white count less than 4000/μL (4.0 × 10^9/L) or greater than 30,000/μL (30.0 × 10^9/L),[13] and blood blasts above 1 percent of total leukocytes[11,19] predict more rapid progression of disease. More elaborate staging protocols may be useful in comparing concurrent and sequential clinical trial results (see "Course and Prognosis" below). In an individual patient under the care of a clinician experienced in the disease, following disease progression is a very important additional factor even in patients deemed at higher risk by formulaic techniques, especially before introducing stem cell transplantation with its morbidity and potential mortality.

ANDROGENS AND GLUCOCORTICOIDS FOR ANEMIA

Severe anemia may improve with androgen therapy in some patients.[383] Testosterone, oxymetholone, and fluoxymesterone have been used but have virilizing effects. In addition, they have the potential for hepatic injury and other side effects. Danazol, 600 to 800 mg/day orally for up to 6 months, can be used. The drug is tapered to the minimum effective dose or discontinued if no significant response occurs. Improvement may be limited to a decreased frequency of red cell transfusion. Androgens often are used after splenectomy if anemia returns and requires transfusion of red cells. They are more effective in splenectomized patients or those with less splenic enlargement. Patients undergoing androgen therapy should have periodic assessment of liver size by physical examination, measurement of liver function tests, and, if appropriate, ultrasonographic imaging to detect liver injury (e.g., peliosis) or tumors.[384] Evaluation of male patients for prostatic enlargement or cancer is prudent before starting androgen therapy. Patients with significant hemolytic anemia may benefit from glucocorticoid therapy. Prednisone 25 mg/m^2 per day orally can be tried. If tolerated, the dose can be continued for 1 to 2 months and then tapered gradually. In children, high-dose glucocorticoid therapy reportedly ameliorates marrow fibrosis and improves hematopoiesis.[385,386]

RECOMBINANT HUMAN ERYTHROPOIETIN FOR ANEMIA

Serum erythropoietin levels usually are appropriate to the severity of anemia in patients with myelofibrosis.[387] Thus, use of erythropoietin as a general approach to the treatment of anemia has been disappointing. In patients, selected by their inappropriately low serum erythropoietin levels (<125 U/L) for the degree of anemia, protracted beneficial effects can result.[388,389]

DRUG THERAPY FOR MYELOPROLIFERATION, SPLENOMEGALY, OR CYTOPENIAS

A variety of drugs have been used for treatment of massive splenomegaly, thrombocytosis, or constitutional symptoms.

Hydroxyurea

Hydroxyurea has become the most commonly used and preferred agent for exaggerated accumulation of platelets, occasionally leukocytes, troublesome areas of extramedullary hematopoiesis, and symptomatic splenomegaly.[390–392] Hydroxyurea can decrease the size of the spleen and liver, decrease or eliminate constitutional symptoms of night sweats or weight loss, and lead to an increase in hemoglobin concentration, a decrease of platelet counts, and, occasionally, a decrease in the degree of marrow fibrosis. Patients with myelofibrosis often do not have the marrow tolerance to chemotherapy of patients with other chronic myeloproliferative diseases. Hydroxyurea can be administered in doses of 0.5 to 1.0 g/day or 1.0 to 2.0 g orally two to three times per week, depending on the level of pretreatment blood cell counts. Patients should be evaluated for dose adjustment at least every week for 1 month and, if appropriate, extended to every 2 weeks for 2 months. Thereafter, monthly evaluation of dose may be appropriate. Although alkylating agents, especially busulfan and other cytotoxic agents, have been used successfully, they have largely been replaced by hydroxyurea. Use of alkylating agents has resurfaced with the suggestion that melphalan may be useful as first-line therapy.[393]

JAK2 V617F Kinase Inhibitors

Because *JAK2* mutations and the resulting effects on JAK-STAT signaling are thought to be a key factor in the clonal expansion leading to primary myelofibrosis in at least 50 percent of patients, an effort to synthesize and test inhibitors of the mutant JAK2 protein product is underway.[394] Early studies of the JAK2 kinase inhibitor TG101209, an oral, bioavailable small molecule, and a potent inhibitor of JAK2 kinase, have shown its ability to inhibit JAK2 V617F-dependent phosphorylation of STAT 3 and 5, inhibit colony growth of cells harboring *JAK2* and *MPL* mutations, and to have therapeutic effects in a nude mouse model of JAK2 V617F-induced myeloproliferative disease.[395] Several JAK2 inhibitors (INCB018424, TG101348, XL019) have been administered to small numbers of patients with primary myelofibrosis.[396–398] Their effects are somewhat different. The most striking and consistent effect with each agent is a decrease in spleen size. They may also suppress blood cell counts, and thrombocytopenia can be dose-limiting. The reduction in large spleen size and decrease in the effects of markedly elevated inflammatory cytokines have improved the quality of life of some patients. In the case of one agent, the response rate was similar in those with and without an apparent *JAK2* mutation. This effect may be explained by the drug's ability to inhibit JAK1 and 2 isoforms, the former having a role in cytokine elaboration. These agents promise to decrease morbidity and possibly mortality. Further larger and more detailed studies in patients with primary myelofibrosis should be forthcoming and help to determine (1) if these agents ameliorate disease manifestations in a high proportion of patients, (2) the duration of their beneficial effects, (3) whether patient survival is improved with their use, and (4) what adverse effects to expect during prolonged administration.

Thalidomide and Lenalidomide

Thalidomide is poorly tolerated at optimal doses of approximately 800 mg/day. Most patients receive about half that amount and are tapered to the lowest effective dose. One study of 14 patients found the drug was not beneficial and had high toxicity rates.[399] Other studies found some decrease in spleen size and improvement in blood hemoglobin and platelet counts in a minority of patients receiving up to 600 mg/day.[400,401] In subsequent studies, lower doses of thalidomide (50 mg/day) coupled with prednisone were more tolerable and resulted in improvement of anemia and thrombocytopenia in about half of patients, with sustained improvement in some patients after treatment was stopped.[402] The thalidomide congener lenalidomide may supersede thalidomide use. Lenalidomide has provided responses in a significant minority of patients.[403–406] The drug can result in marked improvement in hemoglobin concentration or avoidance of a requirement for transfusion (22% of patients treated), improvement in platelet count (50%), and decrease in spleen size (33%). Neutropenia and thrombocytopenia were the most troubling side effects.[403] The drug has also been useful in patients with primary myelofibrosis who have a 5q– cytogenetic abnormality.[404,405]

Cyclosporine, Etanercept, Imatinib Mesylate, Tipifarnib

Cyclosporine has been used to achieve a serum level of 100 to 200 ng/mL in severely anemic patients with evidence of immune abnormalities (positive Coombs test, antinuclear antibodies).[407] Three of six patients responded with an increased hemoglobin concentration. Cyclosporine has been used with apparent success in a single patient with myelofibrosis and red cell aplasia.[408]

Tumor necrosis factor alpha has been proposed as a target to inhibit its possible effects in the pathogenesis of primary myelofibrosis.[409] Of 20 patients treated with soluble tumor necrosis factor alpha receptor (etanercept), 12 had improvement in constitutional symptoms (fever, night sweats, fatigue, weight loss), and 4 had improved blood counts and decreased spleen size.[410,411]

Imatinib mesylate for treatment of myelofibrosis has been examined on empirical grounds and has been largely ineffective in influencing the disease course.[411,412] Modest doses have not been well tolerated, and responses have been infrequent and insubstantial.

The farnesyl transferase inhibitor tipifarnib is not well tolerated.[413] Although it may decrease spleen size, it has shown no advantages over hydroxyurea.

Interferons

Interferon-α and interferon-γ act synergistically to inhibit myeloproliferation.[414] The former has been used extensively for treatment of CML prior to the availability of mutant tyrosine kinase (BCR-ABL) inhibitors (see Chap. 90). Interferon-α has not been used extensively in primary myelofibrosis but has been useful for treatment of splenic enlargement, bone pain, and thrombocytosis in selected patients.[415] Trials comparing interferon therapy with hydroxyurea or other therapy have not been reported.[416] Hydroxyurea is easier to use (oral versus parenteral) and has less frequent and severe side effects than interferon, especially in older patients. A newer preparation polyethylene glycol conjugated interferon-α may prove more practical and tolerable for use in patients with myelofibrosis.

Serosal Implants

Cytarabine Ascites resulting from peritoneal hematopoietic implants has been treated with intraperitoneal cytarabine.[417] Intrasplenic cytarabine administered via a splenic artery catheter has resulted in significant improvement in a patient (see also "Radiotherapy" below).[418]

■ IMMUNE-RELATED FIBROSIS

Intravenous Immunoglobulin

Although autoimmune or systemic lupus erythematosus-related myelofibrosis has responded to glucocorticoids or intravenous immune globulin[239,242] and a variety of other fibrotic disorders occasionally respond,[419] primary myelofibrosis does not have a sustained response to such therapy because the fundamental lesion is the hematopoietic multipotential cell neoplasm, megakaryocytosis, severe megakaryocytic dysmorphia, and cytokine release with resultant fibrogenesis and, sometimes, osteogenesis.

■ BISPHOSPHONATES FOR BONE DISEASE

Debilitating bone pain can be a vexing problem in some patients with osteosclerosis and periostitis. Dramatic improvement in bone pain and hematopoiesis after etidronate 6 mg/kg per day on alternate months[420] or clodronate 30 mg/kg per day for several months, during which marked improvement was still present 33 months later,[421] highlight the potential usefulness of this family of drugs for bone symptoms.[422]

■ RADIOTHERAPY

Radiotherapy can be useful for patients with primary myelofibrosis in several situations. For example, in the presence of (1) severe splenic pain (splenic infarctions) or (2) massive splenic enlargement with contraindication to splenectomy (e.g., thrombocytosis), repeated doses of 0.5 to 2 Gy to the spleen can ameliorate the pain.[423] Splenic radiation can result in further cytopenias or worsening cytopenias, especially thrombocytopenia, an abscopal effect on marrow production, perhaps because of the circulation of large numbers of CD34+ cells exposed in the spleen. Other situations in which radiation may be useful are (3) ascites resulting from myeloid metaplasia of the peritoneum,[424] (4) focal areas of severe bone pain (periostitis or the osteolysis of a myeloid sarcoma),[260,423,425] and (5) extramedullary fibrohematopoietic tumors,[145,423] especially of the epidural space.[179] Low-dose radiation to the liver for symptomatic hepatomegaly and ascites provides only short-term relief.[423,426] Low-dose radiotherapy to the lung has been used successfully to palliate the effects of pulmonary hypertension thought to result from extensive extramedullary hematopoiesis in the organ. Low-dose radiotherapy has relieved signs of respiratory insufficiency, especially hypoxemia.[214]

SPLENECTOMY

Splenectomy has been important in the management of primary myelofibrosis.[427] The major indications for splenectomy include (1) painful enlarged spleen (~50% of patients), (2) excessive transfusion requirements or refractory hemolytic anemia (~25% of patients), (3) portal hypertension (~15% of patients), and (4) severe thrombocytopenia (~10% of patients).

Patients who have a prolonged bleeding time or coagulation times are at serious risk for hemorrhage with surgery and should not undergo the procedure unless the abnormalities can be corrected by platelet transfusion and factor replacement therapy. Evidence of low-grade intravascular coagulation, such as elevated D-dimer levels, may require prophylactic heparin therapy and platelet transfusion should excessive bleeding occur.

Removal of the spleen in patients with primary myelofibrosis may be difficult. Usually the spleen is adherent to neighboring serosal surfaces and structures (e.g., inferior surface of left hemidiaphragm) and has numerous collateral vessels and very dilated splenoportal arteries and veins. Immediate postoperative mortality is a function of surgical experience and skill and of the rapidity of recognition of postoperative complications. In experienced hands, perioperative mortality is approximately 10 percent. Postoperative morbidity from hemorrhage, subphrenic hematoma, subphrenic abscess, injury to the tail of the pancreas, pancreatic fistulas, or portal vein stump or mesenteric vessel thrombosis occurs in approximately 30 percent of patients. Infection, especially, pneumonia occurs in approximately 10 percent of patients. Later postoperative changes include liver enlargement (sometimes massive), extramedullary hematopoietic tumors, thrombocytosis, and a decrease in teardrop-shaped red cells. Leukemic blast transformation occurs in approximately 15 percent of patients after splenectomy. Hydroxyurea or aspirin and anagrelide may be useful for exaggerated thrombocytosis (see Chap. 87). The morbidity and mortality from splenectomy and the modest extension of life have led to increasing conservatism regarding its use. However, splenectomy can improve the condition for which it was performed in about 50 percent of patients. Median survival after splenectomy is about 18 months.

PORTAL-SYSTEMIC VASCULAR SHUNT SURGERY

Circulatory dynamic studies are performed at the time of surgery in patients undergoing operation for portal hypertension and bleeding varices or refractory ascites. In patients in whom the hepatic wedge pressure elevations result from markedly increased blood flow from the spleen to the liver, the preferred treatment procedure for portal hypertension is splenectomy. In patients who have portal hypertension resulting from intrahepatic block or hepatic vein thrombosis and who have a hepatic venous pressure gradient well above the upper limits of normal (6 torr), a splenorenal shunt can be performed[428] or, to avoid abdominal surgery, a transjugular intrahepatic portosystemic shunt can be used.[429,430] Variceal sclerotherapy or variceal ligation has been used to treat bleeding varices resulting from portal hypertension.

HEMATOPOIETIC STEM CELL TRANSPLANTATION

Marrow transplantation is the only curative approach to primary myelofibrosis. Marrow transplantation therapy has been used increasingly in younger patients with a poor prognosis (e.g., severe anemia and leukopenia or exaggerated leukocytosis) who have a histocompatible sibling.[431–438] The median age in most studies is about 45 years, whereas the median age of all patients is about 65 to 70 years. Patients engraft at a rate similar to the rate of patients with hematologic diseases without marrow fibrosis (see Chap. 21). The decision to use full-conditioning allogeneic transplantation is a function of the patient's age (<50 years), the severity of the blood cell and marrow abnormalities, and the likelihood of a protracted indolent course without transplantation. Younger patients, especially those younger than age 50 years, with a DNA-based matched sibling donor, progressive disease, and poor prognostic findings, such as hemoglobin less than 10 g/dL, blast cells greater than 1 percent of blood cells, unfavorable cytogenetics (e.g., abnormalities involving chromosomes 5, 7, or 17 or cells with three or more abnormalities) are usually considered for transplantation. Although a large spleen may slightly delay the expression of donor granulopoiesis, on average the results in patients with a spleen is the same as those who had prior splenectomy.[436,439] In addition, the latter procedure incurs significant risk of morbidity or mortality. Studies of this question continue.

Patients younger than age 50 years who are transplanted with stem cells from a matched sibling donor have a lower posttransplantation mortality and have better outcomes than those older than age 50 years.[413] Transplant-related mortality using full conditioning regimens is about 35–40 percent and 5-year survival is about 50 percent in patients under 50 years.

Donor lymphocyte infusion in patients who have lost donor dominance of hematopoiesis and a return of myelofibrosis can result in regression of fibrosis and return to normal hematopoiesis for at least 6 and 20 months at the time of reporting.[440,441]

In JAK2-positive patients, real-time polymerase chain reaction analysis can permit a sensitive determination of residual JAK2-positive cells after transplantation. In a study of patients receiving low-intensity conditioning, 17 of 21 patients became JAK2-negative and in one case donor lymphocyte infusion eliminated JAK2-positive cells.[442]

The option of nonmyeloablative transplantation in older patients is gaining favor.[435,436,443–446] Several reports of lower posttransplantation mortality and salutary outcomes have led some to consider this approach as the preferred one in patients older than 45 years of age, and perhaps in younger patients as well. One study showed that the outcome of nonmyeloablative transplantation was dramatically better than myeloablative transplant.[435] The study compared 17 patients receiving a myeloablative conditioning regimen and 10 receiving nonmyeloablative conditioning. The median age was 50 years (age range: 5–63 years) at transplantation. After a median followup of 55 months, 20 patients were alive. The transplantation-related mortality was 10 percent in the nonmyeloablative group and 30 percent in the myeloablative group. There was no difference in survival for high- or low-risk patients or between sibling and unrelated donor transplantations. This study confirmed prior smaller comparisons of myeloablative and nonmyeloablative stem cell transplantation.[447]

Given the small sample sizes in studies, there are still unresolved questions about the optimal approach to transplantation for primary myelofibrosis. Among these are the timing of transplantation in patients with stable disease, the optimal pretransplantation conditioning program, the preference of reduced conditioning versus full conditioning in young patients, and the use of blood versus marrow donor stem cells.

Autologous blood stem cells mobilized with granulocyte colony-stimulating factor (G-CSF) and administered after busulfan conditioning to 21 patients with primary myelofibrosis age 45 to 75 years produced clinical benefit, including improved erythropoiesis, improved platelet counts, and decreased splenic size in a plurality of patients. The 2-year actuarial survival rate was 61 percent.[448]

COURSE AND PROGNOSIS

The rate of disease progression has been associated with at least 16 variables measured at the time of diagnosis. Shorter survival has been associated with (1) older age, (2) severity of anemia, (3) exaggerated leukocytosis (>25 × 10^9/L) or leukopenia (<4.0 × 10^9/L), (4) constitutional symptoms of fever, sweating, or weight loss at the time of diagnosis, (5) proportion of blast cells in the blood (≥1%), (6) male gender, (7) severity of thrombocytopenia, (8) proportion of CD34+ cells in the blood, (9) the presence of the V617F mutation in *JAK2*, (10) monocytosis, (11) a decreased proliferating cell nuclear antigen index and a decreased apoptotic index by *in situ* end labeling, (12) degree of liver enlargement, (13) extent of marrow fibrosis, (14) postsplenectomy spleen histology, (15) *WT1* expression in CD34+ cells, and (16) certain clonal cytogenetic abnormalities, especially involving chromosomes 5, 7, or 17 or with three or more abnormalities. Abnormalities such as 13q or 20q did not affect patient survival compared to those patients without cytogenetic alterations. Each retrospective study has found a different subset of these factors to be significant prognostic factors. The most consistent predictive variables appear to be advanced age, severity of anemia, and certain clonal cytogenetic abnormality at the time of diagnosis, each of which represents a poor prognostic indicator.[7,11–13,15,77,273,274,294,296,449–454]

In a study of more than 1000 consecutive cases of myelofibrosis at 7 centers, among which the median survival was 69 months, variables (1) through (5) in the paragraph above proved to be the most useful in dividing patients into 4 risk-factor categories. Shorter survival was observed in patients who were older than age 65 years, had a hemoglobin concentration less than 10 g/dL, a leukocyte count greater than 25 × 10^9/L (25,000/μL), a blood blast cell count equal to or greater than 1 percent, and constitutional symptoms. The patients were assigned to a risk group based on the number of risk factors present. If no risk factors were present, risk was low; if one factor was present, risk was low-intermediate; if two risk factors were present, risk was high-intermediate; and if three or more risk factors were present, risk was high. The application of these variables could distinguish among patients with low risk with a survival of 135 months, low-intermediate risk with a survival of 95 months, high-intermediate risk with a survival of 48 months, and high risk with a survival of 27 months.[455] Overall, the 5-year survival of patients with primary myelofibrosis is approximately 40 percent of the survival expected for healthy age- and sex-matched controls.[456]

The major causes of death are infection, hemorrhage, postsplenectomy mortality, and acute leukemic transformation.[457–461] Acute leukemia occasionally is preceded by the development of myeloid sarcomas.[34,259,427,461,462] Evolution of the disease to acute lymphocytic leukemia or lymphoma may occur.[463,464] An increased risk of progression to leukemia has been reported in splenectomized patients.[465] Progression to acute leukemia is associated with a blast count greater than 3 percent and a platelet count less than 100,000/μL (100 × 10^9/L) at the time of diagnosis. Treatment with erythropoietin or androgens is associated with increased risk of progression to acute leukemia, as well.[466] New drug combinations using JAK2 inhibitors may provide improved efficacy for the treatment of AML evolving in patients with primary myelofibrosis. Rare spontaneous remissions of apparent primary myelofibrosis are documented.[467,468]

Primary myelofibrosis in infants and children has a more varied pathobiology than in adults. Patients have been followed for decades without requiring significant treatment,[469] and spontaneous remission has been described.[470] Because of its variable course, conservative management may be appropriate while the course of the disease is followed.

REFERENCES

1. Heuck G: Zwei Fälle von Leukämie mit eigenthümlichem Blut-resp Knochenmarksbefund. *Virchows Arch (Pathol Anat)* 78:475, 1879.
2. Silverstein MN: *Agnogenic Myeloid Metaplasia*. Publishing Science, Boston, 1975.
3. Mesa RA, Verstovsek S, Cervantes F, et al: Primary myelofibrosis (PMF), post polycythemia vera myelofibrosis (post-PV MF), post essential thrombocythemia myelofibrosis (post-ET MF), blast phase PMF (PMF-BP): Consensus on terminology by the international working group for myelofibrosis research and treatment (IWG-MRT). *Leuk Res* 31:737, 2007.
4. Lichtman MA: Is it chronic idiopathic myelofibrosis, myelofibrosis with myeloid metaplasia, chronic megakaryocytic-granulocytic myelosis, or chronic megakaryocytic leukemia? Further thoughts on the nosology of the clonal myeloid disorders. *Leukemia* 19:1139, 2005.
5. James C, Ugo V, Le Couédic JP, et al: A unique clonal JAK2 mutation leading to constitutive signalling causes polycythaemia vera. *Nature* 434:1144, 2005.
6. Baxter EJ, Scott LM, Campbell PJ, et al: Acquired mutation of the tyrosine kinase JAK2 in human myeloproliferative disorders. *Lancet* 365:1054, 2005.
7. Barosi G: Myelofibrosis with myeloid metaplasia. *Hematol Oncol Clin North Am* 17:1211, 2003.
8. Ward HP, Block MH: The natural history of agnogenic myeloid metaplasia (AMM) and a critical evaluation of its relationship with myeloproliferative syndrome. *Medicine (Baltimore)* 50:357, 1971.
9. Varki A, Lottenberg R, Griffith R, et al: The syndrome of idiopathic myelofibrosis. *Medicine (Baltimore)* 62:353, 1983.
10. Barosi G: Myelofibrosis with myeloid metaplasia. *Hematol Oncol Clin North Am* 17:1211, 2003.
11. Okamura T, Kinukawa N, Niho Y, Mizoguichi H: Primary chronic myelofibrosis: Clinical and prognostic evaluation in 336 Japanese patients. *Int J Hematol* 73:194, 2001.
12. Cervantes F, Pereira A, Esteve J, et al: Idiopathic myelofibrosis: Initial features, evolutionary pattern and survival in a series of 106 patients. *Med Clin North Am* 109:651, 1997.
13. Dupriez B, Morel P, Demory JL, et al: Prognostic factors in agnogenic myeloid metaplasia: A report on 195 cases with a new scoring system. *Blood* 88:1013, 1996.
14. Rupoli S, DaLio L, Sisti S, et al: Primary myelofibrosis: A detailed analysis of the clinicopathologic variables influencing survival. *Ann Hematol* 68:205, 1994.
15. Ozen S, Ferhanoglu B, Senocak M, Tüzüner N: Idiopathic myelofibrosis (agnogenic myeloid metaplasia). *Leuk Res* 21:125, 1997.
16. Landgren O, Goldin LR, Kristinsson SY, et al: Increased risks of polycythemia vera, essential thrombocythemia, and myelofibrosis among 24,577 first-degree relatives of 11,039 patients with myeloproliferative neoplasms in Sweden. *Blood* 112:2199, 2008.
17. Shalev O, Goldfarb A, Ariel I, et al: Myelofibrosis in young adults. *Acta Haematol* 70:396, 1983.
18. Sekhar M, Prentice HG, Poyat U, et al: Idiopathic myelofibrosis in children. *Br J Haematol* 93:394, 1996.
19. Cervantes F, Barosi G, Demory JL, et al: Myelofibrosis with myeloid metaplasia in young individuals: Disease characteristics, prognostic factors and identification of risk groups. *Br J Haematol* 102:684, 1998.
20. Sieff CA, Malleson P: Familial myelofibrosis. *Arch Dis Child* 55:888, 1980.
21. Sheikha A: Fatal familial infantile myelofibrosis. *J Pediatr Hematol Oncol* 26:164, 2004.
22. Rossbach HC: Familial infantile myelofibrosis as an autosomal recessive disorder: Preponderance among children from Saudi Arabia. *Pediatr Hematol Oncol* 23:453, 2006.
23. Cohn SL, Cohn RA, Chou P, et al: Infantile myelofibrosis with nephromegaly secondary to myeloid metaplasia. *Clin Pediatr (Phila)* 30:59, 1991.
24. Mallouh AA, Sa'di AR: Agnogenic myeloid metaplasia in children. *Am J Dis Child* 146:965, 1992.
25. Cervantes F, Barosi G, Hernández-Boluda J-C, et al: Myelofibrosis with myeloid metaplasia in adult individuals 30 years old or younger: Presenting features, evolution and survival. *Eur J Haematol* 66:324, 2001.
26. Segel GB, Lichtman MA: Familial (inherited) leukemia, lymphoma, and myeloma. *Blood Cells Mol Dis* 32:246, 2004.
27. Rumi E: Familial chronic myeloproliferative disorders: The state of the art. *Hematol Oncol* 26:131, 2008.
28. Kaufman S, Briere J, Bernard J: Familial myeloproliferative syndromes: Study of 6 families and review of literature. *Nouv Rev Fr Hematol* 20:1, 1978.
29. Péres-Encinas M, Bello JL, Perez-Crespo S, et al: Familial myeloproliferative syndrome. *Am J Hematol* 46:225, 1994.
30. Kutty J, Ridell B: Epidemiology of the myeloproliferative disorders: Essential thrombocythaemia, polycythemia vera, and idiopathic myelofibrosis. *Pathol Biol* 49:164, 2001.
31. McNally RJ, Rowland D, Roman E, Cartwright RA: Age and sex distributions of haematological malignancies in the U.K. *Hematol Oncol* 15:173, 1997.
32. Ridell B, Carneskog J, Wedel H, et al: Incidence of chronic myeloproliferative disorders in the city of Gotesborg, Sweden 1983–1992. *Eur J Haematol* 65:267, 2000.
33. Phekoo KJ, Richards MA, Møller H, Schey SA: The incidence and outcome of myeloid malignancies in 2,112 adult patients in southeast England. *Haematologica* 91:1400, 2006.

34. Mesa RA, Silverstein MN, Jacobsen SJ, et al: Population-based incidence and survival figures in essential thrombocythemia and agnogenic myeloid metaplasia: An Olmstead County Study 1976–1995. *Am J Hematol* 61:10, 1999.
35. Aksoy M, Erdem S, Dincol G: Two rare complications of chronic benzene poisoning: Myeloid metaplasia and paroxysmal nocturnal hemoglobinuria. *Blut* 30:255, 1975.
36. Hu H: Benzene-associated myelofibrosis. *Ann Intern Med* 106:171, 1987.
37. Tondel M, Perrson B, Carstensen J: Myelofibrosis and benzene exposure. *Occup Med* 45:31, 1995.
38. Anderson RE, Hoshino T, Yamamoto T: Myelofibrosis with myeloid metaplasia in survivors of the atomic bomb in Hiroshima. *Ann Intern Med* 60:1, 1964.
39. Jacobson RS, Salo A, Fialkow PS: Agnogenic myeloid metaplasia: A clonal proliferation of hematopoietic stem cells with secondary myelofibrosis. *Blood* 51:189, 1978.
40. Kahn A, Bernard JF, Cottreau D, et al: A deficient G-6-PD variant with hemizygous expression in blood cells of a woman with primary myelofibrosis. *Humangenetik* 30:41, 1975.
41. Sato Y, Suda T, Suda J, et al: Multilineage expression of haemopoietic precursors with an abnormal clone in idiopathic myelofibrosis. *Br J Haematol* 64:657, 1986.
42. Kreipe H, Jaquet K, Falgner J, et al: Clonal granulocytes and bone marrow cells in the cellular phase of agnogenic myeloid metaplasia. *Blood* 78:1814, 1991.
43. Tsukamoto N, Morita K, Maehara T, et al: Clonality in chronic myeloproliferative disorders defined by X-chromosome linked probes. *Br J Haematol* 86:253, 1994.
44. Buschle M, Janssen JWG, Drexler H, et al: Evidence for pluripotent stem cell origin of idiopathic myelofibrosis: Clonal analysis of a case characterized by a N-*ras* gene mutation. *Leukemia* 2:658, 1988.
45. Lebowitz P, Papac R, Ghosh PK: Impaired retinoblastoma susceptibility (Rb) gene expression in agnogenic myeloid metaplasia. *Blood* 76(Suppl 1):236A, 1990.
46. Reeder TL, Bailey RJ, Dewald GW, Tefferi A: Both B and T lymphocytes may be clonally involved in myelofibrosis with myeloid metaplasia. *Blood* 101:1981, 2003.
47. Popat U, Frost A, Liu E, et al: High levels of circulating CD34 cells, dacryocytes, clonal hematopoiesis, and JAK2 mutation differentiate myelofibrosis with myeloid metaplasia from secondary myelofibrosis associated with pulmonary hypertension. *Blood* 107:3486, 2006.
48. Delhommeau F, Dupont S, Tonetti C, et al: Evidence that the JAK2 G1849T (V617F) mutation occurs in a lymphomyeloid progenitor in polycythemia vera and idiopathic myelofibrosis. *Blood* 109:71, 2007.
49. James C, Mazurier F, Dupont S, et al: The hematopoietic stem cell compartment of JAK2V617F-positive myeloproliferative disorders is a reflection of disease heterogeneity. *Blood* 112:2429, 2008.
50. Wendling F, Varlet P, Charon M, Tambourin P: MPLV: A retrovirus complex inducing an acute myeloproliferative leukemic disorder in adult mice. *Virology* 149:242, 1986.
51. Kaushansky K: Thrombopoietin. *N Engl J Med* 339:746, 1998.
52. Yan X-Q, Lacey D, Hill D, et al: A model of myelofibrosis and osteosclerosis in mice induced by overexpressing thrombopoietin (mpl ligand). *Blood* 88:402, 1996.
53. Villeval JL, Cohen-Solal K, Tuliez M, et al: High thrombopoietin production by hematopoietic cells induces a fatal myeloproliferative syndrome in mice. *Blood* 90:4396, 1997.
54. Chagraoui H, Komura E, Tulliez M, et al: Prominent role of TGF-beta 1 in thrombopoietin-induced myelofibrosis in mice. *Blood* 100:3495, 2002.
55. Chagraoui H, Tulliez M, Smayra T, et al: Stimulation of osteoprotegerin production is responsible for osteosclerosis in mice overexpressing TPO. *Blood* 101:2983, 2003.
56. Vannucchi AM, Bianchi L, Cellai C, et al: Development of myelofibrosis in mice genetically impaired for GATA-1 expression (GATA-1(low) mice). *Blood* 100:1123, 2002.
57. Vannucchi AM, Migliaccio AR, Paoletti F, et al: Pathogenesis of myelofibrosis with myeloid metaplasia: Lessons from mouse models of the disease. *Semin Oncol* 32:365, 2005.
58. Garimella R, Kacena MA, Tague SE, et al: Expression of bone morphogenetic proteins and their receptors in the bone marrow megakaryocytes of GATA-1(low) mice: A possible role in osteosclerosis. *J Histochem Cytochem* 55:745, 2007.
59. Levine RL, Gilliland DG: Myeloproliferative disorders. *Blood* 112:2190, 2008.
60. Levine RL, Wadleigh M, Cools J, et al: Activating mutation in the tyrosine kinase JAK2 in polycythemia vera, essential thrombocythemia, and myeloid metaplasia with myelofibrosis. *Cancer Cell* 7:387, 2005.
61. Kilpivaara O, Levine RL: JAK2 and MPL mutations in myeloproliferative neoplasms: Discovery and science. *Leukemia* 22:1813, 2008.
62. Wernig G, Mercher T, Okabe R, et al: Expression of Jak2V617F causes a polycythemia vera-like disease with associated myelofibrosis in a murine bone marrow transplant model. *Blood* 107:4274, 2006.
63. Lacout C, Pisani DF, Tulliez M, et al: JAK2V617F expression in murine hematopoietic cells leads to MPD mimicking human PV with secondary myelofibrosis. *Blood* 108:1652, 2006.
64. Zaleskas VM, Krause DS, Lazarides K, et al: Molecular pathogenesis and therapy of polycythemia induced in mice by JAK2 V617F. *PLoS ONE* 1:e18, 2006.
65. Kralovics R, Guan Y, Prchal JT: Acquired uniparental disomy of chromosome 9p is a frequent stem cell defect in polycythemia vera. *Exp Hematol* 30:229, 2002.
66. Tiedt R, Hao-Shen H, Sobas MA, et al: Ratio of mutant JAK2-V617F to wild-type Jak2 determines the MPD phenotypes in transgenic mice. *Blood* 111:3931, 2008.
67. Larsen TS, Pallisgaard N, Møller MB, Hasselbalch HC: The JAK2 V617F allele burden in essential thrombocythemia, polycythemia vera and primary myelofibrosis—Impact on disease phenotype. *Eur J Haematol* 79:508, 2007.
68. Pikman Y, Lee BH, Mercher T, et al: MPLW515L is a novel somatic activating mutation in myelofibrosis with myeloid metaplasia. *PLoS Med* 3:e270, 2006.
69. Pardanani AD, Levine RL, Lasho T, et al: MPL515 mutations in myeloproliferative and other myeloid disorders: A study of 1182 patients. *Blood* 108:3472, 2006.
70. Tefferi A: JAK and MPL mutations in myeloid malignancies. *Leuk Lymphoma* 49:388, 2008.
71. Abu-Duhier FM, Goodeve AC, Care RS, et al: Mutational analysis of class III receptor tyrosine kinases (C-KIT, C-FMS, FLT3) in idiopathic myelofibrosis. *Br J Haematol* 120:464, 2003.
72. Kawamata N, Ogawa S, Yamamoto G, et al: Genetic profiling of myeloproliferative disorders by single-nucleotide polymorphism oligonucleotide microarray. *Exp Hematol* 36(11):1477, 2008.
73. Andrieux J, Demory JL, Dupriez B, et al: Dysregulation and overexpression of HMGA2 in myelofibrosis with myeloid metaplasia. *Genes Chromosomes Cancer* 39:82, 2004.
74. Bogani C, Ponziani V, Guglielmelli P, et al: Myeloproliferative Disorders Research Consortium. Hypermethylation of CXCR4 promoter in CD34+ cells from patients with primary myelofibrosis. *Stem Cells* 26:1920, 2008.
75. Rosti V, Massa M, Vannucchi AM, et al: The expression of CXCR4 is down-regulated on the CD34+ cells of patients with myelofibrosis with myeloid metaplasia. *Blood Cells Mol Dis* 38:280, 2007.
76. Ciurea SO, Merchant D, Mahmud N, et al: Pivotal contributions of megakaryocytes to the biology of idiopathic myelofibrosis. *Blood* 110:986, 2007.
77. Guglielmelli P, Zini R, Bogani C, et al: Molecular profiling of CD34+ cells in idiopathic myelofibrosis identifies a set of disease-associated genes and reveals the clinical significance of Wilms' tumor gene 1 (WT1). *Stem Cells* 25:165, 2007.
78. Massa M, Rosti V, Ramajoli I, et al: Circulating CD34+, CD133+, and vascular endothelial growth factor receptor 2-positive endothelial progenitor cells in myelofibrosis with myeloid metaplasia. *J Clin Oncol* 23:5688, 2005.
79. Giraudier S, Chagraoui H, Komura E, et al: Overexpression of FKBP51 in idiopathic myelofibrosis regulates the growth factor independence of megakaryocyte progenitors. *Blood* 100:2932, 2002.
80. Wang JC, Chen C, Lou LH, et al: Blood thrombopoietin, IL-6, and IL-11 levels in patients with agnogenic myeloid metaplasia. *Leukemia* 11:1827, 1997.
81. Moliterno AR, Hankins WD, Spivak JL: Impaired expression of the thrombopoietin receptor by patients with polycythemia vera. *N Engl J Med* 338:572, 1998.
82. Temerinac S, Klippel S, Strunck E, et al: Cloning of PRV-1, a novel member of the uPAR receptor superfamily, which is overexpressed in polycythemia rubra vera. *Blood* 95:2569, 2000.
83. Liu E, Jelinek J, Pastore YD, et al: Discrimination of polycythemia and thrombocytoses by novel, simple, accurate clonality assays and comparison of PRV-1 expression and BFU-E response to erythropoietin. *Blood* 101:3294, 2003.
84. Prockop DJ, Kivirikko KI, Tuderman L, et al: The biosynthesis of collagen and its disorders. *N Engl J Med* 301:13, 1979.
85. Bauermeister DE: Quantitation of bone marrow reticulin: A normal range. *Am J Clin Pathol* 56:24, 1971.
86. Ivànyi JL, Mahunka M, Papp A, Telek B: Prognostic significance of bone marrow reticulum fibers in idiopathic myelofibrosis: Evolution of clinicopathological parameters in a scoring system. *Haematologica* 26:75, 1994.
87. McCarthy DM: Annotation: Fibrosis of the bone marrow: Content and causes. *Br J Haematol* 59:1, 1985.
88. Apaja-Sarkkinen M, Autio-Harmainen H, Alavaikko M, et al: Immunohistochemical study of basement membrane proteins and type III procollagen in myelofibrosis. *Br J Haematol* 63:571, 1986.
89. Hasselbalch H, Junker P, Lisse I, et al: Serum markers for type IV collagen and type III procollagen in the myelofibrosis-osteomyelosclerosis syndrome and other chronic myeloproliferative disorders. *Am J Hematol* 23:101, 1986.
90. Reilly JT: Pathogenesis of idiopathic myelofibrosis: Role of growth factors. *J Clin Pathol* 45:461, 1992.
91. Charron D, Robert L, Couty MC, Binet JL: Biochemical and histological analysis of bone marrow collagen in myelofibrosis. *Br J Haematol* 41:151, 1979.
92. Podolak-Dawidziak M, Wróbel T, Jelen M: Serum concentration of the amino terminal peptide of type III procollagen (PIIINP) in patients with myeloproliferative disorders (MPD). *Pol Arch Med Wewn* 99:24, 1998.
93. Gay S, Gay RE, Prohal JT: Immunohistological studies of bone marrow collagen, in *Myelofibrosis and the Biology of Connective Tissue*, edited by P Berk, H Castro-Malaspina, LR Wasserman, p 291. Alan R. Liss, New York, 1984.
94. Hasselbalch H, Junker P, Horslev-Patersen K, et al: Procollagen type III amino-terminal peptide in serum in idiopathic myelofibrosis and allied conditions. *Am J Hematol* 33:18, 1990.
95. Reilly JT, Nash JRG, Mackie MJ, McVerry BA: Endothelial cell proliferation in myelofibrosis. *Br J Haematol* 60:625, 1985.
96. Baglin TP, Crocker MA, Timmins A, et al: Bone marrow hypervascularity in patients with myelofibrosis identified by infrared thermography. *Clin Lab Haematol* 13:341, 1991.
97. Bock O, Neuse J, Hussein K, et al: Aberrant collagenase expression in chronic idiopathic myelofibrosis is related to the stage of disease but not to the JAK2 mutation status. *Am J Pathol* 169:471, 2006.
98. Bock O, Höftmann J, Theophile K, et al: Bone morphogenetic proteins are overexpressed in the bone marrow of primary myelofibrosis and are apparently induced by fibrogenic cytokines. *Am J Pathol* 172:951, 2008.
99. Dolan G, Forrest P, Eastham J, et al: Serum laminin, procollagen terminal peptide III and thrombocyte platelet derived growth factor concentrations in idiopathic myelofibrosis. *Br J Haematol* 77(Suppl 1):73, 1991.

100. Reilly JT, Nash JRG, Mackie MJ, McVerry BA: Immunoenzymatic detection of fibronectin in normal and pathological haemopoietic tissue. *Br J Haematol* 59:497, 1985.
101. Hasselbalch H, Clemmensen I: Plasma fibronectin in idiopathic myelofibrosis and related chronic myeloproliferative disorders. *Scand J Clin Lab Invest* 47:429, 1987.
102. Soini Y, Kamel D, Apaja-Sarkkinen M, et al: Tenascin immunoreactivity in normal and pathological bone marrow. *J Clin Pathol* 46:218, 1993.
103. Reilly JT, Nash JRG: Vitronectin (serum spreading factor): Its localization in normal and fibrotic tissue. *J Clin Pathol* 41:1269, 1988.
104. Le Bousse-Kerdilès MC, Martyré MC, et al: Involvement of the fibrogenic cytokines, TGF-β and bFGF, in the pathogenesis of idiopathic myelofibrosis. *Pathol Biol* 49:153, 2001.
105. Rameshwar P, Oh HS, Yook C, Chang VT: Substance P-fibronectin cytokine interactions in myeloproliferative disorders with bone marrow fibrosis. *Acta Haematol* 109:1, 2003.
106. Wang JC, Wong C, Kao WW: Immunoreactive prolylhydroxylase in patients with primary and secondary myelofibrosis. *Br J Haematol* 65:171, 1987.
107. Barosi G, Costa A, Liberato LN, et al: Serum procollagen III peptide level correlates with disease activity in myelofibrosis with myeloid metaplasia. *Br J Haematol* 72:16, 1989.
108. Hochweiss S, Fruchtman S, Hahn EG, et al: Increased serum procollagen III aminoterminal peptide in myelofibrosis. *Am J Hematol* 15:343, 1983.
109. Hasselbalch H, Junker P, Lisse I, et al: Circulating hyaluronan in the myelofibrosis/osteomyelosclerosis syndrome and other myeloproliferative disorders. *Am J Hematol* 36:1, 1991.
110. Thiele J, Kvasnicka HM, Fischer R, Diehl V: Clinicopathological impact of the interactivity between megakaryocytes and myeloid stroma in chronic myeloproliferative disorders: A concise update. *Leuk Lymphoma* 24:463, 1997.
111. Schmitt A, Drouin A, Masse J-M, et al: Polymorphonuclear neutrophil and megakaryocyte mutual involvement in myelofibrosis pathogenesis. *Leuk Lymphoma* 43:719, 2002.
112. Frey BM, Rafii S, Teterson M, et al: Adenovector-mediated expression of human thrombopoietin cDNA in immune-compromised mice: Insights into the pathophysiology of osteomyelofibrosis. *J Immunol* 160:691, 1998.
113. Rameshwar P, Chang VT, Thacker UF, Gascón P: Systemic transforming growth factor-beta in patients with bone marrow fibrosis-pathophysiological implications. *Am J Hematol* 59:133, 1998.
114. Rosenfeld M, Keating A, Bowen-Pope BF, et al: Responsiveness of the in vitro hematopoietic microenvironment to platelet-derived growth factor. *Leuk Res* 9:427, 1985.
115. Bernabei PA, Arcangeli A, Casini M, et al: Platelet-derived growth factor(s) mitogenic activity in patients with myeloproliferative disease. *Br J Haematol* 63:353, 1986.
116. Thiele J, Rompick V, Wagner S, Fischer R: Vascular architecture and collagen type IV in primary myelofibrosis and polycythemia vera. *Br J Haematol* 80:227, 1992.
117. Johnston JB, Dalal BI, Israels SJ, et al: Deposition of transforming growth factor-β in the marrow in myelofibrosis, and the intracellular localization and secretion of TGF-β by leukemic cells. *Am J Clin Pathol* 103:574, 1995.
118. Martré M-C: TGF-β and megakaryocytes in the pathogenesis of myelofibrosis in myeloproliferative disorders. *Leuk Lymphoma* 20:39, 1995.
119. Martré M-C, LeBousse-Kerdiles M-C, Romquin N, et al: Elevated levels of basic fibroblast growth factor in megakaryocytes and platelets from patients with idiopathic myelofibrosis. *Br J Haematol* 97:441, 1997.
120. Dalley A, Smith JM, Reilly JT, MacNeil S: Investigation of calmodulin and basic fibroblast growth factor (bFGF) in idiopathic myelofibrosis: Evidence for a role of extracellular calmodulin in fibroblast proliferation. *Br J Haematol* 93:856, 1996.
121. Nathan C: Secretory products of macrophages. *J Clin Invest* 79:319, 1987.
122. Burstein SA, Malpass TW, Yee E, et al: Platelet factor-4 excretion in myeloproliferative disease: Implication for the aetiology of myelofibrosis. *Br J Haematol* 57:383, 1984.
123. Wang JC, Novetsky A, Chen C, et al: Plasm matrix metalloproteinase and tissue inhibitor of metalloproteinase in patients with agnogenic myeloid metaplasia or idiopathic primary myelofibrosis. *Br J Haematol* 119:709, 2002.
124. Kvasnica HM, Thiele J, Amend T, Fischer R: Three-dimensional reconstruction of histiologic structures in human bone marrow from serial sections of trephine biopsies. *Anal Quant Cytol Histol* 16:159, 1994.
125. Reilly JT, Nash JR, Mackie MJ, et al: Endothelial cell proliferation in myelofibrosis. *Br J Haematol* 60:625, 1985.
126. Charbord P: Increased vascularity of bone marrow in myelofibrosis. *Br J Haematol* 62:595, 1986.
127. VanDyke D, Anger HO, Parker H, et al: Markedly increased bone blood flow in myelofibrosis. *J Nucl Med* 12:506, 1971.
128. Hotta T, Utsumi M, Katoh T, et al: Granulocytic and stromal progenitors in the bone marrow of patient with primary myelofibrosis. *Scand J Haematol* 34:251, 1985.
129. Greenberg BR, Woo L, Veomett JC, et al: Cytogenetics of bone marrow fibroblastic cells in idiopathic chronic myelofibrosis. *Br J Haematol* 66:487, 1987.
130. Caughman W, Stern R, Haynes H: Neutrophilic dermatosis of myeloproliferative disorders: Atypical forms of pyoderma gangrenosum and Sweet's syndrome associated with myeloproliferative disorders. *J Am Acad Dermatol* 9:751, 1983.
131. Gibson LE, Dicken CH, Flach DB: Neutrophilic dermatoses and myeloproliferative disease: Report of two cases. *Mayo Clin Proc* 60:735, 1985.
132. Su WPD, Alegre VA, White WL: Myelofibrosis discovered after diagnosis of Sweet's syndrome. *Int J Dermatol* 29:201, 1990.
133. Kanel KT, Kroboth FJ, Swartz WM: Pyoderma gangrenosum with myelofibrosis. *Am J Med* 82:1031, 1987.
134. Loewy G, Matthew A, Distenfeld A: Skin manifestations of agnogenic myeloid metaplasia. *Am J Hematol* 45:167, 1994.
135. Patel BM, Perniciaro C, Gertz MA: Cutaneous extramedullary hematopoiesis. *J Am Acad Dermatol* 32:805, 1995.
136. Rogalski C, Paasch U, Friedrich T, et al: Cutaneous extramedullary hematopoiesis in idiopathic myelofibrosis. *Int J Dermatol* 41:883, 2002.
137. Thiele J, Kvasnicka HM, Zankovich R, Diehl V: Early-stage idiopathic (primary) myelofibrosis—Current issues of diagnostic features. *Leuk Lymphoma* 43:1035, 2002.
138. Buhr T, Büsche G, Choritz H, et al: Evolution of myelofibrosis in chronic idiopathic myelofibrosis as evidenced in sequential bone marrow biopsy specimens. *Am J Clin Pathol* 119:152, 2003.
139. Thiele J, Kvasnicka HM: Chronic myeloproliferative disorders with thrombocythemia comparative study of two classification systems (PSSG, WHO) on 839 patients. *Ann Hematol* 82:148, 2003.
140. King BF, Kopecky KK, Baker MK, et al: Extramedullary hematopoiesis in the adrenal glands: CT characteristics. *J Comput Assist Tomogr* 11:342, 1987.
141. Wat NM, Tse KK, Chan FL, Lam KS: Adrenal extramedullary hematopoiesis. *Br J Haematol* 100:725, 1998.
142. Gibbins J, Pankhurst T, Murray J, et al: Extramedullary haematopoiesis in the kidney: A case report and review of literature. *Clin Lab Haematol* 27:391, 2005.
143. Schunuelle P, Waldherr R, Lehmann KJ, et al: Idiopathic myelofibrosis with extramedullary hematopoiesis in the kidneys. *Clin Nephrol* 52:256, 1999.
144. Ablett MJ, Vosylius P: Perirenal extramedullary haematopoiesis in myelofibrosis demonstrated on computed tomography. *Br J Haematol* 124:406, 2004.
145. Shaver RW, Clore FC: Extramedullary hemopoiesis in myeloid metaplasia. *AJR Am J Roentgenol* 137:874, 1981.
146. Williams ME, Innes DJ, Hutchison WT, et al: Extramedullary hematopoiesis: A cause of severe generalized lymphadenopathy in agnogenic myeloid metaplasia. *Arch Intern Med* 145:1308, 1985.
147. Fianza A, Alberici E, Toretta L: Rapidly growing extramedullary hemopoiesis in lymph nodes. *Haematologica* 86:784, 2001.
148. Sharma BK, Pounder RE, Cruse JP, et al: Extramedullary haemopoiesis in the small bowel. *Gut* 27:873, 1986.
149. MacKinnon S, McNicol AM, Lee FD, et al: Myelofibrosis complicated by intestinal extramedullary haemopoiesis and acute small bowel obstruction. *J Clin Pathol* 39:677, 1986.
150. Soloman D, Goodman H, Jacobs P: Rectal stenosis due to extramedullary hematopoiesis. *Clin Radiol* 49:726, 1994.
151. Sunderland K, Barratt J, Pidcock M: Extramedullary hemopoiesis arising in the gut mimicking carcinoma of the cecum. *Pathology* 26:62, 1994.
152. Brooks JJ, Krugman DT, Danjanor I: Myeloid metaplasia presenting as a breast mass. *Am J Surg Pathol* 4:281, 1980.
153. Martinelli G, Santini D, Bazzocchi F, et al: Myeloid metaplasia of the breast: A lesion which clinically mimics carcinoma. *Virchows Arch* 401:203, 1983.
154. Zonderland HM, Michiels JJ, Ten Kate FJW: Mammographic and sonographic demonstration of extramedullary hematopoiesis of the breast. *Clin Radiol* 44:64, 1991.
155. Navarro M, Crespo C, Pérez L, et al: Massive intrahepatic extramedullary hematopoiesis in myelofibrosis. *Abdom Imaging* 25:184, 2000.
156. Lee IJ, Kim SH, Kim DS, et al: Intrahepatic extramedullary hematopoiesis mimicking a hypervascular hepatic neoplasm on dynamic- and SPIO-enhanced MRI. *Korean J Radiol* 9(Suppl):S34, 2008.
157. Yusen RD, Kollef MH: Acute respiratory failure due to extramedullary hematopoiesis. *Chest* 108:1170, 1995.
158. Schwarz C, Bittner R, Kirsch A, et al: A 62-year-old woman with bilateral pleural effusions and pulmonary infiltrates caused by extramedullary hematopoiesis. *Respiration* 78:110, 2009.
159. García-Manero G, Schuster S, Patrick H, Martinez J: Pulmonary hypertension in patients with myelofibrosis secondary to myeloproliferative diseases. *Am J Hematol* 60:130, 1999.
160. Yang X, Bhuiya T, Esposito M: Sclerosing extramedullary tumor. *Ann Diagn Pathol* 6:183, 2002.
161. Oren I, Goldman A, Haddad N, et al: Ascites and pleural effusion a secondary to extramedullary hematopoiesis. *Am J Med Sci* 318:286, 1999.
162. Miyata T, Masuzawa M, Katsuoka K, Higashihara M: Cutaneous extramedullary hematopoiesis in a patient with idiopathic myelofibrosis. *J Dermatol* 35:456, 2008.
163. Mizoguchi M, Kawa Y, Minami T, et al: Cutaneous extramedullary hematopoiesis in myelofibrosis. *J Am Acad Dermatol* 22:351, 1990.
164. Heinicke MH, Zarrabi MH, Gorevic PD: Arthritis due to synovial involvement by extramedullary haematopoiesis in myelofibrosis with myeloid metaplasia. *Ann Rheum Dis* 42:196, 1983.
165. Leoni F, Fabbri R, Pascarella A, et al: Extramedullary hematopoiesis in thyroid multinodular goiter preceding clinical evidence of agnogenic myeloid metaplasia. *Histopathology* 28:559, 1996.
166. Kwak H-S, Lee J-M: CT findings of extramedullary hematopoiesis in the thorax, liver, and kidneys in a patient with myelofibrosis. *J Korean Med Sci* 15:460, 2000.
167. Humphrey PA, Vollmer RT: Extramedullary hematopoiesis in the prostate. *Am J Surg Pathol* 15:486, 1991.
168. Macumber C, Young GAR, Selby WS: Myelofibrosis presenting as splenic tumor. *Dig Dis Sci* 44:1817, 1999.
169. Balogh K, O'Hara CJ: Myeloid metaplasia masquerading as a urethral caruncle. *J Urol* 135:789, 1986.

170. Oesterling JE, Keating JP, Leroy AJ, et al: Idiopathic myelofibrosis with myeloid metaplasia involving the renal pelvis, ureters and bladder. *J Urol* 147:1360, 1992.
171. La Fianza A, Torretta L, Spinazzola A: Extramedullary hematopoiesis in chronic myelofibrosis encasing the pelvicaliceal system and perirenal spaces: CT findings. *Urol Int* 75:281, 2005.
172. Perazella MA, Buller GK: Nephrotic syndrome associated with agnogenic myeloid metaplasia. *Am J Nephrol* 14:223, 1994.
173. Brown JA, Gomez-Leon G: Subdural hemorrhage secondary to extramedullary hematopoiesis in postpolycythemic myeloid metaplasia. *Neurosurgery* 14:588, 1984.
174. Cornfield DB, Shipkin P, Alluvia A, et al: Intracranial myeloid metaplasia: Diagnosis by CT and Fe52 scans and treatment by cranial irradiation. *Am J Hematol* 15:273, 1983.
175. Lundh B, Brandt L, Cronqvist S, et al: Intracranial myeloid metaplasia in myelofibrosis. *Scand J Haematol* 28:91, 1982.
176. Pless M, Rizzo JFIII, Shang J: Orbital apex syndrome: A rare presentation of extramedullary hematopoiesis. *J Neurooncol* 57.37, 2002.
177. Cameron WR, Ronnert M, Brun A: Extramedullary hematopoiesis of CNS in postpolycythemic myeloid metaplasia. *N Engl J Med* 305:765, 1981.
178. Chan SWW, Datta NN, Thomas TMM, Chan KW: Intracranial chloroma in myelofibrosis. *Surg Neurol* 59:55, 2003.
179. Haidar S, Ortiz-Neira C, Shroff M, et al: Intracranial involvement in extramedullary hematopoiesis: Case report and review of the literature. *Pediatr Radiol* 35:630, 2005.
180. Goh DH, Lee SH, Cho DC, et al: Chronic idiopathic myelofibrosis presenting as cauda equina compression due to extramedullary hematopoiesis: A case report. *J Korean Med Sci* 22:1090, 2007.
181. Cook G, Sharp RA: Spinal cord compression due to extramedullary haemopoiesis in myelofibrosis. *J Clin Pathol* 47:464, 1994.
182. Horwood E, Dowson H, Gupta R, et al: Myelofibrosis presenting as spinal cord compression. *J Clin Pathol* 56:154, 2003.
183. Scott IC, Poynton CH: Polycythaemia rubra vera and myelofibrosis with spinal cord compression. *J Clin Pathol* 61:681, 2008.
184. Ohtsubo M, Hayaski K, Fukushima T, et al: Intracranial extramedullary haematopoiesis in postpolycythemia myelofibrosis. *Br J Radiol* 67:299, 1994.
185. Urman M, O'Sullivan RA, Nugent RA, Lentle BC: Intracranial extramedullary hematopoiesis. *Clin Nucl Med* 16:431, 1991.
186. Lanir A, Aghai E, Simon JS, et al: MR imaging in myelofibrosis. *J Comput Assist Tomogr* 10:634, 1986.
187. Koch BL, Bisset GS, Bisset RR, Zimmer MB: Intracranial extramedullary hematopoiesis: MR findings with pathologic correlation. *AJR Am J Roentgenol* 162:1419, 1994.
188. Bartlett RP, Greipp PR, Tefferi A, et al: Extramedullary hematopoiesis manifesting as a symptomatic pleural effusion. *Mayo Clin Proc* 70:1165, 1995.
189. Oren I, Goldman A, Haddad N, et al: Ascites and pleural effusion secondary to extramedullary hematopoiesis. *Am J Med Sci* 318:286, 1999.
190. Lioté F, Yeni P, Teillet-Thiebaud F, et al: Ascites revealing peritoneal and hepatic extramedullary hematopoiesis with peliosis in agnogenic myeloid metaplasia. *Am J Med* 90:111, 1991.
191. Vilaseca J, Arnau JM, Tallada N, et al: Agnogenic myeloid metaplasia presenting as massive pericardial effusion due to extramedullary hematopoiesis. *Acta Haematol* 73:239, 1985.
192. Haedersdal C, Hasselbalch H, Devantier A, et al: Pericardial haematopoiesis with tamponade in myelofibrosis. *Scand J Haematol* 34:270, 1985.
193. Imam TH, Doll DC: Acute cardiac tamponade associated with pericardial extramedullary hematopoieses in agnogenic myeloid metaplasia. *Acta Haematol* 98:42, 1997.
194. Nagler A, Brenner B, Argov S, et al: Postsplenectomy pericardial effusion in two patients with myeloid metaplasia. *Arch Intern Med* 146:600, 1986.
195. Pedio G, Krause M, Jansova I: Megakaryocytes in ascitic fluid in a case of agnogenic myeloid metaplasia [letter]. *Acta Cytol* 29:89, 1985.
196. Silverman JF: Extramedullary hematopoietic ascitic fluid cytology in myelofibrosis. *Am J Clin Pathol* 84:125, 1985.
197. Stephenson RW, Britt DA, Schumann GB: Primary cytodiagnosis of peritoneal extramedullary hematopoiesis. *Diagn Cytopathol* 2:241, 1986.
198. Hocking WG, Lazar GS, Lipsett JA, et al: Cutaneous extramedullary hematopoiesis following splenectomy for idiopathic myelofibrosis. *Am J Med* 76:956, 1984.
199. Partanen S, Ruutu T, Jubonen E, et al: Effect of splenectomy on circulating haematopoietic progenitors in myelofibrosis. *Scand J Haematol* 37:87, 1986.
200. Hirose Y, Masaki Y, Shimoyama K, et al: Granulocytic sarcoma of megakaryoblastic differentiation in the lymph nodes terminating as acute megakaryocytic leukemia in a case of chronic idiopathic myelofibrosis persisting 16 years. *Eur J Haematol* 67:194, 2001.
201. Chan ACL, Kwong Y-L, Lam CCK: Granulocytic sarcoma megakaryoblastic differentiation complicating chronic idiopathic myelofibrosis. *Hum Pathol* 27:417, 1996.
202. Oishi N, Swisher SN, Stormont JM, et al: Portal hypertension in myeloid metaplasia. *Arch Surg* 81:80, 1960.
203. Rosenbaum DL, Murphy GW, Swisher SN: Hemodynamic studies of the portal circulation in myeloid metaplasia. *Am J Med* 41:360, 1966.
204. Jacobs P, Maze S, Tayob F, et al: Myelofibrosis, splenomegaly, and portal hypertension. *Acta Haematol* 74:45, 1985.
205. Dubois A, Dauzat M, Pignodel C, et al: Portal hypertension in lymphoproliferative and myeloproliferative disorders: Hemodynamic and histological correlations. *Hepatology* 17:246, 1993.
206. Degott C, Carpon JP, Bettan L, et al: Myeloid metaplasia, perisinusoidal fibrosis, and nodular regenerative hyperplasia of the liver. *Liver* 5:276, 1985.
207. Bioulac-Sage P, Roux D, Quinton A, et al: Ultrastructure of sinusoids in patients with agnogenic myeloid metaplasia. *J Submicrosc Cytol* 18:815, 1986.
208. Roux D, Merlio JP, Quinton A, et al: Agnogenic myeloid metaplasia, portal hypertension and sinusoidal abnormalities. *Gastroenterology* 92:1067, 1987.
209. Tsao MS: Hepatic sinusoidal fibrosis in agnogenic myeloid metaplasia. *Am J Clin Pathol* 91:302, 1989.
210. Pereira A, Bruguera M, Cervantes F, Rozman C: Liver involvement at diagnosis of primary myelofibrosis: A clinicopathological study of twenty-two cases. *Eur J Haematol* 40:355, 1988.
211. Valla d, Casadevall N, Huisse MG, et al: Etiology of portal vein thrombosis in adults. *Gastroenterology* 94:1063, 1988.
212. Lee W-C, Lin H-C, Tsay S-H, et al: Esophageal variceal ligation for esophageal variceal hemorrhage in a patient with portal and primary pulmonary hypertension complicating myelofibrosis. *Dig Dis Sci* 46.915, 2001.
213. Yusen RD, Kollef MH: Acute respiratory failure due to extramedullary hematopoiesis. *Chest* 108:1170, 1995.
214. Steensma DP, Hook CC, Stafford SL, Tefferi A: Low-dose, single fraction, whole-lung radiotherapy for pulmonary hypertension associated with myelofibrosis and myeloid metaplasia. *Br J Haematol* 118:813, 2002.
215. Cortelezzi A, Gritti G, et al: Pulmonary arterial hypertension in primary myelofibrosis is common and associated with an altered angiogenic status. *Leukemia* 22:646, 2008.
216. Popat U, Frost A, Liu EL, et al: Myelofibrosis is frequently seen in patients with primary pulmonary hypertension and is associated with polyclonal hematopoiesis and normal CD34 count. *Blood* 102:919A, 2003.
217. Boivin P, Bernard JF, Hakim J, et al: Anomalies immunitaires au cours de splenomegalies myeloides myelosclerose. *Acta Haematol* 51:91, 1974.
218. Lang JM, Oberling F, Mayer S, et al: Autoimmunity in primary myelofibrosis. *Biomedicine* 25:39, 1976.
219. Barge J, Slabodshy-Brousse N, Bernard JF: Histoimmunology of myelofibrosis: A study of 100 cases. *Biomedicine* 29:73, 1978.
220. Vellenga E, Mulder N, The T, et al: A study of the cellular and humoral immune response in patients with myelofibrosis. *Clin Lab Haematol* 4:239, 1982.
221. Rondeau E, Solal-Celigny P, Dhermy D, et al: Immune disorders in agnogenic myeloid metaplasia: Relations to myelofibrosis. *Br J Haematol* 53:467, 1983.
222. Gordon B: Immunological abnormalities in myelofibrosis. *Prog Clin Biol Res* 154:455, 1984.
223. Khumbanonda M, Horowitz HI, Eyster ME: Coombs' positive hemolytic anemia in myelofibrosis with myeloid metaplasia. *Am J Med Sci* 258:89, 1969.
224. Mohite U, Pathare A, Al Kindi S, et al: Autoimmune haemolytic anemia as the presenting manifestation of agnogenic myeloid metaplasia. *Haematologica* 32:495, 2002.
225. Kornblihtt LI, Vassalllu PS, Heller PG, et al: Primary myelofibrosis in a patient who developed primary biliary cirrhosis, autoimmune hemolytic anemia and fibrillary glomerulonephritis. *Ann Hematol* 87:1019, 2008.
226. Schreiber ZA: Immune thrombocytopenia in postpolythemic myelofibrosis. *Am J Hematol* 54:146, 1997.
227. Seelen MAJ, De Meijer PHEM, Posthuma EF, Meinders AE: Myelofibrosis and thrombocytopenic purpura. *Ann Hematol* 75:129, 1997.
228. Wang JC, Wang A: Plasma soluble interleukin-2 receptor in patients with primary myelofibrosis. *Br J Haematol* 86:380, 1994.
229. Leoni P, Rupoli S, Salvi A, et al: Antibodies against terminal galactosyl alpha(1–3) galactose epitopes in patients with idiopathic myelofibrosis. *Br J Haematol* 85:313, 1993.
230. Bernhardt B, Valleta M: Lupus anticoagulant in myelofibrosis. *Am J Med Sci* 272:229, 1976.
231. Cappio FC, Vigliani R, Novarino A, et al: Idiopathic myelofibrosis: A possible role for immune-complexes in the pathogenesis of bone marrow fibrosis. *Br J Haematol* 49:17, 1981.
232. Akikusa B, Komatsu T, Kondo Y, et al: Amyloidosis complicating idiopathic myelofibrosis. *Arch Pathol Lab Med* 111:525, 1987.
233. Hasselbalch H, Nielsen H, Berild D, et al: Circulating immune complexes in myelofibrosis. *Scand J Haematol* 34:177, 1985.
234. Gordon BR, Coleman M, Kohen P, et al: Immunologic abnormalities in myelofibrosis with activation of the complement system. *Blood* 58:904, 1981.
235. Ferhanoglu B, Erzin Y, Baslar Z, Tüzüner HAN: Secondary amyloidosis in the course of idiopathic myelofibrosis. *Leuk Res* 21:897, 1997.
236. Tefferi A, Kantarjian HM, Pardanani AD, et al: The clinical phenotype of myelofibrosis encompasses a chronic inflammatory state that is favorably altered by INCB018424, a selective inhibitor of JAK1/2.*Blood* 112:968, 2008.
237. El Mouzan MI, Ahmed MAM, Saleh MAF, et al: Myelofibrosis and pancytopenia in systemic lupus erythematosus. *Am J Med* 81:935, 1986.
238. Matsouka CH, Lioouris J, Andrianokis A: Systemic lupus erythematosus and myelofibrosis. *Clin Rheumatol* 8:402, 1989.
239. Paquette RL, Meshkinpour A, Rosen PJ: Autoimmune myelofibrosis. A steroid-responsive cause of bone marrow fibrosis associated with systemic lupus erythematosus. *Medicine (Baltimore)* 73:145, 1994.
240. Ramakrishna R, Kyle PW, Day PJ, Mansharan A: Evan's syndrome, myelofibrosis and systemic lupus erythematosus: Role of procollagens in myelofibrosis. *Pathology* 27:255, 1995.

241. Kiss E, Gál I, Simkovics E, et al: Myelofibrosis in systemic lupus erythematosus. *Leuk Lymphoma* 39:661, 2000.
242. Aharon A, Levy Y, Bar-Dayan Y, et al: Successful treatment of early secondary myelofibrosis in SLE with IVIG. *Lupus* 6:408, 1997.
243. Von Knorring J, Selroos OW, Wegelius O: Myeloid metaplasia in disseminated vascular disease. *Acta Med Scand* 195:137, 1974.
244. Connelly TJ, Abruzzo JL, Schwab RH: Agnogenic myeloid metaplasia with polyarteritis. *J Rheumatol* 9:954, 1982.
245. Arellano-Rodrigo E, Esteve J, Giné E, et al: Idiopathic myelofibrosis associated with ulcerative colitis. *Leuk Lymphoma* 43:1481, 2002.
246. Ben-Chetrit E, Gross DJ, Ikon E, et al: The association between auto-immunity and agnogenic myeloid metaplasia. *Scand J Haematol* 31:410, 1983.
247. Hernández-Beluda JC, Jiménez M, Rosiñol L, Cervantes F: Idiopathic myelofibrosis associated with primary biliary cirrhosis. *Leuk Lymphoma* 43:673, 2002.
248. Marie I, Levesque H, Cailleux N, et al: An uncommon association: Sjögren syndrome and autoimmune myelofibrosis. *Rheumatology* 38:370, 1999.
249. Hasselbalch H, Jans H, Nielsen PL: A distinct subtype of idiopathic myelofibrosis with bone marrow features mimicking hairy cell leukemia: Evidence of an autoimmune pathogenesis. *Am J Hematol* 25:225, 1987.
250. Thiele J, Chen Y-S, Kvasnicka H-M, et al: Evolution of fibro-osteosclerotic bone marrow lesions in primary (idiopathic) osteomyelofibrosis—A histomorphometric study on sequential trephine biopsies. *Leuk Lymphoma* 14:163, 1994.
251. Thiele J, Hoeppner B, Zankovich R, Fischer R: Histomorphometry of bone marrow biopsies in primary osteomyelofibrosis-sclerosis (agnogenic myeloid metaplasia): Correlation between clinical and morphological features. *Virchows Arch* 415:191, 1989.
252. Guermazi A, De Kerviler E, Cazals-Hatem D, et al: Imaging findings in myelofibrosis. *Eur J Radiol* 9:1366, 1999.
253. Thiele J, Kvasnicka HM, Fischer R: Histochemistry and morphometry on bone marrow biopsies in chronic myeloproliferative disorders: Aids to diagnosis and classification. *Ann Hematol* 78:496, 1999.
254. Poulsen LW, Melsen F, Bendix KA: Histomorphometric study of haematologic disorders with respect to marrow fibrosis and osteosclerosis. *Acta Pathol Microbiol Immunol Scand* 106:495, 1998.
255. Coindre JM, Reiffers J, Goussot JF, et al: Histomorphometric analysis of sclerotic bone from idiopathic myeloid metaplasia. *J Pathol* 144:163, 1984.
256. Diamond T, Smith A, Schnier R, Manoharan A: Syndrome of myelofibrosis and osteosclerosis: A series of case reports and review of the literature. *Bone* 3:498, 2002.
257. Parfitt AM, Drezner MK, Glorieux FH, et al: Bone histomorphometry: Standardization of nomenclature, symbols, and units. *J Bone Miner Res* 2:595, 1987.
258. Cassi E, DePaoli A, Tosi A, et al: Pure osteolytic lesions in myelofibrosis: Report of 2 cases. *Haematologica* 70:178, 1985.
259. Fayemi AO, Gerber MA, Cohen I, et al: Myeloid sarcoma. *Cancer* 32:253, 1973.
260. Yu JS, Greenway G, Resnick D: Myelofibrosis associated with prominent periosteal bone apposition. *Clin Imaging* 18:89, 1994.
261. Cervantes F, Alvarez-Larrán A, Arellano-Rodrigo E, et al: Frequency and risk factors for thrombosis in idiopathic myelofibrosis: Analysis in a series of 155 patients from a single institution. *Leukemia* 20:55, 2006.
262. Barosi G, Cazzoli M, Frassoni F: Erythropoiesis in myelofibrosis with myeloid metaplasia: Recognition of different classes of patients by erythrokinetics. *Br J Haematol* 48:263, 1981.
263. Barosi G, Berzuinic C, Liberato LN, et al: A prognostic classification of myelofibrosis with myeloid metaplasia. *Br J Haematol* 70:397, 1988.
264. Thiele J, Kvasnicka H-M, Werden C, et al: Idiopathic primary osteomyelofibrosis. *Leuk Lymphoma* 22:303, 1996.
265. Njoku OS, Lewis SM, Catovsky D, et al: Anaemia in myelofibrosis: Its value in prognosis. *Br J Haematol* 54:79, 1983.
266. Howarth JE, Waters HM, Hyde K, Geary CG: Detection of erythroid hypoplasia in myelofibrosis using erythrokinetic studies. *J Clin Pathol* 42:1250, 1989.
267. Thiele J, Windecker R, Kvasnicka HM, et al: Erythropoiesis in primary (idiopathic) osteomyelofibrosis. *Am J Hematol* 46:36, 1994.
268. Bird GW, Wingham J, Richardson SG: Myelofibrosis, autoimmune haemolytic anaemia and Tn-polyagglutinability. *Haematologica* 18:99, 1985.
269. Kuo CY, VanVoolen GA, Morrison AN: Primary and secondary myelofibrosis: Its relationship to the PNH-like defect. *Blood* 40:875, 1972.
270. Veer A, Kosciolek BA, Bauman AW, et al: Acquired hemoglobin H disease in idiopathic myelofibrosis. *Am J Hematol* 6:199, 1979.
271. Barosi G, Baraldi A, Cassola M, et al: Red cell aplasia in myelofibrosis with myeloid metaplasia. *Cancer* 52:1290, 1983.
272. Silverstein MN, Elveback LR: Leukocyte alkaline phosphatase in agnogenic myeloid metaplasia. *Am J Clin Pathol* 61:307, 1974.
273. Douer D, Fabian I, Cline MJ: Circulation pluripotent haemopoietic cells in patients with myeloproliferative disorders. *Br J Haematol* 54:373, 1983.
274. Barosi G, Viarengo G, Pecci A, et al: Diagnostic and clinical relevance of the number of circulating CD34+ cells in myelofibrosis with myeloid metaplasia. *Blood* 98:3249, 2001.
275. Partanen S, Ruutu T, Vuopio P: Circulating haematopoietic progenitors in myelofibrosis. *Scand J Haematol* 29:325, 1982.
276. Wang JC, Cheung CP, Ahmed F, et al: Circulating granulocyte and macrophage progenitor cells in primary and secondary myelofibrosis. *Br J Haematol* 54:301, 1983.
277. Kornberg A, Fibach E, Treves A, et al: Circulating erythroid progenitors in patients with "spent" polycythaemia vera and myelofibrosis with myeloid metaplasia. *Br J Haematol* 52:573, 1982.
278. Colovi MD, Wiernik PH, Jankovi GM, et al: Circulating haematopoietic progenitor cells in primary and secondary myelofibrosis: Relation to collagen and reticulin fibrosis. *Eur J Haematol* 62:155, 1999.
279. Tinggaard-Pedersen N, Laursen B: Megakaryocytes in cubital venous blood in patients with chronic myeloproliferative diseases. *Scand J Haematol* 30:50, 1983.
280. Cervantes F, Hernandez-Boluda JC, Villamor N, et al: Assessment of peripheral blood lymphocyte subsets in idiopathic myelofibrosis. *Eur J Haematol* 65:104, 2000.
281. Marquetty C, Labro-Bryskier MT, Perianin A, et al: Impaired metabolic activity of phagocytosis neutrophils in agnogenic osteomyelofibrosis with splenomegaly. *Am J Med* 16:243, 1984.
282. Perianin A, Labro-Bryskier MT, Marquetty C, et al: Glutathione reductase and nitroblue tetrazolium reduction deficiencies in neutrophils of patients with primary idiopathic myelofibrosis. *Clin Exp Immunol* 57:244, 1984.
283. Briard D, Brouty-Boye D, Giron-Michel Jet al: Impaired NK cell differentiation of blood-derived CD34+ progenitors from patients with myeloid metaplasia with myelofibrosis. *Clin Immunol* 106:201, 2003.
284. Murphy S, Davis JL, Walsh PN, et al: Template bleeding time and clinical hemorrhage in myeloproliferative disease. *Arch Intern Med* 138:1251, 1978.
285. Malpass TW, Savage B, Hanson SR, et al: Correlation between bleeding time and depletion of platelet dense granule ADP in patients with myelodysplastic and myeloproliferative disorders. *J Lab Clin Med* 103:894, 1984.
286. Cunietti E, Gandini R, Marcaro G, et al: Defective platelet aggregation and increased platelet turnover in patients with myelofibrosis and other myeloproliferative diseases. *Scand J Haematol* 26:339, 1981.
287. Schafer AL: Deficiency of platelet lipoxygenase activity in myeloproliferative disorders. *N Engl J Med* 306:381, 1982.
288. Shafer AL: Bleeding and thrombosis in the myeloproliferative disorders. *Blood* 64:1, 1984.
289. Barbui T, Cortelazzo S, Viero P, et al: Thrombohaemorrhagic complications in 101 cases of myeloproliferative disorders: Relationship to platelet number and function. *Eur J Cancer Clin Oncol* 19:1593, 1983.
290. Thiele J, Lorenzen J, Manich B, et al: Apoptosis (programmed cell death) in idiopathic (primary) osteo-/myelofibrosis. *Acta Haematol* 97:137, 1997.
291. Thiele J, Holgado S, Choritz H, et al: Chronic megakaryocyte-granulocytic myelosis—An electron microscope study including freeze-fracture. *Virchows Arch A* 375:129, 1977.
292. Mesa RA, Hanson CA, Rajkumar SV, et al: Evaluation and clinical correlations of bone marrow angiogenesis in myelofibrosis with myeloid metaplasia. *Blood* 15:3374, 2000.
293. Hussein K, Van Dyke DL, Tefferi A: Conventional cytogenetics in myelofibrosis: Literature review and discussion. *Eur J Haematol* 2009.
294. Tam CS, Abruzzo LV, Lin KI, et al: The role of cytogenetic abnormalities as a prognostic marker in primary myelofibrosis: Applicability at the time of diagnosis and later during disease course. *Blood* 30:113, 2009.
295. Nakamura H, Sadamori N, Mine M, et al: Effects of short-term liquid culture of peripheral blood mononuclear cells with recombinant human granulocyte or granulocyte-macrophage colony-stimulating factor in cytogenetic studies of myelofibrosis with myeloid metaplasia. *Leukemia* 6:853, 1992.
296. Reilly JT, Snowden JA, Spearing RL, et al: Cytogenetic abnormalities and their prognostic significance in idiopathic myelofibrosis. *Br J Haematol* 98:96, 1997.
297. Tefferi A, Mesa RA, Schroeder G, et al: Cytogenetic findings and their clinical relevance in myelofibrosis with myeloid metaplasia. *Br J Haematol* 113:763, 2001.
298. Tefferi A, Meyer RG, Wyatt WA, et al: Comparison of peripheral blood interphase cytogenetics with bone marrow karyotype analysis in myelofibrosis with myeloid metaplasia. *Br J Haematol* 115:316, 2001.
299. Sinclair EJ, Forrest EC, Reilly JT, et al: Fluorescence in situ hybridization analysis of 25 cases of idiopathic myelofibrosis and two cases of secondary idiopathic: Monoallelic loss of RB1, D13S319 and D13S25 loci associated with cytogenetic deletion and translocation involving 13q14. *Br J Haematol* 113:365, 2001.
300. Reilly JT: Cytogenetic and molecular genetic aspects of idiopathic myelofibrosis. *Acta Haematol* 108:113, 2002.
301. Andrieux J, Demory JL, Morel P, et al: Frequency of structural abnormalities of the long arm of chromosome 12 in myelofibrosis with myeloid metaplasia. *Cancer Genet Cytogenet* 137:68, 2002.
302. Dingli D, Grand FH, Mahaffey V, et al: Der(6)t(1;6)(q21–23;p21.3): A specific cytogenetic abnormality in myelofibrosis with myeloid metaplasia. *Br J Haematol* 130:229, 2005.
303. Forrester RH, Louro JM: Philadelphia chromosome abnormality in agnogenic myeloid metaplasia. *Ann Intern Med* 64:622, 1966.
304. Weda F, Takashima T, Suzuki M, Kadoya M: MR diagnosis of myelofibrosis. *Radiat Med* 12:135, 1994.
305. Amano Y, Onda M, Amano M, Kumazaki T: Magnetic resonance imaging of myelofibrosis. STIR and gadolinium-enhanced MR images. *Clin Imaging* 21:264, 1997.
306. Schirrmeister H, Bommer M, Buck A, Reske SN: The bone scan ion osteosclerosis. *J Bone Miner Res* 16:2361, 2001.
307. Gilbert HS, Ginsberg H, Fagerstrom R, Brown WV: Characterization of hypocholesterolemia in myeloproliferative diseases. *Am J Med* 71:595, 1981.
308. Naggar L, Jaeger P, Burckhardt P, et al: Hypocalcemia and myelofibrosis: An unrecognized association. *Schweiz Med Wochenschr* 116:1771, 1986.
309. Voss A, Schmidt K, Hasselbalch H, Junker P: Hypercalcemia in idiopathic myelofibrosis. *Am J Hematol* 39:231, 1992.

310. Wang JC, Chen C, Lou L-H, Mora M: Blood thrombopoietin, IL-6 and IL-11 levels in patients with agnogenic myeloid metaplasia. *Leukemia* 11:1827, 1997.
311. Elliott MA, Yoon S-Y, Kao P, et al: Simultaneous measurement of serum thrombopoietin and expression of megakaryocyte c-MPL with clinical and laboratory correlates for myelofibrosis with myeloid metaplasia. *Eur J Haematol* 68:175, 2002.
312. Wang JC, Hashmi G: Elevated thrombopoietin levels in patients with myelofibrosis may not be due to enhanced production of thrombopoietin by bone marrow. *Leuk Res* 27:13, 2003.
313. Wang J, Wang A: Plasma soluble interleukin-2 receptor in patients with primary myelofibrosis. *Br J Haematol* 86:180, 1994.
314. DiRaimondo F, Azzaro MP, Palumbo GA, et al: Elevated vascular endothelial growth factor (VEGF) serum levels in idiopathic myelofibrosis. *Leukemia* 15:976, 2001.
315. Dekmezian R, Kantarjian HM, Heating MJ, et al: The relevance of reticulin stain-measured fibrosis at diagnosis in chronic myelogenous leukemia. *Cancer* 59:1739, 1987.
316. Steensma DP, Hanson C, Letendre L, Teffari A: Myelodysplasia with fibrosis: A distinct entity? *Leuk Res* 25:829, 2001.
317. Thiele J, Zankovich R, Steinberg T, et al: Primary (essential) thrombocythemia versus initial hyperplastic stages of agnogenic myeloid metaplasia with thrombocytosis. *Acta Haematol* 81:192, 1989.
318. Thiele J, Kvasnicka HM, Zancovich R, Diehl V: Relevance of bone marrow features in the differential diagnosis between essential thrombocythemia and early stage idiopathic myelofibrosis. *Haematologica* 85:1126, 2000.
319. Hasselbach H, Jans H, Nielsen PL: A distinct subtype of idiopathic myelofibrosis with bone marrow features mimicking hairy cell leukemia. Evidence of an autoimmune pathogenesis. *Am J Hematol* 25:225, 1979.
320. O'Reilly RA: Splenomegaly at a United States County Hospital: Diagnostic evaluation of 170 patients. *Am J Med Sci* 312:160, 1996.
321. Pullarkat V, Bass RD, Gong JZ, et al: Primary autoimmune myelofibrosis: Definition of a distinct clinicopathologic syndrome. *Am J Hematol* 72:8, 2003.
322. Harrison JS, Corcoran KE, Joshi D, et al: Peripheral monocytes and CD4+ cells are potential sources for increased circulating levels of TGF-beta and substance P in autoimmune myelofibrosis. *Am J Hematol* 81:51, 2006.
323. Popat U, Frost A, Liu E, et al: High levels of circulating CD34 cells, dacrocytes, clonal hematopoiesis, and JAK2 mutation differentiate myelofibrosis with myeloid metaplasia from secondary myelofibrosis associated with pulmonary hypertension. *Blood* 107:3486, 2006.
324. Fortunato A, Mazzone A, Ricevuti G: Myelofibrosis caused by cancer: Presentation of a clinical case with a very difficult diagnosis. *Minerva Med* 76:1051, 1985.
325. Yablonski-Peretz T, Sulkes A, Polliack A, et al: Secondary myelofibrosis with metastatic breast cancer simulating agnogenic myeloid metaplasia: Report of a case and review of the literature. *Med Pediatr Oncol* 13:92, 1985.
326. Ishimura J, Fukushi M: Scintigraphic evaluation of secondary myelofibrosis associated with prostatic cancer before hormonal therapy. *Clin Nucl Med* 15:330, 1990.
327. Smart HE, Canney PA, Kerr DJ: Myelofibrosis associated with metastatic seminoma. *Clin Oncol* 4:132, 1992.
328. Takahashi T, Akihama T, Yamaguchi A, et al: Lysozyme secreting tumor: A case of gastric cancer associated with myelofibrosis due to disseminated bone marrow metastasis. *Jpn J Med* 26:58, 1987.
329. Rubins JM: The role of myelofibrosis in malignant leukoerythroblastosis. *Cancer* 51:308, 1983.
330. Hashim MSK, Kordofani AYA, El Dabi MA: Tuberculosis and myelofibrosis in children. *Ann Trop Paediatr* 17:61, 1997.
331. Viallard J-F, Parrens M, Boiron J-M, et al: Reversible myelofibrosis induced by tuberculosis. *Clin Infect Dis* 34:1641, 2002.
332. Sawers AH, Davson J, Braganza J, et al: Systemic mastocytosis, myelofibrosis and portal hypertension. *J Clin Pathol* 35:617, 1982.
333. Reisberg IR, Oyakawa S: Mastocytosis with malabsorption, myelofibrosis, and massive ascites. *Am J Gastroenterol* 82:54, 1987.
334. Kanbe N, Kurosawa M, Nagata H, et al: Production of fibrogenic cytokines by cord blood-derived cultured human mast cells. *J Allergy Clin Immunol* 106:S85, 2000.
335. Berton A, Levi-Schaffer F, Emonard H, et al: Activation of fibroblasts in collagen lattices by mast cell extracts: A model of fibrosis. *Clin Exp Allergy* 30:485, 2000.
336. Brenner B, Green J, Rosenbaum H, et al: Severe pancytopenia due to marked marrow fibrosis associated with angioimmunoblastic lymphadenopathy. *Acta Haematol* 74:43, 1985.
337. Varma N, Vaiphei K, Varma S: Angiosarcoma presenting with leucoerythroblastic anaemia bone marrow fibrosis and massive splenomegaly. *Br J Haematol* 110:503, 2000.
338. Meckenstock G, Wehmeier A, Schaefer HE, et al: Lymphoid myelofibrosis associated with high grade B cell lymphoma of the liver. *Leuk Lymphoma* 26:197, 1997.
339. Abe Y, Ohshima K, Shiratsuchi M, et al: Cytotoxic T-cell lymphoma presenting as secondary myelofibrosis with high levels of PDGF and TGF-β. *Eur J Haematol* 66:210, 2001.
340. Weirich G, Sandherr M, Fellbaum C, et al: Molecular evidence of bone marrow involvement in advanced case of T$\gamma\delta$ lymphoma with secondary myelofibrosis. *Hum Pathol* 29:761, 1998.
341. Subramanian R, Basu D, Dutta TK: Significance of bone marrow fibrosis in multiple myeloma. *Pathology* 39:512, 2007.
342. Schmidt U, Ruwe M, Leder LD: Multiple myeloma with bone marrow biopsy features simulating concomitant chronic idiopathic myelofibrosis. *Nouv Rev Fr Hematol* 37:159, 1995.
343. Abildgaard N, Bendix-Hanse K, Kristensen JE, et al: Bone marrow fibrosis and disease activity in multiple myeloma monitored by the autoterminal propeptide of procollagen III in serum. *Br J Haematol* 99:641, 1997.
344. Kim CD, Kim SH, Kim YL, et al: Bone marrow immunoscintigraphy (BMIS): A new and important tool for the assessment of marrow fibrosis in renal osteodystrophy? *Adv Perit Dial* 14:183, 1998.
345. Bachmeyer C, Blum L, Cadranel JF, Delfraissy JF: Myelofibrosis in a patient with pachydermoperiostosis. *Clin Exp Dermatol* 30:646, 2005.
346. Nurden AT, Nurden P: The gray platelet syndrome: Clinical spectrum of the disease. *Blood Rev* 21:21, 2007.
347. Sadoun A, Lacotte L, Delwail V, et al: Allogeneic bone marrow transplantation for hypereosinophilic syndrome with advanced myelofibrosis. *Bone Marrow Transplant* 19:741, 1997.
348. Vasquez L, Caballero D, Del Cañizo C, et al: Allogeneic peripheral blood cell transplantation for hypereosinophilic syndrome with myelofibrosis. *Bone Marrow Transplant* 25:217, 2000.
349. Filho FDR, Ferreira VDA, Mendes FDO, et al: Bone marrow fibrosis (pseudo-myelofibrosis) in kala-azar. *Rev Soc Bras Med Trop* 33:363, 2000.
350. Seelen MAJ, De Meijer PHEM, Posthuma EFM, Meinders AE: Myelofibrosis and idiopathic thrombocytopenic purpura. *Ann Hematol* 75:129, 1997.
351. Chang JC, Naqvi T: Thrombotic thrombocytopenic purpura associated with bone marrow metastasis and secondary myelofibrosis in cancer. *Oncologist* 8:375, 2003.
352. Hatake K, Ohtsuki T, Uwai M, et al: Tretinoin induces bone marrow collagenous fibrosis in acute promyelocytic leukemia. *Br J Haematol* 93:646, 1996.
353. Labotka RJ, Morgan RR: Myelofibrosis with neuroblastoma. *Med Pediatr Oncol* 10:21, 1982.
354. Karcher DS, Pearson CE, Butler WM, et al: Giant lymph node hyperplasia involving the thymus with associated nephrotic syndrome and myelofibrosis. *Am J Clin Pathol* 77:100, 1982.
355. Kamien B, Harris L: Twin troubles—Rickets causing myelofibrosis. *J Paediatr Child Health* 43:573, 2007.
356. Stéphan JL, Galambrun C, Dutour A, Freycon F: Myelofibrosis: An unusual presentation of vitamin D-deficient rickets. *Eur J Pediatr* 158:828, 1999.
357. Gruner BA, DeNapoli TS, Elshihabi S, et al: Anemia and hepatosplenomegaly as presenting features in a child with rickets and secondary myelofibrosis. *J Pediatr Hematol Oncol* 25:813, 2003.
358. Stéphan JL, Galambrun C, Dutour A, Freycon F: Myelofibrosis: An unusual presentation of vitamin D-deficient rickets. *Eur J Pediatr* 158:828, 1999.
359. Sartoris DJ, Resnick D: Myelofibrosis arising in treated histiocytosis X. *Eur J Pediatr* 144:200, 1985.
360. Fukuno K, Tsurumi H, Yoshikawa T, et al: A variant of acute promyelocytic leukemia with marked myelofibrosis. *Int J Hematol* 74:322, 2001.
361. Mori A, Wada H, Okada M, et al: Acute promyelocytic leukemia with marrow fibrosis at initial presentation. Possible involvement of transforming growth factor-β_1. *Acta Haematol* 103:220, 2000.
362. Shah-Reddy I, Subramanian L, Narang S: Myelofibrosis and true histiocytic lymphoma. *Tumori* 71:509, 1985.
363. Jennings WH, Li CY, Kiely JM: Concomitant myelofibrosis with agnogenic myeloid metaplasia and malignant lymphoma. *Mayo Clin Proc* 58:617, 1983.
364. Epstein RJ, Joshua DE, Kronenberg H: Idiopathic myelofibrosis complicated by lymphoma: Report of two cases. *Acta Haematol* 73:40, 1985.
365. Kaufman S, Iuclea S, Reif R: Idiopathic myelofibrosis complicated by chronic lymphatic leukaemia. *Clin Lab Haematol* 9:81, 1987.
366. Nieto LH, Sanchez JMR, Arguelles HA, et al: A case of chronic lymphocytic leukemia overwhelmed by rapidly progressive idiopathic myelofibrosis. *Haematologica* 85:973, 2000.
367. Subramanian VP, Gomez GA, Han T, et al: Coexistence of myeloid metaplasia with myelofibrosis and hairy-cell leukemia. *Arch Intern Med* 145:164, 1985.
368. Sotlar K, Bache A, Stellmacher F, et al: Systemic mastocytosis associated with chronic idiopathic myelofibrosis: A distinct subtype of systemic mastocytosis associated with a clonal hematological non-mast cell lineage disorder carrying the activating point mutations KITD816V and JAK2V617F. *J Mol Diagn* 10:58, 2008.
369. Ji SQ, Zhu M, Wang YZ: Primary macroglobulinemia with myelofibrosis: Report of a case. *Chin Med J* 100:83, 1987.
370. Humphrey CA, Morris TCM: The intimate relationship of myelofibrosis and myeloma. *Br J Haematol* 73:269, 1989.
371. Meerkin D, Ashkenazi Y, Gottschalk-Sabag S, Hershko C: Plasma cell dyscrasia with myelofibrosis. *Cancer* 73:625, 1994.
372. Kakkar N, Vashishta RK, Banerjee AK, et al: Primary pulmonary malignant teratoma with yolk sac element associated with hematologic neoplasia. *Respiration* 63:52, 1996.
373. Berner Y, Berrebi A: Myeloproliferative disorders and nonmyelomatous paraprotein: A study of five patients and review of the literature. *Isr J Med Sci* 22:109, 1986.
374. Ellis JT, Peterson P: Myelofibrosis in the myeloproliferative disorders. *Prog Clin Biol Res* 154:19, 1984.
375. Najean Y, Rain JD, Dresch C, et al: Risk of leukaemia, carcinoma and myelofibrosis in ^{32}P- or chemotherapy-treated patients with polycythaemia vera. *Leuk Lymphoma* 22(Suppl 1):111, 1996.
376. Najean Y, Rain JD: Treatment of polycythemia vera: Use of ^{32}P alone or in combination with maintenance therapy using hydroxyurea in 461 patients greater than 65 years of age. *Blood* 89:2319, 1997.

377. Randi ML, Barbone E, Fabris F, et al: Post-polycythemia myeloid metaplasia. *J Med* 25:363, 1994.
378. Lukowicz DF, Myers TJ, Grasso JA, et al: Sideroblastic anemia terminating in myelofibrosis. *Am J Hematol* 13:253, 1982.
379. Hasselbalch H, Berild D: Transition of myelofibrosis to polycythaemia vera. *Scand J Haematol* 30:161, 1983.
380. Talarico L, Wolf BC, Kumar A, Weintraub LR: Reversal of bone marrow fibrosis and subsequent development of polycythemia vera in patients with myeloproliferative disorders. *Am J Hematol* 30:248, 1989.
381. Jallades L, Hayette S, Tigaud I, et al: Emergence of therapy-unrelated CML on a background of BCR-ABL-negative JAK2V617F-positive chronic idiopathic myelofibrosis. *Leuk Res* 32:1608, 2008.
382. Hussein K, Bock O, Seegers A, et al: Myelofibrosis evolving during imatinib treatment of a chronic myeloproliferative disease with coexisting BCR-ABL translocation and JAK2 V617F mutation. *Blood* 109:4106, 2007.
383. Cervantes F, Alvarez-Larrán A, Domingo A, et al: Efficacy and tolerability of danazol as a treatment for the anaemia of myelofibrosis with myeloid metaplasia: Long-term results in 30 patients. *Br J Haematol* 129:771, 2005.
384. Makdisi WJ, Cherian R, Vanveldhuizen PJ, et al: Fatal peliosis of the liver and spleen in a patient with agnogenic myeloid metaplasia treated with danazol. *Am J Gastroenterol* 90:317, 1995.
385. Ozsoylu S, Ruacan S: High-dose intravenous corticosteroid treatment in childhood idiopathic myelofibrosis. *Acta Haematol* 75:49, 1986.
386. Cetingül N, Yener E, Oztop S, et al: Agnogenic myeloid metaplasia in childhood: A report of two cases and efficiency of intravenous high dose methylprednisolone treatment. *Acta Paediatr Jpn* 36:697, 1994.
387. Barois G, Liberato LN, Guarnone R: Serum erythropoietin in patients with myeloid metaplasia. *Br J Haematol* 83:365, 1993.
388. Cervantes F, Alvarez-Larrán A, Hernández-Boluda JC, et al: Erythropoietin treatment of the anaemia of myelofibrosis with myeloid metaplasia: Results in 20 patients and review of the literature. *Br J Haematol* 127:399, 2004.
389. Cervantes F, Alvarez-Larrán A, Hernández-Boluda JC, et al: Darbepoetin-alpha for the anaemia of myelofibrosis with myeloid metaplasia. *Br J Haematol* 134:184, 2006.
390. Lofvenberg E, Wahlin A: Management of polycythaemia vera, essential thrombocythaemia and myelofibrosis with hydroxyurea. *Eur J Haematol* 41:375, 1988.
391. Lofvenberg E, Wahlin A, Roos G, Ost A: Reversal of myelofibrosis by hydroxyurea. *Eur J Haematol* 44:33, 1990.
392. Manoharan A: Management of myelofibrosis with intermittent hydroxyurea. *Br J Haematol* 71:252, 1991.
393. Petti MC, Latagliata R, Spadea T, et al: Melphalan treatment in patients with myelofibrosis with myeloid metaplasia. *Br J Haematol* 116:576, 2002.
394. Wilks AF: The JAK kinases: Not just another kinase drug discovery target. *Semin Cell Dev Biol* 19:319, 2008.
395. Pardanani A, Hood J, Lasho T, et al: TG101209, a small molecule JAK2-selective kinase inhibitor potently inhibits myeloproliferative disorder-associated JAK2V617F and MPLW515L/K mutations. *Leukemia* 21:1658, 2007.
396. Verstovsek S, Kantarjian HM, Pardanani AD, et al: The JAK inhibitor , INCB018424, demonstrates durable and marked clinical responses in primary myelofibrosis (PMF) and post-polycythemia/essential thrombocythemia myelofibrosis (PV/ET-MF). *Blood* 112:622, 2008.
397. Pardanani AD, Gotlib J Jamieson C, et al: A phase I study of TG101348, an orally bioavailable JAK-2 selective inhibitor, in patients with myelofibrosis. *Blood* 112:43, 2008.
398. Shah, NP, Olszynski P, Sokol, L, et al: A phase I study of XL019, a selective JAK2 inhibitor, in patients with primary myelofibrosis polycythemia vera, or post-essential thrombocythemia myelofibrosis. *Blood* 112:441, 2008.
399. Merup M, Kutti J, Birgerård G, et al: Negligible clinical effects of thalidomide in patient with myelofibrosis with myeloid metaplasia. *Med Oncol* 19:79, 2002.
400. Piccaluga PP, Visani G, Pileri SA, et al: Clinical efficacy and antiangiogenic activity of thalidomide in myelofibrosis with myeloid metaplasia. A pilot study. *Leukemia* 16:1609, 2002.
401. Strupp C, Germing U, Scherer A, et al: Thalidomide for treatment of idiopathic myelofibrosis. *Eur J Haematol* 72:52, 2004.
402. Mesa RA, Lliott MA, Schroeder G, Tefferi A: Durable responses to thalidomide-based drug therapy for myelofibrosis with myeloid metaplasia. *Mayo Clin Proc* 79:883, 2004.
403. Tefferi A, Cortes J, Verstovsek S, et al: Lenalidomide therapy in myelofibrosis with myeloid metaplasia. *Blood* 108:1158, 2006.
404. Santana-Davila R, Tefferi A, Holtan SG, et al: Primary myelofibrosis is the most frequent myeloproliferative neoplasm associated with del(5q): Clinicopathologic comparison of del(5q)-positive and -negative cases. *Leuk Res* 32:1927, 2008.
405. Tefferi A, Lasho TL, Mesa RA, et al: Lenalidomide therapy in del(5)(q31)-associated myelofibrosis: Cytogenetic and JAK2V617F molecular remissions. *Leukemia* 21:1827, 2007.
406. Cervantes F, Mesa R, Barosi G: New and old treatment modalities in primary myelofibrosis. *Cancer J* 13:377, 2007.
407. Centanara E, Guarone R, Ippoliti G, Barosi G: Cyclosporine-A in severe refractory anemia of myelofibrosis with myeloid metaplasia: A preliminary report. *Haematologica* 83:622, 1998.
408. Nemoto Y, Tsutani H, Imamura S, et al: Successful treatment of acquired myelofibrosis with pure red cell aplasia. *Br J Haematol* 104:420, 1999.
409. Tsimberidou A-M, Giles FJ: TNF-α targeted therapeutic approaches in patients with hematologic malignancies. *Expert Rev Anticancer Ther* 2:277, 2002.
410. Steensma DP, Mesa RA, Li C-Y, et al: Etanercept, a soluble tumor necrosis factor receptor, palliates constitutional symptoms in patients with myelofibrosis with myeloid metaplasia: Results of a pilot study. *Blood* 99:2252, 2002.
411. Mesa RA: The therapy of myelofibrosis: Targeting pathogenesis. *Int J Hematol* 76 Suppl 2:296, 2002.
412. Tefferi A, Mesa RA, Gray LA, et al: Phase 2 trial of imatinib mesylate in myelofibrosis with myeloid metaplasia. *Blood* 99:3854, 2002.
413. Mesa RA, Camoriano JK, Geyer SM, et al: A phase II trial of tipifarnib in myelofibrosis: Primary, post-polycythemia vera and post-essential thrombocythemia. *Leukemia* 21:1964, 2007.
414. Carlo-Stella C, Cazzola M, Gasner A, et al: Effects of recombinant alpha and gamma interferons on the in vitro growth of circulating hematopoietic progenitors from patients with myelofibrosis and myeloid metaplasia. *Blood* 70:1014, 1987.
415. Sacchi S: The role of α-interferon in essential thrombocythaemia, polycythaema vera and myelofibrosis with myeloid metaplasia (MMM): A concise update. *Leuk Lymphoma* 19:13, 1995.
416. Bachleitner-Hofmann T, Gisslinger H: The role of interferon-α in the treatment of idiopathic myelofibrosis. *Ann Hematol* 78:533, 1999.
417. Stahl RL, Hoppstein L, Davidson TG: Intraperitoneal chemotherapy with cytosine arabinoside in agnogenic myelofibrosis with myeloid metaplasia and ascites due to peritoneal extramedullary hematopoiesis. *Am J Hematol* 43:156, 1993.
418. Camba L, Aldrighetti L, Ciceri F, et al: Locoregional intrasplenic chemotherapy for hypersplenism in myelofibrosis. *Br J Haematol* 114:638, 2001.
419. Amital H, Rewald E, Levy Y, et al: Fibrosis regression induced by intravenous gammaglobulin treatment. *Ann Rheum Dis* 62:175, 2003.
420. Sivera P, Cesano L, Guerrasio A, et al: Clinical and hematological improvement induced by etidronate in a patient with idiopathic myelofibrosis and osteosclerosis. *Br J Haematol* 86:397, 1994.
421. Froom P, Elmalah I, Braester A, et al: Clodronate in myelofibrosis: A case report. *Am J Med Sci* 323:115, 2002.
422. Assous N, Foltz V, Fautrel B, et al: Bone involvement in myelofibrosis: Effectiveness of bisphosphonates. *Joint Bone Spine* 72:591, 2005.
423. Elliott MA, Tefferi A: Splenic irradiation in myelofibrosis with myeloid metaplasia: A review. *Blood Rev* 13:163, 1999.
424. Jacobs P, Wood L, Robson S: Refractory ascites in the chronic myeloproliferative syndrome. *Am J Hematol* 37:128, 1991.
425. Jacobs P, Sellars S: Granulocytic sarcoma preceding leukaemic transformation in myelofibrosis. *Postgrad Med J* 61:1069, 1985.
426. Teffari A, Jimenez T, Gray LA, et al: Radiation therapy for symptomatic hepatomegaly in myelofibrosis with myeloid metaplasia. *Eur J Haematol* 66:37, 2001.
427. Mesa RA, Nagorney DS, Schwager S, et al: Palliative goals, patient selection, and perioperative platelet management: Outcomes and lessons from 3 decades of splenectomy for myelofibrosis with myeloid metaplasia at the Mayo Clinic. *Cancer* 107:361, 2006.
428. Tefferi A, Barrett SM, Silverstein NM, Nagorney DM: Outcome of portal-systemic shunt surgery for portal hypertension associated with intrahepatic obstruction in patients with agnogenic myeloid metaplasia. *Am J Hematol* 46:325, 1994.
429. Angermayr B, Cejna M, Schoder M, et al: Transjugular intrahepatic portosystemic shunt for treatment of portal hypertension due to extramedullary hematopoiesis in idiopathic myelofibrosis. *Blood* 99:4246, 2002.
430. Belohlavek J, Schwarz J, Jirásek A, et al: Idiopathic myelofibrosis complicated by portal hypertension treated with a transjugular intrahepatic portosystemic shunt (TIPS). *Wien Klin Wochenschr* 113:208, 2001.
431. Guardiola P, Anderson JE, Bandini G, et al: Allogeneic stem cell transplantation for agnogenic myeloid metaplasia: A European Group for Blood and Marrow Transplantation, Société Française de Greffe de Moelle, Gruppo Italiano per il Trapianto Midollo Osseo, and Fred Hutchinson Cancer Center Collaborative Study. *Blood* 93:2831, 1999.
432. Deeg HJ, Appelbaum FR: Stem-cell transplantation for myelofibrosis. *N Engl J Med* 334:775, 2001.
433. McCarty JM: Transplant strategies for idiopathic myelofibrosis. *Semin Hematol* 41(Suppl 3):23, 2004.
434. Mittal P, Saliba RM, Giralt SA, et al: Allogeneic transplantation: A therapeutic option for myelofibrosis, chronic myelomonocytic leukemia, and Philadelphia-negative BCR-ABL-negative chronic myelogenous leukemia. *Bone Marrow Transplant* 33:1005, 2004.
435. Papageorgiou SG, Castleton A, Bloor A, Kottaridis PD: Allogeneic stem cell transplantation as treatment for myelofibrosis. *Bone Marrow Transplant* 38:721, 2006.
436. Barosi G, Bacigalupo A: Allogeneic hematopoietic stem cell transplantation for myelofibrosis. *Curr Opin Hematol* 13:74, 2006.
437. Kerbauy DM, Gooley TA, Sale GE, et al: Hematopoietic cell transplantation as curative therapy for idiopathic myelofibrosis, advanced polycythemia vera, and essential thrombocythemia. *Biol Blood Marrow Transplant* 13:355, 2007.
438. Rondelli D: Allogeneic hematopoietic stem cell transplantation for myelofibrosis. *Haematologica* 93:1449, 2008.
439. Li Z, Deeg HJ: Pros and cons of splenectomy in patients with myelofibrosis undergoing stem cell transplantation. *Leukemia* 15:465, 2001.

440. Byrne JL, Beshti H, Clark D, et al: Induction of remission after donor leucocyte infusion for the treatment of relapsed chronic idiopathic myelofibrosis following allogeneic transplantation: Evidence for a "graft vs. myelofibrosis" effect. *Br J Haematol* 108:430, 2000.
441. Cervantes F, Rovira M, Urbano-Ispizua A, et al: Complete remission of idiopathic myelofibrosis following donor lymphocyte infusion after failure of allogeneic transplantation: Demonstration of a graft-versus-myelofibrosis effect. *Bone Marrow Transplant* 26:697, 2000.
442. Kröger N, Badbaran A, Holler E, et al: Monitoring of the JAK2-V617F mutation by highly sensitive quantitative real-time PCR after allogeneic stem cell transplantation in patients with myelofibrosis. *Blood* 109:1316, 2007.
443. Devine SM, Hoffman R, Verma A, et al: Allogeneic blood cell transplantation following reduced-intensity conditioning is effective therapy for older patients with myelofibrosis with myeloid metaplasia. *Blood* 99:2255, 2002.
444. Hessling J, Kroger N, Werner M, et al: Dose-reduced conditioning regimen followed by allogeneic stem cell transplantation in patients with myelofibrosis with myeloid metaplasia. *Br J Haematol* 119:769, 2002.
445. Merup M, Lazarevic V, Nahi H, et al: Different outcome of allogeneic transplantation in myelofibrosis using conventional or reduced-intensity conditioning regimens. *Br J Haematol* 135:367, 2006.
446. Greyz N, Miller WE, Andrey J, Masson J: Long-term remission of myelofibrosis following nonmyeloablative allogenic peripheral blood progenitor cell transplantation in older age. *Bone Marrow Transplant* 34:833, 2004.
447. Hoffman R, Prchal JT, Samuelson S, et al: Philadelphia chromosome-negative myeloproliferative disorders: Biology and treatment. *Biol Blood Marrow Transplant* 13(Suppl 1):64, 2007.
448. Anderson JE, Tefferi A, Craig F, et al: Myeloablation and autologous peripheral blood stem cell rescue results in hematologic and clinical responses in patients with myeloid metaplasia with myelofibrosis. *Blood* 98:586, 2001.
449. Visini G, Finelli C, Castelli U, et al: Myelofibrosis with myeloid metaplasia: Clinical and haematological parameters predicting survival in a series of 133 patients. *Br J Haematol* 75:4, 1990.
450. Cervantes F: Prognostic and current practice in treatment of myelofibrosis and myeloid metaplasia: An update anno 2000. *Pathol Biol (Paris)* 49:148, 2001.
451. Mesa RA, Li C-Y, Schroeder G, Tefferi A: Clinical correlates of splenic histology and splenic karyotype in myelofibrosis with myeloid metaplasia. *Blood* 97:3665, 2001.
452. Kvasnicka HM, Thiele J, Regn C, et al: Prognostic impact of apoptosis and proliferation in idiopathic (primary) myelofibrosis. *Ann Hematol* 78:65, 1999.
453. Elliott MA, Verstovsek S, Dingli D, et al: Monocytosis is an adverse prognostic factor for survival in younger patients with primary myelofibrosis. *Leuk Res* 31:1503, 2007.
454. Campbell PJ, Griesshammer M, Döhner K, et al: V617F mutation in JAK2 is associated with poorer survival in idiopathic myelofibrosis. *Blood* 107:2098, 2006.
455. Cervantes F, Dupriez B, Pereira A, et al: A new prognostic scoring system for primary myelofibrosis based on a study of the International Working Group for Myelofibrosis Research and Treatment. *Blood* 113:2895, 2009.
456. Rozman C, Giralt M, Feliu E, et al: Life expectancy of patients with chronic non-leukemic myeloproliferative disorders. *Cancer* 67:2658, 1991.
457. Silverstein MN, Brown AL, Linman JW: Idiopathic myeloid metaplasia, its evolution into acute leukemia. *Arch Intern Med* 132:709, 1973.
458. Marcus RE, Hibbin JA, Matutes E, et al: Megakaryoblastic transformation of myelofibrosis with expression of the c-*sis* oncogene. *Am J Hematol* 36:186, 1986.
459. Hernandez JM, SanMiguel JF, Gonzalez M, et al: Development of acute leukaemia after idiopathic myelofibrosis. *J Clin Pathol* 45:427, 1992.
460. Palphilon DH, Creamer P, Keeling DH, et al: Restoration of active haemopoiesis in a patient with myelofibrosis and subsequent termination in acute myeloblastic leukaemia: Case report and review of the literature. *Eur J Haematol* 38:279, 1987.
461. Chan ACL, Kwong Y-L, Lam CCK: Granulocytic sarcoma of megakaryoblastic differentiation complicating chronic idiopathic myelofibrosis. *Hum Pathol* 27:417, 1996.
462. Barnes HM, Prchal JT, Scott CW: Extramedullary blast transformation in the central nervous system in idiopathic myelofibrosis. *Am J Hematol* 11:305, 1981.
463. Polliack A, Prokocimer M, Matzner Y, et al: Lymphoblastic leukemic transformation (lymphoblastic crisis) in myelofibrosis and myeloid metaplasia. *Am J Hematol* 9:211, 1980.
464. Yinon A, Kopolovic J, Dollberg L, Hershko C: Evolution of malignant lymphoma in agnogenic myeloid metaplasia. *Oncology* 45:373, 1988.
465. Barosi G, Ambrosetti A, Centra A: Splenectomy and risk of blast transformation in myelofibrosis with myeloid metaplasia. *Blood* 91:3630, 1998.
466. Huang J, Li CY, Mesa RA, et al: Risk factors for leukemic transformation in patients with primary myelofibrosis. *Cancer* 112:2726, 2008.
467. Shreiner DP: Spontaneous hematologic remission in agnogenic myeloid metaplasia. *Am J Med* 60:1014, 1976.
468. Rani MV, Shreiner DP: Spontaneous "remission" of agnogenic myeloid metaplasia and termination in acute myeloid leukemia. *Arch Intern Med* 141:1481, 1981.
469. Altura RA, Headv DR, Wang WC: Long-term survival of infants with idiopathic myelofibrosis. *Br J Haematol* 109:459, 2000.
470. Sah A, Minford A, Parapia LA: Spontaneous remission of juvenile idiopathic myelofibrosis. *Br J Haematol* 112:1083, 2001.

PART XI

Malignant Lymphoid Diseases

CHAPTER 92

CLASSIFICATION OF MALIGNANT LYMPHOID DISORDERS

Thomas J. Kipps and Huan-You Wang

SUMMARY

This chapter outlines the category of neoplastic or preneoplastic lymphocyte and plasma cell disorders. It introduces a framework for evaluating neoplastic lymphocyte and plasma cell disorders, outlines clinical syndromes associated with such disorders, and presents a road map to the chapters in the text that discuss each of these disorders in greater detail. Chapter 80 outlines the diseases caused by nonneoplastic disorders of lymphocytes and plasma cells.

CLASSIFICATION

Lymphocyte and plasma cell malignancies compose a wide spectrum of different morphologic and clinical syndromes (Table 92–1). Lymphocyte neoplasms can originate from cells that are at a stage prior to T- and B-lymphocyte differentiation from a primitive stem cell or from cells at stages of maturation after stem cell differentiation. Thus, acute lymphoblastic leukemias arise from an early lymphoid progenitor cell that may give rise to cells with either B or T cell phenotypes (see Chap. 93). On the other hand, chronic lymphocytic leukemia arises from a more mature B-lymphocyte progenitor (see Chap. 94) and myeloma from progenitors at even later stages of B-lymphocyte maturation (see Chap. 109). Variability in expression of a lymphopoietic progenitor cell disorder may result in the spectrum of lymphocytic diseases, such as a B-lymphocyte or T-lymphocyte lymphoma, and different types of diseases, such as hairy cell leukemia (see Chap. 95), prolymphocytic leukemia (see Chap. 94), natural killer cell large granular lymphocytic leukemia (see Chap. 96),[1] myeloma, and plasmacytoma (see Chap. 109). Hodgkin lymphoma also is derived from a neoplastic B cell that has highly mutated immunoglobulin genes that are no longer expressed into protein (see Chap. 99).

To provide a unified international basis for clinical and investigative work in this field, the International Lymphoma Study Group proposed a classification termed the *revised European-American lymphoma* (REAL) classification (see Chap. 97),[2] which was modified in 2001 by the World Health Organization (WHO).[3] The REAL/WHO classification scheme makes use of the pathologic, immunophenotypic, genetic, and clinical features of a given lymphocyte tumor to delineate them into separate disease entities (see Table 92–1 and Chap. 98).[4] For some of these entities, the neoplastic lymphocytes have distinctive cytogenetic abnormalities, which can be identified using molecular techniques that increasingly are being used in clinical pathology laboratories.[5,6]

The REAL/WHO classification recognizes a basic distinction between nodular lymphocyte-predominant Hodgkin lymphoma and classic Hodgkin lymphoma, reflecting the differences in clinical presentation and behavior, morphology, phenotype, and molecular features (see Chap. 99).[3] Studies have identified features that can be used to distinguish classical Hodgkin lymphoma from anaplastic large cell lymphoma and, to a lesser extent, between nodular lymphocyte-predominant Hodgkin lymphoma and T-cell/histiocyte-rich large B-cell lymphoma.

Acronyms and abbreviations that appear in this chapter include: α/β TCR, T-cell-receptor genes encoding the α and β chains of the T-cell receptor (see Chap. 78); *ALK*, gene encoding anaplastic lymphoma kinase; *BCL2*, gene encoding B-cell chronic lymphocytic leukemia (CLL)/lymphoma 2; *BCL6*, gene encoding B-cell chronic lymphocytic leukemia (CLL)/lymphoma 6; cIg, cytoplasmic immunoglobulin; EBV, Epstein-Barr virus; γ/δ TCR, T-cell-receptor genes encoding the γ and δ chains of the T-cell receptor (see Chap. 78); HL, Hodgkin lymphoma; HLA, human leukocyte antigen; HTLV-1, human T-cell leukemia virus type 1; Ig, immunoglobulin; IgR, immunoglobulin gene rearrangement (see Chap. 77); IL, interleukin; MALT, mucosa-associated lymphoid tissue; *MUM1*, gene encoding multiple myeloma oncogene 1; neg., negative; NK cell, natural killer cell; *NPM*, gene encoding nucleophosmin; *PAX5*, paired box gene 5; POEMS, polyneuropathy, organomegaly, endocrinopathy, monoclonal gammopathy, and skin changes; REAL, revised European-American lymphoma; R-S, Reed-Sternberg; sIg, surface immunoglobulin (see Chap. 77); sIgD, surface IgD; sIgM, surface IgM; TAL1, gene encoding T-cell acute leukemia-1; TCR, T-cell receptor; TdT, terminal deoxynucleotidyl transferase; WHO, World Health Organization.

CLINICAL BEHAVIOR

Lymphomas of similar histology can have widely different spectra of associated clinical symptoms and clinical aggressiveness, making the categorization of lymphoid tumors impossible using a generic grading system based on morphology alone. For example, the neoplastic cells in mantle cell lymphoma appear smaller and more differentiated than those of anaplastic large-cell lymphomas. However, the validation studies for the REAL classification revealed that patients with mantle cell lymphoma or anaplastic large cell lymphomas have a 5-year survival rate of approximately 30 percent and approximately 80 percent, respectively.[7,8] Generally, T-cell lymphomas/leukemias have a more aggressive clinical behavior than B-cell lymphomas of comparable histology. The tendency for more aggressive disease also applies to lymphoid tumors derived from natural killer cells. A helpful distinction is to divide the lymphoid tumors into one of two categories, namely, indolent lymphomas versus aggressive lymphomas, based upon on the characteristics of the disease at the time of presentation and the patients' life expectancy if the disease is left untreated.[9,10] Clinical studies have verified that the different disease categories defined in the REAL/WHO classification each can be segregated into one or the other of these two major categories (Tables 92–2 and 92–3).[7] Analyses of gene expression patterns using microarray technology (see Chap. 10) have enabled identification of subcategories within some of the disease categories defined by the REAL/WHO classification that have different tendencies for disease progression, survival, and/or response rates to standard therapies (see Chap. 98).[11–17]

ASSOCIATED CLINICAL SYNDROMES

ABNORMAL PRODUCTION OF IMMUNOGLOBULIN

When B lymphocytes undergo neoplastic transformation and clonal proliferation, they can secrete monoclonal proteins inappropriately (see Chaps. 107 and 108). If the monoclonal protein is immunoglobulin (Ig) M, IgA, or a member of certain subclasses of IgG (e.g., IgG_3), its presence may increase the viscosity of the blood, impairing blood flow through the microcirculation (see Chaps. 109 and 111). This process may be impeded further by the associated homotypic erythrocyte

TABLE 92–1. Classification of Lymphoma and Lymphoid Leukemia by World Health Organization

Neoplasm	Morphology	Phenotype*	Genotype†
		B-Cell Neoplasms	
Immature B-Cell Neoplasms			
Lymphoblastic leukemia (see Chap. 93)	Medium to large cells with finely stippled chromatin and scant cytoplasm	TdT+, sIg–, CD10+, CD13+/–, CD19+, CD20–, CD22+, CD34+/–, CD33+/–, CD45+/–, CD79a+	t(1;19), t(9;22), and defects at 11q23-defects associated with poor prognosis
Lymphoblastic lymphoma (see Chap. 93)	Medium-size cells with high nuclear to cytoplasmic ratio	See above	See above
Mature B-cell Neoplasms			
Leukemias			
Chronic lymphocytic leukemia (see Chap. 94)	Small cells with round, dense nuclei	sIg+(dim), CD5+, CD10–, CD19+, CD20+(dim), CD22+(dim), CD23+, CD38+/–, CD45+, FMC-7–	IgR, trisomy 12 (~30%), del at 13q14 (~50%), 11q– (15%)
Prolymphocytic leukemia (see Chap. 94)	≥55% prolymphocytes	sIg+(bright), CD5+/–, CD10–, CD19+, CD22+, CD23+/–, CD45+	IgR, trisomy 12 (~30%)
Hairy cell leukemia (see Chap. 95)	Small cells with cytoplasmic projections	sIg+(bright), CD5–, CD10–, CD11c+(bright), CD19+, CD20+, CD25+, CD45+, CD103+, Annexin A+	IgR
Lymphomas			
Small lymphocytic lymphoma (see Chap. 94)	Small round cells	sIg+(dim), CD5+, CD19+, dim CD20+, CD23+, CD45+	IgR, trisomy 12 (~30%), del at 13q14 (~40%), 11q– (~15%)
Lymphoplasmacytic lymphoma (see Chap. 111)	Small cells with plasmacytoid differentiation	cIg+, CD5–, CD10–, CD19+, CD20+/– Plasma cell population: CD38+, CD138+, cIgM+	IgR, 6q– in 50% of marrow-based cases [the t(9;14) was proved to be wrong]
Mantle cell lymphoma (see Chap. 102)	Small- to medium-sized cells	sIgM+, sIgD+, CD5+, CD10–, CD19+, CD20+, CD23–, Cyclin D1+, FMC-7+	IgR, t(11;14)(q13;q32) (~100% by FISH), involving *BCL1* and IgH
Follicular lymphoma (follicle center lymphoma; see Chap. 101)	Small, medium, or large cells with cleaved nuclei	sIg, CD5–, CD10+, CD19+, bright CD20+, CD23–/+, CD38+, CD45+	IgR, t(14;18)(q32;q21) (~85%) involving *BCL2* and IgH
Marginal zone B-cell lymphoma (see Chap. 103)	Small or large monocytoid cells	sIgM+, sIgD–, cIg+ (~50%), CD5–, CD10–, CD11c+/–, CD19+, CD20+, CD23–, CD43+/–	IgR, commonly with trisomy 3 and/or t(11;18)(q21;q21) involving *API2*, *MLT*, or t(1;14)(p22;q32) involving *BCL10*
Mucosa-associated lymphoid tissue (MALT) type (see Chap. 103)	See above	See above	See above
Nodal type	See above	See above	See above
Splenic type	Small to large monocytoid and/or villous lymphocytes	sIgM+, sIgD–, CD5+/–, CD19+, CD20+, CD23–	IgR
Diffuse large B-cell lymphoma (see Chap. 100)	Large, irregular cells that can resemble centroblasts, immunoblasts, multilobate cells, or even RS-like cells	sIgM+, sIgD+/–, CD5–/+, CD10–/+, CD19+, CD20+, CD45+, PAX5+	IgR, 3q27 abnormalities and/or t(3;14)(q27;q32) involving *BCL6* (~40%) or t(14;18)(q32;q21) (~25%) involving *BCL2*
Primary mediastinal (thymic) large B-cell lymphoma (see Chap. 100)	Same as above	sIg–, CD5–, CD10–/+, CD15–, CD19+, CD20+, CD22+, CD30+/–, CD45+, CD79a+	Gain of 9q24 (75%), gain 2p15 (50%) Lack of rearrangements of *BCL2*, *BCL6*, or *MYC*
Burkitt lymphoma (see Chap. 104)	Medium-sized, round cells with abundant cytoplasm	sIgM+, CD5–, CD10+, CD19+, CD20+, CD23–, CD45+	t(8;14)(q24;q32), t(2;8)(q11;q24), or t(8;22)(q24;q11), involving Ig loci and *C-MYC* at 8q24
Burkitt-like lymphoma (see Chap. 104)	Medium-sized, round cells with abundant cytoplasm	Same as above except sIg–, cIg+/–, and CD10–	Same as above except more typically expresses high levels of *BCL2* and ~30% have *BCL2* rearrangements

(continued)

TABLE 92–1. Classification of Lymphoma and Lymphoid Leukemia by World Health Organization (Continued)

Neoplasm	Morphology	Phenotype*	Genotype†
Plasma cell neoplasms			
Myeloma (see Chap. 109)	Plasma cells with occasional plasmablasts	cIg+, sIg–, CD5–, CD10–, CD19–, CD20–, CD38+(bright), CD45–/+, CD56+, CD117+/–(bright), CD138+(bright)	IgR, commonly with complex karyotypes and/or t(6;14)(p25;q32) involving *MUM1*. t(11;14)(q23;q32) can be found in 15–25% of cases
Plasma cell leukemia (see Chap. 109)	Plasmablastic cells with prominent nucleoli	Same as above except usually CD56–	Same as above
Plasmacytoma (see Chap. 109)	Plasma cells	Same as plasma cell myeloma	Same as above
Waldenström macroglobulinemia (see Chap. 111)	Lymphocytes, plasmacytoid cells, and plasma cells	CD5+/–, CD10–, CD19+, CD20+, CD22+, CD38+/–	IgR, complex karyotypes common
Hodgkin Lymphoma (HL)			
Nodular lymphocyte predominant HL (see Chap. 97)	"Popcorn cells" with nuclei resembling those of centroblasts	BCL6+, CD19+, CD20+, CD22+, CD45+, CD79a+, CD15–, and rarely CD30+/–, Bob1+, Oct2+, PAX5+	IgR, with high-level expression of *BCL6*
Classic HL (see Chap. 97)			
Nodular sclerosis HL	R-S cells and lacunar cells dispersed in reactive lymphoid nodules	R-S cells typically are CD15+, CD20–/+, CD30+, CD45–, CD79a–, PAX5+(dim)	R-S cells generally express *PAX5* and *MUM1*, variable expression of *BCL6*, and have IgR without functional Ig
Lymphocyte-rich HL	Few R-S cells with occasional "popcorn" appearance dispersed in lymphoid nodules	Same as above	Same as above
Mixed cellularity HL	R-S cells dispersed among plasma cells, epithelioid histiocytes, eosinophils, and T cells	R-S cells typically are CD15+, CD20–/+, CD30+, CD45–, CD79a–	R-S cells generally express *PAX5* and *MUM1*, variable expression of *BCL6*, and have IgR without functional Ig
Lymphocyte-depleted HL	Prominent numbers of R-S cells with effacement of the nodal structure	Same as above	Same as above
T-Cell Neoplasms			
Immature T-Cell Neoplasms			
Lymphoblastic leukemia (see Chap. 93)	Medium to large cells with finely stippled chromatin and scant cytoplasm	TdT+, CD2+/–, cytoplasmic CD3+, CD1a+/–, CD5+/–, CD7+, CD10–/+, CD4+/CD8+ or CD4–/CD8–, CD34+/–	Abnormalities in *TCR* loci at 14q11 (TCR-α), 7q34 (TCR-β), or 7p15 (TCR-γ), and/or t(1;14)(p32–34; q11) involving *TAL1*
Lymphoblastic lymphoma (see Chap. 93)	Same as above	Same as above	Same as above
Mature T-Cell Neoplasms			
Leukemias			
T-cell prolymphocytic leukemia (see Chap. 106)	Small- to medium-size cells with cytoplasmic protrusions or blebs	TdT–, CD2+, CD3+, CD5+, CD7+, CD4+ and CD8– is more common than CD4– and CD8+, but can be CD4+ and CD8+	α/β TCR rearrangement, inv14(q11;q32)(~75–80%)
T-cell large granular lymphocytic leukemia (see Chap. 96)	Abundant cytoplasm and sparse azurophilic granules	CD2+, CD3+, CD4 –/+, CD5+, CD7+, CD8+/–, CD16+/–, CD56–, CD57+/–	α/β TCR rearrangement, γ/δ rearrangement can be seen
Lymphomas			
Extranodal T/NK-cell lymphoma, nasal type ("angiocentric lymphoma"; see Chaps. 96 and 106)	Angiocentric and angiodestructive growth	CD2+, cytoplasmic CD3+, CD4–, CD5–/+, CD7+, CD8–, CD56+, EBV+	TCR rearrangements usually neg., EBV present by *in situ* hybridization
Cutaneous T-cell lymphoma (mycosis fungoides; see Chap. 105)	Small to large cells with cerebriform nuclei	CD2+, CD3+, CD4+, CD5+, CD7+/–, CD8–, CD25–, CD26+	α/β TCR rearrangements

(continued)

TABLE 92–1. Classification of Lymphoma and Lymphoid Leukemia by World Health Organization (Continued)

Neoplasm	Morphology	Phenotype*	Genotype†
		T-Cell Neoplasms	
Sézary syndrome (see Chap. 105)	Same as above	Same as above	Same as above
Angioimmunoblastic T-cell lymphoma[34]	Small- to medium-size immunoblasts with clear to pale cytoplasm around follicles and high endothelial venules	CD3+/–, CD4+, CD10+, CXCL13+, PD-1+, EBV+	α/β TCR rearrangement (75–90%), IgR (25–30%), trisomy 3 or 5 noted
Peripheral T-cell lymphoma (not otherwise unspecified; see Chap. 106)	Highly variable	CD2+, CD3+, CD5+, CD7–, CD4+CD8– more often than CD4–CD8+, which is more often than CD4+CD8+	α/β TCR rearrangement
Subcutaneous panniculitis-like T-cell lymphoma[35]	Variably sized atypical cells with hyperchromasia infiltrating fat lobule	CD2+, CD3+, CD4–, CD5+, CD7–, CD8+, and cytoxic molecules (perforin, granzyme B, and TIA1)	α/β TCR rearrangement
Enteropathy-associated T-cell lymphoma[36]	Small to large atypical lymphocytes	CD2+, CD3+, CD5–, CD7+, CD8–/+, CD4–, CD103+	β TCR rearrangement
Hepatosplenic T-cell lymphoma[37–39]	Small- to medium-size cells with condensed chromatin and round nuclei	CD2+, CD3+, CD4–, CD5+, CD7+/–, CD8+/–	γ/δ TCR rearrangement, rarely α/β TCR rearrangement, isochromosome 7q
Adult T-cell leukemia/lymphoma (see Chap. 93)	Highly pleomorphic with multilobed nuclei	CD2+, CD3+, CD5+, CD7–, CD25+, CD4+CD8– more often than CD4–CD8+	α/β TCR rearrangement, integrated HTLV-1
Anaplastic large-cell lymphoma[40–42]	Large pleomorphic cells with "horseshoe"-shaped nuclei, prominent nucleoli, and abundant cytoplasm	TdT–, ALK1+, CD2+/–, CD3–/+, CD4–/+, CD5–/+, CD7+/–, CD8–/+, CD13–/+, CD25+/–, CD30+, CD33–/+, CD45+, HLA-DR+, TIA+/–	TCR rearrangement, t(2;5)(p23;q35) resulting in nucleophosmin–anaplastic lymphoma kinase fusion protein (*NPM/ALK*); other translocations involving 2p23 are also seen
Primary cutaneous CD30+ anaplastic large cell lymphoma[43–44]	Anaplastic large cells as above in cutaneous nodules	TdT–, CD2–/+, CD3+/–, CD4+, CD5–/+, CD7+/–, CD25+/–, CD30+, CD45+	TCR rearrangement but without t(2;5)(p23;q35), therefore, ALK1 neg.
		Natural Killer Cell Neoplasms	
Large granular lymphocytic leukemia (see Chap. 96)	Abundant cytoplasm and sparse azurophilic granules	TdT–, CD2+, CD3–, CD4–, CD5–/+, CD7+, CD8–/+, CD11b+, CD16+, CD56+, CD57+/–	No TCR rearrangement
Aggressive NK-cell leukemia[1]	Same as above	Same as above	No TCR rearrangement, EBV present
Extranodal NK-cell lymphoma, nasal-type ("angiocentric lymphoma")[1,45–46]	Angiocentric and angiodestructive growth	CD2+, cytoplasmic CD3ε+, CD4–, CD5–/+, CD7+, CD8–, CD56+	No TCR rearrangement, EBV present

IgR, immunoglobulin gene rearrangement; neg., negative; NK, natural killer; TCR, T-cell receptor; R-S, Reed-Sternberg. Also see acronyms and abbreviations at the beginning of this chapter.

*The immunophenotype revealed by immunohistochemistry and/or flow cytometry of surface antigens that typically are found for neoplastic cells of a given disorder are listed. If a CD antigen is indicated (see Chap. 15), then most of the neoplastic cells express that particular surface protein that is expressed by most tumor cells. CD antigens that have a minus (–) sign suffix are characteristically not expressed by the neoplastic cells of that disease entity. CD antigens that have a +/– sign suffix are not expressed by the neoplastic cells of all patients with that entity or are expressed at low or variable levels on the tumor cells. Antigens that have a –/+ sign suffix are expressed at very low levels or by the tumor cells of a minority of patients.

†The common genetic features associated with a given type of neoplasm are indicated. The numbers in parentheses provide the approximate proportion of cases that have the defined phenotype or genetic abnormality.

aggregation (pathologic rouleaux) that often occurs in blood with a high concentration of immunoglobulin protein. Collectively, this situation may result in the hyperviscosity syndrome, manifested clinically by headache, dizziness, diplopia, stupor, retinal venous engorgement, or frank coma (see Chap. 111).[18,19]

Monoclonal immunoglobulin proteins also can interact with cell surfaces and impair granulocyte or platelet function, or they can interact with coagulation proteins to impair their function in hemostasis (see Chap. 121). Excessive excretion of immunoglobulin light chains can lead to several types of renal tubular dysfunction and renal insufficiency (see Chaps. 108 and 109). IgM deposited in glomerular tufts also can lead to renal disease (see Chap. 111). Cryoglobulins (or immunoglobulins that precipitate at temperatures below 37°C) can result in Raynaud syndrome, skin ulcerations, purpura, digital infarction, and gangrene (see Chap. 53). These manifestations result from immune complex formation, complement activation, and precipitation of cryoglobulins in cutaneous blood vessels. Excessive production of monoclonal immunoglobulin or immunoglobulin fragments in myeloma (see Chap. 109) or in heavy-chain disease (see Chap. 112) may lead to formation of amyloid, resulting in primary amyloidosis (see Chap. 110).

Production of autoreactive antibodies spontaneously or in relationship to a B-lymphocyte neoplasm may lead to autoimmune hemolytic anemia (see Chap. 53), autoimmune thrombocytopenia (see Chap. 119), or, rarely, autoimmune neutropenia (see Chap. 65). Autoantibodies

TABLE 92–2. Indolent Lymphomas

Disseminated Lymphomas/Leukemias
Chronic lymphocytic leukemia
Hairy cell leukemia
Lymphoplasmacytic lymphoma
Splenic marginal zone B-cell lymphoma (with or without villous lymphocytes)
Plasma cell myeloma/plasmacytoma
Nodal Lymphomas
Follicular lymphoma
Nodal marginal zone B-cell lymphoma (with or without monocytoid B cells)
Small lymphocytic lymphoma
Extranodal Lymphomas
Extranodal marginal zone B-cell lymphoma of mucosa-associated lymphoid tissue (MALT) type

TABLE 92–3. Aggressive Lymphomas

Immature B-Cell Neoplasms
B-lymphoblastic leukemia/lymphoma
Mature B-Cell Neoplasms
Burkitt lymphoma/Burkitt cell leukemia
Diffuse large B-cell lymphoma
Follicular lymphoma grade III
Mantle cell lymphoma
Immature T-Cell Neoplasms
T-lymphoblastic lymphoma/leukemia
Peripheral T- and Natural Killer (NK) Cell Neoplasms
T-cell prolymphocytic leukemia/lymphoma
Aggressive NK cell leukemia/lymphoma
Adult T-cell lymphoma/leukemia (associated with HTLV-1 [human T-cell leukemia virus type 1])
Extranodal NK/T cell lymphoma
Enteropathy-associated T-cell lymphoma
Hepatosplenic T-cell lymphoma
Subcutaneous panniculitis-like T-cell lymphoma
Peripheral T-cell lymphomas, not otherwise specified
Angioimmunoblastic T-cell lymphoma
Anaplastic large cell lymphoma, primary, systemic

directed against tissues are implicated in the etiopathogenesis of diseases such as autoimmune thyroiditis, adrenalitis, encephalitis, and conditions with other organ involvement. Peripheral neuropathies as a result of demyelinization can occur in patients with monoclonal immunoglobulin (see Chaps. 108, 109, and 111). The neural injury often is related to antibody activity against myelin-associated glycoproteins or absorption by nerve tissue.[19] Rarely, the polyneuropathy is associated with organomegaly, endocrinopathy, a monoclonal protein and skin changes or with the polyneuropathy, organomegaly, endocrinopathy, monoclonal gammopathy, and skin changes (POEMS) syndrome (see Chap. 109).[20]

MARROW AND OTHER TISSUE INFILTRATION

Well-differentiated malignant B lymphocytes, such as those found in the early stages of chronic lymphocytic leukemia or macroglobulinemia, may infiltrate the marrow extensively, causing minimal impairment of hemopoiesis. Eventually, however, massive infiltration of marrow by malignant B lymphocytes can suppress normal hemopoiesis, resulting in varying combinations of anemia, neutropenia, and/or thrombocytopenia (see Chap. 94). Malignant B-lymphocyte proliferation or infiltration may result in any combination of splenomegaly and lymphadenopathy of either superficial or deep lymph nodes. Many B-cell lymphomas tend to involve isolated lymph node groups (see Chaps. 99 and 100), whereas B-cell chronic lymphocytic leukemia and most low-grade lymphomas tend to involve many superficial and deep lymph node-bearing areas and the spleen (see Chaps. 94–96). Prolymphocytic leukemia and hairy cell leukemia, two uncommon B-lymphocyte malignancies, are prone to infiltrate the marrow and spleen, sometimes causing massive enlargement of the latter (see Chaps. 94 and 95).

LYMPHOKINE-INDUCED DISORDERS

In addition to the consequences of monoclonal immunoglobulin and tumor proliferation, some lymphoid malignancies may elaborate cytokines that contribute to the disease morbidity. Patients with cutaneous T-cell lymphomas have elevated plasma levels of T-helper type 2 (Th2)-associated cytokines (see Chaps. 78 and 105), which may account for the relatively high incidence of eosinophilia (see Chap. 106) and eosinophilic pneumonia observed in patients with this disease.[21] In addition, the neoplastic plasma cells in myeloma may secrete various cytokines and osteoclast activating factors that stimulate osteoclast proliferation and activity leading to extensive osteolysis, severe bone pain, and pathologic fractures (see Chap. 109).[22] Dysregulated extrarenal production of calcitriol, the active metabolite of vitamin D, appears to underlie the hypercalcemia associated with Hodgkin lymphoma and other lymphomas (see Chaps. 97 and 99).[23]

SYSTEMIC SYMPTOMS

Large-cell lymphoma, poorly differentiated lymphoma, and Hodgkin lymphoma frequently are associated with fever, night sweats, weight loss, and anorexia (see Chaps. 97, 99, and 100). Patients with lymphomas or Hodgkin lymphoma have an increased incidence of localized or disseminated herpes zoster,[24] and 10 percent or more of these patients may be affected at some time during the course of their illness. Pruritus is common in Hodgkin lymphoma,[25] and its severity parallels disease activity (see Chap. 99). Systemic symptoms may be present in Hodgkin lymphoma in the absence of obvious, bulky lymph node or splenic tumors, whereas in well-differentiated small cell lymphomas, such as chronic lymphocytic leukemia or Waldenström macroglobulinemia, fever, night sweats, and significant weight loss are uncommon despite generalized lymphadenopathy and splenomegaly. Rather, fever in patients with chronic lymphocytic leukemia or macroglobulinemia usually is secondary to infectious disease (see Chaps. 94 and 111).

METABOLIC SIGNS

Lymphoid malignancies are associated with the most dramatic metabolic disturbances associated with cancers (see Chap. 97). Some lymphomas and lymphocytic leukemias may have an extremely high proliferative rate, a high death fraction of cells, and, therefore, an enormous turnover of nucleoproteins, sometimes causing hyperuricemia and extreme hyperuricosuria. Burkitt lymphoma or acute lymphoblastic leukemia is particularly likely to cause an extreme degree of hyperuricemia, sometimes leading to renal failure prior to cytotoxic therapy (see Chaps. 93 and 104). Also, because these and other lymphocytic malignancies are sensitive to cytotoxic drugs and glucocorticoids, cytotoxic therapy may cause a *tumor lysis syndrome*, characterized by extreme hyperuricemia, hyperuricosuria, hyperkalemia, and/or hyperphosphatemia.[26,27] Precipitation of uric acid in the renal tubules and collecting system can lead to acute obstructive nephropathy and renal failure unless precautions are taken, such as pretreatment with allopurinol, hydration, and alkalization of the urine.[28] For extreme cases, or in cases in which allopurinol cannot be administered (e.g., drug allergy), the drug rasburicase may be required for treatment of hyperuricemia (see Chap. 104).[29]

Hypercalcemia and calciuria are common complications of myeloma because of osteolysis. Hypercalcemia also may occur during the course of lymphomas (see Chap. 96) or myeloma (see Chap. 109). This situation may be caused by several mechanisms, including tumor cell production of interleukin (IL)-1, ectopic parathyroid hormone elaboration, excessive bone resorption, and impaired bone formation.[30]

EXTRANODAL INVOLVEMENT

T-cell leukemias and lymphomas, in addition to causing lymph node and spleen enlargement, may involve the skin, mediastinum, or central nervous system. As the name implies, cutaneous T-cell lymphomas have malignant cells that home to the skin,[31] sometimes producing a severe desquamating erythroderma, as in Sézary syndrome, or small (<2 cm) subcutaneous nodules, as in primary cutaneous CD30-positive T-cell lymphoproliferative disease or anaplastic large cell lymphoma,[32] or a variety of nodular infiltrative lesions, as in mycosis fungoides or adult T-cell leukemia/lymphoma associated with human T-cell leukemia virus type 1 (HTLV-1; see Chap. 105).[33] T-cell acute lymphoblastic leukemia and lymphoblastic lymphoma frequently cause mediastinal enlargement (see Chap. 93). These diseases frequently involve testicles and the leptomeninges and other structures that are transverse to the subarachnoid space, such as the cranial and peripheral nerves.

B-cell lymphomas frequently may involve the salivary glands, endocrine glands, joints, heart, lung, kidney, bowel, bone, or, less frequently, other extranodal sites (see Chap. 97). These diseases may begin as an extranodal tumor, or the tumor may develop during the course of the disease. Marginal zone B-cell lymphoma of mucosa-associated lymphoid tissue (MALT) type frequently involves the stomach and salivary glands, although the disease may be encountered in any extranodal site distinguished by the presence of a columnar or cuboidal epithelium.

REFERENCES

1. Liang X, Graham DK: Natural killer cell neoplasms. *Cancer* 112:1425, 2008.
2. Harris NL, Jaffe ES, Stein H, et al: A revised European-American classification of lymphoid neoplasms: A proposal from the International Lymphoma Study Group. *Blood* 84:1361, 1994.
3. Chan JK: The new World Health Organization classification of lymphomas: The past, the present and the future. *Hematol Oncol* 19:129, 2001.
4. Segal GH, Kjeldsberg CR: Practical lymphoma diagnosis: An approach to using the information organized in the REAL proposal. Revised European-American Lymphoid Neoplasm. *Anat Pathol* 3:147, 1998.
5. Spagnolo DV, Ellis DW, Juneja S, et al: The role of molecular studies in lymphoma diagnosis: A review. *Pathology* 36:19, 2004.
6. Strauchen JA: Immunophenotypic and molecular studies in the diagnosis and classification of malignant lymphoma. *Cancer Invest* 22:138, 2004.
7. A clinical evaluation of the International Lymphoma Study Group classification of non-Hodgkin's lymphoma. The Non-Hodgkin's Lymphoma Classification Project. *Blood* 89:3909, 1997.
8. Fisher RI, Miller TP, Grogan TM: New REAL clinical entities. *Cancer J Sci Am* 4(Suppl 2):S5, 1998.
9. Pileri SA, Ascani S, Sabattini E, et al: The pathologist's view point. Part I—Indolent lymphomas. *Haematologica* 85:1291, 2000.
10. Pileri SA, Ascani S, Sabattini E, et al: The pathologist's view point. Part II—Aggressive lymphomas. *Haematologica* 85:1308, 2000.
11. Alizadeh AA, Eisen MB, Davis RE, et al: Distinct types of diffuse large B-cell lymphoma identified by gene expression profiling. *Nature* 403:503, 2000.
12. Rosenwald A, Alizadeh AA, Widhopf G, et al: Relation of gene expression phenotype to immunoglobulin mutation genotype in B cell chronic lymphocytic leukemia. *J Exp Med* 194:1639, 2001.
13. Davis RE, Staudt LM: Molecular diagnosis of lymphoid malignancies by gene expression profiling. *Curr Opin Hematol* 9:333, 2002.
14. Pileri SA, Ascani S, Leoncini L, et al: Hodgkin's lymphoma: The pathologist's viewpoint. *J Clin Pathol* 55:162, 2002.
15. Copur MS, Ledakis P, Bolton M: Molecular profiling of lymphoma. *N Engl J Med* 347:1376, 2002.
16. Lossos IS, Czerwinski DK, Alizadeh AA, et al: Prediction of survival in diffuse large-B-cell lymphoma based on the expression of six genes. *N Engl J Med* 350:1828, 2004.
17. Ramaswamy S: Translating cancer genomics into clinical oncology. *N Engl J Med* 350:1814, 2004.
18. Stone MJ: Waldenström's macroglobulinemia: Hyperviscosity syndrome and cryoglobulinemia. *Clin Lymphoma Myeloma* 9:97, 2009.
19. Decaux O, Laurat E, Perlat A, et al: Systemic manifestations of monoclonal gammopathy. *Eur J Intern Med* 20:457, 2009.
20. Silberman J, Lonial S: Review of peripheral neuropathy in plasma cell disorders. *Hematol Oncol* 26:55, 2008.
21. Lee CH, Mamelak AJ, Vonderheid EC: Erythrodermic cutaneous T cell lymphoma with hypereosinophilic syndrome: Treatment with interferon alfa and extracorporeal photopheresis. *Int J Dermatol* 46:1198, 2007.
22. Roodman GD: Pathogenesis of myeloma bone disease. *Leukemia* 23:435, 2009.
23. Gupta R, Neal JM: Hypercalcemia due to vitamin D-secreting Hodgkin's lymphoma exacerbated by oral calcium supplementation. *Endocr Pract* 12:227, 2006.
24. Johnson RW, Wasner G, Saddier P, Baron R: Herpes zoster and postherpetic neuralgia: Optimizing management in the elderly patient. *Drugs Aging* 25:991, 2008.
25. Hiramanek N: Itch: A symptom of occult disease. *Aust Fam Physician* 33:495, 2004.
26. Tiu RV, Mountantonakis SE, Dunbar AJ, Schreiber MJ Jr: Tumor lysis syndrome. *Semin Thromb Hemost* 33:397, 2007.
27. Cheson BD: Etiology and management of tumor lysis syndrome in patients with chronic lymphocytic leukemia. *Clin Adv Hematol Oncol* 7:263, 2009.
28. Tosi P, Barosi G, Lazzaro C, et al: Consensus conference on the management of tumor lysis syndrome. *Haematologica* 93:1877, 2008.
29. Cammalleri L, Malaguarnera M: Rasburicase represents a new tool for hyperuricemia in tumor lysis syndrome and in gout. *Int J Med Sci* 4:83, 2007.
30. Roodman GD: Mechanisms of bone lesions in multiple myeloma and lymphoma. *Cancer* 80:1557, 1997.
31. Lansigan F, Choi J, Foss FM: Cutaneous T-cell lymphoma. *Hematol Oncol Clin North Am* 22:979, 2008.
32. Chuang SS, Hsieh YC, Ye H, Hwang WS: Lymphohistiocytic anaplastic large cell lymphoma involving skin: A diagnostic challenge. *Pathol Res Pract* 205:283, 2009.
33. Hwang ST, Janik JE, Jaffe ES, Wilson WH: Mycosis fungoides and Sézary syndrome. *Lancet* 371:945, 2008.
34. Iannitto E, Ferreri AJ, Minardi V, et al: Angioimmunoblastic T-cell lymphoma. *Crit Rev Oncol Hematol* 68:264, 2008.
35. Willemze R, Jansen PM, Cerroni L, et al: Subcutaneous panniculitis-like T-cell lymphoma: Definition, classification, and prognostic factors: An EORTC Cutaneous Lymphoma Group Study of 83 cases. *Blood* 111:838, 2008.
36. Zettl A, deLeeuw R, Haralambieva E, Mueller-Hermelink HK: Enteropathy-type T-cell lymphoma. *Am J Clin Pathol* 127:701, 2007.
37. Minauchi K, Nishio M, Itoh T, et al: Hepatosplenic alpha/beta T cell lymphoma presenting with cold agglutinin disease. *Ann Hematol* 86:155, 2007.
38. Rosh JR, Gross T, Mamula P, et al: Hepatosplenic T-cell lymphoma in adolescents and young adults with Crohn's disease: A cautionary tale? *Inflamm Bowel Dis* 13:1024, 2007.
39. Beyer M, Steinhoff M, Anagnostopoulos I, et al: Hepatosplenic T-cell lymphomas and therapy with TNF-alpha-blocking biologics: A risk for psoriasis patients? *J Dtsch Dermatol Ges* 7:191, 2009.
40. Nguyen JT, Condron MR, Nguyen ND, et al: Anaplastic large cell lymphoma in leukemic phase: Extraordinarily high white blood cell count. *Pathol Int* 59:345, 2009.
41. Wu L, Wang Y, Fu SL, et al: Anaplastic large cell lymphoma with primary involvement of skeletal muscle: A rare case report and review of the literature. *Pediatr Hematol Oncol* 26:142, 2009.
42. Muzzafar T, Wei EX, Lin P, et al: Flow cytometric immunophenotyping of anaplastic large cell lymphoma. *Arch Pathol Lab Med* 133:49, 2009.
43. Martin JM, Ricart JM, Monteagudo C, et al: Primary cutaneous CD30+ anaplastic large-cell lymphomas mimicking keratoacanthomas. *Clin Exp Dermatol* 32:668, 2007.
44. Yamane N, Kato N, Nishimura M, et al: Primary cutaneous CD30+ anaplastic large-cell lymphoma with generalized skin involvement and involvement of one peripheral lymph node, successfully treated with low-dose oral etoposide. *Clin Exp Dermatol* 34: E56, 2009.
45. Chang BH, Stork L, Fan G: A unique case of adolescent CD56-negative extranodal NK/T-cell lymphoma, nasal type. *Pediatr Dev Pathol* 11:50, 2008.
46. Zhang YC, Sha Z, Yu JB, et al: Gastric involvement of extranodal NK/T-cell lymphoma, nasal type: A report of 3 cases with literature review. *Int J Surg Pathol* 16:450, 2008.

CHAPTER 93
ACUTE LYMPHOBLASTIC LEUKEMIA

Ching-Hon Pui

SUMMARY

Acute lymphoblastic leukemia (ALL) is a malignant disorder that originates in a single B- or T-lymphocyte progenitor. Proliferation and accumulation of blast cells in the marrow result in suppression of hematopoiesis and, thereafter, anemia, thrombocytopenia, and neutropenia. Lymphoblasts can accumulate in various extramedullary sites, especially the meninges, gonads, thymus, liver, spleen, and lymph nodes. The disease is most common in children but can be seen in individuals of any age. ALL has many subtypes and can be classified by immunologic, cytogenetic, and molecular genetic methods. These methods can identify biologic subtypes, requiring treatment approaches that differ in their use of specific drugs or drug combinations, dosages of drug, or duration of treatment required to achieve optimal results. For example, cases of childhood ALL having a hyperdiploid karyotype respond well to extended treatment with methotrexate and mercaptopurine, whereas cases with Philadelphia chromosome and *BCR-ABL1* fusion benefit from intensive treatment that includes tyrosine kinase inhibitor and transplantation of allogeneic hematopoietic stem cells in adults. The relative lack of therapeutic success in adult ALL is partly related to a high frequency of cases having unfavorable genetic abnormalities and partly related to poor tolerance to intensive treatment. Nearly 90 percent of children and 40 percent of adults can expect long-term, leukemia-free survival–and probable cure–with contemporary treatment. Currently, emphasis is placed not only on improving the cure rate but also on improving quality of life by preventing acute and late treatment-related complications, such as second malignancies, cardiotoxicity, and endocrinopathy.

DEFINITION AND HISTORY

Acute lymphoblastic leukemia (ALL) is a neoplastic disease that results from multistep somatic mutations in a single lymphoid progenitor cell at one of several discrete stages of development. The immunophenotype of leukemic cells at diagnosis reflects the level of differentiation achieved by the dominant clone. The clonal origin of ALL has been established by cytogenetic analysis, by analysis of restriction fragments in female patients who are heterozygous for polymorphic X chromosome-linked genes, and by analysis of rearrangements of T-cell receptor or immunoglobulin genes.[1] Leukemic cells divide more slowly and require more time to synthesize DNA than do normal hematopoietic counterparts.[2] However, leukemic cells accumulate relentlessly because of their altered response to growth and death signals.[3,4] They compete successfully with normal hematopoietic cells, resulting in anemia, thrombocytopenia, and neutropenia. At diagnosis, leukemic cells not only have replaced normal marrow cells but also have disseminated to various extramedullary sites.

Acronyms and abbreviations that appear in this chapter include: ALL, acute lymphoblastic leukemia; *ATM*, ataxia-telangiectasia mutated gene; CD, cluster of differentiation; CNAs, copy number abnormalities; CNS, central nervous system; CSF, cerebrospinal fluid; EFS, event-free survival; HLA, human leukocyte antigen; Ig, immunoglobulin; RB, retinoblastoma protein; RT-PCR, reverse transcriptase polymerase chain reaction; SEER, Surveillance, Epidemiology, and End Results.

Velpeau[5] is generally credited with the earliest report of leukemia in 1827. Virchow,[6] Bennett,[7] and Craigie[8] recognized the condition as a distinct entity by 1845. In 1847, Virchow coined the term *leukemia*, applying it to two distinct types of the disease—splenic and lymphatic—that could be distinguished from each other based on splenomegaly and enlarged lymph nodes and on the morphologic similarities of the leukemic cells to those normally found in these organs.[9] Ehrlich's introduction of staining methods in 1891 allowed further distinction of leukemia subtypes.[10] Splenic and myelogenous leukemias soon were recognized as the same disease. By 1913, leukemia could be classified as acute or chronic, and as lymphatic or myelogenous.[11] The greater prevalence of ALL in children, especially those ages 1 to 5 years, was recognized in 1917.[12]

Shortly after leukemia was recognized as a discrete disease entity, physicians began using chemicals as palliative therapy. The first advance was the use of a 4-amino analogue of folic acid (aminopterin), prompted by Farber's observation that folic acid might have accelerated the proliferation of leukemic cells. Strikingly, for the first time, complete clinical and hematologic remissions that lasted for several months were seen in children.[13] A year after the report of aminopterin-induced clinical remissions, a newly isolated adrenocorticotrophic hormone was reported to induce prompt, though brief, remissions in patients with leukemia.[14] Almost concurrently, Elion and colleagues[15] synthesized antimetabolites that interfere with synthesis of purine and pyrimidine. Their findings led to the introduction of mercaptopurine, 6-thioguanine, and allopurinol into clinical use. From 1950 to 1960, many new antileukemic agents and occasional cures were introduced. Pinkel and colleagues at St. Jude Children's Research Hospital, in 1962, devised a "total therapy" approach, consisting of four treatment phases: remission induction; intensification or consolidation; therapy for subclinical central nervous system (CNS) leukemia (or preventive meningeal treatment); and prolonged continuation therapy. By the early 1970s, as many as 50 percent of children could enjoy long-term event-free survival (EFS) by this innovative strategy.[16] During the same period, a better understanding of the genetics of human histocompatibility and wider use of human leukocyte antigen (HLA) typing culminated in the successful use of hematopoietic stem cell transplantation for treatment of patients in whom leukemia relapsed.[17] In the early 1980s, Riehm and his coworkers introduced a so-called reinduction or delayed intensification treatment during early continuation therapy, consisting mainly of repetition of the initial remission induction and early intensification phases, and further improved the EFS to approximately 70 percent.[18] Parallel to the advance in treatment is the improved understanding of the biology of ALL. The recognition of ALL as a heterogeneous group of diseases—clinically, immunologically, and genetically[19,20]—set the stage for risk-directed therapy.

Treatment of ALL has progressed incrementally, beginning with the development of effective therapy for CNS disease, followed by intensification of early treatment, especially for patients at high risk of relapse. The current cure rates of nearly 90 percent for children (Fig. 93–1) and 40 percent for adults attest to the steady progress made in treating this disease.[21] Rapid evolution and convergence of multiple genome-wide platforms to identify the total complement of genetic and epigenetic alterations almost certainly will lead to the identification of new targets for specific treatment.[22] A clear precedent is the development of imatinib mesylate, which targets leukemias with the *BCR-ABL1* fusion.[23]

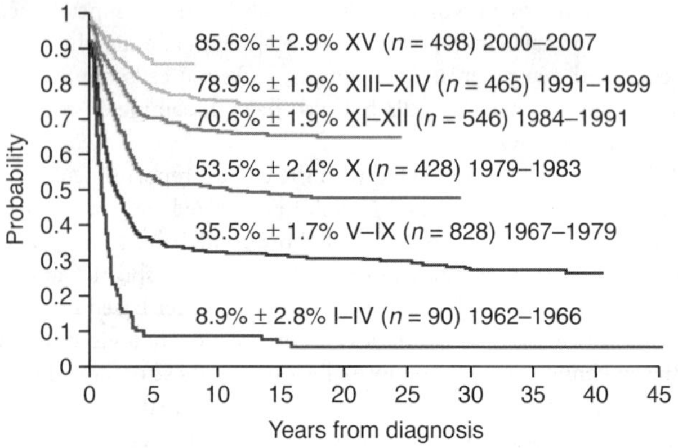

FIGURE 93–1. Kaplan-Meier analysis of event-free survival for 2855 children with ALL treated in 15 consecutive total-therapy studies at St. Jude Children's Research Hospital. Early intensification of systemic and intrathecal chemotherapy with a risk assignment based on sequential measurements of minimal residual disease in the 2000s has boosted the event-free survival estimate to 85.6% ± 2.9% (SE). *(From CH Pui, unpublished data.)*

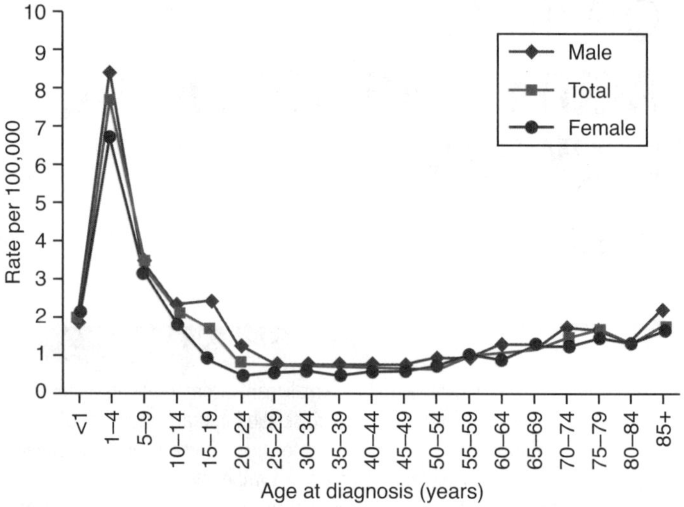

FIGURE 93–2. Age-specific incidence rates for ALL by sex. *(From SEER data, 2001–2005.[22])*

ETIOLOGY AND PATHOGENESIS

Initiation and progression of ALL are driven by successive mutations that alter cellular functions, including an enhanced ability of self-renewal, a subversion of control of normal proliferation, a block in differentiation, and an increased resistance to death signals (apoptosis).[3,4] Environmental agents, such as ionizing radiation and chemical mutagens, have been implicated in the induction of ALL in some patients. However, in most cases, no etiologic factors are discernible. In the favored theory, leukemogenesis reflects the interaction between host pharmacogenetics (susceptibility) and environmental factors, a model that requires confirmation in well-designed population and molecular epidemiologic studies.

INCIDENCE

The age-adjusted incidence rate of ALL was 1.6 per 100,000 men and women per year in the United States, based on cases diagnosed in 2001 to 2005 from 17 Surveillance, Epidemiology, and End Results (SEER) geographic areas.[24] It is estimated that 5430 cases (3220 males and 2210 females) were diagnosed with ALL in 2008 in the United States.[23] This number represents approximately 12 percent of all cases of leukemias. The median age at diagnosis for ALL is 13 years and approximately 61 percent are diagnosed before the age of 20 years.[24] ALL is the most common malignancy diagnosed in patients younger than age 15 years, accounting for 23 percent of all cancers and 76 percent of all leukemias in this age group. Only 20 percent of adult acute leukemias are ALL. Age-specific incidence patterns are characterized by a peak between the ages of 2 and 4 years, followed by falling rates during later childhood, adolescence, and young adulthood (Fig. 93–2).[24] Incidence rises again in the sixth decade and reaches a second, smaller peak in the elderly. The sharp incidence peak of ALL during early childhood has been observed only since the 1930s in the United Kingdom and the United States.[25] In the United States, the peak first appeared in children of European descent, and subsequently was seen in children of African descent in the 1960s. The age peak is absent in many developing or underdeveloped countries, suggesting a leukemogenic contribution from factors associated with industrialization. Except for a slight predominance for females in infancy, ALL affects males of European descent more often than females in all age groups (Fig. 93–2). The frequency distribution is similar among those of African descent.[24] In most age groups, the incidence of ALL is higher in those of European descent than in those of African descent, especially among children age 2 to 3 years.

The incidence of ALL differs substantially in different geographic areas. Rates are higher among populations in northern and western Europe, North America, and Oceania, with lower rates in Asian and African populations.[26] In Europe, the highest rates of ALL among males are found in Spain and the highest rates among females in Denmark. In the United States, the highest rates for both sexes are among Latinos in Los Angeles.

RISK FACTORS

Genetic Syndromes

The precise pathogenetic events leading to the development of ALL are unknown. Only a minority (5%) of cases are associated with inherited, predisposing genetic syndromes. Children with Down syndrome have a 10 to 30 times greater risk of leukemia; acute megakaryoblastic leukemia predominates in patients younger than age 3 years, and ALL is predominant in older age groups. ALL in patients with Down syndrome is a heterogeneous disorder, comprising subtypes with the well-recognized genetic abnormalities found in the general population, such as hyperdiploidy greater than 50 and t(12;21)[*ETV6-RUNX1*], and those more commonly associated with Down syndrome such as +X, del(9) and *CEBPD* rearrangement.[27] Recent studies showed that *P2RY8-CRLF2* fusion and activating *JAK* mutations together contribute to leukemogenesis in approximately half of the cases of Down syndrome patients with ALL.[28,28a] Autosomal recessive genetic diseases associated with increased chromosomal fragility and a predisposition to ALL include ataxia-telangiectasia, Nijmegen breakage syndrome, and Bloom syndrome.[29] Patients with ataxia-telangiectasia have a 70 times greater risk of leukemia and a 250 times greater risk of lymphoma, particularly of the T-cell phenotype.[30] The causative gene, termed *ATM* (ataxia-telangiectasia mutated), encodes a protein involved in DNA repair, regulation of cell proliferation, and apoptosis. Laboratory studies supporting the diagnosis of ataxia-telangiectasia include an elevated serum concentration of α-fetoprotein, presence of characteristic chromosomal aberrations, absent or reduced intranuclear serine protein kinase ATM, and increased *in vitro* radiosensitivity.[31] A high prevalence of germ-line truncating and missense *ATM* gene alterations in children with sporadic T-cell ALL suggests a pathogenetic role of *ATM* in lymphoid malignancies.[30]

Although impaired immune surveillance contributes to the increased risk of Epstein-Barr virus-related malignancies in patients with acquired immunodeficiencies, no compelling evidence indicates defective immunity contributes to the predisposition to ALL in patients with ataxia-telangiectasia or other congenital immunodeficiency syndromes.

Environmental Factors

In utero (but not postnatal) exposure to diagnostic x-rays confers a slightly increased risk of ALL, which correlates positively with the number of exposures.[32] The evidence is weak for an association between the development of ALL and nuclear fallout; exposure to occupational, natural terrestrial, or cosmic ionizing radiation exposure; or paternal radiation exposure prior to conception. There has been concern that exposure to low-energy electromagnetic fields produced by a residential power supply may be associated with the development of childhood ALL. Case-control studies suggested a slightly increased risk of leukemia at very high levels of exposure; assuming the association is real, only approximately 1 percent of leukemias could be attributed to the exposure.[33] Pesticide exposure (occupational or home use) and parental cigarette smoking before or during pregnancy, administration of vitamin K to neonates, maternal alcohol consumption during pregnancy, and increased consumption of dietary nitrites have each been suggested causes. However, each of these associations is controversial, and most have been refuted after careful, controlled investigation. High birth weight has been associated with an increased risk of leukemia before the age of 5 years with fair consistency,[34] and the birth weight is likely a marker for an endogenous factor, such as insulin-like growth factor.

Host Pharmacogenetics

Subtle genetic polymorphisms of xenobiotic-metabolizing enzymes, DNA repair pathways, and cell-cycle checkpoint functions might interact with environmental, dietary, maternal, and other external factors to affect the development of ALL.[4] Although the number of investigations and sample sizes are limited, data exist to support a causal role for polymorphisms in genes encoding detoxifying enzymes (e.g., glutathione *S*-transferase, NAD(P)H:quinone oxidoreductase), folate-metabolizing enzymes (serine hydroxymethyltransferase and thymidylate synthase), cytochrome P450, methylenetetrahydrofolate reductase, and cell-cycle inhibitors in the development of adult and childhood ALL.[35–39] However, all these associations must be confirmed by larger studies with careful attention to ethnic and geographic diversity in the frequency of polymorphisms. Using genome-wide analysis, germline single-nucleotide polymorphisms (SNPs) of *ARID5B* gene have been associated with childhood hyperdiploid B-cell precursor ALL,[39a] a clear example of host genetic variations affecting the susceptibility to the development of childhood ALL.

Development of ALL **in Utero**

Retrospective identification of leukemia-specific fusion genes (e.g., *MLL-AF4, ETV6-RUNX1* [also known as *TEL-AML1*]), hyperdiploidy, or clonotypic rearrangements of immunoglobulin or T-cell receptor loci in the archived neonatal blood spots (Guthrie cards), and development of concordant leukemia in identical twins indicate clearly some leukemias have a prenatal origin.[40,41] In identical twins with the t(4;11)/*MLL-AF4*, the concordance rate is nearly 100 percent, and the latency period is short (a few weeks to a few months). These findings suggest this fusion gene alone either is leukemogenic or requires only a small number of cooperative mutations to cause leukemia. By contrast, the lower concordance rate in twins with the *ETV6-RUNX1* fusion or T-cell phenotype and the longer postnatal latency period suggest additional postnatal events are required for leukemic transformation in this subtype.[40] This theory is supported by the identification of rare cells expressing *ETV6-RUNX1* fusion transcripts in approximately 1 percent of cord blood samples from newborns, a frequency 100 times higher than the incidence of ALL defined by this fusion transcript.[40] A recent study further established the presence of a preleukemic clone with the *ETV6-RUNX1*.[42] Hyperdiploid ALL, another common subtype of childhood ALL, also appears to arise before birth but requires postnatal events for full malignant transformation.[41] The observations of a peak age of development of childhood ALL of 2 to 5 years, an association of industrialization and modern or affluent societies with increased prevalence of ALL, and the occasional clustering of childhood leukemia cases have fueled two parallel infection-based hypotheses to account for postnatal events. The "delayed-infection" hypothesis suggests that some susceptible individuals with a prenatally acquired preleukemic clone had low or no exposure to common infections early in life because they lived in an affluent hygienic environments.[40] Such infectious insulation predisposes the immune system of these individuals to aberrant or pathologic responses after subsequent or delayed exposure to common infections at an age commensurate with increased lymphoid cell proliferation. The "population-mixing" hypothesis predicts that clusters of childhood ALL result from exposure of susceptible (nonimmune) individuals to common but fairly nonpathologic infections after population mixing with carriers.[43] However, clearly not all childhood cases develop *in utero*. For example, t(1;19)/*E2A-PBX1* (also known as *TCF3-PBX1*) ALL appears to have a postnatal origin in most cases.[44] Cases of adult ALL most certainly arise over a protracted time.

■ ACQUIRED GENETIC CHANGES

Acquired genetic abnormalities are a hallmark of ALL, and more than three-fourths of all cases have recurring cytogenetic or molecular lesions with prognostic and therapeutic relevance (Table 93–1).[4]

TABLE 93–1. Frequencies of Common Genetic Aberrations in Childhood and Adult Acute Lymphoblastic Leukemia

Abnormality	Children (%)	Adults (%)
Hyperdiploidy (>50 chromosomes)	23–29	6–7
Hypodiploidy (<45 chromosomes)	1	2
t(1;19)(q23;p13.3) [*TCF3-PBX1*]	4 in white, 12 in black	2–3
t(9;22)(q34;q11.2) [*BCR-ABL1*]	2–3	25–30
t(4;11)(q21;q23) [*MLL-AF4*]	2	3–7
t(8;14)(q23;q32.3)	2	4
t(12;21)(p13;q22) [*ETV6-RUNX1*]	20–25	0–3
NOTCH1 mutations*	7	15
HOX11L2 overexpression*	20	13
LYL1 overexpression*	9	15
TAL1 overexpression*	15	3
HOX11 overexpression*	7	30
MLL-ENL fusion	2	3
Abnormal 9p	7–11	6–30
Abnormal 12p	7–9	4–6
del(7p)/del(7q)/monosomy 7	4	6–11
+8	2	10–12
Intrachromosomal amplification of chromosome 21 (iAMP21)	2	?

*Abnormalities found in T-cell ALL.

Chromosomal changes include abnormalities in the number (ploidy) and structure of chromosomes. The latter comprise translocations (the most frequent abnormality), inversions, deletions, point mutations, and amplifications. Although the frequency of particular genetic subtypes differs between childhood and adult cases, the general mechanisms underlying the induction are similar. Mechanisms include aberrant expression of oncoproteins and chromosomal translocations that generate fusion genes encoding transcription factors or active kinases.

Primary genetic rearrangement by itself is insufficient to induce overt leukemia. Cooperative mutations are necessary for leukemic transformation and include genetic and epigenetic changes in key growth regulatory pathways. Earlier searches for cooperating lesions focused on specific genes and used relatively low-resolution approaches. The candidate gene approach has identified deletion of the *CDKN2A/CDKN2B* tumor-suppressor locus[45] and mutations of *NOTCH1* in T-cell ALL.[46] Current searches applying genome-wide microarray and high-throughput sequencing methodologies have identified a high frequency of common genetic alterations in both B-cell precursor ALL and T-cell ALL. Using SNP microarray, a mean of 6.46 DNA copy number abnormalities (CNAs) per case was identified, suggesting that gross genomic instability is not a feature for most ALL cases.[47] There was a wide variation in the number of CNAs across leukemic subtypes. Interestingly, infant ALL cases with *MLL* rearrangement had less than 1 CNA per case, suggesting that few additional genetic lesions are required for leukemogenesis in these cases. By contrast, *ETV6-RUNX1* and *BCR-ABL1* cases had more than 6 CNAs per case, with some having more than 20 lesions, a finding consistent with the concept that the initiating events occur early in childhood and additional lesions are required for subsequent development of ALL. Strikingly, in one study, more than 40 percent of B-cell precursor ALL cases had mutations in genes encoding regulators of normal lymphoid development. The most frequent target was the lymphoid transcription factor *PAX5* (mutated in approximately 30% of cases), which encode a paired-domain protein required for the pro–B-cell to pre–B-cell transition and B-lineage fidelity. The second most frequently involved gene was *IKZF1* (mutated in almost 30% of the cases), encoding the IKAROS zinc finger DNA-binding protein that is required for the earliest lymphoid differentiation. *IKZF1* was deleted in the vast majority of cases of *BCR-ABL1* ALL cases and chronic myeloid leukemia in lymphoid blast crisis (but not chronic phase).[48] Approximately half of *BCR-ABL1* ALL cases and chronic myeloid leukemia also had deletions of *CDKN2A/B* and *PAX5*. This finding further supports the concept that multiple signaling pathways need to be disrupted to induce leukemia. A subgroup of ALL with very poor outcome was strongly associated with the presence of *IKZF1* deletions.[49,50] Together, these findings suggest that *IKZF1* directly contributes to treatment resistance in ALL.

Gene expression profiling with DNA microarrays allows nearly all T-cell cases to be grouped according to multistep oncogenic pathways.[51] Gene expression studies also show that overexpression of FLT3, a receptor tyrosine kinase important for development of hematopoietic stem cells, is a secondary event in almost all cases with either *MLL* rearrangements or hyperdiploidy.[52–54] The finding has provided an impetus for clinical testing of FLT3 inhibitors in ALL. Other genome-wide interrogations of both leukemic cells and germ-line genetic variation have identified other genetic variations with prognostic or therapeutic relevance and may lead to the development of specific treatment.[55–57]

Epigenetic changes, including hypermethylation of tumor-suppressor genes and hypomethylation of oncogenes and abnormalities in posttranscriptional control mechanisms, such as those involving microRNA, are common findings in cancer. These changes are reversible and do not alter the DNA sequence, yet they can alter gene expression in subtle ways that encourage malignant transformation and progression. The analysis of epigenetic alterations has begun to apply to the development of new biomarkers for risk assignment or disease monitoring, and to the design of alternative treatment in ALL.[58] Evidence indicates that the methylation of multiple genes in ALL is associated with a worse outcome. Surprisingly, methylation of genes was as prominent in childhood as in adult ALL. The differences in the response of children and adults appears not to be related to quantitative methylation but to the specific genes and the specific pathways deactivated. Preliminary studies of hypomethylating agents (e.g., 5-azacytidine and decitabine) are being tested in patients refractory or resistant to current drug programs.[58]

CLINICAL FEATURES

SIGNS AND SYMPTOMS

The clinical presentation of ALL varies. Symptoms may appear insidiously or acutely. The presenting features generally reflect the degree of marrow failure and the extent of extramedullary spread (Table 93–2).[60–64] Approximately half of patients present with fever, which often is induced by pyrogenic cytokines (e.g., interleukin-1, interleukin-6, and tumor

TABLE 93–2. Presenting Clinical Features in Children and Adults with Acute Lymphoblastic Leukemia

Feature	Children	Adult
Age (years)		
<1	2	–
1–9	72–78	–
10–19	20–26	–
20–39	–	55
40–59	–	36
≥60	–	9
Male	56–57	62
Symptoms		
Fever	57	33–56
Fatigue	50	?
Bleeding	43	33
Bone or joint pain	25	25
Lymphadenopathy		
None	30	51
Marked (>3 cm)	15	11
Hepatomegaly		
None	34	65
Marked (below umbilicus)	17	?
Splenomegaly		
None	41	56
Marked (below umbilicus)	17	?
Mediastinal mass	8–10	15
CNS leukemia	3	8
Testicular leukemia	1	0.3

NOTE: Data are expressed as a percent of adult or childhood cases.

SOURCE: Data presented in Pui CH[60] and Möricke A, Reiter A, Zimmermann M, et al,[61] for childhood ALL; and in Chessells JM, Hall E, Prentice HG, et al,[62] Hoelzer DF,[63] and Larson RA, Dodge RK, Burns CP, et al,[64] for adult ALL.

necrosis factor) released from leukemic cells.[65] In these patients, fever resolves within 72 hours after the start of antileukemic therapy.

Fatigue and lethargy are common manifestations of anemia in patients with ALL. In older patients, anemia-related dyspnea, angina, and dizziness may be the dominant presenting features.[63] More than 25 percent of patients, especially young children, may have a limp, bone pain, arthralgia, or an unwillingness to walk because of leukemic infiltration of the periosteum, bone, or joint or because of expansion of the marrow cavity by leukemic cells. Children with prominent bone pain often have nearly normal blood counts, which can contribute to delayed diagnosis. In a small proportion of patients, marrow necrosis can result in severe bone pain and tenderness, fever, and a very high level of serum lactate dehydrogenase.[66] Arthralgia and bone pain are less severe in adults. Less common signs and symptoms include headache, vomiting, altered mental function, oliguria, and anuria. Occasionally, patients present with a life-threatening infection or bleeding (e.g., intracranial hematoma). In the experience at St. Jude Children's Research Hospital, intracranial hemorrhage occurs mainly in patients with an initial leukocyte count greater than 400×10^9/L.[67] Very rarely, ALL produces no signs or symptoms and is detected during routine examination.

PHYSICAL FINDINGS

Among the frequently evident findings are pallor, petechiae, and ecchymosis in the skin and mucous membranes, and bone tenderness as a result of leukemic infiltration or hemorrhage that stretches the periosteum. Liver, spleen, and lymph nodes are the most common sites of extramedullary involvement, and the degree of organomegaly is more pronounced in children than in adults. An anterior mediastinal (thymic) mass is present in 8 to 10 percent of childhood cases and in 15 percent of adult cases (Fig. 93–3). A bulky, anterior mediastinal mass can compress the great vessels and trachea and possibly lead to the superior vena cava syndrome or the superior mediastinal syndrome. Patients with this syndrome present with cough, dyspnea, orthopnea, dysphagia, stridor, cyanosis, facial edema, increased intracranial pressure, and sometimes syncope. Patients who present with orthopnea, upper-body edema, great vessel compression and mainstem bronchus compression are at risk of anesthesia-related complications.[68]

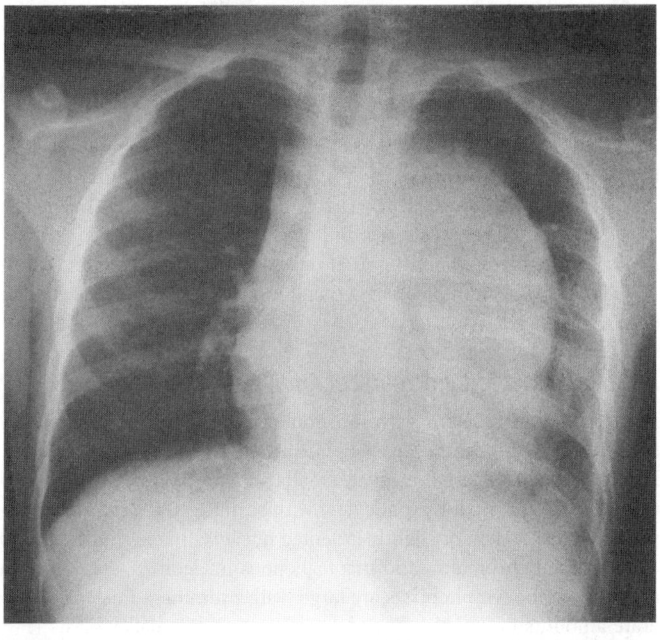

FIGURE 93–3. Chest radiograph of a 12-year-old black male with T-cell ALL and an anterior mediastinal mass.

Painless enlargement of the scrotum can be a sign of testicular leukemia-cell infiltration or hydrocele, the latter resulting from lymphatic obstruction. Both conditions can be readily diagnosed by ultrasonography. Overt testicular disease is relatively rare, generally seen in infants or adolescents with T-cell leukemia and/or hyperleukocytosis, and does not require radiation therapy.[69] Other uncommon presenting features include ocular involvement (leukemic infiltration of the orbit, optic nerve, retina, iris, cornea, or conjunctiva), subcutaneous nodules (leukemia cutis), enlarged salivary glands (Mikulicz syndrome), cranial nerve palsy, and priapism (resulting from leukostasis of the corpora cavernosa and dorsal veins or sacral nerve involvement). Epidural spinal cord compression at presentation is a rare but serious finding that requires immediate treatment to prevent permanent paraparesis or paraplegia. In some pediatric patients, infiltration of tonsils, adenoids, appendix, or mesenteric lymph nodes leads to surgical intervention before leukemia is diagnosed.

LABORATORY FEATURES

Anemia, neutropenia, and thrombocytopenia are common in patients with newly diagnosed ALL. The severity reflects the degree of marrow replacement by leukemic lymphoblasts (Table 93–3).[60–64] Presenting leukocyte counts range widely, from 0.1 to 1500×10^9/L (median: $10–12 \times 10^9$/L). Hyperleukocytosis ($>100 \times 10^9$ white cells/L) occurs in 11 to 13 percent of white children, but occurs more often in black children (23%) and adults (16%) because they are more likely to have T-cell ALL. Profound neutropenia ($<0.5 \times 10^9$/L) is found in 20 to 40 percent of patients, rendering them at high risk for infection. Approximately 90 percent of the patients have circulating leukemic blast cells at diagnosis. Hypereosinophilia, generally reactive, may precede the diagnosis of ALL by several months.[70] Some patients, principally male, have ALL with the t(5;14)(q31;q32) chromosomal abnormality and a hypereosinophilic syndrome (pulmonary infiltration, cardiomegaly, and congestive heart failure). These patients often do not have circulating leukemic blasts or other cytopenias and have a relatively low percentage of blasts in the marrow.[71] Activation of the interleukin-3 gene on chromosome 5 by the enhancer element of the immunoglobulin heavy-chain gene on chromosome 14 is thought to play a central role in leukemogenesis and the associated eosinophilia in these cases.[71] In patients with anemia, a strong inverse relationship exists between the hemoglobin level and age at diagnosis.[62] Occasionally, a child with ALL has a hemoglobin level as low as 1 g/dL.

Decreased platelet counts often are seen at diagnosis (median: 48–52 $\times 10^9$/L). This finding differs from immune thrombocytopenia because the decreased platelet counts almost always are accompanied by anemia, leukocyte abnormalities, or both.[72] Severe bleeding is uncommon, even when platelet counts are as low as 20×10^9/L, provided infection and fever are absent.[73] Occasional patients, principally male, present with thrombocytosis ($>400 \times 10^9$/L).[74] Pancytopenia followed by a period of spontaneous hematopoietic recovery may precede the diagnosis of ALL in rare cases.[75] Coagulopathy, usually mild, can be seen in 3 to 5 percent of patients, most of whom have T-cell ALL, and is only rarely associated with clinical bleeding.[63,76] The level of serum lactate dehydrogenase is increased in most patients with ALL and is well correlated with the size of the leukemic infiltrate.[77] Increased levels of serum uric acid are common in patients with a large leukemic cell burden, a finding that reflects an increased rate of purine catabolism. Patients with massive renal involvement can have increased levels of creatinine, urea nitrogen, uric acid, and phosphorus. Occasionally, patients with T-cell ALL present

TABLE 93–3. Presenting Laboratory Features in Children and Adults with Acute Lymphoblastic Leukemia

Feature	Percent of Total: Children (White/Black)	Percent of Total: Adults
Cell lineage		
T cell	15/24	
B-cell precursor	85/76	
Leukocyte count (× 10^9/L)		
<10	47–49/34	41
10–49	28–31/29	31
50–99	8–12/14	12
>100	11–13/23	16
Hemoglobin concentration (g/dL)		
<8	48/58	28
8–10	24/22	26
>10	28/20	46
Platelet count (× 10^9/L)		
<50	46/40	52
50–100	23/20	22
>100	31/40	26
CNS status*		
CNS1	67–79/60	92–95
CNS2	5–24/27	?
CNS3	3/3	5–8
Traumatic lumbar puncture with blasts	6–7/10	?
Leukemic blasts in marrow (%)		
<90	33/46	29
>90	67/54	71
Leukemic blasts in blood		
Present	87/90	92
Absent	13/10	8

*CNS-1: no blast cells in cerebrospinal fluid sample; CNS-2: <5 leukocytes/μL with blast cells in an atraumatic sample; CNS-3: ≥5 leukocytes/μL with blast cells in an atraumatic sample or the presence of a cranial nerve palsy; and traumatic lumbar puncture with blasts (≥10 erythrocytes/μL with blasts). Data on CNS2 and traumatic lumbar puncture with blasts not available in adults.

SOURCE: Data presented in Pui CH[60] and Möricke A, Reiter A, Zimmermann M, et al[61] for childhood ALL; and in Chessells JM, Hall E, Prentice HG, et al,[62] Hoelzer DF,[63] and Larson RA, Dodge RK, Burns CP, et al,[64] for adult ALL.

with acute renal failure, despite a relatively small leukemic infiltrate.[78] Rarely, patients present with hypercalcemia resulting from release of parathyroid hormone-like protein from lymphoblasts and leukemic infiltration of bone. The t(17;19)(q22;p13.3) with *E2A-HLF* fusion, found in 0.5 percent of B-cell precursor ALL, is typically associated with adolescent age group, disseminated coagulopathy, hypercalcemia, and dismal prognosis.[79] Liver dysfunction as a result of leukemic infiltration occurs in 10 to 20 percent of patients, usually is mild, and has no important clinical or prognostic consequences.[59] However, recognition of patients carrying or infected with hepatitis B virus is important because prompt lamivudine therapy can prevent serious complications from the virus reactivation after immunosuppressive treatment.[80] Serum immunoglobulin levels (mostly IgA and IgM classes) are modestly decreased in approximately one-third of children with ALL. The reduction reflects the decreased number and impaired function of normal lymphocytes.[81] Urinalysis may show microscopic hematuria and the presence of uric acid crystals.

Chest radiography is needed to detect enlargement of the thymus or mediastinal nodes, with or without pleural effusion (see Fig. 93–3). Although bony abnormalities, such as metaphyseal banding, periosteal reactions, osteolysis, osteosclerosis, and osteopenia, can be found in 50 percent of patients, especially children with low leukocyte counts at presentation, skeletal roentgenography is not necessary for case management. Spinal roentgenography is useful in patients with suspected vertebral collapse.

Examination of the cerebrospinal fluid (CSF) is an essential diagnostic procedure. Leukemic blasts can be identified in as many as one-third of pediatric patients and approximately 5 percent of adult patients at diagnosis of ALL; most of these patients lack neurologic symptoms.[82] Traditionally, CNS leukemia is defined by the presence of at least 5 leukocytes per microliter of CSF (with leukemic blast cells apparent in a cytocentrifuged sample) or by the presence of cranial nerve palsies. However, with the omission of prophylactic cranial irradiation in contemporary clinical trials, the presence of any leukemic blast cells in the CSF is associated with increased risk of CNS relapse and is an indication to intensify intrathecal therapy.[83] Different opinions exist regarding when the first lumbar puncture should be performed. Many leukemia therapists perform the procedure at diagnosis but do not instill chemotherapeutic agents intrathecally in the event a second diagnostic test is needed to verify the presence of leukemic cells. Others delay the examination because of concern that circulating leukemic cells from the blood will "seed" the CNS. Several studies show that contamination of the CSF by leukemic cells as a result of traumatic lumbar puncture at diagnosis is associated with an inferior treatment outcome in children with ALL.[83–85] In view of this finding, intrathecal therapy is administered with the diagnostic lumbar puncture in all patients with confirmed leukemia (e.g., the presence of circulating leukemic cells) at St. Jude Children's Research Hospital. The risk of traumatic lumbar puncture can be decreased by administering platelet transfusions to thrombocytopenic patients and by having the most experienced clinician perform the procedure after the patient is under deep sedation or general anesthesia.[83,86]

DIAGNOSIS AND CELL CLASSIFICATION

Examination of marrow aspirate is preferable for diagnosis of ALL because as much as 10 percent of patients lack circulating blasts at the time of diagnosis and because marrow cells are better than blood cells for genetic studies. Fibrosis or tightly packed marrow can lead to difficulties with marrow aspiration that necessitate biopsy. In patients with marrow necrosis, multiple marrow aspirations are sometimes needed to obtain diagnostic tissue.

Morphologic and Cytochemical Analysis

Diagnosis of ALL begins with morphologic analysis of Romanowsky-stained (Wright-Giemsa or May-Grünwald-Giemsa) marrow films. Lymphoblasts tend to be relatively small (ranging from the same size to twice the size of small lymphocytes) with scanty, often light-blue cytoplasm; a round, cleft, or slightly indented nucleus; fine to slightly coarse and clumped chromatin; and inconspicuous nucleoli (Fig. 93–4A). In some cases, the lymphoblasts are large, with prominent nucleoli, moderate amounts of cytoplasm, and an admixture of smaller blasts (Fig. 93–4B). Cytoplasmic granules are found in the lymphoblasts of some patients with ALL (Fig. 93–4C). The granules usually are amphophilic

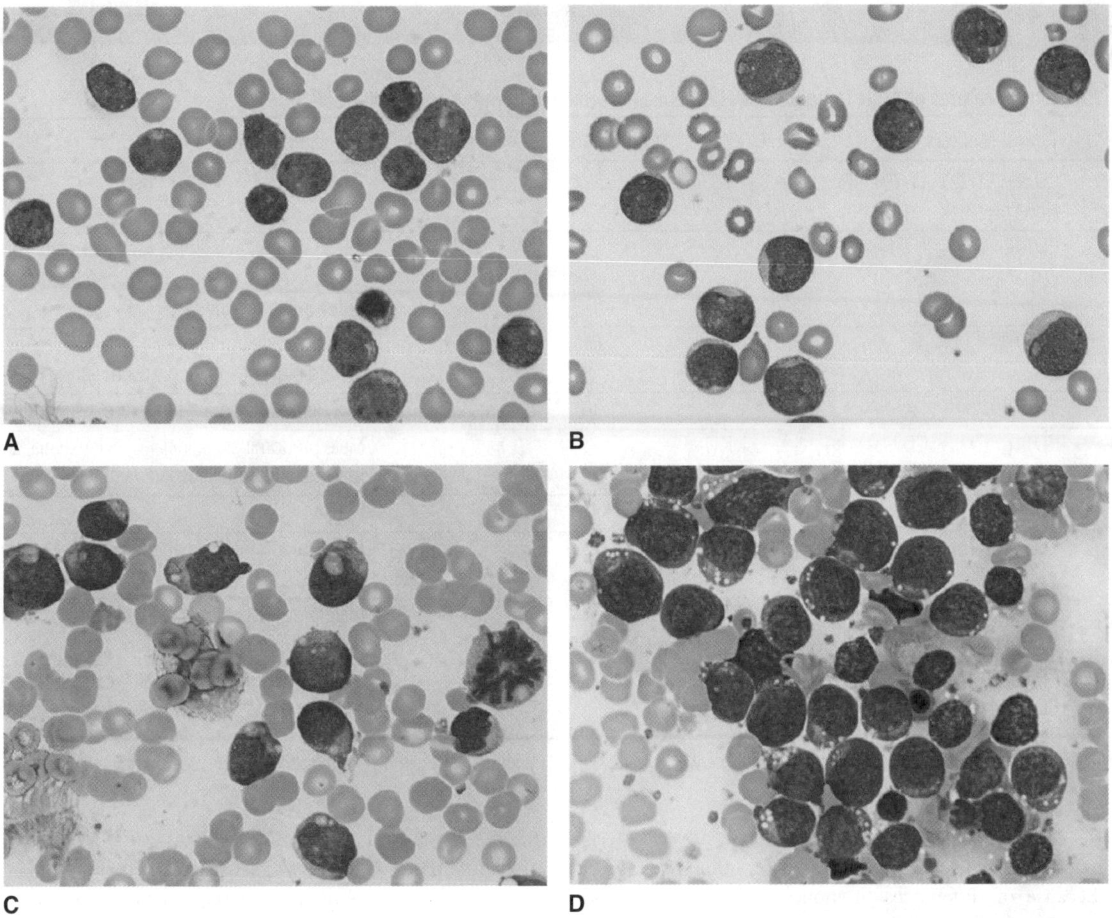

FIGURE 93–4. **A.** Typical lymphoblasts with scanty cytoplasm, regular nuclear shape, fine chromatin, and indistinct nucleoli. **B.** ALL with large blasts showing prominent nucleoli, moderate amounts of cytoplasm, and an admixture of smaller blasts. **C.** ALL with cytoplasmic granules. Fuchsia granules are present in the cytoplasm of many blasts. Such granules may lead to a misdiagnosis of acute myeloid leukemia; however, the granules are negative for myeloperoxidase and myeloid-pattern Sudan black B staining. **D.** B-cell ALL lymphoblasts. The blasts in this phenotype are characterized by intensely basophilic cytoplasm, regular cellular features, and cytoplasmic vacuolation (Images **A–D.** Wright-Giemsa stain; original magnification ×1000).

(which stain fuchsia), readily distinguishable from the primary myeloid granules (which stain deep purple), and demonstrated to be mitochondria in some cases by electron microscopy. B-cell blasts in ALL are characterized by intensely basophilic cytoplasm, regular cellular features, prominent nucleoli, and cytoplasmic vacuolation (Fig. 93–4D).

Analysis of only a Romanowsky-stained film is insufficient to differentiate ALL and acute myeloid leukemia. The cytochemical stains used to discriminate between the two leukemias are the Sudan black stain and the stains for myeloperoxidase and the nonspecific esterases, including α-naphthyl butyrate and α-naphthyl acetate esterase. Stains for these esterases generally do not react with leukemic lymphoblasts. Occasionally, a low level of myeloperoxidase is detected in marrow samples from ALL patients because of the presence of residual normal myeloid precursors.

Immunologic Classification

Because leukemic lymphoblasts lack specific morphologic and cytochemical features, immunophenotyping is an essential part of the diagnostic evaluation. The antibodies that distinguish clusters of differentiation (CD) groups recognize the same cellular antigen but not necessarily the same epitope (see Chap. 15). Most leukocyte antigens lack specificity; hence, a panel of antibodies is needed to establish the diagnosis and to distinguish among the different immunologic subclasses of leukemic cells. The panel used at St. Jude Children's Research Hospital includes antibodies to at least one highly sensitive marker (CD19 for B-cell lineage, CD7 for T-cell lineage, and CD13 or CD33 for myeloid cells) and antibodies to a highly specific marker (cytoplasmic CD79a and CD22 for B-cell lineage, cytoplasmic CD3 for T-cell lineage, and cytoplasmic myeloperoxidase for myeloid cells).[21] These analysis methods enable a firm diagnosis in 99 percent of cases.

Although ALL can be further subclassified according to the recognized steps of normal maturation within the B-cell lineage (pro-B, early pre-B, pre-B, transitional pre-B, and mature B cells) or T-cell lineage (pre-T, mid, and late thymocyte) pathways, the only distinctions of therapeutic importance are those between T-cell, mature B, and other B-cell lineage (B-cell precursor type) immunophenotypes.[21] In some studies, cases of B-cell precursor ALL were subdivided into CD10-positive (common ALL) and CD10-negative (pre-pre-B, pro-B, or CD10-negative B-cell precursor types) leukemias, whereas cases of T-cell lineage ALL were further classified as pre-T (or pro-T) and mature T-cell leukemias.[87,88] Despite their prognostic implications, these refined categories of ALL have not been used in treatment assignment. A distinct subset of T-cell ALL that retain stem cell-like features, termed *early T-cell precursor ALL*, has been identified and associated with a dire prognosis with conventional chemotherapy.[88] Table 93–4 summarizes the salient presenting features of several recognized immunologic subtypes of ALL.

TABLE 93–4. Presenting Features of Acute Lymphoblastic Leukemia According to Immunologic Subtype

Subtype	Typical Markers	Childhood (%)	Adult (%)	Associated Features
B-cell precursor	CD19+, CD22+, CD79a+, cIg±, sIgμ–, HLA-DR+			
Pro-B	CD10–	5	11	Infant or adult age group, high leukocyte count, initial CNS leukemia, pseudodiploidy, *MLL* rearrangement, unfavorable prognosis
Early pre-B	CD10+	63	52	Favorable age group (1–9 years), low leukocyte count, hyperdiploidy (>50 chromosomes)
Pre-B	CD10±, cIg+	16	9	High leukocyte count, black race, pseudodiploidy
B cell	CD19+, CD22+, CD79a+, cIg+, sIgμ+, sIgK+, or sIg+	3	4	Male predominance, initial CNS leukemia, abdominal masses, often renal involvement
T lineage	CD7+, cCD3+			
T cell	CD2+, CD1±, CD4±, CD8±, HLA-DR–, TdT±	10	18	Male predominance, hyperleukocytosis, extramedullary disease
Pre-T	CD2–, CD1–, CD4–, CD8–, HLA-DR±, TdT+	1	6	Male predominance, hyperleukocytosis, extramedullary disease, unfavorable prognosis
Early T-cell precursor	CD1–, CD8–, CD5^{weak}, CD13+, CD33+, CD11b+, CD117+, CD65+, HLA-DR+	2	?	Male predominance, age >10 years, dismal prognosis

cCD3, cytoplasmic CD3; cIg, cytoplasmic immunoglobulin; CNS, central nervous system; sIg, surface immunoglobulin; TdT, terminal deoxynucleotidyl transferase.

Myeloid-associated antigens may be expressed on otherwise typical lymphoblasts. Because of differences in monoclonal antibodies and immunophenotyping techniques, the frequencies of myeloid-associated antigen expression range from 5 to 30 percent in childhood cases and from 10 to 50 percent in adult cases.[64,89] The pattern of myeloid-associated antigen expression is correlated with certain genetic features of blast cells. CD15, CD33, and CD65 are expressed in ALL cases with a rearranged *MLL* gene, and CD13 and CD33 are expressed in cases with the *ETV6-RUNX1*.[89] There is a subset of cases that coexpress both lymphoid and myeloid markers but do not cluster with T-cell, B-cell precursor, or acute myeloid leukemia in gene expression profiling. These cases may not respond to myeloid-directed therapy but attain remission with ALL-directed induction treatment.[90] The presence of myeloid-associated antigens lacks prognostic significance in contemporary treatment programs but can be useful in immunologic monitoring of patients for minimal residual leukemia.[91]

Genetic Classification

ALL arises from a lymphoid progenitor cell having sustained multiple specific genetic damages that lead to malignant transformation and proliferation. Thus, genetic classification of blast cells is expected to yield more relevant biologic information than that obtained by other means. Approximately 75 percent of adult and childhood cases can be readily classified into prognostically or therapeutically relevant subgroups based on the modal chromosome number (or DNA content estimated by flow cytometry), specific chromosomal rearrangements, and molecular genetic changes.[3,4,21,46,92–94] Table 93–5 summarizes the prominent clinical and biologic features of cases with the most common genetic abnormalities.

Two ploidy groups (hyperdiploidy >50 chromosomes and hypodiploidy <44 chromosomes) have clinical relevance. Hyperdiploidy, which is seen in approximately 25 percent of childhood cases and in 6 to 7 percent of adult cases, is associated with a favorable prognosis that may reflect an increased cellular accumulation of methotrexate and its polyglutamates, an increased sensitivity to therapeutic antimetabolites, and a marked propensity of these cells to undergo apoptosis.[95–97] By contrast, hypodiploidy is associated with an exceptionally poor prognosis.[93,94,98] Flow cytometric determination of cellular DNA content is a useful adjunct to cytogenetic analysis because it is automated, rapid, and inexpensive, and its measurements are not affected by the mitotic index of the cell population; results can be obtained in almost all cases. Flow cytometric studies can sometimes identify a small but drug-resistant subpopulation of near-haploid cells that may have been missed by standard cytogenetic analysis.

Phenotype-specific reciprocal translocations are the most biologically and clinically significant karyotypic changes in ALL. Some translocations identified in cases of B-cell and T-cell ALL arise from mistakes in the normal recombination mechanisms that generate antigen receptor genes. Such rearrangements can mobilize the promoter/enhancer element of the immunoglobulin heavy- or light-chain gene or the T-cell antigen receptor β/γ or α/δ gene to sites adjacent to a variety of transcription factor genes. More often, the genetic rearrangements result from the fusions of two genes encoding different transcription factors.[3,4,92–94] These chimeric transcription factors encode active kinases and altered transcription factors that regulate genes involved in the differentiation, self-renewal, proliferation, and drug resistance of hematopoietic stem cells.[3,4]

Specific cytogenetic findings are correlated with presenting clinical features, blast-cell phenotypes, and clinical outcome (see Table 93–5). However, compelling reasons exist to focus on molecular genetic lesions. First, molecular analyses can identify several important submicroscopic genetic alterations not visible by standard karyotyping procedures, such as the *ETV6-RUNX1* fusion, intrachromosomal amplification of chromosome 21, deletions of tumor-suppressor genes, and mutations of protooncogenes.[3,4,92,99,100] Second, cases with clinically important genetic rearrangements can be missed because of technical errors (e.g., karyotyping residual normal metaphase cells rather than leukemic metaphase cells). Hence, fluorescence *in situ* hybridization (FISH) and reverse

TABLE 93–5. Clinical and Biologic Features Associated with the Most Common Genetic Subtypes of Acute Lymphoblastic Leukemia

		Estimated Event-Free Survival (%)	
Subtype	Associated Features	Children	Adults
Hyperdiploidy (>50 chromosomes)	Predominant B-cell precursor phenotype; low leukocyte count; favorable age group (1–9 years) and prognosis in children	80–90 at 5 years	30–50 at 5 years
Hypodiploidy (<45 chromosomes)	Predominant B-cell precursor phenotype; increased leukocyte count; poor prognosis	30–40 at 3 years	10–20 at 3 years
t(12;21)(p13;q22) [*ETV6-RUNX1*]	CD13±/CD33± B-cell precursor phenotype; pseudodiploidy; age 1–9 years; favorable prognosis	90–95 at 5 years	Unknown
t(1;19)(q23;p13.3) [*TCF3-PBX1*]	CD10±/CD20–/CD34– pre-B phenotype; pseudodiploidy; increased leukocyte count; black race; CNS leukemia; prognosis depends on treatment	82–90 at 5 years	20–40 at 3 years
t(9;22)(q34;q11.2) [*BCR-ABL1*]	Predominant B-cell precursor phenotype; older age; increased leukocyte count; improved early outcome with tyrosine kinase inhibitor treatment	80–90 at 3 years	~60 at 1 year
t(4;11)(q21;23) with *MLL-AF4* fusion	CD10±/CD15±/CD33±/CD65± B-cell precursor phenotype; infant and older adult age groups; hyperleukocytosis; CNS leukemia; dismal outcome	32–40 at 5 years	10–20 at 3 years
t(8;14)(q24;q32.3)	B-cell phenotype; L3 morphology; male predominance; bulky extramedullary disease; favorable prognosis with short-term intensive chemotherapy including high-dose methotrexate, cytarabine, and cyclophosphamide	75–85 at 5 years	50–55 at 4 years
NOTCH 1 mutations	T-cell phenotype; favorable prognosis	90 at 5 years	50 at 4 years
HOX11 overexpression	CD10+ T-cell phenotype; favorable prognosis with chemotherapy alone	90 at 5 years	80 at 3 years
Intrachromosomal amplification of chromosome 21	B-cell precursor phenotype; low white blood cell count; intensified treatment required to avert a poor prognosis	30 at 5 years	?

SOURCE: Data presented in Pui CH, Robison LL, Look AT,[4] Möricke A, Reiter A, Zimmermann M, et al,[61] Schultz et al,[212] Yanada et al,[218] Faderl et al,[295] and Mrózek et al.[296]

transcriptase polymerase chain reaction (RT-PCR) assays are used frequently. The application of microarray-based genome-wide analysis of gene expression and DNA copy number, complemented by transcriptional profiling, resequencing and epigenetic approaches, has identified specific genetic alterations with biologic and therapeutic implications. For example, genetic expression profiling studies have classified T-cell ALL cases into several distinct genetic subgroups: *HOX11L2*, *LYL1* plus *LMO2*, *TAL1* plus *LMO1* or *LMO2*, *HOX11*, and *MLL-ENL*. The last two subgroups are associated with a favorable outcome.[51] Notably, the genome-wide studies identified a subgroup of very high-risk B-cell precursor ALL with genetic profile similar to that of cases with *BCR-ABL1* fusion, characterized by *IKZF1* deletion.[49,50]

DIFFERENTIAL DIAGNOSIS

The initial manifestations of ALL can mimic a variety of disorders. The acute onset of petechiae, ecchymoses, and bleeding can suggest idiopathic thrombocytopenic purpura. The latter disorder often is associated with a recent viral infection, large platelets in blood films, normal hemoglobin concentration, and absence of leukocyte abnormalities in blood or marrow. Patients with ALL or aplastic anemia can present with pancytopenia and complications associated with marrow failure. However, in aplastic anemia, hepatosplenomegaly and lymphadenopathy are rare, and the skeletal changes associated with leukemia are absent. The results of marrow aspiration or biopsy usually distinguish between the two diseases, although the diagnosis can be difficult in a patient who has hypocellular marrow that is later replaced by lymphoblasts. In one study, transient pancytopenia preceded ALL in 2 percent of all pediatric cases.[75] During the preleukemic phase in these patients, polymerase chain reaction (PCR) analysis demonstrated monoclonality. This finding suggests hypoplasia resulted from inhibition of normal hematopoiesis by leukemic cells.[101] ALL should be considered in the differential diagnosis of patients with hypereosinophilia, which can be a presenting feature of leukemia or can precede its diagnosis by several months.[70] Occasionally, hematogones in a regenerative marrow may mimic leukemic blast cells and require flow cytometry examination with optimal combinations of antibodies to distinguish.[102]

Infectious mononucleosis and other viral infections, especially those associated with thrombocytopenia or hemolytic anemia, can be confused with leukemia. Detection of reactive lymphocytes or serologic evidence of Epstein-Barr virus infection helps establish the diagnosis. Patients with acute infectious lymphocytosis, pertussis, or parapertussis can have marked lymphocytosis. However, even when leukocyte counts are as high as $50 \times 10^9/L$, the affected cells are mature lymphocytes rather than lymphoblasts. Bone pain, arthralgia, and occasionally arthritis mimic juvenile rheumatoid arthritis, rheumatic fever, other collagen diseases, or osteomyelitis. The marrow should be examined if glucocorticoid treatment is planned for presumed rheumatoid diseases.

In children, ALL should be distinguished from small, round cell tumors involving the marrow, including neuroblastoma, rhabdomyosarcoma, and retinoblastoma. Generally, in patients with solid tumors, a primary lesion may be found by standard diagnostic studies. Disseminated tumor cells often present in characteristic aggregates, and immunophenotypic characteristics of lymphoblasts are absent.

THERAPY

SUPPORTIVE CARE

Optimal management of patients with ALL requires careful attention to supportive care, including immediate treatment or prevention of metabolic and infectious complications (see Chap. 22) and rational use of blood products (see Chaps. 140 and 141). Other important supportive care measures, such as use of indwelling catheters,[103] amelioration of nausea and vomiting, pain control, and continuous psychosocial support for the patient and family, are essential.

Metabolic Complications

Hyperuricemia and hyperphosphatemia with secondary hypocalcemia are frequently encountered at diagnosis, even before chemotherapy is initiated, especially in patients with B-cell or T-cell ALL or precursor B-cell leukemia with high leukemic cell burden. Patients should be given intravenous fluids; allopurinol or rasburicase (recombinant urate oxidase) to treat hyperuricemia; and a phosphate binder, such as aluminum hydroxide, calcium carbonate (if the serum calcium concentration is low), lanthanum carbonate, or sevelamer to treat hyperphosphatemia. Allopurinol, a relatively inexpensive drug, is usually used if the uric acid is less than 7.0 mg/dL. It has a high frequency of allergic skin reactions and should be stopped as soon as the risk of hyperuricemia from the destruction of a large leukemic cell burden has passed. Rasburicase works very rapidly and is extremely effective, especially for very elevated uric acid levels (>7.0 mg/dL), often with one infusion (a far smaller dose than the company recommends). By inhibiting *de novo* purine synthesis in leukemic blast cells, allopurinol can reduce the peripheral blast cell count before chemotherapy.[104] Allopurinol can decrease both the anabolism and catabolism of mercaptopurine by depleting intracellular phosphoribosyl pyrophosphate and by inhibiting xanthine oxidase. If mercaptopurine and allopurinol are given together orally, the dosage of mercaptopurine generally must be reduced. Allopurinol can cause skin rashes but seldom causes severe allergic reactions.

Rasburicase breaks down uric acid to allantoin, a readily excreted metabolite that is 5 to 10 times more soluble than uric acid. Rasburicase is more effective than allopurinol, and it facilitates phosphorus excretion, partly because of rasburicase's potent uricolytic effect (which obviates the need to alkalinize urine) and partly because of improved renal function with its use.[105,106] However, rasburicase is contraindicated in patients with glucose-6-dehydrogenase deficiency because hydrogen peroxide, a by-product of uric acid breakdown, can cause methemoglobinemia or hemolytic anemia.

Hyperleukocytosis

For patients with extreme leukocytosis (leukocyte count $>400 \times 10^9$/L), either leukapheresis or exchange transfusion (in small children) can be used to reduce the burden of leukemic cells. In theory, either treatment should reduce the complications associated with leukostasis, but the short- and long-term benefits of the procedures are questionable.[67] Emergency cranial irradiation, once advocated by some leukemia therapists, probably has no role in the treatment of these patients.[107] Preinduction therapy with low-dose glucocorticoids, with addition of vincristine and cyclophosphamide in cases of B-cell ALL, is a favored means of ameliorating hyperleukocytosis. Pioneered by French investigators, this method, when used in conjunction with urate oxidase, has largely eliminated tumor lysis syndrome and the need for hemodialysis in patients with B-cell ALL.[108]

Infection Control

Infections are common in febrile patients with newly diagnosed ALL. Therefore, any patient presenting with fever, especially a patient with neutropenia, should be given broad-spectrum antibiotics until infection is excluded. Remission induction therapy can increase susceptibility to infection by exacerbating myelosuppression, immunosuppression, and mucosal breakdown. At least 50 percent of patients undergoing induction therapy experience infections. Special precautions should be taken to reduce the risk of infection during this critical phase of treatment, including reverse protective isolation and air filtration; elimination of contact with people with infections; refraining from eating certain food products, such as raw cheese, uncooked vegetables, or unpeeled fruits; and use of antiseptic mouthwash or sitz baths, especially for patients with mucositis. Although one recent study showed no benefit for a "neutropenic diet" in adults receiving induction treatment for acute myeloid leukemia,[109] similar studies have yet to be performed in patients undergoing remission induction for ALL. Administration of granulocyte colony-stimulating factor can hasten recovery from neutropenia and reduce the complications of intensive chemotherapy, but does not improve the event-free survival rate for children or adults.[110,111] One study suggested growth factor increased the risk of therapy-related acute myeloid leukemia in the context of epipodophyllotoxin-based therapy.[112] Use of intensified remission induction, especially in combination with high-dose dexamethasone, apparently has resulted in an increased risk of disseminated fungal infection and death in induction.[113] Chapter 22 addresses diagnosis and treatment of infections in immunocompromised host.

Usually, all patients with ALL are given trimethoprim-sulfamethoxazole, 2 to 3 days per week, as prophylactic therapy for *Pneumocystis carinii (Pneumocystis jiroveci)* pneumonia. Prophylaxis is started after 2 weeks of remission induction and continues until 6 weeks after completion of all chemotherapy. Alternative treatments for patients who cannot tolerate trimethoprim-sulfamethoxazole include aerosolized pentamidine and atovaquone (which should be taken with food or a milky drink).[114,115] Live-virus vaccine should not be administered during immunosuppressive therapy. Siblings and other children who have frequent contact with patients can receive routine immunizations, including inactivated poliomyelitis vaccine. Susceptible patients exposed to varicella virus should receive zoster immunoglobulin within 96 hours of exposure. Such treatment usually prevents or mitigates the clinical manifestations of varicella.

Hematologic Support

ALL or its treatment can lead to thrombocytopenia. Hemorrhagic manifestations are common but usually are limited to the skin and mucous membranes. Although rare, bleeding in the CNS, lungs, or gastrointestinal tract can be life-threatening. Patients with extremely high leukocyte counts ($>400 \times 10^9$/L) at diagnosis are more likely to develop such complications.[67] Coagulopathy attributable to disseminated intravascular coagulation, hepatic dysfunction, or chemotherapy is usually mild.[63,76] Patients receiving induction treatment, including L-asparaginase and a glucocorticoid, generally are in a hypercoagulable state.[116] Platelet transfusions should be given therapeutically for overt bleeding and may be used prophylactically when platelet counts are less than 10×10^9/L.[117] Children generally do not have active bleeding during remission induction therapy with prednisone, vincristine, and L-asparaginase, even when platelet counts are less than 10×10^9/L. A higher threshold for prophylactic platelet transfusions should be considered for active toddlers and patients with fever or infection. Transfusion of packed-leukocyte-poor red cells is indicated in patients with anemia and marrow suppression but should be delayed until the leukocyte count is reduced in patients with extreme hyperleukocytosis.[67] Transfusion should be given slowly in patients with profound but chronic anemia to prevent development of congestive heart failure. Granulocyte transfusions are needed only rarely for patients with absolute neutropenia and documented Gram-negative septicemia or disseminated fungal infection, which responds poorly to antimicrobial treatment. All blood products should be irradiated to prevent graft-versus-host disease.

ANTILEUKEMIC THERAPY

Because ALL is a heterogeneous disease with many distinct subtypes, a uniform approach to therapy is not appropriate. Assessing the probability of relapse is necessary to avert undertreatment or overtreatment. No consensus exists on the risk criteria and the terminology for defining prognostic subgroups. Usually, childhood ALL cases are divided into standard-risk, high- (intermediate- or average-) risk, and very-high-risk groups, although the United States' Children's Oncology Group advocates four categories, including low risk, to accommodate patients with a very low risk of relapse. Adult cases are generally divided into two risk groups. Often infant or elderly ALL are considered special subgroups of ALL that require different treatment. One recent study showed improved outcome for infant ALL, using hybrid treatment protocol with elements to treat both ALL and acute myeloid leukemia, and reducing dose intensity in the very young infants.[118] Even though the median age of ALL in adults is greater than 60 years, very few studies have been performed in those older than 60 years of age and their management remains a therapeutic challenge.[119,120] Some successes have been achieved with the use of dose-reduced regimens and the addition of imatinib for patients with Philadelphia-chromosome–positive ALL.[121] Because cure can rarely be achieved in patients older than age 70 years, maintenance of a good quality of life is a major goal for this age group.

B-Cell ALL

The most effective contemporary treatment regimens for B-cell ALL are drug combinations that include cyclophosphamide given over a relatively short time (3–6 months). The first major breakthrough in this disease was reported by French investigators, who achieved a 68 percent event-free survival rate in their LMB84 study featuring high-dose cyclophosphamide, high-dose methotrexate, vincristine, doxorubicin, and conventional doses of cytarabine.[108] In the LMB89 study, the same group reported a cure rate of 87 percent, which was achieved by using increased doses of methotrexate (to 8 g/m^2 per dose) and cytarabine (3 g/m^2 per dose) and by adding etoposide for patients with a large leukemic cell burden.[122] This excellent result has been confirmed in a randomized international study.[123] Successful treatments also have been developed by the Berlin-Frankfurt-Münster consortium, which uses a multiagent regimen that incorporates cyclophosphamide, high-dose methotrexate (1 g/m^2 per dose), etoposide, ifosfamide, doxorubicin, dexamethasone, and cytarabine (3 g/m^2 per dose).[124] Whether etoposide or ifosfamide contributed to the improved results requires further study.

Effective CNS therapy is an essential component of successful regimens for B-cell ALL and generally consists of methotrexate and cytarabine administered both systematically and intrathecally. Cranial irradiation does not appear to be necessary even for patients presenting with CNS leukemia.[123] B-cell ALL rarely, if ever, recurs after the first year; therefore, prolonged continuation therapy is not necessary.

The treatment approach used for childhood ALL has been applied to B-cell ALL in adults. Because of its demonstrated efficacy in B-cell lymphoma, rituximab (anti-CD20) has been incorporated in front-line clinical trials for adults with B-cell ALL, yielding promising results approaching those of childhood cases.[125,126]

Precursor B-Cell and T-Cell ALL

Treatment for leukemias affecting the precursor B-cell and T-cell lineages consists of three standard phases: remission induction, intensification (consolidation), and prolonged continuation therapy. CNS-directed therapy, which overlaps other treatments, is started early and is given for different lengths of time, depending on the patient's risk of relapse and the intensity of the primary systemic regimen.

Remission Induction The first goal of therapy for patients with leukemia is inducing a complete remission and restoring normal hematopoiesis. The induction regimen typically includes a glucocorticoid (prednisone, prednisolone, or dexamethasone), vincristine, and L-asparaginase for children or an anthracycline for adults.[21,119,120] Children with high- or very-high-risk ALL, and nearly all young adults with ALL, receive four or more drugs during remission induction in contemporary clinical trials. Improvements in chemotherapy and supportive care have resulted in complete remission rates of approximately 98 percent for children and 85 to 90 percent for adults. When a complete clinical remission is induced, patients have various degrees of residual leukemia, and some can still have as many as 10 billion leukemic cells.[127] Because the extent of residual disease is well correlated with long-term outcome,[91,128–130] the concept of a "molecular" or "immunologic" remission, defined as leukemic involvement of less than 0.01 percent of nucleated marrow cells,[127] is beginning to supplant the traditional perception of remission, which is based solely on microscopic criteria.

Attempts have been made to intensify induction therapy based on the premise that more rapid and complete reduction of the leukemic cell burden forestalls the development of drug resistance. However, results of several studies have suggested intensive induction therapy is unnecessary for children with standard-risk ALL, provided patients receive postinduction intensification therapy.[131,132] Intensive induction can lead to increased early morbidity and mortality.[113,133] More intensive induction regimens with additional cyclophosphamide, high-dose cytarabine, or high-dose anthracycline also have been tested in adults with ALL and have yielded no clear benefit,[134–136] partly because of the low tolerance of adults to drug toxicity. However, in one recent study, the use of high-dose dexamethasone (10 mg/m^2 per day) instead of prednisone (60 mg/m^2 per day) during remission induction significantly improved treatment outcome for children with ALL, especially those with T-cell ALL and good prednisone response, despite a higher induction death rate.[113] Conceivably, intensified remission induction with other relatively nonmyelosuppressive drugs can also improve treatment outcome.

Although dexamethasone provided better control of systemic and CNS disease than did prednisone in two randomized studies of childhood ALL,[137,138] one small study showed that an augmented dose of prednisolone produced results comparable with those achieved with dexamethasone.[139] Similarly, the pharmacodynamics of asparaginase differ by formulation and three forms are available: one derived from *Erwinia chrysanthemi*, another prepared from *Escherichia coli*, and a third made of a polyethylene glycol form of the *E. coli* product (pegaspargase).[140] In terms of leukemic control, the dose intensity and duration of asparaginase treatment (i.e., the amount of asparagine depletion) are far more important than the type of asparaginase used. The dosages of the three preparations are based on their half-lives. Pegaspargase, which has the longest half-life, usually is administered at 2500 IU/m^2 every other week for 1 to 2 doses in cases of newly diagnosed ALL. By contrast, the *Erwinia* preparation, which has the shortest half-life, is administered at 20,000 IU/m^2 three times per week for 6 to 12 doses. The doses of *E. coli* L-asparaginase range from 5000 to 10,000 IU/m^2, administered two to three times per week for 6 to 12 doses. Compared with *E. coli* asparaginase, *Erwinia* asparaginase was associated with inferior antileukemic response but fewer toxic effects, a finding now attributed to use of inadequate doses of the *Erwinia* drug.[141,142] Different preparations of the *E. coli* enzyme also have different pharmacologic and pharmacokinetic properties.[143] These differences mandate dosage adjustment to avoid excessive toxicity.[133,144] Notably, antibodies to *E. coli* asparaginase cross-reacted with pegaspargase, and the use of the latter form of asparaginase at the recommended dose was not very effective in patients who had previously received *E. coli* asparaginase, regardless of clinical hypersensitivity.[145]

Because of lower immunogenicity, improved efficacy, and less frequent administration,[145–148] pegaspargase has replaced the native product as the first-line treatment for children in the United States, and is also increasingly used in other childhood and adult ALL trials around the world. Of the various anthracyclines (daunorubicin, doxorubicin, and mitoxantrone) given to adults with ALL, none has proved superior to any other; however, daunorubicin is used most commonly.

Intensification (Consolidation) Therapy When normal hematopoiesis is restored, patients in remission become candidates for intensification therapy. Such treatment, administered shortly after remission induction, refers to high doses of multiple agents not used during the induction phase or to readministration of the induction regimen. Although there is no dispute on the importance of this treatment in childhood ALL, consensus is scarce on the best regimen and duration of treatment. More commonly used regimens for childhood ALL include high-dose methotrexate with or without mercaptopurine,[149,150] high-dose L-asparaginase given for an extended period,[146,151] or a combination of dexamethasone, vincristine, L-asparaginase, and doxorubicin, followed by thioguanine, cytarabine, and cyclophosphamide.[131,149] This phase of therapy has improved outcome, even for patients with low-risk ALL.[152] Patients with *ETV6-RUNX1* have an especially good outcome in clinical trials featuring intensive postremission treatment with glucocorticoids, vincristine, and asparaginase.[153,154] A very high dose of methotrexate (5 g/m^2) appears to improve the treatment outcome of patients with T-cell ALL.[149,155] This finding is consistent with data indicating T-cell lineage blasts accumulate methotrexate polyglutamates (active metabolites of the parent compound) less avidly than do B-cell precursors[95]; therefore, higher serum levels of the drug are needed for an adequate therapeutic effect.[156] The conventional dose of methotrexate (1 g/m^2) may be too low for many patients with B-cell precursor ALL.[150] To this end, our study showed that among B-lineage ALL, blasts with either *ETV6-RUNX1* or *TCF3-PBX1* gene fusion accumulate significantly lower methotrexate polyglutamates compared to those with hyperdiploidy or other genetic abnormalities.[157] This finding suggested that patients with *ETV6-RUNX1* or *TCF3-PBX1* gene fusion benefit from a higher dose of methotrexate.

Based on pediatric studies, intensive consolidation therapy has become a standard in the treatment of adult ALL even though early studies failed to show the benefit of this phase of treatment.[158–160] Various drugs have been used for intensification, including high-dose methotrexate, high-dose cytarabine, cyclophosphamide, and asparaginase. Increasingly, intensification treatment is risk adapted and subtype specific. In the German 06/93 study, high-dose methotrexate was used for patients with standard-risk B-cell precursor ALL, high-dose methotrexate and high-dose cytarabine for high-risk B-cell precursor ALL, and cyclophosphamide for T-cell ALL.[161] The hyper-CVAD (cyclophosphamide, vincristine, Adriamycin, dexamethasone) regimen of the MD Anderson Cancer Center alternates the combination of cyclophosphamide, vincristine, doxorubicin (Adriamycin), and dexamethasone, with high-dose methotrexate and high-dose cytarabine for four courses each.[162] In adults, methotrexate dose should probably be limited to 1.5 to 2 g/m^2 because higher doses may lead to excessive toxicities, delayed subsequent treatment, and reduced compliance.[119] In the Cancer and Leukemia Group B study, a five-drug remission induction was followed by early and late intensification courses with eight drugs.[64] These three studies and the Medical Research Council of the United Kingdom Acute Lymphoblastic Leukaemia Trial XII study[163] suggested the benefit of early intensive consolidation therapy, especially in young adults. In adult T-cell ALL, the benefit is derived from cyclophosphamide and cytarabine. In other adult cases of standard-risk and high-risk ALL, the benefit is derived from high-dose cytarabine.[163,164] More striking perhaps are the markedly improved results in two German multicenter trials using high-dose cytarabine, mitoxantrone, and allogeneic hematopoietic stem cell transplantation in cases bearing the t(4;11), which generally confers an adverse prognosis.[165] Several ongoing trials are testing the efficacy of asparaginase intensification in young adult ALL because this drug clearly improves outcome in childhood ALL[165a] and is better tolerated during consolidation treatment than during remission induction.

Continuation Therapy Excluding cases of mature B-cell leukemia, continuation therapy for 2 to 3 years is an integral part of pediatric and adult regimens. Attempts to shorten the duration of treatment have led to inferior outcomes in both childhood and adult ALL,[159,166,167] although apparently two-thirds of childhood cases could be cured with only 12 months of treatment.[168] However, which subgroups of childhood ALL can be cured with abbreviated therapy is unclear. In a meta-analysis of 42 trials, a third year of continuation therapy reduced the likelihood of relapse during the third year, but no advantage to prolonging treatment beyond 3 years was observed.[169] Early studies demonstrated that the third year of continuation therapy benefits boys but not girls.[170,171] Hence, most studies discontinue all therapy for girls after 2 to 2.5 years of treatment. It is uncertain whether with improved contemporary treatment boys still require prolonged continuation treatment. Whether adults with ALL require prolonged continuation therapy is also unclear. In most adult trials, continuation therapy is given for 2 years. Attempts to intensify continuation treatment failed to improve outcome in adults.[172] Adults often show poor compliance to intensive continuation treatment because of toxicities and social reasons.[119]

A combination of methotrexate administered weekly and mercaptopurine administered daily constitutes the usual continuation regimen for ALL. Accumulation of higher intracellular concentrations of the active metabolites of methotrexate and mercaptopurine and administration of this combination to the limits of tolerance (as indicated by low leukocyte counts) have been associated with improved clinical outcome.[173–176] Many investigators advocate that drug dosage be adjusted to maintain leukocyte counts below $3 \times 10^9/L$ and neutrophil counts between 0.5 and $1.5 \times 10^9/L$ to ensure adequate dose intensity during the continuation treatment in childhood ALL,[4] a practice rarely done in adults.[119] In one study, the dose intensity of mercaptopurine was the most important pharmacologic factor influencing treatment outcome.[177] However, overzealous use of mercaptopurine is counterproductive, as such use results in neutropenia and interruption of chemotherapy, reducing overall dose intensity. The effect of mercaptopurine is better when the drug is administered in the evening.[178] Mercaptopurine should not be given with milk or milk products containing xanthine oxidase, which can degrade the drug.[179] Although the merits of oral and parenteral administration of methotrexate continue to be debated, the latter route circumvents problems of decreased bioavailability and poor compliance, especially in adolescents.[180] Prolonged oral administration of methotrexate in divided doses has proved inferior to intermittent intravenous infusions at higher doses.[181] By contrast, mercaptopurine is most effective when it is given orally on a daily basis; weekly intravenous administration at a higher dose is ineffective.[137,146,182,183] Antimetabolite treatment should not be withheld because of isolated increases of liver enzymes, because such liver function abnormalities are tolerable and reversible.[184]

A few patients (1/300) have an inherited homozygous deficiency of thiopurine *S*-methyltransferase, the enzyme that catalyzes the *S*-methylation (inactivation) of mercaptopurine. In these patients, standard doses of mercaptopurine have potentially fatal hematologic side effects. The drug should be given in much smaller doses (e.g., 10-fold reduction).[185] Approximately 10 percent of the patients are heterozygous for the enzyme deficiency and have intermediate levels of thiopurine methyltransferase.[186] This subgroup can be treated safely with only moderate reductions in mercaptopurine dosage and appears to have better clinical outcomes than do patients with the homozygous wild-type phenotype. Importantly, patients with this enzyme deficiency are at risk for therapy-related leukemia and radiation-related brain tumors.[187,187a,188] Whether reducing the mercaptopurine dosage reduces the risk of therapy-related leukemia in these patients is unknown. Identification of the genetic basis of this autosomal codominant trait has enabled molecular diagnosis in these cases.[189] To this end, emphasis has been placed on the study of inherited differences in drug metabolism and disposition resulting from genetic polymorphisms in drug-metabolizing enzymes and in drug transporters, receptors, and targets.[3,190,191] Ultimately, therapy can be designed according to the genetic constitution of the host and the leukemic cells.

Because thioguanine is more potent than mercaptopurine in model systems and leads to higher concentrations of thioguanine nucleotides in cells and cytotoxic concentrations in cerebrospinal fluid,[192] several randomized trials have been performed to compare the effectiveness of these two drugs.[193–195] Thioguanine, given at a daily dose of 40 mg/m^2 or more, produced superior antileukemic responses to mercaptopurine, but was associated with profound thrombocytopenia, an increased risk of death, and unacceptable rate of hepatic venoocclusive disease.[193–195] Although the lower activity of thiopurine methyltransferase was associated with the complications,[196] this measure could not reliably identify patients at risk. Consequently, mercaptopurine, remains the drug of choice for ALL, although thioguanine could still be tested in short-term courses during the intensification phase of therapy.

In a meta-analysis, intermittent pulses of vincristine and a glucocorticoid improved the efficacy of antimetabolite-based continuation regimens[169] and have been widely adopted in the treatment of childhood ALL. However, in one randomized trial featuring intensive reinduction, the addition of six pulses of vincristine and dexamethasone during early continuation treatment failed to improve outcome of children with intermediate-risk ALL.[197] Another integral component of many protocols is reinduction therapy introduced relatively soon after the first remission. This treatment, which relies on the same drugs used during the initial phase of induction therapy, has improved outcomes for children and adults with ALL.[131,164] A second reinduction phase during continuation treatment may further improve the outcome of patients with standard- or high-risk ALL.[151,198] In the latter study, additional pulses of vincristine and prednisone after reinduction treatment did not improve outcome.[198] This result suggests the benefit of double-delayed intensification resulted from either the increased dose intensity of other agents such as asparaginase or anthracycline or the timing or scheduling of the intensification regimen. The finding also suggests glucocorticoid and vincristine pulses may not be needed after reinduction therapy. In older children and adults, prolonged glucocorticoid therapy may lead to increased risk of osteonecrosis.

Therapy of the CNS The CNS is a common sanctuary for leukemic cells and requires presymptomatic therapy. In the 1970s, the cornerstone of ALL therapy was cranial irradiation (2400 cGy) plus methotrexate administered intrathecally after complete remission was induced. The concern that cranial irradiation could cause second cancer, late neurocognitive deficits, and endocrinopathy stimulated efforts to replace cranial irradiation with early intensification by intrathecal and systemic chemotherapy. Two early clinical trials tested the feasibility of complete omission of prophylactic cranial irradiation in the treatment of childhood ALL.[199,200] Although the cumulative risk of an isolated CNS relapse were relatively low (4% and 3%), the event-free survival rates were only 68.4 percent and 60.7 percent.[199,200] In another study, prophylactic cranial irradiation appeared to improve outcome in T-cell ALL with leukocyte count >100 × 10^9/L.[201] Thus, virtually all childhood study groups continue to rely on prophylactic cranial irradiation for up to 20 percent of patients.[83] A radiation dose of 1200 cGy appeared to provide adequate protection against CNS relapse, even in high-risk patients (e.g., those with T-cell ALL and leukocyte counts >100 × 10^9/L).[149] A study at St. Jude Children's Research Hospital again tested the feasibility of total omission of prophylactic cranial irradiation in the context of risk-adapted intrathecal and systemic chemotherapy.[202] The 5-year survival rate for the 498 patients enrolled was 93.5 percent and the cumulative risk of an isolated CNS relapse rate was only 2.7 percent, a promising result, suggesting that prophylactic cranial irradiation can be safely omitted in the context of the effective intrathecal and systemic chemotherapy. Another study by the Dutch Childhood Oncology Group showed that prophylactic cranial irradiation can be safely omitted from all children with ALL.[202a]

Systemic treatment including high-dose methotrexate, intensive asparaginase, and dexamethasone, as well as optimal intrathecal therapy, is important to control CNS leukemia.[83] Triple intrathecal therapy with methotrexate, cytarabine, and hydrocortisone is more effective than intrathecal methotrexate in preventing CNS relapse.[203] Because the presence of ALL blasts in the cerebrospinal fluid, even from traumatic lumbar puncture, is associated with an increased risk of CNS relapse and poor event-free survival,[83–85] intrathecal therapy should be intensified in patients with this feature. To avoid traumatic lumbar puncture, the diagnostic lumbar puncture should be performed by an experienced clinician while the patient is immobile under general anesthesia or deep sedation, and followed immediately by intrathecal treatment to avoid the need for another lumbar puncture within the next few days.[204] Patients should remain in a prone position for at least 30 minutes after the procedure. Platelets should be administered to patients with thrombocytopenia (i.e., platelet count <100 × 10^9/L) and circulating leukemic cells at diagnosis to reduce the risk of traumatic lumbar puncture with blasts in cerebrospinal fluid.[204] With CNS prophylaxis and high-dose systemic therapy most adults with ALL remain free of CNS disease. CNS disease at the time of leukemia relapse in adults occurs in approximately 10 percent of cases. The frequency of CNS recurrence is about the same whether CNS radiation therapy is used or whether intrathecal cytotoxic therapy is used. A common approach is to use intrathecal methotrexate, cytarabine, and hydrocortisone. Systemic high-dose methotrexate and cytarabine add to the CNS therapy. The outcome after CNS relapse is poor, analogous to the outcome after marrow relapse. Survival after CNS relapse is usually less than 1 year in adults. Concern over the long-term side effects of CNS irradiation has led to the use of intrathecal and high-dose systemic chemotherapy for CNS control in adult ALL.[162]

Stem Cell Transplantation Hematopoietic stem cell transplantation during first remission remains controversial. In adult ALL, long-term disease-free survival rates range from 35 to 40 percent with chemotherapy alone and from 45 to 75 percent with allogeneic transplantation.[205–209] However, interpretation of these results is difficult because of the lack of true randomization. Even so, results of both the adult and pediatric studies suggest allogeneic transplantation benefits some high-risk patients.[205–210] Because of their unfavorable prognosis, patients with the Philadelphia-chromosome–positive ALL and those with a poor initial response to induction therapy commonly were recommended to undergo allogeneic stem cell transplantation during the first remission.[205–210] However, the advent of improved chemotherapy has decreased the survival advantage of transplantation in children with Philadelphia-chromosome–positive ALL.[211] The use of a tyrosine kinase inhibitor has further improved the early treatment results,[212] casting doubt on the use of transplantation in first remission in childhood cases. Allogeneic transplantation appeared to improve the outcome of adults with the t(4;11),[165] but not that of children or infants with the same genotype.[213] Allogeneic transplantation has not been superior to chemotherapy in adults with standard-risk ALL. More recently, reduced intensity-conditioning allografting yielded promising leukemia-free survival in a study of adult ALL.[213a] Thus, the indications for allogeneic transplantation in first remission should be reevaluated as chemotherapy and transplantation continue to improve. Autologous transplantation failed to improve outcome in adult ALL, mainly because of high rate of relapse (~50%). The main advantage of autologous transplant is a short total duration of therapy, which is counterbalanced by more late effects because of the use of total-body irradiation.[206,214]

Targeted Therapies The best example of targeted therapy is the use of tyrosine kinase inhibitor imatinib in Philadelphia-chromosome–positive ALL. Used as a single agent, it can induce complete remission in elderly patients.[215,216] In combination with chemotherapy, it not only induced a higher complete remission rate but also a higher rate of molecular remission (~50%) in adults.[217,218] Although the need of transplantation in childhood cases is uncertain, this treatment modality is still the treatment of choice in adult cases.[218] The use of imatinib allows higher proportion of adult cases suitable for transplantation. Recent data indicated that the outcome depends on minimal residual disease before and after transplantation. In patients with residual disease after transplantation, rapid response to imatinib was associated with a superior survival.[219] It is uncertain whether and when to discontinue imatinib after the patient is treated with chemotherapy or transplantation. A second generation of more potent tyrosine kinase inhibitors (dasatinib, nilotinib) has been developed.[220] Phase I and phase II clinical trials of these agents showed significant activity in patients with relapsed and refractory ALL, as well as in elderly patients.[221–224] Leukemia cell expression of CD20 is associated with an inferior outcome in adult,[225] but not childhood, ALL.[226] Pilot trials using anti-CD20 antibody has yielded some promising results in adult with CD20-positive B-cell precursor ALL.[227,228] Other promising investigational drugs include nelarabine and forodesine for T-cell ALL.[229]

COURSE AND PROGNOSIS

RELAPSE

Relapse is defined as the reappearance of leukemic cells at any site in the body. Most relapses occur during treatment or within the first 2 years after its completion, although initial relapses have been observed 10 or more years after diagnosis.[230] Molecular studies suggest that in some cases, especially those with the *ETV6-RUNX1* fusion, subsequent mutations of the residual preleukemic clone that were not eradicated during initial treatment account for the "late relapse."[231,232] The marrow remains the most common site of relapse in ALL. Anemia, leukocytosis, leukopenia, thrombocytopenia, enlargement of the liver or spleen, bone pain, fever, or a sudden decrease in tolerance to chemotherapy may signal the onset of marrow relapse. In contemporary programs of childhood ALL treatment, the rates of CNS and testicular relapse have decreased to 3 percent or less.[61,146,202] Leukemic relapse occasionally occurs at other extramedullary sites, including the eye, ear, ovary, uterus, bone, muscle, tonsil, kidney, mediastinum, pleura, and paranasal sinus.

Marrow relapse, with or without extramedullary involvement, portends a poor outcome for most patients. Factors indicating an especially poor prognosis include relapse while on therapy or after a short initial remission, T-cell immunophenotype, the presence of the Philadelphia chromosome, and an isolated hematologic relapse.[233–235] Prolonged second remissions (>3 years) can be achieved with chemotherapy in as many as half of patients with late relapses (i.e., >6 months after cessation of therapy) but in only approximately 10 percent of those with early relapse.[233–235] The presence of minimal residual disease after reinduction treatment also portends a very poor prognosis.[236,237] In patients who develop hematologic relapse while on therapy or shortly thereafter, and in those with a high level of minimal residual disease after remission induction for relapse, allogeneic hematopoietic stem cell transplantation is the treatment of choice.[238–240] Autologous transplantation as postinduction treatment offers no substantial advantage over chemotherapy.[241,242] For patients without histocompatible related donors, transplantation of stem cells from cord blood or marrow from matched unrelated donors has yielded encouraging results.[243–245] Outcome may be further improved by a new strategy using a reduced intensity of conditioning regimen and selection of donor-derived alloreactive natural killer cells for haploidentical transplantation.[246,247] For patients with ALL relapses after allogeneic transplantation, a second transplant or donor T-lymphocyte infusion occasionally results in sustained remission.[248]

Although extramedullary relapse is frequently an isolated clinical finding, many occurrences are associated with minimal residual disease in the marrow. CNS relapses are associated with higher level of minimal residual disease in the marrow than testicular relapses.[249] Importantly, submicroscopic marrow involvement at a level of 10^{-4} or higher at the time of overt extramedullary relapse confers a very poor outcome.[249] Hence, patients with extramedullary relapse and minimal residual disease in marrow require intensive treatment to prevent subsequent hematologic relapse. The efficacy of retrieval therapy in children with an isolated CNS relapse depends partly on duration of first complete remission and partly on whether CNS irradiation was previously performed. The strategy of delaying cranial or craniospinal irradiation for 6 to 12 months to allow initial intensification of systemic chemotherapy has yielded long-term second event-free survival of 70 to 80 percent in children with isolated CNS relapse.[250,251] In one study, 12 months of intensive systemic chemotherapy and reduced dose cranial irradiation (18 Gy) resulted in an excellent 4-year event-free survival rate among children with precursor B-cell ALL who had not received cranial irradiation during initial treatment and who had an initial remission duration of 18 months or more.[252] Notably, in this study, a favorable age group of 1 to 9.9 years plus a low presenting leukocyte count ($<50 \times 10^9$/L) at diagnosis of ALL was an independent favorable prognostic factor. For patients, especially those with T-cell ALL, in whom relapse develops during therapy and who had previously undergone cranial irradiation, the remission rate generally does not exceed 30 percent.[250,251] Adults with isolated CNS relapse fare much more poorly than children. Some investigators have selected hematopoietic stem cell transplantation as a treatment option for these high-risk cases.[253,254] However, no firm evidence indicates an advantage of either autologous or allogeneic transplantation over intensive chemotherapy.

One-third of patients with early testicular relapse and two-thirds of patients with late testicular recurrence became long-term survivors after salvage chemotherapy and testicular irradiation.[235,255–258] In one study, some patients with late isolated testicular relapses were successfully treated with chemotherapy that included very high-dose methotrexate, without the addition of radiation therapy.[259] The optimal treatment and prognosis for patients with relapse at unusual extramedullary sites also are unclear. However, the same principles that apply to the clinical management of CNS or testicular relapse probably apply to this subgroup.

TREATMENT SEQUELAE

Despite the increasing intensity of curative treatment for childhood ALL, judicious use of supportive care has reduced the rate of early death from 8 percent in the early 1970s to less than 2 percent in the 1990s.[21] Currently, the induction mortality ranges between 2 percent and 11 percent in adult ALL, with increasing age associated with higher death rate.[119,120,260] Most deaths are caused by bacterial or fungal infections. The death rate among elderly patients receiving remission induction therapy can be as high as 30 percent because of increased hematologic and nonhematologic toxicities (e.g., hepatotoxicity and cardiotoxicity).[63] This poor tolerance of chemotherapy and consequent reduction of dose intensity largely account for the generally poor clinical outcome in elderly patients.

TABLE 93–6. Side Effects Associated with Antileukemic Therapy

Treatment	Acute Complications	Delayed Complications
Prednisone (or prednisolone)	Hyperglycemia, hypertension, changes in mood or behavior, acne, increased appetite, weight gain, peptic ulcer, hepatomegaly, myopathy	Avascular necrosis of bone, osteopenia, growth retardation
Dexamethasone	Same as prednisone, except for increased changes in mood or behavior and myopathy but less salt retention	Same as prednisone
Vincristine	Peripheral neuropathy, constipation, chemical cellulitis, seizures, hair loss	None
Daunorubicin, idarubicin, doxorubicin, or epirubicin	Nausea and vomiting, hair loss, mucositis, marrow suppression, chemical cellulitis, increased skin pigmentation	Cardiomyopathy (with high cumulative dose)
L-Asparaginase	Nausea and vomiting, allergic reactions (manifested as rashes, bronchospasm, severe pain at intramuscular injection site), hyperglycemia, pancreatitis, liver dysfunction, thrombosis, encephalopathy	None
Mercaptopurine	Nausea and vomiting, mucositis, marrow suppression, solar dermatitis, liver dysfunction: increased hematologic toxicity in persons lacking thiopurine methyltransferase	Osteoporosis (long-term use), acute myeloid leukemia in persons with thiopurine methyltransferase deficiency
Methotrexate	Nausea and vomiting, liver dysfunction, marrow suppression, mucositis (resulting from high-dose treatment), solar dermatitis	Leukoencephalopathy, osteopenia (resulting from long-term use)
Etoposide, teniposide	Nausea and vomiting, hair loss, mucositis, marrow suppression, allergic reactions (bronchospasm, urticaria, angioedema, hypotension)	Acute myeloid leukemia
Cytarabine	Nausea and vomiting, fever, skin rashes, mucositis, marrow suppression, liver dysfunction, conjunctivitis (resulting from high-dose treatment)	Decreased fertility (with high cumulative dose)
Cyclophosphamide	Nausea and vomiting, hemorrhagic cystitis, marrow suppression, syndrome of inappropriate secretion of antidiuretic hormone, hair loss	Bladder cancer or acute myeloid leukemia (rare), decreased fertility (with high cumulative dose)
Rituximab	Infusion reactions, mucocutaneous reactions, cardiac arrhythmias, lymphopenia	Reaction of virus infections, progressive multifocal leukoencephalopathy from JC virus infection
Intrathecal methotrexate	Headache, fever, seizure, marrow suppression, mucositis (in patients with renal dysfunction)	Encephalopathy or myelopathy (with high cumulative dose)
Brain irradiation	Hair loss, postirradiation somnolence syndrome (6–10 weeks after treatment)	Seizure, mineralizing microangiopathy, growth hormone deficiency, thyroid dysfunction, obesity, osteopenia, brain tumors, basal cell carcinoma, parotid gland carcinoma, hair loss, cataract (rare), dental abnormalities

Table 93–6 summarizes common side effects associated with antileukemic therapy. Hyperglycemia develops in 10 to 20 percent of children during induction therapy with prednisone, vincristine, and L-asparaginase and has no long-term consequence nor prognostic implication; in some cases, short-term insulin treatment is required.[261] Adolescent age, obesity, a family history of diabetes mellitus, and Down syndrome are associated with increased susceptibility to hyperglycemia.[261,262] This induction regimen can cause a hypercoagulable state[263] leading to cerebral thromboses, peripheral vein thromboses, or both, in as many as 5 percent of patients. Cerebral thrombosis should be distinguished from transient ischemic lesions (posterior reversible encephalopathy syndrome), which are associated with acute hypertension and severe constipation.[264] These lesions are located at the watershed areas between the major cerebral arteries and generally are reversible. Cerebral thrombosis can be readily distinguished from transient ischemic lesions by magnetic resonance imaging or computed tomography (Fig. 93–5). Occasionally, cerebral thrombosis may not be apparent by diagnostic imaging until a few days after the onset of symptoms and signs.

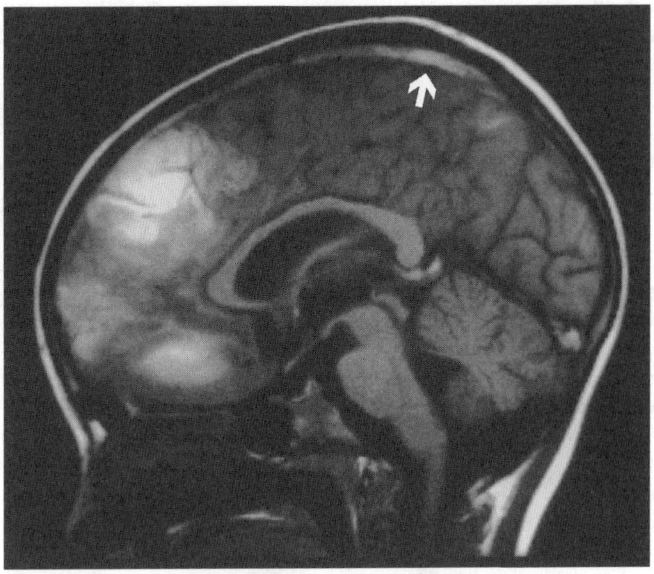

FIGURE 93–5. T1-weighted magnetic resonance image without contrast demonstrates a clot in the superior sagittal sinus (*arrow*) and several frontal lobe hematomas.

Emphasis on the intensive use of methotrexate and glucocorticoids has led to an increased frequency of neurotoxicity,[264,265] and osteonecrosis,[266] underscoring the need for judicious use of even seemingly benign agents. Many long-term survivors of childhood ALL, especially those who received high cumulative doses of glucocorticoid, methotrexate, or cranial irradiation, have developed severe osteoporosis.[267–269] Such development highlights the need for early identification of bone lesions and the introduction of therapy to prevent fractures. Treatment with anthracyclines can produce severe cardiomyopathy, especially when anthracyclines are given in high cumulative and peak doses to young girls.[270] Prolonged infusion did not appear to reduce late cardiotoxicity compared to bolus administration.[271] The existence of a safe cumulative dose of anthracycline is controversial.[272] Cardiac abnormalities are persistent and progressive years after anthracycline therapy.[273] In one study, dexrazoxane prevented or reduced anthracycline-induced cardiotoxicity without interfering with antileukemic activity.[274] In current clinical trials, only limited doses of anthracyclines are used, even for high-risk cases, to decrease the risk of subsequent cardiomyopathy.

Cranial irradiation has been implicated as the cause of numerous late sequelae in children, including second cancer, neurocognitive deficits, and endocrine abnormalities that can lead to obesity, short stature, precocious puberty, and osteoporosis.[275–279] In general, these complications are seen in girls more often than in boys and in young children more often than in older children. Our group's long-term followup study of survivors of childhood ALL revealed a greater than 10 percent cumulative risk of second neoplasms after 30 years of observation, and a higher-than-average mortality rate among patients who had received cranial irradiation.[276,277] Patients who had been irradiated also had a high unemployment rate and, among women, a low marital rate. Many children with profound deficiencies of growth hormone are receiving hormone replacement therapy, which permits attainment of acceptable final heights without an increased chance of relapse.[280] The most devastating complication is the development of brain tumors and acute myeloid leukemia. Children who undergo cranial irradiation at age 6 years or younger are most susceptible to development of brain tumors.[281] Intensive use of antimetabolites before and during cranial irradiation also increases the risk of brain tumor.[188] The median latency period for high-grade brain tumor is 9 years; it is 20 years for low-grade tumors (e.g., meningioma).[276,281]

Acute myeloid leukemia has been linked to intensive treatment with the epipodophyllotoxins (teniposide and etoposide). The risk of disease apparently depends on treatment schedule, concomitant use of other agents (e.g., L-asparaginase, alkylating agents, perhaps antimetabolites), and host pharmacogenetics.[187,282] The long-term survival rate for patients with this complication is very low, even when the patients undergo allogeneic stem cell transplantation.[187] No evidence indicates an increased incidence of cancer or birth defects among the offspring of adult survivors of childhood ALL.[283–285]

PROGNOSTIC FACTORS

The cornerstone of the modern therapeutic approach to childhood ALL has been careful assessment of the risk of relapse so that only high-risk or very-high-risk patients are treated with intensive therapy. Less-toxic treatments (usually antimetabolites) are reserved for low-risk or standard-risk patients. By contrast, almost all adult patients are candidates for intensive therapy. Of the many variables that influence prognosis, treatment is the most important.[21,202] Some of the factors that emerged as useful prognostic indicators have disappeared as treatment has improved; others have shown predictive strength in one or several trials, but not in others. For example, T-cell and B-cell ALL, once associated with a very poor prognosis, now have long-term response rates of 70 to 85 percent in children[4,21,61,146,202] and 50 to 60 percent in adults[119,120,260] as a result of effective intensive chemotherapy.

Age and leukocyte count continue to be used for risk classification in almost every pediatric clinical trial involving precursor B-cell ALL. In a workshop sponsored by the National Cancer Institute, participants agreed on a presenting age of between 1 and 9 years and a leukocyte count of less than 50 × 10^9/L as the minimum criteria for low-risk ALL.[286] These criteria apply only to precursor B-cell ALL and not to T-cell ALL. Among adults, the outcome of therapy worsens with increasing age and leukocyte count. Age younger than 35 years and leukocyte count less than 30 × 10^9/L are considered favorable prognostic indicators (Table 93–7).[119,129,260] However, no clear guidelines exist for assigning prognostic value to particular increments of age or leukocyte counts. In general, age younger than 60 years is considered a practical guide for selecting candidates who might benefit from intensive therapy, including allogeneic transplantation.[287] Any decision to begin aggressive treatment in patients older than age 60 years must be weighed against the risk of increased morbidity and mortality.

TABLE 93–7. Adverse Prognostic Factors in Adult ALL

Factors	B-Cell Precursor	T Cell
Age (years)*	>35	>35
Leukocyte count (×10^9/L)	>30	>100
Immunophenotype	Pro-B (CD10–)	Pre-T
Genetics	t(9;22) [*BCR-ABL1*]	*HOX11L2* expression ?
	t(4;11) [*MLL-AF4*]	*ERG* expression ?
	Hypodiploidy ?	
Treatment response	Delayed remission (>4 weeks)	Delayed remission (>4 weeks)
	Minimal residual disease >10^{-4} after induction	Minimal residual disease >10^4 after induction

*Continuous factor with increasing age associated with progressively worse outcome.

Male sex has long been recognized as an adverse prognostic factor in childhood ALL but has less influence in adult ALL. Its prognostic significance was abolished in a number of childhood studies in which overall outcome was improved.[4,21,61,146,202] Black race conferred a poor outcome in the national clinical trials,[288,289] but in a single-institution study with equal access to effective treatment regimens, race had no prognostic significance.[290]

Primary genetic abnormalities have important prognostic significance. Hyperdiploidy (>50 chromosomes) and *ETV6-RUNX1* fusion—seen primarily in children ages 1 to 9 years—are associated with a favorable prognosis.[4,21] *MLL* rearrangements, which occur in 70 to 80 percent of infants younger than age 1 year and in 10 percent of adults, and Philadelphia chromosome with *BCR-ABL1* fusion, which is found in 3 percent of children but in 25 to 30 percent of adult patients, historically confer a poor outcome.[3,4,21] Interestingly, a marked influence of age on the prognosis of genetic subtypes of ALL is observed. For example, Philadelphia-chromosome–positive ALL is associated with a poor outcome in adolescents but a relatively favorable outcome in children ages 1 to 9 years old who have a low leukocyte count at presentation.[210] Once associated with a dismal outcome, the early treatment outcome of Philadelphia-chromosome–positive ALL in both children and adults has improved substantially with the advent of tyrosine kinase inhibitors.[212,215–219] Among patients with *MLL*-rearranged ALL, infants younger than age 1 year fare considerably worse than older children.[213] The basis of these differences may be related to some combination of

TABLE 93–8. Risk Classification System in St. Jude Total Therapy Study XVI

Risk Group	Feature
Standard	B-cell precursor phenotype in patients ages 1–9 years with a presenting leukocyte count <50 × 10^9/L, *ETV6-RUNX1* fusion, or hyperdiploidy (>50 chromosomes or DNA index >1.16)
	Must not have CNS-3 status, testicular leukemia, t(9;22), t(1;19), rearranged *MLL* gene, hypodiploidy, or ≥0.01% leukemia cells in marrow after 6-week remission induction
High	T-cell ALL and all cases of B-cell precursor ALL that do not meet the criteria for standard or very-high-risk ALL
Very high	Early T-cell precursor, initial induction failure, or ≥1% leukemic cells in marrow after 6-week remission induction

secondary genetic events, the development stage of the target cell undergoing malignant transformation, and the pharmacogenetics or pharmacokinetic features of the patient. In T-cell ALL, *NOTCH1* or *FBXW7* mutation identifies a subgroup of childhoold or adult cases with a favorable outcome.[290a,290b]

A useful adjunct in risk assessment is the response to early treatment, as measured by the rate of clearance of leukemic cells from the blood or marrow with the use of flow cytometric detection of aberrant immunophenotype or analysis by PCR of clonal antigen–receptor gene rearrangements.[91,127–129,202,291,292] This measure accounts for the drug sensitivity or resistance of leukemic cells and the pharmacodynamics of the drugs, which is affected by the pharmacogenetics of the host. Because current techniques allow us to measure minimal residual disease in all patients, and it is the most important prognostic factor,[91,202] this factor has been used for definitive risk assessment at St. Jude (Table 93–8). The expectation is that alteration of treatment intensity according to the level of minimal residual disease will improve the long-term outcome of patients with ALL. The level of minimal residual leukemia is also a strong predictor of treatment outcome in patients at the time of second remission and before allogeneic stem cell transplantation for relapsed leukemia.[236,237,293] We now monitor patients with T-cell ALL with blood samples instead of marrow aspirates because both sources yield comparable levels of residual leukemia.[294]

REFERENCES

1. Gale RE, Wainscoat JS: Clonal analysis using X-linked DNA polymorphisms. *Br J Haematol* 85:2, 1993.
2. Saunders EF, Lampkin BC, Mauer AM: Variation of proliferative activity in leukemic cell populations of patients with acute leukemia. *J Clin Invest* 46:1356, 1967.
3. Pui CH, Relling MV, Downing JR: Acute lymphoblastic leukemia. *N Engl J Med* 350:1535, 2004.
4. Pui CH, Robison LL, Look AT: Acute lymphoblastic leukemia. *Lancet* 371:1030, 2008.
5. Velpeau A: Sur la resorption du pus et sur l'alteration du sang dans les maladies, Clinique de persection nenemant. Premier observation. *Rev Med* 26:216, 1827.
6. Virchow R: Weisses blut. *Notiz Geg Natur Heilk* 36:152, 1845.
7. Bennett JH: Case of hypertrophy of the spleen and liver in which death took place from suppuration of the blood. *Edinburgh Med Surg J* 64:413, 1845.
8. Craigie D: Case of disease of the spleen, in which death took place in consequence of the presence of purulent matter in the blood. *Edinburgh Med Surg J* 64:400, 1845.
9. Virchow R: Weisses Blut und Milztumoren. Part II. Med Z, 1847, 16, 9. *Virchows Arch Path Anat Physiol* 1:565, 1847.
10. Ehrlich P: Farbenanalytische untersuchungen zur histologie und klinick des blutes. *Berl Hirschwald* 137, 1891.
11. Reschad H, Schilling-Torgau V: Ueber eine neue Leukämie durch echte Uebergangsformen (Splenozytenleuämie) und ihre bedeutung für dies, selbständigkeit dieser Zellen. *Munchener Med Wochenschr* 60:1981, 1913.
12. Ward G: The infective theory of acute leukemia. *Br J Child Dis* 14:10, 1917.
13. Farber S, Diamond LK, Mercer RD, et al: Temporary remissions in acute leukemia in children produced by folic acid antagonist, 4-aminopteroylglumatic acid (aminopterin). *N Engl J Med* 238:787, 1948.
14. Farber S: The effect of ACTH in acute leukemia in childhood, in *Proceedings of the First Clinical Conference on the Use of ACTH*, edited by JR Mote, p 325. Blakiston, Philadelphia, 1950.
15. Elion GB, Hitchings GH, Vanderwerff H: Antagonists of nucleic acid derivatives; purines. *J Biol Chem* 192:505, 1951.
16. Pinkel D, Hernandez K, Borella L, et al: Drug dosage and remission duration in childhood lymphocytic leukemia. *Cancer* 27:247, 1971.
17. Thomas ED, Buckner CD, Rudolph RH, et al: Allogeneic marrow grafting for hematological malignancy using HLA-matched donor-recipient pairs. *Blood* 38:267, 1971.
18. Riehm H, Gadner H, Henze G, et al: The Berlin childhood acute lymphoblastic leukemia therapy study, 1970–1976. *Am J Pediatr Hematol Oncol* 2:299, 1980.
19. Sen L, Borella L: Clinical importance of lymphoblasts with T markers in childhood acute leukemia. *N Engl J Med* 292:828, 1975.
20. Williams DL, Look AT, Melvin SL, et al: New chromosomal translocations correlate with specific immunophenotypes of childhood acute lymphoblastic leukemia. *Cell* 36:101, 1984.
21. Pui CH, Evans WE: Treatment of acute lymphoblastic leukemia. *N Engl J Med* 354:166, 2006.
22. Mullighan CG, Downing JR: Global genomic characterization of acute lymphoblastic leukemia. *Semin Hematol* 46:3, 2009.
23. Druker BJ: Translation of the Philadelphia chromosome into therapy for CML. *Blood* 112:4808, 2008.
24. Ries LAG, Melbert D, Krapcho M, et al. (eds): *SEER Cancer Statistics Review*, 1975–2005, National Cancer Institute. Bethesda, MD, http://seer.cancer.gov/csr/1975_2005, based on November 2007 SEER data submission, posted to the SEER web site, 2008.
25. Sandler DP, Ross JA: Epidemiology of acute leukemia in children and adults. *Semin Oncol* 24:3, 1997.
26. Parkin DM, Muir CS, Whelan SL, et al: *Cancer Incidence in Five Continents*, vol 6, no 120. IARC Scientific Publication, Lyon, 1992.
27. Forestier E, Izraeli S, Beverloo B, et al: Cytogenetic features of acute lymphoblastic and myeloid leukemias in pediatric patients with Down syndrome: An iBFM-SG study. *Blood* 111:1575, 2008.
28. Mullighan CG, Zhang J, Harvey RC, et al: JAK mutations in high-risk childhood acute lymphoblastic leukemia. *Proc Natl Acad Sci U S A* 106:9414, 2009.
28a. Mullighan CG, Collins-Underwood JR, Phillips LA, et al: Rearrangement of *CRLF2* in B-progenitor- and Down syndrome-associated acute lymphoblastic leukemia. *Nat Genet* 41:1243, 2009.
29. Vanasse GJ, Concannon P, Willerford DM: Regulated genomic instability and neoplasia in the lymphoid lineage. *Blood* 94:3997, 1999.
30. Liberzon E, Avigad S, Stark B, et al: Germ-line ATM gene alterations are associated with susceptibility to sporadic T-cell acute lymphoblastic leukemia in children. *Genes Chromosomes Cancer* 39:161, 2004.
31. Sun X, Becker-Catania SG, Chen HH, et al: Early diagnosis of ataxia-telangiectasia using radiosensitivity testing. *J Pediatr* 140:724, 2002.
32. Doll R, Wakeford R: Risk of childhood cancer from fetal irradiation. *Br J Radiol* 70:130,1997.
33. Draper G, Vincent T, Kroll ME, Swanson J. Childhood cancer in relation to distance from high voltage power lines in England and Wales: A case-control study. *BMJ* 330:1290, 2005.
34. Hjalgrim LL, Rostgaard K, Hjalgrim H, et al: Birth weight and risk for childhood leukemia in Denmark, Sweden, Norway, and Iceland. *J Natl Cancer Inst* 96:1549, 2004.
35. Davies SM, Bhatia S, Ross JA, et al: Glutathione S-transferase genotypes, genetic susceptibility, and outcome of therapy in childhood acute lymphoblastic leukemia. *Blood* 100:67, 2002.
36. Lanciotti M, Dufour C, Corral L, et al: Genetic polymorphism of NAD(P)H:quinine oxidoreductase is associated with an increased risk of infant acute lymphoblastic leukemia without MLL gene rearrangements. *Leukemia* 19:214, 2005.
37. Wiemels JL, Smith RN, Taylor GM, et al: Methylenetetrahydrofolate reductase (MTHFR) polymorphisms and risk of molecularly defined subtypes of childhood acute leukemia. *Proc Natl Acad Sci U S A* 98:4004, 2001.
38. Skibola CF, Smith MT, Hubbard A, et al: Polymorphisms in the thymidylate synthase and serine hydroxymethyltransferase genes and risk of adult acute lymphocytic leukemia. *Blood* 99:3786, 2002.
39. Healy J, Bélanger H, Beaulieu P, et al. Promoter SNPs in G_1/S checkpoint regulators and their impact on the susceptibility to childhood leukemia. *Blood* 109:683, 2007.
39a. Trevino LR, Yang W, French D, et al: Germline genomic variants associated with childhood acute lymphoblastic leukemia. *Nat Genet* 41:1001, 2009.
40. Greaves M: Infection, immune responses and the aetiology of childhood leukaemia. *Nat Rev Cancer* 6:193, 2006.
41. Maia AT, Tussiwand R, Cazzaniga G, et al: Identification of preleukemic precursors of hyperdiploid acute lymphoblastic leukemia in cord blood. *Genes Chromosomes Cancer* 40:38, 2004.
42. Hong D, Gupta R, Ancliff P, et al: Initiating and cancer-propagating cells in TEL-AML1-associated childhood leukemia. *Science* 319:336, 2008.
43. Kinlen LJ: Infection, immune factors in cancer: The role of epidemiology. *Oncogene* 23:6341, 2004.

44. Wiemels JL, Leonard BC, Wang Y, et al: Site-specific translocation and evidence of postnatal origin of the t(1;19) E2A-PBX1 fusion in childhood acute lymphoblastic leukemia. *Proc Natl Acad Sci U S A* 99:15101, 2002.
45. Sherr CJ: The INK4a/ARF network in tumour suppression. *Nat Rev Mol Cell Biol* 2:731, 2001.
46. Weng P, Ferrando AA, Lee W, et al: Activating mutations of NOTCH1 in human T cell acute lymphoblastic leukemia. *Science* 306:269, 2004.
47. Mullighan CG, Goorha S, Radtke I, et al: Genome-wide analysis of genetic alterations in acute lymphoblastic leukemia. *Nature* 446:758, 2007.
48. Mullighan CG, Miller CB, Radtke I, et al: BCR-ABL1 lymphoblastic leukemia is characterized by the deletion of Ikaros. *Nature* 453:110, 2008.
49. Mullighan CG, Su X, Zhang J, et al: Deletion of IKZF1 and prognosis in acute lymphoblastic leukemia. *N Engl J Med* 360:470, 2009.
50. Den Boer ML, van Slegtenhorst M, De Menezes RX, et al: A subtype of childhood acute lymphoblastic leukaemia with poor treatment outcome: A genome-wide classification study. *Lancet Oncol* 10:125, 2009.
51. Ferrando AA, Look AT: Gene expression profiling in T-cell acute lymphoblastic leukemia. *Semin Hematol* 40:274, 2003.
52. Armstrong SA, Staunton JE, Silverman LB, et al: MLL translocations specify a distinct gene expression profile that distinguishes a unique leukemia. *Nat Genet* 30:41, 2002.
53. Yeoh EJ, Ross ME, Shurtleff SA, et al: Classification, subtype discovery, and prediction of outcome in pediatric acute lymphoblastic leukemia by gene expression profiling. *Cancer Cell* 1:133, 2002.
54. Armstrong SA, Kung AL, Mabon ME, et al: Inhibition of FLT3 in MLL: Validation of a therapeutic target identified by gene expression based classification. *Cancer Cell* 3:173, 2003.
55. Cheok MH, Yang W, Pui CH, et al: Treatment-specific changes in gene expression discriminate *in vivo* drug response in human leukemia cells. *Nat Genet* 34:85, 2003.
56. Holleman A, Cheok MH, Den Boer ML, et al: Gene-expression patterns in drug-resistant acute lymphoblastic leukemia cells and response to treatment. *N Engl J Med* 351:533, 2004.
57. Yang JJ, Cheng C, Yang W, et al: Genome-wide interrogation of germline genetic variation associated with treatment response in childhood acute lymphoblastic leukemia. *JAMA* 301:393, 2009.
58. Garcia-Manero G, Yang H, Kuang SQ, et al: Epigenetics of acute lymphoblastic leukemia. *Semin Hematol* 46:24, 2009.
59. Pui C-H, Crist WM: Acute lymphoblastic leukemia, in *Childhood Leukemia*, edited by C-H Pui, p 288. Cambridge University Press, New York, 1999.
60. Pui CH: Acute lymphoblastic leukemia, in *Childhood Leukemias*, 2nd ed, edited by CH Pui, p 439. Cambridge University Press, New York, 2006.
61. Möricke A, Reiter A, Zimmermann M, et al: Risk-adjusted therapy of acute lymphoblastic leukemia can decrease treatment burden and improve survival: Treatment results of 2169 unselected pediatric and adolescent patients enrolled in the trial ALL-BFM 95. *Blood* 111:4477, 2008.
62. Chessells JM, Hall E, Prentice HG, et al: The impact of age on outcome in lymphoblastic leukemia; MRC UKALL X and XA compared: A report from the MRC Paediatric and Adult Working Parties. *Leukemia* 12:463, 1998.
63. Hoelzer DF: Diagnosis and treatment of adult acute lymphoblastic leukemia, in *Neoplastic Diseases of the Blood*, 3rd ed, edited by PH Wiernik, GP Canellos, JP Dutcher, RA Kyle, p 295. Churchill Livingstone, New York, 1996.
64. Larson RA, Dodge RK, Burns CP, et al: A five-drug remission induction regimen with intensive consolidation for adults with acute lymphoblastic leukemia: Cancer and Leukemia Group B study 8811. *Blood* 85:2025, 1995.
65. Dinarello CA, Bunn PA Jr: Fever. *Semin Oncol* 24:288, 1997.
66. Pui C-H, Stass S, Green A: Bone marrow necrosis in children with malignant disease. *Cancer* 56:1522, 1985.
67. Lowe EJ, Pui C-H, Hancock ML, et al: Early complications in children with acute lymphoblastic leukemia presenting with hyperleukocytosis. *Pediatr Blood Cancer* 45:10, 2005.
68. Anghelescu DL, Burgoyne LL, Liu T, et al: Clinical and diagnostic imaging predict anesthetic complications in children presenting with malignant mediastinal masses. *Paediatr Anaesth* 17:1090, 2007.
69. Hijiya N, Liu W, Sandlund JT, et al: Overt testicular disease at diagnosis of childhood acute lymphoblastic leukemia: Lack of therapeutic role of local irradiation. *Leukemia* 19:1399, 2005.
70. Brito-Babapulle F: The eosinophilias, including the idiopathic hypereosinophilic syndrome. *Br J Haematol* 121:203, 2003.
71. Huang MS, Hasserjian RP: Case 19-2004: A 12-year-od boy with fatigue and eosinophilia. *N Engl J Med* 350:2604, 2004.
72. Dubansky AS, Boyett JM, Falletta J, et al: Isolated thrombocytopenia in children with acute lymphoblastic leukemia: A rare event in a Pediatric Oncology Group study. *Pediatrics* 84:1068, 1989.
73. Beutler E: Platelet transfusions: The 20,000/microL trigger. *Blood* 81:1411, 1993.
74. Blatt J, Penchansky L, Horn M: Thrombocytosis as a presenting feature of acute lymphoblastic leukemia in childhood. *Am J Hematol* 31:46, 1989.
75. Hasle H, Heim S, Schroeder H, et al: Transient pancytopenia preceding acute lymphoblastic leukemia (pre-ALL). *Leukemia* 9:605, 1995.
76. Ribeiro RC, Pui CH: The clinical and biological correlates of coagulopathy in children with acute leukemia. *J Clin Oncol* 4:1212, 1986.
77. Pui C-H, Dodge RK, Dahl GV, et al: Serum lactic dehydrogenase level has prognostic value in childhood acute lymphoblastic leukemia. *Blood* 66:778, 1985.
78. Jones DP, Stapleton FB, Kalwinsky D, et al: Renal dysfunction and hyperuricemia at presentation and relapse of acute lymphoblastic leukemia. *Med Pediatr Oncol* 18:283, 1990.
79. Inukai T, Hirose K, Inaba T, et al: Hypercalcemia in childhood acute lymphoblastic leukemia: Frequent implication of parathyroid hormone-related peptide and E2A-HLF from translocation 17;19. *Leukemia* 21:288, 2007.
80. Liang R: How I treat and monitor viral hepatitis B infection in patients receiving intensive immunosuppressive therapies or undergoing hematopoietic stem cell transplantation. *Blood* 113:3147, 2009.
81. Welch JC, Lilleyman JS: Immunoglobulin concentrations in untreated lymphoblastic leukemia. *Pediatr Hematol Oncol* 12:545, 1995.
82. Pui CH, Mahmoud HH, Rivera GK, et al: Early intensification of intrathecal chemotherapy virtually eliminates central nervous system relapse in children with acute lymphoblastic leukemia. *Blood* 92:411, 1998.
83. Pui CH, Howard SC: Current management and challenges of malignant disease in the CNS in paediatric leukaemia. *Lancet Oncol* 9:257, 2008.
84. Gajjar A, Harrison PL, Sandlund JT, et al: Traumatic lumbar puncture at diagnosis adversely affects outcome in childhood acute lymphoblastic leukemia. *Blood* 96:3381, 2000.
85. Bürger B, Zimmermann M, Mann G, et al: Diagnostic cerebrospinal fluid examination in children with acute lymphoblastic leukemia: Significance of low leukocyte counts with blasts or traumatic lumbar puncture. *J Clin Oncol* 21:184, 2003.
86. Howard SC, Gajjar AJ, Cheng C, et al: Risk factors for traumatic and bloody lumbar puncture in children with acute lymphoblastic leukemia. *JAMA* 288:2001, 2002.
87. Béné MC, Bernier M, Castoldi G, et al: Impact of immunophenotyping on management of acute leukemias. *Haematologica* 84:1024, 1999.
88. Coustan-Smith E, Mullighan CG, Onciu M, et al: Early T-cell precursor leukaemia: A subtype of very high-risk acute lymphoblastic leukaemia. *Lancet Oncol* 10:147, 2009.
89. Pui CH, Rubnitz JE, Hancock ML, et al: Reappraisal of the clinical and biologic significance of myeloid-associated antigen expression in childhood acute lymphoblastic leukemia. *J Clin Oncol* 16:3768, 1998.
90. Rubnitz JE, Onciu M, Pounds S, et al: Acute mixed lineage leukemia in children: The experience of St. Jude Children's Research Hospital. *Blood* 113:5083, 2009.
91. Campana D: Minimal residual disease in acute lymphoblastic leukemia. *Semin Hematol* 46:100, 2009.
92. Meijerink JP, Den Boer ML, Pieters R: New genetic abnormalities and treatment response in acute lymphoblastic leukemia. *Semin Hematol* 46:16, 2009.
93. Moorman AV, Harrison CJ, Buck GA, et al: Karyotype is an independent prognostic factor in adult acute lymphoblastic leukemia (ALL): Analysis of cytogenetic data from patients treated on the Medical Research Council (MRC) UKALLXII/Eastern Cooperative Oncology Group (ECOG) 2993 trial. *Blood* 109:3189, 2007.
94. Pullarkat V, Slovak ML, Kopecky KJ, et al: Impact of cytogenetics on the outcome of adult acute lymphoblastic leukemia: Results of Southwest Oncology Group 9400 study. *Blood* 111:2563, 2008.
95. Synold TW, Relling MV, Boyett JM, et al: Blast cell methotrexate-polyglutamate accumulation *in vivo* differs by lineage, ploidy, and methotrexate dose in acute lymphoblastic leukemia. *J Clin Invest* 94:1996, 1994.
96. Kaspers GJ, Smets LA, Pieters R, et al: Favorable prognosis of hyperdiploid common acute lymphoblastic leukemia may be explained by sensitivity to antimetabolites and other drugs: Results of an *in vitro* study. *Blood* 85:751, 1995.
97. Ito C, Kumagai M, Manabe A, et al: Hyperdiploid acute lymphoblastic leukemia with 51 to 65 chromosomes: A distinct biological entity with a marked propensity to undergo apoptosis. *Blood* 93:315, 1999.
98. Nachman JB, Heerema NA, Sather H, et al: Outcome of treatment in children with hypodiploid acute lymphoblastic leukemia. *Blood* 110:1112, 2007.
99. Moorman AV, Richards SM, Robinson HM, et al: Prognosis of children with acute lymphoblastic leukemia (ALL) and intrachromosomal amplification of chromosome 21 (iAMP21). *Blood* 109:2327, 2007.
100. Paulsson K, Horvat A, Strömbeck B, et al: Mutations in FLT3, NRAS, KRAS, and PTPN11 are frequent and possibly mutually exclusive in high hyperdiploid childhood acute lymphoblastic leukemia. *Genes Chromosomes Cancer* 47:26, 2008.
101. Morely AA, Brisco MJ, Rice M, et al: Leukaemia presenting as marrow hypoplasia: Molecular detection of the leukaemic clone at the time of initial presentation. *Br J Haematol* 98:940, 1997.
102. McKenna RW, Washington LT, Aquino DB, et al: Immunophenotypic analysis of hematogones (B-lymphocyte precursors) in 662 consecutive bone marrow specimens by 4-color flow cytometry. *Blood* 98:2498, 2001.
103. Baskin JL, Pui CH, Reiss U, et al: Management of occlusion and thrombosis associated with long-term indwelling central venous catheters. *Lancet* 374:159, 2009.
104. Masson E, Synold TW, Relling MV, et al: Allopurinol inhibits *de novo* purine synthesis in lymphoblasts of children with acute lymphoblastic leukemia. *Leukemia* 10:56, 1996.
105. Pui C-H, Mahmoud HH, Wiley JM, et al: Recombinant urate oxidase for the prophylaxis or treatment of hyperuricemia in patients with leukaemia or lymphoma. *J Clin Oncol* 19:697, 2001.
106. Coiffier B, Altman A, Pui CH, et al: Guidelines for the management of pediatric and adult tumor lysis syndrome: An evidence-based review. *J Clin Oncol* 26:2767, 2008.

107. Nelson SC, Bruggers CS, Kurtzberg J, Friedman HS: Management of leukemic hyperleukocytosis with hydration, urinary alkalinization, allopurinol. Are cranial irradiation and invasive cytoreduction necessary? *Am J Pediatr Hematol Oncol* 15:351, 1993.
108. Patte C, Philip T, Rodary C, et al: High survival rate in advanced-stage B-cell lymphomas and leukemias without CNS involvement with a short intensive polychemotherapy: Results from the French Pediatric Oncology Society of a randomized trial of 216 children. *J Clin Oncol* 9:123, 1991.
109. Gardner A, Mattiuzzi G, Faderl S, et al: Randomized comparison of cooked and noncooked diets in patients undergoing remission induction therapy for acute myeloid leukemia. *J Clin Oncol* 26:5684, 2008.
110. Pui CH, Boyett JM, Hughes WT, et al: Human granulocyte colony-stimulating factor after induction chemotherapy in children with acute lymphoblastic leukemia. *N Engl J Med* 336:1781, 1997.
111. Larson RA, Dodge RK, Linker CA, et al: A randomized controlled trial of filgrastim during remission induction and consolidation chemotherapy for adults with acute lymphoblastic leukemia: CALGB study 9111. *Blood* 92:1556, 1998.
112. Relling MV, Boyett JM, Blanco JG, et al: Granulocyte-colony stimulating factor and the risk of secondary myeloid malignancy. *Blood* 101:3862, 2003.
113. Schrappe M, Zimmermann M, Möricke A, et al: Dexamethasone in induction can eliminate one third of all relapses in childhood acute lymphoblastic leukemia (ALL): Results of an international randomized trial in 3655 patients (Trial AIEOP-BFM ALL 2000) [abstract 7]. *Blood* 112(11):9, 2008.
114. Weinthal J, Frost JD, Briones G, Cairo MS: Successful *Pneumocystis carinii* pneumonia prophylaxis using aerosolized pentamidine in children with acute leukemia. *J Clin Oncol* 12:136, 1994.
115. Madden RM, Pui CH, Hughes WT, et al: Prophylaxis of *Pneumocystis carinii* pneumonia with atovaquone in children with leukemia. *Cancer* 109:1654, 2007.
116. Pui CH, Jackson CW, Chesney C, et al: Sequential changes in platelet function and coagulation in leukemic children treated with L-asparaginase, prednisone, vincristine. *J Clin Oncol* 1:380, 1983.
117. Heckman KD, Weiner GJ, Davis CS, et al: Randomized study of prophylactic platelet transfusion threshold during induction therapy for adult acute leukemia: 10,000/microL versus 20,000/microL. *J Clin Oncol* 15:1143, 1997.
118. Pieters R, Schrappe M, De Lorenzo P, et al: A treatment protocol for infants younger than 1 year with acute lymphoblastic leukaemia (Interfant-99): An observational study and a multicentre randomised trial. *Lancet* 370:240, 2007.
119. Gökbuget N, Hoelzer D: Treatment of adult acute lymphoblastic leukemia. *Semin Hematol* 46:64, 2009.
120. Rowe JM: Optimal management of adults with ALL. *Br J Haematol* 144:468, 2009.
121. Ottmann OG, Wassmann B, Pfeifer H, et al: Imatinib compared with chemotherapy as front-line treatment of elderly patients with Philadelphia chromosome-positive acute lymphoblastic leukemia (Ph+ALL). *Cancer* 109:2068, 2007.
122. Patte C, Auperin A, Michon J, et al: The Société Francaise d'Oncologie Pédiatrique LMB89 protocol: Highly effective multiagent chemotherapy tailored to the tumor burden and initial response in 561 unselected children with B-cell lymphomas and L3 leukemia. *Blood* 97:3370, 2001.
123. Cairo MS, Gerrard M, Sposto R, et al: Results of a randomized international study of high-risk central nervous system B non-Hodgkin lymphoma and B acute lymphoblastic leukemia in children and adolescents. *Blood* 109:2736, 2007.
124. Woessmann W, Seidemann K, Mann G, et al: The impact of the methotrexate administration schedule and dose in the treatment of children and adolescents with B-cell neoplasms: A report of the BFM Group Study NHL-BFM95. *Blood* 105:948, 2005.
125. Thomas DA, Faderl S, O'Brien S, et al: Chemoimmunotherapy with hyper-CVAD plus rituximab for the treatment of adult Burkitt and Burkitt-type lymphoma or acute lymphoblastic leukemia. *Cancer* 106:1569, 2006.
126. Oriol A, Ribera JM, Bergua J, et al: High-dose chemotherapy and immunotherapy in adult Burkitt lymphoma: Comparison of results in human immunodeficiency virus-infected and noninfected patients. *Cancer* 113:117, 2008.
127. Pui CH, Campana D: New definition of remission in childhood acute lymphoblastic leukemia. *Leukemia* 14:783, 2000.
128. Borowitz MJ, Devidas M, Hunger S, et al: Clinical significance of minimal residual disease in childhood acute lymphoblastic leukemia and its relationship to other prognostic factors: A Children's Oncology Group study. *Blood* 111:5477, 2008.
129. Bruggemann M, Raff T, Flohr T, et al: Clinical significance of minimal residual disease quantification in adult patients with standard-risk acute lymphoblastic leukemia. *Blood* 107:1116, 2006.
130. Holowiecki J, Krawczyk-Kulis M, Giebel S, et al: Status of minimal residual disease after induction predicts outcome in both standard and high-risk Ph-negative adult acute lymphoblastic leukaemia. The Polish Adult Leukemia Group ALL 4-2002 MRD study. *Br J Haematol* 142:227, 2008.
131. Gaynon PS, Trigg ME, Heerema NA, et al: Children's Cancer Group trials in childhood acute lymphoblastic leukemia: 1983–1995. *Leukemia* 14:2223, 2000.
132. Harms DO, Janka-Schaub GE: Co-operative study group for childhood acute lymphoblastic leukemia (COALL): Long-term follow-up trials 82, 85, 89 and 92. *Leukemia* 14:2234, 2000.
133. Liang DC, Hung IJ, Yang CP, et al: Unexpected mortality from the use of *E. coli* L-asparaginase during remission induction therapy for childhood acute lymphoblastic leukemia: A report from the Taiwan Pediatric Oncology Group. *Leukemia* 13:155, 1999.
134. Annino L, Vegna ML, Camera A, et al: Treatment of adult acute lymphoblastic leukemia (ALL): Long-term follow-up of the GIMEMA ALL 0288 randomized study. *Blood* 99:863, 2002.
135. Hallböök H, Simonsson B, Ahlgren T, et al: High-dose cytarabine in upfront therapy for adult patients with acute lymphoblastic leukaemia. *Br J Haematol* 118:748, 2002.
136. Takeuchi J, Kyo T, Naito K, et al: Induction therapy by frequent administration of doxorubicin with four other drugs, followed by intensive consolidation and maintenance therapy for adult acute lymphoblastic leukemia: The JALSG-ALL93 study. *Leukemia* 16:1259, 2002.
137. Bostrom BC, Sensel MR, Sather HN, et al: Dexamethasone versus prednisone and daily oral versus weekly intravenous mercaptopurine for patients with standard-risk acute lymphoblastic leukemia: A report from the Children's Cancer Group. *Blood* 101:3809, 2003.
138. Mitchell CD, Richards SM, Kinsey SE, et al: Benefit of dexamethasone compared with prednisolone for childhood acute lymphoblastic leukaemia: Results of the UK Medical Research Council ALL97 randomized trial. *Br J Haematol* 129:734, 2005.
139. Igarashi S, Manabe A, Ohara A, et al: No advantage of dexamethasone over prednisolone for the outcome of standard- and intermediate-risk childhood acute lymphoblastic leukemia in the Tokyo Children's Cancer Study Group L95-14 protocol. *J Clin Oncol* 23:6489, 2005.
140. Asselin BL, Whitin JC, Coppola DJ, et al: Comparative pharmacokinetic studies of three asparaginase preparations. *J Clin Oncol* 11:1780, 1993.
141. Duval M, Suciu S, Ferster A, et al: Comparison of *Escherichia coli*-asparaginase with *Erwinia*-asparaginase in the treatment of childhood lymphoid malignancies: Results of a randomized European Organisation for Research and Treatment of Cancer—Children's Leukemia Group phase 3 trial. *Blood* 99:2734, 2002.
142. Moghrabi A, Levy DE, Asselin B, et al: Results of the Dana-Farber Cancer Institute ALL Consortium Protocol 95-01 for children with acute lymphoblastic leukemia. *Blood* 109:896, 2007.
143. Vieira Pinheiro JP, Boos J: The best way to use asparaginase in childhood acute lymphatic leukaemia—Still to be defined? *Br J Haematol* 125:117, 2004.
144. Ahlke E, Nowak-Göttl U, Schulze-Westhoff P, et al: Dose reduction of asparaginase under pharmacokinetic and pharmacodynamic control during induction therapy in children with acute lymphoblastic leukaemia. *Br J Haematol* 96:675, 1997.
145. Hak LJ, Relling MV, Cheng C, et al: Asparaginase pharmacodynamics differ by formulation among children with newly diagnosed acute lymphoblastic leukemia. *Leukemia* 18:1072, 2004.
146. Silverman LB, Gelber RD, Dalton VK, et al: Improved outcome for children with acute lymphoblastic leukemia: Results of Dana-Farber Consortium Protocol 91-01. *Blood* 97:1211, 2001.
147. Douer D, Yampolsky H, Cohen LJ, et al: Pharmacodynamics and safety of intravenous pegaspargase during remission induction in adults aged 55 years or younger with newly diagnosed acute lymphoblastic leukemia. *Blood* 1009:2744, 2007.
148. Wetzler M, Sanford BL, Kurtzberg J, et al: Effective asparagine depletion with pegylated asparaginase results in improved outcomes in adult acute lymphoblastic leukemia: Cancer and Leukemia Group B Study 9511. *Blood* 109:4164, 2007.
149. Schrappe M, Reiter A, Ludwig WD, et al: Improved outcome in childhood acute lymphoblastic leukemia despite reduced use of anthracyclines and cranial radiotherapy: Results of trial ALL-BFM 90. German-Austrian-Swiss ALL-BFM Study Group. *Blood* 95:3310, 2000.
150. Evans WE, Relling MV, Rodman JH, et al: Conventional compared with individualized chemotherapy for childhood acute lymphoblastic leukemia. *N Engl J Med* 338:499, 1998.
151. Nachman JB, Sather HN, Sensel MG, et al: Augmented post-induction therapy for children with high-risk acute lymphoblastic leukemia and a slow response to initial therapy. *N Engl J Med* 338:1663, 1998.
152. Chessells JM, Bailey C, Richards SM: Intensification of treatment and survival in all children with lymphoblastic leukaemia: Results of UK Medical Research Council Trial UKALL X. Medical Research Council Working Party on Childhood Leukaemia. *Lancet* 345:143, 1995.
153. Pui CH, Sandlund JT, Pei D, et al: Improved outcome for children with acute lymphoblastic leukemia: Results of Total Therapy Study XIIIB at St. Jude Children's Research Hospital. *Blood* 104:2690, 2004.
154. Loh ML, Goldwasser MA, Silverman LB, et al: Prospective analysis of TEL/AML1-positive patients treated on Dana-Farber Cancer Institute Consortium Protocol 95-01. *Blood* 107:4508, 2006.
155. Pui CH, Sallan S, Relling MV, et al: International Childhood Acute Lymphoblastic Leukemia Workshop: Sausalito, CA, 30 November–1 December 2000. *Leukemia* 15:707, 2001.
156. Galpin AJ, Schuetz JD, Masson E, et al: Differences in folylpolyglutamate synthetase and dihydrofolate reductase expression in human B-lineage versus T-lineage leukemic lymphoblasts: Mechanisms for lineage differences in methotrexate polyglutamylation and cytotoxicity. *Mol Pharmacol* 52:155, 1997.
157. Kager L, Cheok M, Yang W, et al: Folate pathway gene expression differs in subtypes of acute lymphoblastic leukemia and influences methotrexate pharmacodynamics. *J Clin Invest* 115:110, 2005.
158. Ellison RR, Mick R, Cuttner J, et al: The effects of postinduction intensification treatment with cytarabine and daunorubicin in adult acute lymphocytic leukemia: A prospective randomized clinical trial by Cancer and Leukemia Group B. *J Clin Oncol* 9:2002, 1991.

159. Cassileth PA, Andersen JW, Bennett JM, et al: Adult acute lymphocytic leukemia: The Eastern Cooperative Oncology Group experience. *Leukemia* 6(Suppl 2):178, 1992.
160. Stryckmans P, deWitte TH, Marie JP, et al: Therapy of adult ALL: Overview of 2 successive EORTC studies: (ALL-2 & ALL-3). *Leukemia* 6(Suppl 2):199, 1992.
161. Gökbuget N, Hoelzer D, Arnold R, et al: Treatment of adult ALL according to protocols of the German Multicenter Study Group for Adult ALL (GMALL). *Hematol Oncol Clin North Am* 14:1307, 2000.
162. Kantarjian HM, Thomas D, O'Brien S, et al: Long-term follow-up results of hyperfractionated cyclophosphamide, vincristine, doxorubicin, and dexamethasone (Hyper-CVAD), or dose-intensive regimen, in adult acute lymphocytic leukemia. *Cancer* 101:2788, 2004.
163. Durrant IJ, Prentice HG, Richards SM: Intensification of treatment for adults with acute lymphoblastic leukaemia: Results of U.K. Medical Research Council randomized trial UKALL XA. Medical Research Council Working Party on Leukaemia in Adults. *Br J Haematol* 99:84, 1997.
164. Hoelzer D, Gökbuget N: New approaches in acute lymphoblastic leukemia in adults: Where do we go? *Semin Oncol* 27:540, 2000.
165. Ludwig WD, Rieder H, Bartram CR, et al: Immunophenotypic and genotypic features, clinical characteristics, and treatment outcome of adult pro-B acute lymphoblastic leukemia: Results of the German multicenter trials GMALL 03/87 and 04/89. *Blood* 92:1898, 1998.
165a. Storring JM, Minden MD, Kao S, et al: Treatment of adults with BCR-ABL negative acute lymphoblastic leukaemia with a modified paediatric regimen. *Br J Harmol* 146:76, 2009.
166. Riehm H, Gadner H, Henze G, et al: Results and significance of six randomized trials in four consecutive ALL-BFM studies. *Haematol Blood Transfus* 33:439, 1990.
167. Cuttner J, Mick R, Budman DR, et al: Phase III trial of brief intensive treatment of adult acute lymphocytic leukemia comparing daunorubicin and mitoxantrone: A CALGB study. *Leukemia* 5:425, 1991.
168. Toyoda Y, Manabe A, Tsuchida M, et al: Six months of maintenance chemotherapy after intensified treatment for acute lymphoblastic leukemia of childhood. *J Clin Oncol* 18:1508, 2000.
169. Childhood ALL Collaborative Group: Duration and intensity of maintenance chemotherapy in acute lymphoblastic leukaemia: Overview of 42 trials involving 12,000 randomised children. *Lancet* 347:1783, 1996.
170. Sather H, Miller D, Nesbit M, et al: Differences in prognosis for boys and girls with acute lymphoblastic leukaemia. *Lancet* 1:739, 1981.
171. The Medical Research Council's Working Party on Leukaemia in Childhood: Duration of chemotherapy-in-childhood acute lymphoblastic leukaemia. *Med Pediatr Oncol* 10:511, 1982.
172. Mandelli F, Annino L, Rotoli B: The GIMEMA ALL0183 trial: Analysis of 10-year follow-up. GIMEMA Cooperation Group, Italy. *Br J Haematol* 92:665, 1996.
173. Lennard L, Lilleyman JS, Van Loon J, Weinshilboum RM: Genetic variation in response to 6-mercaptopurine for childhood acute lymphoblastic leukaemia. *Lancet* 336:225, 1990.
174. Whitehead VM, Vuchich MJ, Lauer SJ, et al: Accumulation of high levels of methotrexate polyglutamates in lymphoblasts from children with hyperdiploid (greater than 50 chromosomes) B-lineage acute lymphoblastic leukemia: A Pediatric Oncology Group Study. *Blood* 80:1316, 1992.
175. Schmiegelow K, Schroder H, Gustafsson G, et al: Risk of relapse in childhood acute lymphoblastic leukemia is related to RBC methotrexate and mercaptopurine metabolites during maintenance chemotherapy. Nordic Society for Pediatric Hematology and Oncology. *J Clin Oncol* 13:345, 1995.
176. Chessells JM, Harrison G, Lilleyman JS, et al: Continuing (maintenance) therapy in lymphoblastic leukaemia: Lessons from MRC UKALL X. Medical Research Council Working Party in Childhood Leukaemia. *Br J Haematol* 98:945, 1997.
177. Relling MV, Hancock ML, Boyett JM, et al: Prognostic importance of 6-mercaptopurine dose intensity in acute lymphoblastic leukemia. *Blood* 93:2817, 1999.
178. Schmiegelow K, Glomstein A, Kristinsson J, et al: Impact of morning versus evening schedule for oral methotrexate and 6-mercaptopurine on relapse risk for children with acute lymphoblastic leukemia. Nordic Society for Pediatric Hematology and Oncology (NOPHO). *J Pediatr Hematol Oncol* 19:102, 1997.
179. Rivard GE, Lin KT, Leclerc JM, David M: Milk could decrease the bioavailability of 6-mercaptopurine. *Am J Pediatr Hematol Oncol* 11:402, 1989.
180. Lancaster D, Lennard L, Lilleyman JS: Profile of non-compliance in lymphoblastic leukaemia. *Arch Dis Child* 76:365, 1997.
181. Mahoney DH, Shuster J, Nitschke R, et al: Intermediate-dose intravenous methotrexate with intravenous mercaptopurine is superior to repetitive low-dose oral methotrexate with intravenous mercaptopurine for children with lower-risk B-lineage acute lymphoblastic leukemia: A Pediatric Oncology Group Phase III trial. *J Clin Oncol* 16:246, 1998.
182. Vilmer E, Suciu S, Ferster A, et al: Long-term results of three randomized trials (58831, 58832, 58881) in childhood acute lymphoblastic leukemia: A CLCG-EORTC report. Children Leukemia Cooperative Group. *Leukemia* 14:2257, 2000.
183. Kamps WA, Bökkerink JP, Hakvoort-Cammel FG, et al: BFM-oriented treatment for children with acute lymphoblastic leukemia without cranial irradiation and treatment reduction for standard risk patients: Results of DCLSG protocol ALL-8 (1991–1996). *Leukemia* 16:1099, 2002.
184. Farrow AC, Buchanan GR, Zwiener RJ, et al: Serum aminotransferase elevation during and following treatment of childhood acute lymphoblastic leukemia. *J Clin Oncol* 15:1560, 1997.
185. Evans WE, Horner M, Chu YQ, et al: Altered mercaptopurine metabolism, toxic effects, and dosage requirement in a thiopurine methyltransferase-deficient child with acute lymphocytic leukemia. *J Pediatr* 119:985, 1991.
186. Relling MV, Hancock ML, Rivera GK, et al: Mercaptopurine therapy intolerance and heterozygosity at the thiopurine S-methyltransferase gene locus. *J Natl Cancer Inst* 91:2001, 1999.
187. Pui CH, Relling MV: Topoisomerase II inhibitor-related acute myeloid leukaemia. *Br J Haematol* 109:13, 2000.
187a. Schmiegelow K, Al-Modhwahi I, Andersen MK, et al: Methotrexate/6-mercaptopurine maintenance therapy influences the risk of a second malignant neoplasm after childhood acute lymphoblastic leukemia: Results from the NOPHOALL-92 study. *Blood* 113:6077, 2009.
188. Relling MV, Rubnitz JE, Rivera GK, et al: High incidence of secondary brain tumours after radiotherapy and antimetabolites. *Lancet* 354:34, 1999.
189. Yates CR, Krynetski EY, Loennechen T, et al: Molecular diagnosis of thiopurine S-methyltransferase deficiency: Genetic basis for azathioprine and mercaptopurine intolerance. *Ann Intern Med* 126:608, 1997.
190. Relling MV, Dervieux T: Pharmacogenetics and cancer therapy. *Nat Rev Cancer* 1:99, 2001.
191. Evans WE, Relling MV: Moving towards individualized medicine with pharmacogenomics. *Nature* 429:464, 2004.
192. Jacobs SS, Stork LC, Bostrom BC, et al: Substitution of oral and intravenous thioguanine for mercaptopurine in a treatment regimen for children with standard risk acute lymphoblastic leukemia: A collaborative children's oncology group/national cancer institute pilot trial (CCG-1942). *Pediatr Blood Cancer* 49:250, 2007.
193. Harms DO, Gobel U, Spaar HJ, et al: Thioguanine offers no advantage over mercaptopurine in maintenance treatment of childhood ALL: Results of the randomized trial COALL-92. *Blood* 102:2736, 2003.
194. Stork LC, Sather H, Hutchinson RJ, et al: Comparison of mercaptopurine (MP) with thioguanine (TG) and IT methotrexate (ITM) with IT "triples" (ITT) in children with SR-ALL: Results of CCG-1952. *Blood* 100:156a, 2002.
195. Vora A, Mitchell CD, Lennard L, et al: Toxicity and efficacy of 6-thioguanine versus 6-mercaptopurine in childhood lymphoblastic leukaemia: A randomised trial. *Lancet* 368:1339, 2006.
196. Lennard L, Richards S, Cartwright CS, et al: The thiopurine methyltransferase genetic polymorphism is associated with thioguanine-related veno-occlusive disease of the liver in children with acute lymphoblastic leukemia. *Clin Pharmacol Ther* 80:375, 2006.
197. Conter V, Valsecchi MG, Silvestri D, et al: Pulses of vincristine and dexamethasone in addition to intensive chemotherapy for children with intermediate-risk acute lymphoblastic leukemia: A multicentre randomized trial. *Lancet* 369:123, 2007.
198. Lange BJ, Bostrom BC, Cherlow JM, et al: Double-delayed intensification improves event-free survival for children with intermediate-risk acute lymphoblastic leukemia: A report from the Children's Cancer Group. *Blood* 99:825, 2002.
199. Vilmer E, Suciu S, Ferster A, et al: Long-term results of three randomized trials (58831, 58832, 58881) in childhood acute lymphoblastic leukemia: A CLCG-EORTC report. *Leukemia* 14:2257, 2000.
200. Manera R, Ramirez I, Mullins J, Pinkel D: Pilot studies of species-specific chemotherapy of childhood acute lymphoblastic leukemia using genotype and immunophenotype. *Leukemia* 14:1354, 2000.
201. Conter V, Schrappe M, Aric M, et al: Role of cranial radiotherapy for childhood T-cell acute lymphoblastic leukemia with high WBC count and good response to prednisone. Associazione Italiana Ematalogia Oncologia Pediatrica and the Berlin-Frankfurt-Munster groups. *J Clin Oncol* 15:2786, 1997.
202. Pui CH, Campana D, Pei D, et al: Treating childhood acute lymphoblastic leukemia without prophylactic cranial irradiation. *N Engl J Med* 360:2730, 2009.
202a. Veerman AJ, Kamps WA, ven den Berg H, et al: Dexamethasone-based therapy for childhood acute lymphoblastic leukaemia: Results of the prospective Dutch Childhood Oncology Group (DCOG) protocol ALL-9 (1997–2004). *Lancet Oncol* 10:957, 2009.
203. Matloub Y, Lindemulder S, Gaynon PS, et al: Intrathecal triple therapy decreases central nervous system relapse but fails to improve event-free survival when compared to intrathecal methotrexate: Results of the Children's Cancer Group (CCG) 1952 study for standard-risk acute lymphoblastic leukemia. A report from the Children's Oncology Group. *Blood* 108:1165, 2006.
204. Howard SC, Gajjar AJ, Cheng C, et al: Risk factors for traumatic lumbar puncture in children with acute lymphoblastic leukemia. *JAMA* 288:2001, 2002.
205. Hunault M, Harousseau JL, Delain M, et al: Better outcome of adult acute lymphoblastic leukemia after early genoidentical allogeneic bone marrow transplantation (BMT) than after late high-dose therapy and autologous BMT: A GOELAMS trial. *Blood* 104:3028, 2004.
206. Thomas X, Boiron JM, Huguet F, et al: Outcome of treatment in adults with acute lymphoblastic leukemia: Analysis of the LALA-94 trial. *J Clin Oncol* 22:4075, 2004.
207. Kiehl MG, Kraut L, Schwerdtfeger R, et al: Outcome of allogeneic hematopoietic stem-cell transplantation in adult patients with acute lymphoblastic leukemia: No difference in related compared with unrelated transplant in first complete remission. *J Clin Oncol* 22:2816, 2004.
208. Rowe JM, Buck G, Burnett AK, et al: Induction therapy for adults with acute lymphoblastic leukemia: Result of more than 1500 patients from the international ALL trial: MRC UKALL XII/RCOG E2993. *Blood* 106:3760, 2005.
209. Mark DJ, Perez WS, He W, et al: Unrelated donor transplants in adults with Philadelphia-negative acute lymphoblastic leukemia in first complete remission. *Blood* 112:426, 2008.

210. Aricò M, Valsecchi MG, Camitta B, et al: Outcome of treatment in children with Philadelphia chromosome-positive acute lymphoblastic leukemia. *N Engl J Med* 342:998, 2000.
211. Arico M, Schrappe M, Hunger S, et al: Clinical outcome of 640 children with newly diagnosed Philadelphia chromosome-positive acute lymphoblastic leukemia treated between 1995 and 2005 [abstract 568]. *Blood* 112:213, 2008.
212. Schultz KR, Bowman WP, Aledo A, et al: Improved early event free survival with imatinib in Philadelphia chromosome-positive acute lymphoblastic leukemia: A Children's Oncology Group Study. *J Clin Oncol* 27:5715, 2009.
213. Pui CH, Gaynon PS, Boyett JM, et al: Outcome of treatment in childhood acute lymphoblastic leukaemia with rearrangements of the 11q23 chromosomal region. *Lancet* 359:1909, 2002.
213a. Bachanova V, Verneris MR, DeFor T, et al: Prolonged survival in adults with acute lymphoblastic leukemia after reduced-intensity conditioning with cord blood or sibling donor transplantation. *Blood* 113:2902, 2009.
214. Ribera JM, Oriol A, Bethencourt C, et al: Comparison of intensive chemotherapy, allogeneic or autologous stem cell transplantation as post-remission treatment for adult patients with high-risk actue lymphoblastic leukemia. Results of the PETHEMA ALL-93 trial. *Haematologica* 90:1346, 2005.
215. Ottmann OG, Wassmann B, Pfeifer H, et al: Imatinib compared with chemotherapy as front-line treatment of elderly patients with Philadelphia chromosome-positive acute lymphoblastic leukemia (Ph+ALL). *Cancer* 109:2068, 2007.
216. Vignetti M, Fazi P, Cimino G, et al: Imatinib plus steroids induces complete remissions and prolonged survival in elderly Philadelphia chromosome-positive acute lymphoblastic leukemia patients without additional chemotherapy: Results of the GIMEMA LAL0201-B protocol. *Blood* 109:3676, 2007.
217. Thomas DA, Faderl S, Cortes J, et al: Treatment of Philadelphia chromosome-positive acute lymphocytic leukemia with hyper-CVAD and imatinib mesylate. *Blood* 103:4396, 2004.
218. Yanada M, Takeuchi J, Sugiura I, et al: High complete remission rate and promising outcome by combination of imatinib and chemotherapy for newly diagnosed BCR-ABL-positive acute lymphoblastic leukemia: A phase II study by the Japan Adult Leukemia Study Group. *J Clin Oncol* 24:460, 2006.
219. Wassermann B, Pfeifer H, Stadler M, et al: Early molecular response to posttransplantation imatinin determines outcome in MRD+ Philadelphia-positive acute lymphoblastic leukemia (PH+ALL). *Blood* 106:458, 2005.
220. Pui CH, Jeha S: New therapeutic strategies for the treatment of acute lymphoblastic leukemia. *Nat Rev Drug Discov* 6:149, 2007.
221. Talpaz M, Shah NP, Kantarjian H, et al: Dasatinib in imatinib-resistant Philadelphia chromosome-positive Philadelphia chromosome-positive leukemias. *N Engl J Med* 354:2531, 2006.
222. Kantarjian H, Giles F, Wunderle L, et al: Nilotinib in imatinib-resistant CML and Philadelphia chromosome-positive ALL. *N Engl J Med* 354:2542, 2006.
223. Ravandi F, Thomas D, Kantarjian H, et al: Phase II Study of Combination of the HyperCVAD Regimen with Dasatinib in Patients with Philadelphia Chromosome (Ph) or BCR-ABL Positive Acute Lymphoblastic Leukemia (ALL) and Lymphoid Blast Phase Chronic Myeloid Leukemia (CML-LB). *Blood* 110:2814a, 2007.
224. Foa R, Vignetti M, Vitale A, et al: Dasatinib as Front-Line Monotherapy for the Induction Treatment of Adult and Elderly Ph+ Acute Lymphoblastic Leukemia (ALL) Patients: Interim Analysis of the GIMEMA Prospective Study LAL1205. *Blood* 110:7a, 2007.
225. Thomas DA, O'Brien S, Jorgensen JL, et al: Prognostic significance of CD20 expression in adults with de novo precursor B-lineage acute lymphoblastic leukemia. *Blood* 113:6330, 2009.
226. Jeha S, Behm F, Pei D, et al: Prognostic significance of CD20 expression in childhood B-cell precursor acute lymphoblastic leukemia. *Blood* 108:3302, 2006.
227. Thomas D, Kantarjian H, Faderl S, et al: Update of the Modified Hyper-CVAD Regimen with or without Rituximab as Frontline Therapy of Adults with Acute Lymphocytic Leukemia (ALL) or Lymphoblastic Lymphoma (LL). *Blood* 110:2824a, 2007.
228. Gökbuget N, Hoelzer D: Rituximab in the treatment of adult ALL. *Ann Hematol* 85:117, 2006.
229. Ravandi F, Gandhi V: Novel purine nucleoside analogues for T-cell-lineage acute lymphoblastic leukaemia and lymphoma. *Expert Opin Investig Drugs* 15:1601, 2006.
230. Vora A, Frost L, Goodeve A, et al: Late relapsing childhood lymphoblastic leukemia. *Blood* 92:2334, 1998.
231. Konrad M, Metzler M, Panzer S, et al: Late relapses evolve from slow-responding subclones in t(12;21)-positive acute lymphoblastic leukemia: Evidence for the persistence of a preleukemic clone. *Blood* 101:3635, 2003.
232. Mullighan GC, Phillips LA, Su X, et al: Genomic analysis of the clonal origins of relapsed acute lymphoblastic leukemia. *Science* 322:1377, 2008.
233. Rivera GK, Zhou Y, Hancock ML, et al: Bone marrow recurrence after initial intensive treatment for childhood acute lymphoblastic leukemia. *Cancer* 103:368, 2005.
234. Chessells JM, Veys P, Kempski H, et al: Long-term follow-up of relapsed childhood acute lymphoblastic leukaemia. *Br J Haematol* 123:396, 2003.
235. Nguyen K, Devidas M, Cheng SC, et al: Factors influencing survival after relapse from acute lymphoblastic leukemia: A Children's Oncology Group study. *Leukemia* 22:2142, 2008.
236. Coustan-Smith E, Gajjar A, Hijiya N, et al: Clinical significance of minimal residual disease in childhood acute lymphoblastic leukemia. *Leukemia* 18:499, 2004.
237. Paganin M, Zecca M, Fabbri G, et al: Minimal residual disease is an important predictive factor of outcome in children with relapsed "high-risk" acute lymphoblastic leukemia. *Leukemia* 22:2193, 2008.
238. Peters C, Schraduer A, Schrappe M, et al: Allogeneic haematopoietic stem cell transplantation in children with acute lymphoblastic leukemia: The BFM/IBFM/EBMT concepts. *Bone Marrow Transplant* 35(Suppl 1):S9, 2005.
239. Doney K, Hagglund H, Leisenring W, et al: Predictive factors for outcome of allogeneic hematopoietic cell transplantation for adult acute lymphoblastic leukemia. *Biol Blood Marrow Transplant* 9:472, 2003.
240. Fielding AK, Richards SM, Lazarus HM et al: Does imatinib change the outcome in Philadelphia chromosome positive acute lymphoblastic leukaemia in adult? Data from the UKALLXII/ECOG2993 study [abstract 8]. *Blood* 110:10a, 2007.
241. Borgmann A, Schmid H, Hartmann R, et al: Autologous bone-marrow transplants compared with chemotherapy for children with acute lymphoblastic leukaemia in a second remission: A matched-pair analysis. The Berlin-Frankfurt-Munster Study Group. *Lancet* 346:873, 1995.
242. Weisdorf DJ, Billett AL, Hannan P, et al: Autologous versus unrelated donor allogeneic marrow transplantation for acute lymphoblastic leukemia. *Blood* 90:2962, 1997.
243. Laughlin MJ, Eapen M, Rubinstein P, et al: Outcomes after transplantation of cord blood or bone marrow from unrelated donors in adults with leukemia. *N Engl J Med* 351:2265, 2004.
244. Rocha V, Labopin M, Sanz G, et al: Transplants of umbilical-cord blood or bone marrow from unrelated donors in adults with acute leukemia. *N Engl J Med* 351:2276, 2004.
245. Borgmann A, von Stackelberg A, Hartmann R, et al: Unrelated donor stem cell transplantation compared with chemotherapy for children with acute lymphoblastic leukemia in a second remission: A matched-pair analysis. *Blood* 101:3835, 2003.
246. Leung W, Iyengar R, Turner V, et al: Determinants of antileukemia effects of allogeneic NK cells. *J Immunol* 172:644, 2004.
247. Triplett B, Handgretinger R, Pui CH, Leung W: KIR-incompatible hematopoietic-cell transplantation for poor prognosis infant acute lymphoblastic leukemia. *Blood* 107:1238, 2006.
248. Bosi A, Laszlo D, Labopin M, et al: Second allogeneic bone marrow transplantation in acute leukemia: Results of a survey by the European Cooperative Group for Blood and Marrow Transplantation. *J Clin Oncol* 19:3675, 2001.
249. Hagedorn N, Acquaviva C, Fronkova E, et al: Submicroscopic bone marrow involvement in isolated extramedullary relapses in childhood acute lymphoblastic leukemia: A more precise definition of "isolated" and its possible clinical implications, a collaborative study of the Resistant Disease Committee of the international BFM study group. *Blood* 110:4022, 2007.
250. Ribeiro RC, Rivera GK, Hudson M, et al: An intensive re-treatment protocol for children with an isolated CNS relapse of acute lymphoblastic leukemia. *J Clin Oncol* 13:333, 1995.
251. Ritchey AK, Pollock BH, Lauer SJ, et al: Improved survival of children with isolated CNS relapse of acute lymphoblastic leukemia: A Pediatric Oncology Group study. *J Clin Oncol* 17:3745, 1999.
252. Barredo J, Devidas M, Lauer SJ, et al: Isolated CNS relapse of acute lymphoblastic leukemia treated with intensive systemic chemotherapy and delayed CNS radiation: A Pediatric Oncology Group study. *J Clin Oncol* 24:3142, 2006.
253. Weisdorf DJ, Billett AL, Hannan P, et al: Autologous versus unrelated donor allogeneic marrow transplantation for acute lymphoblastic leukemia. *Blood* 90:2962, 1997.
254. Messina C, Valsecchi MG, Aricò M, et al: Autologous bone marrow transplantation for treatment of isolated central nervous system relapse of childhood acute lymphoblastic leukemia. *Bone Marrow Transplant* 21:9, 1998.
255. Buchanan GR, Boyett JM, Pollock BH, et al: Improved treatment results in boys with overt testicular relapse during or shortly after initial therapy for acute lymphoblastic leukemia: A Pediatric Oncology Group study. *Cancer* 68:48, 1991.
256. Wofford MM, Smith SD, Shuster JJ, et al: Treatment of occult or late overt testicular relapse in children with acute lymphoblastic leukemia: A Pediatric Oncology Group study. *J Clin Oncol* 10:624, 1992.
257. Finklestein JZ, Miller DR, Feusner J, et al: Treatment of overt isolated testicular relapse in children on therapy for acute lymphoblastic leukemia. A report from the Children's Cancer Group. *Cancer* 73:219, 1994.
258. Grundy RG, Leiper AD, Stanhope R, Chessells JM: Survival and endocrine outcome after testicular relapse in acute lymphoblastic leukaemia. *Arch Dis Child* 76:190, 1997.
259. van den Berg H, Langeveld NE, Veenhof CH, Behrendt H: Treatment of isolated testicular recurrence of acute lymphoblastic leukemia without radiotherapy. Report from the Dutch Late Effects Study Group. *Cancer* 79:2257, 1997.
260. Ravandi F, Faderl S, Kebriaei P, Kantarjian H: Modern treatment programs for adults with acute lymphoblastic leukemia. *Curr Hematol Malig Rep* 2:169, 2007.
261. Roberson JR, Raju S, Shelso J, et al: Diabetic Ketoacidosis during therapy for childhood acute lymphoblastic leukemia. *Pediatr Blood Cancer* 50:1207, 2008.
262. Pui CH, Burghen GA, Bowman WP, Aur RJA: Risk factors for hyperglycemia in children with leukemia receiving L-asparaginase and prednisone. *J Pediatr* 99:46, 1981.
263. Pui CH, Chesney CM, Weed J, Jackson CW: Altered von Willebrand factor molecule in children with thrombosis following asparaginase-prednisone-vincristine therapy for leukemia. *J Clin Oncol* 3:1266, 1985.
264. Laningham FH, Kun LE, Reddick, et al: Childhood central nervous system leukemia: Historical perspectives, current therapy, and acute neurological sequelae. *Neuroradiology* 49:873, 2007.

265. Waber D, Carpentieri SC, Klar N, et al: Cognitive sequelae in children treated for acute lymphoblastic leukemia with dexamethasone or prednisone. *J Pediatr Hematol Oncol* 22:206, 2000.
266. Kadan-Lottick NS, Dinu I, Wasilewski-Masker K, et al: Osteonecrosis in adult survivors of childhood cancer: A report from the childhood cancer survivor study. *J Clin Oncol* 26:3038, 2008.
267. Rai SN, Hudson MM, McCammon E, et al: Implementing an intervention to improve bone mineral density in survivors of childhood acute lymphoblastic leukemia: BONEII, a prospective placebo-controlled double-blind randomized interventional longitudinal study design. *Contemp Clin Trials* 29:711, 2008.
268. Thomas IH, Donohue JE, Ness KK, et al: Bone mineral density in your adult survivors of acute lymphoblastic leukemia. *Cancer* 113:3248, 2008.
269. Mandel K, Atkinson S, Barr RD, Pencharz P: Skeletal morbidity in childhood acute lymphoblastic leukemia. *J Clin Oncol* 22:1215, 2004.
270. Grenier MA, Lipshultz SE: Epidemiology of anthracycline cardiotoxicity in children and adults. *Semin Oncol* 25:72, 1998.
271. Levitt GA, Dorup I, Sorensen K, Sullivan I: Does anthracycline administration by infusion in children affect late cardiotoxicity? *Br J Haematol* 124:463, 2004.
272. Nysom K, Holm K, Lipsitz SR, et al: Relationship between cumulative anthracycline dose and late cardiotoxicity in childhood acute lymphoblastic leukemia. *J Clin Oncol* 16:545, 1998.
273. Lipshultz S, Lipsitz SR, Sallan SE, et al: Chronic progressive cardiac dysfunction years after doxorubicin therapy for acute lymphoblastic leukemia. *J Clin Oncol* 23:2629, 2005.
274. Lipshultz SE, Rifai N, Dalton VM, et al: The effect of dexrazoxane on myocardial injury in doxorubicin-treated children with acute lymphoblastic leukemia. *N Engl J Med* 351:145, 2004.
275. Oeffinger KC, Mertesn AC, Sklar CA, et al: Chronic health conditions in adult survivors of childhood cancer. *N Engl J Med* 355:1572, 2006.
276. Pui CH, Cheng C, Leung W, et al: Extended follow-up of long-term survivors of childhood acute lymphoblastic leukemia. *N Engl J Med* 349:640, 2003.
277. Hijiya N, Hudson MM, Lensing S, et al: Cumulative incidence of secondary neoplasms as a first event after childhood acute lymphoblastic leukemia. *JAMA* 297:1207, 2007.
278. Geenen MM, Cardous-Ubbink MC, Kremer LCM, et al: Medical assessment of adverse health outcomes in long-term survivors of childhood cancer. 297:2705, 2007.
279. Waber DP, Turek J, Catania L, et al: Neuropsychological outcomes from a randomized trial of triple intrathecal chemotherapy compared with 18 Gy cranial radiation as CNS treatment in acute lymphoblastic leukemia: Findings from Dana-Farber Cancer Institute ALL Consortium Protocol 95–01. *J Clin Oncol* 25:4914, 2007.
280. Leung W, Rose SR, Zhou Y, et al: Outcomes of growth hormone replacement therapy in survivors of childhood acute lymphoblastic leukemia. *J Clin Oncol* 20:2959, 2002.
281. Walter AW, Hancock ML, Pui CH, et al: Secondary brain tumors in children treated for acute lymphoblastic leukemia at St. Jude Children's Research Hospital. *J Clin Oncol* 16:3761, 1998.
282. Pui CH, Ribeiro RC, Hancock ML, et al: Acute myeloid leukemia in children treated with epipodophyllotoxins for acute lymphoblastic leukemia. *N Engl J Med* 325:1682, 1991.
283. Hawkins MM, Draper GJ, Winter DL: Cancer in the offspring of survivors of childhood leukaemia and non-Hodgkin lymphomas. *Br J Cancer* 71:1335, 1995.
284. Kenney LB, Nicholson HS, Brasseux C, et al: Birth defects in offspring of adult survivors of childhood acute lymphoblastic leukemia. A Children's Cancer Group/National Institutes of Health Report. *Cancer* 78:169, 1996.
285. Sankila R, Olsen JH, Anderson H, et al: Risk of cancer among offspring of childhood-cancer survivors. Association of the Nordic Cancer Registries and the Nordic Society of Paediatric Haematology and Oncology. *N Engl J Med* 338:1339, 1998.
286. Smith M, Arthur D, Camitta B, et al: Uniform approach to risk classification and treatment assignment for children with acute lymphoblastic leukemia. *J Clin Oncol* 14:18, 1996.
287. Larson RA: Management of acute leukemia in older patients. *Semin Hematol* 43:126, 2006.
288. Bhatia S, Sather HN, Heerema NA, et al: Racial and ethnic differences in survival of children with acute lymphoblastic leukemia. *Blood* 100:1957, 2002.
289. Kadan-Lottick NS, Ness KK, Bhatia S, Gurney JG: Survival variability by race and ethnicity in childhood acute lymphoblastic leukemia. *JAMA* 290:2008, 2003.
290. Pui CH, Sandlund JT, Pei D, et al: Results of therapy for acute lymphoblastic leukemia in black and white children. *JAMA* 290:2001, 2003.
290a. Breit S, Stanulla M, Flohr T, et al: Activating *NOTCH1* mutations predict favorable early treatment response and long-term outcome in childhood precursor T-cell lymphoblastic leukemia. *Blood* 108:1151, 2009.
290b. Asnafi V, Buzyn A, Le NS, et al: *NOTCH1/FBXW7* mutation identifies a large subgroup with favorable outcome in adult T-cell acute lymphoblastic leukemia (T-ALL): A Group for Research on Adult Acute Lymphoblastic Leukemia (GRAALL) study. *Blood* 113:3918, 2009.
291. Bruggemann M, Raff T, Flohr T, et al: Clinical significance of minimal residual disease quantification in adult patients with standard-risk acute lymphoblastic leukemia. *Blood* 107:1116, 2006.
292. Raff T, Gokbuget N, Luschen S, et al: Molecular relapse in adult standard-risk ALL patients detected by prospective MRD monitoring during and after maintenance treatment: Data from the GMALL 06/99 and 07/03 trials. *Blood* 109:910, 2007.
293. Bader P, Kreyenberg H, Henze GHR, et al: Prognostic value of minimal residual disease quantification before allogeneic stem-cell transplantation in relapsed childhood acute lymphoblastic leukemia: The ALL-REZ BFM Study Group. *J Clin Oncol* 27:377, 2008.
294. Coustan-Smith E, Sancho J, Hancock ML, et al: Use of peripheral blood instead of bone marrow to monitor residual disease in children with acute lymphoblastic leukemia. *Blood* 100:2399, 2002.
295. Faderl S, Jeha S, Kantarjian HM: The biology and therapy of adult acute lymphoblastic leukemia. *Cancer* 98:1337, 2003.
296. Mrózek K, Heerema NA, Bloomfield CD: Cytogenetics in acute leukemia. *Blood Rev* 18:115, 2004.

CHAPTER 94
CHRONIC LYMPHOCYTIC LEUKEMIA AND RELATED DISEASES

Thomas J. Kipps

SUMMARY

Chronic lymphocytic leukemia (CLL) is a neoplastic disease characterized by the accumulation of a monoclonal population of small, mature-appearing CD5+ B lymphocytes in the blood, marrow, and lymphoid tissues. The causes of this disease are unknown, although genetic factors have been found to play a role. The median age of onset is approximately 67 years and men are affected twice as often as women. Lymphadenopathy occurs in approximately 80 percent and splenomegaly in approximately 50 percent of patients at the time of diagnosis. The leukemic cells from most CLL patients have clonal chromosomal abnormalities, of which del 13q14-23.1 is the most common, followed in frequency by trisomy 12, del 11q22.3-q23.1, del 6q21-q23, del 17p13.1, and 14q abnormalities. There is a wide variation in the rate of clinical progression. Many patients are asymptomatic at the time of diagnosis and are observed without treatment until they develop symptoms or evidence of disease progression. Chlorambucil and prednisone had been the mainstay of treatment for approximately 45 years. Deoxyadenosine analogues, such as fludarabine; newer alkylating agents, such as bendamustine; and monoclonal antibodies, notably alemtuzumab and rituximab, alone or in combination with purine analogues, alkylating agents, or glucocorticoids, have improved treatment response rates. Nonmyeloablative hematopoietic stem cell transplantation can be used selectively for some patients and experimental immune-gene therapy may be available in the future. The advanced age of most patients and associated comorbidities requires careful analysis to ensure that therapy will likely provide a net benefit to the patient. Prolymphocytic leukemia is the involvement of blood and marrow with a less-mature-appearing clonal population of lymphocytes, most of which have a lymphoblast appearance. The immune phenotype may be that of a B cell or, less frequently, a T cell. The disease is more aggressive than CLL. Rearrangements and mutations in the ataxia-telangiectasia mutated gene and in T-cell leukemia-1 and related genes apparently contribute to the pathogenesis of T-cell prolymphocytic leukemia. Approximately one-third of patients have erythroderma. Treatment with deoxyadenosine analogues can be effective in a subset of patients with this disease. Investigation into the use of new agents, stem cell transplantation, and/or monoclonal antibodies, such as alemtuzumab, is ongoing, as there are no established cures for T-cell prolymphocytic leukemia.

Acronyms and abbreviations that appear in this chapter include: ATM gene, ataxia-telangiectasia mutated gene; BCL-1, B-cell leukemia 1; β_2M, β_2-microglobulin; CAP, cyclophosphamide, doxorubicin, and prednisone without vincristine; CCP, cladribine in combination with cyclophosphamide and prednisone; CHOP, cyclophosphamide, doxorubicin, vincristine, and prednisone; CLL, chronic lymphocytic leukemia; CR, complete remission; CRi, complete remission with incomplete resolution of cytopenias; CVP, cyclophosphamide, vincristine, and prednisone; DiSC, differential staining cytotoxicity; FC, fludarabine, cyclophosphamide; FCR, fludarabine, cyclophosphamide, and rituximab; FDA, U.S. Food and Drug Administration; FISH, fluorescence *in situ* hybridization; GFR, glomerular filtration rate; GM-CSF, granulocyte-macrophage colony-stimulating factor; HCV, type C hepatitis virus; HTLV-I, human T-cell lymphotropic virus type I; Ig, immunoglobulin; IgHV, immunoglobulin heavy chain variable region; IV, intravenous; LDT, lymphocyte doubling time; Mcl-1, myeloid cell leukemia-1; MRD, minimal residual disease; nPR, nodular partial remission; OR, overall response; PCR, polymerase chain reaction; PCR regimen, chemotherapy regimen using pentostatin, cyclophosphamide, and rituximab; PLL, prolymphocytic leukemia; PR, partial remission; SDF-1, stromal derived factor-1 alpha; SMZL, splenic marginal zone lymphoma; TGF-β, transforming growth factor beta; TK, thymidine kinase; TNF-α, tumor necrosis factor alpha; YAC, yeast artificial chromosome.

DEFINITION AND HISTORY

Chronic lymphocytic leukemia (CLL) is a neoplastic disease characterized by the accumulation of small, mature-appearing lymphocytes in the blood, marrow, and lymphoid tissues. The first descriptions of patients with CLL were published in the early nineteenth century.[1–3] In the 1840s, Virchow described two forms of chronic leukemia that probably correspond to CLL and chronic myelogenous leukemia.[3–5] Patients with the former were noted to have mild-to-moderate splenic enlargement, lymphadenopathy, and large numbers of small agranular cells in the blood that resembled those found in enlarged lymph nodes.[4] Virchow considered this type of leukemia to be principally related to disease of the lymph nodes rather than of the spleen. In 1893, Kundrat introduced the term *lymphosarcoma* to describe an indolent disease that affected lymph nodes.[6] Histochemical staining techniques introduced by Ehrlich at the turn of the twentieth century[7] made it possible for pathologists to distinguish between myeloid and lymphocytic leukemias. These methods enabled Türk in 1903 to establish a relationship of the leukemic cells in CLL to those in lymphosarcoma.[8] He proposed the term *lymphomatoses* to describe several lymphoproliferative disorders, including CLL. Owing to its indolent nature, CLL was considered a "benign" lymphomatosis.

In 1924, Minot and Isaacs described the natural history of 98 patients with CLL,[9] challenging the notion that CLL was a "benign" process. These investigators noted that although gamma radiation could reduce lymph node enlargement or splenomegaly, it apparently did not prolong survival. Radioactive phosphorus later was found effective in reducing lymph node size.[10] However, this approach also was noted to be of limited therapeutic value because of its marrow toxicity and its inability to reverse disease-related cytopenias or to improve survival.[10] In 1954, Tivey found a median survival among 585 patients with CLL of approximately 3 years from onset of symptoms.[11] Soon thereafter, alkylating agents,[12] and later glucocorticoids,[13] were found to be effective therapy for CLL. These agents became the mainstays of treatment.

In 1967, Dameshek hypothesized that CLL was an accumulative disease of immunologically incompetent lymphocytes.[14] In the early 1970s, the leukemic cells from most cases of CLL were found to express surface immunoglobulin, indicating that the neoplastic cells were of B-cell origin.[15] Subsequent studies demonstrated that the CLL cells of female patients who were heterozygous for glucose-6-phosphate dehydrogenase (G6PD) expressed only one G6PD allele,[16] indicating that the leukemia cells arose from a single B-cell clone. Consistent with this notion, the CLL cells from any one patient were found to express only one type of immunoglobulin light chain[17] and idiotype,[18–20] indicating their uniformity in the expression of immunoglobulin, consistent with clonal expansion of cells.

Rai and colleagues introduced a clinical staging system for patients with CLL in 1975,[21] delineating the adverse implication of anemia or thrombocytopenia on patient survival. In 1999, it was recognized that patients with leukemia cells that express unmutated immunoglobulin variable region genes in general have more aggressive disease than do patients whose leukemia cells use mutated antibody genes.[22,23] Nevertheless, gene expression analyses revealed that the leukemia cells of patients with CLL share a common distinctive gene expression profile regardless of immunoglobulin mutation status and that only a handful of genes were differentially expressed between these two subtypes.[24,25]

In the late 1980s, purine analogues, such as fludarabine or 2-chlorodeoxyadenosine (cladribine), were found to be effective in the treatment of CLL. The United States Food and Drug Administration (FDA) approved alemtuzumab (campath-1H) for treatment of patients with refractory disease in 2001 and for initial therapy in 2007, and approved bendamustine hydrochloride for use in the treatment of CLL in 2008. In the fall of 2009, the FDA approved ofatumumab (Arzerra) for treatment of patients with disease refractory to fludarabine and alemtuzumab. New treatment modalities are being examined, including passive or active immunotherapy or nonmyeloablative chemotherapy with marrow transplantation, as the disease still is not considered curable with current monoclonal antibody or chemotherapy.

EPIDEMIOLOGY

CLL has an average incidence of 2.7 persons per 100,000 in the United States. Its incidence ranges from <1 to 5.5 per 100,000 people worldwide.[26,27] The risk of developing CLL increases progressively with age and is 2.8 times higher for older men than for older women.[28] Because of its relative indolence, this disease accounts for approximately 0.8 percent of all cancers and nearly 30 percent of all leukemias at any point in time. It is the most prevalent adult leukemia in Western societies. Generally, the neoplastic lymphocytes are of the B-cell lineage. In less than 2 percent of cases, however, the neoplastic cells are of T-cell origin and are included in the category T-cell prolymphocytic leukemia.

The incidence of CLL in men is twice that of women.[29,30] One retrospective study of women noted a trend toward reduced risk of this leukemia with increasing parity, prompting speculation that pregnancy lowers the risk for CLL.[31] Also, for unknown reasons female patients tend to have a longer survival than male patients.[32–35] However, hormones have not been demonstrated to play any role in the development or progression of this disease. Moreover, the use of hormone replacement therapy for postmenopausal symptoms in women does not apparently influence the relative risk for developing CLL.[36]

Genetic factors apparently contribute to the development of CLL. Although CLL is the most common adult leukemia in Western societies, it is relatively rare in Asia. In Korea, the estimated incidence of this disease is only 1.5 percent of that in the United States.[37] Similarly, CLL is relatively uncommon in China and rare in Japan[38–40]; it accounts for less than 6 percent of all leukemias in Japan.[41] A very low incidence of B-cell CLL is noted even among Japanese immigrants to the United States.[38,42] Likewise, the incidence of CLL in Israel is significantly higher among European immigrants than among those from Africa or Asia.[43]

ETIOLOGY AND PATHOGENESIS

ENVIRONMENTAL FACTORS

No single environmental risk factor has been found to be predictive for CLL. One study noted an increase in CLL in some rural communities, suggesting that environmental agent(s) associated with farming may play a role.[44] Also, a few studies have noted an increase in CLL among persons chronically exposed to electromagnetic fields.[45–47] Another study found an increased incidence in CLL among persons exposed to agent orange.[48] However, other studies have not found an association between the incidence of CLL and exposure to pesticides, sunlight, or known carcinogens.[49–52]

Studies of Japanese atom bomb survivors found increased incidence of leukemias such as chronic myelogenous leukemia (see Chap. 90),[53] but not CLL, which is an uncommon leukemia among persons of Japanese ancestry (see "Epidemiology" on this page). The view that ionizing radiation did not increase the incidence of CLL was supported by subsequent limited studies on persons exposed to ionizing radiation.[54,55] However, more epidemiologic data on populations that have a higher incidence of CLL than the Japanese suggest that exposure to ionizing radiation may increase the risk for disease development, albeit to a lesser extent than that noted for other leukemias.[56] Another study lacking a comparator cohort suggested that there was an increased incidence of aggressive CLL among Ukrainian survivors of the Chernobyl nuclear power plant accident in 1986.[57] However, another report on the 15-country nuclear workers cohort study found little evidence for an associated between exposure to low amounts of external radiation and CLL mortality.[58] Nevertheless, these accounts have challenged the long held view that ionizing radiation does not contribute to the development of CLL.[59]

Some studies found a relatively high prevalence of infection with type C hepatitis virus (HCV) in patients with CLL compared with that of the general population,[60–62] suggesting a possible pathogenic role. However, CLL has been found prevalent in certain populations that have a negligible incidence of HCV infection[63] and patients may develop CLL who do not have any trace of having been exposed to HCV,[64] indicating that infection with HCV is not necessary for development of leukemia. CLL cells are resistant to infection with Epstein-Barr virus, except in unusual cases,[65] making it appear unlikely that Epstein-Barr virus plays a pathogenic role.

HEREDITARY FACTORS

Although most cases of CLL are sporadic, multiple cases of leukemia may be found within a single family. There are numerous reports of families with multiple members having CLL.[66–72] First-degree relatives of patients with CLL are more than three times at risk for having this disorder or other lymphoid malignancies than is the general population.[69] Afflicted individuals within such families often present at a younger age than patients with sporadic CLL, suggesting that genetic factors in familial CLL may contribute to early leukemogenesis.[73,74]

The familial risk for CLL also might be found associated with other indolent lymphoproliferative disorders. For example, first-degree relatives of patients with lymphoplasmacytic lymphoma or Waldenström macroglobulinemia (see Chap. 111) have a greater than threefold risk of developing CLL.[75]

The genetic factors that contribute to the increased incidence of CLL in certain families are unknown. One study noted that the leukemic cells of affected family members oftentimes expressed immunoglobulin heavy-chain variable region genes (IgHV) of the same immunoglobulin heavy chain variable-region gene subgroup.[76] However, each patient's leukemia cells have distinctive IgHV rearrangements,[70,76] even those of monozygous twins,[77] indicating that they originate from disparate somatic events. Studies have associated the risk of developing aggressive CLL with polymorphisms in the gene encoding CD5 (located at 11q13),[78] CD38 (located at 4p15),[79,80] or tumor necrosis factor alpha (TNF-α) (located at 6p21.3),[81] and a gene(s) mapping to 13q21.33-q22.2.[82] Although an early study found no apparent association between human leukocyte antigen (HLA) haplotype and disease susceptibility,[83] other studies have identified certain HLA haplotypes that are more common among patients with CLL than in matched control populations.[84] Moreover, a genome-wide linkage analyses of 206 families with familial CLL for single nucleotide polymorphisms associated with susceptibility for CLL identified disease-risk loci at 6p22.1 (corresponding to the HLA locus), as well as at 2q21.2, and 18q21.1.[85] Another genome-wide association study identified CLL risk loci at 2q13, 2q37.1, 6p25.3, 11q24.1, 15q23, and 19q13.32,[86] while yet another study found disease-susceptibility associated with single nucleotide polymorphisms in or around genes encoding proteins involved in apoptosis or immune regulatory pathways, namely *CCNH* (located at 5q13.3), *APAF1* (located at 12q23), *IL16* (located at 15q26.3), *CASP8* (located at 2q33.1), *NOS2A* (located at 17q11.1), and *CCR7* (located at 17q21.2).[87]

CYTOGENESIS

The leukemic cells of most patients express pan–B-cell surface antigens, such as CD19 and CD20 (see Chap. 15), indicating that they are derived from the B-lymphocyte lineage (see Chap. 76). The level at which the CD20 antigen typically is expressed, however, is substantially lower than that found on normal circulating B cells.[88,89] CLL B cells also express CD27,[90] a member of the tumor-necrosis factor receptor family that also is most commonly expressed on memory B cells.[91]

Studies using gene microarray analyses have provided evidence for the notion that CLL cells are derived from antigen-experienced, memory-type B cells.[92] Indeed, regardless of whether CLL cells use unmutated or mutated immunoglobulin genes, they share common expression levels of many genes and have gene expression profiles that are distinct from that of other B-cell malignancies or normal, nonmalignant adult blood B cells, or even neonatal core blood B cells that also coexpress CD5.[24,25] Furthermore, the gene expression patterns observed in CLL appear to be most compatible with that of antigen-experienced, nonnaïve B cells typically found within the marginal zone of the spleen.[25] Studies performed in mice made transgenic for the immunoglobulin genes that frequently are expressed in CLL suggest that certain immunoglobulins may drive differentiation of B cells into cells that can populate the splenic marginal zone.[93] Coupled with the noted restriction in the repertoire of immunoglobulins expressed in this disease,[94] there is mounting evidence that implicate the antigen-experienced, memory-type B cell as the normal, nonmalignant counterpart to the CLL B cell.

IMMUNOGLOBULIN EXPRESSION

The leukemic cells from over 90 percent of patients express low levels of monoclonal surface immunoglobulin with either κ or λ light chains. Sixty percent of cases express κ light chains, while the other 40 percent express λ light chains.[95–97] Of the heavy-chain isotypes, over half of all cases have surface immunoglobulin (Ig) M and IgD (55 percent), a quarter have IgM exclusive of IgD, and approximately 7 percent have immunoglobulin isotypes other than IgM or IgD (usually IgG or IgA). Less than 5 percent of cases express IgD without detectable IgM. Both IgM and IgM/IgD expressing CLL frequently express cross-reactive idiotypes (see Chap. 77) that commonly are found on IgM autoantibodies.[98]

The immunoglobulins expressed in B-cell CLL often have reactivity for self-antigens, most notably for the constant region of human IgG.[99] An important feature of these autoantibodies is their "polyreactivity," or binding activity for two or more seemingly disparate self-antigens. Because of this, several investigators have used the term *natural autoantibodies* to describe these autoantibodies. Such polyreactivity is a characteristic of some antibodies produced by early immature B cells,[100] which subsequently are deleted or experience further immunoglobulin gene rearrangements and/or mutation. Despite their apparent lack of specificity, such autoantibodies are dependent upon selected immunoglobulin gene rearrangements and nonstochastic pairing of immunoglobulin heavy and light chains,[101–103] indicating that polyreactivity is a selected binding specificity.

The immunoglobulin expressed by CLL B cells may play a role in leukemogenesis.[104–106] For example, an allele of *IGHV1–69*, called 51p1, is expressed at high frequency and without somatic mutation in CLL[107] (see Chap. 77). Moreover, CLL B cells that express 51p1 have restricted use of certain amino acid sequences within the third complementarity determining region that are not commonly observed in nonmalignant B cells, including normal B cells that use the 51p1 allele of *IGHV1–69*[108–110] (see Chap. 77). This restriction is not a feature of polyreactive antibodies *per se* or of antibodies expressed by B cells during fetal development.[102,111] Furthermore, there is nonrandom pairing between certain immunoglobulin heavy chains and light chains encoded by particular immunoglobulin light chain variable regions. One striking example of this restriction is the noted pairing between immunoglobulin heavy chains encoded by *IGHV1–69*, D3–16, and J_H3, with light chains encoded by one κ light chain variable region gene, designated A27, which is expressed by leukemia cells of approximately 1.3 percent of all patients with CLL.[112] Moreover, the immunoglobulin light chain expressed by CLL cells expressing virtually identical heavy chain variable regions appears predicated by the sequence of the immunoglobulin heavy chain third complementarity determining region (HCDR3).[113,114] The restricted use of immunoglobulins by the leukemia B cells and nonstochastic pairing of immunoglobulin light and heavy chains in this disease argues strongly that there is selection in this disease for expression of immunoglobulins with a certain binding activity, conceivably for some self or ubiquitous environmental antigen(s). Because immunoglobulins constitute an important receptor governing the proliferation, survival or death of B cells (see Chaps. 76 and 77), it is conceivable that the immunoglobulins expressed in CLL play a critical role in the early expansion or survival of the nascent leukemia cell clone.

MONOCLONAL B-CELL LYMPHOCYTOSIS

Studies using sensitive flow cytometry have found populations of B cells with the phenotype of CLL cells in the blood of healthy individuals (see Chap. 81).[115] These cells coexpress CD5 and CD19, and have low-level expression CD20 and CD79b (see Chap. 15). Evaluation of first-degree relatives of CLL patients revealed that 14 percent (8 of 59) of healthy individuals with two or more affected family members had circulating B cells with these "CLL–B-cell" characteristics.[116] Moreover, high-sensitivity flow cytometry techniques have allowed for identification of monoclonal or oligoclonal B-cell populations of various phenotypes in more than 5 to 12 percent of healthy individuals older than age 60 years, independent of whether they have lymphocytosis.[115,117]

Termed *monoclonal B-cell lymphocytosis*,[118] this condition may portend development of CLL, especially in individuals with CLL-phenotype monoclonal B-cell lymphocytosis. Such clonal expansions of B cells appear more frequently in men than in women (with a male-to-female ratio of nearly 2:1) and are more common in people ages 60 to 89 years than in younger adults. Because these demographics correspond to the noted predominance of CLL in men and the aged, there is speculation that these clonal B-cell expansions represent cell populations that potentially could evolve into CLL. Indeed, longitudinal studies suggest that patients with CLL-phenotype monoclonal B-cell lymphocytosis may develop frank CLL that eventually will require treatment at the rate of approximately 1.1 percent per year.[115] This condition might be to CLL as essential monoclonal gammopathy is to myeloma, in that each year a comparable proportion of patients with essential monoclonal gammopathy may develop frank plasma cell myeloma (see Chaps. 108 and 109).

ANIMAL MODELS OF CLL

There are several mouse models in which the animals spontaneously develop disease similar to human CLL.[119] For example, mice made transgenic for the human *TCL1* gene under the control of a tissue-specific μ immunoglobulin enhancer (Eμ-TCL1) develop clonal B-cell expansions that are similar to those observed in patients with monoclonal B-cell lymphocytosis.[120] These animals develop detectable clonal expansions of CD5+ B-cell populations in the peritoneum at about 2 to 4 months of age that become evident in the spleen by 5 months of age and then in the marrow by 6 to 8 months of age. Elder mice eventually develop a CLL-like disease in the blood at 8 to 12 months of age, each animal developing a monoclonal outgrowth of B cells that share many features in common with those human CLL B cells, including the coexpression of CD5 and pan-B surface antigens and low-level expression of surface immunoglobulin.[120,121] These cells infiltrate the blood and secondary lymphoid tissues, causing lymphocytosis, splenomegaly, and lymphadenopathy. The pathology of involved lymph nodes appears similar to that of patients with CLL. Similarly, transgenic mice with B cells that overexpress human *BCL-2* and a mutant tumor necrosis factor (TNF) receptor-associated factor (TRAF2) also develop a lymphoproliferative disease that resembles CLL.[122]

Studies indicate that the clonal expansions of B cells that express high-levels of *TCL1* undergo high rates of leukemia cell turnover, which might permit generation of secondary and tertiary mutations that could factor in the pathogenesis of frank leukemia.[123] When these animals were mated with other transgenic mice that express high levels of a B-cell survival factor, namely B-cell activating factor belonging to the TNF family (BAFF or CD257), the progeny expressed high levels of both *TCL1* and CD257 and developed a CLL-like disease at an accelerated rate.[123] The rapid development of leukemia in these animals supports the notion that the leukemia cells in these animals might experience high rates of spontaneous cell death, which can conceal relatively high rates of leukemia cell proliferation (see "Leukemia Cell Accumulation: Growth Kinetics" on page 1436).

Mice made transgenic for *TCL1* using different tissue-specific promoters/enhancers develop other types of lymphoid malignancies.[124,125] Overexpression of the *TCL1* gene *per se* does not cause CLL. Rather, overexpression of *TCL1* by B cells at particular stages of development, combined with other factors, such as stimulation via surface immunoglobulin receptors and/or secondary mutations, appear required for development of a monoclonal B-cell leukemia that resembles CLL.

Finally, another important animal model posited to represent human CLL is that of New Zealand Black (NZB)[126] strain.[119] Aged mice of this strain can develop clonal expansions of B cells that share many features in common with CLL B cells. A genome-wide linkage search of the NZB loci associated with the propensity to develop such B-cell clonal expansions identified three loci on mouse chromosomes 14, 18, and 19.[127] Particularly noteworthy was the locus identified on chromosome 14, which has apparent orthology with human 13q14 that is deleted in approximately half of all case of human CLL (see "Cytogenetic Abnormalities: Chromosome 13 Anomalies" on this page). Moreover, this locus was found to contain the gene encoding the mouse counterpart for human microRNA16–1 (*miR16–1*), for which NZB mice have a genetic polymorphism that results in the production of relatively low amounts of this microRNA in lymphoid tissues. The finding that this genetic polymorphism is associated with the propensity to develop CD5 B-cell clonal expansions in this mouse model provides strong support for the model developed from the analyses of the genetic lesions in human CLL. This model posits that altered expression microRNAs, such as *miR16–1*, is a molecular lesion that plays an important role in the pathogenesis and possible progression of CLL (see "Cytogenetic Abnormalities" at the top of this page).

CYTOGENETIC ABNORMALITIES

Detection of chromosomal abnormalities initially was hampered by the inability to induce leukemic cell proliferation. These cells generally do not grow spontaneously in cell culture and are much more refractory to activation by mitogens or to transformation by Epstein-Barr virus than normal B cells.[14,128] The normal karyotypes noted in some samples could reflect an outgrowth of normal bystander lymphocytes.

Using Q-banding and/or G-banding techniques (see Chap. 11), and improved methods for inducing leukemia cell proliferation *in vitro*, the leukemic cells from more than half of all CLL patients are found to have clonal chromosomal abnormalities.[129–132] Interphase cytogenetics using fluorescence *in situ* hybridization (FISH) has increased the sensitivity for detecting translocations, deletions, or chromosome trisomy.[133–135] Using these techniques, del 13q14-23.1 is the most common chromosomal abnormality in CLL, followed in order by trisomy 12, del 11q22.3-q23.1, del 6q21-q23, deletions at 17p13.1 typically involving deletions/mutations of the *TP53* (also known as *P53*) tumor-suppressor gene,[134,136,137] and 14q abnormalities. Deletions or duplications account for most of the observed genetic defects, as chromosomal translocations are not commonly observed in CLL in the absence of *ex vivo* stimulation.[138] New techniques including use of comparative genomic hybridization, amplotyping by arbitrarily primed polymerase chain reaction, or microsatellite allelotyping may be combined with FISH for detecting additional genetic abnormalities in CLL.[139,140]

Chromosome 13 Anomalies

Deletions in the long arm of chromosome 13 are the most common genetic abnormality in CLL, occurring in approximately half of all CLL cases. These deletions generally occur in the absence of detectable chromosome translocations. Nevertheless, those CLL cells with translocations often are noted to have ones involving the long arm of chromosome 13 with any one of several different chromosomes.[141] Because these translocations generally result in deletions at 13q14, deletions at 13q14 appear to be the contributing genetic lesion, rather than the translocation *per se*.

Deletions in the long arm of chromosome 13 typically occur at 13q14.3 in a region that is telomeric to the retinoblastoma gene *RB1* and centromeric to and including the D13S25 marker.[142–146] There are several genes in this region, designated *DLEU1*, *DLEU2*, *RFP2*, *KCNRG*, *DLEU6*, *DLEU7*, and *DLEU8*.[147,148] A highly conserved alternative first exon of the *LEU2* gene, which originates within a G+C region in the vicinity of the D13S272 marker, gives rise to a transcript encoding a new member of the ras superfamily, designated *ARLTS1*, for adenosine diphosphate (ADP)-ribosylation factor-like tumor-suppressor gene 1.[147] This gene may function like a tumor-suppressor gene in CLL, as well as in other types of cancer, such as those involving the colon or breast.

Also found in this region are genes encoding microRNA (miR genes), namely *miR15* and *miR16–1*.[149] These miR genes belong to a large family of highly conserved noncoding genes scattered throughout the genome that play important roles in development, autoimmune disease, and cancer.[150–152] miRs are transcribed as short hairpin precursors (approximately 70 nucleotides) and are processed into active 21- to 22-nucleotide RNAs by Dicer, a ribonuclease that recognizes target messenger RNAs via base-pairing interactions. These active miRNA in turn can inhibit gene expression, by either causing the degradation or blocking the translation of target messenger RNA, and thereby regulate gene expression in development and disease.

Detailed deletion and expression analysis revealed that *miR15* and *miR16–1* are located within a 30-kb region of loss in CLL, and that both genes are deleted or downregulated in the majority (approximately 68%) of CLL cases.[149] Loss of *miR15* and/or *miR16–1* might contribute to leukemogenesis and account for the frequent deletions that are observed at 13q14.3 in CLL. These microRNAs were the first to be discovered to play a role in the development of cancer.

Chromosome 12 Anomalies

Approximately 20 percent of all patients have CLL cells with trisomy 12, either as the sole genetic abnormality or in combination with other chromosomal abnormalities.[153–155] The leukemia cells with trisomy 12 have duplicated one chromosome 12, while retaining the other homologue.[156] It appears that this genetic lesion is not recessive, as would be the case for the loss of a tumor suppressor gene, but rather provides for a gene dosage effect. More studies on partial trisomy 12 are consistent with this notion, suggesting that trisomy 12 reflects a gene dosage effect of some genes located between 12q13 and 12q22.[153] Leukemia cells with trisomy 12 tend to have a higher frequency of DNA aneuploidy and to express higher levels of CD19, CD20, CD22, CD24, CD25, CD27, CD79b, CD38, surface Ig, and lower levels of CD43, relative to CLL cells lacking trisomy 12, even though the genes encoding many of these surface proteins are not located on chromosome 12 (see Chap. 15).[135,157–160]

Trisomy 12 often is detected in only a subset of the leukemia cells from any one patient.[161,162] Trisomy 12 may not be detectable at diagnosis but is more commonly seen in the leukemia cells of patients with advanced disease or Richter transformation.[129,163–165] Finally, studies suggest that the leukemia cell subset with trisomy 12 may expand during disease progression.[142] Collectively, these studies suggest that trisomy 12 may not a primary factor in leukemogenesis, but is acquired during disease evolution.

Chromosome 11 Anomalies

Approximately 20 percent of patients may have leukemia cells with deletions detectable by FISH in the long arm of chromosome 11, termed *11q–*.[166–168] Array comparative genomic hybridization may detect additional cases that have deletions in the long arm of chromosome 11.[169] Patients with 11q– tend to be younger in age (less than 55 years) and to have more aggressive disease and a greater tendency for developing bulky cervical lymphadenopathy than patients without such genetic changes.[167,170] Furthermore, CLL cells with 11q– have been noted to have higher expression levels of CD38, FMC7, CD25, and surface immunoglobulin, and lower level expression of CD11a/CD18, CD11c/CD18, CD31, CD48, and CD58 than do CLL cells that lack 11q–, arguing that such cells may have a distinctive biology.[159,171] One gene array study comparing CLL cells that have 11q– with CLL cells lacking this deletion found differential expression of nearly 30 genes, with 11q– cases having significant overexpression of *ATF5* and underexpression of *CDC16*, *PCDH8*, *SLAM*, *MNDA*, and *ATF2*, relative to cases without 11q–.[172] Finally, cases with 11q– have distinct microRNA signatures and characteristic low-level expression of *miR-29* and *miR-181*, two microRNAs that appear to downregulate expression of the important protooncogene *TCL1* implicated in the pathogenesis of CLL.[173]

Deletions on chromosome 11 commonly cluster between 11q14–24, particularly at 11q22.3-q23.1, in a region defined by yeast artificial chromosome (YAC) clones 801e11, 975h6, and 755b11.[166,167] An important gene found within this region is *ATM*, for ataxia-telangiectasia mutated. Upon DNA damage, the normal gene product of *ATM* plays an important role in the activation of the tumor-suppressor gene-product *P53*, which induces cell-cycle arrest and DNA repair or cell death,[174] and is required for leukemia cell sensitivity to many anticancer drugs commonly used in the treatment of CLL (e.g., chlorambucil or fludarabine monophosphate). The ATM gene can be found lost through deletion or mutation in leukemia cells of patients with relatively aggressive disease that is resistant to many standard therapies.[166,167,175–178] Some CLL patients carry one defective copy of this gene in the germ-line DNA, suggesting that mutations in ATM may be involved in the pathogenesis of aggressive CLL.[176,179] However, more studies implicate that genes other than ATM might be involved in the pathogenesis of cases harboring the 11q– cytogenetic abnormality.

Chromosome 6 Anomalies

Another recurring chromosome abnormality involves the short arm of chromosome 6, but the genes altered have not been identified.[143,180,181] The abnormalities on chromosome 6 typically involve deletions at 6q23, but can also involve deletions at 6q25–27 and/or 6q21.[182–186] Patients with abnormalities between 6q21 and 6q24 generally have higher proportions of blood prolymphocytes, higher than average expression of CD38, and more aggressive disease than patients with normal cytogenetics or isolated deletions at 13q14.3.[187]

The leukemia cells of several patients have been found to harbor deletions in the long arm of chromosome 6 at 6p24–25, which also have been associated with atypical leukemia cell morphology.[188] However, the frequency of such deletions appears much less than that of deletions in and around 6q23.

Chromosome 17 Anomalies

Interphase FISH can detect deletions in the short arm of chromosome 17 at 17p13.1 in approximately 10 percent of all patients.[189] The critical gene in the region that typically is deleted is *TP53*. *TP53* encodes *P53*, a 53-kDa nuclear phosphoprotein that plays an important role in the induction of proteins responsible for cell-cycle arrest and apoptosis of cells damaged by genotoxic stress, such as that affected by ionizing radiation.[190] The leukemia cells harboring deletions at 17p13.1 often have allelic loss of *TP53* and/or single-base inactivating mutations in the highly conserved exons 5, 7, or 8 of the retained *TP53* allele.[191]

Patients who have CLL cells with 17p– and/or *TP53* mutations generally have more advanced disease, a higher leukemia-cell proliferative rate, a shorter survival, and greater resistance to first-line therapy.[192–196] Moreover, leukemia cell deletions and/or mutations of *TP53* constitute an independent marker for poor survival.[197] The proportions of leukemia cells that harbor deletions at 17p13.1 in any one patient may increase over time, particularly following treatment with alkylating agents or purine analogs (see "Therapeutic Agents" on page 1448).[198] Also, the neoplastic cells from nearly half of the patients with Richter transformation or B-cell prolymphocytic leukemia may have inactivating mutations in *TP53*.[198,199] It appears that *TP53* gene mutations are acquired in the course of the disease and result in leukemic cells that have enhanced resistance to standard anticancer drugs and ionizing radiation.[192]

Chromosome 14 Anomalies

Located on chromosome 14, at band 14q32, are the genes encoding the immunoglobulin heavy chain (see Chap. 77). This band is the site of translocations in B-cell malignancies, with breakpoints often occurring within or near the immunoglobulin heavy-chain J segment minigenes or the immunoglobulin heavy-chain isotype switch regions.[200] Band q11.2 of chromosome 14 also contains genes encoding the α chain and the δ chain of the human T-cell receptor (see Chap. 78). Leukemic cells with inversions of chromosome 14, inv[14] (q11q32), most often are derived from the T-cell lineage and express T-cell differentiation antigens.[201–203] These lesions are common in T-cell prolymphocytic leukemia. Translocations at either of these loci are postulated to reflect an aberrant immunoglobulin or T-cell receptor gene rearrangement that in turn activates a protooncogene located on the other chromosome involved in the translocation.

t(14;18) Rarely, the leukemic cells in B-cell CLL can have t(14;18) translocations that more commonly are found in low-grade nodular

B-cell lymphomas (see Chap. 101).[204–207] This translocation juxtaposes the immunoglobulin heavy chain genes with *BCL-2*.

t(14;19)(q32;q13.1) Although an initial report of t(14;19) translocations in CLL found this translocation in 3 of 30 cases,[208] cytogenetic analyses of 4487 patients with indolent lymphoproliferative diseases, including those with CLL, revealed only six cases to have t(14;19).[209] Only 23 CLL cases have been reported to have t(14;19) to date. Such translocations generally involve the isotype switch regions of IgA on chromosome 14 and result in increased transcription of BCL-3, a gene near the breakpoint on chromosome 19 that encodes a protein of the I-κB family of transcription factors.[209,210] There is a striking association of t(14;19) with trisomy 12. The presence of this and other CLL-associated features argues that patients with t(14;19) do not have a lymphoproliferative disease distinct from that of CLL. Rather, t(14;19) may be an acquired cytogenetic abnormality that occurs during the evolution of preexisting CLL.

t(11;14)(q13;q32) Translocations involving chromosome 14, at band 14q32, and chromosome 11, at band 11q13, or t(11;14)(q13;q32) first were described in CLL.[211–214] The translocation juxtaposes the heavy-chain immunoglobulin genes with a protooncogene, designated *BCL-1*, for B-cell leukemia 1,[214,215] which subsequently was identified as *PRAD1*, a gene encoding cyclin D_1.[216,217] Overexpression of PRAD1 can contribute to cell transformation[218] and may play a role in the development of some cases of B-cell CLL.[218] However, among lymphoid malignancies, the highest incidence of t(11;14) and/or PRAD1 overexpression is noted in mantle zone cell lymphoma.[219–223] Because the neoplastic B cells of mantle cell lymphoma can share many phenotypic features with the leukemic B cells in CLL (see Chaps. 92 and 102), cases of CLL that previously were thought to have t(11;14)(q13;q32) instead may have represented the leukemic phase of mantle cell lymphoma.[221,222,224–226]

Chromosome 18 Anomalies

Approximately 5 percent of CLL patients may have leukemic cells that have aberrant immunoglobulin gene rearrangements with the *BCL-2* located on the long arm of chromosome 18, at 18q21.[204,205,227] In contrast to *BCL-2* gene rearrangements in nodular B-cell lymphomas, the rearrangements in B-cell CLL generally occur at breakpoints in the 5′ end of the *BCL-2* gene and involve the κ or λ immunoglobulin light-chain genes on chromosomes 2 or 22, respectively.[227] Independent of *BCL-2* gene rearrangement, however, the leukemic cells from nearly all patients with B-cell CLL express high levels of the bcl-2 protein that are comparable to that noted for lymphoma cells carrying the t(14;18)(q32;q21) translocation.[228,229] This is associated with hypomethylation of the *BCL-2* locus.[230] Using pulse-field gel electrophoresis to examine for *BCL-2* gene rearrangements in DNA fragments of 50,000 to 10,000 kilobases, one study found that each of nine CLL cases had somatic rearrangements that would not have been detected by conventional techniques.[231] This suggests that there might be previously undetected genetic abnormalities in CLL involving chromosome 18 that could account in part for the high-level expression of the *BCL-2* in such cases.

LEUKEMIA CELL ACCUMULATION

Growth Kinetics

In the spleen, proliferation of CLL cells apparently occurs preferentially in the white pulp zones, even in cases in which both the white and red pulp are extensively infiltrated.[232] However, CLL cells in the blood incorporate extremely low amounts of ^{3}H-thymidine *in vitro*[233] and are mainly in the G_0 stage of the cell cycle, as assessed by flow cytometry.[234] Because most CLL cells are not proliferating, the life span of CLL lymphocytes appears long. Consistent with this, human CLL B cells can survive for many weeks after transfer into mice with severe combined immune deficiency.[235] Studies on patients who ingested heavy water to evaluate the growth kinetics of CLL cells *in vivo*, however, revealed that the leukemic cells of each patient had birth rates ranging from 0.1 percent to greater than 1.0 percent of the entire clone per day.[236] Such high leukemia-cell birth rates were noted even in patients with apparently stable blood lymphocyte counts. This conflicts with the notion that CLL is a static disease. Instead it suggests that the blood lymphocyte count for any one patient is defined by a more dynamic process, in which leukemia cells are generated and die at appreciable rates.

"Proliferation Centers"

The lymph nodes of patients with CLL characteristically are diffusely infiltrated with monomorphic, small, round lymphocytes that efface the normal node architecture. There can be small clusters of prolymphocyte–appearing cells that form aggregates called "proliferation centers" or "pseudofollicles" that are scattered through the lymph node. The cells in such pseudofollicles appear distinctive in that they express relatively high levels of CD20 and other B-cell surface antigens.[237] One study failed to find leukemia cells with the distinctive surface antigen phenotype of "proliferation-center" B cells in the blood of patients with CLL.[238] The abundance of such proliferation centers varies between the lymph nodes of different patients.[239] However, the relative number of such "pseudofollicles" does not have a clear relationship with the extent of lymphocytosis, stage, prior treatment history, or tendency toward progression.[238–240]

Resistance to Apoptosis

CLL B cells express high levels of the antiapoptotic protein bcl-2.[241] In addition, the neoplastic B cells of patients with CLL also characteristically express high levels of other antiapoptotic proteins, such as bcl-x_L, mcl-1, and bag-1,[242] and low levels of the proapoptotic protein bax or bcl-x_s.[243] Bcl-2 and bax proteins form homodimers and heterodimers that influence the susceptibility to apoptosis.[244,245] Moreover, it appears that the relative ratio of bcl-2 and/or bcl-x_L to bax in leukemia cells is related to their resistance to drugs *in vitro*[246–249] and possibly also *in vivo*. Studies suggest that the high-level expression of bcl-2 in leukemia cells is partly a result of loss of microRNAs *miR-15a* and *miR-16–1*, which are deleted or downregulated in the majority of cases of CLL.[250]

The sensitivity of CLL cells to undergoing spontaneous or drug-induced apoptosis may be influenced by the leukemia cell microenvironment. CLL cells often undergo apoptosis *in vitro* under culture conditions that can support the survival and growth of human B-cell lines. However, CLL B cells can survive for long periods *ex vivo* when cultured with marrow stromal cells.[251,252] Similarly, CLL cells can survive for protracted periods *in vitro* when cultured with *nurse-like cells*,[253] which are nonleukemic accessory cells that can differentiate from $CD14^+$ blood mononuclear cells when cocultured with CLL B cells.[254] Cells with the distinctive phenotype and morphology of nurse-like cells can be found in the secondary lymphoid tissues of patients with CLL,[254] where they presumably function to inhibit apoptosis of leukemia cells *in vivo*. Follicular dendritic cells also may protect CLL cells from undergoing cell death.[255] The ability of marrow stromal cells, nurse-like cells, and follicular dendritic cells to inhibit spontaneous apoptosis of CLL cells apparently requires cell–cell contact, and likely involves several distinctive ligand-receptor interactions.

CLL Cell Trafficking

CLL cells recirculate from the blood through secondary lymphoid tissues and back into the systemic circulation in response to certain chemokines, such as stromal-derived factor 1 alpha (SDF-1α or CXCL13), CCL21, and/or CCL19.[256] CLL cells have receptors for such chemokines and can manifest chemotaxis toward a chemokine gradient.[257–259] Production of such chemokines as CXCL13 by nurse-like cells could recruit leukemia cells from the blood into secondary lymphoid tissues, where the leukemia cells in turn could receive survival stimuli from nurse-like cells and/or other stroma elements. Moreover, production of CXCL13 by marrow stromal cells also could account for the accumulation of leukemia cells in the marrow, which invariably is infiltrated by leukemia cells in untreated patients with CLL.

Because chemokine receptors are down-modulated in response to the relevant chemokine, leukemia cells within lymphoid compartments potentially could be replaced by newly arriving leukemia cells and then reenter the systemic circulation. The leukemia cells in the blood that fail to reenter such protective compartments might undergo spontaneous cell death and potentially account for the appearance of "smudge" cells that typically are found in the blood films of patients with this disease. Furthermore, the relative number and activity of such stromal elements might be a limiting factor governing tumor progression.

IMMUNOLOGIC DEFECTS

Immune Deficiency

Patients with CLL typically develop immune deficiency.[260] Over time patients experience a progressive decline in serum immunoglobulin levels, resulting in hypogammaglobulinemia. In addition, patients may develop low complement levels,[261] functional defects in bystander T cells,[262] altered leukemia cell expression of major histocompatibility complex antigens,[263,264] and impaired granulocytic function.[265] The immune deficiency associated with CLL often is compounded by the immune suppressive effects of CLL therapy.[266] CLL patients have an increased risk for opportunistic infections and recurrent virus infection, such as those caused by herpes zoster[267,268] and cytomegalovirus.[269] Furthermore, patients with CLL have a higher risk for skin cancers, such as squamous cell carcinoma and basal cell carcinoma, than do age-matched controls.[270]

The leukemia cells themselves may contribute to the immunodeficiency noted in patients with this disease. Leukemia B cells elaborate immune suppressive cytokines, such as transforming growth factor beta (TGF-β),[271,272] and release soluble surface molecules, such as CD27[90,273,274] that can interfere with cognate intercellular interactions that are required for immune activation. High levels of TGF-β also may account for the reversal in the ratio of CD4 to CD8 T cells that often is noted in the patients with CLL.[275] CLL B cells have little stimulatory activity in autologous or even allogeneic mixed lymphocyte culture.[276,277] Aside from TGF-β, this in part is related to the surface phenotype of the leukemic B cells. Important accessory molecules required for cognate B-cell ↔ T-cell interactions, such as CD80 (see Chaps. 15 and 78), are absent or present at low levels on the leukemic cell surface. This makes leukemic cells poor antigen-presenting cells but possible effective inducers of T-cell anergy (see Chap. 78).

CLL B cells also are effective in down-modulating expression of the CD40-ligand (CD154), a surface glycoprotein that ordinarily is expressed on CD4+ T cells following immune activation.[278,279] Because CD154 plays a critical role in the development of an immune response,[280] such down-modulation may be responsible for the immune deficiency that is acquired in CLL. Given the role of CD154 in T-cell induction of immunoglobulin class switching, this acquired functional defect in CD154 may account for the acquired deficiency of CLL patients to produce IgG of each of the various subclasses.[281] Indeed, the acquired immune deficiency of patients with CLL has features in common with that of persons with inherited functional defects in the gene encoding CD154 and/or other inherited immune deficiencies (see Chap. 82). These shared features include the frequent development of intermittent and intercurrent systemic autoimmunity despite profound immune deficiency. Patients with congenital lack of CD154 or other immune deficiencies develop autoimmune hemolytic anemia (see Chap. 53) or immune thrombocytopenic purpura (see Chap. 119).[282,283] These also are the most common autoimmune diseases that develop in patients with CLL.[284,285]

Autoimmunity

Patients with CLL are prone to developing systemic autoimmune disease. The most common autoimmune disorders result from autoantibodies that are directed against hematopoietic cell antigens, such as those found on red blood cells or platelets,[284,285] although other types of autoimmune disorder also appear more common among CLL patients than in the general population.[286–288] In some cases, the autoantibody is produced by the neoplastic B-cell clone,[289] but most often the autoantibodies are produced by bystander nonneoplastic B cells,[98] reflecting a disease-associated dysregulation in humoral immune tolerance to self antigens. Patients with CLL also may develop pure red blood cell aplasia[290] or neutropenia[284] secondary to the development of autoantibodies against marrow hematopoietic progenitor cells. Although patients with rheumatoid arthritis have been reported to have an increased prevalence of CLL compared to that of the general population,[291] CLL patients in general do not appear to have an increased incidence of pathologic autoimmunity other than that directed against hematopoietic cells.[284,285] The mechanism(s) accounting for the development of autoimmunity may be similar to those involved in development of autoimmune hemolytic anemia or immune thrombocytopenia in patients with certain inherited immune deficiency disorders.[283]

CLINICAL FEATURES

PATIENT POPULATION

At diagnosis, most patients are older than 60 years of age, and 90 percent are older than age 50 years. The median age at diagnosis is approximately 67 years.[26] The disease is rare in persons younger than 25 years of age. There is a 2:1 male-to-female incidence and prevalence of CLL.

GENERAL SYMPTOMS

More than 25 percent of patients are asymptomatic at diagnosis. Such patients generally are detected because of the discovery of nontender lymphadenopathy or an unexplained absolute lymphocytosis. Otherwise, patients may have only mild symptoms of reduced exercise tolerance, fatigue, or malaise. Patients may experience such symptoms even when they apparently lack major organ involvement or anemia. Because of the advanced age of the affected population, patients sometimes present with an exacerbation of another underlying medical condition, such as pulmonary, cerebrovascular, or coronary artery disease.

Some cases may present with chronic rhinitis secondary to nasal involvement of CLL cells.[292] In rare cases, patients may present with a sensorimotor polyneuropathy associated with IgM antibody to various gangliosides.[130] For unknown reasons, patients may note exaggerated responses to insect bites, particularly to those of mosquitoes.[293,294]

Patients who present with more advanced disease may experience weight loss, recurrent infections, bleeding secondary to thrombocytopenia, and/or symptomatic anemia. However, night sweats and fevers (the so-called B symptoms) are uncommon and should prompt evaluation for complicating infectious disease. Indeed, patients with CLL are more prone to viral or bacterial infections secondary to impaired T-cell immunity or hypogammaglobulinemia, respectively.

LYMPHADENOPATHY

Nearly 80 percent of all CLL patients have nontender lymphadenopathy at diagnosis, most commonly involving the cervical, supraclavicular, or axillary lymph nodes. Lymph node enlargement can range from being minimal to massive, the latter potentially causing local disfiguration or organ dysfunction. Some patients may develop symptoms of upper airway obstruction because of oral-pharyngeal lymphadenopathy. However, it is unusual for the lymphadenopathy in CLL to cause obstruction of vascular or lymphatic channels. Lymphedema of the extremities is rare, even in the setting of massive axillary and cervical adenopathy, and superior vena cava obstruction is so uncommon that it should alert the clinician to the possibility of a secondary pulmonary neoplasm. Computerized axial tomography of the abdomen can detect intraabdominal lymph node enlargement in a large number of patients. However, such information has yet to be incorporated into clinical staging schemes. Large retroperitoneal adenopathy can result in ureteral obstruction and hydronephrosis. Rarely, patients may develop periportal lymph node enlargement that results in biliary tract obstruction. Occasional patients may experience acute, painful swelling in previously nontender, chronically enlarged lymph nodes secondary to acute lymphadenitis resulting from infection with herpes simplex virus.[295,296]

SPLENOMEGALY AND HEPATOMEGALY

Approximately half of all CLL patients present with mild to moderate splenomegaly. Occasionally, this may cause symptoms of early satiety and/or abdominal fullness. Sometimes, splenic enlargement may result in hypersplenism, contributing to anemia and thrombocytopenia. However, in CLL such cytopenias are more commonly secondary to extensive marrow involvement with CLL and/or intermittent expression of autoantibodies.[284,297–300] Less frequently, patients develop hepatomegaly secondary to leukemic cell infiltration of the liver. Derangement of hepatic function secondary to visceral involvement is usually mild, and cholestatic jaundice is unusual in the absence of nodal disease causing biliary tract obstruction.

EXTRANODAL INVOLVEMENT

Organ infiltration with leukemic cells is detected at autopsy but is not commonly symptomatic. For example, leukemic cell infiltration of the renal parenchyma can be detected in more than half of all patients examined postmortem. However, CLL only rarely is associated with impaired renal function. Leukemic cell infiltration, however, may become symptomatic when it develops in certain locations, such as in the retroorbit, where it can produce proptosis. Lymph tissue also may develop in the scalp, subconjuctivae, prostate, gonads, or pharynx, the latter sometimes causing symptoms of upper airway obstruction. Infiltration of the pericardium by leukemia cells can produce a constrictive pericarditis[301] or result in cardiac tamponade.[302]

Occasionally, the leukemic cells infiltrate the lung parenchyma, producing nodular or miliary pulmonary infiltrates that can be detected on chest radiograph. This may be associated with pulmonary function test abnormalities. The respiratory tract mucosa also may be involved. Leukemic infiltration of the pleura may result in hemorrhagic or chylous pleural effusions.[303–305]

The gastrointestinal tract also may be infiltrated with leukemic cells, causing abnormal mucosal thickening. This may result in ulceration, gastrointestinal bleeding, or malabsorption. The latter may cause dietary deficiencies of essential nutrients, such as folate. Finding iron deficiency should alert the physician to evaluate for gastrointestinal bleeding that might be due to mucosal ulcerations or to a secondary gastrointestinal malignancy.

Leukemic cell infiltration of the central nervous system is unusual but may produce headache, meningitis, cranial nerve palsy, obtundation, or coma.[306] The development of neurologic changes in CLL, however, also may be caused by infections with unusual organisms, including fungi, *Cryptococcus neoformans, Listeria monocytogenes,* or other pathogens that generally only afflict an immune compromised host (see Chap. 22).

LABORATORY FEATURES

BLOOD FINDINGS

The diagnosis of CLL requires a sustained monoclonal lymphocytosis greater than 5000/μL (5×10^9/L). At diagnosis, the absolute lymphocyte count generally exceeds 10,000/μL (10×10^9/L), and is sometimes greater than 100,000/μL (100×10^9/L). Morphologically, the leukemic cells are phenocopies of normal blood small lymphocytes (Fig. 94–1). Typically these cells have scant, bluish cytoplasm upon Wright-Giemsa staining, moderately condensed and mature-appearing nuclei, and an mean corpuscular volume of 170 fl. A few cells can have prominent nucleoli (Fig. 94–1C). During the preparation of the blood film, many CLL lymphocytes are disrupted and appear as smudge cells (Fig. 94–1A and B). Occasional patients have leukemia cells with intracytoplasmic globules (Fig. 94–1D) or crystalline rod-shaped inclusions (Fig. 94–1E), which may be comprised mostly of immunoglobulin or immunoglobulin light or heavy chains.[307,308]

Patients with CLL may develop anemia secondary to leukemic marrow infiltration (Fig. 94–1F), the myelosuppressive effect of chemotherapy and inhibiting cytokines, autoimmunity directed against red cell antigens (see Chap. 53), hypersplenism (see Chap. 55), and/or a poor nutritional status that leads to deficiency of folic acid, vitamin B_{12}, or iron (see Chaps. 41 and 42). The nature of the blood findings will vary depending on the factor(s) responsible for the anemia.

Most typically, the red cells are normocytic and normochromic. Approximately 15 percent of patients present with normocytic anemia. In the setting of extreme lymphocytosis, the packed red cell volume may be overestimated unless care is taken to exclude from the measurement the expanded buffy coat containing the leukemic cells. Approximately 20 percent of all CLL patients have a positive Coombs test at some time during their disease because of the production of IgG anti-red cell autoantibodies by bystander nonleukemic B cells. Autoimmune hemolytic anemia, however, develops in only approximately 8 percent of CLL patients.

During the most advanced disease stage, patients have thrombocytopenia as a result of marrow replacement and hypersplenism. At any stage, however, patients can develop immune thrombocytopenia as a result of antiplatelet antibodies. Generally, the platelet morphology is not remarkable.

MARROW FINDINGS

The marrow invariably is infiltrated with leukemic lymphocytes. There are four patterns of marrow involvement.[309–311] In approximately one-third of patients, the marrow has an interstitial, or lacy, pattern, which is associated with a better prognosis and/or early stage disease. Approximately 10 percent of patients present with a nodular pattern of marrow involvement, and approximately 25 percent have a mixed nodular-interstitial pattern. These patterns also are associated with a better prognosis. A quarter of the patients present with extensive marrow replacement, producing a diffuse pattern that is associated with advanced clinical stage and/or more aggressive disease.[311,312]

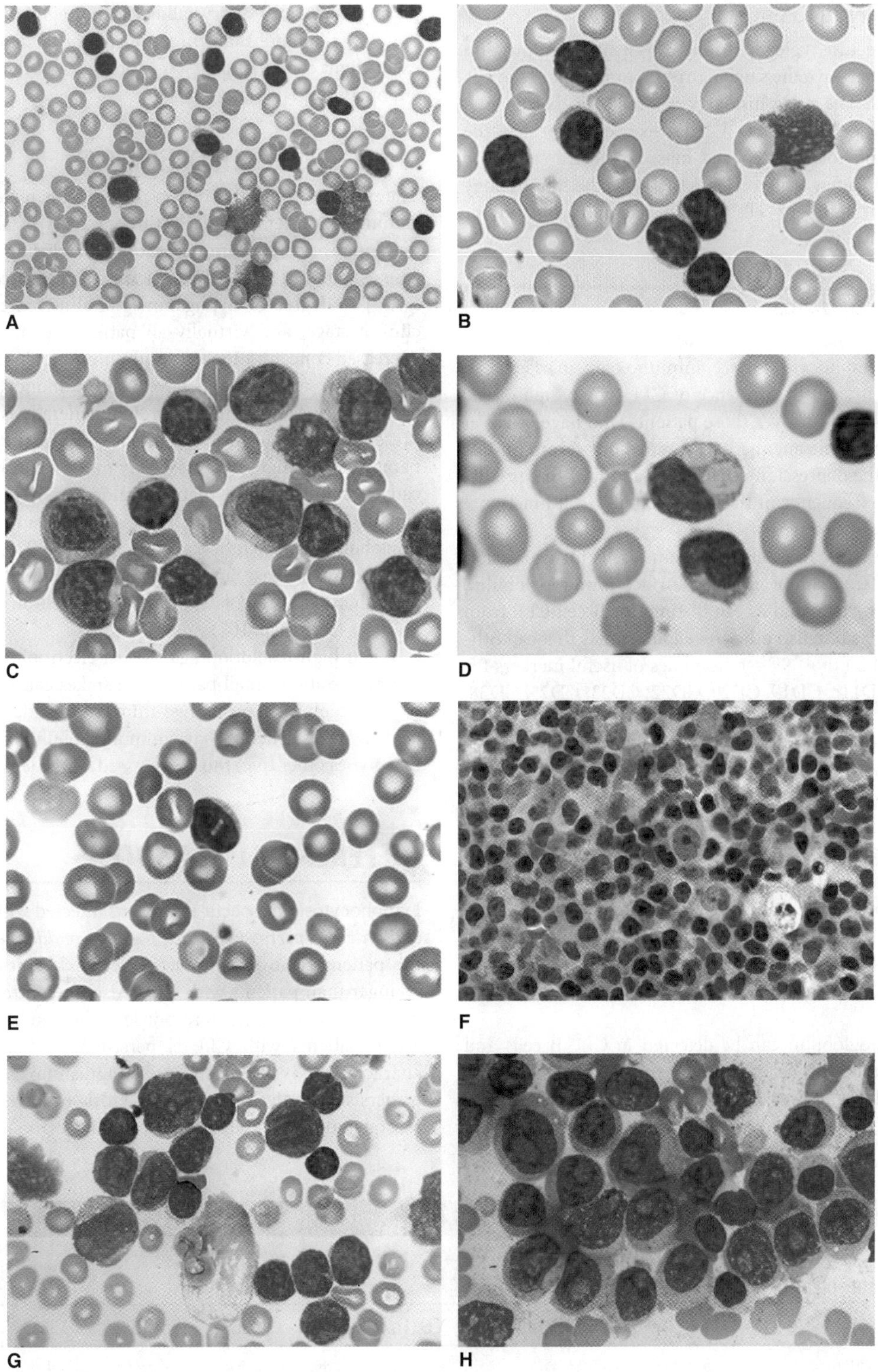

FIGURE 94–1. A. Blood film. Chronic lymphocytic leukemia (CLL). Classical picture of increased lymphocyte count composed of predominately small lymphocytes with scant cytoplasm. Two of 18 lymphocytes are larger with less-dense nuclear chromatin pattern. This degree of variability is consistent with classical CLL. Note also three smudge cells, amorphous cell remnants, a constant feature of CLL. On average about 1 in 5 to 10 lymphocytes are destroyed during blood film preparation as a result of mechanical fragility from the shear forces generated in blood film preparation. **B.** Blood film. CLL. Higher magnification than in **A**. Classical small lymphocytes with a thin rim of cytoplasm, dense chromatin, and generally unapparent nucleoli. Note smudge cell. **C.** Blood film. Variant CLL. Somewhat larger proportion of medium- and larger- sized lymphocytes admixed with small lymphocytes. **D.** Blood film. CLL. Small lymphocyte is shown with intracytoplasmic globules. A small proportion of CLL patients have occasional cells with intracellular inclusions of one sort or another. They may consist of IgA, IgG, or IgM immunoglobulin or immunoglobulin light chains, usually λ type and are more often apparent in marrow than blood.[307,308] **E.** Blood film. CLL. Crystalline rod-shaped inclusion are shown overlying the nucleus. This is likely crystalline immunoglobulin or immunoglobulin light chain. **F.** Marrow biopsy section. CLL. Marrow replaced by a monotonous infiltrate of small lymphocytes with reduction of erythropoiesis and granulopoiesis. Rare large cells are seen, one with a prominent nucleolus. **G.** Blood film. Prolymphocytic leukemia. Note variation in lymphocyte size but with the majority of leukemic lymphocytes being larger, some with clefts, and some with overt nucleoli. **H.** Marrow film. Prolymphocytic leukemia. Note infiltrate of large lymphocytes, most with prominent, large nucleoli. *(Used with permission from* Lichtman's Atlas of Hematology, *www.accessmedicine.com.)*

LYMPH NODE FINDINGS

The lymph node architecture typically is effaced by a diffuse infiltration of small lymphocytes that have the same morphology as that of the circulating leukemic cells. The node histology is similar to that of low-grade small lymphocytic lymphoma. As the disease progresses, the nodes may coalesce and form large fixed masses. In rare cases, the lymph node can contain a few scattered cells that have the morphology and phenotype of Reed-Sternberg cells typically seen in Hodgkin lymphoma (see Chap. 99).[313]

IMMUNOLOGIC STUDIES

Several tests are recommended as part of the laboratory evaluation of patients with CLL. Lymphocyte surface immunologic markers can determine monoclonality and the presence of CLL-type lymphocytes. The direct Coombs test can uncover those patients who have or are at risk for an immune hemolytic anemia. Measurement of serum immunoglobulin quantifies the depression of IgG, IgA, and IgM that predisposes to infection. The frequency of the concomitant T-cell functional defect increases in advanced stages of CLL.

Flow cytometry analyses can evaluate leukemic cells for expression of B-cell or T-cell differentiation antigens, surface immunoglobulin, and κ or λ light chains. Such studies can distinguish B-cell CLL from not only T-cell leukemias but also other B-cell leukemias that can otherwise mimic B-cell CLL (Table 94–1). Examples of useful markers for this are CD5, CD10, CD11c, CD19, CD20, CD22, CD23, CD25, CD38, and CD103 (see Chap. 15).[97,314–317]

CLL cells typically are CD5+, CD10–, CD19+, CD20 (dull), CD23+, CD103–, have low-level expression of surface immunoglobulin, and have low-level or absent expression of membrane CD22 and CD79b. The latter marker identifies an extracellular epitope of the B-cell receptor β chain (see Chap. 77). FMC7, a monoclonal antibody that binds an epitope of CD20 formed when this surface antigen is present at high density,[318] typically does not react with CLL cells, reflecting the low-level expression of CD20 by the leukemia cells of most patients with CLL. Because low-level expression of CD20 is a distinctive characteristic of CLL cells, FMC7 still is used to discriminate CLL from other B-cell malignancies.[319]

Cytoplasmic immunoglobulin can be detected in CLL B cells and may be a valuable adjunct in B-cell phenotyping.[320] Compared to normal cells, CLL B cells have a lower density of surface immunoglobulin but a higher content of cytoplasmic immunoglobulin. Rarely, intracytoplasmic inclusions of crystalloid immunoglobulin have been seen (see Fig. 94–1E). More than three-fourths of patients with CLL may have excess light chains in the Golgi complex and the cisternae of the rough endoplasmic reticulum.[321–323]

PROTEIN ELECTROPHORESIS

The most common finding on serum protein electrophoreses is hypogammaglobulinemia. Nearly three-fourths of all B-cell CLL patients develop severe hypogammaglobulinemia during the course of their disease. Reduction in the serum levels of IgM precedes that of IgG and IgA. The degree of hypogammaglobulinemia correlates loosely with clinical stage, and virtually all patients with advanced disease have decreased concentrations of serum immunoglobulin.

Five percent of patients have a serum monoclonal immunoglobulin paraprotein. The serum paraprotein generally is the same type as that present on the leukemic cell surface. When the concentration of IgM paraprotein is high, hyperviscosity may ensue, and the clinical picture can be confused with that of Waldenström macroglobulinemia (see Chap. 111). In some cases, there is defective and/or unbalanced immunoglobulin chain synthesis by the leukemic B-cell clone, resulting in μ heavy-chain disease and/or immunoglobulin light-chain proteinuria (see Chap. 112). The latter can be detected on urine immunoelectrophoresis (see Chap. 107).

When high-resolution agarose gel electrophoresis is combined with immunofixation, small paraprotein spikes can be identified in the sera or urine samples of nearly two-thirds of all patients.[17,324–326] These paraprotein spikes generally have immunoglobulin heavy chains that belong to isotypes other than those expressed by the leukemic B-cell clone.[17]

DIFFERENTIAL DIAGNOSIS

Lymphocytosis can occur in persons infected with various viruses, such as *Bordetella pertussis* or *Toxoplasma gondii* (see Chap. 81). However, the patients who usually encounter such illness generally are much younger than patients with CLL. Also, in contrast to the reactive lymphocytosis that occurs in response to these infections, the lymphocytosis of patients with CLL is persistent and monoclonal. The latter characteristic is important in distinguishing CLL from unusual cases of persistent polyclonal lymphocytosis of B cells that sometimes can masquerade as B-cell CLL.[327,328] Flow cytometry analyses of blood

TABLE 94–1. Immunophenotype of Chronic B-Cell Leukemias/Lymphomas

Disease Entity	sIg	CD5	CD10	CD11c	CD19	CD20	CD22	CD23	CD25	CD103
Chronic lymphocytic leukemia	+/–	++	–	–/+	+	+/–	–/+	++	–/+	–
Prolymphocytic leukemia	++	+/–	–	–/+	+	+/–	+	+/–	–	–
Hairy cell leukemia	+	–	–	++	+	+	++	–/+	+	++
Mantle cell lymphoma	+	++	–	–	+	+	+	–	–	–
Splenic marginal zone lymphoma	+	–/+	–	+/–	+	+	+/–	–	–	–
Lymphoplasmacytoid lymphoma	–/+	–/+	–	–	+	+/–	+/–	–/+	+/–	–
Follicular center lymphoma	+	–	+	–	+	++	+	–/+	–	–

sIg, surface immunoglobulin.

– Leukemia cells do not express the surface antigen; + leukemia cells from most cases express the surface antigen; +/–, low-level expression; –/+, most cases either do not express the antigen or express it at very low levels; ++, high-level expression of the surface antigen in nearly all cases.

mononuclear cells generally can differentiate between reactive lymphocytosis, polyclonal B-cell lymphocytosis, and monoclonal lymphocytosis secondary to lymphoproliferative disease.[329]

PROLYMPHOCYTIC LEUKEMIA

Prolymphocytic leukemia is a subacute variant of CLL in which more than half of the blood leukemic cells are large lymphocytes, termed *prolymphocytes*. These cells can be distinguished from the leukemic cells in CLL by size and morphology.[330] Prolymphocytes measure 10 to 15 *m*m in diameter (see Fig. 94–1G), whereas CLL cells generally have the size of small resting lymphocytes (7–10 *m*m in diameter). Also, prolymphocytes in the blood or marrow have round or indented nuclei, each possessing a single prominent thick-rimmed nucleolus and chromatin that is more dense than that of a lymphoblast but less dense than that of a typical mature lymphocyte or a CLL B cell. The cytoplasm generally is pale blue and agranular, except for occasional intracytoplasmic inclusions that are visible by electron, and sometimes light, microscopy.[331] By scanning electron microscopy, these prolymphocytes often have more surface microvilli than do leukemic cells from patients with B-cell CLL. They may involve lymph nodes, generally producing a pseudonodular pattern of infiltration that is distinct from that of the diffuse pattern typical of CLL.[332] In contrast to the leukemic B cells in CLL, prolymphocytes typically express high levels of surface immunoglobulin and stain brightly with SN8, a monoclonal antibody specific for CD79b (see Chaps. 15 and 77).[333,334] Also, the neoplastic cells in prolymphocytic leukemia typically have low expression of CD5 relative to that observed on CLL cells.[335] These and other features that distinguish CLL from prolymphocytic leukemia are presented in Table 94–1. Other features of this disease are discussed in "B-Cell Prolymphocytic Leukemia" and "T-Cell Prolymphocytic Leukemia" below.

HAIRY CELL LEUKEMIA

The clinical and laboratory features that assist in distinguishing CLL from hairy cell leukemia and its variants, hairy cell leukemia variant, and splenic lymphoma with villous lymphocytes,[336] are presented in Table 94–1. These diseases are discussed in Chaps. 92 and 95.

The neoplastic B cells in hairy cell leukemia are larger than CLL cells (mean corpuscular volume 400 fl) and have more abundant cytoplasm, often with fine filamentous "hairy" projections. These cells are strongly positive for tartrate-resistant isozyme 5 of acid phosphatase activity. In contrast to CLL B cells, the neoplastic cells in hairy cell leukemia express high levels of CD11c, the α^X chain of the β_2 integrins, and CD103, the α^E subunit of the β_7 integrins (see Chap. 95).

LYMPHOMAS

Lymphomas can have circulating neoplastic cells, sometimes producing a blood lymphocytosis that may be mistaken for CLL. Those lymphomas that most closely can resemble B-cell CLL are discussed below.

Small Lymphocytic Lymphoma

Low-grade small lymphocytic B-cell lymphoma is closely related to B-cell CLL in its biology and clinical features. The neoplastic cells in small lymphocytic lymphoma with blood involvement are the same morphologically as the leukemic cells in CLL. Moreover, the histology of the involved lymph nodes in CLL and small lymphocytic lymphoma are indistinguishable.[337] Similar to the B cells in CLL, the neoplastic B cells in small lymphocytic lymphoma express immunoglobulins that bear autoantibody-associated cross-reactive idiotypes and that are encoded by nonmutated immunoglobulin genes.[95,338] Finally, the neoplastic B cells in both diseases express many of the same surface antigens, including CD5.[339] For these reasons, the distinction between these diseases is primarily clinical, in that CLL invariably is associated with a blood lymphocytosis (greater than 5000/μL (5×10^9/L), whereas small lymphocytic lymphoma invariably is associated with lymph node involvement. Also, although patients with CLL invariably have marrow lymphocytosis, the marrow in small lymphocytic lymphoma need not be involved. When the marrow is involved, the pattern in small lymphocytic lymphoma typically is nodular, rather than interstitial or diffuse.[311]

Mantle Cell Lymphoma

Mantle cell lymphoma (previously called centrocytic lymphoma, mantle zone lymphoma, or intermediate lymphoma) in the Working Formulation is an intermediate-grade B-cell lymphoma (see Chaps. 92, 98, and 102). In contrast to the diffuse lymph node involvement typical in CLL, the histology of lymph nodes in mantle cell lymphoma typically is one of reactive germinal centers surrounded by well-defined, expanded mantle zones of monoclonal B cells.[340] However, heavily involved lymph nodes may lose this architecture and appear diffusely infiltrated, assuming histology similar to that of lymph nodes involved in CLL.

The neoplastic B cells in mantle cell lymphoma express many of the same surface antigens as do CLL B cells, including CD5 (see Table 94–1). However, in contrast to CLL B cells, mantle cell lymphoma cells generally do not express CD23. Mantle cell lymphoma cells also tend to express higher levels of CD79a and CD79b than CLL cells.[335,341]

In contrast to CLL cells, mantle cell lymphoma generally have t(11;14) translocations involving *BCL-1* and immunoglobulin heavy-chain gene complex, resulting in overexpression of cyclin D1.[342,343] The BCL-1 rearrangements of mantle cell lymphoma can be detected via FISH analyses on the neoplastic cells.[344]

Splenic Marginal Zone Lymphoma

Splenic marginal zone lymphoma (SMZL) is an indolent lymphoproliferative disease that accounts for approximately 1 percent of all lymphomas (see Chap. 103). Patients with SMZL typically present with marked splenomegaly, and often have a moderate lymphocytosis of monoclonal B cells that appear as atypical "villous lymphocytes."[345,346] This disorder commonly is called *splenic lymphoma with villous lymphocytes*. The neoplastic B cells in this disease have a mature B-cell phenotype and express IgM and IgD, but typically lack expression of CD23, CD43, CD10, Bcl-6, and cyclin D_1 (see Table 94–1). In contrast to CLL, which has moderate expression of CD5 and weak or negative expression of CD79b, the neoplastic B cells in SMZL have weak or negative expression of CD5 and moderate expression of CD79b.[335,347] Genetic studies have revealed abnormalities in a number of chromosomes, however, 7q31–33 allelic loss appears to be characteristic.[348] The loss of 7q31 spans from 7q31.33 to 7q33 located between sequence tagged site-markers SHGC-3275 and D7S725, a region distinct from that commonly deleted in myelodysplastic disease or acute myeloid leukemia (see Chaps. 88 and 89).

The spleen in SMZL is characterized by a nodular infiltrate in the white pulp that also can extend into the red pulp (see Chap. 5). Within the white pulp, the infiltrate has a biphasic morphology comprising an inner zone of small lymphocytes and a peripheral (marginal) zone of larger lymphoid cells. Usually the splenic lymph nodes and marrow are also involved by a vaguely nodular infiltrate that has similar characteristics. On the other hand, the spleen in CLL typically has diffuse effacement of white pulp architecture and lacks readily identifiable marginal zones.[349]

Lymphomas of Follicular Center Cell Origin

Low-grade lymphomas of follicular center cell origin also can involve the blood. There is often marked adenopathy and occasionally massive splenomegaly. The leukemic cells are small and typically have cleaved nuclei with well-delineated nucleoli. Follicular center small cleaved cell lymphomas express the CD10 (CALLA) antigen. In contrast to CLL, these cells often express high levels of surface immunoglobulin and generally express neither mouse rosette receptors nor the CD5 antigen (see Table 94–1). The cells are FMC7-positive. Biopsy of a lymph node will confirm nodular or diffuse small cleaved cell (poorly differentiated lymphocytic) lymphoma. These diseases are discussed in Chap. 101.

LYMPHOPLASMACYTIC LEUKEMIAS

Plasmacytoid lymphocytes can be seen on the blood films and are always present in the marrow of patients with Waldenström macroglobulinemia (see Chap. 111). These cells have abundant, often basophilic, cytoplasm with mature lymphoid nuclei. By flow cytometry analysis these cells express pan–B-lymphocyte surface antigens CD19, CD20, and CD24 (see Chap. 15) and are monoclonal, as defined by immunoglobulin light-chain expression. Similar to CLL B cells, these cells often express CD5 and CD11b. However, they can be distinguished from CLL cells by their expression of the CD10 (CALLA) and/or CD9 antigens and by their lymphoplasmacytic morphology (see Chaps. 92 and 98).

Patients with plasma cell myeloma may develop plasma cell leukemia. The leukemic cells can be distinguished from those in B-cell CLL by their plasmacytic morphology, their expression of CD38, PCA-1, CD56, and CD85, and their low-level or lack of expression of CD19, CD20, CD24, CD72, and HLA-DR (see Table 94–1). Plasma cell myeloma is discussed in Chap. 109.

T-CELL CHRONIC LYMPHOPROLIFERATIVE DISORDERS

T-cell variants of CLL constitute a heterogeneous group of disorders that must be distinguished from B-cell CLL. T-cell chronic lymphoproliferative diseases are much less common. Several have counterparts in the various B-cell leukemias and are discussed in other chapters, including T-cell prolymphocytic leukemia (discussed in "B-Cell Prolymphocytic Leukemia" and "T-Cell Prolymphocytic Leukemia" below) and T-cell lymphoma (see Chap. 106). A subset of large granular lymphocytic leukemias represents another T-cell chronic leukemia that is discussed in Chap. 96.

These diseases can be distinguished from lymphoproliferative disorders of B cells or natural killer cells by immunophenotype. The leukemic cells from all T-cell malignancies lack expression of monoclonal surface immunoglobulin or B-cell restricted surface differentiation antigens, such as CD19 or CD20 (see Chap. 15), and generally lack immunoglobulin light-chain gene rearrangements (see Chap. 77). Characteristically, chronic T-cell leukemias have rearrangement and expression of the genes encoding the T-cell receptor for antigen (see Chap. 78) and express the CD3 surface antigens (see Chaps. 15 and 78). The latter is a property exclusive to lymphocytes of the T-cell lineage and can be used to distinguish large granular lymphocytic leukemia of T cell versus natural killer cell origin (see Chaps. 96 and 106).

THERAPY, COURSE, AND PROGNOSIS

CLINICAL STAGING

Wide variability exists in the rate of disease progression and the incidence of disease-related complications among patients with CLL. Because of this, the life expectancies of patients with newly diagnosed CLL can vary tremendously. Staging helps to define prognosis and to decide when to initiate therapy.

TABLE 94–2. RAI Clinical Staging System

Revised Staging System	Original Staging System	Clinical Features at Diagnosis	Median Survival, Years*
Low risk	0	Blood and marrow lymphocytosis	12
	I	Lymphocytosis and enlarged lymph nodes	11
Intermediate risk	II	Lymphocytosis and enlarged spleen and/or liver	8
High risk	III	Lymphocytosis and anemia (hemoglobin below 11 g/dL)	5
	IV	Lymphocytosis and thrombocytopenia (platelets below 100,000/μL)	7

*Survival data updated as per Wierda et al.[443]

Two major staging systems have been developed, each having established value in helping to predict survival.[350] Rai and colleagues introduced the first widely used staging system in 1975.[21] This staging system designated five clinical stages using 0 and Roman numerals I through IV. Patients in stages 0 and I have a favorable prognosis, whereas patients in stages III and IV have a relatively short survival (Table 94–2). The prognosis of patients in stage II is intermediate. Although confirmed to have useful predictive value,[351] the number of stages was considered excessive by some investigators. Accordingly, in 1981, Binet and colleagues proposed a three-stage classification system that considered the total lymphoid mass.[352] The most advanced stage, stage C, describes all patients who have anemia and/or thrombocytopenia as a result of impaired marrow function (Table 94–3). The remaining patients are divided into stages A or B, based upon the number of enlarged lymphoid areas (of which there are five: cervical, axillary, or inguinofemoral lymph nodes, and liver or spleen). Patients in groups A or B have less than three or greater than or equal to three areas of lymphoid enlargement, respectively (Table 94–3). Most physicians use either the Binet or the Rai staging system. Generally, disease progression follows a stepwise pattern from earlier to later stages.

In 1987, Rai reorganized his original staging system into three categories: low-risk (stage 0), intermediate-risk (stages I and II), and high-risk (stages III and IV) patients.[353] Low-risk patients have a projected median survival of greater than 150 months (see Table 94–2). In contrast, intermediate- and high-risk patients have median survivals of approximately 90 months and 19 months, respectively. Both the Binet classification and modified Rai classification have proven utility in helping to access disease outcome.[353] Despite the advent of new prognostic markers, these staging systems still have independent prognostic value.[354]

OTHER PROGNOSTIC INDICATORS

In addition to the widely accepted staging systems of Rai and Binet, there are additional indicators that can help identify high-risk patients who may benefit from closer followup. With the exception of a short lymphocyte doubling time, standard guidelines have yet to incorporate these parameters into making the decision of when to initiate therapy.[355]

TABLE 94–3. Binet Clinical Staging System

Stage	Clinical Features at Diagnosis	Median Survival, Years*
A	Blood and marrow lymphocytosis and less than 3 areas§ of palpable lymphoid-tissue enlargement	12
B	Blood and marrow lymphocytosis and 3 or more areas of palpable lymphoid-tissue enlargement	9
C	Same as B with anemia (hemoglobin below 11 g/dL in men or 10 g/dL in women) or thrombocytopenia (platelets less than 100,000/μL)	7

*Survival data updated as per Wierda et al.[443]

§An area is defined as the cervical, axillary, or inguinofemoral lymph nodes, or the liver and spleen. The liver and spleen together count as one area, as do the right and left cervical lymph nodes. However, bilateral enlargement of the axillary lymph nodes or the inguinofemoral lymph nodes each count as two areas. Thus, the number of enlarged lymphoid areas can range from one to five.

This awaits the outcome of clinical trials to determine the value of early treatment based on these parameters in lieu of standard treatment indications.

Leukemic Cell Doubling Time

The lymphocyte doubling time (LDT) is a useful metric for disease progression.[356] The LDT is defined as the number of months it takes for the absolute lymphocyte count to double in number. Patients with short LDTs of 12 months or less have a significantly shorter overall and treatment-free survival than do patients with longer LDTs.[357] Independent of stage, the median survival for patients with a doubling time less than 12 months is significantly shorter than that of patients who had leukemia cell doubling times of greater than 1 year.[357,358]

However, use of the LDT requires followup evaluations of patients and is inherently retrospective. Also, blood lymphocyte counts can be influenced by factors other than disease progression, requiring more than just two or three longitudinal evaluations over time. In addition, patients might have progressive disease that is discordant from the rate of the progression in lymphocytosis. For example, some patients might have relative stable absolute lymphocyte counts, but be found on heavy water labeling to have CLL cells that have a birth rate of 0.1 percent to more than 1 percent of the total leukemia clone per day.[236] A nationwide study is being conducted by the CLL Research Consortium to assess the clinical significance of a high-CLL-cell birth rate and its relationship with LDT and other prognostic parameters. In any case, the significance of the LDT should take into consideration the entire context of the patient's clinical presentation.

Immunoglobulin Gene Mutation Status

CLL B cells can be segregated into at least two groups that differ in the extent to which their expressed immunoglobulin heavy chain variable region genes (IgHV) have undergone somatic mutation.[109,359] About half of all cases have leukemia cells that express nonmutated IgHV genes, whereas the rest express IgHV genes with levels of base substitutions that distinguish them from their germ-line counterparts. The latter resemble more the cases of CLL that express IgA or IgG.[360–363] The extent to which IgHV genes are mutated does not vary within any one leukemia cell population,[364] even when examined over a period of years.[365] It appears certain that leukemia cells that express mutated Ig genes do not evolve from cases that originally expressed unmutated Ig genes.

The mutational status of the immunoglobulin genes expressed by CLL cells can be used to segregate patients into two subsets that have significantly different tendencies for disease progression.[22,23] CLL cells that express nonmutated IgHV genes may have trisomy 12 and atypical morphology more often than those that expressed mutated IgHV genes, which, in turn, more frequently tend to have abnormalities involving 13q14.[366] Furthermore, patients with leukemia cells that express unmutated IgHV genes have a greater tendency for disease progression than those who have leukemia cells that express IgHV genes with less than 98 percent nucleic acid sequence homology with their germ-line counterparts,[22,23] a observation confirmed on subsequent studies.[367–370] Although the immunoglobulin mutation status does not appear to influence the relative response to treatment, patients with CLL cells that expressed unmutated IgHV genes appear to have significantly shorter remission duration than do matched patients who have leukemia cells that express mutated immunoglobulin genes[197,371]

One noted exception to this appears to be represented by patients who have leukemia cells that use a particular immunoglobulin gene, designated *IGHV3–21*. This gene can have somatic mutations when expressed by CLL B cells. However, patients who have CLL cells that use a mutated *IGHV3–21* gene together with a λ immunoglobulin light chain encoded *IGHV3–21* apparently have a risk for aggressive disease similar to that of patients who have leukemia cells that express unmutated IgHV genes.[105,114]

CD38

The leukemia cells of patients with aggressive disease often express CD38, a 45-kDa transmembrane glycoprotein protein that can synthesize cyclic ADP-ribose from nicotinamide adenine dinucleotide and hydrolyze cyclic ADP-ribose to ADP-ribose (see Chaps. 15 and 75).[23] Several studies have corroborated the notion that CD38 is, indeed, an indicator of relatively poor prognosis,[369,372–374] even independent of clinical stage.[367] However, one study concluded that CD38 did not have prognostic significance in a multivariate analysis of other commonly used staging criteria, except in early stage patients.[375] One study involving more than 160 patients who were sampled on two separate occasions at intervals ranging from 4 to 40 months found that the expression level of CD38 varied by less than 10 percent between the first and second sample.[376] However, other studies have noted that expression of CD38 could vary in any one patient during the course of the disease,[367] and appears regulated by the leukemia microenvironment.[377] Nonetheless, high-level leukemia cell expression of CD38 remains associated with an adverse prognosis,[372,378–380] although it might not have the same power to predict outcome as does expression of unmutated IgHV or other markers, such as the zeta-associated protein of 70 kDa (ZAP-70).[381,382]

Confounding this issue further is the observation that patients with CD38-negative leukemia cells might later be found to have leukemia cells that express this surface antigen, suggesting that expression of CD38 might be a secondary event in CLL associated with disease evolution.[373] Although, some studies did not observe an invariant association between expression of CD38 and tendency toward disease progression[383] or between readily identifiable subgroups based on surface antigen phenotype.[384]

The controversy in the use of CD38 as a prognostic indicator in part could be a result of differences in the technique used for distinguishing cases considered "positive" versus "negative" for CD38. As with ZAP-70, the distribution of CD38 expression levels on different leukemia populations does not define two discrete subsets.[385] For this reason, it is necessary to define "positive" cases based upon whether they have 30 percent or more labeled leukemia cells with a fluorescence intensity that is above a defined threshold for "positive" cells. This threshold can vary depending upon the background fluorescence intensities of the isotype-control-stained leukemia cells and the relative brightness of the fluorochrome-conjugated anti-CD38 monoclonal antibody.

Gene Expression Arrays

CLL cells that use unmutated IgHV express many genes in common with CLL cells that express mutated IgHV.[24,25] CLL has a common gene expression signature that serves to distinguish such leukemia cells from other B-cell malignancies except for small lymphocytic lymphoma and from normal cord blood or adult blood B cells. This formed the basis for an international effort to use gene expression profiles to help segregate hematologic malignancies into diagnostic groups.[386]

Zeta-Associated Protein of 70 kDa

CLL cells that use unmutated IgHV genes can be distinguished from those that express mutated IgHV genes through the differential expression of a relatively small subset of genes.[24,25,386] One of these genes encodes ZAP-70. ZAP-70 is a 70-kDa cytoplasmic protein tyrosine kinase that ordinarily is expressed only in natural killer cells and T cells, in which it originally was identified as being able to associate with CD247, the CD3 ζ chain (CD3ζ-chain) of the T-cell-receptor complex (see Chaps. 15 and 78). In contrast to CLL cells that have mutated Ig receptors, CLL cells that use unmutated IgHV genes express ZAP-70 RNA.[24] Subsequent studies found that CLL B cells that had unmutated IgHV genes generally expressed levels of ZAP-70 protein that were comparable to those expressed by normal blood T cells.[387,388] In contrast, CLL B cells that expressed mutated IgHV genes generally do not express detectable levels of ZAP-70 protein. Leukemia cell expression of ZAP-70 can be used as a surrogate marker for immunoglobulin mutational status,[388,389] which can segregate patients who have significantly different tendencies for disease progression.

Using sensitive flow cytometry techniques, the distribution of ZAP-70 expression levels by different leukemia populations does not define two discrete subsets. For this reason, it is necessary to define "positive" cases based upon whether they have 20 percent or more labeled leukemia cells with a fluorescence intensity that is above a defined fluorescence threshold for "positive" cells,[388] a cutoff that has apparent clinical significance.[390] This threshold can vary depending upon the background fluorescence intensities of the isotype-control-stained leukemia cells and the relative brightness of the fluorochrome-conjugated anti–ZAP-70 monoclonal antibody.

Although CLL cells that express unmutated IgHV genes generally also express ZAP-70, this is not always the case. Conversely, there are CLL cells that have ZAP-70 despite expressing mutated immunoglobulin IgHV genes. In one large multiinstitution study,[390] those patients with ZAP-70-positive CLL cells had median time from diagnosis to initial therapy of 2.8 years if the leukemia cells expressed unmutated IgHV genes, and 4.2 years if their leukemia cells express mutated IgHV genes (Fig. 94–2). These two subgroups were not significantly different. However, the median time from diagnosis to initial treatment in each of these groups was significantly shorter than the time in patients with ZAP-70–negative CLL cells who had either mutated or unmutated IgHV genes ($P < 0.001$). The median time from diagnosis to initial therapy among patients who did not have ZAP-70 was 11.0 years in those with a mutated IgHV genes and 7.1 years in those with an unmutated IgHV genes ($P < 0.001$). It appears that the expression of ZAP-70 may be a stronger predictor of the need for early treatment in patients with CLL than is IgHV mutation status.

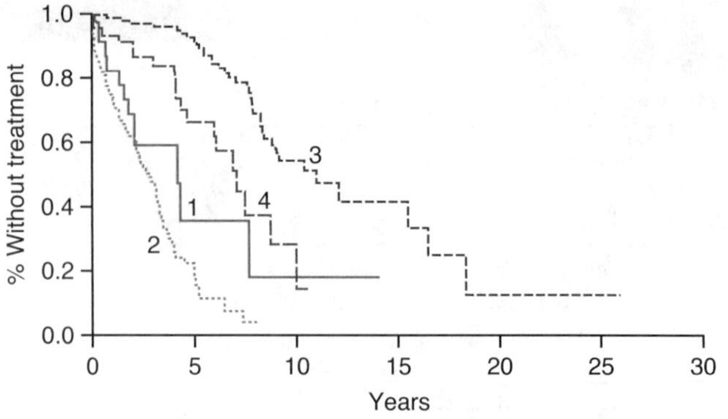

Group	0–5	5–10	10–15	15–25	20–25	25–30
1 ··········ZAP+/mutated	11/24	1/2	0/1	0/0	0/0	0/0
2 ··········ZAP+/unmutated	77/117	6/11	0/0	0/0	0/0	0/0
3 ··········ZAP^Neg/mutated	8/119	23/82	3/18	3/5	0/1	1/1
4 ··········ZAP^Neg/unmutated	12/47	7/17	0/1	0/0	0/0	0/0

(# events/# at risk)

FIGURE 94–2. Relationship between ZAP-70 and IgHV mutational status and time from diagnosis to initial therapy. Kaplan-Meier curves depicting the proportion of untreated patients over time from diagnosis of different groups of cases segregated with respect to IgHV mutational status and whether they did (ZAP+) or did not (ZAP^{Neg}) express ZAP-70.

Additional studies found that ZAP-70 has functional significance in CLL.[387,391] ZAP-70 can enhance the signaling capacity of the surface Ig expressed in CLL, a function that apparently is independent of its kinase activity.[392,393] This might allow ZAP-70+ CLL cells to derive more stimulation from self and/or environmental antigens that interact with the highly selected Ig used in this disease. With repeated exposure to such antigens, the leukemia B cells might derive greater stimulation, leading to increased proliferation and/or resistance to apoptosis. If so, then the expression of ZAP-70 might be more closely tied to the propensity for early disease progression than the mutation status of the expressed IgHV. Consistent with this notion are clinical surveys that find CLL cell expression of ZAP-70 a stronger predictor of aggressive disease than is leukemia cell expression of CD38 or unmutated IgHV.[381]

Other Prognostic Marker Genes

Similar to ZAP-70, several other genes with potential prognostic power have been identified by gene-expression profiling, most notably lipoprotein lipase (LPL)[394–396] and a disintegrin and metalloprotease 29 (ADAM-29).[397–399] Furthermore, a high ratio of LPL relative to ADAM-29 has a strong correlation with expression of unmutated IgHV and adverse clinical outcome.[397] The difference in median gene-expression levels between indolent and aggressive cases is more apparent than is the difference in protein expression, suggesting expression of LPL is under posttranscriptional regulation. Also, the expression level of LPL apparently can be influenced by surface Ig receptor ligation.[400] Nevertheless, because LPL is expressed at low-to-negligible levels by other blood mononuclear cells, its expression in CLL cells can be measured using quantitative reverse-transcriptase polymerase chain reaction (RT-PCR) on blood mononuclear cells or even on lysed whole-blood samples.[401]

Several other genes have been identified as being expressed at higher levels by leukemia cells that use unmutated IgHV versus those that use mutated IgHV. These include activation-induced cytidine deaminase (AID),[402] a kinase anchor protein (gravin) 12 (AKAP12),[399] carnitine palmitoyltransferase 1A gene (CPT1A), dystrophin muscular dystrophy

(DMD) gene,[394,403] Fc receptor-like 2 (FCRL2),[404] nuclear receptor interacting protein 1 (NRIP1),[399] paternally expressed gene 10 (PEG10),[405] septin-10 (SEPT10),[406] sarcoglycan-epsilon (SGCE),[405] seven in absentia homolog 1 (SIAH1),[394,405] CLL upregulated gene 1 (CLLU1),[407] and spastic paraplegia 20 gene (SPG20).[399] Also, expression of the antiapoptotic transcription factor TWIST2 appears selectively silenced by promoter methylation in patients with mutated IgHV genes.[408] Although the expression level of each of these genes has been associated with mutation status, treatment-free or overall survival, the use of such markers has not been validated for routine use in a clinical setting.

Cytogenetics

Survival of patients with abnormal karyotypes is significantly shorter than that of comparably staged patients with normal karyotypes.[409–411] Multiple abnormalities in association with trisomy 12 carry a worse prognosis than trisomy 12 alone.[409,412–414] However, patients who have trisomy 12 as the only cytogenetic abnormality fare worse than those with a normal karyotype or those with isolated abnormalities involving 13q14.[415,416] Patients who have structural abnormalities of chromosomes 14 or 6 also generally have a more adverse clinical course than those with a normal karyotype.[167,411,417] Finally, patients with complex leukemia-cell karyotypes[418] or complex genetics by single nucleotide polymorphism array analysis[419] tend to have an adverse prognosis.

Prospective clinical trials also indicate certain chromosomal deletions identified by FISH are associated with relatively poor response to standard chemotherapy (Fig. 94–3). Patients with leukemia cells that have trisomy 12,[420] deletions at 11q23,[167,421] or deletions at 17p13[422] have an inferior prognosis.[415,423] Döhner and colleagues defined five different categories of patients:[411] 17p deletion, 11q deletion, 12q trisomy, normal karyotype, and 13q deletion as the sole abnormality. Median overall survival was 32, 79, 114, 111, and 133 months, respectively. Disease progression differed significantly between the subgroups: median treatment-free survival was 9, 13, 33, 49, and 92 months, respectively. This model has been confirmed by other studies.[370,423,424]

Deletions at 17p13.1 are commonly associated with defects in *TP53*,[425,426] which encodes *P53*, a protein that plays a critical role in the cytotoxic activity of most forms of chemotherapy.[427] Patients who have leukemia cells that harbor deletions at 17p generally have an adverse prognosis.[196,411] However, perhaps because not all leukemia cells that have deletions at 17p also have loss of *P53* function,[426] about one-quarter of patients who have leukemia cells with detectable del(17p) might respond well to standard combination chemoimmunotherapy and/or have a relatively indolent clinical course.[428]

It also should be noted that FISH analyses at diagnosis might not be able to identify subgroups of patients who have different tendencies for disease progression. Indeed, many cytogenetic abnormalities appear acquired during the course of the disease,[429–431] and might result from leukemia cell turnover induced by other factors that are independent of the deletions observed. For example, the proportion of cases noted to have CLL cells with del(17p) or del(11q) at diagnosis appears only to be approximately 4 percent or 10 percent, respectively. On the other hand, patients with disease refractory to standard chemotherapy agents, such as fludarabine (see "Therapy" on the next page), are noted to have much higher incidences of having CLL cells with del(17p) or del(11q) at 27 percent or 32 percent, respectively. This apparently reflects selection of leukemia cells that have lost the function of *P53* with chemotherapy.[432] Moreover, frequencies of karyotypic evolution range from 11 percent to 62 percent during a median followup ranging from 1 month to 12 years.[184,373,430,431,433] This makes it worthwhile to repeat the FISH analyses prior to subsequent treatment for patients who relapse after initial therapy.

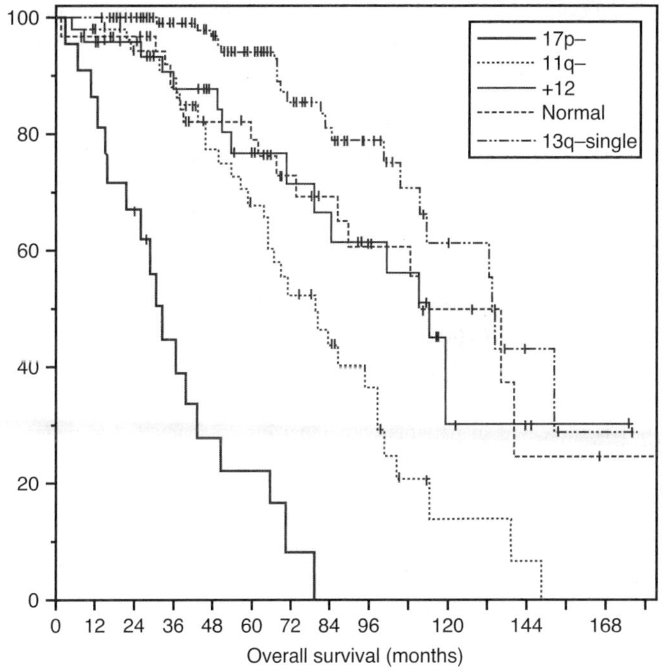

FIGURE 94–3. Prognostic relevance of genomic aberrations in chronic lymphocytic leukemia (CLL). Estimated survival probabilities from the date of diagnosis in 325 CLL patients divided into five categories defines in a hierarchical model of genomic aberrations in CLL. The median survival times for the 17p deletion (n = 23), 11q deletion (n = 56), 12p trisomy (n = 47), normal karyotype (n = 57), and 13q deletions (as single abnormality, n = 117) groups were 32, 79, 114, 111, 133 months, respectively. *(Reproduced with permission from Zenz T, Dohner H, Stilgenbaer S.[918])*

MICRORNAS

Analyses of the relative expression levels of hundreds of different microRNA in CLL and normal B cells by gene-expression array found that the microRNA expression profiles can distinguish normal from neoplastic B cells. Moreover, CLL cells with adverse prognostic markers (e.g., expression of ZAP-70 and unmutated IgHV) have microRNA gene-expression profiles that are distinct from that of leukemia cells lacking such adverse prognostic features.[434] In fact, one unique signature of 13 microRNA genes could differentiate cases of CLL with low-level expression of ZAP-70 from those having high levels of ZAP-70 and cases with mutated IgHV from those with unmutated IgHV. This same signature also can distinguish between cases that differ in clinical behavior. The differential expression of these microRNAs can be used to distinguish between the two different sets of CLL patients who have disparate risks for early disease progression and might provide insights into new targets for therapy. More studies have identified differences in expression levels of a subset of microRNAs between leukemia cell samples that have different cytogenetic abnormalities identified by FISH,[435] suggesting that some of the noted changes in gene expression between cases with differing cytogenetic abnormalities may be a result of posttranscriptional control of gene expression because of certain microRNAs.

SERUM FACTORS

Provided the patient has normal renal function, there are several serum proteins that become elevated in patients with aggressive disease. Moreover, the relative level of each of these proteins has been found to correlate with the kinetics of tumor progression and/or tumor burden.

Important caveats to consider in the use of any of these serum markers is that their levels can increase over time with increasing tumor burden and can be altered by factors unrelated to CLL, such as impaired renal clearance.[436] It should be recognized that certain treatments, diseases, or renal dysfunction could affect the relative level of each of these factors, potentially compromising their use as predictive markers. This is evident, for example, in patients treated with granulocyte-macrophage colony-stimulating factor (GM-CSF).[437] GM-CSF may increase the serum levels of beta-2-microglobulin (β_2M) and thymidine kinase (TK) independent of disease progression.[438]

Serum Beta-2-Microglobulin

β_2M ordinarily is a membrane protein that is noncovalently associated with the α chain of class I HLAs (see Chap. 138). The serum level of β_2M is increased in patients with renal insufficiency.[436] For patients with CLL who have normal renal function, the serum β_2M generally correlates with clinical stage, extent of leukemia-infiltration of the marrow, and bulky disease.[439–442] A high β_2M serum level is an adverse risk factor in evidence-based prognostic normograms,[443] and is associated with poor response to standard chemotherapy.[444]

Thymidine Kinase

Thymidine kinase (TK) is a cellular enzyme used in metabolic pathways for DNA synthesis. The predominant isoform, TK1, is found in dividing cells, but is absent in resting cells. Soluble TK (sTK) can be detected in patients with CLL, particularly in patients with advanced-staged and/or rapidly progressive disease.[442,445–447] Unfortunately, assays for sTK are neither readily available nor standardized for routine clinical use.

Other Serum Markers

High levels of several other serum proteins have been found associated with extensive tumor burden and/or survival. These include soluble CD23 (sCD23),[448,449] matrix metalloproteinase-9 (MMP-9),[450] interleukin-8,[451] interleukin-6,[452] soluble CD44 (sCD44),[453] soluble vascular cell adhesion molecule-1 (sVCAM-1),[454] or soluble CD27 (sCD27).[273,455] Lactate dehydrogenase also is generally elevated in patients with aggressive disease and in nearly all patients with Richter transformation.[32,456] Progressive disease more typically is associated with a greater suppression of T-cell function and a more marked decline in serum IgA.[457] Hypercalcemia is rare in patients with CLL[458] and may indicate Richter transformation[459,460] (see "Richter Transformation" on page 1460).

BLOOD AND MARROW HISTOLOGY

The morphology of the leukemia cells in the blood can have prognostic significance. Atypical morphology with numerous larger prolymphocytic cells or cleaved lymphocytes correlates with poor prognosis,[461–464] and often is associated with trisomy 12.[465] On the other hand, the presence of numerous smudge cells on the blood film is a characteristic associated with a relatively good prognosis.[466]

Biopsy of the marrow can reveal characteristic patterns of leukemia cell infiltration, defined as nodular, interstitial, mixed, or diffuse.[467,468] A diffuse replacement of the marrow is associated with a worse prognosis than a nodular or interstitial pattern.[309–311,440] The marrow biopsy is more reliable than the aspirate in distinguishing patients with favorable disease (nodular and/or interstitial) versus nonfavorable disease (diffuse) independent of clinical stage.[467] In addition, marrow biopsy appears more sensitive than the aspirate in detecting marrow infiltration of leukemia cells.[469] However, both the aspirate and biopsy appear to have independent prognostic value.[467,470] Evaluation of the marrow is considered desirable, especially for patients prior to therapy.[471]

TABLE 94–4. Indications for Therapy in CLL

Anemia
Thrombocytopenia
Disease-related symptoms
Markedly enlarged or painful spleen
Symptomatic lymphadenopathy
Blood lymphocyte count doubling time <6 months
Prolymphocytic transformation
Richter transformation

INDICATIONS FOR THERAPY

The current criteria for initiating therapy have not changed dramatically from the criteria established 1996 National Cancer Institute-designated working group (Table 94–4),[355,471] despite the advent of more powerful prognostic markers and chemoimmunotherapy, which apparently is providing a first-time survival benefit.[472] Clinical studies are in progress or being planned to evaluate the potential benefit of early therapy in newly diagnosed patients who have adverse prognostic markers. Until the outcomes of such studies are known, it is recommended that patients should not be treated solely on the basis of prognostic marker(s), except in clinical trials.[473]

In general practice, newly diagnosed patients with asymptomatic early stage disease (Rai 0 to I, Binet A), should be monitored without therapy unless they have evidence of progressive disease. Studies from the French Cooperative Group on CLL,[474] the Cancer and Leukemia Group B (CALGB),[475] and the Medical Research Council (MRC) in the United Kingdom revealed that the treatment of patients with early stage disease does not prolong survival. In fact the early stage patients treated in one study with alkylating agents had an increased frequency of fatal epithelial cancers and poorer survival than did nontreated patients.[474] Clinical trials are necessary to evaluate for the potential benefit of early intervention therapy based on the use of these newer prognostic markers. Also, whereas most patients with Rai stage III/IV or Binet stage B/C disease benefit from the initiation of treatment, some of these patients also can be monitored without therapy until they have evidence for progressive or symptomatic disease.

Features of progressive disease include (a) evidence of progressive marrow failure causing worsening anemia and/or thrombocytopenia; (b) progressive lymphocytosis with an increase of greater than 50 percent over a 2-month period, or LDT of less than 6 months; (c) massive or progressive lymphadenopathy; or (d) massive (i.e., >6 cm below the left costal margin) or progressive splenomegaly. LDT can be obtained by linear regression analysis of the white blood cell count obtained at intervals of 2 weeks over an observation period of 2 to 3 months. Patients with initial blood lymphocyte counts of less than 30,000/μL may require a longer observation period to determine the LDT. Also, factors contributing to lymphocytosis or lymphadenopathy other than CLL (e.g., infections) should be excluded. Other disease-related complications also require therapeutic intervention. These include intractable autoimmune anemia and/or thrombocytopenia or symptomatic disease. The latter includes (a) unintentional weight loss greater than or equal to 10 percent within the previous 6 months, (b) significant fatigue (i.e., Eastern Cooperative Oncology Group performance status of ≥2; inability to work or perform usual activities), (c) fevers greater than or equal to 38.0° C for 2 or more weeks without other evidence of infection, or (d) night sweats for 1 or more months without evidence of infection.

The symptoms associated with leukocyte aggregates that develop in patients with acute leukemia rarely occur in patients with CLL. The absolute lymphocyte count should not be used as the sole indicator for treatment. Also, hypogammaglobulinemia or monoclonal or oligoclonal paraproteinemia should not be the sole basis for initiating anti-leukemia therapy. However, patients with significant hypogammaglobulinemia who have recurrent infections can benefit from monthly infusions of intravenous immunoglobulin or prophylactic antibiotics.

WHEN TO INITIATE THERAPY FOR RECURRENT DISEASE

The criteria for instituting therapy in patients who have had prior therapy are the same as those used to initiating frontline therapy.[355] Patients who have resistant disease, a short time to progression after the first treatment (e.g., less than 6 months), and/or leukemia cells with del(17p) often do not respond to standard chemotherapy and have a relatively short survival. Such patients should be offered enrollment in investigative clinical protocols.

RESPONSE CRITERIA

Following treatment, patients can be classified as having a complete remission (CR), partial remission (PR), nonresponse (NR), or progressive disease.[355,476] Patients who fulfill all criteria for a CR except for persistent anemia, thrombocytopenia, or neutropenia that apparently is unrelated to CLL, but to drug toxicity, can be classified as having a CR with incomplete marrow recovery (CRi). By definition, patients who achieve a CRi do not have a marrow after treatment that shows leukemia cell infiltration, which by itself could contribute to the noted cytopenia. Preliminary studies suggest that patients with a CRi have a prognosis similar to that of patients who achieve a PR. In clinical trials, CRi patients should be monitored prospectively to determine whether their outcome differs from that of patients with detectable residual disease or with noncytopenic CR.

CR requires all of the following criteria, as assessed at least 2 months after completion of therapy: (a) lack of significant lymphadenopathy (e.g., lymph nodes >1 cm in diameter by physical examination); (b) lack of hepatomegaly or splenomegaly by physical examination; (c) lack of disease-associated constitutional symptoms; (d) an absolute neutrophil count of greater than or equal to 1500/μL; (e) a platelet count of greater than or equal to 100,000/μL; (f) and a hemoglobin greater than or equal to 11.0 g/dL without requiring transfusions. For clinical trials, it is recommended that patients undergo a marrow aspirate and biopsy at least 2 months after the last treatment. The marrow should be free of CLL cells, as assessed via flow cytometry and/or immunohistochemistry. Some patients, who otherwise have features of a CR, have lymphoid nodules in the marrow after therapy and were designated as having a nodular partial response. Such nodules should be assessed by immunohistochemistry to determine whether or not they are comprised primarily of lymphocytes other than CLL cells. If the marrow is found to be hypocellular, a repeat marrow biopsy should be performed after 4 to 6 weeks, provided that the blood counts have recovered. In some cases, it is desirable to postpone the marrow biopsy until the patient satisfies all the other criteria for a CR. However, this time interval for this delay should not exceed 6 months after the last treatment.

PR requires the following for a minimum of 2 months: (a) a reduction in the absolute blood lymphocyte count by greater than 50 percent; (b) a decrease in lymph node size by greater than 50 percent; (c) a decrease in palpable splenomegaly (if present) by greater than or equal to 50 percent; (d) an absolute neutrophil count of greater than or equal to 1500/μL or greater than 50 percent improvement over that noted prior to therapy; (e) a platelet count of greater than 100,000/μL or greater than 50 percent improvement over that noted prior to therapy; and (f) a hemoglobin or greater than 11.0 g/dL or greater than 50 percent improvement over that noted prior to therapy in the absence of transfusions. There should not be any noted increase in lymph nodes over that noted prior to therapy.

Patients are classified as having progressive disease[476] during treatment if they develop (a) new lymphadenopathy; (b) an increase in lymphadenopathy by greater than or equal to 50 percent; (c) an increase in the liver or spleen size by greater than 50 percent or the appearance of hepatomegaly or splenomegaly while on therapy; (d) an increase in the absolute lymphocyte count by greater than or equal to 50 percent; or (e) transformation to a more aggressive histology (e.g., Richter syndrome), which should be established by lymph node biopsy.

Refractory Disease

A patient is defined as having a relapse if they achieved a CR or PR, but experienced disease progression 12 or more months after completing therapy. On the other hand, a patient who experiences disease progression within 6 months of completing therapy is considered to have disease that is refractory to such therapy.

Minimal Residual Disease

Improved leukemia-cell detection methods can reveal patients in CR who have residual leukemia cells, termed *minimal residual disease* (MRD).[477] Although eradication of all leukemia cells appears a desired therapeutic endpoint, the risk-to-benefit ratio of additional therapy to achieve this endpoint in patients who have achieved a CR is unknown. Prospective clinical trials are needed to define whether additional treatment intended solely to eradicate MRD provides a significant benefit to clinical outcome.

Some of the techniques for assessing MRD, such as multiparameter flow cytometry, have undergone a critical evaluation and have become fairly standard.[478] Either four-color flow cytometry (MRD flow) or allele-specific oligonucleotide polymerase chain reaction (PCR) appears reliable and capable of detecting one CLL cell in 10,000 leukocytes. Using such techniques, patients can be defined as having a clinical remission in the absence of MRD when they have blood or marrow with less than one CLL cell per 10,000 leucocytes. Although the blood generally can be used for making this assessment, patients treated with monoclonal antibodies can have few if any detectable CLL cells in the blood, but readily detectable CLL cells in marrow, for 3 or more months after therapy. Another approach is to use PCR to examine for either signature immunoglobulin gene rearrangements of the leukemia cell clone[479–482] or for other genes that are expressed exclusively by the leukemia cells, such as CLL upregulated gene 1 (CLLU-1).[483] Regardless of the methods used, patients who experience eradication of MRD apparently have a longer treatment-free survival than do patients who have achieved a CR but have persistent MRD.[104,484,485] Studies are in progress to evaluate whether treatment intended to eradicate MRD is associated with prolonged survival.

Influence of Cytogenetics on the Type of Therapy

Patients with leukemia cells that have del(17p) have an inferior prognosis and appear resistant to standard chemotherapy.[192,422,486–488] Such patients often have leukemia cells that lack functional *P53*.[489] Despite their relative resistance to standard chemotherapy, patients with leukemia cells that have del(17p) might respond to therapy with alemtuzumab, either alone or in combination with other antileukemia agents.[490–492]

The ATM gene, located on 11q22, encodes a protein that functions upstream of *P53* in the response to genotoxic stress. Patients with CLL cells that harbor ATM mutations generally have an adverse prognosis.[488,493] The inactivation of the ATM gene generally occurs as a consequence of somatic mutation, but can also be present in the germ line, suggesting a predisposition of heterozygous ATM mutation carriers to develop CLL.[176,179] Patients with CLL cells that have del(11q) have significantly lower response rates to single-agent chemotherapy, such as that involving chlorambucil or fludarabine monophosphate. However, the response of such patients to treatment with a combination drug regimen using an alkylating agent, such as cyclophosphamide, with a purine analogue, such as fludarabine monophosphate, did not differ significantly from that of patients who have CLL cells that lack such deletions,[494] suggesting that combination chemotherapy is more effective than single-agent therapy in this subgroup of patients. A poorer response of this subgroup compared to other patients was not as apparent in a subsequent intragroup study.[495] However, the latter study was not powered to observe for such differences.

Other therapies are being evaluated for treatment of patients who have CLL cells with del(17p) or del(11q). These include combination chemoimmunotherapy regimens, such as those involving fludarabine, cyclophosphamide, rituximab, and alemtuzumab (CFAR),[496] oxaliplatin, fludarabine, cytarabine, and rituximab (OFAR),[497] high-dose methylprednisolone and rituximab,[498] or novel agents, such as lenalidomide,[499] BH3 mimnetics,[500,501] and flavopiridol (Alvocidib).[502]

Another strategy for treatment of drug refractory CLL with del(17p) is to circumvent loss of *P53* through activation of P73, a member of the *P53* family.[503–505] Activation of CLL cells via CD40-ligation can be achieved via gene transfer of the ligand for CD40, namely CD154.[274] This strategy has been used to modify leukemia cells *ex vivo* for subsequent use as an autologous cellular vaccine in patients with CLL.[506,507] However, patients treated with autologous leukemia cells expressing CD154 can experience acute effects of such treatment that might be secondary to innate immune effector mechanisms.[508,509] Moreover, CD154 also can induce CLL-cell expression of P73, even in leukemia cells that lack functional *P53*.[510] Induction and activation of P73 is associated with enhanced sensitivity to many anticancer drugs. Leukemia cells lacking functional *P53* can be rendered sensitive to drugs such as fludarabine monophosphate *in vitro*. This forms the basis for a clinical trial involving immune-gene therapy of patients with CLL that is drug refractory or lacking in functional *P53*. Such patients are treated with autologous CLL cells modified to express a recombinant CD154 and then subsequently given chemoimmunotherapy. Conceivably, this and similar approaches might allow us to circumvent the problems associated with drug-resistant disease.

Influence of Age on the Type of Therapy

Although patients older than age 65 years represent the largest group of CLL patients they are underrepresented in clinical trials. The average age of patients presenting to referral centers is the mid-to-late fifties, which is substantially younger than most patients with CLL, which has an average age of onset approaching 70 years of age. Treatment regimens found safe and well tolerated in clinical trials might prove too toxic for elderly patients treated in the community. In addition to having a more limited myeloid reserve and age-related decline in immune function, elderly patients have comorbidities associated with other chronic illnesses. Moreover, age-related decline in renal or hepatic function may extend the half-life of many antileukemia drugs, thus mandating consideration for dose reduction.

To identify elderly patients who are at high risk for therapy-related complications, the German CLL Study Group adopted a Cumulative Illness Rating Scale,[511] which was adopted from a rating system used successfully to assess the burden of comorbidity on elderly cancer patients.[512] Patients who are medically fit with no or just mild comorbidities and a normal life expectancy were designated "GO GO," whereas patients who were medically less fit with multiple or severe comorbidities and an unknown life expectancy were designated as "SLOW GO." Patients who were frail and had fatal comorbidities and a very short life expectancy were designated as "NO GO."

Several treatment regimens have been developed and tested in elderly patients that should be considered when developing a treatment plan for "GO GO" or "SLOW GO" patients.[511,513–520] These treatment regimens generally involve reduced doses of drugs that are used in treatment regimens for younger patients. Even so, many of these studies observed relatively high rates of grades 3 and 4 myelosuppression and/or infections in the patients treated. Although "GO GO" patients generally fare better with therapy than "SLOW GO" patients, caution still should be exercised when treating elderly "GO GO" patients with agents that are likely to induce myelosuppression. For patients designated as "NO GO", consideration should be given for withholding antileukemia treatment unless felt necessary for palliation.

THERAPEUTIC AGENTS

Deoxyadenosine Analogues

Fludarabine Fludarabine (9-β-D-arabinofuranosyl-2-fluoradenine, F-ara-A) is a fluorinated monophosphate derivative of an adenosine analogue that has activity in the treatment of CLL.[521] Given as a 30-minute intravenous infusion at a dose of 25 mg/m^2 daily for 5 days at 4-week intervals, this drug can induce hematologic complete and partial responses in a high percentage of patients.[104] An oral form of fludarabine has been developed that may have comparable activity.[522,523]

Multicenter trials typically have observed overall response rates to parenteral fludarabine of approximately 45 percent, including 10 percent with complete responses, in previously treated patients. Furthermore, overall response rates of approximately 70 percent, including 38 percent with complete responses, are achieved when fludarabine is given as frontline therapy.[524–527] Fludarabine, as a single agent, appears more effective in CLL than some combination chemotherapy regimens, such as CAP (cyclophosphamide 750 mg/m^2 and doxorubicin 50 mg/m^2 on day 1, and prednisone 50 mg/m^2 per day on days 1 to 5).[528] Moreover, remission duration appears significantly longer in patients achieving a response with fludarabine than in those who respond to such combination regimens. However, a subsequent randomized phase III study comparing first-line therapy with fludarabine to chlorambucil in 193 elderly patients with a median age of 70 years failed to reveal a significant difference in progression-free survival time (19 months with fludarabine and 18 months with chlorambucil) or survival (46 months in the fludarabine-treated group versus 64 months in the chlorambucil arm), despite demonstrating higher overall and complete remission rates in the fludarabine-treated group.[520]

Long-term followup studies indicate that even those patients who achieved complete response to fludarabine ultimately will have recurrent disease.[527] The median time to progression of responders was 33 months for those who had not received prior chemotherapy, and 21 months for those who had. The median times to progression were 27 months for patients with a partial response and 30 to 37 months for those achieving a complete response. Although multicenter clinical trials have confirmed the activity of single-agent fludarabine in CLL,[524–526] treatment of patients with this drug has not been shown to improve overall survival.

Approximately one-third of patients who have not received prior therapy and nearly half of those who are refractory to treatment with chlorambucil will not achieve even a partial response to treatment with fludarabine. Logistic regression analysis in one study identified four factors that were associated with poorer response to fludarabine:

Rai stages III–IV disease, prior therapy, older age, and low albumin levels.[529] *In vitro* drug-sensitivity testing using a differential staining cytotoxicity (DiSC) assay may have predictive value in identifying patients with fludarabine-response disease.[530,531] In addition, patients who do not show evidence for a response to the first two cycles of therapy are unlikely to achieve a partial or complete response to subsequent cycles of treatment. For this reason, patients who fail to show any clinical benefit from two cycles of treatment should be considered for alternative types of therapy to minimize toxicity.

The major toxicities are hematologic and immunologic. Neutropenia is noted in approximately two-thirds of treated patients with advanced disease, although this usually is not dose limiting. Patients also may experience reversible neurologic toxicity, even after receiving the standard dose of fludarabine.[532] Highly responsive patients may experience the tumor lysis syndrome.[533,534]

The major morbidity associated with fludarabine is immune suppression. Fludarabine produces a pronounced decrease in the number of blood T cells, especially CD4+ T cells, that often persists for more than a year after therapy.[535,536] Treated patients apparently have an increased incidence of infection with opportunistic organisms, including herpes simplex, herpes zoster, *L. monocytogenes*, and *Pneumocystis jiroveci* (formerly called *Pneumocystis carinii*).[529,536,537]

Patients treated with fludarabine have been noted to have an increased incidence of new-onset autoimmune diseases, such as autoimmune hemolytic anemia, immune thrombocytopenia, and pure red cell aplasia.[538] However, it is controversial whether this defines a causal relationship.[539] Tumor lysis syndrome can be another therapy-related complication.[533,534] Finally, CLL patients treated with fludarabine also may develop transfusion-associated graft-versus-host disease,[540,541] possibly reflecting the overall impairment to the host immune system that is induced by this drug. Despite the associated immune suppression, treatment with fludarabine does not appear to increase the risk for secondary malignancies in patients with CLL.[542]

Pharmacokinetics Within minutes after intravenous infusion, fludarabine is converted to the active metabolite, 2-fluoro-ara-A. This metabolite has a terminal half-life of approximately 20 hours. Renal clearance represents approximately 40 percent of the total-body clearance, which can also be achieved via hemodialysis in patients who experience acute renal failure after drug therapy.[543] Patients with moderate renal impairment (glomerular filtration rate [GFR] of between 17 and 41 mL/min/m^2) will achieve a similar plasma concentration of 2-fluoro-ara-A after receiving 20 percent reduced-dose fludarabine as do patients with normal renal function who received the full dose. Fludarabine should not be administered to patients with a GFR of less than 17 mL/min/m^2, which for an average patient of 1.7 m^2 is approximately 30 mL/min.

Cladribine Cladribine (2-chlorodeoxyadenosine [2CdA], Leustatin) is a deoxyadenosine analogue that also has activity in CLL.[544] Different dosage schedules or administration routes have proved effective, although the response rates do not appear to be superior to those achieved with fludarabine. Monthly courses of cladribine given via intravenous infusion over 2 hours at 0.12 mg/kg, daily for 5 consecutive days, have resulted in overall response rates of approximately 40 percent to 60 percent in patients who were previously treated with alkylating agents.[545] Higher overall response rates are observed in previously untreated patients. Although one study found that patients refractory to fludarabine still could respond to cladribine,[546] subsequent studies have found that patients with advanced CLL refractory to fludarabine therapy were not likely to benefit from treatment with cladribine.[547]

Cladribine also appears effective when administered orally.[548] Overall response rates of 75 percent were noted in previously nontreated CLL patients given cladribine at 10 mg/m^2 per day for 5 consecutive days of each 28-day course[549] or at 10 mg/m^2 per day orally for 3 consecutive days for each 21-day course.[548]

Treatment with cladribine has not been shown to prolong survival. The median duration of partial remissions is approximately 9 months, and nonresponding patients have a relatively short median survival of approximately 4 months. DiSC assays[530] have been reported to have predictive value in assessing a given patient's potential response to therapy.[550] However, the most evident predictor of a good response was a rapid decrease of blood lymphocyte counts following the first course of therapy. As with fludarabine, patients who fail to show any clinical benefit from two cycles of cladribine should be considered for alternative types of therapy to minimize toxicity.

The toxicities of treatment with cladribine are similar to those with fludarabine. Thrombocytopenia is a common dose-limiting toxicity, as is general myelosuppression. As with fludarabine, treated patients experience long-lasting reductions in the levels of blood T cells and have impaired cellular immunity to viral infections. Systemic fungal infections and opportunistic infections are a common cause of morbidity and mortality. In rare cases, patients treated with cladribine can experience tumor lysis syndrome.[551]

Pharmacokinetics After intravenous administration, cladribine has an average half-life in the plasma of approximately 7 hours, but distributes extensively through the body tissues, including the cerebrospinal fluid, which achieves concentrations of approximately 25 percent that are found in the plasma. Both serum creatinine and total bilirubin are significant predictors of drug clearance,[552] and only approximately 20 percent of the administered drug is excreted unchanged in the urine. The cladribine dose has to be adjusted or held for patients with impaired renal or hepatic function.

Pentostatin Pentostatin (deoxycoformycin, Nipent) is a purine analogue synthesized by *Streptomyces antibioticus* that structurally is related to adenosine.[553] This drug inhibits adenosine deaminase, an enzyme important in lymphocyte purine metabolism. Pentostatin generally is administered intravenously at a dosage of 4 mg/m^2 weekly for 3 weeks, then 4 mg/m^2 every other week for 6 weeks, followed by once a month for 6 months.[554] Alternative dosing regimens using pentostatin at 2 mg/m^2 per day for 5 days every 28 days, with the dosage adjusted up or down by 0.5 mg/m^2 in subsequent cycles on the basis of activity or hematologic toxicity, have been associated with improved response rates.[555] Alone or in combination with other agents (see "Combination Therapy" on page 1451), pentostatin has activity in CLL that appears comparable to that of fludarabine.[556]

Clearance More than 90 percent of the administered drug is excreted unchanged in the urine.[557] There is a good correlation between the measure creatinine clearance and pentostatin plasma clearance. For this reason, the dose of this drug should be adjusted for patients with impaired renal function.[557]

Alkylating Agents

Chlorambucil Since its introduction in 1952, chlorambucil (Leukeran) has been the main alkylating agent used for CLL. Although chlorambucil is useful in the palliative therapy of patients with advanced-stage disease, it does not appear to improve survival and should not be used for asymptomatic patients with early stage disease.[474]

Given orally, it generally is well tolerated, without the side effects such as cystitis, alopecia, or gastrointestinal distress, that sometimes may be seen with other alkylating agents. There seems to be relative sparing of the myeloid and megakaryocytic series. Generally, patients are started on a daily oral dose of 2 to 4 mg. This can be advanced to 6 to 8 mg per day if the patient does not experience intolerable hematologic toxicity.

Alternatively, patients can be treated intermittently with a total oral dose of approximately 0.4 to 0.7 mg/kg. This dose can be given on day 1 or divided into four equal daily doses and given on days 1 through 4. The cycle is repeated every 2 to 4 weeks, depending on the time to marrow recovery. Pulse chlorambucil is as effective as continuous administration and is less myelotoxic.[558] Complete response rates of 15 percent and partial response rates of 65 percent are common.[559]

High-dose chlorambucil has been studied for patients with advanced-stage CLL.[560] Chlorambucil was given for less than 6 months at a fixed dose of 15 mg per day until the patient achieved a complete response, or grade 3 toxicity. This treatment was noted in one single-institution study to effect a higher complete and partial response rate (89.5%) than that achieved with cyclophosphamide, doxorubicin, vincristine, and prednisone (CHOP; e.g., 6 monthly cycles of doxorubicin at 25 mg/m^2 on day 1, vincristine 1 mg/m^2 on day 1, cyclophosphamide 30 mg/m^2 per day, and prednisone 40 mg/m^2 per day on days 1 to 5). However, significant myelotoxicity was observed.

Bendamustine Bendamustine (Treanda) is a relatively new alkylating agent that has activity in CLL. Although this agent was synthesized with the intent of combining the alkylating properties of mechlorethamine with the purine antimetabolite properties of benzimidazole, the activity of bendamustine appears to stem from its capacity to act as an alkylating agent.[561] Phase I/II trials with bendamustine at 70 to 100 mg/m^2 given intravenously on each of two consecutive days every 4 weeks demonstrated overall response rates of 56 to 93 percent and complete response rates of 7 to 29 percent in patients with relapsed/refractory CLL.[562–565] A phase III trial comparing the activity of chlorambucil versus bendamustine in the initial therapy of 319 patients with CLL demonstrated significantly higher response rates in patients treated with bendamustine.[566] For this study, patients were randomized to receive either chlorambucil (at a dose of 0.8 mg/kg on days 1 and 15, or as divided doses on days 1 and 2 and 15 and 16, every 4 weeks) or bendamustine at a dose of 100 mg/m^2 on days 1 and 2 every 4 weeks. Depending on tolerance and response, patients received up to six cycles of therapy. Complete and partial responses were observed in 68 percent of the bendamustine-treated group and in 31 percent of the chlorambucil-treated group. Moreover, median progression-free survival was 21.6 months for the bendamustine-treated subgroup and 8.3 months for the chlorambucil-treated subgroup (P <0.0001). Because of these findings, the FDA approved bendamustine for use in the initial therapy of CLL in 2008.[567]

Myelosuppression is the major toxicity incurred by patients treated with bendamustine. In the registration phase III study, 23 percent of treated patients developed grade 3 and 12 percent developed grade 4 neutropenia or thrombocytopenia.[566] This has prompted consideration for using a reduced dose of bendamustine at 70 mg/m^2 on days 1 and 2 of each cycle instead of the 100 mg/m^2 per day dose, particularly for treatment of previously treated patients or elderly patients who might have limited myeloid reserve. For patients who experience grade 3 or greater hematologic toxicity following treatment, it is recommended that the dose be reduced to 50 mg/m^2 on days 1 and 2 of each cycle. If grade 3 hematologic toxicity recurs, then further reduction of the dose to 25 mg/m^2 on days 1 and 2 should be considered. In the event of grade 4 hematologic toxicity or clinically significant grade 2 or higher nonhematologic toxicity, then treatment should be delayed until such toxicity has resolved, or at the discretion of the treating physician.

Pharmacokinetics Bendamustine is primarily metabolized by hydrolysis to metabolites with low cytotoxic activity. Its half-life in the plasma following intravenous administration is approximately 40 minutes. More than 90 percent of the metabolized drug is excreted in the feces. Despite this noted pharmacology, bendamustine is not recommended for treatment of patients with a GFR of less than 23 mL/min/m^2.

Cyclophosphamide Cyclophosphamide is as active as chlorambucil in CLL.[568] Patients can be started on daily oral doses of 50 to 100 mg. Alternatively, patients can be treated intermittently with 500 to 750 mg/m^2 given intravenously or orally every 3 to 4 weeks, depending on the time to marrow recovery. Because intermittent or daily oral cyclophosphamide predisposes to hemorrhagic cystitis, it should be taken as a single dose in the morning rather than at bedtime. Patients should be encouraged to drink at least 2 to 3 L of fluid per day.

Alemtuzumab (Campath-1H)

Alemtuzumab (Campath-1H, MabCampath, or Campath) is humanized monoclonal antibody specific for human CD52, a glycosylphosphatidylinositol-anchored surface protein found on most lymphocytes (see Chap. 15).[569] This antibody can mediate complement-mediated lysis,[570] antibody-dependent cell-mediated cytotoxicity,[571] and direct growth-inhibition of most lymphocytes,[572] including CLL B cells.[573] This antibody was found active in the treatment of CLL when given to patients either via an intravenous[574,575] or subcutaneous route of administration.[576] Of particular interest, this antibody appears capable of clearing leukemia cells with deletions at 17p13,[490] which typically are resistant to standard anti-leukemia drugs.

Alemtuzumab in the Treatment of Relapse/Refractory CLL In May 2001, alemtuzumab received accelerated approval by the FDA for treatment of patients who had received prior alkylating drugs and who had failed prior treatment with fludarabine. This was based upon evidence obtained from an overall response rate of 33 percent and complete response rate of 2 percent in patients who were refractory to fludarabine treatment regimens.[577–579] The multicenter trial enrolled 93 patients who had relapsed disease following treatment with fludarabine.[578] These patients received 3 mg, increased to 10 mg, and then to 30 mg when infusion-related reactions were tolerated.[578] Treatment was continued at 30 mg administered intravenously 3 times per week for a maximum of 12 weeks. Infusion-related toxicity was experienced in 75 (81%), consisting of rigors (90% overall, with 14% having grade 3 or 4), fever (85%, with 14% grade 3 or higher), nausea (53%), and rash (33%). Except for rash, infusion-related toxicity diminished with each successive administration. A major toxicity was immune suppression. Fifty-one (55%) of the patients experienced infections during or after treatment with microorganisms commonly observed in the immune-compromised patient, in particular cytomegalovirus (CMV) (see Chap. 22). A total of 9 deaths occurred during or within 30 days of treatment, of which 5 were secondary to infection. Thirty-one (33%) patients responded, although only 2 patients (2%) achieved a complete response by 1996 National Cancer Institute designated Working Group criteria.[471] Six patients (7%) achieved a CRi, 5 (5%) experienced a nodular partial remission (nPR), and 29 (31%) achieved a PR. Patients with bulky lymph nodes (diameter ≥5 cm) or a performance status of greater than or equal to 2 failed to achieve a beneficial therapeutic outcome. The median duration of response was 8.7 months and median survival after therapy was 16 months. Other studies reported overall response rates of 31 to 54 percent and complete response rates of 0 to 35 percent following 12 to 16 weeks of intravenous alemtuzumab in patients who had relapsed disease and/or disease refractory to fludarabine.[485,575–577,590,919]

Similar thrice weekly dosing regimens have been used for subsequent studies.[580] Patients typically are given successively increasing doses 1 mg, 3 mg, 10 mg, and then 30 mg per injection to mitigate the infusional reactions of fever, chills, and/or rash, which generally are more pronounced during the initial administrations of this antibody. Grade 4 neutropenia is not uncommon, but is not an indication to discontinue treatment. Clinicians also should be cautious of prematurely terminating treatment at 4 to 6 weeks in patients whose disease responds to treatment. Although resolution of lymphocytosis occurs early in most patients, the marrow is unlikely to be clear of disease during the first several weeks of treatment. Also, although this monoclonal antibody has significant activity against leukemia cells in the blood and marrow, it appears less effective in clearing cells in secondary lymphoid tissues,[581,582] where they might be protected from apoptosis by nurse-like cells and other stromal elements.[253] Patients with bulky lymphadenopathy (greater than 5 cm in diameter) appear unlikely to achieve a complete response to therapy with alemtuzumab. In addition, treatment with alemtuzumab reduces the absolute numbers of blood natural killer cells and T lymphocytes to levels that are less than 25 percent of pretreatment values for more than 9 months following treatment.[583] Treated patients have an increased susceptibility to opportunistic infections (especially CMV), and should receive concomitant antimicrobial therapy in prophylaxis against infection (see Chap. 22).[584,585]

Alemtuzumab in the Initial Therapy of CLL FDA approval of alemtuzumab in 2001 was contingent upon the manufacturer's commitment to perform a phase III clinical trial examining the efficacy and safety of alemtuzumab relative to standard therapy.[586] This formed the basis for the large, open-label, international, multicenter randomized trial, designated CAM 307, which was designed to test whether alemtuzumab yielded a longer progression-free survival duration than did single-agent chlorambucil when given as initial therapy for CLL. Two-hundred ninety-seven patients with progressive and/or symptomatic disease were randomized (1:1) to receive either chlorambucil at 40 mg/m^2 every 28 days, for up to 12 months, or intravenous alemtuzumab at 30 mg three times per week, for up to 12 weeks.[587] The 149 patients treated with alemtuzumab had a CR rate of 24 percent, an overall response (OR) rate of 83 percent, and time-to-progression requiring alternative treatment of 23.3 months, which were significantly superior to the CR rate of 2 percent, OR rate of 55 percent, and time-to-progression of 14.7 months observed in the 148 patients treated with chlorambucil.[587] Furthermore, 11 of the 36 alemtuzumab-treated patients who achieved a CR achieved an MRD-negative CR. Adverse events profiles of the two treatment cohorts were similar, except that alemtuzumab-treated patients had infusion-related toxicity and a higher incidence of CMV infections than the chlorambucil-treated group. Because of these findings the FDA approved intravenous alemtuzumab for use in the initial therapy of patients with CLL in September 2007.[586]

Subcutaneous Administration of Alemtuzumab To mitigate the problems associated with intravenous alemtuzumab, such as fever, chills, and/or rash, alemtuzumab also has been administered subcutaneously at 30 mg three times per week for 6 or more weeks.[576] Several subsequent clinical trials involving use of subcutaneous alemtuzumab have been performed, demonstrating the clinical activity of thrice weekly subcutaneous administration of 30 mg alemtuzumab in the initial or second-line treatment of patients with CLL.[588–590]

However, a comparison pharmacokinetic study found that the blood concentrations of alemtuzumab achieved following subcutaneous administration were significantly lower than those observed following intravenous administration of the same amount of antibody.[591] Moreover, this study found that the cumulative dose of intravenous alemtuzumab required to reach 1.0 mcg/mL ranged from 13 mg to 316 mg (mean: 90 mg), whereas the cumulative dose of subcutaneous alemtuzumab to reach 1.0 mcg/mL was 146 mg to 1106 mg (mean: 551 mg).[591] This appears clinically relevant as higher blood concentrations of alemtuzumab apparently correlate with improved clinical responses and/or eradication of MRD following treatment.[592] Administration of alemtuzumab via the subcutaneous route should require longer treatment durations and/or greater amounts of alemtuzumab to achieve comparable clinical responses as those observed with intravenous alemtuzumab. Unfortunately, head-to-head randomized phase III trials comparing the relative efficacy of subcutaneous versus intravenous administration of alemtuzumab have not been performed. The FDA has yet to approve the use of subcutaneous alemtuzumab in the treatment of CLL.

Despite the lack of FDA approval, many clinicians favor administration of alemtuzumab via the subcutaneous route because of its relative ease of use. Compared to intravenous delivery, subcutaneous delivery of alemtuzumab is associated with fewer administration-associated adverse events. Adverse events following subcutaneous administration of alemtuzumab include grade 1 or 2 local bruising and/or discomfort at the site of injection (usually the abdomen). Nevertheless, the hematologic toxicity observed following treatment with intravenous alemtuzumab also is observed following subcutaneous administration. In the largest multi-institution study, involving 109 patients with relapsed CLL who received 30 mg of subcutaneous alemtuzumab three times per week for up to 12 weeks, there were 120 total treatment interruptions in 65 patients. Twenty-seven percent of interruptions were because of neutropenia, 36 percent were because of infection, 3 percent were because of anemia, and 8 percent were because of thrombocytopenia. Treatment was stopped altogether in 65 patients because of insufficient response (43%), infection (29%), hematologic toxicity (14%), or other causes (12%). Moreover, 58 (56%), 59 (57%), and 51 (49%) of the patients experienced grade 3 or 4 neutropenia, thrombocytopenia, or anemia, respectively.[590] Sixteen patients (16%) had reactivation of CMV and 30 patients (29%) had grade 3 or 4 non-CMV infections during or after treatment. It was noted, however, that patient population studied already was at high risk for infections; 35 (32%) of the patients had grade 3 or 4 infections within the 6 months prior to enrollment in the study.[590] Despite the subcutaneous route of administration, the overall response rates and time-to-progression of the patients treated on this trial appeared comparable to those experienced by patients treated with intravenous alemtuzumab.

Alemtuzumab in Consolidation Therapy Because alemtuzumab appears most active in clearing leukemia cells from the blood and marrow that are resistant to standard chemotherapy,[490] several studies have evaluated the use of alemtuzumab in consolidation therapy following treatment with other agents.[593–597]

To evaluate the benefit of alemtuzumab consolidation therapy, patients who responded to initial treatment with fludarabine or fludarabine and cyclophosphamide were randomized to observation or treatment with alemtuzumab administered intravenously at 30 mg three times per week for 12 weeks.[594] However, this study was stopped after accrual of 21 patients because of the increased incidence of severe infections observed in the 11 patients who were treated with alemtuzumab. Conceivably, the short interval between initial treatment and consolidation therapy with alemtuzumab (e.g., less than 2 months) was a factor in the relatively high incidence of infection observed in the alemtuzumab-treated patients.[596] Nevertheless, the alemtuzumab-treated patients enjoyed a longer progression-free survival than the observation group. After a median period of 48 months, the progression-free survival was significantly prolonged for patients who received alemtuzumab consolidation therapy compared to those patients who had no further treatment.[597] In any case, the improvement in long-term outcome of the treated patients provides incentive for conducting additional studies on the relative risk versus benefits of alemtuzumab consolidation after initial therapy.

Rituximab (Rituxan)

Rituximab is an monoclonal antibody specific for CD20 that initially was found effective in the treatment of follicular lymphoma. Infusion of this rituximab at 375 mg/m^2 per week for 4 weeks can induce responses in nearly half of patients treated with relapsed follicular lymphoma.[598,599]

Although CD20 is expressed at low levels by CLL B cells relative to the cells in follicular lymphoma, several clinical trials have demonstrated this monoclonal antibody to have a therapeutic benefit in patients with CLL (Table 94–5). When used as a single agent at the standard dose of 4 weekly injections of 375 mg/m,^{2} rituximab generally can induce only partial responses in less than a third of symptomatic patients.[600,601] Higher response rates may be achieved at higher doses. In one study, thrice weekly infusions of 375 mg/m^2 induced overall response rates of 45% in patients previously treated with chemotherapy[602] (Table 94–5). In another study, response correlated with dose: 22% for patients treated at 500 to 825 mg/m,^{2}43% for those treated at 1000 to 1500 mg/m,^{2} and 75% for those treated at the highest dose of 2250 mg/m.[2603] These higher doses may overcome soluble inhibitors to the CD20 monoclonal antibody that are found in the sera of most patients with CLL.[603,604] Nevertheless, the responses observed with even high doses of single-agent rituximab generally are only partial, limited mainly to the lymph nodes, and typically are associated with median times to disease progression of less than 8 months.[603]

TABLE 94–5. Rituximab Treatment Regimens

Rituximab Treatment	Prior Therapy	No. Patients Evaluable	% CR	% OR	Median TTP (mo.)	Reference
375 mg/m^2 IV qwk × 4	Yes	30	0	13	N/A	McLaughlin et al.[599]
375 mg/m^2 IV qwk × 4	Yes	28	0	25	5	Huhn et al.[920]
500–825 mg/m^2 IV qwk × 4	Yes	24	0	21	N/A	O'Brien et al.[603]
1.0–1.5 g/m^2 IV qwk × 4	Yes	7	0	43	N/A	O'Brien et al. [603]
2.25 g/m^2 IV qwk × 4	Yes	8	0	75	N/A	O'Brien et al.[603]
375 mg/m^2 IV TIW qwk × 4	Mixed	29	4	52	11	Byrd et al.[602]
375 mg/m^2 IV qwk × 4 then q6mo. for 2 y	Yes	44	9	58	19	Hainsworth et al.[601]; Hainsworth[921]

CR, complete response; IV, intravenously; OR, overall response; TIW, three times per week; TTP, time to progression.

Toxicity with the first dose (375 mg/m^2) can be as high as 94 percent of patients but was grade 1 or 2 in most, predominantly fever and chills.[603] Rare patients have experienced tumor lysis syndrome.[605] More commonly, patients can experience a decline in the blood neutrophil count following treatment, sometimes resulting in neutropenia.[606] Finally, patients with leukemia cell counts exceeding 50 × 10^9/L at the time of initial treatment may experience a cytokine-release syndrome thought in part a result of release of TNF-α or interleukin-6.[607] Such patients experience fever, chills, nausea, vomiting, hypotension, and/or dyspnea during the initial infusion of rituximab. When severe, there may be signs of mild disseminated intravascular coagulation within 12 hours after the initiation of treatment (see Chap. 130). The severity of and risk for infusion-related reactions abate with successive infusions. Problems related to the initial treatment can be mitigated by slowing the rate of infusion and by splitting the first dose, giving 100 mg rituximab on the first day and then the remainder of the 375 mg/m^2 dose on day 2.

Glucocorticoids

Glucocorticoids are effective as single agents in CLL, especially for patients with autoimmune hemolytic anemia or immune thrombocytopenia (see Chaps. 53 and 119). Even for nonautoimmune manifestations, prednisone, as a single agent, can control the disease temporarily in approximately 10 percent of patients.[558] Generally, prednisone is given orally at a dose of 40 to 60 mg/day for 1 week and then tapered and stopped after another week. Thereafter, prednisone is given every month for 5 days at 60 mg/day.

Partial responses may be achieved by treatment with intravenous high-dose methylprednisolone at 1 g/m^2 per day for 5 days at monthly intervals for 3 to 7 months.[608,609] This treatment has apparent activity even in patients with CLL lacking functional *P53*.[610] Concomitant therapy with H_2 antagonists and prophylactic antibiotics can reduce the rate of treatment-related complications, which also include fluid retention, hyperglycemia, and immune suppression.

Other Agents

Cytosine Arabinoside High-dose cytosine arabinoside has modest activity in advanced-stage CLL.[611] It is administered intravenously at a dosage of 3 g/m^2 delivered over 2 hours. This may be repeated one to three times every 12 hours to complete one cycle.

Cytosine arabinoside[612] also has been used successfully to treat patients with relapsed or refractory disease as part of a regimen that includes other agents, such as the oxaliplatin, fludarabine monophosphate, ara-C, and rituximab regimen (the OFAR regimen; see "Combination Therapy" below),[497] or the fludarabine monophosphate, ara-C, Novantrone (mitoxantrone), and dexamethasone regimen (the "FAND" regimen).[613]

Etoposide Patients who failed alkylator-based chemotherapy have been noted to achieve partial responses with oral etoposide, lasting 2 to 18 months.[614] Etoposide was administered as a single drug at a dosage of 50 mg/m^2 per day for 21 days in a 28-day cycle. Myelosuppression was the most common and serious dose-limiting effect. Etoposide at 100 mg/m^2 together with cladribine at 0.12 mg/kg/day given intravenously on days 1 through 5 of each 4-week cycle was used to treat patients with relapsed or refractory patients with CLL or other indolent lymphomas. Seven of 20 such patients who received three or more cycles of this regimen achieved a CR (1 patient) or PR to therapy and had a median overall survival time of 22 months (range: 3–30).[615] As expected myelosuppression and infections were the major toxicity of this regimen.

Mitoxantrone Mitoxantrone (Novantrone), a topoisomerase II inhibitor, has apparent activity in CLL.[616] Most clinical studies have used this agent on day 1 of each cycle at 6 to 10 mg/m^2 in combination with other antileukemia agents, such as cyclophosphamide and/or fludarabine,[165,617] cladribine,[618–622] bendamustine,[623] cytosine arabinoside,[624] and/or rituximab[620,625] (see "Combination Therapy" below).

■ COMBINATION THERAPY

Chlorambucil and Prednisone

The standard regimen for treating patients who warrant the initiation of chemotherapy has been the combination of oral chlorambucil and prednisone. Each cycle consists of chlorambucil at 0.4 to 0.7 mg/kg on day 1, with prednisone at 80 mg per day on days 1 through 5. This course is repeated every 2 to 4 weeks, depending on the time to marrow recovery. The dosage of chlorambucil may be divided and given over 2 days. It is raised or lowered based upon the response and the degree of myelosuppression. When the white cell count declines below 10,000/μL the dose of chlorambucil should be reduced to maintain the white cell count between 5000/μL and 10,000/μL. The addition of prednisone to chlorambucil may provide a therapeutic advantage over chlorambucil alone.[559] However, more studies have challenged this notion.[626,627] Nevertheless, responses to the combination of chlorambucil and prednisone occur in approximately 80 percent (complete remissions in 15% plus partial remissions in 65%) of patients.[558,628–630] However, this regimen appears less active than other combination therapy regimens that include newer agents, such as the deoxyadenosine analogues and monoclonal antibodies.

Fludarabine-Containing Regimens

Fludarabine/Cyclophosphamide Combinations of fludarabine, at 20 to 30 mg/m^2 daily for 3 days, and cyclophosphamide, at 200 to 300 mg/m^2 daily for 3 days, given every 28 days can result in favorable clinical responses in extensively pretreated patients.[631] The daily administration of fludarabine at 25 to 30 mg/m^2 for 3 days and cyclophosphamide at 300 mg/m^2 for 3 days induced complete responses after 4 to 6 courses in 30 to 35 percent in previously untreated patients,[632–635] complete response rates that appear higher than that achieved using single agent fludarabine.[636] This was corroborated by subsequent randomized phase III trials comparing the responses to fludarabine versus fludarabine and cyclophosphamide in 375 patients younger than 66 years of age.[494] Patients were randomized to receive either intravenous fludarabine at 25 mg/m^2 for 5 days of each 28-day cycle or intravenous fludarabine at 30 mg/m^2 for 3 days in combination with cyclophosphamide 250 mg/m^2 for 3 days of each 28-day cycle. After 6 courses of therapy, the patients treated with fludarabine and cyclophosphamide (FC) achieved a significantly higher CR rate (24%), OR rate (94%), and longer progression-free survival (48 months) than patients treated with fludarabine alone (7% CR, 83% OR, and 20 months progression-free survival, respectively).[494]

The main complications of this regimen are related to immune suppression and myelosuppression, which can be dose-limiting and severe, particularly in heavily pretreated patients. For this reason, fludarabine commonly is given for 3 days per 28-day cycle at only 25 mg/m^2 along with cyclophosphamide at 250 mg/m.^{2}

Fludarabine/Cyclophosphamide/Rituximab Treatment with rituximab concomitant with fludarabine and cyclophosphamide (FCR) appears highly effective (Tables 94–6 and 94–7). When given at 375 mg/m^2 on day 1 of course 1 and then at 500 mg/m^2 on day 1 of courses 2 to 6, rituximab when used with fludarabine/cyclophosphamide induced complete responses in 25 percent and overall responses in 73 percent of previously treated patients.[637] Moreover, 32 percent of the patients who achieved a complete response did not have evidence for minimal residual disease in the marrow by molecular testing. Higher response rates are observed in previously untreated patients. In one single-institution study of 224 patients, the complete response rate was 70 percent, the nodular partial response rate 10 percent, and the partial response rate 15 percent, for an overall response rate of 95 percent.[580] As with the fludarabine/cyclophosphamide regimen, the major toxicity was related to myelosuppression, with grade 3 to 4 neutropenia occurring during 52 percent of the courses in previously untreated patients.

TABLE 94–6. Chemoimmunotherapy Treatment Regimens for Patients with Frontline Chronic Lymphocytic Leukemia

Treatment Group/Regimen	No. Patients Evaluable	% CR	% OR	PFS at 24 Months	Reference
Sequential F – 25 mg/m^2 IV d 1–5, course 1–6; *after 2 mo. observation, then* R – 375 mg/m^2 IV weekly × 4	53	28	77	45%	Cancer and Leukemia Group B (CALGB) 9712[641]
Or					
Concurrent F – 25 mg/m^2 IV d 1–5, course 1–6; R – 375 mg/m^2 IV d 1, 4, course 1; d 1, course 2–6 *after 2 mo. observation, then* R – 375 mg/m^2 IV weekly × 4	51	47	90	67%	
F – 25 mg/m^2 IV d 2–4, course 1; d 1–3, course 2–6 C – 250 mg/m^2 IV d 2–4, course 1; d 1–3, course 2–6 R – 375–500 mg/m^2 IV d 1, course 1–6	224	70	95	68%	Keating et al.[580]
P – 2 mg/m^2 IV d 1, course 1–6 C – 600 mg/m^2 IV d 1, course 1–6; R – 375 mg/m^2 IV d 1, course 2–6	64	41	91	61%	Kay et al.[649]
F – 25 mg/m^2 IV d 1–3; course 1–6 C – 250 mg/m^2 IV d 1–3; q28d; course 1–6 R – 375 mg/m^2 IV d 0, course 1; 500 mg/m^2 d 1, course 1–6	390	52	95	76%	Hallek et al.[638]
Or					
F – 25 mg/m^2 IV d 1–3; q28d; course 1–6; C – 250 mg/m^2 IV d 1–3; q28d; course 1–6	391	27	88	62%	

C, cyclophosphamide; CR, complete remission; d, day; IV, intravenously; F, fludarabine; No., number; OR, overall response; P, pentostatin; PD, progressive disease; PFS, progression free survival; R, rituximab.

TABLE 94–7. Chemoimmunotherapy Treatment Regimens for Patients with Pretreated Chronic Lymphocytic Leukemia

Treatment Group/Regimen	No. Patients Evaluable	% CR	% OR	Median TTP (mo.)	Reference
F – 25 mg/m² IV d 2–4, course 1; d 1–3, course 2–6 C – 250 mg/m² IV d 1, 4, course 1; d1, course 2–6 R – 375 mg/m² d 1, course 1; 500 mg/m² d1, course 2–6	177	25	73	N/A	Wierda et al.[637]
P – 4 mg/m² IV d 1, course 1–6 C – 600 mg/m² IV d 1, course 1–6; R – 375 mg/m² IV d 1, course 2–6	32	25	75	N/A	Lamanna et al.[648]
F – 25 mg/m² IV d 1–3, course 1–6 C – 250 mg/m² IV d 1–3; course 1–6 R – 375 mg/m² IV, course 1; 500 mg/m² IV, course 2–6	274	24	70	31	Robak et al.[922]
Or					
F – 25 mg/m² IV d 1–3, course 1–6 C – 250 mg/m² IV d 1–3; course 1–6	272	13	58	21	
C – 250 mg/m² IV d 3–5; course 1–6 F – 25 mg/m² IV d 3–5; course 1–6 A – 30 mg/m² IV d 1, 3, 5; course 1–6 R – 375–500 mg/m² IV d 2; course 1–6	28	4	46	16	Wierda, et al[923]
F – 30 mg/m² d 1–3; course 1–6 A – 30 mg/m² d 1–3; course 1–6	36	30	83	13	Elter et al.[924]
F – 25 mg/m² IV d 1–3 A – 30 mg IV TIW × 12 wks	6	17	83	N/A	Kennedy et al.[579]
A – 30 mg IV TIW × 24 wks. *then if there is PD or SD add* F – 40 mg/m² PO d 1–3; course 1; d 1–3, course 2–6	8	0	2	N/A	UKCLL02[925]

A, alemtuzumab; C, cyclophosphamide; CR, complete remission; d, day; IV, intravenously F, fludarabine; N/A, not applicable; No., number; OR, overall response; P, pentostatin; PD, progressive disease; PO, oral; R, rituximab; SD, stable disease; TIW, thrice weekly; TTP, time to tumor progression.

A large multicenter phase III trial established the superiority of FCR over FC (see Table 94–6).[638] Eight-hundred seventeen patients were randomly assigned to received either FC (intravenous fludarabine at 25 mg/m² and cyclophosphamide 250 mg/m² on days 1–3 every 28 days) or FCR (FC plus rituximab at 375 mg/m² on day 1 of the first cycle and then 500 mg/m² on day 1 of cycles 2–6). Both treatment arms were well balanced with respect to age, stage, and prognostic factors. Patients treated with FCR had a significantly higher CR rate (44.5%) and OR rate (95%) than did patients treated with FC, who had CR rates and OR rates of 22.9 percent and 88 percent, respectively. Moreover, after an average followup of 25.5 months, patients treated with FCR had a significantly longer progression-free survival (42.8 months) than did patients treated with FC (32.3 months).[638]

The major toxicity observed with either FCR or FC was hematologic. Severe hematologic toxicity was observed in 55 percent of patients treated with FCR versus 39 percent for patients treated with FC.[638] FCR-treated patients had a significantly higher incidence of grade 3 and 4 neutropenia (33.6%) than did FC-treated patients (20.9%), but not thrombocytopenia (FCR group 7.4% vs. FC group 10.8%) or anemia (FCR group 5.4% vs. FC group 6.8%). The incidence of grade 3 or 4 infections did not differ significantly between the two treatment groups (18.8% for the FCR group and 14.8% for the FC group). Treatment-related mortality did not differ significantly between the two groups (2% of the FCR-treated group vs. 1.5% in the FC-treated group).

In an attempt to mitigate the myelotoxicity observed with the standard FCR treatment regimen and to develop a regimen more suitable for treatment patients who have limited myeloid reserve, a phase II study was developed to examine the clinical response to a modified FCR regimen that used lower doses of fludarabine and cyclophosphamide, but higher doses of rituximab (the so-called FCR-lite regimen).[639] Fifty untreated patients received 375 mg/m² rituximab on day 1 and intravenous fludarabine (at 20 mg/m²) and cyclophosphamide (at 150 mg/m²) on days 2, 3, and 4 of the first 28-day cycle of therapy. The patients subsequently received rituximab at 500 mg/m² on day 1, followed by intravenous fludarabine (at 20 mg/m²) and cyclophosphamide (at 150 mg/m²) on days 2 and 3 for each of the remaining five 28-day cycles. After 6 cycles of therapy, rituximab was given as maintenance therapy at 500 mg/m² once every 3 months until relapse.[639] The use of rituximab in maintenance therapy confounds the ability to compare the outcome of this trial with the outcome of studies using the conventional FCR regimen. It also makes it difficult to use the criteria recommended to assess the response to therapy.[355,471] Nevertheless, a high response rate was observed, with 77 percent and 100 percent of the treated patients being designated as having achieved complete remission or response to therapy, respectively. The median duration of complete response was 22.3 months. Furthermore, the patients treated on this study had a lower incidence of grade 3 or 4 neutropenia (13%) than did patients of other studies who were treated with conventional FCR.

Fludarabine/Rituximab Combined treatment with rituximab and standard doses of fludarabine generally appears well tolerated and more effective than treatment with single-agent fludarabine. In one study, previously untreated patients were given fludarabine at standard doses of 25 mg/m^2 on days 1–5, 29–33, 57–61, and 85–89 together with rituximab at 375 mg/m^2 on days 57, 85, 113, and 151; the overall response rate was 85 percent, with more than 25 percent achieving a complete response.[640] In a larger multiinstitution study, previously untreated patients were randomized to receive 6 monthly courses of fludarabine followed 2 months later by rituximab consolidation therapy or 6 courses of fludarabine concurrently with rituximab followed by rituximab consolidation therapy (see Table 94–6).[641] Overall and complete responses were higher in the latter group, which received more rituximab. Patients in this group achieved a complete response rate of 47 percent and overall response rates of 90 percent. The toxicities of treatment were similar to that noted for patients treated with single-agent fludarabine. In multivariate analyses controlling for pretreatment characteristics, long-term followup of the patients who received fludarabine and rituximab revealed that this group had a significantly better progression-free survival and overall survival than patients treated with fludarabine alone.[472]

Fludarabine Regimens with Mitoxantrone Treatment with mitoxantrone, given at 10 mg/m^2 on the first day of each cycle, together with fludarabine, given at 30 mg/m^2 on days 1 through 3 of a 28-day cycle, achieved an overall response rates of 80 percent in previously untreated patients and 60 percent in patients who were refractory to therapy with alkylating agents.[631] A subsequent study yielded response rates of 83 percent in previously untreated patients, 87 percent in patients previously treated with alkylating agents, 50 percent in patients whose disease was not refractory to fludarabine at the start of therapy, and 25 percent in patients whose disease was refractory to fludarabine.[165] Of note, only 20 percent of previously untreated patients who received this regimen achieved a complete response, a response rate that appeared not significantly different from that of single-agent fludarabine. It appears that the use of this regimen does not have a significant advantage over fludarabine alone.

The regimen of fludarabine at 25 mg/m^2 given on days 1 through 3 of a 28-day cycle together with cyclophosphamide at 200 mg/m^2 on days 1 through 3 and mitoxantrone, given at 10 mg/m^2 on the first day of each cycle, yielded complete responses of 50 percent (and overall responses of 78%) after a median of 3 cycles in patients who had relapsed or who were resistant to standard therapy.[617] Myelosuppression was the major dose-limiting toxicity. In a study of 69 patients who were younger than age 65 years and who had not received prior therapy, patients received the same amounts of fludarabine and cyclophosphamide on days 1 through 3 with a reduced dose of mitoxantrone at 6 mg/m^2 on day 1 of each cycle, which was repeated at 4-week intervals for up to 6 cycles of therapy.[621] The overall response, MRD-negative complete response, MRD-positive CR, nPR, and partial response rates were 90 percent, 26 percent, 38 percent, 14 percent, and 12 percent, respectively. Ten percent of the treated patients developed grade 3 or 4 neutropenia. Factors associated with favorable responses included low-level leukemia cell expression of ZAP-70 and CD38, low serum lactate dehydrogenase levels, and/or leukemia cell expression of mutated immunoglobulin heavy chain variable region genes.[621]

A pilot study involving 30 previously untreated, symptomatic patients younger than age 70 years evaluated the activity of the mitoxantrone (M), fludarabine (F), and cyclophosphamide (C) regimen when used in conjunction with rituximab (R). Treatment consisted of fludarabine at 25 mg/m^2 per day on days 2 to 4, cyclophosphamide at 250 mg/m^2 per day on days 2 to 4, mitoxantrone 6 mg/m^2 on day 2, and rituximab at 375 mg/m^2 on day 1 for the first cycle. For cycles 2 to 6, FCM started on day 1 together with rituximab 500 mg/m^2. Cycles were repeated every 4 to 6 weeks. CR was achieved in 83 percent of 30 patients, nPR in 10 percent, and PR in 3 percent. The overall response rate was 96 percent. Sixteen of 24 CR patients (67%) achieved an MRD-negative CR as assessed via flow cytometry, 13 of which (62% of the total) were MRD-negative, as assessed using the polymerase chain reaction to detect clonal immunoglobulin gene rearrangements. With a median followup of 38.5 months, the median time to treatment failure had not been reached.[642]

Fludarabine Regimens Containing Cisplatin or Oxaliplatin (OFAR Regimen) Cisplatin, administered at 100 mg/m^2 via continuous intravenous infusion over 4 days, has been used in combination with fludarabine given at 30 mg/m^2 via bolus intravenous infusion on days 3 and 4 of a 28-day cycle.[643] These two drugs, alone or in combination with cytosine arabinoside at 500 mg/m^2 on day 4 of the cycle, did not appear to offer significant benefit over that of single-agent fludarabine for the treatment of patients refractory to alkylating agents. Its use as a salvage regimen is under investigation. Myelosuppression was the major dose-limiting toxicity.

The combination regimen involving use of oxaliplatin, fludarabine, cytarabine,[612] and rituximab (OFAR) has activity in patients with relapsed/refractory CLL or Richter transformation.[497] A phase I/II study determined the optimal dose of oxaliplatin at 25 mg/m^2 given intravenously on days 1 to 4 of each 28-day cycle. Intravenous fludarabine (at 30 mg/m^2) and cytarabine (1 g/m^2) are given on days 2 and 3 of each cycle along with rituximab, given at 375 mg/m^2 on day 3 of cycles 1 and then day 1 of each subsequent cycle. Patients received pegfilgrastim (6 mg) on day 6 of each cycle of therapy. Encouraging responses to OFAR were observed in the 20 patients with Richter syndrome and 30 patients with relapse/refractory disease with overall response rates of 50 percent and 33 percent, respectively.[497]

Fludarabine/Prednisone Concomitant use of prednisone with fludarabine does not improve the response rate but does increase the risk for opportunistic infection, resulting in poorer outcome than use of fludarabine alone.[527,529] Because of this, fludarabine/prednisone combinations are not recommended for patients with CLL.

Fludarabine/Chlorambucil Fludarabine has been used in combination with chlorambucil.[644] Chlorambucil was given orally on day 1 at 15 or 20 mg/m^2, and fludarabine was administered intravenously on days 1 to 5 at 10, 15, or 20 mg/m^2, every 28 days. With chlorambucil at 15 mg/m^2 given on day 1, the maximum tolerated dose for fludarabine was 20 mg/m^2. Although responses were observed, treatment with this combination has not been shown to be significantly better than that with fludarabine alone.[644]

Pentostatin-Containing Regimens

Combination therapy with pentostatin (Nipent) appears to yield response frequencies similar to that of fludarabine-containing regimens that use otherwise similar agents.[556] Treatment of previously treated patients with pentostatin at 4 mg/m^2 and cyclophosphamide at 600 mg/m^2 given on day 1 of each 21-day course achieved complete and overall response rates of 17 percent and 74 percent, respectively, in fludarabine-refractory patients.[645] Also, treatment of patients who had no prior treatment, or who were in sensitive first relapse, with pentostatin at 2 to 4 mg/m^2 on day 1 of each cycle together with oral chlorambucil 30 mg/m^2 and prednisone 80 mg/day on days 1 to 5 of each 14-day cycle yielded complete and overall response rates of 45 percent and 87 percent, respectively.[646] However, as with fludarabine-containing regimens that incorporate concomitant use of glucocorticoids, severe (grade 3 or 4) infections were observed in 31 percent of treated patients, suggesting that this regimen is particularly immunosuppressive.

Pentostatin administered with cyclophosphamide and rituximab (the "PCR regimen") is an effective regimen for patients with relapsed

CLL. Initial studies suggested that the activity of pentostatin or pentostatin and cyclophosphamide was enhanced by the coadministration of rituximab.[647] In a study of 46 previously treated patients with CLL (n = 32) or indolent lymphomas (n = 14), patients received pentostatin at 4 mg/m^2, cyclophosphamide at 600 mg/m^2, and rituximab at 375 mg/m^2 on day 1 of each 21-day treatment cycle (see Table 94–6).[648] Patients received sulfamethoxazole-trimethoprim and acyclovir as prophylactic antimicrobial therapy and filgrastim beginning on day 2 of each cycle for 10 consecutive days or until the total neutrophil count was more than 1.0×10^9/L (1000/μL) for 2 consecutive days. The most common grade 3 or higher toxicity was hematologic, with grade 3 or 4 neutropenia, anemia, or thrombocytopenia occurring in 24 (53%), 4 (9%), and 7 (46%) patients, respectively.[648] Only 23 (72%) of the 32 patients with CLL were able to receive the six planned cycles of chemotherapy, the remaining 9 patients having to discontinue treatment because of infections or other comorbidities that developed or were exacerbated during therapy. Nevertheless, clinical responses were observed in 24 (75%) of the 32 CLL patients treated, with 8 (25%), 1 (3%), and 15 (47%) achieving a CR, nPR, and PR, respectively.[648] Responding patients had a estimated median duration of response of 25 months and a median time to next treatment of 40 months.

Pentostatin administered with cyclophosphamide and rituximab appears more effective when used in patients who have not received prior therapy. Pentostatin (at 2 mg/m^2 given on day 1 of each 21-day cycle) together with cyclophosphamide (600 mg/m^2 on day 1) and rituximab (given at 100 mg/m^2 on day 1 and 375 mg/m^2 on days 3 and 5 of the first cycle) were used to treat 64 previously untreated CLL patients, who received up to 6 cycles of therapy along with prophylactic antimicrobial therapy with sulfamethoxazole-trimethoprim and acyclovir, in addition to filgrastim on day 3 of each treatment cycle for 10 consecutive days or until the total neutrophil count was more than 1.0 $\times 10^9$/L (1000/μL) for 2 consecutive days (see Table 94–6).[649] The most common grade 3 or greater toxicity was hematologic, with neutropenia occurring in 26 patients (41%), thrombocytopenia occurring in 13 patients (21%), and anemia requiring red blood cell transfusions occurring in 4 patients (6%). The most common grade 3 or greater nonhematologic toxicities included nausea (n = 6), infection (n = 6), vomiting (n = 4), and fever without neutropenia (n = 4). The overall response rate with this treatment was 91%, with 26 (41%) of the patients achieving a CR, 14 (22%) achieving a nPR, and 18 (28%) achieving a PR. The estimated median duration of response was 34 months. The relative leukemia cell expression level of myeloid cell leukemia-1 (Mcl-1), an antiapoptotic protein of the bcl-2 family (see Chap. 12) prior to therapy appeared to influence the response to such regimens; patients with high CLL cell expression of Mcl-1 had significantly reduced proportions of complete responses and shorter progression-free survival than patients with CLL cells that had low-to-negligible expression of Mcl-1 (19% vs. 57%, P = 0.01; 18.7 vs. 50.8 months, P = 0.02, respectively).[650]

Cladribine-Containing Regimens

A large multicenter trial evaluated the toxicity and response to therapy with cladribine and prednisone (2-CdA+P) versus chlorambucil and prednisone (Chl+P).[651] Two-hundred twenty-nine previously untreated patients were randomized to receive either cladribine at 0.12 mg/kg per day in a 2-hour intravenous infusion together with prednisone at 30 mg/m^2 per day for 5 days (126 patients) or chlorambucil at 12 mg/m^2 per day together with prednisone at 30 mg/m^2 per day for 7 days (103 patients). The patients received 3 courses of therapy at intervals of 28 days or longer because of treatment-related myelosuppression. Patients treated with 2-CdA+P had higher CR rates (47%) and OR rates (87%) than did patients treated with Chl+P, who had CR and OR rates of 12 percent and 57 percent, respectively.[651] However, serious infections were more common in the 2-CdA+P–treated group (56%) than in patients treated with Chl+P (40%). Long-term followup of these patients and of patients allowed to crossover to the other regimen upon treatment failure revealed no difference in overall survival of patients treated initially with 2-CdA+P versus those treated with Chl+P.[652]

The response to cladribine in combination with cyclophosphamide and prednisone (CCP) has been evaluated in 19 patients with CLL.[653] Patients received cladribine at 0.1 mg/kg per day as a subcutaneous bolus injection on days 1 to 3 with intravenous cyclophosphamide 500 mg/m^2 on day 1 and oral prednisone 40 mg/m^2 on days 1 to 5 of a 28-day cycle for a maximum of 6 cycles. Overall response rates of 84 percent were observed, with 4 patients (21%) achieving a complete clinical and hematologic response and 12 (63%) achieving a partial response. In another phase II study, 27 previously untreated patients with CLL received 6 cycles of intravenous cyclophosphamide (1 g/m^2) plus oral prednisone (100 mg/m^2 per day for 5 days) followed by 2 to 6 cycles of 2-chlorodeoxyadenosine (5 mg/m^2 per day for 5 days).[654] This regimen yielded complete and overall response rates of 33 percent and 96 percent, respectively. The major toxicities were treatment-related myelosuppression and immune suppression. Such toxicities became even more apparent when this regimen was used in large multicenter trials, in which the myelosuppression and immune suppression became dose limiting, resulting in posttreatment complications, including fatalities that resulted from infections.[655]

Response rates to 3 courses of cladribine at 4 mg/m^2 per day and cyclophosphamide 350 mg/m^2 per day for 3 days every 4 weeks in patients with refractory or recurrent CLL appeared inferior to those achieved in comparable patients treated with the combination of fludarabine and cyclophosphamide.[656] However, in another study, response rates comparable to that of fludarabine and cyclophosphamide (e.g., complete responses in 30% and overall responses in more than 80%) were observed in previously untreated patients treated with 3 to 6 courses of cladribine at 0.12 mg/kg for 3 consecutive days and cyclophosphamide at 650 mg/m^2 on day 1 of each 4-week course.[657] Although this regimen produced a relatively high response rate in patients with previously untreated CLL who had deletions at 17p13.1, the response duration and survival were not satisfactory.[658] Although addition of mitoxantrone to this regimen did enhance complete response rates, it did not improve overall response rates or progression-free survival and was associated with increased myelotoxicity.[622]

Incorporation of rituximab into treatment regimens with either cladribine or cladribine and cyclophosphamide apparently improves the effectiveness of therapy without substantially adding to treatment-related toxicity, except for infusion-related reactions associated with the initial administrations of rituximab.[659] Eighteen previously treated patients received rituximab at 375 mg/m^2 on day 1 and cladribine at a dose of 0.12 mg/kg per day in a 2-hour intravenous infusion on days 2 to 6 of each 28-day cycle (the RC regimen). In addition, 28 previously treated patients received rituximab at 375 mg/m^2 on day 1 and cladribine at a dose of 0.12 mg/kg per day in a 2-hour intravenous infusion and cyclophosphamide 250 mg/m^2 per day on days 2 to 4 of each 28-day cycle (the RCC regimen). The median number of courses administered was 3 (range: 1–6). Serious grade 3 or 4 toxicity was primarily hematologic and similar to that observed in patients treated with cladribine or cladribine and cyclophosphamide without rituximab. The overall response rates of patients treated with the RC regimen or the RCC regimen were 67 percent or 95 percent, respectively. The median progression-free survival of responders to the RC/RCC regimens was 12 months (range: 4–46).[659]

High-Dose Methylprednisolone and Rituximab

The combination of high-dose methylprednisolone and rituximab (HDMP + R) appears highly active in the treatment of patients with refractory CLL,[498] as well as in patients who had not received prior therapy.[660] A major advantage of this regimen is that it does not employ agents that can cause significant myelosuppression. Fourteen patients with fludarabine-refractory CLL received 1 g/m^2 per day of intravenous methylprednisolone for 5 days on days 1 to 5 of each 28-day cycle together with rituximab at 375 mg/m^2 weekly for the 4 weeks of each cycle.[498] Following three 4-week cycles of therapy, the treated patients experienced a complete remission rate of 36 percent and an overall response rate of 79 percent. The median time to progression was 15 months and the median time to next treatment was 22 months. The acute adverse events were generally grade 1 or 2 and transient. These adverse events were similar to those associated with use of high-dose methylprednisolone, namely fluid retention, dyspepsia, hyperglycemia, and mood changes. The major toxicity was immune suppression, which appeared mitigated by concomitant use of antimicrobials for prophylaxis against infection.

To mitigate glucocorticoid-induced immune suppression, the numbers of days of treatment with high-dose methylprednisolone was reduced to 3 days in a regimen examined for activity in patients who had not received prior therapy.[660] Twenty-eight patients with a median age of 68 years received initial therapy with 3 days of high-dose methylprednisolone on days 1 to 3 of each 28-day cycle together with rituximab and prophylactic antimicrobial therapy. After 3 cycles of therapy, the overall response rate was 96 percent and 9 patients (32%) achieved a CR, two having no evidence for MRD by flow cytometry.[660] Six patients with a CR, but with MRD, elected to receive consolidation with alemtuzumab; 5 of these patients achieved an MRD-negative CR. With more than 3 years of followup the median progression-free survival was 30.3 months and an overall survival was 96 percent, with only 39 percent of patients requiring additional therapy.

Cyclophosphamide, Vincristine, and Prednisone

The combination of cyclophosphamide, vincristine, and prednisone (CVP) is effective in previously untreated patients and in some patients with refractory CLL.[661] The dosages are cyclophosphamide 300 to 400 mg/m^2, orally, daily for 5 days, vincristine 1 to 2 mg intravenously on day 1, and prednisone 40 mg/m^2 orally per day for 5 days. The cycle is repeated every 3 to 4 weeks. Approximately 25 percent of patients achieve a complete remission, and approximately 50 percent obtain a partial remission when treated with this regimen.[661] No differences were noted in response rates or survival of CLL patients treated in randomized trials with either CVP versus chlorambucil and prednisone[630] or chlorambucil alone.[662]

Patients previously treated with chlorambucil and prednisone may respond to CVP. Prolonged therapy over a 12- to 18-month period may prolong survival.[628] In one series, Rai stages III and IV patients had a median survival of 4.2 years following 18 months of therapy, with the median survival of complete responders being more than 60 months. This may be compared historically with the 19-month median survival reported for stages III and IV patients in the mid-1970s.[21] However, treatment with CVP does not appear to offer advantages over treatment with deoxyadenosine analogues such as fludarabine.

Cyclophosphamide, Doxorubicin, Vincristine, and Prednisone

The addition of doxorubicin to CVP chemotherapy (CHOP) has been evaluated in patients with advanced CLL.[663] These patients were treated with CVP, and half also received doxorubicin 25 mg/m^2 on day 1. Adding doxorubicin to the chemotherapeutic regimen increased the median survival from less than 2 years to more than 4 years in one study. However, the mean survival of patients treated with CHOP was similar to that of patients who received CVP over an 18-month period. Vincristine does not appear to add substantially to the CHOP regimen. In a randomized multicenter clinical trial, patients with stage B or C CLL were treated with CHOP or with cyclophosphamide, doxorubicin, and prednisone without vincristine (CAP). The rates of partial response and overall response were, respectively, 64 percent and 75 percent for the CHOP-treated patients, and 65 percent and 72 percent for the CAP-treated patients.[664] However, these response rates compare unfavorably with that of a third group of comparably staged CLL who were treated only with fludarabine, this group achieving partial or overall response rates in this same study of 75 percent and 94 percent respectively.

SPLENECTOMY

Splenectomy may ameliorate the cytopenias associated with advanced-stage CLL, particularly thrombocytopenia.[665–667] In one study, patients who underwent splenectomy for thrombocytopenia and/or anemia had a trend toward improved 3-year actuarial survival (31% ± 9%) over matched subjects who did not undergo splenectomy (12% ± 7%).[666] Preoperative performance status appeared to be the best predictor of perioperative and postoperative survival. Laparoscopic and hand-assisted laparoscopic surgery can be used to remove enlarged spleens[668,669] or accessory spleens,[670] thereby reducing the blood loss and required length of hospitalization from that required for standard splenectomy.

Splenectomy also can be effective in mitigating intractable or recurrent disease-associated autoimmune hemolytic anemia and/or thrombocytopenia, providing for sustained improvement in the majority of patients who undergo this procedure (see Chaps. 53 and 119).[668,671]

RADIATION THERAPY

Systemic irradiation was the first therapeutic modality used in CLL that was found to effect some degree of patient improvement.[9] However, it soon was recognized that the therapeutic benefit was short-lived and often resulted in severe marrow suppression.[672]

Irradiation remains a useful technique for localized treatment to ameliorate symptoms caused by nerve impingement, vital organ compromise, painful bone lesions, or bulky disfigurement. Delivery of 200 Gy can result in rapid shrinkage of lymph nodes or masses.

Splenic irradiation is useful in patients with painful splenomegaly,[673] especially in patients considered poor candidates for surgical splenectomy.[674] Patients may experience systemic improvement after splenic irradiation, possibly as a result of irradiation of leukemic cells circulating through the spleen. However, the low rate of response and the short remission duration argue that splenic irradiation should be combined with other therapeutic approaches.[675]

Endolymphatic radiotherapy[676] and extracorporeal irradiation of blood[677] appear to provide limited improvement in lymphocyte counts but do not appear to improve patient survival. Extracorporeal photochemotherapy also has been tried in B-cell CLL but was found ineffective.[678]

LEUKAPHERESIS

Intensive leukapheresis may reduce organomegaly and improve hemoglobin and platelet levels.[679] The measure has been advocated for patients with marrow failure who are refractory to standard therapy.[680] In addition, leukapheresis has been used successfully to treat patients with extreme lymphocytosis to ameliorate clinical symptoms associated with leukostasis and lower the risk for incurring adverse reactions to subsequent antileukemia therapy.[681] This procedure also has been used successfully to ameliorate lymphocytosis and disease-related complications in pregnant patients with CLL, obviating the use of other antileukemia treatments until after delivery.[682]

SUPPORTIVE MEASURES

Platelet transfusions may be required for patients with active bleeding who have drug or disease-related thrombocytopenia (see Chap. 119). Similarly, patients with symptomatic anemia as a result of autoimmune hemolytic anemia (see Chap. 53) or leukemia cell infiltration of the marrow may require transfusions with leukocyte-depleted pack red blood cells (see Chap. 139).

Erythropoietin

Treatment of patients who develop anemia as a disease-related complication may benefit from treatment with recombinant human erythropoietin.[683–686] The patients most likely to experience improvement are those found to have relatively low levels of erythropoietin.[687] Nevertheless, patients with normal erythropoietin levels and anemia secondary to leukemia cell infiltration of the marrow, still may benefit from treatment starting with thrice weekly injections of epoetin alfa (Procrit or Epogen) at 150 IU/kg or weekly injections of darbepoetin alfa (Aranesp) at 0.45 mcg/kg. Patients who do not respond after 4 to 6 weeks of therapy may respond to increased doses of erythropoietin. Those not responding to this increased dose after four weeks are unlikely to benefit from continued erythropoietin therapy. It should be noted that although use of recombinant erythropoietin may obviate or reduce the frequency of blood transfusions,[687] it also can be associated with serious therapy-related complications, such as skin reactions,[688] polycythemia,[689] or thromboembolic disease.[690]

INVESTIGATIONAL THERAPIES

Marrow or Blood Hematopoietic Stem Cell Transplantation

Autologous Hematopoietic Stem Cell Transplantation Several studies have examined the benefit of high-dose chemotherapy with stem cell rescue in patients with CLL (see Chap. 21). Complicating autologous stem cell transplantation is the high probability that stem cell collections are contaminated with CLL cells, even in patients who have been treated to minimal residual disease.[691–694] This has prompted investigation into more effective purging techniques to remove unwanted leukemia cells prior to transplantation. Nevertheless, a few studies with small numbers of patients have shown that complete clinical responses can be achieved in CLL.[695–697] However, long-term followup of treated patients have provided little evidence of a plateau in the survival curves, suggesting that, at best, autologous stem cell transplantation may only prolong disease-free survival.[694,698]

Allogeneic Hematopoietic Stem Cell Transplantation Transplantation with allogeneic hematopoietic stem cells is being evaluated for younger patients with poor-prognosis CLL.[484,699–703] Treatment-related morbidity rates in some series have been high, occurring in approximately half the treated patients.[700] Aggressive treatment may eradicate the leukemia cells to the levels that cannot be detected using sensitive molecular techniques to detect clonal immunoglobulin gene rearrangements.[484] Patients who relapse following allogeneic hematopoietic stem cell transplantation may respond to infusions of donor leukocytes, demonstrating the effectiveness of a graft-versus-leukemia effect.[702,703]

A long-term followup study was performed on 82 patients who had fludarabine-refractory CLL were subsequently conditioned with 2 Gy total-body irradiation alone or combined with fludarabine followed by hematopoietic stem cell transplantation from related (n = 52) or unrelated (n = 30) donors.[704] These patients had CR rates and OR rates of 55 percent and 70 percent, respectively. The 5-year incidences of nonrelapse mortality, progression/relapse, overall survival, and progression-free survival were 23 percent, 38 percent, 50 percent, and 39 percent, respectively. Among 25 patients who achieved a CR, 8 percent relapsed and 8 percent died as a result of nonrelapse mortality, whereas 84 percent have remained alive and in CR. Among 14 responding patients who were tested and who had no evidence for MRD, 2 died as a result of nonrelapse mortality, 2 relapsed, and 10 remained negative for MRD. At 5 years, 76 percent of living patients were well without additional therapy, whereas 24 percent continued to receive immunosuppression for chronic graft-versus-host disease. In a risk-stratification model, patients who had lymphadenopathy less than 5 cm and no comorbidities had a 5-year overall survival of 71 percent.[704] Collectively, these studies provide encouraging evidence that transplantation may be curative in a subset of patients with CLL,[705,706] including patients who have leukemia cells that harbor deletions at 17p.13.1.[707]

Nonmyeloablative Allogeneic Stem Cell Transplantation Because patients who receive allogeneic cells appear to benefit from a graft-versus-leukemia response, several groups are investigating the use of nonmyeloablative allogeneic stem cell transplantation for patients with CLL that is refractory to standard therapy.[706,708–714] Patients are treated with moderate conditioning regimens, such as low-dose total-body irradiation or fludarabine-cyclophosphamide combinations, prior to receiving allogeneic stem cells from related or unrelated donors. More recently, investigators also have evaluated the use of unrelated cord-blood hematopoietic stem cells as donor cells for allogeneic transplantation of patients with CLL.[715] Generally, complete chimerism, as well as best response, is not achieved immediately after transplantation, but may take over 3 months to develop. Initial treatment-related mortality is lower than that observed for patients treated with standard allogeneic stem cell transplantation, although patients still have a high risk for serious morbidity or mortality secondary to chronic graft-versus-host disease (see Chap. 21). This risk appears to increase following donor leukocyte infusion. Nevertheless, patients with refractory CLL can experience eradication of minimal residual disease several weeks following transplant, providing evidence for a graft-versus-leukemia effect.[694,706,710–712]

Other Agents and Biologics

Flavopiridol (Alvocidib) Flavopiridol is a cyclin-dependent kinase inhibitor that has activity in CLL.[716] This agent apparently can induce leukemia-cell apoptosis independent of functional *P53* or activation of cellular caspases.[717] Evaluation of the pharmacokinetics allowed for development of regimens that appear acutely effective in inducing leukemia-cell apoptosis,[718] an effect that has resulted in fulminant tumor lysis, requiring close medical supervision and occasional hemodialysis, and acute fatalities. A phase I study of flavopiridol in 52 patients with recurrent and/or high-risk CLL yielded partial responses in 40 percent of treated patients.[719]

Lenalidomide (Revlimid) Lenalidomide is an immunomodulating drug derived from thalidomide that has apparent activity in CLL.[720] This drug does not appear directly cytotoxic for leukemia cells, but might disrupt the survival signals that the leukemia cell requires from its microenvironment. In any case, two phase II studies demonstrated that lenalidomide could induce complete and partial remissions in patients who previously had been treated with other agents, most typically a fludarabine-containing regimen.[499,721] However, for unknown reasons, patients with CLL appear more sensitive to lenalidomide than patients with other conditions. This has resulted in CLL patients experiencing unacceptable toxicity when treated at doses of lenalidomide typically used for treatment of myeloma.[722] This has resulted in development of clinical trials evaluating use of low-dose lenalidomide in patients with CLL. Another potential adverse effect of lenalidomide when used to treat patients with CLL is that it also can cause a "tumor flare," which can result in paradoxical enlargement of lymph nodes during the initial course of therapy.[723] However, this does not appear to represent clinical progression in the setting of therapy, as the enlargement of the nodes is self-limiting and/or responsive to low-dose glucocorticoids. Tumor flare does not necessarily constitute a basis for discontinuing treatment.

Ofatumumab (Arzerra) Ofatumumab is a humanized anti-CD20 monoclonal antibody that binds to a different epitope of CD20 than does rituximab and that has should promising activity in early clinical trials.[724] Results of a multi-institutional phase II study evaluating the activity of this antibody in the treatment of patients with relapse/refractory disease showed promising results. Fifty-nine patients who were refractory to fludarabine and alemtuzumab and 79 patients who were refractory to fludarabine and considered inappropriate candidates for alemtuzumab because of bulky adenopathy received 8 weekly intravenous infusions of 2000 mg ofatumumab, followed by 4 monthly infusions of 2000 mg of ofatumumab after having received an initial starting dose of 300 mg. An overall response rate of 58% was observed in the double-refractory group and of 47% in the group refractory to fludarabine with bulky disease. Because of these results, the FDA approved ofatumumab in October of 2009 for use in treating patients with CLL refractory to fludarabine and alemtuzumab.

Active Immune Therapy and Gene Therapy

Cellular vaccines involving leukemia cells that are modified to enhance their capacity to induce an immune response or dendritic cells pulsed with putative leukemia-associated antigens are under investigation (see Chap. 25).[725–728] Another strategy is to modify the leukemia cell through transduction of an adenovirus encoding the ligand for CD40 (CD154; see Chap. 27). Ligation of CD40 can induce CLL cells to express immune costimulatory molecules that are required for stimulation of allogeneic or autologous T cells. Because CLL cells stimulated in this fashion can induce generations of autologous cytotoxic T cells and anti-leukemia antibodies,[274] methods for ligating CD40 have been incorporated into strategies for treating this disease. Treatment of patients with autologous leukemia cells transduced with Ad-CD154 showed promising results in a phase I clinical study.[506,729]

DISEASE COMPLICATIONS

Infection

Infection is a major cause of morbidity and mortality in CLL.[266,730] Patients generally develop worsening hypogammaglobulinemia and often have an impaired antibody response to microbes and hypogammaglobulinemia, making them highly susceptible to recurrent infection. *Streptococcus pneumoniae, Staphylococcus aureus, Streptococcus pyogenes, Escherichia coli,* and the herpes zoster-varicella virus account for most infections, and the lungs, skin, and urinary tract are the sites most affected.[730] Fungal, mycobacterial, and cryptococcal infections are uncommon. However, as noted above, patients treated with purine analogues, such as fludarabine, apparently have an increased incidence of infection with other opportunistic organisms, including herpes simplex, cytomegalovirus, herpes zoster, *L. monocytogenes, P. jiroveci* (formerly called *P. carinii*), and mycobacteria.[529,536,537,731,732] Multivariate analysis identified that disease activity and prior therapy are stronger risk factors than hypogammaglobulinemia for developing serious infections.[733]

Infections usually respond well to antibiotics in CLL patients with early stage disease. However, at later stages, the response is less satisfactory and more often associated with systemic complications. For such patients it often is necessary to administer antibiotics for prolonged periods to eradicate soft-tissue or urinary tract infection. Patients may be immunized with nonviable vaccines, such as those used to immunize patients against influenza or *S. pneumoniae.* However, the response to immunization is often poor. The use of live vaccines is contraindicated because of the risk of the attenuated pathogen being virulent in the immune-compromised host.

Patients with advanced-stage disease, hypogammaglobulinemia, and low levels of specific antibodies to pneumococcal capsular polysaccharide appear to be at greatest risk for severe or multiple infections.[734,735] Immunoglobulin deficiency is the factor that correlates best with the frequency, severity, and pattern of infection.[730] For this reason, investigators have examined the utility of administering intravenous gammaglobulin at 240 to 400 mg/kg every 3 to 4 weeks to patients with severe hypogammaglobulinemia associated with recurrent infections. Such therapy can decrease the frequency of bacterial infections,[736] even when given at the lower dose of 240 mg/kg every 4 weeks.[737]

Many of the treatments for CLL are immune suppressive and can enhance the risk for opportunistic infections. Patients treated with alemtuzumab can experience reactivation of CMV, which can be treated effectively by oral ganciclovir.[269] Patients treated with deoxyadenosine analogues such as fludarabine have a higher risk for complications related to virus infections, such as those caused by herpes zoster.[738] To mitigate this problem, some treatment regimens incorporate use of oral acyclovir at 400 mg twice daily for patients undergoing therapy.[739]

Systemic Autoimmune Disease

CLL patients have an increased risk of autoimmune disease, in particular autoimmune hemolytic anemia and immune thrombocytopenia.[740] Prednisone at a dosage of 1 mg/kg per day is used to treat autoimmune hemolytic anemia or immune thrombocytopenia and can be tapered slowly to the minimum dosage necessary. Case reports suggest that rituximab may be effective in patients refractory to glucocorticoids.[741] These diseases, and various treatment regimens for refractory disease, are discussed in Chaps. 53 and 119.

Second Malignancies

Patients with CLL have an increased risk of second malignancies.[730,742–744] The most frequent second tumors are melanoma, soft-tissue sarcoma, and colorectal, lung, and basal cell skin carcinoma. Patients with CLL also apparently experience higher recurrence rates of basal cell carcinoma after Mohs surgery than the general population[745] and have a higher incidence of developing Merkel cell carcinoma.[746] Patients with CLL also are at risk for developing more aggressive and/or metastatic squamous cell skin carcinomas than the general population.[747]

Multiple myeloma occurs at 10 times the expected rate in patients with CLL[748] but evidently does not arise from the same malignant B-cell clone.[749–751] Patients also rarely can develop diffuse large B-cell lymphomas that do not appear to be associated with transformation of the original clone,[752] although such cases might be considered to represent Richter transformation[753] (see "Richter Transformation" on the next page). Treatment with purine nucleoside analogues, such as fludarabine, pentostatin, or cladribine, appears to increase the risk for developing secondary lymphoproliferative diseases.[754]

Both untreated and treated CLL patients can develop acute myelogenous leukemia or myelodysplastic syndrome.[755,756] The concurrence of acute myelogenous leukemia or myelodysplastic syndrome and untreated CLL may represent two separate disease processes. Therapy-related acute myelogenous leukemia may develop after treatment with single-agent deoxyadenosine analogues, such as fludarabine or cladribine.[757–759] Also, a relatively high incidence of myelodysplasia and/or acute leukemia is noted for patients following autologous stem cell transplantation who received treatment with fludarabine and cyclophosphamide.[760]

Pure Red Cell Aplasia

Patients with CLL or small lymphocytic lymphoma may develop pure red cell aplasia that is unrelated to therapy.[761–763] This condition needs to be differentiated from other causes of anemia, such as autoimmune hemolytic anemia, leukemia-cell infiltration of marrow, which may require a different therapeutic approach. This condition is thought to be an immunologically mediated,[764] although some cases have been found related to infection with B19 parvovirus.[765,766] For CLL patients who develop pure red cell aplasia presumed secondary to pathogenic autoantibodies, the combination of cyclosporine and prednisone appears superior to prednisone alone.[767] Also, there are case reports of improvement in patients with pure red cell aplasia following treatment with rituximab.[768]

RICHTER TRANSFORMATION

Definition and History

In 1928, Maurice N. Richter described an aggressive lymphoma that developed in a patient with CLL.[769] Now described as Richter transformation, this transition from an indolent leukemia to an aggressive, large B-cell, high-grade lymphoma can occur at any time in the course of CLL, occurring in approximately 3 percent of all patients at median interval of 2 years following the initial diagnosis of CLL.[456,753,770–772]

Etiology and Pathogenesis

Nucleic acid sequence analyses of the immunoglobulin genes expressed by the original leukemic cells and the high-grade lymphomas of patients with Richter transformation demonstrated that such lymphomas can arise from the original CLL clone.[773,774] Although it is suggested that such lymphomas primarily are derived from CLL cells that express unmutated immunoglobulin genes,[775] CLL cells that express mutated immunoglobulin genes also may develop into aggressive lymphomas that express clonally related immunoglobulin genes.[771,773] In approximately a quarter of all cases of apparent Richter transformation, however, the lymphoma cells use immunoglobulin genes that are distinct from those of the original CLL clone.[774–777] Conceivably, some of these cases may represent cases of coincident B-cell malignancies that develop in patients with preexisting CLL.[778,779]

The chromosomal abnormalities in the lymphoma cells of patients with Richter transformation are typically complex and commonly include del 8p, del 9p, del 11q (11q23), 12(+), del 13q, 14q(+), del 17p, del 20,[163,198,456,771,780,781] and/or translocations involving chromosome 12.[780,782] Trisomy 12 and chromosome 11 abnormalities are more frequent in patients with Richter syndrome than in the overall population of patients with CLL. In some cases the lymphoma cells have inactivating mutations or deletions in the *P53* tumor-suppressor gene, the ataxia-telangiectasia mutated[783] gene, p16INK4A, the retinoblastoma (*RB*) gene, or p21, increased copy number of *C-MYC*, and/or loss or decreased expression of p27 or *A-MYB*.[165,781] In some cases the lymphoma cells have microsatellite instability that was not seen in the original leukemia cell population.[784] One case was noted to have a 12q13 translocation with chromosome 6 involving the high-mobility group (non-histone chromosomal) protein isoform I-C (HMGI-C) gene, which was expressed by the large-cell lymphoma cell.[782] These genetic lesions often are not found in the original leukemia clone even when the lymphoma cells share expression of the same immunoglobulin genes, suggesting that many such changes are acquired as secondary/tertiary events in disease evolution.[780,781]

Retrospective studies on potential predictors of CLL patients who might develop Richter transformation have identified three independent risk factors: (1) high-level expression of CD38 by leukemia B cells, (2) absence of leukemia-cell deletion at 13q14, and (3) leukemia cell expression of certain IgHV genes, most notably *IGHV4-39*.[785] Another risk factor for development of Richter transformation is bulky lymphadenopathy.[753] How these factors contribute to the development of Richter transformation is not known, but could be a result of their relationship with cell turnover and/or the propensity of the leukemia clone to undergo relatively high rates of somatic mutation and clonal evolution.

Clinical and Laboratory Features

The most common clinical and laboratory features associated with Richter transformation (with their respective incidence indicated in parentheses) include: (1) elevation of serum lactate dehydrogenase (82%); (2) rapid lymph node enlargement (64%); (3) systemic symptoms of fever and/or weight loss (59%); (4) a monoclonal gammopathy on serum protein electrophoresis (44%); and (5) extranodal disease (41%).[456] Patients also may have abdominal symptoms because of increasing hepatosplenomegaly or neurologic symptoms secondary to central nervous system involvement.[786–788] Occasional patients may present with an extranodal mass lesion.[619,789,790] Patients with Richter transformation often have bulky retroperitoneal adenopathy and massive splenomegaly.

Not all patients with CLL that have rapid lymph node enlargement have Richter transformation. Infection with herpes simplex virus can cause acute lymphadenitis.[791] Excisional lymph node biopsy of affected lymph nodes demonstrates zonal necrosis caused by herpes simplex infection that can be distinguished from the large cell lymphoma of patients with Richter transformation. Such cases usually respond well to appropriate antiviral therapy.

For this reason, the diagnosis of Richter transformation generally requires lymph node or marrow biopsy. Involved lymph nodes typically are effaced by large immunoblastic cells with abundant basophilic cytoplasm and irregular nuclei with prominent nucleoli.[337] The typical morphology is similar to that of diffuse large B-cell lymphoma, immunoblastic variant, according to the World Health Organization classification (see Chaps. 92 and 98).[792] However, descriptions of the lymphoma cells in tissue vary from this to that of a diffuse and monotonous collection of centroblasts or centroblasts intermingled with immunoblasts, similar to what the REAL (Revised European-American Lymphoma) classification currently describes as diffuse large B-cell lymphoma, centroblastic variant.[771] In rare cases, plasmablastic lymphoma cells predominate.[793] Regardless of the histology, the lymphoma cells in Richter transformation typically lack or have weak expression of CD5 and/or IgD, even cases that are clonally related to an original CLL clone that does express these surface antigens.

Occasional cases of Richter transformation have histology resembling that of Hodgkin lymphoma (see Chap. 99), termed *Richter syndrome with Hodgkin lymphoma features*.[794–803] These cases account for less than a fifth of all cases of Richter transformation, occurring in approximately 0.5 percent of all patients with CLL.[165,358] In such cases, the involved lymph nodes have histological and immune-phenotypic features of Hodgkin lymphoma (see Chap. 98, Figs. 98-34 through 37), including typical Hodgkin/Reed-Sternberg cells that may express CD15 and/or CD30. Studies on the expressed immunoglobulin genes using single cell polymerase chain reaction techniques found that Hodgkin/Reed-Sternberg cells were derived from the same clone as the CLL cells in two of three cases examined.[804] In contrast, another similar study found that the Hodgkin/Reed-Sternberg cells in two cases had immunoglobulin gene rearrangements that were distinct from those of the original CLL clone.[803] Nevertheless, other studies suggest that the Hodgkin/Reed-Sternberg cells in most cases of may be derived from the original CLL clone.[797] Infection with Epstein-Barr virus is implicated as playing a possible pathogenic role in those cases in which the

Hodgkin/Reed-Sternberg cells are not related to the original CLL clone.[795,803] Such cases have been argued to represent a possible complication of therapy with purine analogues or other agents that may impair immune surveillance.[800,801,803]

Therapy, Course, and Prognosis

Regimens similar to those used to treat high-grade lymphomas, such as diffuse large cell lymphoma, commonly are used to treat patients with Richter syndrome (see Chap. 100). Although occasional patients have achieved long-term remissions following intensive multiagent chemotherapy,[788] most patients at best achieve only a partial remission and have a very poor prognosis. Historically, patients with Richter transformation have median survival of 5 months from diagnosis.[456]

Various combination therapies are under investigation,[772] including regimens incorporating fractionated cyclophosphamide, vincristine, liposomal daunorubicin, and dexamethasone (hyper-CVAD) plus rituximab and GM-CSF alternating with methotrexate and cytarabine plus rituximab and GM-CSF.[805]

Encouraging responses have been observed with a combination regimen involving use of oxaliplatin, fludarabine, cytarabine,[612] and rituximab (OFAR), which induced overall responses rates of approximately 50 percent in the 20 patients with Richter transformation who received this regimen.[497] This regimen is generally less myelotoxic than other aggressive salvage therapies. Nevertheless, patients should receive pegfilgrastim following each cycle of therapy and be monitored closely for cytopenias (neutropenia, thrombocytopenia, or anemia). Treated patients might require blood product support, particularly during the post-treatment nadir, which occurs 9–11 days after each treatment cycle.

Patients with apparent Richter syndrome with characteristics similar to that of Hodgkin lymphoma may respond favorably to therapy for Hodgkin lymphoma (see Chap. 99).[802] However, most patients with such characteristics have refractory disease and a clinical course similar to that of patients with classic Richter transformation.[796]

CLL/PLL AND PROLYMPHOCYTIC TRANSFORMATION

In nearly 15 percent of B-cell CLL patients, the population of leukemic cells consists of a mixture of small lymphocytes and prolymphocytes, the latter cell type accounting for between 10 and 50 percent of the lymphoid cells.[806,807] These patients have been termed to have CLL/PLL (prolymphocytic leukemia), although this term is not in frequent use. These patients have a degree of lymphadenopathy and age distribution similar to that of patients with CLL but more pronounced splenomegaly. In 80 percent of CLL/PLL cases, the proportion of prolymphocytes remains stable, and survival does not differ from that of CLL patients with comparable clinical-stage disease.[808] Such patients generally do not have blood prolymphocyte counts above 15,000/μL or massive splenomegaly.

The remaining patients with CLL/PLL will undergo a prolymphocytic transformation. This is characterized by a decrease in the proportion of leukemic cells able to form rosettes with mouse erythrocytes, increases in the proportions of blood lymphocytes with prolymphocyte morphology and immunophenotype, and progressive splenomegaly. One study noted the leukemic cells in transformation apparently acquired the t(6;12) translocation that commonly is associated with PLL.[809] Patients with this transformation respond poorly to standard chemotherapy, and survival is limited. In one study, the mean survival of patients after transformation to PLL was 9 months.[810]

ACUTE LYMPHOBLASTIC LEUKEMIA

Rarely, patients with CLL may develop acute lymphoblastic leukemia.[811] Studies of a few of the dozen cases reported indicate that the acute leukemia can arise from the same B-cell clone as that of the CLL cells.[812–815] Blastic transformation has been associated with a seven- to eightfold increase in the expression of *C-MYC* and immunoglobulin genes.[815] Leukemic blast cells generally express terminal deoxynucleotidyl transferase and high levels of surface immunoglobulin and HLA-DR.

PROGNOSIS

There are no established cures for CLL, and spontaneous remissions are extremely rare.[816,817] Nevertheless, the prognosis can vary substantially between different patients, depending upon clinical stage and the presence or absence of disease features that have been associated with disease progression and/or a more adverse clinical outcome (see "Clinical Staging" and "Other Prognostic Indicators" on page 1442). Studies suggest that regimens incorporating use of rituximab are improving survival,[472] which should be considered when assessing prognosis based upon algorithms developed from outcomes data of patients treated prior to the advent of monoclonal antibody therapy.

Age and Gender

Gender and patient age influence prognosis.[443] For unknown reasons female patients tend to have a longer survival than male patients.[32–35] Also the male-to-female ratio is greater in patients diagnosed at younger ages (e.g. younger than age 65 years).[35] Patient age had been argued to be an independent prognostic factor.[32,415,818,819] Although the absolute survival of younger patients is longer than that of the aged, their survival is shorter relative to that of age-matched controls.[32,34,820] Moreover, CLL-related deaths occur with a higher frequency in younger patients. Overall, the 5-year survival rate in the United States is 83 percent for those younger than age 65 years and 68 percent for those older than age 65 years.[26] However, a large study from the U.S. National Cancer Data Base revealed that the 5-year relative survival was 69.5 percent, 72.2 percent, 63.1 percent, and 41.7 percent for age groups younger than 40, 40 to 59, 60 to 79, and 80+ years, respectively, indicating that the 5-year survival does not vary significantly between these different age groups.[28] It appears that CLL, and not comorbid disease, caused the greatest percentage of deaths, even among the aged.

Another study also found that younger and older patients have a similar overall median survival probability but had different distributions of causes of deaths.[358] CLL-unrelated deaths and secondary malignancies predominated in the older age group, whereas the direct effects of leukemia were prevalent in the younger age group. At diagnosis, younger and older patients displayed a similar distribution of clinical features, except for a significantly higher male-to-female ratio in younger patients (2.85 vs. 1.29; $p < 0.0001$). Both groups had an elevated rate of second malignancies (8.3% vs. 10.7%), whereas the occurrence of Richter syndrome was significantly higher in younger patients (5.9% vs. 1.2%; $p < 0.00001$). Two subsets of young CLL patients with a different prognostic outcome could be identified. One group, comprising 40 percent of the patients younger than age 55 years, had long-lasting stable disease without treatment and an actuarial survival probability of 94 percent at 12 years from diagnosis. The remaining patients had progressive disease and a median survival probability of 5 years after therapy.[358] A key feature of patients with the more adverse prognosis is evidence for disease progression.[821]

Prognostic Nomogram and Index for Overall Survival Prognostic nomograms have been developed that can assist in predicting survival of untreated[443] patients (Fig. 94–4), or of patients treated with various chemotherapy or immunochemotherapy regimens.[444] Newer prognostic factors, such as leukemia-cell expression of unmutated IgHV genes, ZAP-70, or chromosome abnormalities identified by Interphase FISH, were not considered in these nomograms, which instead rely on clinical

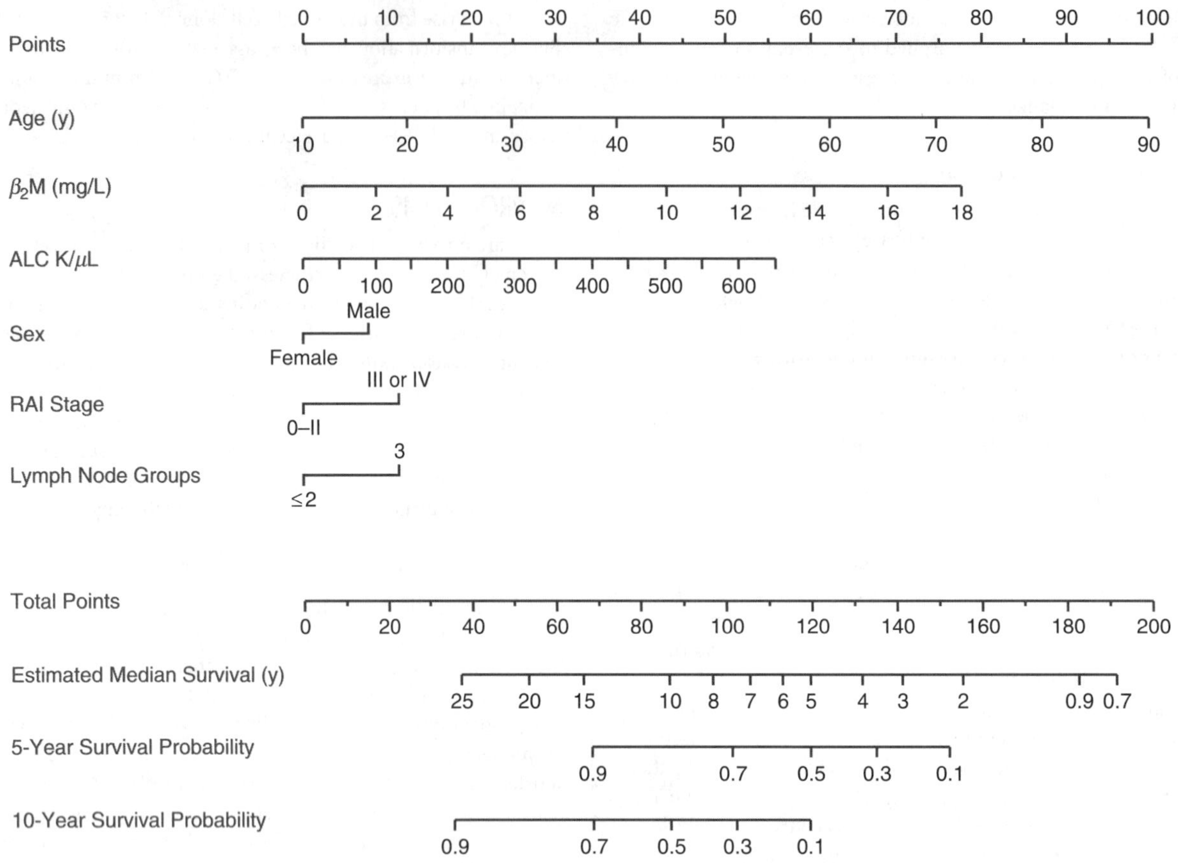

FIGURE 94–4. Nomogram for survival of untreated patients with CLL. The points identified on the top scale for each independent covariate in the top part of the figure are added together to determine the total prognosis score, which then is used on the total points scale (shown in the bottom part of the figure) to identify the estimated median survival time (years) and the probability of 5- and 10-year survival. *(Reproduced with permission from Wierda WG et al.[443] Copyright © the American Society of Hematology.)*

information that is readily available to the practicing clinician. The nomogram for untreated patients uses six independent covariates that were identified in a multivariate Cox proportional hazards assessment of outcomes data obtained on 1674 untreated patients who presented to M.D. Anderson between 1981 and 2004 for evaluation of CLL (see Table 94–8). The developed nomogram allows one to total the points identified on the top scale for each independent covariate (Table 94–9 at the top of the next page). The total point score is then identified on a total points scale that can be used to stratify patients into either a low-risk, intermediate-risk, or high-risk subgroup that have different median survival and different probabilities for achieving 5- and 10-year survival (see Table 94–8). The contribution of each covariate to the total score was greatest for age, serum β_2-microglobulin level, and absolute lymphocyte count, followed by sex, Rai stage (III or IV), and the presence of three palpable lymph node groups. Based upon the cumulative score, patients can be stratified into either low-risk, intermediate-risk, or high-risk categories that have different median times to survival (Fig. 94-5).

TABLE 94–8. Overall Survival Probability and Relative Risk of Death According to Risk Group (N = 1617)

Risk Group	Index Score	No. of Patients	5-y OS (SE)	10-y OS (SE)	RR	95% CI
Low	1–3	194	0.97 (0.01)	0.80 (0.05)	1.00	Reference
Intermediate	4–7	1236	0.80 (0.01)	0.52 (0.03)	3.89	2.42–6.26
High	≥8	187	0.55 (0.04)	0.26 (0.06)	10.48	6.27–17.53

CI, confidence interval; OS, overall survival; RR, relative risk; SE, standard error.

Reproduced with permission from Wierda WG et al.[443]

B-CELL PROLYMPHOCYTIC LEUKEMIA

HISTORY AND DEFINITION

B-cell PLL is a clinical and morphologic variant of CLL that first was described as a distinct entity in 1973.[822] It is a subacute lymphoid leukemia with an incidence that is approximately 10 percent that of CLL. The diagnosis of PLL requires that at least 55 percent of the circulating leukemic lymphocytes have a prolymphocytic morphology.[806] Such cells are larger than resting lymphocytes and have a high nuclear-to-cytoplasmic ratio, a basophilic cytoplasm devoid of granules, moderately condensed chromatin, and a single prominent nucleolus. In 80 percent of such cases, the prolymphocytes are neoplastic B cells, whereas the remaining cases are derived from mature T cells.[823,824]

ETIOLOGY AND PATHOGENESIS

The etiology is unknown. There is a 4:1 male-to-female predominance, suggesting that males are much more

TABLE 94–9. Prognostic Index Based on Presence of Risk Factors

	Point Contribution			
Characteristic	0	1	2	3
Age, y	–	<50	50–65	>65
β_2M, mg/L	<ULN	1–2 × ULN	>2 × ULN	N/A
ALC, × 10^9/L	<20	20–50	>50	N/A
Sex	Female	Male	N/A	N/A
Rai Stage	0–II	III–IV	N/A	N/A
No. of involved nodal groups	≤2	3	N/A	N/A

ALC, absolute lymphocyte count; β_2M, β_2-microglobulin; LDH, lactate dehydrogenase; ULN, upper limit of normal.

Index score is the sum total of the point for each of the six characteristics. An index score of 1–3 = low risk; 4–7 = intermediate risk; ≥8 = high risk. To convert β_2M from mg/L to nM/L, multiply mg/L by 85.

Reproduced with permission from Wierda WG et al.[443] Copyright © the American Society of Hematology.

susceptible to developing this disease. Also, B-cell PLL can evolve from B-cell CLL.[807] Factors that contribute to the pathogenesis or progression of CLL may operate in B-cell PLL.

Cytogenetics

The karyotype of the leukemia cells from many patients displays the 14q+ abnormality.[825] Trisomy 12 is another recurrent abnormality.[826,827] Deletions of the long arm of chromosome 6 (6q-) and rearrangement affecting chromosomes 1 and 12 are occasionally observed. One study observed a t(6;12)(q15;p13) chromosomal anomaly in several independent cases, leading the investigators to postulate that this anomaly is distinctive for a subset of patients with PLL.[809] The (2;13)(q35;q14) translocation that commonly is associated with pediatric rhabdomyosarcoma also has been identified.[828]

The most common abnormalities identified using cytogenetics and FISH analysis are deletion 13q14 (46%), trisomy 12 (21%), and 14q32 rearrangements (21%).[829] In contrast to most CLL, there appears to be preferential loss of *RB1* at the D13S25 locus, suggesting that allelic loss of the *RB1* gene may factor in the pathogenesis of some B-cell PLL.[830] Loss of heterozygosity at 17p13.3 associated with inactivating mutations in the *TP53* gene is observed in as many as three-quarters of the cases examined.[193,831,832] The high frequency of *P53* mutations in B-cell PLL is in marked contrast to what is observed in B-cell CLL and may account for the relative resistance of B-cell PLL to therapy. In addition, some cases of B-cell PLL have t(2;8) translocations involving the *C-MYC* gene that are similar to those observed in Burkitt lymphoma (see Chap. 104).[833] Such mutations may account for the aggressive clinical course of PLL relative to that of CLL.

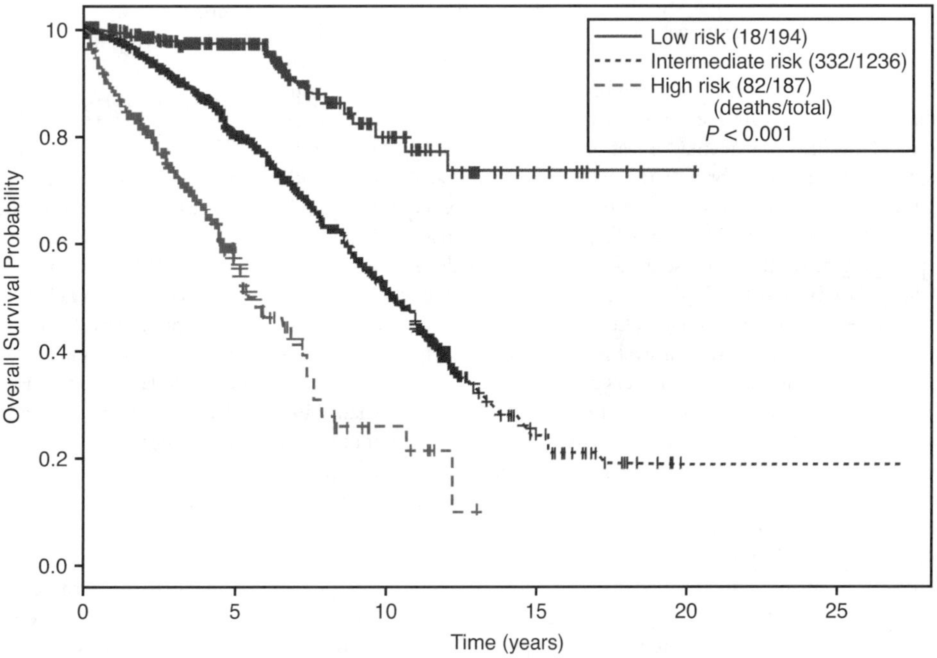

FIGURE 94–5. Kaplan-Meier estimates for overall survival by index score (n = 1617). *(Reproduced with permission from Wierda WG, et al.[443] Copyright © the American Society of Hematology.)*

Cytogenesis

B-cell PLL is derived from mature B cells that have undergone immunoglobulin gene rearrangement (see Chap. 77). These cells invariably have monoclonal immunoglobulin gene rearrangements and express many of the same B-cell surface antigens as do leukemic cells in CLL. In many cases, the disease may evolve from preexistent CLL. The immunoglobulins expressed by PLL B cells bear autoantibody-associated cross-reactive idiotypes, suggesting a biased use of immunoglobulin variable region genes similar to that of leukemic cells in CLL.[834] Moreover, there appear to be a biased use of IgHV-3 and IgHV-4 gene families, with *IGHV3-23*, *IGHV4-59*, and *IGHV4-34* genes accounting for more than half the IgHV used by most cases studied.[835] However, sequence analyses indicate the PLL B cells from at least half of the patients express nonmutated variable region genes, whereas the remaining cases express mutated variable region genes.[835,836] The presence of such somatic mutations suggests that the B-cell PLL cells from at least some individuals may be derived from a postgerminal center B cell (see Chaps. 5 and 77). Regardless of mutational status, leukemia B-cell expression of ZAP-70 ranged from 1 to 91 percent, being either greater than or equal to 20 percent in 57 percent of cases.[835]

CLINICAL FEATURES

More than 50 percent of the patients are older than 70 years of age at diagnosis. Presenting symptoms include fatigue, weakness, weight loss, an acquired bleeding tendency, or early satiety with abdominal discomfort because of splenomegaly. Splenomegaly is massive in nearly two-thirds of the patients. The liver also may be enlarged. Nevertheless, patients typically have minimal palpable lymphadenopathy.

In rare cases, patients may present with leukemic meningitis,[837,838] leukemic pleural effusion,[839] or malignant ascites.[840] A few patients develop cardiopulmonary complications as a result of leukostasis associated with extreme leukocytosis.[841]

LABORATORY FEATURES

More than three-fourths of the patients have blood lymphocyte counts greater than 100,000/μL.[332,339] Greater than 55 percent of the blood lymphocytes have a prolymphocyte morphology, which is larger in size than resting lymphocytes and features prominent nucleoli (see Fig. 94–1G).

The marrow commonly is infiltrated diffusely with neoplastic prolymphocytes (see Fig. 94–1H). At autopsy, these cells can be found to have infiltrated most other organs.[826] At presentation, patients commonly have a normochromic and normocytic anemia, with blood hemoglobin less than 11 g/dL and/or blood platelet counts below 100,000/μL. As in CLL, patients commonly have hypogammaglobulinemia.[842] However, many patients have a monoclonal gammopathy on serum protein electrophoresis.

PLL B cells express B-cell differentiation antigens similar to those of B-cell CLL; however, expression of CD5 is variable.[806] Even in cases that have evolved from CD5+ CLL B cells, the leukemia cells have low to negligible expression of CD5 (see Table 94–1). Also, in contrast to CLL B cells, PLL B cells generally express very high levels of surface immunoglobulin, usually IgM with or without IgD,[843] and react strongly with the antibody FMC7. In addition, PLL B cells generally express high levels of CD22 and often are negative for CD23. Finally, in contrast to CLL B cells, PLL B cells generally stain brightly with SN8, a monoclonal antibody specific for CD79b (see Chaps. 15 and 77).[333,334]

THERAPY, COURSE, AND PROGNOSIS

At presentation, patients commonly have advanced-stage disease that requires treatment. Most patients present with prominent splenomegaly and hyperleukocytosis and have rapid progression soon after diagnosis. Nevertheless, some patients may have a more indolent course.[844] As such, the indications for therapy are similar to those used for patients with CLL. These indications include disease-related symptoms, symptomatic splenomegaly, progressive marrow failure, or a blood prolymphocyte count of more that 200,000/μL.

Treatments for patients with PLL are similar to those described for patients with CLL. Alkylating agents similar to those used in CLL are commonly used. However, chlorambucil or cyclophosphamide, in combination with prednisone and/or vincristine, typically yield response rates of less than 20 percent.[806] Treatment with high-dose glucocorticoids appears less effective for patients with B-cell PLL than for those with CLL.[608] Partial and complete responses have been observed in approximately half the patients treated with intensive combination chemotherapy regimens similar to those used to treat high-grade lymphomas (see Chap. 100), such as CHOP. Unfortunately, responses are relatively short lasting. Although occasional patients may respond to salvage regimens,[845,846] the long-term survival is generally poor. The use of rituximab in the treatment of PLL appears promising.[847]

The deoxyadenosine analogues are active in this disease. Cladribine given at 0.1 mg/kg per day for 7 days by continuous infusion every 28 to 35 days has been noted to induce complete and partial remission in approximately half of the patients with *de novo* B-cell PLL.[848–850] Similarly, fludarabine at a dose of 30 mg/m^2 over 30 minutes daily for 5 days every 4 weeks produced complete and partial remissions in nearly 40 percent of the patients treated.[851] In another study, the response rates to fludarabine were similar to that noted for patients with CLL.[852] Rapid response to fludarabine may be complicated by the tumor lysis syndrome.[853,854] Pentostatin also appears effective, although less so than fludarabine. Twenty patients with B-cell PLL were treated with pentostatin (2′-deoxycoformycin) at a dosage of 4 mg/m^2 intravenously once a week for 3 weeks, then every other week for three doses. The major hematologic toxicity of this regimen was thrombocytopenia. Although 45 percent achieved a partial remission, no patients achieved a complete response. The median duration of the remission was 9 months. Patients with B-cell PLL had a higher rate of response and duration of remission (12 months) than those with PLL of T-cell origin.[855] However, pentostatin also has some activity in T-cell PLL.[856]

Splenectomy may ameliorate symptoms, but only transiently.[665] Splenic irradiation, with 1000 to 1600 Gy delivered to the splenic bed, has been advocated as a primary therapy for this disease,[857,858] especially for symptomatic patients who are considered poor candidates for chemotherapy and/or splenectomy.[859]

Case reports indicate that interferon-α can be effective in inducing cytoreduction in PLL.[860–862] There is one report of a patient who achieved a 5-year survival following a complete response to interferon-α following splenic irradiation.[863] However, generally interferon-α appears less effective than chemotherapy. Spontaneous remissions are extremely rare.[864]

T-CELL PROLYMPHOCYTIC LEUKEMIA

DEFINITION AND HISTORY

In 1989, the French-American-British (FAB) Cooperative Group distinguished five subgroups of T-cell leukemia, namely: T-cell CLL; T-cell PLL; human T-lymphotropic virus type I-positive (HTLV-I+) adult T-cell leukemia/lymphoma; and Sézary syndrome.[865] When a new entity called large granular lymphocytic leukemia was defined (see Chap. 96), the existence of T-cell CLL as a distinct entity became a topic of debate.[866–869] Because of this the World Health Organization commissioned a panel of experts to draft a new classification of the hematologic malignancies.[870] At a meeting in November 1997, this panel proposed a categorization of peripheral T-cell malignancies that largely was based on the REAL classification (see Chap. 92).[871] However, because of its aggressive clinical behavior, T-cell CLL was reclassified under the heading of T-cell PLL, without regard to subtle differences in morphology.[872] Even together they account for less than 5 percent of all chronic lymphoid leukemias.

ETIOLOGY AND PATHOGENESIS

The etiology is not established. There is a 3:2 male-to-female predominance, suggesting that males are more susceptible to developing this disease. In contrast to the relatively low incidence of CLL in Japan, the incidence of T-cell PLL is five to six times higher in the southern islands of Japan than in Western societies.[41]

Infection with HTLV-I has been speculated to play a role in the development of at least some cases of T-cell PLL. Evidence for HTLV-I can be found in the leukemia cells of patients with T-cell PLL, suggesting a causal relationship.[873] However, another study involving 36 patients with T-cell PLL from an area that was nonendemic for HTLV-I failed to reveal any evidence for HTLV-I or human T-lymphotropic virus type II (HTLV-II) DNA or transcripts in the leukemia cells.[874] The association of HTLV-I and T-cell PLL cells may be coincidental in areas with high rates of HTLV-I infection. Alternatively, there may be multiple mechanisms involved in leukemogenesis, some involving HTLV-I in endemic areas.[873]

Consistent with this hypothesis, the cytogenetic features of T-cell PLL appear to vary depending upon the patient population studied. In the United States and Europe, inv(14q), del(11q), translocations involving 11q23, i(8q), trisomy 8q, and rearranged Xq28 are the most common nonrandom chromosomal abnormalities in T-PLL.[875–878] Moreover, abnormalities of the short arm of chromosome 12 (12p) and/or chromosome 5 (5p) and deletions at 13q14.3 are often observed.[878–880] In contrast, chromosome 14 and 8 abnormalities are infrequently noted in the T-cell PLL cells of Japanese patients,[881] suggesting that T-cell PLL is a heterogeneous disorder.

Genetics

Use of comparative genomic hybridization to detect chromosomal imbalances in T-cell PLL of patients in Europe found that the chromosomal regions most often overrepresented were 8q (75%), 5p (62%), and 14q (37%), as well as 6p and 21 (both 25%).[878] On the other hand, chromosomal regions most often underrepresented were 8p and 11q (75%), 13q (37%), and 6q, 7q, 16q, 17p, and 17q (25%). Less common cytogenetic rearrangements are der(6)t(X;6), (p14;q25), der(13)t(13;14)(q22;q11), t(5;13)(q34;p11), r(17)(p13q21), and t(17;20)(q21;q13).[882]

The alterations on chromosomes 5, 6, 8, 11, 13, 14, 17, and/or 21 apparently cluster into discrete regions that may contain genes that are deleted or amplified during leukemogenesis or disease progression. For example, the loss of genetic material on the short arm of chromosome 8 (8p) apparently clusters into two regions. The first region is telomeric to the YAC 899e2, which contains the fibroblast growth factor receptor-1 gene (*FGFR1*) and appears to cluster within a 1.5 megabase YAC 807a2. The second region is more centromeric with breakpoints on either side of YAC 806e9, flanked by YAC 940f10 distally and YAC 910d7 proximally, the latter containing the *MOZ* gene.[876] Furthermore, the deletions on the long arm of chromosome 13 (13q) most commonly involve deletion of D13S25 at 13q14.3.[880] Deletions on the short arm of chromosome 17 (17p) typically involve 17p13.1 with deletion of the *TP53* tumor-suppressor gene.[883] The regions on chromosomes 11 and 14 involve genes at 11q22.3–23.1 and 14q32.1, respectively, that apparently are altered in most cases of T-cell PLL, as discussed in subsections on ATM gene[783] and T-cell leukemia 1 (*TCL1*) and related genes below.[884,885]

Ataxia-Telangiectasia Mutated[783] Gene Patients with ataxia-telangiectasia have a high risk of developing T-cell PLL. Ataxia-telangiectasia is an autosomal recessive disorder characterized by cerebellar ataxia, oculocutaneous telangiectasia, immune deficiency, genome instability, and predisposition to malignancies, particularly T-cell malignancies. The responsible gene, called *ataxia-telangiectasia mutated*,[783] maps to chromosomal region 11q22.3–23.1, is 150 kb in length, consists of 66 exons, and encodes a nuclear phosphoprotein of approximately 350 kDa.[174] Patients with ataxia-telangiectasia develop clonal expansions of T-cells that often progress to T-cell PLL, suggesting that ATM is a predisposing factor. Furthermore, inactivating mutations in ATM are observed in both alleles of T-cell PLL cells from patients who do not have ataxia-telangiectasia.[886–888] Moreover, ATM mutations appear associated with T-cell PLL and are infrequent in other T-cell malignancies, such as T-cell acute lymphocytic leukemia.[889] These findings suggest that ATM functions as a tumor-suppressor gene in T-cell PLL.

T-Cell Leukemia 1 and Related Genes Studies of t(X;14)(q28;q11) chromosomal rearrangements in T-cell PLL have implicated two genes, designated *MTCP1* or *TCL1*, in the pathogenesis of this disease.[875,890–892] These genes encode two homologous proteins, designated p13(MTCP1) and p14(TCL1), with highly similar tertiary structure[893] that often are deregulated in T-cell PLL. In addition, clonal T-cell expansions similar to that of T-cell PLL that develop in patients with ataxia-telangiectasia also have aberrant expression of these genes and/or harbor translocations involving the 14q32.1 or Xq28 regions, where the TCL1 and MTCP1 are respectively located.[894] Mice transgenic for MTCP1 under the control of CD2 regulatory elements spontaneously develop T-cell leukemias that share many features in common with T-cell PLL.[895] Similarly, mice transgenic for *TCL1* under transcriptional control of a T-cell specific promoter developed T-cell leukemias very similar in histology and biology to T-cell PLL.[124] The proteins encoded by these genes may play an important role in the pathogenesis of this disease.

CLINICAL FEATURES

Presenting symptoms include fatigue, weakness, weight loss, and early satiety with abdominal discomfort caused by splenomegaly.[866,869,896] On presentation, patients generally have blood lymphocyte counts in excess of $10 \times 10^3/\mu L$, marrow infiltration, and splenomegaly. In contrast to B-cell PLL, lymphadenopathy is a common finding in T-cell PLL.

About one-third of patients have cutaneous involvement on the torso, arms, and face, which generally is present at the time of diagnosis.[897] Skin manifestations include a diffuse infiltrated erythema; infiltration localized to the face and ears; nodules; and erythroderma, producing a non-scaling, papular, nonpruritic rash. Some cases present with a cutaneous infiltration mimicking a cellulitis that is resistant to antibiotic therapy.[898] Occasional cases may present with primary ocular findings, such as panuveitis.[899]

LABORATORY FEATURES

Biopsy of erythematous skin lesions generally shows a perivascular or periappendageal dermal infiltrate of lymphoid cells with a prolymphocytic morphology.[897]

Neoplastic T cells invariably can be found infiltrating the marrow, often in an interstitial pattern, with varying degrees of involvement.

The leukemia cells express the T-cell differentiation antigens CD2, CD3, CD5, and CD7, but not CD1, HLA-DR, or terminal transferase, reflecting a mature T-cell phenotype (see Chaps. 76 and 78). In more than 75 percent of cases, the leukemia cells have a helper T-cell phenotype as they express CD4, but not CD8.[900] Approximately 15 percent of cases have leukemia cells that express CD8 but not CD4.[866,872,901] In less than 10 percent of the cases, the leukemic T cells express both CD4 and CD8,[902] which is a less-mature phenotype, implying derivation from a more primitive T cell (see Chaps. 5 and 76). Monoclonal gene rearrangements in the genes encoding the α and β chains of the T-cell receptor can be detected in the leukemia-cell genomic DNA (see Chap. 78).

DIFFERENTIAL DIAGNOSIS

The lymphocytosis of T-cell PLL can be distinguished readily from that of B-cell leukemias by immune-phenotypic analyses. The cells are either CD4 or CD8 positive and negative for the alternative marker; about 25 percent of cases coexpress CD4 and CD8, a virtually singular feature of this tumor. CD2, CD3, CD7, and CD52 are also usually highly expressed. This contrasts distinctly with cell surface antigens in the B cell leukemias (see Table 94–2)

Polyclonal T-Cell Lymphocytosis

T-cell PLL should be distinguished from other lymphoproliferative processes that can present with T-cell lymphocytosis, such as the reactive T-cell lymphocytosis that can occur in infectious mononucleosis (see Chap. 84). Lymphocytosis caused by polyclonal T-cell expansion generally consists of both CD4+/CD8– and CD4–/CD8+ T cells and lacks clonal T-cell receptor gene rearrangements (see Chap. 78). Southern analyses for T-cell receptor gene rearrangements or evaluation for expression of T-cell receptor variable region genes can help distinguish T-cell PLL from this entity.

Large Granular Lymphocytic Leukemia

The leukemic cells in this disorder have the distinctive morphology of large granular lymphocytes (see Chap. 96). These cells have abundant cytoplasm that contains many azurophilic granules. Two major subtypes are defined. In the more common type, the leukemic cells are derived from the T-cell lineage and generally express the CD3 surface antigen. This disorder formerly was called Tγ-CLL. In the other subtype, the leukemic cells are derived from natural killer cells and lack expression of CD3. These diseases are discussed in Chaps. 96 and 106.

Adult T-Cell Leukemia/Lymphoma

Adult T-cell leukemia/lymphoma is endemic to the southwest of Japan and the Caribbean region. Most patients have lymphadenopathy, hypercalcemia, and high white blood cell counts. Skin involvement, lytic bone lesions, and hepatomegaly are common. The leukemic cells have polylobed or convoluted nuclei. The diagnosis can be confirmed by demonstration of antibodies to HTLV-I.

Mycosis Fungoides and Sézary Syndrome

Cutaneous T-cell lymphomas (Sézary syndrome and mycosis fungoides) have a helper CD4+ T-cell phenotype and often have blood involvement. This disease is discussed in Chap. 105.

Sézary-cell leukemia is a mature T-cell leukemia with characteristic cerebriform nuclei, whereas Sézary syndrome involves a mature T-cell lymphoma with a similar nuclear morphology. However, the distinction between T-cell PLL and Sézary-cell leukemia is not straightforward. The leukemia cells in either disease can have similar immune phenotypes and cytogenetic abnormalities.[903] Moreover, clinical manifestations are similar, as is the overall clinical course. This has led some investigators to consider Sézary-cell leukemia as a variant form of T-cell PLL.[903,904]

T-Cell CLL

The major feature distinguishing T-cell CLL from T-cell PLL was the morphology of the leukemia cells.[869] However, because T-cell CLL and T-cell PLL share so many other clinical and laboratory features, the distinction of T-cell CLL as a separate entity is currently not considered to have clinical utility. Instead, more attention should be given to distinguishing T-cell PLL with the usual CD4+/CD8− phenotype from exceptional cases of T-cell PLL/T-cell CLL that have a CD4−/CD8+ phenotype, generally lack prolymphocytic morphology, and have an even more aggressive clinical course than typical T-cell PLL.[872,901]

THERAPY

The disease is aggressive and generally refractory to conventional alkylator-based chemotherapy, with a median survival of about 7.5 months.[866]

Treatment with deoxyadenosine analogues yields higher response rates, although it has not been determined whether these drugs provide a survival benefit. Two reports describe treatment of T-cell PLL with cladribine.[905,906] Pentostatin given intravenously at 4 mg/m^2 weekly for the first 4 weeks and then every 2 weeks until maximal responses is effective in inducing complete or partial responses in about half of patients with T-cell PLL.[856]

Patients with extensive cutaneous involvement may benefit from treatments that commonly are used for mycosis fungoides, such as topical glucocorticoids, mechlorethamine, carmustine, ultraviolet light B, psoralen ultraviolet A, or total skin electron beam therapy.[907] These treatments are discussed in Chap. 105. However, systemic therapy is warranted for patients with T-cell PLL, and this generally obviates local therapy.

Alemtuzumab binds to the CD52 antigen, which is expressed on T-cell PLL cells.[908] Clinical trials have found that alemtuzumab induced responses in more than two-thirds of heavily pretreated relapsed/refractory patients with T-cell PLL.[909] Alemtuzumab is particularly effective in clearing malignant lymphocytes from the blood and marrow. In some cases, treatment may result in loss of expression of CD52 by leukemic T-cell population.[910] The major toxicity relates to problems of immune suppression, increasing the susceptibility for opportunistic infections and reactivation of viruses. These can be minimized by careful monitoring and the use of prophylactic antimicrobial therapy.[911]

Treatment of patients with T-cell PLL with high-dose chemoradiotherapy and allogeneic stem cell transplantation from HLA-matched sibling donors has resulted in anecdotal success.[912,913]

COURSE AND PROGNOSIS

In one large study, median survival was 3 years for patients with PLL and 8 years for those with CLL.[808] Patients with T-cell PLL, however, may have an even poorer prognosis than those with B-cell PLL and have a median survival of only approximately 7 months.[824,914–916] However, some patients may experience an initial indolent clinical course with stable moderate leukocytosis.[917] Also, it is not yet certain how these survival times may be affected by the advent of monoclonal antibody therapy and other new modalities of treatment for this disease.

REFERENCES

1. Velpeau A: Sur la resorption du pusuaet sur l'alteration du sang dans les maladies clinique de persection nenemant. Premier observation. *Rev Med* 2:216, 1827.
2. Fuller H: Particulars of a case in which enormous enlargment of the spleen and liver, together with dilation of all the blood vessels of the body, were found coincident with a peculiarly altered condition of the blood. *Lancet* 2:43, 1846.
3. Virchow R: Weisses Blut. *Froriep's Notizen* 36:151, 1845.
4. Virchow R: Weisses Blut und Milztumoren. I. *Med Z* 15:157, 1846.
5. Virchow R: Weisses Blut und Milztumoren. II. *Med Z* 16:9, 1847.
6. Kundrat H: Über Lympho-Sarkomatosis. *Wien Med Wochenschr* 6:211, 1893.
7. Ehrlich P: *Farbenanalytische Untersuchungen zur Histologie und Klinik des Blutes*. Hirschwald, Berlin, 1891.
8. Türk W: Ein System der Lymphomatosen. *Wien Klin Wochenschr* 16:1073, 1903.
9. Minot GR, Isaacs R: Lymphatic leukemia; age incidence, duration and benefit derived from irradiation. *Boston Med Surg* 191:1, 1924.
10. Reinhard EH, Neely CL, Samples DM: Radioactive phosphorus in the treatment of chronic leukemias: Long term results over a period of 15 years. *Ann Intern Med* 50:942, 1959.
11. Tivey H: The prognosis for survival in chronic granulocytic and lymphocytic leukemia. *AJR Am J Roentgenol* 72:68, 1954.
12. Galton DAG, Isreals LG, Nabarro JDN, et al: Clinical trials of p(di-2-chloroethyl-amino)-phenybutyric acid (CD 1348) in malignant lymphoma. *Br Med J* 2:1172, 1955.
13. Shaw RK, Boggs DR, Silberman HR, et al: A study of prednisone therapy in chronic lymphocytic leukemia. *Blood* 17:182, 1961.
14. Dameshek W: Chronic lymphocytic leukemia—An accumulative disease of immunolgically incompetent lymphocytes. *Blood* 29:Suppl:566, 1967.
15. Rubin AD, Schultz E: Surface immunoglobulins on lymphocytes in leukemia. *N Engl J Med* 287:989, 1972.
16. Fialkow PJ, Najfeld V, Reddy AL, et al: Chronic lymphocytic leukaemia: Clonal origin in a committed B-lymphocyte progenitor. *Lancet* 2:444, 1978.
17. Preud'homme JL, Seligmann M: Surface bound immunoglobulins as a cell marker in human lymphoproliferative diseases. *Blood* 40:777, 1972.
18. Salsano F, Froland SS, Natvig JB, Michaelsen TE: Same idiotype of B-lymphocyte membrane IgD and IgM. Formal evidence for monoclonality of chronic lymphocytic leukemia cells. *Scand J Immunol* 3:841, 1974.
19. Fu SM, Winchester RJ, Feizi T, et al: Idiotypic specificity of surface immunoglobulin and the maturation of leukemic bone-marrow-derived lymphocytes. *Proc Natl Acad Sci U S A* 71:4487, 1974.
20. Schroer KR, Briles DE, Van Boxel JA, Davie JM: Idiotypic uniformity of cell surface immunoglobulin in chronic lymphocytic leukemia. Evidence for monoclonal proliferation. *J Exp Med* 140:1416, 1974.
21. Rai KR, Sawitsky A, Cronkite EP, et al: Clinical staging of chronic lymphocytic leukemia. *Blood* 46:219, 1975.
22. Hamblin TJ, Davis Z, Gardiner A, et al: Unmutated Ig V(H) genes are associated with a more aggressive form of chronic lymphocytic leukemia. *Blood* 94:1848, 1999.
23. Damle RN, Wasil T, Fais F, et al: Ig V gene mutation status and CD38 expression as novel prognostic indicators in chronic lymphocytic leukemia. *Blood* 94:1840, 1999.
24. Rosenwald A, Alizadeh AA, Widhopf G, et al: Relation of gene expression phenotype to immunoglobulin mutation genotype in B cell chronic lymphocytic leukemia. *J Exp Med* 194:1639, 2001.

25. Klein U, Tu Y, Stolovitzky GA, et al: Gene expression profiling of B cell chronic lymphocytic leukemia reveals a homogeneous phenotype related to memory B cells. *J Exp Med* 194:1625, 2001.
26. Redaelli A, Laskin BL, Stephens JM, et al: The clinical and epidemiological burden of chronic lymphocytic leukaemia. *Eur J Cancer Care* 13:279, 2004.
27. StatBite: Estimated new cases for the four major leukemias, 2008. *J Natl Cancer Inst* 101:371, 2009.
28. Diehl LF, Karnell LH, Menck HR: The American College of Surgeons Commission on Cancer and the American Cancer Society. The National Cancer Data Base report on age, gender, treatment, and outcomes of patients with chronic lymphocytic leukemia. *Cancer* 86:2684, 1999.
29. Cartwright RA, Gurney KA, Moorman AV: Sex ratios and the risks of haematological malignancies. *Br J Haematol* 118:1071, 2002.
30. Dores GM, Anderson WF, Curtis RE, et al: Chronic lymphocytic leukaemia and small lymphocytic lymphoma: Overview of the descriptive epidemiology. *Br J Haematol* 139:809, 2007.
31. Adami HO, Tsaih S, Lambe M, et al: Pregnancy and risk of non-Hodgkin's lymphoma: A prospective study. *Int J Cancer* 70:155, 1997.
32. Lee JS, Dixon DO, Kantarjian HM, et al: Prognosis of chronic lymphocytic leukemia: A multivariate regression analysis of 325 untreated patients. *Blood* 69:929, 1987.
33. Catovsky D, Fooks J, Richards S: Prognostic factors in chronic lymphocytic leukaemia: The importance of age, sex and response to treatment in survival. A report from the MRC CLL 1 trial. MRC Working Party on Leukaemia in Adults. *Br J Haematol* 72:141, 1989.
34. Montserrat E, Gomis F, Vallespi T, et al: Presenting features and prognosis of chronic lymphocytic leukemia in younger adults [see comments]. *Blood* 78:1545, 1991.
35. Molica S: Sex differences in incidence and outcome of chronic lymphocytic leukemia patients. *Leuk Lymphoma* 47:1477, 2006.
36. Cerhan JR, Vachon CM, Habermann TM, et al: Hormone replacement therapy and risk of non-Hodgkin lymphoma and chronic lymphocytic leukemia. *Cancer Epidemiol Biomarkers Prev* 11:1466, 2002.
37. Ahn YO, Koo HH, Park BJ, et al: Incidence estimation of leukemia among Koreans. *J Korean Med Sci* 6:299, 1991.
38. Haenszel W, Kurihara M: Studies of Japanese migrants. I. Mortality from cancer and other diseases among Japanese in the United States. *J Natl Cancer Inst* 40:43, 1968.
39. Nishiyama H, Mokuno J, Inoue T: Relative frequency and mortality rate of various types of leukemia in Japan. *Gann* 60:71, 1969.
40. Zheng W, Linet MS, Shu XO, et al: Prior medical conditions and the risk of adult leukemia in Shanghai, People's Republic of China. *Cancer Causes Control* 4:361, 1993.
41. Tamura K, Sawada H, Izumi Y, et al: Chronic lymphocytic leukemia (CLL) is rare, but the proportion of T-CLL is high in Japan. *Eur J Haematol* 67:152, 2001.
42. Yanagihara ET, Blaisdell RK, Hayashi T, Lukes RJ: Malignant lymphoma in Hawaii-Japanese: A retrospective morphologic survey. *Hematol Oncol* 7:219, 1989.
43. Bartal A, Bentwich Z, Manny N, Izak G: Ethnical and clinical aspects of chronic lymphocytic leukemia in Israel: A survey on 288 patients. *Acta Haematol* 60:161, 1978.
44. Waterhouse D, Carman WJ, Schottenfeld D, et al: Cancer incidence in the rural community of Tecumseh, Michigan: A pattern of increased lymphopoietic neoplasms. *Cancer* 77:763, 1996.
45. Floderus B, Persson T, Stenlund C, et al: Occupational exposure to electromagnetic fields in relation to leukemia and brain tumors: A case-control study in Sweden. *Cancer Causes Control* 4:465, 1993.
46. Stone R: Polarized debate: EMFs and cancer [news]. *Science* 258:1724, 1992.
47. Feychting M, Forssen U, Floderus B: Occupational and residential magnetic field exposure and leukemia and central nervous system tumors. *Epidemiology* 8:384, 1997.
48. Marwick C: Link found between Agent Orange and chronic lymphocytic leukaemia. *BMJ* 326:242, 2003.
49. Zahm SH, Weisenburger DD, Babbitt PA, et al: Use of hair coloring products and the risk of lymphoma, multiple myeloma, and chronic lymphocytic leukemia [see comments]. *Am J Public Health* 82:990, 1992.
50. Inskip PD, Kleinerman RA, Stovall M, et al: Leukemia, lymphoma, and multiple myeloma after pelvic radiotherapy for benign disease. *Radiat Res* 135:108, 1993.
51. Rushton L, Romaniuk H: A case-control study to investigate the risk of leukaemia associated with exposure to benzene in petroleum marketing and distribution workers in the United Kingdom. *Occup Environ Med* 54:152, 1997.
52. Adami J, Gridley G, Nyren O, et al: Sunlight and non-Hodgkin's lymphoma: A population-based cohort study in Sweden. *Int J Cancer* 80:641, 1999.
53. Preston DL, Kusumi S, Tomonaga M, et al: Cancer incidence in atomic bomb survivors. Part III. Leukemia, lymphoma and multiple myeloma, 1950–1987. *Radiat Res* 137:S68, 1994.
54. Cronkite EP: An historical account of clinical investigations on chronic lymphocytic leukemia in the Medical Research Center, Brookhaven National Laboratory. *Blood Cells* 12:285, 1987.
55. Neugut AI, Ahsan H, Robinson E, Ennis RD: Bladder carcinoma and other second malignancies after radiotherapy for prostate carcinoma. *Cancer* 79:1600, 1997.
56. Richardson DB, Wing S, Schroeder J, et al: Ionizing radiation and chronic lymphocytic leukemia. *Environ Health Perspect* 113:1, 2005.
57. Abramenko I, Bilous N, Chumak A, et al: Chronic lymphocytic leukemia patients exposed to ionizing radiation due to the Chernobyl NPP accident—With focus on immunoglobulin heavy chain gene analysis. *Leuk Res* 32:535, 2008.
58. Vrijheid M, Cardis E, Ashmore P, et al: Ionizing radiation and risk of chronic lymphocytic leukemia in the 15-country study of nuclear industry workers. *Radiat Res* 170:661, 2008.
59. Hamblin TJ: Have we been wrong about ionizing radiation and chronic lymphocytic leukemia? *Leuk Res* 32:523, 2008.
60. La Civita L, Zignego AL, Monti M, et al: Type C hepatitis and chronic lymphocytic leukaemia. *Eur J Cancer* 32A:1819, 1996.
61. Bianco E, Marcucci F, Mele A, et al: Prevalence of hepatitis C virus infection in lymphoproliferative diseases other than B-cell non-Hodgkin's lymphoma, and in myeloproliferative diseases: An Italian Multi-Center case-control study. *Haematologica* 89:70, 2004.
62. Molica S, Mirabelli R, Misuraca D: Characteristics and outcome of B-cell chronic lymphocytic leukemia in hepatitis C virus-positive patients. *Leuk Lymphoma* 47:2421, 2006.
63. McColl MD, Singer IO, Tait RC, et al: The role of hepatitis C virus in the aetiology of non-Hodgkins lymphoma—A regional association? *Leuk Lymphoma* 26:127, 1997.
64. Luppi M, Grazia Ferrari M, Bonaccorsi G, et al: Hepatitis C virus infection in subsets of neoplastic lymphoproliferations not associated with cryoglobulinemia. *Leukemia* 10:351, 1996.
65. Avila-Carino J, Lewin N, Tomita Y, et al: B-CLL cells with unusual properties. *Int J Cancer* 70:1, 1997.
66. Gunz FW: The epidemiology and genetics of the chronic leukaemias. *Clin Haematol* 6:3, 1977.
67. Conley CL, Misiti J, Laster AJ: Genetic factors predisposing to chronic lymphocytic leukemia and to autoimmune disease. *Medicine (Baltimore)* 59:323, 1980.
68. Linet MS, Van Natta ML, Brookmeyer R, et al: Familial cancer history and chronic lymphocytic leukemia. A case-control study. *Am J Epidemiol* 130:655, 1989.
69. Cuttner J: Increased incidence of hematologic malignancies in first-degree relatives of patients with chronic lymphocytic leukemia. *Cancer Invest* 10:103, 1992.
70. Shah AR, Maeda K, Deegan MJ, et al: A clinicopathologic study of familial chronic lymphocytic leukemia. *Am J Clin Pathol* 97:184, 1992.
71. Yuille MR, Houlston RS, Catovsky D: Anticipation in familial chronic lymphocytic leukaemia. *Leukemia* 12:1696, 1998.
72. Goldin LR, Slager SL: Familial CLL: Genes and environment. *Hematology Am Soc Hematol Educ Program* 339, 2007.
73. Yuille MR, Matutes E, Marossy A, et al: Familial chronic lymphocytic leukaemia: A survey and review of published studies. *Br J Haematol* 109:794, 2000.
74. Rawstron A, Hillmen P, Houlston R: Clonal lymphocytes in persons without known chronic lymphocytic leukemia (CLL): Implications of recent findings in family members of CLL patients. *Semin Hematol* 41:192, 2004.
75. Kristinsson SY, Bjorkholm M, Goldin LR, et al: Risk of lymphoproliferative disorders among first-degree relatives of lymphoplasmacytic lymphoma/Waldenstrom macroglobulinemia patients: A population-based study in Sweden. *Blood* 112:3052, 2008.
76. Shen A, Humphries C, Tucker P, Blattner F: Human heavy-chain variable region gene family nonrandomly rearranged in familial chronic lymphocytic leukemia. *Proc Natl Acad Sci U S A* 84:8563, 1987.
77. Brok-Simoni F, Rechavi G, Katzir N, Ben-Bassat I: Chronic lymphocytic leukaemia in twin sisters: Monozygous but not identical [letter]. *Lancet* 1:329, 1987.
78. Perez-Chacon G, Contreras-Martin B, Cuni S, et al: Polymorphism in the CD5 gene promoter in B-cell chronic lymphocytic leukemia and mantle cell lymphoma. *Am J Clin Pathol* 123:646, 2005.
79. Aydin S, Rossi D, Bergui L, et al: CD38 gene polymorphism and chronic lymphocytic leukemia: A role in transformation to Richter syndrome? *Blood* 111:5646, 2008.
80. Jamroziak K, Szemraj Z, Grzybowska-Izydorczyk O, et al: CD38 gene polymorphisms contribute to genetic susceptibility to B-cell chronic lymphocytic leukemia: Evidence from two case-control studies in Polish Caucasians. *Cancer Epidemiol Biomarkers Prev* 18:945, 2009.
81. Jevtovic-Stoimenov T, Kocic G, Pavlovic D, et al: Polymorphisms of tumor-necrosis factor-alpha – 308 and lymphotoxin-alpha + 250: Possible modulation of susceptibility to apoptosis in chronic lymphocytic leukemia and non-Hodgkin lymphoma mononuclear cells. *Leuk Lymphoma* 49:2163, 2008.
82. Ng D, Toure O, Wei MH, et al: Identification of a novel chromosome region, 13q21.33-q22.2, for susceptibility genes in familial chronic lymphocytic leukemia. *Blood* 109:916, 2007.
83. Jones HP, Whittaker JA: Chronic lymphatic leukaemia: An investigation of HLA antigen frequencies and white cell differential counts in patients, relatives and controls. *Leuk Res* 15:543, 1991.
84. Montes-Ares O, Moya-Quiles MR, Montes-Casado M, et al: Human leucocyte antigen-C in B chronic lymphocytic leukaemia. *Br J Haematol* 135:517, 2006.
85. Sellick GS, Goldin LR, Wild RW, et al: A high-density SNP genome-wide linkage search of 206 families identifies susceptibility loci for chronic lymphocytic leukemia. *Blood* 110:3326, 2007.
86. Di Bernardo MC, Crowther-Swanepoel D, Broderick P, et al: A genome-wide association study identifies six susceptibility loci for chronic lymphocytic leukemia. *Nat Genet* 40:1204, 2008.
87. Enjuanes A, Benavente Y, Bosch F, et al: Genetic variants in apoptosis and immunoregulation-related genes are associated with risk of chronic lymphocytic leukemia. *Cancer Res* 68:10178, 2008.
88. Marti GE, Faguet G, Bertin P, et al: CD20 and CD5 expression in B-chronic lymphocytic leukemia. *Ann N Y Acad Sci* 651:480, 1992.

89. Almasri NM, Duque RE, Iturraspe J, et al: Reduced expression of CD20 antigen as a characteristic marker for chronic lymphocytic leukemia. *Am J Hematol* 40:259, 1992.
90. Ranheim EA, Cantwell MJ, Kipps TJ: Expression of CD27 and its ligand, CD70, on chronic lymphocytic leukemia B cells. *Blood* 85:3556, 1995.
91. Weller S, Braun MC, Tan BK, et al: Human blood IgM "memory" B cells are circulating splenic marginal zone B cells harboring a prediversified immunoglobulin repertoire. *Blood* 104:3647, 2004.
92. Klein U, Dalla-Favera R: New insights into the phenotype and cell derivation of B cell chronic lymphocytic leukemia. *Curr Top Microbiol Immunol* 294:31, 2005.
93. Widhopf GF 2nd, Brinson DC, Kipps TJ, Tighe H: Transgenic expression of a human polyreactive Ig expressed in chronic lymphocytic leukemia generates memory-type B cells that respond to nonspecific immune activation. *J Immunol* 172:2092, 2004.
94. Ghia P, Caligaris-Cappio F: The origin of B-cell chronic lymphocytic leukemia. *Semin Oncol* 33:150, 2006.
95. Kipps TJ, Robbins BA, Tefferi A, et al: CD5-positive B-cell malignancies frequently express cross-reactive idiotypes associated with IgM autoantibodies. *Am J Pathol* 136:809, 1990.
96. Geisler CH, Larsen JK, Hansen NE, et al: Prognostic importance of flow cytometric immunophenotyping of 540 consecutive patients with B-cell chronic lymphocytic leukemia. *Blood* 78:1795, 1991.
97. Legac E, Chastang C, Binet JL, et al: Proposals for a phenotypic classification of B-chronic lymphocytic leukemia, relationship with prognostic factors. *Leuk Lymphoma* 5S:53, 1991.
98. Kipps TJ, Carson DA: Autoantibodies in chronic lymphocytic leukemia and related systemic autoimmune diseases. *Blood* 81:2475, 1993.
99. Caligaris-Cappio F: B-chronic lymphocytic leukemia: A malignancy of anti-self B cells. *Blood* 87:2615, 1996.
100. Wardemann H, Yurasov S, Schaefer A, et al: Predominant autoantibody production by early human B cell precursors. *Science* 301:1374, 2003.
101. Martin T, Duffy SF, Carson DA, Kipps TJ: Evidence for somatic selection of natural autoantibodies. *J Exp Med* 175:983, 1992.
102. Martin T, Crouzier R, Weber JC, et al: Structure-function studies on a polyreactive (natural) autoantibody. Polyreactivity is dependent on somatically generated sequences in the third complementarity-determining region of the antibody heavy chain. *J Immunol* 152:5988, 1994.
103. Wardemann H, Hammersen J, Nussenzweig MC: Human autoantibody silencing by immunoglobulin light chains. *J Exp Med* 200:191, 2004.
104. Keating MJ, Chiorazzi N, Messmer B, et al: Biology and treatment of chronic lymphocytic leukemia. *Hematology Am Soc Hematol Educ Program* 153, 2003.
105. Tobin G, Soderberg O, Thunberg U, Rosenquist R: V(H)3–21 gene usage in chronic lymphocytic leukemia—Characterization of a new subgroup with distinct molecular features and poor survival. *Leuk Lymphoma* 45:221, 2004.
106. Messmer BT, Albesiano E, Efremov DG, et al: Multiple distinct sets of stereotyped antigen receptors indicate a role for antigen in promoting chronic lymphocytic leukemia. *J Exp Med* 200:519, 2004.
107. Kipps TJ, Tomhave E, Pratt LF, et al: Developmentally restricted immunoglobulin heavy chain variable region gene expressed at high frequency in chronic lymphocytic leukemia. *Proc Natl Acad Sci U S A* 86:5913, 1989.
108. Johnson TA, Rassenti LZ, Kipps TJ: Ig VH1 genes expressed in B cell chronic lymphocytic leukemia exhibit distinctive molecular features. *J Immunol* 158:235, 1997.
109. Fais F, Ghiotto F, Hashimoto S, et al: Chronic lymphocytic leukemia B cells express restricted sets of mutated and unmutated antigen receptors. *J Clin Invest* 102:1515, 1998.
110. Potter KN, Orchard J, Critchley E, et al: Features of the overexpressed V1–69 genes in the unmutated subset of chronic lymphocytic leukemia are distinct from those in the healthy elderly repertoire. *Blood* 101:3082, 2003.
111. Schroeder HW Jr, Mortari F, Shiokawa S, et al: Developmental regulation of the human antibody repertoire. *Ann N Y Acad Sci* 764:242, 1995.
112. Widhopf GF 2nd, Rassenti LZ, Toy TL, et al: Chronic lymphocytic leukemia B cells of more than 1% of patients express virtually identical immunoglobulins. *Blood* 104:2499, 2004.
113. Widhopf GF 2nd, Goldberg CJ, Toy TL, et al: Nonstochastic pairing of immunoglobulin heavy and light chains expressed by chronic lymphocytic leukemia B cells is predicated on the heavy chain CDR3. *Blood* 111:3137, 2008.
114. Ghia EM, Jain S, Widhopf GF, 2nd, et al: Use of IGHV3–21 in chronic lymphocytic leukemia is associated with high-risk disease and reflects antigen-driven, post-germinal center leukemogenic selection. *Blood* 111:5101, 2008.
115. Rawstron AC, Bennett FL, O'Connor SJ, et al: Monoclonal B-cell lymphocytosis and chronic lymphocytic leukemia. *N Engl J Med* 359:575, 2008.
116. Rawstron AC, Yuille MR, Fuller J, et al: Inherited predisposition to CLL is detectable as subclinical monoclonal B-lymphocyte expansion. *Blood* 100:2289, 2002.
117. Nieto WG, Almeida J, Romero A, et al: Increased frequency (12%) of circulating chronic lymphocytic leukemia-like B-cell clones in healthy subjects using a highly sensitive multicolor flow cytometry approach. *Blood* 114:33, 2009.
118. Marti G, Abbasi F, Raveche E, et al: Overview of monoclonal B-cell lymphocytosis. *Br J Haematol* 139:701, 2007.
119. Scaglione BJ, Salerno E, Balan M, et al: Murine models of chronic lymphocytic leukaemia: Role of microRNA-16 in the New Zealand Black mouse model. *Br J Haematol* 139:645, 2007.
120. Bichi R, Shinton SA, Martin ES, et al: Human chronic lymphocytic leukemia modeled in mouse by targeted TCL1 expression. *Proc Natl Acad Sci U S A* 99:6955, 2002.
121. Yuille MR, Condie A, Stone EM, et al: TCL1 is activated by chromosomal rearrangement or by hypomethylation. *Genes Chromosomes Cancer* 30:336, 2001.
122. Zapata JM, Krajewska M, Morse HC 3rd, et al: TNF receptor-associated factor (TRAF) domain and Bcl-2 cooperate to induce small B cell lymphoma/chronic lymphocytic leukemia in transgenic mice. *Proc Natl Acad Sci U S A* 101:16600, 2004.
123. Enzler T, Kater AP, Zhang W, et al: Chronic lymphocytic leukemia of E{micro}-TCL1 transgenic mice undergoes rapid cell-turnover that can be offset by extrinsic CD257 to accelerate disease progression. *Blood* 114(20):4469, 2009.
124. Virgilio L, Lazzeri C, Bichi R, et al: Deregulated expression of TCL1 causes T cell leukemia in mice. *Proc Natl Acad Sci U S A* 95:3885, 1998.
125. Hoyer KK, French SW, Turner DE, et al: Dysregulated TCL1 promotes multiple classes of mature B cell lymphoma. *Proc Natl Acad Sci U S A* 99:14392, 2002.
126. Barak V, Ginzburg M, Kalickman I, Polliack A: Serum soluble interleukin-2 receptor levels are associated with clinical disease status and histopathological grade in non-Hodgkin's lymphoma and chronic lymphocytic leukemia. *Leuk Lymphoma* 7:431, 1992.
127. Raveche ES, Salerno E, Scaglione BJ, et al: Abnormal microRNA-16 locus with synteny to human 13q14 linked to CLL in NZB mice. *Blood* 109:5079, 2007.
128. Rickinson AB, Finerty S, Epstein MA: Interaction of Epstein-Barr virus with leukaemic B cells *in vitro*. I. Abortive infection and rare cell line establishment from chronic lymphocytic leukaemic cells. *Clin Exp Immunol* 50:347, 1982.
129. Sole F, Woessner S, Perez-Losada A, et al: Cytogenetic studies in seventy-six cases of B-chronic lymphoproliferative disorders. *Cancer Genet Cytogenet* 93:160, 1997.
130. Hilgenfeld E, Padilla-Nash H, Schrock E, Ried T: Analysis of B-cell neoplasias by spectral karyotyping (SKY). *Curr Top Microbiol Immunol* 246:169, 1999.
131. Morgan R, Chen Z, Richkind K, et al: PHA/IL2: An efficient mitogen cocktail for cytogenetic studies of non-Hodgkin lymphoma and chronic lymphocytic leukemia. *Cancer Genet Cytogenet* 109:134, 1999.
132. Buhmann R, Kurzeder C, Rehklau J, et al: CD40L stimulation enhances the ability of conventional metaphase cytogenetics to detect chromosome aberrations in B-cell chronic lymphocytic leukaemia cells. *Br J Haematol* 118:968, 2002.
133. Tanaka K, Arif M, Eguchi M, et al: Interphase fluorescence in situ hybridization overcomes pitfalls of G-banding analysis with special reference to underestimation of chromosomal aberration rates. *Cancer Genet Cytogenet* 115:32, 1999.
134. Chena C, Arrossagaray G, Scolnik M, et al: Interphase cytogenetic analysis in Argentinean B-cell chronic lymphocytic leukemia patients: Association of trisomy 12 and del(13q14). *Cancer Genet Cytogenet* 146:154, 2003.
135. Goorha S, Glenn MJ, Drozd-Borysiuk E, Chen Z: A set of commercially available fluorescent in-situ hybridization probes efficiently detects cytogenetic abnormalities in patients with chronic lymphocytic leukemia. *Genet Med* 6:48, 2004.
136. Dohner H, Stilgenbauer S, Dohner K, et al: Chromosome aberrations in B-cell chronic lymphocytic leukemia: Reassessment based on molecular cytogenetic analysis. *J Mol Med* 77:266, 1999.
137. Barnabas N, Shurafa M, Van Dyke DL, et al: Significance of p53 mutations in patients with chronic lymphocytic leukemia: A sequential study of 30 patients. *Cancer* 91:285, 2001.
138. Sen F, Lai R, Albitar M: Chronic lymphocytic leukemia with t(14;18) and trisomy 12. *Arch Pathol Lab Med* 126:1543, 2002.
139. Odero MD, Soto JL, Matutes E, et al: Comparative genomic hybridization and amplotyping by arbitrarily primed PCR in stage A B-CLL. *Cancer Genet Cytogenet* 130:8, 2001.
140. Novak U, Tobler A, Fey MF: Allelotyping in B-cell chronic lymphocytic leukemia (B-CLL). *Leuk Lymphoma* 45:887, 2004.
141. Gardiner AC, Corcoran MM, Oscier DG: Cytogenetic, fluorescence *in situ* hybridisation, and clinical evaluation of translocations with concomitant deletion at 13q14 in chronic lymphocytic leukaemia. *Genes Chromosomes Cancer* 20:73, 1997.
142. Garcia-Marco JA, Price CM, Catovsky D: Interphase cytogenetics in chronic lymphocytic leukemia. *Cancer Genet Cytogenet* 94:52, 1997.
143. Crossen PE: Genes and chromosomes in chronic B-cell leukemia. *Cancer Genet Cytogenet* 94:44, 1997.
144. Bouyge-Moreau I, Rondeau G, Avet-Loiseau H, et al: Construction of a 780-kb PAC, BAC, and cosmid contig encompassing the minimal critical deletion involved in B cell chronic lymphocytic leukemia at 13q14.3. *Genomics* 46:183, 1997.
145. Corcoran MM, Rasool O, Liu Y, et al: Detailed molecular delineation of 13q14.3 loss in B-cell chronic lymphocytic leukemia. *Blood* 91:1382, 1998.
146. Stilgenbauer S, Nickolenko J, Wilhelm J, et al: Expressed sequences as candidates for a novel tumor suppressor gene at band 13q14 in B-cell chronic lymphocytic leukemia and mantle cell lymphoma. *Oncogene* 16:1891, 1998.
147. Bullrich F, Fujii H, Calin G, et al: Characterization of the 13q14 tumor suppressor locus in CLL: Identification of ALT1, an alternative splice variant of the LEU2 gene. *Cancer Res* 61:6640, 2001.
148. Mabuchi H, Fujii H, Calin G, et al: Cloning and characterization of CLLD6, CLLD7, and CLLD8, novel candidate genes for leukemogenesis at chromosome 13q14, a region commonly deleted in B-cell chronic lymphocytic leukemia. *Cancer Res* 61:2870, 2001.
149. Calin GA, Dumitru CD, Shimizu M, et al: Frequent deletions and down-regulation of micro- RNA genes miR15 and miR16 at 13q14 in chronic lymphocytic leukemia. *Proc Natl Acad Sci U S A* 99:15524, 2002.
150. Croce CM, Calin GA: MiRNAs, cancer, and stem cell division. *Cell* 122:6, 2005.
151. Tili E, Michaille JJ, Costinean S, Croce CM: MicroRNAs, the immune system and rheumatic disease. *Nat Clin Pract Rheumatol* 4:534, 2008.

152. Garzon R, Calin GA, Croce CM: MicroRNAs in Cancer. *Annu Rev Med* 60:167, 2009.
153. Dierlamm J, Michaux L, Criel A, et al: Genetic abnormalities in chronic lymphocytic leukemia and their clinical and prognostic implications. *Cancer Genet Cytogenet* 94:27, 1997.
154. Hjalmar V, Kimby E, Matutes E, et al: Trisomy 12 and lymphoplasmacytoid lymphocytes in chronic leukemic B-cell disorders. *Haematologica* 83:602, 1998.
155. Acar H, Connor MJ: Detection of trisomy 12 and centromeric alterations in CLL by interphase- and metaphase-FISH. *Cancer Genet Cytogenet* 100:148, 1998.
156. Einhorn S, Burvall K, Juliusson G, et al: Molecular analyses of chromosome 12 in chronic lymphocytic leukemia. *Leukemia* 3:871, 1989.
157. Hjalmar V, Hast R, Kimby E: Cell surface expression of CD25, CD54, and CD95 on B- and T-cells in chronic lymphocytic leukaemia in relation to trisomy 12, atypical morphology and clinical course. *Eur J Haematol* 68:127, 2002.
158. Schlette E, Medeiros LJ, Keating M, Lai R: CD79b expression in chronic lymphocytic leukemia. Association with trisomy 12 and atypical immunophenotype. *Arch Pathol Lab Med* 127:561, 2003.
159. Quijano S, Lopez A, Rasillo A, et al: Association between the proliferative rate of neoplastic B cells, their maturation stage, and underlying cytogenetic abnormalities in B-cell chronic lymphoproliferative disorders: Analysis of a series of 432 patients. *Blood* 111:5130, 2008.
160. Quijano S, Lopez A, Rasillo A, et al: Impact of trisomy 12, del(13q), del(17p), and del(11q) on the immunophenotype, DNA ploidy status, and proliferative rate of leukemic B-cells in chronic lymphocytic leukemia. *Cytometry B Clin Cytom* 74:139, 2008.
161. Garcia-Marco J, Matutes E, Morilla R, et al: Trisomy 12 in B-cell chronic lymphocytic leukaemia: Assessment of lineage restriction by simultaneous analysis of immunophenotype and genotype in interphase cells by fluorescence in situ hybridization. *Br J Haematol* 87:44, 1994.
162. Mould S, Gardiner A, Corcoran M, Oscier DG: Trisomy 12 and structural abnormalities of 13q14 occurring in the same clone in chronic lymphocytic leukaemia. *Br J Haematol* 92:389, 1996.
163. Brynes RK, McCourty A, Sun NC, Koo CH: Trisomy 12 in Richter's transformation of chronic lymphocytic leukemia. *Am J Clin Pathol* 104:199, 1995.
164. Shahidi H, Leslie WT, Wool NL, Gregory SA: Transformation of chronic lymphocytic leukemia to immunoblastic lymphoma (Richter's syndrome). *Med Pediatr Oncol* 29:146, 1997.
165. Tsimberidou AM, Keating MJ, Giles FJ, et al: Fludarabine and mitoxantrone for patients with chronic lymphocytic leukemia. *Cancer* 100:2583, 2004.
166. Stilgenbauer S, Liebisch P, James MR, et al: Molecular cytogenetic delineation of a novel critical genomic region in chromosome bands 11q22.3–923.1 in lymphoproliferative disorders. *Proc Natl Acad Sci U S A* 93:11837, 1996.
167. Dohner H, Stilgenbauer S, James MR, et al: 11q deletions identify a new subset of B-cell chronic lymphocytic leukemia characterized by extensive nodal involvement and inferior prognosis. *Blood* 89:2516, 1997.
168. Karhu R, Knuutila S, Kallioniemi OP, et al: Frequent loss of the 11q14–24 region in chronic lymphocytic leukemia: A study by comparative genomic hybridization. Tampere CLL Group. *Genes Chromosomes Cancer* 19:286, 1997.
169. Gunn SR, Hibbard MK, Ismail SH, et al: Atypical 11q deletions identified by array CGH may be missed by FISH panels for prognostic markers in chronic lymphocytic leukemia. *Leukemia* 23:1011, 2009.
170. Joshi AD, Dickinson JD, Hegde GV, et al: Bulky lymphadenopathy with poor clinical outcome is associated with ATM downregulation in B-cell chronic lymphocytic leukemia patients irrespective of 11q23 deletion. *Cancer Genet Cytogenet* 172:120, 2007.
171. Sembries S, Pahl H, Stilgenbauer S, et al: Reduced expression of adhesion molecules and cell signaling receptors by chronic lymphocytic leukemia cells with 11q deletion. *Blood* 93:624, 1999.
172. Mittal AK, Hegde GV, Aoun P, et al: Molecular basis of aggressive disease in chronic lymphocytic leukemia patients with 11q deletion and trisomy 12 chromosomal abnormalities. *Int J Mol Med* 20:461, 2007.
173. Pekarsky Y, Santanam U, Cimmino A, et al: Tcl1 expression in chronic lymphocytic leukemia is regulated by miR-29 and miR-181. *Cancer Res* 66:11590, 2006.
174. Lavin MF, Khanna KK: ATM: The protein encoded by the gene mutated in the radiosensitive syndrome ataxia-telangiectasia. *Int J Radiat Biol* 75:1201, 1999.
175. Starostik P, Manshouri T, O'Brien S, et al: Deficiency of the ATM protein expression defines an aggressive subgroup of B-cell chronic lymphocytic leukemia. *Cancer Res* 58:4552, 1998.
176. Bullrich F, Rasio D, Kitada S, et al: ATM mutations in B-cell chronic lymphocytic leukemia. *Cancer Res* 59:24, 1999.
177. Bevan S, Catovsky D, Marossy A, et al: Linkage analysis for ATM in familial B cell chronic lymphocytic leukaemia. *Leukemia* 13:1497, 1999.
178. Eclache V, Caulet-Maugendre S, Poirel HA, et al: Cryptic deletion involving the ATM locus at 11q22.3 approximately q23.1 in B-cell chronic lymphocytic leukemia and related disorders. *Cancer Genet Cytogenet* 152:72, 2004.
179. Stankovic T, Weber P, Stewart G, et al: Inactivation of ataxia telangiectasia mutated gene in B-cell chronic lymphocytic leukaemia. *Lancet* 353:26, 1999.
180. Michaux L, Wlodarska I, Rack K, et al: Translocation t(1;6)(p35.3;p25.2): A new recurrent aberration in "unmutated" B-CLL. *Leukemia* 19:77, 2005.
181. Russel J, Dutta U, Wand D, et al: The 9p24.3 breakpoint of a constitutional t(6;9)(p12;p24) in a patient with chronic lymphocytic leukemia maps close to the putative promoter region of the DMRT2 gene. *Cytogenet Genome Res* 125:81, 2009.
182. Offit K, Louie DC, Parsa NZ, et al: Clinical and morphologic features of B-cell small lymphocytic lymphoma with del(6)(q21q23). *Blood* 83:2611, 1994.
183. Glassman AB, Harper-Allen EA, Hayes KJ, et al: Chromosome 6 abnormalities associated with prolymphocytic acceleration in chronic lymphocytic leukemia. *Ann Clin Lab Sci* 28:24, 1998.
184. Finn WG, Kay NE, Kroft SH, et al: Secondary abnormalities of chromosome 6q in B-cell chronic lymphocytic leukemia: A sequential study of karyotypic instability in 51 patients. *Am J Hematol* 59:223, 1998.
185. Amiel A, Mulchanov I, Elis A, et al: Deletion of 6q27 in chronic lymphocytic leukemia and multiple myeloma detected by fluorescence in situ hybridization. *Cancer Genet Cytogenet* 112:53, 1999.
186. Fink SR, Paternoster SF, Smoley SA, et al: Fluorescent-labeled DNA probes applied to novel biological aspects of B-cell chronic lymphocytic leukemia. *Leuk Res* 29:253, 2005.
187. Cuneo A, Rigolin GM, Bigoni R, et al: Chronic lymphocytic leukemia with 6q- shows distinct hematological features and intermediate prognosis. *Leukemia* 18:476, 2004.
188. Cuneo A, Roberti MG, Bigoni R, et al: Four novel non-random chromosome rearrangements in B-cell chronic lymphocytic leukaemia: 6p24–25 and 12p12–13 translocations, 4q21 anomalies and monosomy 21. *Br J Haematol* 108:559, 2000.
189. Amiel A, Arbov L, Manor Y, et al: Monoallelic p53 deletion in chronic lymphocytic leukemia detected by interphase cytogenetics. *Cancer Genet Cytogenet* 97:97, 1997.
190. Coates PJ, Lorimore SA, Wright EG: Cell and tissue responses to genotoxic stress. *J Pathol* 205:221, 2005.
191. Thornton PD, Gruszka-Westwood AM, Hamoudi RA, et al: Characterisation of TP53 abnormalities in chronic lymphocytic leukaemia. *Hematol J* 5:47, 2004.
192. el Rouby S, Thomas A, Costin D, et al: P53 gene mutation in B-cell chronic lymphocytic leukemia is associated with drug resistance and is independent of MDR1/MDR3 gene expression. *Blood* 82:3452, 1993.
193. Lens D, De Schouwer PJ, Hamoudi RA, et al: P53 abnormalities in B-cell prolymphocytic leukemia. *Blood* 89:2015, 1997.
194. Cordone I, Masi S, Mauro FR, et al: P53 expression in B-cell chronic lymphocytic leukemia: A marker of disease progression and poor prognosis. *Blood* 91:4342, 1998.
195. Callet-Bauchu E, Salles G, Gazzo S, et al: Translocations involving the short arm of chromosome 17 in chronic B-lymphoid disorders: Frequent occurrence of dicentric rearrangements and possible association with adverse outcome. *Leukemia* 13:460, 1999.
196. Shaw GR, Kronberger DL: TP53 deletions but not trisomy 12 are adverse in B-cell lymphoproliferative disorders. *Cancer Genet Cytogenet* 119:146, 2000.
197. Byrd JC, Stilgenbauer S, Flinn IW: Chronic lymphocytic leukemia. *Hematology Am Soc Hematol Educ Program* 163, 2004.
198. Bea S, Lopez-Guillermo A, Ribas M, et al: Genetic imbalances in progressed B-cell chronic lymphocytic leukemia and transformed large-cell lymphoma (Richter's syndrome). *Am J Pathol* 161:957, 2002.
199. Gaidano G, Ballerini P, Gong JZ, et al: P53 mutations in human lymphoid malignancies: Association with Burkitt lymphoma and chronic lymphocytic leukemia. *Proc Natl Acad Sci U S A* 88:5413, 1991.
200. Croce CM: Molecular biology of lymphomas. *Semin Oncol* 20:31, 1993.
201. Zech L, Gahrton G, Hammarstrom L, et al: Inversion of chromosome 14 marks human T-cell chronic lymphocytic leukaemia. *Nature* 308:858, 1984.
202. Hecht F, Morgan R, Hecht BK, Smith SD: Common region on chromosome 14 in T-cell leukemia and lymphoma. *Science* 226:1445, 1984.
203. Larramendy ML, Peltomaki P, Salonen E, Knuutila S: Chromosomal abnormality limited to T4 lymphocytes in a patient with T-cell chronic lymphocytic leukaemia. *Eur J Haematol* 45:52, 1990.
204. Jonveaux P, Hillion J, Bennaceur AL, et al: T(14;18) and bcl-2 gene rearrangement in a B-chronic lymphocytic leukaemia. *Br J Haematol* 81:620, 1992.
205. Raghoebier S, van Krieken JH, Kluin-Nelemans JC, et al: Oncogene rearrangements in chronic B-cell leukemia. *Blood* 77:1560, 1991.
206. Kern W, Haferlach T, Schnittger S, Schoch C: Detection of t(14;18)(q32;q21) in B-cell chronic lymphocytic leukemia. *Arch Pathol Lab Med* 129:410, 2005.
207. Put N, Meeus P, Chatelain B, et al: Translocation t(14;18) is not associated with inferior outcome in chronic lymphocytic leukemia. *Leukemia* 23:1201, 2009.
208. Ueshima Y, Bird ML, Vardiman JW, Rowley JD: A 14;19 translocation in B-cell chronic lymphocytic leukemia: A new recurring chromosome aberration. *Int J Cancer* 36:287, 1985.
209. Michaux L, Mecucci C, Stul M, et al: BCL3 rearrangement and t(14;19)(q32;q13) in lymphoproliferative disorders. *Genes Chromosomes Cancer* 15:38, 1996.
210. McKeithan TW, Takimoto GS, Ohno H, et al: BCL3 rearrangements and t(14;19) in chronic lymphocytic leukemia and other B-cell malignancies: A molecular and cytogenetic study. *Genes Chromosomes Cancer* 20:64, 1997.
211. Crossen PE: Cytogenetic and molecular changes in chronic B-cell leukemia. *Cancer Genet Cytogenet* 43:143, 1989.
212. Pittman S, Catovsky D: Prognostic significance of chromosome abnormalities in chronic lymphocytic leukaemia. *Br J Haematol* 58:649, 1984.
213. Meeker TC, Grimaldi JC, O'Rourke R, et al: An additional breakpoint region in the BCL-1 locus associated with the t(11;14)(q13;q32) translocation of B-lymphocytic malignancy. *Blood* 74:1801, 1989.
214. Erikson J, Finan J, Tsujimoto Y, et al: The chromosome 14 breakpoint in neoplastic B cells with the t(11;14) translocation involves the immunoglobulin heavy chain locus. *Proc Natl Acad Sci U S A* 81:4144, 1984.

215. Davey MP, Bertness V, Nakahara K, et al: Juxtaposition of the T-cell receptor alpha-chain locus (14q11) and a region (14q32) of potential importance in leukemogenesis by a 14;14 translocation in a patient with T-cell chronic lymphocytic leukemia and ataxia-telangiectasia. *Proc Natl Acad Sci U S A* 85:9287, 1988.
216. Motokura T, Bloom T, Kim HG, et al: A novel cyclin encoded by a bcl1-linked candidate oncogene [see comments]. *Nature* 350:512, 1991.
217. Seto M, Yamamoto K, Iida S, et al: Gene rearrangement and overexpression of PRAD1 in lymphoid malignancy with t(11;14)(q13;q32) translocation. *Oncogene* 7:1401, 1992.
218. Hinds PW, Dowdy SF, Eaton EN, et al: Function of a human cyclin gene as an oncogene. *Proc Natl Acad Sci U S A* 91:709, 1994.
219. Rimokh R, Berger F, Cornillet P, et al: Break in the BCL1 locus is closely associated with intermediate lymphocytic lymphoma subtype. *Genes Chromosomes Cancer* 2:223, 1990.
220. Ambinder RF, Griffin CA: Biology of the lymphomas: Cytogenetics, molecular biology, and virology. *Curr Opin Oncol* 3:806, 1991.
221. Brito-Babapulle V, Ellis J, Matutes E, et al: Translocation t(11;14)(q13;q32) in chronic lymphoid disorders. *Genes Chromosomes Cancer* 5:158, 1992.
222. Williams ME, Swerdlow SH, Rosenberg CL, Arnold A: Characterization of chromosome 11 translocation breakpoints at the bcl-1 and PRAD1 loci in centrocytic lymphoma. *Cancer Res* 52:5541s-5544s, 1992.
223. Swerdlow SH, Saboorian MH, Pelstring RJ, Williams ME: Centrocytic lymphoma: A morphometric study with comparison to other small cleaved follicular center cell lymphomas and genotypic correlates. *Am J Pathol* 142:329, 1993.
224. Einhorn S, Meeker T, Juliusson G, et al: No evidence of trisomy 12 or t(11;14) by molecular genetic techniques in chronic lymphocytic leukemia cells with a normal karyotype. *Cancer Genet Cytogenet* 48:183, 1990.
225. Rechavi G, Katzir N, Brok-Simoni F, et al: A search for bcl1, bcl2, and c-myc oncogene rearrangements in chronic lymphocytic leukemia. *Leukemia* 3:57, 1989.
226. Newman RA, Peterson B, Davey FR, et al: Phenotypic markers and BCL-1 gene rearrangements in B-cell chronic lymphocytic leukemia: A Cancer and Leukemia Group B study. *Blood* 82:1239, 1993.
227. Adachi M, Tefferi A, Greipp PR, et al: Preferential linkage of bcl-2 to immunoglobulin light chain gene in chronic lymphocytic leukemia. *J Exp Med* 171:559, 1990.
228. Schena M, Larsson LG, Gottardi D, et al: Growth- and differentiation-associated expression of bcl-2 in B-chronic lymphocytic leukemia cells. *Blood* 79:2981, 1992.
229. Pezzella F, Tse AG, Cordell JL, et al: Expression of the bcl-2 oncogene protein is not specific for the 14;18 chromosomal translocation. *Am J Pathol* 137:225, 1990.
230. Hanada M, Delia D, Aiello A, et al: Bcl-2 gene hypomethylation and high-level expression in B-cell chronic lymphocytic leukemia. *Blood* 82:1820, 1993.
231. Laytragoon-Lewin N, Kashuba V, Mellstedt H, Klein G: Bcl-2 rearrangement detected by pulsed-field gel electrophoresis (PFGF) in B-chronic lymphocytic leukemia (CLL) cells. *Int J Cancer* 76:909, 1998.
232. Lampert IA, Wotherspoon A, Van Noorden S, Hasserjian RP: High expression of CD23 in the proliferation centers of chronic lymphocytic leukemia in lymph nodes and spleen. *Hum Pathol* 30:648, 1999.
233. Zimmerman TS, Godwin HA, Perry S: Studies of leukocyte kinetics in chronic lymphocytic leukemia. *Blood* 31:277, 1968.
234. Andreeff M, Darzynkiewicz Z, Sharpless TK, et al: Discrimination of human leukemia subtypes by flow cytometric analysis of cellular DNA and RNA. *Blood* 55:282, 1980.
235. Kobayashi R, Picchio G, Kirven M, et al: Transfer of human chronic lymphocytic leukemia to mice with severe combined immune deficiency. *Leuk Res* 16:1013, 1992.
236. Messmer BT, Messmer D, Allen SL, et al: *In vivo* measurements document the dynamic cellular kinetics of chronic lymphocytic leukemia B cells. *J Clin Invest* 115:755, 2005.
237. Naresh KN: Proliferation center cells in the lymph nodes of B-cell chronic lymphatic leukemia express relatively higher levels of CD20. *Hum Pathol* 31:775, 2000.
238. Asplund SL, McKenna RW, Howard MS, Kroft SH: Immunophenotype does not correlate with lymph node histology in chronic lymphocytic leukemia/small lymphocytic lymphoma. *Am J Surg Pathol* 26:624, 2002.
239. Ben-Ezra J, Burke JS, Swartz WG, et al: Small lymphocytic lymphoma: A clinicopathologic analysis of 268 cases. *Blood* 73:579, 1989.
240. Gupta D, Lim MS, Medeiros LJ, Elenitoba-Johnson KS: Small lymphocytic lymphoma with perifollicular, marginal zone, or interfollicular distribution. *Mod Pathol* 13:1161, 2000.
241. Schimmer AD, Munk-Pedersen I, Minden MD, Reed JC: Bcl-2 and apoptosis in chronic lymphocytic leukemia. *Curr Treat Options Oncol* 4:211, 2003.
242. Kitada S, Andersen J, Akar S, et al: Expression of apoptosis-regulating proteins in chronic lymphocytic leukemia: Correlations with *in vitro* and *in vivo* chemoresponses. *Blood* 91:3379, 1998.
243. Gottardi D, Alfarano A, De Leo AM, et al: In leukaemic CD5+ B cells the expression of BCL-2 gene family is shifted toward protection from apoptosis. *Br J Haematol* 94:612, 1996.
244. Korsmeyer SJ: Bcl-2 initiates a new category of oncogenes: Regulators of cell death. *Blood* 80:879, 1992.
245. Coulie PG: Human tumour antigens recognized by T cells: New perspectives for anti-cancer vaccines? *Mol Med Today* 3:261, 1997.
246. McConkey DJ, Chandra J, Wright S, et al: Apoptosis sensitivity in chronic lymphocytic leukemia is determined by endogenous endonuclease content and relative expression of BCL-2 and BAX. *J Immunol* 156:2624, 1996.
247. Pepper C, Bentley P, Hoy T: Regulation of clinical chemoresistance by bcl-2 and bax oncoproteins in B-cell chronic lymphocytic leukaemia. *Br J Haematol* 95:513, 1996.
248. Aguilar-Santelises M, Rottenberg ME, Lewin N, et al: Bcl-2, Bax and p53 expression in B-CLL in relation to *in vitro* survival and clinical progression. *Int J Cancer* 69:114, 1996.
249. Thomas A, El Rouby S, Reed JC, et al: Drug-induced apoptosis in B-cell chronic lymphocytic leukemia: Relationship between p53 gene mutation and bcl-2/bax proteins in drug resistance. *Oncogene* 12:1055, 1996.
250. Cimmino A, Calin GA, Fabbri M, et al: MiR-15 and miR-16 induce apoptosis by targeting BCL2. *Proc Natl Acad Sci U S A* 102:13944, 2005.
251. Panayiotidis P, Jones D, Ganeshaguru K, et al: Human bone marrow stromal cells prevent apoptosis and support the survival of chronic lymphocytic leukaemia cells in vitro. *Br J Haematol* 92:97, 1996.
252. Lagneaux L, Delforge A, Bron D, et al: Chronic lymphocytic leukemic B cells but not normal B cells are rescued from apoptosis by contact with normal bone marrow stromal cells. *Blood* 91:2387, 1998.
253. Burger JA, Tsukada N, Burger M, et al: Blood-derived nurse-like cells protect chronic lymphocytic leukemia B cells from spontaneous apoptosis through stromal cell-derived factor-1. *Blood* 96:2655, 2000.
254. Tsukada N, Burger JA, Zvaifler NJ, Kipps TJ: Distinctive features of "nurselike" cells that differentiate in the context of chronic lymphocytic leukemia. *Blood* 99:1030, 2002.
255. Pedersen IM, Kitada S, Leoni LM, et al: Protection of CLL B cells by a follicular dendritic cell line is dependent on induction of Mcl-1. *Blood* 100:1795, 2002.
256. Burger JA, Kipps TJ: Chemokine receptors and stromal cells in the homing and homeostasis of chronic lymphocytic leukemia B cells. *Leuk Lymphoma* 43:461, 2002.
257. Burger JA, Burger M, Kipps TJ: Chronic lymphocytic leukemia B cells express functional CXCR4 chemokine receptors that mediate spontaneous migration beneath bone marrow stromal cells. *Blood* 94:3658, 1999.
258. Trentin L, Agostini C, Facco M, et al: The chemokine receptor CXCR3 is expressed on malignant B cells and mediates chemotaxis. *J Clin Invest* 104:115, 1999.
259. Till KJ, Lin K, Zuzel M, Cawley JC: The chemokine receptor CCR7 and alpha4 integrin are important for migration of chronic lymphocytic leukemia cells into lymph nodes. *Blood* 99:2977, 2002.
260. Winkelstein A, Jordan PS: Immune deficiencies in chronic lymphocytic leukemia and multiple myeloma. *Clin Rev Allergy* 10:39, 1992.
261. Schlesinger M, Broman I, Lugassy G: The complement system is defective in chronic lymphatic leukemia patients and in their healthy relatives. *Leukemia* 10:1509, 1996.
262. Rossi E, Matutes E, Morilla R, et al: Zeta chain and CD28 are poorly expressed on T lymphocytes from chronic lymphocytic leukemia. *Leukemia* 10:494, 1996.
263. Veenstra H, Jacobs P, Dowdle EB: Abnormal association between invariant chain and HLA class II alpha and beta chains in chronic lymphocytic leukemia. *Cell Immunol* 171:68, 1996.
264. Nuckel H, Rebmann V, Durig J, et al: HLA-G expression is associated with an unfavorable outcome and immunodeficiency in chronic lymphocytic leukemia. *Blood* 105:1694, 2005.
265. Itala M, Vainio O, Remes K: Functional abnormalities in granulocytes predict susceptibility to bacterial infections in chronic lymphocytic leukaemia. *Eur J Haematol* 57:46, 1996.
266. Tsiodras S, Samonis G, Keating MJ, Kontoyiannis DP: Infection and immunity in chronic lymphocytic leukemia. *Mayo Clin Proc* 75:1039, 2000.
267. Bower JH, Hammack JE, McDonnell SK, Tefferi A: The neurologic complications of B-cell chronic lymphocytic leukemia. *Neurology* 48:407, 1997.
268. Hermouet S, Sutton CA, Rose TM, et al: Qualitative and quantitative analysis of human herpesviruses in chronic and acute B cell lymphocytic leukemia and in multiple myeloma. *Leukemia* 17:185, 2003.
269. Laurenti L, Piccioni P, Cattani P, et al: Cytomegalovirus reactivation during alemtuzumab therapy for chronic lymphocytic leukemia: Incidence and treatment with oral ganciclovir. *Haematologica* 89:1248, 2004.
270. Levi F, Randimbison L, Te VC, La Vecchia C: Non-Hodgkin's lymphomas, chronic lymphocytic leukaemias and skin cancers. *Br J Cancer* 74:1847, 1996.
271. Lotz M, Ranheim E, Kipps TJ: Transforming growth factor beta as endogenous growth inhibitor of chronic lymphocytic leukemia B cells. *J Exp Med* 179:999, 1994.
272. Lagneaux L, Delforge A, Bron D, et al: Heterogenous response of B lymphocytes to transforming growth factor-beta in B-cell chronic lymphocytic leukaemia: Correlation with the expression of TGF-beta receptors. *Br J Haematol* 97:612, 1997.
273. van Oers MH, Pals ST, Evers LM, et al: Expression and release of CD27 in human B-cell malignancies. *Blood* 82:3430, 1993.
274. Kato K, Cantwell MJ, Sharma S, Kipps TJ: Gene transfer of CD40-ligand induces autologous immune recognition of chronic lymphocytic leukemia B cells. *J Clin Invest* 101:1133, 1998.
275. Matutes E, Wechsler A, Gomez R, et al: Unusual T-cell phenotype in advanced B-chronic lymphocytic leukaemia. *Br J Haematol* 49:635, 1981.
276. Fu SM, Chiorazzi N, Kunkel HG: Differentiation capacity and other properties of the leukemic cells of chronic lymphocytic leukemia. *Immunol Rev* 48:23, 1979.
277. Ranheim EA, Kipps TJ: Activated T cells induce expression of B7/BB1 on normal or leukemic B cells through a CD40-dependent signal. *J Exp Med* 177:925, 1993.
278. Cantwell M, Hua T, Pappas J, Kipps TJ: Acquired CD40-ligand deficiency in chronic lymphocytic leukemia. *Nat Med* 3:984, 1997.
279. Kneitz C, Goller M, Wilhelm M, et al: Inhibition of T cell/B cell interaction by B-CLL cells. *Leukemia* 13:98, 1999.

280. Grewal IS, Flavell RA: The CD40 ligand: At the center of the immune universe? *Immunol Res* 16:59, 1997.
281. Lacombe C, Gombert J, Dreyfus B, et al: Heterogeneity of serum IgG subclass deficiencies in B chronic lymphocytic leukemia. *Clin Immunol* 90:128, 1999.
282. Martin-Villa JM, Corell A, Ramos-Amador JT, et al: Higher incidence of autoantibodies in X-linked chronic granulomatous disease carriers: Random X-chromosome inactivation may be related to autoimmunity. *Autoimmunity* 31:261, 1999.
283. Etzioni A: Immune deficiency and autoimmunity. *Autoimmun Rev* 2:364, 2003.
284. Hamblin TJ, Oscier DG, Young BJ: Autoimmunity in chronic lymphocytic leukaemia. *J Clin Pathol* 39:713, 1986.
285. Duhrsen U, Augener W, Zwingers T, Brittinger G: Spectrum and frequency of autoimmune derangements in lymphoproliferative disorders: Analysis of 637 cases and comparison with myeloproliferative diseases. *Br J Haematol* 67:235, 1987.
286. Hill PA, Firkin F, Dwyer KM, et al: Membranoproliferative glomerulonephritis in association with chronic lymphocytic leukaemia: A report of three cases. *Pathology* 34:138, 2002.
287. Rosado MF, Morgensztern D, Abdullah S, et al: Chronic lymphocytic leukemia-associated nephrotic syndrome caused by focal segmental glomerulosclerosis. *Am J Hematol* 77:205, 2004.
288. Ziakas PD, Giannouli S, Psimenou E, et al: Membranous glomerulonephritis in chronic lymphocytic leukemia. *Am J Hematol* 76:271, 2004.
289. Ruzickova S, Pruss A, Odendahl M, et al: Chronic lymphocytic leukemia preceded by cold agglutinin disease: Intraclonal immunoglobulin light-chain diversity in V(H)4–34 expressing single leukemic B cells. *Blood* 100:3419, 2002.
290. Bhavnani M: Cyclosporin A treatment of pure red cell aplasia associated with B-CLL [letter; comment]. *Br J Haematol* 79:137, 1991.
291. Taylor HG, Nixon N, Sheeran TP, Dawes PT: Rheumatoid arthritis and chronic lymphatic leukaemia. *Clin Exp Rheumatol* 7:529, 1989.
292. Amir R, Dowdy YG, Goldberg AN: Chronic rhinitis: A manifestation of chronic lymphocytic leukemia. *Am J Otolaryngol* 20:328, 1999.
293. Weed RI: Exaggerated delayed hypersensitivity to mosquito bites in chronic lymphocytic leukemia. *Blood* 26:257, 1965.
294. Barzilai A, Shpiro D, Goldberg I, et al: Insect bite-like reaction in patients with hematologic malignant neoplasms. *Arch Dermatol* 135:1503, 1999.
295. Higgins JP, Warnke RA: Herpes lymphadenitis in association with chronic lymphocytic leukemia. *Cancer* 86:1210, 1999.
296. Mariette X, Molina JM, Asli B, Brouet JC: A patient with chronic lymphoid leukemia and recurrent necrotic herpetic lymphadenitis. *Am J Med* 107:403, 1999.
297. Rustagi PK, Han T, Ziolkowski L, et al: Granulocyte antibodies in leukaemic chronic lymphoproliferative disorders. *Br J Haematol* 66:461, 1987.
298. Lischner M, Prokocimer M, Zolberg A, Shaklai M: Autoimmunity in chronic lymphocytic leukaemia. *Postgrad Med J* 64:590, 1988.
299. Chablani AT, Badakere SS, Bhatia HM: Incidence of antibodies to nuclear antigens, platelets & circulating immune complexes in leukaemias. *Indian J Med Res* 88:348, 1988.
300. Koerner TA, Weinfeld HM, Bullard LS, Williams LC: Antibodies against platelet glycosphingolipids: Detection in serum by quantitative HPTLC-autoradiography and association with autoimmune and alloimmune processes. *Blood* 74:274, 1989.
301. Habboush HW, Dhundee J, Okati DA, Davies AG: Constrictive pericarditis in B cell chronic lymphatic leukaemia. *Clin Lab Haematol* 18:117, 1996.
302. Giannini O, Schonenberger-Berzins R: Fulminant cardiac tamponade in chronic lymphocytic leukaemia. *Ann Oncol* 8:1168, 1997.
303. Sivakumaran M, Qureshi H, Chapman CS: Chylous effusions in CLL. *Leuk Lymphoma* 18:365, 1995.
304. Zeidman A, Yarmolovsky A, Djaldetti M, Mittelman M: Hemorrhagic pleural effusion as a complication of chronic lymphocytic leukemia. *Haematologia (Budap)* 26:173, 1995.
305. Miyahara M, Shimamoto Y, Sano M, et al: Immunoglobulin gene rearrangement in T-cell-rich reactive pleural effusion of a patient with B-cell chronic lymphocytic leukemia. *Acta Haematol* 96:41, 1996.
306. Elliott MA, Letendre L, Li CY, et al: Chronic lymphocytic leukaemia with symptomatic diffuse central nervous system infiltration responding to therapy with systemic fludarabine. *Br J Haematol* 104:689, 1999.
307. Cawley JC, Barker CR, Britchford RD, Smith JL: Intracellular IgA immunoglobulin crystals in chronic lymphocytic leukaemia. *Clin Exp Immunol* 13:407, 1973.
308. Peters O, Thielemans C, Steenssens L, et al: Intracellular inclusion bodies in 14 patients with B cell lymphoproliferative disorders. *J Clin Pathol* 37:45, 1984.
309. Montserrat E, Marques-Pereira JP, Gallart MT, Rozman C: Bone marrow histopathologic patterns and immunologic findings in B-chronic lymphocytic leukemia. *Cancer* 54:447, 1984.
310. Pangalis GA, Roussou PA, Kittas C, et al: Patterns of bone marrow involvement in chronic lymphocytic leukemia and small lymphocytic (well differentiated) non-Hodgkin's lymphoma. Its clinical significance in relation to their differential diagnosis and prognosis. *Cancer* 54:702, 1984.
311. Pangalis GA, Boussiotis VA, Kittas C: Malignant disorders of small lymphocytes. Small lymphocytic lymphoma, lymphoplasmacytic lymphoma, and chronic lymphocytic leukemia: Their clinical and laboratory relationship. *Am J Clin Pathol* 99:402, 1993.
312. Pangalis GA, Roussou PA, Kittas C, et al: B-chronic lymphocytic leukemia. Prognostic implication of bone marrow histology in 120 patients experience from a single hematology unit. *Cancer* 59:767, 1987.
313. Kanzler H, Küppers R, Helmes S, et al: Hodgkin and Reed-Sternberg-like cells in B-cell chronic lymphocytic leukemia represent the outgrowth of single germinal-center B-cell-derived clones: Potential precursors of Hodgkin and Reed-Sternberg cells in Hodgkin's disease. *Blood* 95:1023, 2000.
314. Baldini L, Cro L, Cortelezzi A, et al: Immunophenotypes in "classical" B-cell chronic lymphocytic leukemia. Correlation with normal cellular counterpart and clinical findings. *Cancer* 66:1738, 1990.
315. Sarfati M, Fournier S, Christoffersen M, Biron G: Expression of CD23 antigen and its regulation by IL-4 in chronic lymphocytic leukemia. *Leuk Res* 14:47, 1990.
316. Batata A, Shen B: Immunophenotyping of subtypes of B-chronic (mature) lymphoid leukemia. A study of 242 cases. *Cancer* 70:2436, 1992.
317. De Rossi G, Zarcone D, Mauro F, et al: Adhesion molecule expression on B-cell chronic lymphocytic leukemia cells: Malignant cell phenotypes define distinct disease subsets. *Blood* 81:2679, 1993.
318. Serke S, Schwaner I, Yordanova M, et al: Monoclonal antibody FMC7 detects a conformational epitope on the CD20 molecule: Evidence from phenotyping after Rituxan therapy and transfectant cell analyses. *Cytometry B Clin Cytom* 46:98, 2001.
319. Delgado J, Matutes E, Morilla AM, et al: Diagnostic significance of CD20 and FMC7 expression in B-cell disorders. *Am J Clin Pathol* 120:754, 2003.
320. Pianezze G, Gentilini I, Casini M, et al: Cytoplasmic immunoglobulins in chronic lymphocytic leukemia B cells. *Blood* 69:1011, 1987.
321. Yasuda N, Kanoh T, Shirakawa S, Uchino H: Intracellular immunoglobulin in lymphocytes from patients with chronic lymphocytic leukemia: An immunoelectron microscopic study. *Leuk Res* 6:659, 1982.
322. Newell DG, Hannam-Harris A, Karpas A, Smith JL: The differential ultrastructural localization of immunoglobulin heavy and light chains in human haematopoietic cell lines. *Br J Haematol* 50:445, 1982.
323. Newell DG, Harris AH, Smith JL: The ultrastructural localization of immunoglobulin in chronic lymphocytic lymphoma cells: Changes in light and heavy chain distribution induced by mitogen stimulation. *Blood* 61:511, 1983.
324. Deegan MJ, Abraham JP, Sawdyk M, Van Slyck EJ: High incidence of monoclonal proteins in the serum and urine of chronic lymphocytic leukemia patients. *Blood* 64:1207, 1984.
325. Sinclair D, Dagg JH, Dewar AE, et al: The incidence, clonal origin and secretory nature of serum paraproteins in chronic lymphocytic leukaemia. *Br J Haematol* 64:725, 1986.
326. Pangalis GA, Moutsopoulos HM, Papadopoulos NM, et al: Monoclonal and oligoclonal immunoglobulins in the serum of patients with B-chronic lymphocytic leukemia. *Acta Haematol* 80:23, 1988.
327. Gordon DS, Jones BM, Browning SW, et al: Persistent polyclonal lymphocytosis of B lymphocytes. *N Engl J Med* 307:232, 1982.
328. Wilkinson LS, Tang A, Gjedsted A: Marked lymphocytosis suggesting chronic lymphocytic leukemia in three patients with hyposplenism. *Am J Med* 75:1053, 1983.
329. Batata A, Shen B: Diagnostic value of clonality of surface immunoglobulin light and heavy chains in malignant lymphoproliferative disorders. *Am J Hematol* 43:265, 1993.
330. Melo JV, Wardle J, Chetty M, et al: The relationship between chronic lymphocytic leukaemia and prolymphocytic leukaemia. III. Evaluation of cell size by morphology and volume measurements. *Br J Haematol* 64:469, 1986.
331. Robinson DS, Melo JV, Andrews C, et al: Intracytoplasmic inclusions in B prolymphocytic leukaemia: Ultrastructural, cytochemical, and immunological studies. *J Clin Pathol* 38:897, 1985.
332. Bearman RM, Pangalis GA, Rappaport H: Prolymphocytic leukemia: Clinical, histopathological, and cytochemical observations. *Cancer* 42:2360, 1978.
333. Moreau EJ, Matutes E, A'Hern RP, et al: Improvement of the chronic lymphocytic leukemia scoring system with the monoclonal antibody SN8 (CD79b). *Am J Clin Pathol* 108:378, 1997.
334. Zomas AP, Matutes E, Morilla R, et al: Expression of the immunoglobulin-associated protein B29 in B cell disorders with the monoclonal antibody SN8 (CD79b). *Leukemia* 10:1966, 1996.
335. Cabezudo E, Carrara P, Morilla R, Matutes E: Quantitative analysis of CD79b, CD5 and CD19 in mature B-cell lymphoproliferative disorders. *Haematologica* 84:413, 1999.
336. Matutes E, Morilla R, Owusu-Ankomah K, et al: The immunophenotype of splenic lymphoma with villous lymphocytes and its relevance to the differential diagnosis with other B-cell disorders. *Blood* 83:1558, 1994.
337. Dick FR, Maca RD: The lymph node in chronic lymphocytic leukemia. *Cancer* 41:283, 1978.
338. Pratt LF, Rassenti L, Larrick J, et al: Immunoglobulin gene expression in small lymphocytic lymphoma with little or no somatic hypermutation. *J Immunol* 143:699, 1989.
339. Medeiros LJ, Strickler JG, Picker LJ, et al: "Well-differentiated" lymphocytic neoplasms. Immunologic findings correlated with clinical presentation and morphologic features. *Am J Pathol* 129:523, 1987.
340. Ellison DJ, Turner RR, van Antwerp R, et al: High-grade mantle zone lymphoma. *Cancer* 60:2717, 1987.
341. Bell PB, Rooney N, Bosanquet AG: CD79a detected by ZL7.4 separates chronic lymphocytic leukemia from mantle cell lymphoma in the leukemic phase. *Cytometry B Clin Cytom* 38:102, 1999.
342. Elnenaei MO, Jadayel DM, Matutes E, et al: Cyclin D1 by flow cytometry as a useful tool in the diagnosis of B-cell malignancies. *Leuk Res* 25:115, 2001.

343. Ruchlemer R, Parry-Jones N, Brito-Babapulle V, et al: B-prolymphocytic leukaemia with t(11;14) revisited: A splenomegalic form of mantle cell lymphoma evolving with leukaemia. *Br J Haematol* 125:330, 2004.
344. Matutes E, Carrara P, Coignet L, et al: FISH analysis for BCL-1 rearrangements and trisomy 12 helps the diagnosis of atypical B cell leukaemias. *Leukemia* 13:1721, 1999.
345. Dogan A, Isaacson PG: Splenic marginal zone lymphoma. *Semin Diagn Pathol* 20:121, 2003.
346. Franco V, Florena AM, Iannitto E: Splenic marginal zone lymphoma. *Blood* 101:2464, 2003.
347. Giannouli S, Paterakis G, Ziakas PD, et al: Splenic marginal zone lymphomas with peripheral CD5 expression. *Haematologica* 89:113, 2004.
348. Andersen CL, Gruszka-Westwood A, Ostergaard M, et al: A narrow deletion of 7q is common to HCL, and SMZL, but not CLL. *Eur J Haematol* 72:390, 2004.
349. Kansal R, Ross CW, Singleton TP, et al: Histopathologic features of splenic small B-cell lymphomas. A study of 42 cases with a definitive diagnosis by the World Health Organization classification. *Am J Clin Pathol* 120:335, 2003.
350. Skinnider LF, Tan L, Schmidt J, Armitage G: Chronic lymphocytic leukemia. A review of 745 cases and assessment of clinical staging. *Cancer* 50:2951, 1982.
351. Phillips EA, Kempin S, Passe S, et al: Prognostic factors in chronic lymphocytic leukaemia and their implications for therapy. *Clin Haematol* 6:203, 1977.
352. Binet JL, Auquier A, Dighiero G, et al: A new prognostic classification of chronic lymphocytic leukemia derived from a multivariate survival analysis. *Cancer* 48:198, 1981.
353. Rai KR: A critical analysis of staging in CLL, in *Chronic Lymphocytic Leukemia: Recent Progress and Future Direction*, edited by RP Gale, KR Rai, pp 253–264. Alan R. Liss, Inc., New York, 1987.
354. Vasconcelos Y, Davi F, Levy V, et al: Binet's staging system and VH genes are independent but complementary prognostic indicators in chronic lymphocytic leukemia. *J Clin Oncol* 21:3928, 2003.
355. Hallek M, Cheson BD, Catovsky D, et al: Guidelines for the diagnosis and treatment of chronic lymphocytic leukemia: A report from the International Workshop on Chronic Lymphocytic Leukemia updating the National Cancer Institute-Working Group 1996 guidelines. *Blood* 111:5446, 2008.
356. Molica S, Alberti A: Prognostic value of the lymphocyte doubling time in chronic lymphocytic leukemia. *Cancer* 60:2712, 1987.
357. Montserrat E, Sanchez-Bisono J, Vinolas N, Rozman C: Lymphocyte doubling time in chronic lymphocytic leukaemia: Analysis of its prognostic significance. *Br J Haematol* 62:567, 1986.
358. Mauro FR, Foa R, Giannarelli D, et al: Clinical characteristics and outcome of young chronic lymphocytic leukemia patients: A single institution study of 204 cases. *Blood* 94:448, 1999.
359. Schroeder HW Jr, Dighiero G: The pathogenesis of chronic lymphocytic leukemia: Analysis of the antibody repertoire. *Immunol Today* 15:288, 1994.
360. Friedman DF, Moore JS, Erikson J, et al: Variable region gene analysis of an isotype-switched (IgA) variant of chronic lymphocytic leukemia. *Blood* 80:2287, 1992.
361. Ebeling SB, Schutte ME, Logtenberg T: Molecular analysis of VH and VL regions expressed in IgG-bearing chronic lymphocytic leukemia (CLL): Further evidence that CLL is a heterogeneous group of tumors. *Blood* 82:1626, 1993.
362. Hashimoto S, Dono M, Wakai M, et al: Somatic diversification and selection of immunoglobulin heavy and light chain variable region genes in IgG+ CD5+ chronic lymphocytic leukemia B cells. *J Exp Med* 181:1507, 1995.
363. Matolcsy A, Casali P, Nador RG, et al: Molecular characterization of IgA- and/or IgG-switched chronic lymphocytic leukemia B cells. *Blood* 89:1732, 1997.
364. Kipps TJ, Tomhave E, Chen PP, Carson DA: Autoantibody-associated kappa light chain variable region gene expressed in chronic lymphocytic leukemia with little or no somatic mutation. Implications for etiology and immunotherapy. *J Exp Med* 167:840, 1988.
365. Schettino EW, Cerutti A, Chiorazzi N, Casali P: Lack of intraclonal diversification in Ig heavy and light chain V region genes expressed by CD5+IgM+ chronic lymphocytic leukemia B cells: A multiple time point analysis. *J Immunol* 160:820, 1998.
366. Oscier DG, Thompsett A, Zhu D, Stevenson FK: Differential rates of somatic hypermutation in V(H) genes among subsets of chronic lymphocytic leukemia defined by chromosomal abnormalities. *Blood* 89:4153, 1997.
367. Hamblin TJ, Orchard JA, Ibbotson RE, et al: CD38 expression and immunoglobulin variable region mutations are independent prognostic variables in chronic lymphocytic leukemia, but CD38 expression may vary during the course of the disease. *Blood* 99:1023, 2002.
368. Krober A, Seiler T, Benner A, et al: V(H) mutation status, CD38 expression level, genomic aberrations, and survival in chronic lymphocytic leukemia. *Blood* 100:1410, 2002.
369. Lin K, Sherrington PD, Dennis M, et al: Relationship between p53 dysfunction, CD38 expression, and IgV(H) mutation in chronic lymphocytic leukemia. *Blood* 100:1404, 2002.
370. Oscier DG, Gardiner AC, Mould SJ, et al: Multivariate analysis of prognostic factors in CLL: Clinical stage, IGVH gene mutational status, and loss or mutation of the p53 gene are independent prognostic factors. *Blood* 100:1177, 2002.
371. Lin KI, Tam CS, Keating MJ et al: Relevance of the immunoglobulin VH somatic mutation status in patients with chronic lymphocytic leukemia treated with fludarabine, cyclophosphamide, and rituximab (FCR) or related chemoimmunotherapy regimens. *Blood* 113:3168, 2009.
372. Durig J, Naschar M, Schmucker U, et al: CD38 expression is an important prognostic marker in chronic lymphocytic leukaemia. *Leukemia* 16:30, 2002.
373. Chevallier P, Penther D, Avet-Loiseau H, et al: CD38 expression and secondary 17p deletion are important prognostic factors in chronic lymphocytic leukaemia. *Br J Haematol* 116:142, 2002.
374. Morabito F, Mangiola M, Stelitano C, et al: Peripheral blood CD38 expression predicts time to progression in B-cell chronic lymphocytic leukemia after first-line therapy with high-dose chlorambucil. *Haematologica* 87:217, 2002.
375. Domingo-Domenech E, Domingo-Claros A, Gonzalez-Barca E, et al: CD38 expression in B-chronic lymphocytic leukemia: Association with clinical presentation and outcome in 155 patients. *Haematologica* 87:1021, 2002.
376. D'Arena G, Nunziata G, Coppola G, et al: CD38 expression does not change in B-cell chronic lymphocytic leukemia. *Blood* 100:3052, 2002.
377. Patten PE, Buggins AG, Richards J, et al: CD38 expression in chronic lymphocytic leukemia is regulated by the tumor microenvironment. *Blood* 111:5173, 2008.
378. Ghia P, Guida G, Stella S, et al: The pattern of CD38 expression defines a distinct subset of chronic lymphocytic leukemia (CLL) patients at risk of disease progression. *Blood* 101:1262, 2003.
379. Hayat A, O'Brien D, O'Rourke P, et al: CD38 expression level and pattern of expression remains a reliable and robust marker of progressive disease in chronic lymphocytic leukemia. *Leuk Lymphoma* 47:2371, 2006.
380. Hus I, Bojarska-Junak A, Dmoszynska A, et al: ZAP-70 and CD38 expression are independent prognostic factors in patients with B-cell chronic lymphocytic leukaemia and combined analysis improves their predictive value. *Folia Histochem Cytobiol* 46:147, 2008.
381. Rassenti LZ, Jain S, Keating MJ, et al: Relative value of ZAP-70, CD38, and immunoglobulin mutation status in predicting aggressive disease in chronic lymphocytic leukemia. *Blood* 112:1923, 2008.
382. Morilla A, Gonzalez de Castro D, Del Giudice I, et al: Combinations of ZAP-70, CD38 and IGHV mutational status as predictors of time to first treatment in CLL. *Leuk Lymphoma* 49:2108, 2008.
383. Thunberg U, Johnson A, Roos G, et al: CD38 expression is a poor predictor for VH gene mutational status and prognosis in chronic lymphocytic leukemia. *Blood* 97:1892, 2001.
384. Hulkkonen J, Vilpo L, Hurme M, Vilpo J: Surface antigen expression in chronic lymphocytic leukemia: Clustering analysis, interrelationships and effects of chromosomal abnormalities. *Leukemia* 16:178, 2002.
385. Degan M, Rupolo M, Bo MD, et al: Mutational status of IgVH genes consistent with antigen-driven selection but not percent of mutations has prognostic impact in B-cell chronic lymphocytic leukemia. *Clin Lymphoma* 5:123, 2004.
386. Kohlmann A, Kipps TJ, Rassenti LZ, et al: An international standardization programme towards the application of gene expression profiling in routine leukaemia diagnostics: The Microarray Innovations in Leukemia study prephase. *Br J Haematol* 142:802, 2008.
387. Chen L, Widhopf G, Huynh L, et al: Expression of ZAP-70 is associated with increased B-cell receptor signaling in chronic lymphocytic leukemia. *Blood* 100:4609, 2002.
388. Crespo M, Bosch F, Villamor N, et al: ZAP-70 expression as a surrogate for immunoglobulin-variable-region mutations in chronic lymphocytic leukemia. *N Engl J Med* 348:1764, 2003.
389. Wiestner A, Rosenwald A, Barry TS, et al: ZAP-70 expression identifies a chronic lymphocytic leukemia subtype with unmutated immunoglobulin genes, inferior clinical outcome, and distinct gene expression profile. *Blood* 101:4944, 2003.
390. Rassenti LZ, Huynh L, Toy TL, et al: ZAP-70 compared with immunoglobulin heavy-chain gene mutation status as a predictor of disease progression in chronic lymphocytic leukemia. *N Engl J Med* 351:893, 2004.
391. Chen L, Apgar J, Huynh L, et al: ZAP-70 directly enhances IgM signaling in chronic lymphocytic leukemia. *Blood* 105:2036, 2005.
392. Gobessi S, Laurenti L, Longo PG, et al: ZAP-70 enhances B-cell-receptor signaling despite absent or inefficient tyrosine kinase activation in chronic lymphocytic leukemia and lymphoma B cells. *Blood* 109:2032, 2007.
393. Chen L, Huynh L, Apgar J, et al: ZAP-70 enhances IgM signaling independent of its kinase activity in chronic lymphocytic leukemia. *Blood* 111:2685, 2008.
394. Bilban M, Heintel D, Scharl T, et al: Deregulated expression of fat and muscle genes in B-cell chronic lymphocytic leukemia with high lipoprotein lipase expression. *Leukemia* 20:1080, 2006.
395. Heintel D, Kienle D, Shehata M, et al: High expression of lipoprotein lipase in poor risk B-cell chronic lymphocytic leukemia. *Leukemia* 19:1216, 2005.
396. Huttmann A, Klein-Hitpass L, Thomale J, et al: Gene expression signatures separate B-cell chronic lymphocytic leukaemia prognostic subgroups defined by ZAP-70 and CD38 expression status. *Leukemia* 20:1774, 2006.
397. Oppezzo P, Vasconcelos Y, Settegrana C, et al: The LPL/ADAM29 expression ratio is a novel prognosis indicator in chronic lymphocytic leukemia. *Blood* 106:650, 2005.
398. Nuckel H, Huttmann A, Klein-Hitpass L, et al: Lipoprotein lipase expression is a novel prognostic factor in B-cell chronic lymphocytic leukemia. *Leuk Lymphoma* 47:1053, 2006.
399. van't Veer MB, Brooijmans AM, Langerak AW, et al: The predictive value of lipoprotein lipase for survival in chronic lymphocytic leukemia. *Haematologica* 91:56, 2006.
400. Pallasch CP, Schwamb J, Konigs S, et al: Targeting lipid metabolism by the lipoprotein lipase inhibitor orlistat results in apoptosis of B-cell chronic lymphocytic leukemia cells. *Leukemia* 22:585, 2008.

401. Van Bockstaele F, Pede V, Janssens A, et al: Lipoprotein lipase mRNA expression in whole blood is a prognostic marker in B cell chronic lymphocytic leukemia. *Clin Chem* 53:204, 2007.
402. Heintel D, Kroemer E, Kienle D, et al: High expression of activation-induced cytidine deaminase (AID) mRNA is associated with unmutated IGVH gene status and unfavourable cytogenetic aberrations in patients with chronic lymphocytic leukaemia. *Leukemia* 18:756, 2004.
403. Nikitin EA, Malakho SG, Biderman BV, et al: Expression level of lipoprotein lipase and dystrophin genes predict survival in B-cell chronic lymphocytic leukemia. *Leuk Lymphoma* 48:912, 2007.
404. Li FJ, Ding S, Pan J, et al: FCRL2 expression predicts IGHV mutation status and clinical progression in chronic lymphocytic leukemia. *Blood* 112:179, 2008.
405. Kainz B, Shehata M, Bilban M, et al: Overexpression of the paternally expressed gene 10 (PEG10) from the imprinted locus on chromosome 7q21 in high-risk B-cell chronic lymphocytic leukemia. *Int J Cancer* 121:1984, 2007.
406. Benedetti D, Bomben R, Dal-Bo M, et al: Are surrogates of IGHV gene mutational status useful in B-cell chronic lymphocytic leukemia? The example of Septin-10. *Leukemia* 22:224, 2008.
407. Buhl AM, Jurlander J, Geisler CH, et al: CLLU1 expression levels predict time to initiation of therapy and overall survival in chronic lymphocytic leukemia. *Eur J Haematol* 76:455, 2006.
408. Raval A, Lucas DM, Matkovic JJ, et al: TWIST2 demonstrates differential methylation in immunoglobulin variable heavy chain mutated and unmutated chronic lymphocytic leukemia. *J Clin Oncol* 23:3877, 2005.
409. Han T, Henderson ES, Emrich LJ, Sandberg AA: Prognostic significance of karyotypic abnormalities in B cell chronic lymphocytic leukemia: An update. *Semin Hematol* 24:257, 1987.
410. Escudier SM, Pereira-Leahy JM, Drach JW, et al: Fluorescent in situ hybridization and cytogenetic studies of trisomy 12 in chronic lymphocytic leukemia. *Blood* 81:2702, 1993.
411. Dohner H, Stilgenbauer S, Benner A, et al: Genomic aberrations and survival in chronic lymphocytic leukemia. *N Engl J Med* 343:1910, 2000.
412. Juliusson G, Robert KH, Ost A, et al: Prognostic information from cytogenetic analysis in chronic B-lymphocytic leukemia and leukemic immunocytoma. *Blood* 65:134, 1985.
413. Tefferi A, Bartholmai BJ, Witzig TE, et al: Clinical correlations of immunophenotypic variations and the presence of trisomy 12 in B-cell chronic lymphocytic leukemia. *Cancer Genet Cytogenet* 95:173, 1997.
414. AbdelSalam M, El Sissy A, Samra MA, et al: The impact of trisomy 12, retinoblastoma gene and P53 in prognosis of B-cell chronic lymphocytic leukemia. *Hematology* 13:147, 2008.
415. Juliusson G, Oscier DG, Fitchett M, et al: Prognostic subgroups in B-cell chronic lymphocytic leukemia defined by specific chromosomal abnormalities. *N Engl J Med* 323:720, 1990.
416. Montserrat E, Bosch F, Rozman C: B-cell chronic lymphocytic leukemia: Recent progress in biology, diagnosis, and therapy. *Ann Oncol* 8 Suppl 1:93, 1997.
417. Oscier DG, Stevens J, Hamblin TJ, et al: Correlation of chromosome abnormalities with laboratory features and clinical course in B-cell chronic lymphocytic leukaemia. *Br J Haematol* 76:352, 1990.
418. Mayr C, Speicher MR, Kofler DM, et al: Chromosomal translocations are associated with poor prognosis in chronic lymphocytic leukemia. *Blood* 107:742, 2006.
419. Kujawski L, Ouillette P, Erba H, et al: Genomic complexity identifies patients with aggressive chronic lymphocytic leukemia. *Blood* 112:1993, 2008.
420. Robert KH, Gahrton G, Friberg K, et al: Extra chromosome 12 and prognosis in chronic lymphocytic leukaemia. *Scand J Haematol* 28:163, 1982.
421. Neilson JR, Auer R, White D, et al: Deletions at 11q identify a subset of patients with typical CLL who show consistent disease progression and reduced survival. *Leukemia* 11:1929, 1997.
422. Dohner H, Fischer K, Bentz M, et al: P53 gene deletion predicts for poor survival and non-response to therapy with purine analogs in chronic B-cell leukemias. *Blood* 85:1580, 1995.
423. Glassman AB, Hayes KJ: The value of fluorescence in situ hybridization in the diagnosis and prognosis of chronic lymphocytic leukemia. *Cancer Genet Cytogenet* 158:88, 2005.
424. Dewald GW, Brockman SR, Paternoster SF, et al: Chromosome anomalies detected by interphase fluorescence in situ hybridization: Correlation with significant biological features of B-cell chronic lymphocytic leukaemia. *Br J Haematol* 121:287, 2003.
425. Dicker F, Herholz H, Schnittger S, et al: The detection of TP53 mutations in chronic lymphocytic leukemia independently predicts rapid disease progression and is highly correlated with a complex aberrant karyotype. *Leukemia* 23:117, 2009.
426. Zenz T, Habe S, Denzel T, et al: Detailed analysis of p53 pathway defects in fludarabine-refractory chronic lymphocytic leukemia (CLL): Dissecting the contribution of 17p deletion, TP53 mutation, p53-p21 dysfunction, and miR34a in a prospective clinical trial. *Blood* 114:2589, 2009.
427. Alsafadi S, Tourpin S, Andre F, et al: P53 family: At the crossroads in cancer therapy. *Curr Med Chem* 16(32):4328, 2009.
428. Tam CS, Shanafelt TD, Wierda WG, et al: *De novo* deletion 17p13.1 chronic lymphocytic leukemia shows significant clinical heterogeneity: The M. D. Anderson and Mayo Clinic experience. *Blood* 114:957, 2009.
429. Cuneo A, Bigoni R, Rigolin GM, et al: Late appearance of the 11q22.3–23.1 deletion involving the ATM locus in B-cell chronic lymphocytic leukemia and related disorders. Clinico-biological significance. *Haematologica* 87:44, 2002.
430. Shanafelt TD, Witzig TE, Fink SR, et al: Prospective evaluation of clonal evolution during long-term follow-up of patients with untreated early-stage chronic lymphocytic leukemia. *J Clin Oncol* 24:4634, 2006.
431. Stilgenbauer S, Sander S, Bullinger L, et al: Clonal evolution in chronic lymphocytic leukemia: Acquisition of high-risk genomic aberrations associated with unmutated VH, resistance to therapy, and short survival. *Haematologica* 92:1242, 2007.
432. Mackus WJ, Kater AP, Grummels A, et al: Chronic lymphocytic leukemia cells display p53-dependent drug-induced Puma upregulation. *Leukemia* 19:427, 2005.
433. Oscier D, Fitchett M, Herbert T, Lambert R: Karyotypic evolution in B-cell chronic lymphocytic leukaemia. *Genes Chromosomes Cancer* 3:16, 1991.
434. Calin GA, Ferracin M, Cimmino A, et al: A MicroRNA signature associated with prognosis and progression in chronic lymphocytic leukemia. *N Engl J Med* 353:1793, 2005.
435. Visone R, Rassenti LZ, Veronese A, et al: Karyotype specific microRNA signature in chronic lymphocytic leukemia. *Blood* 114(18):3872, 2009.
436. Acchiardo S, Kraus AP Jr, Jennings BR: Beta 2-microglobulin levels in patients with renal insufficiency. *Am J Kidney Dis* 13:70, 1989.
437. de Nully Brown P, Hansen MM: GM-CSF treatment in patients with B-chronic lymphocytic leukemia. *Leuk Lymphoma* 32:365, 1999.
438. Itala M, Pelliniemi TT, Remes K: GM-CSF raises serum levels of beta 2-microglobulin and thymidine kinase in patients with chronic lymphocytic leukaemia. *Br J Haematol* 94:129, 1996.
439. Di Giovanni S, Valentini G, Carducci P, Giallonardo P: Beta-2-microglobulin is a reliable tumor marker in chronic lymphocytic leukemia. *Acta Haematol* 81:181, 1989.
440. Molica S, Levato D, Cascavilla N, et al: Clinico-prognostic implications of simultaneous increased serum levels of soluble CD23 and beta2-microglobulin in B-cell chronic lymphocytic leukemia. *Eur J Haematol* 62:117, 1999.
441. Spati B, Child JA, Kerruish SM, Cooper EH: Behaviour of serum beta 2-microglobulin and acute phase reactant proteins in chronic lymphocytic leukaemia. A multicentre study. *Acta Haematol* 64:79, 1980.
442. Hallek M, Wanders L, Ostwald M, et al: Serum beta(2)-microglobulin and serum thymidine kinase are independent predictors of progression-free survival in chronic lymphocytic leukemia and immunocytoma. *Leuk Lymphoma* 22:439, 1996.
443. Wierda WG, O'Brien S, Wang X, et al: Prognostic nomogram and index for overall survival in previously untreated patients with chronic lymphocytic leukemia. *Blood* 109:4679, 2007.
444. Wierda WG, O'Brien S, Wang X, et al: Characteristics associated with important clinical end points in patients with chronic lymphocytic leukemia at initial treatment. *J Clin Oncol* 27:1637, 2009.
445. Hallek M, Langenmayer I, Nerl C, et al: Elevated serum thymidine kinase levels identify a subgroup at high risk of disease progression in early, nonsmoldering chronic lymphocytic leukemia. *Blood* 93:1732, 1999.
446. Magnac C, Porcher R, Davi F, et al: Predictive value of serum thymidine kinase level for Ig-V mutational status in B-CLL. *Leukemia* 17:133, 2003.
447. Matthews C, Catherwood MA, Morris TC, et al: Serum TK levels in CLL identify Binet stage A patients within biologically defined prognostic subgroups most likely to undergo disease progression. *Eur J Haematol* 77:309, 2006.
448. Sarfati M, Chevret S, Chastang C, et al: Prognostic importance of serum soluble CD23 level in chronic lymphocytic leukemia. *Blood* 88:4259, 1996.
449. Saka B, Aktan M, Sami U, et al: Prognostic importance of soluble CD23 in B-cell chronic lymphocytic leukemia. *Clin Lab Haematol* 28:30, 2006.
450. Molica S, Vitelli G, Levato D, et al: Increased serum levels of matrix metalloproteinase-9 predict clinical outcome of patients with early B-cell chronic lymphocytic leukaemia. *Eur J Haematol* 70:373, 2003.
451. Wierda WG, Johnson MM, Do KA, et al: Plasma interleukin 8 level predicts for survival in chronic lymphocytic leukaemia. *Br J Haematol* 120:452, 2003.
452. Lai R, O'Brien S, Maushouri T, et al: Prognostic value of plasma interleukin-6 levels in patients with chronic lymphocytic leukemia. *Cancer* 95:1071, 2002.
453. Molica S, Vitelli G, Levato D, et al: Elevated serum levels of soluble CD44 can identify a subgroup of patients with early B-cell chronic lymphocytic leukemia who are at high risk of disease progression. *Cancer* 92:713, 2001.
454. Christiansen I, Sundstrom C, Totterman TH: Elevated serum levels of soluble vascular cell adhesion molecule-1 (sVCAM-1) closely reflect tumour burden in chronic B-lymphocytic leukaemia. *Br J Haematol* 103:1129, 1998.
455. Molica S, Vitelli G, Levato D, et al: CD27 in B-cell chronic lymphocytic leukemia. Cellular expression, serum release and correlation with other soluble molecules belonging to nerve growth factor receptors (NGFr) superfamily. *Haematologica* 83:398, 1998.
456. Robertson LE, Pugh W, O'Brien S, et al: Richter's syndrome: A report on 39 patients. *J Clin Oncol* 11:1985, 1993.
457. Everaus H, Luik E, Lehtmaa J: Active and indolent chronic lymphocytic leukaemia—Immune and hormonal peculiarities. *Cancer Immunol Immunother* 45:109, 1997.
458. Vlasveld LT, Pauwels P, Ermens AA, et al: Parathyroid hormone-related protein (PTH-rP)-associated hypercalcemia in a patient with an atypical chronic lymphocytic leukemia. *Neth J Med* 54:21, 1999.
459. Beaudreuil J, Lortholary O, Martin A, et al: Hypercalcemia may indicate Richter's syndrome: Report of four cases and review. *Cancer* 79:1211, 1997.

460. Schoevaerdts D, Mineur P, Hennaux V, Sibille C: Hypercalcemia, chronic lymphocytic leukemia and multiple myeloma: Uncommon association. *Acta Clin Belg* 54:217, 1999.
461. Dominis M, Jaksic B: Clinical relevance of peripheral blood lymphocyte morphology and lymph node histology in chronic lymphocytic leukemia. *Blood Cells* 12:297, 1987.
462. Vallespi T, Montserrat E, Sanz MA: Chronic lymphocytic leukaemia: Prognostic value of lymphocyte morphological subtypes. A multivariate survival analysis in 146 patients. *Br J Haematol* 77:478, 1991.
463. Oscier DG, Matutes E, Copplestone A, et al: Atypical lymphocyte morphology: An adverse prognostic factor for disease progression in stage A CLL independent of trisomy 12. *Br J Haematol* 98:934, 1997.
464. Schwarz J, Mikulenkova D, Cermakova M, et al: Prognostic relevance of the FAB morphological criteria in chronic lymphocytic leukemia: Correlations with IgVH gene mutational status and other prognostic markers. *Neoplasma* 53:219, 2006.
465. Matutes E, Oscier D, Garcia-Marco J, et al: Trisomy 12 defines a group of CLL with atypical morphology: Correlation between cytogenetic, clinical and laboratory features in 544 patients. *Br J Haematol* 92:382, 1996.
466. Nowakowski GS, Hoyer JD, Shanafelt TD, et al: Using smudge cells on routine blood smears to predict clinical outcome in chronic lymphocytic leukemia: A universally available prognostic test. *Mayo Clin Proc* 82:449, 2007.
467. Montserrat E, Villamor N, Reverter JC, et al: Bone marrow assessment in B-cell chronic lymphocytic leukaemia: Aspirate or biopsy? A comparative study in 258 patients. *Br J Haematol* 93:111, 1996.
468. Geisler CH, Hou-Jensen K, Jensen OM, et al: The bone-marrow infiltration pattern in B-cell chronic lymphocytic leukemia is not an important prognostic factor. Danish CLL Study Group. *Eur J Haematol* 57:292, 1996.
469. Sah SP, Matutes E, Wotherspoon AC, et al: A comparison of flow cytometry, bone marrow biopsy, and bone marrow aspirates in the detection of lymphoid infiltration in B cell disorders. *J Clin Pathol* 56:129, 2003.
470. Jarque I, Larrea L, Gomis F, et al: Bone marrow assessment in B-cell chronic lymphocytic leukaemia: Aspirate or biopsy? *Br J Haematol* 95:754, 1996.
471. Cheson BD, Bennett JM, Grever M, et al: National Cancer Institute–sponsored Working Group guidelines for chronic lymphocytic leukemia: Revised guidelines for diagnosis and treatment. *Blood* 87:4990, 1996.
472. Byrd JC, Rai K, Peterson BL, et al: Addition of rituximab to fludarabine may prolong progression-free survival and overall survival in patients with previously untreated chronic lymphocytic leukemia: An updated retrospective comparative analysis of CALGB 9712 and CALGB 9011. *Blood* 105:49, 2005.
473. Binet JL, Caligaris-Cappio F, Catovsky D, et al: Perspectives on the use of new diagnostic tools in the treatment of chronic lymphocytic leukemia. *Blood* 107:859, 2006.
474. Dighiero G, Maloum K, Desablens B, et al: Chlorambucil in indolent chronic lymphocytic leukemia. French Cooperative Group on Chronic Lymphocytic Leukemia. *N Engl J Med* 338:1506, 1998.
475. Shustik C, Mick R, Silver R, et al: Treatment of early chronic lymphocytic leukemia: Intermittent chlorambucil versus observation. *Hematol Oncol* 6:7, 1988.
476. Eksioglu-Demiralp E, Alpdogan O, Aktan M, et al: Variable expression of CD49d antigen in B cell chronic lymphocytic leukemia is related to disease stages. *Leukemia* 10:1331, 1996.
477. Sayala HA, Rawstron AC, Hillmen P: Minimal residual disease assessment in chronic lymphocytic leukaemia. *Best Pract Res Clin Haematol* 20:499, 2007.
478. Rawstron AC, Villamor N, Ritgen M, et al: International standardized approach for flow cytometric residual disease monitoring in chronic lymphocytic leukaemia. *Leukemia* 21:956, 2007.
479. Schultze JL, Donovan JW, Gribben JG: Minimal residual disease detection after myeloablative chemotherapy in chronic lymphatic leukemia. *J Mol Med* 77:259, 1999.
480. Magnac C, Sutton L, Cazin B, et al: Detection of minimal residual disease in B chronic lymphocytic leukemia (CLL). *Hematol Cell Ther* 41:13, 1999.
481. Stolz F, Panzer S, Panzer-Grumayer ER: Multiplex PCR reaction for the detection and identification of immunoglobulin kappa deleting element rearrangements in B-lineage leukaemias. *Br J Haematol* 106:486, 1999.
482. Bottcher S, Ritgen M, Pott C, et al: Comparative analysis of minimal residual disease detection using four-color flow cytometry, consensus IgH-PCR, and quantitative IgH PCR in CLL after allogeneic and autologous stem cell transplantation. *Leukemia* 18:1637, 2004.
483. Josefsson P, Geisler CH, Leffers H, et al: CLLU1 expression analysis adds prognostic information to risk prediction in chronic lymphocytic leukemia. *Blood* 109:4973, 2007.
484. Provan D, Bartlett-Pandite L, Zwicky C, et al: Eradication of polymerase chain reaction-detectable chronic lymphocytic leukemia cells is associated with improved outcome after bone marrow transplantation. *Blood* 88:2228, 1996.
485. Moreton P, Kennedy B, Lucas G, et al: Eradication of minimal residual disease in B-cell chronic lymphocytic leukemia after alemtuzumab therapy is associated with prolonged survival. *J Clin Oncol* 23:2971, 2005.
486. Wattel E, Preudhomme C, Hecquet B, et al: P53 mutations are associated with resistance to chemotherapy and short survival in hematologic malignancies. *Blood* 84:3148, 1994.
487. Sturm I, Bosanquet AG, Hermann S, et al: Mutation of p53 and consecutive selective drug resistance in B-CLL occurs as a consequence of prior DNA-damaging chemotherapy. *Cell Death Differ* 10:477, 2003.
488. Byrd JC, Gribben JG, Peterson BL, et al: Select high-risk genetic features predict earlier progression following chemoimmunotherapy with fludarabine and rituximab in chronic lymphocytic leukemia: Justification for risk-adapted therapy. *J Clin Oncol* 24:437, 2006.
489. Fridman JS, Lowe SW: Control of apoptosis by p53. *Oncogene* 22:9030, 2003.
490. Stilgenbauer S, Dohner H: Campath-1H-induced complete remission of chronic lymphocytic leukemia despite p53 gene mutation and resistance to chemotherapy. *N Engl J Med* 347:452, 2002.
491. Lozanski G, Heerema NA, Flinn IW, et al: Alemtuzumab is an effective therapy for chronic lymphocytic leukemia with p53 mutations and deletions. *Blood* 103:3278, 2004.
492. Grever MR, Lucas DM, Johnson AJ, Byrd JC: Novel agents and strategies for treatment of p53-defective chronic lymphocytic leukemia. *Best Pract Res Clin Haematol* 20:545, 2007.
493. Austen B, Powell JE, Alvi A, et al: Mutations in the ATM gene lead to impaired overall and treatment-free survival that is independent of IGVH mutation status in patients with B-CLL. *Blood* 106:3175, 2005.
494. Eichhorst BF, Busch R, Hopfinger G, et al: Fludarabine plus cyclophosphamide versus fludarabine alone in first-line therapy of younger patients with chronic lymphocytic leukemia. *Blood* 107:885, 2006.
495. Flinn IW, Neuberg DS, Grever MR, et al: Phase III trial of fludarabine plus cyclophosphamide compared with fludarabine for patients with previously untreated chronic lymphocytic leukemia: US Intergroup Trial E2997. *J Clin Oncol* 25:793, 2007.
496. Tsimberidou AM, Tam C, Abruzzo LV, et al: Chemoimmunotherapy may overcome the adverse prognostic significance of 11q deletion in previously untreated patients with chronic lymphocytic leukemia. *Cancer* 115:373, 2009.
497. Tsimberidou AM, Wierda WG, Plunkett W, et al: Phase I-II study of oxaliplatin, fludarabine, cytarabine, and rituximab combination therapy in patients with Richter's syndrome or fludarabine-refractory chronic lymphocytic leukemia. *J Clin Oncol* 26:196, 2008.
498. Castro JE, Sandoval-Sus JD, Bole J, et al: Rituximab in combination with high-dose methylprednisolone for the treatment of fludarabine refractory high-risk chronic lymphocytic leukemia. *Leukemia* 22:2048, 2008.
499. Ferrajoli A, Lee BN, Schlette EJ, et al: Lenalidomide induces complete and partial remissions in patients with relapsed and refractory chronic lymphocytic leukemia. *Blood* 111:5291, 2008.
500. Balakrishnan K, Wierda WG, Keating MJ, Gandhi V: Gossypol, a BH3 mimetic, induces apoptosis in chronic lymphocytic leukemia cells. *Blood* 112:1971, 2008.
501. Paoluzzi L, Gonen M, Bhagat G, et al: The BH3-only mimetic ABT-737 synergizes the antineoplastic activity of proteasome inhibitors in lymphoid malignancies. *Blood* 112:2906, 2008.
502. Phelps MA, Lin TS, Johnson AJ, et al: Clinical response and pharmacokinetics from a phase I study of an active dosing schedule of flavopiridol in relapsed chronic lymphocytic leukemia. *Blood* 113:2637, 2009.
503. Pietsch EC, Sykes SM, McMahon SB, Murphy ME: The p53 family and programmed cell death. *Oncogene* 27:6507, 2008.
504. Tomasini R, Tsuchihara K, Wilhelm M, et al: TAp73 knockout shows genomic instability with infertility and tumor suppressor functions. *Genes Dev* 22:2677, 2008.
505. Sampath D, Calin GA, Puduvalli VK, et al: Specific activation of microRNA106b enables the p73 apoptotic response in chronic lymphocytic leukemia by targeting the ubiquitin ligase, Itch for degradation. *Blood* 113:3744, 2009.
506. Wierda WG, Cantwell MJ, Woods SJ, et al: CD40-ligand (CD154) gene therapy for chronic lymphocytic leukemia. *Blood* 96:2917, 2000.
507. Fukuda T, Chen L, Endo T, et al: Antisera induced by infusions of autologous Ad-CD154-leukemia B cells identify ROR1 as an oncofetal antigen and receptor for Wnt5a. *Proc Natl Acad Sci U S A* 105:3047, 2008.
508. Chu P, Deforce D, Pedersen IM, et al: Latent sensitivity to Fas-mediated apoptosis after CD40 ligation may explain activity of CD154 gene therapy in chronic lymphocytic leukemia. *Proc Natl Acad Sci U S A* 99:3854, 2002.
509. Dicker F, Kater AP, Fukuda T, Kipps TJ: Fas-ligand (CD178) and TRAIL synergistically induce apoptosis of CD40-activated chronic lymphocytic leukemia B cells. *Blood* 105:3193, 2005.
510. Dicker F, Kater AP, Prada CE, et al: CD154 induces p73 to overcome the resistance to apoptosis of chronic lymphocytic leukemia cells lacking functional p53. *Blood* 108:3450, 2006.
511. Eichhorst B, Goede V, Hallek M: Treatment of elderly patients with chronic lymphocytic leukemia. *Leuk Lymphoma* 50:171, 2009.
512. Extermann M, Overcash J, Lyman GH, et al: Comorbidity and functional status are independent in older cancer patients. *J Clin Oncol* 16:1582, 1998.
513. Robertson LE, O'Brien S, Kantarjian H, et al: A 3-day schedule of fludarabine in previously treated chronic lymphocytic leukemia. *Leukemia* 9:1444, 1995.
514. Marotta G, Bigazzi C, Lenoci M, et al: Low-dose fludarabine and cyclophosphamide in elderly patients with B-cell chronic lymphocytic leukemia refractory to conventional therapy. *Haematologica* 85:1268, 2000.
515. Shvidel L, Shtalrid M, Bairey O, et al: Conventional dose fludarabine-based regimens are effective but have excessive toxicity in elderly patients with refractory chronic lymphocytic leukemia. *Leuk Lymphoma* 44:1947, 2003.
516. Fabbri A, Lenoci M, Gozzetti A, et al: Low-dose oral fludarabine plus cyclophosphamide in elderly patients with chronic lymphoproliferative disorders. *Hematol J* 5:472, 2004.

517. Catovsky D, Richards S, Matutes E, et al: Assessment of fludarabine plus cyclophosphamide for patients with chronic lymphocytic leukaemia (the LRF CLL4 Trial): A randomised controlled trial. *Lancet* 370:230, 2007.
518. Forconi F, Fabbri A, Lenoci M, et al: Low-dose oral fludarabine plus cyclophosphamide in elderly patients with untreated and relapsed or refractory chronic lymphocytic leukaemia. *Hematol Oncol* 26:247, 2008.
519. Shanafelt TD, Lin T, Geyer SM, et al: Pentostatin, cyclophosphamide, and rituximab regimen in older patients with chronic lymphocytic leukemia. *Cancer* 109:2291, 2007.
520. Eichhorst BF, Busch R, Stilgenbauer S, et al: First line therapy with fludarabine compared to chlorambucil does not result in a major benefit for elderly patients with advanced chronic lymphocytic leukemia. *Blood* 114:3382, 2009.
521. Keating MJ, O'Brien S, Plunkett W, et al: Fludarabine phosphate: A new active agent in hematologic malignancies. *Semin Hematol* 31:28, 1994.
522. Boogaerts MA, Van Hoof A, Catovsky D, et al: Activity of oral fludarabine phosphate in previously treated chronic lymphocytic leukemia. *J Clin Oncol* 19:1252, 2001.
523. Rossi JF, van Hoof A, de Boeck K, et al: Efficacy and safety of oral fludarabine phosphate in previously untreated patients with chronic lymphocytic leukemia. *J Clin Oncol* 22:1260, 2004.
524. Gjedde SB, Hansen MM: Salvage therapy with fludarabine in patients with progressive B-chronic lymphocytic leukemia. *Leuk Lymphoma* 21:317, 1996.
525. Angelopoulou MA, Poziopoulos C, Boussiotis VA, et al: Fludarabine monophosphate in refractory B-chronic lymphocytic leukemia: Maintenance may be significant to sustain response. *Leuk Lymphoma* 21:321, 1996.
526. Sorensen JM, Vena DA, Fallavollita A, et al: Treatment of refractory chronic lymphocytic leukemia with fludarabine phosphate via the group C protocol mechanism of the National Cancer Institute: Five-year follow-up report. *J Clin Oncol* 15:458, 1997.
527. Keating MJ, O'Brien S, Lerner S, et al: Long-term follow-up of patients with chronic lymphocytic leukemia (CLL) receiving fludarabine regimens as initial therapy. *Blood* 92:1165, 1998.
528. Johnson S, Smith AG, Loffler H, et al: Multicentre prospective randomised trial of fludarabine versus cyclophosphamide, doxorubicin, and prednisone (CAP) for treatment of advanced-stage chronic lymphocytic leukaemia. The French Cooperative Group on CLL. *Lancet* 347:1432, 1996.
529. O'Brien S, Kantarjian H, Beran M, et al: Results of fludarabine and prednisone therapy in 264 patients with chronic lymphocytic leukemia with multivariate analysis-derived prognostic model for response to treatment. *Blood* 82:1695, 1993.
530. Mason JM, Drummond MF, Bosanquet AG, Sheldon TA: The DiSC assay. A cost-effective guide to treatment for chronic lymphocytic leukemia? *Int J Technol Assess Health Care* 15:173, 1999.
531. Bosanquet AG, Johnson SA, Richards SM: Prognosis for fludarabine therapy of chronic lymphocytic leukaemia based on *ex vivo* drug response by DiSC assay. *Br J Haematol* 106:71, 1999.
532. Cohen RB, Abdallah JM, Gray JR, Foss F: Reversible neurologic toxicity in patients treated with standard-dose fludarabine phosphate for mycosis fungoides and chronic lymphocytic leukemia [see comments]. *Ann Intern Med* 118:114, 1993.
533. Ramachandran A, Majumdar G: Acute tumour lysis syndrome after oral fludarabine in a patient with chronic lymphocytic leukaemia. *Hematol J* 5:528, 2004.
534. Hussain K, Mazza JJ, Clouse LH: Tumor lysis syndrome (TLS) following fludarabine therapy for chronic lymphocytic leukemia (CLL): Case report and review of the literature. *Am J Hematol* 72:212, 2003.
535. Wijermans PW, Gerrits WB, Haak HL: Severe immunodeficiency in patients treated with fludarabine monophosphate. *Eur J Haematol* 50:292, 1993.
536. Anaissie E, Kontoyiannis DP, Kantarjian H, et al: Listeriosis in patients with chronic lymphocytic leukemia who were treated with fludarabine and prednisone. *Ann Intern Med* 117:466, 1992.
537. Bergmann L, Fenchel K, Jahn B, et al: Immunosuppressive effects and clinical response of fludarabine in refractory chronic lymphocytic leukemia. *Ann Oncol* 4:371, 1993.
538. Hamblin TJ, Orchard JA, Myint H, Oscier DG: Fludarabine and hemolytic anemia in chronic lymphocytic leukemia. *J Clin Oncol* 16:3209, 1998.
539. Keating MJ: Chronic lymphocytic leukemia. *Semin Oncol* 26:107, 1999.
540. Briz M, Cabrera R, Sanjuan I, et al: Diagnosis of transfusion-associated graft-versus-host disease by polymerase chain reaction in fludarabine-treated B-chronic lymphocytic leukaemia. *Br J Haematol* 91:409, 1995.
541. Briones J, Pereira A, Alcorta I: Transfusion-associated graft-versus-host disease (TA-GVHD) in fludarabine-treated patients: Is it time to irradiate blood component? *Br J Haematol* 93:739, 1996.
542. Cheson BD, Vena DA, Barrett J, Freidlin B: Second malignancies as a consequence of nucleoside analog therapy for chronic lymphoid leukemias. *J Clin Oncol* 17:2454, 1999.
543. Kielstein JT, Stadler M, Czock D, et al: Dialysate concentration and pharmacokinetics of 2F-Ara-A in a patient with acute renal failure. *Eur J Haematol* 74:533, 2005.
544. Robak T: The place of cladribine in the treatment of chronic lymphocytic leukemia: A 10-year experience in Poland. *Ann Hematol* 84:63, 2005.
545. Robak T, Blasinka-Morawiec M, Krykowski E, et al: Intermittent 2-hour intravenous infusions of 2-chlorodeoxyadenosine in the treatment of 110 patients with refractory or previously untreated B-cell chronic lymphocytic leukemia. *Leuk Lymphoma* 22:509, 1996.
546. Juliusson G, Elmhorn-Rosenborg A, Liliemark J: Response to 2-chlorodeoxyadenosine in patients with B-cell chronic lymphocytic leukemia resistant to fludarabine [see comments]. *N Engl J Med* 327:1056, 1992.
547. Byrd JC, Peterson B, Piro L, et al: A phase II study of cladribine treatment for fludarabine refractory B cell chronic lymphocytic leukemia: Results from CALGB Study 9211. *Leukemia* 17:323, 2003.
548. Karlsson K, Stromberg M, Liliemark J, et al: Oral cladribine for B-cell chronic lymphocytic leukaemia: Report of a phase II trial with a 3-d, 3-weekly schedule in untreated and pretreated patients, and a long-term follow-up of 126 previously untreated patients. *Br J Haematol* 116:538, 2002.
549. Juliusson G, Christiansen I, Hansen MM, et al: Oral cladribine as primary therapy for patients with B-cell chronic lymphocytic leukemia. *J Clin Oncol* 14:2160, 1996.
550. Bosanquet AG, Copplestone JA, Johnson SA, et al: Response to cladribine in previously treated patients with chronic lymphocytic leukaemia identified by *ex vivo* assessment of drug sensitivity by DiSC assay. *Br J Haematol* 106:474, 1999.
551. Anchisi S, Zulian GB, Dietrich PY, Alberto P: Cladribine and tumour lysis syndrome. *Eur J Cancer* 31A:131, 1995.
552. Kearns CM, Blakley RL, Santana VM, Crom WR: Pharmacokinetics of cladribine (2-chlorodeoxyadenosine) in children with acute leukemia. *Cancer Res* 54:1235, 1994.
553. Dillman RO: A new chemotherapeutic agent: Deoxycoformycin (pentostatin). *Semin Hematol* 31:16, 1994.
554. Dillman RO: Pentostatin (Nipent) in the treatment of chronic lymphocyte leukemia and hairy cell leukemia. *Expert Rev Anticancer Ther* 4:27, 2004.
555. Johnson SA, Catovsky D, Child JA, et al: Phase I/II evaluation of pentostatin (2′-deoxycoformycin) in a five day schedule for the treatment of relapsed/refractory B-cell chronic lymphocytic leukaemia. *Invest New Drugs* 16:155, 1998.
556. Sauter C, Lamanna N, Weiss MA: Pentostatin in chronic lymphocytic leukemia. *Expert Opin Drug Metab Toxicol* 4:1217, 2008.
557. Lathia C, Fleming GF, Meyer M, et al: Pentostatin pharmacokinetics and dosing recommendations in patients with mild renal impairment. *Cancer Chemother Pharmacol* 50:121, 2002.
558. Sawitsky A, Rai KR, Glidewell O, Silver RT: Comparison of daily versus intermittent chlorambucil and prednisone therapy in the treatment of patients with chronic lymphocytic leukemia. *Blood* 50:1049, 1977.
559. Han T, Ezdinli EZ, Shimaoka K, Desai DV: Chlorambucil vs. combined chlorambucil-corticosteroid therapy in chronic lymphocytic leukemia. *Cancer* 31:502, 1973.
560. Jaksic B, Brugiatelli M, Krc I, et al: High dose chlorambucil versus Binet's modified cyclophosphamide, doxorubicin, vincristine, and prednisone regimen in the treatment of patients with advanced B-cell chronic lymphocytic leukemia. Results of an international multicenter randomized trial. International Society for Chemo-Immunotherapy, Vienna. *Cancer* 79:2107, 1997.
561. Leoni LM, Bailey B, Reifert J, et al: Bendamustine (Treanda) displays a distinct pattern of cytotoxicity and unique mechanistic features compared with other alkylating agents. *Clin Cancer Res* 14:309, 2008.
562. Kath R, Blumenstengel K, Fricke HJ, Hoffken K: Bendamustine monotherapy in advanced and refractory chronic lymphocytic leukemia. *J Cancer Res Clin Oncol* 127:48, 2001.
563. Aivado M, Schulte K, Henze L, et al: Bendamustine in the treatment of chronic lymphocytic leukemia: Results and future perspectives. *Semin Oncol* 29:19, 2002.
564. Bergmann MA, Goebeler ME, Herold M, et al: Efficacy of bendamustine in patients with relapsed or refractory chronic lymphocytic leukemia: Results of a phase I/II study of the German CLL Study Group. *Haematologica* 90:1357, 2005.
565. Lissitchkov T, Arnaudov G, Peytchev D, Merkle K: Phase-I/II study to evaluate dose limiting toxicity, maximum tolerated dose, and tolerability of bendamustine HCl in pre-treated patients with B-chronic lymphocytic leukaemia (Binet stages B and C) requiring therapy. *J Cancer Res Clin Oncol* 132:99, 2006.
566. Knauf WU, Lissichkov T, Aldaoud A, et al: Phase III randomized study of bendamustine compared with chlorambucil in previously untreated patients with chronic lymphocytic leukemia. *J Clin Oncol* 27:4378, 2009.
567. Traynor K: Treanda approved for chronic lymphocytic leukemia. *Am J Health Syst Pharm* 65:793, 2008.
568. Huguley CMJ: Treatment of chronic lymphocytic leukemia. *Cancer Treat Rev* 4:261, 1977.
569. Isaacs JD, Watts RA, Hazleman BL, et al: Humanised monoclonal antibody therapy for rheumatoid arthritis. *Lancet* 340:748, 1992.
570. Heit W, Bunjes D, Wiesneth M, et al: *Ex vivo* T-cell depletion with the monoclonal antibody Campath-1 plus human complement effectively prevents acute graft-versus-host disease in allogeneic bone marrow transplantation. *Br J Haematol* 64:479, 1986.
571. Dyer MJ, Hale G, Hayhoe FG, Waldmann H: Effects of CAMPATH-1 antibodies *in vivo* in patients with lymphoid malignancies: Influence of antibody isotype. *Blood* 73:1431, 1989.
572. Rowan W, Tite J, Topley P, Brett SJ: Cross-linking of the CAMPATH-1 antigen (CD52) mediates growth inhibition in human B- and T-lymphoma cell lines, and subsequent emergence of CD52-deficient cells. *Immunology* 95:427, 1998.
573. Hale G, Dyer MJ, Clark MR, et al: Remission induction in non-Hodgkin lymphoma with reshaped human monoclonal antibody CAMPATH-1H. *Lancet* 2:1394, 1988.
574. Osterborg A, Fassas AS, Anagnostopoulos A, et al: Humanized CD52 monoclonal antibody Campath-1H as first-line treatment in chronic lymphocytic leukaemia. *Br J Haematol* 93:151, 1996.

575. Osterborg A, Dyer MJ, Bunjes D, et al: Phase II multicenter study of human CD52 antibody in previously treated chronic lymphocytic leukemia. European Study Group of CAMPATH-1H Treatment in Chronic Lymphocytic Leukemia. *J Clin Oncol* 15:1567, 1997.
576. Bowen AL, Zomas A, Emmett E, et al: Subcutaneous CAMPATH-1H in fludarabine-resistant/relapsed chronic lymphocytic and B-prolymphocytic leukaemia. *Br J Haematol* 96:617, 1997.
577. Rai KR, Freter CE, Mercier RJ, et al: Alemtuzumab in previously treated chronic lymphocytic leukemia patients who also had received fludarabine. *J Clin Oncol* 20:3891, 2002.
578. Keating MJ, Flinn I, Jain V, et al: Therapeutic role of alemtuzumab (Campath-1H) in patients who have failed fludarabine: Results of a large international study. *Blood* 99:3554, 2002.
579. Kennedy B, Rawstron A, Carter C, et al: Campath-1H and fludarabine in combination are highly active in refractory chronic lymphocytic leukemia. *Blood* 99:2245, 2002.
580. Keating MJ, O'Brien S, Albitar M, et al: Early results of a chemoimmunotherapy regimen of fludarabine, cyclophosphamide, and rituximab as initial therapy for chronic lymphocytic leukemia. *J Clin Oncol* 23:4079, 2005.
581. Wierda WG: Current and investigational therapies for patients with CLL. *Hematology Am Soc Hematol Educ Program* 285, 2006.
582. James DF, Kipps TJ: Alemtuzumab in chronic lymphocytic leukemia. *Future Oncol* 3:29, 2007.
583. Lundin J, Porwit-MacDonald A, Rossmann ED, et al: Cellular immune reconstitution after subcutaneous alemtuzumab (anti-CD52 monoclonal antibody, CAMPATH-1H) treatment as first-line therapy for B-cell chronic lymphocytic leukaemia. *Leukemia* 18:484, 2004.
584. O'Brien SM, Keating MJ, Mocarski ES: Updated guidelines on the management of cytomegalovirus reactivation in patients with chronic lymphocytic leukemia treated with alemtuzumab. *Clin Lymphoma Myeloma* 7:125, 2006.
585. Elter T, Vehreschild JJ, Gribben J, et al: Management of infections in patients with chronic lymphocytic leukemia treated with alemtuzumab. *Ann Hematol* 88:121, 2009.
586. Demko S, Summers J, Keegan P, Pazdur R: FDA drug approval summary: Alemtuzumab as single-agent treatment for B-cell chronic lymphocytic leukemia. *Oncologist* 13:167, 2008.
587. Hillmen P, Skotnicki AB, Robak T, et al: Alemtuzumab compared with chlorambucil as first-line therapy for chronic lymphocytic leukemia. *J Clin Oncol* 25:5616, 2007.
588. Lundin J, Kimby E, Bjorkholm M, et al: Phase II trial of subcutaneous anti-CD52 monoclonal antibody alemtuzumab (Campath-1H) as first-line treatment for patients with B-cell chronic lymphocytic leukemia (B-CLL). *Blood* 100:768, 2002.
589. Karlsson C, Lundin J, Kimby E, et al: Phase II study of subcutaneous alemtuzumab without dose escalation in patients with advanced-stage, relapsed chronic lymphocytic leukaemia. *Br J Haematol* 144:78, 2009.
590. Stilgenbauer S, Zenz T, Winkler D, et al: Subcutaneous alemtuzumab in fludarabine-refractory chronic lymphocytic leukemia: Clinical results and prognostic marker analyses from the CLL2H study of the German Chronic Lymphocytic Leukemia Study Group. *J Clin Oncol* 27:3994, 2009.
591. Hale G, Rebello P, Brettman LR, et al: Blood concentrations of alemtuzumab and antiglobulin responses in patients with chronic lymphocytic leukemia following intravenous or subcutaneous routes of administration. *Blood* 104:948, 2004.
592. Elter T, Molnar I, Kuhlmann J, et al: Pharmacokinetics of alemtuzumab and the relevance in clinical practice. *Leuk Lymphoma* 49:2256, 2008.
593. Montillo M, Cafro AM, Tedeschi A, et al: Safety and efficacy of subcutaneous Campath-1H for treating residual disease in patients with chronic lymphocytic leukemia responding to fludarabine. *Haematologica* 87:695; discussion 700, 2002.
594. Wendtner CM, Ritgen M, Schweighofer CD, et al: Consolidation with alemtuzumab in patients with chronic lymphocytic leukemia (CLL) in first remission—Experience on safety and efficacy within a randomized multicenter phase III trial of the German CLL Study Group (GCLLSG). *Leukemia* 18:1093, 2004.
595. Montillo M, Tedeschi A, Miqueleiz S, et al: Alemtuzumab as consolidation after a response to fludarabine is effective in purging residual disease in patients with chronic lymphocytic leukemia. *J Clin Oncol* 24:2337, 2006.
596. Hainsworth JD, Vazquez ER, Spigel DR, et al: Combination therapy with fludarabine and rituximab followed by alemtuzumab in the first-line treatment of patients with chronic lymphocytic leukemia or small lymphocytic lymphoma: A phase 2 trial of the Minnie Pearl Cancer Research Network. *Cancer* 112:1288, 2008.
597. Schweighofer CD, Ritgen M, Eichhorst BF, et al: Consolidation with alemtuzumab improves progression-free survival in patients with chronic lymphocytic leukaemia (CLL) in first remission: Long-term follow-up of a randomized phase III trial of the German CLL Study Group (GCLLSG). *Br J Haematol* 144:95, 2009.
598. Maloney DG, Grillo-Lopez AJ, White CA, et al: IDEC-C2B8 (Rituximab) anti-CD20 monoclonal antibody therapy in patients with relapsed low-grade non-Hodgkin's lymphoma. *Blood* 90:2188, 1997.
599. McLaughlin P, Grillo-Lopez AJ, Link BK, et al: Rituximab chimeric anti-CD20 monoclonal antibody therapy for relapsed indolent lymphoma: Half of patients respond to a four-dose treatment program. *J Clin Oncol* 16:2825, 1998.
600. Itala M, Geisler CH, Kimby E, et al: Standard-dose anti-CD20 antibody rituximab has efficacy in chronic lymphocytic leukaemia: Results from a Nordic multicentre study. *Eur J Haematol* 69:129, 2002.
601. Hainsworth JD, Litchy S, Barton JH, et al: Single-agent rituximab as first-line and maintenance treatment for patients with chronic lymphocytic leukemia or small lymphocytic lymphoma: A phase II trial of the Minnie Pearl Cancer Research Network. *J Clin Oncol* 21:1746, 2003.
602. Byrd JC, Murphy T, Howard RS, et al: Rituximab using a thrice weekly dosing schedule in B-cell chronic lymphocytic leukemia and small lymphocytic lymphoma demonstrates clinical activity and acceptable toxicity. *J Clin Oncol* 19:2153, 2001.
603. O'Brien SM, Kantarjian H, Thomas DA, et al: Rituximab dose-escalation trial in chronic lymphocytic leukemia. *J Clin Oncol* 19:2165, 2001.
604. Manshouri T, Do KA, Wang X, et al: Circulating CD20 is detectable in the plasma of patients with chronic lymphocytic leukemia and is of prognostic significance. *Blood* 101:2507, 2003.
605. Yang H, Rosove MH, Figlin RA: Tumor lysis syndrome occurring after the administration of rituximab in lymphoproliferative disorders: High-grade non-Hodgkin's lymphoma and chronic lymphocytic leukemia. *Am J Hematol* 62:247, 1999.
606. Voog E, Morschhauser F, Solal-Celigny P: Neutropenia in patients treated with rituximab. *N Engl J Med* 348:2691; discussion 2691, 2003.
607. Winkler U, Jensen M, Manzke O, et al: Cytokine-release syndrome in patients with B-cell chronic lymphocytic leukemia and high lymphocyte counts after treatment with an anti-CD20 monoclonal antibody (rituximab, IDEC-C2B8). *Blood* 94:2217, 1999.
608. Thornton PD, Hamblin M, Treleaven JG, et al: High dose methyl prednisolone in refractory chronic lymphocytic leukaemia. *Leuk Lymphoma* 34:167, 1999.
609. Bosanquet AG, McCann SR, Crotty GM, et al: Methylprednisolone in advanced chronic lymphocytic leukaemia: Rationale for, and effectiveness of treatment suggested by DiSC assay. *Acta Haematol* 93:73, 1995.
610. Thornton PD, Matutes E, Bosanquet AG, et al: High dose methylprednisolone can induce remissions in CLL patients with p53 abnormalities. *Ann Hematol* 82:759, 2003.
611. Robertson LE, Hall R, Keating MJ, et al: High-dose cytosine arabinoside in chronic lymphocytic leukemia: A clinical and pharmacologic analysis. *Leuk Lymphoma* 10:43, 1993.
612. Brunet C, Bardin N, Oukhouya O, et al: A case report: CD8 expression in B-cell chronic lymphocytic leukemia (B-CLL). Prognostic significance of the aberrant CD8 expression. *Hematol Cell Ther* 40:279, 1998.
613. Mauro FR, Foa R, Meloni G, et al: Fludarabine, ara-C, Novantrone and dexamethasone (FAND) in previously treated chronic lymphocytic leukemia patients. *Haematologica* 87:926, 2002.
614. Shaklai S, Bairey O, Blickstein D, et al: Severe myelotoxicity of oral etoposide in heavily pretreated patients with non-Hodgkin's lymphoma or chronic lymphatic leukemia. *Cancer* 77:2313, 1996.
615. Robak T, Szmigielska-Kaplon A, Blonski JZ, et al: Activity of cladribine combined with etoposide in heavily pretreated patients with indolent lymphoid malignancies. *Chemotherapy* 51:247, 2005.
616. Bellosillo B, Colomer D, Pons G, Gil J: Mitoxantrone, a topoisomerase II inhibitor, induces apoptosis of B-chronic lymphocytic leukaemia cells. *Br J Haematol* 100:142, 1998.
617. Bosch F, Ferrer A, Lopez-Guillermo A, et al: Fludarabine, cyclophosphamide and mitoxantrone in the treatment of resistant or relapsed chronic lymphocytic leukaemia. *Br J Haematol* 119:976, 2002.
618. Robak T, Gora-Tybor J, Lech-Maranda E, et al: Cladribine in combination with mitoxantrone and cyclophosphamide(CMC) in the treatment of heavily pre-treated patients with advanced indolent lymphoid malignancies. *Eur J Haematol* 66:188, 2001.
619. Rogalinska M, Blonski JZ, Hanausek M, et al: 2-Chlorodeoxyadenosine alone and in combination with cyclophosphamide and mitoxantrone induce apoptosis in B chronic lymphocytic leukemia cells *in vivo*. *Cancer Detect Prev* 28:433, 2004.
620. Emmanouilides C, Territo M, Menco H, et al: Mitoxantrone-cyclophosphamide-rituximab: An effective and safe combination for indolent NHL. *Hematol Oncol* 21:99, 2003.
621. Bosch F, Ferrer A, Villamor N, et al: Fludarabine, cyclophosphamide, and mitoxantrone as initial therapy of chronic lymphocytic leukemia: High response rate and disease eradication. *Clin Cancer Res* 14:155, 2008.
622. Robak T, Blonski JZ, Gora-Tybor J, et al: Cladribine alone and in combination with cyclophosphamide or cyclophosphamide plus mitoxantrone in the treatment of progressive chronic lymphocytic leukemia: Report of a prospective, multicenter, randomized trial of the Polish Adult Leukemia Group (PALG CLL2). *Blood* 108:473, 2006.
623. Koppler H, Heymanns J, Pandorf A, Weide R: Bendamustine plus mitoxantrone—a new effective treatment for advanced chronic lymphocytic leukaemia: Results of a phase I/II study. *Leuk Lymphoma* 45:911, 2004.
624. Scaramucci L, Niscola P, Buffolino S, et al: Repeated rituximab maintenance courses in fludarabine-failed young patients with chronic lymphocytic leukaemia responding to FAND chemotherapy. *Hematol J* 5:186, 2004.
625. Weide R, Pandorf A, Heymanns J, Koppler H: Bendamustine/mitoxantrone/rituximab (BMR): A very effective, well tolerated outpatient chemoimmunotherapy for relapsed and refractory CD20-positive indolent malignancies. Final results of a pilot study. *Leuk Lymphoma* 45:2445, 2004.
626. Catovsky D, Richards S, Fooks J, Hamblin TJ: CLL Trials in the United Kingdom. *Leuk Lymphoma* 5(Supp):105, 1991.

627. Montserrat E, Fontanilles M, Estapé J: Treatment of chronic lymphocytic leukemia: A preliminary report of Spanish (Pethema) trials. *Leuk Lymphoma* 5(Supp):89, 1991.
628. Keller JW, Knospe WH, Raney M, et al: Treatment of chronic lymphocytic leukemia using chlorambucil and prednisone with or without cycle-active consolidation chemotherapy. A Southeastern Cancer Study Group Trial. *Cancer* 58:1185, 1986.
629. Montserrat E, Alcala A, Alonso C, et al: A randomized trial comparing chlorambucil plus prednisone vs cyclophosphamide, melphalan, and prednisone in the treatment of chronic lymphocytic leukemia stages B and C. *Nouv Rev Fr Hematol* 30:429, 1988.
630. Raphael B, Andersen JW, Silber R, et al: Comparison of chlorambucil and prednisone versus cyclophosphamide, vincristine, and prednisone as initial treatment for chronic lymphocytic leukemia: Long-term follow-up of an Eastern Cooperative Oncology Group randomized clinical trial. *J Clin Oncol* 9:770, 1991.
631. O'Brien S, Kantarjian H, Beran M, et al: Fludarabine and granulocyte colony-stimulating factor (G-CSF) in patients with chronic lymphocytic leukemia. *Leukemia* 11:1631, 1997.
632. O'Brien SM, Kantarjian HM, Cortes J, et al: Results of the fludarabine and cyclophosphamide combination regimen in chronic lymphocytic leukemia. *J Clin Oncol* 19:1414, 2001.
633. Schmitt B, Wendtner CM, Bergmann M, et al: Fludarabine combination therapy for the treatment of chronic lymphocytic leukemia. *Clin Lymphoma* 3:26, 2002.
634. Tothova E, Kafkova A, Fricova M, et al: Fludarabine combined with cyclophosphamide is highly effective in the treatment of chronic lymphocytic leukemia. *Neoplasma* 50:433, 2003.
635. Tam CS, Wolf MM, Januszewicz EH, et al: Fludarabine and cyclophosphamide using an attenuated dose schedule is a highly effective regimen for patients with indolent lymphoid malignancies. *Cancer* 100:2181, 2004.
636. Rai KR, Peterson BL, Appelbaum FR, et al: Fludarabine compared with chlorambucil as primary therapy for chronic lymphocytic leukemia. *N Engl J Med* 343:1750, 2000.
637. Wierda W, O'Brien S, Wen S, et al: Chemoimmunotherapy with fludarabine, cyclophosphamide, and rituximab for relapsed and refractory chronic lymphocytic leukemia. *J Clin Oncol* 23:4070, 2005.
638. Hallek M, Fingerie-Rowson G, Fink AM, et al. Immunochemotherapy with fludarabine (F), cyclophosphamide©, and rituximab® (FCR) versus fludarabine and cyclophosphamide (FC) improves response rates and progression-free survival (PFS) of previously untreated patients (pts) with advanced chronic lymphocytic leukemia (CLL). *Blood* 112:Abstract 325, 2008.
639. Foon KA, Boyiadzis M, Land SR, et al: Chemoimmunotherapy with low-dose fludarabine and cyclophosphamide and high dose rituximab in previously untreated patients with chronic lymphocytic leukemia. *J Clin Oncol* 27:498, 2009.
640. Schulz H, Klein SK, Rehwald U, et al: Phase 2 study of a combined immunochemotherapy using rituximab and fludarabine in patients with chronic lymphocytic leukemia. *Blood* 100:3115, 2002.
641. Byrd JC, Peterson BL, Morrison VA, et al: Randomized phase 2 study of fludarabine with concurrent versus sequential treatment with rituximab in symptomatic, untreated patients with B-cell chronic lymphocytic leukemia: Results from Cancer and Leukemia Group B 9712 (CALGB 9712). *Blood* 101:6, 2003.
642. Faderl S, Wierda W, O'Brien S, et al: Fludarabine, cyclophosphamide, mitoxantrone plus rituximab (FCM-R) in frontline CLL <70 Years. *Leuk Res* [Epub ahead of print Jul 29], 2009.
643. Giles FJ, O'Brien SM, Santini V, et al: Sequential cis-platinum and fludarabine with or without arabinosyl cytosine in patients failing prior fludarabine therapy for chronic lymphocytic leukemia: A phase II study. *Leuk Lymphoma* 36:57, 1999.
644. Elias L, Stock-Novack D, Head DR, et al: A phase I trial of combination fludarabine monophosphate and chlorambucil in chronic lymphocytic leukemia: A Southwest Oncology Group study. *Leukemia* 7:361, 1993.
645. Weiss MA, Maslak PG, Jurcic JG, et al: Pentostatin and cyclophosphamide: An effective new regimen in previously treated patients with chronic lymphocytic leukemia. *J Clin Oncol* 21:1278, 2003.
646. Oken MM, Lee S, Kay NE, et al: Pentostatin, chlorambucil and prednisone therapy for B-chronic lymphocytic leukemia: A phase I/II study by the Eastern Cooperative Oncology Group study E1488. *Leuk Lymphoma* 45:79, 2004.
647. Tsiara SN, Kapsali HD, Chaidos A, et al: Treatment of resistant/relapsing chronic lymphocytic leukemia with a combination regimen containing deoxycoformycin and rituximab. *Acta Haematol* 111:185, 2004.
648. Lamanna N, Kalaycio M, Maslak P, et al: Pentostatin, cyclophosphamide, and rituximab is an active, well-tolerated regimen for patients with previously treated chronic lymphocytic leukemia. *J Clin Oncol* 24:1575, 2006.
649. Kay NE, Geyer SM, Call TG, et al: Combination chemoimmunotherapy with pentostatin, cyclophosphamide, and rituximab shows significant clinical activity with low accompanying toxicity in previously untreated B chronic lymphocytic leukemia. *Blood* 109:405, 2007.
650. Awan FT, Kay NE, Davis ME, et al: Mcl-1 expression predicts progression-free survival in chronic lymphocytic leukemia patients treated with pentostatin, cyclophosphamide, and rituximab. *Blood* 113:535, 2009.
651. Robak T, Blonski JZ, Kasznicki M, et al: Cladribine with prednisone versus chlorambucil with prednisone as first-line therapy in chronic lymphocytic leukemia: Report of a prospective, randomized, multicenter trial. *Blood* 96:2723, 2000.
652. Robak T, Blonski JZ, Kasznicki M, et al: Comparison of cladribine plus prednisone with chlorambucil plus prednisone in patients with chronic lymphocytic leukemia. Final report of the Polish Adult Leukemia Group (PALG CLL1). *Med Sci Monit* 11:PI71, 2005.
653. Laurencet FM, Zulian GB, Guetty-Alberto M, et al: Cladribine with cyclophosphamide and prednisone in the management of low-grade lymphoproliferative malignancies. *Br J Cancer* 79:1215, 1999.
654. Tefferi A, Li CY, Reeder CB, et al: A phase II study of sequential combination chemotherapy with cyclophosphamide, prednisone, and 2-chlorodeoxyadenosine in previously untreated patients with chronic lymphocytic leukemia. *Leukemia* 15:1171, 2001.
655. Laurencet F, Ballabeni P, Rufener B, et al: The multicenter trial SAKK 37/95 of cladribine, cyclophosphamide and prednisone in the treatment of chronic lymphocytic leukemias and low-grade non-Hodgkin's lymphomas. *Acta Haematol* 117:40, 2007.
656. Montillo M, Tedeschi A, O'Brien S, et al: Phase II study of cladribine and cyclophosphamide in patients with chronic lymphocytic leukemia and prolymphocytic leukemia. *Cancer* 97:114, 2003.
657. Robak T, Blonski JZ, Kasznicki M, et al: Cladribine combined with cyclophosphamide is highly effective in the treatment of chronic lymphocytic leukemia. *Hematol J* 3:244, 2002.
658. Robak T, Blonski JZ, Wawrzyniak E, et al: Activity of cladribine combined with cyclophosphamide in frontline therapy for chronic lymphocytic leukemia with 17p13.1/TP53 deletion: Report from the Polish Adult Leukemia Group. *Cancer* 115:94, 2009.
659. Robak T, Smolewski P, Cebula B, et al: Rituximab plus cladribine with or without cyclophosphamide in patients with relapsed or refractory chronic lymphocytic leukemia. *Eur J Haematol* 79:107, 2007.
660. Castro JE, James DF, Sandoval-Sus JD, et al: Rituximab in combination with high-dose methylprednisolone for the treatment of chronic lymphocytic leukemia. *Leukemia* 23:1779, 2009.
661. Oken MM, Kaplan ME: Combination chemotherapy with cyclophosphamide, vincristine, and prednisone in the treatment of refractory chronic lymphocytic leukemia. *Cancer Treat Rep* 63:441, 1979.
662. A randomized clinical trial of chlorambucil versus COP in stage B chronic lymphocytic leukemia. The French Cooperative Group on Chronic Lymphocytic Leukemia. *Blood* 75:1422, 1990.
663. French Cooperative Group: Prognostic and therapeutic advances in CLL management: The experience of the French Cooperative Group. French Cooperative Group on Chronic Lymphocytic Leukemia. *Semin Hematol* 24:275, 1987.
664. Friedenberg WR, Anderson J, Wolf BC, et al: Modified vincristine, doxorubicin, and dexamethasone regimen in the treatment of resistant or relapsed chronic lymphocytic leukemia. An Eastern Cooperative Oncology Group study. *Cancer* 71:2983, 1993.
665. Coad JE, Matutes E, Catovsky D: Splenectomy in lymphoproliferative disorders: A report on 70 cases and review of the literature. *Leuk Lymphoma* 10:245, 1993.
666. Seymour JF, Cusack JD, Lerner SA, et al: Case/control study of the role of splenectomy in chronic lymphocytic leukemia. *J Clin Oncol* 15:52, 1997.
667. Ruchlemer R, Wotherspoon AC, Thompson JN, et al: Splenectomy in mantle cell lymphoma with leukaemia: A comparison with chronic lymphocytic leukaemia. *Br J Haematol* 118:952, 2002.
668. Hill J, Walsh RM, McHam S, et al: Laparoscopic splenectomy for autoimmune hemolytic anemia in patients with chronic lymphocytic leukemia: A case series and review of the literature. *Am J Hematol* 75:134, 2004.
669. Smith L, Luna G, Merg AR, et al: Laparoscopic splenectomy for treatment of splenomegaly. *Am J Surg* 187:618, 2004.
670. Velanovich V, Shurafa M: Laparoscopic excision of accessory spleen. *Am J Surg* 180:62, 2000.
671. Dearden C: Disease-specific complications of chronic lymphocytic leukemia. *Hematology Am Soc Hematol Educ Program* 450, 2008.
672. Rubin P, Bennett JM, Begg C, et al: The comparison of total body irradiation vs chlorambucil and prednisone for remission induction of active chronic lymphocytic leukemia: An ECOG study. Part I: Total body irradiation-response and toxicity. *Int J Radiat Oncol Biol Phys* 7:1623, 1981.
673. Byhardt RW, Brace KC, Wiernik PH: The role of splenic irradiation in chronic lymphocytic leukemia. *Cancer* 35:1621, 1975.
674. Aabo K, Walbom-Jorgensen S: Spleen irradiation in chronic lymphocytic leukemia (CLL): Palliation in patients unfit for splenectomy. *Am J Hematol* 19:177, 1985.
675. Chisesi T, Capnist G, Dal Fior S: Splenic irradiation in chronic lymphocytic leukemia. *Eur J Haematol* 46:202, 1991.
676. Chiappa S, Bonadonna G, Uslenghi C, et al: The role of endolymphatic radiotherapy in the treatment of chronic lymphatic leukaemia. *Br J Cancer* 20:480, 1966.
677. Chanana AD, Cronkite EP, Rai KR: The role of extracorporeal irradiation of blood in treatment of leukemia. *Int J Radiat Oncol Biol Phys* 1:539, 1976.
678. Wieselthier JS, Rothstein TL, Yu TL, et al: Inefficacy of extracorporeal photochemotherapy in the treatment of B-cell chronic lymphocytic leukemia: Preliminary results. *Am J Hematol* 41:123, 1992.
679. Marti GE, Folks T, Longo DL, Klein H: Therapeutic cytapheresis in chronic lymphocytic leukemia. *J Clin Apher* 1:243, 1983.
680. Cooper IA, Ding JC, Adams PB, et al: Intensive leukapheresis in the management of cytopenias in patients with chronic lymphocytic leukaemia (CLL) and lymphocytic lymphoma. *Am J Hematol* 6:387, 1979.
681. Cukierman T, Gatt ME, Libster D, et al: Chronic lymphocytic leukemia presenting with extreme hyperleukocytosis and thrombosis of the common femoral vein. *Leuk Lymphoma* 43:1865, 2002.

682. Ali R, Ozkalemkas F, Ozkocaman V, et al: Successful labor in the course of chronic lymphocytic leukemia (CLL) and management of CLL during pregnancy with leukapheresis. *Ann Hematol* 83:61, 2004.
683. Osterborg A, Brandberg Y, Molostova V, et al: Randomized, double-blind, placebo-controlled trial of recombinant human erythropoietin, epoetin Beta, in hematologic malignancies. *J Clin Oncol* 20:2486, 2002.
684. Ludwig H, Rai K, Blade J, et al: Management of disease-related anemia in patients with multiple myeloma or chronic lymphocytic leukemia: Epoetin treatment recommendations. *Hematol J* 3:121, 2002.
685. Straus DJ: Epoetin alfa as a supportive measure in hematologic malignancies. *Semin Hematol* 39:25, 2002.
686. Pangalis GA, Siakantaris MP, Angelopoulou MK, et al: Downstaging Rai stage III B-chronic lymphocytic leukemia patients with the administration of recombinant human erythropoietin. *Haematologica* 87:500, 2002.
687. Mauro FR, Gentile M, Foa R: Erythropoietin and chronic lymphocytic leukemia. *Rev Clin Exp Hematol*. Suppl 1:21, 2002.
688. Jabr FI, Taher A: Recurrent skin reaction secondary to darbepoetin alfa for two months in a patient with chronic lymphocytic leukemia. *Am J Hematol* 82:245, 2007.
689. Al-Tourah AJ, Tsang PW, Skinnider BF, Hoskins PJ: Paraneoplastic erythropoietin-induced polycythemia associated with small lymphocytic lymphoma. *J Clin Oncol* 24:2388, 2006.
690. Bennett CL, Silver SM, Djulbegovic B, et al: Venous thromboembolism and mortality associated with recombinant erythropoietin and darbepoetin administration for the treatment of cancer-associated anemia. *JAMA* 299:914, 2008.
691. Gribben JG, Neuberg D, Barber M, et al: Detection of residual lymphoma cells by polymerase chain reaction in peripheral blood is significantly less predictive for relapse than detection in bone marrow. *Blood* 83:3800, 1994.
692. Gahn B, Schafer C, Neef J, et al: Detection of trisomy 12 and Rb-deletion in CD34+ cells of patients with B-cell chronic lymphocytic leukemia. *Blood* 89:4275, 1997.
693. Gahn B, Schafer C, Neef J, et al: Detection of trisomy 12 in CD34+ progenitor cells in a patient with B-cell chronic lymphocytic leukemia by fluorescence *in situ* hybridization. *Ann Oncol* 8 Suppl 2:55, 1997.
694. Gribben JG: Stem-cell transplantation in chronic lymphocytic leukaemia. *Best Pract Res Clin Haematol* 20:513, 2007.
695. Dreger P, von Neuhoff N, Kuse R, et al: Early stem cell transplantation for chronic lymphocytic leukaemia: A chance for cure? *Br J Cancer* 77:2291, 1998.
696. Pavletic ZS, Bierman PJ, Vose JM, et al: High incidence of relapse after autologous stem-cell transplantation for B-cell chronic lymphocytic leukemia or small lymphocytic lymphoma. *Ann Oncol* 9:1023, 1998.
697. Sutton L, Maloum K, Gonzalez H, et al: Autologous hematopoietic stem cell transplantation as salvage treatment for advanced B cell chronic lymphocytic leukemia. *Leukemia* 12:1699, 1998.
698. Paneesha S, Milligan DW: Stem cell transplantation for chronic lymphocytic leukaemia. *Br J Haematol* 128:145, 2005.
699. Khouri I, Champlin R: Allogenic bone marrow transplantation in chronic lymphocytic leukemia. *Ann Intern Med* 125:780, 1996.
700. Michallet M, Archimbaud E, Bandini G, et al: HLA-identical sibling bone marrow transplantation in younger patients with chronic lymphocytic leukemia. European Group for Blood and Marrow Transplantation and the International Bone Marrow Transplant Registry. *Ann Intern Med* 124:311, 1996.
701. Mehta J, Powles R, Singhal S, et al: T cell-depleted allogeneic bone marrow transplantation from a partially HLA-mismatched unrelated donor for progressive chronic lymphocytic leukemia and fludarabine-induced bone marrow failure. *Bone Marrow Transplant* 17:881, 1996.
702. Mehta J, Powles R, Singhal S, et al: Clinical and hematologic response of chronic lymphocytic and prolymphocytic leukemia persisting after allogeneic bone marrow transplantation with the onset of acute graft-versus-host disease: Possible role of graft-versus-leukemia. *Bone Marrow Transplant* 17:371, 1996.
703. Rondon G, Giralt S, Huh Y, et al: Graft-versus-leukemia effect after allogeneic bone marrow transplantation for chronic lymphocytic leukemia. *Bone Marrow Transplant* 18:669, 1996.
704. Sorror ML, Storer BE, Sandmaier BM, et al: Five-year follow-up of patients with advanced chronic lymphocytic leukemia treated with allogeneic hematopoietic cell transplantation after nonmyeloablative conditioning. *J Clin Oncol* 26:4912, 2008.
705. Banerji V, Johnston JB, Seftel MD: The role of hematopoietic stem cell transplantation in Chronic Lymphocytic Leukemia. *Transfus Apher Sci* 37:57, 2007.
706. Sorror ML, Storer BE, Maloney DG, et al: Outcomes after allogeneic hematopoietic cell transplantation with nonmyeloablative or myeloablative conditioning regimens for treatment of lymphoma and chronic lymphocytic leukemia. *Blood* 111:446, 2008.
707. Schetelig J, van Biezen A, Brand R, et al: Allogeneic hematopoietic stem-cell transplantation for chronic lymphocytic leukemia with 17p deletion: A retrospective European Group for Blood and Marrow Transplantation analysis. *J Clin Oncol* 26:5094, 2008.
708. van Besien K, Keralavarma B, Devine S, Stock W: Allogeneic and autologous transplantation for chronic lymphocytic leukemia. *Leukemia* 15:1317, 2001.
709. Maloney DG, Sandmaier BM, Mackinnon S, Shizuru JA: Non-myeloablative transplantation. *Hematology Am Soc Hematol Educ Program* 392, 2002.
710. Schetelig J, Thiede C, Bornhauser M, et al: Evidence of a graft-versus-leukemia effect in chronic lymphocytic leukemia after reduced-intensity conditioning and allogeneic stem-cell transplantation: The Cooperative German Transplant Study Group. *J Clin Oncol* 21:2747, 2003.
711. Dreger P, Brand R, Hansz J, et al: Treatment-related mortality and graft-versus-leukemia activity after allogeneic stem cell transplantation for chronic lymphocytic leukemia using intensity-reduced conditioning. *Leukemia* 17:841, 2003.
712. Khouri IF, Lee MS, Saliba RM, et al: Nonablative allogeneic stem cell transplantation for chronic lymphocytic leukemia: Impact of rituximab on immunomodulation and survival. *Exp Hematol* 32:28, 2004.
713. Thomson KJ, Mackinnon S: Role of allogeneic transplantation in low-grade lymphoma and chronic lymphocytic leukemia. *Curr Opin Hematol* 13:273, 2006.
714. Gribben JG: Stem cell transplantation in chronic lymphocytic leukemia. *Biol Blood Marrow Transplant* 15:53, 2008.
715. Rodrigues CA, Sanz G, Brunstein CG, et al: Analysis of risk factors for outcomes after unrelated cord blood transplantation in adults with lymphoid malignancies: A study by the Eurocord-Netcord and lymphoma working party of the European group for blo od and marrow transplantation. *J Clin Oncol* 27:256, 2009.
716. Chen R, Keating MJ, Gandhi V, Plunkett W: Transcription inhibition by flavopiridol: Mechanism of chronic lymphocytic leukemia cell death. *Blood* 106:2513, 2005.
717. Hussain SR, Lucas DM, Johnson AJ, et al: Flavopiridol causes early mitochondrial damage in chronic lymphocytic leukemia cells with impaired oxygen consumption and mobilization of intracellular calcium. *Blood* 111:3190, 2008.
718. Byrd JC, Lin TS, Dalton JT, et al: Flavopiridol administered using a pharmacologically derived schedule is associated with marked clinical efficacy in refractory, genetically high-risk chronic lymphocytic leukemia. *Blood* 109:399, 2007.
719. Phelps MA, Lin TS, Johnson AJ, et al: Clinical response and pharmacokinetics from a phase 1 study of an active dosing schedule of flavopiridol in relapsed chronic lymphocytic leukemia. *Blood* 113:2637, 2009.
720. Chanan-Khan A, Porter CW: Immunomodulating drugs for chronic lymphocytic leukaemia. *Lancet Oncol* 7:480, 2006.
721. Chanan-Khan A, Miller KC, Musial L, et al: Clinical efficacy of lenalidomide in patients with relapsed or refractory chronic lymphocytic leukemia: Results of a phase II study. *J Clin Oncol* 24:5343, 2006.
722. Andritsos LA, Johnson AJ, Lozanski G, et al: Higher doses of lenalidomide are associated with unacceptable toxicity including life-threatening tumor flare in patients with chronic lymphocytic leukemia. *J Clin Oncol* 26:2519, 2008.
723. Moutouh-de Parseval LA, Weiss L, DeLap RJ, et al: Tumor lysis syndrome/tumor flare reaction in lenalidomide-treated chronic lymphocytic leukemia. *J Clin Oncol* 25:5047, 2007.
724. Coiffier B, Lepretre S, Pedersen LM, et al: Safety and efficacy of ofatumumab, a fully human monoclonal anti-CD20 antibody, in patients with relapsed or refractory B-cell chronic lymphocytic leukemia: A phase 1–2 study. *Blood* 111:1094, 2008.
725. Wahl U, Nossner E, Kronenberger K, et al: Vaccination against B-cell chronic lymphocytic leukemia with trioma cells: Preclinical evaluation. *Clin Cancer Res* 9:4240, 2003.
726. Kokhaei P, Rezvany MR, Virving L, et al: Dendritic cells loaded with apoptotic tumour cells induce a stronger T-cell response than dendritic cell-tumour hybrids in B-CLL. *Leukemia* 17:894, 2003.
727. Reichardt VL, Brossart P: DC-based immunotherapy of B-cell malignancies. *Cytotherapy* 6:62, 2004.
728. Kater AP, van Oers MH, Kipps TJ: Cellular immune therapy for chronic lymphocytic leukemia. *Blood* 110:2811, 2007.
729. Wierda WG, Kipps TJ: Gene therapy and active immune therapy of hematologic malignancies. *Best Pract Res Clin Haematol* 20:557, 2007.
730. Robertson TI: Complications and causes of death in B cell chronic lymphocytic leukaemia: A long term study of 105 patients. *Aust N Z J Med* 20:44, 1990.
731. Morra E, Nosari A, Montillo M: Infectious complications in chronic lymphocytic leukaemia. *Hematol Cell Ther* 41:145, 1999.
732. Vavricka SR, Halter J, Hechelhammer L, Himmelmann A: *Pneumocystis carinii* pneumonia in chronic lymphocytic leukaemia. *Postgrad Med J* 80:236, 2004.
733. Hensel M, Kornacker M, Yammeni S, et al: Disease activity and pretreatment, rather than hypogammaglobulinaemia, are major risk factors for infectious complications in patients with chronic lymphocytic leukaemia. *Br J Haematol* 122:600, 2003.
734. Griffiths H, Lea J, Bunch C, et al: Predictors of infection in chronic lymphocytic leukaemia (CLL). *Clin Exp Immunol* 89:374, 1992.
735. Itala M, Helenius H, Nikoskelainen J, Remes K: Infections and serum IgG levels in patients with chronic lymphocytic leukemia. *Eur J Haematol* 48:266, 1992.
736. Intravenous immunoglobulin for the prevention of infection in chronic lymphocytic leukemia. A randomized, controlled clinical trial. Cooperative Group for the Study of Immunoglobulin in Chronic Lymphocytic Leukemia. *N Engl J Med* 319:902, 1988.
737. Egerer G, Hensel M, Ho AD: Infectious complications in chronic lymphoid malignancy. *Curr Treat Options Oncol* 2:237, 2001.
738. Perkins JG, Flynn JM, Howard RS, Byrd JC: Frequency and type of serious infections in fludarabine-refractory B-cell chronic lymphocytic leukemia and small lymphocytic lymphoma: Implications for clinical trials in this patient population. *Cancer* 94:2033, 2002.
739. Wierda WG: Immunologic monitoring in chronic lymphocytic leukemia. *Curr Oncol Rep* 5:419, 2003.
740. Ward JH: Autoimmunity in chronic lymphocytic leukemia. *Curr Treat Options Oncol* 2:253, 2001.
741. Paydas S: Fludarabine-induced hemolytic anemia: Successful treatment by rituximab. *Hematol J* 5:81, 2004.

742. Greene MH, Hoover RN, Fraumeni JFJ: Subsequent cancer in patients with chronic lymphocytic leukemia—A possible immunologic mechanism. *J Natl Cancer Inst* 61:337, 1978.
743. Quaglino D, Lusvarghi E, Piccinini L, et al: The association between chronic lymphocytic leukaemia and a solid tumor: A survey study of 258 cases of chronic lymphocytic leukaemia covering an eleven year period. *Haematologica* 61:456, 1976.
744. Kyasa MJ, Hazlett L, Parrish RS, et al: Veterans with chronic lymphocytic leukemia/small lymphocytic lymphoma (CLL/SLL) have a markedly increased rate of second malignancy, which is the most common cause of death. *Leuk Lymphoma* 45:507, 2004.
745. Mehrany K, Weenig RH, Pittelkow MR, et al: High recurrence rates of Basal cell carcinoma after Mohs surgery in patients with chronic lymphocytic leukemia. *Arch Dermatol* 140:985, 2004.
746. Barroeta JE, Farkas T: Merkel cell carcinoma and chronic lymphocytic leukemia (collision tumor) of the arm: A diagnosis by fine-needle aspiration biopsy. *Diagn Cytopathol* 35:293, 2007.
747. Mehrany K, Weenig RH, Lee KK, et al: Increased metastasis and mortality from cutaneous squamous cell carcinoma in patients with chronic lymphocytic leukemia. *J Am Acad Dermatol* 53:1067, 2005.
748. Quaglino D, Paterlini P, De Pasquale A, et al: Association of chronic lymphocytic leukaemia and multiple myeloma: Report of a case and review of the literature. *Haematologica* 67:576, 1982.
749. Hoffman KD, Rudders RA: Multiple myeloma and chronic lymphocytic leukemia in a single individual. *Arch Intern Med* 137:232, 1977.
750. Jeha MT, Hamblin TJ, Smith JL: Coincident chronic lymphocytic leukemia and osteosclerotic multiple myeloma. *Blood* 57:617, 1981.
751. Pedersen-Bjergaard J, Petersen HD, Thomsen M, et al: Chronic lymphocytic leukaemia with subsequent development of multiple myeloma. Evidence of two B-lymphocyte clones and of myeloma-induced suppression of secretion of an M-component and of normal immunoglobulins. *Scand J Haematol* 21:256, 1978.
752. Maeshima AM, Taniguchi H, Nomoto J, et al: Secondary CD5+ diffuse large B-cell lymphoma not associated with transformation of chronic lymphocytic leukemia/small lymphocytic lymphoma (Richter syndrome). *Am J Clin Pathol* 131:339, 2009.
753. Rossi D, Gaidano G: Richter syndrome: Molecular insights and clinical perspectives. *Hematol Oncol* 27:1, 2009.
754. Maddocks-Christianson K, Slager SL, Zent CS, et al: Risk factors for development of a second lymphoid malignancy in patients with chronic lymphocytic leukaemia. *Br J Haematol* 139:398, 2007.
755. Lai R, Arber DA, Brynes RK, et al: Untreated chronic lymphocytic leukemia concurrent with or followed by acute myelogenous leukemia or myelodysplastic syndrome. A report of five cases and review of the literature. *Am J Clin Pathol* 111:373, 1999.
756. Coso D, Costello R, Cohen-Valensi R, et al: Acute myeloid leukemia and myelodysplasia in patients with chronic lymphocytic leukemia receiving fludarabine as initial therapy. *Ann Oncol* 10:362, 1999.
757. Kroft SH, Tallman MS, Shaw JM, et al: Myelodysplasia following treatment of chronic lymphocytic leukemia (CLL) with 2-chlorodeoxyadenosine (2-CdA). *Leukemia* 11:170, 1997.
758. Frewin RJ, Provan D, Smith AG: Myelodysplasia occurring after fludarabine treatment for chronic lymphocytic leukaemia. *Clin Lab Haematol* 19:151, 1997.
759. Lam CC, Ma ES, Kwong YL: Therapy-related acute myeloid leukemia after single-agent treatment with fludarabine for chronic lymphocytic leukemia. *Am J Hematol* 79:288, 2005.
760. Milligan DW, Kochethu G, Dearden C, et al: High incidence of myelodysplasia and secondary leukaemia in the UK Medical Research Council Pilot of autografting in chronic lymphocytic leukaemia. *Br J Haematol* 133:173, 2006.
761. Cobcroft R: Pure red cell aplasia associated with small lymphocytic lymphoma. *Br J Haematol* 113:260, 2001.
762. Vlachaki E, Tselios K, Charalambidou S, et al: Pure red cell aplasia complicating B cell small lymphocytic lymphoma: A case report. *Int J Hematol* 88:341, 2008.
763. D'Arena G, Cascavilla N: Chronic lymphocytic leukemia-associated pure red cell aplasia. *Int J Immunopathol Pharmacol* 22:279, 2009.
764. Ding W, Zent CS: Diagnosis and management of autoimmune complications of chronic lymphocytic leukemia/small lymphocytic lymphoma. *Clin Adv Hematol Oncol* 5:257, 2007.
765. Itala M, Kotilainen P, Nikkari S, et al: Pure red cell aplasia caused by B19 parvovirus infection after autologous blood stem cell transplantation in a patient with chronic lymphocytic leukemia. *Leukemia* 11:171, 1997.
766. Sharma P, Singh T, Mishra D, Gaiha M: Parvovirus B-19 induced acute pure red cell aplasia in patients with chronic lymphocytic leukemia and neurofibromatosis type-1. *Hematology* 11:257, 2006.
767. Chikkappa G, Pasquale D, Zarrabi MH, et al: Cyclosporine and prednisone therapy for pure red cell aplasia in patients with chronic lymphocytic leukemia. *Am J Hematol* 41:5, 1992.
768. Narra K, Borghaei H, Al-Saleem T, et al: Pure red cell aplasia in B-cell lymphoproliferative disorder treated with rituximab: Report of two cases and review of the literature. *Leuk Res* 30:109, 2006.
769. Richter MN: Generalized reticular cell sarcoma of lymph nodes associated with lymphatic leukemia. *Am J Pathol* 4:285, 1928.
770. Long JC, Aisenberg AC: Richter's syndrome. A terminal complication of chronic lymphocytic leukemia with distinct clinicopathologic features. *Am J Clin Pathol* 63:786, 1975.
771. Nakamura N, Abe M: Richter syndrome in B-cell chronic lymphocytic leukemia. *Pathol Int* 53:195, 2003.
772. Tsimberidou AM, Keating MJ: Richter syndrome: Biology, incidence, and therapeutic strategies. *Cancer* 103:216, 2005.
773. Cherepakhin V, Baird SM, Meisenholder GW, Kipps TJ: Common clonal origin of chronic lymphocytic leukemia and high-grade lymphoma of Richter's syndrome. *Blood* 82:3141, 1993.
774. Bessudo A, Kipps TJ: Origin of high-grade lymphomas in Richter syndrome. *Leuk Lymphoma* 18:367, 1995.
775. Timar B, Fulop Z, Csernus B, et al: Relationship between the mutational status of VH genes and pathogenesis of diffuse large B-cell lymphoma in Richter's syndrome. *Leukemia* 18:326, 2004.
776. Matolcsy A, Inghirami G, Knowles DM: Molecular genetic demonstration of the diverse evolution of Richter's syndrome (chronic lymphocytic leukemia and subsequent large cell lymphoma). *Blood* 83:1363, 1994.
777. Nakamura N, Kuze T, Hashimoto Y, et al: Analysis of the immunoglobulin heavy chain gene of secondary diffuse large B-cell lymphoma that subsequently developed in four cases with B-cell chronic lymphocytic leukemia or lymphoplasmacytoid lymphoma (Richter syndrome). *Pathol Int* 50:636, 2000.
778. Ratnavel RC, Dunn-Walters DK, Boursier L, et al: B-cell lymphoma associated with chronic lymphatic leukaemia: Two cases with contrasting aggressive and indolent behaviour. *Br J Dermatol* 140:708, 1999.
779. Kaufmann H, Ackermann J, Nosslinger T, et al: Absence of clonal chromosomal relationship between concomitant B-CLL and multiple myeloma—A report on two cases. *Ann Hematol* 80:474, 2001.
780. Chena C, Cerretini R, Noriega MF, et al: Cytogenetic, FISH, and molecular studies in a case of B-cell chronic lymphocytic leukemia with karyotypic evolution. *Eur J Haematol* 69:309, 2002.
781. Lee JN, Giles F, Huh YO, et al: Molecular differences between small and large cells in patients with chronic lymphocytic leukemia. *Eur J Haematol* 71:235, 2003.
782. Santulli B, Kazmierczak B, Napolitano R, et al: A 12q13 translocation involving the HMGI-C gene in richter transformation of a chronic lymphocytic leukemia. *Cancer Genet Cytogenet* 119:70, 2000.
783. Belhiba H, Casse C, Katmeh S, Bourdon J: [Prostatic involvement in leukemia. Report of a case] Les localisations prostatiques des leucemies. A propos d'un cas. *Prog Urol* 2:650, 1992.
784. Fulop Z, Csernus B, Timar B, et al: Microsatellite instability and hMLH1 promoter hypermethylation in Richter's transformation of chronic lymphocytic leukemia. *Leukemia* 17:411, 2003.
785. Rossi D, Cerri M, Capello D, et al: Biological and clinical risk factors of chronic lymphocytic leukaemia transformation to Richter syndrome. *Br J Haematol* 142:202, 2008.
786. Foucar K, Rydell RE: Richter's syndrome in chronic lymphocytic leukemia. *Cancer* 46:118, 1980.
787. Trump DL, Mann RB, Phelps R, et al: Richter's syndrome: Diffuse histiocytic lymphoma in patients with chronic lymphocytic leukemia. A report of five cases and review of the literature. *Am J Med* 68:539, 1980.
788. Harousseau JL, Flandrin G, Tricot G, et al: Malignant lymphoma supervening in chronic lymphocytic leukemia and related disorders. Richter's syndrome: A study of 25 cases. *Cancer* 48:1302, 1981.
789. Milkowski DA, Worley BD, Morris MJ: Richter's transformation presenting as an obstructing endobronchial lesion. *Chest* 116:832, 1999.
790. Fernandez-Suntay JP, Gragoudas ES, Ferry JA, et al: High-grade uveal B-cell lymphoma as the initial feature in Richter syndrome. *Arch Ophthalmol* 120:1383, 2002.
791. Joseph L, Scott MA, Schichman SA, Zent CS: Localized herpes simplex lymphadenitis mimicking large-cell (Richter's) transformation of chronic lymphocytic leukemia/small lymphocytic lymphoma. *Am J Hematol* 68:287, 2001.
792. Harris NL, Jaffe ES, Diebold J, et al: Lymphoma classification—from controversy to consensus: The R.E.A.L. and WHO Classification of lymphoid neoplasms. *Ann Oncol* 11 Suppl 1:3, 2000.
793. Robak T, Urbanska-Rys H, Strzelecka B, et al: Plasmablastic lymphoma in a patient with chronic lymphocytic leukemia heavily pretreated with cladribine (2-CdA): An unusual variant of Richter's syndrome. *Eur J Haematol* 67:322, 2001.
794. Brecher M, Banks PM: Hodgkin's disease variant of Richter's syndrome. Report of eight cases. *Am J Clin Pathol* 93:333, 1990.
795. Rubin D, Hudnall SD, Aisenberg A, et al: Richter's transformation of chronic lymphocytic leukemia with Hodgkin's-like cells is associated with Epstein-Barr virus infection. *Mod Pathol* 7:91, 1994.
796. Giles FJ, O'Brien SM, Keating MJ: Chronic lymphocytic leukemia in (Richter's) transformation. *Semin Oncol* 25:117, 1998.
797. Pescarmona E, Pignoloni P, Mauro FR, et al: Hodgkin/Reed-Sternberg cells and Hodgkin's disease in patients with B-cell chronic lymphocytic leukaemia: An immunohistological, molecular and clinical study of four cases suggesting a heterogeneous pathogenetic background. *Virchows Arch* 437:129, 2000.
798. O'Sullivan MJ, Kaleem Z, Bolger MJ, et al: Composite prolymphocytoid and Hodgkin transformation of chronic lymphocytic leukemia. *Arch Pathol Lab Med* 124:907, 2000.
799. Isikdogan A, Ayyildiz O, Buyukbayram H, Muftuoglu E: Hodgkin's disease variant of Richter's transformation: A case report. *Med Oncol* 19:109, 2002.

800. Robak T, Szmigielska-Kaplon A, Smolewski P, et al: Hodgkin's type of Richter's syndrome in familial chronic lymphocytic leukemia treated with cladribine and cyclophosphamide. *Leuk Lymphoma* 44:859, 2003.
801. Nemets A, Ben Dor D, Barry T, et al: Variant Richter's syndrome: A rare case of classical Hodgkin's lymphoma developing in a patient with chronic lymphocytic leukemia treated with fludarabine. *Leuk Lymphoma* 44:2151, 2003.
802. Alliot C, Tabuteau S, Desablens B: Hodgkin's disease variant of Richter's syndrome: Complete remission of the both malignancies after 14 years. *Hematology* 8:229, 2003.
803. de Leval L, Vivario M, De Prijck B, et al: Distinct clonal origin in two cases of Hodgkin's lymphoma variant of Richter's syndrome associated with EBV infection. *Am J Surg Pathol* 28:679, 2004.
804. Ohno T, Smir BN, Weisenburger DD, et al: Origin of the Hodgkin/Reed-Sternberg cells in chronic lymphocytic leukemia with "Hodgkin's transformation." *Blood* 91:1757, 1998.
805. Tsimberidou AM, Kantarjian HM, Cortes J, et al: Fractionated cyclophosphamide, vincristine, liposomal daunorubicin, and dexamethasone plus rituximab and granulocyte-macrophage-colony stimulating factor (GM-CSF) alternating with methotrexate and cytarabine plus rituximab and GM-CSF in patients with Richter syndrome or fludarabine-refractory chronic lymphocytic leukemia. *Cancer* 97:1711, 2003.
806. Melo JV, Catovsky D, Galton DA: The relationship between chronic lymphocytic leukaemia and prolymphocytic leukaemia. I. Clinical and laboratory features of 300 patients and characterization of an intermediate group. *Br J Haematol* 63:377, 1986.
807. Melo JV, Catovsky D, Galton DA: The relationship between chronic lymphocytic leukaemia and prolymphocytic leukaemia. II. Patterns of evolution of "prolymphocytoid" transformation. *Br J Haematol* 64:77, 1986.
808. Melo JV, Catovsky D, Gregory WM, Galton DA: The relationship between chronic lymphocytic leukaemia and prolymphocytic leukaemia. IV. Analysis of survival and prognostic features. *Br J Haematol* 65:23, 1987.
809. Sadamori N, Han T, Minowada J, et al: Possible specific chromosome change in prolymphocytic leukemia. *Blood* 62:729, 1983.
810. Ghani AM, Krause JR, Brody JP: Prolymphocytic transformation of chronic lymphocytic leukemia. A report of three cases and review of the literature. *Cancer* 57:75, 1986.
811. Zarrabi MH, Grunwald HW, Rosner F: Chronic lymphocytic leukemia terminating in acute leukemia. *Arch Intern Med* 137:1059, 1977.
812. Brouet JC, Preud'homme JL, Seligmann M, Bernard J: Blast cells with monoclonal surface immunoglobulin in two cases of acute blast crisis supervening on chronic lymphocytic leukaemia. *Br Med J* 4:23, 1973.
813. McPhedran P, Heath CWJ: Acute leukemia occurring during chronic lymphocytic leukemia. *Blood* 35:7, 1970.
814. Frenkel EP, Ligler FS, Graham MS, et al: Acute lymphocytic leukemic transformation of chronic lymphocytic leukemia: Substantiation by flow cytometry. *Am J Hematol* 10:391, 1981.
815. Torelli UL, Torelli GM, Emilia G, et al: Simultaneously increased expression of the c-myc and mu chain genes in the acute blastic transformation of a chronic lymphocytic leukaemia. *Br J Haematol* 65:165, 1987.
816. Büchi G, Termine G, Zappalà C, et al: Spontaneous complete remission of CLL. Report of a case studied with monoclonal antibodies. *Acta Haematol* 70:198, 1983.
817. Bernard M, Drenou B, Pangault C, et al: Spontaneous phenotypic and molecular blood remission in a case of chronic lymphocytic leukaemia. *Br J Haematol* 107:213, 1999.
818. Mandelli F, De Rossi G, Mancini P, et al: Prognosis in chronic lymphocytic leukemia: A retrospective multicentric study from the GIMEMA group. *J Clin Oncol* 5:398, 1987.
819. Jaksic B, Vitale B, Hauptmann E, et al: The roles of age and sex in the prognosis of chronic leukaemias. A study of 373 cases. *Br J Cancer* 64:345, 1991.
820. Molica S, Mauro FR, Callea V, et al: A gender-based score system predicts the clinical outcome of patients with early B-cell chronic lymphocytic leukemia. *Leuk Lymphoma* 46:553, 2005.
821. Molica S, Levato D, Dattilo A: Natural history of early chronic lymphocytic leukemia. A single institution study with emphasis on the impact of disease-progression on overall survival. *Haematologica* 84:1094, 1999.
822. Catovsky D, Galetto J, Okos A, et al: Prolymphocytic leukaemia of B and T cell type. *Lancet* 2:232, 1973.
823. Katayama I, Aiba M, Pechet L, et al: B-lineage prolymphocytic leukemia as a distinct clinicopathologic entity. *Am J Pathol* 99:399, 1980.
824. Robak T, Robak P: Current treatment options in prolymphocytic leukemia. *Med Sci Monit* 13:RA69, 2007.
825. Pittman S, Catovsky D: Chromosome abnormalities in B-cell prolymphocytic leukemia: A study of nine cases. *Cancer Genet Cytogenet* 9:355, 1983.
826. Stone RM: Prolymphocytic Leukemia. *Hematol Oncol Clin North Am* 4:457, 1990.
827. Sole F, Woessner S, Espinet B, et al: Cytogenetic abnormalities in three patients with B-cell prolymphocytic leukemia. *Cancer Genet Cytogenet* 103:43, 1998.
828. Adami F, Sancetta R, Trentin L, et al: The pediatric rhabdomyosarcoma translocation (2;13)(q35;q14) in B-prolymphocytic leukemia [letter]. *Leukemia* 7:1676, 1993.
829. Aoun P, Blair HE, Smith LM, et al: Fluorescence in situ hybridization detection of cytogenetic abnormalities in B-cell chronic lymphocytic leukemia/small lymphocytic lymphoma. *Leuk Lymphoma* 45:1595, 2004.
830. Dungarwalla M, Matutes E, Dearden CE: Prolymphocytic leukaemia of B- and T-cell subtype: A state-of-the-art paper. *Eur J Haematol* 80:469, 2008.
831. De Angeli C, Cuneo A, Aguiari G, et al: 5′ region and exon 7 mutations of the TP53 gene in two cases of B-cell prolymphocytic leukemia. *Cancer Genet Cytogenet* 107:137, 1998.
832. Bacher U, Kern W, Schoch C, et al: Discrimination of chronic lymphocytic leukemia (CLL) and CLL/PL by cytomorphology can clearly be correlated to specific genetic markers as investigated by interphase fluorescence in situ hybridization (FISH). *Ann Hematol* 83:349, 2004.
833. Lens D, Coignet LJ, Brito-Babapulle V, et al: B cell prolymphocytic leukaemia (B-PLL) with complex karyotype and concurrent abnormalities of the p53 and c-MYC gene. *Leukemia* 13:873, 1999.
834. Shokri F, Mageed RA, Richardson P, Jefferis R: Immunophenotypic and idiotypic characterisation of the leukaemic B-cells from patients with prolymphocytic leukaemia: Evidence for a selective expression of immunoglobulin variable region (IGV) gene products. *Leuk Res* 17:669, 1993.
835. Del Giudice I, Davis Z, Matutes E, et al: IgVH genes mutation and usage, ZAP-70 and CD38 expression provide new insights on B-cell prolymphocytic leukemia (B-PLL). *Leukemia* 20:1231, 2006.
836. Davi F, Maloum K, Michel A, et al: High frequency of somatic mutations in the VH genes expressed in prolymphocytic leukemia. *Blood* 88:3953, 1996.
837. Hoffman MA, Valderrama E, Fuchs A, et al: Leukemic meningitis in B-cell prolymphocytic leukemia. A clinical, pathologic, and ultrastructural case study and a review of the literature. *Cancer* 75:1100, 1995.
838. Pastor E, Grau E, Real E: Leukemic meningitis in a patient with B-cell prolymphocytic leukemia [letter]. *Haematologica* 82:511, 1997.
839. Andrieu V, Encaoua R, Carbon C, et al: Leukemic pleural effusion in B-cell prolymphocytic leukemia. *Hematol Cell Ther* 40:275, 1998.
840. Shimoni A, Shvidel L, Shtalrid M, et al: Prolymphocytic transformation of B-chronic lymphocytic leukemia presenting as malignant ascites and pleural effusion [letter]. *Am J Hematol* 59:316, 1998.
841. Dietrich PY, Pedraza E, Casiraghi O, et al: Cardiac arrest due to leucostasis in a case of prolymphocytic leukaemia. *Br J Haematol* 78:122, 1991.
842. Takenaka T, Nakamine H, Nishihara T, et al: Prolymphocytic leukemia with IgM hypogammaglobulinemia. *Am J Clin Pathol* 80:237, 1983.
843. Caligaris-Cappio F, Janossy G: Surface markers in chronic lymphoid leukemias of B cell type. *Semin Hematol* 22:1, 1985.
844. Shvidel L, Shtalrid M, Bassous L, et al: B-cell prolymphocytic leukemia: A survey of 35 patients emphasizing heterogeneity, prognostic factors and evidence for a group with an indolent course. *Leuk Lymphoma* 33:169, 1999.
845. Lambertenghi-Deliliers G, Maiolo AT, Annaloro C, et al: Complete remission in prolymphocytic leukemia with 4-demethoxydaunorubicin and arabinosyl cytosine. *Cancer* 54:199, 1984.
846. Swift JF, Wold HG, Gandara DR, et al: Prolymphocytic leukemia. Serial responses to therapy. *Cancer* 54:978, 1984.
847. Mourad YA, Taher A, Chehal A, Shamseddine A: Successful treatment of B-cell prolymphocytic leukemia with monoclonal anti-CD20 antibody. *Ann Hematol* 83:319, 2004.
848. Barton K, Larson RA, O'Brien S, Ratain MJ: Rapid response of B-cell prolymphocytic leukemia to 2-chlorodeoxyadenosine [letter]. *J Clin Oncol* 10:1821, 1992.
849. Saven A, Lee T, Schlutz M, et al: Major activity of cladribine in patients with *de novo* B-cell prolymphocytic leukemia. *J Clin Oncol* 15:37, 1997.
850. Lorand-Metze I, Oliveira GB, Aranha FJ: Treatment of prolymphocytic leukemia with cladribine. *Ann Hematol* 76:85, 1998.
851. Kantarjian HM, Childs C, O'Brien S, et al: Efficacy of fludarabine, a new adenine nucleoside analogue, in patients with prolymphocytic leukemia and the prolymphocytoid variant of chronic lymphocytic leukemia. *Am J Med* 90:223, 1991.
852. List AF, Kummet TD, Adams JD, Chun HG: Tumor lysis syndrome complicating treatment of chronic lymphocytic leukemia with fludarabine phosphate. *Am J Med* 89:388, 1990.
853. Smith RE, Stoiber TR: Acute tumor lysis syndrome in prolymphocytic leukemia. *Am J Med* 88:547, 1990.
854. Cannon LM, Spilove L, Rhodes R, et al: Acute tumor lysis syndrome complicating fludarabine treatment of prolymphocytic leukemia. *Conn Med* 57:651, 1993.
855. Döhner H, Ho AD, Thaler J, et al: Pentostatin in prolymphocytic leukemia: Phase II trial of the European Organization for Research and Treatment of Cancer Leukemia Cooperative Study Group. *J Natl Cancer Inst* 85:658, 1993.
856. Dearden C, Matutes E, Catovsky D: Deoxycoformycin in the treatment of mature T-cell leukaemias. *Br J Cancer* 64:903, 1991.
857. Muncunill J, Villa S, Domingo A, et al: Splenic irradiation as primary therapy for prolymphocytic leukaemia. *Br J Haematol* 76:305, 1990.
858. Yamamoto K, Hamaguchi H, Nagata K, et al: Splenic irradiation for prolymphocytic leukemia: Is it preferable as an initial treatment or not? *Jpn J Clin Oncol* 28:267, 1998.
859. Singh AK, Bates T, Wetherley-Mein G: A preliminary study of low-dose splenic irradiation for the treatment of chronic lymphocytic and prolymphocytic leukaemias. *Scand J Haematol* 37:50, 1986.
860. Terashima T, Ohtake K, Ogawa T: Prolymphocytic leukemia treated with natural and recombinant alpha-interferon. *Am J Hematol* 35:56, 1990.
861. Delannoy A, Balligand JL, Ledant T: Interferon and B-cell prolymphocytic leukaemia [letter]. *Br J Haematol* 66:579, 1987.
862. Jacobs P, le Roux I, Wood L, Bolding E: Interferon response in B-cell prolymphocytic leukemia [letter]. *Br J Haematol* 65:375, 1987.

863. Vivaldi P, Garuti R, Rubertelli M, Mazzon C: Prolymphocytic leukemia: A very satisfactory response to treatment with recombinant interferon alpha. *Haematologica* 77:169, 1992.
864. Blecher TE: "Spontaneous" complete remission in a case of prolymphocytic leukemia [letter]. *Br J Haematol* 63:395, 1986.
865. Bennett JM, Catovsky D, Daniel MT, et al: Proposals for the classification of chronic (mature) B and T lymphoid leukaemias. French-American-British (FAB) Cooperative Group. *J Clin Pathol* 42:567, 1989.
866. Matutes E, Brito-Babapulle V, Swansbury J, et al: Clinical and laboratory features of 78 cases of T-prolymphocytic leukemia. *Blood* 78:3269, 1991.
867. Matutes E, Catovsky D: CLL should be used only for the disease with B-cell phenotype [letter; comment]. *Leukemia* 7:917, 1993.
868. Foon KA, Gale RP: Is there a T-cell form of chronic lymphocytic leukemia? [editorial; see comments]. *Leukemia* 6:867, 1992.
869. Hoyer JD, Ross CW, Li CY, et al: True T-cell chronic lymphocytic leukemia: A morphologic and immunophenotypic study of 25 cases [see comments]. *Blood* 86:1163, 1995.
870. Pileri SA, Milani M, Fraternali-Orcioni G, Sabattini E: From the R.E.A.L. Classification to the upcoming WHO scheme: A step toward universal categorization of lymphoma entities? *Ann Oncol* 9:607, 1998.
871. Harris NL, Jaffe ES, Stein H, et al: A revised European-American classification of lymphoid neoplasms: A proposal from the International Lymphoma Study Group [see comments]. *Blood* 84:1361, 1994.
872. Ascani S, Leoni P, Fraternali Orcioni G, et al: T-cell prolymphocytic leukaemia: Does the expression of CD8+ phenotype justify the identification of a new subtype? Description of two cases and review of the literature. *Ann Oncol* 10:649, 1999.
873. Kojima K, Sawada T, Ikezoe T, et al: Defective human T-lymphotrophic virus type I provirus in T-cell prolymphocytic leukaemia. *Br J Haematol* 105:376, 1999.
874. Pawson R, Schulz TF, Matutes E, Catovsky D: The human T-cell lymphotropic viruses types I/II are not involved in T prolymphocytic leukemia and large granular lymphocytic leukemia. *Leukemia* 11:1305, 1997.
875. Maljaei SH, Brito-Babapulle V, Hiorns LR, Catovsky D: Abnormalities of chromosomes 8, 11, 14, and X in T-prolymphocytic leukemia studied by fluorescence in situ hybridization. *Cancer Genet Cytogenet* 103:110, 1998.
876. Sorour A, Brito-Babapulle V, Smedley D, et al: Unusual breakpoint distribution of 8p abnormalities in T-prolymphocytic leukemia: A study with YACS mapping to 8p11-p12. *Cancer Genet Cytogenet* 121:128, 2000.
877. Pekarsky Y, Hallas C, Croce CM: Molecular basis of mature T-cell leukemia. *JAMA* 286:2308, 2001.
878. Costa D, Queralt R, Aymerich M, et al: High levels of chromosomal imbalances in typical and small-cell variants of T-cell prolymphocytic leukemia. *Cancer Genet Cytogenet* 147:36, 2003.
879. Salomon-Nguyen F, Brizard F, Le Coniat M, et al: Abnormalities of the short arm of chromosome 12 in T cell prolymphocytic leukemia. *Leukemia* 12:972, 1998.
880. Brito-Babapulle V, Baou M, Matutes E, et al: Deletions of D13S25, D13S319 and RB-1 mapping to 13q14.3 in T-cell prolymphocytic leukaemia. *Br J Haematol* 114:327, 2001.
881. Kojima K, Taniwaki M, Yoshino T, et al: Trisomy 12 and t(14;18) in B-cell chronic lymphocytic leukemia. *Int J Hematol* 67:199, 1998.
882. Zver S, Kokalj Vokac N, Zagradisnik B, et al: T cell prolymphocytic leukemia with new chromosome rearrangements. *Acta Haematol* 111:168, 2004.
883. Brito-Babapulle V, Hamoudi R, Matutes E, et al: P53 allele deletion and protein accumulation occurs in the absence of p53 gene mutation in T-prolymphocytic leukaemia and Sézary syndrome. *Br J Haematol* 110:180, 2000.
884. Bradshaw PS, Condie A, Matutes E, et al: Breakpoints in the ataxia telangiectasia gene arise at the RGYW somatic hypermutation motif. *Oncogene* 21:483, 2002.
885. Croce CM, Isobe M, Palumbo A, et al: Gene for alpha-chain of human T-cell receptor: Location on chromosome 14 region involved in T-cell neoplasms. *Science* 227:1044, 1985.
886. Stilgenbauer S, Schaffner C, Litterst A, et al: Biallelic mutations in the ATM gene in T-prolymphocytic leukemia. *Nat Med* 3:1155, 1997.
887. Yuille MA, Coignet LJ, Abraham SM, et al: ATM is usually rearranged in T-cell prolymphocytic leukaemia [published erratum appears in Oncogene 16(22):2955, 1998]. *Oncogene* 16:789, 1998.
888. Stoppa-Lyonnet D, Soulier J, Laugé A, et al: Inactivation of the ATM gene in T-cell prolymphocytic leukemias. *Blood* 91:3920, 1998.
889. Luo L, Lu FM, Hart S, et al: Ataxia-telangiectasia and T-cell leukemias: No evidence for somatic ATM mutation in sporadic T-ALL or for hypermethylation of the ATM-NPAT/E14 bidirectional promoter in T-PLL. *Cancer Res* 58:2293, 1998.
890. Madani A, Choukroun V, Soulier J, et al: Expression of p13MTCP1 is restricted to mature T-cell proliferations with t(X;14) translocations. *Blood* 87:1923, 1996.
891. Gritti C, Choukroun V, Soulier J, et al: Alternative origin of p13MTCP1-encoding transcripts in mature T-cell proliferations with t(X;14) translocations. *Oncogene* 15:1329, 1997.
892. De Schouwer PJ, Dyer MJ, Brito-Babapulle VB, et al: T-cell prolymphocytic leukaemia: Antigen receptor gene rearrangement and a novel mode of MTCP1 B1 activation. *Br J Haematol* 110:831, 2000.
893. Hoh F, Yang YS, Guignard L, et al: Crystal structure of p14TCL1, an oncogene product involved in T-cell prolymphocytic leukemia, reveals a novel beta-barrel topology. *Structure* 6:147, 1998.
894. Thick J, Metcalfe JA, Mak YF, et al: Expression of either the TCL1 oncogene, or transcripts from its homologue MTCP1/c6.1B, in leukaemic and non-leukaemic T cells from ataxia telangiectasia patients. *Oncogene* 12:379, 1996.
895. Gritti C, Dastot H, Soulier J, et al: Transgenic mice for MTCP1 develop T-cell prolymphocytic leukemia. *Blood* 92:368, 1998.
896. Matutes E, Catovsky D: Similarities between T-cell chronic lymphocytic leukemia and the small-cell variant of T-prolymphocytic leukemia [letter; comment]. *Blood* 87:3520, 1996.
897. Mallett RB, Matutes E, Catovsky D, et al: Cutaneous infiltration in T-cell prolymphocytic leukaemia. *Br J Dermatol* 132:263, 1995.
898. Serra A, Estrach MT, Martí R, et al: Cutaneous involvement as the first manifestation in a case of T-cell prolymphocytic leukaemia. *Acta Derm Venereol* 78:198, 1998.
899. Dhar-Munshi S, Alton P, Ayliffe WH: Masquerade syndrome: T-cell prolymphocytic leukemia presenting as panuveitis. *Am J Ophthalmol* 132:275, 2001.
900. Catovsky D, Wechsler A, Matutes E, et al: The membrane phenotype of T-prolymphocytic leukaemia. *Scand J Haematol* 29:398, 1982.
901. Hui PK, Feller AC, Pileri S, et al: New aggressive variant of suppressor/cytotoxic T-CLL. *Am J Clin Pathol* 87:55, 1987.
902. Kluin-Nelemans HC, Gmelig-Meyling FH, Kootte AM, et al: T-cell prolymphocytic leukemia with an unusual phenotype CD4+ CD8+. *Cancer* 60:794, 1987.
903. Brito-Babapulle V, Maljaie SH, Matutes E, et al: Relationship of T leukaemias with cerebriform nuclei to T-prolymphocytic leukaemia: A cytogenetic analysis with in situ hybridization. *Br J Haematol* 96:724, 1997.
904. Pawson R, Matutes E, Brito-Babapulle V, et al: Sézary cell leukaemia: A distinct T cell disorder or a variant form of T prolymphocytic leukaemia? *Leukemia* 11:1009, 1997.
905. Uike N, Choi I, Tokoro A, et al: Adult T-cell leukemia-lymphoma successfully treated with 2-chlorodeoxyadenosine. *Intern Med* 37:411, 1998.
906. Palomera L, Domingo JM, Agullo JA, Soledad-Romero M: Complete remission in T-cell prolymphocytic leukemia with 2-chlorodeoxyadenosine. *J Clin Oncol* 13:1995.
907. Zackheim HS: Cutaneous T cell lymphoma: Update of treatment. *Dermatology* 199:102, 1999.
908. Ravandi F, O'Brien S: Alemtuzumab. *Expert Rev Anticancer Ther* 5:39, 2005.
909. Dearden C: The role of alemtuzumab in the management of T-cell malignancies. *Semin Oncol* 33:S44, 2006.
910. Birhiray RE, Shaw G, Guldan S, et al: Phenotypic transformation of CD52(pos) to CD52(neg) leukemic T cells as a mechanism for resistance to CAMPATH-1H. *Leukemia* 16:861, 2002.
911. Dearden C: Alemtuzumab in peripheral T-cell malignancies. *Cancer Biother Radiopharm* 19:391, 2004.
912. Collins RH, Piñeiro LA, Agura ED, Fay JW: Treatment of T prolymphocytic leukemia with allogeneic bone marrow transplantation. *Bone Marrow Transplant* 21:627, 1998.
913. Murase K, Matsunaga T, Sato T, et al: Allogeneic bone marrow transplantation in a patient with T-prolymphocytic leukemia with small-intestinal involvement. *Int J Clin Oncol* 8:391, 2003.
914. Tsai LM, Tsai CC, Hyde TP, et al: T-cell prolymphocytic leukemia with helper-cell phenotype and a review of the literature. *Cancer* 54:463, 1984.
915. Pawson R, Richardson DS, Pagliuca A, et al: Adult T-cell leukemia/lymphoma in London: Clinical experience of 21 cases. *Leuk Lymphoma* 31:177, 1998.
916. López-Guillermo A, Cid J, Salar A, et al: Peripheral T-cell lymphomas: Initial features, natural history, and prognostic factors in a series of 174 patients diagnosed according to the R.E.A.L. Classification. *Ann Oncol* 9:849, 1998.
917. Garand R, Goasguen J, Brizard A, et al: Indolent course as a relatively frequent presentation in T-prolymphocytic leukaemia. Groupe Français d'Hématologie Cellulaire. *Br J Haematol* 103:488, 1998.
918. Zenz T, Dohner H, Stilgenbauer S: Genetics and risk-stratified approach to therapy in chronic lymphocytic leukemia. *Best Pract Res Clin Haematol* 20:439, 2007.
919. Ferrajoli A, O'Brien SM, Cortes JE, et al: Phase II study of alemtuzumab in chronic lymphoproliferative disorders. *Cancer* 98:773, 2003.
920. Huhn D, von Schilling C, Wilhelm M, et al: Rituximab therapy of patients with B-cell chronic lymphocytic leukemia. *Blood* 98:1326, 2001.
921. Hainsworth JD: Prolonging remission with rituximab maintenance therapy. *Semin Oncol* 31:17, 2004.
922. Robak T, Moiseev SI, Dmoszynska A, et al: Rituximab, fludarabine, and cyclophosphamide (R-FC) prolongs progression free survival in relapsed or refractory chronic lymphocytic leukemia (CLL) compared with FC alone: Final results from the International Randomized Phase III REACH Trial. *Blood* 112:Abstract 1, 2008.
923. Wierda W, O'Brien S, Ferrajoli A, et al: Salvage therapy with combined cyclophosphamide©, fudarabine (F), alemtuzumab (A), and rituximab® (CFAR) for heavily pretreated patients with CLL. *Blood* 106:Abstract 719, 2005.
924. Elter T, Borchmann P, Schulz H, et al: Fludarabine in combination with alemtuzumab is effective and feasible in patients with relapsed or refractory B-cell chronic lymphocytic leukemia: Results of a phase II trial. *J Clin Oncol* 23:7024, 2005.
925. Sayala HA, Moreton P, Jones RA, et al: Interim report of the UKCLL02 trial: A phase II study of subcutaneous alemtuzumab plus fudarabine in patients with fudarabine refractory CLL (On behalf of the NCRI CLL Trials SubGroup). *Blood* 106:Abstract 2120, 2005.

CHAPTER 95
HAIRY CELL LEUKEMIA

Darren Sigal and Alan Saven

SUMMARY

Hairy cell leukemia is an uncommon neoplastic disorder of B lymphocytes that has a much higher prevalence in men than in women. The patient usually presents with bicytopenia or pancytopenia. Absolute neutropenia and monocytopenia are nearly constant features. The blood and marrow biopsy contain hairy cells, which are lymphocytes that have prominent cytoplasmic projections and give the disease its name. Splenomegaly, sometimes massive, is a nearly constant feature. The liver and abdominal lymph nodes may be enlarged. The immunophenotype of the hairy cells, CD11c+, CD19+, CD20+, CD22+, CD25+, and CD103+, confirms the diagnosis. Disease complications include standard or opportunistic infections. Approximately 10 percent of patients may not require immediate treatment. For patients requiring treatment, cladribine is the drug of choice because of the very high complete remission rate and prolonged duration of remission in a high proportion of patients. Pentostatin also is effective in this disease. Interferon-α, rituximab, anti-CD22 recombinant immunotoxin (BL22), or splenectomy can be useful in selected patients unresponsive to cladribine or pentostatin. The patient with hairy cell leukemia can expect a very long duration of survival with current therapy. The 5-year event-free survival rate after treatment is approximately 90 percent of patients initially treated with cladribine.

DEFINITION AND HISTORY

Hairy cell leukemia (HCL) is an uncommon chronic lymphoproliferative disorder characterized by circulating B lymphocytes that display prominent cytoplasmic projections. The neoplastic B cells infiltrate the marrow and spleen. Afflicted individuals often are males who present with bicytopenia or pancytopenia, splenomegaly, or recurrent, serious infections. In 1958, Bouroncle and colleagues[1] recognized the disorder as a distinct clinicopathologic entity and referred to it as *leukemic reticuloendotheliosis*. Eight years later, Schreck and colleagues[2] reported on the same disease, describing "peculiar cells that had numerous short villi on phase contrast microscopy, which they referred to as 'hairy cells.'" The disease designation *hairy cell leukemia* has since gained official recognition. In 1972, Giblett and colleagues[3] made the seminal observation that one-third of children with severe combined immunodeficiency syndrome were deficient in the purine catabolic enzyme adenosine deaminase. Adenosine deaminase catalyzes the irreversible deamination of adenosine to inosine and of 2′-deoxyadenosine to 2′-deoxyinosine. Cohen and investigators[4] reported that the intracellular accumulation of deoxyadenosine triphosphate was responsible for the lymphopenia seen in severe combined immune deficiency. Later, Carson and colleagues[5] reported that 2-chlorodeoxyadenosine (cladribine), a chlorine-substituted purine deoxynucleoside, was the most potent among a panel of substituted purine analogues screened for *in vitro* cytotoxicity. In 1990, investigators at Scripps Clinic, La Jolla, California, first reported on 12 patients with HCL treated with a single 7-day course of cladribine administered at 0.1 mg/kg per day by continuous intravenous infusion.[6] Of the 12 patients, 11 achieved a complete response and 1 a partial response.

Acronyms and abbreviations that appear in this chapter include: DFS, disease-free survival; G-CSF, granulocyte colony-stimulating factor; HCL, hairy cell leukemia; HCLv, hairy cell leukemia variant; IL, interleukin; MRD, minimal residual disease; SMZL, splenic marginal zone lymphoma; TRAP, tartrate-resistant acid phosphatase.

EPIDEMIOLOGY

There are about 600 new cases of hairy cell leukemia diagnosed annually, which represents approximately 2 percent of all new cases of leukemia in the United States. HCL is predominantly a disease of men, with a 4:1 male-to-female predominance. The median age at presentation is 52 years, lower than most other types of adult leukemia. The disease has not been described in children or teenagers. Ashkenazi Jewish males are more frequently affected than are men in other ethnic groups.

ETIOLOGY AND PATHOGENESIS

Some studies suggest that prior exposure to radiation[7] and organic solvents[8] is more frequent among HCL patients. These finding have not been confirmed in other studies[8,9] and whether any environmental factors influence the incidence of HCL has not been established. Some investigators have speculated on an etiologic role for the Epstein-Barr virus in the development of HCL,[10] but the proposal has been disputed.[11]

Hairy cell leukemia, like all clonal (malignant) lymphoid diseases, arises from a sequence of mutations in a single lymphocyte progenitor cell. These genetic events confer a growth and survival advantage on the cells in the clone. The precise genetic transforming cellular changes are not known. The ontogeny of the normal counterpart of the hairy cell is uncertain. Initially, hairy cells were presumed, erroneously, to derive from monocytes. Hairy cells develop pseudopods, are motile, perform phagocytosis, induce the development of a fibronectin matrix in their microenvironments,[12,13] and display Fc receptors,[14] all characteristics shared by monocytes. The discovery of immunoglobulin heavy- and light-chain gene rearrangements clearly established hairy cells as B lymphocytes.[15]

The presence of *BCL-6* mutations and the *hairy* border itself both confer the genotype and phenotype of an activated, late-stage B lymphocyte. Hairy cells display the activation antigens, CD11c and CD22, but not the early B-cell markers, CD21 and CD24.[16,17] The cells coexpress hairy cell leukemia-associated antigen (HC2) and plasma cell antigen-1 (PCA-1), developmental landmarks found transiently on preplasma cell B lymphocytes and on plasma cells, respectively.[18] Hairy cells do not undergo affinity maturation and are not plasma cells.[19] These findings indicate that the hairy cell's normal homologue is between the activated B lymphocyte and the plasma cell in the hierarchy of B-cell ontogeny.

A shared normal progenitor cell has been suggested for the lymphocytes of HCL, hairy cell leukemia variant (HCLv), and splenic marginal zone lymphoma (SMZL) (see "Differential Diagnosis" below).[20,21] However, the normal cell counterpart for SMZL has been identified as the monocytoid B-lymphocyte, which is distinct from the normal cell counterpart of the hairy cell.[22] With similar rates of unmutated immunoglobulin heavy chains and VH4-34 usage, SMZL and HCLv have a closer ancestral bond to each other than to HCL.[23] A hairy cell progenitor probably most closely approximates a B cell activated by T-cell independent mechanisms. This process produces antigen-specific antibodies of all isotypes, except immunoglobulin (Ig)E, preferentially produces the IgG_3 subclass, and colocalizes with macrophages in the splenic red pulp, all consistent with observations found in HCL.[24]

CLINICAL FEATURES

SYMPTOMS AND SIGNS

On initial presentation, 25 percent of patients complain of fatigue and weakness; 25 percent of early satiety or abdominal fullness from splenomegaly; 25 percent are detected as a result of an incidental finding of splenomegaly or abnormal blood counts on a periodic health examination or for an unrelated condition; and 25 percent have an opportunistic infection.[25,26] The development of severe, sometimes life-threatening infections is one of the most frequent serious complications of HCL (see "Microbiology" below). This complication has decreased in frequency since the advent of successful therapy. Easy bruising results from thrombocytopenia as well as platelet dysfunction.[25,27]

Splenomegaly, which may be massive, is found in 90 percent of patients.[12,28] Hepatomegaly can occur. Palpable superficial lymphadenopathy is uncommon and is usually localized when found. However, as a result of the routine use of computerized axial tomography scans in the evaluation of patients with lymphoproliferative disorders, significant deep adenopathy has been found to be present in up to one-third of patients with HCL.[29,30] In 3 percent of patients, the disease manifests as a painful bony lesion (osteolytic) in the axial skeleton or long bones, most commonly involving the proximal femur.[31]

Unusual clinical manifestations include signs and symptoms of cutaneous vasculitis, leukocytoclastic angiitis, erythema nodosum, pulmonary infiltrates, polyarthritis, or Raynaud phenomenon.[32–34] Polyarthritis, skin lesions, or vasculitis may be the initial or an early manifestation of the disease. Signs of pleural or ascitic fluid rarely result from hairy cell involvement of those serosal surfaces.[33]

LABORATORY FEATURES

BLOOD

At the time of diagnosis, pancytopenia occurs in 50 percent of patients; the remaining half usually have bicytopenia.[25,33,35] Anemia is present in about three-quarters of patients and about one-third of patients have a hemoglobin of less than 9.0 g/dL. About two-thirds of patients have a platelet count of less than 100×10^9/L, and as many as one-third of all patients have a platelet count of less than 50×10^9/L.[33] More than 80 percent of patients have absolute neutropenia and monocytopenia with approximately 40 percent having an absolute neutrophil count of less than 0.5×10^9/L.[33,35] Along with impaired interferon-α production,[36] the neutropenia and monocytopenia[37–39] predispose patients to relatively common and opportunistic infections.[25] Occasional patients have elevated leukocyte counts as a result of circulating hairy cells.[25,26,35,37] The cytopenias are the result of the combined effects of hypersplenism and hairy cell infiltration of the marrow.[26,33,37,38] Hairy cell secretion of tumor necrosis factor-α, an inhibitor of hematopoiesis, can result in marked cytopenias even with insignificant marrow involvement with hairy cells.[40]

Hairy cells are mononuclear cells with eccentric or central nuclei.[41,42] Nuclear morphology is variable: round, ovoid, reniform, or convoluted. Nuclear forms tend to have a reticular chromatin pattern. Hairy cells have variable amounts of cytoplasm that is blue-gray in appearance, exhibiting thin cytoplasmic projections (Fig. 95–1).

MARROW

The marrow biopsy usually demonstrates hairy cell infiltrates. Marrow involvement may be diffuse or focal. In some cases, the infiltrate is so subtle that it is difficult to discern. This pattern of HCL infiltration usually involves an hypocellular marrow with scant infiltration by hairy cells, admixed with residual hematopoietic tissue.[41–43] The hairy cells in the marrow aspirate tend to have a slightly coarser reticular chromatin-staining pattern than the hairy cells found in the blood. Hairy cells have monotonous round, oval, or spindle-spaced nuclei that are separated by abundant quantities of pale-staining cytoplasm in a fine fibrillar network. The separation of individual hairy cells is characteristic and referred to as the "fried-egg" appearance. Because of marked marrow reticulin fibrosis, the marrow frequently is difficult or impossible to aspirate (Fig. 95–2). Hairy cells express CD44, a nonintegrin receptor, which may be responsible for hairy cell homing to the glycosaminoglycan and hyaluronan tissue matrix present in the marrow, the engagement of which stimulates fibronectin synthesis, with resultant fibrosis.[42,44]

CYTOGENETICS AND GENETICS

A wide variety of clonal cytogenetic abnormalities have been described.[45,46] Chromosome 5 is involved in clonal aberrations in approximately 40 percent of patients with HCL, most commonly as trisomy 5 or as pericentric inversions and interstitial deletions involving band 5q13.[47] The 5q13.3 breakpoint has been studied and putative candidate tumor-suppressor genes have been described.[46] Mutations in p53 and *BCL* (25% of patients) have been noted, but their role in disease onset or progression is not clear. The cells overexpress cyclin D1, not as a result of the 11;14 translocation characteristic of mantle-cell lymphoma, but as a result of some other unexplained stimulation.[42]

MICROBIOLOGY

Viral, bacterial, fungal, or protozoal agents may be isolated at the time of infection. Before the introduction of successful therapy, concomitant infections were very common, sometimes involving several pathogens. *Staphylococcus aureus*, *Streptococcus pneumoniae*, *Escherichia coli*, and *Pseudomonas aeruginosa* were common bacterial agents involved. Opportunistic organisms isolated in febrile HCL patients have included *Mycobacterium kansasii*, cytomegalovirus, *Pneumocystis carinii*, *Aspergillus* spp., *Histoplasma* spp., *Cryptococcus* spp., *Listeria* spp., and *Toxoplasma gondii*, among others.[25,33,48] Atypical mycobacterial infection was about 10-fold that seen in other types of lymphoproliferative disorders. The success of therapy has made these once common events very uncommon.

HISTOPATHOLOGY OF SPLEEN, LIVER, AND LYMPH NODES

As the main motility-inducing integrin on hairy cells, $\alpha_V\beta_3$ targets splenic vitronectin, lymph node laminin, and liver collagen, enabling hairy cell infiltration.[49,50] The splenic microenvironment actively promotes hairy cell survival and proliferation.[20]

The spleen, virtually always enlarged, has a median weight of 1300 g.[38] On section, the spleen has a dark-red, smooth surface. On light microscopy, the hairy cells typically involve the splenic red pulp. Later, the white pulp atrophies. Blood-filled spaces lined by hairy cells that disrupt the normal splenic sinus architecture are characteristic (see Fig. 95–2).[51] These blood-filled spaces are referred to as *pseudosinuses* or *blood lakes*.

Hepatic infiltration is both sinusoidal and portal.[51] Lymph node involvement is marked by both sinusoidal and interstitial involvement.[52]

TARTRATE-RESISTANT ACID PHOSPHATASE

The hairy cell cytoplasm usually stains strongly positive for tartrate-resistant acid phosphatase (TRAP; see Fig. 95–1). Isoenzyme 5 acid phosphatase, present in the hairy cell cytoplasm, resists decolorization by tartrate.[53,54] TRAP staining of blood white cell concentrates (buffy

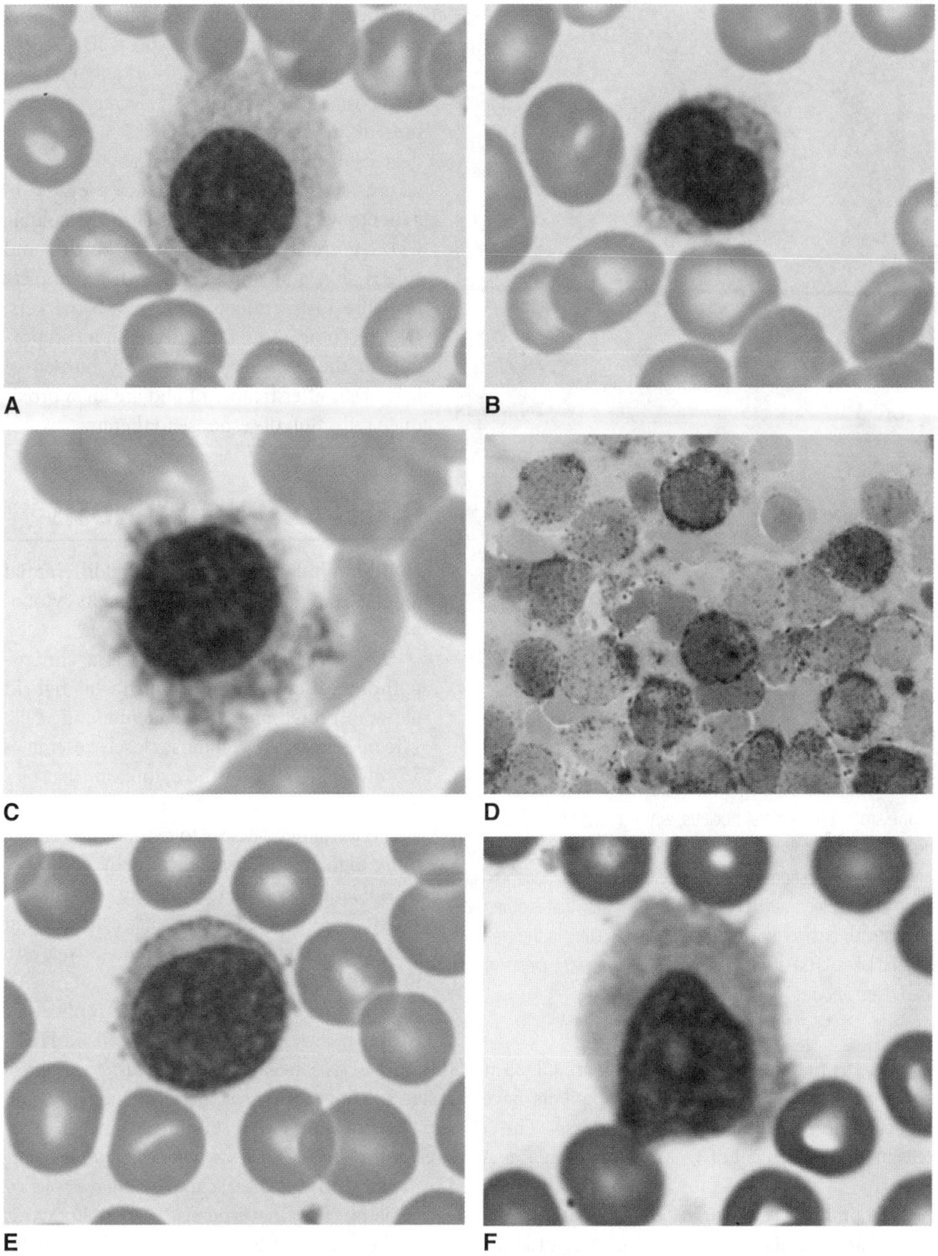

FIGURE 95–1. Cytologic findings in hairy cell leukemia. **A.** Typical hairy cell. The cell is slightly larger than a mature lymphocyte with a round nucleus that has a smooth nuclear contour and lacks a prominent nucleolus. Chromatin is partially condensed and evenly dispersed. Cytoplasm is abundant, gray-blue, agranular, and has a textured appearance. The cytoplasmic margins are irregular with a frayed appearance. Wright stain. **B.** A common variation in the appearance of hairy cells is the nuclear contour that can be oval, reniform (as illustrated), or even lobated. The cell otherwise has features of hairy cell leukemia. Wright stain. **C.** Although rarely a dominant finding, occasional cells are usually present that show the hairy projections embodied in the name of the disease. Wright stain. **D.** The neoplastic cells of hairy cell leukemia consistently show bright positivity for acid phosphatase that is not extinguished by tartrate treatment (tartrate-resistant acid phosphatase). Acid phosphatase stain with tartrate. **E.** Splenic marginal zone lymphoma, also known as splenic lymphoma with villous lymphocytes. The neoplastic cells superficially resemble those in hairy cell leukemia, but have irregularly distributed chromatin, often smudgy, less abundant cytoplasm, which is more basophilic and lacks the textured appearance of the cells in hairy cell leukemia. Rather than the frayed cytoplasmic margins typical of hairy cells, villous lymphocytes generally have a sparse number of irregularly distributed coarse cytoplasmic projections. Wright stain. **F.** Hairy cell leukemia variant. The cells in this rare disorder are generally larger than typical hairy cells. The nuclear chromatin is irregularly distributed and some cells have a single large nucleolus. The cytoplasm can closely resemble that seen in typical hairy cell leukemia. Wright stain. Table 95–1 indicates the CD-surface marker distinctions among the various morphologic cell types shown here with surface projections. *(Robert W. Sharpe, MD, Department of Pathology, Scripps Clinic, LaJolla, CA, generously provided these images.)*

coat) films are positive in 90 percent of cases. Weak to moderate TRAP staining may occur in other diseases, including prolymphocytic leukemia and lymphoma.[55]

ELECTRON MICROSCOPY

In HCL, electron microscopy shows circumferential cytoplasmic projections with fewer and blunter microvilli than seen in splenic lymphoma with circulating B lymphocytes in which the projections tend to be more polarized at one end of the cell.[19,56,57] Ribosome-lamellar complexes can be found in the cytoplasm of hairy cells by transmission electron microscopy in 50 percent of patients (Fig. 95–3).[53] This cytoplasmic inclusion is a cylindrical structure composed of a central hollow space and an outer sheath of multiple parallel lamellae, with ribosomal-like granules in the interlamellar space.[58] These complexes have also been described in other lymphoproliferative disorders.[59]

IMMUNOPHENOTYPIC PROFILE

Hairy cells are mature B cells expressing the pan-B-cell antigens CD19, CD20, and CD22, but not CD21, an antigen lost in the later stages of B-cell development.[16,17,60] Most distinctively, hairy cells express high levels of CD11c, CD22, CD25, and CD103 (Fig. 95–4).[61] The CD11c antigen, the 150-kDa α chain of the 150/95 β_2-integrin that ordinarily is expressed on monocytes and neutrophils,[61,62] stains very potently, with an intensity 30-fold greater than chronic lymphocytic leukemia.[63]

HCL was the first B-cell lymphoproliferative disorder identified that expressed CD25, the interleukin (IL)-2 receptor.[13] CD103 (Bly-7) is the most specific marker for HCL, without any expression on chronic lymphocytic leukemia (CLL) cells.[60] CD103 is also expressed on intraepithelial T lymphocytes as the α^E subunit of the $\alpha^E\beta_7$-integrin.[64]

CD22 is expressed more intensely on hairy cells than in other B-cell chronic lymphoproliferative disorders. CD22 stains 50 times more intensely in HCL than in CLL, in which only weak expression is seen. Weak expression of CD10 (the CALLA antigen) is seen in 26 percent of cases, and weak expression of CD5 is seen in 5 percent of cases. CD5 is the anomalous T-cell antigen strongly expressed on chronic lymphocytic leukemia cells.[60]

Multiparameter immunofluorescence analysis is especially useful for identifying hairy cells because the analysis permits identification of cells coexpressing CD11c, CD25, and CD103 antigens with a pan-B-cell antigen such as CD19, CD20, or CD22.[60] Using flow

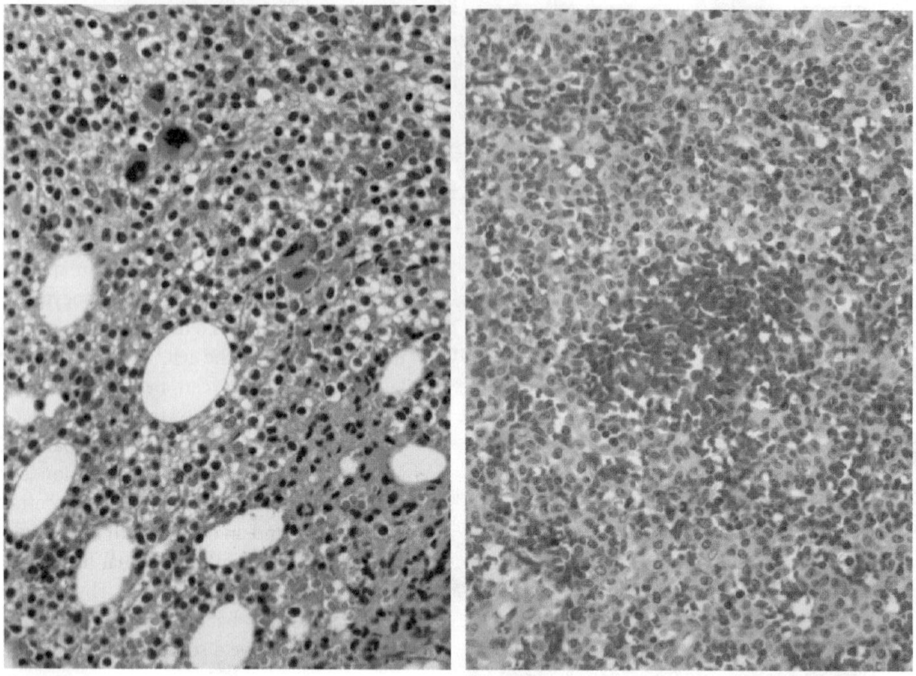

A B

FIGURE 95–2. Histologic findings in hairy cell leukemia. **A.** Marrow. Hairy cell leukemia typically infiltrates the marrow in a diffuse pattern that infiltrates adipose tissue. The infiltrate is monotonous with cells having similar sized nuclei with partially condensed chromatin and lacking prominent nucleoli. Cytoplasm is abundant and pale when stained with hematoxylin and eosin (H&E). This staining pattern results in a striking pale zone around the central nucleus, which resembles a fried egg; hence, the descriptive term "fried-egg pattern" is used for the hairy cell marrow infiltrate. Reticulin staining will usually show a fine meshwork of fibronectin responsible for the difficulty in marrow aspirations of most hairy cell leukemia patients. H&E stain, ×400. **B.** Spleen. Hairy cell leukemia involves the red pulp of the spleen with a histologic appearance that is otherwise similar to the marrow. The neoplastic proliferation disrupts the vascular architecture of the red pulp resulting in the creation of blood-filled spaces lined by hairy cells and referred to as "blood lakes." H&E stain. *(Robert W. Sharpe, MD, Department of Pathology, Scripps Clinic, LaJolla, CA, generously provided these images.)*

cytometry to examine blood lymphocytes, 148 (92%) of 161 patients with HCL had identifiable circulating hairy cells, in some patients representing less than 1 percent of lymphocytes. In contrast, careful morphologic evaluation of blood lymphocytes revealed hairy cells in only 80 percent of patients.[60]

A series of adhesion receptors are strongly expressed on hairy cells. In addition to CD11c and CD103, noted above, CD41d, CD49e, and CD44, which mediate binding to matrix (e.g., fibronectin), are overexpressed.[42]

IMMUNOHISTOCHEMISTRY

Immunohistochemistry performed on marrow biopsy samples can help aid in the diagnosis of HCL and is useful for detecting minimal residual disease following systemic therapies. Most monoclonal antibodies used to detect hairy cells in the blood, including anti-CD103 antibodies, require the marrow be processed by frozen section because the antigens are destroyed by fixation and standard processing.[65] In contrast, the CD20 antibody (L26) and another monoclonal antibody (DBA.44) can be used to stain hairy cells in paraffin sections of the marrow.[66,67] L26 staining is membranous and accentuates the ruffled, abundant cytoplasm of hairy cells, whereas DBA.44, an undefined antigen, stains in both a cytoplasmic granular and a membranous pattern.

CHEMICAL ABNORMALITIES

Abnormal liver function tests occur in 19 percent, azotemia in 27 percent, and hypergammaglobulinemia, possibly monoclonal, in 18 percent of patients.[32] Hypogammaglobulinemia is rare, unlike in CLL. Hairy cells express IL-2 receptor on the cell membrane. Markedly elevated levels of serum soluble IL-2 receptor are present in patients with HCL.[68] The levels decrease with successful therapy. Increased serum levels of soluble CD22 are elevated in patients with HCL.[69] The level of the soluble CD22 correlates with hairy cell burden and spleen size, and normalizes with a complete response to treatment.[69] These two markers, IL-2 receptor and CD22, decrease in proportion to the decrease in the body burden of hairy cells after treatment and are an approximate reflection of response to therapy.

DIFFERENTIAL DIAGNOSIS

HCL should be considered in the differential diagnosis of any disorder resulting in cytopenias and splenomegaly (Table 95–1).

Hairy cell leukemia-variant is a clinicopathologic entity representing a hybrid between prolymphocytic leukemia and HCL. The nucleus of the cell most closely resembles a prolymphocyte and the cytoplasm that of a hairy cell (see Fig. 95–1).[70] HCLv cells generally have higher nuclear to cytoplasmic ratios, more highly condensed chromatin, and more conspicuous central nucleoli than seen in classic HCL.[71] Afflicted individuals who present with massive splenomegaly frequently are in the leukemia phase, and results of TRAP staining are either negative or only very weakly positive. The circulating cells in HCLv usually are CD25-negative and CD103-negative. In the *blastic* variant of HCL, patients have massive splenomegaly, peripheral adenopathy, and cytopenias.[72] The cells are positive with TRAP staining and negative for myeloperoxidase. A newer entity, *hairy B-cell lymphoproliferative disorder*, has been described in Japan.[73] In this disease, patients have splenomegaly without lymphadenopathy. They have persistent lymphocytosis (consisting of abnormal lymphocytes with long microvilli) that is polyclonal, CD25-negative, and only weakly TRAP stain-positive.

Splenic lymphoma with circulating villous lymphocytes, a marginal zone lymphoma, is a closely related disorder that can be difficult to distinguish from HCL. Like patients with HCL, patients with SMZL can present with massive splenomegaly without lymphadenopathy. However, unlike HCL, lymphocytosis is more common.[74] In this disorder, the lymphocytes have more basophilic cytoplasm, and the cytoplasmic projections tend to be polar and more subtle (see Fig. 95–1). Circulating plasmacytoid cells are frequently noted.[19] TRAP staining is either negative or very weakly positive.[53,75] Immunophenotypic analysis identifies cells with strong staining for CD11c, but cells frequently are CD103-negative. Monocytopenia is absent. Sections of spleen show predominant involvement in the white pulp resembling a low-grade lymphoma.[75]

B-cell prolymphocytic leukemia can be confused with HCL. Both disorders occur more often in men and are associated with very enlarged spleens. B-cell prolymphocytic leukemia lymphocytes are only focally TRAP-positive, whereas HCL and HCLv demonstrate strongly positive TRAP staining. In B-cell prolymphocytic leukemia, lymphocyte blood cell counts are typically higher and the leukemia cells are generally CD11c-negative.[76]

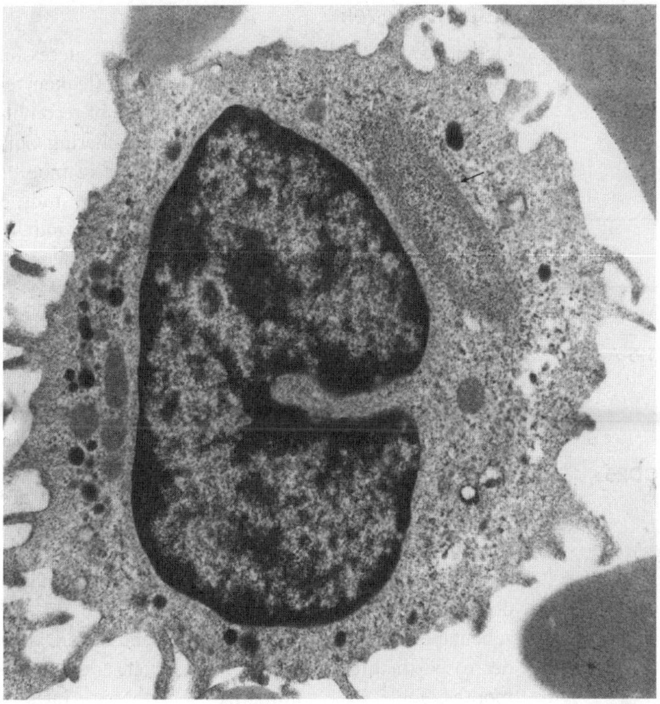

FIGURE 95–3. Transmission electron microscope image of a hairy cell. Nuclear shape is reniform. Heterochromatin is largely confined to areas below the nuclear membrane. Most of the nucleus is filled with euchromatin. The cytoplasm has scattered mitochondria. Occasional micropinocytotic vesicles. The *arrow* points to a characteristic ribosome-lamellar complex, cut longitudinally. The cell membrane shows the characteristic cytoplasmic (hairy) projections. *(From* Lichtman's Atlas of Hematology, *www.accessmedicine.com. Used with permission.)*

Several diseases that present with bi- or tricytopenia and splenomegaly may initially mimic the features of hairy cell leukemia. The most notable is autoimmune myelofibrosis and primary myelofibrosis (see Chap. 91: "Differential Diagnosis").

THERAPY

TREATMENT INDICATIONS

Ninety percent of patients with HCL require treatment at presentation or sometime during the course of the disease. Standard hematologic parameters for initiating therapy in HCL include anemia (hemoglobin <10 g/dL), thrombocytopenia (platelet count $<100 \times 10^9$/L), and neutropenia (absolute neutrophil count $<1.0 \times 10^9$/L), especially when these cytopenias worsen progressively, or are associated with an infection. Other, less-common indications for initiating treatment are symptomatic splenomegaly, leukocytosis with a high proportion of hairy cells (white blood cell count $>20 \times 10^9$/L), bulky or painful lymphadenopathy, vasculitis, bone involvement, or a combination of these factors.

Ten percent of patients, usually elderly males with smaller spleens, normal blood counts, and a lower hairy cell burden, generally do not require treatment for protracted intervals.[77]

PURINE ANALOGUES

Cladribine (2-Chlorodeoxyadenosine)

Cladribine is the treatment of choice for HCL given that single courses of cladribine induce long-lasting complete responses in the vast majority of patients following only a single 7-day infusion (Table 95–2). Relapse rates for complete responders are low, and patients who relapse can be successfully retreated with cladribine. The recommended dose of cladribine is 0.1 mg/kg per day by continuous intravenous infusion for 7 days.[6] Successful administration of subcutaneous,[78] oral,[79] and a weekly intravenous administration of cladribine[80] have been reported.

Response Pattern Long-term followup of 349 evaluable patients who had received cladribine revealed 319 (91%) achieved complete responses and 22 (7%) partial responses; the overall response rate was 98 percent.[81] The overall median duration of response followup was 52 months. Ninety patients (26%) relapsed at a median of 29 months. The time-to-treatment failure rate at 48 months for all 341 responders was 19 percent, 16 percent for complete responders, and 54 percent for partial responders. Of 53 evaluable patients treated with cladribine at first relapse, 33 (62%) achieved complete responses and 14 (26%) achieved partial responses. Thus, patients who relapse can be successfully retreated with cladribine. A followup study of 207 assessable patients with at least 7 years of followup after cladribine treatment revealed that 196 (95%) achieved complete responses and 11 (5%) partial responses after a single course of cladribine. The overall survival rate was 97 percent at 108 months and the median first-response duration for all responders was 98 months.[82]

Side Effects Fever is the principal toxicity of cladribine therapy in HCL, occurring in 42 percent of patients treated. Fever is related to the disappearance of hairy cells and appears most marked in patients with the greatest pretreatment HCL burden, as judged by spleen size. Infections unrelated to a central catheter used to deliver the cladribine are uncommon. Herpes zoster is the most frequently reported late infection.[81] Cladribine also is immunosuppressive, causing a decrease of CD4+ lymphocytes for an extended period of time.[83]

Pentostatin (2′-Deoxycoformycin)

Pentostatin is a very good, second-line drug in the therapy of HCL for the small number of patients intolerant to or unresponsive to cladribine. The standard dose of pentostatin for patients with HCL is 4 mg/m^2 every other week for 3 to 6 months until maximum response is achieved as judged by the blood and marrow hairy cell prevalence, spleen size, and improvement in blood counts.

Characteristics and Response Pattern Pentostatin is a natural product of *Streptomyces antibioticus.* It irreversibly binds to adenosine deaminase. Pentostatin was first shown to have activity in a single patient with HCL in 1984.[84] In the Intergroup Study, which was organized by the National Cancer Institute and reported in 1995, 313 patients with HCL were randomized to either interferon-α_{2A}, 3 mU/m^2 subcutaneously three times per week, which was the principal drug to treat HCL at that time, or pentostatin, 4 mg/m^2 intravenously every 2 weeks.[85] Of 159 patients randomized to interferon, 17 (11%) achieved a complete response and 43 (27%) a partial response; the overall response rate was 38 percent. Of the 154 patients randomized to pentostatin, 117 (76%) achieved a complete response and 4 (3%) a partial response; the overall response rate was 79 percent. Response rates were significantly higher and relapse-free survival was significantly longer for patients who received pentostatin than it was for those who received interferon. The crossover design of the study complicated assessment of differences in overall survival. A long-term followup study of 241 HCL patients who received pentostatin in the Intergroup Study revealed that of 154 patients treated with interferon as initial therapy, 87 crossed over to receive pentostatin after the patients did not respond to initial therapy.[86] The median duration of followup was 9.3 years. The estimated 5- and 10-year survival rates for all patients were 90 percent and 81 percent, respectively. Survival curves for patients initially treated with

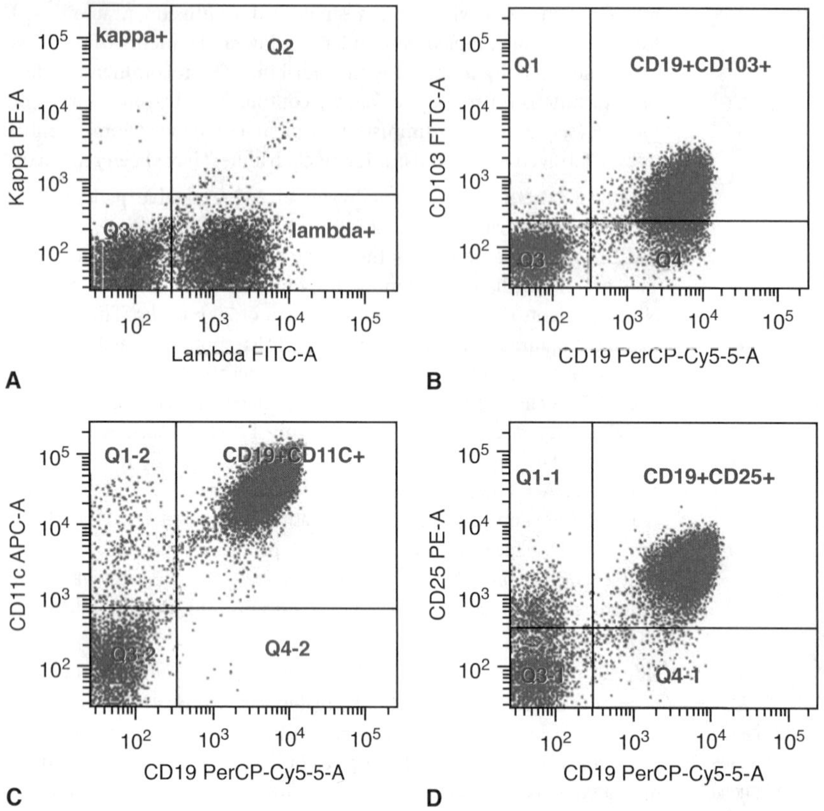

FIGURE 95–4. Flow cytometry in hairy cell leukemia. Hairy cell leukemia has a characteristic immunophenotypic profile that generally permits distinction from other B-cell neoplasms. Hairy cells show immunoglobulin light chain restriction **(A)** with moderate to bright expression of surface immunoglobulin. Hairy cells consistently show **(B)** expression of CD103, **(C)** bright CD11c, and **(D)** CD25, coupled with increased side scatter, reflecting cytoplasmic complexity unusual for lymphocytes. The flow cytometric findings have supplanted TRAP staining as the primary laboratory method for confirmation of the diagnosis of hairy cell leukemia.

pentostatin and then crossed over were similar. The mortality rate and incidence of second malignancies were not higher than expected in the general population. Table 95–2 summarizes the response rates of several pentostatin clinical trials.

Side Effects Pentostatin-induced toxicities include fever, nausea, vomiting, photosensitivity, and keratoconjunctivitis.[87,88] Severe myelosuppression may occur soon after initiation of pentostatin therapy, especially in patients with preexisting myelosuppression.[89,90] Severe infections, including disseminated herpes zoster, *E. coli*, *Haemophilus influenzae*, pneumococcus, and fungal infections, were observed early after initiation of pentostatin.[88] Pentostatin should not be given to patients with active and uncontrolled infections, a poor performance status, or impaired renal function.[91] Pentostatin is strongly immunosuppressive.[92] During pentostatin therapy and for at least 1 year thereafter, CD4 and CD8 lymphocytes can decrease to less than 200 cells/mL.

INTERFERON

Although interferon-α is an active agent against HCL, it does not induce the same high complete-response rates seen with the purine nucleoside analogues. Accordingly, use of interferon-α for treatment of HCL should be reserved for patients who have active infections and, thus, cannot undergo therapy with purine nucleoside analogues initially because of their associated immunosuppression,[48,83] or for patients who have not responded to previous systemic therapy with a cladribine and pentostatin.[93]

Response Pattern

Quesada and colleagues[94] first reported on the successful use of partially purified human interferon-α (leukocyte) in patients with HCL in 1984. In 1986, use of recombinant interferon-α_{2B} interferon (Intron A, Schering Corporation, Kenilworth, NY), at 2 mU/m^2 for 12 months was reported in 64 patients with HCL.[95] In the study, 3 (5%) patients achieved a complete response and 45 (70%) a partial response. Twelve months of interferon-α therapy is optimal because treatment for longer periods does not increase response rates or lower relapse rates, but does increase toxicity.[96,97] Recombinant interferon-α_{2A} (Roferon, Hoffmann-La Roche, Nutley, NJ), which has a cysteine residue at position 23 (α_{2B} has an arginine residue), induced similar response rates when administered to 30 patients with HCL.[98] Median time-to-treatment failure after discontinuation of interferon was 18 to 25 months.[99] The standard dose recommendation for interferon-α_{2B} is 2 mU/m^2 administered subcutaneously three times per week for 12 months. The standard dose recommendation for interferon-α_{2A} is 3 mU/m^2 subcutaneously given daily for 6 months and then decreased to three times per week for an additional 6 months. Table 95–2 summarizes the response rates of several interferon clinical trials.

Side Effects

The most common side effect of interferon is a flu-like syndrome consisting of fever myalgia, and malaise. Acetaminophen often ameliorates these symptoms. An unexpectedly high incidence of second neoplasms in patients after treatment of HCL with interferon-α_{2B} has been reported.[100] Of 69 patients followed for a median of 91 months, 13 patients (19%) developed a second neoplasm; 6 were of hematopoietic origin and 7 were adenocarcinoma. Epidemiologic studies, however, have not established a significantly increased risk of a second malignancy in patients with HCL.[33]

RITUXIMAB

Because hairy cells express the B-cell antigen CD20, rituximab (Rituxan, Biogen Idec, Cambridge, MA), a chimeric humanized mouse anti-CD20 monoclonal antibody, represented a rational therapeutic approach. Rituximab has a role in HCL patients who relapse after cladribine therapy with a response duration of less than 18 months and who demonstrate a significantly hypoplastic marrow or a prior severe opportunistic infection.

Response Pattern

Twenty-four HCL patients who relapsed after treatment with cladribine were treated with rituximab at 375 mg/m^2 intravenously for 4 weeks.[101] Of the 24 patients, 3 (13%) achieved a complete remission and 3 (13%) had a partial response. The principal toxicity was culture-negative febrile neutropenia. At a median followup of 14.6 months, two responders had relapsed. In another study, 15 patients with relapsed or refractory HCL after nucleoside analogues were treated with rituximab, 375 mg/m^2 weekly for 8 weeks.[102] Of the 15 patients, 8 (53%) achieved a complete response, and 4 (26%) had a partial response. Of the 12 responders followed for a median of 32 months, 5 patients progressed. Toxicity was minimal. Combinations of rituximab with a purine analogue have been evaluated as initial therapy and at the time of relapse.[103,104]

TABLE 95–1. Differential Diagnosis of Hairy Cell Leukemia

Parameters	HCL	HCL-Variant	Splenic Lymphoma with Villous Lymphocytes
Blood			
Morphology			
Nuclear shape	Ovoid, reniform	Round	Round
Chromatin	Reticular ± nucleolus	Coarse with central nucleolus	Coarse ± nucleolus
Cytoplasm	Blue-gray, abundant	Blue-gray, abundant	Basophilic, scant to moderate
Monocytopenia	+	–	–
TRAP stain	+++	±	±
Aspirated marrow*	–	+	+
Splenic involvement	Red pulp	Red pulp	White pulp
Flow cytometry			
CD22	+++	++	++
CD11c	+++	++	+
CD25	++	–	±
CD103	++	±	–

–, absent; ±, absent to weakly positive; +, positive; ++, strongly positive; +++, very strongly positive.

*Refers to ease of aspiration of marrow. "–" means usually difficult.

ANTI-CD22 RECOMBINANT IMMUNOTOXIN BL22

Recombinant immunotoxin BL22 is effective for treatment of HCL resistant to cladribine.[105] BL22 contains the variable domain of an anti-CD22 monoclonal antibody fused to a fragment of a *Pseudomonas* exotoxin. Of 16 patients resistant to cladribine, 11 achieved a complete remission and 2 had a partial remission with BL22, for an overall response rate of 81 percent. During a median followup of 16 months, 3 of the 11 complete responders relapsed and 2 of the 16 patients developed a reversible hemolytic–uremic syndrome. Although BL22 is a targeted approach, future use of this agent in HCL might be limited given the potentially life-threatening nature of it toxicity.

SPLENECTOMY

Splenectomy was one of the principal treatments of HCL before the introduction of interferon-α and then the purine analogues, because splenectomy could rapidly reverse blood cytopenias. Ninety percent of patients improved in at least one hematologic parameter, and approximately 50 percent achieved normalization of blood counts.[106,107] Thrombocytopenia was mitigated in 75 percent of patients, usually within days of splenectomy. Splenic size alone is not always predictive of the potential response to splenectomy.[38] The present indications for splenectomy are active and uncontrolled infection, the resolution of which can be rapid and striking because of the salutary effect of the postsplenectomy increase in neutrophils and monocytes coupled with appropriate antimicrobials. The postsplenectomy increase in platelets can eliminate or decrease thrombocytopenic bleeding. Massive, symptomatic splenomegaly, if very troubling to the patient (pain, dragging sensation), may also be an indication for splenectomy. Splenic rupture, an occasional occurrence in HCL, as in any situation, requires removal of the spleen.

RELAPSES AFTER PURINE ANALOGUE THERAPY

In the absence of prospective, randomized clinical trial results in this HCL patient population, the following treatment algorithm is suggested.[101] Patients are retreated at relapse only when they demonstrate significant cytopenias, as defined in "Treatment Indications" above. For patients who achieved a prior cladribine-induced response of greater than 18 months' duration, a repeat course of cladribine generally is recommended because retreatment with cladribine in such patients results in an 88 percent response rate.[87] Second courses of cladribine within a 12-month interval are avoided to prevent the potential for cumulative myelotoxicity. Pentostatin also is a therapeutic alternative in this patient cohort.[108] Nonpurine analogue therapy is recommended for HCL patients who relapse after prior cladribine with a response duration of less than 18 months and who have a significantly hypoplastic marrow or a previous severe opportunistic infection. In these patients, splenectomy, interferon, and rituximab are reasonable therapeutic options.

MINIMAL RESIDUAL DISEASE

Long-term followup studies have documented durable remissions extending beyond 11 years for HCL patients treated with a single 7-day course of cladribine.[87,102,109] Unfortunately, a plateau in the relapse rate has not occurred, suggesting all long-term responders are at risk for late relapse. An explanation for this may be the prevalence of minimal residual disease (MRD) in these patients. Complete responses in HCL studies have historically relied on standard morphologic assessment and TRAP staining. More sensitive immunohistochemical techniques using DBA.44 and L26 monoclonal antibodies have detected MRD in 20 to 50 percent of HCL patients who received cladribine and met standard criteria for a complete response.[110,111] Combination therapy with rituximab and cladribine has eliminated MRD in 90 percent of patients when used at the time of diagnosis.[97] However, a consensus has not been reached on the significance of MRD in HCL.[112,113] Nineteen patients from the Scripps Clinic cladribine database (median disease-free survival: 16 years) who remained in a continuous complete hematologic remission after a single 7-day course of cladribine underwent repeat marrow biopsy. Nine (47%) patients were without MRD, suggesting that some HCL patients may be cured. Ten (53%) had MRD or gross morphologic disease, indicating that patients with residual disease may not progress for many years. Thus the decision to use combination therapy to treat residual disease is not clear cut and may require development of sensitive criteria for evidence of progression.[114]

IRRADIATION

Lytic bone lesions, especially in the proximal femur, can be managed with low-dose irradiation at 1500 to 3000 rads.[115]

GRANULOCYTE COLONY-STIMULATING FACTOR

The first use of recombinant granulocyte colony-stimulating factor (G-CSF) in HCL patients was reported in 1988.[116] Because cladribine treatment of HCL is complicated by neutropenic fever in 42 percent of patients, investigators at the Scripps Clinic treated 35 HCL patients (with comparison to 105 historical controls) with priming G-CSF followed by cladribine and then G-CSF again to determine if G-CSF would reduce neutropenia and febrile episodes.[117] Although G-CSF increased the absolute neutrophil count in patients with HCL and shortened the duration of severe neutropenia after cladribine, the percentage of febrile patients,

TABLE 95–2. Interferon and Purine Nucleoside Analogue Treatment Results in Hairy Cell Leukemia

References	Patients (No.)	Previously Untreated (No.)	Responses: Complete (No.)	Responses: Partial (No.)	Median Disease-Free Survival (months)
Interferon					
Berman et al[97]	23	10	0	16	24
Quesada et al[98]	30	7	9	17	>10
Ratain et al[99]	68	8	9	42	25
Foon et al[118]	14	5	1	12	NR
Rai et al[119]	25	25	7	6	NR
Golomb et al[120]	195	NR	7	152	NR
Grever et al[121]	159	159	17	43	20
Total	514	214 (42%)	50 (10%)	288 (56%)	
Purine Nucleoside Analogues					
A. Pentostatin					
Flinn et al[86]	154	154	117*	5*	>120
Cassileth et al[89]	50	19	32	10	>39
Else et al[108]	187	76†	153	28†	120
Grem et al[122]	66	NR	43	17	>6
Kraut et al[123]	23	10	20	1	13.5
Ho et al[124]	33	33	11	15	>11.5
Total	513	292 (57%)	376 (73%)	76 (15%)	
B. Cladribine					
Saven et al[82]	349	179	319	22	98‡
Else et al[108]	41	18†	31	6†	120
Chadha et al[109]	85	60	67	13	>115
Estey et al[126]	46	27	36	5	>30§
Juliusson et al[127]	16	3	12	0	12
Hoffman et al[128]	49	21	37	12	>55
Total	586	308 (53%)	502 (86%)	58 (10%)	

NR, not reported.

*Data from Grever M, Kopecky K, Foucar MK, et al.[121]

†Data from Else EM, Kurzrock R, Kantarjian HM, et al.[126]

‡Data from Goodman GR, Burian C, Koziol JA, Saven A.[81]

§Data from Seymour J, Kurzrock R, Freireich EJ, et al.[83]

number of febrile days, and frequency of admissions for antibiotics were not statistically different in the two groups. Thus, the routine use of G-CSF following treatment with cladribine does not appear necessary in the absence of severe neutropenia.

COURSE AND PROGNOSIS

The advent of cladribine therapy has resulted in approximately a 90 to 92 percent rate of complete remission and approximately 6 to 8 percent rate of partial response. Prior to the use of interferon and purine nucleoside analogues in the treatment of HCL, patients with HCL had median survivals of 53 months.[75] Purine nucleoside analogue therapy, notably cladribine, has increased overall survival rates at 4 years to greater than 95 percent.[87] Remission durations of longer than 10 years are commonplace. Moreover, relapsed patients have a relatively high response to second courses of cladribine or another agent (see "Cladribine [2-Chlorodeoxyadenosine]" above for further details). Serious infections with a variety of usual and opportunistic organisms, once the cause of death in more than half of patients, are now uncommon. Regardless of the curative potential of purine nucleoside analogue therapy, most patients with HCL can anticipate a long survival.

REFERENCES

1. Bouroncle BA, Wiseman BK, Doan CA: Leukemic reticuloendotheliosis. *Blood* 13:609, 1958.

2. Schrek R, Donnelly WJ: "Hairy" cells in blood in lymphoreticular neoplastic disease and "flagellated" cells of normal lymph nodes. *Blood* 27:199, 1966.
3. Giblett ER, Anderson JE, Cohen F, et al: Adenosine deaminase deficiency in two patients with severely impaired cellular immunity. *Lancet* 2:1067, 1972.
4. Cohen A, Hirshhorn R, Horowitz SD, et al: Deoxyadenosine triphosphate as a potentially toxic metabolite in adenosine deaminase deficiency. *Proc Natl Acad Sci U S A* 75:472, 1978.
5. Carson DA, Wasson DB, Kaye J, et al: Deoxycytidine kinase-mediated toxicity of deoxyadenosine analogs toward malignant human lymphoblasts *in vitro* and toward murine L1210 leukemia *in vivo*. *Proc Natl Acad Sci U S A* 77:6865, 1980.
6. Piro LD, Carrera CJ, Carson DA, Beutler E: Lasting remissions in hairy cell leukemia induced by a single infusion of 2-chlorodeoxyadenosine. *N Engl J Med* 322:1117, 1990.
7. Stewart DJ, Keating MJ: Radiation exposure as a possible etiologic factor in hairy cell leukemia. *Cancer* 46:1577, 1980.
8. Oleske D, Golomb HM, Farber MD, Levy PS: A case-control inquiry into the etiology of hairy cell leukemia. *Am J Epidemiol* 121:675, 1985.
9. Clavel J, Mandereau L, Conso F: Occupational exposure to solvents and hairy cell leukaemia. *Occup Environ Med* 55:59, 1998.
10. Wolf BC, Martin AW, Neiman RS, et al: The detection of Epstein-Barr virus in hairy cell leukemia cells by *in situ* hybridization. *Am J Clin Pathol* 136:717, 1990.
11. Chang KL, Chen YY, Weiss LM: Lack of evidence of Epstein-Barr virus in hairy cell leukemia and monocytoid B-cell lymphoma. *Hum Pathol* 24:58, 1993.
12. Golomb HM: Hairy cell leukemia. An unusual lymphoproliferative disease: A study of 24 patients. *Cancer* 42:946, 1978.
13. Burthem J, Cawley JC: The marrow fibrosis of hairy-cell leukemia is caused by the synthesis and assembly of a fibronectin matrix by the hairy cells. *Blood* 83:497, 1994.
14. Jaffe ES, Shevach EM, Frank MM, et al: Leukemic reticuloendotheliosis: presence of a receptor for cytophilic antibody. *Am J Med* 57:108, 1974.
15. Korsmeyer SJ, Greene WC, Cossman J, et al: Rearrangement and expression of immunoglobulin genes and expression of Tac antigen in hairy cell leukemia. *Proc Natl Acad Sci U S A* 80:4522, 1983.
16. Knapp W DB, Gilks WR, et al: *White Cell Differentiation Antigens*. Oxford University Press, Oxford, 1989.
17. Posnett DN, Wang CY, Chiorazzi N, et al: An antigen characteristic of hairy cell leukemia cells is expressed on certain activated B cells. *J Immunol* 133:1635, 1984.
18. Anderson KC, Boyd AW, Fisher DC, et al: Hairy cell leukemia: A tumor of preplasma cells. *Blood* 65:620, 1985.
19. Wagner SD, Martinelli V, Luzzatto L: Similar patterns of V kappa gene usage but different degrees of somatic mutation in hairy cell leukemia, prolymphocytic leukemia, Waldenström's macroglobulinemia, and myeloma. *Blood* 83:3647, 1994.
20. Chiu A, Xu W, He B, et al: Splenic sinusoids stimulate the survival and proliferation of hairy cell leukemia B cells through BAFF, APRIL, and heparin-sulphate proteoglycans. *Blood* 108:4959, 2006.
21. Catovsky D, O'Brien M, Melo JV, et al: Hairy cell leukemia variant: An intermediate disease between hairy cell leukemia and B prolymphocytic leukemia. *Semin Oncol* 11:362, 1984.
22. Burke JS, Sheibani K: Hairy cells and monocytoid B lymphocytes: Are they related? *Leukemia* 1:298, 1987.
23. Hockley S, Giannouli S, Morilla A, et al: Different IGH rearrangement and somatic hypermutation patterns in hairy-cell leukemia, hairy-cell leukemia variant, and splenic marginal zone lymphoma. *Blood* 110:2082, 2007.
24. Burthem J, Zuzel M, Cawley JC: What is the nature of the hairy cell and why should we be interested? *Br J Haematol* 97:511, 1997.
25. Flandrin G, Sigaux F, Sebahoun G, Bouffette P: Hairy cell leukemia: Clinical presentation and follow-up of 211 patients. *Semin Oncol* 11:458, 1984.
26. Catovsky D: Hairy cell leukemia and prolymphocytic leukemia. *Clin Haematol* 6:245, 1977.
27. Levine PH, Katayama I: The platelet in leukemic reticuloendotheliosis. Functional and morphological evidence of a qualitative disorder. *Cancer* 36:1353, 1975.
28. Katayama I, Finkel HE: Leukemic reticuloendotheliosis. A clinicopathologic study with review of the literature. *Am J Med* 57:115, 1974.
29. Hakimian D, Tallman MS, Hogan DK, et al: Prospective evaluation of internal adenopathy in a cohort of 43 patients with hairy cell leukemia. *J Clin Oncol* 12:268, 1994.
30. Mercieca J, Matutes E, Moskovic E: Massive abdominal lymphadenopathy in hairy cell leukaemia: A report of 12 cases. *Br J Haematol* 82:547, 1992.
31. Quesada JR, Keating MJ, Libshitz HI, Llamas L: Bone involvement in hairy cell leukemia. *Am J Med* 74:228, 1983.
32. Dorsey JK, Penick GD: The association of hairy cell leukemia with unusual immunologic disorders. *Arch Intern Med* 142:902, 1982.
33. Kraut EH: Clinical manifestations and infectious complications of hairy-cell leukaemia. *Best Pract Res Clin Haematol* 16:33, 2003.
34. Remková A, Halcín A, Stenová E, et al: Acute vasculitis as a first manifestation of hairy cell leukemia. *Eur J Intern Med* 18:238, 2007.
35. Goyette RE: Hairy cell leukemia, in *Hematology: A Comprehensive Guide to the Diagnosis and Treatment of Blood Disorders*, edited by RE Goyette, p 576. PMIC, Los Angeles, 1997.
36. Siegal FP, Shodell M, Shah K, et al: Impaired interferon alpha response in hairy cell leukemia is corrected by therapy with 2-chloro-2′-deoxyadenosine: Implications for susceptibility to opportunistic infections. *Leukemia* 8:1474, 1994.
37. Turner A, Kjeldsberg CR: Hairy cell leukemia: A review. *Medicine (Baltimore)* 57:477, 1978.
38. Golomb HM, Vardiman JW: Response to splenectomy in 65 patients with hairy cell leukemia: An evaluation of spleen weight and marrow involvement. *Blood* 61:349, 1983.
39. Seshadri RS, Brown EJ, Zipursky A: Leukemic reticuloendotheliosis. A failure of monocyte production. *N Engl J Med* 295:181, 1976.
40. Lindemann A, Ludwig WD, Oster W: High-level secretion of tumor necrosis factor-alpha contributes to hematopoietic failure in hairy cell leukemia. *Blood* 73:880, 1989.
41. Bartl R, Frisch B, Hill W: Marrow histology in hairy cell leukemia. *Am J Clin Pathol* 79:531, 1983.
42. Zuzel M, Cawley JC: The biology of hairy cells. *Best Pract Res Clin Haematol* 16:1, 2003.
43. Burke JS: The value of the bone-marrow biopsy in the diagnosis of hairy cell leukemia. *J Clin Pathol* 70:876, 1978.
44. Aziz KA, Till KJ, Zuzel M, Cawley JC: Involvement of CD44-hyaluronan interaction in malignant cell homing and fibronectin synthesis in hairy cell leukemia. *Blood* 96:3161, 2000.
45. Sambani C, Trafalis DT, Mitsoulis-Mentzikoff C, et al: Clonal chromosome rearrangements in hairy cell leukemia: Personal experience and review of literature. *Cancer Genet Cytogenet* 129:138, 2001.
46. Haglund U, Juliusson G, Stellan B, Gahrton G: Hairy cell leukemia is characterized by clonal chromosome abnormalities clustered to specific regions. *Blood* 83:2637, 1994.
47. Wu X, Ivanova G, Merup M, et al: Molecular analysis of the human chromosome 5q13.3 region in patients with hairy cell leukemia and identification of tumor suppressor gene candidates. *Genomics* 60:161, 1999.
48. Kraut EH, Neff JC, Bouroncle BA, et al: Immunosuppressive effects of pentostatin. *J Clin Oncol* 8:848, 1990.
49. Burthem J, Baker PK, Hunt JA, Cawley JC: The function of c-fms in hairy-cell leukemia: Macrophage colony-stimulating factor stimulates hairy-cell movement. *Blood* 83:1381, 1994.
50. Burthem J, Baker PK, Cawley JC: Hairy cell interactions with extracellular matrix: Expression of specific integrin receptors and their role in the cell's response to specific adhesive proteins. *Blood* 84:873, 1994.
51. Nanba K, Soban EJ, Bowling MC, Berard CW: Splenic pseudosinuses and hepatic angiomatous lesions: Distinctive features of hairy cell leukemia. *Am J Clin Pathol* 67:415, 1977.
52. Vardiman JW, Golomb HM: Autopsy findings in hairy cell leukemia. *Semin Oncol* 11:370, 1984.
53. Yam LT, Janckila AJ, Li CY, Lam WKW: Cytochemistry of tartrate resistant acid phosphatase: Fifteen years' experience. *Leukemia* 1:285, 1987.
54. Li CY, Yam LT, Lam KW: Studies of acid phosphatase isoenzymes in human leukocytes: Demonstration of isoenzyme specificity. *J Histochem Cytochem* 18:901, 1970.
55. Drexler HG, Gaedicke G, Minowade J: Isoenzyme studies in human leukemia-lymphoma cell lines: II. Acid phosphatase. *Leuk Res* 9:537, 1985.
56. Katayama I, Li CY, Yam LT: Ultrastructural characteristics of the "hairy cells" of leukemic reticuloendotheliosis. *Am J Pathol* 361:370, 1972.
57. Melo JV, Robinson DS, Gregory C, Catovsky D: Splenic B cell lymphoma with "villous" lymphocytes in the peripheral blood: A disorder distinct from hairy cell leukemia. *Leukemia* 1:294, 1987.
58. Rosner MC, Golomb HM: Ribosome-lamella complex in hairy cell leukemia. Ultrastructure and distribution. *Lab Invest* 42:236, 1980.
59. Brunning RD, Parkin J: Ribosome-lamella complexes in neoplastic hematopoietic cells. *Am J Pathol* 79:565, 1975.
60. Robbins BA, Ellison DJ, Spinosa JC, et al: Diagnostic application of two-color flow cytometry in 161 cases of hairy cell leukemia. *Blood* 82: 1277, 1993.
61. Visser L, Shaw A, Slupsky J, et al: Monoclonal antibodies reactive with hairy cell leukemia. *Blood* 74:320, 1989.
62. Schwarting R, Stein H, Wang CY: The monoclonal antibodies alpha SHCL-1 (alpha Leu-14) and alpha S-HCL-3 (alpha Leu-M5) allow the diagnosis of hairy cell leukemia. *Blood* 65:974, 1985.
63. Hanson CA, Gribbin TE, Schnitzer B, et al: CD11c (LEU-M5) expression characterizes a B-cell chronic lymphoproliferative disorder with features of both chronic lymphocytic leukemia and hairy cell leukemia. *Blood* 76:2360, 1990.
64. Cepek KL, Parker CM, Madara JL, et al: Integrin alpha E beta 7 mediates adhesion of T lymphocytes to epithelial cells. *J Immunol* 150:3459, 1993.
65. Thaler J, Denz H, Dietze O, et al: Immunohistological assessment of marrow biopsies from patients with hairy cell leukemia: Changes following treatment with alpha-2-interferon and deoxycoformycin. *Leuk Res* 13:377, 1989.
66. Stroup R, Sheibani K: Antigenic phenotypes of hairy cell leukemia and monocytoid B-cell lymphoma. An immunohistochemical evaluation of 66 cases. *Hum Pathol* 23:172, 1992.
67. Hounieu H, Chittal SM, al Saati T, et al: Hairy cell leukemia. Diagnosis of marrow involvement in paraffin-embedded sections with monoclonal antibody DBA.44. *Am J Clin Pathol* 98:26, 1992.
68. Steis RG, Marcon L, Clark J, et al: Serum soluble IL-2 receptor as a tumor marker in patients with hairy cell leukemia. *Blood* 77:1304, 1988.
69. Matsushita K, Margulies I, Onda M, et al: Soluble CD22 as a tumor marker for hairy cell leukemia. *Blood* 112:2272, 2008.
70. Sainati L, Matutes E, Mulligan S, et al: A variant form of hairy cell leukemia resistant to alpha-interferon: Clinical and phenotype characteristics of 17 patients. *Blood* 76:157, 1990.
71. Cawley JC, Burns GF, Hayhoe RGH: A chronic lymphoproliferative disorder with distinctive features: A distinct variant of hairy cell leukemia. *Leuk Res* 4:547, 1980.

72. Diez-Martin JL, Li CY, Banks PM: Blastic variant of hairy cell leukemia. *Am J Clin Pathol* 87:576, 1987.
73. Machii T, Yamaguchi M, Inoue R, et al: Polyclonal B-cell lymphocytosis with features resembling hairy cell leukemia-Japanese variant. *Blood* 89:2008, 1997.
74. Sun T, Susin M, Brody J: Splenic lymphoma with circulating villous lymphocytes: Report of seven cases and review of the literature. *Am J Clin Pathol* 45:39, 1994.
75. Yam LT, Li CY, Lam KW: Tartrate-resistant acid phosphatase isoenzyme in the reticulum cells of leukemic reticuloendotheliosis. *N Engl J Med* 284:357, 1971.
76. Slovak ML, Weiss LM, Nathwan BN: Cytogenetic studies of composite lymphomas: Monocytoid B-cell lymphoma and other B-cell non-Hodgkin's lymphomas. *Hum Pathol* 24:1086, 1993.
77. Golomb HM, Catovsky D, Golde DW: Hairy cell leukemia: A clinical review of 71 cases. *Ann Intern Med* 89:677, 1978.
78. Juliusson G, Heldal D, Hippe E, et al: Subcutaneous injections of 2-chlorodeoxyadenosine for symptomatic hairy cell leukemia. *J Clin Oncol* 13:989, 1995.
79. Juliusson G, Christiansen I, Hansen MM, et al: Oral cladribine as primary therapy for patients with B-cell chronic lymphocytic leukemia. *J Clin Oncol* 14:2160, 1996.
80. Robak T, Jamroziak K, Gora-Tybor J, et al: Cladribine in a weekly versus daily schedule for untreated active hairy cell leukemia: final report from the Polish Adult Leukemia Group (PALG) of a prospective, randomized, multicenter trial. *Blood* 109:3672, 2007.
81. Goodman GR, Burian C, Koziol JA, Saven A: Extended follow-up of patients with hairy cell leukemia after treatment with cladribine. *J Clin Oncol* 21:891, 2003.
82. Saven A, Burian C, Koziol JA, Piro LD: Long-term follow-up of patients with hairy cell leukemia after cladribine treatment. *Blood* 92:1918, 1998.
83. Seymour J, Kurzrock R, Freireich EJ, Estey EH: 2-Chlorodeoxyadenosine induces durable remissions and prolonged suppression of CD4+ lymphocyte counts in patients with hairy cell leukemia. *Blood* 83:2906, 1994.
84. Spiers ASD, Parekh SJ: Complete remission in hairy cell leukemia achieved with pentostatin. *Lancet* 1:1080, 1984.
85. Grever M, Kopecky K, Foular K: Randomization comparison of pentostatin versus interferon alpha-2a in previously untreated patients with hairy cell leukemia. *J Clin Oncol* 13:974, 1995.
86. Flinn IW, Kopecky KJ, Foucar MK, et al: Long-term follow-up of remission duration, mortality, and second malignancies in hairy cell leukemia patients treated with pentostatin. *Blood* 96:2981, 2000.
87. Spiers ASD, Parekh SJ, Bishop MB: Hairy cell leukemia: Induction of complete remission with pentostatin (2′-deoxycoformycin). *J Clin Oncol* 2:1336, 1984.
88. Johnston JB, Glazer RI, Pugh L, Israels LG: The treatment of hairy cell leukemia with 2′-deoxycoformycin. *Br J Haematol* 63:525, 1986.
89. Cassileth PA, Cheuvant B, Spiers ASD, et al: Pentostatin induces durable remissions in hairy cell leukemia. *J Clin Oncol* 9:243, 1991.
90. Ho AD, Thaler J, Stryckmans P, et al: Pentostatin in refractory chronic lymphocytic leukemia: A phase II trial of the European Organization for Research and Treatment of Cancer. *J Natl Cancer Inst* 82:1416, 1990.
91. Spiers ASD, Moore D, Cassileth PA, et al: Remissions in hairy cell leukemia with pentostatin (2′-deoxycoformycin). *N Engl J Med* 316: 825, 1987.
92. Urba WJ, Baseler MW, Kopp WC, et al: Deoxycoformycin-induced immunosuppression in patients with hairy cell leukemia. *Blood* 73:38, 1989.
93. Seymour JF, Estey EH, Keating MJ, Kurzrock R: Response to interferon-a in patients with hairy cell leukemia relapsing after treatment with 2-chlorodeoxyadenosine. *Leukemia* 9:929, 1995.
94. Quesada JR, Reuben J, Manning JT, et al: Alpha-interferon for induction of remission in hairy cell leukemia. *N Engl J Med* 310:15, 1984.
95. Golomb HM, Jacobs A, Fefer A, et al: Alpha-2 interferon therapy of hairy cell leukemia: A multicenter study of 64 patients. *J Clin Oncol* 4: 900, 1986.
96. Golomb HM, Ratain MJ, Fefer A, et al: Randomized study of the duration of treatment with interferon alfa-2b in patients with hairy cell leukemia. *J Natl Cancer Inst* 80:369, 1988.
97. Berman E, Heller G, Kempin S, et al: Incidence of response and long-term follow-up in patients with hairy cell leukemia with recombinant alpha-2a. *Blood* 75:839, 1990.
98. Quesada JR, Hersh E M, Manning J, et al: Treatment of hairy cell leukemia with recombinant alpha-interferon. *Blood* 68:493, 1986.
99. Ratain MJ, Golomb HM, Vardiman JW, et al: Relapse after interferon alpha-2b therapy for hairy cell leukemia: Analysis of diagnostic variables. *J Clin Oncol* 6:1714, 1988.
100. Kampmeier P, Spielberger R, Dickstein J, et al: Increased incidence of second neoplasms in patients treated with interferon a-2b for hairy cell leukemia: A clinicopathologic assessment. *Blood* 83:2931, 1994.
101. Nieva J, Bethel K, Saven A: Phase 2 study of rituximab in the treatment of cladribine-failed patients with hairy cell leukemia. *Blood* 102:810, 2003.
102. Thomas DA, O'Brian S, Bueso-Ramos C, et al: Rituximab in relapsed or refractory hairy cell leukemia. *Blood* 102:3906, 2003.
103. Else M, Osuji N, Forconi F, et al: The role of rituximab in combination with pentostatin or cladribine for the treatment of recurrent/refractory hairy cell leukemia. *Cancer* 110:2240, 2007.
104. Ravandi F, Jorgensen JL, O'Brien S, et al: Eradication of minimal residual disease in hairy cell leukemia. *Blood* 107:4658, 2006.
105. Kreitman RJ, Wilson WH, Bergeron K, et al: Efficacy of the anti-CD22 recombinant immunotoxin BL22 in chemotherapy-resistant hairy-cell leukemia. *N Engl J Med* 345:241, 2001.
106. Mintz U, Golomb HM: Splenectomy as initial therapy in twenty-six patients with leukemic reticuloendotheliosis (hairy cell leukemia). *Cancer Res* 39:2366, 1979.
107. Jansen J, Hermans J: Splenectomy in hairy cell leukemia: A retrospective multicenter analysis. *Cancer* 47:2066, 1981.
108. Else M, Dearden CE, Matutes E, et al: Long-term follow-up of 228 hairy cell leukemia patients treated with pentostatin or cladribine with 15.4 years median time from diagnosis. *Blood* 112:731, 2008.
109. Chadha P, Rademaker AW, Mendiratta P, et al: Treatment of hairy cell leukemia with 2-chlorodeoxyadenosine (2-CdA): long-term follow-up of the Northwestern University experience. *Blood* 106:241, 2005.
110. Ellison DJ, Sharpe RW, Robbins BA, et al: Immunomorphologic analysis of bone marrow biopsies after treatment with 2-chlorodeoxyadenosine for hairy cell leukemia. *Blood* 84:4310, 1994.
111. Hakimian D, Tallman MS, Kiley C, Peterson L: Detection of minimal residual disease by immunostaining of bone marrow biopsies after 2-chlorodeoxyadenosine for hairy cell leukemia. *Blood* 82:1798, 1993.
112. Tallman MS, Hakimian D, Kopecky KJ, et al: Minimal residual disease in patients with hairy cell leukemia in complete remission treated with 2-chlorodeoxyadenosine or 2′-deoxycoformycin and prediction of early relapse. *Clin Cancer Res* 5:1665, 1999.
113. Matutes E, Meeus P, McLennan K, Catovsky D: The significance of minimal residual disease in hairy cell leukaemia treated with deoxycoformycin: a long-term follow-up study. *Br J Haematol* 98:375, 1997.
114. Sigal D, Sharpe R, Burian C, Saven A: Potential curability of cladribine in selected patients with hairy cell leukemia. *J Clin Oncol* 26:702s, 2008.
115. Lembersky BC, Ratain MJ, Golomb HM: Skeletal complications in hairy cell leukemia: Diagnosis and therapy. *J Clin Oncol* 6:1280, 1988.
116. Glaspy JA, Baldwin GC, Robertson PA, et al: Therapy for neutropenia in hairy cell leukemia with recombinant human granulocyte colony-stimulating factor. *Ann Intern Med* 109:789, 1988.
117. Saven A, Burian C, Adusumalli J, Koziol JA: Filgrastim for cladribine-induced neutropenic fever in patients with hairy cell leukemia. *Blood* 93:2471, 1999.
118. Foon KA, Maluish AE, Abrams PG, et al: Recombinant leukocyte alpha interferon therapy for advanced hairy cell leukemia. Therapeutic and immunologic results. *Am J Med* 80:351, 1986.
119. Rai K, Mick R, Ozer H, et al: Alpha-interferon therapy in untreated active hairy cell leukemia: A Cancer and Leukemia Group B (CALGB) study [abstract]. *Proc Am Soc Clin Oncol* 6:159, 1987.
120. Golomb H, Fefer A, Golde D, et al: Update of a multi-institutional study of 195 patients (pts) with hairy cell leukemia (HCL) treated with interferon alfa-2b (IFN) [abstract]. *Proc Am Soc Clin Oncol* 6:215, 1990.
121. Grever M, Kopecky K, Foucar MK, et al: Randomized comparison of pentostatin versus interferon alfa-2a in previously untreated patients with hairy cell leukemia: An Intergroup Study. *J Clin Oncol* 13:974, 1995.
122. Grem J, King S, Cheson B, et al: Pentostatin in hairy cell leukemia: Treatment by the special exception mechanism. *J Natl Cancer Inst* 81:448, 1989.
123. Kraut EH, Bouroncle BA, Grever MR: Pentostatin in the treatment of advanced hairy cell leukemia. *J Clin Oncol* 7:168, 1989.
124. Ho AD, Thaler J, Mandelli F, et al: Response to pentostatin in hairy-cell leukemia refractory to interferon-alpha: the European Organization for Research and Treatment of Cancer Leukemia Cooperative Group. *J Clin Oncol* 7:1533, 1989.
125. Else M, Ruchlemer R, Osuji N, et al: Long remissions in hairy cell leukemia with purine analogs: A report of 219 patients with a median follow-up of 12.5 years. *Cancer* 104:2442, 2005.
126. Estey EM, Kurzrock R, Kantarjian HM, et al: Treatment of hairy cell leukemia with 2-chlorodeoxyadenosine (2-CdA). *Blood* 79:882, 1992.
127. Juliusson G, Liliemark J: Rapid recovery from cytopenia in hairy cell leukemia after treatment with 2-chloro-2′-deoxyadenosine (CdA): Relation to opportunistic infections. *Blood* 79:888, 1992.
128. Hoffman MA, Janson D, Rose E, Rai KR: Treatment of hairy cell leukemia with cladribine: Response, toxicity and long-term follow-up. *J Clin Oncol* 15:1138, 1997.

CHAPTER 96
LARGE GRANULAR LYMPHOCYTIC LEUKEMIA

Thomas P. Loughran and Marshall E. Kadin

SUMMARY

Clonal diseases of larger granular lymphocytes (LGLs) can arise from either T cells or natural killer (NK) cells. Although T-LGL and NK-LGL cells have a similar morphology, they have distinctive surface antigen phenotypes and represent two discrete diseases with different clinical features and clinical outcomes. T-LGL leukemia is defined as a clonal proliferation of CD3+ LGL; NK-LGL leukemia is defined as a clonal proliferation of CD3– LGL. The clinical presentation of NK-LGL leukemia is different from that of T-LGL leukemia. Patients with NK-LGL leukemia usually are younger, more often have systemic B symptoms, and typically have more massive hepatosplenomegaly. Lymphadenopathy and gastrointestinal tract involvement are common. Examination of the blood film is important in making the diagnosis of T-LGL leukemia because approximately 25 percent of patients do not have an increased total lymphocyte count. Most patients with T-LGL leukemia have chronic neutropenia, and approximately half have neutrophil counts less than 500/μL (0.5×10^9/L). In contrast, less than one-fifth of patients with NK-LGL have severe neutropenia. Anemia is observed in 50 percent and 100 percent of cases of T-LGL and NK-LGL leukemia, respectively. Patients with T-LGL leukemia frequently have humoral immune abnormalities, such as elevated rheumatoid factor, and red cell aplasia may occur. Morbidity and mortality usually result as the consequence of recurrent and sometimes lethal infections secondary to severe chronic neutropenia. In contrast to the chronic course of T-LGL leukemia, NK-LGL leukemia has an acute presentation and poor clinical outcome. Most patients die within 2 months of diagnosis from disseminated disease with multiorgan failure despite aggressive combination chemotherapy.

DEFINITION AND HISTORY

Large granular lymphocytic (LGL) leukemia was initially described in 1985 as a clonal disorder involving blood, marrow, liver, and spleen.[1] LGLs comprise 10 to 15 percent of normal blood mononuclear cells and may be of either CD3– (natural killer [NK] cell) or CD3+ (T-cell) lineage. LGL leukemia is of two types: *T-LGL leukemia* and *NK-LGL leukemia*, reflecting different cellular origins.[2,3] T-LGL leukemia is defined as a clonal proliferation of CD3+ LGL; NK-LGL leukemia is defined as a clonal proliferation of CD3– LGL. T-cell receptor gene rearrangement studies are useful for confirming the clonality of T-LGL leukemia. NK cell leukemia also is a clonal disease, as demonstrated by cytogenetics.[4] However, NK cells and NK cell leukemia lack convenient clonal markers, such as antigen receptor gene rearrangements.

Acronyms and abbreviations that appear in this chapter include: CD, cluster of differentiation; CMV, cytomegalovirus; CTL, cytotoxic T lymphocytes; HLA, human leukocyte antigen; HTLV, human T-cell leukemia virus; KIR, killer immunoglobulin-like receptor; LGL, large granular lymphocyte; NK, natural killer cell; NK-LGL, natural killer cell large granular lymphocyte; PI3K, phosphatidylinositol 3′-kinase; STAT, signal transducer and activator of transcription; TCR, T-cell receptor; T-LGL, T-cell large granular lymphocyte.

ETIOLOGY AND PATHOGENESIS

The etiology of T-LGL leukemia is unknown. Infection with human T-cell leukemia virus (HTLV)-II has been detected in two patients.[5] However, most patients are not infected with members of this retroviral family, including the two more recently discovered HTLV viruses, HTLV-III and HTLV-IV.[6] Nevertheless, serologic findings show frequent reactivity to the BA-21 epitope of the p21e *env* protein of HTLV-I, suggesting that a cellular or retroviral protein with homology to BA-21 may be important in pathogenesis.[5] Evidence implicates cytomegalovirus (CMV) as the inciting antigen in the rare CD4+ subset of LGL leukemia.[7] Epstein-Barr virus infection has been implicated in the pathogenesis of NK-LGL leukemia.[8] Leukemic LGL show many characteristics of antigen-activated cytotoxic T lymphocytes (CTLs), suggesting that an initial step in LGL expansion is an antigen-driven mechanism.[9–11] Normal CTLs are regulated through apoptosis. Leukemic LGL constitutively express high levels of Fas (CD95) and Fas ligand (CD178), yet are resistant to Fas-mediated death.[12] Constitutive activation of survival signaling pathways is a central pathogenetic mechanism in LGL leukemia. Evidence for importance of signal transducer and activator of transcription (STAT)-3/Mcl-1, phosphatidylinositol 3′-kinase (PI3K)/AKT, and sphingolipid signaling leading to apoptotic resistance have all been demonstrated.[13–15] Utilizing a network modeling approach, it was found that interleukin-15 and platelet-derived growth factor are the two key mediators controlling interactions amongst these survival pathways.[16] Disease manifestations such as neutropenia are related, at least in part, to circulating CD178 in these patients.[17] Targeting of normal tissue by leukemic LGL may also play a role in disease pathogenesis. Lysis of endothelial cells resulting from activation of NK receptors via signaling partners DAP10 and DAP12 might explain development of pulmonary hypertension observed in some patients with LGL leukemia.[18]

CLINICAL FEATURES

Table 96–1 summarizes the clinical features of T-LGL leukemia. Rheumatoid arthritis might be a prominent feature of LGL leukemia, sometimes resulting in a clinical picture resembling that of Felty syndrome (see Chap. 65).[19] The clinical presentation of NK-LGL leukemia is different from that of T-LGL leukemia. Patients with NK-LGL leukemia usually are younger, more often have systemic B symptoms, which are classified as fever over 38°C for at least 3 days, unintended weight loss of greater than 10 percent of body weight, and drenching sweats, usually at night, and typically have more massive hepatosplenomegaly. Lymphadenopathy and gastrointestinal tract involvement are common.[20] Pulmonary hypertension has developed in occasional cases.[18]

LABORATORY FEATURES

■ HEMATOLOGIC FINDINGS

Examination of the blood film is important in making the diagnosis of T-LGL leukemia because approximately 25 percent of patients do not have an increased total lymphocyte count.[3] LGL can be identified by morphology, although immunophenotyping is necessary to distinguish whether the LGLs are of T-cell or NK-cell lineage (Fig. 96–1). The median LGL count of patients with T-LGL leukemia, however, is 4200/μL (4.2×10^9/L). Patients with NK-LGL leukemia generally have much higher LGL counts, sometimes exceeding 50,000/μL (50.0×10^9/L).

TABLE 96–1. Clinical Features of CD3-Positive Large Granular Lymphocytic Leukemia

Feature	Percent of Cases
Recurrent infections	~30
B symptoms (fever, sweats, weight loss)	~25
Splenomegaly	~35
Hepatomegaly	~12
Lymphadenopathy	~2

TABLE 96–2. Serologic Findings in CD3-Positive Large Granular Lymphocytic Leukemia

Feature	Percent of Patients
Rheumatoid factor	~60
Circulating immune complexes	~50
Antinuclear antibody	~40
Antineutrophil antibody	~40
Polyclonal hypergammaglobulinemia	~25
Positive direct antiglobulin (Coombs) test	~15
Monoclonal gammopathy	~8

Most patients (84%) with T-LGL leukemia have chronic neutropenia, and approximately 48 percent have neutrophil counts less than 500/μL (0.5 × 10^9/L).[3] In contrast, 18 percent of patients with NK-LGL have severe neutropenia.[3] Anemia is observed in 50 percent and 100 percent of cases of T-LGL and NK-LGL leukemia, respectively. Red cell aplasia (see Chap. 35) and Coombs-positive hemolytic anemia (see Chap. 53) are seen with T-LGL leukemia.[1,2,] LGL leukemia is the most commonly associated disease in patients with red cell aplasia.[21] The role of large granular lymphocytes in the suppression of erythropoiesis in a patient with LGL leukemia was established by showing that the suppression of LGL leukemia cells *in vivo* or the removal of these cells *in vitro* restored erythropoiesis by releasing the inhibition of an erythroid progenitor at a level between the burst-forming unit– and colony-forming unit–erythroid.[22] The role of cells with T-cell antigens also was established by the response to antithymocyte globulin.[23] An occasional patient seemed to have suppression of erythropoiesis by a humoral immune mechanism.[23] A rare case of both amegakaryocytic thrombocytopenia and red cell aplasia has occurred and responded to immunotherapy.[24] Anemia associated with NK-LGL leukemia is most likely a result of marrow infiltration. Thrombocytopenia and coagulopathy are features of NK-LGL leukemia.[3] Moderate thrombocytopenia occurring with T-LGL leukemia can resemble immune thrombocytopenic purpura (see Chap. 119).[1]

IMMUNOPHENOTYPING

Immunophenotyping can be used to distinguish T-LGL leukemia from NK-LGL leukemia. T-leukemic LGLs usually are CD3+, CD4–, CD8+, CD16+, CD56–, CD57+, and often human leukocyte antigen (HLA)-DR+. Less commonly, leukemic LGLs express CD4 with variable CD8 expression.[25] Leukemic T-LGL usually express the T-cell receptor (TCR) $\alpha\beta$+ heterodimer, although cases with similar clinical features have been described that express the $\gamma\delta$ TCR heterodimer.[26] In contrast to normal LGL of T-cell origin, leukemic LGL express significantly lower levels of CD5 and show abnormal killer immunoglobulin-like receptor (KIR) expression.[27] NK-leukemic LGL usually are CD3–, CD4–, CD8–, CD16+, CD56+, and CD57–.[8]

Twenty cases of a $\gamma\delta$ T-cell LGL variant of $\alpha\beta$ T-cell LGL leukemia have been described.[26] When compared to cases with the $\alpha\beta$ T-cell subtype, which represents the majority of T-cell LGL leukemias, the clinical findings were similar in the two groups insofar as age and sex distribution, frequency of recurrent infections, and the association with autoimmune diseases, especially rheumatoid arthritis. Approximately 50 percent of the $\gamma\delta$ T-cell LGL leukemia cells expressed CD3+ CD8+/CD16+/CD57+. The clinical course was relatively indolent; 85 percent of patients were alive at 3 years. Fifty percent of patients with $\gamma\delta$ T-cell LGL leukemia required treatment, and about half of those responded. $\gamma\delta$ and $\alpha\beta$ T-cell LGL leukemia are each best considered an antigen-driven T-cell lymphoproliferation.[26]

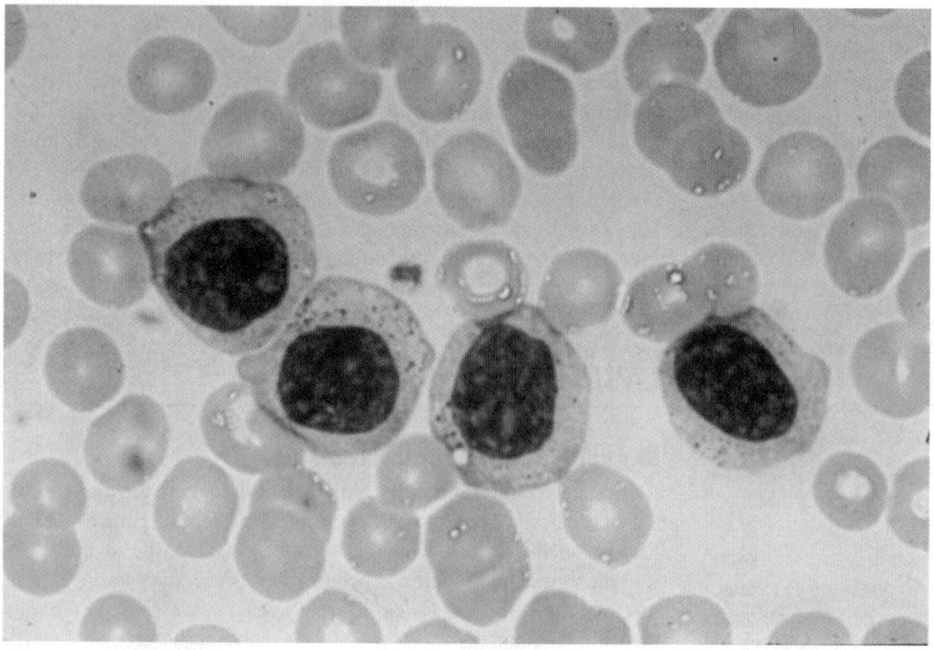

FIGURE 96–1. Four LGL in blood film have abundant pale blue cytoplasm containing large azurophilic granules and a single nucleus with clumped chromatin and one or two pale nucleoli (Giemsa stain). *(Used with permission from Bruce Cheson, MD.)*

IMMUNE ABNORMALITIES

Patients with T-LGL leukemia frequently have humoral immune abnormalities, including positive tests for rheumatoid factor (sometimes with rheumatoid arthritis), antinuclear antibodies, antineutrophil cytoplasmic antibodies, polyclonal hypergammaglobulinemia, hypogammaglobulinemia, circulating immune complexes, autoimmune hemolytic anemia, autoimmune thrombocytopenic purpura, and immune red cell aplasia (Table 96–2). These patients also may have defects in cellular immunity, such as diminished NK activity.[1] Immune function has not been evaluated in most patients with NK-LGL leukemia.

B-CELL MALIGNANCIES

Coexisting clonal B-cell disorders have been found in about one-quarter of patients with LGL-leukemia.[28] These were principally essential monoclonal gammopathy and chronic lymphocytic leukemia, with one case of follicular lymphoma. The coassociation of B-cell neoplasms with T-cell LGL leukemia was interpreted as the result of either a common antigen that drives clonal B and T cells, or a B-cell malignancy serving as the stimulus for lymphocyte expansion representing deviant antitumor surveillance.[26]

HISTOPATHOLOGIC FEATURES

The marrow biopsy in T-LGL may contain nodules of B lymphocytes and scattered LGL, which are better seen in the aspirate. Various superimposed findings may reflect secondary immune diseases such as granulocyte maturation arrest and absence of red cell precursors (red cell aplasia). T-LGL leukemia invariably affects the spleen, where the major findings are leukemic cell infiltration of the red pulp cords and sinuses, plasma cell hyperplasia, and prominent germinal centers (Fig. 96–2).[1,29] Hepatic sinusoids and portal areas are infiltrated by LGL. Lymph nodes usually are not involved but can have expanded paracortical areas containing plasma cells and LGL.

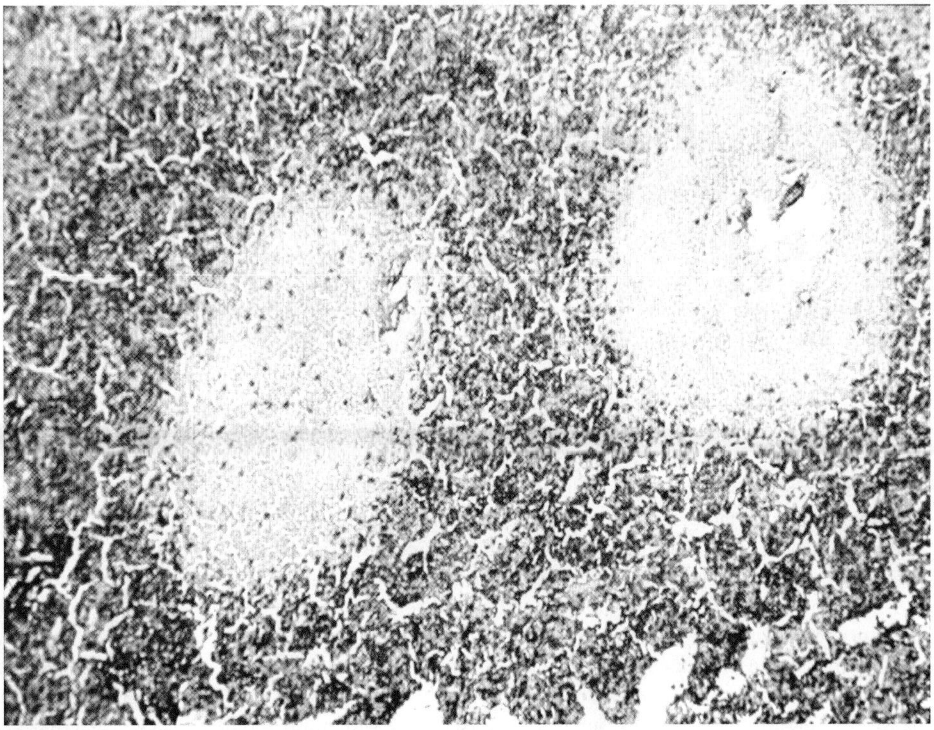

FIGURE 96–2. Spleen in LGL leukemia. CD8+ LGL cells in red pulp surrounding unstained B-cell follicles.

DIFFERENTIAL DIAGNOSIS

The diagnosis of T-LGL leukemia should be considered in patients with chronic or cyclic neutropenia[30] and in patients with pure red cell aplasia or rheumatoid arthritis who have increased concentrations of LGL. HIV infection can lead to a mildly increased concentration of LGL cells; however, the LGLs are not monoclonal.[31] Some patients may have elevated numbers of CD3− LGL, but lack the clinical features of NK-LGL leukemia and have a chronic clinical course.[32] X-chromosome inactivation studies have shown that some patients have clonal expansion of LGL.[33] NK cells from these patients express a restricted KIR phenotype of activating receptors. This finding is in contrast to the diversified KIR repertoire seen in normal NK cells (see Chap. 79 for more information on NK biology and KIR receptors).[34,35] This restricted KIR phenotype suggests a clonal origin and may have diagnostic utility. Of interest, sera from these patients with chronic NK lymphocytosis also have frequent reactivity to BA-21.[36] Table 96–3

TABLE 96–3. Comparative Features of Large Granular Lymphocytic Leukemia

Variable	T-Cell LGL Leukemia (Indolent Variant)	T-Cell LGL Leukemia (Aggressive Variant)	NK-LGL Leukemia (Aggressive)	Chronic NK Lymphocytosis
Median age (years)	60	40	40	60
Male-to-female ratio	1	2	1	7
Phenotype	CD3+CD57+CD16+TCR$\alpha\beta$	CD3+CD56+CD16+TCR$\alpha\beta$	CD3−CD16+CD56+	CD3−CD16+CD56+
Clinical features	One-third asymptomatic Two-thirds symptomatic Cytopenias, splenomegaly, occasionally rheumatoid arthritis	Symptomatic, usually with B symptoms (fever, sweats, weight loss) Lymphadenopathy, hepatosplenomegaly	Symptomatic, usually with B symptoms (fever, sweats, weight loss) Lymphadenopathy, hepatosplenomegaly	Most patients are asymptomatic; approximately 40% with symptoms (cytopenias, vasculitis, neuropathy, splenomegaly)
Treatment approach	Observation or immunosuppressive therapy if required	Acute lymphoblastic leukemia-type therapy	Acute lymphoblastic leukemia-type therapy	Observation or immunosuppressive therapy if required
Prognosis	Relatively good	Poor	Very poor	Relatively good

summarizes the differential features of T-LGL leukemia, NK-LGL leukemia, and chronic NK lymphocytosis.

THERAPY, COURSE, AND PROGNOSIS

Morbidity and mortality usually result as consequences of neutropenia.[3] Optimum treatment for correction of neutropenia is not defined. Treatment with oral low-dose methotrexate, cyclosporine, or oral cyclophosphamide has been efficacious in small series.[37–39] In one series, HLA-DR4 genotype predicted hematologic response to cyclosporine.[40] Clinical improvement is associated with reductions in plasma levels of CD178.[17] A report of four patients treated with fludarabine monophosphate indicated that each achieved a therapeutic benefit.[41] Although treatment with glucocorticoids has ameliorated the neutropenia of some patients, neutropenia generally recurs as the medication is tapered. Splenectomy is of limited benefit. Experience with recombinant growth factors is too limited to draw conclusions.[42,43]

Treatment with prednisone, cyclophosphamide, or cyclosporine is usually effective in correcting pure red cell aplasia associated with T-LGL leukemia.[3] Alemtuzumab (Campath-1H) has been effective in refractory red cell aplasia.[44]

In contrast to the chronic course of T-LGL leukemia, NK-LGL leukemia has an acute presentation and poor clinical outcome. Most patients die within 2 months of diagnosis from disseminated disease with multiorgan failure despite aggressive combination chemotherapy.[20] Patients with chronic NK lymphocytosis usually do not require treatment.

A registry has been formed to better define the natural history of LGL leukemia. Clinical trials are also being administered through the registry. For more information, the registry can be contacted at tloughran@psu.edu.

REFERENCES

1. Loughran TP Jr, Kadin ME, Starkebaum G, et al: Leukemia of large granular lymphocytes: Association with clonal chromosomal abnormalities and auto-immune neutropenia, thrombocytopenia and hemolytic anemia. *Ann Intern Med* 102:169, 1985.
2. Sokol L, Loughran TP Jr: Large granular lymphocyte leukemia. *Oncologist* 11:263, 2006.
3. Lamy T, Loughran TP Jr: Clinical features of LGL leukemia. *Semin Hematol* 40:185, 2003.
4. Taniwaki M, Tagawa S, Nishigaki H, et al: Chromosomal abnormalities define clonal proliferation in CD3– large granular lymphocyte leukemia. *Am J Hematol* 33:32, 1990.
5. Loughran TP Jr, Hadlock KG, Perzova R, et al: Epitope mapping of HTLV envelope seroreactivity in LGL leukemia. *Br J Haematol* 101:318, 1998.
6. Duong YT, Jia H, Lust JA, et al: Short communication: Absence of evidence of HTLV-3 and HTLV-4 in patients with large granular lymphocyte (LGL) leukemia. *AIDS Res Hum Retroviruses* 24:1503, 2008.
7. Rodriguez-Caballero A, Garcia-Montero A, Barcena P, et al: Expanded cells in monoclonal TCR-$\alpha\beta^+$/$CD4^+$/NKa^+/$CD8^{-/+dim}$ T-LGL lymphocytosis recognize hCMV antigens. *Blood* 112:4609, 2008.
8. Kawa-Ha K, Ishihara S, Ninomiya T, et al: CD3-negative lymphoproliferative disease of granular lymphocytes containing Epstein-Barr viral DNA. *J Clin Invest* 84:51, 1989.
9. Wlodarski MW, O'Keefe C, Howe EC, et al: Pathologic clonal cytotoxic T-cell responses: Nonrandom nature of the T-cell-receptor restriction in large granular lymphocyte leukemia. *Blood* 106:2769, 2005.
10. Yang J, Epling-Burnette PK, Painter JS, et al: Antigen activation and impaired Fas-induced death-inducing signaling complex formation in T-large-granular lymphocyte leukemia. *Blood* 111:1610, 2008.
11. Wlodarski MW, Nearman Z, Jankowska A, et al: Phenotypic differences between healthy effector CTL and leukemic LGL cells support the notion of antigen-triggered clonal transformation in T-LGL leukemia. *J Leukoc Biol* 83:589, 2008.
12. Lamy T, Liu JH, Landowski TH, et al: Dysregulation of CD95/CD95 ligand-apoptotic pathway in CD95+ LGL leukemia. *Blood* 92:4771, 1998.
13. Epling-Burnette PK, Liu JH, Catlett-Falcone R, et al: Inhibition of STAT3 signaling leads to apoptosis of leukemic large granular lymphocytes and decreased Mcl-1 expression. *J Clin Investig* 107:3, 351, 2001.
14. Schade AE, Powers JJ, Wlodarski MW, Maciejewski JP: Phosphatidylinositol-3-phosphate kinase pathway activation protects leukemic large granular lymphocytes from undergoing homeostatic apoptosis. *Blood* 107:4834, 2006.
15. Shah, MV, Zhang R, Irby R, et al: Molecular profiling of LGL leukemia reveals role of sphingolipid signaling in survival of cytotoxic lymphocytes. *Blood* 112:770, 2008.
16. Zhang R, Shah MV, Yang J, et al: Network model of survival signaling in large granular lymphocyte leukemia. *Proc Natl Acad Sci U S A* 105:16308, 2008.
17. Liu JH, Wei S, Lamy T, et al: Chronic neutropenia mediated by Fas ligand. *Blood* 95:3119, 2000.
18. Chen X, Bai F, Sokol L, Zhou J, et al: A critical role for DAP10 and DAP12 in CD8+ T cell-mediated tissue damage in large granular lymphocyte leukemia. *Blood* 113:3226, 2009.
19. Loughran TP Jr, Starkebaum G, Kidd P, Neiman P: Clonal proliferation of large granular lymphocytes in rheumatoid arthritis. *Arthritis Rheum* 31:31, 1988.
20. Cheung MM, Chan JK, Wong KF: Natural killer cell neoplasms: A distinctive group of highly aggressive lymphomas/leukemias. *Semin Hematol* 40:221, 2003.
21. Lacy MQ, Kurtin PJ, Tefferi A, et al: Pure red cell aplasia: Association with large granular lymphocyte leukemia and the prognostic value of cytogenetic abnormalities. *Blood* 87:3000, 1996.
22. Abkowitz JL, Kadin ME, Powell JS, Adamson JW: Pure red cell aplasia: Lymphocyte inhibition of erythropoiesis. *Br J Haematol* 63:59, 1986.
23. Abkowitz JL, Powell JS, Nakamura JM, et al: Pure red cell aplasia: Response to therapy with anti-thymocyte globulin. *Am J Hematol* 23:363, 1986.
24. Lai DW, Loughran TP Jr, Maciejewski JP, et al: Acquired amegakaryocytic thrombocytopenia and pure red cell aplasia associated with an occult large granular lymphocyte leukemia. *Leuk Res* 32:823, 2008.
25. Lima M, Almeida J, dos Anjos Teixeira M, et al: TCR$\alpha\beta$+/CD4+ large granular lymphocytosis, a new clonal T-cell lymphoproliferative disorder. *Am J Pathol* 163:763, 2003.
26. Bourgault-Rouxel AS, Loughran TP Jr, Zambello R, et al: Clinical spectrum of gammadelta+ T cell LGL leukemia: Analysis of 20 cases. *Leuk Res* 32:45, 2008.
27. Lundell R, Hartung L, Hill S, et al: T-cell large granular lymphocyte leukemias have multiple phenotypic abnormalities involving pan-T-cell antigens and receptors for MHC molecules. *Am J Clin Pathol* 124:937, 2005.
28. Viny AD, Lichtin A, Pohlman B, et al: Chronic B-cell dyscrasias are an important clinical feature of T-LGL leukemia. *Leuk Lymphoma* 49:932, 2008.
29. Agnarsson BA, Loughran TP Jr, Starkebaum G, Kadin ME: The pathology of large granular lymphocyte leukemia. *Hum Pathol* 20:643, 1989.
30. Loughran TP Jr, Hammond WP: Adult onset cyclic neutropenia is a "benign" neoplasm associated with clonal proliferation of large granular lymphocytes. *J Exp Med* 164:2089, 1986.
31. Zambello R, Trentin L, Agostini C, et al: Persistent polyclonal lymphocytosis in HIV-1 infected patients. *Blood* 81:3015, 1993.
32. Tefferi A, Li CY, Witzig TE, et al: Chronic natural killer cell lymphocytosis: A descriptive clinical study. *Blood* 84:2721, 1994.
33. Boudewijns M, van Dongen J, Langerak A: The human androgen receptor x-chromosome inactivation assay for clonality diagnostics of killer cell proliferations. *J Mol Diagn* 9:337, 2007.
34. Zambello R, Falco M, Della Chiesa M, et al: Expression and function of KIR and natural cytotoxicity receptors in NK-type lymphoproliferative diseases of granular lymphocytes. *Blood* 102:1797, 2003.
35. Epling-Burnette PK, Painter JS, Chaurasia P, et al: Dysregulated NK receptor expression in patients with lymphoproliferative disease of granular lymphocytes. *Blood* 103:3431, 2004.
36. Loughran TP Jr, Hadlock KG, Yang Q, et al: Seroreactivity to an envelope protein of human T-cell leukemia/lymphoma virus in patients with CD3– (NK) lymphoproliferative disease of granular lymphocytes. *Blood* 90:1977, 1997.
37. Loughran TP Jr, Kidd PG, Starkebaum G: Treatment of large granular lymphocyte leukemia with oral low-dose methotrexate. *Blood* 84:2164, 1994.
38. Sood R, Stewart CC, Aplan PD, et al: Neutropenia associated with T-cell large granular lymphocyte leukemia: Long-term response to cyclosporine therapy despite persistence of abnormal cells. *Blood* 91:3372, 1998.
39. Osuji N, Matutes E, Tjonnfjord G, et al: T-cell large granular lymphocyte leukemia: A report on the treatment of 29 patients and a review of the literature. *Cancer* 107:570, 2006.
40. Battiwalla M, Melenhorst J, Saunthararajah Y, et al: HLA-DR4 predicts haematological response to cyclosporine in T-cell large granular lymphocyte lymphoproliferative disorders. *Br J Haematol* 123:449, 2003.
41. Sternberg A, Eagleton H, Pillai N, et al: Neutropenia and anaemia associated with T-cell large granular lymphocyte leukaemia responds to fludarabine with minimal toxicity. *Br J Haematol* 120:699, 2003.
42. Thomssen C, Nissen C, Gratwohl A, et al: Agranulocytosis associated with T-gamma-lymphocytosis: No improvement of peripheral blood granulocyte count with human-recombinant granulocyte-macrophage colony-stimulating factor (GM-CSF). *Br J Haematol* 71:157, 1989.
43. Kaneko T, Ogawa Y, Hirata Y, et al: Agranulocytosis associated with granular lymphocyte leukaemia: Improvement of peripheral blood granulocyte count with human recombinant granulocyte colony-stimulating factor (G-CSF). *Br J Haematol* 74:121, 1990.
44. Ru X, Liebman HA: Successful treatment of refractory pure red cell aplasia associated with lymphoproliferative disorders with the anti-CD52 monoclonal antibody alemtuzumab (Campath-1H). *Br J Haematol* 123:278, 2003.

CHAPTER 97

GENERAL CONSIDERATIONS OF LYMPHOMA: EPIDEMIOLOGY, ETIOLOGY, HETEROGENEITY, AND PRIMARY EXTRANODAL DISEASE

Kenneth A. Foon and Marshall A. Lichtman

SUMMARY

The lymphomas are a heterogeneous group of malignancies that originate in a single lymphocyte that has undergone transforming mutations that confer on it a growth and survival advantage in comparison to its normal cellular counterparts. The neoplasm usually originates in a lymph node, or lymphatic tissue in other sites (extranodal lymphoma), and can be localized or widespread at the time of diagnosis. Men are usually affected more frequently than women and the disease increases logarithmically with age. Classification systems have considered the likely lymphoid progenitor that corresponds to the phenotype (immunotype) and genotype of the malignant cells in the clone. By identifying whether the involved lymphocytes have (1) surface features of B, T , or natural killer (NK) cells, (2) the complete pattern of the CD antigens on their surface, the appearance of the histopathology in the tissue section, specific cytogenetic findings, especially translocations (e.g., t[11;14]), and immunocytochemical markers (e.g., cyclin D1), the specific tissue location (e.g., mucosa-associated lymphatic tissue), the unique pathologic diagnosis can usually be made. Although most lymphomas are without an evident cause, *human T-cell leukemia/lymphoma virus I* (HTLV-1), Epstein-Barr virus, hepatitis C virus, and human herpes virus-8 infections, as well as infections with the bacteria *Helicobacter pylori* and, perhaps, *Chlamydophila psittaci* either are established as causal (e.g., HTLV-1) or have very strong associations with lymphoma incidence (hepatitic C virus), suggesting their role in causation. HIV is permissive in that by inducing severe immunodeficiency it sets the stage for a Epstein-Barr virus-induced or human herpes virus-8–induced lymphoma. These relationships may vary by geographical area. Several occupational and industrial exposures are suspected of being related to lymphoma incidence, for example, organochlorines, phenoxyacid herbicides, and others, but these associations have not been established with scientific certainty. At present, the estimated attributable risk of lymphoma from all suspected exogenous factors together is relatively small in proportion to the number of annual cases, leaving most cases without an apparent cause. There are wide discrepancies in the incidence of specific lymphoma subtypes in different geographic regions (e.g., follicular lymphoma very common in the United States and very uncommon in East Asia). Primary extranodal lymphoma may involve virtually any tissue or organ. Depending on the site, important functional abnormalities may ensue (e.g., bilateral adrenal gland replacement and hypoadrenocorticism, hypothalamic-pituitary involvement and diabetes insipidus). Some combination of surgical excision, radiotherapy, and multidrug chemotherapy and lymphocyte-specific monoclonal antibody therapy is used in treatment depending on the site and histopathology.

Abbreviations and acronyms used in this chapter include: MALT lymphoma, marginal zone B-cell lymphoma of mucosa-associated lymphatic tissue; NK, natural killer; REAL, revised European-American classification of lymphoid neoplasm; SEER, Surveillance, Epidemiology, and End Results; WHO, World Health Organization.

DEFINITION AND HISTORY

Lymphomas are a heterogeneous group of malignancies of B cells, T cells, and, rarely, natural killer (NK) cells that usually originate in the lymph nodes, but which may originate in any organ of the body. Lymphoma previously was referred to as *lymphosarcoma* and its two major subtypes designated *reticulum cell sarcoma* and *giant follicular lymphoma* (Brill-Symmers disease).[1–5] In 1966, Rappaport[6] published a classification system based on the patterns of lymphoma cell growth, size, and shape that attempted to correlate morphology with clinical outcome. The classification proved to have some inaccuracies, such as the term *histiocytic lymphoma* to describe lymphoid tumors of large transformed lymphocytes that were not derived from the monocyte-macrophage lineage. Nonetheless, the Rappaport classification was an important milestone and became the most widely used classification in the United States. In 1974, Lukes and Collins proposed another classification system, which incorporated morphology with immunologic subtype, that was endorsed by the Committee on Nomenclature.[7] Another scheme, the Kiel classification, introduced by Karl Lennert and colleagues, had been more popular in Europe.[8] By the 1970s at least six classifications of lymphoma had been published, and the major ones included two in the United States, one in continental Europe, and one in the United Kingdom. There was no success in reaching a consensus classification that could be used worldwide. A National Cancer Institute study showed that there was poor reproducibility among different pathologists looking at the same slides and trying to classify the case of lymphoma using any existing scheme. In 1982, a Working Formulation sponsored by the National Cancer Institute attempted to reconcile the large number of competing classifications then in use.[9] The Working Formulation was clinically useful and gained wide popularity. It divided the specific subtypes among high-grade, intermediate-grade, and low-grade lymphomas, focusing in part on expected rate of progression, and not just on the phenotype of the case in question. With advances in our understanding of the immune system and lymphocyte progenitor developmental sequences, and the availability of monoclonal antibodies for subtyping lymphoid cells and lymphocyte gene profiling, a new classification schema became possible that represented a classification of lymphomas in the classical sense, related to cell type, tissue of origin, immunophenotype, and, later, genotype.

In 1994, a revised European-American classification of lymphoid neoplasms (the REAL classification) was proposed by the International Lymphoma Study Group (see Chaps. 92 and 98).[10] This group distinguished three major categories of lymphoid malignancies, which included B-cell, T-cell, and Hodgkin lymphoma. Lymphomas were defined by morphologic, immunologic, and genetic techniques. Many of the lymphomas were associated with distinct clinical presentations, and cases that did not fit into defined entities were left unclassified. Further subclassification[11] divided each of the B-cell and T-cell lineages into (1) indolent lymphomas (low risk of rapid progression), (2) aggressive lymphomas (intermediate risk of progression), and (3) very aggressive lymphomas (high risk of progression). In 1995, a collaborative project of the European Association for Haematopathology and the Society for Hematopathology began to revise the REAL classification. In 2001, they published the World Health Organization (WHO) classification of Tumors of the Haematopoietic and Lymphoid Tissues that is used in this chapter and represents the current worldwide consensus classification of malignancies that arise in a lymphocyte. In 2008, the WHO updated this classification (see Chaps. 92 and 98).[12]

EPIDEMIOLOGY

Approximately 66,000 new cases of non-Hodgkin lymphoma (NHL) were projected to be diagnosed and approximately 19,000 persons in the United States were expected to die of lymphoma in 2008.[13] These numbers represent 4.5 percent of the annual incidence of all cancers and 3 percent of annual cancer-related deaths. The most recent age-adjusted incidence rates per 100,000 population provided by Surveillance, Epidemiology, and End Results (SEER) Program of the United States National Cancer Institute are: 25.6 for white males, 18.4 for black males, 17.5 for white females, and 13.1 for black females. The increased risk for men is similar to that found in other countries, although the incidence of NHL in the United States is approximately threefold that of several underdeveloped countries and twofold that of several comparable industrialized countries.[14] The risk of developing lymphoma is less in the United States among persons of African descent in comparison to those of European descent. A logarithmic increase in incidence in NHL among men and women occurs with increasing age (Fig. 97–1).

Follicular lymphoma represents approximately 30 percent of NHL cases in the United States, but is very uncommon in many developing countries and in Asia, especially in Japan and China.[14,15] The United States has a higher incidence of all lymphomas than does Japan, whereas the incidence of extranodal lymphoma is higher in Japan.[14,15] Burkitt lymphoma occurs most frequently in tropical Africa, whereas T-cell leukemia/lymphoma is most common in southwest Japan, the southeastern United States, northeastern South America, and the Caribbean basin.

The incidence of NHL increased dramatically in the last half of the 20th century. The increase has been documented in countries in Europe, Asia, and in the United States.[14,15] From 1973 to 1990, inclusive, the increase in the United States was slightly more than 80 percent, or approximately 4 to 5 percent per year (Fig. 97–2). The increase in incidence probably started after World War II, but the best data in the United States were acquired after 1972. The increase had affected men and women, all age groups except children, and most histologic types examined. The increased incidence per year reached a plateau in the early 1990s, if total lymphoma cases were examined. There still appears to have been an increased incidence among women and older men during some of this later period.[15] There has been no explanation for the increased frequency of NHL in the many countries around the world over the period of time under consideration. The immunodeficiency virus was not prevalent in the human population when the increase was first apparent, although in later years HIV-related lymphoma may have played a small part in increasing incidence rates. Orbital adnexal lymphoma and mantle cell lymphoma are exceptions and each has increased at approximately 6 percent a year in the most recent surveys.[16,17]

Several occupations and industries and several potentially hazardous exposures, such as pesticides, herbicides, dyes, engine exhausts, and solvents, have been found in one study or another to be more frequent in lymphoma patients than "matched" healthy comparison groups.[15,18,19] The results often have been inconsistent from study to study. Expert opinion indicates that no workplace exposure has been conclusively linked to lymphoma.[20] Farming or living in a community in which farming is prevalent has been a frequent association with higher lymphoma incidence.[15,18,19]

An increased risk of lymphoma in the siblings of patients with lymphoma or related hematolymphopoietic malignancies has been reported repeatedly, as has nonsyndromic familial clustering.[21–24] Nonsyndromic familial lymphoma refers to apparently healthy family members, unlike syndromic familial lymphoma in which immunodeficiency syndromes are the predisposing phenotype (e,g., Wiskott-Aldrich syndrome; see "Immunosuppression" below) The familial cases occur in different generations and among enough family members to strongly suggest that a predisposition gene (unidentified) is resulting in an incidence above that in the population at large. Li-Fraumeni syndrome is such an example, involving germ line mutations in p53. Alternatively, it is possible that family members inherit a susceptibility to an environmental lymphomagen (unidentified).

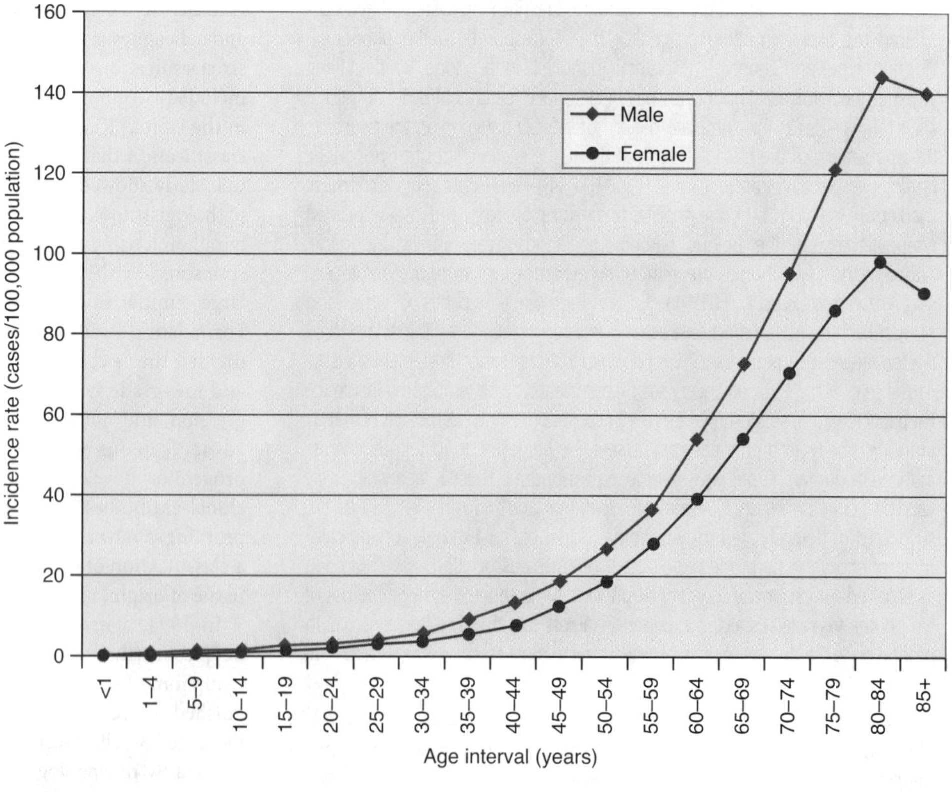

FIGURE 97–1. The graph depicts the rate of increase with age in lymphoma incidence among American males and females. This pattern is true for Americans of European or of African descent. *(Data from the National Cancer Institute, Surveillance, Epidemiology, and End Results Program website of the National Cancer Institute, http://seer.cancer.gov, Table 19.6 , Non-Hodgkin Lymphoma, Incidence by Age.)*

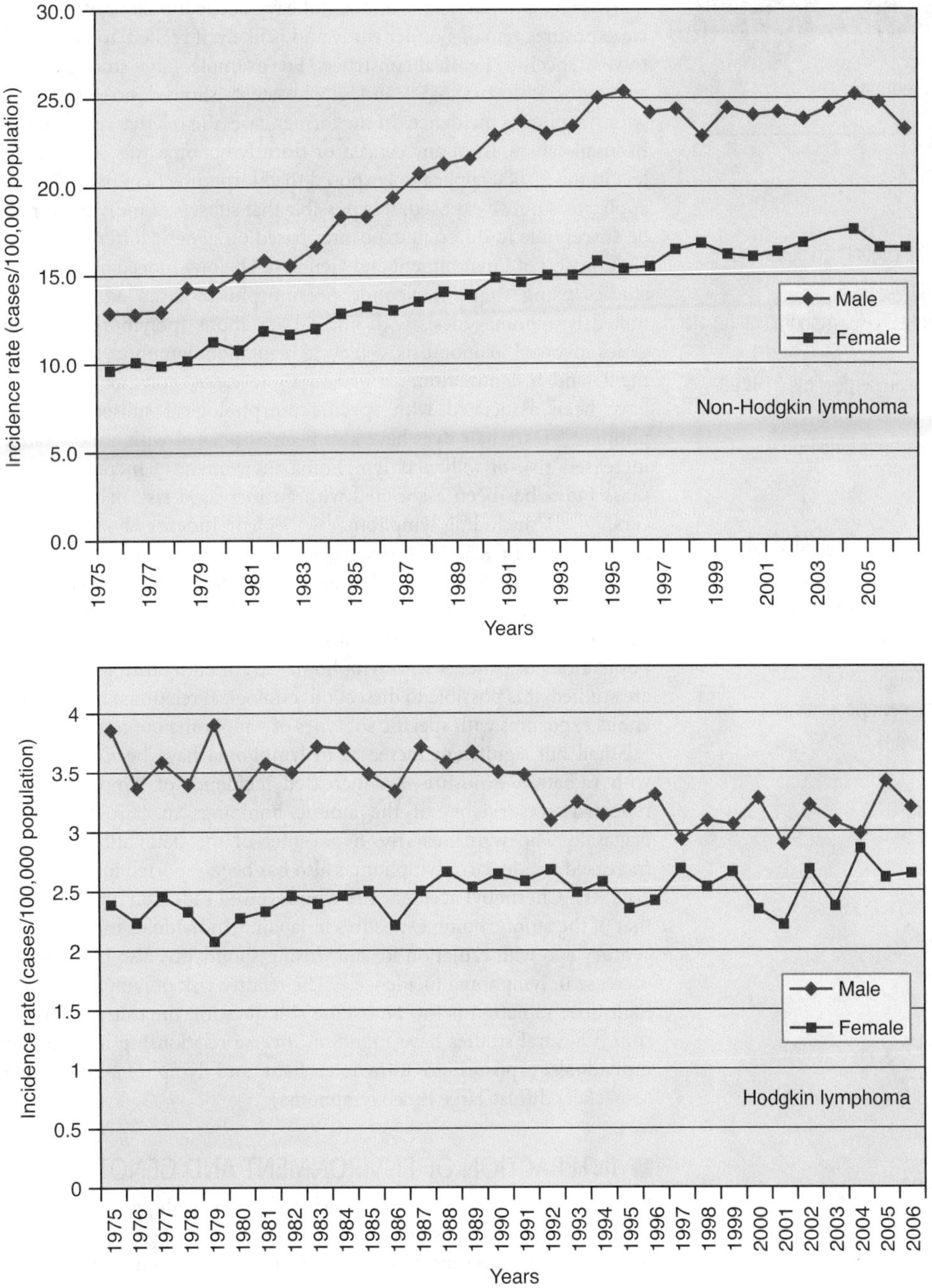

FIGURE 97–2. Incidence of non-Hodgkin and Hodgkin lymphoma by calendar year. The incidence of non-Hodgkin lymphoma approximately doubled from the early 1970's to the mid-1990's in the United States and in other industrialized countries that tracked incidence of specific cancers. No satisfactory explanation has been uncovered for this change. The so-called "epidemic" of lymphoma ended in the mid-1990's and the incidence curves have been "flat" over the last 10 years or so. The increase in incidence was present in Americans of European and African descent and among men and women. In stark contrast and serving as an internal control, the incidence of Hodgkin lymphoma is essentially unchanged over that period of time. *(Data from the Surveillance, Epidemiology, and End-Result Program website of the National Cancer Institute, http://seer.cancer.gov, Tables 9.4 [Hodgkin lymphoma] and 19.4 [non-Hodgkin lymphoma].)*

ETIOLOGY AND PATHOGENESIS

■ HISTOPATHOLOGICAL HETEROGENEITY

Unlike other cancers, the malignancy referred to as "lymphoma" can take on nearly 40 phenotypes.[12] Table 97–1 lists most of the phenotypes considered distinguishable by pathologists using light microscopy, immunophenotyping, immunohistochemistry or immunocytochemistry, and cytogenetic analysis. Approximately 88 percent of lymphomas originate in a cell that carries features most consistent with normal B lymphocytes (B-cell CD surface antigens or immunoglobulin gene rearrangement). The remaining cases are lymphomas in which the phenotype and, where applicable, the genotype are most closely related to T cells or NK cells (T-cell receptor chain rearrangements or specific immunophenotypes). This heterogeneity is problematic for histopathologic diagnosis, classifying patients in clinical trials, and in the approach to therapy; it also makes studies of epidemiology and etiology more difficult. To understand acquired (environmental) or genetic causes of the type of lymphoma in question, the latter studies, to be insightful, should stratify the study group by specific histopathologic diagnosis. This requirement can be difficult if one is studying uncommon phenotypes.

The histopathologic diversity of lymphoma is the result of the complexity of the immune system; its wide distribution through many organs with highly specialized sites, such as mucosa-associated lymphatic tissue (MALT); its differentiation into T-lymphocyte, B-lymphocyte, and NK-lymphocytic lineages; its complex maturation through many progenitor cell levels; the concomitant sequential alterations in expression of immune complex genes and the myriad opportunities for transforming mutations; and the transforming effects of mutations in the several genes encoding immunoglobulin chains or the T-cell receptor. Thus, studies in prevalent subtypes of lymphoma such as follicular and diffuse large B-cell lymphomas are more common than in uncommon or rare subtypes. In addition, epidemiologic or etiologic findings relevant to one subtype may not be relevant to another subtype or to lymphoma in general.

■ ENVIRONMENTAL FACTORS

An increased incidence of lymphoma has been observed, especially among farmers and gardeners.[14,15,18–20] The increased incidence in agricultural workers may be attributed to exposure to a variety of agents, including organochlorines, organophosphates, and phenoxyacid herbicides.[14,15] Despite many studies, an association with lymphoma incidence with herbicide or pesticide exposure has not reached the level of scientific certainty.[15] Indeed, evidence indicates that modest exposure to herbicides by adults who use such products in and around their homes is not likely to

TABLE 97–1. Histologic Subtypes and Relative Frequency of the Non-Hodgkin Lymphomas

A. B-cell lymphomas (~88% of all NHL)
   1. Diffuse large B-cell lymphomas (30%)
      T-cell rich large B-cell lymphoma
      Primary diffuse large B-cell lymphoma of the central nervous system
      Primary cutaneous diffuse large B-cell lymphoma
      Epstein-Barr virus (EBV)-positive diffuse large B-cell lymphoma of the elderly
      Diffuse large B-cell lymphoma arising in human herpesvirus (HHV)-8–associated multicentric Castleman disease
      Diffuse large B-cell lymphomas with features simulating Hodgkin lymphoma
   2. Follicular lymphoma (25%)
   3. Extranodal marginal zone lymphoma of mucosa-associated lymphatic tissue (MALT lymphoma) (7.0%)
   4. Small lymphocytic lymphoma-chronic lymphocytic leukemia (7.0%)
   5. Mantle cell lymphoma (5.0%)
   6. Primary mediastinal (thymic) large B-cell lymphoma (3.0%)
   7. Lymphoplasmacytic lymphoma-Waldenström macroglobulinemia (<2%)
   8. Nodal marginal zone B-cell lymphoma (<1.5%)
   9. Splenic marginal zone lymphoma (<1%)
   10. Extranodal marginal zone B-cell lymphoma (<1%)
   11. Intravascular large B-cell lymphoma (<1%)
   12. Primary effusion lymphoma (<1%)
   13. Primary cutaneous follicle center lymphoma (1%)
   14. Burkitt lymphoma–Burkitt leukemia (1.5%)
   15. Plasmablastic lymphoma <1.0%
   16. Lymphomatoid granulomatosis (<1%)

B. T-and NK-cell lymphomas (~12% of all NHL)
   1. Extranodal T or NK lymphoma
   2. Enteropathy-associated T-cell lymphoma
   3. Hepatosplenic T-cell lymphoma
   4. Subcutaneous panniculitis-like T-cell lymphoma
   5. Cutaneous T-cell lymphoma (Sézary syndrome and mycosis fungoides)
   6. Primary cutaneous gamma-delta T-cell lymphoma
   7. Anaplastic large-cell lymphoma
   8. Angioimmunoblastic T-cell lymphoma
   9. Primary T-cell lymphoma unspecified

C. Immunodeficiency-associated lymphoproliferative disorders (see Table 97–2 for inherited diseases associated with immunodeficiencies and lymphoma)
   1. HIV-associated lymphoma
   2. Posttransplantation lymphoproliferative disorder
   3. Lymphoma associated with a primary immune disorder

SOURCE: This table is compiled from information presented in the World Health Organization Classification of Tumors of Hematopoietic and Lymphoid Tissues.[12] The parenthetical percentages are approximate but give some sense of the relative distribution of subtypes. The frequency of lymphoma varies depending on the geographical area under consideration. The frequencies cited here are approximate and related to those observed in the United States, the United Kingdom, or Western Europe. Some very rare subtypes are not listed.

increase lymphoma risk,[15a] although heavy occupational or other similar exposures remains under study and is likely, if related, to be so only to very specific chemical constructs. For example, large studies of two pesticides, chlorpyrifos[15b] and glyphosate[15c] showed no association with lymphoma incidence. In the former case, the relative risk of death from all causes, from any cancer, or from lymphoma was significantly less in the 22,000 applicators exposed to chlorpyrifos than in the 33,000 applicators not so exposed. It is possible that subsets of individuals may be susceptible to different exposures based on genetic differences. (see "Interaction of Environment and Genotype" below) Indeed, preliminary studies using single nucleotide polymorphism–based analysis have linked lymphomagenesis with normal variations (polymorphisms) in genes involved in apoptosis, cell cycle regulation, lymphocyte development, and inflammation.[15d,15e,15f] In some cases, polymorphic genes have been associated with specific morphological subsets of lymphoma.[15g] Dark hair dyes have also been associated with a moderately increased risk of follicular lymphoma in women.[15h] Increased body mass index has been associated with an increased risk of many cancers,[15i,15j,15k] including lymphoma.[15k,15l,15m,15n] Indexes above 30 to 35 kg/m^2 (normal = 8.5–25 kg/m^2) have been associated with an increased risk. The risk factors discussed in this section have not been found uniformly in all studies of their association with lymphoma and should be considered provisional associations at this time. In addition, as larger populations of patients with lymphoma, stratified by histological type, are studied, it is possible to dissect out etiological relationships of exogenous exposures with specific subtypes of lymphoma but not others.

Small but significant increases in lymphoma have been associated with radiation exposure. An increased incidence of lymphoma was reported in survivors of the atomic bombings in Hiroshima and Nagasaki who were near the hypocenter of the detonation.[25–28] An increased incidence of lymphomas also has been reported for individuals at the Chernobyl accident site who received radiation equivalent to that of the atomic bomb exposures in Japan.[29] Individuals treated a half century ago with radiation for ankylosing spondylitis also had a small increase in lymphoma incidence.[30] The relative risk of lymphoma with high-dose radiation is low and some still question the causal relationship.[31] Several studies have found an inverse relationship between an individuals exposure to ultraviolet light and lymphoma incidence (especially diffuse large B-cell lymphoma).[32]

INTERACTION OF ENVIRONMENT AND GENOTYPE

Using a relatively large population of patients with lymphoma and matched controls, among whom an association between exposure to organochlorines and the incidence of lymphoma was found, polymorphic immune gene variations were a significant factor in the relationship of this exposure to lymphoma incidence.[33] Associations between all exposures and NHL risk were limited to the same genotypes for interferon-γ, *IFNG* (C-1615T) TT, and interleukin-4, *IL4* (5′-UTR, Ex1–168C→T) CC. Associations between PCB180 in plasma and dust and NHL risk were limited to the same genotypes for interleukin-16, *IL16* (3′-UTR, Ex22+871A→G) AA, interleukin-8, *IL8* (T-251A) TT, and interleukin-10, *IL10* (A-1082G) AG/GG. This result indicates that the relation between organochlorine exposure and NHL risk may be modified by particular variants in immune genes, supporting the concept of a gene-environment interaction for induction of NHL.

INFECTIOUS AGENTS

Human T-Cell Leukemia/Lymphoma Virus I

The most compelling evidence for a viral etiology of lymphoma is adult T-cell leukemia/lymphoma.[34] A C-type RNA tumor virus, isolated from patients, has been designated human T-cell leukemia/lymphoma virus-I (HTLV-1).[35] HTLV-1 is an acquired retrovirus that is not related to other known animal retroviruses. HTLV-1 can immortalize lymphoid cells in culture and induce malignancy in an infected human host. Incidence of infection with HTLV-1 in endemic areas is very high, yet few of these infected patients develop adult T-cell leukemia/lymphoma. HTLV-1 also leads to a neurologic disorder called *tropical spastic paraparesis*.[36] Host determinants affect transformation of lymphocytes by HTLV-1, and these may be genetic factors.[35] Development of adult T-cell leukemia/lymphoma is associated with infection by the virus.[37] Serum specimens from Japanese patients with adult T-cell leukemia/lymphoma are positive for HTLV-1, as are serum samples from adult T-cell leukemia/lymphoma patients in the Caribbean, where adult T-cell leukemia/lymphoma is endemic.[38] The highest prevalence of adult T-cell leukemia/lymphoma in Japan is in the southern island of Kyushi, where 10 to 15 percent of the population has antibody to HTLV-1.[39] On the Japanese islands where adult T-cell leukemia/lymphoma is rare, the rate is less than 1 percent. These and additional data from the Caribbean, the southeastern United States, South America, and Africa indicate that adult T-cell leukemia/lymphoma clusters in regions where HTLV-1 is prevalent.[37,38] How these regions are linked is not known. One hypothesis is that HTLV-1 was brought to the Americas from Africa by the slave trade and then to the southern islands of Japan by trade with Japan and Africa.[38,40]

Host susceptibility, a shared environmental exposure, or both contribute to HTLV-1 infection. The prevalence of HTLV-1 antibodies in close family members is three to four times higher than in the corresponding normal population.[40,41] In some instances, cell cultures of antibody-positive, clinically normal patients yield HTLV-1 isolates.[41] Blood donors are routinely screened for antibodies to HTLV-1 to prevent transmission by this route.

Epstein-Barr Virus

Some B-cell lymphomas, including Burkitt lymphoma, posttransplantation lymphoma, and HIV-associated lymphomas (immunodeficiency-related Burkitt lymphoma, primary central nervous system lymphoma, primary effusion lymphoma, the immunoblastic-plasmacytoid type of diffuse large B-cell lymphoma, and oral cavity plasmablastic lymphoma) may be caused by Epstein-Barr virus (EBV; see Chaps. 100 and 104).[42] EBV is a DNA virus in the herpes virus family that first was described in cultured lymphoblasts from patients with African Burkitt lymphoma.[43] EBV binds to the CD21 antigen (also the receptor for the C3d component of complement) on B lymphocytes.[44] It is capable of transforming B lymphocytes into lymphoblastoid cells that may proliferate perpetually in cell culture.[45] EBV is present in greater than 95 percent of cases of endemic Burkitt lymphoma and in approximately 20 percent of cases of nonendemic Burkitt lymphoma.[46,47] Malaria is holoendemic in regions where endemic Burkitt lymphoma exists.[48] A three-step process in the development of this lymphoma has been proposed:[49,50] (1) EBV initiates a polyclonal proliferation of B cells; (2) malaria stimulates further the proliferating B cells; and (3) the transforming B cells incur specific reciprocal translocations of chromosome 8 with chromosome 2, 14, or 22, resulting in a clonal expansion of B lymphocytes.

Extranodal NK/T-cell lymphoma, nasal type is mostly endemic to East Asia and is usually associated with EBV infection (see Chaps. 84 and 106). The EBV genome is typically detected in the lymphoma cells.[51,52] Geographic localization of extranodal NK/T-cell lymphoma matches the endemic distribution of EBV, suggesting the role of EBV in lymphomagenesis.

Human Herpesvirus-8

Human herpesvirus-8 (HHV-8) is associated with Kaposi sarcoma, Castleman disease, and primary effusion lymphoma, found most commonly in immunodeficient individuals infected with HIV.[42,53–56] HHV-8 is not a ubiquitous virus. It is mainly endemic in areas where classical or Kaposi sarcoma is of high prevalence, including the Mediterranean basin and East and Central Africa. In the latter areas, the HHV-8 seroprevalence can reach 80 percent in the adult population.[55] In the homosexual population (mainly in the United States and Europe), HHV-8 is principally transmitted during repeated sexual contacts, whereas in Africa it is mainly transmitted from mother to child and among siblings. Saliva seems to play a major role in HHV-8 transmission.[55] Posttransplantation primary effusion lymphoma is associated with HHV-8.[56]

Hepatitis Virus B and C

Hepatitis B and C have been implicated in the pathogenesis of lymphoproliferative diseases. In one study, 334 newly diagnosed lymphoma patients and 1014 controls had a serologic evaluation for the presence of prior hepatitis virus B or C infection.[57] The results suggested that hepatitis B seropositivity was significantly higher in patients with diffuse large B-cell lymphoma and follicular lymphoma, and seropositivity for hepatitis C was significantly higher in diffuse large B-cell lymphoma patients. A similar result was found in another study in Taiwan, an area with a high frequency of hepatitis B virus infection.[58] In two other studies, seropositivity for hepatitis C was significantly higher in patients with B-cell lymphomas.[59,60] Hepatitis C virus has a predilection for B cells. Hepatitis C virus RNA levels are significantly higher in B cells than CD4+ or CD8+ T cells or other cells in infected patients, and the virus is associated with immunopathologic reactions, such as cryoglobulinemia, and, not infrequently, clonality of infected B lymphocytes.[61] A significantly higher frequency of elevated free serum immunoglobulin light chains was present in hepatitis C–infected patients with NHL than in infected patients without lymphoma.[61] Hepatitic C virus infection may be associated with the onset of diffuse large B-cell lymphoma, marginal zone lymphoma, and lymphoplasmcytic lymphoma, but not follicular lymphoma.[59]

Helicobacter pylori

Helicobacter pylori can cause marginal zone B-cell lymphoma of mucosa-associated lymphatic tissue (synonym: MALT lymphomas) of the stomach and probably causes some of the higher-grade lymphomas, either from transformation of a MALT or *de novo* large cell lymphoma.[62–64] This spiral Gram-negative bacillus is the first bacterium demonstrated to cause a human neoplasm. It had been thought that the stomach was sterile because of the acid environment, but *H. pylori* had evolved to tolerate the environment, perhaps in part, because it secretes urease, an enzyme that converts urea to ammonia, making the microenvironment around the organism less acidic. Although the stomach has no endogenous lymphoid tissue, the latter develops in response to the organism, and ultimately the chronic inflammatory reaction can result in the transformation and selection of a mutant lymphocyte with a growth and survival advantage leading to a lymphoma (see Chap. 103).

Chlamydophila psittaci

Ocular adnexal lymphomas are the most common tumor of the eye. The majority of ocular adnexal lymphomas are extranodal, mucosa-associated lymphoid tissue lymphomas and have been linked to *Chlamydophila psittaci* infection in several reports. In one study, this organism was detected in lymphoma tissue in 75 percent of cases.[65] DNA was detected in conjunctional swabs and/or blood mononuclear cells from 50 percent of patients. Mononuclear phagocytes were the carriers of *C. psittaci* in this population of patients.[66] Confirmatory reports of the association of *C. psittaci* with adnexal ocular lymphoma have been published.[67,68] Epidemiologic data suggest that ocular adnexal lymphomas are associated with household animals and chronic conjunctivitis and are consistent with *C. psittaci* exposure. Although several studies show a strong association between the organism and ocular adnexal lymphoma, there are several studies that either find a weak association[68,69] or do not find the association.[70–72] Reconciliation of this discrepancy may be achieved, if the proposal that the relationship may differ in different geographical regions and that several different organisms may be associated with lymphoma in this site are correct.[73,74]

Other Bacteria

Other bacterial infestations have been found in association with lymphomas of mucosa-associated lymphatic tissue. *Campylobacter jejuni* and *Borrelia burgdorferi* have been connected to the onset of immunoproliferative disease of the small intestine disease and B-cell lymphoma of the skin.[75]

IMMUNOSUPPRESSION

Inherited

A number of the rare immunodeficiency syndromes tabulated in Table 97–2[76–98] result from gene mutations leading to deficiencies in cellular or humoral immunity or both. These syndromes have a paradoxically

TABLE 97–2. Inherited Syndromes Predisposing to Lymphoma

Syndrome	Altered Genes: Inheritance	Altered Genes: Description	Mechanism	Leukemia Type	References
DNA repair defects					
Ataxia telangiectasia	R	*ATM* homozygotes Dominant-negative missense mutations	Genomic instability Increased translocations in T cells formed at the time of V(D)J recombination	T-cell lymphoma, T-cell ALL, T-cell PLL, B-cell lymphoma	76, 77
Bloom	R	*BLM*	Genomic instability	ALL, lymphoma	78, 79
Nijmegen breakage	R	*NBS1*	Genomic instability Altered telomere maintenance	Lymphoid tumors, especially B-cell lymphoma	80, 81
Tumor-suppressor gene defect					
Li-Fraumeni*	D	*p53*	Defect in tumor suppressor	CLL, ALL, Hodgkin and Burkitt lymphoma	82, 83
Immunodeficiency states					
Common variable immuno-deficiency	R and D	Defect in CD40 signaling	Failure of B-cell maturation	Burkitt, MALT, other B-cell lymphomas, Hodgkin lymphoma	84, 85
Severe combined immunodeficiency disease (SCID)	R	*ADA*	Defective T- + B-cell function	B-cell lymphoma	86
Wiskott-Aldrich	X	*WASP*	Signaling and apoptosis	Hodgkin and non-Hodgkin lymphoma	87, 88
X-linked immunodeficiency with normal or increased IgM	X	*CD40L*	CD40 ligand defect on T cell	Hodgkin and non-Hodgkin lymphoma	89, 90
X-linked lymphoproliferative syndrome (XLP)	X	*SAP*	Defect in immune signaling	EBV-related B-cell lymphoma	91
Apoptotic defect					
Autoimmune lymphoproliferative syndrome (ALPS)	D	*APT (FAS)*	Germ-line heterozygous *FAS* mutations; defective apoptosis	Lymphoma	92, 93
Unknown defect					
Dubowitz	R	Unknown	Unknown	ALL, lymphoma	94
Poland	D	May not be inherited	Unknown	ALL, lymphoma	95–97
WT	D	Unknown	Unknown	ALL, Castleman disease	98

ALL, acute lymphocytic leukemia; CLL, chronic lymphocytic leukemia; D, dominant; EBV, Epstein-Barr virus; MALT, mucosa-associated lymphatic tissue lymphoma; R, recessive; T-PLL, T prolymphocytic leukemia; X, X-linked.

*Li-Fraumeni or Li-Fraumeni–like syndrome has been described in which a gene other than *p53* is mutated. *hCHK2* in particular has been described as etiologic.[206,207] We have not included these variants in the table because we are uncertain if lymphoma is one of the cancers for which susceptibility is increased.

SOURCE: Modified from Segel GB, Lichtman MA.[24]

high frequency of autoantibodies but, more relevant to this discussion, an increased probability of developing a lymphoma. Because these syndromes are so uncommon, reliable assessment of the increased risk of lymphoma often has to be inferred. The increased risk of approximately 0.5 to 10 percent of patients, depending on the immunodeficiency disease in question, is several orders of magnitude above the risk in the general population (age-adjusted incidence rate in the United States younger than 65 years of age: males = 0.011% and females = 0.008%). With the exception of common variable immunodeficiency, the syndromes present in childhood and because several are X-chromosome-linked, males are affected more commonly than females. The lymphomas induced may result from a susceptibility to Epstein-Barr virus and the lymphoproliferation may initially be polyclonal before evolving to a monoclonal tumor. Extranodal involvement appears to be more common than in persons with lymphoma who are immunocompetent. The initial manifestations of the immunodeficiency are usually infections or autoimmune abnormalities, such as immune cytopenias, and lymphoma is a later complication. We have included Li-Fraumeni syndrome in this cluster for convenience of presentation. This germ-line predisposition syndrome does not have an immunodeficiency phenotype as do all the other entries in Table 97–2. Rather, it is a nonsyndromic familial cancer syndrome transmitting susceptibility to mutations in *p53*. The cancers that occur in these families include lymphoma.

Acquired

A variety of types of immunosuppressed individuals develop lymphoma. Chap. 83 discusses AIDS-related lymphoma. Posttransplantation lymphoproliferative diseases generally display B-cell lineage derivation, involvement of extranodal sites, aggressive histology and clinical behavior, and frequent association with EBV infection. The occurrence of immunoglobulin (Ig) V mutations in the overwhelming majority of posttransplantation lymphoproliferative disease indicates that malignant transformation targets germinal center B cells and their descendants, both in EBV-positive and EBV-negative cases.[99–101] Posttransplantation T-cell lymphomas may occur and often arise in extranodal sites, such as skin or central nervous system.[102,103]

The incidence and severity of lymphomas have increased with the introduction of immunosuppressive agents such as cyclosporine. The incidence of lymphomas has also increased in recipients of mismatched T-cell–depleted marrow hematopoietic stem cell grafts.

AUTOIMMUNITY

Some autoimmune disorders are risk factors for lymphoma. An increased incidence of malignant lymphocytic diseases is present in patients with systemic lupus erythematosus, Sjögren syndrome, autoimmune thyroid disease, and, perhaps, rheumatoid arthritis.[104,105] Among nearly 30,000 participants aggregated from 12 case-controlled studies, Sjögren syndrome was associated with a 6.5-fold increased risk of NHL (especially diffuse large B-cell and follicular lymphomas) and a 1000-fold increased risk of parotid gland marginal zone lymphoma. Systemic lupus erythematosus was associated with a 2.7-fold increased risk of NHL (especially diffuse large B-cell and marginal zone B-cell lymphomas).[105] Autoimmune hemolytic anemia was associated with diffuse large B-cell NHL. T-cell NHL risk was increased for patients with celiac disease and psoriasis. Results for rheumatoid arthritis were heterogeneous among studies.[105] Hashimoto thyroiditis is associated with an increased risk of thyroid marginal zone lymphoma, but may also have a higher risk of nonthyroidal marginal zone lymphoma.[106] Sarcoidosis is an inflammatory (granulomatous) disorder that may predispose to lymphoma.[107]

CHROMOSOMAL TRANSLOCATIONS ASSOCIATED WITH HISTOPATHOLOGIC SUBTYPE

Chromosomal abnormalities involving all chromosomes may occur in lymphomas (see Chap. 11). Lymphoid malignancies have a high frequency of translocation-inducing fusion genes. Usually they are of two types: one involving oncogenes that are activated by juxtaposing with immunoglobulin (*IgH*) or T-cell receptor (*TCR*) genes, or by formation of chimeric genes that constitutively activate mutant kinases or mutant transcription factors. The molecular alterations leading to translocations involving nonimmune genes are not known, whereas there is strong evidence that mistakes in V(D)J recombinase activity are responsible for those translocations involving *IgH* or the *TCR* genes.[108]

As in translocations associated with childhood acute lymphocytic leukemia (ALL) and adult chronic myelogenous leukemia (CML) and acute myelogenous leukemia (AML), translocations involving t(14;18)(*IgH;BCL-2*) are found in healthy persons. Presumably, additional genetic events are required for transformation of a lymphocyte to occur. Alternatively, cells containing these translocations may be entering an apoptotic process, destined to be eliminated.[108]

FOLLICULAR LYMPHOMA

Approximately 85 percent of follicular lymphomas carry the chromosomal translocation t(14;18)(q32;q21) in which the *BCL-2* oncogene on chromosome 18q21 is brought in continuity with the immunoglobulin heavy-chain loci on 14q32.[109] The expression of the BCL-2 protein is increased.[110] The accumulation of the BCL-2 protein permits accumulation of long-lived centrocytes, as BCL-2 protein inhibits its programmed cell depth (apoptosis), leading to a longer cell life (see Chap. 101).[111] The *BCL-2* rearrangement can be detected by the polymerase chain reaction (see Chap. 101).

BURKITT LYMPHOMA

In Burkitt lymphoma, the common genetic abnormality is the translocation of the *MYC* oncogene from chromosome 8 to either the Ig heavy-chain region on chromosome 14, t(8;14)(q24;q32) or, less commonly, the κ region on chromosome 2, t(2;8)(p13;q24) or the region on chromosome 22, t(8;22)(q24;q11). In the African endemic cases, the breakpoint on chromosome 14 includes the heavy-chain joining region, suggesting translocation occurs before complete Ig gene rearrangement in an early B cell (Chap. 104). In nonendemic cases, the translocation involves the Ig heavy-chain switch region, suggesting translocation occurs at a later stage of B-cell development.[112] EBV genomes are demonstrated in the tumor cells in most of the African cases, in approximately one third of the cases associated with AIDS,[113,114] but less frequently in non-African, nonimmune-deficient cases (see Chap. 104).

ANAPLASTIC LARGE CELL LYMPHOMA

The translocation t(2;5)(p23;q35) of anaplastic large cell lymphoma (ALCL) involves the nucleophosmin *(NPM)* gene at 5p35 and the ALCL tyrosine kinase *(ALK)* gene at 2p23,[115] leading to expression of the novel fusion protein p80.[115] This translocation has been identified in approximately 50 percent of systemic cases and may be higher in children with ALCL.[117,118] The t(2;5) translocation is not common in primary cutaneous ALCL (see Chap. 100).[119]

MARGINAL ZONE LYMPHOMA OF MUCOSA-ASSOCIATED LYMPHATIC TISSUE

t(11;18)(*API2-MALT1*), t(1;14)(*IGH-BCL10*), t(14;18)(*IGH-MALT1*), and t(3;14)(*IGH-FOXP1*) occur in marginal zone B-cell lymphoma of mucosa-associated lymphatic tissue of different sites. The first three chromosome translocations are specifically associated with the marginal zone lymphoma of mucosa-associated lymphatic tissue lymphomas and the oncogenic products of these translocations target the nuclear factor-κB pathway (see Chap. 103).[75]

MANTLE CELL LYMPHOMA

t(11;14)(q13;q32) is present in the cells of most cases of mantle cell lymphoma. The diagnosis of mantle cell lymphoma is now dependent upon the identification of the 11;14 translocation that results in cyclin D1 upregulation. Fluorescence *in situ* hybridization (FISH) is the most useful test to identify the juxtaposition of the *CCND1* and *IGH* genes in mantle cell lymphoma (see Chap. 102).[120]

CLINICAL FEATURES

HISTORY AND PHYSICAL EXAMINATION

A complete history and physical examination are important to provide evidence for the distribution of palpable lymphadenopathy, evidence of extranodal disease, or a functional disturbance of an organ system. It is important to ascertain whether the patient suspected of having lymphoma has fever (i.e., temperature >38°C [>100.4°F] for 3 consecutive days), night sweats, or metabolic wasting resulting in loss of more than 10 percent of body weight within the preceding 6 months. The presence of such "B" symptoms has unfavorable prognostic significance.

An examination should be made of all lymph node areas. Involved nodes typically are nontender, firm, and rubbery. The throat should be examined for involvement of the oropharyngeal lymphoid tissue (Waldeyer ring). The aggressive lymphomas more likely involve extranodal sites, such as the skin and central nervous system (CNS); see "Primary Extranodal Lymphoma" below. Liver and spleen size should be assessed as well as palpation of the abdomen for evidence of enlargement of deep nodes (e.g., paraaortic, iliac).

STAGING

Table 97–3 lists the staging procedures that are often used. Generally, staging laparotomy is not indicated. Sensitive imaging procedures have all but replaced surgical examination of the abdomen as a staging procedure. Surgery may be indicated for diagnosis and excision of intraabdominal or intrathoracic extranodal disease, or to treat low-grade lymphomas of the gastrointestinal tract. The role of surgery for large intraabdominal masses (>10 cm) is controversial and is no longer recommended in general.

Although the Ann Arbor staging classification (Table 97–4) is not optimal for staging lymphoma,[121] it still is considered the gold standard and impacts patient survival. The staging system was created for Hodgkin lymphoma, which spreads principally by contiguity from lymph node areas (see Chap. 99), rather than principally hematogenously, as does non-Hodgkin lymphoma. For this reason, more than 80 percent of patients with low-grade lymphoma and more than 50 percent of patients with intermediate- or high-grade lymphoma present with stage III or IV disease. However, staging is critically important for patients who appear to be in stages I and II and whose treatment may be radiation therapy if they have low-risk follicle-center lymphomas or by a combination of radiation therapy and limited cycles of chemotherapy if they have an intermediate- or high-risk lymphoma. The current lymphoma staging and prognostic indicators are discussed in the chapters on individual lymphomas, especially Chap. 100 on diffuse large B-cell lymphoma.

TABLE 97–3. Staging Procedures for Lymphoma

Initial studies
History and physical examination
Biopsy specimen
Pathologic diagnosis
Flow cytometry
Immunohistochemistry
Cytogenetic analysis
CT/PET scans of neck, chest, abdomen, and pelvis
Additional studies
Immunoglobulin and T-cell-receptor gene rearrangement studies
Polymerase chain reaction for *BCL-1* and *BCL-2*
Ultrasonography and MRI to clarify abnormalities
CT scan or MRI of brain if neurologic signs or symptoms
Analysis of cerebrospinal fluid if neurologic signs or symptoms
Gastrointestinal studies (imaging and endoscopy) if Waldeyer ring involvement

CT, computed tomography; MRI, magnetic resonance imaging; PET, positron emission tomography.

PRIMARY EXTRANODAL LYMPHOMA

Lymphomas involving extranodal sites most commonly occur simultaneously with nodal involvement, either at the time of diagnosis or sometime during the course of the disease. Extranodal involvement that occurs as the only initial evidence of lymphoma after staging

TABLE 97–4. Ann Arbor Staging System

Stage I*	Restricted to one lymph node-bearing area
Stage II*	Two or more areas of nodal involvement on one side of the diaphragm
Stage III*	Lymphatic involvement on both sides of the diaphragm
Stage IV	Liver, marrow involvement, or extensive extranodal disease
Symptom status A	Absence of fevers, sweats, or weight loss
Symptom status B	Unexplained fevers >38°C (100.4°F), drenching night sweats, weight loss of >10% of body weight in the preceding 6 months
Clinical stage	Assigned stage based only on history, physical findings, and laboratory and imaging studies
Pathologic stage	Assigned stage based only on areas of biopsy-proven involvement
Substage E	Localized, extranodal disease

*The spleen is considered a single nodal area.

procedures is referred to as *primary extranodal lymphoma*. The presence of a tumor or mass outside of the lymph nodes is usually not considered lymphoma until a biopsy is done and the histopathology clarifies the situation. On the other hand, solitary extranodal lymphomas can occur in virtually any organ or tissue and should be considered in the differential diagnosis of a solitary mass lesion anywhere. The histopathology of primary extranodal lymphoma is usually either marginal zone lymphoma of mucosa-associated lymphatic tissue or diffuse large B-cell lymphoma. Follicular lymphoma and several other histologic subtypes of lymphoma may occur also. Therapy is usually some combination of surgical excision, radiotherapy, multidrug chemotherapy and a lymphocyte-directed monoclonal antibody, often rituximab-cyclophosphamide, hydroxydoxorubicin, vincristine (Oncovin), and prednisone (R-CHOP), depending on the location involved and the lymphoma histopathological subtype present.

An unanswered pathogenetic question about primary extranodal lymphoma is the propensity to appear in both of a paired organ simultaneously, such as ovarian, testicular, breast, ocular, adrenal, renal, and ureteral bilateral extranodal lymphoma. It is also curious that several of these sites (e.g., kidney) are virtually devoid of any aggregates of lymphatic tissue. If the transformed lymphocyte arises outside these tissues, it has some type of tropism for both paired organs. If it arises in one of the pair, the same explanation may exist. It seems improbable that a transforming event would occur in each organ simultaneously (separate clones).

■ CENTRAL NERVOUS SYSTEM

Primary lymphomas originating in and confined to the leptominges,[122] brain,[123] or spinal cord[124] are uncommon. They almost always are an aggressive histological subtype, usually diffuse large B-cell lymphoma.[125] Spinal cord compression typically presents with back pain, followed by extremity weakness, paresis, and paralysis. Leptomeningeal spread may present with cranial nerve palsies and signs of meningeal irritation, for example, headache and stiff neck. Intracerebral mass lesions may present with headaches, lethargy, papilledema, focal neurologic signs, or seizures. Intracerebral lymphoma increased dramatically after the onset of the human immunodeficiency virus epidemic as a result of the association with AIDS-related aggressive lymphomas (see Chap. 83). The incidence of intracerebral lymphoma has slowed in AIDS patients because of more successful antiviral therapy.

Primary pituitary (or hypothalamic) extranodal lymphoma may result in hypopituitarism. Diabetes insipidus or anterior pituitary failure may occur. The lesion may invade the sella turcica or other neighboring bone and nervous tissue.[126–128]

■ EYE

Ophthalmic lymphoma, the most common orbital malignancy, which includes lymphoma localized to the eyelid, conjunctiva, lacrimal sac, lacrimal gland, orbit, or intraocular space. This location accounts for approximately 7 percent of all extranodal lymphomas.[129] The most frequent subtype is extranodal marginal zone lymphoma of mucosa-associated lymphatic tissue. Bilateral involvement is not unusual. The most common site of ocular lesions is the periorbital soft tissues, particularly the conjunctival mucosal surfaces and the area surrounding the lacrimal gland.[130] These lesions typically have a low-risk of progression and commonly have the histology of a marginal zone lymphoma of mucosa-associated lymphatic tissue or follicular center cell lymphoma and may be associated with *C. psittaci* (see "Infectious Agents" above). In a Danish study, approximately 50 percent of orbital and ocular adnexal lymphomas were of the marginal zone lymphoma of mucosa-associated lymphatic tissue subtype; diffuse large B-cell lymphoma was the most common intraocularly.[129,131] Lymphoma arising in the lacrimal sac was usually diffuse large B-cell lymphoma. There has been a striking increase in incidence rates for lymphoma of the eye over the past 30 years.[16,132] Patients with marginal zone lymphoma of mucosa-associated lymphatic tissue of the eye may relapse or have progression of disease after initial therapy and relapses can be found at extraocular sites.[131] Overall survival, however, was not significantly worse for patients with relapse. The frequency of translocations involving the *MALT1* and *IGH* gene loci is low in ocular region marginal zone lymphoma of mucosa-associated lymphatic tissue (~5%), but may predict increased risk of relapse.[131]

The therapy for ocular lymphoma is usually radiation, which may be curative in the majority of patients.[133]Anecdotal reports of responses to rituximab or rituximab postradiation suggest that rituximab may have a therapeutic role in low-grade lymphomas involving the eye. In the rare situation where diffuse large B-cell lymphoma involves the periorbital soft tissue, treatment is determined by the distribution of the disease.

Intraocular lymphomas are a rare presentation of lymphoma of the eye.[134] Most cases are large B-cell lymphomas, but they often have an indolent pattern. The diagnosis is established by a vitrectomy. There is an approximately 50 percent chance that the disease will be bilateral. Also, the disease frequently is associated with brain or leptomeningeal involvement. The mainstay of therapy is radiation, but most patients experience relapse within the eye or brain. Chemotherapeutic agents typically do not penetrate the eye or brain. Most patients are offered palliation with radiation and glucocorticoids, but recurrence is typical. These tumors behave much like large B-cell lymphomas of the brain, and consideration of more aggressive therapy is reasonable.

■ PARANASAL SINUSES

Localized non-Hodgkin lymphoma involving the nasal cavity and/or paranasal sinuses may be diffuse B-cell lymphoma, T-cell lymphoma, or natural killer (NK)/T-cell lymphoma.[135–140] The nasal cavity is the predominant site of involvement in T-cell and NK/T-cell lymphoma, whereas sinus involvement without nasal disease is common in B-cell lymphoma. Systemic B symptoms are more frequently observed in NK/T-cell lymphoma. Based on *in situ* hybridization studies, there is a strong association of Epstein-Barr virus with NK/T-cell lymphoma. These lymphomas may involve the frontal, maxillary, ethmoid, and sphenoid sinuses and typically involve bone. They present with local pain, upper airway obstruction, rhinorrhea, facial swelling, or epistaxis. They may extend into the periorbital area causing proptosis, visual loss, or diplopia. These lymphomas typically are diffuse large B-cell lymphomas in the United States and Western Europe and more often T- and NK-cell lymphomas in Asia.

■ SKIN

The three main types of cutaneous B-cell lymphomas are primary cutaneous marginal zone B-cell lymphoma, primary cutaneous follicular center lymphoma, and primary cutaneous large B-cell lymphoma (leg type) as defined in the World Health Organization–European Organization for Research and Treatment of Cancer.[141] Primary cutaneous marginal zone B-cell and primary cutaneous follicle center lymphoma are indolent types with an excellent prognosis that should be treated primarily with nonaggressive therapies. Primary cutaneous large B-cell lymphoma (leg type) is a diffuse dermal infiltrate of neoplastic B cells with extension to both the papillary dermis and the subcutaneous fat.[142,143] It is an aggressive lymphoma that should be treated primarily with aggressive chemotherapy. The cutaneous lymphomas may present as a solitary soft-tissue mass and mimic a soft-tissue sarcoma until biopsy clarifies the diagnosis. When it involves the leg, it has been called cutaneous diffuse large B-cell lymphoma, leg type (see Chap. 100). Chap. 105 discusses classical T-cell cutaneous lymphomas.

CHEST AND LUNG

Primary pulmonary lymphoma may present as a pulmonary nodule or mass and may be associated with hilar lymph node enlargement. The histopathology is usually marginal zone B-cell lymphoma of the mucosa-associated lymphoid tissue or diffuse large B-cell lymphoma. Rarely lymphomatoid granulomatosis has been present.[144,145] Lung biopsy is usually required to make a definitive diagnosis. Pleural effusions may occur as a result of either central lymphatic obstruction or pleural seeding.

Primary chest wall lymphoma may present as local pain or may be accompanied by fever, sweating, and dyspnea. These masses usually require excision for biopsy. They may be associated with pleural effusion and involvement of neighboring ribs.[146]

Primary endobronchial lymphoma is a rare occurrence and may follow lung transplantation. It can lead to airway obstruction as an early sign.

HEART

Primary cardiac lymphoma may involve the heart or pericardium or both. Patients may present with dyspnea, edema, arrhythmia, or pericardial effusion. The effusion may result in cardiac tamponade. Lymphomatous masses may be found in the right atrium (most common), pericardium, right ventricle, left atrium, or left ventricle. Most cases are a B-cell lymphoma; less than 5 percent are of T-cell lineage.[147–149]

GASTROINTESTINAL TRACT

Gastrointestinal lymphoma is the most common form of extranodal lymphoma, accounting for one-third of cases. The most commonly involved site is the stomach, followed by the small bowel, ileum, cecum, colon, and rectum. Lymphoma of the stomach typically causes dyspeptic symptoms and sometimes anorexia or early satiety. Hemorrhage is unusual but if present suggests a high-grade lymphoma. Diagnosis typically is made by gastroscopic biopsy.[150] *H. pylori* infection has been implicated in the pathogenesis of mucosa-associated lymphatic tissue gastric lymphoma.[151] At gastroscopy, mild to severe gastritis is common. Multiple biopsies are important to obtaining adequate material to determine the presence of *H. pylori*. Mucosa-associated lymphatic tissue lymphoma is common, but diffuse large B-cell lymphoma also may arise *de novo* or may be found in the background of a mucosa-associated lymphatic tissue lymphoma.[150] If both subtypes of lymphoma are present, the treatment should be directed at the large B-cell lymphoma.

In the bowel, the small intestine, rectum, and colon may be involved, in that order of frequency.[152] The intestinal location most often involved is the ileocecal region followed by small bowel, large bowel, and multiple intestinal sites.[152] Primary esophageal lymphoma is rare.[153] Primary colonic lymphoma is associated with symptoms of diarrhea, lower gastrointestinal bleeding, and nausea and vomiting secondary to low-grade obstruction. The most common disease location is the cecum, followed by the right colon, and the sigmoid colon.[154]

Rare cases of lymphoma may be confined to the liver. Right upper quadrant pain is the most common symptom. In about half of cases there is a history of previous inflammatory liver disease, such as hepatitis C.[155–158]

Primary extranodal lymphoma of the pancreas may present with abdominal pain, nausea, vomiting, obstructive jaundice, and weight loss, and very rarely signs of pancreatitis.[159–161]

The gallbladder may be the site of primary extranodal lymphoma and may present with right upper quadrant pain or other symptoms and signs consistent with cholecystitis.[162,163] It may extend into the bile ducts with jaundice and other signs of bile duct obstruction.[164]

GENITOURINARY

Testicular

Primary lymphoma of the testes typically presents as a painless enlargement of the testis in an older man. A hydrocele may also be present.[165–168] The histologic type usually is a diffuse large B-cell lymphoma. At presentation, two thirds of cases are localized to the testicle or to the testicle and pelvic or abdominal lymph nodes. After orchiectomy has established the diagnosis, patients are staged with a special focus on the remaining testicle. If sonography of the remaining testicle demonstrates a solid mass, it should be assumed to be lymphoma. Patients presenting with testicular lymphoma have a poorer prognosis compared to patients with other presentations of diffuse large B-cell lymphoma.[167] Patients experience relapse in either the CNS or the opposite testicle.

Ovary

Primary lymphoma of the ovary is often bilateral and presents as an abdominal mass with abdominal pain or palpation of a mass on physical examination.[169–173]

Uterus, Cervix, Genitalia

Cases of lymphoma limited to the uterus,[174–176] uterine cervix,[177,178] vagina, or vulva[179] can occur. Uterine and cervical lymphoma usually presents with an abdominal mass or vaginal bleeding. Lymphoma can develop within a uterine leiomyoma.[176]

Kidney

Lymphomatous involvement of both kidneys usually presents with renal failure, which can be reversed with either radiation or multidrug chemotherapy. Bilateral enlargement of the kidneys without obstruction and other organ or nodal involvement and absence of other causes of renal failure are characteristic of primary renal lymphoma.[180–184] The origins of the lymphoma are perplexing as the kidney is thought to be devoid of lymphoid tissue. Both careful staging and postmortem examination have verified the absence of lymphoma in other sites. An increased association of renal cell carcinoma and primary renal lymphoma may exist.[184] Rarely, the lymphomatous involvement, although still solely extranodal, involves only the perirenal space.[185]

Ureter, Bladder, Prostate

Bilateral ureteral involvement with obstructive renal failure may occur.[186] Primary lymphoma of the bladder may rarely extend to the kidney. Usually it is localized and responds well to treatment.[187–189] Primary extranodal lymphoma may involve the prostate.[190,191]

SPLEEN

Primary splenic lymphoma is rare.[192,193] Concomitant marrow involvement is present in most cases. When primary to the spleen, the lymphoma may be principally confined to the red pulp and is usually consistent histopathologically with diffuse large B-cell lymphoma.[193] In the absence of lymph node involvement or splenic white pulp involvement at the time of diagnosis or during the course of the disease, it can be considered an "extranodal" splenic lymphoma.[192]

BONE

Primary bone lymphoma may involve any bone but usually affects the long bones.[194–196] The presentation is usually bone pain and the lesions are usually lytic when imaged.[194] When the skull is involved the lymphoma may invade the central nervous system.[196]

BREAST

The clinical presentation of primary lymphoma of the female breast often mimics carcinoma of the breast. A small proportion of cases may be bilateral. The pathologic diagnosis is diffuse large B-cell lymphoma in approximately 85 percent of cases. BCL-2 expression is frequently present in the tumor cells. Small lymphocytic lymphoma, follicular lymphoma, and marginal zone lymphoma of mucosa-associated lymphoid tissue may also be the histopathologic diagnosis.[197,198] Staging may uncover either nodal involvement, marrow involvement or other extranodal sites with lymphoma in as many as half of cases. Approximately 10 percent of cases of primary breast lymphoma relapse in the central nervous system.[197,198]

ENDOCRINE GLANDS

Primary adrenal lymphoma usually present bilaterally and thus may lead to adrenal insufficiency. In the latter case, the presenting symptoms may be fatigue, asthenia, and other signs of hypoadrenocorticism.[199–202] Primary thyroid lymphoma often occurs in a gland afflicted by Hashimoto thyroiditis. Thus, it occurs more frequently in women than men. The patient may present with an enlarged thyroid (goiter) or have symptoms as a result of tracheal compression.[203–205] The histopathology may be diffuse large B-cell lymphoma or marginal zone B-cell lymphoma of mucosa-associated lymphatic tissue. Primary pituitary lymphoma is discussed under "Central Nervous System" above.

REFERENCES

1. Oberling C: Les reticulosarcomes et les reticuloendotheliosarcomes de la moelle ossue se (sarcomes d'Ewing). *Bull Assoc Fr Etude Cancer* 17:259, 1928.
2. Roulet F: Das primare Retothelsarkom der Lymphknoten. *Virchows Arch A Pathol Anat Histol* 277:15, 1930.
3. Ewing J: Endothelioma of lymph nodes. *J Med Res* 28:1, 1913.
4. Brill NE, Baehr G, Rosenthal N: Generalized giant lymph follicle hyperplasia of lymph nodes and spleen: A hitherto undescribed type. *JAMA* 84:668, 1925.
5. Symmers D: Follicular lymphadenopathy with splenomegaly: A newly recognized disease of the lymphatic system. *Arch Pathol Lab Med* 3:816, 1927.
6. Rappaport H: Tumors of the hematopoietic system, in *Atlas of Tumor Pathology*, sec 3, fasc 8, p 97. US Armed Forces Institute of Pathology, Washington, DC, 1966.
7. Lukes RJ, Craver LF, Hall TC, et al: Report of the nomenclature committee. *Cancer Res* 26:1311, 1966.
8. Lennert K, Mohri N, Stein H, Kaiserling E: The histopathology of malignant lymphoma. *Br J Haematol* 31(Suppl):193, 1975.
9. The Non-Hodgkin's Lymphoma Pathologic Classification Project: National Cancer Institute sponsored study of classifications of non-Hodgkin's lymphomas: Summary and description of a Working Formulation for clinical usage. *Cancer* 49:2112, 1982.
10. Harris NL, Jaffe ES, Stein H, et al: A revised European-American classification of lymphoid neoplasms: A proposal from the International Lymphoma Study Group. *Blood* 84:1361, 1994.
11. Hiddemann W, Longo DL, Coiffier B, et al: Lymphoma classification—The gap between biology and clinical management is closing. *Blood* 88:4085, 1996.
12. SH Swerdlow, Campo E, Harris NL, et al: *World Health Organization Classification of Tumors of Hematopoietic and Lymphoid Tissues*, 4th ed. IARC, Lyon, France, 2008.
13. Jemal A, Siegel R, Ward E, et al: Cancer statistics 2008. *CA Cancer J Clin* 58:71, 2008.
14. Chiu BC, Weisenburger DD: An update of the epidemiology of non-Hodgkin's lymphoma. *Clin Lymphoma* 4:161, 2003.
15. Alexander DD, Mink PJ, Adami HO, et al: The non-Hodgkin lymphomas: A review of the epidemiologic literature. *Int J Cancer* 120 Suppl 12:1, 2007.

15a. Hartge P, Colt JS, Severson RK, et al: Residential herbicide use and risk of non-Hodgkin lymphoma. *Cancer Epidemiol Biomarkers Prev* 14:934, 2005.

15b. Lee WJ, Alavanja MC, Hoppin JA, et al: Mortality among pesticide applicators exposed to chlorpyrifos in the Agricultural Health Study. *Environ Health Perspect* 115:528, 2007.

15c. De Roos AJ, Blair A, Rusiecki JA, et al: Alavanja MC. Cancer incidence among glyphosate-exposed pesticide applicators in the Agricultural Health Study. *Environ Health Perspect* 113:49, 2005.

15d. Lan Q, Morton LM, Armstrong B, et al: Genetic variation in caspase genes and risk of non-Hodgkin lymphoma: a pooled analysis of 3 population-based case-control studies. *Blood* 114:264, 2009.

15e. Morton LM, Purdue MP, Zheng T, et al: Risk of non-Hodgkin lymphoma associated with germline variation in genes that regulate the cell cycle, apoptosis, and lymphocyte development. *Cancer Epidemiol Biomarkers Prev* 18:1259, 2009.

15f. Wang SS, Purdue MP, Cerhan JR, et al: Common gene variants in the tumor necrosis factor (TNF) and TNF receptor superfamilies and NF-kB transcription factors and non-Hodgkin lymphoma risk. *PLoS One* 4:e5630, 2009.

15g. Purdue MP, Lan Q, Wang SS, Kricker A, et al: A pooled investigation of Toll-like receptor gene variants and risk of non-Hodgkin lymphoma. *Carcinogenesis* 30:275,2009.

15h. Zhang Y, Sanjose SD, Bracci PM, et al: Personal use of hair dye and the risk of certain subtypes of non-Hodgkin lymphoma. *Am J Epidemiol* 167:1321, 2008.

15i. Becker S, Dossus L, Kaaks R: Obesity related hyperinsulinaemia and hyperglycaemia and cancer development. *Arch Physiol Biochem* 115:86, 2009.

15j. Renehan AG, Roberts DL, Dive C: Obesity and cancer: pathophysiological and biological mechanisms. *Arch Physiol Biochem* 114:71, 2008.

15k. Renehan AG, Tyson M, Egger M, et al: Body-mass index and incidence of cancer: a systematic review and meta-analysis of prospective observational studies. *Lancet* 371:569, 2008.

15l. Willett EV, Morton LM, Hartge P, et al: Interlymph Consortium. Non-Hodgkin lymphoma and obesity: a pooled analysis from the InterLymph Consortium. *Int J Cancer* 122:2062, 2008.

15m. Maskarinec G, Erber E, Gill J, et al: Overweight and obesity at different times in life as risk factors for non-Hodgkin's lymphoma: the multiethnic cohort. *Cancer Epidemiol Biomarkers Prev* 17:196, 2008.

15n. Chiu BC, Soni L, Gapstur SM, et al: Obesity and risk of non-Hodgkin lymphoma (United States). *Cancer Causes Control* 18:677, 2007.

16. Moslehi R, Devesa SS, Schairer C, Fraumeni JF Jr: Rapidly increasing incidence of ocular non-Hodgkin lymphoma. *J Natl Cancer Inst* 98:936, 2006.
17. Zhou Y, Wang H, Fang W, et al: Incidence trends of mantle cell lymphoma in the United States between 1992 and 2004. *Cancer* 113:791, 2008.
18. Schenk M, Purdue MP, Colt JS, et al: Occupation/industry and risk of non-Hodgkin's lymphoma in the United States. *Occup Environ Med* 66:23, 2009.
19. Karunanayake CP, McDuffie HH, Dosman JA, et al: Occupational exposures and non-Hodgkin's lymphoma: Canadian case-control study. *Environ Health* 7:44, 2008.
20. Blair A: Occupational exposures and non-Hodgkin lymphoma: Where do we stand? *Occup Environ Med* 63:1, 2006.
21. Linet MS, Pottern LM: Familial aggregation of hematopoietic malignancies and risk of non-Hodgkin's lymphoma. *Cancer Res* 52(19 Suppl):5468s, 1992.
22. McDuffie HH, Pahwa P, Karunanayake CP, et al: Clustering of cancer among families of cases with Hodgkin lymphoma (HL), multiple myeloma (MM), non-Hodgkin's lymphoma (NHL), soft tissue sarcoma (STS) and control subjects. *BMC Cancer* 9:70, 2009.
23. Lu Y, Sullivan-Halley J, Cozen W, et al: Family history of haematopoietic malignancies and non-Hodgkin's lymphoma risk in the California Teachers Study. *Br J Cancer* 100:524, 2009.
24. Segel GB, Lichtman MA: Familial (inherited) leukemia, lymphoma, and myeloma. *Blood Cells Mol Dis* 32:246, 2004.
25. Beebe GW, Kato H, Land C: Studies of the mortality of A-bomb survivors. Mortality and radiation dose 1950–1974. *Radiat Res* 75:138, 1978.
26. Anderson RE, Nishiyama H, Yohei I, et al: Pathogenesis of radiation related leukemia and lymphoma. Speculations based primarily on experience of Hiroshima and Nagasaki. *Lancet* 1:1060, 1972.
27. Shimizu Y, Kato H, Schull WJ: Risk of cancer among atomic bomb survivors. *J Radiat Res (Tokyo)* 32(Suppl 2):54, 1991.
28. Richardson DB, Sugiyama H, Wing S, et al: Positive associations between ionizing radiation and lymphoma mortality among men. *Am J Epidemiol* 169:969, 2009.
29. Kesminiene A, Evrard AS, Ivanov VK, et al: Risk of hematological malignancies among Chernobyl liquidators. *Radiat Res* 170:721, 2008.
30. Court-Brown WM, Doll R: *Leukemia and aplastic anemia in patients irradiated for ankylosing spondylitis*. Medical Research Council Special Report Series, no 295. Her Majesty's Stationery Office, London, 1957.
31. Ron E: Ionizing radiation and cancer risk: Evidence from epidemiology. *Radiat Res* 150(5 Suppl):S30, 1998.
32. Boffetta P, van der Hel O, Kricker A, et al: Exposure to ultraviolet radiation and risk of malignant lymphoma and multiple myeloma—A multicentre European case-control study. *Int J Epidemiol* 37:1080, 2008.
33. Colt JS, Rothman N, Severson RK, et al: Organochlorine exposure, immune gene variation, and risk of non-Hodgkin lymphoma. *Blood* 113:1899, 2009.
34. Murata K, Yamada Y: The state of the art in the pathogenesis of ATL and new potential targets associated with HTLV-1 and ATL. *Int Rev Immunol* 26:249, 2007.

35 Poiesz BJ, Ruscetti FW, Gazdar AF, et al: Detection and isolation of type C retrovirus particles from fresh and cultured lymphocytes of a patient with cutaneous T-cell lymphoma. *Proc Natl Acad Sci U S A* 77:7415, 1980.

36. Jacobson S, Raine CS, Mingioli ES, et al: Isolation of an HTLV-I-like retrovirus from patients with tropical spastic paraparesis. *Nature* 331:540, 1988.
37. Snoda S: Relationship of HTLV-I-related adult T-cell leukemia and HTLV-I-associated myelopathy to distinct HLA haplotypes. *Jikken Igaku* 5:769, 1987.

38. Wong-Staal F, Gallo RC: The family of human T-lymphotropic leukemia viruses: HTLV-I as the cause of adult T cell leukemia and HTLV-III as the cause of acquired immunodeficiency syndrome. *Blood* 65:253,1985.
39. Blattner WA, Kalyanaraman VS, Robert-Guroff M, et al: The human type-C retrovirus HTLV, in blacks from the Caribbean region, and relationship to adult T-cell leukemia/lymphoma. *Int J Cancer* 30:257, 1982.
40. Robert-Guroff M, Kalyanaraman VS, Blattner WA, et al: Evidence for human T-cell lymphoma-leukemia virus infection of family members of human T cell lymphoma-leukemia virus positive T-cell leukemia-lymphoma patients. *J Exp Med* 157:248, 1983.
41. Sarin PS, Aoki T, Shibata A, et al: High incidence of human type-C retrovirus (HTLV) in family members of a HTLV-positive Japanese T-cell leukemia patient. *Proc Natl Acad Sci U S A* 80:2370, 1983.
42. Carbone A, Cesarman E, Spina, M, et al: HIV-associated lymphomas and gamma-herpes viruses. *Blood* 113:1213, 2009.
43 Epstein MA, Achang BG, Barr YH: Virus particles in cultured lymphoblasts from Burkitt's lymphoma. *Lancet* 1:702, 1964.
44. Nemerow GR, Wolfert R, McNaughton ME, Cooper NR: Identification and characterization of the Epstein-Barr virus receptor on human B lymphocytes and its relation to the C3d complement receptor (CR2). *J Virol* 55:347, 1985.
45. Henle W, Diehl V, Kohn G, et al: Herpes-type virus and chromosome marker in normal leucocytes after growth with irradiated Burkitt cells. *Science* 157:1064, 1967.
46. Anderson M, Klein G, Ziegler J, Henle W: Association of Epstein-Barr viral genomes with American Burkitt lymphoma. *Nature* 260:357, 1976.
47. Potter M, Mushinski JF: Oncogenes in B neoplasia. *Cancer Invest* 2:285, 1984.
48. Morrow RH Jr: Epidemiological evidence for the role of falciparum malaria in the pathogenesis of Burkitt's lymphoma, in *Burkitt's Lymphoma: A Human Cancer Model*, edited by G Lenoir, T O'Conor, CLM Olweny, p 177. ARC Scientific, Lyon, France, 1985.
49. Klein G: Lymphoma development in mice and humans: Diversity of initiation is followed by convergent cytogenetic evolution. *Proc Natl Acad Sci U S A* 76:2442, 1979.
50. Klein G: Specific chromosomal translocations and the genesis of B-cell-derived tumors in mice and men. *Cell* 19:311, 1983.
51. Suzuki R, Takeuchi K, Ohshima K, et al: Extranodal NK/T-cell lymphoma: Diagnosis and treatment cues. *Hematol Oncol* 26:66, 2008.
52. Aozasa K, Takakuwa T, Hongyo T, et al: Nasal NK/T-cell lymphoma: Epidemiology and pathogenesis. *Int J Hematol* 87:110, 2008.
53. Gessain A: Human herpesvirus 8 (HHV-8): Clinical and epidemiological aspects and clonality of associated tumors. *Bull Acad Natl Med* 192:1189, 2008.
54. Laurent C, Meggetto F, Brousset P: Human herpesvirus 8 infections in patients with immunodeficiencies. *Hum Pathol* 39:983, 2008.
55. Sullivan RJ, Pantanowitz L, Casper C, et al: HIV/AIDS: Epidemiology, pathophysiology, and treatment of Kaposi sarcoma-associated herpesvirus disease: Kaposi sarcoma, primary effusion lymphoma, and multicentric Castleman disease. *Clin Infect Dis* 47:1209, 2008.
56. Dotti G, Fiocchi R, Motta T, et al: Primary effusion lymphoma after heart transplantation: A new entity associated with human herpesvirus-8. *Leukemia* 13:664, 1999.
57. Okan V, Yilmaz M, Bayram A, et al: Prevalence of hepatitis B and C viruses in patients with lymphoproliferative disorders. *Int J Hematol* 88:403, 2008.
58. Chen MH, Hsiao LT, Chiou TJ, et al: High prevalence of occult hepatitis B virus infection in patients with B cell non-Hodgkin's lymphoma. *Ann Hematol* 87:475, 2008.
59. de Sanjose S, Benavente Y, Vajdic CM, Hepatitis C and non-Hodgkin lymphoma among 4784 cases and 6269 controls from the International Lymphoma Epidemiology Consortium. *Clin Gastroenterol Hepatol* 6:451, 2008.
60. Schollkopf C, Smedby KE, Hjalgrim H, et al: Hepatitis C infection and risk of malignant lymphoma. *Int J Cancer* 122:1885, 2008.
61. Inokuchi M, Ito T, Uchikoshi M, et al: Infection of B cells with hepatitis C virus for the development of lymphoproliferative disorders in patients with chronic hepatitis C. *J Med Virol* 81:619, 2009.
62. Isaacson PG, Spencer J: Gastric lymphoma and *Helicobacter pylori. Important Adv Oncol* 111, 1996.
63. Nakamura S, Yao T, Aoyagi K, et al: *Helicobacter pylori* and primary gastric lymphoma: A histopathologic and immunohistochemical analysis of 237 patients. *Cancer* 79:3, 1997.
64. Isaacson PG: Update on MALT lymphomas. *Best Pract Res Clin Haematol* 18:57, 2005.
65. Ferreri AJ, Dolcetti R, Dognini GP, et al: Chlamydophila psittaci is viable and infectious in the conjunctiva and peripheral blood of patients with ocular adnexal lymphoma: Results of a single-center prospective case-control study. *Int J Cancer* 123:1089, 2008.
66. Yoo C, Ryu MH, Huh J, et al: *Chlamydia psittaci* infection and clinicopathologic analysis of ocular adnexal lymphomas in Korea. *Am J Hematol* 82:821, 2007.
67. Ponzoni M, Ferreri AJ, Guidoboni M, et al: Chlamydia infection and lymphomas: Association beyond ocular adnexal lymphomas highlighted by multiple detection methods. *Clin Cancer Res* 14:5794, 2008.
68. Chan CC, Shen D, Mochizuki M, et al: Detection of *Helicobacter pylori* and *Chlamydia pneumoniae* genes in primary orbital lymphoma. *Trans Am Ophthalmol Soc* 104:62, 2006.
69. Gracia E, Froesch P, Mazzucchelli L, et al: Low prevalence of *Chlamydia psittaci* in ocular adnexal lymphomas from Cuban patients. *Leuk Lymphoma* 48:104, 2007.
70. Zhang GS, Winter JN, Variakojis D, et al: Lack of an association between *Chlamydia psittaci* and ocular adnexal lymphoma. *Leuk Lymphoma* 48:577, 2007.
71. Yakushijin Y, Kodama T, Takaoka I, et al: Absence of chlamydial infection in Japanese patients with ocular adnexal lymphoma of mucosa-associated lymphoid tissue. *Int J Hematol* 85:223, 2007.
72. Vargas RL, Fallone E, Felgar RE, et al: Is there an association between ocular adnexal lymphoma and infection with *Chlamydia psittaci*? The University of Rochester experience. *Leuk Res* 30:547, 2006.
73. Chanudet E, Zhou Y, Bacon CM, et al: *Chlamydia psittaci* is variably associated with ocular adnexal MALT lymphoma in different geographical regions. *J Pathol* 209:344, 2006.
74. Verma V, Shen D, Sieving PC, Chan CC: The role of infectious agents in the etiology of ocular adnexal neoplasia. *Surv Ophthalmol* 53:312, 2008.
75. Du MQ: MALT lymphoma: Recent advances in aetiology and molecular genetics. *J Clin Exp Hematop* 47:31, 2007.
76. Meyn MS: Ataxia-telangiectasia, cancer and the pathology of the ATM gene. *Clin Genet* 55:289, 1999.
77. Perlman S, Becker-Catania S, Gatti RA: Ataxia-telangiectasia: Diagnosis and treatment. *Semin Pediatr Neurol* 10:173, 2003.
78. Kaneko H, Kondo N: Clinical features of Bloom syndrome and function of the causative gene, BLM helicase. *Expert Rev Mol Diagn* 4:393, 2004.
79. Kaneko H, Inoue R, Fukao T, et al: Two Japanese siblings with Bloom syndrome gene mutation and B-cell lymphoma. *Leuk Lymphoma* 27:539, 1997.
80. Dembowska-Baginska B, Perek D, Brozyna A, et al: Non-Hodgkin lymphoma (NHL) in children with Nijmegen Breakage syndrome (NBS). *Pediatr Blood Cancer* 52:186, 2009.
81. Krüger L, Demuth I, Neitzel H, et al: Cancer incidence in Nijmegen breakage syndrome is modulated by the amount of a variant NBS protein. *Carcinogenesis* 28:107, 2007.
82. Malkin D, Li FP, Strong, LC, Fraumeni JF et al: Germline p53 mutations in a familial syndrome of breast cancer sarcomas, and other neoplasms. *Science* 250:1233, 1990.
83. Srivastava S, Zou Z, Pirollo K, et al: Germ-line transmission of a mutated p53 gene in a cancer-prone family with Li-Fraumeni Syndrome. *Nature* 348:747, 1990.
84. Cunningham-Rundles C, Bodian C: Common variable immunodeficiency: Clinical and immunological features of 248 patients. *Clin Immunol* 92:34,1999.
85. Chua I, Quinti I, Grimbacher B: Lymphoma in common variable immunodeficiency: Interplay between immune dysregulation, infection and genetics. *Curr Opin Hematol* 15:368, 2008.
86. Mustillo P, Bajwa RP, Termuhlen AM, et al: Tumor immune surveillance defect of X-linked severe combined immunodeficiency is not Epstein-Barr virus specific. *Pediatr Blood Cancer* 51:706, 2008.
87. Rengan R, Ochs HD: Molecular biology of the Wiskott-Aldrich syndrome. *Rev Immunogenet* 2:243, 2000.
88. Shcherbina A, Candotti F, Rosen FS, Remold-O'Donnell E: High incidence of lymphomas in a subgroup of Wiskott-Aldrich syndrome patients. *Br J Haematol* 121:529, 2003.
89. Rangel-Santos A, Wakim VL, Jacob CM, et al: Molecular characterization of patients with X-linked Hyper-IgM syndrome: Description of two novel CD40L mutations. *Scand J Immunol* 69:169, 2009.
90. Winkelstein JA, Marino MC, Ochs H, et al: The X-linked hyper-IgM syndrome: Clinical and immunologic features of 79 patients. *Medicine (Baltimore)* 82:373, 2003.
91. Macginnitie AJ, Geha R: X-linked lymphoproliferative disease: Genetic lesions and clinical consequences. *Curr Allergy Asthma Rep* 2:361, 2002.
92. Strauss SE, Jaffe ES, Puck JM, et al: The development of lymphomas in families with autoimmune lymphoproliferative syndrome with germ-line fas mutations and defective lymphocyte apoptosis. *Blood* 98:194, 2001.
93. Holzelova E, Vonarbourg C, Stolzenberg M-C, et al: Autoimmune lymphoproliferative syndrome with somatic FAS mutations. *N Engl J Med* 351:1409, 2004.
94. Grobe H: Dubowitz syndrome and acute lymphatic leukemia. *Monatsschr Kinderheilkd* 131:467, 1983.
95. Fokin AA, Robicsek F: Poland syndrome revisited. *Ann Thorac Surg* 74:2218, 2002.
96. Parikh PM, Karandikar SM, Koppikar S, et al: Poland syndrome with acute lymphoblastic leukemia in an adult. *Med Pediatr Oncol* 16:290, 1988.
97. Sackey K, Odone V, George SL, Murphy SB: Poland syndrome associated with childhood non-Hodgkin lymphoma. *Am J Dis Child* 138:600, 1984.
98. Vergin C, Cetingul N, Kavakli K, et al: A patient with WT syndrome and Castleman disease. *Acta Paediatr Jpn* 37:108, 1995.
99. Capello D, Rossi D, Gaidano G: Post-transplant lymphoproliferative disorders: Molecular basis of disease histogenesis and pathogenesis. *Hematol Oncol* 23:61, 2005.
100. Dolcetti R: B lymphocytes and Epstein-Barr virus: The lesson of post-transplant lymphoproliferative disorders. *Autoimmun Rev* 7:96, 2007.
101. Taylor AL, Marcus R, Bradley JA: Post-transplant lymphoproliferative disorders (PTLD) after solid organ transplantation. *Crit Rev Oncol Hematol* 56:155, 2005.
102. Lok C, Viseux V, Denoeux JP, Bagot M: Post-transplant cutaneous T-cell lymphomas. *Crit Rev Oncol Hematol* 56:137, 2005.
103. Jamali FR, Otrock ZK, Soweid AM, et al: An overview of the pathogenesis and natural history of post-transplant T-cell lymphoma *Leuk Lymphoma* 48:1780, 2007 (corrected and republished article originally printed in *Leuk Lymphoma*, 48:1237, 2007).
104. Kinlen LJ: Incidence of cancer in rheumatoid arthritis and other disorders after immunosuppressive therapy. *Am J Med* 78(Suppl 1A):44, 1985.
105. Ekstrom Smedby K, Vajdic CM, Falster M, et al: Autoimmune disorders and risk of non-Hodgkin lymphoma subtypes: A pooled analysis within the InterLymph Consortium. *Blood* 111:4028, 2008.
106. Troch M, Woehrer S, Streubel B, et al: Chronic autoimmune thyroiditis (Hashimoto's thyroiditis) in patients with MALT lymphoma. *Ann Oncol* 19:1336, 2008.

107. Ji J, Shu X, Li X, Sundquist K, et al: Cancer risk in hospitalized sarcoidosis patients: A follow-up study in Sweden. *Ann Oncol* 20:1121, 2009.
108. Brassesco MS: Leukemia/lymphoma-associated gene fusions in normal individuals. *Genet Mol Res* 7:782, 2008.
109. Ong ST, Le Beau MM: Chromosomal abnormalities and molecular genetics of non-Hodgkin's lymphoma. *Semin Oncol* 25:447, 1998.
110. Korsmeyer SJ: Bcl-2 initiates a new category of oncogenes: Regulators of cell death. *Blood* 80:879, 1992.
111. Hockenbery D, Zutter M, Hickey W, et al: BCL2 protein is topographically restricted in tissues characterized by apoptotic cell death. *Proc Natl Acad Sci U S A* 88:6961, 1991.
112. Neri A, Barriga F, Knowles D, et al: Different regions of the immunoglobulin heavy-chain locus are involved in chromosomal translocations in distinct pathogenetic forms of Burkitt lymphoma. *Proc Natl Acad Sci U S A* 85:2748, 1988.
113. Hamilton-Dutoit S, Pallesen G, Franzmann M, et al: AIDS-related lymphoma. Histopathology, immunophenotype, and association with Epstein-Barr virus as demonstrated by in situ nucleic acid hybridization. *Am J Pathol* 138:149, 1991.
114. Ballerini P, Gaidano G, Gong J, et al: Multiple genetic lesions in AIDS-related non-Hodgkin's lymphoma. *Blood* 81:166, 1993.
115. Filippa DA, Ladanyi M, Wollner N, et al: CD30 (Ki-1)-positive malignant lymphomas: Clinical, immunophenotypic, histologic, and genetic characteristics and differences with Hodgkin's disease. *Blood* 87:2905, 1996.
116. Morris SW, Kirstein MN, Valentine MB, et al: Fusion of a kinase gene, ALK, to a nucleolar protein gene, NPM, in non-Hodgkin's lymphoma. *Science* 263:1281, 1994.
117. Lopategui JR, Sun L-H, Chan JKC, et al: Low frequency association of the t(2;5)(p23;q35) chromosomal translocation with CD30+ lymphomas from American and Asian patients. *Am J Pathol* 146:323, 1995.
118. Downing JR, Shurtleff SA, Zielenska M, et al: Molecular detection of the (2;5) translocation of non-Hodgkin's lymphoma by reverse transcriptase polymerase chain reaction. *Blood* 85:3416, 1995.
119. DeCoteau JF, Butmarc JR, Kinney MC, Kadin ME: The t(2;5) chromosomal translocation is not a common feature of primary cutaneous CD30+ lymphoproliferative disorders: Comparison with anaplastic large-cell lymphoma of nodal origin. *Blood* 87:3437, 1996.
120. Campbell LJ: Cytogenetics of lymphomas. *Pathology* 37:493, 2005.
121. Carbone PP: Report on the committee on Hodgkin's disease staging classification. *Cancer Res* 31:1860, 1971.
122. Merlin E, Chabrier S, Verkarre V, et al: Primary leptomeningeal ALK+ lymphoma in a 13-year-old child. *J Pediatr Hematol Oncol* 30:963, 2008.
123. Pollack IF, Lunsford LD, Flickinger JC, et al: Prognostic factors in the diagnosis and treatment of primary central nervous system lymphomas. *Cancer* 63:939, 1989.
124. Epelbaum R, Haim N, Ben-Shahar M, et al: Non-Hodgkin's lymphoma presenting with spinal epidural involvement. *Cancer* 58:2120, 1986.
125. Paul T, Challa S, Tandon A, et al: Primary central nervous system lymphomas: Indian experience, and review of literature. *Indian J Cancer* 45:112, 2008.
126. Layden BT, Dubner S, Toft DJ, et al: Primary CNS lymphoma with bilateral symmetric hypothalamic lesions presenting with panhypopituitarism and diabetes insipidus. *Pituitary* 2009 (Epub).
127. Moshkin O, Muller P, Scheithauer BW, et al: Primary pituitary lymphoma: A histological, immunohistochemical, and ultrastructural study with literature review. *Endocr Pathol* 20:46, 2009.
128. Kozáková D, Machálečková K, Brtko P, et al: Primary B-cell pituitary lymphoma of the Burkitt type: Case report of the rare clinic entity with typical clinical presentation. *Cas Lek Cesk* 147:569, 2008.
129. Sjö LD: Ophthalmic lymphoma: Epidemiology and pathogenesis. *Acta Ophthalmol* 87(Thesis 1):1, 2009.
130. Conners JM: Problems in lymphoma management: Special sites of presentation. *Oncology* 12:188, 1998.
131. Sjö LD, Heegaard S, Prause JU, et al: Extranodal marginal zone lymphoma in the ocular region: Clinical, immunophenotypical, and cytogenetical characteristics. *Invest Ophthalmol Vis Sci* 50:516, 2009.
132. Sjö LD, Ralfkiaer E, Prause JU: Increasing incidence of ophthalmic lymphoma in Denmark from 1980 to 2005. *Invest Ophthalmol Vis Sci* 49:3283, 2008.
133. Esik O, Ikeda H, Mukai K, Kaneko A: A retrospective analysis of different modalities for treatment of primary orbital non-Hodgkin's lymphomas. *Radiother Oncol* 38:13, 1996.
134. Whitcup SM, de Smet MD, Rubin BI, et al: Intraocular lymphoma: Clinical and histopathologic diagnosis. *Ophthalmology* 100:1399, 1993.
135. Kim GE, Koom WS, Yang WI, et al: Clinical relevance of three subtypes of primary sinonasal lymphoma characterized by immunophenotypic analysis. *Head Neck* 26:584, 2004.
136. Abbondanzo SL, Wenig BM: Non-Hodgkin's lymphoma of the sinonasal tract: A clinicopathologic and immunophenotypic study of 120 cases. *Cancer* 75:1281, 1995.
137. Frierson HF, Mills SE, Innes DJ: Non-Hodgkin's lymphomas of the sinonasal region: Histologic subtypes and their clinicopathologic features. *Am J Clin Pathol* 81:721, 1984.
138. Oprea C, Cainap C, Azoulay R, et al: Primary diffuse large B-cell non-Hodgkin lymphoma of the paranasal sinuses: A report of 14 cases. *Br J Haematol* 131:468, 2005.
139. Sands NB, Tewfik MA, Hwang SY, Desrosiers M: Extranodal T-cell lymphoma of the sinonasal tract presenting as severe rhinitis: Case series. *J Otolaryngol Head Neck Surg* 37:528, 2008.
140. Shohat I, Berkowicz M, Dori S, et al: Primary non-Hodgkin's lymphoma of the sinonasal tract. *Oral Surg Oral Med Oral Pathol Oral Radiol Endod* 97:328, 2004.
141. Willemze R: Primary cutaneous B-cell lymphoma: Classification and treatment. *Curr Opin Oncol* 18:425, 2006.
142. Zhao J, Han B, Shen T, et al: Primary cutaneous diffuse large B-cell lymphoma (leg type) after renal allograft: Case report and review of the literature. *Int J Hematol* 89:113, 2009.
143. Levy A, Randall MB, Henson T: Primary cutaneous B-cell lymphoma, leg type restricted to the subcutaneous fat arising in a patient with dermatomyositis. *Am J Dermatopathol* 30:578, 2008.
144. Hu YH, Hsiao LT, Yang CF, et al: Prognostic factors of Chinese patients with primary pulmonary non-Hodgkin's lymphoma: The single-institute experience in Taiwan. *Ann Hematol* 88:839, 2009.
145. Kennedy JL, Nasthwani BN, Burke JS, et al: Pulmonary lymphomas and other pulmonary lymphoid lesions: A clinicopathologic and immunologic study of 64 patients. *Cancer* 56:539, 1985.
146. Tabatabai A, Hashemi M, Ahmadinejad M, et al: Primary chest wall lymphoma with no history of tuberculous pyothorax: Diagnosis and treatment. *J Thorac Cardiovasc Surg* 136:1472, 2008.
147. Ikeda H, Nakamura S, Nishimaki H, et al: Primary lymphoma of the heart: Case report and literature review. *Pathol Int* 54:187, 2004.
148. Antoniades L, Eftychiou C, Petrou PM, et al: Primary cardiac lymphoma: Case report and brief review of the literature. *Echocardiography* 26:214, 2009.
149. Legault S, Couture C, Bourgault C, et al: Primary cardiac Burkitt-like lymphoma of the right atrium. *Can J Cardiol* 25:163, 2009.
150. Psyrri A, Papageorgiou S, Economopoulos T: Primary extranodal lymphomas of stomach: Clinical presentation, diagnostic pitfalls and management. *Ann Oncol* 19:1992, 2008.
151. Mbulaiteye SM, Hisada M, El-Omar EM: *Helicobacter pylori* associated global gastric cancer burden. *Front Biosci* 14:1490, 2009.
152. Lee J, Kim WS, Kim K, et al: Intestinal lymphoma: Exploration of the prognostic factors and the optimal treatment. *Leuk Lymphoma* 45:339, 2004.
153. Zhu Q, Xu B, Xu K, et al: Primary non-Hodgkin's lymphoma in the esophagus. *J Dig Dis* 9:241, 2008.
154. Gonzalez QH, Heslin MJ, Dávila-Cervantes A, et al: Primary colonic lymphoma. *Am Surg* 74:214, 2008.
155. Chan WK, Tse EW, Fan YS, et al: Positron emission tomography/computed tomography in the diagnosis of multifocal primary hepatic lymphoma. *J Clin Oncol* 26:5479, 2008.
156. Asagi A, Miyake Y, Ando M, et al: A case of primary malignant lymphoma of the liver treated by R-CHOP therapy. *Nippon Shokakibyo Gakkai Zasshi* 106:389, 2009.
157. Doi H, Horiike N, Hiraoka A, et al: Primary hepatic marginal zone B cell lymphoma of mucosa-associated lymphoid tissue type: Case report and review of the literature. *Int J Hematol* 88:418, 2008.
158. Kaneko F, Yokomori H, Sato A, et al: A case of primary hepatic non-Hodgkin's lymphoma with chronic hepatitis C. *Med Mol Morphol* 41:171, 2008 (erratum in: *Med Mol Morphol* 41:243, 2008).
159. Lin H, Li SD, Hu XG, Li ZS: Primary pancreatic lymphoma: Report of six cases. *World J Gastroenterol* 12:5064, 2006.
160. Sata N, Kurogochi A, Endo K, et al: Follicular lymphoma of the pancreas: A case report and proposed new strategies for diagnosis and surgery of benign or low-grade malignant lesions of the head of the pancreas. *JOP* 8:44, 2007.
161. Liakakos T, Misiakos EP, Tsapralis D, et al: A role for surgery in primary pancreatic B-cell lymphoma: A case report. *J Med Case Reports* 2:167, 2008.
162. Mitropoulos FA, Angelopoulou MK, Siakantaris MP, et al: Primary non-Hodgkin's lymphoma of the gall bladder. *Leuk Lymphoma* 40:123, 2000.
163. Jelic TM, Barreta TM, Yu M, et al: Primary, extranodal, follicular non-Hodgkin lymphoma of the gallbladder: Case report and a review of the literature. *Leuk Lymphoma* 45:381, 2004.
164. Ferluga D, Luzar B, Gadzijev EM: Follicular lymphoma of the gallbladder and extrahepatic bile ducts. *Virchows Arch* 442:136, 2003.
165. Vural F, Cagirgan S, Saydam G, et al: Primary testicular lymphoma. *J Natl Med Assoc* 99:1277, 2007.
166. Vitolo U, Ferreri AJ, Zucca E: Primary testicular lymphoma. *Crit Rev Oncol Hematol* 65:183, 2008.
167. Zucca EC, Conconi A, Mughal TI, et al: Patterns of outcome and prognostic factors in primary large-cell lymphoma of the testis in a survey by the International Extranodal Lymphoma Study Group. *J Clin Oncol* 21:20, 2003.
168. Fonseca RH, Habermann TM, Colgan JP, et al: Testicular lymphoma is associated with a high incidence of extranodal recurrence. *Cancer* 88:154, 2000.
169. Elharroudi T, Ismaili N, Errihani H, Jalil A: Primary lymphoma of the ovary. *J Cancer Res Ther* 4:195, 2008.
170. Ray S, Mallick MG, Pal PB, et al: Extranodal non-Hodgkin's lymphoma presenting as an ovarian mass. *Indian J Pathol Microbiol* 51:528, 2008.
171. Muñoz Martín AJ, Pérez Fernández R, Viñuela Beneítez MC, et al: Primary ovarian Burkitt lymphoma. *Clin Transl Oncol* 10:673, 2008.
172. Pectasides D, Iacovidou I, Psyrri A, et al: Primary ovarian lymphoma: Report of two cases and review of the literature. *J Chemother* 20:513, 2008.
173. Crawshaw J, Sohaib SA, Wotherspoon A, Shepherd JH: Primary non-Hodgkin's lymphoma of the ovaries: Imaging findings. *Br J Radiol* 80:e155, 2007.

174. Hamadani M, Kharfan-Dabaja M, Kamble R, et al: Marginal zone B-cell lymphoma of the uterus: A case report and review of the literature. *J Okla State Med Assoc* 99:154, 2006.
175. Latteri MA, Cipolla C, Gebbia V, et al: Primary extranodal non-Hodgkin lymphomas of the uterus and the breast: Report of three cases. *Eur J Surg Oncol* 21:432, 1995.
176. Merz H, Lange K, Koch BU, et al: Primary extranodal CD8 positive epitheliotropic T-cell lymphoma arising in a leiomyoma of the uterus. *BJOG* 110:527, 2003.
177. Gabriele A, Gaudiano L: Primary malignant lymphoma of the cervix. A case report. *J Reprod Med* 48:899, 2003.
178. Hanprasertpong J, Hanprasertpong T, Thammavichit T, et al: Primary non-Hodgkin's lymphoma of the uterine cervix. *Asian Pac J Cancer Prev* 9:363, 2008.
179. Sungurtekin U, Lacin S, Ayhan S: Primary genital non-Hodgkin lymphoma. *Aust N Z J Obstet Gynaecol* 38:346, 1998.
180. Diskin CJ, Stokes TJ, Dansby LM, et al: Acute renal failure due to a primary renal B-cell lymphoma. *Am J Kidney Dis* 50:885, 2007.
181. Kuo CC, Li WY, Huang CC, et al: Primary renal lymphoma. *Br J Haematol* 144:628, 2009.
182. James TC, Shaikh H, Escuadro L, Villano JL: Bilateral primary renal lymphoma. *Br J Haematol* 143:1, 2008.
183. Lopez R: Acute renal failure due to a primary renal B-cell lymphoma. *Am J Kidney Dis* 52:808, 2008.
184. Kunthur A, Wiernik PH, Dutcher JP: Renal parenchymal tumors and lymphoma in the same patient: Case series and review of the literature. *Am J Hematol* 81:271, 2006.
185. Mai KT, Burns BB, Isotalo P, et al: Primary extranodal perirenal malignant lymphoma. *Can J Urol* 5:599, 1998.
186. Kubota Y, Kawai A, Tsuchiya T, et al: Bilateral primary malignant lymphoma of the ureter. *Int J Clin Oncol* 12:482, 2007.
187. Terzic T, Radojevic S, Cemerikic-Martinovic et al: Primary non-Hodgkin lymphoma of urinary bladder with nine years later renal involvement and absence of systemic lymphoma: A case report. *Med Oncol* 25:248, 2008.
188. Hughes M, Morrison A, Jackson R: Primary bladder lymphoma: Management and outcome of 12 patients with a review of the literature. *Leuk Lymphoma* 46:873, 2005.
189. Horasanli K, Kadihasanoglu M, Aksakal OT, et al: A case of primary lymphoma of the bladder managed with multimodal therapy. *Nat Clin Pract Urol* 5:167, 2008.
190. Bostwick DG, Iczkowski KA, Amin MB, et al: Malignant lymphoma involving the prostate: Report of 62 cases. *Cancer* 83:732, 1998.
191. Jhavar S, Agarwal JP, Naresh KN, et al: Primary extranodal mucosa associated lymphoid tissue (MALT) lymphoma of the prostate. *Leuk Lymphoma* 41:445, 2001.
192. Kehoe J, Straus DJ: Primary lymphoma of the spleen: Clinical features and outcome after splenectomy. *Cancer* 62:1433, 1988.
193. Kashimura M, Noro M, Akikusa B, et al: Primary splenic diffuse large B-cell lymphoma manifesting in red pulp. *Virchows Arch* 453:501, 2008.
194. Bakhshi S, Singh P, Thulkar S: Bone involvement in pediatric non-Hodgkin's lymphomas. *Hematology* 13:348, 2008.
195. Catlett JP, Williams SA, O'Connor SC, et al: Primary lymphoma of bone: An institutional experience. *Leuk Lymphoma* 49:2125, 2008.
196. Agrawal A, Sinha A: Lymphoma of frontotemporal region with massive bone destruction and intracranial and intraorbital extension. *J Cancer Res Ther* 4:203, 2008.
197. Giardini RP, Piccolo C, Rilke F: Primary non-Hodgkin's lymphomas of the female breast. *Cancer* 69:725, 1992.
198. Validire P, Capovilla M, Asselain B, et al: Primary breast non-Hodgkin's lymphoma: A large single center study of initial characteristics, natural history, and prognostic factors. *Am J Hematol* 84:133, 2009.
199. Hernández Marín B, Díaz Muñoz de la Espada VM, Alvarez Alvarez R, et al: Adrenal failure caused by primary adrenal non-Hodgkin lymphoma: A case report and review of the literature. *An Med Interna* 25:131, 2008.
200. Nishiuchi T, Imachi H, Fujiwara M, et al: A case of non-Hodgkin's lymphoma primary arising in both adrenal glands associated with adrenal failure. *Endocrine* 35:34, 2009.
201. Gu B, Ding Q, Xia G, et al: Primary bilateral adrenal non-Hodgkin's lymphoma associated with normal adrenal function. *Urology* 73:752, 2009.
202. Zhou J, Ye D, Wu M, et al: Bilateral adrenal tumor: Causes and clinical features in eighteen cases. *Int Urol Nephrol* 41:547, 2009.
203. Skacel M, Ross CW, Hsi ED: A reassessment of primary thyroid lymphoma: High-grade MALT-type lymphoma as a distinct subtype of diffuse large B-cell lymphoma. *Histopathology* 37:10, 2000.
204. Derringer GA, Thompson LD, Frommelt RA, et al: Malignant lymphoma of the thyroid gland: A clinicopathologic study of 108 cases. *Am J Surg Pathol* 24:623, 2000.
205. Hwang YC, Kim TY, Kim WB, et al: Clinical characteristics of primary thyroid lymphoma in Koreans. *Endocr J* 56:399, 2009.
206. Bell DW, Varley JM, Szydlo TE, et al: Heterozygous germ line hCHK2 mutations in Li-Fraumeni syndrome. *Science* 24:2528, 1999.
207. Varley J: TP53, hChk2, and the Li-Fraumeni syndrome. *Methods Mol Biol* 222:117, 2003.

CHAPTER 98

PATHOLOGY OF MALIGNANT LYMPHOMAS

Randy D. Gascoyne and Brian F. Skinnider

SUMMARY

The classification of malignant lymphomas has been a contentious issue during the past fifty years, undergoing numerous changes during its evolution. The recent World Health Organization (WHO) classification of lymphoid neoplasms has gained worldwide acceptance by both pathologists and oncologists. It provides a list of distinct diseases that are defined by a combination of morphologic, phenotypic, genetic, and clinical features, and attempts to correlate each disease with a cell of origin. Because the classification of lymphomas requires the integration of such diverse information, the diagnosis has become more complex compared to other solid malignancies. As a result, several ancillary studies have become useful in the diagnosis of lymphomas, which requires special handling of biopsy material in which a diagnosis of lymphoma is suspected.

The WHO classification identifies three major categories of lymphoid malignancies: B-cell neoplasms, T- and natural killer (NK) cell neoplasms, and Hodgkin lymphoma. Two major categories are identified within the B-cell and T-/NK cell neoplasms: precursor neoplasms and peripheral or mature neoplasms. Unlike previous lymphoma classifications, the WHO classification does not group different lymphomas by clinical outcome or histologic grade. It recognizes that each disease has distinctive clinical features and response to treatment and may have a spectrum of clinical aggressiveness that may correlate with histologic grade or gene expression patterns. The WHO classification recognizes that several of the diseases it describes are heterogenous and likely include two or more distinct diseases that cannot be identified based on current data, and remains open to incorporate new data as they become available. One such source of new data for classifying lymphoma is the study of gene expression profiling by complement DNA microarray technology, which is providing new insights into the classification of diseases such as diffuse large B-cell lymphoma and chronic lymphocytic leukemia. Proteomics approaches will add further texture to the molecular taxonomy of lymphoma classification.

HISTORICAL ASPECTS OF LYMPHOMA CLASSIFICATION

During much of the 20th century, the classification of malignant lymphoma was fraught with controversy, with consensus reached during the past decade. A detailed discussion of the history of lymphoma classification is beyond the scope of this chapter and can be found elsewhere.[1]

Acronyms and abbreviations that appear in this chapter include: ABC, activated B-cell; ALCL, anaplastic large cell lymphoma; ALK, anaplastic lymphoma kinase; EBV, Epstein-Barr virus; FISH, fluorescence *in situ* hybridization; GCB, germinal center B cell; Ig, immunoglobulin; IGH, immunoglobulin heavy chain; LP, lymphocyte predominant; MALT, mucosa-associated lymphoid tissue; NF-κB, nuclear factor-κB; NK, natural killer; PCR, polymerase chain reaction; PTCL, peripheral T-cell lymphoma; REAL, revised European-American lymphoma; TNF, tumor necrosis factor; WHO, World Health Organization.

From Thomas Hodgkin's description in 1832 of what became known as Hodgkin lymphoma[2] to the first half of the 20th century, several types of lymphomas with distinctive morphologic and clinical features were described using a variety of terms, including lymphoma, lymphosarcoma, reticulum cell sarcoma, and giant follicular lymphoma.[1] However, many of the terms were not used uniformly, resulting in significant misunderstanding, particularly between pathologists and clinicians. Starting in the 1930s, several attempts were made to classify lymphomas and provide some uniformity of diagnosis. Classifications included the American Registry of Pathology classification based on morphologic and clinical features in 1934,[3] and the Gall and Mallory classification in 1942,[4] based primarily on morphologic features. These classifications culminated in the Rappaport classification, initially published in 1956, which divided lymphomas based on growth pattern, cell type, and stage of differentiation.[5,6] Most importantly, this classification demonstrated clinical relevance, showing that lymphomas with a nodular pattern had a better prognosis than diffuse lymphomas.

In the 1960s and 1970s, an explosion of studies on the immune system had a profound effect on our understanding of lymphocyte biology and had a consequent effect on our understanding of malignant lymphomas. Normal lymphocytes now could be classified into distinct lineages (B, T, and natural killer [NK]) which could be determined by expression of lineage-specific surface antigens and eventually by genetic analysis of B- and T-cell receptors.[7,8] Several new lymphoma classification schemes were developed to incorporate the new immunologic data, the most important being the Kiel classification[9] (used primarily in Europe) and the Lukes and Collins classification[10] (used primarily in North America). By the 1970s, at least five classification schemes were widely used in different parts of the world. At the same time, clinical studies were beginning to show that some patients with aggressive lymphomas could be cured with combination chemotherapy.[11] Oncologists needed to interpret results of clinical trials performed in different institutions, a situation made difficult by the use of different classification schemes that were not easily translated among themselves.

The problem was addressed by the United States National Cancer Institute, which convened a large group of investigators to determine which classification scheme was best at predicting clinical outcome of lymphoma. None of the classification schemes was identified as predicting clinical outcome better than the other schemes. Therefore, pathologists were advised to continue using one of the six classification schemes studied, and a "Working Formulation" was developed so that oncologists could translate clinical data derived in different institutions using different classification schemes.[12] Lymphomas were divided into 10 categories based solely on morphologic features. To help clinicians deal with a large number of lymphoma subtypes, the lymphomas were further grouped into three clinical prognostic groups (clinical grades). Although the Working Formulation was not intended to be a stand-alone classification scheme, it was used as such by many institutions, particularly in North America.

However, increasing phenotypic and genotypic data enabled defining several distinctive lymphoma subtypes. The Working Formulation lumped different lymphomas into broad categories that were obscuring the distinctive features of the newly described entities. The Working Formulation categories were based solely on morphologic features and were not able to incorporate new immunologic and molecular genetic data that were recognizing new types of lymphomas, including mantle cell lymphomas, marginal zone lymphomas, and peripheral T-cell lymphomas.

In the 1980s and 1990s, several new lymphoma entities based on new immunologic and molecular genetic data were identified. Although attempts were made to incorporate these new entities into the existing classification schemes,[13] problems with uniformity between different institutions persisted. A desire to eliminate the continued confusion ultimately led to a new approach to lymphoma classification proposed by the

TABLE 98–1. The WHO Classification of Lymphoid Neoplasms

Precursor lymphoid neoplasms
- B lymphoblastic leukemia/lymphoma, NOS
- B lymphoblastic leukemia/lymphoma with recurrent genetic abnormalities
 - B lymphoblastic leukemia/lymphoma with t(9;22)(q34;q11.2); *BCR-ABL1*
 - B lymphoblastic leukemia/lymphoma with t(v;11q23); MLL rearranged
 - B lymphoblastic leukemia/lymphoma with t(12;21)(p13;q22); *TEL-AML1*
 - B lymphoblastic leukemia/lymphoma with hyperdiploidy
 - B lymphoblastic leukemia/lymphoma with hypodiploidy
 - B lymphoblastic leukemia/lymphoma with t(5;14)(q31;q32); *IL3-IGH*
 - B lymphoblastic leukemia/lymphoma with t(1;19)(q23;p13.3); *E2A-PBX1*
- T lymphoblastic leukemia/lymphoma

Mature B-cell neoplasms
- Chronic lymphocytic leukemia/small lymphocytic lymphoma
- B-cell prolymphocytic leukemia
- Splenic B-cell marginal zone lymphoma
- Hairy cell leukemia
- Splenic B-cell lymphoma/leukemia, unclassifiable
- Lymphoplasmacytic lymphoma
- Heavy chain diseases
- Plasma cell neoplasms
- Extranodal marginal zone lymphoma of mucosa-associated lymphoid tissue (MALT lymphoma)
- Nodal marginal zone lymphoma
- Follicular lymphoma
- Primary cutaneous follicle center lymphoma
- Mantle cell lymphoma
- Diffuse large B-cell lymphoma (DLBCL), NOS
 - T-cell/histiocyte-rich large B-cell lymphoma
 - Primary DLBCL of the CNS
 - Primary cutaneous DLBCL, leg type
 - EBV-positive DLBCL of the elderly
- DLBCL associated with chronic inflammation
- Lymphomatoid granulomatosis
- Primary mediastinal (thymic) large B-cell lymphoma
- Intravascular large B-cell lymphoma
- ALK-positive large B-cell lymphoma

- Plasmablastic lymphoma
- Large B-cell lymphoma arising in HHV-8–associated multicentric Castleman disease
- Primary effusion lymphoma
- Burkitt lymphoma
- B-cell lymphoma, unclassifiable, with features intermediate between DLBCL and Burkitt lymphoma
- B-cell lymphoma, unclassifiable, with features intermediate between DLBCL and classical Hodgkin lymphoma

Mature T- and NK cell neoplasms
- T-cell prolymphocytic leukemia
- T-cell large granular lymphocytic leukemia
- Chronic lymphoproliferative disorder of NK cells
- Aggressive NK cell leukemia
- EBV-positive T-cell lymphoproliferative diseases of childhood
- Adult T-cell leukemia/lymphoma
- Extranodal NK/T-cell lymphoma, nasal type
- Enteropathy-associated T-cell lymphoma
- Hepatosplenic T-cell lymphoma
- Subcutaneous panniculitis-like T-cell lymphoma
- Mycosis fungoides
- Sézary syndrome
- Primary cutaneous CD30-positive T-cell lymphoproliferative disorders
- Primary cutaneous peripheral T-cell lymphoma, rare subtypes
- Peripheral T-cell lymphoma, NOS
- Angioimmunoblastic T-cell lymphoma
- Anaplastic large cell lymphoma, ALK positive
- Anaplastic large cell lymphoma, ALK negative

Hodgkin lymphoma
- Nodular lymphocyte predominant Hodgkin lymphoma
- Classical Hodgkin lymphoma
 - Nodular sclerosis Hodgkin lymphoma
 - Mixed cellularity Hodgkin lymphoma
 - Lymphocyte-rich classical Hodgkin lymphoma
 - Lymphocyte depleted Hodgkin lymphoma

ALK, anaplastic lymphoma kinase; CNS, central nervous system; EBV, Epstein-Barr virus; HHV, human herpesvirus; NK, natural killer; NOS, not otherwise specified.

International Lymphoma Study Group that used all available information, including morphology, immunophenotype, genetic and clinical features, to define a list of distinctive entities that could be uniformly diagnosed by hematopathologists. The proposal was published in 1994 and was known as the revised European-American lymphoma (REAL) classification.[14] The REAL classification identified "real" diseases that hematopathologists were recognizing in their daily practice. The authors also attempted to correlate lymphoma classification to normal lymphocyte biology by postulating a cell of origin for each lymphoma. Importantly, this classification identified entities that had distinctive clinical features and could be reproducibly diagnosed by expert hematopathologists.[15]

WORLD HEALTH ORGANIZATION CLASSIFICATION

In the late 1990s, a new World Health Organization (WHO) classification for lymphoproliferative disorders was being developed, based on the REAL classification. First published in 2001 (and revised in 2008), the WHO classification represented a consensus between an international group of more than 50 experienced hematopathologists, including contributions from a clinical advisory committee of hematologists and oncologists experienced in treating lymphomas.[16] The WHO classification (Table 98–1) identified several major categories including precursor lymphoid neoplasms, mature B-cell neoplasms, mature, T- and NK cell neoplasms, and Hodgkin lymphoma.

Distinctive lymphoma entities were identified based upon a combination of morphologic, immunophenotypic, genetic, and clinical features. The 2008 WHO classification includes several provisional entities and categories of unclassifiable neoplasms with features intermediate between two distinct entities. This allows the classification to retain flexibility so that new data that further identify distinct diseases within these entities can be incorporated. In distinction from the Working Formulation, lymphomas were not classified based on clinical outcome. The WHO classification agreed that each type of lymphoma that was identified by pathologic and clinical features could have a spectrum of clinical aggressiveness, and that lumping distinct entities into groups based on clinical outcome would inhibit the development of targeted therapeutic approaches. Therefore, the WHO classification represents a complete change from the Working Formulation, with the emphasis on pathologic classification rather than classification based on survival characteristics.

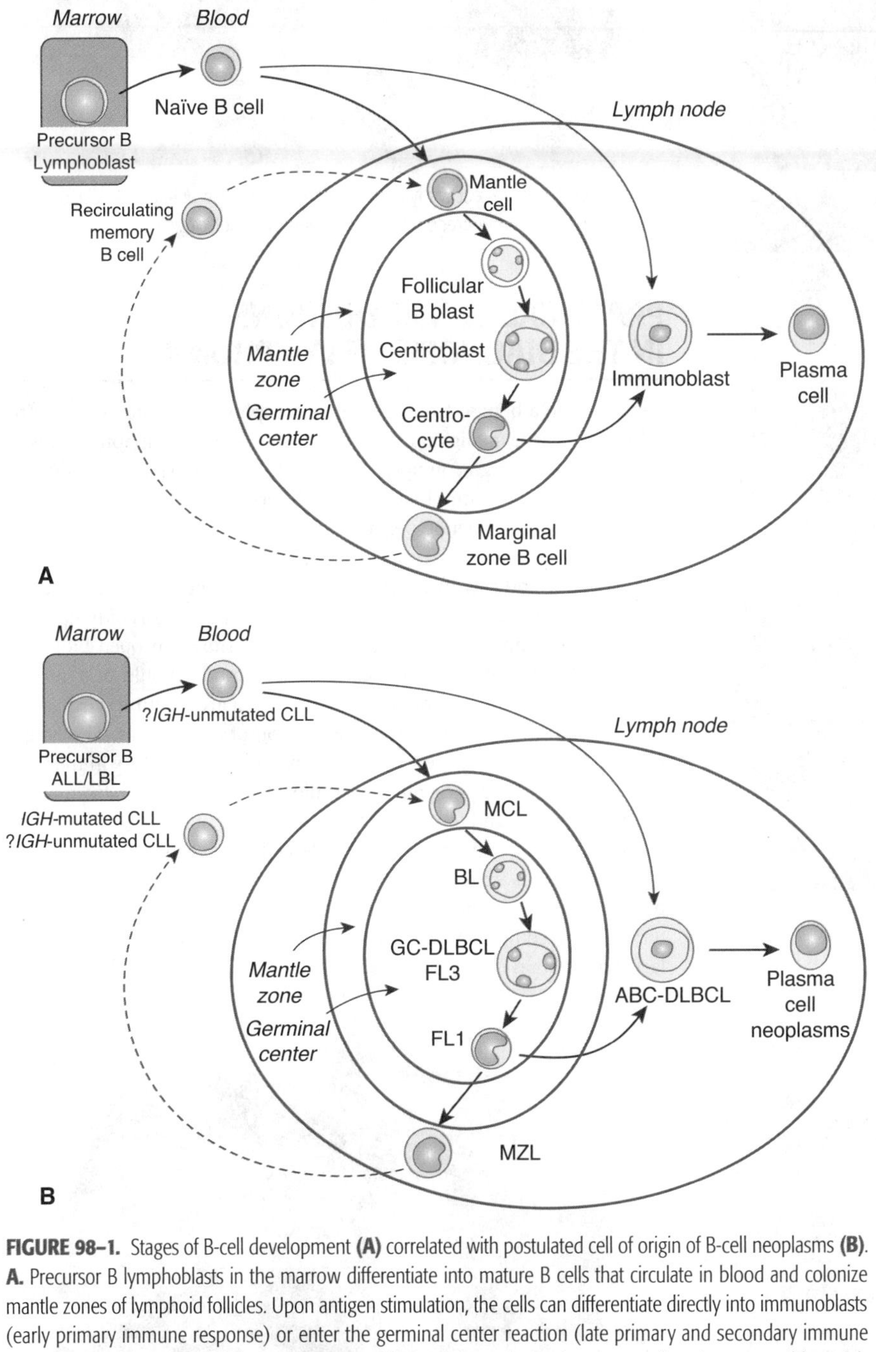

FIGURE 98–1. Stages of B-cell development **(A)** correlated with postulated cell of origin of B-cell neoplasms **(B)**. **A.** Precursor B lymphoblasts in the marrow differentiate into mature B cells that circulate in blood and colonize mantle zones of lymphoid follicles. Upon antigen stimulation, the cells can differentiate directly into immunoblasts (early primary immune response) or enter the germinal center reaction (late primary and secondary immune responses). In the germinal center, cells undergo blast transformation and progress to form large centroblasts, followed by small centrocytes. These cells differentiate into either antibody-secreting plasma cells through an immunoblast stage or memory B cells that can recirculate or localize to the marginal zones of lymphoid follicles. **B.** B-cell neoplasms correlate with different stages of development. ABC-DLBCL, activated B-cell-type diffuse large B-cell lymphoma; ALL/LBL, acute lymphoblastic leukemia/lymphoblastic lymphoma; BL, Burkitt lymphoma; CLL, chronic lymphocytic leukemia; FL1, follicular lymphoma, grade 1; FL3, follicular lymphoma, grade 3; GC-DLBCL, germinal center type diffuse large B-cell lymphoma; MCL, mantle cell lymphoma; MZL, marginal zone lymphoma.

Genome-wide expression studies have been instrumental in further delineating distinctive subtypes of lymphomas of clinical relevance. Using complementary DNA microarray technology, the expression of thousands of genes at the messenger RNA level can be studied simultaneously and compared to other tumor samples.[17] The technique is quickly proving to be a very promising approach to further classifying lymphomas. Such studies have (1) defined more than one distinct entity in what was previously characterized as a morphologically homogeneous entity, (2) identified distinct gene expression patterns that each encompass a disease that may demonstrate morphologic heterogeneity, and (3) identified new surface molecules and signaling pathways that could provide targets for new therapeutic approaches. The impact of the new gene expression profiles is detailed in the sections on separate lymphomas below.

The WHO classification attempts to correlate each lymphoma to normal lymphocyte biology by postulating a cell of origin for each neoplasm. This correlation is particularly well suited for B-cell lymphomas in which several distinct stages of normal B-cell development can be identified (Fig. 98–1A) but is not as satisfying for T- or NK-cell neoplasms (see Chaps. 78 and 79). Briefly, B-cell development begins in the marrow with precursor B lymphoblasts that differentiate into naïve B cells that circulate the blood (see Chap. 77). The lymph node is the primary site where B cells encounter antigen, where naïve B cells colonize primary follicles and in mantle zones of secondary follicles (Figs. 98–2 to 98–6). Upon antigen stimulation, these cells undergo blast transformation and enter the germinal center reaction in the late primary immune response and the secondary immune response. In the germinal center, cells downregulate *BCL2* (Fig. 98–7) and initially transform into intermediate-sized cells (follicular B blasts), then into large centroblasts, and finally into small centrocytes (Fig. 98–3).[18] Cells that survive the germinal center upregulate *BCL2* and either differentiate into short-lived plasma cells through an immunoblast stage or differentiate into memory cells that populate follicular marginal zones or recirculate in the blood. Several B-cell lymphomas can be correlated with these stages of development (Fig. 98–1B) and are mentioned in the sections on separate lymphomas below.

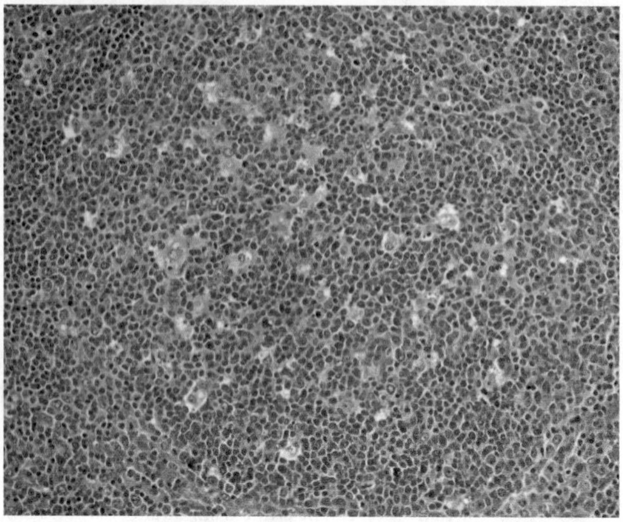

FIGURE 98–2. Reactive germinal center in a normal lymph node.

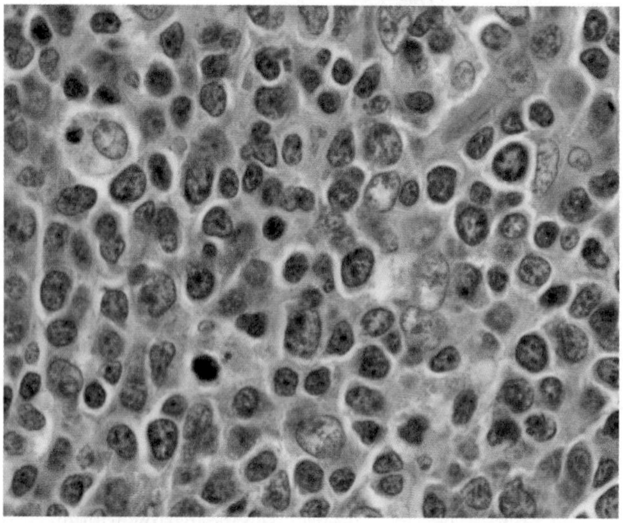

FIGURE 98–3. Spectrum of cells within the germinal center in a normal lymph node, ranging from small lymphocytes to larger cells with nucleoli.

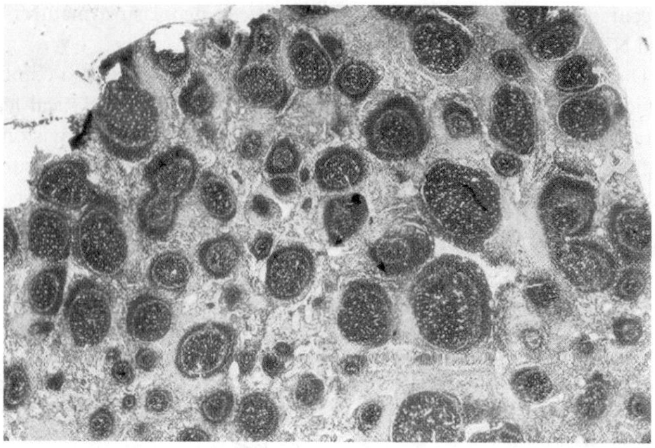

FIGURE 98–5. Same reactive lymph node stained with an antibody to CD20 (B-cell marker), showing B cells predominantly localized to the follicles.

PRACTICAL CONSIDERATIONS IN THE DIAGNOSIS OF LYMPHOMA

Determining a benign from malignant lymphoid infiltrate often can be difficult because malignant lymphocytes in many lymphomas closely resemble their benign counterparts. Therefore, diagnosis commonly rests on demonstrating a combination of an abnormal architectural pattern, an abnormal immunophenotype, and evidence of lymphoid monoclonality. As a result, several ancillary special studies have become instrumental in the diagnosis and classification of lymphoma, requiring special handling of the biopsy material (Table 98–2). Whenever a diagnosis of lymphoma is considered clinically, the surgeon should perform an open biopsy of the largest involved lymph node. The lymph node should be removed intact whenever possible, because assessment of architecture is extremely important in the diagnosis and classification of lymphomas. The lymph node should be sent immediately to the pathology laboratory in the fresh state, at which time the pathologist allocates the tissue for fixation for routine histology and for special studies.

Automated flow cytometry on single-cell suspensions prepared from tissue samples is extremely helpful in demonstrating B-cell monotypia by surface light-chain restriction. It also determines the expression pattern of surface markers helpful in subclassifying lymphomas, particularly lymphomas of small B cells.[19] A wide variety of antibodies that can

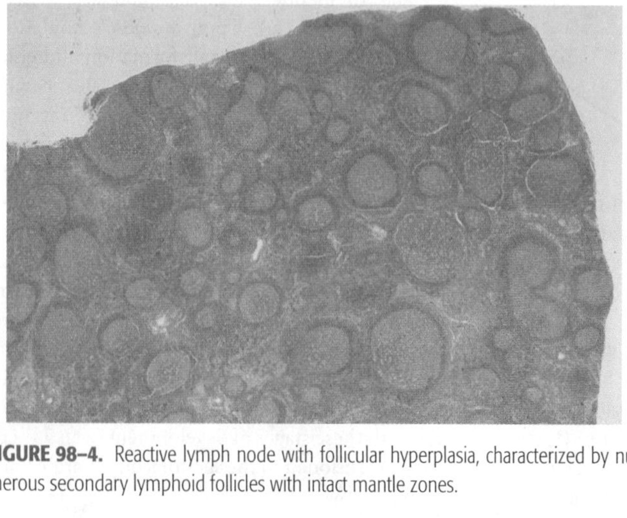

FIGURE 98–4. Reactive lymph node with follicular hyperplasia, characterized by numerous secondary lymphoid follicles with intact mantle zones.

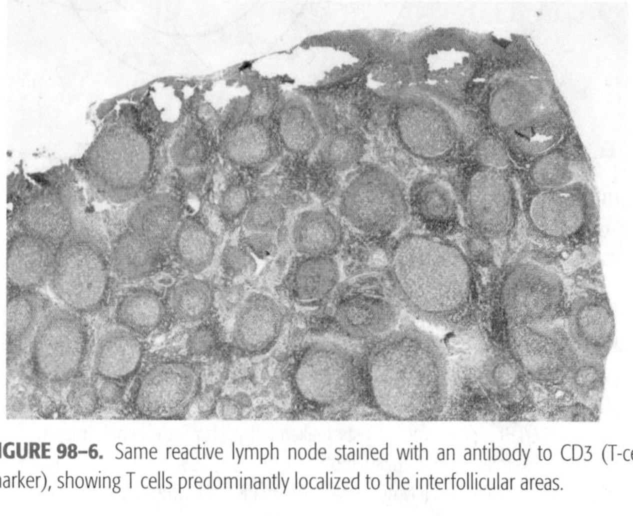

FIGURE 98–6. Same reactive lymph node stained with an antibody to CD3 (T-cell marker), showing T cells predominantly localized to the interfollicular areas.

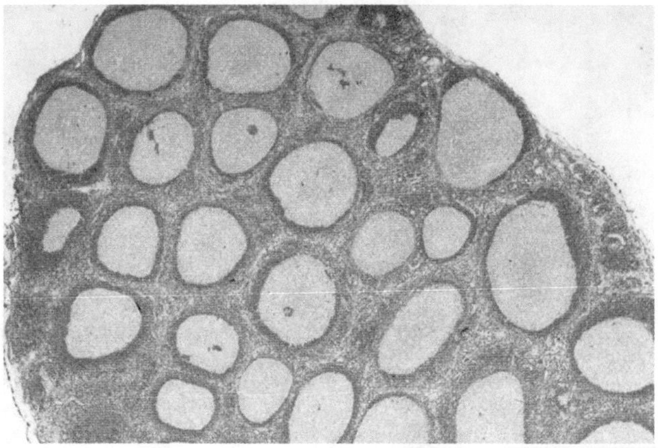

FIGURE 98–7. Same reactive lymph node stained with an antibody to the antiapoptotic protein Bcl-2. Note the negative staining of the germinal centers where most of the cells will die during the maturation process.

be used on formalin-fixed tissue now are available, allowing accurate diagnosis and subclassification of lymphoma in most cases.[20]

Molecular genetic techniques to determine B- or T-cell monoclonality or lymphoma-specific chromosomal translocations include polymerase chain reaction (PCR), Southern blot, fluorescence *in situ* hybridization (FISH), and cytogenetic analysis.[21] Although PCR and FISH now can be performed on formalin-fixed tissue, interpretable results might not be obtained because of DNA degradation caused by fixation. These tests are optimally performed on fresh tissue. Results from molecular genetic testing should be interpreted in conjunction with the morphologic and immunophenotypic data, as some benign reactive lymphoid proliferations show evidence of lymphoid monoclonality.[22]

TABLE 98–2. Routine and Ancillary Studies for Lymphoma Diagnosis

Method	Applications	Type of Tissue Needed
Routine histology	Examination of routine sections allows diagnosis of lymphoma in certain situations. In the remaining cases, the diagnosis requires the use of ancillary studies	Formalin-fixed
Immunohistochemistry	Immunophenotyping for lymphoma classification; can demonstrate B-cell monotypia (light-chain restriction) and unique antigen expression in some cases	Formalin-fixed
Flow cytometry	Demonstration of B-cell monotypia by surface immunoglobulin light chain restriction; immunophenotyping for lymphoma classification	Fresh tissue (single-cell suspensions)
Polymerase chain reaction analysis	Demonstration of B- and T-cell clonality by immunoglobulin and T-cell receptor analyses; demonstration of lymphoma specific translocations (example, *BCL2* gene rearrangements)	Frozen tissue; can be performed on paraffin tissue, but may not yield amplifiable DNA in some cases
Cytogenetics	Demonstration of clonality; demonstration of lymphoma-specific translocations	Sterile fresh tissue
Fluorescent *in situ* hybridization	Demonstration of lymphoma-specific translocations	Fresh tissue; can be performed on paraffin tissue, but yield is variable

The diagnosis of lymphoma has become more complex than the diagnosis of other malignancies because diagnosis of lymphoma rests on correlation of morphologic features with immunophenotype and genetic data in many cases. Because of the complexity of diagnosis and the relative infrequency of lymphoma in general pathology practice, a second review by a hematopathologist with expertise in lymphoma pathology is recommended. The second review can have a significant impact on the clinical management of patients.[23]

Whereas open biopsy of an involved lymph node is the most useful diagnostic procedure, core needle biopsies and fine needle aspiration can play a role in limited situations. Core needle biopsy might be helpful in the diagnosis of deep-seated disease in the abdomen or retroperitoneum, and the patient may avoid a laparotomy. However, a definitive diagnosis by core biopsy is not always possible, necessitating an open biopsy. Fine-needle aspiration is not helpful in primary diagnosis of lymphoma,[24,25] but it may be helpful in detecting recurrence of a previously diagnosed lymphoma or in ruling out a nonhematolymphoid lesion causing lymphadenopathy. Although flow cytometry can be used in conjunction with cytologic examination to provide additional information for lymphoma diagnosis and classification, tissue biopsy generally is required before commencement of therapy.

PRECURSOR B- AND T-CELL LYMPHOMAS/LEUKEMIAS

Lymphoblastic leukemia/lymphoma represents a malignancy of lymphoblasts, either of B or T lineage. They can present in the marrow (leukemia) or with predominant tissue involvement (lymphoma), but they are considered single-disease entities. Most cases of acute lymphoblastic leukemias are of B lineage, whereas most cases of lymphoblastic lymphoma are of T lineage, with the mediastinum being a common site of involvement (see Chap. 93). The morphologic features are the same regardless of site or lineage, consisting of small- to intermediate-size cells with finely dispersed nuclear chromatin, inconspicuous nucleoli, and scant cytoplasm (Fig. 98–8). Assessment of lineage and distinction from minimally differentiated acute myeloid leukemia require immunophenotypic data and may require molecular genetic analysis of B- and T-cell receptors. Lymphoblastic neoplasms are distinguished from other lymphomas by the expression of terminal deoxynucleotide transferase, which is specifically expressed at the lymphoblast stage of development.

The 2008 WHO classification includes several categories of B-lymphoblastic leukemia/lymphoma characterized by recurrent genetic abnormalities.[16] Many of these are associated with distinct clinical or pathologic features, have prognostic implications, or are considered biologically distinct entities.

MATURE B-CELL NON-HODGKIN LYMPHOMAS

■ CHRONIC LYMPHOCYTIC LEUKEMIA/SMALL LYMPHOCYTIC LYMPHOMA

Chronic lymphocytic leukemia is a neoplasm of mature B lymphocytes characterized by blood and marrow involvement and commonly associated

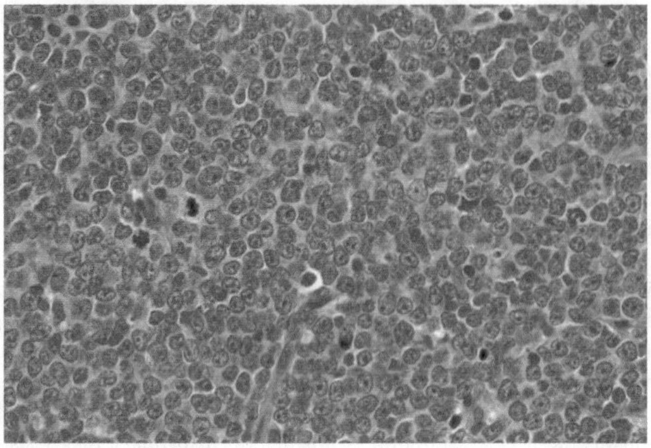

FIGURE 98–8. Lymphoblastic lymphoma of T-cell type, characterized by a diffuse proliferation of medium-sized cells with finely distributed chromatin and high mitotic activity.

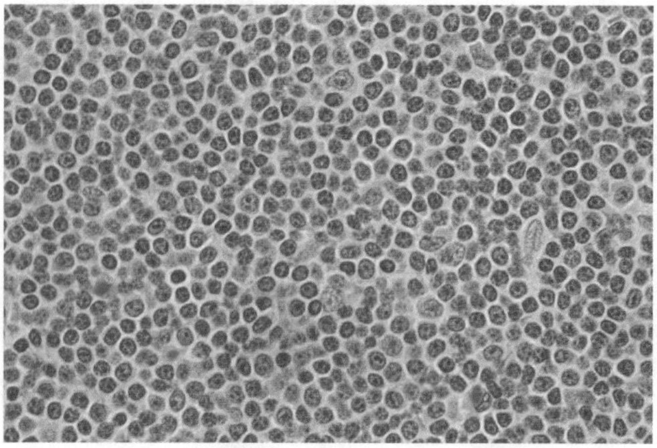

FIGURE 98–10. Small lymphocytic lymphoma, characterized by small lymphocytes with mature chromatin pattern. Note that individual lymphocytes in small lymphocytic lymphoma are morphologically indistinguishable from benign lymphocytes.

with lymph node involvement (see Chap. 94). Small lymphocytic lymphoma is the nonleukemic form of the disease (see Chaps. 94 and 97). Lymph nodes involved by chronic lymphocytic leukemia show a diffuse infiltrate of small mature lymphocytes admixed with prolymphocytes and paraimmunoblasts, which characteristically form ill-defined nodules known as *proliferation* or *growth centers* (Figs. 98–9 and 98–10). The B cells have a characteristic immunophenotype, demonstrating expression of CD5 and CD23 and dim expression of CD20 and restricted light chain. Studies have divided chronic lymphocytic leukemia into two distinct subtypes with distinct clinical behavior (see Chap. 94). The type with the more favorable prognosis expresses mutated immunoglobulin heavy chain variable region genes (*IGH* genes), whereas the other subtype expresses unmutated *IGH* genes. The *IGH* gene mutation status is reflected in differences in gene expression.[26,27] The gene encoding the zeta-associated protein of 70 kDa (ZAP-70) is one of these genes, which generally is expressed by leukemia cells that express unmutated *IGH* genes and hence can be used to discriminate between the two subtypes.[28] Certain cytogenetic abnormalities also correlate with clinical aggressiveness.[29]

Some cases of chronic lymphocytic leukemia/small lymphocytic lymphoma demonstrate plasmacytic features but are distinct from an entity known as *lymphoplasmacytic lymphoma*, which is characterized by a prominent component of plasmacytic lymphocytes and plasma cells (Fig. 98–11). These cases typically do not express CD5, less often involve blood, and often are associated with a monoclonal immunoglobulin (Ig) M serum protein that can cause hyperviscosity or cryoglobulinemia (Waldenström macroglobulinemia). Although lymphoplasmacytic lymphoma has been suggested to be frequently associated with the cytogenetic alteration t(9;14)(p13;q32), the true frequency of this association remains controversial.

■ MANTLE CELL LYMPHOMA

Mantle cell lymphoma most commonly involves lymph nodes, but it can involve extranodal sites, including the gastrointestinal tract, as a clinical variant known as *lymphomatous polyposis* (Fig. 98–12). It typically is composed of a uniform population of small to medium lymphocytes with irregular nuclei and a virtual absence of large transformed cells (Fig. 98–13).[30,31] It most commonly has a diffuse growth pattern, but it can show a nodular or, more rarely, a mantle zone pattern (Fig. 98–14). The postulated cell of origin is the B cell of the inner mantle zone. The lymphoma cells coexpress CD5, as does chronic lymphocytic leukemia, but mantle cell lymphoma can be distinguished by lack of CD23 expression and expression of cyclin D1 (Fig. 98–15).

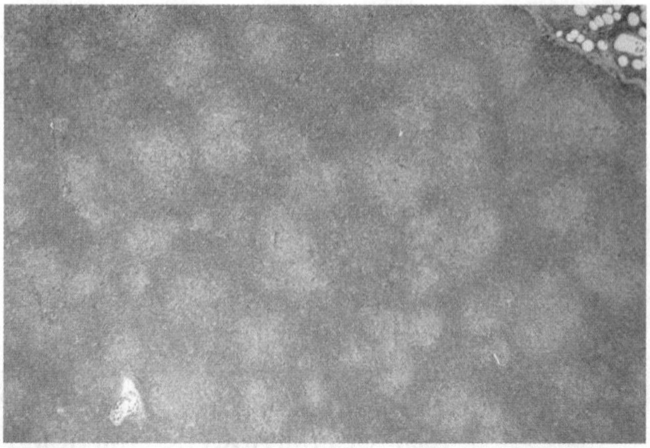

FIGURE 98–9. Small lymphocytic lymphoma with vague nodular appearance imparted by proliferation centers.

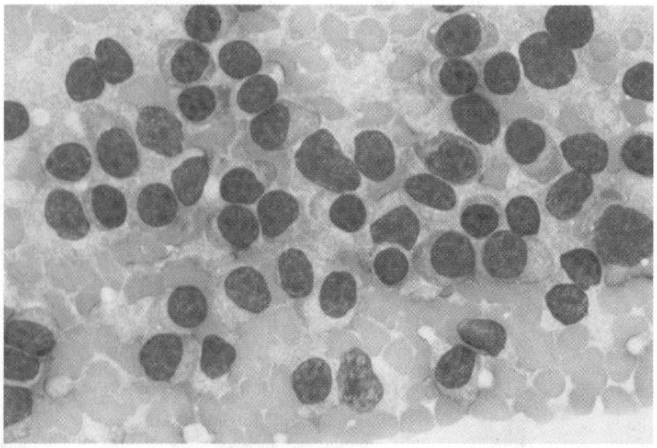

FIGURE 98–11. Imprint preparation of lymphoplasmacytic lymphoma demonstrating small lymphocytes and cells with plasmacytoid features (eccentric nuclei and bluish cytoplasm).

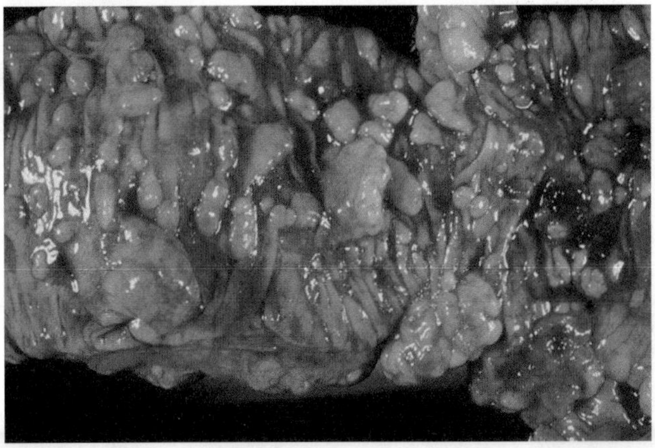

FIGURE 98–12. Large bowel involved with mantle cell lymphoma (multiple lymphomatous polyposis).

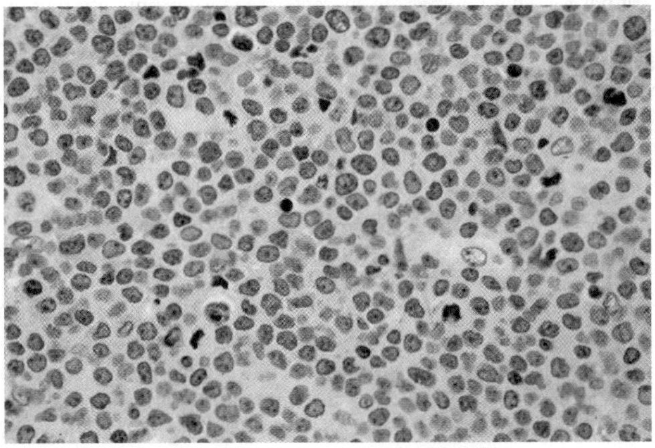

FIGURE 98–13. Mantle cell lymphoma with a diffuse pattern, characterized by a monomorphous infiltrate of small irregular lymphocytes with numerous mitotic figures.

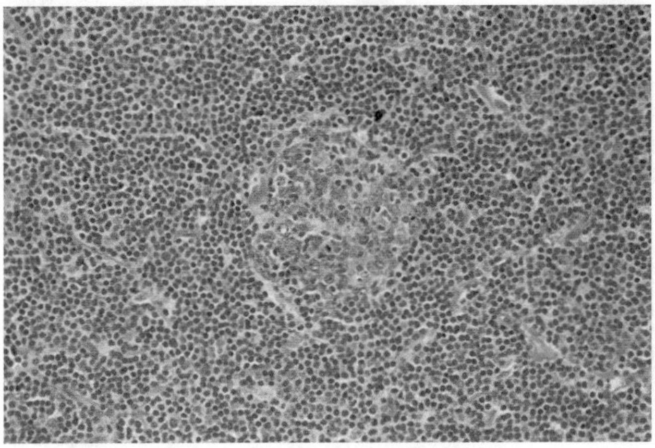

FIGURE 98–14. Mantle cell lymphoma with a mantle-zone pattern, characterized by monomorphous small lymphocytes surrounding a benign germinal center.

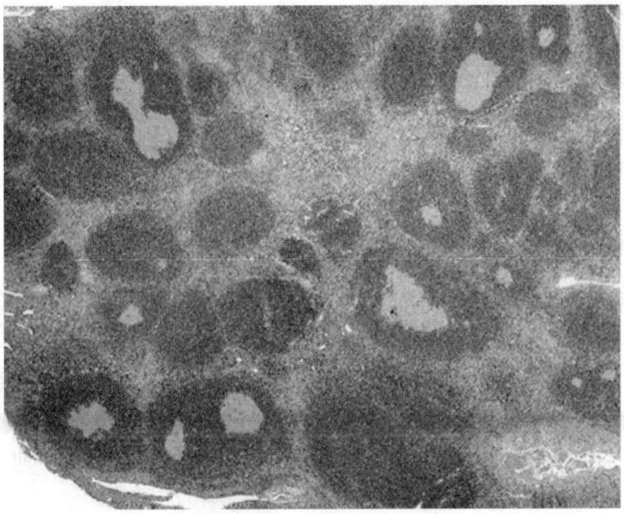

FIGURE 98–15. Mantle cell lymphoma with mantle-zone pattern stained with antibody to cyclin D1.

Cyclin D1 expression results from the chromosomal translocation t(11;14)(q13;q32) characteristic of mantle cell lymphoma. Although many pathologists would not diagnose mantle cell lymphoma without evidence of t(11;14) or cyclin D1 expression, gene expression data demonstrate a subset of mantle cell lymphomas that are cyclin D1-negative.[32] Some of these cyclin D1-negative cases have chromosomal translocations involving the *CCND2* gene, which encodes for the cyclin D2 protein.[33] Overall, patients with mantle cell lymphoma have a median survival of approximately 3 years, but gene expression data that determined tumor cell proliferation were able to identify patient subsets that differed in median survival by more than 5 years (see Chap. 102).[32]

FOLLICULAR LYMPHOMA

Follicular lymphoma is a proliferation of cells that correspond to normal germinal center cells[34] retaining expression of germinal center markers (BCL6, CD10) and demonstrates a follicular architecture (Fig. 98–16) imparted by nodular aggregates of CD21-positive follicular dendritic cells (see Chap. 101). Follicular lymphomas are composed of

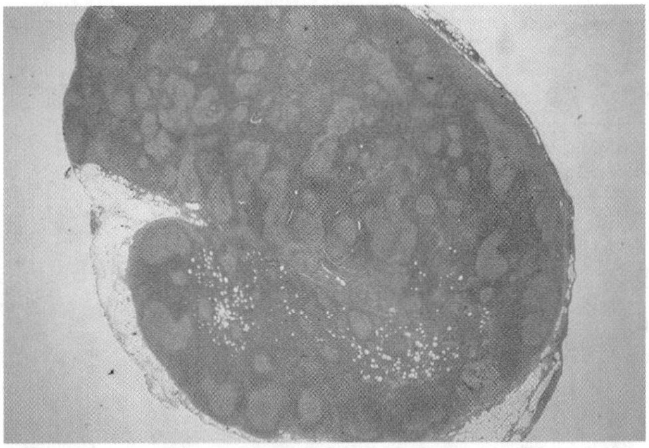

FIGURE 98–16. Grade 2 follicular lymphoma (low-power magnification), characterized by crowded follicles throughout the entire lymph node.

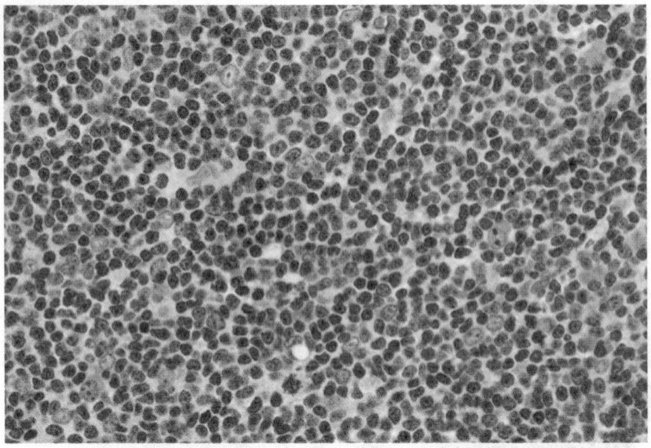

FIGURE 98–17. Center of a neoplastic follicle in grade 1 follicular lymphoma with almost exclusively small centrocytes.

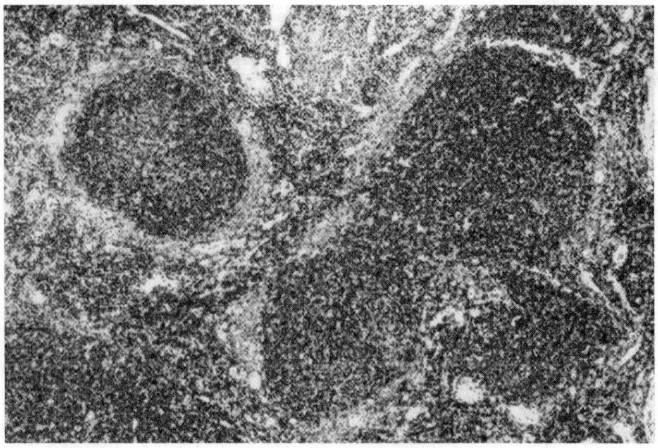

FIGURE 98–19. Positive BCL2 immunostain of a follicular lymphoma (contrast with Fig. 98–7).

a variable mixture of centrocytes (small cleaved cells) and centroblasts (large noncleaved cells). They can be divided into three grades (grades 1–3) based on the number of centroblasts present. The most common is grade 1 (<5 centroblasts per high-power microscopic field), previously known as *follicular small cleaved cell lymphoma* (Fig. 98–17). Both grade 1 and grade 2 tumors are indolent, and distinction between them is not required. Grade 3 follicular lymphoma (>15 centroblasts per high-power microscopic field) can be further divided into grade 3A (mixture of centroblasts and centrocytes) (Fig. 98–18) and grade 3B (solid sheets of centroblasts). Data have shown some molecular genetic differences between 3A and 3B cases, but further study is required because no significant clinical impact has been demonstrated.[35–37] Follicular lymphoma can have an accompanying diffuse component, and identification of a diffuse area of large cells (diffuse large B-cell lymphoma) indicates transformation to a more aggressive disease. Approximately 90 percent of follicular lymphoma demonstrate the t(14;18)(q32;q21) involving rearrangement of the *BCL2* gene, leading to the constitutive expression of the antiapoptotic BCL2 protein. Although BCL2 protein expression does not help distinguish follicular lymphoma from other lymphomas, it is a helpful feature in distinguishing it from reactive follicles that are BCL2-negative (Fig. 98–19).

MARGINAL ZONE B-CELL LYMPHOMAS

Marginal zone lymphomas are characterized by a proliferation of predominantly small lymphocytes, commonly with abundant pale cytoplasm (called *monocytoid B cells)* and plasmacytic features (see Chap. 103). The postulated cell of origin of these lymphomas is the postgerminal center B-cell of the marginal zone at various anatomic sites. Marginal zone lymphomas can be divided into three distinct types based on site of presentation: (1) extranodal marginal zone lymphomas of mucosa-associated lymphoid tissue (MALT), (2) splenic marginal zone lymphomas,[38] and (3) nodal marginal zone lymphomas (Fig. 98–20).[39] This classification is supported by distinctive cytogenetic abnormalities in each entity. Extranodal lymphomas of the MALT type are the most common and arise in mucosal sites subject to long-standing chronic inflammation (Fig. 98–21), including chronic infection, the prototypical example being chronic *Helicobacter pylori* infection of the stomach.[40] At early stages of development, many of these lymphomas respond to treatment with antibiotics to eradicate *H. pylori*, whereas later changes, including cases with chromosomal translocations activating genes involved in nuclear factor-κB (NF-κB) signaling,[41] lead to antigen-independent growth (see Chap. 97).

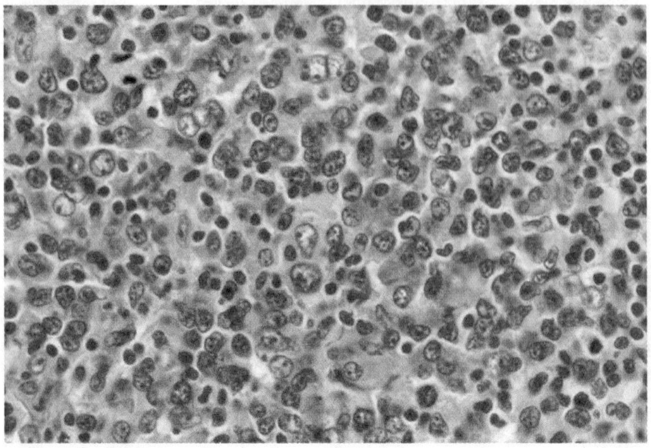

FIGURE 98–18. Grade 3A follicular lymphoma with >15 centroblasts per high-power field.

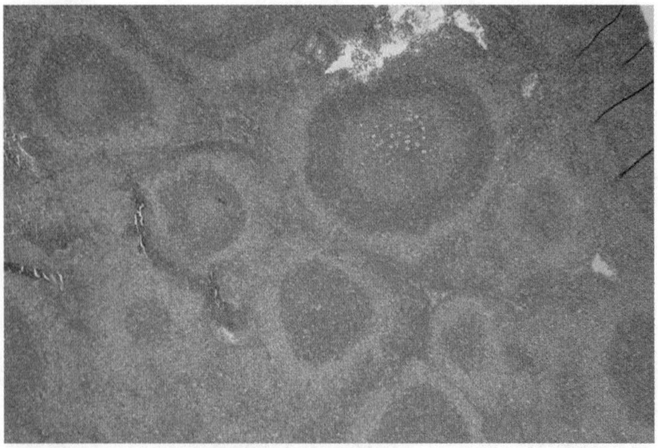

FIGURE 98–20. Lymph node involved by marginal zone B-cell lymphoma, in which the benign germinal centers and mantle zones are surrounded by expanded pale marginal zones.

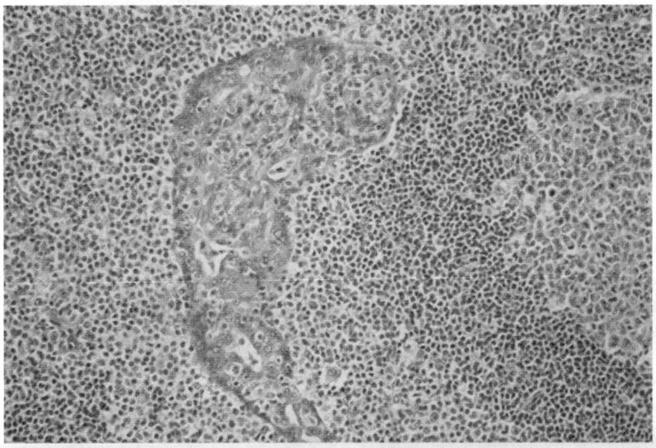

FIGURE 98–21. Salivary gland involved by MALT lymphoma, showing a diffuse infiltrate of small lymphocytes with pale cytoplasm, infiltrating an enlarged salivary gland duct (lymphoepithelial lesion).

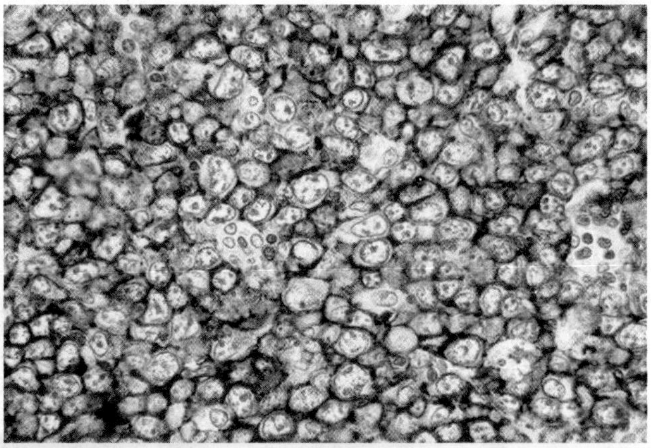

FIGURE 98–23. Diffuse large B-cell stained with antibody to CD20 (B-cell marker).

DIFFUSE LARGE B-CELL LYMPHOMA

Diffuse large B-cell lymphoma is characterized by a diffuse infiltrate of large B cells that can resemble centroblasts or immunoblasts (Figs. 98–22 and 98–23). The 2008 WHO classification identifies several types of large B-cell lymphoma, the most common type being diffuse large B-cell lymphoma, not otherwise specified, which constitutes 25 to 30 percent of all non-Hodgkin lymphomas (see Chap. 100).

Gene expression data have shown that diffuse large B-cell lymphoma is a heterogeneous entity consisting of at least three entities having distinct gene expression profiles based on cell of origin: (1) cases with an expression profile similar to germinal center B cells (GCBs), (2) cases expressing genes typical of activated B cells (ABCs), and (3) cases with a different pattern referred to as "unclassifiable" that are neither GCB type nor ABC type (Fig. 98–24).[42–44] Importantly, clinical differences were apparent, with GCB-type cases having a significantly better prognosis compared to the other two types, even when clinical prognostic markers are considered (see Chap. 100). Gene-expression profiling has identified potential therapeutic targets, indicating the ABC-type shows a pattern of NF-κB activation that plays a role in the proliferation and survival of the cells.[45] This finding may provide novel therapeutic targets for these lymphomas. It has been suggested that division of diffuse large B-cell lymphoma into clinically distinct groups may be determined by the expression profile of a limited number of genes using routine immunohistochemistry.[46] However, such an approach to classification is limited by problems of reproducibility of immunohistochemical staining and interpretation.[47] Newer gene-expression profiling studies confirm the clinical significance of these cell-of-origin distinctions in the current era of therapy (including anti-CD20 antibody therapy) and identified nonneoplastic cells in the microenvironment as important contributors to patient survival.[48]

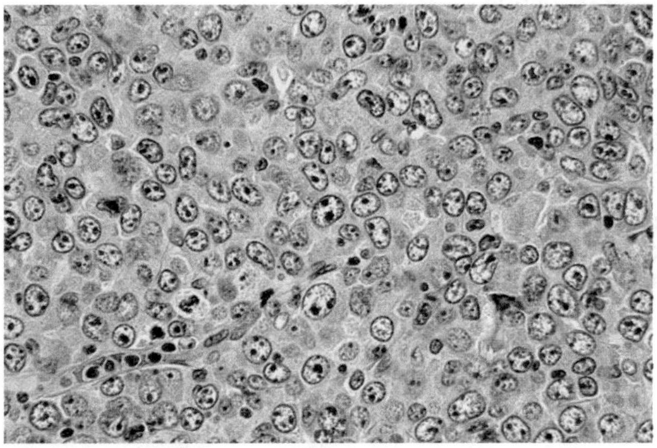

FIGURE 98–22. Diffuse large B-cell lymphoma.

Mediastinal large B-cell lymphoma is a distinct subtype of diffuse large B-cell lymphoma that has been separately identified in the WHO classification.[49] Patients with mediastinal lymphomas typically are younger than those with conventional diffuse large B-cell lymphomas, with presentation in the mediastinum. The histology shows large cells with abundant cytoplasm associated with diffuse fibrosis (Fig. 98–25). Gene expression studies have demonstrated an expression profile, distinct from conventional diffuse large B-cell lymphoma, that shares some features with classic Hodgkin lymphoma (Fig. 98–26).[50,51] Indeed, the 2008 WHO classification recognizes that some cases of mediastinal lymphomas can have features that are intermediate between diffuse large B-cell lymphoma and classical Hodgkin lymphoma.[16]

BURKITT LYMPHOMA

Burkitt lymphoma is a highly aggressive lymphoma characterized histologically by a diffuse infiltrate of intermediate-size cells with a high mitotic rate (see Chap. 104). The lymphomas commonly have a significant spontaneous cell death (apoptosis), which results in a "starry sky" appearance caused by numerous macrophages that have engulfed the apoptotic debris (known as *tingible body macrophages*; Figs. 98–27 and 98–28). The postulated cell of origin is the early follicular B blast cell of the germinal center. Virtually all cases of Burkitt lymphoma are characterized by chromosomal translocations involving the *MYC* gene on chromosome 8. The *MYC* gene most commonly is translocated to the *IGH* gene on chromosome 14, resulting in t(8;14)(q24;q32), but it also can involve the light-chain genes on chromosomes 2p12 (κ) and 22q11 (λ). A diagnosis of Burkitt lymphoma can be suggested based on morphologic examination alone, but should be supported by immunophenotypic data (positive for CD20, CD10, and BCL6; negative or focally weakly positive for BCL2; growth fraction near 100% as determined by Ki-67 stain) and confirmed by molecular testing for *MYC* translocations whenever possible.

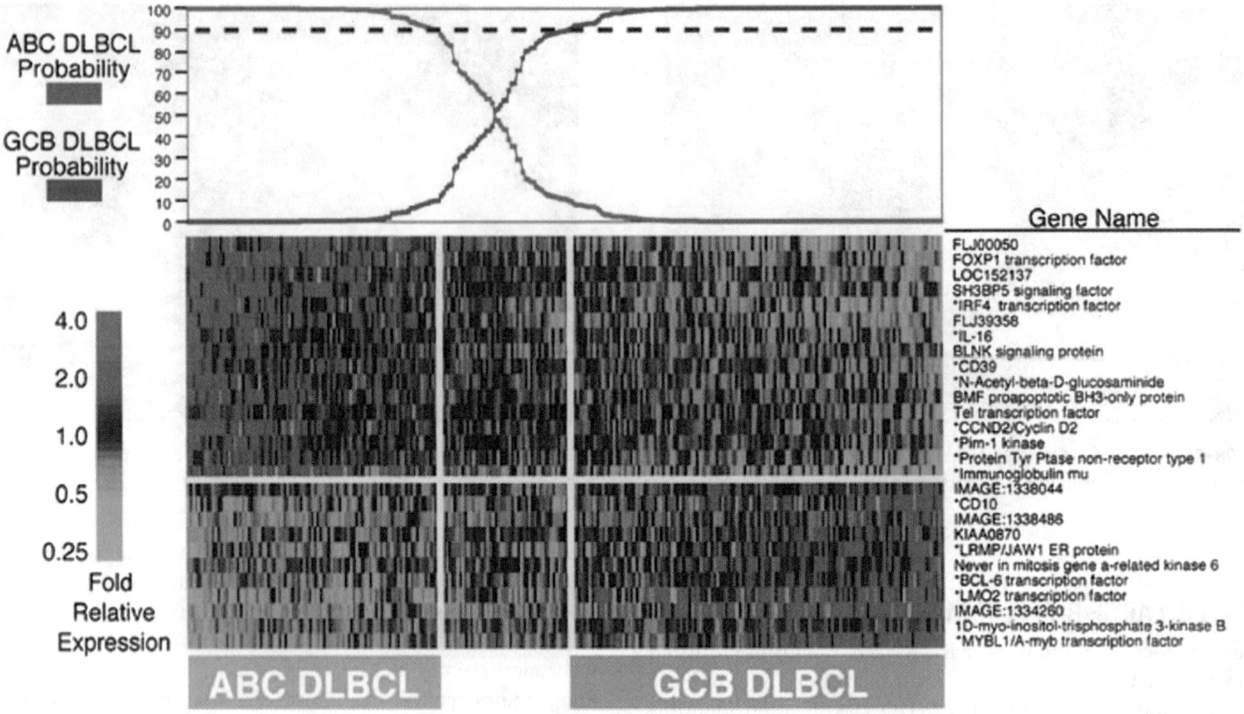

FIGURE 98–24. Gene expression profiling diffuse large B-cell lymphoma, showing the subgroup discriminator used divide cases into germinal center B-cell-like (GCB) and activated B-cell-like (ABC). Each vertical column represents an individual patient and each horizontal row a unique gene. Red is relative overexpression of a gene and green relative underexpression. Using a probability of subgroup assignment of 90%, approximately 15% of cases are left unclassified (cases between the vertical yellow bars that are neither GCB or ABC). This approach allows one to analyze thousands of genes from a single patient in one experiment, and forms the basis of the new molecular classification of lymphoma. *(Reproduced from Wright G, Tan B, Rosenwald A, et al: A gene expression-based method to diagnose clinically distinct subgroups of diffuse large B cell lymphoma.* Proc Natl Acad Sci U S A *100:9991, 2003 by permission of the National Academy of Sciences, USA.)*

Gene-expression studies show that Burkitt lymphoma has a consistent gene-expression signature, but that there is not always correlation between the diagnosis based on gene-expression profiling and the diagnosis based on standard diagnostic testing.[52,53] To reflect this, the 2008 WHO classification recognizes a provisional entity of B-cell lymphoma, unclassifiable, with features intermediate between diffuse large B-cell lymphoma and Burkitt lymphoma.[16] Further study of such cases may allow for more definitive classification of these intermediate cases.

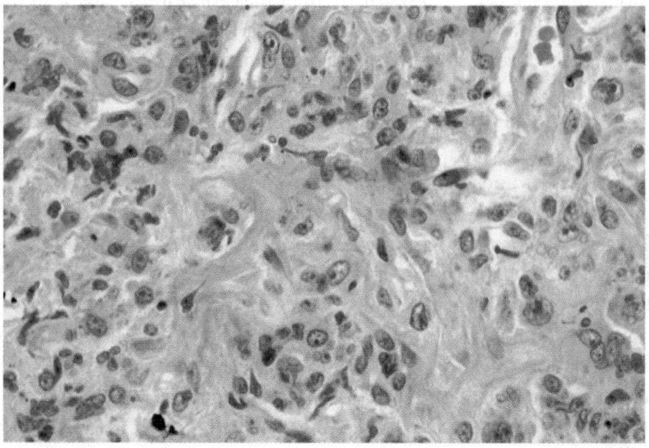

FIGURE 98–25. Primary mediastinal large B-cell lymphoma with sclerosis.

MATURE T-CELL AND NK CELL NON-HODGKIN LYMPHOMAS

T cells and NK cells share several immunophenotypic and functional features; therefore, these neoplasms are grouped together in the WHO classification (see Chap. 106). These lymphomas make up 10 to 15 percent of non-Hodgkin lymphomas in Western countries, with a higher incidence in Asia. The two most common types of mature T-cell lymphoma in adults are (1) peripheral T-cell lymphoma (PTCL), not otherwise specified, and (2) angioimmunoblastic T-cell lymphoma. Anaplastic large cell lymphoma (ALCL) represents a unique subtype of T-cell lymphoma particularly common in children.

PTCLs typically grow in a diffuse pattern that effaces normal nodal architecture or, more rarely, show expansion of the interfollicular areas. They show a diverse cytologic spectrum, with most cases showing a mixture of large- to intermediate-size cells and occasional cases showing predominantly small cells (Figs. 98–29 and 98–30). Cell type has no prognostic relevance. A reactive background consisting of eosinophils, plasma cells, and macrophages may be present, in which case the diagnosis of Hodgkin lymphoma may be entertained. Immunophenotypic data cannot prove clonality as in B-cell lymphomas, but evidence of an aberrant T-cell phenotype supports a diagnosis of T-cell lymphoma. Molecular techniques to demonstrate clonal rearrangement of T-cell receptor genes can be helpful in confirming the diagnosis. As currently defined, PTCL is a heterogeneous entity that can be further classified in the future based on gene expression patterns. Angioimmunoblastic T-cell lymphoma is uncommon and typically presents with systemic symptoms and polyclonal hypergammaglobulinemia.

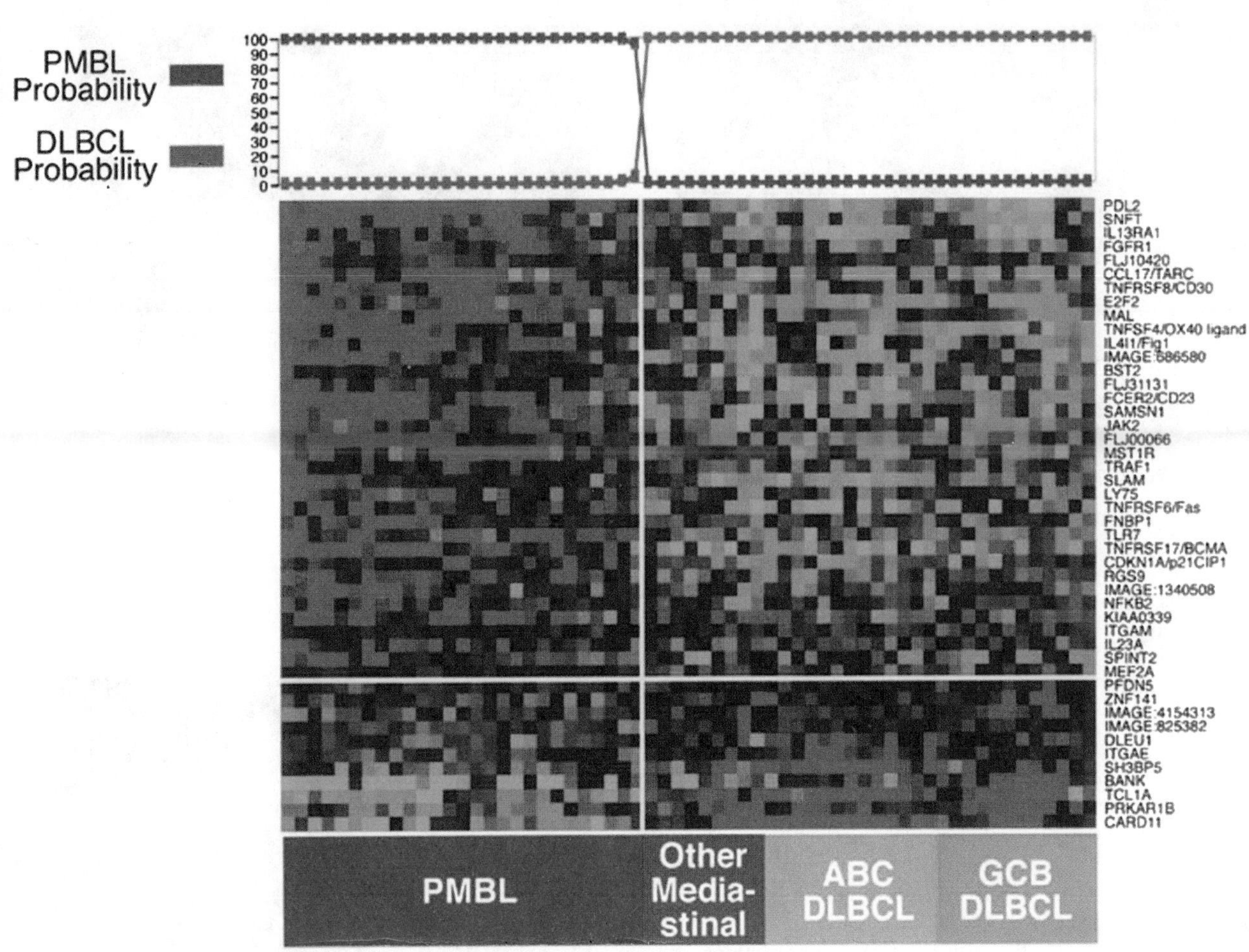

FIGURE 98–26. Gene-expression profiling of primary mediastinal large B-cell lymphoma (PMBCL), contrasting the expression profile with nodal diffuse large B-cell lymphomas (DCBCL). This figure shows numerous genes that are overexpressed in PMBCL (red). Many of these genes are shared with classical Hodgkin lymphoma, suggesting a biologic overlap between these two diseases. Cases listed as "Other Mediastinal" refer to those cases of DLBCL with mediastinal involvement, but not felt to be typical of PMBCL. This is borne out by the gene-expression data, showing that these cases are more closely related to DLBCL rather than PMBCL. *(Reproduced from Rosenwald A, Wright G, Leroy K, Yu X, et al: Molecular Diagnosis of Primary Mediastinal B Cell Lymphoma Identifies a Clinically Favorable Subgroup of Diffuse Large B Cell Lymphoma Related to Hodgkin Lymphoma.* J Exp Med *198:851, 2003, by permission of the Rockefeller University Press.)*

ALCL can show significant morphologic variability but typically is composed of large pleomorphic cells characterized by the presence of "hallmark" cells with horseshoe- or kidney-shaped nuclei and a perinuclear eosinophilic region (Fig. 98–31).[54] Early involvement of lymph nodes can be limited to the sinuses, with obliteration of nodal architecture in later stages. ALCL is characterized by uniform, strong

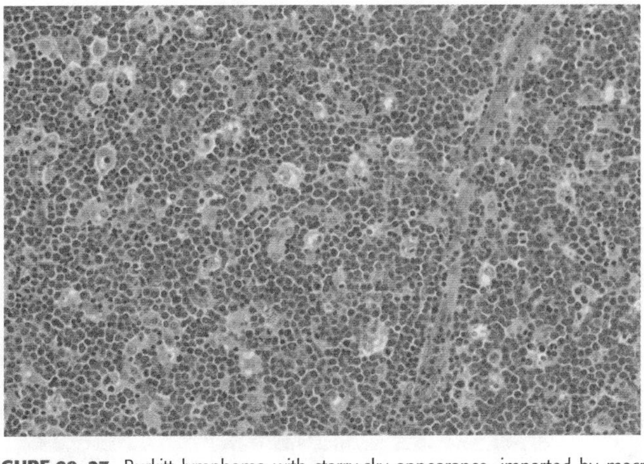

FIGURE 98–27. Burkitt lymphoma with starry-sky appearance, imparted by macrophages that have engulfed apoptotic debris of dying tumor cells.

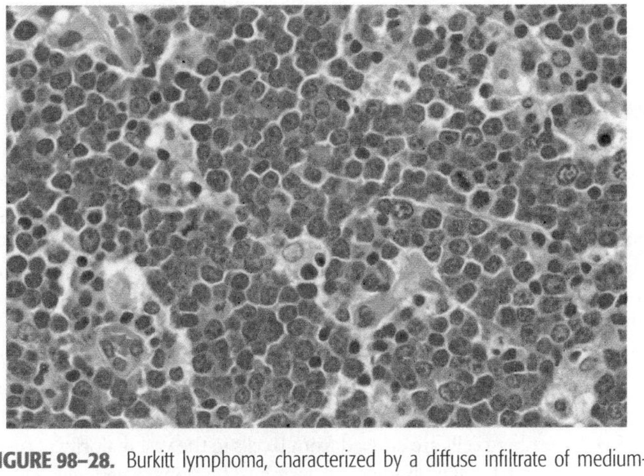

FIGURE 98–28. Burkitt lymphoma, characterized by a diffuse infiltrate of medium-sized cells with small nucleoli and a high mitotic activity.

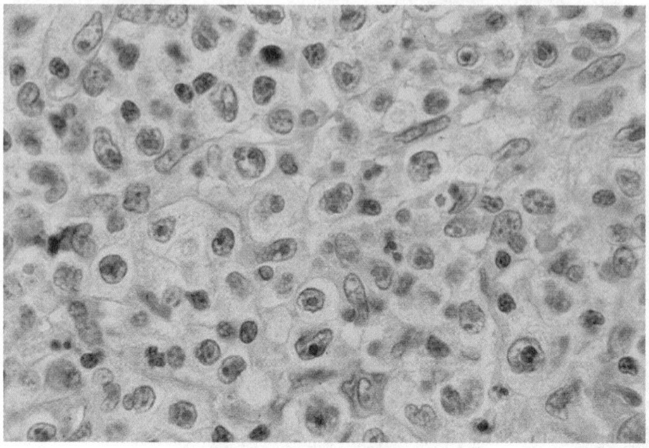

FIGURE 98–29. Peripheral T-cell lymphoma, unspecified, composed predominantly of large cells.

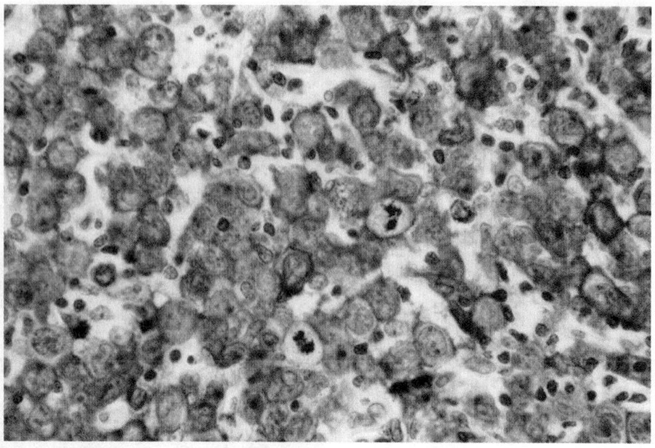

FIGURE 98–30. Peripheral T-cell lymphoma stained with antibody to CD3 (T-cell marker).

expression of CD30 (Fig. 98–32). The majority of cases express one or more T-cell antigens and demonstrate clonal T-cell receptor gene rearrangement.[54] ALCL is divided into two entities based on the expression of anaplastic lymphoma kinase (ALK; Fig. 98–33). ALK-positive ALCL is most often seen in the first three decades of life and has a favorable prognosis compared to ALK-negative ALCL.[55,56] Expression of ALK is the result of chromosomal translocations involving the *ALK* gene on chromosome 2p23, the most common translocation being the t(2;5)(p23;q35) involving the nucleophosmin gene on chromosome 5.[57] ALK-negative ALCL is recognized as a provisional entity that is distinct from ALK-positive ALCL and PTCL, not otherwise specified.[58]

Other types of mature T-/NK cell lymphomas are uncommon and include enteropathy-associated T-cell lymphoma (an aggressive T-cell lymphoma typically arising in the small bowel from a background of celiac disease) and extranodal NK/T-cell lymphoma, nasal type (an aggressive Epstein-Barr virus [EBV]-associated neoplasm commonly involving the nasal cavity). A detailed description of these specific lymphoma subtypes is beyond the scope of this chapter and can be found in the WHO classification.[16]

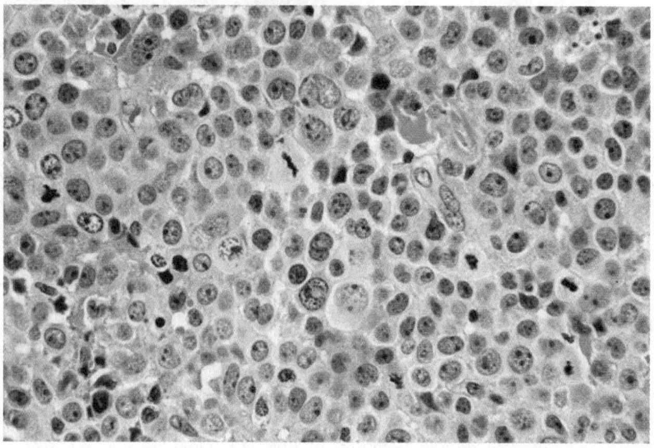

FIGURE 98–31. Anaplastic large cell lymphoma, T-cell type, containing a population of large cells with wreath-shaped nuclei and an eosinophilic perinuclear accentuation.

HODGKIN LYMPHOMA

Hodgkin lymphoma consists of two distinct clinicopathologic entities: *classical Hodgkin lymphoma* (including four subtypes) and *nodular lymphocyte predominant Hodgkin lymphoma* (see Chap. 99).

■ CLASSICAL HODGKIN LYMPHOMA

The neoplastic cell of classical Hodgkin lymphoma is the Reed-Sternberg cell, first described more than 100 years ago.[59,60] It is a large cell with two or more nuclei or nuclear lobes, each of which contains a large eosinophilic nucleolus (Fig. 98–34). The presence of Reed-Sternberg cells alone is insufficient for a diagnosis of Hodgkin lymphoma, because cells with similar morphology can be seen in a variety of non-Hodgkin lymphomas and benign reactive conditions.[61] For a diagnosis of Hodgkin lymphoma, diagnostic Reed-Sternberg cells must be found in an appropriate background consisting of a variable polymorphous reactive infiltrate of inflammatory and accessory cells.[62]

Reed-Sternberg cells are derived from B cells in the vast majority of cases of classical Hodgkin lymphoma, as determined by clonal rearrangement of

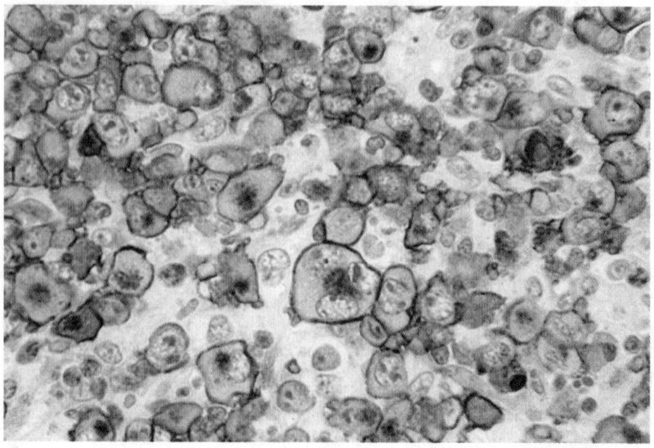

FIGURE 98–32. Anaplastic large cell lymphoma stained with antibody to CD30.

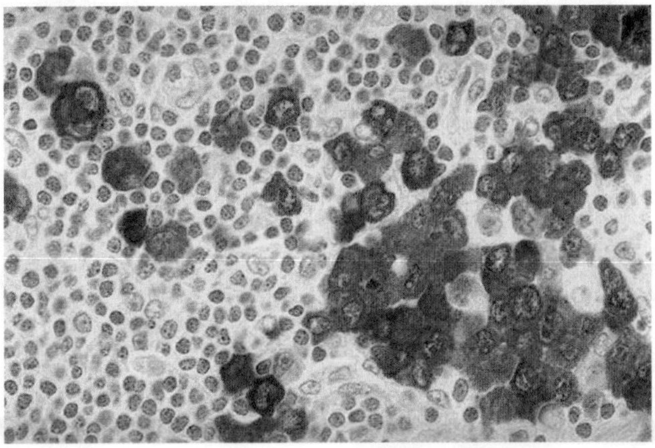

FIGURE 98–33. Anaplastic large cell lymphoma stained with antibody to ALK (anaplastic lymphoma kinase).

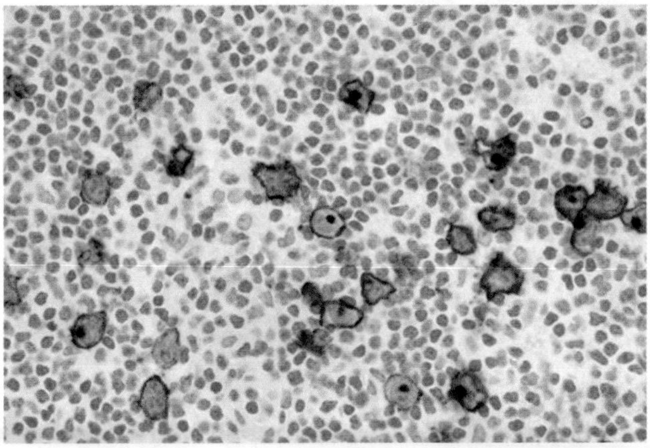

FIGURE 98–35. Classical Hodgkin lymphoma stained with antibody to CD30.

IG heavy-chain genes.[63] However, Reed-Sternberg cells have lost most of their B-lineage antigens, including expression of *IG*. Reed-Sternberg cells express CD30 in almost all cases of classical Hodgkin lymphoma and express CD15 in the majority (Figs. 98–35 and 98–36).[62] They typically are negative for CD45 (leukocyte common antigen) and positive for B-cell marker CD20 in 20 to 40 percent of cases, usually of variable intensity in a minority of cells. Classical Hodgkin lymphoma is associated with EBV in 20 to 40 percent of cases and is thought to play a role in the pathogenesis of these cases.[64] Reed-Sternberg cells express many cytokines and several members of the tumor necrosis factor (TNF) receptor family (e.g., CD40, CD30).[65] The cytokines are thought to play a role in the recruitment of reactive infiltrate and to contribute to Reed-Sternberg cell proliferation and survival. The TNF receptor family members can be activated by ligands expressed by the surrounding reactive infiltrate, leading to proliferation and survival.

The most common subtype of classical Hodgkin lymphoma is the nodular sclerosis variant. The variant is characterized by the presence of broad collagen bands dividing the tumor into nodules and by the presence of "lacunar" cells, mononuclear Reed-Sternberg variants that typically show retraction artifact so that the cells appear to be in lacunae (Fig. 98–37). These cells are found within a reactive infiltrate that typically includes prominent eosinophils and lymphocytes. Different grading schemes have been proposed for nodular sclerosis Hodgkin lymphoma, but no prognostic relevance is clear.[66,67]

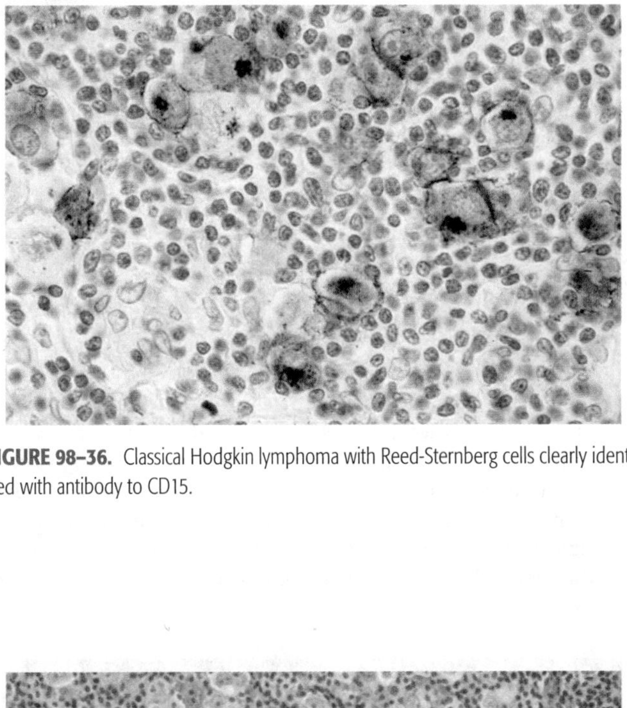

FIGURE 98–36. Classical Hodgkin lymphoma with Reed-Sternberg cells clearly identified with antibody to CD15.

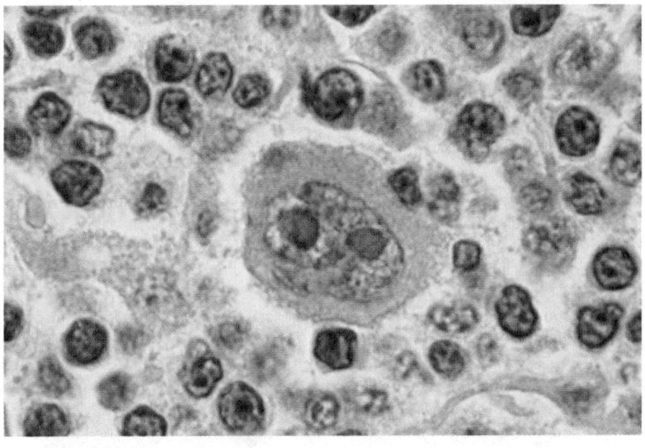

FIGURE 98–34. Diagnostic Reed-Sternberg cell in Hodgkin lymphoma.

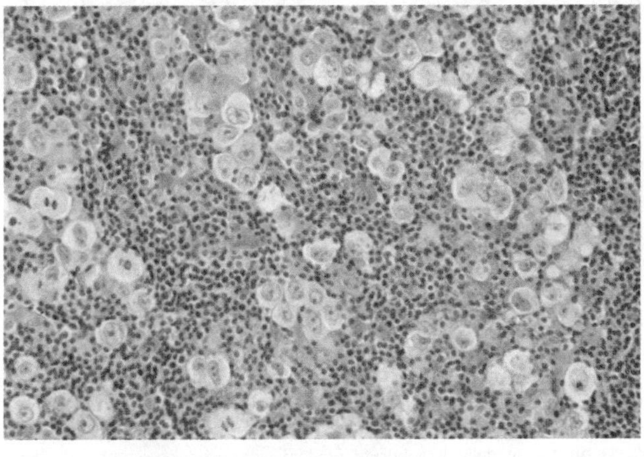

FIGURE 98–37. Classical Hodgkin lymphoma, nodular sclerosis type with characteristic lacunar cells.

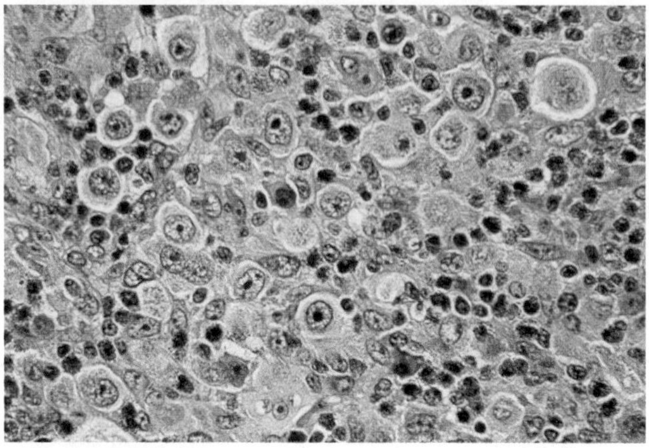

FIGURE 98–38. Mixed cellularity Hodgkin lymphoma.

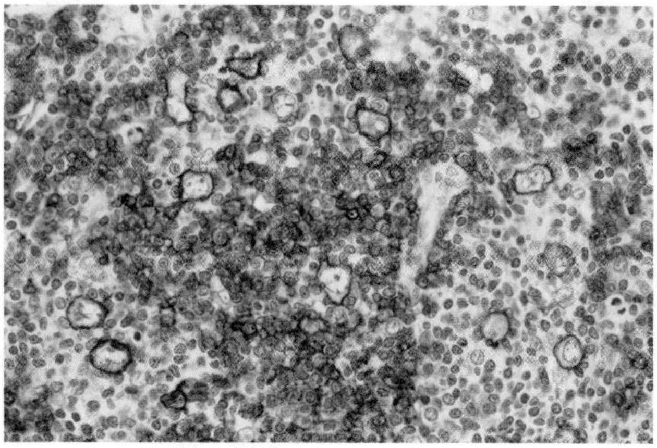

FIGURE 98–40. Nodular lymphocyte predominance Hodgkin lymphoma stained with antibody CD20. Note the positive staining of the LP cells (popcorn cells).

The second most common subtype is the mixed cellularity variant, which is characterized by Reed-Sternberg cells in a mixed inflammatory background without the broad collagen bands seen in nodular sclerosis (Fig. 98–38). Mixed cellularity cases are more commonly associated with EBV compared to the nodular sclerosis variant.

The lymphocyte-rich and lymphocyte-depleted subtypes of classical Hodgkin lymphoma are the least common, each representing approximately 5 percent of all cases. The lymphocyte-rich variant has a small number of Reed-Sternberg cells in a background of small lymphocytes with absent or rare eosinophils and neutrophils, typically in a nodular pattern. It is easily confused with nodular lymphocyte predominant Hodgkin lymphoma, so immunohistochemical staining to determine the immunophenotype of the Reed-Sternberg cells is required to make the distinction.[68,69] It can rarely have a diffuse growth pattern.

In the past, the lymphocyte-depleted variant had been divided into reticular and diffuse fibrosis types. The diffuse fibrosis variant is characterized by a hypocellular infiltrate with prominent diffuse nonbirefringent sclerosis accompanied by rare Reed-Sternberg cells and a minor reactive inflammatory component. The reticular variant showed an increased number of large atypical cells, commonly with bizarre multinucleated cells, with a minor reactive component. It now is recognized that the vast majority of these cases are cases of ALCL or diffuse large B-cell lymphomas, and as such the diagnosis of the reticular variant of lymphocyte-depleted Hodgkin lymphoma is rare and should be made only in the presence of definitive supportive immunophenotypic data.

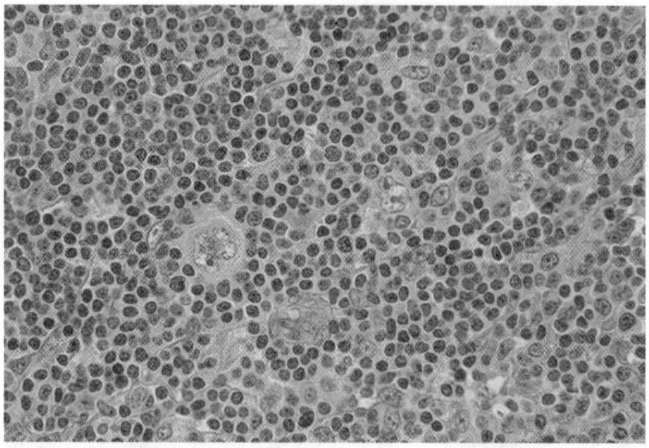

FIGURE 98–39. Nodular lymphocyte predominance Hodgkin lymphoma showing characteristic LP cells (popcorn cells) in a background of small benign lymphocytes.

NODULAR LYMPHOCYTE-PREDOMINANT HODGKIN LYMPHOMA

Nodular lymphocyte-predominant Hodgkin lymphoma has several pathologic and clinical features that are distinct from classical Hodgkin lymphoma.[70] This variant previously was called *lymphocytic and/or histiocytic predominance Hodgkin lymphoma* in the Lukes and Butler classification. The malignant cell population is the lymphocyte predominant (LP) cells. These cells are large cells with a single nucleus that contains multilobated or folded features. They often are referred to as "popcorn" cells because they resemble popped kernels of corn (Fig. 98–39). Nucleoli typically are smaller than the nucleoli seen in classic Reed-Sternberg cells. They differ from Reed-Sternberg cells in classical Hodgkin lymphoma in that they retain expression of CD45 and B-lineage markers (CD20, IG) and are negative for CD15 and CD30 (Fig. 98–40).[71] As the name implies, the cells have a complete or partial nodular architectural pattern with a background consisting primarily of lymphocytes. Histiocytes are also a common feature, but neutrophils and eosinophils are absent or rare.

REFERENCES

1. Magrath IT: Historical perspective: The evolution of modern concepts of biology and management, in *The Non-Hodgkin's Lymphomas*, 2nd ed, edited by IT Magrath, p 47. Arnold, London, 1997.
2. Hodgkin T: On some morbid appearances of the absorbent glands and spleen. *Trans Med Soc Lond* 17:68, 1832.
3. Callendar GR: Tumors and tumor-like conditions of the lymphocyte, the myelocyte, the erythrocyte, and the reticulum cell. *Am J Pathol* 10:443, 1934.
4. Gall EA, Mallory TB: Malignant lymphoma: A clinicopathologic survey of 618 cases. *Am J Pathol* 18:381, 1942.
5. Rappaport H, Winter W, Hicks E: Follicular lymphoma: A re-evaluation of its position in the scheme of malignant lymphoma, based on a survey of 253 cases. *Cancer* 9:792, 1956.
6. Rappaport H: *Tumors of the Hematopoietic System, Fasc 8*. Armed Forces Institute of Pathology, Washington, DC, 1966.
7. Arnold A, Cossman J, Bakhshi A, et al: Immunoglobulin-gene rearrangements as unique clonal markers in human lymphoid neoplasms. *N Engl J Med* 309:1593, 1983.
8. Aisenberg AC, Krontiris TG, Mak TW, Wilkes BM: Rearrangement of the gene for the beta chain of the T-cell receptor in T-cell chronic lymphocytic leukemia and related disorders. *N Engl J Med* 313:529, 1985.

9. Gerard-Marchant R, Hamlin I, Lennert K, et al: Classification of nonHodgkin's lymphoma. *Lancet* ii:406, 1974.
10. Lukes RJ, Collins RD: Immunologic characterization of human malignant lymphomas. *Cancer* 34(Suppl 4):1488, 1974.
11. Schein PS, Chabner BA, Canellos GP, et al: Potential for prolonged disease-free survival following combination chemotherapy of non-Hodgkin's lymphoma. *Blood* 43:181, 1974.
12. National Cancer Institute sponsored study of classifications of non-Hodgkin's lymphomas: Summary and description of a working formulation for clinical usage. The Non-Hodgkin's Lymphoma Pathologic Classification Project. *Cancer* 49:2112, 1982.
13. Stansfeld AG, Diebold J, Noel H, et al: Updated Kiel classification for lymphomas. *Lancet* 1:292, 1988.
14. Harris NL, Jaffe ES, Stein H, et al: A revised European-American classification of lymphoid neoplasms: A proposal from the International Lymphoma Study Group. *Blood* 84:1361, 1994.
15. A clinical evaluation of the International Lymphoma Study Group classification of non-Hodgkin's lymphoma. By the Non-Hodgkin's Lymphoma Classification Project. *Blood* 89:3909, 1997.
16. Swerdlow SH, Campo E, Harris NL, et al: *WHO Classification of Tumours of Haematopoietic and Lymphoid Tissues*. IARC Press, Lyon, 2008.
17. Liang P, Pardee AB: Analyzing differential gene expression in cancer. *Nat Rev Cancer* 3:869, 2003.
18. MacLennan IC: Germinal centers. *Annu Rev Immunol* 12:117, 1994.
19. Jennings CD, Foon KA: Recent advances in flow cytometry: Application to the diagnosis of hematologic malignancy. *Blood* 90:2863, 1997.
20. Frizzera G, Wu CD, Inghirami G: The usefulness of immunophenotypic and genotypic studies in the diagnosis and classification of hematopoietic and lymphoid neoplasms. An update. *Am J Clin Pathol* 111(Suppl 1):S13, 1999.
21. Mauvieux L, Macintyre EA: Practical role of molecular diagnostics in non-Hodgkin's lymphomas. *Baillieres Clin Haematol* 9:653, 1996.
22. Collins RD: Is clonality equivalent to malignancy: Specifically, is immunoglobulin gene rearrangement diagnostic of malignant lymphoma? *Hum Pathol* 28:757, 1997.
23. Lester JF, Dojcinov SD, Attanoos RL, et al: The clinical impact of expert pathological review on lymphoma management: A regional experience. *Br J Haematol* 123:463, 2003.
24. Hajdu SI, Melamed MR: Limitations of aspiration cytology in the diagnosis of primary neoplasms. *Acta Cytol* 28:337, 1984.
25. Pontifex AH, Haley L: Fine-needle aspiration cytology in lymphomas and related disorders. *Diagn Cytopathol* 5:432, 1989.
26. Klein U, Tu Y, Stolovitzky GA, et al: Gene expression profiling of B cell chronic lymphocytic leukemia reveals a homogeneous phenotype related to memory B cells. *J Exp Med* 194:1625, 2001.
27. Rosenwald A, Alizadeh AA, Widhopf G, et al: Relation of gene expression phenotype to immunoglobulin mutation genotype in B cell chronic lymphocytic leukemia. *J Exp Med* 194:1639, 2001.
28. Wiestner A, Rosenwald A, Barry TS, et al: ZAP-70 expression identifies a chronic lymphocytic leukemia subtype with unmutated immunoglobulin genes, inferior clinical outcome, and distinct gene expression profile. *Blood* 101:4944, 2003.
29. Dohner H, Stilgenbauer S, Benner A, et al: Genomic aberrations and survival in chronic lymphocytic leukemia. *N Engl J Med* 343:1910, 2000.
30. Weisenburger DD, Armitage JO: Mantle cell lymphoma: An entity comes of age. *Blood* 87:4483, 1996.
31. Argatoff LH, Connors JM, Klasa RJ, et al: Mantle cell lymphoma: A clinicopathologic study of 80 cases. *Blood* 89:2067, 1997.
32. Rosenwald A, Wright G, Wiestner A, et al: The proliferation gene expression signature is a quantitative integrator of oncogenic events that predicts survival in mantle cell lymphoma. *Cancer Cell* 3:185, 2003.
33. Gesk S, Klapper W, Martin-Subero JI, et al: A chromosomal translocation in cyclin D1-negative/cyclin D2-positive mantle cell lymphoma fuses the CCND2 gene to the IGK locus. *Blood* 108;1109, 2006.
34. Jaffe ES, Shevach EM, Frank MM, et al: Nodular lymphoma: Evidence for origin from follicular B lymphocytes. *N Engl J Med* 290:813, 1974.
35. Bosga-Bouwer AG, van Imhoff GW, Boonstra R, et al: Follicular lymphoma grade 3B includes 3 cytogenetically defined subgroups with primary t(14;18) 3q27, or other translocations: t(14;18) and 3q27 are mutually exclusive. *Blood* 101:1149, 2003.
36. Hans CP, Weisenburger DD, Vose JM, et al: A significant diffuse component predicts for inferior survival in grade 3 follicular lymphoma, but cytologic subtypes do not predict survival. *Blood* 101:2363, 2003.
37. Ott G, Katzenberger T, Lohr A, et al: Cytomorphologic, immunohistochemical, and cytogenetic profiles of follicular lymphoma: 2 types of follicular lymphoma grade 3. *Blood* 99:3806, 2002.
38. Thieblemont C, Felman P, Callet-Bauchu E, et al: Splenic marginal zone lymphoma: A distinct clinical and pathological entity. *Lancet Oncol* 4:95, 2003.
39. Nathwani BN, Drachenberg MR, Hernandez AM, et al: Nodal monocytoid B-cell lymphoma (nodal marginal-zone B-cell lymphoma). *Semin Hematol* 36:128, 1999.
40. Zucca E, Bertoni F, Roggero E, Cavalli F: The gastric marginal zone B cell lymphoma of MALT type. *Blood* 96:410, 2000.
41. Bertoni F, Cotter FE, Zucca E: Molecular genetics of extranodal marginal zone (MALT-type) B-cell lymphoma. *Leuk Lymphoma* 35:57, 1999.
42. Alizadeh AA, Eisen MB, Davis RE, et al: Distinct types of diffuse large B-cell lymphoma identified by gene expression profiling. *Nature* 403:503, 2000.
43. Rosenwald A, Wright G, Chan WC, et al: The use of molecular profiling to predict survival after chemotherapy for diffuse large-B-cell lymphoma. *N Engl J Med* 346:1937, 2002.
44. Wright G, Tan B, Rosenwald A, et al: A gene expression-based method to diagnose clinically distinct subgroups of diffuse large B cell lymphoma. *Proc Natl Acad Sci U S A* 100:9991, 2003.
45. Davis RE, Brown KD, Siebenlist U, Staudt LM: Constitutive nuclear factor kappaB activity is required for survival of activated B cell-like diffuse large B cell lymphoma cells. *J Exp Med* 194:1861, 2001.
46. Hans CP, Weisenburger DD, Greiner TC, et al: Confirmation of the molecular classification of diffuse large B-cell lymphoma by immunohistochemistry using a tissue microarray. *Blood* 103:275, 2004.
47. De Jong D, Rosenwald A, Chhanabhai M, et al: Immunohistochemical prognostic markers in diffuse large B-cell lymphoma: Validation of tissue microarray as a prerequisite for broad clinical applications—A study from the Lunenburg Lymphoma Biomarker Consortium. *J Clin Oncol* 25:805, 2007.
48. Lenz G, Wright G, Dave SS, et al: Stromal gene signatures in large B-cell lymphomas. *N Engl J Med* 359:2313, 2008.
49. van Besien K, Kelta M, Bahaguna P: Primary mediastinal B-cell lymphoma: A review of pathology and management. *J Clin Oncol* 19:1855, 2001.
50. Rosenwald A, Wright G, Leroy K, et al: Molecular diagnosis of primary mediastinal B cell lymphoma identifies a clinically favorable subgroup of diffuse large B cell lymphoma related to Hodgkin lymphoma. *J Exp Med* 198:851, 2003.
51. Savage KJ, Monti S, Kutok JL, et al: The molecular signature of mediastinal large B-cell lymphoma differs from that of other diffuse large B-cell lymphomas and shares features with classical Hodgkin lymphoma. *Blood* 102:3871, 2003.
52. Dave SS, Fu K, Wright GW, et al: Molecular diagnosis of Burkitt's lymphoma. *N Engl J Med* 354:2431, 2006.
53. Hummel M, Bentink S, Berger H, et al: A biologic definition of Burkitt's lymphoma from transcriptional and genomic profiling. *N Engl J Med* 354:2419, 2006.
54. Stein H, Foss HD, Durkop H, et al: CD30(+) anaplastic large cell lymphoma: A review of its histopathologic, genetic, and clinical features. *Blood* 96:3681, 2000.
55. Gascoyne RD, Aoun P, Wu D, et al: Prognostic significance of anaplastic lymphoma kinase (ALK) protein expression in adults with anaplastic large cell lymphoma. *Blood* 93:3913, 1999.
56. Benharroch D, Meguerian-Bedoyan Z, Lamant L, et al: ALK-positive lymphoma: A single disease with a broad spectrum of morphology. *Blood* 91:2076, 1998.
57. Duyster J, Bai RY, Morris SW: Translocations involving anaplastic lymphoma kinase (ALK). *Oncogene* 20:5623, 2001.
58. Savage KJ, Harris NL, Vose JM, et al: ALK-negative anaplastic large cell lymphoma (ALCL) is clinically and immunophenotypically different from both ALK-positive ALCL and peripheral T-cell lymphoma, not otherwise specified: report from the International Peripheral T-Cell Lymphoma Project. *Blood* 111:5496, 2008.
59. Sternberg C: Uber eine Eigenartige unter dem Bilde der Pseudoleukamie verlaufende Tuberculose des lymphatischen Apparates. *Z Heilk* 19:21, 1898.
60. Reed DM: On the pathologic changes in Hodgkin's disease, with especial reference to its relation to tuberculosis. *Johns Hopkins Hosp Rep* 10:133, 1902.
61. Strum SB, Park JK, Rappaport H: Observation of cells resembling Sternberg-Reed cells in conditions other than Hodgkin's disease. *Cancer* 26:176, 1970.
62. Harris NL: Hodgkin's disease: Classification and differential diagnosis. *Mod Pathol* 12:159, 1999.
63. Kuppers R, Rajewsky K: The origin of Hodgkin and Reed/Sternberg cells in Hodgkin's disease. *Annu Rev Immunol* 16:471, 1998.
64. Jarrett RF, MacKenzie J: Epstein-Barr virus and other candidate viruses in the pathogenesis of Hodgkin's disease. *Semin Hematol* 36:260, 1999.
65. Skinnider BF, Mak TW: The role of cytokines in classical Hodgkin lymphoma. *Blood* 99:4283, 2002.
66. MacLennan KA, Bennett MH, Tu A, et al: Relationship of histopathologic features to survival and relapse in nodular sclerosing Hodgkin's disease. A study of 1659 patients. *Cancer* 64:1686, 1989.
67. Ferry JA, Linggood RM, Convery KM, et al: Hodgkin disease, nodular sclerosis type. Implications of histologic subclassification. *Cancer* 71:457, 1993.
68. von Wasielewski R, Werner M, Fischer R, et al: Lymphocyte-predominant Hodgkin's disease. An immunohistochemical analysis of 208 reviewed Hodgkin's disease cases from the German Hodgkin Study Group. *Am J Pathol* 150:793, 1997.
69. Anagnostopoulos I, Hansmann ML, Franssila K, et al: European Task Force on Lymphoma project on lymphocyte predominance Hodgkin disease: Histologic and immunohistologic analysis of submitted cases reveals 2 types of Hodgkin disease with a nodular growth pattern and abundant lymphocytes. *Blood* 96:1889, 2000.
70. Mason DY, Banks PM, Chan J, et al: Nodular lymphocyte predominance Hodgkin's disease. A distinct clinicopathological entity. *Am J Surg Pathol* 18:526, 1994.
71. Chan WC: Cellular origin of nodular lymphocyte-predominant Hodgkin's lymphoma: Immunophenotypic and molecular studies. *Semin Hematol* 36:242, 1999.

CHAPTER 99
HODGKIN LYMPHOMA

Sandra J. Horning

SUMMARY

Classic Hodgkin lymphoma, characterized by multinucleated Hodgkin and Reed-Sternberg cells residing in a mixed infiltrate of nonneoplastic cells, is derived from mature B-cells at the germinal center stage of differentiation. Hodgkin and Reed-Sternberg cells contain monoclonal immunoglobulin gene rearrangements but have lost much of the B-cell specific expression program and have acquired inappropriate gene products. Multiple signaling pathways and transcription factors are deregulated in Hodgkin lymphoma. Although transforming events are incompletely understood, recurrent genetic lesions involve the JAK-STAT and nuclear factor κB pathways. Epstein-Barr virus, which is an important environmental factor in well-described subsets of Hodgkin lymphoma, also leads to nuclear factor κB activation. The inflammatory microenvironment promotes survival and allows escape of Hodgkin and Reed-Sternberg cells from immune attack. Morphologic and immunophenotypic features distinguish the four subtypes of classical Hodgkin lymphoma, accounting for 95 percent of cases, and nodular lymphocyte predominance Hodgkin lymphoma. Hodgkin lymphoma spreads in a predictable, contiguous manner and is classified into four stages, I to IV. Hodgkin lymphoma is treated with the intent to cure the disease in all stages, and long-term survival exceeds 85 percent for all stages. Doxorubicin-containing chemotherapy plays a major role in treatment of all stages of the disease whereas, because of concerns for late toxicities, radiotherapy is used selectively. A valuable diagnostic test for assessment of disease and response to treatment, 18-fluorodeoxyglucose positron emission tomography, is being assessed as a measure of response-adapted treatment. High-dose therapy and autologous transplantation is effective in patients who have relapsed, and several promising new biologic agents are available. Consideration for late treatment effects guides therapy and followup in Hodgkin lymphoma, which disproportionately affects adolescents and young adults. Major treatment challenges include the maintenance of high cure rates with fewer short-term and long-term complications, biomarker identification of the small refractory subgroup, and integration of biologic therapies in the treatment of a frequently curable tumor.

Acronyms and abbreviations that appear in this chapter include: ABVD, Adriamycin (doxorubicin), bleomycin, vinblastine, dacarbazine; BEACOPP, bleomycin, etoposide, Adriamycin (doxorubicin), cyclophosphamide, vincristine, procarbazine, prednisone; BEAM, bischloroethylnitrosourea (carmustine), etoposide, Ara C (cytarabine), melphalan; CBV, cyclophosphamide, bischloroethylnitrosourea (carmustine), etoposide; COPP, cyclophosphamide, vincristine, procarbazine, prednisone; CT, computed tomography; EBV, Epstein-Barr virus; EBVP, epirubicin, bleomycin, vinblastine, prednisone; EORTC, European Organization for the Research and Treatment of Cancer; FDG, 18-fluorodeoxyglucose; GHSG, German Hodgkin Study Group; HLA, human leukocyte antigen; IL, interleukin; LMP, latent membrane protein; MOPP, mechlorethamine (nitrogen mustard), Oncovin (vincristine), procarbazine, prednisone; MVPP, nitrogen mustard, vinblastine, procarbazine, prednisone; NF-κB, nuclear factor-κB; PET, positron emission tomography; RANKL, receptor activator of nuclear factor κB; STAT, signal transducer and activator of transcription.

DEFINITION AND HISTORY

Classic Hodgkin lymphoma is a neoplasm of lymphoid tissue, in most cases derived from germinal center B cells, defined by the presence of the malignant Hodgkin and Reed-Sternberg cells with a characteristic immunophenotype and appropriate cellular background. Classic Hodgkin lymphoma accounts for 95 percent of cases and contains four histologic subtypes (nodular sclerosis, mixed cellularity, lymphocyte-rich and lymphocyte-depleted), distinguished on the basis of microscopic appearance and relative proportions of Hodgkin Reed-Sternberg cells, lymphocytes and fibrosis (Table 99–1). Nodular lymphocyte-predominant represents the other major category, which is distinguished by Hodgkin and Reed-Sternberg variants termed lymphocytic and histiocytic cells that, unlike classic Hodgkin lymphoma, express typical B-lineage markers.

HISTORICAL ASPECTS

In his historic 1832 paper entitled *On Some Morbid Appearances of the Absorbent Glands and Spleen*, Thomas Hodgkin described the clinical histories and gross postmortem findings of seven cases of the disease that was later to bear his name.[1] In 1856, Samuel Wilks independently described 10 cases of "a peculiar enlargement of the lymphatic glands frequently associated with disease of the spleen," including four of Hodgkin's original cases.[2] Upon discovering Hodgkin's original report, he used the appellation "Hodgkin's Disease" in a subsequent series of 15 cases published in 1865.[2] Thirteen years after Hodgkin's original paper, the first cases of leukemia were described. Cases in which the neoplastic cells remained confined to the lymphatic system were described by Dreschfield (1892)[3] and Kundrat (1893)[4]; the latter gave the name *lymphosarcoma* to these cases. The description of additional members of the lymphoma–leukemia complex continued up to the present time.

Carl Sternberg (1898)[5] and Dorothy Reed (1902)[6] are credited with the first definitive and thorough descriptions of Hodgkin lymphoma, although a number of investigators from England, Germany, and France had previously recognized the characteristic multinucleated giant cells. In 1926, Fox examined microscopic sections from the gross specimens preserved in the Gordon Museum of Guy's Hospital in London of three of Hodgkin's original cases.[7] It is remarkable that the preserved microanatomy allowed him to confirm the histopathologic diagnosis in two of these cases. Jackson and Parker made the first serious effort at the histopathologic classification of Hodgkin lymphoma, correlating their findings with prognosis.[8] A second advance was made in 1966 when Lukes, Butler, and Hicks proposed a classification that related well to clinical presentation and course.[9] Their proposal was slightly modified into the Rye classification, in which four histopathologic subtypes were described: lymphocyte-predominant, nodular sclerosis, mixed cellularity and lymphocyte-depleted. In the World Health Organization Classification of Lymphoid Neoplasms, the nodular lymphocyte-predominant subtype is clearly distinguished from classical Hodgkin lymphoma.[10] The "lymphocyte-rich" subtype of classical Hodgkin lymphoma was introduced in 1999 (see Chap. 98).

Peters described a clinical staging system in 1950, emphasizing the diagnostic evaluation of the anatomic extent of disease.[11] In 1952, Kinmouth introduced lower-extremity lymphangiography that allowed roentgenologic visualization of the pelvic and retroperitoneal lymph nodes and was found to be far more sensitive than palpation or other radiographic methods.[12] The frequency of unsuspected splenic involvement was revealed in a group of 65 patients subjected to laparotomy and splenectomy with biopsy of splenic hilar, paraaortic and mesenteric nodes, and liver at Stanford University.[13] These diagnostic procedures led to improved understanding of the mode of dissemination of disease

TABLE 99–1. Classification of Hodgkin Lymphoma

Histological Subtype	Immunophenotype
Nodular lymphocyte-predominant	CD20+ CD30– CD15– Ig+
Classical	CD20–* CD30+ CD15+ Ig–
Nodular sclerosis	
Mixed cellularity	
Lymphocyte-rich	
Lymphocyte-depleted	

*infrequently positive.

and correlated well with prognosis, culminating in the modern concepts of staging codified at the Rye, New York, conference in 1965,[14] and further refined at the Workshop on the Staging of Hodgkin's Disease in Ann Arbor, Michigan, in 1971.[15]

Pusey (1902)[16] and Senn (1903)[17] were the first to report dramatic regressions of lymphadenopathy with exposure to X-rays newly discovered by Roentgen in 1896. Based upon the nearly inevitable recurrence in untreated areas, Gilbert proposed the systematic treatment of both involved and uninvolved areas in 1939.[18] Peters (1950) is given credit for the first demonstration of the curative potential of radiotherapy in her classic paper.[11] The development of megavoltage radiotherapy (doses >4000 cGy), as reported by Kaplan in 1962,[19] permitted the delivery of tumoricidal doses to virtually all lymphoid regions in the body within acceptable limits of normal tissue tolerance.

The chemotherapy of Hodgkin lymphoma originated as a byproduct of the wartime work on the mustard gases.[20,21] Following the initial work with the nitrogen mustards, antimetabolites were synthesized and a number of alkaloids and antibiotics extracted from various plant, fungus, and microbial sources became available for clinical use. DeVita and colleagues introduced the first highly effective combination chemotherapy, MOPP (nitrogen mustard, vincristine [Oncovin], procarbazine, and prednisone), based on experimental studies indicating the desirability of combining agents with non-overlapping toxicities.[22] Combination chemotherapy extended the curative potential for Hodgkin lymphoma to advanced disease. The ABVD (doxorubicin [Adriamycin], bleomycin, vinblastine, dacarbazine) regimen introduced by Bonadonna and colleagues represented another major advance.[23] Based on a more favorable safety profile and greater efficacy, ABVD replaced MOPP, as discussed below.

EPIDEMIOLOGY

The estimated incidence of Hodgkin lymphoma in the United States was 8510 cases in 2009. It is more common in Americans of European descent (age-adjusted incidence 3.3/100,000) than in Americans of African descent (2.9/100,000).[24] The disease has a median age of onset of 38 years with a bimodal incidence with peaks at ages 15 to 34 and in those older than age 60 years.[25,26] Three distinct forms of Hodgkin lymphoma have been described: a rare childhood form (ages 0–14 years), a young adult form (15–34 years), and an older adult form (55–74 years). Data from the Surveillance, Epidemiology and End Results (SEER) program of the National Cancer Institute analyses show variation in age-specific incidence rates with a smaller second peak in Americans of European descent whereas the second peak is more prominent in Americans of Hispanic descent.[27] Except for Americans of Asian descent, for whom the incidence has increased by 5.2 percent per year, the incidence of Hodgkin lymphoma has been stable in the United States from 1993 to 2000. The nodular sclerosis subtype predominates in young adults, whereas the mixed cellularity subtype is more common in the pediatric population and at older ages. There is a male predominance at all ages (~1.2:1) and this is most marked in childhood cases (85% males).

Early studies associated an increased risk of Hodgkin lymphoma in the young adult population with high socioeconomic status.[25] Living in a rental home, sharing a bedroom, and attending daycare or nursery school and early parity in women have been associated with reduced risk. The relationship of incidence to neighborhood socioeconomic status was demonstrated in California for younger but not for older patients.[26] Although associations with occupational exposure, such as exposure to pesticides, and lifestyle factors such as cigarette smoking have been reported, the aggregate data do not indicate consistent causal relationships with exogenous chemicals or toxins. A personal or family history of an autoimmune disorder, particularly sarcoidosis, has been associated with an increased risk of Hodgkin lymphoma.[28] Shared etiologic factors with multiple sclerosis have been suggested but these are thought to be of minor importance.

The geographic patterns vary for the three major age groups: the incidence of Hodgkin lymphoma is greater in childhood in less-developed countries, whereas the incidence peaks in young adulthood and is associated with more favorable histologic subtypes in developed countries.[29] Presence of the Epstein-Barr virus (EBV) in Hodgkin and Reed-Sternberg cells is more common in less-developed countries and in pediatric and older adult cases. The worldwide incidence of the disease is much lower in the Asian population, whether residing in the Far East or in the United States, although the reported rate in Vancouver, Canada, among immigrants of Chinese descent was higher than among Chinese residing in Hong Kong.[30,31] Together these data suggest a complex interaction among possible socioeconomic, environmental, immunologic, genetic, and infectious factors in the incidence of Hodgkin lymphoma.

POSSIBLE INFECTIOUS ETIOLOGY

The demographic features have long supported the "hygiene hypothesis" that one or more subtypes of Hodgkin lymphoma represent delayed exposure to an infectious etiology. In 1966, MacMahon proposed that the first age peak in young adults was infectious in nature, whereas that seen in the second peak resulted from causes similar to other lymphomas.[25] As noted above, socioeconomic status correlates with the first, but not the second, peak.[26] Several reports of clustering of Hodgkin lymphoma at the time of diagnosis suggested the possibility of infectious transmission.[32] The weaknesses of the retrospective methodology in these studies have been critically assessed, and further statistical analyses indicate that these likely occurred by chance alone.

A threefold increased risk of Hodgkin lymphoma in young adults is conferred by a prior history of serologically confirmed infectious mononucleosis. In addition, elevations in titers of EBV, the etiologic agent of infectious mononucleosis, have been reported in people diagnosed with Hodgkin lymphoma.[33,34] A large population study showed that people who developed the disease had abnormally high titers of EBV viral capsid antigen and early antigen in prediagnostic sera.[35] In two subsequent reports, a significantly increased risk of Hodgkin lymphoma after serologically verified infectious mononucleosis and limited to EBV-positive cases was reported in young adults.[36,37] The median incubation time was approximately 4.1 years.

EBV genomes have been detected in 30 to 50 percent of Hodgkin lymphoma tissues in developed countries, and EBV-associated cases are more common in the cases with mixed cellularity histology, Hispanic ethnicity, and age-greater-than-60-years subgroups.[38,39] Several studies report a high incidence of EBV association, 85 to 100 percent, in pediatric Hodgkin lymphoma in which geographic, ethnic, and racial factors have been implicated in the association.[40] EBV within Hodgkin and Reed-Sternberg cells is typical in human immunodeficiency virus (HIV)-infected individuals with Hodgkin lymphoma,[41] and the incidence of Hodgkin lymphoma is 10 to 20 times higher than the general population in patients with HIV. In contrast to non-Hodgkin lymphoma, the incidence of Hodgkin lymphoma in the HIV-infected population has increased despite less-severe immunosuppression in the era of highly active antiretroviral therapy.[42,43]

■ GENETIC BASIS

Genetic susceptibility and familial aggregation appear to play a role in the incidence of Hodgkin lymphoma. The increased risk of the disease among identical, but not fraternal, twins provides the strongest evidence for a genetic association.[44] Hodgkin lymphoma-prone families, with or without other forms of cancer, have been described in the literature and it is estimated that 4.5 percent of cases are familial.[45–47] The standard incidence ratio for age-specific familial risk from the Swedish Cancer Registry was higher for Hodgkin lymphoma (4.8) than any other neoplasm.[48] Relative risk for familial disease is stronger in individuals greater than 40 years, males, and siblings, and a shared risk with chronic lymphocytic leukemia and non-Hodgkin lymphoma has been described.[47] An increased incidence in same sex siblings (8- to 12-fold) versus opposite sex siblings (1.3- to 1.4-fold) in the Swedish registry is consistent with older data and has been interpreted in support of an environmental influence or a pseudoautosomal susceptibility gene located on a sex chromosome.[49–51]

Immunoregulatory genes within or near the major histocompatibility complex that may govern susceptibility to viral infections have been postulated to influence susceptibility to Hodgkin lymphoma, an hypothesis that is supported by the demonstration of lifelong, depressed cellular immunity in Hodgkin lymphoma patients and their healthy relatives.[52] Several groups described specific human leukocyte antigen (HLA) susceptibility or resistance regions, but these data have been relatively weak and sometimes inconsistent. Data implicate HLA related to EBV status in Hodgkin lymphoma, with HLA*A02 associated with a reduced risk and HLA*A01 associated with an increased risk of EBV-positive disease.[53]

ETIOLOGY AND PATHOGENESIS

■ ORIGIN OF THE REED-STERNBERG CELL

The histologic diagnosis of Hodgkin lymphoma is based on the recognition of the Reed-Sternberg cell in an appropriate cellular background. The classic Reed-Sternberg cell has a bilobed nucleus with prominent eosinophilic nucleoli separated by a clear space from the thickened nuclear membrane (see Fig. 99–1 and see also Chap. 98, Fig. 98–35). Mononuclear variants (Hodgkin cells) have similar nuclear characteristics and may represent Reed-Sternberg cells cut in a plane that shows only one lobe of the nucleus. Reed-Sternberg cells are not pathognomonic for Hodgkin lymphoma; they may be seen in reactive and other neoplastic conditions. Study of the Reed-Sternberg cell has been complicated by the fact that the neoplastic cells are sparsely interspersed among a reactive mixed nonclonal cell population of lymphocytes, eosinophils, histiocytes, plasma cells, and neutrophils. Difficulty in the characterization of the neoplastic cells, which account for only approximately 1 to 2 percent of the cellular composition, led to controversy regarding the etiology and pathogenesis of Hodgkin lymphoma for more than 150 years. Molecular analyses of single cells facilitated discovery that classical Hodgkin lymphoma, in the large majority of cases, and nodular lymphocyte-predominant Hodgkin lymphoma are clonal disorders derived from germinal center B cells.[54] The need to survive negative selection in the germinal center, the determination of genetic alterations and constitutive activity of key signaling pathways, and the involvement of EBV in a subset of cases have led to hypotheses for the means by which Hodgkin and Reed-Sternberg cells undergo malignant transformation. Application of additional genomic technology promises to clarify the molecular changes underlying malignant transformation and cellular proliferation.

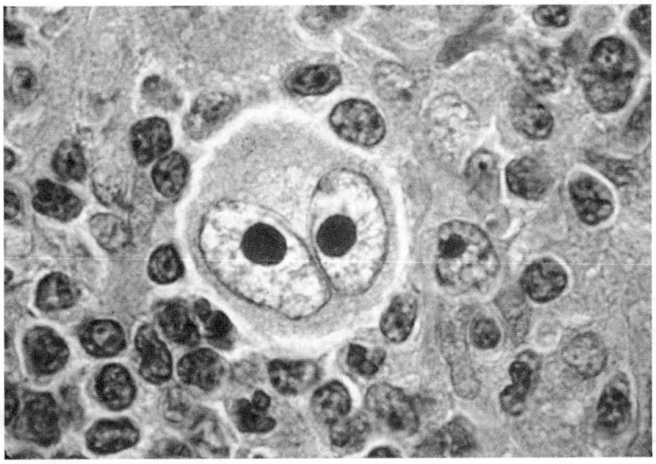

FIGURE 99–1. High magnification of lymph node section in a patient with Hodgkin lymphoma. A Reed-Sternberg cell is in the center of the field with the classical findings of giant size compared to background lymphocytes, binucleation, and prominent eosinophilic nucleoli.

Antigen Receptor Rearrangements

Reed-Sternberg cells and their mononuclear variants demonstrate inconsistent lineage-specific antigen expression that is unlike any other cell of the hematopoietic system. The origin of these cells was eventually determined through isolation of single cells by micromanipulation of histologic sections and analysis for immunoglobulin variable gene rearrangements.[54,55] Nearly all Hodgkin and Reed-Sternberg cells have rearranged and somatically mutated immunoglobulin VH genes, indicating a germinal center or postgerminal center origin of classic Hodgkin and Reed-Sternberg cells.[56–58] Extrapolating from the fact that a subset of these cells carries crippling mutations, it is possible that Hodgkin and Reed-Sternberg cells originate from a preapoptotic germinal center B-cell with unfavorable mutations that has escaped negative selection. Rare cases of classical Hodgkin lymphoma with a clonal T-cell receptor gene rearrangement have been observed.[59] In contrast, single-cell analyses of nodular lymphocyte-predominance Hodgkin lymphoma demonstrated clonal immunoglobulin gene rearrangements with ongoing mutations, an intraclonal diversity consistent with a germinal center origin of lymphocyte and histiocytic cells.[60–62]

Reprogramming of Hodgkin and Reed-Sternberg Cells

Hodgkin and Reed-Sternberg cells show a global loss of their B-cell phenotype, retaining only B-cell features associated with their interaction with T cells and their antigen-presenting function.[63] Furthermore, Hodgkin and Reed-Sternberg cells express markers of other lineages, including T cells, dendritic cells, cytotoxic cells, and myeloid cells.[64]

The lack of expression of numerous B-cell genes is the result of loss of transcription factor expression (OCT2, BOB1, PU.1) and epigenetic silencing.[65–67] The main B-cell lineage commitment factor, PAX5, is typically expressed, but its target genes are downregulated.[68,69] Reduced expression of target genes likely reflects the fact that B-cell genes are regulated by coordinated action of multiple transcription factors.

The heterogeneity of expression of myeloid, T-cell, dendritic cell, and other genes by Hodgkin and Reed-Sternberg cells is the result of many factors. Early B-cell factor 1 levels are low, de-repressing the expression of T-cell and myeloid genes and lowering transcription of B-cell–specific genes.[64] Notch 1, which plays a key role in promoting T-cell differentiation and inhibiting B-cell development, is expressed in Hodgkin and Reed-Sternberg cells.[70] Notch 1 also contributes to the expression of GATA2, a transcription factor required for proliferation and survival of hematopoietic stem cells.[71] The hematopoietic stem cell regulator polycomb G proteins are also expressed by Hodgkin and Reed-Sternberg cells and are thought to contribute to the expression of markers of different hematopoietic lineages.[72] The signal transducer and activation of transcription factors (STAT) 5A and 5B are implicated in Hodgkin and Reed-Sternberg reprogramming as they upregulate CD30 and downregulate B-cell–receptor expression.[73] Together, these factors cause a global loss of the B-cell phenotype and aberrant expression of genes of other cell lineages.

Genetic Alterations and Signaling Pathways

Because Hodgkin and Reed-Sternberg cells lack expression of functional B-cell surface receptors, rescue from apoptosis is probably an important mechanism of survival.[54,74] The most prevalent genetic lesions in Hodgkin and Reed-Sternberg cells involve two signaling pathways: Janus kinase (JAK)-STAT and nuclear factor-κB (NF-κB). Hodgkin and Reed-Sternberg cells have frequent gains in JAK2 and inactivation of the negative regulator of JAK-STAT signaling, suppressor of cytokine signaling 1, resulting in enhanced cytokine signaling.[75,76] Genetic alterations in NF-κB include gains and amplifications of the NF-κB transcription factor REL in about half of cases of Hodgkin lymphoma.[77] Somatic mutations of the gene encoding the inhibitor of NF-κB (IκBα) occur in approximately 20 percent of cases.[78,79] Inactivating mutations and deletions of the gene encoding A20, a negative regulator of NF-κB, have been found in approximately 40 percent of cases, nearly all of which were EBV-negative.[80]

Autocrine and paracrine signaling events also contribute to constitutive activation of the JAK-STAT pathway and NF-κB transcription.[73] STAT factors are activated by autocrine means through expression of interleukins 13 and 21 and their receptors by Hodgkin and Reed-Sternberg cells and augmented by NF-κB activity.[81–83] Receptor tyrosine kinases expressed in these cells may also contribute to STAT activation. The tumor necrosis factor receptor family, which includes CD30, CD40, transmembrane activator and calcium modulator and cyclophilin ligand interactor (TACI), B-cell maturation antigen (BCMA), and receptor activator of nuclear factor-κB (RANK), is involved in NF-κB signaling through interactions with the Hodgkin lymphoma microenvironment or in an autocrine fashion.[84,85]

Multiple-receptor tyrosine kinases are aberrantly expressed in Hodgkin and Reed-Sternberg, including platelet-derived growth factor receptor-α. In addition, deregulated and constitutive activation of the phosphoinositide 3-kinase (PI3K)-AKT and extracellular signal-regulated kinase (ERK) pathways are implicated in Hodgkin and Reed-Sternberg cells. The activator protein 1 (AP1) transcription factors also appear to play a role, inducing target genes such as galectin 1 and CD30 in Hodgkin and Reed-Sternberg cells.

Several factors point to the pathogenetic role of EBV in approximately 40 percent of classical Hodgkin lymphoma. The viral proteins latent membrane protein 1 (LMP1) and latent membrane protein 2 (LMP2), in particular, appear to have hijacked signaling pathways to promote the survival of EBV-infected Hodgkin and Reed-Sternberg cells. LMP1 induces constitutive NF-κB signaling by mimicking the CD40 receptor and can activate JAK-STAT, PI3K, and AP1 signaling. LMP2 functions as a surrogate for the B-cell receptor. The role of EBV in the pathogenesis of Hodgkin lymphoma also is supported by the findings that (1) there is an inverse relationship between expression of multiple receptor tyrosine kinases and EBV expression, (2) there is an ability of EBV to rescue crippled germinal center B cells in the laboratory, (3) mutations preventing any B-cell receptor expression are in EBV-positive Hodgkin and Reed-Sternberg cells, and (4) there is a inverse relationship between mutations reducing the expression of the NF-κB regulator A20 and EBV-positive Hodgkin and Reed-Sternberg cells.

Overall, genetic alterations involving the JAK-STAT and NF-κB signaling pathways and further activation via autocrine or paracrine mechanisms interact to support the growth and survival of Hodgkin lymphoma cells. In the EBV-positive subset of patients, viral genes can provide the pathogenetic function of genetic lesions found in EBV-negative cases.

■ ROLE OF THE MICROENVIRONMENT

The survival of Hodgkin and Reed-Sternberg cells appear to be dependent on their microenvironment, which represents 95 to 99 percent of the cellular composition of the tumor. Hodgkin and Reed-Sternberg cells attract T cells, B cells, neutrophils, plasma cells, eosinophils and mast cells by secretion of chemokines (see Fig. 99–2). For instance, CCL5, CCL17, and CCL22 attract T-helper 2 and T-regulatory cells. Other chemokines attract eosinophils and mast cells and interleukin-8 attracts neutrophils. These chemokines may also have direct effects on Hodgkin and Reed-Sternberg cells. T cells represent the largest and probably most important population. CD4+ T cells trigger CD40 signaling and CD4+ T-regulatory cells have potent immunosuppressive activity against infiltrating cytotoxic T cells. Other interactions include activation of TACI and BCMA through their ligand production by neutrophils and activation of CD30 through CD30 ligand-expressing mast cells and eosinophils. Connective tissue cells and their products can be involved in complex interactions, such as the stimulation of fibroblasts via factors expressed by Hodgkin and Reed-Sternberg cells and the consequent secretion by these fibroblasts of eotaxin and CCL5, which attract eosinophils and T-regulatory cells to the Hodgkin lymphoma microenvironment.

The differentiation of CD4+ T cells to T-regulatory cells and the immunosuppressive features of the Hodgkin lymphoma microenvironment have received much attention. A hallmark of these changes is the shift from an antitumor, cytotoxic T-helper 1 response to a protumor, humoral T-helper 2 response. Hodgkin and Reed-Sternberg cells produce a number of immunosuppressive factors such as interleukin-10, transforming growth factor-β, galectin 1, and prostaglandin E_2. Hodgkin and Reed-Sternberg cells express programmed cell death protein 1 (PD1) ligand that binds and inhibits T-cell cytotoxic function.

CLINICAL FEATURES

■ PRESENTING MANIFESTATIONS

History and Physical Examination

Constitutional symptoms, some of which confer a less-favorable prognosis, accompany the diagnosis of Hodgkin lymphoma in approximately 30 percent of cases. Fever in excess of 38°C, drenching night

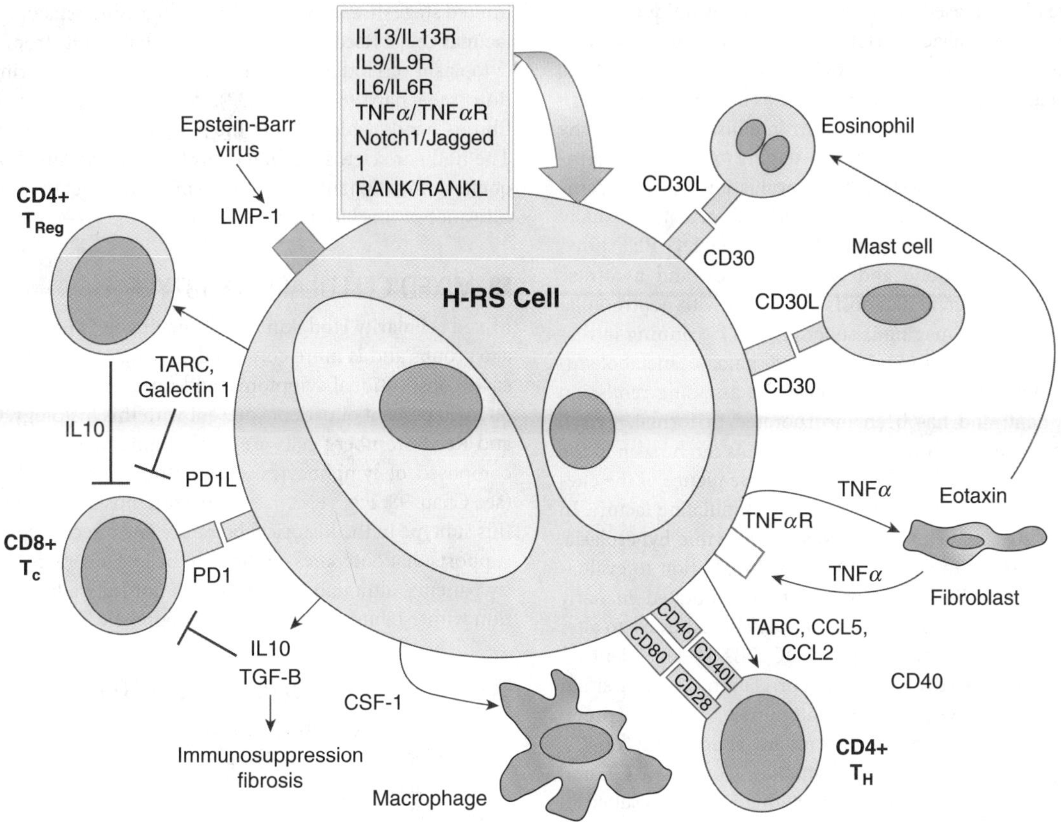

FIGURE 99–2. The Reed-Sternberg cell and its environment. In a network of highly complex interactions, Reed-Sternberg cells elaborate chemokines that attract a variety of cells, which cascade their influence on the microenvironment. R-S cells express ligands that play a role in autocrine and paracrine interactions and also produce a number of immunosuppressive factors (e.g., galectin 1) that directly contribute to a pro-tumor, humoral T helper 2 environment (see section on Role of the Micronenvironment for further details).

sweats, and weight loss exceeding 10 percent of baseline body weight during the 6 months preceding diagnosis are designated as symptomatic "B" disease. Fevers are usually of low grade and irregular. Rarely, a cyclic pattern of high fevers for 1 to 2 weeks alternating with afebrile periods of similar duration is present at diagnosis. This latter classic Pel-Ebstein fever is virtually diagnostic of the disease.[86,87] Generalized pruritus, often accompanied by marked excoriation, may be present at diagnosis; it is not prognostically significant. Pain in involved lymph nodes immediately after the ingestion of alcohol is a curious complaint that is nearly specific to Hodgkin lymphoma. It occurs in fewer than 10 percent of patients and has no prognostic significance.[88] The etiology of these symptoms has been the subject of speculation, but remains largely unexplained. Patients with extensive intrathoracic disease may present with cough, chest pain, dyspnea, and, rarely, hemoptysis. Infrequently, patients present with bone pain, including the constellation of back pain accompanied by signs and symptoms of spinal cord compression.

Detection of an unusual mass or swelling in the superficial, supradiaphragmatic lymph nodes (60–70% cervical and supraclavicular, 15–20% axillary) is the most common presentation of Hodgkin lymphoma. Only 15 to 20 percent of patients have subdiaphragmatic disease at presentation.[89] Lymphadenopathy is usually nontender and has a "rubbery" consistency. By inspection, a diffuse, puffy swelling rather than a discrete mass may be apparent in the supraclavicular, infraclavicular, or anterior chest wall regions. Infrequently, compression of the superior vena cava will result in facial swelling and engorgement of the veins in the neck and upper chest. Auscultation of the chest may reveal a pleural effusion. Rarely, a significant pericardial effusion is present at diagnosis. Palpation is an insensitive method for the detection of intraabdominal adenopathy or organ enlargement but this type of examination should be focused on the size of the liver and spleen and masses in the upper retroperitoneal area.

Paraneoplastic Findings

A number of rare paraneoplastic syndromes have been described in Hodgkin lymphoma at the time of diagnosis. These include vanishing bile duct syndrome and idiopathic cholangitis with clinical jaundice, the nephrotic syndrome with anasarca, autoimmune hematologic disorders (e.g., immune thrombocytopenia or hemolytic anemia), and neurologic signs and symptoms.[90–92] Although parenchymal involvement of the central nervous system or meningeal involvement is rare in Hodgkin lymphoma, paraneoplastic syndromes include subacute cerebellar degeneration, myelopathy progressive multifocal encephalopathy, and limbic encephalitis.[90,93]

RADIOGRAPHIC FEATURES

Intrathoracic disease is present at diagnosis in two-thirds of patients. Mediastinal adenopathy is common in Hodgkin lymphoma, particularly in young women with the nodular sclerosis subtype.[94] Although computed tomography (CT) of the chest is standard, a chest radiograph has been used traditionally to describe mediastinal mass size.[95] Hilar adenopathy, pulmonary parenchymal involvement, pleural effusions, pericardial effusions, and chest wall masses may be appreciated by chest CT; these are more common in the presence of extensive mediastinal disease. CT of the abdomen and pelvis is routinely employed in the diagnostic evaluation of Hodgkin lymphoma. Although technologic advances have greatly increased the resolution of this technique and the subsequent detection of celiac, portal, splenic hilar, and mesenteric lymph nodes, the correlation with histologic involvement of the spleen, determined by laparotomy staging in the past, has been disappointing.

Whole-body ^{18}F-fluorodeoxyglucose positron emission tomography (FDG-PET) has become standard in the staging of Hodgkin lymphoma.[96] FDG-PET correlates well with CT evaluation and may demonstrate additional areas of disease, although this information usually results in few changes in stage or initial therapy.[97,98] FDG-PET, however, is more sensitive to bone and hepatic disease and a diffuse increase in signal can be seen at diagnosis in patients with neutrophilia at presentation. FDG-PET imaging is superior to CT scanning in distinguishing active residual disease (increased glucose metabolism) from inactive residual tissue, a major problem in assessing remission status after treatment, and has been incorporated in formal revised response guidelines.[99] False-positive FDG-PET scans can be seen in the marrow during or at the end of treatment as a consequence of the chemotherapy effect or use of hematopoietic colony-stimulating factors. In followup, false-positive studies may be caused by thymic hyperplasia, granulomatous disease, or infectious disorders. In addition to evaluation of residual masses, FDG-PET has been incorporated in early response monitoring for risk stratification and, in clinical trials, to alter therapy.[100–102] The predictive accuracy of FDG-PET is dependent on expertise of the imaging staff and clinical correlation. In most situations, but particularly in FDG-PET, avid anatomic sites that were previously uninvolved or those without concomitant abnormality on CT scan, usually require tissue biopsy confirmation. Combined CT and FDG-PET technology is now standard for staging and has resulted in improved anatomic definition of sites with increased signal.

CLINICAL AND PATHOLOGIC CORRELATION

NODULAR LYMPHOCYTE PREDOMINANCE SUBTYPE

There is a strong correlation between age at onset, the anatomic extent of disease and histologic subtype of Hodgkin lymphoma. Approximately 5 to 10 percent of patients present with nodular lymphocyte-predominant, which is considered to be a unique subtype. Progressive transformation of germinal centers may precede or follow nodular lymphocyte-predominance Hodgkin lymphoma in other sites.[103,104] The cellular composition is predominantly benign B lymphocytes with or without histiocytes. The characteristic multilobated, CD20+ lymphocyte and histiocytic cells are relatively abundant (see Chap. 98, Fig. 98–40). Patients most commonly present with stage I disease (70%) in peripheral lymph node sites, particularly in the axillae, and there is a 4:1 male predominance.[105] The nodular lymphocyte-predominance Hodgkin lymphoma subtype is associated with large cell non-Hodgkin lymphoma as a composite tumor or a large cell lymphoma may occur at a later date.[106,107] The large cell variant T-cell–rich B-cell lymphoma may be difficult to distinguish from nodular lymphocyte-predominance Hodgkin lymphoma and may occur concurrently or subsequently (see Chap. 100).[108]

NODULAR SCLEROSIS SUBTYPE

Classical Hodgkin lymphoma, defined by its phenotype of CD30+, CD15+, and CD20– Hodgkin and Reed-Sternberg cells, has four subtypes of which the nodular sclerosis subtype constitutes 40 to 70 percent. Nodular sclerosis subtype is noted for its distinctive histologic features and frequent involvement of the lower cervical, supraclavicular, and mediastinal lymph nodes in adolescents and young adults, particularly females. Approximately 70 percent of patients present with limited stage disease. One of the distinguishing histologic features is the lacunar cell, a Reed-Sternberg variant that results from retraction of the cytoplasm of Hodgkin and Reed-Sternberg cells during formalin fixation (see Chap. 98, Fig. 98–38). Another is the thickened capsule and fibrous bands which divide the lymphoid tissue into cellular nodules. The nodular sclerosis subtype has been subclassified based on the frequency of malignant cells and normal lymphocytes but the clinical significance of this has been disputed.

MIXED CELLULARITY SUBTYPE

Mixed cellularity Hodgkin lymphoma involves both pediatric and older age groups and is more commonly associated with advanced stage disease, constitutional symptoms, and immunodeficiency. Approximately 30 to 50 percent of patients present with this histology. Classic Hodgkin and Reed-Sternberg cells are easily found amid a cellular background composed of lymphocytes, eosinophils, plasma cells, and histiocytes (see Chap. 98, Fig. 98–39). A worse prognosis has been characteristic of this subtype in the historical literature and a recent epidemiologic study supports that outcomes continue to be less favorable for mixed cellularity patients, although this result was not fully adjusted for the association with established unfavorable prognostic factors.[109]

LYMPHOCYTE DEPLETION SUBTYPE

There are two rare subtypes of classical Hodgkin lymphoma. Lymphocyte-depletion Hodgkin lymphoma has two morphologic subtypes: reticular and diffuse fibrosis. The reticular variant contains abundant pleomorphic neoplastic cells whereas the diffuse fibrosis variant has a prominent fibroblastic proliferation with few normal lymphocytes. Hodgkin and Reed-Sternberg cells are sparse. Lymphocyte-depletion presents in the older age group with symptomatic, extensive disease. Peripheral and mediastinal adenopathy is much less common than in other cases of Hodgkin lymphoma.[110] Presentation with fever of unknown origin, jaundice, hepatosplenomegaly, or pancytopenia is not uncommon. This subtype is also associated with the acquired immunodeficiency syndrome.

LYMPHOCYTE-RICH SUBTYPE

The lymphocyte-rich subtype was introduced by the World Health Organization classification in 1999 (see Table 99–1) following an expert pathology review of cases of nodular lymphocyte-predominant.[111] The two subtypes differ subtly on morphologic grounds, but the major difference is that the Hodgkin and Reed-Sternberg cells in lymphocyte-rich have the classic CD30+ CD20– immunophenotype. The presenting features are very similar although patients with the lymphocyte-rich subtype tend to be older compared with nodular lymphocyte-predominant Hodgkin lymphoma patients.[111] A higher rate of multiple relapses and a more favorable prognosis upon relapse is characteristic of nodular lymphocyte-predominant Hodgkin lymphoma.

ANATOMIC DISTRIBUTION OF DISEASE

In approximately 70 percent of patients, Hodgkin lymphoma presents in the cervical nodes; in 12 percent, in the axillary nodes; and in 9 percent, in the inguinal nodes.[112] A small minority of patients presents with exclusive subdiaphragmatic disease. In an historical series of 285 consecutive, unselected, and untreated patients evaluated at Stanford University, involvement of abdominal lymph nodes and spleen was documented in 272 of these patients upon laparotomy, a surgical diagnostic procedure in which the intraabdominal and pelvic lymph nodes are biopsied, the spleen is removed and examined pathologically in thin slices, the liver is biopsied by needle and wedge technique, and the marrow is biopsied. The frequency of splenic involvement at laparotomy in untreated patients averaged 37 percent in 17 published series.[112] Involvement of the spleen was strongly dependent on histologic subtype: it was involved in 60 percent of mixed cellularity and lymphocyte-depleted cases compared with 34 percent of nodular lymphocyte-predominant and nodular sclerosis cases. Hepatic and marrow disease were invariably associated with splenic involvement.

Two different theories, the "contiguity" theory of Kaplan and Rosenberg[113] and the "susceptibility" theory of Smithers,[114] have been proposed for the mode of spread of Hodgkin lymphoma. In support of the former, most cases of Hodgkin lymphoma appear to spread via lymphatic channels to contiguous lymphatic structures in a predictable, nonrandom pattern. Controversy has surrounded the mode of spread to the spleen, which lacks afferent lymphatics. When four or more lymph node regions were involved, the possibility of spread by hematogenous distribution appeared more likely.[115] Disseminated disease is more common in mixed cellularity and lymphocyte-depleted cases, consistent with the presence of reported vascular invasion.[116] Whereas vascular invasion is controversial, it is more common in the spleen than in lymph nodes and connotes a poor prognosis.[117,118]

STAGING

Hodgkin lymphoma is classified using the four-stage Ann Arbor classification as indicated in Table 99–2.[15] Clinical stage refers to the results of physical, imaging, and laboratory examination, while pathologic stage refers to the use of additional biopsy procedures. The classification is further characterized by the presence or absence of constitutional symptoms. Extranodal disease, representing extracapsular extension of lymph node disease that could be incorporated in a standard radiotherapy field, is distinguished from disseminated, stage IV disease. The correlation of this staging classification system with prognosis was extensively verified when radiotherapy served as the principle treatment for all but stage IV disease. Additional prognostic information such as mediastinal bulk, other bulky nodal masses, and the extent of subdiaphragmatic nodal disease was included in a modification of the Ann Arbor system, known as the Cotswold classification in 1989.[119]

Prognostic factors and recommended staging procedures for untreated patients have evolved with changes in therapy. Exploratory laparotomy and splenectomy, which historically advanced about one-third of clinical stages I and II patients to pathologic stages III and IV, but reducing fewer than one-fourth of clinical stage III patients to pathologic stage I or II, is no longer performed.[120] Computed tomography of the chest, abdomen, and pelvis and FDG-PET provide sensitive delineation of involved sites with the exception of the spleen and marrow, and the use of chemotherapy in all stages of disease has reduced the critical nature of detecting subclinical disease.

Marrow involvement occurs in approximately 12 percent of new patients and is more common in patients of older age, advanced stage, less-favorable histology, or those with constitutional symptoms or immunodeficiency. Because the marrow is almost never involved in young, asymptomatic patients with favorable clinical stage I or II presentations, marrow biopsy may be omitted in their staging procedure.

TABLE 99–2. Ann Arbor Staging System for Hodgkin Lymphoma

Stage	
I.	Involvement of a single lymph node region (I) or a single extralymphatic organ or site (I_E)
II.	Involvement of two or more lymph node regions on the same side of the diaphragm alone (II) or with involvement of limited, contiguous extralymphatic organ or tissue (II_E)
III.	Involvement of lymph node regions on both sides of the diaphragm (III), which may include the spleen (III_S) or limited, contiguous extralymphatic organ or site (III_E) or both (III_{ES})
IV.	Multiple or disseminated foci of involvement of one or more extralymphatic organs or tissues, with or without associated lymph node involvement
Modifying Features	
A.	Asymptomatic
B.	Drenching night sweats; fever >38°C; loss of more than 10% body weight in 6 months
X.	Bulky disease: mass >10 cm; >0.33 mediastinal mass ratio
E.	Involvement of a single, contiguous or proximal extranodal site

Mediastinal mass ratio is the ratio of the maximal width of a mediastinal mass relative to the maximal width of the mediastinum, as measured by CT imaging.

LABORATORY FEATURES

There are no diagnostic laboratory features of Hodgkin lymphoma. A complete blood count may reveal one or another of granulocytosis,[121] eosinophilia,[122] lymphocytopenia,[123] thrombocytosis,[124] or anemia.[125] The anemia is usually the result of chronic disease, but rarely may be caused by hemolysis secondary to high fever[126] or associated with a positive direct antiglobulin (Coombs) test.[127] Thrombocytopenia may occur as a result of marrow involvement, hypersplenism or an immune mechanism.[128–130] Immune neutropenia can occur in Hodgkin lymphoma.[131] Cytopenias are particularly common in advanced-stage disease and the lymphocyte-depleted subtype. Elevation of the erythrocyte sedimentation rate is most common in advanced disease and correlates with constitutional symptoms.[132,133] The degree of sedimentation rate elevation correlates with prognosis, particularly in limited-stage disease.[134] Although nonspecific, it may be useful to follow it, as it may herald recurrent disease. Serum lactate dehydrogenase levels are elevated in 35 percent of patients at diagnosis.[135,136] The alkaline phosphatase may be elevated in Hodgkin lymphoma, nonspecifically in limited disease, or in association with involvement of liver, bone, or marrow in advanced disease.[137] Hypercalcemia is unusual in Hodgkin lymphoma and appears to be secondary to synthesis of increased levels of 1,25-dihydroxyvitamin D by Hodgkin lymphoma cells.[138] A variety of other abnormalities have been reported, including hypoglycemia[139,140] resulting from an autoantibody to insulin receptors and hyponatremia resulting from inappropriate secretion of antidiuretic hormone.[141]

Anemia, granulocytosis, lymphopenia and low serum albumin constitute four of seven adverse prognostic factors identified in advanced Hodgkin lymphoma by an international consortium.[142] Similar to the non-Hodgkin lymphomas, serum β_2-microglobulin levels correlate with tumor burden and prognosis in Hodgkin lymphoma.[143] Serum levels of cytokines including soluble CD30, interleukin (IL)-6, IL-10, and the IL-2 receptor, have been reported to correlate with constitutional symptoms and advanced disease.[144–147] Examination of pleural fluid in Hodgkin lymphoma may reveal transudative, exudative or chylous properties. Because cytology rarely yields diagnostic Hodgkin and Reed-Sternberg cells, the etiology is most often considered to be one of central lymphatic obstruction. Laboratory abnormalities, including abnormal liver function tests associated with marked enlargement of porta hepatis nodes and biliary obstruction or intrahepatic cholestasis, may be prominent in rare presentations of Hodgkin lymphoma.[148] The nephrotic syndrome is a rare presentation of Hodgkin lymphoma.[149]

DIFFERENTIAL DIAGNOSIS

Clinically enlarged lymph nodes may be associated with a variety of infectious, inflammatory, autoimmune, and neoplastic disorders. Biopsy of unexplained, persistent, or recurrent adenopathy should be reviewed by an experienced hematopathologist. The most likely diagnosis is either Hodgkin lymphoma or a non-Hodgkin lymphoma. Distinction from primary mediastinal B-cell lymphoma may be difficult based on both clinical and histologic features; evidence indicates that this disorder is genetically akin to classic Hodgkin lymphoma, and this "gray zone" lymphoma has a provisional category in the new World Health Organization classification.[10,150,151] Mixed cellularity Hodgkin lymphoma may demonstrate varied cellular and stromal composition and should be distinguished from peripheral T-cell lymphoma and T-cell–rich, B-cell lymphoma can be difficult to distinguish from nodular lymphocyte-predominant Hodgkin lymphoma.[108] Immune markers of Hodgkin and Reed-Sternberg cells, such as CD30, CD20, and CD15, are invaluable for differential diagnosis (see Chap. 98, Figs. 98–36 and 98–41). Nonneoplastic conditions that simulate Hodgkin lymphoma include viral infections, particularly infectious mononucleosis. Depleted nodes of any histology may resemble the diffuse fibrosis variant of lymphocyte-depleted, including the depleted phase of lymph nodes from HIV-infected patients. The diagnosis in an extranodal site depends upon the organ involved and whether there is a known diagnosis of Hodgkin lymphoma. Diagnostic Hodgkin and Reed-Sternberg cells are not required in liver and marrow because the foci of involvement are so small. Of course, the rare presentations of Hodgkin lymphoma, such as those in the central nervous system, liver, or as a fever of unknown origin may lead to an extensive differential diagnosis.

THERAPY

HISTORICAL PERSPECTIVE

Hodgkin lymphoma first became a curable neoplasm through the systematic study of the spread of the disease and the use of higher dose, extended field radiotherapy delivery with supervoltage techniques.[152] When used alone, radiotherapy doses to involved fields usually ranged from 3500 to 4400 cGy with prophylactic doses of 3000 to 3500 cGy to uninvolved tissues. The mantle, paraaortic region, and pelvis constitute the classic radiotherapy regions. With increased recognition of late effects, radiation therapy has been modified to reduce field size to areas of known or bulky disease and dose has also been lowered in combination with chemotherapy. Furthermore, initial disease reduction with chemotherapy results in less radiation exposure to the neck, female breast, heart, and lungs, all of which should result in fewer late complications. Advances in radiotherapy technique deliver more precise dose distribution, sparing normal tissues. The first modern combination chemotherapy program was The MOPP regimen devised by DeVita and colleagues.[22] The national mortality figures for Hodgkin lymphoma decreased by more than 60 percent in the decade that followed the introduction of MOPP chemotherapy.[153] Bonadonna and colleagues developed an important alternative regimen for the treatment of Hodgkin lymphoma. ABVD, which was effective in the treatment of patients who had failed MOPP[154,155] and offered a more favorable toxicity profile as discussed below. ABVD subsequently became the preferred primary chemotherapy regimen, alone or in combination with radiotherapy.[156,157] Of the multiple alternative chemotherapy regimens introduced for the treatment of advanced Hodgkin lymphoma, only the bleomycin, etoposide, doxorubicin, cyclophosphamide, vincristine, prednisone, procarbazine (BEACOPP) combination developed by Diehl and colleagues has demonstrated superior cure rates in multiple phase III studies.[158] Table 99–3 describes the drugs, doses, and schedules of combination chemotherapy programs effective in the management of Hodgkin lymphoma.

FAVORABLE, LIMITED-STAGE DISEASE

In North America, favorable, limited-stage disease is typically defined as asymptomatic stage I or II supradiaphragmatic disease with no bulky sites. A more restrictive definition is used in Europe based on the number of Ann Arbor sites, erythrocyte sedimentation rate, age and extranodal sites, as well as bulky disease (Table 99–4).[158] Approximately 35 percent of stages I and II patients meet this more limited definition of favorable disease. For many years, extended-field (subtotal lymphoid) radiotherapy, usually administered after staging laparotomy, was the treatment of choice for early stage, favorable Hodgkin lymphoma. A change in that standard was compelled by the observation that the overall mortality rate from other causes, particularly second cancers, exceeded deaths resulting from Hodgkin lymphoma at 15 to 20 years.[159] Early studies from Stanford University demonstrated that involved-field radiotherapy plus chemotherapy produced results equivalent or superior to wide-field radiotherapy.[160,161] Subsequently, several randomized trials demonstrated the superiority of involved-field radiotherapy plus anthracycline-containing chemotherapy compared to extended-field radiotherapy in early stage favorable Hodgkin lymphoma.[162–165]

The next series of clinical trials were designed to test the optimal number of cycles of chemotherapy and the volume and dose of radiotherapy when both modalities are used in limited Hodgkin lymphoma. The Milan Tumor Institute described greater than 95 percent disease control with four cycles of ABVD and radiotherapy, with no advantage seen for extended- versus involved-field radiotherapy.[166] Similarly, no advantage to more extensive radiation in combination with chemotherapy was observed in a German Hodgkin Study Group (GHSG) study.[167] A comparison of two versus four cycles of ABVD chemotherapy paired with 20 Gy or 30 Gy radiotherapy was made in a four-arm trial conducted by the GHSG. The final results of this trial have not been published, but multiple published interim analyses show freedom from progression rates in excess of 95 percent for all four treatment arms.[168] In a subsequent trial, the GHSG evaluated four cycles of ABVD, AV, ABV, or AVD plus 30 Gy involved-field radiotherapy. Final results of this study are awaited, but the AV and ABV arms were closed early because of poorer results. With the goal of avoiding radiotherapy and its late effects, current studies are assessing interim FDG-PET scanning as a means of identifying patients (PET-negative) for whom radiotherapy can be omitted. In addition to these efforts, there is considerable interest in the use of chemotherapy alone in limited-stage Hodgkin lymphoma.

Only a limited number of studies evaluated chemotherapy alone in favorable, early stage Hodgkin lymphoma. A North American study in selected limited-stage patients tested a radiotherapy-containing strategy, based on risk factors, against ABVD alone.[169] At 5 years, the progression-free survival significantly favored the radiotherapy-containing approach but the absolute difference, 87 versus 93 percent, was modest and no survival differences have been observed to date. A single institution study of ABVD versus ABVD plus radiotherapy demonstrated no significant progression-free survival difference between the treatment

TABLE 99–3. Combination Chemotherapy for Hodgkin Lymphoma

Drug	Dose mg/m^2	Route	Schedule (days administered)	Cycle Length (days)
COPP				28
cyclophosphamide	650	IV	1,8	
vincristine	1.4*	IV	1,8	
procarbazine	100	PO	1–14	
prednisone	40	PO	1–14	
ABVD				28
doxorubicin	25	IV	1,15	
bleomycin	10	IV	1,15	
vinblastine	6	IV	1,15	
dacarbazine	375	IV	1,15	
COPP/ABVD				28
Alternate cycles of COPP with ABVD				
BEACOPP (Standard)				21
bleomycin	10	IV	8	
etoposide	100	IV	1–3	
doxorubicin	25	IV	1	
cyclophosphamide	650	IV	1	
vincristine	1.4*	IV	8	
procarbazine	100	PO	1–7	
prednisone	40	PO	1–14	
BEACOPP (Escalated)				21
bleomycin	10	IV	8	
etoposide	200	IV	1–3	
doxorubicin	35	IV	1	
cyclophosphamide	1250	IV	1	
vincristine	1.4*	IV	8	
procarbazine	100	PO	1–7	
prednisone	40	PO	1–14	
(G-CSF)	(+)	SQ	8+	
BEACOPP (14-day)				14
Standard BEACOPP given every 14 days with growth factor support.				
STANFORD V				12 weeks
nitrogen mustard	6	IV	day 1 on wk 1,5,9	
doxorubicin	25	IV	day 1 on wk 1,3,5,7,9,11	
vinblastine	6	IV	day 1 on wk 1,3,5,7,9,11	
vincristine	1.4*	IV	day 1 on wk 2,4,6,8,10,12	
bleomycin	5	IV	day 1 on wk 2,4,6,8,10,12	
etoposide	60 × 2	IV	day 1 & 2 on wk 3,7,11	
prednisone	40	PO	day 1 on wk 1–10, taper	
G-CSF for dose reduction, delay				

*capped at 2 mg.

arms, but this trial accrued relatively small numbers of patients.[170] In a European trial, the epirubicin, bleomycin, vinblastine, prednisone (EBVP) regimen was tested against the same chemotherapy plus 20- or 30-Gy involved-field radiotherapy.[171] Inferiority of the EBVP combination resulted in the trial's early closure. Other studies comparing chemotherapy alone with combined modality treatment have included limited- and advanced-stage patients and both adults and children.[172,173] Together these studies show a modest (≤12%) progression-free survival benefit for combined modality treatment compared with ABVD-containing chemotherapy. The high cure rate with current limited chemotherapy and low-dose radiotherapy strategies creates a high standard to be achieved using a longer course of chemotherapy alone. Long-term followup of these clinical trials to include overall survival and the profile of late effects are needed to determine the optimal therapeutic strategy for favorable, early stage Hodgkin lymphoma.

Several subsets of limited-stage patients deserve further mention. Classical clinical stage I Hodgkin lymphoma patients presenting with inguinofemoral disease may be treated with brief chemotherapy and involved-field radiotherapy. More extensive subdiaphragmatic presentations of Hodgkin lymphoma are best managed with a full course of chemotherapy alone or combined modality therapy. Historically, about half of patients with masses greater than one-third of the chest diameter relapsed after radiotherapy alone,[95,174] and their management is described in the following section. Similarly, stages I to IIB patients are generally managed with chemotherapy or combined modality treatment. Nodular lymphocyte-predominant Hodgkin lymphoma presents as asymptomatic, limited-stage disease in most (~80%) patients.[111] Peripheral lymph nodes in the neck, axilla, or groin are commonly involved as stage IA disease. The European Task Force on lymphoma reported a 96 percent complete response rate and 99 percent and 94 percent 8-year disease-specific survival for stages I and II disease, respectively.[111] Because of the low likelihood of occult disease in nodular lymphocyte-predominant Hodgkin lymphoma and the tendency for the disease to remain localized for years, regional radiation therapy is considered the treatment of choice. Analyses from the GHSG demonstrate that outcomes with limited radiation therapy are comparable to the use of more extensive radiation and combined modality regimens.[175]

LOCALLY EXTENSIVE LIMITED-STAGE HODGKIN LYMPHOMA

Extensive mediastinal Hodgkin lymphoma, defined as a mass greater than one-third the maximum intrathoracic diameter on a standing posteroanterior chest radiograph of greater than 10 cm by CT, is frequently accompanied by extranodal

TABLE 99–4. Prognostic Factors for Hodgkin Lymphoma

Limited Stage		Advanced Stage
EORTC	GHSG	International Collaborative Study
Adverse Prognostic Factors		Adverse Prognostic Factors
MMR ≥0.35	MMR ≥0.35	Age ≥45 years
ESR >30 if symptomatic	ESR >30 if asymptomatic	Stage IV
ESR >50 if asymptomatic	ESR >50 if asymptomatic	Male sex
>3 Ann Arbor sites	>2 Ann Arbor sites	White blood count $>15 \times 10^9$/l
Age ≥50	Extranodal disease	Lymphocyte count $<0.6 \times 10^9$/L or <8%
	Massive splenic disease	Albumin <4 g/dl
		Hemoglobin <10.5 g/dl
Presence of any factor is considered unfavorable. Two-thirds of limited stage patients have one or more adverse factors.		Factors summed to yield the international prognostic score. 75% of patients have a score of 1–3.

EORTC, European Organization for the Research and Treatment of Cancer; GHSG, German Hodgkin Study Group; MMR, mediastinal mass ratio, which is the ratio of the maximal width of a mediastinal mass relative to the maximal width of the mediastinum, as measured by CT imaging; ESR, erythrocyte sedimentation rate.

extension to lung, pericardium, and chest wall. Pleural effusions may also be seen. The use of combined chemotherapy and radiation (combined modality therapy) results in freedom from relapse in approximately 80 percent of such patients. Application of radiotherapy after chemotherapy also reduces radiotherapy exposure to normal heart and lung tissue. The optimal chemotherapy regimen and its duration, the radiation dose and volume for combined treatment have been the subjects of investigation. In the Milan study of 232 patients treated with subtotal lymphoid irradiation sandwiched between six courses of chemotherapy, the ABVD–radiation therapy combination was significantly superior to the MOPP–radiation therapy combination as measured by both freedom from progression and survival.[176,177] Subsequently, the Milan group reported the efficacy of four cycles of ABVD and involved-field radiotherapy in stages I to II patients, many of whom had massive mediastinal disease.[166] The 12-week Stanford V program, which includes modified mantle radiotherapy, provided greater than 90 percent durable remissions in patients with massive mediastinal disease.[178] The GHSG reported no difference in progression-free survival between ABVD–radiation therapy with standard BEACOPP–radiation therapy in the HD11 study of intermediate Hodgkin lymphoma patients, a proportion of whom had extensive mediastinal disease.[179] No differences between four or six cycles of ABVD and six cycles of BEACOPP, each followed by 30-Gy involved-field radiotherapy, were reported in the H9U study conducted by the European Organization for the Research and Treatment of Cancer (EORTC)/Groupe d'Etude des Lymphomes de l'Adulte (GELA).[171] The GHSG HD14 study has reported an advantage in progression-free survival for two cycles of escalated BEACOPP and two cycles of ABVD plus radiation therapy compared to four cycles of ABVD–radiation therapy, in a specified interim analysis; no survival benefit was seen.[180] At 3 years, 90 percent of ABVD–radiation therapy patients were disease-free compared to 96 percent treated with the BEACOPP–ABVD–radiation therapy regimen. No survival differences were observed. Other investigators are exploring the role of interim PET to dictate the use of radiation therapy after chemotherapy, even in bulky mediastinal disease. With such high rates of therapeutic success, it will be increasingly important to weigh risks and benefits with more intensive treatment.

ADVANCED DISEASE

ABVD became the standard therapy for advanced Hodgkin lymphoma by proving to be superior to the MOPP chemotherapy and equal to, but less toxic than, hybrid or alternating combinations with MOPP.[156,157,181–183] Specifically, the incidence of secondary myelodysplasia, leukemia and sterility was less with ABVD. The GHSG developed the BEACOPP regimen (see Table 99–3) based upon mathematical modeling that indicated a moderate increase in chemotherapy dose intensity would result in a significant increase in the cure rate. In the original HD9 study, BEACOPP was given in "standard" and "escalated" versions, the latter facilitated by granulocyte colony-stimulating factor use, and was compared with the cyclophosphamide, vincristine (Oncovin), procarbazine, prednisone (COPP)–ABVD regimen.[158] Patients with initial tumors equal to or greater than 5 cm or residual radiographic disease received 36-Gy radiotherapy after chemotherapy. The 5- and 10-year results demonstrated a significant progression-free and overall survival advantage for escalated BEACOPP compared to COPP–ABVD.[158,184] The results, cure rates in excess of 80 percent for escalated BEACOPP, are the best ever recorded for a large phase III trial in advanced Hodgkin lymphoma. The superiority of escalated BEACOPP was observed regardless of the clinical international prognostic score.[185] Despite these outcomes, BEACOPP has not been universally accepted as the new standard in advanced Hodgkin lymphoma because of concerns about the acute toxicity, which includes greater need for hospitalization and transfusion, and late toxicity, which includes male and female sterility and an increased risk of secondary leukemia.[158,186] In addition, approximately two-thirds of patients received radiotherapy in the HD9 study. Two randomized clinical trials from Italy subsequently confirmed the superiority of BEACOPP over ABVD for the endpoint of progression-free survival (Table 99–5).[187,188] In the first trial, the four escalated plus two standard cycles regimen of BEACOPP was compared to ABVD and another multidrug regimen; all patients were to receive consolidation radiotherapy for bulky or residual disease. BEACOPP yielded significantly superior progression-free survival compared to ABVD although no difference in overall survival was observed.[187] In the second study, patients were randomized to ABVD versus four cycles of standard and four cycles of escalated BEACOPP with preplanned retreatment and high-dose therapy and autologous transplantation for treatment failures.[188] This study also showed a significantly higher progression-free survival for the BEACOPP arm but no difference in overall survival. In each of the three cited trials, the hazard ratio with BEACOPP was approximately 0.5. Standards of care in advanced Hodgkin lymphoma continue to be debated given the lack of a survival benefit with the BEACOPP program, which benefits approximately 15 percent of patients while exposing 100 percent of patients to more toxicity. In addition, results of an international study comparing the hybrid four escalated and four standard BEACOPP regimen with ABVD in patients with a high international prognostic score as defined below are pending.[182]

Efforts to reduce the risk of treatment-related morbidity of escalated BEACOPP have included studying the combination of four cycles of escalated and four cycles of standard BEACOPP and eliminating the

TABLE 99–5. Selected Randomized Clinical Therapeutic Trials in Hodgkin's Lymphoma

Study (Number of patients)	Treatment	Failure-Free Survival (%)	Overall Survival (%)	Follow-up (years)
Limited stage, favorable and unfavorable				
Milan (140)	4 ABVD + IFRT	94	96	12
	4 ABVD + STLI	93	94	
		p = NS	p = NS	
NCIC-ECOG (399)	RT-containing	93	96	5
	4-6 ABVD	87	94	
		p = 0.006	p = NS	
Limited stage, favorable				
EORTC/GELA H9F(783)	6 EBVP + 20-IFRT	88	98	4
	6 EBVP + 30-IFRT	85	100	
	6 EBVP	69	98	
		p ≤0.001	p = 0.241	
GHSG HD10 (1370)	2 ABVD + 30-IFRT	No difference to date*		4
	2 ABVD + 20-IFRT			
	4 ABVD + 30-IFRT			
	4 ABVD + 30-IFRT			
Limited stage, unfavorable				
EORTC/GELA H9U (808)	6 ABVD + 30-IFRT	91	95	4
	4 ABVD + 30-IFRT	87	94	
	4 BEACOPP + 30-IFRT	90	93	
		p = NS	p = NS	
GHSG HD11 (1422)	4 ABVD + 30-IFRT	No difference to date*		2.5
	4 ABVD + 20-IFRT			
	4 BEACOPP + 30-IFRT			
	4 BEACOPP+ 20-IFRT			
Advanced stage				
GHSG HD9 (1201)	8 COPP/ABVD + RT	69	83	5
	8 BEACOPP + RT	76	88	
	8 $BEACOPP_{esc}$ + RT	87	91	
		p <0.002	p <0.002	

ABVD,doxorubicin, bleomycin, vinblastine, dacarbazine; BEACOPP, bleomycin, etoposide, doxorubicin, cyclophosphamide, vincristine, procarbazine, prednisone; COPP, cyclophosphamide, vincristine, procarbazine, prednisone; EBVP, epirubicin, bleomycin, vinblastine, prednisone; ECOG, Eastern Cooperative Oncology Group; EORTC, European Organization for the Research and Treatment of Cancer; GELA, Groupe d'Etude des Lymphomes de l'Adulte; GHSG, German Hodgkin Study Group; IFRT, involved field radiotherapy; NCIC, National Cancer Institute of Canada; RT, radiotherapy; STLI, subtotal lymphoid irradiation.

*Interim analysis; **Interim analysis

radiation therapy. In the subsequent GHSG HD12 no significant differences in progression-free survival were observed for patients treated with or without consolidative radiotherapy, and the four standard plus four escalated regimen performed as well as eight cycles of escalated BEACOPP.[189] Numerous investigations are underway to determine if interim PET scans can direct more-intensive treatment with escalated BEACOPP to the subgroup that benefits.[102] Likewise, interim and end-of-treatment PET scans are being used to direct the use of consolidative radiotherapy.[190,191] Although there is great enthusiasm regarding this approach to direct subsequent treatment, it is notable that the majority of patients remaining PET-positive after four cycles of escalated BEACOPP appear to be cured by the planned therapy, in contrast to findings with ABVD.[190]

The Stanford group took an alternate approach to bulky and advanced Hodgkin lymphoma by abbreviating the duration of therapy and reducing cumulative drug doses.[178] Whereas this approach was highly successful in institutional and phase II cooperative group trials, results elsewhere have been mixed to date.[178,192,193] Inferior progression-free survival was observed in an Italian phase III trial comparing Stanford V to ABVD or a multidrug regimen.[194] However, the overall survivals were not different. Radiotherapy was administered per physician preference rather than the original protocol prescription, and, in some cases, responses were judged as early as 8 weeks.[194] The United Kingdom trials group compared Stanford V–radiation therapy with ABVD–radiation therapy and found the progression-free survival outcomes at 5 years to be similar—74 and 76 percent in the two arms.[195] Overall survivals were also similar: 92 percent for Stanford V versus 90 percent for ABVD. More pulmonary toxicity was observed with ABVD. The Intergroup study in North America also compared ABVD to the Stanford V chemotherapy and radiotherapy program in locally extensive and advanced Hodgkin lymphoma, but the results of this phase III trial are not yet available.

The use of radiotherapy as a consolidation to combination chemotherapy in advanced Hodgkin lymphoma is controversial. Encouraging data from single institutions in adults and children were not borne out in randomized trials, some of which were criticized as underpowered. Furthermore, chemotherapy regimens have evolved over the time span of these studies. The application of 30-Gy involved-field radiotherapy to patients in complete remission after MOPP–ABV was studied in an adequately powered phase III trial.[196] No significant difference in failure-free survival was observed. Of note, all patients in partial remission received 40 Gy on this study and their outcome was not different from complete remission patients. The GHSG HD12 study randomized patients to observation or consolidation radiotherapy, with the incorporation of a central review panel, following BEACOPP with no difference in outcome in final analysis.[189] Both recent Italian studies comparing ABVD with BEACOPP routinely incorporated consolidation radiation therapy for residual or bulky disease.[187,188] The HD15 study limited the use of radiotherapy to patients with positive PET scans after four cycles of chemotherapy. With this approach, only 12 percent of patients received radiotherapy and the cure rates among PET-negative patients, who did not receive radiotherapy, was 96 percent after 1 year.[191] In sum, the data do not support the routine use of radiotherapy following a full course of chemotherapy in advanced Hodgkin lymphoma. However, the role of this potent treatment in patients with an early incomplete response or following a brief course of chemotherapy is likely to be more significant.[178,190]

RECURRENT DISEASE

Historically, patients who relapsed after a full course of chemotherapy had a low chance for cure with second-line treatment, with the duration of initial remission a significant predictor of subsequent response and relapse-free survival. High-dose therapy and autologous blood stem cell transplantation improved the outlook for such patients and is routinely employed in first relapse for most patients younger than age 65 years, based on institutional and phase III trial experience.[197,198] Cure rates with transplantation range from 40 to 60 percent with transplant-related mortality less than 5%.[199–201] High-dose regimens include BEAM (carmustine, etoposide, cytarabine, melphalan), CBV (cyclophosphamide, carmustine, etoposide), and augmented CBV regimens. Total-body irradiation is rarely employed but consolidation radiotherapy may play a role in some cases. The superiority of any single regimen has not been definitively established; however, the use of high-dose sequential therapy coupled with tandem autologous transplantation is being tested in randomized trials.[202,203] In most cases, second-line chemotherapy with ICE (ifosfamide, carboplatin, etoposide), DHAP (dexamethasone, cytarabine, cisplatin), or IGEV (ifosfamide, gemcitabine, vinorelbine) is used to achieve a minimal disease state prior to stem cell mobilization and transplantation.[204] Prognostic factors for the success of transplantation, including the response to secondary treatment, have been described by several groups.

As treatment has evolved to limited chemotherapy and low-dose radiotherapy or chemotherapy alone in early stage Hodgkin lymphoma, the management of the small number of patients with recurrence has done likewise. The GHSG reported on the outcome of 42 of 1129 patients with recurrence after two cycles of ABVD and involved-field radiotherapy. With varied management, the 3-year freedom-from-treatment failure rate was 52 percent.[205] Among 23 patients with relapse after ABVD alone and 10 patients after combined ABVD and radiotherapy who participated in the National Cancer Institute of Canada (NCIC)/Eastern Cooperative Oncology Group (ECOG) trial in early stage Hodgkin lymphoma, freedom-from-second-progression rates exceeded 90 percent in both groups, with patients receiving a variety of treatments, including radiation therapy, chemotherapy, combined modality, and high-dose therapy with transplantation.[206]

Treatment failures following autologous transplantation present a challenge, with longevity directly related to the time to relapse after transplant. Allogeneic transplantation in multiply recurrent Hodgkin lymphoma has been limited by significant transplant-related mortality, although long-term disease control has been observed in a small subset together with anecdotal evidence of a graft-versus-Hodgkin antitumor effect. Nonmyeloablative transplantation conditioning regimens reduce transplant-related mortality but disease recurrence continues to present a major challenge, with failure-free survivals in the 20 to 30 percent range.[207,208]

The anti-CD20 antibody rituximab achieves high response rates in nodular lymphocyte-predominant Hodgkin lymphoma and can be used as retreatment or as an extended-treatment regimen.[209,210] Monoclonal antibodies directed against the CD30 antigen are well tolerated in classical Hodgkin lymphoma but have limited therapeutic value.[211] However, the antibody-drug conjugate SGN-35, which combines the anti-CD30 antibody linked to the tubulin inhibitor monomethylauristatin E, has resulted in significant responses in heavily treated patients in two phase I clinical trials.[212,213] Important trials of SGN-35 are in progress.

COURSE AND PROGNOSIS

The goal of treatment is to cure the greatest number of patients with minimal complications. Improvements in management have resulted in high cure rates in a majority of those patients who are younger than age 65 years. Survival expectations at 10 years for patients diagnosed from 2006 to 2010 exceed 90 percent for patients to age 44 years, 80 percent for patients to age 54 years, and 70 percent for patients to age 64 years.[214] These outstanding results have been achieved by refining the use of radiotherapy and chemotherapy and improved outcomes for secondary treatments. However, the late effects of treatment for Hodgkin lymphoma remain a concern for cured patients, and a small subset of patients has refractory disease.

CLINICAL PROGNOSTIC FACTORS

A number of complex prognostic factor schemes have been developed for limited Hodgkin lymphoma treated with radiotherapy alone (see Table 99–4). Massive mediastinal disease and constitutional symptoms were consistently identified as independent predictors of relapse, whereas only older age was predictive of inferior survival. European and Canadian investigators incorporated gender, age, erythrocyte sedimentation rate (ESR), number of Ann Arbor disease sites, stage, and histology into stratifications for favorable, very favorable, and unfavorable disease categories. The EORTC defines four or more nodal sites, ESR greater than 50 in asymptomatic patients or ESR greater than 40 in symptomatic patients, and histology as indicators of intermediate disease, whereas the GHSG designates any one of the following: massive mediastinal disease, extranodal disease, ESR greater than 50 if asymptomatic and greater than 30 if symptomatic, and three or more nodal sites as intermediate disease (see Table 99–4). It is important to be aware of the variable eligibility criteria when interpreting the literature in early stage Hodgkin lymphoma and to note that these clinical variables are currently used to group patients for clinical investigations. The international prognostic score, based on seven factors (see Table 99–4), is used in advanced disease.[185] Each factor reduced the freedom from progression by approximately 7 percent. Only 7 percent of patients were in the worst prognostic group (five to seven factors) and the freedom from progression in this subset was 42 percent at 5 years. Consensus with regard to prognostic factors promotes uniformity in clinical trial design and provides a rationale for alternate approaches in high-risk subsets. The superiority of escalated BEACOPP was seen across the spectrum of the international prognostic score, but approximately 30 percent of high-risk (four to seven factors) patients experience treatment failure.[184] Alternately, the improvement in progression-free survival with BEACOPP over ABVD in an Italian study was limited to higher-risk patients.[187] Age has been a consistent adverse prognostic marker regardless of tumor burden, but recent gains eliminate this adverse factor up to approximately age 55 years.[215,216] Although less-intensive treatment may explain inferior results in a subset of patients, results in older patients are worse, even when the intensity of therapy is controlled.[215] The BEACOPP regimen was associated with unacceptable toxicity and demonstrated no advance over ABVD for patients older than age 65 years.[217]

FDG-PET imaging at the completion of treatment provides a high degree of negative predictive value, ranging from 81 to 100 percent.[218] The positive predictive value at the end of chemotherapy is more variable and is related to disease extent and use of radiotherapy.[191,219,220] There is great interest in FDG-PET scans after one to three cycles of chemotherapy, as several studies indicate that negative results predict treatment success whereas positive results predict a high likelihood of treatment failure.[100,101,221] Numerous ongoing phase III clinical trials are designed to alter treatment based on early PET results with a goal of achieving high cure rates and minimizing toxicity. PET status prior to autologous transplantation has emerged as a dominant prognostic factor also.[222–224]

Patients with primary progressive Hodgkin lymphoma have the least-favorable prognosis. Fortunately, newer treatment approaches have reduced the proportion of patients in this category. Among patients referred for transplantation, sensitivity to standard-dose second-line chemotherapy predicts for better survival: responding patients had an event-free survival of 60 percent versus 19 percent for those without a response.[224] In addition to PET status and clinical response to secondary treatment, prognostic factors for the success of transplantation include time to relapse, disease extent at relapse, constitutional symptoms at relapse, and anemia.[199,200,225]

Clinical prognostic factors are surrogates for the underlying cellular and molecular biology of Hodgkin lymphoma. Serum levels of cytokines, including soluble CD30, a probable marker of tumor burden, and IL-10, a measure of immunosuppression related to the microenvironment, are associated with adverse prognosis independent of clinical features.[226] The chemokine CCL17, secreted by Hodgkin and Reed-Sternberg cells, is elevated in patients' sera and is being studied as a marker of response.[227,228] Multiple, but not all, investigators found BCL-2 expression to be of prognostic significant.[229–232] CD20 expression by Hodgkin and Reed-Sternberg cells has been associated with less-favorable outcomes, but this has not been confirmed in other series.[233,234] Lack of HLA class II expression, which may allow immune escape of Hodgkin and Reed-Sternberg cells, was found to be an independent prognostic factor.[235] The prognostic significance of the EBV association varies with age, conferring an adverse outcome in older individuals.[236,237] Furthermore, single nucleotide polymorphisms in HLA-A2 have been associated with risk of EBV-positive Hodgkin lymphoma.[53] A number of studies have focused on the inflammatory microenvironment of Hodgkin lymphoma. Increased numbers of T-regulatory cells have correlated with favorable outcomes and decreased numbers of markers for cytotoxic T cells have correlated with adverse outcomes in several series.[238–240] Together, these findings suggest an important interplay between characteristics of Hodgkin and Reed-Sternberg cells and the inflammatory environment.

COMPLICATIONS OF TREATMENT

The treatment of Hodgkin lymphoma is associated with important acute and chronic side effects. Although the acute complications of chemotherapy and radiotherapy may be troublesome, they are relatively easily managed. Late-treatment effects in the form of sterility, second malignancy, and cardiopulmonary disease are more serious and are known to contribute to shortened longevity for cured patients.[241,242] Excess mortality from second malignancy and cardiac disease increase with time and are currently the leading causes of death for Hodgkin lymphoma patients. As treatment has evolved, the risks of radiation-related complications has lessened but long latency periods and uncertainty regarding associations with lower doses make it difficult to predict individual risks. Recognition and understanding of these problems helps to shape primary treatment choice and facilitate optimal followup for survivors.

Acute leukemia and myelodysplasia were the initial second malignancies to be observed after successful treatment for Hodgkin lymphoma with MOPP chemotherapy.[243] The risk following MOPP was proportional to the cumulative dose of alkylating agents and was associated with recurring abnormalities of chromosomes 5 and 7.[244,245] Actuarial risks of approximately 5 percent with relative risks in excess of 100 have been reported over a 7- to 10-year period with alkylating agent-based therapies. The risk of secondary leukemia is greater in patients older than age 35 years. Prognosis for secondary leukemia is poor with survivals of less than 1 year.[247] The risk of acute leukemia is significantly less after ABVD chemotherapy,[157] although it is not absent. A large international study observed a significant reduction in excess absolute risk after 1984, presumably as a consequence of change in primary therapy.[247] However, acute leukemia may complicate Hodgkin lymphoma treatment with higher doses of etoposide and doxorubicin, such as in the BEACOPP regimen.[186,248] This form of leukemia tends to occur earlier and be associated with balanced translocations of chromosome 11. Patients who have received second-line therapies and autologous transplantation are at highest risk for myelodysplasia and secondary leukemia.

There is an increased relative risk of non-Hodgkin lymphomas after treatment for Hodgkin lymphoma.[249,250] These are diffuse, aggressive B-cell lymphomas that may occur early or late after treatment. There is no clear relationship to the type of primary treatment. The incidence of secondary lymphoma in a series of 5406 patients treated on GHSG protocols was 0.9 percent; prognosis was worse if lymphoma developed within 3 months of primary therapy.[251] Although prognosis was relatively poor in this series, the data antedated the routine use of rituximab in treatment regimens. It is not clear how non-Hodgkin lymphomas relate to treatment-related immunodeficiency, predisposition to B-cell malignancy, or a shared common cell of origin. Marginal zone lymphomas with identical B-cell receptor genes also have been identified.[252] Diffuse large B-cell lymphoma and its variants are most frequent in nodular lymphocyte-predominant Hodgkin lymphoma, where they have been found to be genetically related.[253]

An increased risk of solid cancers after treatment for Hodgkin lymphoma has long been recognized, and with time, these have emerged to account for 75 to 80 percent of all cases of second malignancy.[250,254,255] The risk is related to radiotherapy exposure, with tumors occurring in or at the edges of the radiation field. The most common solid tumors are breast, lung, and gastrointestinal malignancies. The latency for developing second cancers is an important consideration, as these typically develop after at least 10 years and continue to pose excess risk for as long as 30 years after treatment. Breast cancer is increased in women treated before age 30 years and is markedly increased in children and adolescents.[256–258] Case-control studies have examined the relationship of radiation dose to the breast and the risk of cancer, finding a 3.2-fold increased risk with doses greater than 4 Gy and an eightfold risk for doses greater than 40 Gy.[259,260] Elimination of routine axillary radiation, which is now standard, results in a 2.7-fold reduction in risk and it is anticipated that risks may further decline with current low-dose or nodal radiotherapy.[261] Cofactors are important for defining the risks of second breast cancer, which are highest for women younger than age 30 years when irradiated and for those who continue to have normal menses.[260,261]

Lung cancer risk is greatest among patients who are older than 45 years of age when treated. Tobacco exposure has a multiplying effect and alkylating agent exposure also contributes to risk. Among patients with chest irradiation, a tobacco history, and alkylating chemotherapy, the lung cancer risk was 49-fold higher than in patients who had none of these exposures.[262] Alkylating agent chemotherapy independently increases risk of lung cancer with dose–response associations reported in population-based studies.[262–264]

Estimates of relative risks of cardiac mortality in Hodgkin lymphoma survivors range from 2.2- to sevenfold.[241,242,265,266] Mediastinal radiotherapy is associated with an increased risk of cardiac disease. An increased risk of death from coronary artery disease and acute myocardial infarction has been identified in adults and children.[257,267,268] Other types of cardiac disease are often asymptomatic including valvular disease, conduction defects, and cardiomyopathy.[269,270] The risks of radiation-related heart disease do not appear to be influenced significantly by the addition of chemotherapy. The onset of increased risk is within 5 to 10 years. As risk is associated with the dose and volume of radiotherapy and the latency is 5 to 10 or more years, the hazards associated with current lower dose and smaller fields remain to be assessed.[265] Established cardiac risk factors, including hypertension, hypercholesterolemia, and smoking, significantly contribute to the subsequent risk of cardiac disease after therapy, offering opportunities to reduce individual risks.[271] Risks of cardiac disease after chemotherapy alone have not been extensively studied but a British report indicated an elevated risk of cardiac mortality of 7.8 following ABVD alone, which rose to 12.1 when given with mediastinal irradiation.[272] These results provide a cautionary note, but more data are needed and these results do not address cumulative exposures that are lower with modern therapy.

Noncoronary vascular complications have been reported after neck irradiation, with associations to dose greater than 36 Gy and cofactors of hypertension, diabetes and hypercholesterolemia.[273,274] In a retrospective cohort study, the standardized incidence ratio for was 2.2 for stroke and 3.1 for transient ischemic attack.[274] However, it is important to note that modern approaches to Hodgkin lymphoma therapy use lower radiation doses, smaller fields, and planning techniques that limit dose inhomogeneity and hot spots commonly seen in the neck area with older techniques.

Approximately 90 percent of males are permanently sterilized by six cycles of MOPP chemotherapy.[275] The risk is related to the cumulative dose of alkylating agents such that two to three cycles of MOPP result in azoospermia in approximately 50 percent of patients.[276] Female fertility after alkylating agent-based treatment is related to age at treatment as well as cumulative alkylating agent dose.[277,278] The ABVD combination is associated with temporary amenorrhea and azoospermia with full recovery noted in 50 to 90 percent of patients.[279,280] A case-control study found no significant reduction in fertility among women treated with ABVD.[281] In contrast, no men had normospermia following treatment with BEACOPP and amenorrhea occurred in more than 50 percent of women.[282,283] Several authors have described pregnancy outcome following treatment for Hodgkin lymphoma. No increase in birth defects or complications of pregnancy has been seen.[278]

Thyroid dysfunction is common after neck irradiation, reaching a risk of 47 percent at 26 years in the Stanford series.[284] Thus, patients at risk should be monitored in during followup observation. Rarely, hyperthyroidism, Graves ophthalmopathy or thyroid neoplasms occur after neck radiotherapy.[284] Lhermitte sign, a transient complaint of an "electric shock" sensation produced by head flexion, is a common sequela of mantle radiotherapy.[285] The incidence of radiation pneumonitis depends on the volume of lung irradiated and the total dose. Symptoms include cough, dyspnea, and fever. Although prospective assessment of pulmonary function demonstrates reduction of lung volumes following mantle radiotherapy, recovery is seen in 12 to 24 months and symptomatic radiation pneumonitis is unusual.[286,287]

Full-dose radiation therapy interferes with normal growth and development in children. Current therapy programs use low-dose or no radiotherapy for all stages of disease. Overwhelming sepsis is a rare event in patients who have been splenectomized and treated for Hodgkin lymphoma, particularly children.[288,289] Vaccination against encapsulated organisms 10 to 14 days prior to the onset of treatment is advised. However, it must be recognized that neither vaccines nor antibiotic prophylaxis may provide adequate protection. Fatigue is commonly reported in Hodgkin lymphoma survivors and has been related to pulmonary function and peak oxygen uptake.[269,290]

With the high rates of cure currently attained in the management of Hodgkin lymphoma, reduction in late effects and quality of life assume even greater importance. Patient education is essential to promote healthy behaviors to reduce modifiable risk factors. In addition, early detection and prevention strategies for second cancers and cardiac disease should be considered in high-risk patients. However, the choice and efficacy of diagnostic testing, and their optimal timing and frequency, require further study.[291] Most of the documented late effects relate to outdated chemotherapy and radiotherapy, and that modeling, as well as recent data, indicate that lesser exposures significantly reduce second cancer risk.[261,292] Modern therapies will likely further reduce the risks of late complications. It continues to be important to follow long-term survivors, and the contribution of genetic and environmental factors is an important ongoing area of inquiry.

REFERENCES

1. Hodgkin T: On some morbid appearances of the absorbent glands and spleen. *Med Chir Trans* 17:68, 1832.
2. Wilks S: Cases of lardaceous disease and some allied affections, with remarks. *Guys Hosp Rep* 17:103, 1856.
3. Dreschfield J: Clinical lecture on acute Hodgkin's (or pseudoleucocythemia). *BMJ* 1:893, 1892.
4. Kundrat H: Uber Lympho-sarkomatosis. *Wien Wochenschr* 6:211, 1893.
5. Sternberg C: Uber eine eigenartige unter dem Bilde der Pseudoleukamie verlaufende Tuberculose des lymphatischen Appartes. *Z Heilk* 19:21, 1898.
6. Reed D: On the pathological changes in Hodgkin's disease, with especial reference to its relation to tuberculosis. *Johns Hopkins Hosp Rep* 10:133, 1902.
7. Fox H: Remarks on the presentation of microscopical preparations made from some of the original tissue described by Thomas Hodgkin. *Ann Med Hist* 8:370, 1926.
8. Jackson H, Parker F: *Hodgkin's Disease and Allied Disorders*. Oxford University Press, New York, 1947.
9. Lukes RJ, Butler JJ, Hicks EB: Natural history of Hodgkin's disease as related to its pathologic picture. *Cancer* 19:317, 1966.
10. Stein H: Hodgkin lymphoma, in *WHO Classification of Tumours of Haematopoietic and Lymphoid Tissues*, 4th ed. International Agency for Research on Cancer, Eds SH Swerdlow, E Campo, NL Harris, ES Jaffe, SA Pileri, H Stein, J Thiele, JW Vardiman, p 321, Lyon, France, 2008.
11. Peters M: A study of survivals in Hodgkin's disease treated radiologically. *Am J Roentgenol* 63:299, 1950.
12. Kinmouth J: Lymphangiography in man: Method of outlining lymphatic trunks and operation. *Clin Sci* 11:13, 1952.
13. Glatstein E, Guernsey JM, Rosenberg SA, et al: The value of laparotomy and splenectomy in the staging of Hodgkin's disease. *Cancer* 24:709, 1969.
14. Rosenberg S: Report of the committee on the staging of Hodgkin's disease. *Cancer Res* 26:1310, 1966.
15. Carbone P, Kaplan H, Musshoff K: Report of the committee on the Hodgkin's disease staging. *Cancer Res* 31:1860, 1971.
16. Pusey W: Cases of sarcoma and of Hodgkin's disease treated by exposures to x-rays: A preliminary report. *JAMA* 38:166, 1902.
17. Senn N: Therapeutical value of Roentgen ray in treatment of pseudoleukemia. *NY Med J* 77:665, 1903.
18. Gilbert R: Radiotherapy in Hodgkin's disease (malignant granulomatosis): Anatomic and clinical foundations, governing principles, results. *Am J Roentgenol* 41:198, 1939.
19. Kaplan H: The radical radiotherapy of regionally localized Hodgkin's disease. *Radiology* 78:553, 1962.
20. Goodman L, Wingtrobe M, Dameshek W: Nitrogen mustard therapy: Use of methyl bis(b-chloroethyl)amine hydrochloride and tris-(b-chloroethyl)amine hydrochloride for Hodgkin's disease, lymphosarcoma, leukemia, and certain allied and miscellaneous disorders. *JAMA* 132:126, 1946.
21. Jacobson L, Spurr C, Baron EG: Nitrogen mustard therapy: Use of methyl bis(b-chloroethyl)amine hydrochloride on neoplastic disorders of the hematopietic system. *JAMA* 132:263, 1946.
22. DeVita V, Serpick A, Carbone P: Combination chemotherapy in the treatment of advanced Hodgkin's disease. *Ann Intern Med* 73:881, 1970.
23. Bonadonna G, Zucali R, Monfardini S, et al: Combination chemotherapy of Hodgkin's disease with Adriamycin, bleomycin, vinblastine, and imidazole carboxamide versus MOPP. *Cancer* 36:252, 1975.
24. Surveillance, Epidemiology and End Results (SEER) Program (www.seer.cancer.gov) SEER*Stat Database. National Cancer Institute, DCCPS, Surveillance Research Program, Cancer Statistics Branch, based on the November 2005 SEER data submission.
25. MacMahon B: Epidemiology of Hodgkin's disease. *Cancer Res* 26:1189, 1966.
26. Clarke C, Glaser S, Keegan T, et al: Neighborhood socioeconomic status and Hodgkin's lymphoma incidence in California. *Cancer Epidemiol Biomarkers Prev* 14:1441, 2005.
27. Surveillance, Epidemiology, and End Results Program, National Cancer Institute, 2009. http://seer.cancer.gov/csr/1975_2006/browse_csr.php?section=9&page=sect_09_table.01.html.

28. Landgren O, Engels EA, Pfeiffer RM, et al: Autoimmunity and susceptibility to Hodgkin lymphoma: A population-based case-control study in Scandinavia. *J Natl Cancer Inst* 98:1321, 2006.
29. Grufferman S, Delzell E: Epidemiology of Hodgkin's disease. *Epidemiol Rev* 6:76, 1984.
30. Au WY, Gascoyne RD, Gallagher RE, et al: Hodgkin's lymphoma in Chinese migrants to British Columbia: A 25-year survey. *Ann Oncol* 15:626, 2004.
31. Katanoda K, Yako-Suketomo H: Comparison of time trends in Hodgkin and non-Hodgkin lymphoma incidence (1973–97) in East Asia, Europe and USA, from cancer incidence in five continents Vol. IV-VIII. *Jpn J Clin Oncol* 38:391, 2008.
32. Vianna NJ, Greenwald P, Davies JN: Extended epidemic of Hodgkin's disease in high-school students. *Lancet* 1:1209, 1971.
33. Rosdahl N, Larsen SO, Clemmesen J: Hodgkin's disease in patients with previous infectious mononucleosis: 30 years' experience. *Br Med J* 2:253, 1974.
34. Kvale G, Hoiby EA, Pedersen E: Hodgkin's disease in patients with previous infectious mononucleosis. *Int J Cancer* 23:593, 1979.
35. Mueller N, Evans A, Harris N: Altered antibody titers to Epstein-Barr virus before the diagnosis of Hodgkin's disease. *N Engl J Med* 320:689, 1989.
36. Hjalgrim H, Askling J, Rostgaard K, et al: Characteristics of Hodgkin's lymphoma after infectious mononucleosis. *N Engl J Med* 349:1324, 2003.
37. Alexander FE, Lawrence DJ, Freeland J, et al: An epidemiologic study of index and family infectious mononucleosis and adult Hodgkin's disease (HD): Evidence for a specific association with EBV+ve HD in young adults. *Int J Cancer* 107:298, 2003.
38. Glaser SL, Lin RJ, Stewart SL, et al: Epstein-Barr virus-associated Hodgkin's disease: Epidemiologic characteristics in international data. *Int J Cancer* 70:375, 1997.
39. Armstrong AA, Alexander FE, Cartwright R, et al: Epstein-Barr virus and Hodgkin's disease: Further evidence for the three disease hypothesis. *Leukemia* 12:1272, 1998.
40. Ambinder RF, Browning PJ, Lorenzana I, et al: Epstein-Barr virus and childhood Hodgkin's disease in Honduras and the United States. *Blood* 81:462, 1993.
41. Herndier BG, Sanchez HC, Chang KL, et al: High prevalence of Epstein-Barr virus in the Reed-Sternberg cells of HIV-associated Hodgkin's disease. *Am J Pathol* 142:1073, 1993.
42. Powles T, Robinson D, Stebbing J, et al: Highly active antiretroviral therapy and the incidence of non-AIDS-defining cancers in people with HIV infection. *J Clin Oncol* 27:884, 2009.
43. Biggar RJ, Jaffe ES, Goedert JJ, et al: Hodgkin lymphoma and immunodeficiency in persons with HIV/AIDS. *Blood* 108:3786, 2006.
44. Mack TM, Cozen W, Shibata DK, et al: Concordance for Hodgkin's disease in identical twins suggesting genetic susceptibility to the young-adult form of the disease. *N Engl J Med* 332:413, 1995.
45. Ferraris AM, Racchi O, Rapezzi D, et al: Familial Hodgkin's disease: A disease of young adulthood? *Ann Hematol* 74:131, 1997.
46. Chang ET, Smedby KE, Hjalgrim H, et al: Family history of hematopoietic malignancy and risk of lymphoma. *J Natl Cancer Inst* 97:1466, 2005.
47. Goldin LR, Pfeiffer RM, Gridley G, et al: Familial aggregation of Hodgkin lymphoma and related tumors. *Cancer* 100:1902, 2004.
48. Hemminki K, Li X, Czene K: Familial risk of cancer: Data for clinical counseling and cancer genetics. *Int J Cancer* 108:109, 2004.
49. Grufferman S, Cole P, Smith PG, et al: Hodgkin's disease in siblings. *N Engl J Med* 296:248, 1977.
50. Altieri A, Hemminki K: The familial risk of Hodgkin's lymphoma ranks among the highest in the Swedish Family-Cancer Database. *Leukemia* 20:2062, 2006.
51. Horwitz MS, Mealiffe ME: Further evidence for a pseudoautosomal gene for Hodgkin's lymphoma: Reply to "The familial risk of Hodgkin's lymphoma ranks among the highest in the Swedish Family-Cancer Database" by Altieri A and Hemminki K. *Leukemia* 21:351, 2007.
52. Cimino G, Lo CF, Cartoni C, et al: Immune-deficiency in Hodgkin's disease (HD): A study of patients and healthy relatives in families with multiple cases. *Eur J Cancer Clin Oncol* 24:1595, 1988.
53. Niens M, Jarrett RF, Hepkema B, et al: HLA-A*02 is associated with a reduced risk and HLA-A*01 with an increased risk of developing EBV+ Hodgkin lymphoma. *Blood* 110:3310, 2007.
54. Küppers R, Rajewsky K, Zhao M, et al: Hodgkin disease: Hodgkin and Reed-Sternberg cells picked from histological sections show clonal immunoglobulin gene rearrangements and appear to be derived from B cells at various stages of development. *Proc Natl Acad Sci U S A* 91:10962, 1994.
55. Küppers R, Roers A, Kanzler H: Molecular single cell studies of normal and transformed lymphocytes. *Cancer Surv* 30:45, 1997.
56. Kanzler H, Kuppers R, Hansmann ML, et al: Hodgkin and Reed-Sternberg cells in Hodgkin's disease represent the outgrowth of a dominant tumor clone derived from (crippled) germinal center B cells. *J Exp Med* 184:1495, 1996.
57. Bargou RC, Emmerich F, Krappmann D, et al: Constitutive nuclear factor-kappaB-RelA activation is required for proliferation and survival of Hodgkin's disease tumor cells. *J Clin Invest* 100:2961, 1997.
58. Jox A, Zander T, Kuppers R, et al: Somatic mutations within the untranslated regions of rearranged Ig genes in a case of classical Hodgkin's disease as a potential cause for the absence of Ig in the lymphoma cells. *Blood* 93:3964, 1999.
59. Muschen M, Rajewsky K, Brauninger A, et al: Rare occurrence of classical Hodgkin's disease as a T cell lymphoma. *J Exp Med* 191:387, 2000.
60. Braeuninger A, Küppers R, Strickler JG, et al: Hodgkin and Reed-Sternberg cells in lymphocyte predominant Hodgkin disease represent clonal populations of germinal center-derived tumor B cells 94(25):14211. *Proc Natl Acad Sci U S A* 94:9337, 1997.
61. Ohno T, Stribley JA, Wu G, et al: Clonality in nodular lymphocyte-predominant Hodgkin's disease. *N Engl J Med* 337:459, 1997.
62. Marafioti T, Hummel M, Anagnostopoulos I, et al: Origin of nodular lymphocyte-predominant Hodgkin's disease from a clonal expansion of highly mutated germinal-center B cells. *N Engl J Med* 337:453, 1997.
63. Schwering I, Brauninger A, Klein U, et al: Loss of the B-lineage-specific gene expression program in Hodgkin and Reed-Sternberg cells of Hodgkin lymphoma. *Blood* 101:1505, 2003.
64. Mathas S, Janz M, Hummel F, et al: Intrinsic inhibition of transcription factor E2A by HLH proteins ABF-1 and Id2 mediates reprogramming of neoplastic B cells in Hodgkin lymphoma. *Nat Immunol* 7:207, 2006.
65. Ushmorov A, Leithauser F, Sakk O, et al: Epigenetic processes play a major role in B-cell-specific gene silencing in classical Hodgkin lymphoma. *Blood* 107:2493, 2006.
66. Stein H, Marafioti T, Foss HD, et al: Down-regulation of BOB.1/OBF.1 and Oct2 in classical Hodgkin disease but not in lymphocyte predominant Hodgkin disease correlates with immunoglobulin transcription. *Blood* 97:496, 2001.
67. Re D, Muschen M, Ahmadi T, et al: Oct-2 and Bob-1 deficiency in Hodgkin and Reed Sternberg cells. *Cancer Res* 61:2080, 2001.
68. Cobaleda C, Schebesta A, Delogu A, et al: Pax5: The guardian of B cell identity and function. *Nat Immunol* 8:463, 2007.
69. Foss HD, Reusch R, Demel G, et al: Frequent expression of the B-cell-specific activator protein in Reed-Sternberg cells of classical Hodgkin's disease provides further evidence for its B-cell origin. *Blood* 94:3108, 1999.
70. Jundt F, Acikgoz O, Kwon SH, et al: Aberrant expression of Notch1 interferes with the B-lymphoid phenotype of neoplastic B cells in classical Hodgkin lymphoma. *Leukemia* 22:1587, 2008.
71. Kumano K, Chiba S, Shimizu K, et al: Notch1 inhibits differentiation of hematopoietic cells by sustaining GATA-2 expression. *Blood* 98:3283, 2001.
72. Dukers DF, van Galen JC, Giroth C, et al: Unique polycomb gene expression pattern in Hodgkin's lymphoma and Hodgkin's lymphoma-derived cell lines. *Am J Pathol* 164:873, 2004.
73. Scheeren FA, Diehl SA, Smit LA, et al: IL-21 is expressed in Hodgkin lymphoma and activates STAT5: Evidence that activated STAT5 is required for Hodgkin lymphomagenesis. *Blood* 111:4706, 2008.
74. Marafioti T, Hummel M, Foss HD, et al: Hodgkin and Reed-Sternberg cells represent an expansion of a single clone originating from a germinal center B-cell with functional immunoglobulin gene rearrangements but defective immunoglobulin transcription. *Blood* 95:1443, 2000.
75. Joos S, Kupper M, Ohl S, et al: Genomic imbalances including amplification of the tyrosine kinase gene JAK2 in CD30+ Hodgkin cells. *Cancer Res* 60:549, 2000.
76. Weniger MA, Melzner I, Menz CK, et al: Mutations of the tumor suppressor gene SOCS-1 in classical Hodgkin lymphoma are frequent and associated with nuclear phospho-STAT5 accumulation. *Oncogene* 25:2679, 2006.
77. Barth TF, Martin-Subero JI, Joos S, et al: Gains of 2p involving the REL locus correlate with nuclear c-Rel protein accumulation in neoplastic cells of classical Hodgkin lymphoma. *Blood* 101:3681, 2003.
78. Cabannes E, Khan G, Aillet F, et al: Mutations in the IkBa gene in Hodgkin's disease suggest a tumour suppressor role for IkappaBalpha. *Oncogene* 18:3063, 1999.
79. Emmerich F, Theurich S, Hummel M, et al: Inactivating I kappa B epsilon mutations in Hodgkin/Reed-Sternberg cells. *J Pathol* 201:413, 2003.
80. Schmitz R, Hansmann ML, Bohle V, et al: TNFAIP3 (A20) is a tumor suppressor gene in Hodgkin lymphoma and primary mediastinal B cell lymphoma. *J Exp Med* 206:981, 2009.
81. Lamprecht B, Kreher S, Anagnostopoulos I, et al: Aberrant expression of the Th2 cytokine IL-21 in Hodgkin lymphoma cells regulates STAT3 signaling and attracts Treg cells via regulation of MIP-3alpha. *Blood* 112:3339, 2008.
82. Baus D, Pfitzner E: Specific function of STAT3, SOCS1, and SOCS3 in the regulation of proliferation and survival of classical Hodgkin lymphoma cells. *Int J Cancer* 118:1404, 2006.
83. Kapp U, Yeh WC, Patterson B, et al: Interleukin 13 is secreted by and stimulates the growth of Hodgkin and Reed-Sternberg cells. *J Exp Med* 189:1939, 1999.
84. Fiumara P, Snell V, Li Y, et al: Functional expression of receptor activator of nuclear factor kappaB in Hodgkin disease cell lines. *Blood* 98:2784, 2001.
85. Chiu A, Xu W, He B, et al: Hodgkin lymphoma cells express TACI and BCMA receptors and generate survival and proliferation signals in response to BAFF and APRIL. *Blood* 109:729, 2007.
86. Pel PK: Zur symptomatolgie der sogennanten pseudoleukamie. II. Pseudokeukamie oder chronisches Ruckfallsfieber? *Berl Klin Wochenschr* 24:844, 1887.
87. Ebstein WV: Das chronische Ruckfallsfieber, eine neu infectionskrankheit. *Berl Klin Wochenschr* 24:565, 1887.
88. Atkinson K, Austin DE, McElwain TJ, et al: Alcohol pain in Hodgkin's disease. *Cancer* 37:895, 1976.
89. Rueffer U, Sieber M, Josting A, et al: Prognostic factors for subdiaphragmatic involvement in clinical stage I-II supradiaphragmatic Hodgkin's disease: A retrospective analysis of the GHSG. *Ann Oncol* 10:1343, 1999.
90. Cavalli F: Rare syndromes in Hodgkin's disease. *Ann Oncol* 9 Suppl 5:S109, 1998.

91. Barta SK, Yahalom J, Shia J, et al: Idiopathic cholestasis as a paraneoplastic phenomenon in Hodgkin's lymphoma. *Clin Lymphoma Myeloma* 7:77, 2006.
92. Audard V, Larousserie F, Grimbert P, et al: Minimal change nephrotic syndrome and classical Hodgkin's lymphoma: Report of 21 cases and review of the literature. *Kidney Int* 69:2251, 2006.
93. Gerstner ER, Abrey LE, Schiff D, et al: CNS Hodgkin lymphoma. *Blood* 112:1658, 2008.
94. Filly R, Bland N, Castellino RA: Radiographic distribution of intrathoracic disease in previously untreated patients with Hodgkin's disease and non-Hodgkin's lymphoma. *Radiology* 120:277, 1976.
95. Mauch P, Gorshein D, Cunningham J, et al: Influence of mediastinal adenopathy on site and frequency of relapse in patients with Hodgkin's disease. *Cancer Treat Rep* 66:809, 1982.
96. Juweid ME: Utility of positron emission tomography (PET) scanning in managing patients with Hodgkin lymphoma. *Hematology Am Soc Hematol Educ Program* 259, 510–1, 2006.
97. Jerusalem G, Warland V, Najjar F, et al: Whole-body 18F-FDG PET for the evaluation of patients with Hodgkin's disease and non-Hodgkin's lymphoma. *Nucl Med Commun* 20:13, 1999.
98. Bangerter M, Moog F, Buchmann I, et al: Whole-body 2-[18F]-fluoro-2-deoxy-D-glucose positron emission tomography (FDG-PET) for accurate staging of Hodgkin's disease. *Ann Oncol* 9:1117, 1998.
99. Juweid ME, Stroobants S, Hoekstra OS, et al: Use of positron emission tomography for response assessment of lymphoma: Consensus of the Imaging Subcommittee of International Harmonization Project in Lymphoma. *J Clin Oncol* 25:571, 2007.
100. Gallamini A, Hutchings M, Rigacci L, et al: Early interim 2-[18F]fluoro-2-deoxy-D-glucose positron emission tomography is prognostically superior to international prognostic score in advanced-stage Hodgkin's lymphoma: A report from a joint Italian-Danish study. *J Clin Oncol* 25:3746, 2007.
101. Hutchings M, Loft A, Hansen M, et al: FDG-PET after two cycles of chemotherapy predicts treatment failure and progression-free survival in Hodgkin lymphoma. *Blood* 107:52, 2006.
102. Dann EJ, Bar-Shalom R, Tamir A, et al: Risk-adapted BEACOPP regimen can reduce the cumulative dose of chemotherapy for standard and high-risk Hodgkin lymphoma with no impairment of outcome. *Blood* 109:905, 2007.
103. Poppema S, Kaiserling E, Lennert K: Nodular paragranuloma and progressively transformed germinal centers. Ultrastructural and immunohistologic findings. *Virchows Arch B Cell Pathol* 31:211, 1979.
104. Burns BF, Colby TV, Dorfman RF: Differential diagnostic features of nodular L & H Hodgkin's disease, including progressive transformation of germinal centers. *Am J Surg Pathol* 8:253, 1984.
105. Hansmann ML, Zwingers T, Boske A, et al: Clinical features of nodular paragranuloma (Hodgkin's disease, lymphocyte predominance type, nodular). *J Cancer Res Clin Oncol* 108:321, 1984.
106. Miettinen M, Franssila KO, Saxen E: Hodgkin's disease, lymphocytic predominance nodular. Increased risk for subsequent non-Hodgkin's lymphomas. *Cancer* 51:2293, 1983.
107. Sundeen JT, Cossman J, Jaffe ES: Lymphocyte predominant Hodgkin's disease nodular subtype with coexistent "large cell lymphoma." Histological progression or composite malignancy [see comments]? *Am J Surg Pathol* 12:599, 1988.
108. Rudiger T, Gascoyne RD, Jaffe ES, et al: Workshop on the relationship between nodular lymphocyte predominant Hodgkin's lymphoma and T cell/histiocyte-rich B cell lymphoma. *Ann Oncol* 13 Suppl 1:44, 2002.
109. Allemani C, Sant M, De Angelis R, et al: Hodgkin disease survival in Europe and the U.S.: Prognostic significance of morphologic groups. *Cancer* 107:352, 2006.
110. Neiman RS, Rosen PJ, Lukes RJ: Lymphocyte-depletion Hodgkin's disease. A clinicopathological entity. *N Engl J Med* 288:751, 1973.
111. Diehl V, Sextro M, Franklin J, et al: Clinical presentation, course, and prognostic factors in lymphocyte-predominant Hodgkin's disease and lymphocyte-rich classical Hodgkin's disease: Report from the European Task Force on Lymphoma Project on Lymphocyte-Predominant Hodgkin's Disease. *J Clin Oncol* 17:776, 1999.
112. Kaplan HS: *Hodgkin's Disease*. Harvard University Press, Cambridge, MA, 1980.
113. Rosenberg SA, Kaplan HS: Evidence for an orderly progression in the spread of Hodgkin's disease. *Cancer Res* 26:1225, 1966.
114. Smithers DW: Spread of Hodgkin's disease. *Lancet* 1:1262, 1970.
115. Hutchison GB: Anatomic patterns by histologic type of localized Hodgkin's disease of the upper torso. *Lymphology* 5:1, 1972.
116. Rappaport H, Berard CW, Butler JJ, et al: Report of the Committee on Histopathological Criteria Contributing to Staging of Hodgkin's Disease. *Cancer Res* 31:1864, 1971.
117. Naeim F, Waisman J, Coulson WF: Hodgkin's disease: The significance of vascular invasion. *Cancer* 34:655, 1974.
118. Kirschner RH, Abt AB, O'Connell MJ, et al: Vascular invasion and hematogenous dissemination of Hodgkin's disease. *Cancer* 34:1159, 1974.
119. Lister TA, Crowther D, Sutcliffe SB, et al: Report of a committee convened to discuss the evaluation and staging of patients with Hodgkin's disease: Cotswolds meeting [published erratum appears in *J Clin Oncol* 8(9):1602, 1990] [see comments]. *J Clin Oncol* 7:1630, 1989.
120. Kaplan HS, Dorfman RF, Nelsen TS, et al: Staging laparotomy and splenectomy in Hodgkin's disease: Analysis of indications and patterns of involvement in 285 consecutive, unselected patients. *Natl Cancer Inst Monogr* 36:291, 1973.
121. Simmons AV, Spiers AS, Fayers PM: Haematological and clinical parameters in assessing activity in Hodgkin's disease and other malignant lymphomas. *Q J Med* 42:111, 1973.
122. Tauro GP: Hodgkin's disease associated with raised eosinophil counts. *Med J Aust* 2:604, 1966.
123. MacLennan KA, Hudson BV, Jelliffe AM, et al: The pretreatment peripheral blood lymphocyte count in 1100 patients with Hodgkin's disease: The prognostic significance and the relationship to the presence of systemic symptoms. *Clin Oncol* 7:333, 1981.
124. Ultmann JE, Cunningham JK, Gellhorn A: The clinical picture of Hodgkin's disease. *Cancer Res* 26:1047, 1966.
125. MacLennan KA, Vaughan HB, Easterling MJ, et al: The presentation haemoglobin level in 1103 patients with Hodgkin's disease (BNLI report no. 21). *Clin Radiol* 34:491, 1983.
126. Storgaard L, Karle H: Fever and haemolysis in Hodgkin's diseases. *Acta Med Scand* 197:311, 1975.
127. Jones SE: Autoimmune disorders and malignant lymphoma. *Cancer* 31:1092, 1973.
128. Sonnenblick M, Kramer R, Hershko C: Corticosteroid responsive immune thrombocytopenia in Hodgkin's disease. *Oncology* 43:349, 1986.
129. Cohen JR: Idiopathic thrombocytopenic purpura in Hodgkin's disease: A rare occurrence of no prognostic significance. *Cancer* 41:743, 1978.
130. Kedar A, Khan AB, Mattern JQ, et al: Autoimmune disorders complicating adolescent Hodgkin's disease. *Cancer* 44:112, 1979.
131. Hunter JD, Logue GL, Joyner JT: Autoimmune neutropenia in Hodgkin's disease. *Arch Intern Med* 142:386, 1982.
132. Le Bourgeois J, Tubiana M: The erythrocyte sedimentation rate as a monitor for relapse in patients with previously treated Hodgkin's disease. *Int J Radiat Oncol Biol Phys* 2:241, 1977.
133. Haybittle JL, Hayhoe FG, Easterling MJ, et al: Review of British National Lymphoma Investigation studies of Hodgkin's disease and development of prognostic index. *Lancet* 1:967, 1985.
134. Tubiana M, Henry AM, van dW, et al: A multivariate analysis of prognostic factors in early stage Hodgkin's disease. *Int J Radiat Oncol Biol Phys* 11:23, 1985.
135. Schilling RF, McKnight B, Crowley JJ: Prognostic value of serum lactic dehydrogenase level in Hodgkin's disease. *J Lab Clin Med* 99:382, 1982.
136. Friedenberg WR, Gatlin PF, Mazza JJ, et al: Prognostic value of serum lactic dehydrogenase level in Hodgkin's disease [letter]. *J Lab Clin Med* 103:489, 1984.
137. Aisenberg AC, Kaplan MM, Rieder SV: Serum alkaline phosphatase at the onset of Hodgkin's disease. *Cancer* 26:318, 1970.
138. Mercier RJ, Thompson JM, Harman GS, et al: Recurrent hypercalcemia and elevated 1,25-dihydroxyvitamin D levels in Hodgkin's disease. *Am J Med* 84:165, 1988.
139. Braund WJ, Naylor BA, Williamson DH, et al: Autoimmunity to insulin receptor and hypoglycaemia in patient with Hodgkin's disease. *Lancet* 1:237, 1987.
140. Walters EG, Tavare JM, Denton RM, et al: Hypoglycaemia due to an insulin-receptor antibody in Hodgkin's disease. *Lancet* 1:241, 1987.
141. Eliakim R, Vertman E, Shinhar E: Syndrome of inappropriate secretion of antidiuretic hormone in Hodgkin's disease. *Am J Med Sci* 291:126, 1986.
142. Hasenclever D, Diehl V: A prognostic score for advanced Hodgkin's disease. International Prognostic Factors Project on Advanced Hodgkin's Disease. *N Engl J Med* 339:1547, 1998.
143. Dimopoulos MA, Cabanillas F, Lee JJ, et al: Prognostic role of serum beta 2-microglobulin in Hodgkin's disease. *J Clin Oncol* 11:1108, 1993.
144. Nadali G, Vinante F, Ambrosetti A, et al: Serum levels of soluble CD30 are elevated in the majority of untreated patients with Hodgkin's disease and correlate with clinical features and prognosis. *J Clin Oncol* 12:793, 1994.
145. Kurzrock R, Redman J, Cabanillas F, et al: Serum interleukin 6 levels are elevated in lymphoma patients and correlate with survival in advanced Hodgkin's disease and with B symptoms. *Cancer Res* 53:2118, 1993.
146. Pizzolo G, Chilosi M, Vinante F, et al: Soluble interleukin-2 receptors in the serum of patients with Hodgkin's disease. *Br J Cancer* 55:427, 1987.
147. Sarris AH, Kliche KO, Pethambaram P, et al: Interleukin-10 levels are often elevated in serum of adults with Hodgkin's disease and are associated with inferior failure-free survival. *Ann Oncol* 10:433, 1999.
148. Lieberman DA: Intrahepatic cholestasis due to Hodgkin's disease. An elusive diagnosis. *J Clin Gastroenterol* 8(3 Pt 1):304, 1986.
149. Routledge RC, Hann IM, Jones PH: Hodgkin's disease complicated by the nephrotic syndrome. *Cancer* 38:1735, 1976.
150. Savage KJ, Monti S, Kutok JL, et al: The molecular signature of mediastinal large B-cell lymphoma differs from that of other diffuse large B-cell lymphomas and shares features with classical Hodgkin lymphoma. *Blood* 102:3871, 2003.
151. Rosenwald A, Wright G, Leroy K, et al: Molecular diagnosis of primary mediastinal B cell lymphoma identifies a clinically favorable subgroup of diffuse large B cell lymphoma related to Hodgkin lymphoma. *J Exp Med* 198:851, 2003.
152. Kaplan HS, Rosenberg SA: The treatment of Hodgkin's disease. *Med Clin North Am* 50:1591, 1966.
153. Feuer EJ, Kessler LG, Baker SG, et al: The impact of breakthrough clinical trials on survival in population based tumor registries. *J Clin Epidemiol* 44:141, 1991.
154. Santoro A, Bonadonna G: Prolonged disease-free survival in MOPP-resistant Hodgkin's disease after treatment with Adriamycin, bleomycin, vinblastine and dacarbazine (ABVD). *Cancer Chemother Pharmacol* 2:101, 1979.

155. Santoro A, Bonfante V, Bonadonna G: Salvage chemotherapy with ABVD in MOPP-resistant Hodgkin's disease. *Ann Intern Med* 96:139, 1982.
156. Canellos GP, Anderson JR, Propert KJ, et al: Chemotherapy of advanced Hodgkin's disease with MOPP, ABVD, or MOPP alternating with ABVD. *N Engl J Med* 327:1478, 1992.
157. Duggan DB, Petroni GR, Johnson JL, et al: Randomized comparison of ABVD and MOPP/ABV hybrid for the treatment of advanced Hodgkin's disease: Report of an intergroup trial. *J Clin Oncol* 21:607, 2003.
158. Diehl V, Franklin J, Pfreundschuh M, et al: Standard and increased-dose BEACOPP chemotherapy compared with COPP-ABVD for advanced Hodgkin's disease. *N Engl J Med* 348:2386, 2003.
159. Hancock SL, Hoppe RT, Horning SJ, et al: Intercurrent death after Hodgkin disease therapy in radiotherapy and adjuvant MOPP trials. *Ann Intern Med* 109:183, 1988.
160. Rosenberg SA, Kaplan HS: The evolution and summary results of the Stanford randomized clinical trials of the management of Hodgkin's disease: 1962–1984. *Int J Radiat Oncol Biol Phys* 11:5, 1985.
161. Horning SJ, Hoppe RT, Hancock SL, et al: Vinblastine, bleomycin, and methotrexate: An effective adjuvant in favorable Hodgkin's disease. *J Clin Oncol* 6:1822, 1988.
162. Noordijk EM, Carde P, Hagenbeek A, et al: Combination of radiotherapy and chemotherapy is advisable in all patients with clinical stage I-II Hodgkin's disease. Six year results of the EORTC-GPMC controlled clinical trials "H7-VF," "H7-F," and "H7-UF" [abstract]. *Int J Radiat Oncol Biol Phys* 77:173, 1997.
163. Press OW, LeBlanc M, Lichter AS, et al: Phase III randomized intergroup trial of subtotal lymphoid irradiation versus doxorubicin, vinblastine, and subtotal lymphoid irradiation for stage IA to IIA Hodgkin's disease. *J Clin Oncol* 19:4238, 2001.
164. Tesch H, Sieber M, Ruffer J, et al: Two cycles ABVD plus radiotherapy is more effective than radiotherapy alone in early stage HD: Interim analysis of the HD7 trial of the GHSG clinic of internal medicine, University of Cologne. *Proc Am Soc Hematol* 92 Suppl I0:485a, 1998.
165. Ferme C, Eghbali H, Meerwaldt JH, et al: Chemotherapy plus involved-field radiation in early-stage Hodgkin's disease. *N Engl J Med* 357:1916, 2007.
166. Bonadonna G, Bonfante V, Viviani S, et al: ABVD plus subtotal nodal versus involved-field radiotherapy in early-stage Hodgkin's disease: Long-term results. *J Clin Oncol* 22:2835, 2004.
167. Engert A, Schiller P, Josting A, et al: Involved-field radiotherapy is equally effective and less toxic compared with extended-field radiotherapy after four cycles of chemotherapy in patients with early-stage unfavorable Hodgkin's lymphoma: Results of the HD8 trial of the German Hodgkin's Lymphoma Study Group. *J Clin Oncol* 21:3601, 2003.
168. Diehl V, Brillant C, Engert A, et al: Reduction of combined modality treatment intensity in early stage Hodgkin's lymphoma: Interim analysis of the HD 10 trial of the GHSG. *ASH Annual Meeting Abstracts* 104:1307, 2004.
169. Meyer R, Gospodarowicz M, Connors JM, et al: A randomized phase III comparison of single-modality ABVD with a strategy that includes radiation therapy in patients with early-stage Hodgkin's disease: The HD-6 trial of the National Cancer Institute of Canada Clinical Trials Group (Eastern Cooperative Oncology Group Trial JHD06). *Blood* 102:Abstract 81, 2003.
170. Straus DJ, Portlock CS, Qin J, et al: Results of a prospective randomized clinical trial of doxorubicin, bleomycin, vinblastine, and dacarbazine (ABVD) followed by radiation therapy (RT) versus ABVD alone for stages I, II, and IIIA nonbulky Hodgkin disease. *Blood* 104:3483, 2004.
171. Noordijk E, Thomas J, Ferme C, et al: First results of the EORTC-GELA H9 randomized trials: The H9-F trial and H9u trial in patients with favorable or unfavorable early stage Hodgkin's lymphoma. *Proc Am Soc Clin Oncol* 23:6505A, 2005.
172. Laskar S, Gupta T, Vimal S, et al: Consolidation radiation after complete remission in Hodgkin's disease following six cycles of doxorubicin, bleomycin, vinblastine, and dacarbazine chemotherapy: Is there a need? *J Clin Oncol* 22:62, 2004.
173. Nachman JB, Sposto R, Herzog P, et al: Randomized comparison of low-dose involved-field radiotherapy and no radiotherapy for children with Hodgkin's disease who achieve a complete response to chemotherapy. *J Clin Oncol* 20:3765, 2002.
174. Hoppe RT, Coleman CN, Cox RS, et al: The management of stage I-II Hodgkin's disease with irradiation alone or combined modality therapy: The Stanford experience. *Blood* 59:455, 1982.
175. Nogova L, Reineke T, Eich HT, et al: Extended field radiotherapy, combined modality treatment or involved field radiotherapy for patients with stage IA lymphocyte-predominant Hodgkin's lymphoma: A retrospective analysis from the German Hodgkin Study Group (GHSG). *Ann Oncol* 16:1683, 2005.
176. Santoro A, Bonadonna G, Valagussa P, et al: Long-term results of combined chemotherapy-radiotherapy approach in Hodgkin's disease: Superiority of ABVD plus radiotherapy versus MOPP plus radiotherapy. *J Clin Oncol* 5:27, 1987.
177. Bonfante V, Santoro A, Viviani S, et al: ABVD in the treatment of Hodgkin's disease. *Semin Oncol* 19(2 Suppl 5):38; discussion 44, 1992.
178. Horning SJ, Hoppe RT, Breslin S, et al: Stanford V and radiotherapy for locally extensive and advanced Hodgkin's disease: Mature results of a prospective clinical trial. *J Clin Oncol* 20:630, 2002.
179. Klimm B, Engert A, Brillant C, et al: Comparison of BEACOPP and ABVD chemotherapy in intermediate stage Hodgkin's lymphoma: Results of the fourth interim analysis of the HD11 trial of the GHSG. *Proc Am Soc Clin Oncol* 23:6507A, 2005.
180. Borchmann P, Engert A, Pluetschow A, et al: Dose-intensified combined modality treatment with 2 cycles of BEACOPP escalated followed by 2 cycles of ABVD and involved field radiotherapy (IF-RT) is superior to 4 cycles of ABVD and IFRT in patients with early unfavourable Hodgkin lymphoma (HL): An analysis of the German Hodgkin Study Group (GHSG) HD14 trial. *ASH Annual Meeting Abstracts* 112:367, 2008.
181. Canellos GP, Niedzwiecki D: Long-term follow-up of Hodgkin's disease trial. *N Engl J Med* 346:1417, 2002.
182. Viviani S, Bonadonna G, Santoro A, et al: Alternating versus hybrid MOPP and ABVD combinations in advanced Hodgkin's disease: Ten-year results. *J Clin Oncol* 14:1421, 1996.
183. Connors JM, Klimo P, Adams G, et al: Treatment of advanced Hodgkin's disease with chemotherapy—Comparison of MOPP/ABV hybrid regimen with alternating courses of MOPP and ABVD: A report from the National Cancer Institute of Canada clinical trials group. *J Clin Oncol* 15:1638, 1997.
184. Engert A, Diehl V, Franklin J, et al: Escalated-dose BEACOPP in the treatment of patients with advanced-stage Hodgkin's lymphoma: 10 years of follow-up of the GHSG HD9 Study. *J Clin Oncol* 27:4548, 2009.
185. Hasenclever D, Diehl V: A prognostic score for advanced Hodgkin's disease. International Prognostic Factors Project on Advanced Hodgkin's Disease. *N Engl J Med* 339:1506, 1998.
186. Leone G, Pagano L, Ben-Yehuda D, et al: Therapy-related leukemia and myelodysplasia: Susceptibility and incidence. *Haematologica* 92:1389, 2007.
187. Federico M, Luminari S, Iannitto E, et al: ABVD compared with BEACOPP compared with CEC for the initial treatment of patients with advanced Hodgkin's lymphoma: Results from the HD2000 Gruppo Italiano per lo Studio dei Linfomi Trial. *J Clin Oncol* 27:805, 2009.
188. Gianni AM, Rambaldi A, Zinzani PL, et al: Comparable 3-year outcome following ABVD or BEACOPP first-line chemotherapy, plus pre-planned high-dose salvage, in advanced Hodgkin lymphoma (HL): A randomized trial of the Michelangelo, GITIL and IIL cooperative groups. *J Clin Oncol* 26:Abstract 8506, 2008.
189. Diehl V, Haverkamp H, Mueller R, et al: Eight cycles of BEACOPP escalated compared with 4 cycles of BEACOPP escalated followed by 4 cycles of BEACOPP baseline with or without radiotherapy in patients in advanced stage Hodgkin lymphoma (HL): Final analysis of the HD12 trial of the German Hodgkin Study Group (GHSG). *J Clin Oncol* 27:15s (abstract 8544), 2009.
190. Markova J, Kobe C, Skopalova M, et al: FDG-PET for assessment of early treatment response after four cycles of chemotherapy in patients with advanced-stage Hodgkin's lymphoma has a high negative predictive value. *Ann Oncol* 20:1270, 2009.
191. Kobe C, Dietlein M, Franklin J, et al: Positron emission tomography has a high negative predictive value for progression or early relapse for patients with residual disease after first-line chemotherapy in advanced-stage Hodgkin lymphoma. *Blood* 112:3989, 2008.
192. Horning SJ, Williams J, Bartlett NL, et al: E1492: Assessment of the Stanford V regimen and consolidative radiotherapy for bulky and advanced Hodgkin's disease. *J Clin Oncol* 18:972, 2000.
193. Aversa SM, Salvagno L, Soraru M, et al: Stanford V regimen plus consolidative radiotherapy is an effective therapeutic program for bulky or advanced-stage Hodgkin's disease. *Acta Haematol* 112:141, 2004.
194. Chisesi T, Federico M, Levis A, et al: ABVD versus Stanford V versus MEC in unfavourable Hodgkin's lymphoma: Results of a randomised trial. *Ann Oncol* 13 Suppl 1:102, 2002.
195. Johnson PWM, Horwich A, Jack A, et al: Randomised comparison of the Stanford V (SV) regimen and ABVD in the treatment of advanced Hodgkin lymphoma (HL): Results from a UK NCRI Lymphoma Group Study, ISRCTN 64141244. *ASH Annual Meeting Abstracts* 112:370, 2008.
196. Aleman BM, Raemaekers JM, Tirelli U, et al: Involved-field radiotherapy for advanced Hodgkin's lymphoma. *N Engl J Med* 348:2396, 2003.
197. Linch DC, Winfield D, Goldstone AH, et al: Dose intensification with autologous bone-marrow transplantation in relapsed and resistant Hodgkin's disease: Results of a BNLI randomised trial. *Lancet* 341:1051, 1993.
198. Schmitz N, Pfistner B, Sextro M, et al: Aggressive conventional chemotherapy compared with high-dose chemotherapy with autologous haemopoietic stem-cell transplantation for relapsed chemosensitive Hodgkin's disease: A randomised trial. *Lancet* 359:2065, 2002.
199. Horning SJ, Chao NJ, Negrin RS, et al: High-dose therapy and autologous hematopoietic progenitor cell transplantation for recurrent or refractory Hodgkin's disease: Analysis of the Stanford University results and prognostic indices. *Blood* 89:801, 1997.
200. Nademanee A, O'Donnell MR, Snyder DS, et al: High-dose chemotherapy with or without total body irradiation followed by autologous bone marrow and/or peripheral blood stem cell transplantation for patients with relapsed and refractory Hodgkin's disease: Results in 85 patients with analysis of prognostic factors. *Blood* 85:1381, 1995.
201. Stiff PJ, Unger JM, Forman SJ, et al: The value of augmented preparative regimens combined with an autologous bone marrow transplant for the management of relapsed or refractory Hodgkin disease: A Southwest Oncology Group phase II trial. *Biol Blood Marrow Transplant* 9:529, 2003.
202. Josting A, Sieniawski M, Glossmann JP, et al: High-dose sequential chemotherapy followed by autologous stem cell transplantation in relapsed and refractory aggressive non-Hodgkin's lymphoma: Results of a multicenter phase II study. *Ann Oncol* 16:1359, 2005.

203. Fung HC, Stiff P, Schriber J, et al: Tandem autologous stem cell transplantation for patients with primary refractory or poor risk recurrent Hodgkin lymphoma. *Biol Blood Marrow Transplant* 13:594, 2007.
204. Santoro A, Magagnoli M, Spina M, et al: Ifosfamide, gemcitabine, and vinorelbine: A new induction regimen for refractory and relapsed Hodgkin's lymphoma. *Haematologica* 92:35, 2007.
205. Sieniawski M, Franklin J, Nogova L, et al: Outcome of patients experiencing progression or relapse after primary treatment with two cycles of chemotherapy and radiotherapy for early-stage favorable Hodgkin's lymphoma. *J Clin Oncol* 25:2000, 2007.
206. Macdonald DA, Ding K, Gospodarowicz MK, et al: Patterns of disease progression and outcomes in a randomized trial testing ABVD alone for patients with limited-stage Hodgkin lymphoma. *Ann Oncol* 18:1680, 2007.
207. Burroughs LM, O'Donnell PV, Sandmaier BM, et al: Comparison of outcomes of HLA-matched related, unrelated, or HLA-haploidentical related hematopoietic cell transplantation following nonmyeloablative conditioning for relapsed or refractory Hodgkin lymphoma. *Biol Blood Marrow Transplant* 14:1279, 2008.
208. Sureda A, Robinson S, Canals C, et al: Reduced-intensity conditioning compared with conventional allogeneic stem-cell transplantation in relapsed or refractory Hodgkin's lymphoma: An analysis from the Lymphoma Working Party of the European Group for Blood and Marrow Transplantation. *J Clin Oncol* 26:455, 2008.
209. Horning SJ, Bartlett NL, Breslin S, et al: Results of a prospective phase II trial of limited and extended rituximab treatment in nodular lymphocyte predominant Hodgkin's disease (NLPHD). *ASH Annual Meeting Abstracts* 110:644, 2007.
210. Schulz H, Rehwald U, Morschhauser F, et al: Rituximab in relapsed lymphocyte-predominant Hodgkin Lymphoma: Long-term results of a phase 2 trial of the German Hodgkin Lymphoma Study Group (GHSG). *Blood* 111:109, 2008.
211. Forero-Torres A, Leonard JP, Younes A, et al: A phase II study of SGN-30 (anti-CD30 mAb) in Hodgkin lymphoma or systemic anaplastic large cell lymphoma. *Br J Haematol* 146:171, 2009.
212. Younes A, Forero-Torres A, Bartlett NL, et al: Multiple complete responses in a phase 1 dose-escalation study of the antibody-drug conjugate SGN-35 in patients with relapsed or refractory CD30-positive lymphomas. *ASH Annual Meeting Abstracts* 112:1006, 2008.
213. Bartlett N, Forero-Torres A, Rosenblatt JD, et al: Complete remissions with weekly dosing of SGN-35, a novel antibody-drug conjugate (ADC) targeting CD30, in a phase I dose-escalation study in patients with relapsed or refractory Hodgkin lymphoma or systemic anaplastic large cell lymphoma. *J Clin Oncol* 27:15S (abstract 8500), 2009.
214. Brenner H, Gondos A, Pulte D: Survival expectations of patients diagnosed with Hodgkin's lymphoma in 2006–2010. *Oncologist* 14:806, 2009.
215. Evens AM, Sweetenham JW, Horning SJ: Hodgkin lymphoma in older patients: An uncommon disease in need of study. *Oncology (Williston Park)* 22:1369, 2008.
216. Brenner H, Gondos A, Pulte D: Ongoing improvement in long-term survival of patients with Hodgkin disease at all ages and recent catch-up of older patients. *Blood* 111:2977, 2008.
217. Ballova V, Ruffer JU, Haverkamp H, et al: A prospectively randomized trial carried out by the German Hodgkin Study Group (GHSG) for elderly patients with advanced Hodgkin's disease comparing BEACOPP baseline and COPP-ABVD (study HD9elderly). *Ann Oncol* 16:124, 2005.
218. Kobe C, Dietlein M, Franklin J, et al: Positron emission tomography has a high negative predictive value for progression or early relapse for patients with residual disease after first line chemotherapy in advanced-stage Hodgkin lymphoma. *Blood* 112:3989, 2008.
219. Advani R, Maeda L, Lavori P, et al: Impact of positive positron emission tomography on prediction of freedom from progression after Stanford V chemotherapy in Hodgkin's disease. *J Clin Oncol* 25:3902, 2007.
220. Sher DJ, Mauch PM, Van Den Abbeele A, et al: Prognostic significance of mid- and post-ABVD PET imaging in Hodgkin's lymphoma: The importance of involved-field radiotherapy. *Ann Oncol* 20:1848, 2009.
221. Mikhaeel NG, Mainwaring P, Nunan T, et al: Prognostic valude of interim and post treatment FDG-PET scanning in Hodgkin lymphoma. *Ann Oncol* 13:21, 2002.
222. Svoboda J, Andreadis C, Elstrom R, et al: Prognostic value of FDG-PET scan imaging in lymphoma patients undergoing autologous stem cell transplantation. *Bone Marrow Transplant* 38:211, 2006.
223. Jabbour E, Hosing C, Ayers G, et al: Pretransplant positive positron emission tomography/gallium scans predict poor outcome in patients with recurrent/refractory Hodgkin lymphoma. *Cancer* 109:2481, 2007.
224. Moskowitz CH, Kewalramani T, Nimer SD, et al: Effectiveness of high dose chemoradiotherapy and autologous stem cell transplantation for patients with biopsy-proven primary refractory Hodgkin's disease. *Br J Haematol* 124:645, 2004.
225. Josting A, Engert A, Diehl V, et al: Prognostic factors and treatment outcome in patients with primary progressive and relapsed Hodgkin's disease. *Ann Oncol* 13 Suppl 1:112, 2002.
226. Casasnovas RO, Mounier N, Brice P, et al: Plasma cytokine and soluble receptor signature predicts outcome of patients with classical Hodgkin's lymphoma: A study from the Groupe d'Etude des Lymphomes de l'Adulte. *J Clin Oncol* 25:1732, 2007.
227. Niens M, Visser L, Nolte IM, et al: Serum chemokine levels in Hodgkin lymphoma patients: Highly increased levels of CCL17 and CCL22. *Br J Haematol* 140:527, 2008.
228. Weihrauch MR, Manzke O, Beyer M, et al: Elevated serum levels of CC thymus and activation-related chemokine (TARC) in primary Hodgkin's disease: Potential for a prognostic factor. *Cancer Res* 65:5516, 2005.
229. Brink AA, Oudejans JJ, van den Brule AJ, et al: Low p53 and high bcl-2 expression in Reed-Sternberg cells predicts poor clinical outcome for Hodgkin's disease: Involvement of apoptosis resistance? *Mod Pathol* 11:376, 1998.
230. Rassidakis GZ, Medeiros LJ, Vassilakopoulos TP, et al: BCL-2 expression in Hodgkin and Reed-Sternberg cells of classical Hodgkin disease predicts a poorer prognosis in patients treated with ABVD or equivalent regimens. *Blood* 100:3935, 2002.
231. Vassallo J, Metze K, Traina F, et al: The prognostic relevance of apoptosis-related proteins in classical Hodgkin's lymphomas. *Leuk Lymphoma* 44:483, 2003.
232. Montalban C, Garcia JF, Abraira V, et al: Influence of biologic markers on the outcome of Hodgkin's lymphoma: A study by the Spanish Hodgkin's Lymphoma Study Group. *J Clin Oncol* 22:1664, 2004.
233. Portlock CS, Donnelly GB, Qin J, et al: Adverse prognostic significance of CD20 positive Reed-Sternberg cells in classical Hodgkin's disease. *Br J Haematol* 125:701, 2004.
234. Tzankov A, Krugmann J, Fend F, et al: Prognostic significance of CD20 expression in classical Hodgkin lymphoma: A clinicopathological study of 119 cases. *Clin Cancer Res* 9:1381, 2003.
235. Diepstra A, van Imhoff GW, Karim-Kos HE, et al: HLA class II expression by Hodgkin Reed-Sternberg cells is an independent prognostic factor in classical Hodgkin's lymphoma. *J Clin Oncol* 25:3101, 2007.
236. Diepstra A, van Imhoff GW, Schaapveld M, et al: Latent Epstein-Barr virus infection of tumor cells in classical Hodgkin's lymphoma predicts adverse outcome in older adult patients. *J Clin Oncol* 27:3815, 2009.
237. Keegan TH, Glaser SL, Clarke CA, et al: Epstein-Barr virus as a marker of survival after Hodgkin's lymphoma: A population-based study. *J Clin Oncol* 23:7604, 2005.
238. Kelley TW, Pohlman B, Elson P, et al: The ratio of FOXP3+ regulatory T cells to granzyme B+ cytotoxic T/NK cells predicts prognosis in classical Hodgkin lymphoma and is independent of bcl-2 and MAL expression. *Am J Clin Pathol* 128:958, 2007.
239. Alvaro T, Lejeune M, Salvado MT, et al: Outcome in Hodgkin's lymphoma can be predicted from the presence of accompanying cytotoxic and regulatory T cells. *Clin Cancer Res* 11:1467, 2005.
240. Alvaro-Naranjo T, Lejeune M, Salvado-Usach MT, et al: Tumor-infiltrating cells as a prognostic factor in Hodgkin's lymphoma: A quantitative tissue microarray study in a large retrospective cohort of 267 patients. *Leuk Lymphoma* 46:1581, 2005.
241. Ng AK, Bernardo MP, Weller E, et al: Long-term survival and competing causes of death in patients with early-stage Hodgkin's disease treated at age 50 or younger. *J Clin Oncol* 20:2101, 2002.
242. Hoppe RT: Hodgkin's disease: Complications of therapy and excess mortality. *Ann Oncol* 8 Suppl 1:115, 1997.
243. Arseneau JC, Sponzo RW, Levin DL, et al: Nonlymphomatous malignant tumors complicating Hodgkin's disease. Possible association with intensive therapy. *N Engl J Med* 287:1119, 1972.
244. Kaldor JM, Day NE, Clarke EA, et al: Leukemia following Hodgkin's disease. *N Engl J Med* 322:7, 1990.
245. Levine EG, Bloomfield CD: Leukemias and myelodysplastic syndromes secondary to drug, radiation, and environmental exposure. *Semin Oncol* 19:47, 1992.
246. Josting A, Wiedenmann S, Franklin J, et al: Secondary myeloid leukemia and myelodysplastic syndromes in patients treated for Hodgkin's disease: A report from the German Hodgkin's Lymphoma Study Group. *J Clin Oncol* 21:3440, 2003.
247. Schonfeld SJ, Gilbert ES, Dores GM, et al: Acute myeloid leukemia following Hodgkin lymphoma: A population-based study of 35,511 patients. *J Natl Cancer Inst* 98:215, 2006.
248. Diehl V: Advanced Hodgkin's disease: ABVD is better, yet is not good enough! *J Clin Oncol* 21:583, 2003.
249. van LF, Somers R, Taal BG, et al: Increased risk of lung cancer, non-Hodgkin's lymphoma, and leukemia following Hodgkin's disease. *J Clin Oncol* 7:1046, 1989.
250. Tucker MA, Coleman CN, Cox RS, et al: Risk of second cancers after treatment for Hodgkin's disease. *N Engl J Med* 318:76, 1988.
251. Rueffer U, Josting A, Franklin J, et al: Non-Hodgkin's lymphoma after primary Hodgkin's disease in the German Hodgkin's Lymphoma Study Group: Incidence, treatment, and prognosis. *J Clin Oncol* 19:2026, 2001.
252. Schmitz R, Renne C, Rosenquist R, et al: Insights into the multistep transformation process of lymphomas: IgH-associated translocations and tumor suppressor gene mutations in clonally related composite Hodgkin's and non-Hodgkin's lymphomas. *Leukemia* 19:1452, 2005.
253. Huang JZ, Weisenburger DD, Vose JM, et al: Diffuse large B-cell lymphoma arising in nodular lymphocyte predominant Hodgkin lymphoma: A report of 21 cases from the Nebraska Lymphoma Study Group. *Leuk Lymphoma* 45:1551, 2004.
254. Boivin JF, Hutchison GB, Lyden M, et al: Second primary cancers following treatment of Hodgkin's disease. *J Natl Cancer Inst* 72:233, 1984.
255. Henry AM: Second cancers after radiotherapy and chemotherapy for early stages of Hodgkin's disease. *J Natl Cancer Inst* 71:911, 1983.
256. Shapiro CL, Mauch PM: Radiation-associated breast cancer after Hodgkin's disease: Risks and screening in perspective [editorial; comment]. *J Clin Oncol* 10:1662, 1992.
257. Hancock SL, Donaldson SS, Hoppe RT: Cardiac disease following treatment of Hodgkin's disease in children and adolescents. *J Clin Oncol* 11:1208, 1993.
258. Bhatia S, Robison LL, Oberlin O, et al: Breast cancer and other second neoplasms after childhood Hodgkin's disease. *N Engl J Med* 334:745, 1996.

259. Travis LB, Hill D, Dores GM, et al: Cumulative absolute breast cancer risk for young women treated for Hodgkin lymphoma. *J Natl Cancer Inst* 97:1428, 2005.
260. van Leeuwen FE, Klokman WJ, Stovall M, et al: Roles of radiation dose, chemotherapy, and hormonal factors in breast cancer following Hodgkin's disease. *J Natl Cancer Inst* 95:971, 2003.
261. De Bruin ML, Sparidans J, van't Veer MB, et al: Breast cancer risk in female survivors of Hodgkin's lymphoma: Lower risk after smaller radiation volumes. *J Clin Oncol* 27:4239, 2009.
262. Travis LB, Gospodarowicz M, Curtis RE, et al: Lung cancer following chemotherapy and radiotherapy for Hodgkin's disease. *J Natl Cancer Inst* 94:182, 2002.
263. Swerdlow AJ, Schoemaker MJ, Allerton R, et al: Lung cancer after Hodgkin's disease: A nested case-control study of the relation to treatment. *J Clin Oncol* 19:1610, 2001.
264. Swerdlow AJ, Barber JA, Hudson GV, et al: Risk of second malignancy after Hodgkin's disease in a collaborative British cohort: The relation to age at treatment. *J Clin Oncol* 18:498, 2000.
265. Eriksson F, Gagliardi G, Liedberg A, et al: Long-term cardiac mortality following radiation therapy for Hodgkin's disease: Analysis with the relative seriality model. *Radiother Oncol* 55:153, 2000.
266. Hancock SL, Donaldson SS, Hoppe RT: Cardiac disease following treatment of Hodgkin's disease in children and adolescents [see comments]. *J Clin Oncol* 11:1208, 1993.
267. Hancock SL, Hoppe RT, Horning SJ, et al: Intercurrent death after Hodgkin disease therapy in radiotherapy and adjuvant MOPP trials [published erratum appears in *Ann Intern Med* 114:810, 1991]. *Ann Intern Med* 109:183, 1988.
268. Boivin JF, Hutchison GB, Lubin JH, et al: Coronary artery disease mortality in patients treated for Hodgkin's disease. *Cancer* 69:1241, 1992.
269. Adams MJ, Lipsitz SR, Colan SD, et al: Cardiovascular status in long-term survivors of Hodgkin's disease treated with chest radiotherapy. *J Clin Oncol* 22:3139, 2004.
270. Heidenreich PA, Hancock SL, Lee BK, et al: Asymptomatic cardiac disease following mediastinal irradiation. *J Am Coll Cardiol* 42:743, 2003.
271. Aleman BM, van den Belt-Dusebout AW, De Bruin ML, et al: Late cardiotoxicity after treatment for Hodgkin lymphoma. *Blood* 109:1878, 2007.
272. Swerdlow AJ, Higgins CD, Smith P, et al: Myocardial infarction mortality risk after treatment for Hodgkin disease: A collaborative British cohort study. *J Natl Cancer Inst* 99:206, 2007.
273. Hull MC, Morris CG, Pepine CJ, Mendenhall NP: Valvular dysfunction and carotid, subclavian, and coronary artery disease in survivors of Hodgkin lymphoma treated with radiation therapy. *JAMA* 290:2831, 2003.
274. De Bruin ML, Dorresteijn LD, van't Veer MB, et al: Increased risk of stroke and transient ischemic attack in 5-year survivors of Hodgkin lymphoma. *J Natl Cancer Inst* 101:928, 2009.
275. Chapman RM, Sutcliffe SB, Rees LH, et al: Cyclical combination chemotherapy and gonadal function. Retrospective study in males. *Lancet* 1:285, 1979.
276. da Cunha MF, Meistrich ML, Fuller LM, et al: Recovery of spermatogenesis after treatment for Hodgkin's disease: Limiting dose of MOPP chemotherapy. *J Clin Oncol* 2:571, 1984.
277. Chapman RM, Sutcliffe SB, Malpas JS: Cytotoxic-induced ovarian failure in women with Hodgkin's disease. I. Hormone function. *JAMA* 242:1877, 1979.
278. Horning SJ, Hoppe RT, Kaplan HS, et al: Female reproductive potential after treatment for Hodgkin's disease. *N Engl J Med* 304:1377, 1981.
279. Anselmo AP, Cartoni C, Bellantuono P, et al: Risk of infertility in patients with Hodgkin's disease treated with ABVD vs MOPP vs ABVD/MOPP. *Haematologica* 75:155, 1990.
280. Viviani S, Santoro A, Ragni G, et al: Gonadal toxicity after combination chemotherapy for Hodgkin's disease. Comparative results of MOPP vs ABVD. *Eur J Cancer Clin Oncol* 21:601, 1985.
281. Hodgson DC, Pintilie M, Gitterman L, et al: Fertility among female Hodgkin lymphoma survivors attempting pregnancy following ABVD chemotherapy. *Hematol Oncol* 25:11, 2007.
282. Sieniawski M, Reineke T, Nogova L, et al: Fertility in male patients with advanced Hodgkin Lymphoma treated with BEACOPP: A report of the German Hodgkin Study Group (GHSG). *Blood* 111:71, 2008.
283. Behringer K, Breuer K, Reineke T, et al: Secondary amenorrhea after Hodgkin's lymphoma is influenced by age at treatment, stage of disease, chemotherapy regimen, and the use of oral contraceptives during therapy: A report from the German Hodgkin's Lymphoma Study Group. *J Clin Oncol* 23:7555, 2005.
284. Hancock SL, Cox RS, McDougall IR: Thyroid diseases after treatment of Hodgkin's disease. *N Engl J Med* 325:599, 1991.
285. Carmel RJ, Kaplan HS: Mantle irradiation in Hodgkin's disease. An analysis of technique, tumor eradication, and complications. *Cancer* 37:2813, 1976.
286. Smith LM, Mendenhall NP, Cicale MJ, et al: Results of a prospective study evaluating the effects of mantle irradiation on pulmonary function. *Int J Radiat Oncol Biol Phys* 16:79, 1989.
287. Horning SJ, Adhikari A, Rizk N, et al: Effect of treatment for Hodgkin's disease on pulmonary function: Results of a prospective study. *J Clin Oncol* 12:297, 1994.
288. Donaldson SS, Kaplan HS: Complications of treatment of Hodgkin's disease in children. *Cancer Treat Rep* 66:977, 1982.
289. Rosner F, Zarrabi MH: Late infections following splenectomy in Hodgkin's disease. *Cancer Invest* 1:57, 1983.
290. Knobel H, Havard Loge J, Brit Lund M, et al: Late medical complications and fatigue in Hodgkin's disease survivors. *J Clin Oncol* 19:3226, 2001.
291. Carver JR, Shapiro CL, Ng A, et al: American Society of Clinical Oncology clinical evidence review on the ongoing care of adult cancer survivors: Cardiac and pulmonary late effects. *J Clin Oncol* 25:3991, 2007.
292. Hodgson DC, Koh ES, Tran TH, et al: Individualized estimates of second cancer risks after contemporary radiation therapy for Hodgkin lymphoma. *Cancer* 110:2576, 2007.

CHAPTER 100

DIFFUSE LARGE B-CELL LYMPHOMA

Michael Boyiadzis and Kenneth A. Foon

SUMMARY

Diffuse large B-cell lymphomas (DLBCLs) are a heterogeneous group of tumors consisting of large, transformed B cells, accounting for approximately 25 to 30 percent of lymphoma cases. Incidence increases with age; the median age at presentation is in the seventh decade. The disease typically presents as a nodal or extranodal mass with rapid tumor growth associated with systemic symptoms. Approximately 50 to 60 percent of patients will present in an advanced stage. DLBCL is potentially curable with combination chemotherapy. For localized disease, six cycles of rituximab, cyclophosphamide, doxorubicin, vincristine, and prednisone (R-CHOP) or three cycles of R-CHOP plus involved field radiation therapy is recommended, and for advanced DLBCL, six cycles of R-CHOP is appropriate. Whether dose adjusted rituximab, etoposide, prednisone, vincristine, cyclophosphamide, and doxorubicin (R-EPOCH) or dose-intensified R-CHOP is superior to standard R-CHOP is currently under investigation. High-dose chemotherapy with autologous stem cell transplantation is effective in relapsed or refractory DLBCL. Allogeneic stem cell transplantation should be considered, usually, as part of a clinical trial.

Acronyms and abbreviations that appear in this chapter include: ABC, activated B-cell–like; ACVBP, doxorubicin (Adriamycin), cyclophosphamide, vindesine, bleomycin, prednisone; ALLO-HSCT, allogeneic hematopoietic stem cell transplantation; ASCT, autologous stem cell transplantation; BEAM, high-dose carmustine, etoposide, cytarabine, and melphalan; CDE, cyclophosphamide, doxorubicin, etoposide; CHOP, cyclophosphamide, doxorubicin, vincristine, prednisone; CHOPE or CHOEP, CHOP plus etoposide; CNOP, cyclophosphamide, mitoxantrone, vincristine, prednisone; CNS, central nervous system; CR, complete remission; CVAD, cyclophosphamide, doxorubicin, vincristine, dexamethasone; CytaBOM, cytarabine, bleomycin, vincristine, methotrexate (with leucovorin rescue); DFS, disease-free survival; DLBCL, diffuse large B-cell lymphoma; DSHNHL, Deutsche (German) High-Grade Non-Hodgkin's Lymphoma Study Group; EBV, Epstein-Barr virus; EFS, event-free survival; EPOCH, etoposide, prednisone, vincristine, cyclophosphamide, doxorubicin; ESHAP, etoposide, methylprednisolone, cytarabine, cisplatin; FDG, fluoro-2-deoxyglucose; GCB, germinal center B-cell–like; GELA, Group d'Etade des Lymphomes de l'Adulte study; GVHD, graft-versus-host disease; ICE, ifosfamide, carboplatin, etoposide; I-CHOP, intensified CHOP; IFRT, involved-field radiation therapy; Ig, immunoglobulin; IL, interleukin; IVLBCL, intravascular large B-cell lymphoma; LDH, lactate dehydrogenase; MACOP-B, high-dose methotrexate, doxorubicin, cyclophosphamide, vincristine, prednisone, bleomycin; m-BACOD, moderate-dose methotrexate, bleomycin, doxorubicin, cyclophosphamide, vincristine, dexamethasone; MOPP, mechlorethamine, vincristine, procarbazine, prednisone; OS, overall survival; PFS, progression-free survival; ProMACE, prednisone, methotrexate, doxorubicin, cyclophosphamide, etoposide; PTLD, posttransplantation lymphoproliferative disorder; R-CHOP, rituximab plus CHOP; R-EPOCH, rituximab plus EPOCH; R-ICE, rituximab plus ICE; VACOP-B, vincristine, doxorubicin, cyclophosphamide, etoposide, prednisone, and bleomycin; WHO, World Health Organization.

DIFFUSE LARGE B-CELL LYMPHOMA

DEFINITION AND HISTORY

Diffuse large B-cell lymphomas (DLBCLs) are a heterogeneous group of aggressive lymphomas of large, transformed B cells. Consideration of morphology, biology, and clinical expression result in the subsets that are considered distinct disease entities as shown in Table 100–1 as proposed by the panel on classification of lymphoid tumors of the World Health Organization (WHO).[1] The disease can arise *de novo* or may transform from a low-grade lymphoma, such as small lymphocytic lymphoma or follicular lymphoma. The history of the evolution of lymphoma diagnostic categories and their subtypes is discussed in Chaps. 97 and 98.

EPIDEMIOLOGY

DLBCL is the most common B-cell lymphoid neoplasm in the United States and Europe and accounts for approximately 28 percent of all mature B-cell lymphomas.[2,3] Incidence varies by ethnicity: Americans of European descent have higher rates than Americans of African descent. Like most other lymphomas there is a male predominance. The most common presentation is in late middle-aged and older persons; the median age at diagnosis is approximately 65 years. Because lymphoma incidence rates have increased over the period from after the second world war to the mid-1990s, numerous exogenous factors have been examined to see if one or more have played a role. Specific chemical representations of herbicides (e.g., phenoxyacids), pesticides (e.g., organochlorines), dark hair dyes, body mass index, tobacco use, alcohol use, and inflammatory states are among those that have been evaluated. At this time no association with an inhalant, contactant, or ingestant has reached a level of scientific certainty as producing an increased relative risk of DLBCL.[3A]

ETIOLOGY AND PATHOGENESIS

DLBCL is a molecularly heterogeneous disease with multiple complex chromosomal translocations and genetic abnormalities as identified by cytogenetics and gene expression profiling. The disease is derived from B cells that have undergone somatic mutation in the immunoglobulin (Ig) genes in the lymph node germinal center. *BCL6* gene rearrangements may be specific for DLBCL.[4] Approximately 40 percent of cases in immunocompetent hosts and approximately 20 percent of HIV-related cases display *BCL6* rearrangements.[5–7] Chromosomal translocations involving band 3q27 lead to a truncated *BCL6* gene within its 5′ flanking region. This situation commonly occurs within the first exon or first intron, leading to complete removal or truncation of the promoter sequences; the coding sequence is left intact.[8] In a small number of cases, the breakpoint is not located in the immediate proximity of the *BCL6* gene. Increased expression of *BCL6* occurs from a process termed *promoter substitution* by which heterologous promoters are juxtaposed to the *BCL6* coding domain. This process occurs through reciprocal translocations between 3q27 and chromosomal partner sites, including 14q32 (IgH), 2p11 (Igκ), and 22q11 (Igλ).[8,9]

The BCL6 protein mediates the specific binding of several transcription factors to DNA. It also may be involved in induction of germinal-center-associated functions, given that it is expressed in germinal center B cells but not in plasma cells. Therefore, downregulation of *BCL6* may be necessary for terminal differentiation of B cells to memory B cells and plasma cells.[10]

Approximately 30 percent of DLBCLs have the t(14;18) translocation involving the Ig heavy-chain gene and *BCL2*. The *BCL2* gene rearrangements may occur in DLBCL in two conditions: a transformation of a previous follicular lymphoma or in DLBCL with a germinal center gene

TABLE 100–1. Diffuse Large B-Cell Lymphoma: Variants and Subtypes

I. Diffuse large B-cell lymphoma, not otherwise specified (NOS)[22,28]
  A. Common morphologic variants[1]
    1. Centroblastic
    2. Immunoblastic
    3. Anaplastic
  B. Rare morphologic variants
  C. Molecular subgroups[28–30]
    1. Germinal center B-cell–like
    2. Activated B-cell–like
  D. Immunohistochemical subgroups[1]
    1. CD5-positive DLBCL
    2. Germinal center B-cell–like
    3. Nongerminal center B-cell–like
II. Diffuse large B-cell lymphoma subtypes
  A. T-cell/histiocyte-rich large B-cell lymphoma[153–155]
  B. Primary DLBCL of the CNS[166–168]
  C. Primary cutaneous DLBCL, leg type[160–163]
  D. EBV-positive DLBCL of the elderly[169,170]
III. Other lymphomas of large B cells
  A. Primary mediastinal (thymic) large B-cell lymphoma[14,120,121,124]
  B. Intravascular large B-cell lymphoma[130,135]
  C. DLBCL associated with chronic inflammation[171–174]
  D. Lymphomatoid granulomatosis[127–128]
  E. ALK-positive DLBCL[164–165]
  F. Plasmablastic lymphoma (see Chap. 83)[175,176]
  G. Large B-cell lymphoma arising in HHV8-associated multicentric Castleman disease (see Chap. 83)[177,178]
  H. Primary effusion lymphoma (see Chap. 83)[179,180]
IV. Borderline cases
  A. B-cell lymphoma, unclassifiable, with features intermediate between diffuse large B-cell lymphoma and Burkitt lymphoma
  B. B-cell lymphoma, unclassifiable, with features intermediate between diffuse large B-cell lymphoma and classical Hodgkin lymphoma

ALK, anaplastic lymphoma kinase; DLBCL, diffuse large B-cell lymphoma; EBV, Epstein-Barr virus; HHV, human herpes virus.

expression profile. The presence of *p53* mutation in combination with *BCL2* denotes that the tumor is derived from a histologic transformation of a prior follicular lymphoma.[11]

Normally, mutations in the variable region of the Ig genes allow antibody diversity in germinal center B cells. However, aberrant somatic hypermutation occurs in more than 50 percent of cases of DLBCL. This alteration targets multiple loci, including the protooncogenes *PIM1*, *MYC*, *RhoH/TTF* (*ARHH*), and *PAX5*.[9] The c-*MYC* gene rearrangement occurs in 5 to 15 percent of patients with DLBCL.

Gene-expression profiling studies have distinguished three molecular subtypes of DLBCL known as (1) germinal center B-cell–like (GCB), (2) activated B-cell–like (ABC), and (3) primary mediastinal B-cell lymphoma (see Chap. 98).[12–15] GCB DLBCLs may arise from normal germinal center B cells, ABC DLBCLs may arise from postgerminal center B cells that are arrested during plasmacytic differentiation, and primary mediastinal B-cell lymphomas may arise from thymic B cells. These DLBCL subtypes arise by distinct pathogenetic mechanisms, as judged by high-resolution, genome-wide copy-number analysis coupled with gene-expression profiling.[16] An amplicon on chromosome 19 was detected in 26 percent of ABC cases but in only 3 percent of GCB and primary mediastinal B-cell lymphoma cases. A highly upregulated gene in this amplicon was *SPIB*, which encodes an ETS family transcription factor. Deletion of the *INK4a/ARF* tumor-suppressor locus and trisomy 3 occurred almost exclusively in ABC subtypes and was associated with inferior outcome for patients with this subtype. *FOXP1* emerged as a potential oncogene in ABC DLBCL that was upregulated by trisomy 3 and by more focal high-level amplifications. In GCB DLBCL, amplification of the oncogenic miR-17–92 microRNA cluster and deletion of the tumor-suppressor *PTEN* were recurrent, but these events did not occur in ABC-type DLBCL.

CLINICAL FEATURES

Signs and Symptoms

Patients with DLBCL typically present with a rapidly enlarging, symptomatic, lymphatic masses. The typical presentation is of a rapidly enlarging lymph node in the neck or an abdominal mass. B symptoms (drenching night sweats, fever, weight loss) are observed in approximately 30 percent of patients. Extranodal disease occurs in approximately 40 percent of patients, most commonly involving the gastrointestinal tract.[17,18] Other sites that may be affected include the testis, bone, thyroid, salivary glands, skin, liver, breast, nasal cavity, paranasal sinuses, and central nervous system (CNS). DLBCL can be highly invasive, with local compression of vessels (e.g., superior vena cava syndrome) or airways (e.g., tracheobronchial compression) requiring urgent treatment.

Unusual symptoms and presentations may occur with some subtypes of DLBCL, such as intravascular large B-cell lymphoma, which may present with unexplained fever, or pleural cavity lymphoma, which may present with pleural effusions. Approximately 50 to 60 percent of patients present with disseminated DLBCL (stage III or IV), whereas 40 percent have more localized disease (stage I or II). Marrow involvement occurs in approximately 15 percent of patients. Discordant disease in which the lymph nodes are involved with DLBCL but the marrow contains a low-grade lymphoma may occur. This combination is not associated with a poorer prognosis but increases the risk of late relapse. CNS dissemination may occur after testicular or paranasal sinuses involvement.[19] Elevated serum lactic dehydrogenase (LDH) level and marrow involvement are other findings associated with CNS involvement. Patients at high risk for CNS dissemination should undergo an examination of spinal fluid for cells and protein content. Patients with involvement of the Waldeyer ring have an increased risk of gastrointestinal lymphoma.

LABORATORY FEATURES

Blood and Marrow

Lymphoma involvement of the marrow occurs in approximately 10 to 20 percent of cases of DLBCL. Lymphoma cells were present in the blood in about one-third of those cases with marrow involvement, based on examination of blood films. Presumably these percentages would increase if a more sensitive assay was used, such as flow cytometry. Marrow involvement may lead to anemia, and in severe cases to moderate degrees of leucopenia and thrombocytopenia. Of course, this may worsen as effects of cytotoxic therapy ensue.

Cell Immunophenotype

The malignant cells have surface monoclonal Ig of either κ or λ light-chain type. The most commonly expressed surface Ig is IgM. Less commonly, the cells are negative for surface Ig.[20] The lymphoma cells generally express the pan-B-cell antigens, CD19, CD20, CD22, PAX5, and CD79a. They also express CD45 and, less commonly, CD10 or CD5.[20,21] The CD5+ lymphomas may be more aggressive with a worse prognosis.[22] CD10+ DLBCL may be difficult to distinguish from Burkitt lymphoma or from follicular lymphoma when it is composed of many large cells (i.e., higher-grade follicular lymphoma).[23] When a mature CD10+ B-cell phenotype is identified by flow cytometry, distinction between these possibilities should be further evaluated by morphology.

Histopathology

The lymph node is usually effaced by a diffuse infiltrate of large lymphocytes. The cytologic patterns may be varied and are referred to as centroblastic, immunoblastic, and anaplastic depending on the size, the number of nucleoli, the basophilia of the cytoplasm, and the presence of bizarre and pleomorphic nuclei. Other rare morphologic variants occur, for example, with a myxoid or fibrillary appearances. Although on histologic sections, the diffuse growth pattern of DLBCL can be distinguished from the nodular growth pattern of follicular lymphoma, this distinction is often not possible in fine-needle aspirate, body fluid, blood, or marrow specimens (see Chap. 98, Figs. 98–23 and 98–24). In addition, follicular lymphoma and DLBCL overlap in their genotype as the translocation t(14;18)(q32;q21) is identified in approximately 20 percent of DLBCL and most cases of follicular lymphoma (see Chap. 101).

The cells in DLBCL undergo Ig variable-region gene rearrangement and are commonly somatically mutated. Isotype switch variants may occur.[24] Adhesion molecules such as LFA-1 (leukocyte function-associated antigen-1; CD16/CD18) and CD44 are expressed in 50 to 75 percent of cases of DLBCL. CD44 is expressed in highly aggressive subsets of DLBCL and is associated with disseminated disease and a poor prognosis.[25]

PROGNOSTIC FACTORS

International Prognostic Index

In 1993, a model was proposed to assign a prognosis to patients with aggressive lymphoma undergoing treatment with doxorubicin-containing chemotherapeutic regimens termed the *international prognostic index* (IPI).[26,27] The model used clinical data, including (1) tumor stage, (2) serum LDH level, (3) number of extranodal disease sites involved, (4) performance status, and (5) patient age. This model resulted in the IPI, which is used to forecast the behavior of aggressive lymphoma (Table 100–2). For patients younger than age 60 years, an age-adjusted IPI has been proposed in which all the factors of the IPI are used, except for age and presence of extranodal sites. The 5-year survival rates for patients age 60 years or younger with IPI scores of 0, 1, 2, and 3 were 83, 69, 46, and 32 percent, respectively (Table 100–3 and Fig. 100–1).[26]

TABLE 100–2. International Prognostic Factor Index for Non-Hodgkin Lymphoma

Risk Factors
Age >60 years
Serum lactic dehydrogenase greater than twice normal
Performance status ≥2
Stage III or IV
Extranodal involvement at >1 site

Each factor accounts for 1 point, for a total score that ranges from 0 to 3 for patients <61 years of age. The latter age-adjusted index includes all variables except for age and extranodal sites. For patients ≥61 years of age, a total score ranges from 0 to 5 and includes each variable shown in this table.

Gene-Expression Profiling

Gene-expression profiling has also been used to delineate groups of patients with DLBCL who may differ in their response to therapy and prognosis (Fig. 100–2).[28,29] Six genes identified by gene-expression analysis and detected by quantitative real-time polymerase chain reaction can identify three prognostic groups in patients with DLBCL (Fig. 100–3).[30,31] The six genes that were used in this model occur in the germinal center B-cell signature *(LMO2, BCL6)*, activated B-cell signature (*BCL2, CCND2, SCYA3*), and lymph node signature (*FN1*). In this study, expression of *LMO2*, *BCL6*, and *FN1* correlated with prolonged survival, whereas expression of *BCL2*, *CCND2*, and *SCYA3* correlated with short survival.

Serum Lactic Dehydrogenase and β_2-Microglobulin

Patients with an elevated β_2-microglobulin level and high serum LDH have a poor prognosis, with a 26 percent survival compared to 81 percent survival in patients without elevation of these markers.[32]

BCL6 Protein Expression

Approximately 70 percent of DLBCL cases are of germinal center origin, as demonstrated by BCL6 protein overexpression. Patients with a germinal center B-cell pattern have a more favorable prognosis than do patients with the postgerminal center gene-expression pattern.[33] The

TABLE 100–3. Outcome According to Risk Group Defined by the International Prognostic Index

International Index	No. of Risk Factors	Complete Response Rate (%)	Relapse-Free Survival (%)		Survival (%)	
Age-Adjusted International Prognostic Index, Patients >60 Years of Age						
			2-Year	5-Year	2-Year	5-Year
Low	0 or 1	87	79	70	84	73
Low-intermediate	2	67	66	50	66	51
High-intermediate	3	55	59	49	54	43
High	4 or 5	44	58	40	34	26
Age-Adjusted International Index, Patients <61 Years of Age						
			2-Year	5-Year	2-Year	5-Year
Low	0	92	88	86	90	83
Low-intermediate	1	78	74	66	79	69
High-intermediate	2	57	62	53	59	46
High	3	46	61	58	37	32

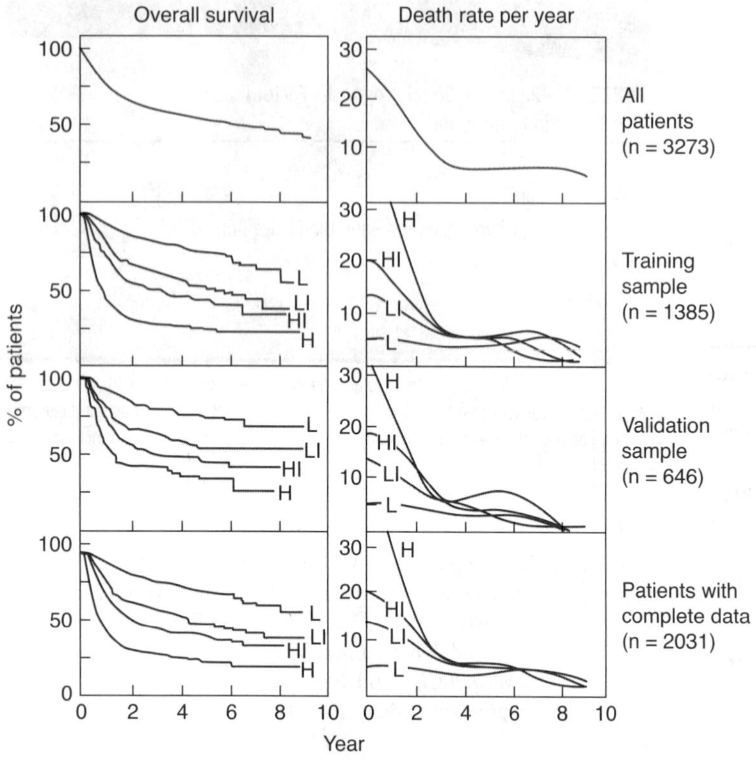

FIGURE 100–1. (*Left panels*) Kaplan-Meier survival curves for the four risk groups. (*Right panels*) Death rates during the study period. Only 2031 of the 3273 patients had sufficient relevant information for classification according to the international index. H, high risk; HI, high-intermediate risk; L, low risk; LI, low-intermediate risk.

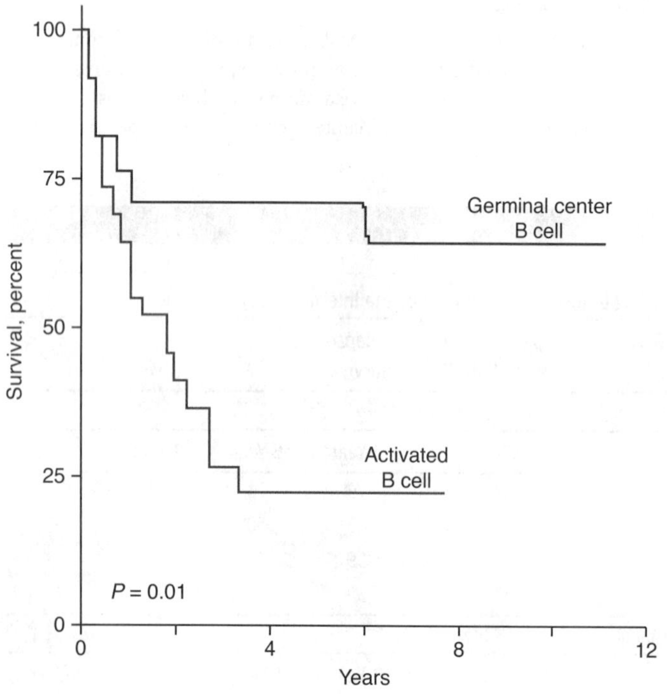

FIGURE 100–2. Overall survival in a group of patients with diffuse large B-cell lymphoma whose cell of origin was determined by gene-expression profiling. Survival of patients with diffuse large B-cell lymphoma whose malignant cells were thought to arise from a germinal center B cell was significantly better than in patients whose cell of origin arose from activated B cells.

BCL2 gene rearrangement or BCL2 protein expression is associated with a poor prognosis,[34] whereas the presence of *BCL6* denotes a better prognosis.[28–30]

Lymphoma Cell Survivin

Survivin, a member of the inhibitor-of-apoptosis gene family, is not expressed in normal tissue but is expressed in 60 percent of patients with DLBCL and is associated with a poor prognosis.[35]

Infiltrating CD4+ T Cells

The high number of infiltrating CD4+ T cells in DLBCL is associated with a better prognosis.[36] However, T-cell-histiocyte-rich B-cell lymphoma is not a favorable phenotype.

Cyclin D3 Expression, p53 Gene Mutation, Serum Vascular Endothelial Growth Factor, Cytokine Elaboration

Cyclin D3 expression, *p53* gene mutation, and expression of serum vascular endothelial growth factor or elevation in plasma cytokines such as interleukin (IL)-2, IL-10, and IL-6 has been associated with a poor prognosis.

Positron Emission Tomography

Fluorine-18-fluorodeoxyglucose-positron emission tomography (FDG-PET) is used for staging and following patients with DLBCL. FDG-PET was reported to be a useful tool to predict outcomes of therapy.[37–39] However, a meta-analysis of 13 studies that included 311 patients with DLBCL found discrepancies in the ability of this modality to prognosticate.[40] This meta-analysis concluded that FDG-PET remains an unproven test for clinical practice, proposing that it should be reserved for research settings when regimens and imaging conditions are standardized.

THERAPY

General Considerations

DLBCL is potentially curable with combination chemotherapy (see Figure 100–4). The dose administered during the first 12 weeks of therapy determines survival; therefore, reduction of chemotherapy doses should be avoided, if at all possible. Before therapy is instituted, several factors should be considered, including the patient's clinical stage, symptoms, and the IPI. In addition, response should be evaluated according to the defined criteria. Other considerations, such as the patient's age and comorbid conditions, are important before a therapeutic intervention is selected. Future trials and therapies may be individualized according to subgroups of DLBCL based on gene expression patterns.

Early Stage Diffuse Large B-Cell Lymphoma (Stages I and II)

Localized disease occurs in approximately 25 percent of patients. In the early 1980s, the standard of care was radiation therapy.[41] Historically, the 5-year disease-free survival with radiation therapy in stage I disease was 50 percent and in stage II disease was approximately 20 percent. Combining chemotherapy with radiation therapy improved the outcome.[42–47] The addition of chemotherapy prior to radiation resulted in improved control of local and disseminated disease. The role of chemotherapy alone has been studied in several randomized trials.

A Southwest Oncology Group study randomly assigned 401 patients with stage I and nonbulky stage II disease to receive either eight cycles of cyclophosphamide, hydroxydaunorubicin, Oncovin (vincristine), and

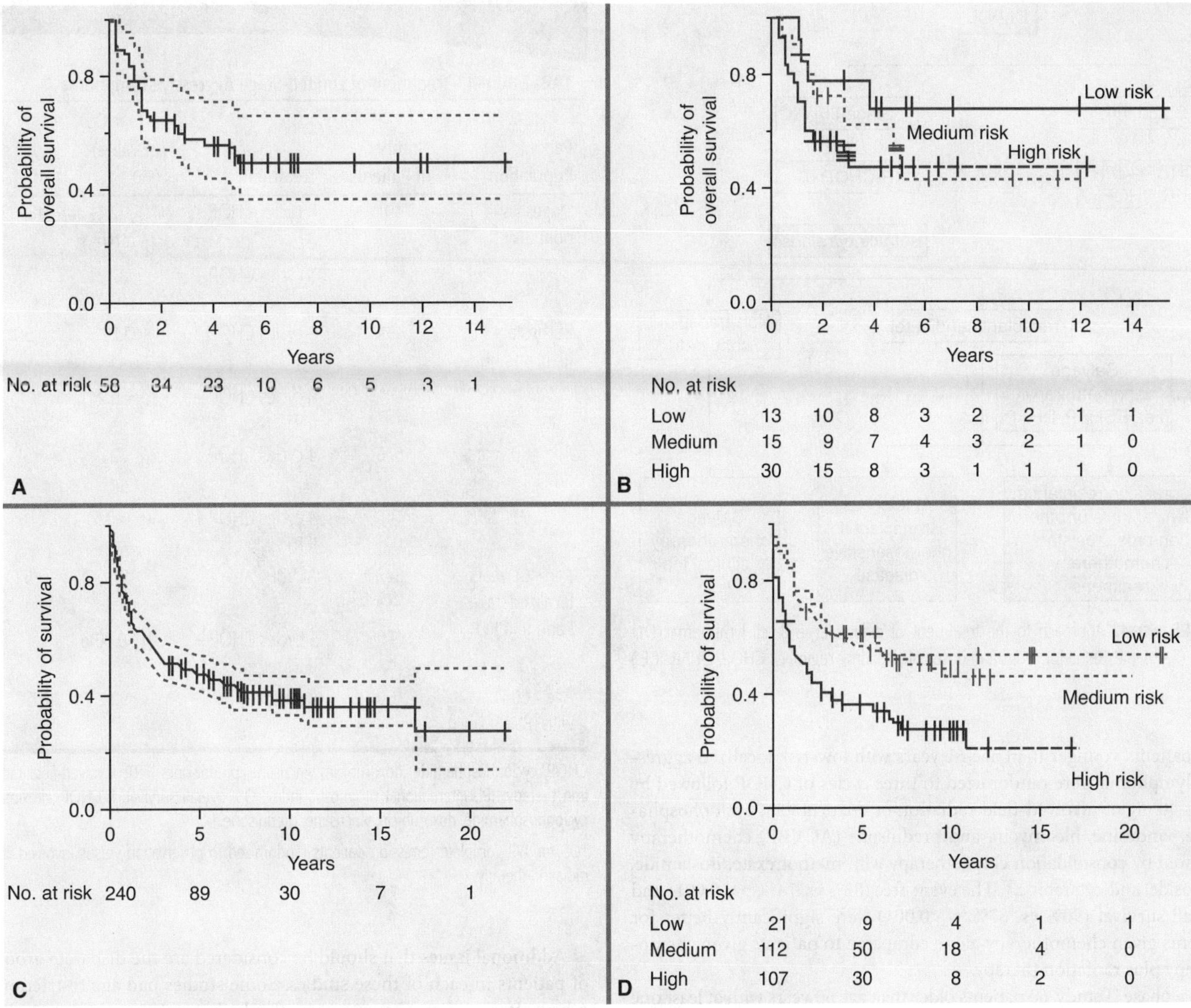

FIGURE 100–3. A. Kaplan-Meier estimates of overall survival in all 58 patients with diffuse large B-cell lymphoma (DLBCL).[19] **B.** Kaplan-Meier estimates of overall survival in the 58 patients after subdivision into three groups (low, medium, and high risk of death) based on the six-gene model for prediction. *Dotted lines* represent 95% confidence intervals. According to log likelihood estimates, $P = 0.02$ for the model as a continuous variable and $P = 0.31$ for the model as a class. **C, D.** Similar analyses of the data on the 240 patients with DLBCL.[44] $P < 0.001$ for the model based on a continuous variable and for the model based on the three discrete groups shown in the figure.

prednisone (CHOP) chemotherapy or three cycles of CHOP plus involved-field radiotherapy (Table 100–4).[48] The 5-year overall and progression-free survival rates of the patients treated with the combined modality were significantly better (82% and 72%, respectively, p = 0.02) compared to patients treated with chemotherapy alone (77% and 64%, respectively, p = 0.03). Cardiac toxicity was greater in patients treated with 8 cycles of CHOP without radiation therapy. A subanalysis using modified IPI criteria showed that patients with poor risk factors had a worse overall survival. The failure-free survival curves overlapped at 7 years and the overall survival (OS) curves overlapped at 9 years. The treatment advantage of CHOP plus involved-field radiation for the first 7 years diminished as a result of lymphoma recurrence between 5 and 10 years.[49]

In an Eastern Cooperative Group (ECOG) trial involving 399 patients with bulky stage I (mediastinal or retroperitoneal mass, or a mass >10 cm), stage IE, stage II, or stage IIE disease, patients were randomized to receive either eight cycles of CHOP alone or eight cycles of CHOP with involved-field radiation.[50] Patients in complete remission received 30 Gy of involved-field radiation or no therapy. Patients with partial remission received 40 Gy to the involved field and radiation to the contiguous noninvolved regions. Among 172 complete remission (CR) patients, the 6-year disease-free survival (DFS) was 73 percent for low-dose involved-field radiation versus 56 percent for CHOP followed by observation only (p = 0.05) without a survival difference between the two arms. At 6 years, failure-free survival was 63 percent in patients in partial remission (PR) and conversion to CR with high-dose radiation therapy did not influence outcome. For the patient in CR after eight cycles of CHOP, low-dose involved-field radiation prolonged DFS and provided local control, but did not influence survival. The majority of PR patients were event free at 6 years despite residual radiographic abnormalities.

In a Group d'Etade des Lymphomes de l'Adulte (GELA) study, 576 patients older than age 60 years with stages I and II disease and an IPI score of 0 were randomized to four cycles of CHOP with or without involved-field radiation (40 Gy).[51] The 5-year event-free survival was 61 percent for patients treated with CHOP compared to 64 percent for patients treated with CHOP plus involved-field radiation, and the overall survival was 72 and 68 percent, respectively. In another GELA study,

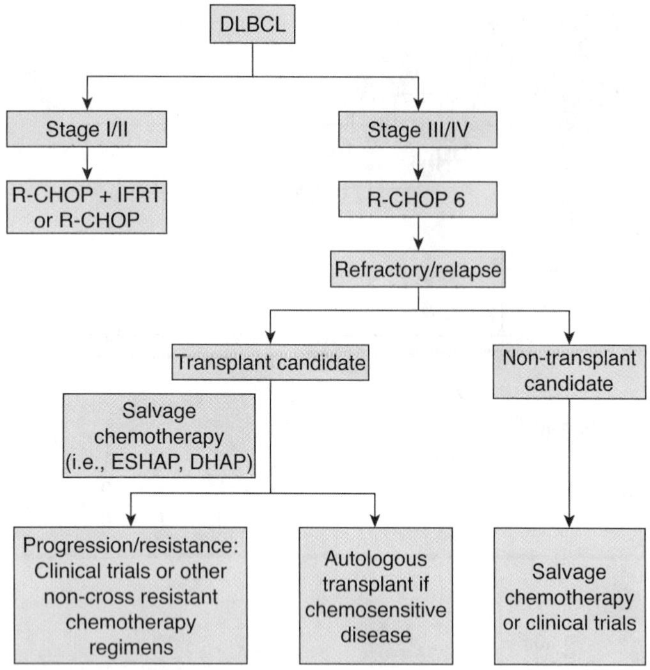

FIGURE 100–4. Approach to the treatment of diffuse large B-cell lymphoma (DLBCL). (See Table 100–3 for drugs and doses of multidrug regimens CHOP, DHAP, ICE.)

TABLE 100–4. Treatment of Limited-Stage Aggressive Lymphoma

Patient Population	Number of Patients	Treatment	5-Year OS (p value) (%)	Ref.
Stages I and II, nonbulky	401	8 cycles CHOP	72	48, 49
		vs.	(p = 0.05)	
		3 cycles CHOP + IFRT	82	
Bulky stages I, IE, II, and IIE	399	8 cycles CHOP	73*	50
		vs.	87	
		8 cycles CHOP + IFRT	(p = 0.24)	
Age >60 years, IPI O	576	4 cycles CHOP	72	51
		vs.	68	
		4 cycles CHOP + IFRT	(p = 0.5)	
Age <61 years, localized stages I and II, IPI O	647	ACVBP	90	52
		vs.	87	
		3 cycles CHOP + IFRT	(p <0.001)	
Age >60 years with IPI >O	60	R-CHOP + IFRT	92	58

CHOP, cyclophosphamide, doxorubicin, vincristine, prednisone; IFRT, involved-field radiation therapy; IPI, international prognostic index; OS, overall survival; R-CHOP, rituximab, cyclophosphamide, doxorubicin, vincristine, prednisone.

*OS for 172 complete remission patients randomized to observation versus involved-field radiation therapy.

647 patients younger than age 61 years with low-risk localized aggressive lymphoma were randomized to three cycles of CHOP followed by 30 to 40 Gy of involved-field radiation or doxorubicin, cyclophosphamide, vindesine, bleomycin, and prednisone (ACVBP) chemotherapy followed by consolidation chemotherapy with methotrexate, ifosfamide, etoposide, and cytarabine.[52] The event-free (82% vs. 74%, p = 0.001) and overall survival (90% vs. 87%, p <0.001) were significantly better for patients given chemotherapy alone compared to patients given chemotherapy plus radiation therapy.

In a phase II study, 60 patients older than age 60 years with at least one adverse risk factor as defined by the IPI received rituximab on days −7, 1, 22, and 43, and CHOP on days 3, 24, and 45.[53] This therapy was followed by 40 to 46 Gy involved-field radiation. Progression-free survival (PFS) was 95 percent at 2 years and 88 percent at 4 years, and OS was 95 percent at 2 years and 92 percent at 4 years. PFS and OS for historical controls not treated with rituximab was 78 percent and 88 percent at 4 years, respectively. The addition of rituximab to three cycles of CHOP plus involved-field radiation met prespecified study criteria of efficacy.

Systemic chemotherapy has improved the outcome in patients with localized aggressive lymphoma. These studies bring into question the role of involved-field radiation. Early data suggested a significant OS benefit for CHOP plus involved-field radiation compared to CHOP alone,[48] but followup data revealed overlap of the failure-free survival curves at 7 years and the OS curves at 9 years.[54] A randomized study in patients younger than age 61 years with an IPI of zero showed an OS advantage for patients who received dose-intense ACVBP compared to those who received three cycles of CHOP plus involved-field radiation.[52] Two other randomized studies using either four or eight cycles of CHOP versus the same cycles of CHOP plus involved-field radiation suggested that there was no survival advantage if radiation was included.[50,51] A phase II study of 60 patients younger than age 60 years with an IPI greater than zero who were treated with three cycles of R-CHOP plus involved-field radiation had a 4-year OS of 92 percent, which was superior to any of the randomized studies.[52]

Additional issues that should be considered are the disparate groups of patients in each of these studies. Some studies had age restrictions, others were restricted to patients with a high-risk IPI, and other studies included only patients with a low-risk IPI. Likely, low-risk patients with localized disease will do very well with any of these therapy options, and the critical question is how to approach the moderate-risk and high-risk patients. Rituximab has changed the therapeutic paradigm in advanced DLBCL and likely will impact therapy in localized disease as suggested in a phase II study.[53] Randomized studies will be required to address these issues, including whether high-dose, intensive chemotherapy without radiation therapy should be the treatment of choice in patients younger than age 61 years based on the results of one study.[52] High-dose intensive chemotherapy is not used in advanced DLBCL and cannot be recommended outside of the clinical research setting. Until further data from randomized studies is available, either six cycles of rituximab, cyclophosphamide, doxorubicin, vincristine, and prednisone (R-CHOP) or three cycles of R-CHOP plus involved-fields radiation therapy in localized DLBCL is recommended.

Advanced Stage Diffuse Large B-cell Lymphoma (Bulky Stages I and II or III and IV)

Combination chemotherapy (mechlorethamine, vincristine, procarbazine, prednisone [MOPP]) proved so successful for treatment of Hodgkin lymphoma that this approach was used for treatment of DLBCL with CHOP and cyclophosphamide, vincristine, procarbazine, and prednisone (C-MOPP; synonym: COPP).[54] Between 1972 and 1975, reports of complete remission with long-lasting progression-free survival marked the beginning of cures in patients with DLBCL. Cyclophosphamide 750 mg/m^2 IV, doxorubicin 50 mg/m^2 IV, vincristine 1.4 mg/m^2 with a maximum of 2 mg, and prednisone 100 mg orally administered daily for days 1 through 5 of each cycle (CHOP) became the most popular regimen in the United States for treatment of DLBCL (Table 100–5). Cycles are repeated every 21 days. CHOP has been administered in other modified regimens with a day 1 and day 8 schedule and variable doses of prednisone. Patients receive four to six cycles, and those who achieve complete remission subsequently receive two more cycles. Most complete responders achieve durable relapse-free survival, depending on the prognostic factors.

Based on the success of CHOP chemotherapy, several combination chemotherapy regimens were developed. Many showed dramatic improvement in the response rates in phase II clinical trials, with up to 80 percent complete remissions and 60 percent prolonged disease-free survival.[55,56] Phase II trials of m-BACOD (moderate-dose methotrexate, bleomycin, doxorubicin, cyclophosphamide, vincristine, dexamethasone), ProMACE (prednisone, methotrexate, doxorubicin, cyclophosphamide, etoposide)/CytaBOM (cytarabine, bleomycin, vincristine, methotrexate), and MACOP-B (high-dose methotrexate, doxorubicin, cyclophosphamide, vincristine, prednisone, bleomycin) showed superior responses compared to the results with CHOP chemotherapy.[57] However, the significant responses that were demonstrated in single-institutional studies could not be repeated in multiinstitutional studies and were not as significant when reanalyzed after 2 years of observation. A prospective randomized study that compared m-BACOD with CHOP showed no difference in the complete remission rates, disease-free survival, or overall survival.[58] Because of these conflicting data, a four-arm phase III study was conducted and enrolled patients in a randomized prospective trial comparing CHOP, m-BACOD, MACOP-B, and ProMACE/CytaBOM.[59] This landmark trial enrolled 897 patients with intermediate- or high-grade lymphoma, of whom 85 percent had diffuse or follicular large-cell lymphoma. In the trial, each of these regimens produced equivalent results. The disease-free survival was 35 to 40 percent of patients: a 4-year survival of 36 percent in the patients who received CHOP, 34 percent in the m-BACOD group, 45 percent in those treated with ProMACE/CytaBOM, and 39 percent in the MACOP-B group ($p = 0.14$). CHOP chemotherapy was the safest regimen, with only 1 percent fatality from drug toxicity compared to 6 percent fatality in the MACOP-B arms. The improved complete response rates in the single-institution phase II clinical trial largely resulted from enrollment of patients with favorable IPI scores. The more intensive regimens offered no improvement in the remission rate, disease-free survival, and overall survival. The IPI was developed in part to allow comparison of the subgroups of patients in the different clinical trials so that accurate assessments of the chemotherapy regimens could be made. However, long-term followup and studies conducted in very young patients have shown advantages to regimens different from CHOP in selected groups of patients.[60]

Other regimens that were developed but which did not show improvement over CHOP chemotherapy include the CVAD regimen (infusional CHOP),[61] CHOPE (CHOP plus etoposide; also known as CHOEP) in escalating doses along with growth factors,[62] and infusional CDE (cyclophosphamide, doxorubicin, etoposide) along with growth factors.[63] In one phase III study of 143 patients with aggressive lymphoma, randomized patients were to receive six cycles of either CHOP or intensified CNOP (cyclophosphamide, mitoxantrone, vincristine, prednisone; i.e., CHOP with doxorubicin replaced by mitoxantrone). The response rate, 5-year progression-free survival, and overall survival did not differ between the two groups. Intensified CNOP was associated with more leukopenia, febrile episodes, and secondary leukemia.[64]

Thus for patients with a good IPI score (0–2), current therapeutic regimens are effective, whereas for patients with poor prognostic factors (IPI 3–5), current therapy seems to be inadequate. One regimen was designed by the United States National Cancer Institute based on *in vitro* data that showed tumor cells had relatively less resistance with prolonged low concentration exposure to vincristine, doxorubicin, and etoposide than with brief higher concentration exposure.[65] These investigators designed a regimen that included etoposide, because of its single-agent activity and its *in vitro* synergy, with prednisone, vincristine, cyclophosphamide, and doxorubicin (EPOCH). They administered vincristine, etoposide, and doxorubicin as a continuous intravenous infusion over 96 hours. EPOCH was initially evaluated in 131 patients with relapsed or refractory lymphoma and demonstrated a 74 percent overall response rate and tolerable toxicity.[66] Pharmacokinetics demonstrated interpatient variability and suggested the need for dose adjustment in individual patients.[67] This led to incorporation of a dose-adjustment strategy based on hematopoietic nadir.[68] Fifty patients with previously untreated DLBCL were treated with dose-adjusted EPOCH and demonstrated complete responses of 92 percent with PFS and OS of 70 and 73 percent, respectively. In another trial, 72 patients with untreated DLBCL were treated with dose-adjusted EPOCH and rituximab with 5-year PFS and OS of 79 percent and 80 percent, respectively.[69] Based on. historical controls, the addition of rituximab only benefited BCL2–positive patients.

In a 2 × 2 factorial design by the German (Deutsch) High-Grade Non-Hodgkin's Lymphoma Study Group (DSHNHL), the question of whether the addition of etoposide to the CHOP regimen or the reduction of treatment intervals from 3 to 2 weeks would improve outcome of young good prognosis patients.[70] They concluded that CHOEP (cyclophosphamide, doxorubicin, vincristine, prednisone, and etoposide) was significantly better than CHOP with respect to the primary endpoint of event-free survival, while the reduction of treatment intervals from 3 to 2 weeks resulted in a significantly better OS. When the three intensified regimens—CHOP every 2 weeks (CHOP-14), CHOE (cyclophosphamide, doxorubicin, vincristine, and etoposide) every 3 weeks (CHOE-21), and CHOEP given every 2 weeks (CHOEP-14)—were compared with standard CHOP every three weeks (CHOP-21) regimen, CHOEP-21 improved EFS while CHOEP-14 improved event-free survival (EFS), CR rates and OS over baseline CHOP-21. Consequently, CHOEP-14 became the preferred chemotherapy regimen for young patients with a good prognosis by this group of investigators.

The Monoclonal AntibodyTherapeutic International Trial (MInT) Group trial addressed the role of rituximab in young patients.[71] A total of 824 patients with a good prognosis with an age-adjusted IPI of 0 or 1 and stage II to IV disease or stage I with bulky disease were randomized to receive 6 cycles of a CHOP-like regimens or the same regimen plus rituximab given on day 1 of each chemotherapy cycle. Patients with bulky disease received additional radiotherapy to the those areas. After a median observation time of 2 years, the addition of rituximab increased EFS from 61 percent to 80 percent ($p = 0.000000007$) and OS from 86 percent to 95 percent ($p = 0.0002$). These results suggest that 6 cycles of rituximab with a CHOP-like regimen is the best therapy for young patients with good-prognosis DLBCL. Subset analysis suggested that patients with IPI of zero and no bulky disease represent a very favorable subgroup with a 2-year EFS of 90 percent, whereas patients with an age-adjusted IPI of 1 and/or bulky disease represent a less-favorable subgroup with only 77 percent 2-year EFS. The 2-year OS was 97 percent and 90 percent, respectively.

The Dutch-Belgian Hemato-Oncology Cooperative Group tested intensified 12-week CHOP (I-CHOP) compared with standard 24-week CHOP in intermediate-risk DLBCL.[72] The low-intermediate-risk patients had improved OS (67% vs. 52%, $p = 0.05$), DFS (58% vs. 45%, $p = 0.06$), and EFS (41% vs. 30%, $p = 0.21$) when they were treated with I-CHOP compared with standard CHOP. High-intermediate-risk patients did not benefit from I-CHOP. Their data suggest I-CHOP

TABLE 100–5. Combination Chemotherapy for Intermediate- and High-Grade Lymphoma

Regimen	Dose	Route	Days of Treatment	Interval between Treatment Cycles (Days)	Cycles
R-CHOP-21					
Rituximab	375 mg/m^2	IV	1	21	6–8
Cyclophosphamide	750 mg/m^2	IV	1		
Doxorubicin	50 mg/m^2	IV	1		
Vincristine	1.4 mg/m^2	IV	1		
Prednisone	100 mg/day	PO	1–5		
CHOP-14					
Cyclophosphamide	750 mg/m^2	IV	1	14	6–8
Doxorubicin	50 mg/m^2	IV	1		
Vincristine	1.4 mg/m^2	IV	1		
Prednisone	100 mg/day	PO	1–5		
I-CHOP					
Cyclophosphamide	1000 mg/m^2	IV	1	14	6
Doxorubicin	70 mg/m^2	IV			
Vincristine	2 mg	IV	1		
Prednisone	100 mg	PO	1–5		
CHOPE-21					
Cyclophosphamide	750 mg/m^2	IV	1	21	6–8
Doxorubicin	50 mg/m^2	IV	1		
Vincristine	2 mg/m^2	IV	1		
Etoposide	100 mg/m^2	IV	1–3		
Prednisone	100 mg/day	PO	1–5		
Dose-Adjusted R-EPOCH*					
Rituximab	375 mg/m^2	IV	1	21	6–8
Etoposide	50 mg/m^2/day	CIV	1–4 (96 hours)		
Doxorubicin	10 mg/m^2/day	CIV	1–4 (96 hours)		
Vincristine	0.4 mg/day	CIV	1–4 (96 hours)		
Cyclophosphamide	750 mg/m^2/day	IV	5		
Prednisone	60 mg/m^2/day	PO	1–5		
ESHAP (for relapsed lymphoma)					
Etoposide	40 mg/m^2	IV	1–4	21	
Methylprednisone	500 mg/m^2	IV	1–5		
Cytarabine	2 mg/m^2	IV	5		
Cisplatin	25 mg/m^2	CIV	1–4		
DHAP (for relapsed l lymphoma)					
Dexamethasone	40 mg/m^2	PO or IV	1–4	21	
Cisplatin	100 mg/m^2	CIV	1		
Cytarabine	2 mg/m^2	IVq12h × 2 doses	2		
R±ICE (for relapsed lymphoma)					
Rituximab	375 mg/m^2	IV	1	14	
Mesna	5000 mg/m^2	IV	l (day 2)		
Carboplatin	AUC = 5 (maximum 800 mg)	IV	1 (day 2)		
Etoposide	100 mg/m^2	IV	1–3		
Neulasta	6 mg	SQ	1 (day 4)		

AUC, area under the curve; CIV, continuous intravenous infusion; I-CHOP, intensified-CHOP; IV, intravenously; PO, by mouth; SQ, subcutaneously.

*Doses of etoposide, doxorubicin, and cyclophosphamide are increased 20% over the dose in the previous cycle if the nadir of the absolute neutrophil count in the previous cycle was ≥0.5 × 10^9/L.

The reader is advised to verify drugs, doses, and administration schedules of these regimens.

might be preferable to standard CHOP in younger patients with low-intermediate-risk DLBCL.

R-CHOP continues to be the standard of care for younger patients with DLBCL. Six cycles of R-CHOP is recommended. In a large European study named the "Rituximab with CHOP over age 60 years" (RICOVER-60) trial of elderly patients (discussed in "Chemotherapy in Patients Older Than Age 60 Years" below) there was no benefit to eight cycles of R-CHOP-14 over six cycles of R-CHOP-14.[73] Whether dose-adjusted R-EPOCH or dose-intensified R-CHOP or R-CHOEP for any subgroup of patients will prove to be superior to standard R-CHOP will require prospective randomized studies.

Chemotherapy in Patients Older Than Age 60 Years

More than half of patients diagnosed with DLBCL are older than age 60 years. Although many of these patients are as healthy as younger adults and may be treated in a similar fashion as younger patients, some older patients either are too frail or are not willing to accept highly aggressive therapeutic interventions. Patients older than age 60 years with a low or low-intermediate IPI have a worse relapse-free and overall survival rate than younger patients. This status may result from the less-aggressive therapeutic interventions often administered or from comorbid diseases (e.g., diabetes, renal, pulmonary, and cardiac disease).[74] Death may result from an unrelated comorbid condition or treatment-related complications. Several studies have attempted to modify therapy specifically for older patients.[75,76]

In an attempt to decrease the toxicity of chemotherapy in elderly patients, a randomized trial compared standard CHOP to weekly CHOP in which the dose of CHOP chemotherapy was divided into thirds and each dose was given once per week for 3 weeks, rather than one dose given every 3 weeks.[77] Patients who received the weekly dose had no difference in rates of complete response and progression-free survival, but they had a worse overall survival compared to the group that received standard CHOP therapy. The DSHNHL study showed that older patients might benefit from treatment with a higher dose of CHOP chemotherapy.[70,78] In a randomized trial of six cycles of standard CHOP-21 compared to six cycles of CHOP-14 along with growth factor support and radiotherapy to bulky disease, the complete response rate was 63 percent versus 77 percent for CHOP-21 and CHOP-14, respectively. In patients with elevated serum LDH, the complete response was 49 percent versus 70 percent, respectively. In the older patients, addition of etoposide did not improve the response rate.[78] This result contrasts with the results of the same study in younger patients, in whom the addition of etoposide (CHOPE) resulted in an improved response rate. Several studies have compared treatment with CHOP to treatment with an alternative regimen substituting mitoxantrone for doxorubicin.[79–81] These studies indicted that treatment with CHOP was superior. A Scandinavian study randomized 455 patients to treatment with CHOP versus CHOP plus or minus growth factor support. The complete remission rate (60% vs. 43%), time to treatment failure, and overall survival rate were higher in patients treated with the CHOP regimen.[79] These results were similar to a Dutch study that demonstrated the complete remission rate (49% vs. 31%) and the 3-year overall survival rate (42% vs. 26%) were higher in patients treated with CHOP.[80]

The GELA conducted a randomized trial in 399 patients ages 60 to 80 years with newly diagnosed DLBCL[82,83] who were treated with eight cycles of CHOP-21 or the same chemotherapy plus eight infusions of rituximab. The combination of CHOP and rituximab significantly improved complete response rate from 63 to 76 percent, EFS from 38 to 57 percent, as well as OS from 57 to 70 percent compared to CHOP-21. There were no differences in toxicity, with treatment-related mortality of 6 percent in both arms.

In an ECOG trial, 632 older patients were treated with six to eight cycles of CHOP-21 and randomized to the same chemotherapy plus five infusions of rituximab.[84] The results confirmed the positive results of the GELA trial for the addition of rituximab to CHOP for time to treatment failure and OS in this elderly patient population. A second randomization in this trial suggested that patients who received rituximab with CHOP did not benefit from maintenance rituximab therapy.

In the RICOVER-60 study, 1222 elderly patients were randomized to six or eight cycles of CHOP-14 or six to eight cycles of R-CHOP-14.[73] Six cycles of R-CHOP-14 significantly improved EFS, PFS, and OS over six cycles of CHOP-14. There was no benefit to eight cycles of R-CHOP-14 over six cycles of R-CHOP-14.

Based on the data from these three studies, six cycles of R-CHOP is the optimal treatment for older patients with DLBCL. Superiority of R-CHOP-14 over R-CHOP-21 has not been addressed to date. It is generally recommended to support older patients with G-CSF.[79,85,86]

Role of High-Dose Chemotherapy and Autologous Stem Cell Transplantation in Initial Therapy

High-dose chemotherapy with autologous stem cell transplantation (ASCT) has been effective in relapsed or refractory aggressive lymphomas. However, conflicting results of ASCT as part of initial treatment have been reported.[87–93] A meta-analysis evaluated the role of high-dose chemotherapy with ASCT as part of initial treatment.[94] Fifteen randomized control trials including 3079 patients were eligible for this meta-analysis. Overall treatment-related mortality was 6 percent in the ASCT group, which was not significantly different than with conventional chemotherapy. Thirteen studies including 2018 patients showed significantly higher CR rates in the group receiving ASCT ($p = 0.004$). However, ASCT did not have an effect on overall survival, when compared to conventional chemotherapy. Subgroup analysis of prognostic groups according to IPI did not show any survival difference between ASCT and chemotherapy alone in 12 trials. Event-free survival also showed no significant difference between ASCT and conventional chemotherapy.

High-dose chemotherapy and ASCT is not recommended for newly diagnosed DLBCL; a subgroup of patients with poor prognostic features may benefit from such aggressive therapy and it should be considered principally in the context of a clinical trial. Abbreviated courses of chemotherapy prior to transplantation are not beneficial, and patients should receive a full course of standard chemotherapy and achieve a maximum response prior to transplantation.

Recurrent and Refractory Diffuse Large B-Cell Lymphoma

Chemotherapy Despite major advances in initial treatment of advanced DLBCL a substantial proportion of patients are either refractory or will relapse after chemotherapy. Relapse usually occurs within the first 2 to 3 years after diagnosis, but is uncommon after 4 years of diagnosis.[95] Cure of relapsed or refractory patients may first require response to a differently configured regimen followed by ASCT. Several such regimens have been evaluated in refractory and relapsed DLBCL with response rates up to 60 percent; none of these regimens has been proven to be the preferred regimen. In addition, the use of single agents, such as etoposide,[96] cisplatin,[97] mitoxantrone,[98] lenalidomide,[99] and paclitaxel,[100] result in response rates from 20 to 40 percent; however, responses to monotherapy are generally not long lasting.

A prospective phase II study of etoposide, vincristine, and doxorubicin given over 96 hours with bolus cyclophosphamide and oral prednisone (EPOCH) was examined in 131 patients with relapsed or resistant lymphoma.[66] In 125 assessable patients, 29 (23%) achieved complete responses and 60 (48%) achieved partial responses. Among 42 patients with resistant disease, 57 percent responded, and in 28 patients with relapsed lymphomas, 89 percent responded with 54 percent complete responses. With a median followup of 76 months, the overall and event-free survivals were 17.5 and 7 months, respectively. In 33 patients with sensitive aggressive disease who did not receive ASCT, EFS was 19 percent at 36 months.

The addition of rituximab to the ifosfamide-carboplatin-etoposide (ICE) chemotherapy regimen (R-ICE) increased the CR rate of patients with relapsed or primary refractory DLBCL under consideration for ASCT.[101] The CR rate was 53 percent, significantly better than the 27 percent CR rate ($p = 0.01$) achieved among 147 similar consecutive historical control patients with DLBCL treated with ICE. Progression-free survival for patients who underwent transplantation after R-ICE was marginally better than those of 95 consecutive historical control patients who underwent transplantation after ICE (54% vs. 43%).

A prospective study of 122 patients with relapsed and refractory adult lymphoma patients evaluated the role of etoposide, methylprednisolone, cytarabine, and cisplatin (ESHAP).[102] Forty-five patients (37%) attained a complete remission and 33 (27%) attained a partial remission, for a total response rate of 64 percent. The median duration of CR was 20 months, with 28 percent in CR at 3 years. The overall median survival duration was 14 months; the survival rate at 3 years was 31 percent. Overall time to treatment failure found 10 percent of all patients to be alive and disease free at 40 months.

Autologous Stem Cell Transplantation The role of ASCT in relapsed DLBCL was demonstrated in a randomized trial of 109 patients who responded to subsequent chemotherapy and were randomly assigned to receive four courses of chemotherapy plus radiotherapy (54 patients) or radiotherapy plus intensive chemotherapy and ASCT (55 patients).[103] At 5 years, the event-free survival was 46 percent in the transplantation group and 12 percent in the chemotherapy/radiotherapy group ($p = 0.001$), and the rate of overall survival was 53 and 32 percent, respectively ($p = 0.038$). Patients with relapsed or primary refractory DLBCL who achieve CR before ASCT, generally, have better outcomes than those who achieve only PR. Disease sensitivity at the time of ASCT has remained the most significant prognostic variable for predicting treatment outcome. Patients who undergo ASCT when the disease is resistant to the initial induction therapy have less than a 10 to 20 percent probability of DFS.

Allogeneic Hematopoietic Stem Cell Transplantation Allogeneic hematopoietic stem cell transplantation (ALLO-HSCT) has also been used in patients with DLBCL. The European Bone Marrow Transplant Group performed a case-controlled study by matching 101 ALLO-HSCT patients with 101 ASCT patients.[104] The PFS was similar in both types of transplants (49% for ALLO-HSCT vs. 46% for ASCT). The overall relapse and progression rate for the ALLO-HSCT patients was 23 percent compared with 38 percent in the ASCT patients. This difference was not statistically significant. Nine patients who had undergone ASCT died from early procedure-related toxicity and 17 patients who had undergone ALLO-HSCT died from early procedure-related toxicity. To reduce the treatment-related mortality associated with ALLO-HSCT, nonmyeloablative preparative regimens were developed to minimize the toxicity associated with standard high-dose chemotherapy, achieve sufficient engraftment to prevent graft rejection and exploit the graft-versus-tumor effect of ALLO-HSCT. In a prospective study, 31 patients with DLBCL and 1 patient with Burkitt lymphoma received ALLO-HSCT following 2 Gy total-body irradiation with or without fludarabine.[105] Twenty-four patients had undergone prior ASCT. With a median followup of 45 months, 3-year OS and PFS was 45 percent and 35 percent, respectively. Three-year cumulative incidences of relapse and nonrelapse mortality were 41 percent and 25 percent, respectively. Cumulative incidences of acute graft-versus-host disease (GVHD) grades II to IV, grades III to IV, and chronic GVHD were 53, 19, and 47 percent, respectively. In another study, 48 consecutive patients with relapsed or refractory DLBCL (30 patients with *de novo* disease and 18 patients with transformed follicular lymphoma) underwent transplantation with an alemtuzumab-containing regimen.[106] The PFS and OS rates at 4 years was 48 and 47 percent, respectively. Seventeen percent of patients developed grade II to IV acute GVHD, and 13 percent experienced extensive chronic GVHD. Four-year estimated nonrelapse mortality was 32 percent, and relapse risk was 33 percent. Although these results are promising, ALLO-HSCT cannot be recommended before ASCT except in the context of a clinical trial.

Radioimmunotherapy as Monotherapy Radioimmunotherapy as monotherapy is not recommended for DLBCL but its role as part of a conditioning regimen prior to ASCT has been studied. A phase II trial evaluated the safety and efficacy of combining ^{90}Y-ibritumomab tiuxetan with high-dose carmustine, cytarabine, etoposide, and melphalan (BEAM) and ASCT in patients with lymphoma who were considered ineligible for total-body irradiation because of older age or prior radiotherapy.[107] The addition of ^{90}Y-ibritumomab tiuxetan to BEAM with ASCT was feasible and the toxicity and tolerability profile similar to that observed with BEAM alone. Similarly, ^{131}I-tositumomab (up to 0.75 Gy) was combined with BEAM followed by ASCT for the treatment of chemotherapy-resistant relapsed or refractory lymphoma. Short-term and long-term toxicities were similar to that in patients previously treated with BEAM alone, with an overall survival rate of 55 percent and an event-free survival rate of 39 percent.[108]

Summary of Approach to Patients with Relapsed Disease Patients with relapsed disease should receive multidrug chemotherapy. If chemosensitivity is demonstrated and no contraindications are present, ASCT should be performed. If patients are elderly or have comorbid conditions the goal should be palliation. Radiotherapy can be used to alleviate symptoms at a particular site of involvement in patients with relapsed DLBCL and single agent therapy can be used but with low expected response rates and duration of responses.

Therapy for Specific Subtypes and Clinical Presentations

Primary Testicular Lymphoma Primary testicular lymphoma represents 1 to 2 percent of all lymphomas, with an estimated incidence of 0.26 per 100,000 males per year.[109] Even though lymphomas account for only 1 to 7 percent of all testicular malignancies, they represent the most common testicular tumor in men older than 50 years of age. Histologically, 80 to 90 percent of primary testicular lymphomas are DLBCL, with a mean age at diagnosis of 68 years (range: 21–98).[110,111] Most patients present with stage I-II with isolated involvement of the right or left testis equal in frequency; 6 percent of lymphomas have bilateral involvement. Primary testicular lymphoma shows a tendency to disseminate to several extranodal sites, including the contralateral testis, CNS, skin, Waldeyer ring, lung, pleura, and soft tissues. Treatment using radiation therapy alone provides suboptimal disease control, even for patients with stage I disease. Chemotherapy without anthracyclines was shown to produce inferior results compared with regimens with anthracyclines. Thus, chemotherapy with anthracycline-containing regimens (e.g., R-CHOP) is the recommended therapy after orchiectomy. The median OS is 4.4 years for testicular DLBCL. Given the observed propensity for CNS relapses, CNS prophylaxis with high-dose methotrexate should be considered. Radiation therapy to the contralateral testis should be administered.[109,112,113] Chapter 97 discusses extranodal lymphomas of all sites.

Lymphoma during Pregnancy Lymphoma is the fourth most frequent malignancy diagnosed during pregnancy, occurring in approximately 1 in 6000 deliveries.[114] Reports of therapeutic interventions in pregnant patients with lymphoma are limited, and management and outcome issues are largely composed of small retrospective studies and case reports. Treatment during pregnancy, whether radiation therapy or chemotherapy, is potentially teratogenic. Fetal exposure to antineoplastic agents may include impaired growth, diminished neurologic and/or intellectual function, decreased gonadal and reproductive function, mutagenesis of germ-line tissue, and carcinogenesis.[115] The risks of treatment to the fetus are greatest during the first trimester as in all other cases in which multidrug regimens are used. Therapeutic abortion is a consideration under these circumstances. CHOP during the second and third trimesters may be administered relatively safely with much less risk of significant adverse fetal outcomes.[116,117] The prognosis of patients who receive optimal chemotherapy is similar to that of nonpregnant patients.[118]

Only a few cases of rituximab administration during pregnancy have been reported, most of them for the treatment of nonmalignant disorders such as autoimmune diseases. Patients with supradiaphragmatic stage I disease may be considered for localized radiotherapy as a temporary measure until the second trimester, when chemotherapy holds less risk for the fetus.[119] Patients close to delivery should be treated with full-dose chemotherapy as soon after pregnancy as possible.

PRIMARY MEDIASTINAL LARGE B-CELL LYMPHOMA

DEFINITION

Primary mediastinal large B-cell lymphoma arises in the mediastinal lymphatic structures, probably from a thymic B-cell precursor.

EPIDEMIOLOGY

This variant type of DLBCL accounts for approximately 3 percent of lymphomas, and is most commonly seen in young and middle-aged adults, with about two-thirds of cases in females.

CLINICAL FEATURES

Signs and Symptoms

The clinical presentation is typically an anterior mediastinal mass that is locally invasive of neighboring tissues including the lungs and may lead to airway obstruction and superior vena cava syndrome in approximately 40 percent of patients.[120] Occasional nearby regional nodes, especially the cervical chain, may become involved. Distant nodal involvement at presentation is more suggestive of typical DLBCL with mediastinal involvement. Relapses tend to be extranodal, including the liver, gastrointestinal tract, kidneys, ovaries, and central nervous system. Marrow involvement is very unusual.

LABORATORY FINDINGS

Primary mediastinal B-cell lymphoma and Hodgkin lymphoma have shared gene-expression profiles, raising questions about biologic relationships.[14,121] Sometimes bizarre multinucleated cells may mimic Reed-Sternberg cells along with other morphologic similarities to Hodgkin lymphoma. Fibrotic bands may intersperse with the tumor cells, sometimes referred to as primary B-cell mediastinal lymphoma with sclerosis (see Chap. 98, Fig. 98–26). Immunohistochemistry may be helpful in the differential diagnosis since primary mediastinal lymphoma lacks the CD30 and CD15 antigens characteristic of Hodgkin lymphoma, and it expresses the B-cell–associated antigens CD19, CD20, CD22, and CD79a.[122] Other markers that can distinguish it from sarcomas, melanoma, thymoma, and seminoma include the melanocytic marker HMB-45, keratin, and placental leukocyte alkaline phosphatase. Rarely, anaplastic large cell lymphoma presents primarily in the mediastinum with the characteristic immunophenotype L26, CD3+, dot-like paranuclear staining with CD30 (Ki-1) antigen, and epithelial membrane antigen positivity.[123]

THERAPY

Several regimens have been evaluated in primary mediastinal large B-cell lymphoma. A retrospective study compared the outcomes of 426 patients who had fibrotic tumor reactions (sclerosis) and previously untreated disease using CHOP-like regimens, third-generation (MACOP-B, VACOP-B [etoposide, doxorubicin, cyclophosphamide, vincristine, prednisone, and bleomycin], ProMACE CytaBOM) regimens, or high-dose chemotherapy with autologous hematopoietic stem cell transplantation.[124] With chemotherapy, the CR rates were 49, 51, and 53 percent with first-generation, third-generation, and high-dose chemotherapy treatments, respectively. All patients who achieved CR and PR had radiation therapy to the mediastinum. The final CR rates were 61 percent for CHOP-like regimens, 79 percent for MACOP-B and other regimens, and 75 percent for high-dose chemotherapy/autologous hematopoietic stem cell transplantation. Projected 10-year progression-free survival rates were 35, 67, and 78 percent, respectively, and projected 10-year overall survival rates were 44, 71, and 77 percent, respectively.

In another retrospective study of 138 patients with primary mediastinal B-cell lymphoma the effectiveness of two chemotherapy regimens (CHOP vs. MACOP-B/VACOP-B) and the role of mediastinal involved-field radiotherapy as consolidation were evaluated.[125] CR was 51 percent in the CHOP group and 80 percent in MACOP-B/VACOP-B. Event-free survival was 40 percent with CHOP and 76 percent in the MACOP-B/VACOP-B group. The addition of involved-field radiation therapy improved the outcome, regardless of the type of chemotherapy used.

The incorporation of rituximab in dose-adjusted EPOCH resulted in 100 percent overall survival and 91 percent event-free survival, compared to 78 percent overall survival and 67 percent event-free survival observed with dose-adjusted EPOCH without rituximab.[126] Although outcomes appear to be superior for more intensive therapies over CHOP-type regimens in retrospective studies, they have not been compared in prospective randomized trials with R-CHOP. In addition, the exact role and long-term effects of radiotherapy in these patients is not well established, and it should be reserved for patients that have residual disease in the mediastinum after initial treatment with chemotherapy.

LYMPHOMATOID GRANULOMATOSIS

DEFINITION

Lymphomatoid granulomatosis is a rare lymphoproliferative disorder characterized by angiocentric and angiodestructive Epstein-Barr virus (EBV)-positive B-cell proliferation associated with extensive reactive T-cell infiltration.[1]

EPIDEMIOLOGY

Approximately two-thirds of cases occur in males. The median age of presentation is in the fifth decade of life, although pediatric cases occur.

CLINICAL FINDINGS

The most common sites of involvement are the lungs (90%). Other common sites of involvement include the skin (25–50%), kidney (30–40%), liver (29%), and the CNS (26%). The spleen and the lymph nodes are less often involved.[127] Nearly all patients are symptomatic at presentation. The distribution of disease leads to cough, dyspnea, and sometimes chest pain. Fever, weight loss, and joint pain are very frequent. Abdominal pain and diarrhea as a result of gastrointestinal involvement and various neurologic signs, including diplopia, ataxia, mental status changes, and others may be evident. Skin involvement can be morphologically diverse (e.g., ulcerations, plaques, maculopapules) but are usually accompanied by subcutaneous nodules.

LABORATORY FINDINGS

Imaging Studies

The pulmonary lesions are usually bilateral, nodules in the lower half of the lung. They may cavitate. Nodules may also be found in the brain and kidney and sometimes other locales.

Histopathology

The grading of lymphomatoid granulomatosis relates to the proportion of EBV-positive B cells relative to the reactive lymphocytes in the background.[1] Grade 1 lesions contain a polymorphous lymphoid infiltrate without cytologic atypia. Large transformed lymphoid cells are absent or rare. Infrequent EBV-positive cells are identified by *in situ* hybridization with an EBV-encoded RNA probe. Grade 2 lesions contain occasional large lymphoid cells or immunoblasts in a polymorphous background. *In situ* hybridization for EBV readily identifies EBV-positive cells, which are present at 5 to 20/high-power field. Grade 3 lesions still show an inflammatory background, but contain large atypical B cells that are CD20-positive. By *in situ* hybridization, EBV-positive cells are numerous (>50/high-power field).

TREATMENT AND PROGNOSIS

The clinical prognosis is variable in lymphomatoid granulomatosis with a median survival of two years[128]; poor prognostic findings include neurologic involvement and higher pathologic grade. The disease is uncommon and the optimal treatment regimen is unclear, but generally consists of a glucocorticoid and combination chemotherapy. In a prospective study, patients with grades I and II disease were treated with interferon-α, and those with grade III received dose-adjusted R-EPOCH chemotherapy.[129] Among 27 patients with grade I/II, 56 percent were in continuous CR for a median of 52 months. Among the grade III patients who received dose-adjusted R-EPOCH, 40 percent achieved CR and at a median follow up of 46 months; OS and PFS was 69 and 82 percent, respectively.

INTRAVASCULAR LARGE B-CELL LYMPHOMA

DEFINITION

Intravascular large B-cell lymphoma is a rare type of extranodal large B-cell lymphoma characterized by selective growth of lymphoma cells within the lumina of vessels, sparing the large arteries and veins.[1]

EPIDEMIOLOGY

This tumor usually occurs in adults in the sixth and seventh decade. It occurs equally in men and women.

CLINICAL FINDINGS

The clinical manifestations of this lymphoma are extremely variable and most symptoms are related to the organs affected. Two major patterns of clinical presentation have been recognized: the first is in European countries with brain and skin involvement and the second in the Asian countries where patients present with multiorgan failure, hepatosplenomegaly, pancytopenia and hemophagocytic syndrome.[130–134] B symptoms (fever, drenching sweats, and weight loss) are common in both types. An isolated cutaneous variant almost unique to Western countries has been identified in females and is associated with a better prognosis.[130] In the latter case, the skin lesions range from single to striking clusters of nodules and tumors. They may be painful and appear as violaceous plaques, erythematous nodules, or tumors that may ulcerate. These lesions commonly appear on the arms and legs, abdomen and breasts, but may occur anywhere.

LABORATORY FINDINGS

Laboratory findings are not specific. Increased LDH levels and β_2-microglobulin levels are observed in most patients. Elevated erythrocyte sedimentation rate and abnormalities in hepatic, renal, and thyroid function are also common.[135] Tumor cells express B-cell–associated antigens and occasionally express CD5.

TREATMENT

Anthracycline-based chemotherapy has been used for type of lymphoma. Retrospective studies have shown that addition of rituximab to chemotherapy improved clinical outcomes.[136,137] One study analyzed 106 patients who received chemotherapy either with rituximab (R-chemotherapy, n = 49) or without rituximab (chemotherapy, n = 57). The CR rate was 82 percent for patients in the R-chemotherapy group compared to 51 percent in the chemotherapy group (p = 0.001). PFS and OS rates at 2 years after diagnosis were 56 and 66 percent, respectively, in the R-chemotherapy group, compared with 27 and 46 percent for patients in the chemotherapy group (p = 0.001 for PFS and p = 0.01 for OS). For patients with CNS involvement, more intensive chemotherapy with drugs such as methotrexate and cytarabine that reach the CNS are required. One approach might be R-CHOP with high-dose methotrexate. A second issue is the high incidence of CNS relapse following initial response to chemotherapy. Currently, prophylactic high-dose methotrexate following initial treatment with R-CHOP cannot be recommended, but this approach should be evaluated in prospective clinical studies.

POSTTRANSPLANT LYMPHOPROLIFERATIVE DISORDERS

DEFINITION

Posttransplant lymphoproliferative disorders (PTLD) result from lymphoid or plasmacytic proliferations that develop in the setting of solid organ or marrow transplantation. Although PTLD represent an uncommon complication in transplant patients, they are a significant cause of morbidity and mortality.[138]

EPIDEMIOLOGY

The incidence of PTLD is approximately 1 to 2 percent of solid-organ transplant recipients, which is 30 to 50 times higher than the incidence of lymphoproliferative diseases in the immunocompetent general population.[139] There is a clear association between PTLD and the type of organ transplanted. Among the most commonly transplanted solid organs, cardiac-lung and intestinal transplantation have the highest incidence of PTLD.[140] The highest incidence occurs in the first year of transplantation. The incidence of PTLD after blood or marrow transplantation ranges from 0.5 to 1 percent.

PATHOGENESIS

The major risk factors that have been identified for the development of PTLD include EBV-positive serology pretransplantation, type of organ transplanted, and intensity of immunosuppressive regimen used.[141–143] The onset of posttransplant lymphoma in most patients is related to B-cell proliferation induced by infection with EBV in the setting of chronic immunosuppression. The genome of the virus can be detected in the cells of the majority of cases.[144] However, in approximately 20 to 30 percent of cases, the involved tissue is negative for the virus.[145] Involvement of the lymph node, gastrointestinal tract, lungs, and liver are common in all allograft types. The majority of PTLD in solid-organ transplant recipients are of host origin and only a minority of donor origin. In contrast, the majority of PTLD in hematopoietic stem cell allografts are of donor origin. Involvement of the grafted organ occurs in approximately 30 percent of patients and may lead to organ damage and fatal complications.[146]

TREATMENT

Management of PTLD is not uniform. A wide variety of approaches, including decrease in immunosuppressive drugs, antiviral therapy, interferon, intravenous immunoglobulin, adoptive therapies with EBV-specific cytotoxic T lymphocytes, chemotherapy, radiation, and rituximab therapy, have been reported. If feasible, reduction of immunosuppression is the first step in the treatment of these patients. Many cases of polyclonal PTLD may resolve completely with a reduction in immunosuppressive therapy.[147] Patients with late PTLD and more aggressive monoclonal PTLD are less likely to respond.[148] Rituximab has shown promising results in the treatment of CD20+ PTLD. In a multicenter prospective trial, 43 patients with previously untreated B-cell PTLD, not responding to tapering of immunosuppression, were treated with 4 weekly injections of rituximab at 375 mg/m^2.[149] The overall response rate was 44 percent, whereas the overall survival was 86 and 67 percent at 80 days and 1 year, respectively. The only baseline factor predicting response at day 80 was a normal level of serum LDH. A retrospective study evaluated the efficacy and safety of chemotherapy salvage therapies in adult recipients of solid-organ transplants with a second progression of PTLD after initial therapy with rituximab.[150] CHOP therapy achieved a favorable overall response rate of 70 percent in this setting, indicating that PTLD generally remains chemotherapy-sensitive after progression following the initial use of rituximab.

A prospective trial evaluated a stepwise treatment approach beginning with reduction of immunosuppression, then interferon-α, and finally chemotherapy with ProMACE-CytaBOM plus granulocyte-monocyte colony-stimulating factor.[151] Sixteen eligible patients began treatment with reduced immunosuppression. The response rate to reduced immunosuppression was 0 of 16 CR and 1 of 16 PR (6%). Six of the 16 patients (38%) had documented rejection of the transplanted organ during the period of reduced immunosuppression. Eight of the 16 patients had documented progressive disease during the period of reduced immunosuppression. Thirteen patients underwent treatment with interferon. The response rate was 2 of 13 (15%) CR and 2 of 13 (15%) PR. Seven eligible patients proceeded to ProMACE-CytaBOM chemotherapy. The response rate to chemotherapy was 5 of 7 (67%) CR. Four of the five CRs had remission durations of more than 2 years. The median survival for the treatment cohort as a whole was 19 months, with a range of 5 days to 60+ months. Overall survival was 50 percent at 2 years, 44 percent at 4 years, and 24 percent at 8 years.

The following sequence is generally recommended. If possible, the first step is reduction in immunosuppression, followed by four weekly cycles of rituximab if reduction of the immunosuppression is ineffective. If both steps are ineffective, then six cycles of R-CHOP is recommended.

T-CELL–HISTIOCYTE-RICH LARGE B-CELL LYMPHOMA

DEFINITION

T-cell–histiocyte-rich large B-cell lymphoma is characterized by effacement of the architecture of the lymph node by a lymphohistiocytic infiltrate with a diffuse or vaguely nodular growth pattern.[1,152] There are a limited number of large atypical B cells occurring singly or in small clusters with a predominant background infiltrate composed of T cells and histiocytes, the latter usually of the nonepithelioid type.

EPIDEMIOLOGY

This pattern of disease accounts for less than 5 percent of all cases of DLBCL and occurs at a younger age on average. The median age of onset is in the fourth decade, compared to the sixth decade for DLBCL.[153–156] A male predominance is noted in most series, in contrast to DLBCL, which occurs equally in men and women.

CLINICAL FINDINGS

This variant more often presents with advanced stage disease, and often in multiple extranodal sites, and with an elevated LDH, as compared to DLBCL.[152,154,155] The lymphoma infiltrates the spleen, liver, and marrow with greater frequency than does DLBCL. Marrow involvement occurs in approximately one-third of the cases, a frequency considerably higher than in DLBCL and patients are more likely to develop "B" symptoms than patients with DLBCL.[154,157]

TREATMENT AND COURSE

When treated with CHOP-like regimens, most series suggest that the outcome for these patients is similar to patients with typical DLBCL.[154,156–159] Complete response rates to regimens based on CHOP chemotherapy are approximately 60 percent, with 3-year and 5-year overall survival rates estimated at 50 to 64 percent and 45 to 58 percent, respectively. Two case-control analyses have been performed comparing T-cell–histiocyte-rich large B-cell lymphoma and DLBCL and no differences in overall survival was observed.[154,156] Based on these data, this subtype of large B-cell lymphoma should be treated in the same fashion as traditional DLBCL. Six cycles of R-CHOP for advanced disease would be an reasonable initial approach to therapy.

PRIMARY CUTANEOUS DIFFUSE LARGE B-CELL LYMPHOMA, LEG TYPE

DEFINITION

This lymphoma is a primary cutaneous DLBCL composed solely of large transformed B cells with a predilection for the skin of the leg.[1]

EPIDEMIOLOGY

Primary cutaneous DLBCL, leg type constitute approximately 4 percent of all primary cutaneous B-cell lymphomas.[1,160] The median age at the time of presentation is 60 to 70 years.

CLINICAL FINDINGS

These lymphomatous tumors affect the skin of the legs in most cases, but approximately 10 percent arise at other sites.[161–163] Multiple tumors, sometimes ulcerating, are associated with poorer prognosis. There are frequent relapses and extracutaneous dissemination.

LABORATORY FINDINGS

The B cells are usually positive for CD20 and usually express BCL2 and FOX-P1. Fluorescence *in situ* hybridization of the lymphoma cells often finds translocations involving *MYC, BCL6*, or *IGH* genes. Amplification of the *BCL2* gene presumably explains the high frequency of BCL2 overexpression in the absence of a t(14;18), not seen in this variant of lymphoma. The gene-expression profile of these lymphoma cells is often the same as activated B-cell like DLBCL.

TREATMENT

Anthracycline-containing chemotherapy with rituximab should be considered as initial therapy. The incorporation of rituximab improves the response rates and overall survival.[161–163] However, because of the advanced age of the patient at diagnosis this might not be feasible and patients may receive local radiation therapy or less-aggressive chemotherapy, depending on the presence of frailty or other comorbidities.

ANAPLASTIC LYMPHOMA KINASE-POSITIVE LARGE B-CELL LYMPHOMA

DEFINITION

Anaplastic lymphoma kinase (ALK)-positive large B-cell lymphoma is an uncommon neoplasm of large immunoblast-like B cells that are stain for nuclear and or cytoplasmic ALK protein. The lymphoma cells may undergo plasmablastic differentiation.[1]

EPIDEMIOLOGY

The average age of presentation is in the fourth decade with a male predilection. Most patients present with advanced stage disease.

CLINCAL FINDINGS

Patients usually present with widespread disease. The most common affected nodal areas are in the neck and mediastinum. Common extranodal involvement include the liver, spleen, bone, and gastrointestinal tract.[164,165]

LABORATORY FINDINGS

The lymphoma cells are large immunoblasts with a large central nucleolus. In some cases the histopathologic appearance will show maturation to plasmablastic cells. The lymphoma cells stain for the ALK protein, usually with a granular cytoplasmic appearance but nuclear staining may also occur. These cells are usually CD3, CD20, CD30, CD79a negative. MUC1 mucin, a high-molecular-weight transmembrane glycoprotein, also known as epithelial membrane antigen and CD138 are usually strongly expressed by these cells. Monoclonal (light-chain restricted) IgA or IgG is present in the cytoplasm. Occasional cases may have a t(2;17)(p23;q23) that results in a clathrin-ALK fusion protein.

TREATMENT AND COURSE

The clinical course of ALK-positive large B-cell lymphoma is aggressive with a median survival time of 24 months. These tumors are usually negative for CD20, making the utility of rituximab uncertain. Anthracycline-based chemotherapy is often inadequate and more intensive therapies should be considered.[164,165]

HUMAN IMMUNODEFICIENCY RELATED DIFFUSE LARGE B-CELL LYMPHOMA VARIANTS

Primary effusion lymphoma, plasmablastic lymphoma, and large B-cell lymphoma arising in human herpesvirus 8-associated multicentric Castleman disease usually develop in the setting of acquired immunodeficiency induced by HIV and are discussed in Chap. 83.

REFERENCES

1. Swerdlow SH, World Health Organization, International Agency for Research on Cancer: *WHO Classification of Tumours of Haematopoietic and Lymphoid Tissues*. World Health Organization International Agency for Research on Cancer, Lyon, France 2008.
2. Fisher SG, Fisher RI: The epidemiology of non-Hodgkin's lymphoma. *Oncogene* 23:38, 2004.
3. Morton LM, Wang SS, Devesa SS, et al: Lymphoma incidence patterns by WHO subtype in the United States, 1992–2001. *Blood* 107:1, 2006.

3a. Alexander, DD; Mink, PJ; Adami, HO et al: The non-Hodgkin lymphomas: A review of the epidemiologic literature *International Journal of Cancer* 120:1-39, 2007

4. Ye BH, Lista F, Lo Coco F, et al: Alterations of a zinc finger-encoding gene, BCL-6, in diffuse large-cell lymphoma. *Science* 262:5134, 1993.
5. Dalla-Favera R, Migliazza A, Chang CC, et al: Molecular pathogenesis of B cell malignancy: The role of BCL-6. *Curr Top Microbiol Immunol* 246, 1999.
6. Gaidano G, Lo Coco F, Ye BH, et al: Rearrangements of the BCL-6 gene in acquired immunodeficiency syndrome-associated non-Hodgkin's lymphoma: Association with diffuse large-cell subtype. *Blood* 84:2, 1994.
7. Lo Coco F, Ye BH, Lista F, et al: Rearrangements of the BCL6 gene in diffuse large cell non-Hodgkin's lymphoma. *Blood* 83:7, 1994.
8. Ye BH, Chaganti S, Chang CC, et al: Chromosomal translocations cause deregulated BCL6 expression by promoter substitution in B cell lymphoma. *EMBO J* 14:24, 1995.
9. Kaneita Y, Yoshida S, Ishiguro N, et al: Detection of reciprocal fusion 5′-BCL6/partner-3′ transcripts in lymphomas exhibiting reciprocal BCL6 translocations. *Br J Haematol* 113:3, 2001.
10. Chang CC, Ye BH, Chaganti RS, et al: BCL-6, a POZ/zinc-finger protein, is a sequence-specific transcriptional repressor. *Proc Natl Acad Sci U S A* 93:14, 1996.
11. Lo Coco F, Gaidano G, Louie DC, et al: p53 mutations are associated with histologic transformation of follicular lymphoma. *Blood* 82:8, 1993.
12. Alizadeh AA, Eisen MB, Davis RE, et al: Distinct types of diffuse large B-cell lymphoma identified by gene expression profiling. *Nature* 403:6769, 2000.
13. Rosenwald A, Wright G, Chan WC, et al: The use of molecular profiling to predict survival after chemotherapy for diffuse large-B-cell lymphoma. *N Engl J Med* 346:25, 2002.
14. Rosenwald A, Wright G, Leroy K, et al: Molecular diagnosis of primary mediastinal B cell lymphoma identifies a clinically favorable subgroup of diffuse large B cell lymphoma related to Hodgkin lymphoma. *J Exp Med* 198:6, 2003.
15. Wright G, Tan B, Rosenwald A, et al: A gene expression-based method to diagnose clinically distinct subgroups of diffuse large B cell lymphoma. *Proc Natl Acad Sci U S A* 100:17, 2003.
16. Lenz G, Wright GW, Emre NC, et al: Molecular subtypes of diffuse large B-cell lymphoma arise by distinct genetic pathways. *Proc Natl Acad Sci U S A* 105:36, 2008.
17. Aviles A, Neri N, Huerta-Guzman J: Large bowel lymphoma: An analysis of prognostic factors and therapy in 53 patients. *J Surg Oncol* 80:2, 2002.
18. Paryani S, Hoppe RT, Burke JS, et al: Extralymphatic involvement in diffuse non-Hodgkin's lymphoma. *J Clin Oncol* 1:11, 1983.
19. van Besien K, Ha CS, Murphy S, et al: Risk factors, treatment, and outcome of central nervous system recurrence in adults with intermediate-grade and immunoblastic lymphoma. *Blood* 91:4, 1998.
20. Doggett RS, Wood GS, Horning S, et al: The immunologic characterization of 95 nodal and extranodal diffuse large cell lymphomas in 89 patients. *Am J Pathol* 115:2, 1984.
21. Stein H, Lennert K, Feller AC, Mason DY: Immunohistological analysis of human lymphoma: Correlation of histological and immunological categories. *Adv Cancer Res* 42:67, 1984.
22. Yamaguchi M, Seto M, Okamoto M, et al: *De novo* CD5+ diffuse large B-cell lymphoma: A clinicopathologic study of 109 patients. *Blood* 99:3, 2002.
23. Craig FE, Foon KA: Flow cytometric immunophenotyping for hematologic neoplasms. *Blood* 111:8, 2008.
24. Ottensmeier CH, Stevenson FK: Isotype switch variants reveal clonally related subpopulations in diffuse large B-cell lymphoma. *Blood* 96:7, 2000.

25. Stauder R, Eisterer W, Thaler J, Gunthert U: CD44 variant isoforms in non-Hodgkin's lymphoma: A new independent prognostic factor. *Blood* 85:10, 1995.
26. A predictive model for aggressive non-Hodgkin's lymphoma. The International Non-Hodgkin's Lymphoma Prognostic Factors Project. *N Engl J Med* 329:14, 1993.
27. A clinical evaluation of the International Lymphoma Study Group classification of non-Hodgkin's lymphoma. The Non-Hodgkin's Lymphoma Classification Project. *Blood* 89:11, 1997.
28. Hans CP, Weisenburger DD, Greiner TC, et al: Confirmation of the molecular classification of diffuse large B-cell lymphoma by immunohistochemistry using a tissue microarray. *Blood* 103:1, 2004.
29. Shipp MA, Ross KN, Tamayo P, et al: Diffuse large B-cell lymphoma outcome prediction by gene-expression profiling and supervised machine learning. *Nat Med* 8:1, 2002.
30. Alizadeh AA, Eisen MB, Davis RE, et al: Distinct types of diffuse large B-cell lymphoma identified by gene expression profiling. *Nature* 403:503, 2000.
31. Lossos IS, Czerwinski DK, Alizadeh AA, et al: Prediction of survival in diffuse large-B-cell lymphoma based on the expression of six genes. *N Engl J Med* 350:18, 2004.
32. Swan F Jr, Velasquez WS, Tucker S, et al: A new serologic staging system for large-cell lymphomas based on initial beta 2-microglobulin and lactate dehydrogenase levels. *J Clin Oncol* 7:10, 1989.
33. Lossos IS, Jones CD, Warnke R, et al: Expression of a single gene, BCL-6, strongly predicts survival in patients with diffuse large B-cell lymphoma. *Blood* 98:4, 2001.
34. Gascoyne RD, Adomat SA, Krajewski S, et al: Prognostic significance of Bcl-2 protein expression and Bcl-2 gene rearrangement in diffuse aggressive non-Hodgkin's lymphoma. *Blood* 90:1, 1997.
35. Adida C, Haioun C, Gaulard P, et al: Prognostic significance of survivin expression in diffuse large B-cell lymphomas. *Blood* 96:5, 2000.
36. Ansell SM, Stenson M, Habermann TM, Jelinek DF, Witzig TE: Cd4+ T-cell immune response to large B-cell non-Hodgkin's lymphoma predicts patient outcome. *J Clin Oncol* 19:3, 2001.
37. Gallamini A, Hutchings M, Rigacci L, et al: Early interim 2-[18F]fluoro-2-deoxy-D-glucose positron emission tomography is prognostically superior to international prognostic score in advanced-stage Hodgkin's lymphoma: A report from a joint Italian-Danish study. *J Clin Oncol* 25:24, 2007.
38. Haioun C, Itti E, Rahmouni A, et al: [18F]fluoro-2-deoxy-D-glucose positron emission tomography (FDG-PET) in aggressive lymphoma: An early prognostic tool for predicting patient outcome. *Blood* 106:4, 2005.
39. Zijlstra JM, Hoekstra OS, Raijmakers PG, et al: 18FDG positron emission tomography versus 67Ga scintigraphy as prognostic test during chemotherapy for non-Hodgkin's lymphoma. *Br J Haematol* 123:3, 2003.
40. Terasawa T, Lau J, Bardet S, et al: Fluorine-18-fluorodeoxyglucose positron emission tomography for interim response assessment of advanced-stage Hodgkin's lymphoma and diffuse large B-cell lymphoma: A systematic review. *J Clin Oncol* 27:11, 2009.
41. Chen MG, Prosnitz LR, Gonzalez-Serva A, Fischer DB: Results of radiotherapy in control of stage I and II non-Hodgkin's lymphoma. *Cancer* 43:4, 1979.
42. Jones SE, Miller TP, Connors JM: Long-term follow-up and analysis for prognostic factors for patients with limited-stage diffuse large-cell lymphoma treated with initial chemotherapy with or without adjuvant radiotherapy. *J Clin Oncol* 7:9, 1989.
43. Longo DL, Glatstein E, Duffey PL, et al: Treatment of localized aggressive lymphomas with combination chemotherapy followed by involved-field radiation therapy. *J Clin Oncol* 7:9, 1989.
44. Monfardini S, Banfi A, Bonadonna G, et al: Improved five year survival after combined radiotherapy-chemotherapy for stage I-II non-Hodgkin's lymphoma. *Int J Radiat Oncol Biol Phys* 6:2, 1980.
45. Nissen NI, Ersboll J, Hansen HS, et al: A randomized study of radiotherapy versus radiotherapy plus chemotherapy in stage I-II non-Hodgkin's lymphomas. *Cancer* 52:1, 1983.
46. Tondini C, Zanini M, Lombardi F, et al: Combined modality treatment with primary CHOP chemotherapy followed by locoregional irradiation in stage I or II histologically aggressive non-Hodgkin's lymphomas. *J Clin Oncol* 11:4, 1993.
47. Vokes EE, Ultmann JE, Golomb HM, et al: Long-term survival of patients with localized diffuse histiocytic lymphoma. *J Clin Oncol* 3:10, 1985.
48. Miller TP, Dahlberg S, Cassady JR, et al: Chemotherapy alone compared with chemotherapy plus radiotherapy for localized intermediate- and high-grade non-Hodgkin's lymphoma. *N Engl J Med* 339:1, 1998.
49. Miller TP, Leblanc M, Spier C, et al: CHOP alone compared to CHOP plus radiotherapy foe early stage aggressive non-Hodgkin's lymphomas: Update of the Southwest Oncology Group (SWOG) randomized trial. *Blood* 98:11, 2001.
50. Horning SJ, Weller E, Kim K, et al: Chemotherapy with or without radiotherapy in limited-stage diffuse aggressive non-Hodgkin's lymphoma: Eastern Cooperative Oncology Group study 1484. *J Clin Oncol* 22:15, 2004.
51. Bonnet C, Fillet G, Mounier N, et al: CHOP alone compared with CHOP plus radiotherapy for localized aggressive lymphoma in elderly patients: A study by the Groupe d'Etude des Lymphomes de l'Adulte. *J Clin Oncol* 25:7, 2007.
52. Reyes F, Lepage E, Ganem G, et al: ACVBP versus CHOP plus radiotherapy for localized aggressive lymphoma. *N Engl J Med* 352:12, 2005.
53. Persky DO, Unger JM, Spier CM, et al: Phase II study of rituximab plus three cycles of CHOP and involved-field radiotherapy for patients with limited-stage aggressive B-cell lymphoma: Southwest Oncology Group study 0014. *J Clin Oncol* 26:14, 2008.
54. DeVita VT Jr, Canellos GP, Chabner B, et al: Advanced diffuse histiocytic lymphoma, a potentially curable disease. *Lancet* 1:7901, 1975.
55. Gaynor ER, Ultmann JE, Golomb HM, Sweet DL: Treatment of diffuse histiocytic lymphoma (DHL) with COMLA (cyclophosphamide, Oncovin, methotrexate, leucovorin, cytosine arabinoside): A 10-year experience in a single institution. *J Clin Oncol* 3:12, 1985.
56. Schein PS, DeVita VT Jr, Hubbard S, et al: Bleomycin, Adriamycin, cyclophosphamide, vincristine, and prednisone (BACOP) combination chemotherapy in the treatment of advanced diffuse histiocytic lymphoma. *Ann Intern Med* 85:4, 1976.
57. Fisher RI, DeVita VT Jr, Hubbard SM, et al: Diffuse aggressive lymphomas: Increased survival after alternating flexible sequences of proMACE and MOPP chemotherapy. *Ann Intern Med* 98:3, 1983.
58. Gordon LI, Harrington D, Andersen J, et al: Comparison of a second-generation combination chemotherapeutic regimen (m-BACOD) with a standard regimen (CHOP) for advanced diffuse non-Hodgkin's lymphoma. *N Engl J Med* 327:19, 1992.
59. Fisher RI, Gaynor ER, Dahlberg S, et al: Comparison of a standard regimen (CHOP) with three intensive chemotherapy regimens for advanced non-Hodgkin's lymphoma. *N Engl J Med* 328:14, 1993.
60. Linch DC, Smith P, Hancock BW, et al: A randomized British National Lymphoma Investigation trial of CHOP vs. a weekly multi-agent regimen (PACEBOM) in patients with histologically aggressive non-Hodgkin's lymphoma. *Ann Oncol* 11 Suppl 1:87, 2000.
61. Gaynor ER, Unger JM, Miller TP, et al: Infusional CHOP chemotherapy (CVAD) with or without chemosensitizers offers no advantage over standard CHOP therapy in the treatment of lymphoma: A Southwest Oncology Group Study. *J Clin Oncol* 19:3, 2001.
62. Bartlett NL, Petroni GR, Parker BA, et al: Dose-escalated cyclophosphamide, doxorubicin, vincristine, prednisone, and etoposide (CHOPE) chemotherapy for patients with diffuse lymphoma: Cancer and Leukemia Group B studies 8852 and 8854. *Cancer* 92:2, 2001.
63. Sparano JA, Weller E, Nazeer T, et al: Phase 2 trial of infusional cyclophosphamide, doxorubicin, and etoposide in patients with poor-prognosis, intermediate-grade non-Hodgkin lymphoma: An Eastern Cooperative Oncology Group trial (E3493). *Blood* 100:5, 2002.
64. Pangalis GA, Vassilakopoulos TP, Michalis E, et al: A randomized trial comparing intensified CNOP vs. CHOP in patients with aggressive non-Hodgkin's lymphoma. *Leuk Lymphoma* 44:4, 2003.
65. Lai GM, Chen YN, Mickley LA, Fojo AT, Bates SE. P-glycoprotein expression and schedule dependence of Adriamycin cytotoxicity in human colon carcinoma cell lines. *Int J Cancer* 49:5, 1991.
66. Gutierrez M, Chabner BA, Pearson D, et al: Role of a doxorubicin-containing regimen in relapsed and resistant lymphomas: An 8-year follow-up study of EPOCH: *J Clin Oncol* 18:21, 2000.
67. Wilson WH, Bates SE, Fojo A, et al: Controlled trial of dexverapamil, a modulator of multidrug resistance, in lymphomas refractory to EPOCH chemotherapy. *J Clin Oncol* 13:8, 1995.
68. Wilson WH, Grossbard ML, Pittaluga S, et al: Dose-adjusted EPOCH chemotherapy for untreated large B-cell lymphomas: A pharmacodynamic approach with high efficacy. *Blood* 99:8, 2002.
69. Wilson WH, Dunleavy K, Pittaluga S, et al: Phase II study of dose-adjusted EPOCH and rituximab in untreated diffuse large B-cell lymphoma with analysis of germinal center and post-germinal center biomarkers. *J Clin Oncol* 26:16, 2008.
70. Pfreundschuh M, Trumper L, Kloess M, et al: Two-weekly or 3-weekly CHOP chemotherapy with or without etoposide for the treatment of elderly patients with aggressive lymphomas: Results of the NHL-B2 trial of the DSHNHL. *Blood* 104:3, 2004.
71. Pfreundschuh M, Trumper L, Osterborg A, et al: CHOP-like chemotherapy plus rituximab versus CHOP-like chemotherapy alone in young patients with good-prognosis diffuse large-B-cell lymphoma: A randomised controlled trial by the MabThera International Trial (MInT) Group. *Lancet Oncol* 7:5, 2006.
72. Verdonck LF, Notenboom A, de Jong DD, et al: Intensified 12-week CHOP (I-CHOP) plus G-CSF compared with standard 24-week CHOP (CHOP-21) for patients with intermediate-risk aggressive non-Hodgkin lymphoma: A phase 3 trial of the Dutch-Belgian Hemato-Oncology Cooperative Group (HOVON). *Blood* 109:7, 2007.
73. Pfreundschuh M, Schubert J, Ziepert M, et al: Six versus eight cycles of bi-weekly CHOP-14 with or without rituximab in elderly patients with aggressive CD20+ B-cell lymphomas: A randomised controlled trial (RICOVER-60). *Lancet Oncol* 9:2, 2008.
74. Goss PE: Non-Hodgkin's lymphomas in elderly patients. *Leuk Lymphoma* 10:3, 1993.
75. Bessell EM, Burton A, Haynes AP, et al: A randomised multicentre trial of modified CHOP versus MCOP in patients aged 65 years and over with aggressive non-Hodgkin's lymphoma. *Ann Oncol* 14:2, 2003.
76. Zinzani PL, Storti S, Zaccaria A, et al: Elderly aggressive-histology non-Hodgkin's lymphoma: First-line VNCOP-B regimen experience on 350 patients. *Blood* 94:1, 1999.
77. Meyer RM, Browman GP, Samosh ML, et al: Randomized phase II comparison of standard CHOP with weekly CHOP in elderly patients with non-Hodgkin's lymphoma. *J Clin Oncol* 13:9, 1995.
78. Wunderlich A, Kloess M, Reiser M, et al: Practicability and acute haematological toxicity of 2- and 3-weekly CHOP and CHOEP chemotherapy for aggressive non-Hodgkin's lymphoma: Results from the NHL-B trial of the German High-Grade Non-Hodgkin's Lymphoma Study Group (DSHNHL). *Ann Oncol* 14:6, 2003.
79. Osby E, Hagberg H, Kvaloy S, et al: CHOP is superior to CNOP in elderly patients with aggressive lymphoma while outcome is unaffected by filgrastim treatment: Results of a Nordic Lymphoma Group randomized trial. *Blood* 101:10, 2003.

80. Sonneveld P, de Ridder M, van der Lelie H, et al: Comparison of doxorubicin and mitoxantrone in the treatment of elderly patients with advanced diffuse non-Hodgkin's lymphoma using CHOP versus CNOP chemotherapy. *J Clin Oncol* 13:10, 1995.
81. Tirelli U, Errante D, Van Glabbeke M, et al: CHOP is the standard regimen in patients > or = 70 years of age with intermediate-grade and high-grade non-Hodgkin's lymphoma: Results of a randomized study of the European Organization for Research and Treatment of Cancer Lymphoma Cooperative Study Group. *J Clin Oncol* 16:1, 1998.
82. Coiffier B, Lepage E, Briere J, et al: CHOP chemotherapy plus rituximab compared with CHOP alone in elderly patients with diffuse large-B-cell lymphoma. *N Engl J Med* 346:4, 2002.
83. Feugier P, Van Hoof A, Sebban C, et al: Long-term results of the R-CHOP study in the treatment of elderly patients with diffuse large B-cell lymphoma: A study by the Groupe d'Etude des Lymphomes de l'Adulte. *J Clin Oncol* 23:18, 2005.
84. Habermann TM, Weller EA, Morrison VA, et al: Rituximab-CHOP versus CHOP alone or with maintenance rituximab in older patients with diffuse large B-cell lymphoma. *J Clin Oncol* 24:19, 2006.
85. Morrison VA, Picozzi V, Scott S, et al: The impact of age on delivered dose intensity and hospitalizations for febrile neutropenia in patients with intermediate-grade non-Hodgkin's lymphoma receiving initial CHOP chemotherapy: A risk factor analysis. *Clin Lymphoma* 2:1, 2001.
86. Sonnen R, Schmidt WP, Kuse R, Schmitz N: Treatment results of aggressive B non-Hodgkin's lymphoma in advanced age considering comorbidity. *Br J Haematol* 119:3, 2002.
87. Haioun C, Lepage E, Gisselbrecht C, et al: Benefit of autologous bone marrow transplantation over sequential chemotherapy in poor-risk aggressive non-Hodgkin's lymphoma: Updated results of the prospective study LNH87-2. Groupe d'Etude des Lymphomes de l'Adulte. *J Clin Oncol* 15:3, 1997.
88. Kluin-Nelemans HC, Zagonel V, Anastasopoulou A, et al: Standard chemotherapy with or without high-dose chemotherapy for aggressive non-Hodgkin's lymphoma: Randomized phase III EORTC study. *J Natl Cancer Inst* 93:1, 2001.
89. Santini G, Salvagno L, Leoni P, et al: VACOP-B versus VACOP-B plus autologous bone marrow transplantation for advanced diffuse non-Hodgkin's lymphoma: Results of a prospective randomized trial by the non-Hodgkin's Lymphoma Cooperative Study Group. *J Clin Oncol* 16:8, 1998.
90. Verdonck LF, van Putten WL, Hagenbeek A, et al: Comparison of CHOP chemotherapy with autologous bone marrow transplantation for slowly responding patients with aggressive non-Hodgkin's lymphoma. *N Engl J Med* 332:16, 1995.
91. Gisselbrecht C, Lepage E, Molina T, et al: Shortened first-line high-dose chemotherapy for patients with poor-prognosis aggressive lymphoma. *J Clin Oncol* 20:10, 2002.
92. Haioun C, Lepage E, Gisselbrecht C, et al: Survival benefit of high-dose therapy in poor-risk aggressive non-Hodgkin's lymphoma: Final analysis of the prospective LNH87-2 protocol—a Groupe d'Etude des lymphomes de l'Adulte study. *J Clin Oncol* 18:16, 2000.
93. Kaiser U, Uebelacker I, Abel U, et al: Randomized study to evaluate the use of high-dose therapy as part of primary treatment for "aggressive" lymphoma. *J Clin Oncol* 20:22, 2002.
94. Greb A, Bohlius J, Schiefer D, et al: High-dose chemotherapy with autologous stem cell transplantation in the first line treatment of aggressive non-Hodgkin lymphoma (NHL) in adults. *Cochrane Database Syst Rev* 1:CD004024, 2008.
95. Lee AY, Connors JM, Klimo P, et al: Late relapse in patients with diffuse large-cell lymphoma treated with MACOP-B: *J Clin Oncol* 15:5, 1997.
96. Schmoll H: Review of etoposide single-agent activity. *Cancer Treat Rev* 9 Suppl:21, 1982.
97. Shipp MA, Takvorian RC, Canellos GP: High-dose cytosine arabinoside. Active agent in treatment of non-Hodgkin's lymphoma. *Am J Med* 77:5, 1984.
98. Bajetta E, Buzzoni R, Valagussa P, Bonadonna G: Mitoxantrone: An active agent in refractory non-Hodgkin's lymphomas. *Am J Clin Oncol* 11:2, 1988.
99. Wiernik PH, Lossos IS, Tuscano JM, et al: Lenalidomide monotherapy in relapsed or refractory aggressive non-Hodgkin's lymphoma. *J Clin Oncol* 26:30, 2008.
100. Rizzieri DA, Sand GJ, McGaughey D, et al: Low-dose weekly paclitaxel for recurrent or refractory aggressive non-Hodgkin lymphoma. *Cancer* 100:11, 2004.
101. Kewalramani T, Zelenetz AD, Nimer SD, et al: Rituximab and ICE as second-line therapy before autologous stem cell transplantation for relapsed or primary refractory diffuse large B-cell lymphoma. *Blood* 103:10, 2004.
102. Velasquez WS, McLaughlin P, Tucker S, et al: ESHAP—An effective chemotherapy regimen in refractory and relapsing lymphoma: A 4-year follow-up study. *J Clin Oncol* 12:6, 1994.
103. Philip T, Guglielmi C, Hagenbeek A, et al: Autologous bone marrow transplantation as compared with salvage chemotherapy in relapses of chemotherapy-sensitive non-Hodgkin's lymphoma. *N Engl J Med* 333:23, 1995.
104. Chopra R, Goldstone AH, Pearce R, et al: Autologous versus allogeneic bone marrow transplantation for non-Hodgkin's lymphoma: A case-controlled analysis of the European Bone Marrow Transplant Group Registry data. *J Clin Oncol* 10:11, 1992.
105. Rezvani AR, Norasetthada L, Gooley T, et al: Non-myeloablative allogeneic haematopoietic cell transplantation for relapsed diffuse large B-cell lymphoma: A multicentre experience. *Br J Haematol* 143:3, 2008.
106. Thomson KJ, Morris EC, Bloor A, et al: Favorable long-term survival after reduced-intensity allogeneic transplantation for multiple-relapse aggressive non-Hodgkin's lymphoma. *J Clin Oncol* 27:3, 2009.
107. Krishnan A, Nademanee A, Fung HC, et al: Phase II trial of a transplantation regimen of yttrium-90 ibritumomab tiuxetan and high-dose chemotherapy in patients with non-Hodgkin's lymphoma. *J Clin Oncol* 26:1, 2008.
108. Vose JM, Bierman PJ, Enke C, et al: Phase I trial of iodine-131 tositumomab with high-dose chemotherapy and autologous stem-cell transplantation for relapsed non-Hodgkin's lymphoma. *J Clin Oncol* 23:3, 2005.
109. Zucca E, Conconi A, Mughal TI, et al: Patterns of outcome and prognostic factors in primary large-cell lymphoma of the testis in a survey by the International Extranodal Lymphoma Study Group. *J Clin Oncol* 21:1, 2003.
110. Gundrum JD, Mathiason MA, Derek BM, et al: Primary testicular diffuse large B-cell lymphoma: a population-based study on the incidence, natural history, and survival comparison with primary nodal counterpart before and after the introduction of rituximab. *J Clin Onco* 27:5227, 2009.
111. Pingali S, Go RS, Gundrum JD, Wright L, Gay G: Adult testicular lymphoma in the United States (1985–2004): Analysis of 3,669 cases from the National Cancer Data Base (NCDB). *Journal of Clinical Oncology* 26 (15S):19503, 2008.
112. Fonseca R, Habermann TM, Colgan JP, et al: Testicular lymphoma is associated with a high incidence of extranodal recurrence. *Cancer* 88:1, 2000.
113. Visco C, Medeiros LJ, Mesina OM, et al: Non-Hodgkin's lymphoma affecting the testis: Is it curable with doxorubicin-based therapy? *Clin Lymphoma* 2:1, 2001.
114. Pentheroudakis G, Pavlidis N: Cancer and pregnancy: Poena magna, not anymore. *Eur J Cancer* 42:2, 2006.
115. Pereg D, Koren G, Lishner M: Cancer in pregnancy: Gaps, challenges and solutions. *Cancer Treat Rev* 34:4, 2008.
116. Pereg D, Koren G, Lishner M: The treatment of Hodgkin's and non-Hodgkin's lymphoma in pregnancy. *Haematologica* 92:9, 2007.
117. Aviles A, Diaz-Maqueo JC, Torras V, et al: Non-Hodgkin's lymphomas and pregnancy: Presentation of 16 cases. *Gynecol Oncol* 37:3, 1990.
118. Zuazu J, Julia A, Sierra J, et al: Pregnancy outcome in hematologic malignancies. *Cancer* 67:3, 1991.
119. Resnik R: Cancer during pregnancy. *N Engl J Med* 341:2, 1999.
120. van Besien K, Kelta M, Bahaguna P: Primary mediastinal B-cell lymphoma: A review of pathology and management. *J Clin Oncol* 19:6, 2001.
121. Savage KJ, Monti S, Kutok JL, et al: The molecular signature of mediastinal large B-cell lymphoma differs from that of other diffuse large B-cell lymphomas and shares features with classical Hodgkin lymphoma. *Blood* 102:12, 2003.
122. Perrone T, Frizzera G, Rosai J: Mediastinal diffuse large-cell lymphoma with sclerosis. A clinicopathologic study of 60 cases. *Am J Surg Pathol* 10:3, 1986.
123. Nakagawa A, Nakamura S, Koshikawa T, et al: Clinicopathologic study of primary mediastinal non-lymphoblastic non-Hodgkin's lymphomas among the Japanese. *Acta Pathol Jpn* 43:1–2,1993.
124. Zinzani PL, Martelli M, Bertini M, et al: Induction chemotherapy strategies for primary mediastinal large B-cell lymphoma with sclerosis: A retrospective multinational study on 426 previously untreated patients. *Haematologica* 87:12, 2002.
125. Todeschini G, Secchi S, Morra E, et al: Primary mediastinal large B-cell lymphoma (PMLBCL): Long-term results from a retrospective multicentre Italian experience in 138 patients treated with CHOP or MACOP-B/VACOP-B: *Br J Cancer* 90:2, 2004.
126. Dunleavy K, Pittaluga S, Janik J, et al: Primary mediastinal large B-cell lymphoma (PMBL) outcome is significantly improved by the addition of rituximab to dose adjusted (DA)-EPOCH and overcomes the need for radiation. *Annals of Oncology* 59(Suppl 5):929, 2005.
127. Katzenstein AL, Carrington CB, Liebow AA: Lymphomatoid granulomatosis: A clinicopathologic study of 152 cases. *Cancer* 43:1, 1979.
128. Gitelson E, Al-Saleem T, Smith MR: Review: Lymphomatoid granulomatosis: Challenges in diagnosis and treatment. *Clin Adv Hematol Oncol* 7:1, 2009.
129. Dunleavy K, Janik J, Cohen J, et al: 16. Clinical-pathological correlations: 079 Study of the treatment and biology of lymphomatoid granulomatosis (LYG); a rare EBV lymphoproliferative disorder. *Ann Oncol* 16:v59, 2005.
130. Ferreri AJ, Campo E, Seymour JF, et al: Intravascular lymphoma: Clinical presentation, natural history, management and prognostic factors in a series of 38 cases, with special emphasis on the "cutaneous variant." *Br J Haematol* 127:2, 2004.
131. Ferreri AJ, Dognini GP, Campo E, et al: Variations in clinical presentation, frequency of hemophagocytosis and clinical behavior of intravascular lymphoma diagnosed in different geographical regions. *Haematologica* 92:4, 2007.
132. Murase T, Nakamura S: An Asian variant of intravascular lymphomatosis: An updated review of malignant histiocytosis-like B-cell lymphoma. *Leuk Lymphoma* 33:5–6,1999.
133. Murase T, Nakamura S, Kawauchi K, et al: An Asian variant of intravascular large B-cell lymphoma: Clinical, pathological and cytogenetic approaches to diffuse large B-cell lymphoma associated with haemophagocytic syndrome. *Br J Haematol* 111:3, 2000.
134. Shimazaki C, Inaba T, Nakagawa M: B-cell lymphoma-associated hemophagocytic syndrome. *Leuk Lymphoma* 38:1, 2000.
135. Ponzoni M, Ferreri AJ, Campo E, et al: Definition, diagnosis, and management of intravascular large B-cell lymphoma: Proposals and perspectives from an international consensus meeting. *J Clin Oncol* 25:21, 2007.
136. Ferreri AJ, Dognini GP, Govi S, et al: Can rituximab change the usually dismal prognosis of patients with intravascular large B-cell lymphoma? *J Clin Oncol* 26:31, 2008.
137. Shimada K, Matsue K, Yamamoto K, et al: Retrospective analysis of intravascular large B-cell lymphoma treated with rituximab-containing chemotherapy as reported by the IVL study group in Japan. *J Clin Oncol* 26:19, 2008.
138. Oton AB, Wang H, Leleu X, et al: Clinical and pathological prognostic markers for survival in adult patients with post-transplant lymphoproliferative disorders in solid transplant. *Leuk Lymphoma* 49:9, 2008.

139. Adami J, Gabel H, Lindelof B, et al: Cancer risk following organ transplantation: A nationwide cohort study in Sweden. *Br J Cancer* 89:7, 2003.
140. Tsao L, Hsi ED: The clinicopathologic spectrum of posttransplantation lymphoproliferative disorders. *Arch Pathol Lab Med* 131:8, 2007.
141. Cockfield SM, Preiksaitis JK, Jewell LD, Parfrey NA: Post-transplant lymphoproliferative disorder in renal allograft recipients. Clinical experience and risk factor analysis in a single center. *Transplantation* 56:1, 1993.
142. Swinnen LJ, Costanzo-Nordin MR, Fisher SG, et al: Increased incidence of lymphoproliferative disorder after immunosuppression with the monoclonal antibody OKT3 in cardiac-transplant recipients. *N Engl J Med* 323:25, 1990.
143. Walker RC, Paya CV, Marshall WF, et al: Pretransplantation seronegative Epstein-Barr virus status is the primary risk factor for posttransplantation lymphoproliferative disorder in adult heart, lung, and other solid organ transplantations. *J Heart Lung Transplant* 14:2, 1995.
144. Hanto DW: Classification of Epstein-Barr virus-associated posttransplant lymphoproliferative diseases: Implications for understanding their pathogenesis and developing rational treatment strategies. *Annu Rev Med* 46:381, 1995.
145. Leblond V, Davi F, Charlotte F, et al: Posttransplant lymphoproliferative disorders not associated with Epstein-Barr virus: A distinct entity? *J Clin Oncol* 16:6, 1998.
146. Kew CE 2nd, Lopez-Ben R, Smith JK, et al: Posttransplant lymphoproliferative disorder localized near the allograft in renal transplantation. *Transplantation* 69:5, 2000.
147. Rees L, Thomas A, Amlot PL: Disappearance of an Epstein-Barr virus-positive posttransplant plasmacytoma with reduction of immunosuppression. *Lancet* 352:9130, 1998.
148. Tsai DE, Hardy CL, Tomaszewski JE, et al: Reduction in immunosuppression as initial therapy for posttransplant lymphoproliferative disorder: Analysis of prognostic variables and long-term follow-up of 42 adult patients. *Transplantation* 71:8, 2001.
149. Choquet S, Leblond V, Herbrecht R, et al: Efficacy and safety of rituximab in B-cell post-transplantation lymphoproliferative disorders: Results of a prospective multicenter phase 2 study. *Blood* 107:8, 2006.
150. Trappe R, Riess H, Babel N, et al: Salvage chemotherapy for refractory and relapsed posttransplant lymphoproliferative disorders (PTLD) after treatment with single-agent rituximab. *Transplantation* 83:7, 2007.
151. Swinnen LJ, LeBlanc M, Grogan TM, et al: Prospective study of sequential reduction in immunosuppression, interferon alpha-2B, and chemotherapy for posttransplantation lymphoproliferative disorder. *Transplantation* 86:2, 2008.
152. Achten R, Verhoef G, Vanuytsel L, De Wolf-Peeters C: T-cell/histiocyte-rich large B-cell lymphoma: A distinct clinicopathologic entity. *J Clin Oncol* 20:5, 2002.
153. Abramson JS: T-cell/histiocyte-rich B-cell lymphoma: Biology, diagnosis, and management. *Oncologist* 11:4, 2006.
154. Aki H, Tuzuner N, Ongoren S, et al: T-cell-rich B-cell lymphoma: A clinicopathologic study of 21 cases and comparison with 43 cases of diffuse large B-cell lymphoma. *Leuk Res* 28:3, 2004.
155. Bouabdallah R, Mounier N, Guettier C, et al: T-cell/histiocyte-rich large B-cell lymphomas and classical diffuse large B-cell lymphomas have similar outcome after chemotherapy: A matched-control analysis. *J Clin Oncol* 21:7, 2003.
156. Boudova L, Torlakovic E, Delabie J, et al: Nodular lymphocyte-predominant Hodgkin lymphoma with nodules resembling T-cell/histiocyte-rich B-cell lymphoma: Differential diagnosis between nodular lymphocyte-predominant Hodgkin lymphoma and T-cell/histiocyte-rich B-cell lymphoma. *Blood* 102:10, 2003.
157. Greer JP, Macon WR, Lamar RE, et al: T-cell-rich B-cell lymphomas: Diagnosis and response to therapy of 44 patients. *J Clin Oncol* 13:7, 1995.
158. McBride JA, Rodriguez J, Luthra R, et al: T-cell-rich B large-cell lymphoma simulating lymphocyte-rich Hodgkin's disease. *Am J Surg Pathol* 20:2, 1996.
159. Rodriguez J, Pugh WC, Cabanillas F: T-cell-rich B-cell lymphoma. *Blood* 82:5, 1993.
160. Willemze R, Jaffe ES, Burg G, et al: WHO-EORTC classification for cutaneous lymphomas. *Blood* 105:10, 2005.
161. Grange F, Beylot-Barry M, Courville P, et al: Primary cutaneous diffuse large B-cell lymphoma, leg type: Clinicopathologic features and prognostic analysis in 60 cases. *Arch Dermatol* 143:9, 2007.
162. Grange F, Maubec E, Bagot M, et al: Treatment of cutaneous B-cell lymphoma, leg type, with age-adapted combinations of chemotherapies and rituximab. *Arch Dermatol* 145:3, 2009.
163. Kodama K, Massone C, Chott A, Metze D, Kerl H, Cerroni L: Primary cutaneous large B-cell lymphomas: Clinicopathologic features, classification, and prognostic factors in a large series of patients. *Blood* 106:7, 2005.
164. Beltran B, Castillo J, Salas R, et al: ALK-positive diffuse large B-cell lymphoma: Report of four cases and review of the literature. *J Hematol Oncol* 2:11, 2009.
165. Reichard KK, McKenna RW, Kroft SH: ALK-positive diffuse large B-cell lymphoma: Report of four cases and review of the literature. *Mod Pathol* 20:3, 2007.
166. Paul T, Challa S, Tandon A,et al: Primary central nervous system lymphomas: Indian experience, and review of literature. *Indian J Cancer* 45:112, 2008.
167. Abrey LE, Yahalom J, DeAngelis LM: Treatment for primary CNS lymphoma: The next step. *J Clin Oncol* 18:3144, 2000.
168. Tun HW, Personett D, Baskerville KA, et al: Pathway analysis of primary central nervous system lymphoma. *Blood* 111:3200, 2008.
169. Wong HH, Wang J: Epstein-Barr virus positive diffuse large B-cell lymphoma of the elderly. *Leuk Lymphoma* 50:335, 2009.
170. Oyama T, Yamamoto K, Asano N, et al: Age-related EBV-associated B-cell lymphoproliferative disorders constitute a distinct clinicopathologic group: A study of 96 patients. *Clin Cancer Res* 13:5124, 2007.
171. Baecklund E, Iliadou A, Askling J, et al: Association of chronic inflammation, not its treatment, with increased lymphoma risk in rheumatoid arthritis. *Arthritis Rheum* 54:692, 2006.
172. Smedby KE, Hjalgrim H, Askling J, et al: Autoimmune and chronic inflammatory disorders and risk of non-Hodgkin lymphoma by subtype. *J Natl Cancer Inst* 98:51, 2006.
173. Rothman N, Skibola CF, Wang SS, et al: Genetic variation in TNF and IL10 and risk of non-Hodgkin lymphoma: A report from the InterLymph Consortium. *Lancet Oncol* 7:27, 2006.
174. Smedby KE, Baecklund E, Askling J: Malignant lymphomas in autoimmunity and inflammation: A review of risks, risk factors, and lymphoma characteristics. *Cancer Epidemiol Biomarkers Prev* 15:2069, 2006.
175. Rafaniello Raviele P, Pruneri G, Maiorano E: Plasmablastic lymphoma: A review. *Oral Dis* 15:38, 2009.
176. Ustun C, Reid-Nicholson M, Nayak-Kapoor A, et al: Plasmablastic lymphoma: CNS involvement, coexistence of other malignancies, possible viral etiology, and dismal outcome. *Ann Hematol* 88:351, 2009.
177. Malnati MS, Dagna L, Ponzoni M, Lusso P: Human herpesvirus 8 (HHV-8/KSHV) and hematologic malignancies. *Rev Clin Exp Hematol* 7:375, 2003.
178. Katano H, Sata T: Human herpesvirus 8 virology, epidemiology and related diseases. *Jpn J Infect Dis* 53:137, 2000.
179. Chen YB, Rahemtullah A, Hochberg E: Primary effusion lymphoma. *Oncologist* 12:569, 2007.
180. O'Hara AJ, Vahrson W, Dittmer DP: Gene alteration and precursor and mature microRNA transcription changes contribute to the miRNA signature of primary effusion lymphoma. *Blood* 111:2347, 2008.

CHAPTER 101
FOLLICULAR LYMPHOMA

Oliver W. Press

SUMMARY

Follicular Lymphoma is an indolent, neoplastic disorder of germinal center-derived B lymphocytes that afflicts approximately 14,000 people in the United States each year. It typically presents as a disseminated disorder with painless, diffuse lymphadenopathy and marrow infiltration, often with associated hepatosplenomegaly and circulating lymphoma cells in the blood. A characteristic translocation, t(14;18), is found in the cells of 85 percent of patients, which deregulates BCL2 protein expression and inhibits apoptosis of affected B cells. The cells typically express monoclonal surface immunoglobulin, CD10, CD19, CD20, CD22, CD45, and CD79a on their cell surface, but not CD5 or CD23. Patients are often asymptomatic at the time of presentation, and may live for many years in good health without therapy. On the other hand, most patients eventually develop progressive lymphadenopathy, causing symptoms mandating intervention. Many treatment regimens are effective at inducing remissions, including single-agent rituximab or chlorambucil; or several multidrug programs, such as rituximab, cyclophosphamide, vincristine, and prednisone (R-CVP); rituximab, cyclophosphamide, doxorubicin, vincristine, and prednisone (R-CHOP); rituximab, fludarabine, mitoxantrone, and dexamethasone (R-FND); and radiolabeled monoclonal antibodies. None of these therapies, however, is considered curative and most patients eventually relapse with recurrent disease. The role of autologous and allogeneic hematopoietic cell transplantation is controversial. Histologic transformation to aggressive lymphoma occurs in 30 to 40 percent of patients, usually leading to death within 1 to 2 years of transformation.

DEFINITION AND HISTORY

Follicular lymphoma (FL) is an indolent lymphoid neoplasm that is derived from mutated germinal center B cells and exhibits a nodular or follicular histologic pattern. It is typically composed of a mixture of small, cleaved follicle center cells (centrocytes) and large noncleaved follicle center cells (centroblasts). The disease has masqueraded under multiple previous monikers, including "nodular lymphoma" in the Rappaport classification, and "follicle center cell lymphoma" in the Working Formulation.[1] The current World Health Organization (WHO) classification proposes the terms *follicular lymphoma, grades 1, 2, and 3*, to differentiate cases based on the numbers of centroblasts per high-power microscopic field (see "Lymph Node Morphology and Lymphocyte Immunophenotype" below).[1]

Abbreviations and acronyms that appear in this chapter include: ADCC, antibody-dependent cellular cytotoxicity; AML, acute myelocytic leukemia; CDC, complement-dependent cytotoxicity; CHOP, cyclophosphamide, doxorubicin, vincristine, prednisone; CR, complete remission; CVP, cyclophosphamide, vincristine, prednisone; FCM, fludarabine, cyclophosphamide, mitoxantrone; FDG, fluoro-2-deoxyglucose; FL, follicular lymphoma; FND, fludarabine, mitoxantrone (Novantrone), dexamethasone; GELF, Groupe d'Etudes des Lymphomes Folliculaires; GM-CSF, granulocyte-macrophage colony-stimulating factor; Gy, gray; HLA, histocompatibility locus antigen; IFN, interferon; Ig, immunoglobulin; IPI, international prognostic index; KLH, keyhole limpet hemocyanin; LDH, lactate dehydrogenase; NHL, non-Hodgkin lymphoma; ORR, overall response rate; OS, overall survival; PACE, cisplatin, doxorubicin, cyclophosphamide, etoposide; PCR, polymerase chain reaction; PET, positron emission tomography; PFS, progression-free survival; PR, partial remission; ProMACE/MOPP, prednisone, methotrexate, doxorubicin, cyclophosphamide, etoposide, mechlorethamine, vincristine, procarbazine, prednisone; R-CHOP, rituximab plus CHOP; R-CVP, rituximab plus CVP; REAL, revised European-American lymphoma; RIT, radioimmunotherapy; WHO, World Health Organization.

EPIDEMIOLOGY

FL accounts for approximately 20 to 25 percent of adult non-Hodgkin lymphomas (NHL) in the United States, with an annual incidence of approximately 14,000 new cases per year.[2,3] FL is most common in North America and Western Europe, and much less frequent in Eastern Europe, Asia, Africa, and in Americans of African descent.[1] The median age at diagnosis is 59 years, and the male-to-female ratio is 1:1.7. The disease is rare in persons younger than age 20 years, and pediatric cases appear to represent a separate disease entity that is typically localized, lacks the t(14;18) translocation and BCL2 expression, and has a very good prognosis.[4]

CLINICAL FEATURES

SYMPTOMS AND SIGNS

Patients with FL usually present with painless diffuse lymphadenopathy. Less frequently, patients may have vague abdominal complaints, including pain, early satiety, and increasing girth, which are caused by a large abdominal mass. Approximately 10 percent of patients present with B symptoms (fever, drenching night sweats, or loss of 10 percent of the body weight). The disease usually is widespread at presentation, with involvement of multiple lymph node–bearing sites, liver, and spleen. The marrow is involved in 40 to 70 percent of patients at diagnosis. FL may occasionally present with primary involvement of extranodal sites, such as the skin, gastrointestinal tract, ocular adnexa, and breast, but CNS disease is rare, unless histologic transformation to diffuse large B-cell lymphoma has occurred.[1]

STAGING THE DISEASE

Evaluation of FL involves performance of a medical history, physical examination (with attention to the lymph nodes in Waldeyer ring and size and involvement of liver and spleen), laboratory testing (including a complete blood count, examination of the blood film and a differential white cell count, lactic dehydrogenase [LDH], β_2-microglobulin, comprehensive metabolic panel, serum uric acid level), lymph node biopsy, marrow aspiration and biopsy, flow cytometric analysis of blood, marrow and lymph node cells, and computed tomography of the chest, abdomen, and pelvis.[5] Excisional lymph node biopsies are strongly preferred for the initial histologic diagnosis of FL, although in cases in which nodal masses are inaccessible, generous needle core biopsies may suffice. The diagnosis should not be established merely on the basis of flow cytometry of the blood or marrow, or on cytologic examination of aspiration needle biopsies of lymph node or other tissue.[5] Hepatitis B serology should be assessed if rituximab therapy is contemplated, as hepatitis reactivation with rituximab may occasionally be fatal. In selected circumstances, additional computed tomography (CT) scans of the neck, positron emission tomography (PET)/CT imaging, measurement of the cardiac ejection fraction, serum protein electrophoresis, quantitative immunoglobulins, and hepatitis C testing may be useful. Patients in whom chemotherapy is contemplated should receive counseling regarding contraception, fertility issues, and sperm or egg banking.[6] Although fluoro-2-deoxy-glucose (FDG)-PET has become popular, it has significant limitations in evaluation of FL. In one study, 7 of 28 patients whose initially positive PET/CT converted to negative after therapy had persistently positive marrow biopsies, indicating PET scans do not reliably detect complete remissions in this disease.[7,8]

LABORATORY FEATURES

LYMPH NODE MORPHOLOGY AND LYMPHOCYTE IMMUNOPHENOTYPE

FL exhibits a predominantly nodular lymph node pattern, however, the neoplastic follicles are distorted and as the disease progresses, the malignant follicles efface the nodal architecture (see Chap. 98, Fig. 98–17), commonly resulting in the development of areas of diffuse involvement, which may predominate histologically. The WHO has developed a three-grade system of classifying FL according to the proportion of centroblasts detected microscopically: grade 1 lymphomas have 0 to 5 centroblasts, grade 2 lymphomas have 6 to 15 centroblasts, and grade 3 lymphomas have more than 15 centroblasts per high-power microscopic field (Fig. 101–1).[1] Grade 3 FL is further subdivided into grade 3A, in which some small centrocytes are present despite the predominance of centroblasts, and grade 3B, in which solid sheets of centroblasts are exclusively present and centrocytes are entirely absent.[1] Some, but not all, studies suggest that grades 1 and 2 lymphomas follow a more indolent course than grade 3 FL, and many authorities suggest that these lower grades should be treated more conservatively than grade 3 FL.[5] Other studies indicate a similar natural history for grades 1, 2, and 3A.[9] Nearly all authorities now agree, however, that grade 3B FL behaves aggressively and should be treated with anthracycline-containing regimens (e.g., rituximab, cyclophosphamide, doxorubicin, vincristine, prednisone [R-CHOP]) similar to diffuse large B-cell lymphoma.[1] FL cells of all grades typically express monoclonal surface immunoglobulin, are positive for *BCL-2*, *BCL6*, and CD10, and express the pan-B-cell surface antigens CD19, CD20, CD22, and CD79a, but do not express CD5, CD23, CD11c, or CD43.

CYTOGENETICS

The classic cytogenetic finding detected in FL is the t(14;18)(q32;q21) translocation that juxtaposes the *BCL-2* gene on band q21 of chromosome 18 with the immunoglobulin (Ig) heavy-chain gene on band 32 of chromosome 14 (Fig. 101–2).[10] The Ig enhancer element results in amplified expression of the translocated gene product and, thus, overexpression of BCL-2 protein leading to inhibition of apoptosis of affected B cells. Quantitative real-time polymerase chain reaction (PCR) assays on blood and marrow can determine the number of t(14;18)-expressing cells and may be useful in predicting the outcome of therapy. The t(14;18) translocation is found in about 85 percent of patients in the United States, but the translocation is present in a significantly lower percentage of Asian patients afflicted with FL. Detection of the t(14;18) translocation in lymphoid cells is neither necessary nor sufficient for the diagnosis of FL. Small numbers of B cells harboring the t(14;18) translocation can be detected in the blood of 25 to 75 percent of healthy individuals, as well as in reactive lymph nodes and tonsils if a very sensitive nested or reverse-transcription

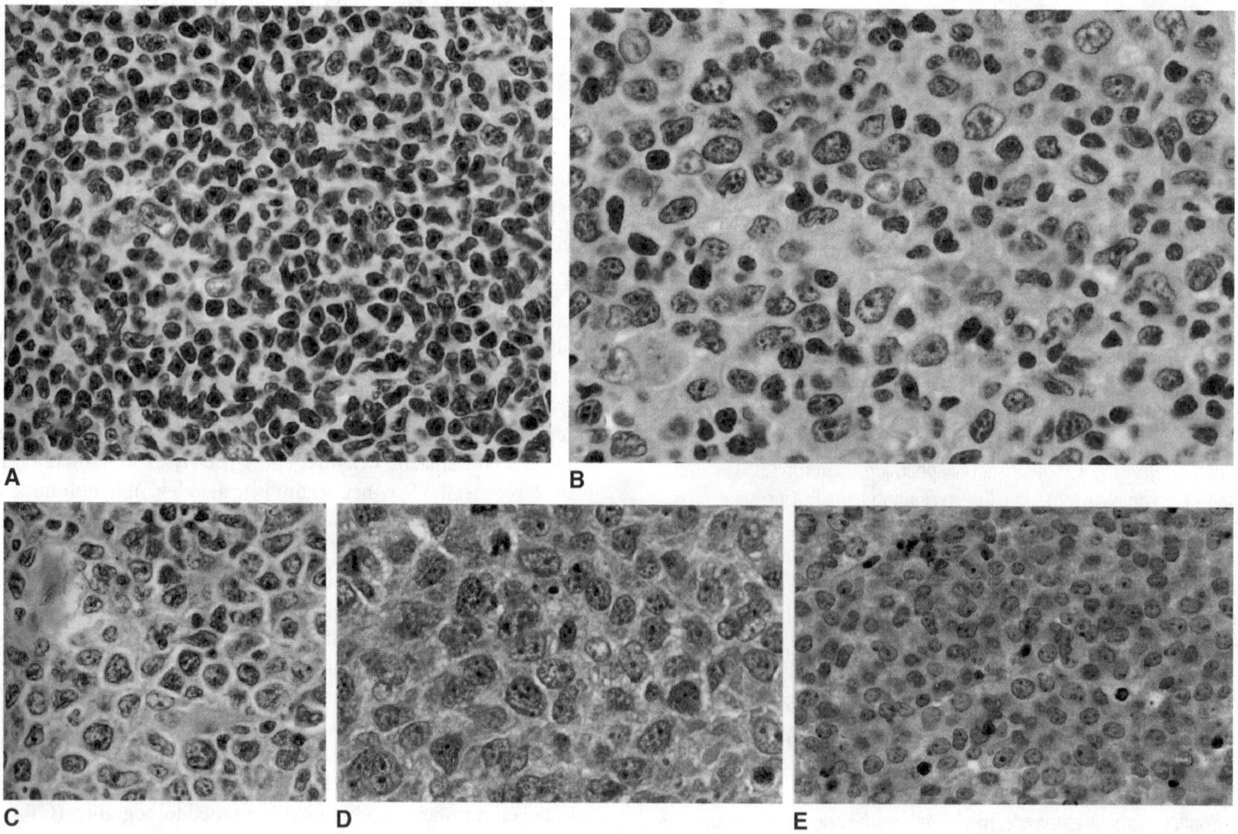

FIGURE 101–1. Follicular lymphoma grading is based on the relative proportions of small cells (centrocytes) and centroblasts (centroblasts). **A.** Grade 1 (0–5 centroblasts/high-powered field); **B.** grade 2 (6–15 centroblasts/high-powered field); **C.** grade 3A (>15 centroblasts/high-powered field). **D** and **E.** Grade 3B. See text for further definitions of grades 1, 2, 3A, and 3B. *(Reproduced with permission from Harris NL, Nathwani BN, Swerdlow SH, et al.[1])*

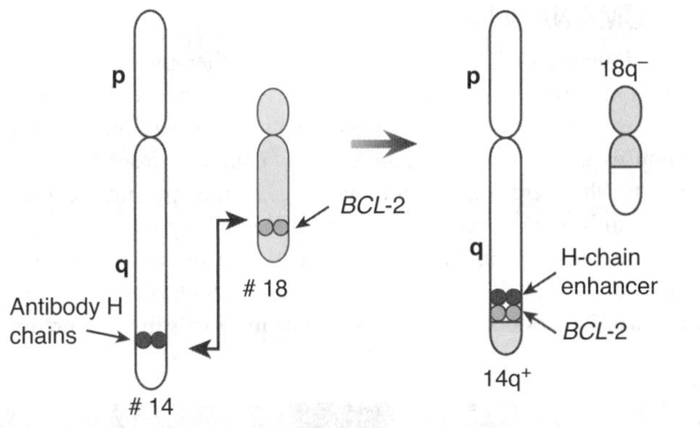

FIGURE 101–2. The t(14;18)(q32;q21) translocation juxtaposes the *BCL-2* gene on band q21 of chromosome 18 with the immunoglobulin heavy-chain gene on band 32 of chromosome 14.

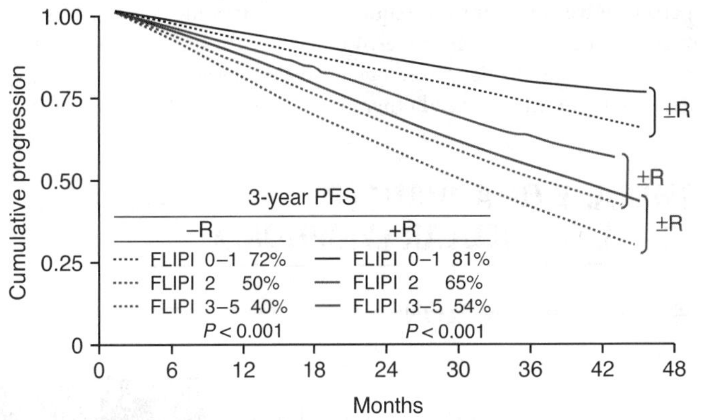

FIGURE 101–3. Progression-free survival of 827 patients with FL stratified by the Follicular Lymphoma International Prognostic Index (FLIPI) into low risk (0–1 risk factors, 40% of patients, *black lines*), intermediate risk (2 risk factors, 33% of patients, *blue lines*), or high risk (3–5 risk factors, 27% of patients, *red lines*). Of the 827 patients, 267 were treated with chemotherapy regimens without rituximab (*dotted lines*) and 560 were treated with rituximab-containing regimens (*solid lines*). *(Reproduced with permission from Federico M, Guglielmi C, Luminari S, et al.[13])*

polymerase chain reaction (RT-PCR) assay is employed.[1] Additional cytogenetic abnormalities are found in 90 percent of patients with FL, most commonly, loss of 1p, 6q, 10q, and 17p, and gains of 1, 6p, 7, 8, 12q, X, and 18q/dup. The significance of these additional abnormalities is currently the subject of intense investigation. The finding of multiple cytogenetic abnormalities is commonly associated with higher histologic grade and with the probability of transformation to aggressive lymphoma.

PROGNOSTIC FACTORS

■ CLINICAL AND LABORATORY VARIABLES

An international working group developed an international prognostic index (IPI) based on five independent variables (age, stage, LDH level, performance status, and number of extranodal sites) that affected overall survival of aggressive lymphoma patients treated with anthracycline-based combination chemotherapy.[11] The IPI was subsequently applied retrospectively to FL and found to be predictive of both overall and progression-free survival for FL (as well as diffuse large B-cell lymphoma). Nevertheless, the IPI was considered to be suboptimal for segregating indolent lymphoma patients into prognostic categories because only 10 to 15 percent of patients with FL fall into the poor risk category using this index. To redress this deficiency, a French cooperative group conducted a detailed prognostic factor analysis of 4167 patients with FL diagnosed between 1985 and 1992 for whom prolonged followup was available to assess overall survival.[12] Five adverse prognostic factors were detected: age (>60 years vs. ≤60 years), Ann Arbor stage (III–IV vs. I–II), hemoglobin level (<120 g/L vs. ≥120 g/L), number of nodal areas (>4 vs. ≤4), and serum LDH level (high vs. normal). Three risk groups were defined: low risk (0–1 adverse factors, 36% of patients), intermediate risk (2 factors, 37% of patients, hazard ratio [HR] of 2.3), and poor risk (≥3 adverse factors, 27% of patients, HR = 4.3). The Follicular Lymphoma International Prognostic Index (FLIPI) discriminated outcomes for FL better than the IPI, both in the original cohort[12] and in later studies evaluating patients treated with modern combined rituximab-chemotherapy regimens (Fig. 101–3).[13] In addition to the variables defined in the IPI and FLIPI indices, high β_2-microglobulin level,[14] the presence of bulky tumors, and male sex have been identified in some studies as associated with poor outcome for FL patients.

■ GENE EXPRESSION PROFILING

The most sophisticated method of assessing the prognosis of FL has utilized genomic scale gene-expression profiling to assess 191 biopsy specimens obtained from patients with untreated FL for whom long-term followup was available.[15] Two gene-expression signatures were identified that allowed construction of a survival predictor that enabled segregation of patients into four quartiles with disparate median lengths of survival (13.6, 11.1, 10.8, and 3.9 years), independent of clinical prognostic variables. One signature (immune-response 1) was associated with a good prognosis and included genes encoding T-cell markers (e.g., *CD7, CD8B1, ITK, LEF1,* and *STAT4*) as well as genes that are highly expressed in macrophages (e.g., *ACTN1* and *TNFSF13B*). The immune-response-2 signature was associated with a poor prognosis and included genes known to be preferentially expressed in macrophages, dendritic cells, or both (e.g., *TLR5, FCGR1A, SEPT10, LGMN,* and *C3AR1*). Flow cytometry and cell sorting confirmed that these signatures reflected gene expression by nonmalignant tumor-infiltrating immune cells (CD19-negative cells) and not by the FL cells themselves (CD19-positive cells). The length of survival correlated with the molecular features of the nonmalignant immune cells present in the tumor at diagnosis and presumably reflected the robustness of the immune response mounted against the tumor.

THERAPY OF LIMITED STAGE I-II FOLLICULAR LYMPHOMA

■ RADIOTHERAPY

Patients with stage I or II FL represent only 10 to 30 percent of all cases in most series.[1,3] Standard management for stage I or limited contiguous stage II FL involves the administration of involved field radiotherapy (35 to 40 Gy).[5] Adjuvant chemotherapy does not appear to improve survival in this setting, though some studies suggest that combined chemoradiotherapy may improve progression-free survival.[16] A retrospective review of 177 patients with stage I or II and grade 1 or 2 FL reported a median survival of 14 years following radiation therapy as a single modality.[17] Approximately 50 percent of the patients were relapse-free at 5 to 10 years.

■ OBSERVATION

Excellent survival has also been observed in patients with early stage FL who received no initial therapy.[18] In a group of 43 selected patients, 56 percent were free from the requirement for treatment for at least 10 years and 86 percent were alive 10 years after diagnosis. Based on this study, many authorities have concluded that "watchful waiting" is an acceptable alternative to radiotherapy for stage I or II FL.

THERAPY OF ADVANCED STAGE FOLLICULAR LYMPHOMA

OBSERVATION ALONE

Many patients with FL, particularly grades 1 or 2, will exhibit an indolent, asymptomatic course despite the absence of therapy. Because there is no conclusive evidence that survival of FL patients is improved by immediate institution of therapy, or that conventional management (other than allogeneic stem cell transplantation) can cure the disease, a "watch-and-wait" approach is often recommended for patients with extensive stage II or stage III or IV FL. In one study, survival was 82 percent at 5 years and 73 percent at 10 years after an initial strategy of observation alone, and the median time until therapy was required was 3 years.[19] Spontaneous regressions occurred in 23 percent of untreated patients. No differences in survival were observed in a trial of 309 patients randomized to initial watchful waiting or to chlorambucil.[20] In another trial, patients were randomized to either watchful waiting or to immediate aggressive combination chemotherapy with ProMACE/MOPP (prednisone, methotrexate, doxorubicin, cyclophosphamide, etoposide, mechlorethamine, vincristine, procarbazine, prednisone) chemotherapy followed by total nodal irradiation.[21] The overall survival rates for the two groups were similar, although the disease-free survival rate was naturally higher in the patients treated with combined modality therapy. Criteria established by the Groupe d'Etudes des Lymphomes Folliculaires (GELF) are useful to identify patients who may benefit from intervention rather than "watchful waiting." These criteria suggest that treatment is likely to be required for patients with a maximum diameter of any site of disease greater than 7 cm, more than three nodal sites greater than 3 cm in diameter, systemic B symptoms, a spleen size greater than 16 cm, pleural effusions, local compressive symptoms, circulating lymphoma cells, or cytopenias as a result of the lymphoma.[5,22]

SINGLE-AGENT CHEMOTHERAPY

FL patients can be palliated effectively with a variety of single chemotherapy agents (Table 101–1). Responses to single-agent therapy, such as chlorambucil, a nucleoside analogue, or bendamustine, range from 70 to 90 percent and may last for several years.[20,23]

COMBINATION CHEMOTHERAPY

In randomized trials, single-agent alkylating therapy was compared to treatment with cyclophosphamide, vincristine, and prednisone (CVP) (see Table 101–1). Patients treated with CVP had more complete responses and shorter median time to complete response than did patients who were treated with single-agent therapy, but did not have significantly longer overall survival rates.[24] Similarly, intensive combination regimens that included doxorubicin also demonstrated excellent responses for patients with FL, but no evidence indicates such treatment with CHOP (cyclophosphamide, doxorubicin, vincristine, and prednisone

TABLE 101–1. Therapeutic Regimens for Follicular Lymphoma

Agent(s)	Dose	Route	Day(s) of Treatment	Repeat Cycle at Day
Single agents				
Chlorambucil	0.08–0.12 mg/kg	PO	Daily	
	or 0.4–1.0 mg/kg	PO	1	28
Cyclophosphamide	50–100 mg/m^2	PO	Daily	
	or 300 mg/m^2	PO	1–5	28
Fludarabine	25 mg/m^2/day	IV	1–5	28
Pentostatin	4 mg/m^2	IV	1	14
Cladribine	0.1 mg/kg/day	IV (continuous)	1–7	28
	or 0.14 mg/kg/day	IV (2 h)	1–5	28
Bendamustine	100–120 mg/m^2/day	IV	1, 2	21 or 28
Rituximab	375 mg/m^2/day	IV	1, 8, 15, 22	
Combination therapy				
Stanford CVP				
Cyclophosphamide	400 mg/m^2	PO	1–5	21
Vincristine	1.4 mg/m^2 (maximum 2 mg)	IV	1	21
Prednisone	100 mg/m^2	PO	1–5	21
R-CVP				
Rituximab	375 mg/m^2	IV	1	21
Cyclophosphamide	1000 mg/m^2	IV	1	21
Vincristine	1.4 mg/m^2 (maximum 2 mg)	IV	1	21
Prednisone	100 mg	PO	1–5	21
R-CHOP				
Rituximab	375 mg/m^2	IV	1	21
Cyclophosphamide	750 mg/m^2	IV	1	21
Doxorubicin	50 mg/m^2	IV	1	
Vincristine	1.4 mg/m^2	IV	1	
Prednisone	100 mg	PO	1–5	
FND				
Fludarabine	25 mg/m^2	IV	1–3	28
Mitoxantrone	10 mg/m^2	IV	1	
Dexamethasone	20 mg	IV or PO	1–5	
CF				
Cyclophosphamide	600–1000 mg/m^2	IV	1	
Fludarabine	20 mg/m^2	IV	1–5	21–28

without rituximab) prolongs survival.[25] In recent years, fludarabine-containing regimens have become popular because of their high response rates and favorable toxicity profiles. Approximately 90 to 100 percent of FL patients respond to regimens such as FND (fludarabine, mitoxantrone, and dexamethasone) or fludarabine plus cyclophosphamide, with complete response rates of greater than 50 percent being reported in some studies.[26,27] However, purine nucleoside analogues are toxic to hematopoietic stem cells, and may cause protracted cytopenias and difficulty harvesting blood stem cells. Consequently, many lymphoma specialists are reluctant to use fludarabine or cladribine early in the disease course for fear that these drugs will make subsequent attempts at salvage therapy problematic as a consequence of cytopenias.

MONOCLONAL ANTIBODY THERAPY

Rituximab is a human–mouse chimeric monoclonal antibody that binds to the CD20 antigen that is expressed on nearly all normal and malignant B cells but not on any other human tissues. After binding to B cells, rituximab induces cell death via antibody-dependent cellular cytotoxicity (ADCC), complement-fixation (complement-dependent cytotoxicity [CDC]), induction of apoptosis, and by facilitating cross-presentation of lymphoma-associated antigens by dendritic cells.[28] Rituximab was approved by the FDA for therapy of indolent lymphomas based on the results of a pivotal trial that evaluated 166 patients for whom previous treatment had failed.[29] Four weekly infusions of rituximab were administered at a dose of 375 mg/m.[2] The response rate was 48 percent, including a 6 percent complete response rate and a median time to progression of approximately 1 year.[29] A second response to rituximab may be achieved in 40 percent of patients who relapse after an initial remission to rituximab.[30] The response rate to first-line therapy with rituximab in newly diagnosed FL is approximately 70 to 75 percent with a complete remission rate of 18 to 27 percent.[31,32] Extended courses of rituximab or "rituximab maintenance" therapy have become popular. Various schedules are employed, including administration of four doses of 375 mg/m^2 every 6 months for 2 years, one dose every 3 months for 2 years, or one dose every 2 months for four doses.[33–36] In one study, 38 patients with FL received rituximab as initial and maintenance therapy, experiencing an overall response rate of 76 percent, with a complete response rate of 37 percent and a median progression-free survival of 34 months.[37] Several humanized anti-CD20 monoclonal antibodies have been engineered to exhibit superior ADCC (e.g., ocrelizumab, GA101) or CDC (e.g., ofatumumab) and are undergoing clinical trials to determine if they are superior to rituximab. In addition, monoclonal antibodies targeting other B-cell targets are also in development, including epratuzumab (anti-CD22), lumiliximab (anti-CD23), dacetuzumab (anti-CD40), galiximab (anti-CD80), and apolizumab (anti–HLA-DRβ).

RITUXIMAB PLUS CHEMOTHERAPY

The introduction of rituximab into treatment protocols for FL has revolutionized the management of this disease. Multiple randomized controlled clinical trials have now documented the superiority of combining rituximab with chemotherapy compared to the use of chemotherapy alone in terms of overall response rates (ORR), complete response (CR) rates, event-free survival (EFS), progression-free survival (PFS), and overall survival (OS; Table 101–2). In one study, induction therapy consisting of 8 cycles of R-CVP was compared to 8 cycles of CVP without rituximab in 321 patients with newly diagnosed FL (Fig. 101–4).[38] R-CVP was superior to CVP alone in terms of ORR (81% vs. 57%), CR rate (41% vs. 10%), time to progression (32 months vs. 15 months), time to treatment failure (27 months vs. 7 months), and OS (83% vs. 77% at 4 years, p = 0.029).[38,39] Similarly, R-CHOP was compared to CHOP for first-line treatment of 428 patients with

TABLE 101–2. Selected Randomized Studies of Chemotherapy Alone vs. Rituximab Plus Chemotherapy for First-Line Therapy of Follicular Lymphoma

Study	Treatment	Median Followup (months)	Overall Response Rate (percent)	Complete Remission (percent)	Median TTP, TTF, or EFS* (months)	Overall Survival (percent)
Marcus[38]	CVP, 159	53	57	10	15	77
	R-CVP, 162		81	41	34	83
					p < 0.0001	p = 0.0290
Hiddemann[40]	CHOP, 205	18	90	17	29	74
	R-CHOP, 223		96	20	NR	87
					p < 0.001	p = 0.016
Herold[41]	MCP, 96	47	75	25	26	74
	R-MCP, 105		92	50	NR	87
					p < 0.0001	p = 0.0096
Salles[43]	CHVP-IFN, 183	42	73	63	46%	84
	R-CHVP-IFN, 175		84	79	67%	91
					p < 0.0001	p = 0.029
Hochster[44]	CVP, 117	36	NA	NA	15	91
	CVP + Rituximab maintenance, 120				61	75 at 42 mo.
						p = 0.03 one sided

EFS, event-free survival; NA, not available; NR, not reported; TTF, time to treatment failure; TTP, time to progression.

*One of these endpoints was used in one or another study, but the results are internally consistent within each study shown.

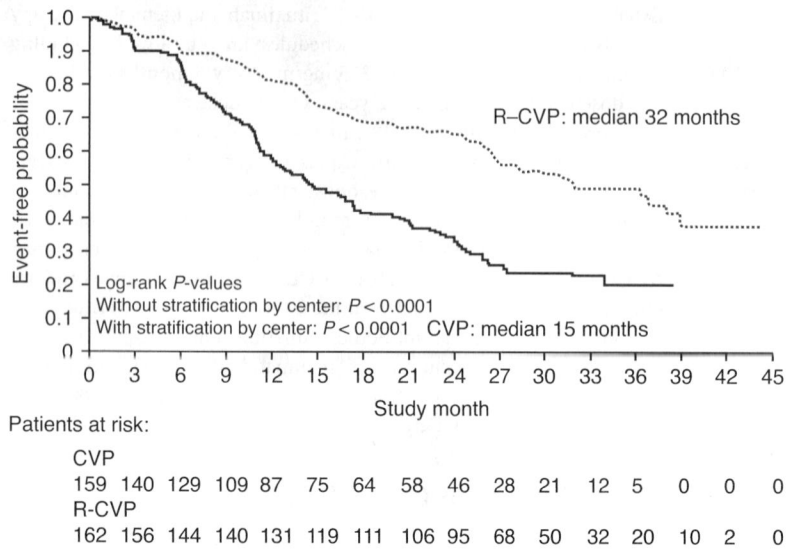

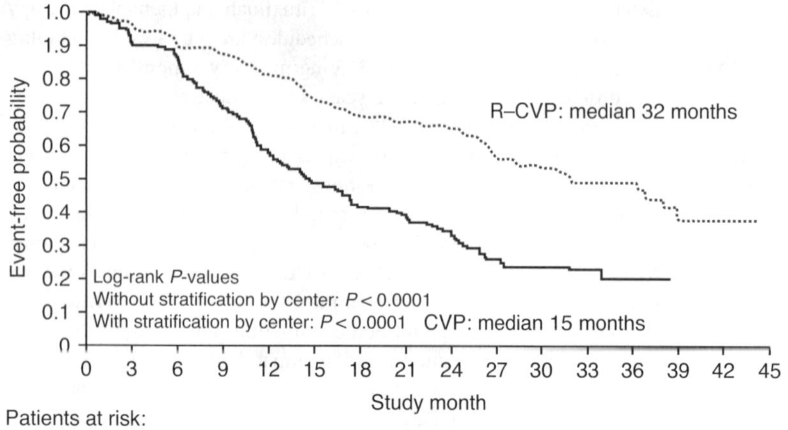

Patients at risk:

CVP															
	159	140	129	109	87	75	64	58	46	28	21	12	5	0	0	0
R-CVP															
	162	156	144	140	131	119	111	106	95	68	50	32	20	10	2	0

FIGURE 101–4. Time to disease progression, relapse, or death after a median followup of 30 months among 321 patients with grade 1 or 2 FL assigned to chemotherapy with CVP or with R-CVP. *Solid line* represents CVP; *dotted line*, R-CVP. *(Reproduced with permission from Marcus R, Imrie K, Belch A, et al.[38])*

advanced stage FL. R-CHOP exhibited a superior ORR (96% vs. 90%), time to treatment failure ($p < 0.001$), duration of response ($p = 0.001$), and OS ($p = 0.016$) compared to CHOP alone.[40] Similar benefits have also been reported for the addition of rituximab to MCP (mitoxantrone, chlorambucil, and prednisolone) and CHVP + IFN (cyclophosphamide, doxorubicin, etoposide, prednisolone and interferon) in front-line therapy and for CHOP and FCM (fludarabine, cyclophosphamide, mitoxantrone) for relapsed FL.[36,41–43] Maintenance rituximab (375 mg/m^2 for 4 doses every 6 months for 2 years) has also been tested in previously untreated patients who were given CVP for 8 cycles before randomization.[44] In this study, PFS was significantly longer for the group given maintenance rituximab (56% after 4 years) compared to the observation group (33% after 4 years, $p < 0.0000001$). Differences in PFS were most significant in favor of maintenance rituximab for patients with a high initial tumor burden and minimal residual disease after CVP. Overall survival after 4 years was also superior for maintenance rituximab (88% for maintenance rituximab vs. 72% for observation, $p = 0.03$ [one sided]). The roles of rituximab in remission induction as well as maintenance were also studied in 465 patients with relapsed FL randomized first to either induction therapy with CHOP or R-CHOP, and then randomized to either maintenance rituximab given every 3 months for 2 years or no maintenance therapy.[36] The addition of rituximab to CHOP induction improved the ORR (85% vs. 72%), CR rate (30% vs. 16%), and median PFS (33 months vs. 20 months). Furthermore, rituximab maintenance further improved the median PFS (52 months from second randomization vs. 15 months without maintenance) and OS (85% vs. 77% after 3 years from second randomization).

RADIOIMMUNOTHERAPY

Radiolabeled monoclonal antibodies targeting lymphoma-associated cell surface antigens, including idiotypic immunoglobulin, CD20, CD22, and HLA-DR, have emerged as effective and safe therapeutic agents for patients with FL.[45–48] Two radioimmunoconjugates targeting the CD20 antigen, ^{131}iodine-tositumomab (Bexxar) and ^{90}yttrium-ibritumomab tiuxetan (Zevalin), have been approved by the FDA for relapsed, refractory, and transformed indolent lymphomas.[49–51] Radioimmunotherapy is an attractive therapeutic option for lymphomas because (1) many high-quality antibodies are available targeting pan-B-cell antigens expressed at high levels on lymphoma cells, (2) lymphomas are exquisitely sensitive to radiotherapy, and (3) cross-fire radiotherapy from β particles emitted by decaying radionuclides on targeted lymphoma cells can kill neighboring antigen-negative tumor cells (or inaccessible cells deep in tumor clumps), which would escape killing by nonradioactive antibodies. Several trials have demonstrated overall response rates of 50 to 80 percent and complete response rates of 15 to 40 percent in patients with relapsed or refractory indolent lymphoma treated with either ^{131}iodine-tositumomab or ^{90}yttrium-ibritumomab tiuxetan.[49,51,52] In a randomized study comparing treatment of patients with relapsed FL with either ^{90}Y-ibritumomab tiuxetan or rituximab, the ORR (86% vs. 55%) and the CR rate (30% vs. 15%) were both statistically superior in the group treated with the radioimmunoconjugate.[51] Similarly, ^{131}I-tositumomab was compared with unlabeled tositumomab in a randomized trial of relapsed indolent lymphoma and both the ORR (55% vs. 19%) and the CR rate (33% vs. 8%) were higher in patients receiving the radiolabeled antibody.[53]

Six phase II studies have studied front-line radioimmunotherapy (RIT) for patients with newly diagnosed FL, either as a single agent or in combination with various chemotherapy regimens, including CVP, CHOP, and fludarabine. In all six studies, outstanding ORR rates (90–100%) and CR rates (50–96%) were observed with first-line RIT, with median progression-free survivals in excess of 5 years in several of the studies (Fig. 101–5).[54–56] A phase III randomized study evaluated the utility of consolidation therapy with ^{90}Y-ibritumomab tiuxetan for patients with FL in remission after front-line chemotherapy.[57] In this trial, 414 patients in either partial or complete remission after a variety of chemotherapy induction regimens (chlorambucil, CVP, CHOP, fludarabine or rituximab combinations) were randomized to either consolidation with RIT or to no consolidation. Radioimmunotherapy dramatically improved the median progression-free survival in the total patient population (36.5 months vs. 13.3 months, $p < 0.0001$), and this advantage was observed regardless of whether patients were in partial remission (PR; 29.3 months vs. 6.2 months, $p < 0.0001$) or CR (53.9 months vs. 29.5 months, $p = 0.015$) at the time of consolidation. Furthermore, RIT consolidation converted 77 percent of patients who were in PR after induction chemotherapy to CR following RIT.

The major toxicity of radioimmunotherapy is myelosuppression, with cytopenic nadirs occurring 4 to 7 weeks after treatment and requiring 2 to 4 weeks for recovery. Growth factor administration and transfusions are required in approximately 20 percent of patients. Human antimouse antibodies (HAMA) may develop in the serum of approximately 1 percent of patients treated with ^{90}Y-labeled ibritumomab and in 10 percent of patients treated with ^{131}I-labeled tositumomab. A potential long-term concern with both radiolabeled antibody formulations is the potential development of myelodysplasia and acute leukemia as late complications. Hypothyroidism may also occur as a delayed toxicity of ^{131}I-labeled tositumomab in approximately 10 percent of patients.

INTERFERON-α_2

Interferon (IFN)-α_2 has been studied in 10 large phase III studies evaluating its utility in both the induction phase of treatment and for maintenance therapy. A meta-analysis of 1922 newly diagnosed patients with FL treated in these trials concluded that the addition of IFN-α_2 to induction chemotherapy did not significantly influence response rates, but did

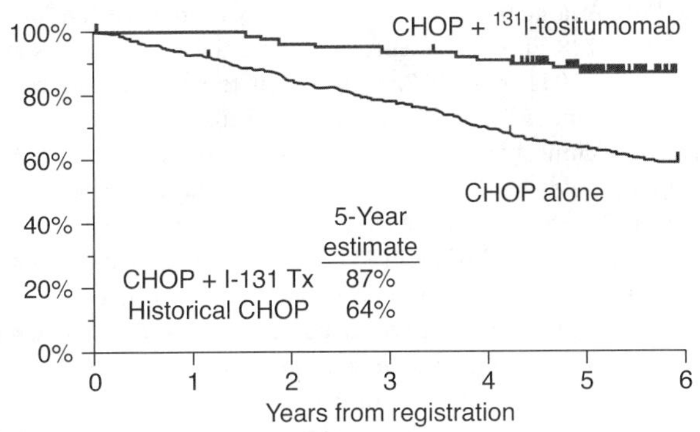

FIGURE 101–5. Comparison of the overall survival (OS) of 90 patients with advanced stage FL treated with six cycles of CHOP (cyclophosphamide, doxorubicin, vincristine, prednisone) chemotherapy followed by ^{131}I-tositumomab radioimmunotherapy with the OS of 356 similar patients treated with CHOP without radioimmunotherapy. Five-year estimates of OS with each regimen are shown. *(Reproduced with permission from Press OW, Unger JM, Braziel RM, et al.[55])*

show a significant difference in favor of IFN-α_2 with regard to survival.[58] Results differed greatly from trial to trial and further analyses were carried out in order to define the circumstances in which IFN-α_2 prolonged OS. The survival advantage was seen when IFN-α_2 was given (1) in conjunction with relatively intensive initial chemotherapy ($p = 0.00005$), (2) at a dose ≥5 million units ($p = 0.000002$), (3) at a cumulative dose ≥36 million units per month ($p = 0.000008$), and (4) when given with induction chemotherapy rather than as maintenance therapy ($p = 0.004$).[58] With regard to remission duration, there was also a significant difference in favor of IFN-α_2, irrespective of the intensity of chemotherapy used, IFN dose, or whether IFN was given as a maintenance strategy or with chemotherapy. Despite these salutary findings, interferon is rarely employed to treat FL in the United States because of its unfavorable toxicity profile (asthenia, fatigue, flu-like symptoms, cytopenias) and because of the perception that rituximab confers similar or superior advantages with much less toxicity.

IDIOTYPE VACCINES

The idiotypic immunoglobulin protein expressed on the surface of B lymphoma cells represents a true tumor-specific antigen and is an ideal target for immunotherapeutic strategies.[59–61] Several groups have reported favorable phase II trials using idiotypic vaccines produced either by rescue hybridoma fusions or recombinant DNA approaches. The idiotypic immunoglobulin in most of the vaccines is coupled to keyhole limpet hemocyanin (KLH) and administered with sargramostim (granulocyte-macrophage colony-stimulating factor) to enhance immunogenicity. Specific immune responses are generated in approximately 50 percent of immunized FL patients who are in complete remission at the time of vaccination. Patients exhibiting immune responses to the vaccine experience longer remission durations and superior survival compared to patients failing to mount immune responses to the vaccine. Three phase III randomized trials have been conducted using idiotypic vaccination following either CVP, PACE [cisplatin, doxorubicin (Adriamycin), cyclophosphamide, etoposide], or rituximab therapy. Two of the trials have been reported in preliminary abstract form, but neither has demonstrated a therapeutic benefit.[59] The third trial has stopped accruing patients but has not yet been reported.

HEMATOPOIETIC STEM CELL TRANSPLANTATION

The role of high-dose chemoradiotherapy and hematopoietic stem cell transplantation in the management of patients with FL remains highly controversial. Proponents of autologous stem cell transplantation of indolent NHL note the favorable outcome of a collaborative study of 121 adult patients conducted by St. Bartholomew's Hospital and the Dana-Farber Cancer Institute, where an apparent plateau in the remission duration curve of 48 percent was observed with a median followup of 13.5 years.[62] Survival was longer in patients transplanted in second remission compared to those transplanted later in their disease course. The value of autologous stem cell transplantation was also tested in a randomized trial of 89 patients with relapsed FL (Fig. 101–6). Transplanted patients experienced a marked advantage in PFS and a marginal OS advantage compared to patients randomized to continued conventional salvage chemotherapy without transplantation.[63] When used as part of initial therapy for high-risk patients, randomized studies demonstrate a prolongation of PFS, but no improvement in OS.[64,65] Adverse outcomes associated with autologous stem cell transplantation include treatment-related mortality (3–5%) and a substantial increase in the incidence of secondary myelodysplasia and acute myelogenous leukemia, occurring in 7 to 19 percent of patients, particularly if total body irradiation is employed in the conditioning regimen.

The application of allogeneic marrow or blood stem cell transplantation for the treatment of indolent NHL has been hampered by difficulties identifying histocompatibility locus antigen-matched donors, high rates of morbidity and mortality, and the advanced age of many patients with indolent NHL. Although allogeneic transplantation affords long-term PFS for approximately 40 to 50 percent of patients with relapsed FL, transplant-related mortality rates range from 20 percent to 40 percent.[66] Therefore, careful patient selection and informed consent are essential. When allogeneic and autologous stem cell transplantation are compared, the long-term survival rates are comparable.[66,67] Autologous stem cell transplantation is associated with a greater likelihood of dying

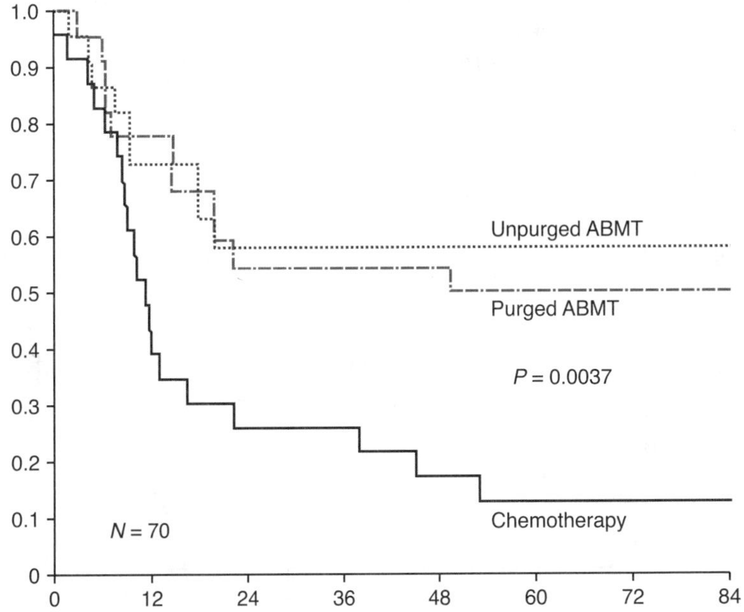

FIGURE 101–6. Progression-free survival of 70 patients with relapsed FL randomized to either conventional chemotherapy (*solid line*), or to high-dose chemoradiotherapy with autologous marrow transplantation using either marrow purged to remove tumor cells (*long dashes*) or unpurged marrow (*short dashes*). ABMT, autologous bone marrow transplantation. *(Reproduced with permission from Schouten HC, Qian W, Kvaloy S, et al.[63])*

from recurrent disease, and allogeneic stem cell transplantation results in a higher frequency of death from graft-versus-host disease, infection, and venoocclusive disease. Nonmyeloablative and reduced-intensity allogeneic transplantation conditioning regimens have been developed to exploit the benefit of a graft-versus-lymphoma effect while minimizing transplant-related morbidity and mortality. Preliminary results of this approach are very encouraging, with 52 to 85 percent OS and 43 to 83 percent PFS after 3 to 5 years with 15 to 43 percent nonrelapse mortality.[68,69]

TRANSFORMED FOLLICULAR LYMPHOMA

Approximately 30 to 40 percent of patients with FL undergo documented transformation to a more aggressive histology, usually diffuse large B-cell lymphoma, with an annual rate of transformation of approximately 3 percent (Fig. 101–7A). Clinically, histologic transformation is characterized by the sudden explosive growth of a single lymph node site (or extranodal mass). Anthracycline-based chemotherapy (e.g., R-CHOP) is the most appropriate therapy for patients experiencing transformation, however, the prognosis is poor despite such aggressive management. Whereas 50 to 65 percent of patients presenting with *de novo* diffuse large B-cell lymphoma are cured with R-CHOP chemotherapy, less than 10 percent of patients with diffuse large B-cell lymphoma arising by transformation from FL with be cured by this regimen (Fig. 101–7B). Most series report median survivals of 6 to 20 months for patients undergoing transformation.[19,70–72] Because of the poor outcome of R-CHOP chemotherapy alone, many authorities advise high-dose chemoradiotherapy and either autologous or allogeneic stem cell transplantation following induction of remission with R-CHOP. Selected series suggest that long-term PFS is achievable in approximately 20 to 30 percent of patients undergoing autologous or nonmyeloablative allogeneic transplantation for transformed FL.[68,73]

A PRAGMATIC APPROACH TO THERAPY OF FOLLICULAR LYMPHOMA

There is currently little consensus among lymphoma experts with regard to the optimal management of patients with either front-line or relapsed FL. A large prospective cohort study monitored the "patterns of care" for 2728 FL patients enrolled across the United States at 265 sites between 2004 and 2007.[2] The initial therapeutic strategy was observation alone in 18 percent of patients; rituximab monotherapy in 14 percent; a clinical trial in 6 percent; radiation therapy in 6 percent; chemotherapy alone in 3 percent; and chemotherapy plus rituximab in 52 percent. R-CHOP was employed in 55 percent of patients receiving chemoimmunotherapy, R-CVP in 23 percent, rituximab plus fludarabine-based regimens in 16 percent, and other drugs in 6 percent of cases. The results of this study support the contention that there is no single standard of care for the treatment of *de novo* FL.

Recognizing the absence of a consensus in the management of FL, at this time all patients with FL should be considered for entry into clinical trials to define the best regimens and to allow evaluation of the multitude of available promising new drugs and antibodies. Patients who are ineligible for trials or who decline enrollment should receive individualized treatment. Patients with localized stage I or II disease should be offered local radiotherapy. Elderly patients with asymptomatic, advanced stage disease are best monitored with observation alone, particularly if their disease is of low volume and if they have multiple coexistent medical illnesses. Patients who are symptomatic, have cytopenias, massive splenomegaly, effusions, or bulky adenopathy should be treated with rituximab plus chemotherapy. Several regimens are acceptable including R-CVP and R-CHOP, with the latter regimen being most appropriate for young patients with aggressive presentations and rapidly growing bulky adenopathy and B symptoms. The roles of maintenance rituximab and consolidative radioimmunotherapy following initial induction chemoimmunotherapy of newly diagnosed patients are under active investigation. Management of FL following relapse depends on the patient's initial treatment and the resultant remission duration. If the first remission lasts many years, the initial treatment regimen may again be used. If the initial remission is short, an alternative second-line regimen should be selected from among the many available options, including R-CVP, R-CHOP, R-FND, radioimmunotherapy, and bendamustine. Patients with a good performance status, who experience very short response durations, should be considered for autologous or allogeneic stem cell transplantation. Patients who undergo histologic transformation should receive R-CHOP and be offered the option of stem cell transplantation.

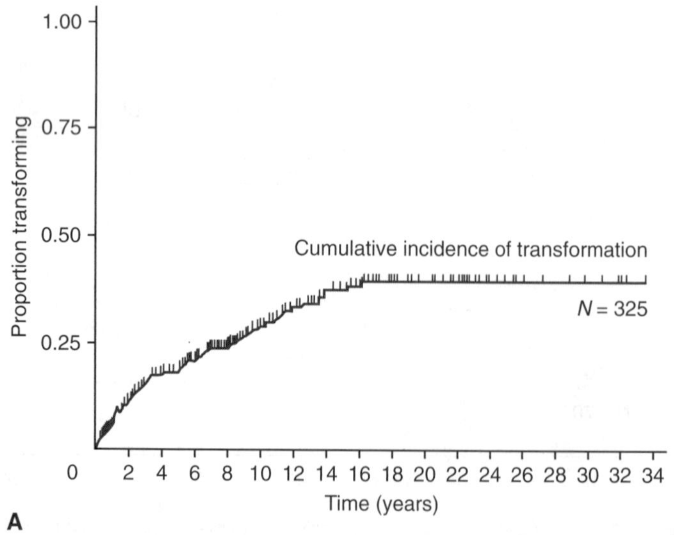

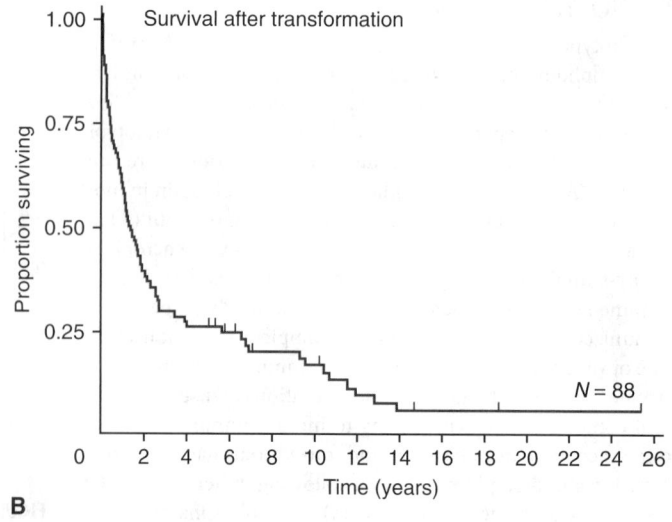

FIGURE 101–7. A. Transformation of FL to an histologic pattern compatible with rapid progression of disease. The line depicts the cumulative incidence of histologic transformation to a histologic pattern compatible with more rapid progression (e.g., diffuse large B-cell lymphoma) in 325 patients followed from the date of diagnosis of FL. **B.** The proportion of patients with FL surviving after transformation to a less-favorable histologic pattern. The graph shows the survival of the 88 patients from the date of their transformation to aggressive lymphoma. *(Redrawn from Montoto S, Davies AJ, Matthews J, et al.[70])*

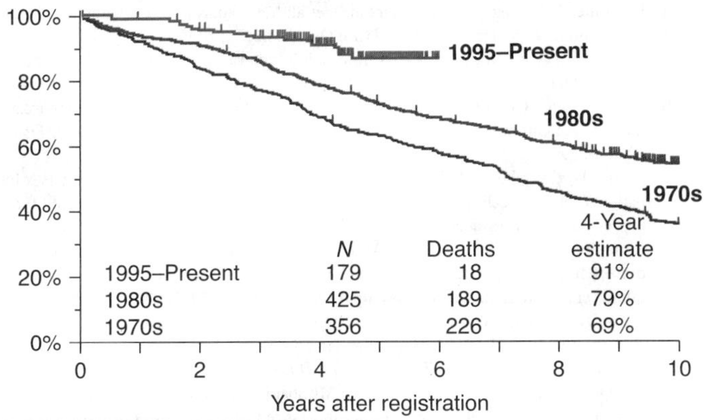

FIGURE 101–8. Improved survival of patients with follicular lymphoma treated by the Southwest Oncology Group. *(Reproduced in modified form with permission from Fisher RI, LeBlanc M, Press OW, et al.*[74]*)*

COURSE AND PROGNOSIS

FL has been considered an indolent but incurable disease for which the median survival of approximately 10 years is minimally affected by medical interventions. This attitude is no longer valid, and survival of FL patients has been progressively increasing over the past 20 years (Fig. 101–8).[74–76] Much of the improvement in survival appears attributable to the introduction of rituximab, better salvage therapies (fludarabine, bendamustine, radioimmunotherapy), improved supportive care measures, and the wider implementation of stem cell transplantation. Controversy persists over whether any of the grades of FL are curable with standard chemoimmunotherapy regimens, although advocates for the curability of grade 2 (follicular mixed, small-cleaved, and large cell) and grade 3 (follicular large cell) FL using anthracycline-containing regimens exist. Further clinical research will settle these disputes and permit formulation of a consensus standard of care for the management of both newly diagnosed and relapsed FL.

REFERENCES

1. Harris NL, Nathwani BN, Swerdlow SH, et al: Follicular lymphoma, in *WHO Classification of Tumours of Haematopoietic and Lymphoid Tissues*, edited by SH Swerdlow, E Campo, NL Harris, ES Jaffe, SA Pileri, H Stein, J Thiele, JW Vardiman. International Agency for Research on Cancer, Lyon, 2008.
2. Friedberg JW, Taylor MD, Cerhan JR, et al: Follicular lymphoma in the United States: First report of the National LymphoCare Study. *J Clin Oncol* 27:1202, 2009.
3. Groves FD, Linet MS, Travis LB, Devesa SS: Cancer surveillance series: Non-Hodgkin's lymphoma incidence by histologic subtype in the United States from 1978 through 1995. *J Natl Cancer Inst* 92:1240, 2000.
4. Swerdlow SH, Campo E, Harris NL, et al: *WHO Classification of Tumours of Haematopoietic and Lymphoid Tissues*. International Agency for Research on Cancer, Lyon, 2008.
5. Zelenetz AD, Advani RH, Byrd JC, et al: Non-Hodgkin's lymphomas. *J Natl Compr Canc Netw* 6:356, 2008.
6. Lee SJ, Schover LR, Partridge AH, et al: American Society of Clinical Oncology recommendations on fertility preservation in cancer patients. *J Clin Oncol* 24:2917, 2006.
7. Czuczman MS, Grillo-Lopez AJ, McLaughlin P, et al: Clearing of cells bearing the bcl-2 [t(14;18)] translocation from blood and marrow of patients treated with rituximab alone or in combination with CHOP chemotherapy. *Ann Oncol* 12:109, 2001.
8. Rambaldi A, Lazzari M, Manzoni C, et al: Monitoring of minimal residual disease after CHOP and rituximab in previously untreated patients with follicular lymphoma. *Blood* 99:856, 2002.
9. Miller TP, LeBlanc M, Grogan TM, Fisher RI: Follicular lymphomas: Do histologic subtypes predict outcome? *Hematol Oncol Clin North Am* 11:893, 1997.
10. Reed JC: Bcl-2-family proteins and hematologic malignancies: History and future prospects. *Blood* 111:3322, 2008.
11. A predictive model for aggressive non-Hodgkin's lymphoma. The International Non-Hodgkin's Lymphoma Prognostic Factors Project. *N Engl J Med* 329:987, 1993.
12. Solal-Celigny P, Roy P, Colombat P, et al: Follicular lymphoma international prognostic index. *Blood* 104:1258, 2004.
13. Federico M, Bellei M, Pro B, et al: Revalidation of FLIPI in patients with follicular lymphoma registered in the F2 study and treated upfront with immunochemotherapy. *Proc Am Soc Clin Oncol* 25:443s, 2007.
14. Federico M, Guglielmi C, Luminari S, et al: Prognostic relevance of serum beta2 microglobulin in patients with follicular lymphoma treated with anthracycline-containing regimens. A GISL study. *Haematologica* 92:1482, 2007.
15. Dave SS, Wright G, Tan B, et al: Prediction of survival in follicular lymphoma based on molecular features of tumor-infiltrating immune cells. *N Engl J Med* 351:2159, 2004.
16. Besa PC, McLaughlin PW, Cox JD, Fuller LM: Long term assessment of patterns of treatment failure and survival in patients with stage I or II follicular lymphoma. *Cancer* 75:2361, 1995.
17. Mac Manus MP, Hoppe RT: Is radiotherapy curative for stage I and II low-grade follicular lymphoma? Results of a long-term follow-up study of patients treated at Stanford University. *J Clin Oncol* 14:1282, 1996.
18. Advani R, Rosenberg SA, Horning SJ: Stage I and II follicular non-Hodgkin's lymphoma: Long-term follow-up of no initial therapy. *J Clin Oncol* 22:1454, 2004.
19. Horning SJ, Rosenberg SA: The natural history of initially untreated low grade non Hodgkin's lymphomas. *N Engl J Med* 311:1471, 1984.
20. Ardeshna KM, Smith P, Norton A, et al: Long-term effect of a watch and wait policy versus immediate systemic treatment for asymptomatic advanced-stage non-Hodgkin lymphoma: A randomised controlled trial. *Lancet* 362:516, 2003.
21. Young RC, Longo DL, Glatstein E, et al: The treatment of indolent lymphomas: Watchful waiting v aggressive combined modality treatment. *Semin Hematol* 25:11, 1988.
22. Brice P, Bastion Y, Lepage E, et al: Comparison in low-tumor-burden follicular lymphomas between an initial no-treatment policy, prednimustine, or interferon alfa: A randomized study from the Groupe d'Etude des Lymphomes Folliculaires. Groupe d'Etude des Lymphomes de l'Adulte. *J Clin Oncol* 15:1110, 1997.
23. Friedberg JW, Cohen P, Chen L, et al: Bendamustine in patients with rituximab-refractory indolent and transformed non-Hodgkin's lymphoma: Results from a phase II multicenter, single-agent study. *J Clin Oncol* 26:204, 2008.
24. Lister TA, Cullen MH, Beard ME, et al: Comparison of combined and single-agent chemotherapy in non-Hodgkin's lymphoma of favourable histological type. *Br Med J* 1:533, 1978.
25. Dana BW, Dahlberg S, Nathwani BN, et al: Long-term follow-up of patients with low-grade malignant lymphomas treated with doxorubicin-based chemotherapy or chemoimmunotherapy. *J Clin Oncol* 11:644, 1993.
26. Flinn IW, Byrd JC, Morrison C, et al: Fludarabine and cyclophosphamide with filgrastim support in patients with previously untreated indolent lymphoid malignancies. *Blood* 96:71, 2000.
27. McLaughlin P, Hagemeister FB, Romaguera JE, et al: Fludarabine, mitoxantrone, and dexamethasone: An effective new regimen for indolent lymphoma. *J Clin Oncol* 14:1262, 1996.
28. Maloney D, Smith B, Rose A: Rituximab: Mechanism of action and resistance. *Semin Oncol* 29:2, 2002.
29. McLaughlin P, Grillo-Lopez AJ, Link BK, et al: Rituximab chimeric anti-CD20 monoclonal antibody therapy for relapsed indolent lymphoma: Half of patients respond to a four-dose treatment program. *J Clin Oncol* 16:2825, 1998.
30. Davis TA, Grillo-Lopez AJ, White CA, et al: Rituximab anti-CD20 monoclonal antibody therapy in non-Hodgkin's lymphoma: Safety and efficacy of re-treatment. *J Clin Oncol* 18:3135, 2000.
31. Colombat P, Salles G, Brousse N, et al: Rituximab (anti-CD20 monoclonal antibody) as single first-line therapy for patients with follicular lymphoma with a low tumor burden: Clinical and molecular evaluation. *Blood* 97:101, 2001.
32. Hainsworth JD: Rituximab as first-line systemic therapy for patients with low-grade lymphoma. *Semin Oncol* 27:25, 2000.
33. Hainsworth JD: Rituximab as first-line and maintenance therapy for patients with indolent non-Hodgkin's lymphoma: Interim follow-up of a multicenter phase II trial. *Semin Oncol* 29:25, 2002.
34. Hainsworth J: First-line and maintenance treatment with rituximab for patients with indolent non-Hodgkin's lymphoma. *Semin Oncol* 30:9, 2003.
35. Ghielmini M, Schmitz SF, Cogliatti S, et al: Effect of single-agent rituximab given at the standard schedule or as prolonged treatment in patients with mantle cell lymphoma: A study of the Swiss Group for Clinical Cancer Research (SAKK). *J Clin Oncol* 23:705, 2005.
36. van Oers MH, Klasa R, Marcus RE, et al: Rituximab maintenance improves clinical outcome of relapsed/resistant follicular non-Hodgkin lymphoma in patients both with and without rituximab during induction: Results of a prospective randomized phase 3 intergroup trial. *Blood* 108:3295, 2006.
37. Hainsworth JD, Litchy S, Burris HA 3rd, et al: Rituximab as first-line and maintenance therapy for patients with indolent non-Hodgkin's lymphoma. *J Clin Oncol* 20:4261, 2002.
38. Marcus R, Imrie K, Belch A, et al: CVP chemotherapy plus rituximab compared with CVP as first-line treatment for advanced follicular lymphoma. *Blood* 105:1417, 2005.
39. Marcus R, Imrie K, Solal-Celigny P, et al: Phase III study of R-CVP compared with cyclophosphamide, vincristine, and prednisone alone in patients with previously untreated advanced follicular lymphoma. *J Clin Oncol* 26:4579, 2008.

40. Hiddemann W, Kneba M, Dreyling M, et al: Frontline therapy with rituximab added to the combination of cyclophosphamide, doxorubicin, vincristine, and prednisone (CHOP) significantly improves the outcome for patients with advanced-stage follicular lymphoma compared with therapy with CHOP alone: Results of a prospective randomized study of the German Low-Grade Lymphoma Study Group. *Blood* 106:3725, 2005.
41. Herold M, Haas A, Srock S, et al: Rituximab added to first-line mitoxantrone, chlorambucil, and prednisolone chemotherapy followed by interferon maintenance prolongs survival in patients with advanced follicular lymphoma: An East German Study Group Hematology and Oncology Study. *J Clin Oncol* 25:1986, 2007.
42. Forstpointner R, Dreyling M, Repp R, et al: The addition of rituximab to a combination of fludarabine, cyclophosphamide, mitoxantrone (FCM) significantly increases the response rate and prolongs survival as compared with FCM alone in patients with relapsed and refractory follicular and mantle cell lymphomas: Results of a prospective randomized study of the German Low-Grade Lymphoma Study Group. *Blood* 104:3064, 2004.
43. Salles G, Mounier N, de Guibert S, et al: Rituximab combined with chemotherapy and interferon in follicular lymphoma patients: Results of the GELA-GOELAMS FL2000 study. *Blood* 112:4824, 2008.
44. Hochster HS, Weller E, Gascoyne RD, et al: Maintenance rituximab after CVP results in superior clinical outcome in advanced follicular lymphoma (FL): Results of the E1496 phase III trial from the Eastern Cooperative Oncology Group and the Cancer and Leukemia Group B [abstract 349]. *Blood* 106:106a, 2005.
45. Press OW: Evidence mounts for the efficacy of radioimmunotherapy for B-cell lymphomas. *J Clin Oncol* 26:5147, 2008.
46. DeNardo GL, DeNardo SJ, Goldstein DS, et al: Maximum-tolerated dose, toxicity, and efficacy of (131)I-Lym-1 antibody for fractionated radioimmunotherapy of non-Hodgkin's lymphoma. *J Clin Oncol* 16:3246, 1998.
47. Pantelias A, Pagel J, Hedin N, et al: Comparative biodistributions of pretargeted radioimmunoconjugates targeting CD20, CD22 and DR molecules on human B cell lymphomas. *Blood* 109:4980, 2007.
48. Goldenberg DM, Sharkey RM: Advances in cancer therapy with radiolabeled monoclonal antibodies. *Q J Nucl Med Mol Imaging* 50:248, 2006.
49. Kaminski MS, Estes J, Zasadny KR, et al: Radioimmunotherapy with iodine (131)I tositumomab for relapsed or refractory B-cell non-Hodgkin lymphoma: Updated results and long-term follow-up of the University of Michigan experience. *Blood* 96:1259, 2000.
50. Witzig TE, Flinn IW, Gordon LI, et al: Treatment with ibritumomab tiuxetan radioimmunotherapy in patients with rituximab-refractory follicular non-Hodgkin's lymphoma. *J Clin Oncol* 20:3262, 2002.
51. Witzig TE, Gordon LI, Cabanillas F, et al: Randomized controlled trial of yttrium-90-labeled ibritumomab tiuxetan radioimmunotherapy versus rituximab immunotherapy for patients with relapsed or refractory low-grade, follicular, or transformed B-cell non-Hodgkin's lymphoma. *J Clin Oncol* 20:2453, 2002.
52. Witzig TE: The use of ibritumomab tiuxetan radioimmunotherapy for patients with relapsed B-cell non-Hodgkin's lymphoma. *Semin Oncol* 27:74, 2000.
53. Davis TA, Kaminski MS, Leonard JP, et al: The radioisotope contributes significantly to the activity of radioimmunotherapy. *Clin Cancer Res* 10:7792, 2004.
54. Kaminski MS, Tuck M, Estes J, et al: ^{131}I-tositumomab therapy as initial treatment for follicular lymphoma. *N Engl J Med* 352:441, 2005.
55. Press OW, Unger JM, Braziel RM, et al: Phase II trial of CHOP chemotherapy followed by tositumomab/iodine I-131 tositumomab for previously untreated follicular non-Hodgkin's lymphoma: Five-year follow-up of Southwest Oncology Group Protocol S9911. *J Clin Oncol* 24:4143, 2006.
56. Leonard JP, Coleman M, Kostakoglu L, et al: Abbreviated chemotherapy with fludarabine followed by tositumomab and iodine I 131 tositumomab for untreated follicular lymphoma. *J Clin Oncol* 23:5696, 2005.
57. Morschhauser F, Radford J, Van Hoof A, et al: Phase III trial of consolidation therapy with yttrium-90-ibritumomab tiuxetan compared with no additional therapy after first remission in advanced follicular lymphoma. *J Clin Oncol* 26:5156, 2008.
58. Rohatiner AZ, Gregory WM, Peterson B, et al: Meta-analysis to evaluate the role of interferon in follicular lymphoma. *J Clin Oncol* 23:2215, 2005.
59. Houot R, Levy R: Vaccines for lymphomas: Idiotype vaccines and beyond. *Blood Rev* 23:137, 2009.
60. Hsu FJ, Caspar CB, Czerwinski D, et al: Tumor-specific idiotype vaccines in the treatment of patients with B-cell lymphoma—Long-term results of a clinical trial. *Blood* 89:3129, 1997.
61. Kwak LW, Campbell MJ, Czerwinski DK, et al: Induction of immune responses in patients with B-cell lymphoma against the surface-immunoglobulin idiotype expressed by their tumors. *N Engl J Med* 327:1209, 1992.
62. Rohatiner AZ, Nadler L, Davies AJ, et al: Myeloablative therapy with autologous bone marrow transplantation for follicular lymphoma at the time of second or subsequent remission: Long-term follow-up. *J Clin Oncol* 25:2554, 2007.
63. Schouten HC, Qian W, Kvaloy S, et al: High-dose therapy improves progression-free survival and survival in relapsed follicular non-Hodgkin's lymphoma: Results from the randomized European CUP trial. *J Clin Oncol* 21:3918, 2003.
64. Lenz G, Dreyling M, Schiegnitz E, et al: Myeloablative radiochemotherapy followed by autologous stem cell transplantation in first remission prolongs progression-free survival in follicular lymphoma: Results of a prospective, randomized trial of the German Low-Grade Lymphoma Study Group. *Blood* 104:2667, 2004.
65. Deconinck E, Foussard C, Milpied N, et al: High-dose therapy followed by autologous purged stem-cell transplantation and doxorubicin-based chemotherapy in patients with advanced follicular lymphoma: A randomized multicenter study by GOELAMS. *Blood* 105:3817, 2005.
66. van Besien K, Loberiza FR Jr, Bajorunaite R, et al: Comparison of autologous and allogeneic hematopoietic stem cell transplantation for follicular lymphoma. *Blood* 102:3521, 2003.
67. Bierman PJ, Sweetenham JW, Loberiza FR Jr, et al: Syngeneic hematopoietic stem-cell transplantation for non-Hodgkin's lymphoma: A comparison with allogeneic and autologous transplantation—The Lymphoma Working Committee of the International Bone Marrow Transplant Registry and the European Group for Blood and Marrow Transplantation. *J Clin Oncol* 21:3744, 2003.
68. Rezvani AR, Storer B, Maris M, et al: Nonmyeloablative allogeneic hematopoietic cell transplantation in relapsed, refractory, and transformed indolent non-Hodgkin's lymphoma. *J Clin Oncol* 26:211, 2008.
69. Khouri IF, McLaughlin P, Saliba RM, et al: Eight-year experience with allogeneic stem cell transplantation for relapsed follicular lymphoma after nonmyeloablative conditioning with fludarabine, cyclophosphamide, and rituximab. *Blood* 111:5530, 2008.
70. Montoto S, Davies AJ, Matthews J, et al: Risk and clinical implications of transformation of follicular lymphoma to diffuse large B-cell lymphoma. *J Clin Oncol* 25:2426, 2007.
71. Al-Tourah AJ, Gill KK, Chhanabhai M, et al: Population-based analysis of incidence and outcome of transformed non-Hodgkin's lymphoma. *J Clin Oncol* 26:5165, 2008.
72. Oviatt DL, Cousar JB, Collins RD, et al: Malignant lymphomas of follicular center cell origin in humans. V. Incidence, clinical features, and prognostic implications of transformation of small cleaved cell nodular lymphoma. *Cancer* 53:1109, 1984.
73. Williams CD, Harrison CN, Lister TA, et al: High-dose therapy and autologous stem-cell support for chemosensitive transformed low-grade follicular non-Hodgkin's lymphoma: A case-matched study from the European Bone Marrow Transplant Registry. *J Clin Oncol* 19:727, 2001.
74. Fisher RI, LeBlanc M, Press OW, et al: New treatment options have changed the survival of patients with follicular lymphoma. *J Clin Oncol* 23:8447, 2005.
75. Swenson WT, Wooldridge JE, Lynch CF, Forman-Hoffman VL, et al: Improved survival of follicular lymphoma patients in the United States. *J Clin Oncol* 23:5019, 2005.
76. Liu Q, Fayad L, Cabanillas F, et al: Improvement of overall and failure-free survival in stage IV follicular lymphoma: 25 years of treatment experience at The University of Texas M.D. Anderson Cancer Center. *J Clin Oncol* 24:1582, 2006.

CHAPTER 102
MANTLE CELL LYMPHOMA

Jorge E. Romaguera and Peter W. McLaughlin

SUMMARY

Mantle cell lymphoma (MCL) is a subtype of non-Hodgkin lymphoma that is characterized by widespread disease in most patients at the time of diagnosis. The lymphoma cells usually contain a translocation between chromosomes 11 and 14, juxtaposing the gene encoding the immunoglobulin heavy chain and the gene encoding cyclin D1. The cells overexpress cyclin D1, which can be identified with immunocytochemistry, providing a relatively easy marker for diagnosis. The disease has a lower rate of complete remission, duration of response, and overall survival after conventional chemotherapy when compared with other lymphomas. More aggressive, multidrug therapy, usually including cytarabine and rituximab, has improved outcome, and the median survival has increased to about 5 years. Consolidation therapy with autologous stem cell transplantation is also used. New chemotherapeutic agents and radioimmunotherapy may add further to advances in treatment.

DEFINITION AND HISTORY

Mantle cell lymphoma (MCL) is a lymphoma subtype that usually is characterized by cells carrying an immunophenotype similar to lymphocytes in the mantle zone of normal germinal follicles, secretory immunoglobulin (sIg) M+, sIgD+, CD5+, CD20+, CD10–, CD43+, and the cytogenetic abnormality t(11;14) (q13;q32) in the tumor cells, resulting in the overexpression of cyclin D1. MCL had been previously named intermediate lymphocytic lymphoma, centrocytic lymphoma, lymphocytic lymphomas with intermediate differentiation, and marginal zone lymphoma. In 1992, a proposal was made to replace the previous designations by the term "mantle cell lymphoma" because of the morphologic and immunophenotypic similarity of the tumor cells to the lymphocytes found in the mantle zone of secondary germinal centers and the resting B lymphocytes of primary germinal centers.[1] In 1994, the term *mantle cell lymphoma* was incorporated into the revised European-American classification of the International Lymphoma Study Group.[2] MCL remains a distinctive subtype of lymphoma in the World Health Organization classification of malignant lymphopoietic disorders.[3]

Acronyms and abbreviations that appear in this chapter include: ATM, ataxia-telangiectasia mutation; bcl-1, b-cell lymphoma 1; CDK, cyclin D kinase; CHOP, cyclophosphamide, doxorubicin, vincristine, prednisone; CLL, chronic lymphocytic leukemia; CR, complete response; Cru, complete response unconfirmed; DFS, disease-free survival; DHAP, dexamethasone, high-dose cytarabine, cisplatin; E2F, elongation factor 2; EFS, event-free survival; FFS, failure-free survival; LDH, lactate dehydrogenase; MCL, mantle cell lymphoma; MIPI, mantle cell international prognostic index; mRNA, messenger RNA; mTOR, mammalian target of rapamycin; NF-κB, nuclear factor-κB; ORR, objective response rate; OS, overall survival; PFS, progression-free survival; PI3K, phosphoinositol 3 kinase; RB1, retinoblastoma 1; R-HDS, rituximab high-dose sequential therapy; SCT, stem cell transplantation; SLL, small lymphocytic leukemia; TTF, time to treatment failure.

EPIDEMIOLOGY

MCL was thought to represents approximately 6 percent of all non-Hodgkin lymphomas,[4] although a lower incidence was reported in a recent analysis.[5] In the latter report, MCL represented approximately 3 percent of all lymphoma cases reported in the United States between 1992 and 2004. The overall annual incidence rate was 0.55 cases per 100,000 persons. Between 1992 and 2004, the age-adjusted annual incidence more than doubled from about 0.3 to 0.7 cases per 100,000. The incidence in males is nearly two and one-half times that in females and the incidence increases with age, but this lymphoma subtype is infrequent before age 50 years. The median age at presentation is about 68 years.[5] There is no known causal agent associated with MCL.

ETIOLOGY AND PATHOGENESIS

GENETIC ALTERATIONS

As in all lymphomas, genetic mutations result in a cell that after transformation gains a proliferative and survival advantage over normal lymphocytes and undergo clonal expansion to form the tumor. The t(11;14) is the primary event in the pathogenesis of mantle cell lymphoma, facilitating the deregulation of the cell cycle at the G1-S phase transition.[6] The need for additional genetic events in the progression of MCL has been supported by clinical observations. For example, low numbers of cells carrying the t(11;14) translocation have been found in the blood of 1 to 2 percent of healthy individuals without any evidence of disease.[7] Cytogenetic studies have identified secondary genetic alterations that may be involved in the pathogenesis and progression of MCL and have shown that MCL has one of the highest levels of genomic instability among the malignant lymphoid neoplasms.[8] These genetic anomalies include losses in chromosomes 1p13-p31, 2q13, 6q23-27, 8p21, 9p21, 10p14-15, 11q22-23, 13q11-13, 13q14-34, 17p13, and 22q12; gains in chromosomes 3q25, 4p12-13, 7p21-22, 8q21, 9q22, 10p11-12, 12q13, and 18q11q23; and high copy-number amplifications of certain chromosomal regions. Dysregulation occurs not only in the cell cycle but also in the DNA damage response as well as in cell survival pathways.[6] The blastoid cytologic variant is associated with the most genetic alterations.[9]

BIOLOGIC PATHWAYS AND POTENTIAL THERAPEUTIC TARGETS

Figure 102–1 depicts a proposed pathway of progression of MCL. These altered molecular pathways in MCL provide insight into its resistance to conventional treatment and its poor prognosis. Dysregulation of the lymphoma cells' progression through the cell cycle is a hallmark of MCL. The overexpressed cyclin D1 complexes with CDK4, which results in at least two important downstream effects. The complex of cyclin D1 and CDK4 (or CDK6) leads to phosphorylation of the retinoblastoma gene *RB1*, with the net result (via release of elongation factor 2 [E2F] transcription factors) of progression of the lymphoma cells into S phase. The cyclin D1–CDK4 complex may also neutralize the ability of the CDK inhibitor p27 to induce G1 cell-cycle arrest.

The *ATM* (ataxia-telangiectasia mutant) gene is mutated in approximately 40 percent of patients with MCL. *ATM* inactivation facilitates genomic instability in lymphoma cells through impaired response to DNA damage. Phosphoinositol 3 kinase (PI3K), which is influenced by *ATM*, is a key kinase in this pathway. The PI3K-Akt pathway is important in this setting because it is upstream of mTOR (mammalian target of rapamycin), which is, in turn, upstream of cyclin D1, p27, and other proteins.

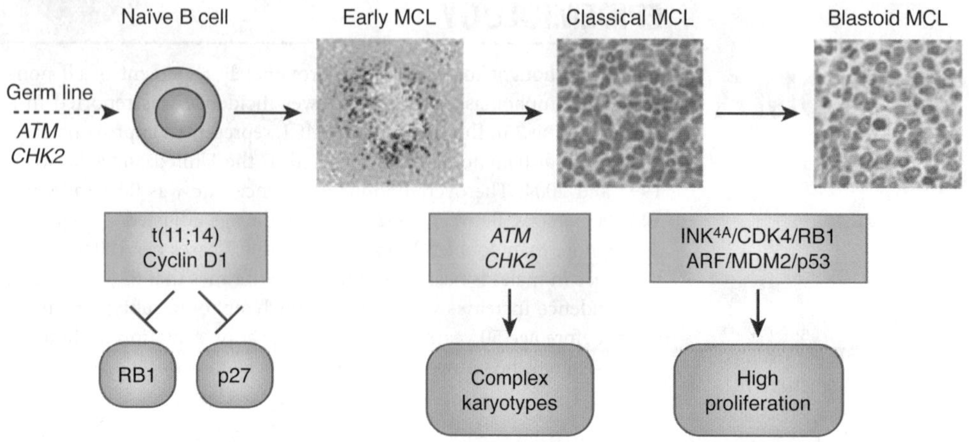

FIGURE 102–1. Proposed model of molecular pathogenesis in the development and progression of MCL. The presence of ataxia-telangiectasia mutated (*ATM*) or cell-cycle checkpoint kinase 2 (*CHK2*) inactivating mutations in the germ line of some patients suggests that they may facilitate the development of the tumor. The t(11;14) translocation occurs in an immature B cell and leads to the constitutive deregulation of cyclin D1 and early expansion of tumor B cells in the mantle zone areas of lymphoid follicles. Acquired inactivation of DNA damage response pathways may facilitate additional genetic alterations and the development of classical mantle cell lymphoma (MCL). Further genetic alterations may target genes of the cell cycle and senescence regulatory pathways, leading to more proliferative and aggressive variants of MCL. *(Courtesy of Jares P, Colomer D, Campo E*[6] *and with permission of* Nature Reviews: Cancer.*)*

Chromosomal 17p abnormalities are observed in up to 26 percent of MCL cases[10] and are associated with p53 mutations, which correlate with poor prognosis,[11] most likely as a result of impairment of the DNA damage response.

CLINICAL FEATURES

The typical presentation is that of an older patient with lymphadenopathy in several sites (e.g., cervical, axillary, inguinal). The patient may be asymptomatic but a significant proportion may have fever, night sweats, or weight loss (Table 102–1).[12] The liver may be enlarged and the spleen is enlarged in 40 percent of patients at the time of diagnosis. In 25 percent of the cases, there is symptomatic gastrointestinal involvement; at its most extreme, this condition is known as *polyposis coli* (see Chap. 98, Fig. 98–13). Gastrointestinal symptoms may include abdominal pain and diarrhea, signs of small-bowel obstruction, hematochezia, or, uncommonly, protein-losing enteropathy, intestinal malabsorption, chylous ascites, an abdominal mass, or an acute abdomen as a result of bowel perforation. The intestinal polyps usually appear in the ileocecal region. The macroscopic appearance of polyps is not specific to mantle cells lymphoma. Biopsy and histopathologic evaluation and immunocytochemistry are required to identify the characteristic cells and immunophenotype of lymphomatous mantle cells to make a specific diagnosis. Gastrointestinal involvement can be detected in 90 percent of cases; half of these can be diagnosed only by pan-endoscopy and microscopic evaluation of random biopsies.[13] The highest yield is from a colonoscopy with biopsy.

LABORATORY FEATURES

BLOOD AND MARROW

Approximately 50 percent of patients present with blood and marrow involvement, sometimes with an overt leukemic phase, but more often with subtle involvement as detected by flow cytometry of blood or marrow for the malignant lymphocyte immunophenotype.

BIOPSY

Histologically, MCL presents most commonly as a diffuse effacement of the lymph nodes, less commonly as a nodular pattern, and rarely as a mantle zone pattern, defined as greater than 90 percent of the follicles presenting with preservation of the germinal center (Fig. 102–2) (see also Chap. 98, Figs. 98–14 and 98–15).[14] There are four cytologic variants, including a marginal zone-like variant; a small cell variant, resembling chronic lymphocytic leukemia; a blastoid cell variant (with intermediate-size blasts); and a pleomorphic variant with medium-to-large cells, with the last two patterns being associated with a more aggressive clinical course.[3]

Immunophenotyping reveals lymphocytes that express B-cell antigens CD19 and CD20, plus aberrant expression of the T-cell antigen CD5, and negative staining for CD23.

CYTOGENETIC FEATURES

The reciprocal chromosomal translocation t(11;14)(q13;q32), which involves the cyclin D1 genes (e.g., *CCND1, PRAD1, bcl*-1) on chromosome 11 and the Ig heavy-chain locus on chromosome 14, occurs in practically all cases. Because of the high level of genetic instability of cells in MCL additional chromosome abnormalities are common, especially deletions of sequences in chromosome 1, 2, 6, 8, 10, 11, 13, or 17 or gain in sequences in chromosomes 3, 4, 7, 8, 9, 10, 12, or 18. Chromosome 17p abnormalities (p53 mutations) occur in a quarter of patients.

IMMUNOHISTOCHEMICAL FINDINGS

The chromosomal translocation t(11;14) results in overexpression of the *CCND1* gene, which encodes cyclin D1, a cell-cycle protein not normally expressed in lymphoid cells. Almost all cases of MCL show overexpression of cyclin D1 messenger ribonucleic acid (mRNA) (see Chap. 98, Fig. 98–16). The rare cases that are negative for cyclin D1 usually overexpress cyclin D2 or D3.[6] MCL cells stain strongly for the antiapoptotic molecule BCL-2 and are negative for the germinal center markers CD10 and BCL-6.[14]

DIFFERENTIAL DIAGNOSIS

The immunophenotype of MCL has some similarities to that of chronic lymphocytic leukemia (CLL) or small lymphocytic lymphoma (SLL) in that the lymphoma cells express surface IgM and IgD and the B-cell–associated antigens CD19 and CD20, and have aberrant expression of the T-cell antigen CD5. The intensity of staining for B-cell antigens and Ig is greater in MCL than in CLL or SLL. In contrast to CLL or SLL, MCL cells are positive for FMC7 and typically do not express CD23. Like follicular lymphoma, MCL is positive for CD20 and BCL-2, but in contrast to follicular lymphoma, MCL is negative for CD10 and BCL-6.[14] This finding occurs because most cases do not originate in the germinal center but rather arise from naïve cells in the mantle zone of the follicle. More importantly, almost all cases of MCL overexpress cyclin D1, and no other lymphoma shows overexpression of cyclin D1.

TABLE 102–1. Patient Characteristics at Presentation (304 Cases)

Characteristic	Number
Age (years)	
<60	123
>60	178
Sex	
Male	230
Female	71
Stage	
I–II	23
III–IV	267
Status (WHO)	
0–1	233
≥2	43
LDH	
Elevated	56
Normal	140
IPI	
0–1	15
≥2	75
Marrow involvement	
Yes	207
No	81
B symptoms	
Yes	107
No	155
Extranodal involvement	
Yes	161
No	16

LDH, lactate dehydrogenase; IPI, international prognostic index; WHO, World Health Organization.
SOURCE: Data from Tiemann M, Schrader C, Klapper W, et al.[12]

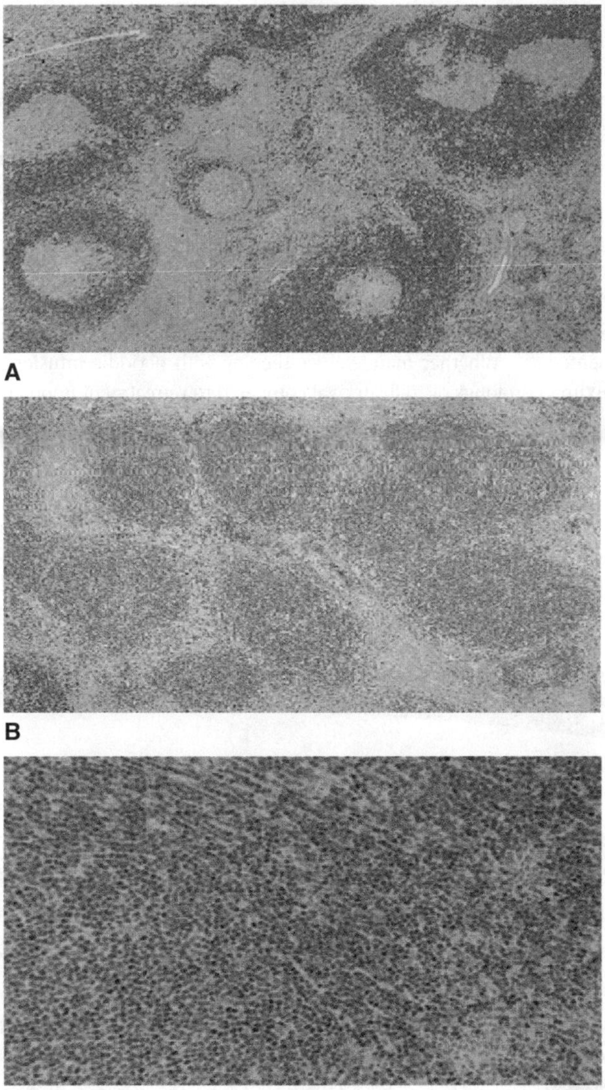

A

B

C

FIGURE 102–2. Cyclin D-1 staining reveals several histopathologic patterns in the lymph node biopsy of patients with mantle cell lymphoma. **A.** Mantle zone pattern. More than 90 percent of the follicles have reactive germinal centers surrounded by mantles of neoplastic lymphoid cells. This is an uncommon occurrence, representing less than 6 percent of lymph node patterns. **B.** Nodular pattern. In this example, less than 90 percent of follicles have reactive germinal centers. Distinct visualization of follicles. **C.** Diffuse pattern. Effacement of the architecture of the lymph node and replacement by malignant lymphoid cells. *(Used with permission from L. Jeffrey Medeiros, MD.)*

THERAPY

INITIAL THERAPY

MCL is still considered incurable. Because of the presence of advanced disease at presentation, most patients require systemic therapy. Current strategies involve intensification of therapy with or without consolidation with stem cell transplantation (SCT).

Therapy for Stage I–II Disease

Localized disease is rare. There is no consensus on the best therapeutic approach; a retrospective review of 17 patients who received involved-field radiotherapy with or without chemotherapy reported a 5-year progress-free survival (PFS) of 68 percent and overall survival (OS) of 71 percent.[15]

Doxorubicin-Containing Chemotherapy

MCL is responsive to doxorubicin-containing chemotherapy, but the complete remission rates are only 30 to 40 percent, the duration of response is 10 to12 months, and the median survival 3 to 4 years,[16] all of which are lower when compared with other lymphoma subtypes.

Fludarabine Alone or in Combination

Fludarabine has been tested in a small number of untreated MCL patients and has achieved an overall response rate of 41 percent with a complete remission rate of 29 percent.[17] The median OS in this study was 2 years. Fludarabine therapy may limit the ability to collect later autologous stem cells, if needed.

The Importance of Rituximab

The anti-CD20 monoclonal antibody rituximab is the most important recent addition to the therapy of lymphomas, including MCL. Rituximab alone produces a 38 percent response in patients with untreated MCL, with a median duration of response of 1.2 years and with very little hematologic or nonhematologic toxicity, and can be utilized in selected patients who would otherwise not tolerate cytotoxic therapy, thus prolonging and improving the quality of life.[18] Rituximab improves both the response and duration of response when combined in the initial treatment and after relapse.[19–22] If the response to initial therapy is less than complete, the role of additional doses of rituximab is not established.[23] Meta-analysis data also suggest that rituximab can improve the overall survival.[22] In patients with blood involvement, the first dose of rituximab should be delivered with caution because of the risk of tumor lysis syndrome or cytokine-release syndrome. If necessary, the first cycle can be given without rituximab in order to avoid these potential complications. The role of rituximab as an agent of *in vivo* purging of malignant cells in the blood and marrow prior to autologous transplantation has been documented.[24,25] Whether maintenance therapy with periodic infusions of rituximab prolongs overall survival compared to retreatment upon clinical or molecular recurrence is yet to be determined.

The Importance of Cytarabine

Several studies suggest that cytarabine adds significantly to the response. These include, among others, a study where dexamethasone, cytarabine (ara-c), cisplatin (DHAP) was able to further cytoreduce tumors that were not responding to cyclophosphamide, hydroxydoxorubicin (Adriamycin), vincristine (Oncovin), and prednisone (CHOP),[26] prior to autologous SCT, as well as a trial,[27] in which high doses of cytarabine significantly improved results of an autologous SCT-containing regimen when compared with prior historical treatment without cytarabine. In the latter study, rituximab was also added to the initial therapy, but rituximab alone cannot account for the impressive results. High doses of cytarabine are also an important component of the intense nontransplantation regimens.[28]

Intense Chemotherapy with and without Stem Cell Transplantation

Several reports have either intensified conventional therapy and/or incorporated consolidation high-dose chemotherapy followed by SCT as part of initial therapy. As seen in Table 102–2, the more intense chemotherapy combinations have produced better rates of complete remission and duration of response.[29–31] Whether consolidation with SCT is needed as part of initial therapy is not clear, as intense chemoimmunotherapy regimens omitting consolidation with SCT have achieved similar results.[31]

TABLE 102–2. Reports of Therapy for Untreated Mantle Cell Lymphoma Studies Including More Than 20 Patients

Study	Regimen	Age (years)	No. of Patients	CR/CRu (%)	Outcome	Median Followup Time (months)
Howard et al[23]	CHOP-R	31–69	40	48	Median PFS, 16.5 months	25
*Lenz et al[19]	CHOP-R	37–78	62	34	Median TTF, 21 months	18
Neelapu et al[29]	EPOCH-R	22–73	26	92	Median EFS, 22 months	46
Kahl et al[30]	Modified R-hyper-CVAD†	40–81	22	64	50% 3-year PFS	37
Fayad et al[31]	Hyper-CVAD-R+methotrexate-cytarabine-R	41–65	65	89	60% 5-year FFS	58
Magni et al[24]	R-HDS–autoSCT	23–65	28	100	10-year EFS of 57% for low risk, 34% for high risk MIPI	NA
Khouri et al[32]	Hyper-CVAD–autoSCT	38–66	33	100	43% 5-year DFS	49
Vandenberghe et al[33]	Chemo–autoSCT	24–70	195‡	67	33% 5-year PFS	44
§Geisler et al[27]	Maxi-CHOP–cytarabine autoSCT	38–65	160	90	56% 6-year EFS	41
Lefrere et al[26]	CHOP/DHAP-autoSCT	33–64	28	89	Median EFS 51 months	NA
Dreyling et al[34]	CHOP/interferon	35–65	122	28	25% 3-year PFS	25
	CHOP/autoSCT			81	54% 3-year PFS	
Evens et al[35]	CTAP/VMAC/autoSCT	39–63	25	76	54% 5-year EFS	66
Vigouroux et al[36]	CHOP/DHAP/autoSCT	40–63	30	87	40% 5-year PFS	55
Thieblemont et al[37]	Doxorubicin-containing + rituximab + DHAP/auto SCT	29–65	29	71	Median FFS 42 months	31
van 't Veer et al[38]	R-CHOP + Cytarabine/autoSCT	32–66	87	64	36% 4-year FFS	42
de Guibert et al[39]	R-DHAP/autoSCT	47–74	24	92	65% 3-year FFS	28

autoSCT, autologous stem cell transplantation; CHOP, cyclophosphamide, doxorubicin, vincristine, prednisone; CR, complete remission; Cru, complete remission unconfirmed; DFS, disease free survival; DHAP, dexamethasone, high-dose cytarabine, cisplatin; EFS, event-free survival; EPOCH, etoposide, prednisone, vincristine, cyclophosphamide, doxorubicin; FFS, failure-free survival; hyper-CVAD, fractionated cyclophosphamide, vincristine, doxorubicin, dexamethasone; MIPI, Mantle Cell International Prognostic Index; NA, not available; ORR, objective response rate; PFS, progression-free survival; PR, partial response; R, rituximab; TTF, time to treatment failure.

*Prospective, randomized study statistically superior to CHOP without rituximab.

†Maintenance rituximab q 6 months × 2 years.

‡Fifteen percent underwent transplantation at relapse.

§Patients with molecular recurrence treated with rituximab and not counted as events.

Risk of Central Nervous System Disease

There is no consensus on the risk of central nervous system (CNS) disease in patients with MCL or the need to give CNS prophylaxis. Studies have reported an incidence of CNS of 4 percent and a 5-year actuarial risk of 26 percent.[40–42] Possible risk factors mentioned in these studies include the presence of blastoid cytology and an elevated lymphoma cell proliferative rate.

Minimal Residual Disease

Current molecular techniques allow for detection of 1 in 10^4 to 1 in 10^6 lymphoma cells, although the methodology utilized is not uniform among laboratories. A report[25] suggested a correlation between molecular recurrence and clinical recurrence, a fact utilized in a trial as a basis for preemptive treatment with rituximab[27] before any clinical evidence of recurrence was evident. Other clinical researchers have not seen the correlation, perhaps related to differences in the sensitivity of their molecular tests.[43]

THERAPY FOR RECURRENT AND REFRACTORY DISEASE

The inherent resistance of MCL to conventional doses of chemotherapy is evident at relapse. Table 102–3 summarizes most of the reported single-agent and combination chemotherapy trials. Among the studied salvage therapies, several successful ones have exploited biologic insights. For example, the first-generation proteosome inhibitor bortezomib has shown a 31 percent response rate as single-agent therapy and has been approved by the FDA for this purpose. Bortezomib is thought to exert its effect in part indirectly through alterations in p27, cyclin D1, and nuclear factor-κB (NF-κB). Temsirolimus is a promising mTOR inhibitor that has also shown a 38 percent overall response rate in this situation. Another drug, lenalidomide, belongs to a different class of agents (immunomodulators) and has shown a 53 percent overall response rate with 13 percent complete remissions.[57] Conversely, single-agent therapy with the cyclin D kinase inhibitor flavopiridol has not been effective, probably as a result of its schedule dependency. Research using flavopiridol in combination chemotherapy with a specific schedule suggests this could be a promising approach.[66]

TABLE 102–3. Response Rates as a Result of Different Salvage Therapies for Relapsed or Refractory Mantle Cell Lymphoma

Study	Regimen	No. of Patients	CR/CRu (%)	PR (%)	ORR (%)
Foran et al[18]	Rituximab	35	14	23	37
Gressin et al[44]	VAD ± chlorambucil	30	43	30	73
Foran et al[17]	Fludarabine	17	29	12	41
Kaufmann et al[45]	Rituximab + thalidomide	16	31	50	81
Dang et al[46]	Ontak	8	12.5	25	37.5
Cohen et al[47]	Cyclophosphamide + fludarabine	30	30	33	63
Goy et al[48]	Bortezomib	29	21	21	42
O'Connor et al[49]	Bortezomib	11	9	36	45
McLaughlin et al[50]	Fludarabine + mitoxantrone + dexamethasone	5	20	80	100
Seymour et al[51]	Fludarabine + cisplatin + cytarabine	8			88
Forstpointner et al[20]	Fludarabine + cyclophosphamide + mitoxantrone	24	0	46	46
Forstpointner et al[20]	Fludarabine + cyclophosphamide + mitoxantrone + rituximab	24	29	29	58
Rummel et al[52]	Bendamustine + rituximab	16	50	25	75
Fisher et al[53]	Bortezomib	141	8	25	33
Robak et al[54]	2-CdA + rituximab or rituximab/cyclophosphamide	9	22	45	67
O'Connor et al[55]	Epothilone ixabepilone	15	0	1	7
Robinson et al[56]	Bendamustine + rituximab	12	59	33	92
Wiernik et al[57]	Lenalidomide	15	13	40	53
Witzig et al[58]	Temsirolimus	34	3	35	38
Ansell et al[59]	Low-dose temsirolimus	27	4	37	41
Inwards et al[60]	Cladribine	24	21	25	46
Coleman et al[61]	PEP-C (prednisone, cyclophosphamide, etoposide, procarbazine)	22	46	36	82
Rodriguez et al[62]	Gemcitabine, oxaliplatin, rituximab	14	64	14	78
Weide et al[63]	Bendamustine, mitoxantrone, rituximab	57	35	54	87
Lin et al[64]	Flavopiridol	10	0	0	0
Kouroukis et al[65]	Flavopiridol	28	0	11	11

CR, complete remission; Cru, complete remission unconfirmed; DFS, disease-free survival; ORR, objective response rate; PR, partial response.

Among conventional chemotherapy options, regimens include nucleoside analogues, particularly the R-FCM regimen (rituximab, fludarabine, cyclophosphamide, and mitoxantrone).[20] The bifunctional alkylating agent bendamustine in combination with rituximab has moved quickly as an initial therapy option, and in one study showed as much efficacy as R-CHOP with less toxicity in a multiinstitutional prospective randomized trial.[65]

However, because second and later remissions are brief, SCT deserves consideration after cytoreduction with salvage chemotherapy. Unfortunately, recurrent/refractory MCL recurs after high-dose chemotherapy followed by rescue of autologous stem cell infusion.[33–39] The current consensus is that the best results with the longest duration of disease control after relapse is consolidation of a response, preferably a complete response, with allogeneic SCT, based on evidence of graft-versus-lymphoma activity in MCL. A reduced intensity allograft can achieve PFS and event-free survival (EFS) rates of 40 to 80 percent and OS rates of 55 to 86 percent after a median followup of 2 to 3 years, with 5 to 30 percent acute graft-versus-host disease and 0 to 24 percent treatment-related mortality.[68–72]

Radioimmunotherapy Plus Chemotherapy

MCL is very sensitive to radiotherapy, but because the disease is advanced at presentation in a great majority of patients, conventional involved-field radiotherapy usually has no role. However, a systemic approach with radioimmunotherapy is an option worth exploring. ^{131}I-tositumomab used as a part of initial therapy, before chemotherapy, has been reported.[73] In 25 patients, the overall response was 88 percent and the complete remission (CR) rate was 50 percent, with a molecular remission of 46 percent, all just after one dose of the radioimmunoconjugate and before the start of the CHOP chemotherapy. The median event-free survival was 21.6 months.

In the relapsed/refractory setting, single-agent ibritumomab tiutexan-^{90}yttrium has resulted in a 41 percent overall response rate (ORR; 29% CR/Cru [complete response unconfirmed]) but with a short time to progression of 5 months.[74] In another use of radioimmunotherapy in the relapsed/refractory setting, the approach was to cytoreduce the tumor and consolidate with high doses of cyclophosphamide and etoposide, followed by myeloablative doses of ^{131}I-tositumomab.[75] This resulted in a 100 percent ORR (91% CR) and a 3-year PFS of 61 percent. Other clinical researchers have explored the use of standard doses of ibritumomab tiutexan-^{90}yttrium as part of the preparative regimen for autologous SCT in 41 patients with relapsed MCL and reported a 2-year OS and PFS of 90 percent and 70 percent after a median followup of 18.4 months.[76]

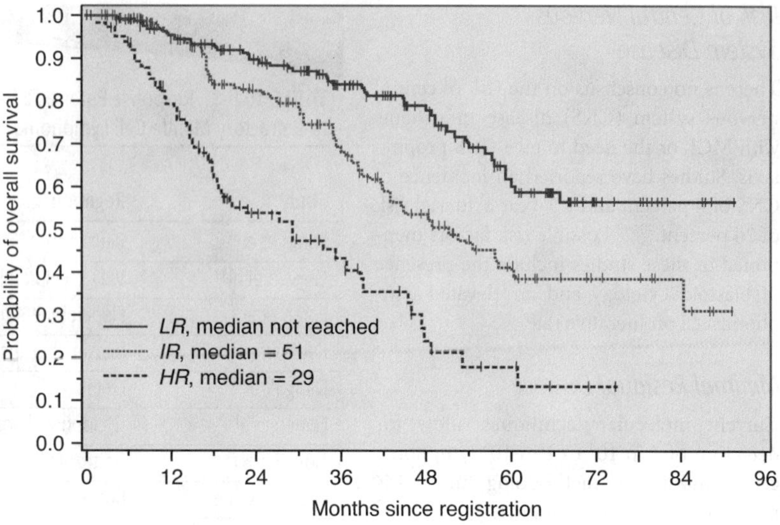

Numbers of patients at risk

LR	180	153	131	99	69	39	15	4
IR	145	116	83	57	37	19	9	5
HR	84	58	29	19	8	5	1	0

FIGURE 102–3. Overall survival according to the Mantle Cell International Prognostic Index (MIPI). *LR* indicates low risk, prognostic score less than 5.7; *IR* indicates intermediate risk, prognostic score 5.7 or more but less than 6.2; and *HR* indicates high risk, prognostic score 6.2 or more. The prognostic score is calculated as $[0.03535 \times \text{age (years)}] + 0.6978 \text{ (if ECOG} > 1) + [1.367 \times \log_{10}(\text{LDH/ULN})] + [0.9393 \times \log_{10}(\text{WBC count})]$. ECOG, Eastern Cooperative Oncology Group performance status score; LDH, lactate dehydrogenase; ULN, upper limits of normal; WBC, white blood cell. *(Reproduced with permission from Hoster E, Dreyling M, Klapper W, et al.[82])*

COURSE AND PROGNOSIS

Prospects for patients with this incurable lymphoma have improved over the past decade as a result of advances in therapy, as well as improvement in diagnostic tools and supportive therapy. In addition, newer therapies have been made available and have altered the overall survival of those patients in whom the disease recurs. A study reported an improvement in overall median survival from 2.7 years in the 1975 to 1986 era to 5.8 years in the 1996 to 2004 era.[77] In this study, the authors concluded that addition of doxorubicin, stem cell transplantation, and rituximab, as well as improved patient care, accounted for the longer survival. Another retrospective study of patients treated without intense initial chemotherapy and with watchful waiting for those with stable disease reported a median overall survival of 5 years.[78] The question of whether intense therapy or a conservative approach results in a longer overall survival requires additional studies and a longer followup to be answered. It requires the correct identification of the subgroups within MCL that have a better or worse prognosis. Only then can studies be accurately compared and significant advances in the management of MCL be made. Most of the reported prognostic variables and models are retrospective and were devised with patients who received therapy in the form of a doxorubicin-containing regimen with or without rituximab. Among the reported prognostic variables, molecular profiling has determined a group of genes associated with proliferation that can identify patient subsets that differ by more than 5 years in median survival.[79] An immunohistochemical test for the proliferation antigen Ki67 has also shown prognostic value when retrospectively examined in MCL patients treated with a variety of regimens, mostly doxorubicin-containing.[80] A five-gene model to predict survival in MCL using frozen or formalin-fixed, paraffin-embedded tissue has been devised.[81] Other variables reported to be of prognostic importance are the pretreatment serum level of β_2-microglobulin[28] and lactic dehydrogenase (LDH),[12,28] blastoid cytology,[12] age,[12,28] Ann Arbor stage,[4] extranodal presentation,[12] and constitutional symptoms,[12] among others. A prognostic model called the Mantle Cell International Prognostic Index (MIPI) has been introduced, which uses four independent prognostic factors: age, performance status, LDH, and leukocyte count.[82] Figure 102–3 shows survival curves utilizing this model. Patients were classified according to the MIPI into low-risk (44% of patients, median OS not reached), intermediate-risk (35%, 51 months), and high-risk groups (21%, 29 months). Retrospective applications of this model suggest some correlation with prognosis.[24,83]

With new therapies based on knowledge of biology in MCL, as well as new prognostic models that can be used to tailor therapy and compare among studies, the prospects look good for continuing improvement in the effects of therapy of MCL.

REFERENCES

1. Banks PM, Chan J, Cleary ML, et al: Mantle cell lymphoma. A proposal for unification of morphologic, immunologic, and molecular data. *Am J Surg Pathol* 16:637, 1992.
2. Harris NL, Jaffe ES, Stein H, et al: A revised European-American classification of lymphoid neoplasms: A proposal from the International Lymphoma Study Group. *Blood* 84:1361, 1994.
3. Swerdlow SH, Campo E, Harris NL, et al: *WHO Classification of Tumours of Haematopoietic and Lymphoid Tissues* (4th ed). International Agency for Research on Cancer, Lyon, France, 2008.
4. The Non-Hodgkin's Lymphoma Classification Project. A clinical evaluation of the International Lymphoma Study Group classification of non-Hodgkin's lymphoma. *Blood* 89:3909, 1997.
5. Zhou Y, Wang H, Fang W, et al: Incidence trends of mantle cell lymphoma in the United States between 1992 and 2004. *Cancer* 113:791, 2008.
6. Jares P, Colomer D, Campo E: Genetic and molecular pathogenesis of mantle cell lymphoma: Perspectives for new targeted therapeutics. *Nat Rev Cancer* 7:750, 2007.
7. Hirt C, Schuler F, Dolken L, et al: G. Low prevalence of circulating t(11;14)(q13;q32)-positive cells in the peripheral blood of healthy individuals as detected by real-time quantitative PCR. *Blood* 104:904, 2004.

8. Salaverria I, Perez-Galan P, Colomer D, et al: Mantle cell lymphoma: From pathology and molecular pathogenesis to new therapeutic perspectives. *Haematologica* 91:11, 2006.
9. Ott, G, Kalla J, Ott MM, et al: Blastoid variants of mantle cell lymphoma: Frequent bcl-1 rearrangements at the major translocation cluster region and tetraploid chromosome clones. *Blood* 89:1421, 1997.
10. Cuneo A, Bigoni R, Rigolin GM, et al: Cytogenetic profile of lymphoma of follicle mantle lineage: Correlation with clinicobiologic features. *Blood* 93:1372, 1999.
11. Greiner TC, Moynihan MJ, Chan WC, et al: Mutations in mantle cell lymphoma are associated with variant cytology and predict a poor prognosis. *Blood* 87:4302, 1996.
12. Tiemann M, Schrader C, Klapper W, et al: European MCL Network: Histopathology, cell proliferation indices and clinical outcome in 304 patients with mantle cell lymphoma (MCL): A clinicopathological study from the European MCL Network. *Br J Haematol* 131:29, 2005.
13. Romaguera JE, Medeiros LJ, Hagemeister FB, et al: Frequency of gastrointestinal involvement and its clinical significance in mantle cell lymphoma. *Cancer* 97:586, 2003. Erratum in: *Cancer* 97:3131, 2003.
14. Weisenburger DD, Armitage JO: Mantle cell lymphoma—An entity comes of age. *Blood* 87:4483, 1996.
15. Leitch HA, Gascoyne RD, Chhanabhai M, et al: Limited-stage mantle-cell lymphoma. *Ann Oncol* 10:1555, 2003.
16. Fisher RI, Dahlberg S, Nathwani BN, et al: A clinical analysis of two indolent lymphoma entities: Mantle cell lymphoma and marginal zone lymphoma (including mucosa-associated lymphoid tissue and monocytoid B-cell categories): A Southwest Oncology Group study. *Blood* 85:1075, 1995.
17. Foran JM, Rohatiner AZ, Coiffier B, et al: Multicenter phase II study of fludarabine phosphate for patients with newly diagnosed lymphoplasmacytoid lymphoma, Waldenström's macroglobulinemia, and mantle-cell lymphoma. *J Clin Oncol* 17:546, 1999.
18. Foran JM, Rohatiner AZ, Cunningham D, et al: European phase II study of rituximab (chimeric anti-CD20 monoclonal antibody) for patients with newly diagnosed mantle-cell lymphoma and previously treated mantle-cell lymphoma, immunocytoma, and small B-cell lymphocytic lymphoma. *J Clin Oncol* 18:317, 2000. Erratum in: *J Clin Oncol* 18:2006, 2000.
19. Lenz G, Dreyling M, Hoster E, et al: Immunochemotherapy with rituximab and cyclophosphamide, doxorubicin, vincristine, and prednisone significantly improves response and time to treatment failure, but not long-term outcome in patients with previously untreated mantle cell lymphoma: Results of a prospective randomized trial of the German Low Grade Lymphoma Study Group (GLSG) *J Clin Oncol* 23:1984, 2005.
20. Forstpointner R, Dreyling M, Repp R, et al: German Low-Grade Lymphoma Study Group. The addition of rituximab to a combination of fludarabine, cyclophosphamide, mitoxantrone (FCM) significantly increases the response rate and prolongs survival as compared with FCM alone in patients with relapsed and refractory follicular and mantle cell lymphomas: Results of a prospective randomized study of the German Low-Grade Lymphoma Study Group. *Blood* 104:3064, 2004.
21. Ghielmini M, Schmitz SF, Cogliatti S, et al: Swiss Group for Clinical Cancer Research. Effect of single-agent rituximab given at the standard schedule or as prolonged treatment in patients with mantle cell lymphoma: A study of the Swiss Group for Clinical Cancer Research (SAKK). *J Clin Oncol* 23:705, 2005.
22. Schulz H, Bohlius JF, Trelle S, et al: Immunochemotherapy with rituximab and overall survival in patients with indolent or mantle cell lymphoma: A systematic review and meta-analysis. *J Natl Cancer Inst* 99:706, 2004.
23. Howard OM, Gribben JG, Neuberg DS, et al: Rituximab and CHOP induction therapy for newly diagnosed mantle-cell lymphoma: Molecular complete responses are not predictive of progression-free survival. *J Clin Oncol* 20:1288, 2002.
24. Magni M, Di Nicola M, Carlo-Stella C, et al: High-dose sequential chemotherapy and *in vivo* rituximab-purged stem cell autografting in mantle cell lymphoma: A 10-year update of the R-HDS regimen. *Bone Marrow Transplant* 43:509, 2009.
25. Pott C, Schrader C, Gesk S, et al: Quantitative assessment of molecular remission after high-dose therapy with autologous stem cell transplantation predicts long-term remission in mantle cell lymphoma. *Blood* 107:2271, 2006.
26. Lefrère F, Delmer A, Levy V, et al: Sequential chemotherapy regimens followed by high-dose therapy with stem cell transplantation in mantle cell lymphoma: An update of a prospective study. *Haematologica* 10:1275, 2004.
27. Geisler CH, Kolstad A, Laurell A, et al: Nordic Lymphoma Group. Long-term progression-free survival of mantle cell lymphoma after intensive front-line immunochemotherapy with in vivo-purged stem cell rescue: A nonrandomized phase 2 multicenter study by the Nordic Lymphoma Group. *Blood* 112:2687, 2008.
28. Romaguera JE, Fayad LE, Rodriguez MA, et al: High rate of durable remissions after treatment of newly diagnosed aggressive mantle-cell lymphoma with rituximab plus hyper-CVAD alternating with rituximab plus high-dose methotrexate and cytarabine. *J Clin Oncol* 23:7013, 2005.
29. Neelapu SS, Kwak LW, Kobrin CB, et al: Vaccine-induced tumor-specific immunity despite severe B-cell depletion in mantle cell lymphoma. *Nat Med* 11:986, 2005.
30. Kahl BS, Longo WL, Eickhoff JC, et al: Wisconsin Oncology Network. Maintenance rituximab following induction chemoimmunotherapy may prolong progression-free survival in mantle cell lymphoma: A pilot study from the Wisconsin Oncology Network. *Ann Oncol* 17:1418, 2006.
31. Fayad L, Thomas D, Romaguera J: Update of the M. D. Anderson Cancer Center experience with hyper-CVAD and rituximab for the treatment of mantle cell and Burkitt-type lymphomas. *Clin Lymphoma Myeloma* 8(Suppl 2):S57, 2007.
32. Khouri IF, Saliba RM, Okoroji GJ, et al: Long-term follow-up of autologous stem cell transplantation in patients with diffuse mantle cell lymphoma in first disease remission: The prognostic value of beta$_2$-microglobulin and the tumor score. *Cancer* 98:2630, 2003.
33. Vandenberghe E, Ruiz de Elvire C, Loberiza FR, et al: Outcome of autologous transplantation for mantle cell lymphoma: A study by the European Blood and Bone Marrow Transplant and Autologous Blood and Marrow Transplant Registries. *Br J Haematol* 120:793, 2003.
34. Dreyling M, Lenz G, Hoster E, et al: Early consolidation by myeloablative radiochemotherapy followed by autologous stem cell transplantation in first remission significantly prolongs progression-free survival in mantle cell lymphoma: Results of a prospective randomized trial of the European MCL Network. *Blood* 105:2677, 2005.
35. Evens AM, Winter JN, Hou N, et al: A phase II clinical trial of intensive chemotherapy followed by consolidative stem cell transplant: Long-term follow-up in newly diagnosed mantle cell lymphoma. *Br J Haematol* 140:385, 2008.
36. Vigouroux S, Gaillard F, Moreau P, et al: High-dose therapy with autologous stem cell transplantation in first response in mantle cell lymphoma. *Haematologica* 90:1580, 2005.
37. Thieblemont C, Antal D, Lacotte-Thierry L, et al: Chemotherapy with rituximab followed by high-dose therapy and autologous stem cell transplantation in patients with mantle cell lymphoma. *Cancer* 104:1434, 2005.
38. van 't Veer MB, de Jong D, Mackenzie M, et al: High-dose ara-C and beam with autograft rescue in R-CHOP responsive mantle cell lymphoma patients. *Br J Haematol* 144:524, 2009.
39. de Guibert S, Jaccard A, Bernard M, et al: Rituximab and DHAP followed by intensive therapy with autologous stem-cell transplantation as first-line therapy for mantle cell lymphoma. *Haematologica* 91:425, 2006.
40. Valdez R, Kroft SH, Ross CW, et al: Cerebrospinal fluid involvement in mantle cell lymphoma. *Mod Pathol* 15:1073, 2002.
41. Oinonen R, Franssila K, Elonen E: Central nervous system involvement in patients with mantle cell lymphoma. *Ann Hematol* 78:145, 1999.
42. Ferrer A, Bosch F, Villamor N, et al: Central nervous system involvement in mantle cell lymphoma. *Ann Oncol* 19:135, 2008.
43. Freedman AS, Neuberg D, Gribben JG, et al: High-dose chemoradiotherapy and anti-B-cell monoclonal antibody-purged autologous bone marrow transplantation in mantle-cell lymphoma: No evidence for long-term remission. *J Clin Oncol* 16:13, 1998.
44. Gressin R, Legouffe E, Leroux D, et al: Treatment of mantle-cell lymphomas with the VAD +/− chlorambucil regimen with or without subsequent high-dose therapy and peripheral blood stem-cell transplantation. *Ann Oncol* 8(Suppl 1):103, 1997.
45. Kaufmann H, Raderer M, Wöhrer S, et al: Antitumor activity of rituximab plus thalidomide in patients with relapsed/refractory mantle cell lymphoma. *Blood* 104:2269, 2004.
46. Dang NH, Fayad L, McLaughlin P, et al: Phase II trial of the combination of denileukin diftitox and rituximab for relapsed/refractory B-cell non-Hodgkin lymphoma. *Br J Haematol* 138:502, 2007.
47. Cohen BJ, Moskowitz C, Straus D, et al: Cyclophosphamide/fludarabine (CF) is active in the treatment of mantle cell lymphoma. *Leuk Lymphoma* 42:1015, 2001.
48. Goy A, Younes A, McLaughlin P, et al: Phase II study of proteasome inhibitor bortezomib in relapsed or refractory B-cell non-Hodgkin's lymphoma. *J Clin Oncol* 23:667, 2005.
49. O'Connor OA, Wright J, Moskowitz C, et al: Phase II clinical experience with the novel proteasome inhibitor bortezomib in patients with indolent non-Hodgkin's lymphoma and mantle cell lymphoma. *J Clin Oncol* 23:676, 2005.
50. McLaughlin P, Hagemeister FB, Romaguera JE, et al: Fludarabine, mitoxantrone, and dexamethasone: An effective new regimen for indolent lymphoma. *J Clin Oncol* 14:1262, 1996.
51. Seymour JF, Grigg AP, Szer J, et al: Cisplatin, fludarabine, and cytarabine: A novel, pharmacologically designed salvage therapy for patients with refractory, histologically aggressive or mantle cell non-Hodgkin's lymphoma. *Cancer* 94:585, 2002.
52. Rummel MJ, Al-Batran SE, Kim SZ, et al: Bendamustine plus rituximab is effective and has a favorable toxicity profile in the treatment of mantle cell and low-grade non-Hodgkin's lymphoma. *J Clin Oncol* 23:3383, 2005.
53. Fisher RI, Bernstein SH, Kahl BS, et al: Multicenter phase II study of bortezomib in patients with relapsed or refractory mantle cell lymphoma. *J Clin Oncol* 24:4867, 2006.
54. Robak T, Smolewski P, Cebula B, et al: Rituximab combined with cladribine or with cladribine and cyclophosphamide in heavily pretreated patients with indolent lymphoproliferative disorders and mantle cell lymphoma. *Cancer* 107:1542, 2006.
55. O'Connor OA, Portlock C, Moskowitz C, et al: A multicentre phase II clinical experience with the novel aza-epothilone Ixabepilone (BMS247550) in patients with relapsed or refractory indolent non-Hodgkin lymphoma and mantle cell lymphoma. *Br J Haematol* 143:201, 2008.
56. Robinson KS, Williams ME, van der Jagt RH, et al: Phase II multicenter study of bendamustine plus rituximab in patients with relapsed indolent B-cell and mantle cell non-Hodgkin's lymphoma. *J Clin Oncol* 26:4473, 2008.
57. Wiernik PH, Lossos IS, Tuscano JM, et al: Lenalidomide monotherapy in relapsed or refractory aggressive non-Hodgkin's lymphoma. *J Clin Oncol* 26:4952, 2008.
58. Witzig TE, Geyer SM, Ghobrial I, et al: Phase II trial of single-agent temsirolimus (CCI-779) for relapsed mantle cell lymphoma. *J Clin Oncol* 23:5347, 2005.
59. Ansell SM, Inwards DJ, Rowland KM Jr, et al: Low-dose, single-agent temsirolimus for relapsed mantle cell lymphoma: A phase 2 trial in the North Central Cancer Treatment Group. *Cancer* 113:508, 2008.

60. Inwards DJ, Fishkin PA, Hillman DW, et al: Long-term results of the treatment of patients with mantle cell lymphoma with cladribine (2-CDA) alone (95–80–53) or 2-CDA and rituximab (N0189) in the North Central Cancer Treatment Group. *Cancer* 113:108, 2008.
61. Coleman M, Martin P, Ruan J, et al: Low-dose metronomic, multidrug therapy with the PEP-C oral combination chemotherapy regimen for mantle cell lymphoma. *Leuk Lymphoma* 49:447, 2008.
62. Rodríguez J, Gutierrez A, Palacios A, et al: Rituximab, gemcitabine and oxaliplatin: An effective regimen in patients with refractory and relapsing mantle cell lymphoma. *Leuk Lymphoma* 48:2172, 2007.
63. Weide R, Hess G, Köppler H, et al: German Low Grade Lymphoma Study Group. High anti-lymphoma activity of bendamustine/mitoxantrone/rituximab in rituximab pretreated relapsed or refractory indolent lymphomas and mantle cell lymphomas. A multicenter phase II study of the German Low Grade Lymphoma Study Group (GLSG). *Leuk Lymphoma* 48:1299, 2007.
64. Lin TS, Howard OM, Neuberg DS, et al: Seventy-two hour continuous infusion flavopiridol in relapsed and refractory mantle cell lymphoma. *Leuk Lymphoma* 43:793, 2002.
65. Kouroukis CT, Belch A, Crump M, et al: National Cancer Institute of Canada Clinical Trials Group. Flavopiridol in untreated or relapsed mantle-cell lymphoma: Results of a phase II study of the National Cancer Institute of Canada Clinical Trials Group. *J Clin Oncol* 21:1740, 2003.
66. Christian BA, Grever MR, Byrd JC, et al: Flavopiridol in the treatment of chronic lymphocytic leukemia. *Curr Opin Oncol* 19:573, 2007.
67. Rummel MJ, von Gruenhagen U, Niederle N, et al: On behalf of the StiL. Bendamustine plus rituximab versus CHOP plus rituximab in the first-line treatment of patients with indolent and mantle cell lymphomas—First interim results of a randomized phase III study of the StiL (Study Group Indolent Lymphomas, Germany). *Blood* 110:385, 2007.
68. Khouri IF, Lee MS, Saliba RM, et al: Nonablative allogeneic stem-cell transplantation for advanced/recurrent mantle-cell lymphoma. *J Clin Oncol* 21:4407, 2003.
69. Corradini P, Dodero A, Farina L, et al: Allogeneic stem cell transplantation following reduced-intensity conditioning can induce durable clinical and molecular remissions in relapsed lymphomas: Pre-transplant disease status and histotype heavily influence outcome. *Leukemia* 21:2316, 2007.
70. Armand P, Kim HT, Ho VT, et al: Allogeneic transplantation with reduced-intensity conditioning for Hodgkin and non-Hodgkin lymphoma: Importance of histology for outcome. *Biol Blood Marrow Transplant* 14:418, 2008.
71. Robinson SP, Goldstone AH, Mackinnon S, et al: Lymphoma Working Party of the European Group for Blood and Bone Marrow Transplantation. Chemoresistant or aggressive lymphoma predicts for a poor outcome following reduced-intensity allogeneic progenitor cell transplantation: An analysis from the Lymphoma Working Party of the European Group for Blood and Bone Marrow Transplantation. *Blood* 100:4310, 2002.
72. Maris MB, Sandmaier BM, Storer BE, et al: Allogeneic hematopoietic cell transplantation after fludarabine and 2 Gy total body irradiation for relapsed and refractory mantle cell lymphoma. *Blood* 104:3535, 2004.
73. Zelenetz A, Donnelly G, Pandit-Tarkar N, et al: Sequential rituximab tositumomab/131 tositumomab followed by CHOP chemotherapy is a safe and highly effective regimen. *Ann Oncol* 16(Suppl5):54, 2005.
74. Oki Y, Pro B, Delpassand E et al: A phase II study of Yttrium^{90} ibritumomab tiuxetan (Zevalin) for treatment of patients with relapsed and refractory mantle cell lymphoma. *Blood* 104:720, 2004.
75. Gopal AK, Rajendran JG, Petersdorf SH, et al: High-dose chemo-radioimmunotherapy with autologous stem cell support for relapsed mantle cell lymphoma. *Blood* 99:3158, 2002.
76. Krishnan A, Nademanee A, Fung HC, et al: Phase II trial of a transplantation regimen of yttrium-90 ibritumomab tiuxetan and high-dose chemotherapy in patients with non-Hodgkin's lymphoma. *J Clin Oncol* 26:90, 2008.
77. Herrmann A, Hoster E, Zwingers T, et al: Improvement of overall survival in advanced stage mantle cell lymphoma. *J Clin Oncol* 27:511, 2009.
78. Martin P, Chadburn A, Christos P, et al: Intensive treatment strategies may not provide superior outcomes in mantle cell lymphoma: Overall survival exceeding 7 years with standard therapies. *Ann Oncol* 19:1327, 2008.
79. Rosenwald A, Wright G, Wiestner A, et al: The proliferation gene expression signature is a quantitative integrator of oncogenic events that predicts survival in mantle cell lymphoma. *Cancer Cell* 3:185, 2003.
80. Determann O, Hoster E, Ott G, et al: European Mantle Cell Lymphoma Network and the German Low Grade Lymphoma Study Group. Ki-67 predicts outcome in advanced-stage mantle cell lymphoma patients treated with anti-CD20 immunochemotherapy: Results from randomized trials of the European MCL Network and the German Low Grade Lymphoma Study Group. *Blood* 111:2385, 2008.
81. Hartmann E, Fernàndez V, Moreno V, et al: Five-gene model to predict survival in mantle-cell lymphoma using frozen or formalin-fixed, paraffin-embedded tissue. *J Clin Oncol* 26:4966, 2008.
82. Hoster E, Dreyling M, Klapper W, et al: A new prognostic index (MIPI) for patients with advanced-stage mantle cell lymphoma. German Low Grade Lymphoma Study Group (GLSG); European Mantle Cell Lymphoma Network. *Blood* 111:558, 2008.
83. Martin P, Chadburn A, Christos P, et al: Outcome of deferred initial therapy in mantle-cell lymphoma. *J Clin Oncol* 27:1209, 2009.

CHAPTER 103

MARGINAL ZONE B-CELL LYMPHOMAS

Emanuele Zucca

SUMMARY

Marginal zone B-cell lymphomas comprise three distinct clinicopathologic entities with variable clinical presentations, namely, the extranodal marginal zone lymphomas also known as mucosa-associated lymphatic tissue (MALT) lymphoma, the nodal marginal zone lymphoma, and the splenic marginal zone lymphoma. The extranodal type is the most common, accounting for approximately 7.5 percent of all cases of non-Hodgkin lymphoma.

The marginal zone B cells usually have small- to medium-size, irregular nuclei with dispersed chromatin, and inconspicuous nucleoli, resembling centrocytes and express surface immunoglobulins, pan-B antigens (CD19, CD20, and CD79a) and marginal zone-associated antigens (CD35 and CD21), but lack CD5, CD10, CD23, and cyclin D1 expression. Recurrent karyotype abnormalities have been described. All marginal zone lymphoma types present gains of chromosomes 3 and 18 at a higher frequency in comparison with other B-cell lymphomas. Rearrangements and deletions affecting chromosome 7q are most common in primary splenic lymphoma. In extranodal marginal zone lymphoma, three disparate translocations [t(11;18)(q21;q21), t(1;14)(p22;q32), and t(14;18)(q32;q21)], despite involving different genes, appear to affect the same signalling pathway, resulting in the activation of nuclear factor-kappa B (NF-κB), a transcription factor with a central role in immunity, inflammation, and apoptosis. These translocations are not present in splenic and nodal marginal zone lymphomas. Deletions or mutations of the tumor necrosis factor-α–induced protein 3 gene (TNFAIP3, A20, a negative regulator of the NF-κB pathway) on chromosome 6q was described in all subtypes of marginal zone lymphoma and are likely to represent another pathogenetic mechanism that can lead to NF-κB activation. The most common site of MALT lymphoma is the stomach, although primary involvement may occur at many other sites, including small intestine, lung, salivary gland, thyroid, skin, and other tissues. Most MALT lymphomas arise at sites normally devoid of lymphoid tissue, often preceded by a chronic inflammatory condition (infections or autoimmune disorders), such as Sjögren syndrome, Hashimoto thyroiditis, or, in the case of gastric MALT lymphoma, infection with *Helicobacter pylori*. Other infectious agents may have a pathogenetic role (*Borrelia burgdorferi* in cutaneous localizations, *Chlamydophila psittaci* in the ocular adnexa, and *Campylobacter jejuni* in the small intestine). Hepatitis C virus is associated with a subset of nodal and splenic marginal zone lymphomas. Appropriate antibiotic therapy eradicating *H. pylori* infection can lead to the regression of gastric MALT lymphoma in approximately 75 percent of cases. Patients who do not respond to antibiotic therapy may be considered for involved-field radiotherapy. Chemotherapy and immunotherapy with rituximab can be effective in patients with disseminated disease. Patients with splenic or nodal marginal zone lymphoma and hepatitis C virus infection may achieve a lymphoma remission after treatment of viral infection. Once hepatitis C virus infection is ruled out, most patients with nodal or splenic lymphoma can be managed initially with a wait-and-see policy. When treatment is needed, splenectomy is the treatment of choice for the splenic lymphomas. Chemotherapy may be considered for patient who have contraindication to splenectomy and for those with nodal marginal zone lymphoma. Alkylating agents and purine analogues have been reported to be active and can be used as single agent or in combination. Rituximab, alone or in combination with chemotherapy, is also very active.

Acronyms and abbreviations that appear in this chapter include: *BCL2*, B-cell lymphoma/leukemia-2 gene; *BCL10*, B-cell lymphoma/leukemia-10 gene; CD, cluster of differentiation; CHOP, cyclophosphamide, doxorubicin, vincristine, prednisone; CVP, cyclophosphamide, vincristine, prednisone; HCV, hepatitis C virus; Ig, immunoglobulin; LDH, lactate dehydrogenase; MALT, mucosa-associated lymphoid tissue; MALT-1, mucosa-associated lymphoid tissue translocation gene 1; MZL, marginal zone lymphoma; NF-κB, nuclear factor-kappa B; TNFAIP3, A20, tumor necrosis factor-α–induced protein 3 gene; WHO, World Health Organization.

DEFINITION AND CLASSIFICATION

The World Health Organization (WHO) classification of tumors of hematopoietic and lymphoid tissues comprises three separate marginal zone lymphoma (MZL) entities, namely, the extranodal marginal zone B-cell lymphoma of mucosa-associated lymphoid tissue (currently known as MALT lymphoma), the nodal marginal zone B-cell lymphoma (previously named monocytoid lymphoma), and the splenic marginal zone B-cell lymphoma (with or without circulating villous lymphocytes).[1–3] The term *marginal zone lymphoma* means that extranodal MZL, nodal MZL, and splenic MZL are believed to derive from B cells normally present in the marginal zone, which is the outer part of the mantle zone of B-cell follicles. The morphology of MZL cells is heterogeneous, including centrocyte-like B-cell cells with irregularly shaped nuclei, cells resembling monocytoid cells, and small B lymphocytes. Any of these cytologic aspects can predominate, or they can coexist within the same case. A salient feature of extranodal MZL is the presence of a variable number of lymphoepithelial lesions defined by evident invasion and partial destruction of mucosal glands by the lymphoma B cells. A number of nonneoplastic reactive T cells is often present. Scattered transformed large blast cells are also usually found.[1]

The B cells of MZLs show the immunophenotype of the normal marginal zone B cells present in spleen, Peyer patches, and in lymph nodes. Therefore, the tumor B cells express surface immunoglobulins and pan-B antigens (CD19, CD20, and CD79a), express the marginal zone-associated antigens CD35 and CD21, and lack CD5, CD10, CD23, and cyclin D_1 expression. The tumor cells of extranodal MZL typically express immunoglobulin (Ig) M, less often IgA or IgG, whereas splenic zone lymphoma is typically IgD-positive. Indeed, the splenic marginal zone lymphoma is morphologically distinct and is characterized by small round lymphocytes that are present in the mantle and marginal zones of the splenic white pulp, usually with a central residual germinal center, and infiltrate the red pulp.[1–3] Chapter 98 provides a more detailed description of the histologic and immunophenotypical characteristics of MZL.

EPIDEMIOLOGY AND PATHOGENESIS

Marginal zone lymphomas are distinct B-cell neoplasms with variable clinical presentations. Primary splenic and nodal MZL are rare, each comprising approximately 1 to 2 percent of lymphomas, whereas the extranodal MZL of MALT type is not uncommon, representing approximately 7.5 percent of the cases of non-Hodgkin lymphoma.[4]

Extranodal marginal zone B-cell lymphoma (MALT lymphoma) usually arises in mucosal sites where lymphocytes are not normally present and where a MALT is acquired in the context of chronic inflammation processes. A continual antigenic stimulation is, therefore, considered to be the background where abnormal B-cell clones acquiring successive genetic abnormalities can progressively replace the normal B-cell population of the inflammatory tissue and give rise to the MZL.[5] The acquisition of MALT is indeed induced by a series of agents, which appear to be different in each organ. The onset of MALT lymphomas in the stomach is preceded by the acquisition of MALT as a result of *Helicobacter pylori* infection and there is a compelling evidence for a pathogenetic role of this infection in gastric lymphoma.[5] *H. pylori* was identified by epidemiologic studies in the early 1990s as involved in gastric MALT lymphoma pathogenesis, and this recognition was supported by the repeated demonstration of tumor regressions in patients with early stage *H. pylori*-positive gastric MALT lymphoma treated with anti-*Helicobacter* antibiotic therapy.[6–12] Other bacterial infections have been found to be possibly implicated in the pathogenesis of MZLs arising in the skin (*Borrelia burgdorferi*),[13] in the ocular adnexa (*Chlamydophila psittaci*),[14] and in the small intestine (*Campylobacter jejuni*).[15] There is, however, a great and incompletely explained geographic variation in the strength of these associations. An increased risk of developing MALT lymphoma has been also reported in individuals affected by autoimmune disorders, especially Sjögren syndrome and systemic lupus erythematosus.[16]

Several recurrent chromosomal translocations have been described in extranodal MZLs.[17–21] These translocations show a different anatomical distribution and they appear mutually exclusive. Three of them [t(11;18)(q21;q21), t(1;14)(p22;q32), and t(14;18)(q32;q21)] are the most characterized, and, interestingly, they all appear to affect the same signalling pathway, activating nuclear factor-kappa B (NF-κB), a transcription factor with a central role in immunity, inflammation, and apoptosis.[22,23]

The t(11;18)(q21;q21), occurs in 15 to 40 percent of cases and results in the reciprocal fusion of cellular inhibitor of apoptosis protein 2 (cIAP2) on 11q21 with MALT1 on 18q21.[17,24] This translocation is more common in patients with primary gastric MZL that does not respond to anti-*Helicobacter* antibiotic therapy and in more advanced cases.[25]

The t(1;14)(p22;q32) translocation is detected in only 1 to 2 percent of extranodal MZL cases, and it determines an overexpression of the *BCL10* gene.[18] The t(14;18)(q32;q21), described in approximately 20 percent of extranodal MZL cases, appears cytogenetically identical to the t(14;18)(q32;q21) of follicular lymphoma, but the translocation in MZL deregulates the *MALT1* gene instead of the *BCL2* gene.[19] Other nonrandom chromosomal alterations have been described in extranodal MZL, but their role in lymphomagenesis is still unknown.[20,21]

Extranodal marginal zone B-cell lymphomas, together with the splenic and the nodal subtypes, present gains of chromosomes 3 and 18 at a higher frequency in comparison with other B-cell tumors.[26,27] Rearrangements and deletions affecting chromosome 7q, alongside gains of chromosomes 3 and 18 are the most common abnormalities in primary splenic lymphoma.[3,28–30] Gains of 3q and 18q, are also the most common alterations in nodal MZL.[29] In contrast, the recurrent translocations of extranodal MZL are not present in splenic and nodal MZL.

Homozygous deletions of the chromosomal band 6q23, involving the tumor necrosis factor-α–induced protein 3 gene (TNFAIP3, A20) were described in MZL (either extranodal, nodal, or splenic), and in other lymphoma types, suggesting a role for A20 as a tumor suppressor gene.[31–33] Indeed, this gene is a negative regulator of the NF-κB pathway, which is activated by the t(11;18), t(1;14) and t(14;18) translocations. Hence A20 inactivation, by either somatic mutation and/or deletion seems to be a common genetic aberration across all MZL subtypes, which may be another important pathogenetic mechanism that contributes to lymphomagenesis by inducing constitutive NF-κB activation.

CLINICAL FEATURES OF EXTRANODAL MARGINAL ZONE LYMPHOMA

The most common site of MALT lymphoma is the stomach, encompassing at least one-third of all cases. Extranodal MZLs may also arise at many other sites, including the salivary gland, the thyroid, the upper airways, the lung, the ocular adnexa (lachrymal gland, conjunctiva, eyelid, orbital soft tissue), the breast, the liver, the urogenital system, the skin and other soft tissues, and even the dura.[34] Primary intestinal involvement is typical of a particular and rare subtype of MALT lymphoma, the immunoproliferative small intestinal disease.[1]

As a general rule, the presenting symptoms of extranodal MZLs are related to the primary location. Elevated lactate dehydrogenase (LDH) or β_2-microglobulin levels, as well as constitutional B symptoms, are extremely rare at presentation.[10,35] MALT lymphoma can remain localized for a prolonged period within the tissue of origin, but regional lymph nodes can sometimes be infiltrated and dissemination at multiple sites is not uncommon, occurring in up to one-fourth of cases.[36–39] Marrow involvement is reported in 10 to 15 percent of cases. When dissemination is confined to multiple mucosal sites (i.e., lymph nodes and marrow are not involved), it does not appear to adversely affect the outcome. Most patients have indeed a favorable outcome with overall survival usually higher than 80 percent at 5 years.[36–39]

Nongastric MALT lymphoma patients may have a tendency to progress more often,[40] but whether different sites have a different natural history remains an open question. The frequency of involvement of any specific site, even in large multicenter series, is not high enough to clearly determine whether the anatomic localization has prognostic relevance. In a radiotherapy study, gastric and thyroid MALT lymphomas had the best outcome, whereas distant failures were more common for other sites.[41] In general, despite frequent relapses, MALT lymphomas at any sites most often maintain an indolent course.[36] Histologic transformation to large-cell lymphoma is reported in approximately 10 percent of the cases, most often as a late event and independent from dissemination.[37,39]

TREATMENT OF PRIMARY *H. PYLORI*-POSITIVE GASTRIC MARGINAL ZONE LYMPHOMA

The most common presenting symptoms of gastric MALT lymphoma are nonspecific upper gastrointestinal complaints that often lead to an endoscopy, usually revealing nonspecific gastritis or peptic ulcer with mass lesions being unusual. Diagnosis is based on the histopathologic evaluation of the gastric biopsies.[42] The presence *H. pylori* must be determined by histochemistry or, alternatively, urea breath test. In addition to routine histology and immunohistochemistry, fluorescence *in situ* hybridization analysis or use of polymerase chain reaction for detection of t(11;18) may be useful for identifying patients that are unlikely to respond to antibiotic therapy. The initial staging procedures should include a gastroduodenal endoscopy with multiple biopsies taken from each region of the stomach, duodenum, gastroesophageal junction, and from any abnormal-appearing site. Endoscopic ultrasound is recommended to evaluate the regional lymph nodes and gastric wall infiltration. Other recommended laboratory and radiologic studies include complete blood counts, basic biochemical studies, including LDH and β_2-microglobulin, computed tomography of the chest, abdomen, and pelvis, and a marrow aspirate and biopsy (Table 103–1). The role of positron emission tomographic scan is controversial and still investigational.

TABLE 103–1. Recommended Minimum Staging Procedures for Extranodal Marginal Zone Lymphoma

- History (duration and presence of local or systemic symptoms)
- Physical examination (careful evaluation of all lymph node regions, inspection of the upper airways and tonsils, clinical evaluation of the size of liver and spleen, detection of any palpable mass)
- Laboratory tests, including complete blood cell counts and examination of a blood film, LDH, evaluation of renal and liver function
- Standard posteroanterior and lateral chest radiographs
- Abdominal and pelvic computed tomography imaging
- Search for *H. pylori* infection (biopsy histology or breath test) is needed in gastric lymphoma. Other chronic infections that may have a pathogenetic role should also be investigated when lymphoma presents at certain sites (i.e., *B. burgdorferi* in cutaneous localizations, *C. psittaci* in the ocular adnexa, and *C. jejuni* in the small bowel).
- Marrow biopsy
- Additional investigations may include:
  1. *For gastric lymphoma:* gastroduodenal endoscopy with multiple gastric biopsies from all the visible lesions and the noninvolved areas and gastric endoscopic ultrasound
  2. *For intestinal presentation:* esophagogastroduodenoscopy, small-bowel studies and colonoscopy
  3. *For pulmonary lesions:* bronchoscopy and bronchoalveolar lavage

TABLE 103–2. Standard Anti-*Helicobacter* Treatments Based on Consensus Guidelines

Triple therapy
- Proton-pump inhibitor (standard dose, twice daily)
- Clarithromycin (500 mg twice daily)
- Amoxicillin (1000 mg twice daily) or metronidazole (500 mg twice daily) for 14 days

Quadruple therapy
- Proton-pump inhibitor (standard dose twice daily)
- Metronidazole 500 mg three times daily
- Tetracycline 500 mg four times daily
- Bismuth subcitrate 120 mg four times daily for 14 days

Quadruple therapy is an alternative first choice treatment in areas with a high prevalence (>15–20%) of clarithromycin resistance, or in patients who have previously received a macrolide antibiotic. Bismuth-containing quadruple therapy is the best second-choice treatment. Proton-pump inhibitor plus amoxicillin or tetracycline and metronidazole are recommended if bismuth is not available.

SOURCE: Based on data provided in Fuccio L, Laterza L, Zagari RM, et al[43]; Malfertheiner P, Megraud F, O'Morain C, et al[44]; Chey WD, Wong BC.[45]

Eradication of *H. pylori* with antibiotics plus proton-pump inhibitor regimens should be the sole initial treatment of localized (i.e., confined to the stomach) *H. pylori*-positive gastric MALT lymphoma. Several effective anti-*H. pylori* programs are available and the choice should be based on the current guidelines (Table 103–2).[43–45]

It is expected that following 2 weeks of antibiotic treatment, *H. pylori* will be eradicated in approximately 80 percent of the patients.[45] In case of unsuccessful eradication, second-line therapy should be attempted with alternative triple- or quadruple-therapy regimens of proton-pump inhibitor plus antibiotics.[43–45]

H. pylori eradication results in complete regression of gastric MALT lymphoma in approximately 50 to 75 percent of cases.[5,46,47] Most, but not all, responses are durable.[46,48] Unfortunately, the interpretation of residual lymphoid infiltrate in posttreatment gastric biopsies can be very difficult and there are no uniform criteria for the definition of histologic remission.[42,49] Moreover, several studies of postantibiotic molecular followup showed long-term persistence of monoclonal B cells after histologic regression of the lymphoma in about half of the studied cases.[50]

Consequently, histologic evaluation of repeat biopsies remains an essential followup procedure. Strict followup is recommended, with multiple biopsies taken 2 to 3 months after treatment to document that the lymphoma is not progressing and that *H. pylori* eradication has been achieved and, subsequently, at least twice per year for 2 years (and then once a year) to monitor the histologic regression of the lymphoma.[51] In case of persistent but stable (minimal) residual disease, a wait-and-see policy seems to be safe.[46,48] The long-term risk of transformation into aggressive lymphoma is lower in MALT lymphoma than in other indolent subtypes, particularly for the primary gastric presentation, but the risk has not yet been quantified.[37,39,46,48] Moreover, several cases have, been reported of gastric adenocarcinoma developed in patients with gastric MALT lymphoma. In a Dutch tumor-registry study, the risk of gastric adenocarcinoma among patients diagnosed with gastric MALT lymphoma was sixfold higher than in the general population.[52] This finding supports a policy of careful long-term systemic followup even in patients with persistent complete remission of gastric MALT lymphoma after cure of *H. pylori* infection.

TREATMENT OF *H. PYLORI*–INDEPENDENT GASTRIC MARGINAL ZONE LYMPHOMA

There is no clear consensus for the treatment of patients with gastric MALT lymphoma requiring further treatment beyond *H. pylori* eradication or with extensive disease.

Factors that suggest resistance to antibiotic therapy include invasion beyond the submucosa and the presence of the translocation t(11:18). Patients who do not respond or have only a partial response to antibiotic therapy may be considered for surgery or radiotherapy. Because gastric MALT lymphoma is multifocal, the surgical procedure is a total gastrectomy with its associated complications.[5] Surgery has not been shown to achieve superior results in comparison with organ-preserving strategies.[53] On the contrary, excellent disease control using involved-field radiotherapy alone has been reported by several institutions in patients with stages I and II MALT lymphoma of the stomach without evidence of *H. pylori* infection or with persistent lymphoma after antibiotic eradication. The modern development of advanced radiotherapy planning techniques, such as three-dimensional conformal radiotherapy and intensity-modulated radiotherapy, has reduced the toxicity that is related to the irradiation of normal gastric mucosa and of nontarget organs, and excellent results have been achieved using fairly moderate doses (30–40 Gy given in 4 weeks to the stomach and perigastric nodes).[54,55]

Patients with systemic disease should be considered for systemic chemotherapy and/or immunotherapy with anti-CD20 monoclonal antibodies, as described below for the nongastric MZL. Systemic treatment may also be considered when radiotherapy is difficult to deliver for whatever reason. Lymphoma with diffuse large-cell infiltration should be treated according to the recommendations for diffuse large B-cell lymphoma.

TREATMENT OF NONGASTRIC EXTRANODAL MARGINAL ZONE LYMPHOMA

Multiorgan involvement is not uncommon and complete staging procedures are recommended (see Table 103–1).[56] Besides standard lymphoma evaluation procedures, the investigations should focus on the specific organs involved; additional investigations may include esophagogastroduodenoscopy, small-bowel studies and colonoscopy for intestinal presentation, and bronchoscopy and bronchoalveolar lavage in the presence of lung lesions. Particular attention should be given to the demonstration of chronic infections that may have a pathogenetic role (*B. burgdorferi* in cutaneous localizations, *C. psittaci* in the ocular adnexa, and *C. jejuni* in the small intestine).

Retrospective series included patients treated with surgery, radiotherapy, and chemotherapy, alone or in combination. In most patients, good disease control and excellent cause-specific and overall survival has been demonstrated, independent of the treatment modality selected.[36–39,41]

The optimal management of nongastric disease is not clearly established and should be "patient-tailored," taking into account the site, the stage and the clinical characteristics of the individual patient.

In general, the treatment used for *H. pylori*-negative cases can be applied to non-gastric MALT lymphoma. Radiation therapy is considered the treatment of choice for localized lesions.[55] Indeed, MALT lymphomas at different sites have been successfully eradicated with involved-field radiation therapy encompassing the involved organ alone with doses of approximately 30 to 36 Gy.[54,55]

Analogous to other indolent lymphomas, asymptomatic patients with disseminated disease may be initially followed with a watchful waiting policy. However, the extranodal involvement itself is often representing an indication for treatment. Patients with symptomatic systemic disease or those where irradiation may be difficult (e.g., patients with liver involvement or with multiple lung lesions) should be considered for systemic chemotherapy and/or immunotherapy with anti-CD20 monoclonal antibodies. However, only a few compounds and regimens have been tested specifically in MALT lymphomas.

Alkylating agents (chlorambucil or cyclophosphamide) have been reported to be useful and have been used as single agent or in combination.[57–59] Some antitumor activity has also been shown for the purine analogues fludarabine and cladribine, which might, however, be associated with an increased risk of secondary myelodysplastic syndrome,[59,60] and of a combination regimen of chlorambucil, mitoxantrone, and prednisone.[61] Another potentially active agent is the proteasome inhibitor bortezomib but its toxicity profile may not be optimal.[62,63] Aggressive anthracycline-containing chemotherapy should be reserved for patients with a high tumor burden.[35,64]

Phase II studies have shown activity of the anti-CD20 monoclonal antibody rituximab in either gastric or nongastric localizations, with a response rate of approximately 70 percent,[65,66] and may represent an additional option for the treatment of systemic disease. The efficacy of the combination of rituximab with chlorambucil is being explored in a randomized study.

Antibiotic treatment can be effective in patients with lymphoma of the ocular adnexa despite the evident geographical variability of its association with *C. psittaci* infection and the possibility that other etiopathogenic agents could be involved.[67]

Specific problems are encountered in the management of immunoproliferative small intestinal disease; its natural course is usually prolonged, often over many years, including a potentially reversible early phase, when antibiotic treatment may lead to lymphoma regression. In the advanced disease, anthracycline-containing regimens should be used, combined with nutritional support plus antibiotics to control diarrhea and malabsorption.[68]

CLINICAL FEATURES AND TREATMENT OF PRIMARY SPLENIC MARGINAL ZONE LYMPHOMA (WITH OR WITHOUT CIRCULATING VILLOUS LYMPHOCYTES)

The very rare splenic MZL comprises less than 1 percent of all lymphomas.[4] More than half of the cases present circulating villous lymphocytes with characteristic fine, short cytoplasm polar projections. When these are more than 20 percent of the lymphocytes count, the term *splenic lymphoma with villous lymphocytes* is commonly used.[3]

Most patients are older than 50 years of age, and there is a similar incidence in males and females. The disease can present with massive splenomegaly, which produces abdominal discomfort and pain, and diagnosis can be made following a splenectomy performed to establish the cause of unexplained spleen enlargement. However, diagnosis can also follow investigations for anemia and/or thrombocytopenia, which in splenic MZL are present in one-quarter of cases, more often related to splenic sequestration than to marrow infiltration, and constantly associated with lymphocytosis. B symptoms are not common. Autoimmune hemolytic anemia or other autoimmune phenomena can be found in up to 15 percent of patients. Up to one-third of cases have liver involvement. The splenic hilar lymph nodes appear involved in approximately 25 percent of cases, whereas peripheral lymph node involvement is typically absent.[69–71]

Despite relevant geographical variations, hepatitis C virus (HCV) seems to be involved in lymphomagenesis. Analogous to the *H. pylori* infection in the gastric MZL, it appears that HCV may be responsible of an antigen-driven stimulation of the lymphoma clone.[72,73]

Indeed, patients with splenic MZL and HCV infection may achieve a lymphoma remission after treatment of HCV infection with interferon-α (alone or in combination with ribavirin), although this treatment has no antitumor effect on HCV-negative splenic MZL.[72,73]

Once HCV infection is ruled out, most patients can be initially managed with a wait-and-see policy, and they do not seem to have a worse outcome.[69,71] When treatment is needed, it is usually because of large, symptomatic splenomegaly or cytopenias. Splenectomy appears to be the treatment of choice; it allows a reduction/disappearance of circulating tumor lymphocytes and recovery of the lymphoma-associated cytopenia.[71] The benefit of splenectomy often persists for several years. The time to next treatment can be longer than 5 years. Adjuvant chemotherapy after splenectomy may result in higher rate of complete responses; however, there is no evidence of a survival benefit.[71]

Chemotherapy alone may be considered for the patient who requires treatment but has contraindication to splenectomy and for the patient with clinical progression after removal of the spleen. Alkylating agents have been reported to be active and can be used as single agent or in combination (as in the cyclophosphamide, vincristine, prednisone [CVP] or cyclophosphamide, doxorubicin, vincristine, and prednisone [CHOP] regimens). The purine analogue fludarabine is also effective and can be used alone or in combination with cyclophosphamide.[30]

Rituximab, alone or in combination with chemotherapy, is also very useful[71] and rituximab, alone, can be the treatment of choice in elderly patients and in those with impaired renal function.[30]

Patients with disseminated disease can be observed in advanced stages of either splenic or nodal or extranodal MZLs and a precise diagnosis can be very difficult in cases presenting with concomitant splenic, extranodal and nodal involvement.[71] In a retrospective French series of 124 patients with non–MALT-type MZLs from Lyon,[69] four clinical subtypes were observed: splenic (48% of cases), nodal (30%), disseminated (splenic and nodal, 16%), and leukemic (not splenic or nodal, 6%). Even when the disease is restricted to the cases presenting with splenomegaly, nearly all patients have marrow involvement, often accompanied by involvement of blood. Because of the high frequency of marrow or liver involvement, most all cases are classified as Ann Arbor stage IV disease. Serum paraproteinemia is observed in approximately 20 percent of cases and is most frequently of IgM type, posing the problem of the differential diagnosis with lymphoplasmacytic lymphoma (Waldenström macroglobulinemia), which often presents with clinical features similar to those of splenic MZL (splenomegaly, marrow lymphoplasmacytic infiltration, anemia); marked hyperviscosity and hypergammaglobulinemia, however, are uncommon in splenic MZL.[69] The clinical course is most usually indolent. In the Lyon study, the subgroup of patients with splenic lymphoma had the more favorable outcome with a median survival of more than 9 years.[69] Histologic transformation is rare, often associated with B symptoms, disease dissemination, and poorer outcome.[35]

CLINICAL FEATURES AND TREATMENT OF NODAL MARGINAL ZONE LYMPHOMA

Nodal MZL is also associated with HCV infection in some epidemiologic studies.[73] This type of lymphoma is a disease of older people, with the median age at presentation in the sixth decade, and affects both sexes, with a slight female predominance.[74] The disease can present with localized—most often in the neck—or disseminated adenopathy. Marrow is involved at presentation in less than half of cases. Transformation to high-grade lymphoma has been described in some cases. In a French series of non-MALT marginal zone B-cell lymphomas,[69] the nodal cases comprised 30 percent of patients and showed more aggressive behavior. No prospective studies have been conducted thus far and there is no consensus regarding the best treatment. Individual cases are managed differently according to the lesion histology (number of large cells) and clinical features (site and stage) of the individual patient. Treatment options may include single-agent chlorambucil or fludarabine or combination chemotherapy regimens (such as the CVP or CHOP). Rituximab may also have some efficacy and can be combined with chemotherapy. Anti-HCV treatment may induce lymphoma regression in some HCV-infected patients.[35,73] Autologous transplantation has been used in younger patients with adverse prognostic factors or increased large cell number.[69]

REFERENCES

1. Isaacson PG, Chott A, Nakamura S, Muller-Hermelink HK, et al: Extranodal marginal zone B-cell lymphoma of mucosa-associated lymphoid tissue (MALT lymphoma), in *WHO Classification of Tumours of Haematopoietic and Lymphoid Tissues*, edited by S Swerdlow, E Campo, NL Harris, ES Jaffe, SA Pileri, H Stein, J Thiele, JW Vardiman, p 214. IARC, Lyon, 2008.
2. Campo E, Pileri SA, Jaffe ES, et al: Nodal marginal zone B-cell lymphoma, in *WHO Classification of Tumours of Haematopoietic and Lymphoid Tissues*, edited by S Swerdlow, E Campo, NL Harris, ES Jaffe, SA Pileri, H Stein, J Thiele, JW Vardiman, p 218. IARC, Lyon, 2008.
3. Isaacson PG, Piris MA, Berger F, et al: Splenic B-cell marginal zone lymphoma, in *WHO Classification of Tumours of Haematopoietic and Lymphoid Tissues*, edited by S Swerdlow, E Campo, NL Harris, ES Jaffe, SA Pileri, H Stein, J Thiele, JW Vardiman, p 185. IARC, Lyon, 2008.
4. The Non-Hodgkin's Lymphoma Classification Project: A clinical evaluation of the International Lymphoma Study Group classification of non-Hodgkin's lymphoma. *Blood* 89:3909, 1997.
5. Zucca E, Bertoni F, Roggero E, Cavalli F: The gastric marginal zone B-cell lymphoma of MALT type. *Blood* 96:410, 2000.
6. Wotherspoon AC, Doglioni C, Diss TC, et al: Regression of primary low-grade B-cell gastric lymphoma of mucosa-associated lymphoid tissue type after eradication of *Helicobacter pylori*. *Lancet* 342:575, 1993.
7. Roggero E, Zucca E, Pinotti G, et al: Eradication of *Helicobacter pylori* infection in primary low- grade gastric lymphoma of mucosa-associated lymphoid tissue. *Ann Intern Med* 122:767, 1995.
8. Bayerdorffer E, Neubauer A, Rudolph B, et al: Regression of primary gastric lymphoma of mucosa-associated lymphoid tissue type after cure of *Helicobacter pylori* infection. MALT Lymphoma Study Group. *Lancet* 345:1591, 1995.
9. Neubauer A, Thiede C, Morgner A, et al: Cure of *Helicobacter pylori* infection and duration of remission of low-grade gastric mucosa-associated lymphoid tissue lymphoma. *J Natl Cancer Inst* 89:1350, 1997.
10. Pinotti G, Zucca E, Roggero E, et al: Clinical features, treatment and outcome in a series of 93 patients with low-grade gastric MALT lymphoma. *Leuk Lymphoma* 26:527, 1997.
11. Steinbach G, Ford R, Glober G, et al: Antibiotic treatment of gastric lymphoma of mucosa-associated lymphoid tissue. An uncontrolled trial. *Ann Intern Med* 131:88, 1999.
12. Ruskone-Fourmestraux A, Lavergne A, Aegerter PH, et al: Predictive factors for regression of gastric MALT lymphoma after anti-*Helicobacter pylori* treatment. *Gut* 48:297, 2001.
13. Roggero E, Zucca E, Mainetti C, et al: Eradication of *Borrelia burgdorferi* infection in primary marginal zone B-cell lymphoma of the skin. *Hum Pathol* 31:263, 2000.
14. Ferreri AJ, Guidoboni M, Ponzoni M, et al: Evidence for an association between *Chlamydia psittaci* and ocular adnexal lymphomas. *J Natl Cancer Inst* 96:586, 2004.
15. Lecuit M, Abachin E, Martin A, et al: Immunoproliferative small intestinal disease associated with *Campylobacter jejuni*. *N Engl J Med* 350:239, 2004.
16. Ekstrom Smedby K, Vajdic CM, Falster M, et al: Autoimmune disorders and risk of non-Hodgkin lymphoma subtypes: A pooled analysis within the InterLymph Consortium. *Blood* 111:4029, 2008.
17. Murga Penas EM, Hinz K, Roser K, et al: Translocations t(11;18)(q21;q21) and t(14;18)(q32;q21) are the main chromosomal abnormalities involving MLT/MALT1 in MALT lymphomas. *Leukemia* 17:2225, 2003.
18. Willis TG, Jadayel DM, Du MQ, et al: Bcl10 is involved in t(1;14)(p22;q32) of MALT B cell lymphoma and mutated in multiple tumor types. *Cell* 96:35, 1999.
19. Streubel B, Lamprecht A, Dierlamm J, et al: T(14;18)(q32;q21) involving IGH and MALT1 is a frequent chromosomal aberration in MALT lymphoma. *Blood* 101:2335, 2003.
20. Streubel B, Vinatzer U, Lamprecht A, et al: T(3;14)(p14.1;q32) involving IGH and FOXP1 is a novel recurrent chromosomal aberration in MALT lymphoma. *Leukemia* 19:652, 2005.
21. Vinatzer U, Gollinger M, Mullauer L, et al: Mucosa-associated lymphoid tissue lymphoma: Novel translocations including rearrangements of ODZ2, JMJD2C, and CNN3. *Clin Cancer Res* 14:6426, 2008.
22. Isaacson PG, Du MQ: MALT lymphoma: From morphology to molecules. *Nat Rev Cancer* 4:644, 2004.
23. Farinha P, Gascoyne RD: Molecular pathogenesis of mucosa-associated lymphoid tissue lymphoma. *J Clin Oncol* 23:6370, 2005.
24. Hosokawa Y, Suzuki H, Suzuki Y, et al: Antiapoptotic function of apoptosis inhibitor 2-MALT1 fusion protein involved in t(11;18)(q21;q21) mucosa-associated lymphoid tissue lymphoma. *Cancer Res* 64:3452, 2004.
25. Liu H, Ye H, Ruskone-Fourmestraux A, et al: T(11;18) is a marker for all stage gastric MALT lymphomas that will not respond to *H. pylori* eradication. *Gastroenterology* 122:1286, 2002.
26. Dierlamm J, Pittaluga S, Wlodarska I, et al: Marginal zone B-cell lymphomas of different sites share similar cytogenetic and morphologic features. *Blood* 87:299, 1996.
27. Callet-Bauchu E, Baseggio L, Felman P, et al: Cytogenetic analysis delineates a spectrum of chromosomal changes that can distinguish non-MALT marginal zone B-cell lymphomas among mature B-cell entities: A description of 103 cases. *Leukemia* 19:1818, 2005.
28. Andersen CL, Gruszka-Westwood A, Atkinson S, et al: Recurrent genomic imbalances in B-cell splenic marginal-zone lymphoma revealed by comparative genomic hybridization. *Cancer Genet Cytogenet* 156:122, 2005.
29. Mollejo M, Camacho FI, Algara P, et al: Nodal and splenic marginal zone B cell lymphomas. *Hematol Oncol* 23:108, 2005.
30. Matutes E, Oscier D, Montalban C, et al: Splenic marginal zone lymphoma proposals for a revision of diagnostic, staging and therapeutic criteria. *Leukemia* 22:487, 2008.
31. Honma K, Tsuzuki S, Nakagawa M, et al: TNFAIP3 is the target gene of chromosome band 6q23.3-q24.1 loss in ocular adnexal marginal zone B cell lymphoma. *Genes Chromosomes Cancer* 47:1, 2008.
32. Novak U, Rinaldi A, Kwee I, et al: The NF-{kappa}B negative regulator TNFAIP3 (A20) is inactivated by somatic mutations and genomic deletions in marginal zone lymphomas. *Blood* 113:4918, 2009.
33. Compagno M, Lim WK, Grunn A, et al: Mutations of multiple genes cause deregulation of NF-kappaB in diffuse large B-cell lymphoma. *Nature* 459:717, 2009.
34. Thieblemont C, Coiffier B: MALT lymphoma: Sites of presentations, clinical features and staging procedures, in *MALT Lymphomas*, edited by E Zucca, F Bertoni, p 60. Landes Bioscience, Georgetown, TX, 2004.

35. Thieblemont C: Clinical presentation and management of marginal zone lymphomas. *Hematology Am Soc Hematol Educ Program 2005*, p 307.
36. Zucca E, Conconi A, Pedrinis E, et al: Nongastric marginal zone B-cell lymphoma of mucosa-associated lymphoid tissue. *Blood* 101:2489, 2003.
37. Thieblemont C, Berger F, Dumontet C, et al: Mucosa-associated lymphoid tissue lymphoma is a disseminated disease in one third of 158 patients analyzed. *Blood* 95:802, 2000.
38. Raderer M, Wohrer S, Streubel B, et al: Assessment of disease dissemination in gastric compared with extragastric mucosa-associated lymphoid tissue lymphoma using extensive staging: A single-center experience. *J Clin Oncol* 24:3136, 2006.
39. de Boer JP, Hiddink RF, Raderer M, et al: Dissemination patterns in non-gastric MALT lymphoma. *Haematologica* 93:201, 2008.
40. Thieblemont C, Bastion Y, Berger F, et al: Mucosa-associated lymphoid tissue gastrointestinal and nongastrointestinal lymphoma behavior: Analysis of 108 patients. *J Clin Oncol* 15:1624, 1997.
41. Tsang RW, Gospodarowicz MK, Pintilie M, et al: Localized mucosa-associated lymphoid tissue lymphoma treated with radiation therapy has excellent clinical outcome. *J Clin Oncol* 21:4157, 2003.
42. Copie-Bergman C, Wotherspoon A: MALT lymphoma pathology, initial diagnosis, and posttreatment evaluation, in *Extranodal Lymphomas Pathology and Management*, edited by F Cavalli, H Stein, E Zucca, p 114. Informa UK, London, 2008.
43. Fuccio L, Laterza L, Zagari RM, et al: Treatment of *Helicobacter pylori* infection. *BMJ* 337:a1454, 2008.
44. Malfertheiner P, Megraud F, O'Morain C, et al: Current concepts in the management of Helicobacter pylori infection: The Maastricht III Consensus Report. *Gut* 56:772, 2007.
45. Chey WD, Wong BC: American College of Gastroenterology guideline on the management of *Helicobacter pylori* infection. *Am J Gastroenterol* 102:1808, 2007.
46. Stathis A, Chini C, Bertoni F, et al: Long-term outcome following *Helicobacter pylori* eradication in a retrospective study of 105 patients with localized gastric marginal zone B-cell lymphoma of MALT type. *Ann Oncol* 20:1086, 2009.
47. Hancock B, Qian W, Linch D, et al: Chlorambucil versus observation after anti-*Helicobacter* therapy in gastric MALT lymphomas: Results of the international randomised LY03 trial. *Br J Haematol* 144:367, 2009.
48. Fischbach W, Goebeler ME, Ruskone-Fourmestraux A, et al: Most patients with minimal histological residuals of gastric MALT lymphoma after successful eradication of *Helicobacter pylori* can be managed safely by a watch and wait strategy: Experience from a large international series. *Gut* 56:1685, 2007.
49. Bertoni F, Zucca E. State-of-the-art therapeutics: Marginal-zone lymphoma. *J Clin Oncol* 23:6415, 2005.
50. Bertoni F, Conconi A, Capella C, et al: Molecular follow-up in gastric mucosa-associated lymphoid tissue lymphomas: Early analysis of the LY03 cooperative trial. *Blood* 99:2541, 2002.
51. Zucca E, Dreyling M. Gastric marginal zone lymphoma of MALT type: ESMO clinical recommendations for diagnosis, treatment and follow-up. *Ann Oncol* 19(Suppl 2):ii70, 2008.
52. Capelle LG, de Vries AC, Looman CW, et al: Gastric MALT lymphoma: Epidemiology and high adenocarcinoma risk in a nation-wide study. *Eur J Cancer* 44:2470, 2008.
53. Koch P, Probst A, Berdel WE, et al: Treatment results in localized primary gastric lymphoma: Data of patients registered within the German multicenter study (GIT NHL 02/96). *J Clin Oncol* 23:7050, 2005.
54. Yahalom J: MALT lymphomas: A radiation oncology viewpoint. *Ann Hematol* 80 Suppl 3:B100, 2001.
55. Tsang RW, Gospodarowicz MK: Radiation therapy for localized low-grade non-Hodgkin's lymphomas. *Hematol Oncol* 23:10, 2005.
56. Raderer M, Vorbeck F, Formanek M, et al: Importance of extensive staging in patients with mucosa-associated lymphoid tissue (MALT)-type lymphoma. *Br J Cancer* 83:454, 2000.
57. Ben Simon GJ, Cheung N, McKelvie P, et al: Oral chlorambucil for extranodal, marginal zone, B-cell lymphoma of mucosa-associated lymphoid tissue of the orbit. *Ophthalmology* 113:1209, 2006.
58. Levy M, Copie-Bergman C, Traulle C, et al: Conservative treatment of primary gastric low-grade B-cell lymphoma of mucosa-associated lymphoid tissue: Predictive factors of response and outcome. *Am J Gastroenterol* 97:292, 2002.
59. Zinzani PL, Stefoni V, Musuraca G, et al: Fludarabine-containing chemotherapy as frontline treatment of nongastrointestinal mucosa-associated lymphoid tissue lymphoma. *Cancer* 100:2190, 2004.
60. Jager G, Hofler G, Linkesch W, Neumeister P: Occurrence of a myelodysplastic syndrome (MDS) during first-line 2-chloro-deoxyadenosine (2-CDA) treatment of a low-grade gastrointestinal MALT lymphoma. Case report and review of the literature. *Haematologica* 89:ECR01, 2004.
61. Wohrer S, Drach J, Hejna M, et al: Treatment of extranodal marginal zone B-cell lymphoma of mucosa-associated lymphoid tissue (MALT lymphoma) with mitoxantrone, chlorambucil and prednisone. *Ann Oncol* 14:1758, 2003.
62. Conconi AR, Lopez-Guillermo A, Martinelli G, et al: Activity of Bortezomib in MALT Lymphomas: A IELSG Phase II Study (abstract #368). *Ann Oncol* 19:iv191, 2008.
63. Troch M, Jonak C, Mullauer L, et al: A phase II study of bortezomib in patients with MALT lymphoma. *Haematologica* 94:738, 2009.
64. Raderer M, Wohrer S, Streubel B, et al: Activity of rituximab plus cyclophosphamide, doxorubicin/mitoxantrone, vincristine and prednisone in patients with relapsed MALT lymphoma. *Oncology* 70:411, 2006.
65. Conconi A, Martinelli G, Thieblemont C, et al: Clinical activity of rituximab in extranodal marginal zone B-cell lymphoma of MALT type. *Blood* 102:2741, 2003.
66. Martinelli G, Laszlo D, Ferreri AJ, et al: Clinical activity of rituximab in gastric marginal zone non-Hodgkin's lymphoma resistant to or not eligible for anti-*Helicobacter pylori* therapy. *J Clin Oncol* 23:1979, 2005.
67. Ferreri AJ, Dolcetti R, Du MQ, et al: Ocular adnexal MALT lymphoma: An intriguing model for antigen-driven lymphomagenesis and microbial-targeted therapy. *Ann Oncol* 19:835, 2008.
68. Al-Saleem T, Al-Mondhiry H: Immunoproliferative small intestinal disease (IPSID): A model for mature B-cell neoplasms. *Blood* 105:2274, 2005.
69. Berger F, Felman P, Thieblemont C, et al: Non-MALT marginal zone B-cell lymphomas: A description of clinical presentation and outcome in 124 patients. *Blood* 95:1950, 2000.
70. Chacon JI, Mollejo M, Munoz E, et al: Splenic marginal zone lymphoma: Clinical characteristics and prognostic factors in a series of 60 patients. *Blood* 100:1648, 2002.
71. Thieblemont C, Felman P, Callet-Bauchu E, et al: Splenic marginal-zone lymphoma: A distinct clinical and pathological entity. *Lancet Oncol* 4:95, 2003.
72. Hermine O, Lefrere F, Bronowicki JP, et al: Regression of splenic lymphoma with villous lymphocytes after treatment of hepatitis C virus infection. *N Engl J Med* 347:89, 2002.
73. Arcaini L, Paulli M, Boveri E, et al: Splenic and nodal marginal zone lymphomas are indolent disorders at high hepatitis C virus seroprevalence with distinct presenting features but similar morphologic and phenotypic profiles. *Cancer* 100:107, 2004.
74. Nathwani BN, Anderson JR, Armitage JO, et al: Marginal zone B-cell lymphoma: A clinical comparison of nodal and mucosa-associated lymphoid tissue types. Non-Hodgkin's Lymphoma Classification Project. *J Clin Oncol* 17:2486, 1999.

CHAPTER 104
BURKITT LYMPHOMA

Jonathan W. Friedberg and Archibald S. Perkins

SUMMARY

Burkitt lymphoma is one of the highly aggressive lymphomas. It was the first tumor to be etiologically associated with (1) a virus, specifically Epstein-Barr virus, (2) a specific chromosomal translocation involving chromosome 8, and (3) one of the first cancers shown to be curable by chemotherapy alone. It presents in three clinically distinct forms: endemic, sporadic, and immunodeficiency associated. Burkitt lymphoma is an uncommon form of lymphoma in adults, with an incidence of approximately 1200 patients per year in the United States. It represents a highly curable malignancy in the modern therapeutic era. Over the last decade, the definition of Burkitt lymphoma has evolved significantly, largely as a consequence of improvements in immunohistochemical, cytogenetic, and molecular diagnostic techniques, and an increased understanding of the molecular basis of this disease. Modern techniques have more clearly defined Burkitt lymphoma at the molecular level. A group of patients have an ambiguous diagnosis between Burkitt lymphoma and diffuse large B-cell lymphoma, now defined by the World Health Organization, many of whom have a very poor prognosis. With intensive chemotherapeutic regimens, the majority of patients with Burkitt lymphoma are cured. Future studies are needed to best define therapy in older patients, and in the setting of relapsed or refractory disease.

DEFINITION AND HISTORY

Burkitt lymphoma (BL) may present in three distinct forms: endemic (African), sporadic, and immunodeficiency associated.[1–4] The endemic form (eBL) typically presents in the jaw or maxilla, and is associated with Epstein-Barr virus (EBV) infection at an early age. Although there are reports dating to as early as 1910, it was Denis Burkitt who is credited with describing this lymphoma as a common tumor in children of Uganda.[5] Further studies by Burkitt and others led to associations with EBV and malaria,[6] as well as environmental factors.[7] Subsequently, tumors of a similar histopathologic appearance were identified in nonendemic regions, and these were found to occur in older individuals with only occasional association with EBV; presentation was typically abdominal rather than orofacial.[8] A third class of BL was identified in immunosuppressed patients, typically HIV-positive. Evidence for involvement of the *MYC* gene came with the identification of recurrent translocations involving the long arm of chromosome 8 in BL,[9] that all involved *MYC*.

Abbreviations and acronyms used in this chapter: AID, activation-induced cytosine deamination; BL, Burkitt lymphoma; CNS, central nervous system; CODOX-M/IVAC, cyclophosphamide, doxorubicin, vincristine, methotrexate, ifosfamide, etoposide and high-dose cytarabine, with intrathecal cytarabine and methotrexate; EBER, Epstein-Barr virus-encoded RNA; eBL, endemic Burkitt lymphoma; EBNA, Epstein-Barr nuclear antigen; EBV, Epstein-Barr virus; FISH, fluorescence *in situ* hybridization; GC, germinal center; HAART, highly active antiretroviral therapy; hyper-CVAD, fractionated cyclophosphamide, vincristine, doxorubicin, dexamethasone; NHL, non-Hodgkin lymphoma; WHO, World Health Organization.

EPIDEMIOLOGY

The endemic form is found in eastern equatorial Africa, with a peak age incidence at 4 to 7 years, and is nearly twice as frequent in boys as in girls. It accounts for 20 percent of cancers in newborns to 14-year-olds, and for the majority of non-Hodgkin lymphomas (NHLs) in all ages.[7] Infection by EBV (first identified in BL cells)[10] is found in nearly 100 percent of patients with eBL, and higher titers are linked to increase risk of eBL.[11] Although not as close, there is also an association with malaria[12] and certain other environmental factors.[13] Sporadic BL, defined as cases outside of endemic African regions, accounts for 1 to 2 percent of NHL, is higher in males than in females, and has a median age of 30 years. Immunosuppression-related Burkitt lymphoma increased in incidence during the AIDS epidemic; however, with improved antiretroviral therapy, the incidence has been decreased again in the United States and countries with access to effective therapy for HIV.

ETIOLOGY AND PATHOGENESIS

The unifying feature of all three types of BL is activation of the *MYC* gene via immunoglobulin (Ig) translocation leading to high levels of MYC protein, which activates transcription of a plethora of genes involved in cell growth. Translocations are thought to occur via double-strand breaks that occur during normal class-switch reaction and somatic hypermutation, which, in turn, depend on activation-induced cytosine deamination (AID).[14] AID-induced somatic point mutation of growth-regulatory genes (such as *MYC*) may also play an important role.[15] In a tumor with *MYC* deregulation, essentially 100 percent of viable cells are in cycle and express Ki-67.[16]

In endemic BL, EBV infection likely plays a role prior to the *MYC* translocation event, inducing proliferation via Epstein-Barr nuclear antigen (EBNA)-2 and inhibiting apoptosis (via EBNA3A- and EBNA3C-induced epigenetic silencing proapoptotic protein BIM, a key defender of MYC-induced tumorigenesis).[17] The exact role of malaria in eBL is not clear, but it may also stimulate B cells via direct action[18] and/or via T-cell–specific immunosuppression.[19]

Immunosuppression-associated BL occurs predominantly in HIV-positive patients, and its occurrence is independent of immune status. However, with severe HIV immunosuppression and high EBV viral loads, patients become more susceptible to EBV-associated lymphoproliferative disorders (often polyclonal), as is seen in immunosuppressed allograft patients.[20] These findings suggest that EBV-induced transformation does not result in BL; rather BL emerges in the setting of chronic antigen stimulation (via opportunistic infections, e.g., malaria) of a hyperstimulated but overall intact immune system.[17]

CLINICAL FEATURES

The endemic (African) form often presents as a jaw or facial bone tumor. It may spread to extranodal sites, especially to the marrow and meninges. Almost all cases are EBV positive. The nonendemic or American form presents as an abdominal mass in approximately 65 percent of cases, often with ascites. Extranodal sites, such as the kidneys, gonads, breast, marrow, and central nervous system (CNS) may be involved. Involvement of the marrow and CNS is much more common in the nonendemic form. Patients with more than 25 percent marrow involvement with malignant cells often are referred to as having *acute Burkitt cell leukemia*. In addition, in contrast to the endemic form, only 15 percent of the nonendemic cases are EBV positive.

TABLE 104–1. Murphy Staging System for Burkitt Lymphoma

Stage I: Single nodal or extranodal site excluding mediastinum or abdomen
Stage II: Single extranodal tumor with regional nodal involvement
Two extranodal tumors on one side of diaphragm
Primary gastrointestinal tumor with or without associated mesenteric nodes
Two or more nodal areas on one side of diaphragm
Stage IIR: Completely resected intraabdominal disease
Stage III: Two single extranodal tumors on opposite sides of diaphragm
All primary intrathoracic tumors
All paraspinal or epidural tumors
All extensive primary intraabdominal disease
Two or more nodal areas on opposite sides of diaphragm
Stage IIIA: Localized, nonresectable abdominal disease
Stage IIIB: Widespread multiorgan abdominal disease
Stage IV: Initial CNS or marrow involvement (<25%)

SOURCE: Adapted with permission from Perkins AS, Friedberg JW.[21]

Immunodeficiency-related cases often involve the lymph nodes and are associated with EBV in 30 percent of the cases. Staging using the system modified for childhood BL (Murphy staging system, Table 104–1) is often used rather than the Ann Arbor system (see Chap. 97), given that BL is largely an extranodal lymphoma.[21]

LABORATORY FEATURES

BLOOD AND MARROW

Patients with bulky disease may have Burkitt cells in marrow and blood with accompanying suppression of normal blood counts. Rare cases, often males, may present principally with marrow and blood involvement, so-called Burkitt cell leukemia (see Chap. 93).

The serum lactic dehydrogenase is often elevated as a reflection of the high cell turnover, especially in patients with bulky disease.

HISTOPATHOLOGY AND CYTOLOGY

BL is characterized by monomorphic medium-size cells with round nuclei, multiple nucleoli, and basophilic cytoplasm.[22] Burkitt cells have a very high proliferative rate and frequent mitotic figures. BL has a diffuse pattern of growth comprised of intermediate-sized B cells (12 μM) with high nuclear-to-cytoplasmic ratio. Nuclear contours are round to oval without cleaves or folds, a key feature in the distinction from diffuse large cell lymphoma. Nucleoli are typically multiple, small-to-intermediate in size, and the nuclear chromatin is relatively immature, being finely granular. The rate of proliferation, as determined with Ki-67 staining, is at or above 95 percent. These cells are characterized by a high rate of spontaneous apoptosis leading to the characteristic "starry sky" pattern in marrow and lymph nodes—a monomorphic diffuse background of lymphoma cells that is interspersed with reactive macrophages engulfing cellular debris (Fig. 104–1). Characteristic features of BL on cytology are the strongly basophilic cytoplasm (a consequence of the abundant polyribosomes), and the presence of lipid-filled cytoplasmic vesicles, some of which overlie the nucleus.

IMMUNOPHENOTYPE

BL cells are mature B cells, positive for CD19, CD20, CD22, and CD79a, and have monotypic surface IgM; they lack CD5 and CD23. BL cells also show immunologic similarity to germinal center cells of B-cell follicles rather than activated B cells, being positive for BCL6, CD10, Tcl1, and CD38, and negative for Mum-1, CD44, CD138, and Bcl-2. However, germinal center cells markers are not specific for BL, since a significant proportion of diffuse large B-cell lymphoma also has this germinal center cell signature.

EPSTEIN-BARR VIRUS STUDIES

Although EBV is associated with 98 percent of eBL, it is also seen in 20 percent of sporadic cases, and in 30 to 40 percent of HIV-associated cases.[23] This can be detected using *in situ* hybridization for EBV-encoded RNA (EBER). Although EBV likely plays a key role in B-cell stimulation during a prelymphoma stage, the role for EBV after lymphoma development is unclear, as is whether EBV positivity is clinically meaningful. In EBV-positive endemic cases, CD21 (the EBV receptor) is expressed and is negative in most EBV-negative nonendemic BL cases. HIV is associated with BL: 30 to 40 percent of these cases will have EBV-positive

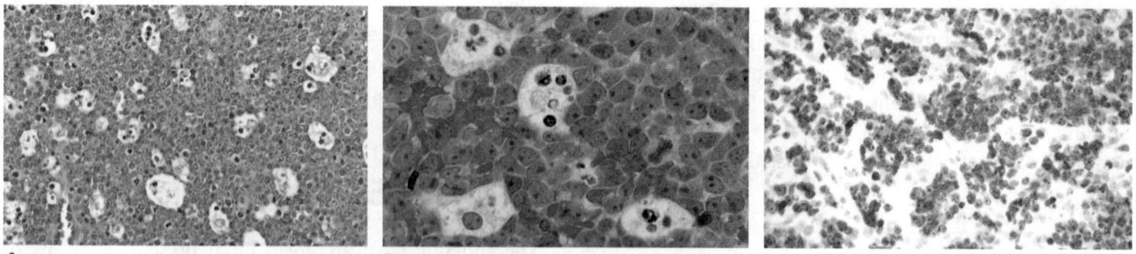

A B C

FIGURE 104–1. A. Lymph node biopsy section. Replaced by monomorphic population of medium-sized lymphoma cells (Burkitt cells) with interspersed macrophages engorged with cellular debris as a result of the high cell turnover rate (high rate of apoptosis and cell proliferation). **B.** Marrow section. (Higher magnification than in **A.**) Replaced by monomorphic population of medium-sized lymphoma cells (Burkitt cells) with interspersed macrophages engorged with cellular debris as a result of the high cell turnover rate. The interspersed macrophages embedded in the solid monomorphic infiltrate of Burkitt cells generate the "starry sky appearance," a descriptor commonly used in lymph node and marrow sections in Burkitt lymphoma. The macrophages are frequently referred to as "tingible body macrophages," a term derived from a description of phagocytized nuclear debris of small lymphocytes by macrophages in germinal centers of normal lymph nodes more than 100 years ago. **C.** Ki-67 immunoperoxidase stain of Burkitt lymphoma showing the very high prevalence of cells in the mitotic cycle (virtually all nuclei show the reddish-brown reaction product of the stain). The Ki-67 monoclonal antibody identifies a nuclear protein expressed throughout the cell cycle and is a marker of cell proliferative activity (see "Histopathology and Cytology" above). *(Used with permission from* Lichtman's Atlas of Hematology, *www.accessmedicine.com.)*

lymphoma cells. In HIV-infected individuals, a variant of BL with plasmacytoid appearance may be present and shares features with classic BL and diffuse large B-cell lymphoma. In contrast to primary effusion lymphomas and diffuse large B-cell lymphoma, EBV-positive, HIV-associated BL does not express LMP1 nor EBNA2. Blood involvement is less common in HIV-positive than in HIV-negative cases. BL is associated with HIV infection but not other forms of immunosuppression.

CYTOGENETICS

All cases of BL have a translocation between the long arm of chromosome 8, the site of the *MYC* protooncogene (8q24), and one of three translocation partners: the Ig heavy-chain region on chromosome 14; the κ light-chain locus on chromosome 2; or the λ light-chain locus on chromosome 22. The translocations involving *MYC* can be detected by fluorescence *in situ* hybridization (FISH) using so-called *MYC* "break apart" probes: a set of two fluorescently tagged DNA probes of two different colors that hybridize to the upstream and downstream side of the gene. In an unperturbed gene, they hybridize together within interphase cells giving a composite color, whereas with translocation, the two fluors are separated. A key feature of BL is the relative simplicity of their karyotype: In a good proportion of cases, the *MYC* translocation is the sole abnormality. This distinguishes it from diffuse large B-cell lymphoma. However, in one-third of BL cases, alterations at the p53 gene at 17p can be found. This likely contributes to tumorigenesis by causing loss of p53-mediated apoptosis, which high levels of MYC are known to activate. Whether this portends a distinct prognosis relative to cases with normal 17p is not known.

DIFFERENTIAL DIAGNOSIS

The majority of BL cases, even in the adult, possess all of the criteria for the diagnosis: high mitotic rate in an appropriate morphologic and immunophenotypic setting, together with a Ig-positive MYC translocation. However, a reasonable minority of cases do not fit neatly into the diagnosis of either BL or diffuse large B-cell lymphoma.[24] Typically, this arises because of the absence of key morphologic features of BL in a lesion that otherwise resembles BL: a nonmonomorphic nuclear morphology; fewer tingible body macrophages than is typical; or an abnormal immunophenotype. To date, the diagnostic "touchstone" for this group of lesions, if such exists, has been pathology, particularly the cellular morphology and rate of Ki-67 positivity as discussed above (see also Chaps. 92 and 98).[25]

ATYPICAL BURKITT LYMPHOMA AND THE ROLE OF GENE EXPRESSION STUDIES

Gene expression analysis has been applied to the diagnosis of BL, specifically to help refine the diagnosis of cases within the BL/diffuse large B-cell lymphoma overlap zone. A core group of eight cases of pediatric BL who fulfilled all World Health Organization (WHO) criteria for BL were studied.[26] Tumors that matched this expression pattern were termed "molecular BL" (mBL), while those that lacked this pattern were called non-mBL, with an intermediate group also being identified. Key characteristics of the mBL group were lower cytogenetic complexity and *MYC* translocations involving immunoglobulin genes, rather than non-Ig partners (the former resulting in high levels of MYC expression, a hallmark of BL), as well as lack of expression of genes in the nuclear factor-κB (NF-κB) pathway. A BL signature was also identified that included highly expressed target genes of MYC, as well as markers of germinal center B cells.[27] In a second study, a lower expression of target genes of the NF-κB pathway was also found. Based on molecular expression, they identified a set of high-grade B-cell neoplasms with the BL signature that had been diagnosed as diffuse large B-cell lymphoma. These patients, which had been treated with a cyclophosphamide, hydroxydaunomycin, vincristine (Oncovin), prednisone (CHOP)-like regimen rather than high-dose therapy, faired poorly, and may have benefited from the higher intensity regimen.[27]

The molecular markers for Burkitt lymphoma identified by the gene array studies were in large part surrogate markers for high levels of *MYC* expression. Immunohistologic staining with three markers, Tcl1, CD38, and CD44, can identify tumors with a translocation at *MYC*: Tcl1+/CD38+/CD44– is 100 percent specific and approximately 80 percent sensitive. Whereas most cases with this immunophenotype are BL, these markers were not effective at distinguishing MYC-positive diffuse large B-cell lymphoma from BL.[27a]

THERAPY

GENERAL CONSIDERATIONS

BL is a highly aggressive tumor; however, therapy with multiagent chemotherapeutic programs results in excellent long-term remission rates and long-term survival of up to 85 percent of children. Applying the same chemotherapy regimens to adults has shown dramatically improved response rates.[28–30] Risk stratification allows patients with limited disease to be treated with less-intensive therapy than more advanced cases and still achieve very high responses. Patients with limited-stage disease have an excellent prognosis, with greater than 90 percent cure rates. These patients should not be undertreated. Patients with extensive disease can achieve 80 percent long-term survival. The regimens employ multiple non–cross-resistant drugs used over a short period. These drugs include high-dose cyclophosphamide, methotrexate, vincristine, prednisone, high-dose methotrexate, high-dose cytarabine, etoposide, and sometimes ifosfamide. CNS prophylaxis therapy, either intrathecal or systemic, is given in almost all patients with BL. Radiation therapy does not play a role in the treatment of BL, and use of radiation therapy for limited stage diseases is of no additional benefit.[31,32]

TUMOR LYSIS SYNDROME

The tumor lysis syndrome is a serious metabolic complication of rapidly growing tumors, of which BL is a classic example. The syndrome is the result of the rapid destruction of tumor cells, highly sensitive to chemotherapy, and can result in hyperuricemia, hyperkalemia, hyperphosphatemia, secondary hypocalcemia, metabolic acidosis, and renal failure. In tumors such as BL the cell death rate (and proliferative rate) may be so substantial in patients with bulky disease that the tumor lysis syndrome may occur before therapy, so-called spontaneous tumor lysis.[33] The latter is a highly morbid phenomenon with a poor prognosis for a salutary outcome from therapy and a complication with a high death rate. It occurs in patients with a high body burden of tumor, usually with abdominal disease, a common situation in BL. Its principal manifestation is the combination of hyperuricemia and azotemia. In BL a critical part of therapy is recognizing incipient or overt spontaneous tumor lysis rapidly or preventing chemotherapy-induced tumor lysis. The lactic dehydrogenase has been used as a surrogate marker for risk of tumor lysis with a serum level twice the upper limit of normal for the laboratory in question being the threshold for urgent concern. The usual prophylactic therapy for this situation is carefully monitored hydration of at least 3 L of saline per day and either allopurinol or rasburicase to decrease serum uric acid concentration and thereby hyperuricosuria. Rasburicase acts more quickly than allopurinol and should be used if risk is considered high or if evidence of spontaneous tumor lysis is present initially.[34,35] Continuous venovenous hemofiltration has also been very useful in allowing concomitant full-dose chemotherapy and preventing tumor lysis and renal failure.[36,37]

SPECIFIC REGIMENS

The specific regimens that have been developed to treat BL are generally adapted from pediatric experience; Table 104–2 depicts representative trial results, including adult patients. There are no studies directly comparing these regimens, and comparison among the single-arm studies is difficult because of lack of uniform diagnostic criteria, staging, and the heterogeneous patient populations studied. In general, shorter durations of chemotherapy (i.e., 6 months) are as good as longer (18 months) periods of treatment. Other studies have shown a dramatically improved response with use of 4 cycles of chemotherapy as opposed to 15 cycles. BL has a high proliferative rate, so subsequent chemotherapy cycles should be started as soon as hematologic recovery occurs. Waiting for a fixed period between cycles may lead to regrowth of resistant tumor cells between cycles. Cyclophosphamide, doxorubicin, vincristine, methotrexate, ifosfamide, etoposide and high-dose cytarabine, with intrathecal cytarabine and methotrexate (CODOX-M/IVAC) is among the most commonly used regimens in the United States for adults with Burkitt lymphoma, based upon an initial favorable publication from the National Cancer Institute indicating extremely high response rates.[28] Two subsequent, small, phase 2 trials have used this regimen with minor modifications, and have successfully enrolled greater numbers of older patients, demonstrating cure rates of approximately 64 percent.[38,39] These cure rates are substantially less than the initial report by Magrath and coworkers,[32] but still better than historical data with standard-dose regimens. Mead and colleagues published results of a modification of this regimen in patients with aggressive lymphomas and high proliferative rate as measured by Ki-67 fraction.[40] Burkitt lymphoma was strictly defined as the following: germinal center phenotype, BCL-2 negative, *MYC* rearrangement positive, and absence of the t(14;18) or abnormalities at chromosome 3q27. Overall survival of the subgroup defined as Burkitt lymphoma was 67 percent in this group of older patients. Treatment-related mortality was 8 percent. Outcomes were similar among all age groups with the exception of patients older than age 65 years who clearly had an inferior prognosis. These results likely reflect the true outcome of this regimen in practice.

Another regimen commonly used for the therapy of BL is fractionated cyclophosphamide, vincristine, doxorubicin, and dexamethasone (hyper-CVAD) alternating with high-dose methotrexate and cytarabine.[41] The outcome of patients at a single institution (M.D. Anderson Cancer Center) with BL treated with this regimen in combination with the monoclonal antibody rituximab resulted in an overall survival of 89 percent with only one death. No additive toxicity was observed.[42,43] Rituximab has also been combined with CODOX-M/IVAC, with promising initial results.[44]

No clear advantage of autologous stem cell transplantation in patients with BL has been observed, although incorporating planned autologous transplantation into the initial therapeutic algorithm has been used with reasonable results.[45]

Historically, patients with HIV have been managed with less-intensive chemotherapy because of the concern of immunosuppression-related morbidity. In the highly active antiretroviral therapy (HAART) era, HIV-positive patients with BL should be treated similarly to nonimmunocompromised patients. The rate of treatment failure in HIV-positive patients with BL was significantly lower with a highly aggressive protocol when compared with patients who were treated with less-aggressive chemotherapy. In addition, patients tolerated the aggressive protocol reasonably well, particularly when HAART therapy was incorporated into the regimen.[46]

TABLE 104–2. Outcome of Burkitt Lymphoma in Published Larger Studies

Citation	Regimen	No.	2-Year Outcome
Hoelzer[49]	Short duration/dose intensive; pediatric NHL based	35	51% (estimated survival)
Magrath[32]	CODOX-M/IVAC	54	89% (actual survival)
Mead[40]	CODOX-M/IVAC	58	64% (progression-free survival)
Rizzieri[29]	Short duration/dose intensive	92	Cohort 1: 54% (estimated survival); Cohort 2: 50% (estimated survival)
Thomas[42]	Hyper-CVAD with rituximab	31	89% (estimated survival)

CODOX-M/IVAC, cyclophosphamide, doxorubicin, vincristine, methotrexate, ifosfamide, etoposide and high-dose cytarabine, with intrathecal cytarabine and methotrexate; hyper-CVAD, fractionated cyclophosphamide, vincristine, doxorubicin, and dexamethasone.

COURSE AND PROGNOSIS

To better define optimal therapy and outcome of adults with BL, an international effort has focused on the group of patients with adult patients with BL.[47] Authors of 12 large treatment series (10 prospective; 2 retrospective) provided outcome information of patients enrolled on their clinical trials who were older than age 40 years. In this pooled analysis, patients older than age 40 years were underrepresented in the published literature, and had significantly inferior outcomes in 10 of the 12 series. Despite this, the majority of adult patients were cured using these regimens.

According to data from the National Cancer Institute's Surveillance, Epidemiology, and End Results program, up to 30 percent of BL diagnosis in the United States includes an "older" group of patients, age 60 years or older. Treatment options may be limited for this group of patients, as many older patients may not tolerate high-dose methotrexate and are not candidates for autologous transplantation. Although the relatively small number of patients older than age 60 years treated with the hyper-CVAD–rituximab regimen had favorable outcome,[37] these were probably highly selected patients with no comorbidities. Novel therapeutics with lower toxicity profiles are needed for this group of patients.

For patients with relapsed or refractory disease, autologous transplantation is best reserved for patients inadequately treated initially, as a consolidation procedure. Patients who relapse after appropriate therapy for BL tend to have highly treatment-resistant disease. These patients can be retreated with chemotherapy and considered for allogeneic stem cell transplantation because autologous transplantation is often not beneficial in these patients.[48] The majority of these patients have poor outcomes.

REFERENCES

1. Cheson BD: Adult Burkitt lymphoma: Too soon to declare victory. *Oncology (Williston Park)* 22:1518, 2008.
2. Sehn LH: Management of Burkitt lymphoma: A continuing challenge. *Oncology (Williston Park)* 22:1519, 2008.

3. Harris NL, Swerdlow S, Campo E, et al: The World Health Organization Classification of lymphoid neoplasms: What's new? *Ann Oncol* 19:iv119, 2008.
4. Johnson NA, Savage KJ, Ben-Neriah S, et al: Lymphomas with concurrent t(14;18) translocations are underreported and clinical outcome depends on the myc partner. *Blood* 112:299, 2008.
5. Burkitt D: A sarcoma involving the jaws in African children. *Br J Surg* 46:218, 1958.
6. Wright DH: Burkitt's lymphoma: A review of the pathology, immunology, and possible etiologic factors. *Pathol Annu* 6:337–363, 1971.
7. Orem J, Mbidde EK, Lambert B, et al: Burkitt's lymphoma in Africa, a review of the epidemiology and etiology. *Afr Health Sci* 7:166, 2007.
8. Magrath I: The pathogenesis of Burkitt's lymphoma. *Adv Cancer Res* 55:133, 1990.
9. Manolov G, Manolova Y. Marker band in one chromosome 14 from Burkitt lymphomas. *Nature* 237:33, 1972.
10. Epstein MA, Achong BG, Barr YM: Virus Particles in Cultured Lymphoblasts from Burkitt's Lymphoma. *Lancet* 1:702, 1964.
11. de-Thé G, Geser A, Day NE, et al: Epidemiological evidence for causal relationship between Epstein-Barr virus and Burkitt's lymphoma from Ugandan prospective study. *Nature* 274:756, 1978.
12. Geser A, Brubaker G, Draper CC: Effect of a malaria suppression program on the incidence of African Burkitt's lymphoma. *Am J Epidemiol* 129:740, 1989.
13. Aya T, Kinoshita T, Imai S, et al: Chromosome translocation and c-MYC activation by Epstein-Barr virus and *Euphorbia tirucalli* in B lymphocytes. *Lancet* 337:1190, 1991.
14. Dorsett Y, Robbiani DF, Jankovic M, et al: A role for AID in chromosome translocations between c-myc and the IgH variable region. *J Exp Med* 204:2225, 2007.
15. Bhatia K, Huppi K, Spangler G, et al: Point mutations in the c-Myc transactivation domain are common in Burkitt's lymphoma and mouse plasmacytomas. *Nat Genet* 5:56, 1993.
16. Braziel RM, Arber DA, Slovak ML, et al: The Burkitt-like lymphomas: A Southwest Oncology Group study delineating phenotypic, genotypic, and clinical features. *Blood* 97:3713, 2001.
17. Thorley-Lawson DA, Allday MJ: The curious case of the tumour virus: 50 years of Burkitt's lymphoma. *Nat Rev Microbiol* 6:913, 2008.
18. Donati D, Zhang LP, Chene A, et al: Identification of a polyclonal B-cell activator in Plasmodium falciparum. *Infect Immun* 72:5412, 2004.
19. Ho M, Webster HK, Green B, et al: Defective production of and response to IL-2 in acute human falciparum malaria. *J Immunol* 141:2755, 1988.
20. Biggar RJ, Chaturvedi AK, Goedert JJ, Engels EA: AIDS-related cancer and severity of immunosuppression in persons with AIDS. *J Natl Cancer Inst* 99:962, 2007.
21. Perkins AS, Friedberg JW: Burkitt lymphoma in adults. *Hematology Am Soc Hematol Educ Program*341, 2008.
22. Yano T, van Krieken JH, Magrath IT, et al: Histogenetic correlations between subcategories of small noncleaved cell lymphomas. *Blood* 79:1282, 1992.
23. Brady G, MacArthur GJ, Farrell PJ: Epstein-Barr virus and Burkitt lymphoma. *J Clin Pathol* 60:1397, 2007.
24. Harris NL, Horning SJ: Burkitt's lymphoma—The message from microarrays. *N Engl J Med* 354:2495, 2006.
25. Bertrand P, Bastard C, Maingonnat C, et al: Mapping of MYC breakpoints in 8q24 rearrangements involving non-immunoglobulin partners in B-cell lymphomas. *Leukemia* 21:515, 2007.
26. Hummel M, Bentink S, Berger H, et al: A biologic definition of Burkitt's lymphoma from transcriptional and genomic profiling. *N Engl J Med* 354:2419, 2006.
27. Dave SS, Fu K, Wright GW, et al: Molecular diagnosis of Burkitt's lymphoma. *N Engl J Med* 354:2431, 2006.
27a. Rodig SJ, Vergilio JA, Shahsafaei A, Dorfman DM: Characteristic expression patterns of TCL1, CD38, and CD44 identify aggressive lymphomas harboring a MYC translocation. *Am J Surg Pathol* 32:113, 2008.
28. Magrath I, Adde M, Shad A, et al: Adults and children with small non-cleaved-cell lymphoma have a similar excellent outcome when treated with the same chemotherapy regimen. *J Clin Oncol* 14:925, 1996.
29. Rizzieri DA, Johnson JL, Niedzwiecki D, et al: Intensive chemotherapy with and without cranial radiation for Burkitt leukemia and lymphoma: Final results of Cancer and Leukemia Group B Study 9251. *Cancer* 100:1438, 2004.
30. Soussain C, Patte C, Ostronoff M, et al: Small noncleaved cell lymphoma and leukemia in adults. A retrospective study of 65 adults treated with the LMB pediatric protocols. *Blood* 85:664, 1995.
31. Link MP, Donaldson SS, Berard CW, et al: Results of treatment of childhood localized non-Hodgkin's lymphoma with combination chemotherapy with or without radiotherapy. *N Engl J Med* 322:1169, 1990.
32. Magrath IT, Haddy TB, Adde MA: Treatment of patients with high grade non-Hodgkin's lymphomas and central nervous system involvement: Is radiation an essential component of therapy? *Leuk Lymphoma* 21:99, 1996.
33. Hsu HH, Chan YL, Huang CC: Acute spontaneous tumor lysis presenting with hyperuricemic acute renal failure: Clinical features and therapeutic approach. *J Nephrol* 17:50, 2004.
34. Hummel M, Reiter S, Adam K, et al: Effective treatment and prophylaxis of hyperuricemia and impaired renal function in tumor lysis syndrome with low doses of rasburicase. *Eur J Haematol* 80:331, 2008.
35. Goldman SC, Holcenberg JS, Finklestein JZ et al: A randomized comparison between rasburicase and allopurinol in children with lymphoma or leukemia at high risk for tumor lysis. *Blood* 97:2998, 2001.
36. Saccente SL, Kohaut EC, Berkow RL: Prevention of tumor lysis syndrome using continuous veno-venous hemofiltration. *Pediatr Nephrol* 9:569, 1995.
37. Choi KA, Lee JE, Kim YG, et al: Efficacy of continuous venovenous hemofiltration with chemotherapy in patients with Burkitt lymphoma and leukemia at high risk of tumor lysis syndrome. *Ann Hematol* 88:639, 2009.
38. Lacasce A, Howard O, Lib S, et al: Modified Magrath regimens for adults with Burkitt and Burkitt-like lymphomas: Preserved efficacy with decreased toxicity. *Leuk Lymphoma* 45:761, 2004.
39. Mead GM, Sydes MR, Walewski J, et al: An international evaluation of CODOX-M and CODOX-M alternating with IVAC in adult Burkitt's lymphoma: Results of United Kingdom Lymphoma Group LY06 study. *Ann Oncol* 13:1264, 2002.
40. Mead GM, Barrans SL, Qian W, et al: A prospective clinicopathologic study of dose-modified CODOX-M/IVAC in patients with sporadic Burkitt lymphoma defined using cytogenetic and immunophenotypic criteria (MRC/NCRI LY10 trial). *Blood* 112:2248, 2008.
41. Thomas DA, Cortes J, O'Brien S, et al: Hyper-CVAD program in Burkitt's-type adult acute lymphoblastic leukemia. *J Clin Oncol* 17:2461, 1999.
42. Thomas DA, Faderl S, O'Brien S, et al: Chemoimmunotherapy with hyper-CVAD plus rituximab for the treatment of adult Burkitt and Burkitt-type lymphoma or acute lymphoblastic leukemia. *Cancer* 106:1569, 2006.
43. Fayad L, Thomas D, Romaguera J: Update of the M.D. Anderson Cancer Center experience with hyper-CVAD and rituximab for the treatment of mantle cell and Burkitt-type lymphomas. *Clin Lymphoma Myeloma* 8 Suppl 2:S57, 2007.
44. Abramson JS, Barnes JA, Toomey CE, et al: Rituximab added to CODOX-M/IVAC is highly effective in HIV-negative and HIV-positive Burkitt lymphoma. *Blood* 112:1229, 2008.
45. Song KW, Barnett MJ, Gascoyne RD, et al: Haematopoietic stem cell transplantation as primary therapy of sporadic adult Burkitt lymphoma. *Br J Haematol* 133:634, 2006.
46. Hoffmann C, Wolf E, Wyen C, et al: AIDS-associated Burkitt or Burkitt-like lymphoma: Short intensive polychemotherapy is feasible and effective. *Leuk Lymphoma* 47:1872, 2006.
47. Kelly JL, Toothaker SR, Ciminello L, et al: Outcomes of patients with Burkitt lymphoma older than age 40 treated with intensive chemotherapeutic regimens. *Clin Lymphoma Myeloma* 9:307, 2009.
48. Grigg AP, Seymour JF: Graft versus Burkitt's lymphoma effect after allogeneic marrow transplantation. *Leuk Lymphoma* 43:889, 2002.
49. Hoelzer D, Ludwig WD, Thiel E, et al: Improved outcome in adult B-cell acute lymphoblastic leukemia. *Blood* 87:495, 1996.

CHAPTER 105
CUTANEOUS T-CELL LYMPHOMA (MYCOSIS FUNGOIDES AND SÉZARY SYNDROME)

Larisa J. Geskin

SUMMARY

Cutaneous T-cell lymphoma (CTCL) is a heterogeneous group of malignant lymphomas that share the propensity for malignant T lymphocytes that express cutaneous lymphocyte antigen (CLA) to infiltrate the skin. Mycosis fungoides (MF) is the most common variant of CTCL, representing 50 percent of all cases. Sézary syndrome (SS) is a leukemic variant of MF, affecting approximately 5 percent of patients with MF. MF and SS are the most common malignant proliferations of mature memory T lymphocytes of the helper phenotype (CD4+CD45RO+), which renders patients immunocompromised even at the earliest stages of the disease. Advanced stages are associated with severe immune suppression. Diagnosis is established by skin biopsy, followed by staging work up which includes radiologic imaging and pathologic evaluation of the lymph nodes, internal organs, blood, and marrow, as appropriate according to presenting manifestations of the disease.

MF is divided into early and advanced stages for therapeutic and prognostic reasons. There are numerous therapeutic options available. However, no therapy has been definitively shown to improve survival. In early stages, the disease follows an indolent course and has favorable prognosis. In advanced stages, the prognosis is poor. Considering the overall protracted course of the disease, its indolent character, immunocompromised status of the patients, and absence of definitive therapy, aggressive multiagent chemotherapy contributing to immunosuppression should be reserved for end-stage palliation. The goal of therapy for MF and SS is to induce long-term remissions without further compromising a patient's immune system or quality of life.

DEFINITION AND HISTORY

Mycosis fungoides (MF) and Sézary syndrome (SS) are the most common malignant proliferations of mature memory T lymphocytes of the helper phenotype (CD4+CD45RO+).[1] In 1806, Baron Jean-Louis Alibert described a patient who presented with skin patches that grew into plaques and mushroom-like tumors and first coined the term *mycosis fungoides*.[2] In 1938, Sézary and Bouvrain described a syndrome of pruritus, generalized exfoliative erythroderma, and abnormal hyperconvoluted lymphoid cells in the blood.[3] Today this condition is referred to as *Sézary syndrome*, a condition seen in a subset of patients with MF.

Prior to the 1970s, cutaneous lymphomas were believed to be cutaneous counterparts of the systemic lymphomas. In 1975, Lutzner and associates[4] suggested the term *cutaneous T-cell lymphoma* (CTCL), recognizing that these cutaneous lymphomas have significant similarities of malignant cell morphology and phenotype and represent separate entities different from their systemic counterpart. This definition has helped to distinguish cutaneous lymphomas from systemic disease; however, it also led to inappropriate use of an umbrella term *CTCL* interchangeably with MF. The World Health Organization (WHO)-European Organization for Research and Treatment of Cancer (EORTC) classification was developed and accepted in 2005[5] to resolve differences between various classifications (Table 105–1). CTCL staging and classification scheme combining WHO and EORTC approaches were recently revised.[6]

Acronyms and abbreviations used in this chapter include: CD, cluster of differentiation; CLA, cutaneous lymphocyte antigen; CTCL, cutaneous T-cell lymphoma; EBT, electron beam therapy; EORTC, European Organization for Research and Treatment of Cancer; Ig, immunoglobulin; MF, mycosis fungoides; NCCN, National Comprehensive Cancer Network; NK, natural killer; PUVA, psoralen ultraviolet A; SS, Sézary syndrome; Th2, T-helper type 2; TNMB, tumor, node, metastasis, blood; UV, ultraviolet light; WHO, World Health Organization.

EPIDEMIOLOGY

MF is twice as common in males as in females. The median age at diagnosis is 55 years. Americans of African descent have a higher incidence of MF and a poorer prognosis than Americans of European descent. MF occurs least often in Asians and Hispanics. Evidence for a genetic predisposition (germ-line transmission of susceptibility) in patients with CTCL is inconclusive. Approximately 1000 new cases of MF are reported annually in the United States, composing approximately 1.5 percent of all lymphomas. The mortality rate is 0.064 per 100,000 persons per year but varies widely according to the stage of disease. Stage I mortality is not different from the mortality of age-matched controls. However, stage IV has a 27 percent 5-year survival and 10 percent 15-year survival.[7,8] Median survival in Sézary syndrome (end-stage MF) is 1.5 years. The mortality rate of MF in the United States has been declining, possibly because of earlier diagnosis of the disease.[9,10]

ETIOLOGY AND PATHOGENESIS

The etiologies of MF and Sézary syndrome are unknown. Human T-cell lymphotropic virus (HTLV)-I originally was isolated from patients thought to have CTCL.[11] Seroepidemiologic studies, however, suggest that HTLV-I is associated with adult T-cell leukemia/lymphoma.[12] Less than 1 percent of patients with CTCL in the United States have serologic evidence for prior infection with HTLV-I. In a series of CTCL patients from Italy, a new retrovirus, called *HTLV-V*, was isolated.[13] The significance of this finding is not clear. No specific known viruses were linked to the etiology of CTCL, although clinical presentation and immunological abnormalities observed in these patients do not exclude a possibility of an involvement by a novel infectious agent.[14]

A "persistent antigen stimulation" hypothesis has been proposed as an initial event after MF was observed to be a disease of mature CD4+ memory cells, but the antigen is not known.[15,16] MF also may be viewed as a disease of immune deregulation. Tumor progression is associated with decreased antigen-specific T-cell responses and impaired cell-mediated cytotoxicity.[17–19] On the other hand, improved survival is associated with intact cell-mediated immunity.[20] Progression of MF is associated with progressive T-helper type 2 (Th2) skewing and increased production of Th2 cytokines.[21,22] This alteration accounts for many of the immune abnormalities associated with advanced MF, such as hypereosinophilia, increased serum immunoglobulin (Ig) A and IgE, impaired natural killer (NK) cell function, and impaired cellular immunity.[23] Late-stage MF and Sézary syndrome is associated with

TABLE 105–1. World Health Organization–European Organization for Research and Treatment of Cancer Classification of Primary Cutaneous T-Cell and Natural Killer Cell Lymphomas

I. Mycosis Fungoides
  A. MF variants and subtypes
    1. Folliculotropic MF
    2. Pagetoid reticulosis
    3. Granulomatous slack skin
II. Sézary Syndrome
III. Adult T-Cell Leukemia/Lymphoma
IV. Primary Cutaneous CD30+ Lymphoproliferative Disorders
  A. Primary cutaneous anaplastic large cell lymphoma
  B. Lymphomatoid papulosis
V. Subcutaneous Panniculitis-Like T-Cell Lymphoma
VI. Extranodal Natural Killer/T-Cell Lymphoma, Nasal Type
VII. Primary Cutaneous Peripheral T-Cell Lymphoma, Unspecified
  A. Primary cutaneous aggressive epidermotropic CD8+ T-cell lymphoma (provisional)
  B. Cutaneous $\gamma\delta$ T-cell lymphoma (provisional)
  C. Primary cutaneous CD4+ small/medium-sized pleomorphic T-cell lymphoma (provisional)
VIII. Precursor Hematologic Neoplasm
  A. CD4+/CD56+ hematodermic neoplasm (blastic NK-cell lymphoma)

declining immunocompetence, resulting in severe life-threatening infections, and a high incidence of secondary malignancies. The latter increase is not attributable to prior treatment with carcinogenic agents alone.[24]

Environmental factors have been implicated in etiology of CTCL in Europe,[25] but have not been confirmed by epidemiologic studies in the United States.

CLINICAL FEATURES

The clinical presentation of MF is highly variable. Cutaneous manifestations of the disease result from skin infiltration of malignant cutaneous lymphocyte antigen (CLA)-positive lymphocytes and depend on the extent of skin involvement. Patients initially may present with "chronic dermatitis" that is resistant to therapy, which can be misdiagnosed as spongiotic dermatitis (so-called eczema), "psoriasis-like dermatitis," or other chronic, nonspecific dermatoses, usually associated with pruritus. Histologically, diagnosis may be difficult, especially at the early stages of the disease and in its erythrodermic form, as the abnormal atypical infiltrate can be minimal and can be masked by normal inflammatory infiltrates in the skin, or it can be misinterpreted as normal inflammatory infiltrate because of its mature CD4+ phenotype.

MF may progress through distinct stages of skin involvement, ranging from patch (Fig. 105–1A) to plaque (Fig. 105–1B) to tumor (Fig. 105–1C), but it may never progress or lesions may arise *de novo*. For descriptive purposes, the skin manifestations of MF are divided into patch stage (patch-only disease), plaque stage (both patches and plaques), and tumor stage (more than one tumor present, usually in the context of patches and plaques). A *patch* is defined as a flat lesion with various degrees of erythema and fine scaling; it may be atrophic or poikilodermatous (Fig. 105–2A), containing areas of hyperpigmentation, hypopigmentation, atrophy, and telangiectasias. A *plaque* is a demarcated erythematous, brownish, or violaceous lesion of at least 1-mm elevation with a variable amount of scale. Tumors are elevated at least 5 mm above the skin surface and may resemble a plaque or be dome shaped without significant scaling. Tumors almost universally are present in the setting of preexisting patches and plaques (Fig. 105–1C). A rare variant of MF, so-called *MF d'emblée*, is an aggressive form of MF with a poor prognosis, in which tumors of MF arise *de novo* without preexisting patches or plaques.

Distribution of the lesions depends on the clinical stage at presentation. In earlier stages, the lesions have a predilection for folds and non–sun-exposed body areas ("bathing trunk" distribution). In later stages, such as the tumor stage and erythroderma (generalized skin involvement), the lesions can affect the face, including development of ectropion, and other exposed areas, such as palms and soles (keratoderma; Fig. 105–2B). Tumors may be generalized, and ulceration is common. Progression through the stages is variable but commonly occurs over several years.[26] Lesions usually

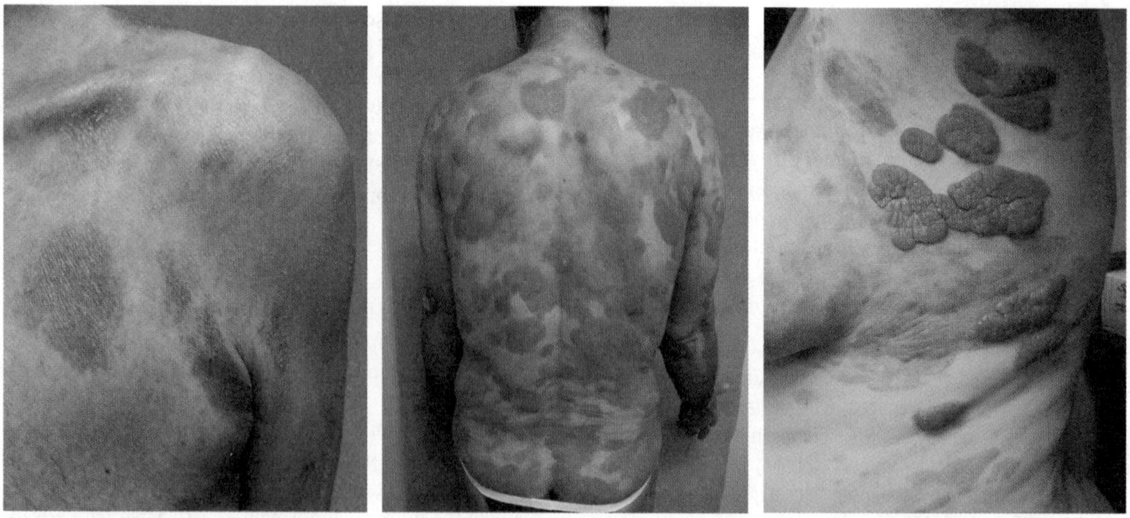

A B C

FIGURE 105–1. Mycosis fungoides. **A.** Erythematous atrophic patches with fine scale. **B.** Extensive patches and thicker plaques. **C.** Tumors on the background of preexisting patches and plaques.

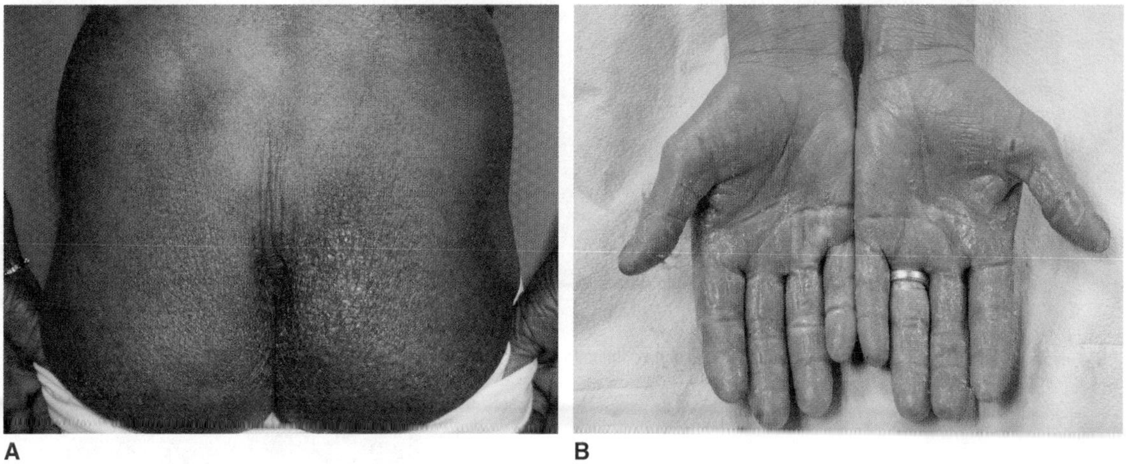

FIGURE 105–2. Mycosis fungoides. A. Poikiloderma. B. Keratoderma.

are associated with pruritus, which may range from mild to severe, leading to insomnia, weight loss, depression, and suicidal ideations. Pruritus is one of the most important quality-of-life issues for these patients.

Erythrodermic skin involvement occurs in 5 percent of patients with MF. Manifestations range from very faint to severe, with significant scaling, keratoderma, painful fissures of the hands and feet, nail dystrophy, and nail loss leading to the patient's inability to walk and maintain daily activities. Severely inflamed skin is a breeding ground for bacteria and other pathogens, with resulting fevers, chills, and septicemia. Extremity peripheral edema may be significant in the later stages and lead to cardiovascular compromise.

Depending on the stage of presentation, these patients may present with nodal involvement and/or visceral metastases. The clinical presentation usually reflects the site and severity of involvement and ranges from completely asymptomatic to severe pain, organ malfunction, or at the end-stage disease multiorgan failure.

LABORATORY FINDINGS

The diagnosis of CTCL usually is established by correlating clinical and pathologic findings.

HISTOPATHOLOGY

Early lesions may show polymorphous infiltration (containing mixed inflammatory cells) compatible with several benign dermatoses. Classically, MF lesions show superficial band-like (lichenoid) lymphocytic infiltrate (Fig. 105–3A). The lymphocytes may range from small to large, with characteristic convoluted (cerebriform) nuclei. The hallmark of the malignant infiltrate in MF is epidermotropism (presence of lymphocytes in the epidermis without spongiosis) with formation of the epidermal clusters of lymphocytes around Langerhans cells termed *Pautrier microabscesses* (Fig. 105–3B). Atypical lymphocytes line up along the dermoepidermal junction and are surrounded by a halo artifact (Fig. 105–3C), which is an important feature of early disease.[27] Superficial dermal collagen may be thickened, so called ropey collagen. In more advanced stages, the infiltrate is less polymorphic, with a predominance of larger atypical cells extending deeper into the dermis; epidermotropism may be lost. Transformation to large T-cell lymphoma (CD30+ or CD30−) may occur and carries a poor prognosis in the setting of MF.[28–30]

IMMUNOPHENOTYPING

Immunophenotyping plays an important role in diagnosis. The cells usually are CD3+CD4+CD45RO+CD8− , a phenotype associated with mature helper-inducer T lymphocytes (Fig. 105–4A and B).[31–33] These cells function as helper T lymphocytes in *in vitro* assays.[34] The CD7 antigen, expressed by more than 85 percent of normal circulating T lymphocytes, may be absent from the circulating Sézary cells[35] and skin-infiltrating lymphocytes (Fig. 105–4C). The cells may express T-cell activation markers, such as HLA-DR (human leukocyte antigen-D related) or CD25 (interleukin [IL]-2 receptor) and have loss of CD26

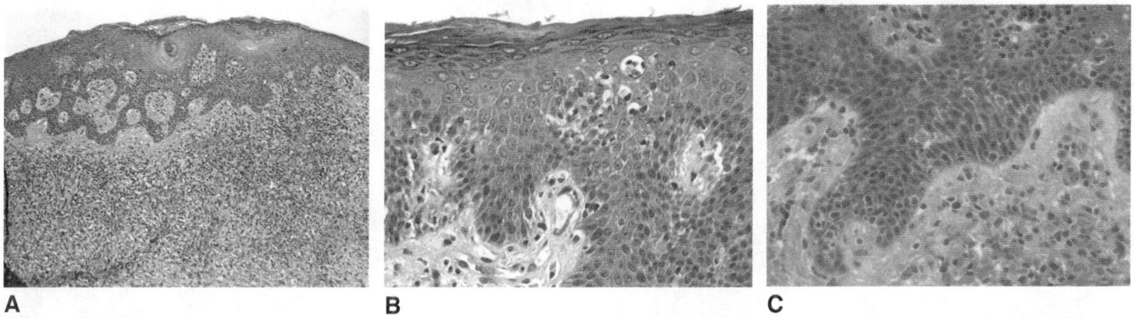

FIGURE 105–3. Mycosis fungoides. Skin biopsies stained with hematoxylin and eosin. A. Lichenoid (band-like) lymphocytic infiltrate in the superficial dermis. B. Epidermotropic atypical lymphocytes lining the dermoepidermal junction in the absence of spongiosis-forming Pautrier microabscesses. Note, halo artifact around lymphocytes at the dermato-epidermal junction. C. Atypical lymphocytes in the epidermis.

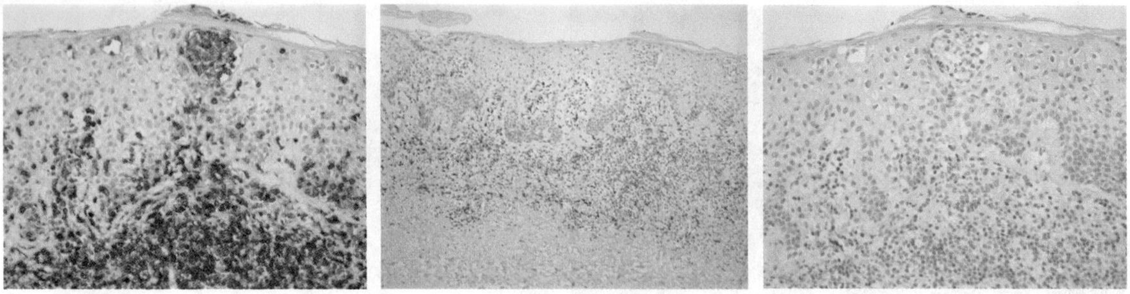

A B C

FIGURE 105–4. Mycoses fungoides. Immunohistochemistry. **A.** CD4+ lichenoid infiltrate in the superficial dermis. Note Pautrier microabscess in the epidermis. **B.** Few CD8+ cells are present. **C.** Loss of maturation marker CD7.

expression.[36,37] Loss of CD26 expression on CD4+ cells is considered to be one of the most important markers for malignant T lymphocytes.

CYTOCHEMISTRY

Like most malignant T cells, the MF cells stain for acid phosphatase, α-naphthyl acetate esterase, and β-glucuronidase. The cells are generally negative for peroxidase, alkaline phosphatase, and esterase. Periodic acid-Schiff–positive granules are present in some cases. Rearrangement of the TCRVβ gene can be identified. In rare instances, the classic clinical presentation of MF may be associated with an aberrant CD4 phenotype or may have CD4– CD8+ T-cell phenotype.[38,39]

BLOOD FINDINGS

Blood involvement is manifested by atypical lymphocytes with convoluted (cerebriform) nuclei on the blood film. The blood film requires very careful inspection by light microscopy since the abnormal nuclear shape is subtle (Fig. 105–5) compared with electron micrographic studies (Fig. 105–6). The presence of these atypical lymphocytes is not exclusive to MF/SS, as low numbers of similar cells can be found in some benign dermatoses and in the blood of patients on immunosuppressive drugs. Assessment of the blood film by light microscopy is subjective, but usually is consistent within the same observer. Flow cytometry is used to quantify blood involvement more accurately. Because there are no known specific markers for Sézary cells, surrogate indicators such as loss of normal maturation molecules CD7 and, more specifically, CD26 on CD3+ or CD4+ lymphocytes, are used. An abnormal phenotype with increased overall numbers of CD4+ cells, with loss of at least 40 percent CD7 and at least 30 percent CD26 molecules, are considered to be significant and, together with demonstration of clonality, are ranked as B2, high tumor burden blood involvement.[6] B2 leukemic blood involvement carries prognostic significance (Tables 105–2 and 105–3) and places the patient, even without lymph nodal involvement, into stage IVA1 category. Patients with erythroderma and low tumor burden in peripheral blood (B1, Table 105–2) are also upgraded to stage IIIB.

CYTOGENETIC FINDINGS

Cytogenetic abnormalities are not consistently identified, but loss of heterozygosity on 10q and microsatellite instability may be seen in advanced-stage disease.[40] A possible association exists with homozygous deletion of *PTEN* and *CDKN2A*, tumor-suppressor genes on the short arm of chromosomes 10 and 9, respectively. These may be silenced with progression of disease.[41,42]

STAGING

MF is classified according to the widely accepted modified *tumor, node, metastasis, blood (TNMB) classification*, originally adopted in 1975 by

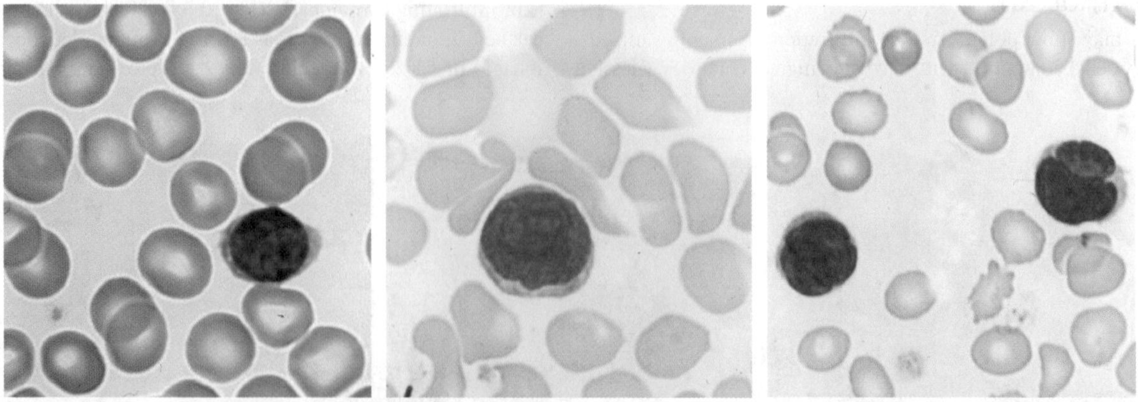

A B C

FIGURE 105–5. Blood lymphocytes. **A.** Normal small lymphocyte. **B.** Sézary cell. Note the nuclear swirls and the light microscopic appearance of the Sézary cell nucleus. Without careful inspection in cases of lymphocytosis, Sézary cells can be mistaken for small lymphocytes as seen in chronic lymphocytic leukemia. **C.** Blood lymphocytes from a patient with mycosis fungoides and disseminated disease involving marrow and blood. Note clefted appearance of the nucleus. *(Used with permission from* Lichtman's Atlas of Hematology, *www.accessmedicine.com.)*

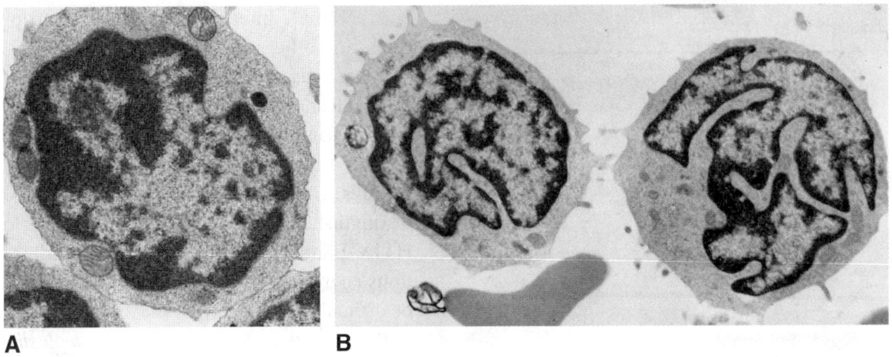

FIGURE 105–6. Transmission electron micrographs of lymphocytes. **A.** Normal lymphocyte. **B.** Two lymphocytes from a patient with Sézary cells in the blood. The latter have the striking cerebriform nuclear abnormalities characteristic of Sézary cells. *(Used with permission from* Lichtman's Atlas of Hematology, *www.accessmedicine.com.)*

the Mycosis Fungoides Cooperative Study Group[43,44] and recently revised to match modern developments in the field.[6] Accurate determination of the stage in MF and SS is of outmost importance because of it prognostic significance and its critical role in different therapeutic choices (Fig. 105–7). Cutaneous lesions are classified using the *T staging system* (Table 105–2). The area of the skin and type of the lesions were found to correlate with patient survival and are important prognostic predictors. Prognosis varies according to tumor burden. The presence of tumors (T3) may indicate a worse prognosis than erythroderma (T4).[8]

The extent of extracutaneous disease usually reflects the extent of skin involvement. In early disease, significant involvement of lymph nodes and blood is unlikely. However, lymphadenopathy is present in approximately half of patients and increases with progressive cutaneous involvement.[45,46] Lymph nodes are assigned the *N category* in the TNMB staging of MF (see Table 105–2). Computed tomography scans are used to assess pretreatment involvement of intra-abdominal lymph nodes.[47–49]

Histopathologic examination of affected lymph nodes may show partial or complete effacement of normal architecture, with a monomorphic infiltrate of MF cells. However, in most cases, the nodal architecture is not effaced, and dermatopathic changes with varying numbers of atypical lymphocytes in the T-cell paracortical areas of the node are frequently present. Even the presence of dermatopathic changes alone in the lymph nodes carries prognostic significance (see Tables 105–2 and 105–3).[26,50] Abnormal lymph nodes should have an excisional biopsy regardless of the T stage.[51]

Metastatic disease is the most significant prognostic predictor (see Tables 105–2 and 105–3). Patients with visceral involvement that includes liver, spleen, pleura, and lung have a median survival of less than 1 year.[52] Blood involvement may be an important predictor of progression and survival.[53] The number of circulating Sézary cells increases with advancing disease, and the cells are particularly prominent in patients with generalized erythroderma. However, even in early disease, a high frequency of clonal T cells in the blood may be detected using a highly sensitive polymerase chain reaction technique, suggesting that early systemic disease is common.[54] Blood involvement is rated as *B category* in the TNMB staging (see Table 105–2). For staging

TABLE 105–2. TNMB Classification of Mycosis Fungoides

T: Skin
T1: Limited patches, papules, or plaques covering <10% of the skin surface (T1a = patch only; T1b = plaques ± patches)
T2: Generalized patches, papules, or plaques covering 10% of the skin surface (T2a = patch only; T2b = plaques ± patches)
T3: At least one tumor (≥1 cm in diameter)
T4: Generalized erythroderma over at least 80% body surface area
N: Lymph nodes
N0: No clinically abnormal peripheral lymph nodes; biopsy not required
N1: Clinically abnormal peripheral lymph nodes; histopathology Dutch grade 1 or NCI LN0 to 2
N2: Clinically abnormal peripheral lymph nodes; histopathology Dutch grade 2 or NCI LN3
N3: Clinically abnormal peripheral lymph nodes; histopathology Dutch grades 3–4 or NCI LN4
NX: Clinically abnormal peripheral lymph nodes; no histologic confirmation
M: Visceral organs
M0: No visceral organ involvement
M1: Visceral organ involvement; requires histologic confirmation and specify organ
B: Blood
B0: Atypical circulating cells not present (<5%); specify "a" if flow cytometry is negative for clonal T lymphocytes or "b" if positive for clonal T lymphocytes
B1: Atypical circulating cells present (>5%, minimal blood involvement); specify "a" if flow cytometry is negative for clonal T lymphocytes or "b" if positive for clonal T lymphocytes
B2: Leukemia (≥1000 cells/μL, CD4 to CD8 ratio of 10 or higher, evidence of a T-cell clone in the blood)

CTCL, cutaneous T-cell lymphoma.

NOTE: T indicates the size of the tumor and whether it has invaded nearby tissue. N indicates the regional lymph nodes that are involved. M indicates distant metastasis. B indicates whether there are tumor cells in the blood.

TABLE 105–3. Revised Staging of Mycosis Fungoides and Sézary Syndrome[6]

	T	N	M	B
IA	1	0	0	0, 1
IB	2	0	0	0, 1
IIA	1, 2	1, 2	0	0, 1
IIB	3	0–2	0	0, 1
III	4	0–2	0	0, 1
IIIA	4	0–2	0	0
IIIB	4	0–2	0	1
IVA1	1–4	0–2	0	2
IVA2	1–4	3	0	0–2
IVB	1–4	0–3	1	0–2

See Table 105–2 for definitions of T1–T4, N0–N3, and M0–M1.

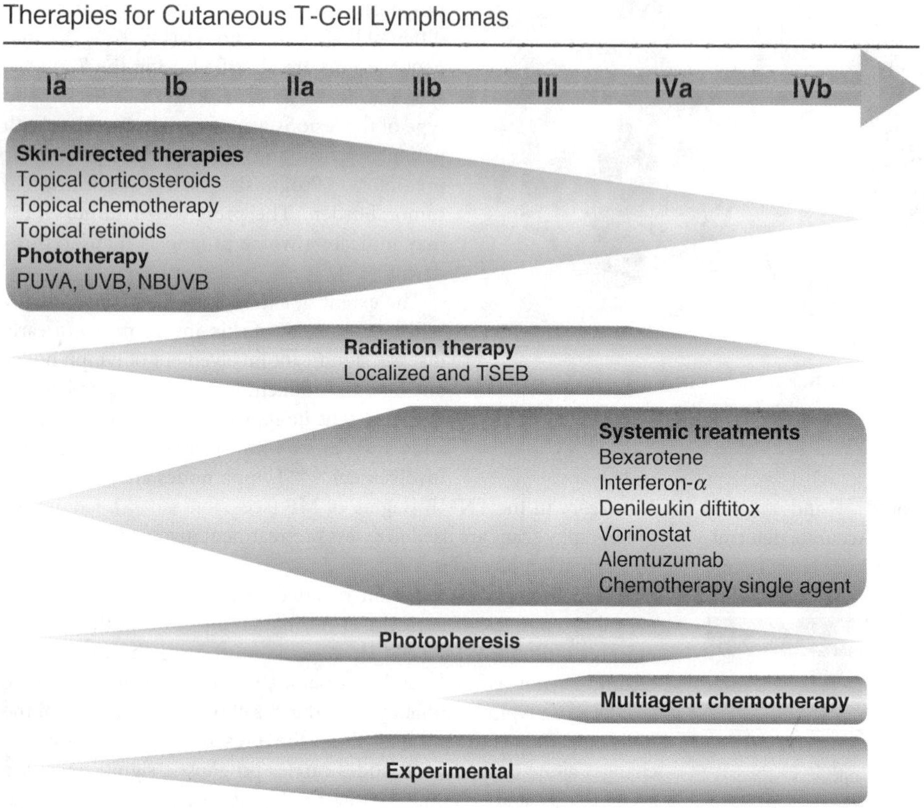

FIGURE 105–7. Cutaneous T-cell lymphoma treatment algorithm. NBUVB, narrowband ultraviolet B; PUVA, psoralen ultraviolet A; TSEB, total-skin electron beam; UVB, ultraviolet B.

purposes, the B2 blood rating is equivalent to nodal involvement.[55,56] Leukemic blood involvement without lymph node involvement is classified as stage IVA1 disease in the revised criteria (Table 105–3). The B2 rating is defined as a Sézary cell count of 1000 cells/μL or more; or (1) a CD4 to CD8 ratio of 10 or higher caused by an increase in circulating T cells and/or (2) an aberrant loss or expression of pan–T-cell markers by flow cytometry (>40% CD4+ and CD7- or >30% CD4+ and CD26-). Malignant cells also can be detected using sensitive techniques such as cytogenetics or T-cell receptor (TCR) gene rearrangement studies.[57–61] Patients with blood involvement have a higher likelihood of lymphadenopathy and visceral involvement. Marrow infiltration is infrequently detected by biopsy despite circulating malignant cells; it is identified at autopsy in 30 to 40 percent of cases. The cytologic appearance of the malignant cells in visceral organs is similar to that of the malignant cells in the skin.[62]

In the erythrodermic subset of MF, three T4 subsets can be identified (Table 105–4). In general, Sézary syndrome, considered to be a triad of exfoliative erythroderma, generalized lymphadenopathy, and leukemia, historically had the worst prognosis among the forms of MF.

DIFFERENTIAL DIAGNOSIS

Diagnosis of MF is based on a constellation of findings, which include clinical presentation, skin and lymph node biopsies (if indicated), and blood evaluation. A number of benign dermatoses can mimic MF or Sézary syndrome, and may even have TCR gene rearrangements.[63–66] Such benign conditions include psoriasis and psoriasiform dermatoses (e.g., pityriasis rubra pilaris, seborrheic dermatitis, contact dermatitis, and eczema), intertrigo, tinea, drug eruptions, and other conditions.

Cutaneous and systemic lymphomas other than MF should be considered in the differential diagnosis. Smoldering adult T-cell leukemia/lymphoma has a number of clinical features similar to MF, but it usually can be distinguished by the presence of antibodies to HTLV-I and by other associated findings unusual in MF. However, this distinction may be difficult.[67,68]

Pagetoid reticulosis *(Woringer-Kolopp disease)* is a rare skin disorder that consists of solitary or localized cutaneous plaques. It affects young males almost exclusively. It has a benign course, and the prognosis is excellent.[69–71] It is an epidermal process, with the majority of atypical lymphocytes found within hyperplastic epidermis.[72] Although the disease usually is indolent and localized, some patients present with a disseminated form referred to as the *Ketron-Goodman variant.*[73] The histologic findings are similar to those found in Woringer-Kolopp disease, with predominantly epidermal involvement by malignant cells and a poor prognosis.[73] This variant is a disease of an activated T-lymphocyte that only occasionally expresses the helper T-cell CD4 antigen.[74,75] Like MF, the neoplastic cells have TCR gene rearrangements.

Other variants of CTCL, such as alopecia mucinosa, folliculotropic MF, and adnexatropic CTCL, should be considered in the differential diagnosis. The diagnosis is made by skin biopsy. CD30+ (Ki-1) and CD30– lymphomas can mimic tumors of MF; they present as erythematous or violaceous nodules that ulcerate. The critical issue is to differentiate primary cutaneous CD30+ lymphoproliferative disorder from CD30+ large cell transformation of MF and from secondary cutaneous involvement as a result of CD30+ nodal lymphoma. The course of CD30+ lymphomas of the skin is indolent, they carry a favorable prognosis and tend to regress spontaneously, whereas transformed MF and nodal lymphoma carry poor prognosis. In rare instances, these lymphomas progress to systemic involvement and have the same prognosis as nodal CD30+ lymphomas.[76,77] Lymphomatoid papulosis is a benign counterpart of CD30+ lymphoproliferative disorders of the skin with excellent prognosis. It usually presents as crops of recurrent pruritic or painful erythematous papules or nodules, which ulcerate and heal spontaneously; it usually runs a chronic course.[78] It may be associated with other malignancies, mainly MF and other lymphomas, in up to 10 percent of the cases. Therefore close observation and followup are recommended for patients with lymphomatoid papulosis. Low-dose oral methotrexate is a drug of choice for this disorder.

THERAPY

A variety of therapeutic modalities produce remissions in most patients with MF. Cure is uncommon and possible only in early disease. In general, MF therapy is divided into (1) skin-directed therapy and (2) systemic therapy (Table 105–5). Skin-directed therapy is the mainstream therapy in early disease but can be used as an adjunct in systemic disease. Therapeutic decisions may be difficult and heavily depend on the stage at presenta-

TABLE 105–4. Classification of Erythrodermic Cutaneous T-Cell Lymphoma

Erythrodermic Subset (T4)	Preexisting MF	Blood
Sézary syndrome	Rarely	Leukemia: B2
Erythrodermic mycosis fungoides	Always	Normal or minimally abnormal: B0–B1
Erythrodermic cutaneous T-cell lymphoma, not otherwise specified	Absent	Normal or minimally abnormal: B0–B1

tion. Revised practice guidelines are available on National Comprehensive Cancer Network (NCCN) website (www.nccn.org).[79] See Fig. 105–7 for an overview of the treatment algorithm for MF and SS.

SKIN-DIRECTED THERAPIES

Topical Glucocorticoids

These agents are effective during early stages of MF. They are limited to temporary short-term use because of suppression of collagen synthesis (skin atrophy), striae formation, skin fragility, and secondary infections.

TABLE 105–5. Therapeutic Option for Mycosis Fungoides and Sézary Syndrome

Skin-Directed Therapy	Systemic Therapy
Topical therapy	Immunomodulators
Topical glucocorticoids	Interferon-α
Nitrogen mustard (mechlorethamine)	Extracorporeal photophoresis (ECP)
	Antibodies/fusion proteins
Carmustine (BCNU, nitrosourea)	Denileukin diftitox (ONTAK, DAB_{389}–IL-2)
Retinoids (bexarotene, tretinoin)	Alemtuzumab (Campath)
Topical tacrolimus (Protopic)	Retinoids
Imiquimod (Aldara)	Oral bexarotene (Targretin)
Light therapy	Acitretin (Soriatane)
UVB and PUVA	Isotretinoin (Accutane)
Photodynamic therapy	Histone deacetylase inhibitors
Electron beam	Vorinostat (Zolinza)
Localized	Romidepsin (Istodax)
Total-skin	Chemotherapy (alone or in combinations)
	Oral prednisone, methotrexate, doxorubicin, cyclophosphamide; chlorambucil; pentostatin, cladribine, fludarabine, pralatrexate, several others

PUVA, psoralen and ultraviolet radiation of the A spectrum; UVB, ultraviolet radiation of the B spectrum.

The class of topical preparation used depends on the area and the site of involvement. Ultrapotent topical glucocorticoids should not be used on the face, neck, or intertriginous areas. When used in these locations there is a risk of development of glucocorticoid-induced acne, glaucoma and cataracts, and severe skin atrophy. Use of potent glucocorticoids for extensive periods of time (>2 weeks) may result in severe poikiloderma, leading to skin breakdown and consequent risk of infection.

Topical glucocorticoids are rarely used as monotherapy, but may be effective as additional modality for symptomatic relieve of pruritus.

Topical Tacrolimus (Protopic)

Topical tacrolimus has been approved for use in atopic dermatitis. It is as effective as mid- to low-potency glucocorticoids for use on facial skin and intertriginous areas in patients with MF. A major advantage of tacrolimus compared with steroids is that it does not suppress collagen synthesis and therefore does not cause skin atrophy.[80] However, because the use of calcineurin inhibitors in CTCL is controversial, tacrolimus use should be limited to short-term use on small areas.

Topical Nitrogen Mustard

This drug is used predominantly in patients with early cutaneous stages of disease. In more advanced stages, this approach is used to supplement other therapies. The major advantage of topical therapy is its relatively low toxicity. Disadvantages include the inconvenience of daily application to large areas of skin, allergic reactions in up to half of cases,[81] the potential for development of skin cancer,[82] and the inability to cure the disease. Nitrogen mustard 10 mg diluted in 60 mL of tap water or 60 g of a water-miscible cream or an anhydrous ointment, which may have less allergic sensitization, is administered daily using a cotton swab or small paint brush. Therapy is continued for up to 12 months in responders. Frequency then is reduced to every other day for an additional 1 to 2 years. Therapy is discontinued after 3 years or when cutaneous lesions disappear completely.

Topical Carmustine

Carmustine (BCNU) is not currently widely used for treatment of MF because of its severe irritant reactions and its absorption from the skin that results in systemic toxicity. The preparation ranges from 20 to 40 mg/dL in petrolatum ointment. It is applied at night and washed off in the morning. Monitoring includes biweekly complete blood counts to identify marrow suppression. Carmustine causes irreversible skin thinning, telangiectasias, and hyperpigmentation.[83]

Topical Retinoids

Bexarotene (Targretin) 1 percent gel topical retinoid (rexinoid) is most commonly used for MF. It is a small lipophilic molecule that is related to vitamin A. It readily crosses the cytoplasmic membrane and binds to nuclear receptors (retinoid X receptors), resulting in changes in gene expression mediated through specific intracellular receptors. Complete responses of 20 percent and overall responses of 60 percent are reported.[84,85] It is applied in a thin layer to the patches and plaques twice daily. The major toxicity is irritation at the site. Topical bexarotene is FDA approved for treatment of MF patients who are refractory to at least one other topical therapy. Oral administration of bexarotene is associated with severe birth defects. Considering potential absorption of the drug from the skin surface, bexarotene should not be given to pregnant women.

Phototherapy

Several means of phototherapy currently are available for treatment of MF. They include ultraviolet radiation (UV) of the A (UVA) and B

(UVB) spectra. UVB therapy and narrow-band UVB both are effective in the treatment of early disease (mainly patches and very thin plaques). Phototherapy may result in complete clearing of the lesions. Therapy should be instituted at least three times per week. On average, 4 to 8 weeks are required to achieve the response. Maintenance therapy is required after a response occurs and consists of once weekly UVB irradiation for the long-term. The main side effects are related to acute burning and long-term use association with slight increase in the incidence of skin cancers.[86–88]

Phototherapy involving UVA radiation is used with psoralen and is referred to as *PUVA*. Psoralen is a phototoxic furocoumarin activated by UVA light. In its active form, psoralen binds covalently and irreversibly to DNA. UVA light penetrates only the upper part of the dermis. Therefore, psoralen activated by UVA light affects cells primarily in the epidermis and papillary dermis. A 60 percent complete remission rate and long-term remissions (>10 years) have been reported with PUVA; patients with generalized erythroderma and tumors have lower response rates than do patients with plaques.[89–91] Psoralen usually is given at a dose of 0.6 mg/kg orally, 2 hours before the UVA light therapy. Treatments initially are given three times per week. Maintenance therapy may be given every 2 to 4 weeks for an indefinite period. Adverse effects of PUVA therapy include mild nausea, pruritus, and sunburn-like changes, with atrophy and dry skin. PUVA is not cross-resistant with other treatment modalities. Disadvantages of PUVA therapy are the necessity to visit the doctor's office frequently (from three times a week to once a month) and its expense. Home PUVA boxes are available and may be programmed by the physician to administer PUVA at home. Long-term side effects include an increased incidence of skin cancers and melanoma.[92]

Photodynamic Therapy

Photodynamic therapy is a new type of photochemotherapy that utilizes two properties of porphyrins: their selective accumulation in the tumor (e.g., 5-aminolevulinic acid) and their ability to generate cytotoxic oxygen species at the tumor site after red-light irradiation. 5-Aminolevulinic acid is a natural porphyrin precursor and upon irradiation is converted in the tumor to the highly photoactive endogenous protoporphyrin IX. Red-light irradiation is safe and penetrates deep in the tissue, allowing for treatment of thick tumors. Photodynamic therapy is especially useful in patients with limited skin area involved by few tumors. The main problem with the treatment is that the pain induced during irradiation limits its use for larger areas.[93,94]

Electron Beam Therapy

Electron beam therapy (EBT) is highly effective form of treatment of MF and can be used as a localized therapy to specific sites or lesions, or as radiation of the entire skin surface (total-skin electron beam therapy). It significantly penetrates only into the upper dermis, systemic effects are minimal, and the complete remission rate is 80 percent.[95–97] Twenty percent of patients remain relapse free at 3 years. The relapse rate depends on the stage of the disease, and usually is short-lived (may be as short as 2–3 weeks) in patients with erythroderma or numerous tumors. Typically, treatment is 4 Gy per week to a total dose of 36 Gy in 8 to 9 weeks. The advantage of EBT is the high frequency of durable complete responses without systemic toxicity. Disadvantages are alopecia, atrophy, edema, dermatitis, and increased risk of cutaneous malignancy. Up to three courses of EBT can be safely administered when used in a highly fractionated fashion (1 Gy per dose). Lower doses of electron beam have been reported as effective, although with slightly higher relapse rates.[98]

Imiquimod (Aldara)

Imiquimod is a new topical immunomodulator that is extremely effective in the treatment of condylomata acuminata, actinic keratoses, basal cell carcinomas, keratoacanthomas, and other cutaneous malignancies. The mode of action is not known but is thought to be related to induction of tumor necrosis factor-α and interferons resulting in activation of Th1-type immune response and rejection of cancer or virally infected cells. Several groups reported the effectiveness of imiquimod in early patch MF.[99,100] It should be used three times per week for 3 months. Long-term followup data is not available at this time.

SYSTEMIC THERAPY

Oral Retinoids

Bexarotene (Targretin) is an FDA-approved X-receptor-selective retinoid ("rexinoid") for therapy of MF. It is a first-line systemic agent for patients without contraindications to retinoids. At the currently FDA-approved dose of 300 mg/m^2 per day, overall response rate to bexarotene monotherapy in clinical trials ranged from 45 to 57 percent with at least 2 percent complete responses.[101,102] Higher doses are associated with higher response rates and shorter time to response, but also with higher incidence of adverse events. All patients on bexarotene develop central hypothyroidism and hyperlipidemia (most significantly hypertriglyceridemia), requiring coadministration of the thyroid supplements and lipid-lowering agents. Other adverse events include headaches, possibly as a result of pseudotumor cerebri, leucopenia, and pruritus. The majority of side effects are laboratory in nature and dose-dependent; bexarotene is usually well tolerated by the patients. Its use is recommended beginning with refractory or persistent stage IA disease; bexarotene is considered to be a first-line drug in more advanced stages (NCCN guidelines). Standard procedures for management of patients on bexarotene therapy are reviewed in reference 103. Bexarotene is safe to use long-term for maintenance therapy. Bexarotene and other retinoids are labeled pregnancy category X, and must not be given to a pregnant woman or a woman who intends to become pregnant.

Other retinoids have been used for treatment of MF and SS, including isotretinoin, acitretin, etretinate (not available in the United States), and all-*trans* retinoic acid. The activity of these compounds in MF/SS was demonstrated only in case series or small open-label pilot studies, but there are no prospective studies formally evaluating these drugs.[104]

Histone Deacetylase Inhibitors

Two novel histone deacetylase inhibitors (vorinostat and romidepsin) have been approved by the FDA for use in patients with CTCL.[105,105a] Vorinostat (Zolinza) was evaluated in open-label phase IIb clinical trial and was shown to have an overall response rate of 30 percent. Notably, cutaneous manifestations alone were used as endpoints for evaluation of response rates in this clinical trial. No complete responses were observed on the clinical trial. Median time to recurrence in patients with advanced disease was 56 days. Median time to progression was 4.9 months overall, and 9.8 months for stage IIB or higher responders. Overall, 32 percent of patients had pruritus relief. The most common drug-related adverse events were diarrhea (49%), fatigue (46%), nausea (43%), and anorexia (26%); most were grade 2 or lower, but those grade 3 or higher included fatigue (5%), pulmonary embolism (5%), thrombocytopenia (5%), and nausea (4%). Romidepsin (Istodax) was evaluated in two international multicenter open-label phase II clinical studies involving a total of 167 patients. In pooled analysis, the overall response rate was 35 percent with a median response duration of 14 months in one study, and 11 months in the other study. Six percent of those studied had complete responses.[105a] Side effects included nausea (67%), fatigue (49%), anorexia (37%), electrocardiograph T-wave changes (29%), anemia (26%), dysgeusia (23%), neutropenia (22%), and leukopenia (20%). Serious adverse events were observed in 2 percent of patients and included supraventricular and ventricular arrhythmias and infection.

Interferon-α

Interferon-α can be used as a single agent or combined with other systemic therapies. The response rate when interferon-α is used as a monotherapy is 50 to 70 percent at doses beginning at 3 to 5×10^6 U/day or three times per week.[106] Toxicity includes acute flu-like symptoms and fatigue.

Extracorporeal Photopheresis

PUVA can be delivered by an extracorporeal technique.[107,108] White cells are collected by leukapheresis, exposed to a photoactivating drug, and irradiated with UVA. The cells then are reinfused into the patient. The effect may be both a direct cytotoxic effect on the tumor cells and an immunologic effect by activating lymphocytes against the tumor cells. Photopheresis typically is administered every 2 to 4 weeks until clearance of disease. Side effects are minimal and may be related to fluid shifts during the procedure.[92]

Monoclonal Antibodies

Alemtuzumab (Campath-1H) is a humanized IgG_1 monoclonal antibody that targets the CD52 antigen. Response rates of 50 percent in a small cohort of patients have been reported.[109,110] Low-dose alemtuzumab is safe and effective in very elderly Sézary syndrome patients.[111] Alemtuzumab effectively depletes leukemic cells from the blood of these patients. Subcutaneous administration of low doses, as needed, have been effective in Sézary syndrome patients.[112]

Recombinant Fusion Proteins

Denileukin diftitox (ONTAK) is an IL-2 diphtheria toxin fusion protein. The safety and efficacy of denileukin diftitox in patients with MF was examined in a phase III trial of 71 patients who had not responded to a median of five prior therapies. This trial led to preliminary FDA-approval of the drug in 1999. Denileukin diftitox was administered in two doses: 9 mcg/kg per day or 18 mcg/kg per day for 5 consecutive days. The overall response rate was 30 percent of patients, with 10 percent of those treated achieving a complete remission.[113] There was no dose–response relationship, but patients with more advanced disease (stage IIB or higher) had a greater likelihood of response at the higher dose ($P = 0.07$). The median time to response was 6 weeks, and the duration of response in this trial was approximately 7 months.

A larger phase III randomized, double-blind, placebo-controlled trial was conducted and led to full FDA approval in October 2008.[114] The objective response rate was 37 percent on 9 mcg/kg per day and 46 percent on 18 mcg/kg per day, which was statistically significant ($p = 0.002$). Patients receiving 18 mcg/kg per day had progression-free survival of 971+ days and a duration of response of 220 days. Time to response was 92 days; time to treatment failure was 169 days. Importantly, 45 percent of best responses occurred in cycle 4 and beyond, suggesting that appropriate trial of the drug is necessary to achieve optimal responses. All complete remissions occurred from four cycles and beyond.[114]

Side effects are numerous, including a capillary leak syndrome. Other side effects are infection, hepatitis, increased fluid retention, rash, shortness of breath, and flu-like symptoms such as chills, fever, weakness, bone and muscle pain, headache, nausea, and vomiting. Cardiac arrhythmias and thrombotic emergencies have been reported occasionally. Usually, adverse events are the most severe during the first two cycles with the severity of the side effects tapering down as the treatments continue.

Chemotherapy

Pralatrexate (FOLOTYN) is a novel antifolate analogue indicated for the treatment of patients with relapsed or refractory peripheral T-cell lymphoma (PTCL). It was evaluated in a pivotal phase II nonrandomized open-label international study, the largest prospective study in patients with relapsed or refractory PTCL. The trial enrolled 115 patients, 111 of whom received 30 mg/m^2 of pralatrexate intravenously weekly for 6 of 7 weeks, supplemented with B_{12} and folic acid; 109 patients were evaluable for efficacy. Patients were heavily pretreated and failed prior therapies, including CHOP and autologous stem cell transplant. The objective response rate (ORR) was 27 percent (n = 29) with a complete response (CR) of 10 percent (n = 11), and a partial response (PR) of 17 percent (n = 18); 23 patients (21%) had stable disease. Majority of responses (69%) were observed after the first cycle. Long-term responses (>1 year) have been observed. Adverse events included mucosal inflammation (Gr 3 = 17%, Gr 4 = 4%) and thrombocytopenia (Gr 3 = 14%, Gr 4 = 19%).[114a] The largest experience with single-agent chemotherapy is with alkylating agents, including nitrogen mustard 0.4 mg/ kg given intravenously every 4 to 6 weeks, cyclophosphamide, or chlorambucil. Response rates of 60 percent, with 15 percent complete remissions, have been reported.[115,116] Similar results are obtained with methotrexate 2.5 to 10 mg/day orally[117]; bleomycin 7.5 to 15 mg intramuscularly given twice weekly; and doxorubicin 60 mg/m^2 intravenously given once per month.[118,119] Pegylated doxorubicin used in advanced MF has resulted in an overall response of 88 percent.[120] Purine analogues, including fludarabine and pentostatin, have response rates as high as 50 percent.[121–123] Gemcitabine has a similar response rate.[124] Neither single-agent nor multiagent therapy cures MF. Chemotherapy with a single agent and polychemotherapy result in a higher incidence of transformation to large cell lymphoma, which carries a worse prognosis than the original diagnosis.[125,126] Because responses to therapy are generally higher after combination therapy, single-agent chemotherapy is used rarely. However, use of multiagent chemotherapy results in increased immunosuppression and increased risk of serious infections, leading to death in majority of patients who develop this complication.[127] Combination therapy produces objective responses in greater than 80 percent of patients and complete responses in approximately 25 percent of cases.[91,128] Duration of remission varies, with a median of approximately 1 year. No long-term disease-free survival has been reported. A number of novel agents are currently in clinical trials, including a new promising purine nucleoside analogue, purine nucleoside phosphorylase inhibitor forodesine, the thalidomide derivative lenalidomide.

Combined Modality Therapy

Several multidrug regimens reportedly improve clinical response in patients with MF, including combination of extracorporeal photophoresis with low-dose interferon-α and oral bexarotene; prednisone and fludarabine; and PUVA and oral bexarotene.[96,129]

Because in general MF is an indolent malignancy of T cells with excellent prognosis in early stages, the treatment should be conservative, with skin-directed therapies (nitrogen mustard, topical glucocorticoids, topical bexarotene) combined with light therapy, low-dose interferon, low-dose methotrexate, or other single-agent chemotherapy. The survival of patients treated with aggressive chemotherapy is not different from the survival of patients treated conservatively, but aggressive chemotherapy results in greater toxicity. Because no curative

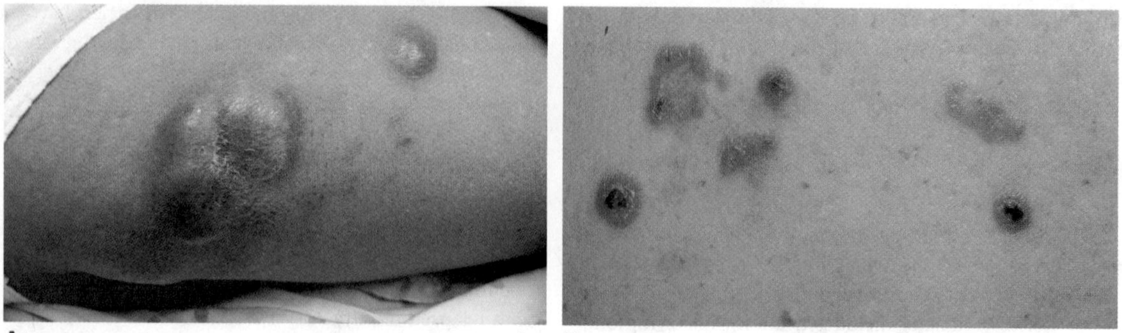

A B

FIGURE 105–8. CD30+ lymphoproliferative disorders. **A.** Primary cutaneous anaplastic large cells lymphoma. Large cutaneous tumors on the anterior thigh. **B.** Lymphomatoid papulosis. Numerous small erythematous papules and small nodules. Some with necrotic centers in crops. Some lesions show spontaneous regression.

therapy exists, the goal of therapy is to prevent progression to more advanced stages and to preserve the patient's quality of life for as long as possible.

COURSE AND PROGNOSIS

Prognosis largely depends on the stage at presentation. Fifty percent of deaths among patients with MF result from infections. Septicemia and bacterial pneumonia are common; they usually are caused by *Staphylococcus* or *Pseudomonas* and develop from cutaneous lesions.[26] Herpes virus infections occur in up to 10 percent of patients with advanced MF. Progressive MF with widespread visceral involvement late in the course of the disease is the next most common cause of death.

PRIMARY CUTANEOUS ANAPLASTIC LARGE CELL LYMPHOMA

■ CLINICAL FINDINGS

CD30+ cutaneous lymphoproliferative disorders are the second most common CTCLs after MF and represent approximately 25 percent of CTCL cases.[78] There is a spectrum of CD30+ lymphoproliferative disorders, including lymphomatoid papulosis and primary cutaneous ALCL as its malignant counterpart. It is defined by the presence of skin involvement without evidence of extracutaneous disease for at least 6 months after presentation (Fig. 105–8A).[3] Secondary involvement of lymph nodes may not necessarily be associated with a worse prognosis.[4] In some cases, distinction between lymphomatoid papulosis and primary cutaneous ALCL cannot be made because of discrepancy between clinical features and histologic appearance. These cases are referred to as *borderline lesions*, and their classification should take into consideration their clinical behavior and appearance.

Other CD30+ cutaneous lymphoproliferative disorders include large cell transformation of MF, systemic ALCL, cutaneous NK/T-cell lymphoma, and Hodgkin lymphoma. Making the distinction among these cases is critical because management and prognosis are significantly different (see "Treatment" below). The descriptive term *anaplastic* could be omitted from the name of this lymphoma because these lymphomas may have an anaplastic, immunoblastic, or pleomorphic cell morphology. Regardless of pathologic type, these CD30+ large cell lymphomas have a similar clinical course, treatment, and prognosis.[78,130–132]

CD30+ primary cutaneous ALCL can occur at any age, with the peak incidence in patients in their sixties, with a slight male predominance.[76,133] Primary cutaneous ALCL can occur anywhere on the body. The lesions are brownish to violaceous nodules or tumors, ranging in number from solitary (most commonly) to numerous with generalized involvement. They may regress spontaneously. Histopathologically, at least 75 percent of the large cells should express CD30. Most cases are CD4+, with loss of pan–T-cell markers CD2, CD3, and CD5. In rare cases, the cells are CD8+CD30+. In contrast to systemic ALCL, primary cutaneous large cell lymphoma is negative for CD15 and epithelial membrane antigen.[134] In addition, primary cutaneous large cell lymphoma usually does not express anaplastic lymphoma kinase (ALK)-1 or the t(2;5) chromosomal translocation.[135,136] Presence of ALK-1 in cutaneous lesions without systemic involvement does not carry a worse prognosis.

LYMPHOMATOID PAPULOSIS

Lymphomatoid papulosis is the benign counterpart of primary cutaneous ALCL. It is characterized by crops of erythematous, dome-shaped papules or nodules that may ulcerate spontaneously (see Fig. 105–8B). It regresses over a few months with minor sequela such as scarring or atrophy (see Fig. 105–8B). The three main histologic types of lymphomatoid papulosis are A, B, and C. In type A, the infiltrate usually is wedge shaped with ulcer formation. The large atypical cells of type A resemble immunoblasts of Reed-Sternberg cells. These cells are surrounded by neutrophils and eosinophils. Type B cells resemble MF, with lichenoid lymphocytic infiltrate of cells with cerebriform nuclei and some epidermotropism. Type C cells resemble ALCL, with sheets of large CD30+ cells in the infiltrate. The histologic distinction between lymphomatoid papulosis and the corresponding condition may be difficult, and clinical correlation is required.[137] In rare cases, lymphomatoid papulosis evolves into more aggressive primary cutaneous large cell lymphoma. In addition, a higher incidence of lymphoid and nonlymphoid malignancies is observed in patients with lymphomatoid papulosis.[138]

■ TREATMENT

Lymphomatoid papulosis is extremely responsive to low-dose methotrexate therapy, requiring 10 to 15 mg weekly, with noticeable clinical response within a month. Other treatment options include PUVA therapy, retinoids, topical and systemic glucocorticoids, and intralesional and systemic interferon-α.[78,130,137] Treatment of primary cutaneous large cell lymphoma depends on the extent of skin involvement. In cases of solitary lesions, radiotherapy should be the initial treatment modality. A combination of PUVA and interferon-α may be considered. Combination chemotherapy should be reserved for resistant cases.[30,78,130] A new anti-CD30 antibody is in clinical trials to evaluate its efficacy and safety; the interim results are encouraging.

REFERENCES

1. Lorincz AL: Cutaneous T-cell lymphoma (mycosis fungoides). *Lancet* 347:871, 1996.
2. Alibert J: Description des maladies de la peau observeés à l'Hôpital Saint-Louis et exposition des meilleures méthodes suivies pour leur traitement. Barrois l'aîné et fils, 1806.
3. Sezary A, Bouvrain Y: Erythrodermie avec présence de cellules monstrueses dans le derme et dans lang circulant. *Bull Soc Fr Dermatol Syphiligr* 45, 1938.
4. Lutzner M, Edelson R, Schein P, et al: Cutaneous T-cell lymphomas: The Sézary syndrome, mycosis fungoides, and related disorders. *Ann Intern Med* 83:534, 1975.
5. Willemze R, Jaffe ES, Burg G, et al: WHO-EORTC classification for cutaneous lymphomas. *Blood* 105:3768, 2005.
6. Olsen E, Vonderheid E, Pimpinelli N, et al: Revisions to the staging and classification of mycosis fungoides and Sézary syndrome: A proposal of the International Society for Cutaneous Lymphomas (ISCL) and the cutaneous lymphoma task force of the European Organization of Research and Treatment of Cancer (EORTC). *Blood* 110:1713, 2007.
7. Criscione VD, Weinstock MA: Incidence of cutaneous T-cell lymphoma in the United States, 1973–2002. *Arch Dermatol* 143:854, 2007.
8. Kim YH, Liu HL, Mraz-Gernhard S, et al: Long-term outcome of 525 patients with mycosis fungoides and Sézary syndrome: Clinical prognostic factors and risk for disease progression. *Arch Dermatol* 139:857, 2003.
9. Weinstock MA, Reynes JF: The changing survival of patients with mycosis fungoides: A population-based assessment of trends in the United States. *Cancer* 85:208, 1999.
10. Weinstock MA, Gardstein B: Twenty-year trends in the reported incidence of mycosis fungoides and associated mortality. *Am J Public Health* 89:1240, 1999.
11. Poiesz BJ, Ruscetti FW, Gazdar AF, et al: Detection and isolation of type C retrovirus particles from fresh and cultured lymphocytes of a patient with cutaneous T-cell lymphoma. *Proc Natl Acad Sci U S A* 77:7415, 1980.
12. Wong-Staal F, Gallo RC: The family of human T-lymphotropic leukemia viruses: HTLV-I as the cause of adult T cell leukemia and HTLV-III as the cause of acquired immunodeficiency syndrome. *Blood* 65:253, 1985.
13. Fine RM. HTLV-V: A new human retrovirus associated with cutaneous T-cell lymphoma (mycosis fungoides). *Int J Dermatol* 27:473, 1988.
14. Yawalkar N, Ferenczi K, Jones DA, et al: Profound loss of T-cell receptor repertoire complexity in cutaneous T-cell lymphoma. *Blood* 102:4059, 2003.
15. Burg G, Dummer R, Haeffner A, et al: From inflammation to neoplasia: Mycosis fungoides evolves from reactive inflammatory conditions (lymphoid infiltrates) transforming into neoplastic plaques and tumors. *Arch Dermatol* 137:949, 2001.
16. Tan RS, Butterworth CM, McLaughlin H, et al: Mycosis fungoides—A disease of antigen persistence. *Br J Dermatol* 91:607, 1974.
17. Hoppe RT, Medeiros LJ, Warnke RA, Wood GS: CD8-positive tumor-infiltrating lymphocytes influence the long-term survival of patients with mycosis fungoides. *J Am Acad Dermatol* 32:448, 1995.
18. Seo N, Tokura Y, Matsumoto K, et al: Tumour-specific cytotoxic T lymphocyte activity in Th2-type Sézary syndrome: Its enhancement by interferon-gamma (IFN-gamma) and IL-12 and fluctuations in association with disease activity. *Clin Exp Immunol* 112:403, 1998.
19. Yoo EK, Cassin M, Lessin SR, Rook AH: Complete molecular remission during biologic response modifier therapy for Sézary syndrome is associated with enhanced helper T type 1 cytokine production and natural killer cell activity. *J Am Acad Dermatol* 45:208, 2001.
20. Vonderheid EC, Ekbote SK, Kerrigan K, et al: The prognostic significance of delayed hypersensitivity to dinitrochlorobenzene and mechlorethamine hydrochloride in cutaneous T cell lymphoma. *J Invest Dermatol* 110:946, 1998.
21. Dummer R, Geertsen R, Ludwig E, et al: Sézary syndrome, T-helper 2 cytokines and accessory factor-1 (AF-1). *Leuk Lymphoma* 28:515, 1998.
22. Vowels BR, Cassin M, Vonderheid EC, Rook AH: Aberrant cytokine production by Sézary syndrome patients: Cytokine secretion pattern resembles murine Th2 cells. *J Invest Dermatol* 99:90, 1992.
23. Rook AH, Heald P: The immunopathogenesis of cutaneous T-cell lymphoma. *Hematol Oncol Clin North Am* 9:997, 1995.
24. Smoller BR: Risk of secondary cutaneous malignancies in patients with long-standing mycosis fungoides. *J Am Acad Dermatol* 1994;31:295.
25. Morales-Suarez-Varela MM, Olsen J, Johansen P, et al: Occupational risk factors for mycosis fungoides: A European multicenter case-control study. *J Occup Environ Med* 46:205, 2004.
26. Epstein EH Jr, Levin DL, Croft JD Jr, Lutzner MA: Mycosis fungoides. Survival, prognostic features, response to therapy, and autopsy findings. *Medicine (Baltimore)* 51:61, 1972.
27. Naraghi ZS, Seirafi H, Valikhani M, et al: Assessment of histologic criteria in the diagnosis of mycosis fungoides. *Int J Dermatol* 42:45, 2003.
28. Sigel JE, Hsi ED: Immunohistochemical analysis of CD30-positive lymphoproliferative disorders for expression of CD95 and CD95L. *Mod Pathol* 13:446, 2000.
29. Duncan LM: Cutaneous lymphoma. Understanding the new classification schemes. *Dermatol Clin* 17:569, 1999.
30. Liu HL, Hoppe RT, Kohler S, et al: CD30+ cutaneous lymphoproliferative disorders: The Stanford experience in lymphomatoid papulosis and primary cutaneous anaplastic large cell lymphoma. *J Am Acad Dermatol* 49:1049, 2003.
31. Haynes BF, Metzgar RS, Minna JD, Bunn PA: Phenotypic characterization of cutaneous T-cell lymphoma. Use of monoclonal antibodies to compare with other malignant T cells. *N Engl J Med* 304:1319, 1981.
32. Kung PC, Berger CL, Goldstein G, et al: Cutaneous T cell lymphoma: Characterization by monoclonal antibodies. *Blood* 57:261, 1981.
33. Schroff RW, Foon KA, Billing RJ, Fahey JL: Immunologic classification of lymphocytic leukemias based on monoclonal antibody-defined cell surface antigens. *Blood* 59:207, 1982.
34. Broder S, Edelson RL, Lutzner MA, et al: The Sézary syndrome: A malignant proliferation of helper T cells. *J Clin Invest* 58:1297, 1976.
35. Haynes BF, Hensley LL, Jegasothy BV: Phenotypic characterization of skin-infiltrating T cells in cutaneous T-cell lymphoma: Comparison with benign cutaneous T-cell infiltrates. *Blood* 60:463, 1982.
36. Jones D, Dang NH, Duvic M, et al: Absence of CD26 expression is a useful marker for diagnosis of T-cell lymphoma in peripheral blood. *Am J Clin Pathol* 115:885, 2001.
37. Bernengo MG, Novelli M, Quaglino P, et al: The relevance of the CD4+ CD26- subset in the identification of circulating Sézary cells. *Br J Dermatol* 144:125, 2001.
38. Lu D, Patel KA, Duvic M, Jones D: Clinical and pathological spectrum of CD8-positive cutaneous T-cell lymphomas. *J Cutan Pathol* 29:465, 2002.
39. Santucci M, Pimpinelli N, Massi D, et al: Cytotoxic/natural killer cell cutaneous lymphomas. Report of EORTC Cutaneous Lymphoma Task Force Workshop. *Cancer* 97:610, 2003.
40. Scarisbrick JJ, Woolford AJ, Russell-Jones R, Whittaker SJ: Loss of heterozygosity on 10q and microsatellite instability in advanced stages of primary cutaneous T-cell lymphoma and possible association with homozygous deletion of PTEN: *Blood* 95:2937, 2000.
41. Navas IC, Algara P, Mateo M, et al: p16(INK4a) is selectively silenced in the tumoral progression of mycosis fungoides. *Lab Invest* 82:123, 2002.
42. Navas IC, Ortiz-Romero PL, Villuendas R, et al: p16(INK4a) gene alterations are frequent in lesions of mycosis fungoides. *Am J Pathol* 156:1565, 2000.
43. Bunn PA Jr, Lamberg SI: Report of the Committee on Staging and Classification of Cutaneous T-Cell Lymphomas. *Cancer Treat Rep* 63:725, 1979.
44. Lamberg SI, Bunn PA Jr: Cutaneous T-cell lymphomas. Summary of the Mycosis Fungoides Cooperative Group-National Cancer Institute Workshop. *Arch Dermatol* 115:1103, 1979.
45. Green SB, Byar DP, Lamberg SI: Prognostic variables in mycosis fungoides. *Cancer* 47:2671, 1981.
46. Lamberg SI, Green SB, Byar DP, et al: Clinical staging for cutaneous T-cell lymphoma. *Ann Intern Med* 100:187, 1984.
47. Fuks ZY, Castellino RA, Carmel JA, et al: Lymphography in mycosis fungoides. *Cancer* 34:106, 1974.
48. Hamminga L, Mulder JD, Evans C, et al: Staging lymphography with respect to lymph node histology, treatment, and follow-up in patients with mycosis fungoides. *Cancer* 47:692, 1981.
49. Toro JR, Stoll HL Jr, Stomper PC, Oseroff AR: Prognostic factors and evaluation of mycosis fungoides and Sézary syndrome. *J Am Acad Dermatol* 37:58, 1997.
50. Bunn PA Jr, Huberman MS, Whang-Peng J, et al: Prospective staging evaluation of patients with cutaneous T-cell lymphomas. Demonstration of a high frequency of extracutaneous dissemination. *Ann Intern Med* 93:223, 1980.
51. Breneman DL, Raju US, Breneman JC, et al: Lymph node grading for staging of mycosis fungoides may benefit from examination of multiple excised lymph nodes. *J Am Acad Dermatol* 48:702, 2003.
52. Zackheim HS, Amin S, Kashani-Sabet M, McMillan A: Prognosis in cutaneous T-cell lymphoma by skin stage: Long-term survival in 489 patients. *J Am Acad Dermatol* 40:418, 1999.
53. Scarisbrick JJ, Whittaker S, Evans AV, et al: Prognostic significance of tumor burden in the blood of patients with erythrodermic primary cutaneous T-cell lymphoma. *Blood* 97:624, 2001.
54. Muche JM, Lukowsky A, Asadullah K, et al: Demonstration of frequent occurrence of clonal T cells in the peripheral blood of patients with primary cutaneous T-cell lymphoma. *Blood* 90:1636, 1997.
55. Vonderheid EC, Pena J, Nowell P: Sézary cell counts in erythrodermic cutaneous T-cell lymphoma: Implications for prognosis and staging. *Leuk Lymphoma* 47:1841, 2006.
56. Vonderheid EC, Bernengo MG, Burg G, et al: Update on erythrodermic cutaneous T-cell lymphoma: Report of the International Society for Cutaneous Lymphomas. *J Am Acad Dermatol* 46:95, 2002.
57. Bergman R: How useful are T-cell receptor gene rearrangement studies as an adjunct to the histopathologic diagnosis of mycosis fungoides? *Am J Dermatopathol* 21:498, 1999.

58. Cherny S, Mraz S, Su L, et al: Heteroduplex analysis of T-cell receptor gamma gene rearrangement as an adjuvant diagnostic tool in skin biopsies for erythroderma. *J Cutan Pathol* 28:351, 2001.
59. Delfau-Larue MH, Dalac S, Lepage E, et al: Prognostic significance of a polymerase chain reaction-detectable dominant T-lymphocyte clone in cutaneous lesions of patients with mycosis fungoides. *Blood* 92:3376, 1998.
60. Poszepczynska-Guigne E, Bagot M, Wechsler J, et al: Minimal residual disease in mycosis fungoides follow-up can be assessed by polymerase chain reaction. *Br J Dermatol* 148:265, 2003.
61. Wood GS, Tung RM, Haeffner AC, et al: Detection of clonal T-cell receptor gamma gene rearrangements in early mycosis fungoides/Sézary syndrome by polymerase chain reaction and denaturing gradient gel electrophoresis (PCR/DGGE). *J Invest Dermatol* 103:34, 1994.
62. Long JC, Mihm MC: Mycosis fungoides with extracutaneous dissemination: A distinct clinicopathologic entity. *Cancer* 34:1745, 1974.
63. Smith DI, Vnencak-Jones CL, Boyd AS: T-lymphocyte clonality in benign lichenoid keratoses. *J Cutan Pathol* 29:623, 2002.
64. Nihal M, Mikkola D, Horvath N, et al: Cutaneous lymphoid hyperplasia: A lymphoproliferative continuum with lymphomatous potential. *Hum Pathol* 34:617, 2003.
65. Holm N, Flaig MJ, Yazdi AS, Sander CA: The value of molecular analysis by PCR in the diagnosis of cutaneous lymphocytic infiltrates. *J Cutan Pathol* 29:447, 2002.
66. Shieh S, Mikkola DL, Wood GS: Differentiation and clonality of lesional lymphocytes in pityriasis lichenoides chronica. *Arch Dermatol* 137:305, 2001.
67. Zucker-Franklin D: The role of human T cell lymphotropic virus type I tax in the development of cutaneous T cell lymphoma. *Ann N Y Acad Sci* 941:86, 2001.
68. Kikuchi A, Ohata Y, Matsumoto H, et al: Anti-HTLV-1 antibody positive cutaneous T-cell lymphoma. *Cancer* 79:269, 1997.
69. Palmer RA, Keefe M, Slater D, Whittaker SJ: Case 4: Pagetoid reticulosis (Woringer-Kolopp type) or unilesional mycosis fungoides (MF). *Clin Exp Dermatol* 27:345, 2002.
70. Wood GS, Weiss LM, Hu CH, et al: T-cell antigen deficiencies and clonal rearrangements of T-cell receptor genes in pagetoid reticulosis (Woringer-Kolopp disease). *N Engl J Med* 318:164, 1988.
71. Cohen EL: Woringer-Kolopp disease (pagetoid reticulosis). *Clin Exp Dermatol* 3:447, 1978.
72. Scarabello A, Fantini F, Giannetti A, Cerroni L: Localized pagetoid reticulosis (Woringer-Kolopp disease). *Br J Dermatol* 147:806, 2002.
73. Nakada T, Sueki H, Iijima M: Disseminated pagetoid reticulosis (Ketron-Goodman disease): Six-year follow-up. *J Am Acad Dermatol* 47:S183, 2002.
74. Fierro MT, Novelli M, Savoia P, et al: CD45RA+ immunophenotype in mycosis fungoides: Clinical, histological and immunophenotypical features in 22 patients. *J Cutan Pathol* 28:356, 2001.
75. Haghighi B, Smoller BR, LeBoit PE, et al: Pagetoid reticulosis (Woringer-Kolopp disease): An immunophenotypic, molecular, and clinicopathologic study. *Mod Pathol* 13:502, 2000.
76. Bekkenk MW, Geelen FA, van Voorst Vader PC, et al: Primary and secondary cutaneous CD30(+) lymphoproliferative disorders: A report from the Dutch Cutaneous Lymphoma Group on the long-term follow-up data of 219 patients and guidelines for diagnosis and treatment. *Blood* 95:3653, 2000.
77. Bekkenk MW, Vermeer MH, Jansen PM, et al: Peripheral T-cell lymphomas unspecified presenting in the skin: Analysis of prognostic factors in a group of 82 patients. *Blood* 102:2213, 2003.
78. Willemze R, Meijer CJ: Primary cutaneous CD30-positive lymphoproliferative disorders. *Hematol Oncol Clin North Am* 17:1319, vii, 2003.
79. Horwitz SM, Olsen EA, Duvic M, et al: Review of the treatment of mycosis fungoides and Sézary syndrome: A stage-based approach. *J Natl Compr Canc Netw* 6:436, 2008.
80. Reitamo S, Rissanen J, Remitz A, et al: Tacrolimus ointment does not affect collagen synthesis: Results of a single-center randomized trial. *J Invest Dermatol* 111:396, 1998.
81. Vonderheid EC, Van Scott EJ, Johnson WC, et al: Topical chemotherapy and immunotherapy of mycosis fungoides: Intermediate-term results. *Arch Dermatol* 113:454, 1977.
82. Du Vivier A, Vonderheid EC, Van Scott EJ, Urbach F: Mycosis fungoides, nitrogen mustard and skin cancer. *Br J Dermatol* 99:61, 1978.
83. Zackheim HS, Epstein EH Jr, Grekin DA: Treatment of mycosis fungoides with topical BCNU: *Cancer Treat Rep* 63:623, 1979.
84. Kempf W, Kettelhack N, Duvic M, Burg G: Topical and systemic retinoid therapy for cutaneous T-cell lymphoma. *Hematol Oncol Clin North Am* 17:1405, 2003.
85. Martin AG: Bexarotene gel: A new skin-directed treatment option for cutaneous T-cell lymphomas. *J Drugs Dermatol* 2:155, 2003.
86. Baron ED, Stevens SR: Phototherapy for cutaneous T-cell lymphoma. *Dermatol Ther* 16:303, 2003.
87. Ramsay DL, Lish KM, Yalowitz CB, Soter NA: Ultraviolet-B phototherapy for early-stage cutaneous T-cell lymphoma. *Arch Dermatol* 128:931, 1992.
88. Samson Yashar S, Gielczyk R, Scherschun L, Lim HW: Narrow-band ultraviolet B treatment for vitiligo, pruritus, and inflammatory dermatoses. *Photodermatol Photoimmunol Photomed* 19:164, 2003.
89. Gilchrest BA: Methoxsalen photochemotherapy for mycosis fungoides. *Cancer Treat Rep* 63:663, 1979.
90. Herrmann JJ, Roenigk HH Jr, Hurria A, et al: Treatment of mycosis fungoides with photochemotherapy (PUVA): Long-term follow-up. *J Am Acad Dermatol* 33:234, 1995.
91. Roenigk HH Jr, Kuzel TM, Skoutelis AP, et al. Photochemotherapy alone or combined with interferon alpha-2a in the treatment of cutaneous T-cell lymphoma. *J Invest Dermatol* 95:198S, 1990.
92. Geskin L: ECP versus PUVA for the treatment of cutaneous T-cell lymphoma. *Skin Therapy Lett* 12:1, 2007.
93. Orenstein A, Haik J, Tamir J, et al: Photodynamic therapy of cutaneous lymphoma using 5-aminolevulinic acid topical application. *Dermatol Surg* 26:765; discussion 769, 2000.
94. Edstrom DW, Porwit A, Ros AM: Photodynamic therapy with topical 5-aminolevulinic acid for mycosis fungoides: Clinical and histological response. *Acta Derm Venereol* 81:184, 2001.
95. Jones GW, Kacinski BM, Wilson LD, et al: Total skin electron radiation in the management of mycosis fungoides: Consensus of the European Organization for Research and Treatment of Cancer (EORTC) Cutaneous Lymphoma Project Group. *J Am Acad Dermatol* 47:364, 2002.
96. Duvic M, Apisarnthanarax N, Cohen DS, et al: Analysis of long-term outcomes of combined modality therapy for cutaneous T-cell lymphoma. *J Am Acad Dermatol* 49:35, 2003.
97. Hoppe R: Total skin electron beam therapy in the management of mycosis fungoides, in *The Role of High Energy Electrons in the Treatment of Cancer*, edited by M Vaeth, p 80. S Karger, Basel, Switzerland, 1991.
98. Kamstrup MR, Specht L, Skovgaard GL, Gniadecki R: A prospective, open-label study of low-dose total skin electron beam therapy in mycosis fungoides. *Int J Radiat Oncol Biol Phys* 71:1204, 2008.
99. Do JH, McLaughlin SS, Gaspari AA: Topical imiquimod therapy for cutaneous T-cell lymphoma. *Skinmed* 2:316, 2003.
100. Dummer R, Urosevic M, Kempf W, et al: Imiquimod induces complete clearance of a PUVA-resistant plaque in mycosis fungoides. *Dermatology* 207:116, 2003.
101. Duvic M, Hymes K, Heald P, et al: Bexarotene is effective and safe for treatment of refractory advanced-stage cutaneous T-cell lymphoma: Multinational phase II-III trial results. *J Clin Oncol* 19:2456, 2001.
102. Duvic M, Martin AG, Kim Y, et al: Phase 2 and 3 clinical trial of oral bexarotene (Targretin capsules) for the treatment of refractory or persistent early-stage cutaneous T-cell lymphoma. *Arch Dermatol* 137:581, 2001.
103. Assaf C, Bagot M, Dummer R, et al: Minimizing adverse side-effects of oral bexarotene in cutaneous T-cell lymphoma: An expert opinion. *Br J Dermatol* 155:261, 2006.
104. Zhang C, Duvic M: Treatment of cutaneous T-cell lymphoma with retinoids. *Dermatol Ther* 19:264, 2006.
105. Olsen EA, Kim YH, Kuzel TM, et al: Phase IIb multicenter trial of vorinostat in patients with persistent, progressive, or treatment refractory cutaneous T-cell lymphoma. *J Clin Oncol* 25:3109, 2007.
105a. Piekarz RL, Frye R, Turner M, et al: Phase II multi-institutional trial of the histone deacetylase inhibitor romidepsin as monotherapy for patients with cutaneous T-cell lymphoma. *J Clin Oncol* 27:5410, 2009.
106. Olsen EA: Interferon in the treatment of cutaneous T-cell lymphoma. *Dermatol Ther* 16:311, 2003.
107. Edelson R, Berger C, Gasparro F, et al: Treatment of cutaneous T-cell lymphoma by extracorporeal photochemotherapy. Preliminary results. *N Engl J Med* 316:297, 1987.
108. Knobler R, Girardi M: Extracorporeal photochemoimmunotherapy in cutaneous T cell lymphomas. *Ann N Y Acad Sci* 941:123, 2001.
109. Kennedy GA, Seymour JF, Wolf M, et al: Treatment of patients with advanced mycosis fungoides and Sézary syndrome with alemtuzumab. *Eur J Haematol* 71:250, 2003.
110. Lundin J, Hagberg H, Repp R, et al: Phase 2 study of alemtuzumab (anti-CD52 monoclonal antibody) in patients with advanced mycosis fungoides/Sézary syndrome. *Blood* 101:4267, 2003.
111. Alinari L, Geskin L, Grady T, et al: Subcutaneous alemtuzumab for Sézary syndrome in the very elderly. *Leuk Res* 32:1299, 2008.
112. Bernengo MG, Quaglino P, Comessatti A, et al: Low-dose intermittent alemtuzumab in the treatment of Sézary syndrome: Clinical and immunologic findings in 14 patients. *Haematologica* 92:784, 2007.
113. Olsen E, Duvic M, Frankel A, et al: Pivotal phase III trial of two dose levels of denileukin diftitox for the treatment of cutaneous T-cell lymphoma. *J Clin Oncol* 19:376, 2001.
114. Negro-Vilar A, Dziewanowska Z, Groves ES, et al: Efficacy and safety of denileukin diftitox (Dd) in a phase III, double-blind, placebo-controlled study of CD25+ patients with cutaneous T-cell lymphoma (CTCL). *J Clin Oncol* 25:8026, 2007.
114a. O'Connor OA, Horwitz S, Hamlin P, et al: Phase II-I-II study of two different doses and schedules of pralatrexate, a high-affinity substrate for the reduced folate carrier, in patients with relapsed or refractory lymphoma reveals marked activity in T-cell malignancies. *J Clin Oncol* 27:4357, 2009.
115. Van Scott EJ, Grekin DA, Kalmanson JD, et al: Frequent low doses of intravenous mechlorethamine for late-stage mycosis fungoides lymphoma. *Cancer* 36:1613, 1975.
116. Van Scott EJ, Auerbach R, Clendenning WE: Treatment of mycosis fungoides with cyclophosphamide. *Arch Dermatol* 85:499, 1962.
117. Zackheim HS, Kashani-Sabet M, Hwang ST: Low-dose methotrexate to treat erythrodermic cutaneous T-cell lymphoma: Results in twenty-nine patients. *J Am Acad Dermatol* 34:626, 1996.
118. Spigel SC, Coltman CA Jr: Therapy of mycosis fungoides with bleomycin. *Cancer* 32:767, 1973.
119. Levi JA, Diggs CH, Wiernik PH: Adriamycin therapy in advanced mycosis fungoides. *Cancer* 39:1967, 1977.

120. Wollina U, Dummer R, Brockmeyer NH, et al: Multicenter study of pegylated liposomal doxorubicin in patients with cutaneous T-cell lymphoma. *Cancer* 98:993, 2003.
121. Foss FM: Activity of pentostatin (Nipent) in cutaneous T-cell lymphoma: Single-agent and combination studies. *Semin Oncol* 27:58, 2000.
122. Kurzrock R: Therapy of T cell lymphomas with pentostatin. *Ann N Y Acad Sci* 941:200, 2001.
123. Quaglino P, Fierro MT, Rossotto GL, et al: Treatment of advanced mycosis fungoides/Sézary syndrome with fludarabine and potential adjunctive benefit to subsequent extracorporeal photochemotherapy. *Br J Dermatol* 150:327, 2004.
124. Zinzani PL, Baliva G, Magagnoli M, et al: Gemcitabine treatment in pretreated cutaneous T-cell lymphoma: Experience in 44 patients. *J Clin Oncol* 18:2603, 2000.
125. Vonderheid EC: Treatment of cutaneous T cell lymphoma: 2001. *Recent Results Cancer Res* 160:309, 2002.
126. Abd-el-Baki J, Demierre MF, Li N, Foss FM: Transformation in mycosis fungoides: The role of methotrexate. *J Cutan Med Surg* 6:109, 2002.
127. Kaye FJ, Bunn PA Jr, Steinberg SM, et al: A randomized trial comparing combination electron-beam radiation and chemotherapy with topical therapy in the initial treatment of mycosis fungoides. *N Engl J Med* 321:1784, 1989.
128. Rosen ST, Foss FM: Chemotherapy for mycosis fungoides and the Sézary syndrome. *Hematol Oncol Clin North Am* 9:1109, 1995.
129. Vonderheid EC: Treatment planning in cutaneous T-cell lymphoma. *Dermatol Ther* 16:276, 2003.
130. Kadin ME, Carpenter C: Systemic and primary cutaneous anaplastic large cell lymphomas. *Semin Hematol* 40:244, 2003.
131. Willemze R, Beljaards RC: Spectrum of primary cutaneous CD30 (Ki-1)-positive lymphoproliferative disorders. A proposal for classification and guidelines for management and treatment. *J Am Acad Dermatol* 28:973, 1993.
132. Bergman R, Marcus-Farber BS, Manov L, et al: Clinicopathologic reassessment of non-mycosis fungoides primary cutaneous lymphomas during 17 years. *Int J Dermatol* 41:735, 2002.
133. Tomaszewski MM, Moad JC, Lupton GP: Primary cutaneous Ki-1(CD30) positive anaplastic large cell lymphoma in childhood. *J Am Acad Dermatol* 40:857, 1999.
134. Gorczyca W, Tsang P, Liu Z, et al: CD30-positive T-cell lymphomas co-expressing CD15: An immunohistochemical analysis. *Int J Oncol* 22:319, 2003.
135. Jaffe ES: Anaplastic large cell lymphoma: The shifting sands of diagnostic hematopathology. *Mod Pathol* 14:219, 2001.
136. DeCoteau JF, Butmarc JR, Kinney MC, Kadin ME: The t(2;5) chromosomal translocation is not a common feature of primary cutaneous CD30+ lymphoproliferative disorders: Comparison with anaplastic large-cell lymphoma of nodal origin. *Blood* 87:3437, 1996.
137. El Shabrawi-Caelen L, Kerl H, Cerroni L: Lymphomatoid papulosis: Reappraisal of clinicopathologic presentation and classification into subtypes A, B, and C: *Arch Dermatol* 140:441, 2004.
138. Wang HH, Myers T, Lach LJ, et al: Increased risk of lymphoid and nonlymphoid malignancies in patients with lymphomatoid papulosis. *Cancer* 86:1240, 1999.

CHAPTER 106

MATURE T-CELL AND NATURAL KILLER CELL LYMPHOMAS

Oscar B. Goodman Jr. and Nam H. Dang

SUMMARY

Mature T-cell lymphomas comprise a biologically heterogeneous group of diseases defined by their histopathologic and clinical characteristics. They account for approximately 10 to 15 percent of all lymphoid malignancies. There is considerable variation in incidence worldwide with respect to race and region. Although the reason for this is not known, in some instances specific viral infections are linked to selected subtypes. In general, these lymphomas are biologically more aggressive and less responsive to conventional chemotherapy than their B-cell counterparts, but have a highly variable course. With the exception of anaplastic large cell lymphoma, the role of intensive chemotherapy remains largely undefined,[1] prompting many to examine the potential utility of targeted therapies in these diseases.

CLASSIFICATION

The classification of mature T-cell and natural killer (NK)-cell lymphomas has undergone reorganization over the last 15 years. Initially, the working formulation, based on morphology, did not define lymphomas based on cell of origin.[2] In 1994, the revised European-American classification of lymphoid neoplasm (REAL) was developed by the International Lymphoma Study Group, and although largely descriptive, incorporated cell lineages and clinical features and was the first classification to designate T-cell lymphomas.[3] The REAL classification further divided T-cell lymphomas into two groups based on the extent of maturation, the precursor T-cell lymphomas, and peripheral T-cell lymphomas. T-cell lymphomas were further subdivided by clinical behavior and risk (low, intermediate, and high risk).

Abbreviations and acronyms used in this chapter include: ADCC, antibody-dependent cell-mediated cytotoxicity; AILD, angioimmunoblastic lymphadenopathy with dysproteinemia; AITL, angioimmunoblastic T-cell lymphoma; ALCL, anaplastic large cell lymphoma; CHOP, cyclophosphamide, hydroxydaunorubicin (doxorubicin), vincristine (Oncovin), prednisone; CR, complete remission; EBV, Epstein-Barr virus; HTLV, human T-lymphotropic virus; IPI, international prognostic index; LGL, larger granular lymphocyte; MACOP-B, high-dose methotrexate, doxorubicin, cyclophosphamide, vincristine, prednisone, bleomycin; mAb, monoclonal antibody; NK, natural killer; PCR, polymerase chain reaction; PR, partial remission; PTCL, peripheral T-cell lymphoma; RANKL, receptor activator of nuclear factor-κB ligand; RANTES, regulated upon activation, normal T-cell expressed and secreted; REAL, revised European-American classification of lymphoid neoplasm; TARC, thymus and activation-regulated chemokine; TCR, T-cell receptor; VEPA, vincristine, cyclophosphamide, prednisolone, and doxorubicin; VEPA-M, VEPA plus methotrexate; WHO, World Health Organization.

In 2001, the European Association for Haematopathology and the Society for Hematopathology jointly revised the REAL classification, creating the World Health Organization (WHO) classification of Tumors of the Haematopoietic and Lymphoid in use today and further described in Chaps. 92 and 98. There are 14 major disease categories of mature T-cell and NK cell neoplasms, defined on the basis of anatomical disease distribution and the putative cell of origin (Table 106–1).[4] Chap. 105 discusses the cutaneous T-cell lymphomas, mycosis fungoides, Sézary syndrome, and primary cutaneous CD30-positive T-cell lymphoproliferative disorders.

LEUKEMIC MATURE T-CELL AND NATURAL KILLER CELL NEOPLASMS

T-CELL PROLYMPHOCYTIC LEUKEMIA

Epidemiology

T-cell prolymphocytic leukemia (T-PLL) represents less than 1 percent of all lymphomas and approximately 20 percent of all prolymphocytic leukemias, the remainder being of B-cell origin (see Chap. 94). This disease has a male predilection with a 3:2 male-to-female ratio. Human T-cell lymphotropic virus (HTLV)-1 infection has been implicated in at least some cases of T-PLL, particularly in southwestern Japan where HTLV-1 infection is endemic.[5,6] In these cases, despite HTLV seronegativity, genomic integration of defective HTLV-1 provirus can be detected by polymerase chain reaction (PCR).

Clinical Features

This is a rare disease characterized by massive splenomegaly and leukocytosis. The clinical course is typically fulminant as there is no standard therapy. In T-PLL, prolymphocytes constitute more than 55 percent of the white blood cells. In addition to the characteristic appearance of the prolymphocytes, cells in the T-PLL exhibit convoluted nuclei, with leukemia cutis seen in approximately one-third of cases. In T-PLL, the prolymphocytes typically express the pan T-markers CD2, CD3, CD5, and CD7. The majority of cases express a CD4+CD8– immunophenotype, consistent with a malignant cell of T-helper origin, but gain or loss of CD8 or CD4, respectively, may also be seen. The most common cytogenetic abnormalities involve chromosome 14.[7]

Therapy

T-PLL is relatively resistant to conventional chemotherapy, as demonstrated by a study involving 78 patients with T-PLL.[8] Thirty-two patients had received alkylating agents and nine (28%) experienced transient partial remission (PR). Five of 15 patients (33%) responded to CHOP (cyclophosphamide, hydroxydaunorubicin [doxorubicin], vincristine [Oncovin], prednisone), with one complete remission (CR) lasting 3 months. However, of the 31 patients treated with pentostatin, 15 had responses, 3 complete, lasting 8, 10, and 12 months, and 12 partial, of which 8 were in 15 patients treated with pentostatin as initial therapy. Based on these data, pentostatin and cladribine represent the current preferred cytotoxic chemotherapy for T-PLL, although their efficacy is limited.

Alemtuzumab (CAMPATH-1H), a humanized immunoglobulin (Ig) $G_1\kappa$ monoclonal antibody (mAb) to the panlymphocytic antigen CD52, has demonstrated some activity. In a study involving 39 patients with T-PLL of whom 37 had chemorefractory disease, 76 percent of patients responded to CAMPATH-1H administered three times weekly intravenously. Patient dose escalation up to 30 mg, three times weekly, resulted in a complete response in 60 percent of patients.[9]

TABLE 106–1. WHO Classification of Mature T- and NK-Cell Neoplasms

Leukemic neoplasms:
T-cell prolymphocytic leukemia
T-cell large granular lymphocytic leukemia
Aggressive NK-cell leukemia
Nodal neoplasms:
Adult T-cell leukemia/lymphoma
Anaplastic large cell lymphoma
Peripheral T-cell lymphoma, unspecified
Angioimmunoblastic T-cell lymphoma
Extranodal neoplasms:
Hepatosplenic T-cell lymphoma
Nasal NK/T-cell lymphoma
Enteropathy-type T-cell lymphoma
Subcutaneous panniculitis T-cell lymphoma
Cutaneous neoplasms
Mycosis fungoides
Sézary syndrome
Primary cutaneous CD-30 positive T-cell lymphoproliferative disorders

CD, cluster of differentiation; NK, natural killer; WHO, World Health Organization.

Both myeloablative and low-intensity conditioning allogeneic stem cell transplantation has been used in patients with T-PLL, with a number of good responses.[10–13] Although the numbers are small, long-term complete responses were observed, accompanied by graft-versus-host disease (GVHD) in all cases, suggesting a potent graft-versus-leukemia response.

T-CELL LARGE GRANULAR LYMPHOCYTIC LEUKEMIA

Epidemiology, Etiology, and Pathogenesis

T-cell large granular lymphocytic (LGL) leukemia accounts for approximately 2 to 5 percent of all mature T-cell/NK cell neoplasms.[14] Most cases (85%) diagnosed in Western countries are indolent, and occur at a median age of 60 years (see Chap. 96). An aggressive variant comprising the remainder occurs in younger patients and is more common in Asia and South America. The etiology and pathogenesis of T-cell LGL is not well understood, but chronic antigenic activation of CD8+ T cells has been proposed to initiate the expansion of the LGL compartment.[15,16]

Clinical Features

The majority of patients will present with a constellation of signs and symptoms including cytopenias in association with recurrent bacterial infections, splenomegaly (20–50%), or rheumatoid arthritis (25–33%), reflective of concomitant immune system dysregulation.[17] T-cell LGL is often indistinguishable from Felty syndrome,[18] and thus they appear to be intimately related disorders. Splenomegaly results from the direct invasion of the splenic red pulp by neoplastic cells.[19]

Laboratory Features

Neutropenia is the most common cytopenia and is found in 80 percent of patients, with nearly half of patients presenting with grade IV neutropenia (neutrophil count <500/μL), typically associated with infection.[14] Multiple mechanisms account for neutropenia, including antineutrophil antibody-dependent cytotoxicity (ADCC), a maturation arrest mediated by destruction by the neoplastic cells or enhanced FAS-dependent apoptosis of neutrophils.[20,21] Anemia is seen in nearly half of patients with T-cell LGL leukemia, with pure red cell aplasia seen in approximately 15 percent of patients.[22] Thrombocytopenia, seen in approximately 20 percent of patients, results from inhibition of megakaryopoiesis, immune destruction or splenic sequestration.[14] The diagnosis of T-cell LGL leukemia is typically suspected based on clinical presentation and may be confirmed by performing PCR T-cell receptor rearrangement studies. Clonal populations of leukemic LGL cells exhibiting a CD3+CD8+CD57+ immunophenotype may be observed using flow cytometry, but are not necessary to establish the diagnosis.[23]

Therapy

Treatment of T-cell LGL leukemia is largely guided by the patient's signs and symptoms, with recurrent infections in the setting of neutropenia, or other symptomatic cytopenias triggering therapy. No phase III randomized clinical trials have been performed and so treatment is based on retrospective data from smaller studies. Although monotherapy with prednisone (1 mg/kg per day) may be efficacious, it is not usually sufficient to induce a sustained remission, and thus is typically given with low-dose oral methotrexate (10 mg/m^2 weekly) then tapered after 1 month of therapy. With this approach, the majority of patients achieve a CR. Alternatively, oral cyclosporine (5–10 mg/kg daily) or oral cyclophosphamide (100 mg orally daily) may be used. After normalization of cytopenias, these agents should be tapered down and maintained at the lowest possible dose to minimize toxicity.[23] Currently, this approach is being evaluated prospectively by the Eastern Cooperative Oncology Group (ECOG 5998 trial). Durable responses have also been observed with purine nucleoside analogues.[24]

A number of targeted therapeutic approaches are also being investigated. The humanized anti-CD2 mAb siplizumab (MEDI-507, MedImmune, Gaithersburg, MD), is available in two phase I dose-escalation studies in patients with relapsed or refractory CD2+ T-cell lymphoma-leukemia, including T-cell LGL leukemia. Given the expression of CD52 by malignant cells, alemtuzumab is also being examined as a therapy.[25] Given the constitutive activation of the renin–angiotensin system–mitogen-activated protein kinase pathway, tipifarnib, an oral farnesyltransferase inhibitor is also being evaluated in a phase II trial through the Office of Rare Diseases.

AGGRESSIVE NATURAL KILLER-CELL LYMPHOMA

Epidemiology, Etiology, and Pathogenesis

Aggressive NK-cell leukemia is a rare disease, accounting for less than 1 percent of all T-cell lymphomas (see Chap. 96). They are typically accompanied by an atypical lymphocytosis in the blood. Younger patients (median age: 39 years) of Asian ethnicity are affected most commonly. The Epstein-Barr virus (EBV) has been implicated in its pathogenesis.[26] The most common observed cytogenetic abnormalities are deletions of 17p13 and 6q21–25.[27] 17p13 is the site of the p53 gene. Isochromosome(i)7 (q10) also occurs. Genes corresponding to 6q21–25 and i(7)(q10) are unknown.

Clinical Features

Typically, the presentation is fulminant with cytopenias, hepatosplenomegaly, and disseminated intravascular coagulation.[28] NK-cell leukemias can readily be distinguished from their T-cell counterparts by their immunophenotype, which is typically CD2+ CD3–CD56+, and are usually negative for CD57.[17] There is also an indolent NK-cell leukemia, not currently classified as a separate entity by the WHO, which presents as a chronic leukemia with an isolated atypical lymphocytosis in the absence of systemic symptoms.[17]

Therapy

Conventional cytotoxic chemotherapy usually is ineffective for aggressive NK-cell leukemias.[29] Induction chemotherapy using acute lymphocytic leukemia-like regimens that include central nervous system prophylaxis, followed by high-dose chemotherapy and allogeneic stem cell transplantation, is appropriate (see Chap. 93).[30] For relapsed or refractory disease, clinical trials should be considered. Like T-cell LGL leukemias, the neoplastic cells are CD2+, and the CD2 antibody siplizumab may represent a rational therapeutic strategy. In a multicenter phase I trial that enrolled 16 patients, one of the two objective responses observed was in a patient with NK-cell leukemia.[31]

NODAL MATURE T-CELL NEOPLASMS

■ ADULT T-CELL LEUKEMIA/LYMPHOMA

Epidemiology

Adult T-cell leukemia/lymphoma is a viral-associated lymphoproliferative syndrome initially characterized in 1977 and later identified in other countries including the United States and Caribbean islands.[32,33] Considerable evidence implicates HTLV-1, a retrovirus, in the pathogenesis of this disease.[34] Disease incidence is highest in southwestern Japan, and also endemic in South America, equatorial Africa, and the Caribbean region, paralleling the prevalence of HTLV-1 infection. Among HTLV-1 carriers, the lifetime risk of developing adult T-cell leukemia/lymphoma is approximately 2.5 to 4 percent.[35,36] HTLV-1 infection is more common in females and it is transmitted by sexual and blood-borne routes. The mean age of patients with adult T-cell leukemia/lymphoma is 62 years, with a male-to-female ratio of 1.2:1.[37]

Clinical Features

Neoplastic cells suppress B-cell immunoglobulin secretion by a complex mechanism involving induction of suppressor cells after activation of normal suppressor cell precursors.[38] Opportunistic infections are common in patients with adult T-cell leukemia/lymphoma, even indolent forms.[39] *Pneumocystis carinii* infections and cryptococcal meningitis are common, as well as bacterial and other fungal infections.

Clinically, the disease may present with both a leukemic and lymphomatous component involving marrow, blood, and lymph nodes, either initially or developing during the disease course. Clinical presentations are variable, including an aggressive acute syndrome with leukemia, a lymphoma without lymphocytosis, a chronic process with a modest leukemic phase, and a smoldering condition.[40] Presenting features include lymphadenopathy, hepatosplenomegaly, leukemia cutis, cerebrospinal fluid involvement, hypercalcemia (with or without lytic bone lesions), and interstitial lung disease. Onset of symptoms typically is acute, with rapidly developing cutaneous lesions, hypercalcemia, or both.[32] Hypercalcemia in adult T-cell leukemia/lymphoma results from the paraneoplastic production of parathyroid hormone-related protein by osteoclasts, with osteoclastogenesis mediated by malignant T cells. Neoplastic cells derived from patients with hypercalcemia, but not from those with normal calcium levels, express receptor activator of nuclear factor-κB (RANKL), a factor that promotes the differentiation of hematopoietic stem cells to osteoclasts. *In vitro*, direct contact between the neoplastic T cell and the stem cell is required, implicating a membranous rather than soluble form of RANKL.[1]

Patients with hypercalcemia typically present with weakness, lethargy, confusion, polyuria, and polydipsia. The median survival is less than 1 year, with lymphomatous disease having a slightly better prognosis than the acute leukemic form. A multivariate analysis of 126 patients with acute (13%) and lymphomatous (87%) subtypes of adult T-cell leukemia/lymphoma performed by the International Peripheral T-Cell Lymphoma Project indicated that the international prognostic index (IPI) was the only independent predictor of overall survival.[37]

In addition to the acute and lymphomatous forms, chronic and smoldering forms of adult T-cell leukemia/lymphoma occur, typically presenting with predominance of skin lesions and a lack of visceral, marrow, and blood involvement. Survival rates for these subtypes exceed 2 years. The proportion of adult T-cell leukemia/lymphoma cells in the blood of patients with smoldering disease is low (<5%), with minimal lymphadenopathy, hepatosplenomegaly, and marrow infiltration. Patients have developed aggressive adult T-cell leukemia/lymphoma after years of indolent disease. Patients with smoldering adult T-cell leukemia/lymphoma are more likely to have a normal karyotype.

Cutaneous involvement occurs in approximately two-thirds of patients. The appearance of skin lesions varies, in some cases appearing as discrete tumors, whereas in others there are small nodules that may be confluent. Other patients present with plaques, papules, nonspecific erythematous patches, or erythroderma. Histologically, focal epidermal infiltration with lymphoma cells or Pautrier microabscesses is seen in most patients with cutaneous involvement. Pautrier microabscesses, thought to be pathognomonic of mycosis fungoides, may also occur in patients with adult T-cell leukemia/lymphoma (see Chap. 105). The cutaneous presentation of HTLV-1 infection at times can be clinically similar to that of mycoses fungoides, but diagnostically distinguishable as most cases of mycosis fungoides show no antibodies to the structural proteins of HTLV-1. However, HTLV-1 seropositivity is not entirely specific for adult T-cell leukemia/lymphoma as patients with cutaneous T-cell lymphoma may harbor the Tax sequence of HTLV-1, encoding the regulatory protein $p40^{Tax}$.[41]

Lymph node enlargement occurs in nearly all patients, although the nodes initially may be small. Many patients have generalized lymphadenopathy, and most have retroperitoneal adenopathy. Hilar adenopathy is common, but a mediastinal mass is rare. The patient's marrow may be infiltrated with leukemia cells. Additional extranodal sites of disease include the lung, liver, skin, gastrointestinal tract, and central nervous system, which can manifest itself as cord myelopathy and spastic paraparesis. In addition, adult T-cell leukemia/lymphoma can be associated with several histologic subtypes, including (1) diffuse, poorly differentiated small cell lymphoma, (2) mixed large and small cell lymphoma, and (3) large cell immunoblastic lymphoma. No apparent correlation exists between clinical course and lymph node histopathology.

Laboratory Features

The neoplastic cells are pleomorphic, have highly lobulated nuclei with condensed nuclear chromatin, inconspicuous nucleoli, and exhibit a mature helper T-lymphocyte immunophenotype, expressing CD2, CD3, and CD4 antigens (Fig. 106–1).[42] In approximately 20 percent of cases, nuclear lobulation is less pronounced, and the cells may be difficult to distinguish from Sézary cells (see Fig. 105–6A and –B). The antigen CD25, the p55 subunit of the interleukin (IL)-2 receptor, is also frequently expressed,[43] suggesting an opportunity for targeted therapy. Clonal rearrangements of the T-cell receptor (TCR) β-chain are typically present.[44–46]

When a leukemic phase is present, the leukocyte count ranges from 5000 to 100,000/μL (5–100 × 10^9/L). Not all patients have blood involvement at diagnosis, although circulating leukemia cells eventually are identified in most cases. Anemia and thrombocytopenia are

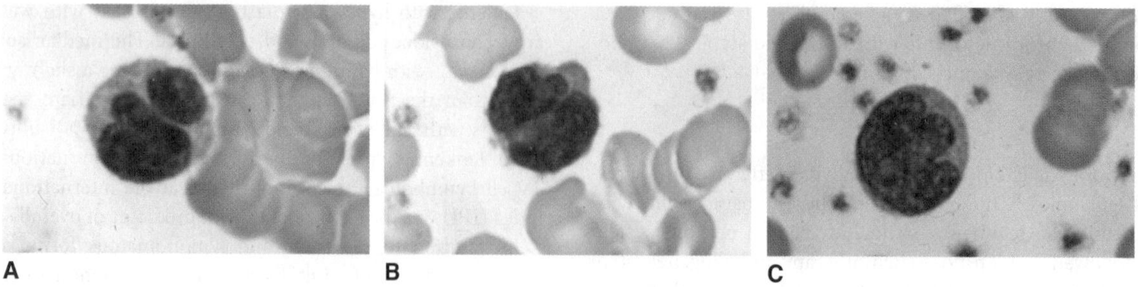

FIGURE 106–1. Blood film from a patient from the Caribbean region with adult T-cell leukemia-lymphoma. **A–C.** Note highly lobulated and clefted nuclei in lymphocytes, findings characteristic of this disease. *(Reproduced from* Lichtman's Atlas of Hematology, *www.accessmedicine.com, with permission.)*

uncommon at presentation. Radionuclide bone scans of patients with the acute adult T-cell leukemia/lymphoma syndrome typically show a diffuse increased uptake throughout the skeleton, most prominent in the joints and skull. These scans are referred to as *superscans* and are unusual in other patients with malignant lymphomas. Isolated lytic bone lesions also may occur.

Therapy

Although initial anthracycline-based combination chemotherapy results in responses approximately 70 percent of the time, only one-third of patients achieve a CR. Based on the International Peripheral T-Cell Lymphoma Project analysis of patients with adult T-cell leukemia/lymphoma, there was no overall survival benefit for those patients receiving an anthracycline-containing regimen.[37] Despite its limited efficacy, cytotoxic chemotherapy remains the mainstay of therapy for this disease. In Japan, a randomized phase III trial of vincristine, cyclophosphamide, prednisolone, and doxorubicin (VEPA) versus VEPA plus methotrexate (VEPA-M)[47,48] resulted in a complete response rate of 37 percent (11/30) in patients treated with VEPA-M and 17 percent (4/24) in patients treated with VEPA. Median survival, however, was 6 months. A phase II Japanese study tested LSG 15 administered with granulocyte colony-stimulating factor support to patients with treatment-naïve aggressive adult T-cell leukemia/lymphoma. The eight-drug regimen (vincristine, cyclophosphamide, doxorubicin, prednisone, ranimustine, vindesine, etoposide, and carboplatin) was administered to 96 previously untreated patients. For the 93 eligible patients, the overall response rate was 81 percent, with 35 percent complete responses and 45 percent partial responses. The median survival was 13 months.[49] A combination trial of pentostatin, vincristine, doxorubicin, etoposide, and prednisolone resulted in 28 percent complete responses (17/60) and 24 percent (14/60) partial responses. Median survival, however, was only 7.4 months.[50] Irinotecan is a modestly active drug in adult T-cell leukemia/lymphoma, with a response rate of 30 percent (5/13) in a phase II trial, with one complete responder. Major toxicities included leucopenia (83%), nausea (69%), and diarrhea (62%).[51]

Encouraging responses have been observed in patients who received passive immunotherapy or radioimmunotherapy using monoclonal antibodies specific for antigens expressed by the neoplastic T cells, such as CD25.[52,53] Even in pretreated patients, complete responses to denileukin diftitox have been observed.[54] Of 15 patients with adult T-cell leukemia/lymphoma who received α-interferon and zidovudine (AZT), 11 of whom had previously received anthracycline-containing chemotherapy regimens, 7 patients had progressive disease and 8 were in remission. Partial responses lasting 2 to 44+ months (median duration: 10 months) occurred in 10 (67%) patients; 4 (26%) patients had primary refractory disease, and 1 patient was not evaluable. Eight patients died 3 to 41 months from diagnosis. Median survival for all 15 patients was 18 months; median survival for nonresponders was 6 months, and the 6 patients with partial responses were alive 8 to 82 months from diagnosis, with 55 percent of all patients alive at 4 years.[55] Allogeneic stem cell transplantation in 10 patients resulted in a median disease-free survival of greater than 17 months, although the transplantation-related mortality was 40 percent.[56]

ANAPLASTIC LARGE CELL LYMPHOMA

Epidemiology, Etiology, and Pathogenesis

Anaplastic large cell lymphoma (ALCL) accounts for 2 to 8 percent of all T-cell lymphomas. ALCL has a bimodal age distribution, being fairly common in children and adolescents. The cells from these patients were first noted to react with an anti–Ki-1 antibody (anti-CD30).[57] The disease may be either anaplastic lymphoma kinase (ALK) positive (60–70%) or negative (30–40%)[58,59]; in the former, a nonrandom t(2;5)(p23;q35) translocation causes fusion of the *NPM* and *ALK* genes.[60] The resultant *NPM-ALK* fusion gene encodes the 80-kDa chimeric protein NPM-ALK (p80) that functions as an oncogene in ALK-positive ALCL. Thus, ALK immunoreactivity is a highly specific marker for this disease.[58,59,61] Either T or null immunophenotypes may be observed in ALCL. The T-cell variant expresses pan-T antigens CD2, CD2, CD4, CD5, and CD7, whereas the null variant lacks both T and B antigens, but usually expresses cytotoxic molecules such as granzyme B and perforin, and has rearranged TCR genes, suggesting a T-cell origin.[62,63]

The phosphatidylinositol 3-kinase-Akt and STAT3 pathways, involved in cell proliferation and apoptosis, are activated by NPM-ALK and NPM-ALK and contribute to malignant transformation *in vitro* and *in vivo*.[64–68] A small percentage of ALK-positive large cell lymphomas demonstrate alternative *ALK* fusion gene partners, producing variant ALK fusion proteins.[59,69] The cutaneous form of primary CD30+ ALCL is defined as a separate entity by the WHO classification.[70]

Genomic and proteomic cluster analyses strongly suggest that ALK-positive and ALK-negative ALCL are two distinct disease entities. There is evidence of CEBPB, PTPN12, SERPINA1, and BCL6 overexpression in the former, and CCR7, CNTFR, IL-21, and IL-22 overexpression in the latter.[71] Based on comparative genomic hybridization and fluorescence *in situ* hybridization for TP53 and ATM loci, gains of 17p and 17q24-qter, and losses of 4q13-q21 and 11q14 were more common in ALK-positive tumors, whereas gains of 1q and 6p21 were preferentially observed in ALK-negative tumors.[72]

Clinical Features

ALCL has an aggressive clinical course, frequently presenting with systemic symptoms, advanced disease, and extranodal localization. The T-cell phenotype has a predilection for cutaneous involvement with sparing of marrow and extranodal sites.[73,74] Compared to ALK-negative patients, ALK-positive patients tend to be younger and have better performance statuses and lower serum lactate dehydrogenase (LDH) levels.[75] Nodal presentation is equally common in both groups, but an increased incidence of extranodal involvement is observed in the ALK-negative group.[76] Ninety percent of children with this disease are ALK positive.[61,75]

The International Peripheral T-Cell Lymphoma Project reported that the prognosis for patients with ALK positive ALCL is superior to that with ALK-negative ALCL: 5-year failure-free survivals are 60 percent and 36 percent, respectively ($P = 0.015$), and 5-year overall survival rates are 70 percent and 49 percent, respectively ($P = 0.016$).[77] CD56 expression has been shown to be a favorable, independent prognostic factor.[76]

Seldom does ALCL involve the central nervous system. Approximately 20 percent of patients have morphologic evidence of marrow involvement based on routine morphologic examination, but this rate of involvement doubles when immunohistochemical techniques such as anti-CD30 and anti-ALK antibodies are used.[78] Marrow involvement is an unfavorable prognostic factor in ALCL. In general, remission rates and survival with cytotoxic chemotherapy are better for ALCL than for other peripheral T-cell lymphomas.[73,74]

Laboratory Features

ALCL cells tend to grow cohesively and are found preferentially invading lymph node sinuses.[79] There are three morphologic variants based on the size of the neoplastic and admixed reactive cells:[80] the "common type," representing most cases, is characterized by large pleomorphic tumor cells; the "small cell variant," representing 5 to 10 percent of cases, has a dominant population of small- to medium-size tumor cells mixed with large anaplastic cells that stain for CD30 and ALK; and the "lymphohistiocytic variant," representing 5 to 10 percent of cases, is closely related to the small cell variant and contains small neoplastic cells mixed with large anaplastic cells and a large number of histiocytes (see Chap. 98, Figs. 98–32 to 98–34).[81]

Treatment

In general, ALCL, an aggressive lymphoma, is the most chemosensitive of the T-cell lymphomas with rates of survival and response similar to diffuse-large B cell lymphomas. Given the high incidence of ALCL in the pediatric population, intensive anthracycline-based chemotherapy regimens have been studied in children.[82,83] Similarly, most adult patients are treated with doxorubicin-based regimens, resulting in a 70 percent rate of complete response and a 5-year survival rate of 60 percent.[73,74] Patients randomized to doxorubicin, bleomycin, vinblastine, and dacarbazine (ABVD) or high-dose methotrexate, doxorubicin, cyclophosphamide, vincristine, prednisone, bleomycin (MACOP-B) had equivalent results.[84] High-dose chemotherapy with autologous stem cell rescue has shown promising results, but the number of patients studied was limited.[85–89] Case series suggest a potential role for therapy in the form of an allogeneic transplantation in patients who relapse, but patient numbers are small in these series, with fewer than 20 patients undergoing transplantation.[90–92] Nonetheless, disease-free survival was observed even in patients with active, refractory ALCL, suggesting a graft-versus-ALCL effect.

■ PERIPHERAL T-CELL LYMPHOMA, UNSPECIFIED

Epidemiology, Etiology, and Pathogenesis

The peripheral T-cell lymphomas that do not fit into any of the currently recognized histopathologic categories are designated *peripheral T-cell lymphoma, unspecified* (PTCL) and are the most common of the T-cell neoplasms, represent approximately 50 percent of the total cases of T-cell lymphoma, excluding adult T-cell leukemia/lymphoma.[93] It is more common in Asia. The majority of cases arises in lymph nodes and includes mixtures of small and large atypical lymphoid cells, typically with an inflammatory background. Epithelioid histiocytes may be a prominent cellular component, hence these so-called *lymphoepithelioid cell lymphomas* (previously referred to as a *Lennert lymphoma*) are now classified as a morphologic variant of peripheral T-cell lymphoma, unspecified (see Chap. 98, Figs. 98–30 and 98–31).[94]

Clinical Features

In general, patients with PTCL are considered to have a more aggressive disease than patients with diffuse large B-cell lymphoma. Patients typically present with bulky lymphadenopathy and have a higher incidence of B symptoms, extranodal involvement, elevated LDH level, and stage 4 disease.[93] Pruritus, peripheral eosinophilia, and the hemophagocytic syndrome may accompany PTCL.[95–97]

Compared to diffuse large B-cell lymphoma, PTCL has a higher portion of adverse risk factors and overall poorer prognosis.[98–101] The prognostic index for PTCL is based on a retrospective analysis of 385 cases of PTCL, and is similar to the international prognostic index except that marrow involvement replaces stage.[102]

Laboratory Features

The immunophenotype typically is that of a mature T cell expressing either a CD4 or CD8 phenotype. Deletion of any of the pan–T-cell antigens is frequently seen. Rearrangements of the TCR genes are common, and the most common phenotype is the CD4+ $\alpha\beta$. Based on complementary DNA and oligonucleotide microarray analysis of 23 PTCL cases, overexpression of genes associated with proliferation, or a proliferation signature, appears to be associated with poor prognosis, but this needs prospective validation. Genes comprising this signature include *CCNA, CCNB, PCNA*, and *TOP2A*.[103]

Therapy

Patients with PTCL typically are treated with doxorubicin-containing regimens that can achieve CRs and, rarely, result in long-term disease-free survival. Overall, both response rate and survival are lower than those in patients with diffuse large B-cell lymphoma.[104,105] Based on a retrospective analysis of a PTCL cohort, use of an initial anthracycline-containing regimen did not improve survival outcomes, indicating the relative chemoresistance of this T-cell lymphoma subtype.[106] In a retrospective analysis of 44 T-cell lymphoma specimens, the majority of which were PTCL, lymphoma cell expression of CYP3A correlated with a lower rate of complete response, and contributed to primary resistance to anthracyclines and topoisomerase II inhibitors *in vitro*.[107] Nonetheless, a role for early high-dose chemotherapy with autologous stem cell rescue in PTCL is suggested by the finding that outcomes for transplanted PTCL patients are similar to those of patients with diffuse large B-cell lymphoma.[108–110] A retrospective Spanish study using autologous stem cell transplantation as consolidation therapy for patients with PTCL in first remission reported a 5-year overall survival of 68 percent and progression-free survival of 63 percent.[111] A multivariate analysis found that the only factor associated with a shorter overall survival and progression free survival was the presence of more than two risk factors from the prognostic index for PTCL risk system.[103] Allogeneic transplantation has not been well studied in this disease, and transplant-related mortality is significant.[112]

Other approaches to treatment include cyclosporine, pentostatin, and retinoids.[113–115] Responses have been reported, but none of these therapies stands out as a major new breakthrough for treatment of PTCL, unspecified. Targeted therapies such as denileukin diftitox, zanolimumab, siplizumab, and alemtuzumab may be of benefit in PTCL. These are discussed in the section on targeted therapy.

ANGIOIMMUNOBLASTIC T-CELL LYMPHOMA

Epidemiology, Etiology, and Pathogenesis

Angioimmunoblastic T-cell lymphoma (AITL) represents approximately 1 percent of all cases of lymphoma. Angioimmunoblastic lymphadenopathy with dysproteinemia (AILD) was initially described in 1974,[116] and many cases evolve into AITL.[117] The median patient age at diagnosis is approximately 65 years, with a slight male predominance.[118]

AITL is considered a separate entity among lymphoma subtypes. Both a secondary form, evolving from AILD, and a *de novo* form may occur. Histologically, a loss of lymphoid architecture with a pleomorphic cellular infiltrate and proliferation of small arborizing blood vessels are observed. Small lymphocytes, plasma cells, immunoblasts, histiocytes, and often eosinophils infiltrate the involved lymph node. As a result, the normal lymphoid architecture may be obliterated, with loss of the germinal center and extensive intranodal neovascularization. The malignant cells are CD4+ $\alpha\beta$ T cells with TCR β and γ rearrangements[119–121] and express CD10 approximately 90 percent of the time, a marker specific for AITL.[122] The normal counterpart of AITL is suspected to be the follicular helper cell based on genomic profiling revealing the expression of specific markers such as CXCL13. Furthermore, a subset of CD30-negative PTCL had a similar gene expression profile, suggesting that these may be more similar to AITL than PTCL.[123]

Scattered EBV+ B cells are almost always present and reflect the accompanying immunodeficient state. Abnormal karyotypes, frequently involving the X chromosome and chromosomes 1, 3, and 5 can be found; complex karyotype are a negative prognostic factor.[124] Most patients with AITL have an unfavorable prognosis if they have an IPI score greater than 2.

Clinical Features

Patients with AILD are also at risk of developing B-cell lymphomas.[119,125] Patients typically present with B symptoms (fever, drenching sweats, and weight loss), generalized lymphadenopathy, rash, polyclonal hypergammaglobulinemia, blood eosinophilia, autoimmune hemolytic anemia (direct Coombs positive), and an infection.

Hypereosinophilic Syndrome Blood eosinophilia occurs in approximately 15 percent of all T-cell lymphomas.[126] There is a strong association between hypereosinophilic syndrome and a clonal expansion of a T-lymphocyte population; approximately 20 percent of patients with this syndrome exhibit a clonal population of T-cells that overexpress IL-5, the principal eosinophilopoietin.[127,128] Patients with hypereosinophilia associated with an clonal T-cell population are at increased risk of developing T-cell lymphomas in a frequency approaching 25 percent after 3 to 8 years of onset of hypereosinophilia.[128] IL-5 is involved in eosinophil production, activation, chemotaxis, and survival, and is the most frequent cytokine involved in eosinophilia associated with T-cell lymphoproliferative disorders. In 20 cases of AITL and 30 cases of PTCL studied, intratumoral eosinophilia was quantified and compared to levels of IL-5, regulated upon activation, normal T-cell expressed and secreted (RANTES), eotaxin, and thymus and activation-regulated chemokine (TARC).[129] Of these 50 cases, 68 percent of the evaluable cases were IL-5 positive, correlating with the presence of eosinophilia ($p = 0.044$). Intratumoral IL-5 was expressed predominantly by lymphoma cells. Although the majority of cases expressed RANTES (58%) and eotaxin (62%), expression of these cytokines did not correlate with the presence of eosinophilia. Although a minority of tumors (30%) expressed TARC, principally in nonlymphoid cells, degree of expression correlated with frequency of eosinophils ($p = 0.0003$). The majority (13/15) of TARC-positive lymphomas, however, were also positive for IL-5.

Therapies

Most patients with AITL are treated with doxorubicin-based regimens. The complete response rate is similar to the rate of other PTCL (approximately 50%), and there is no evidence that intensive regimens improve survival outcomes.[130] Some patients, particularly those patients with a more benign form of the disease, may be managed with glucocorticoid monotherapy.[131] Based on multivariate analysis male sex, mediastinal lymphadenopathy, and anemia are negative prognostic factors.[130] Responses to low-dose methotrexate and cyclosporine have also been reported.[132–134]

PREDOMINANTLY EXTRANODAL NK AND T-CELL LYMPHOMAS

EXTRANODAL NK/T-CELL LYMPHOMA

Epidemiology, Etiology, and Pathology

Extranodal NK/T-cell lymphoma of the nasal type previously was referred to as lethal midline granuloma, malignant granuloma, and angiocentric lymphoma, and is always associated with EBV infection of the neoplastic cells.[135] It involves midline facial structures and is an uncommon subtype, representing approximately 1 percent of total cases of lymphoma.[28,136,137] The disease is subclassified as nasal and extranasal in distribution; the nasal form is approximately five times more common than the extranasal form. Extranasal location confers a poor prognosis with a median survival of 6 months, versus 5 years for localized nasal disease.[138] Although rarely affecting Americans of European descent, especially those of Spanish descent, Native Americans, and Americans of Asian descent,[139,140] the disease typically afflicts middle-aged men, with a median age of 50 years at diagnosis, but may also affect children.[141,142]

Clinical Features

Typically, patients present with an obstructing, hemorrhagic nasal mass, which may invade adjacent structures, including the nasal sinuses, and nasopharynx, and as a result, cranial nerve palsies may be present. Hematogenous spread to the skin, gastrointestinal tract, and testes tends to occur later in the disease course.[143–145]

Laboratory Findings

The histopathology shows angiocentric plesiomorphic small- or medium-size atypical lymphoid cells with vascular invasion and ischemic tissue necrosis. The malignant cells are generally EBV positive and express the pan–T-cell antigens CD2 and CD7, whereas CD3 is often absent.

Therapy

Primary disease is treated with combined local radiation therapy and a chemotherapy regimen that includes doxorubicin. Compared to patients with T-cell or B-cell phenotypes, those with NK/T-cell lymphoma (51 patients, 45.1%) had more frequent involvement of the nasal cavity alone, a higher risk of skin dissemination, more frequently developed the hemophagocytic syndrome. Patients in a Chinese study received CHOP, CEOP (cyclophosphamide, epirubicin, vincristine, prednisone) or ProMACE (prednisone, methotrexate, doxorubicin, cyclophosphamide, etoposide) plus CytaBOM (cytarabine, bleomycin, vincristine, methotrexate with leucovorin rescue) with or without radiation.[146] Analyzed retrospectively, the CR rate for NK/T-cell disease was 56 percent compared to 70 percent and 76 percent for T-cell and B-cell phenotypes, respectively. The 5-year actuarial disease-free survival rates were 25.1 percent for NK/T-cell disease, compared to 41.9 percent and 40.9 percent for T-cell and B-cell phenotypes, respectively. The median overall survival was 12.5 months for NK/T-cell phenotype, 93.4 months for T-cell phenotype and 17 months for B-cell phenotype. In another study, patients with localized nasal NK/T-cell lymphoma received four cycles of CHOP and involved field radiotherapy, with an overall response rate of 58 percent and an estimated overall 3-year survival of 59 percent. Only 35 percent of patients completed the planned sequential chemoradiotherapy because of disease progression during chemotherapy, suggesting that CHOP-like regimens are suboptimal in the initial management of localized nasal NK/T-cell lymphoma[143]

Following chemoradiotherapy, patients are monitored with nasal endoscopy to look for local recurrence, along with EBV serologies. High-dose chemotherapy with autologous stem cell rescue has been used successfully as a salvage therapy.[148] Case reports of successful allogeneic transplantation exist, but patient numbers are very small.[149–152]

■ ENTEROPATHY-TYPE T-CELL LYMPHOMA

Epidemiology, Etiology, and Pathogenesis

Enteropathy-type intestinal T-cell lymphoma (EATCL) accounts for less than 1 percent of all cases of lymphoma, but accounts for nearly 25 percent of all primary intestinal lymphomas. This is a disease of adults who often, but not always, have antecedent gluten-sensitive enteropathy (celiac disease)[3,153,154]; a lack of response to a gluten-free diet typically precedes that of lymphoma.[155] Accordingly, the disease incidence is higher in areas where celiac disease is common. The median patient age at diagnosis is 55 years with a male-to-female ratio of 3:1.

The tumors are composed of small, medium, large, or anaplastic lymphocytes.[3] The neoplastic cells are CD3-, CD7-, and CD103-positive, sometimes CD8-positive, and CD4-negative.[156] The TCR-β genes are rearranged, [153,154] although in a minority of cases the cells express the $\gamma\delta$ receptor.[3]

Clinical Features

The disease most commonly involves the jejunum or ileum, but other regions of the gastrointestinal tract may be affected. As a result of the malabsorption accompanying the disease, frequent presenting signs and symptoms include weight loss, diarrhea, nausea, and vomiting, accompanied by abdominal pain and bowel obstruction.[154] Patients typically present with jejunal or ileal ulcers, which may be multiple and may have perforated. Most patients are diagnosed at surgery. The course can be fulminant; death often occurs during treatment secondary to the consequences of intestinal perforation. Postmortem examination reveals chemotherapy refractory malignant ulcers, most often in the jejunum.

Therapy

Combination chemotherapy with an anthracycline-based regimen is commonly recommended; however, many of the patients cannot tolerate chemotherapy. A report of 27 patients with intestinal T-cell lymphoma, the majority of whom had EATCL or EATC-like lymphoma, of whom 14 patients were treated with multiagent chemotherapy, only 7 (50%) completed therapy. Twenty of these 27 patients died, and 17 died within 6 months from diagnosis. The overall median survival was 4 months, and patients with stage I disease had better survival rates than other patients.[158] A British single-institution study reported 31 patients with EATCL, 24 of whom received intensive weekly anthracycline-based chemotherapy. Most of the patients could not complete the course of chemotherapy, and there were a large number of complications related to the anatomy of the disease, such as gastrointestinal bleeding, small bowel perforation, and enterocolic fistulae. Twelve patients required either enteral or parental feeding. The overall response rate was 58 percent, with 10 complete responses and 4 partial responses. Relapses occur at a median interval of 6 months, with a median survival of approximately 1 year. The 5-year relapse failure-free survival was 19 percent and actuarial 5-year survival was 20 percent, with most patients dying from disease progression.[154]

■ HEPATOSPLENIC T-CELL LYMPHOMA

Epidemiology, Etiology, Pathogenesis, and Clinical Findings

Hepatosplenic T-cell lymphoma represents less than 1 percent of all lymphomas and was previously described as hepatosplenic $\gamma\delta$ T-cell lymphoma. The tumor cells have a sinus or sinusoidal localization in the liver and spleen,[159] as well as in the marrow. Skin lesions may be found, but are rare. The neoplastic cells are CD3+ T cells that are CD4- and CD8-negative, although rarely CD8 is positive; CD56 and TCR-δ are positive in the majority of cases.[159] The phenotype is consistent with immature $\gamma\delta$ T cells. The disease typically occurs in young males who present with isolated hepatosplenomegaly without lymphadenopathy,[160] frequently accompanied by cytopenias, B symptoms, and elevated serum LDH. Clonal rearrangement of the TCR-γ gene usually present, and in most cases the lymphoma cells have an isochromosome 7q [I(7)(q10)] along with trisomy 8, which also may be seen in the $\alpha\beta$ variant of this disease.[161–164] These findings suggest that i(7q) serves as marker specific for hepatosplenic T-cell lymphoma, and may play a role in its pathogenesis.

Therapy

The majority of patients respond to initial therapy with a doxorubicin-containing multidrug regimen, but of relatively short duration. Forty-five patients with hepatosplenic T-cell lymphoma, most of whom were treated with alkylating agents, CHOP or CHOP-like therapies, second- or third-generation regimens for high-grade lymphomas, and autologous or allogeneic marrow or peripheral stem cell transplantation. Complete responses were achieved in 5 patients (11%), and relapses were common and early in the treatment course. Although transient clinical improvement was seen in the majority of patients undergoing therapy, early relapses were common, and 36 patients (80%) died from the disease; only 4 patients (9%) survived. The patients in this study had a median survival of only 8 months (range: 0–42 months). The role of high-dose therapy with autologous stem cell rescue and other aggressive forms of therapy is unknown, but 2 of 4 patients who were still alive in this series received allogeneic stem cell transplantation.[160] A retrospective review of 15 patients with this type of lymphoma identified four negative prognostic findings: male gender, failure to achieve a CR, history of immunocompromise, and absence of a gene rearrangement in the T-cell receptor γ chain.[165]

■ SUBCUTANEOUS PANNICULITIS-LIKE T-CELL LYMPHOMA

Pathogenesis and Clinical Features

Subcutaneous panniculitis-like T-cell lymphoma is a rare disorder presenting with subcutaneous, often painful nodules.[166,167] The lesions consist of atypical lymphoid cells, and reactive histiocytes with admixed adipose tissue often associated with coagulation necrosis. In most cases, the tumor is composed of CD8+ $\alpha\beta$ T cells, but CD4– $\gamma\delta$ T cells are seen in a minority of cases, a marker for more aggressive disease. These cells are mature cytotoxic T cells that express TIA-1, granzymes, and perforin genes.

The lesions typically begin in the extremities and may spontaneously regress for a number of years but eventually progress.[166] They may ulcerate, and patients may have systemic symptoms. The hemophagocytic syndrome may be prominent in this disease, either at the time of initial presentation or later in its course.[167,168]

Therapy

Responses to combination chemotherapy have been reported but are usually of short duration.[166,169,170] Responses to glucocorticoids, interferon-α, zidovudine, and cyclosporine also have been reported.[169,171,172] Therapy for this disease remains controversial. Although standard chemotherapy may be effective, complete responses are rare. Single patient cases of successful allogeneic stem cell transplantation have been reported, but the rarity of this disease hampers further investigation of this modality.[173,174] The use of denileukin diftitox in two patients has been reported with evidence of activity, and bexarotene restored a clinical response in one of the patients after disease progression.[175]

TABLE 106–2. Summary of T-Cell–Specific Cell-Surface Markers

Antigen	Normal Cell Distribution	Function
CD2	T, NK, dendritic cells, thymocytes	Cell-adhesion ligand for CD58 on antigen-presenting cell
CD3	T	T-cell receptor complex
CD4	T	HLA-class II coreceptor
CD25	T	55-kDa low-affinity IL-2 receptor (IL-2R) polypeptide chain
CD26	T, NK, epithelial	Dipeptidyl peptidase IV
CD30	T, B	TNF receptor superfamily member
CD52	T, B, NK, monocytes, macrophages	Unknown

CD, cluster of differentiation; HLA, human leukocyte antigen; NK, natural killer; TNF, tumor necrosis factor.

SOURCE: Reproduced with permission from Goodman OB, Dang NH: Novel antibody approaches for T-cell lymphomas. *Clin Lymphoma Myeloma* 8(Suppl 5):S193, 2008.

CELL-SURFACE ANTIGENS AS THERAPY TARGETS: MATURE T-CELL AND NATURAL KILLER CELL LYMPHOMAS

Since the approval of rituximab, the CD20-directed targeted mAb, in 1997, the concept of targeted therapy for the treatment of lymphomas has seen dramatic advances. The inherent poor prognosis of these diseases and the variety of potential therapeutic targets present on NK and T cells have spurred the development and clinical evaluation of several new mAbs for use in treating these diseases. Many of the signaling pathways targeted by these mAbs are intimately involved in T-cell activation and function aberrantly in T-cell lymphomas, potentially contributing to the growth of the neoplastic T-cells. These T-cell surface antigens are often present on the neoplastic cells, rendering them susceptible to targeted therapies. These antigens are fairly specific for the T-cell lineage, potentially minimizing toxicity against other tissues. Moreover, combination with standard cytotoxic chemotherapy has yielded some promising results.

■ T-CELL SURFACE TARGETS FOR ANTIBODY THERAPY

Neoplastic cellular signaling is initiated on the cell surface as a result of TCR engagement and depends on other costimulatory molecules (Table 106–2), transducing downstream mitogenic events. Because neoplastic T-cell division and survival are exquisitely dependent on these signaling events, these costimulatory molecules represent potential therapeutic targets.

CD2

This costimulatory molecule is a transmembrane approximately 50-kDa glycoprotein expressed on dendritic cells,[176] NK cells, thymocytes, and mature T cells.[177] A member of the immunoglobulin (Ig) superfamily, it functions primarily to further localize the activated T cell in proximity to an antigen-presenting cell by binding CD58 (leukocyte function-associated antigen [LFA]-3) and CD59. Upon T-cell activation, both the number of surface CD2 molecules as well at the stability of the dimeric complex formed with CD58 are enhanced, resulting in the formation of a high-affinity intercellular bridge.[178] As a result of CD2–CD58 ligation, the Wiskott-Aldrich syndrome protein (WASP)[179] and the protein tyrosine kinase $p56^{lck}$ associate with the intracytoplasmic domain of CD2,[180] resulting in actin polymerization with further strengthening of intercellular adhesion, and enhanced T-cell activation.[179] Of therapeutic importance, engagement of CD2 by either LFA-3 or a mAb can directly trigger T-cell apoptosis and tachyphylaxis of TCR signaling. Thus, targeting CD2 with a mAb both attenuates mitogenic TCR signaling by reducing the avidity of the intercellular bridge with the antigen-presenting cell, as well as by selectively promoting apoptosis of the neoplastic T cell.

CD3

This antigen is an integral component of the TCR complex, comprising five invariant polypeptide chains: γ, δ, ε, ζ, and η. The CD3 polypeptides are in a stable complex with the α and β chains of the T-cell receptor.[181] The extracellular domain CD3 comprises the γ, δ, and ε chains, with extracellular immunoglobulin-like domains, a transmembrane domain, and a short intracytoplasmic domain. The first generation of antibodies that targeted the T-cell antigen, such as muromonab-CD3 (Orthoclone OKT3), triggered T-cell activation as a result of crosslinking of the TCR with the Fc receptor, which lead to T-cell activation and the associated massive release of cytokines, such as tumor necrosis factor (TNF), and associated toxicity, including hypotension, hypoglycemia, and capillary leak syndrome.[182] These side effects had limited the utility of CD3 therapeutic targeting in T-cell lymphoma. The selective anti-CD3 antibody visilizumab with a mutated FcR region has been engineered, which retains its CD3 selectiveness but fails to activate the TCR and therefore is associated with significantly less cytokine release.[183]

CD4

This molecule is an immunoglobulin superfamily member that facilitates the recognition of human leukocyte antigen class II polypeptides as a TCR coreceptor. It is normally expressed on regulatory and helper T cells, monocytes, macrophages, and dendritic cells,[184] and is also expressed by neoplastic T cells in cutaneous T-cell lymphomas as well as PTCL. Targeting this molecule results in potent inhibition of TCR signaling. Both TCR-dependent and TCR-independent mechanisms have been purported. Targeting CD4 with the mAb OKT4C results in the subsequent attenuation of TCR signaling.[185] One proposed mechanism by which this occurs is the uncoupling of the TCR from the CD4-associated and costimulatory protein tyrosine kinase $p56^{lck}$, which upon association with the inhibitory adapters SHIP-1 and DOK,[186] results in attenuation of T-cell receptor signaling. In addition, targeting CD4 results in antibody-mediated apoptosis via monocyte Fc-γreceptor.[187]

CD25

This is the 55-kDa low-affinity IL-2 receptor (IL-2R) polypeptide chain. Unlike the β(p75) and γ(p64) polypeptides, which together with CD25 comprise the high-affinity IL-2R, CD25 is rapidly upregulated following IL-2 binding. Thus, this antigen is expressed primarily on activated T cells and the mAbs function as IL-2R receptor antagonists. The CD25 antigen is selectively upregulated in cutaneous T-cell lymphoma (CTCL). Based on prospective immunohistochemical analysis of skin biopsy specimens, 24 of 113 (22%) patients with CTCL express CD25 on >20 percent of the neoplastic lymphocytes.[188] The expression of CD25 correlates with histologic grade and stage, as well as response to the CD25-targeted therapy denileukin diftitox (ONTAK). Within a given patient, there appears to be upregulation in T cells in cutaneous lesions relative to those in lymph nodes specifically in the cutaneous lesions.[189] T-cell receptor activation also results in the expression of the costimulatory molecule CD40L, an effect which can be abrogated by the CD25-specific mAb daclizumab, suggesting that CD40L induction may result from IL-2R activation.[190]

CD26

This marker is a 110-kDa type II transmembrane protein normally expressed by a variety of epithelial cells, as well as by activated T and NK cells. Its extracellular dipeptidyl peptidase IV enzymatic activity is enhanced on activated T cells. Its known substrates include various chemokines, including RANTES, the macrophage inflammatory chemokine LD78β, the interferon-inducible chemokines IP10, SDF-1, interferon-inducible T-cell α chemoattractant, and collagen. Its extracellular domain also has a number of binding partners, including adenosine deaminase and caveolin. By inducing cell-cycle arrest at the G_1-S checkpoint, the anti-CD26 1F7 mAb exhibits antitumor activity in the CD30+ T-ALCL cell line Karpas 299.[191] In mature T- and NK-cell lymphomas, there is variable expression in LGL-T,[192] and high levels of expression in more aggressive T-cell lymphomas, such as hepatosplenic gamma-delta T-cell lymphoma[193] and T-cell ALCL.[194] A phase I trial involving humanized anti-CD26 mAb will be conducted with relapsed CD26-positive tumors, including patients with T-cell lymphomas.

CD30 (Ki-1)

This TNF-receptor superfamily member is a type I transmembrane glycoprotein with a 595-amino-acid extracytoplasmic domain normally bound by CD30 ligand (CD153) and by mAbs such as SGN30. The expression of CD30 in normal tissues is largely restricted to interfollicular B and T cells and centroblasts.[195] Originally discovered in 1982 on the surface of Reed-Sternberg cells,[196] it is now known to be expressed on a number of malignant cells of both B- and T-cell origin, including ALCL, immunoblastic B-cell lymphoma, myeloma, and cutaneous T-cell lymphomas.[197] The extracellular domain of this molecule is shed as soluble CD30, as a result of cleavage by TNF-α converting enzyme,[198] a zinc metalloprotease. Serum levels of sCD30 correlate with lymphoma activity. The accumulation of sCD30 is inhibited by hydroxamic acid-derived protease inhibitors, which may improve the efficacy of CD30-directed therapies.[199]

CD52

Discovered in 1983 in a screen for an antibody capable of depleting human T cells from marrow via complement fixation,[200] CD52 is a glycosylphosphatidylinositol-linked glycoprotein with unknown function. It is present on the surface of B cells, T cells, NK cells, monocytes, and macrophages, but notably absent from cells of myeloid, erythroid, and megakaryocytoid lineages. In general, CD52 transcription is downregulated in T-cell lymphomas when compared with normal T lymphocytes,[201] consistent with the lower response rates seen with this agent.[202] However, a significant number of these lymphomas do express CD52 leading to the possibility of tailoring therapy based on CD52 expression status. Because this antigen is present on normal T and B lymphocytes, profound lymphopenia with associated immunosuppression has also limited the use of CD52-targeted mAb therapy in T-cell lymphoma, as well as other diseases. The mAb targeting the CD52 antigen results in cellular apoptosis, complement-dependent cytotoxicity, and ADCC.

THERAPEUTIC MONOCLONAL ANTIBODIES

Zanolimumab

Zanolimumab (HM6G.2, HuMax-CD4, $hIgG_1\kappa$ antibody) is a fully humanized mAb directed against CD4 (see Table 106–3). It has both cytotoxic and antiproliferative effects through multiple mechanisms, including direct inhibition of TCR signaling, ADCC, and long-term Fc-dependent downregulation of CD4.[186] Its activity has been evaluated in two separate but otherwise identical clinical trials for patients with refractory CD4-positive CTCL, one for early stage patients, and one for advanced stage patients.[203] Zanolimumab was administered on a weekly schedule for 16 weeks. Three different doses were used: 280 mg (early and advanced stage), 560 mg (early stage), and 980 mg (advanced stage). For patients with mycoses fungoides, there appeared to be a dose response that paralleled the trough serum concentrations, with the greatest percentage of objective responders (75%) seen at the highest dose, while for patients with Sézary syndrome, responses occurred 20 to 25 percent of the time and independent of serum concentrations,[203] suggesting that its effects in Sézary syndrome were less specific, possibly as a result of off-target or downstream effects.

Another open-label clinical trial examined the use of zanolimumab in relapsed or refractory PTCL. Twenty-one patients received weekly 980-mg doses of zanolimumab for 12 consecutive weeks. There were five (24%) objective responders with two complete responses seen, one in a patient with PTCL and in another with angioimmunoblastic T-cell lymphoma. The latter response was durable, with no relapse observed at 252 days.[204] These data suggest that zanolimumab is broadly active in T-cell lymphoma.

Siplizumab

Siplizumab (MEDI-507) is a humanized mAb directed against the extracellular domain of CD2. It has been evaluated in a single phase I open-label dose-escalation trial in patients with refractory CD2-positive (minimum 30% of neoplastic cells by immunohistochemistry) adult T-cell leukemia. At the last update, 13 patients were enrolled with diagnoses of adult T-cell leukemia/lymphoma (n = 7), cutaneous T-cell lymphoma (n = 2), PTCL (n = 1), and LGL (n = 3).[205] Siplizumab (dose range: 0.4–1.2 mg/kg) was administered to 4 patient cohorts (3 patients per cohort) on a biweekly schedule for a total of 8 doses over 16 weeks. Administration occurred over 2 to 3 days, depending on the dose, with

TABLE 106–3. Trials of Monoclonal Antibodies in NK/T-Cell Lymphomas

Target	Drug(s)	Species	Diseases Treated	Reference(s)
CD4	Zanolimumab	Human	PTCL	203
CD2	Siplizumab	Human	ATLL, PTCL, LGL-T	204
			LGL-NK, PTCL	205
CD3	Visilizumab	Human	Not reported	206
CD25	Daclizumab	Human	PTCL, ATLL	207
CD30	MDX 060	Human	ALCL	222, 223
	SGN30	Chimeric	ALCL	31, 197
CD52	Alemtuzumab	Human	T-PLL	249
	CHOP + alemtuzumab		AITCL, ALCL, EATCL, PTCL	213, 214, 217
	FAC + alemtuzumab		PTCL	219
	EPOCH + alemtuzumab		Any TCL- chemotherapy-naïve	217

AITCL, angioimmunoblastic T-cell lymphoma; ALCL, anaplastic large cell lymphoma; ATLL, adult T-cell leukemia/lymphoma; CD, cluster of differentiation; CHOP, cyclophosphamide, doxorubicin, vincristine, prednisone; EPOCH, etoposide, prednisone, vincristine, cyclophosphamide, doxorubicin; FAC, 5-fluorouracil, Adriamycin, cyclophosphamide; LGL, larger granular lymphocyte; NK, natural killer cell; PTCL, peripheral T-cell lymphoma; T, T cell; TCL, T-cell lymphoma; T-PLL, T-cell prolymphocytic leukemia.

SOURCE: Reproduced with permission from Goodman OB, Dang NH: Novel antibody approaches for T-cell lymphomas. *Clin Lymphoma Myeloma* 8(Suppl 5):S193, 2008.

a median of two courses per patient. There were no dose-limiting toxicities, and the highest dose administered was 1.2 mg/kg per week, with planned additional cohorts of 2.4 mg/kg, 3.4 mg/kg, and 4.8 mg/kg. Five patients were removed from the trial because of progression and three because of cytomegalovirus antigenemia; the protocol has now been amended to allow treatment for the virus while on study. There were >90 percent declines in both blood CD4+ and CD8+ T-cell counts, as well as a 79 percent decline in NK-cell count, hence transient lymphopenia was the principal adverse event, observed in 7 of 9 patients with adverse events. There were two serious adverse events deemed unrelated to treatment: indwelling catheter sepsis and febrile neutropenia. There were three confirmed PRs (two adult T-cell leukemia/lymphoma, one LGL-T). No immunogenicity was observed up to the 0.8 mg/kg dose.[205]

In a multicenter phase I trial for patients with CD-2 positive, T-cell lymphoma, 16 patients with PTCL (n = 9), cutaneous T-cell lymphoma (n = 6), and NK-LGL (n = 1) were enrolled[31] and treated with 0.7 mg/kg (n = 3), 3.4 mg/kg (n = 10). There were two responses observed, one PR in an NK-LGL patient at 3.4 mg/kg and one CR in a PTCL patient at 3.4 mg/kg. There were two single cases of dose-limiting toxicities observed for which cohort expansion did not reveal additional dose-limiting toxicities: erythematous confluent dermatitis at 3.4 mg/kg and pulmonary edema at 4.8 mg/kg. There was one case of tumor lysis syndrome constituting a treatment-related serious adverse event at 3.4 mg/kg. Significant peripheral T-cell depletion was observed.[31]

Alemtuzumab

Alemtuzumab (CAMPATH-1H) is a humanized $IgG_1\kappa$ mAb to CD52. It is approved for use in chronic lymphocytic leukemia as both initial therapy[207] and for refractory patients.[208] The first suggestion of activity in T-cell lymphomas came with the observation that of 39 patients with T-PLL of whom 37 had chemorefractory disease, 76 percent of patients responded to CAMPATH-1H administered three times weekly, intravenously, with dose escalation up to a dose of 30 mg three times weekly, and 60 percent had complete responses.[9] A prospective phase II open label multicenter trial conducted in Europe enrolled 22 patients with advanced mycosis fungoides or Sézary syndrome.[209] The study endpoints were response rate, toxicity including infectious complications, and impact on itching. Eighty-six percent of the patients had stages III and IV disease. Response rates were documented by disease site with an overall response rate of 55 percent in both skin and lymph nodes, and 86 percent in blood. Notably, all of the responses in lymph nodes were complete, while 31 percent of the patients with skin involvement were complete responders. Grade 3 toxicities included infusion-related fevers (5%) and rigors (18%), as well as fatigue (9%); there were no grade 4 toxicities. Eighteen percent of the patients had grade IV neutropenia after 8 to 12 weeks of treatment, and one patient had grade IV thrombocytopenia. Fifty percent of 22 evaluable patients had infectious complications, with 1 case of fatal aspergillosis, 1 case of fatal mycobacterial pneumonia, and 4 cases of treatable cytomegalovirus reactivation. There was one case of systemic herpes simplex virus reactivation that resolved with foscarnet therapy. Three patients had fever of unknown origin and one had febrile neutropenia. A similar study in Sweden and Germany enrolled 14 heavily pretreated patients with stages III and IV disease, and an overall response rate of 36 percent was observed.[210] However, a fatal opportunistic infection rate of 36 percent was observed, highlighting the lymphopenia observed with pan-lymphocytic targeting. There were also two cases of hemophagocytic syndrome associated with EBV reactivation.[211]

Given alemtuzumab's hematologic and infectious toxicity profile, lower doses of alemtuzumab have been evaluated. Fourteen patients with Sézary syndrome were treated on two cohorts with intrapatient dose escalation and intercohort deescalation of the alemtuzumab dose from a final dose of 15 mg (n = 4) in cohort one to 10 mg (n = 10) in cohort two.[212] Four doses of alemtuzumab were administered at the final dose on an alternating day schedule. Retreatment occurred every time circulating Sézary cell counts exceeded 2000/mm^3. A median 95 percent reduction in Sézary cell count was observed. There were 12 responders (86% of patients treated), with 3 complete responders, one confirmed by skin and blood TCR assays, all of whom were in the low-dose cohort. The median time to treatment failure was 12 months. Infectious complications occurred in all four patients in the 15-mg dosing cohort, but in none of the patients receiving 10 mg ($p = 0.001$).[212] Thus, these data argue that intermittent low-dose alemtuzumab has considerable activity and is less toxic.

Alemtuzumab has been combined with conventional chemotherapy in the initial treatment of PTCL. An Italian prospective phase II open label multicenter trial examined the combination of alemtuzumab with CHOP chemotherapy for the front-line treatment of T-cell lymphoma.[213] Eight cycles of CHOP on a 28-day schedule were administered along with a two-phase dosing schedule of alemtuzumab at a dose of 30 mg every 4 weeks either for 12 weeks (three cycles) or 28 weeks (seven cycles). Of the 24 evaluable patients, 17 (71%) achieved a CR and 1 had a PR. Complete responses were achieved by all patients with AITCL (6/6), ALCL (3/3), and EATCL (1/1), while half of the patients with PTCL did so (7 of 14). Subset analysis was conducted on the 15 patients evaluable for CD52 status; however, the study was underpowered to demonstrate differences between these groups. Nonetheless, 2 of 4 patients with a CD52– phenotype progressed, while 2 of 4 achieved a CR. Of the CD52+ patients, 8 of 11 (73%) achieved a CR. Neutropenia was the most common hematologic toxicity, occurring in 59 of 176 (34%) of CHOP-C cycles. Despite prophylaxis against *Pneumocystis carinii*, varicella-zoster virus, herpes simplex virus, and antibacterial prophylaxis for patients with grade IV neutropenia, infectious complications were common, with 15 of 176 cases demonstrating cytomegalovirus reactivation, 2 cases of invasive aspergillosis after three to four cycles of CHOP-C, and 1 case of progressive multifocal leukoencephalopathy posttreatment, resulting in dementia.[213]

In another phase II trial, 20 patients with newly diagnosed PTCL received dose-dense CHOP plus intravenous alemtuzumab 10 mg on day 1 and 20 mg on day 2 in the first 3-week cycle, then 30 mg on day 1 in subsequent cycles, based on 3-week intervals. The overall response rate was 80 percent, with 13 complete responders (65.0%), 3 partial responses (15.0%), and an estimated 1-year event-free survival of 43.3 percent. The regimen was very toxic; grade IV neutropenia was observed in 18 patients (90.0%), with febrile neutropenia in 11 patients (55.0%). Five patients (25%) experienced cytomegalovirus reactivation, while three patients developed cytomegalovirus diseases. There were two treatment-related deaths, prompting closure of the study.[214]

Two alemtuzumab phase III trials, ACT1 and ACT2, combining CHOP with alemtuzumab as primary treatment for patients with PTCL have been opened by the European Intergroup.

Another phase II trial combined alemtuzumab with fludarabine, cyclophosphamide, and doxorubicin for patients with PTCL.[215] There were 23 newly diagnosed patients and 11 relapsed or refractory patients. Of the newly diagnosed patients, an overall response rate of 75 percent was observed with a 43 percent CR rate and a median overall survival of 21 months. Of the relapsed or refractory patients, the overall response rate was 36 percent with no complete responders. Fifty-eight percent of the patients sustained grades III to IV neutropenia, and 44 percent had grades III to IV thrombocytopenia. There was a 15 percent grades III to IV infectious complication rate. The data resulted in the continuation of the study for front-line treatment of PTCL. The EPOCH regimen (etoposide, prednisone, vincristine, cyclophosphamide, and doxorubicin) is a useful regimen in T-cell lymphoma, with a response rate of 85 percent and a CR rate of 50 percent seen in a mixed cohort of treatment-naïve (n = 14) and pretreated (n = 7) patients.[216] Although overall response rates did not differ based on treatment status, a CR rate of 61.5 percent was observed for treatment-naïve patients, versus 28.5 percent for pretreated patients. Thus the combination of EPOCH + alemtuzumab has been tested in a phase I dose-escalation study in chemotherapy-naïve patients (n = 17) with CD52-positive T-cell lymphomas. Patients received an alemtuzumab dose of 30 mg (n = 8), with subsequent dose escalation to 60 mg (n = 3) and 90 mg (n = 3). Five patients (29%) achieved a CR.[217] Marrow aplasia as a dose-limiting toxicity was observed in two-thirds of patients from both the 60- and 90-mg cohorts. Grade IV lymphopenia was seen in all but 1 patient, and infectious complications were seen in 11 patients (65%).

Alemtuzumab in combination with chemotherapy has also been assessed in patients with relapsed PTCL. A phase II prospective study was undertaken in 16 patients with relapsed PTCL (n = 7) and extranodal NK-cell lymphoma (n = 7). Patients received alemtuzumab (total of 70 mg per cycle) in combination with cisplatin, cytarabine, and dexamethasone. The overall response rate was 50 percent, but was 83 percent (three CR, three PR) in patients with PTCL, but only 13 percent with those with extranodal NK-cell lymphoma (one PR). Autologous stem cells were harvested in all but one patient. The median overall survival was 6 months, with responders surviving longer than nonresponders (P = 0.038). There was significant toxicity with grade IV neutropenia observed in 14 of 16 (83%) patients, with 4 treatment-related deaths (25%). The amended phase II trial has reduced alemtuzumab to 40 mg per cycle.[218]

Visilizumab

Visilizumab (HuM291) is a humanized anti-CD3 mAb of the immunoglobulin G_2 isotype directed against the invariant ε chain of the TCR.[183] It has been engineered to lack an ability to bind to type II Fcγ receptor, resulting in no activation of resting T cells as was seen with earlier anti-CD3 antibody prototypes.[219,2220] Its use is most advanced in the field of glucocorticoid-refractory GVHD, with response rates of 32 percent seen 6 weeks postadministration in a phase II multicenter trial.[221] A single dose of antibody was administered to 44 patients, with repeat dosing because of recurrent acute GVHD in 2 patients, 1 at 18 days and another 49 days following the initial dose. Plasma EBV DNA titers were followed for 6 weeks after initial administration and exceeded 1000 copies per milliliter in 19 patients (43%), who were effectively treated with rituximab administered weekly until EBV DNA levels declined to less than 1000 copies, for up to four doses. Seven subjects received a single dose of rituximab, while 10 subjects received multiple doses. No fatal cases of posttransplantation lymphoproliferative disorder were observed.[221]

To date, there are no published reports of the use of this antibody in T-cell lymphomas. A phase I multidose escalation trial of visilizumab for patients with refractory CD3-positive T-cell lymphomas was undertaken and completed at Stanford University.[206] In all, approximately 12 to 15 patients were enrolled, and the results have not been reported.

CD30-Targeted Therapies

MDX-060 MDX-060 is a humanized mAb directed against CD30. A phase I/II dose-escalation trial enrolled 72 heavily pretreated (median: 4 prior regimens) patients, 9 with T-cell lymphoma (7 ALCL, 2 unspecified), and the remainder with Hodgkin lymphoma.[222] Two of the patients with ALCL (29%) had complete responses, with responses or stable disease seen at all dose levels (1, 5, 10, and 15 mg/kg) except the initial dose level of 0.1 mg/kg. Overall, the antibody was well tolerated, with pulmonary toxicity (dyspnea and acute respiratory distress syndrome) being the most common grade III/IV toxicity thought to be related to the infusion, occurring in 3 of 72 (4%) patients. A larger phase II with a target enrollment of 45 patients with ALCL has been completed[223] with pending results.

SGN-30 SGN-30 is a chimeric mAb. *In vitro* binding assays have demonstrated that specific binding of SGN-30 is restricted to activated T cells, and CD30+ cancer-cell lines. In a phase I multidose escalation study involving predominantly heavily pretreated patients, dosages of 2 mg/kg, 4 mg/kg, 8 mg/kg, and 12 mg/kg were each administered to 24 patients (6 patients per group) on a weekly schedule for 6 consecutive weeks. Overall treatment was well tolerated with no dose-limiting toxicity observed. There was one CR and no PR observed. The most commonly observed toxicities were asthenia, fever, and nausea, all observed in 3 of 24 (12.5%) patients. In the 8-mg/kg dosing group, there was one CR (a patient with cutaneous ALCL). Four patients exhibited human antichimeric antibodies.[197] A phase II trial utilizing a dose of 12 mg/kg enrolled 19 patients, of whom 17 were evaluable.[224] The overall response rate was 58 percent, with five CRs (three of whom had mycoses fungoides) and five PRs (all were ALCL patients). One patient with mycoses fungoides had stable disease. Overall, SGN-30 was well tolerated with grades III to IV toxicities restricted to pruritus and rash in one patient (6%) each, probably unrelated to drug. Although the data are limited, there does appear to be significant activity of this agent, and more studies are needed. There is also the potential for additional dose escalation of SGN-30.

Daclizumab Daclizumab is a humanized mAb targeting the CD25 chain of the IL-2 receptor that functions as a competitive inhibitor of IL-2. In a phase I trial, 35 heavily pretreated patients with CD25-positive malignancies, 6 of whom had T-cell leukemia/lymphoma, were treated with escalating doses of a daclizumab LMB-2 (*Pseudomonas* exotoxin A) conjugate. The maximum tolerated dose was 40 mcg/kg on alternating days, and the dose-limiting toxicity was transaminitis. There was one CR and seven PR, of which one responder was a patient with cutaneous T-cell lymphoma, and another a patient with adult T-cell leukemia/lymphoma. All responses were seen at a dose >20 mcg/kg. The maximum tolerated dose was 40 mcg/kg with dose-limiting toxicity observed at 63 mcg/kg of transaminitis and cardiomyopathy. Overall, liver function abnormalities and fevers were the most common toxicities.[225]

Results with denileukin diftitox (ONTAK), a cytotoxic fusion protein that also targets CD25,[226] suggest that daclizumab may also be of benefit in CD25-negative T-cell lymphoma. In a phase II study that enrolled 27 patients with relapsed/refractory T-cell lymphoma, the majority of whom had PTCL, objective responses were seen in patients with CD25-positive (8/13 patients) as well as CD25-negative tumors (5/11 patients), suggesting that this target may be of general relevance to this disease.[227] Overall, therapy was well-tolerated with no grade IV toxicities. The most common grade III toxicity was transaminitis (6/27 patients). Although there are no published data describing the use of daclizumab in CD25-negative T-cell lymphoma, these data support further investigation of daclizumab in this patient population.

OTHER TREATMENT MODALITIES INCLUDING CHEMOTHERAPY

CONVENTIONAL CHEMOTHERAPY

With the exception of ALCL, treating T-cell lymphomas with conventional anthracycline-based chemotherapeutic regimens has resulted in limited success. Low overall response rates, short progression-free survival, and resistant disease underscore the inherent chemorefractoriness of T-cell lymphomas compared to their B-cell counterparts. Of 134 cases of PTCL diagnosed at three centers from 1973 to 1986, 80 patients had been treated with intensive regimens such as CHOP with or without bleomycin, CAP-BOP (cyclophosphamide, doxorubicin, procarbazine, bleomycin, vincristine, prednisone), COMLA (cyclophosphamide, vincristine, methotrexate, cytosine arabinoside), and MACOP-B.[228] For all patients, the median survival was 17 months, and the 4-year survival was 28 percent. Of the 80 patients who received intensive combination chemotherapy, 50 percent achieved a CR, with 4-year disease-free survival being 41 percent. The 4-year overall survival of the intensively treated group was 45 percent. Fifty percent of the intensively treated patients had stage IV disease, and 4-year disease-free survival for that group was only 10 percent.

At the Mayo Clinic, 78 patients with PTCL were treated with anthracycline-containing regimens, including CHOP, ProMACE-CytaBOM, and m-BACOD (methotrexate, bleomycin, doxorubicin, cyclophosphamide, vincristine, dexamethasone).[229] The median overall survival was 22 months (range: 1 to 105+ months). The IPI was highly prognostic, with median survivals for high-risk, high-intermediate risk, low-intermediate, and low-risk patients of 6 months, 15 months, 24 months, and not reached, respectively (P <0.001). Among the various T-cell subtypes there were no significant differences in response rates or overall survival. The Non-Hodgkin's Lymphoma Classification Project included 96 cases of non-ALCL PTCL comprising 7 percent of all non-Hodgkin lymphoma cases. The majority (70%) of these patients had received doxorubicin-containing regimens. The 5-year overall survival was 26 percent, and the failure-free survival was 20 percent.[93]

Of the T-cell lymphomas, ALCL appears to confer relative chemosensitivity and is predictive of improved outcomes with cytotoxic chemotherapy. A European study evaluated 288 PTCL patients (60 cases of T-ALCL and 228 cases of non-ALCL PTCL) treated with anthracycline-containing regimens such as NCVB (mitoxantrone, cyclophosphamide, vindesine, bleomycin, prednisone), ACVB (doxorubicin, cyclophosphamide, vindesine, bleomycin, prednisone) and m-BACOD, followed by consolidation and maintenance therapies or autologous stem cell transplantation. Overall there was a 54 percent complete response rate, with 72 percent of patients with ALCL achieving a complete response versus only 49 percent for those with non-ALCL T-cell lymphomas. Five-year overall survival rates mirrored the complete response rates: 41 percent for all patients, and 64 percent and 35 percent for ALCL and non-ALCL PTCL, respectively. Multivariate analysis revealed five prognostic factors: (1) age older than 60 years, (2) performance status, (3) elevated LDH, (4) advanced stage, and (5) non-ALCL PTCL.[74] Similarly a Spanish study evaluated 174 patients with T-cell lymphomas. Thirty were ALCL and the remainder consisted of PTCL-unspecified (95 cases), AITL (22 cases), angiocentric intestinal T-cell lymphoma (12 cases), and hepatosplenic $\gamma\delta$ T-cell lymphoma (1 case). Most patients received doxorubicin-containing regimens. Rates of complete response were 69 percent for ALCL cases and 45 percent for other PTCL subtypes, with a median survival of 65 months for ALCL and 20 months for other PTCL subtypes, and 4-year survival probabilities of 62 percent and 32 percent, respectively.[230]

Sixty-eight T-cell lymphoma patients treated from 1984 to 1995 were studied. Patients received anthracycline-containing regimens such as CHOP-bleomycin alternating with DHAP (dexamethasone, cisplatin, cytarabine), CHOP-bleomycin alternating with OPEN (vincristine, etoposide, mitoxantrone, prednisone), CHOP-bleomycin alternating with CMED (cyclophosphamide, etoposide, methotrexate, dexamethasone), or alternating triple therapy consisting of ASHAP (cytarabine, doxorubicin, cisplatin, methylprednisolone), MBACOS (doxorubicin, cyclophosphamide, vincristine, bleomycin, methylprednisolone, methotrexate), and MINE (mesna, ifosfamide, mitoxantrone, etoposide). The complete response rate was 65 percent, the 5-year failure-free survival rate was 38 percent, and overall survival result was 38 percent. ALCL patients had a better outcome.[231] In addition, late relapses were common in non-ALCL patients.

Included in Non-Hodgkin's Lymphoma Classification Project were 33 T-null (indeterminant)-ALCL patients. Compared to the non–T-ALCL PTCL group, patients were significantly younger, less likely to have advance stage disease or marrow involvement, more likely to have a favorable IPI score, and, importantly, have greater survival results. The estimated 5-year overall survival for all T-null-ALCL patients in this series was 75 percent and the failure-free survival was 56 percent, and most (81%) of these patients had been treated for curative intent with doxorubicin-containing regimens. The status of ALK expression was neither predictive of response nor survival.[232] In contrast, a study that evaluated 57 patients with systemic T-null-ALCL treated with intensive anthracycline-based chemotherapy reported 5-year overall survival rate of 57 percent (56% for 32 cases of T-ALCL and 83% for 25 cases of null-ALCL).[75] Expression of ALK in this study predicted survival; the 5-year overall survival was 93 percent and the 5-year failure-free survival was 88 percent, while the 5-year overall survival was 37 percent and the 5-year failure-free survival was 37 percent for the ALK- cases (P <0.005). Finally, a retrospective study involving patients with systemic T-null-ALCL who for the most part received doxorubicin-containing regimens demonstrated an overall survival of 71 percent for the ALK-positive subgroup versus 15 percent for the ALK-negative subgroup. Similarly, 10-year disease-free survival rates were 82 percent for the ALK+ patients and 28 percent for the ALK– patients.[61] Studies evaluating treatment for other specific T-cell lymphoma subtypes that are non-ALCL generally have reported disappointing response, duration of response, and survival rates, and are included in the disease-specific treatment sections.

PRALATREXATE

Pralatrexate is a second-generation 10-deazaaminopterin antifolate. Compared to its predecessor methotrexate, it is more effectively internalized by its receptor, the reduced folate carrier type one (RFC-1), thereby achieving higher intercellular concentrations and is more effectively retained in the cell as a result of its more extensive polyglutamylation.[233,234] Pralatrexate was evaluated and found to be more active than methotrexate *in vitro* and *in vivo* using a variety of lymphoma cell lines and tumor xenografts, and activity correlated with RFC-1 expression.[235] Based on the experience, 16 patients were treated with a biweekly dose of 135 mg/m^2, with high rates of grade III/IV mucositis observed (6/16, 37.5%) as a dose-limiting toxicity. One patient with PTCL had a CR, prompting the treatment of four additional patients with chemorefractory T-cell lymphomas, all of whom had a CR. In a phase I/II trial, patients were given vitamin B_{12} and folic acid replacement to correct methylmalonic acid and homocysteine levels, and treated with a weekly dose of 30 mg/m^2. This approach resulted in thrombocytopenia replacing mucositis as the dose-limiting toxicity. Although only 1 of 18 patients with B-cell lymphoma responded, of the 20 evaluable T-cell lymphoma patients, 10 (50%) responded, with 9 complete responders.[234,236,237] These data led the FDA to grant pralatrexate orphan drug and fast-track designation in T-cell lymphomas, and led to a large phase II trial to evaluate the safety and efficacy of pralatrexate in patients with relapsed or refractory T-cell lymphoma. Enrolling 115 patients, the Pralatrexate in Patients with Relapsed or Refractory Peripheral T-cell Lymphoma Study represented the largest prospective trial of patients with T-cell lymphoma. In general, patients were heavily pretreated, receiving a median of three prior lines of systemic therapy. The primary endpoint of the study was objective response, and of the 109 evaluable patients, 29 (23%) patients responded, with median duration of response estimated to be greater than 9 months as a secondary endpoint.[238]

ROMIDEPSIN

Romidepsin (depsipeptide, FR-901228) is a pan-histone deacetylase (HDAC) inhibitor derived as fermentation product of *Chromobacterium violaceum* with a cyclic peptide that is structurally distinct from other known HDAC inhibitors. It was originally identified in a high-throughput screen for compounds capable of reversing the malignant phenotype of H-ras transformed NIH-3T3 cells. In a phase I study, objective responses were observed in patients with refractory T-cell lymphomas, including a complete response in a patient with PTCL.[239] An open-label phase II trial was undertaken for patients with progressive or relapsed cutaneous T-cell lymphoma or PTCL. Patients received romidepsin 14 mg/m^2 as a 4-hour infusion on days 1, 8, and 15 every 28 days. Of the 43 patients with PTCL, the mean number of prior therapies was 3.9 (range: 1–12) and the mean number of cycles of treatment was 6.8 (range: 1–37). The overall response rate was 39 percent, with 16 percent of the patients achieving a complete response. The overall median duration of response was 8.3 months (range: 1.6 months to 4.8+ years). Adverse events related to treatment were mild and included most commonly nausea (86%, all grades 1–2), asthenia (79%, all grades 1–2), thrombocytopenia (70%, with 7% grades 3–4), and granulocytopenia (63% with 5% grades 3–4).[240,241]

HIGH-DOSE CHEMOTHERAPY AND TRANSPLANTATION

Several groups have examined the impact of high-dose chemotherapy on T-cell lymphomas. In a retrospective analysis of 36 patients with relapsed or refractory PTCL who received high-dose chemotherapy and autologous (29 patients) or allogeneic (7 patients) hematopoietic transplantation,[109] the 3-year overall survival rate was 36 percent and progression-free survival rate was 28 percent. The 3-year probabilities of survival for the autologous and allogeneic groups were 39 percent and 29 percent, respectively, whereas the progression-free survival rates at 3 years were 32 percent and 14 percent, respectively. The pretransplantation serum LDH level was the most important prognostic factor for both overall survival and progression-free survival results. An IPI score of ≤ 1 was predictive of increased overall survival but progression-free survival rates did not differ. At a median followup of 43 months, 13 patients (36%) were still alive with no evidence of disease. These data were comparable to published studies on high-dose chemotherapy for relapsed or refractory B-cell lymphomas, and suggested that stem cell transplantation should be considered for selected patients with T-cell lymphomas. In a study of 41 patients with relapsed intermediate or high-grade lymphomas (17 cases of T-cell and 24 cases of B-cell lymphomas) who underwent high-dose therapy and autologous transplantation for salvage therapy, comparable results were obtained for B- and T-cell lymphomas.[108] Although not statistically significant, the T-cell patients had a slightly higher CR rate (59% compared to 42%), and the duration of remission was similar overall (median time to progression of 30 months, with no late relapses). The 2-year overall survival rates for both groups were similar, being 35 percent for T-cell lymphomas and 30 percent for B-cell lymphomas, as were the 2-year rates of disease-free survival (28% for the T-cell group and 17% for the B-cell group). Predictors of poor outcome for both groups of patients were poor performance status, bulky tumor, and high serum LDH levels. A study involving 40 patients with relapsed T-cell lymphomas from Norway and Sweden also examined the role of high-dose therapy with autologous stem cell transplantation.[110] All patients had chemosensitive disease and had received anthracycline-containing regimens, primarily CHOP, VACOP-B (etoposide, doxorubicin, cyclophosphamide, vincristine, prednisone, bleomycin), or MACOP-B prior to transplantation. At the time of stem cell transplant, 17 patients were in first PR or CR, and 23 were in second or third PR or CR. The conditioning regimens used were BEAM (high-dose carmustine, etoposide, cytarabine, and melphalan) in 15 patients, BEAC (carmustine, etoposide, cytarabine, cyclophosphamide) in 14 patients, BEAC without etoposide and total-body irradiation in 1 patient, cyclophosphamide and total-body radiation in 8 patients, and melphalan and mitoxantrone in 2 patients. Although there were 3 (7.5%) treatment-related deaths, 32 patients (80%) achieved a CR after transplantation. Relapses occurred in 16 patients, all within 2 years following transplantation. The 3-year overall, event-free, and relapse-free survival rates were 58 percent, 48 percent, and 56 percent, respectively. As expected given its chemosensitivity, patients with ALCL had better outcomes than did those with other histologies (79% vs. 44%, respectively). Overall, these data appeared similar to historical data reported for stem cell transplantation performed for relapsed high-grade B-cell lymphomas.[242]

PURINE ANALOGUES

The purine analogues pentostatin (deoxycoformycin), fludarabine, and cladribine (2-chlorodeoxyadenosine) are a group of structurally similar drugs that are active agents in the therapy of T-cell lymphomas. T-cells have high levels of adenosine deaminase, a key enzyme involved in purine metabolism, and as adenosine deaminase inhibitors, these drugs produce DNA damage and impairment of DNA repair. As single agents, the purine analogues are relatively well tolerated, producing mild myelosuppression, although the latter adverse effect is more severe with cladribine than with pentostatin. Of note is the fact that these agents produce lymphopenia and immunosuppression, occasionally resulting in the development of opportunistic infections.

Several studies have demonstrated that pentostatin has activity in T-cell lymphoma therapy. Investigators demonstrated that pentostatin has activity in mature T-cell malignancies. One hundred forty-five patients with mature T-cell tumors, most of whom had disease considered relapsed/refractory to anthracycline-containing regimens or alkylating agents, received pentostatin-based chemotherapy. The overall response rate was 32 percent and the median overall duration of response was 6 months, ranging from 3 to 66 months.[113] For the 55 patients with T-PLL, 5 achieved a CR and 20 achieved a PR, lasting from 3 to 16 months (median: 6 months), for an overall response rate of 45 percent. Two of 5 patients with LGL leukemia also achieved a CR, one lasting 18 months and the other lasting 12 months. However, other subsets of T-cell disease in this study had lower response rates to pentostatin. Two of 25 patients with adult T-cell leukemia/lymphoma achieved a CR, one lasting 33 months and the other died of an opportunistic infection while still in CR 5 months after stopping drug treatment; another patient achieved a PR lasting 5 months. The overall response rate was 12 percent. Twenty-seven patients with PTCL were treated, with 5 responses, none complete, resulting in an overall response rate of 19 percent. The durations of response ranged from 3 to 28 months, with a median of 9 months. Response rates of previously untreated patients compared to those for patients previously treated with one or more regimens did not differ significantly (35% vs. 29%, respectively); histologic subtype was the single most important factor influencing results.

Fourteen patients with relapsed noncutaneous T-cell lymphomas were treated with pentostatin.[243] One patient (7%) had a CR and six (43%) had partial responses, with the median progression-free survival result for responders being 6 months (range: 2–15 months). A significant reduction in circulating CD26+ T lymphocytes was observed in treated patients, possibly related to immunosuppression, predisposing them to opportunistic infections. One patient with PR had reactivation of genital herpes that cleared upon pentostatin discontinuation with recovery of CD26+ T-cell levels. Because CD4+CD26+ T lymphocytes are memory helper T cells, the selective loss of CD26+ T cells in lymphoma patients treated with pentostatin has important clinical implications, and may partly explain the relatively high incidence of opportunistic infections.

Another study also demonstrated 2-chlorodeoxyadenosine (2-CDA) activity in T-cell lymphomas, as 22 patients with such varied diagnoses as T-LGL, T-PLL, T-cell chronic lymphocytic leukemia (T-CLL), and PTCL who were treated with 2-CDA had a response rate of 41 percent. Four responders (18%) had CRs (one T-PLL, one patient with mycosis fungoides, two T-LGL) while five patients (23%) had PRs (two T-CLL, one Sézary syndrome, two PTCL). All patients with PR and one CR patient developed relapses at a median of 7 months (range: 5 to 26 months), while three patients with CR remained in remission at 30+, 36+, and 54+ months. The median overall survival was 12 months, and the main toxicities were fever and infection.[244] The combination of fludarabine, mitoxantrone, and dexamethasone has produced one CR that lasted 15 months after treatment cessation in a patient with aggressive subcutaneous panniculitis-like T-cell lymphoma.[245]

GEMCITABINE

Gemcitabine is a novel pyrimidine antimetabolite with clinical activity and a low toxicity profile in solid tumors and selected T-cell hematologic malignancies. A phase II study involving 44 previously treated patients with either mycosis fungoides (n = 30) or PTCL with exclusive skin involvement (n = 14) treated with gemcitabine reported 5 (11.5%) CRs and 26 (59%) PRs, for an overall response rate of 70.5 percent.[246] Two of 14 (14.5%) PTCL patients had CRs and 8 of 14 (57%) achieved PR, similar to response rates seen for mycosis fungoides patients. The median duration of CR was 15 months (range: 6 to 22 months) and of PR was 10 months (range: 2 to 15 months). Another multicenter phase II trial treated 32 untreated patients, 5 of whom had PTCL with skin involvement, the remainder having cutaneous T-cell lymphoma. Gemcitabine at a dose of 1200 mg/m^2 was administered on days 1, 8, and 15 of each 28-day cycle for 6 cycles. All patients with PTCL responded, with one CR and four PRs. Treatment was well-tolerated with mild hematologic toxicity.[247] Gemcitabine was also found to be effective and well tolerated therapy for relapsed or refractory T-cell malignancies in another study involving 10 patients with various histologies.[248] There were two CR and four PR, for an overall response rate of 60 percent, with a median duration of response of 13.5 months.

REFERENCES

1. Escalon MP, Liu NS, Yang Y, et al: Prognostic factors and treatment of patients with T-cell non-Hodgkin lymphoma: The M.D. Anderson Cancer Center experience. *Cancer* 103:2091, 2005.
2. Robb-Smith AH: U.S. National Cancer Institute working formulation of non-Hodgkin's lymphomas for clinical use. *Lancet* 2:432, 1982.
3. Harris NL, Jaffe ES, Stein H, et al: A revised European-American classification of lymphoid neoplasms: A proposal from the International Lymphoma Study Group. *Blood* 84:1361, 1994.
4. Jaffe ES, Krenacs L, Raffeld M: Classification of T-cell and NK-cell neoplasms based on the REAL classification. *Ann Oncol* 8 Suppl 2:17, 1997.
5. Kojima K, Hara M, Sawada T, et al: Human T-lymphotropic virus type I provirus and T-cell prolymphocytic leukemia. *Leuk Lymphoma* 38:381, 2000.
6. Kojima K, Sawada T, Ikezoe T, et al: Defective human T-lymphotrophic virus type I provirus in T-cell prolymphocytic leukaemia. *Br J Haematol* 105:376, 1999.
7. Maslak P: T-cell prolymphocytic leukemia. *ASH Image Bank* 100213, 2001.
8. Matutes E, Brito-Babapulle B, Swansbury J, et al: Clinical and laboratory features of 78 cases of T-prolymphocytic leukemia. *Blood* 78:3269, 1991.
9. Dearden CE, Matutes E, Cazin B, et al: High remission rate in T-cell prolymphocytic leukemia with CAMPATH-1H. *Blood* 98:1721, 2001.
10. Okamura K, Ikeda T, Shimakura Y, et al: [Allogeneic bone marrow transplantation for chemotherapy-resistant T-prolymphocytic leukemia.] *Rinsho Ketsueki* 46:527, 2005.
11. Murase K, Matsunaga T, Sato T, et al: Allogeneic bone marrow transplantation in a patient with T-prolymphocytic leukemia with small-intestinal involvement. *Int J Clin Oncol* 8:391, 2003.
12. Garderet L, Bittencourt H, Kaliski A, et al: Treatment of T-prolymphocytic leukemia with nonmyeloablative allogeneic stem cell transplantation. *Eur J Haematol* 66:137, 2001.
13. Collins RH, Pineiro LA, Agura ED, Fay JW: Treatment of T prolymphocytic leukemia with allogeneic bone marrow transplantation. *Bone Marrow Transplant* 21:627, 1998.
14. Lamy T, Loughran TP Jr: Clinical features of large granular lymphocyte leukemia. *Semin Hematol* 40:185, 2003.
15. Epling-Burnette PK, Loughran TP Jr: Survival signals in leukemic large granular lymphocytes. *Semin Hematol* 40:213, 2003.
16. Zambello R, Trentin L, Facco M, et al: Analysis of the T cell receptor in the lymphoproliferative disease of granular lymphocytes: Superantigen activation of clonal CD3+ granular lymphocytes. *Cancer Res* 55:6140, 1995.
17. Lamy T, Loughran TP: Large granular lymphocyte leukemia. *Cancer Control* 5:253, 1998.
18. Semenzato G, Pandolfi F, Chisesi T, et al: The lymphoproliferative disease of granular lymphocytes. A heterogeneous disorder ranging from indolent to aggressive conditions. *Cancer* 60:2971, 1987.
19. Osuji N, Matutes E, Catovsky D, et al: Histopathology of the spleen in T-cell large granular lymphocyte leukemia and T-cell prolymphocytic leukemia: A comparative review. *Am J Surg Pathol* 29:935, 2005.
20. Berliner N, Horwitz M, Loughran TP Jr: Congenital and acquired neutropenia. *Hematology Am Soc Hematol Educ Program* 63, 2004.

21. Loughran TP Jr, Clark EA, Price TH, Hammond WP: Adult-onset cyclic neutropenia is associated with increased large granular lymphocytes. *Blood* 68:1082, 1986.
22. Loughran TP Jr: Clonal diseases of large granular lymphocytes. *Blood* 82:14, 1993.
23. Sokol L, Loughran TP Jr: Large granular lymphocyte leukemia. *Oncologist* 11:263, 2006.
24. Witzig TE, Weitz JJ, Lundberg JH, Tefferi A: Treatment of refractory T-cell chronic lymphocytic leukemia with purine nucleoside analogues. *Leuk Lymphoma* 14:137, 1994.
25. Osuji N, Gel Giudice I, Matutes E, et al: CD52 expression in T-cell large granular lymphocyte leukemia—Implications for treatment with alemtuzumab. *Leuk Lymphoma* 46:723, 2005.
26. Chan JK, Sin VC, Wong KF, et al: Nonnasal lymphoma expressing the natural killer cell marker CD56: A clinicopathologic study of 49 cases of an uncommon aggressive neoplasm. *Blood* 89:4501, 1997.
27. Siu LL, Chan JK, Kwong YL: Natural killer cell malignancies: Clinicopathologic and molecular features. *Histol Histopathol* 17:539, 2002.
28. Cheung MM, Chan JK, Wong KF: Natural killer cell neoplasms: A distinctive group of highly aggressive lymphomas/leukemias. *Semin Hematol* 40:221, 2003.
29. Ruskova A, Thula R, Chan G: Aggressive natural killer-cell leukemia: Report of five cases and review of the literature. *Leuk Lymphoma* 45:2427, 2004.
30. Okamura T, Kishimoto T, Inoue M, et al: Unrelated bone marrow transplantation for Epstein-Barr virus-associated T/NK-cell lymphoproliferative disease. *Bone Marrow Transplant* 31:105, 2003.
31. Casale DA, Bartlett NL, Hurd DD, et al: A phase I open label dose escalation study to evaluate MEDI-507 in patients with CD2-positive T-cell lymphoma/leukemia. *Blood* 108:771A, 2006.
32. Uchiyama T, Yodoi J, Sagawa K, et al: Adult T-cell leukemia: Clinical and hematologic features of 16 cases. *Blood* 50:481, 1977.
33. Bunn PA Jr, Schechter GP, Jaffe E, et al: Clinical course of retrovirus-associated adult T-cell lymphoma in the United States. *N Engl J Med* 309:257, 1983.
34. Franchini G, Nicot C, Johnson JM: Seizing of T cells by human T-cell leukemia/lymphoma virus type 1. *Adv Cancer Res* 89:69, 2003.
35. Tajima K: The 4th nation-wide study of adult T-cell leukemia/lymphoma (ATL) in Japan: Estimates of risk of ATL and its geographical and clinical features. The T- and B-cell Malignancy Study Group. *Int J Cancer* 45:237, 1990.
36. Shuh M, Beilke M: The human T-cell leukemia virus type 1 (HTLV-1): New insights into the clinical aspects and molecular pathogenesis of adult T-cell leukemia/lymphoma (ATLL) and tropical spastic paraparesis/HTLV-associated myelopathy (TSP/HAM). *Microsc Res Tech* 68:176, 2005.
37. Suzumiya J, Ohshima K, Tamura K, et al: The international prognostic index predicts outcome in aggressive adult T-cell leukemia/lymphoma: Analysis of 126 patients from the International Peripheral T-Cell Lymphoma Project. *Ann Oncol* 20:715, 2009.
38. Aisenberg AC, Krontiris TG, Mak TW, et al: Rearrangement of the gene for the beta chain of the T-cell receptor in T-cell chronic lymphocytic leukemia and related disorders. *N Engl J Med* 313:529, 1985.
39. Moriyama K, Muranishi H, Nishimura J, et al: Immunodeficiency in preclinical smoldering adult T-cell leukemia. *Jpn J Clin Oncol* 18:363, 1988.
40. Shimoyama M: Diagnostic criteria and classification of clinical subtypes of adult T-cell leukaemia-lymphoma. A report from the Lymphoma Study Group (1984–87). *Br J Haematol* 79:428, 1991.
41. Pancake BA, Wassef EH, Zucker-Franklin D: Demonstration of antibodies to human T-cell lymphotropic virus-I tax in patients with the cutaneous T-cell lymphoma, mycosis fungoides, who are seronegative for antibodies to the structural proteins of the virus. *Blood* 88:3004, 1996.
42. Waldmann TA, Greene WC, Sarin PS, et al: Functional and phenotypic comparison of human T cell leukemia/lymphoma virus positive adult T cell leukemia with human T cell leukemia/lymphoma virus negative Sézary leukemia, and their distinction using anti-Tac. Monoclonal antibody identifying the human receptor for T cell growth factor. *J Clin Invest* 73:1711, 1984.
43. Maeda K, Takahashi M: Characterization of skin infiltrating cells in adult T-cell leukaemia/lymphoma (ATLL): Clinical, histological and immunohistochemical studies on eight cases. *Br J Dermatol* 121:603, 1989.
44. Flug F, Pelicci PG, Bonetti F, et al: T-cell receptor gene rearrangements as markers of lineage and clonality in T-cell neoplasms. *Proc Natl Acad Sci U S A* 82:3460, 1985.
45. Waldmann TA, Davis MM, Bongiovanni KF, Korsmeyer SJ: Rearrangements of genes for the antigen receptor on T cells as markers of lineage and clonality in human lymphoid neoplasms. *N Engl J Med* 313:776, 1985.
46. Bertness V, Kirsch I, Hollis G, et al: T-cell receptor gene rearrangements as clinical markers of human T-cell lymphomas. *N Engl J Med* 313:534, 1985.
47. Shimoyama M, Ota K, Kikuchi M, et al: Major prognostic factors of adult patients with advanced T-cell lymphoma/leukemia. *J Clin Oncol* 6:1088, 1988.
48. Shimoyama M, Ota K, Kikuchi M, et al: Chemotherapeutic results and prognostic factors of patients with advanced non-Hodgkin's lymphoma treated with VEPA or VEPA-M. *J Clin Oncol* 6:128, 1988.
49. Yamada Y, Tomonaga M, Fukuda H, et al: A new G-CSF-supported combination chemotherapy, LSG15, for adult T-cell leukaemia-lymphoma: Japan Clinical Oncology Group Study 9303. *Br J Haematol* 113:375, 2001.
50. Tsukasaki K, Tobinai K, Shimoyama M, et al: Deoxycoformycin-containing combination chemotherapy for adult T-cell leukemia-lymphoma: Japan Clinical Oncology Group Study (JCOG9109). *Int J Hematol* 77:164, 2003.
51. Tsuda H, Takatsuki K, Ohno R, et al: Treatment of adult T-cell leukaemia-lymphoma with irinotecan hydrochloride (CPT-11). CPT-11 Study Group on Hematological Malignancy. *Br J Cancer* 70:771, 1994.
52. Waldmann TA, White JD, Carrasquillo JA, et al: Radioimmunotherapy of interleukin-2R alpha-expressing adult T-cell leukemia with yttrium-90-labeled anti-Tac. *Blood* 86:4063, 1995.
53. Waldmann TA, Goldman CK, Bongiovanni KF, et al: Therapy of patients with human T-cell lymphotrophic virus I-induced adult T-cell leukemia with anti-Tac, a monoclonal antibody to the receptor for interleukin-2. *Blood* 72:1805, 1988.
54. Evens AM, Ziegler SL, Gupta R, et al: Sustained hematologic and central nervous system remission with single-agent denileukin diftitox in refractory adult T-cell leukemia/lymphoma. *Clin Lymphoma Myeloma* 7:472, 2007.
55. Matutes E, Taylor GP, Cavenagh J, et al: Interferon alpha and zidovudine therapy in adult T-cell leukaemia lymphoma: Response and outcome in 15 patients. *Br J Haematol* 113:779, 2001.
56. Utsunomiya A, Miyazaki Y, Takatsuka Y, et al: Improved outcome of adult T cell leukemia/lymphoma with allogeneic hematopoietic stem cell transplantation. *Bone Marrow Transplant* 27:15, 2001.
57. Stein H, Mason DY, Gerdes J, et al: The expression of the Hodgkin's disease associated antigen Ki-1 in reactive and neoplastic lymphoid tissue: Evidence that Reed-Sternberg cells and histiocytic malignancies are derived from activated lymphoid cells. *Blood* 66:848, 1985.
58. Pulford K, Lamant L, Morris SW, et al: Detection of anaplastic lymphoma kinase (ALK) and nucleolar protein nucleophosmin (NPM)-ALK proteins in normal and neoplastic cells with the monoclonal antibody ALK1. *Blood* 89:1394, 1997.
59. Falini B, Gigema B, Fizzotti M, et al: ALK expression defines a distinct group of T/null lymphomas ("ALK lymphomas") with a wide morphological spectrum. *Am J Pathol* 153:875, 1998.
60. Rimokh R, Magaud JP, Berger F, et al: A translocation involving a specific breakpoint (q35) on chromosome 5 is characteristic of anaplastic large cell lymphoma ("Ki-1 lymphoma"). *Br J Haematol* 71:31, 1989.
61. Falini B, Pileri S, Zinzani PL, et al: ALK+ lymphoma: Clinico-pathological findings and outcome. *Blood* 93:2697, 1999.
62. Krenacs L, Wellmann A, Sorbara L, et al: Cytotoxic cell antigen expression in anaplastic large cell lymphomas of T- and null-cell type and Hodgkin's disease: Evidence for distinct cellular origin. *Blood* 89:980, 1997.
63. Foss HD, Anagnostopoulos I, Araujo I, et al: Anaplastic large-cell lymphomas of T-cell and null-cell phenotype express cytotoxic molecules. *Blood* 88:4005, 1996.
64. Slupianek A, Nieborowska-Skorska M, Hoser G, Morrione A: Role of phosphatidylinositol 3-kinase-Akt pathway in nucleophosmin/anaplastic lymphoma kinase-mediated lymphomagenesis. *Cancer Res* 61:2194, 2001.
65. Kuefer MU, Look AT, Pulford K, et al: Retrovirus-mediated gene transfer of NPM-ALK causes lymphoid malignancy in mice. *Blood* 90:2901, 1997.
66. Duyster J, Bai RY, Morris SW: Translocations involving anaplastic lymphoma kinase (ALK). *Oncogene* 20:5623, 2001.
67. Bai RY, Ouyang T, Miething C, et al: Nucleophosmin-anaplastic lymphoma kinase associated with anaplastic large-cell lymphoma activates the phosphatidylinositol 3-kinase/Akt antiapoptotic signaling pathway. *Blood* 96:4319, 2000.
68. Zhang Q, Raghunath PN, Xue L, et al: Multilevel dysregulation of STAT3 activation in anaplastic lymphoma kinase-positive T/null-cell lymphoma. *J Immunol* 168:466, 2002.
69. Benharroch D, Meguerian-Bedoyan Z, Lamant L, et al: ALK-positive lymphoma: A single disease with a broad spectrum of morphology. *Blood* 91:2076, 1998.
70. DeCoteau JF, Bulmarc JR, Kinney MC, Kadin ME: The t(2;5) chromosomal translocation is not a common feature of primary cutaneous CD30+ lymphoproliferative disorders: Comparison with anaplastic large-cell lymphoma of nodal origin. *Blood* 87:3437, 1996.
71. Lamant L, de Reynies A, Duplantier MM, et al: Gene-expression profiling of systemic anaplastic large-cell lymphoma reveals differences based on ALK status and two distinct morphologic ALK+ subtypes. *Blood* 109:2156, 2007.
72. Salaverria I, Bea S, Lopez-Guillermo A, et al: Genomic profiling reveals different genetic aberrations in systemic ALK-positive and ALK-negative anaplastic large cell lymphomas. *Br J Haematol* 140:516, 2008.
73. Tilly H, Gaulard P, Lepage E, et al: Primary anaplastic large-cell lymphoma in adults: Clinical presentation, immunophenotype, and outcome. *Blood* 90:3727, 1997.
74. Gisselbrecht C, Gaulard P, Lepage E, et al: Prognostic significance of T-cell phenotype in aggressive non-Hodgkin's lymphomas. Groupe d'Etudes des Lymphomes de l'Adulte (GELA). *Blood* 92:762, 1998.
75. Gascoyne RD, Aoun P, Wu D, et al: Prognostic significance of anaplastic lymphoma kinase (ALK) protein expression in adults with anaplastic large cell lymphoma. *Blood* 93:3913, 1999.
76. Suzuki R, Kagami Y, Takeuchi K, et al: Prognostic significance of CD56 expression for ALK-positive and ALK-negative anaplastic large-cell lymphoma of T/null cell phenotype. *Blood* 96:2993, 2000.
77. Savage KJ, Harris NL, Vose JM, et al: ALK- anaplastic large-cell lymphoma is clinically and immunophenotypically different from both ALK+ ALCL and peripheral T-cell lymphoma, not otherwise specified: Report from the International Peripheral T-Cell Lymphoma Project. *Blood* 111:5496, 2008.
78. Fraga M, Brousset P, Schlaifer D, et al: Bone marrow involvement in anaplastic large cell lymphoma. Immunohistochemical detection of minimal disease and its prognostic significance. *Am J Clin Pathol* 103:82, 1995.

79. Morris SW, Kirstein MN, Valentine MB, et al: Fusion of a kinase gene, ALK, to a nucleolar protein gene, NPM, in non-Hodgkin's lymphoma. *Science* 263:1281, 1994.
80. Kadin ME: Anaplastic large cell lymphoma and its morphological variants. *Cancer Surv* 30:77, 1997.
81. Falini B: Anaplastic large cell lymphoma: Pathological, molecular and clinical features. *Br J Haematol* 114:741, 2001.
82. Brugieres L, Deley MC, Pacquement H, et al: CD30(+) anaplastic large-cell lymphoma in children: Analysis of 82 patients enrolled in two consecutive studies of the French Society of Pediatric Oncology. *Blood* 92:3591, 1998.
83. Massimino M, Gasparini M, Giardini R: Ki-1 (CD30) anaplastic large-cell lymphoma in children. *Ann Oncol* 6:915, 1995.
84. Zinzani PL, Martelli M, Magagnoli M, et al: Anaplastic large cell lymphoma Hodgkin's-like: A randomized trial of ABVD versus MACOP-B with and without radiation therapy. *Blood* 92:790, 1998.
85. Fanin R, Silvestri F, Geromin A, et al: Primary systemic CD30 (Ki-1)-positive anaplastic large cell lymphoma of the adult: Sequential intensive treatment with the F-MACHOP regimen (+/– radiotherapy) and autologous bone marrow transplantation. *Blood* 87:1243, 1996.
86. Fanin R, Silvestri F, Geromin A, et al: Sequential intensive treatment with the F-MACHOP regimen (+/– radiotherapy) and autologous stem cell transplantation for primary systemic CD30 (Ki-1)-positive anaplastic large cell lymphoma in adults. *Leuk Lymphoma* 24:369, 1997.
87. Fanin R, Ruiz de Elvira MC, Sperotto A, et al: Autologous stem cell transplantation for T and null cell CD30-positive anaplastic large cell lymphoma: Analysis of 64 adult and paediatric cases reported to the European Group for Blood and Marrow Transplantation (EBMT). *Bone Marrow Transplant* 23:437, 1999.
88. Deconinck E, Lamy T, Foussard C, et al: Autologous stem cell transplantation for anaplastic large-cell lymphomas: Results of a prospective trial. *Br J Haematol* 109:736, 2000.
89. Vranovsky A, Ladicka M, Lakota J: Autologous stem cell transplantation in first-line treatment of high-risk aggressive non-Hodgkin's lymphoma. *Neoplasma* 55:107, 2008.
90. Woessmann W, Peters C, Lenhard M, et al: Allogeneic haematopoietic stem cell transplantation in relapsed or refractory anaplastic large cell lymphoma of children and adolescents—A Berlin-Frankfurt-Munster group report. *Br J Haematol* 133:176, 2006.
91. Chen CH, Chen SW, Shen WL, et al: Successful allogeneic stem cell transplantation for an adult with refractory anaplastic lymphoma kinase-positive anaplastic large cell lymphoma. *Int J Hematol* 85:105, 2007.
92. Cesaro S, Pillon M, Visintin G, et al: Unrelated bone marrow transplantation for high-risk anaplastic large cell lymphoma in pediatric patients: A single center case series. *Eur J Haematol* 75:22, 2005.
93. Rudiger T, Weisenburger DD, Anderson JR, et al: Peripheral T-cell lymphoma (excluding anaplastic large-cell lymphoma): Results from the Non-Hodgkin's Lymphoma Classification Project. *Ann Oncol* 13:140, 2002.
94. Kim H, Jacobs C, Warnke RA, Dorfman RF: Malignant lymphoma with a high content of epithelioid histiocytes: A distinct clinicopathologic entity and a form of so-called "Lennert's lymphoma." *Cancer* 41:620, 1978.
95. Saragoni A, Falini B, Medri L, et al: [Peripheral T-cell lymphoma associated with hemophagocytic syndrome: A recently identified entity. Clinico-pathologic and immunohistochemical study of 2 cases.] *Pathologica* 82:359, 1990.
96. King PD, Diaz-Arias AA, Birkby WF, Loy TS: Reactive hemophagocytic syndrome simulating acute hepatitis. A case due to hepatic peripheral T-cell lymphoma. *J Clin Gastroenterol* 19:234, 1994.
97. Aubriet S, Zenone T, Kanitakis J, Vital Durand D: [Peripheral T-cell lymphoma 9 months after hemophagocytic syndrome with a favorable outcome after splenectomy.] *Rev Med Interne* 20:718, 1999.
98. Lippman SM, Miller TP, Spier CM, et al: The prognostic significance of the immunotype in diffuse large-cell lymphoma: A comparative study of the T-cell and B-cell phenotype. *Blood* 72:436, 1988.
99. Armitage JO, Vose JM, Linder J, et al: Clinical significance of immunophenotype in diffuse aggressive non-Hodgkin's lymphoma. *J Clin Oncol* 7:1783, 1989.
100. Shimizu K, Hamajima N, Ohnishi K, et al: T-cell phenotype is associated with decreased survival in non-Hodgkin's lymphoma. *Jpn J Cancer Res* 80:720, 1989.
101. Shimoyama M, Oyama A, Tajima K, et al: Differences in clinicopathological characteristics and major prognostic factors between B-lymphoma and peripheral T-lymphoma excluding adult T-cell leukemia/lymphoma. *Leuk Lymphoma* 10:335, 1993.
102. Gallamini A, Stelitano C, Calvi R, et al: Peripheral T-cell lymphoma unspecified (PTCL-U): A new prognostic model from a retrospective multicentric clinical study. *Blood* 103:2474, 2004.
103. Cuadros M, Dave SS, Jaffe ES, et al: Identification of a proliferation signature related to survival in nodal peripheral T-cell lymphomas. *J Clin Oncol* 25:3321, 2007.
104. Greer JP, York JC, Cousar JB, et al: Peripheral T-cell lymphoma: A clinicopathologic study of 42 cases. *J Clin Oncol* 2:788, 1984.
105. Coiffier B, Berger F, Byron PA, Maguad JP: T-cell lymphomas: Immunologic, histologic, clinical, and therapeutic analysis of 63 cases. *J Clin Oncol* 6:1584, 1988.
106. Armitage J, Vose J, Weisenburger D: International peripheral T-cell and natural killer/T-cell lymphoma study: Pathology findings and clinical outcomes. *J Clin Oncol* 26:4124, 2008.
107. Rodríguez-Antona C, Leskelä S, Zajac M, et al: Expression of CYP3A4 as a predictor of response to chemotherapy in peripheral T-cell lymphomas. *Blood* 110:3345, 2007.
108. Vose JM, Peterson C, Bierman PJ, et al: Comparison of high-dose therapy and autologous bone marrow transplantation for T-cell and B-cell non-Hodgkin's lymphomas. *Blood* 76:424, 1990.
109. Rodriguez J, Munsell M, Yazji S, et al: Impact of high-dose chemotherapy on peripheral T-cell lymphomas. *J Clin Oncol* 19:3766, 2001.
110. Blystad AK, Enblad G, Kvaloy S, et al: High-dose therapy with autologous stem cell transplantation in patients with peripheral T cell lymphomas. *Bone Marrow Transplant* 27:711, 2001.
111. Rodriguez J, Conde E, Gutierrez A, et al: The results of consolidation with autologous stem-cell transplantation in patients with peripheral T-cell lymphoma (PTCL) in first complete remission: The Spanish Lymphoma and Autologous Transplantation Group experience. *Ann Oncol* 18:652, 2007.
112. Kahl C, Leithauser M, Wolff D, et al: Treatment of peripheral T-cell lymphomas (PTCL) with high-dose chemotherapy and autologous or allogeneic hematopoietic transplantation. *Ann Hematol* 81:646, 2002.
113. Mercieca J, Matutes E, Dearden C, et al: The role of pentostatin in the treatment of T-cell malignancies: Analysis of response rate in 145 patients according to disease subtype. *J Clin Oncol* 12:2588, 1994.
114. Cooper DL, Braveman IM, Sarris AH, et al: Cyclosporine treatment of refractory T-cell lymphomas. *Cancer* 71:2335, 1993.
115. Cheng AL, Su IJ, Chen CC, et al: Use of retinoic acids in the treatment of peripheral T-cell lymphoma: A pilot study. *J Clin Oncol* 12:1185, 1994.
116. Frizzera G, Moran EM, Rappaport H: Angio-immunoblastic lymphadenopathy with dysproteinaemia. *Lancet* 1:1070, 1974.
117. Brice P, Calvo F, d'Agay MF, et al: Peripheral T cell lymphoma following angioimmunoblastic lymphadenopathy. *Nouv Rev Fr Hematol* 29:371, 1987.
118. Siegert W, Nerl C, Agthe A, et al: Angioimmunoblastic lymphadenopathy (AILD)-type T-cell lymphoma: Prognostic impact of clinical observations and laboratory findings at presentation. The Kiel Lymphoma Study Group. *Ann Oncol* 6:659, 1995.
119. Willenbrock K, Roers A, Seidl C, et al: Analysis of T-cell subpopulations in T-cell non-Hodgkin's lymphoma of angioimmunoblastic lymphadenopathy with dysproteinemia type by single target gene amplification of T cell receptor- beta gene rearrangements. *Am J Pathol* 158:1851, 2001.
120. Weiss LM, Strickler JG, Dorgman RF, et al: Clonal T-cell populations in angioimmunoblastic lymphadenopathy and angioimmunoblastic lymphadenopathy-like lymphoma. *Am J Pathol* 122:392, 1986.
121. Feller AC, Griesser H, Schilling CV, et al: Clonal gene rearrangement patterns correlate with immunophenotype and clinical parameters in patients with angioimmunoblastic lymphadenopathy. *Am J Pathol* 133:549, 1988.
122. Attygalle A, Al-Jehani R, Diss TC, et al: Neoplastic T cells in angioimmunoblastic T-cell lymphoma express CD10. *Blood* 99:627, 2002.
123. de Leval L, Rickman DS, Thielen C, et al: The gene expression profile of nodal peripheral T-cell lymphoma demonstrates a molecular link between angioimmunoblastic T-cell lymphoma (AITL) and follicular helper T (TFH) cells. *Blood* 109:4952, 2007.
124. Schlegelberger B, Himmler A, Bartles H, et al: Significance of cytogenetic findings for the clinical outcome in patients with T-cell lymphoma of angioimmunoblastic lymphadenopathy type. *J Clin Oncol* 14:593, 1996.
125. Smith JL, Hodges E, Quin CT, et al: Frequent T and B cell oligoclones in histologically and immunophenotypically characterized angioimmunoblastic lymphadenopathy. *Am J Pathol* 156:661, 2000.
126. Murata, K, Yamada Y, Kamihira S, et al: Frequency of eosinophilia in adult T-cell leukemia/lymphoma. *Cancer* 69:966 1992.
127. Simon, HU, Plötz SG, Dummer R, Blaser K: Abnormal clones of T cells producing interleukin-5 in idiopathic eosinophilia. *N Engl J Med* 341:1112 1999.
128. Vaklavas C, Tefferi A, Butterfield J, et al: "Idiopathic" eosinophilia with an Occult T-cell clone: Prevalence and clinical course. *Leuk Res* 31:691 2007.
129. Thielen C, Radermacher V, Trimeche M, et al: TARC and IL-5 expression correlates with tissue eosinophilia in peripheral T-cell lymphomas. *Leuk Res* 32:1431 2008.
130. Mourad N, Mounier N, Briere J, et al: Clinical, biologic, and pathologic features in 157 patients with angioimmunoblastic T-cell lymphoma treated within the Groupe d'Etude des Lymphomes de l'Adulte (GELA) trials. *Blood* 111:4463, 2008.
131. Siegert W, Agthe A, Griesser H, et al: Treatment of angioimmunoblastic lymphadenopathy (AILD)-type T-cell lymphoma using prednisone with or without the COP-BLAM/IMVP-16 regimen. A multicenter study. Kiel Lymphoma Study Group. *Ann Intern Med* 117:364, 1992.
132. Takemori N, Kodiara J, Toyoshima N, et al: Successful treatment of immunoblastic lymphadenopathy-like T-cell lymphoma with cyclosporin A. *Leuk Lymphoma* 35:389, 1999.
133. Quintini G, Lannitto E, Barbera V, et al: Response to low-dose oral methotrexate and prednisone in two patients with angio-immunoblastic lymphadenopathy-type T-cell lymphoma. *Hematol J* 2:393, 2001.
134. Gerlando Q, Barbera V, Ammatuna E, et al: Successful treatment of angioimmunoblastic lymphadenopathy with dysproteinemia-type T-cell lymphoma by combined methotrexate and prednisone. *Haematologica* 85:880, 2000.
135. Chan JK, Ng CS, Ngan KC, et al: Angiocentric T-cell lymphoma of the skin. An aggressive lymphoma distinct from mycosis fungoides. *Am J Surg Pathol* 12:861, 1988.
136. Liang X, Graham DK: Natural killer cell neoplasms. *Cancer* 112:1425, 2008.
137. Chan JK: Natural killer cell neoplasms. *Anat Pathol* 3:77, 1998.

138. Au WY, Weisenburger DD, Intragumtomchai T, et al: Clinical differences between nasal and extranasal natural killer/T-cell lymphoma: A study of 136 cases from the International Peripheral T-Cell Lymphoma Project. *Blood* 113:3931, 2009.
139. Liang R, Loke SL, Ho FC, et al: Histologic subtypes and survival of Chinese patients with non-Hodgkin's lymphomas. *Cancer* 66:1850, 1990.
140. Quintanilla-Martinez L, Franklin JL, Guerrero I, et al: Histological and immunophenotypic profile of nasal NK/T cell lymphomas from Peru: High prevalence of p53 overexpression. *Hum Pathol* 30:849, 1999.
141. Liang R, Todd D, Chan TK, et al: Nasal lymphoma. A retrospective analysis of 60 cases. *Cancer* 66:2205, 1990.
142. Kato N, Yasukawa K, Onozuka T, et al: Nasal and nasal-type T/NK-cell lymphoma with cutaneous involvement. *J Am Acad Dermatol* 40:850, 1999.
143. Chiang AK, Tao Q, Srivastava G, Ho FC: Nasal NK- and T-cell lymphomas share the same type of Epstein-Barr virus latency as nasopharyngeal carcinoma and Hodgkin's disease. *Int J Cancer* 68:285, 1996.
144. Gutierrez MI, Spangler G, Kingma D, et al: Epstein-Barr virus in nasal lymphomas contains multiple ongoing mutations in the EBNA-1 gene. *Blood* 92:600, 1998.
145. Gaal K, Weiss LM, Chen WG, et al: Epstein-Barr virus nuclear antigen (EBNA)-1 carboxy-terminal and EBNA-4 sequence polymorphisms in nasal natural killer/T-cell lymphoma in the United States. *Lab Invest* 82:957, 2002.
146. Cheung MM, Chan JK, Lau WH, et al: Primary non-Hodgkin's lymphoma of the nose and nasopharynx: Clinical features, tumor immunophenotype, and treatment outcome in 113 patients. *J Clin Oncol* 16:70, 1998.
147. Kim WS, Song SY, Ahn YC, et al: CHOP followed by involved field radiation: Is it optimal for localized nasal natural killer/T-cell lymphoma? *Ann Oncol* 12:349, 2001.
148. Liang R, Chen F, Lee CK, et al: Autologous bone marrow transplantation for primary nasal T/NK cell lymphoma. *Bone Marrow Transplant* 19:91, 1997.
149. Kako S, Izutsu K, Oshima K, et al: Regression of the tumor after withdrawal of cyclosporine in relapsed extranodal natural killer/T cell lymphoma following allogeneic hematopoietic stem cell transplantation. *Am J Hematol* 82:937, 2007.
150. Yagi T, Fujino H, Hirai M, et al: Esophageal actinomycosis after allogeneic peripheral blood stem cell transplantation for extranodal natural killer/T cell lymphoma, nasal type. *Bone Marrow Transplant* 32:451, 2003.
151. Kimura S, Horie A, Hiki Y, et al: Nephrotic syndrome with crescent formation and massive IgA deposition following allogeneic bone marrow transplantation for natural killer cell leukemia/lymphoma. *Blood* 101:4219, 2003.
152. Nawa Y, Takenaka K, Shinagawa K, et al: Successful treatment of advanced natural killer cell lymphoma with high-dose chemotherapy and syngeneic peripheral blood stem cell transplantation. *Bone Marrow Transplant* 23:1321, 1999.
153. Isaacson PG, O'Connor NT, Spencer J, et al: Malignant histiocytosis of the intestine: A T-cell lymphoma. *Lancet* 2:688, 1985.
154. Gale J, Simmonds PD, Mead GM, et al: Enteropathy-type intestinal T-cell lymphoma: Clinical features and treatment of 31 patients in a single center. *J Clin Oncol* 18:795, 2000.
155. Trier JS: Celiac sprue. *N Engl J Med* 325:1709, 1991.
156. Katoh A, Ohshima K, Kanda M, et al: Gastrointestinal T cell lymphoma: Predominant cytotoxic phenotypes, including alpha/beta, gamma/delta T cell and natural killer cells. *Leuk Lymphoma* 39:97, 2000.
157. Murray A, Cuevas EC, Jones DB, Wright DH: Study of the immunohistochemistry and T cell clonality of enteropathy-associated T cell lymphoma. *Am J Pathol* 146:509, 1995.
158. Chott A, Dragosics B, Radaszkiewicz T: Peripheral T-cell lymphomas of the intestine. *Am J Pathol* 141:1361, 1992.
159. Farcet JP, Gaulard P, Marolleau JP, et al: Hepatosplenic T-cell lymphoma: Sinusal/sinusoidal localization of malignant cells expressing the T-cell receptor gamma delta. *Blood* 75:2213, 1990.
160. Weidmann E: Hepatosplenic T cell lymphoma. A review on 45 cases since the first report describing the disease as a distinct lymphoma entity in 1990. *Leukemia* 14:991, 2000.
161. Wang CC, Tien HF, Lin MT, et al: Consistent presence of isochromosome 7q in hepatosplenic T gamma/delta lymphoma: A new cytogenetic-clinicopathologic entity. *Genes Chromosomes Cancer* 12:161, 1995.
162. Kanavaros P, Farcet JP, Gaulard P, et al: Recombinative events of the T cell antigen receptor delta gene in peripheral T cell lymphomas. *J Clin Invest* 87:666, 1991.
163. Jonveaux P, Daniel MT, Martel V, et al: Isochromosome 7q and trisomy 8 are consistent primary, non-random chromosomal abnormalities associated with hepatosplenic T gamma/delta lymphoma. *Leukemia* 10:1453, 1996.
164. Alonsozana EL, Stamberg J, Kumar D, et al: Isochromosome 7q: The primary cytogenetic abnormality in hepatosplenic gamma delta T cell lymphoma. *Leukemia* 11:1367, 1997.
165. Falchook GS, Vega F, Dang NH, et al: Hepatosplenic gamma-delta T-cell lymphoma: Clinicopathological features and treatment. *Ann Oncol* 20:1080, 2009.
166. Go RS, Wester SM: Immunophenotypic and molecular features, clinical outcomes, treatments, and prognostic factors associated with subcutaneous panniculitis-like T-cell lymphoma: A systematic analysis of 156 patients reported in the literature. *Cancer* 101:1404, 2004.
167. Takeshita M, Okamura S, Oshiro Y, et al: Clinicopathologic differences between 22 cases of CD56-negative and CD56-positive subcutaneous panniculitis-like lymphoma in Japan. *Hum Pathol* 35:231, 2004.
168. Paulli M, Berti E: Cutaneous T-cell lymphomas (including rare subtypes). Current concepts. II. *Haematologica* 89:1372, 2004.
169. Wang CY, Su WP, Kurtin PJ: Subcutaneous panniculitic T-cell lymphoma. *Int J Dermatol* 35:1, 1996.
170. Matsue K, Itoh M, Tsukuda K, et al: Successful treatment of cytophagic histiocytic panniculitis with modified CHOP-E. Cyclophosphamide, Adriamycin, vincristine, prednisone, and etoposide. *Am J Clin Oncol* 17:470, 1994.
171. Papenfuss JS, Aoun P, Bierman PJ, Armitage JO: Subcutaneous panniculitis-like T-cell lymphoma: Presentation of 2 cases and observations. *Clin Lymphoma* 3:175, 2002.
172. Springinsfeld G, Guillaume JC, Boeckler P, et al: [Two cases of subcutaneous panniculitis-like T-cell lymphoma (CD4– CD8+ CD56–).] *Ann Dermatol Venereol* 136:264, 2009.
173. Perez-Persona E, Mateos-Mazon JJ, Lopez-Villar O, et al: Complete remission of subcutaneous panniculitic T-cell lymphoma after allogeneic transplantation. *Bone Marrow Transplant* 38:821, 2006.
174. Ichii M, Hatanaka K, Imakita M, et al: Successful treatment of refractory subcutaneous panniculitis-like T-cell lymphoma with allogeneic peripheral blood stem cell transplantation from HLA-mismatched sibling donor. *Leuk Lymphoma* 47:2250, 2006.
175. Hathaway T, Subtil A, Kuo P, Foss F: Efficacy of denileukin diftitox in subcutaneous panniculitis-like T-cell lymphoma. *Clin Lymphoma Myeloma* 7:541, 2007.
176. Crawford K, Stark A, Kitchens B, et al: CD2 engagement induces dendritic cell activation: Implications for immune surveillance and T-cell activation. *Blood* 102:1745, 2003.
177. Dumont C, Deas O, Mollereau B, et al: Potent apoptotic signaling and subsequent unresponsiveness induced by a single CD2 mAb (BTI-322) in activated human peripheral T cells. *J Immunol* 160:3797, 1998.
178. Zhu DM, Dustin ML, Cairo CW, et al: Mechanisms of cellular avidity regulation in CD2-CD58-mediated T cell adhesion. *ACS Chem Biol* 1:649, 2006.
179. Badour K, Zhang J, Shi F, et al: The Wiskott-Aldrich syndrome protein acts downstream of CD2 and the CD2AP and PSTPIP1 adaptors to promote formation of the immunological synapse. *Immunity* 18:141, 2003.
180. Bell GM, Fargnoli J, Bolen JB, et al: The SH3 domain of p56lck binds to proline-rich sequences in the cytoplasmic domain of CD2. *J Exp Med* 183:169, 1996.
181. Manolios N, Letourneur R, Bonifacino JS, Klausner RD: Pairwise, cooperative and inhibitory interactions describe the assembly and probable structure of the T-cell antigen receptor. *EMBO J* 10:1643, 1991.
182. Alegre M, Vandenabeele P, Flamand V, et al: Hypothermia and hypoglycemia induced by anti-CD3 monoclonal antibody in mice: Role of tumor necrosis factor. *Eur J Immunol* 20:707, 1990.
183. Carpenter PA, Appelbaum FR, Corey L, et al: A humanized non-FcR-binding anti-CD3 antibody, visilizumab, for treatment of steroid-refractory acute graft-versus-host disease. *Blood* 99:2712, 2002.
184. Springer TA: Adhesion receptors of the immune system. *Nature* 346:425, 1990.
185. Bank I, Chess L: Perturbation of the T4 molecule transmits a negative signal to T cells. *J Exp Med* 162:1294, 1985.
186. Rider DA, Havenith CE, de Ridder R, et al: A human CD4 monoclonal antibody for the treatment of T-cell lymphoma combines inhibition of T-cell signaling by a dual mechanism with potent Fc-dependent effector activity. *Cancer Res* 67:9945, 2007.
187. Choy EHS, Adjaye J, Forrest L, et al: Chimaeric anti-CD4 monoclonal antibody cross-linked by monocyte Fc gamma receptor mediates apoptosis of human CD4 lymphocytes. *Eur J Immunol* 23:2676, 1993.
188. Talpur R, Jones DM, Alencar AJ, et al: CD25 expression is correlated with histological grade and response to denileukin diftitox in cutaneous T-cell lymphoma. *J Invest Dermatol* 126:575, 2006.
189. Jones D, Ibrahim S, Patel K, et al: Degree of CD25 expression in T-cell lymphoma is dependent on tissue site: Implications for targeted therapy. *Clin Cancer Res* 10:5587, 2004.
190. Snyder JT, Shen J, Azmi H, et al: Direct inhibition of CD40L expression can contribute to the clinical efficacy of daclizumab independently of its effects on cell division and Th1/Th2 cytokine production. *Blood* 109:5399, 2007.
191. Ho L, Aytac U, Stephens LC, et al: *In vitro* and *in vivo* antitumor effect of the anti-CD26 monoclonal antibody 1F7 on human CD30+ anaplastic large cell T-cell lymphoma Karpas 299. *Clin Cancer Res* 7:2031, 2001.
192. Dang NH, Aytac U, Sato K, et al: T-large granular lymphocyte lymphoproliferative disorder: Expression of CD26 as a marker of clinically aggressive disease and characterization of marrow inhibition. *Br J Haematol* 121:857, 2003.
193. Ruiz P, Mailhot S, Delgado P, et al: CD26 expression and dipeptidyl peptidase IV activity in an aggressive hepatosplenic T-cell lymphoma. *Cytometry* 34:30, 1998.
194. Carbone A, Gloghini A, Zagonel V, et al: The expression of CD26 and CD40 ligand is mutually exclusive in human T-cell non-Hodgkin's lymphomas/leukemias. *Blood* 86:4617, 1995.
195. Chiarle R, Podda A, Prolla G, et al: CD30 in normal and neoplastic cells. *Clin Immunol* 90:157, 1999.
196. Schwab U, Stein H, Gerdes J, et al: Production of a monoclonal antibody specific for Hodgkin and Sternberg-Reed cells of Hodgkin's disease and a subset of normal lymphoid cells. *Nature* 299:65, 1982.
197. Bartlett NL, Younes A, Carabasi MH, et al: A phase 1 multidose study of SGN-30 immunotherapy in patients with refractory or recurrent CD30+ hematologic malignancies. *Blood* 111:1848, 2008.
198. Hansen HP, Dietrich S, Kisseleva T, et al: CD30 shedding from Karpas 299 lymphoma cells is mediated by TNF-alpha-converting enzyme. *J Immunol* 165:6703, 2000.

199. Hansen HP, Matthey B, Barth S, et al: Inhibition of metalloproteinases enhances the internalization of anti-CD30 antibody Ki-3 and the cytotoxic activity of Ki-3 immunotoxin. *Int J Cancer* 98:210, 2002.
200. Hale G, Hoang T, Prospero T, et al: Removal of T cells from bone marrow for transplantation: A monoclonal antilymphocyte antibody that fixes human complement. *Blood* 62:873, 1983.
201. Piccaluga PP, Agostinelli C, Righi S, et al: Expression of CD52 in peripheral T-cell lymphoma. *Haematologica* 92:566, 2007.
202. Rodig SJ, Abramson JS, Pinkus GS, et al: Heterogeneous CD52 expression among hematologic neoplasms: Implications for the use of alemtuzumab (CAMPATH-1H). *Clin Cancer Res* 12:7174, 2006.
203. Kim YH, Duvic M, Obitz E, et al: Clinical efficacy of zanolimumab (HuMax-CD4): Two phase 2 studies in refractory cutaneous T-cell lymphoma. *Blood* 109:4655, 2007.
204. d'Amore F, Radford J, Jerkeman M, et al: Zanolimumab (HuMax-CD4™), a fully human monoclonal antibody: Efficacy and safety in patients with relapsed or treatment-refractory non-cutaneous CD4+ T-cell lymphoma. *ASH Annu Meet Abstracts* 110:3409, 2007.
205. Janick JE, Morris M, Stetler-Stevenson M, et al: Phase I trial of siplizumab in CD2-positive lymphoproliferative disease. ASCO Annual Meeting Proceedings, No. 16S (June 1 Supplement). *J Clin Oncol* 23:2533, 2005.
206. *Monoclonal Antibody Therapy in Treating Patients with Advanced or Recurrent Lymphoma*. Available at http://clinicaltrials.gov/ct2/show/NCT00006009. Accessed May 20, 2009.
207. Hillmen P, Skotnicki AB, Robak T, et al: Alemtuzumab compared with chlorambucil as first-line therapy for chronic lymphocytic leukemia. *J Clin Oncol* 25:5616, 2007.
208. Rai KR, Freter CE, Mercier RJ, et al: Alemtuzumab in previously treated chronic lymphocytic leukemia patients who also had received fludarabine. *J Clin Oncol* 20:3891, 2002.
209. Lundin J, Hagberg H, Repp R, et al: Phase 2 study of alemtuzumab (anti-CD52 monoclonal antibody) in patients with advanced mycosis fungoides/Sézary syndrome. *Blood* 101:4267, 2003.
210. Enblad G, Hagberg H, Erlanson M, et al: A pilot study of alemtuzumab (anti-CD52 monoclonal antibody) therapy for patients with relapsed or chemotherapy-refractory peripheral T-cell lymphomas. *Blood* 103:2920, 2004.
211. Reisman RP, Greco MA: Virus-associated hemophagocytic syndrome due to Epstein-Barr virus. *Hum Pathol* 15:290, 1984.
212. Bernengo MG, Quaglino P, Comessatti A, et al: Low-dose intermittent alemtuzumab in the treatment of Sézary syndrome: Clinical and immunologic findings in 14 patients. *Haematologica* 92:784, 2007.
213. Gallamini A, Zaja F, Patti C, et al: Alemtuzumab (Campath-1H) and CHOP chemotherapy as first-line treatment of peripheral T-cell lymphoma: Results of a GITIL (Gruppo Italiano Terapie Innovative nei Linfomi) prospective multicenter trial. *Blood* 110:2316, 2007.
214. Kim JG, Sohn SK, Yee SC, et al: Alemtuzumab plus CHOP as front-line chemotherapy for patients with peripheral T-cell lymphomas: A phase II study. *Cancer Chemother Pharmacol* 60:129, 2007.
215. Weidmann EH, Hess, G, Krause SW, et al: A phase II immunochemotherapy study with alemtuzumab, fludarabine, cyclophosphamide, and doxorubicin (Campath-FCD) in peripheral T-cell lymphomas. ASH Annual Meeting Abstracts. *Blood* 108:2721, 2006.
216. Peng YL, Huang HQ, Lin XB, et al: [Clinical outcomes of patients with peripheral T-cell lymphoma (PTCL) treated by EPOCH regimen.] *Ai Zheng* 23:943, 2004.
217. Janik JE, Dunleavy K, Pittaluga S, et al: A pilot trial of Campath-1H and dose-adjusted EPOCH in CD52-expressing aggressive T-cell malignancies. *ASH Annu Meet Abstr* 106:3348, 2005.
218. Kim SJ, Kim K, Kim BS, et al: Alemtuzumab and DHAP (A-DHAP) is effective for relapsed peripheral T-cell lymphoma, unspecified: Interim results of a phase II prospective study. *Ann Oncol* 20:390, 2009.
219. Cole MS, Stellrecht KE, Shi JD, et al: HuM291, a humanized anti-CD3 antibody, is immunosuppressive to T cells while exhibiting reduced mitogenicity in vitro. *Transplantation* 68:563, 1999.
220. Hsu DH, Shi JD, Homola M, et al: A humanized anti-CD3 antibody, HuM291, with low mitogenic activity, mediates complete and reversible T-cell depletion in chimpanzees. *Transplantation* 68:545, 1999.
221. Carpenter PA, Lowder J, Johnston L, et al: A phase II multicenter study of visilizumab, humanized anti-CD3 antibody, to treat steroid-refractory acute graft-versus-host disease. *Biol Blood Marrow Transplant* 11:465, 2005.
222. Ansell SM, Horwitz SM, Engert A, et al: Phase I/II study of an anti-CD30 monoclonal antibody (MDX-060) in Hodgkin's lymphoma and anaplastic large-cell lymphoma. *J Clin Oncol* 25:2764, 2007.
223. *MDX-060 in Patients with Relapsed or Refractory Classic Systemic or Primary Cutaneous Anaplastic Large Cell Lymphoma*. Available at http://clinicaltrials.gov/ct2/show/NCT00298467. Accessed May 20, 2009.
224. Duvic M, Kim Y, Korman NJ, et al: Zanolimumab, a Fully Human Monoclonal Antibody: Early Results of an Ongoing Clinical Trial in Patients with CD4+ Mycosis Fungoides (MF) Type CTCL (Stage IB-IVB) Who Are Refractory or Intolerant to Targretin and One Other Standard Therapy. *ASH Annu Meet Abstr* 108:2731, 2006.
225. Kreitman RJ, Wilson WH, White JD, et al: Phase I trial of recombinant immunotoxin anti-Tac(Fv)-PE38 (LMB-2) in patients with hematologic malignancies. *J Clin Oncol* 18:1622, 2000.
226. Wong BY, Gregory SA, Dang NH: Denileukin diftitox as novel targeted therapy for lymphoid malignancies. *Cancer Invest* 25:495, 2007.
227. Dang NH, Pro B, Hagemeister FB, et al: Phase II trial of denileukin diftitox for relapsed/refractory T-cell non-Hodgkin lymphoma. *Br J Haematol* 136:439, 2007.
228. Armitage JO, Greer JP, Levine AM, et al: Peripheral T-cell lymphoma. *Cancer* 63:158, 1989.
229. Ansell SM, Habermann TM, Kurtin PJ, et al: Predictive capacity of the International Prognostic Factor Index in patients with peripheral T-cell lymphoma. *J Clin Oncol* 15:2296, 1997.
230. Lopez-Guillermo A, Cid J, Salar A, et al: Peripheral T-cell lymphomas: Initial features, natural history, and prognostic factors in a series of 174 patients diagnosed according to the R.E.A.L. classification. *Ann Oncol* 9:849, 1998.
231. Melnyk A, Rodriguez A, Pugh WC, Cabannillas F: Evaluation of the Revised European-American Lymphoma classification confirms the clinical relevance of immunophenotype in 560 cases of aggressive non-Hodgkin's lymphoma. *Blood* 89:4514, 1997.
232. Weisenburger DD, Anderson JR, Diebold J, et al: Systemic anaplastic large-cell lymphoma: Results from the non-Hodgkin's lymphoma classification project. *Am J Hematol* 67:172, 2001.
233. Matherly LH, Voss MK, Anderson LA, et al: Enhanced polyglutamylation of aminopterin relative to methotrexate in the Ehrlich ascites tumor cell in vitro. *Cancer Res* 45:1073, 1985.
234. O'Connor OA: Pralatrexate: An emerging new agent with activity in T-cell lymphomas. *Curr Opin Oncol* 18:591, 2006.
235. Wang ES, O'Connor O, She Y, et al: Activity of a novel anti-folate (PDX, 10-propargyl 10-deazaaminopterin) against human lymphoma is superior to methotrexate and correlates with tumor RFC-1 gene expression. *Leuk Lymphoma* 44:1027, 2003.
236. O'Connor OA, Hamlin PA, Portlock C, et al: Pralatrexate, a novel class of antifol with high affinity for the reduced folate carrier-type 1, produces marked complete and durable remissions in a diversity of chemotherapy refractory cases of T-cell lymphoma. *Br J Haematol* 139:425, 2007.
237. Mould DR, Sweeney K, Duffull S, et al: A population pharmacokinetic and pharmacodynamic evaluation of pralatrexate in patients with hematologic malignancies. *ASH Annu Meet Abstr* 110:1370, 2007.
238. *Study of Pralatrexate with Vitamin B12 and Folic Acid in Patients with Relapsed or Refractory Peripheral T-Cell Lymphoma*. Available at: http://clinicaltrials.gov/ct2/show/NCT00364923. Accessed: May 20, 2009.
239. Piekarz RL, Robey R, Sandor V, et al: Inhibitor of histone deacetylation, depsipeptide (FR901228), in the treatment of peripheral and cutaneous T-cell lymphoma: A case report. *Blood* 98:2865, 2001.
240. Piekarz R, Wright J, Frye R, et al: Results of a phase 2 NCI multicenter study of romidepsin in patients with relapsed peripheral T-cell lymphoma (PTCL). *ASH Annu Meet Abstr* 112:1567, 2008.
241. *FR901228 in Treating Patients with T-Cell Lymphoma*. Available at http://clinicaltrials.gov/ct2/show/NCT00364923. Accessed May 20, 2009.
242. Philip T, Guglielmi C, Hagenbeek A, et al: Autologous bone marrow transplantation as compared with salvage chemotherapy in relapses of chemotherapy-sensitive non-Hodgkin's lymphoma. *N Engl J Med* 333:1540, 1995.
243. Dang NH, Hagemeister FB, Duvic M, et al: Pentostatin in T-non-Hodgkin's lymphomas: Efficacy and effect on CD26+ T lymphocytes. *Oncol Rep* 10:1513, 2003.
244. O'Brien S, Kurzrock R, Duvic M, et al: 2-Chlorodeoxyadenosine therapy in patients with T-cell lymphoproliferative disorders. *Blood* 84:733, 1994.
245. Au WY, Ng WM, Choy C, Kwong YL: Aggressive subcutaneous panniculitis-like T-cell lymphoma: Complete remission with fludarabine, mitoxantrone and dexamethasone. *Br J Dermatol* 143:408, 2000.
246. Zinzani PL, Baliva G, Magagnoli M, et al: Gemcitabine treatment in pretreated cutaneous T-cell lymphoma: Experience in 44 patients. *J Clin Oncol* 18:2603, 2000.
247. Marchi E, Alinari L, Tani M, et al: Gemcitabine as frontline treatment for cutaneous T-cell lymphoma: Phase II study of 32 patients. *Cancer* 104:2437, 2005.
248. Sallah S, Wan JY, Nguyen NP: Treatment of refractory T-cell malignancies using gemcitabine. *Br J Haematol* 113:185, 2001.
249. Lundin J, Kimby E, Bjorkholm M, et al: Phase II trial of subcutaneous anti-CD52 monoclonal antibody alemtuzumab (Campath-1H) as first-line treatment for patients with B-cell chronic lymphocytic leukemia (B-CLL). *Blood* 100:768, 2002.

CHAPTER 107

PLASMA CELL NEOPLASMS: GENERAL CONSIDERATIONS

H. Elizabeth Broome

SUMMARY

Plasma cell neoplasms are monoclonal expansions of plasma cells and their precursors. These often can be detected and monitored by evaluating the levels of monoclonal immunoglobulin or immunoglobulin chains in the plasma or urine. Rapidly progressive plasma cell neoplasms often present with evidence of organ dysfunction or have a much higher potential for organ dysfunction. On the other hand, patients with nonprogressive or slowly progressive essential monoclonal gammopathy can live for many years with no evidence of disease except for abnormalities on laboratory tests. Moreover, although monoclonal immunoglobulin protein generally is detected in plasma cell myeloma, other conditions also may result in production of monoclonal immunoglobulin. This chapter summarizes the laboratory studies used to evaluate for monoclonal immunoglobulins or monoclonal immunoglobulin gene rearrangements; delineates laboratory features that can help distinguish plasma cell myeloma from related conditions that may also be associated with a monoclonal immunoglobulin; and provides references to relevant chapters in the textbook that focus on a particular plasma cell or B-cell disorders.

DEFINITION AND HISTORY

PLASMA CELL NEOPLASMS

Plasma cell neoplasms (PCNs) are monoclonal expansions of a single B lymphocyte characterized by plasma cell morphology and monoclonal immunoglobulin gene rearrangement. The vast majority of PCNs produce monoclonal immunoglobulin or immunoglobulin fragments. For such PCNs, the cells within the neoplasm produce the same whole immunoglobulin chain or chain fragment. In a given neoplasm, the monoclonal proteins generally have the same heavy-chain class/isotype (γ, α, μ, δ, or ε), same light-chain class (κ or λ), and same idiotypes (or antigenic determinants of the immunoglobulin variable regions; see Chap. 77).[1] The neoplastic plasma cells also share chromosomal anomalies, if any are present,[2] although clonal evolution may occur as the disease progresses (see Chap. 109). Since Henry Bence Jones[3] first discovered what turned out to be monoclonal light chains in the urine of myeloma patients more than 160 years ago, the monoclonal immunoglobulin molecules (or their constituent chains) produced by plasma cell neoplasms have remained the best examples of tumor-specific antigens in the field of oncology. These proteins usually are called *M* proteins, which at various times in history has stood for *malignant*, *myeloma*, and now *monoclonal* proteins. Table 107–1 lists the diseases associated with M proteins. Some of the diseases are nonprogressive or very slowly progressive, whereas some are malignant and more rapidly progressive, causing disease and organ damage.

Acronyms and abbreviations that appear in this chapter include: CAS, cold agglutinin syndrome; CSF, cerebrospinal fluid; HLA, human leukocyte antigen; Ig, immunoglobulin; IL, interleukin; PCN, plasma cell neoplasm; PCR, polymerase chain reaction; TNF, tumor necrosis factor.

ESSENTIAL MONOCLONAL GAMMOPATHY

Over half of patients with a monoclonal immunoglobulin in their serum have nonprogressive or very slowly progressive essential monoclonal gammopathy, often called monoclonal gammopathy of undetermined significance (MGUS). Clinical and laboratory features consistent with essential monoclonal gammopathy are an M protein level less than 30 g/L, no renal insufficiency, no anemia, normal serum calcium, no bony lesions on skeletal surveys, and less than 10 percent plasma cells in the marrow. A low but significant percentage of patients with essential monoclonal gammopathy develop frank B cell malignancies each year, usually multiple myeloma (see Chap. 108).[4–6]

Table 107–2 lists biologic features of monoclonal gammopathy.

CHRONIC COLD AGGLUTININ SYNDROME

Chronic cold agglutinin syndrome (CAS) is a disease in which elderly patients produce immunoglobulin (Ig) M that binds red cells and causes their agglutination at temperatures below 37°C (see Chap. 53). For more than 90 percent of patients with CAS, this erythrocyte-binding IgM is monoclonal.[7] Flow cytometry of the marrow mononuclear cells typically demonstrates the presence of a low percentage of clonal B cells. A minority of patients with CAS have other evidence of lymphoma (see Chap. 97) or Waldenström macroglobulinemia (see Chap. 111). Without other features diagnostic of a lymphoid malignancy, such as adenopathy, splenomegaly, marrow lymphocytosis, or serum hyperviscosity, these cases of CAS rarely progress to frank malignancy.[8,9] The disorder bears no relationship to acute, postinfectious CAS, in which the offending immunoglobulins are polyclonal and disappear after the inciting infectious agent is eradicated.

CRYOGLOBULINS

Cryoglobulins are complexes of immunoglobulins that precipitate upon exposure to cold (see Chap. 111). Three classes of cryoglobulins are recognized. *Type 1 cryoglobulins* are monoclonal IgM, IgG, or IgA molecules. *Type 2 cryoglobulins* are monoclonal immunoglobulins, usually of the IgM class, with antibody activity against other immunoglobulins, usually IgG. There is an association of type 2 cryoglobulins with hepatitis B and C infection.[10–12] *Type 3 cryoglobulins* are composed of polyclonal immunoglobulins with antiimmunoglobulin activity. Cryoglobulins may cause a variety of pathologic conditions, all related to the formation of immune complexes. They are detected by allowing serum to stand and precipitate or gel at 4°C for 24 to 72 hours.

TRANSIENT M PROTEINS

Transient M proteins occasionally are associated with certain infections and immunosuppression, especially after transplantation (see Chap. 108).[13,14] Patients with any of a variety of congenital immunodeficiencies in which the T-cell arm of immunity is more affected than the B-cell arm may develop transient, low-level monoclonal gammopathies, typically of the IgM class. Monoclonal molecules also have been described in hyperimmunized laboratory animals. They do not progress to malignant disease.[15,16] These transient monoclonal antibodies usually are not high affinity to the presumed cause of inflammation or experimental immunogen.

The age-adjusted incidence rate of myeloma in the United States is approximately 5.6 per 100,000 (7.1 for men and 4.6 for women). The incidence of monoclonal gammopathy is approximately 100 times as

TABLE 107–1. Diseases Associated with M Proteins

Disease	Reference (Chapter)
Non- or slowly progressive	
Essential monoclonal gammopathy	108
Chronic cold agglutinin syndrome	53
Transient (after inflammation)	108
Transient (after marrow transplant)	21, 108
Immunodeficiency (see particularly T cell)	83
Malignant and progressive	
Plasma cell myeloma	109
Solitary plasmacytoma	109
Neoplasms causing amyloidosis or light-chain deposition in tissues	110
Neoplasms causing dermatologic lesions	
Waldenström macroglobulinemia	111
Heavy-chain disease: α, γ, μ, or rarely δ, but no light chains	112
Chronic lymphocytic leukemia and related lymphomas	94

high, and the transient monoclonal gammopathies associated with all the various forms of inflammation and immunodeficiency are approximately 400 times more frequent (see Chaps. 108 and 109). The frequency of all the disorders increases dramatically with age. The monoclonal gammopathies in immunodeficient hosts occur at a much younger age than myeloma or monoclonal gammopathy.

ETIOLOGY AND PATHOGENESIS

GENETIC BACKGROUND

In the mouse, the genetic background of the animal is an important risk factor for developing monoclonal gammopathy or plasmacytomas. Approximately 40 to 60 percent of C57BL/K, C3H, or NZB inbred strains of mice develop M proteins of the IgM class. BALB/c and CBA/Kij, two other inbred stains of mice, have a very low incidence of spontaneous plasma cell neoplasm. Surprisingly, mice of the BALB/c strain are most susceptible to developing plasmacytomas after repeated intraperitoneal injections of mineral oil. NZB mice also are fairly susceptible to induction of plasmacytomas by this method. However, C57BL/Ka mice are resistant. There are at least several genetic aberrations responsible for these differences between inbred strains of mice. One example is a single amino acid substitution at the *Frap* locus in the Balb/c mice that leads to quantitative decreases in protein activity and increases in plasmacytoma susceptibility.[17,17a–20]

Human families with a high incidence of plasma cell neoplasms have been reported.[21] No consistent genetic aberrations have been described in these families. Essential monoclonal gammopathy and myeloma occurs more frequently in relatives of patients with those diseases than in the general population.[22–24] Also, differences in the prevalence of essential monoclonal gammopathy between ethnic groups have been observed. There is a two- to threefold excess risk of essential monoclonal gammopathy and myeloma in Americans of African descent compared to Americans of European descent while the risk of progression from essential monoclonal gammopathy to myeloma was very similar for the two races.[25] These observations indicate the host's genetic background is an important risk factor for development of plasma cell neoplasms in mammals.

Numerous attempts have been made to induce plasmacytomas that secrete antibodies to specific antigens in BALB/c mice. The animals were hyperimmunized with any one of a variety of antigens in mineral oil. Plasmacytomas arose but almost never made antibodies reactive with the injected antigen.[26] Thus, no relationship between chronic antigenic stimulation and development of plasma cell neoplasms is apparent in these animals. However, this is not the case with Aleutian minks infected with the Aleutian disease virus.[27] Many of these animals develop M proteins consisting of antibodies that bind specifically to the infecting virus. In humans, no consistent relationship is observed between prior inflammatory disease and subsequent development of a plasma cell neoplasm. However, monoclonal gammopathies occur at increased frequency in patients with inflammatory and autoimmune diseases.[15,28,29] However, there is no evidence that such monoclonal antibodies bind to an antigen(s) that stimulates development of the inflammatory disease.

CHROMOSOMAL ANOMALIES

Approximately 90 percent of mouse plasmacytomas induced by mineral oil in mice show consistent chromosomal anomalies. In these plasmacytomas, the c-*myc* gene on mouse chromosome 15 is fused with either the immunoglobulin heavy-chain locus on mouse chromosome 12 or the immunoglobulin κ light-chain locus on mouse chromosome 6.[30] The fusion of c-*myc* with an immunoglobulin heavy- or light-chain locus resembles the typical chromosomal anomalies seen in human Burkitt lymphoma.[31,32] However, the biologic behaviors of murine plasmacytomas and human Burkitt lymphoma are radically different.

Certain chromosomal abnormalities in neoplastic cells may be seen repeatedly in patients with myeloma or plasma cell leukemia (late, preterminal stage of myeloma; see Chap. 109).[33] Molecular and fluorescent *in situ* hybridization studies have demonstrated that the myeloma cells from all patients with myeloma have genetic abnormalities, but the low proliferative rate of the myeloma cells means that only approximately 30 to 50 percent have detectable cytogenetic abnormalities in their

TABLE 107–2. Some Biologic Features of Monoclonal Gammopathy

	Myeloma	Monoclonal Gammopathy	Immunodeficiency
Clonal size	Large	Medium	Small
Immunoglobulin production	>30 g/L	<30 g/L	<3 g/L
Time course	Progressive	Persistent	Transient
Abnormal immunoglobulin structure	Frequent	Rare	Never
Bone destruction	Frequent	Never	Never
Mouse models			
Transformed clone	+	+	–
Transplantable generations	<4	–	
Autonomous growth	+	+?	–
Immortality	+	–	–

Modified with permission from Radl.[18]

marrow mononuclear cells at diagnosis. Almost half of the patients with cytogenetic abnormalities have hyperdiploidy with a median chromosome number of 54 caused by nonrandom gains of chromosomes 3, 5, 7, 9, 11, 15, 19, or 21. Hyperdiploidy is associated with better prognosis.[33]

The nonhyperdiploid karyotype cases are associated with a high prevalence of translocations predominantly involving the long arm of chromosome 14 ($14q^+$) at the immunoglobulin heavy-chain locus. Often the donated material is from chromosome 11, generating a t(11;14) (q13;q32) and deregulated expression or cyclin D_1. Cyclin D (D_1, D_2, and D_3) expression is deregulated by this translocation and other, unknown mechanisms in almost all plasma cell myelomas.[34] Approximately 50 to 70 percent of myeloma or plasma cell leukemia cases have abnormalities involving chromosome 1. The anomalies are highly variable, and no consistent deletions, additions, or translocations have been found. Patients with plasma cells that have monosomy 13 (loss of Rb) have shortened survival (see Chap. 109).[35]

Oncogenomic profiling has implicated certain cellular molecular pathways in the multistep transformation of normal plasma cells in essential monoclonal gammopathy and myeloma.[36] Also, the pattern of gene expression in myeloma predicts outcome endpoints such as length of complete remission and event-free survival.[37,38,38a]

MARROW ENVIRONMENT

The majority of normal, polyclonal IgG is produced by plasma cells in the marrow, reflecting the dependence of normal plasma cell function on the normal marrow environment.[39] Similarly, myeloma and other plasma cell dyscrasias mostly grow or survive in the marrow since the normal marrow environment is critical for their pathogenesis and progression. Direct and indirect interactions between the myeloma cells, nonmyeloma cells, and the extracellular matrix in the marrow are critical for the growth, survival, and drug resistance of neoplastic plasma cells. The indirect interactions include secreted cytokines and growth factors that regulate myeloma cells through paracrine and autocrine mechanisms. Direct cell–cell and cell–matrix interaction through adhesion molecules also affect the myeloma cells.

The cellular components of the marrow environment include hematopoietic cells, mesenchymal cells, and immune system cells. All these cell types have progenitors and maturing precursors in the marrow. Members of these different cell types interact to regulate hematopoiesis, bone homeostasis, immunoglobulin production, and the homing of cells to the marrow. The growth and survival of myeloma disrupts the normal interaction of these cell types resulting in bone loss, decreased hematopoiesis, and decreased normal immunoglobulin production.

Under *in vitro* experimental conditions, adhesion of neoplastic plasma cells to marrow stromal cells, adherent cells derived from normal donor marrow, activates many signaling pathways leading to modulation of transcription and the upregulation of cell-cycle-regulating proteins, antiapoptotic proteins, and telomerase activity (reviewed in reference 40). The myeloma cells and marrow stromal cells interact through integrins, cytokines, and growth factors, such as interleukin (IL)-6. IL-6 is a major growth, survival, and drug resistance factor for myeloma cells.[41] IL-6 also causes the myeloma cells to produce vascular endothelial growth factor (VEGF). In a feed-back loop, VEGF contributes to IL-6 production by the marrow stromal cells.[42]

The myeloma cells produce other cytokines that contribute to the pathophysiology of the bone disease, resulting in lytic lesions of bone. The osteolytic lesions weaken the bone matrix, leading to pathologic fractures. The lesions are produced by osteoclasts that are activated by cytokines released by the malignant plasma cells themselves. Formerly called *osteoclast activating factor*, the factor involved now is thought to be a combination of different cytokines, including macrophage inflammatory protein-1α (MIP-1α), receptor activator of nuclear transcription factor-κB ligand (RANKL), osteoprotegerin ligand (CD138), VEGF, tumor necrosis factor-alpha (TNF-α), TNF-β, IL-1β, and/or IL-6 (see Chap. 109).[43–46] Osteoclasts, in turn, modulate myeloma cell growth and survival. A recently FDA-approved drug targeting RANKL shows promise for decreasing bone loss in myeloma.[46a]

LABORATORY FEATURES

MARROW EXAMINATION

Detecting and quantifying the presence of clonal plasma cells in the marrow is important for the diagnosis and monitoring of plasma cell dyscrasias. The percentage of clonal plasma cells in the marrow is a criterion for distinguishing essential monoclonal gammopathy from myeloma (see Chaps. 108, 109) since myeloma typically has a higher percentage of clonal plasma cells in the marrow than essential monoclonal gammopathy.[47] The marrow from patients with plasma cell dyscrasias varies from scattered plasma cells with normal morphology to "sheets" or large nodules of plasma cells with highly abnormal morphology. The abnormal morphology may include multinucleation, "blastic"-type nuclear chromatin, nucleoli, cytoplasmic "irregularities," and inclusions, both cytoplasmic and nuclear (see Chaps. 74, 109). Normal marrow contains up to 2 percent polyclonal plasma cells, but marrow biopsies from myeloma patients may show almost complete replacement of the marrow biopsy with clonal plasma cells. Some reactive marrows, especially from individuals infected with HIV, may show as many as 20 percent or more polyclonal plasma cells. Determining whether the plasma cells are clonal is critical to diagnosis.

The percentage of plasma cells can be determined by microscopic evaluation of marrow aspirate smears, flow cytometry on marrow material (either aspirates or cell suspensions from a biopsy), and by immunohistochemistry of sections from a marrow biopsy or clot (see Chap. 3). Morphologic assessment of the aspirate is the "gold standard" for determining the percentage of plasma cells, but clonality can only be inferred with this method as morphologic abnormalities associated with clonality may be subtle. Flow cytometry and immunohistochemistry allow determination of both the percentage of plasma cells and their clonality. However, depending on the method used, the percentage of plasma cells may vary considerably.

Usually, the percentage of plasma cells by flow cytometry is significantly less than the percentage by aspirate differential. The main reason for this difference is that the samples sent for flow cytometry usually are collected after the samples are used for preparing marrow particle smears for differential counts, and repeated aspirates from the same needle site become more diluted with blood.[48] Another reason for this difference is that processing for flow cytometry appears to negatively affect plasma cell survival or antigen expression relative to other marrow cells.[49] Immunohistochemistry on sections from marrow biopsy or clot with anti-CD138 usually gives a higher percentage of plasma cells than aspirate smear differentials. This difference probably reflects a relative difference between the "aspirability" of plasma cells versus other marrow cells.[50] Immunohistochemical staining of the clot or biopsy for kappa and lambda immunoglobulin light chain can establish clonality. However, immunoglobulin in the plasma and tissues can cause high background staining further complicating interpretation. For this reason, in situ hybridization of immunoglobulin light chain RNA is a complementary technique to immunohistochemistry for detection of light chain clonality in plasma cell dyscrasias.[50a]

Flow cytometry identifies clonal plasma cells by their skewed cytoplasmic light-chain expression and by aberrant antigen expression. Aberrant antigen expression allows flow cytometry detection of minimal levels of clonal plasma cells among normal plasma cells.[48] Typical myeloma cells show surface expression of CD38 (bright), CD56, CD138, CD200, and monoclonal cytoplasmic Ig ($\gamma > \alpha > \mu$; $\kappa > \lambda$). They usually lack surface expression of immunoglobulin, human leukocyte antigen (HLA)-DR, CD19, CD20, and CD27. Myeloma cells often aberrantly express CD20, CD28, and CD117. Normal plasma cells have a similar immunophenotype except that they express CD19 (>70%), CD27, CD81, CD200, and polyclonal cytoplasmic Ig (κ to λ is about 2:1). Also, normal plasma cells do not express CD28 (<15%) or CD56. All the plasma cells in 90 percent of cases of myeloma express CD56 and aberrantly lack CD19.[51] These aberrant antigen profiles allow the use of flow cytometry to monitor for minimal residual disease after treatment down to greater than 0.01 percent of total nucleated cells. Also, aberrant antigen expression on plasma cells from patients with essential monoclonal gammopathy has value for predicting progression to myeloma.[52]

QUANTITATIVE IMMUNOGLOBULIN AND FREE LIGHT-CHAIN ASSAYS

Intact, complete immunoglobulins in serum, urine, or cerebral spinal fluid (CSF) usually are measured by nephelometry. This technique is based on the observation that antigen–antibody complexes form cloudy precipitates. The precipitates can be detected photoelectrically. Varying dilutions of the fluid in question are incubated with antibodies specific for any one of the different immunoglobulin heavy and light chains. After precipitates form, the amount of precipitate is determined by comparison with standard curves produced by precipitating immunoglobulins of known concentration.

A similar nephelometric assay is used to detect immunoglobulin free light chains in serum or urine. Free κ or λ immunoglobulin light chains are not associated with complete immunoglobulin molecules, and there are assays that specifically can detect free light chains, distinguishing them from κ or λ that is part of intact immunoglobulin molecules.[53] Free light-chain concentrations in serum are dependent on the balance between production by plasma cells and renal clearance. Free light chains are cleared rapidly through the renal glomeruli and have a serum half-life of 2 to 4 hours in patients with normal renal function. After filtration through the glomeruli, they are metabolized by the renal proximal tubular cells. Normally, very little of this protein escapes into the urine. Abnormal concentrations of free κ or λ light chain can occur under many circumstances, including immune suppression, immune stimulation, reduced renal clearance, and clonal plasma cell dyscrasias. Sera from patients with nonclonal increases in free light chains have a κ-to-λ ratio that is approximately 2:1. Free light chains with a significantly abnormal κ-to-λ ratio usually indicate clonal plasma cell dyscrasias. Therefore, both the level of free light chains and the ratio of κ to λ free light chains are important for diagnosis.

The International Myeloma Working Group has published guidelines for the use of serum free light-chain analysis.[54] For optimally sensitive detection of plasma cell dyscrasias, this group recommends the combination of serum free light-chain assay, serum protein electrophoresis, and serum immunofixation. This panel of assays negates the need for 24-hour urine studies to diagnose myeloma or other diseases associated with aberrant monoclonal Ig proliferation other than light-chain amyloidosis. Screening for light-chain amyloidosis still requires urine immunofixation electrophoresis if the serum tests, including serum free light-chain, do not reveal evidence for an M protein. Baseline free light-chain concentrations is a major prognostic indicator for every plasma cell neoplasm. For quantitative monitoring of patients with oligosecretory myeloma and most patients with what had previously been called "nonsecretory myeloma," free light-chain is the serum assay of choice for quantitative monitoring. In amyloidosis patients, free light-chain measurements outperform serum protein electrophoresis and immunofixation for monitoring responses to treatment.

PROTEIN ELECTROPHORESIS AND IMMUNOFIXATION

Serum

The most common screening test for an M protein is serum electrophoresis. In this test, a few microliters of serum are spotted onto a support medium, such as cellulose acetate, that has been equilibrated at a basic pH. When an electric current is applied across the support medium, the proteins in the serum migrate toward the anode at a velocity proportional to the ratio of their negative charge to molecular weight. After a migration period of approximately 30 minutes, depending on the precise conditions, the cellulose acetate is taken up, dried, immersed in a stain that detects proteins, such as ponceau SX or Coomassie blue, and examined by eye or densitometry. Figure 107–1 illustrates the procedure and typical results.

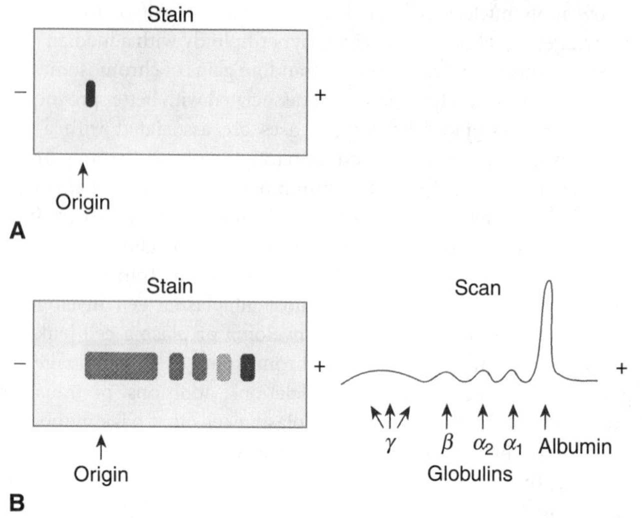

FIGURE 107–1. Normal serum electrophoresis. **A.** Apply serum to support medium. **B.** Electrophoretically separate proteins. Stain, observe, and scan.

Albumin is the most abundant protein in normal serum. This protein migrates as a sharp peak because, except in rare cases, all albumin molecules have exactly the same amino acid sequence and hence the same electrophoretic mobility. In contrast, the γ-globulins comprise immunoglobulins that have billions of different amino acid sequences and varying carbohydrate side chains. Consequently, these proteins migrate in a very broad band that typically contains IgA and IgM in the front (toward the β-globulins) and IgG spread through the entire range of globulins. IgD and IgE normally are secreted at such low levels that they are not detectable by this method. When a plasma cell neoplasm produces an M protein, the electrophoretic pattern is altered (Fig. 107–2).

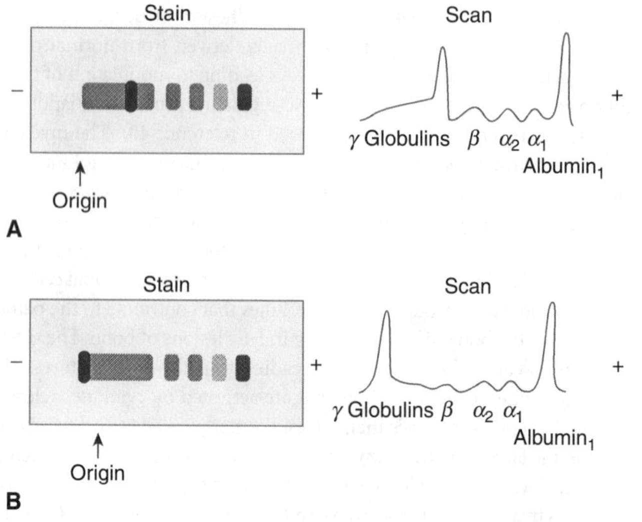

FIGURE 107–2. M protein electrophoresis. **A.** Fast-moving M protein spike. **B.** Slow-moving M protein spike.

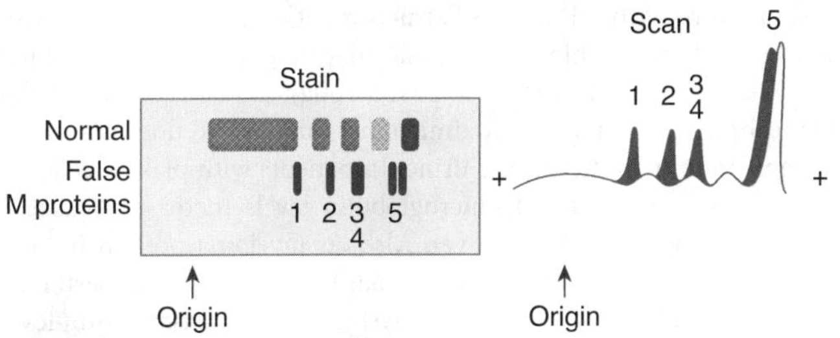

FIGURE 107–3. False M proteins. Band 1 is typical of fibrinogen, which may be confused with M proteins of the IgA or IgM class. If fibrinogen is present, the serum was incompletely clotted or plasma was used. Band 2 is hemoglobin–haptoglobin complexes or high levels of transferrin, which may be seen in intravascular hemolysis or iron deficiency, respectively. Bands 3/4 may be seen with hyperalphaglobulinemia (one of the acute-phase reactants, as is haptoglobin) and with some of the congenital hyperlipoproteinemias. Band 5 is an albumin variant resulting from a rare autosomal trait, bisalbuminemia, or from some drugs, such as penicillin, that bind to albumin and alter its electrophoretic mobility.

A monoclonal immunoglobulin protein may migrate anywhere in the globulin region. IgM and IgA M proteins tend to migrate faster than most IgG molecules. Accordingly, the M protein in Figure 107–2A probably is an IgA or IgM, whereas the spike in Figure 107–2B probably is an IgG molecule. To distinguish these immunoglobulin classes with certainty requires immunofixation electrophoresis. Figure 107–3 illustrates false monoclonal "immunoglobulins."

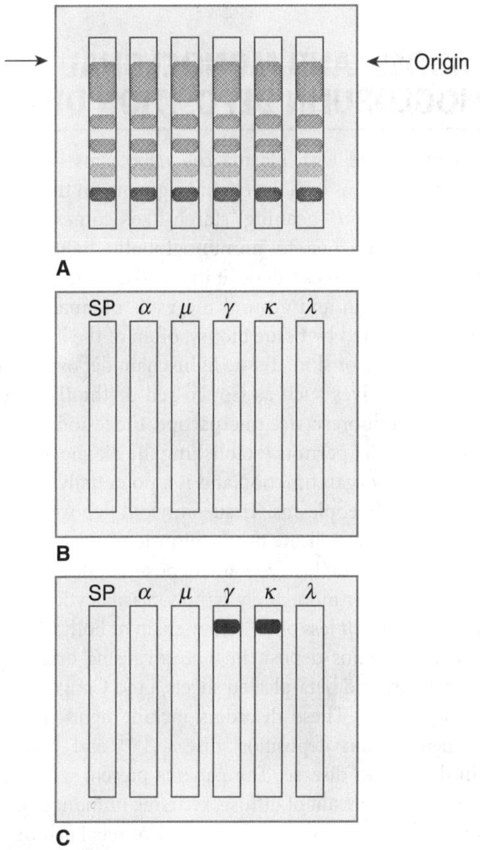

FIGURE 107–4. Immunofixation electrophoresis. **A.** Serum samples are placed in each of several lanes of an agarose gel support medium for protein electrophoresis. **B.** Overlay each lane with antiserum to a specific immunoglobulin heavy or light chain, typically anti-α, -μ, -γ, -κ, or -λ. Allow precipitation to occur. **C.** Wash and stain. Only immunoprecipitates remain in the gel. Nonprecipitated proteins wash out. Results show an IgG $_{\kappa}$M protein.

Figure 107–4 illustrates the principle of immunofixation electrophoresis. This technique is useful for more sensitive detection of M proteins than protein electrophoresis alone. Also, this technique identifies the immunoglobulin heavy-chain class and light-chain type in putative M proteins.

Table 107–3 lists several clinical conditions that generally are associated with a serum protein abnormality that can be detected by electrophoresis, immunoelectrophoresis, or serum free light-chain analysis. Electrophoresis and immunoelectrophoresis also are useful for detecting a variety of serum protein abnormalities other than M proteins.

Spinal Fluid and Urine

Electrophoresis can be performed on concentrated specimens of CSF or urine. Evaluation of CSF allows for detection of a plasmacytoma secreting M protein in the central nervous system. Evaluation of the urine is useful for detecting excessive and unbalanced synthesis of immunoglobulin molecules. Because proteins larger than albumin (or 67 kDa) normally do not pass through the glomeruli, whole immunoglobulins are not present in normal urine. However, free immunoglobulin light chains are only approximately 25 kDa and hence pass freely through the glomerulus. Patients with a circulating M protein who pass whole immunoglobulins in their urine generally have severe renal dys-

TABLE 107–3. Clinical Indications for Electrophoresis of Serum and Urine Proteins

Clinical Indication	Abnormality and Interpretation
Unexplained edema or ascites	Hypoalbuminemia
Suspected liver disease	Hypoalbuminemia frequent; hyperglobulinemia suggests cirrhosis or chronic active hepatitis
Collagen diseases, sarcoidosis	Polyclonal hyperglobulinemia
Collagen diseases, sarcoidosis	Hypogammaglobulinemia or agammaglobulinemia
Chronic lymphocytic leukemia, malignant lymphoma	Hypogammaglobulinemia or, rarely, IgG or IgM M proteins
Unexplained proteinuria	Albumin or a mixture of all serum proteins found with urinary tract infections or the nephrotic syndrome; homogeneous urine proteins that migrate in the globulin region usually indicative of plasma cell neoplasms secreting free light or heavy chains
Evidence of plasma cell myeloma	Serum or urinary monoclonal neoplasms, e.g., bone pain, protein, with reduced normal immunoglobulins, frequent infections, elevated immunoglobulins and sedimentation rate, rouleaux, hypoalbuminemia, proteinuria, hyperviscosity, or osteolytic skeletal lesions
Amyloidosis	Monoclonal serum or urinary proteins frequent
Acquired clotting disorders	M proteins or amyloid bind to some clotting factors, such as I, II, VIII, IX, X, and XI
Acquired neuropathy	M proteins infiltrate peripheral nerves

function, often because of renal amyloidosis secondary to deposition of immunoglobulin chains in the renal parenchyma.

Free light chains that appear in the urine can be detected by sulfosalicylic acid precipitation, electrophoresis of concentrated urine, immunofixation electrophoresis, or free light-chain analysis. Immunofixation and free light-chain analysis also are useful for evaluating whether the immunoglobulin light chains are only κ, only λ, or both. Urine electrophoresis is one of the most important tools for diagnosis and followup of patients with plasma cell neoplasms. The amount of light chain excreted in a fixed amount of time often is proportional to the amount of light chain produced, which in turn is proportional to the number of neoplastic plasma cells. Thus, serial measurements of the amount of immunoglobulin light chain excreted over time are a convenient way to follow tumor mass and the effects of therapy.

Measurements of immunoglobulin light chains in urine do not always correlate with the rate of immunoglobulin light-chain production. Immunoglobulin light chains normally are reabsorbed and metabolized in the proximal tubules of the kidney. As renal damage progresses, the amount of light chains excreted in the urine increases, partly because of deteriorating renal function. For this reason, the best estimate of tumor cell mass in a patient with myeloma is by measuring the M protein in serum. However, mutations of tumor cells that cause them to secrete less immunoglobulin, hydration of the patient, and renal disease also may influence the amount of serum M protein, independent of tumor cell burden.

IMMUNOGLOBULIN GENE REARRANGEMENTS

The most sensitive and specific test to determine whether a lymphoproliferative disorder is monoclonal is by analyzing immunoglobulin gene rearrangements. Because B cells rearrange both immunoglobulin heavy- and light-chain genes to produce unique immunoglobulin genes, the detection of non–germ-line DNA immunoglobulin gene fragments serves as a unique marker for each clonal B-cell disorder (see Chap. 11). Southern blot or polymerase chain reaction (PCR) techniques can detect these clonal gene rearrangements and are useful for evaluating most B-cell lymphoproliferative disorders. Rearrangement of immunoglobulin heavy-chain genes occurs very early in B-cell development and may be detected even in cells that produce no M protein (see Chap. 77). Both monoclonal and oligoclonal rearrangements can be detected by these techniques, making it particularly valuable in the diagnosis of lymphoproliferative disorders in immunodeficient hosts, in whom truly oligoclonal, life-threatening lymphoproliferations occur.[55]

The most sensitive test based on clonal IgH rearrangements is quantitative polymerase chain reaction with allele-specific oligonucleotides (ASOs).[56] This test is the "gold standard" for minimal residual disease detection for most B-cell malignancies, but it is mostly only a research method because of high expense and questions about the necessity for such high levels of sensitivity. To perform the test, the laboratory designs and synthesizes ASO probes after sequencing the VDJ region from a patient's B-cell clone. These ASO probes, together with probes from consensus sequences from the IgH locus, allow sensitive detection of minimal residual disease detection by PCR amplification of genomic DNA from clinical samples collected after treatment.

SERUM β_2-MICROGLOBULIN

β_2-Microglobulin is an invariant protein chain that forms part of many different class I membrane structures coded by the HLAs. Class I structures are present on essentially all nucleated cells, including lymphocytes and plasma cells. In rapidly dividing cell populations, membrane turnover leads to shedding of many molecules, including HLA class I proteins. Because β_2-microglobulin is not covalently linked to the other protein chains of the HLA class I structures, it is released into the extracellular fluid and the blood. The molecular weight of β_2-microglobulin is less than 12,000, allowing it to pass through the normal glomerulus. It is reabsorbed by normal proximal renal tubules and does not appear in significant quantities in the urine. In patients with plasma cell neoplasms, however, serum β_2-microglobulin levels increase because of increased neoplastic cell turnover. Also, as myeloma protein-induced renal damage occurs, reduced glomerular filtration increases serum β_2-microglobulin levels. Renal tubular dysfunction increases serum levels even further. Therefore, serum β_2-microglobulin provides another parameter with which to monitor for neoplastic cell mass, cell turnover, effect on renal function, and response to treatment.[57,58]

SERUM VISCOSITY

Large molecules such as IgM pentamers and IgA dimers can significantly increase serum viscosity. Some IgG molecules, particularly those of the IgG_3 subclass, tend to aggregate and increase serum viscosity.[59] The increased plasma viscosity can cause sludging of capillary flow and disturbances of vision, other central nervous system abnormalities, and some clotting disorders (see Chap. 111). In the laboratory, serum viscosity is measured as resistance to flow through standardized glass tubing compared to distilled water. The test usually is performed at room temperature, but if a patient has cryoglobulins which aggregate increasingly at temperatures below 37°C, then serum viscosity measurements should be performed at 37°C. The relative viscosity of normal serum ranges from 1.1 to 1.8 times that of water. Patients usually do not experience clinical symptoms with serum viscosities of less than four times that of water.

AMYLOIDOSIS AND MONOCLONAL IMMUNOGLOBULIN DEPOSITION DISEASES

Amyloidosis associated with plasma cell neoplasms is caused by the deposition of light chains or light-chain fragments in tissues (see Chap. 110). The name *amyloid*, meaning "starch-like," comes from the polysaccharide groups attached to immunoglobulin light- (and heavy-) chain molecules. Amyloid can deposit in any tissue and often has a predilection for packing in and around the walls of small blood vessels. Amyloid is best detected by tissue biopsy, often of the kidney, liver, rectum, oral cavity, heart, or skin. Tissue light-chain deposition has a regular order and binds dyes such as Congo red or thioflavin B.[60] Under polarized light or a fluorescence microscope, the lesions have a characteristic appearance that permits establishing the diagnosis. Amyloidosis may severely impair organ function and is a potentially serious complication of plasma cell neoplasms. Tissue amyloid deposits may interfere with hemostasis and complicate needle biopsies of internal organs.

Monoclonal light- and heavy-chain deposition diseases occur with plasma cell dyscrasias, or more rarely, lymphoplasmacytic neoplasms, that secrete abnormal light, or less often, heavy chain or both. These abnormal immunoglobulin proteins deposit in tissues causing organ dysfunction but do not form amyloid beta-pleated sheets, bind Congo red, or contain amyloid P-component. These disorders include light-chain deposition disease,[61,62] heavy-chain deposition disease,[63,64] and both light- and heavy-chain deposition disease. The patients present with symptoms of organ dysfunction as a result of diffuse, systemic immunoglobulin deposits, usually including nephrotic syndrome and/or renal failure.

REFERENCES

1. Kubagawa H, Vogler LB, Capra JD, et al: Studies on the clonal origin of multiple myeloma. Use of individually specific (idiotype) antibodies to trace the oncogenic

event to its earliest point of expression in B-cell differentiation. *J Exp Med* 150:792, 1979.
2. Lewis JP, MacKenzie MR: Non-random chromosomal aberrations associated with multiple myeloma. *Hematol Oncol* 2:307, 1984.
3. Bence Jones H: Papers on chemical pathology, lecture 3. *Lancet* 2:269, 1847.
4. Axelsson U: An eleven-year follow-up on 64 subjects with M-components. *Acta Med Scand* 201:173, 1977.
5. Axelsson U, Bachmann R, Hallen J: Frequency of pathological proteins (M-components) om 6,995 sera from an adult population. *Acta Med Scand* 179:235, 1966.
6. Hallen J: Frequency of "abnormal" serum globulins (M-components) in the aged. *Acta Med Scand* 173:737, 1963.
7. Berentsen S, Ulvestad E, Langholm R, et al: Primary chronic cold agglutinin disease: A population based clinical study of 86 patients. *Haematologica* 91:460, 2006.
8. Crisp D, Pruzanski W: B-cell neoplasms with homogeneous cold-reacting antibodies (cold agglutinins). *Am J Med* 72:915, 1982.
9. Frank MM, Atkinson JP, Gadek J: Cold agglutinins and cold-agglutinin disease. *Annu Rev Med* 28:291, 1977.
10. Brouet JC, Clauvel JP, Danon F, et al: Biologic and clinical significance of cryoglobulins. A report of 86 cases. *Am J Med* 57:775, 1974.
11. De Bandt M, Ribard P, Meyer O, et al: Type II IgM monoclonal cryoglobulinemia and hepatitis C virus infection. *Clin Exp Rheumatol* 9:659, 1991.
12. Gorevic PD, Kassab HJ, Levo Y, et al: Mixed cryoglobulinemia: Clinical aspects and long-term follow-up of 40 patients. *Am J Med* 69:287, 1980.
13. Regamey N, Hess V, Passweg J, et al: Infection with human herpesvirus 8 and transplant-associated gammopathy. *Transplantation* 77:1551, 2004.
14. Mitus AJ, Stein R, Rappeport JM, et al: Monoclonal and oligoclonal gammopathy after bone marrow transplantation. *Blood* 74:2764, 1989.
15. Penny R, Hughes S: Repeated stimulation of the reticuloendothelial system and the development of plasma-cell dyscrasias. *Lancet* 1:77, 1970.
16. Rosenblatt J, Hall CA: Plasma-cell dyscrasia following prolonged stimulation of reticuloendothelial system. *Lancet* 1:301, 1970.
17. Bliskovsky V, Ramsay ES, Frap SJ: FKBP12 rapamycin-associated protein, is a candidate gene for the plasmacytoma resistance locus Pctr2 and can act as a tumor suppressor gene. *Proc Natl Acad Sci USA* 100(25):14982–14987, 2003.
17a. K. Zhang, D. Kagan, W. DuBois, R. Robinson et al: Mndal, a new interferon-inducible family member, is highly polymorphic, suppresses cell growth, and may modify plasmacytoma susceptibility. *Blood* 114:2952-2960, 2009.
18. Radl J: Age-related monoclonal gammopathies: Clinical lessons from the aging C57mouse BL. *Immunol Today* 11:234, 1990.
19. Radl J, Hollander CF, van den Berg P, et al: Idiopathic paraproteinaemia. I Studies in an animal model—The ageing C57BL/KaLwRij mouse. *Clin Exp Immunol* 33:395, 1978.
20. Potter M, Pumphrey JG, Bailey DW: Genetics of susceptibility to plasmacytoma induction. I BALB/cAnN (C), C57BL/6N (B6), C57BL/Ka (BK), (C times B6)F1, (C times BK)F1, and C times B recombinant-inbred strains. *J Natl Cancer Inst* 54:1413, 1975.
21. Meijers KA, De Leeu MB, Voormolen-Kalova M: The multiple occurrence of myeloma and asymptomatic paraproteinaemia within one family. *Clin Exp Immunol* 12:185, 1972.
22. Kalff MW Hijmans W: Immunoglobulin analysis in families of macroglobulinaemia patients. *Clin Exp Immunol* 5:479, 1969.
23. Williams RC, Erickson JL, Polesky HF, et al: Studies of monoclonal immunoglobulins (M-components) in various kindreds. *Ann Intern Med* 67:309, 1967.
24. Landgren O, Kristinsson SY, Goldin LR, et al: Risk of plasma-cell and lymphoproliferative disorders among 14,621 first-degree relatives of 4,458 patients with monoclonal gammopathy of undetermined significance (MGUS) in Sweden. *Blood* 114:791, 2009.
25. Landgren O, Gridley G, Turesson I, et al: Risk of monoclonal gammopathy of undetermined significance (MGUS) and subsequent multiple myeloma among African American and white veterans in the United States. *Blood* 107:904, 2006.
26. Cohn M, Notani G, Rice SA: Characterization of the antibody to the C-carbohydrate produced by a transplantable mouse plasmacytoma. *Immunochemistry* 6:111, 1969.
27. Porter DD, Larsen AE, Porter HG: Aleutian disease of mink. *Adv Immunol* 29:261, 1980.
28. Isomaki HA, Hakulinen T, Joutsenlahti U: Excess risk of lymphomas, leukemia and myeloma in patients with rheumatoid arthritis. *J Chronic Dis* 31:691, 1978.
29. Goldenberg GJ, Paraskevas F, Israels LG: The association of rheumatoid arthritis with plasma cell and lymphocytic neoplasms. *Arthritis Rheum* 12:569, 1969.
30. Mushinski JF, Bauer SR, Potter M, et al: Increased expression of myc-related oncogene mRNA characterizes most BALB/c plasmacytomas induced by pristane or Abelson murine leukemia virus. *Proc Natl Acad Sci U S A* 80:1073, 1983.
31. Taub R, Kirsch I, Morton C, et al: Translocation of the c-myc gene into the immunoglobulin heavy chain locus in human Burkitt lymphoma and murine plasmacytoma cells. *Proc Natl Acad Sci U S A* 79:7837, 1982.
32. Dalla-Favera R, Bregni M, Erikson J, et al: Human c-myc onc gene is located on the region of chromosome 8 that is translocated in Burkitt lymphoma cells. *Proc Natl Acad Sci U S A* 79:7824, 1982.
33. Avet-Loiseau H, Attal M, Moreau P, et al: Genetic abnormalities and survival in multiple myeloma: The experience of the Intergroupe Francophone du Myelome. *Blood* 109:3489, 2007.
34. Bergsagel PL, Kuehl WM, Zhan F, et al: Cyclin dysregulation D, an early and unifying pathogenic event in multiple myeloma. *Blood* 106:296, 2005.
35. Perez-Simon JA, Garcia-Sanz R, Tabernero MD, et al: Prognostic value of numerical chromosome aberrations in multiple myeloma: A FISH analysis of 15 different chromosomes. *Blood* 91:3366, 1998.
36. Davies FE, Dring AM, Li C, et al: Insights into the multistep transformation of MGUS to myeloma using microarray expression analysis. *Blood* 102:4504, 2003.
37. Shaughnessy JD Jr, Zhan F, Burington BE, et al: A validated gene expression model of high-risk multiple myeloma is defined by deregulated expression of genes mapping to chromosome 1. *Blood* 109:2276, 2007.
38. Decaux O, Lode L, Magrangeas F, et al: Prediction of survival in multiple myeloma based on gene expression profiles reveals cell cycle and chromosomal instability signatures in high-risk patients and hyperdiploid signatures in low-risk patients: A study of the Intergroupe Francophone du Myelome. *J Clin Oncol* 26:4798, 2008.
38a. Anguiano A, Tuchman SA, Acharya C, et al: Gene expression profiles of tumor biology provide a novel approach to prognosis and may guide the selection of therapeutic targets in multiple myeloma. *J Clin Oncol* 27:4197, 2009.
39. Benner R, Hijmans W, Haaijman JJ: The bone marrow: The major source of serum immunoglobulins, but still a neglected site of antibody formation. *Clin Exp Immunol* 46:1, 1981.
40. Mitsiades CS, Mitsiades NS, Richardson PG, et al: Multiple myeloma: A prototypic disease model for the characterization and therapeutic targeting of interactions between tumor cells and their local microenvironment. *J Cell Biochem* 101:950, 2007.
41. Klein B, Zhang XG, Jourdan M, et al: Interleukin-6 is the central tumor growth factor *in vitro* and *in vivo* in multiple myeloma. *Eur Cytokine Netw* 1:193, 1990.
42. Dankbar B, Padro T, Leo R, et al: Vascular endothelial growth factor and interleukin-6 in paracrine tumor-stromal cell interactions in multiple myeloma. *Blood* 95:2630, 2000.
43. Lichtenstein A, Berenson JR, Norman D, et al: Production of cytokines by bone marrow cells obtained from patients with multiple myeloma. *Blood* 74:1266, 1989.
44. Ashcroft AJ, Davies FE, Morgan GJ: Aetiology of bone disease and the role of bisphosphonates in multiple myeloma. *Lancet Oncol* 4:284, 2003.
45. Han JH, Choi SJ, Kurihara N, et al: Macrophage inflammatory protein-1alpha is an osteoclastogenic factor in myeloma that is independent of receptor activator of nuclear factor kappa ligand B. *Blood* 97:3349, 2001.
46. Nakagawa M, Kaneda T, Arakawa T, et al: Vascular endothelial growth factor (VEGF) directly enhances osteoclastic bone resorption and survival of mature osteoclasts. *FEBS Lett* 473:161, 2000.
46a. Roodman GD, Dougall WC: RANK ligand as a therapeutic target for bone metastases and multiple myeloma. *Cancer Treat Rev* 34(1):92-101, 2008. Epub 2007 Oct 26.
47. Swerdlow S, Campo E, Harris NL, Jaffe, ES, Pileri, SA, Stein H, Thiele J, Vardiman, JW (eds): *WHO Classification of Tumours of Haematopoietic and Lymphoid Tissues.* Fourth ed. International Agency for Research on Cancer (IARC), Geneva, Switzerland, 2008.
48. Rawstron AC, Orfao A, Beksac M, et al: Report of the European Myeloma Network on multiparametric flow cytometry in multiple myeloma and related disorders. *Haematologica* 93:431, 2008.
49. Smock KJ, Perkins SL, Bahler DW: Quantitation of plasma cells in bone marrow aspirates by flow cytometric analysis compared with morphologic assessment. *Arch Pathol Lab Med* 131:951, 2007.
50. Ng AP, Wei A, Bhurani D, et al: The sensitivity of CD138 immunostaining of bone marrow trephine specimens for quantifying marrow involvement in MGUS and myeloma, including samples with a low percentage of plasma cells. *Haematologica* 91:972, 2006.
50a. Beck RC, Tubbs RR, Hussein M, Pettay J, et al: Automated colorimetric in situ hybridization (CISH) detection of immunoglobulin (Ig) light chain mRNA expression in plasma cell (PC) dyscrasias and non-Hodgkin lymphoma. *Diagn Mol Pathol* 12(1):14-20, 2003.
51. Paiva B, Vidriales MB, Cervero J, et al: Multiparameter flow cytometric remission is the most relevant prognostic factor for multiple myeloma patients who undergo autologous stem cell transplantation. *Blood* 112:4017, 2008.
52. Perez-Persona E, Vidriales MB, Mateo G, et al: New criteria to identify risk of progression in monoclonal gammopathy of uncertain significance and smoldering multiple myeloma based on multiparameter flow cytometry analysis of bone marrow plasma cells. *Blood* 110:2586, 2007.
53. Bradwell AR, Carr-Smith HD, Mead GP, et al: Highly sensitive, automated immunoassay for immunoglobulin free light chains in serum and urine. *Clin Chem* 47:673, 2001.
54. Dispenzieri A, Kyle R, Merlini G, et al: International Myeloma Working Group guidelines for serum-free light chain analysis in multiple myeloma and related disorders. *Leukemia* 23:215, 2009.
55. Beral V, Peterman T, Berkelman R, et al: AIDS-associated non-Hodgkin lymphoma. *Lancet* 337:805, 1991.
56. van der Velden VH, Hochhaus A, Cazzaniga G, et al: Detection of minimal residual disease in hematologic malignancies by real-time quantitative PCR: Principles, approaches, and laboratory aspects. *Leukemia* 17:1013, 2003.
57. Cuzick J, Cooper EH, MacLennan IC: The prognostic value of serum beta 2 microglobulin compared with other presentation features in myelomatosis. *Br J Cancer* 52:1, 1985.
58. Rotta M, Storer BE, Sahebi F, et al: Long-term outcome of patients with multiple myeloma after autologous hematopoietic cell transplantation and nonmyeloablative allografting. *Blood* 113:3383, 2009.

59. Capra JD Kunkel HG: Aggregation of gamma-G3 proteins: Relevance to the hyperviscosity syndrome. *J Clin Invest* 49:610, 1970.
60. Kyle RA, Greipp PR: Amyloidosis (AL). Clinical and laboratory features in 229 cases. *Mayo Clin Proc* 58:665, 1983.
61. Pozzi C, D'Amico M, Fogazzi GB, et al: Light chain deposition disease with renal involvement: Clinical characteristics and prognostic factors. *Am J Kidney Dis* 42:1154, 2003.
62. Buxbaum J: Mechanisms of disease: Monoclonal immunoglobulin deposition. Amyloidosis, light chain deposition disease, and light and heavy chain deposition disease. *Hematol Oncol Clin North Am* 6:323, 1992.
63. Aucouturier P, Khamlichi AA, Touchard G, et al: Brief report: Heavy-chain deposition disease. *N Engl J Med* 329:1389, 1993.
64. Kambham N, Markowitz GS, Appel GB, et al: Heavy chain deposition disease: The disease spectrum. *Am J Kidney Dis* 33:954, 1999.

CHAPTER 108
ESSENTIAL MONOCLONAL GAMMOPATHY

Marshall A. Lichtman

SUMMARY

Essential monoclonal gammopathy is defined by two key features: (1) the presence of a monoclonal immunoglobulin in the serum or of monoclonal light chains in the urine and (2) the absence of evidence for an overt malignancy of B lymphocytes or plasma cells (e.g., lymphoma, myeloma or amyloidosis). The prevalence of essential monoclonal gammopathy depends on the demographic features in the population under study. In Americans of European descent, the prevalence increases from approximately 2 percent in individuals 50 years of age to approximately 7 percent in octogenarians. It is two to three times as prevalent in persons of African descent. The condition has been reported in association with a large variety of disorders, especially nonlymphocytic cancers. These coincidences are thought, in most cases, to be the chance concurrence of conditions that have a high prevalence in older persons. Some cases of essential monoclonal gammopathy are symptomatic because the immunoglobulin can interact with plasma proteins or neural tissue and cause serious dysfunction, for example, an acquired bleeding disorder or an incapacitating neuropathy. In such cases, disability may be so great that attempts to remove the immunoglobulin by plasmapheresis and to suppress its production using immune or cytotoxic therapy can be warranted. Because myeloma or lymphoma might emerge at the time the monoclonal immunoglobulin is first detected, periodic evaluation of the patient is required to ascertain if essential monoclonal gammopathy is the appropriate diagnosis. Long-term followup at appropriate intervals is prudent to detect conversion from a stable, asymptomatic condition to a progressive lymphoma or myeloma, which occurs in approximately 1 percent of cases per year. In the absence of a symptomatic gammopathy or evolution to a progressive clonal gammopathy, periodic followup is all that is required.

DEFINITION AND HISTORY

The syndrome of essential monoclonal gammopathy has two important characteristics. The first feature is a plasma immunoglobulin (Ig) or urinary Ig light chain that has the molecular features of the product of a single clone of B lymphocytes or plasma cells: homogeneous electrophoretic migration and a single light-chain type. The second feature is the absence of evidence of an overt neoplastic disorder of B lymphocytes or plasma cells, such as lymphoma, myeloma, or amyloidosis.

The observations that Bence Jones proteinuria can precede the clinical signs of multiple myeloma by many years[1] and that hyperglobulinemia without evidence of multiple myeloma can occur in some patients[2] antedated the concept of monoclonal gammopathy as a syndrome. With the more frequent clinical application of zonal electrophoresis of plasma proteins during the 1950s and 1960s, patients were discovered who had a monoclonal Ig, either without an associated disease or with diseases such as nonlymphoid cancers, infections, and inflammatory disorders, which typically are not associated with a monoclonal proliferation of B lymphocytes.[3–10] The presence of a monoclonal protein in plasma or urine, if it is not associated with a disease, is referred to as *essential monoclonal gammopathy*. Several synonyms for the syndrome have been used, particularly *monoclonal gammopathy* and *benign monoclonal gammopathy*.[6] *Monoclonal gammopathy of unknown significance* has became fashionable as a designation preferable to *benign monoclonal gammopathy* because some patients progress to myeloma, macroglobulinemia, amyloidosis, or a B-cell lymphoma over decades of observation.[10,11] The term *essential monoclonal gammopathy* seems best, because it neither highlights a benign process nor indicates that the risks of subsequent lymphoma or myeloma are unknown; that risk is universally appreciated. It is unnecessary to assign the postscript "of unknown significance" to the numerous well-defined benign neoplasms and adenomas at risk of clonal evolution and progression, such as colonic adenomatous polyps, uterine leiomyomas, monoclonal B-cell lymphocytosis, and clonal sideroblastic anemia, among many others. Biologically, essential monoclonal gammopathy is one of many such well-defined examples of a benign neoplasm with the potential to evolve to a progressive neoplasm.

Table 108–1 presents an immunologic classification of essential monoclonal gammopathy.

Acronyms and abbreviations that appear in this chapter include: CD, cluster of differentiation; HLA, human leukocyte antigen; Ig, immunoglobulin; IL, interleukin.

EPIDEMIOLOGY

Monoclonal gammopathy can occur at any age, but it is unusual before puberty, and its frequency increases with age.[12,13] The frequency of a serum paraprotein using zonal electrophoresis is approximately 1 percent in persons older than age 25 years,[4] approximately 3 percent in those older than age 70 years,[4,9] and approximately 10 percent in those older than age 80 years.[3] A much higher prevalence of monoclonal gammopathy has been reported using more sensitive screening methods, such as isoelectric focusing or immunoblotting.[14,15] Prevalence rates differ in different geographic areas and have been somewhat lower in Minnesota,[13] Iceland,[16] the Netherlands,[17] and Japan.[18] The prevalence rate among Africans[19] and Americans of African descent[13,20–22] is significantly greater than the rate among those of European descent in each comparative age group. Males are more frequently affected than females. Familial occurrence also has been described.[23–25] An increased incidence of monoclonal gammopathy may be associated with several occupational groups, including farmers and industrial workers, but such associations are not firmly established.[26]

ETIOLOGY AND PATHOGENESIS

Monoclonal gammopathy can be compared with any benign tumor, such as a colonic adenomatous polyp, which can remain the same size indefinitely or undergo malignant transformation at an unpredictable future time.

Monoclonal gammopathy is caused by the proliferation of a single B lymphocyte, a plasma cell progenitor, leading to a clonal population that reaches a steady-state at approximately 1 to 5×10^{10} cells. At this cell-population density, marrow lymphocyte or plasma cell prevalence is indistinguishable from that of normal marrow. IgG and IgA monoclonal gammopathy arise from somatically mutated postswitch preplasma cells and may have translocations involving the Ig heavy-chain region on chromosome 14. IgM monoclonal gammopathy arises from a mutated postgerminal center lymphocyte that does not have evidence of isotype switching.[27] Not surprisingly, these origins determine the phenotype of the clonal B-lymphocytic diseases that may evolve. For

TABLE 108–1. Types of Monoclonal Immunoglobulin Synthesized by Abnormal B-Cell Clone

IgG, IgA, IgM,[6–11] IgE,[47] IgD[48,49]
IgG + IgA, IgG + IgM, IgG + IgA + IgM[50–53]
Monoclonal κ or λ light chain (Bence Jones proteinuria)[10,54]

example, IgG or IgA monoclonal gammopathy tend to evolve into myeloma or plasmacytoma (plasma cell phenotypes) and IgM monoclonal gammopathies tend to evolve into lymphomas and Waldenström macroglobulinemia (lymphocytic phenotypes).

The expanded clone secretes monoclonal Ig at a rate per cell sufficient for detection by standard tests. The clonal expansion, however, does not cause osteolysis, hypercalcemia, renal insufficiency, inhibit hematopoietic proliferation and maturation, or impair differentiation of polyclonal B lymphocytes to plasma cells. As such, polyclonal Ig synthesis is normal, and patients do not necessarily incur an increased risk of infection. The cells in the stable (benign) clone do not accumulate further and do not elaborate significant amounts of osteoclast-activating factors that are responsible for bone destruction.

Despite these significant differences from myeloma in the behavior of the neoplastic B cells, cytogenetic abnormalities akin to those seen in myeloma may be present in plasma cells derived from patients with essential monoclonal gammopathy.[27–37] G-banding cytogenetic evaluations usually are normal in patients with monoclonal gammopathy, presumably related to the unavailability of cells in the cell cycle (metaphase). However, clones containing numerical abnormalities (e.g., trisomy or monosomy) and translocations have been identified with fluorescence in situ hybridization of interphase cells (see "Clinical Features: Cytogenetic Analysis" below). The presence of clonal cytogenetics changes does not necessarily predict clonal evolution and progression. Although approximately 25 to 30 percent of patients with myeloma have an antecedent period of essential monoclonal gammopathy and presumably undergo clonal evolution to myeloma,[33,36] the presence of clonal cytogenetic abnormalities does not correlate with such evolution.[27,28,35] Gene expression studies of plasma cells isolated from normal marrow and marrow from patients with essential monoclonal gammopathy have identified several hundred genes that are differently expressed.[38,39] The predominate finding was a gradient of overexpression of 41 of 52 genes studied in plasma cells from normal subjects, from patients with monoclonal gammopathy, and from patients with myeloma, respectively.[39] In addition, myeloma patients could be stratified into those with gene expression profiles that were more or less similar to that of essential monoclonal gammopathy. The group more similar to monoclonal gammopathy constituted approximately 30 percent of myeloma patients, coincidentally the proportion of myeloma patients thought to evolve from a prior monoclonal gammopathy.

The C57BL mouse provides a model of essential monoclonal gammopathy. The frequency of monoclonal gammopathy increases with age in these mice.[40] The gammopathy can be transferred to either irradiated or nonirradiated mice by marrow or spleen cells.[41] The transfer can be accomplished only during the first four consecutive transplantations, and no effect is seen on the survival of the recipient compared with that of appropriate control animals. In contrast, if mouse B-cell lymphoma or myeloma cells are transplanted into normal mice, the engraftment frequency is higher than that of B cells from mice with essential monoclonal gammopathy. Passage from the original recipient to a new recipient is unlimited. Progressive disease develops, and survival of the recipient animals is impaired. Thus, an intrinsic difference exists in the growth potential (degree of malignancy) of these B-cell clones.[33] The frequency of monoclonal gammopathy increases with age, but progression to myeloma in the C57BL mouse is a rare event.[42] Studies in transgenic mice and their litter mates replicate the increased incidence of B cell clones and gammopathy with aging.[43]

Occasionally, monoclonal gammopathy is the result of exaggerated production of natural antibody by a B lymphocyte clone.[44] For example, patients with cold agglutinins may have monoclonal IgM for years. A few monoclonal IgM antibodies act as rheumatoid factors and may form cryoglobulins through complex formation with IgG molecules.

CLINICAL FEATURES

BLOOD CELLS AND MARROW

Blood counts and the marrow examination are normal. Notably anemia is not present and the proportion of plasma cells in marrow is less than 10 percent. Although an increased percent of plasma cells is the most constant morphologic feature of myeloma, the presence of cytologic atypia as judged by frequent binucleate plasma cells and large plasma cell nucleoli are finding more specific for myeloma.[45] Quantitative microscopy of the number of marrow microvessels per high-power field, using immunohistochemistry, indicates microvessel density on average is threefold greater than in normal persons, but far less than in patients with myeloma, although overlap with myeloma can ocur.[46]

CYTOGENETIC ANALYSIS

Hyperdiploidy, assessed by DNA content, is present in about half the cases and hypodiploidy in approximately 10 percent.[32] Use of interphase fluorescence in situ hybridization has uncovered numerical chromosome abnormalities in the plasma cells of more than 50 percent of subjects. Clones containing trisomy or monosomy involving chromosomes 3, 6, 7, 9, 11, 13, 17, and 18 have been identified.[28–31,34,35] Deletions of 13q14 are present in about one-quarter of patients and abnormalities involving 14q32, the site of the Ig heavy-chain genes, in approximately 60 percent of subjects.[28–31] The frequency of these chromosome abnormalities is different when compared to the frequency in patients with lymphoma or myeloma. Moreover, chromosomal changes do not appear to be correlated with progression. Thus, the role of cytogenetic abnormalities in contributing to progression is ill-defined.

MONOCLONAL PROTEIN

Characteristically, individuals are detected by the unexpected identification of a monoclonal protein in plasma or urine in the absence of symptoms or signs (e.g., anemia, marrow plasmacytosis, lymph node enlargement, plasmacytoma, bone lesions, or amyloid deposits) caused by diseases associated with monoclonal proteins.[6–10,44,47–54]

Monoclonal IgG gammopathy occurs in approximately 70 percent of persons and IgM and IgA in approximately 15 to 20 percent and 10 percent, respectively. A few percent of persons may have biclonal or triclonal gammopathy.[6–10,44,47–54]

Most patients with essential monoclonal gammopathy have a monoclonal protein concentration of less than 30 g/L, but exceptions occur. The diagnosis reflects the sum of (1) the monoclonal protein level, (2) the marrow plasma cell concentration (usually <10%), (3) the absence of other features of progressive plasma cell neoplasm (e.g., hypercalcemia, osteolysis, otherwise unexplained anemia, otherwise unexplained renal disease), and (4) the absence of progression on periodic long-term follow up.

A developing consensus favors measurement of serum protein electrophoresis, free light chain (and κ:λ ratio), and immunofixation without urinary Ig measurements to detect monoclonal gammopathies.[55–57] Some pathologists are still reluctant to give up urinary measurements because of the uncommon occurrence of urinary monoclonal light chains in the absence of evidence of an abnormality of serum monoclonal light chains.[58] Followup of these cases has not shown any clinical consequence of these uncommon false-negative serum light-chain measurements.

FUNCTIONAL IMPAIRMENT FROM A MONOCLONAL PROTEIN

Some patients have monoclonal proteins with antibody specificity directed against plasma or cell proteins, resulting in symptomatic pathophysiologic effects, such as immune hemolytic anemia,[59] acquired von Willebrand disease,[60,61] immune neutropenia,[62,63] and other functional manifestations[64–69] (Table 108–2).

Rare patients may have isolated urinary light-chain excretion and renal disease.[70–73]

NEUROPATHIES

Frequency of Occurrence

A significant association exists between the occurrence of neuropathies and essential monoclonal gammopathy.[74–81] Approximately 10 percent of patients with idiopathic neuropathy have a monoclonal Ig, a frequency about eight times that of age-adjusted healthy comparison groups.[74–78] The frequency of neuropathy among patients with monoclonal gammopathy varies depending on the distribution of Ig classes, but is in the range of 3 to 5 percent. IgM monoclonal gammopathy has a significantly higher frequency of neuropathy than does IgG or IgA monoclonal gammopathy.[74,75]

Mechanisms of Nerve Damage

Monoclonal antibodies, especially IgM, can react with peripheral nerve myelin, specifically with myelin-associated glycoprotein, glycolipids, or sulfatides.[79–84] Although various antinerve antibodies are present in approximately 40 percent of patients with neuropathy and IgG monoclonal gammopathy, a similar frequency has been found in such patients without neuropathy.[85] Neuropathy in the absence of reactivity of the monoclonal protein with nerve antigens implies other mechanisms also operate to cause nerve damage.[74,76,83] Deposition of monoclonal protein in the epineurium has been proposed as an alternative mechanism of nerve injury.[86] Also, 25 percent of 16 patients with IgG monoclonal gammopathy and neuropathy had polyclonal, not monoclonal, antibodies against neurofilament protein.[83] In addition, a proportion of patients develop a detectable monoclonal protein after the onset of the neuropathy, sometimes years after.[85]

TABLE 108–2. Functional Abnormalities Associated with Essential Monoclonal Gammopathy

Plasma protein disturbances
Antierythrocyte antibodies,[59] acquired von Willebrand disease,[60,61] immune neutropenia,[62,63] cryoglobulinemia,[10] cryofibrinogenemia,[10] acquired C1 esterase inhibitor deficiency (angioedema),[10] acquired antithrombin,[64] insulin antibodies,[65,66] antiacetylcholine receptor antibodies,[67] "antiphospholipid" antibodies,[68] dysfibrinogenemia[69]
Renal disease[70–73]
Neuropathies[74–78]
Deep venous thrombosis[103,104]

Signs and Symptoms

Patients with essential IgM monoclonal gammopathy and neuropathy can have dysesthesia of the hands and feet, loss of vibration and position sense, atrophy of distal muscles, ataxia, and intention tremor.[81,82,84] The monoclonal antibodies reactive with nerve antigens usually are of the IgM type. Serum often contains antibodies to myelin-associated glycoprotein.[74,75] In contrast, patients with essential IgG or IgA monoclonal gammopathy usually have chronic inflammatory demyelinating polyneuropathy, but a minority have sensory axonal or mixed neuropathy.[75,85,87–89] The neuropathy may be (1) mild with minor motor and/or sensory signs with or without mild functional impairment, (2) moderately disabling but with full range of activities, or (3) severely disabling, interfering with walking, dressing, and eating.[85] The course may be relapsing and remitting or progressive. Essential IgA gammopathy is associated with dysautonomia.[90] The presence or absence of antibody to myelin-associated glycoprotein may have an effect on the specific nature of the neuropathic manifestations.[75,76,81–84]

Diagnostic Findings

Demyelinization is reflected in decreased nerve conduction velocity. Axonal loss is reflected in decreased sensory potentials.[76,80,81,87–91] Electromyography may show denervation of muscles.[76,80] Immunofluorescence studies of sural nerve or of skin biopsies may uncover Ig binding to nerve.[76,81] Morphologic studies of nerve biopsies may show decreased or absent myelinated fibers or axonal degeneration. A rare case of crystal formation in the epineurium has been described.[92]

Management

At least seven treatment approaches have been used to ameliorate the neuropathies: (1) intravenous Ig administration; (2) glucocorticoids alone; (3) immunoadsorption of perfused blood with staphylococcal protein A; (4) plasma exchange or plasmapheresis; (5) immunosuppressive cytotoxic chemotherapy, such as cyclophosphamide, chlorambucil, or fludarabine with or without added glucocorticoids; (6) rituximab (anti-cluster of differentiation [CD]20 antibody) to deplete B cells; and (7) high-dose cytotoxic therapy with autologous hematopoietic stem cell rescue.[74–76,84,85,91,93–102] In some cases, use of plasmapheresis has been followed by cytotoxic therapy in an effort to produce a sustained effect. Plasma exchange has shown benefit in a small clinical trial. The other modalities of treatment await such studies.[74] Response rates to each form of therapy are low and duration of response is variable,[76,85,93–98] but some patients obtain coincidental significant improvement for prolonged periods. A recommendation has been made to start therapy with intravenous Ig, especially in essential monoclonal IgM-associated neuropathy, because of the relative safety of this approach.[74] Mild symptoms and signs may not be an indication for treatment because of the low response rate and the potential noxious effects of therapy.[74]

COINCIDING DISORDERS

Monoclonal gammopathy unrelated to a clinically evident proliferation of B lymphocytes or plasma cells has been observed in association with a wide variety of conditions (Table 108–3).[103–164] Although they are grouped under the designation *monoclonal gammopathy with a coincidental disease*, few such reports have examined whether the coincidence is greater than expected from a control group matched for age and

TABLE 108–3. Disorders Reported in Coincidence with Monoclonal Gammopathy

Axial bone fracture[105]
Connective tissue diseases and autoimmune diseases: Crohn disease, cryoglobulinemia, Hashimoto thyroiditis, lupus erythematosus, myasthenia gravis, pernicious anemia, polymyalgia rheumatica, psoriatic arthritis, rheumatoid arthritis, scleroderma, Sjögren disease[106–115]
Corneal diseases: pseudo–Kayser-Fleischer ring,[116] corneal gammopathy[117]
Cutaneous diseases: Schnitzler syndrome, urticaria, hyperkeratotic spicules, pyoderma gangrenosum (neutrophilic dermatoses), psoriasis, scleromyxedema[118–124]
Diffuse idiopathic skeletal hyperostosis[125]
Endocrine diseases: hyperparathyroidism[126,127]
Gaucher disease, type I[128,129]
Hepatic disease: cirrhosis,[114] hepatitis,[130,131]
Hereditary spherocytosis[132]
Infectious diseases: bacterial endocarditis, *Corynebacterium* species, cytomegalovirus, human immunodeficiency virus, *Mycobacterium tuberculosis*, purpura fulminans[17,114,133–136]
Metabolic disease: hyperlipidemia[137]
Neutropenia, chronic[138]
Osteoporosis[139]
Pituitary macroadenoma[140]
Pregnancy[141]
Pseudomyeloma (severe osteoporosis)[142,143]
Carcinomas: colon, lung, prostate, other[3,5,6,144–147]
Myeloproliferative diseases: acute and chronic myelogenous leukemia, chronic neutrophilic leukemia, polycythemia vera[148–152]
T-cell lymphomas, Hodgkin lymphoma[153–156]
After chemotherapy, radiotherapy, or marrow, kidney, or liver transplantation[157–162]
Miscellaneous diseases[163–165]
Transient, monoclonal, or oligoclonal gammopathies[166–168]
Factitious hyperferremia[169]
Factitious increase in C-reactive protein[170]
Vitamin B_{12} deficiency[106,171]

ethnicity, the two variables having the greatest impact on the incidence of monoclonal gammopathy. Non–B-cell malignancies, including solid tumors,[3,5,6,16,144–147] myeloproliferative disorders,[148–152] and Hodgkin and T-cell lymphomas,[153–156] are associated with monoclonal Ig. These relationships could result from various factors: (1) patients with a monoclonal Ig have an increased risk of developing cancer; (2) the monoclonal Ig is an antibody against some antigen associated with the cancer; (3) the monoclonal Ig is the product of cancer cells; or (4) coincidence. The last possibility is favored by two epidemiologic studies that found the same frequency of monoclonal gammopathy in a matched control group as in cancer patients.[9,16] Furthermore, when the monoclonal Ig is associated with a cancer, it usually persists after successful resection of the tumor.

Chemotherapy, radiotherapy, organ or marrow transplantation,[157–162] and other miscellaneous disorders[5,7,10,20,23,113,114,163–165] are associated with a transient or persistent monoclonal Ig (see Table 108–3). The high prevalence of monoclonal proteins and associated diseases, especially after age 50 years, indicates some of these associations are coincidental. Thus, although surgical correction of hyperparathyroidism is associated with disappearance of the plasma monoclonal protein,[126] statistical studies of this disorder suggest a coincidental relationship in most patients.[127] Gaucher disease type I has a higher-than-expected frequency of polyclonal (~40%) and monoclonal (~20%) gammopathy, and, probably, of myeloma.[128,129] Elaboration of proinflammatory cytokines, growth factors, and chemokines, several involved in B-cell function, is disturbed in type I Gaucher disease. An increase of interleukin (IL)-10 and pulmonary and activation-regulated chemokine is notable. The administration of recombinant glucocerebrosidase therapy may decrease the occurrence and progression of gammopathies.[129]

Some observers propose that in clonal myeloid diseases the monoclonal protein reflects B-cell lineage involvement. In inflammatory, autoimmune, and infectious diseases, the association is viewed as an unusual expansion of a restricted population of B lymphocytes. Following marrow transplantation, the presence of oligoclonal blood B-lymphocyte populations reflects the process of reconstitution of the B-cell population.

LABORATORY FEATURES

PLASMA AND URINARY MONOCLONAL IMMUNOGLOBULINS

The monoclonal protein usually is an IgG; however, IgM, IgA, IgD, and IgE, urinary light chains, double gammopathy involving IgA and IgG or IgM and IgA, and triple gammopathy can occur (see Table 108–1).[144,172] By definition, no findings other than a plasma or urinary monoclonal protein are present that permit diagnosis of B-lymphocyte or plasma cell malignancy.

In monoclonal gammopathy of the IgG type, the concentration of monoclonal Ig usually is less than 3.0 g/dL. In the IgA or IgM type, the concentration usually is less than 2.5 g/dL.[10,172] However, dramatic exceptions to this rule exist. Occasional patients with essential monoclonal gammopathy have concentrations as high as 6.0 g/dL. Some patients have Bence Jones proteinuria as the sole manifestation of monoclonal gammopathy.[1,10] The amount of urinary light chains excreted occasionally is so large (>1.0 g/day) that renal dysfunction develops.[70,73]

Most patients with myeloma or macroglobulinemia have significantly depressed nonmonoclonal Ig levels. For example, patients with IgG myeloma usually have very low IgA and IgM concentrations and reduced polyclonal IgG level. Patients with monoclonal gammopathy usually have normal polyclonal Ig levels; and, if a decrease of their polyclonal Ig levels is present, it is usually not as severe as in myeloma.[10,172,173]

OLIGOCLONAL IMMUNOGLOBULINS

Oligoclonal or monoclonal serum Ig levels have been detected with high-resolution agarose gel electrophoresis in hospitalized patients with acute-phase reactions or polyclonal hyperglobulinemia.[168] Oligoclonal Ig bands are frequently seen in the cerebrospinal fluid and serum of patients with a variety of neurologic conditions, especially multiple sclerosis, when the fluids are analyzed by isoelectric focusing.[174] Patients with AIDS have B-cell activation and aberrancies of B-cell regulation. High-resolution electrophoresis indicates most AIDS patients with advanced disease have monoclonal or oligoclonal serum Ig bands. Persons with AIDS, lymphadenopathy syndrome, or antibody to the human immunodeficiency virus also have oligoclonal or monoclonal Ig bands by standard zonal electrophoresis.[134,135] These monoclonal proteins are typically IgG.

LYMPHOCYTE AND PLASMA CELL PHENOTYPES

The concentration of plasma cells in the marrow is less than 10 percent, and the incorporation of tritiated thymidine into marrow plasma cells is negligible (<1%) in essential monoclonal gammopathy. Marrow plasma cells in monoclonal gammopathy do not express neural cell adhesion molecule (CD56), whereas myeloma cells strongly express this surface protein.[205] Blood T-lymphocyte subset levels are normal in monoclonal gammopathy, whereas CD4+ T-cell levels are lower and CD8+ T-cell levels higher in myeloma and macroglobulinemia.[184,191,193,198] Blood B-cell concentration is normal in monoclonal gammopathy, but often is decreased in myeloma patients. Clonally restricted, idiotype-positive blood B cells are characteristic of myeloma but not of monoclonal gammopathy.[187]

β_2-Microglobulin is the light chain of cell surface human leukocyte antigen (HLA) molecules and is present in low concentrations in normal serum. Its concentration in serum frequently is elevated in myeloma, and the magnitude of the elevation is positively correlated with tumor mass. β_2-Microglobulin concentration is not elevated in essential monoclonal gammopathy.[178,179]

The distinction between stable essential monoclonal gammopathy and emerging (so-called larval myeloma) or low-infiltrate myeloma (so-called smoldering myeloma) with a very low tumor burden is blurred at the margins. This finding has not kept investigators from looking for a distinguishing test. More than 40 variables have been studied as an index for discriminating a stable (benign) from progressive (malignant) clone (Table 108–4). No single test is sufficiently sensitive and specific to be useful in an individual patient. Periodic examination of the patient is the best method for detecting the emergence of myeloma or lymphoma or a related disease. Measurement of the concentration of the serum monoclonal protein, urinary light chains, serum β_2-microglobulin, and hemoglobin concentration at appropriate intervals is required. The marrow should be reexamined if the monoclonal protein level increases or hemoglobin concentration decreases significantly. Practical and sensitive methods for measuring bone density would be an additional useful measure of stability or progression.

TABLE 108–4. Variables Used in an Attempt to Distinguish Essential Monoclonal Gammopathy from Myeloma or Lymphoma

Lymphocytes and Immunoglobulins
Igκ light chain expression[177]
Ig light chains in urine[177]
Polyclonal Ig serum concentration[177]
β_2-microglobulin or C-reactive protein serum concentration[176–180]
Ig-secreting cells in blood[181]
Idiotype-reactive blood T lymphocytes[182,183]
CD4-to-CD8 lymphocyte ratio in blood or marrow[184–186]
Clonally restricted B lymphocytes[187–190]
Immunofluorescence of lymphocytes[191]
Natural killer cell frequency[192]
Plasma Cells
Frequency[6,7,9,10,13,172]
Morphology[193–196]
MB2 antibody reactivity[197]
Proliferative index[180,193,194,198]
Asynchronous replication[199]
DNA content or interphase fluorescent in situ hybridization[28,29,33,193,194]
Gene expression profile [39,235]
Ratio of monoclonal CD19–/CD38+/CD56++ to polyclonal CD19+/CD38++/CD56– cells[200]
Blood or marrow concentration[10,187,189,193,198]
J chains[201]
Acid phosphatase[202]
Multidrug resistance expression[203]
CD19 expression[204]
CD56/neural cell adhesion molecule expression[205]
Proportion of CD19+/CD56– plasma cells in marrow[206]
5′ Nucleotidase[207]
Bone Integrity
Magnetic resonance imaging[208,209]
Dual-energy x-ray absorptiometry[210]
Histomorphometry[211]
Urinary pyridinium-collagen complexes[212]
Miscellaneous
Marrow microvessel density[46]
Neural cell adhesion molecules[213]
Serum IL-1β[214]
Serum IL-6, IL-10, soluble CD16, soluble IL-6 receptor, IL-1β[215–220]
Serum transforming growth factor-β[221]
Urinary deoxypyridinoline excretion rate[221]
Hemoglobin concentration[8,114,144]
Mononuclear cell E-cadherin gene methylation[222]

COURSE, PROGNOSIS, AND THERAPY

Longitudinal studies have reported three major patterns of outcome for patients with essential monoclonal gammopathy.[10,223–225] Approximately 25 percent of patients do not progress. In this group, occasional patients experience increases in monoclonal protein concentration of up to 50 percent of their initial diagnostic value. However, these patients restabilize and do not develop signs of myeloma, macroglobulinemia, amyloidosis, or lymphoma. About half of patients die of an unrelated cause. The remaining 25 to 30 percent of patients develop a plasmacytoma, myeloma, amyloidosis, macroglobulinemia, lymphoma, or chronic lymphocytic leukemia over several decades of observation. The occurrence of a lymphoma or myeloma in the latter group of patients continues to increase slowly without reaching a plateau. Evolution to a progressive clonal B-cell disorder has been observed more than 25 years after the diagnosis of monoclonal gammopathy. The actuarial risk of progressing to a clonal B-cell malignancy for all classes of monoclonal protein is approximately 1 percent per year.[223–226] IgM gammopathy usually progresses to lymphoma, macroglobulinemia, amyloidosis, or chronic lymphocytic leukemia.[227] Although one large study found that IgM monoclonal gammopathy evolved to a progressive clonal lymphoid disorder at a rate of approximately 1.5 percent per year,[228] two other large studies found no significant difference in the rate of progression when patients with IgG or IgM were compared.[229,230] IgG or IgA monoclonal gammopathy evolves principally into myeloma, plasmacytoma, or amyloidosis.[231,232] Several studies have found a somewhat higher progression rate in persons with IgA monoclonal gammopathy.[16,233]

Patients with a higher percentage of plasma cells in the marrow, higher monoclonal Ig levels at the time of diagnosis, lower levels of polyclonal Ig, an elevated erythrocyte sedimentation rate, and a lower relative proportion of CD19+ plasma cells evolve to a progressive clonal B-lymphocyte disease more rapidly.[229–234,238] None of these variables have the specificity and sensitivity to be highly accurate in predicting the behavior of an individual patient. Neither the plasma cell gene expression profile nor the cell population cytogenetic findings are sufficiently specific to predict progression from a stable to an unstable clone based on current studies.[31,235] These findings indicate, not surprisingly, that the qualitative leap is between normal, polyclonal plasma cells (B lymphocytes) and the emergence of a monoclonal population either stable or progressively growing and that the distinctions between the latter two states are subtle, complex, and as yet unidentified. In rare patients, the monoclonal protein appears transiently in relation to a disease (e.g., infection)[165–167] or disappears spontaneously even when not associated with a disease (clonal exhaustion).[3]

Generally, the diagnosis of essential monoclonal gammopathy cannot be made with certainty at the time of the initial evaluation. Periodic reexamination is required to document a stable clinical course. One of the most subtle interfaces is between essential monoclonal gammopathy and smoldering myeloma (see Chap. 109). In the latter, the marrow plasma cell concentration is between 10 and 20 percent or the monoclonal protein concentration is greater than 3 g/dL or both. There is no anemia, increase in serum calcium, or evident bone or kidney disease.[236] Careful observation of patients with presumed essential monoclonal gammopathy should permit identification of those who are better categorized as smoldering myeloma. Although at this time treatment is not recommended for smoldering myeloma until progression, calls for clinical trials to assess whether early treatment may improve outcome have been made.[237] Therapy is not required for essential monoclonal gammopathy without a confirmed diagnosis of myeloma, macroglobulinemia, amyloidosis, or lymphoma with evidence of progressive disease. Therapy may be indicated, however, if the monoclonal protein interferes with the vital function of a normal plasma or tissue constituent or is associated with a disabling neuropathy.

REFERENCES

1. Prentiss RG Jr: Multiple myeloma with diffuse skeletal involvement: Case report. *Mil Surg* 80:294, 1937.
2. Waldenstrom JG: Incipient myelomatosis or essential hyperglobulinemia with fibrinogenopenia: A new syndrome? *Acta Med Scand* 117:216, 1944.
3. Hallen J: Frequency of "abnormal serum globulins" (M-components) in the aged. *Acta Med Scand* 173:737, 1963.
4. Axelsson U, Bachmann R, Hallen J: Frequency of pathological proteins (M-components) in 6995 sera from an adult population. *Acta Med Scand* 179:235, 1966.
5. Migliore PJ, Alexanian R: Monoclonal gammopathy in human neoplasia. *Cancer* 21:1127, 1968.
6. Ritzmann SE, Loukes D, Sakai H, et al: Idiopathic (asymptomatic) monoclonal gammopathies. *Arch Intern Med* 135:95, 1975.
7. Amies A, Ko HS, Pruzanski W: M-components: A review of 1242 cases. *Can Med Assoc J* 114:889, 1976.
8. Lindstrom FD, Dahlstrom V: Multiple myeloma or benign monoclonal gammopathy? A study of differential diagnostic criteria in 44 cases. *Clin Immunol Immunopathol* 10:168, 1978.
9. Salerin JP, Vicariot M, Deroff P, et al: Monoclonal gammopathies in the adult population of Finistère, France. *J Clin Pathol* 35:63, 1982.
10. Kyle RA: Monoclonal gammopathy of undetermined significance and solitary myeloma. *Hematol Oncol Clin North Am* 11:71, 1997.
11. Owen RG, Parapia LA, Higginson J, et al: Clinicopathological correlates of IgM paraproteinemias. *Clin Lymphoma* 1:39, 2000.
12. Ligthart GL, Radl J, Corberand JX, et al: Monoclonal gammopathies in human aging: Increased occurrence with age and correlation with health status. *Mech Ageing Dev* 52:235, 1990.
13. Kyle RA, Rajkumar SV: Epidemiology of the plasma-cell disorders. *Best Pract Res Clin Haematol* 20:637, 2007.
14. Sinclair D, Sheehan T, Parrott DMV, Stott DI: The incidence of monoclonal gammopathy in a population over 45 years old determined by isoelectric focusing. *Br J Haematol* 67:745, 1986.
15. Radl J, Wels J, Hoogeven CM: Immunoblotting with (sub)class specific antibodies reveals a high frequency of monoclonal antibodies in persons thought to be immunodeficient. *Clin Chem* 34:1839, 1988.
16. Ögmundsdóttir HM, Haraldsdóttir V, M Jóhannesson G, et al: Monoclonal gammopathy in Iceland: A population-based registry and follow-up. *Br J Haematol* 118:166, 2002.
17. Ong F, Hermans J, Noordik EM, et al: A population-based registry on paraproteinaemia in the Netherlands. *Br J Haematol* 99:914, 1997.
18. Iwanaga M, Tagawa M, Tsukasaki K, et al: Prevalence of monoclonal gammopathy of undetermined significance: Study of 52,802 persons in Nagasaki City, Japan. *Mayo Clin Proc* 82:1474, 2007.
19. Landgren O, Katzmann JA, Hsing AW, et al: Prevalence of monoclonal gammopathy of undetermined significance among men in Ghana. *Mayo Clin Proc* 82:1468, 2007.
20. Schecter GP, Shoff N, Chan C, et al: The frequency of monoclonal gammopathy in black and white veterans in a hospital population, in *Epidemiology and Biology of Multiple Myeloma*, edited by GI Obrams, M Potter, p 93. Springer-Verlag, New York, 1991.
21. Singh J, Dudley AW, Kulig KA: Increased incidence of monoclonal gammopathy of undetermined significance in blacks and its age-related differences with whites on the basis of a study of 397 men and one woman in a hospital setting. *J Lab Clin Med* 116:785, 1990.
22. Landgren O, Gridley G, Turesson I, et al: Risk of monoclonal gammopathy of undetermined significance (MGUS) and subsequent multiple myeloma among African American and white veterans in the United States. *Blood* 107:904, 2006.
23. Bizzaro N, Pasini P: Familial occurrence of multiple myeloma and monoclonal gammopathy of undetermined significance in siblings. *Haematologica* 75:58, 1990.
24. Lynch HT, Sanger WG, Pirruccello S, et al: Familial multiple myeloma: A family study and review of the literature. *J Natl Cancer Inst* 94:1479, 2001.
25. Ögmundsdóttir HM, Haraldsdóttirm V, Jóhannesson GM, et al: Familiality of benign and malignant paraproteinemias. A population-based cancer-registry study of multiple myeloma families. *Haematologica* 90:66, 2005.
26. Pasqualetti P, Collacciani A, Casole R: Risk of monoclonal gammopathy of undetermined significance. *Am J Hematol* 52:217, 1996.
27. Fonesca R, Bailey RJ, Ahmann GJ, et al: Genomic abnormalities in monoclonal gammopathy of undetermined significance. *Blood* 100:1417, 2002.
28. Zandecki M, Lai JL, Genevieve F, et al: Several cytogenetic subclones may be identified within plasma cells from patients with monoclonal gammopathy of undetermined significance both at diagnosis and during the indolent course of the disease. *Blood* 90:3682, 1997.
29. Avet-Loiseau H, Facon T, Daviet A, et al: 14q32 translocations and monosomy 13 observed in monoclonal gammopathy of undetermined significance delineate a multistep process for the oncogenesis of multiple myeloma. *Cancer Res* 59:4546, 1999.
30. Königsberg R, Ackermann J, Kaufmann H, et al: Deletions of chromosome 13q in monoclonal gammopathy of undetermined significance. *Leukemia* 14:1975, 2000.
31. Schilling G, Dierlamm J, Hossfeld DK: Prognostic impact of cytogenetic aberrations in patients with multiple myeloma or monoclonal gammopathy of unknown significance. *Hematol Oncol* 23:102, 2005.
32. Brousseau M, Leleu X, Gerard J, et al: Hyperdiploidy is a common finding in monoclonal gammopathy of undetermined significance and monosomy 13 is restricted to these hyperdiploid patients. *Clin Cancer Res* 13:6026, 2007.
33. Avet-Loiseau H, Li J-Y, Morineau N: Monosomy 13 is associated with the transition of monoclonal gammopathy of undetermined significance to multiple myeloma. *Blood* 94:2583, 1999.
34. Bernasconi P, Cavigliano PM, Boni M, et al: Long-term follow up with conventional cytogenetics and band 13q14 interphase/metaphase in situ hybridization monitoring in monoclonal gammopathies of undetermined significance. *Br J Haematol* 118:545, 2002.
35. Rasillo A, Tabernero MD, Sanchez ML, et al: Fluorescence in situ hybridization analysis of aneuploidization patterns in monoclonal gammopathy of undetermined significance versus multiple myeloma and plasma cell leukemia. *Cancer* 97:601, 2003.
36. Zojer N, Ludwig H, Fiegi M, et al: Patterns of somatic mutations in VH genes reveal pathways of clonal transformations from MGUS to multiple myeloma. *Blood* 101:4137, 2003.
37. Lloveras E, Sole F, Florensa L, et al: Contribution of cytogenetics and in situ hybridization to the study of monoclonal gammopathy of undetermined significance. *Cancer Genet Cytogenet* 132:25, 2002.
38. Davies FE, Dring AM, Li C, et al: Insights into the multistep transformation of MGUS to myeloma using microarray expression analysis. *Blood* 102:4504, 2003.
39. Zhan F, Hardin J, Kordesmeier B, et al: Global gene expression profiling of multiple myeloma, monoclonal gammopathy of undetermined significance, and normal bone marrow plasma cells. *Blood* 99:1745, 2002.
40. Radl J, Hollander CF: Homogeneous immunoglobulins in sera of mice during aging. *J Immunol* 112:2271, 1974.
41. Radl J, DeGlopper E, Schuit HRE, Zurcher C: Idiopathic paraproteinemia: II. Transplantation of the paraprotein-producing clone from old to young 57B1/KaLwRij mice. *J Immunol* 122:609, 1979.
42. Radl J: Age-related monoclonal gammopathies: Clinical lessons from the aging C57BL mouse. *Immunol Today* 11:234, 1990.
43. van Arkel C, Hopstaken CM, Zurcher C, et al: Monoclonal gammopathies in aging m, x-transgenic mice: Involvement of the B-1 cell lineage. *Eur J Immunol* 27:2436, 1997.
44. George G, Gilburd B, Schoenfeld Y: The emerging concept of pathogenic natural antibodies. *Hum Antibodies* 8:70, 1997.

45. Milla F, Oriol A, Aguilar J, et al: Usefulness and reproducibility of cytomorphic evaluations to differentiate myeloma from monoclonal gammopathies of unknown significance. *Am J Clin Pathol* 115:127, 2001.
46. Rajkumar SV, Mesa RA, Fonesca R, et al: Bone marrow angiogenesis in 400 patients with monoclonal gammopathy of undetermined significance, multiple myeloma, and primary amyloidosis. *Clin Cancer Res* 8:2210, 2002.
47. Ludwig H, Vormittag W: "Benign" monoclonal Ig E gammopathy. *Br Med J* 281:539, 1980.
48. O'Connor ML, Rice DT, Buss DH, Muss HB: Immunoglobulin D benign monoclonal gammopathy. *Cancer* 68:611, 1991.
49. Kinoshita K, Nagai H, Murate T, et al: Ig D monoclonal gammopathy of undetermined significance. *Int J Hematol* 65:169, 1997.
50. Imhof JW, Balliux RE, Mul NAJ, Poen H: Monoclonal and diclonal gammopathies. *Acta Med Scand* 179(Suppl 455):102, 1966.
51. Jensen K, Jensen B, Olesen H: Three M-components in serum from an apparently healthy person. *Scand J Haematol* 4:485, 1967.
52. Kyle RA, Robinson RA, Katzmann JA: The clinical aspects of biclonal gammopathies: Review of 57 cases. *Am J Med* 71:999, 1981.
53. Riddell S, Traczyk Z, Paraskevas F, Israels LG: The double gammopathies: Clinical and immunological studies. *Medicine (Baltimore)* 65:135, 1986.
54. Kyle RA, Greipp PR: "Idiopathic" Bence Jones proteinuria. *N Engl J Med* 306:564, 1982.
55. Hill PG, Forsyth JM, Rai B, Mayne S. Serum free light chains: An alternative to the urine Bence Jones proteins screening test for monoclonal gammopathies. *Clin Chem* 52:1743, 2006.
56. Katzmann JA, Dispenzieri A, Kyle RA, et al: Elimination of the need for urine studies in the screening algorithm for monoclonal gammopathies by using serum immunofixation and free light chain assays. *Mayo Clin Proc* 81:1575, 2006
57. Jagannath S: Value of serum free light chain testing for the diagnosis and monitoring of monoclonal gammopathies in hematology. *Clin Lymphoma Myeloma* 7:518, 2007.
58. Beetham R, Wassell J, Wallage MJ, et al: Can serum free light chains replace urine electrophoresis in the detection of monoclonal gammopathies? *Ann Clin Biochem* 44:516, 2007.
59. Kay NE, Gordon LI, Douglas SD: Autoimmune hemolytic anemia in association with monoclonal IgM(k) with anti-i-activity. *Am J Med* 64:845, 1978.
60. Lamboley V, Zabraniecki L, Sie P, et al: Myeloma and monoclonal gammopathy of uncertain significance associated with acquired von Willebrand's syndrome. Seven new cases with a literature review. *Joint Bone Spine* 69:62, 2002.
61. Agarwal N, Klix MM, Burns CP: Successful management with intravenous immunoglobulins of acquired von Willebrand disease associated with monoclonal gammopathy of undetermined significance. *Ann Intern Med* 6:141:83, 2004.
62. Nocente R, Cammarota G, Gentiloni Silveri N, et al: A case of Sweet's syndrome associated with monoclonal immunoglobulin of IgG-lambda type and p-ANCA positivity. *Panminerva Med* 44:149, 2002.
63. Carrington PA, Walsh SE, Houghton JB: Benign paraproteinemia and immune neutropenia. *Clin Lab Haematol* 2:407, 1989.
64. Gabriel DA, Carr ME, Cook L, Roberts HR: Spontaneous antithrombin in a patient with benign paraprotein. *Am J Hematol* 25:85, 1987.
65. Sluiter WJ, Marrink J, Houwen B: Monoclonal gammopathy with an insulin binding IgG(K) M-component, associated with severe hypoglycaemia. *Br J Haematol* 62:679, 1986.
66. Wasada T, Egueli Y, Takayama S, Yoo K, et al: Insulin autoimmune syndrome associated with benign monoclonal gammopathy. *Diabetes Care* 12:147, 1989.
67. Ahlberg RE, Lefvert AK: Monoclonal gammopathy and antibody activity against the acetylcholine receptor. *Am J Hematol* 29:49, 1988.
68. Disdier P, Swiader L, Aillaud M-F, et al: Ig M monoclonal gammopathy, lymphoid proliferations and lupus anticoagulant. *Am J Med* 102:319, 1997.
69. Dear A, Brennan SO, Sheat MJ, et al: Acquired dysfibrinogenemia caused by monoclonal production of immunoglobulin lambda light chain. *Haematologica* 92:e111, 2007.
70. Maldonado JE, Velosa JA, Kyle RA, et al: Fanconi syndrome in adults: A manifestation of a latent form of myeloma. *Am J Med* 58:354, 1975.
71. Gavarotti P, Fortina F, Costa D, et al: Benign monoclonal gammopathy presenting with severe renal failure. *Scand J Haematol* 36:115, 1986.
72. Maes B, Vanwalleghem J, Kuypers D, et al: IgA antiglomerular basement membrane disease associated with bronchial carcinoma and monoclonal gammopathy. *Am J Kidney Dis* 33:E3, 1999.
73. Hashimoto T, Arakawa K, Ohta Y, et al: Acquired Fanconi syndrome with osteomalacia secondary to monoclonal gammopathy of undetermined significance. *Intern Med* 46:241, 2007.
74. Drappatz J, Batchelor T: Neurologic complications of plasma cell disorders. *Clin Lymphoma* 5:163, 2004.
75. Lozeron P, Adams D: Monoclonal gammopathy and neuropathy. *Curr Opin Neurol* 20:536, 2007.
76. Ropper AH, Gorsin KC: Neuropathies associated with paraproteinemia. *N Engl J Med* 338:1601, 1998.
77. Kissel JT, Mendell JR: Neuropathies associated with monoclonal gammopathies. *Neuromuscul Disord* 6:3, 1996.
78. Vallatt JM, Jauberteau MO, Bordessoule D, et al: Link between peripheral neuropathy and monoclonal dysglobulinemia: A study of 66 cases. *J Neurol Sci* 137:124, 1996.
79. Lee KW, Inghirami G, Spatz L, et al: The B-cells that express anti-MAG antibodies in neuropathy and non-malignant IgM monoclonal gammopathy belong to the CD5 subpopulation. *J Neuroimmunol* 31:83, 1991.
80. Cocito D, Durelli L, Isoardo G: Different clinical, electrophysiological and immunological features of CDIP associated with paraproteinemia. *Acta Neurol Scand* 108:274, 2003.
81. Chassande B, Léger J-M, Younes-Chennoufi AB, et al: Peripheral neuropathy associated with IgM monoclonal gammopathy: Correlation between M-protein antibody activity and clinical/electrophysiological features in 40 cases. *Muscle Nerve* 21:55, 1998.
82. Pestronk A, Li F, Bieser BS, et al: Anti-MAG antibodies. *Neurology* 44:1131, 1994.
83. Stubbs EB Jr, Lawlor MW, Richards MP, et al: Anti-neurofilament antibodies in neuropathy with monoclonal gammopathy of undetermined significance produce experimental motor nerve conduction block. *Acta Neuropathol* 105:109, 2003.
84. Ellie E, Vital A, Steck A, et al: Neuropathy associated with "benign" anti-myelin-associated glycoprotein IgM gammopathy: Clinical, immunological, neurophysiological pathological findings and response to treatment in 33 cases. *J Neurol* 243:34, 1996.
85. Di Troia A, Carpo M, Meucci N, et al: Clinical features and anti-neural reactivity in neuropathy associated with IgG monoclonal gammopathy of undetermined significance. *J Neurol Sci* 164:64, 1999.
86. Vallat JM, Magy L, Richard L, Piaser M, et al: Intranervous immunoglobulin deposits: An underestimated mechanism of neuropathy. *Muscle Nerve* 38:904, 2008.
87. Gorsin KC, Ropper AH: Axonal neuropathy associated with monoclonal gammopathy of undetermined significance. *J Neurol Neurosurg Psychiatry* 62:163, 1997
88. Wilson JR, Stittsworth JD Jr, Fisher MA: Electrodiagnostic patterns in MGUS neuropathy. *Electromyogr Clin Neurophysiol* 41:409, 2001.
89. Nicholas G, Maisonobe T, Le Forestier N, et al: Proposed revised electrophysiological criteria for chronic inflammatory demyelinating polyradiculopathy. *Muscle Nerve* 25:26, 2002.
90. Jonsson V, Schroder HD, Trojaborg W, et al: Autoimmune reactions in patients with M-component and peripheral neuropathy. *J Intern Med* 232:185, 1992.
91. Gorsin KC, Allan G, Ropper AH: Chronic inflammatory demyelinating polyneuropathy: Clinical features and response to treatment in 67 consecutive patients with and without a monoclonal gammopathy. *Neurology* 48:321, 1997.
92. Vital A, Nedelec-Ciceri C, Vital C: Presence of crystalline inclusions in the peripheral nerve of a patient with IgA lambda monoclonal gammopathy of undetermined significance. *Neuropathology* 28:526, 2008.
93. Latov N: Pathogenesis and therapy of neuropathies associated with monoclonal gammopathies. *Ann Neurol* 37(Suppl 1):532, 1995.
94. Sghirlanzoni A, Solari A, Ciano C: Chronic inflammatory demyelinating polyradiculopathy: Long-term course and treatment of 60 patients. *Neurol Sci* 21:31, 2000.
95. Kiprov DD, Miller RG: Paraproteinemia associated with demyelinating polyneuropathy or myositis: Treatment with plasmapheresis and immunosuppressive drugs. *Artif Organs* 9:47, 1985.
96. Gorson KC: Clinical features, evaluation, and treatment of patients with polyneuropathy associated with monoclonal gammopathy of undetermined significance (MGUS). *J Clin Apher* 14:149, 1999.
97. Blume G, Pestronk A, Goodnough LT: Anti-MAG antibody-associated polyneuropathies: Improvement following immunotherapy with monthly plasma exchange and IV cyclophosphamide. *Neurology* 45:1577, 1995.
98. Oksenhendler E, Chevret S, Léger JM, et al: Plasma exchange and chlorambucil in polyneuropathy associated with monoclonal IgM gammopathy. *J Neurol Neurosurg Psychiatry* 59:243, 1995.
99. Lee YC, Came N, Schwarer A, Day B: Autologous peripheral blood stem cell transplantation for peripheral neuropathy secondary to monoclonal gammopathy of unknown significance. *Bone Marrow Transplant* 30:53, 2002.
100. Niermeijer JM, Eurelings M, Lokhorst H, et al: Neurologic and hematologic response to fludarabine treatment in IgM MGUS polyneuropathy. *Neurology* 67:2076, 2006.
101. Finsterer J: Treatment of immune-mediated, dysimmune neuropathies. *Acta Neurol Scand* 112:115, 2005.
102. Renaud S, Fuhr P, Gregor M, et al: High-dose rituximab and anti-MAG-associated polyneuropathy. *Neurology* 66:742, 2006.
103. Kristinsson SY, Fears TR, Gridley G, et al: Deep vein thrombosis following monoclonal gammopathy of undetermined significance (MGUS) and multiple myeloma. *Blood* 112:3582, 2008. .
104. Auwerda JJ, Sonneveld P, de Maat MP, Leebeek FW: Prothrombotic coagulation abnormalities in patients with paraprotein-producing B-cell disorders. *Clin Lymphoma Myeloma* 7:462, 2007.
105. Melton LJ 3rd, Rajkumar SV, Khosla S, et al: Fracture risk in monoclonal gammopathy of undetermined significance. *J Bone Miner Res* 19:25, 2004.
106. Burner E, Swahlen A, Cruchaud A: Nonmalignant monoclonal immunoglobulinemia, pernicious anemia, and gastric carcinoma: A model of immunologic dysfunction. *Am J Med* 60:1019, 1976.
107. Rowland LP, Osserman EF, Scharfman WB, et al: Myasthenia gravis with a myeloma-type gamma-G (IgG) immunoglobulin abnormality. *Am J Med* 46:599, 1969.
108. Ilfeld D, Barzilay J, Vana D, et al: IgG monoclonal gammopathy in four patients with polymyalgia rheumatica [letter]. *Ann Rheum Dis* 44:501, 1985.
109. Nanji AA: Monoclonal gammopathy associated with Crohn's disease during treatment with total parenteral nutrition. *JPEN J Parenter Enteral Nutr* 9:621, 1985.
110. Wallach D, Carado Y, Foldes C, Cottennot F: Dermatomyositis and monoclonal gammopathy. *Ann Dermatol Venereol* 112:783, 1985.
111. McFadden N, Ree K, Syland E, Larse TE: Scleredema adultorum associated with a monoclonal gammopathy and generalized hyperpigmentation. *Arch Dermatol* 123:629, 1987.

112. Oikarinen A, Ala-Kokko L, Palatsi R, et al: Scleroderma and paraproteinemia. *Arch Dermatol* 123:226, 1987.
113. Johnsson V, Svendsen B, Vostrup S, et al: Multiple autoimmune manifestations in monoclonal gammopathy of undetermined significance and chronic lymphocytic leukemia. *Leukemia* 10:327, 1996.
114. Kyle RA: Monoclonal gammopathy of unknown significance (MGUS). *Baillieres Clin Haematol* 8:761, 1995.
115. Kagaya M, Takahashi H: A case of type I cryoglobulinemia associated with a monoclonal gammopathy of undetermined significance (MGUS). *J Dermatol* 32:128, 2005.
116. Probst LE, Hoffman E, Cherian MG, et al: Ocular copper deposition associated with benign monoclonal gammopathy and hypercupremia. *Cornea* 15:94, 1996.
117. Secundo W, Seifert P: Monoclonal corneal gammopathy: Topographic considerations. *Ger J Ophthalmol* 5:262, 1996.
118. de Koning HD, Bodar EJ, van der Meer JW, et al: Schnitzler syndrome: beyond the case reports: review and follow-up of 94 patients with an emphasis on prognosis and treatment. *Semin Arthritis Rheum* 37:137, 2007.
119. Ryan JG, de Koning HD, Beck LA, et al: IL-1 blockade in Schnitzler syndrome: ex vivo findings correlate with clinical remission. *J Allergy Clin Immunol* 121:260, 2008.
120. Wayte JA, Rogers S, Powell FC: Pyoderma gangrenosum, erythema elevatum diutinum and Ig A monoclonal gammopathy. *Australas J Dermatol* 36:21, 1995.
121. Doutre MS, Beylot C, Bioulac P, Bezian JH: Monoclonal IgM and chronic urticaria: Two cases. *Ann Allergy* 58:413, 1987.
122. Samochocki Z, Szudzinski A: Gangrenous pyoderma in monoclonal IgA gammopathy and functional disorders of T lymphocytes. *Przegl Dermatol* 73:409, 1986.
123. Abraham Z, Feuerman EJ: IgA benign monoclonal gammopathy with recurrent self-healing skin tumors. *J Am Acad Dermatol* 21:1303, 1989.
124. Paul C, Fermaud J-P, Flageul B, et al: Hyperkeratotic spicules and monoclonal gammopathy. *J Am Acad Dermatol* 33:346, 1995.
125. Scutellari PN, Antinolfi G: Association between monoclonal gammopathy of undetermined significance (MGUS) and diffuse idiopathic skeletal hyperostosis (DISH). *Radiol Med (Torino)* 108:172, 2004.
126. Schnur MJ, Appel GB, Bilezikian JP: Primary hyperparathyroidism and benign monoclonal gammopathy. *Arch Intern Med* 137:1201, 1977.
127. Rao DS, Antonelli R, Kane KR, et al: Primary hyperparathyroidism and monoclonal gammopathy. *Henry Ford Hosp Med J* 39:41, 1991.
128. Schoenfeld Y, Berliner S, Pinkhas J, Beutler E: The association of Gaucher's disease and dysproteinemias. *Acta Haematol* 64:241, 1980.
129. de Fost M, Out TA, de Wilde FA, et al: Immunoglobulin and free light chain abnormalities in Gaucher disease type I: Data from an adult cohort of 63 patients and review of the literature. *Ann Hematol* 87:439, 2008.
130. Andreone P, Zignego AL, Cursaro C, et al: Prevalence of monoclonal gammopathies in patients with hepatitis C virus infection. *Ann Intern Med* 129:294, 1998.
131. Hamazaaki K, Baba M, Hasegawa H, et al: Chronic hepatitis associated with monoclonal gammopathy of undetermined significance. *Gastroenterol Hepatol* 18:459, 2003.
132. Schafer AL, Miller JB, Lester EP, et al: Monoclonal gammopathy in hereditary spherocytosis: A possible pathogenetic relation. *Ann Intern Med* 88:45, 1978.
133. Danon F, Bussel A, Perol Y: Immunoglobulines monoclonales infections a cytomegalovirus et hémopathies malignes. *Ann Immunol (Paris)* 128A:83, 1977.
134. Papadopoulos NM, Lane HC, Costello R, et al: Oligoclonal immunoglobulins in patients with the acquired immunodeficiency syndrome. *Clin Immunol Immunopathol* 35:43, 1985.
135. Heriot K, Hallquist AE, Tomar RH: Paraproteinemia in patients with acquired immunodeficiency syndrome (AIDS) or lymphadenopathy syndrome (LAS). *Clin Chem* 31:1224, 1985.
136. Kouns DM, Marty AM, Sharpe RW: Oligoclonal bands in serum protein electrophoretograms of individuals with human immunodeficiency virus antibodies. *JAMA* 256:2343, 1986.
137. Johnston JD, Lumb PJ, Wierzbicki AS: Hyperlipidaemia in association with benign paraproteinemia. *Ann Clin Biochem* 34:697, 1997.
138. Papadaki HA, Eliopoulos DG, Ponticoglou C, Eliopoulos GD: Increased frequency of monoclonal gammopathy of undetermined significance in patients with nonimmune chronic idiopathic neutropenia syndrome. *Int J Hematol* 73:339, 2001.
139. Dizdar O, Erman M, Cankurtaran M, et al: Lower bone mineral density in geriatric patients with monoclonal gammopathy of undetermined significance. *Ann Hematol* 87:57, 2008.
140. Tucci A, Bonadonna S, Cattaneo C, et al: Transformation of MGUS to overt multiple myeloma: The possible role of pituitary microadenoma secreting high levels of insulin-like growth factor 1 (IGF-1). *Leuk Lymphoma* 44:543, 2003.
141. Chryssikkopoulos A, Dalamaga AL, Hassiakos D: Monoclonal gammopathy of unknown significance in pregnancy. *Clin Exp Obstet Gynecol* 24:31, 1997.
142. Buonocore E, Solmon A, Kerley HE: Pseudomyeloma. *Radiology* 95:41, 1970.
143. Maldonado JE, Riggs L, Bayrd ED: Pseudomyeloma. *Arch Intern Med* 135:267, 1975.
144. Kyle RA: Monoclonal gammopathy of unknown significance. *Curr Top Microbiol Immunol* 210:375, 1996.
145. Solomon A: Homogeneous (monoclonal) immunoglobulins in cancer. *Am J Med* 63:169, 1977.
146. Colls BM, Lorier MA: Immunocytoma, cancer, and other associations of monoclonal gammopathy: A review of 224 cases. *N Z Med J* 82:221, 1975.
147. Abdul M, Hassein NM: Gammopathy associated with advanced prostate cancer. *Urol Res* 23:185, 1995.
148. Shoenfeld Y, Berliner S, Ayalone A, et al: Monoclonal gammopathy in patients with chronic and acute myeloid leukemia. *Cancer* 54:280, 1984.
149. Berner Y, Berrebi A: Myeloproliferative disorders and nonmyelomatous paraprotein. *Isr J Med Sci* 22:109, 1986.
150. Tosato F, Fossaluzza V, Rossi P, et al: Monoclonal gammopathy of undetermined significance in a case of primary thrombocythemia. *Haematologica* 71:417, 1986.
151. Economopoulos T, Economidou J, Papageorgiou E, et al: Monoclonal gammopathy in chronic myeloproliferative disorders. *Blut* 58:7, 1989.
152. Ito T, Kojima H, Otani K, et al: Chronic neutrophilic leukemia associated with monoclonal gammopathy of unknown significance. *Acta Haematol* 95:140, 1996.
153. Offit K, Macris NT, Hellman G, Rotterdam, HZ: Consecutive lymphoma with monoclonal gammopathy in a married couple. *Cancer* 57:277, 1986.
154. Venencie PY, Winkelmann RK, Puissant A, Kyle RA: Monoclonal gammopathy in Sézary syndrome: Report of three cases and review of the literature. *Arch Dermatol* 120:605, 1984.
155. Kamihira S, Taguchi H, Kinoshita K, Ichimaru M: Monoclonal gammopathy in adult T-cell leukemia/lymphoma: A report of three cases. *Jpn J Clin Oncol* 14:699, 1984.
156. Chisesi I, Capnist G, Barbui T: Two serum IgG M-components of differing light chain types in a case of Hodgkin's disease. *Acta Haematol* 55:250, 1976.
157. Hammarstrom L, Smith CIE: Frequent occurrence of monoclonal gammopathies with an imbalanced light-chain ratio following bone marrow transplantation. *Transplantation* 43:447, 1987.
158. Mitus AJ, Stein R, Rappeport JM, et al: Monoclonal and oligoclonal gammopathy after bone marrow transplantation. *Blood* 74:2764, 1989.
159. Passweg J, Thiel G, Bock HA: Monoclonal gammopathy after intense induction immunosuppression in renal transplant patients. *Nephrol Dial Transplant* 11:2461, 1996.
160. Badley AD, Portela DF, Patel R, et al: Development of monoclonal gammopathy precedes the development of Epstein-Barr virus-induced posttransplant lymphoproliferative disorder. *Liver Transpl Surg* 2:375, 1996.
161. Touchard G, Pasdeloup T, Parpeix J, et al: High prevalence and usual persistence of serum monoclonal immunoglobulins evidenced by sensitive methods in renal transplant recipients. *Nephrol Dial Transplant* 12:1199, 1997.
162. Ho JL, Polde PA, McEniry D, et al: Acquired immunodeficiency syndrome with progressive multifocal leukoencephalopathy and monoclonal B-cell proliferation. *Ann Intern Med* 100:693, 1984.
163. Nagler A, Ben-Arieh Y, Brenner B, et al: Eosinophilic fibrohistiocytic lesion of bone marrow associated with monoclonal gammopathy and osteolytic lesions. *Am J Hematol* 23:277, 1986.
164. Hineman VL, Phyliky RL, Banks PM: Angiofollicular lymph node hyperplasia and peripheral neuropathy: Association with monoclonal gammopathy. *Mayo Clin Proc* 57:379, 1982.
165. Radl J, VandenBerg A: Transitory appearance of homogeneous immunoglobulins—paraproteins—in children with severe combined immunodeficiency before and after transplantation, in *Protides of Biological Fluids*, vol 20, edited by H Peeters, p. 203. Pergamon, Oxford, 1973.
166. DelCarpio J, Espinoza LR, Lauater S, Osterland CK: Transient monoclonal proteins in drug hypersensitivity reactions. *Am J Med* 66:1051, 1979.
167. Keshgegian AA: Prevalence of small monoclonal proteins in the serum of hospitalized patients. *Am J Clin Pathol* 77:436, 1982.
168. VanCamp B, Reynaerts PH, Naets JP, Radl J: Transient IgA_1-λ para-proteinemia during treatment of acute myeloblastic leukemia. *Blood* 55:21, 1980.
169. Bakker AJ, Kothman-Tijkotte MJ: Artifactually high concentration of iron determined in serum from a patient with a monoclonal immunoglobulin. *Clin Chem* 36:1517, 1990.
170. Yu A, Pira U: False increase in serum C-reactive protein caused by monoclonal IgM-lambda: a case report. *Clin Chem Lab Med* 39:983, 2001.
171. Baz R, Alemany C, Green R, Hussein MA: Prevalence of vitamin B_{12} deficiency in patients with plasma cell dyscrasias: a retrospective review. *Cancer* 101:790, 2004.
172. Malacrida V, De-Francesco D, Banfi G, et al: Laboratory investigation of monoclonal gammopathy during 10 years of screening in a general hospital. *J Clin Pathol* 40:793, 1987.
173. Moller-Petersen J, Schmidt EB: Diagnostic value of the concentration of M-component in initial classification of monoclonal gammopathy. *Scand J Haematol* 26:295, 1986.
174. Link H, Kostulas V: Utility of isoelectric focusing of cerebrospinal fluid and serum of agarose evaluated for neurological patients. *Clin Chem* 29:810, 1983.
175. Vuckovic J, Ilic A, Knezevic N, et al: Progress in monoclonal gammopathy of undetermined significance. *Br J Haematol* 97:649, 1997.
176. Bataille R: New insights in the clinical biology of multiple myeloma. *Semin Hematol* 34:23, 1997.
177. Baldini L, Guffanti A, Cesana BM, et al: Role of different hematologic variables in defining the risk of malignant transformation in monoclonal gammopathy. *Blood* 87:92, 1996.
178. Morrell A, Riesen W: Serum β_2-macroglobulin, serum creatinine and bone marrow plasma cells in benign and malignant monoclonal gammopathy. *Acta Haematol* 64:87, 1980.
179. Fine JM, Lambin P, Desjobert H: Serum neopterin and β_2-microglobulin concentrations in monoclonal gammopathies. *Acta Med Scand* 224:179, 1988.
180. French M, Fench P, Remy F, et al: Plasma cell proliferation in monoclonal gammopathy: Relations with other biologic variables—Diagnostic and prognostic significance. *Am J Med* 98:60, 1995.

181. Witzig TE, Gonchoroff NJ, Katzmann JA, et al: Peripheral blood B cell labeling indices are a measure of disease activity in patients with monoclonal gammopathies. *J Clin Oncol* 6:1041, 1988.
182. Yi Q, Eriksson I, He W, et al: Idiotype-specific T lymphocytes in monoclonal gammopathies: Evidence for the presence of CD4+ and CD8+ subsets. *Br J Haematol* 96:338, 1997.
183. Yi Q, Osterborg A, Bergenbrant S, et al: Idiotype-reactive T-cell subsets and tumor load in monoclonal gammopathies. *Blood* 86:3043, 1995.
184. San Miguel JF, Caballero MD, Gonzalez M: T-cell subpopulations in patients with monoclonal gammopathies: Essential monoclonal gammopathy, multiple myeloma and Waldenstrom macroglobulinemia. *Am J Hematol* 20:267, 1985.
185. Halapi E, Werner A, Wahlstrom J, et al: T cell repertoire in patients with multiple myeloma and monoclonal gammopathy of undetermined significance: Clonal CD8+ T cell expansions are found preferentially in patients with a low tumor burden. *Eur J Immunol* 27:2245, 1997.
186. Corso A, Castelli G, Pagnucco G, et al: Bone marrow T-cell subsets in patients with monoclonal gammopathies: Correlation with clinical stage and disease. *Haematologica* 82:43, 1997.
187. Billadeau D, Greipp P, Ahmann G, et al: Detection of B-cells clonally related to the tumor population in multiple myeloma and MGUS. *Curr Top Microbiol Immunol* 194:9, 1995.
188. Miguel-Garcia A, Matutes E, Tarin F, et al: Circulating Ki 67 positive lymphocytes in multiple myeloma and benign monoclonal gammopathy. *J Clin Pathol* 48:835, 1995.
189. Billadeau D, Van Ness B, Kimlinger T, et al: Clonal circulation cells are common in plasma cell proliferative disorders: A comparison of monoclonal gammopathy, smoldering myeloma, and active myeloma. *Blood* 88:289, 1996.
190. Isaksson E, Bjockholm M, Holm G, et al: Blood clonal B-cell excess in patients with monoclonal gammopathy of undetermined significance (MGUS): Association with malignant transformation. *Br J Haematol* 92:71, 1996.
191. Lindstrom FD, Hardy WR, Eberle BJ, Williams RC Jr: Multiple myeloma and benign monoclonal gammopathy: Differentiation by immunofluorescence of lymphocytes. *Ann Intern Med* 78:837, 1973.
192. Sawanoborj M, Suzuki K, Nakagawa Y, et al: Natural killer cell frequency and serum cytokine levels in monoclonal gammopathies: Correlation of bone marrow granular lymphocytes to prognosis. *Acta Haematol* 98:150, 1997.
193. Greipp PR, Kyle RA: Clinical, morphological and cell kinetic differences among multiple myeloma, monoclonal gammopathy of undetermined significance and smoldering myeloma. *Blood* 62:166, 1983.
194. Leo E, Kropff M, Lindemann A, et al: DNA aneuploidy, increased proliferation and nuclear area of plasma cells in monoclonal gammopathy of undetermined significance and multiple myeloma. *Anal Quant Cytol Histol* 17:113, 1995.
195. Pérez-Persona E, Vidriales MB, Mateo G, et al: New criteria to identify risk of progression in monoclonal gammopathy of uncertain significance and smoldering multiple myeloma based on multiparameter flow cytometry analysis of bone marrow plasma cells. *Blood* 110:2586, 2007.
196. Turesson I: Nucleolar size in benign and malignant plasma cell proliferation. *Acta Med Scand* 197:7, 1975.
197. Dehou MF, Schots R, Lacor P, Arras N, et al: Diagnostic and prognostic value of the MB2 monoclonal antibody in paraffin-embedded bone marrow sections of patients with multiple myeloma and monoclonal gammopathy of undetermined significance. *J Clin Pathol* 94:287, 1990.
198. Boccadoro M, Gavarotti P, Fossati G: Low plasma cell 3(H)-thymidine incorporation in MGUS, smoldering myeloma and remission phase myeloma: Reliable identification of patients not requiring therapy. *Br J Haematol* 58:689, 1984.
199. Amiel A, Kirgner I, Gaber E, et al: Replication pattern in cancer: Asynchronous replication in multiple myeloma and in monoclonal gammopathy. *Cancer Genet Cytogenet* 108:32, 1999.
200. Almeida J, Orfao A, Mateo G, et al: Immunophenotype and DNA content characteristics of plasma cells in multiple myeloma and monoclonal gammopathy of undetermined significance. *Pathol Biol* 47:119, 1999.
201. Yasuda N, Kanoh T, Uchino H: J chain synthesis in human myeloma cells: Light and electron microscopic studies. *Clin Exp Immunol* 40:573, 1980.
202. Cassuto JP, Hammore JC, Pastorelli E, et al: Plasma cell acid phosphatase, a discriminative test for benign and malignant monoclonal gammopathies. *Biomedicine* 27:97, 1977.
203. Sonneveld P, Durie BGM, Lokhorst HM, et al: Analysis of multidrug-resistance (MDR-1) glycoprotein and CD56 expression to separate monoclonal gammopathy from multiple myeloma. *Br J Haematol* 83:63, 1993.
204. Zandecki N, Facon T, Bernard F, et al: CD19 and immunophenotype of bone marrow plasma cells in monoclonal gammopathy of undetermined significance. *J Clin Pathol* 48:548, 1995.
205. Ely SA, Knowles DM: Expression of CD56/neural adhesion molecule correlates with the presence of lytic bone lesions in multiple myeloma and distinguishes myeloma from monoclonal gammopathy of undetermined significance and lymphomas with plasmacytoid differentiation. *Am J Pathol* 160:1293, 2002.
206. Sezer O, Heider U, Zavrski I, Possinger K: Differentiation of monoclonal gammopathy of undetermined significance and multiple myeloma using flow cytometric characteristics of plasma cells. *Haematologica* 86:837, 2001.
207. Majumdar G, Heard SE, Singh AK: Use of cytoplasmic 5-prime nucleotidase for differentiating malignant from benign monoclonal gammopathies. *J Clin Pathol* 43:891, 1990.
208. Van de Berg BC, Michaux L, Lecouvet FE, et al: Nonmyelomatous monoclonal gammopathy: Correlation of bone marrow MR images with laboratory findings and spontaneous clinical outcome. *Radiology* 202:249, 1997.
209. Bellaiche L, Laredo J-D, Lioté F, et al: Magnetic resonance appearance of monoclonal gammopathies of unknown significance and multiple myeloma. *Spine* 22:2551, 1997.
210. Laroche M, Attal M, Pouilles JM, et al: Dual-energy x-ray absorption in patients with multiple myeloma and benign gammopathies. *Clin Exp Rheumatol* 14:108, 1996.
211. Bataille R, Chappard D, Basle M: Quantifiable excess of bone resorption in monoclonal gammopathy is an early symptom of malignancy: A prospective study of 87 bone biopsies. *Blood* 87:4762, 1996.
212. Pecherstorfer M, Seibel MJ, Woitge HW, et al: Bone resorption in multiple myeloma and in monoclonal gammopathy of undetermined significance: Quantification by urinary pyridinium cross-links of collagen. *Blood* 90:3743, 1997.
213. Ong F, Kaiser U, Seelen PJ, et al: Serum neural cell adhesion molecule differentiates multiple myeloma from paraproteinemias due to other causes. *Blood* 87:712, 1996.
214. Lacy MQ, Donovan KA, Heimbach JK, et al: Comparison of interleukin-1 beta expression by in situ hybridization in monoclonal gammopathy of undetermined significance and multiple myeloma. *Blood* 93:300, 1999.
215. Greco C, Ameglio F, Alvino S, et al: Selection of patients with monoclonal gammopathy of undetermined significance is mandatory for a reliable use of interleukin-6 and other nonspecific multiple myeloma serum markers. *Acta Haematol* 92:1, 1994.
216. Mathiot C, Mary JY, Tartour E, et al: Soluble CD16 (sCD16), a marker of malignancy in individuals with monoclonal gammopathy of undetermined significance (MGUS). *Br J Haematol* 95:660, 1996.
217. Gaillard JP, Bataille R, Brailly H, et al: Increased and highly stable levels of functional soluble interleukin-6 receptor levels in sera of patients with monoclonal gammopathy. *Eur J Immunol* 23:820, 1993.
218. DuVillard L, Guiguet M, Casasnovas R-O, et al: Diagnostic value of serum IL-6 level in monoclonal gammopathies. *Br J Haematol* 89:243, 1995.
219. Cozzolino F, Torcia M, Aldinucci D, et al: Production of interleukin-1 by bone marrow myeloma cells. *Blood* 74:380, 1989.
220. Donovan KA, Lacy MQ, Kline MP, et al: Contrast in cytokine expression between patients with monoclonal gammopathy of undetermined significance or multiple myeloma. *Leukemia* 12:593, 1998.
221. Diamond T, Levy S, Smith A, et al: Non-invasive markers of bone turnover and plasma cytokines differ in osteoporotic patients with multiple myeloma and monoclonal gammopathies of undetermined significance. *Intern Med* 31:272, 2001.
222. Seidl S, Ackerman J, Kaufmann H, et al: DNA methylation analysis identifies the E-cadherin gene as a potential marker of disease progression in patients with monoclonal gammopathy. *Cancer* 100:2598, 2004.
223. Pasqualetti P, Festucci V, Collacciani A, Casale R: The natural history of monoclonal gammopathy of undetermined significance. *Acta Haematol* 97:174, 1997.
224. Gregersen H, Ibsen JS, Mellemkjaer L, et al: Mortality and causes of death in patients with monoclonal gammopathy of undetermined significance. *Br J Haematol* 112:353, 2001.
225. Kyle RA: A long-term study of the prognosis in monoclonal gammopathy of undetermined significance. *N Engl J Med* 346:564, 2002.
226. Pasqualetti P, Casale R: Risk of malignant transformation in patients with monoclonal gammopathy of undetermined significance. *Biomed Pharmacother* 51:74, 1997.
227. Morra E, Cesana C, Klersy C, et al: Clinical characteristics and factors predicting evolution of asymptomatic IgM monoclonal gammopathies and IgM-related disorders. *Leukemia* 18:1512, 2004.
228. Kyle RA, Therneau TM, Rajkumar SV, et al: Long-term follow-up of IgM monoclonal gammopathy of undetermined significance. *Blood* 102:3759, 2003.
229. Gregersen H, Mellemkjaer L, Ibsen JS, et al: The impact of M-component type and immunoglobulin concentration on risk of malignant transformation in patients with monoclonal gammopathy of undetermined significance. *Haematologica* 86:1172, 2001.
230. Montoto S, Rozman K, Rosinol L, et al: Malignant transformation in IgM monoclonal gammopathy of undetermined significance. *Semin Oncol* 30:178, 2003.
231. Van De Donk N, De Weerdt O, Eureling M, et al: Malignant transformation of monoclonal gammopathy of undetermined significance: Cumulative incidence and prognostic factors. *Leuk Lymphoma* 42:609, 2001.
232. Cesana C, Klersy C, Barbarano L, et al: Prognostic factors for malignant transformation in monoclonal gammopathy of undetermined significance and smoldering multiple myeloma. *J Clin Oncol* 15:1625, 2002.
233. Sackmann F, Pavlovsky MA, Corrado C, et al: Prognostic factors in monoclonal gammopathy of undetermined significance. *Haematologica* 93:153, 2008.
234. Rosiñol L, Cibeira MT, Montoto S, et al: Monoclonal gammopathy of undetermined significance: predictors of malignant transformation and recognition of an evolving type characterized by a progressive increase in M protein size. *Mayo Clin Proc* 82:428, 2007.
235. Zhan F, Barlogie B, Arzoumanian V, et al: Gene-expression signature of benign monoclonal gammopathy evident in multiple myeloma is linked to good prognosis. *Blood* 109:1692, 2007.
236. Kyle RA, Rajkumar SV: Monoclonal gammopathy of undetermined significance and smoldering multiple myeloma. *Hematol Oncol Clin North Am* 21:1093, 2007.
237. Barlogie B, van Rhee F, Shaughnessy JD Jr, et al: Seven year median time to progression with thalidomide for smoldering myeloma: Partial response identifies subset requiring earlier salvage therapy for symptomatic disease. *Blood* 112:3122, 2008.
238. Olteanu H, Wang HY, Chen W, et al: Immunophenotypic studies of monoclonal gammopathy of undetermined significance. *BMC Clin Pathol* 8:13, 2008.

CHAPTER 109
MYELOMA

Frits van Rhee, Elias Anaissie, Edgardo Angtuaco, Twyla Bartel, Joshua Epstein, Bijay Nair, John Shaughnessy, Shmuel Yaccoby, and Bart Barlogie

SUMMARY

Myeloma is a malignancy of terminally differentiated B cells (plasma cells) that produces a complete and/or partial (light chain) monoclonal immunoglobulin protein. Myeloma cells induce, in the context of the extracellular matrix, critical alterations in the marrow microenvironment, which, in turn, evoke cell-survival signals, contributing to resistance to therapy of this genomically complex and generally hypoproliferative tumor. The disease causes clinical symptoms by way of tumor mass effects (e.g., cord compression), cytokine production (e.g., anemia), bone destruction (e.g., pain), protein deposition in visceral organs (e.g., kidney and heart), and immunosuppression (e.g., infection). Clinical manifestations of myeloma vary as a result of the heterogeneous biology, spanning the entire spectrum from indolent to highly aggressive disease with extramedullary features. Magnetic resonance imaging has become an important tool with which to stage the disease and to distinguish solitary plasmacytoma of bone from myeloma and, within the latter category, to document the extent and pattern of marrow involvement, which can be diffuse, micronodular, or macrofocal. Fluorodeoxyglucose positron emission tomography permits functional metabolic imaging of the entire body and, hence, detection of both intramedullary and extramedullary myeloma lesions. Prognosis has been correlated with serum levels of β_2-microglobulin shed from the surface of myeloma cells and C-reactive protein, reflecting endogenous interleukin-6 activity, and with the myeloma cell labeling-index. The molecular analysis of myeloma, using gene expression profiling and other genetic techniques, indicates that myeloma is a heterogeneous disorder comprising at least 7 subentities. Gene expression profiling can identify 15 percent of patients with very aggressive myeloma who have a poor outcome with all current therapies. The immunomodulatory drugs, thalidomide and lenalidomide, and the proteasome inhibitor bortezomib have demonstrated the ability to ameliorate advanced and otherwise refractory disease, by cotargeting both myeloma and stromal cell components, and are now used in combination with melphalan and prednisone as initial therapy. Melphalan-based autologous hematopoietic stem cell transplantation (auto-HSCT) in combination with novel agent can achieve remarkable results in patients with good risk myeloma as defined by favorable gene expression profiles. Such patients can achieve a 10-year survival, exceeding 60 percent of patients. The duration of complete remission in these patients has been sustained, raising the hope that some of these patients are cured.

Acronyms and abbreviations that appear in this chapter include: auto-HSCT, autologous hematopoietic stem cell transplantation; β_2M, β_2-microglobulin; CT, computed tomography; del, deletion; FDG, fluorodeoxyglucose; FISH, fluorescence *in situ* hybridization; GVHD, graft-versus-host disease; GVM, graft-versus-myeloma effect; ISS, International Staging System; LCDD, light-chain deposition disease; MIP, macrophage inflammatory protein; MP, melphalan-prednisone; MRI, magnetic resonance imaging; PET, positron emission tomography; SCID, severe combined immunodeficiency; TGF-β, transforming growth factor-β; VTE, venous thromboembolism.

DEFINITION

Myeloma accounts for approximately 1 percent of all malignancies and 10 percent of hematologic tumors, representing the second most frequently occurring hematologic malignancy in the United States.[1] At any one time, 50,000 people suffer from myeloma, and approximately 15,000 cases are diagnosed each year. The median age at onset is approximately 65 years, although occasionally myeloma occurs as early as the second decade of life. Myeloma is a disease of neoplastic plasma cells that synthesize abnormal amounts of immunoglobulin or immunoglobulin fragments. Clinical manifestations are heterogeneous and include the formation of tumors, monoclonal immunoglobulin production, decreased immunoglobulin secretion by normal plasma cells leading to hypogammaglobulinemia, impaired hematopoiesis resulting in anemia and other cytopenias, osteolytic bone disease, hypercalcemia, and renal dysfunction. Symptoms are caused by tumor mass effects, cytokines released by the myeloma cells or indirectly by marrow stroma and bone cells in response to adhesion of tumor cells, and by the myeloma protein leading to deposition diseases (AL amyloidosis and light-chain deposition disease [LCDD]).

Myeloma belongs to a spectrum of disorders referred to as plasma cell dyscrasias. These include clinically benign conditions, such as essential monoclonal gammopathy and smoldering myeloma (see Chap. 108); rare and biologically intriguing disorders, such as Castleman disease and α-heavy-chain disease (see Chap. 112); macroglobulinemia (see Chap. 111); solitary plasmacytoma with a high potential for cure when arising in soft tissue; and myeloma, a disseminated B-cell malignancy not curable with conventional-dose chemotherapy. All disorders share plasma cell morphologic features, and most are associated with the production of immunoglobulin molecules (see Chap. 77). Although most plasma cell dyscrasias result from the expansion of a single clone of cells, with resultant monoclonal protein secretion, oligoclonal and polyclonal protein abnormalities accompany some conditions, such as Castleman disease or angioimmunoblastic lymphoproliferative disease, now recognized as a T-cell lymphoma (see Chaps. 105 and 106).

ETIOLOGY AND PATHOGENESIS

GENETIC PREDISPOSITION

The etiology of human myeloma is unknown.[2] There have been several reports of families with an increased incidence of myeloma.[3–6] One study found a two- to threefold increased risk of developing essential monoclonal gammopathy or myeloma in first-degree relatives from patients with monoclonal gammopathy or myeloma, implying shared environmental exposures and/or genetic predispositions.[7] Detailed analysis of kinships with myeloma may discover cancer susceptibility loci. In one family, heterozygosity of the *p16* gene seemed to predispose to melanoma, myeloma, and pancreatic cancer.[8] The notion of familial predisposition is supported by racial differences in both essential monoclonal gammopathy and myeloma, with the highest rates reported in blacks, both in the United States and in Africa, with intermediate rates in persons of European descent, and lower rates in persons of Japanese and Spanish (Latino) descent.[9–13] The rate of progression of monoclonal gammopathy to myeloma is 1 percent per year and does not increase over time, which is consistent with a multihit genetic model with essential monoclonal gammopathy as a primary event and myeloma as secondary event.

ENVIRONMENTAL EXPOSURE

Environmental exposure to radiation and chemicals has been associated with an increased incidence of myeloma, although the relationship with chemical exposures has not reached the level of scientific and medical certainty.[14] Studies of atomic bomb survivors showed an increased incidence of myeloma 15 to 20 years after radiation exposure,[15] as well an increased risk of developing monoclonal gammopathy in individuals exposed to more than 0.1 Gy[16] in Nagasaki. Epidemiological studies examining the associations between myeloma and autoimmune diseases or infections are of interest.[17] A retrospective study of more than 4 million American male veterans of military service of European and African descent found elevated risks of developing essential monoclonal gammopathy or myeloma in patients suffering from autoimmune or inflammatory disorders, suggesting that immune-mediated mechanism may play a role in triggering plasma cell dyscrasias.[18] Human herpes virus 8, also called Kaposi sarcoma-associated herpes virus, is involved in the pathogenesis of pleural cavity lymphoma,[19] Kaposi sarcoma,[20] and Castleman disease,[21] and has been identified by some investigators in marrow dendritic cells of myeloma patients.[22–25] These findings, however, have not been confirmed by others.[26–28] The myeloma microenvironment plays an important role in the progression of monoclonal gammopathy to myeloma. For example, patients with high levels of the WNT-signaling inhibitor DKK1 are more likely to progress to myeloma, whereas patients with an immune response to the stem cell antigen SOX2 have a reduced risk.[29]

Hyperdiploid myeloma typically has multiple trisomies of odd-numbered chromosomes 3, 5, 7, 9, 11, 15, 19, and 21, whereas non-hyperdiploid myeloma is associated with immunoglobulin heavy chain (IgH) gene translocations located at chromosome 14q32.[49–51] Interphase fluorescence *in situ* hybridization (FISH)[52,53] and other molecular genetic studies have identified five primary recurrent chromosomal rearrangements involving the *IgH* gene (14q32):[33] (1) 11q13, *cyclin D1*[54–62]; (2) 4p16.3, fibroblast growth factor *FGF-R3*, and *MMSET*[63–68]; (3) 6p21, *cyclin D3*[69]; (4) 16q23, *c-MAF*[70]; and (5) 20q11, *MAF-B*,[71] which account for almost 40 percent of all genetic abnormalities seen in myeloma and are more common in patients without hyperdiploid karyotypes.[72] The juxtaposition of immunoglobulin enhancer elements explains the high constitutive expression of resident oncogenes. These translocations result from errors in IgH switch recombination during B-cell development in germinal centers and have been detected even at the monoclonal gammopathy stage, together with RB1 deletions.[73–77] Hyperdiploidy accounts for the remaining 60 percent of myeloma. Alterations in gene copy number detectable by FISH and comparative genomic hybridization are important for disease progression and prognosis. Such alterations include gain of chromosome 1q, loss of chromosome 1p, deletion 13p and deletion 17p. Gain of the gene *AGO2*,

PATHOGENESIS

■ GENETIC ALTERATION

Most if not all cases of symptomatic myeloma evolve from a benign precursor condition, essential monoclonal gammopathy, also referred to as monoclonal gammopathy of undetermined significance,[30] which is a monoclonal disorder (neoplasm) that can undergo clonal evolution to a progressive disease at the rate of approximately 1 percent of cases per year. It may progress to lymphoma, amyloidosis, or myeloma, often in the latter case through an indolent or smoldering stage. A study of 30 patients transplanted at Walter Reed Army Medical Center found that 27 patients (90%) had prior essential monoclonal gammopathy detectable in samples previously obtained during mandatory blood tests for active medical personnel.[31]

The presence of somatic hypermutations in the immunoglobulin variable region genes of plasma cells of subjects with both monoclonal gammopathy and myeloma strongly suggests that malignant transformation has occurred in a more mature B cell that had traversed the germinal centers of lymph nodes (Fig. 109–1).[32–36] Subsequently, myeloma cells home to, survive in, and expand exclusively within the marrow, until late stages of the disease when extramedullary growth can ensue, at which point it is possible to establish long-term human myeloma cell lines.[37,38] The presence of clonotypic cells in the blood even at diagnosis underscores the importance of hematogenous spread as a means of disease dissemination.[39–48]

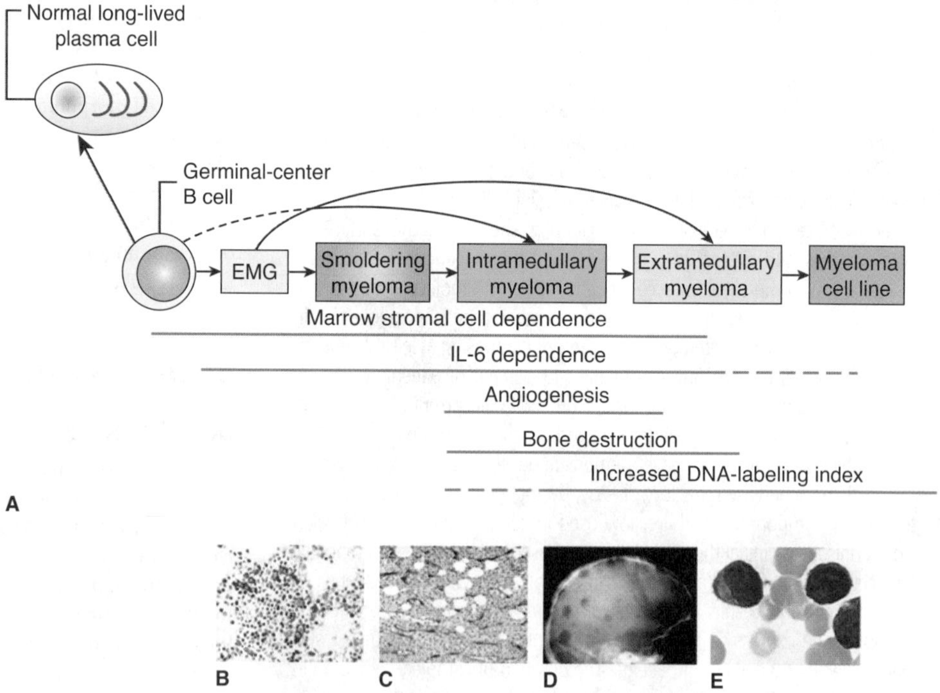

FIGURE 109–1. Stages of myeloma. **A.** Myeloma arises from a normal germinal-center B cell. At least 30 to 50 percent of myeloma cases arise from the benign plasma-cell neoplasm essential monoclonal gammopathy (EMG). It does not always pass through a period of smoldering myeloma. Initially, myeloma is confined to the marrow (intramedullary), but with time the tumor can acquire the ability to grow in extramedullary locations (such as blood, pleural fluid, and skin). Some of these extramedullary myelomas can establish immortalized cell lines *in vitro*. The transition of essential monoclonal gammopathy to intramedullary myeloma is manifest by increased numbers of myeloma cells at multiple foci, and also associated angiogenesis and osteolytic bone destruction. **B.** The low proliferative index in a patient with essential monoclonal gammopathy. Bright red surface staining for syndecan identifies the plasma cells (10%), none of which stain for the brown nuclear proliferation marker Ki67. **C.** A marrow biopsy stained for CD34, identifying the endothelial cells, and emphasizing the increased vascularity in myeloma. **D.** A skull radiograph shows the classic "punched-out" lytic bone lesions. Although the skull lesions are asymptomatic, extensive vertebral involvement causes compression fractures, resulting in pain and loss of height (5 cm on average by the time of diagnosis). **E.** A blood film contains circulating plasma cells in a patient with plasma cell leukemia. *(Reproduced with permission from Kuehl WM, Bergsagel PL: Multiple myeloma: Evolving genetic events and host interactions.* Nat Rev Cancer *2:175, 2002.)*

important in microRNA regulation and expression, located at 8q24 is related to a poor prognosis and suggests that that microRNA activity is important in regulation of myeloma cell growth. Mutational activation of the *NRAS* or *KRAS* oncogenes[78–87] and inactivation of *CDKN2A, CDKN2C, CDKN1B,* and/or *PTEN* tumor-suppressor genes are related to disease progression. Late events involve inactivation of *TP53*[88–95] and secondary translocations of *c-MYC*.[32,78,96–99]

Although universally aneuploid according to DNA flow cytometry[100] and interphase FISH analyses,[52] the hypoproliferative nature of myeloma[101] and its stromal dependence[102] account for the high frequency (65–70%) of normal diploid metaphase karyotypes (originating in normal hematopoietic cells) observed in untreated patients.[103–106] The remaining one-third of untreated myeloma patients often have complex cytogenetic abnormalities involving multiple chromosomes. Although initially thought to represent a major technical shortcoming of standard cytogenetics, the *in vitro* mitotic capacity in the absence of surrounding marrow habitat defines a myeloma entity that is stroma-independent, referred to as "malignant myeloma" with a poor prognosis.[107]

A major breakthrough in our understanding of myeloma has been brought about by gene expression profiling of CD138-positive, purified myeloma cells. At least 7 distinct subgroups can be identified by analyzing purified myeloma cells, using training sets and test sets of patients enrolled on the Total Therapy 2 and Total Therapy 3 protocols (Fig. 109–2).[108] Four groups were characterized by translocations involving the IgH locus and protooncogenes. Translocations t(14;16)(q32;23) and t(14;20)(q32;11) resulted in overexpression of the *MAF* and *MAFB* oncogenes, respectively, occurring in approximately 6 percent of myeloma cases. Dysregulation of MAF and MAFB resulted in alteration of similar downstream signaling pathways explaining the designation of a single MAF/MAFB signaling subgroup. The *DKK1* gene, strongly implicated in the pathogenesis of myeloma bone lesions, is underexpressed in MAF/MAFB myeloma, which has a low incidence of myelomatous focal bone lesions. The t(4;14)(p16;q32) produces the overexpression of the *FGFR3* and *MMSET* genes. The product of the *MMSET* gene plays a critical role in regulating downstream transcriptional events since 25 percent of cases are FGFR3 negative. The MMSET positive subgroup of patients particularly benefits from proteasome inhibition by bortezomib. The t(11;14)(q13;q32) and t(6;14)(p21;q32) activate cyclin D_1 and cyclin D_3 (CD-1 and CD-2 subgroups) in 17 and 2 percent of myeloma patients, respectively. The CD-2 subgroup is characterized by overexpression of CD20, the early B-cell marker VPREB, and the B-cell transcription factor PAX-5. CD-2 myeloma often exhibits a lymphoplasmacytoid morphology and the plasma cells stain for CD20 by flow cytometry or immunohistochemistry. The CD-1 subgroup lacks this morphology. The CD-1 subgroup achieves remission more rapidly, but has an increased frequency of early relapse; nevertheless, because their tumor cells remain sensitive to cytotoxic agents, excellent long-term survivals occur. The hyperdiploidy group defined by gene-expression profiling has karyotypic abnormalities comprising trisomies of odd-numbered chromosomes. Overexpressed genes include the Wnt signaling antagonists *FRZB* and *DKK1* explaining the increased frequency of osteolytic bone disease in this group. Other overexpressed genes include the macrophage inflammatory protein (MIP)-1α chemokine receptor, *NCAM1, TNFSF10,* and several interferon-induced genes. Underexpressed are the campath-1 antigen, CD52, and genes located on chromosome 1, such as the cell-cycle regulator *CKS1B*, which is implicated in poor survival. The group with low bone disease is typified by a paucity of magnetic resonance imaging (MRI)-defined focal bone lesions. Consistent with this is the low expression of FRZB and DKK1. This group has high expression of the interleukin (IL)-6-receptor gene, *CCDN2,* and *CST6.* The proliferative group overexpressed cell-cycle and proliferation-associated genes, and cancer-testes antigens. Other high-risk features of the group include a high proliferation index similar to that of myeloma cell lines and the presence of a very high percentage (~70–85%) of cytogenetic abnormalities. In general terms, the groups with MAF/MAFB and MMSET expression have more aggressive disease because they have a larger proportion of patients with high-risk disease as defined by gene-expression profiling.

CYTOKINES AND CHEMOKINES

Milestones in myeloma biologic research are linked to the discovery of IL-6 as a myeloma growth and survival factor[109–114] and to the recognition of stromal cell dependence of myeloma cells.[35,102,115] A clearer picture is now emerging, where an intense cell-adhesion-mediated crosstalk exists between myeloma cells (endowed with receptors for many growth-promoting cytokines and chemokines, especially IL-6,[116] IL-15,[117,118] insulin-like growth factor-1,[119] and hepatocyte growth factor[120] in various host cell compartments.[121–123] A hallmark of the plasma cell stage of B-cell maturation, CD138 (syndecan-1)[124–127] is shed and often deposited abundantly in the extracellular matrix, trapping growth-promoting and proangiogenic cytokines, and thus contributing to myeloma progression and invasion. Indeed, the poor prognostic implications of soluble syndecan-1 levels are a

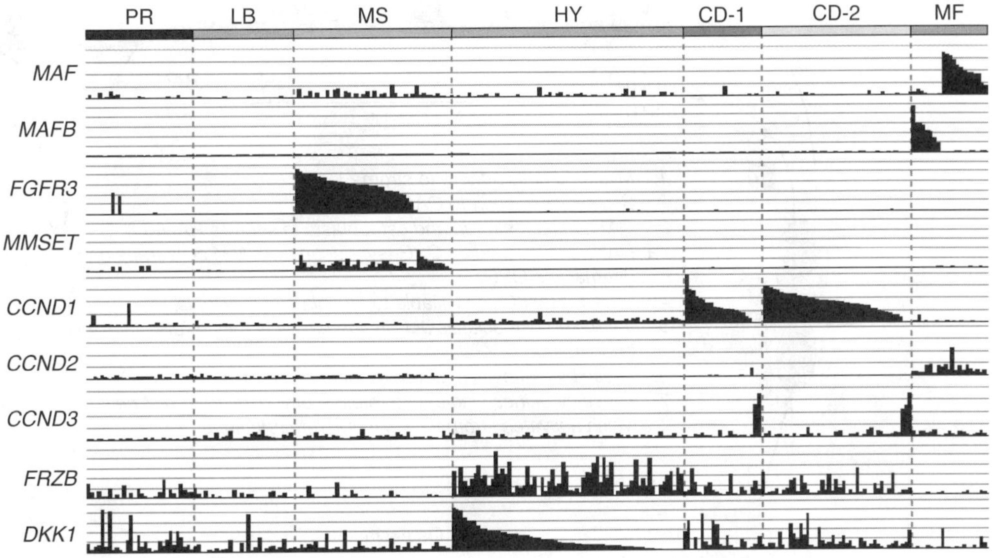

FIGURE 109–2. Myeloma subgroups are typified by unique gene expression profiles. Affymetrix signals (expression level: vertical axis) of the *MAF, MAFB, FGFR3, MMSET, CCND1, CCDN2, CCDN3, FRZB,* and *DDK1* genes are derived from purified plasma cells from 256 newly diagnosed myeloma patients. The gene expression levels are proportional to the height of each bar, representing a single patient sample. Seven subgroups are indicated (PR, proliferation; LB, low bone disease; MS, MMSET; HY, hyperdiploidy; MF, c-MAF and MAFB). Spiked expression of *CCND1, MAF* and *MAFB, FGFR3,* and *MMSET* are strongly associated with specific subgroup designations. *FRZB* and *DKK1* are significantly underexpressed in the LB and MF subgroups.

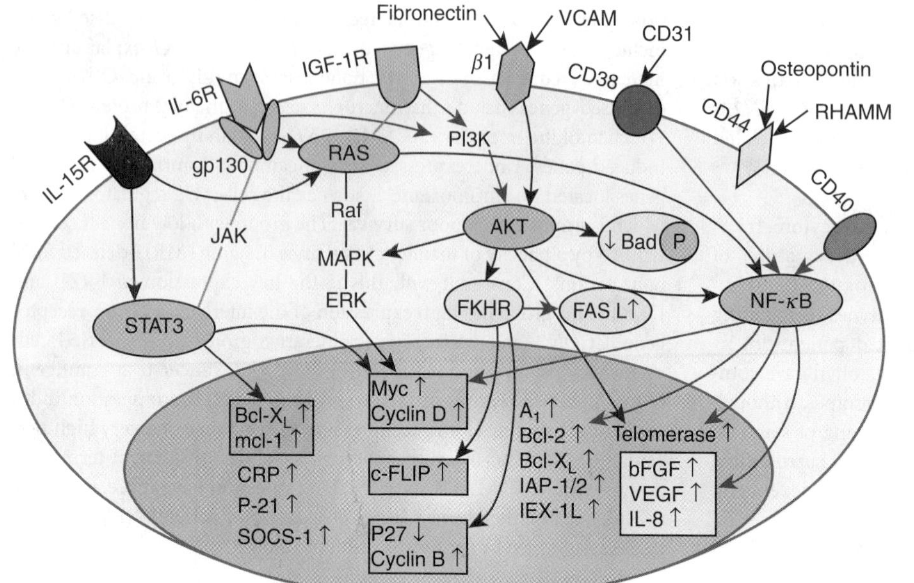

FIGURE 109–3. The microenvironment provides factors engaging receptors present on myeloma cells, which promote their survival and proliferation. bFGF, basic fibroblast growth factor; CRP, C-reactive protein; ERK, extracellular response kinase; gp130, glycoprotein 130; IAP, inhibitors of apoptosis; IEX, immediate early response gene X-1; IGF, insulin-like growth factor; IL, interleukin; JAK, Janus kinase; MAPK, mitogen activated protein kinase; NF-κB, nuclear factor-κB; PI3K, phosphatidylinositol 3′-kinase; RHAMM, receptor for hyaluronan-mediated motility; SOCS-1, suppressor of cytokine synthesis 1; VCAM, vascular cell adhesion molecule; VEGF, vascular endothelial growth factor.

reflection of these relationships.[128–131] Heparanase enhances shedding of syndecan-1 and promotes dissemination of myeloma cells to bone.[132,133]

Homing of cells to the marrow is mediated via several chemokine receptors expressed by myeloma cells—CXCR4, CXCR3, CCR1, CCR2, and CCR5—with receptor expression profiles differing between medullary and extramedullary disease.[134,135]

Growth and survival signals are mediated via phosphatidylinositol 3′-kinase (PI3K)/AKT, signal transducer and activator of transcription (STAT) 3, renin–angiotensin system (RAS)/mitogen-activated protein kinase (MAPK), and nuclear factor-κB (NF-κB)[136–142] pathways (Fig. 109–3). Thus, the interaction of myeloma cell with the marrow microenvironment holds important clues to understanding disease progression and drug resistance and opens new avenues for therapeutic interventions.[143]

BONE METABOLISM

Osteolytic bone lesions are a hallmark of advanced myeloma, eventually developing in 70 to 80 percent of patients and resulting from an imbalance of osteoclast and osteoblast number and function.[144] The underlying mechanisms include osteoclast activation through the receptor activation of NF-κB ligand (RANKL)[145] and the MIP-1α/β chemokine and the IL-3 pathways.[146] Expression of RANKL by stromal cells is drastically increased upon contact with myeloma cells, while its decoy receptor, osteoprotegerin (OPG), is suppressed and additionally inactivated by syndecan-mediated internalization into myeloma cells (Fig. 109–4).[147,148] MIP-1α, originating in myeloma cells,[149,150] directly facilitates maturation of precursor cells into osteoclasts, which are further activated by

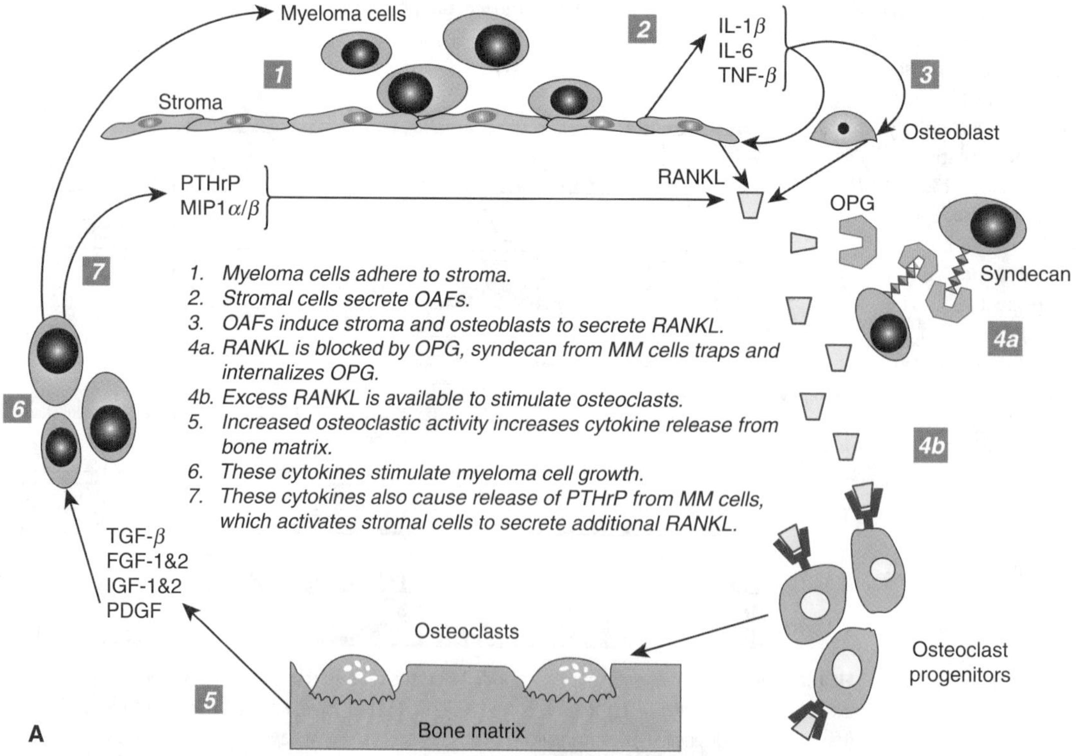

FIGURE 109–4. The mechanism of bone destruction in myeloma. **A.** Bone destruction is caused by activation of osteoclasts but also by blocking of differentiation of mesenchymal precursor cells to mature osteoblasts resulting in increased bone destruction and decreased bone formation. *(Modified with permission from Tricot G: New insights into role of microenvironment in multiple myeloma.* Lancet 355:248, 2000).

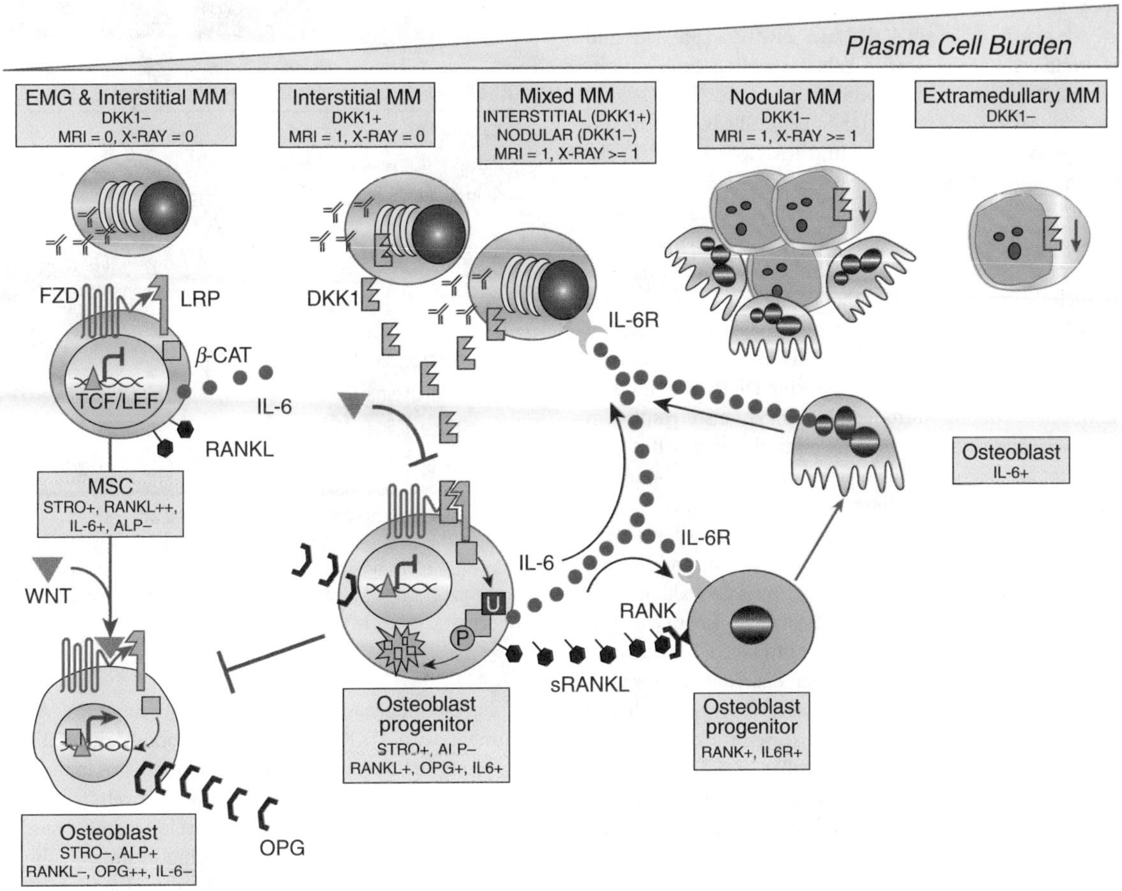

B

FIGURE 109–4. (*continued*) New insights into role of microenvironment in multiple myeloma. **B.** A model integrating the temporal variation in DKK1 expression in the natural history of a subtype of myeloma that interacts closely with cells of the bone microenvironment. During the earliest stages of myeloma (disease progression is depicted from left to right) myeloma plasma cells (cells with blue nucleus and purple cytoplasm) grow in a diffuse-interstitial pattern and do not exhibit MRI- or radiography-defined bone lesions. Myeloma plasma cells at this stage do not express DKK1. Mesenchymal stem cells also termed marrow stromal cells (MSCs), characterized as STRO-1-positive, IL-6-positive, receptor activator of NF-κB ligand (RANKL)-positive, and alkaline phosphatase (ALP)-negative, express the Wnt receptors FZD and LRP5 and respond to Wnt signal by stabilizing cytoplasmic β-catenin, which, in turn, translocates to the nucleus where it interacts with latent TCF/LEF transcription factors to induce target genes resulting in differentiation of MSCs into mature bone-mineralizing osteoblasts, characterized as ALP-positive, osteoprotegerin (OPG)-positive, STRO-1-negative, RANKL-negative, and IL-6-negative. During disease progression, myeloma plasma cells begin synthesizing DKK1. The mechanism by which DKK1 is activated is unknown. Myeloma-derived DKK1, a potent inhibitor of Wnt signaling, binds to the LRP coreceptor on MSCs blocking Wnt signaling, which results in the phosphorylation of β-catenin by GSK3B followed by ubiquination and degradation by the proteasome. The antagonism of Wnt signaling blocks the terminal differentiation of MSCs into osteoblasts. Gregory and colleagues have shown that DKK1 is produced by MSCs and that this induces these cells to reenter the cell cycle (*Gregory C, Singh H, Perry AS, et al: The Wnt signaling inhibitor Dickkopf-1 is required for reentry into the cell of human adult stem cells form bone marrow.* J Bio Chem *278:28067, 2003*). Thus it is possible that the DKK1 made by myeloma plasma cells blocks differentiation and induces proliferation of MSCs. Myeloma plasma cells signal through Wnt and it causes their proliferation (*Qiang Y, Endo Y, Rubin JS, et al: Wnt signaling in B-cell neoplasia.* Oncogene *22:1536, 2003, Derksen P, Tjin E, Meijer HP, et al: Illegitimate ENT signaling promotes proliferation of multiple myeloma cells. PNAS 101:6122, 2004*). It is not clear if the DKK1 may also down regulate Wnt signaling in plasma cells and if this influences myeloma cell proliferation. The osteoblast progenitor cells, but not mature osteoblasts, are a rich source of RANKL (*Atkins GJ, Kostakis P, Pan B, et al: RANKL expression is related to the differentiation state of human osteoblasts.* J Bone Miner Res *18:1088, 2003*), suggesting that the DKK1-mediated block of osteoblast differentiation may also significantly contribute to elevated RANKL in the marrow of myeloma patients. At this stage, plasma cells have an interstitial or mixed interstitial and nodular growth pattern with MRI-defined focal lesions. Although DKK1 expression can be detected in plasma cells that grow interstitially, expression is dramatically reduced or undetectable by immunohistochemistry in cells within focal lesions. During progression, myeloma plasma cells shift from a predominantly interstitial growth pattern (DKK1-positive) to a nodular pattern where large sheets of plasma cells (DKK1-negative) form foci and exhibit aggressive morphologic characteristics (high nuclear-to-cytoplasmic ratio and prominent nucleoli). Downregulation of DKK1 expression accompanies this shift from interstitial to nodular growth. The continued and chronic exposure of the marrow to elevated DKK1 results in overproduction of RANKL and IL-6 by immature osteoblasts and MSCs, and results in the differentiation of osteoclast progenitors into mature bone-resorbing osteoclasts that also produce IL-6. The loss of mature osteoblasts and increase in osteoclasts leads to radiography-detectable lytic bone lesions found exclusively adjacent to nodular plasmacytomas. The downregulation of DKK1 in plasma cells within these nodules is likely a result of direct contact with osteoclasts (*Yaccoby S, Wezeman M, Henderson A, Barlogie B, Epstein J: Role and fate of osteoblasts in myeloma. The 9th International Myeloma Workshop. Salamanca, Spain, May 2003. Abstract #149*). The molecular means by which osteoclasts extinguish the expression of DKK1 in myeloma plasma cells is currently not known. As disease progresses, interstitial growth gives way to a largely nodular growth pattern, and in the terminal stages of disease, plasma cell growth is highly proliferative and can become extramedullary. Plasma cells derived from virtually all extramedullary stages of myeloma are DKK1-negative. EMG, essential monoclonal gammopathy; FGF, fibroblast growth factor; IGF, insulin-like growth factor; IL, interleukin; OAF, osteoclast-activating factors; OPG, osteoprotegerin; PDGF, platelet-derived growth factor; PTHrP, parathyroid hormone-related protein; TGF, transforming growth factor; TNF, tumor necrosis factor.

MIP-1α–induced RANKL expression by stromal cells, resulting in increased bone resorption.[151,152] DKK1 and FRZB, expressed and secreted by myeloma cells, interfere with WNT signaling, thus inhibiting osteoblast maturation and enhance bone destruction.[153]

Some of these pathways can be targeted therapeutically by administration of decoy receptors for RANKL (OPG and RANK-Fc).[147,154] In the severe combined immunodeficiency-human (SCID-hu) model system, administration of these molecules is associated with prevention of osteolytic bone disease and myeloma growth inhibition.[147] A new paradigm has thus emerged of a strong interdependence between myeloma cells and osteoclasts, such that myeloma cells enhance the formation of osteoclasts whose activity, in turn, is essential for the survival and growth of myeloma cells. Increasing the number of osteoblasts in this model via injection of marrow mesenchymal cells, by blocking DKK1 activity with neutralizing antibodies, or by introducing Wnt3a, also results in increased bone mineral density and inhibition of myeloma growth.[155–158] RANKL and OPG not only have been associated with myeloma bone disease, but also with clinical outcome,[159] attesting to the close interrelation between myeloma progression and components of the marrow microenvironment, especially hematopoietic cell-derived osteoclasts and mesenchymal cell-derived osteoblasts.[160] These bone markers, along with serum levels of tartrate-resistant acid phosphatase isoenzyme 5b (TRACP-5b), a novel resorption marker only produced by activated osteoclasts,[161] and elevated levels of bone collagen degradation products, including the N-terminal crosslinking telopeptide of type I collagen (NTX), can predict early progression of bone disease in myeloma.[162,163] Bone alkaline phosphatase (bALP) and osteocalcin (OC), markers of bone formation, are suppressed in myeloma patients. The s-RANKL/OPG ratio is highly correlated with serum levels of TRACP-5b, IL-6, and β_2-microglobulin (β_2M) and urinary excretion of NTX.[159]

ANIMAL MODELS

The two main animal models that have been extensively exploited to study human myeloma biology and therapy are the SCID-hu/SCID-rabbit(rab) mouse systems[164,165] and the 5T murine myeloma model.[166] Human myeloma cell-lines, engrafted in SCID and nonobese diabetic (NOD)/SCID mice, are principally used to explore homing and novel drugs.[167] Murine genetic models have been developed and are valuable in understanding myeloma development and progression.[168,169]

The SCID-hu or the SCID-rab mice models provide microenvironmental support for growth and expansion of human primary myeloma cells. Primary myeloma cells grown in human fetal bone (the SCID-hu model) or rabbit bone (SCID-rab model) implanted in SCID mice manifest and produce typical disease manifestations including increase circulating monoclonal immunoglobulins, induction of osteolytic bone resorption, suppression of bone formation in bone areas adjacent to tumor foci, and stimulation of angiogenesis. Primary myeloma cells grow restrictively in the implanted bones, while myeloma cells from patients with extramedullary disease grow also on the outer surface of the implanted bone in SCID-hu or SCID-rab mice.

The SCID-hu/SCID-rab animal models are being exploited to study important biologic issues in the myeloma pathophysiology and development of novel targeted therapies: (1) mature myeloma cells with a CD138+CD45– or CD138+ phenotype retain self-renewal and transplantation potential[161,165]; (2) blocking activity of the common osteoclastogenic factor, RANKL, reveals that marrow-derived, but not extramedullary, myeloma cell growth is dependent upon osteoclast activity and the marrow microenvironment[170]; (3) myeloma growth and the development of bone destruction are critically linked; (4) therapeutic agents (e.g., bisphosphonates, thalidomide, bortezomib) target components of the marrow microenvironment, such as osteoclasts, osteoblasts, and endothelial cells, and can control the growth of myeloma cells[170–172]; (5) pharmacologic approaches to promote canonical Wnt signaling (e.g., treatment with DKK1-neutralizing antibody or Wnt3a) prevent bone loss, promote bone formation, and suppress myeloma growth, underlining the critical role of Wnt signaling in myeloma pathogenesis[155,158]; (6) targeted therapy against specific myeloma growth and survival factors such as APRIL (a proliferation-inducing ligand),[173] fibroblast activation protein (FAP),[174] and syndecan-1[175] reduced growth of certain primary myeloma cells in the SCID-hu model.

Some of these findings were observed in the 5T murine myeloma model,[176–178] where myeloma growth was associated with angiogenesis and depended on osteoclasts.[179–182] In many of the studies in the SCID-hu and SCID-rab mice, treatment response varied between human samples, reflecting the differences in the disease among patients, and emphasizing the importance of these animal models for studying crucial biologic questions and development of novel interventions for myeloma.

TABLE 109–1. Criteria for Diagnosis of Myeloma*

Major criteria
Plasmacytomas on tissue biopsy
Marrow plasmacytosis with >30% plasma cells
Monoclonal globulin spike on serum electrophoresis >3.5 g/dL for immunoglobulin (Ig) G or >2.0 g/dL for IgA; 1.0 g/24 h of κ or λ light-chain excretion on urine electrophoresis in the absence of amyloidosis
Minor criteria
Marrow plasmacytosis 10–30%
Monoclonal globulin spike present, but less than the levels defined above
Lytic bone lesions
Normal IgM <0.05 g/dL, IgA <0.1 g/dL, or IgG <0.6 g/dL

*The diagnosis of plasma cell myeloma is confirmed when at least one major and one minor criterion or at least *three minor criteria* are documented in *symptomatic* patients with *progressive* disease. The presence of features not specific for the disease, such as the following, supports the diagnosis, particularly if of recent onset: anemia, hypercalcemia, azotemia, bone demineralization, or hypoalbuminemia.

CLINICAL AND LABORATORY FEATURES

Table 109–1 summarizes the commonly accepted diagnostic criteria for myeloma. The International Myeloma Working Group has issued simplified criteria for the classification of myeloma and related disorders.[183–185] For the diagnosis of symptomatic myeloma, neither a minimum serum or urine M-protein level nor a minimal clonal marrow plasmacytosis level was included (Table 109–2). The most critical

TABLE 109–2. Simplified Criteria for the Classification of Myeloma*

M-protein in serum and/or urine
Marrow (clonal) plasma cells* or plasmacytoma
Related organ or tissue impairment (ROTI), end-organ damage, including bone lesions

*If flow cytometry is performed, most plasma cells (>90%) will show a "neoplastic" phenotype.

NOTE: Some patients may have no symptoms but have related organ or tissue impairment.[185]

TABLE 109–3. Diagnostic Criteria for Myeloma Requiring Therapy

Presence of an monoclonal immunoglobulin* in serum and/or urine plus clonal plasma cells in the marrow and /or a documented clonal plasmacytoma
PLUS one or more of the following:†
Calcium elevation (>11.5 mg/dL) [>2.65 mmol/L]
Renal insufficiency (creatinine >2 mg/dL) [177 μmol/L or more]
Anemia (hemoglobin <10 g/dL or 2 g/dL <normal) (hemoglobin <12.5 mmol/L‡ or 1.25mmol/L <normal)
Bone disease (lytic lesions or osteopenia)

*In patients with no detectable monoclonal immunoglobulin, an abnormal serum free-light chain (FLC) ratio on the serum FLC assay can substitute and satisfy this criterion. For patients, with no serum or urine monoclonal immunoglobulin and normal serum FLC ratio, the baseline marrow must have >10% clonal plasma cells; these patients are referred to as having "nonsecretory myeloma." Patients with biopsy-proven amyloidosis and/or systemic light-chain deposition disease (LCDD) should be classified as "myeloma with documented amyloidosis" or "myeloma with documented LCDD," respectively, if they have >30% plasma cells and/or myeloma-related bone disease.

†Must be attributable to the underlying plasma cell disorder.

‡Hemoglobin of 10 g/dL is 12.5 mmol/L [or 100 g/L].[482]

TABLE 109–4. Symptomatic Myeloma

Symptoms and Laboratory Features	Frequency (%)
Bone pain (spine, chest, less common in long bones)	65
Weakness and fatigue	50
Anemia	65
Renal Insufficiency	20
Hypercalcemia	20
Serum monoclonal immunoglobulin (Ig) peak on standard electrophoresis	80
Monoclonal Ig peak on immunofixation of serum or urine	97
Monoclonal IgG	50
Monoclonal IgA	20
Monoclonal light chains only	20
Urinary monoclonal light chains	75
Marrow plasmacytosis >10%	90

criterion of symptomatic disease and, hence, initiation of therapy, is evidence of organ or tissue impairment (end-organ damage) manifested by anemia, hypercalcemia, lytic bone lesions, renal insufficiency, hyperviscosity, amyloidosis, or recurrent infections, referred to as "CRAB" for hyper*c*alcemia, *r*enal failure, *a*nemia, and *b*one lesions (Table 109–3; Fig. 109–5). These signs and symptoms generally result from myeloma cell mass effects or from the proteins or cytokines secreted by myeloma cells or normal accessory cells under the influence of tumor cell products (Table 109–4; Fig. 109–5).

HEMATOLOGIC ABNORMALITIES

The most prominent and diagnostically important finding is a plasmacytosis in the marrow. The appearance of the neoplastic plasma (myeloma) cells by light microscopy may be quite varied. The plasma cells may be indistinguishable from normal by light microscopy on the one hand or may be very abnormal on the other with some combination of giant size, large nucleoli, a high frequency of binucleate or multinucleate cells, inclusion globules of crystallized immunoglobulin, Russell bodies, or other inclusions (see Fig. 109–6). The extent of the plasma cell infiltrate may range from just above the normal upper limit of 8 to 10 percent of marrow cells to a virtual complete replacement of marrow with myeloma cells (see Fig. 109–6). Occasionally, the biopsy specimen may contain a normal proportion of plasma cells but a subsequent biopsy may show an increased proportion. Anemia of variable severity affects more than two-thirds of patients with myeloma.

Myelomatous involvement of the marrow typically causes anemia, the degree of which appears related to tumor mass and degree of marrow infiltration by myeloma cells. Overexpression of FAS-ligand, MIP-1α, and tumor necrosis factor-related apoptosis-inducing ligand by the myeloma cells triggers death signals in immature erythroblasts.[186] Most patients have an inappropriate erythropoietin response for the level of their anemia, which is further accentuated in the presence of renal failure.[187] This blunted erythropoietin response may result from the production of cytokines, such as IL-1 and tumor necrosis factor-β,[188] or to increased serum viscosity levels.[189] Overproduction of IL-6 by marrow stroma, normal accessory cells, and/or myeloma cells may contribute to the anemia by upregulating hepatic production of hepcidin, which blocks release of iron from macrophages and inhibits iron absorption from the intestine.[190]

Thrombocytopenia is uncommon in early phases of myeloma, even with extensive marrow myeloma cell replacement,[191] possibly because of the thrombopoietic activity of IL-6.[192] However, thrombocytopenia may develop subsequent to therapy or from autoimmune mechanisms (such as those accounting for anemia or factor VIII deficiency[193–195]). Concomitant myelodysplastic syndrome should be considered in patients who have had prolonged exposure to alkylating agents.

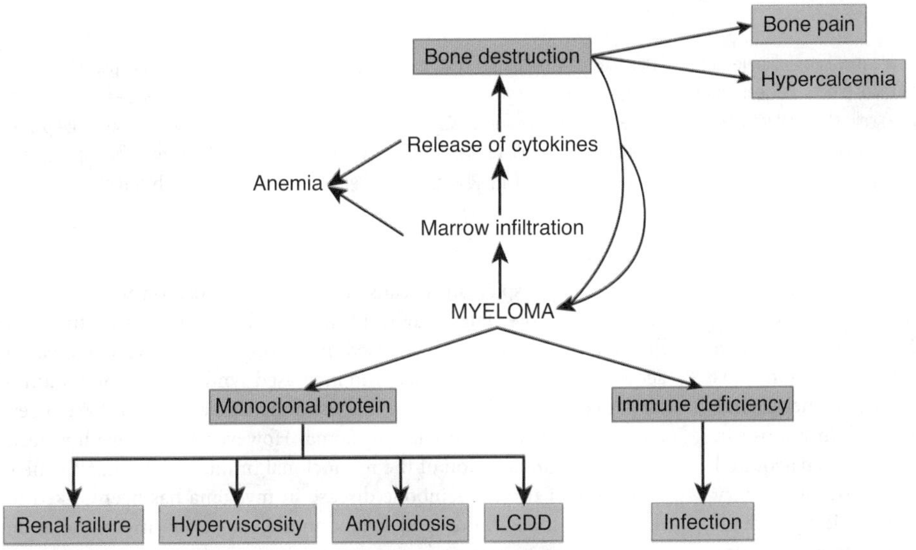

FIGURE 109–5. Disease manifestations in myeloma. LCDD, light-chain deposition disease.

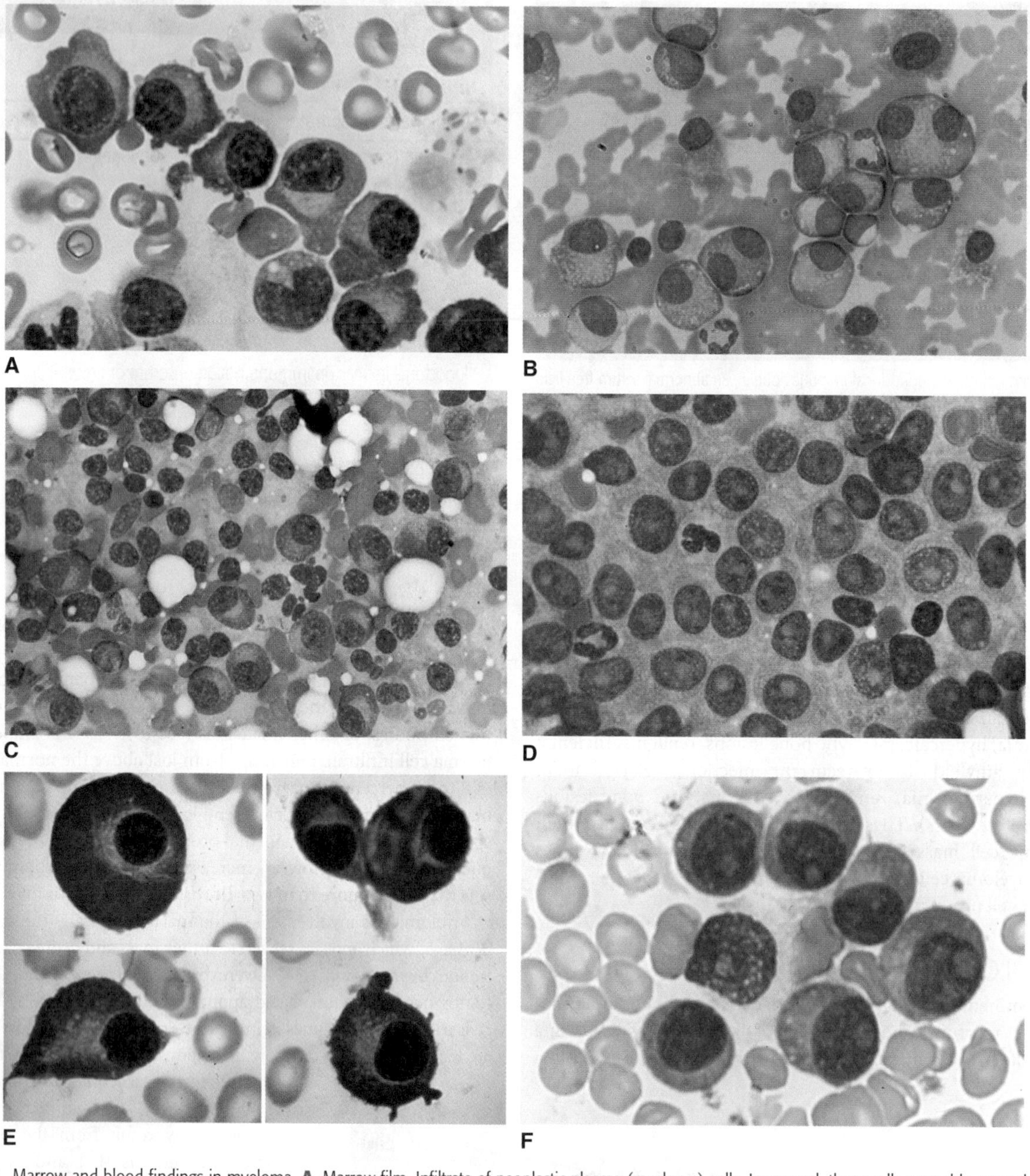

FIGURE 109-6 Marrow and blood findings in myeloma. **A.** Marrow film. Infiltrate of neoplastic plasma (myeloma) cells. In general, these cells resemble normal plasma cells in their appearance with characteristic nuclear:cytoplasmic area ratio, blocky nuclear chromatin pattern, intense cytoplasmic basophilia, and a prominent 'hof" or clear area (Golgi zone). **B.** Marrow film. Infiltrate of malignant plasma (myeloma) cells showing very large cell size and binucleate forms. **C.** Imprint of marrow biopsy. Marked increase of neoplastic plasma (myeloma) cells. **D.** Marrow section. Striking infiltrate of plasmablasts with very large prominent nucleoli. **E.** Marrow film. Examples of "flaming" plasma cells with reddish-purple cytoplasmic coloration, found more commonly in monoclonal IgA synthesizing myeloma cells. **F.** Blood film. Plasma cell leukemia. Striking increase in blood plasmablasts. *(Reproduced with permission from* Lichtman's Atlas of Hematology, *www.accessmedicine.com.)*

Bleeding has been reported in 15 percent of patients with immunoglobulin (Ig) G myeloma and in more than 30 percent of patients with IgA myeloma.[196,197] The antibody portion (Fab) of the myeloma protein may bind to fibrin during clotting and prevent fibrin aggregation. This probably represents the most common coagulopathy in patients with myeloma.[198] Bleeding may also be a result of anoxia and thrombosis in the capillary circulation, of perivascular amyloid, and/or of an acquired coagulopathy,[199] such as factor X deficiency, in the case of primary amyloidosis. Factor X deficiency associated with systemic light-chain amyloid (AL) amyloidosis apparently cannot be traced to an inhibitor *in vitro* (see Chap. 110).[200] Thrombocytosis should alert one to the possibility of hyposplenism because of amyloid deposition in the spleen. Hypercoagulable states may result from defective fibrin structure and fibrinolysis because of increased immunoglobulin levels, increased acquired protein C resistance, and increased synthesis of proinflammatory markers such as IL-6. Lupus anticoagulants also have been reported in association with myeloma. However, these have not been traced to a direct action of the monoclonal immunoglobulin.[201] A new syndrome of thromboembolic disease in myeloma has been linked to the use of thalidomide and lenalidomide, especially in combination with glucocorticoids and/or doxorubicin.[202] A further potential risk factor is concomitant administration of erythropoiesis-stimulating agents. The use of low-molecular-weight heparin, aspirin, or full-dose anticoagulation with Coumadin has been effective in reducing the frequency of thromboembolism, especially during the early phases of therapy when a high disease burden is present.[202]

IMMUNOGLOBULIN ABNORMALITIES

Most patients with myeloma secrete a monoclonal immunoglobulin that can be detected by immunofixation analysis. The immunoglobulins produced by the myeloma cells can be found to have unique immunoglobulin idiotypes (see Chaps. 77 and 107).[41] Approximately 60 percent of myeloma patients have detectable monoclonal IgG (usually >3.5 g/dL), 20 percent have monoclonal IgA (typically >2 g/dL), and 20 percent have only monoclonal immunoglobulin light chains. Excess light-chain proteinuria, however, can accompany IgG, IgA, and, especially, IgD myeloma.

A small proportion of patients have nonsecretory myeloma, in which the neoplastic plasma cells do not secrete detectable amounts of monoclonal immunoglobulin although most cases still contain readily identifiable cytoplasmic immunoglobulin. Myelomas producing monoclonal IgD, IgE, IgM, or more than one immunoglobulin class are rare. The presence of a low concentration of serum monoclonal immunoglobulin should alert to the possibility of the IgD myeloma isotype, especially when associated with excess λ light chains in the serum and light-chain proteinuria as 80 percent of IgD myeloma are of the λ light-chain variety. Suppression of uninvolved immunoglobulin classes is typical for symptomatic myeloma.[203] Even patients with light-chain type myeloma, nonsecretory myeloma, or IgD or IgE myeloma often have depressed levels of normal, polyclonal serum IgG, IgA, and IgM.

The introduction of assays to quantify free κ and free λ light chains in serum has made possible the reclassification of approximately one-half to two-thirds of patients previously thought to have nonsecretory myeloma and can be used to measure the response to therapy.[204,205] The serum "freelite" assay recognizes previously hidden determinants of the light chain using an antibody-based assay (Fig. 109–7). The half-life of free light chains is 2 to 4 hours, and the assay can detect response to therapy in days. Whole immunoglobulins have a half-life of 17 to 21 days, and responses are much slower to become apparent.

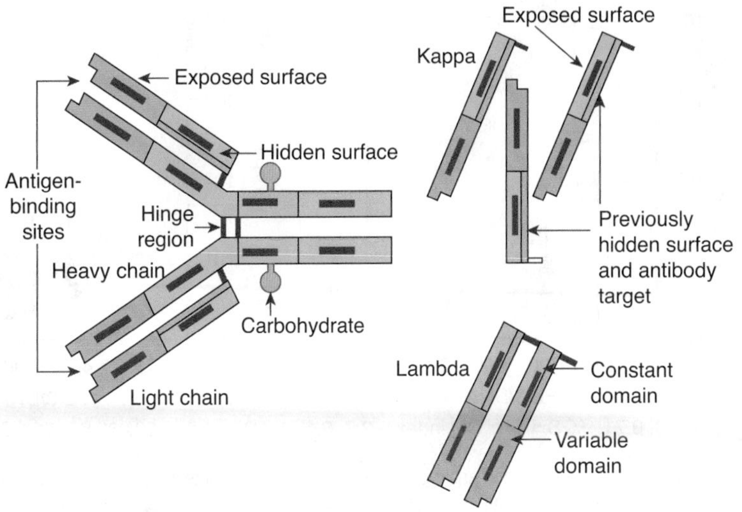

FIGURE 109–7. Principle of the free light-chain assay. Antibody molecule showing heavy and light chains. The free light-chain assay recognized the "hidden" antigenic surface (red) by immunoassay.

Baseline values for serum-free light chains have prognostic value, which is possible because higher levels of serum freelite reflect increased myeloma burden or are associated with IgH translocations.[206–208] Higher freelite chain levels are associated with a greater rate of progression of essential monoclonal gammopathy and smoldering myeloma to symptomatic myeloma.[209,210] In patients, high baseline free light chains, conferred worse overall survival and event-free survival, despite the fact these patients achieved higher near-complete remission rates. Further steep reductions in free light chains after therapy were also associated with inferior overall and event-free survival, presumably reflecting the presence of highly proliferative myeloma cells, which are killed more rapidly by combination chemotherapy. This aggressive type of myeloma is characterized by rapid regrowth after treatment, resulting in early relapse and disease-related death, despite the initial rapid cell kill achieved.[208] The ratio between the κ and λ light chains is now also included in the definition of stringent complete response by the Uniform International Response Criteria.[211]

An analysis of all patients enrolled on Total Therapy 1, 2, and 3 protocols showed that IgA isotype adversely affects outcome in multivariate analysis. IgD was of borderline significance, probably because of its rare occurrence, but was strongly associated with β_2M and lactic dehydrogenase (LDH) serum levels, reflecting tumor burden, as well as the presence of metaphase cytogenetic abnormalities, and assignment to the more aggressive proliferation subgroup on gene-expression profile analysis.[212]

MARROW FINDINGS

The marrow can be evenly infiltrated (diffuse involvement) but commonly displays considerable site-to-site variation in myeloma cell density in a given patient (focal/nodular involvement). Mixed patterns may also occur.[213,214] Patients may also present with a normal, randomly procured marrow aspirate and biopsy, but have multiple plasmacytomas, a condition sometimes referred to as macrofocal myeloma. Cytologically, myeloma cells consist predominantly of plasma cells exhibiting varying degrees of maturity. Low-grade cells typically exhibit a morphology resembling normal plasma cells with clumped chromation, an eccentric nucleus, and perinuclear hof.[215,216] More aggressive forms of myeloma may have larger cells with a centrally located nucleus, which has open chromatin and punched nucleoli, indicating increased transcriptional activity. These cells dominate in plasmablastic myeloma, which is characterized by the presence of readily identifiable mitotic figures.

Osteoclasts are often increased and osteoblasts decreased. Amyloid deposition, recognized on Congo red stain, may be diffuse or focal and sometimes only perivascular. Specialized laboratories can perform qualitative assessment of microvessel density using CD131 or CD34 monoclonal antibodies.[217–219] Secondary myelodysplastic changes typically develop after prolonged treatment with alkylating agents, such as melphalan or nitrosoureas, considered potential leukemogens, although myelodysplastic syndromes can occur concurrently with myeloma in this older patient population (see Chap. 88).[220,221] Pancytopenia in the context of a hypercellular marrow should prompt cytogenetic and interphase FISH studies to detect the most commonly encountered abnormalities associated with therapy-related myelodysplastic syndromes: – 5,5q– ; – 7,7q– ; t(1;7) (q10; p10); +8; del 20q; and involvement of 11q23 or 21q22 induced by topoisomerase II-inhibiting cytotoxic agents.[222]

The frequent presence of DNA aneuploidy and universal light-chain restriction, characteristic of myeloma, has been exploited diagnostically to quantitate marrow involvement by means of two-parameter flow cytometry, employing propidium iodide for nuclear DNA staining and anti-κ and anti-λ light-chain antibodies to label cytoplasmic immunoglobulin (Fig. 109–8).[223]

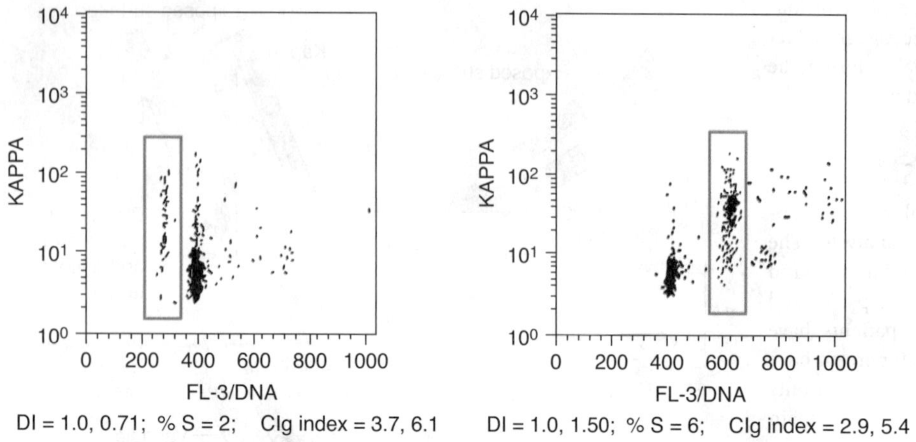

FIGURE 109–8. Flow cytometric analysis of marrow nuclear DNA content (propidium iodide) and cytoplasmic immunoglobulin light-chain content (FITC conjugated anti-κ monoclonal antibody) in two myeloma cases. *Left panel* reveals the presence of a κ-restricted hypodiploid clone (DNA-index 0.71). *Right panel* shows the presence of a κ-restricted hyperdiploid clone (DNA-index 1.5).

Most laboratories perform flow cytometric phenotype studies to capture typically CD138+CD45– mature plasma cells,[112,224] frequently coexpressing CD56+ (neural-cell adhesion molecule [N-CAM]).[225,226] Fewer than 20 percent of cases express CD20+[62] or CD117+ (KIT),[227] which have not been effectively targeted by rituximab or imatinib mesylate. Sensitive flow cytometry analysis can be used to detect and quantify minimal residual disease at a level of 1 residual myeloma cell in 10,000 to 100,000 cells.[228]

Metaphase cytogenetic studies should be performed to identify the one-third of newly diagnosed patients harboring cytogenetic abnormalities, which confer a poor prognosis, especially in cases of hypodiploidy and chromosome 1 abnormalities, as compared to patients with a hyperdiploid karyotype that fare better (Fig. 109–9).[229–235] Interphase FISH studies have been helpful in some series to discern a prognostically less-favorable chromosome deletion 13[236–238] or *P53* deletion.[89] When performed together with metaphase karyotyping, however, FISH-defined deletion 13 does not add prognostically relevant information.[239]

Because mature plasma cells represent the dominant tumor phenotype in most myeloma cases, the proportion of cycling cells is typically exceedingly small.[101,240–243] Thus the plasma cell labeling index, as determined by tritiated thymidine or bromodeoxyuridine techniques, averages 0.5 percent. Fewer than 5 percent of patients display values in excess of 5 percent.[244,245] The bromodeoxyuridine labeling index of marrow has become an important prognostic variable. As values exceed 0.5 percent at diagnosis, the duration of event-free and overall survival are progressively shortened.[246]

RENAL DISEASE

Some form of renal impairment occurs in 30 to 50 percent of myeloma patients at diagnosis, with up to 10 percent of patients requiring hemodialysis during their course of management. Myeloma cast nephropathy is the most common cause of renal impairment and is also referred to as myeloma kidney. Abnormalities of renal function occur when the tubular absorptive capacity for light chains is exhausted, resulting in the formation of tubular casts in the distal nephron formed by the binding of light chains to uromodulin (Tamm-Horsfall protein). These tubular casts obstruct the distal nephron and parts of the ascending loop of Henle and contribute to development of interstitial nephritis.[247] Cast formation is directly related to the rate of light-chain synthesis and typically the amount of total proteinuria approximately matches the amount of light chain and/or immunoglobulin secretion. However, there is considerable variation in the nephrotoxic proclivity of light chains (e.g., λ light chains are more nephrotoxic than the κ type) and some patients may have minimal light-chain secretion and present with renal impairment before other manifestations of myeloma appear.

The second most common cause of nephropathy is hypercalcemia. Concomitant hypercalciuria leads to volume depletion and prerenal azotemia. In addition, hypercalcemia is conducive to calcium deposits in the renal tubules, also producing interstitial nephritis.[248,249] AL amyloidosis associated with light-chain immunoglobulin proteinuria usually presents as the nephrotic syndrome, with very little light-chain secretion in the urine, but can lead, over time, to renal failure (see Chap. 110).[250–252] Amyloid deposits can be found in every part of the kidney, but predominate in the glomeruli, where they can be detected by Congo red staining. AL amyloidosis is more common in patients with λ light-chain myeloma proteins than in patients with κ light-chain myeloma, especially those with λ light-chain proteins that have immunoglobulin variable regions belonging to the λ VI light-chain subgroup. The differential diagnosis of nephrotic syndrome in the myeloma patient should include renal vein thrombosis. Probably underestimated, however, is the frequency of immunoglobulin LCDD, a disease more commonly associated with κ light-chain myeloma proteins, often at barely detectable levels. This also leads to impaired glomerular filtration.[252,253] The light-chain deposits are typically nonfibrillar, and as a result Congo red staining is negative. Immunofixation studies specific for κ or λ light chains may reveal linear involvement of the basement membrane. Acquired adult Fanconi renal syndrome is also caused by κ light chains.

Tumor cell involvement of the kidneys is uncommon but should be suspected in patients with renal enlargement; however, it is more often caused by AL amyloid (see Chap. 110).[250] A complicating factor in the pathogenesis of renal failure in myeloma is the frequent use of nonsteroidal antiinflammatory drugs for pain control, use of nephrotoxic antibiotics, and imaging contrast agents.[254] A further reason for renal function impairment is the administration of bisphosphonates, especially when given rapidly. Consequently, review of renal function prior to each cycle of bisphosphonate therapy is advisable. Nonspecific proteinuria (e.g., albuminuria) may precede the onset of renal failure.

Kidney biopsy can be helpful to diagnose accurately the type of renal disease in myeloma patients. Biopsy specimens should be processed fresh-frozen to allow for immunofixation studies, including electron microscopy and Congo red staining for amyloidosis.

The mainstay of the management of renal impairment in myeloma is supportive care. This approach includes hydration, use of calcitonin and a slow infusion of a single dose of a bisphosphonate to correct hypercalcemia rapidly, and prompt initiation of cytoreductive chemotherapy. The efficacy of removal of light chains by plasma exchange is controversial. A new dialysis filter has been developed that removes light chains with great efficiency, renewing the interest in the application of hemodialysis.

In general, cast nephropathy-induced renal impairment is (partially) reversible in approximately 50 percent of patients. Improvements in renal function are unlikely to occur more than 6 months after diagnosis. The likelihood of significant improvement of renal function in LCDD and amyloidosis is much less.

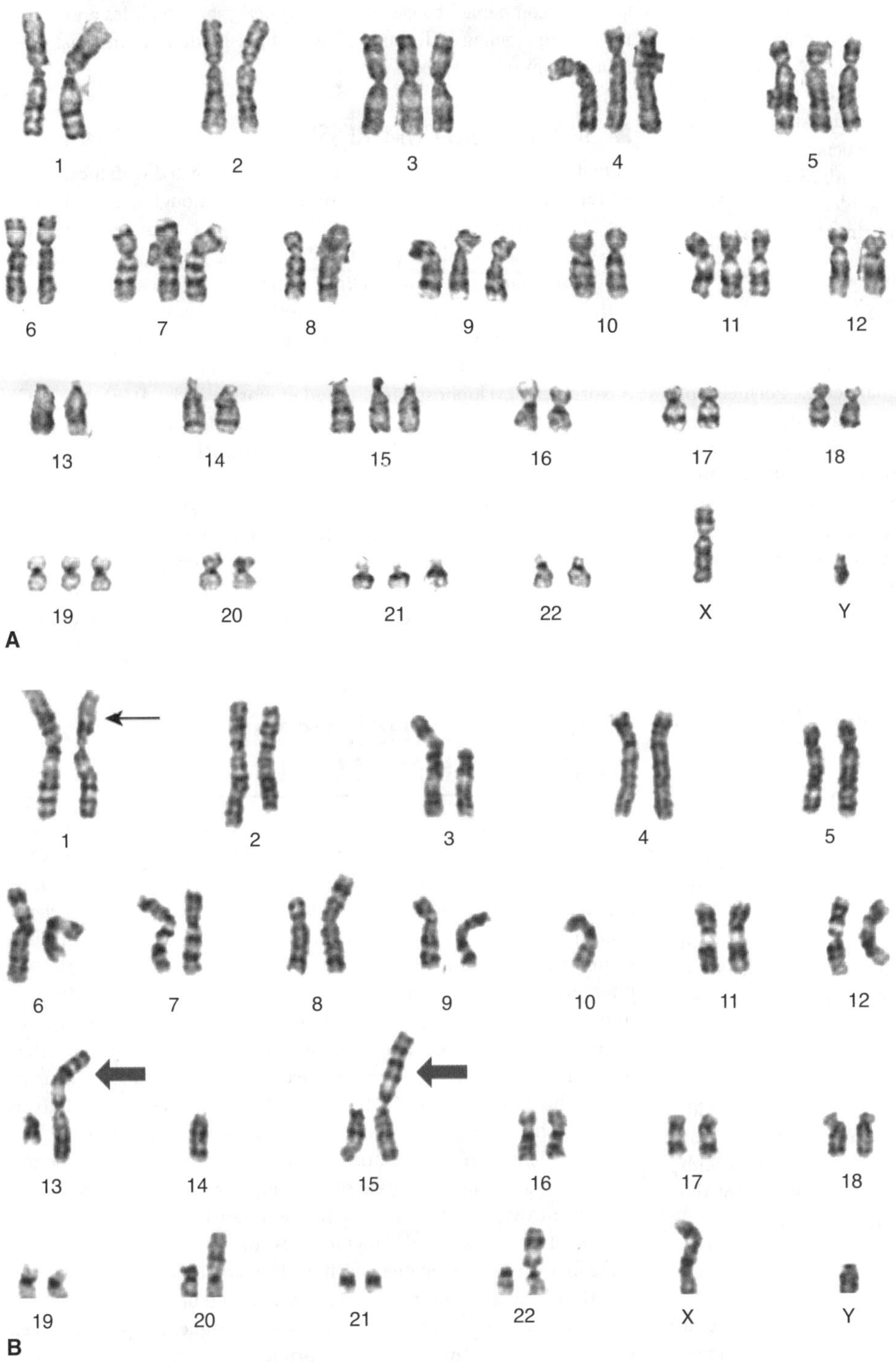

FIGURE 109–9. A. Hyperdiploid karyotype with typical trisomies of uneven chromosomes (3, 5, 7, 9, 11, 15, 19, and 21). **B.** Complex hypodiploid karyotype with abnormalities of chromosome 1q and 1p. There is del(1)(p11p22) and "jumping" translocations of 1q involving der(1;13)(q10;q10) and der(1;15)(q10;q10) (*open arrows*).

■ PAIN

Pain suffered by subjects with myeloma frequently results from vertebral compression fractures at sites of osteopenia or, more typically, from lytic bone lesions, which may also result in pathologic fractures of long bones and ribs. Localized pain can also be induced by regional tumor growth compressing the spinal cord and nerve roots. Painful mass effects also can be provoked by amyloid deposition (see Chap. 110) at various anatomic sites, e.g., the median nerve sheath, as in amyloid-associated carpal tunnel syndrome.[255]

■ INFECTIONS

Infection is a leading cause of morbidity and mortality in myeloma patients. Infection is not only related to dysfunction of the immune system intrinsic to myeloma, but is also influenced by other factors, including type and duration of therapy (e.g., cytotoxic agents, glucocorticoids, autologous/allogeneic hematopoietic stem cell transplantation), age, and coexisting comorbidities. Extensive immunologic abnormalities involving both the innate and adaptive immune system have been reported in myeloma.[256] Hypogammaglobulinemia reflecting suppression of CD19+ B lymphocytes results in susceptibility to encapsulated organisms, such as *Streptococcus pneumoniae* and *Haemophilus influenzae*.

Deficiencies in cellular immune function account for the recurrent infections commonly seen in myeloma.[203,257,258] Dendritic cells are highly specialized antigen-presenting cells central to the induction of cellular and humoral immune response (see Chap. 19). The function of abnormal dendritic cells in myeloma is well recognized. Dendritic cells exhibit an immature phenotype with reduced expression of the important costimulatory molecule B7.1.[259,260] They have a reduced capacity to stimulate antigen specific T cells and present patient-specific idiotype to autologous T cells.[260] A number of cytokines present in the myeloma microenvironment may be responsible for these abnormalities, including transforming growth factor (TGF)-β, IL-6, and IL-10.[259,260] TGF-β and IL-10 can induce tolerance of antigen-specific T cells and skew the immune response to an unproductive Th2-type response. TGF-β may also contribute to the induction of immunosuppressive T-regulatory cells.[261] IL-6 is a paracrine and autocrine growth factor for myeloma cells and inhibits the production of dendritic cells from CD34+ progenitor cells.[260] β_2M shed by myeloma cells is reflective of tumor burden and high levels assign patients to a poor prognostic category in the International Staging System (ISS). β_2M has a number of immunosuppressive effects, including the reduction of IL-2 secretion by dendritic cells and a reduction of costimulatory and adhesion molecules expressed by dendritic cells, which negatively influences the induction of antigen-specific T cells.[262] Dendritic cells may stimulate clonogenic myeloma growth.[263]

Abnormalities in T-cell function include reversed CD4+/CD8+ T-cell ratios, severe disruptions in the T-cell repertoire, and abnormal intracellular signal transduction impairing T-cell activation.[264–266]

Prevention of infection relies on the use of antiviral drugs to prevent herpes simplex virus and varicella-zoster virus reactivation, fluoroquinolones as antimicrobial prophylaxis, and fluconazole to reduce the risk of fungal infections. In patients with persistently low CD4+ counts, *Pneumocystis carinii* prophylaxis should be considered. Infusion of intravenous immunoglobulin has not proven to be beneficial as general prophylaxis, but can be useful for specific patients with recurrent bacterial infection. The Centers for Disease Control guidelines recommend the use of oseltamivir for influenza protection during the winter season in immunocompromised individuals.

NEUROPATHY

Neurologic abnormalities generally are caused by regional myeloma cell growth compressing the spinal cord or cranial nerves. Polyneuropathies are observed with perineuronal or perivascular (*vasa nervorum*) amyloid deposition[255] and can also be seen with osteosclerotic myeloma, sometimes as part of the complete polyneuropathy, organomegaly, endocrinopathy, monoclonal gammopathy, and skin changes (POEMS) syndrome.[267,268] The humoral and cellular mechanisms mediating this peculiar syndrome are unknown, but vascular endothelial growth factor appears to be the central cytokine.

HYPERVISCOSITY

Hyperviscosity occurs in fewer than 10 percent of patients with myeloma.[269–272] Although noted in a higher proportion of patients with Waldenström macroglobulinemia (see Chap. 111),[273] hyperviscosity may be seen more commonly in association with myeloma because of its 10-fold higher incidence than that of macroglobulinemia.[199] Symptoms of hyperviscosity result from circulatory problems, leading to cerebral, pulmonary, renal, and other organ dysfunction (see "Hyperviscosity Syndrome" in Chap. 111). Hyperviscosity often is associated with bleeding.

While there is a general correlation between clinical symptoms and relative serum viscosity, the relationship between serum immunoglobulin levels and symptoms is not consistent from one patient to the next. This may be related to the different physicochemical properties of each of the classes and subclasses of immunoglobulin molecules (see Chap. 77). Because of a greater tendency for IgA to form polymers, patients with IgA myeloma have hyperviscosity more frequently than do patients with IgG myeloma, and almost one-quarter of IgA myeloma patients may have features of the hyperviscosity syndrome.[272] Among patients with IgG myeloma, those with tumors expressing immunoglobulins of the IgG_3 subclass are the most susceptible to developing this syndrome.[274]

EXTRAMEDULLARY DISEASE

Plasma cell leukemia (>2000 myeloma cells/μL of blood) is rare at presentation, but can develop in approximately 5 percent of patients as a terminal disease manifestation.[275–278] Using appropriate tools (CD138+/CD45− or DNA/cytoplasmic immunoglobulin (cIg) flow cytometry), low levels of circulating plasma cells can be detected in the majority of patients. Other extramedullary disease manifestations are observed with increasing frequency as the duration of disease control is extended by high-dose melphalan and modern salvage therapies. Visceral organ involvement of liver, lymph nodes, spleen, kidneys, breasts, pleura, meninges, and cutaneous sites should be suspected in the presence of elevated serum levels of LDH[279,280] and is best confirmed by computed tomography (CT) or positron emission tomography (PET) scanning. Systematic application of CT-PET in the Total Therapy 3 trial revealed the presence of extramedullary disease in 14 of 239 patients (6%), who were untreated.[281] Such extramedullary disease is almost always accompanied by complex cytogenetic abnormalities and a high tumor-cell labeling index as well as by high-grade immunoblastic cell morphology.[234]

SPINAL CORD COMPRESSION

Spinal cord compression has traditionally been treated with local radiotherapy and/or decompressive laminectomy. Although local radiotherapy has curative potential for the management of truly solitary plasmacytoma, its role in palliation has to be assessed in the context of long-term management and in light of the underlying cause. In patients suffering from systemic disease, chemotherapy that includes high-dose dexamethasone pulsing, as part of the combination oral dexamethasone, daily thalidomide, and 4 days of continuous-infusion cisplatin, doxorubicin, cyclophosphamide, and etoposide (DT PACE). DT PACE has been shown to provide effective treatment. In the absence of symptom relief and lack of tumor shrinkage on MRI within 1 week, local radiation should be added.

If cord compression results from vertebral collapse without identifiable plasmacytoma on MRI, radiation may not be beneficial, and decompressive laminectomy should be the treatment of choice. The local doses of radiotherapy to the spinal cord should not exceed 30 Gy, and liberal use of local radiation for the management of rib fractures is discouraged.

INITIAL EVALUATION OF THE PATIENT WITH MYELOMA

Minimal evaluation requirements include evaluation of the complete blood count; examination of the blood film for the presence of rouleaux and circulating myeloma cells; a multichemical scan for the detection of hypercalcemia, renal failure, serum β_2M, C-reactive protein, and elevation of LDH (Table 109–5). Myeloma protein studies should include serum protein electrophoresis to quantitate the serum protein electrophoretic pattern in combination with nephelometric quantitation of immunoglobulin levels, serum-free light-chain assay, and a 24-hour urine collection to quantitate 24-hour total urinary protein and determine specific urinary proteins, for example, light chains with urine electrophoresis. Urinary light chains have also been referred to as "Bence Jones protein," so named because the English physician and chemist, Henry Bence Jones, described some of their physicochemical features in a presumptive case of myeloma reported in the mid-19th century. In 1850, Dr. William MacIntyre reported what he described as a case of "Mollities and Fragilitas Ossium accompanied by urine charged with animal matter," uniformly recognized as the first case report of myeloma with postmortem description of marrow and bones and urine findings. Dr. MacIntyre and his colleague, Dr. Watson, asked Bence Jones to further analyze the urinary protein. Bence Jones confirmed the findings of Drs. MacIntyre and Watson, who had cared for the patient in question, that the urine contained a protein that when acidified precipited on heating and then redissolved as the temperature of the urine was increased toward boiling. It took about 100 years for protein chemistry and immunology to advance sufficiently such that the protein was shown to be either the monoclonal lambda or kappa light chain of an immunoglobulin molecule.

Immunofixation of serum and urine is needed for the immunoglobulin heavy- and light-chain isotype determination. Serum-free light-chain assay is of particular use in the monitoring of patients with a plasma monoclonal immunoglobulin, the diagnosis and monitoring of patients who would otherwise be considered to have nonsecretory myeloma, and patients who only have light-chain proteinuria. Marrow

TABLE 109–5. Assessment of Multiple Myeloma

Complete blood count and differential count; examination of blood film
Chemistry screen, including calcium, creatinine, lactate dehydrogenase, BNP, proBNP
β_2-Microglobulin, C-reactive protein
Serum protein electrophoresis, immunofixation, quantification of immunoglobulins, serum-free light chains
24-h urine collection for protein electrophoresis, immunofixation, quantification of immunoglobulins including light chains
Marrow aspirate and trephine biopsy with metaphase cytogenetics, FISH, immunophenotyping; gene array, and plasma cell labeling index (if available)
Bone survey and MRI; CT-PET (if available)
Echocardiogram with assessment of diastolic function and measurement of interventricular septal thickness; EKG[185]

BNP, brain natriuretic peptide; CT, computed tomography; EKG, electrocardiogram; FISH, fluorescence *in situ* hybridization; MRI, magnetic resonance imaging; PET, positron-emission tomography; proBNP, prohormone B-type natriuretic peptide.

aspiration and biopsy should include genetic studies (FISH, cytogenetics, and gene-expression profiling), flow cytometry, cIgDNA, and plasma cell labeling index. Radiographic examination usually comprises a metastatic bone survey to detect vertebral compression fractures, osteopenia, and impending fractures of long bones and pelvis. MRI and CT-PET are more sensitive than the bone survey, and better capture early bone disease, the extent of bone disease, and extramedullary disease. Both MRI and CT-PET findings have also important prognostic implications.[281,282] Assessment of the heart by echocardiogram and electrocardiogram is useful to detect cardiac amyloidosis and/or LCDD, and, in selected cases, cardiac MRI may be helpful to demonstrate myocardial infiltration. Measurement of brain natriuretic peptide and N-terminal prohormone B-type natriuretic peptide are useful screening tests to detect cardiac dysfunction caused by amyloidosis or LCDD.

STAGING

The Salmon-Durie staging system has been in use for more than 30 years but is being replaced by newer staging systems, which reflect better myeloma biology.[283] The Salmon-Durie system relates myeloma cell mass to the extent of bony disease, hemoglobin and calcium levels, and the monoclonal immunoglobulin levels in serum and urine (Table 109–6). However, measurement of bone disease by skeletal survey in myeloma is observer-dependent and potentially subjective.

The Southwest Oncology Group introduced an ISS based on two widely available parameters, serum β_2M and albumin, and recognizes three stages. Stage I is defined by β_2M <3.5 mg/L and albumin ≥3.5 g/100 mL; stage III is characterized by a β_2M of ≥5.5 mg/L.[284] The intermediate stage II has neither features of stage I or III. β_2M correlates with tumor mass and impairment in renal function, whereas a low albumin reflects the effect of IL-6 produced by the microenvironment of myeloma cells on the liver.[285–287] The different ISS stages were predictive of outcome in an analysis of more than 11,000 patients receiving either standard therapies or melphalan-based high-dose therapy followed by autologous hematopoietic stem cell transplantation (auto-HSCT; Table 109–7, Fig. 109–10). A weakness of the ISS is that it does not take cytogenetics into account, a variable, which was available for few patients.

TABLE 109–6. Assessment of Myeloma Tumor Mass (Salmon-Durie)

I. High tumor mass (stage III) (>1.2 × 10[12] myeloma cells/m²)*
   One of the following abnormalities must be present:
   A. Hemoglobin <8.5 g/dL, hematocrit <25%
   B. Serum calcium >12 mg/dL
   C. Very high serum or urine myeloma protein production rates:
      1. IgG peak >7 g/dL
      2. IgA peak >5 g/dL
      3. Urine light chains >12 g/24 h
   D. >3 lytic bone lesions on bone survey (bone scan not acceptable)
II. Low tumor mass (stage I) (<0.6 × 10[12] myeloma cells/m²)*
   All of the following must be present:
   A. Hemoglobin >10.5 g/dL or hematocrit >32%
   B. Serum calcium normal
   C. Low serum myeloma protein production rates:
      1. IgG peak <5 g/dL
      2. IgA peak <3 g/dL
      3. Urine light chains <4 g/24 h
   D. No bone lesions or osteoporosis
III. Intermediate tumor mass (stage II) (0.6–1.2 × 10[12] myeloma cells/m²)*
   All patients who do not qualify for high or low tumor mass categories are considered to have intermediate tumor mass.
   A. No renal failure (creatinine ≤2 mg/dL)
   B. Renal failure (creatinine >2 mg/dL)

*Estimated number of neoplastic plasma cells.[283]

PROGNOSIS

The prognosis of myeloma is determined by three factors: (1) host, (2) tumor biology and disease burden, and (3) type of therapy applied. Host parameters such as comorbidities, advanced age, frailty, and poor performance status negatively impact overall outcome and increases treatment-related morbidity and mortality. With the advent of new drugs, utilized in combination or incorporated into a high-dose melphalan-based auto-HSCT approaches, some poor prognostic factors can be overcome (see "Management of Newly Diagnosed Myeloma" below).

TABLE 109–7. International Staging System (ISS)

Stage I:	28%	β_2M <3.5 ALB ≥3.5
Stage II:	39%	β_2M <3.5 ALB <3.5 or β_2M 3.5–5.5
Stage III:	33%	β_2M >5.5

%, percent of all patients with myeloma; ALB, serum albumin in g/dL; β_2M, serum β_2-microglobulin in mg/L.[183]

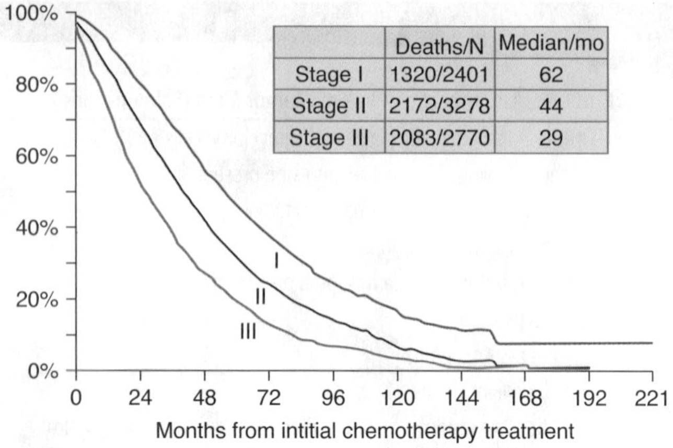

FIGURE 109–10. International Staging System. Survival of previously untreated patients with myeloma according to the International Staging System (ISS). *(Reproduced with permission from Greipp PR, San Muguel J, Durie B, et al: International Staging System for Multiple Myeloma.* J Clin Oncol *23:3412, 2005.)*

Advances in cytogenetics, gene-expression profiling, and imaging (MRI and CT-PET) have greatly increased our understanding of tumor biology and burden. Furthermore, such variables are more powerful prognostic indicators than standard prognostic variables.

The hypoproliferative nature of myeloma[241] and its stromal dependence[288] accounts for the high frequency (approximately two-thirds) of normal diploid metaphase karyotypes, derived from normal hematopoietic cells, observed in untreated patients.[289] The capacity of myeloma cells to grow *in vitro* without the support of the marrow microenvironment (approximately one-third of newly diagnosed patients) defines an entity that is stroma independent and has a poor prognosis.[107] Suppression of abnormal metaphase cytogenetics is critical to long-term survival. Cytogenetic findings associated with poor outcome include hypodiploidy and deletions 13q and 17p13, the locus of the tumor-suppressor gene P53.[229–235,290] Gains of chromosome 1q arm and loss of 1p occur in tandem duplications and jumping translocations of chromosome 1, and signify more aggressive and more advanced myeloma.[50,291–293] Gain of the 1q21 region (amp1q21) increases from approximately 40 percent at diagnosis to 70 percent at relapse and indicates that this abnormality plays a role in disease progression. Both the proportion of cells with 1q21 and the copy number increases at relapse suggesting the existence of a gene-dosage effect involved in drug resistance (Fig. 109–11A).[294] The gene *CKS1B* located at 1q21 controls the G_1 to S transition of the cell cycle and has been linked to shorter progression-free survival after auto-HSCT.[295,296] Combining hypodiploidy and high β_2M has also been used to identify patient populations with a poor outcome.[233,238] In contrast, hyperdiploidy, which accounts for almost half of the patients with abnormal cytogenetics and involves nonrandom gains of chromosomes 3, 5, 7, 9, 11, 15, 19, and 21, is associated with chemosensitive disease and better overall survival. Translocation t(11;14) also confers a better outcome.[297]

Interphase FISH does not depend on cycling cells and increases the detection of abnormal cells to 80 to 90 percent.[51] Interphase FISH can also detect cytogenetically silent translocations, for example, t(4;14), t(14;16), and t(14;20), and can be performed on stored material. The deleterious effects of del 13q are dependent on its frequent association with del 17p and t(4;14).[298] In the Eastern Cooperative Oncology Group trial E9486/9487, three distinct prognostic groups were recognized in patients treated with conventional chemotherapy: a poor prognosis was typified by t(4;14) and/or t(14;16) and/or del 17p; an intermediate prognosis by del 13q but without t(4;14),t(14;16) and del 17p; and a good prognosis group who have t(11;14) or no abnormalities.[299] Similar observations have been reported for del 17p, t(4;14), and t(14;16) in the setting of auto-HSCT.[300–302] FISH data of nearly 1000 patients enrolled on the IFM99 therapeutic trials[296] indicated that del 13q, t(4;14), and del 17p all adversely influenced overall survival and event-free survival. On multivariate analysis, only del 17p and t(4;14) independently predicted event-free survival and overall survival. The overall survival and event-free survival in patients who did not have t(4;14) and del 17p were similar regardless of the presence of del 13q. Furthermore, t(4;14) and del 17p separated distinct groups within each ISS stage. Patients who lacked t(4;14) and del 17p and who had a β_2M of less than 4 mg/L had an excellent 4-year overall survival of 83 percent and benefited from tandem auto-HSCT. Conversely, patients who had either t(4;14) or del 17p combined with a β_2M of less than 4 mg/L had a poor prognosis, with an overall survival of only 19 months after auto-HSCT. These patients should be considered for other treatment options.

The above data suggest that analysis of metaphase cytogenetic abnormalities and FISH can identify patients who do not do well with auto-HSCT or standard therapies. Individual prognostication remains highly variable despite the application of these more sophisticated cytogenetic techniques. The Total Therapy 2 patient dataset revealed that standard prognostic variables and metaphase cytogenetic had limited ability to account for outcome variability with hazard ratios not exceeding 2.0.[53,303,304]

Gene-expression profiling in leukemia and lymphoma has allowed for disease subclassifications, which are clinically important in terms of outcome.[305–309] Since the year 2000 the regular use of gene-expression profiling analysis on newly diagnosed patients allowed for the interpretation of outcome in the context of whole human genomic data. This has allowed for the identification of 70 genes linked to early disease-related death (Fig. 109–11B).[310] Thirty percent of these genes map to chromosome 1, with upregulated genes localizing to chromosome 1q and downregulated genes localizing to chromosome 1p. A high-risk score can be calculated with predicts for inferior overall survival, event-free survival, and shorter remission duration. In multivariate analyses of the two patient datasets, the 70-gene risk score was the dominant measurement predicting prognosis (Figs. 109–11C and D). A 17-gene subset could predict for outcome almost as well as the 70-gene model.[310] The importance of this risk score was confirmed in a study in newly diagnosed patients treated with auto-HSCT, in patients with relapsed myeloma treated in the phase 3 Assessment of Proteasome Inhibition for Extending Remissions (APEX) study comparing bortezomib to high-dose dexamethasone and in the Phase 2 Study of Uncontrolled Multiple Myeloma Managed with Proteasome Inhibition Therapy (SUMMIT) and Clinical Response and Efficacy Study of Bortezomib in the Treatment of Relapsing Multiple Myeloma (CREST) trials for relapsed/refractory myeloma.[311–313] Furthermore, postrelapse survival was significantly shorter in patients treated who had a high-risk score at relapse.[212] Overall, at relapse the percentage of patients with a 70-gene high-risk score may be 75 percent.[310] High-risk patients can be found in all seven subgroups of myeloma, but the proliferative, MMSET, and MAF/MAFB groups are especially enriched for high-risk patients (Fig. 109–12).

A 15-gene model has been developed by the Intergroupe Francophone du Myélome, which identifies high-risk patients by upregulation of genes involved in cell-cycle control, DNA replication and repair, and spindle assembly who have a 3-year overall survival of 43 percent.[314] Conversely, low-risk patients were heterogeneous or displayed hyperdiploid gene signatures and had significantly better 3-year overall survival of 91 percent. A comparison of the University of Arkansas Medical Center 17-gene score with the Intergroupe Francophone du Myélome 15-gene score showed that the former gene score predicted

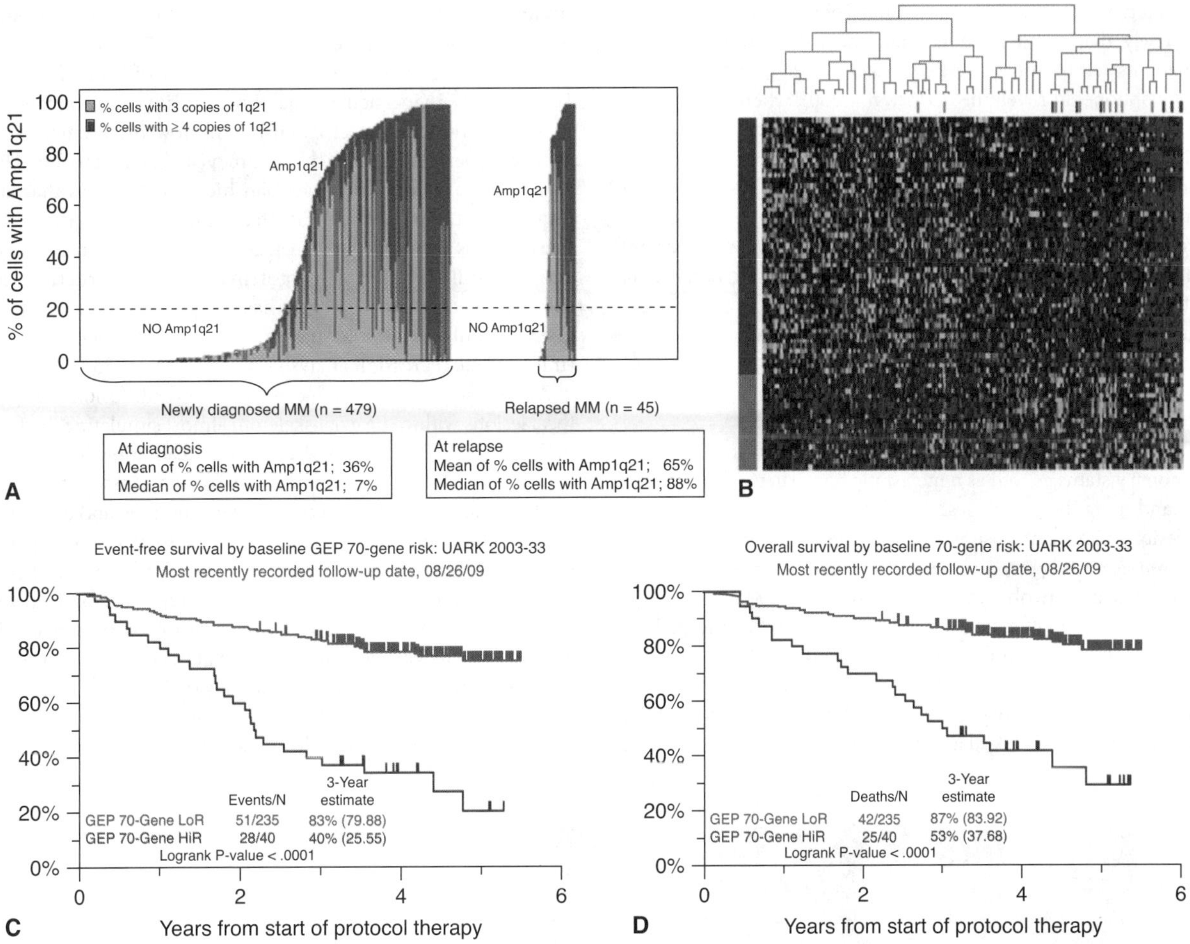

FIGURE 109–11. **A.** The proportion of cells with Amp1q21 at diagnosis and relapse. The proportion of cells with Amp1q21 is indicated by the height of the bar on the y-axis. The proportion of cells with three and with four or more copies of 1q21 in each sample is indicated by blue and purple, respectively. A total of 479 newly diagnosed MM and 45 relapsed MM samples are ordered from the lowest to highest proportion of cells with Amp1q21 from left to right in each group on the x-axis. The mean/median percentages of cells with Amp1q21 at diagnosis and relapse were 36%/65% and 7%/88%, respectively. *(Reproduced with permission from Hanamura I, Stewart J, Huang Y, Zhan F, et al. Frequent gain of chromosome band 1q21 in plasma-cell dyscrasias detected by fluorescence in situ hybridization: incidence increases from MGUS to relapsed myeloma and is related to prognosis and disease progression following tandem stem-cell transplantation.* Blood *108:1724, 2006.)* **B.** Heat maps of the 70 genes illustrate remarkably similar expression patterns among 351 newly diagnosed patients used to identify the 70 genes. Red bars above the patient columns denote patients with disease-related deaths. The 51 genes in rows designated by the red bar on the left (top rows; upregulated) identified patients in the upper quartile of expression at high risk for early disease-related death. The 19 gene rows designated by the green bar (downregulated) identified patients in the lower quartile of expression at high risk of early disease-related death. *(Reproduced with permission from Shaughnessy JD Jr, Zhan F, Burington BE, et al. A validated gene expression model of high-risk multiple myeloma is defined by deregulated expression of genes mapping to chromosome 1.* Blood *109:2276, 2007.)* **C.** Patients treated on Total Therapy 3 with a good risk 70 gene score enjoy superior overall survival. **D.** Patients treated on Total Therapy 3 with a good risk 70 gene score have superior event-free survival.

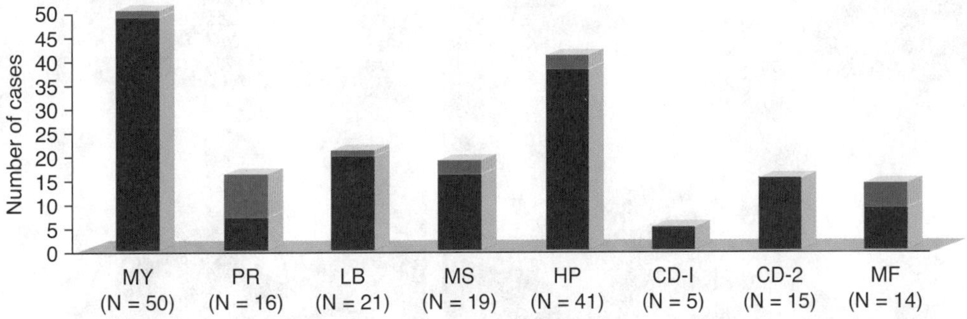

FIGURE 109–12. Patients with high-risk myeloma as defined by the 70-gene risk model can be found in all myeloma subgroups. My, myeloid; PR, proliferation; LB, low bone disease; MS, MMSET; HP, hyperdiploidy; MF, c-MAF/MAFB. The MF, PR, and MS subgroups are most enriched for high-risk patients. MAF, musculoaponeurotic fibrosarcoma oncogene homolog; MAFB, musculoaponeurotic fibrosarcoma oncogene homolog B; MMSET, multiple myeloma SET domain. *(Reproduced with permission from Shaughnessy JD Jr, Zhan F, Burington BE, et al. A validated gene expression model of high-risk multiple myeloma is defined by deregulated expression of genes mapping to chromosome 1.* Blood *109:2276, 2007.)*

outcome in all datasets (Total Therapy 2 and Total Therapy 3 datasets, n = 532; newly diagnosed patients from the Mayo clinic, n = 57; relapsed patients treated on the APEX trial, n = 264; and the Intergroupe Francophone du Myélome dataset, n = 250), whereas the Intergroupe Francophone du Myélome 15-gene score was not able to predict outcome in the Total Therapy 2 and Total Therapy 3 datasets.

Thus, myeloma at the genomic level is a very complex disease with at least seven subgroups, each of which can be divided into high-risk and low-risk groups. Gene-expression profiling data should have an important impact on the interpretation of future clinical trials. Gene microarray data are likely to become available in the near future to the general oncologist and may ultimately assist in selecting therapy for individual patients.

IMAGING STUDIES

Radiographic studies should include a chest radiograph to determine cardiopulmonary status as well as a metastatic bone survey, including a rib series and long bone images. Roentgenographically detectable osteolytic lesions require at least 50 to 70 percent loss of bone mass,[315] and hence represent advanced bone destruction. When seen on CT, these lesions typically involve the marrow space, whereas metastatic disease from other malignancies will more often involve the pedicle and the portion of the vertebral body adjacent to the pedicle (the "vertebral pedicle sign") (Fig. 109–13A and B).[316]

In the initial evaluation of patients with myeloma, MRI studies of the axial skeleton, including the skull and face, the entire spine, pelvis with studies of the shoulders and sternum has allowed detection and characterization of focal intramedullary disease in 60 to 70 percent of patients at time of diagnosis, even before the onset of bone destruction (Fig. 109–13C).[317] In particular, the short-tau inversion recovery (STIR)-weighted MRI can detect extensive marrow involvement resulting in diffuse hyperintensity of the entire visualized marrow. The diffuse hyperintense marrow however can hide focal lesions that are usually unmasked after a few cycles of effective therapy (Fig. 109–13D). Often, these lesions reemerge as the earliest signs of relapse at a time when a patient is still in remission by protein and marrow criteria. The number of MRI-detectable focal lesions has marked adverse prognostic consequences, only second to the presence of cytogenetic abnormalities (multivariate regression analysis) (Fig. 109–13E and F).[282]

A promising MRI technique of whole-body diffusion can highlight the focal lesions within the axial skeleton, almost simulating the focal lesions detected on STIR-weighted MRI studies. In addition, MRI can accurately detect associated spinal compression fractures, assess the potential for fractures caused by large focal lesions of the spine and extremities, characterize the compressive spinal cord effects of expanding focal spine lesions, and help detect sites for biopsies of focal lesions for tissue characterization. Comparison followup studies after therapy help to evaluate the response of the focal lesions and detect early recurrence of disease. MRI can also detect later complications of the disease, such as continuing fractures of the spine, onset of infections such as osteomyelitis, avascular necrosis of the femoral or humeral heads, leptomeningeal disease, and extramedullary spread to the liver and other solid organs.

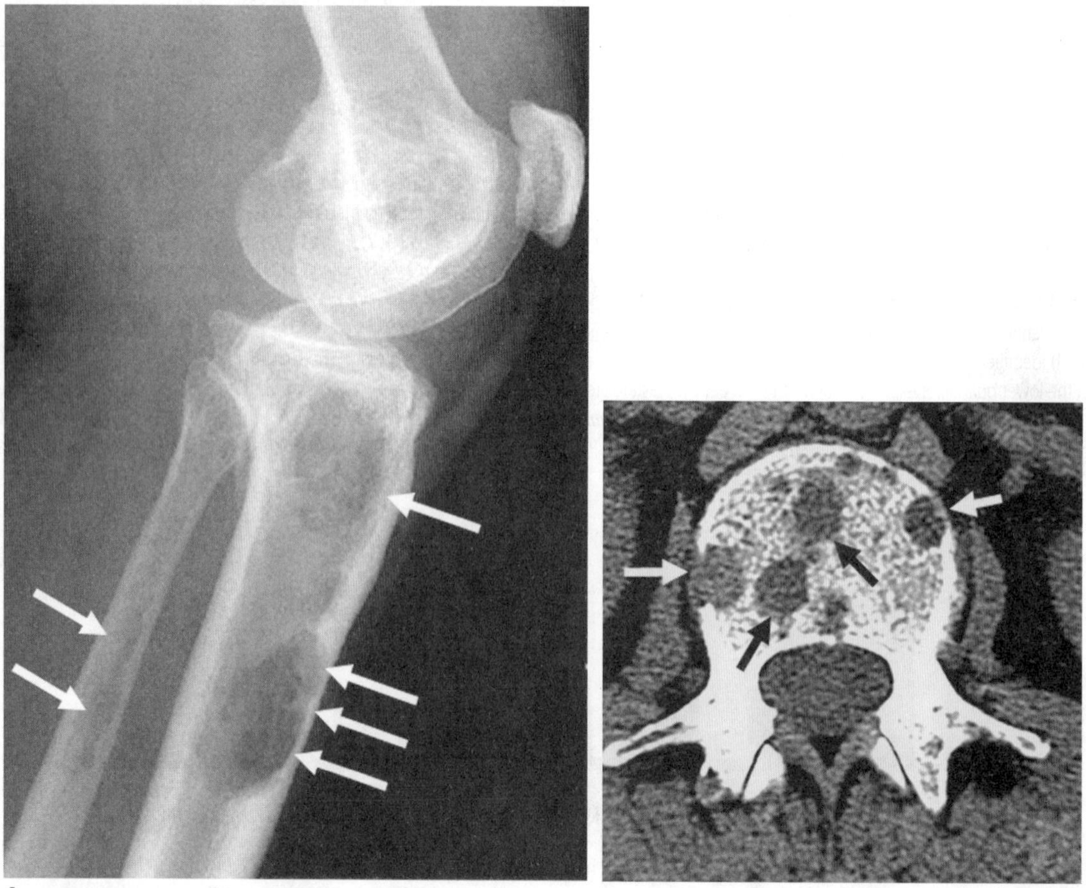

A B

FIGURE 109–13. A. Typical appearance of focal lytic lesions on radiography in a case of myeloma (*arrows*) seen on a lateral view of the tibia and fibula. **B.** CT scan of a lumbar vertebral body shows involvement of the "red marrow" space of the vertebral body.

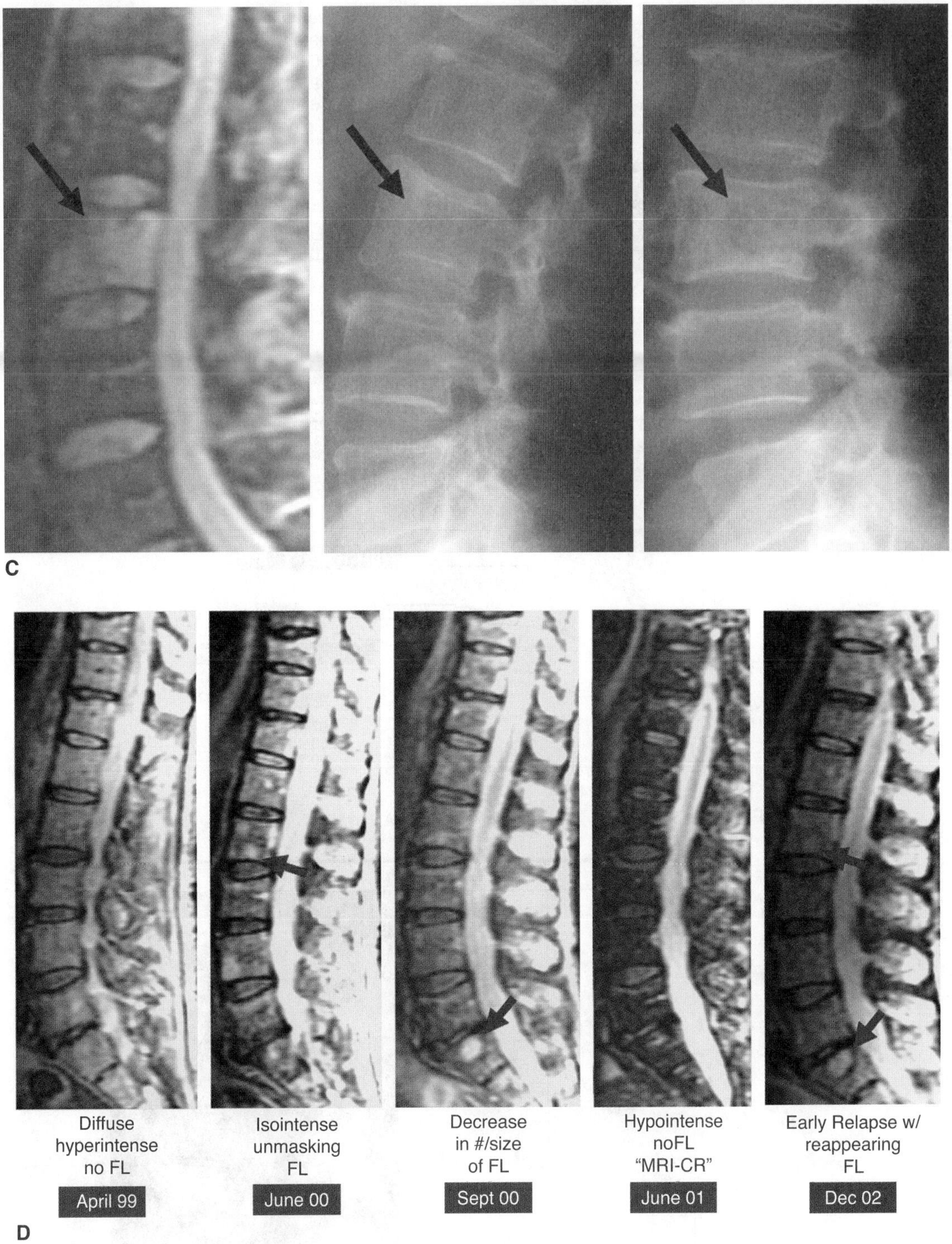

FIGURE 109–13. (*continued*) **C.** MRI detects intramedullary tumor months before radiographic changes are apparent. Short-tau inversion recovery (STIR)-weighted MRI (*left*) demonstrates a focal lesion at L3, not seen on a concurrent radiographic series (*center*), but visible 1 year later (*right*). **D.** STIR-weighted MRI shows diffuse hyperintensity prior to therapy. After initiation of successful therapy, focal lesions were unmasked (*red arrows*), which reduce in size and eventually disappear. The last panel shows relapsing disease with reappearing focal lesions in patient who, at that time, did not have protein or marrow evidence of relapse. FL, focal lesion; MRI-CR, magnetic resonance imaging-computed radiography.

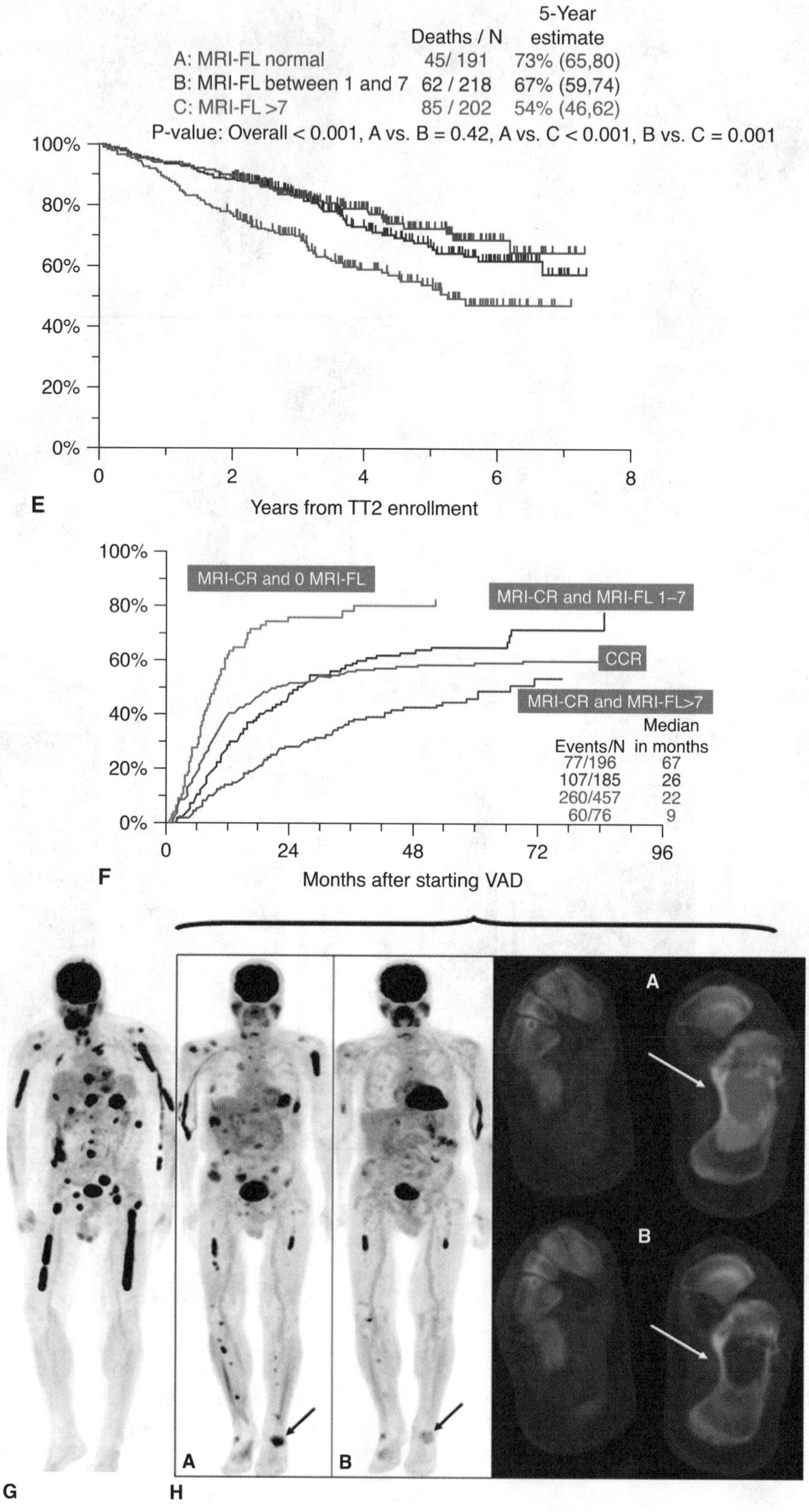

FIGURE 109–13. (*continued*) **E.** Survival after Total Therapy 2 (TT 2) is negatively affected not only by numbers of MRI-defined focal lesions (FL). *(Reproduced with permission from Walker R, Barlogie B, Haessler J, et al: Magnetic resonance imaging in multiple myeloma: diagnostic and clinical implications.* J Clin Oncol *25:1121, 2007.)* **F.** Attainment of MRI-CR lags behind in patients with more than seven MRI-defined focal lesions. CCR, clinical complete response. *(Reproduced with permission from Walker R, Barlogie B, Haessler J, et al: Magnetic resonance imaging in multiple myeloma: diagnostic and clinical implications.* J Clin Oncol *25:1121, 2007.)* **G.** Myeloma patient with extensive macrofocal active disease at baseline. **H.** Panel A demonstrates multifocal active bony myelomatous disease in a patient who is treatment naïve. One of the largest hyper metabolic foci lies within the left calcaneus bone where osteolysis is seen on CT. Panel B is the same patient after the patient has undergone one cycle of treatment, demonstrating a good response to therapy with a decrease in both the number of focal lesions and their metabolic activity.

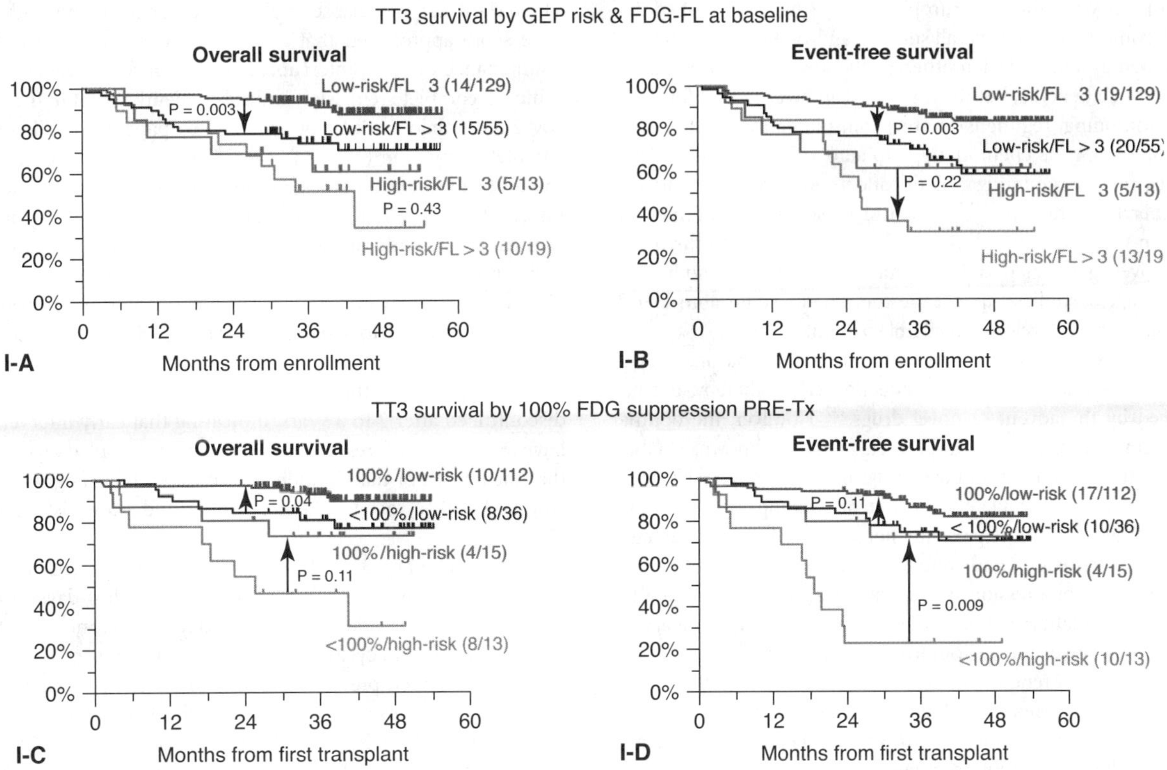

FIGURE 109–13. *(continued)* **I.** Patients who have good risk myeloma based on the 70-gene model and who have ≤3 focal lesions (FL) on PET enjoy superior overall survival (*panel A*) and event-free survival (*panel B*). Patients with high-risk myeloma as defined by the 70-gene model who do not achieve a PET-defined complete response have dismal overall survival (*panel C*) and event-free survival (*panel D*). *(Reproduced with permission from Bartel TB, Haessler J, Brown TL, et al: F18-fluorodeoxyglucose positron emission tomography in the context of other imaging techniques and prognostic factors in multiple myeloma.* Blood *114:2068, 2009.)*

Fluoro-2-deoxyglucose (FDG)-PET scanning is a convenient tool of whole-body imaging when performed in the context of CT scanning. This whole-body approach not only allows detection of bony myelomatous disease, but also provides easier detection of extramedullary disease and possible infection in these patients. Osteolysis, if present, is seen on the CT portion of the examination. An advantage of FDG-PET/CT imaging is early detection of metabolic disease and short-term monitoring of response to therapy (Fig. 109–13G and H). Because PET imaging is dependent upon metabolic uptake, active disease is often identified even before bony destruction occurs on anatomic imaging. Likewise, resolution of active disease is typically immediate on FDG-PET, whereas the abnormalities seen on MRI or CT usually take longer to resolve or never resolve. It has been shown that the number of focal lesions on PET and their metabolic intensity and the presence of extramedullary disease at baseline PET in untreated patients affect survival outcomes.[281] Particularly, in low-risk gene expression-defined patients more than three focal bone lesions on CT-PET independently imparted an inferior overall survival (Fig. 109–13I, panels A and B). Furthermore, failure to completely suppress FDG-PET uptake after induction therapy in high-risk patients was associated with a dismal outcome after auto-HSCT, suggesting that this allows for the identification of patients who require a different treatment approach (Fig. 109–13I, panels C and D). The usefulness of CT-PET is being investigated for predicting response and survival by early therapy-induced FDG suppression as has been shown in malignant lymphoma. Utilizing both MRI and FDG-PET/CT has 100 percent specificity and 100 percent positive predictive value, thereby warranting both imaging techniques in evaluating these patients.[318] Bone densimetric analysis is advised to establish the need for bisphosphonate administration and should be performed annually.[319]

DIFFERENTIAL DIAGNOSIS

If the initial laboratory evaluation indicates the presence of a monoclonal immunoglobulin in serum and or urine, the finding requires further studies to distinguish among (1) essential monoclonal gammopathy; (2) solitary plasmacytoma of bone or soft tissue; (3) indolent myeloma; (4) immunoglobulin deposition diseases, such as primary amyloidosis or LCDD; and (5) symptomatic or progressive myeloma.[185] Table 109–4 lists the important studies that can be done to distinguish among these possibilities. Tables 109–1 through 109–4 indicate the findings of symptomatic myeloma. The International Myeloma Working Group has developed new standardized diagnostic criteria that have been widely adopted.[185]

TREATMENT

■ MANAGEMENT OF NEWLY DIAGNOSED MYELOMA

Every newly diagnosed myeloma patient should be assessed for fitness to undergo auto-HSCT. Although some centers use an age cutoff (usually ≤60–65 years), it is reasonable to take performance status, organ function, and comorbidities into account, rather than age, when deciding whether a patient is eligible. Emerging data from the Arkansas Total Therapy trials suggest that the goal of myeloma therapy has changed from achieving disease control to achieving long-term disease-free survival, if not cure, in the majority of patients. In this context one should adopt a strategic approach to therapy. Enrollment of the patient in clinical trials that include auto-HSCT and that use risk stratification based on cytogenetic or gene-expression data is advisable.

Four prospective randomized European studies have established that auto-HSCT confers superior overall survival and/or event-free survival when compared to standard chemotherapy therapy.[320–323] Three studies did not show such benefits, but these studies can be criticized for using inferior conditioning regimens in the transplantation group, high crossover rates from the chemotherapy to auto-HSCT arm for refractory patients, and the randomization of patients after induction chemotherapy rather than initially.[324–326] Each of these studies commenced enrollment in the 1990s and, thus, were conducted prior to the introduction of novel agents such as thalidomide, lenalidomide, and bortezomib. Nevertheless, studies support the continued role for auto-HSCT in the management of myeloma in eligible patients.

Vincristine, doxorubicin (Adriamycin), and dexamethasone (VAD) had long been used as the standard induction chemotherapy, but has been replaced by the advent of novel drugs.[327] However, the optimal induction therapy prior to auto-HSCT is currently not known. Doublet and especially triplet regimens of novel drugs in combination with dexamethasone can induce complete remission rates comparable to transplantation regimens.[328,329] It is presently not known whether these high, very good, partial remission and complete remission rates translate into improved long-term progression-free survival and overall survival after autologous transplantation. Combinations that include alkylating agents should be avoided since damage to normal hematopoietic stem cells can be incurred, which may render it impossible to collect stem cells for auto-HSCT.[330] Lenalidomide may also hamper the collection of stem cells, although stem cell mobilization with growth factors and chemotherapy may overcome the myelosuppressive effects of lenalidomide.[331–334] An International Myeloma Working Group panel recommends the collection of stem cells within the first six cycles of treatment regimens containing thalidomide, lenalidomide, or bortezomib.[335]

The concept of two sequential (tandem) auto-HSCT was based on the notion that in adult acute leukemia cures were not observed unless a complete remission rate of 40 percent was achieved. Because a single transplantation yields a rate of 20 percent, it was hypothesized that a tandem auto-HSCT would yield a complete remission rate of 40 percent and would result in the cure of at least some patients.[336–339] Seven randomized trials have been published comparing single versus tandem auto-HSCT. One trial was withdrawn as a result of inconsistencies in the dataset.[340] Of the remaining six studies, five report superior event-free survival and two studies report better overall and event-free survival for the tandem transplantation group. Both the Bologna 96 and Intergroupe Francophone du Myélome 94 studies reported that patients who benefitted most from a second transplantation were those who did not achieve at least a very good partial remission after the first transplantation. It has, therefore, been proposed to reserve a second transplantation for this particular subgroup of patients, although in a stringent multivariate analysis of all three Total Therapy trials a second transplantation was important when this parameter was introduced as a time-dependent covariate.[341]

Combination therapy with novel drugs achieve complete remission rates comparable to those obtained with auto-HSCT, which has led to the design of ongoing studies that compare novel agents followed by auto-HSCT with novel agents and, then, auto-HSCT in case of disease relapse. Novel agents seen to be able to overcome some of the cytogenetic adverse prognostic factors such as del 13, t(4;14), and del 17p. It is too early to abandon auto-HSCT as the followup in clinical trials with new agents is too short to determine whether increased complete remission rates translate into durable remissions and event-free survival and overall survival. Complete remission rates as a surrogate marker for eventual outcome may prove to be inadequate. In the Total Therapy 3 study sustaining a complete remission for 3 years rather than mere achievement of the remission was critical for long-term survival. The hazard risk for relapse in Total Therapy 3 patients with a high 70-gene score approached that of patients with low-risk myeloma after maintenance of an uninterrupted remission for 3 years. Patients who achieved complete remission and subsequently lost it in the Total Therapy 2 study had an inferior outcome to patients who never attained complete remission (Fig. 109–14).[342] Data derived from clinical trials should be allowed to mature as long-term followup may yield surprising results. In the tandem auto-HSCT Total Therapy 2 study, patients were initially randomized to thalidomide or no thalidomide during their entire treatment program and improved event-free survival was observed early. However, the curves measuring overall survival for the two groups started to separate at 5 years, achieving statistical significance in favor of the thalidomide group at 10 years. This is unexpected, taking into account that in a sizeable fraction thalidomide had been discontinued after 2 to 3 years, indicating that early interventions may have long-term unforeseen consequences.[343] Detailed analysis revealed that the benefit of thalidomide was confined to a subgroup of patients who had both cytogenetic abnormalities and a low-risk 70-gene score (Fig. 109–15).

In Total Therapy 3, bortezomib, which both targets myeloma cells and the microenvironment, was combined with 4-days of oral dexamethasone, daily thalidomide, and 4 days of continuous-infusion cisplatin, doxorubicin, cyclophosphamide, and etoposide (DT PACE). DT PACE is a regimen previously shown to be highly effective as therapy for relapsed patients.[344] Two cycles of Velcade (bortezomib), doxorubicin (Doxil), dexamethasone (VTD), as part of VTD-PACE, were used as induction and consolidation therapy, respectively, prior to and after melphalan 200 mg/m^2 tandem auto-HSCT (Fig. 109–16). VTD was given for 1 year as maintenance followed by 2 years dexamethasone and thalidomide. The principal findings of Total Therapy 3 are: (1) unprecedented high overall survival, event-free survival, and duration of complete remission when compared to Total Therapy 2 and Total Therapy 1 studies (Fig. 109–17)[345,346]; (2) an anticipated cure fraction in the order of 50 percent in the 85 percent of patients who have a low-risk gene-expression profile (Fig. 109–18); (3) MMSET-type myeloma, characterized by t(4;14) no longer confers a poor prognosis (Fig. 109–19)[347]; (4) del 17p is only an adverse variable in patients with a high-risk gene-expression profile (Fig. 109–20); and (5) high-risk myeloma, defined by the 70-gene risk score, still has a poor outcome (Fig. 109–21).[348] The results of Total Therapy 3 have led to the assignment of newly diagnosed myeloma to two different protocols based on the 70-gene risk score. Total Therapy 4 randomizes low-risk patients to standard Total Therapy 3 versus a lighter version of Total Therapy 3 with the goal of reducing toxicity but retaining the superior efficacy observed in the original Total Therapy 3 study. High-risk patients are assigned to a single-arm Total Therapy 5 study that combines melphalan and VTD-PACE throughout the treatment regimen, thus applying a more dose-dense, but less dose-intense schedule, which relies on drug synergism rather than dose escalation.

THERAPY FOR THE TRANSPLANTATION-INELIGIBLE PATIENT

The traditional age limit for autotransplantation is 65 years, although older patients should be considered for transplantation provided good organ function is present. Physiologic rather than chronologic age is more suitable for determining transplantation eligibility (see Chap. 8). The standard of care for elderly patients for many years has been melphalan and prednisone (MP). However, the introduction of the novel drugs thalidomide, lenalidomide, and bortezomib has changed the treatment paradigm for the elderly patient population. Four randomized controlled trials suggest that melphalan, prednisone, and thalidomide

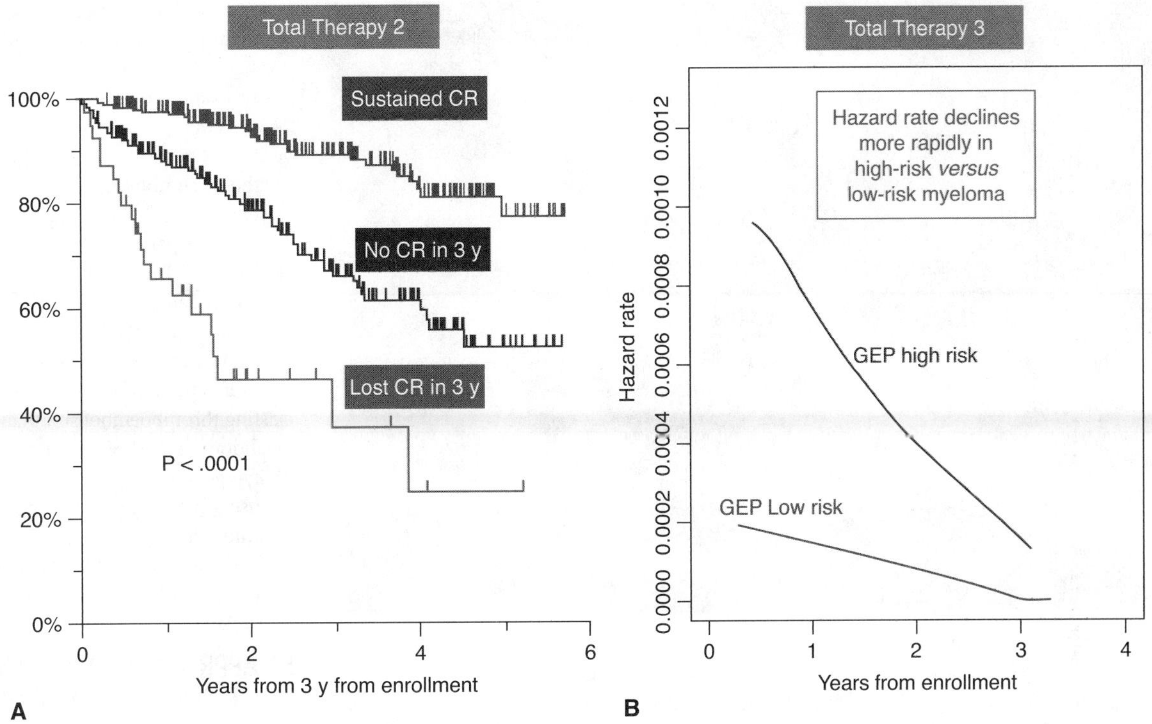

FIGURE 109–14. Complete remission duration rather than complete remission (CR) per se is a more meaningful endpoint in myeloma. **A.** Total Therapy 2 patients who lose a complete response have the worst survival. Patients who maintain their response enjoy the best outcome. **B.** Patients with high-risk myeloma as defined by the 70-gene risk model who remain in uninterrupted CR for 3 years have the same risk of relapse at 3 years as patients with low-risk myeloma. These findings indicate that sustenance of CR is the key to long-term survival in high-risk disease.

(MPT) provide significant benefit compared to MP alone, with four studies showing superior event-free survival and two French studies showing improved overall survival as well.[349–352] Based on these data, MPT has been proposed as the new standard of care for transplantation-ineligible patients. However, all studies showed an increase in adverse events in the MPT arm, including infections, neuropathy, and thromboembolism, suggesting that thromboprophylaxis and antimicrobial prophylaxis is required.[353]

The combination of bortezomib (Velcade), melphalan, and prednisone (VMP) may be an alternative initial regimen in elderly patients. A large Spanish phase I/II trial showed a complete remission and partial remission rate of 32 and 89 percent, respectively, with overall survival at 16 months reaching 91 percent, which was significantly better than MP-treated historical controls (66%).[354] A large randomized phase III study, the Velcade as Initial Standard Therapy in Multiple Myeloma (VISTA) trial, confirmed these findings and observed improved response rates including a complete response rate of 33 percent, superior time to progression (24 vs. 16 months), and better overall survival in the VMP arm. Some adverse cytogenetic features, including del 17p, t(4;14), and t(14;16) were overcome.[355] Bortezomib does have significant side effects, including peripheral neuropathy, transient cytopenias, and herpes zoster reactivation, and the latter necessitates antiviral prophylaxis. The

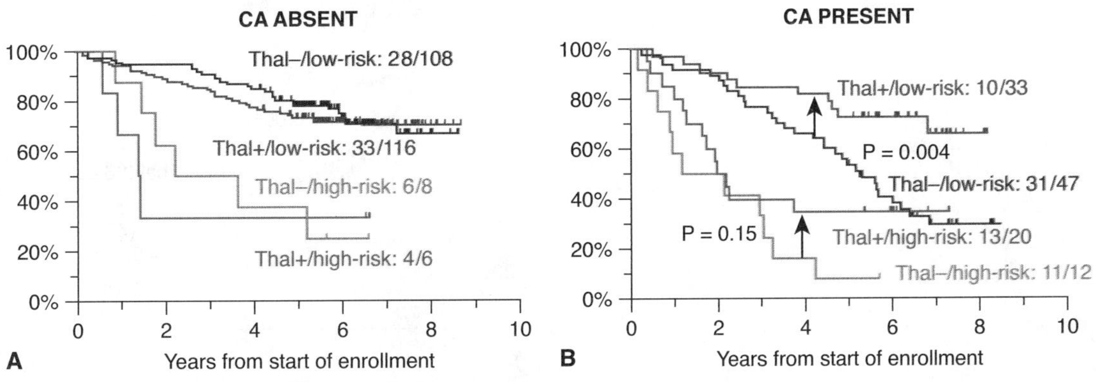

FIGURE 109–15. Long-term followup data of Total Therapy 2 randomizing patients upfront to thalidomide (Thal+) or no thalidomide (Thal–) indicate that patients with cytogenetic abnormalities (CA) and a low-risk 70-gene score are thalidomide beneficiaries (panel **B**). Patients with no cytogenetic abnormalities do not benefit regardless of 70-gene risk assignment (panel **A**).

	TT1	TT2 (+/– THAL)	TT3 (VEL- THAL)
	5 cycles	*4 cycles*	*2 cycles*
INDUCTION	VAD x 4 CTX EDAP	VAD DCEP CAD DCEP	VTD-PACE x 2
TANDEM TRANSPLANTATION	MEL200 x 2	MEL200 x 2	MEL200 x 2
CONSOLIDATION	None	D-PACE x 4	VTD-PACE x 2
MAINTENANCE	IFN indefinitely	IFN + DEX indefinitely	VRD 3 y
Median followup	14 years	7 years	4 years

FIGURE 109–16. Overview of the treatment regimens utilized in the Total Therapy protocols. CAD, Cytoxan, Adriamycin, Dexamethasone; CTX, Cytoxan (cyclophosphamide); DCEP, DEX, Cyclophosphamide, Etoposide, Cisplatin; DPACE, Dex, Cisplatin, Adriamycin, Cyclophosphamide, Etoposide; EDAP, Etoposide, Dexamethasone, Adriamycin, Cisplatin; IFN, Interferon; MEL, Melphalan; TT, Total Therapy; VAD, Velcade (bortezomib), Adriamycin (doxorubicin), Dexamethasone (decadron); VRD, bortezomib, lenalidomide, dexamethasone; VTDPACE, Velcade, Thalidomide, Dexamethasone, Cisplatin, Adriamycin, Cytoxan, Etoposide.

combination of melphalan, prednisone, and lenalidomide may also be useful initial management of older patient. An Italian phase I/II study reported a complete response rate of 24 percent with an event-free survival at 1 year of 92 percent.[356] It is not certain which of these combinations are superior and selection of a particular regimen may be tailored to the patient based on practical considerations. In patients with preexistent polyneuropathy it is probably wise to avoid bortezomib and thalidomide, whereas lenalidomide may be less suitable for patients with renal impairment. In patients with preexisting thromboembolism, thalidomide and lenalidomide are best avoided. The presence of cytogenetic abnormalities would favor the use of VMP or perhaps melphalan, lenalidomide, and prednisone. MPT could be selected because of decreased cost and the convenience of oral administration.

APPROACH TO RELAPSED OR REFRACTORY PATIENTS

A number of options are available for the therapy of relapsing patients. Long-term

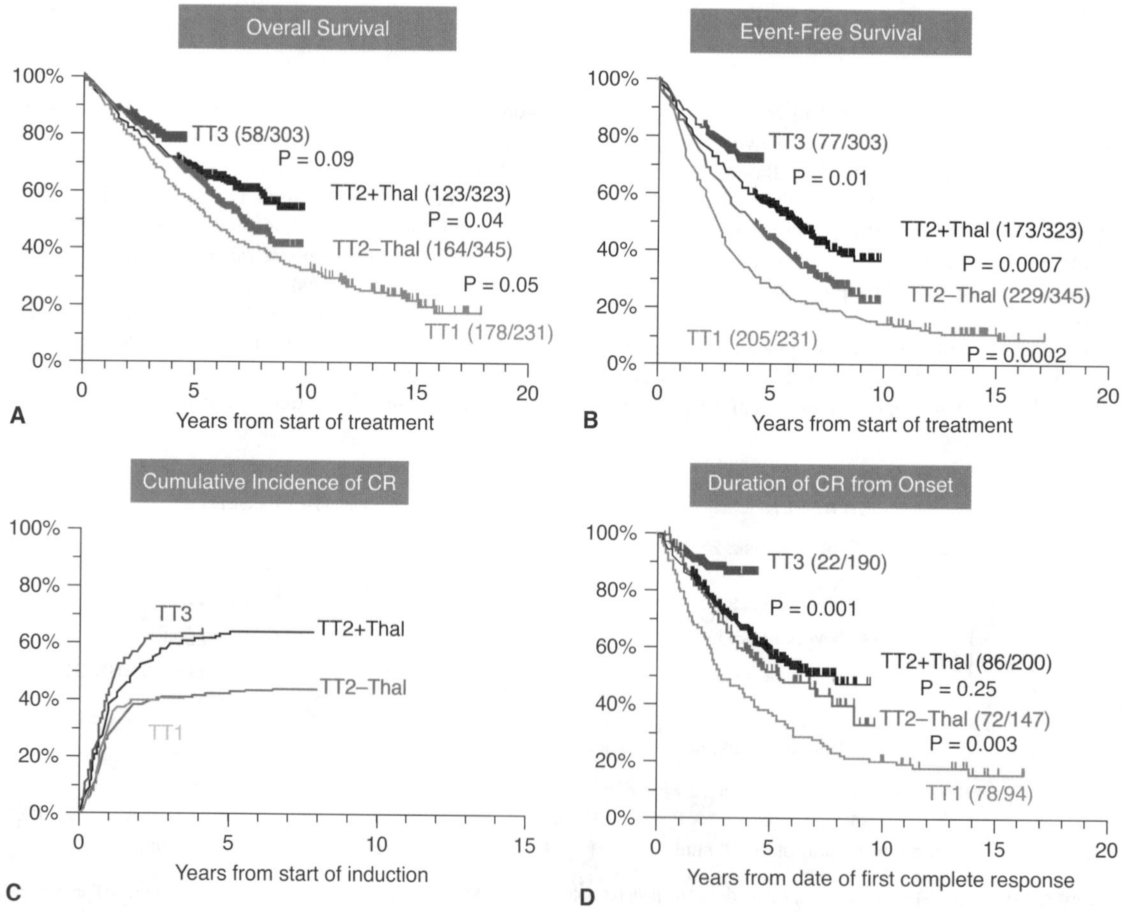

FIGURE 109–17. Improvement in overall survival, event-free survival, and complete response (CR) duration with successive Total Therapy protocols. Note that the CR rate in Total Therapy 3 and in the thalidomide (Thal) arm of Total Therapy 2 is similar, yet patients treated on Total Therapy 3 enjoyed superior overall survival and CR duration.

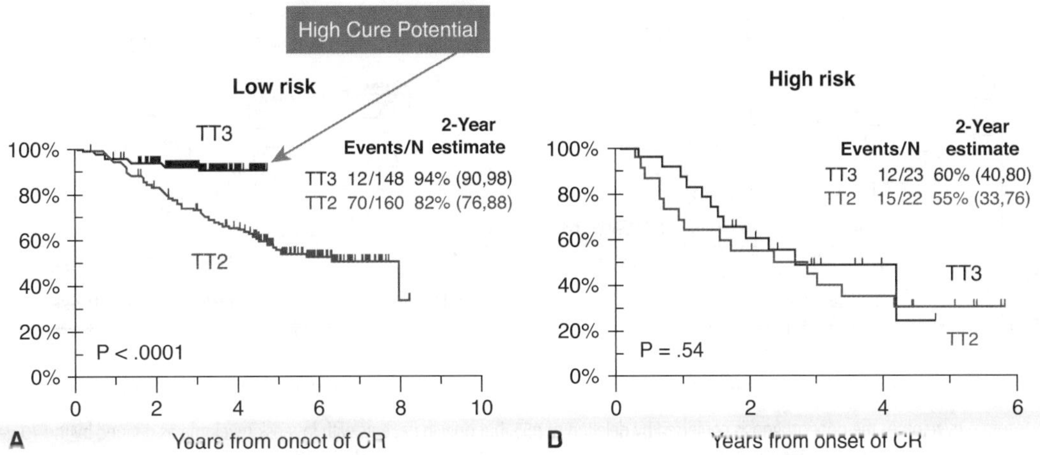

FIGURE 109–18. Patients treated on Total Therapy 3 study who have low-risk myeloma as defined by the 70-gene risk score, comprising 85% of patients, have durable complete remission, boding well for possible cure (panel **A**). No suggest progress has been made in high-risk patients (panel **B**). CR, complete response.

followup of the first thalidomide trial showed that 10 years after initiation of therapy 17 of the original cohort of 169 patients were alive and 10 have had an uninterrupted remission.[357] The combination of thalidomide and dexamethasone was superior to dexamethasone alone in several studies.[358–360] Patients who have had prior thalidomide exposure should probably best be treated with one of the other novel agents. Furthermore, cytogenetic abnormalities predict for a poor long-term response to thalidomide.[357,361] The thalidomide analogue, lenalidomide, is more potent than its predecessor and is not associated with sedation, peripheral neuropathy, and severe constipation. In two large, randomized phase III trials, lenalidomide with high-dose dexamethasone produced a superior response and delayed time-to-progression compared to dexamethasone and placebo.[362,363] The combination of lenalidomide and dexamethasone had activity in both bortezomib-naïve and previously treated patients, in thalidomide-resistant patients, and after prior auto-HSCT. An analysis of the expanded access lenalidomide program, enrolling 1438 patients, showed that the combination of lenalidomide and dexamethasone had an acceptable safety profile with less than 10 percent of patients experiencing pneumonia and deep-vein thrombosis.[364] Two phase II studies, SUMMIT and CREST, demonstrated activity of the bortezomib in relapsed or refractory myeloma patients.[365,366] An update of the 202 patients enrolled in the SUMMIT study showed median times to progression and duration of response of 7 and 13 months, respectively.[367] A similar analysis of the CREST study demonstrated 5-year survivals of 32 and 45 percent in patients treated with 1.0 mg/m^2 and 1.3 mg/m^2 of bortezomib, respectively.[368] The randomized phase III APEX study found a median overall survival of 30 months in the bortezomib group versus 24 months in the dexamethasone group.[369,370] Other regimens have been explored as well, including, for example, bortezomib and pegylated doxorubicin with or without thalidomide, bortezomib combined with thalidomide and dexamethasone, bendamustine with prednisone and thalidomide, lenalidomide with doxorubicin and dexamethasone.[371–375]

The choice of therapy for relapsed or refractory patients depends on a number of factors including time since last therapy, prior exposure to novel agents, alone or in combination, and drug-induced comorbidities, for example, neuropathy, renal malfunction, and loss of patient physiologic reserve. Data derived for the Total Therapy 2 study show that the most import predictor of outcome at the time of relapse was the 70-gene risk score (Fig. 109–22). The 3-year postrelapse survival of patients with a low-risk 70-gene score 71 percent versus only 17 percent for patients with a high-risk 70-gene score. Low-risk relapse will almost always respond to a suitable combination of novel agents. High-risk relapse, usually characterized by rapid if not explosive myeloma growth, has a poor prognosis, requiring immediate reinduction with a potent combination regimen such as VTD-PACE followed by either application of experimental regimens or attempt at salvage transplantation. A salvage transplantation always deserves consideration, especially

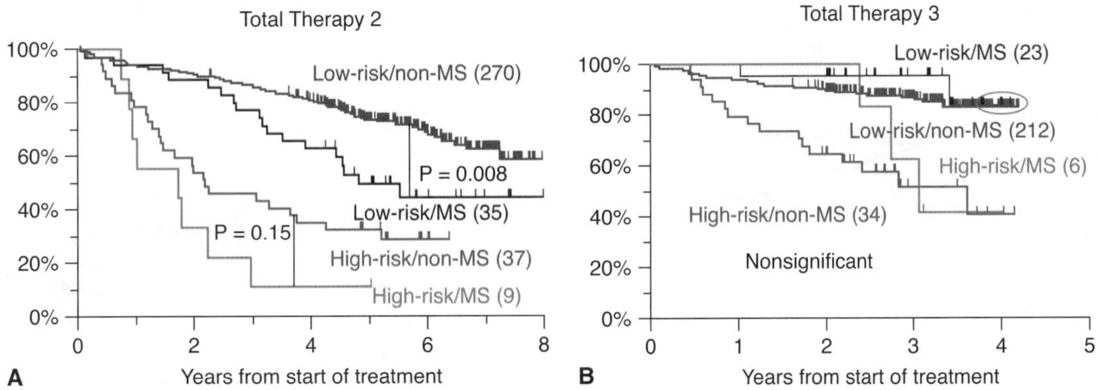

FIGURE 109–19. Incorporation of bortezomib in the Total Therapy 3 protocol (panel **B**) helps to overcome the poor prognosis conferred by the MMSET (MS)-type myeloma, characterized by t(4;14), in the Total Therapy 2 study (panel **A**).

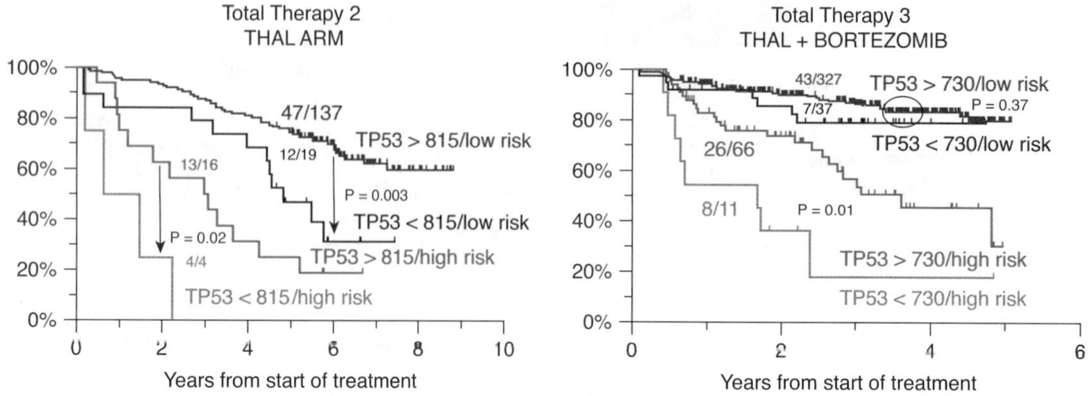

FIGURE 109–20. Bortezomib overcomes the poor prognosis conferred by deletion of p53, but only in patients with low-risk myeloma as defined by the 70-gene risk model (panel **B**). Deletion of p53 is a poor prognostic indicator in Total Therapy 2 regardless of the 70-gene score in both high-risk and low-risk myeloma (panel **A**). THAL, thalidomide.

in patients who have obtained more than 3 years benefit from their initial transplants.[376]

ALLOGENEIC HEMATOPOIETIC STEM CELL TRANSPLANTATION

Allogeneic transplantation was seen as an attractive option to treat myeloma because it has the potential to be curative, provides a donor graft that is not contaminated with myeloma stem cells, and may establish a graft-versus-myeloma (GVM) effect that could eradicate any surviving myeloma cells.[377,378] Furthermore, molecular remissions have been observed, which predict for longer survival.[379,380] However, the early experience with myeloablative allogeneic transplantation has not been encouraging as a result of a high mortality, varying from 30 to 50 percent, despite improvements made in patient selection and supportive care.[381–389] Reduced-intensity conditioning regimens were introduced to

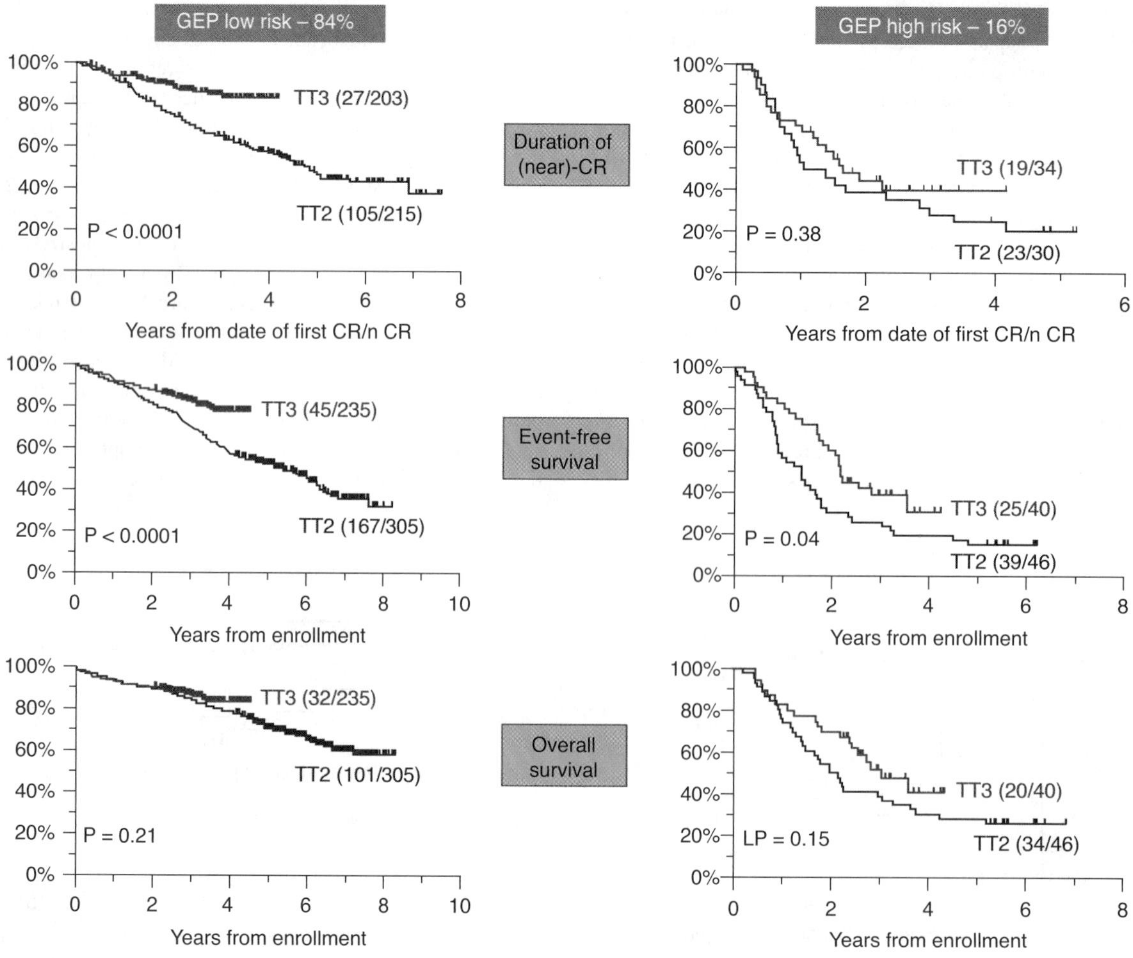

FIGURE 109–21. Comparison of outcome in Total Therapy 2 (TT2) based on 70-gene risk score. Note the enormous improvement with Total Therapy 3 (TT3) versus in the 85% of patients with low-risk myeloma. No such improvement is observed in defined high-risk myeloma, which continues to pose a formidable challenge.

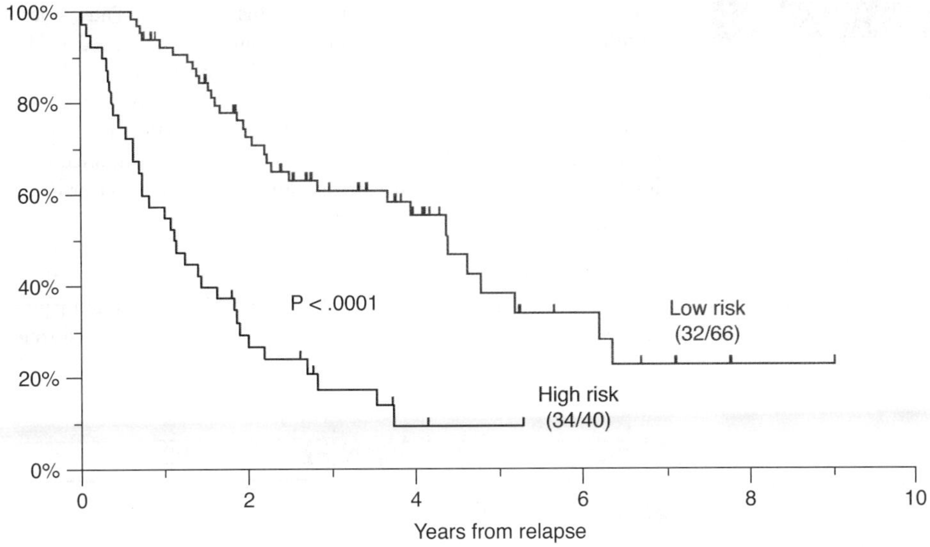

FIGURE 109–22. Patients who relapse on Total Therapy 2 and have a low-risk 70-gene risk score fare considerably better than their counterparts with high-risk myeloma.

reduce transplantation-related mortality and extend the age limit for allografting.[390–395] In order to combine the cytoreductive effect of high-dose therapy with the benefit of the GVM effect, a single auto-HSCT was used initially, followed approximately 3 months later with a reduced intensity allograft, a concept also referred to as a tandem auto-"mini"-allograft. There are no studies comparing tandem auto-HSCT prospectively with tandem auto-"mini"-allografting. Instead, studies rely on "genetic" randomization with patients who have an human leukocyte antigen (HLA)-identical sibling donor being assigned to a tandem auto-"mini"-allograft. Three randomized trials and one single center study detailing the long-term followup of 102 patients have been published.[396–400] All these studies report a significant morbidity and mortality with a posttransplantation mortality of 11 to 18 percent with chronic graft-versus-host disease (GVHD) occurring in 43 to 74 percent of patients. One-third were still on immunosuppression after 5 years and donor lymphocyte transfusions were relatively ineffective.[401] Furthermore, GVHD did not protect from relapse, improve complete remission rate or duration, or prolong overall survival.[396,399,400] The 5-year overall survival varied from 35 to 64 percent, with a plateau being observed in only one study.[396] These data should be compared to the tandem auto-HSCT Total Therapy 2 study and a large French trial, in which the 5-year overall survival was on the order of 65 percent without incurring the transplantation-related mortality of 11 to 18 percent or the long-term morbidity associated with chronic GVHD.[343,402] In Total Therapy 2, nearly two-thirds of patients who had normal metaphase cytogenetics, implying good-risk disease, were alive at 7 years.[343,402] Total Therapy 3 utilized both thalidomide and bortezomib in induction pre- and consolidation and maintenance posttandem auto-HSCT, and early results suggest that overall survival will be superior to Total Therapy 3, especially in the 85 percent of patients with gene-expression profile-defined good-risk disease.[347]

It has been suggested that tandem auto-"mini"-allografting be limited to patients with high-risk disease in whom higher initial morbidity and mortality may be more acceptable. However, most allograft studies in myeloma lack comprehensive characterization of patients in terms of metaphase cytogenetic abnormalities or gene expression. Detection of del 13 and del 17p has been reported to be negative prognostic factors for allografting in myeloma.[403] Also, clonal metaphase cytogenetic abnormalities significantly increase the risk of relapse indicating the escape from the GVM effect.[404,405] Taken together these data suggest that good-risk patients will do exceeding well with current auto-HSCT approaches, especially when combined with novel drugs, which does not justify subjecting these patients to the toxicity associated with allograft procedures. Furthermore, high-risk patients do not benefit from current allograft approaches. Consequently, routine allografting for myeloma cannot be recommended. Allografting should only be undertaken in the context of clinical trials, which aim to reduce chronic GVHD, separate GVM from GVHD, and amplify the GVM effect to improve outcome by ameliorating toxicity and maximizing the antimyeloma effect of immunologic effector cells.[406]

MONITORING DISEASE MARKERS FOR DOCUMENTATION OF RESPONSE AND RELAPSE

The previously widely used criteria for assessing response developed by the European Bone Marrow Transplant Registry, also referred to as the European Bone Marrow Transplant criteria, have been supplanted by a new system for evaluating response, the International Uniform Response Criteria proposed by the International Myeloma Working Group (Table 109–8).[211,407] The new response criteria incorporate the serum-free light-chain assay to allow for assessment of patient previously thought to have hyposecretory or nonsecretory disease. Stricter definitions of complete remission resulted in the inclusion of a category of stringent complete remission in which monoclonal plasma cells are not detectable in the marrow by immunohistochemistry or immunofluorescence and the free light-chain ratio is normal. The previously used near complete remission (only positivity by serum monoclonal immunoglobulin immunofixation) is now included in the new category very good partial response and the previously used minor response category is eliminated.

Survival endpoints include progression-free survival, event-free survival, and disease-free survival. Progression-free survival is the time from start of therapy to myeloma progression or death and includes all patients. It is being used as a surrogate for overall survival. In the case of event-free survival, precise definition of what constitutes an event is required (e.g., significant drug toxicity, death, etc.). Stable disease is no longer used as a measure of treatment efficacy, but rather time-to-progression, which is measured from the start of therapy and, importantly, includes all patients entered into clinical studies. Duration of a response is calculated from the onset of response and only counts the subgroup of responding patients. Long-term followup is recommended to fully evaluate the impact of novel treatment, which is recommended as exemplified by the Total Therapy 2 data in which a difference in overall survival only appeared after 10 years. Other limitations of the new criteria are that response calls are determined by monoclonal immunoglobulin and marrow evaluation. Dynamic changes in skeletal events readily identified by modern imaging techniques such as MRI and CT-PET are excluded from response assessments.

TABLE 109–8. Uniform Response Criteria from the International Myeloma Working Group

Response Subcategory*	Response Criteria
CR	Negative immunofixation of the serum and urine and disappearance of any soft-tissue plasmacytomas and <5% plasma cells in marrow.†
sCR	CR as defined above plus
	Normal FLC ratio and
	Absence of clonal cells in marrow† by immunohistochemistry or immunofluorescence.‡
VGPR	Serum and urine M-component detectable by immunofixation but not on electrophoresis or 90 or greater reduction in serum M-component plus urine M-component <100 mg per 24 h.
PR	>50% reduction of serum M-protein and reduction in 24-h urinary M-protein by >90% or to <200 mg per 24 h.
	If the serum and urine M-protein are unmeasurable, >50% decrease in the difference between involved and uninvolved FLC levels is required in place of the monoclonal Ig criteria.
	If serum and urine monoclonal Ig are unmeasurable, and serum-free light assay is also unmeasurable, >50% reduction in plasma cells is required in place of M-protein, provided baseline marrow plasma cell percentage was >30%.
	In addition to the above listed criteria, if present at baseline, a >50% reduction in the size of soft-tissue plasmacytomas is also required.
	Not meeting criteria for CV, VGPR, PR, or progressive disease.

CR, complete response; FLC, free light chain; PR, partial response; sCR, stringent complete response; SD, stable disease; VGPR, very good partial response.

*All response categories require two consecutive assessments made at anytime before the institution of any new therapy; complete and PR and SD categories also require no known evidence of progressive or new bone lesions if radiographic studies were performed. Radiographic studies are not required to satisfy these response requirements.

†Confirmation with repeat marrow biopsy not needed.

‡Presence/absence of clonal cells is based upon the κ/λ of >4:1 or <1:2. Alternatively, the absence of clonal plasma cells can be defined based on the investigation of phenotypically aberrant plasma cells. The sensitivity level is 10^{3-} (less than on phenotypically aberrant plasma within a total of 1000 plasma cells). Examples of aberrant phenotypes include (1) $CD38+^{dim}$ and $CD56+^{strong}$, CD19– , and CD45– ; (2) $CD38+^{dim}$, CD138+, CD56++, and CD28+; (3) CD138+, CD19– , CD56++, and CD117+.[482]

NOTE: SD is not recommended for use as an indicator of response; stability of disease is best described by providing the time-to-progression estimates.

Disease features can change over the course of the disease, now often spanning more than 10 years. Not infrequently, with successive relapses, clonal evolution occurs, resulting in loss of previously secreted complete immunoglobulin and switch to only light-chain secretion ("Bence Jones escape") or entire loss of immunoglobulin-secretory capacity, often associated with extramedullary spread, best signified by increased LDH levels and lesions found on CT-PET examination. Occasionally, unexplained anemia or pancytopenia accompanies disappearing myeloma protein markers, necessitating prompt marrow examination to detect fulminant relapse.

Many induction regimens currently in use affect tumor cytoreduction rapidly, so that monoclonal immunoglobulin reduction of 50 percent or more is apparent within a few months of therapy. Thus, at least monthly myeloma protein evaluations should be performed during induction. After two to four induction cycles and prior to high-dose melphalan-based auto-HSCT, the disease is restaged, to include marrow examination with cytogenetics and MRI and/or CT-PET of indicator lesions in order to capture whether intramedullary or extramedullary disease has been reduced. Disease monitoring should be performed at least every month for the first year and at a minimum every other month thereafter. Marrow biopsy, including cytogenetic examinations, should be performed at least semiannually, and more frequently in cases in which cytogenetic abnormalities were documented at diagnosis. MRI examination of previously abnormal sites should be performed every 3 to 6 months.

SPECIAL DISEASE MANIFESTATIONS

IGM MYELOMA

A rare diagnostic dilemma concerns the existence of an IgM myeloma entity that is distinct from Waldenström macroglobulinemia (histopathologic diagnosis, immunocytoma).[61,408] Upon examination, plasma cells, rather than the lymphoplasmacytic infiltrate, are seen to dominate the marrow of myeloma, whereas mastocytosis is a hallmark of immunocytoma. DNA-aneuploidy and the presence of lytic bone lesions support a diagnosis of myeloma. Myeloma, also of the IgM isotype, is resistant to purine analogues, which are effective in Waldenström macroglobulinemia.[409,410]

SOLITARY PLASMACYTOMA

Solitary plasmacytoma of bone[411–413] or soft tissue[414,415] requires the absence of indicators of systemic disease, such as marrow plasmacytosis, anemia, or other lytic or soft-tissue lesions. Histologic or cytologic evidence of monoclonal plasma cell infiltration is required. Approximately 50 percent of patients with solitary plasmacytoma have low monoclonal immunoglobulin levels in serum or urine that typically disappear upon institution of effective radiotherapy (40 to 50 Gy), as shown by immunofixation analysis. Persistence of monoclonal protein after therapy may indicate a background of essential monoclonal gammopathy or the presence of multifocal lesions. CT is recommended for a more detailed evaluation of early bone disease not recognized on standard roentgenographic examination.[416] MRI and FDG-PET scanning are powerful tools for detecting plasma cell myeloma involving the marrow in a macrofocal fashion or solitary plasmacytoma.[413,417–420] The detection of a solitary MRI lesion (cytologically proven) in the setting of essential monoclonal gammopathy changes the diagnosis to solitary plasmacytoma. In contrast to most patients with plasma cell myeloma, patients with solitary plasmacytoma or essential monoclonal gammopathy have normal serum immunoglobulin levels.

Multiple solitary plasmacytomas may be seen at the outset as a result of advanced imaging by MRI and PET, or these may develop over time in approximately 5 percent of patients with apparently solitary plasmacytoma (Table 109–9). Random marrow examinations should be negative.

Patients with soft-tissue solitary plasmacytomas can often be cured with appropriate local radiation (dose of at least 4.5 Gy). By contrast, this local treatment approach fails in the majority of patients with solitary plasmacytomas of bone.[421] The development of myeloma in such patients probably reflects multifocal systemic disease present at the outset and hitherto not detectable by standard radiographic imaging but readily by applying MRI[422] and CT-PET.[423]

Local radiation, typically administered with high-dose dexamethasone, also has a palliative role for the treatment of focal lesions as part

TABLE 109–9. Multiple Solitary Plasmacytomas (± Recurrent)

No monoclonal immunoglobulin in serum and/or urine*
More than one localized area of bone destruction or extramedullary tumor of clonal plasma cells which may be recurrent
Normal marrow
Normal skeletal survey and magnetic resonance image of spine and pelvis if done
No related organ or tissue impairment (no end organ damage other than the localized bone lesions)[185]

*A small monoclonal immunoglobulin may sometimes be present.

SOURCE: Reproduced from The International Myeloma Working Group. Criteria for the classification of monoclonal gammopathies, multiple myeloma and related disorders: a report of the International Myeloma Working Group. *Br J Haematol* 121:749, 2003 (Table IX).

of disseminated myeloma. However, especially in newly diagnosed patients, primary systemic therapy controls focal problems, including cord compression, as quickly and effectively as dose local radiation in the large majority of patients. Avoiding radiation to major marrow-containing skeletal regions preserves the ability to procure adequate blood stem cells in necessary quantity.

AL AMYLOIDOSIS

When clinical features of congestive heart failure, nephrotic syndrome, malabsorption, coagulopathy, skin rash (oral mucosal rash, "raccoon's eyes") or neuropathy are present, a careful search for primary amyloidosis should be carried out (see Chap. 110). LCDD may also have a similar clinical presentation. The primary difference between AL amyloidosis and LCDD is the difference in structure of the deposited protein; in AL amyloidosis it is fibrillar versus granular in LCDD. LCDD is usually associated with the κ light-chain subtype, whereas AL amyloidosis is associated with the λ light-chain subtype of myeloma.

Primary AL amyloidosis and immunoglobulin deposition diseases are best characterized functionally as essential monoclonal gammopathy with clinical manifestations because of normal tissue infiltration by these processes, although they can also accompany overt myeloma. Further workup following suspicion on clinical presentation depends on the organ of concern. Cardiac amyloidosis may be associated with low voltage on an electrocardiogram, arrhythmias, increased interventricular septal thickness greater than 12 mm, diastolic dysfunction or speckling on echocardiogram, and elevation of markers, such as B-type natriuretic peptide, N-terminal pro-B-type natriuretic protein, and cardiac troponin T.[424,425] Involvement of the gastrointestinal tract may present with decreased albumin and prealbumin. Renal involvement may present as nonspecific proteinuria with high total protein on 24-hour collection and low monoclonal immunoglobulin. Carpal tunnel syndrome and peripheral neuropathy may be a manifestation of amyloid, and nerve conduction studies may help in this diagnosis. Orthostatic hypotension also should alert to the possibility of systemic amyloidosis as a result of amyloid deposition in *vasa nervorum* of the autonomic nervous system or in adrenal glands resulting in hypoadrenalism. Occasionally, primary amyloidosis presents as tumors either mostly consisting of amyloid or mixed with plasmacytoma. Typically, MRI signals can distinguish plasmacytomas, which show hypointensity on T1-weighted images and hyperintensity on STIR-weighted images, whereas amyloidoma-type lesions remain hypointense.

Appropriate biopsy techniques should be applied to clarify the presence and extent of accompanying amyloidosis or, similarly, LCDD in these patients. The diagnosis of AL amyloid (see Chap. 110) often can be made by fine-needle aspiration of subcutaneous fat or by biopsy of the rectal mucosa,[426] although biopsy of accessible clinically involved tissue is preferable. AL amyloid also may be detectable on marrow biopsy.[252] Staining the tissue with Congo red may reveal perivascular amyloid with its classical apple-green birefringence when viewed under polarized light.[427] Thioflavin T is also a useful stain, producing intense yellow green fluorescence in AL amyloidosis. LCDD require immunofluorescence analysis of unfixed tissue; formalin fixation should be avoided whenever it is suspected.

Even though the tumor load is very low, patients with AL amyloidosis and immunoglobulin deposition disease suffer from the consequences of myeloma secretory products, even at relatively modest amounts, resulting in damage to kidneys, heart, gastrointestinal tract, liver, spleen, and peripheral and autonomic nerves. All current treatment targets the monoclonal plasma cell population and advances have paralleled the advances in treatment of myeloma. Whereas standard melphalan-prednisone has been only marginally effective, high-dose dexamethasone pulsing plus interferon, effecting more rapid and profound responses in myeloma, has also shown encouraging results in AL amyloidosis.[428,429] Similar positive results have been obtained with dexamethasone plus melphalan.[430] The Boston University group has pioneered the use of high-dose melphalan with auto-HSCT (see Fig. 109–16),[431] which is an effective regimen in carefully selected patients. In a study of 312 patients, high-dose melphalan (100–200 mg/m^2) with auto-HSCT resulted in a median survival of 4.6 years with a treatment-related mortality of 13 percent.[432] There was also significant improvement in organ function. The role of allogeneic transplantation in AL amyloidosis is unclear.

Cardiac amyloid remains the most challenging clinical condition and is currently addressed with repeated cycles of dose-reduced melphalan (70–100 mg/m^2) and stem cell support to avoid cardiac catastrophes possibly linked to arrhythmias, caused by fluid overload or cytokines.[433] There is a prevailing misconception that high-dose dexamethasone pulsing, alone or with added thalidomide, even at low doses, is safer and better tolerated than appropriately dosed melphalan with stem cell support. Owing to its hematopoietic stem cell–compromising properties, melphalan, even at 50 to 70 mg/m,[2] is still best administered in the context of autologous stem cell support. Incorporation of the newer agents, such as thalidomide, lenalidomide, and bortezomib, shows promising results in the treatment of patients with AL amyloidosis in combination with other agents such as melphalan, dexamethasone, and cyclophosphamide.

SMOLDERING MYELOMA

Patients with smoldering myeloma have historically been followed without therapy.[434–436] Once the diagnosis is established, through careful monitoring of disease markers over the duration of 2 to 3 months, these patients have been offered, at some institutions, thalidomide plus bisphosphonate therapy.[437] This approach has shown promising results by delaying the onset of progression to symptomatic disease and, in approximately 20 to 30 percent of patients, inducing mostly partial responses.[438] The Southwest Oncology Group has initiated a trial for patients with smoldering myeloma at high risk for early progression (IgA isotype, urinary light chain excretion >1 g/day, and presence of lytic lesions), evaluating thalidomide plus dexamethasone plus zoledronic acid. This secondary prevention trial is aimed at disease control through therapeutic cotargeting of both myeloma cells and the marrow microenvironment.

EMERGENT COMPLICATIONS OF NEW MYELOMA THERAPY

VENOUS THROMBOEMBOLISM

Patients with myeloma are at an increased risk for deep vein thrombosis and pulmonary embolism, particularly when known risk factors are present (history of venous thromboembolism [VTE], immobilization, dehydration others).[353] Genetic predispositions include high levels of homocysteine, and deficiencies of antithrombin III, protein C, and protien S, as well as mutations in the factor V Leiden and/or prothrombin genes. Genetic abnormalities should be suspected with repeated episodes of VTE. The incidence of VTE is highest during the first 3 to 4 months following diagnosis and occurs in approximately 3 to 4 percent of patients receiving either dexamethasone alone or MP, but is much higher when newer agents are combined with dexamethasone and melphalan.[327,349,351] A number of procoagulant abnormalities have been described in myeloma, including endothelial damage, paraprotein interference with fibrin structure, elevated von Willebrand multimers, elevated factor VIII, decreased protein S, and acquired activated protein C resistance.[439,440] A single nucleotide polymorphism analysis discovered 18 polymorphisms associated with thalidomide-induced VTE. These polymorphisms were involved in pathways important for drug transport or metabolism, DNA repair, and cytokine pathways.[441] The precise mechanisms causing VTE remain elusive, but the type of therapy plays an important role.

The incidence of VTE with single-agent thalidomide is approximately 2 to 4 percent in newly diagnosed and in relapsed patients, comparable to that observed with dexamethasone alone or MP, implying that thalidomide alone does not increase the risk of VTE. However, the risk for VTE increases significantly when thalidomide is combined with either dexamethasone, melphalan, doxorubicin, or cyclophosphamide, or with multiagent chemotherapy.[202,353] The combination of MPT causes VTE in 12 to 20 percent of patients who do not receive anticoagulant prophylaxis, whereas the incidence of VTE with thalidomide and dexamethasone in newly diagnosed patients was 14 to 26 percent.[327,349,351,442] Most VTEs occur within the first 60 days of therapy, coinciding with maximum cytoreduction. In the Total Therapy 2 study, 22 percent of patients developed a VTE, 95 percent of which occurred in the first 12 months of therapy.[443] Oral regimens principally promote deep vein thrombosis or pulmonary embolism, whereas infusional regimens can give rise to central line-related thrombosis in approximately 50 percent of patients.[441]

Single-agent lenalidomide does not appear to increase VTE, at least not in the setting of myeloma relapse, but is associated with a marked increased in VTE risk when lenalidomide is combined with dexamethasone.[353] Three risk factors for lenalidomide-associated VTE are higher dexamethasone doses, administration of erythropoietin, and concomitant administration of other agents. When combined with cyclophosphamide, the incidence of lenalidomide-induced VTE was 14 percent.[444] Bortezomib did not seem to increase the risk of VTE, at least not in patients with relapsed or refractory disease.[445]

Prevention of VTE is based on the assessment for known risk factors for VTE: (1) myeloma-related (hyperviscosity, newly diagnosed status); (2) therapy-related (high-dose dexamethasone [≥480 mg/month], doxorubicin, multiagent chemotherapy); (3) individual factors (age, history of VTE, inherited thrombophilia, obesity, immobilization, central venous line, infections, surgery, administration of erythropoietin); and (4) factors related to comorbidities (acute infection, diabetes mellitus, cardiac or renal dysfunction). Therapy-related risk factors weigh highest in the risk-equation of VTE. The following thromboprophylaxis is recommended: (1) acetylsalicylic acid (aspirin) in either a standard dose of 325 mg/day or in a low-dose of 81 mg/day for patients with one or no risk factor or (2) low-molecular-weight heparin (LMWH) once a day, or full-dose warfarin for patients if two or more risk factors or therapy-related risks are present. The recommended duration of prophylaxis in general is 6 to 12 months.[353]

Therapy for VTE should begin with standard therapeutic doses of LMWH. Oral anticoagulation may be considered as a followup. If oral anticoagulation is deemed inappropriate in a given patient, LMWH should be continued as long as the patient is receiving antineoplastic therapy. The optimal duration of therapy is unknown but one study reported a recurrence of VTE of 10 percent in patients who had discontinued anticoagulant therapy,[446] suggesting that long-term prophylaxis may be indicated in some patients. A survival benefit for patients who were anticoagulated for a VTE may suggested an additional effect of anticoagulants on the myelomatous process.[443]

PERIPHERAL NEUROPATHY

Bortezomib-[447,448] and thalidomide-induced[449,450] peripheral neuropathy should be distinguished from other causes such as paraneoplastic neuropathies, antecedent chemotherapy with neurotoxic agents (vincristine or cisplatinum), diabetes mellitus, and AL amyloidosis. Patients with AL amyloidosis of the peripheral nerves are especially sensitive to neurotoxic agents. Clinical findings include bilateral tingling, and numbness in the toes and/or fingers and/or pain ascending in the extremities when neurotoxic drug therapy is continued. Symptoms are typically in a glove-and-stocking distribution. Neurologic examination should evaluate sensory loss, deep tendon reflexes, and distal weakness, especially in the lower extremities. If significant weakness or asymmetry of signs is present, a neurologic consultation must be obtained along with electromyography and nerve conduction studies.

Bortezomib inhibits nuclear factor-κB activation, blocking the transcription of nerve growth factor–mediated neuron survival. Other proposed mechanisms for bortezomib-induced neuropathy include mitochondria and endoplasmic reticulum damage because of activation of the mitochondrial-based apoptotic pathway.[447,451,452] Second-generation, more selective proteasome inhibitors such as carfilzomib have a reduced neurotoxicity.[453] Grade 3 or 4 bortezomib-induced neurotoxicity occurs in approximately 20 percent of newly diagnosed patients and in 30 percent of patients with relapsing disease.[454–456] A 50 percent dose reduction should be made for bortezomib-induced grade 2 neuropathy while grade 3 or 4 requires drug discontinuation. Improvement or resolution of symptoms has been reported in 3 months, whilst in other patients maximum improvement may take 2 years.[365,454,457,458] Emerging results suggest that lenalidomide when combined with bortezomib may have a neuroprotective effect. The same may apply for heat shock protein-90 inhibitors.[459]

Daily thalidomide dose, dose intensity, cumulative dose ≥400 mg, and duration of therapy have all been implicated in the pathogenesis of thalidomide-induced neuropathy, which occurs in up to 75 percent of patients.[449,450,460–465] Dose reduction or cessation of therapy with the option of switching to lenalidomide will usually improve neuropathy, although resolution or improvement of neuropathy can take considerable time as thalidomide appears to induce an axonal-length-dependent neuropathy.[466] Symptomatic treatment for thalidomide- and bortezomib-induced neuropathy usually comprises gabapentin, pregabalin, or tricyclic antidepressants.

OSTEONECROSIS OF THE JAWS

Bisphosphonates are synthetic, stable analogues of inorganic pyrophosphate.[467] They bind to hydroxyapatite, the major calcium-containing bone mineral in areas where osteoclast-induced bone resorption occurs, thus exposing osteoclasts to high bisphosphonate concentrations.[468] The most commonly used bisphosphonates in myeloma are pamidronate and zoledronic acid, both of which induce osteoclast cell death, reducing skeletal events, such as pathologic fractures and hypercalcemia and improving osteoporosis, but without associated increase in overall survival.[469,470] Most experts currently recommend 2 years of bisphosphonate therapy with extended therapy for selected patients with active bone disease.[468,471,472] Osteonecrosis of the jaw (ONJ) is a severe "bone" disease, associated with bisphosphonate therapy that affects the jaws and typically presents as infection with necrotic bone in the mandible or maxilla. ONJ is characterized by the presence of exposed bone in the maxillofacial region that does not heal within 8 weeks. Although asymptomatic at times, ONJ usually presents as pain and/or numbness in the affected area, soft-tissue swelling, drainage, and tooth mobility. The exact cause of ONJ is not known and is likely to be multifactorial. The risk of developing ONJ increases with duration of bisphosphonate exposure and is 5 to 15 percent at 4 years.[473–475] A further predisposing factor for ONJ is invasive dental procedures such as extractions.[6,476] The incidence of ONJ is approximately 5 percent. Approximately 50 percent of affected patients had dental work prior to developing ONJ.[476] A genome-wide single nucleotide polymorphism analysis has shown that a polymorphism in the cytochrome P450–2C polypeptide is associated with an increased risk of developing ONJ on bisphosphonate therapy, although the mechanism underlying this genetic predisposition to ONJ has as yet not been elucidated.[477,478] To prevent ONJ, patients should be referred for dental evaluation prior to commencing intravenous bisphosphonates and should be advised to maintain excellent oral hygiene and avoid dental procedures while receiving these agents.[479] Antibiotic prophylaxis before dental procedures may reduce the incidence of ONJ in patients receiving bisphosphonate therapy.[480] Management is usually conservative (discontinuation of bisphosphonates, limited debridement, antibiotic therapy, and topical mouth rinses).[481] Surgical resection of necrotic bone should be reserved for refractory cases. A series of 97 patients observed healing of ONJ in 75 percent of patients. Patients who had developed spontaneous ONJ have a significantly higher risk of nonhealing and ONJ recurrence.[6]

PERSPECTIVE

Since the last edition of this textbook in 2006, enormous progress has been witnessed in fundamental and therapeutic research in myeloma. Gene-expression profiling has led to the molecular classification of myeloma into several distinct entities, similar to lymphoma and leukemia, which take into account not only the myeloma-based transcriptome, but also the microenvironment-associated gene signature. Gene-expression-defined risk models have been validated in multiple studies and capture with high precision patients in whom current therapies are destined to fail. It is the group of patients with gene-expression-defined high-risk myeloma who are most in need of future innovation. Several new drugs have been added to the therapeutic armamentarium, including bortezomib, thalidomide, and lenalidomide, which when applied in combination with or without dexamethasone, low-dose melphalan, and pegylated doxorubicin, can achieve complete remission rates similar to auto-HSCT. The long-term outcome of treatment with novel drugs is presently not known because of the short duration of followup. The protagonists of new drugs increasingly embrace a "Total Therapy-like" approach and combine multiple agents. The role of auto-HSCT has been questioned by some and clinical trials are being designed or are in progress to compare upfront melphalan-based auto-HSCT with auto-HSCT at the time of relapse. Perhaps the real debate, however, is not between the "transplanters" vis-à-vis the "novelists." At the time of this writing, it is evident that the incorporation of novel drugs into melphalan-based auto-HSCT treatment programs has led to enormous progress in myeloma. Nearly 85 percent of newly diagnosed myeloma patients have gene-expression-defined good risk and fare so well that the prospect of cure has become a reality. The rapid dissemination of DNA microarray-based technology should allow for identification of high-risk patients by the community oncologist in the near future, and enrollment of such patients in innovative trials is encouraged. Pharmacogenomics of both myeloma cells and the tumor microenvironment ultimately should lead to highly sophisticated, individualized, targeted therapies. A large number of new agents are presently in clinical trial, which will hopefully further improve myeloma outcome in the future.

REFERENCES

1. SEER: *Surveillance Epidemiology & End Results* [online]. Available at: http://seer.cancer.gov/csr/1975_2006/results_merged/sect_18_myeloma.pdf.
2. Bataille R, Harousseau JL: Multiple myeloma. *N Engl J Med* 336:1657, 1997.
3. Lynch HT, Sanger WG, Pirruccello S, et al: Familial multiple myeloma: A family study and review of the literature. *J Natl Cancer Inst* 93:1479, 2001.
4. Grosbois B, Jego P, Attal M, et al: Familial multiple myeloma: Report of fifteen families. *Br J Haematol* 105:768, 1999.
5. Bourguet CC, Grufferman S, Delzell E, et al: Multiple myeloma and family history of cancer. A case-control study. *Cancer* 56:2133, 1985.
6. Badros A, Terpos E, Katodritou E, et al: Natural history of osteonecrosis of the jaw in patients with multiple myeloma. *J Clin Oncol* 26:5904, 2008.
7. Vachon CM, Kyle RA, Therneau TM, et al: Increased risk of monoclonal gammopathy in first-degree relatives of patients with multiple myeloma or monoclonal gammopathy of undetermined significance. *Blood* 114:785, 2009.
8. Lynch HT, Ferrara K, Barlogie B, et al: Familial myeloma. *N Engl J Med* 359:152, 2008.
9. Kyle RA, Therneau TM, Rajkumar SV, et al: Prevalence of monoclonal gammopathy of undetermined significance. *N Engl J Med* 354:1362, 2006.
10. Landgren O, Gridley G, Turesson I, et al: Risk of monoclonal gammopathy of undetermined significance (MGUS) and subsequent multiple myeloma among African American and white veterans in the United States. *Blood* 107:904, 2006.
11. Cohen HJ, Crawford J, Rao MK, et al: Racial differences in the prevalence of monoclonal gammopathy in a community-based sample of the elderly. *Am J Med* 104:439, 1998.
12. Iwanaga M, Tagawa M, Tsukasaki K, et al: Prevalence of monoclonal gammopathy of undetermined significance: Study of 52,802 persons in Nagasaki City, Japan. *Mayo Clin Proc* 82:1474, 2007.
13. Ruiz-Delgado GJ, Ruiz-Arguelles GJ: Genetic predisposition for monoclonal gammopathy of undetermined significance. *Mayo Clin Proc* 83:601; author reply 602, 2008.
14. Riedel DA, Pottern LM: The epidemiology of multiple myeloma. *Hematol Oncol Clin North Am* 6:225, 1992.
15. Ichimaru M, Ishimaru T, Mikami M, Matsunaga M: Multiple myeloma among atomic bomb survivors in Hiroshima and Nagasaki, 1950–76: Relationship to radiation dose absorbed by marrow. *J Natl Cancer Inst* 69:323, 1982.
16. Iwanaga M, Tagawa M, Tsukasaki K, et al: Relationship between monoclonal gammopathy of undetermined significance and radiation exposure in Nagasaki atomic bomb survivors. *Blood* 113:1639, 2009.
17. Gramenzi A, Buttino I, D'Avanzo B, et al: Medical history and the risk of multiple myeloma. *Br J Cancer* 63:769, 1991.
18. Brown LM, Gridley G, Check D, Landgren O: Risk of multiple myeloma and monoclonal gammopathy of undetermined significance among white and black male United States veterans with prior autoimmune, infectious, inflammatory, and allergic disorders. *Blood* 111:3388, 2008.
19. Said W, Chien K, Takeuchi S, et al: Kaposi's sarcoma-associated herpesvirus (KSHV or HHV8) in primary effusion lymphoma: Ultrastructural demonstration of herpesvirus in lymphoma cells. *Blood* 87:4937, 1996.
20. Schalling M, Ekman M, Kaaya EE, et al: A role for a new herpes virus (KSHV) in different forms of Kaposi's sarcoma. *Nat Med* 1:707, 1995.
21. Soulier J, Grollet L, Oksenhendler E, et al: Kaposi's sarcoma-associated herpesvirus-like DNA sequences in multicentric Castleman's disease. *Blood* 86:1276, 1995.
22. Rettig MB, Ma HJ, Vescio RA, et al: Kaposi's sarcoma-associated herpesvirus infection of bone marrow dendritic cells from multiple myeloma patients. *Science* 276:1851, 1997.
23. Said JW, Rettig MR, Heppner K, et al: Localization of Kaposi's sarcoma-associated herpesvirus in bone marrow biopsy samples from patients with multiple myeloma [see comments]. *Blood* 90:4278, 1997.

24. Chauhan D, Bharti A, Raje N, et al: Detection of Kaposi's sarcoma herpesvirus DNA sequences in multiple myeloma bone marrow stromal cells. *Blood* 93:1482, 1999.
25. Raje N, Gong J, Chauhan D, et al: Bone marrow and peripheral blood dendritic cells from patients with multiple myeloma are phenotypically and functionally normal despite the detection of Kaposi's sarcoma herpesvirus gene sequences. *Blood* 93:1487, 1999.
26. Tarte K, Olsen SJ, Yang Lu Z, et al: Clinical-grade functional dendritic cells from patients with multiple myeloma are not infected with Kaposi's sarcoma-associated herpesvirus. *Blood* 91:1852, 1998.
27. Yi Q, Ekman M, Anton D, et al: Blood dendritic cells from myeloma patients are not infected with Kaposi's sarcoma-associated herpesvirus (KSHV/HHV-8). *Blood* 92:402, 1998.
28. Tisdale JF, Stewart AK, Dickstein B, et al: Molecular and serological examination of the relationship of human herpesvirus 8 to multiple myeloma: Orf 26 sequences in bone marrow stroma are not restricted to myeloma patients and other regions of the genome are not detected. *Blood* 92:2681, 1998.
29. Spisek R, Kukreja A, Chen LC, et al: Frequent and specific immunity to the embryonal stem cell-associated antigen SOX2 in patients with monoclonal gammopathy. *J Exp Med* 204:831, 2007.
30. Kyle RA, Therneau TM, Rajkumar SV, et al: A long-term study of prognosis in monoclonal gammopathy of undetermined significance. *N Engl J Med* 346:564, 2002.
31. Weiss BM, Abadie J, Verma P, et al: A monoclonal gammopathy precedes multiple myeloma in most patients. *Blood* 113:5418, 2009.
32. Kuehl WM, Bergsagel PL: Multiple myeloma: Evolving genetic events and host interactions. *Nat Rev Cancer* 2:175, 2002.
33. Bergsagel PL, Kuehl WM: Chromosome translocations in multiple myeloma. *Oncogene* 20:5611, 2001.
34. Barlogie B, Epstein J, Selvanayagam P, Alexanian R: Plasma cell myeloma—New biological insights and advances in therapy. *Blood* 73:865, 1989.
35. Hallek M, Bergsagel PL, Anderson KC: Multiple myeloma: Increasing evidence for a multistep transformation process. *Blood* 91:3, 1998.
36. MacLennan I, Chan E: The origin of bone marrow plasma cells, in *Epidemiology and Biology of Multiple Myeloma*, edited by G Obrams, M Potter, p 129. Springer, Berlin, Germany, 1991.
37. Okuno Y, Takahashi T, Suzuki A, et al: Establishment and characterization of four myeloma cell lines which are responsive to interleukin-6 for their growth. *Leukemia* 5:585, 1991.
38. Durie BG, Vela E, Baum V, et al: Establishment of two new myeloma cell lines from bilateral pleural effusions: Evidence for sequential *in vivo* clonal change. *Blood* 66:548, 1985.
39. Bast EJ, van Camp B, Reynaert P, et al: Idiotypic peripheral blood lymphocytes in monoclonal gammopathy. *Clin Exp Immunol* 47:677, 1982.
40. Berenson J, Wong R, Kim K, et al: Evidence for peripheral blood B lymphocyte but not T lymphocyte involvement in multiple myeloma. *Blood* 70:1550, 1987.
41. Mellstedt H, Holm G, Pettersson D, Peest D: Idiotype-bearing lymphoid cells in plasma cell neoplasia. *Clin Haematol* 11:65, 1982.
42. Pilarski LM, Jensen GS: Monoclonal circulating B cells in multiple myeloma. A continuously differentiating, possibly invasive, population as defined by expression of CD45 isoforms and adhesion molecules. *Hematol Oncol Clin North Am* 6:297, 1992.
43. Pilarski LM, Mant MJ, Ruether BA: Pre-B cells in peripheral blood of multiple myeloma patients. *Blood* 66:416, 1985.
44. Ruiz-Arguelles GJ, Katzmann JA, Greipp PR, et al: Multiple myeloma: Circulating lymphocytes that express plasma cell antigens. *Blood* 64:352, 1984.
45. Berenson JR, Lichtenstein AK: Clonal rearrangement of immunoglobulin genes in the peripheral blood of multiple myeloma patients. *Br J Haematol* 73:425, 1989.
46. Corradini P, Boccadoro M, Voena C, Pileri A: Evidence for a bone marrow B cell transcribing malignant plasma cell VDJ joined to C mu sequence in immunoglobulin (IgG)- and IgA-secreting multiple myelomas. *J Exp Med* 178:1091, 1993.
47. Billadeau D, Ahmann G, Greipp P, Van Ness B: The bone marrow of multiple myeloma patients contains B cell populations at different stages of differentiation that are clonally related to the malignant plasma cell. *J Exp Med* 178:1023, 1993.
48. Chen BJ, Epstein J: Circulating clonal lymphocytes in myeloma constitute a minor subpopulation of B cells. *Blood* 87:1972, 1996.
49. Bergsagel PL, Kuehl WM, Zhan F, et al: Cyclin D dysregulation: An early and unifying pathogenic event in multiple myeloma. *Blood* 106:296, 2005.
50. Cremer FW, Bila J, Buck I, et al: Delineation of distinct subgroups of multiple myeloma and a model for clonal evolution based on interphase cytogenetics. *Genes Chromosomes Cancer* 44:194, 2005.
51. Fonseca R, Barlogie B, Bataille R, et al: Genetics and cytogenetics of multiple myeloma: A workshop report. *Cancer Res* 64:1546, 2004.
52. Zandecki M, Lai JL, Facon T: Multiple myeloma: Almost all patients are cytogenetically abnormal. *Br J Haematol* 94:217, 1996.
53. Tabernero D, San Miguel JF, Garcia-Sanz M, et al: Incidence of chromosome numerical changes in multiple myeloma: Fluorescence in situ hybridization analysis using 15 chromosome-specific probes. *Am J Pathol* 149:153, 1996.
54. Raynaud SD, Bekri S, Leroux D, et al: Expanded range of 11q13 breakpoints with differing patterns of cyclin D1 expression in B-cell malignancies. *Genes Chromosomes Cancer* 8:80, 1993.
55. Meeus P, Stul MS, Mecucci C, et al: Molecular breakpoints of t(11;14)(q13;q32) in multiple myeloma. *Cancer Genet Cytogenet* 83:25, 1995.
56. Vaandrager JW, Kluin P, Schuuring E: The t(11;14)(q13;q32) in multiple myeloma cell line KMS12 has its 11q13 breakpoint 330 kb centromeric from the cyclin D1 gene. *Blood* 89:349, 1997.
57. Vasef MA, Medeiros LJ, Yospur LS, et al: Cyclin D1 protein in multiple myeloma and plasmacytoma: An immunohistochemical study using fixed, paraffin-embedded tissue sections. *Mod Pathol* 10:927, 1997.
58. Ronchetti D, Finelli P, Richelda R, et al: Molecular analysis of 11q13 breakpoints in multiple myeloma. *Blood* 93:1330, 1999.
59. Hoyer JD, Hanson CA, Fonseca R, et al: The (11;14)(q13;q32) translocation in multiple myeloma. A morphologic and immunohistochemical study. *Am J Clin Pathol* 113:831, 2000.
60. Janssen JW, Vaandrager JW, Heuser T, et al: Concurrent activation of a novel putative transforming gene, myeov, and cyclin D1 in a subset of multiple myeloma cell lines with t(11;14)(q13;q32). *Blood* 95:2691, 2000.
61. Avet-Loiseau H, Garand R, Lode L, et al: Translocation t(11;14)(q13;q32) is the hallmark of IgM, IgE, and nonsecretory multiple myeloma variants. *Blood* 101:1570, 2003.
62. Robillard N, Avet-Loiseau H, Garand R, et al: CD20 is associated with a small mature plasma cell morphology and t(11;14) in multiple myeloma. *Blood* 102:1070, 2003.
63. Chesi M, Nardini E, Lim RS, et al: The t(4;14) translocation in myeloma dysregulates both FGFR3 and a novel gene, MMSET, resulting in IgH/MMSET hybrid transcripts. *Blood* 92:3025, 1998.
64. Richelda R, Ronchetti D, Baldini L, et al: A novel chromosomal translocation t(4; 14)(p16.3; q32) in multiple myeloma involves the fibroblast growth-factor receptor 3 gene. *Blood* 90:4062, 1997.
65. Intini D, Baldini L, Fabris S, et al: Analysis of FGFR3 gene mutations in multiple myeloma patients with t(4;14). *Br J Haematol* 114:362, 2001.
66. Chesi M, Brents LA, Ely SA, et al: Activated fibroblast growth factor receptor 3 is an oncogene that contributes to tumor progression in multiple myeloma. *Blood* 97:729, 2001.
67. Ronchetti D, Greco A, Compasso S, et al: Deregulated FGFR3 mutants in multiple myeloma cell lines with t(4;14): Comparative analysis of Y373C, K650E and the novel G384D mutations. *Oncogene* 20:3553, 2001.
68. Perfetti V, Coluccia AM, Intini D, et al: Translocation T(4;14)(p16.3;q32) is a recurrent genetic lesion in primary amyloidosis. *Am J Pathol* 158:1599, 2001.
69. Shaughnessy J Jr, Gabrea A, Qi Y, et al: Cyclin D3 at 6p21 is dysregulated by recurrent chromosomal translocations to immunoglobulin loci in multiple myeloma. *Blood* 98:217, 2001.
70. Chesi M, Bergsagel PL, Shonukan OO, et al: Frequent dysregulation of the c-maf proto-oncogene at 16q23 by translocation to an Ig locus in multiple myeloma. *Blood* 91:4457, 1998.
71. Hanamura I, Iida S, Akano Y, et al: Ectopic expression of MAFB gene in human myeloma cells carrying (14;20)(q32;q11) chromosomal translocations. *Jpn J Cancer Res* 92:638, 2001.
72. Fonseca R, Harrington D, Oken MM, et al: Biological and prognostic significance of interphase fluorescence in situ hybridization detection of chromosome 13 abnormalities (delta13) in multiple myeloma: An eastern cooperative oncology group study. *Cancer Res* 62:715, 2002.
73. Dao DD, Sawyer JR, Epstein J, et al: Deletion of the retinoblastoma gene in multiple myeloma. *Leukemia* 8:1280, 1994.
74. Avet-Loiseau H, Facon T, Daviet A, et al: 14q32 translocations and monosomy 13 observed in monoclonal gammopathy of undetermined significance delineate a multistep process for the oncogenesis of multiple myeloma. Intergroupe Francophone du Myelome. *Cancer Res* 59:4546, 1999.
75. Drach J, Angerler J, Schuster J, et al: Interphase fluorescence in situ hybridization identifies chromosomal abnormalities in plasma cells from patients with monoclonal gammopathy of undetermined significance. *Blood* 86:3915, 1995.
76. Zandecki M, Obein V, Bernardi F, et al: Monoclonal gammopathy of undetermined significance: Chromosome changes are a common finding within bone marrow plasma cells. *Br J Haematol* 90:693, 1995.
77. Rasillo A, Tabernero MD, Sanchez ML, et al: Fluorescence in situ hybridization analysis of aneuploidization patterns in monoclonal gammopathy of undetermined significance versus multiple myeloma and plasma cell leukemia. *Cancer* 97:601, 2003.
78. Ernst TJ, Gazdar A, Ritz J, Shipp MA: Identification of a second transforming gene, rasn, in a human multiple myeloma line with a rearranged c-myc allele. *Blood* 72:1163, 1988.
79. Neri A, Murphy JP, Cro L, et al: Ras oncogene mutation in multiple myeloma. *J Exp Med* 170:1715, 1989.
80. Paquette RL, Berenson J, Lichtenstein A, et al: Oncogenes in multiple myeloma: Point mutation of N-ras. *Oncogene* 5:1659, 1990.
81. Portier M, Moles JP, Mazars GR, et al: p53 and RAS gene mutations in multiple myeloma. *Oncogene* 7:2539, 1992.
82. Liu P, Leong T, Quam L, et al: Activating mutations of N- and K-ras in multiple myeloma show different clinical associations: Analysis of the Eastern Cooperative Oncology Group Phase III Trial. *Blood* 88:2699, 1996.
83. Bezieau S, Devilder MC, Avet-Loiseau H, et al: High incidence of N and K-Ras activating mutations in multiple myeloma and primary plasma cell leukemia at diagnosis. *Hum Mutat* 18:212, 2001.

84. Bezieau S, Avet-Loiseau H, Moisan JP, Bataille R: Activating Ras mutations in patients with plasma-cell disorders: A reappraisal. *Blood* 100:1101; author reply 1103, 2002.
85. Corradini P, Ladetto M, Voena C, et al: Mutational activation of N- and K-ras oncogenes in plasma cell dyscrasias. *Blood* 81:2708, 1993.
86. Matozaki S, Nakagawa T, Nakao Y, Fujita T: RAS gene mutations in multiple myeloma and related monoclonal gammopathies. *Kobe J Med Sci* 37:35, 1991.
87. Crowder C, Kopantzev E, Williams K, et al: An unusual H-Ras mutant isolated from a human multiple myeloma line leads to transformation and factor-independent cell growth. *Oncogene* 22:649, 2003.
88. Neri A, Baldini L, Trecca D, et al: p53 gene mutations in multiple myeloma are associated with advanced forms of malignancy. *Blood* 81:128, 1993.
89. Drach J, Ackermann J, Fritz E, et al: Presence of a p53 gene deletion in patients with multiple myeloma predicts for short survival after conventional-dose chemotherapy. *Blood* 92:802, 1998.
90. Schultheis B, Kramer A, Willer A, et al: Analysis of p73 and p53 gene deletions in multiple myeloma. *Leukemia* 13:2099, 1999.
91. Mazars GR, Portier M, Zhang XG, et al: Mutations of the p53 gene in human myeloma cell lines. *Oncogene* 7:1015, 1992.
92. Corradini P, Inghirami G, Astolfi M, et al: Inactivation of tumor suppressor genes, p53 and Rb1, in plasma cell dyscrasias. *Leukemia* 8:758, 1994.
93. Preudhomme C, Facon T, Zandecki M, et al: Rare occurrence of P53 gene mutations in multiple myeloma. *Br J Haematol* 81:440, 1992.
94. Ackermann J, Meidlinger P, Zojer N, et al: Absence of p53 deletions in bone marrow plasma cells of patients with monoclonal gammopathy of undetermined significance. *Br J Haematol* 103:1161, 1998.
95. Teoh G, Urashima M, Ogata A, et al: MDM2 protein overexpression promotes proliferation and survival of multiple myeloma cells. *Blood* 90:1982, 1997.
96. Greil R, Fasching B, Loidl P, Huber H: Expression of the c-myc proto-oncogene in multiple myeloma and chronic lymphocytic leukemia: An *in situ* analysis. *Blood* 78:180, 1991.
97. Sawyer JR, Lukacs JL, Thomas EL, et al: Multicolour spectral karyotyping identifies new translocations and a recurring pathway for chromosome loss in multiple myeloma. *Br J Haematol* 112:167, 2001.
98. Shou Y, Martelli ML, Gabrea A, et al: Diverse karyotypic abnormalities of the c-myc locus associated with c-myc dysregulation and tumor progression in multiple myeloma. *Proc Natl Acad Sci U S A* 97:228, 2000.
99. Avet-Loiseau H, Gerson F, Magrangeas F, et al: Rearrangements of the c-myc oncogene are present in 15% of primary human multiple myeloma tumors. *Blood* 98:3082, 2001.
100. Latreille J, Barlogie B, Dosik G, et al: Cellular DNA content as a marker of human multiple myeloma. *Blood* 55:403, 1980.
101. Latreille J, Barlogie B, Johnston D, et al: Ploidy and proliferative characteristics in monoclonal gammopathies. *Blood* 59:43, 1982.
102. Caligaris-Cappio F, Bergui L, Gregoretti MG, et al: Role of bone marrow stromal cells in the growth of human multiple myeloma. *Blood* 77:2688, 1991.
103. Dewald GW, Kyle RA, Hicks GA, Greipp PR: The clinical significance of cytogenetic studies in 100 patients with multiple myeloma, plasma cell leukemia, or amyloidosis. *Blood* 66:380, 1985.
104. Gould J, Alexanian R, Goodacre A, et al: Plasma cell karyotype in multiple myeloma. *Blood* 71:453, 1988.
105. Sawyer JR, Waldron JA, Jagannath S, Barlogie B: Cytogenetic findings in 200 patients with multiple myeloma. *Cancer Genet Cytogenet* 82:41, 1995.
106. Van Den Berghe H: Chromosomes in plasma-cell malignancies. *Eur J Haematol Suppl* 51:47, 1989.
107. Shaughnessy J, Jacobson J, Sawyer J, et al: Continuous absence of metaphase-defined cytogenetic abnormalities, especially of chromosome 13 and hypodiploidy, ensures long-term survival in multiple myeloma treated with Total Therapy I: Interpretation in the context of global gene expression. *Blood* 101:3849, 2003.
108. Zhan F, Huang Y, Colla S, et al: The molecular classification of multiple myeloma. *Blood* 108:2020, 2006.
109. Kawano M, Hirano T, Matsuda T, et al: Autocrine generation and requirement of BSF-2/IL-6 for human multiple myelomas. *Nature* 332:83, 1988.
110. Klein B, Zhang XG, Jourdan M, et al: Paracrine rather than autocrine regulation of myeloma-cell growth and differentiation by interleukin-6. *Blood* 73:517, 1989.
111. Thomas X, Xiao HQ, Chang R, Epstein J: Circulating B lymphocytes in multiple myeloma patients contain an autocrine IL-6 driven pre-myeloma cell population. *Curr Top Microbiol Immunol* 182:201, 1992.
112. Hata H, Xiao H, Petrucci MT, et al: Interleukin-6 gene expression in multiple myeloma: A characteristic of immature tumor cells. *Blood* 81:3357, 1993.
113. Brandt SJ, Bodine DM, Dunbar CE, Nienhuis AW: Dysregulated interleukin 6 expression produces a syndrome resembling Castleman's disease in mice. *J Clin Invest* 86:592, 1990.
114. Suematsu S, Matsusaka T, Matsuda T, et al: Generation of plasmacytomas with the chromosomal translocation t(12;15) in interleukin 6 transgenic mice. *Proc Natl Acad Sci U S A* 89:232, 1992.
115. Grigorieva I, Thomas X, Epstein J: The bone marrow stromal environment is a major factor in myeloma cell resistance to dexamethasone. *Exp Hematol* 26:597, 1998.
116. Bataille R, Klein B: The bone-resorbing activity of interleukin-6. *J Bone Miner Res* 6:1143, 1991.
117. Hjorth-Hansen H, Waage A, Borset M: Interleukin-15 blocks apoptosis and induces proliferation of the human myeloma cell line OH-2 and freshly isolated myeloma cells. *Br J Haematol* 106:28, 1999.
118. Tinhofer I, Marschitz I, Henn T, et al: Expression of functional interleukin-15 receptor and autocrine production of interleukin-15 as mechanisms of tumor propagation in multiple myeloma. *Blood* 95:610, 2000.
119. Xu F, Gardner A, Tu Y, et al: Multiple myeloma cells are protected against dexamethasone-induced apoptosis by insulin-like growth factors. *Br J Haematol* 97:429, 1997.
120. Borset M, Hjorth-Hansen H, Seidel C, et al: Hepatocyte growth factor and its receptor c-met in multiple myeloma. *Blood* 88:3998, 1996.
121. Anderson KC: Moving disease biology from the laboratory to the clinic. *Semin Oncol* 29:17, 2002.
122. Tricot G: New insights into role of microenvironment in multiple myeloma. *Lancet* 355:248, 2000.
123. Roodman GD: Role of the bone marrow microenvironment in multiple myeloma. *J Bone Miner Res* 17:1921, 2002.
124. Ridley RC, Xiao H, Hata H, et al: Expression of syndecan regulates human myeloma plasma cell adhesion to type I collagen. *Blood* 81:767, 1993.
125. Wijdenes J, Vooijs WC, Clement C, et al: A plasmocyte selective monoclonal antibody (B-B4) recognizes syndecan-1. *Br J Haematol* 94:318, 1996.
126. Dhodapkar MV, Kelly T, Theus A, et al: Elevated levels of shed syndecan-1 correlate with tumour mass and decreased matrix metalloproteinase-9 activity in the serum of patients with multiple myeloma. *Br J Haematol* 99:368, 1997.
127. Dhodapkar MV, Abe E, Theus A, et al: Syndecan-1 is a multifunctional regulator of myeloma pathobiology: Control of tumor cell survival, growth, and bone cell differentiation. *Blood* 91:2679, 1998.
128. Borset M, Hjertner O, Yaccoby S, et al: Syndecan-1 is targeted to the uropods of polarized myeloma cells where it promotes adhesion and sequesters heparin-binding proteins. *Blood* 96:2528, 2000.
129. Aref S, Goda T, El-Sherbiny M: Syndecan-1 in multiple myeloma: Relationship to conventional prognostic factors. *Hematology* 8:221, 2003.
130. Rigolin GM, Tieghi A, Ciccone M, et al: Soluble urokinase-type plasminogen activator receptor (suPAR) as an independent factor predicting worse prognosis and extra-bone marrow involvement in multiple myeloma patients. *Br J Haematol* 120:953, 2003.
131. Seidel C, Sundan A, Hjorth M, et al: Serum syndecan-1: A new independent prognostic marker in multiple myeloma. *Blood* 95:388, 2000.
132. Yang Y, Macleod V, Miao HQ, et al: Heparanase enhances syndecan-1 shedding: A novel mechanism for stimulation of tumor growth and metastasis. *J Biol Chem* 282:13326, 2007.
133. Yang Y, MacLeod V, Bendre M, et al: Heparanase promotes the spontaneous metastasis of myeloma cells to bone. *Blood* 105:1303, 2005.
134. Alsayed Y, Ngo H, Runnels J, et al: Mechanisms of regulation of CXCR4/SDF-1 (CXCL12)-dependent migration and homing in multiple myeloma. *Blood* 109:2708, 2007.
135. Trentin L, Miorin M, Facco M, et al: Multiple myeloma plasma cells show different chemokine receptor profiles at sites of disease activity. *Br J Haematol* 138:594, 2007.
136. Kishimoto T, Akira S, Narazaki M, Taga T: Interleukin-6 family of cytokines and gp130. *Blood* 86:1243, 1995.
137. Chauhan D, Uchiyama H, Akbarali Y, et al: Multiple myeloma cell adhesion-induced interleukin-6 expression in bone marrow stromal cells involves activation of NF-kappa B: *Blood* 87:1104, 1996.
138. Feinman R, Koury J, Thames M, et al: Role of NF-kappaB in the rescue of multiple myeloma cells from glucocorticoid-induced apoptosis by bcl-2. *Blood* 93:3044, 1999.
139. Ge NL, Rudikoff S: Insulin-like growth factor I is a dual effector of multiple myeloma cell growth. *Blood* 96:2856, 2000.
140. Hideshima T, Nakamura N, Chauhan D, Anderson KC: Biologic sequelae of interleukin-6 induced PI3-K/Akt signaling in multiple myeloma. *Oncogene* 20:5991, 2001.
141. Mitsiades N, Mitsiades CS, Poulaki V, et al: Biologic sequelae of nuclear factor-kappaB blockade in multiple myeloma: Therapeutic applications. *Blood* 99:4079, 2002.
142. Pene F, Claessens YE, Muller O, et al: Role of the phosphatidylinositol 3-kinase/Akt and mTOR/P70S6-kinase pathways in the proliferation and apoptosis in multiple myeloma. *Oncogene* 21:6587, 2002.
143. Damiano JS, Cress AE, Hazlehurst LA, et al: Cell adhesion mediated drug resistance (CAM-DR): Role of integrins and resistance to apoptosis in human myeloma cell lines. *Blood* 93:1658, 1999.
144. Bataille R, Chappard D, Marcelli C, et al: Mechanisms of bone destruction in multiple myeloma: The importance of an unbalanced process in determining the severity of lytic bone disease. *J Clin Oncol* 7:1909, 1989.
145. Hofbauer LC, Heufelder AE: Osteoprotegerin and its cognate ligand: A new paradigm of osteoclastogenesis. *Eur J Endocrinol* 139:152, 1998.
146. Lee JW, Chung HY, Ehrlich LA, et al: IL-3 expression by myeloma cells increases both osteoclast formation and growth of myeloma cells. *Blood* 103:2308, 2004.
147. Pearse RN, Sordillo EM, Yaccoby S, et al: Multiple myeloma disrupts the TRANCE/osteoprotegerin cytokine axis to trigger bone destruction and promote tumor progression. *Proc Natl Acad Sci U S A* 98:11581, 2001.
148. Standal T, Seidel C, Hjertner O, et al: Osteoprotegerin is bound, internalized, and degraded by multiple myeloma cells. *Blood* 100:3002, 2002.
149. Choi SJ, Cruz JC, Craig F, et al: Macrophage inflammatory protein 1-alpha is a potential osteoclast stimulatory factor in multiple myeloma. *Blood* 96:671, 2000.

150. Abe M, Hiura K, Wilde J, Moriyama K, et al: Role for macrophage inflammatory protein (MIP)-1alpha and MIP-1beta in the development of osteolytic lesions in multiple myeloma. *Blood* 100:2195, 2002.
151. Han Z, Boyle DL, Chang L, et al: c-Jun N-terminal kinase is required for metalloproteinase expression and joint destruction in inflammatory arthritis. *J Clin Invest* 108:73, 2001.
152. Oyajobi BO, Franchin G, Williams PJ, et al: Dual effects of macrophage inflammatory protein-1alpha on osteolysis and tumor burden in the murine 5TGM1 model of myeloma bone disease. *Blood* 102:311, 2003.
153. Tian E, Zhan F, Walker R, et al: The role of the Wnt-signaling antagonist DKK1 in the development of osteolytic lesions in multiple myeloma. *N Engl J Med* 349:2483, 2003.
154. Body JJ, Greipp P, Coleman RE, et al: A phase I study of AMGN-0007, a recombinant osteoprotegerin construct, in patients with multiple myeloma or breast carcinoma related bone metastases. *Cancer* 97:887, 2003.
155. Yaccoby S, Ling W, Zhan F, et al: Antibody-based inhibition of DKK1 suppresses tumor-induced bone resorption and multiple myeloma growth *in vivo*. *Blood* 109:2106, 2007.
156. Yaccoby S, Wezeman MJ, Zangari M, et al: Inhibitory effects of osteoblasts and increased bone formation on myeloma in novel culture systems and a myelomatous mouse model. *Haematologica* 91:192, 2006.
157. Yaccoby S, Wezeman M, Henderson A, Barlogie B, Epstein J: Role and fate of osteoblasts in myeloma. *Hematol J* 4(Suppl 1) s38, 2003.
158. Qiang YW, Shaughnessy JD Jr, Yaccoby S: Wnt3a signaling within bone inhibits multiple myeloma bone disease and tumor growth. *Blood* 112:374, 2008.
159. Terpos E, Szydlo R, Apperley JF, et al: Soluble receptor activator of nuclear factor kappaB ligand-osteoprotegerin ratio predicts survival in multiple myeloma: Proposal for a novel prognostic index. *Blood* 102:1064, 2003.
160. Bataille R, Chappard D, Marcelli C, et al: Recruitment of new osteoblasts and osteoclasts is the earliest critical event in the pathogenesis of human multiple myeloma. *J Clin Invest* 88:62, 1991.
161. Yaccoby S, Epstein J: The proliferative potential of multiple myeloma plasma cells manifest in the SCID-hu host. *Blood* 94:3576, 1999.
162. Mundy GR: Metastasis to bone: Causes, consequences and therapeutic opportunities. *Nat Rev Cancer* 2:584, 2002.
163. Sezer O, Heider U, Zavrski I, et al: RANK ligand and osteoprotegerin in myeloma bone disease. *Blood* 101:2094, 2003.
164. Yaccoby S, Barlogie B, Epstein J: Primary myeloma cells growing in SCID-hu mice: A model for studying the biology and treatment of myeloma and its manifestations. *Blood* 92:2908, 1998.
165. Yata K, Yaccoby S: The SCID-rab model: A novel *in vivo* system for primary human myeloma demonstrating growth of CD138-expressing malignant cells. *Leukemia* 18:1891, 2004.
166. Vanderkerken K, Asosingh K, Croucher P, Van Camp B: Multiple myeloma biology: Lessons from the 5TMM models. *Immunol Rev* 194:196, 2003.
167. Mitsiades CS, Anderson KC, Carrasco DR: Mouse models of human myeloma. *Hematol Oncol Clin North Am* 21:1051, viii, 2007.
168. Horie Y, Suzuki A, Kataoka E, et al: Hepatocyte-specific Pten deficiency results in steatohepatitis and hepatocellular carcinomas. *J Clin Invest* 113:1774, 2004.
169. Chesi M, Robbiani DF, Sebag M, et al: AID-dependent activation of a MYC transgene induces multiple myeloma in a conditional mouse model of post-germinal center malignancies. *Cancer Cell* 13:167, 2008.
170. Yaccoby S, Pearse RN, Johnson CL, et al: Myeloma interacts with the bone marrow microenvironment to induce osteoclastogenesis and is dependent on osteoclast activity. *Br J Haematol* 116:278, 2002.
171. Yaccoby S, Johnson C, Mahaffey S, et al: Antimyeloma efficacy of thalidomide in the SCID-hu model. *Blood* 100:4162, 2002.
172. Pennisi A, Li X, Ling W, Khan S, et al: The proteasome inhibitor, bortezomib suppresses primary myeloma and stimulates bone formation in myelomatous and nonmyelomatous bones *in vivo*. *Am J Hematol* 84:6, 2009.
173. Yaccoby S, Pennisi A, Li X, et al: Atacicept (TACI-Ig) inhibits growth of TACI (high) primary myeloma cells in SCID-hu mice and in coculture with osteoclasts. *Leukemia* 22:406, 2008.
174. Pennisi A, Li X, Ling W, et al: Inhibitor of DASH proteases affects expression of adhesion molecules in osteoclasts and reduces myeloma growth and bone disease. *Br J Haematol* 145:775, 2009.
175. Yang Y, MacLeod V, Dai Y, et al: The syndecan-1 heparan sulfate proteoglycan is a viable target for myeloma therapy. *Blood* 110:2041, 2007.
176. Radl J: Animal model of human disease. Benign monoclonal gammopathy (idiopathic paraproteinemia). *Am J Pathol* 105:91, 1981.
177. Radl J, Croese JW, Zurcher C, et al: Animal model of human disease. Multiple myeloma. *Am J Pathol* 132:593, 1988.
178. Radl J: Four major mechanisms in the development of monoclonal gammopathies. Postulations and facts, in *Third EURAGE Symposium on Monoclonal Gammopathies: Clinical Significance and Basic Mechanisms*. Brussels, Belgium, 1991.
179. Van Valckenborgh E, De Raeve H, Devy L, et al: Murine 5T multiple myeloma cells induce angiogenesis *in vitro* and *in vivo*. *Br J Cancer* 86:796, 2002.
180. Asosingh K, De Raeve H, Van Riet I, et al: Multiple myeloma tumor progression in the 5T2MM murine model is a multistage and dynamic process of differentiation, proliferation, invasion, and apoptosis. *Blood* 101:3136, 2003.
181. Vanderkerken K, De Leenheer E, Shipman C, et al: Recombinant osteoprotegerin decreases tumor burden and increases survival in a murine model of multiple myeloma. *Cancer Res* 63:287, 2003.
182. Asosingh K, De Raeve H, Menu E, et al: Angiogenic switch during 5T2MM murine myeloma tumorigenesis: Role of CD45 heterogeneity. *Blood* 103:3131, 2004.
183. Greipp P, San Miguel J, Durie B: A new international staging system for multiple myeloma from the International Myeloma Working Group. *Blood* 102:190a, 2003.
184. Kyle RA, Rajkumar SV: Criteria for diagnosis, staging, risk stratification and response assessment of multiple myeloma. *Leukemia* 23:3, 2009.
185. Criteria for the classification of monoclonal gammopathies, multiple myeloma and related disorders: A report of the International Myeloma Working Group. *Br J Haematol* 121:749, 2003.
186. Silvestris F, Cafforio P, Tucci M, Dammacco F: Negative regulation of erythroblast maturation by Fas-L(+)/TRAIL(+) highly malignant plasma cells: A major pathogenetic mechanism of anemia in multiple myeloma. *Blood* 99:1305, 2002.
187. Ludwig H, Pecherstorfer M, Leitgeb C, Fritz E: Recombinant human erythropoietin for the treatment of chronic anemia in multiple myeloma and squamous cell carcinoma. *Stem Cells* 11:348, 1993.
188. Faquin WC, Schneider TJ, Goldberg MA: Effect of inflammatory cytokines on hypoxia-induced erythropoietin production. *Blood* 79:1987, 1992.
189. Singh A, Eckardt KU, Zimmermann A, et al: Increased plasma viscosity as a reason for inappropriate erythropoietin formation. *J Clin Invest* 91:251, 1993.
190. Kawabata H, Tomosugi N, Kanda J, et al: Anti-interleukin 6 receptor antibody tocilizumab reduces the level of serum hepcidin in patients with multicentric Castleman's disease. *Haematologica* 92:857, 2007.
191. Barlogie B, Gale RP: Multiple myeloma and chronic lymphocytic leukemia: Parallels and contrasts. *Am J Med* 93:443, 1992.
192. Kerr R, Stirling D, Ludlam CA: Interleukin 6 and haemostasis. *Br J Haematol* 115:3, 2001.
193. Glueck HI, Hong R: A circulating anticoagulant in gamma-1A-multiple myeloma: Its modification by penicillin. *J Clin Invest* 44:1866, 1965.
194. Wenz B, Friedman G: Acquired factor VIII inhibitor in a patient with malignant lymphoma. *Am J Med Sci* 268:295, 1974.
195. Kelsey PR, Leyland MJ: Acquired inhibitor to human factor VIII associated with paraproteinaemia and subsequent development of chronic lymphatic leukaemia. *Br Med J (Clin Res Ed)* 285:174, 1982.
196. Perkins HA, MacKenzie MR, Fudenberg HH: Hemostatic defects in dysproteinemias. *Blood* 35:695, 1970.
197. Lackner H: Hemostatic abnormalities associated with dysproteinemias. *Semin Hematol* 10:125, 1973.
198. Coleman M, Vigliano EM, Weksler ME, Nachman RL: Inhibition of fibrin monomer polymerization by lambda myeloma globulins. *Blood* 39:210, 1972.
199. Kelsey P, Delamore I: Clinical features of multiple myeloma, in *Multiple Myeloma and Other Paraproteinaemias*, edited by I Delamore, p 117. Churchill Livingstone, Edinburgh, Scotland, 1986.
200. Furie B, Greene E, Furie BC: Syndrome of acquired factor X deficiency and systemic amyloidosis *in vivo* studies of the metabolic fate of factor X. *N Engl J Med* 297:81, 1977.
201. Kunkel LA: Acquired circulating anticoagulants in malignancy. *Semin Thromb Hemost* 18:416, 1992.
202. Zangari M, Siegel E, Barlogie B, Anaissie E, et al: Thrombogenic activity of doxorubicin in myeloma patients receiving thalidomide: Implications for therapy. *Blood* 100:1168, 2002.
203. Broder S, Humphrey R, Durm M, Blackman M, et al: Impaired synthesis of polyclonal (non-paraprotein) immunoglobulins by circulating lymphocytes from patients with multiple myeloma: Role of suppressor cells. *N Engl J Med* 293:887, 1975.
204. Bradwell A, Tang L, Drayson M: Immunoassay for detection of free light chains in serum of patients with nonsecretory myeloma [abstract 4901]. *Blood* 96:271b, 2000.
205. Drayson M, Tang LX, Drew R, et al: Serum free light-chain measurements for identifying and monitoring patients with nonsecretory multiple myeloma. *Blood* 97:2900, 2001.
206. Dispenzieri A, Kyle R, Merlini G, Miguel JS, et al: International Myeloma Working Group guidelines for serum-free light chain analysis in multiple myeloma and related disorders. *Leukemia* 23:215, 2009.
207. Dispenzieri A, Lacy MQ, Katzmann JA, et al: Absolute values of immunoglobulin free light chains are prognostic in patients with primary systemic amyloidosis undergoing peripheral blood stem cell transplantation. *Blood* 107:3378, 2006.
208. van Rhee F, Bolejack V, Hollmig K, et al: High serum-free light chain levels and their rapid reduction in response to therapy define an aggressive multiple myeloma subtype with poor prognosis. *Blood* 110:827, 2007.
209. Rajkumar SV, Kyle RA, Therneau TM, et al: Serum free light chain ratio is an independent risk factor for progression in monoclonal gammopathy of undetermined significance. *Blood* 106:812, 2005.
210. Dispenzieri A, Kyle RA, Katzmann JA, et al: Immunoglobulin free light chain ratio is an independent risk factor for progression of smoldering (asymptomatic) multiple myeloma. *Blood* 111:785, 2008.
211. Durie B, Harousseau J-L, Miguel J, et al: International uniform response criteria for multiple myeloma. *Leukemia* 20:1467, 2006.
212. Nair B, Shaughnessy JD Jr, Zhou Y, et al: Gene expression profiling of plasma cells at myeloma relapse from tandem transplantation trial Total Therapy 2 predicts subsequent survival. *Blood* 113:6572, 2009.

213. Bartl R, Frisch B, Fateh-Moghadam A, et al: Histologic classification and staging of multiple myeloma. A retrospective and prospective study of 674 cases. *Am J Clin Pathol* 87:342, 1987.
214. Waldron J, Jazieh A, Jagannath S, et al: Bone marrow morphology (BMM) adds critical prognostic information to other standard parameters (SP) including cytogenetics among newly diagnosed multiple myeloma (MM) patients receiving total therapy (TT). *Blood* 90:90a, 1997.
215. Greipp PR, Raymond NM, Kyle RA, O'Fallon WM: Multiple myeloma: Significance of plasmablastic subtype in morphological classification. *Blood* 65:305, 1985.
216. Greipp PR, Leong T, Bennett JM, et al: Plasmablastic morphology—An independent prognostic factor with clinical and laboratory correlates: Eastern Cooperative Oncology Group (ECOG) myeloma trial E9486 report by the ECOG Myeloma Laboratory Group. *Blood* 91:2501, 1998.
217. Munshi N, Wilson C, Penn J, et al: Angiogenesis in newly diagnosed multiple myeloma (MM): Poor prognosis with increased microvessel density (MVD) in bone marrow biopsies (BMBX). *Blood* 92:98a, 1998.
218. Bellamy WT, Richter L, Frutiger Y, Grogan TM: Expression of vascular endothelial growth factor and its receptors in hematopoietic malignancies. *Cancer Res* 59:728, 1999.
219. Kumar S, Fonseca R, Dispenzieri A, et al: Bone marrow angiogenesis in multiple myeloma: Effect of therapy. *Br J Haematol* 119:665, 2002.
220. Govindarajan R, Jagannath S, Flick JT, et al: Preceding standard therapy is the likely cause of MDS after autotransplants for multiple myeloma. *Br J Haematol* 95:349, 1996.
221. Tricot G, Barlogie B, Sawyer J: MM-MDS is a poor prognostic marker for outcome after tandem transplants in multiple myeloma (MM). *Proc Am Soc Clin Oncol* 22:765(abstract 2279), 2003.
222. Barlogie B, Tricot G, Haessler J, et al: Cytogenetically defined myelodysplasia after melphalan-based autotransplants for myeloma linked to poor hematopoietic stem cell mobilization: The Arkansas experience in more than 3000 patients treated since 1989. *Blood* 111:94, 2008.
223. Barlogie B, Alexanian R, Dixon D, et al: Prognostic implications of tumor cell DNA and RNA content in multiple myeloma. *Blood* 66:338, 1985.
224. Bataille R, Robillard N, Pellat-Deceunynck C, Amiot M: A cellular model for myeloma cell growth and maturation based on an intraclonal CD45 hierarchy. *Immunol Rev* 194:105, 2003.
225. Van Camp B, Durie BG, Spier C, et al: Plasma cells in multiple myeloma express a natural killer cell-associated antigen: CD56 (NKH-1; Leu-19). *Blood* 76:377, 1990.
226. Epstein J: Myeloma phenotype: Clues to disease origin and manifestation. *Hematol Oncol Clin North Am* 6:249, 1992.
227. Ocqueteau M, Orfao A, Garcia-Sanz R, et al: Expression of the CD117 antigen (c-Kit) on normal and myelomatous plasma cells. *Br J Haematol* 95:489, 1996.
228. Almeida J, Orfao A, Ocqueteau M, Mateo G, et al: High-sensitive immunophenotyping and DNA ploidy studies for the investigation of minimal residual disease in multiple myeloma [see comment]. *Br J Haematol* 107:121, 1999.
229. Tricot G, Barlogie B, Jagannath S, et al: Poor prognosis in multiple myeloma is associated only with partial or complete deletions of chromosome 13 or abnormalities involving 11q and not with other karyotype abnormalities. *Blood* 86:4250, 1995.
230. Tricot G, Sawyer JR, Jagannath S, et al: Unique role of cytogenetics in the prognosis of patients with myeloma receiving high-dose therapy and autotransplants. *J Clin Oncol* 15:2659, 1997.
231. Seong C, Delasalle K, Hayes K, et al: Prognostic value of cytogenetics in multiple myeloma. *Br J Haematol* 101:189, 1998.
232. Desikan R, Barlogie B, Sawyer J, et al: Results of high-dose therapy for 1000 patients with multiple myeloma: Durable complete remissions and superior survival in the absence of chromosome 13 abnormalities. *Blood* 95:4008, 2000.
233. Smadja NV, Bastard C, Brigaudeau C, et al: Hypodiploidy is a major prognostic factor in multiple myeloma. *Blood* 98:2229, 2001.
234. Fassas AB, Spencer T, Sawyer J, et al: Both hypodiploidy and deletion of chromosome 13 independently confer poor prognosis in multiple myeloma. *Br J Haematol* 118:1041, 2002.
235. Jacobson J, Barlogie B, Shaughnessy J, et al: MDS-type abnormalities within myeloma signature karyotype (MM-MDS): Only 13% 1-year survival despite tandem transplants. *Br J Haematol* 122:430, 2003.
236. Konigsberg R, Zojer N, Ackermann J, et al: Predictive role of interphase cytogenetics for survival of patients with multiple myeloma. *J Clin Oncol* 18:804, 2000.
237. Zojer N, Konigsberg R, Ackermann J, et al: Deletion of 13q14 remains an independent adverse prognostic variable in multiple myeloma despite its frequent detection by interphase fluorescence in situ hybridization. *Blood* 95:1925, 2000.
238. Facon T, Avet-Loiseau H, Guillerm G, et al: Chromosome 13 abnormalities identified by FISH analysis and serum beta2-microglobulin produce a powerful myeloma staging system for patients receiving high-dose therapy. *Blood* 97:1566, 2001.
239. Shaughnessy J Jr, Tian E, Sawyer J, et al: Prognostic impact of cytogenetic and interphase fluorescence in situ hybridization-defined chromosome 13 deletion in multiple myeloma: Early results of total therapy II: *Br J Haematol* 120:44, 2003.
240. Durie BG, Salmon SE, Moon TE: Pretreatment tumor mass, cell kinetics, and prognosis in multiple myeloma. *Blood* 55:364, 1980.
241. Drewinko B, Alexanian R, Boyer H, et al: The growth fraction of human myeloma cells. *Blood* 57:333, 1981.
242. Boccadoro M, Massaia M, Dianzani U, Pileri A: Multiple myeloma: Biological and clinical significance of bone marrow plasma cell labelling index. *Haematologica* 72:171, 1987.
243. Greipp PR, Witzig TE, Gonchoroff NJ, et al: Immunofluorescence labeling indices in myeloma and related monoclonal gammopathies. *Mayo Clin Proc* 62:969, 1987.
244. Witzig TE, Gonchoroff NJ, Katzmann JA, et al: Peripheral blood B cell labeling indices are a measure of disease activity in patients with monoclonal gammopathies. *J Clin Oncol* 6:1041, 1988.
245. Greipp PR, Lust JA, O'Fallon WM, et al: Plasma cell labeling index and beta 2-microglobulin predict survival independent of thymidine kinase and C-reactive protein in multiple myeloma. *Blood* 81:3382, 1993.
246. San Miguel JF, Garcia-Sanz R, Gonzalez M, et al: A new staging system for multiple myeloma based on the number of S-phase plasma cells. *Blood* 85:448, 1995.
247. Solomon A, Weiss DT, Kattine AA: Nephrotoxic potential of Bence Jones proteins. *N Engl J Med* 324:1845, 1991.
248. Alexanian R, Barlogie B: Implications of renal failure in multiple myeloma, in *The Kidney in Plasma Cell Dyscrasias*, edited by L Minetti, G D'Amico, C Ponticelli, p 260. Kluwer, Dordrecht, Netherlands, 1988.
249. Alexanian R, Barlogie B, Dixon D: Renal failure in multiple myeloma. Pathogenesis and prognostic implications. *Arch Intern Med* 150:1693, 1990.
250. Kyle RA, Greipp PR: Amyloidosis (AL). Clinical and laboratory features in 229 cases. *Mayo Clin Proc* 58:665, 1983.
251. Zucker-Franklin D: Renal amyloidosis: New perspectives, in *The Kidney in Plasma Cell Dyscrasias*, edited by L Minetti, G D'Amico, C Ponticelli, p 45. Kluwer, Dordrecht, Netherlands, 1988.
252. Buxbaum J: Mechanisms of disease: Monoclonal immunoglobulin deposition. Amyloidosis, light chain deposition disease, and light and heavy chain deposition disease. *Hematol Oncol Clin North Am* 6:323, 1992.
253. Gallo G, Buxbaum J: Monoclonal immunoglobulin deposition disease: Immunopathologic aspects of renal involvement, in *The Kidney in Plasma Cell Dyscrasias*, edited by L Minetti, G D'Amico, C Ponticelli, p 171. Kluwer, Kordrecht, Netherlands, 1988.
254. Reeves WB, Foley RJ, Weinman EJ: Nephrotoxicity from nonsteroidal anti-inflammatory drugs. *South Med J* 78:318, 1985.
255. Hind C, Baltz M, Pepys M: Amyloidosis, in *Multiple Myeloma and Other Paraproteinaemias*, edited by I Delamore, p 234. Churchill Livingstone, Edinburgh, Scotland, 1986.
256. Pratt G, Goodyear O, Moss P: Immunodeficiency and immunotherapy in multiple myeloma. *Br J Haematol* 138:563, 2007.
257. Ullrich S, Zolla-Pazner S: Immunoregulatory circuits in myeloma. *Clin Haematol* 11:87, 1982.
258. Jacobson DR, Zolla-Pazner S: Immunosuppression and infection in multiple myeloma. *Semin Oncol* 13:282, 1986.
259. Brown RD, Pope B, Murray A, et al: Dendritic cells from patients with myeloma are numerically normal but functionally defective as they fail to up-regulate CD80 (B7-1) expression after huCD40LT stimulation because of inhibition by transforming growth factor-beta1 and interleukin-10. *Blood* 98:2992, 2001.
260. Ratta M, Fagnoni F, Curti A, et al: Dendritic cells are functionally defective in multiple myeloma: The role of interleukin-6. *Blood* 100:230, 2002.
261. Rao PE, Petrone AL, Ponath PD: Differentiation and expansion of T cells with regulatory function from human peripheral lymphocytes by stimulation in the presence of TGF-{beta}. *J Immunol* 174:1446, 2005.
262. Xie J, Wang Y, Freeman ME 3rd, et al: Beta 2-microglobulin as a negative regulator of the immune system: High concentrations of the protein inhibit in vitro generation of functional dendritic cells. *Blood* 101:4005, 2003.
263. Kukreja A, Hutchinson A, Dhodapkar K, et al: Enhancement of clonogenicity of human multiple myeloma by dendritic cells. *J Exp Med* 203:1859, 2006.
264. Mariani S, Coscia M, Even J, et al: Severe and long-lasting disruption of T-cell receptor diversity in human myeloma after high-dose chemotherapy and autologous peripheral blood progenitor cell infusion. *Br J Haematol* 113:1051, 2001.
265. Mills KH, Cawley JC: Abnormal monoclonal antibody-defined helper/suppressor T-cell subpopulations in multiple myeloma: Relationship to treatment and clinical stage. *Br J Haematol* 53:271, 1983.
266. Mozaffari F, Hansson L, Kiaii S, et al: Signalling molecules and cytokine production in T cells of multiple myeloma-increased abnormalities with advancing stage. *Br J Haematol* 124:315, 2004.
267. Waldenstrom JG, Adner A, Gydell K, Zettervall O: Osteosclerotic "plasmocytoma" with polyneuropathy, hypertrichosis and diabetes. *Acta Med Scand* 203:297, 1978.
268. Miralles GD, O'Fallon JR, Talley NJ: Plasma-cell dyscrasia with polyneuropathy. The spectrum of POEMS syndrome. *N Engl J Med* 327:1919, 1992.
269. Pruzanski W, Watt JG: Serum viscosity and hyperviscosity syndrome in IgG multiple myeloma. Report on 10 patients and a review of the literature. *Ann Intern Med* 77:853, 1972.
270. Somer T: Hyperviscosity syndrome in plasma cell dyscrasias. *Adv Microcirc* 6:1-55 1975.
271. Preston FE, Cooke KB, Foster ME, et al: Myelomatosis and the hyperviscosity syndrome. *Br J Haematol* 38:517, 1978.
272. Chandy KG, Stockley RA, Leonard RC, et al: Relationship between serum viscosity and intravascular IgA polymer concentration in IgA myeloma. *Clin Exp Immunol* 46:653, 1981.

273. Waldenstrom JG: Incipient myelomatosis or "essential" hyperglobulinaemia with fibrinogenopenia—A new syndrome. *Acta Med Scand* 117:216, 1944.
274. Capra JD, Kunkel HG: Aggregation of gamma-G3 proteins: Relevance to the hyperviscosity syndrome. *J Clin Invest* 49:610, 1970.
275. Bichel J, Effersoe P, Gormsen H, Harboe N: Leukemic myelomatosis (plasma cell leukemia); a review with report of four cases. *Acta Radiol* 37:196, 1952.
276. Noel P, Kyle RA: Plasma cell leukemia: An evaluation of response to therapy. *Am J Med* 83:1062, 1987.
277. Garcia-Sanz R, Orfao A, Gonzalez M, et al: Primary plasma cell leukemia: Clinical, immunophenotypic, DNA ploidy, and cytogenetic characteristics. *Blood* 93:1032, 1999.
278. Guikema JE, Vellenga E, Abdulahad WH, et al: CD27-triggering on primary plasma cell leukaemia cells has anti-apoptotic effects involving mitogen activated protein kinases. *Br J Haematol* 124:299, 2004.
279. Barlogie B, Smallwood L, Smith T, Alexanian R: High serum levels of lactic dehydrogenase identify a high-grade lymphoma like myeloma. *Ann Intern Med* 110:521, 1989.
280. Cherng NC, Asal NR, Kuebler JP, et al: Prognostic factors in multiple myeloma. *Cancer* 67:3150, 1991.
281. Bartel TB, Haessler J, Brown TL, et al: F18-fluorodeoxyglucose positron emission tomography in the context of other imaging techniques and prognostic factors in multiple myeloma. *Blood* 114:2068, 2009.
282. Walker R, Barlogie B, Haessler J, et al: Magnetic resonance imaging in multiple myeloma: Diagnostic and clinical implications. *J Clin Oncol* 25:1121, 2007.
283. Durie BG, Salmon SE: A clinical staging system for multiple myeloma. Correlation of measured myeloma cell mass with presenting clinical features, response to treatment, and survival. *Cancer* 36:842, 1975.
284. Greipp PR, San Miguel J, Durie BG, et al: International staging system for multiple myeloma. *J Clin Oncol* 23:3412, 2005.
285. Bataille R, Grenier J, Sany J: Beta-2-microglobulin in myeloma: Optimal use for staging, prognosis, and treatment—A prospective study of 160 patients. *Blood* 63:468, 1984.
286. Garewal H, Durie BG, Kyle RA, et al: Serum beta 2-microglobulin in the initial staging and subsequent monitoring of monoclonal plasma cell disorders. *J Clin Oncol* 2:51, 1984.
287. Child JA, Norfolk DR, Cooper EH: Serum beta 2-microglobulin in myelomatosis. *Br J Haematol* 63:406, 1986.
288. Podar K, Chauhan D, Anderson KC: Bone marrow microenvironment and the identification of new targets for myeloma therapy. *Leukemia* 23:10, 2009.
289. Arzoumanian V, Hoering A, Sawyer J, et al: Suppression of abnormal karyotype predicts superior survival in multiple myeloma. *Leukemia* 22:850, 2008.
290. Barlogie B, Shaughnessy J, Epstein J, et al: Plasma cell myeloma, in *Williams Hematology*, 7th ed., edited by M Lichtman, E Beutler, T Kipps, U Seligsohn, K Kaushansky, JT Prchal, p 1501. McGraw Hill Medical Publishing, New York, 2005.
291. Sawyer JR, Tricot G, Mattox S, et al: Jumping translocations of chromosome 1q in multiple myeloma: Evidence for a mechanism involving decondensation of pericentromeric heterochromatin. *Blood* 91:1732, 1998.
292. Le Baccon P, Leroux D, Dascalescu C, et al: Novel evidence of a role for chromosome 1 pericentric heterochromatin in the pathogenesis of B-cell lymphoma and multiple myeloma. *Genes Chromosomes Cancer* 32:250, 2001.
293. Sawyer JR, Tricot G, Lukacs JL, et al: Genomic instability in multiple myeloma: Evidence for jumping segmental duplications of chromosome arm 1q. *Genes Chromosomes Cancer* 42:95, 2005.
294. Hanamura I, Stewart J, Huang Y, et al: Frequent gain of chromosome band 1q21 in plasma-cell dyscrasias detected by fluorescence *in situ* hybridization: Incidence increases from MGUS to relapsed myeloma and is related to prognosis and disease progression following tandem stem-cell transplantation. *Blood* 108:1724, 2006.
295. Chang H, Qi X, Trieu Y, et al: Multiple myeloma patients with CKS1B gene amplification have a shorter progression-free survival post-autologous stem cell transplantation. *Br J Haematol* 135:486, 2006.
296. Zhan F, Colla S, Wu X, et al: CKS1B, overexpressed in aggressive disease, regulates multiple myeloma growth and survival through SKP2- and p27Kip1-dependent and -independent mechanisms. *Blood* 109:4995, 2007.
297. Avet-Loiseau H, Daviet A, Brigaudeau C, et al: Cytogenetic, interphase, and multicolor fluorescence in situ hybridization analyses in primary plasma cell leukemia: A study of 40 patients at diagnosis, on behalf of the Intergroupe Francophone du Myelome and the Groupe Francais de Cytogenetique Hematologique. *Blood* 97:822, 2001.
298. Avet-Loiseau H, Attal M, Moreau P, et al: Genetic abnormalities and survival in multiple myeloma: The experience of the Intergroupe Francophone du Myelome. *Blood* 109:3489, 2007.
299. Fonseca R, Blood E, Rue M, et al: Clinical and biologic implications of recurrent genomic aberrations in myeloma. *Blood* 101:4569, 2003.
300. Moreau P, Facon T, Leleu X, et al: Recurrent 14q32 translocations determine the prognosis of multiple myeloma, especially in patients receiving intensive chemotherapy. *Blood* 100:1579, 2002.
301. Gertz MA, Lacy MQ, Dispenzieri A, et al: Clinical implications of t(11;14)(q13;q32), t(4;14)(p16.3;q32), and -17p13 in myeloma patients treated with high-dose therapy. *Blood* 106:2837, 2005.
302. Chang H, Qi C, Yi QL, et al: p53 gene deletion detected by fluorescence in situ hybridization is an adverse prognostic factor for patients with multiple myeloma following autologous stem cell transplantation. *Blood* 105:358, 2005.
303. Haessler J, Shaughnessy J, Zhan F, et al: Benefit of complete response in multiple myeloma limited to high risk subgroup identified by gene expression profiling. *Clin Cancer Res* 13:7073, 2007.
304. Shaughnessy J, Tian E, Sawyer J, et al: High incidence of chromosome 13 deletion in multiple myeloma detected by multiprobe interphase FISH. *Blood* 96:1505, 2000.
305. Alizadeh AA, Eisen MB, Davis RE, et al: Distinct types of diffuse large B-cell lymphoma identified by gene expression profiling. *Nature* 403:503, 2000.
306. Yeoh EJ, Ross ME, Shurtleff SA, et al: Classification, subtype discovery, and prediction of outcome in pediatric acute lymphoblastic leukemia by gene expression profiling [see comment]. *Cancer Cell* 1:133, 2002.
307. Rosenwald A, Wright G, Leroy K, et al: Molecular diagnosis of primary mediastinal B cell lymphoma identifies a clinically favorable subgroup of diffuse large B cell lymphoma related to Hodgkin lymphoma. *J Exp Med* 198:851, 2003.
308. Bullinger L, Dohner K, Bair E, et al: Use of gene-expression profiling to identify prognostic subclasses in adult acute myeloid leukemia [see comment]. *N Engl J Med* 350:1605, 2004.
309. Lossos IS, Czerwinski DK, Alizadeh AA, et al: Prediction of survival in diffuse large-B-cell lymphoma based on the expression of six genes. *N Engl J Med* 350:1828, 2004.
310. Shaughnessy JD Jr, Zhan F, Burington BE, et al: A validated gene expression model of high-risk multiple myeloma is defined by deregulated expression of genes mapping to chromosome 1. *Blood* 109:2276, 2007.
311. Chng WJ, Kuehl WM, Bergsagel PL, Fonseca R: Translocation t(4;14) retains prognostic significance even in the setting of high-risk molecular signature. *Leukemia* 22:459, 2008.
312. Zhan F, Barlogie B, Mulligan G, et al: High-risk myeloma: A gene expression based risk-stratification model for newly diagnosed multiple myeloma treated with high-dose therapy is predictive of outcome in relapsed disease treated with single-agent bortezomib or high-dose dexamethasone. *Blood* 111:968, 2008.
313. Mulligan G, Mitsiades C, Bryant B, et al: Gene expression profiling and correlation with outcome in clinical trials of the proteasome inhibitor bortezomib. *Blood* 109:3177, 2007.
314. Decaux O, Lode L, Magrangeas F, et al: Prediction of survival in multiple myeloma based on gene expression profiles reveals cell cycle and chromosomal instability signatures in high-risk patients and hyperdiploid signatures in low-risk patients: A study of the Intergroupe Francophone du Myelome. *J Clin Oncol* 26:4798, 2008.
315. Resnick D, M Kransdorf: *Bone and Joint Imaging.* Chap 49. Plasma cell dyscrasias. Elsevier, Amsterdam, 2004.
316. Jacobson H, Poppel M, Shapiro J, et al: The vertebral pedicle sign: A roentgen finding to differentiate metastatic carcinoma from multiple myeloma *Am J Roentgenol Radium Ther Nucl Med* 80:817, 1958.
317. Angtuaco EJ, Fassas AB, Walker R, Sethi R, et al: Multiple myeloma: Clinical review and diagnostic imaging. *Radiology* 231:11, 2004.
318. Shortt CP, Gleeson TG, Breen KA, et al: Whole-body MRI versus PET in assessment of multiple myeloma disease activity. *AJR Am J Roentgenol* 192:980, 2009.
319. Abildgaard N, Brixen K, Kristensen JE, et al: Assessment of bone involvement in patients with multiple myeloma using bone densitometry. *Eur J Haematol* 57:370, 1996.
320. Attal M, Harousseau JL, Stoppa AM, et al: A prospective, randomized trial of autologous bone marrow transplantation and chemotherapy in multiple myeloma. Intergroupe Francais du Myelome. *N Engl J Med* 335:91, 1996.
321. Fermand JP, Katsahian S, Divine M, et al: High-dose therapy and autologous blood stem-cell transplantation compared with conventional treatment in myeloma patients aged 55 to 65 years: Long-term results of a randomized control trial from the Group Myelome-Autogreffe. *J Clin Oncol* 23:9227, 2005.
322. Child JA, Morgan GJ, Davies FE, et al: High-dose chemotherapy with hematopoietic stem-cell rescue for multiple myeloma. *N Engl J Med* 348:1875, 2003.
323. Palumbo A, Bringhen S, Petrucci MT, et al: Intermediate-dose melphalan improves survival of myeloma patients aged 50 to 70: Results of a randomized controlled trial. *Blood* 104:3052, 2004.
324. Blade J, Rosinol L, Sureda A, et al: High-dose therapy intensification compared with continued standard chemotherapy in multiple myeloma patients responding to the initial chemotherapy: Long-term results from a prospective randomized trial from the Spanish cooperative group PETHEMA. *Blood* 106:3755, 2005.
325. Barlogie B, Kyle RA, Anderson KC, et al: Standard chemotherapy compared with high-dose chemoradiotherapy for multiple myeloma: Final results of phase III US Intergroup Trial S9321. *J Clin Oncol* 24:929, 2006.
326. Segeren CM, Sonneveld P, van der Holt B, et al: Overall and event-free survival are not improved by the use of myeloablative therapy following intensified chemotherapy in previously untreated patients with multiple myeloma: A prospective randomized phase 3 study. *Blood* 101:2144, 2003.
327. Rajkumar SV, Blood E, Vesole D, et al: Phase III clinical trial of thalidomide plus dexamethasone compared with dexamethasone alone in newly diagnosed multiple myeloma: A clinical trial coordinated by the Eastern Cooperative Oncology Group. *J Clin Oncol* 24:431, 2006.
328. Cavo M, Zamagni E, Tosi P, et al: Superiority of thalidomide and dexamethasone over vincristine-doxorubicin-dexamethasone (VAD) as primary therapy in preparation for autologous transplantation for multiple myeloma. *Blood* 106:35, 2005.
329. Lokhorst HM, Schmidt-Wolf I, Sonneveld P, et al: Thalidomide in induction treatment increases the very good partial response rate before and after high-dose therapy in previously untreated multiple myeloma. *Haematologica* 93:124, 2008.

330. de la Rubia J, Blade J, Lahuerta JJ, et al: Effect of chemotherapy with alkylating agents on the yield of CD34+ cells in patients with multiple myeloma. Results of the Spanish Myeloma Group (GEM) Study. *Haematologica* 91:621, 2006.
331. Popat U, Saliba R, Thandi R, et al: Impairment of filgrastim-induced stem cell mobilization after prior lenalidomide in patients with multiple myeloma. *Biol Blood Marrow Transplant* 15:718, 2009.
332. Kumar S, Dispenzieri A, Lacy MQ, et al: Impact of lenalidomide therapy on stem cell mobilization and engraftment post-peripheral blood stem cell transplantation in patients with newly diagnosed myeloma. *Leukemia* 21:2035, 2007.
333. Mazumder A, Kaufman J, Niesvizky R, et al: Effect of lenalidomide therapy on mobilization of peripheral blood stem cells in previously untreated multiple myeloma patients. *Leukemia* 22:1280; author reply 1281, 2008.
334. Mark T, Stern J, Furst JR, et al: Stem cell mobilization with cyclophosphamide overcomes the suppressive effect of lenalidomide therapy on stem cell collection in multiple myeloma. *Biol Blood Marrow Transplant* 14:795, 2008.
335. Kumar S, Giralt S, Stadtmauer EA, et al: Mobilization in myeloma revisited: IMWG consensus perspectives on stem cell collection following initial therapy with thalidomide-, lenalidomide-, or bortezomib-containing regimens. *Blood* 114:1729, 2009.
336. Barlogie B, Alexanian R, Dicke KA, et al: High-dose chemoradiotherapy and autologous bone marrow transplantation for resistant multiple myeloma. *Blood* 70:869, 1987.
337. Harousseau JL, Milpied N, Laporte JP, et al: Double-intensive therapy in high-risk multiple myeloma. *Blood* 79:2827, 1992.
338. Fermand JP, Levy Y, Gerota J, et al: Treatment of aggressive multiple myeloma by high-dose chemotherapy and total body irradiation followed by blood stem cells autologous graft. *Blood* 73:20, 1989.
339. Alexanian R, Haut A, Khan AU, et al: Treatment for multiple myeloma. Combination chemotherapy with different melphalan dose regimens. *JAMA* 208:1680, 1969.
340. Abdelkefi A, Torjman L, Ben Romdhane N, et al: First-line thalidomide-dexamethasone therapy in preparation for auto-SCT in young patients (<61 years) with symptomatic multiple myeloma. *Bone Marrow Transplant* 43:893, 2009.
341. Hoering A, Crowley J, Shaughnessy JD Jr, et al: Complete remission in multiple myeloma examined as time-dependent variable in terms of both onset and duration in total therapy protocols. *Blood* 114:1299, 2009.
342. Barlogie B, Anaissie E, Haessler J, et al: Complete remission sustained 3 years from treatment initiation is a powerful surrogate for extended survival in multiple myeloma. *Cancer* 113:355, 2008.
343. Barlogie B, Pineda-Roman M, van Rhee F, et al: Thalidomide arm of total therapy 2 improves complete remission duration and survival in myeloma patients with metaphase cytogenetic abnormalities. *Blood* 112:3115, 2008.
344. Lee CK, Barlogie B, Munshi N, et al: DTPACE: An effective, novel combination chemotherapy with thalidomide for previously treated patients with myeloma. *J Clin Oncol* 21:2732, 2003.
345. Barlogie B, van Rhee F, Shaughnessy JD Jr, et al: Making progress in treating multiple myeloma with total therapies: Issue of complete remission and more. *Leukemia* 22:1633, 2008.
346. Barlogie B, Anaissie E, van Rhee F, et al: Incorporating bortezomib into upfront treatment for multiple myeloma: Early results of total therapy 3. *Br J Haematol* 138:176, 2007.
347. Pineda-Roman M, Zangari M, Haessler J, et al: Sustained complete remissions in multiple myeloma linked to bortezomib in total therapy 3: Comparison with total therapy 2. *Br J Haematol* 140:625, 2008.
348. Xiong W, Wu X, Starnes S, et al: An analysis of the clinical and biologic significance of TP53 loss and the identification of potential novel transcriptional targets of TP53 in multiple myeloma. *Blood* 112:4235, 2008.
349. Facon T, Mary JY, Hulin C, et al: Melphalan and prednisone plus thalidomide versus melphalan and prednisone alone or reduced-intensity autologous stem cell transplantation in elderly patients with multiple myeloma (IFM 99–06): A randomised trial. *Lancet* 370:1209, 2007.
350. Hulin C, Facon T, Rodon P, et al: Efficacy of melphalan and prednisone plus thalidomide in patients older than 75 years with newly diagnosed multiple myeloma: IFM 01/01 trial. *J Clin Oncol* 27:3664, 2009.
351. Palumbo A, Bringhen S, Caravita T, et al: Oral melphalan and prednisone chemotherapy plus thalidomide compared with melphalan and prednisone alone in elderly patients with multiple myeloma: Randomised controlled trial. *Lancet* 367:825, 2006.
352. Waage A, Gimsing P, Juliusson J, et al: Thalidomide to newly diagnosed patients with multiple myeloma: A placebo controlled randomised phase 3 trial [abstract]. *Blood* 110:78, 2007.
353. Palumbo A, Rajkumar SV, Dimopoulos MA, et al: Prevention of thalidomide- and lenalidomide-associated thrombosis in myeloma. *Leukemia* 22:414, 2008.
354. Mateos MV, Hernandez JM, Hernandez MT, et al: Bortezomib plus melphalan and prednisone in elderly untreated patients with multiple myeloma: Results of a multicenter phase 1/2 study. *Blood* 108:2165, 2006.
355. San Miguel JF, Schlag R, Khuageva NK, et al: Bortezomib plus melphalan and prednisone for initial treatment of multiple myeloma. *N Engl J Med* 359:906, 2008.
356. Palumbo A, Falco P, Corradini P, et al: Melphalan, prednisone, and lenalidomide treatment for newly diagnosed myeloma: A report from the GIMEMA—Italian Multiple Myeloma Network. *J Clin Oncol* 25:4459, 2007.
357. van Rhee F, Dhodapkar M, Shaughnessy JD Jr, et al: First thalidomide clinical trial in multiple myeloma: A decade. *Blood* 112:1035, 2008.
358. Palumbo A, Giaccone L, Bertola A, et al: Low-dose thalidomide plus dexamethasone is an effective salvage therapy for advanced myeloma. *Haematologica* 86:399, 2001.
359. Dimopoulos MA, Zervas K, Kouvatseas G, et al: Thalidomide and dexamethasone combination for refractory multiple myeloma. *Ann Oncol* 12:991, 2001.
360. Anagnostopoulos A, Weber D, Rankin K, et al: Thalidomide and dexamethasone for resistant multiple myeloma. *Br J Haematol* 121:768, 2003.
361. Barlogie B, Desikan R, Eddlemon P, et al: Extended survival in advanced and refractory multiple myeloma after single-agent thalidomide: Identification of prognostic factors in a phase 2 study of 169 patients. *Blood* 98:492, 2001.
362. Weber DM, Chen C, Niesvizky R, et al: Lenalidomide plus dexamethasone for relapsed multiple myeloma in North America. *N Engl J Med* 357:2133, 2007.
363. Dimopoulos M, Spencer A, Attal M, et al: Lenalidomide plus dexamethasone for relapsed or refractory multiple myeloma. *N Engl J Med* 357:2123, 2007.
364. Chen C, Reece DE, Siegel D, et al: Expanded safety experience with lenalidomide plus dexamethasone in relapsed or refractory multiple myeloma. *Br J Haematol* 146:164, 2009.
365. Richardson PG, Barlogie B, Berenson J, et al: A phase 2 study of bortezomib in relapsed, refractory myeloma. *N Engl J Med* 348:2609, 2003.
366. Jagannath S, Barlogie B, Berenson J, et al: A phase 2 study of two doses of bortezomib in relapsed or refractory myeloma. *Br J Haematol* 127:165, 2004.
367. Richardson PG, Barlogie B, Berenson J, et al: Extended follow-up of a phase II trial in relapsed, refractory multiple myeloma: Final time-to-event results from the SUMMIT trial. *Cancer* 106:1316, 2006.
368. Jagannath S, Barlogie B, Berenson JR, et al: Updated survival analyses after prolonged follow-up of the phase 2, multicenter CREST study of bortezomib in relapsed or refractory multiple myeloma. *Br J Haematol* 143:537, 2008.
369. Richardson PG, Sonneveld P, Schuster MW, et al: Bortezomib or high-dose dexamethasone for relapsed multiple myeloma. *N Engl J Med* 352:2487, 2005.
370. Richardson PG, Sonneveld P, Schuster M, et al: Extended follow-up of a phase 3 trial in relapsed multiple myeloma: Final time-to-event results of the APEX trial. *Blood* 110:3557, 2007.
371. Chanan-Khan AA, Niesvizky R, Hohl RJ, et al: Phase III randomised study of dexamethasone with or without oblimersen sodium for patients with advanced multiple myeloma. *Leuk Lymphoma* 50:559, 2009.
372. Orlowski RZ, Nagler A, Sonneveld P, et al: Randomized phase III study of pegylated liposomal doxorubicin plus bortezomib compared with bortezomib alone in relapsed or refractory multiple myeloma: Combination therapy improves time to progression. *J Clin Oncol* 25:3892, 2007.
373. Pineda-Roman M, Zangari M, van Rhee F, et al: VTD combination therapy with bortezomib-thalidomide-dexamethasone is highly effective in advanced and refractory multiple myeloma. *Leukemia* 22:1419, 2008.
374. Ponisch W, Rozanski M, Goldschmidt H, et al: Combined bendamustine, prednisolone and thalidomide for refractory or relapsed multiple myeloma after autologous stem-cell transplantation or conventional chemotherapy: Results of a phase I clinical trial. *Br J Haematol* 143:191, 2008.
375. Knop S, Gerecke C, Liebisch P, et al: Lenalidomide, Adriamycin, and dexamethasone (RAD) in patients with relapsed and refractory multiple myeloma: A report from the German Myeloma Study Group DSMM (Deutsche Studiengruppe Multiples Myelom). *Blood* 113:4137, 2009.
376. Lee C, Barlogie B, Fassas A, et al: Third autotransplant for the management of 98 patients among 1358 who had received prior tandem autotransplants: Benefit apparent when 2nd to 3rd transplant interval exceeds 3 years. *Blood* (American Socitey of Hematology Annual Meeting Abstracts)104: 540, 2004.
377. Lokhorst HM, Schattenberg A, Cornelissen JJ, et al: Donor leukocyte infusions are effective in relapsed multiple myeloma after allogeneic bone marrow transplantation. *Blood* 90:4206, 1997.
378. Tricot G, Vesole DH, Jagannath S, et al: Graft-versus-myeloma effect: Proof of principle. *Blood* 87:1196, 1996.
379. Bird JM, Russell NH, Samson D: Minimal residual disease after bone marrow transplantation for multiple myeloma: Evidence for cure in long-term survivors. *Bone Marrow Transplant* 12:651, 1993.
380. Corradini P, Voena C, Tarella C, et al: Molecular and clinical remissions in multiple myeloma: Role of autologous and allogeneic transplantation of hematopoietic cells. *J Clin Oncol* 17:208, 1999.
381. Gahrton G, Tura S, Ljungman P, et al: Allogeneic bone marrow transplantation in multiple myeloma. European Group for Bone Marrow Transplantation [comment]. *N Engl J Med* 325:1267, 1991.
382. Reece DE, Shepherd JD, Klingemann HG, et al: Treatment of myeloma using intensive therapy and allogeneic bone marrow transplantation. *Bone Marrow Transplant* 15:117, 1995.
383. Alyea E, Weller E, Schlossman R, et al: Outcome after autologous and allogeneic stem cell transplantation for patients with multiple myeloma: Impact of graft-versus-myeloma effect. *Bone Marrow Transplant* 32:1145, 2003.
384. Bjorkstrand BB, Ljungman P, Svensson H, et al: Allogeneic bone marrow transplantation versus autologous stem cell transplantation in multiple myeloma: A retrospective case-matched study from the European Group for Blood and Marrow Transplantation. *Blood* 88:4711, 1996.
385. Gahrton G, Tura S, Ljungman P, et al: Prognostic factors in allogeneic bone marrow transplantation for multiple myeloma. *J Clin Oncol* 13:1312, 1995.

386. Hunter HM, Peggs K, Powles R, et al: Analysis of outcome following allogeneic haemopoietic stem cell transplantation for myeloma using myeloablative conditioning—Evidence for a superior outcome using melphalan combined with total body irradiation. *Br J Haematol* 128:496, 2005.
387. Varterasian M, Janakiraman N, Karanes C, et al: Transplantation in patients with multiple myeloma: A multicenter comparative analysis of peripheral blood stem cell and allogeneic transplant. *Am J Clin Oncol* 20:462, 1997.
388. Gahrton G, Svensson H, Cavo M, et al: Progress in allogenic bone marrow and peripheral blood stem cell transplantation for multiple myeloma: A comparison between transplants performed 1983–93 and 1994–8 at European Group for Blood and Marrow Transplantation centres. *Br J Haematol* 113:209, 2001.
389. Bensinger WI, Buckner CD, Anasetti C, et al: Allogeneic marrow transplantation for multiple myeloma: An analysis of risk factors on outcome. *Blood* 88:2787, 1996.
390. Giralt S, Estey E, Albitar M, et al: Engraftment of allogeneic hematopoietic progenitor cells with purine analog-containing chemotherapy: Harnessing graft-versus-leukemia without myeloablative therapy. *Blood* 89:4531, 1997.
391. Slavin S, Nagler A, Naparstek E, et al: Nonmyeloablative stem cell transplantation and cell therapy as an alternative to conventional bone marrow transplantation with lethal cytoreduction for the treatment of malignant and nonmalignant hematologic diseases. *Blood* 91:756, 1998.
392. Garban F, Attal M, Rossi JF, et al: Immunotherapy by non-myeloablative allogeneic stem cell transplantation in multiple myeloma: Results of a pilot study as salvage therapy after autologous transplantation. *Leukemia* 15:642, 2001.
393. McSweeney PA, Niederwieser D, Shizuru JA, et al: Hematopoietic cell transplantation in older patients with hematologic malignancies: Replacing high-dose cytotoxic therapy with graft-versus-tumor effects. *Blood* 97:3390, 2001.
394. Michallet M, Bilger K, Garban F, et al: Allogeneic hematopoietic stem-cell transplantation after nonmyeloablative preparative regimens: Impact of pretransplantation and posttransplantation factors on outcome. *J Clin Oncol* 19:3340, 2001.
395. Mohty M, Fegueux N, Exbrayat C, et al: Reduced intensity conditioning: Enhanced graft-versus-tumor effect following dose-reduced conditioning and allogeneic transplantation for refractory lymphoid malignancies after high-dose therapy. *Bone Marrow Transplant* 28:335, 2001.
396. Bruno B, Rotta M, Patriarca F, et al: Nonmyeloablative allografting for newly diagnosed multiple myeloma: The experience of the Gruppo Italiano Trapianti di Midollo. *Blood* 113:3375, 2009.
397. Bruno B, Rotta M, Patriarca F, et al: A comparison of allografting with autografting for newly diagnosed myeloma. *N Engl J Med* 356:1110, 2007.
398. Rosinol L, Perez-Simon JA, Sureda A, et al: A prospective PETHEMA study of tandem autologous transplantation versus autograft followed by reduced-intensity conditioning allogeneic transplantation in newly diagnosed multiple myeloma. *Blood* 112:3591, 2008.
399. Garban F, Attal M, Michallet M, et al: Prospective comparison of autologous stem cell transplantation followed by dose-reduced allograft (IFM99–03 trial) with tandem autologous stem cell transplantation (IFM99–04 trial) in high-risk *de novo* multiple myeloma. *Blood* 107:3474, 2006.
400. Rotta M, Storer BE, Sahebi F, et al: Long-term outcome of patients with multiple myeloma after autologous hematopoietic cell transplantation and nonmyeloablative allografting. *Blood* 113:3383, 2009.
401. Stewart AK: Reduced-intensity allogeneic transplantation for myeloma: Reality bites. *Blood* 113:3135, 2009.
402. Attal M, Harousseau JL, Leyvraz S, et al: Maintenance therapy with thalidomide improves survival in patients with multiple myeloma. *Blood* 108:3289, 2006.
403. Schilling G, Hansen T, Shimoni A, et al: Impact of genetic abnormalities on survival after allogeneic hematopoietic stem cell transplantation in multiple myeloma. *Leukemia* 22:1250, 2008.
404. Lee CK, Zangari M, Fassas A, et al: Clonal cytogenetic changes and myeloma relapse after reduced intensity conditioning allogeneic transplantation. *Bone Marrow Transplant* 37:511, 2006.
405. van Rhee F, Crowley J, Barlogie B: Allografting or autografting for myeloma [comment]. *N Engl J Med* 356:2646; author reply 2646, 2007.
406. van Rhee F: Con: Allogenic transplantation in multiple myeloma. *Clin Adv Hematol Oncol* 4:391, 2006.
407. Blade J, Samson D, Reece D, et al: Criteria for evaluating disease response and progression in patients with multiple myeloma treated by high-dose therapy and haemopoietic stem cell transplantation. Myeloma Subcommittee of the EBMT. European Group for Blood and Marrow Transplant. *Br J Haematol* 102:1115, 1998.
408. Kyle RA, Garton JP: The spectrum of IgM monoclonal gammopathy in 430 cases. *Mayo Clin Proc* 62:719, 1987.
409. Dimopoulos MA, Panayiotidis P, Moulopoulos LA, et al: Waldenström's macroglobulinemia: Clinical features, complications, and management. *J Clin Oncol* 18:214, 2000.
410. Dhodapkar MV, Jacobson JL, Gertz MA, et al: Prognostic factors and response to fludarabine therapy in patients with Waldenström macroglobulinemia: Results of United States intergroup trial (Southwest Oncology Group S9003). *Blood* 98:41, 2001.
411. Corwin J, Lindberg RD: Solitary plasmacytoma of bone vs. extramedullary plasmacytoma and their relationship to multiple myeloma. *Cancer* 43:1007, 1979.
412. Bataille R, Sany J: Solitary myeloma: Clinical and prognostic features of a review of 114 cases. *Cancer* 48:845, 1981.
413. Dimopoulos MA, Moulopoulos A, Delasalle K, Alexanian R: Solitary plasmacytoma of bone and asymptomatic multiple myeloma. *Hematol Oncol Clin North Am* 6:359, 1992.
414. Knowling MA, Harwood AR, Bergsagel DE: Comparison of extramedullary plasmacytomas with solitary and multiple plasma cell tumors of bone. *J Clin Oncol* 1:255, 1983.
415. Whittaker J: Solitary plasmacytoma, in *Multiple Myeloma and Other Paraproteinaemias*, edited by I Delamore, p 193. Churchill Livingstone, New York, 1986.
416. Kyle RA, Schreiman JS, McLeod RA, Beabout JW: Computed tomography in diagnosis and management of multiple myeloma and its variants. *Arch Intern Med* 145:1451, 1985.
417. Daffner RH, Lupetin AR, Dash N, et al: MRI in the detection of malignant infiltration of bone marrow. *AJR Am J Roentgenol* 146:353, 1986.
418. Dohner H, Guckel F, Knauf W, et al: Magnetic resonance imaging of bone marrow in lymphoproliferative disorders: Correlation with bone marrow biopsy. *Br J Haematol* 73:12, 1989.
419. Moulopoulos LA, Dimopoulos MA, Weber D, et al: Magnetic resonance imaging in the staging of solitary plasmacytoma of bone. *J Clin Oncol* 11:1311, 1993.
420. Angtuaco E, Jazieh A, Ferris E, et al: Complete remission by MRI (MR-CR) after tandem autotransplants associated with superior survival [abstract]. *Blood* 92(Suppl 1):97a, 1998.
421. Dimopoulos MA, Moulopoulos LA, Maniatis A, Alexanian R: Solitary plasmacytoma of bone and asymptomatic multiple myeloma. *Blood* 96:2037, 2000.
422. Moulopoulos LA, Maris TG, Papanikolaou N, et al: Detection of malignant bone marrow involvement with dynamic contrast-enhanced magnetic resonance imaging. *Ann Oncol* 14:152, 2003.
423. Durie BG, Waxman AD, D'Agnolo A, Williams CM: Whole-body (18)F-FDG PET identifies high-risk myeloma. *J Nucl Med* 43:1457, 2002.
424. Hind CR, Gibson DG, Lavender JP, Pepys MB: Non-invasive demonstration of cardiac involvement in acquired forms of systemic amyloidosis. *Lancet* 1:1417, 1984.
425. Palladini G, Campana C, Klersy C, et al: Serum N-terminal pro-brain natriuretic peptide is a sensitive marker of myocardial dysfunction in AL amyloidosis. *Circulation* 107:2440, 2003.
426. Libbey CA, Skinner M, Cohen AS: Use of abdominal fat tissue aspirate in the diagnosis of systemic amyloidosis. *Arch Intern Med* 143:1549, 1983.
427. Cooper J: A histochemical construct of the amyloid fibril, in *Amyloidosis E.A.R.S.*, edited by Tribe C, Bacon P, p 31. John Wright and Sons, Ltd, Bristol, England, 1983.
428. Dhodapkar MV, Jagannath S, Vesole D, et al: Treatment of AL-amyloidosis with dexamethasone plus alpha interferon. *Leuk Lymphoma* 27:351, 1997.
429. Dhodapkar MV, Jacobson JL, Gertz MA, et al: Prognostic factors and response to fludarabine therapy in Waldenström's macroglobulinemia: An update of a US intergroup trial (SW0G S9003). *Semin Oncol* 30:220, 2003.
430. Palladini G, Perfetti V, Obici L, et al: Association of melphalan and high-dose dexamethasone is effective and well tolerated in patients with AL (primary) amyloidosis who are ineligible for stem cell transplantation. *Blood* 103:2936, 2004.
431. Dispenzieri A, Kyle RA, Lacy MQ, et al: Superior survival in primary systemic amyloidosis patients undergoing peripheral blood stem cell transplantation: A case-control study. *Blood* 103:3960, 2004.
432. Skinner M, Sanchorawala V, Seldin DC, et al: High-dose melphalan and autologous stem-cell transplantation in patients with AL amyloidosis: An 8-year study. *Ann Intern Med* 140:85, 2004.
433. Comenzo RL, Gertz MA: Autologous stem cell transplantation for primary systemic amyloidosis. *Blood* 99:4276, 2002.
434. Alexanian R: Localized and indolent myeloma. *Blood* 56:521, 1980.
435. Kyle RA, Greipp PR: Smoldering multiple myeloma. *N Engl J Med* 302:1347, 1980.
436. Dimopoulos MA, Moulopoulos A, Smith T, et al: Risk of disease progression in asymptomatic multiple myeloma. *Am J Med* 94:57, 1993.
437. Dhodapkar MV, Singh J, Mehta J, et al: Anti-myeloma activity of pamidronate *in vivo*. *Br J Haematol* 103:530, 1998.
438. Weber DM, Dimopoulos MA, Moulopoulos LA, et al: Prognostic features of asymptomatic multiple myeloma. *Br J Haematol* 97:810, 1997.
439. Zangari M, Saghafifar F, Mehta P, et al: The blood coagulation mechanism in multiple myeloma. *Semin Thromb Hemost* 29:275, 2003.
440. Auwerda JJ, Sonneveld P, de Maat MP, Leebeek FW: Prothrombotic coagulation abnormalities in patients with newly diagnosed multiple myeloma. *Haematologica* 92:279, 2007.
441. Johnson DC, Corthals S, Ramos C, et al: Genetic associations with thalidomide mediated venous thrombotic events in myeloma identified using targeted genotyping. *Blood* 112:4924, 2008.
442. Rajkumar SV, Hayman S, Gertz MA, Dispenzieri A, et al: Combination therapy with thalidomide plus dexamethasone for newly diagnosed myeloma. *J Clin Oncol* 20:4319, 2002.
443. Zangari M, Barlogie B, Cavallo F, et al: Effect on survival of treatment-associated venous thromboembolism in newly diagnosed multiple myeloma patients. *Blood Coagul Fibrinolysis* 18:595, 2007.
444. Morgan GJ, Schey SA, Wu P, et al: Lenalidomide (Revlimid), in combination with cyclophosphamide and dexamethasone (RCD), is an effective and tolerated regimen for myeloma patients. *Br J Haematol* 137:268, 2007.
445. Richardson PG, Blood E, Mitsiades C, et al: A randomized phase 2 study of lenalidomide therapy for patients with relapsed or relapsed and refractory multiple myeloma. *Blood* 108:3458, 2006.
446. Baglin T, Luddington R, Brown K, Baglin C: Incidence of recurrent venous thromboembolism in relation to clinical and thrombophilic risk factors: Prospective cohort study. *Lancet* 362:523, 2003.

447. Argyriou AA, Iconomou G, Kalofonos HP: Bortezomib-induced peripheral neuropathy in multiple myeloma: A comprehensive review of the literature. *Blood* 112:1593, 2008.
448. Richardson PG, Sonneveld P, Schuster MW, et al: Reversibility of symptomatic peripheral neuropathy with bortezomib in the phase III APEX trial in relapsed multiple myeloma: Impact of a dose-modification guideline. *Br J Haematol* 144:895, 2009.
449. Mileshkin L, Stark R, Day B, et al: Development of neuropathy in patients with myeloma treated with thalidomide: Patterns of occurrence and the role of electrophysiologic monitoring. *J Clin Oncol* 24:4507, 2006.
450. Plasmati R, Pastorelli F, Cavo M, et al: Neuropathy in multiple myeloma treated with thalidomide: A prospective study. *Neurology* 69:573, 2007.
451. Pei XY, Dai Y, Grant S: Synergistic induction of oxidative injury and apoptosis in human multiple myeloma cells by the proteasome inhibitor bortezomib and histone deacetylase inhibitors. *Clin Cancer Res* 10:3839, 2004.
452. Landowski TH, Megli CJ, Nullmeyer KD, et al: Mitochondrial-mediated disregulation of Ca2+ is a critical determinant of Velcade (PS-341/bortezomib) cytotoxicity in myeloma cell lines. *Cancer Res* 65:3828, 2005.
453. Dikic I, Crosetto N, Calatroni S, Bernasconi P: Targeting ubiquitin in cancers. *Eur J Cancer* 42:3095, 2006.
454. Badros A, Goloubeva O, Dalal JS, et al: Neurotoxicity of bortezomib therapy in multiple myeloma: A single-center experience and review of the literature. *Cancer* 110:1042, 2007.
455. Caravita T, Petrucci MT, Spagnoli A, et al: Neuropathy in multiple myeloma patients treated with bortezomib: A multicenter experience. *Blood* 110: 4823, 2007.
456. Jagannath S, Durie BG, Wolf J, et al: Bortezomib therapy alone and in combination with dexamethasone for previously untreated symptomatic multiple myeloma. *Br J Haematol* 129:776, 2005.
457. Richardson PG, Briemberg H, Jagannath S, et al: Frequency, characteristics, and reversibility of peripheral neuropathy during treatment of advanced multiple myeloma with bortezomib. *J Clin Oncol* 24:3113, 2006.
458. Chen CI, Kouroukis CT, White D, et al: Bortezomib is active in patients with untreated or relapsed Waldenström's macroglobulinemia: A phase II study of the National Cancer Institute of Canada Clinical Trials Group. *J Clin Oncol* 25:1570, 2007.
459. Mitsiades CS, Mitsiades NS, McMullan CJ, et al: Antimyeloma activity of heat shock protein-90 inhibition. *Blood* 107:1092, 2006.
460. Richardson P, Schlossman R, Jagannath S, et al: Thalidomide for patients with relapsed multiple myeloma after high-dose chemotherapy and stem cell transplantation: Results of an open-label multicenter phase 2 study of efficacy, toxicity, and biological activity. *Mayo Clin Proc* 79:875, 2004.
461. Ghobrial IM, Rajkumar SV: Management of thalidomide toxicity. *J Support Oncol* 1:194, 2003.
462. Bastuji-Garin S, Ochonisky S, Bouche P, et al: Incidence and risk factors for thalidomide neuropathy: A prospective study of 135 dermatologic patients. *J Invest Dermatol* 119:1020, 2002.
463. Briani C, Zara G, Rondinone R, et al: Thalidomide neurotoxicity: Prospective study in patients with lupus erythematosus. *Neurology* 62:2288, 2004.
464. Offidani M, Corvatta L, Marconi M, et al: Common and rare side-effects of low-dose thalidomide in multiple myeloma: Focus on the dose-minimizing peripheral neuropathy. *Eur J Haematol* 72:403, 2004.
465. Tosi P, Zamagni E, Cellini C, et al: Neurological toxicity of long-term (>1 yr) thalidomide therapy in patients with multiple myeloma. *Eur J Haematol* 74:212, 2005.
466. Apfel SC, Zochodne DW: Thalidomide neuropathy: Too much or too long? *Neurology* 62:2158, 2004.
467. Rogers MJ, Gordon S, Benford HL, et al: Cellular and molecular mechanisms of action of bisphosphonates. *Cancer* 88:2961, 2000.
468. Terpos E, Sezer O, Croucher PI, et al: The use of bisphosphonates in multiple myeloma: Recommendations of an expert panel on behalf of the European Myeloma Network. *Ann Oncol* 20:1303, 2009.
469. Rosen LS, Gordon D, Kaminski M, et al: Zoledronic acid versus pamidronate in the treatment of skeletal metastases in patients with breast cancer or osteolytic lesions of multiple myeloma: A phase III, double-blind, comparative trial. *Cancer J* 7:377, 2001.
470. Rosen LS, Gordon D, Kaminski M, et al: Long-term efficacy and safety of zoledronic acid compared with pamidronate disodium in the treatment of skeletal complications in patients with advanced multiple myeloma or breast carcinoma: A randomized, double-blind, multicenter, comparative trial. *Cancer* 98:1735, 2003.
471. Lacy MQ, Dispenzieri A, Gertz MA, et al: Mayo clinic consensus statement for the use of bisphosphonates in multiple myeloma. *Mayo Clin Proc* 81:1047, 2006.
472. Durie BG: Use of bisphosphonates in multiple myeloma: IMWG response to Mayo Clinic consensus statement. *Mayo Clin Proc* 82:516; author reply 517, 2007.
473. Dimopoulos MA, Kastritis E, Anagnostopoulos A, et al: Osteonecrosis of the jaw in patients with multiple myeloma treated with bisphosphonates: Evidence of increased risk after treatment with zoledronic acid. *Haematologica* 91:968, 2006.
474. Zervas K, Verrou E, Teleioudis Z, et al: Incidence, risk factors and management of osteonecrosis of the jaw in patients with multiple myeloma: A single-centre experience in 303 patients. *Br J Haematol* 134:620, 2006.
475. Badros A, Weikel D, Salama A, et al: Osteonecrosis of the jaw in multiple myeloma patients: Clinical features and risk factors. *J Clin Oncol* 24:945, 2006.
476. Clarke BM, Boyette J, Vural E, et al: Bisphosphonates and jaw osteonecrosis: The UAMS experience. *Otolaryngol Head Neck Surg* 136:396, 2007.
477. Sarasquete ME, Garcia-Sanz R, Marin L, et al: Bisphosphonate-related osteonecrosis of the jaw is associated with polymorphisms of the cytochrome P450 CYP2C8 in multiple myeloma: A genome-wide single nucleotide polymorphism analysis. *Blood* 112:2709, 2008.
478. Terpos E, Dimopoulos MA: Genetic predisposition for the development of ONJ. *Blood* 112:2596, 2008.
479. Dimopoulos MA, Kastritis E, Bamia C, et al: Reduction of osteonecrosis of the jaw (ONJ) after implementation of preventive measures in patients with multiple myeloma treated with zoledronic acid. *Ann Oncol* 20:117, 2009.
480. Montefusco V, Gay F, Spina F, et al: Antibiotic prophylaxis before dental procedures may reduce the incidence of osteonecrosis of the jaw in patients with multiple myeloma treated with bisphosphonates. *Leuk Lymphoma* 49:2156, 2008.
481. Khan AA, Sandor GK, Dore E, et al: Canadian consensus practice guidelines for bisphosphonate associated osteonecrosis of the jaw. *J Rheumatol* 35:1391, 2008.
482. Durie B, Harousseau J-L, Miguel J, et al: International uniform response criteria for multiple myeloma. *Leukemia* 20:1467, 2006.

CHAPTER 110
THE AMYLOIDOSES

Vaishali Sanchorawala, Daniel R. Jacobson, David C. Seldin, and Joel N. Buxbaum

SUMMARY

The amyloidoses are disorders caused by extracellular protein misfolding and tissue deposition. A soluble protein secreted into the serum or extracellular space aggregates into insoluble, fibrillar tissue deposits, leading to organ dysfunction. The site and rate of protein deposition determine the clinical presentation. Amyloid deposits contain a single major fibrillar component and many minor associated protein and glycosaminoglycan components. To date, 27 different fibril proteins have been isolated in human amyloidosis; the major form associated with hematologic diseases is made up of immunoglobulin light chains. Light-chain amyloidosis (AL amyloidosis) is caused by a monoclonal plasma cell or lymphoproliferative disorder in which the secreted immunoglobulin, either because of its amino acid sequence or some other structural feature, is predisposed to fibrillogenesis under physiologic conditions. AL amyloidosis is characterized by fatigue, weight loss, purpura, heart failure, proteinuria, renal failure, gastrointestinal dysfunction, neuropathy, and various other symptoms, depending upon the organ(s) involved. Diagnosis of amyloidosis (of any type) is made by biopsy of an affected organ or subcutaneous fat aspiration followed by Congo red staining. In the face of similar clinical features, distinguishing AL amyloidosis from the other systemic amyloidoses, in which AL-specific treatment would be inappropriate, is critical. Chemotherapy reduces the size of the plasma cell clone that produces the amyloidogenic light chain and prolongs survival.

DEFINITION AND HISTORY

Amyloidosis is a term for diseases that have in common the extracellular deposition of insoluble fibrillar proteins in tissues and organs. These diseases are a subset of a growing group of disorders recognized to be caused by misfolding of proteins; these disorders include Alzheimer disease and other neurodegenerative diseases, prion diseases, serpinopathies, and some cases of cystic fibrosis. A unifying feature of the amyloidoses is that the deposits share a common β-pleated sheet structural conformation that confers unique staining properties. The term *amyloid* is attributed to the pathologist Rudolf Virchow (1821–1902), who, in 1854, thought such deposits in autopsy livers were starch-like because of their peculiar staining reaction with iodine and sulfuric acid.[1] One hundred years later "amyloid" was found to be a proteinaceous fibrillar deposit in tissues.[2] Biochemical characterization of the fibril proteins from clinical cases proved the "amyloidoses" to be a spectrum of diseases, often with a fatal outcome because of progressive deposition of amyloid fibrils in major organs. A growing list of treatments are available to target the source of the abnormal protein and, for some types, to inhibit the amyloidogenic protein misfolding process.

Acronyms and abbreviations that appear in this chapter include: AA, amyloid A; Aβ_2M, amyloid β_2-microglobulin; AF, familial amyloid; AL, light-chain amyloid; CPHPC, 6-R-2-carboxy-pyrrolidin-1-yl-6-oxo-hexanoyl pyrrolidine-2-carboxylic acid; HDM/autoSCT, high-dose melphalan and autologous stem cell transplantation; IDOX, 4-iodo-4-deoxydoxorubicin; IEF, isoelectric focusing; IMiDs, immunomodulatory drugs; MIDD, monoclonal immunoglobulin deposition disease; NT-proBNP, N-terminal probrain natriuretic peptide; SAP, serum amyloid P component; TTR, transthyretin; VAD, infusional vincristine, doxorubicin (Adriamycin), and dexamethasone.

CLASSIFICATION AND EPIDEMIOLOGY

In the past, the amyloidoses were classified according to the clinical or pathologic features of the associated diseases. Secondary (amyloid A [AA]) amyloidosis accompanied chronic inflammatory processes. Familial (AF) amyloidosis was recognized by distinctive clinical manifestations within kindreds. All other types, except the type occurring in association with myeloma, were termed *primary*, in the sense that they were idiopathic. The development of methods for dissolving and fractionating amyloid fibrils extracted from tissues permitted the identification of 27 different proteins as amyloid precursors to date (Table 110–1). Classification now is based upon the chemical nature of the fibrillar component of the deposits, for example, immunoglobulin light-chain amyloidosis termed as *AL amyloidosis*. Terms such as *primary*, *secondary*, *senile*, *dialysis-associated*, and *myeloma-associated* have been abandoned in favor of the etiologically based, chemical terminology.[3]

In the localized forms of amyloidosis, the deposits occur at the site of synthesis of the precursor protein. In the systemic amyloidoses, the deposits form in organs at a distance from the precursor-producing cells.

The epidemiologic data on the incidence of amyloidosis is limited. One study based on the National Center for Health Statistics data estimated the incidence of AL amyloidosis as 4.5 per 100,000.[4] AL amyloidosis, like the other plasma cell neoplasms, usually begins after age 40 years and is associated with rapid progression, multisystem involvement, and a short survival. AA amyloidosis is increasingly rare, occurring in less than 1 percent of persons with chronic inflammatory diseases in the United States and Europe, but is more common in Turkey and the Middle East, where it occurs in association with familial Mediterranean fever.[5,6] It may begin within a year after onset of the underlying inflammatory disease or many years later. It is the only type of amyloidosis that occurs in children. Amyloid β_2-microglobulin (Aβ_2M) amyloidosis usually manifests as deposits in the joint synovial, occurs in patients on long-term dialysis, and is also declining in incidence with changes in dialysis techniques.[7]

The inherited amyloidoses are rare in the United States, with an estimated incidence of less than 1 per 100,000.[8] They are autosomal dominant diseases in which a variant plasma protein forms amyloid deposits, generally beginning in mid-life, however, rarely before childhood. Amyloidogenic transthyretin (ATTR) amyloidosis is the most common form of familial amyloidosis and is associated with mutations of the gene encoding transthyretin (TTR). There are nearly 100 types of mutations known to be associated with ATTR amyloidosis.[9] One variant, Val-122-Ile, has a carrier frequency that may be as high as 4 percent among Americans of African descent and is associated with late-onset cardiac amyloidosis.[10] There are also regions with a high incidence of ATTR amyloidosis caused by mutations such as Val-30-Met in Portugal, Sweden, Japan, and other countries. Even wild-type TTR can form fibrils, leading to senile systemic amyloidosis, which predominantly affects the heart, in older patients.[11,12] Other familial amyloidoses, caused by variant apolipoprotein A-I, A-II, gelsolin, fibrinogen Aα, or lysozyme, are reported in only a few families worldwide.

TABLE 110–1. The Modern (Chemical) Classification of Human Amyloidosis

Amyloid Protein	Precursor Protein	Clinical Syndrome(s)
AL	Immunoglobulin light chains or light-chain fragments	Plasma cell disorders
AH	Immunoglobulin heavy chain	Systemic amyloidosis
ATTR	Transthyretin (TTR)	Familial amyloidotic polyneuropathy, familial amyloid cardiomyopathy, senile systemic amyloidosis, isolated vitreous amyloidosis
AA	Apo-SAA	Inflammation-associated, acquired, or inherited (tumor necrosis factor receptor-associated periodic syndrome, TRAPS, and familial Mediterranean fever)
Aβ_2M	β_2-Microglobulin	Dialysis-associated amyloid
AApoAI	Apolipoprotein A-I	Familial amyloidosis involving various organs
AApoAII	Apolipoprotein A-II	Familial renal amyloidosis
AFib	Fibrinogen α chain	Familial renal amyloidosis
ALys	Lysozyme	Familial systemic amyloidosis
ACys	Cystatin C	Hereditary cerebral hemorrhage with amyloidosis, Icelandic type
Aβ	β-Protein precursor	Alzheimer disease, Down syndrome, hereditary cerebral hemorrhage with amyloidosis, Dutch type
AprP	Prion protein	Creutzfeldt-Jakob and Gerstmann-Straüssler-Scheinker diseases
AGel	Gelsolin	Hereditary corneal amyloidosis
AKer	Keratoepithelin	Hereditary corneal amyloidosis
ALac	Lactoferrin	Hereditary corneal amyloidosis
ACal	Calcitonin	Medullary carcinoma of the thyroid (in multiple endocrine neoplasia)
AIAPP	Amylin (islet amyloid polypeptide)	Insulinoma, type II diabetes mellitus
AANF	Atrial natriuretic factor	Isolated atrial amyloidosis
APro	Prolactin	Pituitary amyloid
ACytokeratin	Keratin	Cutaneous amyloidosis
Abri/ADan	Bri/Dan	Familial British and Danish dementia
AIns	Insulin	Iatrogenic
AMed	Lactadherin	Senile aortic
APin	To be named	Pindborg tumor-associated protein

Amyloid Precursor Proteins

The amyloid precursor proteins are usually small, with molecular weights between 4000 and 25,000 daltons. They do not share any detectable amino acid sequence homology, although the secondary structures of many of the proteins have substantial β-pleated sheet structure. The known exceptions include serum amyloid A (SAA) and PrP^c, which contain little or no β folding in the precursor protein despite extensive β-sheet in the deposited fibrils.

The clinical amyloidoses are *in vivo* disorders of protein structure in which the precursor proteins are secreted from the cell in a soluble form, only to become insoluble at some tissue site, ultimately compromising organ function. They represent a part of the total spectrum of protein deposition disorders. *In vivo* the protein aggregates in the intracellular deposition diseases such as Parkinson disease (in which there is cytoplasmic deposition of synuclein and other proteins in Lewy bodies) and Huntington disease (in which there is intranuclear deposition of proteins such as huntingtin rich in poly-Glu tracts) fail to form the regular fibrils seen in the amyloidoses.[14,15] The isolated proteins α-synuclein (Parkinson disease) and huntingtin will form amyloid fibrils when incubated under the appropriate conditions *in vitro*.

Genetic Factors

In some cases, the aberrant secondary structure seen in amyloid reflects a hereditary alteration in sequence that predisposes to fibril formation, as seen in the proteins TTR, lysozyme, fibrinogen, cystatin c, gelsolin, amyloid-β protein precursor (AβPP), and apolipoprotein A-I (ApoAI). In other cases, wild-type molecules are the fibril precursors (TTR, β_2-microglobulin [β_2M], ApoAI). The deposits are primarily extracellular, but fibrillar structures within lysosomes of macrophages and the cisternae of plasma cells in light-chain amyloid (AL) marrow occur.[16]

ETIOLOGY AND PATHOGENESIS

MECHANISMS OF AMYLOID FIBRIL FORMATION

The exact mechanism of fibril formation is unknown and may be different among the various types of amyloid.[13] However, studies indicate there is a common underlying mechanism in which a partially unfolded protein intermediate forms multimers and then higher-order polymers. Some of the factors that contribute to fibrillogenesis include variant or unstable protein structure, extensive β conformation of the precursor protein, proteolytic processing of the precursor protein, association with components of the serum or extracellular matrix (e.g., amyloid P-component, amyloid-enhancing factor, apolipoprotein E, and glycosaminoglycans), and physical properties, including pH of the tissue site.

Accessory Molecules

The role of P component and of the other accessory molecules in amyloid deposition is not clear. Although they do not appear to be required for fibril formation, they may stabilize the fibril, protecting it from proteolysis once it is formed, or enhance the transition from protofibril to fibril. In experimental systems, the rate of amyloid deposition is slower in the absence of P component.[17] Intravenously injected purified P component preferentially binds to amyloid deposits. This property has been exploited clinically, using radiolabeled P component, to localize and quantify the total body burden of amyloid in the so-called SAPscan.[18] The scan has been particularly useful in evaluating liver, spleen, and endocrine deposits, less so in disease involving the heart because of signal-to-noise issues.

Apolipoprotein E (ApoE) is found in all types of amyloid deposits.[19] One ApoE allele (ApoE$_4$) is strongly associated with Alzheimer disease.

$ApoE_4$ also may be a risk factor for other forms of amyloidosis, but its association with other amyloidoses is less-well supported by the epidemiologic evidence. The mechanism of ApoE involvement is not known.

The heparan sulfate proteoglycan perlecan is a basement membrane component intimately associated with all types of tissue amyloid deposits.[20] As with P component and ApoE, its role in amyloidogenesis remains undefined. Compounds known to bind to heparan sulfate proteoglycans, such as anionic sulfonates, decrease fibril deposition in murine models of AA disease and have been suggested as potential therapeutic agents.[21] One such chemical compound, eprodisate, has been demonstrated to slow the progression of AA amyloid renal failure in a randomized phase III clinical trial.[22]

Role of Proteolysis

In some instances, the amyloid precursors undergo proteolysis, which may enhance the kinetics of folding into a prefibrillar structural intermediate. In some of the amyloidoses (e.g., Aβ or AA), a normal proteolytic process may be disturbed, yielding a higher than normal concentration of a prefibrillar molecule. Whether tissue deposition is purely physicochemical or depends upon an interaction equivalent to that between ligand and receptor, in which some component of tissue ground substance is the binding target, is not known. When cleavage occurs relative to deposition in cases in which proteolysis is observed also is not known.

Cellular Origin and Immunoglobulins

AL amyloidosis is usually caused by a plasma cell neoplasm in the marrow, and can occur in isolation or along with myeloma (see Chap. 109). Similar cytogenetic changes have been identified in both plasma cell diseases, suggesting they may have a common molecular pathogenesis.[23] By two-dimensional gel electrophoresis and mass spectrometry, amyloid fibril deposits are composed of intact 23-kDa monoclonal immunoglobulin light chains as well as C-terminal truncated fragments.[24] Although all kappa (κ) and lambda (λ) light-chain subtypes have been identified in amyloid fibrils, λ subtypes predominate, and the λ VI subtype appears to have unique structural properties that predispose it to fibril formation,[25] often in the kidney.[26] AL amyloidosis is usually a rapidly progressive disease with amyloid deposits in multiple tissue sites. AL can also occur in other B lymphoproliferative disorders including Waldenström macroglobulinemia and lymphoma.[27]

The Role of Inflammation

AA amyloidosis is a complication of severe, long-standing inflammation, as occurs in rheumatic diseases or chronic infections such as tuberculosis. The AA amyloid fibrils are usually composed of an 8-kDa, 76-amino-acid amino-terminal portion of the 12-kDa precursor, SAA.[28] SAA is a polymorphic protein encoded by a family of SAA genes, which are acute phase apoproteins synthesized in the liver and transported by high-density lipoprotein (HDL3) in the plasma. Several years of an underlying inflammatory disease causing an elevated SAA usually precedes fibril formation, although infections can produce AA deposition more quickly. AA fibril formation can be accelerated by an amyloid enhancing factor present in high concentration in the spleen (which may be early SAA aggregates or deposits), by basement membrane heparan sulfate proteoglycan, or by seeding with AA or heterologous fibrils.[29]

Factors related to β_2M fibril formation are under investigation. The formerly high prevalence of Aβ_2M disease in patients undergoing long-term dialysis argues against an amyloidogenic variant β_2-microglobulin molecule. Permeability of dialysis membranes may be a factor as the molecular weight of β_2-microglobulin is 11.8 kDa, above the porosity of standard membranes. It has also been hypothesized that dialysis membranes may be bioincompatible and induce proinflammatory mediators that stimulate or modify β_2-microglobulin and contribute to fibril formation.[30]

Familiality (Inheritance) and Aging

In variant familial amyloidotic polyneuropathy or cardiomyopathy ATTR amyloidosis (also called familial amyloidotic polyneuropathy or cardiomyopathy), and all other forms of familial amyloidosis, inherited mutations or polymorphisms in the genes encoding large serum proteins produce amyloid-prone variants. The process of fibrillogenesis has been best studied for TTR, in which variant TTR molecules appear to be prone to dissociation from stable tetramers and to unfolding, leading to misfolding, polymerization, and fibril formation.[31] The role of aging is intriguing, because patients with the variant proteins do not have clinically apparent disease in childhood, despite the lifelong presence of the abnormal protein.[32] Further evidence of an age-related "trigger" is that senile cardiac amyloidosis, caused by the deposition of fibrils derived from normal wild-type TTR, is exclusively a disease of elderly people.[12]

DIAGNOSIS

■ TISSUE BIOPSY

A tissue biopsy demonstrating amyloid fibrils is necessary for the diagnosis of amyloidosis (Fig. 110–1). The least-invasive biopsy is the

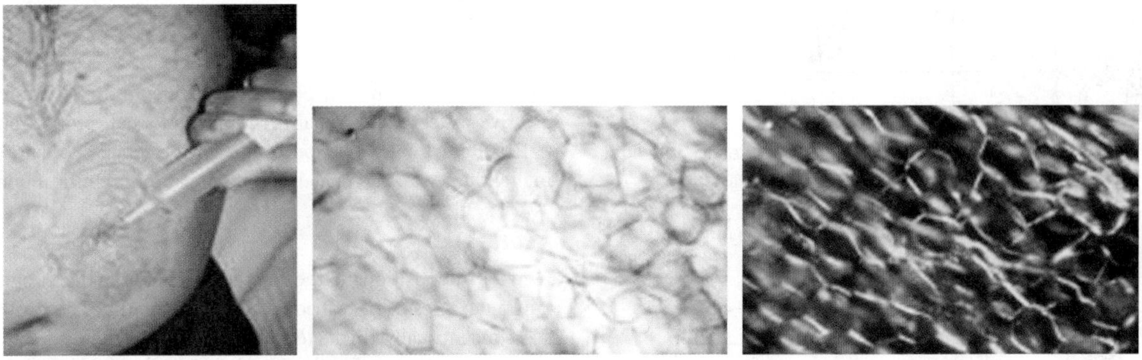

FIGURE 110–1. A. Subcutaneous fat aspirate. **B.** Aspirated fat stained with Congo red and viewed by light microscopy. **C.** Same specimen viewed under polarized light (×200). The staining and birefringence is evident in the walls and connective tissue surrounding the adipose cells.

abdominal fat aspirate, which is positive in 80 to 90 percent of patients with either AL or ATTR amyloidosis and in 60 to 70 percent of patients with AA amyloidosis.[33] It is easy to perform after local injection of anesthetic, and has a low rate of infectious or hemorrhagic complications. If the aspirate is negative but clinical suspicion for disease persists, a more invasive tissue biopsy should be done. Although a biopsy of a clinically involved organ is recommended, almost any tissue biopsy is likely to be positive if the patient has systemic amyloidosis. In a series of 100 patients with AL amyloidosis, 85 percent of 249 tissues biopsied were positive including all samples from the kidney, heart, and liver.[34] Once the diagnosis of amyloidosis is made, a careful evaluation of the entire clinical picture, including manner of presentation, organ system involvement, underlying diseases, and family history should provide a clue to the type of amyloid.

SERUM AND URINE IMMUNOGLOBULIN ASSAY AND MARROW EXAMINATION

Identification of a plasma cell neoplasm distinguishes AL from other types of amyloidosis (Fig. 110–2). More than 90 percent of patients have a serum or urine monoclonal immunoglobulin protein or a free light chain on testing by immunofixation electrophoresis or by a nephelometric assay for free light chains.[35,36] In addition, there is often an increased percentage of plasma cells in the marrow, which are monoclonal on immunohistochemical staining.[37] A monoclonal serum protein by itself is not diagnostic of amyloidosis, as essential monoclonal gammopathy is common in older patients. However, when monoclonal gammopathy is present in a patient with biopsy-proven amyloidosis, the AL type should be strongly suspected.

IMMUNOHISTOCHEMISTRY AND MASS SPECTROMETRY–BASED MICROSEQUENCING

Immunohistochemical staining by light or electron microscopy should be carried out by a laboratory familiar with the techniques and able to perform appropriate controls.[38] Mass spectrometry–based microsequencing of small amounts of protein extracted from fibril deposits is an alternative method to identify the components of the fibrils.[39]

AA amyloidosis should be suspected in patients with renal amyloidosis and a chronic inflammatory condition or infection. AL and

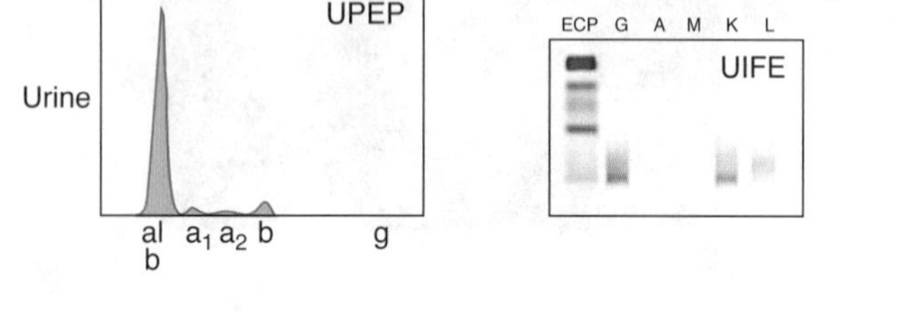

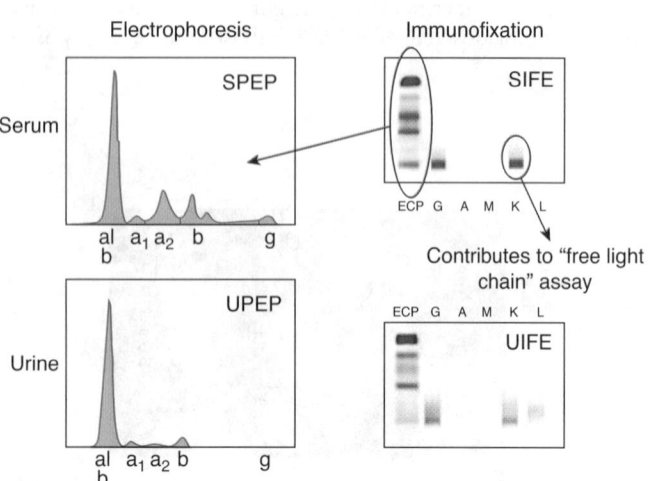

FIGURE 110–2. Protein electrophoresis and immunofixation electrophoresis of serum and urine.

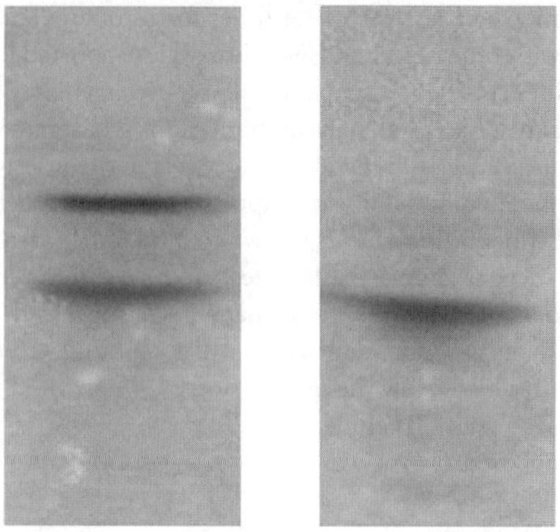

FIGURE 110–3. Isoelectric focusing of serum samples shows bands of both mutant (lane 1) and wild-type TTR (lane 2) protein.

ATTR amyloidosis should be ruled out and confirmation of AA amyloidosis made by immunohistochemical staining for AA protein.

ISOELECTRIC FOCUSING AND POLYMERASE CHAIN REACTION

Familial amyloidosis should be excluded in patients who do not have a plasma cell neoplasm or the AA type of amyloidosis. Although the disease has a dominant inheritance, family history may not be apparent when the disease occurs later in life; also, some cases occur through new mutations. Variant TTR proteins can usually be detected by isoelectric focusing (IEF; Fig. 110–3).[40] An abnormal IEF procedure should be followed by polymerase chain reaction–based sequencing of the TTR exons to determine the precise TTR mutation, and can be used to identify mutations in TTR, fibrinogen, lysozyme, and apolipoproteins when AF is suspected and TTR IEF is negative.

CLINICAL FEATURES

AL AMYLOIDOSIS

The organs most frequently affected in AL amyloidosis are the kidneys and the heart[41–43]; however, virtually any tissue other than the brain can be involved.

Kidney

Kidney involvement usually presents as nephrotic syndrome with progressive worsening of renal function. In a small proportion of patients (~10%), amyloid deposition occurs in the renal vasculature or tubulointerstitium, causing renal dysfunction without significant proteinuria.[44]

Heart

Amyloid deposition in the heart results in rapidly progressive heart failure as a result of restrictive cardiomyopathy. The ventricular walls are concentrically thickened with normal or reduced cavity size. The ventricular ejection fraction can be normal or only slightly decreased, but impaired ventricular filling limits cardiac output.[43] Low voltage on the electrocardiogram is found in a high proportion of patients and is often associated with a pseudoinfract pattern.[43]

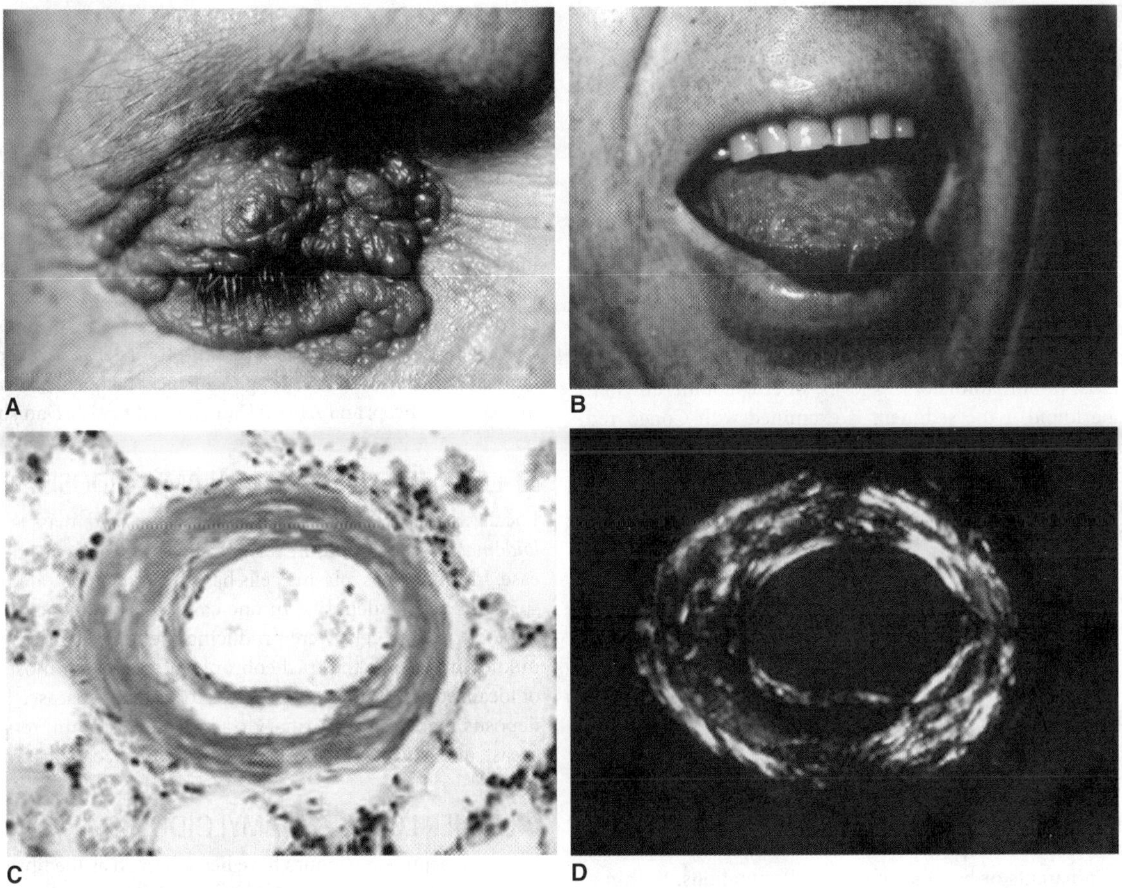

FIGURE 110–4. **A.** Extensive amyloid deposits in the upper and lower palpebrae. **B.** Multiple amyloid deposits in the tongue. **C.** Patient with AL amyloidosis. Marrow small vessel stained with Congo red. Amyloid replacement of vascular wall. **D.** Same image as in **(C)** viewed under polarized light with the polarizing filters set at 90-degree angles. The Congo red-stained material shows birefringence with transmission of apple-green colored light. This is due to the characteristic β-pleated sheet structure of the abnormal amyloid proteins deposited in tissue. In AL amyloidosis, the deposited material is monoclonal immunoglobulin light chains. Corresponding immunohistochemistry stains for κ and λ light chains (not shown) confirmed the presence of a small, monoclonal plasma cell population in this patient's marrow sample, confirming a diagnosis of AL amyloidosis. *(Used with permission from* Lichtman's Atlas of Hematology, *www.accessmedicine.com.)*

Liver

Hepatomegaly is common and can occur as a result of either congestion from right heart failure or amyloid infiltration of the liver. Hepatomegaly from amyloid infiltration can be massive and on physical examination, the liver is typically "rock hard" and nontender. Profound elevation of alkaline phosphatase with only mild elevation of transaminases is characteristic of hepatic amyloidosis as infiltration occurs in the sinusoids.[45]

Nervous System

Autonomic nervous system involvement by AL amyloidosis can lead to orthostatic hypotension, early satiety because of delayed gastric emptying, erectile dysfunction, and intestinal motility issues. Painful, bilateral, symmetric, distal sensory neuropathy that progresses to motor neuropathy is the usual manifestation of peripheral nervous system involvement.

Soft Tissues

Soft tissue involvement is characterized by macroglossia, carpal tunnel syndrome, skin nodules, arthropathy, alopecia, nail dystrophy, submandibular gland enlargement, periorbital purpura, and hoarseness of voice. Although present in a minority of patients, macroglossia is a hallmark feature of AL amyloidosis (Fig. 110–4).

Endocrine Glands

Endocrinopathies such as hypothyroidism and hypoadrenalism are rare, but are reported to occur with AL amyloidosis as a result of amyloid infiltration of the glands.[42]

Coagulation Proteins

Many clotting abnormalities have been described in AL. Factor X may bind to amyloid fibrils, leading to its rapid clearance from the blood, with consequent prolongation of the prothrombin and partial thromboplastin times.[46] Elevated levels of tissue and urine plasminogen activators and a decreased level of tissue plasminogen activator inhibitor, leading to hyperfibrinolytic states, can occur.[47]

AA AMYLOIDOSIS

AA amyloidosis can occur at any age. The primary clinical manifestation is proteinuria and/or renal insufficiency.[5] A study from Finland found AA amyloidosis to be the most common cause of nephrotic syndrome in patients with rheumatoid arthritis.[48] Hepatomegaly, splenomegaly, and autonomic neuropathy frequently occur as the disease progresses; cardiomyopathy occurs rarely. With chronic inflammatory diseases, amyloid progression is slow and survival is often more than 10 years, particularly with treatment for end-stage renal disease. In contrast, untreated infections such as osteomyelitis, tuberculosis, or leprosy can produce a more rapidly progressive amyloid syndrome, which will remit with effective treatment of the infection.

■ Aβ_2M AMYLOIDOSIS

Several distinct rheumatologic conditions are observed in Aβ_2M amyloidosis including carpal tunnel syndrome, persistent joint effusions, spondyloarthropathy, and cystic bone lesions. Carpal tunnel syndrome is usually the first symptom of disease. Persistent joint effusions accompanied by mild discomfort occur in up to 50 percent of patients on dialysis for more than 12 years. Involvement is bilateral and large joints (shoulders, knees, wrists, and hips) are more frequently affected. The synovial fluid is noninflammatory, and β_2-microglobulin amyloid deposits can be found if the sediment is examined with Congo red staining. Spondyloarthropathy with destructive changes of the intervertebral discs and paravertebral erosions have occurred in association with β_2-microglobulin amyloid deposits. Cystic bone lesions sometimes leading to pathologic fractures have been described in the femoral head, acetabulum, humerus, tibial plateau, vertebral bodies, and carpal bones. Although less common, visceral β_2-microglobulin amyloid deposits do occasionally occur in the gastrointestinal tract, heart, tendons, and subcutaneous tissues of the buttocks.

■ ATTR FAMILIAL AMYLOIDOSIS

The clinical features of ATTR amyloidosis overlap AL amyloidosis such that the diseases cannot be reliably distinguished on clinical grounds alone. A family history makes ATTR more likely, but many patients appear to present sporadically, either because of a lack of ascertainment in parents or because of new TTR mutations. Within a family, disease tends to occur with the same symptomatology. For ATTR Val-30-Met, peripheral neuropathy begins in the extremities as sensory neuropathy and progresses to motor neuropathy. This pattern varies with different TTR variants. Autonomic neuropathy is manifest by gastrointestinal symptoms of diarrhea with weight loss and orthostatic hypotension. Patients with TTR T60A and several other mutations have myocardial thickening similar to that caused by AL amyloidosis, although heart failure is less common and the prognosis is better. Vitreous opacities caused by amyloid deposits are pathognomonic of ATTR amyloidosis.

The TTR variant, Val-122-Ile, is a common allele in the African American population and is associated with cardiomyopathy. In a large referral population, 25 percent of black patients with amyloidosis had this TTR variant. It is likely that this disease is underdiagnosed as a result of a lack of physician awareness and the difficulty of distinguishing amyloid and hypertensive cardiomyopathy without an endomyocardial biopsy.[10]

OTHER FORMS OF AMYLOIDOSIS

■ HEREDITARY RENAL AMYLOIDOSES

The hereditary renal amyloidoses (amyloidosis ApoA-I [AApoAI], ApoA-II [AApoAII], amyloidosis fibrinogen α-chain [AFib], amyloidosis lysozyme [ALys]) can resemble AL with renal involvement and should be considered when a renal biopsy shows amyloid deposition.[49] The clinical differentiation between the hereditary renal amyloidoses and AL with a dominant renal presentation often is suggested by the family history and immunoglobulin studies. The definitive diagnosis is made by immunohistologic staining of the biopsy material with antibodies specific for the candidate amyloid precursor proteins.

■ AMYLOIDOSES LOCALIZED TO THE CENTRAL NERVOUS SYSTEM

Little clinical confusion should exist between AL disease and any of the primarily central nervous system amyloidoses because AL deposits are rarely found in the central nervous system, although they may be found in the cerebral vessels. The primary central nervous system amyloidoses include amyloidosis cystatin C (ACys); hereditary cerebral hemorrhage with amyloidosis-Icelandic type, in which the precursor is the protease inhibitor cystatin c; the Aβ amyloidoses, including Dutch-type hereditary cerebral hemorrhage with amyloidosis, Alzheimer disease, and Down syndrome; amyloidosis PrP (APrP), the prionoses including Creutzfeldt-Jakob disease, Gerstmann-Straüssler-Scheinker disease, fatal familial insomnia, bovine spongiform encephalopathy, kuru, and scrapie in goats and sheep; and ABri/ADan, familial British/Danish dementia.[50]

■ LOCALIZED LIGHT-CHAIN AMYLOIDOSIS

Localized amyloid deposits, including amyloid masses termed *amyloidomas*, may be found in various sites in the absence of systemic disease. In some cases, plasma cells have been demonstrated histologically surrounding the deposits. In one case, DNA sequencing revealed that the local plasma cells were producing the deposited light chains.[51] For unknown reasons, the tracheobronchial tree is the most common site of localized AL; it does not progress to systemic disease.[52] Localized AL deposits involving the urinary tract,[53] mediastinum, retroperitoneum, breast, and skin (as either plaques or nodules), can occur.

■ OTHER LOCALIZED AMYLOIDOSES

Four polypeptide hormones have been defined as the fibril precursors in tissue-specific localized amyloidoses: Atrial natriuretic factor amyloidosis (AANF) affects older persons, often with congestive heart failure. The precursor protein is atrial natriuretic factor, a hormone that controls salt and water homeostasis, synthesized by the cardiac atria. The amyloid deposits are confined to the atria and are considered of minor clinical significance.[54] In calcitonin amyloid (ACal), the precursor protein is calcitonin, a calcium regulatory hormone synthesized by the thyroid. Patients with medullary carcinoma of the thyroid may develop localized amyloid deposition in the tumors. The pathogenesis is based on increased local calcitonin production, leading to a high local concentration of the peptide, which polymerizes and results in fibril formation.[55] In pancreatic islet cell amyloid polypeptide amyloidosis (AIAPP), the precursor protein is a polypeptide (IAPP), also known as amylin. IAPP is a protein secreted by the β cells that is in the secretory granules and released in along with insulin. Normally, IAPP modulates insulin activity in skeletal muscle. IAPP amyloid is found in insulinomas and in the pancreas of patients with diabetes mellitus type 2.[56] In prolactin amyloid (Apro), prolactin or its fragments are found in the pituitary amyloid. This deposition occurs in older people and, rarely, in amyloidomas in a patients with prolactin-producing pituitary tumors.[57] Three proteins (gelsolin, keratoepithelin, and lactoferrin) have been found in fibrils from patients with autosomal dominant corneal amyloidosis.[58] Medin, an integral fragment of lactadherin, which is produced in aortic smooth muscle cell, forms the amyloid seen in the aorta of all older humans.[59] Insulin has been found in fibrils at the site of insulin injection.[60] Cytokeratin has been found in amyloidosis localized to the skin.[61]

TREATMENT AND PROGNOSIS

In theory potential treatments of the amyloidoses can be directed at interfering with any of several pathogenetic processes. Production of the precursor can be reduced or its catabolism enhanced; generation of the prefibrillar intermediate can be blocked; interactions between prefibrillar molecules yielding the fibril can be inhibited; deposition can be slowed; or deposits can be actively mobilized. At present, standard treatment of AL involves only one of these strategies, that is, reducing production of the monoclonal light-chain precursor with chemotherapy or, occasionally, radiotherapy or surgery of a localized amyloidogenic plasmacytoma. Equally important are supportive measures that maintain organ function in the absence of specific treatment or while specific therapy is administered.

AL AMYLOIDOSIS

Assessment of Treatment Response

Criteria for hematologic and organ responses for AL amyloidosis were unified and formalized in a consensus report.[62] Complete hematologic response is defined as absence of monoclonal protein in serum and urine by immunofixation electrophoresis, normal serum-free light-chain ratio and marrow biopsy with less than 5 percent plasma cells with no clonal predominance by immunohistochemistry. Hematologic response is associated with a substantial survival advantage, improved quality of life, and improved organ function.[63–65] Improved organ function may be evident 3 to 6 months following treatment, although more delayed responses also occur. Reduction in proteinuria is gradual with continued improvement over 2 or more years.[66] Importantly, a complete clonal hematologic response is not a prerequisite for clinical response and clinical improvement may still occur in patients with a partial clonal response. However, the rate of clinical response is higher in patients with a complete hematologic response than in those with a partial one. In one report, a reduction in serum-free light-chain concentration of greater than 90 percent was associated with a similar high likelihood of clinical improvement and prolonged survival, whether or not patients achieved a complete response after treatment.[67]

High-Dose Melphalan and Autologous Blood Stem Cell Transplantation

High-dose intravenous melphalan chemotherapy (HDM) followed by autologous blood stem cell transplantation (autoSCT) is presently considered the most effective treatment for AL amyloidosis at many centers. Table 110–2 summarizes the results of single and multicenter studies of HDM/autoSCT. Encouraging hematologic and clinical responses have been reported in these studies, and although these are not controlled trials, the rates of complete hematologic response (25–67%) far exceed those observed with cyclic oral melphalan and prednisone, treatment that had been the standard approach, previously. A case-matched control study has suggested the superiority of HDM/autoSCT compared to conventional oral melphalan and prednisone.[68] Dexamethasone has been substituted for prednisone and higher rates of responses have been seen in single-center studies.[69] This regimen has been compared with HDM/autoSCT in a multicenter trial conducted in France that failed to show a survival benefit for HDM/autoSCT.[70] However, in this study, many of the patients randomized to HDM/autoSCT treatment were not actually transplanted, the toxicity on the transplant arm was excessive, and followup was short. Thus, the question of optimal therapy remains open, particularly as transplant techniques are refined, and drug regimens are improved. However, patients should be carefully selected for transplant, as advanced cardiac disease, multiorgan involvement, hypotension, and poor performance status are poor prognostic factors for the outcome of HDM/autoSCT. With these caveats, remarkable outcomes have been seen. Updated results from the Amyloid Treatment and Research Program at Boston University Medical Center demonstrate a median survival of 73 months for 497 patients with AL amyloidosis treated with HDM/autoSCT from 1994 to 2007 (Fig. 110–5). The 5-year survival for this group of patients is 55 percent.

TABLE 110–2. Results of Single and Multicenter Studies of HDM/AUTOSCT in AL Amyloidosis

	No. of Patients	TRM	Hematologic Complete Response	Organ Response
Single-center clinical trials				
Gertz et al, 2007[63]	270	11%	33%	NR
Mollee et al, 2004[108]	20	35%	28%	Renal 46%, cardiac 25%, liver 50%
Schonland et al, 2005[109]	41	7%	50%	40%
Skinner et al, 2004[110]	277	13%	40%	44%
Chow et al, 2005[111]	15	0%	67%	27%
Multicenter clinical trials				
Moreau et al, 1998[112]	21	43%	25%	83%
Gertz et al, 2004[113]	28	14%	NA	75%
Goodman et al, 2006[77]	92	23%	83% (CR + PR)	48%
Vesole et al, 2006[114]	114	18%	36%	Renal 46%, liver 58%, cardiac 47%

CR, complete response; NR, not reported; PR, partial response; TRM, treatment-related mortality.

Special Problems Associated with HDM/AutoSCT in AL Amyloidosis

Several challenges with HDM/autoSCT are unique to patients with AL amyloidosis. Amyloid deposition in the gastrointestinal tract predisposes to gastrointestinal bleeding during periods of cytopenia; this can be exacerbated by amyloid-associated coagulopathies such as factor X deficiency. Anasarca is common in patients with nephrotic syndrome and is exacerbated by granulocyte colony-stimulating factor administration. Hypotension from cardiac disease or autonomic nervous system involvement, atrial and ventricular arrhythmias in patients with amyloid cardiomyopathy, difficulties with endotracheal intubation as a consequence of macroglossia, and spontaneous splenic, hepatic, and esophageal rupture are also problems that can arise during treatment in these patients.

HDM/AutoSCT Following Heart Transplantation

Patients with severe systolic or diastolic heart failure because of amyloid cardiomyopathy are intolerant of chemotherapy and glucocorticoid-containing regimens. Thus, orthotopic heart transplantation may be

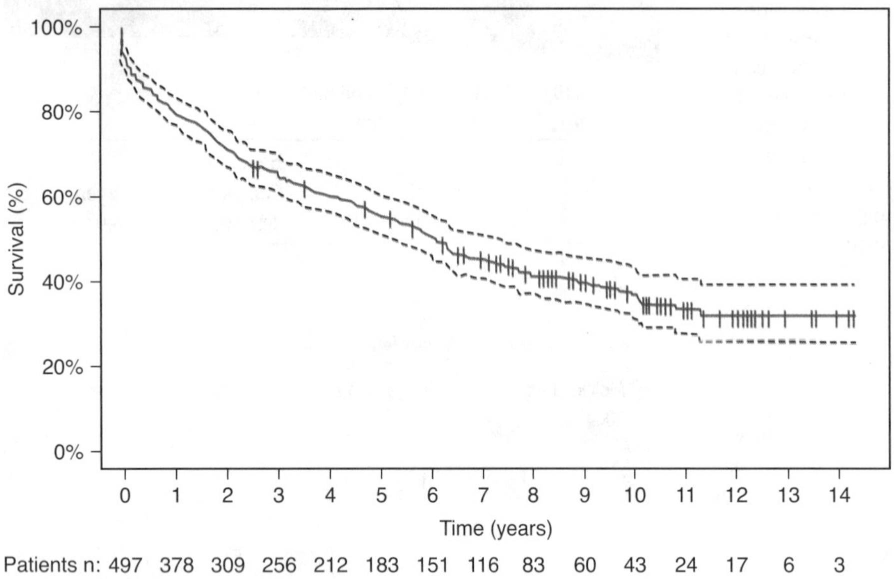

FIGURE 110–5. Overall survival of 497 patients with AL amyloidosis treated with high-dose melphalan and autologous stem cell transplantation at Boston University Medical Center during the period 1994 to 2007.

required as a life-saving procedure. Because of the high likelihood of amyloid recurrence in the transplanted organ,[71] as well as progression in other organs, heart transplantation should be followed by antiplasma cell therapy. Thus, carefully selected patients, without other significant organ involvement, can benefit from a double transplant protocol of heart transplantation followed by HDM/autoSCT.[72,73]

Allogeneic Marrow Transplantation

There is a small experience with allogeneic and syngeneic marrow transplantation for AL amyloidosis. A report by the European Cooperative Group for Blood and Marrow Transplantation describes 19 patients who underwent allogeneic transplantation.[74] The group is heterogeneous as it included 4 syngeneic, 8 reduced-intensity conditioning, and 7 full-dose allogeneic transplants, and 10 were T-cell–depleted grafts. Complete hematologic responses were seen in 10 of the 19 patients. However the followup period was short, the treatment-related mortality was 40 percent, and only 4 patients were alive at 36 months. This report was compiled from registry data from 11 centers. The patient selection and the total number of patients evaluated at these centers as potential allogeneic transplant recipients are not known. Nonetheless, it represents the largest number of patients reported, and it is important for the physician to be aware of the feasibility of allogeneic transplant and the potential for a beneficial graft-versus-tumor effect, as 5 of 7 patients with complete remission had chronic graft-versus-host disease. This approach may deserve further investigation in the context of clinical trials.

Oral Melphalan-Based Regimens

The conventional treatment approach for AL amyloidosis, adopted from experience with myeloma, is to administer low-dose oral melphalan in association with prednisone in a cyclical fashion. Two randomized clinical trials have demonstrated the efficacy of this regimen, however, the impact was modest increasing the median patients survival to only approximately 18 months.[34,75] This form of treatment only rarely results in complete hematologic responses or reversal of amyloid-related organ dysfunction.

Many patients with advanced disease, particularly those with cardiac involvement, are unable to tolerate the fluid retention and worsening congestive heart failure associated with glucocorticoid treatment. The use of oral melphalan as a single agent, administered continuously rather than cyclically, has been studied in patients with cardiac amyloidosis.[76] In 30 such treated patients, 7 of 13 patients evaluable after 3 to 4 months of treatment achieved a partial hematologic response and 3 achieved a complete hematologic response. Six of the patients survived for longer than 1 year. This melphalan treatment was effective in inducing hematologic responses in patients who received total doses of melphalan greater than 300 mg.

High-Dose Dexamethasone-Containing Regimens

A rapid response to therapy is essential in AL amyloidosis to prevent progressive organ failure. In myeloma, infusional vincristine, doxorubicin (Adriamycin), and dexamethasone (VAD) may induce a rapid clonal response. However, this regimen presents potential problems in patients with AL amyloidosis: vincristine can exacerbate autonomic or peripheral neuropathy; doxorubicin can worsen cardiomyopathy; and the intensive high-dose dexamethasone can cause severe fluid retention in patients with renal and cardiac amyloidosis or trigger severe, often fatal, ventricular arrhythmias. At the United Kingdom National Amyloidosis Center, 98 patients with AL amyloidosis were treated with a median of four cycles of standard VAD or cyclophosphamide, vincristine, doxorubicin (Adriamycin), methyl-prednisolone (CVAMP). A hematologic response occurred in 54 percent, an organ response was evident in 42 percent, and the treatment-related mortality was only 7 percent. However, the responses were not durable with evidence of hematologic relapse in 21 percent of patients after a median time of 20 months (range: 7–54 months).[77]

Experience with myeloma has indicated that dexamethasone accounted for most (80%) of the plasma cell reduction achieved with VAD and avoided the potential toxicity of vincristine and doxorubicin (Adriamycin). Pulsed high-dose dexamethasone, as used in the VAD regimen, has been reported to benefit AL patients with varying response rates.[78] A Southwest Oncology Group trial with 87 eligible and analyzable patients found that 53 percent of patients had a hematologic response, and the hematologic response was complete in 24 percent. Organ function improved in 45 percent. The median progression-free survival was 27 months and overall survival 31 months.

The toxicity of dexamethasone used with the same schedule of the VAD regimen in AL patients is substantial. A less toxic schedule (40 mg/day for 4 days every 21 days) induced organ response in 35 percent of patients in a median time of 4 months, without significant toxicity.[79] The combination of melphalan and dexamethasone produced hematologic response in 67 percent in a median time of 4.5 months, with complete remission in 33 percent and functional improvement of the involved organs in 48 percent. Treatment-related mortality was low (4%). Median duration of response was 24 months (range: 12–48 months). Based upon the finding that dexamethasone 1 day a week is less toxic than 4-day pulses in patients with myeloma, this regimen has been employed.

Immunomodulators

So-called immunomodulatory drugs (IMiDs), based upon thalidomide, have been found to modify the marrow microenvironment and cytokine milieu leading to regression of plasma cell neoplasms. Thalidomide itself can induce responses in up to half of patients treated with it alone or in combination with dexamethasone, but it is poorly tolerated in patients with AL amyloidosis, causing severe fatigue, worsening edema, cognitive difficulties, constipation, neuropathy, bradycardia, thromboembolic complications, and worsening of renal function. Side effects prevent dose escalation above 200 to 300 mg/day and frequently led to stopping drug.[80–82]

Thalidomide has also been combined with cyclophosphamide and dexamethasone (CTD regimen) in an oral regimen and has shown to be effective in inducing hematologic responses in 74 percent (complete response: 21%; partial response: 53%) of patients with low treatment-related mortality of 4 percent and median over all survival of 41 months.[83]

Because of the toxicity of thalidomide, there was great enthusiasm for using the second-generation drug lenalidomide for patients with AL amyloidosis. In a small study of 34 patients with AL amyloidosis who either had persistent disease following HDM/autoSCT or who were ineligible for HDM/autoSCT, lenalidomide with dexamethasone produced hematologic responses in 67 percent of patients with significant organ responses.[84] A study from a different center showed a hematologic response in 41 percent of patients and organ response in 23 percent of patients.[85] Of note, the median time to hematologic response in both the studies was 6 months. Lenalidomide has a different toxicity profile than thalidomide. Adverse events of thromboembolic complications, myelosuppression, and immunosuppression are noted with lenalidomide, but neurotoxicity has not been seen. Unappreciated in large studies of patients with myeloma, lenalidomide can exacerbate azotemia in patients with renal amyloidosis.[86]

Proteasome Inhibitors

Proteasome inhibitors appear to be particularly toxic to plasma cells, which are synthesizing massive amounts of immunoglobulin as well as structural and cell-cycle–active proteins. The first general intravenous proteasome inhibitor, bortezomib, has been approved for use in myeloma. The ability of this drug, in combination with dexamethasone, to rapidly reduce the concentration of the circulating monoclonal protein makes this an attractive option also for AL amyloidosis,[87,88] and a multicenter, international phase I/II trial has completed accrual.[89] The median time to hematologic response is on the order of a month, and hematologic responses of 50 to 88 percent are being seen.

Investigational Therapies

Following upon the improved results described with the above agents, a series of combination regimens are entering clinical trials, combining bortezomib with melphalan or lenalidomide and dexamethasone, as well as melphalan or cyclophosphamide and lenalidomide and dexamethasone. The proteasome inhibitors and IMiDs are also being studied as induction or in combination with HDM/autoSCT. Third-generation IMiDs and oral proteasome inhibitors are in development and may be useful for AL amyloidosis.

An iodinated derivative of doxorubicin, 4-iodo-4-deoxydoxorubucin (IDOX), binds with high affinity to amyloid fibrils and promotes their disaggregation *in vitro* and *in vivo* in experimentally induced murine AA amyloidosis.[90] Administration of IDOX to patients with AL amyloidosis showed promising results in a small, uncontrolled series, but its efficacy was unable to be demonstrated in a larger multicenter trial, possibly because the effect size was less than anticipated.[91] Strategies that combine IDOX with chemotherapy to suppress precursor production and promote amyloid resorption is a rational approach that warrants investigation.

Disruption of the interaction between serum amyloid P (SAP) and amyloid is another approach being investigated as a degradation-promoting treatment. Because SAP is present in all types of amyloid deposits, targeting the SAP-amyloid interaction could have broad application. SAP itself is highly resistant to proteolysis, and binding of SAP to amyloid fibrils protects them from proteolysis *in vitro*. SAP exists in a dynamic equilibrium between the circulation, where it is unbound, and tissue, where it is bound to amyloid. It was hypothesized that removal of circulating SAP would drive SAP from tissue amyloid to the circulation and render the tissue amyloid less resistant to proteolysis. R-1-[6-[R-2-carboxy-pyrrolidin-1-yl]-6-oxo-hexanoyl]pyrrolidine-2-carboxylic acid (CPHPC), a palindromic compound that binds with high affinity to SAP, crosslinks two SAP molecules together in a manner that occludes the binding surface of SAP.[92] CPHPC administration depleted SAP from the circulation and from amyloid deposits in murine models, and studies in humans demonstrated rapid SAP clearance from the circulation. However, the impact of CPHPC administration on amyloid deposits *in vivo* is not known and is currently being studied in phase II trials.

Antitumor necrosis factor-α therapy, in the form of etanercept, in 16 patients with advanced AL produced symptomatic improvement in most of them, and half had objective responses, notably in those with macroglossia.[93] However, this approach does not have any impact on the underlying plasma cell neoplasm and therefore, is of limited benefit.

Immunotherapy, both active and passive, is another approach that is being pursued. Dendritic-cell–based idiotype vaccination is well tolerated but has limited clinical impact. AL burden can be markedly reduced in mice by passive immunization with an anti-light-chain murine monoclonal antibody specific for an amyloid-related epitope.[94] A humanized antibody is being produced for a phase I/II clinical trial in patients with AL disease.

Supportive Treatment

Regardless of the specific treatment directed against the plasma cell dyscrasia, supportive care to decrease symptoms and support organ function plays an important role in the management of this disease and requires the coordinated care by specialists in multiple disciplines. The mainstay of the treatment of amyloid cardiomyopathy is sodium restriction and the careful administration of diuretics. Achieving a balance between heart failure and intravascular volume depletion is particularly important especially in patients with autonomic nervous system involvement or nephrotic syndrome. Diuretic resistance is common in patients with severe nephrotic syndrome, and metolazone or spironolactone may be required in conjunction with loop diuretics. β-blockers to control rate and afterload reduction with angiotensin-converting enzyme inhibitors can help selected patients. However, these agents should be used cautiously, starting with a low dose and withdrawal if hypotension develops. Digoxin is contraindicated in patients with amyloid cardiomyopathy because of binding of digoxin to amyloid fibrils and leading to severe digoxin toxicity. Calcium channel blockers can aggravate congestive heart failure in amyloid cardiomyopathy and should generally be avoided. Patients with recurrent syncope may require permanent pacemaker implantation, and ventricular arrhythmias can be treated with amiodarone and, in some patients, implantable defibrillators.

Orthostatic hypotension can be severe and difficult to manage. Fitted waist-high elastic stockings and midodrine are helpful. Fludrocortisone is often problematic because of associated fluid retention. Continuous norepinephrine infusion has been reported to be a successful treatment of severe hypotension refractory to conventional treatment. Supportive treatment for amyloid-associated kidney disease, as for other causes of nephrotic syndrome includes salt restriction, diuretics, and treatment of secondary hyperlipidemia. Adequate protein intake should be maintained. An impact on proteinuria of angiotensin-converting enzyme inhibitors or angiotensin receptor blockers has not been established but it is reasonable to use these agents, if not precluded by hypotension. Both hemodialysis and peritoneal dialysis are used for amyloidosis-associated end-stage renal disease. Diarrhea is a common and incapacitating problem for patients with autonomic nervous system involvement. Loperamide, opioids, and octreotide may decrease diarrhea in some patients. Adequate oral or intravenous feeding is mandatory in patients who are undernourished and protein deficient as a consequence of nephrotic syndrome. Neuropathic pain is difficult to control. Gabapentin, although well tolerated, often fails to relieve pain. Other analgesics may be used as adjuvant agents. Duloxetine may be effective in controlling pain of neuropathy. Nonnephrotoxic analgesics may be used as adjuvant agents. Bleeding in AL amyloidosis is frequent and multifactorial, because of both capillary fragility because of amyloid deposition in vessel walls, as well as coagulopathy caused by adsorption of clotting factors, particularly factor X, by amyloid deposits. Factor X is difficult to replace with plasma and patients with life-threatening bleeding caused by factor X deficiency should be treated with recombinant factor VII.

Biomarkers of Prognosis and Treatment Response

The rate of disease progression is variable in AL amyloidosis and depends on the extent of organ involvement. The presence of clinically apparent cardiac involvement is an important determinant of outcome. The serum concentration of N-terminal probrain natriuretic peptide (NT-proBNP), either alone or in conjunction with levels of cardiac troponins has been shown to be a sensitive marker of AL amyloidosis-associated cardiac dysfunction and a strong predictor of survival following aggressive treatment.[95,96] High circulating levels of free light chains are associated with poor outcome,[97] and greater reductions in levels following treatment of the underlying plasma cell neoplasm are associated with both reduction in NT-proBNP and improved survival.

Therapy of Localized AL Amyloidosis

Treatment of localized AL (most often in the tracheobronchial tree, lungs, or genitourinary tract) has not been studied systematically. Because progression to systemic disease rarely occurs, chemotherapy is not indicated. Localized radiotherapy, aimed at destroying the local collection of plasma cells producing the AL precursor, can be of clinical benefit (Berk and associates, manuscript in preparation). In patients with massive macroglossia, surgical resection has not been effective. Relief can sometimes be achieved with laser techniques, although formal studies of efficacy have not been reported.

AA AMYLOIDOSIS

The major therapy in AA amyloidosis is treatment of the underlying inflammatory or infectious disease. Treatment that suppresses or eliminates the inflammation or infection also decreases the SAA protein. For familial Mediterranean fever, colchicine in a dose of 1.2 to 1.8 mg/day is the appropriate treatment. Colchicine has not been helpful for AA amyloidosis of other causes, or for other amyloidoses. A multicenter trial using a new antiamyloid drug, eprodisate, has been completed and found to significantly delay worsening of renal function in patients with AA amyloidosis.[22] Eprodisate interferes with the interaction of AA amyloid protein and glycosaminoglycans in tissues and thus prevents fibril formation and deposition.

Aβ_2M AMYLOIDOSIS

The treatment for Aβ_2M amyloidosis is difficult because the 11-kDa β_2-microglobulin molecule is too large to pass through a dialysis membrane. However, consistent with a postulated role of copper in initiating Aβ_2M fibrillogenesis, copper-free dialysis membranes appear to reduce the incidence of disease.[98] Furthermore, patients on chronic ambulatory peritoneal dialysis usually have lower plasma levels of β_2-microglobulin than those on hemodialysis and may not develop amyloid deposits as quickly. Symptoms of arthropathy are common and prevalence may approach 100 percent of individuals on dialysis for more than 15 years. Patients who have received kidney transplants after developing Aβ_2M report an improvement in symptoms.

ATTR FAMILIAL AMYLOIDOSIS

Without intervention, survival after ATTR disease onset is 5 to 15 years. Orthotopic liver transplantation, which removes the major source of variant TTR production and replaces it with normal TTR, is the major treatment for ATTR amyloidosis.[99] Liver transplantation arrests disease progression and some improvement in autonomic and peripheral neuropathy can occur.[100] Cardiomyopathy has not improved and in some patients appears to have worsened after liver transplantation.[101] Long-term outcome and the timing of transplantation are being evaluated. An international multicenter randomized placebo-controlled clinical trial is underway to test the efficacy of the nonsteroidal anti-inflammatory drug, diflunisal, for the treatment of TTR amyloidosis. Laboratory studies have suggested that diflunisal stabilizes variant TTRs and prevents unfolding and aggregation.[102]

AL AMYLOIDOSIS AND RELATIONSHIP TO OTHER IMMUNOGLOBULIN DEPOSITION DISEASES

AL is caused by a monoclonal plasma cell or lymphoproliferative disorder. In most patients with a monoclonal plasma cell disorder, whether myeloma or essential monoclonal gammopathy, the secreted monoclonal immunoglobulin (Ig) remains soluble in body fluids. In AL amyloidosis, the physicochemical characteristics of the Ig light chains lead to its deposition as amyloid fibrils and deposits. From 10 to 20 percent of myeloma patients develop clinical evidence of AL,[42] although additional patients have subclinical deposition.

In some patients with clonal plasma cell disorders, nonfibrillar aggregation and deposition of Ig light or heavy chains can occur. These disorders are termed "monoclonal immunoglobulin deposition diseases" (MIDD).[103] The Ig deposits do not bind Congo red, do not contain P component or other components of amyloid fibrils, and, unlike amyloid deposits, do not possess a fibrillar ultrastructure. The kidneys and heart are the most frequent sites for MIDD.[104] The pathologic diagnosis of nonamyloid MIDD depends upon the identification of non-Congophilic Ig deposits in tissues via immunohistochemistry, using specific anti-H and anti-L sera, and the presence of the characteristic ultrastructural appearance of amorphous protein aggregates. MIDD is probably underdiagnosed because appropriate immunohistochemical staining is not routinely performed.

As in AL, once the diagnosis of MIDD is established, determination of whether the patient has myeloma (e.g., serum and urine evaluation for monoclonal protein, marrow aspiration and biopsy, skeletal survey) should be made. Regimens effective for myeloma and AL should be used to reduce end-organ damage because MIDD is a similar monoclonal plasma cell disorder.[105–107]

Treatment of the amyloidoses begins with suspicion of a systemic protein deposition disease based upon the clinical spectrum of amyloid syndromes, and obtaining appropriate biopsies and screening tests to type the amyloid. For difficult cases and for identification of variant serum proteins, amyloid referral centers can provide specialized diagnostic techniques. Effective therapy is at hand for AL, AA, and ATTR amyloidosis and will improve with future innovations. Thus, timely and accurate diagnosis has become essential. An understanding of the biophysical properties of amyloid proteins and of the mechanisms of protein misfolding in a wide variety of diseases will enable the further development of more specific and less toxic antifibril drugs.

REFERENCES

1. Virchow VR: Ueber einem Gehirn and Rueckenmark des Menchen auf gefundene Substanz mit chemischen reaction der Cellulose. *Virchows Arch Pathol Anat* 6:135, 1854.
2. Cohen AS, Calkins E: Electron microscopic observations on a fibrous component in amyloid of diverse origins. *Nature* 183:1202, 1959.
3. Westermark P, Benson MD, Buxbaum JN, et al: A primer of amyloid nomenclature. *Amyloid* 14:179, 2007.
4. Simms RW, Prout MN, Cohen AS: The epidemiology of AL and AA amyloidosis. *Baillieres Clin Rheumatol* 8:627, 1994.
5. Gertz MA, Kyle RA: Secondary systemic amyloidosis: Response and survival in 64 patients. *Medicine (Baltimore)* 70:246, 1991.
6. Livneh A, Langevitz P, Shinar Y, et al: MEFV mutation analysis in patients suffering from amyloidosis of familial Mediterranean fever. *Amyloid* 6:1, 1999.
7. Drueke TB: Beta2-microglobulin and amyloidosis. *Nephrol Dial Transplant* 15 Suppl 1:17, 2000.
8. Benson MD. Amyloidosis, in *The Metabolic and Molecular Bases of Inherited Disease*, 8th ed., vol. IV, edited by CR Scriver, AL Beaudet, WS Sly, D Valle, p 5345. McGraw Hill, New York, 2001.
9. Connors LH, Lim A, Prokaeva T, et al: Tabulation of human transthyretin (TTR) variants, 2003. *Amyloid* 10:160, 2003.
10. Jacobson DR, Pastore RD, Yaghoubian R, et al: Variant-sequence transthyretin (isoleucine 122) in late-onset cardiac amyloidosis in black Americans [see comments]. *N Engl J Med* 336:466, 1997.
11. Kyle RA, Spittell PC, Gertz MA, et al: The premortem recognition of systemic senile amyloidosis with cardiac involvement. *Am J Med* 101:395, 1996.
12. Ng B, Connors LH, Davidoff R, et al: Senile systemic amyloidosis presenting with heart failure: A comparison with light chain–associated amyloidosis. *Arch Intern Med* 165:1425, 2005.
13. Lansbury PT Jr: Evolution of amyloid: What normal protein folding may tell us about fibrillogenesis and disease. *Proc Natl Acad Sci U S A* 96:3342, 1999.
14. Conway KA, Harper JD, Lansbury PT: Accelerated *in vitro* fibril formation by a mutant alpha-synuclein linked to early-onset Parkinson disease. *Nat Med* 4:1318, 1998.
15. Karpuj MV, Garren H, Slunt H, et al: Transglutaminase aggregates huntingtin into nonamyloidogenic polymers, and its enzymatic activity increases in Huntington's disease brain nuclei. *Proc Natl Acad Sci U S A* 96:7388, 1999.
16. Ishihara T, Takahashi M, Koga M, et al: Amyloid fibril formation in the rough endoplasmic reticulum of plasma cells from a patient with localized A lambda amyloidosis. *Lab Invest* 64:265, 1991.
17. Botto M, Hawkins PN, Bickerstaff MC, et al: Amyloid deposition is delayed in mice with targeted deletion of the serum amyloid P component gene. *Nat Med* 3:855, 1997.
18. Hawkins PN, Lavender JP, Pepys MB: Evaluation of systemic amyloidosis by scintigraphy with 123I-labeled serum amyloid P component. *N Engl J Med* 323:508, 1990.
19. Gallo G, Wisniewski T, Choi-Miura NH, et al: Potential role of apolipoprotein-E in fibrillogenesis. *Am J Pathol* 145:526, 1994.
20. Kisilevsky R: The relation of proteoglycans, serum amyloid P and apo E to amyloidosis current status, 2000. *Amyloid* 7:23, 2000.
21. Kisilevsky R, Lemieux LJ, Fraser PE, et al: Arresting amyloidosis in vivo using small-molecule anionic sulphonates or sulphates: Implications for Alzheimer's disease. *Nat Med* 1:143, 1995.
22. Dember LM, Hawkins PN, Hazenberg BP, et al: Eprodisate for the treatment of renal disease in AA amyloidosis. *N Engl J Med* 356:2349, 2007.
23. Hayman SR, Bailey RJ, Jalal SM, et al. Translocations involving the immunoglobulin heavy-chain locus are possible early genetic events in patients with primary systemic amyloidosis. *Blood* 98:2266, 2001.
24. Lavatelli F, Perlman DH, Spencer B, et al. Amyloidogenic and associated proteins in systemic amyloidosis proteome of adipose tissue. *Mol Cell Proteomics* 7:1570, 2008.
25. Solomon A, Frangione B, Franklin EC: Bence Jones proteins and light chains of immunoglobulins. Preferential association of the V lambda VI subgroup of human light chains with amyloidosis AL (lambda). *J Clin Invest* 70:453, 1982.
26. Teng J, Russell WJ, Gu X, et al: Different types of glomerulopathic light chains interact with mesangial cells using a common receptor but exhibit different intracellular trafficking patterns. *Lab Invest* 84:440, 2004.
27. Sanchorawala V, Blanchard E, Seldin DC, et al: AL amyloidosis associated with B-cell lymphoproliferative disorders: Frequency and treatment outcomes. *Am J Hematol* 81:692, 2006.
28. Husby G, Marhang G, Dowton B, et al: Serum amyloid A (SAA): Biochemistry, genetics, and the pathogenesis of AA amyloidosis. *Amyloid: Int J Exp Clin Invest* 1:119, 1994.
29. Johan K, Westermark G, Engstrom U, et al: Acceleration of amyloid protein A amyloidosis by amyloid-like synthetic fibrils. *Proc Natl Acad Sci U S A* 95:2558, 1998.
30. Zingraff J, Drueke T: Beta2-microglobulin amyloidosis: Past and future. *Artif Organs* 22:581, 1998.
31. Hammarstrom P, Wiseman RL, Powers ET, Kelly JW: Prevention of transthyretin amyloid disease by changing protein misfolding energetics. *Science* 299:713, 2003.
32. Suhr OB, Svendsen IH, Ohlsson PI, et al: Impact of age and amyloidosis on thiol conjugation of transthyretin in hereditary transthyretin amyloidosis. *Amyloid* 6:187, 1999.
33. Libbey CA, Skinner M, Cohen AS: Use of abdominal fat tissue aspirate in the diagnosis of systemic amyloidosis. *Arch Intern Med* 143:1549, 1983.
34. Skinner M, Anderson J, Simms R, et al: Treatment of 100 patients with primary amyloidosis: A randomized trial of melphalan, prednisone, and colchicine versus colchicine only. *Am J Med* 100:290, 1996.
35. Abraham RS, Katzmann JA, Clark RJ, et al: Quantitative analysis of serum free light chains. A new marker for the diagnostic evaluation of primary systemic amyloidosis. *Am J Clin Pathol* 119:274, 2003.
36. Akar H, Seldin DC, Magnani B, et al: Quantitative serum free light chain assay in the diagnostic evaluation of AL amyloidosis. *Amyloid* 12:210, 2005.
37. Swan N, Skinner M, O'Hara CJ: Bone marrow core biopsy specimens in AL (primary) amyloidosis. A morphologic and immunohistochemical study of 100 cases. *Am J Clin Pathol* 120:610, 2003.
38. Arbustini E, Verga L, Concardi M, et al: Electron and immuno-electron microscopy of abdominal fat identifies and characterizes amyloid fibrils in suspected cardiac amyloidosis. *Amyloid* 9:108, 2002.
39. Lim A, Wally J, Walsh MT, et al: Identification and location of a cysteinyl posttranslational modification in an amyloidogenic kappa1 light chain protein by electrospray ionization and matrix-assisted laser desorption/ionization mass spectrometry. *Anal Biochem* 295:45, 2001.
40. Connors LH, Ericsson T, Skare J, et al: A simple screening test for variant transthyretins associated with familial transthyretin amyloidosis using isoelectric focusing. *Biochim Biophys Acta* 1407:185, 1998.
41. Falk RH, Comenzo RL, Skinner M: The systemic amyloidoses. *N Engl J Med* 337:898, 1997.
42. Kyle RA: Primary systemic amyloidosis: Clinical and laboratory features in 474 cases. *Semin Hematol* 32:45, 1995.
43. Falk RH: Diagnosis and management of the cardiac amyloidoses. *Circulation* 112:2047, 2005.
44. Dember LM: Emerging treatment approaches for the systemic amyloidoses. *Kidney Int* 68:1377, 2005.
45. Park MA, Mueller PS, Kyle RA, et al: Primary (AL) hepatic amyloidosis: Clinical features and natural history in 98 patients. *Medicine* (Baltimore) 82:291, 2003.
46. Lucas FV, Fishleder AJ, Becker RC, et al: Acquired factor X deficiency in systemic amyloidosis. *Cleve Clin J Med* 54:399, 1987.
47. Sane DC, Pizzo SV, Greenberg CS: Elevated urokinase-type plasminogen activator level and bleeding in amyloidosis: Case report and literature review. *Am J Hematol* 31:53, 1989.
48. Helin HJ, Korpela MM, Mustonen JT, Pasternack AI: Renal biopsy findings and clinicopathologic correlations in rheumatoid arthritis. *Arthritis Rheum* 38:242, 1995.
49. Hawkins PN. Hereditary systemic amyloidosis with renal involvement. *J Nephrol* 16:443, 2003.
50. Revesz T, Ghiso J, Lashley T, et al: Cerebral amyloid angiopathies: A pathologic, biochemical, and genetic view. *J Neuropathol Exp Neurol* 62:885, 2003.
51. Yood RA, Skinner M, Rubinow A, et al: Bleeding manifestations in 100 patients with amyloidosis. *JAMA* 249:1322, 1983.
52. Berk JL, O'Regan A, Skinner M: Pulmonary and tracheobronchial amyloidosis. *Semin Respir Crit Care Med* 23:155, 2002.
53. Tirzaman O, Wahner-Roedler DL, Malek RS, et al: Primary localized amyloidosis of the urinary bladder: A case series of 31 patients. *Mayo Clin Proc* 75:1264, 2000.
54. Looi LM: Isolated atrial amyloidosis: A clinicopathologic study indicating increased prevalence in chronic heart disease. *Hum Pathol* 24:602, 1993.
55. Saad MF, Ordonez NG, Rashid RK, et al: Medullary carcinoma of the thyroid. A study of the clinical features and prognostic factors in 161 patients. *Medicine* (Baltimore) 63:319, 1984.
56. Kahn SE, Andrikopoulos S, Verchere CB: Islet amyloid: A long-recognized but underappreciated pathological feature of type 2 diabetes. *Diabetes* 48:241, 1999.
57. Westermark P, Eriksson L, Engstrom U, et al: Prolactin-derived amyloid in the aging pituitary gland. *Am J Pathol* 150:67, 1997.
58. Klintworth GK: The molecular genetics of the corneal dystrophies—Current status. *Front Biosci* 8:d687, 2003.
59. Haggqvist B, Naslund J, Sletten K, et al: Medin: An integral fragment of aortic smooth muscle cell-produced lactadherin forms the most common human amyloid. *Proc Natl Acad Sci U S A* 96:8669, 1999.
60. Storkel S, Schneider HM, Muntefering H, Kashiwagi S: Iatrogenic, insulin-dependent, local amyloidosis. *Lab Invest* 48:108, 1983.
61. Chang YT, Liu HN, Wang WJ, et al: A study of cytokeratin profiles in localized cutaneous amyloids. *Arch Dermatol Res* 296:83, 2004.
62. Gertz MA, Comenzo R, Falk RH, et al: Definition of organ involvement and treatment response in immunoglobulin light chain amyloidosis (AL): A consensus opinion from the 10th International Symposium on Amyloid and Amyloidosis, Tours, France, 18–22 April 2004. *Am J Hematol* 79:319, 2005.

63. Gertz MA, Lacy MQ, Dispenzieri A, et al: Effect of hematologic response on outcome of patients undergoing transplantation for primary amyloidosis: Importance of achieving a complete response. *Haematologica* 92:1415, 2007.
64. Skinner M, Sanchorawala V, Seldin DC, et al: High-dose melphalan and autologous stem-cell transplantation in patients with AL amyloidosis: An 8-year study. *Ann Intern Med* 140:85, 2004.
65. Seldin DC, Anderson JJ, Sanchorawala V, et al: Improvement in quality of life of patients with AL amyloidosis treated with high-dose melphalan and autologous stem cell transplantation. *Blood* 104:1888, 2004.
66. Dember LM, Sanchorawala V, Seldin DC, et al: Effect of dose-intensive intravenous melphalan and autologous blood stem-cell transplantation on al amyloidosis-associated renal disease. *Ann Intern Med* 134:746, 2001.
67. Sanchorawala V, Seldin DC, Magnani B, et al: Serum free light-chain responses after high-dose intravenous melphalan and autologous stem cell transplantation for AL (primary) amyloidosis. *Bone Marrow Transplant* 36:597, 2005.
68. Dispenzieri A, Kyle RA, Lacy MQ, et al: Superior survival in primary systemic amyloidosis patients undergoing peripheral blood stem cell transplantation: A case-control study. *Blood* 103:3960, 2004.
69. Palladini G, Perfetti V, Obici L, et al: Association of melphalan and high-dose dexamethasone is effective and well tolerated in patients with AL (primary) amyloidosis who are ineligible for stem cell transplantation. *Blood* 103:2936, 2004.
70. Jaccard A, Moreau P, Leblond V, et al: High-dose melphalan versus melphalan plus dexamethasone for AL amyloidosis. *N Engl J Med* 357:1083, 2007.
71. Dubrey SW, Burke MM, Hawkins PN, Banner NR: Cardiac transplantation for amyloid heart disease: The United Kingdom experience. *J Heart Lung Transplant* 23:1142, 2004.
72. Gillmore JD, Goodman HJ, Lachmann HJ, et al: Sequential heart and autologous stem cell transplantation for systemic AL amyloidosis. *Blood* 107:1227, 2006.
73. Lacy MQ, Dispenzieri A, Hayman SR, et al: Autologous stem cell transplant after heart transplant for light chain (Al) amyloid cardiomyopathy. *J Heart Lung Transplant* 27:823, 2008.
74. Schonland SO, Lokhorst H, Buzyn A, et al: Allogeneic and syngeneic hematopoietic cell transplantation in patients with amyloid light-chain amyloidosis: A report from the European Group for Blood and Marrow Transplantation. *Blood* 107:2578, 2006.
75. Kyle RA, Gertz MA, Greipp PR, et al: A trial of three regimens for primary amyloidosis: Colchicine alone, melphalan and prednisone, and melphalan, prednisone, and colchicine. *N Engl J Med* 336:1202, 1997.
76. Sanchorawala V, Wright DG, Seldin DC, et al: Low-dose continuous oral melphalan for the treatment of primary systemic (AL) amyloidosis. *Br J Haematol* 117:886, 2002.
77. Goodman HJ, Gillmore JD, Lachmann HJ, et al: Outcome of autologous stem cell transplantation for AL amyloidosis in the UK. *Br J Haematol* 134:417, 2006.
78. Dhodapkar MV, Hussein MA, Rasmussen E, et al: Clinical efficacy of high-dose dexamethasone with maintenance dexamethasone/alpha interferon in patients with primary systemic amyloidosis: Results of United States Intergroup Trial Southwest Oncology Group (SWOG) S9628. *Blood* 104:3520, 2004.
79. Palladini G, Anesi E, Perfetti V, et al: A modified high-dose dexamethasone regimen for primary systemic (AL) amyloidosis. *Br J Haematol* 113:1044, 2001.
80. Palladini G, Perfetti V, Perlini S, et al: The combination of thalidomide and intermediate-dose dexamethasone is an effective but toxic treatment for patients with primary amyloidosis (AL). *Blood* 105:2949, 2005.
81. Dispenzieri A, Lacy MQ, Rajkumar SV, et al: Poor tolerance to high doses of thalidomide in patients with primary systemic amyloidosis. *Amyloid* 10:257, 2003.
82. Seldin DC, Choufani EB, Dember LM, et al: Tolerability and efficacy of thalidomide for the treatment of patients with light chain–associated (AL) amyloidosis. *Clin Lymphoma* 3:241, 2003.
83. Wechalekar AD, Goodman HJ, Lachmann HJ, et al: Safety and efficacy of risk-adapted cyclophosphamide, thalidomide, and dexamethasone in systemic AL amyloidosis. *Blood* 109:457, 2007.
84. Sanchorawala V, Wright DG, Rosenzweig M, et al: Lenalidomide and dexamethasone in the treatment of AL amyloidosis: Results of a phase 2 trial. *Blood* 109:492, 2007.
85. Dispenzieri A, Lacy MQ, Zeldenrust SR, et al: The activity of lenalidomide with or without dexamethasone in patients with primary systemic amyloidosis. *Blood* 109:465, 2007.
86. Batts ED, Sanchorawala V, Hegerfeldt Y, Lazarus HM: Azotemia associated with use of lenalidomide in plasma cell dyscrasias. *Leuk Lymphoma* 49:1108, 2008.
87. Kastritis E, Anagnostopoulos A, Roussou M, et al: Treatment of light chain (AL) amyloidosis with the combination of bortezomib and dexamethasone. *Haematologica* 92:1351, 2007.
88. Wechalekar AD, Lachmann HJ, Offer M, et al: Efficacy of bortezomib in systemic AL amyloidosis with relapsed/refractory clonal disease. *Haematologica* 93:295, 2008.
89. Reece DE, Rodriguez GP, Chen C, et al: Phase I-II trial of bortezomib plus oral cyclophosphamide and prednisone in relapsed and refractory multiple myeloma. *J Clin Oncol* 26:4777, 2008.
90. Merlini G, Ascari E, Amboldi N, et al: Interaction of the anthracycline 4′-iodo-4′-deoxydoxorubicin with amyloid fibrils: Inhibition of amyloidogenesis. *Proc Natl Acad Sci U S A* 92:2959, 1995.
91. Gertz MA, Lacy MQ, Dispenzieri A, et al: A multicenter phase II trial of 4-iodo-4deoxydoxorubicin (IDOX) in primary amyloidosis (AL). *Amyloid* 9:24, 2002.
92. Pepys MB, Herbert J, Hutchinson WL, et al: Targeted pharmacological depletion of serum amyloid P component for treatment of human amyloidosis. *Nature* 417:254, 2002.
93. Hussein MA, Juturi JV, Rybicki L, et al: Etanercept therapy in patients with advanced primary amyloidosis. *Med Oncol* 20:283, 2003.
94. Hrncic R, Wall J, Wolfenbarger DA, et al: Antibody-mediated resolution of light chain–associated amyloid deposits. *Am J Pathol* 157:1239, 2000.
95. Dispenzieri A, Gertz MA, Kyle RA, et al: Serum cardiac troponins and N-terminal pro-brain natriuretic peptide: A staging system for primary systemic amyloidosis. *J Clin Oncol* 22:3751, 2004.
96. Dispenzieri A, Gertz MA, Kyle RA, et al: Prognostication of survival using cardiac troponins and N-terminal pro-brain natriuretic peptide in patients with primary systemic amyloidosis undergoing peripheral blood stem cell transplantation. *Blood* 104:1881, 2004.
97. Palladini G, Lavatelli F, Russo P, et al: Circulating amyloidogenic free light chains and serum N-terminal natriuretic peptide type B decrease simultaneously in association with improvement of survival in AL. *Blood* 107:3854, 2006.
98. Morgan CJ, Gelfand M, Atreya C, Miranker AD: Kidney dialysis-associated amyloidosis: A molecular role for copper in fiber formation. *J Mol Biol* 309:339, 2001.
99. Lewis WD, Skinner M, Simms RW, et al: Orthotopic liver transplantation for familial amyloidotic polyneuropathy. *Clin Transplant* 8:107, 1994.
100. Bergethon PR, Sabin TD, Lewis D, et al: Improvement in the polyneuropathy associated with familial amyloid polyneuropathy after liver transplantation. *Neurology* 47:944, 1996.
101. Dubrey SW, Davidoff R, Skinner M, et al: Progression of ventricular wall thickening after liver transplantation for familial amyloidosis. *Transplantation* 64:74, 1997.
102. Sekijima Y, Dendle MA, Kelly JW: Orally administered diflunisal stabilizes transthyretin against dissociation required for amyloidogenesis. *Amyloid* 13:236, 2006.
103. Buxbaum J, Gallo G: Nonamyloidotic monoclonal immunoglobulin deposition disease. Light-chain, heavy-chain, and light- and heavy-chain deposition diseases. *Hematol Oncol Clin North Am* 13:1235, 1999.
104. Pozzi C, D'Amico M, Fogazzi GB, et al: Light chain deposition disease with renal involvement: Clinical characteristics and prognostic factors. *Am J Kidney Dis* 42:1154, 2003.
105. Weichman K, Dember LM, Prokaeva T, et al: Clinical and molecular characteristics of patients with non-amyloid light chain deposition disorders, and outcome following treatment with high-dose melphalan and autologous stem cell transplantation. *Bone Marrow Transplant* 38:339, 2006.
106. Salant DJ, Sanchorawala V, D'Agati VD: A case of atypical light chain deposition disease—Diagnosis and treatment. *Clin J Am Soc Nephrol* 2:858, 2007.
107. Hassoun H, Flombaum C, D'Agati VD, et al: High-dose melphalan and auto-SCT in patients with monoclonal Ig deposition disease. *Bone Marrow Transplant* 42:405, 2008.
108. Mollee PN, Wechalekar AD, Pereira DL, et al: Autologous stem cell transplantation in primary systemic amyloidosis: The impact of selection criteria on outcome. *Bone Marrow Transplant* 33:271, 2004.
109. Schonland SO, Perz JB, Hundemer M, et al: Indications for high-dose chemotherapy with autologous stem cell support in patients with systemic amyloid light chain amyloidosis. *Transplantation* 80(Suppl):S160, 2005.
110. Skinner M, Sanchorawala V, Seldin DC, et al: High-dose melphalan and autologous stem-cell transplantation in patients with AL amyloidosis: An 8-year study. *Ann Intern Med* 140:85, 2004.
111. Chow LQ, Bahlis N, Russell J, et al: Autologous transplantation for primary systemic AL amyloidosis is feasible outside a major amyloidosis referral centre: The Calgary BMT Program experience. *Bone Marrow Transplant* 36:591, 2005.
112. Moreau P, Leblond V, Bourquelot P, et al: Prognostic factors for survival and response after high-dose therapy and autologous stem cell transplantation in systemic AL amyloidosis: A report on 21 patients. *Br J Haematol* 101:766, 1998.
113. Gertz MA, Blood E, Vesole DH, et al: A multicenter phase 2 trial of stem cell transplantation for immunoglobulin light-chain amyloidosis (E4A97): An Eastern Cooperative Oncology Group Study. *Bone Marrow Transplant* 34:149, 2004.
114. Vesole DH, Pérez WS, Akasheh M, et al: Plasma Cell Disorders Working Committee of the Center for International Blood and Marrow Transplant Research. High-dose therapy and autologous hematopoietic stem cell transplantation for patients with primary systemic amyloidosis: A Center for International Blood and Marrow Transplant Research Study. *Mayo Clin Proc* 81:880, 2006.

CHAPTER 111
MACROGLOBULINEMIA

Steven P. Treon and Giampaolo Merlini

SUMMARY

Waldenström macroglobulinemia (WM) is a clonal lymphocytic neoplasm resulting in the accumulation, predominantly in the marrow, of immunoglobulin (Ig) M-secreting lymphoplasmacytic cells. Twenty percent of patients have a familial predisposition, indicating an important genetic component. The disease can have long periods of indolence and asymptomatic patients should be followed periodically. Patients with a disease-related hemoglobin level <10g/L, platelet count <100 × 10^9/L, bulky adenopathy or organomegaly, symptomatic hyperviscosity, peripheral neuropathy, amyloidosis, cryoglobulinemia, cold-agglutinin disease, or evidence of disease progression should be considered for therapy. Nucleoside analogues and oral alkylating agents should be avoided in younger patients as a result of an increased risk of secondary malignancies, especially myelodysplasia or acute myelogenous leukemia. Plasmapheresis is useful for symptomatic hyperviscosity, and as a prophylactic measure prior to rituximab administration in patients with high plasma IgM levels. Cyclophosphamide in combination with glucocorticoids and rituximab is appropriate initial treatment. Bortezomib in combination with glucocorticoids and rituximab may be particularly beneficial in those patients with symptomatic hyperviscosity and those needing more immediate disease control.

In relapsed or refractory patients, one can use or reuse a frontline regimen or use bortezomib, alemtuzumab, or autologous stem cell transplantation. In a younger patient with a matched donor, allogeneic stem cell transplantation can be considered.

DEFINITION AND HISTORY

Waldenström macroglobulinemia (WM) is a lymphoid neoplasm resulting from the accumulation, predominantly in the marrow, of a clonal population of lymphocytes, lymphoplasmacytic cells, and plasma cells, which secrete a monoclonal immunoglobulin (Ig) M.[1] WM corresponds to lymphoplasmacytic lymphoma (LPL) as defined in the Revised European-American Lymphoma (REAL) and World Health Organization classification systems.[2,3] Most cases of LPL are WM; less than 5 percent of cases are IgA-secreting, IgG-secreting, or nonsecreting LPL.

In 1944, Jan Waldenström, a Swedish physician-scientist, reported in *Acta Medica Scandinavica* three cases of a disease he presciently thought was related to myeloma but for the absence of bone involvement and the scarcity of plasma cells in the infiltrate of small lymphocytes. He noted the increase in plasma protein concentration, marked increased serum viscosity, exaggerated bleeding and retinal hemorrhages, and virtually every other feature of the disorder in his case descriptions. In collaboration with a colleague, he showed, using ultracentrifugation and electrophoresis, that the abundant abnormal protein had a molecular weight of approximately 1 million and was not an aggregate of smaller proteins. The disease, which he described with such thoroughness, was later named in his honor.

Acronyms and abbreviations used in this chapter include: CD16, FcγRIIIA receptor; CD40L, CD40 ligand; CDR, complement determination region; CHOP, cyclophosphamide, doxorubicin, vincristine, prednisone; GM_1, ganglioside M_1; HCV, hepatitis C virus; Ig, immunoglobulin; IL, interleukin; κ, kappa light chain; λ, lambda light chain; LPL, lymphoplasmacytic lymphoma; MAG, myelin-associated glycoprotein; R-CHOP, cyclophosphamide, doxorubicin, vincristine, prednisone, rituximab; R-CP, cyclophosphamide, prednisone, rituximab; R-CVP, cyclophosphamide, vincristine, prednisone, rituximab; sCD27, soluble CD27; WM, Waldenström macroglobulinemia.

EPIDEMIOLOGY

The age-adjusted incidence rate of WM is 3.4 per 1 million among males and 1.7 per 1 million among females in the United States. It increases in incidence geometrically with age.[4,5] The incidence rate is higher among Americans of European descent. Americans of African descent represent approximately 5 percent of all patients.

Genetic factors play a role in the pathogenesis of WM. Approximately 20 percent of patients are of Eastern European descent, specifically of Ashkenazi-Jewish ethnic background. Familial disease has been reported commonly, including multigenerational clustering of WM and other B-cell lymphoproliferative diseases.[6–10] Approximately 20 percent of 257 sequential patients with WM presenting to a tertiary referral center had a first-degree relative with either WM or another B-cell disorder.[7] Familial clustering of WM with other immunologic disorders, including hypogammaglobulinemia and hypergammaglobulinemia (particularly polyclonal IgM), autoantibody production (particularly to the thyroid), and manifestation of hyperactive B cells has also been reported in relatives without WM.[9,10] Increased expression of the *BCL-2* gene with enhanced B-cell survival may underlie the increased immunoglobulin synthesis in familial WM.[9]

The role of environmental factors is uncertain, but chronic antigenic stimulation from infections and certain drug or chemical exposures have been considered but have not reached a level of scientific certainty. Hepatitis C virus (HCV) infection was not implicated in a study of 100 consecutive patients with WM. No association was found using serologic and molecular diagnostic studies for HCV infection.[11–13]

PATHOGENESIS

CYTOGENETIC FINDINGS

The lymphoid cells of patients with WM have a variety of numerical and structural chromosome abnormalities. Loss of all or part of chromosomes 17, 18, 19, 20, 21, 22, X, and Y have been commonly observed, and gains in chromosomes 3, 4, and 12 also occur.[7,14–19] Chromosome 6q deletions encompassing 6q21–25 have been observed in up to half of WM patients, and at a comparable frequency amongst patients with and without a familial history.[7,19] The presence of 6q deletions may distinguish patients with WM from those with IgM monoclonal gammopathy. The prognostic significance of 6q deletions is disputed.[20,21] Although 6q deletions have been reported in other B-cell malignancies, several candidate tumor-suppressor genes in this region are under investigation in WM patients, including *BLIMP*-1,[22] a master regulatory gene implicated in lymphoplasmacytic differentiation. The absence of an immunoglobulin heavy-chain switch region rearrangements in WM, characteristic of IgM myeloma, distinguish the two diseases.[23]

NATURE OF THE TUMOR CELL

The marrow B-cells in WM undergo maturation from small lymphocytes with large focal deposits of surface immunoglobulins, to lymphoplasmacytic cells, to plasma cells that contain intracytoplasmic immunoglobulins.[24] Clonal B cells are detectable among blood B lym-

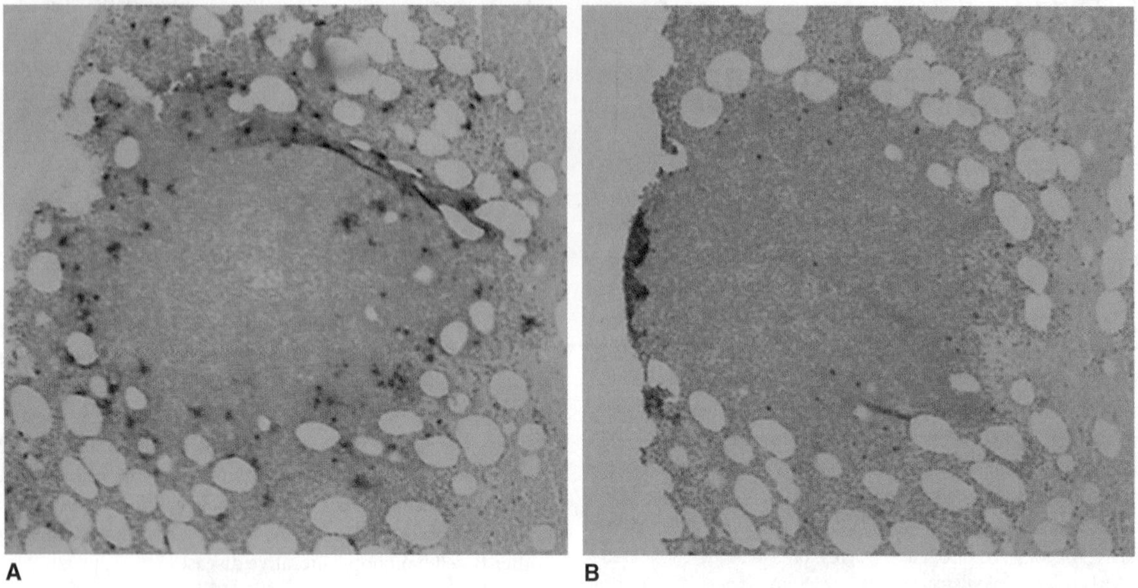

FIGURE 111–1. Marrow clot section. **A.** Tryptase-staining mast cells surrounding a nodule of lymphoplasmacytic cells in a patient with Waldenström macroglobulinemia. **B.** Mast cells in the same section exhibit strong CD40 ligand signaling, which has been shown to support (at least in part) the growth and survival of lymphoplasmacytic cells.

phocytes, and their number increases in patients who fail to respond to therapy or who progress.[25] These lymphocytes have the capacity to mature spontaneously, in culture, to plasma cells. This progression is mediated by an interleukin (IL)-6–dependent process in essential IgM monoclonal gammopathy, but largely an IL-6–independent process in patients with WM.[26] These cells express the monoclonal IgM present in the blood and a variable percentage of them also express surface IgD.

Immunophenotype

The characteristic immunophenotypic profile of the lymphoplasmacytic cells in WM includes the expression of the pan–B-cell markers CD19, CD20, CD22, CD79, and FMC7.2.[27–29] Expression of CD5, CD10, and CD23 may be found in 10 to 20 percent of cases, and does not exclude the diagnosis of WM.[30]

Cellular Phenotype

The phenotype of lymphoplasmacytic cells in WM cell suggests that the clone is a post-germinal center B cell. This proposition is strengthened by the results of the analysis of the nature (silent or amino-acid replacing) and distribution (in framework or complement determination regions [CDR]) of somatic mutations in Ig heavy- and light-chain variable regions found in patients with WM.[31,32] These analyses showed a high rate of replacement mutations, compared with the closest germ line genes, clustering in the CDR regions and without intraclonal variation. Subsequent studies showed a strong preferential usage of VH3/JH4 gene families, no intraclonal variation, and no evidence for any isotype-switched transcripts.[33,34] These data indicate that WM may originate from a IgM^+ and/or IgM^+ IgD^+ memory B cell. Normal IgM^+ memory B cells localize in marrow, where they mature to IgM-secreting cells.[35]

MARROW MICROENVIRONMENT

Increased numbers of mast cells, admixed with aggregates of malignant lymphocytes, are found in the marrow (Fig. 111–1).[29,36] Coculture of autologous mast cells or mast cell lines with lymphoplasmacytic cells result in dose-dependent lymphoid cell proliferation and tumor colony formation, primarily through the effect of CD40 ligand (CD40L) signaling. Furthermore, the malignant lymphoid cells induce the upregulation of CD40L on mast cells derived from WM patients and mast cell lines through the elaboration of soluble CD27 (sCD27).[37]

CLINICAL FEATURES

Table 111–1 presents the clinical and laboratory findings at time of diagnosis of WM in one large institutional study.[7] Unlike most indolent lymphomas, splenomegaly and lymphadenopathy are uncommon (≤15%). Purpura is frequently associated with cryoglobulinemia and in rare circumstances with light-chain (AL) amyloidosis (see Chap. 110). Hemorrhagic and neuropathic manifestations are multifactorial (see "IgM-Related Neuropathy" below). The morbidity associated with WM is caused by the concurrence of two main components: tissue infiltration by neoplastic cells and, importantly, the physicochemical and immunologic properties of the monoclonal IgM. As shown in Table 111–2, the monoclonal IgM can produce clinical manifestations through several different mechanisms related to its physicochemical properties, nonspecific interactions with other proteins, antibody activity, and tendency to deposit in tissues.[38–40]

MORBIDITY MEDIATED BY THE EFFECTS OF IGM

Hyperviscosity Syndrome

The increased plasma IgM levels leads to blood hyperviscosity and its complications.[41] The mechanisms behind the marked increase in the resistance to blood flow and the resulting impaired transit through the microcirculatory system are complex.[41–43] The main determinants are: (1) a high concentration of monoclonal IgMs, which may form aggregates and may bind water through their carbohydrate component; and (2) their interaction with blood cells. Monoclonal IgM increases red cell aggregation (rouleaux formation) and red cell internal viscosity while reducing red cell deformability. The presence of cryoglobulins contributes to increasing blood viscosity, as well as to the tendency to induce erythrocyte aggregation. Serum viscosity is proportional to IgM concentration up to 30 g/L, then increases sharply at higher levels. Increased

TABLE 111–1. Clinical and Laboratory Findings for 356 Consecutive Newly Diagnosed Patients with Waldenström Macroglobulinemia

	Median	Range	Normal Reference Range
Age (years)	58	32–91	NA
Gender (male/female)	215/141		NA
Marrow involvement (% of area on slide)	30	5–95	NA
Adenopathy (% of patients)	15		NA
Splenomegaly (% of patients)	10		NA
IgM (mg/dL)	2620	270–12,400	40–230
IgG (mg/dL)	674	80–2770	700–1600
IgA (mg/dL)	58	6–438	70–400
Serum viscosity (cp)	2.0	1.1–7.2	1.4–1.9
Hematocrit (%)	35	17–45	35–44
Platelet count (× 10^9/L)	275	42–675	155–410
White cell count (× 10^9/L)	6.4	1.7–22	3.8–9.2
β_2-M (mg/dL)	2.5	0.9–13.7	0–2.7
LDH (U/mL)	313	61–1701	313–618

β_2M, β_2-microglobulin; cp, centipoise; LDH, lactic dehydrogenase; NA, not applicable.

SOURCE: Data from patients seen at the Dana Farber Cancer Institute, Boston, MA.

plasma viscosity may also contribute to inappropriately low erythropoietin production, which is the major reason for anemia in these patients.[44] Renal synthesis of erythropoietin is inversely correlated with plasma viscosity.[44] Clinical manifestations are related to circulatory disturbances that can be best appreciated by ophthalmoscopy, which shows distended and tortuous retinal veins, hemorrhages, and papilledema (Fig. 111–2).[45] Symptoms usually occur when the monoclonal IgM concentration exceeds 50 g/L or when serum viscosity is >4.0 centipoises (cp), but there is individual variability, with some patients showing no evidence of hyperviscosity even at 10 cp.[41] The most common symptoms are oronasal mucosal bleeding, visual disturbances because of retinal bleeding, and dizziness that rarely may lead to stupor or coma. Heart failure can be aggravated, particularly in the elderly, owing to increased blood viscosity, expanded plasma volume, and anemia. Inappropriate red cell transfusion can exacerbate hyperviscosity and may precipitate cardiac failure.

Cryoglobulinemia

The monoclonal IgM can behave as a cryoglobulin (type I) in up to 20 percent of patients, but it is symptomatic in 5 percent or less of cases.[46] Cryoprecipitation is mainly dependent on the concentration of monoclonal IgM; for this reason plasmapheresis or plasma exchange are commonly effective in this condition. Symptoms result from impaired blood flow in small vessels and include Raynaud phenomenon, acrocyanosis, and necrosis of the regions most exposed to cold, such as the tip of the nose, ears, fingers, and toes (Fig. 111–3), malleolar ulcers, purpura, and cold urticaria. Renal manifestations are infrequent.

Autoantibody Activity

Monoclonal IgM may exert its pathogenic effects through specific recognition of autologous antigens, the most notable being nerve constituents, immunoglobulin determinants, and red blood cell antigens.

IgM-Related Neuropathy

In a series of 215 patients, peripheral neuropathy was present in 24 percent,[46] although prevalence rates ranging from 5 to 40 percent are reported in other studies.[47,48] Approximately 8 percent of idiopathic neuropathies are associated with a monoclonal gammopathy, with a preponderance of IgM (60%) followed by IgG (30%) and IgA (10%).[49,50] The nerve damage is mediated by diverse pathogenetic mechanisms: (1) IgM antibody activity toward nerve constituents causing demyelinating polyneuropathies; (2) endoneurial granulofibrillar deposits of IgM without antibody activity, associated with axonal polyneuropathy; (3) occasionally by tubular deposits in the endoneurium associated with IgM cryoglobulin; and, rarely, (4) by amyloid deposits or by neoplastic cell infiltration of nerve structures.[51]

Half of the patients with IgM neuropathy have a distinctive clinical syndrome that is associated with antibodies against a minor 100-kDa

TABLE 111–2. Physicochemical and Immunological Properties of the Monoclonal IGM Protein in Waldenström's Macroglobulinemia

Properties of IgM Monoclonal Protein	Diagnostic Condition	Clinical Manifestations
Pentameric structure	Hyperviscosity	Headaches, blurred vision, epistaxis, retinal hemorrhages, leg cramps, impaired mentation, intracranial hemorrhage
Precipitation on cooling	Cryoglobulinemia (type I)	Raynaud phenomenon, acrocyanosis, ulcers, purpura, cold urticaria
Autoantibody activity to myelin-associated glycoprotein, ganglioside M_1, sulfatide moieties on peripheral nerve sheaths	Peripheral neuropathies	Sensorimotor neuropathies, painful neuropathies, ataxic gait, bilateral foot drop
Autoantibody activity to IgG	Cryoglobulinemia (type II)	Purpura, arthralgia, renal failure, sensorimotor neuropathies
Autoantibody activity to red blood cell antigens	Cold agglutinins	Hemolytic anemia, Raynaud phenomenon, acrocyanosis, livedo reticularis
Tissue deposition as amorphous aggregates	Organ dysfunction	Skin: bullous skin disease, papules, Schnitzler syndrome
		Gastrointestinal: diarrhea, malabsorption, bleeding
		Kidney: proteinuria, renal failure (light-chain component)
Tissue deposition as amyloid fibrils (light-chain component most commonly)	Organ dysfunction	Fatigue, weight loss, edema, hepatomegaly, macroglossia, organ dysfunction of involved organs (heart, kidney, liver, peripheral sensory and autonomic nerves)

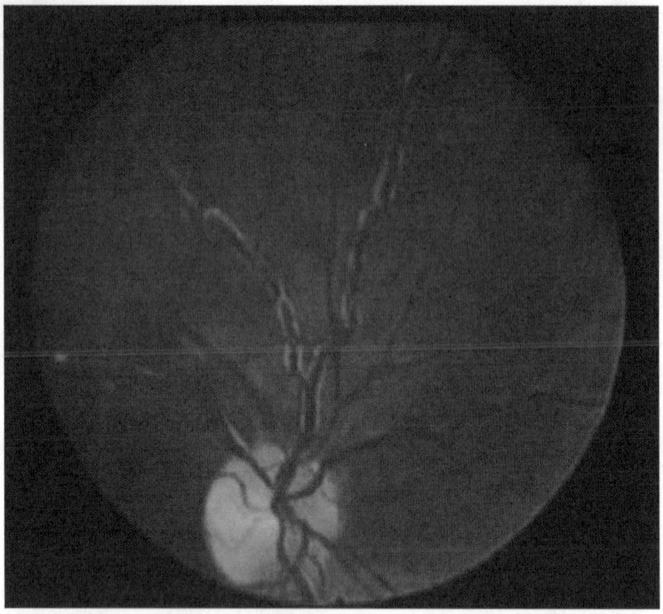

FIGURE 111–2. Funduscopic examination of a patient with Waldenström macroglobulinemia with hyperviscosity-related changes, including dilated retinal vessels, hemorrhages, and "venous sausaging." The white material at the edge of the veins may be cryoglobulin. *(Used with permission from Marvin J. Stone, MD.)*

glycoprotein component of nerve, myelin-associated glycoprotein (MAG). Anti-MAG antibodies are generally monoclonal IgM*κ*, and usually also exhibit reactivity with other glycoproteins or glycolipids that share antigenic determinants with MAG.[52–54] The anti–MAG-related neuropathy is typically distal and symmetrical, affecting both motor and sensory functions; it is slowly progressive with a long period of stability.[48,55]

Most patients present with sensory complaints (paresthesias, aching discomfort, dysesthesias, or lancinating pains), imbalance and gait ataxia, owing to lack proprioception; leg muscles atrophy in advanced stage. Patients with predominantly demyelinating sensory neuropathy in association with monoclonal IgM to gangliosides with disialosyl moieties, such as GD1b, GD3, GD2, GT1b, and GQ1b, have also been reported.[56,57] Anti-GD1b and anti-GQ1b antibodies were associated with sensory ataxic neuropathy.[61] These antiganglioside monoclonal IgMs present core clinical features of chronic ataxic neuropathy sometimes with present ophthalmoplegia and/or red blood cell cold agglutinating activity. The disialosyl epitope is also present on red blood cell glycophorins, thereby accounting for the red cell cold agglutinin activity of anti-Pr2 specificity.[58,59] Monoclonal IgM proteins that bind to gangliosides with a terminal trisaccharide moiety, including ganglioside M_2 (GM_2) and GalNac-GD1A, are associated with chronic demyelinating neuropathy and severe sensory ataxia, unresponsive to glucocorticoids.[60] Antiganglioside IgM proteins may also cross-react with lipopolysaccharides of *Campylobacter jejuni*, whose infection is known to precipitate the Miller-Fisher syndrome, a variant of the Guillain-Barré syndrome.[61] Thus, molecular mimicry may play a role in this condition. Antisulfatide monoclonal IgM proteins, associated with sensory-sensorimotor neuropathy, have been detected in 5 percent of patients with IgM monoclonal gammopathy and neuropathy.[62] Motor neuron disease has been reported in patients with WM and monoclonal IgM with anti-GM_1 and sulfoglucuronyl paragloboside activity.[63] Polyneuropathy, organomegaly, endocrinopathy, M protein, and skin changes (the POEMS syndrome) are rare in patients with WM.[64]

Cold Agglutinin Hemolytic Anemia

Monoclonal IgM may have cold agglutinin activity, that is, it can recognize specific red cell antigens at temperatures below 37°C, producing chronic hemolytic anemia. This disorder occurs in <10 percent of WM patients[65] and is associated with cold agglutinin titers greater than 1:1000 in most cases. The monoclonal component is usually an IgM*κ* and reacts most commonly with red cell I/i antigens, resulting in complement fixation and activation.[66,67] Mild to moderate chronic hemolytic anemia can be exacerbated after cold exposure. Hemoglobin usually remains above 70 g/L. The hemolysis is usually extravascular, mediated by removal of C3b opsonized red cells by the mononuclear phagocyte system, primarily in the liver. Intravascular hemolysis from complement destruction of red blood cell membrane is infrequent. The agglutination of red cells in the skin circulation also causes Raynaud syndrome, acrocyanosis, and livedo reticularis. Macroglobulins with the properties of both cryoglobulins and cold agglutinins with anti-Pr specificity can occur. These properties may have as a common basis the binding of the sialic acid-containing carbohydrate present on red blood cell glycophorins and on Ig molecules. Several other macroglobulins with antibody activity toward autologous antigens (i.e., phospholipids, tissue and plasma proteins, etc.) and foreign ligands have also been described.

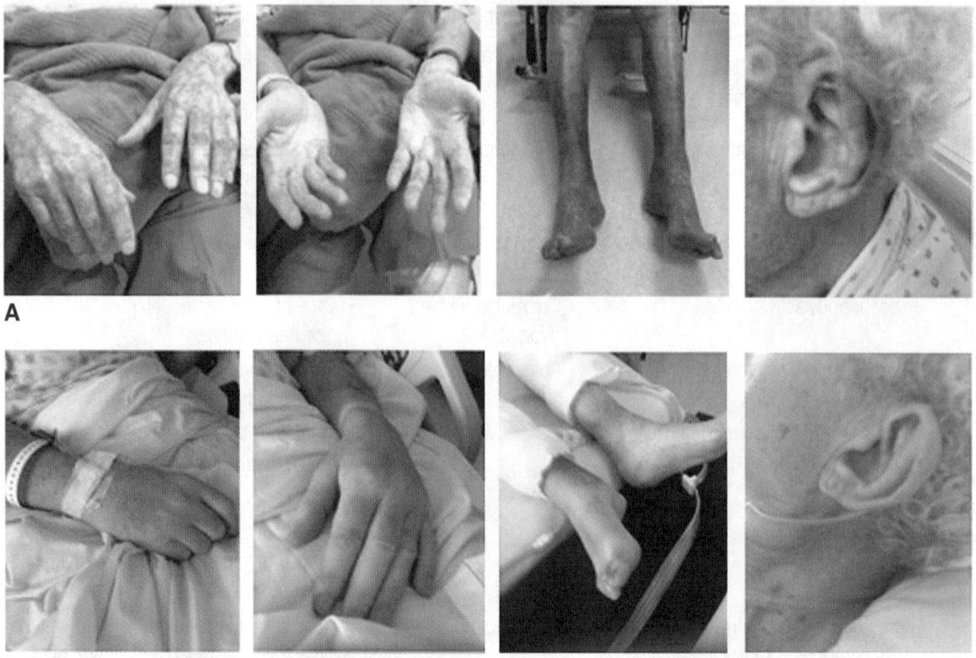

FIGURE 111–3. Cryoglobulinemia manifesting with severe acrocyanosis in a patient with Waldenström macroglobulinemia before **(A)** and following warming and plasmapheresis **(B)**.

IgM Tissue Deposition

The monoclonal protein can deposit in several tissues as amorphous aggregates. Linear deposition of monoclonal IgM along the skin basement membrane is associated with bullous skin disease.[68] Amorphous IgM deposits in the dermis result in IgM storage papules on the extensor surface of the extremities, referred to as macroglobulinemia cutis.[69] Deposition of monoclonal IgM in the lamina propria and/or submucosa of the intestine may be associated with diarrhea, malabsorption, and gastrointestinal bleeding.[70,71] Kidney involvement is less common and less severe in WM than in myeloma, probably because the amount of light chain excreted in the urine is generally lower in WM than in myeloma and because of the absence of contributing factors, such as hypercalcemia. Urinary cast nephropathy, however, has occurred in WM.[72] On the other hand, the IgM macromolecule is more susceptible to being trapped in the glomerular loops where ultrafiltration presumably contributes to its precipitation, forming subendothelial deposits of aggregated IgM proteins that occlude the glomerular capillaries.[73] Mild and reversible proteinuria may result and most patients are asymptomatic. The deposition of monoclonal light chain as fibrillar amyloid deposits (AL amyloidosis) is uncommon in patients with WM.[74] Clinical expression and prognosis are similar to those of other AL amyloidosis patients with involvement of heart (44%), kidneys (32%), liver (14%), lungs (10%), peripheral or autonomic nerves (38%), and soft tissues (18%). The incidence of cardiac and pulmonary involvement is higher in patients with monoclonal IgM than with other immunoglobulin isotypes. The association of WM with reactive amyloidosis has been documented rarely.[75,76] Simultaneous occurrence of fibrillary glomerulopathy, characterized by glomerular deposits of wide noncongophilic fibrils and amyloid deposits, has been described.[77]

■ MANIFESTATIONS RELATED TO TISSUE INFILTRATION BY NEOPLASTIC CELLS

Tissue infiltration by neoplastic cells is uncommon but can involve various organs and tissues, including the liver, spleen, lymph nodes, lungs, gastrointestinal tract, kidneys, skin, eyes, and central nervous system.

Lung

Pulmonary involvement in the form of masses, nodules, diffuse infiltrate, or pleural effusions is uncommon; the overall incidence of pulmonary and pleural findings is approximately 4 percent.[78–80] Cough is the most common presenting symptom, followed by dyspnea and chest pain. Chest radiographic findings include parenchymal infiltrates, confluent masses, and effusions.

Gastrointestinal Tract

Malabsorption, diarrhea, bleeding, or obstruction may indicate involvement of the gastrointestinal tract at the level of the stomach, duodenum, or small intestine.[81–84]

Renal System

In contrast to myeloma, infiltration of the kidney interstitium with lymphoplasmacytoid cell can occur in WM,[85] and renal or perirenal masses are not uncommon.[86]

Skin

The skin can be the site of dense lymphoplasmacytic infiltrates, similar to that seen in the liver, spleen, and lymph nodes, forming cutaneous plaques and, rarely, nodules.[87] Chronic urticaria and IgM gammopathy are the two cardinal features of the Schnitzler syndrome, which is not usually associated initially with clinical features of WM,[88] although evolution to WM is not uncommon. Thus, close followup of these patients is important.

Joints

Invasion of articular and periarticular structures by WM malignant cells is rarely reported.[89]

Eye

The neoplastic cells can infiltrate the periorbital structures, lacrimal gland, and retroorbital lymphoid tissues, resulting in ocular nerve palsies.[90,91]

Central Nervous System

Direct infiltration of the central nervous system by monoclonal lymphoplasmacytic cells as infiltrates or as tumors constitutes the rarely observed Bing-Neel syndrome, characterized clinically by confusion, memory loss, disorientation, and motor dysfunction (reviewed in reference 92).

LABORATORY FINDINGS

■ BLOOD ABNORMALITIES

Anemia is the most common finding in patients with symptomatic WM and is caused by a combination of factors: decrease in red cell survival, impaired erythropoiesis, moderate plasma volume expansion, and blood loss from the gastrointestinal tract. Blood films are usually normocytic and normochromic, and rouleaux formation is often pronounced. Mean red cell volume may be elevated spuriously owing to erythrocyte aggregation. In addition, the hemoglobin estimate can be inaccurate, that is, falsely high, because of interaction between the monoclonal protein and the diluent used in some automated analyzers.[93] Leukocyte and platelet counts are usually within the reference range at presentation, although patients may occasionally present with severe thrombocytopenia. Monoclonal B-lymphocytes expressing surface IgM and late-differentiation B-cell markers are uncommonly detected in blood by flow cytometry. A raised erythrocyte sedimentation rate is almost always present and may be the first clue to the presence of the macroglobulinemia. The clotting abnormality detected most frequently is prolongation of thrombin time. AL amyloidosis should be suspected in all patients with nephrotic syndrome, cardiomyopathy, hepatomegaly, or peripheral neuropathy. Diagnosis requires the demonstration of green birefringence under polarized light of amyloid deposits stained with Congo red.

■ MARROW FINDINGS

Central to the diagnosis of WM is the demonstration, by trephine biopsy, of marrow infiltration by a lymphoplasmacytic cell population characterized by small lymphocytes with evidence of plasmacytoid and plasma cell maturation (Fig. 111–4). The pattern of marrow infiltration may be diffuse, interstitial, or nodular, usually with an intertrabecular pattern of infiltration. A solely paratrabecular pattern of infiltration is unusual and should raise the possibility of follicular lymphoma.[1] The marrow cell immunophenotype should be confirmed by flow cytometry and/or immunohistochemistry. The cell immunoprofile: sIgM+CD19+CD20+CD22+CD79+ is characteristic of WM.[27–29] Up to 20 percent of cases may express either CD5, CD10 or CD23.[30] In these cases, chronic lymphocytic leukemia and mantle cell lymphoma should be considered.[1] "Intranuclear" periodic acid-Schiff–positive inclusions (Dutcher-Fahey bodies)[94] consisting of IgM deposits

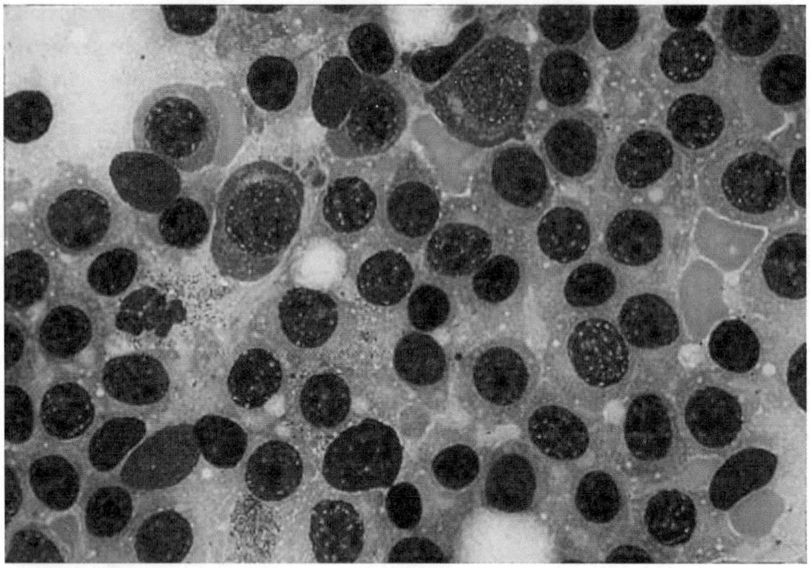

FIGURE 111–4. Marrow film from a patient with Waldenström macroglobulinemia. Note infiltrate of mature lymphocytes, lymphoplasmacytic cells, and plasma cells. *(Used with permission from Marvin J. Stone, MD.)*

in the perinuclear space, and sometimes in intranuclear vacuoles, may be seen occasionally in lymphoid cells. An increased number of mast cells, usually in association with the lymphoid aggregates is commonly found, and their presence may help in differentiating WM from other B-cell lymphomas (see Fig. 111–1).[2,3,36]

IMMUNOLOGIC ABNORMALITIES

High-resolution electrophoresis combined with immunofixation of serum and urine are recommended for identification and characterization of the IgM monoclonal protein. The light chain of the monoclonal IgM is κ in 75 to 80 percent of patients. More than one M component may be present. The concentration of the serum monoclonal protein is very variable but in most cases lies within the range of 15 to 45 g/L. Densitometry should be adopted to determine IgM levels for serial evaluations because nephelometry is unreliable and shows large laboratory variation. The presence of cold agglutinins or cryoglobulins may affect determination of IgM levels and, therefore, testing for cold agglutinins and cryoglobulins should be performed at diagnosis. If present, subsequent serum samples should be analyzed at 37°C for determination of serum monoclonal IgM level. Although Bence Jones proteinuria is frequently present, it exceeds 1 g/24 h in only 3 percent of cases. Whereas IgM levels are elevated in WM patients, IgA and IgG levels are most often depressed and do not recover after successful treatment, suggesting that patients with WM harbor a defect which prevents normal plasma cell development and/or Ig heavy chain rearrangements.[95,96]

SERUM VISCOSITY

Because of its large size (almost 1,000,000 daltons), most IgM molecules are retained within the intravascular compartment and can exert an undue effect on serum viscosity. Consequently, serum viscosity should be measured if the patient has signs or symptoms of hyperviscosity syndrome. Funduscopy remains an excellent indicator of clinically relevant hyperviscosity. Among the first clinical signs of hyperviscosity are the appearance of peripheral and midperipheral dot and blot-like hemorrhages in the retina, which are best appreciated with indirect ophthalmoscopy and scleral depression.[45] In more severe cases of hyperviscosity, dot, blot, and flame-shaped hemorrhages can appear in the macular area along with markedly dilated and tortuous veins with focal constrictions resulting in "venous sausaging," as well as papilledema.

IMAGING

Magnetic resonance imaging (MRI) of the spine in conjunction with computed tomography (CT) of the abdomen and pelvis are useful in evaluating the disease status.[97] Marrow involvement can be documented by MRI studies of the spine in more than 90 percent of patients; CT of the abdomen and pelvis demonstrates enlarged nodes in approximately 40 percent of WM patients.[97]

LYMPH NODE BIOPSY

Lymph node biopsy may show preserved architecture or replacement by infiltration of neoplastic cells with lymphoplasmacytoid, lymphoplasmacytic, or polymorphous cytologic patterns.

POLYMERASE CHAIN REACTION

The residual disease after high-dose chemotherapy with allogeneic or autologous stem-cell rescue can be monitored by polymerase chain reaction–based methods using primers specific for the monoclonal Ig variable regions.

TREATMENT

DECIDING ON INITIATING TREATMENT

As part of the Second International Workshop on Waldenström's macroglobulinemia, a consensus panel was organized to recommend criteria for the initiation of therapy in patients with WM.[98] The panel recommended that initiation of therapy should not be based on the IgM level *per se*, as this may not correlate with the clinical manifestations of WM. The consensus panel did, however, agree that initiation of therapy is appropriate for patients with constitutional symptoms, such as recurrent fever, night sweats, fatigue as a consequence of anemia, or weight loss. Progressive symptomatic lymphadenopathy or splenomegaly provide additional reasons to begin therapy. Anemia with a hemoglobin value of ≤10 g/dL or a platelet count of $\leq 100 \times 10^9$/L owing to marrow infiltration, also justifies treatment. Certain complications, such as hyperviscosity syndrome, symptomatic sensorimotor peripheral neuropathy, systemic amyloidosis, renal insufficiency, or symptomatic cryoglobulinemia, may also be indications for therapy.[98]

INITIAL THERAPY

The International Workshop on Waldenström Macroglobulinemia has formulated recommendations for both initial therapy and therapy for refractory disease based on the best available evidence. The panels considered alkylating agents (e.g., chlorambucil), nucleoside analogues (cladribine or fludarabine), the monoclonal antibody rituximab, as well as combinations as reasonable choices for the initial therapy of WM.[99–101] Individual patient considerations, including the presence of cytopenias, need for more rapid disease control, age, and candidacy for autologous transplant therapy, should be taken into account in making the choice of the drugs to use. For patients who are candidates for autologous stem cell transplantation, which typically is reserved for those patients younger than 70 years of age, the panel recommended that exposure to alkylating agents or nucleoside analogues should be limited. The use of nucleoside analogues should be approached cautiously in patients with

WM as there appears to be an increased risk for the development of disease transformation as well as myelodysplasia and acute myelogenous leukemia.

Alkylating Agents

Oral alkylating drugs, alone and in combination therapy with glucocorticoids, have been extensively evaluated in the treatment of WM. Chlorambucil has been administered on both a continuous (i.e., daily dose schedule) and an intermittent schedule. Patients receiving chlorambucil on a continuous schedule typically receive 0.1 mg/kg per day, whereas on the intermittent schedule patients typically receive 0.3 mg/kg for 7 days, every 6 weeks. In a prospective randomized study, no significant difference in the overall response rate between these schedules was observed,[102] although the median response duration was greater for patients receiving intermittent- versus continuous-dose chlorambucil (46 vs. 26 months). Despite the favorable median response duration in this study for use of the intermittent schedule, no difference in the median overall survival was observed. Moreover, an increased incidence for development of myelodysplasia and acute myelogenous leukemia with the intermittent (3 of 22 patients) versus the continuous (0 of 24 patients) chlorambucil schedule prompted the preference for use of continuous chlorambucil dosing. The use of glucocorticoids in combination with alkylating agent therapy has also been explored. Chlorambucil (8 mg/m^2) plus prednisone (40 mg/m^2) given orally for 10 days, every 6 weeks, resulted in a major response (i.e., reduction of IgM by more than 50%) in 72 percent of patients.[103] Alkylating agent regimens employing melphalan and cyclophosphamide in combination with glucocorticoids have also been examined.[104,105] This approach produced slightly higher overall response rates and response durations, although the benefit of these more complex regimens over chlorambucil remains to be demonstrated. Pretreatment factors associated with shorter survival in the entire population of patients receiving single-agent chlorambucil were age older than 60 years, male sex, hemoglobin less than 10 g/dL, leukocytes less than 4×10^9/L, and platelets less than 150×10^9/L. Organomegaly, signs of hyperviscosity, renal failure, monoclonal IgM level, blood lymphocytosis, and percentage of marrow lymphoid cells were not significantly correlated with survival.[106] Additional factors to be taken into account in considering alkylating agent therapy for patients with WM include necessity for more rapid disease control given the slow response, as well as consideration for preserving stem cells in patients who are candidates for autologous stem cell transplantation therapy.

Nucleoside Analogue Therapy

Cladribine administered as a single agent by continuous intravenous infusion, by 2-hour daily infusion, or by subcutaneous bolus injections for 5 to 7 days has resulted in major responses in 40 to 90 percent of patients who received primary therapy, whereas in the previously treated patients, responses have ranged from 38 to 54 percent.[107–113] Median time to achievement of response in responding patients following cladribine ranged from 1.2 to 5 months. The overall response rate with daily infusion of fludarabine, administered mainly on 5-day schedules, in previously untreated and treated patients ranged from 38 to 100 percent and 30 to 40 percent, respectively,[114–119] similar to the responses to cladribine. Median time to achievement of response for fludarabine (3–6 months) was also similar to cladribine. In general, response rates and durations of responses have been greater for patients receiving nucleoside analogues as initial therapy, although in several studies in which both untreated and previously treated patients were enrolled, no difference in the overall response rate was reported.

Myelosuppression commonly occurs following prolonged exposure to either of the nucleoside analogues. A sustained decrease in both CD4+ and CD8+ T lymphocytes, measured 1 year following initiation of therapy, is notable.[106,108] Treatment-related mortality as a consequence of myelosuppression and/or opportunistic infections attributable to immunosuppression occurred in up to 5 percent of all treated patients in some series with either nucleoside analogue.

Factors predicting for a better response to nucleoside analogues include younger age at start of treatment (<70 years), higher pretreatment hemoglobin (>95 g/L), higher platelet count (>75 × 10^9/L), disease relapsing off therapy, and a long interval between first-line therapy and initiation of a nucleoside analogue in relapsing patients.[106,112,118] There are limited data on the use of an alternate nucleoside analogue in previously treated patients among whom disease relapsed or who had resistance when not on cladribine or fludarabine therapy.[120,121] Three of 4 (75%) patients responded to cladribine after progression following an unmaintained remission to fludarabine, whereas only 1 of 10 (10%) with disease resistant to fludarabine responded to cladribine.[120] A response in 2 of 6 patients (33%) and disease stabilization in the remaining patients to fludarabine, in spite of an inadequate response or progressive disease, following cladribine therapy has been reported.[121]

Harvesting autologous blood stem cells succeeded on the first attempt in 14 of 15 patients who did not receive nucleoside analogue therapy as compared to 2 of 6 patients who received a nucleoside analogue.[122] A sevenfold increase in transformation to an aggressive lymphoma and a threefold increase in the development of myelodysplasia or acute myelogenous leukemia were observed among patients who received a nucleoside analogue versus other therapies for their WM.[123] A meta-analysis of several trials in which patients were treated with nucleoside analogues in WM patients, included patients who had previously received an alkylating agent, and showed a crude incidence of approximately 8 percent for development of disease transformation and of approximately 5 percent for development of myelodysplasia or acute myelogenous leukemia.[124] None of the risk factors—that is, gender, age, family history of WM, or B-cell malignancies, typical markers of tumor burden and prognosis, type of nucleoside analogue therapy (cladribine vs. fludarabine), time from diagnosis to nucleoside analogue use, nucleoside analogue treatment as primary or salvage therapy, or treatment with an oral alkylator (i.e., chlorambucil)—predicted for the occurrence of transformation or development of myelodysplasia or acute myelogenous leukemia in patients treated with a nucleoside analogue.[124]

CD20-Directed Antibody Therapy

Rituximab is a chimeric monoclonal antibody that targets CD20, a widely expressed antigen on lymphoplasmacytic cells in WM.[125] Several retrospective and prospective studies have indicated that rituximab, when used at standard doses (i.e., 4 weekly infusions of 375 mg/m^2) induced major responses in approximately 30 percent of previously treated and untreated patients.[126–132] Even patients who achieved minor responses benefited from rituximab by improved hemoglobin and platelet counts, and reduction of lymphadenopathy and/or splenomegaly. The median time to treatment failure in these studies was found to range from 8 to 27+ months. Patients on an extended rituximab schedule consisting of 4 weekly courses at 375 mg/m^2 per week, repeated 3 months later by another 4-week course have demonstrated major response rates of approximately 45 percent, with time to progression estimates of 16+ to 29+ months.[132,133]

In many WM patients, a transient increase of serum IgM may be noted immediately following initiation of rituximab treatment.[132,134–136] Such an increase does not herald treatment failure and most patients will return to their baseline serum IgM level by 12 weeks. Some patients continue to show a prolonged increase in IgM despite an apparent reduction in their marrow tumor cells. However, patients with baseline serum IgM levels of >50 g/dL or serum viscosity of >3.5 cp may be particularly at risk for a hyperviscosity-related event and plasmapheresis should be considered in these patients in advance of rituximab therapy.[135] Because of the decreased likelihood of response in patients with higher IgM levels, as well as the possibility that serum IgM and blood viscosity levels may abruptly rise, rituximab monotherapy should not be used as sole therapy for the treatment of patients at risk for hyperviscosity symptoms.

Time to response after rituximab is slow and exceeds 3 months on the average. The time to best response in one study was 18 months.[133] Patients with baseline serum IgM levels of <60 g/dL are more likely to respond, regardless of the underlying marrow involvement by tumor cells.[132,133] An analysis of 52 patients who were treated with single-agent rituximab found the objective response rate was significantly lower in patients who had either low serum albumin (<35 g/L) or a serum monoclonal protein greater than 40 g/L. The presence of both adverse prognostic factors was associated with a short time to progression (3.6 months). Patients who had normal serum albumin and relatively low serum monoclonal protein levels derived a substantial benefit from rituximab with a time to progression exceeding 40 months.[137]

A correlation between polymorphisms at position 158 in the FcγRIIIa receptor (CD16), an activating Fc receptor on important effector cells that mediate antibody-dependent cell-mediated cytotoxicity, and rituximab response was observed in WM patients. Individuals may encode either the amino acid valine or phenylalanine at position 158 in the FcγRIIIa receptor. WM patients who carried the valine amino acid (either in a homozygous or heterozygous pattern) had a fourfold higher major response rate (i.e., 50% decline in serum IgM levels) to rituximab versus those patients who expressed phenylalanine in a homozygous pattern.[138]

Combination Therapies

Because rituximab is not myelosuppressive, its combination with chemotherapy has been explored. A regimen of rituximab, cladribine, and cyclophosphamide used in 17 previously untreated patients resulted in a partial response in 94 percent of WM patients, including a complete response in 18 percent.[139] No patient had relapsed with a median followup of 21 months. The combination of rituximab and fludarabine used in 43 patients of whom 32 (75%) were previously untreated, led to an overall response rate of 95.3 percent, with 83 percent of patients achieving a major response (i.e., 50% reduction in disease burden).[140] The median time to progression was 51.2 months in this series, and was longer for those patients who were previously untreated and for those achieving a very good partial remission (i.e., 90% reduction in disease) or better. Hematologic toxicity was common: grade 3 neutropenia and thrombocytopenia observed in 27 and 4 patients, respectively. Two deaths occurred in this study from pneumonia. Secondary malignancies including transformation to aggressive lymphoma and development of myelodysplasia or acute myelogenous leukemia were observed in six patients in this series. The addition of rituximab to fludarabine and cyclophosphamide has also been explored in previously treated patients, of whom 4 of 5 patients had a response.[141] In another combination study, rituximab along with pentostatin and cyclophosphamide given to 13 patients with untreated and previously treated WM or lymphoplasmacytic lymphoma resulted in a major response in 77 percent of patients.[142] The combination of rituximab, dexamethasone, and cyclophosphamide was used as primary therapy to treat 72 patients with WM in whom a major response was observed in 74 percent of patients in this study, and the 2-year progression-free survival was 67 percent.[143] Therapy was well tolerated, although one patient died of interstitial pneumonia.

Two studies have examined cyclophosphamide, doxorubicin, vincristine, prednisone (CHOP) in combination with rituximab (R-CHOP). In a randomized trial involving 69 patients, most of whom had WM, the addition of rituximab to CHOP resulted in a higher overall response rate (94% vs. 67%) and median time to progression (63 vs. 22 months) in comparison to patients treated with CHOP alone.[144] R-CHOP was also used in 13 WM patients, 10 of whom had relapsed or refractory disease.[145] Among 13 evaluable patients, 10 patients achieved a major response (77%), including 3 complete and 7 partial remissions. Two other patients achieved a minor response. In a retrospective study of symptomatic WM patients who received either R-CHOP; rituximab, cyclophosphamide, vincristine, and prednisone (R-CVP); or cyclophosphamide, prednisone, and rituximab (R-CP) and were similar in most pretreatment variables, the overall response rates to therapy were comparable among all three treatment groups—R-CHOP (96%), R-CVP (88%), and R-CP (95%)—although there was a trend for more complete remissions among patients treated with R-CVP and R-CHOP.[146] Adverse events attributed to therapy showed a higher incidence for neutropenic fever and treatment related neuropathy for R-CHOP and R-CVP versus R-CP. The results of this study suggest that in WM, the use of R-CP may provide analogous treatment responses to more intense cyclophosphamide-based regimens while minimizing treatment-related complications.

The use of two cycles of oral cyclophosphamide along with subcutaneous cladribine to 37 patients with previously untreated WM led to a partial response in 84 percent of patients and the median duration of response was 36 months.[139] Fludarabine in combination with intravenous cyclophosphamide resulted in partial responses in 6 of 11 (55%) WM patients with either primary refractory disease or who had relapsed on treatment.[147] The combination of fludarabine plus cyclophosphamide was also evaluated in 49 patients, 35 of whom were previously treated. Seventy-eight percent of the patients achieved a response and median time to treatment failure was 27 months.[148] Hematologic toxicity was frequent and three patients died of treatment-related toxicities. Two important findings in this study were the development of acute leukemia in two patients, histologic transformation to diffuse large B-cell lymphoma in one patient, and two cases of solid malignancies (prostate and melanoma), as well as failure to mobilize stem cells in 4 of 6 patients.

In view of the above data, the consensus panel on therapeutics amended its original recommendations for the therapy of WM to include the use of combination therapy with either (1) nucleoside analogues and alkylating agents, (2) rituximab in combination with nucleoside analogues, (3) rituximab, nucleoside analogues, plus alkylating agents, or (4) rituximab and cyclophosphamide-based therapy as reasonable therapeutics options for the treatment of WM.[100,101]

THERAPY FOR RELAPSED OR REFRACTORY PATIENTS

For patients in relapse or who have refractory disease, the consensus panels recommended the use of an alternative first-line agent as (e.g., alkylating agents, nucleoside inhibitors, or anti-CD20 monoclonal antibodies), with the caveat that for those patients for whom autologous stem cell transplantation is considered, further exposure to stem cell–damaging agents (i.e., alkylating agents and nucleoside analogue drugs) should be avoided, and a non-stem-cell–toxic agent should be considered if stem cells have not been harvested previously.[100,101]

Several novel agents including bortezomib, thalidomide alone or in combination, and alemtuzumab can be considered in the treatment of relapsed or refractory patients. Autologous stem cell transplantation remains an option for the therapy of WM, particularly among younger patients who have had multiple relapses or who have primary refractory disease.

Proteasome Inhibitor

Bortezomib, a stem cell–sparing agent,[149–151] is a proteasome inhibitor that induces apoptosis of primary WM lymphoplasmacytic cells.[152]

Bortezomib may also impair the marrow microenvironmental support for lymphoplasmacytic cells. Among 27 patients, all but 1 patient with relapsed/or refractory disease, who received up to 8 cycles of bortezomib at 1.3 mg/m^2 on days 1, 4, 8, and 11, had their median serum IgM levels decline significantly from 4.7 g/dL to 2.1 g/dL.[153] The overall response rate was 85 percent, with 10 and 13 patients achieving a minor (<25%) and major (<50%) decrease in IgM level. Responses occurred at median of 1.4 months. The median time to progression for all responding patients in this study was 7.9 (range: 3–21.4+) months, and the most common grade III/IV toxicities were sensory neuropathies (22.2%), leukopenia (18.5%), neutropenia (14.8%), dizziness (11.1%), and thrombocytopenia (7.4%). Sensory neuropathies resolved or improved in nearly all patients following cessation of therapy. Twenty-seven patients with both untreated (44%) and previously treated (56%) disease received bortezomib, utilizing the standard schedule until they either demonstrated progressive disease or two cycles beyond a complete response or stable disease. The overall response rate was 78 percent, with major responses observed in 44 percent of patients. Sensory neuropathy occurred in 20 patients following 2 to 4 cycles of therapy.[154] Among the 20 patients developing a neuropathy, 14 patients resolved and 1 patient demonstrated a improvement at 2 to 13 months. Using bortezomib monotherapy in WM, major responses occurred in 6 of 10 (60%) previously treated WM patients,[155] whereas a major response occurred in 1 of 2 patients with WM who were included in a series of relapsed or refractory patients with non-Hodgkin lymphoma.[156] The combination of bortezomib, dexamethasone, and rituximab as primary therapy in patients with WM resulted in an overall response rate of 96 percent, and a major response rate of 83 percent.[157] The incidence of grade 3 neuropathy was approximately 30 percent, but was reversible in most patients following discontinuation of therapy. An increased incidence of herpes zoster was also observed prompting the prophylactic use of antiviral therapy. Alternative schedules for administration of bortezomib (i.e., once weekly at higher doses) in combination with rituximab in patients with WM have achieved overall response rates of 80 to 90 percent.[158,159] Bortezomib-related peripheral neuropathy may be reduced with this schedule.[158]

CD52-Directed Antibody Therapy

Alemtuzumab is a humanized monoclonal antibody that targets CD52, an antigen expressed on marrow lymphoplasmacytic cells in WM patients, as well as on mast cells, which are increased in the marrow of patients with WM and provide growth and survival signals to tumor cells through several tumor necrosis factor ligands (CD40L, APRIL [a proliferation-inducing ligand], B-lymphocyte-stimulating protein).[160] Twenty-eight subjects with the clinicopathologic diagnosis of lymphoplasmacytic lymphoma, including 27 patients with IgM (WM) and one with IgA monoclonal gammopathy were enrolled in a prospective, multicenter study.[161] Five patients were untreated and 23 were previously treated, all of whom had previously received rituximab. Patients received three daily test doses of alemtuzumab (3, 10, and 30 mg IV) followed by 30 mg alemtuzumab IV three times a week for up to 12 weeks. All patients received acyclovir and Bactrim or equivalent prophylaxis for the duration of therapy plus 8 weeks following the last infusion of alemtuzumab. Among 25 patients evaluable for response, the overall response rate was 76 percent, which included 8 (32%) major responders and 11 (44%) minor responders. Hematologic toxicities were common among previously treated (but not untreated) patients and included grade 3 of neutropenia (39%), thrombocytopenia (18%), and anemia (7%). Grade 3 or 4 nonhematologic toxicity for all patients included dermatitis (11%), fatigue (7%), and infection (7%). Cytomegalovirus reactivation and infection occurred among previously treated patients and may have been for the cause of one death. With a median followup of 8.5+ months, 11 of 19 responding patients remain free of progression. High rates of response with the use of alemtuzumab as salvage therapy have also been reported in a small series of heavily pretreated WM patients (with a median of four prior therapies). These patients received up to 12 weeks of therapy (at 30 mg IV three times per week) following initial dose escalation.[162] Among the seven patients receiving alemtuzumab, five patients achieved a partial response and one patient a complete response. Infectious complications were common. Cytomegalovirus reactivation occurred in three patients and required ganciclovir therapy, and three patients were hospitalized for bacterial infections. Opportunistic infection occurred in two patients, and was responsible for their deaths.

Thalidomide and Lenalidomide

Thalidomide as a single agent, and in combination with dexamethasone and clarithromycin, was also examined in patients with WM in view of the success of these regimens in patients with advanced myeloma. Five of 20 (25%) previously untreated and treated patients who received single-agent thalidomide had a major response.[163] Dose escalation from the thalidomide start dose of 200 mg daily was hindered by development of side effects, including the development of peripheral neuropathy in five patients requiring discontinuation or dose reduction. Ten of 12 (83%) previously treated patients had a major response to low doses of thalidomide (50 mg orally daily) in combination with dexamethasone (40 mg orally once a week) and clarithromycin (250 mg orally twice a day).[164] However, in a followup study using a higher thalidomide dose (200 mg orally daily) along with dexamethasone (40 g orally once a week) and clarithromycin (500 mg orally twice a day), only 2 of 10 (20%) previously treated patients responded.[165] Thalidomide and its analogue lenalidomide significantly augmented rituximab-mediated, antibody-dependent, cell-mediated cytotoxicity against lymphoplasmacytic cells.[166] An expansion of natural killer cells occurs with thalidomide use, which in previous studies was shown to be associated with the rituximab response.[167,168] One approach investigated in the treatment of symptomatic patients with WM is the combination of thalidomide with rituximab. Patients in this study received thalidomide at 200 mg daily for 2 weeks, followed by 400 mg daily for 1 year plus four weekly infusions of rituximab at 375 mg/m^2 beginning 1 week after initiation of thalidomide, followed by four additional weekly infusions of rituximab at 375 mg/m^2 beginning at week 13.[169] The overall and major response rates (i.e., ≥50 decrease in IgM) in this study were 72 and 64 percent, respectively. Median serum IgM levels decreased from 3.7 to 1.6 g/dL and, the median hematocrit rose from 33 to 38 percent at best response. The median time to progression for responders was 38 months. Dose reduction of thalidomide was required in all patients and led to discontinuation in 11 patients. Among 11 patients experiencing grade ≥2 neuroparesthesia, 10 demonstrated reduction to grade 1 or less at a median of 6.7 months. Given the high incidence of treatment-related neuropathy, lower doses of thalidomide (i.e., ≤200 mg/day) should be considered in this patient population.

In a phase II study of lenalidomide and rituximab in WM, patients were started on lenalidomide at 25 mg daily on a syncopated schedule in which therapy was administered for 3 weeks, followed by a 1-week pause for an intended duration of 48 weeks.[170] Patients received 1 week of therapy with lenalidomide, after which rituximab (375 mg/m^2) was administered weekly on weeks 2 to 5, and again on weeks 13 to 16. The overall and major response rates in this study were 50 and 25 percent, respectively, and the median time to progression for responders was 18.9 months. In two patients, significant reduction in extramedullary bulky disease was observed. However, an acute decrease in hematocrit occurred during first 2 weeks of lenalidomide therapy in 13 of 16 (81%) patients with a median absolute decrease in hematocrit of 5 percent, resulting in anemia-related complications and hospitalizations in 4 patients. Despite dose reduction, most patients in this study continued to have troublesome anemia with lenalidomide. There was no evidence of hemolysis or more general myelosuppression with lenalidomide in this study. Therefore, the mechanism for lenalidomide-related anemia in WM patients remains to be determined, and the use of this agent among WM patients should be avoided.

HIGH-DOSE THERAPY AND STEM CELL TRANSPLANTATION

The use of autologous stem cell transplantation therapy has also been explored in patients with WM.[171,172] These studies involved eight previously treated WM patients between the ages of 45 and 69 years, who received either melphalan at 200 mg/m^2 (n = 7) or melphalan at 140 mg/m^2 along with total-body irradiation as tumor-suppressive therapy. Stem cells were collected in eight patients, although a second collection procedure was required for two patients who had previous exposure to nucleoside analogue. There was no transplant-related mortality and toxicities were manageable. All eight patients responded, with 7 of 8 patients achieving a major response, and one patient achieving a complete response with durations of response raging from 5+ to 77+ months. A regimen of dexamethasone, BCNU, etoposide, cytarabine, melphalan (DEXA-BEAM) was followed by myeloablative therapy with cyclophosphamide and total-body irradiation and autologous stem cell transplantation in seven WM patients, which included four untreated patients with progression-free survival ranging from 4+ to 30+ months.[173] Three evaluable patients, who were previously treated, also attained a major response in a study in which WM patients received various preparative regimens and showed event-free survivals of 26+, 31, and 108+ months.[174] High-dose chemotherapy followed by autologous stem cell transplantation in 18 patients, previously treated with a median of three (range: 1–5) prior regimens, was well tolerated with an improvement in response status observed for seven patients (six partial to complete remission; one had stabilized disease); one patient had progressive disease.[175] The median event-free survival for all nonprogressing patients was 12 months.

Allogeneic hematopoietic stem cell transplantation was used in 10 previously treated WM patients (ages 35–46 years), who had received a median of three prior therapies, including three patients with progressive disease despite therapy.[175] Two of three patients with progressive disease responded, and an improvement in response status was observed in five patients. The median event-free survival for nonprogressing evaluable patients was 31 months. Three patients died from transplantation-related toxicity. In a retrospective review of WM patients who underwent either autologous or allogeneic transplantation, and among whom were 78 percent of patients in this cohort with two or more previous therapies, 58 percent were resistant to their previous therapy.[176] The relapse rate at 3 years was 29 percent in the allogeneic group and 24 percent in the autologous group. Nonrelapse mortality, however, was 40 percent in the allogeneic group and 11 percent in the autologous group.

Among 202 WM patients who received autologous stem cell transplantation, which included primarily relapsed or refractory patients, the 5-year progression-free and overall survival rate was 61 and 33 percent, respectively.[177] Chemosensitive disease at time of the autologous transplantation was the most important prognostic factor for nonrelapse mortality, response rate, and progression-free and overall survival. Among 106 allogeneic stem cell transplantation patient were 44 patients who received a conventional myeloablative transplantation and 62 patients who received a reduced-intensity conditioning allogeneic transplantation. The 106 patients predominately included those with more advanced disease and was notable for 3-year nonrelapse mortality rate of 33 percent after transplantation.[177] The 5-year progression-free and overall survival rates in this series were 48 and 63 percent, respectively. Among the 106 patients who underwent an allogeneic stem cell transplantation, 48 developed acute, 16 developed limited, and 11 developed extensive chronic graft-versus-host disease. Reduced-intensity conditioning with allogeneic stem cell transplantation induced responses, including complete responses, among patients with advanced WM: 6 complete, 1 near complete, and 4 partial responses among 12 evaluable patients. Autologous, as well as reduced-intensity allogeneic stem cell transplantation have a role in the treatment of relapsed or refractory patients, when patients are carefully selected.

RESPONSE CRITERIA IN WALDENSTRÖM MACROGLOBULINEMIA

Response to treatment of WM has been difficult to interpret because of different response criteria in different studies. A consensus for uniform response criteria in WM has been achieved.[179,180] The category of minor response was adopted at the Third International Workshop of WM, given that clinically meaningful responses were observed with newer biologic agents, and is based on ≥25 to <50 percent decrease in serum IgM level, which is used as a surrogate marker of disease in WM. In distinction, the term major response is used to denote a response of ≥50 percent in serum IgM levels, and includes partial and complete responses.[180] Table 111–3 summarizes the response categories and criteria for progressive disease in WM based on consensus recommendations. An important concern with the use of IgM as a surrogate marker of disease is that it can fluctuate, independent of tumor

TABLE 111–3. Summary of Updated Response Criteria from the 3rd International Workshop on Waldenström Macroglobulinemia[100,180]

Complete response (CR)	Disappearance of monoclonal protein by immunofixation; no histologic evidence of marrow involvement, and resolution of any adenopathy/organomegaly (confirmed by CT scan), along with no signs or symptoms attributable to WM. Reconfirmation of the CR status is required at least 6 weeks apart with a second immunofixation.
Partial response (PR)	A ≥50% reduction of serum monoclonal IgM concentration on protein electrophoresis and a decrease in adenopathy/organomegaly on physical examination or on CT scan. No new symptoms or signs of active disease.
Minor response (MR)	A ≥25% but <50% reduction of serum monoclonal IgM by protein electrophoresis. No new symptoms or signs of active disease.
Stable disease (SD)	A <25% reduction and <25% increase of serum monoclonal IgM by electrophoresis without progression of adenopathy/organomegaly, cytopenias, or clinically significant symptoms because of disease and/or signs of WM.
Progressive disease (PD)	A ≥25% increase in serum monoclonal IgM by protein electrophoresis confirmed by a second measurement or progression of clinically significant findings because of disease (i.e., anemia, thrombocytopenia, leukopenia, bulky adenopathy/organomegaly) or symptoms (unexplained recurrent fever ≥38.4°C, drenching night sweats, ≥10mL/kg loss, or hyperviscosity, neuropathy, symptomatic cryoglobulinemia or amyloidosis) attributable to WM.

TABLE 111–4. Prognostic Scoring Systems in Waldenström Macroglobulinemia

Study	Adverse Prognostic Factors	Number of Groups	Survival
Gobbi et al.[185]	Hgb <9 g/dL	0–1 prognostic factors	Median: 48 months
	Age >70 years	2–4 prognostic factors	Median: 80 months
	Weight loss		
	Cryoglobulinemia		
Morel et al.[186]	Age ≥65 years	0–1 prognostic factors	5-year: 87% of patients
	Albumin <4 g/dL	2 prognostic factors	5-year: 62%
	Number of cytopenias:	3–4 prognostic factors	5-year: 25%
	Hgb <12 g/dL		
	Platelets <150 × 10^9/L		
	WBC <4 × 10^9/L		
Dhodapkar et al.[187]	β_2M ≥3 g/dL	β_2M <3 mg/dL + Hgb ≥12 g/dL	5-year: 87% of patients
	Hgb <12 g/dL	β_2M <3 mg/dL + Hgb <12 g/dL	5-year: 63%
	IgM <4 g/dL	β_2M ≥3 mg/dL + IgM ≥4 g/dL	5-year: 53%
		β_2M ≥3 mg/dL + IgM <4 g/dL	5-year: 21%
Application of International Staging System Criteria for Myeloma to WM Dimopoulos et al.[188]	Albumin ≤3.5 g/dL	Albumin ≥3.5 g/dL + β_2M <3.5 mg/dL	Median: NR
	β_2M ≥3.5 mg/L	Albumin ≤3.5 g/dL + β_2M <3.5 or β_2M 3.5–5.5 mg/dL	Median: 116 months
		β_2M >5.5 mg/dL	Median: 54 months
International Prognostic Scoring System for WM Morel et al.[190]	Age >65 year	0–1 prognostic factors (excluding age)	5 year: 87% of patients
	Hgb <11.5 g/dL	2 prognostic factors (or age >65 years)	5 year: 68%
	Platelets <100 × 10^9/L	3–5 prognostic factors	5 year: 36%
	β_2M >3 mg/L		
	IgM >7 g/dL		

β_2M, β_2-microbloulin; Hgb, hemoglobulin; NR, not reported; WBC, white blood cell count.

cell killing, particularly with newer biologically targeted agents such as rituximab and bortezomib.[128–130,146,172] Rituximab induces a spike or flare in serum IgM levels that can occur when used as monotherapy and in combination with other agents including cyclophosphamide, nucleoside analogues, thalidomide, and lenalidomide, and last for several weeks to months,[132,135,136,146,153,169,170,181] whereas bortezomib can suppress IgM levels independent of tumor cell killing in certain patients.[153,182] Moreover, with selective B-cell depleting agents such as rituximab and alemtuzumab, residual IgM producing plasma cells are spared and continue to persist, thus potentially skewing the relative response and assessment to treatment.[183] Therefore, in circumstances where the serum IgM levels appear out of context with the clinical progress of the patient, a marrow biopsy should be considered so as to clarify the patient's underlying disease burden. Soluble CD27 may serve as an alternative surrogate marker in WM,[37] and may remain a faithful marker of disease in patients experiencing a rituximab-related IgM flare, as well as during plasmapheresis therapy.[184]

COURSE AND PROGNOSIS

WM typically presents as an indolent disease. The median survival reported in several large series has ranged from 5 to 10 years,[185–190] although in a followup of 436 consecutive patients diagnosed with WM, the median overall survival from time of diagnosis was in excess of 10 years.[123] The presence of 6q deletions may have prognostic significance, although this is disputed.[20,21] Age is an important prognostic factor (>65 years),[185,187,190] but is influenced by comorbidities. Anemia that reflects both marrow involvement and the serum level of the IgM monoclonal protein (because of the impact of IgM on intravascular fluid retention) has emerged as a strong adverse prognostic factor with hemoglobin levels of <9 to 12 g/dL associated with decreased survival in several series.[185–187,190] Other cytopenias also may be significant predictors of survival.[186,190] The precise level of cytopenias with prognostic significance has not been determined. Some series have identified a platelet count of <100 to 150 × 10^9/L and a granulocyte count of <1.5 × 10^9/L as independent prognostic factors.[186,187] The number of cytopenias in a given patient has been proposed as a prognostic factor.[186] Serum albumin levels also correlate with survival in WM patients in some studies, using multivariate analyses.[186,188] Elevated serum β_2-microglobulin levels (>3–3.5 g/dL),[187–190] a very high serum IgM M-protein (>7 g/dL),[190] a low serum IgM M-protein (<4 g/dL),[187] and the presence of cryoglobulins[185] decrease overall survival. Several scoring systems have been proposed based on these analyses (Table 111–4).

REFERENCES

1. Owen RG, Treon SP, Al-Katib A, et al: Clinicopathological definition of Waldenström's macroglobulinemia: Consensus Panel Recommendations from the Second International Workshop on Waldenström's macroglobulinemia. *Semin Oncol* 30:110, 2003.
2. Harris NL, Jaffe ES, Stein H, et al: A revised European-American classification of lymphoid neoplasms: A proposal from the International Lymphoma Study Group. *Blood* 84:1361, 1994.
3. Harris NL, Jaffe ES, Diebold J, et al: The World Health Organization classification of neoplastic diseases of the hematopoietic and lymphoid tissues. Report of the Clinical Advisory Committee meeting, Airlie House, Virginia, November, 1997. *Ann Oncol* 10:1419, 1999.
4. Groves FD, Travis LB, Devesa SS, et al: Waldenström's macroglobulinemia: Incidence patterns in the United States, 1988–1994. *Cancer* 82:1078, 1998.
5. Herrinton LJ, Weiss NS: Incidence of Waldenström's macroglobulinemia. *Blood* 82:3148, 1993.
6. Bjornsson OG, Arnason A, Gudmunosson S, et al: Macroglobulinaemia in an Icelandic family. *Acta Med Scand* 203:283, 1978.
7. Treon SP, Hunter ZR, Aggarwal A, et al: Characterization of familial Waldenström's macroglobulinemia. *Ann Oncol* 17:488, 2006.
8. Renier G, Ifrah N, Chevailler A, et al: Four brothers with Waldenström's macroglobulinemia. *Cancer* 64:1554, 1989.
9. Ogmundsdottir HM , Sveinsdottir S, Sigfusson A, et al: Enhanced B cell survival in familial macroglobulinaemia is associated with increased expression of Bcl-2. *Clin Exp Immunol* 117:252, 1999.
10. Linet MS, Humphrey RL, Mehl ES, et al: A case-control and family study of Waldenström's macroglobulinemia. *Leukemia* 7:1363, 1993.
11. Santini GF, Crovatto M, Modolo ML, et al: Waldenström macroglobulinemia: A role of HCV infection? *Blood* 82:2932, 1993.

12. Silvestri F, Barillari G, Fanin R, et al: Risk of hepatitis C virus infection, Waldenström's macroglobulinemia, and monoclonal gammopathies. *Blood* 88:1125, 1996.
13. Leleu X, O'Connor K, Ho A, et al: Hepatitis C viral infection is not associated with Waldenström's macroglobulinemia. *Am J Hematol* 82:83, 2007.
14. Carbone P, Caradonna F, Granata G, et al: Chromosomal abnormalities in Waldenström's macroglobulinemia. *Cancer Genet Cytogenet* 61:147, 1992.
15. Mansoor A, Medeiros LJ, Weber DM, et al: Cytogenetic findings in lymphoplasmacytic lymphoma/Waldenström macroglobulinemia. Chromosomal abnormalities are associated with the polymorphous subtype and an aggressive clinical course. *Am J Clin Pathol* 116:543, 2001.
16. Han T, Sadamori N, Takeuchi J, et al: Clonal chromosome abnormalities in patients with Waldenström's and CLL-associated macroglobulinemia: Significance of trisomy 12. *Blood* 62:525, 1983.
17. Rivera AI, Li MM, Beltran G, Krause JR: Trisomy 4 as the sole cytogenetic abnormality in a Waldenström macroglobulinemia. *Cancer Genet Cytogenet* 133:172, 2002.
18. Wong KF, So CC, Chan JC, et al: Gain of chromosome 3/3q in B-cell chronic lymphoproliferative disorder is associated with plasmacytoid differentiation with or without IgM overproduction. *Cancer Genet Cytogenet* 136:82, 2002.
19. Schop RF, Kuehl WM, Van Wier SA, et al: Waldenström macroglobulinemia neoplastic cells lack immunoglobulin heavy chain locus translocations but have frequent 6q deletions. *Blood* 100:2996, 2002.
20. Ocio EM, Schop RF, Gonzalez B, et al: 6q deletion in Waldenström's macroglobulinemia is associated with features of adverse prognosis. *Br J Haematol* 136:80, 2007.
21. Chang H, Qi C, Trieu Y, et al: Prognostic relevance of 6q deletion in Waldenström's macroglobulinemia: A multicenter study. *Clin Lymphoma Myeloma* 9:36, 2009.
22. Leleu X, Hunter ZR, Xu L, et al: Expression of regulatory genes for lymphoplasmacytic cell differentiation in Waldenström macroglobulinemia *Br J Haematol* 145:59, 2009.
23. Avet-Loiseau H, Garand R, Lode L, et al: 14q32 translocations discriminate IgM multiple myeloma from Waldenström's macroglobulinemia. *Semin Oncol* 30:153, 2003.
24. Preud'homme JL, Seligmann M: Immunoglobulins on the surface of lymphoid cells in Waldenstrom's macroglobulinemia. *J Clin Invest* 51:701, 1972.
25. Smith BR, Robert NJ, Ault KA: In Waldenström's macroglobulinemia the quantity of detectable circulating monoclonal B lymphocytes correlates with clinical course. *Blood* 61:911, 1983.
26. Levy Y, Fermand JP, Navarro S, et al: Interleukin 6 dependence of spontaneous in vitro differentiation of B cells from patients with IgM gammopathy. *Proc Natl Acad Sci U S A* 87:3309, 1990.
27. Owen RG, Barrans SL, Richards SJ, et al: Waldenström macroglobulinemia. Development of diagnostic criteria and identification of prognostic factors. *Am J Clin Pathol* 116:420, 2001.
28. Feiner HD, Rizk CC, Finfer MD, et al: IgM monoclonal gammopathy/Waldenström's macroglobulinemia: A morphological and immunophenotypic study of the bone marrow. *Mod Pathol* 3:348, 1990.
29. San Miguel JF, Vidriales MB, Ocio E, et al: Immunophenotypic analysis of Waldenström's macroglobulinemia. *Semin Oncol* 30:187, 2003.
30. Hunter ZR, Branagan AR, Manning R, et al: CD5, CD10, CD23 expression in Waldenström's macroglobulinemia. *Clin Lymphoma* 5:246, 2005.
31. Wagner SD, Martinelli V, Luzzatto L: Similar patterns of V kappa gene usage but different degrees of somatic mutation in hairy cell leukemia, prolymphocytic leukemia, Waldenström's macroglobulinemia, and myeloma. *Blood* 83:3647, 1994.
32. Aoki H, Takishita M, Kosaka M, Saito S: Frequent somatic mutations in D and/or JH segments of Ig gene in Waldenström's macroglobulinemia and chronic lymphocytic leukemia (CLL) with Richter's syndrome but not in common CLL. *Blood* 85:1913, 1995.
33. Shiokawa S, Suehiro Y, Uike N, et al: Sequence and expression analyses of mu and delta transcripts in patients with Waldenström's macroglobulinemia. *Am J Hematol* 68:139, 2001.
34. Sahota SS, Forconi F, Ottensmeier CH, et al: Typical Waldenström macroglobulinemia is derived from a B-cell arrested after cessation of somatic mutation but prior to isotype switch events. *Blood* 100:1505, 2002.
35. Paramithiotis E, Cooper MD: Memory B lymphocytes migrate to bone marrow in humans. *Proc Natl Acad Sci U S A* 94:208, 1997.
36. Tournilhac O, Santos DD, Xu L, et al: Mast cells in Waldenström's macroglobulinemia support lymphoplasmacytic cell growth through CD154/CD40 signaling. *Ann Oncol* 17:1275, 2006.
37. Ho A, Leleu X, Hatjiharissi E, et al: CD27-CD70 interactions in the pathogenesis of Waldenström's macroglobulinemia. *Blood* 112:4683, 2008.
38. Merlini G, Farhangi M, Osserman EF: Monoclonal immunoglobulins with antibody activity in myeloma, macroglobulinemia and related plasma cell dyscrasias. *Semin Oncol* 13:350, 1986.
39. Farhangi M, Merlini G: The clinical implications of monoclonal immunoglobulins. *Semin Oncol* 13:366, 1986.
40. Marmont AM, Merlini G: Monoclonal autoimmunity in hematology. *Haematologica* 76:449, 1991.
41. Mackenzie MR, Babcock J: Studies of the hyperviscosity syndrome. II: Macroglobulinemia. *J Lab Clin Med* 85:227, 1975.
42. Gertz MA, Kyle RA: Hyperviscosity syndrome. *J Intensive Care Med* 10:128, 1995.
43. Kwaan HC, Bongu A: The hyperviscosity syndromes. *Semin Thromb Hemost* 25:199, 1999.
44. Singh A, Eckardt KU, Zimmermann A, et al: Increased plasma viscosity as a reason for inappropriate erythropoietin formation. *J Clin Invest* 91:251, 1993.
45. Menke MN, Feke GT, McMeel JW, et al: Hyperviscosity-related retinopathy in Waldenström's macroglobulinemia. *Arch Ophthalmol* 124:1601, 2006.
46. Merlini G, Baldini L, Broglia C, et al: Prognostic factors in symptomatic Waldenström's macroglobulinemia. *Semin Oncol* 30:211, 2003.
47. Dellagi K, Dupouey P, Brouet JC, et al: Waldenström's macroglobulinemia and peripheral neuropathy: A clinical and immunologic study of 25 patients. *Blood* 62:280, 1983.
48. Nobile-Orazio E, Marmiroli P, Baldini L, et al: Peripheral neuropathy in macroglobulinemia: Incidence and antigen-specificity of M proteins. *Neurology* 37:1506, 1987.
49. Nemni R, Gerosa E, Piccolo G, Merlini G: Neuropathies associated with monoclonal gammopathies. *Haematologica* 79:557, 1994.
50. Ropper AH, Gorson KC: Neuropathies associated with paraproteinemia. *N Engl J Med* 338:1601, 1998.
51. Vital A: Paraproteinemic neuropathies. *Brain Pathol* 11:399, 2001.
52. Latov N, Braun PE, Gross RB, et al: Plasma cell dyscrasia and peripheral neuropathy: Identification of the myelin antigens that react with human paraproteins. *Proc Natl Acad Sci U S A* 78:7139, 1981.
53. Chassande B, Leger JM, Younes-Chennoufi AB, et al: Peripheral neuropathy associated with IgM monoclonal gammopathy: Correlations between M-protein antibody activity and clinical/electrophysiological features in 40 cases. *Muscle Nerve* 21:55, 1998.
54. Weiss MD, Dalakas MC, Lauter CJ, et al: Variability in the binding of anti-MAG and anti-SGPG antibodies to target antigens in demyelinating neuropathy and IgM paraproteinemia. *J Neuroimmunol* 95:174, 1999.
55. Latov N, Hays AP, Sherman WH: Peripheral neuropathy and anti-MAG antibodies. *Crit Rev Neurobiol* 3:301, 1988.
56. Dalakas MC, Quarles RH: Autoimmune ataxic neuropathies (sensory ganglionopathies): Are glycolipids the responsible autoantigens? *Ann Neurol* 39:419, 1996.
57. Eurelings M, Ang CW, Notermans NC, et al: Antiganglioside antibodies in polyneuropathy associated with monoclonal gammopathy. *Neurology* 57:1909, 2001.
58. Ilyas AA, Quarles RH, Dalakas MC, et al: Monoclonal IgM in a patient with paraproteinemic polyneuropathy binds to gangliosides containing disialosyl groups. *Ann Neurol* 18:655, 1985.
59. Willison HJ, O'Leary CP, Veitch J, et al: The clinical and laboratory features of chronic sensory ataxic neuropathy with anti-disialosyl IgM antibodies. *Brain* 124:1968, 2001.
60. Lopate G, Choksi R, Pestronk A: Severe sensory ataxia and demyelinating polyneuropathy with IgM anti-GM_2 and GalNAc-GD1A antibodies. *Muscle Nerve* 25:828, 2002.
61. Jacobs BC, O'Hanlon GM, Breedland EG, et al: Human IgM paraproteins demonstrate shared reactivity between *Campylobacter jejuni* lipopolysaccharides and human peripheral nerve disialylated gangliosides. *J Neuroimmunol* 80:23, 1997.
62. Nobile-Orazio E, Manfredini E, Carpo M, et al: Frequency and clinical correlates of antineural IgM antibodies in neuropathy associated with IgM monoclonal gammopathy. *Ann Neurol* 36:416, 1994.
63. Gordon PH, Rowland LP, Younger DS, et al: Lymphoproliferative disorders and motor neuron disease: An update. *Neurology* 48:1671, 1997.
64. Pavord SR, Murphy PT, Mitchell VE: POEMS syndrome and Waldenström's macroglobulinaemia. *J Clin Pathol* 49:181, 1996.
65. Crisp D, Pruzanski W: B-cell neoplasms with homogeneous cold-reacting antibodies (cold agglutinins). *Am J Med* 72:915, 1982.
66. Pruzanski W, Shumak KH: Biologic activity of cold-reacting autoantibodies (first of two parts). *N Engl J Med* 297:538, 1977.
67. Pruzanski W, Shumak KH: Biologic activity of cold-reacting autoantibodies (second of two parts). *N Engl J Med* 297:583, 1977.
68. Whittaker SJ, Bhogal BS, Black MM: Acquired immunobullous disease: A cutaneous manifestation of IgM macroglobulinaemia. *Br J Dermatol* 135:283, 1996.
69. Daoud MS, Lust JA, Kyle RA, Pittelkow MR: Monoclonal gammopathies and associated skin disorders. *J Am Acad Dermatol* 40:507, 1999.
70. Gad A, Willen R, Carlen B, et al: Duodenal involvement in Waldenström's macroglobulinemia. *J Clin Gastroenterol* 20:174, 1995.
71. Case records of the Massachusetts General Hospital. Weekly clinicopathological exercises. Case 3–1990. A 66-year-old woman with Waldenström's macroglobulinemia, diarrhea, anemia, and persistent gastrointestinal bleeding. *N Engl J Med* 322:183, 1990.
72. Isaac J, Herrera GA: Cast nephropathy in a case of Waldenström's macroglobulinemia. *Nephron* 91:512, 2002.
73. Morel-Maroger L, Basch A, Danon F, et al: Pathology of the kidney in Waldenström's macroglobulinemia. Study of sixteen cases. *N Engl J Med* 283:123, 1970.
74. Gertz MA, Kyle RA, Noel P: Primary systemic amyloidosis: A rare complication of immunoglobulin M monoclonal gammopathies and Waldenström's macroglobulinemia. *J Clin Oncol* 11:914, 1993.
75. Moyner K, Sletten K, Husby G, Natvig JB: An unusually large (83 amino acid residues) amyloid fibril protein AA from a patient with Waldenström's macroglobulinaemia and amyloidosis. *Scand J Immunol* 11:549, 1980.
76. Gardyn J, Schwartz A, Gal R, et al: Waldenström's macroglobulinemia associated with AA amyloidosis. *Int J Hematol* 74:76, 2001.
77. Dussol B, Kaplanski G, Daniel L, et al: Simultaneous occurrence of fibrillary glomerulopathy and AL amyloid. *Nephrol Dial Transplant* 13:2630, 1998.

78. Rausch PG, Herion JC: Pulmonary manifestations of Waldenström macroglobulinemia. *Am J Hematol* 9:201, 1980.
79. Fadil A, Taylor DE: The lung and Waldenström's macroglobulinemia. *South Med J* 91:681, 1998.
80. Kyrtsonis MC, Angelopoulou MK, Kontopidou FN, et al: Primary lung involvement in Waldenström's macroglobulinaemia: Report of two cases and review of the literature. *Acta Haematol* 105:92, 2001.
81. Kaila VL, el Newihi HM, Dreiling BJ, et al: Waldenström's macroglobulinemia of the stomach presenting with upper gastrointestinal hemorrhage. *Gastrointest Endosc* 44:73, 1996.
82. Yasui O, Tukamoto F, Sasaki N, et al: Malignant lymphoma of the transverse colon associated with macroglobulinemia. *Am J Gastroenterol* 92:2299, 1997.
83. Rosenthal JA, Curran WJ Jr, Schuster SJ: Waldenström's macroglobulinemia resulting from localized gastric lymphoplasmacytoid lymphoma. *Am J Hematol* 58:244, 1998.
84. Recine MA, Perez MT, Cabello-Inchausti B, et al: Extranodal lymphoplasmacytoid lymphoma (immunocytoma) presenting as small intestinal obstruction. *Arch Pathol Lab Med* 125:677, 2001.
85. Veltman GA, van Veen S, Kluin-Nelemans JC, et al: Renal disease in Waldenström's macroglobulinaemia. *Nephrol Dial Transplant* 12:1256, 1997.
86. Moore DF Jr, Moulopoulos LA, Dimopoulos MA: Waldenström macroglobulinemia presenting as a renal or perirenal mass: Clinical and radiographic features. *Leuk Lymphoma* 17:331, 1995.
87. Mascaro JM, Montserrat E, Estrach T, et al: Specific cutaneous manifestations of Waldenström's macroglobulinaemia. A report of two cases. *Br J Dermatol* 106:17, 1982.
88. Schnitzler L, Schubert B, Boasson M, et al: Urticaire chronique, lésions osseuses, macroglobulinémie IgM: Maladie de Waldenström? *Bull Soc Fr Dermatol Syphiligr* 81:363, 1974.
89. Roux S, Fermand JP, Brechignac S, et al: Tumoral joint involvement in multiple myeloma and Waldenström's macroglobulinemia—Report of 4 cases. *J Rheumatol* 23:2175, 1996.
90. Orellana J, Friedman AH: Ocular manifestations of multiple myeloma, Waldenström's macroglobulinemia and benign monoclonal gammopathy. *Surv Ophthalmol* 26:157, 1981.
91. Ettl AR, Birbamer GG, Philipp W: Orbital involvement in Waldenström's macroglobulinemia: Ultrasound, computed tomography and magnetic resonance findings. *Ophthalmologica* 205:40, 1992.
92. Civit T, Coulbois S, Baylac F, et al: [Waldenström's macroglobulinemia and cerebral lymphoplasmacytic proliferation: Bing and Neel syndrome. Apropos of a new case.] *Neurochirurgie* 43:245, 1997.
93. McMullin MF, Wilkin HJ, Elder E: Inaccurate haemoglobin estimation in Waldenström's macroglobulinaemia. *J Clin Pathol* 48:787, 1995.
94. Dutcher TF, Fahey JL: The histopathology of macroglobulinemia of Waldenström. *J Natl Cancer Inst* 22:887, 1959.
95. Treon SP, Branagan AR, Hunter Z, et al: IgA and IgG hypogammaglobulinemia persists in most patients with Waldenström's macroglobulinemia despite therapeutic responses, including complete remissions. *Blood* 2004; 104: 306b.
96. Treon SP, Hunter Z, Ciccarelli BT, et al: IgA and IgG hypogammaglobulinemia is a constitutive feature in most Waldenström's macroglobulinemia patients and may be related to mutations associated with common variable immunodeficiency disorder (CVID) *Blood* 112:3749, 2008.
97. Moulopoulos LA, Dimopoulos MA, Varma DG, et al: Waldenström macroglobulinemia: MR imaging of the spine and CT of the abdomen and pelvis. *Radiology* 188:669, 1993.
98. Kyle RA, Treon SP, Alexanian R, et al: Prognostic markers and criteria to initiate therapy in Waldenström's macroglobulinemia: Consensus Panel Recommendations from the Second International Workshop on Waldenström's macroglobulinemia. *Semin Oncol* 30:116, 2003.
99. Gertz M, Anagnostopoulos A, Anderson KC, et al: Treatment recommendations in Waldenström's macroglobulinemia: Consensus Panel Recommendations from the Second International Workshop on Waldenström's macroglobulinemia. *Semin Oncol* 30:121, 2003.
100. Treon SP, Gertz MA, Dimopoulos MA, et al: Update on treatment recommendations from the Third International Workshop on Waldenström's Macroglobulinemia. *Blood* 107:3442, 2006.
101. Dimopoulos MA, Gertz MA, Kastritis E, et al: Update on treatment recommendations from the Fourth International Workshop on Waldenström's Macroglobulinemia. *J Clin Oncol* 2009; 27: 120–6.
102. Kyle RA, Greipp PR, Gertz MA, et al: Waldenström's macroglobulinaemia: A prospective study comparing daily with intermittent oral chlorambucil. *Br J Haematol* 108:737, 2000.
103. Dimopoulos MA, Alexanian R: Waldenström's macroglobulinemia. *Blood* 83:1452, 1994.
104. Petrucci MT, Avvisati G, Tribalto M, et al: Waldenström's macroglobulinaemia: Results of a combined oral treatment in 34 newly diagnosed patients. *J Intern Med* 226:443, 1989.
105. Case DC Jr, Ervin TJ, Boyd MA, Redfield DL: Waldenström's macroglobulinemia: Long-term results with the M-2 protocol. *Cancer Invest* 9:1, 1991.
106. Facon T, Brouillard M, Duhamel A, et al: Prognostic factors in Waldenström's macroglobulinemia: A report of 167 cases. *J Clin Oncol* 11:1553, 1993.
107. Dimopoulos MA, Kantarjian H, Weber D, et al: Primary therapy of Waldenström's macroglobulinemia with 2-chlorodeoxyadenosine. *J Clin Oncol* 12:2694, 1994.
108. Delannoy A, Ferrant A, Martiat P, et al: 2-Chlorodeoxyadenosine therapy in Waldenström's macroglobulinaemia. *Nouv Rev Fr Hematol* 36:317, 1994.
109. Fridrik MA, Jager G, Baldinger C, et al: First-line treatment of Waldenström's disease with cladribine. Arbeitsgemeinschaft Medikamentose Tumortherapie. *Ann Hematol* 74:7, 1997.
110. Liu ES, Burian C, Miller WE, Saven A: Bolus administration of cladribine in the treatment of Waldenström macroglobulinaemia. *Br J Haematol* 103:690, 1998.
111. Hellmann A, Lewandowski K, Zaucha JM, et al: Effect of a 2-hour infusion of 2-chlorodeoxyadenosine in the treatment of refractory or previously untreated Waldenström's macroglobulinemia. *Eur J Haematol* 63:35, 1999.
112. Betticher DC, Hsu Schmitz SF, Ratschiller D, et al: Cladribine (2-CDA) given as subcutaneous bolus injections is active in pretreated Waldenström's macroglobulinaemia. Swiss Group for Clinical Cancer Research (SAKK). *Br J Haematol* 99:358, 1997.
113. Dimopoulos MA, Weber D, Delasalle KB, et al: Treatment of Waldenström's macroglobulinemia resistant to standard therapy with 2-chlorodeoxyadenosine: Identification of prognostic factors. *Ann Oncol* 6:49, 1995.
114. Dimopoulos MA, O'Brien S, Kantarjian H, et al: Fludarabine therapy in Waldenström's macroglobulinemia. *Am J Med* 95:49, 1993.
115. Foran JM, Rohatiner AZ, Coiffier B, et al: Multicenter phase II study of fludarabine phosphate for patients with newly diagnosed lymphoplasmacytoid lymphoma, Waldenström's macroglobulinemia, and mantle-cell lymphoma. *J Clin Oncol* 17:546, 1999.
116. Thalhammer-Scherrer R, Geissler K, Schwarzinger I, et al: Fludarabine therapy in Waldenström's macroglobulinemia. *Ann Hematol* 79:556, 2000.
117. Dhodapkar MV, Jacobson JL, Gertz MA, et al: Prognostic factors and response to fludarabine therapy in patients with Waldenström macroglobulinemia: Results of United States intergroup trial (Southwest Oncology Group S9003). *Blood* 98:41, 2001.
118. Zinzani PL, Gherlinzoni F, Bendandi M, et al: Fludarabine treatment in resistant Waldenström's macroglobulinemia. *Eur J Haematol* 54:120, 1995.
119. Leblond V, Ben Othman T, Deconinck E, et al: Activity of fludarabine in previously treated Waldenström's macroglobulinemia: A report of 71 cases. Groupe Cooperatif Macroglobulinemie. *J Clin Oncol* 16:2060, 1998.
120. Dimopoulos MA, Weber DM, Kantarjian H, et al: 2-Chlorodeoxyadenosine therapy of patients with Waldenström macroglobulinemia previously treated with fludarabine. *Ann Oncol* 5:288, 1994.
121. Lewandowski K, Halaburda K, Hellmann A: Fludarabine therapy in Waldenström's macroglobulinemia patients treated previously with 2-chlorodeoxyadenosine. *Leuk Lymphoma* 43:361, 2002.
122. Popat U, Saliba R, Thandi R, et al: Impairment of filgrastim-induced stem cell mobilization after prior lenalidomidein patients with multiple myeloma. *Biol Blood Marrow Transplant*. 15:718, 2009.
123. Leleu XP, Manning R, Soumerai JD, et al: Increased incidence of transformation and myelodysplasia/acute leukemia in patients with Waldenström macroglobulinemia treated with nucleoside analogs. *J Clin Oncol* 27:250, 2009.
124. Leleu X, Tamburini J, Roccaro A, et al: Balancing risk versus benefit in the treatment of Waldenström's macroglobulinemia patients with nucleoside analogue based therapy. *Clin Lymphoma Myeloma* 9:71, 2009.
125. Treon SP, Kelliher A, Keele B, et al: Expression of serotherapy target antigens in Waldenström's macroglobulinemia: Therapeutic applications and considerations. *Semin Oncol* 30:248, 2003.
126. Treon SP, Shima Y, Preffer FI, et al: Treatment of plasma cell dyscrasias with antibody-mediated immunotherapy. *Semin Oncol* 26(Suppl 14):97, 1999.
127. Byrd JC, White CA, Link B, et al: Rituximab therapy in Waldenström's macroglobulinemia: Preliminary evidence of clinical activity. *Ann Oncol* 10:1525, 1999.
128. Weber DM, Gavino M, Huh Y, et al: Phenotypic and clinical evidence supports rituximab for Waldenström's macroglobulinemia. *Blood* 94:125a, 1999.
129. Foran JM, Rohatiner AZ, Cunningham D, et al: European phase II study of rituximab (chimeric anti-CD20 monoclonal antibody) for patients with newly diagnosed mantle-cell lymphoma and previously treated mantle-cell lymphoma, immunocytoma, and small B-cell lymphocytic lymphoma. *J Clin Oncol* 18:317, 2000.
130. Treon SP, Agus DB, Link B, et al: CD20-Directed antibody-mediated immunotherapy induces responses and facilitates hematologic recovery in patients with Waldenström's macroglobulinemia. *J Immunother* 24:272, 2001.
131. Gertz MA, Rue M, Blood E, et al: Multicenter phase 2 trial of rituximab for Waldenström macroglobulinemia (WM): An Eastern Cooperative Oncology Group Study (E3A98). *Leuk Lymphoma* 45:2047, 2004.
132. Dimopoulos MA, Zervas C, Zomas A, et al: Treatment of Waldenström's macroglobulinemia with rituximab. *J Clin Oncol* 20:2327, 2002.
133. Treon SP, Emmanouilides C, Kimby E, et al: Extended rituximab therapy in Waldenström's Macroglobulinemia. *Ann Oncol* 16:132, 2005.
134. Donnelly GB, Bober-Sorcinelli K, Jacobson R, Portlock CS: Abrupt IgM rise following treatment with rituximab in patients with Waldenström's macroglobulinemia. *Blood* 98:240b, 2001.
135. Treon SP, Branagan AR, Hunter Z, et al: Paradoxical increases in serum IgM and viscosity levels following rituximab in Waldenström's macroglobulinemia. *Ann Oncol* 15:1481, 2004.

136. Ghobrial IM, Fonseca R, Greipp PR, et al: Initial immunoglobulin M "flare" after rituximab therapy in patients with Waldenström macroglobulinemia: An Eastern Cooperative Oncology Group Study. *Cancer* 101:2593, 2004.
137. Dimopoulos MA, Anagnostopoulos A, Zervas C, et al: Predictive factors for response to rituximab in Waldenström's macroglobulinemia. *Clin Lymphoma* 5:270, 2005.
138. Treon SP, Hansen M, Branagan AR, et al: Polymorphisms in FcγRIIIA (CD16) receptor expression are associated with clinical responses to rituximab in Waldenström's macroglobulinemia. *J Clin Oncol* 23:474, 2005.
139. Weber DM, Dimopoulos MA, Delasalle K, et al: 2-chlorodeoxyadenosine alone and in combination for previously untreated Waldenström's macroglobulinemia. *Semin Oncol* 30:243, 2003.
140. Treon SP, Branagan AR, Ioakimidis L, et al: Long term outcomes to fludarabine and rituximab in Waldenström's macroglobulinemia. *Blood* 113:3673, 2009.
141. Tam CS, Wolf MM, Westerman D, et al: Fludarabine combination therapy is highly effective in first-line and salvage treatment of patients with Waldenström's macroglobulinemia. *Clin Lymphoma Myeloma* 6:136, 2005.
142. Hensel M, Villalobos M, Kornacker M, et al: Pentostatin/cyclophosphamide with or without rituximab: An effective regimen for patients with Waldenström's macroglobulinemia/lymphoplasmacytic lymphoma. *Clin Lymphoma Myeloma* 6:131, 2005.
143. Dimopoulos MA, Anagnostopoulos A, Kyrtsonis MC, et al: Primary treatment of Waldenström's macroglobulinemia with Dexamethasone, Rituximab and Cyclophosphamide. *J Clin Oncol* 25:3344, 2007.
144. Buske C, Hoster E, Dreyling MH, et al: The addition of rituximab to front-line therapy with CHOP (R-CHOP) results in a higher response rate and longer time to treatment failure in patients with lymphoplasmacytic lymphoma: Results of a randomized trial of the German Low-Grade Lymphoma Study Group (GLSG). *Leukemia* 23:153, 2009.
145. Treon SP, Hunter Z, Branagan A: CHOP plus rituximab therapy in Waldenström's macroglobulinemia. *Clin Lymphoma Myeloma* 5:273, 2005.
146. Ioakimidis L, Patterson CJ, Hunter ZR, et al: Comparative outcomes following CP-R, CVP-R and CHOP-R in Waldenström's macroglobulinemia. *Clin Lymphoma Myeloma* 9:62, 2009.
147. Dimopoulos MA, Hamilos G, Efstathiou E, et al: Treatment of Waldenström's macroglobulinemia with the combination of fludarabine and cyclophosphamide. *Leuk Lymphoma* 44:993, 2003.
148. Tamburini J, Levy V, Chateilex C, et al: Fludarabine plus cyclophosphamide in Waldenström's macroglobulinemia: Results in 49 patients. *Leukemia* 19:1831, 2005.
149. Jagannath S, Durie BG, Wolf J, et al: Bortezomib therapy alone and in combination with dexamethasone for previously untreated symptomatic multiple myeloma. *Br J Haematol* 129:776, 2005.
150. Oakervee HE, Popat R, Curry N, et al: PAD combination therapy (PS-341/bortezomib, doxorubicin and dexamethasone) for previously untreated patients with multiple myeloma. *Br J Haematol* 129:755, 2005.
151. Harousseau JL, Attal M, Leleu X, et al: Bortezomib plus dexamethasone as induction treatment prior to autologous stem cell transplantation in patients with newly diagnosed multiple myeloma. Preliminary results of an IFM phase II study. *Blood* 104:416a, 2004.
152. Mitsiades CS, Mitsiades N, McMullan CJ, et al: The proteasome inhibitor bortezomib (PS-341) is active against Waldenström's macroglobulinemia. *Blood* 102:181a, 2003.
153. Treon SP, Hunter ZR, Matous J, et al: Multicenter clinical trial of bortezomib in relapsed/refractory Waldenström's macroglobulinemia: Results of WMCTG trial 03–248. *Clin Cancer Res* 13:3320, 2007.
154. Chen CI, Kouroukis CT, White D, et al: Bortezomib is active in patients with untreated or relapsed Waldenström's macroglobulinemia: A phase II study of the National Cancer Institute of Canada Clinical Trials Group. *J Clin Oncol* 25:1570, 2007.
155. Dimopoulos MA, Anagnostopoulos A, Kyrtsonis MC, et al: Treatment of relapsed or refractory Waldenström's macroglobulinemia with bortezomib. *Haematologica* 90:1655, 2005.
156. Goy A, Younes A, McLaughlin P, et al: Phase II study of proteasome inhibitor bortezomib in relapsed or refractory B-cell non-Hodgkin's lymphoma. *J Clin Oncol* 23:657, 2005.
157. Treon SP, Ioakimidis L, Soumerai JD, et al: Primary therapy of Waldenström's macroglobulinemia with bortezomib, dexamethasone and rituximab. *J Clin Oncol* 27:3830, 2009.
158. Ghobrial IM, Matous J, Padmanabhan S, et al: Phase II trial of combination of bortezomib and rituximab in relapsed and/or refractory Waldenström's macroglobulinemia. *Blood* 112:832, 2008.
159. Agathocleous A, Rule S, Johson P: Preliminary results of a phase I/II study of weekly or twice weekly bortezomib in combination with rituximab in patients with follicular lymphoma, mantle cell lymphoma, and Waldenström's macroglobulinemia. *Blood* 110:754a, 2007.
160. Santos DD, Hatjiharissi E, Tournilhac O, et al: CD52 is expressed on human mast cells and is a potential therapeutic target in Waldenström's macroglobulinemia and mast cell disorders. *Clin Lymphoma Myeloma* 6:478, 2006.
161. Hunter ZR, Boxer M, Kahl B, et al: Phase II study of alemtuzumab in lymphoplasmacytic lymphoma: Results of WMCTG trial 02–079. Proc Am Soc *Clin Oncol* (Part 1 Suppl. S) 24:427s, 2006.
162. Owen RG, Rawstron AC, Osterborg A, et al: Activity of alemtuzumab in relapsed/refractory Waldenström's macroglobulinemia. *Blood* 2003; 102: 644a.
163. Dimopoulos MA, Zomas A, Viniou NA, et al: Treatment of Waldenström's macroglobulinemia with thalidomide. *J Clin Oncol* 19:3596, 2001.
164. Coleman C, Leonard J, Lyons L, et al: Treatment of Waldenström's macroglobulinemia with clarithromycin, low-dose thalidomide and dexamethasone. *Semin Oncol* 30:270, 2003.
165. Dimopoulos MA, Zomas K, Tsatalas K, et al: Treatment of Waldenström's macroglobulinemia with single agent thalidomide or with combination of clarithromycin, thalidomide and dexamethasone. *Semin Oncol* 30:265, 2003.
166. Hayashi T, Hideshima T, Akiyama M, et al: Molecular mechanisms whereby immunomodulatory drugs activate natural killer cells: Clinical application. *Br J Haematol* 128:192, 2005.
167. Davies FE, Raje N, Hideshima T, et al: Thalidomide and immunomodulatory derivatives augment natural killer cell cytotoxicity in multiple myeloma. *Blood* 98:210, 2001.
168. Janakiraman N, McLaughlin P, White CA, et al: Rituximab: Correlation between effector cells and clinical activity in NHL. *Blood* 92:337a, 1998.
169. Treon SP, Soumerai JD, Branagan AR, et al: Thalidomide and rituximab in Waldenström's macroglobulinemia. *Blood* 112:4452, 2008.
170. Treon SP, Soumerai JD, Branagan AR, et al: Lenalidomide and rituximab in Waldenström's macroglobulinemia. *Clin Cancer Res* 15:355, 2008.
171. Desikan R, Dhodapkar M, Siegel D, et al: High-dose therapy with autologous haemopoietic stem cell support for Waldenström's macroglobulinaemia. *Br J Haematol* 105:993, 1999.
172. Munshi NC, Barlogie B: Role for high dose therapy with autologous hematopoietic stem cell support in Waldenström's macroglobulinemia. *Semin Oncol* 30:282, 2003.
173. Dreger P, Glass B, Kuse R, et al: Myeloablative radiochemotherapy followed by reinfusion of purged autologous stem cells for Waldenström's macroglobulinaemia. *Br J Haematol* 106:115, 1999.
174. Anagnostopoulos A, Dimopoulos MA, Aleman A, et al: High-dose chemotherapy followed by stem cell transplantation in patients with resistant Waldenström's macroglobulinemia. *Bone Marrow Transplant* 27:1027, 2001.
175. Tournilhac O, Leblond V, Tabrizi R, et al: Transplantation in Waldenström's macroglobulinemia—The French Experience. *Semin Oncol* 30:291, 2003.
176. Anagnostopoulos A, Hari PN, Perez WS, et al: Autologous or allogeneic stem cell transplantation in patients with Waldenström's macroglobulinemia. *Biol Blood Marrow Transplant* 12:845, 2006.
177. Kyriakou H, on behalf of the Lymphoma Working Party of the European Group for Blood and Bone Marrow Transplantation: Haematopoietic stem cell transplantation for Waldenström's macroglobulinemia. Proceedings of the 5th International Workshop on Waldenström's macroglobulinemia, Stockholm, Sweden 2008 (Abstract 146).
178. Maloney D: Evidence for GVWM following mini-allo in Waldenström's macroglobulinemia. Proceedings of the 5th International Workshop on Waldenström's macroglobulinemia, Stockholm, Sweden 2008 (Abstract 147).
179. Weber D, Treon SP, Emmanouilides C, et al: Uniform response criteria in Waldenström's macroglobulinemia: Consensus panel recommendations from the Second International Workshop on Waldenström's Macroglobulinemia. *Semin Oncol* 30:127, 2003.
180. Kimby E, Treon SP, Anagnostopoulos A, et al: Update on recommendations for assessing response from the Third International Workshop on Waldenström's Macroglobulinemia. *Clin Lymphoma Myeloma* 6:380, 2006.
181. Nichols GL, Savage DG: Timing of rituximab/fludarabine in Waldenström's macroglobulinemia may avert hyperviscosity. *Blood* 104:237b, 2004.
182. Strauss SJ, Maharaj L, Hoare S, et al: Bortezomib therapy in patients with relapsed or refractory lymphoma: Potential correlation of *in vitro* sensitivity and tumor necrosis factor alpha response with clinical activity. *J Clin Oncol* 24:2105, 2006.
183. Varghese AM, Rawstron AC, Ashcroft J, et al: Assessment of bone marrow response in Waldenström's macroglobulinemia. *Clin Lymphoma Myeloma* 9:53, 2009.
184. Ciccarelli BT, Yang G, Hatjiharissi E, et al: Soluble CD27 is a faithful marker of disease burden and is unaffected by the rituximab induced IgM flare, as well as plasmapheresis in patients with Waldenström's macroglobulinemia. *Clin Lymphoma Myeloma* 9:56, 2009.
185. Gobbi PG, Bettini R, Montecucco C, et al: Study of prognosis in Waldenström's macroglobulinemia: A proposal for a simple binary classification with clinical and investigational utility. *Blood* 83:2939, 1994.
186. Morel P, Monconduit M, Jacomy D, et al: Prognostic factors in Waldenström macroglobulinemia: A report on 232 patients with the description of a new scoring system and its validation on 253 other patients. *Blood* 96:852, 2000.
187. Dhodapkar MV, Jacobson JL, Gertz MA, et al: Prognostic factors and response to fludarabine therapy in patients with Waldenström macroglobulinemia: Results of United States intergroup trial (Southwest Oncology Group S9003). *Blood* 98:41, 2001.
188. Dimopoulos M, Gika D, Zervas K, et al: The international staging system for multiple myeloma is applicable in symptomatic Waldenström's macroglobulinemia. *Leuk Lymphoma* 45:1809, 2004.
189. Anagnostopoulos A, Zervas K, Kyrtsonis M, et al: Prognostic value of serum beta 2-microglobulin in patients with Waldenström's macroglobulinemia requiring therapy. *Clin Lymphoma Myeloma* 7:205, 2006.
190. Morel P, Duhamel A, Gobbi P, et al: International prognostic scoring system for Waldenström macroglobulinemia. *Blood* 113:4163, 2009.

CHAPTER 112
HEAVY-CHAIN DISEASE

Dietlind L. Wahner-Roedler and Robert A. Kyle

SUMMARY

The heavy-chain diseases (HCDs) are B-cell lymphoplasma cell proliferative disorders in which neoplastic cells produce monoclonal immunoglobulins (Ig) consisting of truncated heavy chains without attached light chains. The complex abnormalities of HCD proteins and the usual lack of normal light chains are a result of several distinct gene alterations, including somatic mutations, deletions, and insertions. HCDs involving the three main Ig classes have been described: α-HCD is the most common and has the most uniform presentation; γ- and μ-HCDs have variable clinical presentations and histopathologic features. The diagnosis is established from immunofixation of serum, urine, or secretory fluids in the case of α-HCD or from immunohistologic analysis of the proliferating lymphoplasmacytic cells in nonsecretory disease. Treatment of α-HCD consists of antibiotics. If there is no response to antibiotics or if aggressive non-Hodgkin lymphoma is diagnosed, chemotherapy is indicated. Treatment of γ- and μ-HCDs depends on the underlying clinicopathologic features rather than on the presence of the abnormal protein. Table 112–1 summarizes the features of the HCDs.

γ-HEAVY-CHAIN DISEASE

DEFINITION AND HISTORY

γ-Heavy-chain disease (HCD) is not a specific pathologic process but is a biochemical expression of a mutant B-cell clone. The "disease" should be considered a serologically determined entity with a great variety of clinical and histopathologic features. It is defined by the recognition of monoclonal deleted γ chains devoid of light chains.

The first case of γ-HCD was described in 1964 by Franklin and colleagues,[1] who observed a homogeneous band between γ and β globulin in an African American patient with generalized lymphadenopathy. Comparison of the proteins in the urine to those in the serum showed that they were the same, a suggestion of the presence of a low-molecular-weight serum γ-globulin, which then was shown to be a fragment of a γ heavy chain (HC). Since this first description, approximately 130 patients with γ-HCD have been described in the literature.[2–4]

EPIDEMIOLOGY

γ-HCD has been described throughout the world. Although initially γ-HCD was reported to occur equally in men and women,[3] there was a clear predominance of women in a newer described series of 23 patients.[4] The median age at diagnosis in that series was 68 years (range: 42–87 years).

ETIOLOGY AND PATHOGENESIS

The etiology of γ-HCD is unknown.

Acronyms and abbreviations that appear in this chapter include: C_H1 (2, 3, 4), constant region 1 (2, 3, 4); D, diversity; HC, heavy chain; HCD, heavy-chain disease; Ig, immunoglobulin; IPSID, immunoproliferative small intestinal disease; J, joining; V, variable.

CLINICAL FEATURES

Originally, γ-HCD was considered to be a lymphomatous illness. However, it has become clear that γ-HCD has various clinical and pathologic features that can be divided into three broad categories, as described below.

Disseminated Lymphoproliferative Disease

Disseminated lymphoproliferative disease is present in most patients at the time of diagnosis, and various series have reported it in 57 to 66 percent of patients.[3–5] On physical examination at the time of diagnosis in two different series,[3,4] lymphadenopathy was present in 56 percent and 62 percent of patients, splenomegaly in 38 percent and 52 percent, and hepatomegaly in 8 percent and 37 percent.

Localized Proliferative Disease

In approximately 25 percent of patients, the lymphoproliferative process is localized. Localized disease may be extramedullary or may involve only the marrow.[3,4] Cutaneous involvement is the most frequently reported extramedullary presentation.[3,4] Patients presenting with extramedullary plasmacytoma of the thyroid or parotid gland or an oropharyngeal mass[4] and hypertrophic spinal pachymeningitis have been described.[6]

No Apparent Proliferative Disease

No proliferative lymphoplasmacytic disease is apparent in 9 percent to 17 percent of patients with γ-HCD. In most of these patients, an underlying autoimmune disorder has been reported. Autoimmune disorders with or without underlying lymphoid proliferation include rheumatoid arthritis, autoimmune cytopenias, systemic lupus erythematosus, Sjögren syndrome, myasthenia gravis, thyroiditis, and vasculitis.[4]

LABORATORY FEATURES

Molecular Biology and Genetics

Most γ-HCD proteins are dimers of truncated HCs devoid of light chains. The molecular weight of the monomeric unit varies from 27,000 to 49,000. The length of the truncated γ chain varies, but usually it is one-half to three-fourths the length of the normal γ chain. Structural analysis of the defective monoclonal γ-HC of 23 patients with γ-HCD showed several characteristic features (Fig. 112–1). The proteins usually begin with a normal variable region. In most cases, this sequence is short and interrupted by a large deletion encompassing the remainder of the variable region, although four of the HCs shown in Fig. 112–1 appear to have retained most or all of their variable (V), diversity (D), and joining (J) sequences. In all γ-HCD proteins, the entire constant region 1 (C_H1) domain is also deleted, with normal sequence beginning at the hinge or occasionally at the C_H2 domain. C_H1 is responsible for light-chain binding. In the absence of an associated light chain, the C_H1 domain binds to heat shock protein 78 (HC binding protein), and the HC undergoes proteasomal degradation rather than secretion.

In two cases of γ-HCD (OMM and RIV), genomic sequence data are available (Fig. 112–2). The presence of large deletions in the switch/C_H1 regions of these two γ-HCD genes explains why the corresponding HCD proteins lack C_H1. Because the normal C_H1 acceptor splice site is deleted, the donor splice of the leader, or the J region, is spliced directly to the next available functional acceptor splice site at the beginning of the hinge or C_H2 domain.

Protein Findings

The serum protein electrophoretic pattern is extremely variable. A monoclonal peak is detected in 60 to 86 percent of patients.[3,4] When

TABLE 112–1. Summary of Features of the Heavy-Chain Diseases

Feature	Type of Heavy-Chain Disease α	γ	μ
Year described	1968	1964	1969
Incidence	Rare	Very rare	Very rare
Age at diagnosis	Young adult (<30 years)	Older adult (60–70 years)	Older adult (50–60 years)
Demographics	Mediterranean region	Worldwide	Worldwide
Structurally abnormal monoclonal protein	IgA	IgG	IgM
MGUS phase	No	Rarely	Rarely
Urine monoclonal light chain	No	No	Yes
Urine abnormal heavy chain	Small amounts	Often present	Infrequent
Sites involved	Small intestine, mesenteric lymph nodes	Lymph nodes, marrow, spleen	Lymph nodes, marrow, liver, spleen
Pathology	Extranodal marginal zone lymphoma (MALT or IPSID)	Lymphoplasmacytoid lymphoma	Small lymphocytic lymphoma, CLL
Associated diseases	Infection, malabsorption	Autoimmune diseases	None
Therapy	Antibiotics, chemotherapy	Chemotherapy	Chemotherapy

CLL, chronic lymphocytic leukemia; Ig, immunoglobulin; IPSID, immunoproliferative small intestinal disease; MALT, mucosa-associated lymphoid tissue; MGUS, monoclonal gammopathy of undetermined significance.

SOURCE: Adapted from Witzig TE, Wahner-Roedler DL: Heavy chain disease. *Curr Treat Options Oncol* 3:247, 2002. Used with permission.

present, it is most commonly in the β_1 or β_2 region. The median value of the monoclonal spike at diagnosis in 19 patients was 1.59 g/dL (range: 0.40–3.91 g/dL).[4] The diagnosis is established by immunofixation of the serum or a concentrated urine specimen. A modified immunoselection technique for the diagnosis of HCD has been described.[28] In one case of γ-HCD, low concentrations of free HCs in serum were detected by capillary zone electrophoresis coupled with immunosubtraction.[29] The amount of HCD protein in the urine usually is small (<1 g/24 h) but may reach 20 g/24 h. An occasional patient with Bence Jones proteinuria has been described.[4]

No standard has been established to identify the subclass of the HC fragment. In reported cases in which the HC fragment subclass has been studied, different methods have been used, ranging from Ouchterlony in the earlier cases to indirect immunofluorescence staining, immunoblotting, amino acid sequence, immunoselection, and enzyme-linked immunosorbent assay.[30] Immunoglobulin (Ig) G subclass distribution shows a lower-than-expected incidence of IgG_2. The most common subclass is IgG_1, which occurs in 65 percent of cases. IgG_3 has been identified in 27 percent of patients, IgG_4 in 5 percent, and IgG_2 in 3 percent.[3] Although biclonal gammopathy has been reported in 1 percent to 8 percent of all patients with serum monoclonal components, the association between γ-HCD and another monoclonal protein is much higher. In a series of 23 patients with γ-HCD, 7 percent had an IgM-λ intact monoclonal Ig.[4] No association between γ-HCD and monoclonal IgA has been described, although the IgG-IgA association was the most frequent in several series of biclonal gammopathies. One patient described in the literature was unique in that the serum contained two deleted γ chains of different subclasses (IgG_1 and IgG_2).[31]

Hematologic Abnormalities

Anemia is frequent. It is usually normochromic, normocytic, and moderate. Coombs-positive autoimmune hemolytic anemia has been reported in several cases and may be associated with thrombocytopenia. The total and differential leukocyte counts are usually normal. Lymphocytosis may occur, and an occasional patient presents with chronic lymphocytic leukemia. In some cases, rare circulating plasmacytoid lymphocytes or plasma cells have been noted. Plasma cell leukemia has been reported in two patients.[32,33]

Marrow aspirates and biopsy specimens often show an increase of plasma cells, lymphocytes, or plasmacytoid lymphocytes, similar to the marrow findings in Waldenström macroglobulinemia. The typical marrow features of myeloma or chronic lymphocytic leukemia are rare. Marrow changes consistent with a myeloproliferative disorder have been noted in a few patients.[4]

Other Features

Bone lesions are rare in γ-HCD. Cytogenetic studies have seldom been reported. No unique abnormalities or characteristics of lymphoma have been found.

Pathology

In contrast to α-HCD, γ-HCD has no consistent morphologic pattern. The most frequent histopathologic finding is a pleomorphic malignant lymphoplasmacytic proliferation in marrow and lymph nodes. These lymphocytoid plasma cells express pan–B-cell markers and cytoplasmic γ-HC without light chains and are negative for CD5 and CD10.[34]

Non-Hodgkin lymphoma without any consistent morphologic type was diagnosed in 18 (38 percent) of 47 patients in whom lymph nodes were examined. A lymphoplasmacytic proliferation was present in 36 percent and hyperplastic nodes and plasmacytoma in 11 percent each; there was one case of Hodgkin lymphoma and one of probable Hodgkin lymphoma.[5] Plasmacytic infiltration may be found in the salivary glands or thyroid.[3,4]

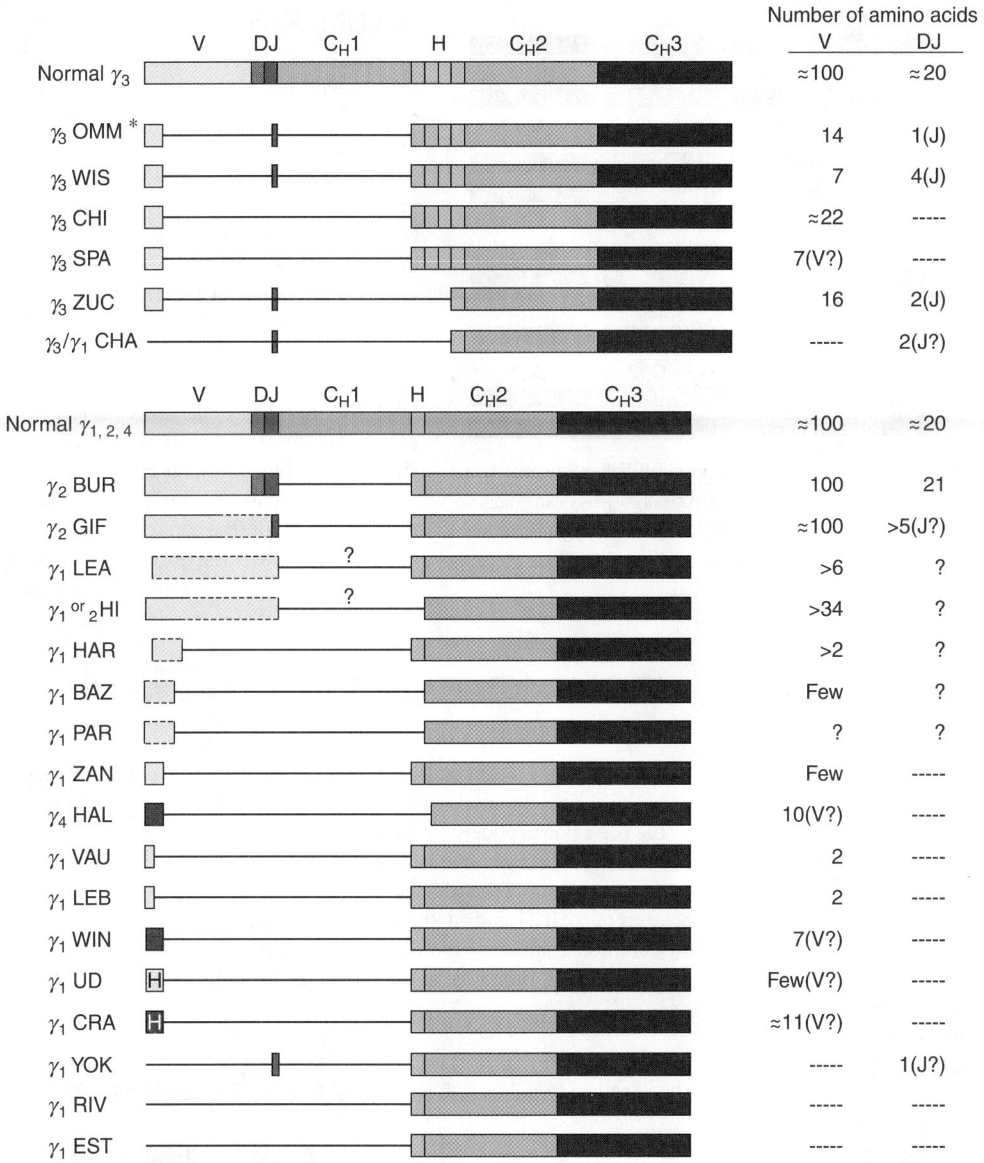

FIGURE 112–1. Structure of various deleted γ-heavy-chain disease (HCD) proteins compared with that of normal chains. *Structure shown is a primary synthetic product synthesized by the HCD cells. Serum protein was modified after synthesis and did not contain any amino acids before the hinge. [H], indicates heterogeneous amino acid sequences; [H], unusual and heterogeneous amino acid sequences; ■, unusual amino acid sequences; boxes, coding regions; lines, deletions; dashed lines, likely structures for which sequence data are missing; ?, probable missing domain based on molecular weight and partial protein structure analysis; V, variable region; D, diversity segment; J, joining region; H, hinge region; C_H1, C_H2, C_H3, constant regions of heavy chains. OMM,[7] WIS,[14] CHI,[15] SPA,[16] ZUC,[17] CHA,[18] BUR,[9] GIF,[10] LEA,[11] HI,[12] HAR,[11] BAZ,[19] PAR,[20] ZAN,[21] HAL,[22] VAU,[23] LEB,[23] WIN,[13] UD,[24] CRA,[25] YOK,[26] RIV,[8] EST.[27]

DIFFERENTIAL DIAGNOSIS

All patients presenting with a lymphoplasma cell proliferative disorder should be evaluated for γ-HCD.

THERAPY

Because γ-HCD is a heterogeneous condition, the choice of therapy depends on the clinical picture. In an asymptomatic patient with a monoclonal γ-HC of undetermined significance, no therapy is indicated. Any associated autoimmune disease should be managed with standard therapy. In symptomatic patients with a low-grade lymphoplasmacytic malignancy, a trial of chlorambucil may be beneficial. Melphalan and prednisone can be used if the proliferation is predominantly plasmacytic. A trial of cyclophosphamide, vincristine, and prednisone with or without doxorubicin is reasonable for patients with evidence of a progressive lymphoplasma cell proliferative process or high-grade non-Hodgkin lymphoma. One patient achieved a complete response after six courses of fludarabine.[35] Successful treatment of γ-HCD with low-dose etoposide has been reported.[36] CD20 expression has been analyzed in only seven cases and was detected in six of the seven, including one in which CD20 expression appeared transient.[4,37–39] Rituximab monotherapy was given in two cases, resulting in clinical responses in both.[4,37] In another case, a combination of rituximab with chemotherapy had an antitumor effect in lymphoplasmacytic-type γ-HCD.[38] In localized extramedullary plasmacytomas treated with radiation[3] or surgical removal (or both), complete clinical and serologic remission has been achieved.

COURSE AND PROGNOSIS

The clinical course of γ-HCD is extremely variable and ranges from an asymptomatic, benign, or transient process to a rapidly progressive neoplasm leading to death within a few weeks. Patients with the features of monoclonal gammopathy of undetermined significance have remained clinically well for 2 to 7 years of followup.[4,40] Spontaneous disappearance of the γ-HCD protein has been reported.[3] The median duration of survival in a series of 23 patients was 7.4 years (range: 1 month to more than 21 years).[4]

The amount of serum γ-HCD protein usually parallels the severity of the associated malignant process. Disappearance of the monoclonal component from serum and urine associated with apparent complete response has been induced by chemotherapy,[35] radiotherapy,[3] or surgical removal of a localized process. In some instances, however, the γ-HCD protein does not vary in parallel with the associated process, and relapse can occur without the reappearance of the pathologic protein.[3]

α-HEAVY-CHAIN DISEASE

DEFINITION AND HISTORY

α-HCD is a proliferative disorder of B-lymphoid cells involving the IgA secretory immune system, especially the gastrointestinal tract. It is defined by the recognition of internally deleted monoclonal α chains devoid of light chains.

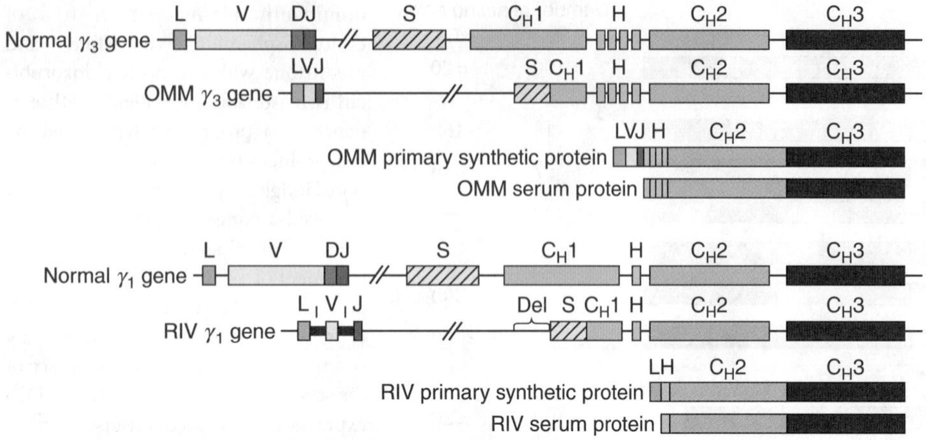

FIGURE 112–2. Structure of two genes coding for γ-heavy-chain-disease proteins compared with that of normal γ_3 and γ_1 genes. Boxes indicate coding regions; ▨, switch region; ▬, inserted noncoding sequence; lines, intervening (noncoding) sequences; L, leader region; V, variable region; D, diversity segment; J, joining region; S, switch region; H, hinge region; C_H1, C_H2, C_H3, constant regions of heavy chains; I, inserted sequence; Del, deleted sequence. OMM,[7] RIV.[8]

In the first case description of α-HCD, in 1968 by Seligman and colleagues,[41] an Arab woman had severe malabsorption resulting from a lymphoplasmacytic infiltrate in the small bowel. Since then, more than 400 cases have been reported.

EPIDEMIOLOGY

The majority of reported cases have been from northern Africa, Israel, and surrounding Middle Eastern countries. A common variable for patients with α-HCD is a low socioeconomic status. In a study of the distribution of monoclonal gammopathies in Tunisia published in 1990, 17 percent of 198 cases were attributed to α-HCD.[42] In a later study of 270 cases observed between 1992 and 2000 at the university hospital of Sfax in Tunisia, only 2.2 percent were attributed to α-HCD,[43] a finding that might be partially explained by improved socioeconomic conditions. Similarly, a persistent decrease in the incidence of immunoproliferative small intestinal disease (IPSID) since 1986 as a result of improving sanitation has been reported from Iran[44] and Greece.[45] α-HCD has a predilection for young adults. The prevalence of the disease is slightly higher in males than in females.

ETIOLOGY AND PATHOGENESIS

The cause of α-HCD is unknown. The disease might be considered a model showing the complex interactions of the environment with genetic factors and the infection–immunity–cancer interrelationships originating from the same proliferating clone. Although the mechanisms leading to the development of a clonal population synthesizing the structurally abnormal IgA are still speculative, the lymphoplasmacytic infiltration of the intestinal mucosa is likely a response of the alimentary tract immune system to protracted luminal antigenic stimulation. A causal relationship between infection and pathogenesis is supported by the observation that α-HCD can respond to broad-spectrum antibiotics. Using molecular strategies, *Campylobacter jejuni* was detected in 5 of 7 patients with α-HCD.[46] However, no specific microorganism has been found in other clinical studies. The putative agent may be present only at the onset of the disease and absent at diagnosis.

CLINICAL FEATURES

In most cases, patients who have α-HCD present with the digestive form. The disease is characterized by malabsorption manifested by diarrhea, weight loss, and abdominal pain. Ascites, tetany, edema, and clubbing may be present. Hepatosplenomegaly and peripheral lymphadenopathy are infrequent. Fever is uncommon. Amenorrhea, alopecia, and growth retardation in children and adolescents correlate with the duration and the severity of the malabsorptive process. α-HCD may be confined to the respiratory tract, but this is extremely rare, as is a lymphomatous form characterized by generalized lymphadenopathy. α-HCD has been reported in a patient with a goiter from a plasmacytoma of the thyroid[47] and in a patient with polyneuropathy, organomegaly, endocrinopathy, monoclonal protein, and skin lesions (POEMS).[48]

LABORATORY FEATURES

Molecular Biology and Genetics

Most α-HCD proteins consist of multiple polymers. The molecular weight of the basic monomeric unit varies from 29,000 to 34,000. The length of the basic polypeptide subunit differs from patient to patient and in most instances is between one-half and three-fourths that of a normal α chain. Sequence data are available for several α-HCD proteins (Fig. 112–3). In all cases of α-HCD studied, the α-HCD protein belonged to the α_1 subclass. Common features of the defective α chain include deleted V regions, missing C_H1 domains, and the absence of light chains. Most of the

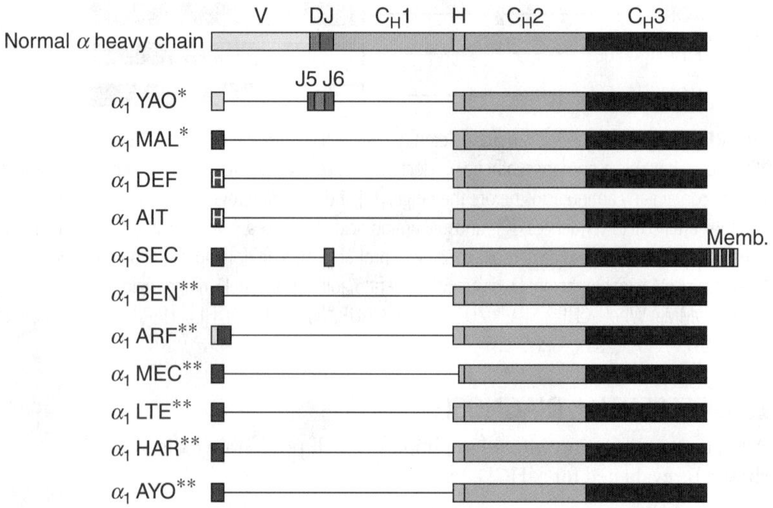

FIGURE 112–3. Structure of various α-heavy-chain disease proteins compared with that of normal chain. *Structures shown are primary synthetic products synthesized by the HCD cells. Serum proteins were modified after synthesis and did not contain any amino acids before the hinge. **Structures shown are deduced amino acid sequences determined by complementary DNA sequencing. H, indicates unusual and heterogeneous amino acid sequences; ■, unusual amino acid sequences; boxes, coding regions; lines, deletion; V, variable region; D, diversity segment; J, joining region; H, hinge region; C_H1, C_H2, C_H3, constant regions of heavy chains; Memb., membrane exon. YAO,[51] MAL,[50] DEF,[52] AIT,[53] SEC,[49] BEN,[54] ARF,[54] MEC,[54] LTE,[54] HAR,[54] AYO.[54]

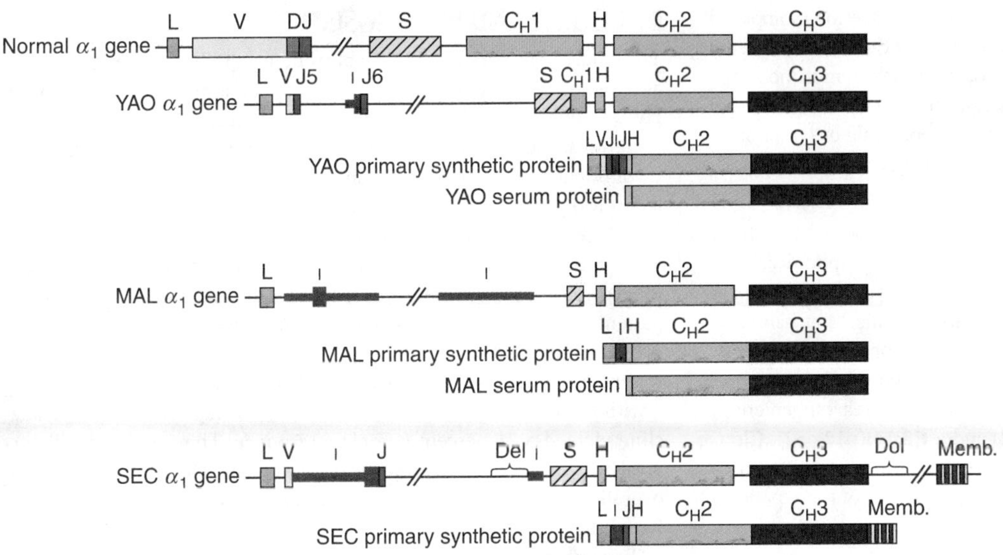

FIGURE 112–4. Structure of three genes coding for different α_1-heavy-chain disease proteins compared with that of normal α_1 gene. Boxes indicate coding regions; ▨, switch region; ■, inserted coding sequence; ■, inserted noncoding sequence; lines, intervening (noncoding) sequences; L, leader region; V, variable region; D, diversity segment; J, joining region; S, switch region; H, hinge region; C_H1, C_H2, C_H3, constant regions of heavy chains; I, inserted sequence; Del, deleted sequence; Memb., membrane exon. YAO,[51] MAL,[50] SEC.[49]

proteins have short, non–Ig-related sequences of unknown origin at the amino terminus. The complete sequences of the genes encoding three α-HCD proteins are shown in Fig. 112–4. These three genes show striking similarity in their position and extent of the two main deletions, which encompass sequences in the V/J and the switch/C_H1 region.

Protein Findings

In contrast to other monoclonal gammopathies, the characteristic sharp spike of a monoclonal gammopathy is not found on serum protein electrophoresis in α-HCD. In about half of cases, an abnormal broad band is found in the α_2- or β-globulin region, which is probably related to polymerization of the α chains. In the other half of cases, serum protein electrophoresis shows no evidence of an abnormal protein. Identification of the α-HCD protein depends on immunoselection or immunofixation. The pathologic protein may easily escape detection by immunoelectrophoresis when its serum concentration is low. In most patients, the α-HCD protein can be found in the serum. During the course of the disease, the progressive diminution of mature plasma cells and their replacement by immature immunoblasts likely is followed by a progressive decrease in the serum concentration of α-HCD protein. α-HCD protein hyposecretion also may be found during the early stage of the disease.

In most cases, the α-HCD protein also is found in the jejunal secretions.[55] α-HCD protein has been found in the intestinal or gastric fluid in a few cases when it was undetectable in serum and urine. The concentration of α-HCD protein in the urine is low. Bence Jones proteinuria has never been documented.

Synthesis of the α-HCD protein by the proliferating cells has been demonstrated by immunohistochemical or immunocytochemical methods and by biosynthesis studies *in vitro*.[56] These techniques are helpful in the recognition of nonsecreting forms of α-HCD.

Hematologic and Metabolic Abnormalities

Mild to moderate anemia is often found. Hypokalemia, hypocalcemia, hypomagnesemia, and hypoalbuminemia are common. The intestinal isoenzyme fraction of the alkaline phosphatase level may be increased. Results of tests to indicate malabsorption are usually positive.

Imaging Procedures

Abnormal radiographic findings of the small intestine include hypertrophic and pseudopolypoid mucosal folds, occasionally associated with strictures and filling defects. The extent of the disease should be evaluated with computed tomography.

Endoscopy

α-HCD intestinal lesions nearly always affect the duodenum and jejunum, and therefore endoscopy with biopsy is a useful tool in the workup of patients in whom α-HCD is suspected. Several endoscopic patterns have been defined. The infiltrated pattern is the most specific, followed by the nodular pattern. Other primary lesions (ulcerations, mosaic pattern, and mucosal fold thickening alone) are nonspecific.

Pathology

In the digestive form of α-HCD, the proliferation involves the whole length or at least the proximal half of the small intestine and adjacent mesenteric lymph nodes. Gastric and colorectal mucosae that belong to the IgA secretory system may be involved.

The disease progresses in three histopathologic stages.[57] In stage A, a mature plasmacytic or lymphoplasmacytic infiltration of the mucosal lamina propria is noted. Villous atrophy is variable. Stage B is characterized by the presence of atypical plasmacytic or lymphoplasmacytic cells and more or less atypical immunoblast-like cells extending at least to the submucosa. Subtotal or total villous atrophy is present. Stage C corresponds to an immunoblastic lymphoma. Similar to the changes described in the small intestine, three histologic stages (A, B, C) have been described in the mesenteric lymph nodes. Involvement of liver, spleen, and peripheral lymph nodes is uncommon. The histologic lesions may progress at any given site from stage A to stage B or from stage B to stage C. However, different stages can be found at the same time in different organs or even at different sites in the same organ. Thus, accurate pathologic staging of α-HCD requires a laparotomy with sampling of multiple sites in all patients with α-HCD in whom no stage C lesions are found on peroral biopsy. This recommendation is based on the observation that mesenteric lymph nodes may harbor malignant lymphoma when the intestinal mucosa reveals only a benign-appearing cellular infiltrate that one might be tempted to treat with antibiotics alone.[58] Salem and Estephan[59] published a staging system based on anatomical spread of the disease, which they suggested to be complementary to the Galian staging system; however, most use the Galian staging system for determining prognosis and therapeutic strategies.

In the past, confusion existed over whether Mediterranean lymphoma and α-HCD were different conditions. In 1976, a consensus panel concluded that α-HCD and Mediterranean lymphoma constitute a spectrum of disease, and the term *immunoproliferative small intestinal disease* (IPSID) came into use. This term is applied to small intestinal lesions whose pathologic features are identical to those of α-HCD regardless of the type of immunoglobulin synthesized.[55,60] The pattern of α-HCD pathologic lesions often includes clear lymphoepithelial lesions composed of centrocytic-like cells. This indicates that α-HCD can be considered a subtype of lymphoma arising from mucosa-associated lymph node tissue.[61] The pathologic changes in the few cases of the respiratory form of α-HCD are poorly documented. In a case of lymph node or lymphomatous form, lymph node biopsy showed diffuse plasmacytic lymphoma.

Cytogenetics

Cytogenetic abnormalities have been found in the lymphoid cells of patients with α-HCD. The clonal proliferation in this disease appears to be associated with frequent alterations of chromosome 14 at band q32 resulting from translocations that differ from those observed in the vast majority of other non-Hodgkin lymphomas. Abnormal karyotypes were reported in 3 of 4 patients.[62] Two patients had a rearrangement of 14q32 resulting from a t(9;14)(p11;q32) and a t(2;14)(p12;q32). Cloning and sequencing of the der(14) breakpoint of a chromosome translocation involving the 14q32 immunoglobulin locus in 1 of these patients suggested that the translocation originated from a local pairing of the 2 chromosomes, 9 and 14.[63] One case showed complex rearrangements, including t(5;9). No abnormalities were found in the intestinal tumor of the fourth case with immunoblastic lymphoma.

DIFFERENTIAL DIAGNOSIS

The digestive form of α-HCD must be differentiated from non-Hodgkin lymphoma, although this is an uncommon diagnosis in the age range typical of α-HCD. Other causes of malabsorption need to be considered, especially celiac disease. Enteric presentation of γ-HCD, variable immunodeficiency, and acquired immunodeficiency syndrome with clinicopathologic features simulating IPSID must be excluded.

THERAPY

Patients with stage A lesions limited to the bowel and to the mesenteric lymph nodes should be treated initially with oral antibiotics. In the absence of a documented parasite, tetracycline, metronidazole, or ampicillin is appropriate. Patients with stage B or C lesions or stage A lesions without improvement after a 6-month course of antibiotic treatment should be given chemotherapy. The treatment regimens are those commonly used to treat non-Hodgkin lymphoma. There have been few controlled clinical trials. In a prospective randomized study, a doxorubicin-based regimen (cyclophosphamide, doxorubicin hydrochloride, vincristine, and prednisone) provided a higher response rate than a non–doxorubicin-containing protocol (cyclophosphamide, vincristine, procarbazine, and prednisone) or total abdominal irradiation.[64] Similar results were noted in a retrospective study.[65] Good results have been reported with cyclophosphamide, doxorubicin, teniposide, and prednisone, sometimes alternating with bleomycin, vinblastine, and doxorubicin[66] and with cyclophosphamide, epidoxorubicin, vincristine, prednisolone, ifosfamide, methotrexate, etoposide (VP-16), and dexamethasone.[67] Surgical resection should be considered for focal or bulky transmural lymphomatous tumors and extramedullary plasmacytoma. Autologous hematopoietic stem cell transplantation has been recommended for patients with advanced or refractory disease,[55] but to our knowledge there are no reports in the literature demonstrating the utility of this approach. Previous trials have not incorporated immunotherapy with rituximab, an anti-CD20 monoclonal antibody, in the management of IPSID. As expected, the centrocyte-like cells are CD20-positive, but the plasma cells are not. In light of the extreme plasma cell differentiation and the plasmacytic nature of large-cell IPSID lymphoma, there is interest in investigating the value of treating patients with IPSID with newer multiple myeloma therapies, including proteasome inhibitors, at least in refractory cases (see Chap. 97).[58]

COURSE AND PROGNOSIS

The course of α-HCD is variable but generally progressive in the absence of therapy. Followup should include a periodic search for α-HCD protein in serum and urine and, if negative, in the intestinal secretions. Bowel radiography, ultrasonography, and esophagogastroduodenojejunal endoscopy should be performed. A second-look laparotomy may be necessary.[55] Relapses may occur after treatment at any stage of the disease. The long-term prognosis for patients with α-HCD remains imprecise because of the lack of large series with prolonged followup. In a small prospective Tunisian study,[66] including 8 patients with stage A disease and 15 with stages B and C, the survival of the total group was 90 percent at 2 years. A series from Turkey[68] reported 5-year treatment results of 23 patients with IPSID, including 5 with secretion of α chains. In patients with stage A disease, tetracycline yielded a 71 percent complete response. The 5-year overall survival rate for the entire group was 70 percent. However, the median overall survival for 3 patients with immunoblastic lymphoma was only 7 months.

Thirteen patients were studied who had IPSID associated with α-HCD.[69] Six patients, two with high-grade lymphoma and four with low-grade disease, received chemotherapy or radiotherapy or both. One patient died at 76 months, and five were alive at an average of 92 months. Five patients with low-grade disease received conservative therapy (antibiotics and in some cases prednisone). All five patients were alive at an average of 40 months after presentation. Three of these five patients achieved remission at 5, 6, and 27 months. Two of the five patients had persistent disease at 20 and 25 months. Two patients did not receive treatment and died of high-grade lymphoma.

Another study[70] described 6 patients who had α-HCD with lymphoma. All patients responded poorly to chemotherapy; the median duration of survival was 10.5 months.

A subsequent study[71] described 12 patients with secretory and nonsecretory IPSID. Six patients presented with stage A disease. Four patients responded to antibiotic or glucocorticoid therapy. In two patients, stage A disease evolved into stage C. Three patients presented with stage B disease. Two of these patients responded completely to chemotherapy, and the third refused treatment and died after 16 months. Three patients with stage C disease at diagnosis received aggressive combination chemotherapy and remained in complete remission with a median followup of 2.2 years.

Preliminary results suggest that flow cytometric analysis of S-phase fraction[72] and certain immunomarkers, such as syndecan, bcl6, and p53,[73] may be useful prognostic indicators in the clinical management of patients with IPSID. Patients with a poor prognosis have a higher fraction of cells in S phase, lower syndecan-1 expression, and higher bcl6 expression than those with a good prognosis.

μ-HEAVY-CHAIN DISEASE

DEFINITION AND HISTORY

μ-HCD is a proliferative disorder of B lymphocytes defined by the recognition of monoclonal deleted μ-HCs. In the first reported case, in 1969 by Forte and colleagues,[74] the patient had chronic lymphocytic leukemia. Since then, about 34 additional cases have been reported.[75–78]

EPIDEMIOLOGY

μ-HCD is extremely rare. In a series of 27 patients, the majority were white (76%) and male (55%). The median age at diagnosis in 27 patients was 57.5 years (range: 15–80 years).[75]

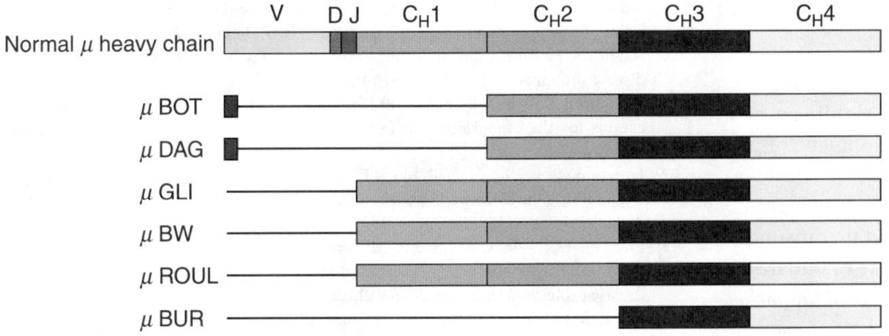

FIGURE 112–5. Structure of various deleted μ-heavy-chain disease proteins compared with that of normal chain. ■, indicates unusual amino acid sequences; boxes, coding regions; lines, deletions; V, variable region; D, diversity segment; J, joining region; C_H1, C_H2, C_H3, C_H4, constant regions of heavy chains. BOT,[82] DAG,[83] GLI,[81] BW,[80] ROUL,[78] BUR.[84]

■ ETIOLOGY AND PATHOGENESIS

The cause of μ-HCD is unknown.

■ CLINICAL FEATURES

The most common presenting symptoms of patients with μ-HCD are those of a lymphoproliferative malignancy. An associated lymphoplasma cell proliferative disorder was noted in 22 of 27 patients at some time during the disease and designated as chronic lymphocytic leukemia, non-Hodgkin lymphoma, Waldenström macroglobulinemia, or multiple myeloma.[75] μ-HCD protein has been described in one patient each with systemic lupus erythematosus, hepatic cirrhosis, hepatosplenomegaly with ascites, pulmonary infection, splenomegaly with pancytopenia,[75] and myelodysplasia.[76] Three cases of μ-HCD associated with amyloidosis have been reported.[79]

Splenomegaly and hepatomegaly are common in μ-HCD and were noted in 21 of 22 and 15 of 21 patients, respectively.[75] Peripheral lymphadenopathy is less frequent and was described in 10 of 25 patients.[75]

■ LABORATORY FEATURES

Molecular Biology and Genetics

The molecular weight of the μ-HCD protein determined in eight patients ranged from 26,500 to 158,000. The higher molecular weights are thought to be the result of polymerization of the μ-chain fragments. The μ-HCD fragments from six patients were subjected to detailed chemical analysis. Figure 112–5 depicts the structure of these six μ-HCD proteins compared with that of normal μ-HC. The V_H domain is absent in all cases. The normal sequence began with C_H1 in three cases, C_H2 in two cases, and C_H3 in one case. There are sequence data for only one gene coding for a μ-HCD protein (Fig. 112–6).

Protein Findings

A monoclonal spike was found on serum protein electrophoresis in less than half of a series of patients with μ-HCD (8 of 19).[75] The diagnosis of μ-HCD is made by documentation of the abnormal HC. Immunofixation of both serum and urine should be done. When these procedures yield ambiguous results, two-dimensional gel electrophoresis is a useful additional tool. The combination of capillary immunotyping electrophoresis and high-resolution two-dimensional electrophoresis has been used successfully for the detection of μ-HCD in one patient,[85] whereas in another capillary zone electrophoresis failed to detect the μ-HCD protein.[86]

Three of 33 reported patients with μ-HCD had a biclonal gammopathy. Hypogammaglobulinemia was noted in 10 of 22 patients.[75] Hypergammaglobulinemia with a polyclonal pattern in the γ-globulin fraction was described in one case.[76] In contrast to γ- and α-HCD in which there usually is no detectable monoclonal light chain in the serum and urine, Bence Jones proteinuria was found in more than half the cases of μ-HCD (14 of 22 patients).[75] μ-HCD protein was found in the urine of only two patients.[75] Three cases of nonsecretory μ-HCD have been reported.[87–89] μ-HCs were documented by immunofluorescence on the cell surface of proliferating lymphocytes in one case and in marrow plasma cells of the two others.

Hematologic Abnormalities

Anemia is frequent, but lymphocytosis and thrombocytopenia are uncommon. One patient had a positive direct antiglobulin test.[76] Examination of the marrow usually shows an increase in lymphocytes, plasma cells, or plasmacytoid lymphocytes. Plasmacytosis was noted in 18 of 20 cases; in 13 of these, vacuolated plasma cells were found.[75] The presence of vacuolated plasma cells in the marrow of a patient with a lymphoplasmacytic proliferative disorder should always suggest the possibility of μ-HCD.

Other Features

Lytic bone lesions were described in 3 of 15 patients,[75] and osteoporosis was mentioned in 3 others. No cytogenetic studies have been reported.

Pathology

In a literature review including 27 documented cases of μ-HCD, 22 patients (81%) had an associated lymphoplasma cell proliferative disorder designated as chronic lymphocytic leukemia, lymphoma, Waldenström macroglobulinemia, or myeloma.[75]

■ DIFFERENTIAL DIAGNOSIS

The differential diagnosis of μ-HCD includes all lymphoplasma cell proliferative disorders. Without a suspicion for the disease, μ-HCD is difficult to diagnose. The finding of Bence Jones proteinuria in a patient with a lymphoproliferative disorder and vacuolated plasma cells in the marrow deserves further investigation for possible μ-HCD.

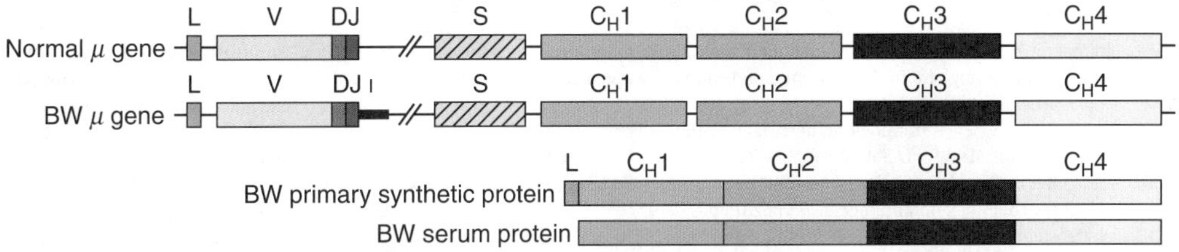

FIGURE 112–6. Structure of a gene coding for a μ-heavy-chain disease protein compared with that of normal μ gene. Boxes indicate coding regions; ▨, switch region; ▬, inserted noncoding sequence; L, leader region; V, variable region; D, diversity segment; J, joining region; S, switch region; C_H1, C_H2, C_H3, C_H4, constant regions of heavy chains; I, inserted sequence. BW.[80]

THERAPY

There is no specific therapy for μ-HCD. The finding of a μ-HCD protein in the serum of an apparently normal patient should be considered to represent monoclonal gammopathy of undetermined significance, and the patient should be followed closely for the development of a symptomatic lymphoplasma cell proliferative disorder. Once this develops, chemotherapy is indicated. Various agents have been used. Initially, a combination of cyclophosphamide, vincristine, and prednisone with or without doxorubicin is a reasonable choice. The use of fludarabine has been reported in two patients with μ-HCD; one had an "apparent hematologic response,"[90] and the other had a partial response.[77] Vincristine, cyclophosphamide, prednisolone, and doxorubicin (Adriamycin) in combination with rituximab led to complete resolution of tumoral lesions in one patient with μ-HCD.[91]

COURSE AND PROGNOSIS

The course of μ-HCD is variable. Because of the rarity of the disease, no large series of patients treated systematically in a single center has been reported. The median duration of survival from the time of diagnosis is 24 months (range: <1 month–11 years).[75] Because several of the reported patients had findings consistent with μ-HCD before recognition of the μ-HCD protein, the course is probably longer than reported in most patients. In one patient, the hematologic data became normal and the μ-HC disappeared after 2 years without specific treatment.[92]

REFERENCES

1. Franklin EC, Lowenstein J, Bigelow B, Meltzer M: Heavy chain disease: A new disorder of serum gamma-globulins: Report of the first case. *Am J Med* 37:332, 1964.
2. Fermand JP, Brouet JC: Heavy-chain diseases. *Hematol Oncol Clin North Am* 13:1281, 1999.
3. Fermand JP, Brouet JC, Danon F, Seligmann M: Gamma heavy chain "disease": Heterogeneity of the clinicopathologic features: Report of 16 cases and review of the literature. *Medicine (Baltimore)* 68:321, 1989.
4. Wahner-Roedler DL, Witzig TE, Loehrer LL, Kyle RA: Gamma-heavy chain disease: Review of 23 cases. *Medicine (Baltimore)* 82:236, 2003.
5. Wester SM, Banks PM, Li CY: The histopathology of gamma heavy-chain disease. *Am J Clin Pathol* 78:427, 1982.
6. Yunokawa K, Hagiyama Y, Mochizuki Y, et al: Hypertrophic spinal pachymeningitis associated with heavy-chain disease: Case report. *J Neurosurg Spine* 7:459, 2007.
7. Alexander A, Anicito I, Buxbaum J: Gamma heavy chain disease in man: Genomic sequence reveals two noncontiguous deletions in a single gene. *J Clin Invest* 82:1244, 1988.
8. Guglielmi P, Bakhshi A, Cogne M, et al: Multiple genomic defects result in an alternative RNA splice creating a human gamma H chain disease protein. *J Immunol* 141:1762, 1988.
9. Prelli F, Frangione B: Franklin's disease: Ig gamma 2 H chain mutant BUR. *J Immunol* 148:949, 1992.
10. Cooper SM, Franklin EC, Frangione B: Molecular defect in a gamma-2 heavy chain. *Science* 176:187, 1972.
11. Frangione B, Franklin EC, Smithies O: Unusual genes at the aminoterminus of human immunoglobulin variants. *Nature* 273:400, 1978.
12. Terry WD, Ohms J: Implications of heavy chain disease protein sequences for multiple gene theories of immunoglobulin synthesis. *Proc Natl Acad Sci U S A* 66:558, 1970.
13. Hauke G, Schiltz E, Bross KJ, et al: Unusual sequence of immunoglobulin L-chain rearrangements in a gamma heavy chain disease patient. *Scand J Immunol* 36:463, 1992.
14. Frangione B, Rosenwasser E, Prelli F, Franklin EC: Primary structure of human gamma 3 immunoglobulin deletion mutant: Gamma 3 heavy-chain disease protein Wis. *Biochemistry* 19:4304, 1980.
15. Frangione B: A new immunoglobulin variant: Gamma3 heavy chain disease protein CHI. *Proc Natl Acad Sci U S A* 73:1552, 1976.
16. Frangione B, Franklin EC: Correlation between fragmented immunoglobulin genes and heavy chain deletion mutants. *Nature* 281:600, 1979.
17. Wolfenstein-Todel C, Frangione B, Prelli F, Franklin EC: The amino acid sequence of "heavy chain disease" protein ZUC: Structure of the Fc fragment of immunoglobulin G3. *Biochem Biophys Res Commun* 71:907, 1976.
18. Arnaud P, Wang AC, Gianazza E, et al: Gamma heavy chain disease protein CHA: Immunological and structural studies. *Mol Immunol* 18:379, 1981.
19. Smith LL, Barton BP, Garver FA, et al: Physicochemical and immunochemical properties of gamma l heavy chain disease protein BAZ. *Immunochemistry* 15:323, 1978.
20. Rabin BS, Moon J: Clinical findings in a case of newly defined gamma heavy chain disease protein. *Clin Exp Immunol* 14:563, 1973.
21. Franklin EC, Prelli F, Frangione B: Human heavy chain disease protein WIS: Implications for the organization of immunoglobulin genes. *Proc Natl Acad Sci U S A* 76:452, 1979.
22. Frangione B, Lee L, Haber E, Bloch KJ: Protein Hal: Partial deletion of a "γ" immunoglobulin gene(s) and apparent reinitiation at an internal AUG codon. *Proc Natl Acad Sci U S A* 70:1073, 1973.
23. Franklin EC, Kyle R, Seligmann M, Frangione B: Correlation of protein structure and immunoglobulin gene organization in the light of two new deleted heavy chain disease proteins. *Mol Immunol* 16:919, 1979.
24. Sala P, Tonutti E, Pizzolitto S, et al: Immunochemical and structural characterization of an IgG1 heavy chain disease. *Ric Clin Lab* 19:59, 1989.
25. Franklin EC, Frangione B: The molecular defect in a protein (CRA) found in gamma-1 heavy chain disease, and its genetic implications. *Proc Natl Acad Sci U S A* 68:187, 1971.
26. Nabeshima Y, Ikenaka T: N- and C-terminal amino acid sequences of a gamma-heavy chain disease protein YOK. *Immunochemistry* 13:245, 1976.
27. Biewenga J, Frangione B, Franklin EC, van Loghem E: A gamma l heavy-chain disease protein (EST) lacking the entire VH and CH1 domains. *Scand J Immunol* 11:601, 1980.
28. Sun T, Peng S, Narurkar L: Modified immunoselection technique for definitive diagnosis of heavy-chain disease. *Clin Chem* 40:664, 1994.
29. Luraschi P, Infusino I, Zorzoli I, et al: Heavy chain disease can be detected by capillary zone electrophoresis. *Clin Chem* 51:247, 2005.
30. Lee MT, Parwani A, Humphrey R, et al: Gamma heavy chain disease in a patient with diabetes and chronic renal insufficiency: Diagnostic assessment of the heavy chain fragment. *J Clin Lab Anal* 22:146, 2008.
31. Lebreton JP, Fontaine M, Rousseaux J, et al: Deleted IgG1 and IgG2 H chains in a patient with an IgG subclass imbalance. *Clin Exp Immunol* 47:206, 1982.
32. Keller H, Spengler GA, Skvaril F, et al: [Heavy chain disease: A case of IgG-heavy-chain-fragment and IgM-type K-paraproteinemia with plasma cell leukemia (German)]. *Schweiz Med Wochenschr* 100:1012, 1970.
33. Woods R, Blumenschein GR, Terry WD: A new type of human gamma heavy chain disease protein: Immunochemical and physical characteristics. *Immunochemistry* 7:373, 1970.
34. Grogan TM, Muller-Hermelink HK, Van Camp B, et al: Plasma cell neoplasms, in *World Health Organization Classification of Tumours: Pathology and Genetics of Tumours of Haematopoietic and Lymphoid Tissues*, edited by ES Jaffe, NL Harris, H Stein, JW Vardiman, p 154. IARC Press, Lyon, France, 2001.
35. Agrawal S, Abboudi Z, Matutes E, Catovsky D: First report of fludarabine in gamma-heavy chain disease. *Br J Haematol* 88:653, 1994.
36. Ishikawa K, Hirai M, Tsutsumi H, et al: [Successful treatment of heavy-chain disease with etoposide (Japanese)]. *Nippon Ronen Igakkai Zasshi* 34:221, 1997.
37. Munshi NC, Digumarthy S, Rahemtullah A: Case records of the Massachusetts General Hospital: Case 13–2008: A 46-year-old man with rheumatoid arthritis and lymphadenopathy. *N Engl J Med* 358:1838, 2008.
38. Takano H, Nagata K, Mikoshiba M, et al: Combination of rituximab and chemotherapy showing anti-tumor effect in gamma heavy chain disease expressing CD20. *Am J Hematol* 83:938, 2008.
39. Jacobson E, Sharp G, Rimmer J, MacPherson B: A 59-year-old woman with immunotactoid glomerulopathy, heavy-chain disease, and non-Hodgkin lymphoma. *Arch Pathol Lab Med* 128:689, 2004.
40. Galanti LM, Doyen C, Vander Maelen C, et al: Biological diagnosis of a gamma-1-heavy chain disease in an asymptomatic patient. *Eur J Haematol* 54:202, 1995.
41. Seligmann M, Danon F, Hurez D, et al: Alpha-chain disease: A new immunoglobulin abnormality. *Science* 162:1396, 1968.
42. Makni S, Zouari R, Barbouch MR, et al: [Monoclonal gammopathies in Tunisia (French)]. *Rev Fr Transfus Hemobiol* 33:31, 1990.
43. Mseddi-Hdiji S, Haddouk S, Ben Ayed M, et al: [Monoclonal gammopathies in Tunisia: Epidemiological, immunochemical and etiological analysis of 288 cases (French)]. *Pathol Biol (Paris)* 53:19, 2005.
44. Lankarani KB, Masoompour SM, Masoompour MB, et al: Changing epidemiology of IPSID in southern Iran. *Gut* 54:311, 2005.
45. Economidou I, Manousos ON, Triantafillidis JK, et al: Immunoproliferative small intestinal disease in Greece: Presentation of 13 cases including two from Albania. *Eur J Gastroenterol Hepatol* 18:1029, 2006.
46. Lecuit M, Abachin E, Martin A, et al: Immunoproliferative small intestinal disease associated with *Campylobacter jejuni*. *N Engl J Med* 350:239, 2004.
47. Tracy RP, Kyle RA, Leitch JM: Alpha heavy-chain disease presenting as goiter. *Am J Clin Pathol* 82:336, 1984.
48. Kim SK, Park IK, Park BH, et al: A case report: Isolated α heavy chain monoclonal gammopathy in a patient with polyneuropathy, organomegaly, endocrinopathy, monoclonal gammopathy and skin change syndrome. *Int J Clin Pract Suppl* 147:26, 2005.
49. Cogne M, Preud'homme JL: Gene deletions force nonsecretory alpha-chain disease plasma cells to produce membrane-form alpha-chain only. *J Immunol* 145:2455, 1990.

50. Tsapis A, Bentaboulet M, Pellet P, et al: The productive gene for alpha-H chain disease protein MAL is highly modified by insertion-deletion processes. *J Immunol* 143:3821, 1989.
51. Bentaboulet M, Mihaesco E, Gendron MC, et al: Genomic alterations in a case of alpha heavy chain disease leading to the generation of composite exons from the JH region. *Eur J Immunol* 19:2093, 1989.
52. Wolfenstein-Todel C, Mihaesco E, Frangione B: "Alpha chain disease" protein def: Internal deletion of a human immunoglobulin A1 heavy chain. *Proc Natl Acad Sci U S A* 71:974, 1974.
53. Wolfenstein-Todel C, Mihaesco E, Frangione B: Variant of a human immunoglobulin: "alpha chain disease" protein AIT. *Biochem Biophys Res Commun* 65:47, 1975.
54. Fakhfakh F, Dellagi K, Ayadi H, et al: Alpha heavy chain disease alpha mRNA contain nucleotide sequences of unknown origins. *Eur J Immunol* 22:3037, 1992.
55. Rambaud JC, Halphen M, Galian A, Tsapis A: Immunoproliferative small intestinal disease (IPSID): Relationships with alpha-chain disease and "Mediterranean" lymphomas. *Springer Semin Immunopathol* 12:239, 1990.
56. Tashiro T, Sato H, Takahashi T, et al: Non-secretory alpha chain disease involving stomach, small intestine and colon. *Intern Med* 34:255, 1995.
57. Galian A, Lecestre MJ, Scotto J, et al: Pathological study of alpha-chain disease, with special emphasis on evolution. *Cancer* 39:2081, 1977.
58. Al-Saleem T, Al-Mondhiry H: Immunoproliferative small intestinal disease (IPSID): A model for mature B-cell neoplasms. *Blood* 105:2274, 2005.
59. Salem PA, Estephan FF: Immunoproliferative small intestinal disease: Current concepts. *Cancer J* 11:374, 2005.
60. Martin IG, Aldoori MI: Immunoproliferative small intestinal disease: Mediterranean lymphoma and alpha heavy chain disease. *Br J Surg* 81:20, 1994.
61. Isaacson PG: Gastrointestinal lymphoma. *Hum Pathol* 25:1020, 1994.
62. Berger R, Bernheim A, Tsapis A, et al: Cytogenetic studies in four cases of alpha chain disease. *Cancer Genet Cytogenet* 22:219, 1986.
63. Pellet P, Tsapis A, Brouet JC: Alpha heavy chain disease of patient MAL: Structure of the non-functional rearranged alpha gene translocated on chromosome 9. *Eur J Immunol* 20:2731, 1990.
64. Khojasteh A, Saalabian MJ, Haghshenass M: Randomized comparison of abdominal irradiation (AI) vs CHOP vs C-MOPP for the treatment of immunoproliferative small intestinal disease (IPSID) associated lymphoma (AL) [abstract]. *Proc Annu Meeting Am Soc Clin Oncol* 2:207, 1983.
65. Salimi M, Spinelli JJ: Chemotherapy of Mediterranean abdominal lymphoma: Retrospective comparison of chemotherapy protocols in Iranian patients. *Am J Clin Oncol* 19:18, 1996.
66. Ben-Ayed F, Halphen M, Najjar T, et al: Treatment of alpha chain disease: Results of a prospective study in 21 Tunisian patients by the Tunisian-French Intestinal Lymphoma Study Group. *Cancer* 63:1251, 1989.
67. Hubmann R, Kaiser W, Radaszkiewicz T, et al: Malabsorption associated with a high-grade-malignant non-Hodgkin's lymphoma, alpha-heavy-chain disease and immunoproliferative small intestinal disease. *Z Gastroenterol* 33:209, 1995.
68. Akbulut H, Soykan I, Yakaryilmaz F, et al: Five-year results of the treatment of 23 patients with immunoproliferative small intestinal disease: A Turkish experience. *Cancer* 80:8, 1997.
69. Price SK: Immunoproliferative small intestinal disease: A study of 13 cases with alpha heavy-chain disease. *Histopathology* 17:7, 1990.
70. Shih LY, Liaw SJ, Dunn P, Kuo TT: Primary small-intestinal lymphomas in Taiwan: Immunoproliferative small-intestinal disease and nonimmunoproliferative small-intestinal disease. *J Clin Oncol* 12:1375, 1994.
71. Malik IA, Shamsi Z, Shafquat A, et al: Clinicopathological features and management of immunoproliferative small intestinal disease and primary small intestinal lymphoma in Pakistan. *Med Pediatr Oncol* 25:400, 1995.
72. Demirer T, Uzunalimoglu O, Anderson T, et al: Flow cytometric measurement of proliferation-associated nuclear antigen P105 and DNA content in immuno-proliferative small intestinal disease (IPSID). *J Surg Oncol* 58:25, 1995.
73. Vaiphei K, Kumari N, Sinha SK, et al: Roles of syndecan-1, bcl6 and p53 in diagnosis and prognostication of immunoproliferative small intestinal disease. *World J Gastroenterol* 12:3602, 2006.
74. Forte FA, Prelli F, Yount W, et al: Heavy chain disease of the μ type: Report of the first case [abstract]. *Blood* 34:831, 1969.
75. Wahner-Roedler DL, Kyle RA: Mu-heavy chain disease: Presentation as a benign monoclonal gammopathy. *Am J Hematol* 40:56, 1992.
76. Witzens M, Egerer G, Stahl D, et al: A case of mu heavy-chain disease associated with hyperglobulinemia, anemia, and a positive Coombs test. *Ann Hematol* 77:231, 1998.
77. Yanai M, Maeda A, Watanabe N, et al: Successful treatment of mu-heavy chain disease with fludarabine monophosphate: A case report. *Int J Hematol* 79:174, 2004.
78. Cogne M, Aucouturier P, Brizard A, et al: Complete variable region deletion in a mu heavy chain disease protein (ROUL): Correlation with light chain secretion. *Leuk Res* 17:527, 1993.
79. Kinoshita K, Yamagata T, Nozaki Y, et al: Mu-heavy chain disease associated with systemic amyloidosis. *Hematology* 9:135, 2004.
80. Bakhshi A, Guglielmi P, Siebenlist U, et al: A DNA insertion/deletion necessitates an aberrant RNA splice accounting for a mu heavy chain disease protein. *Proc Natl Acad Sci U S A* 83:2689, 1986.
81. Franklin EC, Frangione B, Prelli F: The defect in mu heavy chain disease protein GLI. *J Immunol* 116:1194, 1976.
82. Barnikol-Watanabe S, Mihaesco E, Mihaesco C, et al: The primary structure of mu-chain-disease protein BOT: Peculiar amino-acid sequence of the N-terminal 42 positions. *Hoppe Seylers Z Physiol Chem* 365:105, 1984.
83. Mihaesco C, Ferrara P, Guillemot JC, et al: A new extra sequence at the amino terminal of a mu heavy chain disease protein (DAG). *Mol Immunol* 27:771, 1990.
84. Lebreton JP, Ropartz C, Rousseaus J, et al: Immunochemical and biochemical study of a human Fcmu-like fragment (mu-chain disease). *Eur J Immunol* 5:179, 1975.
85. Maisnar V, Tichy M, Stulik J, et al: Capillary immunotyping electrophoresis and high resolution two-dimensional electrophoresis for the detection of mu-heavy chain disease. *Clin Chim Acta* 389:171, 2008.
86. Marien G, Verhoef G, Bossuyt X: Detection of heavy chain disease by capillary zone electrophoresis. *Clin Chem* 51:1302, 2005.
87. Gordon J, Hamblin TJ, Smith JL, et al. A human B-cell lymphoma synthesizing and expressing surface mu-chain in the absence of detectable light chain. *Blood* 58:552, 1981.
88. Guglielmo P, Granata P, Di Raimondo F, et al: "Mu" heavy chain type "non-excretory" myeloma. *Scand J Haematol* 29:36, 1982.
89. Leglise MC, Briere J, Abgrall JF, Hurez D. Non-secretory myeloma of heavy mu-chain type [French]. *Nouv Rev Fr Hematol* 25:103, 1983.
90. Preud'homme JL, Bauwens M, Dumont G, et al: Cast nephropathy in mu heavy chain disease. *Clin Nephrol* 48:118, 1997.
91. Maeda A, Mori M, Torii S, et al: Multiple extranodal tumors in mu-heavy chain disease. *Int J Hematol* 84:286, 2006.
92. Wetter O, Schmidt CG, Linder KH, Leene W: [Heavy chain disease: Humoral and cellular findings in six patients with mu chain disease (German; author's transl)]. *J Cancer Res Clin Oncol* 94:207, 1979.

PART XII

Hemostasis and Thrombosis

CHAPTER 113
MEGAKARYOPOIESIS AND THROMBOPOIESIS

Kenneth Kaushansky

SUMMARY

Each day the adult human produces approximately 1×10^{11} platelets, a level of production that can increase 10- to 20-fold in times of increased demand and an additional 5- to 10-fold under the stimulation of exogenous thrombopoietin-mimetic drugs. Production of platelets depends on the proliferation and differentiation of hematopoietic stem and progenitor cells to cells committed to the megakaryocyte lineage, their maturation to large, polyploid megakaryocytes, and their final fragmentation into platelets. The external influences that impact megakaryopoiesis and thrombopoiesis are a supportive marrow stroma consisting of endothelial and other cells, matrix glycosaminoglycans, and a family of protein hormones and cytokines, including thrombopoietin, stem cell factor, and stromal cell-derived factor-1. The role of the cytokines essential for these processes has been defined, insights into the two most unusual aspects of thrombopoiesis—endomitosis and proplatelet formation—have been gathered, and reagents to specifically modify platelet production have been generated. This chapter focuses on the development of megakaryocytes, their precursors and their progeny, and the hematopoietic growth factors and transcriptionally active molecules that control the survival, proliferation, and differentiation of these cells.

KINETICS OF THROMBOPOIESIS

The circulatory life span of a platelet is approximately 10 days in humans with normal platelet counts, but somewhat shorter in patients with moderate (7 days) to severe (5 days) thrombocytopenia, as a higher proportion of the total-body platelet mass is consumed in the day-to-day function of maintaining vascular integrity.[1] Based on a "normal" level of 200,000 platelets/μL, a blood volume of 5 L, and a half-life of 10 days, 1×10^{11} platelets per day are produced. If 1 megakaryocyte produces approximately 1000 platelets, approximately 1×10^8 megakaryocytes are generated in the marrow each day.

Several independent lines of evidence indicate the transit time from megakaryocyte progenitor cell to release of platelets into the circulation ranges from 4 to 7 days. For example, following platelet apheresis, the platelet count falls, recovers substantially by day 4, and completely recovers by day 7.[2] In most physiologic and pathologic states, the platelet count is inversely related to plasma thrombopoietin levels. For example, liver failure is associated with moderate thrombocytopenia as a result of splenomegaly and thrombopoietin deficiency. Within the first week following orthotopic liver transplantation, the platelet count rises substantially, with kinetics matching those of thrombopoietin infusion.[3,4] These findings indicate expansion of the megakaryocyte mass takes from 3 to 4 days following a thrombopoietin stimulus in humans and, coupled with the approximate 12 hours required for platelet release,[5] results in a relatively brisk response to thrombocytopenia.

Acronyms and abbreviations that appear in this chapter include: CAMT, congenital amegakaryocytic thrombocytopenia; FGF, fibroblast growth factor; GP, glycoprotein; HPS, Hermansky-Pudlak syndrome; IFN, interferon; ITP, immune thrombocytopenic purpura; IL, interleukin; MAPK, mitogen-activated protein kinase; P4P, polyphosphate-4-phosphatase; PI3K, phosphoinositol 3 kinase; RACK, RhoA kinase; SDF, stromal cell-derived factor; TGF, transforming growth factor.

CELLULAR PHYSIOLOGY OF THROMBOPOIESIS

Platelets form by fragmentation of megakaryocyte membrane extensions termed *proplatelets*, in a process that consumes nearly the entire cytoplasmic complement of membranes, organelles, granules, and soluble macromolecules. Although at first controversial, as the process was initially observed only *in vitro, in situ* microscopic studies have identified proplatelet formation and fragmentation in living animals.[6] Each megakaryocyte is estimated to give rise to 1000 to 3000 platelets[7] before the residual nuclear material is engulfed and eliminated by marrow macrophages.[8] The continuum of megakaryocyte development is arbitrarily divided into four stages. The major criteria differentiating these stages are the quality and quantity of the cytoplasm and the size, lobulation, and chromatin pattern of the nucleus (Table 113–1).

MEGAKARYOBLAST

Stage I megakaryocytes, also termed *megakaryoblasts*, account for approximately 20 percent of all cells destined to form platelets. These cells in human marrow are 8 to 24 μm in spherical diameter (i.e., the actual size *in vivo*, as opposed to the apparent size of a cell on a flattened marrow smear), contain a relatively large, minimally indented nucleus with loosely organized chromatin and multiple nucleoli, and scant basophilic cytoplasm containing a small Golgi complex, a few mitochondria and α granules, and abundant free ribosomes (Fig. 113–1).

Surface Adhesion Molecule Expression

Although elegant experiments clearly demonstrated that the gene for integrin α_{IIb} is expressed as early as the erythroid-megakaryocytic progenitor stage[9] and possibly in the common myeloid progenitor, the cell surface protein becomes demonstrable and functionally important only at the early stages of megakaryocyte development. Integrin $\alpha_{IIb}\beta_3$ is an integral transmembrane protein of two subunits, but only the α subunit is megakaryocyte-lineage specific. Absence of integrin $\alpha_{IIb}\beta_3$ leads to Glanzmann thrombasthenia resulting from failure of the defective platelets to engage fibrinogen and other adhesive ligands during hemostasis (see Chap. 121). Megakaryocytes and platelets contain in their cytoplasmic membranes about twice the amount of integrin $\alpha_{IIb}\beta_3$ as is present on the cell surface. The granule compartment serves as a mobilizable pool that is exteriorized upon platelet activation. During the early and midstages of megakaryocyte development, the granule content of integrin rises. Moreover, as developing megakaryocytes do not synthesize but contain fibrinogen in their α-granules and cells from patients with Glanzmann thrombasthenia do not, integrin $\alpha_{IIb}\beta_3$ clearly begins to function, at least at the level of fibrinogen binding and uptake, long before platelet formation.

The glycoprotein (GP) Ib-IX complex is expressed only slightly after the appearance of integrin $\alpha_{IIb}\beta_3$.[10] Although endothelial cells reportedly express GPIb,[11] its levels are very low; otherwise, GPIb is a second megakaryocyte-specific protein. Glycoprotein V also is expressed in complex with GPIb and GPIX, in a ratio of 1:2:2.[12] However, the genetic elimination of GPV has little effect on platelet adhesion,[13] and unlike GPIb and GPIX, no mutations of GPV are associated with Bernard-Soulier disease (see Chap. 121).[14] Therefore, GPV does not appear to be

TABLE 113–1. Maturation Stages of Megakaryocytes

Term	Size (μM)	Morphology
Megakaryoblast (stage I)	>10	Lobed nucleus, basophilic cytoplasm
Basophilic megakaryocyte (stage II)	>20	Horseshoe-shaped nucleus, basophilic cytoplasm, azurophilic granules around centrosome
Granular megakaryocyte (stage III)	>25–50	Large multilobed nucleus, acidophilic cytoplasm, numerous azurophilic granules
Mature megakaryocyte (stage IV)	>25–50	Pyknotic nucleus, groups of 10–12 azurophilic granules

required for the GPIb-V-IX complex to function as a von Willebrand factor receptor. Rather, GPV is a target of thrombin, potentially playing a role in platelet activation.[15]

Demarcation Membranes

Another feature of the megakaryoblast is the initial development of demarcation membranes, which begin as invaginations of the plasma membrane and ultimately develop into a highly branched interconnected system of channels that course through the cytoplasm. The demarcation membrane system is in open communication with the extracellular space, based on studies using electron dense tracers.[16] Biochemical analysis indicates the composition of these membranes is very similar to the plasma membrane at each stage of megakaryocyte development. Over the 72 hours required for stage III/IV cells to develop from megakaryoblasts, the demarcation membrane system grows substantially. The purpose of the demarcation membrane system has been disputed for several decades. As the term implies, many believed the demarcation membrane system acts to compartmentalize the megakaryocyte cytoplasm into "platelet territories," which ultimately fragment into mature platelets along the cleavage planes so formed. In contrast, the current belief is that these membranes provide the material necessary for development of proplatelet processes, structures that form in stage IV megakaryocytes and give rise upon fragmentation to mature platelets.[17]

Endomitosis

One of the most characteristic features of megakaryocyte development is endomitosis, a unique form of mitosis in which the DNA is repeatedly replicated in the absence of nuclear or cytoplasmic division. The resultant cells are highly polyploid. Endomitosis begins in megakaryoblasts (Fig. 113–2) following the many standard cell divisions required to expand the number of megakaryocytic precursor cells and is completed by the end of stage II megakaryocyte development.[18] During the endomitotic phase, each cycle of DNA synthesis produces an exact doubling of all the chromosomes, resulting in cells containing DNA content from 8 to 128 times the normal chromosomal complement in a single, highly lobated nucleus. Although poorly understood for many years, the ability to produce large numbers of normal megakaryocytes in culture has started to shed light on this enigmatic process. Endomitosis is not simply the absence of mitosis but rather consists of recurrent cycles of aborted mitoses.[19] Cell-cycle kinetics in endomitotic cells also are unusual, characterized by a short G_1 phase, a relatively normal DNA synthesis phase, a short G_2 phase, and a very short endomitosis phase.[20] During the endomitosis phase, megakaryocytic chromosomes condense, the nuclear membrane breaks down, and multiple (at advanced stages) mitotic spindles form upon which the replicated chromosomes assemble. However, following initial chromosomal separation, individual chromosomes fail to complete their normal migration to opposite poles of the cell, the spindle dissociates, the nuclear membrane reforms around the entire chromosomal complement, and the cell again enters G_1 phase.

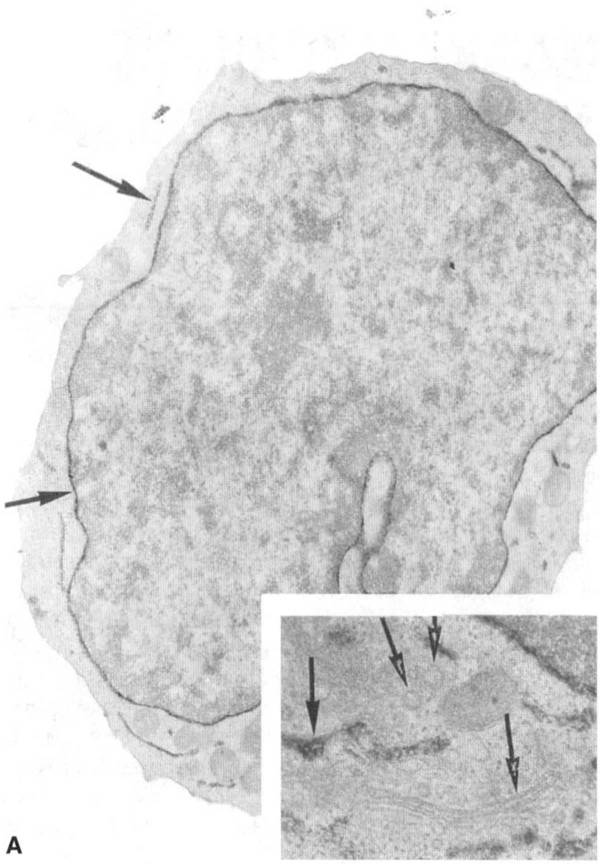

A

FIGURE 113–1. Electron micrograph of a normal human megakaryoblast stained for platelet peroxidase. The small cell (<9 μm) exhibits dense platelet peroxidase in the perinuclear space and endoplasmic reticulum (*arrows*) (magnification ×12,150). (*Inset*) Enlargement of the Golgi zone. The Golgi saccules and vesicles are devoid of platelet peroxidase (*open arrows*), whereas the endoplasmic reticulum contains platelet peroxidase activity (*closed arrow*) (magnification ×25,000). *(Courtesy of Dr. J. Breton-Gorius.)*

Regulation of Gene Expression

The promoters for integrin α_{IIb}, GPIb, GPVI, GPIX, and platelet factor-4 genes have been the focus of several studies and are active at the megakaryoblast stage of development. Consensus sequences for both GATA-1 and members of the Ets family of transcription factors (e.g., Fli-1) are present in the 5′ flanking regions of these genes, deletion of which reduces or eliminates reporter gene expression,[21–24] at least in mature hematopoietic cells. MafB also enhances GATA-1 and Ets activity during megakaryoblast differentiation,[25] induced by activation of ERK1/2, one of the primary downstream events of thrombopoietin stimulation.[26]

Another target of GATA-1 in megakaryocytes is polyphosphate-4-phosphatase (P4P), which was first identified by subtraction cloning between normal and GATA-1 knockdown megakaryocytes.[27] One of the unexplained features of megakaryocytes in GATA-1 knockdown mice is that, rather than massive cell death as seen in GATA-1–deficient

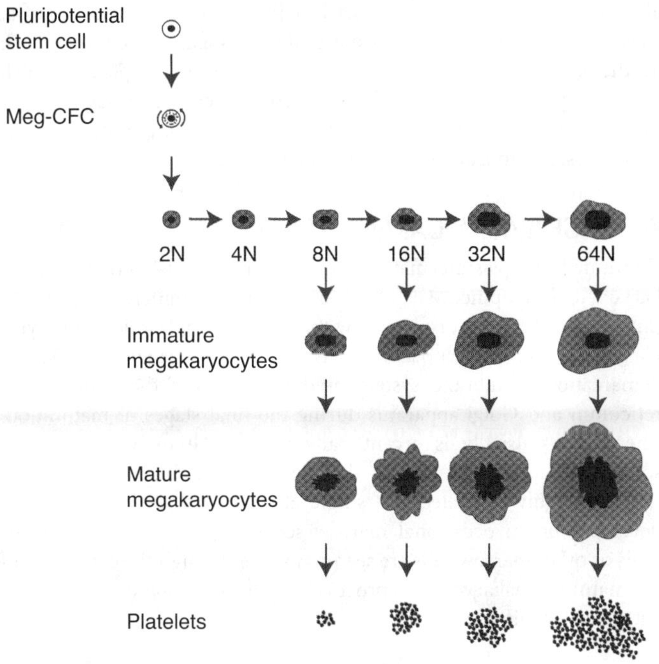

FIGURE 113–2. Origin and development of megakaryocytes. The pluripotential stem cell produces a progenitor committed to megakaryocyte differentiation (colony-forming unit–megakaryocyte [CFU-MK]), which can undergo mitosis. Eventually the CFU-MK stops mitosis and enters endomitosis. During endomitosis, neither cytoplasm nor nucleus divides, but DNA replication proceeds and gives rise to immature polyploid progenitors, which then enlarge and mature into morphologically identifiable, mature megakaryocytes that shed platelets. This figure does not necessarily imply that endomitosis and platelet formation are sequential but they can occur simultaneously. Meg-CFC, megakaryocyte colony-forming cells.

erythroid progenitors,[28] the aberrantly developing megakaryoblasts in GATA-1 knockdown marrow are highly abundant and proliferate *in vitro* far more than control cells.[29] P4P catalyzes hydrolysis of the D-4 position phosphate of $PI_{3,4}P$ and $PI_{3,4,5}P$. These membrane phospholipids are products of phosphoinositol 3 kinase (PI3K) action on membrane phospholipids, and they play an important role in the proliferative and survival response to megakaryocyte growth factors. When reintroduced into the knockdown mice, P4P diminishes the exuberant growth characteristic of the knockdown cells.[27] These findings are similar to the phenotype of cells from PTEN or SHIP knockout mice, enzymes that hydrolyze the D-3 and D-5 positions of $PI_{3,4,5}P$.

Another transcription factor vital for megakaryoblast differentiation is RUNX1 (also termed CBFA2 and AML1), the gene responsible for thrombocytopenia seen in familial platelet disorder/predisposition to acute myelogenous leukemia (see Chap. 119).[30] In this disorder, haploinsufficiency of RUNX1 is associated with thrombocytopenia. As its genetic elimination in mice leads to significant maturation defects in the megakaryocyte lineage,[31] the human disorder almost certainly results from this genetic alteration. During normal megakaryoblast differentiation, RUNX1 levels rise and, conversely, fall during erythroid differentiation. In response to phosphorylation by ERK1/2, RUNX1, in complex with CBFβ and together with GATA-1, induces integrin α_{IIb} and integrin α_2 expression in megakaryoblast-like cells,[32] providing the beginnings of a molecular explanation for megakaryocyte development.

Cytokine Dependency

The cytokines, hormones, and chemokines that affect the survival and proliferation of megakaryoblasts include thrombopoietin, interleukin (IL)-3, stem cell factor (also termed mast cell growth factor, steel factor, and *c-kit* ligand), and stromal cell-derived factor (SDF)-1. Thrombopoietin is the most critical (for additional details, see the more extensive discussion in "Hormones and Cytokines" below), as genetic elimination of the *TPO* gene in mice leads to circulating platelet levels approximately 10 percent of normal. Homozygous or complex heterozygous mutation of the gene encoding the thrombopoietin receptor cMpl leads to congenital amegakaryocytic thrombocytopenia, in which platelet levels are approximately 10 percent of normal because of a near absence of megakaryocytic progenitors and megakaryoblasts (see Chap. 119). The importance of stem cell factor to megakaryoblast development is revealed by experimental findings both *in vitro* and *in vivo*. Genetic reduction in expression of stem cell factor or its receptor *c-kit* leads to a 50 percent reduction in circulating platelet levels.[33] The cytokine acts in synergy with thrombopoietin to enhance megakaryocyte production in semisolid and suspension culture systems.[34] Evidence that IL-3 contributes to normal or accelerated megakaryopoiesis *in vivo* is weak. Genetic elimination of the IL-3 gene fails to affect platelet counts, even when combined with thrombopoietin receptor deficiency,[35] but the cytokine can induce growth of marrow progenitors into colonies containing immature megakaryocytes *in vitro* in the absence of thrombopoietin.[36] The chemokine SDF-1 appears to play a role in megakaryocyte proliferation. *In vitro*, SDF-1 acts in synergy with thrombopoietin to support the survival and proliferation of megakaryocyte progenitors.[37] The combination of fibroblast growth factor (FGF)-4 and SDF-1 restores megakaryopoiesis in *TPO* and c-*mpl* null mice.[38]

SIGNAL TRANSDUCTION

The survival and proliferation of megakaryoblasts depends on at least two thrombopoietin-induced signaling pathways: PI3K and mitogen-activated protein kinase (MAPK; see Chap. 14). In the presence of chemical inhibitors of PI3K, the favorable effects of thrombopoietin on megakaryocyte progenitor survival and proliferation are eliminated,[39] although constitutively activating this pathway is not sufficient for thrombopoietin-induced growth. MAPK is another important signaling pathway stimulated by thrombopoietin. Using purified marrow megakaryocytic progenitors and model cell lines, several groups showed that inhibition of MAPK blocks megakaryoblast maturation[26,40–42] because of its effect of activating Ets transcription factors.

STAGE II MEGAKARYOCYTES

Stage II megakaryocytes contain a lobulated nucleus and more abundant, but less intensely basophilic, cytoplasm. Ultrastructurally, the cytoplasm contains more abundant α granules and organelles. The demarcation membrane system begins to expand at this stage of development. Stage II megakaryocytes measure up to 30 μm in diameter, constitute approximately 25 percent of marrow megakaryocytes, and are the stage of development during which endomitosis is most prominent, generating cells displaying ploidy values of 8N to 64N.

Endomitosis

Whereas megakaryoblasts are generally thought to be able to expand by cell division, at an early stage of their maturation, the cells begin to undergo endomitosis, in which cells diverge from the normal cell cycle during mid- to late anaphase. Like normally mitotic cells, endomitotic megakaryocytes condense their chromatin into chromosomes, form a spindle, dissolve the nuclear membrane, and assemble the chromosomes on a metaphase plate, then the chromosomes begin to separate during early anaphase. However, rather than the dividing chromosomes migrating to opposite poles of the cell to allow the formation of a cleavage furrow, the chromosomes quickly decondense, the nuclear membrane reforms around the entire chromosomal complement, and the endomitotic cells reenter G_1 and then S phase. A number of attempts to understand this process at the biochemical level have involved leukemic cell lines. Alterations in cyclin B, cdc2, cell-cycle kinase inhibitors, and aurora kinases have been claimed to be responsible for endomitosis.[43,44] Unfortunately, although these hypotheses possibly explain the polyploidy in various leukemic cell lines, the hypotheses have not been substantiated in studies of normal endomitotic megakaryocytes.[19,45,46] Endomitosis departs from a normal mitotic cell cycle at the late anaphase stage, when furrow invagination aborts short of cell abscission.[47] Additional studies indicate that disordered localization of the small G protein RhoA, and the reduced function of its kinase, RACK, may be responsible for this property.[47,48]

Cytoplasmic Development

Early in megakaryocyte development, the cytoplasm acquires a rich network of microfilaments and microtubules. Toward stages III and IV, the proteins accumulate in the cell periphery, creating an organelle poor peripheral zone. Biochemically, the megakaryocyte cytoskeleton is composed of actin, α-actinin, filamin, nonmuscle myosin (including the product of the *MYH9* gene), mutated in several giant platelet thrombocytopenic syndromes[49] (see Chap. 119), β_1-tubulin, talin, and several other actin-binding proteins. Like platelets, megakaryocytes can respond to external stimuli by changing shape, transporting organelles around the cytoplasm, and secreting granules. These functions are dependent on the microfilament and microtubule systems of the cell. In addition, microtubules play a vital role during the later stages of platelet formation.[50]

Regulation of Gene Expression

As discussed earlier, GATA-1 is vital for committing primitive multipotent progenitors to the erythroid–megakaryocyte pathway. However, the transcription factor also is critical later in megakaryopoiesis, for cytoplasmic development. The first convincing evidence that GATA proteins affect megakaryocyte development came from overexpression studies of *GATA-1* in a leukemic cell line, in which the transcription factor led to partial megakaryocytic differentiation.[51] Reduction in *GATA-1* expression also impairs cytoplasmic development in murine megakaryocytes, reducing demarcation membranes and platelet-specific granules.[29]

Platelet Granule Formation

Although more prominent in later stages of differentiation (Fig. 113–3), platelet-specific α granules first begin to form adjacent to the Golgi apparatus as 300- to 500-nm round or oval organelles in stage II megakaryocytes. Three distinct compartments are recognized in α granules: (1) a central, electron-dense nucleoid, containing fibrinogen, platelet factor-4, β-thromboglobulin, transforming growth factor (TGF)-β_1, vitronectin, and tissue plasminogen activator-like plasminogen activator; (2) a peripheral zone, containing tubules and von Willebrand factor (arranged much like that seen in endothelial cell Weibel-Palade bodies); and (3) the granule membrane, containing many of the critical platelet receptors for cell rolling (P-selectin), firm adhesion (GPIb-V-IX), and aggregation (integrin $\alpha_{IIb}\beta_3$). Proteins present in α granules arise from *de novo* megakaryocyte synthesis (e.g., GPIb-V-IX, GPIV, integrin $\alpha_{IIb}\beta_3$, von Willebrand factor, P-selectin, β-thromboglobulin, platelet-derived growth factor), nonspecific pinocytosis of environmental proteins (albumin and immunoglobulin G), or cell surface membrane receptor-mediated uptake from the environment (e.g., fibrinogen, fibronectin, factor V). Insights into platelet granule formation have come from a molecular understanding of Hermansky-Pudlak Syndrome (HPS). In this disorder, characterized by oculocutaneous albinism and a qualitative platelet bleeding disorder, a complex of at least eight proteins form in various granule associated complexes such as the biogenesis of lysosome-related organelles complexes, which affect δ granule formation.[52] These complexes are thought to be involved in cargo transport of a number of subcellular granules, such as lysosomes, melanosomes, and platelet δ granules.

STAGE III/IV MEGAKARYOCYTES

Continued cytoplasmic maturation characterizes stage III/IV megakaryocyte development (Fig. 113–4). Cells are extremely large (40–60 μm in diameter) and display a low nuclear-to-cytoplasmic ratio. Cytoplasmic basophilia disappears as cells progress from stage III to IV. The demarcation membrane system gradually replaces the endoplasmic reticulum and Golgi apparatus during the final stages of maturation. The nucleus usually is eccentrically placed. Although the nucleus sometimes appears as several distinct nuclei in biopsy sections, it remains highly lobulated but single at all stages of megakaryocyte development. In occasional marrow sections (Fig. 113–4C), neutrophils or other marrow cells are seen transiting through the cytoplasm of the mature megakaryocyte, a process termed *emperipolesis*, and is of no pathologic significance.

Proplatelet Formation

Careful microscopic studies have localized marrow megakaryocytes to the abluminal surface of sinusoidal endothelial cells. In specially prepared specimens, the megakaryocytes can be seen issuing long, slender cytoplasmic processes between endothelial cells and into the sinusoidal lumen, structures termed *proplatelet processes* (Fig. 113–5).[53] The processes have been reproduced *in vitro* and *in vivo*.[6] The processes consist of a β-tubulin cytoskeleton and highway, transporting organelles and platelet constituents from the megakaryocyte to the terminal projection, the nascent platelet.[17]

Membrane Composition

Most of the specific characteristics of platelet membranes are present at stages III and IV of megakaryocyte development. Megakaryocyte membrane lipid composition progressively changes through development, achieving approximately four times the content of phospholipids and cholesterol as found in immature cells. Megakaryocytes contain about the same amounts of membrane neutral and phospholipid as platelets, but contain relatively more phosphatidylinositol and less phosphatidylserine and arachidonic acid.

Regulation of Gene Expression

One transcription factor that plays an important role in the final stages of megakaryocyte maturation is NF-E2. Initially described as an erythroid-specific, heterodimeric protein belonging to the basic leucine zipper family of transcription factors, NF-E2 is composed of a ubiquitously expressed p18 subunit, and a 45 kDA protein (p45) expressed only in erythroid cells and megakaryocytes.[54,55] NF-E2 binds to tandem AP-1–like motifs, such as those seen in the second deoxyribonuclease (DNAse) hypersensitive site of the β-globin locus control region, and is required for β-globin expression.[56] However, genetic elimination of p45 failed to significantly affect erythropoiesis. Rather, p45-deficient mice display prominent alterations in megakaryocyte development and severe thrombocytopenia,[57] leading to death from widespread hemorrhage soon after birth. Examination of the animals reveals modest expansion of marrow megakaryocytes but failure of the cells to produce platelets because of defects in cytoplasmic maturation, including substantial reductions in platelet granules and demarcation membranes.

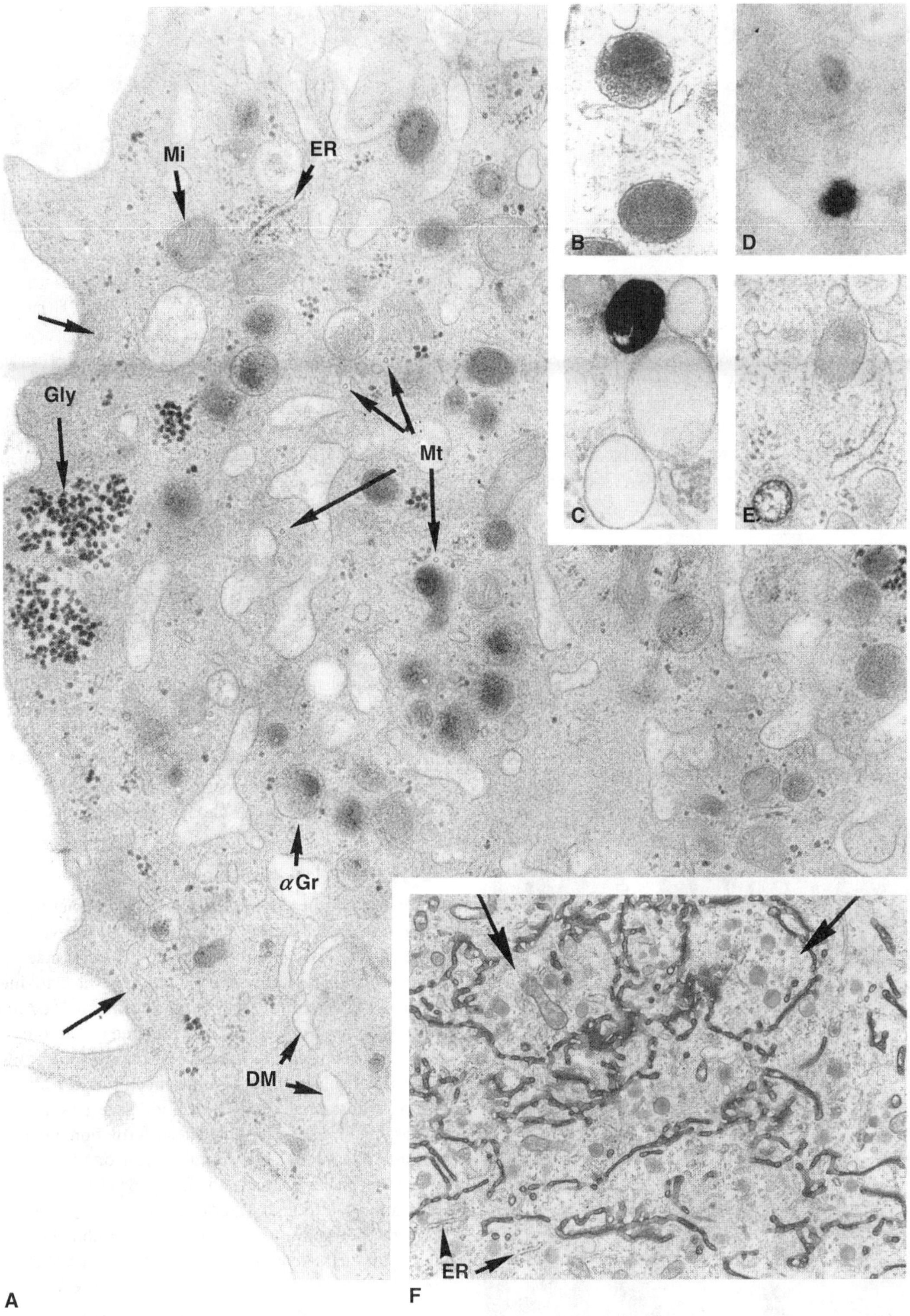

FIGURE 113–3. **A.** Ultrastructure of the cytoplasm of a mature megakaryocyte. The majority of the granules are α granules (αGr) exhibiting dense nucleoid. Demarcation membranes (DM) are slightly dilated. Transverse sections of microtubules (Mt) are dispersed. At the periphery, a longitudinal microtubule runs under the cell membrane (*arrows*). Dense aggregates of glycogen (Gly), small cisternae of endoplasmic reticulum (ER), and free ribosomes are seen (magnification ×30,320). **B.** Morphology of an α granule. Dense nucleoid is located at the *top*. In a clear zone at the opposite pole, four transverse sections of tubular structures are adjacent to the granule membrane (magnification ×37,200). **C.** Dense body can be distinguished from α granule by the black deposit when calcium is added to the fixative (magnification ×37,200). **D.** Cytochemical detection of acid phosphatase using β-glycophosphate as substrate and cerium as a trapping agent. Dense cerium–phosphate precipitates are present in lysosomal granules, whereas α granules are unreactive (magnification ×37,200). **E.** Microperoxisome visualized using alkaline diaminobenzidine. Note the small size of a reactive granule compared to the α granule. **F.** Distribution of a dense tracer filling the lumen of the demarcation membrane system in a maturing megakaryocyte (*arrows*). In contrast to the demarcation membrane system, which is open to the extracellular space, the endoplasmic reticulum (ER) is not labeled (magnification ×9700). *(Courtesy of Dr. Janine Breton-Gorius.)*

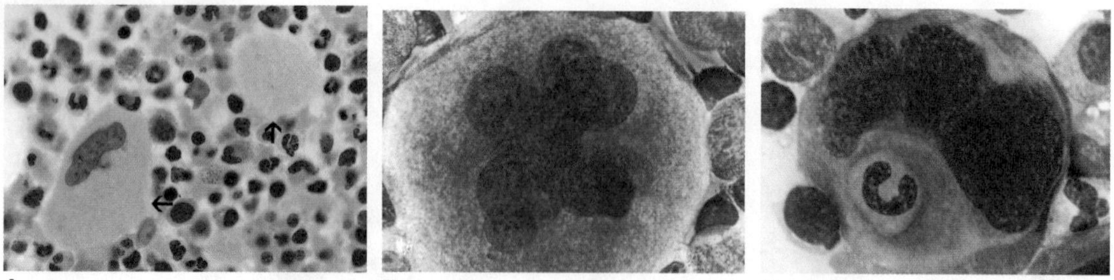

FIGURE 113–4. Megakaryocyte morphology. **A.** Normal human marrow biopsy. Two megakaryocytes are evident. In one case the section is through the cell at the level of the nuclei (*horizontal arrow*), and in the other it is through the cytoplasm above or below the nucleus (*vertical arrow*). **B.** Normal human marrow aspirate. Mature (stage III) megakaryocyte with a multilobated nucleus and abundant cytoplasm. **C.** Normal human marrow aspirate. Mature megakaryocyte with a neutrophil embedded in the cytoplasm. Many ultrastructural studies have confirmed that this appearance represents marrow cells entering the canalicular system of megakaryocyte cytoplasm through its opening to the exterior of the cell (emperipolesis). *(Used with permission from* Lichtman's Atlas of Hematology, *www.accessmedicine.com.)*

Thus, the loss of either GATA-1 or NF-E2 results in failure of late aspects of cellular maturation. As p45 NF-E2 is induced by GATA-1/FOG,[58] the lack of cytoplasmic development in GATA-deficient mice likely is an indirect effect.

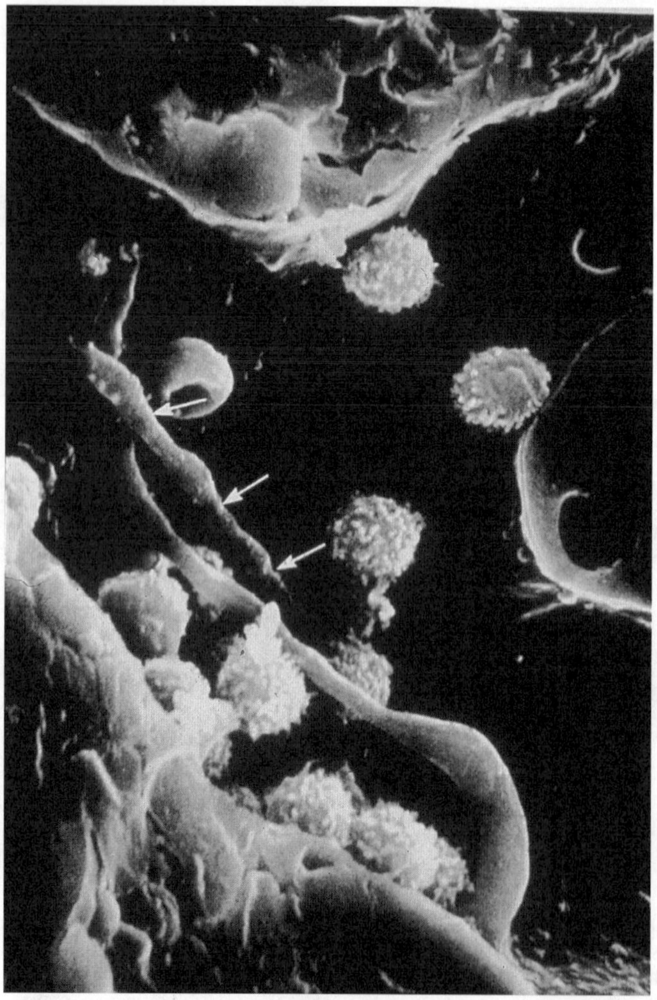

FIGURE 113–5. Megakaryocyte proplatelet processes in the marrow sinusoid. Scanning electron micrograph showing the luminal view of the confluence of two marrow sinusoids with two proplatelet processes protruding through the lining endothelial cells. One of the processes has intermittent constrictions (*arrows*), indicating potential sites for platelet formation. Other cells depicted include lymphocytes and erythrocytes (magnification ×3000). *(From Becker RP, De Bruyn P,[54] with permission.)*

Nearly all studies of megakaryopoiesis have focused on the marrow. The final stages of megakaryocyte fragmentation also are proposed to occur in the lung, at least for some cells, a theory based on the finding that platelet levels in pulmonary venous blood exceed those found in the pulmonary artery.[59] Whether this process represents the migration and fragmentation of intact megakaryocytes in the lung or merely the final size reduction of large fragments of megakaryocyte cytoplasm that also are released into the blood is not clear. Some data exist supporting the notion that lung megakaryocytes contribute to blood platelet production.[60] However, in mice administered high doses of thrombopoietin, with platelet counts as high as 4 million/μm^3, neither intact megakaryocytes nor denuded nuclei were found in the lungs of these animals.[61] One study found that canine lungs contain 2.5 megakaryocytes per cm^2.[62] Extrapolation of these data suggest human lungs contain approximately 6000 megakaryocytes, only enough to account for a small proportion (<0.1%) of daily platelet production.

PLATELET FORMATION

Numerous studies have indicated thrombopoietin is the primary regulator of megakaryocyte maturation.[36,63] However, despite the importance of the hormone for generation of fully mature megakaryocytes from which platelets arise, elimination of the cytokine during the final stages of platelet formation is not detrimental.[64] Although proplatelet formation is possible under serum-free conditions,[65] most investigators have reported the presence of plasma and/or an integrin ligand-containing substratum (e.g., fibronectin or vitronectin) stimulates the process substantially.[64,66] These findings suggest external signals probably are required for normal platelet formation. One report suggests the thrombin–antithrombin complex with or without high-density lipoprotein particles mediates the favorable effect of plasma on proplatelet formation,[67] although other data suggest prothrombin and its conversion to thrombin by megakaryocytes inhibit the process.[68] Although the cytokine(s) required for this process is not known, activation of protein kinase C-α clearly is necessary for the process to occur.[66]

Platelet formation involves massive reorganization of megakaryocyte cytoskeletal components, including actin and tubulin, during a highly active, motile process in which the termini of the process branch and issue platelets.[5] The size of the individual platelets formed is of interest. Unfortunately, little is known about this aspect of platelet formation except that tubulin is proposed to act as a measuring device for the proper site to pinch off platelets from proplatelet processes. The mechanism of platelet formation clearly must be affected in some way by the transcription factor GATA-1, the glycoprotein Ib-IX complex, the Wiskott-Aldrich syndrome protein, and platelet myosin, as defects in each of these genes leads to unusually large or small platelets (see Chap.

119).[69,70] Finally, localized cytoplasmic membrane proteolysis, a sublethal form of apoptosis, likely plays a role in initiating the final stages of platelet formation.[71]

EXTRINSIC REGULATION OF MEGAKARYOCYTE PRODUCTION

HORMONES AND CYTOKINES

Several cytokines, first identified using alternate hematopoietic activity assays, affect megakaryocyte development. IL-3, granulocyte-macrophage colony-stimulating factor, and stem cell factor support the proliferation of megakaryocytic progenitors in plasma-containing cultures.[72–74] In 1994, several groups reported the purification and/or cloning of thrombopoietin.[75] This cytokine clearly is the primary regulator of megakaryopoiesis but cannot explain thrombopoiesis in its entirety.

Interleukin-3

IL-3 is a 25- to 30-kDa protein produced almost exclusively by T lymphocytes.[76] The mature human protein contains 133 amino acids, but N-linked carbohydrate modification accounts for the larger than expected Mr of the cytokine. Granulocyte-macrophage colony-stimulating factor is an 18- to 30-kDa protein also produced by T lymphocytes. However, endothelial cells, monocytes, and fibroblasts also produce the protein and, like IL-3, granulocyte-macrophage colony-stimulating factor is highly modified with both N-linked and O-linked carbohydrate.[77] Although the two proteins display essentially no primary sequence homology, their tertiary structures are highly related,[78] and the receptors for the two cytokines share a common subunit.[79] However, the physiologic relevance of IL-3 and granulocyte-macrophage colony-stimulating factor for steady-state thrombopoiesis is uncertain. Administration of the cytokines to mice or humans has only minimal effects on thrombopoiesis, and genetic elimination of either has no impact on megakaryopoiesis, even when combined with elimination of other thrombopoietic cytokines.[80,81]

IL-6 and Related Cytokines

IL-6, cloned by several groups using multiple assays (hepatocyte growth, myeloma cell growth, immunoglobulin secretion, antiviral activity), enhances megakaryocyte maturation. IL-6 is a 26-kDa polypeptide produced by T lymphocytes, fibroblasts, macrophages, and stromal cells in response to inflammatory stimuli.[82] The mature protein is composed of 184 amino acids, contains two disulfide bonds, and displays both N-linked and O-linked carbohydrate modification. Although IL-6 alone fails to affect *in vitro* megakaryopoiesis, it augments the number of megakaryocyte colonies obtained in the presence of IL-3 or stem cell factor[83] and exerts primarily a differentiating effect.[84,85] Administration of IL-6 to mice or nonhuman primates or patients results in a modest thrombocytosis.[86–88] These findings suggest IL-6 contributes to megakaryopoiesis *in vivo*, a conclusion supported by its production by tumor cells in selected cases of paraneoplastic thrombocytosis.[89] However, genetic elimination of the cytokine fails to significantly affect basal platelet production.[90] Evidence suggests the cytokine affects platelet production indirectly[91] by stimulating thrombopoietin production.

IL-6 acts through a heterodimeric receptor, composed of a signaling subunit, termed GP130, and an affinity-converting subunit, termed IL-6Rα. GP130 also acts as the signaling subunit for several other cytokines, including IL-11 and leukemia inhibitory factor. Therefore, the finding that these cytokines also stimulate megakaryopoiesis in a manner similar to that of IL-6 is not surprising. IL-11 and leukemia inhibitory factor act in synergy with IL-3 or stem cell factor to augment megakaryocyte formation. IL-11 is a 23-kDa polypeptide, initially cloned from a gibbon marrow stromal cell line, whose activity can support the proliferation of an IL-6 responsive myeloma cell line.[92,93] Leukemia inhibitory factor displays a wide range of activities,[94] including (1) inducing the acute phase hepatic response, (2) inducing an adrenergic-to-cholinergic switch in neurons, (3) inhibiting lipoprotein lipase in adipocytes, and (4) maintaining pluripotentiality in embryonic cells.

Like IL-6, IL-11 and leukemia inhibitory factor enhance megakaryocytic maturation *in vitro*[95,96] and augment the effects of IL-3 and stem cell factor on primitive hematopoietic cells. Consistent with the *in vitro* findings, administration of either recombinant IL-11 or leukemia inhibitory factor to rodents, nonhuman primates, or humans produces modest thrombocytosis.[97–100] Despite the *in vitro* and *in vivo* findings, genetic elimination of either leukemia inhibitory factor or the IL-11 receptor has no effect on thrombopoiesis,[101] even when combined with elimination of the thrombopoietin receptor.[102]

Stem Cell Factor

In contrast to the hematopoietic cytokine family, stem cell factor is more closely related to other hematopoietic proteins that utilize protein tyrosine kinase receptors, such as macrophage colony-stimulating factor and the flt-3 ligand.[103] Nevertheless, stem cell factor stimulates megakaryocyte colony growth when used in combination with other cytokines.[104] Moreover, genetic elimination of its receptor *c-kit* reduces megakaryocyte production[105] and the rebound thrombocytosis that occurs following immunosuppressive therapy.[106,107]

Stem cell factor was first identified using several different biologic assays (in addition to this term, the cytokine has been dubbed *c-kit* ligand, mast cell growth factor, and steel factor).[108] Later studies indicate the cytokine acts primarily on primitive cells of the hematopoietic, melanogenic, and germ cell lineages. Stem cell factor is a dimeric protein composed of two identical noncovalently linked polypeptides. The soluble form monomer contains 165 residues,[109] derived by proteolytic cleavage of a membrane-bound splice form of the molecule.[110] The membrane bound form is more active than the soluble cytokine, as intracellular signaling in response to membrane-bound stem cell factor is prolonged in receptor-bearing cells.[111] Moreover, a naturally occurring mutant allele of the gene (Sl^d), which allows production of the soluble but not the membrane-bound form of the cytokine, results in a phenotype nearly identical to deletion of the entire locus,[112] again pointing to the importance of the membrane-bound form present on marrow stromal cells.

FLT-3 Ligand

The flt-3 ligand initially was identified as a ligand for a novel member of the protein tyrosine kinase family of receptors.[103] This growth factor also affects megakaryocyte formation. Like stem cell factor, to which it is most closely related, flt-3 ligand is found in both soluble and membrane-bound forms, is a noncovalently linked dimer, and affects primarily primitive hematopoietic cells.[113] Although several studies have shown that flt-3 ligand used alone does not support megakaryocyte colony formation, some studies suggest it works in synergy with other megakaryocyte stimulatory agents to augment the proliferation of megakaryocytic progenitor cells in culture.[114,115] Administration of flt-3 ligand to mice expands the number of marrow and splenic progenitor cells that can give rise to megakaryocytes *in vitro*.[116] However, genetic elimination of either flt-3 ligand or its receptor does not produce a platelet phenotype.

Thrombopoietin

The term *thrombopoietin* was first coined in 1958 to describe the primary regulator of platelet production.[117] A major impetus to the discovery of thrombopoietin in 1986 was the identification of the myeloproliferative leukemia virus (MPLV), which induces a vast expansion of hematopoietic cells.[118] The responsible viral oncogene was characterized in 1990,[119] and its cellular homologue c-*Mpl* was cloned in 1992.[120] Based on the presence of two copies of the hematopoietic cytokine receptor motif[121] and the ability of a fusion of cMpl and the IL-4 receptor to signal in factor dependent cells,[122] c-*Mpl* clearly encoded a growth factor receptor, but its ligand was not known. Using three distinct strategies, four separate groups were able to clone complementary DNA for the corresponding hormone and report their results in 1994 (reviewed in ref. 75). The gene for thrombopoietin encodes a 36-kDa polypeptide,[123] which also is predicted to be extensively posttranslationally modified, resulting in an approximately 50- to 70-kDa protein.

Thrombopoietin bears striking homology to erythropoietin, the primary regulator of erythropoiesis, within the amino-terminal half of the predicted polypeptide. The two proteins are more closely related than any other two cytokines within the hematopoietic cytokine family, sharing 20 percent identical amino acids, an additional 25 percent conservative substitutions, and identical positions of three of the four cysteine residues. Unlike any of the other cytokines in the family, thrombopoietin contains a 181-residue carboxyl-terminal extension, which bears homology to no known proteins. Two functions have been assigned to this region: it prolongs the circulatory half-life of the hormone,[3] and it aids in its secretion from the cells that normally synthesize the hormone.[124]

The biologic activities of thrombopoietin have been demonstrated *in vitro* and *in vivo*, in mice, rats, dogs, nonhuman primates, and man. Incubation of marrow cells with thrombopoietin stimulates megakaryocyte survival and proliferation, alone and in combination with other cytokines.[34] *In vivo*, thrombopoietin stimulates platelet production in a log-linear manner to levels 10-fold higher than baseline[3,61,125] without affecting the blood red or white cell counts. In addition, because of its affect on hematopoietic stem cells (see Chap. 16), the number of erythroid and myeloid progenitors and mixed myeloid progenitors in marrow and spleen also are increased,[126,127] an effect that is particularly impressive when the hormone is administered following myelosuppressive therapy.[126,128,129] This effect likely results from the synergy between thrombopoietin and the other hematopoietic cytokines circulating at high levels in this condition.

Based on genetic studies, thrombopoietin clearly is the primary regulator of thrombopoiesis. Elimination of either the c-*Mpl* or *Tpo* gene leads to profound thrombocytopenia in mice as a result of a greatly reduced number of megakaryocyte progenitors, mature megakaryocytes, and the reduced polyploidy of the remaining megakaryocytes.[130] A similar result occurs in humans. Patients with congenital amegakaryocytic thrombocytopenia (CAMT) display numerous homozygous or mixed heterozygous nonsense or severe missense mutations of the thrombopoietin receptor *c-Mpl* (see Chap. 119).[131,132] The effect of thrombopoietin on hematopoietic stem cells is particularly revealed by consideration of children with CAMT. Within 5 years of birth, nearly every patient with CAMT develops aplastic anemia as a result of stem cell exhaustion.

The thrombopoietin gene displays an unusual 5′ flanking structure. Unlike the majority of genes that initiate translation of the encoded polypeptide with the first ATG codon present in the messenger ribonucleic acid (mRNA), thrombopoietin translation initiates at the eighth ATG codon located within the third exon of a full-length transcript.[133] However, since the eighth ATG of thrombopoietin mRNA is embedded in the short, open reading frame of the seventh ATG, its translation is particularly inefficient because of the mechanism of ribosomal initiation.[134] As such, little thrombopoietin protein is produced for any given amount of mRNA. Although this molecular arrangement has no known physiologic consequences, it forms the basis for an unusual form of disease, a disorder of translation efficiency. Four cases of autosomal dominant familial thrombocytosis have been linked to mutations in the region surrounding the initiation codon. In two families, a single mutation in different nucleotides of the intron 3 splice donor sequence results in alternate splicing of the primary thrombopoietin transcript, eliminating the seventh and eighth ATG codons, creating a new amino-terminus by fusing of the fifth open reading frame with the thrombopoietin coding sequence. This novel thrombopoietin mRNA is efficiently translated, resulting in supraphysiologic levels of hormone production and nonclonal expansion of thrombopoiesis.[135,136] In another mutant thrombopoietin allele, deletion of a single nucleotide within the seventh open reading frame leads to its fusion with the thrombopoietin coding sequence and now enhanced translation of thrombopoietin from the seventh ATG codon.[137] A fourth mutation has been described within the seventh open reading frame, leading to premature termination of that short peptide, preventing its interference with translation initiation from the usual eighth initiation codon,[138] again enhancing thrombopoietin production (reviewed in ref. 139). Of note, while reactive thrombocytosis is not thought to lead to hypercoagulability (see Chap. 120), several patients in these pedigrees developed thromboses, raising the physiologic question of why should chronic stimulation of platelets with enhanced levels of thrombopoietin lead to hypercoagulability.

The physiologic regulation of thrombopoietin production has received much attention. Experimental induction of immune-mediated thrombocytopenia results in relatively rapid restoration of platelet levels, followed by a brief period of rebound thrombocytosis.[140] In these experimental cases and in most naturally occurring cases of thrombocytopenia, plasma hormone concentrations vary inversely with platelet counts, rising to maximal levels within 24 hours of onset of profound thrombocytopenia.[141] Two nonmutually exclusive models have been advanced to explain these findings. In the first model, thrombopoietin production is constitutive, but its consumption, and hence the level remaining in the blood to affect megakaryopoiesis, is determined by the mass of c-Mpl receptors present on platelets and megakaryocytes accessible to the plasma.[142] In this way, states of thrombocytosis result in increased thrombopoietin consumption (by the expanded platelet mass of c-Mpl receptors), reducing megakaryopoiesis. Conversely, thrombocytopenia reduces blood thrombopoietin destruction, resulting in elevated blood levels of the hormone that drive megakaryopoiesis and platelet recovery. This model is based on one of the mechanisms regulating macrophage colony-stimulating factor levels.[143] The invariable levels of thrombopoietin-specific mRNA present in the liver and kidney of experimental animals and patients with thrombocytopenia or thrombocytosis support this model.[144,145] Moreover, thrombopoietin knockout mice display a gene dosage effect.[146] Platelet levels in heterozygous mice are intermediate between that seen in wild-type and nullizygous animals, suggesting active regulation of the remaining thrombopoietin allele cannot compensate for the mild (60% of normal) thrombocytopenia induced by the loss of one allele.

A second model suggests thrombopoietin expression is a regulated event. Very low platelet levels can induce thrombopoietin-specific mRNA production. Several studies show that thrombopoietin mRNA levels are modulated in response to moderate to severe thrombocytopenia, at least in the marrow.[145,147] The signal(s) responsible for this form of thrombopoietin regulation is being uncovered, but is, at least in part, mediated by transcriptional enhancement.[148] CD40 ligand, platelet-derived growth factor, fibroblast growth factor, TGF-β, platelet factor-4, and thrombospondin modulate thrombopoietin production from marrow stromal cells.[149,150]

The human thrombopoietin gene 5′ flanking region lacks a TATA box or CAAT motif and directs transcription initiation at multiple sites over a 50-nucleotide region.[151] Reporter gene analysis in a hepatocyte cell line identified an Ets2 transcription factor-binding motif responsible for high-level expression of the gene. The 5′ flanking region also includes SP-1, AP-2, and nuclear factor-κB binding sites,[152] although the contribution of these transcription factors to thrombopoietin gene expression, either under steady-state or inflammatory conditions, has not been studied.

Stromal Cell-Derived Factor-1

Chemokines are members of a rapidly growing class of molecules that play multiple roles in blood cell physiology.[153] Initially defined as substances that induce leukocyte chemotaxis, four classes of the 8- to 12-kDa polypeptides have been recognized, based on the spacing of cysteine residues close to the amino-terminus of the proteins. An equally rapidly growing family of chemokine receptors also has been discovered, classified by the subfamily of chemokines they serve. All chemokine receptors are members of the seven-transmembrane family of receptors that signal through heterotrimeric G proteins.

Most work has been conducted with the CC and CXC subfamilies of chemokines, molecules that display modest inhibitory effects on cell proliferation when used alone and potent effects when used in combination on hematopoietic progenitors at all levels of development.[154] On many levels, the CXC chemokine SDF-1 and its receptor CXCR4 are notable exceptions to the many features shared by most members of the chemokine and chemokine receptor families. For example, although all the other genes for the known CXC chemokines reside on the long arm of human chromosome 14, SDF-1 localizes to the long arm of chromosome 10.[155] Moreover, most chemokine receptors can be activated by multiple ligands. For example, the chemokine MIP (macrophage inflammatory protein)-1α can bind and activate CCR1 and CCR5, and IL-8 can bind both CXCR1 and CXCR2.[156] In contrast, as the phenotype of genetic elimination of both CXCR4 and SDF-1 are almost identical,[157,158] CXCR4 appears to be the only receptor for SDF-1, and SDF-1 is the only ligand for CXCR4.

The marrow stroma is the primary source of SDF-1, and most of the cell types known to express CXCR4 are hematopoietic in origin. One of the major phenotypes in SDF-1– or CXCR4-deficient neonatal mice is marrow aplasia, thought to be secondary to failure of perinatal hematopoietic stem cell homing (see Chap. 16).[159] In addition, megakaryocytes display CXCR4[160] and migrate in response to an SDF-1 concentration gradient.[161] Several groups have shown that SDF-1 augments thrombopoietin-induced megakaryocyte growth in suspension culture.[37,160] Later studies have shown the synergy between SDF-1 and other stimuli on megakaryocyte growth extends to cell surface adhesion.[38]

Transforming Growth Factor-β

In addition to the many positive regulators of megakaryopoiesis, several substances down-modulate their development. Five isoforms of TGF-β have been identified, all disulfide-linked homodimers each containing 112 residues.[162] TGF-β_1 is the predominant type of TGF found in hematopoietic tissues. Platelet α granules are a particularly rich source of the cytokine. In general, transforming growth factors are inhibitors of hematopoiesis,[163,164] particularly of megakaryocyte development.[165,166] The best understood TGF-β growth inhibitory effects are exerted on cell-cycle progression. After binding to one of five receptors, two pathways that block cell cycle progression are activated. pRb is hypophosphorylated,[167] antagonizing the effects of G_1 phase cyclin-dependent kinases, and cell-cycle inhibitors, including p27 and $p15^{INK}$, are upregulated, affecting cell-cycle progression.[168,169] In contrast to these negative effects of TGF-β on cell proliferation, the cytokine enhances megakaryocyte differentiation.

INTERFERON-α

A second class of cytokines that negatively impact thrombopoiesis are the interferons (IFNs), proteins first defined by their ability to induce an antiviral state in mammalian cells.[170] Biochemical fractionation has revealed three classes of IFNs: IFN-α, a family of 17 distinct but highly homologous molecules; IFN-β, a single molecule more distantly related to the various isoforms of IFN-α; and IFN-γ, a unique molecule that shares functional properties but not structure with the others. IFNs exert profound inhibitory effects on hematopoiesis.[171]

The genes for the IFN-α/β subfamily cluster on the short arm of chromosome 9 and encode 165- to 172-residue polypeptides, of which 35 percent are invariant across the family of IFN-α molecules. IFNs of the α/β type are produced by transcriptional upregulation in fibroblasts and leukocytes in response to viruses and other infectious agents and to inflammatory cytokines. Once bound to the IFN receptors, a cascade of kinases and intracellular mediators are triggered, initiated by JAKs (Janus family kinases), STAT (signal transducer and activator of transcription) factors, and p38 MAPK (see Chap. 14), resulting in changes in gene transcription.

IFN-α inhibits megakaryopoiesis, the clinical use of which is responsible for modest to severe thrombocytopenia in a significant number of patients undergoing therapy for chronic viral hepatitis.[172,173] The mechanisms responsible for the inhibitory effect of IFN-α are multifactorial. Some studies suggest a direct inhibitory effect of IFN-α on growth factor-induced proliferation pathways. For example, the cytokine augments double-stranded RNA-activated protein kinase activity, inhibiting translation initiation factor-2, implicating reduction of the growth factor-induced protein synthesis necessary for growth factor response.[174] IFN-β induces expression of the cell-cycle inhibitor $p27^{kip1}$, arresting cells in G_0/G_1.[175] Other studies have demonstrated IFN-α induces a SOCS (suppressor of cytokine signaling)-1–based feedback mechanism that cross-reacts and depresses thrombopoietin signaling.[176] Thus, in addition to the multiple positive mediators of megakaryopoiesis, several cytokines block the process and can lead to thrombocytopenia.

MEGAKARYOCYTE MICROENVIRONMENT

Chapter 4 details the role of the marrow microenvironment in hematopoiesis. This chapter discusses only aspects particularly vital for megakaryocyte growth. The cellular concentration within the marrow is estimated to be 10^9/mL. Consequently, cell–cell and cell–matrix interactions will occur.[177] A particularly important interaction for thrombopoiesis is between the marrow sinusoidal endothelial cell and the mature megakaryocyte. Studies using *in situ* videomicroscopy indicate that proplatelet processes extend through the sinusoids into the vascular lumen, where the shear stress of flowing blood liberates single platelets.[6] Marrow stromal cells influence hematopoiesis in a number of other ways, perhaps the most prominent through production of several cytokines that positively or negatively affect megakaryocyte growth.[145,178–180] Stromal cells are the origin of a number of extracellular matrix proteins and glycomucins that either directly affect hematopoietic cells or indirectly affect hematopoietic cells by binding growth factors and presenting them in a functional context.[181,182] Stromal cells also bear ligands for Notch proteins, cell surface receptors that are critical mediators of cell fate decisions.[183] Notch and its ligands Delta and Jagged play important roles as regulators of hematopoietic progenitor cell proliferation[184] and play a potential role in influencing the lineage fate choice between erythropoiesis and megakaryopoiesis.[185] Cell–cell interactions mediated by integrins present on hematopoietic cells and counterreceptors on stromal cells are very important for megakaryopoiesis,[186] both by bringing hematopoietic cells into close proximity to stromal cells producing soluble or cell-bound cytokines and more directly by triggering or augmenting intracellular signaling, promoting entry into the cell cycle, and preventing programmed cell death.

THERAPEUTIC MANIPULATION OF THROMBOPOIESIS BY NATURALLY OCCURRING CYTOKINES

Thrombocytopenia is a major clinical problem with multiple origins (see Chap. 119). Primary marrow diseases, certain infections, and solid tumors with a high propensity for marrow metastases directly affect platelet production. Nearly all leukemias, advanced lymphomas, and myelomas ultimately cause thrombocytopenia by this mechanism. Hypersplenism and thrombopoietin deficiency contribute to platelet sequestration and reduced platelet production in patients with hepatic failure. Consumptive coagulopathies, initiated by infection, tumors, or severe injury, can be responsible for severe thrombocytopenia. In other patients, autoimmune thrombocytopenia arises during the course of disease or is a primary disease. However, the most common cause of significant thrombocytopenia is iatrogenic: the use of potentially curative or palliative chemotherapy or radiation therapy in patients with malignancy. An estimated 300,000+ persons yearly worldwide undergo courses of chemotherapy adequate to produce clinically significant thrombocytopenia. Recovery from the marrow suppressive effects of most chemotherapeutic agents occurs within 1 to 3 weeks following discontinuation of therapy. However, some agents, including mitomycin C or nitrosoureas, can produce prolonged periods of marrow suppression. Moreover, the widespread use of IFN-α for chronic hepatitis C infection adds large numbers of patients who experience thrombocytopenia as a dose-limiting toxicity. Tumor- or treatment-related thrombocytopenia often delays much needed additional therapy, may necessitate potentially complicated platelet transfusions (see Chap. 141), and cause significant morbidity and occasional mortality. Given the increased understanding of the humoral basis for megakaryopoiesis and thrombopoiesis, numerous attempts have been made to manipulate these processes for therapeutic benefit.

INTERLEUKIN-11

IL-11 augments the growth of megakaryocytic progenitors in the presence of IL-3[187,188] and acts to promote megakaryocyte maturation rather than proliferation.[189,190] The preclinical effects of IL-11 were evaluated in mice, rats, and subhuman primates and revealed moderate activity in normal animals and following cytoreductive therapy.[98,191,192]

The first clinical trials of IL-11 were reported in abstract form in 1993 and 1994.[193,194] Randomized clinical trials were reported a few years later.[195–197] Most studies reported IL-11 ameliorated drug-induced thrombocytopenia. For example, IL-11 administered to patients with advanced stages of breast cancer undergoing multiple courses of anthracycline-based chemotherapy significantly reduced the need for platelet transfusions by 27 percent. However, use of the drug in patients undergoing autologous stem cell transplantation did not enhance platelet recovery or other indices of hematopoiesis. Although chemical evidence of an acute-phase response was noted in many of the patients treated in these studies, the drug was generally well tolerated, even though fluid retention has been a significant side effect, often necessitating concomitant use of diuretics. IL-11 (oprelvekin, Neumega) was approved by the Food and Drug Administration in 1998 for use in patients undergoing chemotherapy who have evidence of previous drug-induced thrombocytopenia (see Chap. 119).

INTERFERON-α

As noted earlier in this chapter (see "Hormones and Cytokines" above), IFN suppresses hematopoiesis and thrombopoiesis by multiple mechanisms. As a consequence, IFN-α has been used to reduce platelet counts in patients with many forms of myeloproliferative disease. The first reported clinical trial was performed in patients with a mixture of these disorders. The trial found the mean platelet count decreased significantly from 1050×10^9/L to 340×10^9/L.[198] Long-term therapy with IFN also was shown to be effective and safe.[199] From these and other studies, IFN (2–5 million units 3 times per week) clearly effectively reduces the platelet count toward normal in most patients with myeloproliferative disease. More aggressive regimens (2–6 million units daily) result in complete hematologic remissions but with no evidence that the clonal disorder responsible has been affected.[200] Not surprisingly, reduced energy level, weight loss, myalgia, and depression have been consistently reported, forcing discontinuation of the drug in approximately one-third of patients taking low to moderate doses of various forms of IFN-α.[201] Of some concern and possibly related to its effects on the immune system, a significant number of patients treated with IFN for thrombocytosis have developed antibodies to the administered drug, with subsequent reduced efficacy.[202]

THROMBOPOIETIN

Clinically, the most important activity of thrombopoietin likely is its effects on megakaryopoiesis, potentially ameliorating the thrombocytopenia that occurs in natural and iatrogenic states of marrow failure. In this regard, a number of promising results in preclinical trials of the cytokine were reported.[126,128,129,203] In general, in rodent, dog, and nonhuman primates, almost every model of myelosuppression or immune-mediated platelet destruction has responded favorably to parenteral administration of thrombopoietin. In addition to the favorable effects on platelet recovery, many of these studies also reported enhanced recovery or hematopoietic progenitors of all lineages, accelerated recovery of erythrocytes or leukocytes, or both. The only exception to these generally favorable results has been reported in animal models of stem cell transplantation, where negligible to minimal acceleration of blood cell recovery was found, unless the stem cell donor was treated with the hormone.[204,205]

A number of clinical trials in patients with cancer undergoing cytotoxic therapy have been conducted. Results were varied, with the hormone helpful in many patients,[206–208] but not in all clinical situations.[209,210] In general, the hormone has been useful in patients who were administered moderately aggressive chemotherapeutic regimens that produce clinically important thrombocytopenia. However, the hormone has not been helpful in the setting of high-dose, prolonged cytotoxic therapy, as in the treatment of acute myelogenous leukemia, or in stem cell transplantation, unless, as in the animal studies, it is administered to the stem cell donor.[211] Thrombopoietin also reportedly increases platelet levels in patients with immune-mediated thrombocytopenia.[212] The timing of drug administration can significantly impact both the total amount of drug required and its efficacy.[213] For example, administration of one dose of drug before and once following myelosuppressive therapy was as effective as any other multidose regimen. This regimen resulted in significant reductions in nadir platelet counts and the need for platelet transfusion during chemotherapy cycles supplemented with thrombopoietin. Nevertheless, use of a modified form of recombinant thrombopoietin is associated with antibody formation to the drug, which cross-reacts with and neutralizes the native hormone, resulting in thrombocytopenia.[214] Although this effect has not been reported with a nonmodified recombinant thrombopoietin, most efforts using thrombopoietin in patients with thrombocytopenia are focusing on small peptide or organic mimics that bind to and activate the thrombopoietin receptor (reviewed in ref. 218).[215–217] Both types of thrombopoietin mimetic agents have been tested in clinical trials (see Chap. 119). Two lead indications have been tested; primary immune thrombocytopenia (ITP) and IFN-induced thrombocytopenia in patients being treated for chronic hepatitis C infection. The results of these trials have been very promising. For example, in a randomized control phase III clinical trial of a peptibody bearing 4 copies of a c-Mpl receptor stimulating peptide on an immunoglobulin scaffold, 84 percent of heavily pretreated patients with ITP responded to treatment, with rates being slightly lower or higher depending on whether they had previously undergone splenectomy.[219] Likewise, the administration of a small, orally available organic thrombopoietin mimetic to patients with ITP resulted in 81 percent of patients achieving a platelet count above 50 × 10^9/L.[220] These studies have led to FDA approval of the two thrombopoietin agonists for use in patients with ITP. The same molecule was administered to patients with modest hepatic insufficiency undergoing IFN/ribavirin therapy for hepatitis C; 75 percent of such patients were able to complete 3 months of therapy without IFN dose reduction, compared to 6 percent of patients given placebo.[221] Although these results require confirmation, it is clear that thrombopoietin mimetics will play an important role in the treatment of thrombocytopenia.

REFERENCES

1. Hanson SR, Slichter SJ: Platelet kinetics in patients with bone marrow hypoplasia: Evidence for a fixed platelet requirement. *Blood* 66:1105, 1985.
2. Dettke M, Hlousek M, Kurz M, et al: Increase in endogenous thrombopoietin in healthy donors after automated plateletpheresis. *Transfusion* 38:449, 1998.
3. Harker LA, Marzec UM, Hunt P, et al: Dose-response effects of pegylated human megakaryocyte growth and development factor on platelet production and function in nonhuman primates. *Blood* 88:511, 1996.
4. O'Malley CJ, Rasko JE, Basser RL, et al: Administration of pegylated recombinant human megakaryocyte growth and development factor to humans stimulates the production of functional platelets that show no evidence of *in vivo* activation. *Blood* 88:3288, 1996.
5. Italiano JE Jr, Lecine P, Shivdasani RA, Hartwig JH: Blood platelets are assembled principally at the ends of proplatelet processes produced by differentiated megakaryocytes. *J Cell Biol* 147:1299, 1999.
6. Junt T, Schulze H, Chen Z, et al. Dynamic visualization of thrombopoiesis within bone marrow. *Science* 317:1767, 2007.
7. Harker LA, Finch CA: Thrombokinetics in man. *J Clin Invest* 48:963, 1969.
8. Radley JM, Haller CJ: Fate of senescent megakaryocytes in the bone marrow. *Br J Haematol* 53:277, 1983.
9. Tronik-Le Roux D, Roullot V, Schweitzer A, et al: Suppression of erythro-megakaryocytopoiesis and the induction of reversible thrombocytopenia in mice transgenic for the thymidine kinase gene targeted by the platelet glycoprotein alpha IIb promoter. *J Exp Med* 181:2141, 1995.
10. Debili N, Robin C, Schiavon V, et al: Different expression of CD41 on human lymphoid and myeloid progenitors from adults and neonates. *Blood* 97:2023, 2001.
11. Wu G, Essex DW, Meloni FJ, et al: Human endothelial cells in culture and in vivo express on their surface all four components of the glycoprotein Ib/IX/V complex. *Blood* 90:2660, 1997.
12. Hickey MJ, Hagen FS, Yagi M, Roth GJ: Human platelet glycoprotein V: Characterization of the polypeptide and the related Ib-V-IX receptor system of adhesive, leucine-rich glycoproteins. *Proc Natl Acad Sci U S A* 90:8327, 1993.
13. Kahn ML, Diacovo TG, Bainton DF, et al: Glycoprotein V-deficient platelets have undiminished thrombin responsiveness and do not exhibit a Bernard-Soulier phenotype. *Blood* 94:4112, 1999.
14. Lopez JA, Andrews RK, Afshar-Kharghan V, Berndt MC: Bernard-Soulier syndrome. *Blood* 91:4397, 1998.
15. Ramakrishnan V, DeGuzman F, Bao M, et al: A thrombin receptor function for platelet glycoprotein Ib-IX unmasked by cleavage of glycoprotein V. *Proc Natl Acad Sci U S A* 98:1823, 2001.
16. Breton-Gorius J, Reyes F: Ultrastructure of human bone marrow cell maturation. *Int Rev Cytol* 46:251, 1976.
17. Italiano JE Jr, Shivdasani RA: Megakaryocytes and beyond: The birth of platelets. *J Thromb Haemost* 1:1174, 2003.
18. Ebbe S, Stohlman F Jr: Megakaryocytopoiesis in the rat. *Blood* 26:20, 1965.
19. Vitrat N, Cohen-Solal K, Pique C, et al: Endomitosis of human megakaryocytes are due to abortive mitosis. *Blood* 91:3711, 1998.
20. Odell TT Jr, Reiter RS: Generation cycle of rat megakaryocytes. *Exp Cell Res* 53:321, 1968.
21. Lemarchandel V, Ghysdael J, Mignotte V, et al: GATA and Ets *cis*-acting sequences mediate megakaryocyte-specific expression. *Mol Cell Biol* 13:668, 1993.
22. Bastian LS, Kwiatkowski BA, Breininger J, et al: Regulation of the megakaryocytic glycoprotein IX promoter by the oncogenic Ets transcription factor Fli-1. *Blood* 93:2637, 1999.
23. Ramachandran B, Surrey S, Schwartz E: Megakaryocyte-specific positive regulatory sequence 5′ to the human PF4 gene. *Exp Hematol* 23:49, 1995.
24. Furihata K, Kunicki TJ: Characterization of human glycoprotein VI gene 5′ regulatory and promoter regions. *Arterioscler Thromb Vasc Biol* 22:1733, 2002.
25. Sevinsky JR, Whalen AM, Ahn NG: Extracellular signal-regulated kinase induces the megakaryocyte GPIIb/CD41 gene through MafB/Kreisler. *Mol Cell Biol* 24:4534, 2004.
26. Rojnuckarin P, Drachman JG, Kaushansky K: Thrombopoietin-induced activation of the mitogen-activated protein kinase (MAPK) pathway in normal megakaryocytes: Role in endomitosis. *Blood* 94:1273, 1999.
27. Vyas P, Norris FA, Joseph R, et al: Inositol polyphosphate 4-phosphatase type I regulates cell growth downstream of transcription factor GATA-1. *Proc Natl Acad Sci U S A* 97:13696, 2000.
28. Pevny L, Simon MC, Robertson E, et al: Erythroid differentiation in chimaeric mice blocked by a targeted mutation in the gene for transcription factor GATA-1. *Nature* 349:257, 1991.
29. Shivdasani RA, Fujiwara Y, McDevitt MA, Orkin SH: A lineage-selective knockout establishes the critical role of transcription factor GATA-1 in megakaryocyte growth and platelet development. *EMBO J* 16:3965, 1997.
30. Song WJ, Sullivan MG, Legare RD, et al: Haploinsufficiency of CBFA2 causes familial thrombocytopenia with propensity to develop acute myelogenous leukaemia. *Nat Genet* 23:166, 1999.
31. Ichikawa M, Asai T, Saito T, et al: AML-1 is required for megakaryocytic maturation and lymphocytic differentiation, but not for maintenance of hematopoietic stem cells in adult hematopoiesis. *Nat Med* 10:299, 2004.
32. Elagib KE, Racke FK, Mogass M, et al: RUNX1 and GATA-1 coexpression and cooperation in megakaryocytic differentiation. *Blood* 101:4333, 2003.
33. Ebbe S, Phalen E, Stohlman F Jr: Abnormalities of megakaryocytes in W-WV mice. *Blood* 42:857, 1973.
34. Broudy VC, Lin NL, Kaushansky K: Thrombopoietin (c-mpl ligand) acts synergistically with erythropoietin, stem cell factor, and interleukin-11 to enhance murine megakaryocyte colony growth and increases megakaryocyte ploidy *in vitro*. *Blood* 85:1719, 1995.
35. Gainsford T, Roberts AW, Kimura S, et al: Cytokine production and function in c-mpl–deficient mice: No physiologic role for interleukin-3 in residual megakaryocyte and platelet production. *Blood* 91:2745, 1998.
36. Kaushansky K, Broudy VC, Lin N, et al: Thrombopoietin, the Mp1 ligand, is essential for full megakaryocyte development. *Proc Natl Acad Sci U S A* 92:3234, 1995.
37. Hodohara K, Fujii N, Yamamoto N, Kaushansky K: Stromal cell-derived factor-1 (SDF-1) acts together with thrombopoietin to enhance the development of megakaryocytic progenitor cells (CFU-MK). *Blood* 95:769, 2000.
38. Avecilla ST, Hattori K, Heissig B, et al: Chemokine-mediated interaction of hematopoietic progenitors with the bone marrow vascular niche is required for thrombopoiesis. *Nat Med* 10:64, 2004.
39. Geddis AE, Fox NE, Kaushansky K: Phosphatidylinositol 3-kinase is necessary but not sufficient for thrombopoietin-induced proliferation in engineered Mpl-bearing cell lines as well as in primary megakaryocytic progenitors. *J Biol Chem* 276:34473, 2001.
40. Miyazaki R, Ogata H, Kobayashi Y: Requirement of thrombopoietin-induced activation of ERK for megakaryocyte differentiation and of p38 for erythroid differentiation. *Ann Hematol* 80:284, 2001.
41. Pettiford SM, Herbst R: The protein tyrosine phosphatase HePTP regulates nuclear translocation of ERK2 and can modulate megakaryocytic differentiation of K562 cells. *Leukemia* 17:366, 2003.
42. Dorsey JF, Cunnick JM, Mane SM, Wu J: Regulation of the Erk2-Elk1 signaling pathway and megakaryocytic differentiation of Bcr-Abl(+) K562 leukemic cells by Gab2. *Blood* 99:1388, 2002.
43. Zhang Y, Nagata Y, Yu G, et al: Aberrant quantity and localization of Aurora-B/AIM-1 and survivin during megakaryocyte polyploidization and the consequences of Aurora-B/AIM-1-deregulated expression. *Blood* 103:3717, 2004.
44. Matsumura I, Tanaka H, Kawasaki A, et al: Increased D-type cyclin expression together with decreased cdc2 activity confers megakaryocytic differentiation of a human thrombopoietin-dependent hematopoietic cell line. *J Biol Chem* 275:5553, 2000.
45. Carow CE, Fox NE, Kaushansky K: Kinetics of endomitosis in primary murine megakaryocytes. *J Cell Physiol* 188:291, 2001.
46. Geddis AE, Kaushansky K: Megakaryocytes express functional aurora kinase B in endomitosis. *Blood 104:1017*, 2004.
47. Geddis AE, Fox NE, Tkachenko E, Kaushansky K. Endomitotic megakaryocytes that form a bipolar spindle exhibit cleavage furrow ingression followed by furrow regression. *Cell Cycle* 6:455, 2007.
48. Lordier L, Jalil A, Aurade F, et al: Megakaryocyte endomitosis is a failure of late cytokinesis related to defects in the contractile ring and Rho/Rock signaling. *Blood* 112:3164, 2008.
49. Seri M, Cusano R, Gangarossa S, et al: Mutations in MYH9 result in the May-Hegglin anomaly, and Fechtner and Sebastian syndromes. The May-Hegglin/Fechtner Syndrome Consortium. *Nat Genet* 26:103, 2000.
50. Hartwig J, Italiano J Jr: The birth of the platelet. *J Thromb Haemost* 1:1580, 2003.
51. Visvader JE, Elefanty AG, Strasser A, Adams JM: GATA-1 but not SCL induces megakaryocytic differentiation in an early myeloid line. *EMBO J* 11:4557, 1992.
52. Huizing M, Parkes JM, Helip-Wooley A, White JG, Gahl WA: Platelet alpha granules in BLOC-2 and BLOC-3 subtypes of Hermansky-Pudlak syndrome. *Platelets* 18:150, 2007.
53. Tavassoli M, Aoki M: Localization of megakaryocytes in the bone marrow. *Blood Cells* 15:3, 1989.
54. Becker RP, De Bruyn P: The transmural passage of blood cells into myeloid sinusoids and the entry of platelets into sinusoidal circulation; a scanning electron microscope investigation. *Am J Anat* 145:183–205, 1975.

55. Andrews NC, Erdjument-Bromage H, Davidson MB, et al: Erythroid transcription factor NF-E2 is a haematopoietic-specific basic-leucine zipper protein. *Nature* 362:722, 1993.
56. Bean TL, Ney PA: Multiple regions of p45 NF-E2 are required for beta-globin gene expression in erythroid cells. *Nucleic Acids Res* 25:2509, 1997.
57. Shivdasani RA, Rosenblatt MF, Zucker-Franklin D, et al: Transcription factor NF-E2 is required for platelet formation independent of the actions of thrombopoietin/MGDF in megakaryocyte development. *Cell* 81:695, 1995.
58. Querfurth E, Schuster M, Kulessa H, et al: Antagonism between C/EBPbeta and FOG in eosinophil lineage commitment of multipotent hematopoietic progenitors. *Genes Dev* 14:2515, 2000.
59. Howell WH DD: The production of blood platelets in the lungs. *J Exp Med* 65:177, 1939.
60. Slater DN, Trowbridge EA, Martin JF: The megakaryocyte in thrombocytopenia: A microscopic study which supports the theory that platelets are produced in the pulmonary circulation. *Thromb Res* 31:163, 1983.
61. Kaushansky K, Lok S, Holly RD, et al: Promotion of megakaryocyte progenitor expansion and differentiation by the c-Mpl ligand thrombopoietin. *Nature* 369:568, 1994.
62. Kaufman RM, Airo R, Pollack S, et al: Origin of pulmonary megakaryocytes. *Blood* 25:767, 1965.
63. Harker LA, Marzec UM, Kelly AB: Effects of Mpl ligands on platelet production and function in nonhuman primates. *Stem Cells* 16(Suppl 2):107, 1998.
64. Choi ES, Nichol JL, Hokom MM, et al: Platelets generated *in vitro* from proplatelet-displaying human megakaryocytes are functional. *Blood* 85:402, 1995.
65. Norol F, Vitrat N, Cramer E, et al: Effects of cytokines on platelet production from blood and marrow CD34+ cells. *Blood* 91:830, 1998.
66. Rojnuckarin P, Kaushansky K: Actin reorganization and proplatelet formation in murine megakaryocytes: The role of protein kinase C alpha. *Blood* 97:154, 2001.
67. Ishida Y, Yano K, Ito T, et al: Purification of proplatelet formation (PPF) stimulating factor: Thrombin/antithrombin III complex stimulates PPF of megakaryocytes in vitro and platelet production *in vivo*. *Thromb Haemost* 85:349, 2001.
68. Hunt P, Hokom MM, Wiemann B, et al: Megakaryocyte proplatelet-like process formation *in vitro* is inhibited by serum prothrombin, a process which is blocked by matrix-bound glycosaminoglycans. *Exp Hematol* 21:372, 1993.
69. Geddis AE, Kaushansky K: Inherited thrombocytopenias: Toward a molecular understanding of disorders of platelet production. *Curr Opin Pediatr* 16:15, 2004.
70. Eckly A, Strassel C, Freund M, et al: Abnormal megakaryocyte morphology and proplatelet formation in mice with megakaryocyte-restricted MYH9 inactivation. *Blood* 113(14):3182, 2009.
71. De Botton S, Sabri S, Daugas E, et al: Platelet formation is the consequence of caspase activation within megakaryocytes. *Blood* 100:1310, 2002.
72. Quesenberry PJ, Ihle JN, McGrath E: The effect of interleukin 3 and GM-CSA-2 on megakaryocyte and myeloid clonal colony formation. *Blood* 65:214, 1985.
73. Kaushansky K, O'Hara PJ, Berkner K, et al: Genomic cloning, characterization, and multilineage growth-promoting activity of human granulocyte-macrophage colony-stimulating factor. *Proc Natl Acad Sci U S A* 83:3101, 1986.
74. Briddell RA, Bruno E, Cooper RJ, et al: Effect of c-kit ligand on in vitro human megakaryocytopoiesis. *Blood* 78:2854, 1991.
75. Kaushansky K: Thrombopoietin: The primary regulator of platelet production. *Blood* 86:419, 1995.
76. Yang YC, Ciarletta AB, Temple PA, et al: Human IL-3 (multi-CSF): Identification by expression cloning of a novel hematopoietic growth factor related to murine IL-3. *Cell* 47:3, 1986.
77. Wong GG, Witek JS, Temple PA, et al: Human GM-CSF: Molecular cloning of the complementary DNA and purification of the natural and recombinant proteins. *Science* 228:810, 1985.
78. Feng Y, Klein BK, Vu L, et al: 1H 13C, and 15N NMR resonance assignments, secondary structure, and backbone topology of a variant of human interleukin-3. *Biochemistry* 34:6540, 1995.
79. Lopez AF, Eglinton JM, Gillis D, et al: Reciprocal inhibition of binding between interleukin 3 and granulocyte-macrophage colony-stimulating factor to human eosinophils. *Proc Natl Acad Sci U S A* 86:7022, 1989.
80. Scott CL, Robb L, Mansfield R, et al: Granulocyte-macrophage colony-stimulating factor is not responsible for residual thrombopoiesis in Mpl null mice. *Exp Hematol* 28:1001, 2000.
81. Chen Q, Solar G, Eaton DL, de Sauvage FJ: IL-3 does not contribute to platelet production in c-Mpl–deficient mice. *Stem Cells* 16(Suppl 2):31, 1998.
82. Kishimoto T: The biology of interleukin-6. *Blood* 74:1, 1989.
83. Quesenberry PJ, McGrath HE, Williams ME, et al: Multifactor stimulation of megakaryocytopoiesis: Effects of interleukin 6. *Exp Hematol* 19:35, 1991.
84. Williams N, De Giorgio T, Banu N, et al: Recombinant interleukin 6 stimulates immature murine megakaryocytes. *Exp Hematol* 18:69, 1990.
85. Mei RL, Burstein SA: Megakaryocytic maturation in murine long-term bone marrow culture: Role of interleukin-6. *Blood* 78:1438, 1991.
86. Ishibashi T, Kimura H, Shikama Y, et al: Interleukin-6 is a potent thrombopoietic factor *in vivo* in mice. *Blood* 74:1241, 1989.
87. Asano S, Okano A, Ozawa K, et al: *In vivo* effects of recombinant human interleukin-6 in primates: Stimulated production of platelets. *Blood* 75:1602, 1990.
88. van Gameren MM, Willemse PH, Mulder NH, et al: Effects of recombinant human interleukin-6 in cancer patients: A phase I–II study. *Blood* 84:1434, 1994.
89. Blay JY, Favrot M, Rossi JF, Wijdenes J: Role of interleukin-6 in paraneoplastic thrombocytosis. *Blood* 82:2261, 1993.
90. Bernad A, Kopf M, Kulbacki R, et al: Interleukin-6 is required *in vivo* for the regulation of stem cells and committed progenitors of the hematopoietic system. *Immunity* 1:725, 1994.
91. Kaser A, Brandacher G, Steurer W, et al: Interleukin-6 stimulates thrombopoiesis through thrombopoietin: Role in inflammatory thrombocytosis. *Blood* 98:2720, 2001.
92. Du X, Williams DA: Interleukin-11: Review of molecular, cell biology, and clinical use. *Blood* 89:3897, 1997.
93. Gough NM: Molecular genetics of leukemia inhibitory factor (LIF) and its receptor. *Growth Factors* 7:175, 1992.
94. Hilton DJ: LIF: Lots of interesting functions. *Trends Biochem Sci* 17:72, 1992.
95. Debili N, Masse JM, Katz A, et al: Effects of the recombinant hematopoietic growth factors interleukin-3, interleukin-6, stem cell factor, and leukemia inhibitory factor on the megakaryocytic differentiation of CD34+ cells. *Blood* 82:84, 1993.
96. Teramura M, Kobayashi S, Hoshino S, et al: Interleukin-11 enhances human megakaryocytopoiesis in vitro. *Blood* 79:327, 1992.
97. Metcalf D, Nicola NA, Gearing DP: Effects of injected leukemia inhibitory factor on hematopoietic and other tissues in mice. *Blood* 76:50, 1990.
98. Neben TY, Loebelenz J, Hayes L, et al: Recombinant human interleukin-11 stimulates megakaryocytopoiesis and increases peripheral platelets in normal and splenectomized mice. *Blood* 81:901, 1993.
99. Farese AM, Myers LA, MacVittie TJ: Therapeutic efficacy of recombinant human leukemia inhibitory factor in a primate model of radiation-induced marrow aplasia. *Blood* 84:3675, 1994.
100. Gordon MS, McCaskill-Stevens WJ, Battiato LA, et al: A phase I trial of recombinant human interleukin-11 (Neumega rhIL-11 growth factor) in women with breast cancer receiving chemotherapy. *Blood* 87:3615, 1996.
101. Nandurkar HH, Robb L, Tarlinton D, et al: Adult mice with targeted mutation of the interleukin-11 receptor (IL11Ra) display normal hematopoiesis. *Blood* 90:2148, 1997.
102. Gainsford T, Nandurkar H, Metcalf D, et al: The residual megakaryocyte and platelet production in c-Mpl–deficient mice is not dependent on the actions of interleukin-6, interleukin-11, or leukemia inhibitory factor. *Blood* 95:528, 2000.
103. Lyman SD, James L, Vanden Bos T, et al: Molecular cloning of a ligand for the flt3/flk-2 tyrosine kinase receptor: A proliferative factor for primitive hematopoietic cells. *Cell* 75:1157, 1993.
104. Avraham H, Vannier E, Cowley S, et al: Effects of the stem cell factor, c-kit ligand, on human megakaryocytic cells. *Blood* 79:365, 1992.
105. Ebbe S, Phalen E, Stohlman F Jr: Abnormalities of megakaryocytes in S1-S1d mice. *Blood* 42:865, 1973.
106. Arnold J, Ellis S, Radley JM, Williams N: Compensatory mechanisms in platelet production: The response of Sl/Sld mice to 5-fluorouracil. *Exp Hematol* 19:24, 1991.
107. Hunt P, Zsebo KM, Hokom MM, et al: Evidence that stem cell factor is involved in the rebound thrombocytosis that follows 5-fluorouracil treatment. *Blood* 80:904, 1992.
108. Broudy VC: Stem cell factor and hematopoiesis. *Blood* 90:1345, 1997.
109. Langley KE, Bennett LG, Wypych J, et al: Soluble stem cell factor in human serum. *Blood* 81:656, 1993.
110. Cheng HJ, Flanagan JG: Transmembrane kit ligand cleavage does not require a signal in the cytoplasmic domain and occurs at a site dependent on spacing from the membrane. *Mol Biol Cell* 5:943, 1994.
111. Miyazawa K, Williams DA, Gotoh A, et al: Membrane-bound Steel factor induces more persistent tyrosine kinase activation and longer life span of c-kit gene-encoded protein than its soluble form. *Blood* 85:641, 1995.
112. Flanagan JG, Chan DC, Leder P: Transmembrane form of the kit ligand growth factor is determined by alternative splicing and is missing in the Sld mutant. *Cell* 64:1025, 1991.
113. Lyman SD, Jacobsen SE: c-kit ligand and Flt3 ligand: Stem/progenitor cell factors with overlapping yet distinct activities. *Blood* 91:1101, 1998.
114. Ramsfjell V, Borge OJ, Veiby OP, et al: Thrombopoietin, but not erythropoietin, directly stimulates multilineage growth of primitive murine bone marrow progenitor cells in synergy with early acting cytokines: Distinct interactions with the ligands for c-kit and FLT3. *Blood* 88:4481, 1996.
115. Piacibello W, Garetto L, Sanavio F, et al: The effects of human FLT3 ligand on in vitro human megakaryocytopoiesis. *Exp Hematol* 24:340, 1996.
116. Brasel K, McKenna HJ, Morrissey PJ, et al: Hematologic effects of flt3 ligand in vivo in mice. *Blood* 88:2004, 1996.
117. Kelemen E CI, Tanos B: Demonstration and some properties of human thrombopoietin in thrombocythemic sera. *Acta Haematol* 20:350, 1958.
118. Wendling F, Varlet P, Charon M, Tambourin P: MPLV: A retrovirus complex inducing an acute myeloproliferative leukemic disorder in adult mice. *Virology* 149:242, 1986.
119. Souyri M, Vigon I, Penciolelli JF, et al: A putative truncated cytokine receptor gene transduced by the myeloproliferative leukemia virus immortalizes hematopoietic progenitors. *Cell* 63:1137, 1990.
120. Vigon I, Mornon JP, Cocault L, et al: Molecular cloning and characterization of MPL, the human homolog of the v-Mpl oncogene: Identification of a member of the hematopoietic growth factor receptor super-family. *Proc Natl Acad Sci U S A* 89:5640, 1992.
121. Cosman D: The hematopoietin receptor superfamily. *Cytokine* 5:95, 1993.
122. Skoda RC, Seldin DC, Chiang MK, et al: Murine c-Mpl: A member of the hematopoietic growth factor receptor superfamily that transduces a proliferative signal. *EMBO J* 12:2645, 1993.
123. Lok S, Kaushansky K, Holly RD, et al: Cloning and expression of murine thrombopoietin cDNA and stimulation of platelet production *in vivo*. *Nature* 369:565, 1994.

124. Linden HM, Kaushansky K: The glycan domain of thrombopoietin enhances its secretion. *Biochemistry* 39:3044, 2000.
125. Basser RL, Rasko JE, Clarke K, et al: Thrombopoietic effects of pegylated recombinant human megakaryocyte growth and development factor (PEG-rHuMGDF) in patients with advanced cancer. *Lancet* 348:1279, 1996.
126. Kaushansky K, Broudy VC, Grossmann A, et al: Thrombopoietin expands erythroid progenitors, increases red cell production, and enhances erythroid recovery after myelosuppressive therapy. *J Clin Invest* 96:1683, 1995.
127. Farese AM, Hunt P, Boone T, MacVittie TJ: Recombinant human megakaryocyte growth and development factor stimulates thrombocytopoiesis in normal nonhuman primates. *Blood* 86:54, 1995.
128. Akahori H, Shibuya K, Obuchi M, et al: Effect of recombinant human thrombopoietin in nonhuman primates with chemotherapy-induced thrombocytopenia. *Br J Haematol* 94:722, 1996.
129. Neelis KJ, Hartong SC, Egeland T, et al: The efficacy of single-dose administration of thrombopoietin with coadministration of either granulocyte/macrophage or granulocyte colony-stimulating factor in myelosuppressed rhesus monkeys. *Blood* 90:2565, 1997.
130. Gurney AL, Carver-Moore K, de Sauvage FJ, Moore MW: Thrombocytopenia in c-Mpl–deficient mice. *Science* 265:1445, 1994.
131. van den Oudenrijn S, Bruin M, Folman CC, et al: Mutations in the thrombopoietin receptor, Mpl, in children with congenital amegakaryocytic thrombocytopenia. *Br J Haematol* 110:441, 2000.
132. Ballmaier M, Germeshausen M, Schulze H, et al: c-mpl mutations are the cause of congenital amegakaryocytic thrombocytopenia. *Blood* 97:139, 2001.
133. Sohma Y, Akahori H, Seki N, et al: Molecular cloning and chromosomal localization of the human thrombopoietin gene. *FEBS Lett* 353:57, 1994.
134. Morris D: *cis*-Acting mRNA structures in gene-specific translational control, in *Post-Transcriptional Gene Regulation*, edited by JB Harford, DR Morris, p 165. Wiley-Liss, New York, 1997.
135. Wiestner A, Schlemper RJ, Van der Maas AP, Skoda RC: An activating splice donor mutation in the thrombopoietin gene causes hereditary thrombocythaemia. *Nat Genet* 18:49, 1998.
136. Jorgensen MJ, Raskind WH, Wolff JF, et al: Familial thrombocytosis associated with overproduction of thrombopoietin due to a novel splice donor site mutation. *Blood* 92:205a, 1998.
137. Kondo T, Okabe M, Sanada M, et al: Familial essential thrombocythemia associated with one-base deletion in the 5′-untranslated region of the thrombopoietin gene. *Blood* 92:1091, 1998.
138. Ghilardi N, Wiestner A, Kikuchi M, et al: Hereditary thrombocythaemia in a Japanese family is caused by a novel point mutation in the thrombopoietin gene. *Br J Haematol* 107:310, 1999.
139. Cazzola M, Skoda RC: Translational pathophysiology: A novel molecular mechanism of human disease. *Blood* 95:3280, 2000.
140. Odell TT Jr, McDonald TP, Detwiler TC: Stimulation of platelet production by serum of platelet-depleted rats. *Proc Soc Exp Biol Med* 108:428, 1961.
141. Nichol JL, Hokom MM, Hornkohl A, et al: Megakaryocyte growth and development factor. Analyses of in vitro effects on human megakaryopoiesis and endogenous serum levels during chemotherapy-induced thrombocytopenia. *J Clin Invest* 95:2973, 1995.
142. Kuter DJ, Rosenberg RD: The reciprocal relationship of thrombopoietin (c-Mpl ligand) to changes in the platelet mass during busulfan-induced thrombocytopenia in the rabbit. *Blood* 85:2720, 1995.
143. Bartocci A, Mastrogiannis DS, Migliorati G, et al: Macrophages specifically regulate the concentration of their own growth factor in the circulation. *Proc Natl Acad Sci U S A* 84:6179, 1987.
144. Emmons RV, Reid DM, Cohen RL, et al: Human thrombopoietin levels are high when thrombocytopenia is due to megakaryocyte deficiency and low when due to increased platelet destruction. *Blood* 87:4068, 1996.
145. McCarty JM, Sprugel KH, Fox NE, et al: Murine thrombopoietin mRNA levels are modulated by platelet count. *Blood* 86:3668, 1995.
146. de Sauvage FJ, Carver-Moore K, Luoh SM, et al: Physiological regulation of early and late stages of megakaryocytopoiesis by thrombopoietin. *J Exp Med* 183:651, 1996.
147. Sungaran R, Markovic B, Chong BH: Localization and regulation of thrombopoietin mRNa expression in human kidney, liver, bone marrow, and spleen using in situ hybridization. *Blood* 89:101, 1997.
148. McIntosh B, Kaushansky K: Marrow stromal production of thrombopoietin is regulated by transcriptional mechanisms in response to platelet products. *Exp Hematol* 36:799, 2008.
149. Solanilla A, Dechanet J, El Andaloussi A, et al: CD40-ligand stimulates myelopoiesis by regulating flt3-ligand and thrombopoietin production in bone marrow stromal cells. *Blood* 95:3758, 2000.
150. Sungaran R, Chisholm OT, Markovic B, et al: The role of platelet alpha-granular proteins in the regulation of thrombopoietin messenger RNA expression in human bone marrow stromal cells. *Blood* 95:3094, 2000.
151. Kamura T, Handa H, Hamasaki N, Kitajima S: Characterization of the human thrombopoietin gene promoter. A possible role of an Ets transcription factor, E4TF1/GABP. *J Biol Chem* 272:11361, 1997.
152. Chang MS, McNinch J, Basu R, et al: Cloning and characterization of the human megakaryocyte growth and development factor (MGDF) gene. *J Biol Chem* 270:511, 1995.
153. Rollins BJ: Chemokines. *Blood* 90:909, 1997.
154. Broxmeyer HE, Mantel CR, Aronica SM: Biology and mechanisms of action of synergistically stimulated myeloid progenitor cell proliferation and suppression by chemokines. *Stem Cells* 15(Suppl 1):69, discussion 15(Suppl 1):78, 1997.
155. Shirozu M, Nakano T, Inazawa J, et al: Structure and chromosomal localization of the human stromal cell-derived factor 1 (SDF1) gene. *Genomics* 28:495, 1995.
156. Luster AD: Chemokines—Chemotactic cytokines that mediate inflammation. *N Engl J Med* 338:436, 1998.
157. Nagasawa T, Hirota S, Tachibana K, et al: Defects of B-cell lymphopoiesis and bone-marrow myelopoiesis in mice lacking the CXC chemokine PBSF/SDF-1. *Nature* 382:635, 1996.
158. Ma Q, Jones D, Borghesani PR, et al: Impaired B-lymphopoiesis, myelopoiesis, and derailed cerebellar neuron migration in CXCR4- and SDF-1-deficient mice. *Proc Natl Acad Sci U S A* 95:9448, 1998.
159. Aiuti A, Webb IJ, Bleul C, et al: The chemokine SDF-1 is a chemoattractant for human CD34+ hematopoietic progenitor cells and provides a new mechanism to explain the mobilization of CD34+ progenitors to peripheral blood. *J Exp Med* 185:111, 1997.
160. Wang JF, Liu ZY, Groopman JE: The alpha-chemokine receptor CXCR4 is expressed on the megakaryocytic lineage from progenitor to platelets and modulates migration and adhesion. *Blood* 92:756, 1998.
161. Hamada T, Mohle R, Hesselgesser J, et al: Transendothelial migration of megakaryocytes in response to stromal cell-derived factor 1 (SDF-1) enhances platelet formation. *J Exp Med* 188:539, 1998.
162. Daopin S, Piez KA, Ogawa Y, Davies DR: Crystal structure of transforming growth factor-beta 2: An unusual fold for the superfamily. *Science* 257:369, 1992.
163. Keller JR, Mantel C, Sing GK, et al: Transforming growth factor beta 1 selectively regulates early murine hematopoietic progenitors and inhibits the growth of IL-3-dependent myeloid leukemia cell lines. *J Exp Med* 168:737, 1988.
164. Dybedal I, Jacobsen SE: Transforming growth factor beta (TGF-beta), a potent inhibitor of erythropoiesis: Neutralizing TGF-beta antibodies show erythropoietin as a potent stimulator of murine burst-forming unit erythroid colony formation in the absence of a burst-promoting activity. *Blood* 86:949, 1995.
165. Ishibashi T, Miller SL, Burstein SA: Type beta transforming growth factor is a potent inhibitor of murine megakaryocytopoiesis *in vitro*. *Blood* 69:1737, 1987.
166. Kuter DJ, Gminski DM, Rosenberg RD: Transforming growth factor beta inhibits megakaryocyte growth and endomitosis. *Blood* 79:619, 1992.
167. Laiho M, DeCaprio JA, Ludlow JW, et al: Growth inhibition by TGF-beta linked to suppression of retinoblastoma protein phosphorylation. *Cell* 62:175, 1990.
168. Polyak K, Kato JY, Solomon MJ, et al: p27Kip1, a cyclin-Cdk inhibitor, links transforming growth factor-beta and contact inhibition to cell cycle arrest. *Genes Dev* 8:9, 1994.
169. Teofili L, Martini M, Di Mario A, et al: Expression of p15(ink4b) gene during megakaryocytic differentiation of normal and myelodysplastic hematopoietic progenitors. *Blood* 98:495, 2001.
170. Theofilopoulos AN, Baccala R, Beutler B, Kono DH: Type I interferons (/) in immunity and autoimmunity. *Annu Rev Immunol* 23:307, 2005.
171. Broxmeyer HE, Cooper S, Rubin BY, Taylor MW: The synergistic influence of human interferon-gamma and interferon-alpha on suppression of hematopoietic progenitor cells is additive with the enhanced sensitivity of these cells to inhibition by interferons at low oxygen tension *in vitro*. *J Immunol* 135:2502, 1985.
172. Fattovich G, Giustina G, Favarato S, Ruol A: A survey of adverse events in 11,241 patients with chronic viral hepatitis treated with alfa interferon. *J Hepatol* 24:38, 1996.
173. Dusheiko G: Side effects of alpha interferon in chronic hepatitis C. *Hepatology* 26(Suppl 1):112S, 1997.
174. Jaster R, Tschirch E, Bittorf T, Brock J: Interferon-alpha inhibits proliferation of Ba/F3 cells by interfering with interleukin-3 action. *Cell Signal* 11:769, 1999.
175. Kuniyasu H, Yasui W, Kitahara K, et al: Growth inhibitory effect of interferon-beta is associated with the induction of cyclin-dependent kinase inhibitor p27Kip1 in a human gastric carcinoma cell line. *Cell Growth Differ* 8:47, 1997.
176. Wang Q, Miyakawa Y, Fox N, Kaushansky K: Interferon-alpha directly represses megakaryopoiesis by inhibiting thrombopoietin-induced signaling through induction of SOCS-1. *Blood* 96:2093, 2000.
177. Long MW: Blood cell cytoadhesion molecules. *Exp Hematol* 20:288, 1992.
178. Toksoz D, Zsebo KM, Smith KA, et al: Support of human hematopoiesis in long-term bone marrow cultures by murine stromal cells selectively expressing the membrane-bound and secreted forms of the human homolog of the steel gene product, stem cell factor. *Proc Natl Acad Sci U S A* 89:7350, 1992.
179. Yang L, Yang YC: Regulation of interleukin (IL)-11 gene expression in IL-1 induced primate bone marrow stromal cells. *J Biol Chem* 269:32732, 1994.
180. Linenberger ML, Jacobson FW, Bennett LG, et al: Stem cell factor production by human marrow stromal fibroblasts. *Exp Hematol* 23:1104, 1995.
181. Gordon MY, Riley GP, Watt SM, Greaves MF: Compartmentalization of a haematopoietic growth factor (GM-CSF) by glycosaminoglycans in the bone marrow microenvironment. *Nature* 326:403, 1987.
182. Roberts R, Gallagher J, Spooncer E, et al: Heparan sulphate bound growth factors: A mechanism for stromal cell mediated haemopoiesis. *Nature* 332:376, 1988.
183. Artavanis-Tsakonas S, Matsuno K, Fortini ME: Notch signaling. *Science* 268:225, 1995.
184. Karanu FN, Murdoch B, Miyabayashi T, et al: Human homologues of Delta-1 and Delta-4 function as mitogenic regulators of primitive human hematopoietic cells. *Blood* 97:1960, 2001.
185. Lam LT, Ronchini C, Norton J, et al: Suppression of erythroid but not megakaryocytic differentiation of human K562 erythroleukemic cells by notch-1. *J Biol Chem* 275:19676, 2000.

186. Fox NE, Kaushansky K: Engagement of integrin a4b1 enhances thrombopoietin-induced megakaryopoiesis. *Exp Hematol* 33:94, 2005.
187. Bruno E, Briddell RA, Cooper RJ, Hoffman R: Effects of recombinant interleukin 11 on human megakaryocyte progenitor cells. *Exp Hematol* 19:378, 1991.
188. Neben S, Turner K: The biology of interleukin 11. *Stem Cells* 11(Suppl 2):156, 1993.
189. Burstein SA, Mei RL, Henthorn J, et al: Leukemia inhibitory factor and interleukin-11 promote maturation of murine and human megakaryocytes in vitro. *J Cell Physiol* 153:305, 1992.
190. Yonemura Y, Kawakita M, Masuda T, et al: Synergistic effects of interleukin 3 and interleukin 11 on murine megakaryopoiesis in serum-free culture. *Exp Hematol* 20:1011, 1992.
191. Yonemura Y, Kawakita M, Masuda T, et al: Effect of recombinant human interleukin-11 on rat megakaryopoiesis and thrombopoiesis *in vivo*: Comparative study with interleukin-6. *Br J Haematol* 84:16, 1993.
192. Schlerman FJ, Bree AG, Kaviani MD, et al: Thrombopoietic activity of recombinant human interleukin 11 (rHuIL 11) in normal and myelosup-pressed nonhuman primates. *Stem Cells* 14:517, 1996.
193. Gordon MS SG, Battiato L, et al : The in vivo effects of subcutaneously (SC) administered recombinant human interleukin-11 (Neumega rhIL-11 growth factor; rhIL-11) in women with breast cancer (BC). *Blood* 82(Suppl 1):498a, 1993.
194. Champlin RE MR, Kaye JA, et al: Recombinant human interleukin eleven (rhIL-11) following autologous BMT for breast cancer. *Blood* 84(suppl 1):395a, 1994.
195. Tepler I, Elias L, Smith JW 2nd, et al: A randomized placebo-controlled trial of recombinant human interleukin-11 in cancer patients with severe thrombocytopenia due to chemotherapy. *Blood* 87:3607, 1996.
196. Isaacs C, Robert NJ, Bailey FA, et al: Randomized placebo-controlled study of recombinant human interleukin-11 to prevent chemotherapy-induced thrombocytopenia in patients with breast cancer receiving dose-intensive cyclophosphamide and doxorubicin. *J Clin Oncol* 15:3368, 1997.
197. Vredenburgh JJ, Hussein A, Fisher D, et al: A randomized trial of recombinant human interleukin-11 following autologous bone marrow transplantation with peripheral blood progenitor cell support in patients with breast cancer. *Biol Blood Marrow Transplant* 4:134, 1998.
198. Tichelli A, Gratwohl A, Berger C, et al: Treatment of thrombocytosis in myeloproliferative disorders with interferon alpha-2a. *Blut* 58:15, 1989.
199. Gisslinger H, Ludwig H, Linkesch W, et al: Long-term interferon therapy for thrombocytosis in myeloproliferative diseases. *Lancet* 1:634, 1989.
200. Sacchi S, Gugliotta L, Papineschi F, et al: Alfa-interferon in the treatment of essential thrombocythemia: Clinical results and evaluation of its biological effects on the hematopoietic neoplastic clone. Italian Cooperative Group on ET. *Leukemia* 12:289, 1998.
201. Taylor PC, Dolan G, Ng JP, et al: Efficacy of recombinant interferon-alpha (rIFN-alpha) in polycythaemia vera: A study of 17 patients and an analysis of published data. *Br J Haematol* 92:55, 1996.
202. Tornebohm-Roche E, Merup M, Lockner D, Paul C: Alpha-2a interferon therapy and antibody formation in patients with essential thrombocythemia and polycythemia vera with thrombocytosis. *Am J Hematol* 48:163, 1995.
203. Hokom MM, Lacey D, Kinstler OB, et al: Pegylated megakaryocyte growth and development factor abrogates the lethal thrombocytopenia associated with carboplatin and irradiation in mice. *Blood* 86:4486, 1995.
204. Fibbe WE, Heemskerk DP, Laterveer L, et al: Accelerated reconstitution of platelets and erythrocytes after syngeneic transplantation of bone marrow cells derived from thrombopoietin pretreated donor mice. *Blood* 86:3308, 1995.
205. Molineux G, Hartley C, McElroy P, et al: Megakaryocyte growth and development factor accelerates platelet recovery in peripheral blood progenitor cell transplant recipients. *Blood* 88:366, 1996.
206. Fanucchi M, Glaspy J, Crawford J, et al: Effects of polyethylene glycol conjugated recombinant human megakaryocyte growth and development factor on platelet counts after chemotherapy for lung cancer. *N Engl J Med* 336:404, 1997.
207. Vadhan-Raj S, Murray LJ, Bueso-Ramos C, et al: Stimulation of megakaryocyte and platelet production by a single dose of recombinant human thrombopoietin in patients with cancer. *Ann Intern Med* 126:673, 1997.
208. Basser RL, Underhill C, Davis I, et al: Enhancement of platelet recovery after myelosuppressive chemotherapy by recombinant human megakaryocyte growth and development factor in patients with advanced cancer. *J Clin Oncol* 18:2852, 2000.
209. Archimbaud E, Ottmann OG, Yin JA, et al: A randomized, double-blind, placebo-controlled study with pegylated recombinant human megakaryocyte growth and development factor (PEG-rHuMGDF) as an adjunct to chemotherapy for adults with *de novo* acute myeloid leukemia. *Blood* 94:3694, 1999.
210. Bolwell B, Vredenburgh J, Overmoyer B, et al: Phase 1 study of pegylated recombinant human megakaryocyte growth and development factor (PEG-rHuMGDF) in breast cancer patients after autologous peripheral blood progenitor cell (PBPC) transplantation. *Bone Marrow Transplant* 26:141, 2000.
211. Somlo G, Sniecinski I, Ter Veer A, et al: Recombinant human thrombopoietin in combination with granulocyte colony-stimulating factor enhances mobilization of peripheral blood progenitor cells, increases peripheral blood platelet concentration, and accelerates hematopoietic recovery following high-dose chemotherapy. *Blood* 93:2798, 1999.
212. Nomura S, Dan K, Hotta T, et al: Effects of pegylated recombinant human megakaryocyte growth and development factor in patients with idiopathic thrombocytopenic purpura. *Blood* 100:728, 2002.
213. Vadhan-Raj S, Patel S, Bueso-Ramos C, et al: Importance of predosing of recombinant human thrombopoietin to reduce chemotherapy-induced early thrombocytopenia. *J Clin Oncol* 21:3158, 2003.
214. Li J, Yang C, Xia Y, et al: Thrombocytopenia caused by the development of antibodies to thrombopoietin. *Blood* 98:3241, 2001.
215. Kimura T, Kaburaki H, Tsujino T, et al: A non-peptide compound which can mimic the effect of thrombopoietin via c-Mpl. *FEBS Lett* 428:250, 1998.
216. de Serres M, Yeager RL, Dillberger JE, et al: Pharmacokinetics and hematological effects of the PEGylated thrombopoietin peptide mimetic GW395058 in rats and monkeys after intravenous or subcutaneous administration. *Stem Cells* 17:316, 1999.
217. Broudy VC, Lin NL: AMG531 stimulates megakaryopoiesis *in vitro* by binding to Mpl. *Cytokine* 25:52, 2004.
218. Kaushansky K: Hematopoietic growth factor mimetics. *Ann N Y Acad Sci* 938:131, 2001.
219. Kuter DJ, Bussel JB, Lyons RM, et al: Efficacy of romiplostim in patients with chronic immune thrombocytopenic purpura: A double-blind randomised controlled trial. *Lancet* 371:395, 2008.
220. Bussel JB, Cheng G, Saleh MN, et al: Eltrombopag for the treatment of chronic idiopathic thrombocytopenic purpura. *N Engl J Med* 357:2237, 2007.
221. McHutchison JG, Dusheiko G, Shiffman ML, et al: Eltrombopag for thrombocytopenia in patients with cirrhosis associated with hepatitis C. *N Engl J Med* 357:2227, 2007.

CHAPTER 114

PLATELET MORPHOLOGY, BIOCHEMISTRY, AND FUNCTION

Susan S. Smyth, Sidney Whiteheart,
Joseph E. Italiano Jr., and Barry S. Coller

SUMMARY

The approximately 1 trillion platelets that circulate in an adult human are small anucleate cell fragments adapted to adhere to damaged blood vessels, to aggregate one with another, and to facilitate the generation of thrombin. These actions contribute to hemostasis by producing a platelet plug and then reinforcing the plug by the action of thrombin converting fibrinogen to fibrin strands. To accomplish these tasks, platelets have surface receptors that can bind adhesive glycoproteins; these include the GPIb/IX/V complex, which supports platelet adhesion by binding von Willebrand factor, especially under conditions of high shear, and the integrin $\alpha_{IIb}\beta_3$ (GPIIb/IIIa) receptor, which is platelet specific and mediates platelet aggregation by binding fibrinogen and/or von Willebrand factor. Other receptors for adhesive glycoproteins ($\alpha_2\beta_1$ [GPIa/IIa], GPVI, and perhaps others for collagen; $\alpha_5\beta_1$ [GPIc*/IIa] for fibronectin; and $\alpha_6\beta_1$ [GPIc/IIa] for laminin) also contribute to platelet adhesion, but their precise contributions are less-well defined. Activated platelets express both surface P-selectin, which mediates interactions with leukocytes, and CD40 ligand, which activates a number of proinflammatory cells, and release chemokines and a soluble form of CD40 ligand, thus initiating an inflammatory reaction. Platelet coagulant activity results from the exposure of negatively charged phospholipids on the surface of platelets and the generation of platelet microparticles, along with release and activation of platelet factor V and perhaps exposure of specific receptors for activated coagulation factors. Platelets change shape with activation as a result of a complex reorganization of the platelet membrane skeleton and cytoskeleton. With activation, platelets undergo release of α granule, dense body, and lysosomal contents. The activation process involves a number of receptors for agonists such as adenosine diphosphate (ADP), epinephrine, thrombin, collagen, thromboxane A_2, vasopressin, serotonin, platelet-activating factor, lysophosphatidic acid, sphingosine-1-phosphate, and thrombospondin, as well as several signal transduction pathways, including phosphoinositide metabolism, arachidonic acid release and conversion into thromboxane A_2, and phosphorylation of a number of different target proteins. Increases in intracellular calcium result from, and further contribute to, platelet activation. Platelet activation results in a change in the conformation of the $\alpha_{IIb}\beta_3$ receptor, leading to high-affinity ligand binding and platelet aggregation.

Activated platelets express both surface P-selectin, which mediates interactions with leukocytes, and CD40 ligand, which activates a number of proinflammatory cells, and release chemokines and a soluble form of CD40 ligand, thus initiating an inflammatory reaction. Platelet coagulant activity results from the exposure of negatively charged phospholipids on the surface of platelets and the generation of platelet microparticles, along with release and activation of platelet factor V and perhaps exposure of specific receptors for activated coagulation factor. Platelets also act as storehouses for a variety of molecules that affect platelet function, inflammation, innate immunity, cell proliferation, vascular tone, fibrinolysis, and wound healing; these agents are actively released upon platelet activation. Other vasoactive and platelet activating substances are newly synthesized when platelets are activated. Through cooperative biochemical interactions, platelets can communicate with, and are affected by, other blood cells and endothelial cells.

Quantitative and qualitative disorders of platelets cause hemorrhagic diatheses (see Chaps. 119–122). In pathologic states, uncontrolled platelet thrombus formation can lead to vasoocclusion and ischemic tissue necrosis, as, for example, in myocardial infarction and stroke (see Chap. 135). Platelets may also facilitate tumor growth and metastasis.

Acronyms and abbreviations that appear in this chapter include: ADMIDAS, adjacent to metal ion-dependent adhesion site; AP3, activator protein 3; APP, amyloid precursor protein; CIB, calcium and integrin binding protein; COX, cyclooxygenase; DAG, diacylglycerol; DTS, dense tubular system; FAK, focal adhesion kinase; GP, glycoprotein; GPI, glycosyl phosphatidylinositol; ITAM, immunoreceptor tyrosine-based activation motif; ITIM, immunoreceptor tyrosine-based inhibitory motif; LPS, lipopolysaccharide; MIDAS, metal ion–dependent adhesion site; NO, nitric oxide; PAF, platelet-activating factor; PAR, protease-activated receptor; PDGF, platelet-derived growth factor; PG, prostaglandin; PLC, phospholipase C; SR, sarcoplasmic reticulum; TGF, transforming growth factor; TLR, toll-like receptor; TLT, TREM-like transcript-1; TREM, triggering receptors express on myeloid cells; VEGF, vascular endothelial growth factor; VWF, von Willebrand factor.

PLATELET MORPHOLOGY AND BIOCHEMISTRY

LIGHT MICROSCOPIC APPEARANCE

On films made from blood anticoagulated with the strong calcium chelating agent ethylenediaminetetraacetic acid (EDTA) and stained with Wright stain, platelets appear as small bluish-gray, oval-to-round shaped cell fragments with several purple-red granules (see Chap. 2). The mean diameter of platelets varies in different individuals, ranging from approximately 1.5 to 3.0 μm, approximately one-third to one-fourth that of erythrocytes. There is also considerable variability in the size of platelets in a single individual, with occasional platelets in normal blood samples having diameters greater than one-third the diameter of erythrocytes. Overall, platelet size appears to follow a log normal distribution with an average volume of approximately 7 fL.[1] When unanticoagulated blood is used to prepare blood films, platelets undergo variable activation and spreading, and thus platelet aggregates are commonly seen; platelets from such specimens may demonstrate three or four very long finger-like processes extending out from the body of the platelet (filopodia), and some platelets may be devoid of granules.

ELECTRON MICROSCOPIC APPEARANCE AND BIOCHEMISTRY

Electron microscopy reveals a fuzzy coat (glycocalix) extending 14 to 20 nm from the platelet surface, which is thought to be composed of membrane glycoproteins (GPs), glycolipids, mucopolysaccharides, and adsorbed plasma proteins (Fig. 114–1).[2] Platelets move in an electric field because of their net negative surface charge; sialic acid residues attached to proteins and lipids are major contributors to this negative charge in platelets and most other cells.[3] The electrostatic repulsion created by the negative surface charge may help prevent resting platelets from attaching to each other or to negatively charged endothelial cells.

Indentations on the platelet surface are openings of the open canalicular system, which is an elaborate channel system composed of invaginations of the plasma membrane that extend throughout the platelet

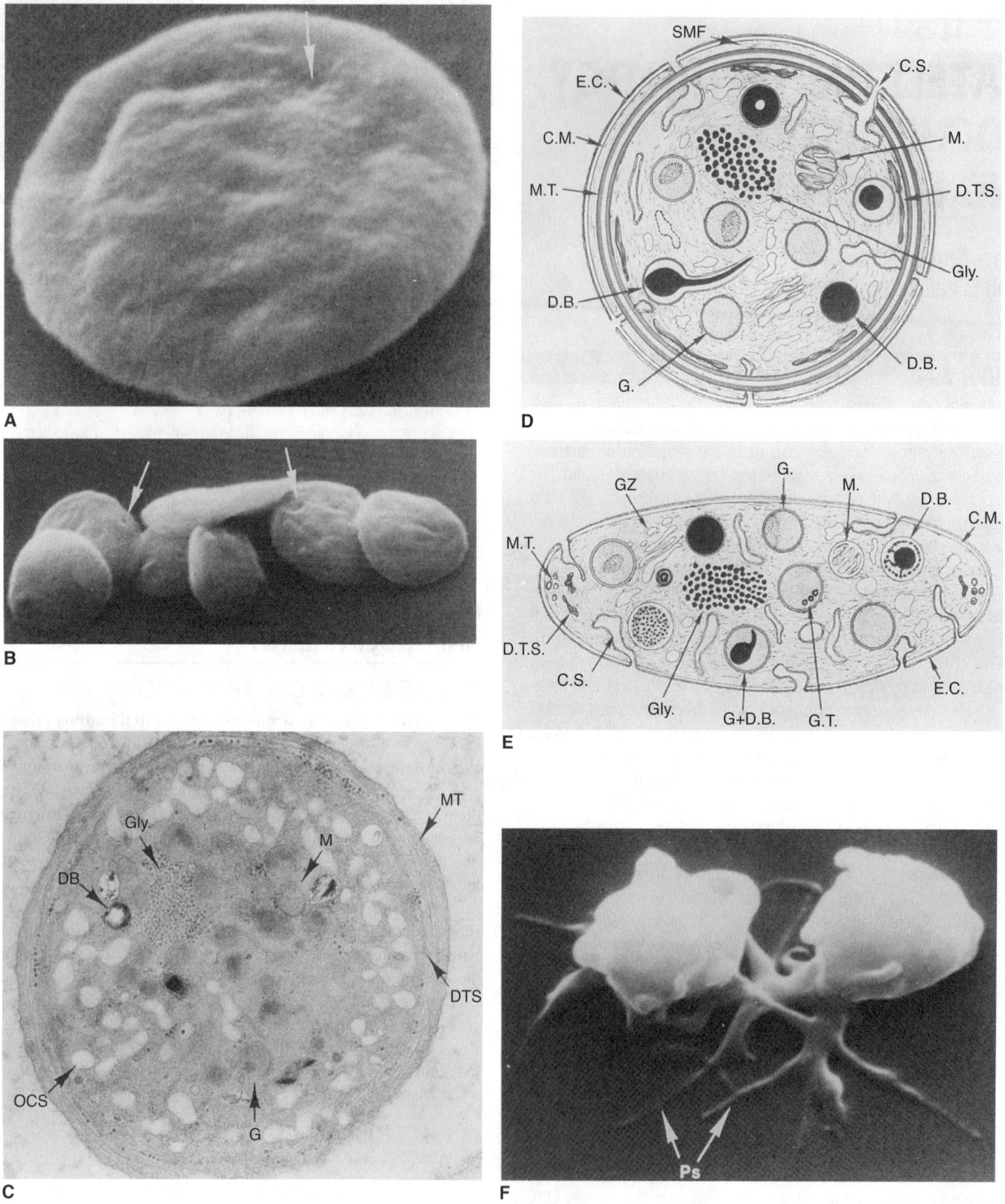

FIGURE 114–1. A, B. Discoid platelets. The lentiform shape of blood platelets is well preserved in samples fixed in glutaraldehyde and critical point dried for study in the scanning electron microscope. The indentations apparent on the otherwise smooth surfaces of the platelets (*arrows*) indicate sites where channels of the open canalicular system (OCS) communicate with the cell exterior. (**A:** ×13,200; **B:** ×35,000.) **C–E.** Ultrastructural features observed in thin sections of discoid platelets cut in the equatorial plane (**C** and **D**) or cross section (**E**). Components include the exterior coat (E.C.), trilaminar unit membrane (C.M.), and submembrane area containing the specialized filaments of the membrane skeleton (SMF). The plasma membrane indentations form the walls of the channels of the surface-connected open canalicular system (C.S. and OCS). The circumferential band of microtubules (M.T.) is seen as a continuous band beneath the plasma membrane on the equatorial section and as small open cylinders at the ends of the platelet on the cross section. Glycogen granules (Gly) are prominent punctate structures in the cytoplasm, and residual Golgi zones (GZ) can also be identified. Organelles include mitochondria (M), dense granules (here termed *dense bodies* [D.B.]), and α granules (G), many of which have regions of electron density (nucleoids). The dense tubular system (DTS and D.T.S.), the platelet equivalent of the sarcoplasmic reticulum, sequesters calcium. (**C:** ×30,000.) **F.** Platelet shape change. Platelets were exposed to adenosine diphosphate (ADP) and then fixed and examined by scanning electron microscopy. The platelets lose their discoid shape and become spiny spheres with long extensions, variably referred to as *filopodia* or *pseudopodia* (Ps). (×17,000) *(Reproduced with permission from White JG.[1569])*

(see Fig. 114–1 and "Membrane Systems" below). The contents of platelet granules can gain access to the outside when the granules fuse with either the plasma membrane or any region of the open canalicular system. Similarly, glycoproteins contained within granule membranes then join the plasma membrane after granule fusion with either the plasma membrane or the open canalicular system.

The Plasma Membrane

The plasma membrane is a trilaminar unit composed of a bilayer of phospholipids in which cholesterol, glycolipids, and glycoproteins are embedded.[2,4] Platelets prepared by the freeze-fracture technique demonstrate more intramembranous particles embedded in the outer platelet membrane leaflet than in the inner leaflet, which is the reverse of findings in erythrocytes; this observation presumably reflects the many external receptors that mediate platelet interactions. The plasma membrane contains the sodium- and calcium-adenosine triphosphatase (ATPase) pumps that control the intracellular ionic environment of the platelet. Approximately 57 percent of platelet phospholipids are contained in the plasma membrane (Table 114–1). The phospholipids are asymmetrically organized in the plasma membrane; the negatively charged phospholipids are almost exclusively present in the inner leaflet, whereas the others are more evenly distributed between the inner and outer leaflets.[5] The negatively charged phospholipids, especially phosphatidylserine, are able to accelerate several steps in the coagulation sequence and so their presence in the inner leaflet of resting platelets, separated from the plasma coagulation factors, is a control mechanism for preventing inappropriate coagulation.[6,7] During platelet activation induced by select agonists, the aminophospholipids may become exposed on the platelet surface or on the surface of microparticles (see "Platelet Coagulant Activity" below), triggering cell-surface-based coagulation reactions.[6–9]

The phospholipid asymmetry in resting platelets may be maintained by an ATP-dependent aminophospholipid translocase that actively moves phosphatidylserine and phosphatidylethanolamine from the outer to the inner leaflet.[6,10] Interactions of negatively charged phospholipids with cytoskeletal or other cytoplasmic elements may also contribute to the asymmetry.[6,7,11,12]

Lipid rafts are dynamic, cholesterol- and sphingolipid-rich membrane microdomains that are important in signaling and intracellular trafficking. In platelets, the cholesterol/phospholipid molar ratio is twofold higher in rafts than in bulk membranes, with sphingomyelin accounting for the majority of total raft lipids.[13] Platelet lipid rafts contain the marker proteins flotillin (1 and 2) and stomatin and the ganglioside GM_1; they are also notable for being devoid of caveolin. Other proteins such as CD36, CD63, CD9, $\alpha_{IIb}\beta_3$, and glucose transporter GLUT-3 are present in rafts prepared from resting platelets.[13] Upon activation GPVI, Fc gamma chain, FcγRIIa, and GPIb/IX/V partition into the lipid rafts,[14,15] as do c-SRC,[16] phosphatidic acid, and phosphoinositol (PI)3-kinase products.[17,18] Factor XI binds to extracellularly oriented lipid rafts and undergoes activation.[19] The calcium entry channel hTRPc1 is associated with lipid rafts in platelets and, upon platelet activation, contributes to calcium entry that is regulated by the state of intracellular calcium stores (store-mediated calcium entry).[20] The detrimental effects of chilling platelets are thought to be caused, at least in part, by the temperature-dependent coalescence of platelet lipid rafts.[21]

Table 114–1 outlines the lipid composition of platelet membranes. The enrichment of selected phospholipids with arachidonic acid furnishes a store of substrate for conversion to thromboxane A_2 (TXA_2; see "Signaling Pathways in Platelet Activation and Aggregation" below), a vital mediator of platelet aggregation.

The glycoproteins in the plasma membrane are discussed below.

TABLE 114–1. Platelet Lipids

I. 17% Dry Weight, Primarily in Membranes
II. Membranes
  A. Protein 57%
  B. Lipid 35%
  C. Carbohydrate 8%
III. Membrane Lipids
  A. Phospholipid 75%
  B. Neutral lipid 20%
  C. Glycolipid 5%
IV. Phospholipids
  A. Phosphatidylcholine (PC) 38%
  B. Phosphatidylethanolamine (PE) 27%
  C. Sphingomyelin 17%
  D. Phosphatidylserine 10%
  E. Phosphatidylinositol 5%
V. Membrane Phospholipid Asymmetry (percentage of each phospholipid in the exterior leaflet)
  A. Uncharged phospholipids
    1. Phosphatidylcholine 45%
    2. Sphingomyelin 93%
  B. Negatively charged phospholipids
    1. Phosphatidylethanolamine 20%
    2. Phosphatidylinositol 16%
    3. Phosphatidylserine 9%
VI. Neutral Lipids
  A. Cholesterol 95%
  B. Cholesterol: phospholipid = 0.5 on molar basis
VII. Glycolipids
  A. Gangliosides [0.5% of total lipids; 6% of total sialic acid; primarily hematoside (GM3)]
  B. Neutral glycolipids (64% lactosyl ceramide)
  C. Ceramides (A and B)
VIII. Arachidonic Acid (29;4)
  A. 42% of fatty acids in PI
  B. 32% of fatty acids in PE
  C. 23% of fatty acids in PS

SOURCE: Adapted with permission from Coller BS.[1573]

Cytoskeletal Elements

The discoid shape of the resting platelet is maintained by a well-defined and highly specialized cytoskeleton. This system of molecular struts and girders preserves the shape and integrity of the platelet as it encounters high shear forces in the circulation. The platelet cytoskeleton is operationally defined as proteins that are insoluble in the presence of the nonionic detergent Triton X-100 under defined ionic conditions. The three major cytoskeletal elements are the spectrin membrane skeleton, the marginal microtubule coil, and the actin cytoskeleton.

Membrane Skeleton The plasma membrane and open canalicular system of the resting platelet are supported by a highly structured cytoskeletal

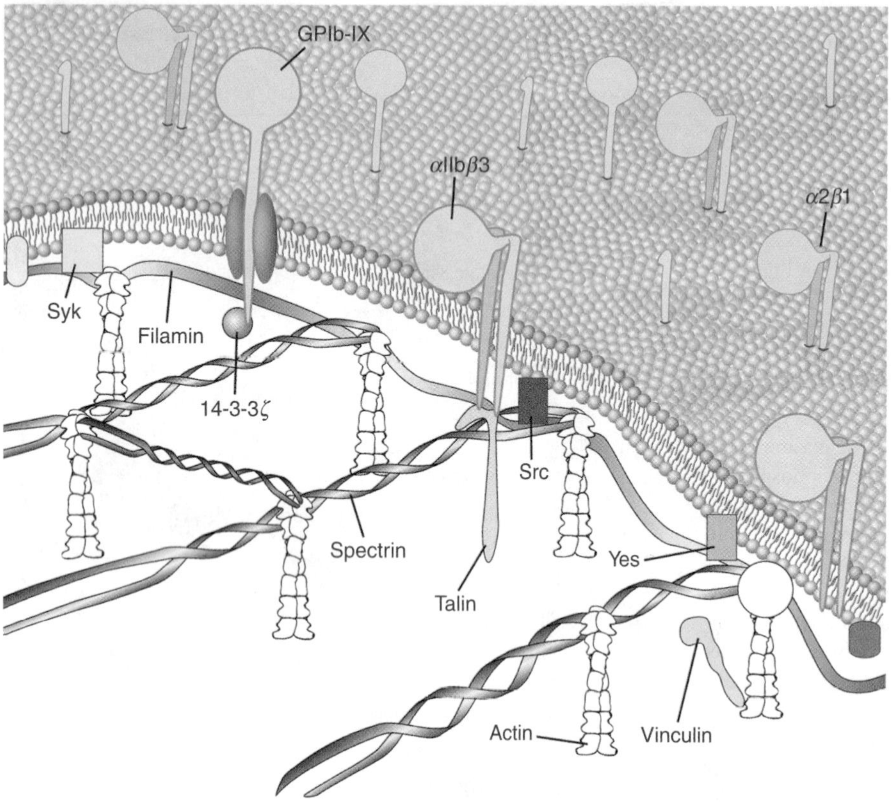

FIGURE 114–2. Diagrammatic depiction of established and hypothetical connections between select platelet transmembrane glycoproteins and the underlying membrane skeleton. Although evidence exists for direct interactions between $\alpha_{IIb}\beta_3$ with talin and Src and between GPIbα with 14-3-3ζ and filamin, the remainder of the interactions are only hypothetical and are based on the recovery of proteins in the membrane skeleton fraction of solubilized platelets. *(Adapted from Fox JEB,[504] with permission.)*

system (Figs. 114–1 and 114–2). This two-dimensional network, located just beneath the plasma membrane has remarkable structural resemblance to its red blood cell counterpart (see Chap. 45). Thus, both involve the self-assembly of elongated spectrin strands that interconnect through their binding to actin filaments, generating triangular pores. Platelets contain approximately 2000 molecules of spectrin.[22–25] The spectrin network coats the cytoplasmic surfaces of both the plasma membrane and the open canalicular system. In contrast to the erythrocyte membrane skeletons, however, in which spectrin molecules connect on short actin filaments, in platelets, spectrin joins into a network by binding to the ends of actin filaments in close apposition to the plasma membrane. As a result, the spectrin lattice is assembled into a continuous network by its association with actin filaments. Moreover, tropomodulins, which are abundant in erythrocytes, are not expressed at significant levels in platelets and thus are unlikely to play a role in capping the pointed ends of actin filaments. Instead, these ends appear to be free in resting platelets. Finally, the protein adducin is abundantly expressed in platelets and appears to cap the majority of the barbed ends of the filaments making up the resting platelet cytoskeleton.[26] This serves to target them to the spectrin-based membrane skeleton, as the affinity of spectrin for adducin-actin complexes is greater than for either adducin or actin alone.[27–29]

The platelet spectrin–actin filament network is fortified by interactions with filamin A (actin binding protein), a noncovalent dimer of two identical molecular weight 280,000 units which fastens GPIb/IX/V complexes to the sides of actin filaments (see "Actin Filaments" below). By interacting with both the transmembrane glycoprotein GPIbα and the actin immediately below the membrane, filamin A connects these components to the spectrin network and the resulting membrane cytoskeleton probably contributes to the platelet's discoid shape. In addition, the association of GPIbα with the membrane skeleton restricts the expansion of the spectrin network and probably helps to organize receptors into linear arrays on the platelet surface, thus enhancing receptor cooperation (see Fig. 114–2).[30] Filamin also binds to the cytoplasmic domains of the β_3 subunits of integrin receptors and this keeps the receptor in a low-affinity state.[31–33] Other proteins that have been found in the membrane skeleton include talin, vinculin, dystrophin-related protein, molecules implicated in signal transduction, and several isoenzymes of protein kinase C.[30]

Talin has been implicated in controlling $\alpha_{IIb}\beta_3$ activation by binding to the cytoplasmic domain of β_3 when phosphorylated and/or cleaved by calpain (see "$\alpha_{IIb}\beta_3$" below; Fig. 114–3).[34–38] Migfilin (filamin-binding LIM protein-1) is a 373-amino-acid protein of molecular weight 50,000 that can displace filamin from the β_3 cytoplasmic domain, thus facilitating talin binding and $\alpha_{IIb}\beta_3$ activation.[31] Moreover, joining $\alpha_{IIb}\beta_3$ to the membrane skeleton via a β_3 linkage creates the possibility for an actin–myosin contraction process to supply sufficient force to $\alpha_{IIb}\beta_3$ to induce conformational changes in the receptor that result in high-affinity ligand binding.[39] The protein vimentin (Mr 58,000), which is an important component of intermediate filaments, is present in platelets and contributes to the membrane cytoskeleton. When platelets are activated, vitronectin–plasminogen-activator inhibitor-1 (PAI-1) complexes bind to surface vimentin where they are strategically located to inhibit fibrinolysis.[40] With platelet activation, $\alpha_{IIb}\beta_3$ and $\alpha_2\beta_1$ join the cytoskeleton. Thus, the cytoskeleton may affect whether receptors are free to move in the plane of the membrane; it may also have a role in moving certain receptors from the surface to the interior of platelets and vice versa via the open canalicular system.[30,41] The membrane skeleton may also be important in platelet spreading after adhesion.

Microtubules One of the most distinguishing features of the resting platelet is its marginal microtubule coil (see Fig. 114–1). Located below the plasma membrane, it plays an important role in platelet formation from megakaryocytes and maintaining the platelet's discoid shape.[2,42–44] Microtubules are the largest cytoskeletal filaments (25 nm) and are comprised of hollow polarized polymers composed of 13 protofilaments made up of $\alpha\beta$ tubulin dimers (each 110,000 kDa) that associate with several high-molecular-weight proteins (microtubule-associated proteins).[44–46] Motor proteins of the dynein and kinesin families are also associated with microtubules.[47–49] In cells, $\alpha\beta$ tubulin subunits are in dynamic equilibrium with assembled microtubules such that reversible cycles of assembly and disassembly of microtubules are frequently observed. The critical concentration for tubulin polymerization is 5 μM, which is well below the tubulin concentration in platelets (70 μM) and thus 60 percent of platelet tubulin is present as polymer.[46,50,51] On cross section, approximately 8 to 12 separate hollow structures are observed at the tapered ends of the platelet (see Fig. 114–1). Direct visualization of microtubule assembly in resting mouse platelets indicates that the circumferential coil in platelets is composed of at least eight actively polymerizing microtubules.[52] Microtubule dynamics allows for necessary changes in platelet shape that occur during the platelet life span and with activation.

Platelets contain four different tubulin isoforms (β_1, β_2, β_4, β_5), but β_1 is dominant and is specific for megakaryocytes and platelets. Targeted gene deletion of β_1-tubulin in mice results in thrombocytopenia and abnormal platelet and microtubule morphology.[44] β_1-Tubulin–deficient platelets are spherical in shape, probably as a result of having defective marginal bands with fewer (~2–3) than normal (~8) microtubule coils.[53] A heterozygous genetic alteration of human β_1 tubulin (Q43P) has been described in association with macrothrombocytopenia (see Chap. 121),[54] but it is not certain that it is causal. A heterozygous β_1-tubulin mutation (R207H) in a strategically located region of the molecule has been reported in association with macrothrombocytopenia (see Chap. 121).[55]

Actin Filaments Actin is the most abundant of all the platelet proteins, with 2 million molecules expressed per platelet (0.5 mM).[56] Like tubulin, actin is in a dynamic monomer–polymer equilibrium, with 40 percent of the actin subunits polymerized to form 2000 to 5000 linear actin filaments in resting platelets (Fig. 114–4).[25] The rest of the actin in the platelet cytoplasm is maintained in storage as a 1:1 complex with β_4-thymosin; this stored actin is converted to filaments during platelet activation to drive cell spreading.[57] Thus, actin filaments crisscross the interior of the cell, interconnected at various points into a rigid

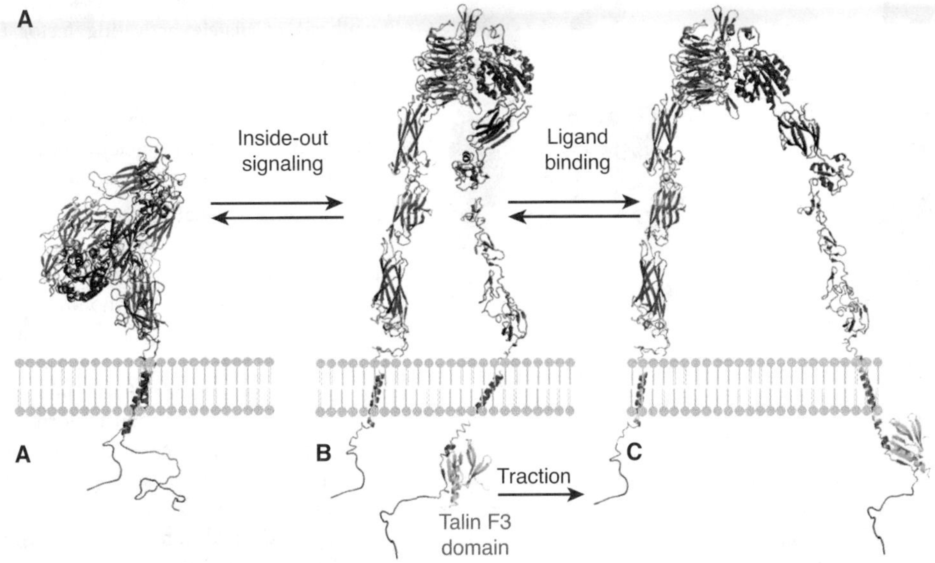

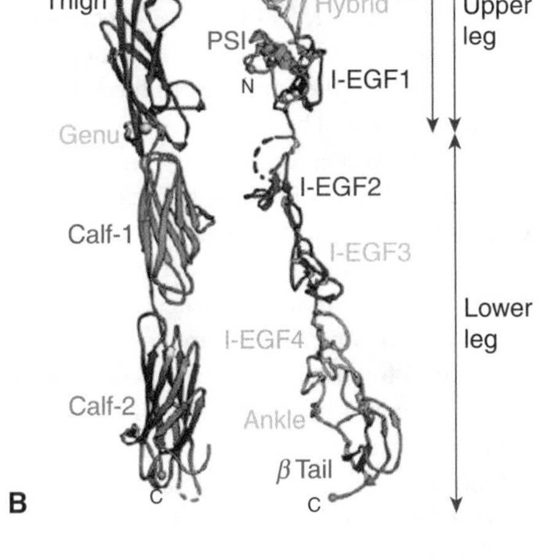

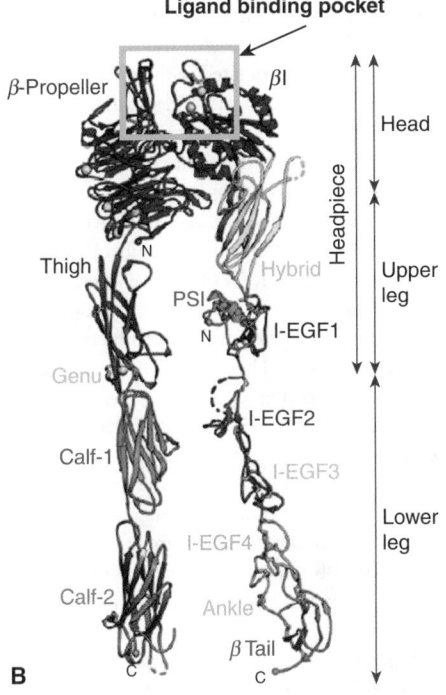

FIGURE 114–3. $\alpha_{IIb}\beta_3$ Integrin structure and activation. **A.** Model for $\alpha_{IIb}\beta_3$ integrin inside-out activation and outside-in signaling. The α-subunit is in *blue* and the β-subunit is in *red*. The bent, inactive receptor is depicted in (*A*). Under resting conditions, the β_3 cytoplasmic domain appears to interact with filamin. Cellular stimulation both induces migfilin to displace filamin from the β_3 cytoplasmic domain and initiates a conformational change in talin that alters the interactions between the talin head and rod domains and exposes the talin head domain. The FERM F3 domain in the head then binds to the β_3 cytoplasmic domain, which unclasps the α-subunit cytoplasmic and transmembrane domains from their complex with the β_3 cytoplasmic and transmembrane domains. Kindlin-3 binding to the β_3 cytoplasmic domain may facilitate talin binding and appears to be required for the conversion to the high-affinity state. The binding of talin then leads to separation of the ectodomain subunit tails and may diminish the interaction of the integrin headpiece with the tails. Although small ligands can bind to the receptor without headpiece extension, the large glycoprotein ligands may require extension to facilitate access to the ligand-binding site. Extension (*B*) may occur spontaneously after leg separation, or may result from traction force exerted on the β_3 cytoplasmic domain via talin's association with the cytoskeleton and actin–myosin contractile force. Ligand binding to the integrin is associated with a swing out motion of the β_3 hybrid domain from the βA(I) domain (*C*), which results in both increased ligand affinity via alterations in the ADMIDAS (adjacent to metal ion-dependent adhesion site) and MIDAS (metal ion-dependent adhesion site) regions of β_3 and greater leg separation. This conformational change may initiate outside-in signaling. The ligated integrins may then cluster (not shown). The structure in panel (*A*) is based on the crystal structure of the ectodomain (PDB 3FCS)[39] and the nuclear magnetic resonance (NMR) structure of the transmembrane and cytoplasmic domains (PDB 2K9J)[696] connected to unstructured cytosolic domains.[33] The structure in (*B*) is based on the same ectodomain crystal structure, but with extension at the genus of the subunits (PDB 3FCS),[39] and the NMR structures of the separated transmembrane and cytoplasmic domains (PDBs 2K1A and 2RMZ),[696] connected to unstructured cytosolic domains. The structure in (*C*) is based on crystal structure of the liganded receptor (PDB 2VDN) headpiece,[657] the extended structure of ectodomain (PDB3FCS),[39] and the monomeric transmembrane structures (PDBs 2K1A and 2RMZ) connected to unstructured cytosolic tails.[36,1570] *(Adapted with permission from Lau TL, Kim C, Ginsberg MH, et al.[696] Figure courtesy of Dr. Ana Negri.)* **B.** Domain structure of $\alpha_{IIb}\beta_3$. The individual domains and the ligand-binding pocket are identified in the model of the extended integrin. I-EGF, integrin epidermal growth factor; PSI, plexins, semaphorins, integrins. *(Reproduced with permission from Zhu J, Luo BH, Xiao T, et al.[39]) (continued)*

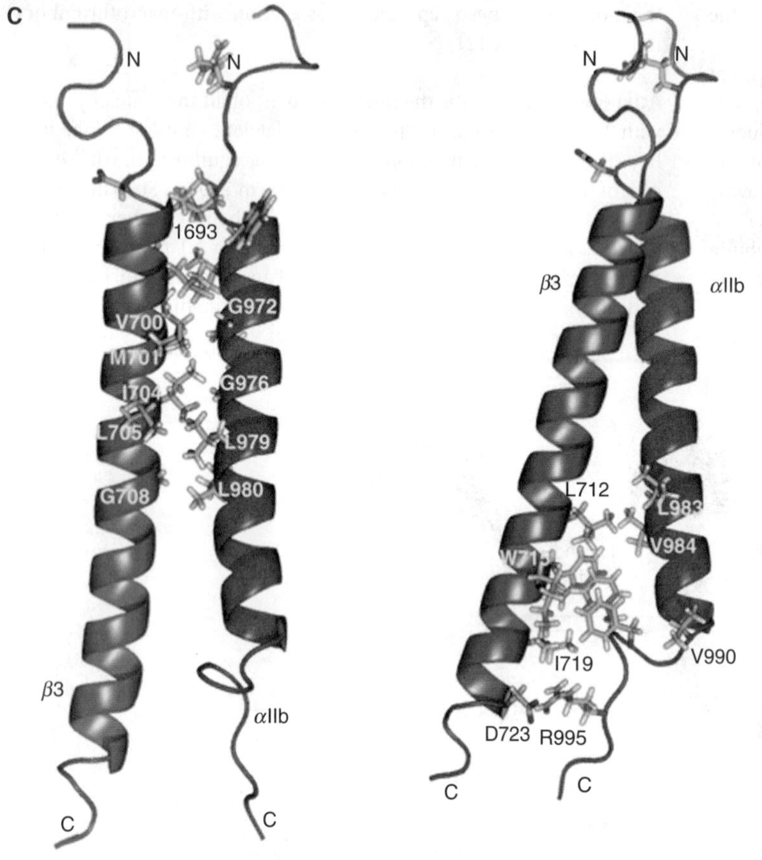

FIGURE 114–3. Continued. **C.** The integrin transmembrane complex. Selected views of the NMR structure of the α_{IIb} (*red*) and β_3 (*blue*) transmembrane complex. The *left panel* depicts contacts involved in the outer membrane clasp and the *right panel* depicts the contacts involved in the inner membrane clasp. Note that after the α_{IIb} helical region ends at V990, the next 5 residues (GFFKR) reenter the membrane; the two aromatic F residues make hydrophobic contacts with β_3 and α_{IIb} R995 makes a salt bridge with β_3 D723. *(Reproduced with permission from Lau TL, Kim C, Ginsberg MH, et al.[696])*

cytoplasmic network by abundantly expressed actin crosslinking proteins, including filamin and α-actinin.[58–60] Filamin exists in solution as homodimers of subunits that themselves are elongated strands composed primarily of 24 repeats, each approximately 100 amino acids in length, that are folded into immunoglobulin (Ig) G-like β barrels.[61,62] There are three filamin genes and they are located on the X chromosome and on chromosomes 3 and 7.[63,64] Filamin A (X chromosome) and filamin B (chromosome 3) are expressed in platelets, with filamin A accounting for approximately 90 percent of total filamin.

Filamin is a prototypical scaffolding protein that attracts binding partners, including the small guanosine triphosphatase (GTPase), RalA, Rac, Rho, and Cdc-42,[65] and positions them adjacent to the plasma membrane.[66] Approximately 90 percent of the filamin in resting platelets interacts with the cytoplasmic tail of the GPIbα subunit of the GPIb-IX-V complex via a binding site in filamin's second rod domain (repeats 17–20).[67,68] This interaction has three consequences. First, it positions filamin's self-association domain and associated partner proteins at the plasma membrane while presenting filamin's actin-binding sites into the cytoplasm. Second, because a large fraction of filamin is also bound to actin, it aligns the GPIb-IX-V complexes into rows on the plasma membrane surface of the platelet over the underlying actin filaments. Third, because the filamin linkages between actin filaments and the GPIb-IX-V complex pass through the pores of the spectrin lattice, it restrains the molecular movement of the spectrin strands in this lattice and holds the lattice in compression. The filamin-GPIbα connection is essential for the formation and release of discoid platelets by megakaryocytes, as platelets lacking this connection are produced in lower numbers and the ones that are produced are abnormally large and fragile. Platelets deficient in GPIb (Bernard-Soulier syndrome; see Chap. 121) are giant in size, perhaps as a result of abnormalities in organizing the cytoskeleton.

Organelles

Peroxisomes Peroxisomes are very small organelles present in platelets. They are thought to contribute to lipid metabolism, especially plasmalogen synthesis, and may participate in the synthesis of platelet-activating factor (PAF).[69] They contain acyl-coenzyme A (CoA):dihydroxyacetone phosphate acyltransferase, which catalyzes the first step in the synthesis of ether phospholipids. Deficiencies of this enzymatic activity have been identified in the cerebrorenal Zellweger syndrome and the platelet activity can be used to diagnose the disorder.[70,71]

Mitochondria and Platelet Energetics Platelets contain approximately four to seven mitochondria of relatively small size; like in other tissues, they are involved in oxidative energy metabolism.[72,73] Control of mitochondrial BCL-2 family proteins, including BCL-XL and BAK, directly affects a platelet's life span and alterations in these proteins can produce thrombocytopenia (see Chaps. 113 and 119).[74] Abnormalities of mitochondrial enzymes, including the reduced form of nicotinamide adenine dinucleotide (NADH) coenzyme Q reductase (complex I), have been implicated in the pathophysiology of aging and several neurodegenerative disorders, including Alzheimer disease, schizophrenia, and some forms of Parkinson disease. Assays of platelet mitochondrial enzyme levels have been used in these studies.[75–80] In addition, hyperglycemia-induced mitochondrial superoxide generation may contribute to the enhanced platelet aggregation observed in diabetes.[81] Loss of the mitochondrial inner leaflet potential has been associated with surface expression of platelet procoagulant activity and coated platelet formation[82–85] (see "Platelet Coagulant Activity" below).

Platelets have sizable stores of glycogen that can often be seen by electron microscopy (see Fig. 114–1). Glycogen can be broken down into glucose-1-phosphate, and platelets can also take up glucose from their surrounding medium. Platelet glycolysis rates significantly exceed those of erythrocytes and skeletal muscle.[86] Oxidative metabolism probably contributes to energy production in resting platelets, but it has been estimated that less than 1 percent of the pyruvate produced by glycolysis actually enters the citric acid cycle. The remainder is either converted to lactate or remains as pyruvate; both leave the platelet.[87] Platelet mitochondria are capable of oxidation of fatty acids, but its importance to energy production is unclear.[88–91] Platelets can actively metabolize acetate, which has been exploited to improve platelet storage conditions.[91,92] Amino acids may also act as energy sources and feed into the citric acid cycle, but their contributions are uncertain.

As in all cells, ATP consumption by platelets is partially devoted to maintaining ionic and osmotic homeostasis.[93,94] In addition, the continuous polymerization and depolymerization of actin involves conversion of ATP to adenosine diphosphate (ADP), and this may account for as much as 40 percent of the ATP consumption in resting platelets.[95] The continuous polymerization and depolymerization of tubulin that occurs in the coil of resting platelet involves conversion of guanosine triphosphate (GTP) to guanosine diphosphate (GDP), and thus consumes

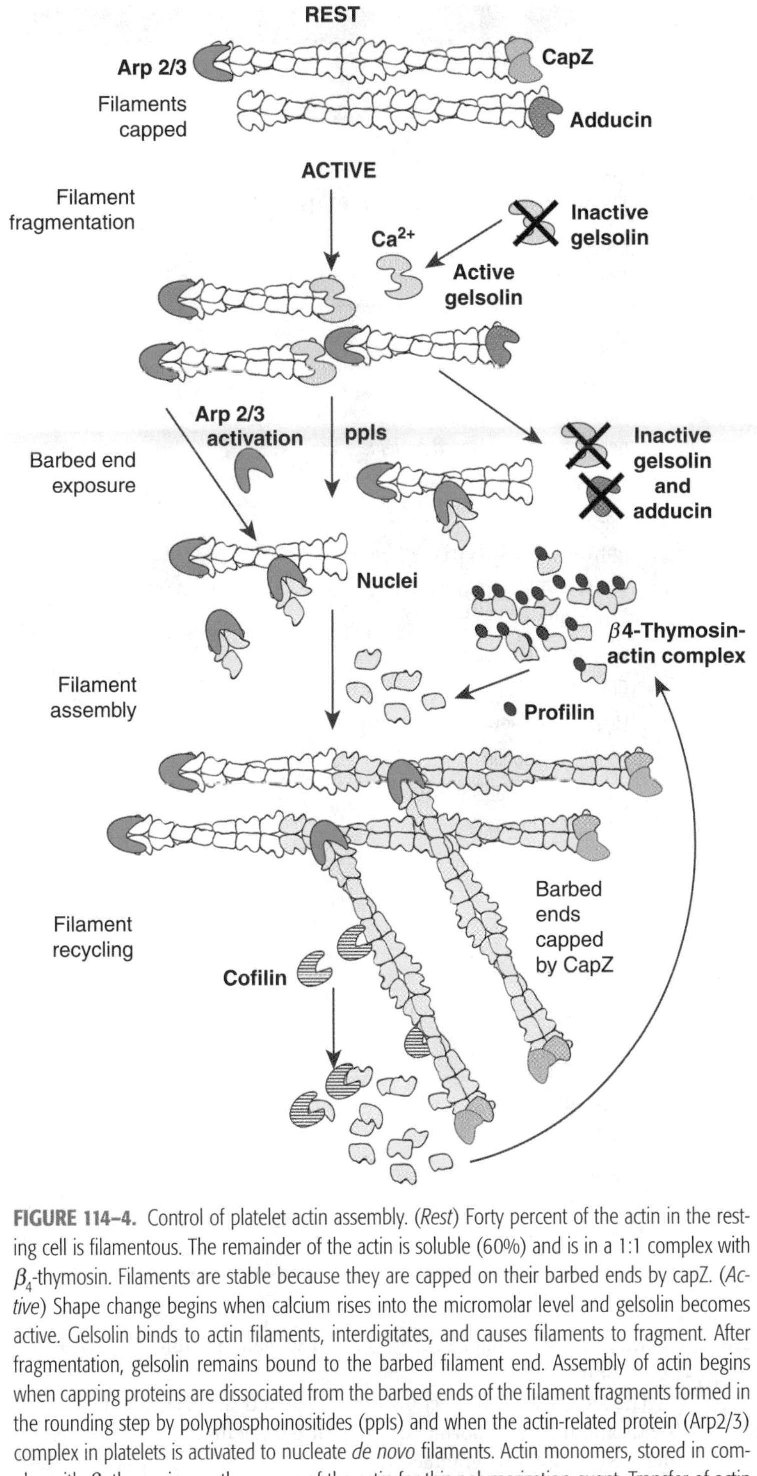

FIGURE 114–4. Control of platelet actin assembly. (*Rest*) Forty percent of the actin in the resting cell is filamentous. The remainder of the actin is soluble (60%) and is in a 1:1 complex with β_4-thymosin. Filaments are stable because they are capped on their barbed ends by capZ. (*Active*) Shape change begins when calcium rises into the micromolar level and gelsolin becomes active. Gelsolin binds to actin filaments, interdigitates, and causes filaments to fragment. After fragmentation, gelsolin remains bound to the barbed filament end. Assembly of actin begins when capping proteins are dissociated from the barbed ends of the filament fragments formed in the rounding step by polyphosphoinositides (ppls) and when the actin-related protein (Arp2/3) complex in platelets is activated to nucleate *de novo* filaments. Actin monomers, stored in complex with β_4-thymosin, are the source of the actin for this polymerization event. Transfer of actin from β_4-thymosin to the barbed ends of actin filaments is facilitated by profilin. Once assembly is complete, capZ recaps the barbed filament ends. *(Adapted with permission from Hartwig JH.[46])*

energy.[52] Continuing dephosphorylation and rephosphorylation of phosphatidylinositols, which are important in signal transduction, has been estimated to consume as much as 7 percent of the total ATP produced.[96] Protein phosphorylation also occurs as an ongoing process, but its fractional use of ATP is not clear in resting cells. Platelet stimulation leads to a marked increase in both glycolytic activity and oxidative ATP production, perhaps because of the abrupt decrease in ATP that occurs with platelet activation or the increase in cytoplasmic pH.[89] The increased ATP appears to be utilized, at least in part, for phosphatidylinositide and protein phosphorylation.

Depleting platelets of their metabolic pool of ATP and ADP decreases their responses to stimuli, but the effects are not uniform: shape change is only minimally affected, whereas there is an increasingly significant effect on aggregation, α-granule and dense granule (also termed *dense bodies*) secretion, arachidonic acid liberation, and lysosome secretion.[97–100]

Lysosomes Lysosomes are produced from the endosomal membrane system through a complex mechanism involving membrane and protein sorting and trafficking.[101] Platelet lysosomes contain acid hydrolases typical of these organelles (e.g., β-glucuronidase, cathepsins, aryl sulfatase, β-hexosaminidase, β-galactosidase, endoglucosidase [heparitinase], β-glycerophosphatase, elastase, and collagenase).[72] With activation, platelets secrete some of these enzymes; however, lysosomal contents are more slowly and less completely released than are those from α granules and dense granules.[97,98,102] Thus, stronger agonists are required to induce lysosomal enzyme release than release from the other granules. Proteins present in lysosomal membranes (e.g., lysosome-associated membrane protein [LAMP]-1, LAMP-2, and CD63 [LAMP-3]) are present in platelets, and their appearance on the plasma membrane serves as markers of high-level platelet activation.[103,104] The elastase and collagenase activities released from platelet lysosomes may contribute to vascular damage at sites of platelet thrombus formation.[105] The heparitinase may be able to cleave heparin-like molecules from the surface of endothelial cells, and the resulting soluble molecules appear to inhibit growth of smooth muscle cells.[106]

Dense Granules Platelets contain approximately three to eight electron-dense organelles, 20 to 30 nm in diameter (see Fig. 114–1).[2,107] The intrinsic electron density of dense granules when viewed as unstained whole mounts derives from their high content of calcium (Table 114–2)[2,72]; the granules are also dense when viewed by transmission electron microscopy because they are highly osmophilic.[107] Dense granules contain high concentrations of serotonin, which is taken up from plasma by a plasma membrane carrier and then trapped in the dense granules.[107] Trapping of serotonin may occur as a result of the lower pH (~6.1) maintained in dense granules as a result of the action of an H+ pumping ATPase on the dense body membrane.[107] ADP and ATP are also highly concentrated in dense granules.[72] There is more ADP than ATP in the dense granules (ATP-to-ADP = 2:3), which is the reverse of their relative concentrations in the cytoplasm (ATP-to-ADP = 8:1). As there is little connection between the pools of adenine nucleotides in the cytoplasm and the dense granules, they have been respectively designated as the *metabolic* and *storage pools* of adenine nucleotides.[72] Storage of adenine nucleotides at such a high concentration in dense granules appears to be achieved by stacking the ATP and ADP purine rings vertically in aggregates that are stabilized by the interactions of calcium ions with the polyphosphate groups.[108,109] The planar hydroxyindole rings of serotonin may also enter these stacks, providing a molecular basis for the trapping mechanism. Trapping of serotonin must differ from that of adenine nucleotides, however, because dense granule serotonin exchanges readily with external serotonin.[72] Transport and delivery of platelet-derived serotonin may play an important role in a variety of biologic phenomena, including vasospasm, platelet coagulant activity, and liver regeneration.[110]

TABLE 114–2. Platelet Granule and Cytoplasmic Contents

Dense granules I[1574]	
ADP	653 mM
ATP	436 mM
Calcium	2181 mM
Serotonin	65 mM
Pyrophosphate	326 mM
GDP	
Magnesium	

α Granules[120,129,132]

Platelet-specific proteins:
 Platelet factor 4 (PF4)
 β-Thromboglobulin (β-TG) family (platelet basic protein, low-affinity PF4, β-thromboglobulin, and β-thromboglobulin-F)
 Multimerin

Adhesive glycoproteins:
 Fibrinogen
 von Willebrand factor (VWF)
 VWF propeptide
 Fibronectin
 Thrombospondin-1
 Vitronectin

Coagulation factors:
 Factor V
 Protein S
 Factor XI

Mitogenic factors:
 Platelet-derived growth factor (PDGF)
 Transforming growth factor-β (TGF-β)
 Endothelial cell growth factor
 Epidermal growth factor (EGF)
 Insulin-like growth factor I

Angiogenic factors:
 Multiple inducers and inhibitors (see text)

Fibrinolytic inhibitors:
 α_2-Plasmin inhibitor (α_2-PI)
 Plasminogen activator inhibitor-1 (PAI-1)
Albumin
Immunoglobulins
Granule membrane-specific proteins:
 P-selectin (CD62P)
 CD63 (LAMP-3)
 GMP 33

Other secreted or released proteins[120,132]
 Protease nexin I
 Gas6
 Amyloid β-protein precursor (protease nexin II)
 Tissue factor pathway inhibitor (TFPI)
 Factor XIII
 α_1-Protease inhibitor
 Cl-inhibitor
 High-molecular-weight kininogen
 α_2-Macroglobulin
 Vascular permeability factor
 Interleukin (IL)-1β
 Histidine-rich glycoprotein

Chemokines:
 MIP-Iα (CCL3)
 RANTES (CCL5)
 MCP-3 (CCL7)
 GROα (CXCL1)
 PF4 (CXCL4)
 ENA-78 (CXCL5)
 NAP-2 (CXCL7)
 IL-8 (CXCL8)
 TARC (CCL17)

The membrane of dense granules contains glycoproteins that are also found on the plasma membrane and the membranes of α granules and lysosomes, including CD36, LAMP-2, CD63, P-selectin, integrin $\alpha_{IIb}\beta_3$, and GPIb/IX. Abnormalities of eight different genes have been implicated in the Hermansky-Pudlak syndrome (see Chap. 121), which is characterized by a deficiency of dense granules, and so these genes are presumed to participate in dense body formation. As with lysosomes, dense granules are thought to derive from endosomes, via different types of multivesicular bodies. The eight genes associated with Hermansky-Pudlak syndrome are thought to affect sorting and/or trafficking of membrane structures through participation in protein complexes that mediate these phenomena.[111,112] These complexes include three biogenesis of lysosome-related organelles complexes (BLOCs) and the activator protein 3 (AP3) complex.[101] Similarly, the product of the *LYST* gene, which is abnormal in some patients with Chédiak-Higashi syndrome (who also have abnormal dense granules), is proposed to associate with the dense granule

membrane (see Chap. 121).[113] The *LYST* gene product is part of the AP3 complex.[101]

The prolongation of bleeding time in patients with Hermansky-Pudlak syndrome and the abnormalities in their platelet function *in vitro* suggest that released dense granule contents contribute to platelet activation through a positive feedback mechanism. Release of ADP, which is a potent platelet activator (Fig. 114–5), and serotonin, a weaker agonist (see "Signaling Pathways in Platelet Activation and Aggregation" below), probably account for most of the positive feedback effects on platelet aggregation. ATP is a partial antagonist of ADP-induced activation, but as ATP is rapidly catabolized to ADP in plasma ($T_{1/2}$ = 1.5 minutes), and ADP is rapidly catabolized to AMP ($T_{1/2}$ = 4 minutes) and then to adenosine,[72] a platelet inhibitor,[114] it is difficult to predict the overall effect of ATP release. Adding to the complexity *in vivo* is the presence of an ecto-ATP diphosphohydrolase (ATPDase) (CD39; ecto-ADPase) present on endothelial and lymphoid cells, which can metabolize ATP and ADP to adenosine monophosphate (AMP) and thus probably limits the

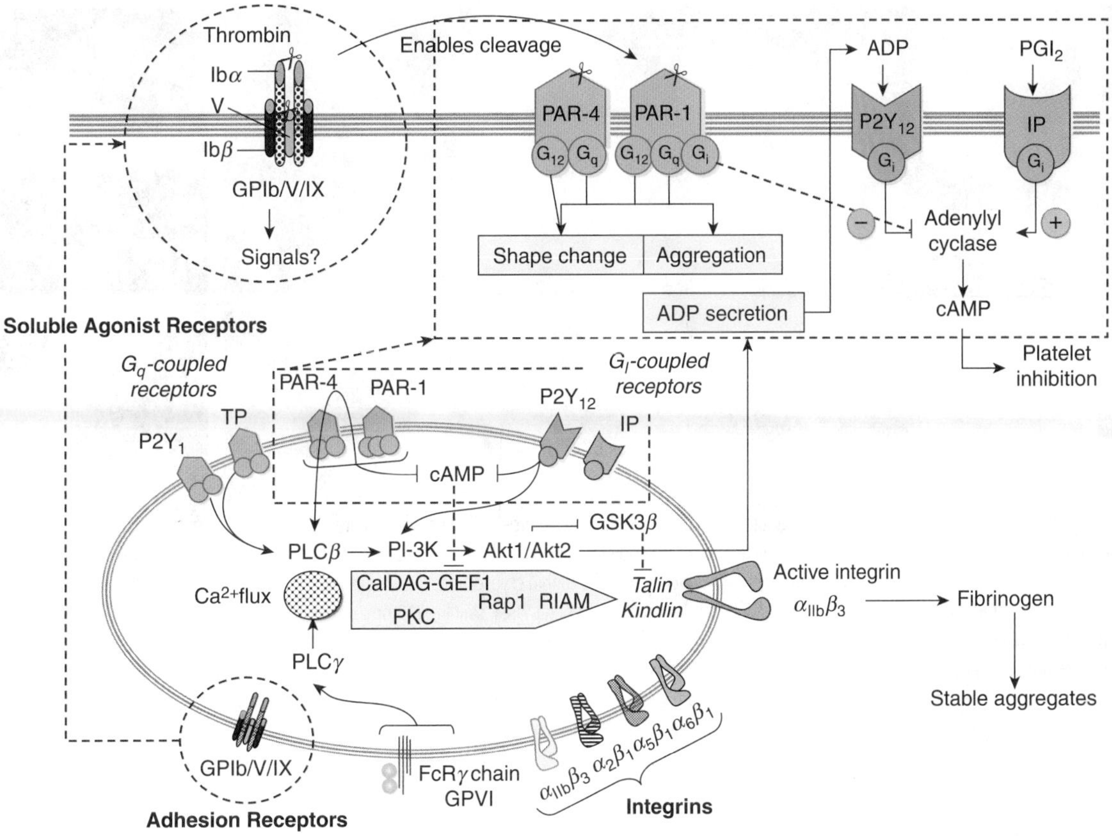

FIGURE 114–5. Role of G-protein-coupled receptors in platelet activation. Under basal conditions, prostacyclin produced by endothelial cells inhibits platelet activation by binding to its platelet receptor IP and increasing cyclic adenosine monophosphate (cAMP). When the endothelium is denuded, collagen interaction with GPVI can initiate signaling via the FcRγ chain. In addition, the glycoprotein (GP) Ib/V/IX complex can mediate adhesion of platelets to the newly exposed or deposited von Willebrand factor. This, in turn, can lead to platelet activation directly by a pathway not shown. GPIb/V/IX can also contribute to platelet activation by thrombin by facilitating the cleavage of protease-activated receptor (PAR)-1. PAR-1 can also be cleaved and activated via collagen-induced release and activation of pro-MMP-1 to MMP-1. In concert with PAR-4, cleaved PAR-1 initiates intracellular signaling pathways through molecular switches from the G_q, G_{12}, and G_i protein families. This results in ADP secretion and subsequent activation of both $P2Y_{12}$, and $P2Y_1$. A number of signals can also initiate the synthesis of thromboxane A_2, which can exit from the platelet and activate the same or other platelets by binding to its own receptor, TP. Ultimately, activation of phospholipase C (PLC) β and γ, and released calcium (Ca^{2+}) initiate a series of steps that terminate in talin and kindlin binding to the cytoplasmic domain of β_3 and activation of the glycoprotein (GP) $\alpha_{IIb}\beta_3$ receptor to its high-affinity ligand-binding state. CalDAG-GEF1, calcium and diacylglycerol-regulated guanine-nucleotide exchange factor 1; PKC, protein kinase C; RIAM, Rap1-GTP-interacting adapter molecule. *(Reproduced with permission from Smyth SS, Woulfe DS, Weitz JI, et al.[157])*

amount of ADP present.[115] ATP released from platelets may also serve as a high energy phosphate source for platelet ecto-protein kinases, which can phosphorylate several proteins, including CD36 (GPIV).[116–119]

α Granules An important platelet function is storage and release of a variety of bioactive substances packaged in α granules. α Granules are the most abundant granule type of platelets, numbering approximately 50 to 80 per platelet.[120,121] They are approximately 200 nm in diameter on cross section and demonstrate internal variation in electron density, often with an eccentric area of accentuated electron density, termed a *nucleoid*, in which β-thromboglobulin, platelet factor 4, and proteoglycans are concentrated (see Fig. 114–1).[122] The more electron-lucent areas contain tubular elements in which von Willebrand factor (VWF), multimerin, and factor V are preferentially localized.[2] Proteomic analysis of proteins released from activated human platelets has identified more than 300 proteins, most of which are stored within α granules.[123–125] The list of α-granule proteins includes adhesive proteins, coagulation factors, protease inhibitors, chemokines, and angiogenesis regulatory proteins. Some of the most important proteins present in α granules are listed in Table 114–2 and described in detail below. Platelets contain distinct subpopulations of α granules that undergo differential release of their contents during activation. For example, some α granules contain proangiogenic proteins, such as vascular endothelial growth factor (VEGF), whereas others contain antiangiogenic factors, such as endostatin (Fig. 114–6).[126] These two subclasses of α granules can be differentially induced to undergo degranulation by exposure of human platelets to agonists specific for either proteinase-activated receptor (PAR)-1 or PAR-4. Fibrinogen and von Willebrand factor are localized in separate α granules,[127] and glass activation of platelets results in the selective release of the fibrinogen-containing granules.

The α granule acquires its protein content by both biosynthesis (predominantly at the megakaryocyte level) and endocytosis (at both the megakaryocyte and circulating platelet levels). Small amounts of virtually all plasma proteins are nonspecifically taken up into α granules, and thus the plasma levels of these proteins determine their platelet levels.[128,129] For example, the α-granule pool of immunoglobulins contains most of the platelet immunoglobulin; therefore, total platelet immunoglobulin is more affected by changes in plasma immunoglobulin levels than by changes in surface immunoglobulin (see Chap. 119).[128,129]

The cell biologic pathways that regulate α-granule assembly are not fully understood, but several studies suggest that multivesicular bodies play a crucial intermediary role in α-granule biogenesis.[111,130] These

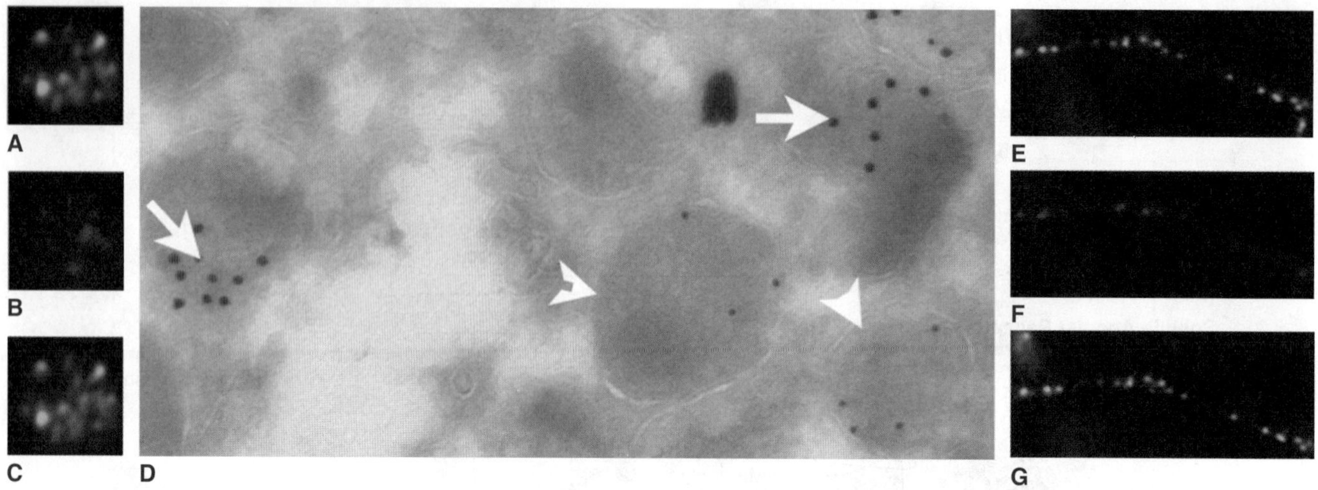

FIGURE 114–6. Platelets contain separate and distinct α-granule populations. **A–C.** Specific pro- and antiangiogenic regulators organize into separate, distinct α-granules in resting platelets. Double immunofluorescence microscopy of resting platelets using antibodies against vascular endothelial growth factor (VEGF) **(A)** and endostatin **(B)** and an overlay **(C)**. **D.** Localization of proteins in resting, human platelets using immunoelectron microscopy of ultrathin cryosections. Double immunogold labeling on platelet sections was performed with the use of anti-VEGF antibody and antiendostatin antibodies. Large gold particles representing anti-VEGF staining (15 nm, *arrows*) are evident on one population of α granules and small gold particles (5 nm) representing endostatin staining are abundantly present on a different population of α granules (*arrowheads*). **E–G.** Pro- and antiangiogenic regulatory proteins are also segregated into separate, distinct α granules in megakaryocyte proplatelets. Megakaryocytes generate platelets by remodeling their cytoplasm into long proplatelet extensions, which serve as assembly lines for platelet production. Distinct α granules are visualized along proplatelets. Shown is a double-immunofluorescence microscopy experiment of proplatelets using antibodies against VEGF **(E)** and endostatin **(F)**, and an overlay **(G)**. *(Adapted with permission from Italiano JE Jr, Richardson JL, Patel-Hett S, et al.[126])*

membranous sacs, containing numerous small vesicles, develop from budding vesicles in the Golgi complex within megakaryocytes and can interact with endocytic vesicles. They are abundant in immature megakaryocytes and decrease in number with cellular maturation, suggesting that they are the precursors of α granules and/or dense granules. Multivesicular bodies may also function as a sorting hub to rout proteins into distinct classes of α granules.

The platelet-specific proteins (platelet factor 4 and the β-thromboglobulin family) are present in α granules at concentrations that are approximately 20,000 times higher than their plasma concentrations (when each is expressed as a fraction of total protein in platelets or plasma, respectively; see Table 114–2).[131,132] These Mr 7000 to 11,000 proteins bind to heparin, but with varying affinities. They also share amino acid sequence homology with each other and with other members of the "intercrine-cytokine" family of molecules, such as interleukin (IL)-8 (neutrophil-activating peptide 1 [NAP1]), which are active in inflammation, cell growth, and malignant transformation (Fig. 114–7).[133–135]

Platelet factor 4 (PF4) is a CXC chemokine (CXCL4) that does not contain the Glu-Leu-Arg (ELR) conserved sequence.[136,137] It binds to heparin with high affinity and can neutralize heparin's anticoagulant activity.[131,138–140] PF4–heparin complexes are the target antigen in heparin-induced thrombocytopenia, and so are of great medical relevance. PF4 tetramers complex with a proteoglycan carrier.[141,142] Specific PF4 lysine residues (amino acids 61, 62, 65, and 66) have been implicated in its binding to heparin, and X-ray crystallography indicates that these lysines are on the surface of the PF4 tetramer and interact with negatively charged heparin molecules that wind around this core.[143–145]

After PF4 is released from platelets, it also binds to heparin-like molecules on the surface of endothelial cells.[144] Heparin administration can mobilize this endothelial-bound pool of PF4 into the circulation.[144] PF4-heparin complexes and PF4–heparin-like molecule complexes on endothelial cells have also been implicated as the key target antigens in heparin-induced thrombocytopenia with thrombosis.[146,147] PF4 also binds to hepatocytes, which take it up and catabolize it.[148] PF4 is a weak neutrophil and fibroblast attractant.[136,149] It inhibits angiogenesis, perhaps through inhibition of endothelial cell proliferation.[150] A large number of other activities have been ascribed to PF4, including histamine release from basophils[151]; inhibition of both tumor growth[152] and megakaryocyte maturation[153–155]; reversal of immunosuppression[149,156]; enhancement of fibroblast attachment to substrata[157]; potentiation of platelet aggregation[158]; inhibition of contact activation[159]; and enhancement of both polymorphonuclear leukocyte responsiveness to the activating peptide f-Met-Leu-Phe and monocyte responsiveness to lipopolysaccharide.[160,161]

The β-thromboglobulin family of proteins are CXC chemokines that contain the conserved Glu-Leu-Arg (ELR) sequence.[136] They include platelet basic protein, low-affinity PF4 (connective tissue-activating peptide III [CTAP-III]), β-thromboglobulin, and β-thromboglobulin-F (NAP2, CXCL7) (see Table 114–2 and Fig. 114–7).[132,162–164] All of these proteins share the same carboxy terminus but differ in the length of their amino termini, presumably as a result of proteolytic digestion of the parent molecule, platelet basic protein (see Fig. 114–7). These proteins bind to heparin but with lower affinity than PF4, and thus neutralize heparin less well. Unlike PF4, they are cleared from the circulation by the kidney rather than the liver.[165] CTAP-III is a weak fibroblast mitogen, and β-thromboglobulin is a chemoattractant for fibroblasts.[136] β-Thromboglobulin-F NAP2 (CXCL7) binds to CXCR2 and is chemotactic for granulocytes and activates them to undergo endocytosis.[136,137,164] Platelet α granules also contain additional chemokines (see Table 114–2) that can variably activate leukocytes and platelets.[137]

The biochemistry of the adhesive glycoproteins contained in α granules and others variably present in plasma and extracellular matrix is described in Table 114–3 and in other chapters (see Chaps. 115 and 126 for fibrinogen and Chap. 127 for VWF). Their relative concentrations in α granules vary significantly. Their localization in platelet α granules allows them to achieve high local concentrations when released from platelets at the site of vascular injury.

Multimerin comprises a family of disulfide-linked homomultimers, ranging in molecular weight from 450,000 to many millions.[166] The Mr 450,000 multimer is thought to be a trimer of a single subunit of either

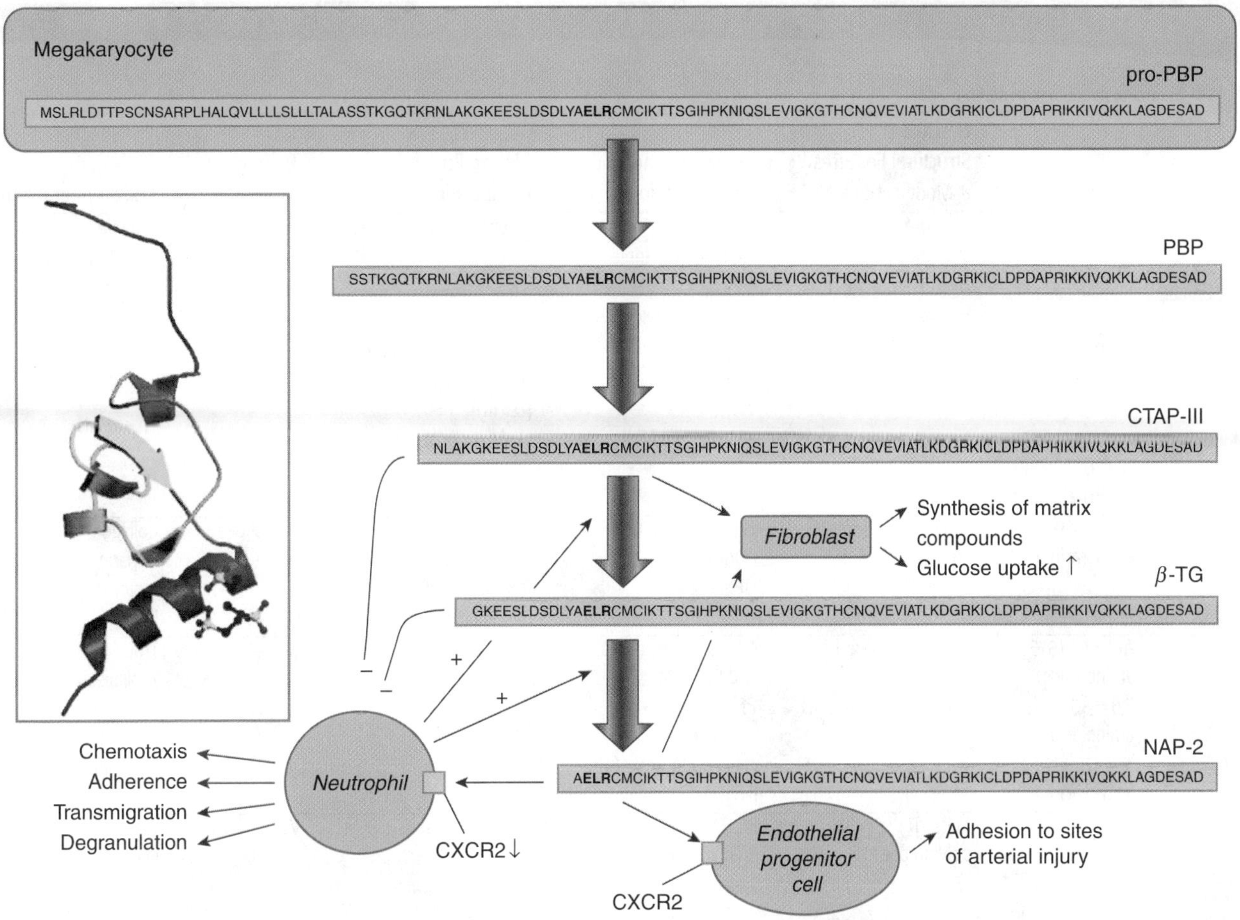

FIGURE 114–7. Amino acid sequences of the differentially truncated peptide forms of the platelet-specific β-thromboglobulin family of proteins, also known as the cytokine CXCL7. Starting with pro-PBP in megakaryocytes, sequential proteolytic modification (*blue arrows*) generates different CXCL7 peptides with different biologic functions that are indicated by *short red arrows*. Neutrophil-activating peptide-2 (NAP-2) is the chemotactically most active form of CXCL7. Further truncation removing the ELR domain (*bold ELR*) results in loss of activity. The insert depicts the tertiary structure of connective tissue activating peptide-III (CTAP-III), complexed with the heparin analogue polyvinylsulfonic acid (ball-and-stick structure adjacent to the helix), as given by protein database (PDB). *(Reproduced with permission from Gleissner CA, von Hundelshausen P, Ley K: Platelet chemokines in vascular disease.* Art Thromb Vasc Biol *28:1920, 2008.)*

Mr 167,000[167] or Mr 155,000[166] that is synthesized in megakaryocytes and endothelial cells and stored in the electron-lucent region of α granules in platelets and dense-core granules in endothelial cells.[168] It colocalizes with VWF in platelets, but not endothelial cells. Although multimerin's multimeric structure is similar to that of VWF, the deduced amino acid sequence of its subunit is not homologous to that of VWF.[166] The prepromultimerin subunit contains 1228 amino acids. It undergoes glycosylation and proteolysis during synthesis. It is composed of a number of domains, including an amino-terminal region that includes an RGD sequence, coiled-coil sequences, epidermal growth factor–like domains, and a carboxy-terminal globular head similar to that found in the complement protein C1q. Multimerin binds both factor V and factor Va, and all of the biologically active factor V in platelets is bound to multimerin.[122] With thrombin activation of platelets, factor V separates from multimerin, and the higher-molecular-weight multimerin multimers bind to platelets. Multimerin does not circulate in plasma at an appreciable concentration, but it may act as an adhesive extracellular matrix protein.

Fibrinogen is concentrated in α granules as judged by the ratio of platelet-to-plasma fibrinogen. Megakaryocytes do not appear to synthesize fibrinogen; instead, it is taken up from plasma by a process that involves the $\alpha_{IIb}\beta_3$ receptor.[169] Because fibrinogen molecules that contain altered sequences in the γ chain are not stored in α granules, even when the molecules are heterodimeric (i.e., contain one normal and one abnormal γ chain), it is possible that uptake requires simultaneous binding of a single fibrinogen molecule to two different $\alpha_{IIb}\beta_3$ receptors via the γ-chain carboxy-terminal sequence (see "$\alpha_{IIb}\beta_3$ (GPIIb/IIIa; Fibrinogen Receptor; CD41/CD61)" below and Chap. 121).[169,170]

The VWF stored in platelet α granules contributes to hemostasis because in certain pathologic states it correlates better with bleeding symptoms than does plasma VWF (see Chap. 127). VWF is in megakaryocytes and endothelial cells (see Chaps. 117 and 127). The multimeric structure of platelet VWF is thought to reflect endothelial VWF more nearly than plasma VWF, since higher Mr multimers are present (see Chap. 127).

Fibronectin is present in α granules, but no clear role in platelet function under normal conditions has been identified for this adhesive protein. In mouse models, fibronectin has been paradoxically reported to both support platelet thrombus formation in mice that lack both fibrinogen and VWF and inhibit platelet aggregation and thrombus formation[171,172]; the former effect may be mediated by insoluble fibronectin fibrils, whereas the latter may be mediated by soluble fibronectin.[173]

Vitronectin, which gets its name from its propensity to bind to glass, also binds to PAI-1, the urokinase receptor (uPAR), collagen, and

TABLE 114–3. Adhesive Glycoproteins

Protein	Subunit, κDa	Unusual 1° Structural Features & Modifications	Domain Homologies & Binding Regions	Mature Protein Composition	Mature Protein M_r	Known Interactions
Collagens	95–180	Gly-Pro-X repeating sequence Hydroxylysine Hydroxyproline	RGD Right-handed triple helix	Tropocollagen = 3 chains		Variable Thrombospondin
Type I	α_1(I) α_2(I)		DGEA† VWFC	$[\alpha_1(I)]_2\alpha_2(I)$ (major component) $[\alpha_1(I)]_3$		Fibronectin von Willebrand factor
Type III	α_1(III)		VWFC	$[\alpha_1(III)]_3$		
Type VI	α_1(VI) α_2(VI) α_3(VI)		3 VWFA 3 VWFA 12 VWFA	$\alpha_1(VI)\alpha_2(VI)\alpha_3(VI)$		
von Willebrand factor	220 (2050 amino acids)	Large propeptide (741 amino acids); A, B, C, D, E repeats	$\alpha_{IIb}\beta_3$ – RGD 1789–1791 I Domains GPIb – 230–310	Dimer = protomer Multimers of protomers from 2 to ~40 via disulfide bonds	880,000–~20,000,000	Collagen Heparin Factor VIII Fibrin
Fibrinogen	Aα = 63 (625 amino acids) Bβ = 56 (461 amino acids) γ = 47 (427 amino acids)	Alternately spliced γ chains Phosphorylation of Aα	2 RGDs in Aα (95–97 and 572–574) $\alpha_V\beta_3$ – RGD 572–574 $\alpha_{IIb}\beta_3$–C-terminal γ-chain dodecamer (400–411)	2 Aα, 2 Bβ, 2 γ via disulfide bonds	340,000	Thrombospondin ?Collagen Staphylococci Factor XIII Thrombin
Vitronectin	1 chain = 75 (458 amino acids) 2 chain = 65+10 via disulfide bonds	Met→Thr polymorphism	RGD Somatomedin B 2 Hemopexin	Same as subunits	75,000 and 65,000+ 10,000	Glass Plastic Heparin Serine protease: serpin complexes PAI-1 uPAR Factor XIII
Fibronectin	220 (2355 amino acids)	Types I, II, and III repeats Alternately spliced forms	RGD (1493–1495)	Heterodimer via disulfide bonds	440,000	Fibrin Heparin Collagen DNA Staphylococci
Thrombospondin 1	180 (1150 amino acids)		RGD (?functional) VTCG† α_1(I) Collagen Epidermal growth factor Malaria antigen	Trimer via disulfide bonds	450,000	Calcium Plasminogen Collagen Fibrinogen Histidine-rich glycoprotein Fibronectin Laminin Heparin
Osteopontin	32 (298 amino acids)	Phosphorylation Sulfation	RGD			Hydroxyapatite Plaque components
Laminin	A = 400 B_1 = 215 (1765 amino acids) B_2 = 205 (1576 amino acids)		YIGSR† RGD (?functional) EGF	A, B_1, B_2, via disulfide bonds	850,000	Collagen type IV Nidogen/entactin Osteonectin Heparin sulfate C1q Plasminogen Plasmin
Multimerin	155 or 167 kDa	Large prepro-peptide (1228 amino acids)	RGD in N-terminal region EGF		450,000–~5,000,000	Factor V

EGF, epidermal growth factor; PAI-1, plasminogen activator-1; RDG, arginine-glycine-aspartic acid sequence; uPAR, urine-type plasminogen activator receptor; VWFA, VWFC, von Willebrand factor A and C repeats.

Known Platelet Receptors	Electron Microscopy Structure	Plasma Concentration, mcg/mL	Platelet Concentration,* mcg/mL	Ratio Platelet/ Plasma	Sites of Synthesis
$\alpha_2\beta_1$ (GPIa/IIa;CD49b/CD29; VLA-2) GPVI GPIV (CD36)?	Tropocollagen = rodlike coil, 15 × 3000; other forms have variable degrees of fibril formation	–	–	–	Fibroblasts
GPIb (CD42b, c) $\alpha_{IIb}\beta_3$ (GPIIb/IIIa; CD41/CD61)	Elliptical, nodular coil, length 5000, but with some 11,000 Å	10	34	3.4	Endothelial cells Megakaryocytes
$\alpha_{IIb}\beta_3$ (GPIIb/IIIa; CD41/CD61) $\alpha_V\beta_3$ (CD51/CD61)	Trinodular, asymmetrical; 475 Å diameter	3000	7300	2.4	Hepatocytes
$\alpha_{IIb}\beta_3$ (GPIIb/IIIa; CD41/CD61) $\alpha_V\beta_3$ (CD51/CD61)		350	800	2.3	?Hepatocytes
$\alpha_5\beta_1$ (GPIc*/IIa (CD49e/CD29; VLA-5) $\alpha_{IIb}\beta_3$ (GPIIb/IIIa; CD41/CD61)	Extended antiparallel dimeric structure	300	315	1.1	Hepatocytes Fibroblasts ?Endothelial cells Megakaryocytes Monocytes, etc.
GPIV (CD36) $\alpha_{IIb}\beta_3$ (GPIIb/IIIa; CD41/CD61)? Integrin associated protein (CD47)	3 Asymmetrical dumbbells, joined near smaller globular domains	0.16	4900	30,625	Megakaryocytes Many cultured cells
$\alpha_V\beta_3$		–	–	–	Bone ?Other cells
$\alpha_6\beta_1$ (GPIc/IIa; CD49/CD29; VLA-6)	Cross-like structure	–	–	–	Fibroblasts Many other cell types
Unknown	Unknown	–	–	–	Megakaryocytes Endothelial cells

*Assumes 10^{11} platelets per mL of packed platelets.

†DGEA, VTCG, and YIGSR are other amino acid sequences involved in function.

heparin; it also forms ternary complexes with serine proteases and serpins in the coagulation and complement systems. It is present in platelets at levels that suggest it is concentrated,[174] but it does not appear to be synthesized in megakaryocytes. The binding of PAI-1 with vitronectin stabilizes PAI-1 in its active conformation, and it has been proposed that only the approximately 5 percent of PAI-1 complexed with vitronectin in platelet α granules is active.[40] Mice deficient in vitronectin have been reported to be protected from, or have a predisposition to develop, thrombosis, depending on the method of inducing thrombosis.[175–177]

Thrombospondin-1 is unique among the adhesive glycoproteins in blood in that it is present almost exclusively inside the platelet.[178–180] It constitutes approximately 20 percent of the released platelet proteins. Thrombospondin-1 is synthesized by megakaryocytes, cultured endothelial cells, and other cultured cells.[181,182] Although $\alpha_{IIb}\beta_3$, GPIb/IX, $\alpha_V\beta_3$, proteoglycans, integrin-associated protein (CD47 or IAP), and CD36 (GPIV) have all been implicated as receptors for thrombospondin,[183–189] CD47 appears to be most important in initiating platelet activation by thrombospondin (see "Signaling Pathways in Platelet Activation and Aggregation" below).[187,188,190] The phosphorylation state of CD36 (GPIV) may affect its ability to bind thrombospondin.[185] Thrombospondin contains an Arg-Gly-Asp (RGD) sequence, which may contribute to its binding to platelets, but other regions are probably also involved.[179] The conformation of thrombospondin varies with the calcium concentration of the surrounding environment. Thrombospondin can interact with many other adhesive glycoproteins, including fibronectin and fibrinogen,[191–193] and it is a component of the extracellular matrix.[194] Thrombospondin appears to stabilize platelet aggregates that are formed[195]; it may also act as a negative regulator of angiogenesis, modulate fibrinolysis, and contribute to activation of latent transforming growth factor (TGF)-β1 released from platelets.[196,197,197a]

Platelets contribute approximately 20 percent of the factor V present in whole blood, with nearly all of it in α granules.[198–200] Human platelet factor V appears to be taken up from plasma rather than being synthesized in megakaryocytes, which is in stark contrast to the situation in mice. When stored in α granules, factor V associates with multimerin.[201,202] Platelet-derived factor V appears to undergo unique posttranslational modifications and proteolytic activation, resulting in resistance to protein C-catalyzed inactivation.[203–205] Evidence from patients with inhibitors and deficiencies of plasma and platelet factor V indicates that platelet-derived factor V has an important role in hemostasis.[200,206,207] Platelets undergo microvesiculation when activated, and the microvesicles, which are rich in factor V, are potent promoters of coagulation.[208]

Protein S (see Chap. 116), plasminogen activator inhibitor-1 (see Chap. 136), and α_2-plasmin inhibitor (see Chap. 136) are also contained in α granules and can be released from platelets. Similarly, tissue factor pathway inhibitor (see Chap. 116), α_1-protease inhibitor, and C-1 inhibitor (see Chap. 116) are also found in α granules.

Gas6 is a 75-kDa vitamin K–dependent protein that contains γ-carboxyglutamic acids and is similar in structure to protein S.[209,210] Gas6 was originally isolated as a growth arrest–specific gene from quiescent fibroblasts, but subsequently was found to enhance platelet aggregation and secretion in response to several agonists.[211] Mice deficient in Gas6 have abnormalities in platelet aggregation and are protected from experimental thrombosis.[211] Gas6 is present in α granules and secreted with platelet activation. Platelets also express Mer, a tyrosine kinase receptor for Gas6, and mice deficient in Mer demonstrate both abnormalities in platelet aggregation and protection from thrombosis, but not to the same extent as mice deficient in Gas6.[212,213] Other Gas6 receptors in the same family as Mer also appear to contribute to platelet thrombus stability.[212–216]

Platelet-derived growth factor (PDGF) is a disulfide-linked dimeric molecule of molecular weight 30,000 that is mitogenic for smooth muscle cells.[217] Platelet α granules contain a mixture of the homodimer PDGF-BB (30%) and the heterodimer PDGF-AB (70%); the different forms appear to have different functional activities.[218] PDGF may play a role in normal cell proliferation, as well as in the development of atherosclerosis, tumor growth, wound repair, and fibroproliferative responses.[219–221] After it was discovered in platelets and named platelet-derived growth factor, other tissues were found to produce the same factor; thus, despite its name, PDGF is not exclusively derived from platelets. PDGF is structurally related to the transforming protein p28^{sis} of simian sarcoma virus,[222,223] and it is a true epiphany that linked viral oncogenesis to normal pathways of cell growth. The PDGF receptor is in the tyrosine kinase family.[224] Recombinant human PDGF-BB is used topically to improve healing of foot ulcerations in diabetics.[225]

Platelets contain high concentrations of VEGF, an important stimulator of angiogenesis, and can release VEGF after stimulation *in vitro* and during the hemostatic response to a bleeding time wound.[226–228] Megakaryocytes express messenger RNA (mRNA) of the three VEGF isoforms (121, 165, and 189 amino acids),[229] and by immunoblot VEGF protein bands of apparent molecular weights 34,000 and 44,000 are identifiable in platelets.[230] Platelets and megakaryocytes also express the gene transcript for the VEGF receptor termed *KDR*.[231] Another endothelial growth factor structurally related to VEGF, VEGF-C, has also been identified in platelets.[232] Platelet levels of VEGF have been reported to be increased in malignancies, and so elevated levels of platelet VEGF may be a cancer biomarker.[126,233] Platelet VEGF has also been postulated to play in role in tumor growth[234] and proliferative retinopathy in sickle cell disease.[235,236]

Epidermal growth factor has also been identified in platelets, but the kinetics of its release upon thrombin or collagen stimulation differs from that of other granule proteins.[237]

Platelets contain the highest levels of all peripheral tissues of amyloid precursor protein (APP), which contains the sequence for the self-aggregating 40- to 43-amino-acid residue peptide, Aβ, that has been strongly implicated in the pathogenesis of Alzheimer disease.[238–240] The isoforms containing the Kunitz protease inhibitor domain (APP 770 and APP 751) predominate in platelets. Although synthesized as a membrane protein, platelet APP is cleaved by α-, β-, and γ-secretase activities, producing all of the fragments produced by neurons, as well as the soluble sAPPα, sAPPβ, and Aβ peptides, and the corresponding remaining C-terminal membrane-associated fragments.[241,242] Calpain, which is present in platelets, can also cleave platelet APP.[243] Approximately 90 percent of platelet APP is soluble and stored in α granules, but full-length APP surface expression is increased threefold by thrombin stimulation.[244] Platelets are the major source of plasma sAPPs and Aβ.[241,245] APPs released by platelets are potent inhibitors of factors XIa[246] and IXa,[247,248] and also can inhibit platelet aggregation induced by ADP or epinephrine. In contrast, Aβ appears to enhance ADP-induced platelet aggregation and support platelet adhesion. It is possible, but not certain, that plasma Aβ contributes to brain Aβ in Alzheimer disease.[239] Patients with Alzheimer disease are reported to have altered platelet APP metabolism.[249–254]

Factor XIII is present in the cytoplasm of platelets; it differs from plasma factor XIII in having only the "a" subunits (see Chap. 115).[255–258] Platelet factor XIII accounts for approximately 50 percent of total blood factor XIII,[255,256] and platelet factor XIII may contribute to the plasma pool.[259] Upon platelet activation, factor XIII redistributes to the platelet periphery where it associates with the cytoskeleton and crosslinks filamin and vinculin in a transglutaminase reaction.[260] It may also crosslink thymosin β_4 to fibrin after thrombin stimulation[261] and, in concert with calpain, decreases integrin $\alpha_{IIb}\beta_3$ adhesive function in thrombus formation on collagen.[262] Transglutaminase-mediated conjugation of serotonin to α-granule proteins after platelet stimulation with collagen and thrombin results in the generation of a subpopulation of platelets that are coated with fibrinogen, thrombospondin, factor V, VWF, and fibronectin, either directly through ligand-receptor interactions or through interactions between the serotonin conjugates and platelet surface fibrinogen or thrombospondin ("coated" platelets).[263,264]

Platelet α granules contain a high concentration of TGF-β_1, a 25,000 molecular weight homodimeric protein that promotes the growth of certain cells and inhibits the growth of others.[265–268] For example, TGF-β can increase thrombopoietin production by marrow stromal cells. In turn, thrombopoietin induces both increased megakaryocyte production and megakaryocyte expression of TGF-β receptors. The interaction of TGF-β with these receptors then results in inhibition of megakaryocyte maturation.[269] TGF-β_1 also induces synthesis of extracellular matrix proteins, PAI-1, and metalloproteinases. It has been implicated in wound healing, malignancy, and tissue fibrosis.[270] In addition, TGF-β_1 has been reported to enhance platelet aggregation through a nontranscriptional effect.[271] Migration of endothelial cells is inhibited by TGF-β_1, but it acts as a chemoattractant for monocytes and fibroblasts. TGF-β exists in three isoforms (TGF-β_1, TGF-β_2, and TGF-β_3), but platelets contain only TGF-β_1. TGF-β_1 released from platelets can stimulate smooth muscle cells to express and release VEGF, thus perhaps supporting reendothelialization after vascular injury.[272]

TGF-β_1 released from platelets is inactive (latent) because it is complexed with the remaining portion of its precursor protein (latency-associated peptide [LAP]). LAP, in turn, is covalently coupled to another protein, the latent TGF-β-binding protein-1 (LTBP-1), which localizes the complex to the extracellular matrix.[273] Activation of latent TGF-β_1 is a complex process that is thought to involve a conformational change in LAP that results in altering its ability to shield the active site in TGF-β_1.[273] Activation of latent TGF-β_1 can be achieved by several different mechanisms, including acidification; proteolysis by plasmin, a furin-like enzyme, or other enzymes; interaction with integrin $\alpha_V\beta_6$; interaction with thrombospondin-1 or a small peptide derived from thrombospondin-1; or exposure to stirring or shear.[179,197,273–275] The physiologic activator(s), however, remains unclear. The ability of thrombospondin-1 to activate TGF-β_1 is of especial interest because both TGF-β_1 and thrombospondin-1 are present in α granules. However, data from mice suggest only a minor role for platelet thrombospondin in either TGF-β_1 packaging or activation.[276–278] Only a very small percentage of the TGF-β_1 released from platelets with thrombin stimulation becomes activated, but this amount is sufficient to activate synthesis of plasminogen activator inhibitor-1.[274–276,279] Active TGF-β can bind to three different cell surface proteins, a proteoglycan (β-glycan), and two serine/threonine kinases.[270,280]

Platelets may also release proteins that affect the uptake of oxidized low-density lipoproteins by macrophages, furnishing another potential link between platelet activation and atherosclerosis.[281]

Exosomes In addition to the contents of α granules, activated platelets release both microparticles (see "Platelet Coagulant Activity" below), which are derived from the plasma membrane, and exosomes, which are internal membrane multivesicular bodies.[282] Exosomes are smaller than microparticles (40–100 nm vs. 100–1000 nm), enriched in CD63 and tetraspanins (see "Platelet Membrane Glycoproteins, Platelet Adhesion," and "Platelet Aggregation" below) and relatively deficient in membrane proteins such as GPIb/IX and platelet-endothelial cell adhesion molecule (PECAM)-1. Unlike microparticles, exosomes are not highly procoagulant as judged by their inability to bind prothrombin or factor X, or to present negatively charged phospholipids on their surface. They may, however, contain nicotinamide adenine dinucleotide (phosphate) (NAD(P)H) oxidase activity, which has the potential to generate reactive oxygen species that contribute to endothelial cell apoptosis in sepsis.[283]

Ribosomes, Messenger RNA, and Protein Translation Platelets contain only a relatively small number of ribosomes, have just remnants of a Golgi apparatus (see Fig. 114–1), and have only a small amount of mRNA.[284,285] Because they lack nuclei, they cannot synthesize mRNA, but mRNAs for a number of protein transcripts are present on functional platelet polysomes.[217] Application of the polymerase chain reaction to platelet mRNA permitted the molecular biologic analysis of platelet membrane glycoproteins and select plasma proteins that are synthesized in platelets, such as VWF.[215,216] Although not quantitatively abundant, transcription profiling has identified close to 3000 transcripts in platelets (see "Platelet Proteome, Transcriptome, and Secretome" below).[286]

The ability of platelets to synthesize proteins provides a mechanism for them to act as a link between hemostasis, inflammation, and innate immunity. Platelets have several unique extranuclear mechanisms to translate mRNA into protein after platelet activation.[287] The "signal-dependent" pathway for protein translation involves mammalian target of rapamycin (mTOR) and redistribution of mRNA and the mRNA-binding protein eukaryotic initiation factor 4E (eIF4E).[288] This mechanism is initiated by the engagement of platelet integrins, which promote cytoskeletal reorganization and the redistribution of eIF4E from the membrane skeleton and cytoplasm to the cytoskeletal core where mRNA transcripts are concentrated. The signal-dependent pathway results in synthesis of B-cell lymphoma 3 (BCL-3) following platelet activation. The newly synthesized BCL-3, in turn, regulates clot retraction.[289]

Activated platelets also synthesize IL-1β and tissue factor. Synthesis of these proteins occurs through a process that is distinct from translation involving mTOR and eIF4E, and instead requires the splicing of pre-mRNA present in mature platelets.[290,291] Spliceosome factors and pre-mRNA are transported from the megakaryocyte cell body to proplatelets during thrombogenesis. Splicing of pre-mRNA to mature RNA provides platelets with a mechanism to alter their proteomic profile in the absence of a nuclei and without new transcription.

Membrane Systems

Open Canalicular System The surface-connected open canalicular system is an elaborate series of conduits that begin as indentations of the plasma membrane and tunnel throughout the interior of the platelet.[2,292] Tracer studies demonstrate that the open canalicular system is contiguous with the exterior of the platelet, even though elements of the open canalicular system may appear as closed vesicles or vacuoles by electron microscopy of sectioned platelets.[2,292,293]

The open canalicular system may serve several functions. It provides a mechanism for entry of external elements into the interior of the platelet. It also provides a potential route for the release of granule contents to the outside, eliminating the need for granule fusion with the plasma membrane itself.[293,294] This latter function is especially important because, under most circumstances, platelet granules appear to move to the center of the platelet upon platelet activation rather than to the periphery.[2,295] Controversy remains, however, regarding the relative frequency with which secretion occurs via the open canalicular system versus direct fusion with the plasma membrane.[2,296]

The open canalicular system also represents an extensive internal store of membrane. Both filopodia formation and platelet spreading after adhesion require a dramatic increase in surface plasma membrane compared to the plasma membrane of resting platelets, and it is not possible for new membrane to be synthesized during the short time-course of these phenomena. Thus, the membrane of the open canalicular system most likely contributes to the increase in plasma membrane under these conditions; the membranes of α granules, dense granules, and, to a lesser extent, lysosomes may also contribute, but only if the stimulus is sufficient to induce the fusion of these organelles with the plasma membrane (release reaction). Finally, the membrane of the open canalicular system may serve as a storage site for plasma membrane glycoproteins. For example, under certain conditions, platelet activation by thrombin leads to a consistent, selective loss of GPIb/IX from the platelet surface and data from electron microscopy indicate that the GPIb/IX becomes sequestered in the open canalicular system.[41,297,298] Plasmin may produce a similar phenomenon.[41,299] Platelet activation leads to an increase in surface $\alpha_{IIb}\beta_3$, and although much of this $\alpha_{IIb}\beta_3$ receptor is thought to derive from α-granule membranes, at least some may come from $\alpha_{IIb}\beta_3$ in the membranes of dense granules and the open canalicular system.[41,300] Similarly, GPVI, the $P2Y_1$ ADP receptor, and the thromboxane A_2 receptor, and perhaps other receptors, are present in the open canalicular system and can be recruited to the platelet surface with activation.[301,302]

Dense Tubular System/Sarcoplasmic Reticulum The dense tubular system (DTS) is a closed-channel network of residual endoplasmic reticulum characterized histocytochemically by the presence of peroxidase activity.[2,303–305] The channels of the DTS are less extensive than those of the open canalicular system and tend to cluster in regions in close approximation to the open canalicular system.[2] The DTS is analogous to the sarcoplasmic reticulum (SR) of muscle because it can sequester ionized calcium (Ca^{2+}) and release it when platelets are activated, leading to shape change, granule centralization, and secretion.[306–309] Calreticulin, a calcium-binding protein found in the DTS/SR, probably helps to sequester calcium.[310,311] Release of Ca^{2+} from the DTS/SR involves the binding of inositol 1,4,5 trisphosphate (IP3), a messenger molecule formed during signal transduction, to IP3 type II receptors on the DTS/SR membrane (Fig. 114–8).[312,313] Cyclic AMP inhibits Ca^{2+} release from the DTS/SR, either by enhancing the calcium pumping mechanism[314] or by inhibiting release induced by IP3.[315] NO inhibits Ca^{2+} uptake by the DTS/SR at high concentrations and stimulates uptake at low concentrations by effects on the calcium ATPase(s) SERCA26 and SERCA3.[316,317] Depletion of intracellular calcium stores activates store-operated calcium entry (SOCE) into platelets (reviewed in reference 308). The depletion of Ca^{2+} from the DTS/SR is sensed by stromal interaction molecule 1 (STIM1), a transmembrane protein with a Ca^{2+} binding motif (EF hand) in the DTS/SR.[318–320] Loss of Ca^{2+} binding to STIM1 results in translocation and activation of Orai1, a calcium release–activated calcium (CRAC) channel in the plasma membrane,[321,322] that allows Ca^{2+} entry into the platelet. Although mice with defects in STIM1 and Orai1 have demonstrated abnormalities in platelet function,[318–320] humans with mutations in these proteins have had immune dysfunction, but no overt hemostatic or thrombotic abnormalities.[323–325] The human canonical transient receptor potential 1 (hTRPC1) has also been implicated in regulating platelet SOCE, but mice deficient in this protein do not have a defect in platelet Ca^{2+} entry.[326–328]

The DTS membrane is also probably a major site of prostaglandin (PG) and thromboxane synthesis[307,329]; in fact, the peroxidase activity used to identify the dense tubular system is an enzymatic component of PG synthesis.[329,330]

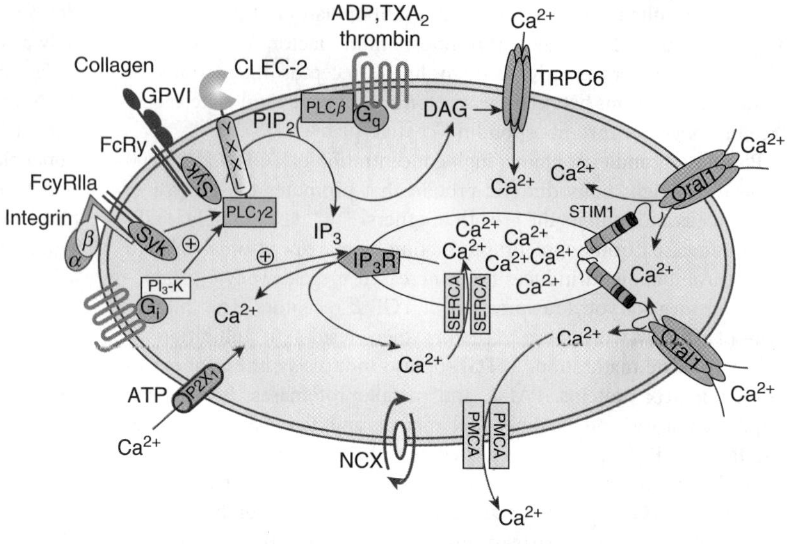

FIGURE 114–8. Platelet calcium homeostasis. Upon receptor activation different phospholipase (PL) C isoforms hydrolyze phosphatidylinositol-4,5-bisphosphate (PIP_2) to inositol-1,4,5-trisphosphate (IP_3) and diacylglycerol (DAG). IP_3 releases Ca^{2+} from the intracellular stores in the dense tubular system/sarcoplasmic reticulum (DTS/SR). The transmembrane protein STIM1 senses the reduction in Ca^{2+} through a decrease in Ca^{2+} occupancy of its EF hand domain, and then opens Orai1 Ca^{2+} channels in the plasma membrane, a process called *store-operated calcium entry* (SOCE), whereas DAG mediates non-SOCE through canonical transient receptor potential channel 6 (TRPC6). Additionally, a direct receptor-operated calcium (ROC) channel, $P2X_1$, and a Na^+/Ca^{2+} exchanger (NCX) contribute to the elevation in Ca^{2+} in the platelet cytoplasm. The counteracting mechanisms to replenish DTS/SR Ca^{2+} stores involve Ca^{2+} ATPases (SERCAs). Plasma membrane Ca^{2+} ATPases (PMCAs) pump Ca^{2+} through the plasma membrane out of the cell. Because of controversies about the localization and role of TRPC1 in the literature, this protein is not depicted in the figure. ADP, adenosine diphosphate; ATP, adenosine triphosphate; CLEC-2, C-type lectin-like receptor 2; FcγRIIa, Fc γ receptor IIa; FcRγ, Fc receptor γ chain; GPVI, glycoprotein VI; IP_3R, IP_3-receptor; PI_3-K, phosphatidylinositol 3-kinase; Syk, spleen tyrosine kinase; TXA_2, thromboxane A_2. *(Adapted with permission from Varga-Szabo D, Braun A, Nieswandt B.[309])*

■ PLATELET PROTEOME, TRANSCRIPTOME, AND SECRETOME

A number of proteomic and genomic approaches have been used to catalog the proteins and mRNAs expressed by platelets.[331] Proteomic analyses of intact platelets,[332–335] platelet membranes,[336,337] platelet lipid rafts,[338] platelet granules,[123,339] released microparticles,[340] and the proteins secreted upon activation[124] have identified hundreds of platelet proteins and defined alternatively spliced forms of the proteins.[340a] A central resource for platelet proteomics, including data on protein interactions and phosphorylation is available at http://plateletweb.bioapps.biozentram.uni-wuerzburg.de.[340b,340c] Additional proteomic studies have probed the changes in protein phosphorylation that occur during platelet activation.[341–344] Microarray[125,345,346] and serial analysis of gene expression (SAGE) techniques[337,347] have identified nearly 2000 mRNAs that are expressed in platelets and in precursor megakaryocytes. These studies have confirmed previous data regarding platelet/megakaryocyte-specific protein expression and have identified many new proteins that were not previously known to be associated with platelets. Although these techniques are still being refined, and isolation of pure populations of platelets remains challenging, analyzing large numbers of proteins and mRNA transcripts can provide important information that cannot be obtained using previous methods. As an example, by combining proteomic and genomic catalogues with databases of protein–protein interactions, new interactome maps can be generated.[347]

To date, more than 300 proteins and small molecules have been shown to be secreted from activated platelets.[124] This "secretome" can be classified by granular source or proposed function. Dense core granules are the source of small molecules (i.e., ADP, serotonin, and calcium) that are critical for platelet activation. α Granules contain adhesive glycoproteins, platelet-specific proteins, and factors affecting cell growth, inflammation, and wound repair (as discussed in "Dense Granules and α Granules" above). Platelets also release lysosomal enzymes (i.e., cathepsins and hexosaminidase). Functionally, the "secretome" can be divided into even more categories, including adhesive proteins (e.g., fibrinogen, VWF, and thrombospondin-1, which are released from α granules and function in aggregation), mitogens (e.g., insulin-like growth factor [IGF]-1, VEGF, and basic fibroblast growth factor [bFGF], which promote wound healing and vessel regrowth), and chemokines and cytokines (e.g., RANTES [regulated on activation, normal T-cell expressed, presumed secreted], IL-8, and MIP1α, which activate passing neutrophils and monocytes and lead to a range of inflammatory responses). Thus, platelet secretion is pivotal in establishing the microenvironment at the site of blood vessel injury, including vessel injury associated with inflammation and wounds.

PLATELET GENOMICS

Variations in the coding sequences of platelet glycoproteins were identified as part of the effort to identify the antigens responsible for alloimmune neonatal purpura and posttransfusion purpura (see Chaps. 119 and 138).[331,348] In the process, these studies pioneered in the discovery of what is now termed *single nucleotide polymorphisms*. Subsequent population studies established the considerable variability that exists in the frequency of single nucleotide polymorphisms in many different platelet proteins in different populations.[349–351] Variability in platelet function, in particular the response to agonist activation, has been correlated with some of these single nucleotide polymorphisms.[349,350] Moreover, those associated with apparently enhanced function have been analyzed as potential markers of increased risk of cardiovascular disease. Although a number of such associations have been made, the data are complex and the evidence is incomplete, providing insights into key signaling pathways.[349,350,350a] Other studies have attempted to separate large populations of apparently normal individuals according to the sensitivity of their platelets to agonist activation, and then use genetic mapping techniques to identify genes that may contribute to the differences in platelet sensitivity.[352] These studies are still in their early stages, but hold considerable promise for defining important pathways in platelet activation. Additionally, ongoing genome-wide association studies are likely to reveal new information that may ultimately result in an improved understanding of the interplay between genomic variability and platelet function.

PLATELET PHYSIOLOGY AND BIOCHEMISTRY

OVERVIEW OF PLATELET ADHESION, AGGREGATION, AND PLATELET THROMBUS FORMATION

The hemostatic system is under elaborate control mechanisms lest the response either be inadequate to meet the hemorrhagic challenge or result in inappropriate thrombosis in response to trivial provocation. Evolutionary pressures have probably favored a more active hemostatic system as individuals with more active hemostatic systems were more likely to avoid death from hemorrhage prior to attaining sexual maturity or in association with childbirth. Our active hemostatic system may be less-well adapted to our modern age, which is characterized by long life spans and progressive vascular disease, given that the deposition of a platelet-fibrin thrombus on a damaged atherosclerotic plaque is the cause of most myocardial infarctions and many strokes.

The platelet's major function is to seal openings in the vascular tree. It is appropriate, therefore, that the initiating signal for platelet deposition and activation is exposure of underlying portions of the blood vessel wall that are normally concealed from circulating platelets by an intact endothelial lining (Table 114–4 and Fig. 114–9).[353] Additional parameters that probably control the platelet response are: (1) the depth of injury, with deeper damage exposing more platelet-reactive materials and tissue factor[354–357] (see Chap. 115); (2) the vascular bed, with the blood vessels serving mucocutaneous tissues especially dependent on platelets for hemostasis, in contrast to the vascular beds in muscles and joints, which rely more on the coagulation mechanism; (3) the age of the individual, as the composition of the blood vessel wall probably changes with age; (4) the hematocrit, as increased numbers of erythrocytes enhance platelet interactions with the blood vessel wall by forcing platelets to the periphery of the bloodstream (as the erythrocytes disproportionately occupy the axial region), by imparting radially directed energy to platelets as the erythrocytes engage in flip-flop motions, and perhaps by releasing the platelet activator ADP at sites of vascular injury[358–360]; and (5) the speed of blood flow and the size of the blood vessel, which will determine the number of platelets passing by a single point in a given time interval, the amount of time a platelet has to interact with the blood vessel wall or other platelets, the rate of dilution of platelet activating agents, and the forces tending to pull a platelet from the vessel wall or another platelet (shear rate).[355,358,360,361] The vasospastic response that accompanies vascular injury, to which platelets contribute by release of thromboxane A_2 and serotonin, probably plays a key role in decreasing hemorrhage and facilitating platelet and fibrin deposition via its effect on blood flow.

Platelet thrombi appear to rapidly recruit tissue factor from the blood; the tissue factor is associated with small lipid-containing vesicles and may derive from leukocyte membranes that contain PSGL-1, a ligand for the P-selectin expressed on the surface of activated platelets.[362,363] An alternatively spliced form of tissue factor circulating in blood may also associate with platelet thrombi.[364] Some investigators have reported the presence of tissue factor in platelet α granules, leading to surface expression when platelets are activated, but others have not been able to identify platelet tissue factor.[365,366] Activated platelets may generate tissue factor through a process that requires pre-mRNA splicing.[367,368] Additionally, interactions between activated platelets and leukocytes may affect tissue factor expression, localization, and function. Activated platelets expressing P-selectin recruit neutrophils and monocytes by binding to PSGL-1 (Fig. 114–10). Generation of

TABLE 114–4. Components of the Blood Vessel Wall That Are Hemostatically Active

I.	Subendothelium
	von Willebrand factor
	Collagen (types IV, V, and VI)
	Fibronectin
	Thrombospondin
	Laminin
	Vitronectin
	Fibrinogen (fibrin)
II.	Media
	Collagen (types I and III)
III.	Adventitia
	Collagen (types I and III)
	Tissue factor

SOURCE: Adapted with permission from Coller BS.[355]

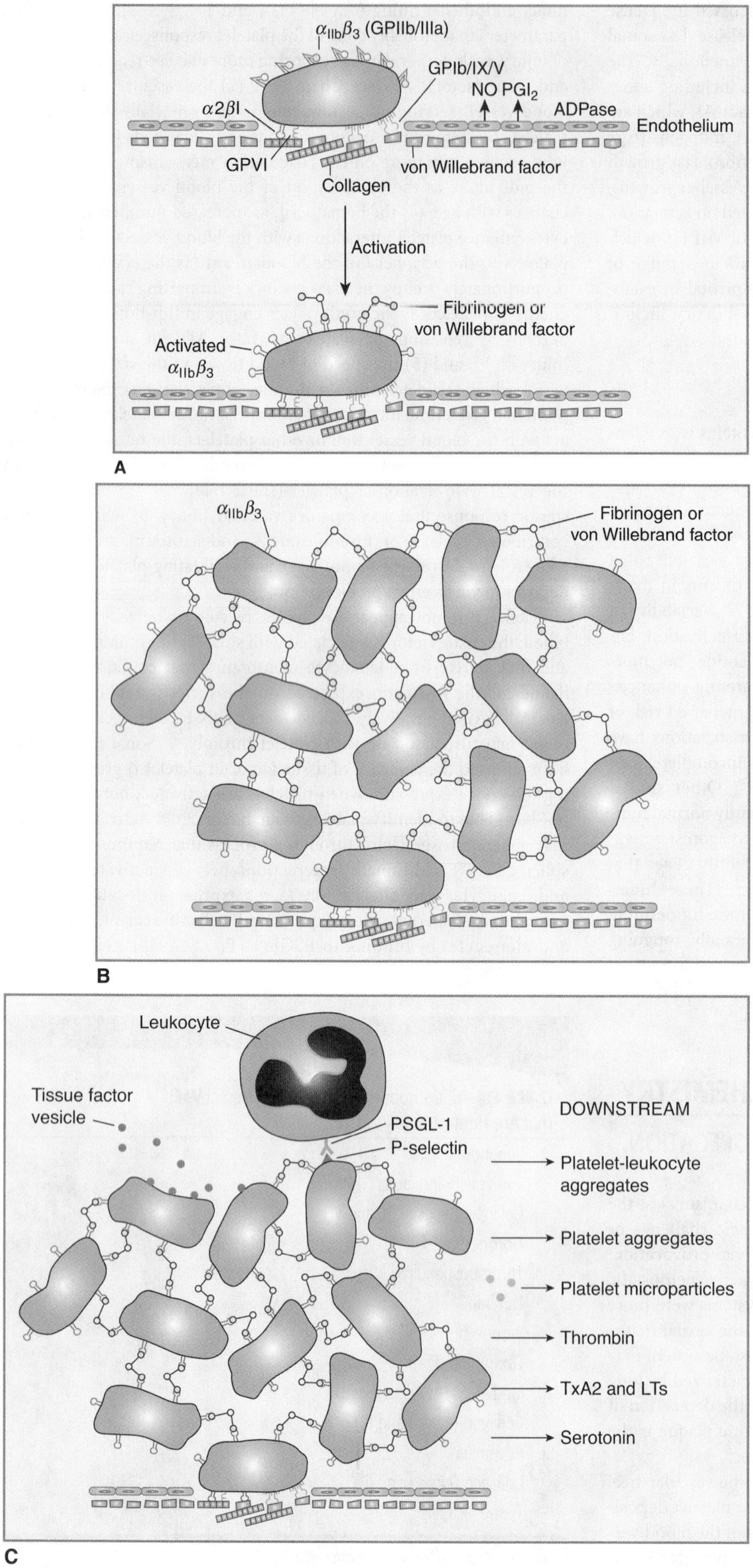

FIGURE 114–9. Platelet adhesion, activation, aggregation, and platelet–leukocyte interactions. **A.** Endothelial cells limit platelet deposition because they separate platelets from the adhesive proteins in the subendothelial area, produce two inhibitors of platelet function (nitric oxide [NO] and prostacyclin [PGI_2]), and contain a potent enzyme (CD39) that can digest adenosine diphosphate (ADP) released from platelets. Platelet adhesion is initiated by loss of endothelial cells (or, in the case of an atherosclerotic lesion, rupture or erosion of the plaque), which exposes adhesive glycoproteins such as collagen and von Willebrand factor in the subendothelium. Other adhesive glycoproteins probably also are exposed (see Table 114–4). In addition, von Willebrand factor and perhaps other adhesive glycoproteins in plasma deposit in the damaged area, in part by binding to collagen. Platelets adhere to the subendothelium via receptors that bind to the adhesive glycoproteins. Glycoprotein (GP) Ib binding to von Willebrand factor plays a prominent role, but $\alpha_2\beta_1$ (GPIa/IIa) and GPVI binding to collagen and other platelet receptors (see Table 114–5) probably also play a role. After platelets adhere, they undergo an activation process that leads to a conformational change in $\alpha_{IIb}\beta_3$ receptors involving headpiece extension and leg separation (see Fig. 114–5), resulting in their ability to bind with high-affinity select multivalent adhesive proteins, most prominently fibrinogen and von Willebrand factor, including the von Willebrand factor that binds to collagen in the subendothelial area. **B.** Platelet aggregation occurs when the multivalent adhesive glycoproteins bind simultaneously to $\alpha_{IIb}\beta_3$ receptors on two different platelets, resulting in receptor crosslinking. Clustering of the receptors probably also contributes to the stability of the aggregates (not shown). **C.** After platelets adhere and aggregate, they help to initiate coagulation by binding tissue factor-containing vesicles circulating in the plasma, exposing negatively charged phospholipids on their surface (not shown), releasing platelet factor V (not shown), and releasing procoagulant microparticles. Activated platelets also express P-selectin on their surface, which leads to recruitment of leukocytes via interactions between platelet P-selectin and P-selectin glycoprotein ligand-1 (PSGL-1) expressed on the surface of leukocytes. Other interactions between platelets and leukocytes are detailed in Figures 114–10 and 114–11. Thrombus formation is a dynamic cyclical process, with platelets repeatedly adhering, aggregating, and then breaking off and embolizing downstream. Platelet–leukocyte aggregates, platelet aggregates, platelet microparticles, thrombin, thromboxane A_2 (TXA_2), leukotrienes (LTs), and serotonin probably all go downstream and affect the microvasculature. Ultimately the vessel either becomes fully occluded or loses its thrombogenic reactivity, that is, it becomes passivated.

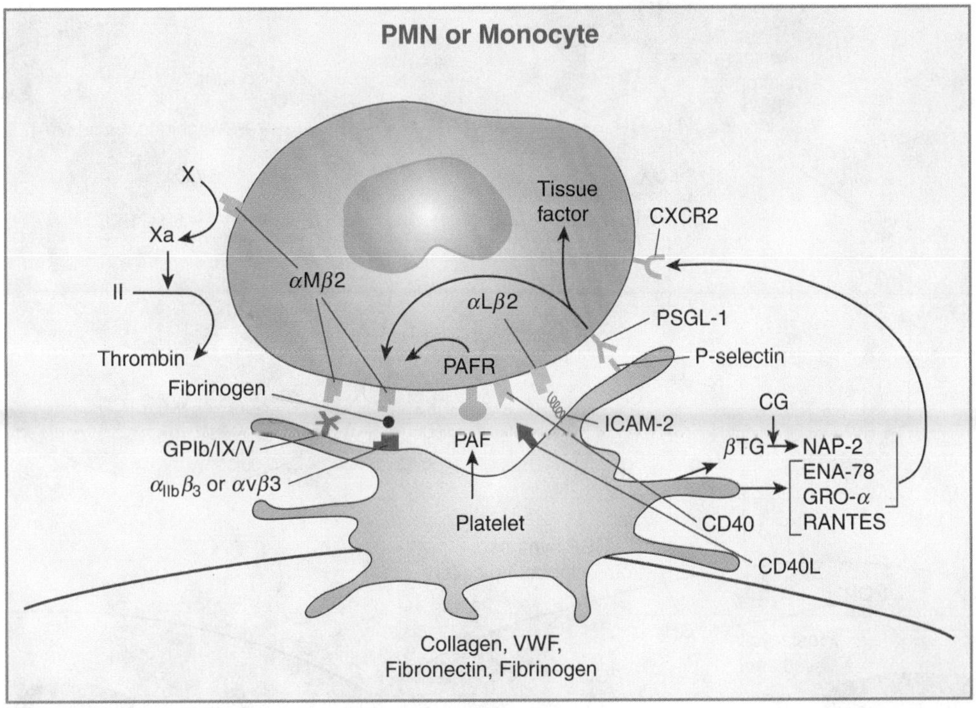

FIGURE 114–10. Platelet–leukocyte interactions. A number of interactions can occur between platelets and leukocytes, including neutrophils and monocytes. The interaction between platelet P-selectin and leukocyte P-selectin glycoprotein ligand-1 (PSGL-1) probably is the most important initial interaction (and can lead to tissue factor synthesis by monocytes), but fibrinogen binding simultaneously to activated $\alpha_M\beta_2$ on leukocytes and either $\alpha_{IIb}\beta_3$ or $\alpha_V\beta_3$ on platelets may play a role under certain circumstances. Platelets can release platelet-activating factor (PAF), which can interact with a PAF receptor (PAFR) on leukocytes, leading to $\alpha_M\beta_2$ activation and binding of fibrinogen and factor X. Leukocyte $\alpha_M\beta_2$ can also interact with platelet junctional adhesion molecule-3 (JAM-3) or GPIb. Platelets can release chemokines (e.g., ENA-78, GRO-α, and RANTES [regulated on activation, normal T-cell expressed, presumed secreted]), and β-thromboglobulin (βTG) released by platelets can be converted by leukocyte cathepsin G (CG) into the potent chemotactic CXC chemokine neutrophil-activating protein (NAP)-2. Some of the chemokines, in turn, activate leukocytes by binding to the chemokine receptor CXCR2. Platelets also contain the potent immune-stimulating molecule CD40 ligand (CD40L), and both express it on the platelet surface and release it into the circulation upon platelet activation. The interaction between thrombospondin and CD36 molecules on both platelets and some leukocytes and the presence of CD40 on platelets are not shown. PMN, polymorphonuclear cell; VWF, von Willebrand factor.

P-selectin–containing microparticles from platelets and binding of platelets and/or the platelet-derived microparticles to leukocytes can lead to the initiation of the synthesis of tissue factor by leukocytes as well as the "deencryption" of leukocyte tissue factor. The latter phenomenon results in greater tissue factor activity per unit of tissue factor antigen, and may result from the simultaneous expression of surface phosphatidylserine or as a result of release of the oxidoreductase enzyme protein disulfide isomerase (PDI).[369,370] All of these mechanisms may contribute to the initiation of coagulation on the surface of the platelet thrombus.[369,371–373] In addition, the proximity of platelets, leukocytes, and endothelial cells facilitates transcellular metabolism, resulting in the generation of vasoactive agents that none of the cells can produce by itself (Fig. 114–11).

The blood shear rate differentially affects platelet adhesion to surfaces; VWF-dependent adhesion is most important at higher shear rates, probably because high shear rates cause conformational changes in VWF and/or platelet GPIb.[359,360,374–379] Shear rates, which reflect the differences in flow velocity as a function of distance from the blood vessel wall, vary considerably throughout the vasculature, being highest in small arterioles and lowest in large arteries and veins; very high rates are observed at the tips of severely stenotic atherosclerotic arteries.[360,361,379] Very high shear rates can cause platelets to aggregate via a mechanism that involves VWF binding to GPIb/IX followed by intracellular signaling, leading to activation of $\alpha_{IIb}\beta_3$.[380–383] Platelets contribute more significantly to arterial thrombi than to venous thrombi, perhaps as a result of differences in the shear rates in the different beds.[355]

The subendothelial layer immediately subjacent to the endothelium contains a large number of adhesive proteins[353,355] (see Table 114–4), and the platelet has receptors for many of these (see Tables 114–3 and 114–5). GPIb/IX is a receptor complex that is particularly important in mediating adhesion to VWF immobilized in the subendothelium, and this receptor appears to dominate the adhesion process at high shear (see Chap. 127).[360,383] GPIb/IX may also mediate adhesion via interactions with proteins other than VWF as loss of GPIb/IX has a more profound effect on thrombus formation than loss of VWF in model systems.[384,385] Three different sources of VWF may contribute to the subendothelial VWF: synthesis by endothelial cells, deposition from plasma, and release from platelet α granules.[377,386] Constitutively deposited subendothelial VWF appears to associate with type VI collagen,[387] but it can bind to multiple collagen types. Plasma VWF binds via its A3 domain to types I and III collagens when they are exposed by deep injury in the blood vessel wall and adherent VWF may be able to recruit additional VWF from the circulation or released from adjacent endothelial cells.[359,360,375,388] The interaction between GPIbα and VWF does not itself cause firm adhesion; rather, it results in tethering and slow translocation, probably because the bonds between VWF and GPIbα both form rapidly and dissociate rapidly.[353,360,375,377] Adhesion initiated by GPIbα-VWF interactions are stabilized by interactions between VWF and $\alpha_{IIb}\beta_3$.[353,360,377,389] The metalloproteinase

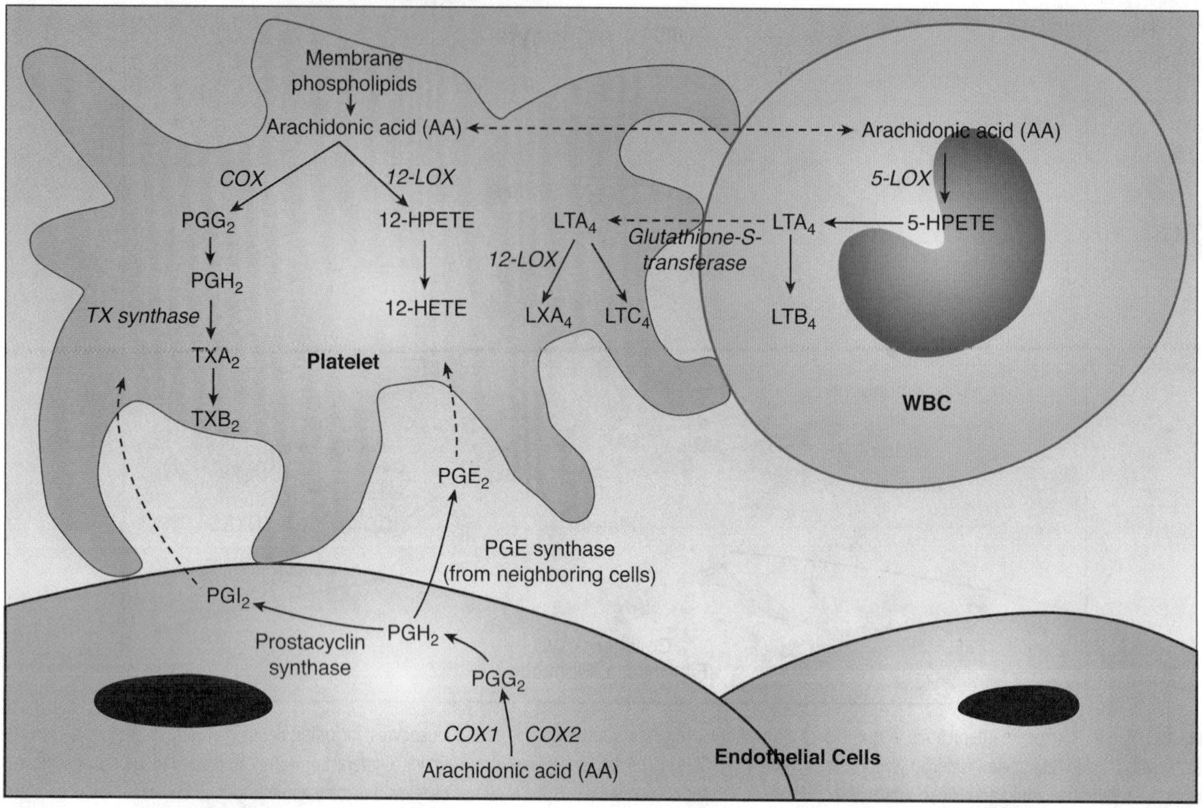

FIGURE 114–11. Select aspects of transcellular eicosanoid metabolism. At sites of platelet-white blood cell (WBC) interactions, free arachidonic acid (AA) can be generated by both activated platelets and leukocytes and exchanged between the cells. In the platelet, cyclooxygenase 1 (COX-1), the target for aspirin, generates the major AA metabolite prostaglandin (PG) G_2, the precursor for PGH_2 that, in turn, is converted by thromboxane (TX) synthase to TXA_2. TXA_2 and PGH_2 promote platelet activation and inflammation through binding to thromboprostanoid (TP) receptors. TXA_2 is rapidly converted to TXB_2. Platelets also express platelet-type 12-lipoxygenase (LOX) that converts AA to the relatively unstable intermediate 12-hydroperoxy-5,8,10,14-eicosatetraenoic acid (12-HPETE), which is subsequently converted to 12-hydroxyeicosatetraenoic acid (12-HETE). Platelets from most mammalian species do not possess 5-LOX and, therefore, cannot generate leukotriene A_4 (LTA_4) from AA. However, LTA_4 produced by leukocytes can be transferred to interacting platelets, where it can be metabolized by glutathione-S-transferase to LTC_4 or by platelet 12-LOX to the antiinflammatory mediator lipoxin (LXA_4). In endothelial cells, AA can also be released from membrane phospholipids, but unlike in the platelet, it is sequentially metabolized by COX-1 or COX-2 and prostacyclin synthase to PGI_2, which inhibits platelet activation by effects on the platelet inhibitory prostanoid (IP) receptor. Endothelial cells can also serve as a source of PGH_2 that is metabolized by PGE synthase to PGE_2. At high concentrations, PGE_2 inhibits platelet activation, and at lower concentrations ($<10^{-6}$ M), it activates platelets through the EP3 receptor. *(Illustration generated by Matt Hazard, Teaching and Academic Support Center, the University of Kentucky.)*

ADAMTS-13 (a disintegrin and metalloproteinase with thrombospondin domain 13) can modulate the size of VWF multimers by cleaving the VWF subunit and because increased multimer size enhances the ability of VWF to interact with platelets, it can affect platelet deposition and thrombus formation.[390]

Intravital microscopy and *ex vivo* flow chamber studies indicate that discoid platelets that show minimal or no evidence of activation can form the initial layers of platelet aggregates when laminar flow is disrupted by a stenotic lesion, but that stable thrombus development requires the generation and/or release of soluble activators.[361] Membrane tethers, which can undergo restructuring and stabilization, are important in achieving interactions with matrix proteins and other platelets.

The biologic contributions of the interactions between the $\alpha_6\beta_1$ (GPIc/IIa) receptor and laminin, the $\alpha_5\beta_1$ (GPIc*/IIa) receptor and fibronectin, and the $\alpha_V\beta_3$ receptor and vitronectin or other matrix proteins in initiating platelet adhesion remain unknown, but there is some experimental support for the role of the first two in mice.[391] The $\alpha_{IIb}\beta_3$ integrin can function as an adhesion receptor for immobilized fibrinogen even in the absence of platelet activation,[392,393] but platelet activation is required for $\alpha_{IIb}\beta_3$-mediated adhesion to VWF and fibronectin,[393] and for platelet thrombus formation. Platelets may interact directly with exposed collagen, including types I, III, and VI via GPVI and $\alpha_2\beta_1$ (GPIa/IIa), or perhaps one or more of the many other receptors implicated in platelet-collagen interactions (e.g., CD36 [GPIV], p65).[391,394–405] The interaction of platelets with collagen is most evident at relatively low shear rates. GPVI may be more important in binding to intact collagen fibrils and $\alpha_2\beta_1$ may be more important in binding to collagen that has been exposed to proteases and adopted a spiraled structure.[405,406] The density of $\alpha_2\beta_1$ receptors on platelets in fact, affects the efficiency of platelet thrombus formation on collagen-coated surfaces.[407–410] In addition, fibrinogen, fibronectin, and VWF, whether released from platelets or circulating in plasma, may also bind to collagen. In turn, these proteins may then interact with platelet $\alpha_{IIb}\beta_3$, $\alpha_5\beta_1$ (GPIc*/II), and/or GPIb/IX, completing a sandwich mechanism initiated by collagen exposure.[360,397]

Depending on the vascular bed, available adhesive glycoproteins, and shear conditions, it is likely that various combinations of platelet receptors, including GPIbα, $\alpha_2\beta_1$ (GPIa/IIa), GPVI, and $\alpha_{IIb}\beta_3$ act in concert to transform the tethering and slow translocation of platelets initiated by GPIbα interacting with VWF into stable platelet adhesion.

For platelet plug formation to occur, platelets must undergo activation as well as adhesion. Adhesion to VWF via GPIb/IX can itself initiate activation via signaling through interactions with FcRγ-chain, FcγRIIA, or ζ14-3-3.[353,359,360,377,383,400,405,411] Table 114–6 and Figure 114–12 list physiologic and pathologic platelet activators, which are divided into strong and weak agents. Most of these activators are released or synthesized at the site of vascular injury, resulting in a local response. In addition, cooperative biochemical interactions between erythrocytes and platelets may enhance platelet activation.[412]

It has been speculated that vascular injury results in release of ADP from erythrocytes, thus leading to platelet activation. Adhesion of platelets to subendothelial structures, in particular VWF at high shear, may itself lead to platelet activation, including generation of TXA_2, release of ADP and serotonin, and activation of the $\alpha_{IIb}\beta_3$ receptors on the luminal side of the platelet so that they adopt their high-affinity ligand-binding conformation(s).[377] These positive feedback mechanisms insure an adequate hemostatic response. Depending on the nature of the surface to which they adhere, platelets also undergo variable spreading reactions and become anchored by a process that at least partially involves $\alpha_{IIb}\beta_3$ ligation and clustering, leading to "outside-in" signaling, cytoskeletal reorganization, and tyrosine phosphorylation; these reactions also contribute to initiating the release reaction.[413–419] When exposed to collagen, some platelets directly adhere and others adhere only after being recruited to the surface by platelet–platelet interactions with the already adherent platelets.[416]

The activated luminal $\alpha_{IIb}\beta_3$ receptors on adherent platelets may then bind VWF, fibrinogen, or perhaps other adhesive glycoproteins, and await the interaction with another platelet, which itself may have undergone activation of its $\alpha_{IIb}\beta_3$ receptors as a result of exposure to released ADP and TXA_2. Alternatively, a platelet may become activated and bind VWF or fibrinogen while still circulating, in which case the platelet–ligand complex may bind directly to an activated $\alpha_{IIb}\beta_3$ receptor on the luminal surface. The binding of adhesive ligands to platelet receptors then repeats itself, resulting in the recruitment of additional layers of platelets, and ultimately the formation of a hemostatic plug. Intravital videomicroscopy of the mesenteric and cremasteric circulations of mice after endothelial cell damage demonstrates that, at least in these vascular beds, platelet thrombus formation is initially a very dynamic process, with many platelets depositing but then embolizing.[420] The thrombus grows relatively slowly compared to what its growth would be if all of the platelets that deposited remained attached to the surface.[421–423] The process is similar in the carotid artery of the mouse, which is a considerably larger blood vessel, but still less than 1 mm.[424]

A number of mechanisms stabilize platelet aggregates as demonstrated by increased embolization of platelets during *in vivo* thrombus formation when specific proteins are inhibited or deleted through gene targeting. These include absence of fibrinogen (presumably limiting fibrin formation),[423] leptin,[425–427] CD40 ligand,[428] growth arrest-specific gene 6 product (Gas6) and its receptors (Axl, Sky, and Mer),[213–216,429] Eph kinases and ephrins,[430] factor XII,[431] plasminogen activator inhibitor-1 and vitronectin,[177] and inhibition of select regions of fibrinogen.[424] Precisely how each of these contributes to thrombus stability remains to be established.

The aggregated platelets can facilitate thrombin generation by one or more different mechanisms, including recruitment of bloodborne tissue factor, synthesis or activation of tissue factor, formation of procoagulant microvesicles, exposure of activated factor V, exposure of negatively charged phospholipids, and perhaps activation of the contact system (see "Platelet Coagulant Activity" below). The thrombin thus generated further activates platelets, leading to more extensive degranulation; it also further activates coagulation and initiates the deposition of fibrin strands that reinforce the platelet thrombus and serve as sites for additional VWF deposition.[432] Thrombin also helps to consolidate the plug by initiating platelet-mediated clot retraction (see "Signaling Pathways in Platelet Activation and Aggregation" below). Finally, thrombin affects the surface membrane receptors, downregulating GPIb/IX and upregulating $\alpha_{IIb}\beta_3$, perhaps facilitating the transition from platelet adhesion to platelet aggregation.[41,297,298,433]

Release of vasoactive and mitogenic agents, as well as chemokines, from platelets contributes to the inflammatory response, as does the appearance of P-selectin on the surface of activated platelets and endothelial cells, as P-selectin recruits neutrophils to the damaged region (see "Platelet–Leukocyte Interactions, Platelet–Tissue Factor Interactions, and the Role of Platelets in Inflammation and Infection" below).[434–436] Platelets themselves will roll on endothelial cells that have been activated to expose P-selectin on their surface,[436,437] and both GPIbα and platelet PSGL-1 have been implicated as counterreceptors for endothelial cell P-selectin.[383,438,439] Platelets also express CD40 ligand on their surface, as well as on the surface of microparticles derived from activated platelets.[440] CD40 ligand can interact with CD40 on lymphocytes, monocytes, and endothelial cells, leading to cell activation and enhanced inflammatory and immune responses. In addition, activated platelets release a soluble form of CD40 ligand that has been implicated in thrombus formation. Plasma levels of soluble CD40 ligand may also serve as a marker of platelet activation, vascular disease, and a predisposition to develop restenosis after percutaneous coronary intervention.[441–446] Finally, after contributing to hemostasis and initiating an inflammatory response, platelet-fibrin thrombi eventually resolve, most likely by a combination of embolization, fibrinolysis, and macrophage removal of debris.

Several inhibitory factors serve to balance platelet activation and thus prevent excessive platelet deposition (Table 114–7). The dilutional effects of flowing blood are probably most important; thus, alterations in the surface of the blood vessel that produce local areas of stasis in which platelets and coagulation factors may concentrate are prothrombogenic.[355,358] Endothelial cells can synthesize two potent inhibitors of platelet activation, prostacyclin and nitric oxide (NO; see "Inhibitory Pathways in Platelets" below and Chap. 117).[447–450] Basal synthesis of prostacyclin probably is too low to influence formation of platelet aggregates, but activated endothelial cells produce more prostacyclin. Activated platelets can also facilitate prostacyclin synthesis via production and release of endoperoxide intermediates and compounds that can activate endothelial prostacyclin production via receptor-mediated mechanisms. In addition, activated platelets can release microparticles that can transfer arachidonic acid to endothelial cells.[451] Thus, generation of prostacyclin at sites of vascular injury or inflammation may provide a mechanism to limit platelet accumulation. NO, which is synthesized by endothelial cells, is a potent inhibitor of *ex vivo* platelet adhesion and aggregation. Data from animal models suggest that a deficiency of NO predisposes animals to thrombosis,[448,450,452,453] although there may be minimal, or even paradoxical, effects in some models of thrombosis due, perhaps in part, to the antifibrinolytic effect of NO.[454,455] Alternatively, it has been proposed that NO may produce a biphasic response on platelets, enhancing secretion at low concentrations and inhibiting platelet function at higher concentrations.[456,457] NO synthesis is probably enhanced at sites of injury as a result of release from activated platelets, so it may well contribute to platelet inhibition, especially as its antiplatelet effects synergizes with prostacyclin.[448,450] Endothelial cells and lymphocytes also have CD39, an ecto-ATP diphosphohydrolase (ecto-ADPase) that can digest ATP and ADP to AMP, and thus limit the effects of released ADP.[115,119] They also have CD73, which can convert AMP into the platelet inhibitor adenosine. Under certain conditions, leukocytes appear to interact biochemically

TABLE 114–5. Important Platelet Surface Proteins

Gene Family	Common Name	Platelet Chain Designation	Integrin Designation	VLA† Designation	CD† Designation		M_r Nonreduced		M_r Reduced
Integrin	Fibrinogen/ receptor		$\alpha_{IIb}\beta_3$		$\alpha_{IIb}\beta_3$-CD41a	α_{IIb}	145,000	$\alpha_{IIb}\alpha$	125,000
					α_{IIb}-CD4lb			$\alpha_{IIb}\beta$	23,000
					β_3-CD61	β_3	90,000		114,000
	Collagen receptor	GPIa/IIa	$\alpha_2\beta_1$	VLA-2	α_2-CD49b	α_2	150,000		
					β_1-CD29	β_1	138,000		148,000
	Fibronectin receptor	GPIc*/IIa	$\alpha_5\beta_1$	VLA-5	α_5-CD49e	α_5	140,000		
					β_1-CD29	β_1	138,000		148,000
	Laminin receptor	GPIc/IIa	$\alpha_6\beta_1$	VLA-6	α_6-CD49f	α_6	140,000		
					β_1-CD29	β_1	138,000		148,000
	Vitronectin receptor	α_V/GPIIIa	$\alpha_V\beta_3$		α_V-CD51	α_V	150,000	α_V	125,000
					β_3-CD61			α_V	25,000
						β_3	90,000		114,000
Leucine-rich repeat glycoproteins	von Willebrand factor receptor	GPIb/IX			Ib/IX-CD42	GPIb	170,000	GPIbα	145,000
					Ibα-CD42b			GPIbβ	22,000
					Ibβ-CD42c				
					IX-CD42a	GPIX	17,000		17,000
		GPV				GPV	82,000		82,000
Immunoglobulin family cell adhesion molecules	PECAM-I				CD31		130,000		
	Fcγ-RII				CD32		40,000		
	HLA-Class 1								
	ICAM-2				CD102				59,000
	GPVI						62,000		65,000
	IAP				CD47		50,000		
Selectins	P-Selectin (GMP 140; PADGEM)				CD62P		140,000		
Tetraspanins	p24				CD9		24,000		
					CD63				
	PETA-3				CD151		27,000		
	Lamp 3 (granulophysin)				CD63		53,000		
Miscellaneous	GPIV				CD36		88,000		
	Lamp 1				CD107a		110,000		
	Lamp 2				CD107b		120,000		
	67 kDa Laminin receptor						67,000		
	ADP P2X1 receptor						70,000		
	Leukosialin, sialophorin				CD43		90,000		
Seven transmembrane domain (G protein-linked)	PAR-1						70,000		
	PAR-4								
	Thromboxane A_2 receptor								55,000
	α_2-Adrenergic receptor								64,000
	Vasopressin receptor						125,000		
	ADP $P2Y_1$ receptor								
	ADP $P2Y_{12}$ receptor								

Fib, fibrinogen; Fn, fibronectin; GP, glycoprotein; HLA, human leukocyte antigen; IAP, integrin-associated protein; ICAM, intercellular adhesion molecule; Lamp, lysosome-associated membrane protein; PAR, protease-activated receptor; PECAM, platelet-endothelial cell adhesion molecule; PSGL-1, P-selectin glycoprotein ligand-1; TSP, thrombospondin; TX, thromboxane; Vn, vitronectin; VWF, von Willebrand factor.

Amino Acids	Carbo-hydrate	Lipid	Phosphorylated	Chromo-some	Ligands	Platelet Specific	Function	Molecules on Platelet Surface (S) or Internal (I)
α_{IIb} 1039	+	–	–	17	Fib, VWF, Fn, Vn, ?TSP	+	Adhesion, aggregation,	(S) 80,000
						+	protein trafficking	(I) 40,000
β_3 762	+	–	+	17				
α_2 1152				5	Collagen	–	Adhesion	(S) 1000
β_1 778				10		–		
α_5 1008				12	Fn	–	Adhesion	(S) 1000
β_1 778				10				
α_6 1067				2	Laminin	–	Adhesion	(S) 1,000
β_3 778				10				
α_V 1048				2	Vn, Fib, VWF Fn, ?TSP, Osp	–	?Adhesion, ?protein trafficking	(S) 100
GPIIIa 762	+	–		17				
GPIbα 610(8)*	+	–		1	VWF, Thrombin	+?	Adhesion (high shear),	(S) 25,000
GPIbβ 181(1)*	+	+	–	22		+?	?thrombin activation	(S) 25,000
GPIX 160(1)*	+	+	+	3		+?		(S) 25,000
GPV 544(15)*	+	+	+	3		+?		(S) 12,500
PECAM-1 738	+	?	+	17	Heparin	–	?Adhesion	(S) 8000
FcγRII 324	+		+	1	Immune complexes	–	Immune complex binding	(S) ~1000
HLA	+			6	–		Histocompatibility	(S)
ICAM-2 274				17	LFA-1	–	Platelet-leukocyte adhesion	(S) 2600
GPVI 316	+	–		?	Collagen	+	Activation	(S) ~2000
IAP 287	+			3	TSP	–	Activation	
P-Selectin 830	+	+	+	1	Sialyl-Le^x PSGL-1		Platelet-leukocyte adhesion	(I) 20,000
CD9 228	+				?	–	Activation	(S) 40,000
CD151 253	+	–	–	11	?	–	Activation	(I) ~2000
Lamp 3 238	+							(I) 10,000
GPIV 471	+		+	7	Collagen, TSP	–	Adhesion	(S) 20,000
Lamp 1 389	+			13	?	–	?	(I) 1200
Lamp 2 381	+			X	?			
67 kDa ?295				X	Laminin	–	Adhesion	
P2X$_1$ 399	+			17	ATP, ADP	–	Activation	(S) 13–130
CD43 400	+		+	16	ICAM-1	–	Adhesion	
PAR-1 425				5	Thrombin	–	Activation	(S) ~1800
PAR-4 385	+		+	19	Thrombin	–	Activation	
TXA$_2$ 343				19	PGH$_2$/thromboxane A$_2$	–	Activation	~200
α_2-Adrenergic 450				10	Epinephrine	–	Activation	~250
Vasopressin 418				?x	Vasopressin	–	Activation	~75
P2Y$_1$ 373	+			3	ADP	–	Activation	
P2Y$_{12}$ 342				3	ADP	+	Activation	

*Number of leucine-rich repeats.

†CD, cluster of differentiation (see Chap. 15); VLA, very-late antigen.

TABLE 114–6. Physiologic and Pathologic Platelet Activators

Strong
Adhesion to collagen and perhaps other elements exposed in normal blood vessels after vascular damage
Adhesion to elements exposed in atherosclerotic blood vessels after plaque rupture
Thrombin
High concentrations of collagen *in vitro*
Adenosine diphosphate (ADP)
Weak
Epinephrine
Thromboxane A_2/prostaglandin H_2
Serotonin
Platelet-activating factor
Vasopressin
Thrombospondin-1
Other
Shear
Thrombolytic agents (plasmin)

SOURCE: Adapted with permission from Coller BS.[355]

with platelets to limit platelet activation,[458] but cathepsin G released from activated leukocytes can activate platelets.[459,460]

Because thrombin is such a potent activator of platelets, the control mechanisms that limit thrombin production also can be considered control mechanisms for platelet aggregation (see Chap. 116). Platelets can also become desensitized to stimulation by some agonists if they have previously been exposed to low concentrations of that agonist (homologous desensitization). It is possible that in the penumbra of released platelet agonists, some platelets become inhibited by this mechanism.[461–463]

The $\alpha_{IIb}\beta_3$ receptor occupies a central role in determining the extent of platelet aggregation, in part because it is present at an extraordinarily high density on the platelet surface (receptors are probably less than 20 nm apart).[419,464–467] This permits it to rapidly initiate platelet aggregation. On the other hand, the receptor is not in its high-affinity ligand-binding state on resting platelets but rather needs to be activated by agonists, including ADP, serotonin, thrombin, collagen, and TXA_2, that are localized to sites of vascular injury.[415,465,466] As a result, platelets can circulate in plasma containing high concentrations of the $\alpha_{IIb}\beta_3$ ligands fibrinogen and VWF without ongoing platelet thrombus formation.

Thus, platelet adhesion is controlled by the exposure of the subendothelium, with the platelet GPIb/IX receptor for immobilized VWF and the $\alpha_{IIb}\beta_3$ receptor for immobilized fibrinogen always competent to interact with these adhesive ligands.[378,392,393,468] ADAMTS-13 may be an important regulator of thrombus formation via its effects on VWF multimer size.[390] In contrast, the ability of $\alpha_{IIb}\beta_3$ to mediate platelet aggregation by binding fluid-phase VWF[469] or fibrinogen[465,466,470,471] is under the control of an elaborate activation mechanism that limits the response to sites of vascular injury.

The agonists that activate the $\alpha_{IIb}\beta_3$ receptor are likely to work in combination *in vivo*. In fact, the mixture of agonists present is likely to change as the process unfolds, with collagen perhaps more important at the beginning, thrombin more important later on, and the other agonists in varying mixtures throughout. The platelet activation effects of multiple agonists may be additive or synergistic, depending on the mechanism(s) involved (see "Signaling Pathways in Platelet Activation and Aggregation" below).[472,473] For example, although epinephrine is a relatively weak platelet agonist itself, it probably plays an important role by enhancing the platelet's response to other agonists, including the ability to overcome aspirin-induced inhibition of platelet thrombus formation.[474] Changes in epinephrine levels that can accompany cigarette smoking or vascular collapse, as during myocardial infarction, may therefore have significant effects on platelet thrombus formation.[474–476] Platelets can also be activated by shear stresses *ex vivo*; while the *in vivo* significance of this phenomenon remains unknown, it offers another potential link between the blood vessel narrowing produced by atherosclerotic vascular disease and platelet activation.[360,381,382,477]

PLATELET ENERGY METABOLISM

Platelets have sizable stores of glycogen that can often be seen on electron microscopy (see Fig. 114–1). Glycogen can be broken down into glucose-1-phosphate, and platelets can also take up glucose from their surrounding medium. Both sources of glucose can be converted to glucose-6-phosphate, which can then enter glycolysis or the hexose monophosphate shunt. Platelet glycolysis rates significantly exceed those of erythrocytes and skeletal muscle.[86] Oxidative metabolism

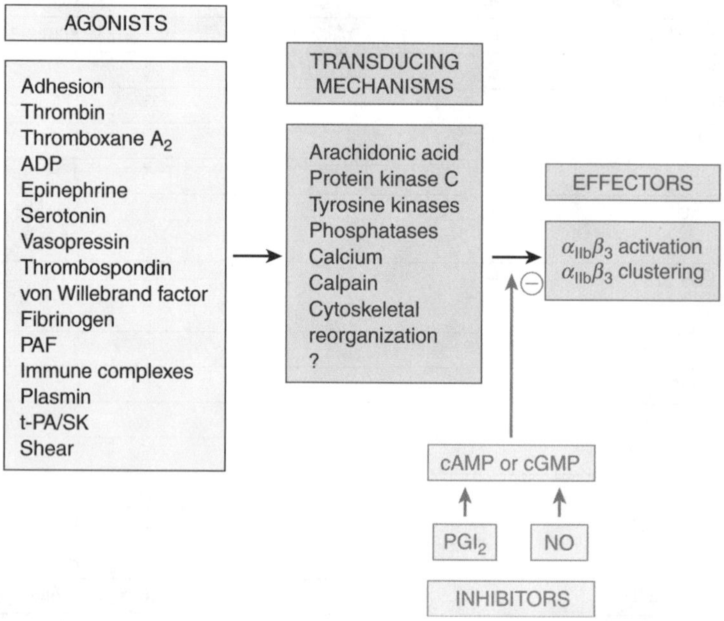

FIGURE 114–12. Platelet activation and aggregation. Many different agents and phenomena can initiate platelet activation, and a select group is listed as agonists. Virtually all of these agonists are released, synthesized, present, or occur at sites of vascular injury, providing both geographic and temporal restriction of the response. These agonists can initiate aggregation either alone or in combination with one or more other agonists. Not shown are a number of different signal transduction mechanisms have been defined that convert the agonist signal into a change in the conformation of the $\alpha_{IIb}\beta_3$ receptor and related changes that result in ligand binding, receptor clustering, and platelet aggregation. Not shown are a number of additional receptor–ligand interactions that enhance the stability of platelet aggregates. Two inhibitors produced by endothelial cells, PGI_2 (prostacyclin) and NO (nitric oxide), inhibit signal transduction via increases in cAMP (cyclic adenosine monophosphate) and cGMP (cyclic guanosine monophosphate), respectively. Not shown is endothelial ADPase (CD39) that inhibits ADP-induced platelet activation. ADP, adenosine diphosphate; PAF, platelet-activating factor; SK, streptokinase; t-PA, tissue-type plasminogen activator.

TABLE 114–7. Factors That Prevent or Inhibit Platelet Activation

Flowing blood
Prostacyclin (PGI_2)
Nitric oxide (NO)
Endothelial cell CD39 (ATP diphosphohydrolase; ecto-ADPase)
Platelet refractoriness
Leukocyte–platelet interactions*
Inhibitors of thrombin generation and thrombin action

*Both activating and inhibitory interactions.

SOURCE: Adapted with permission from Coller BS.[355]

probably contributes to energy production in resting platelets, but it has been estimated that less than 1 percent of the pyruvic acid produced by glycolysis actually enters the citric acid cycle, the remainder terminating in lactate or pyruvate, which leave the platelet.[87] Platelet mitochondria are capable of β oxidation of fatty acids, but it is not clear how much this process contributes to energy production.[88–91] Platelets can actively metabolize acetate, and this ability has been exploited to improve platelet storage conditions.[91,92] Amino acids may also act as energy sources and feed into the citric acid cycle, but the contribution of this process to platelet energy metabolism is uncertain.

As in all cells, ATP consumption by platelets is partially devoted to maintaining ionic and osmotic homeostasis.[93,94] In addition, the continuous polymerization and depolymerization of actin involves conversion of ATP to ADP, which may account for as much as 40 percent of the ATP consumption in resting platelets.[95] The inositol phosphates, which are important in signal transduction, undergo continual dephosphorylation and rephosphorylation; these reactions are estimated to consume as much as 7 percent of the total ATP produced.[96] Protein phosphorylation also occurs as an ongoing event, but its fractional use of ATP is not clear.

Depleting platelets of the metabolic pool of ATP and ADP decreases their ability to respond to stimuli, but the effect is not uniform: thus, shape change is only minimally affected, whereas there are increasingly significant inhibitory effects on platelet aggregation, α-granule and dense granule secretion, arachidonic acid liberation, and lysosome secretion.[97–100]

Platelet stimulation is accompanied by a marked increase in both glycolytic activity and oxidative ATP production, perhaps through a feedback mechanism in response to the abrupt decrease in ATP that occurs with platelet activation or as a result of the increase in cytoplasmic pH.[89] The increased ATP appears to be utilized, at least in part, in phosphoinositide phosphorylation and protein phosphorylation.

PLATELET SHAPE CHANGE, SPREADING, CONTRACTION, SECRETION, AND CLOT RETRACTION

Overview

The cytoskeleton establishes the platelet structure and its ability to respond to stimuli through changes in shape and force generation; as such, the platelet cytoskeleton can be considered analogous to an animal's bones and muscles. Table 114–8 lists the major components of the platelet contractile system. These elements are thought to contribute to platelet shape change, secretion, and clot retraction after platelet activation.

When exposed to a variety of agonists, platelets undergo dramatic changes in shape within seconds. Shape change follows a reproducible sequence of events during which the resting platelet cytoskeleton is dismantled and reorganized. The first noticeable change following activation is the dismantling of the microtubule coil and conversion from discs to spheres. Filopodia and lamellipodia, generated by new actin filament assembly, then extend from the plasma membrane. At the same time, intracellular organelles and granules, and the dismantled microtubule coil, are compressed into the center of the platelet. Once shape change is finished, the actin cytoskeleton is used as a platform for contraction, and contractile tension is exerted between platelets and between platelets and the adjacent fibrin strands.

Platelet Shape Change

Platelet shape change occurs in response to many different agonists. It involves loss of the platelet's normal discoid shape (~1.5–2.5 μm diameter and ~0.5–0.9 μm width) and transformation to a spiny sphere with long, thin filopodia extending several μm out from the platelet and ending in points that are as small as 0.1 μm in diameter (see Fig. 114–1).[2,478] In the aggregometer, it has been generally assumed that the initial decrease in light transmission immediately after adding certain agonists is a reflection of platelets undergoing shape change,[479] but this interpretation has been challenged by the suggestion that microaggregation rather than shape change accounts for this phenomenon.[480] Although the reason platelets undergo shape change is unclear, one possibility is that it reduces electrostatic repulsion between two negatively charged platelets or between a platelet and a negatively charged surface or cell without the need to reduce surface charge density. Thus, after changing shape, the tip of a platelet filopodium can more easily approach and make contact with a surface or a cell because the great bulk of the repulsive surface charge is now at a distance from the tip.[3]

A change in platelet shape from disc to sphere is the first event that is observed as the platelet is activated. Agonist binding to select receptors activates phospholipase Cβ, which hydrolyzes membrane-bound phosphatidylinositol-4,5-bisphosphate to inositol-1,4,5-triphosphate (IP_3) and diacylglycerol. IP_3 then binds to receptors on the DTS/SR, generating a rise in cytosolic calcium concentrations to 5 to 10 μM (see Fig. 114–8). Although calcium can influence the activity of many actin-binding proteins, one of the major proteins that is activated is gelsolin, which is present in platelets at a concentration of approximately 5 μM. Actin filaments in resting platelets are relatively stable because their barbed ends (the end from which they can grow by adding additional actin monomers), are capped with the protein CapZ and α,γ-adducins (see Fig. 114–4). Calcium-activated gelsolin both severs existing actin filaments and caps the newly created barbed ends. This increases the number of actin filaments by an estimated 10-fold, and substitutes gelsolin for CapZ and α,γ-adducins as the actin filament capping protein.[481] Severing of actin filaments that interact with the planar lattice composed of filamin A (actin-binding protein), GPIb/IX, and spectrin in the membrane cytoskeleton releases the constraints on the spectrin network. This allows the membrane skeleton to swell (but not produce filopodia; Fig. 114–13) by incorporating into the plasma membrane the membranes from the open canalicular system, and later the membranes from the granules that release their contents.

The protrusive force for lamellipodia and filopodia formation comes from new actin polymerization, such that there is a doubling of actin filament content. This burst of actin filament assembly is powered by the generation of barbed-end nucleation sites after receptor activation. These nucleation sites are generated *de novo* by the activation of the Arp2/3 complex or by the exposure of the barbed ends of preexisting filaments.[482] Because barbed ends have a higher affinity for actin molecules than do the actin-sequestering proteins, they have the capacity to initiate actin filament polymerization.

TABLE 114–8. Platelet Cytoskeletal Proteins*

Protein	Properties
Actin[1575]	Mr = 42,000 20–30% of total platelet protein (0.55 M; 2×10^6 per platelet) β and γ forms present at a ratio of 5:1 Monomeric actin (G-actin) bound to calcium-ATP (or ADP) Polymerization requires energy (ATP→ADP) and produces F-actin F-actin filaments: two strands of intertwined helices with polarity based on ability to interact with myosin fragment ("pointed" and "barbed" ends) Steady-state polymerization: monomers lost from pointed end while others join barbed end ("treadmilling")
Profilin[1576]	Mr = 15,200 Forms 1:1 reversible complex with actin monomer Prevents actin polymerization May help "recharge" actin monomers with ATP
Gelsolin[1577]	Mr = 81,000 (5 μM; 2×10^4 per platelet) Binds to barbed end of F-actin filaments Severs actin filaments Facilitates nucleation Produces shorter filaments with gel→sol transformation
Thymosin β_4[517,518]	Mr = 5000 (0.55 M; 2×10^6 per platelet) Binds actin monomer Inhibits actin polymerization
Tropomyosin[1578]	Mr = 28,000; rod-shaped dimer of 35-nm length Binds to groove on actin filaments (6 actins: 1 tropomyosin) Not all actin filaments have bound tropomyosin
Caldesmon[1579]	Mr = 80,000; asymmetric Binds to actin, tropomyosin, myosin, and calmodulin May control actin filament bundling and actomyosin ATPase
Filamin A (X) and B (3) (Actin-binding protein)[30,46,481,504,1580,1581]	Filamin A/B = 10/1 Mr = 260,000 subunit; tail-to-tail dimer; elongated 162-nm flexible rod composed of 24 immunoglobulin-like domains; phosphorylated 2–3% of platelet protein Binds actin with 1 actin-binding protein molecule per 14 actin molecules Binds GPIbα and integrin β subunit cytoplasmic domains and links GPIb/IX to actin Binds small GTPases ralA, ras, rho, cdc-42, as well as kinases and phosphatases, and exchange factors Trio and Toll Crosslinks actin filaments to form a gel Dephosphorylation leads to loss of activity
Migfilin[31,702]	Mr = 50,000; binds kindlin-2 and VASP (vasodilator-stimulated phosphoprotein) Can displace filamin from β_3 cytoplasmic domain, facilitating binding of talin
Talin[37,1582,1583]	Mr = 235,000 3% of platelet protein Binds to β_3-integrin cytoplasmic tail to activate $\alpha_{IIb}\beta_3$; also binds vinculin and α-actinin; cleaved and activated by calpain
α-Actinin[1576]	Mr = 100,000 and 102,000; dimer Binds actin at 1:10 stoichiometry; binds Ca^{2+} Forms gel with F-actin; cooperates with actin-binding protein; promotes actin polymerization
Vinculin[523,1584,1585]	Mr = 130,000 Binds to talin; may link actin to membrane proteins at adhesion sites
Myosin II[1586,1587]	Mr = 480,000 ($2 \times 200{,}000$; $2 \times 20{,}000$; $2 \times 16{,}000$) 2–5% of platelet protein; 325×111-nm filaments Myosin light chain (Mr = 20,000); phosphorylated; required for ATPase activity
Myosin light-chain kinase[1588]	Mr = 105,000 Phosphorylates myosin light chain and activates actomyosin ATPase leading to contraction
Calmodulin[1589]	Mr = 17,000 Binds four calciums and activates myosin light-chain kinase
CapZ[46,481]	Mr = 36,000 and 32,000 (5 μM; 2×10^4 per platelet) Heterodimer Binds barbed ends of actin filaments
Cofilin[46,481]	Mr = 20,000 Accelerates depolymerization of actin filaments
Fimbrin (L-plastin)	Mr = 68,000 Bundles actin filaments Found in microvilli
VASP[46,481]	Mr = 50,000 Tetrameric Binds profilin, vinculin, zyxin
GTPases[46,492,504]	Cdc42–filopodia Rho–stress fibers Rac–lamellipodia and ruffles Rap1b–$\alpha_{IIb}\beta_3$ control
Tyrosine kinases	pp60src pp125Fak–$\alpha_{IIb}\beta_3$ signaling pp72syk–GPVI signaling
Adaptor proteins	14-3-3ζ–binds to GPIbα Pleckstrin–phosphorylated on activation
PI kinases	PI-3 kinase PI_4P-5 kinase
Spectrin	α,β heterodimers form head to head tetramers Bind to actin filaments
α,γ Adducins	Cap barbed ends of actin filaments and bind to spectrin Phosphorylated with platelet activation and cleaved by calpain

*See Fox[504]; Daniel[1590]; Furman, Gardner, and Goldschmidt-Clermont,[515]; Hartwig[46]; and Hartwig, Barkalow, and Azim.[481]

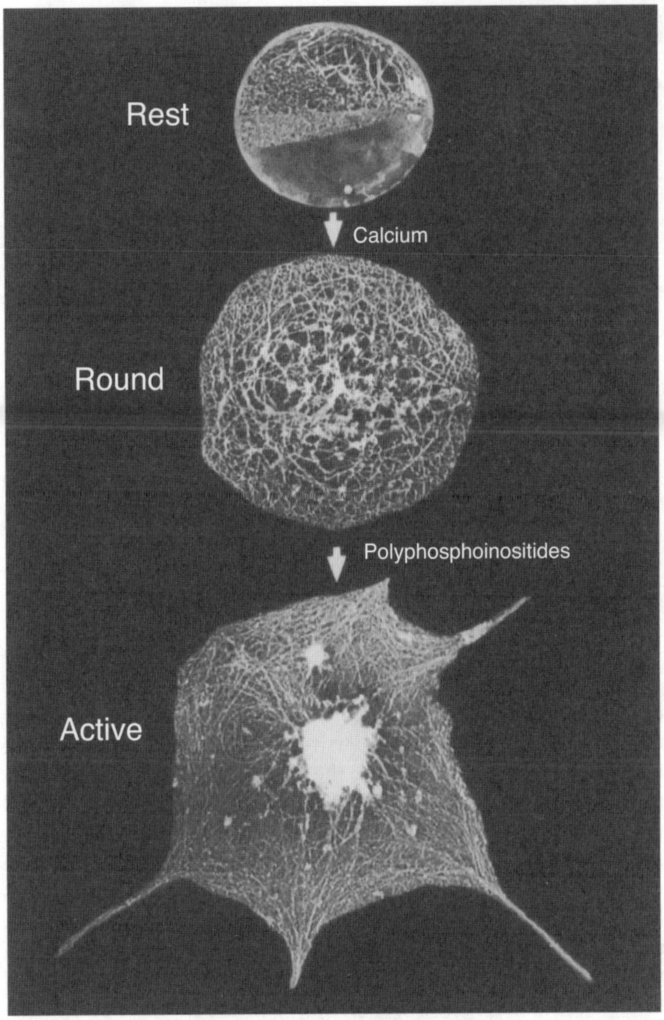

FIGURE 114–13. Control of platelet shape change. Resting platelets are small discs. Platelets convert from discs in two steps. In the first step, a calcium transient activates platelet gelsolin. Gelsolin binds, severs, and caps actin filaments. Fragmentation of endogenous filaments causes the cell to become spherical. In the second step, spherical cells protrude lamellae and filopods. Actin filament assembly drives the protrusion of cellular processes. *(Adapted with permission from Hartwig JH, Barkalow K, Azim A, et al.[481])*

Platelets contain two proteins whose main function is to bind and sequester actin monomers (see Fig. 114–4). The first is profilin, which is present at a concentration of 50 μM. Profilin can sequester actin monomers from the pointed ends of actin filaments, but not the barbed ends. Profilin also functions as a major transfer factor in actin filament polymerization. The second, and more abundant protein involved in sequestration of actin monomers and stimulation of the polymerization of actin is thymosin-β_4. With a platelet concentration of 55 μM, it is equimolar to actin. Thymosin-β_4 binds actin molecules with an affinity that is greater than that of the pointed end of the actin filament, allowing it to compete effectively for molecules from the pointed end. Thymosin-β_4 has a lower affinity for actin monomer than actin has for the barbed end of the filament, resulting in filament assembly when barbed ends are free. Thymosin-β_4 maintains a large pool of unpolymerized actin, and 60 percent of the total actin in the platelet is bound to thymosin-β_4. The affinity of thymosin-β_4 for actin monomer is regulated by the nucleotide that is bound to actin.[483]

The platelet actin assembly reaction that follows the addition of agonists starts when free barbed ends are formed (see Fig. 114–4). Barbed ends are generated by the uncapping of filament ends and the *de novo* assembly of filaments by the Arp2/3 complex. Platelets contain high concentrations of barbed-end capping proteins that regulate the accessibility of these ends to regulate actin dynamics. Platelets contain 5 μM each of gelsolin[484] and capZ,[485] and 3 μM adducin.[486] Uncapping of the actin filaments appears to be accomplished by the inactivation of capping proteins by phosphoinositides that are produced during platelet activation, including phosphatidylinositol-3,4-bisphosphate ($PI_{3,4}P_2$), $PI_{4,5}P_2$, and $PI_{3,4,5}P_3$.[481] The uncapped actin filaments act as nuclei onto which actin monomers (which are maintained in an available pool by association with thymosin-β_4) can assemble on the barbed ends of the filaments. Profilin accelerates actin polymerization by facilitating the transfer of actin from the actin–thymosin-β_4 complex to the barbed ends of the actin filaments. In addition to exposing new filament ends as a source of nuclei, new nucleation sites are generated by activation by the Arp2/3 complex. The Arp2/3 complex mimics the pointed ends of actin filaments and stimulates barbed-end assembly of actin filaments. The Arp2/3 complex is made up of seven polypeptides, two of which have actin-related sequences, Arp2 and Arp3.[487,488] Platelets contain high concentrations of the Arp2/3 complex (2–10 μM). Approximately 30 percent of the Arp2/3 complex is bound to the resting platelet cytoskeleton. Once platelets are activated, the Arp2/3 complex redistributes to the cytoskeleton, increasing three-fold and concentrating in the lamellipodia zone of actin filament assembly. Several signaling pathways regulate the activity of the Arp2/3 complex, including Wiskott-Aldrich syndrome protein (WASP) family members. Mutations in the WASP gene result in Wiskott-Aldrich syndrome, an inherited X-linked recessive disorder characterized by thrombocytopenia and T-cell immunodeficiency (see Chap. 121).

Simultaneous with these changes, the peripheral microtubule coil becomes constricted and fragmented, and is ultimately compressed into the center of the cell. As the filopodia form, the platelet's granules and organelles move to the center, surrounded by the microtubule coil, resulting in an increase in electron density. Activation of myosin II via phosphorylation of myosin light chain kinase, contributes to the inward contractile force by its interaction with the actin fibers.

Platelet Spreading and Surface-Induced Activation

After platelets adhere to surfaces, they undergo variable degrees of spreading and activation. The patterns of spreading and activation depend primarily on the protein surface on which they spread, with collagen consistently inducing the most activation.[399,489] In addition to the nature of the surface, the protein density, especially in the case of fibrinogen, can dramatically affect the signaling systems that are activated in the adherent platelets.[490]Activation can result in release of granule contents and exposure of activated $\alpha_{IIb}\beta_3$ receptors on the luminal surface of the platelets, where they are strategically located to bind adhesive glycoprotein ligands that can recruit additional platelets.[491] If the surface density of platelets is sufficient, the platelets can also enter into lateral associations, which appear to depend on $\alpha_{IIb}\beta_3$.[416] In general, platelet spreading results in the development of broad lamellipodia rather than spike-like filopodia (see Fig. 114–1).[481,492] The different morphologies of platelet spreading reflect differences in the organization of the network of actin filaments. Ultrastructural examination of lamellipodia reveals them to be replete with actin filaments that are organized into orthogonal networks. This organization is established by the actin filament crosslinking protein filamin A. In contrast, filopodia contain long actin filaments that are organized as tight bundles. These structural differences reflect the different signals initiated by the adhesion process, and both phosphoinositides and the small GTPase molecules Rac and Cdc42 appear to be particularly important in this process.[46] In platelets, Rac is activated by thrombin receptor ligation and it

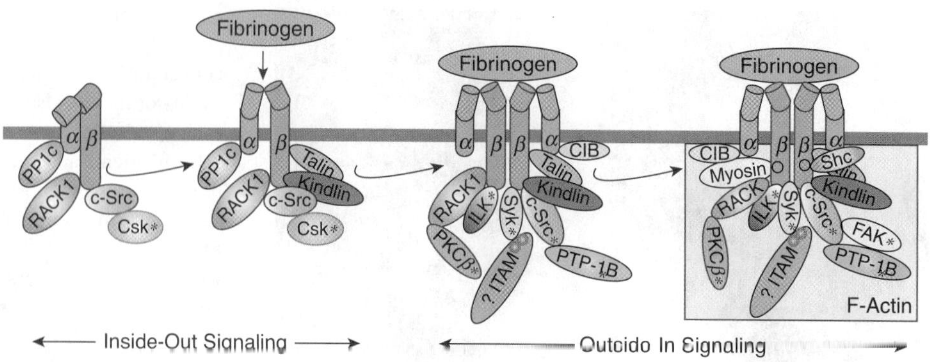

FIGURE 114–14. Protein interactions with the cytoplasmic domains of $\alpha_{IIb}\beta_3$ regulate inside-out and outside-in signaling. Shown are some, but not all, of the proteins reported to associate with the $\alpha_{IIb}\beta_3$ cytoplasmic domains, many in a dynamic fashion. Some are associated within resting platelets, whereas others are recruited to, or dissociate from, the integrin during inside-out or outside-in signaling, leading to F-actin assembly. In addition, several proteins with enzymatic function become activated (*asterisks*) after fibrinogen binding to $\alpha_{IIb}\beta_3$. Not shown are the many additional adapter molecules, enzymes, and substrates that may become recruited through more indirect interactions. CIB, calcium and integrin-binding 1; Csk, c-Src tyrosine kinase; ILK, integrin-linked kinase; ITAM, a yet-to-be identified protein with one or more immunoreceptor tyrosine activation motifs; PKCβ, protein kinase Cβ; PP1c, protein phosphatase 1c; RACK1, receptor for activated C kinase 1; Syk, spleen tyrosine kinase. *(Reproduced with permission from Coller BS, Shattil SJ.[419])*

stimulates actin filament uncapping.[493] Proteins that have been implicated in organizing the tips of the filopodia where the actin bundles attach to the plasma membrane are the small GTPase Cdc42, the exchange protein WASP, vinculin, vasodilator-stimulated phosphoprotein (VASP), zyxin, and profiling.[311] Pleckstrin, a platelet protein that is phosphorylated during platelet activation, appears to participate in this process by binding to phosphoinositides and affecting Rac via an exchange factor.[494,495] Platelets from mice deficient in pleckstrin have a defect in granule secretion, $\alpha_{IIb}\beta_3$ activation, and aggregation mediated by protein kinase C. Thrombin can overcome this abnormality via a pathway involving phosphoinositide 3-kinase (PI3K).[496] Signaling after adhesion results from the assembly of protein complexes on the cytoplasmic surfaces of the receptor(s) involved in the adhesion process, including focal adhesion kinase (FAK), which is activated by integrin ligation and colocalizes with a number of cytoskeletal proteins. Deletion of FAK in megakaryocytes and platelets results in defects in platelet spreading.[497] These complexes then initiate local cytoskeletal rearrangements as well as the generation of signaling molecules that act throughout the platelet to produce a variety of effects, including the translation of new proteins.[415,418,419,498] The nature and extent of the signaling may determine whether the adherent platelets recruit additional platelets or white blood cells. In particular, the conversion of spread platelets to a microvesiculated procoagulant form is associated with the recruitment of neutrophils.[499] Additionally, spread platelets can assemble fibronectin matrix on their surface, which may be important in stabilizing platelet–platelet interactions.[500]

Membrane glycoproteins are affected by cytoskeletal rearrangements associated with platelet shape change and spreading. Activation of platelets in suspension under certain conditions results in movement of GPIb/IX receptors from the surface of platelets to the open canalicular system.[297,298] With adherent platelets, the GPIb internalization is much slower.[311] The initial effect of activation on $\alpha_{IIb}\beta_3$ is an increase in receptors on the plasma membranes as the $\alpha_{IIb}\beta_3$ receptors in α granules, and perhaps dense granules and the open canalicular system, join the plasma membrane. Inside-out activation of $\alpha_{IIb}\beta_3$ from its inactive to active conformation is associated with cytoskeletal changes, in particular, the binding of talin to the β_3-integrin cytoplasmic domain (see Figs. 114–3 and 114–14).[34,37,501,502] Tyrosine kinases, including FAK[413,503] and Src,[503] may play a role in this process, along with cortactin, an 85-kDa protein that is phosphorylated on tyrosine, and small GTP-binding proteins such as Rho, Rac, and Cdc42.[22,481,492,504] When the attachment of $\alpha_{IIb}\beta_3$ to the cytoskeleton includes actin and myosin, the force produced by the cytoskeleton on $\alpha_{IIb}\beta_3$ may supply the energy to produce the conformational changes that lead to higher ligand-binding affinity.[39] After activation, more $\alpha_{IIb}\beta_3$ molecules become associated with the cytoskeleton, and this presumably reflects the interaction with talin and other cytoskeletal proteins and ligand-induced $\alpha_{IIb}\beta_3$ clustering, resulting in the development of protein complexes, including cytoskeletal proteins, on the cytoplasmic surface of the receptor (Fig. 114–14).[37,415,505] When ligand-coated beads are added to adherent platelets and bind to $\alpha_{IIb}\beta_3$ receptors, the beads are transported to the center of the platelets, indicating that the cytoskeleton can move $\alpha_{IIb}\beta_3$ receptors that have ligand attached to them.[506,507]

Platelets contain calpains, which are calcium-dependent, sulfhydryl, neutral proteases composed of two subunits that preferentially cleave cytoskeletal proteins, in particular filamins and talin,[492,508] but have also been reported to cleave the cytoplasmic domain of β_3, and a number of molecules involved in signaling, including kinases and phosphatases (see "Calcium-Dependent Proteases [Calpains]" below). Mu-calpain requires micromolar calcium and m-calpain required millimolar calcium for activation. It has been proposed that calpains are involved in cytoskeletal reorganization upon platelet activation, and specifically, perhaps, to binding of ligand to $\alpha_{IIb}\beta_3$ via cleavage of the integrin β_3 cytoplasmic tail and talin.[37,509–511] Calpain cleavage of the integrin β_3 cytoplasmic tail may switch the function of the integrin from promoting platelet spreading to mediating clot retraction.[512] Calpains have also been implicated in platelet spreading, microparticle formation, and the generation of platelet coagulant activity.[492,510,513] Mice lacking mu-calpain have reduced platelet aggregation and clot retraction, but normal bleeding time.[514]

Platelet Contraction and Secretion

The contractile mechanism involving actin and myosin is thought to facilitate granule secretion, but the details remain obscure.[107,515] In fact, mice with nearly complete disruption of the platelet heavy-chain myosin gene *Myh9* have a defect in secretion, but only in response to low concentrations of select agonists.[516] The cytoskeleton of resting platelets consists of the membrane skeleton described above, which lies just beneath the membrane, and a lacy cytoplasmic actin filament network composed of 2000 to 5000 linear actin polymers, which also contains α-actin, filamins (actin-binding proteins) A and B, tropomyosin, vinculin, and caldesmon.[22,46,63,504,517–521] The contractile response is also thought to be initiated by an increase in cytosolic calcium, which results in the formation of a calcium–calmodulin complex that then activates myosin light-chain kinase; phosphatases and cyclic adenosine monophosphate (cAMP) kinase can modulate this response (see "Signaling Pathways in Platelet Activation and Aggregation" below). After the initial platelet shape change, actin becomes organized centrally into thick filamentous masses, where it probably associates with phosphorylated myosin filaments.[522,523] The centralization of organelles within a contractile ring correlates with secretion.[2] There is controversy, however, as to whether platelets secrete their granular contents by fusion with the open canalicular system in the center of the platelet or by direct fusion with the plasma membrane.[2,296]

An intricate pathway of protein–protein interactions has been proposed for platelet secretion in which granules tether and dock to the inner leaflet of the plasma membrane, after which fusion of the two opposing lipid bilayers mediates cargo release.[524] Docking and tethering are thought to be, in part, mediated by small GTP-binding proteins of the Rab family. Platelets have been reported to contain at least 11 Rabs, although only a few are functionally relevant. Rab27a and b are important for both granule biogenesis and secretion,[525] while Rab 4 appears to have a role in secretion.[526] The α-granule-associated Rab6 is phosphorylated upon thrombin stimulation in a protein kinase C (PKC) dependent manner and phosphorylation seems to increase its GTP-loading.[527]

Platelet granule–plasma membrane fusion is analogous to exocytosis in neurons, where detailed studies have shown the importance of a core set of integral membrane proteins called *soluble* N-*ethylmaleimide-sensitive factor attachment protein receptors* (SNAREs).[528] It is generally accepted that vesicle/granule-target membrane fusion is governed by the binding of a SNARE from the cargo-containing granule or vesicle (v-SNARE), with a heteromeric protein complex in the target membrane (t-SNAREs). The resulting, *trans*-bilayer complex is minimally sufficient for membrane fusion.[529] In human platelets, the v-SNAREs are vesicle-associated membrane protein (VAMP)-2/synaptobrevin, VAMP-3/cellubrevin, VAMP-7/TI-VAMP, and VAMP-8/endobrevin, with the latter being most abundant.[530–534] There are two classes of t-SNAREs: the soluble *N*-ethylmaleimide-sensitive factor attachment protein (SNAP)-23/25/29 type and the syntaxin type. Human platelets contain syntaxins 2, 4, 7, and 11,[530–534] as well as SNAP-23, -25, and -29.[535,536] Functional studies using *in vitro* assays and genetically altered mice, have established that VAMP-8 is the primary v-SNARE required for secretion from all three classes of platelet granules.[530,533] VAMP-2 or VAMP-3 can also play a role at higher levels of stimulation. As for t-SNAREs, SNAP-23 and syntaxin 2 are required for each secretion event. Syntaxin 4 appears to also play a role, but only in α-granule and lysosome release.[537–540]

Although the SNARE proteins are sufficient to mediate membrane fusion, they do so inefficiently and thus require accessory proteins to control where and when they interact. Many of these regulators may be sensitive to second messengers such as diacylglycerol (DAG) and Ca^{2+}, whereas others are substrates for kinases, such as PKC. The Munc18 family (a, b, and c) control syntaxins and have been shown to be critical for platelet secretion.[541–543] Studies show that Munc18a and c are phosphorylated by PKC upon platelet activation and that this affects Munc18/syntaxin binding affinity.[542,543]At least two members of the Munc13 family are present in platelets (Munc13-1 and Munc13-4; Schraw TD, Ren Q, and Whiteheart SW, unpublished data).[544] Munc13-4 appears to be important for dense granule release and functions through its interactions with Rab27.[545,546] Munc13s have Ca^{2+} and DAG binding sites and thus may be regulated by the secondary messengers generated during platelet activation.

Munc13-4 has drawn particular attention because of its involvement in familial hemophagocytic lymphohistiocytosis and Griscelli syndrome. Munc13-4 is mutated in type 3 FHL[547] and interacts with the protein mutated in type 2 Griscelli syndrome, namely Rab27a.[548] One feature common to both diseases is the inability of T cells to properly organize the cytotoxic synapse required for toxin secretion and target cell killing.[547] For familial hemophagocytic lymphohistiocytosis patients, it is not clear whether they have bleeding-time defects as they generally receive marrow transplants very early in life.

Clot Retraction

When blood initially clots in the test tube, the fibrin mesh extends throughout, trapping virtually all of the serum in a gel-like state. If platelets are present, within minutes to hours, the clot retracts, extruding a very large fraction of the serum.[549] This process is thought to mimic *in vivo* phenomena that result in consolidation of thrombi and perhaps enhancement of wound healing. Clot retraction has also been implicated in decreasing the efficiency of thrombolysis, which may partially account for the resistance of platelet-rich thrombi to fibrinolytic agents.[550] The platelet requirement for clot retraction is indisputable as is a requirement for $\alpha_{IIb}\beta_3$ and a contractile mechanism involving actin and myosin.[551,552] In fact, nearly complete selective disruption of the myosin *Myh9* gene in mouse megakaryocytes gives rise to a phenotype characterized by macrothrombocytopenia; absence of clot retraction; reduced secretion in response to low concentrations of agonists, but not high concentrations; prolonged bleeding time; and protection from thrombus formation.[516] The mice do not, however, have evidence of spontaneous bleeding.[516] Myosin activation involves phosphorylation of the myosin light chain, a process that is governed by calcium-regulated myosin light-chain kinase activity and Rho kinase-regulated myosin phosphatase activity. Calpain-cleavage of the cytoplasmic tail of integrin β_3 may promote RhoA activity and serve a molecular switch to convert platelet spreading to clot retraction.[512] Despite these data, no model describing the details of the clot retraction process has gained acceptance.[553] Proposed mechanisms include movement of platelet filopodia along fibrin strands, tugging of fibrin strands by filopodia, and internalization of fibrin by the action of the membrane skeleton.[551–556]

Platelet $\alpha_{IIb}\beta_3$ is required for clot retraction, as demonstrated by studies of patients with Glanzmann thrombasthenia (see Chap. 121) and studies of normal platelets in the presence of agents that block either the $\alpha_{IIb}\beta_3$ receptor[554,557–562] or the fibrinogen γ-chain C-terminal sequence that mediates interactions with the $\alpha_{IIb}\beta_3$ receptor.[563] Clot retraction correlates temporally with an $\alpha_{IIb}\beta_3$-dependent decrease in protein tyrosine phosphorylation, presumably via activation of one or more phosphatases,[564] and may require both $\alpha_{IIb}\beta_3$-mediated mitogen-activated protein kinase (MAPK) activation[565] and translation of proteins such as Bcl-3, with the latter facilitated by ligand binding to $\alpha_{IIb}\beta_3$.[289] Results with $\alpha_{IIb}\beta_3$ antagonists demonstrate, however, differences in their ability to inhibit clot retraction that do not correlate with their ability to block fibrinogen binding to platelets,[554,562] and patients with Glanzmann thrombasthenia differ in the extent of their defect in clot retraction. Some $\alpha_{IIb}\beta_3$ mutations, such as β_3 L262P, interfere with interactions with fibrinogen but do not prevent interactions with fibrin and clot retraction.[566] Of particular note, fibrinogen lacking the γ-chain C-terminal sequence (400–411) that mediates binding to platelet $\alpha_{IIb}\beta_3$, as well as the two RGD-containing regions in fibrinogen, is still capable of supporting clot retraction.[567,568] It is well established that when fibrinogen converts to fibrin, new sites become exposed on the surface of the molecule. Therefore, one possible explanation for this paradox is that additional or alternative $\alpha_{IIb}\beta_3$ binding sequences in the fibrinogen γ-chain (e.g., 316–322, 370–383, or other regions) may be able to mediate clot retraction.[569,570] It is also possible that GPIb/IX contributes to clot retraction by virtue of the binding of GPIbα to the thrombin and/or VWF bound to the fibrin.[571,572] Thus, although $\alpha_{IIb}\beta_3$ is required for clot retraction, the process is not a simple reflection of fibrinogen binding to $\alpha_{IIb}\beta_3$.

■ PLATELET COAGULANT ACTIVITY

In resting platelets, the negatively charged phospholipids, including phosphatidylserine, are almost exclusively present in the inner leaflet. Among the mechanisms proposed to account for this asymmetry are unidirectional enzymatic movement by an aminophospholipid translocase (flippase) and/or association between the negatively charged phospholipids and elements in the cytoplasm, including cytoskeletal elements and their accompanying proteins.[10,12,573,574] When platelets are activated by strong agonists, there is a redistribution of negatively charged phospholipids to the outer leaflet of the platelet plasma membrane and this movement has been ascribed to one or more enzymes that can alter phospholipid distribution in the membrane. Platelets contain a calcium-activated plasma membrane "scramblase" enzyme (phospholipid scramblase 1) of predicted molecular weight approximately 35,000 that in model systems reverses the asymmetric distribution of negatively charged phospholipids in membrane bilayers, but the role of this enzyme *in vivo* is uncertain as the platelets of mice lacking this enzyme can redistribute their negatively charged phospholipids upon activation.[573,575–578] A highly homologous enzyme, phospholipid scramblase 3 has also been identified in platelets and other cells but its role is also uncertain.[577] A "floppase" activity, which promotes outward-directed lipid transport, has been postulated in platelets, and while the multidrug resistance protein 1 (ABCC1) has been suggested to account for this activity in erythrocytes,[579] no specific molecule with this function has yet been identified in platelets.[580] A floppase would also be a candidate for reversing the phospholipid asymmetry with platelet activation. Because platelet activation with strong agonists also results in the formation of microparticles, which are particularly rich in surface-exposed negatively charged phospholipids, it is possible that the molecular reorganization of the membrane that produces microparticles also results in surface exposure of negatively charged phospholipids on both the microparticles and the residual platelet membrane. Microparticles also are rich in factor Va and thus actively support thrombin generation.[8,451,581]

Microparticle formation can be induced *in vitro* by activation of platelets with ionophore A23187, complement C5b-9, or the combination of thrombin and collagen; by adding tissue factor to recalcified platelet-rich plasma; or by high shear stress.[451,582–587] Incubation of platelets with sera from patients with heparin-induced thrombocytopenia can also produce microparticles,[588,589] perhaps accounting, in part, for the thrombosis that is sometimes associated with this disorder (see Chap. 119). Elevations of cytosolic Ca^{2+}, calpain activation, cytoskeletal reorganization, protein phosphorylation, and phospholipid translocation are all implicated in microparticle formation. Inhibition of $\alpha_{IIb}\beta_3$, and perhaps $\alpha_V\beta_3$, decreases tissue factor-induced platelet coagulant activity and microparticle formation in the presence or absence of fibrin,[590] whereas inhibition of GPIb inhibits tissue factor-induced microparticle formation only in the presence of fibrin.[591]

The biologic relevance of platelet microparticles is supported by the finding of increased circulating levels of platelet microparticles in patients with activated coagulation and fibrinolysis, diabetes mellitus, sickle cell anemia, human immunodeficiency virus infection, unstable angina, heparin-induced thrombocytopenia with thrombosis, and respiratory distress syndrome.[451,592] Microparticles can bind to fibrin thrombi via one or more of the receptors present on their surface, including $\alpha_{IIb}\beta_3$, GPIb/IX, P-selectin, and perhaps PSGL-1.[593]

Microparticles bind factors VIII, Va, and Xa, allowing them to form both the factor Xase and prothrombinase complexes on their surface.[451] They can also bind protein S and facilitate inactivation of factors Va and VIIIa which could serve an anticoagulant function.[594,595] In addition, microparticles can activate platelets by supplying arachidonic acid. In a similar manner, they can activate endothelial cells and monocytes, resulting in enhanced monocyte attachment to endothelial cells, a potential contributor to atherosclerosis.[451]

Evidence supporting the importance of platelet microparticle formation to platelet coagulant activity has been gathered from observations of patients who have significant bleeding diatheses in association with defects in platelet microparticle formation (Scott syndrome; see Chap. 121).[596–598] Platelets from the most intensively studied patient had an impaired ability to accelerate the activation of both factor X and prothrombin. In addition, this patient's platelets exhibited both abnormal factor V binding and abnormal exposure of negatively charged phospholipids. In flow chamber studies, her platelets did not support normal fibrin deposition. The defect in microparticle formation appears to be the primary abnormality, given that the patient's erythrocytes also failed to undergo normal vesiculation in response to the calcium ionophore A23187.[596,599] Although an abnormality in the scramblase enzyme was considered a possible cause of this patient's abnormalities, no mutation was identified in phospholipid scramblase 1.[580,600,601] A heterozygous missense mutation in ABCA1 combined with reduced mRNA expression of both normal and mutant alleles was reported in the lymphocytes of one patient with Scott syndrome.[602]

Platelet activation leading to increased platelet coagulant activity shares several features with cell apoptosis, including surface exposure of negatively charged phospholipids and membrane blebbing leading to microparticle formation. Platelets contain the apoptosis-related proteins procaspase-3 and procaspase-9, as well as the caspase activators APAF-1 and cytochrome c.[603–605] There are conflicting data, however, regarding the relative roles of caspases and calpains in the development of platelet coagulant activity.[580,603] Mitochondrial alterations may link platelet apoptotic phenomena with the development of procoagulant activity.[83] During apoptotic and necrotic cell death, high levels of calcium promote the opening of the mitochondrion's permeability transition pore, which, in turn, results in loss of mitochondrial membrane potential and rupture of the mitochondrial outer membrane. Thrombin plus convulxin stimulation of platelets reduces the mitochondrial membrane potential and enhances procoagulant activity. Cyclophilin D is a critical component of the permeability transition pore, and in its absence, phosphatidylserine exposure and thrombin generation are impaired. Although platelet activation and initiation of apoptosis both result in exposure of phosphatidylserine, it has been suggested that phosphatidylserine exposure associated with apoptosis is mediated by yet another enzyme, perhaps the ABC1 ATP-binding protein.[606] This pathway was intact in the lymphocytes of a patient with Scott syndrome.

Although conflicting data exist on whether resting platelets contain tissue factor, activated platelets can synthesize tissue factor by splicing pre-mRNA into mature mRNA and then translating the tissue factor protein.[291,368] Additionally, platelet thrombi can recruit tissue factor from blood by binding leukocyte-derived, tissue factor-containing microparticles or by binding an alternatively spliced, soluble form of tissue factor.[268,271,452–455] The interaction between PSGL-1 on the surface of leukocyte-derived microparticles and P-selectin on the surface of activated platelets appears to play an important role in the binding of microparticles to platelet thrombi.[455] Interactions between platelets and leukocytes, and perhaps leukocyte-derived microparticles, reportedly enhance ("deencrypt" or decrypt) tissue factor activity, probably by supplying negatively charged phopholipids[369] and/or the oxidoreductase enzyme PDI.[370]

Platelet dense granules contain polyphosphate, a linear polymer of inorganic phosphate, which is released during platelet activation and promotes clot formation. Polyphosphates accelerate factor V activation[607] and alter the structure of fibrin clots. In the presence of polyphosphates, fibrin clots have thicker fibers and are more resistant to fibrinolysis.[608]

Incontrovertible evidence exists that platelets accelerate thrombin formation, but the precise mechanisms involved remain controversial.[596,597,609–611] The effect of platelets on activation of factor X by factors IXa and VIIIa and the activation of prothrombin by factors Xa and Va have been extensively studied.[597,611] Both reactions are accelerated by platelets, most dramatically when the platelets have been activated by thrombin or other agonists. Platelets also are able to accelerate factor VIII activation by thrombin.[583] It is likely that factor VIIIa on platelets acts as a binding site for factor IXa, and that factor Va on platelets acts as a binding site for factor Xa.[584] The effector cell protease receptor-1 (EPR-1) or a similar molecule may act as another binding site for Xa on activated platelets.[585] A separate receptor for factor IXa may also exist, and it has been suggested that only approximately 10 percent of activated platelets expose on average approximately 6000 factor IXa binding sites per platelet.[612] The concept that only a subpopulation of platelets develops a procoagulant phenotype with activation is supported by data from the percentage of activated platelets demonstrating high levels of factors Va and Xa ("coated" platelets).[263,264,611,613] It remains unclear, however, whether factors VIIIa and Va bind to specific receptors on platelets or whether they bind nonspecifically to negatively charged phospholipids, most particularly phosphatidylserine, that join the outer leaflet of the platelet plasma membrane bilayer when platelets are activated.[573,584,596,609,611] The assembly of the factor IXa/factor VIIIa/platelet complex increases the catalytic efficiency of factor X activation (k_{cat}/K_m) by a factor of 2.4×10^6.[611] Prothrombin binds to approximately 20,000 sites on activated platelets with a kDa equal to its plasma concentration (~0.15 μm).[614] The $\alpha_{IIb}\beta_3$ integrin binds prothrombin via an RGD-dependent mechanism, and may contribute to the localization of prothrombin to the surface of unactivated and activated platelets.[615] Factor XI has been shown to bind to both GPIbα and the apolipoprotein E receptor 2 (ApoER2, LRP8), a member of the low-density lipoprotein (LDL) family of receptors; and GPIbα has been shown to complex with ApoER2.[615a,615b,615c,615d] Dimeric factor XI may need to interact with both receptors simultaneously, as has also been proposed for the binding of both β2-glycoprotein I-anti-β2-glycoprotein I antibody complexes and protein C.[615c,615d]

The binding of activated coagulation factors to the surface of platelets appears to protect them from inactivation by inhibitors in plasma and platelets.[200] For example, the presence of platelet microparticles confers resistance to the anticoagulant effect of activated protein C, an observation with both theoretical and practical implications.[616] The relatively large platelet pool of factor V,[198,617] which appears to be complexed to multimerin,[166] and the ability of platelet proteases to activate it[204,205,618] also probably contribute to platelet coagulant activity. The bleeding diathesis in patients with Quebec platelet syndrome, who have proteolysis of their platelet α-granule factor V, supports the potential importance of platelet factor V in normal hemostasis (see Chap. 121), as do the studies of another patient with abnormal platelet factor V.[597] Further support comes from data on the hemostatic effectiveness of transfused platelets containing factor V in patients with inhibitors to plasma factor V.[207,611,619]

In addition to its hemostatic effects, platelet coagulant activity may play an important role in innate immunity. Thus, factor V-mediated thrombin generation protects against certain infections, such as group A streptococci. Reducing either plasma or platelet factor V levels increases mortality in mice infected with group A streptococci, perhaps because coagulation prevents the dissemination of bacteria.[620]

In addition to the platelet's role in accelerating the activation of factor X and prothrombin, there are other connections between platelets and the coagulation system, including: (1) the presence of fibrinogen in α granules and perhaps on the surface of platelets, where it is strategically located for interactions with locally generated thrombin[169,200]; (2) the presence of intracellular VWF and the binding of extracellular VWF to platelets (via GPIb/X and $\alpha_{IIb}\beta_3$), with the potential colocalization of factor VIII attached to the VWF (see Chap. 127); (3) activation of factor XI by thrombin on the platelet surface,[621,622] with the dimeric structure of factor XI allowing it to interact both with the platelet and factor IX simultaneously[623]; (4) a factor XI-like protein associated with platelet membranes, which may be an alternatively spliced form of factor XI lacking exon V; the level of this factor appears to correlate better with hemorrhagic symptoms than does the level of plasma factor XI[200,624]; (5) the presence of cytoplasmic factor XIII (see Chap. 115); (6) the presence of inhibitors of coagulation (α_1-protease inhibitor, C-1 inhibitor, tissue factor pathway inhibitor, the thrombin inhibitor protease nexin I, and the factors IXa and XIa inhibitor protease nexin II or β-amyloid precursor protein)[200,247]; and (7) promotion of factor XII activation by ADP-treated platelets.[200]

PLATELET MEMBRANE GLYCOPROTEINS, PLATELET ADHESION, AND PLATELET AGGREGATION

Platelet membrane glycoproteins mediate the interactions between the platelet and its external environment. Receptors can receive signals from outside the platelet and send signals inside. In addition, receptors can receive signals from inside the platelet that affect their external domains. Platelet glycoprotein receptors are derived from several different receptor families (integrins, leucine-rich glycoproteins, immunoglobulin cell adhesion molecules, selectins, quadraspanins, and seven transmembrane domain receptors; see Table 114–5). One member of the integrin family, $\alpha_{IIb}\beta_3$, is virtually unique to platelets, whereas the leucine-rich glycoproteins GPIb/IX and GPV appear to have highly restricted expression, including primarily platelets and cytokine-activated endothelial cells.[625,626] All of the other receptors are expressed more widely on other cell types.

Integrins

Integrin receptors are heterodimeric complexes composed of an α subunit containing three or four divalent cation-binding domains and a β subunit rich in disulfide bonds. Both subunits are transmembrane glycoproteins and are coded by different genes. There are at least 18 α subunits and 8 β subunits.[464,627–629] Three major families of integrin receptors are recognized based on the β subunit: β_1, β_2, and β_3. Integrins are widely distributed on different cell types, and each integrin demonstrates unique ligand-binding properties. Integrin receptors mediate interactions between cells and between proteins and cells; they are also involved in protein trafficking in cells. Integrin receptors can also transduce messages from outside the cell to inside the cell, and from inside the cell to outside the cell.

$\alpha_{IIb}\beta_3$ (GPIIb/IIIa; Fibrinogen Receptor; CD41/CD61) The $\alpha_{IIb}\beta_3$ complex, a member of the β_3 integrin receptor family, is the dominant platelet receptor, with 80,000 to 100,000 receptors present on the surface of a resting platelet (see Fig. 114–3).[464,465,471,627,630] Another 20,000 to 40,000 receptors are present inside platelets, primarily in α-granule membranes, but also in dense granules and membranes lining the open canalicular system; these receptors are able to join the plasma membrane when platelets are activated and undergo the release reaction.[631–633] On average, $\alpha_{IIb}\beta_3$ receptors are less than 20 nm apart on the platelet surface and thus are among the most densely expressed adhesion/aggregation receptors present on any cell type.

On resting platelets, $\alpha_{IIb}\beta_3$ has low affinity for fibrinogen in solution, but when platelets are activated with ADP, epinephrine, thrombin, or other agonists, $\alpha_{IIb}\beta_3$ binds fibrinogen relatively strongly.[465,466,470] The signal transduction mechanisms that mediate activation are discussed below. Activation induces changes in the $\alpha_{IIb}\beta_3$ receptor itself that are responsible for the change in fibrinogen-binding affinity,[634,635] but changes in the microenvironment surrounding $\alpha_{IIb}\beta_3$ may also be involved. The $\alpha_{IIb}\beta_3$ receptors in α granules appear to cycle to and from the plasma membrane.[636] This recycling helps to explain the ability of $\alpha_{IIb}\beta_3$ to take up fibrinogen from plasma and transport it to α granules, where it is concentrated.[169,174]

Data from other integrin receptors identified a cell recognition sequence composed of RGD in the ligand fibronectin,[637,638] and this same sequence is important in ligand binding to $\alpha_V\beta_3$ and $\alpha_{IIb}\beta_3$. Fibrinogen contains one RGD sequence near the carboxy terminus of each of the two Aα chains (amino acids 572 to 574) and another at amino acids 95 to 97.[639] In addition, the carboxy-terminal 12-amino-acid region of each of the two γ chains (amino acids 400 to 411) contains a sequence that includes Lys-Gln-Ala-Gly-Asp-Val, which appears to be the most important in the binding of fibrinogen to platelets.[393,640–642] von Willebrand factor contains an RGD sequence in its carboxy-terminal domain and that region mediates the binding to $\alpha_{IIb}\beta_3$.[375,378] Small, synthetic peptides containing the RGD or γ-chain sequence inhibit the binding of fibrinogen to platelets, and these observations have been exploited to produce therapeutic agents (tirofiban and eptifibatide) to inhibit platelet thrombus formation (see Chap. 135). Similarly, monoclonal antibodies that inhibit binding of ligands to $\alpha_{IIb}\beta_3$ have been developed and a mouse/human chimeric Fab fragment of one of them has been developed into a drug (abciximab) that is an effective antiplatelet agent (see Chap. 135).

The binding of fibrinogen to $\alpha_{IIb}\beta_3$ appears to be a multistep process:[465,643–648] (1) the initial interaction is most likely via the γ-chain carboxy-terminal region(s) and divalent cation-dependent[393,641,642,649]; (2) subsequent interactions enhance the binding and internalization of the fibrinogen,[650] render it irreversible, even when divalent cations are removed[651]; (3) binding of fibrinogen induces changes in the receptor that can be recognized by antibodies (ligand-induced binding sites [LIBS])[241]; (4) binding of fibrinogen to $\alpha_{IIb}\beta_3$ induces changes in fibrinogen (receptor-induced binding sites [RIBS]) that can be recognized by antibodies and may involve exposure of the Aα chain Arg-Gly-Asp-Phe (RGDF) sequence at amino acids 95 to 98[652,653]; and (5) fibrinogen binding induces receptor clustering.[505,654]

By electron microscopy, the receptors appear to have a globular head of 8 to 12 nm and two 18-nm long tails representing the carboxy-terminal regions of each subunit, including their hydrophobic transmembrane domains.[655,656] Crystallographic, electron microscopic, and biochemical data from $\alpha_{IIb}\beta_3$ and the related integrin receptor $\alpha_V\beta_3$ indicate that the unactivated receptors are in a bent conformation and that activation involves both extension of the receptor head and a swing out motion in the β_3 subunit (see Fig. 114–3)[39,657–663]; thus, the published electron micrographs of $\alpha_{IIb}\beta_3$ are probably of the extended (activated) forms of the receptor.

$\alpha_{IIb}\beta_3$ shares the same basic structural features of all integrin receptors (see Table 114–5).[419] The α subunit, α_{IIb}, is a transmembrane protein with four characteristic divalent cation binding sites (see Fig. 114–3). The mature protein contains 1008 amino acids,[464,627,664] with one transmembrane domain; during processing it is cleaved into a heavy chain and a light chain connected by a disulfide bond. The β subunit, β_3, contains 762 amino acids and is rich in cysteine residues, with a characteristic cysteine-rich region near its transmembrane domain.[464,627,665] The α_{IIb} and β_3 cytoplasmic tails consist of 20 and 47 amino acids, respectively. The genes coding for α_{IIb} and β_3 are very close to each other on chromosome 17 at q21.32, but are not so close as to share common regulatory domains.[666,667] Both proteins are synthesized in megakaryocytes and join to form a calcium-dependent, noncovalent complex in the rough endoplasmic reticulum.[627,668] Calnexin probably serves as a chaperone for α_{IIb},[669] but it is unclear which chaperone(s) are involved in β_3 folding and/or $\alpha_{IIb}\beta_3$ complex formation. The $\alpha_{IIb}\beta_3$ complex subsequently undergoes further processing in the Golgi apparatus, where the carbohydrate structures undergo maturation and the pro-GPIIb molecule is cleaved into its heavy and light chains by furin or a similar enzyme.[627,670,671] Approximately 15 percent of the mass of both α_{IIb} and β_3 is composed of carbohydrate.[672] The mature $\alpha_{IIb}\beta_3$ complex is then transported to the plasma membrane or the membranes of α granules or dense granules. If α_{IIb} and β_3 do not form a proper complex, either because of a structural abnormality in either subunit or the failure to synthesize one of the subunits, the subunit(s) that are synthesized are rapidly degraded and so are not expressed on the membrane surface (see Chap. 121). Degradation of α_{IIb} appears to involve retrotranslocation from the endoplasmic reticulum into the cytoplasm, ubiquitination, and proteolysis by the megakaryocyte proteosome.[669]

Both α_{IIb} and β_3 are composed of a series of domains (see Fig. 114–3). The amino-terminal region of α_{IIb} contains a seven-blade β-propeller domain, and each blade is composed of four β strands connected by loops. The propeller interacts with the βA (I like) domain of β_3, forming the globular head region observed in electron micrographs. The four calcium ions bound by the propeller domain interact with β hairpin loops in blades 4 to 7 that extend away from the interface with β_3. In addition, there is a unique α_{IIb} cap subdomain made up of four loops from blades 1 to 3 that are unique to α_{IIb} and contribute to its ligand-binding specificity. The remainder of the extracellular components of α_{IIb} are made up of a thigh, genu (knee-like), and two calf domains,[39] much like the structure of the related α_V subunit.[660,662] The cytoplasmic domain of α_{IIb} interacts with the cytoplasmic domain of β_3 and the interaction is important in controlling activation of the $\alpha_{IIb}\beta_3$ receptor.[471,673–676] The cytoplasmic domain of α_{IIb} has a GFFKR sequence near the membrane that is thought to control inside-out activation of the $\alpha_{IIb}\beta_3$ receptors because mutations or deletions in this region result in the receptor adopting a conformation with high affinity for fibrinogen.[471,677–679] A number of studies using mutagenesis and nuclear magnetic resonance spectroscopy identified different structures for the transmembrane and cytoplasmic domains, and differences in the relative roles of heterodimeric and homodimeric associations.[676,680–683] Disrupting the conformation of this region also results in a constitutively high affinity receptor,[36,684] supporting the conclusion that inside-out activation of $\alpha_{IIb}\beta_3$ requires separation of the transmembrane and cytoplasmic domains.

The β_3 subunit domains are not linearly arranged because the first domain (PSI [plexins, semaphorins, and integrins]) was subjected to the insertion of a hybrid domain, which itself was subjected to the insertion of a βA (I-like) domain; the latter domain is homologous to the VWF A domain and integrin I domains, both of which bind ligands (see Fig. 114–3).[657,685] The double insertion in the PSI domain explains why there is a "long-range" disulfide bond extending form C13 to C435; thus even though the βA domain makes contact with the α_{IIb} propeller (via Arg261 and other residues that interact with two rings of hydrophobic residues in the α_{IIb} "cage"), it is not the amino-terminus of the molecule. The PSI domain contains Leu33, which defines Pl^{A1} (HPA-1a) specificity, as opposed to the alloantigen Pl^{A2} (HPA-1b), which is produced by a Pro33 polymorphism (see Chap. 138). The β_3 leg is composed of four integrin epidermal growth factor domains that are rich in disulfide bonds. This region interacts with the α_{IIb} stalk region and the globular head in the bent, unactivated receptor, but not in the activated receptor.[39,657] Mutations in the integrin epidermal growth factor domains, including cysteine residues, can activate the receptor, as can the binding of monoclonal antibodies.[686–689] The importance of the normal disulfide bond pairings in β_3 is further supported by data demonstrating that certain reducing agents can cause activation of $\alpha_{IIb}\beta_3$, fibrinogen binding, and platelet aggregation,[690,691] and an enzyme capable of catalyzing the exchange of thiol groups and disulfide in proteins (PDI) has been identified on the surface of platelets and in platelet releasates.[690,692–694] Moreover, regions in β_3 itself have the same consensus sequence (CGXC) present in PDI that is thought to mediate the catalysis.[695] One model suggests that $\alpha_{IIb}\beta_3$ can achieve a low level of activation without alterations in disulfide bonds, but that maximal activation requires PDI or similar activity along with a source of thiols such as plasma glutathione or a membrane NAD(P)H oxidoreductase system.[690] It is still unclear, however, whether disulfide bond alterations contribute to activation *in vivo* under physiologic or pathologic conditions.

Transmembrane domain structures of α_{IIb} and β_3 have been proposed based on nuclear magnetic resonance and structural modeling studies.[681,682,696–700] The α_{IIb} transmembrane helix is shorter than the β_3 helix and so they traverse the membrane at an angle of approximately 25 degrees. The association of the α_{IIb} and β_3 ectodomains near the site of entry into the membrane results in the transmembrane helices being directly juxtaposed in the region of the membrane closest to the ectodomain (outer membrane clasp). Near the cytoplasmic end of the membrane the helices are held together by an inner membrane clasp composed of the α_{IIb} residues immediately after the end of the helix (^{991}GFFKR^{995}), with the membrane re-immersion of F992 and F993 filling the gap and interacting with β_3 W715 and I719, and α_{IIb} R995 creating a salt bridge with β_3 723 and perhaps β_3 726. Of note, these regions are conserved in many other integrins receptors and so the basic mechanism may be common to many of the receptors.

Inside-out signaling is accomplished by the talin F3 domain binding to the β_3 cytoplasmic domain and disrupting the inner membrane clasp (see Figs. 114–3 and 114–14).[37,415,502,673–675,677–680,684,701,701a] This may be facilitated by migfilin displacing filamin from the β_3 cytoplasmic domain as the latter interaction may prevent talin binding.[31,702] Talin binding results in dissociation of the transmembrane helices and reorganization of the cytoplasmic region of β_3 into a more extended helix. $\alpha_{IIb}\beta_3$ ectodomain chain separation, headpiece extension, and β_3 swing out then follow, either spontaneously or as a result of the traction force generated by the cytoskeleton on β_3 through talin. Outside-in signaling is presumed to be initiated by loss of ectodomain interactions between the membrane-proximal regions of α_{IIb} and β_3, perhaps as a result of ligand binding producing even greater β_3 swing out, resulting in disruption of the outer membrane clasp and subsequent dissociation of the transmembrane helices. This potentially may facilitate the interaction of the cytoplasmic domains with cytoskeletal elements and signaling molecules.

The β_3 tail also contains two NXXY motifs and Y747 and Y759 within these motifs are phosphorylated upon platelet aggregation, thus producing docking sites for signaling molecules.[419] Studies in mice and in recombinant systems demonstrate a role for the sites in clot retraction and platelet aggregate stability.[703,704]

A number of proteins have been shown to bind to the cytoplasmic domains of α_{IIb} and/or β_3, either directly or through interactions with other proteins, including signaling molecules (Src, Shc, FAK, paxillin, and ILK, all of which bind to β_3), cytoskeletal proteins kindlin3 (kindlin, skelemin, α-actin, and myosin, which bind to β_3, and filamin and talin, which bind to α_{IIb} and/or β_3), and other proteins (β_3-endonexin and CD98 binding to β_3 and calcium and integrin binding protein [CIB] and calreticulin binding to α_{IIb}) (see Fig. 114–13).[471,502,675,701,705–719] These interactions are important in mediating inside-out signaling and outside-in signaling.[419] Force on the β_3 cytoplasmic domain by actin-myosin action may supply the energy for the conformational change in $\alpha_{IIb}\beta_3$ from bent to extended.[39] The latter was previously termed the ligand-associated metal binding site (LIMBS) based on the crystal structure of $\alpha_V\beta_3$.[662,663]

The junction between the α_{IIb} propeller and the β_3 βA (I-like) domain is the site of ligand binding to $\alpha_{IIb}\beta_3$ (see Fig. 114–14). This region of β_3 contains three divalent cation binding sites: metal ion-dependent adhesion site (MIDAS), adjacent to MIDAS (ADMIDAS), and SyMBS (synergy metal binding site).[39] The latter was previously termed LIMBS based on the crystal structure of $\alpha_V\beta_3$.[662,663]

The crystal structure of $\alpha_V\beta_3$ demonstrated that an RGD peptide bound primarily via interactions between the Arg in the peptide and two Asp residues (D150 and D218) in α_V and between the Asp in the peptide and the MIDAS cation.[663] The binding pocket in $\alpha_{IIb}\beta_3$ is similar but differs in that only one Asp in α_{IIb} (D224) is available to interact with an Arg (or Lys as in the fibrinogen γ-chain peptide), the distance between D224 in α_{IIb} and the MIDAS cation is longer, and a cap subdomain of the α_{IIb} propeller contributes Phe160 to a hydrophobic exosite in combination with Tyr190.[39,657] As a result, the pocket is able to accommodate the longer fibrinogen γ-chain C-terminal peptide better, with the peptide's Asp and C-terminal Val carboxyls interacting with the MIDAS and ADMIDAS cations, respectively.[649] It also explains why $\alpha_{IIb}\beta_3$ can bind peptides containing the longer Lys residue (KGD peptides).[720] Crystal structures are also available for the $\alpha_{IIb}\beta_3$ receptor with the drugs eptifibatide and tirofiban, which are effective antithrombotic agents because of their ability to block ligand binding to $\alpha_{IIb}\beta_3$, and demonstrate specificity for $\alpha_{IIb}\beta_3$ compared to $\alpha_V\beta_3$.[657] The basis of the specificity of these agents involves in part their interaction with the α_{IIb}-specific exosite and the greater length between their positive and negative charges.[657] The third $\alpha_{IIb}\beta_3$ antagonist drug, abciximab, is a chimeric murine monoclonal antibody Fab fragment.[659] Its epitope has been localized to a region on β_3 very close to the MIDAS, suggesting that it works by steric interference with ligand binding, disruption of the binding pocket, or both mechanisms.[659]

Two major conformational changes in $\alpha_{IIb}\beta_3$ have been described in association with activation: headpiece extension and β_3 hybrid and PSI domain swing-out (see Fig. 114–3).[39,657] Headpiece extension can contribute to ligand binding by enhancing access to the binding site; it can also contribute to platelet aggregation by extending the receptor out further from the platelet surface,[721] thus facilitating the ability of fibrinogen to bridge between platelets. The β_3 hybrid and PSI domain swing-out motion appears to enhance ligand binding, but the precise mechanism is unclear.[649] Swing-out is associated with movement of the ADMIDAS metal ion and the α_1-β_1 loop toward the MIDAS and the latter movement allows two backbone nitrogens in the α_1-β_1 loop to interact with a ligand carboxyl oxygen, thus reinforcing the binding to the MIDAS metal ion.[39,649] Mutations that produce swing-out of the hybrid and PSI domains result in constitutive ligand binding to $\alpha_{IIb}\beta_3$.[722]

Binding of fibrinogen to platelet $\alpha_{IIb}\beta_3$ leads to platelet aggregation, presumably via crosslinking of $\alpha_{IIb}\beta_3$ molecules on two different platelets by fibrinogen.[656] The dimeric and relatively rigid structure of fibrinogen, and the location of the binding sites at the ends of the γ chains, are all consistent with such a model as the two binding sites on a single fibrinogen molecule are probably more than 45 nm apart. Soon after fibrinogen binds, it can be dissociated from the platelet by chelating the divalent cations, but the binding becomes irreversible within an hour.[651] Fibrinogen binding alone is insufficient for platelet aggregation, but the events necessary after fibrinogen binding, which probably include ligand- and/or cytoskeletal-mediated receptor clustering, are not well understood.[2,651,723,724] After ligands bind to $\alpha_{IIb}\beta_3$, "outside-in" signaling through $\alpha_{IIb}\beta_3$ can occur, resulting in a number of phosphorylation events, changes in the platelet cytoskeleton, platelet spreading, and even initiation of protein translation.[415,498,725]

In addition to fibrinogen, several other proteins can bind to $\alpha_{IIb}\beta_3$ on activated platelets, including VWF, fibronectin, vitronectin, thrombospondin, and prothrombin[183,615,726]; each of these contains an RGD sequence in the region implicated in the initial interaction with platelets. There are subtle differences in the binding of each of these ligands, however, with regard to divalent cation preference and competent activating agents.[634] The binding of all of these other ligands can also be inhibited by RGD-containing peptides, indicating a common requirement for the interaction between the RGD sequence in the protein and the RGD-binding site in $\alpha_{IIb}\beta_3$.[727,728]

Platelet aggregation measured in the aggregometer *ex vivo* depends upon fibrinogen binding to $\alpha_{IIb}\beta_3$. It is less clear whether fibrinogen is the most important ligand supporting platelet aggregation *in vivo* because studies performed in model systems under flowing conditions indicate that VWF is the major ligand at higher shear rates.[469] Even in the aggregometer, VWF can partially substitute for fibrinogen if the fibrinogen concentration is very low.[729] *In vivo*, mice deficient in both VWF and fibrinogen still make platelet thrombi in response to vascular injury.[171,423,730] Although fibronectin was initially implicated in supporting the development of such thrombi, mice deficient in fibrinogen, VWF, and fibronectin have paradoxically increased platelet aggregation and thrombus formation, suggesting that fibronectin may play an inhibiting role in thrombus formation under certain circumstances.[172]

Although unactivated platelets do not bind soluble fibrinogen (or other adhesive glycoproteins) to an appreciable extent, they can adhere to fibrinogen immobilized on a surface.[392,393] This activation-independent adhesion may be a result of alterations in the structure of fibrinogen when it is immobilized on a surface.[653,731] Alternatively, there may always be a few $\alpha_{IIb}\beta_3$ receptors that are transiently in the proper conformation to bind fibrinogen, and immobilization may result in high local density of fibrinogen and favorable kinetics for adhesion. Finally, it is possible that even low-affinity fibrinogen interactions with $\alpha_{IIb}\beta_3$ are sufficient to initiate $\alpha_{IIb}\beta_3$ interactions with the cytoskeleton such that actin-myosin-induced contraction provides the energy required for the conformational changes needed to achieve higher-affinity binding.[39]

Fibrinogen and/or fibrin have been identified on the surface of damaged blood vessels; thus it is possible that $\alpha_{IIb}\beta_3$ mediates platelet adhesion under those circumstances.[732] In contrast, $\alpha_{IIb}\beta_3$ on unactivated platelets does not appear to be able to mediate adhesion to VWF or fibronectin[393]; if platelets are activated, however, $\alpha_{IIb}\beta_3$ can support adhesion to these glycoproteins.[727] In models of platelet accumulation under flowing conditions, $\alpha_{IIb}\beta_3$ acts in synergy with GPIb/IX, von Willebrand factor, and fibrinogen at the apex of thrombi, where shear forces are greatest.[389,405,411] The $\alpha_{IIb}\beta_3$ integrin has also been implicated in platelet spreading after adhesion,[414,416,491] and it is necessary for clot retraction (see above) and the uptake of plasma fibrinogen into platelet α granules.[169,174]

Less-well-defined roles for $\alpha_{IIb}\beta_3$ have been suggested in the binding of plasminogen,[733] calcium transport across the platelet membrane (see "Calcium" below),[734–736] IgE binding to platelets leading to parasite cytotoxicity,[737] and interactions with the *Borrelia* species spirochetes that cause Lyme disease,[738] *Hantavirus*,[739] and other pathogens.[739a] $\alpha_{IIb}\beta_3$ also mediates factor XIIIa binding to platelets, but this is primarily as a result of factor XIII's association with fibrinogen.[256] XIIIa and calpain have also been implicated in limiting platelet–platelet interactions after activation by adhesion to collagen.[740]

$\alpha_2\beta_1$ (GPIa/IIa; Collagen Receptor; VLA-2; CD49b/CD29) Integrin $\alpha_2\beta_1$ (GPIa/IIa) is widely distributed on different cell types and can mediate adhesion to collagen.[396–398,741–744] The α_2 subunit (GPIa) contains a region of 191 amino acids inserted in the amino-terminal β-propeller region (I domain) that is homologous to similar regions in other proteins that are known to interact with collagen, including VWF and cartilage matrix protein.[745] This region has a MIDAS and crystallographic data of the α_2 I domain in complex with a collagen-related peptide containing the type I collagen sequence GFOGER (where O indicates hydroxyproline) demonstrated that the glutamic acid in the peptide coordinates a Mg^{2+} in the MIDAS.[746–748]

Both $\alpha_2\beta_1$ and GPVI appear to participate in platelet interactions with collagen (see "Collagen: GPVI and $\alpha_2\beta_1$" below).[744,749,750] Bleeding defects have been described in patients with decreased levels of $\alpha_2\beta_1$ and GPVI, but the precise contributions of the decreases in these receptors is uncertain (see Chap. 121). Although $\alpha_2\beta_1$ is capable of supporting adhesion to collagen without exogenous activators, like $\alpha_{IIb}\beta_3$, it appears to be able to increase its affinity for ligand in response to inside-out activation.[751] Potential initiators of $\alpha_2\beta_1$ activation include signaling after GPVI interaction with collagen and GPIb-mediated adhesion to VWF.[746,752,753] Thus, one possible scenario is that following GPIb-mediated adhesion to VWF and collagen adhesion and activation mediated by GPVI, $\alpha_2\beta_1$ may promote firm adhesion to collagen, stabilize thrombus growth on collagen, and promote procoagulant activity.[403,754] In addition, the affinity of $\alpha_2\beta_1$ may also be modulated by alterations in disulfide bonds because inhibition of platelet protein disulfide isomerase and sulfhydryl blocking agents inhibit $\alpha_2\beta_1$-mediated platelet adhesion to type I collagen and to the related peptide GFOGER.[690,755] The state of the collagen may also influence whether $\alpha_2\beta_1$ or GPVI mediates the interaction with collagen, because GPVI appears to mediate adhesion to fibrillar collagen whereas $\alpha_2\beta_1$ preferentially adheres to collagen that has been treated with proteases.[405,406]

Ligand binding to $\alpha_2\beta_1$ is enhanced in the presence of magnesium or manganese and is inhibited by calcium, and thus the conditions in human blood, where calcium is abundant and magnesium is only present at low levels, do not provide optimal cation concentrations for the receptor's function.[397] Integrin $\alpha_2\beta_1$ can, however, mediate platelet adhesion to collagen in heparinized blood.[397,398] Regions of collagen type I have been implicated as potential binding sites for $\alpha_2\beta_1$[756]; the peptide sequence 502 to 516 of collagen type I α_1 chain, which contains a Gly-Glu-Arg (GER) sequence, may be of particular importance,[757] but other regions of the collagen molecule may also be important.[758] In type III collagen, amino acids 522 to 528 of fragment α_1 (III) CB4 contain a binding region for $\alpha_2\beta_1$.[759]

Three different alleles for the α_2 gene, which differ at nucleotides 807 (T or C) and 1648 (G or A), have been described.[349] The 807 substitution does not affect the amino acid sequence, but the 1648 substitution causes a change from Glu to Lys, resulting in the Br^b and Br^a alloantigens (HPA-5a and HPA-5b; see Chap. 138). Allele 1 (T-G) is present in 39 percent of individuals, allele 2 (C-G) in 53 percent, and allele 3 (C-A) in 7 percent.[408,760] Individuals with allele 1 have higher $\alpha_2\beta_1$ platelet density than individuals with allele 2, and individuals with allele 3 have the lowest density. The density of $\alpha_2\beta_1$ correlates with platelet deposition on collagen under flow. The association of these polymorphisms with cardiovascular disease morbidity and mortality, including the risk of developing myocardial infarction[761,762] and stroke,[763] has been extensively studied without firm conclusions, although there is some suggestion that they may be associated with cardiovascular risk.[349,350,764–766]

Integrin $\alpha_2\beta_1$ is probably linked to the membrane skeleton.[767] Its ligand specificity appears to be determined by the cell on which it is expressed, because on endothelial cells it functions as a laminin receptor as well as a collagen receptor.[768,769] Engagement of $\alpha_2\beta_1$ is capable of initiating platelet protein synthesis.[498] $\alpha_2\beta_1$ is implicated in megakaryocyte development and platelet formation from megakaryocytes. In particular, loss of activated $\alpha_2\beta_1$ receptors on the surface of megakaryocytes as a result of interacting with collagen is implicated in the transition from the marrow to the peripheral circulation.[751]

$\alpha_5\beta_1$ (GPIc*/IIa; Fibronectin Receptor; VLA-5; CD49e/CD29) The β_1 integrin $\alpha_5\beta_1$ is a receptor that is expressed on a wide variety of different cells and mediates adhesion to fibronectin.[629,637,638] It is important in interactions with extracellular matrix, and data from cells other than platelets indicate a role for this receptor in developmental biology and metastasis formation. The RGD sequence in fibronectin is crucial for cell adhesion, but other regions in fibronectin probably also contribute.

RGD-containing peptides can inhibit cell adhesion mediated by $\alpha_5\beta_1$. As with other integrin receptors, the adhesion depends on the presence of divalent cations. Integrin $\alpha_5\beta_1$ is competent to mediate adhesion of resting platelets to fibronectin,[770,771] but its affinity may be modulated by activation.[772] The biologic role of this receptor on platelets is not clear. Although it may be involved in hemostasis and/or thrombosis, it is also possible that its function is restricted to megakaryocyte binding to marrow matrix, as it seems to serve this function on other hematopoietic precursors.[773] Integrin $\alpha_5\beta_1$ is not the only fibronectin receptor on platelets, because with appropriate activation, $\alpha_{IIb}\beta_3$ can also bind fibronectin.[183,629]

$\alpha_6\beta_1$ (GPIc/IIa; Laminin Receptor; VLA-6; CD49f/CD29) Platelet adhesion to laminin, which is found in basement membranes and extracellular matrix, can be mediated by the $\alpha_6\beta_1$ integrin receptor.[629,774,775] This adhesion is best demonstrated with magnesium and manganese, calcium does not support adhesion. This receptor is competent on resting platelets, but its role in platelet physiology is not clear. It appears to be able to signal in platelets via PI3-kinase to induce morphologic changes.[776] A 67,000-kDa laminin receptor has also been identified on platelets; this receptor is present on other cells as well.[777]

$\alpha_V\beta_3$ (Vitronectin Receptor; CD51/CD61) The $\alpha_V\beta_3$ receptor shares the same β_3 subunit as $\alpha_{IIb}\beta_3$ (GPIIb/IIIa) (see Fig. 114–3).[628,629,665,778,779] The α_V and α_{IIb} subunits have 36 percent sequence identity.[780] Integrin $\alpha_V\beta_3$ differs dramatically, however, from $\alpha_{IIb}\beta_3$ in its platelet surface density, as there are only approximately 50 to 100 $\alpha_V\beta_3$ receptors per platelet.[781] The crystal structure of the external domains of $\alpha_V\beta_3$ alone and in complex with a peptide containing the RGD cell recognition sequence found in a number of ligands have been solved at high resolution.[662,663] Such RGD peptides inhibit ligand binding to $\alpha_V\beta_3$. The most important findings were: (1) the receptor adopts a bent conformation in which the globular headpiece composed of the N-terminal β-propeller region of α_V and the βA (I-like) domain of β_3, lies near the legs of the α_V and β_3 subunits, and (2) the RGD peptide binds to the headpiece with the Arg (R) making contact with α_V and the Asp (D) making contact with the MIDAS domain in β_3. Current evidence suggests that the bent conformation is the inactive one and that activation results in extension of the headpiece and pivoting between the β_3 βA and hybrid domains in association with leg separation.[657,658,778,779] The $\alpha_V\beta_3$ receptor can mediate adhesion to vitronectin, but only in the presence of magnesium or manganese, not calcium.[781] It can also mediate interactions with fibrinogen, VWF, prothrombin, and thrombospondin.[184,782–785] Platelet stimulation can activate $\alpha_V\beta_3$, analogous to activation of $\alpha_{IIb}\beta_3$ and $\alpha_2\beta_1$. Activated $\alpha_V\beta_3$ may uniquely mediate adhesion to osteopontin, a protein found in high concentrations in atherosclerotic plaque.[786] The receptor's role in platelet physiology is not defined, but it may contribute to the development of platelet coagulant activity.[590]

The $\alpha_V\beta_3$ receptor is also present on endothelial cells,[640,784] osteoclasts,[787] smooth muscle cells, and other cells; it has been implicated in bone resorption,[788–790] endothelial–matrix interactions,[640,784] lymphoid cell apoptosis,[791] neovascularization,[792] tumor angiogenesis,[792–794] and intimal hyperplasia after vascular injury.[795–797]

The presence or absence of $\alpha_V\beta_3$ on the platelets of patients with Glanzmann thrombasthenia can help localize the abnormality to either α_{IIb} (if $\alpha_V\beta_3$ is present in normal or increased amounts) or β_3 (if $\alpha_V\beta_3$ is reduced or absent) (see Chap. 121).

Leucine-Rich Repeat Glycoprotein Receptors

GPIb/GPIX/V (CD42) GPIb is composed of GPIbα (CD42b) (610 amino acids) disulfide-bonded to GPIbβ (CD42c) (122 amino acids).[374,383,625,798–801] GPIb appears to exist on the surface of platelets in a 1:1 complex with GPIX (160 amino acids) and a 2:1 complex with GPV (Fig. 114–15). The GPIbα gene is on the short arm of chromosome 17 and the GPIbβ gene is on the long arm of chromosome 22. The GPIX gene is on the long arm of chromosome 3.[802–804] GPIX is required for efficient surface expression of GPIb,[805] but beyond that, its function is unknown. GPIb/IX is expressed on megakaryocytes and platelets; there is controversy as to whether GPIb/IX is expressed on endothelial cells, either constitutively or after cytokine activation.[626,806–812] The promoters for GPIb/IX lack TATA or CAAT boxes, but contain binding sites for the GATA and ETS families of transcription factors, which, along with the expression of the cofactor FOG (friend of GATA-1), may account for the limited expression of GPIb/IX.[813–821]

A genetic polymorphism in GPIbα affects the number of repeating 13-amino-acid units (1, 2, 3, or 4) and produces changes in the molecular weight of GPIbα.[822] The two-repeat variant is most common, but there is considerable ethnic variation in the frequency of the different numbers of repeats. This molecular weight polymorphism has been linked to the Sib and Ko alloantigens, which have been localized to a T→M variation at amino acid 145 of GPIbα, with M associated with either three or four repeats and T associated with either one or two repeats (see Chap. 138).[760] Some, but not all reports suggest an association between the alleles with the larger number of repeats and vascular disease.[349,350,760,823–825] Two other GPIbα polymorphisms have been described: (1) C or T at position –5 from the ATG start codon (RS system), and (2) a nucleotide dimorphism at the third bases of the codon for Arg 358.[799,826,827] A C at position –5 is present in only 8 to 17 percent of individuals, and more closely resembles the sequence surrounding the ATG start codon (Kozak sequence) considered optimal for translation. In fact, this polymorphism is associated with higher levels of platelet surface GPIb, and may be a risk factor for ischemic vascular disease.[828–836] GPIb has been implicated as a target antigen in autoimmune thrombocytopenia and in quinine and quinidine-induced thrombocytopenia (see Chap. 119).

GPIbα has a large number of *O*-linked carbohydrate chains terminating in sialic acid residues,[837] and the latter contribute significantly to the negative charge of the platelet membrane.[3] Electron micrographic analysis indicates that GPIb exists as a long flexible rod (~60 nm) with two globular domains of approximately 9 and 16 nm.[838] Thus, GPIb probably extends much further out from the platelet's surface than does $\alpha_{IIb}\beta_3$, which may account for its primacy in platelet adhesion, as well as the increased risk of cardiovascular disease in individuals with longer GPIb molecules because of an increased number of 13-amino-acid repeats. The long extension may also make it susceptible to conformational changes induced by shear forces.[625] The extracellular region of GPIbα is readily cleaved by a variety of proteases, including platelet calpains and ADAM17 (tumor necrosis factor-a converting enzyme; TACE),[839,839a] yielding a soluble fragment named *glycocalicin* that circulates in normal plasma at 1 to 3 mcg/mL.[840] It is likely that ADAM17 TACE is primarily responsible for the production of glycocalicin *in vivo* since mice with defects in TACE have markedly reduced levels of glycocalicin.[839a] Levels of plasma glycocalicin correlate with platelet production and thus has been used to differentiate thrombocytopenia as a result of decreased platelet production from thrombocytopenia caused by increased platelet destruction.[841–847]ADAM17 may also contribute to activation-dependent proteolytic shedding of GPV.[847a]

GPIbβ and GPIX have free sulfhydryl groups in their cytoplasmic domains that undergo palmitoylation, at least in part, further anchoring the protein to the membrane.[848,849] The penultimate serine residue at the C-terminus of GPIbα is phosphorylated, providing an attachment site for the signal-complex protein 14-3-3ζ.[850] Similarly, GPIbβ can undergo phosphorylation of Ser 166 in its cytoplasmic domain as a result of protein kinase A activation via cAMP, providing another

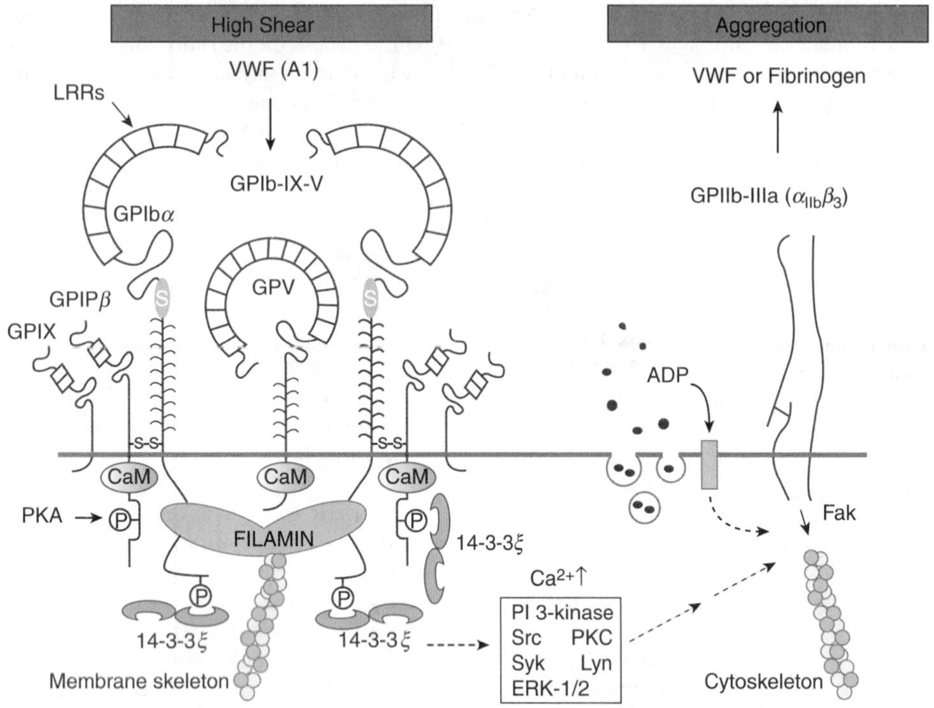

FIGURE 114–15. Schematic of the GPIb/IX/V complex and associated proteins. The complex consists of four polypeptide chains, each of which is encoded by its own gene. The arrangement is hypothetical but is based on the stoichiometry of two copies each of GPIbα, GPIbβ, and GPIX for every copy of GPV, and the demonstration that GPV associates predominantly with GPIbα. The N-terminal region of GPIbα, composed of leucine-rich repeats (LRRs) can bind a number of different ligands, with von Willebrand factor (VWF; via its A1 domain) and thrombin the best characterized and most established as important in platelet physiology. The mucin-like region is very rich in carbohydrate and provides GPIbα with an extended conformation, making it the receptor that probably extends furthest from the surface of the platelet. Thrombin can cleave GPV. A variety of proteins, particularly calpain, can cleave GPIbα near its insertion into the membrane. The cleavage product glycocalicin circulates in plasma. In the cytoplasmic domain, the complex associates with several proteins, including 14-3-3ζ, calmodulin (CaM), and filamin (actin-binding protein). It is through the association with the latter protein that the complex is linked to a submembrane structure of short actin filaments known as the platelet membrane skeleton (see Fig. 114–2). Phosphorylation of GPIbα and β by protein kinase A (PKA) may control the association with 14-3-3ζ. The Fc receptor γ-chain (FcRα chain) probably also is associated with the complex, although the stoichiometry is not established, and may participate in signaling. A number of intermediate signaling molecules and ADP may participate in activating the $\alpha_{IIb}\beta_3$ receptor after VWF binding to GPIb/IX/V. *(Reproduced with permission from Andrews RK, Gardiner EE, Shen Y, et al.[1572])*

binding site for 14-3-3ζ (see Fig. 114–15).[851–853] The cytoplasmic domain of GPIbα connects GPIb to filamin A (actin binding protein), thus connecting GPIb to the platelet cytoskeleton.[376,767,854] Alterations in the cytoskeleton can affect GPIb functional activity.[855–857] GPIbα associates with 14-3-3ζ, which can bind PI3-kinase and has been implicated in GPIb-mediated intracellular signaling that results in $\alpha_{IIb}\beta_3$ activation.[376,858,858a] GPIb also appears to be in close proximity to FcγRIIA and the Fc receptor γ-chain, two receptors that can initiate signaling via tyrosine phosphorylation of their cytoplasmic immunoreceptor tyrosine-based activation motif (ITAM) sequences by Src family kinases and recruitment of the tyrosine kinase syk.[859–862]

GPIbα has eight leucine-rich repeats in the amino-terminal region of its extracellular domain, whereas GPIbβ and GPIX have one each.[374,798,804] These repeats are consensus sequences of 24 amino acids with 7 regularly spaced leucines; well-defined disulfide loop sequences flank the repeats.[625] Similar leucine-rich repeats are present in a variety of other proteins.

The crystal structure of the N-terminus of GPIbα (amino acid residues 1–305) alone, and in complex with the A1 domain of VWF provides important information on the interactions between these proteins (Fig. 114–16). This region of GPIbα adopts a curved shape made up of an N-terminal β-hairpin flanking sequence (finger) containing a C4–C17 disulfide loop (H1–D18), eight leucine-rich repeats (K19–W204), a β-switch region (V227–S241), and a C-terminal sulfated anionic region (D269–D287), with Y276, Y278, and Y279 undergoing posttranslation sulfation.[863–865] The VWF A1 domain interacts with the concave face of GPIbα with two areas of tight interactions, at the N-terminal β-hairpin plus first leucine-rich repeat (with VWF A1 domain loops $\alpha_1\beta_2$, $\beta_3\alpha_2$, and $\alpha_3\beta_4$), and a more extensive interaction at leucine-rich repeats 5 to 8 plus the β-switch region (with VWF A1 domain helix α_3, loop $\alpha_3\beta_4$, and strand β_3). The structure of the VWF A1 domain when not bound to GPIbα differs from that of the bound VWF A1 in that the $\alpha_1\beta_2$ loop protrudes in a way that would prevent interaction with GPIbα.[865] This observation and others related to differences in the ability of different-size fragments of VWF and GPIbα to interact indicate that other regions of both proteins probably contribute to both the binding and activation of the receptor. The crystal structure of GPIbα with the naturally occurring mutation M239V in the β-hairpin region that results in platelet-type (pseudo-) von Willebrand disease (see Chap. 121) has also been obtained[864] and demonstrates a more stable β-hairpin conformation, which probably accounts for the approximately sixfold increase in binding affinity, primarily through an increase in the association rate. Other natural and site-directed mutations causing the platelet-type von Willebrand disease pattern of enhanced VWF binding (G233V, V234G, D235V, K237V) also affect the β-hairpin region. A number of Bernard-Soulier syndrome mutations that cause loss of VWF binding to GPIbα localize to the concave face of leucine-rich repeats 5, 6, and 7 (L129P, A156V, and L179del) and to the sides of leucine-rich repeat 2 (C65R and L57P).[863]

A molecular model for GPIbβ has been proposed based on homology to the Nogo receptor and GPIbα.[866] Four conserved disulfide bonds are predicted (C1–C7, C5–C14, C68–C93, and C70–C116), along with the unpaired C122, which crosslinks to GPIbα. The molecule presents a hydrophobic surface, which was predicted to interact with the hydrophobic face of GPIbα, and a more hydrophilic β sheet face that may participate in VWF binding.

Plasma VWF will not bind to GPIb under static conditions unless the antibiotic ristocetin or the snake venom botrocetin is added. The mechanism by which ristocetin induces VWF binding to GPIb is unclear, but effects on VWF, as well as on platelet surface charge, have been described, and dimerization of ristocetin molecules has also been implicated.[386,625,867,868] Botrocetin initially binds to VWF, exposing the VWF A1 domain, but after the A1 domain makes contact with GPIbα, the botrocetin slides along the A1 domain and makes contact with GPIbα, resulting in a decrease in the off-rate of the reaction.[869,870]

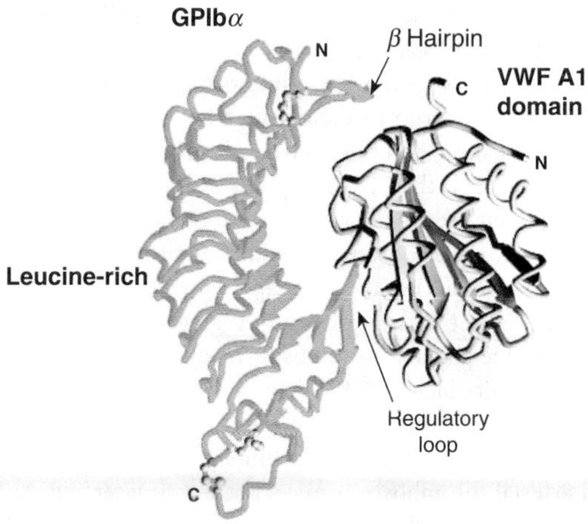

FIGURE 114–16. Structure of the complex between the N-terminus of GPIbα and the A1 domain of von Willebrand factor (VWF). The amino-terminal region of GPIbα folds into a concave surface produced by the leucine rich repeats, and the A1 domain of VWF fits into this structure. Flanking the cysteine-rich repeats in GPIbα are an N-terminal β-hairpin region and a C-terminal regulatory loop. The latter is important in controlling access of the VWF A1 domain to the GPIb binding site. *(Adapted with permission from Dumas JJ, Kumar R, McDonagh T, et al.[865])*

Peptide studies implicate the anionic, sulfated tyrosine region of GPIbα contributes to the binding of botrocetin-treated VWF.[625,870]

Unlike $\alpha_{IIb}\beta_3$, which requires intact, activated platelets to bind to VWF, GPIb-mediated VWF binding does not require platelet activation or even platelet metabolic integrity as fixed platelets are readily agglutinated in the presence of VWF and either ristocetin or botrocetin.[386] This observation forms the basis of the assay of plasma VWF activity (see Chap. 127).

Platelets will adhere to VWF when the latter is immobilized on a surface, even in the absence of ristocetin or botrocetin.[377,386,468,871] Under these circumstances, the VWF is believed to undergo a conformational change that allows for direct interactions. It may not, however, be necessary to propose a change in VWF conformation because the interaction between VWF and GPIb appears to have both high association and dissociation rates, permitting tethering and translocation on a surface coated with a high density of VWF, but minimal interaction in fluid phase.[375] Similarly, VWF associated with fibrin can interact with platelet GPIb without ristocetin or botrocetin.[432,872] The C1C2 domains of VWF appear to contain a fibrin-binding site.[572]

Shear stress is an important factor in GPIb-mediated adhesion of platelets to immobilized VWF and subendothelial surfaces.[374,377,468,871,873,874] Platelets deficient in GPIb or platelets in which GPIb has been blocked with monoclonal antibodies[468,873] adhere poorly to subendothelial surfaces at all shear rates, but the defect in blood from patients with von Willebrand disease is manifest primarily at higher shear rates.[377,378,468] In what may be a related phenomenon, subjecting platelets to high shear stresses can induce platelet aggregation, which is mediated by VWF binding to GPIb, followed by platelet activation and $\alpha_{IIb}\beta_3$-dependent platelet aggregation.[380,382,875] Whether the shear rates generated *in vivo* in stenotic blood vessels are of sufficient magnitude and duration to produce a similar degree of platelet activation is unknown. It is also uncertain as to whether the effect of shear is acting on GPIb, on VWF, or on both,[374,375,382,625] but shear-induced changes in the structure of VWF, leading to a more extended conformation, have been defined.[876] GPIb forms catch bonds with VWF, meaning that increasing force first prolongs and then shortens bond lifetimes.[877]

GPIb also functions as a binding site for thrombin.[625,878,879] The regions between amino acids 216 and 240 and amino acids 269 and 287 were proposed as thrombin-binding sites based on biochemical data, with the latter region demonstrating similarity to hirudin, a thrombin-binding protein.[625,880] Sulfation of the three tyrosine residues in the latter region is particularly important for thrombin binding.[376]

Two somewhat different crystal structures of the interactions between thrombin and the negatively charged tail region of GPIb have been reported, but in both cases two molecules of thrombin bind to each GPIb molecule using different regions on thrombin (exosites I and II).[881–884] This raises the possibility that free thrombin or thrombin adherent to fibrin can cluster GPIb/IX/V complexes.

The functional significance of the binding of thrombin to platelet GPIb is not established, but GPIb has been proposed as the high-affinity binding site for thrombin.[878,885] If true, it appears that not all GPIb molecules serve this function because there are only approximately 50 high-affinity thrombin-binding sites and approximately 25,000 GPIb molecules per platelet.[878,879] One possible explanation is that only the subpopulation of GPIb molecules in lipid rafts are able to function in activating platelets.[15] Platelets lacking GPIb (Bernard-Soulier syndrome) do, in fact, have blunted responses to thrombin (see Chap. 121). One possible model is that binding of thrombin to GPIb facilitates its effect on one or more of the other thrombin receptors, and there is experimental support for this hypothesis.[886,887]

GPIb has also been demonstrated to interact with P-selectin in a cation-independent manner.[376,383,438] Although GPIb shares a number of features with the P-selectin ligand, PSGL-1 (both are sialomucins and have analogous anionic/sulfated tyrosine sequences) the interaction between GPIb and P-selectin appears to be more like the interaction between P-selectin and heparin.[376,383] In inflamed mesenteric venules in animals, platelets are observed to roll on the activated endothelium[888] and so it is possible that platelet GPIb interacts with endothelial P-selectin in this interaction.[376] PSGL-1, a well-documented ligand for P-selectin on leukocytes, has also been identified on the surface of platelets,[439] and may also contribute to this interaction.

GPIbα binds high-molecular-weight kininogen and factor XII, and both of these interfere with thrombin-induced platelet activation.[889,890] Factor XI also binds to GPIbα, where it undergoes activation by thrombin.[891] Activated $\alpha_M\beta_2$, an integrin receptor on leukocytes, also can bind to GPIbα via the I-domain of $\alpha_M\beta_2$,[892] and this interaction has been proposed to play an important role in transmigration of leukocytes through platelet thrombi at sites of vascular injury.

Glycoprotein V, the third member of the GPIb/IX/V complex, has a molecular weight of 82,000 and is composed of 544 amino acids, including 15 leucine-rich repeats.[893–896] GPV appears to form a noncovalent complex with GPIb/IX, but because the number of GPV molecules on the surface of platelets is approximately 50 percent of the number of GPIb and GPIX molecules,[897] it has been suggested that the basic unit consists of two GPIb molecules, two GPIX molecules, and one GPV molecule.[383,625,799] GPV is deficient in platelets from patients with Bernard-Soulier syndrome (see Chap. 121), but GPV is not required for surface expression of the GPIb/IX complex.[898] A soluble fragment of molecular weight 69,000 is cleaved from GPV by thrombin, but cleavage does not correlate with thrombin-induced platelet activation.[899] Platelets from mice lacking GPV appear to respond more actively to thrombin and ADP than wild-type mice, raising the possibility that GPV inhibits platelet activation.[900] The platelets from these mice also adhere to immobilized VWF and can bind VWF in the presence of botrocetin, indicating that GPV is not required for the interaction between VWF and the GPIb/IX/V complex.[900] It has been proposed that removing a portion of GPV by thrombin proteolysis allows thrombin access to GPIbα, thus facilitating its ability to activate platelets. In support of this model, thrombin's ability to activate platelets doesn't require proteolytic activity if GPV is absent, suggesting a direct nonproteolytic effect mediated via GPIbα.[901]

Immunoglobulin Family of Cell Surface Adhesion Receptors and Their Associated Membrane Proteins

PECAM-1 (CD31) PECAM-1 is a transmembrane glycoprotein of the immunoglobulin gene family with six immunoglobulin-like domains of the C2 group and a molecular weight of 130,000.[902,903] In addition to platelets and endothelial cells, it is expressed on monocytes, myeloid cells, and some lymphocyte subsets. There are approximately 8000 PECAM-1 molecules on the surface of platelets.[904] PECAM promotes homophilic interactions via a homophilic-binding domain in the immunoglobin-like repeats. The cytoplasmic tail of PECAM is 118 amino acids in length and contains serine, threonine, and tyrosine phosphorylation sites.

Early studies demonstrated that antibodies that crosslinked PECAM-1 molecules on the platelet surface enhanced platelet adhesion and aggregate formation,[905] suggesting that PECAM-1 might be a costimulatory agonist, working in concert with platelet $\alpha_{IIb}\beta_3$.[905] More recent evidence indicates that PECAM, in fact, is a member of a family of inhibitory receptors, the immunoreceptor tyrosine-based inhibitory motif (ITIM) family. Ig-ITIM proteins contain the XYXXL consensus sequence that, upon phosphorylation, recruits and activates phosphatases, such as SHP-1 and SHP-2,[906] via their SH2 domains. PECAM contains two ITIM domains and appears to negatively regulate collagen-induced platelet activation mediated by the ITAM-bearing GPVI/FcRγ-chain complex and GPIb/IX/V signaling. Platelets from mice lacking PECAM-1 are hyperresponsive to subthreshold doses of collagen, and when compared to wild-type mice, form larger platelet thrombi on VWF and in experimental settings *in vivo*.

In endothelial cells, PECAM-1 is localized to the contact areas between endothelial cells, where it is likely to be involved in controlling transmigration of leukocytes.[907] It appears to be capable of both homotypic and heterotypic adhesive interactions, with the latter perhaps mediated by glycosaminoglycan interactions with a region in the second immunoglobulin domain.[908] An antibody to PECAM-1 decreased neutrophil accumulation and myocardial infarct size in a rat model of ischemia–reperfusion injury.[909]

TREM-Like Transcript-1 TREM-like transcript-1 (TLT-1) is a receptor whose external domain is homologous to those in the family termed triggering receptors express on myeloid cells (TREMs). Like those receptors, it contains a single V-set immunoglobulin domain, but its cytoplasmic domain is much longer and carries a canonical ITIM capable of becoming phosphorylated and binding the Src homology-containing protein, tyrosine phosphate-1 (SHP-1).[910] The phosphatase can then dephosphorylate signaling molecules, leading to inhibition of platelet activation. PECAM-1 has a similar ability to bind SHP-1. TLT-1 appears to be restricted in expression to platelets and megakaryocytes. It is primarily in α-granule membranes in unactivated platelets and joins the plasma membrane when platelets are activated.

GPVI GPVI is an Mr 62,000 transmembrane glycoprotein of 316 amino acids (Fig. 114–17).[395,629,911,912] It belongs to the immunoglobulin superfamily, and is the major platelet signaling receptor for collagen (Fig. 114–17). GPVI on the platelet surface exists in a complex with FcRγ-chain. Because the latter is a dimer, two GPVI molecules associate with one FcRγ-chain, forming a high-affinity complex.[911] The GPVI extracellular region contains two immunoglobulin C2-like domains and its transmembrane domain contains an Arg residue that is essential for association with the FcRγ-chain. The 51-amino-acid cytoplasmic domain contains a proline-rich sequence that binds SH3 (Src homology 3) domains of Src family tyrosine kinases. GPVI signals through the FcR γ-chain, which contains an ITAM. An unpaired thiol in the cytoplasmic tail of GPVI can undergo oxidation after ligand binding, resulting in homodimer formation, and this may be required for signaling.[913] When GPVI binds collagen, the ITAM domain of the FcR γ-chain becomes phosphorylated by the Src kinases Fyn and/or Lyn, resulting in the formation of large complex of signal-transducing proteins.[801,914] (For a discussion of the role of GPVI as a receptor for collagen, see "Signaling Pathways in Platelet Activation and Aggregation" below.) GPVI is required for stable platelet thrombus formation on collagen surfaces *in vitro*. However, mice lacking GPVI have a relatively mild phenotype and are protected from thrombosis in some but not all experimental models. GPVI and FcR γ-chain appear to play important roles in ferric chloride-mediated arterial thrombosis in mice, but not in laser-induced thrombosis, perhaps because the former but not the latter injury elicits collagen exposure along the damaged vessel. Inherited and acquired defects in human platelet GPVI have been reported (see Chap. 121) and the associated bleeding disorders have been variably described as mild to severe.[915] Two alternatively spliced forms and several polymorphisms have been identified for GPVI, but their functional relevance has not been clearly established.

Fc Receptor γ-Chain The Fc receptor γ (FcRγ)-chain[916] exists as a homodimer of molecular weight 20,000 that physically and functionally associates with GPVI[917] and GPIb/IX[860] (see Figs. 114–12, 114–14, and 114–17). In mouse platelets, the absence of FcRγ chain results in lack of surface expression of GPVI. The FcRγ-chain, along with FcγRIIA, are the only known platelet proteins with immune-receptor tyrosine-containing activation motifs (ITAMs).[914] Phosphorylation of the ITAM domain serves to recruit proteins with Src homology 2 (SH2) domains, which are essential for collagen-mediated signaling through the GPVI/ FcR γ-chain pathway.[801,914,918] The FcR γ-chain may also contribute to GPIb/IX-mediated intracellular signaling after VWF binding.[383,860,862]

Fcγ Receptor IIA (FcγRIIA; CD32) The FcγRIIA is a low-affinity immunoglobulin receptor of molecular weight 40,000 that is widely distributed on hematopoietic cells.[629] Three different mRNA transcripts (A, B, and C) make similar FcγRIIA molecules[919] and these are preferentially expressed on different cells. FcγRIIA contains an ITAM domain and thus may be important for signaling by its associated proteins, including GPIb and select integrins, as well as through direct stimulation by immune complexes. Crosslinking of FcγRIIA initiates tyrosine phosphorylation, phosphoinositol metabolism, activation of phospholipase C (PLC)γ_2, calcium signaling, and cytoskeletal rearrangements.[746,747] FcγRIIA appears to be in close proximity to the GPIb-IX-V complex,[477] and signal transduction that accompanies VWF binding to GPIb may be mediated at least in part through FcγRIIA.[691,753] FcγRIIA may also be important in mediating integrin $\alpha_{IIb}\beta_3$ outside-in signaling.[920]

The FcγRIIA on platelets may bind immune complexes generated in certain diseases.[921,922] It may also provide a second binding site for antibodies that bind to platelets via their antibody-binding site (see "CD9" below). This second interaction can potentially lead to bridging between platelets, with the antibody binding to an antigen on one platelet and an FcγRIIA receptor on another platelet.[923] It is also possible that antibodies can bind to both an antigen and an FcγRIIA on a single platelet. These interactions can lead to platelet activation through engagement of FcγRIIA, followed by crosslinking of FcγRIIA receptors, which can lead to tyrosine phosphorylation, phosphoinositol metabolism, activation of phospholipase Cγ_2, calcium signaling, and cytoskeletal rearrangements.[924,925] This type of interaction appears to play an important role in heparin-induced thrombocytopenia (see Chap. 119). Cooperation between FcγRIIA and C1q receptor was reported.[926]

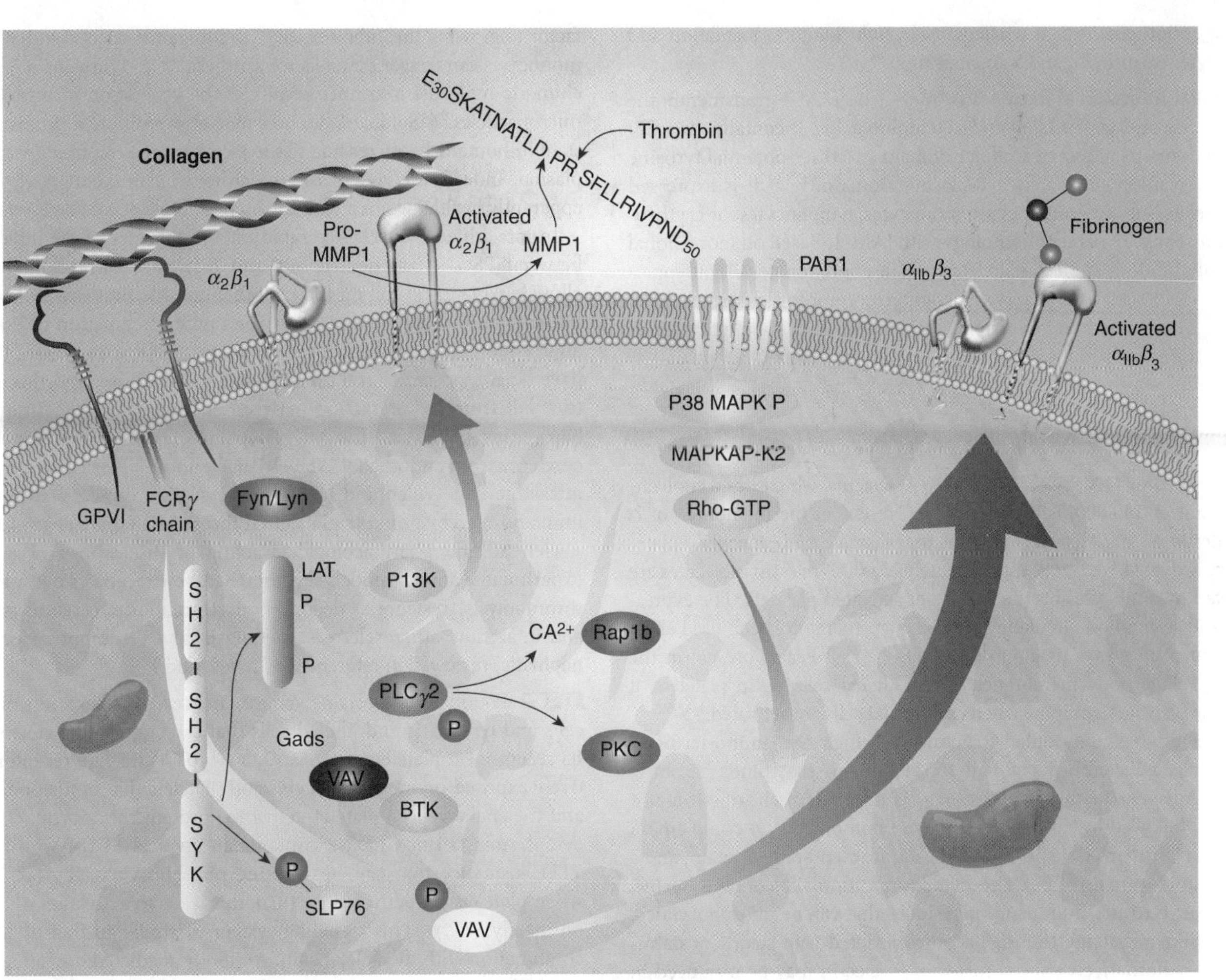

FIGURE 114–17. Collagen and thrombin activation of platelets. The platelet collagen receptor GPVI is physically and functionally coupled to the immunoreceptor tyrosine-based activation motif (ITAM)-containing FcRγ chain. Upon collagen binding to GPVI, GPVI dimerizes as a result of oxidation of intracytoplasmic thiol groups (not shown) and then tyrosine motifs within the FcRγ chain are phosphorylated (P) by the Src family kinases Fyn and/or Lyn. This action initiates a chain of events that includes recruitment of the tyrosine kinase Syk, which is phosphorylated and activated by Fyn and Lyn, and phosphorylation of adaptor proteins LAP and SLP76. A cascade of signaling molecules is formed, including Gads, VAV, Bruton tyrosine kinase (BTK), and PLCγ_2 that results in downstream activation of protein kinase C (PKC) and phosphoinositol-3-kinase (PI3K). Ultimately integrins $\alpha_2\beta_1$ and $\alpha_{IIb}\beta_3$ are converted to a high-affinity ("active") state. Activation of $\alpha_2\beta_1$ promotes firm adhesion to collagen and reinforces intracellular signaling pathways. Pro-matrix metalloproteinase (MMP) 1 is cleaved to active MMP1 following platelet binding to collagen. MMP1 can, in turn, activate the thrombin receptor PAR-1 by cleaving its N-terminal region and creating a tethered ligand that can bind to another region on the molecule. Activation of PAR-1 initiates mitogen-activated protein kinase (MAPK)-mediated and Rho-GTPase-mediated signaling that can reinforce collagen-induced platelet activation. *(Illustration by Matt Hazard, Teaching and Academic Support Center, The University of Kentucky.)*

FcγRIIA expression on platelets shows considerable variation among individuals (~600 to 1500 molecules per platelet), and this variation correlates with FcγRIIA-mediated function.[922] This variation in receptor density may explain individual differences in immune-mediated disorders such as heparin-induced thrombocytopenia with thrombosis.[927] An H131R polymorphism within FcγRIIA affects the binding of different IgG subclasses.[928,929] The H131R polymorphism may also have clinical significance because the R131 allele is associated with increased binding of activation-dependent antibodies to platelets.[930] A variety of associations have been identified between the H131ER polymorphism and different aspects of heparin-induced thrombocytopenia and immune thrombocytopenia, but the data differ from study to study and no consensus has yet emerged.[931–936]

ICAM-2 (CD102) Intracellular adhesion molecule-2 (ICAM-2), a member of the immunoglobulin family of receptors, is an endothelial cell ligand for the β_2-integrin $\alpha_L\beta_2$ (LFA-1) on lymphocytes and myeloid cells.[937] Approximately 2600 ICAM-2 molecules are present on platelets, distributed on the membrane surface and open canalicular system.[937] Platelet ICAM-2 may contribute to platelet-leukocyte interactions (see "Platelet–Leukocyte Interactions, Platelet–Tissue Factor Interactions, and the Role of Platelets in Inflammation and Infection" below).

FcεRI Platelets express the high-affinity IgE receptor FcεRI and appear to participate in both defense against parasitic diseases, including malaria, and allergic phenomena.[938–941]

Junctional Adhesion Molecule-1 (JAM-1; F11) JAM-1 (F11) was identified on platelets by the ability of a monoclonal antibody directed against the receptor to initiate platelet activation via crosslinking to FcγRIIA.[942–946] The protein, a member of the immunoglobulin superfamily, contains two immunoglobulin domains.[946,947] It is capable of mediating platelet activation through several pathways, including association with FcγRIIA.[948] Although its precise role in platelet physiology is unknown, it is able to interact with the $\alpha_L\beta_1$ receptor on leukocytes, and in endothelial cells it participates in tight junction formation and leukocyte recruitment and transmigration.[947]

Junctional Adhesion Molecule-3 (JAM-3) The JAM-3 transmembrane protein has an Mr of 43,000 and 279 amino acids. It contains two C2-type Ig domains in its extracellular domain and three potential tyrosine phosphorylation sites in its cytoplasmic domain.[947,949] It is expressed on platelets but not granulocytes, monocytes, lymphocytes, or erythrocytes. It shares 32 percent homology with JAM-1. Based on monoclonal antibody binding studies, platelets contain approximately 1600 copies of JAM-3. Platelet JAM-3 acts as a counterreceptor for leukocyte $\alpha_M\beta_2$ and $\alpha_X\beta_2$ receptors and contributes to platelet–leukocyte interactions under some conditions.[949] Its precise role in platelet physiology is uncertain.

Lectin-Containing Receptors

P-Selectin (GMP140; PADGEM; CD62P) P-selectin, which has a molecular weight of 140,000, is a glycoprotein present in the membrane of α granules in resting platelets that joins the plasma membrane when platelets are activated.[434–436,950] Approximately 13,000 P-selectin molecules are detected by antibodies on the surface of activated platelets. The expression of P-selectin on circulating platelets has, therefore, been used as an indicator of *in vivo* activation of platelets.[104,634] It is also present in the Weibel-Palade body membranes of endothelial cells; as in platelets, it joins the plasma membrane when endothelial cells are activated.[434,950]

P-selectin has a modular structure in which the amino-terminal region has a calcium-dependent lectin domain that binds carbohydrates. Adjacent to the lectin domain is an epidermal growth factor domain, followed by nine repeats that are homologous to complement regulatory proteins ("sushi" domains), a transmembrane domain, and a cytoplasmic domain.[435,950] The cytoplasmic domain contains serine, threonine, tyrosine, and histidine residues that can be phosphorylated. In addition, a cysteine residue becomes acylated with stearic or palmitic acid. Alternatively spliced forms of P-selectin may be produced in which sushi domains are omitted. The selectin family also includes E-selectin (ELAM-1; CD62E), which is expressed on the surface of activated endothelial cells, and L-selectin (LAM-1; CD62L), which is expressed only on myeloid and lymphoid cells.[951]

Soluble P-selectin is present in plasma from humans and mice. Alternative splicing generates a soluble form of human P-selectin that lacks the transmembrane domain.[952] In mice, at least a portion of soluble P-selectin is derived from proteolytic cleavage of surface P-selectin by an unidentified protease.[953]

Recognition of ligand by P-selectin requires specific carbohydrate and protein structures. Fucose and sialic acid are important carbohydrate components, with sialyl-3-fucosyl-*N*-acetyllactosamine (sLe^x [sialyl Lewis X]; CD15S) a preferred ligand structure.[954–957] Myeloid and tumor cell sulfatides may also act as ligands for P-selectin.[958,959] P-selectin glycoprotein ligand-1 (PSGL-1), a mucin-like transmembrane glycoprotein homodimer (molecular weight 220,000) expressed on neutrophils, monocytes, lymphocytes, and to a small extent on platelets is an important ligand for P-selectin.[439,960–962] Both sulfation of tyrosine residues contained in an anionic region and branched fucosylation of *O*-linked carbohydrates are required for optimal binding to P-selectin.

P-selectin can mediate the attachment of neutrophils and monocytes to platelets and endothelial cells. Thus, neutrophils and monocytes may be recruited to sites of vascular injury where platelets deposit and become activated (see "Platelet–Leukocyte Interactions, Platelet–Tissue Factor Interactions, and the Role of Platelets in Inflammation and Infection" below). Platelet P-selectin can also recruit procoagulant monocyte-derived microparticles containing both PSGL-1 and tissue factor to growing thrombi *in vivo*.[963] Binding of P-selectin to PSGL-1 on monocytes can trigger tissue factor synthesis[964] and infusing a P-selectin chimeric molecule into mice results in the generation of procoagulant microparticles.[965] Soluble P-selectin may also promote a prothrombotic state in humans by increasing tissue factor-expressing microparticles in plasma. Indeed, the risk of future cardiovascular events is elevated in apparently healthy women with the highest levels of soluble P-selectin.[966]

In intact blood vessels, the rapid on and off rates of the interactions between PSGL-1 on neutrophils and P-selectin on endothelial cells allow leukocytes to roll on the endothelium, the first step in leukocyte transmigration (see Chap. 66).[967] The rapid upregulation of P-selectin after endothelial cell activation allows for a quick response. Platelets have been reported to roll on activated endothelium, and this appears to result from an interaction between endothelial P-selectin and perhaps either platelet GPIbα[376,888] or platelet PSGL-1.[437,439] Upon their corelease from endothelial Weibel-Palade bodies, P-selectin may tether ultralarge von Willebrand factor to the surface of activated endothelium and thereby promote platelet GPIbα-mediated platelet rolling.[968]

Genetic and pharmacologic targeting of P-selectin or PSGL-1 in experimental animal models suggests that these receptors may modulate thrombolysis, restenosis, deep venous thrombosis, cerebral ischemia and infarction, atherosclerosis, metastasis, and thrombotic glomerulonephritis (reviewed in references 372, 969, and 970).

CLEC-2 Podoplanin is a sialoglycoprotein present on a variety of tumor cells and lymphatic endothelial cells that can aggregate platelets.[971–973] Its receptor on platelets is CLEC-2, a c-type lectin-like receptor selectively exposed on megakaryocytes and platelets that binds podoplanin and the snake venom platelet-activating protein rhodocytin.[974,975] The cytoplasmic tail of CLEC-2 contains an atypical ITAM with a single YITL sequence that can be tyrosine phosphorylated by Src kinases when platelets are activated. In turn, this leads to activation of Syk and ultimately PLCγ_2. This signaling system is similar to that of GPVI in combination with the FcRγ-chain. Antibody-mediated down regulation of CLEC-2 on mouse platelets results in decreased platelet aggregation, prolonged bleeding time, and protection from experimental thrombosis.[975a] In experimental tumor models, inhibiting the podoplanin/CLEC-2 system reduces metastases. A role for platelets in lymphatic development has been postulated but no direct data yet bear on this hypothesis. HIV-1 can also bind to CLEC-2. A search for an endogenous vascular ligand for CLEC-2 is ongoing.

Tetraspanins

Tetraspanins are a family of four-transmembrane-domain-containing proteins that have conserved cysteine residues that form crucial disulfide bonds. The extracellular and intracellular loops in these proteins contain many motifs known to mediate interactions with other proteins.[976] Although the specific function(s) of tetraspanins is yet unclear, these proteins are able to associate with several membrane proteins and have been reported to modulate integrin function. Oligomers of tetraspanins are known to facilitate the formation of larger complexes of membrane proteins that could serve as scaffolds for several platelet signaling events.[977] CD9 is the most abundant platelet tetraspanin (~40,000 molecules per platelet), followed by CD151, Tspan9, and CD63.[978] The levels of TSSC6 are not known.

CD9 (5H9; BA2; P24; GIG2; MIC3; MRP-1; BTCC-1; DRAP-27; TSPAN29) CD9 is a 228-amino-acid tetraspanin that is present on platelets endothelial cells, smooth muscle cells, cultured fibroblasts, some lymphoblasts, eosinophils, basophils, and other cells.[979–981] It colocalizes with $\alpha_{IIb}\beta_3$ on the inner surface of α granules in resting platelets and on pseudopods of activated platelets.[982] Binding of monoclonal antibodies specific for CD9 to platelets results in platelet aggregation by triggering phosphatidylinositol metabolism via a mechanism that also requires binding to the platelet FcγRIIA receptor.[983–985] The platelet activation induced by the binding of such antibodies requires external calcium and results in an association between CD9 and $\alpha_{IIb}\beta_3$.[986]

CD63 (Granulophysin; LAMP-3) CD63 (molecular weight 53,000) appears to be present in both lysosomal and dense granule membranes in platelets.[103,987] CD63 is also present in Weibel-Palade bodies in endothelial cells, the lysosomal membranes of a variety of other cells, as well as the membranes of melanosomes. It appears on the surface membrane when platelets are activated, making it a useful marker for platelet activation.[103,104] CD63 is markedly reduced or absent from the dense granules of patients with Hermansky-Pudlak syndrome,[987] who have oculocutaneous albinism and a defect in platelet dense granules (see Chap. 121). The amino acid sequence of CD63 has been deduced from complementary DNA cloning.[988]

CD151 (GP27; MER2; RAPH; SFA1; PETA-3; TSPAN24) CD151, a glycoprotein of molecular weight 27,000 is present on platelets, endothelial cells, and many other cells.[989–991] Antibodies to CD151, like those to CD9, can initiate platelet aggregation by binding to both CD151and FcγRIIA.[989] The role of CD151 in platelet physiology remains to be firmly established but it may participate with FcγRIIA as a signal transduction complex.[989] CD151 appears to functionally associate with $\alpha_{IIb}\beta_3$ and, in mice, loss of CD151 impairs platelet aggregation and clot retractions.[992]

TSSC6 (PHMX; PHEMX FLJ17158; FLJ97586; MGC22455; TSPAN32) TSSC6 is a 340-amino-acid tetraspanin that is expressed in marrow, spleen, thymus, and several hematopoietic cell types.[993] It is present in platelets and has been reported to interact with $\alpha_{IIb}\beta_3$. Mice deficient in TSSC6 show a slightly prolonged bleeding time and a significantly increased rebleeding.[977] Platelets lacking TSSC6 show impaired aggregation and clot retraction.

Glycosyl Phosphatidylinositol-Anchored Proteins (CD55; CD59; CD109; Prion Protein)

At least five separate platelet proteins are attached to the membrane through a glycosyl phosphatidylinositol (GPI) link. These include proteins involved in complement regulation (CD55, decay accelerating factor, and CD59, membrane inhibitor of reactive lysis)[994]; CD109, a molecular weight 170,000 protein that carries both ABO oligosaccharides and an alloantigen (Gov) involved in neonatal isoimmune thrombocytopenia[995]; and a molecular weight 500,000 protein of unknown identity. Patients with paroxysmal nocturnal hemoglobinuria have abnormalities in the GPI anchor and thus variably lack all of the GPI-linked proteins. The diagnosis of paroxysmal nocturnal hemoglobinuria can be established by assessing platelet expression of these proteins.[996–998] Patients with paroxysmal nocturnal hemoglobinuria have been reported to have platelet function abnormalities,[996] raising the possibility that one or more of these proteins has a role in platelet function, but no specific platelet function roles have yet been assigned to the proteins. Of particular interest is the presence of the normal prion protein, which is a molecular weight 27,000 to 30,000 GPI-linked protein that is both upregulated and shed from the platelet surface with platelet activation.[999–1002] In fact, platelets contain the majority of the prion protein present in normal blood.

Tyrosine Kinase Receptors

Eph Kinases and Ephrin Ligands Eph-kinase receptors comprise the largest family of cell surface-associated tyrosine kinases with 14 members identified in mammals. Eph kinases have a conserved structure consisting of an N-terminal extracellular ephrin-binding domain, two fibronectin type II repeats, and intracellular kinase, sterile α motif (SAM), and PDZ binding domains. A total of eight ephrins have been identified that serve as cell surface ligands for the Eph kinases. In general, Eph A kinases recognize ephrins that contain a GPI anchor (ephrin A family), whereas Eph B kinases bind to ligands with a transmembrane domain (ephrin B family). The Eph receptors and the ephrins appear to signal bidirectionally at sites of cell-to-cell contact. Platelets contain two Eph kinases, EphA4 and EphB1, and ephrin B1.[1003] Messenger RNA for ephrinA3 has also been detected in platelets, but confirmation of the presence of ephrinA3 protein in platelets is lacking. Forced clustering of either Eph kinases or ephrins in platelets promotes cytoskeletal reorganization, adhesion, granule secretion, and Rap1b activation in concert with other platelet stimuli.[1003,1004] Eph kinase–ephrin interactions may stabilize platelet aggregates and thrombus formation after platelet–platelet contact has occurred.[1005]

Thrombopoietin Receptor (c-mpl; CD110) The thrombopoietin receptor (c-mpl; molecular weight 80–84,000) is expressed at low levels on platelets (~25–224 per platelet) and binds thrombopoietin with high affinity (Kd ~0.50 nM).[1006–1009] Steady-state plasma levels of thrombopoietin are in part maintained by platelets and megakaryocytes, which bind thrombopoietin via the thrombopoietin receptor and then internalize and degrade the growth factor. Although its major functions are to support the survival and expansion of hematopoietic stem cells and to stimulate megakaryocyte growth and maturation (see Chap. 113), thrombopoietin also is able to sensitize platelets to activation by agonists.[1010–1015] Mutations of the receptor have been associated with inherited thrombocytopenia (see Chap. 119) and myeloproliferative disorders (see Chaps. 85–87).[1016,1017] It can also contribute to hematopoiesis through effects on other progenitors in other cell lineages.

Scavenger Receptors CD36 (GPIV) CD36 (GPIV) is a molecular weight 88,000 glycoprotein that is highly, but variably, expressed on platelets (~20,000 copies per platelet).[186,1018–1022] The nucleotide sequence of CD36 (GPIV) complementary DNA encodes a protein of 471 residues with a molecular weight of 53,000 and 10 potential N-linked glycosylation sites.[1023] It is unusual in having two putative transmembrane domains and two short cytoplasmic tails. The cytoplasmic regions may associate with intracellular tyrosine kinases of the Src family and undergo phosphorylation.[1024] Antibodies to CD36 (GPIV) have been reported to produce neonatal alloimmune thrombocytopenia (see Chap. 119).[1025] Biochemical data suggest that it may form dimers and multimers.[1026] Increased platelet surface expression of CD36 (GPIV) has been described in patients with myeloproliferative disorders.[1027] CD36 (GPIV) is also expressed on phagocytic cells (with the exception of neutrophils), fat and muscle cells, cardiac myocytes, and microvascular endothelial cells. The phosphorylation status of the extracellular region of the protein may control its ligand-binding properties,[185] offering a potential explanation for some of the variable results obtained under different conditions.[185,186,1028]

CD36 (GPIV) plays an important role in long-chain fatty acid transport in the heart, fat, and muscle, and may contribute to atherosclerosis and insulin sensitivity.[1029,1030] Oxidized low-density lipoproteins (LDLs), which can be produced by the effects of endothelial cell or platelet NO on LDLs, bind to CD36 (GPIV) and, perhaps in concert with scavenger receptor-A, can increase platelet reactivity to agonists via signal transduction mediated in part by Src kinases and a mitogen-activated protein kinase.[1031–1033] The variability in platelet CD36 (GPIV) expression may account for the variability in platelet hyperreactivity in response to elevated levels of oxidized LDLs. CD36 (GPIV) can also mediate microparticle binding to platelets, which augments platelet-mediated thrombosis in model systems.[1034] Thus, CD36 (GPIV) has been reported to contribute to atherogenesis, diabetes, the metabolic syndrome, angiogenesis, and inflammation.[1035–1038] It has been proposed as a platelet receptor for thrombospondin[1039] and collagen,[1040,1041] but the functional significance of these interactions remains unclear because individuals who lack CD36 (GPIV) on an inherited basis (Nak^a-negative) do not have a bleeding disorder (see Chap. 121).[1042] CD36 (GPIV) may play a role in the thrombospondin-mediated interaction reported between platelets and sickle erythrocytes,[1043] apoptosis, innate immunity, and in the binding of *Plasmodium falciparum*–infected erythrocytes to endothelial cells and monocytes.[1021,1023]

Scavenger Receptor-BI (CLA-I) The class B scavenger receptor (SR)-BI (CLA-I) is related to CD36 (GPIV) and is expressed on platelets, endothelial cells, and hepatocytes.[1022] It transports the cholesteryl esters from high-density lipoprotein cholesterol and facilitates bidirectional flux of free cholesterol between cells and lipoproteins. Oxidized, but not unoxidized, high-density lipoprotein can inhibit platelet aggregation via binding to SR-BI.[1044] SR-BI has many other lipid ligands, however, and it is uncertain how these interact under physiologic conditions.

Miscellaneous

CD40 Ligand (CD40L; CD154) and CD40 CD40 ligand (CD40L; CD154) is a trimeric transmembrane protein (molecular weight 33,000) of the tumor-necrosis factor family (TNF) that localizes to α granules in resting platelets and rapidly appears on the surface of platelets upon activation. Within minutes to hours of platelet activation, an 18,000-dalton fragment of CD40L is released from the platelet surface, perhaps mediated in part by matrix metalloproteinase (MMP-2) bound to $\alpha_{IIb}\beta_3$.[1045] This soluble form of CD40L circulates as a trimer. The bulk of soluble CD40L in plasma is derived from activated platelets and, hence, can serve as a marker for platelet activation *in vivo*. Elevated levels of soluble CD40L are observed in acute coronary syndromes, following percutaneous coronary intervention, in the setting of coronary artery bypass surgery, and in peripheral vascular disease[443] (reviewed in references 444 and 1046). Moreover, elevated levels of soluble CD40L are associated with recurrent cardiovascular events in the setting of acute coronary syndromes[443,1047] and restenosis following percutaneous coronary intervention.[446] CD40L and, to a lesser extent its counterreceptor CD40, have been implicated in the progression of atherosclerosis in animal models.

The extracellular portion of CD40L binds to CD40 a molecular weight 48,000 transmembrane receptor. Approximately 600 to 1000 copies of CD40 are present on both resting and activated platelets,[445] and while CD40L has been reported to initiate platelet activation via binding to CD40,[1048] the functional significance of CD40–CD40L interactions in platelet physiology remains to be determined. CD40L also contains a KGD sequence (RGD in mice) that has been implicated in binding to $\alpha_{IIb}\beta_3$. In mice, CD40L–$\alpha_{IIb}\beta_3$ interactions appear to stabilize thrombus growth,[445] perhaps by activating receptor-mediated signaling.[441] Additionally, $\alpha_{IIb}\beta_3$ antagonists block the release of soluble CD40L from activated platelets. Both platelet-associated and soluble CD40L may stimulate leukocytes to release proinflammatory cytokines; CD40L may also inhibit endothelial cell migration after vascular injury.[1049] The inhibitory affects of CD40L on reendothelialization may partially explain why elevated levels of soluble CD40L are associated with higher rates of clinical restenosis.[446] Finally, platelet CD40L may modulate adaptive immunity by serving as a costimulatory signal for antigen presenting cells.[1050,1051]

Fas Ligand, LIGHT, and TRAIL Fas ligand (FasL), LIGHT (homologous to *l*ymphotoxins, exhibits *i*nducible expression, and competes with herpes simplex virus *g*lycoprotein D for *h*erpes virus entry mediator, a receptor expressed by *T* lymphocytes), and TNF-related apoptosis-inducing ligand (TRAIL), along with CD40L, belong to the TNF family of cytokines.[1052] With activation, platelets express FasL, LIGHT, and TRAIL on their surface and release soluble forms of these receptors,[1052–1054] analogous to activation-dependent CD40L platelet expression and release. The receptor Fas (Apo-1, CD95), is expressed on a wide variety of normal and malignant cells. Engagement of Fas by FasL initiates signaling that results in apoptosis, and this process is important in embryonic development, cellular hemostasis, and immune regulation.[1052] The surface-expressed FasL on platelets is biologically active and can initiate apoptosis. The soluble form of FasL may act as an inhibitor of apoptosis induced by surface-expressed FasL.[1052] Similarly, platelet-derived LIGHT is biologically active and can initiate inflammatory responses in monocytes and endothelial cells.[1054]

LAMP-1 and LAMP-2 (CD107a, CD107b) LAMP-1 and LAMP-2 are lysosome-associated membrane proteins that are approximately 30 percent homologous. They are integral membrane glycoproteins of molecular weights 110,000 and 120,000, respectively, that are contained within lysosomal membranes.[1055] When platelets undergo the release reaction, they join the plasma membrane. Each protein has two extracellular disulfide-bonded loops containing 36 to 38 amino acids. The loops are separated by a region rich in proline and serine that shares homology with the hinge region of IgA. There are multiple N-linked glycosylation sites on each glycoprotein and they contain more than 60 percent carbohydrate. Among the carbohydrate residues are polylactosaminoglycans that may possess sialylated Lewis^x structures, which are thought to interact with selectins (see "Lectin-Containing Receptors" above).

C1q Receptors Platelets have several receptors for C1q, a molecular weight 460,000 glycoprotein composed of six globular domains attached to a short collagen-like triple helix.[1056–1058] One is for the collagen-like domain (cC1qR, molecular weight 60,000–67,000 nonreduced and 72,000–75,000 reduced), and another is for the globular domain (gC1qR, molecular weight 28,000–33,000).[1059,1060] A third receptor of molecular weight 126,000 enhances phagocytosis.[1061] C1q circulates with C1r and C1s as a calcium-dependent complex, but interaction with immune complexes leads ultimately to dissociation of the complex and release of free C1q, with its collagen-like domain exposed. cC1qR has sequence homology to calreticulin and can modulate platelet–collagen interactions at low collagen concentrations. It may also localize immune complexes, and when crosslinked by aggregated C1q, it can initiate platelet activation, aggregation, secretion, and expression of platelet coagulant activity.[1062] Thus, the binding of C1q monomers to platelets inhibits collagen-induced platelet aggregation but has little effect on platelet adhesion to collagen.[1063] C1q multimers support platelet adhesion and can induce aggregation via activation of $\alpha_{IIb}\beta_3$.[1062] C1q can also augment platelet aggregation induced by aggregated IgG.[926] The gC1qR may self associate to form a doughnut-shaped ternary complex.[1064] In addition to binding C1q, this receptor can bind *Staphylococcus aureus* protein A on endothelial cells, where it functions as a receptor for high-molecular-weight kininogen.[1060] It may, therefore, participate in contact activation.

GMP-33 (Thrombospondin N-Terminal Fragment) A molecular weight 33,000 α-granule membrane protein was initially identified as an activation-dependent protein that joins the plasma membrane when platelets undergo the release reaction. Approximately 4000 antibody molecules directed against GMP-33 bind to unactivated platelets, and 19,000 bind to activated platelets.[1065] Subsequent studies identified this antigen as a membrane-associated fragment from the N-terminal of thrombospondin.[1066]

Leukosialin, Sialophorin (CD43) Leukosialin, a glycoprotein of molecular weight 90,000, may act as a ligand for ICAM-1.[1067] It is expressed on myeloid and some lymphoid cells. Abnormalities in leukosialin have been described in Wiskott-Aldrich syndrome (see Chap. 121).

Toll-Like Receptors 1, 2, 4, and 6 Toll-like receptors (TLRs) are involved in innate immunity by virtue of their ability to sense products of protozoa, fungi, viruses, and bacteria, including endotoxin (lipopolysaccharide [LPS]), and then activate intracellular signaling pathways to initiate the inflammatory response.[1068] TLRs 1, 2, 4, and 6 have been identified in platelets and in platelet-rich coronary thrombi. TLR-2 has been implicated in detecting the anchor motif of bacterial lipoproteins, and it has been proposed that a complex of vitronectin, TLR-2, and β3-containing integrins may participate in the recognition process.[1068a] All of the components of the LPS signaling complex, including relatively high levels of TLR-4[1069] and CD14, MD2, and MyD88 (myeloid differentiation factor 88), have been identified in platelets.[1070] LPS binding to platelets stimulates secretion and potentiates agonist activation by signaling through the TLR-4 complex.[1070] LPS binding to platelet TLR-4 causes release of CD40L[1071] and modulates the release of cytokines by platelets.[1072,1073] In experimental animal models, TLR-4 may mediate LPS-induced thrombocytopenia.[1069] The interactions of LPS, produced by Gram-negative bacteria including toxigenic *Escherichia coli*, with platelet TLR-4 has been proposed to contribute to the pathophysiology of hemolytic uremic syndrome (see Chap. 119).[1071] Ligand binding to platelet TLR-4 also promotes platelet–neutrophil interactions, neutrophil activation, and the formation of neutrophil extracellular traps, which capture and sequester bacteria from the circulation.[1074]

Peroxisome Proliferator-Activated Receptors Peroxisome proliferator-activated receptors (PPARs) belong to a nuclear hormone receptor family of ligand-activated transcription factors.[1075] PPARγ is one of the three PPAR family members and is widely expressed in white adipose tissue, macrophages, B and T lymphocytes, smooth muscle cells, fibroblasts, and endothelial cells. It has been implicated in metabolism, insulin responsiveness, adipocyte differentiation, immune function, and inflammation. The thiazolidinedione class of insulin-sensitizing drugs used to treat type 2 diabetic patients act by binding PPARγ. Both PPARβ/δ and PPARγ are present in platelets. PPARγ agonists decrease thrombin-induced platelet aggregation and release of ATP, thromboxane, and CD40L.[1075] Thus, PPARγ appears to downregulate platelet activation. Activated platelets release PPARγ complexed with the retinoid X receptor.[1076] Treatment with select thiazolidinediones is associated with reductions in markers of platelet activation, including aggregation and P-selectin expression. PPARβ ligands synergize with NO to inhibit platelet function.[1077,1078]

Matrix Metalloproteinases Platelets contain a number of MMPs, as well as MMP activators and inhibitors.[1079] MMP-1 can be activated by collagen and, in turn, cleave PAR-1 at a site two amino acids N-terminal to the site of thrombin cleavage.[1080] This cleavage, like thrombin's, activates PAR-1 by activating a tethered ligand. Thus, MMP-1 can augment collagen-induced platelet activation mediated by GPVI and $\alpha_2\beta_1$. MMP-2 has been implicated in enhancing platelet aggregation. It exists in an inactive form in resting platelets and it is cleaved into its active form when platelets are activated, probably by MTI-MMP.[1045] It then moves to the surface via binding to $\alpha_{IIb}\beta_3$ and may then go on to cleave CD40 ligand. Other related proteins in platelets include MMP-1, 3, 9, and 14, ADAM-10 and 17, and TIMP 1, 2, and 3. Platelets also contain ADAMTS-13, which cleaves VWF, thus controlling hemostasis and thrombosis (see Chap. 127).

PLATELETS AND THROMBOLYSIS

The interactions between platelets and the fibrinolytic system are complex, and Table 114–9 contains a partial listing of reported findings.[1081–1085] Both profibrinolytic[196,733,1086–1092] and antifibrinolytic[1093–1101] effects of platelets have been described, and so it is difficult to predict the net effect. Because platelet-rich thrombi are known to resist thrombolysis in animal models, the antifibrinolytic effects of platelets appear to predominate *in vivo*.[1102]

TABLE 114–9. Platelets and Thrombolysis

Profibrinolytic effects of platelets
Tissue-type plasminogen activator (t-PA) and single-chain urokinase-type t-PA identified on or in platelets.
Unactivated platelets bind plasminogen, and binding is enhanced by thrombin.
Thrombospondin, a plasminogen-binding protein, is expressed on the surface of platelets after activation.
Activation of plasminogen by t-PA is enhanced by platelets.
Clot lysis is enhanced by platelets in some model systems.
Antifibrinolytic effects of platelets
Plasminogen activator inhibitor-1 and α_2-antiplasmin are present in platelet granules.
Platelets release a protein that stimulates cells to release a fibrinolysis inhibitor.
Platelets contain factor XIII, which can crosslink fibrin, making it resist fibrinolysis, and can crosslink α_2-antiplasmin to fibrin, enhancing its antifibrinolytic effects.
Platelet $\alpha_{IIb}\beta_3$ can bind plasma factor XIIIa directly or indirectly, localizing it to the site of thrombus formation.
Platelets facilitate clot retraction, which diminishes the efficiency of fibrinolysis.
Platelet-activating effects of thrombolytic agents
Streptokinase and t-PA activate platelets *in vivo* and *in vitro*.
Plasmin, at high doses, can aggregate platelets.
Thrombolytic agents may paradoxically generate the potent platelet agonist thrombin or release it from thrombi.
Thrombolytic agents may blunt the prostacyclin increase that accompanies acute thrombosis.
Platelet-inhibiting effects of thrombolytic agents
Plasmin, at low doses, can inhibit platelet activation and aggregation.
Platelets can be disaggregated by t-PA by selective lysis of platelet-bound fibrinogen.
Plasmin can cause redistribution and/or cleavage of platelet glycoprotein Ib.
Inhibition of platelet aggregation by the depletion of plasma fibrinogen, if severe, and generation of fibrin(ogen) degradation products.
Proteolysis of plasma von Willebrand factor.
Prolongation of the bleeding time.

SOURCE: Adapted with permission from Coller BS.[355]

The effects of fibrinolytic agents on platelets are similarly complex. For example, there is considerable evidence that fibrinolytic agents can activate platelets soon after administration,[1103–1109] via either a direct effect of plasmin,[1110–1113] perhaps acting on PAR-4[1114] or an indirect effect through the paradoxical generation of thrombin.[1083,1115–1118] Interpretation of the latter studies are complicated by the ability of tissue plasminogen activator to release fibrinopeptides from fibrinogen, one of the biomarkers used to assess thrombin activation.[1119]

Stimulation of platelets by thrombolytic agents may prolong the time required for reperfusion of thrombosed blood vessels and may contribute to reocclusion after successful reperfusion.[355,1081] In animal models and in humans, potent antiplatelet agents can, in fact, speed reperfusion, abolish reocclusion, and diminish the size of myocardial infarcts.[1120–1122] In human studies, the benefits of combining $\alpha_{IIb}\beta_3$ antagonists with fibrinolytic agents in enhancing coronary thrombolysis have been counterbalanced by an increase in major hemorrhage.[1123] Combining a potent $\alpha_{IIb}\beta_3$ antagonist with a reduced dose of a fibrinolytic agent in acute ST-elevation myocardial infarction when patients are rapidly treated with percutaneous coronary intervention has demonstrated evidence for more rapid reperfusion, but clinical benefit has been variable and bleeding has been increased.[1124,1125] In experimental models of stroke, paradoxically, early treatment with $\alpha_{IIb}\beta_3$ antagonists reduces the hemorrhage associated with thrombolytic therapy, perhaps by preventing platelet aggregation in the microcirculation and the release of agents that can damage the vasculature and diminish its integrity.[105,1126,1127] In human studies, however, a potent $\alpha_{IIb}\beta_3$ antagonist given alone did not improve clinical outcomes.[1128,1129]

With prolonged use of thrombolytic agents, inhibition of platelet function can occur via a variety of mechanisms.[299,1106,1109,1130–1140] These effects may contribute to some of the hemorrhagic phenomena and prolonged bleeding times observed with this therapy. One proposed mechanism is that the thrombolytic agents make platelets refractory to further stimulation by agonists.

PLATELET–LEUKOCYTE INTERACTIONS, PLATELET–TISSUE FACTOR INTERACTIONS, AND THE ROLE OF PLATELETS IN INFLAMMATION AND INFECTION

Leukocytes can bind to activated platelets and in model systems transmigrate through a platelet monolayer (reviewed in reference 1141; see Figs. 114–9 to 114–11). Animal models and studies of human tissue demonstrate that within hours after vascular injury, leukocytes become enmeshed in platelet thrombi and/or transiently form a monolayer on top of adherent or aggregated platelets.[1142,1143] These interactions may be important at sites of vascular injury or inflammation where leukocytes have been shown to deposit on adherent and aggregated platelets. Platelet recruitment of leukocytes has been associated with a number of systemic and inflammatory processes in animal models, including the development of intimal hyperplasia after vascular injury,[1144] ischemia–reperfusion injury, alloimmunity-mediated transplant rejection,[1145] obesity,[1146] and acute lung injury.[1147] By depositing chemokines such as RANTES (CCL5) on activated endothelium[1148,1149] or by direct interactions with leukocytes,[1150] platelets may also enhance leukocyte recruitment to inflamed or atherosclerotic endothelium and thereby promote the development and progression of atherosclerosis.

Many mechanisms of platelet–leukocyte interactions have been defined, but the initial interaction appears to be mediated primarily by the interaction between P-selectin (CD62P) expressed on the surface of activated platelets and PSGL-1 on the surface of neutrophils and monocytes.[950,954,1151–1155] P-selectin–PSGL-1 interactions are characterized by rapid on and off rates that promote tethering and rolling of leukocytes along adherent platelets. These transient interactions are stabilized by subsequent contacts mediated, in large part, by activation of leukocyte β_2 integrins. Platelet surface-immobilized and released chemokines promote firm leukocyte adhesion and arrest by acting through G-protein-coupled receptors to activate leukocyte β_2 integrins. Platelets can synthesize and release PAF, which can activate leukocyte $\alpha_M\beta_2$. The CC chemokine RANTES (CCL5) and the CXC chemokines (ENA-78, GRO-α), released by activated platelets can also activate leukocytes. The chemokine neutrophil-activating peptide-2 (NAP-2) can be produced by the action of leukocyte cathepsin G on β-thromboglobulin secreted by platelets (see Fig. 114–7).[137,1156] Activated $\alpha_M\beta_2$ on leukocytes can interact with platelet GPIbα[438] as well as with platelet-bound fibrinogen via a region(s) on the γ chain (amino acids 190–202,[1157] and 377–395[1158]). Thrombospondin may serve as a bridging molecule between CD36 (GPIV) receptors, which are expressed on both platelets and mononuclear cells.[1159] Platelets also have ICAM-2 on their surface, which is a ligand for the leukocyte integrin receptor $\alpha_L\beta_2$; although this ligand–receptor interaction appears to have only a minor role in platelet–leukocyte adhesion, it may be more important in leukocyte tethering.[1156] Platelet JAM-3 has also been suggested as a counterreceptor for leukocyte $\alpha_M\beta_2$.[949]

Transcellular metabolism of eicosanoids can result in production of unique products (see "Prostaglandin H_2/Thromboxane A_2 and Other Arachidonic Acid Metabolites: Thromboxane Prostanoid Receptor" below, Fig. 114–11, and Chap. 117) and leukocytes can modify platelet activation.[1160] In a complementary fashion the intimate relationship between leukocytes and platelets allows the latter to contribute to the inflammatory response, including the release of chemokines that can activate leukocytes; PDGF, which can affect fibroblast and smooth muscle cells; TGF-β_1, which both stimulates and inhibits cellular growth; and PF-4, which can prime neutrophils and has antiangiogenic activity. Platelets synthesize the cytokine IL-1β an important mediator of the inflammatory response.[1161] Platelets also contain FcγIIA receptors that can localize IgG and immune complexes, resulting in complement activation. Platelets also express CD40L on their surface after activation, and this molecule can interact with CD40, a member of the tumor necrosis factor receptor family, on leukocytes and endothelial cells, leading to their activation and their elaboration of a number of proinflammatory molecules (see "CD40 Ligand (CD40L; CD154) and CD40" above).[440,1162,1163] Platelet CD40L also promotes procoagulant activity in endothelial cells.[1164] Finally, platelet–leukocyte interactions can promote the generation of reactive oxygen species, but platelets can also generate signals to stop the production of reactive oxygen species.[1165]

Platelet–leukocyte interactions may be important in the initiation of coagulation and fibrin formation through a P-selectin–dependent pathway. In fact, platelet–leukocyte aggregates facilitate thrombin generation to a greater extent than either platelets or leukocytes alone.[1166,1167] Coincubation of platelets and leukocytes generates tissue factor activity, in part, through P-selectin–PSGL-1 interactions. The induction of tissue factor activity involves both *de novo* protein synthesis and exposure ("deencryption") of latent tissue factor. The latter may occur by P-selectin–mediated production of tissue factor containing microparticles from leukocytes. Real-time imaging of platelet thrombus formation *in vivo* indicates that tissue factor accumulates in growing thrombi before leukocytes become associated with the thrombus. The accumulation of tissue factor and fibrin formation in thrombi depend on both platelet P-selectin and PSGL-1. These observations, coupled with the finding of bloodborne tissue factor antigen in the circulation,[362] has led to a model in which platelet P-selectin recruits tissue factor–containing leukocyte microparticles to platelet-rich thrombi.[363] Neutrophil-derived microparticles express active integrin $\alpha_M\beta_2$, which can interact with platelets by binding to GPIbα. This, in turn, can initiate platelet P-selectin expression, which will enhance the interactions with neutrophil microparticles containing the counterreceptor PSGL-1.[1168] In mice, increases in soluble P-selectin levels promote a procoagulant state associated with elevated levels of leukocyte-derived microparticles,[1169] and a P-selectin–immunoglobulin chimeric molecule can increase levels of leukocyte-derived microparticles *in vitro* and normalize the bleeding time in hemophilia A mice.[965]

Several clinical observations support a potential role for platelet–leukocyte interactions in vascular disease, including the presence of circulating platelet–leukocyte aggregates in patients with unstable angina[1170] and after coronary artery angioplasty[1171]; in the latter situation, the presence of such aggregates appears to confer a worse prognosis for ischemic vascular complications.[1171] Circulating platelet–leukocyte aggregates are perhaps the most sensitive indicator of systemic platelet activation, reflecting the expression of P-selectin on the surface of platelets.[1172] Polymorphisms of PSGL-1 involving variable numbers of tandem repeats demonstrated that the longer PSGL-1 molecules were better able to form platelet–leukocyte aggregates; in some, but not all studies, the longer molecules were associated with increased risk of some forms of thrombotic vascular disease.[1173–1178]

Platelets can contribute to both innate and adaptive immunity in several ways. Bacterial endotoxin binding to toll-like receptors can activate platelets (see "Toll-Like Receptors 1, 2, 4, and 6" above), enhance platelet-neutrophil interactions, and promote bacterial trapping by stimulating the production of neutrophil extracellular traps (NETs) composed of DNA, histones, and enzymes that degrade pathogens.[1074] The production of these traps confers resistance to a variety of pathogens, including Gram-positive (*S. aureus*, *Streptococcus pneumoniae*, and Group A streptococci) and Gram-negative (*Salmonella typhimurium*, *Shigella flexneri*, and *E. coli*) bacteria. Thrombocytopenia is often present in association with bloodborne bacterial infections (sepsis) and the severity of the thrombocytopenia mirrors the severity of the infection. Platelet factor V contributes to resistance to Group A streptococcal infection[620] by promoting thrombin generation and fibrin deposition, which may help to wall off the bacteria.[620] Platelets also influence the function of lymphocytes.[1179] They enhance cytolytic T-cell proliferation and antibody production by B cells. Platelets can inhibit the responses of helper T cells, and via release of TGF-β_1, increase T-regulatory cells. Finally, platelets can bind to malarial-infected erythrocytes and both suppress the growth of the parasites and destroy the intraerythrocytic malarial parasites.[941]

SIGNALING PATHWAYS IN PLATELET ACTIVATION AND AGGREGATION

Overview

Platelets generally circulate in a quiescent state, but are poised to be activated in response to a variety of agonists that become available at sites of vascular injury or ruptured atherosclerotic plaques. Table 114–10 lists a number of different phenomena that occur with platelet activation. Agonists differ in their intrinsic ability to produce these phenomena, and added complexity derives from differences in dose responses to each agonist and the synergistic effects of agonists used in combination. Agonists are diverse (see Table 114–6) and include small and large soluble molecules, enzymes, and immobilized adhesive glycoproteins. They can be classified as either "strong" or "weak," depending on whether full activation, including the release reaction, can be initiated without the augmenting effect of platelet aggregation itself (see Table 114–6). Low doses of strong agonists behave like weak agonists. Most agonists are released, synthesized, or formed at the site of vascular injury and this undoubtedly serves to localize the response.

Agonists bind to receptors of two general categories: seven-transmembrane G-protein-coupled receptors and receptors that can initiate phosphorylation of target proteins (see Figs. 114–5 and 114–12). In both cases, a sequence of signaling events ultimately leads to platelet activation. Table 114–10 lists physiologic responses of platelets to agonists, with all of them leading to the activation of the $\alpha_{IIb}\beta_3$ receptor to a high-affinity ligand-binding state and subsequent platelet aggregation. Moreover, binding of ligands to platelets and platelet aggregation itself further propagates signals that are required for stabilization of the platelet aggregates and clot retraction. In this section, the major agonists, receptors, and signaling pathways involved in early stages of platelet activation that lead to shape change, granule secretion, and platelet aggregation, as well as postaggregation signaling events, are described.

TABLE 114–10. Phenomena Associated with Platelet Activation

Increased platelet cytosolic calcium
Shape change
Change in $\alpha_{IIb}\beta_3$ to high-affinity ligand-binding conformation(s)
Generation of arachidonic acid metabolites (e.g., thromboxane A_2)
Phosphorylation of select platelet proteins
Platelet aggregation
Induction of platelet coagulant activity
Release of α-granule contents
Release of dense granule contents
Release of lysosomal contents
Surface expression of proteins contained in lysosomal membranes
Surface expression of proteins contained in α-granule membranes (e.g., P-selectin)
Recruitment of microvesicles containing tissue factor from blood
Recruitment of circulating neutrophils and monocytes via P-selectin

Agonist-Induced Platelet Activation

Many platelet agonists initiate platelet activation by binding to seven-transmembrane heterotrimeric, G-protein-coupled receptors (see Fig. 114–5). When such receptors are activated, the Gα subunit exchanges GDP for GTP and dissociates from the β/γ complex. The free Gα subunit, and in some cases, the β/γ complex can activate some relatively common downstream pathways and initiate positive feedback loops. Activation of these pathways is usually intertwined. One common pathway involves the activation of one or more isozymes of phospholipase C (PLC), leading to phosphoinositide hydrolysis. Three classes of PLC (β, γ, and δ) have been described, and multiple isozymes exist within each class.[1180] The best-studied PLCs in platelets include PLCβ and PLCγ_2. PLCβ is often activated downstream of the seven-transmembrane G-protein-coupled receptor family, whereas PLCγ_2 can be activated by phosphorylation on tyrosine, which is a downstream signal from other types of agonist receptors. PLC of either type hydrolyzes phospholipids between the glycerol backbone and the phosphate moiety; the PLCβ class is relatively specific for phosphoinositides, whereas PLCγ can cleave other types of phospholipids as well. The hydrolysis of one particular phosphoinositide, phosphatidylinositol 4,5-bisphosphate (PIP_2), by either class of PLC is critical in platelet function, as it results in the formation of two important products, IP_3 and DAG. IP_3 binds to specific receptors on the DTS/SR, causing a release of intracellular Ca^{2+} (see Fig. 114–7). Increases in intracellular Ca^{2+} are important for activation of a number of signaling enzymes and proteins involved in cytoskeletal reorganization (see "Calcium" below). Increases in calcium are also important in granule fusion and the release reaction. DAG binds to PKC and participates in its conversion to an active enzyme. For many agonists, activation of one or more of the multiple isozymes of PKC is an obligatory step in the conversion of $\alpha_{IIb}\beta_3$ to a high-affinity fibrinogen receptor and subsequent platelet aggregation.[717,1181,1182] One consequence of PKC activation is to cause the release of ADP from dense granules. Released ADP acts at its own seven-transmembrane G-protein-coupled receptor(s) to potentiate the action of numerous agonists. The precise mechanism(s) by which PKC causes $\alpha_{IIb}\beta_3$ activation, however, remains unclear.

Activation of a number of receptors also leads to the activation of phospholipase A_2 (PLA_2), which releases arachidonic acid from membrane lipid stores. Arachidonic acid is rapidly converted to PG products, PGH_2 and TXA_2, which are themselves potent activators of platelet aggregation (see "Prostaglandin H_2/Thromboxane A_2 and Other Arachidonic Acid Metabolites: Thromboxane Prostanoid Receptor" below).

ADP: $P2Y_1$, $P2Y_{12}$, and $P2X_1$ Purine Receptors for ADP and ATP Platelets express receptors for both ADP and ATP. Both nucleotides are present in platelet dense granules and are secreted when platelets are activated by adequate concentrations of most, if not all, agonists. Another source of these nucleotides is the red blood cell; damaged red blood cells, or those subjected to high shear stress, may release ADP and ATP, increasing their local concentrations. ADP is an especially important physiologic agonist, not only because it can induce platelet aggregation independent of other agonists, but because secreted ADP contributes significantly to the full aggregation response induced by many other agonists. This has been convincingly demonstrated in experimental systems in which secreted ADP is rapidly degraded or inhibited. Moreover, submaximal concentrations of ADP synergize with other agonists, and this has been most well studied with epinephrine (see "Epinephrine: α_{2a} Adrenergic Receptors" below). ADP induces or contributes to a variety of responses in platelets: shape change, granule release, TXA_2 production, activation of $\alpha_{IIb}\beta_3$, and platelet aggregation.[1183,1184] Recent pharmacologic and cloning and sequencing studies suggest that ADP exerts its full effect on platelets through at least two different receptors. These receptors, $P2Y_1$ and $P2Y_{12}$, are G-protein coupled, and are responsible for most of the physiologic effects of ADP.[1185]

The platelet $P2Y_{12}$ receptor, which is the target of the thienopyridine class of drugs (ticlopidine, clopidogrel, and prasugrel) that are used in the treatment of acute coronary syndromes and peripheral vascular disease, as well as to prevent thrombosis following percutaneous vascular interventions, has been cloned and sequenced. It couples to $G\alpha i$[1186–1188] to inhibit adenylyl cyclases, a class of enzymes that produce cAMP, which in turn activates type A protein kinases that inhibit platelet activation by a variety of effects. VASP is phosphorylated in response to $P2Y_{12}$-mediated activation of protein kinase A and so the extent of VASP phosphorylation in response to a combination of ADP and an agent that stimulates cAMP formation can be used as a marker for receptor blockade (see "Nitric Oxide" below).[1189] Decreases in cAMP level alone are likely insufficient to activate platelets,[1190,1191] and ADP-activation of platelets requires synergistic effects between the signaling pathways of the $P2Y_1$ and $P2Y_{12}$ receptors (and perhaps the $P2X_1$ ATP receptor discussed below). Studies of $P2Y_{12}$ knockout mice demonstrate that $P2Y_{12}$ contributes to multiple steps during thrombosis, including platelet adhesion and activation, thrombus growth, and thrombus stability.[1192] Platelets obtained from $P2Y_{12}$-deficient mice respond only weakly to ADP and less vigorously than normal to other agonists such as collagen and thrombin.[1193] A minor $P2Y_{12}$ haplotype (H2) is associated with enhanced ADP-induced platelet aggregation, as well as resistance to the antiplatelet effects of clopidogrel.[1194,1195]

The platelet $P2Y_1$ receptor, the other G-protein-coupled ADP receptor on platelets, also has been cloned and sequenced and, like most heterotrimeric G-protein-coupled receptors, is predicted to span the membrane seven times.[1196] Data from experiments with inhibitors of $P2Y_1$ and mice lacking $P2Y_1$ suggest that stimulation of this receptor is necessary, but insufficient, to induce platelet aggregation. Thus, platelets from $P2Y_1$-null mice are unable to change shape or aggregate in response to ADP; however, ADP activation does cause a decrease in cAMP via its effects on $P2Y_{12}$.[1197,1198] $P2Y_1$ couples to heterotrimeric G-proteins containing $G\alpha q$. The importance of $G\alpha q$ can be inferred from the observation that platelets from mice that do not express $G\alpha q$ do not aggregate in response to ADP and that patients with abnormalities in $G\alpha q$ have a bleeding disorder and abnormal platelet function (see Chap. 121).[1199] Activation of PLCβ and subsequent phosphoinositide hydrolysis has been linked to both shape change and platelet activation.

$P2X_1$, the third purine nucleotide receptor on platelets, is a member of the P2X family of ligand-gated ion channels rather than a G-protein-coupled receptor.[1200] This receptor is predicted to span the plasma membrane twice and is largely extracellular.[1201] Although $P2X_1$ has been described as both an ATP and an ADP receptor, the bulk of current evidence suggests that it is an ATP receptor that is antagonized by ADP.[1202,1203] Because ATP antagonizes the $P2Y_{12}$ receptor, the overall contribution of $P2X_1$, which is stimulated by ATP, to platelet activation, is not clear. Nonetheless, ATP is released from platelets upon stimulation with agonists such as collagen[1204] and ATP binding to $P2X_1$ causes a rapid Ca^{2+} influx.[1205] However, Ca^{2+} influx induced by stimulation of this receptor alone appears to be insufficient to induce platelet shape change or aggregation.[1190] It does, however, synergize with the P2Y platelet ADP receptors.[1205] This synergy is likely a result of the specific downstream signaling events evoked by ATP stimulation of this receptor, which include Ca^{2+} influx and extracellular signal-regulated kinase (ERK) 2 activation.[1204] Support for a biologically important role for this receptor comes from data in both mice with targeted deletions of $P2X_1$, which have impaired *in vivo* thrombus formation,[1206] and mice that overexpress $P2X_1$, which have a prothrombotic phenotype.[1207] A variant of $P2X_1$ P($2X_1$del), which lacks 17 amino acids, has been described in megakaryocyte-like cell lines,[1208] but its functional role is uncertain.[1202,1203]

Several antiplatelet agents inhibit ADP-induced platelet activation. Thus, metabolites of ticlopidine, clopidogrel, and prasugrel inhibit the $P2Y_{12}$ receptor[1209] (see Chap. 135), whereas soluble CD39 catabolizes ADP and ATP.[1210]

Epinephrine: α_{2a} Adrenergic Receptors When added to platelet-rich plasma, epinephrine uniquely initiates a first phase of aggregation without first inducing shape change; after a plateau period, a second wave of aggregation occurs. The ability of epinephrine to synergize with other agonists, such as ADP, is well documented, but there is controversy as to whether epinephrine, in the absence of released ADP or TXA_2, is sufficient to initiate platelet aggregation.[1211–1213] Epinephrine can cause an elevation in intracellular calcium, even in aspirin-treated platelets,[1211] possibly by opening an external channel or causing release of calcium from membrane sources[1212,1213]; it does not appear to mobilize intracellular calcium or generate measurable amounts of IP_3. Analysis of the purified epinephrine receptor and its nucleotide sequence identified it as a seven-transmembrane G-protein-coupled, α_{2a} adrenergic receptor of molecular weight 64,000.[1214,1215] It couples to $G\alpha i$ family members, primarily $G\alpha z$, to inhibit adenylyl cyclase and thus prevent formation of cAMP.[1216] The reduction in cAMP caused by epinephrine is probably insufficient, however, to initiate platelet aggregation, and it is likely that other effectors are required for platelet activation.[1217–1220] Platelets from a patient with a chronic bleeding disorder contained reduced amounts of $G\alpha i_1$ and displayed impaired epinephrine-induced aggregation, suggesting that $G\alpha i_1$ may also contribute to epinephrine-mediated responses.[1221] Polymorphisms of the α_{2a} adrenergic receptor have been associated with enhanced platelet reactivity and signaling.[1222,1223]

The physiologic and pathologic significance of epinephrine-induced platelet activation remain unclear, but there is a possibility that sympathetic stimulation may contribute to enhanced platelet activation.[1224] In particular, in animal models, infusion of epinephrine can enhance platelet thrombus formation and can overcome the inhibition produced by aspirin.[1225,1226] Increased sympathetic tone may thus account for the resistance to antiplatelet agents during acute coronary syndromes.[1227]

Prostaglandin H_2/Thromboxane A_2 and Other Arachidonic Acid Metabolites: Thromboxane Prostanoid Receptor The metabolism of arachidonic acid (AA) to TXA_2 is a fundamental pathway contributing to agonist-induced platelet activation and aggregation (see Fig. 114–11). Many agonists stimulate the release of arachidonic acid from phosphatidylcholine (PC) and phosphatidylethanolamine (PE) in the plasma membrane.[1228] Most AA is released by the action of PLA_2, but some is also released by the concerted actions of PLC and DAG kinase, followed by PLA_2 and perhaps by the action of PLC followed by the action of DAG lipase. PLA_2 is a cytosolic enzyme, with multiple isoforms in platelets.[1229] PLA_2 acts on the C2 position of triacylglycerols such as PC and PE to form free AA and the resulting lysophospholipid. PLA_2 also converts phosphatidic acid into lysophosphatidic acid, which is also a platelet agonist. Some PLA_2 isozymes are activated by the rise in intracellular platelet Ca^{2+} that occurs during agonist-stimulated activation, whereas other isozymes are activated in a Ca^{2+}-independent manner. Studies in mice[1230] and in a patient with recurrent small intestinal ulcers and platelet dysfunction[1231] have identified cytosolic $PLA_2\alpha$ as the principal phospholipase responsible for the liberation of the AA that is essential for eicosanoid biosynthesis in platelets. Ligand binding to integrin $\alpha_{IIb}\beta_3$ activates cytosolic $PLA_2\alpha$ perhaps through one or more intermediary proteins.[1232]

AA is subsequently metabolized by cyclooxygenases (COXs) to generate PG and thromboxanes and by lipoxygenases (LOXs) to generate leukotrienes (LTs) and hydroxyeicosatetraenoic acids (HPETEs). The main COXs in platelets, COX-1, metabolizes AA to PGG_2, which is subsequently converted to PGH_2.[1233,1234] Thromboxane synthase next converts PGH_2 to TXA_2, which is spontaneously and rapidly converted to the inactive metabolite, TXB_2.[1235] TXA_2 and its precursor, PGH_2, can both stimulate platelet thromboxane receptors to induce platelet aggregation.[1235–1237] An inducible COX, COX-2, is present in many cells involved in mediating the inflammatory response and megakaryocytes, but only trace amounts are present in normal platelets.[1238,1239] COX inhibitors such as aspirin inhibit platelet function by inhibiting COX-1 and decreasing TXA_2 production.[1235] It has been hypothesized that some patients whose platelets are resistant to aspirin inhibition may have increased amounts of COX-2, which is not as readily inhibited by aspirin as COX-1.[1236] Selective COX-2 inhibitor drugs have been associated with increased risk of thrombosis and this has been ascribed to their inhibition of prostacyclin production without the compensatory inhibition of thromboxane production via COX-1.[1240]

TXA_2 is a potent platelet agonist that exerts its effects via interaction with specific members of the thromboxane prostanoid receptor (TP) family of G-protein-coupled receptors. There are two TP isoforms in human platelets (TPα and TPβ), which arise from alternative splicing of exon 3 of the TP gene; TPβ, but not TPα, undergoes agonist-induced internalization.[1241] Although both TPα and TPβ mRNA can be detected in platelet lysates, it appears that TPα is the dominant form.[1242] The TXA_2 receptor has been localized to the platelet plasma membrane,[1243] and on SDS-polyacrylamide gel electrophoresis it migrates as a broad band of apparent molecular weight 55,000 to 57,000[1244,1245] because of variability in glycosylation.[1242] Pharmacologic studies suggest the existence of two distinct TXA_2 receptor subtypes based on differing affinities for agonist ligands. The low-affinity binding sites may mediate platelet aggregation and granule secretion, whereas the high-affinity sites seem to be associated with platelet shape change.[1246] Studies of TP-deficient mice demonstrate that this gene locus is responsible for most, if not all, the biologic effects attributed to TXA_2.[1247] Bleeding times in these mice are prolonged, confirming the importance of this pathway in normal hemostasis. Platelet aggregation to collagen, but not ADP, is delayed, demonstrating the importance of TXA_2 production to the collagen response in platelets. TXA_2 pathways activate Gαq,[1199,1248] Gα_{12} and Gα_{13},[1249,1250] Gα_{11},[1251] and Gαi$_2$.[1252,1253] Activation of Gαq is essential for aggregation and secretion whereas the G$\alpha_{12/13}$-pathways contribute to shape change and aggregation.[1254–1256] It is unclear whether TP directly couples to Gαi[1257] or activates this pathway indirectly via released ADP.[1253,1254] A significant portion of PGH_2/TXA_2-induced platelet aggregation is actually mediated by secreted ADP, as ADP scavenger systems inhibit aggregation induced by a stable PGH_2/TXA_2 analogue either partially (30%)[1258] or totally.[1257]

AA can also be converted to leukotrienes and lipoxins by the sequential actions of LOXs and other enzymes. Platelets from most animal species lack 5-LOX, but possess 12-LOX. AA liberated by cytosolic $PLA_2\alpha$ can therefore be oxygenated by 12-LOX to generate 12-hydro(pero)xyeicosatetraenoic acid (12-HPETE), an unstable intermediate that is reduced by glutathione peroxidase or other mechanisms to generate 12-hydroxyeicosatetraenoic acid (HETE). The generation of 12-HPETE in platelets is slower and more sustained than the generation of thromboxane.[1259] Platelets from mice deficient in the platelet-type 12 LOX are hypersensitive to stimulation by ADP, suggesting an inhibitory role for this pathway in platelet activation by ADP.[1260] 12-LOX activity in platelets can be regulated by signaling through the GPVI collagen receptor.[1261] Because they lack 5-LOX, platelets do not generate LTB_4, nor do they appear to possess LTB_4 receptors.[1262] However, they participate in leukotriene and lipoxin generation through transcellular metabolism involving leukocytes. Leukocyte metabolism of AA, some of which may be derived from platelets, by 5-LOX generates LTA_4, which is then released and can be transformed by glutathione-S-transferase in platelets to LTC_4.[1263] The generation of LTC_4 by platelets requires P-selectin mediated adhesion to leukocytes.[1264] Leukocyte-derived LTA_4 can also be converted by platelets to the anti-inflammatory metabolite lipoxin (LX)A_4 by the actions of 12-LOX in platelets.[1265]

Thrombin Thrombin is derived from the inactive zymogen, prothrombin, which circulates in plasma. When acted upon by the prothrombinase complex (factor [F] Xa, FVa, Ca^{2+}) assembled on the membrane of activated platelets and other cells, prothrombin is cleaved into thrombin[1266] (see Chap. 115), one of the most potent platelet agonists. The proteolytic activity of thrombin is required for its role as a platelet agonist.[1267] Thrombin activates PAR-1, a seven-transmembrane G-protein-coupled receptor on platelets and other cells,[1268–1270] by cleaving an extracellular 41-amino-acid peptide from the N-terminus of the receptor (see Fig. 114–17). Removal of this peptide results in a new amino-terminus, which acts as a "tethered ligand," by binding to another region of PAR-1 to activate the receptor and initiate signal transduction. Short peptides modeled after the "tethered ligand" region (e.g., SFLLRN) also activate PAR-1 signaling. The 41-amino-acid cleavage product of PAR-1 can also induce platelet aggregation by a poorly defined mechanism.[1271] PAR-1 can also be cleaved to an active form by MMP-1 when platelets are stimulated with collagen, but the cleavage site is two amino acids N-terminal to the thrombin cleavage.[1080]

Cloning of PAR-1 and gene deletion experiments in mice led to the discovery of additional members of the PAR family:[1270,1272,1273] PAR-1 and PAR-4 are the main thrombin signaling receptors on human platelets; PAR-3 and PAR-4 mediate thrombin activation on mouse platelets; and PAR-2 is a receptor for trypsin and other proteases. Short endogenous peptide sequences that function as selective agonists have been identified for PAR-1 (SFLLR), PAR2 (SLIGK), and PAR4 (GYPGQV). On human platelets, a full response to thrombin requires both PAR-1 and PAR-4.[1273,1274] The receptors display distinct kinetics of activation and desensitization; PAR-1 mediates a substantial portion of thrombin signaling, but PAR-4 contributes at high doses of thrombin.[1274–1277] PAR-3 and PAR-4 serve as thrombin receptors on mouse platelets,[1272] where PAR-4 is the primary signaling molecule[1278] and PAR-3 functions as a cofactor for the cleavage and activation of PAR-4 by thrombin.[1279] Deficiency of either PAR-4 or PAR-3 results in a bleeding defect and protection from experimental thrombosis in mice.[1278,1280] An oral PAR-1 antagonist (SCH530348) is under development as an antithrombotic agent (see Chap. 135).[1281]

When platelets are exposed to a subaggregating concentration of thrombin, they become relatively insensitive to subsequent stimulation with an aggregating concentration of thrombin, a process termed *homologous desensitization*. This involves rapid receptor internalization and alterations in the thrombin receptor signaling systems.[1282] Trafficking of the thrombin receptor to lysosomes is dictated by the amino acid sequence in the cytoplasmic tail of PAR-1[1283] and requires phosphorylation. In comparison with PAR-1, activation-dependent internalization of PAR-4 occurs to a lesser extent and termination of PAR-4 signaling occurs more slowly,[1276] resulting in distinct patterns of signaling through each receptor.

Thrombin can bind to GPIbα, and platelets from patients lacking the GPIb/IX complex (Bernard-Soulier syndrome) have decreased thrombin-induced platelet aggregation (see Chap. 121). A region on GPIbα with three sulfated tyrosines and a large number of anionic amino acids, with homology to the high-affinity thrombin-inhibitor hirudin, contains the thrombin-binding site. Crystal structures of the extracellular, amino-terminal domain of GPIbα bound to thrombin indicate that two thrombin molecules interact with each GPIbα.[882,883] This bivalent interaction may allow thrombin to serve as a bridge linking GPIbα receptors on the same or adjacent platelets. Although the physiologic role of GPIb in thrombin signaling is not completely established, thrombin binding may promote signaling through receptor multimerization and/or enhanced PAR cleavage.

Tachykinins: Substance P and Endokinins A and B The tachykinin neurotransmitter substance P induces platelet aggregation and the release reaction at micromolar concentrations and enhances aggregation induced by other agonists at lower concentrations.[1284] Platelets express two seven-transmembrane G-protein-coupled receptors for substance P (NK_1 and NK_2) and NK_1 has been implicated in mediating the response to substance P.[1285] In addition, an amidated peptide from the C-terminus of the related tachykinins endokinins A and B (GKASQFFGLM-NH_2) initiates platelet aggregation. Substance P has also been identified in platelets and platelets secrete substance P when activated.

Chemokines: Chemokine Receptors CCR1, CCR3, CCR4, CXCR1, and CXCR4 Based on monoclonal antibody binding and/or mRNA expression studies, platelets and/or megakaryocytes have been reported to express the seven-transmembrane G-protein-coupled chemokine receptors CCR1, CCR3, CCR4, CXCR1, and CXCR4 (reviewed in references 137 and 1286). These receptors may play a role in megakaryopoiesis and platelet production. In addition, a number of chemokines, in particular platelet factor 4 (CXCL4), CXCL12, CCL13, and CCL22 have been variably found to be able to either augment platelet activation and aggregation induced by other agonists, or to actually fully initiate platelet adhesion, activation, and aggregation. Because high concentrations of the chemokines relative to plasma concentrations are required to demonstrate these effects, it is unclear what role these receptors play in platelet physiology, but it is possible that local chemokine levels are higher in areas of inflammation.

Lipid Mediators (Platelet-Activating Factor, Lysophosphatidic Acid, and Sphingosphine-1-Phosphate) PAF (a mixture of 1-*O*-hexadecyl-2-acetyl-sn-glycero-3-phosphocholine and 1-*O*-octadecyl-2-acetyl-sn-glycero-3-phosphocholine[1287]) is a phospholipid ether produced by platelets, leukocytes, and other cells. PAF is a potent platelet agonist and mediator of inflammation. Cellular responses to PAF are mediated by a specific seven-transmembrane G-protein-coupled receptor.[1288,1289] PAF induces G-protein-dependent inhibition of adenylyl cyclase and activation of PLC,[1290] which cause phosphoinositide turnover, leading to the activation of PKC and an increase in intracellular Ca^{2+}.[1289] PAF also indirectly activates PLA_2, which causes release of arachidonic acid from the platelet membrane.[1291] All of these effects contribute to the overall platelet response to PAF. PAF is catabolized by PAF acetyl hydrolase and this enzyme may play an important role in inflammation and atherosclerosis.[1292]

LDLs activate human platelets, and oxidized LDLs are more potent platelet activators. One active component in oxidized LDLs is oxidized phosphatidylcholine ($oxPC_{36}$), which increases with diet-induced hyperlipidemia. $oxPC_{36}$ signals through CD36 (GPIV)[1032] via phosphorylation of the mitogen-activated protein (MAP) kinases p38 and c-Jun N-terminal kinase (JNK).[1033] Platelet activation by oxidized LDL in the absence of hyperlipidemia may also require scavenger receptor A.[1293] Increases in levels of $oxPC_{36}$ with hyperlipidemia may provide an explanation for observations that atherogenic mice have a prothrombotic phenotype as indicated *in vivo* by decreased tail-bleed time and propensity to thrombosis in response to either ferric chloride or photochemical injury, and *in vitro* by increased platelet aggregation.[1032,1294]

Activated platelets likely contribute to lysophosphatidic acid (LPA) generation in blood[1295] via lysophospholipase D (lysoPLD)-catalyzed hydrolysis of a lysophosphophosphatidylcholine (LPC).[1296] Autotaxin, initially identified as a tumor-cell derived motility factor, appears to be responsible for the majority of lysoPLD activity in serum; it is also responsible for the formation of LPA from LPC.[1297] Mild oxidation of LDL generates LPA, and the LPA component of oxidized LDL in the lipid-rich thrombogenic core of atherosclerotic lesions exposed during plaque rupture may be an important platelet activator.[1298]

In human platelets, LPA elicits shape-change,[1299] platelet-monocyte aggregate formation,[1300] and fibronectin-matrix assembly[1301]; it also potentiates ADP-induced platelet aggregation. LPA signaling pathways couple to Rho activation,[1299] Src kinase activity, and calcium entry[1302] with little activation of Gαq-dependent pathways.[1303] Some of the platelet responses to LPA in whole blood are attenuated by $P2Y_1$ and $P2Y_{12}$ receptor antagonists, suggesting that released ADP may play an important role in mediating aspects of LPA's responses.[1302] The platelet receptor(s) responsible for LPA signaling are not known.

Sphingosine 1-phosphate (S1P) is a weaker activator of platelets than LPA and requires high concentrations (>10 μM) to induce platelet aggregation,[1304] raising the possibility that a contaminant or a S1P-derived metabolite may account for its biologic activity.[1305] S1P elicits platelet shape change,[1306] activates protein kinases, and stimulates fibronectin matrix assembly.[1301] Paradoxically, S1P has also been reported to inhibit thrombin- and epinephrine-induced platelet aggregation.[1307]

Serotonin Platelets serve as the major serotonin (5-hydroxytryptophan [5HT]) storage site in the circulation because they have the capacity to take it up actively and store it in dense granules. The release of serotonin from dense granules during platelet activation may amplify platelet aggregation and granule release. Serotonergic receptors, which are seven-transmembrane G-protein-coupled receptors, exist in seven main subfamilies termed $5HT_1$ to $5HT_7$.[1308] The receptor that mediates serotonin's effects on platelet function is of the $5HT_{2A}$ subtype and is identical to the $5HT_{2A}$ receptor present in the brain frontal cortex.[1309–1312] The $5HT_2$ receptor-blocking compound ketanserin antagonizes serotonin's stimulatory effects on platelets and neurons.[1313] Two naturally occurring amino acid substitutions have been identified in the receptor.[1314] Platelets from patients heterozygous for the H452Y polymorphism have a blunted calcium response when stimulated with serotonin compared to platelets from patients homozygous for H452.[1314] Silent polymorphisms in the $5HT_{2A}$ gene (T102C in exon 1 and –1438A/G in the promoter region) have been correlated with nonfatal acute myocardial infarctions and enhanced $5HT_{2A}$ receptor-mediated small platelet aggregate formation.[1315] Many studies have been performed correlating platelet serotonin transporter activity and $5HT_{2A}$ receptors with a number of neuropsychiatric disorders.[1316–1320] There is some concern, however, about the correlation between $5HT_{2A}$ receptors on platelets and those in the brain.[1321] Hyperresponsive $5HT_{2A}$ receptors have been implicated in the association between depression and increased risk of cardiovascular events.[1322]

Addition of serotonin in micromolar concentrations to platelets *in vitro* causes elevation of intracellular calcium, phospholipase C activation, protein phosphorylation, and mild aggregation.[1323,1324] In whole blood, serotonin does not itself cause platelet aggregation, but it does enhance aggregation induced by ADP and thrombin.[1325] Serotonin released from platelets can cause vasoconstriction of blood vessels that have suffered endothelial damage,[1326] further promoting thrombus formation. Inhibition of serotonin's action has a favorable effect in animal models of thrombosis and vascular damage, but it is not clear whether the benefit derives from effects on platelet aggregation or vasoconstriction.[1327] Mice deficient in serotonin have prolonged bleeding times, suggesting a physiologic role for serotonin in hemostasis.[1328]

A role for serotonin in linking procoagulant proteins to activated platelets has been described. Serotonin can attach via a transglutaminase-dependent reaction to multiple substrates, including fibrinogen, VWF, thrombospondin, fibronectin, and α_2-antiplasmin. These serotonylated proteins then associate to a subpopulation of activated platelets termed "coated" (COAT) platelets, perhaps via interactions with fibrinogen or thrombospondin.[1328,1329] Tissue transglutaminase in platelets can also catalyze the addition of serotonin to the small G-proteins Rab4 and RhoA in a reaction that renders them constitutively active and promotes α-granule secretion.[1330]

The serotonin transporter SERT, which takes up and releases serotonin, contributes to platelet stores of serotonin. Expression of SERT is required for normal ADP- and thrombin-mediated aggregation of mouse platelets.[1331] Furthermore, SERT activity is enhanced by ligand binding to integrin $\alpha_{IIb}\beta_3$. Case reports have suggested an association between the use of a serotonin reuptake inhibitor (SSRI) and bleeding abnormalities.[1332] Reports conflict as to whether SSRI use may protect from myocardial infarction or reduce the complications of acute thrombosis. In mice, platelet release of serotonin is essential for liver regeneration following partial hepatectomy.[110]

Vasopressin: V_1-Type Receptor Vasopressin interacts with platelets to induce shape change, aggregation, and dense granule release.[1333] These events follow an induced rise in intracellular calcium and phospholipase C activation.[1334] The platelet binding site is classified pharmacologically as a V_1-type receptor,[1335] and radiolabeled vasopressin binds with a Kd of 1 to 10 nM.[1336] Unlike the case with V_2 receptors that activate adenylate cyclase, the V_1 receptors appear to activate phospholipase C,[1337] perhaps via coupling through $G\alpha q11$.[1338] There are fewer than 100 binding sites for vasopressin per platelet,[1339] and there is controversy as to whether physiologic concentrations of vasopressin are sufficiently high to activate platelets directly[1340,1341]; even if vasopressin does not directly activate platelets, it may be able to enhance platelet activation induced by other agonists. Vasopressin V_{1a} receptor antagonists inhibit vasopressin-induced platelet aggregation.[1342,1343]

Angiotensin II: AT1-Type Receptor Platelets express angiotensin II (AngII) AT1-type receptors.[1344] AngII treatment of platelet-rich plasma results in shape change but not platelet aggregation.[1345,1346] Infusion of AngII into normal volunteers results in platelet activation as assessed by plasma β-thromboglobulin levels and platelet surface expression of P-selectin and fibrinogen binding sites.[1347] Certain AT1 receptor antagonists, such as losartan and irbesartan, competitively inhibit TXA_2 receptors on platelets.[1345,1348,1349] AT1 receptor antagonists stimulate NO release from isolated platelets.[1350] In hypertensive rats treated with losartan, platelet function appears to be attenuated,[1351] but data in humans on the effects of administering AT1 receptor antagonists are inconsistent.[1352–1355]

Thrombospondin: Integrin-Associated Protein (CD47) Thrombospondin (TSP), a large disulfide-bonded trimer (subunit molecular weight 160,000), is both a platelet α-granule protein and an extracellular matrix protein present in the subendothelium. TSP is rapidly released from platelets upon thrombin stimulation. In addition to its role as an adhesive protein, TSP also functions as an agonist to stimulate $\alpha_{IIb}\beta_3$-mediated platelet aggregation.[1356,1357] Multiple potential TSP receptors are present on platelets, including CD36 (GPIV), $\alpha_{IIb}\beta_3$, $\alpha_V\beta_3$, and integrin-associated protein (CD47 or IAP). Of these receptors, CD47 is most strongly implicated as the major signaling receptor in response to TSP. CD47 was first discovered as a protein that copurifies with integrins, including $\alpha_{IIb}\beta_3$,[1356] $\alpha_V\beta_3$,[1358] and $\alpha_2\beta_1$.[1359] The sequence of CD47 indicates that it has a single immunoglobulin-like extracellular domain, five membrane-spanning regions, and a short cytoplasmic tail.[190,1357,1358] CD47 probably generates signals independent of integrins and affects integrin function via downstream effects. CD47 couples physically and functionally to the large G-protein, $G\alpha i$,[1360] which is of note as all known large G-proteins couple to receptors with seven rather than five transmembrane-spanning regions. Further downstream signaling probably involves the activation of tyrosine kinases, including Syk, Lyn, and Fak, as well as $PLC\gamma_2$ (see Fig. 114–14).[1356] Studies of mice with targeted deletions of CD47 indicate that it may block the inhibitory effects of NO on platelets,[1361] which may contribute to its role in stimulating platelet adhesion to activated endothelium under low shear rates.[1362]

How other TSP binding sites on platelets contribute to the overall response induced by TSP is not clear. CD36 (GPIV) copurifies with several tyrosine kinases, including Fyn, Lyn, and Yes.[1363] However, whether TSP binding to CD36 (GPIV) activates these kinases and whether they then contribute to the observed platelet response is unknown.

TSP-1 also functions as a reductase for VWF; in α granules it appears to reduce VWF multimer size.[1364,1365] In contrast, TSP-1 also binds to the A3 domain of plasma VWF, where it competes for ADAMTS-13 binding, thus slowing the rate of VWF cleavage, thus favoring large VWF multimers.[1365] TSP-1 also makes a small, but significant, contribution to the conversion of latent TGF-β_1 released from platelets to active TGF-β_1.[278]

Collagen: GPVI and $\alpha_2\beta_1$ Upon vascular injury, collagens in the subendothelium become exposed to flowing blood and promote both platelet attachment and activation, thereby contributing to normal hemostasis. Collagen is also one of the most thrombogenic substances in atherosclerotic plaques, and upon plaque rupture it is believed to contribute to platelet aggregation and thrombus formation, leading to ischemic damage.[1366] The types of collagen present in the subendothelium include I, III, IV, V, VI, VIII, and XIII,[1367] the most abundant being types I and III (>95%). Under conditions that mimic physiologic blood flow, platelets adhere tightly to collagen types I, III, and IV, weakly to types VI, VII, and VIII, and not at all to type V. However, under static conditions, platelets can adhere to types I to VIII.[1042] Collagens are normally acid insoluble fibers, but can form spiral microfibrils when subjected to proteolysis. Differences in the nature of the collagen surface influence its recognition by platelets (see below).[1368]

Collagen-induced platelet activation probably involves multiple receptors, most notably GPVI (see Fig. 114–17) and integrin $\alpha_2\beta_1$, with indirect activation of PAR-1 via activation of MMP-1 (see Fig. 114–17).[1080] GPVI is a molecular weight 62,000 glycoprotein from the immunoglobulin superfamily[395,1369–1371] (see "Platelet Membrane Glycoproteins,

Platelet Adhesion, and Platelet Aggregation" above) that functions in concert with the FcR γ-chain, with the latter initiating intracellular signaling.[629,911,912,1372–1375] Other collagen receptors on platelets include CD36 (GPIV)[1020] and a molecular weight 65,000 protein called GP65.[1376] The I (inserted) domain in the α_2 subunit of $\alpha_2\beta_1$ is homologous to a number of collagen-binding domains in other proteins and mediates adhesion of the receptor to collagen. Integrin $\alpha_2\beta_1$ recognizes spiral microfibrils, but not the acid insoluble form of collagen in which the monomers assume a banded pattern.[1368] The potential interrelation of all of the collagen receptors is unknown, but GPVI appears to be responsible for platelet interactions with insoluble collagens and GPVI and $\alpha_2\beta_1$ work in concert to recognize collagen spiral microfibrils, perhaps by assembling intracellular proteins into complexes.[749,1377,1378]

Glycoprotein VI exists as a dimer in a stable physical complex with the dimeric FcR γ-chain; FcR γ-chain is absent from GPVI-deficient platelets.[911,917] The crystal structure of GPVI revealed a dimeric structure with parallel orientation of the collagen binding domains, separated by a distance (5.5 nm) that matches the orientation of the collagen triple helix.[1375] Molecular docking studies suggested that collagen interacts with a shallow groove on the surface. The addition of either collagen or an antibody that can crosslink GPVI induces tyrosine phosphorylation of the FcR γ-chain.[917] The kinases contributing to this event are probably Fyn and/or Lyn.[801,914,1379] Tyrosine phosphorylation of the ITAM on the FcR γ-chain increases the ITAM's affinity for proteins containing SH2 domains, resulting in the recruitment of such proteins to the FcR γ-chain.[801,914] The nonreceptor tyrosine kinase Syk contains two adjacent SH2 domains and a tyrosine kinase domain. In platelets from normal mice, Syk physically associates with the FcRγ-chain and becomes phosphorylated and activated after collagen stimulation,[917] whereas in platelets from mice lacking FcRγ-chain, collagen is unable to induce Syk phosphorylation and activation.[1372] Similarly, in platelets lacking GPVI or in platelets in which the $\alpha_2\beta_1$ integrin is blocked, collagen induced Syk phosphorylation is also inhibited, demonstrating that GPVI, $\alpha_2\beta_1$, and Syk all participate in the platelet response to collagen. The β subunit of the $\alpha_2\beta_1$ receptor also has tyrosines spaced in a manner reminiscent of an ITAM motif, and thus it is possible that Syk might also associate with this collagen receptor. In addition to Syk,[1380] Src[1381] also becomes tyrosine phosphorylated in response to collagen. Although Src is an abundant kinase in platelets, its role in platelet signaling is unclear, as mice lacking Src do not suffer from any obvious bleeding disorder.[1382] Syk, on the other hand, appears to play a critical role in collagen activation of platelets since platelets from mice lacking Syk do not aggregate or undergo secretion in response to collagen.[1372] Collagen stimulation of platelets also results in tyrosine phosphorylation and activation of PLCγ_2,[1383] and activation of this enzyme causes phosphoinositide hydrolysis, leading to $\alpha_{IIb}\beta_3$ activation. PLCγ_2 activation occurs downstream of Syk, as evidenced by the findings that collagen is unable to activate PLCγ_2 in platelets pretreated with a Syk-selective inhibitor[1377] or in platelets from Syk knockout mice.[1372] It is unknown whether Syk activates PLCγ_2 directly, but the Bruton tyrosine kinase (BTK) might be positioned between Syk and PLCγ_2 because patients lacking BTK not only exhibit the B-cell deficiency X-linked agammaglobulinaemia, but also show reduced platelet responsiveness to collagen and diminished phosphorylation of PLCγ_2.[1384] Signaling via GPVI also activates the other major collagen receptor $\alpha_2\beta_1$,[1385,1386] perhaps via talin binding to the β_1 cytoplasmic domain,[37] elimination of an inhibitory influence of the α_2 cytoplasmic domain,[37] and/or extracellular disulfide exchange.[755]

Intermediate events of GPVI signaling involve the activation of a small G-protein, Rap-1, which has been implicated in integrin activation in platelets and megakaryocytes.[1387] Full GPVI-induced Rap-1 activation appears to involve both release of ADP (acting on the P2Y$_{12}$ ADP receptor) and ADP receptor-independent pathways.[1388] GPVI signaling also results in the activation of at least one negative regulator of platelet function, c-CBL, which is tyrosine phosphorylated and activated downstream of Src kinases. Platelets deficient in c-CBL show enhanced aggregation responses in response to GPVI engagement.[1389] While much of the GPVI-mediated signaling occurs via the associated FcRγ, the cytoplasmic domain of GPVI also contains a highly basic region that binds calmodulin and a proline-rich region that binds Src kinases, which also appear to contribute to GPVI-mediated signaling.[1390]

The $\alpha_2\beta_1$ integrin can also signal in response to collagen, independent of GPVI and induce phosphorylation and activation of many of the same signaling components attributed to the GPVI induced signaling cascade, such as Src, Syk, SLP-76, and PLCγ_2. Other components include plasma membrane calcium ATPase and focal adhesion kinase or FAK.[1391] However, separate studies indicate that $\alpha_2\beta_1$ must be in an active conformation in order to participate in this signaling.[751,1392] Thus it appears that collagen-induced signaling via GPVI activates $\alpha_2\beta_1$, allowing both receptors to participate in the signaling necessary for a full response to collagen.[1392]

The inactive form of MMP-1 (proMMP-1) is associated with $\alpha_2\beta_1$,[1080] as well as $\alpha_{II}\beta_3$.[1393] With collagen activation, MMP-1 becomes activated and then can cleave the N-terminal region of PAR-1, resulting in the generation of a new N-terminal that can insert into the receptor and initiate downstream signaling through the p38 MAPK, Rho-GTP pathway. Of note, the cleavage of PAR-1 by MMP-1 is at a site two amino acids N-terminal to the cleavage site of thrombin (see Fig. 114–17). The combined activation of PAR-1, $\alpha_2\beta_1$, and GPVI may account for the high thrombogenicity of collagen surfaces.

The levels of GPVI and $\alpha_2\beta_1$ expressed on platelets vary among individuals, but it is unclear whether there is a correlation between the levels of expression of each of them.[349,1394–1396] The level of expression of these receptors correlates with the ability of platelets to be stimulated by collagen. GPVI is present on the membranes of the open canalicular system and α granules, but these pools are not detectable on the surface of resting platelets. These pools merge with the plasma membrane pool in stimulated platelets, increasing the apparent surface expression of GPVI by approximately 60 percent.[1397]

CD36 (GPIV) can also bind collagen and antibodies to CD36 (GPIV) partially inhibit platelet adhesion to collagen.[1398,1399] Platelets from patients lacking CD36 (GPIV) responded normally to collagen in one study,[1400] but showed a minor defect in adhesion to collagen under flow conditions in another study.[1401]

Platelets stimulated with collagen exhibit several distinct responses. While elevated cAMP levels normally inhibit platelet aggregation, collagen-stimulated platelets are relatively resistant to inhibition by cAMP.[1402] This may be related to the fact that collagen stimulates the PLCγ isotype, which is insensitive to cAMP-mediated inhibition, whereas other agonists such as thrombin stimulate PLCβ, which is inhibited by cAMP. In addition, phosphatase inhibition decreases collagen-induced, but not thrombin- or ADP-induced platelet aggregation,[1403] suggesting that one or more phosphatases are critical in collagen-induced platelet aggregation.

GPIb/IX/V The GPIb/IX/V complex promotes the initial interactions of platelets with VWF, particularly under conditions of high shear, resulting in platelet tethering. GPIb/IX/V can also initiate signals that activate the $\alpha_{IIb}\beta_3$ receptor, resulting in firm platelet adhesion and aggregation.[383] Some of the first evidence that the GPIb/IX/V complex could serve as a signaling receptor came from studies in which antibodies to $\alpha_{IIb}\beta_3$ partially inhibited ristocetin-induced platelet aggregation.[557] Subsequently, ristocetin-mediated interaction of VWF with platelets was observed to cause PIP_2 metabolism, activation of PKC, and an increase in intracellular Ca^{2+}. Likewise, shear forces initiate signaling through the binding of VWF to GPIb/IX/V.[1404] In heterologous systems such as Chinese hamster ovary (CHO) cells expressing both GPIb/IX and $\alpha_{IIb}\beta_3$, occupancy of GPIb/IX by VWF can lead to activation of $\alpha_{IIb}\beta_3$.[1405,1406] In platelets, the GPIb/IX/V complex associates with signaling proteins with ITAM motifs, such as the FCγRIIA receptor[859] and FcRγ chain[862]; however, engagement of GPIb/IX/V alone is sufficient to activate $\alpha_{IIb}\beta_3$.[1407] The signaling pathway triggered by engagement of GPIb/IX/V is incompletely understood but appears to involve activation of Src[1301,1407,1408] and PI3K, and recruitment of the adaptor proteins SLP-76 and ADAP (SLAP-130).[1407] The result is activation of PLCγ_2,[1409] PKC, and $\alpha_{IIb}\beta_3$. Signaling through the GPIb/IX/V complex also causes release of arachidonic acid and generation of TXA_2. A cyclic guanosine monophosphate (cGMP) and MAPK-dependent pathway for GPIb/IX-mediated activation of $\alpha_{IIb}\beta_3$ has also been reported.[1410] The GPIb/IX/V complex binds several intracellular proteins including filamin (actin-binding protein),[854] calmodulin,[1411] and 14-3-3ζ.[851,1412,1413] 14-3-3ζ binds to both GPIbα and cRaf and this may link GPIb/IX/V signaling to the Raf/MEK (mitogen-activated kinase)/MAPK signaling pathway; moreover, protein exists as a dimer, which may allow it to bridge and dimerize GPIb molecules.[1412] In CHO cells, clustering of GPIb/IX promotes stable adhesion via $\alpha_{IIb}\beta_3$.[1414]

The GPIb/IX/V complex also appears to be involved in transmitting at least one cAMP-dependent inhibitory signal. Thus, elevated cAMP, which activates protein kinase A, induces phosphorylation of GPIbβ on serine 166.[853] Elevated cAMP also normally inhibits agonist-induced platelet actin polymerization. However, in platelets from patients with Bernard-Soulier syndrome, which lack GPIb/IX/V, actin polymerization proceeds normally after collagen stimulation, even when cAMP is elevated, suggesting that cAMP-mediated phosphorylation of GPIbβ may be required for the cAMP-mediated inhibition.[1415]

Glycoprotein V, a molecular weight 82,000 membrane-spanning protein that is a member of the leucine-rich repeat family and complexes with GPIb/IX, is a substrate for thrombin.[1416] GPV-null platelets display enhanced responses to thrombin[1417] and GPV-null mice have accelerated thrombus growth in response to vascular injury.[1418] Proteolytically inactive thrombin selectively activates mouse platelets lacking GPV and induces thrombosis in GPV-deficient but not wild-type mice.[901] Together, these observations suggest that GPV may function as a negative regulator of thrombin signaling through GPIb/IX, and in its absence, thrombin may function as a ligand for GPIb/IX.

Additional Intermediate Signaling Molecules

Calcium Elevation of intracellular Ca^{2+} has a multitude of effects on platelet physiology.[1220,1419] The concentration of Ca^{2+} in resting platelets (100–500 nM) is very low compared to the plasma concentration of Ca^{2+} (~2 mM). Exposure of platelets to most agonists is accompanied by a rapid, transient rise in the intracellular free Ca^{2+} concentration to micromolar levels, followed by a less-rapid return to normal resting levels. The cytoplasmic Ca^{2+} concentration at any given time is a result of the rates of passive Ca^{2+} influx, active Ca^{2+} extrusion across the plasma membrane, and both active release and/or uptake of Ca^{2+} by the DTS/SR (see "Dense Tubular System/Sarcoplasmic Reticulum" above), which is a Ca^{2+} storage depot in platelets analogous to the sarcoplasmic reticulum in muscle. Active Ca^{2+} extrusion and uptake of Ca^{2+} are mediated by several pumps (see Fig. 114–8). The cytosolic pool of Ca^{2+} turns over rapidly because of a plasma membrane Na^+/Ca^{2+} antiporter, whereas the DTS/SR contains a more slowly exchanging pool of Ca^{2+} regulated by a Ca^{2+}/Mg^{2+} ATPase (sarco-/endoplasmic reticulum Ca^{2+}-ATPase 3 [SERCA3]), a pump that also appears to be located in the plasma membrane.[1420] During agonist stimulation, most Ca^{2+} enters the platelet cytosolic compartment through receptor-operated calcium channels (reviewed in reference 1421) in the plasma membrane. Collagen, for example, causes Na^+ entry into platelets, which reverses the Na^+/Ca^{2+} antiporter to promote Ca^{2+} entry, thus contributing to platelet aggregation.[1422] Release of intracellular Ca^{2+} from the DTS/SR also occurs rapidly in response to agonist stimulation, in large part as a result of the IP_3 generated as part of the phosphoinositide cycle.[1421,1423] The release of internal stores of Ca^{2+} results in translocation of STIM1 from the DTS/SR, followed by activation of the plasma membrane Ca^{2+} channel Orai1, leading to SOCE.[308] Calcium entry is also supported by TRPC6 mediating non–SOCE-induced by diacylglycerol.[308,1421] The role of TRPC1 remains to be defined.[20,308] $\alpha_{IIb}\beta_3$ may also participate in Ca^{2+} entry.[1424]

Elevations of Ca^{2+} induce numerous downstream events, including activation of Ca^{2+} sensitive forms of PLA_2[1425] and PKC[1426]; calmodulin-dependent enzymes such as myosin light-chain kinase, which phosphorylates myosin light chain[1427] and promotes cytoskeletal rearrangements required for platelet shape change; and gelsolin, which facilitates actin severing and rearrangement, secretion, and aggregation. In addition, Ca^{2+} probably plays a direct role in controlling the secretory machinery which mediates the membrane fusion events that result in degranulation and the release reaction. Calcium-dependent proteases or calpains also become activated and play an important role in postaggregation events. The Ca^{2+} binding protein CIB[1428] binds to the membrane proximal region of α_{IIb}[1429] and contributes to platelet spreading.[417]

Phosphoinositide 3-Kinases PI3Ks are a family of lipid kinases that phosphorylate the D-3 protein–protein hydroxyl group of the myoinositol ring of phosphoinositides (reviewed in references 1430 and 1431). Class I PI3Ks are heterodimeric p complexes containing both adaptor and catalytic subunits that utilize phosphatidylinositol (Ptdlns), Ptdlns(4)P, and Ptdlns(4,5)P_2 as substrates to form Ptdlns(3)P, Ptdlns(3,4)P_2, and Ptdlns(3,4,5)P_3, respectively. Class Ia (PI3Kα, PI3Kβ, and PI3Kδ) and class Ib (PI3Kγ) have distinct subunits and regulatory features. The catalytic subunit of class Ia PI3K is a molecular weight 110,000 to 120,000 protein; the adaptor subunit, p85 (PI3K p85α), has two SH2 domains, a breakpoint cluster region homology domain, a proline-rich region, and a single SH3 domain. Members of this class of PI3K possess intrinsic serine-threonine protein kinase activity in addition to lipid kinase activity, and they appear to be regulated, at least in part, by binding of the p85 subunit to tyrosine-phosphorylated proteins. Although platelets possess PI3Kα and PI3Kδ the main class Ia member that is thought to contribute to platelet function is PI3Kβ. Class Ib PI3K (PI3Kγ) has been isolated from platelets and neutrophils and contains both regulatory (p101) and (p110γ) subunits; the latter is activated by the β/γ subunit of heterodimeric G proteins. Both isoforms of PI3K appear to associate with the platelet cytoskeleton after agonist activation.

In platelets, 3-phosphorylated phosphoinositides are produced in response to a variety of agonists, including thrombin, TXA_2, LPA, ADP, and collagen, and may mediate early signaling events that precede $\alpha_{IIb}\beta_3$ activation as well as late events involved in stabilizing fibrinogen binding and platelet aggregation.[1430–1432] Thrombin stimulates rapid accumulation of Ptdlns(3,4,5)P_3 and Ptdlns(3,4)P_2,[1433] and late production of Ptdlns(3,4)P_2; the latter requires fibrinogen binding to $\alpha_{IIb}\beta_3$ and calpain activity.[1434] Collagen promotes the association of class Ia P13K via the SH2 domains with tyrosine-phosphorylated forms of FcRγ-chain and the regulatory protein, linker for activation of T cells (LAT), to modulate PI3K.[1435] Platelets from mice lacking PI3K p85α aggregate normally to ADP, thrombin, U46619, and PMA (phorbol myristate acetate), but display impaired responses to collagen and collagen-related peptide (CRP) and diminished tyrosine phosphorylation of the PI3K effectors BTK, Tec, Akt, and PLCγ_2.[1436] FcγRIIA-induced platelet aggregation requires PI3K activity, which is upstream of PLCγ_2 in the pathway.[1437] Genetic deletion of PI3Kβ in mice results in embryonic lethality, but mice possessing a kinase dead form of the enzyme have been generated. Platelets from these mice have defects in G-protein-coupled receptor-, collagen-, and integrin-mediated signaling pathways.[1438] Platelets from mice lacking PI3Kγ isoform aggregate normally to thrombin and collagen but have impaired responses to ADP, and PI3Kγ-deficient mice are protected from ADP-induced thromboembolism.[1439] Platelets from mice expressing a kinase dead form of PI3Kγ have defective G-protein-coupled receptor-induced activation of Rap1 and aggregation, but normal responses through GPVI-activated pathways.[1438] A working model to explain the observations is that PI3Kβ serves as a common intermediary of signals elicited by G-protein-coupled receptor, collagen, and integrin ligation, whereas PI3Kγ primarily affects G-protein-coupled receptor-initiated pathways. Many of the biologic actions of PI3K are mediated by their phospholipid products, which bind to specific sequences in proteins. The pleckstrin homology (PH) domains (~100 amino acids long) present in pleckstrin and other platelet proteins involved in signal transduction, recognize either PI(3,4)P_2 or PI(3,4,5)P_3.[1440] Binding of PI(3,4,5)P_3 to the amino terminal PH domain in PLCγ enhances its activity.[1441] PI(3,4,5)P_3 binding to PH domains in BTK[1442] targets BTK to the plasma membrane, where it is further phosphorylated and activated.[1443] PI(3,4)P_2 or PI(3,4,5)P_3 binding to the PH domains in the serine/threonine kinase Akt (or protein kinase B) changes the conformation of Akt, permitting it to become activated by phosphorylation on serine and threonine by Akt-kinase (PDK1).[1444,1445] Akt activation is biphasic, occurring before and after platelet aggregation.[1434] Two isoforms of Akt are present in human platelets: Akt1 and Akt2.[1446] The Akt isoforms have multiple substrates in platelets. One prominent substrate is glycogen synthase kinase-3β, which is inactivated by Akt-mediated phosphorylation. Glycogen synthase kinase-3β suppresses platelet function and thrombosis in mice.[1447] Akt activation also stimulates NO production and resultant PKG-dependent degranulation.[1448] Finally, Akt has been implicated in activation of a cAMP-dependent phosphodiesterase (PDE3A), which plays a role in reducing platelet cAMP levels after thrombin stimulation.[1449] Each of these Akt-mediated events is expected to contribute to platelet activation. Deficiency of Akt2 in mice impairs platelet aggregation, secretion, and fibrinogen binding in response to low doses of thrombin and U46619, but has minimal effects on collagen signaling.[1450] Akt2-null mice have normal bleeding times, but are protected from experimental thrombosis, as are mice with a deficiency of Akt1.[1451,1452] Interestingly, in platelets containing either kinase dead PI3Kβ or PI3Kγ, activation of Akt by ADP was abolished, and yet under the same condition, aggregation was only modestly affected,[1438] which raises questions about the role of Akt in these events.

Small G Proteins The Ras superfamily of small GTPases are intracellular transducers that act as "on–off" switches to facilitate the response to extracellular stimuli. Platelets contain many members of the Ras subfamily (Ras, Ral, and Rap), the Rho subfamily (Rho, Rac, and Cdc42), the Rab subfamily (Rab 1, 3, 4, 6, 8, 11, 27, 31, and 32),[1453–1456] and the Arf subfamily (Arf1 or 3 and 6).[1457]

Rho family GTPases are regulators of cytoskeletal remodeling: Cdc42 for filopodia formation, Rac for lamellipodia and membrane ruffling, and Rho for focal adhesion and stress fiber formation.[1458,1459] Platelets have Cdc42,[1460] Rac1,[1461] and RhoA.[1454] Resting platelets have very low levels of the GTP-bound forms of these GTPases,[1462–1464] but all are converted to their GTP-bound states upon platelet activation.[1465,1466] Thus, receptor-mediated signaling activates Rho family GTPases. Cdc42 and Rac1 are activated at a very early phase of stimulation (~10 seconds) and reach maximal activation 30 seconds after stimulation with collagen, thrombin, or ADP.[1463–1465,1467] This temporal response is consistent with an early role for these GTPases in filopodia and lamellipodia formation. Integrin-dependent secondary signaling is required for full activation of RhoA,[1462] but not Cdc42 or Rac1,[1463,1465] suggesting a role for RhoA in both early (adhesion/aggregation) and late (clot retraction) stages of platelet activation. More detailed descriptions of each subfamily follows.

Ras Platelets contain at least one Ras (H-Ras).[1468] Despite its intensively studied functions in proliferation, differentiation, and cell survival in nucleated cells,[1469,1470] the exact role of Ras and its signaling in platelets is unclear. Platelets do contain most of the downstream Ras effectors: Raf-1, MEK (MAPK/ERK kinase), and ERK.[1471] Ras and ERK are both known to be activated upon platelet stimulation.[1468]

Rho Inactivation of RhoA with C3 exoenzyme treatment inhibits shape change,[1472–1474] adhesion/aggregation,[1462,1474–1476] and formation of focal adhesion.[1475] Platelets treated with the exoenzyme also show decreased stress fibers formation, a process which is mediated by Rho-kinase (ROCK)-dependent phosphorylation of myosin light chain (MLC).[1462,1472,1476]

Rac In nucleated cells, Rac1 functions in actin remodeling via activation of three downstream effectors; PIP5K Iα (phosphatidylinositol 4-phosphate 5-kinase type Iα), PAK (p21-Cdc42/Rac-activated kinase), and SCAR/WAVE (suppressor of cyclic AMP receptor/WASP-family verprolin-homologous protein).[1477] The roles of Rac1 in lamellipodia formation and aggregation have been examined using platelets from mice lacking Rac1. Rac1 deletion does not affect platelet production[1478–1480] or filopodia formation, but does affect lamellipodia formation upon stimulation with thrombin and collagen.[1478] Aggregation was diminished in $Rac1^{-/-}$ platelets when stimulated with low-dose thrombin or collagen, or when subjected to shear stress under flow condition.[1478,1480]

Cdc42 The assessment of Cdc42 function in platelets is less clear. Wiskott-Aldrich syndrome is caused by a defect in the WASP, which is a downstream effector of Cdc42. However, the platelets from affected individuals have normal shape change, including filopodia formation and Arp2/3 activation[1481] (see Chap. 121). One study suggested that Cdc42 might function in GPVI mediated integrin $\alpha_2\beta_1$ activation and subsequent platelet adhesion on collagen-coated surfaces.[1482]

Rap Rap GTPases participate in cell adhesion, cell–cell junction formation, and the development of cell polarity in nucleated cells.[1483] In platelets Rap1a, Rap1b, and Rap2 are all activated upon platelet stimulation.[1484,1485] Platelets from *Rap1b*$^{-/-}$ mice have a defect in platelet aggregation and decreased integrin $\alpha_{IIb}\beta_3$ activation upon platelet stimulation with ADP or PAR4 peptide.[1486] With the discovery of the important role of CalDAG-GEF1, an exchange factor for Rap1 in platelet function, Rap1's role in integrin signaling has been a major focus of research.[1487] Platelets lacking CalDAG-GEF1 have decreased Rap1b activation and $\alpha_{IIb}\beta_3$ activation.[1488] $\alpha_{IIb}\beta_3$ activation could be completely blocked by treating CalDAG-$GEF1^{-/-}$ platelets with a PKC inhibitor, suggesting that CalDAG-GEF1 and PKC function independently to activate $\alpha_{IIb}\beta_3$.[1489] Studies using CHO cells reconstituted with $\alpha_{IIb}\beta_3$, talin, and Rap1GTP-interacting adapter molecule (RIAM) show that Rap1-GTP-dependent talin recruitment to β_3-integrin by RIAM is required for $\alpha_{IIb}\beta_3$ activation.[1490] The function of Rap2 remains to be determined; CalDAG-GEF1 does not interact with it.[1491]

Ral In nucleated cells, Ral GTPases (RalA and RalB) are thought to function in regulated exocytosis by recruiting a multi-subunit complex termed "exocyst" for targeting secretory vesicles to specific plasma membrane domains.[1492] Both RalA and RalB in platelets are associated with platelet dense granules,[1493] and become rapidly activated in a Ca^{2+}-dependent manner upon platelet activation.[1494] A recombinant Ral-interacting domain of Sec5, a downstream effector of RalA in exocyst complex, inhibits serotonin release from platelet-dense granules, suggesting a role for Ral-exocyst in platelet granule release.[1495]

Rab Rab GTPases are the largest family of small GTPases; 63 members are detected in the human genome.[1496] They are highly compartmentalized to different organelle membranes and function by coordinating vesicle transport, including vesicle formation and tethering to their target compartments.[1496] Rab proteins have been shown to play roles in both granule biogenesis and secretion (see discussion above).

Arf Arf family GTPases, in nucleated cells, function in secretory and cytoskeletal processes. Platelets contain Arf1 or 3 and Arf6. Functional studies of Arf6 show that unlike other platelet GTPases, it is in the GTP-bound state in resting platelets and there is a conversion to the GDP-bound state upon platelet activation.[1457] Inhibitors of this transition disrupt aggregation, secretion, and clot retraction. Further analysis suggests that the Arf6-GTP to Arf6-GDP transition is required for activation of Rho family proteins in platelets.

Calcium-Dependent Proteases (Calpains) After ligand binding, integrin clustering, and platelet aggregation, neutral, cysteine proteases termed *calpains* become activated by a rise in intracellular calcium.[492] The most important and well-studied calpains in platelets are μ-calpain (calpain-1), which is activated by micromolar concentrations of calcium and accounts for 80 percent of the cysteine protease activity in platelets, and m-calpain (calpain-2), which requires millimolar levels of calcium for activation.[1497] Each calpain consists of a common 30,000 molecular weight regulatory subunit paired with a unique catalytic subunit of molecular weight 80,000. Activated μ-calpain cleaves numerous proteins[492] including cytoskeletal proteins (e.g., filamin [actin-binding protein], talin, WASP, and cortactin), tyrosine kinases (e.g., BTK, Src, Syk, and FAK), tyrosine phosphatases (e.g., protein tyrosine phosphatase 1B [PTP1B also called PTPN1], SHP-1, and PTPMEG), as well as other important platelet proteins (e.g., β_3, SNAP-23, Vav, phospholipase C-β (PLC-β), and certain isoforms of PKC.[1497] Cleavage of talin by calpain *in vitro* enables talin to activate $\alpha_{IIb}\beta_3$,[34] but the role of calpain in activation of $\alpha_{IIb}\beta_3$ by talin in intact platelets is uncertain. Calpain also appears to be upstream of, and able to affect, the activation of the small G proteins Rac and RhoA (see "Rac" and "Rho" above). Calpain's full role in platelet secretion has not been defined, although it is clear that the t-SNARE, SNAP-23 is inactivated by calpain-mediate cleavage.[1498] Thus, calpains, through their effects on structural and signaling molecules, affect multiple aspects of platelet function. Mice deficient in μ-calpain demonstrate abnormal platelet aggregation, decreased clot retraction, and reduced tyrosine phosphorylation of several platelet proteins, including the β_3 subunit of $\alpha_{IIb}\beta_3$. These abnormalities in platelet function can be reversed by inhibition of tyrosine phosphatases or by deletion of PTP1B, suggesting that μ-calpain's effects on platelet kinases and phosphatases may be central to its role in platelet function.[1499]

Inside-Out Activation of $\alpha_{IIb}\beta_3$ and Outside-In Signaling by Activated $\alpha_{IIb}\beta_3$

The active state of $\alpha_{IIb}\beta_3$ is defined as the conformation that is competent to bind large, soluble, adhesive proteins such as fibrinogen and VWF with relatively high affinity. Precise regulation of the activation state of $\alpha_{IIb}\beta_3$ is essential for maintenance of normal hemostasis, such that $\alpha_{IIb}\beta_3$ activation only occurs upon vascular injury. Crystallographic and electron microscopic studies suggest that the extracellular portion of both $\alpha_{IIb}\beta_3$ and the related integrin, $\alpha_V\beta_3$, are in a bent conformation when inactive and an extended conformation when activated.[39,658,662] The activation state of $\alpha_{IIb}\beta_3$ is controlled by the cytoplasmic domains of this integrin in concert with specific intracellular binding proteins. Thus, under basal conditions, interactions between the cytoplasmic domains of α_{IIb} and β_3 maintain the receptor in the unactivated state. Interrupting the interactions between the cytoplasmic domains results in long-range conformational changes that convert the extracellular portion of the integrin to an active state.[1500] Interactions between regions of the α_{IIb} and β_3 transmembrane and cytoplasmic domains near the membrane involve upper and lower membrane clasps and a salt bridge between acidic and basic amino acid residues of each subunit[674,679,696,697] (see "$\alpha_{IIb}\beta_3$" section above). Mutations that disrupt these interactions result in $\alpha_{IIb}\beta_3$ activation.[679,696,697] Cytoskeletal restraints appear to further maintain $\alpha_{IIb}\beta_3$ in an inactive conformation, as treatment of platelets with low doses of the actin depolymerizing agents activate the integrin.[501] Upon agonist activation, the binding of the cytoskeletal linking proteins talin and kindlin to β_3 may play a key role in the conversion of $\alpha_{IIb}\beta_3$, as well as several other integrins, to an active conformation.[37] One model suggests that filamin binding to the β_3 cytoplasmic tail maintains the receptor in an inactive state by preventing talin binding. The cytoskeletal adapter protein migfilin can displace filamin from the β_3 subunit and facilitate the binding of talin.[31] Talin itself can exist in a conformation that is either less or more favorable for binding to β_3 at multiple sites. The affinity of talin for β integrins increases in response to PIP_2 binding to talin.[1501] PIP_2 may be generated locally from phosphatidylinositol via the enzyme phosphatidylinositol phosphate kinase type 1γ(PIPKI), which can bind to talin.[1502,1503] Talin is composed of a molecular weight 47,000 head domain and a molecular weight 190,000 rod domain. The head contains a "FERM" domain named for the proteins 4.1, ezrin, radixin, and moesin, that promotes specific interactions with cytoplasmic regions of multiple proteins. The F3 region of the FERM domain, which resembles a phosphotyrosine binding domain,[1504] binds sequentially to membrane distal and proximal regions of β_3 in addition to establishing electrostatic interactions with the lipid head groups, disrupting its interaction with the membrane and α_{IIb}.[4,88,502,696,697,700,1504–1506] This binding site is not available when PIPKI is bound to talin, so presumably any prebound PIPKI would be displaced from talin upon talin interaction with β_3.[1507] After talin binding, the reorganization of the transmembrane and intracytoplasmic domains disrupt the interaction of α_{IIb} and β_3 and this is transmitted to the ectodomain.[696,697,1500] The β_3 cytoplasmic domain can also bind proteins that connect it to the cytoskeleton such as α-actinin, ICAP1, filamin, Src, and skelemin, and so it has been proposed that interactions of the β_3 subunit with the actin-myosin contraction apparatus via the cytoskeleton may supply the energy needed to adopt the extended conformation of $\alpha_{IIb}\beta_3$ with the swing out of the of β_3 hybrid domain away from the of βA (I-like) domain.[39] The rod-like region of talin has also been reported to interact with β_3[1508] and an unknown region of talin has been reported to interact with α_{IIb}.[701] Although these interactions may serve to stabilize or subsequently cluster the integrin, their exact roles are unknown.

Members of the kindlin family of focal adhesion proteins that contain phosphotyrosine binding domains serve as integrin activators,[1509–1511] perhaps functioning to facilitate talin–integrin interactions. Kindlin-2 binds the C-terminus of integrin β_3 in a region containing the conserved TS(752)T sequence and NITY(759) motif, and acts synergically with talin to promote $\alpha_{IIb}\beta_3$ activation in a recombinant expression system.[1510] Whereas kindlin-2 is widely distributed, kindlin-3 expression is limited to hematopoietic cells, including platelets. Genetic deletion of kindlin-3 in mice results in a severe bleeding phenotype and defective activation of $\alpha_{IIb}\beta_3$ on platelets.[1511] Mutations in kindlin-3 have been described in patients with leukocyte adhesion deficiency (LAD)-III, which is characterized by abnormalities in leukocyte and platelet integrin activation and function (see Chap. 121).[1512–1515] In fact, the bleeding symptoms are even more severe than those in Glanzmann thrombasthenia and the platelet aggregation defects are similar. Mutational analysis also identified the NXXY motif (Tyr795) and preceding threonine-region in kindlin binding to integrin β_1.[1516] Finally, based on model systems, it has been proposed that α_{IIb} transmembrane and cytoplasmic domains from adjacent $\alpha_{IIb}\beta_3$ receptors may form homodimers and β_3 transmembrane and cytoplasmic domains may form homotrimers, resulting in stabilization of the activated state and clustering of $\alpha_{IIb}\beta_3$ receptors,[505,1517] but it is not clear that these interactions are favored under biologic conditions.[696,697]

Platelet aggregation is commonly described as progressing through two phases, an initial reversible aggregation phase, which is often the response observed with low concentrations of agonists, followed by a stronger, irreversible phase. The irreversible phase of aggregation correlates with TXA_2 production and platelet secretion of ADP. Fibrinogen binding to $\alpha_{IIb}\beta_3$ and the platelet–platelet contacts that occur during the initial phase of aggregation initiate specific signal transduction events, resulting in positive feedback loops that promote irreversible aggregation, maintain secretion, and initiate later events like clot retraction.[704]

Fibrinogen or VWF binding to the extracellular region of $\alpha_{IIb}\beta_3$ transmits long-range conformational changes to the integrin cytoplasmic domains, perhaps via a pivot action between the β_3 βA (I-like) and hybrid domains[657] that induce signaling from outside the platelet to inside the platelet (outside-in signaling).[684,688] These conformational changes, along with integrin clustering,[654] are likely to be the bases for outside-in signal transduction through $\alpha_{IIb}\beta_3$, perhaps by altering the association of the cytoplasmic domains with one another and initiating recruitment of proteins with enzymatic activity to the cytoplasmic tails, forming complexes capable of generating signaling molecules.

One important signaling molecule that is constitutively associated with the β_3 cytoplasmic tail is the tyrosine kinase, Src.[1518–1520] Src binds to the C-terminus of the integrin in resting platelets via its SH3 domain independent of its catalytic activity.[1518] This pool of Src in unstimulated platelets appears to exist in a minimally active state with its activity suppressed in part by the Src regulator Csk, which phosphorylates Src at Tyr 529. Platelet adhesion to immobilized fibrinogen increases the Src activity associated with $\alpha_{IIb}\beta_3$ in part as a result of the dissociation of Csk and subsequent dephosphorylation of Src 529.[1519] Full Src activation occurs upon $\alpha_{IIb}\beta_3$ clustering and transphosphorylation of Src on Tyr 418. Src activation is required for several subsequent signaling events such as the activation of the tyrosine kinase Syk. Syk, along with Src, is required for platelet spreading on fibrinogen.[1518] Syk binds to unphosphorylated β_3 via its N-terminus.[1521,1522] Some of these events have now been visualized in living platelets.[1523] Negative regulators of Src activation include PECAM-1, which can recruit the protein tyrosine phosphatases SHP-1 and SHP-2 via its ITIMs[1520,1524–1526]; carcinoembryonic antigen-related cell adhesion molecule-1 (CEACAM-1), which also possess ITIMs[1527]; and perhaps G6b-B[337,1528,1529] and TLT-1.[910]

When platelets are aggregated in response to one of multiple agonists, the β_3 cytoplasmic domain becomes phosphorylated on tyrosine.[703,711] Two sites of potential tyrosine phosphorylation exist on the β_3 cytoplasmic domain and both may be used. Several molecules have been identified that bind specifically to the tyrosine-phosphorylated cytoplasmic domain of β_3. A synthetic β_3 cytoplasmic domain peptide containing phosphate groups on the two candidate tyrosines binds to the contractile protein myosin,[703] and this interaction may facilitate the transmission of cytoskeletal tension from inside the platelet to outside and thus initiate clot retraction. Recombinant, mutated β_3 that cannot be phosphorylated is unable to support extensive clot retraction when expressed in a cell line.[703] Other proteins that bind to the diphosphorylated β_3 cytoplasmic domain include the adapter proteins SHC,[712] which also become tyrosine phosphorylated during platelet aggregation.[712] Therefore, it is possible that SHC may link diphosphorylated β_3 to the Ras/Raf/MAPK pathway.[712,1530] Mice containing mutated β_3 molecules that cannot be phosphorylated exhibit a mild bleeding disorder as evidenced by occasional rebleeding of tail cuts. Moreover platelets derived from these mice form abnormally loose thrombi when activated by shear forces.[704] Other β_3 cytoplasmic-domain-binding proteins have been described, including skelemin, a member of a family of proteins that regulate myosin,[709] and talin.

Some signaling events that occur downstream of $\alpha_{IIb}\beta_3$ require only integrin clustering, whereas other events require clustering, ligand binding, and/or platelet aggregation. For example, the tyrosine kinase Syk becomes activated in response to $\alpha_{IIb}\beta_3$ clustering, independent of cytoskeletal assembly, whereas activation of the tyrosine kinase FAK requires integrin clustering, ligand binding to $\alpha_{IIb}\beta_3$, and cytoskeletal assembly.[1531] In studies conducted in cell lines, activation of Syk downstream of $\alpha_{IIb}\beta_3$ leads to phosphorylation of Vav1, a guanine nucleotide exchange factor for Rac, and lamellipodia formation. Syk and Vav1 cooperate to activate JNK, ERK2, and Akt.[1531] These pathways are also likely to be involved in postaggregation events in the platelet.

Proteins other than the well-described $\alpha_{IIb}\beta_3$ ligands fibrinogen and VWF also induce signaling events via binding to $\alpha_{IIb}\beta_3$. One such protein is CD40L, a TNF family member that is expressed on a variety of cells including activated platelets (see "CD40 Ligand (CD40L; CD154) and CD40" above). Platelets are also the major source of a soluble form of CD40L.[442] In addition to binding to its classical receptor, CD40, CD40L also binds to $\alpha_{IIb}\beta_3$ on platelets and induces signaling events[441] that are required for normal arterial thrombus formation in mice.[445] CD40L may also initiate platelet aggregation by binding to CD40 on platelets.[1048]

Inhibitory Pathways in Platelets

Prostaglandins Prostaglandins that inhibit platelet activation include PGE_2, at high concentrations, and PGI_2 (also called prostacyclin), at low concentrations (reviewed in references 1532 and 1533; see Fig. 114–11). In the vasculature, the endothelium produces PGI_2 and PGE_2, which are important in maintaining vascular patency.[1534] Inhibition is initiated by the binding of these PG to their own specific G-protein-coupled receptors.[1535,1536] Prostaglandin receptor occupancy converts the Gα subunit to the GTP bound active form, which then activates adenylyl cyclase. Adenylyl cyclase catalyzes the formation of cAMP. The exact amount of cAMP present in the cell is also determined by its rate of breakdown by phosphodiesterases (PDEs). Biochemical studies and studies from gene targeted mice support a primary role for PDE_{3A} in platelets.[1537–1539] Therefore, agents that inhibit PDE such as theophylline, caffeine, and the drug cilostazol, also elevate cAMP levels in platelets and other cells.[1540] cAMP then activates protein kinase A (PKA), which phosphorylates specific target proteins. PKA inhibits platelet activation by several pathways. One mechanism involves PKA-dependent phosphorylation of VASP as discussed under Nitric Oxide below. A separate mechanism involves the phosphorylation and inhibition of Gα13, which couples to the TXA_2 receptor, thus impairing this activation pathway.[1541] Also, PKA phosphorylates GPIbβ on serine 166, and negatively regulates the ability of GPIb to bind VWF.[1542] In addition, PKA may phosphorylate and inhibit the IP_3 receptor, which represses agonist-induced intracellular Ca^{2+}-mobilization.[1543] Phosphoinositide metabolism is also affected, as the activities of both PLC and PLA_2 are suppressed.[1544] Moreover, PKA also phosphorylates Raf kinase on three sites, which inhibits Raf kinase function in part by inhibiting its binding to the activating protein GTP-bound Ras.[1545,1546] Finally, the small G protein, Rap1b, which contributes to $\alpha_{IIb}\beta_3$ activation,[1387] is phosphorylated by PKA,[1547] although it appears that this phosphorylation event does not inhibit platelet function[1548] and in fact may contribute to Rap1b activation.[1549]

Paradoxically, in contrast to the inhibitory effects of high levels of PGE_2, low levels of PGE_2 ($<10^{-6}$ M) potentiate agonist-induced platelet aggregation by acting via the EP3 receptor to decrease intraplatelet cAMP levels.[1550,1551] Mice lacking the EP3 receptor are protected from

AA-induced thrombosis[1552]; thus it is possible that PGE_2 present in atherosclerotic lesions contributes to atherothrombosis.

Nitric Oxide Nitric oxide is synthesized from L-arginine by NO synthase in endothelial cells, platelets, and other cells. The formation of NO is enhanced at sites of shear stress and by platelet agonists (e.g., thrombin or ADP),[1553] and it readily diffuses into platelets.[1554,1555] Similar to PGI_2 or PGE_2, NO pretreatment of platelets inhibits platelet activation and can reverse platelet aggregation soon after initiation. However, NO works not by elevating cAMP, but instead by increasing cGMP.[1556] NO synthase activity in platelets increases during platelet activation, suggesting that NO production is a normal negative feedback mechanism that limits further platelet aggregation. NO and PGI_2 act together synergistically to inhibit platelet activation.[1557]

Elevation in intracellular cGMP levels activates cGMP-dependent protein kinase (PKG), whose downstream targets include ERK and the TXA_2 receptor.[1558] In mice, the absence of PKG results in enhanced platelet accumulation along damaged vessels after ischemic injury, supporting an important role for PKG in platelet deposition.[1559] VASP, a member of the proline-rich, actin-regulatory Ena/VASP protein family, is phosphorylated in response to elevations in either cAMP or cGMP,[1560] and both PKA and PKG phosphorylate VASP *in vitro*.[1561] A role for VASP in inhibition of platelet function was established in studies of VASP-deficient mice: Platelets obtained from the mice display increased P-selectin expression and $\alpha_{IIb}\beta_3$ activation in response to agonists,[1562] and platelet adhesion at sites of vascular injury or atherosclerosis is enhanced in VASP-deficient mice.[1563] The enhanced platelet adhesion in VASP-null mice is not corrected by NO, suggesting that VASP may be a key negative regulator of platelet function in the cGMP-mediated pathways.

Elevation in intracellular cGMP can also increase cAMP levels via inhibition of phosphodiesterase activity.[1564] This crosstalk between cGMP and cAMP-dependent pathways may synergize to contribute to the inhibitory effects of NO on platelet function.

CD39 (ATP Diphosphohydrolase; Ecto-ADP-ase) Vascular endothelium regulates platelet function by producing prostacyclin and NO, as well as by expressing CD39 NTPDase1, a plasma membrane-associated ecto-nucleotide (ATP diphosphohydrolase; ATPDase; ecto-ADPase; EC 3.6.1.5) that converts extracellular ATP to ADP, and ADP to AMP.[119,1565,1566] CD39 limits the platelet-activating effects of ADP released by damaged tissues, red blood cells, and activated platelets; furthermore, AMP generated by CD39 is degraded by an ecto-5′ nucleotidase (CD73; EC 3.1.3.5) to adenosine, an inhibitor of ADP-induced platelet activation, that increases cAMP binding to the A2a adenosine receptor on platelets.[1567] Adenosine deaminase (EC 3.5.4.4) degrades adenosine to inosine. CD39 is a molecular weight 95,000 cell surface glycoprotein expressed on endothelial cells, subsets of activated natural killer cells, B cells, monocytes, and T cells (see Chap. 117). Small amounts may also be on platelets and erythrocytes. It is present in the lymphocytes in chronic lymphocytic leukemia and this may partially account for the thromboprotection noted in that disorder.[1568] CD39 is localized to lipid raft-like caveolae in the plasma membrane, and the cholesterol content may control enzymatic activity. It contains two putative transmembrane regions separated by an extracellular domain with six glycosylation sites and apyrase-like regions that confer the ATPDase activity. A related molecule, NTPDase2, which is found on the basolateral surface of endothelial cells, the adventitia of some blood vessels, and microvascular pericytes, is relatively selective for ATP, and thus it has the capacity to increase platelet aggregation by enhancing the production of ADP from ATP.[1566] The physiologic roles of the NTPDases are complex because of their production of variably prothrombotic and antithrombotic agents. It has been postulated that recruitment of microparticles enriched in monocyte CD39/NTPDase1 to thrombi could contribute to the limitation of the size of platelet thrombi. A role for CD39/NTPDase1 in ischemia reperfusion and allograft rejection has also been proposed. Mouse models support the potential of modulating graft rejection and thrombosis by using gene therapy to increase CD39/NTPDase1. A soluble recombinant form of CD39 inhibits platelet aggregation and recruitment *in vitro* and may have potential as an antithrombotic agent *in vivo*.[1210]

REFERENCES

1. Holme S, Heaton A, Konchuba A, et al: Light scatter and total protein signal distribution of platelets by flow cytometry as parameters of size. *J Lab Clin Med* 112:223, 1988.
2. White JG: Anatomy and structural organization of the platelet, in *Hemostasis and Thrombosis: Basic Principles and Clinical Practice*, 3rd ed, edited by RW Colman, J Hirsh, VJ Marder, EW Salzman, p 397. JB Lippincott, Philadelphia, 1993.
3. Coller BS: Biochemical and electrostatic considerations in primary platelet aggregation. *Ann N Y Acad Sci* 416:693, 1984.
4. van Joost T, van Ulsen J, Vuzevski VD, et al: Purpuric contact dermatitis to benzoyl peroxide. *J Am Acad Dermatol* 22:359, 1990.
5. Schick PK: Megakaryocyte and platelet lipids, in *Hemostasis and Thrombosis: Basic Principles and Clinical Practice*, 3 ed, edited by RW Colman, J Hirsh, VJ Marder, EW Salzman, p 574. JB Lippincott, Philadelphia, 1993.
6. Heemskerk JW, Bevers EM, Lindhout T: Platelet activation and blood coagulation. *Thromb Haemost* 88:186, 2002.
7. Solum NO: Procoagulant expression in platelets and defects leading to clinical disorders. *Arterioscler Thromb Vasc Biol* 19:2841, 1999.
8. Sims PJ, Faioni EM, Wiedmer T, et al: Complement proteins C5b-9 cause release of membrane vesicles from the platelet surface that are enriched in the membrane receptor for coagulation factor Va and express prothrombinase activity. *J Biol Chem* 263:18205, 1988.
9. Sims PJ, Wiedmer T, Esmon CT, et al: Assembly of the platelet prothrombinase complex is linked to vesiculation on the platelet plasma membrane. Studies in Scott syndrome: An isolated defect in platelet procoagulant activity. *J Biol Chem* 264:137, 1989.
10. Bevers EM, Tilly RHJ, Senden JMG, et al: Exposure of endogenous phosphatidylserine at the outer surface of stimulated platelets is reversed by restoration of aminophospholipid translocase activity. *Biochemistry* 28:2382, 1989.
11. Tuszynski GP, Mauco GP, Koshy A, et al: The platelet cytoskeleton contains elements of the prothrombinase complex. *J Biol Chem* 259:6947, 1984.
12. Comfurius P, Bevers EM, Zwaal RFA: The involvement of cytoskeleton in the regulation of transbilayer movement of phospholipids in human blood platelets. *Biochim Biophys Acta* 815:143, 1985.
13. Bodin S, Tronchere H, Payrastre B: Lipid rafts are critical membrane domains in blood platelet activation processes. *Biochim Biophys Acta* 1610:247, 2003.
14. Locke D, Chen H, Liu Y, et al: Lipid rafts orchestrate signaling by the platelet receptor glycoprotein VI. *J Biol Chem* 277:18801, 2002.
15. Shrimpton CN, Borthakur G, Larrucea S, et al: Localization of the adhesion receptor glycoprotein Ib-IX-V complex to lipid rafts is required for platelet adhesion and activation. *J Exp Med* 196:1057, 2002.
16. Heijnen HF, Van Lier M, Waaijenborg S, et al: Concentration of rafts in platelet filopodia correlates with recruitment of c-Src and CD63 to these domains. *J Thromb Haemost* 1:1161, 2003.
17. Bodin S, Tronchere H, Payrastre B: Lipid rafts are critical membrane domains in blood platelet activation processes. *Biochim Biophys Acta* 1610:247, 2003.
18. Bodin S, Giuriato S, Ragab J, et al: Production of phosphatidylinositol 3,4,5-trisphosphate and phosphatidic acid in platelet rafts: Evidence for a critical role of cholesterol-enriched domains in human platelet activation. *Biochemistry* 40:15290, 2001.
19. Baglia FA, Shrimpton CN, Lopez JA, et al: The glycoprotein Ib-IX-V complex mediates localization of factor XI to lipid rafts on the platelet membrane. *J Biol Chem* 278:21744, 2003.
20. Brownlow SL, Harper AG, Harper MT, et al: A role for hTRPC1 and lipid raft domains in store-mediated calcium entry in human platelets. *Cell Calcium* 35:107, 2004.
21. Lopez JA, del Conde I, Shrimpton CN: Receptors, rafts, and microvesicles in thrombosis and inflammation. *J Thromb Haemost* 3:1737, 2005.
22. Fox JE: The platelet cytoskeleton. *Thromb Haemost* 70:884, 1993.
23. Fox JEB, Boyles JK, Berndt MC, et al: Identification of a membrane skeleton in platelets. *J Cell Biol* 106:1525, 1988.
24. Fox JEB, Reynolds CC, Morrow JS, et al: Spectrin is associated with membrane-bound actin filaments in platelets and is hydrolyzed by the Ca2+-dependent protease during platelet activation. *Blood* 69:537, 1987.
25. Hartwig JH, DeSisto M: The cytoskeleton of the resting human blood platelet: Structure of the membrane skeleton and its attachment to actin filaments. *J Cell Biol* 112:407, 1991.

26. Barkalow K, Italiano JE Jr, Matsuoka Y, et al: A-Adducin dissociates from F-actin filaments and spectrin during platelet activation. *J Cell Biol* 161:557, 2003.
27. Kaiser HW, O'Keefe E, Bennett V: Adducin: Ca++-dependent association with sites of cell–cell contact. *J Cell Biol* 109:557, 1989.
28. Kuhlman PA, Hughes CA, Bennett V, et al: A new function for adducin. Calcium/calmodulin-regulated capping of the barbed ends of actin filaments. *J Biol Chem* 271:7986, 1996.
29. Matsuoka Y, Li X, Bennett V: Adducin: Structure, function, and regulation. *Cell Mol Life Sci* 57:884, 2000.
30. Fox JE: The platelet cytoskeleton. *Thromb Haemost* 70:884, 1993.
31. Ithychanda SS, Das M, Ma YQ, et al: Migfilin, a molecular switch in regulation of integrin activation. *J Biol Chem* 284:4713, 2009.
32. Kiema T, Lad Y, Jiang P, et al: The molecular basis of filamin binding to integrins and competition with talin. *Mol Cell* 21:337, 2006.
33. Calderwood DA, Huttenlocher A, Kiosses WB, et al: Increased filamin binding to beta-integrin cytoplasmic domains inhibits cell migration. *Nat Cell Biol* 3:1060, 2001.
34. Yan B, Calderwood DA, Yaspan B, et al: Calpain cleavage promotes talin binding to the beta 3 integrin cytoplasmic domain. *J Biol Chem* 276:28164, 2001.
35. Ulmer TS, Yaspan B, Ginsberg MH, et al: NMR analysis of structure and dynamics of the cytosolic tails of integrin alpha IIb beta 3 in aqueous solution. *Biochemistry* 40:7498, 2001.
36. Vinogradova O, Velyvis A, Velyviene A, et al: A Structural mechanism of integrin alpha(IIb)beta(3) "inside-out" activation as regulated by its cytoplasmic face. *Cell* 110:587, 2002.
37. Tadokoro S, Shattil SJ, Eto K, et al: Talin binding to integrin beta tails: A final common step in integrin activation. *Science* 302:103, 2003.
38. Tremuth L, Kreis S, Melchior C, et al: A fluorescence cell biology approach to map the second integrin-binding site of talin to a 130-amino acid sequence within the rod domain. *J Biol Chem* 279:22258, 2004.
39. Zhu J, Luo BH, Xiao T, et al: Structure of a complete integrin ectodomain in a physiologic resting state and activation and deactivation by applied forces. *Mol Cell* 32:849, 2008.
40. Podor TJ, Singh D, Chindemi P, et al: Vimentin exposed on activated platelets and platelet microparticles localizes vitronectin and plasminogen activator inhibitor complexes on their surface. *J Biol Chem* 277:7529, 2002.
41. Nurden P, Heilmann E, Pannocchia A, et al: Two-way trafficking of membrane glycoproteins on thrombin-activated human platelets. *Semin Hematol* 31:240, 1994.
42. Cramer EM, Norol F, Guichard J, et al: Ultrastructure of platelet formation by human megakaryocytes cultured with the Mpl ligand. *Blood* 89:2336, 1997.
43. Italiano JE Jr, Lecine P, Shivdasani RA, et al: Blood platelets are assembled principally at the ends of proplatelet processes produced by differentiated megakaryocytes. *J Cell Biol* 147:1299, 1999.
44. Italiano JE, Hartwig JH: Megakaryocyte development and platelet formation, in *Platelets*, edited by AD Michelson, p 23. Academic Press, San Diego, 2007.
45. Crawford N, Scrutton MC: Biochemistry of the blood platelet, in *Haemostasis and Thrombosis*, 3rd ed, edited by AL Bloom, CD Forbes, DP Thomas, EGD Tuddenham, p 89. Churchill Livingstone, Edinburgh, Scotland, 1994.
46. Hartwig JH: Platelet structure, in *Platelets*, 2nd ed, edited by AD Michelson, p 75. Academic Press, San Diego, 2007.
47. Sheetz MP: Microtubule motor complexes moving membranous organelles. *Cell Struct Funct* 21:369, 1996.
48. Miki H, Okada Y, Hirokawa N: Analysis of the kinesin superfamily: Insights into structure and function. *Trends Cell Biol* 15:467, 2005.
49. Pfister KK, Shah PR, Hummerich H, et al: Genetic analysis of the cytoplasmic dynein subunit families. *PLoS Genet* 2:e1, 2006.
50. Kenney DM, Linck RW: The cytoskeleton of unstimulated blood platelets: Structure and composition of the isolated marginal microtubular band. *J Cell Sci* 78:1, 1985.
51. Kenney DM, Linck RW: The cytoskeleton of unstimulated blood platelets: Structure and composition of the isolated marginal microtubular band. *J Cell Sci* 78:1, 1985.
52. Patel-Hett S, Richardson JL, Schulze H, et al: Visualization of microtubule growth in living platelets reveals a dynamic marginal band with multiple microtubules. *Blood* 111:4605, 2008.
53. Italiano JE Jr, Bergmeier W, Tiwari S, et al: Mechanisms and implications of platelet discoid shape. *Blood* 101:4789, 2003.
54. Freson K, De Vos R, Wittevrognel C, et al: The β1-tubulin Q43P functional polymorphism reduces the risk of cardiovascular disease in men by modulating platelet function and structure. *Blood* 106:2356, 2005.
55. Kunishima S, Kobayashi R, Itoh TJ, et al: Mutation of the beta1-tubulin gene associated with congenital macrothrombocytopenia affecting microtubule assembly. *Blood* 113:458, 2009.
56. Nachmias VT, Yoshida K: The cytoskeleton of the blood platelet: A dynamic structure. *Adv Cell Biol* 2:181, 1988.
57. Safer D, Nachmias VT: Beta thymosins as actin binding peptides. *Bioessays* 16:473, 1994.
58. Rosenberg S, Stracher A: Effect of actin-binding protein on the sedimentation properties of actin. *J Cell Biol* 94:51, 1982.
59. Rosenberg S, Stracher A, Lucas RC: Isolation and characterization of actin and actin-binding protein from human platelets. *J Cell Biol* 91:201, 1981.
60. Rosenberg S, Stracher A, Burridge K: Isolation and characterization of a calcium-sensitive alpha-actinin-like protein from human platelet cytoskeletons. *J Biol Chem* 256:12986, 1981.
61. Fucini P, Renner C, Herberhold C, et al: The repeating segments of the F-actin cross-linking gelation factor (ABP-120) have an immunoglobulin-like fold. *Nat Struct Biol* 4:223, 1997.
62. Gorlin JB, Yamin R, Egan S, et al: Human endothelial actin-binding protein (ABP-280, non-muscle filamin): A molecular leaf spring. *J Cell Biol* 111:1089, 1990.
63. Gorlin JB, Henske E, Warren ST, et al: Actin-binding protein (ABP-280) filamin gene (FLN) maps telomeric to the color vision locus (R/GCP) and centromeric to G6PD in Xq28. *Genomics* 17:496, 1993.
64. Takafuta T, Wu G, Murphy GF, et al: Human beta-filamin is a new protein that interacts with the cytoplasmic tail of glycoprotein 1ba. *J Biol Chem* 273:17531, 1998.
65. Ohta Y, Suxuki N, Nakamura S, et al: The small GTPase RalA targets filamin to induce filopodia. *Proc Natl Acad Sci U S A* 96:2122, 1999.
66. Stossel TP, Condeelis J, Cooley L, et al: Filamins as integrators of cell mechanics and signalling. *Nat Rev Mol Cell Biol* 2:138, 2001.
67. Kovacsovics TJ, Hartwig JH: Thrombin-induced GPIb-IX centralization on the platelet surface requires actin assembly and myosin II activation. *Blood* 87:618, 1996.
68. Meyer SC, Zuerbig S, Cunningham CC, et al: Identification of the region in actin-binding protein that binds to the cytoplasmic domain of glycoprotein IBalpha. *J Biol Chem* 272:2914, 1997.
69. van den BH, de Vet EC, Zomer AW: The role of peroxisomes in ether lipid synthesis. Back to the roots of PAF. *Adv Exp Med Biol* 416:33, 1996.
70. Wanders RJ, van Weringh G, Schrakamp G, et al: Deficiency of acyl-CoA:dihydroxyacetone phosphate acyltransferase in thrombocytes of Zellweger patients: A simple postnatal diagnostic test. *Clin Chim Acta* 151:217, 1985.
71. van den BH, Schrakamp G, Hardeman D, et al: Ether lipid synthesis and its deficiency in peroxisomal disorders. *Biochimie* 75:183, 1993.
72. Holmsen H: Platelet secretion and energy metabolism, in *Hemostasis and Thrombosis: Basic Principles and Clinical Practice*, 3rd ed, edited by RW Colman, J Hirsh, VJ Marder, EW Salzman, p 524. JB Lippincott, Philadelphia, 1993.
73. Shuster RC, Rubenstein AJ, Wallace DC: Mitochondrial DNA in anucleate human blood cells. *Biochem Biophys Res Commun* 155:1360, 1988.
74. Mason KD, Carpinelli MR, Fletcher JI, et al: Programmed anuclear cell death delimits platelet life span. *Cell* 128:1173, 2007.
75. Schapira AH: Mitochondrial dysfunction in neurodegenerative disorders. *Biochim Biophys Acta* 1366:225, 1998.
76. Lenaz G, Bovina C, Castelluccio C, et al: Mitochondrial complex I defects in aging. *Mol Cell Biochem* 174:329, 1997.
77. Cardoso SM, Proenca MT, Santos S, et al: Cytochrome c oxidase is decreased in Alzheimer's disease platelets. *Neurobiol Aging* 25:105, 2004.
78. Mancuso M, Filosto M, Bosetti F, et al: Decreased platelet cytochrome c oxidase activity is accompanied by increased blood lactate concentration during exercise in patients with Alzheimer disease. *Exp Neurol* 182:421, 2003.
79. Lenaz G, D'Aurelio M, Merlo PM, et al: Mitochondrial bioenergetics in aging. *Biochim Biophys Acta* 1459:397, 2000.
80. Dror N, Klein E, Karry R, et al: State-dependent alterations in mitochondrial complex I activity in platelets: A potential peripheral marker for schizophrenia. *Mol Psychiatry* 7:995, 2002.
81. Yamagishi SI, Edelstein D, Du XL, et al: Hyperglycemia potentiates collagen-induced platelet activation through mitochondrial superoxide overproduction. *Diabetes* 50:1491, 2001.
82. Dale GL, Friese P: Bax activators potentiate coated-platelet formation. *J Thromb Haemost* 4:2664, 2006.
83. Jobe SM, Wilson KM, Leo L, et al: Critical role for the mitochondrial permeability transition pore and cyclophilin D in platelet activation and thrombosis. *Blood* 111:1257, 2008.
84. Leung R, Gwozdz AM, Wang H, et al: Persistence of procoagulant surface expression on activated human platelets: Involvement of apoptosis and aminophospholipid translocase activity. *J Thromb Haemost* 5:560, 2007.
85. Remenyi G, Szasz R, Friese P, et al: Role of mitochondrial permeability transition pore in coated-platelet formation. *Arterioscler Thromb Vasc Biol* 25:467, 2005.
86. Karpatkin S, Langer RM: Biochemical energetics of simulated platelet plug formation: Effect of thrombin, adenosine diphosphate, and epinephrine on intra- and extracellular adenine nucleotide kinetics. *J Clin Invest* 47:2158, 1968.
87. Akkerman JWN, Gorter G, Schrama L, et al: A novel technique for rapid determination of energy consumption in platelets: Determination of different energy consumption associated with three secretory responses. *Biochem J* 210:145, 1983.
88. Akkerman JWN, Holmsen H: Interrelationships among platelet responses: Studies on the burst in protein liberation, lactate production and oxygen uptake during platelet aggregation and Ca++ secretion. *Blood* 57:956, 1981.
89. Akkerman JWN, Verhgoeven AJM: Energy metabolism and function, in *Platelet Responses and Metabolism,* 3rd ed, edited by H Holmsen, p 69. CRC Press, Boca Raton, FL, 1987.
90. Holmsen H, Farstad M: Energy metabolism, in *Platelet Responses and Metabolism,* 2nd ed, edited by H Holmsen, p 245. CRC Press, Boca Raton, FL, 1987.
91. Guppy M, Abas L, Neylon C, et al: Fuel choices by human platelets in human plasma. *Eur J Biochem* 244:161, 1997.
92. Shimizu T, Murphy S: Roles of acetate and phosphate in the successful storage of platelet concentrates prepared with an acetate-containing additive solution. *Transfusion* 33:304, 1993.

93. Simons ER, Greenberg-Sperssky SM: Transmembrane monovalent cation gradients, in *Platelet Responses and Metabolism*, 3rd ed, edited by H Holmsen, p 31. CRC Press, Boca Raton, FL, 1987.
94. Dean WL: Structure, function and subcellular localization of a human platelet Ca^{++}-ATPase. *Cell Calcium* 10:289, 1989.
95. Daniel JL, Molish IR, Robkin L, et al: Nucleotide exchange between cytosolic ATP and F-actin-bound ADP may be a major ATP-utilizing process in unstimulated platelets. *Eur J Biochem* 156:677, 1986.
96. Verhoeven AJM, Tysnes O-B, Aarbakke GM, et al: Turnover of the phosphomonoester groups of polyphosphoinositol lipids in unstimulated platelets. *Eur J Biochem* 166:3, 1987.
97. Holmsen H, Kaplan KL, Dangelmaier CA: Differential energy requirements for platelet responses: A simultaneous study of aggregation three secretory processes, arachidonate liberation, phosphatidylinositol turnover and phosphatide production. *Biochem J* 208:9, 1982.
98. Verhoeven AJM, Mommersteeg ME, Akkerman JWN: Quantification of energy consumption in platelets during thrombin-induced aggregation and secretion: Tight coupling between platelet responses and the increment in energy consumption. *Biochem J* 221:777, 1984.
99. Holmsen H, Kaplan KL, Dangelmaier CA: Differential requirements for platelet responses: A simultaneous study of dense granule, α-granule and acid hydrolase secretion, arachidonate liberation, phosphatidylinositol turnover and phosphatidate formation. *Biochem J* 208:9, 1982.
100. Akkerman JW, Gorter G, Soons H, et al: Close correlation between platelet responses and adenylate energy charge during transient substrate depletion. *Biochim Biophys Acta* 760:34, 1983.
101. Huizing M, Helip-Wooley A, Westbroek W, et al: Disorders of lysosome-related organelle biogenesis: Clinical and molecular genetics. *Annu Rev Genomics Hum Genet* 9:359, 2008.
102. Ciferri S, Emiliani C, Guglielmini G, et al: Platelets release their lysosomal content in vivo in humans upon activation. *Thromb Haemost* 83:157, 2000.
103. Nieuwenhuis HK, van Osterhout JJG, Rozemuller E, et al: Studies with a monoclonal antibody against activated platelets: Evidence that a secreted 53,000 molecular weight lysosome-like granule protein is exposed on the surface of activated platelets in the circulation. *Blood* 70:838, 1987.
104. Abrams C, Shattil SJ: Immunological detection of activated platelets in clinical disorders. *Thromb Haemost* 65:467, 1991.
105. Zhang ZG, Zhang L, Tsang W, et al: Dynamic platelet accumulation at the site of the occluded middle cerebral artery and in downstream microvessels is associated with loss of microvascular integrity after embolic middle cerebral artery occlusion. *Brain Res* 912:181, 2001.
106. Castellot JJ, Favreau LV, Karnovsky MJ, et al: Inhibition of vascular smooth muscle cell growth by endothelial cell derived heparin. Possible role of a platelet endoglucosidase. *J Biol Chem* 257:11256, 1982.
107. McNicol A, Israels SJ: Platelet dense granules: Structure, function and implications for haemostasis. *Thromb Res* 95:1, 1999.
108. Ugurbil K, Holmsen H, Shulman RG: Adenine nucleotide storage pools and secretion in platelets as studied by 31P nuclear magnetic resonance. *Proc Natl Acad Sci U S A* 76:2227, 1979.
109. Ugurbil K, Fukami MH, Holmsen H: 31P-NMR studies of nucleotide and amine storage in the dense granules of pig platelets. *Biochemistry* 23:4097, 1984.
110. Lesurtel M, Graf R, Aleil B, et al: Platelet-derived serotonin mediates liver regeneration. *Science* 312:104, 2006.
111. Gunay-Aygun M, Huizing M, Gahl WA: Molecular defects that affect platelet dense granules. *Semin Thromb Hemost* 30:537, 2004.
112. Youssefian T, Cramer EM: Megakaryocyte dense granule components are sorted in multivesicular bodies. *Blood* 95:4004, 2000.
113. Nagle DL, Karim MA, Woolf EA, et al: Identification and mutation analysis of the complete gene for Chédiak-Higashi syndrome. *Nat Genet* 14:307, 1996.
114. FitzGerald GA: Dipyridamole. *N Engl J Med* 316:1247, 1987.
115. Marcus AJ, Safier LB, Hajjar KA, et al: Inhibition of platelet function by an aspirin-insensitive endothelial cell ADPase. Thromboregulation by endothelial cells. *J Clin Invest* 88:1690, 1991.
116. Naik UP, Kornecki E, Ehrlich YH: Phosphorylation and dephosphorylation of human platelet surface proteins by an ecto-protein kinase/phosphatase system. *Biochim Biophys Acta* 1092:256, 1991.
117. Kalafatis M, Rand MD, Jenny RJ, et al: Phosphorylation of factor Va and factor VIIIa by activated platelets. *Blood* 81:704, 1993.
118. Hatmi M, Gavaret JM, Elalamy I, et al: Evidence for cAMP-dependent platelet ectoprotein kinase activity that phosphorylates platelet glycoprotein IV (CD36). *J Biol Chem* 271:24776, 1996.
119. Marcus AJ, Broekman MJ, Drosopoulos JH, et al: The endothelial cell ecto-ADPase responsible for inhibition of platelet function is CD39. *J Clin Invest* 99:1351, 1997.
120. Harrison P, Cramer EM: Platelet α granules. *Blood Rev* 7:52, 1993.
121. Reed GL: Platetet secretion, in *Platelets*, 2nd ed, edited by AD Michelson, p 309. Academic Press, San Diego, 2007.
122. Hayward CP, Furmaniak-Kazmierczak E, Cieutat AM, et al: Factor V is complexed with multimerin in resting platelet lysates and colocalizes with multimerin in platelet alpha-granules. *J Biol Chem* 270:19217, 1995.
123. Maynard DM, Heijnen HF, Horne MK, et al: Proteomic analysis of platelet alpha-granules using mass spectrometry. *J Thromb Haemost* 5:1945, 2007.
124. Coppinger JA, Cagney G, Toomey S, et al: Characterization of the proteins released from activated platelets leads to localization of novel platelet proteins in human atherosclerotic lesions. *Blood* 103:2096, 2004.
125. McRedmond JP, Park SD, Reilly DF, et al: Integration of proteomics and genomics in platelets: A profile of platelet proteins and platelet-specific genes. *Mol Cell Proteomics* 3:133, 2004.
126. Italiano JE Jr, Richardson JL, Patel-Hett S, et al: Angiogenesis is regulated by a novel mechanism: Pro- and antiangiogenic proteins are organized into separate platelet alpha granules and differentially released. *Blood* 111:1227, 2008.
127. Sehgal S, Storrie B: Evidence that differential packaging of the major platelet granule proteins von Willebrand factor and fibrinogen can support their differential release. *J Thromb Haemost* 5:2009, 2007.
128. George JN: Platelet immunoglobulin G: Its significance for the evaluation of thrombocytopenia and for understanding the origin of alpha-granule protein. *Blood* 76:859, 1990.
129. George JN: Platelet IgG: Measurement, interpretation, and clinical significance. *Prog Hemost Thromb* 10:97–126:97, 1991.
130. Heijnen HF, Debili N, Vainchencker W, et al: Multivesicular bodies are an intermediate stage in the formation of platelet alpha-granules. *Blood* 91:2313, 1998.
131. Niewiarowski S, Holt JC, Cook JJ: Biochemistry and physiology of secreted platelet proteins, in *Hemostasis and Thrombosis: Basic Principles and Clinical Practice*, 3rd ed, edited by RW Colman, J Hirsh, VJ Marder, EW Salzman, p 546. JB Lippincott, Philadelphia, 1993.
132. Niewiarowski S: Secreted platelet proteins, in *Haemostasis and Thrombosis*, 3rd ed, edited by AL Bloom, CD Forbes, DP Thomas, EGD Tuddenham, p 167. Churchill Livingstone, Edinburgh, Scotland, 1994.
133. Kawahara RS, Deuel TF: Platelet-derived growth factor-inducible gene JE is a member of a family of small inducible genes related to platelet factor 4. *J Biol Chem* 264:679, 1989.
134. Brown KD, Zurawski SM, Mosmann TR, et al: A family of small inducible proteins secreted by leukocytes are members of a new super-family that includes leukocyte and fibroblast-derived inflammatory agents, growth factors, and indicators of various activation processes. *J Immunol* 142:679, 1989.
135. Oppenheim JJ, Zachariae COC, Mukaida N, et al: Properties of the novel proinflammatory supergene "intercrine" cytokine family. *Annu Rev Immunol* 9:617, 1991.
136. Rollins BJ: Chemokines. *Blood* 90:909, 1997.
137. Gear AR, Camerini D: Platelet chemokines and chemokine receptors: Linking hemostasis, inflammation, and host defense. *Microcirculation* 10:335, 2003.
138. Handin RI, Cohen HJ: Purification and binding properties of human platelet factor 4. *J Biol Chem* 58:731, 1976.
139. Loscalzo J, Melnick B, Handin RI: The interaction of platelet factor 4 and glycosaminoglycans. *Arch Biochem Biophys* 240:446, 1985.
140. Rucinski B, Niewiarowski S, Strzyzewski M, et al: Human platelet factor 4 and its C-terminal peptides: Heparin binding and clearance from the circulation. *Thromb Haemost* 63:493, 1990.
141. Barber AG, Kaser-Glanzmann R, Jakabova M, et al: Chromatography of chondroitin sulfate proteoglycan carrier for heparin neutralizing activity (platelet factor 4) released from human blood platelets. *Biochim Biophys Acta* 286:312, 1972.
142. Huang SS, Huang JS, Deuel TF: Proteoglycan carrier of human platelet factor 4: Isolation and characterization. *J Biol Chem* 257:11546, 1982.
143. Cowan SW, Bakshi EN, Machim KJ, et al: Binding of heparin to human platelet factor 4. *Biochem J* 234:485, 1986.
144. Busch C, Dawes J, Pepper DW, et al: Binding of platelet factor 4 to cultured human umbilical vein endothelial cells. *Thromb Res* 19:129, 1980.
145. Clore GM, Gronenborn AM: Three-dimensional structures of alpha and beta chemokines. *FASEB J* 9:57, 1995.
146. Visentin GP, Ford SE, Scott JP, et al: Antibodies from patients with heparin-induced thrombocytopenia/thrombosis are specific for platelet factor 4 complexed with heparin or bound to endothelial cells. *J Clin Invest* 93:81, 1994.
147. Warkentin TE: Heparin-induced thrombocytopenia. *Curr Hematol Rep* 1:63, 2002.
148. Rucinski B, Stewart GJ, DeFeo PA, et al: Uptake and processing of human platelet factor 4 by hepatocytes. *Proc Soc Exp Biol Med* 186:361, 1987.
149. Deuel TF, Senior RM, Change D, et al: Platelet factor 4 is chemotactic for neutrophils and monocytes. *Proc Natl Acad Sci U S A* 78:4854, 1981.
150. Maione TE, Gray GS, Petro J, et al: Inhibition of angiogenesis by recombinant human platelet factor-4 and related peptides. *Science* 247:77, 1990.
151. Brindley LL, Sweet JM, Goetzl EJ: Stimulation of histamine release from human basophils by human platelet factor 4. *J Clin Invest* 72:1218, 1983.
152. Maione TE, Gray GS, Petro J, et al: Inhibition of angiogenesis by recombinant human platelet factor-4 and related peptides. *Science* 247:77, 1990.
153. Gewirtz AM, Calabretta B, Rucinski B, et al: Inhibition of human megakaryocytopoiesis *in vitro* by platelet factor 4 and a synthetic C-terminal PF4 peptide. *J Clin Invest* 83:1477, 1989.
154. Han ZC, Sensebe L, Abgrall JF, et al: Platelet factor 4 inhibits human megakaryocytopoiesis *in vitro*. *Blood* 75:1234, 1990.
155. Lambert MP, Rauova L, Bailey M, et al: Platelet factor 4 is a negative autocrine *in vivo* regulator of megakaryopoiesis: Clinical and therapeutic implications. *Blood* 110:1153, 2007.
156. Katz IR, Thorbecke GJ, Bell MK, et al: Protease-induced immunoregulatory activity of platelet factor 4. *Proc Natl Acad Sci U S A* 83:3491, 1986.

157. Beyth RJ, Culp LA: Complementary adhesive responses of human skin fibroblasts to the cell-binding domain of fibronectin and the heparin sulfate-binding protein, platelet factor 4. *Exp Cell Res* 155:537, 1984.
158. Capitanio AM, Niewiarowski S, Rucinski B, et al: Interaction of platelet factor 4 with human platelets. *Biochim Biophys Acta* 839:161, 1985.
159. Dumenco LL, Everson B, Culp LA, et al: Inhibition of the activation of Hageman factor (Factor XII) by platelet factor 4. *J Lab Clin Med* 112:394, 1988.
160. Engstad CS, Lia K, Rekdal O, et al: A novel biological effect of platelet factor 4 (PF4): Enhancement of LPS-induced tissue factor activity in monocytes. *J Leukoc Biol* 58:575, 1995.
161. Aziz KA, Cawley JC, Zuzel M: Platelets prime PMN via released PF4: Mechanism of priming and synergy with GM-CSF. *Br J Haematol* 91:846, 1995.
162. Castor CW, Miller JW, Walz D: Structural and biological characteristics of connective tissue activating peptide (CTAP III), a major human platelet-derived growth factor. *Proc Natl Acad Sci U S A* 80:765, 1983.
163. Holt JC, Harrie ME, Holt AM, et al: Characterization of human platelet basic protein, a precursor form of low-affinity platelet factor 4 and beta-thromboglobulin. *Biochemistry* 25:1988, 1986.
164. Walz A, Dewald B, von Tscharner V, et al: Effects of the neutrophil-activating peptide NAP-2, platelet basic protein, connective tissue-activating peptide III and platelet factor 4 on human neutrophils. *J Exp Med* 170:1745, 1989.
165. Bastl CP, Musial J, Kloczewiak M, et al: Role of kidney in the catabolic clearance of human platelet antiheparin proteins from rat circulation. *Blood* 57:233, 1981.
166. Hayward CP: Multimerin: A bench-to-bedside chronology of a unique platelet and endothelial cell protein—from discovery to function to abnormalities in disease. *Clin Invest Med* 20:176, 1997.
167. Polgar J, Magnenat E, Wells TN, et al: Platelet glycoprotein Ia* is the processed form of multimerin—Isolation and determination of N-terminal sequences of stored and released forms. *Thromb Haemost* 80:645, 1998.
168. Hayward CP, Cramer EM, Song Z, et al: Studies of multimerin in human endothelial cells. *Blood* 91:1304, 1998.
169. Harrison P: Platelet α-granular fibrinogen. *Platelets* 3:1, 1992.
170. Coller BS, Seligsohn U, West SM, et al: Absence of the γ-Leu 427 (γ') variant in the platelet alpha-granular fibrinogen pool supports the role of glycoprotein IIb/IIIa in mediating fibrinogen uptake in platelets/megakaryocytes. *Blood* 79:3394, 1992.
171. Ni H, Yuen PS, Papalia JM, et al: Plasma fibronectin promotes thrombus growth and stability in injured arterioles. *Proc Natl Acad Sci U S A* 100:2415, 2003.
172. Reheman A, Yang H, Zhu G, et al: Plasma fibronectin depletion enhances platelet aggregation and thrombus formation in mice lacking fibrinogen and von Willebrand factor. *Blood* 113:1809, 2009.
173. Cho J, Mosher DF: Role of fibronectin assembly in platelet thrombus formation. *J Thromb Haemost* 4:1461, 2006.
174. Coller BS, Seligsohn U, West SM, et al: Platelet fibrinogen and vitronectin in Glanzmann thrombasthenia: Evidence consistent with specific roles for glycoprotein IIb/IIIA and $\alpha V\beta 3$ integrins in platelet protein trafficking. *Blood* 78:2603, 1991.
175. Fay WP, Parker AC, Ansari MN, et al: Vitronectin inhibits the thrombotic response to arterial injury in mice. *Blood* 93:1825, 1999.
176. Eitzman DT, Westrick RJ, Nabel EG, et al: Plasminogen activator inhibitor-1 and vitronectin promote vascular thrombosis in mice. *Blood* 95:577, 2000.
177. Konstantinides S, Schafer K, Thinnes T, et al: Plasminogen activator inhibitor-1 and its cofactor vitronectin stabilize arterial thrombi after vascular injury in mice. *Circulation* 103:576, 2001.
178. Baenziger NL, Brodie GN, Majerus PW: A thrombin-sensitive protein of human platelet membranes. *Proc Natl Acad Sci U S A* 68:240, 1971.
179. Lawler J, Hynes RO: The structure of human thrombospondin, an adhesive glycoprotein with multiple calcium-binding sites and homologies with several different proteins. *J Cell Biol* 103:1635, 1986.
180. Adams JC, Lawler J: The thrombospondins. *Int J Biochem Cell Biol* 36:961, 2004.
181. Mosher DF, Doyle MJ, Jaffe EA: Synthesis and secretion of thrombospondin by cultured human endothelial cells. *J Cell Biol* 93:343, 1982.
182. Schwartz BS: Monocyte synthesis of thrombospondin. *J Biol Chem* 264:7512, 1989.
183. Plow EF, McEver RP, Coller BS, et al: Related binding mechanisms for fibrinogen, fibronectin, von Willebrand factor and thrombospondin on thrombin-stimulated human platelets. *Blood* 66:724, 1985.
184. Lawler J, Hynes RO: An integrin receptor on normal and thrombasthenic platelets which binds thrombospondin. *Blood* 74:2022, 1989.
185. Asch AS, Liu I, Briccetti FM, et al: Analysis of CD36 binding domains: Ligand specificity controlled by dephosphorylation of an ectodomain. *Science* 262:1436, 1993.
186. Aiken ML, Ginsberg MH, Byers-Ward V, et al: Effects of OKM5, a monoclonal antibody to glycoprotein IV, on platelet aggregation and thrombospondin surface expression. *Blood* 76:2501, 1990.
187. Chung J, Wang XQ, Lindberg FP, et al: Thrombospondin-1 acts via IAP/CD47 to synergize with collagen in alpha2beta1-mediated platelet activation. *Blood* 94:642, 1999.
188. Chung J, Gao AG, Frazier WA: Thrombospondin acts via integrin-associated protein to activate the platelet integrin $\alpha IIb\beta 3$. *J Biol Chem* 272:14740, 1997.
189. Jurk K, Clemetson KJ, de Groot PG, et al: Thrombospondin-1 mediates platelet adhesion at high shear via glycoprotein Ib (GPIb): An alternative/backup mechanism to von Willebrand factor. *FASEB J* 17:1490, 2003.
190. Gao AG, Lindberg FP, Finn MB, et al: Integrin-associated protein is a receptor for the C-terminal domain of thrombospondin. *J Biol Chem* 271:21, 1996.
191. Leung LLK, Nachman RL: Complex formation of platelet thrombospondin with fibrinogen. *J Clin Invest* 70:542, 1982.
192. Tuszynski GP, Srivastava S, Switalska HI, et al: The interaction of human platelet thrombospondin with fibrinogen. *J Biol Chem* 260:12240, 1985.
193. Elzie CA, Murphy-Ullrich JE: The N-terminus of thrombospondin: The domain stands apart. *Int J Biochem Cell Biol* 36:1090, 2004.
194. Dardik R, Lahav J: Functional changes in the conformation of thrombospondin-1 during complexation with fibronectin or heparin. *Exp Cell Res* 248:407, 1999.
195. Leung LLK: Role of thrombospondin in platelet aggregation. *J Clin Invest* 74:1764, 1984.
196. Silverstein RL, Leung LLK, Harpel PC, et al: Complex formation of platelet thrombospondin with plasminogen. *J Clin Invest* 74:1625, 1984.
197. Schultz-Cherry S, Murphy-Ullrich JE: Thrombospondin causes activation of latent transforming growth factor-beta secreted by endothelial cells by a novel mechanism. *J Cell Biol* 122:923, 1993.
197a. Ahamed J, Janczak CA, Wittkowski KM, Coller BS: *In vitro* and *in vivo* evidence that thrombospondin-1 (TSP-1) contributes to stirring- and shear-dependent activation of platelet-derived TGF-beta1. *PLoS One* 4:e6608, 2009.
198. Tracy PB, Eide LC, Bowie EJW, et al: Radioimmunoassay of factor V in human plasma and platelets. *Blood* 60:59, 1982.
199. Chesney CM, Pifer D, Colman RW: Subcellular localization and secretion of factor V from human platelets. *Proc Natl Acad Sci U S A* 78:5180, 1981.
200. Bouchard BA, Butenas S, Mann KG, et al: Interactions between platelets and the coagulation system, in *Platelets*, edited by AD Michelson, p 229. Academic Press, San Diego, 2002.
201. Camire RM, Pollak ES, Kaushansky K, et al: Secretable human platelet-derived factor V originates from the plasma pool. *Blood* 92:3035, 1998.
202. Yang TL, Pipe SW, Yang A, et al: Biosynthetic origin and functional significance of murine platelet factor V. *Blood* 102:2851, 2003.
203. Kane WH, Mruk JS, Majerus PW: Activation of coagulation factor V by a platelet protease. *J Clin Invest* 70:1092, 1982.
204. Tracy PB, Nesheim ME, Mann KG: Proteolytic alterations of factor Va bound to platelets. *J Biol Chem* 662:669, 1983.
205. Gould WR, Silveira JR, Tracy PB: Unique *in vivo* modifications of coagulation factor V produce a physically and functionally distinct platelet-derived cofactor: Characterization of purified platelet-derived factor V/Va. *J Biol Chem* 279:2383, 2004.
206. Tracy PB, Giles AR, Mann KG, et al: Factor V (Quebec): A bleeding diathesis associated with a qualitative platelet factor V deficiency. *J Clin Invest* 74:1221, 1984.
207. Nesheim ME, Nichols WL, Cole TL, et al: Isolation and study of an acquired inhibitor of human coagulation factor V. *J Clin Invest* 405:415, 1986.
208. Bode AP, Sandberg H, Dombrose FA, et al: Association of factor V activity with membranous vesicles released from human platelets: Requirement for platelet stimulation. *Thromb Res* 39:49, 1985.
209. Manfioletti G, Brancolini C, Avanzi G, et al: The protein encoded by a growth arrest-specific gene (gas6) is a new member of the vitamin K-dependent proteins related to protein S, a negative coregulator in the blood coagulation cascade. *Mol Cell Biol* 13:4976, 1993.
210. Melaragno MG, Fridell YW, Berk BC: The Gas6/Axl system: A novel regulator of vascular cell function. *Trends Cardiovasc Med* 9:250, 1999.
211. Angelillo-Scherrer A, de Frutos P, Aparicio C, et al: Deficiency or inhibition of Gas6 causes platelet dysfunction and protects mice against thrombosis. *Nat Med* 7:215, 2001.
212. Chen C, Li Q, Darrow AL, et al: Mer receptor tyrosine kinase signaling participates in platelet function. *Arterioscler Thromb Vasc Biol* 24:1118, 2004.
213. Gould WR, Baxi SM, Schroeder R, et al: Gas6 receptors Axl, Sky and Mer enhance platelet activation and regulate thrombotic responses. *J Thromb Haemost* 3:733, 2005.
214. Saller F, Burnier L, Schapira M, et al: Role of the growth arrest-specific gene 6 (gas6) product in thrombus stabilization. *Blood Cells Mol Dis* 36:373, 2006.
215. Angelillo-Scherrer A, Burnier L, Flores N, et al: Role of Gas6 receptors in platelet signaling during thrombus stabilization and implications for antithrombotic therapy. *J Clin Invest* 115:237, 2005.
216. Maree AO, Jneid H, Palacios IF, et al: Growth arrest specific gene (GAS) 6 modulates platelet thrombus formation and vascular wall homeostasis and represents an attractive drug target. *Curr Pharm Des* 13:2656, 2007.
217. Deuel TF, Huang SS, Huang JS: Platelet derived growth factor: Purification, characterization and role in normal and abnormal cell growth, in *Biochemistry of Platelets*, edited by DR Phillips, MA Shuman, p 347. Academic Press, London, 1986.
218. Heldin C-H, Westermark B: Platelet-derived growth factor: Three isoforms and two receptor types. *Trends Genet* 5:108, 1989.
219. Ross R: Peptide regulatory factors. Platelet-derived growth factor. *Lancet* 1:1179, 1989.
220. Madtes DK, Raines EW, Ross R: Modulation of local concentrations of platelet-derived growth factor. *Am Rev Respir Dis* 140:1118, 1989.
221. Berk BC, Alexander RW: Vasoactive effects of growth factors. *Biochem Pharmacol* 38:219, 1989.
222. Waterfield MD, Scrace GT, Whittle N, et al: Platelet-derived growth factor is structurally related to the putative transforming protein p28-sis of simian sarcoma virus. *Nature* 304:35, 1983.
223. Doolittle RF, Hunkapiller MW, Hood LE, et al: Simian sarcoma virus onc gene, v-sis, is derived from the gene (or genes) encoding a platelet-derived growth factor. *Science* 22:275, 1983.

224. Williams LT: Signal transduction by the platelet-derived growth factor receptor. *Science* 24:1564, 1989.
225. Nagai MK, Embil JM: Becaplermin: Recombinant platelet derived growth factor, a new treatment for healing diabetic foot ulcers. *Expert Opin Biol Ther* 2:211, 2002.
226. Maloney JP, Silliman CC, Ambruso DR, et al: In vitro release of vascular endothelial growth factor during platelet aggregation. *Am J Physiol* 275:H1054, 1998.
227. Weltermann A, Wolzt M, Petersmann K, et al: Large amounts of vascular endothelial growth factor at the site of hemostatic plug formation *in vivo*. *Arterioscler Thromb Vasc Biol* 19:1757, 1999.
228. Webb NJ, Bottomley MJ, Watson CJ, et al: Vascular endothelial growth factor (VEGF) is released from platelets during blood clotting: Implications for measurement of circulating VEGF levels in clinical disease. *Clin Sci (Lond)* 94:395, 1998.
229. Mohle R, Green D, Moore MA, et al: Constitutive production and thrombin-induced release of vascular endothelial growth factor by human megakaryocytes and platelets. *Proc Natl Acad Sci U S A* 94:663, 1997.
230. Amirkhosravi A, Amaya M, Siddiqui F, et al: Blockade of GPIIb/IIIa inhibits the release of vascular endothelial growth factor (VEGF) from tumor cell-activated platelets and experimental metastasis. *Platelets* 10:285, 1999.
231. Katoh O, Tauchi H, Kawaishi K, et al: Expression of the vascular endothelial growth factor (VEGF) receptor gene, KDR, in hematopoietic cells and inhibitory effect of VEGF on apoptotic cell death caused by ionizing radiation. *Cancer Res* 55:5687, 1995.
232. Wartiovaara U, Salven P, Mikkola H, et al: Peripheral blood platelets express VEGF-C and VEGF which are released during platelet activation. *Thromb Haemost* 80:171, 1998.
233. Salven P, Orpana A, Joensuu H: Leukocytes and platelets of patients with cancer contain high levels of vascular endothelial growth factor. *Clin Cancer Res* 5:487, 1999.
234. Verheul HM, Pinedo HM: Tumor growth: A putative role for platelets? *Oncologist* 3:II, 1998.
235. Solovey A, Gui L, Ramakrishnan S, et al: Sickle cell anemia as a possible state of enhanced anti-apoptotic tone: Survival effect of vascular endothelial growth factor on circulating and unanchored endothelial cells. *Blood* 93:3824, 1999.
236. Cao J, Mathews MK, McLeod DS, et al: Angiogenic factors in human proliferative sickle cell retinopathy. *Br J Ophthalmol* 83:838, 1999.
237. Kiuru J, Viinikka L, Myllyla G, et al: Cytoskeleton-dependent release of human platelet epidermal growth factor. *Life Sci* 49:1997, 1991.
238. Busch AI, Martins RN, Rumble B, et al: The amyloid precursor protein of Alzheimer's disease is released by human platelets. *J Biol Chem* 265:15977, 1990.
239. Li Q, Beyreuther K, Masters CL: Alzheimer's disease, in *Platelets*, 2nd ed, edited by AD Michelson, p 779. Academic Press, San Diego, 2007.
240. Bush AI, Martins RN, Rumble B, et al: The amyloid precursor protein of Alzheimer's disease is released by human platelets. *J Biol Chem* 265:15977, 1990.
241. Li QX, Whyte S, Tanner JE, et al: Secretion of Alzheimer's disease Aβ amyloid peptide by activated human platelets. *Lab Invest* 78:461, 1998.
242. Li Q, Cappai R, Evin G, et al: Products of the Alzheimer's disease amyloid precursor protein generated by β-secretase are present in human platelets, and secreted upon degranulation. *Am J Alzheimers Dis* 13:236, 1998.
243. Li QX, Evin G, Small DH, et al: Proteolytic processing of Alzheimer's disease beta A4 amyloid precursor protein in human platelets. *J Biol Chem* 270:14140, 1995.
244. Li QX, Berndt MC, Bush AI, et al: Membrane-associated forms of the beta A4 amyloid protein precursor of Alzheimer's disease in human platelet and brain: Surface expression on the activated human platelet. *Blood* 84:133, 1994.
245. Van Nostrand WE, Schmaier AH, Farrow JS, et al: Protease nexin-2/amyloid beta-protein precursor in blood is a platelet-specific protein. *Biochem Biophys Res Commun* 175:15, 1991.
246. Scandura JM, Zhang Y, Van Nostrand WE, et al: Progress curve analysis of the kinetics with which blood coagulation factor XIa is inhibited by protease nexin-2. *Biochemistry* 36:412, 1997.
247. Schmaier AH, Dahl LD, Rozemuller AJM, et al: Protease nexin-2/amyloid β protein precursor. A tight-binding inhibitor of coagulation factor IXa. *J Clin Invest* 92:2540, 1993.
248. Schmaier AH, Dahl LD, Hasan AA, et al: Factor IXa inhibition by protease nexin-2/amyloid beta-protein precursor on phospholipid vesicles and cell membranes. *Biochemistry* 34:1171, 1995.
249. Rosenberg RN, Baskin F, Fosmire JA, et al: Altered amyloid protein processing in platelets of patients with Alzheimer disease. *Arch Neurol* 54:139, 1997.
250. Borroni B, Akkawi N, Martini G, et al: Microvascular damage and platelet abnormalities in early Alzheimer's disease. *J Neurol Sci* 203–204:189, 2002.
251. Di Luca M, Pastorino L, Bianchetti A, et al: Differential level of platelet amyloid beta precursor protein isoforms: An early marker for Alzheimer disease. *Arch Neurol* 55:1195, 1998.
252. Baskin F, Rosenberg RN, Iyer L, et al: Platelet APP isoform ratios correlate with declining cognition in AD. *Neurology* 54:1907, 2000.
253. Davies TA, Long HJ, Tibbles HE, et al: Moderate and advanced Alzheimer's patients exhibit platelet activation differences. *Neurobiol Aging* 18:155, 1997.
254. Davies TA, Fine RE, Johnson RJ, et al: Non-age related differences in thrombin responses by platelets from male patients with advanced Alzheimer's disease. *Biochem Biophys Res Commun* 194:537, 1993.
255. McDonagh J, McDonagh RP, Jr, Delage JM, et al: Factor XIII in human plasma and platelets. *J Clin Invest* 48:940, 1969.
256. Devine DV, Bishop PD: Platelet-associated factor XIII in platelet activation, adhesion, and clot stabilization. *Semin Thromb Hemost* 22:409, 1996.
257. Lorand L, Graham RM: Transglutaminases: Crosslinking enzymes with pleiotropic functions. *Nat Rev Mol Cell Biol* 4:140, 2003.
258. Adany R, Bardos H: Factor XIII subunit A as an intracellular transglutaminase. *Cell Mol Life Sci* 60:1049, 2003.
259. Inbal A, Muszbek L, Lubetsky A, et al: Platelets but not monocytes contribute to the plasma levels of factor XIII subunit A in patients undergoing autologous peripheral blood stem cell transplantation. *Blood Coagul Fibrinolysis* 15:249, 2004.
260. Serrano K, Devine DV: Intracellular factor XIII crosslinks platelet cytoskeletal elements upon platelet activation. *Thromb Haemost* 88:315, 2002.
261. Huff T, Otto AM, Muller CS, et al: Thymosin beta4 is released from human blood platelets and attached by factor XIIIa (transglutaminase) to fibrin and collagen. *FASEB J* 16:691, 2002.
262. Kulkarni S, Jackson SP: Platelet factor XIII and calpain negatively regulate integrin alpha IIbbeta 3 adhesive function and thrombus growth. *J Biol Chem* 279:30697, 2004.
263. Szasz R, Dale GL: Thrombospondin and fibrinogen bind serotonin-derivatized proteins on COAT-platelets. *Blood* 100:2827, 2002.
264. Szasz R, Dale GL: COAT platelets. *Curr Opin Hematol* 10:351, 2003.
265. Massague J: TGFbeta in Cancer. *Cell* 134:215, 2008.
266. ten Dijke P, Arthur HM: Extracellular control of TGFbeta signalling in vascular development and disease. *Nat Rev Mol Cell Biol* 8:857, 2007.
267. Rubtsov YP, Rudensky AY: TGFbeta signalling in control of T-cell-mediated self-reactivity. *Nat Rev Immunol* 7:443, 2007.
268. Leask A: TGFbeta, cardiac fibroblasts, and the fibrotic response. *Cardiovasc Res* 74:207, 2007.
269. Sakamaki S, Hirayama Y, Matsunaga T, et al: Transforming growth factor-beta1 (TGF-beta1) induces thrombopoietin from bone marrow stromal cells, which stimulates the expression of TGF- beta receptor on megakaryocytes and, in turn, renders them susceptible to suppression by TGF-beta itself with high specificity. *Blood* 94:1961, 1999.
270. Shi Y, Massague J: Mechanisms of TGF-beta signaling from cell membrane to the nucleus. *Cell* 113:685, 2003.
271. Hoying JB, Yin M, Diebold R, et al: Transforming growth factor beta1 enhances platelet aggregation through a non-transcriptional effect on the fibrinogen receptor. *J Biol Chem* 274:31008, 1999.
272. Kronemann N, Bouloumi A, Bassus S, et al: Aggregating human platelets stimulate expression of vascular endothelial growth factor in cultured vascular smooth muscle cells through a synergistic effect of transforming growth factor-beta(1) and platelet-derived growth factor(AB). *Circulation* 100:855, 1999.
273. Annes JP, Munger JS, Rifkin DB: Making sense of latent TGFbeta activation. *J Cell Sci* 116:217, 2003.
274. Blakytny R, Ludlow A, Martin GE, et al: Latent TGF-beta1 activation by platelets. *J Cell Physiol* 199:67, 2004.
275. Ahamed J, Burg N, Yoshinaga K, et al: *In vitro* and *in vivo* evidence for shear-induced activation of latent transforming growth factor-beta1. *Blood* 112:3650, 2008.
276. Abdelouahed M, Ludlow A, Brunner G, et al: Activation of platelet-transforming growth factor beta-1 in the absence of thrombospondin-1. *J Biol Chem* 275:17933, 2000.
277. Crawford SE, Stellmach V, Murphy-Ullrich JE, et al: Thrombospondin-1 is a major activator of TGF-beta1 *in vivo*. *Cell* 93:1159, 1998.
278. Ahamed J, Janczak CA, Wittkowski KM, Coller BS: *In vitro* and *in vivo* evidence that thrombospondin-1 (TSP-1) contributes to stirring- and shear-dependent activation of platelet-derived TGF-β1. *PLoS ONE* 4:e6608, 2009.
279. Slivka SR, Loskutoff DJ: Platelets stimulate endothelial cells to synthesize type 1 plasminogen activator inhibitor. Evaluation of the role of transforming growth factor beta. *Blood* 77:1013, 1991.
280. Lin HY, Wang XF, Ng-Eaton E, et al: Expression cloning of the TGF-beta type II receptor, a functional transmembrane serine/threonine kinase. *Cell* 68:775, 1992.
281. Fuhrman B, Brook GJ, Aviram M: Proteins derived from platelet alpha granules modulate the uptake of oxidized low density lipoprotein by macrophages. *Biochim Biophys Acta* 1127:15, 1992.
282. Heijnen HF, Schiel AE, Fijnheer R, et al: Activated platelets release two types of membrane vesicles: Microvesicles by surface shedding and exosomes derived from exocytosis of multivesicular bodies and alpha-granules. *Blood* 94:3791, 1999.
283. Janiszewski M, Do Carmo AO, Pedro MA, et al: Platelet-derived exosomes of septic individuals possess proapoptotic NAD(P)H oxidase activity: A novel vascular redox pathway. *Crit Care Med* 32:818, 2004.
284. Ts'ao CH: Rough endoplasmic reticulum and ribosomes in blood platelets. *Scand J Haematol* 8:134, 1971.
285. Booyse FM, Hoveke TP, Rafelson ME Jr: Studies on human platelets. II. Protein synthetic activity of various platelet populations. *Biochim Biophys Acta* 157:660, 1968.
286. Gnatenko DV, Perrotta PL, Bahou WF: Proteomic approaches to dissect platelet function: Half the story. *Blood* 108:3983, 2006.
287. Weyrich AS, Schwertz H, Kraiss LW, et al: Protein synthesis by platelets: Historical and new perspectives. *J Thromb Haemost* 7:241, 2009.
288. Weyrich AS, Dixon DA, Pabla R, et al: Signal-dependent translation of a regulatory protein, Bcl-3, in activated human platelets. *Proc Natl Acad Sci U S A* 95:5556, 1998.
289. Weyrich AS, Denis MM, Schwertz H, et al: MTOR-dependent synthesis of Bcl-3 controls the retraction of fibrin clots by activated human platelets. *Blood* 109:1975, 2007.

290. Denis MM, Tolley ND, Bunting M, et al: Escaping the nuclear confines: Signal-dependent pre-mRNA splicing in anucleate platelets. *Cell* 122:379, 2005.
291. Schwertz H, Tolley ND, Foulks JM, et al: Signal-dependent splicing of tissue factor pre-mRNA modulates the thrombogenicity of human platelets. *J Exp Med* 203:2433, 2006.
292. Behnke O: The morphology of blood platelet membrane systems. *Ser Haematol* 3:3, 1970.
293. White JG: Electron microscopic studies of platelet secretion. *Prog Hemost Thromb* 2:49, 1974.
294. Suzuki H, Yamazaki H, Tanoue K: Immunocytochemical studies on co-localization of alpha-granule membrane alphaIIbbeta3 integrin and intragranular fibrinogen of human platelets and their cell-surface expression during the thrombin-induced release reaction. *J Electron Microsc (Tokyo)* 52:183, 2003.
295. Stenberg PE, Shuman MA, Levine SP, et al: Redistribution of α granules and their contents in thrombin-stimulated platelets. *J Cell Biol* 98:748, 1984.
296. Ginsberg MH, Taylor L, Painter RG: The mechanism of thrombin-induced platelet factor 4 secretion. *Blood* 55:661, 1980.
297. George JN, Pickett EB, Saucerman S, et al: Platelet surface glycoproteins. Studies on resting and activated platelets and platelet membrane microparticles in normal subjects, and observations in patients during adult respiratory distress syndrome and cardiac surgery. *J Clin Invest* 78:340, 1986.
298. Michelson AD: Thrombin-induced down-regulation of the platelet membrane glycoprotein Ib-IX complex. *Semin Thromb Hemost* 18:18, 1992.
299. Michelson AD, Barnard MR: Plasmin-induced redistribution of platelet glycoprotein Ib. *Blood* 76:2005, 1990.
300. Suzuki H, Nakamura S, Itoh Y, et al: Immunocytochemical evidence for the translocation of α-granule membrane glycoprotein IIb/IIIa (integrin αIIbβ3) of human platelets to the surface membrane during the release reaction. *Histochemistry* 97:381, 1992.
301. Suzuki H, Murasaki K, Kodama K, et al: Intracellular localization of glycoprotein VI in human platelets and its surface expression upon activation. *Br J Haematol* 121:904, 2003.
302. Nurden P, Poujol C, Winckler J, et al: Immunolocalization of P2Y1 and TPalpha receptors in platelets showed a major pool associated with the membranes of alpha-granules and the open canalicular system. *Blood* 101:1400, 2003.
303. Breton-Gorius J, Guichard J: Ultrastructural localization of peroxidase activity in human platelets and megakaryocytes. *Am J Pathol* 66:277, 1972.
304. White JG: Interaction of membrane systems in blood platelets. *Am J Pathol* 66:295, 1972.
305. Cramer EM: Platelets and megakaryocytes: Anatomy and structural organization, in *Hemostasis and Thrombosis: Basic Principles in Clinical Practice*, edited by RW Colman, J Hirsh, VJ Marder, AW Clowes, JN George, p 411. Lippincott, Williams & Wilkins, Philadelphia, 2001.
306. Robblee LS, Shepro D, Belamarich FA: Calcium uptake and associated adenosine triphosphate activity of isolated platelet membranes. *J Gen Physiol* 61:462, 1973.
307. Menashi S, Davis C, Crawford N: Calcium uptake associated with an intracellular membrane fraction prepared from human blood platelets by high-voltage, free-flow electrophoresis. *FEBS Lett* 140:298, 1982.
308. Bergmeier W, Stefanini L: Novel molecules in calcium signaling in platelets. *J Thromb Haemost* 7:187, 2009.
309. Varga-Szabo D, Braun A, Nieswandt B: Calcium signaling in platelets. *J Thromb Haemost* 7:1057, 2009.
310. Michalak M, Mariani P, Opas M: Calreticulin, a multifunctional Ca2+ binding chaperone of the endoplasmic reticulum. *Biochem Cell Biol* 76:779, 1998.
311. Hartwig JH: Platelet morphology, in *Thrombosis and Hemorrhage*, 2nd ed, edited by J Loscalzo, AI Schafer, p 207. Williams & Wilkins, Baltimore, MD, 1999.
312. Brownlow SL, Sage SO: Rapid agonist-evoked coupling of type II Ins(1,4,5)P3 receptor with human transient receptor potential (hTRPC1) channels in human platelets. *Biochem J* 375:697, 2003.
313. van Gorp RM, Feijge MA, Vuist WM, et al: Irregular spiking in free calcium concentration in single, human platelets. Regulation by modulation of the inositol trisphosphate receptors. *Eur J Biochem* 269:1543, 2002.
314. Kaser-Glanzmann R, Jakabova M, George JN, et al: Further characterization of calcium accumulating vesicles from human blood platelets. *Biochim Biophys Acta* 542:357, 1978.
315. Tertyshnikova S, Fein A: Inhibition of inositol 1,4,5-trisphosphate-induced Ca2+ release by cAMP- dependent protein kinase in a living cell. *Proc Natl Acad Sci U S A* 95:1613, 1998.
316. Pernollet MG, Lantoine F, Devynck MA: Nitric oxide inhibits ATP-dependent Ca2+ uptake into platelet membrane vesicles. *Biochem Biophys Res Commun* 222:780, 1996.
317. Teijeiro RG, Silveira JR, Sotelo JR, et al: Calcium efflux from platelet vesicles of the dense tubular system. Analysis of the possible contribution of the Ca2+ pump. *Mol Cell Biochem* 199:7, 1999.
318. Grosse J, Braun A, Varga-Szabo D, et al: An EF hand mutation in Stim1 causes premature platelet activation and bleeding in mice. *J Clin Invest* 117:3540, 2007.
319. Dziadek MA, Johnstone LS: Biochemical properties and cellular localisation of STIM proteins. *Cell Calcium* 42:123, 2007.
320. Varga-Szabo D, Braun A, Kleinschnitz C, et al: The calcium sensor STIM1 is an essential mediator of arterial thrombosis and ischemic brain infarction. *J Exp Med* 205:1583, 2008.
321. Braun A, Varga-Szabo D, Kleinschnitz C, et al: Orai1 (CRACM1) is the platelet SOC channel and essential for pathological thrombus formation. *Blood* 113:2056, 2009.
322. Bergmeier W, Oh-Hora M, McCarl CA, et al: R93W mutation in Orai1 causes impaired calcium influx in platelets. *Blood* 113:675, 2009.
323. Feske S, Muller JM, Graf D, et al: Severe combined immunodeficiency due to defective binding of the nuclear factor of activated T cells in T lymphocytes of two male siblings. *Eur J Immunol* 26:2119, 1996.
324. Feske S, Gwack Y, Prakriya M, et al: A mutation in Orai1 causes immune deficiency by abrogating CRAC channel function. *Nature* 441:179, 2006.
325. Picard C, McCarl CA, Papolos A, et al: STIM1 mutation associated with a syndrome of immunodeficiency and autoimmunity. *N Engl J Med* 360:1971, 2009.
326. Redondo PC, Jardin I, Lopez JJ, et al: Intracellular Ca2+ store depletion induces the formation of macromolecular complexes involving hTRPC1, hTRPC6, the type II IP3 receptor and SERCA3 in human platelets. *Biochim Biophys Acta* 1783:1163, 2008.
327. Sage SO, Brownlow SL, Rosado JA: TRP channels and calcium entry in human platelets. *Blood* 100:4245, 2002.
328. Varga-Szabo D, Authi KS, Braun A, et al: Store-operated Ca(2+) entry in platelets occurs independently of transient receptor potential (TRP) C1. *Pflugers Arch* 457:377, 2008.
329. Gerrard JM, White JG, Rao GHR, et al: Localization of platelet prostaglandin production in the platelet dense tubular system. *Am J Pathol* 83:283, 1976.
330. Picot D, Loll PJ, Garavito RM: The X-ray crystal structure of the membrane protein prostaglandin H_2 synthase-1. *Nature* 367:243, 1994.
331. Garcia A, Senis Y, Tomlinson MG, et al: Platelet genomics and proteomics, in *Platelets*, 2nd ed, edited by AD Michelson, p 99. Academic Press, San Diego, 2007.
332. Garcia A, Prabhakar S, Brock CJ, et al: Extensive analysis of the human platelet proteome by two-dimensional gel electrophoresis and mass spectrometry. *Proteomics* 4:656, 2004.
333. Marcus K, Immler D, Sternberger J, et al: Identification of platelet proteins separated by two-dimensional gel electrophoresis and analyzed by matrix assisted laser desorption/ionization-time of flight-mass spectrometry and detection of tyrosine-phosphorylated proteins. *Electrophoresis* 21:2622, 2000.
334. Martens L, Van Damme P, Van Damme J, et al: The human platelet proteome mapped by peptide-centric proteomics: A functional protein profile. *Proteomics* 5:3193, 2005.
335. O'Neill EE, Brock CJ, von Kriegsheim AF, et al: Towards complete analysis of the platelet proteome. *Proteomics* 2:288, 2002.
336. Moebius J, Zahedi RP, Lewandrowski U, et al: The human platelet membrane proteome reveals several new potential membrane proteins. *Mol Cell Proteomics* 4:1754, 2005.
337. Senis YA, Tomlinson MG, Garcia A, et al: A comprehensive proteomics and genomics analysis reveals novel transmembrane proteins in human platelets and mouse megakaryocytes including G6b-B, a novel immunoreceptor tyrosine-based inhibitory motif protein. *Mol Cell Proteomics* 6:548, 2007.
338. Maguire PB, Foy M, Fitzgerald DJ: Using proteomics to identify potential therapeutic targets in platelets. *Biochem Soc Trans* 33:409, 2005.
339. Hernandez-Ruiz L, Valverde F, Jimenez-Nunez MD, et al: Organellar proteomics of human platelet dense granules reveals that 14-3-3zeta is a granule protein related to atherosclerosis. *J Proteome Res* 6:4449, 2007.
340. Garcia BA, Smalley DM, Cho H, et al: The platelet microparticle proteome. *J Proteome Res* 4:1516, 2005.
340a. Power KA, McRedmond JP, de Stefani A, et al: High-throughput proteomics detection of novel splice isoforms in human platelets. *PLoS One* 4:e5001, 2009.
340b. Dittrich M, Birschmann I, Mietner S, et al: Platelet protein interactions: Map, signaling components, and phosphorylation groundstate. *Arterioscler Thromb Vasc Biol* 28:1326, 2008.
340c. Cagney G, McRedmond J: A central resource for platelet proteomics. *Arterioscler Thromb Vasc Biol* 28:1214, 2008.
341. Foy M, Harney DF, Wynne K, et al: Enrichment of phosphotyrosine proteome of human platelets by immunoprecipitation. *Methods Mol Biol* 357:313, 2007.
342. Garcia A, Senis YA, Antrobus R, et al: A global proteomics approach identifies novel phosphorylated signaling proteins in GPVI-activated platelets: Involvement of G6f, a novel platelet Grb2-binding membrane adapter. *Proteomics* 6:5332, 2006.
343. Maguire PB, Wynne KJ, Harney DF, et al: Identification of the phosphotyrosine proteome from thrombin activated platelets. *Proteomics* 2:642, 2002.
344. Zahedi RP, Lewandrowski U, Wiesner J, et al: Phosphoproteome of resting human platelets. *J Proteome Res* 7:526, 2008.
344a. Qureshi AH, Chaoji V, Maiguel D, Faridi MH, et al: Proteomic and phospho-proteomic profile of human platelets in basal, resting state: Insights into integrin signaling. *PLoS One* 4:e7627, 2009.
345. Bugert P, Dugrillon A, Gunaydin A, et al: Messenger RNA profiling of human platelets by microarray hybridization. *Thromb Haemost* 90:738, 2003.
346. Gnatenko DV, Dunn JJ, McCorkle SR, et al: Transcript profiling of human platelets using microarray and serial analysis of gene expression. *Blood* 101:2285, 2003.
347. Dittrich M, Birschmann I, Mietner S, et al: Platelet protein interactions: Map, signaling components, and phosphorylation ground state. *Arterioscler Thromb Vasc Biol* 28:1326, 2008.
348. Newman PJ, Valentin N: Human platelet alloantigens: Recent findings, new perspectives. *Thromb Haemost* 74:234, 1995.
349. Yee DL, Bray PF: Clinical and functional consequences of platelet membrane glycoprotein polymorphisms. *Semin Thromb Hemost* 30:591, 2004.

350. Vijayan KV, Bray PF: Molecular mechanisms of prothrombotic risk due to genetic variations in platelet genes: Enhanced outside-in signaling through the Pro33 variant of integrin beta3. *Exp Biol Med (Maywood)* 231:505, 2006.

350a. Jones CI, Bray S, Garner SF, et al: A functional genomics approach reveals novel quantitative trait loci associated with platelet signaling pathways. *Blood* 114:1405, 2009.

351. Afshar-Kharghan V, Vijayan KV, Bray PF: Platelet polymorphisms, in *Platelets*, 2nd ed, edited by AD Michelson, p 281. Academic Press, San Diego, 2007.

352. Bray PF: Platelet hyperreactivity: Predictive and intrinsic properties. *Hematol Oncol Clin North Am* 21:633, 2007.

353. Ruggeri ZM: Platelets in atherothrombosis. *Nat Med* 8:1227, 2002.

354. Badimon L, Badimon JJ, Turitto VT, et al: Platelet thrombus formation on collagen type I. A model of deep vessel injury. Influence of blood rheology, von Willebrand factor, and blood coagulation. *Circulation* 78:1431, 1988.

355. Coller BS: Platelets in cardiovascular thrombosis and thrombolysis, in *The Heart and Cardiovascular System*, 2nd ed, edited by HA Fozzard, RB Jennings, AM Katz, HE Morgan, E Haber, p 219. Raven Press, New York, 1991.

356. Weiss HJ, Turitto VT, Baumgartner HR, et al: Evidence for the presence of tissue factor activity on subendothelium. *Blood* 73:968, 1989.

357. Wilcox JN, Smith KM, Schwartz SM, et al: Localization of tissue factor in the normal vessel wall and in the atherosclerotic plaque. *Proc Natl Acad Sci U S A* 86:2839, 1989.

358. Goldsmith HL, Turitto VT: Rheological aspects of thrombosis and haemostasis: Basic principles and applications. *Thromb Haemost* 55:415, 1986.

359. de Groot PG, Sixma JJ: Perfusion chambers, in *Platelets*, edited by AD Michelson, p 575. Academic Press, San Diego, 2007.

360. Savage B, Ruggeri ZM: Platelet thrombus formation in flowing blood, in *Platelets*, edited by AD Michelson, p 359. Academic Press, San Diego, 2007.

361. Jackson SP, Nesbitt WS, Westein E: Dynamics of platelet thrombus formation. *J Thromb Haemost* 7:17, 2009.

362. Giesen PL, Rauch U, Bohrmann B, et al: Blood-borne tissue factor: Another view of thrombosis. *Proc Natl Acad Sci U S A* 96:2311, 1999.

363. Furie B, Furie BC: Role of platelet P-selectin and microparticle PSGL-1 in thrombus formation. *Trends Mol Med* 10:171, 2004.

364. Bogdanov VY, Balasubramanian V, Hathcock J, et al: Alternatively spliced human tissue factor: A circulating, soluble, thrombogenic protein. *Nat Med* 9:458, 2003.

365. Engelmann B, Luther T, Muller I: Intravascular tissue factor pathway—A model for rapid initiation of coagulation within the blood vessel. *Thromb Haemost* 89:3, 2003.

366. Mezzano D, Matus V, Saez CG, et al: Tissue factor storage, synthesis and function in normal and activated human platelets. *Thromb Res* 122 Suppl 1:S31, 2008.

367. Schwertz H, Tolley ND, Foulks JM, et al: Signal-dependent splicing of tissue factor pre-mRNA modulates the thrombogenicity of human platelets. *J Exp Med* 203:2433, 2006.

368. Panes O, Matus V, Saez CG, et al: Human platelets synthesize and express functional tissue factor. *Blood* 109:5242, 2007.

369. Osterud B: The role of platelets in decrypting monocyte tissue factor. *Semin Hematol* 38:2, 2001.

370. Reinhardt C, von Bruhl ML, Manukyan D, et al: Protein disulfide isomerase acts as an injury response signal that enhances fibrin generation via tissue factor activation. *J Clin Invest* 118:1110, 2008.

371. Muller I, Klocke A, Alex M, et al: Intravascular tissue factor initiates coagulation via circulating microvesicles and platelets. *FASEB J* 17:476, 2003.

372. Cambien B, Wagner DD: A new role in hemostasis for the adhesion receptor P-selectin. *Trends Mol Med* 10:179, 2004.

373. Scholz T, Temmler U, Krause S, et al: Transfer of tissue factor from platelets to monocytes: Role of platelet-derived microvesicles and CD62P. *Thromb Haemost* 88:1033, 2002.

374. Roth GJ: Developing relationships: Arterial platelet adhesion, glycoprotein Ib, and leucine-rich glycoproteins. *Blood* 77:5, 1991.

375. Ruggeri ZM: Structure and function of von Willebrand factor. *Thromb Haemost* 82:576, 1999.

376. Andrews RK, Shen Y, Gardiner EE, et al: The glycoprotein Ib-IX-V complex in platelet adhesion and signaling. *Thromb Haemost* 82:357, 1999.

377. Ruggeri ZM: Von Willebrand factor, platelets and endothelial cell interactions. *J Thromb Haemost* 1:1335, 2003.

378. Savage B, Ruggeri ZM: Platelet thrombus formation in flowing blood, in *Platelets*, edited by AD Michelson, p 215. Academic Press, San Diego, 2002.

379. Mailhac A, Badimon JJ, Fallon JT, et al: Effect of an eccentric severe stenosis on fibrin(ogen) deposition on severely damaged vessel wall in arterial thrombosis. Relative contribution of fibrin(ogen) and platelets. *Circulation* 90:988, 1994.

380. Moake JL, Turner NA, Stathopoulos NA, et al: Involvement of large plasma von Willebrand factor (vWF) multimers and unusually large vWF forms derived from endothelial cells in shear stress-induced platelet aggregation. *J Clin Invest* 78:1456, 1986.

381. Ikeda Y, Handa M, Kawano K, et al: The role of von Willebrand factor and fibrinogen in platelet aggregation under varying shear stress. *J Clin Invest* 87:1234, 1991.

382. Ruggeri ZM: Mechanisms of shear-induced platelet adhesion and aggregation. *Thromb Haemost* 70:119, 1993.

383. Andrews RK, Lopez JA, Berndt MC: The GPIb-IX-V complex, in *Platelets*, edited by AD Michelson, p 145. Academic Press, San Diego, 2007.

384. Bergmeier W, Piffath CL, Goerge T, et al: The role of platelet adhesion receptor GPIbalpha far exceeds that of its main ligand, von Willebrand factor, in arterial thrombosis. *Proc Natl Acad Sci U S A* 103:16900, 2006.

385. Bergmeier W, Chauhan AK, Wagner DD: Glycoprotein Ibalpha and von Willebrand factor in primary platelet adhesion and thrombus formation: Lessons from mutant mice. *Thromb Haemost* 99:264, 2008.

386. Coller BS: Platelet von Willebrand factor interactions, in *Platelet Glycoproteins*, edited by J George, D Phillips, A Nurden, p 215. Plenum, New York, 1985.

387. Rand JH, Patel ND, Schwartz E, et al: 150-kD von Willebrand factor binding protein extracted from human vascular subendothelium is type VI collagen. *J Clin Invest* 88:253, 1991.

388. Savage B, Sixma JJ, Ruggeri ZM: Functional self-association of von Willebrand factor during platelet adhesion under flow. *Proc Natl Acad Sci U S A* 99:425, 2002.

389. Goto S, Ikeda Y, Saldivar E, et al: Distinct mechanisms of platelet aggregation as a consequence of different shearing flow conditions. *J Clin Invest* 101:479, 1998.

390. Donadelli R, Orje JN, Capoferri C, et al: Size regulation of von Willebrand factor-mediated platelet thrombi by ADAMTS13 in flowing blood. *Blood* 107:1943, 2006.

391. Gruner S, Prostredna M, Schulte V, et al: Multiple integrin-ligand interactions synergize in shear-resistant platelet adhesion at sites of arterial injury *in vivo*. *Blood* 102:4021, 2003.

392. Coller BS: Interaction of normal, thrombasthenic, and Bernard-Soulier platelets with immobilized fibrinogen: Defective platelet-fibrinogen interaction in thrombasthenia. *Blood* 55:169, 1980.

393. Savage B, Ruggeri ZM: Selective recognition of adhesive sites in surface-bound fibrinogen by glycoprotein IIb-IIIa on nonactivated platelets. *J Biol Chem* 266:11227, 1991.

394. Chiang TM, Rinaldy A, Kang AH: Cloning, characterization, and functional studies of a nonintegrin platelet receptor for type I collagen. *J Clin Invest* 100:514, 1997.

395. Clemetson JM, Polgar J, Magnenat E, et al: The platelet collagen receptor glycoprotein VI is a member of the immunoglobulin superfamily closely related to FcalphaR and the natural killer receptors. *J Biol Chem* 274:29019, 1999.

396. Clemetson KJ: Platelet collagen receptors: A new target for inhibition? *Haemostasis* 29:16, 1999.

397. Coller BS, Beer JH, Scudder LE, et al: Collagen-platelet interactions: Evidence for a direct interaction of collagen with platelet GPIa/IIa and an indirect interaction with platelet GPIIb/IIa mediated by adhesive proteins. *Blood* 74:182, 1989.

398. Saelman EU, Nieuwenhuis HK, Hese KM, et al: Platelet adhesion to collagen types I through VIII under conditions of stasis and flow is mediated by GPIa/IIa ($\alpha 2\beta 1$-integrin). *Blood* 83:1244, 1994.

399. Watson SP: Collagen receptor signaling in platelets and megakaryocytes. *Thromb Haemost* 82:376, 1999.

400. Nakamura T, Kambayashi J, Okuma M, et al: Activation of the GP IIb-IIIa complex induced by platelet adhesion to collagen is mediated by both alpha2beta1 integrin and GP VI. *J Biol Chem* 274:11897, 1999.

401. Matsuno K, Diaz-Ricart M, Montgomery RR, et al: Inhibition of platelet adhesion to collagen by monoclonal anti-CD36 antibodies. *Br J Haematol* 92:960, 1996.

402. Nieswandt B, Watson SP: Platelet-collagen interaction: Is GPVI the central receptor? *Blood* 102:449, 2003.

403. Kuijpers MJ, Schulte V, Bergmeier W, et al: Complementary roles of glycoprotein VI and alpha2beta1 integrin in collagen-induced thrombus formation in flowing whole blood *ex vivo*. *FASEB J* 17:685, 2003.

404. Kato K, Kanaji T, Russell S, et al: The contribution of glycoprotein VI to stable platelet adhesion and thrombus formation illustrated by targeted gene deletion. *Blood* 102:1701, 2003.

405. Savage B, Almus-Jacobs F, Ruggeri ZM: Specific synergy of multiple substrate-receptor interactions in platelet thrombus formation under flow. *Cell* 94:657, 1998.

406. Savage B, Ginsberg MH, Ruggeri ZM: Influence of fibrillar collagen structure on the mechanisms of platelet thrombus formation under flow. *Blood* 94:2704, 1999.

407. Kunicki TJ, Orchekowski R, Annis D, et al: Variability of integrin alpha 2 beta 1 activity on human platelets. *Blood* 82:2693, 1993.

408. Kritzik M, Savage B, Nugent DJ, et al: Nucleotide polymorphisms in the alpha2 gene define multiple alleles that are associated with differences in platelet alpha2 beta1 density. *Blood* 92:2382, 1998.

409. Roest M, Sixma JJ, Wu YP, et al: Platelet adhesion to collagen in healthy volunteers is influenced by variation of both alpha(2)beta(1) density and von Willebrand factor. *Blood* 96:1433, 2000.

410. Henrita vZ, Saelman EU, Schut-Hese KM, et al: Platelet adhesion to collagen type IV under flow conditions. *Blood* 88:3862, 1996.

411. Ruggeri ZM, Dent JA, Saldivar E: Contribution of distinct adhesive interactions to platelet aggregation in flowing blood. *Blood* 94:172, 1999.

412. Santos MT, Valles J, Marcus AJ, et al: Enhancement of platelet reactivity and modulation of eicosanoid production by intact erythrocytes. A new approach to platelet activation and recruitment. *J Clin Invest* 87:571, 1991.

413. Shattil S: Regulation of platelet anchorage and signaling by integrin $\alpha IIb\beta 3$. *Thromb Haemost* 70:224, 1993.

414. Weiss HJ, Turitto VT, Baumgartner HR: Further evidence that glycoprotein IIb-IIIa mediates platelet spreading on subendothelium. *Thromb Haemost* 65:202, 1991.

415. Shattil SJ: Signaling through platelet integrin $\alpha IIb\beta 3$: Inside-out, outside-in and sideways. *Thromb Haemost* 82:318, 1999.

416. Patel D, Vaananen H, Jirouskova M, et al: The dynamics of GPIIb/IIIa-mediated platelet-platelet interactions in platelet adhesion/thrombus formation on collagen in vitro as revealed by videomicroscopy. *Blood* 101:929, 2003.

417. Naik UP, Naik MU: Association of CIB with GPIIb/IIIa during outside-in signaling is required for platelet spreading on fibrinogen. *Blood* 102:1355, 2003.

418. Shattil SJ, Newman PJ: Integrins: Dynamic scaffolds for adhesion and signaling in platelets. *Blood* 104:1606, 2004.
419. Coller BS, Shattil SJ: The GPIIb/IIIa (integrin alphaIIbbeta3) odyssey: A technology-driven saga of a receptor with twists, turns, and even a bend. *Blood* 112:3011, 2008.
420. Dubois C, Atkinson B, Furie B, et al: Real-time imaging of platelets during thrombus formation, in *Platelets*, edited by AD Michelson, p 611. Academic Press, San Diego, 2007.
421. Denis CC, Methia N, Frenette PS, et al: A mouse model of severe von Willebrand disease: Defects in hemostasis and thrombosis. *Proc Natl Acad Sci U S A* 95:9524, 1998.
422. Celi A, Merrill-Skoloff G, Gross P, et al: Thrombus formation: Direct real-time observation and digital analysis of thrombus assembly in a living mouse by confocal and widefield intravital microscopy. *J Thromb Haemost* 1:60, 2003.
423. Ni H, Denis CV, Subbarao S, et al: Persistence of platelet thrombus formation in arterioles of mice lacking both von Willebrand factor and fibrinogen. *J Clin Invest* 106:385, 2000.
424. Jirouskova M, Chereshnev I, Vaananen H, et al: Antibody blockade or mutation of the fibrinogen gamma-chain C-terminus is more effective in inhibiting murine arterial thrombus formation than complete absence of fibrinogen. *Blood* 103:1995, 2004.
425. Giandomenico G, Dellas C, Czekay RP, et al: The leptin receptor system of human platelets. *J Thromb Haemost* 3:1042, 2005.
426. Konstantinides S, Schafer K, Koschnick S, et al: Leptin-dependent platelet aggregation and arterial thrombosis suggests a mechanism for atherothrombotic disease in obesity. *J Clin Invest* 108:1533, 2001.
427. Konstantinides S, Schafer K, Neels JG, et al: Inhibition of endogenous leptin protects mice from arterial and venous thrombosis. *Arterioscler Thromb Vasc Biol* 24:2196, 2004.
428. Andre P, Prasad KS, Denis CV, et al: CD40L stabilizes arterial thrombi by a beta3 integrin—dependent mechanism. *Nat Med* 8:247, 2002.
429. Balogh I, Hafizi S, Stenhoff J, et al: Analysis of Gas6 in human platelets and plasma. *Arterioscler Thromb Vasc Biol* 25:1280, 2005.
430. Prevost N, Woulfe DS, Jiang H, et al: Eph kinases and ephrins support thrombus growth and stability by regulating integrin outside-in signaling in platelets. *Proc Natl Acad Sci U S A* 102:9820, 2005.
431. Renne T, Pozgajova M, Gruner S, et al: Defective thrombus formation in mice lacking coagulation factor XII. *J Exp Med* 202:271, 2005.
432. Loscalzo J, Inbal A, Handin RI: Von Willebrand protein facilitates platelet incorporation into polymerizing fibrin. *J Clin Invest* 78:1112, 1986.
433. Michelson AD, Barnard MR: Thrombin-induced changes in platelet membrane glycoproteins Ib, IX, and IIb-IIIa complex. *Blood* 70:1673, 1987.
434. McEver RP, Beckstead JH, Moore KL, et al: GMP-140, a platelet-granule membrane protein, is also synthesized by vascular endothelial cells and is localized in Weibel-Palade bodies. *J Clin Invest* 84:92, 1989.
435. McEver RP: Properties of GMP-140, an inducible granule membrane protein of platelets and endothelium. *Blood Cells* 16:73, 1990.
436. McEver RP: P-selectin/PSGL-1 and other interactions between platelets, leukocytes, and endothelium, in *Platelets*, 2nd ed, edited by AD Michelson, p 231. Academic Press, San Diego, 2007.
437. Frenette PS, Johnson RC, Hynes RO, et al: Platelets roll on stimulated endothelium *in vivo*: An interaction mediated by endothelial P-selectin. *Proc Natl Acad Sci U S A* 92:7450, 1995.
438. Romo GM, Dong JF, Schade AJ, et al: The glycoprotein Ib-IX-V complex is a platelet counterreceptor for P-selectin. *J Exp Med* 190:803, 1999.
439. Frenette PS, Denis CV, Weiss L, et al: P-Selectin glycoprotein ligand 1 (PSGL-1) is expressed on platelets and can mediate platelet-endothelial interactions *in vivo*. *J Exp Med* 191:1413, 2000.
440. Henn V, Slupsky JR, Grafe M, et al: CD40 ligand on activated platelets triggers an inflammatory reaction of endothelial cells. *Nature* 391:591, 1998.
441. Prasad KS, Andre P, He M, et al: Soluble CD40 ligand induces beta3 integrin tyrosine phosphorylation and triggers platelet activation by outside-in signaling. *Proc Natl Acad Sci U S A* 100:12367, 2003.
442. Prasad KS, Andre P, Yan Y, et al: The platelet CD40L/GP IIb-IIIa axis in atherothrombotic disease. *Curr Opin Hematol* 10:356, 2003.
443. Heeschen C, Dimmeler S, Hamm CW, et al: Soluble CD40 ligand in acute coronary syndromes. *N Engl J Med* 348:1104, 2003.
444. Andre P, Nannizzi-Alaimo L, Prasad SK, et al: Platelet-derived CD40L: The switch-hitting player of cardiovascular disease. *Circulation* 106:896, 2002.
445. Andre P, Prasad KS, Denis CV, et al: CD40L stabilizes arterial thrombi by a beta3 integrin-dependent mechanism. *Nat Med* 8:247, 2002.
446. Cipollone F, Ferri C, Desideri G, et al: Preprocedural level of soluble CD40L is predictive of enhanced inflammatory response and restenosis after coronary angioplasty. *Circulation* 108:2776, 2003.
447. Luscher TF: Platelet-vessel wall interaction: Role of nitric oxide, prostaglandins and endothelins. *Baillieres Clin Haematol* 6:609, 1993.
448. Loscalzo J: Nitric oxide insufficiency, platelet activation, and arterial thrombosis. *Circ Res* 88:756, 2001.
449. Mitchell JA, Ali F, Bailey L, et al: Role of nitric oxide and prostacyclin as vasoactive hormones released by the endothelium. *Exp Physiol* 93:141, 2008.
450. Rex S, Freedman JE: Inhibition of platelet function by the endothelium, in *Platelets*, edited by AD Michelson, p 251. Academic Press, San Diego, 2007.
451. Barry OP, FitzGerald GA: Mechanisms of cellular activation by platelet microparticles. *Thromb Haemost* 82:794, 1999.
452. Freedman JE, Loscalzo J, Barnard MR, et al: Nitric oxide released from activated platelets inhibits platelet recruitment. *J Clin Invest* 100:350, 1997.
453. Freedman JE, Sauter R, Battinelli EM, et al: Deficient platelet-derived nitric oxide and enhanced hemostasis in mice lacking the NOSIII gene. *Circ Res* 84:1416, 1999.
454. Iafrati MD, Vitseva O, Tanriverdi K, et al: Compensatory mechanisms influence hemostasis in setting of eNOS deficiency. *Am J Physiol Heart Circ Physiol* 288:H1627, 2005.
455. Ozuyaman B, Godecke A, Kusters S, et al: Endothelial nitric oxide synthase plays a minor role in inhibition of arterial thrombus formation. *Thromb Haemost* 93:1161, 2005.
456. Marjanovic JA, Li Z, Stojanovic A, et al: Stimulatory roles of nitric-oxide synthase 3 and guanylyl cyclase in platelet activation. *J Biol Chem* 280:37430, 2005.
457. Marjanovic JA, Stojanovic A, Brovkovych VM, et al: Signaling-mediated functional activation of inducible nitric-oxide synthase and its role in stimulating platelet activation. *J Biol Chem* 283:28827, 2008.
458. Valles J, Santos MT, Marcus AJE, et al: Down-regulation of human platelet reactivity by neutrophils. Participation of lipoxygenase derivatives and adhesive proteins. *J Clin Invest* 92:1357, 1993.
459. Selak MA: Cathepsin G and thrombin: Evidence for two different platelet receptors. *Biochem J* 297:269, 1994.
460. Molino M, Di Lallo M, Martelli N, et al: Effects of leukocyte-derived cathepsin G on platelet membrane glycoprotein Ib-IX and IIb-IIIa complexes: A comparison with thrombin. *Blood* 82:2442, 1993.
461. Peerschke EI: Ca^{2+} mobilization and fibrinogen binding of platelets refractory to adenosine diphosphate stimulation. *J Lab Clin Med* 106:111, 1985.
462. Murray R, FitzGerald GA: Regulation of thromboxane receptor activation in human platelets. *Proc Natl Acad Sci U S A* 86:124, 1989.
463. Coughlin SR: Protease-activated receptors and platelet function. *Thromb Haemost* 82:353, 1999.
464. Phillips DR, Charo IF, Parise LV, et al: The platelet membrane glycoprotein IIb-IIIa complex. *Blood* 71:831, 1988.
465. Plow EF, Ginsberg MH: Cellular adhesion: GPIIb-IIIa as a prototypic adhesion receptor. *Prog Hemost Thromb* 9:117, 1989.
466. Peerschke EI: The platelet fibrinogen receptor. *Semin Hematol* 22:241, 1985.
467. Plow EF, Pesho MM, Ma YQ: Integrin $\alpha IIb\beta 3$, in *Platelets*, edited by AD Michelson, p 179. Academic Press, San Diego, 2007.
468. Sixma JJ: Interaction of blood platelets with the vessel wall, in *Haemostasis and Thrombosis*, 3rd ed, edited by AL Bloom, CD Forbes, DP Thomas, EGD Tuddenham, p 259. Churchill Livingstone, Edinburgh, Scotland, 1994.
469. Weiss HJ, Hawiger J, Ruggeri ZM, et al: Fibrinogen-independent platelet adhesion and thrombus formation on subendothelium mediated by glycoprotein IIb-IIIa complex at high shear rate. *J Clin Invest* 83:288, 1989.
470. Bennett JS: The platelet-fibrinogen interaction, in *Platelet Membrane Glycoproteins*, edited by JN George, AT Nurden, DR Phillips, p 193. Plenum, New York, 1985.
471. Plow EF, Pesho MM, Ma YQ: Integrin $\alpha IIb\beta 3$, in *Platelets*, edited by AD Michelson, p 165. Academic Press, San Diego, 2007.
472. Steen VM, Holmsen H: Syntergism between thrombin and epinephrine in human platelets: Different dose-response relationships for aggregation and dense granule secretion. *Thromb Haemost* 54:680, 1985.
473. Ware JA, Smith M, Salzman EW: Synergism of platelet-aggregating agents. Role of elevation of cytoplasmic calcium. *J Clin Invest* 80:267, 1987.
474. Folts JD, Rowe GG: Epinephrine potentiation of *in vivo* stimuli reverses aspirin inhibition of platelet thrombus formation in stenosed canine coronary arteries. *Thromb Res* 50:507, 1988.
475. Folts JD, Bonebrake FC: The effects of cigarette smoke and nicotine on platelet thrombus formation in stenosed dog coronary arteries: Inhibition with phentolamine. *Circulation* 65:465, 1989.
476. Hjemdahl P, Chronos NA, Wilson DJ, et al: Epinephrine sensitizes human platelets *in vivo* and *in vitro* as studied by fibrinogen binding and P-selectin expression. *Arterioscler Thromb* 14:77, 1994.
477. Moake JL, Turner NA, Stathopoulos NA, et al: Shear-induced platelet aggregation can be mediated by vWF released from platelets, as well as by exogenous large or unusually large vWF multimers, requires adenosine diphosphate, and is resistant to aspirin. *Blood* 71:1366, 1988.
478. Nachmias VT: Platelet and megakaryocyte shape change: Triggered alterations in the cytoskeleton. *Semin Hematol* 20:261, 1983.
479. Maurer-Spurej E, Devine DV: Platelet aggregation is not initiated by platelet shape change. *Lab Invest* 81:1517, 2001.
480. Born GV, Dearnley R, Foulks JG, et al: Quantification of the morphological reaction of platelets to aggregating agents and of its reversal by aggregation inhibitors. *J Physiol* 280:193, 1978.
481. Hartwig JH, Barkalow K, Azim A, et al: The elegant platelet: Signals controlling actin assembly. *Thromb Haemost* 82:392, 1999.
482. Falet H, Hoffmeister KM, Neujahr R, et al: Importance of free actin filament barbed ends for Arp2/3 complex function in platelets and fibroblasts. *Proc Natl Acad Sci U S A* 99:16782, 2002.
483. Carlier MF, Didry D, Erk I, et al: Tbeta 4 is not a simple G-actin sequestering protein and interacts with F-actin at high concentration. *J Biol Chem* 271:9231, 1996.

484. Lind SE, Yin HL, Stossel TP: Human platelets contain gelsolin. A regulator of actin filament length. *J Clin Invest* 69:1384, 1982.
485. Barkalow K, Hartwig JH: The role of actin filament barbed-end exposure in cytoskeletal dynamics and cell motility. *Biochem Soc Trans* 23:451, 1995.
486. Barkalow KL, Italiano JE Jr, Chou DE, et al: Alpha-adducin dissociates from F-actin and spectrin during platelet activation. *J Cell Biol* 161:557, 2003.
487. Machesky LM, Gould KL: The Arp2/3 complex: A multifunctional actin organizer. *Curr Opin Cell Biol* 11:117, 1999.
488. Mullins RD, Heuser JA, Pollard TD: The interaction of Arp2/3 complex with actin: Nucleation, high affinity pointed end capping, and formation of branching networks of filaments. *Proc Natl Acad Sci U S A* 95:6181, 1998.
489. Heemskerk JW, Vuist WM, Feijge MA, et al: Collagen but not fibrinogen surfaces induce bleb formation, exposure of phosphatidylserine, and procoagulant activity of adherent platelets: Evidence for regulation by protein tyrosine kinase-dependent Ca2+ responses. *Blood* 90:2615, 1997.
490. Jirouskova M, Jaiswal JK, Coller BS. Ligand density dramatically affects integrin {alpha}IIb{beta}3-mediated platelet signaling and spreading. *Blood* 109:5269, 2007.
491. Coller BS, Kutok JL, Scudder LE, et al: Studies of activated GPIIb/IIIa receptors on the luminal surface of adherent platelets. Paradoxical loss of luminal receptors when platelets adhere to high density fibrinogen. *J Clin Invest* 92:2796, 1993.
492. Fox JEB: On the role of calpain and Rho proteins in regulating integrin-induced signaling. *Thromb Haemost* 82:391, 1999.
493. Hartwig JH, Bokoch GM, Carpenter CL, et al: Thrombin receptor ligation and activated Rac uncap actin filament barbed ends through phosphoinositide synthesis in permeabilized human platelets. *Cell* 82:643, 1995.
494. Ma AD, Abrams CS: Pleckstrin homology domains and phospholipid-induced cytoskeletal reorganization. *Thromb Haemost* 82:399, 1999.
495. Lemmon MA, Ferguson KM, Abrams CS: Pleckstrin homology domains and the cytoskeleton. *FEBS Lett* 513:71, 2002.
496. Lian L, Wang Y, Flick M, et al: Loss of pleckstrin defines a novel pathway for PKC-mediated exocytosis. *Blood* 113:3577, 2009.
497. Hitchcock IS, Fox NE, Prevost N, et al: Roles of focal adhesion kinase (FAK) in megakaryopoiesis and platelet function: Studies using a megakaryocyte lineage specific FAK knockout. *Blood* 111:596, 2008.
498. Pabla R, Weyrich AS, Dixon DA, et al: Integrin-dependent control of translation: Engagement of integrin alphaIIbbeta3 regulates synthesis of proteins in activated human platelets. *J Cell Biol* 144:175, 1999.
499. Kulkarni S, Woollard KJ, Thomas S, et al: Conversion of platelets from a proaggregatory to a proinflammatory adhesive phenotype: Role of PAF in spatially regulating neutrophil adhesion and spreading. *Blood* 110:1879, 2007.
500. Cho J, Mosher DF: Role of fibronectin assembly in platelet thrombus formation. *J Thromb Haemost* 4:1461, 2006.
501. Bennett JS, Zigmond S, Vilaire G, et al: The platelet cytoskeleton regulates the affinity of the integrin alpha(IIb)beta(3) for fibrinogen. *J Biol Chem* 274:25301, 1999.
502. Patil S, Jedsadayanmata A, Wencel-Drake JD, et al: Identification of a talin-binding site in the integrin beta(3) subunit distinct from the NPLY regulatory motif of post-ligand binding functions. The talin n-terminal head domain interacts with the membrane-proximal region of the beta(3) cytoplasmic tail. *J Biol Chem* 274:28575, 1999.
503. Shattil SJ, Brugge JS: Protein tyrosine phosphorylation and the adhesive functions of platelets. *Curr Opin Cell Biol* 3:869, 1991.
504. Fox JEB: Platelet cytoskeleton, in *Hemostasis and Thrombosis: Basic Principles and Clinical Practice*, edited by RW Colman, J Hirsh, VJ Marder, AW Clowes, JN George, p 429. Lippincott Williams & Wilkins, Philadelphia, 2001.
505. Li R, Mitra N, Gratkowski H, et al: Activation of integrin alphaIIbbeta3 by modulation of transmembrane helix associations. *Science* 300:795, 2003.
506. Olorundare OE, Simmons SR, Albrecht RM: Cytochalasin D and E: Effects on fibrinogen receptor movement and cytoskeletal reorganization in fully spread, surface-activated platelets: A correlative light and electron microscopic investigation. *Blood* 79:99, 1992.
507. White JG: Induction of patching and its reversal on surface-activated human platelets. *Br J Haematol* 76:108, 1990.
508. Fox JEB, Goll DE, Reynolds CC, et al: Identification of two proteins (actin-binding protein and P235) that are hydrolyzed by endogenous Ca^{++}-dependent protease during platelet aggregation. *J Biol Chem* 260:1060, 1985.
509. Fox JE, Reynolds CC, Phillips DR: Calcium-dependent proteolysis occurs during platelet aggregation. *J Biol Chem* 258:9973, 1983.
510. Fox JE, Taylor RG, Taffarel M, et al: Evidence that activation of platelet calpain is induced as a consequence of binding of adhesive ligand to the integrin, glycoprotein IIb-IIIa. *J Cell Biol* 120:1501, 1993.
511. Xi X, Bodnar RJ, Li Z, et al: Critical roles for the COOH-terminal NITY and RGT sequences of the integrin beta3 cytoplasmic domain in inside-out and outside-in signaling. *J Cell Biol* 162:329, 2003.
512. Flevaris P, Stojanovic A, Gong H, et al: A molecular switch that controls cell spreading and retraction. *J Cell Biol* 179:553, 2007.
513. Dachary-Prigent J, Freyssinet J-M, Pasquet J-M, et al: Annexin V as a probe of aminophospholipid exposure and platelet membrane vesiculation: A flow cytometry study showing a role for free sulfhydryl groups. *Blood* 81:2554, 1993.
514. Azam M, Andrabi SS, Sahr KE, et al: Disruption of the mouse mu-calpain gene reveals an essential role in platelet function. *Mol Cell Biol* 21:2213, 2001.
515. Furman MI, Gardner TM, Goldschmidt-Clermont PJ: Mechanisms of cytoskeletal reorganization during platelet activation. *Thromb Haemost* 70:229, 1993.
516. Leon C, Eckly A, Hechler B, et al: Megakaryocyte-restricted MYH9 inactivation dramatically affects hemostasis while preserving platelet aggregation and secretion. *Blood* 110:3183, 2007.
517. Weber A, Nachmias VT, Pennise CR, et al: Interaction of thymosin-β-4 with muscle and platelet actin. Implications for actin sequestration in resting platelets. *Biochemistry* 31:6179, 1992.
518. Nachmias VT, Yoshida K: The cytoskeleton of the blood platelets: A dynamic structure. *Adv Cyclic Nucleotide Res* 2:181, 1999.
519. Fox JEB, Boyles JK, Reynolds CC, et al: Actin filament content and organization in unstimulated platelets. *J Cell Biol* 98:1985, 1984.
520. Escolar G, Krumwiede M, White JG: Organization of the actin cytoskeleton of resting and activated platelets in suspension. *Am J Pathol* 123:86, 1986.
521. Takafuta T, Wu G, Murphy GF, et al: Human beta-filamin is a new protein that interacts with the cytoplasmic tail of glycoprotein Ibalpha. *J Biol Chem* 273:17531, 1998.
522. Nachmias VT: Cytoskeleton of human platelets at rest and after spreading. *J Cell Biol* 86:795, 1980.
523. Gonnella PA, Nachmias VT: Platelet activation and microfilament bundling. *J Biol Chem* 89:146, 1981.
524. Ren Q, Ye S, Whiteheart SW: The platelet release reaction: Just when you thought platelet secretion was simple. *Curr Opin Hematol* 15:537, 2008.
525. Tolmachova T, Abrink M, Futter CE, et al: Rab27b regulates number and secretion of platelet dense granules. *Proc Natl Acad Sci U S A* 104:5872, 2007.
526. Shirakawa R, Yoshioka A, Horiuchi H, et al: Small GTPase Rab4 regulates Ca2+-induced alpha-granule secretion in platelets. *J Biol Chem* 275:33844, 2000.
527. Fitzgerald ML, Reed GL: Rab6 is phosphorylated in thrombin-activated platelets by a protein kinase C-dependent mechanism: Effects on GTP/GDP binding and cellular distribution. *Biochem J* 342(Pt 2):353, 1999.
528. Sudhof TC, Rothman JE: Membrane fusion: Grappling with SNARE and SM proteins. *Science* 323:474, 2009.
529. Weber T, Zemelman BV, McNew JA, et al: SNAREpins: Minimal machinery for membrane fusion. *Cell* 92:759, 1998.
530. Ren Q, Barber HK, Crawford GL, et al: Endobrevin/VAMP-8 is the primary v-SNARE for the platelet release reaction. *Mol Biol Cell* 18:24, 2007.
531. Bernstein AM, Whiteheart SW: Identification of a cellubrevin/vesicle associated membrane protein 3 homologue in human platelets. *Blood* 93:571, 1999.
532. Lemons PP, Chen D, Bernstein AM, et al: Regulated secretion in platelets: Identification of elements of the platelet exocytosis machinery. *Blood* 90:1490, 1997.
533. Polgar J, Chung SH, Reed GL: Vesicle-associated membrane protein 3 (VAMP-3) and VAMP-8 are present in human platelets and are required for granule secretion. *Blood* 100:1081, 2002.
534. Graham GJ, Ren Q, Dilks JR, et al: Endobrevin/VAMP-8-dependent dense granule release mediates thrombus formation *in vivo*. *Blood* 114:932, 2009.
535. Flaumenhaft R, Croce K, Chen E, et al: Proteins of the exocytotic core complex mediate platelet alpha-granule secretion. Roles of vesicle-associated membrane protein, SNAP-23, and syntaxin 4. *J Biol Chem* 274:2492, 1999.
536. Polgar J, Lane WS, Chung SH, et al: Phosphorylation of SNAP-23 in activated human platelets. *J Biol Chem* 278:44369, 2003.
537. Chen D, Bernstein AM, Lemons PP, et al: Molecular mechanisms of platelet exocytosis: Role of SNAP-23 and syntaxin 2 in dense core granule release. *Blood* 95:921, 2000.
538. Lemons PP, Chen D, Whiteheart SW: Molecular mechanisms of platelet exocytosis: Requirements for alpha-granule release. *Biochem Biophys Res Commun* 267:875, 2000.
539. Chen D, Lemons PP, Schraw T, et al: Molecular mechanisms of platelet exocytosis: Role of SNAP-23 and syntaxin 2 and 4 in lysosome release. *Blood* 96:1782, 2000.
540. Flaumenhaft R, Furie B, Furie BC: Alpha-granule secretion from alpha-toxin permeabilized, MgATP-exposed platelets is induced independently by H+ and Ca2+. *J Cell Physiol* 179:1, 1999.
541. Houng A, Polgar J, Reed GL: Munc18-syntaxin complexes and exocytosis in human platelets. *J Biol Chem* 278:19627, 2003.
542. Reed GL, Houng AK, Fitzgerald ML: Human platelets contain SNARE proteins and a Sec1p homologue that interacts with syntaxin 4 and is phosphorylated after thrombin activation: Implications for platelet secretion. *Blood* 93:2617, 1999.
543. Schraw TD, Lemons PP, Dean WL, et al: A role for Sec1/Munc18 proteins in platelet exocytosis. *Biochem J* 374:207, 2003.
544. Shirakawa R, Higashi T, Tabuchi A, et al: Munc13–4 is a GTP-Rab27-binding protein regulating dense core granule secretion in platelets. *J Biol Chem* 279:10730, 2004.
545. Vu T-KH, Hung DT, Wheaton VI, et al: Molecular cloning of a functional thrombin receptor reveals a novel proteolytic mechanism of receptor activation. *Cell* 64:1057, 1991.
546. Shirakawa R, Higashi T, Kondo H, et al: Purification and functional analysis of a Rab27 effector munc 13-4 using a semi-intact platelet dense-granule secretion assay. *Methods Enzymol* 403:778, 2005.
547. Feldmann J, Callebaut I, Raposo G, et al: Munc13-4 is essential for cytolytic granules fusion and is mutated in a form of familial hemophagocytic lymphohistiocytosis (FHL3). *Cell* 115:461, 2003.
548. Neeft M, Wieffer M, de Jong AS, et al: Munc13-4 is an effector of rab27a and controls secretion of lysosomes in hematopoietic cells. *Mol Biol Cell* 16:731, 2005.

549. Budtz-Olsen OE: *Clot Retraction*. Charles Thomas, Springfield, IL, 1951.
550. Kunitada S, FitzGerald GA, Fitzgerald DJ: Inhibition of clot lysis and decreased binding of tissue-type plasminogen activator as a consequence of clot retraction. *Blood* 79:1420, 1992.
551. Pollard TD, Fujiwara K, Handin R, et al: Contractile proteins in platelet activation and contraction. *Ann N Y Acad Sci* 283:218, 1977.
552. Cohen I, Gerrard JM, White JG: Ultrastructure of clots during isometric contraction. *J Cell Biol* 91:775, 1982.
553. Cohen I: The mechanism of clot retraction, in *Platelet Membrane Glycoproteins*, edited by JN George, AT Nurden, DR Phillips, p 299. Plenum Press, New York, 1985.
554. Carr ME Jr, Carr SL, Hantgan RR, et al: Glycoprotein IIb/IIIa blockade inhibits platelet-mediated force development and reduces gel elastic modulus. *Thromb Haemost* 73:499, 1995.
555. Leistikow EA: Platelet internalization in early thrombogenesis. *Semin Thromb Hemost* 22:289, 1996.
556. Morgenstern E, Daub M, Dierichs R: A new model for *in vitro* clot formation that considers the mode of the fibrin(ogen) contacts to platelets and the arrangement of the platelet cytoskeleton. *Ann N Y Acad Sci* 936:449, 2001.
557. Coller BS, Peerschke EI, Scudder LE, et al: A murine monoclonal antibody that completely blocks the binding of fibrinogen to platelets produces a thrombasthenic-like state in normal platelets and binds to glycoproteins IIb and/or IIIa. *J Clin Invest* 72:325, 1983.
558. Collet JP, Montalescot G, Lesty C, et al: A structural and dynamic investigation of the facilitating effect of glycoprotein IIb/IIIa inhibitors in dissolving platelet-rich clots. *Circ Res* 90:428, 2002.
559. Huang TC, Jordan RE, Hantgan RR, et al: Differential effects of c7E3 Fab on thrombus formation and rt-PA-mediated thrombolysis under flow conditions. *Thromb Res* 102:411, 2001.
560. Braaten JV, Jerome WG, Hantgan RR: Uncoupling fibrin from integrin receptors hastens fibrinolysis at the platelet-fibrin interface. *Blood* 83:982, 1994.
561. Seiffert D, Pedicord DL, Kieras CJ, et al: Regulation of clot retraction by glycoprotein IIb/IIIa antagonists. *Thromb Res* 108:181, 2002.
562. Mousa SA, Khurana S, Forsythe MS: Comparative *in vitro* efficacy of different platelet glycoprotein IIb/IIIa antagonists on platelet-mediated clot strength induced by tissue factor with use of thromboelastography: Differentiation among glycoprotein IIb/IIIa antagonists. *Arterioscler Thromb Vasc Biol* 20:1162, 2000.
563. Jirouskova M, Smyth SS, Kudryk B, et al: A hamster antibody to the mouse fibrinogen gamma chain inhibits platelet-fibrinogen interactions and FXIIIa-mediated fibrin cross-linking, and facilitates thrombolysis. *Thromb Haemost* 86:1047, 2001.
564. Osdoit S, Rosa JP: Fibrin clot retraction by human platelets correlates with alpha(IIb)beta(3) integrin-dependent protein tyrosine dephosphorylation. *J Biol Chem* 276:6703, 2001.
565. Flevaris P, Li Z, Zhang G, et al: Two distinct roles of mitogen-activated protein kinases in platelets and a novel Rac1-MAPK-dependent integrin outside-in retractile signaling pathway. *Blood* 113:893, 2009.
566. Ward CM, Kestin AS, Newman PJ: A Leu262Pro mutation in the integrin beta(3) subunit results in an alpha(IIb)-beta(3) complex that binds fibrin but not fibrinogen. *Blood* 96:161, 2000.
567. Rooney MM, Farrell DH, van Hemel BM, et al: The contribution of the three hypothesized integrin-binding sites in fibrinogen to platelet-mediated clot retraction. *Blood* 92:2374, 1998.
568. Rooney MM, Parise LV, Lord ST: Dissecting clot retraction and platelet aggregation. Clot retraction does not require an intact fibrinogen gamma chain C terminus. *J Biol Chem* 271:8553, 1996.
569. Podolnikova NP, Yakubenko VP, Volkov GL, et al: Identification of a novel binding site for platelet integrins alpha IIb beta 3 (GPIIbIIIa) and alpha 5 beta 1 in the gamma C-domain of fibrinogen. *J Biol Chem* 278:32251, 2003.
570. Remijn JA, Ijsseldijk MJ, de Groot PG: Role of the fibrinogen gamma-chain sequence gamma316–322 in platelet-mediated clot retraction. *J Thromb Haemost* 1:2245, 2003.
571. Dubois C, Steiner B, Kieffer N, et al: Thrombin binding to GPIbalpha induces platelet aggregation and fibrin clot retraction supported by resting alphaIIbbeta3 interaction with polymerized fibrin. *Thromb Haemost* 89:853, 2003.
572. Keuren JF, Baruch D, Legendre P, et al: Von Willebrand factor C1C2 domain is involved in platelet adhesion to polymerized fibrin at high shear rate. *Blood* 103:1741, 2004.
573. Bevers EM, Comfurius P, Dekkers DW, et al: Lipid translocation across the plasma membrane of mammalian cells. *Biochim Biophys Acta* 1439:317, 1999.
574. Pomorski T, Menon AK: Lipid flippases and their biological functions. *Cell Mol Life Sci* 63:2908, 2006.
575. Zhou Q, Zhao J, Stout JG, et al: Molecular cloning of human plasma membrane phospholipid scramblase. A protein mediating transbilayer movement of plasma membrane phospholipids. *J Biol Chem* 272:18240, 1997.
576. Zhou Q, Sims PJ, Wiedmer T: Identity of a conserved motif in phospholipid scramblase that is required for Ca2+-accelerated transbilayer movement of membrane phospholipids. *Biochemistry* 37:2356, 1998.
577. Zhou Q, Zhao J, Wiedmer T, et al: Normal hemostasis but defective hematopoietic response to growth factors in mice deficient in phospholipid scramblase 1. *Blood* 99:4030, 2002.
578. Sahu SK, Gummadi SN, Manoj N, et al: Phospholipid scramblases: An overview. *Arch Biochem Biophys* 462:103, 2007.
579. Dekkers DW, Comfurius P, van Gool RG, et al: Multidrug resistance protein 1 regulates lipid asymmetry in erythrocyte membranes. *Biochem J* 350 Pt 2:531, 2000.
580. Zwaal RF, Comfurius P, Bevers EM: Scott syndrome, a bleeding disorder caused by defective scrambling of membrane phospholipids. *Biochim Biophys Acta* 1636:119, 2004.
581. Thiagarajan P, Tait JF: Collagen-induced exposure of anionic phospholipid in platelets and platelet-derived microparticles. *J Biol Chem* 266:24302, 1991.
582. Miyazaki Y, Nomura S, Miyake T, et al: High shear stress can initiate both platelet aggregation and shedding of procoagulant containing microparticles. *Blood* 88:3456, 1996.
583. Hultin MB: Modulation of thrombin-mediated activation of factor VIII:C by calcium ions, phospholipid, and platelets. *Blood* 66:53, 1985.
584. Nesheim ME, Furmaniak-Kazmierczak E, Henin C, et al: On the existence of platelet receptors for factors V(a) and factor VIII (a). *Thromb Haemost* 70:80, 1993.
585. Bouchard BA, Catcher CS, Thrash BR, et al: Effector cell protease receptor-1, a platelet activation-dependent membrane protein, regulates prothrombinase-catalyzed thrombin generation. *J Biol Chem* 272:9244, 1997.
586. Enjeti AK, Lincz LF, Seldon M: Microparticles in health and disease. *Semin Thromb Hemost* 34:683, 2008.
587. Piccin A, Murphy WG, Smith OP: Circulating microparticles: Pathophysiology and clinical implications. *Blood Rev* 21:157, 2007.
588. Lee DH, Warkentin TE, Denomme GA, et al: A diagnostic test for heparin-induced thrombocytopenia: Detection of platelet microparticles using flow cytometry. *Br J Haematol* 95:724, 1996.
589. Kelton JG: Heparin-induced thrombocytopenia: An overview. *Blood Rev* 16:77, 2002.
590. Reverter JC, Beguin S, Kessels H, et al: Inhibition of platelet-mediated, tissue factor-induced thrombin generation by the mouse/human chimeric 7E3 antibody. Potential implications for the effect of c7E3 Fab treatment on acute thrombosis and "clinical restenosis." *J Clin Invest* 98:863, 1996.
591. Beguin S, Kumar R, Keularts I, et al: Fibrin-dependent platelet procoagulant activity requires GPIb receptors and von Willebrand factor. *Blood* 93:564, 1999.
592. George JN, Pickett EB, Saucerman S, et al: Platelet surface glycoproteins. Studies on resting and activated platelets and platelet membrane microparticles in normal subjects, and observations in patients during adult respiratory distress syndrome and cardiac surgery. *J Clin Invest* 78:340, 1986.
593. Siljander P, Carpen O, Lassila R: Platelet-derived microparticles associate with fibrin during thrombosis. *Blood* 87:4651, 1996.
594. Dahlback B, Wiedmer T, Sims PJ: Binding of anticoagulant vitamin K-dependent protein S to platelet-derived microparticles. *Biochemistry* 31:12769, 1992.
595. Tans G, Rosing J, Thomassen MC, et al: Comparison of anticoagulant and procoagulant activities of stimulated platelets and platelet-derived microparticles. *Blood* 77:2641, 1991.
596. Weiss HJ: Scott syndrome—A disorder of platelet coagulant activity. *Semin Hematol* 31:312, 1994.
597. Weiss HJ, Lages B: Platelet prothrombinase activity and intracellular calcium responses in patients with storage pool deficiency, glycoprotein IIb-IIIa deficiency, or impaired platelet coagulant activity—A comparison with Scott syndrome. *Blood* 89:1599, 1997.
598. Toti F, Satta N, Fressinaud E, et al: Scott syndrome, characterized by impaired transmembrane migration of procoagulant phosphatidylserine and hemorrhagic complications, is an inherited disorder. *Blood* 87:1409, 1996.
599. Zhou Q, Sims PJ, Wiedmer T: Expression of proteins controlling transbilayer movement of plasma membrane phospholipids in the B lymphocytes from a patient with Scott syndrome. *Blood* 92:1707, 1998.
600. Tubman VN, Levine JE, Campagna DR, et al: X-linked gray platelet syndrome due to a GATA1 Arg216Gln mutation. *Blood* 109:3297, 2007.
601. Steinberg MH, Kelton JG, Coller BS: Plasma glycocalicin: An aid in the classification of thrombocytopenic disorders. *N Engl J Med* 317:1037, 1987.
602. Albrecht C, McVey JH, Elliott JI, et al: A novel missense mutation in ABCA1 results in altered protein trafficking and reduced phosphatidylserine translocation in a patient with Scott syndrome. *Blood* 106:542, 2005.
603. Shcherbina A, Remold-O'Donnell E: Role of caspase in a subset of human platelet activation responses. *Blood* 93:4222, 1999.
604. Wolf BB, Goldstein JC, Stennicke HR, et al: Calpain functions in a caspase-independent manner to promote apoptosis-like events during platelet activation. *Blood* 94:1683, 1999.
605. Augereau O, Rossignol R, DeGiorgi F, et al: Apoptotic-like mitochondrial events associated to phosphatidylserine exposure in blood platelets induced by local anaesthetics. *Thromb Haemost* 92:104, 2004.
606. Hamon Y, Broccardo C, Chambenoit O, et al: ABC1 promotes engulfment of apoptotic cells and transbilayer redistribution of phosphatidylserine. *Nat Cell Biol* 2:399, 2000.
607. Smith SA, Mutch NJ, Baskar D, et al: Polyphosphate modulates blood coagulation and fibrinolysis. *Proc Natl Acad Sci U S A* 103:903, 2006.
608. Smith SA, Morrissey JH: Polyphosphate enhances fibrin clot structure. *Blood* 112:2810, 2008.
609. Zwaal RFA, Comfurius P, Bevers EM: Platelet procoagulant activity and microvesicle formation. Its putative role of hemostasis and thrombosis. *Biochim Biophys Acta* 1180:1, 1992.

610. Swords NA, Tracy PB, Mann KG: Intact platelet membranes, not platelet-released microvesicles, support the procoagulant activity of adherent platelets. *Arterioscler Thromb* 13:1613, 1993.
611. Bouchard BA, Butenas S, Mann KG, et al: Interactions between platelets and the coagulation system, in *Platelets*, edited by AD Michelson, p 377. Academic Press, San Diego, 2007.
612. London FS, Marcinkiewicz M, Walsh PN: A subpopulation of platelets responds to thrombin- or SFLLRN-stimulation with binding sites for factor IXa. *J Biol Chem* 279:19854, 2004.
613. Alberio L, Safa O, Clemetson KJ, et al: Surface expression and functional characterization of alpha-granule factor V in human platelets: Effects of ionophore A23187, thrombin, collagen, and convulxin. *Blood* 95:1694, 2000.
614. Scandura JM, Ahmad SS, Walsh PN: A binding site expressed on the surface of activated human platelets is shared by factor X and prothrombin. *Biochemistry* 35:8890, 1996.
615. Byzova TV, Plow EF: Networking in the hemostatic system. Integrin alphaiibbeta3 binds prothrombin and influences its activation. *J Biol Chem* 272:27183, 1997.
615a. Baglia FA, Shrimpton CN, Emsley J, et al: Factor XI interacts with the leucine-rich repeats of glycoprotein Ibα on the activated platelet. *J Biol Chem* 279:49323, 2004.
615b. Pennings MT, Derksen RH, van Lummel M, et al: Platelet adhesion to dimeric beta-glycoprotein I under conditions of flow is mediated by at least two receptors: Glycoprotein Ibα and apolipoprotein E receptor 2. *J Thromb Haemost* 5:369, 2006.
615c. White-Adams TC, Berny MA, Tucker EI, et al: Identification of coagulation factor XI as a ligand for platelet apolipoprotein E receptor 2 (ApoER2). *Arterioscler Thromb Vasc Biol* 29:1602, 2009.
615d. Lisman T: Factor XI binding to platelets: glycoprotein Ibα has an accomplice. *Arterioscler Thromb Vasc Biol* 29:1409, 2009.
616. Taube J, McWilliam N, Luddington R, et al: Activated protein C resistance: Effect of platelet activation, platelet-derived microparticles, and atherogenic lipoproteins. *Blood* 93:3792, 1999.
617. Chiu HC, Schick P, Colman RW: Biosynthesis of coagulation factor V by megakaryocytes. *J Clin Invest* 75:339, 1985.
618. Osterud B, Rapaport SI, Lavine KK: Factor V activity of platelets: Evidence for an activated factor V molecule and for a platelet activator. *Blood* 49:834, 1977.
619. Chediak J, Ashenhurst JB, Garlick I, et al: Successful management of bleeding in a patient with factor V inhibitor by platelet transfusions. *Blood* 56:835, 1980.
620. Sun H, Wang X, Degen JL, et al: Reduced thrombin generation increases host susceptibility to group A streptococcal infection. *Blood* 113:1358, 2009.
621. Baglia FA, Walsh PN: Thrombin-mediated feedback activation of factor XI on the activated platelet surface is preferred over contact activation by factor XIIa or factor XIa. *J Biol Chem* 275:20514, 2000.
622. Oliver JA, Monroe DM, Roberts HR, et al: Thrombin activates factor XI on activated platelets in the absence of factor XII. *Arterioscler Thromb Vasc Biol* 19:170, 1999.
623. Gailani D, Ho D, Sun MF, et al: Model for a factor IX activation complex on blood platelets: Dimeric conformation of factor XIa is essential. *Blood* 97:3117, 2001.
624. Walsh PN: Platelets and factor XI bypass the contact system of blood coagulation. *Thromb Haemost* 82:234, 1999.
625. Lopez JA: The platelet glycoprotein Ib-IX complex. *Blood Coagul Fibrinolysis* 5:97, 1994.
626. Wu G, Essex DW, Meloni FJ, et al: Human endothelial cells in culture and *in vivo* express on their surface all four components of the glycoprotein Ib/IX/V complex. *Blood* 90:2660, 1997.
627. Bennett JS: The molecular biology of platelet membrane proteins. *Semin Hematol* 27:186, 1990.
628. Hynes R: Integrins. Bidirectional, allosteric signaling machines. *Cell* 110:673, 2002.
629. Kasirer-Friede A, Kahn ML, Shattil SJ: Platelet integrins and immunoreceptors. *Immunol Rev* 218:247, 2007.
630. Wagner CL, Mascelli MA, Neblock DS, et al: Analysis of GPIIb/IIIa receptor number by quantification of 7E3 binding to human platelets. *Blood* 88:907, 1996.
631. Woods VL Jr, Wolff LE, Keller DM: Resting platelets contain a substantial centrally located pool of glycoprotein IIb-IIIa complexes which may be accessible to some but not other extracellular proteins. *J Biol Chem* 261:15242, 1986.
632. Cramer ER, Savidge GF, Vainchenker W, et al: α Granule pool of glycoprotein IIb-IIIa in normal and pathologic platelets and megakaryocytes. *Blood* 75:1220, 1990.
633. Youssefian T, Masse JM, Rendu F, et al: Platelet and megakaryocyte dense granules contain glycoproteins Ib and IIb-IIIa. *Blood* 89:4047, 1997.
634. Coller BS: Activation-specific platelet antigens, in *Platelet Immunobiology: Molecular and Clinical Aspects*, edited by TJ Kunicki, JN George, p 166. JB Lippincott, Philadelphia, 1989.
635. Sims PJ, Ginsberg MH, Plow EF, et al: Effect of platelet activation on the conformation of the plasma membrane glycoprotein IIb-IIIa complex. *J Biol Chem* 266:7345, 1991.
636. Wencel-Drake JD: Plasma membrane GPIIb/IIIa. Evidence for a cycling receptor pool. *Am J Clin Pathol* 136:61, 1990.
637. Hynes RO: Integrins: A family of cell surface receptors. *Cell* 48:549, 1987.
638. Ruoslahti E: Fibronectin and its receptors. *Annu Rev Biochem* 57:375, 1988.
639. Doolittle RF, Watt KWK, Cottrell BA, et al: The amino acid sequence of the alpha-chain of human fibrinogen. *Nature* 280:464, 1979.
640. Cheresh DA, Berliner SA, Vicente V, et al: Recognition of distinct adhesive sites on fibrinogen by related integrins on platelets and endothelial cells. *Cell* 58:945, 1989.
641. Farrell DH, Thiagarajan P, Chung DW, et al: Role of fibrinogen α and γ chain sites in platelet aggregation. *Proc Natl Acad Sci U S A* 89:10729, 1992.
642. Farrell DH, Thiagarajan P: Binding of recombinant fibrinogen mutants to platelets. *J Biol Chem* 269:226, 1994.
643. Muller B, Zerwes HG, Tangemann K, et al: Two-step binding mechanism of fibrinogen to alpha IIb beta 3 integrin reconstituted into planar lipid bilayers. *J Biol Chem* 268:6800, 1993.
644. Huber W, Hurst J, Schlatter D, et al: Determination of kinetic constants for the interaction between the platelet glycoprotein IIb-IIIa and fibrinogen by means of surface plasmon resonance. *Eur J Biochem* 227:647, 1995.
645. Goldsmith HL, McIntosh FA, Shahin J, et al: Time and force dependence of the rupture of glycoprotein IIb-IIIa-fibrinogen bonds between latex spheres. *Biophys J* 78:1195, 2000.
646. Litvinov RI, Bennett JS, Weisel JW, et al: Multi-step fibrinogen binding to the integrin (alpha)IIb(beta)3 detected using force spectroscopy. *Biophys J* 89:2824, 2005.
647. Hsieh CF, Chang BJ, Pai CH, et al: Stepped changes of monovalent ligand-binding force during ligand-induced clustering of integrin alphaIIB beta3. *J Biol Chem* 281:25466, 2006.
648. Peerschke EI: Reversible and irreversible binding of fibrinogen to platelets. *Platelets* 8:311, 1997.
649. Springer TA, Zhu J, Xiao T: Structural basis for distinctive recognition of fibrinogen gammaC peptide by the platelet integrin alphaIIbbeta3. *J Cell Biol* 182:791, 2008.
650. Wencel-Drake JD, Boudignon-Proudhon C, Dieter MG, et al: Internalization of bound fibrinogen modulates platelet aggregation. *Blood* 87:602, 1996.
651. Peerschke EIB: Events occurring after thrombin-induced fibrinogen binding to platelets. *Semin Thromb Hemost* 18:34, 1992.
652. Zamarron C, Ginsberg MH, Plow EF: A receptor-induced binding site in fibrinogen elicited by its interaction with platelet membrane glycoprotein IIb-IIIa. *J Biol Chem* 266:17106, 1991.
653. Ugarova TP, Budzynski AZ, Shattil SJ, et al: Conformational changes in fibrinogen elecited by its interaction with platelet membrane glycoprotein GPIIb-IIIa. *J Biol Chem* 268:21080, 1993.
654. Hato T, Pampori N, Shattil SJ: Complementary roles for receptor clustering and conformational change in the adhesive and signaling functions of integrin alphaIIb beta3. *J Cell Biol* 141:1685, 1998.
655. Carrell NA, Fitzgerald LA, Steiner B, et al: Structure of human platelet membrane glycoproteins IIb and IIIa as determined by electron microscopy. *J Biol Chem* 260:1743, 1985.
656. Weisel JW, Nagaswami C, Vilaire G, et al: Examination of the platelet membrane glycoprotein IIb-IIIa complex and its interaction with fibrinogen and other ligands by electron microscopy. *J Biol Chem* 267:16637, 1992.
657. Xiao T, Takagi J, Coller BS, et al: Structural basis for allostery in integrins and binding to fibrinogen-mimetic therapeutics. *Nature* 432:59, 2004.
658. Takagi J, Petre BM, Walz T, et al: Global conformational rearrangements in integrin extracellular domains in outside-in and inside-out signaling. *Cell* 110:599, 2002.
659. Artoni A, Li J, Mitchell B, et al: Integrin $\beta3$ regions controlling binding of murine mAb 7E3: Implications for the mechanism of integrin $\alpha IIb\beta3$ activation. *Proc Natl Acad Sci U S A* 101:13114, 2004.
660. Arnaout M, Goodman S, Xiong J: Coming to grips with integrin binding to ligands. *Curr Opin Cell Biol* 14:641, 2002.
661. Arnaout MA: Integrin structure: New twists and turns in dynamic cell adhesion. *Immunol Rev* 186:125, 2002.
662. Xiong JP, Stehle T, Diefenbach B, et al: Crystal structure of the extracellular segment of integrin alphaVbeta3. *Science* 294:339, 2001.
663. Xiong JP, Stehle T, Zhang R, et al: Crystal structure of the extracellular segment of integrin alpha Vbeta3 in complex with an Arg-Gly-Asp ligand. *Science* 296:151, 2002.
664. Poncz M, Eisman R, Heidenreich R, et al: Structure of the platelet membrane glycoprotein IIb. Homology to the alpha subunits of the vitronectin and fibronectin membrane receptors. *J Biol Chem* 262:8476, 1987.
665. Fitzgerald LA, Steiner B, Rall SC, Jr., et al: Protein sequence of endothelial glycoprotein IIIa derived from a cDNA clone. Identity with platelet glycoprotein IIIa and similarity to "integrin". *J Biol Chem* 262:3936, 1987.
666. Bray PF, Barsh G, Rosa JP, et al: Physical linkage of the genes for platelet membrane glycoproteins IIb and IIIa. *Proc Natl Acad Sci U S A* 85:8683, 1988.
667. Thornton MA, Poncz M, Korostishevsky M, et al: The human platelet alphaIIb gene is not closely linked to its integrin partner beta3. *Blood* 94:2039, 1999.
668. Steiner B, Parise LV, Leung B, et al: Ca(2+) dependent structural transitions of the platelet glycoprotein IIb-IIIa complex. Preparation of stable glycoprotein IIb and IIIa monomers. *J Biol Chem* 266:14986, 1991.
669. Mitchell WB, Li J, French DL, et al: AlphaIIbbeta3 biogenesis is controlled by engagement of alphaIIb in the calnexin cycle via the N15-linked glycan. *Blood* 107:2713, 2006.
670. Duperray A, Troesch A, Berthier R, et al: Biosynthesis and assembly of platelet GPIIb-IIIa in human megakaryocytes: Evidence that assembly between pro-GPIIb and GPIIIa is a prerequisite for expression of the complex on the cell surface. *Blood* 74:1603, 1989.
671. O'Toole TE, Loftus JC, Plow EF, et al: Efficient surface expression of platelet GPIIb-IIIa requires both subunits. *Blood* 74:14, 1989.

672. McEver RP, Baenziger JU, Majerus PW: Isolation and structural characterization of the polypeptide subunits of membrane glycoprotein IIb-IIIa from human platelets. *Blood* 59:80, 1982.
673. Muir TW, Williams MJ, Ginsberg MH, et al: Design and chemical synthesis of a neoprotein structural model for the cytoplasmic domain of a multisubunit cell-surface receptor: Integrin alpha IIb beta 3 (platelet GPIIb-IIIa). *Biochemistry* 33:7701, 1994.
674. Haas TA, Plow EF: The cytoplasmic domain of alphaIIb beta3. A ternary complex of the integrin alpha and beta subunits and a divalent cation. *J Biol Chem* 271:6017, 1996.
675. Vallar L, Melchior C, Plancon S, et al: Divalent cations differentially regulate integrin alphaIIb cytoplasmic tail binding to beta3 and to calcium- and integrin-binding protein. *J Biol Chem* 274:17257, 1999.
676. Kim C, Lau TL, Ulmer TS, et al: Interactions of platelet integrin {alpha}IIb and {beta}3 transmembrane domains in mammalian cell membranes and their role in integrin activation. *Blood* 113:4747, 2009.
677. O'Toole TE, Mandelman D, Forsyth J, et al: Modulation of the affinity of integrin $\alpha IIb\beta 3$ (GPIIb- IIIa) by the cytoplasmic domain of alpha IIb. *Science* 254:845, 1991.
678. O'Toole TE, Katagiri Y, Faull RJ, et al: Integrin cytoplasmic domains mediate inside-out signal transduction. *J Cell Biol* 124:1047, 1994.
679. Hughes PE, Diaz-Gonzalez F, Leong L, et al: Breaking the integrin hinge. A defined structural constraint regulates integrin signaling. *J Biol Chem* 271:6571, 1996.
680. Kim M, Carman CV, Springer TA: Bidirectional transmembrane signaling by cytoplasmic domain separation in integrins. *Science* 301:1720, 2003.
681. Luo BH, Carman CV, Takagi J, et al: Disrupting integrin transmembrane domain heterodimerization increases ligand binding affinity, not valency or clustering. *Proc Natl Acad Sci U S A* 102:3679, 2005.
682. Li W, Metcalf DG, Gorelik R, et al: A push-pull mechanism for regulating integrin function. *Proc Natl Acad Sci U S A* 102:1424, 2005.
683. Partridge AW, Liu S, Kim S, et al: Transmembrane domain helix packing stabilizes integrin alphaIIbbeta3 in the low affinity state. *J Biol Chem* 280:7294, 2005.
684. Leisner TM, Wencel-Drake JD, Wang W, et al: Bidirectional transmembrane modulation of integrin alphaIIbbeta3 conformations. *J Biol Chem* 274:12945, 1999.
685. Xiong JP, Stehle T, Goodman SL, et al: A novel adaptation of the integrin PSI domain revealed from its crystal structure. *J Biol Chem* 279:40252, 2004.
686. Kashiwagi H, Tomiyama Y, Tadokoro S, et al: A mutation in the extracellular cysteine-rich repeat region of the beta3 subunit activates integrins alphaIIbbeta3 and alphaVbeta3. *Blood* 93:2559, 1999.
687. Frelinger AL, III, Du XP, Plow EF, et al: Monoclonal antibodies to ligand-occupied conformers of integrin alpha IIb beta 3 (glycoprotein IIb-IIIa) alter receptor affinity, specificity, and function. *J Biol Chem* 266:17106, 1991.
688. Du X, Gu M, Weisel JW, et al: Long range propagation of conformational changes in integrin alpha IIb beta 3. *J Biol Chem* 268:23087, 1993.
689. Kamata T, Ambo H, Puzon-McLaughlin W, et al: Critical cysteine residues for regulation of integrin alphaIIbbeta3 are clustered in the epidermal growth factor domains of the beta3 subunit. *Biochem J* 378:1079, 2004.
690. Essex DW: The role of thiols and disulfides in platelet function. *Antioxid Redox Signal* 6:736, 2004.
691. Zucker MB, Masiello NC: Platelet aggregation caused by dithiothreitol. *Thromb Haemost* 51:119, 1984.
692. Chen K, Detwiler TC, Essex DW: Characterization of protein disulphide isomerase released from activated platelets. *Br J Haematol* 90:425, 1995.
693. Essex DW, Chen K, Swiatkowska M: Localization of protein disulfide isomerase to the external surface of the platelet plasma membrane. *Blood* 86:2168, 1995.
694. Essex DW: Redox control of platelet function. *Antioxid Redox Signal* 11:1191, 2009.
695. O'Neill S, Robinson A, Deering A, et al: The platelet integrin alpha IIbbeta 3 has an endogenous thiol isomerase activity. *J Biol Chem* 275:36984, 2000.
696. Lau TL, Kim C, Ginsberg MH, et al: The structure of the integrin alphaIIbbeta3 transmembrane complex explains integrin transmembrane signalling. *EMBO J* 28:1351, 2009.
697. Zhu J, Luo BH, Barth P, et al: The structure of a receptor with two associating transmembrane domains on the cell surface: Integrin alphaIIbbeta3. *Mol Cell* 34:234, 2009.
698. Gottschalk KE: A coiled-coil structure of the alphaIIbbeta3 integrin transmembrane and cytoplasmic domains in its resting state. *Structure* 13:703, 2005.
699. Luo BH, Springer TA, Takagi J: A specific interface between integrin transmembrane helices and affinity for ligand. *PLoS Biol* 2:776, 2004.
700. Wegener KL, Partridge AW, Han J, et al: Structural basis of integrin activation by talin. *Cell* 128:171, 2007.
701. Knezevic I, Leisner TM, Lam SC: Direct binding of the platelet integrin alphaIIbbeta3 (GPIIb-IIIa) to talin. Evidence that interaction is mediated through the cytoplasmic domains of both alphaIIb and beta3. *J Biol Chem* 271:16416, 1996.
701a. Anthis NJ, Wegener KL, Feng Y, et al: The structure of an integrin/talin complex reveals the basis of inside-out signal transduction. *Embo J* 28:3623, 2009.
702. He P, Zhang H, Yun CC: IRBIT, inositol 1,4,5-triphosphate (IP3) receptor-binding protein released with IP3, binds Na+/H+ exchanger NHE3 and activates NHE3 activity in response to calcium. *J Biol Chem* 283:33544, 2008.
703. Jenkins AL, Nannizzi-Alaimo L, Silver D, et al: Tyrosine phosphorylation of the beta3 cytoplasmic domain mediates integrin-cytoskeletal interactions. *J Biol Chem* 273:13878, 1998.
704. Law DA, DeGuzmann FR, Heiser P, et al: Integrin cytoplasmic tyrosine motif is required for outside-in alphaIIbbeta3 signalling and platelet function. *Nature* 401:808, 1999.
705. Shattil SJ, O'Toole T, Eigenthaler M, et al: Beta 3-endonexin, a novel polypeptide that interacts specifically with the cytoplasmic tail of the integrin beta 3 subunit. *J Cell Biol* 131:807, 1995.
706. Eigenthaler M, Hofferer L, Shattil SJ, et al: A conserved sequence motif in the integrin beta3 cytoplasmic domain is required for its specific interaction with beta3-endonexin. *J Biol Chem* 272:7693, 1997.
707. Calderwood DA, Zent R, Grant R, et al: The talin head domain binds to integrin {beta} subunit cytoplasmic tails and regulates integrin activation. *J Biol Chem* 274:28071, 1999.
708. Zent R, Fenczik CA, Calderwood DA, et al: Class- and splice variant-specific association of CD98 with integrin beta cytoplasmic domains. *J Biol Chem* 275:5059, 2000.
709. Reddy KB, Gascard P, Price MG, et al: Identification of an interaction between the m-band protein skelemin and beta-integrin subunits. Colocalization of a skelemin-like protein with beta1- and beta3-integrins in non-muscle cells. *J Biol Chem* 273:35039, 1998.
710. Calderwood DA, Shattil SJ, Ginsberg MH: Integrins and actin filaments: Reciprocal regulation of cell adhesion and signaling. *J Biol Chem* 275:22607, 2000.
711. Law DA, Nannizzi-Alaimo L, Phillips DR: Outside-in integrin signal transduction. Alpha IIb beta 3-(GP IIb IIIa) tyrosine phosphorylation induced by platelet aggregation. *J Biol Chem* 271:10811, 1996.
712. Cowan KJ, Law DA, Phillips DR: Identification of shc as the primary protein binding to the tyrosine-phosphorylated beta 3 subunit of alpha IIbbeta 3 during outside-in integrin platelet signaling. *J Biol Chem* 275:36423, 2000.
713. Schaller MD, Otey CA, Hildebrand JD, et al: Focal adhesion kinase and paxillin bind to peptides mimicking beta integrin cytoplasmic domains. *J Cell Biol* 130:1181, 1995.
714. Hannigan GE, Leung-Hagesteijn C, Fitz-Gibbon L, et al: Regulation of cell adhesion and anchorage-dependent growth by a new beta 1-integrin-linked protein kinase. *Nature* 379:91, 1996.
715. Otey CA, Pavalko FM, Burridge K: An interaction between alpha-actinin and the beta 1 integrin subunit *in vitro*. *J Cell Biol* 111:721, 1990.
716. Naik UP, Patel PM, Parise LV: Identification of a novel calcium-binding protein that interacts with the integrin alphaIIb cytoplasmic domain. *J Biol Chem* 272:4651, 1997.
717. Shock DD, Naik UP, Brittain JE, et al: Calcium-dependent properties of CIB binding to the integrin alphaIIb cytoplasmic domain and translocation to the platelet cytoskeleton. *Biochem J* 342:729, 1999.
718. Leung-Hagesteijn CY, Milankov K, Michalak M, et al: Cell attachment to extracellular matrix substrates is inhibited upon downregulation of expression of calreticulin, an intracellular integrin alpha-subunit-binding protein. *J Cell Sci* 107(Pt 3):589, 1994.
719. Rojiani MV, Finlay BB, Gray V, et al: *In vitro* interaction of a polypeptide homologous to human Ro/SS-A antigen (calreticulin) with a highly conserved amino acid sequence in the cytoplasmic domain of integrin alpha subunits. *Biochemistry* 30:9859, 1991.
720. Scarborough RM, Naughton MA, Teng W, et al: Design of potent and specific integrin antagonists. Peptide antagonists with high specificity for glycoprotein IIb-IIIa. *J Biol Chem* 268:1066, 1993.
721. Beer JH, Springer KT, Coller BS: Immobilized Arg-Gly-Asp (RGD) peptides of varying lengths as structural probes of the platelet GPIIb/IIIa receptor. *Blood* 79:117, 1992.
722. Luo BH, Springer TA, Takagi J: Stabilizing the open conformation of the integrin headpiece with a glycan wedge increases affinity for ligand. *Proc Natl Acad Sci U S A* 100:2403, 2003.
723. Heilmann E, Hourdille P, Pruvost A, et al: Thrombin-induced platelet aggregates have a dynamic structure: Time-dependent redistribution of GPIIb/IIIa complexes and secreted adhesive proteins. *Arterioscler Thromb* 11:704, 1991.
724. Isenberg WM, McEver RP, Phillips DR, et al: The platelet fibrinogen receptor: An immunogold-surface replica study of agonist-induced ligand binding and receptor clustering. *J Cell Biol* 104:1655, 1987.
725. Prevost N, Shattil SJ: Outside-in signaling by integrin $\alpha IIb\beta 3$, in *Platelets*, edited by AD Michelson, p 347. Academic Press, San Diego, 2007.
726. Asch E, Podack E: Vitronectin binds to activated human platelets and plays a role in platelet aggregation. *J Clin Invest* 85:1372, 1990.
727. Haverstick DM, Cowan JF, Yamada KM, et al: Inhibition of platelet adhesion to fibronectin, fibrinogen, and von Willebrand factor substrates by a synthetic tetrapeptide derived from the cell-binding domain of fibronectin. *Blood* 66:946, 1985.
728. Plow EF, D'Souza SE, Ginsberg MH: Ligand binding to GPIIb-IIIa: A status report. *Semin Thromb Hemost* 18:324, 1992.
729. Schullek J, Jordan J, Montgomery RR: Interaction of von Willebrand factor with human platelets in the plasma milieu. *J Clin Invest* 73:421, 1984.
730. Ni H, Papalia JM, Degen JL, et al: Control of thrombus embolization and fibronectin internalization by integrin alpha IIb beta 3 engagement of the fibrinogen gamma chain. *Blood* 102:3609, 2003.
731. Moskowitz KA, Kudryk B, Coller BS: Fibrinogen coating density affects the conformation of immobilized fibrinogen: Implications for platelet adhesion and spreading. *Thromb Haemost* 79:824, 1998.
732. Hatton MW, Moar SL, Richardson M: Deendothelialization *in vivo* initiates a thrombogenic reaction at the rabbit aorta surface. Correlation of uptake of fibrinogen and

antithrombin III with thrombin generation by the exposed subendothelium. *Am J Pathol* 135:499, 1989.

733. Miles LA, Ginsberg MH, White JG, et al: Plasminogen interacts with human platelets through two distinct mechanisms. *J Clin Invest* 77:2001, 1986.
734. Peerschke EI, Grant RA, Zucker MB: Decreased association of 45-calcium with platelets unable to aggregate due to thrombasthenia or prolonged calcium deprivation. *Br J Haematol* 46:247, 1980.
735. Powling MJ, Hardisty RM: Glycoprotein IIb-IIIa complex and Ca^{++} influx into stimulated platelets. *Blood* 66:731, 1985.
736. Rybak MEM, Renzulli LA: Effect of calcium channel blockers on platelet GPIIb-IIIa as a calcium channel in liposomes: Comparison with effects on the intact platelet. *Thromb Haemost* 67:131, 1991.
737. Ameisen JC, Joseph M, Caen JP, et al: A role for glycoprotein IIb-IIIa complexes in the binding of IgE to human platelets and platelet IgE-dependent cytolytic function. *Br J Haematol* 64:21, 1986.
738. Coburn J, Barthold SW, Leong JM: Diverse Lyme disease spirochetes bind integrin alpha IIb beta 3 on human platelets. *Infect Immun* 62:5559, 1994.
739. Gavrilovskaya IN, Brown EJ, Ginsberg MH, et al: Cellular entry of hantaviruses which cause hemorrhagic fever with renal syndrome is mediated by beta3 integrins. *J Virol* 73:3951, 1999.

739a. Scibelli A, Roperto S, Manna L, et al: Engagement integrins as a cellular route of invasion by bacterial pathogens. *Vet J* 173:478, 2007.

740. Kulkarni S, Jackson SP: Platelet factor XIII and calpain negatively regulate integrin alphaIIbbeta3 adhesive function and thrombus growth. *J Biol Chem* 279:30697, 2004.
741. Pischel KD, Hemler MD, Huang C, et al: Use of the monoclonal antibody 12F1 to characterize the differentiation antigen VLA-2. *J Immunol* 138:226, 1987.
742. Kunicki DJ, Nugent DJ, Staats SJ, et al: The human fibroblast II extracellular matrix receptor mediates platelet adhesion to collagen and is identical to the platelet glycoprotein Ia-IIa complex. *J Biol Chem* 263:4516, 1988.
743. Staatz WD, Rajpara SM, Wayner EA, et al: The membrane glycoprotein Ia-IIa (VLA-2) complex mediates the Mg^{++}-dependent adhesion of platelets to collagen. *J Cell Biol* 108:1917, 1989.
744. Barnes MJ, Knight CG, Farndale RW: The collagen-platelet interaction. *Curr Opin Hematol* 5:314, 1998.
745. Takada Y, Hemler ME: The primary structure of the VLA-2/collagen receptor $\alpha 2$ subunit (platelet GPIa): Homology to other integrins and the presence of a possible collagen-binding domain. *J Cell Biol* 109:397, 1987.
746. Clemetson KJ: Platelet receptors, in *Platelets*, edited by AD Michelson, p 65. Academic Press, San Diego, 2002.
747. Emsley J, King SL, Bergelson JM, et al: Crystal structure of the I domain from integrin alpha2beta1. *J Biol Chem* 272:28512, 1997.
748. Emsley J, Knight CG, Farndale RW, et al: Structural basis of collagen recognition by integrin alpha2beta1. *Cell* 101:47, 2000.
749. Nieuwenhuis HK, Akkerman JWN, Houdijk WPM, et al: Human blood platelets showing no response to collagen fail to express surface glycoprotein Ia. *Nature* 318:470, 1985.
750. Sarratt KL, Chen H, Zutter MM, et al: GPVI and alpha2beta1 play independent critical roles during platelet adhesion and aggregate formation to collagen under flow. *Blood* 106:1268, 2005.
751. Zou Z, Schmaier AA, Cheng L, et al: Negative regulation of activated {alpha}2 integrins during thrombopoiesis. *Blood* 113:6271, 2009.
752. Schoolmeester A, Vanhoorelbeke K, Katsutani S, et al: Monoclonal antibody IAC-1 is specific for activated alpha2beta1 and binds to amino acids 199 to 201 of the integrin alpha2 I-domain. *Blood* 104:390, 2004.
753. Cruz MA, Chen J, Whitelock JL, et al: The platelet glycoprotein Ib-von Willebrand factor interaction activates the collagen receptor alpha2beta1 to bind collagen: Activation-dependent conformational change of the alpha2-I domain. *Blood* 105:1986, 2005.
754. He L, Pappan LK, Grenache DG, et al: The contributions of the alpha 2 beta 1 integrin to vascular thrombosis *in vivo*. *Blood* 102:3652, 2003.
755. Lahav J, Wijnen EM, Hess O, et al: Enzymatically catalyzed disulfide exchange is required for platelet adhesion to collagen via integrin alpha2beta1. *Blood* 102:2085, 2003.
756. Staatz WD, Walsh JJ, Pexton T, et al: The $\alpha_2\beta_1$ integrin cell surface collagen receptor binds to the $\alpha 1$(I)-CB3 peptide of collagen. *J Biol Chem* 265:4778, 1990.
757. Knight CG, Morton LF, Onley DJ, et al: Identification in collagen type I of an integrin alpha2 beta1-binding site containing an essential GER sequence. *J Biol Chem* 273:33287, 1998.
758. Santoro SA, Walsh JJ, Staatz WD, et al: Distinct determinants on collagen support $\alpha 2\beta 1$ integrin-mediated platelet adhesion and platelet activation. *Cell Regul* 2:905, 1991.
759. Verkleij MW, Ijsseldijk MJ, Heijnen-Snyder GJ, et al: Adhesive domains in the collagen III fragment alpha1(III)CB4 that support alpha2b. *Thromb Haemost* 82:1137, 1999.
760. Bray PF: Integrin polymorphisms as risk factors for thrombosis. *Thromb Haemost* 82:337, 1999.
761. Moshfegh K, Wuillemin WA, Redondo M, et al: Association of two silent polymorphisms of platelet glycoprotein Ia/IIa receptor with risk of myocardial infarction: A case-control study. *Lancet* 353:351, 1999.
762. Santoso S, Kunicki TJ, Kroll H, et al: Association of the platelet glycoprotein Ia C807T gene polymorphism with nonfatal myocardial infarction in younger patients. *Blood* 93:2449, 1999.
763. Carlsson LE, Santoso S, Spitzer C, et al: The alpha2 gene coding sequence T807/A873 of the platelet collagen receptor integrin alpha2beta1 might be a genetic risk factor for the development of stroke in younger patients. *Blood* 93:3583, 1999.
764. von Beckerath N, Koch W, Mehilli J, et al: Glycoprotein Ia gene C807T polymorphism and risk for major adverse cardiac events within the first 30 days after coronary artery stenting. *Blood* 95:3297, 2000.
765. Matsubara Y, Murata M, Maruyama T, et al: Association between diabetic retinopathy and genetic variations in alpha2beta1 integrin, a platelet receptor for collagen. *Blood* 95:1560, 2000.
766. Roest M, Banga JD, Grobbee DE, et al: Homozygosity for 807 T polymorphism in alpha(2) subunit of platelet alpha(2)beta(1) is associated with increased risk of cardiovascular mortality in high-risk women. *Circulation* 102:1645, 2000.
767. Fox JEB: Linkage of a membrane skeleton to integral membrane glycoproteins in human platelets. Identification of one of the glycoproteins as glycoprotein Ib. *J Clin Invest* 76:1673, 1985.
768. Elices MJ, Hemler ME: The integrin VLA-2 can be a laminin as well as a collagen receptor. *Proc Natl Acad Sci U S A* 86:9906, 1989.
769. Kirchhofer D, Languinol R, Ruoslahti E, et al: $\alpha 2\beta 1$ Integrins from different cell types show different binding specificities. *J Biol Chem* 265:615, 1990.
770. Piotrowicz RS, Orchekowski RP, Nugent DJ, et al: Glycoprotein Ic-IIa functions as an activation-independent fibronectin receptor on human platelets. *J Cell Biol* 106:1359, 1988.
771. Wayner EA, Carter WG, Piotrowicz RS, et al: The function of multiple extracellular matrix receptors in mediating cell adhesion to extracellular matrix: Preparation of monoclonal antibodies to the fibronectin receptor that specifically inhibit cell adhesion of fibronectin and react with platelet glycoproteins Ic-IIa. *J Cell Biol* 107:1881, 1988.
772. Garcia AJ, Huber F, Boettiger D: Force required to break alpha5beta1 integrin-fibronectin bonds in intact adherent cells is sensitive to integrin activation state. *J Biol Chem* 273:10988, 1998.
773. Vuillet-Gaugler MH, Breton-Gorius J, Vainchenker W, et al: Loss of attachment to fibronectin with terminal human erythroid differentiation. *Blood* 75:865, 1990.
774. Sonnenberg A, Modderman PW, Hogervorst F: Laminin receptor on platelets is the integrin VLA-6. *Nature* 336:487, 1988.
775. Hindriks G, Ijsseldijk MJ, Sonnenberg A, et al: Platelet adhesion to laminin: Role of $Ca2+$ and $Mg2+$ ions, shear rate, and platelet membrane glycoproteins. *Blood* 79:928, 1992.
776. Chang JC, Chang HH, Lin CT, et al: The integrin alpha6beta1 modulation of PI3K and Cdc42 activities induces dynamic filopodium formation in human platelets. *J Biomed Sci* 12:881, 2005.
777. Tandon NN, Holland EA, Kralisz U, et al: Interaction of human platelets with laminin and identification of the 67 kDa laminin receptor on platelets. *Biochem J* 274:535, 1991.
778. Luo BH, Carman CV, Springer TA: Structural basis of integrin regulation and signaling. *Annu Rev Immunol* 25:619, 2007.
779. Arnaout MA, Goodman SL, Xiong JP: Structure and mechanics of integrin-based cell adhesion. *Curr Opin Cell Biol* 19:495, 2007.
780. Fitzgerald LA, Poncz M, Steiner B, et al: Comparison of cDNA-derived protein sequences of the human fibronectin and vitronectin receptor α subunits and platelet glycoprotein IIb. *Biochemistry* 26:8158, 1987.
781. Coller BS, Cheresh DA, Asch E, et al: Platelet vitronectin receptor expression differentiates Iraqi-Jewish from Arab Patients with Glanzmann thrombasthenia in Israel. *Blood* 77:75, 1991.
782. Kieffer N, Fitzgerald LA, Wolf D, et al: Adhesive properties of the $\beta 3$ integrins. Comparison of GPIIb-IIIa and the vitronectin receptor individually expressed in human melanoma cells. *J Cell Biol* 113:451, 1991.
783. Lam SC, Plow EF, D'Souza SE, et al: Isolation and characterization of a platelet membrane protein related to the vitronectin receptor. *J Biol Chem* 264:3742, 1989.
784. Charo IF, Bekeart LS, Phillips DR: Platelet glycoprotein IIb-IIIa-like proteins mediate endothelial cell attachment to adhesive proteins and the extracellular matrix. *J Biol Chem* 262:9935, 1987.
785. Byzova TV, Plow EF: Activation of alphaVbeta3 on vascular cells controls recognition of prothrombin. *J Cell Biol* 143:2081, 1998.
786. Bennett JS, Chan C, Vilaire G, et al: Agonist-activated alphavbeta3 on platelets and lymphocytes binds to the matrix protein osteopontin. *J Biol Chem* 272:8137, 1997.
787. Beckstead JH, Stenberg PE, McEver RP, et al: Immunohistochemical localization of membrane and alpha-granule proteins in human megakaryocytes: Application to plastic-embedded bone marrow biopsy specimens. *Blood* 67:285, 1986.
788. Davies J, Warwick J, Totty N, et al: The osteoclast functional antigen, implicated in the regulation of bone resorption is biochemically related to the vitronectin receptor. *J Cell Biol* 109:1817, 1989.
789. McHugh KP, Hodivala-Dilke K, Zheng MH, et al: Mice lacking beta3 integrins are osteosclerotic because of dysfunctional osteoclasts. *J Clin Invest* 105:433, 2000.
790. Feng X, Novack DV, Faccio R, et al: A Glanzmann's mutation in beta 3 integrin specifically impairs osteoclast function. *J Clin Invest* 107:1137, 2001.
791. Savill J, Dransfield I, Hogg N, et al: Vitronectin receptor-mediated phagocytosis of cells undergoing apoptosis. *Nature* 343:170, 1990.
792. Brooks PC, Clark RA, Cheresh DA: Requirement of vascular integrin $\alpha V\beta 3$ for angiogenesis. *Science* 264:569, 1994.
793. Varner JA, Cheresh DA: Integrins and cancer. *Curr Opin Cell Biol* 8:724, 1996.

794. Trikha M, Zhou Z, Nemeth JA, et al: CNTO 95, a fully human monoclonal antibody that inhibits alphav integrins, has antitumor and antiangiogenic activity *in vivo*. *Int J Cancer* 110:326, 2004.
795. Choi ET, Engel L, Callow AD, et al: Inhibition of neointimal hyperplasia by blocking $\alpha_v\beta_3$ integrin with a small peptide antagonist G*pen*GRGDSPCA. *J Vasc Surg* 19:125, 1994.
796. Sajid M, Stouffer GA: The role of alpha(v)beta3 integrins in vascular healing. *Thromb Haemost* 87:187, 2002.
797. Stouffer GA, Smyth SS: Effects of thrombin on interactions between beta3-integrins and extracellular matrix in platelets and vascular cells. *Arterioscler Thromb Vasc Biol* 23:1971, 2003.
798. Lopez JH, Chung DW, Fujikawa K, et al: The α and β chains of human platelet glycoprotein Ib are both transmembrane proteins containing a leucine-rich amino acid sequence. *Proc Natl Acad Sci U S A* 85:2135, 1988.
799. Lopez JA, Andrews RK, Afshar-Kharghan V, et al: Bernard-Soulier syndrome. *Blood* 91:4397, 1998.
800. Clemetson KJ, Clemetson JM: Platelet GPIb complex as a target for anti-thrombotic drug development. *Thromb Haemost* 99:473, 2008.
801. Ozaki Y, Asazuma N, Suzuki-Inoue K, et al: Platelet GPIb-IX-V-dependent signaling. *J Thromb Haemost* 3:1745, 2005.
802. Du X, Beutler L, Ruan C, et al: Glycoprotein Ib and glycoprotein IX are fully complexed in the intact platelet membrane. *Blood* 69:1524, 1987.
803. Hickey MJ, Williams SA, Roth GJ: Human platelet GPIX: An adhesive prototype of leucine-rich glycoproteins with flank-center-flank structures. *Proc Natl Acad Sci U S A* 86:6773, 1989.
804. Hickey MJ, Deaven LL, Roth GJ: Human platelet glycoprotein IX. Characterization of cDNA and localization of the gene to chromosome 3. *FEBS Lett* 274:189, 1991.
805. Lopez JA, Leung B, Reynolds CC, et al: Efficient plasma membrane expression of a functional platelet glycoprotein Ib-IX complex requires the presence of its three subunits. *J Biol Chem* 267:12851, 1992.
806. Sprandio JD, Shapiro SS, Thiagarajan P, et al: Cultured human umbilical vein endothelial cells contain a membrane glycoprotein immunologically related to platelet glycoprotein Ib. *Blood* 71:234, 1988.
807. Asch AS, Adelman B, Fujimoto M, et al: Identification and isolation of a platelet GPIb-like protein in human umbilical vein endothelial cells and bovine aortic smooth muscle cells. *J Clin Invest* 81:1600, 1988.
808. Konkle BA, Shapiro SS, Asch AS, et al: Cytokine-enhanced expression of glycoprotein Ib alpha in human endothelium. *J Biol Chem* 265:19833, 1990.
809. Rajagopalan V, Essex DW, Shapiro SS, et al: Tumor necrosis factor-alpha modulation of glycoprotein Ib-alpha expression in human endothelial and erythroleukemia cells. *Blood* 80:153, 1992.
810. Bombeli T, Schwartz BR, Harlan JM: Adhesion of activated platelets to endothelial cells: Evidence for a GPIIbIIIa-dependent bridging mechanism and novel roles for endothelial intercellular adhesion molecule 1 (ICAM-1), alphavbeta3 integrin, and GPIbalpha. *J Exp Med* 187:329, 1998.
811. Tan L, Kowalska MA, Romo GM, et al: Identification and characterization of endothelial glycoprotein Ib using viper venom proteins modulating cell adhesion. *Blood* 93:2605, 1999.
812. Perrault C, Lankhof H, Pidard D, et al: Relative importance of the glycoprotein Ib-binding domain and the RGD sequence of von Willebrand factor for its interaction with endothelial cells. *Blood* 90:2335, 1997.
813. Uzan G, Prenant M, Prandini MH, et al: Tissue-specific expression of the platelet GPIIb gene. *J Biol Chem* 266:8932, 1991.
814. Prandini MH, Uzan G, Martin F, et al: Characterization of a specific erythromegakaryocytic enhancer within the glycoprotein IIb promoter. *J Biol Chem* 267:10370, 1992.
815. Lemarchandel V, Ghysdael J, Mignotte V, et al: GATA and Ets cis-acting sequences mediate megakaryocyte-specific expression. *Mol Cell Biol* 13:668, 1993.
816. Martin F, Prandini MH, Thevenon D, et al: The transcription factor GATA-1 regulates the promoter activity of the platelet glycoprotein IIb gene. *J Biol Chem* 268:21606, 1993.
817. Block KL, Poncz M: Platelet glycoprotein IIb gene expression as a model of megakaryocyte-specific expression. *Stem Cells* 13:135, 1995.
818. Hashimoto Y, Ware J: Identification of essential GATA and Ets binding motifs within the promoter of the platelet glycoprotein Ib alpha gene. *J Biol Chem* 270:24532, 1995.
819. Bastian LS, Yagi M, Chan C, et al: Analysis of the megakaryocyte glycoprotein IX promoter identifies positive and negative regulatory domains and functional GATA and Ets sites. *J Biol Chem* 271:18554, 1996.
820. Tsang AP, Visvader JE, Turner CA, et al: FOG, a multitype zinc finger protein, acts as a cofactor for transcription factor GATA-1 in erythroid and megakaryocytic differentiation. *Cell* 90:109, 1997.
821. Krause DS, Perkins AS: Gotta find GATA a friend. *Nat Med* 3:960, 1997.
822. Lopez JA, Ludwig EW, McCarthy BJ: Polymorphism of human glycoprotein Ibα results from a variable number of repeats of a 13-amino acid sequence in the mucin-like macroglycopeptide region. Structure function implications. *J Biol Chem* 267:10055, 1992.
823. Murata M, Matsubara Y, Kawano K, et al: Coronary artery disease and polymorphisms in a receptor mediating shear stress-dependent platelet activation. *Circulation* 96:3281, 1997.
824. Gonzalez-Conejero R, Lozano ML, Rivera J, et al: Polymorphisms of platelet membrane glycoprotein Ib associated with arterial thrombotic disease. *Blood* 92:2771, 1998.
825. Carlsson LE, Greinacher A, Spitzer C, et al: Polymorphisms of the human platelet antigens HPA-1, HPA-2, HPA-3, and HPA-5 on the platelet receptors for fibrinogen (GPIIb/IIIa), von Willebrand factor (GPIb/IX), and collagen (GPIa/IIa) are not correlated with an increased risk for stroke. *Stroke* 28:1392, 1997.
826. Kaski S, Kekomaki R, Partanen J: Systematic screening for genetic polymorphism in human platelet glycoprotein Ibalpha. *Immunogenetics* 44:170, 1996.
827. Suzuki K, Hayashi T, Akiba J, et al: StyI polymorphism at nucleotide 1610 in the human platelet glycoprotein Ib alpha gene. *Jpn J Hum Genet* 41:419, 1996.
828. Afshar-Kharghan V, Li CQ, Khoshnevis-Asl M, et al: Kozak sequence polymorphism of the glycoprotein (GP) Ibalpha gene is a major determinant of the plasma membrane levels of the platelet GP Ib-IX-V complex. *Blood* 94:186, 1999.
829. Baker RI, Eikelboom J, Lofthouse E, et al: Platelet glycoprotein Ibalpha Kozak polymorphism is associated with an increased risk of ischemic stroke. *Blood* 98:36, 2001.
830. Meisel C, Afshar-Kharghan V, Cascorbi I, et al: Role of Kozak sequence polymorphism of platelet glycoprotein Ibalpha as a risk factor for coronary artery disease and catheter interventions. *J Am Coll Cardiol* 38:1023, 2001.
831. Douglas H, Michaelides K, Gorog DA, et al: Platelet membrane glycoprotein Ibalpha gene -5T/C Kozak sequence polymorphism as an independent risk factor for the occurrence of coronary thrombosis. *Heart* 87:70, 2002.
832. Kenny D, Muckian C, Fitzgerald DJ, et al: Platelet glycoprotein Ib alpha receptor polymorphisms and recurrent ischaemic events in acute coronary syndrome patients. *J Thromb Thrombolysis* 13:13, 2002.
833. Rosenberg N, Zivelin A, Chetrit A, et al: Effects of platelet membrane glycoprotein polymorphisms on the risk of myocardial infarction in young males. *Isr Med Assoc J* 4:411, 2002.
834. Jilma-Stohlawetz P, Homoncik M, Jilma B, et al: Glycoprotein Ib polymorphisms influence platelet plug formation under high shear rates. *Br J Haematol* 120:652, 2003.
835. Carlsson LE, Lubenow N, Blumentritt C, et al: Platelet receptor and clotting factor polymorphisms as genetic risk factors for thromboembolic complications in heparin-induced thrombocytopenia. *Pharmacogenetics* 13:253, 2003.
836. Ozelo MC, Origa AF, Aranha FJ, et al: Platelet glycoprotein Ibα polymorphisms modulate the risk for myocardial infarction. *Thromb Haemost* 92:384, 2004.
837. Tsuji T, Tsunehisa S, Watanabe Y, et al: The carbohydrate moiety of human platelet glycocalicin. *J Biol Chem* 258:6335, 1983.
838. Fox JEB, Aggerbeck LP, Berndt MC: Structure of the glycoprotein Ib-IX complex from platelet membranes. *J Biol Chem* 263:4882, 1988.
839. Solum NO, Hagen I, Filion-Myklebust C, et al: Platelet glycocalicin: Its membrane association in solvent and aqueous media. *Biochim Biophys Acta* 597:235, 1990.
839a. Bergmeier W, Piffath CL, Cheng G, et al: Tumor necrosis factor-α-converting enzyme (ADAM17) mediates GPIbα shedding from platelets *in vitro* and *in vivo*. *Circ Res* 95:677, 2004.
840. Coller BS, Kalomiris EL, Steinberg M, et al: Evidence that glycocalicin circulates in normal plasma. *J Clin Invest* 73:794, 1984.
841. Kurata Y, Hayashi S, Kiyoi T, et al: Diagnostic value of tests for reticulated platelets, plasma glycocalicin, and thrombopoietin levels for discriminating between hyperdestructive and hypoplastic thrombocytopenia. *Am J Clin Pathol* 115:656, 2001.
842. Steinberg MH, Kelton JG, Coller BS: Plasma glycocalicin. An aid in the classification of thrombocytopenic disorders. *N Engl J Med* 317:1037, 1987.
843. Kunishima S, Kobayashi S, Takagi A, et al: Rapid detection of plasma glycocalicin by a latex agglutination test. A useful adjunct in the differential diagnosis of thrombocytopenia. *Am J Clin Pathol* 100:579, 1993.
844. Kunishima S, Kobayashi S, Naoe T: Increased but highly dispersed levels of plasma glycocalicin in patients with disseminated intravascular coagulation. *Eur J Haematol* 56:173, 1996.
845. Beer JH, Buchi L, Steiner B: Glycocalicin: A new assay—the normal plasma levels and its potential usefulness in selected diseases. *Blood* 83:691, 1994.
846. Steffan A, Pradella P, Cordiano I, et al: Glycocalicin in the diagnosis and management of immune thrombocytopenia. *Eur J Haematol* 61:77, 1998.
847. Himmelfarb J, Nelson S, McMonagle E, et al: Elevated plasma glycocalicin levels and decreased ristocetin-induced platelet agglutination in hemodialysis patients. *Am J Kidney Dis* 32:132, 1998.
847a. Rabie T, Strehl A, Ludwig A, et al: Evidence for a role of ADAM17 (TACE) in the regulation of platelet glycoprotein V. *J Biol Chem* 280:14462, 2005.
848. Kalomiris EL, Coller BS: Thiol-specific probes indicate that the alpha chain of platelet glycoprotein Ib is a transmembrane protein with a reactive endofacial sulfhydryl group. *Biochemistry* 24:5430, 1985.
849. Muszbek L, Laposata M: Glycoprotein Ib and glycoprotein IX in human platelets are acylated with palmitic acid through thioester linkages. *J Biol Chem* 264:9716, 1989.
850. Du X, Fox JE, Pei S: Identification of a binding sequence for the 14-3-3 protein within the cytoplasmic domain of the adhesion receptor, platelet glycoprotein Ib alpha. *J Biol Chem* 271:7362, 1996.
851. Calverley DC, Kavanagh TJ, Roth GJ: Human signaling protein 14-3-3zeta interacts with platelet glycoprotein Ib subunits Ibalpha and Ibbeta. *Blood* 91:1295, 1998.
852. Andrews RK, Harris SJ, McNally T, et al: Binding of purified 14-3-3 zeta signaling protein to discrete amino acid sequences within the cytoplasmic domain of the platelet membrane glycoprotein Ib-IX-V complex. *Biochemistry* 37:638, 1998.
853. Wardell MR, Reynolds CC, Berndt MC, et al: Platelet glycoprotein Ib beta is phosphorylated on serine 166 by cyclic AMP-dependent protein kinase. *J Biol Chem* 264:15656, 1989.

854. Andrews RK, Fox JE: Identification of a region in the cytoplasmic domain of the platelet membrane glycoprotein Ib-IX complex that binds to purified actin-binding protein. *J Biol Chem* 267:18605, 1992.
855. Coller BS: Inhibition of von Willebrand factor-dependent platelet function by increased platelet cyclic AMP and its prevention by cytoskeleton-disrupting agents. *Blood* 57:846, 1981.
856. Coller BS: Effects of tertiary amine local anesthetics on von Willebrand factor-dependent platelet function: Alteration of membrane reactivity and degradation of GPIb by a calcium-dependent protease(s). *Blood* 248:1355, 1982.
857. Dong JF, Li CQ, Sae-Tung G, et al: The cytoplasmic domain of glycoprotein (GP) Ibalpha constrains the lateral diffusion of the GP Ib-IX complex and modulates von Willebrand factor binding. *Biochemistry* 36:12421, 1997.
858. Munday AD, Berndt MC, Mitchell CA: Phosphoinositide 3-kinase forms a complex with platelet membrane glycoprotein Ib-IX-V complex and 14-3-3zeta. *Blood* 96:577, 2000.
858a. Mu FT, Cranmer SL, Andrews RK, et al: Functional association of PI3-kinase with platelet glycoprotein Ibα, the major ligand-binding subunit of the glycoprotein Ib-IX-V complex. *J Thromb Haemostas* ePublished, 2009.
859. Sullam PM, Hyun WC, Szollosi J, et al: Physical proximity and functional interplay of the glycoprotein Ib-IX-V complex and the Fc receptor FcgammaRIIA on the platelet plasma membrane. *J Biol Chem* 273:5331, 1998.
860. Falati S, Edmead CE, Poole AW: Glycoprotein Ib-V-IX, a receptor for von Willebrand factor, couples physically and functionally to the Fc receptor γ-chain, Fyn, and Lyn to activate human platelets. *Blood* 94:1648, 1999.
861. Watson SP, Asazuma N, Atkinson B, et al: The role of ITAM- and ITIM-coupled receptors in platelet activation by collagen. *Thromb Haemost* 86:276, 2001.
862. Wu Y, Suzuki-Inoue K, Satoh K, et al: Role of Fc receptor gamma-chain in platelet glycoprotein Ib-mediated signaling. *Blood* 97:3836, 2001.
863. Uff S, Clemetson JM, Harrison T, et al: Crystal structure of the platelet glycoprotein Ib(alpha) N-terminal domain reveals an unmasking mechanism for receptor activation. *J Biol Chem* 277:35657, 2002.
864. Huizinga EG, Tsuji S, Romijn RA, et al: Structures of glycoprotein Ibalpha and its complex with von Willebrand factor A1 domain. *Science* 297:1176, 2002.
865. Dumas JJ, Kumar R, McDonagh T, et al: Crystal structure of the wild-type von Willebrand factor A1-glycoprotein Ibalpha complex reveals conformation differences with a complex bearing von Willebrand disease mutations. *J Biol Chem* 279:23327, 2004.
866. Tang J, Stern-Nezer S, Liu PC, et al: Mutation in the leucine-rich repeat C-flanking region of platelet glycoprotein Ibbeta impairs assembly of von Willebrand factor receptor. *Thromb Haemost* 92:75, 2004.
867. Scott JP, Montgomery RR, Retzinger GS: Dimeric ristocetin flocculates proteins, binds to platelets, and mediates von Willebrand factor-dependent agglutination of platelets. *J Biol Chem* 266:8149, 1991.
868. Berndt MC, Ward CM, Booth WJ, et al: Identification of aspartic acid 514 through glutamic acid 542 as a glycoprotein Ib-IX complex receptor recognition sequence in von Willebrand factor. Mechanism of modulation of von Willebrand factor by ristocetin and botrocetin. *Biochemistry* 31:11144, 1992.
869. Andrews RK, Booth WJ, Gorman JJ, et al: Purification of botrocetin from *Bothrops jararaca* venom. Analysis of the botrocetin-mediated interaction between von Willebrand factor and the human platelet membrane glycoprotein Ib-IX complex. *Biochemistry* 28:8317, 1989.
870. Fukuda K, Doggett T, Laurenzi IJ, et al: The snake venom protein botrocetin acts as a biological brace to promote dysfunctional platelet aggregation. *Nat Struct Mol Biol* 12:152, 2005.
871. Olson JD, Zaleski A, Herrmann D, et al: Adhesion of platelets to purified solid-phase von Willebrand factor: Effect of wall shear rate, ADP, thrombin, and ristocetin. *J Lab Clin Med* 114:6, 1989.
872. Parker RI, Gralnick HR: Fibrin monomer induces binding of endogenous vWF to the glycocalicin portion of platelet glycoprotein Ib. *Blood* 70:1589, 1987.
873. Sakariassen KS, Fressinaud E, Grima JP, et al: Role of platelet membrane glycoproteins and von Willebrand factor in adhesion of platelets to subendothelium and collagen. *Ann N Y Acad Sci* 516:52, 1987.
874. Sakariassen KS, Nievelstein PFEM, Coller BS, et al: The role of platelet membrane glycoproteins Ib and IIb-IIIa in platelet adherence to human artery subendothelium. *Br J Haematol* 63:681, 1986.
875. Ikeda Y, Murata M, Araki Y, et al: Importance of fibrinogen and platelet membrane glycoprotein IIb/IIIa in shear-induced platelet aggregation. *Thromb Res* 51:157, 1988.
876. Siediecki CA, Lestini BJ, Kottke-Marchant KK, et al: Shear-dependent changes in the three-dimensional structure of human von Willebrand factor. *Blood* 88:2939, 1996.
877. Yago T, Lou J, Wu T, et al: Platelet glycoprotein Ibalpha forms catch bonds with human WT vWF but not with type 2B von Willebrand disease vWF. *J Clin Invest* 118:3195, 2008.
878. Jamieson GA: The activation of platelets by thrombin: A model for activation by high and moderate affinity receptor pathways. *Prog Clin Biol Res* 283:137, 1988.
879. Ruggeri Z: The platelet glycoprotein Ib-IX complex. *Prog Hemost Thromb* 10:35, 1991.
880. Katagiri Y, Hayashi Y, Yamamoto K, et al: Localization of von Willebrand factor and thrombin-interactive domains in human platelet glycoprotein Ib. *Thromb Haemost* 63:122, 1990.
881. Vanhoorelbeke K, Ulrichts H, Romijn RA, et al: The GPIbalpha-thrombin interaction: Far from crystal clear. *Trends Mol Med* 10:33, 2004.
882. Celikel R, McClintock RA, Roberts JR, et al: Modulation of alpha-thrombin function by distinct interactions with platelet glycoprotein Ibalpha. *Science* 301:218, 2003.
883. Dumas JJ, Kumar R, Seehra J, et al: Crystal structure of the GpIbalpha-thrombin complex essential for platelet aggregation. *Science* 301:222, 2003.
884. Adams TE, Huntington JA: Thrombin-cofactor interactions: Structural insights into regulatory mechanisms. *Arterioscler Thromb Vasc Biol* 26:1738, 2006.
885. Harmon JT, Jamieson GA: The glycocalicin portion of platelet glycoprotein Ib expresses both high and moderate affinity receptor sites of thrombin. A soluble radioreceptor assay for the injection of thrombin with platelets. *J Biol Chem* 261:13224, 1986.
886. Adam F, Verbeuren TJ, Fauchere JL, et al: Thrombin-induced platelet PAR4 activation: Role of glycoprotein Ib and ADP. *J Thromb Haemost* 1:798, 2003.
887. De Candia E, Hall SW, Rutella S, et al: Binding of thrombin to glycoprotein Ib accelerates the hydrolysis of Par 1 on intact platelets. *J Biol Chem* 276:4692, 2001.
888. Frenette PS, Moyna C, Hartwell DW, et al: Platelet-endothelial interactions in inflamed mesenteric venules. *Blood* 91:1318, 1998.
889. Bradford HN, Dela Cadena RA, Kunapuli SP, et al: Human kininogens regulate thrombin binding to platelets through the glycoprotein Ib-IX-V complex. *Blood* 90:1508, 1997.
890. Bradford HN, Pixley RA, Colman RW: Human factor XII binding to the glycoprotein Ib-IX-V complex inhibits thrombin-induced platelet aggregation. *J Biol Chem* 275:22756, 2000.
891. Baglia FA, Badellino KO, Li CQ, et al: Factor XI binding to the platelet glycoprotein Ib-IX-V complex promotes factor XI activation by thrombin. *J Biol Chem* 277:1662, 2002.
892. Simon DI, Chen Z, Xu H, et al: Platelet glycoprotein Ibα is a counterreceptor for the leukocyte integrin Mac-1 (CD11b/CD18). *J Exp Med* 192:193, 2000.
893. Berndt MC, Phillips DR: Purification and preliminary physiochemical characterization of human platelet membrane glycoprotein V. *J Biol Chem* 256:59, 1981.
894. Zafar RS, Walz DA: Platelet membrane glycoprotein V: Characterization of the thrombin-sensitive glycoprotein from human platelets. *Thromb Res* 53:31, 1989.
895. Shimomura T, Fujimura K, Maehama S, et al: Rapid purification and characterization of human platelet glycoprotein V: The amino acid sequence contains leucine-rich repetitive modules as in glycoprotein Ib. *Blood* 75:2349, 1990.
896. Lanza F, Morales M, De La Salle C, et al: Cloning and characterization of the gene encoding the human platelet glycoprotein V. A member of the leucine-rich glycoprotein family cleaved during thrombin-induced platelet activation. *J Biol Chem* 268:20801, 1993.
897. Modderman PW, Admiraal LG, Sonnenberg A, et al: Glycoproteins V and Ib-IX form a noncovalent complex in the platelet membrane. *J Biol Chem* 267:364, 1992.
898. Dong JF, Gao S, Lopez JA: Synthesis, assembly, and intracellular transport of the platelet glycoprotein Ib-IX-V complex. *J Biol Chem* 273:31449, 1998.
899. McGowan EB, Ding A, Detwiler TC: Correlation of thrombin-induced glycoprotein V hydrolysis and platelet activation. *J Biol Chem* 258:11243, 1983.
900. Ramakrishnan V, Reeves PS, DeGuzman F, et al: Increased thrombin responsiveness in platelets from mice lacking glycoprotein V. *Proc Natl Acad Sci U S A* 96:13336, 1999.
901. Ramakrishnan V, DeGuzman F, Bao M, et al: A thrombin receptor function for platelet glycoprotein Ib-IX unmasked by cleavage of glycoprotein V. *Proc Natl Acad Sci U S A* 98:1823, 2001.
902. Newman PJ, Berndt MC, Gorski J, et al: PECAM-1 (CD31) cloning and relation to adhesion molecules of the immunoglobulin gene superfamily. *Science* 247:1219, 1990.
903. Novinska MS, Rathore V, Newman DK, et al: PECAM-1, in *Platelets*, 2nd ed, edited by AD Michelson, p 221. Academic Press, San Diego, 2007.
904. Metzelaar MJ, Korteweg J, Sixma JJ, et al: Biochemical characterization of PECAM-1 (CD31 antigen) on human platelets. *Thromb Haemost* 66:700, 1991.
905. Varon D, Jackson DE, Shenkman B, et al: Platelet/endothelial cell adhesion molecule-1 serves as a costimulatory agonist receptor that modulates integrin-dependent adhesion and aggregation of human platelets. *Blood* 91:500, 1998.
906. Jackson DE, Ward CM, Wang R, et al: The protein-tyrosine phosphatase SHP-2 binds platelet/endothelial cell adhesion molecule-1 (PECAM-1) and forms a distinct signaling complex during platelet aggregation. Evidence for a mechanistic link between PECAM-1- and integrin-mediated cellular signaling. *J Biol Chem* 272:6986, 1997.
907. Albelda SM, Muller WA, Buck CA, et al: Molecular and cellular properties of PECAM-1 (endoCAM/CD31): A novel vascular cell-cell adhesion molecule. *J Cell Biol* 114:1059, 1991.
908. DeLisser HM, Yan HC, Newman PJ, et al: Platelet/endothelial cell adhesion molecule-1 (CD31)-mediated cellular aggregation involves cell surface glycosaminoglycans. *J Biol Chem* 268:16037, 1993.
909. Gumina RJ, el Schultz J, Yao Z, et al: Antibody to platelet/endothelial cell adhesion molecule-1 reduces myocardial infarct size in a rat model of ischemia-reperfusion injury. *Circulation* 94:3327, 1996.
910. Washington AV, Schubert RL, Quigley L, et al: A TREM family member, TLT-1, is found exclusively in the {alpha}-granules of megakaryocytes and platelets. *Blood* 104:1042, 2004.
911. Moroi M, Jung SM: Platelet glycoprotein VI: Its structure and function. *Thromb Res* 114:221, 2004.

912. Kahn ML: Platelet-collagen responses: Molecular basis and therapeutic promise. *Semin Thromb Hemost* 30:419, 2004.
913. Arthur JF, Gardiner EE, Kenny D, et al: Platelet receptor redox regulation. *Platelets* 19:1, 2008.
914. Watson SP, Asazuma N, Atkinson B, et al: The role of ITAM- and ITIM-coupled receptors in platelet activation by collagen. *Thromb Haemost* 86:276, 2001.
915. Arthur JF, Dunkley S, Andrews RK: Platelet glycoprotein VI-related clinical defects. *Br J Haematol* 139:363, 2007.
916. Gibbins J, Asselin J, Farndale R, et al: Tyrosine phosphorylation of the Fc receptor gamma-chain in collagen- stimulated platelets. *J Biol Chem* 271:18095, 1996.
917. Tsuji M, Ezumi Y, Arai M, et al: A novel association of Fc receptor gamma-chain with glycoprotein VI and their co-expression as a collagen receptor in human platelets. *J Biol Chem* 272:23528, 1997.
918. Chacko GW, Duchemin AM, Coggeshall KM, et al: Clustering of the platelet Fc gamma receptor induces noncovalent association with the tyrosine kinase p72syk. *J Biol Chem* 269:32435, 1994.
919. Qiu WQ, de Bruin D, Brownstein BH, et al: Organization of the human and mouse low-affinity Fc gamma R genes: Duplication and recombination. *Science* 248:732, 1990.
920. Boylan B, Gao C, Rathore V, et al: Identification of FcgammaRIIa as the ITAM-bearing receptor mediating alphaIIbbeta3 outside-in integrin signaling in human platelets. *Blood* 112:2780, 2008.
921. Rosenfeld SI, Looney RJ, Leddy JP, et al: Human platelet Fc receptor for immunoglobulin G. Identification as a 40,000-molecular-weight membrane protein shared by monocytes. *J Clin Invest* 76:2317, 1985.
922. Rosenfeld SI, Ryan DH, Looney RJ, et al: Human Fc gamma receptors: Stable interdonor variation in quantitative expression on platelets correlates with functional responses. *J Immunol* 138:2869, 1987.
923. Anderson GP, van de Winkel JG, Anderson CL: Anti-GPIIb/IIIa (CD41) monoclonal antibody-induced platelet activation requires Fc receptor-dependent cell-cell interaction. *Br J Haematol* 79:75, 1991.
924. Hildreth JE, Derr D, Azorsa DO: Characterization of a novel self-associating Mr 40,000 platelet glycoprotein. *Blood* 77:121, 1991.
925. Gratacap MP, Payrastre B, Viala C, et al: Phosphatidylinositol 3,4,5-trisphosphate-dependent stimulation of phospholipase C-gamma2 is an early key event in FcgammaRIIA-mediated activation of human platelets. *J Biol Chem* 273:24314, 1998.
926. Peerschke EI, Ghebrehiwet B: C1q augments platelet activation in response to aggregated Ig. *J Immunol* 159:5594, 1997.
927. Chong BH, Pilgrim RL, Cooley MA, et al: Increased expression of platelet IgG Fc receptors in immune heparin-induced thrombocytopenia. *Blood* 81:988, 1993.
928. Parren PW, Warmerdam PA, Boeije LC, et al: On the interaction of IgG subclasses with the low affinity Fc gamma RIIa (CD32) on human monocytes, neutrophils, and platelets. Analysis of a functional polymorphism to human IgG2. *J Clin Invest* 90:1537, 1992.
929. Warmerdam PA, Parren PW, Vlug A, et al: Polymorphism of the human Fc gamma receptor II (CD32): Molecular basis and functional aspects. *Immunobiology* 185:175, 1992.
930. Chen J, Dong JF, Sun C, et al: Platelet FcgammaRIIA His131Arg polymorphism and platelet function: Antibodies to platelet-bound fibrinogen induce platelet activation. *J Thromb Haemost* 1:355, 2003.
931. Denomme GA, Warkentin TE, Horsewood P, et al: Activation of platelets by sera containing IgG1 heparin-dependent antibodies: An explanation for the predominance of the Fc gammaRIIa "low responder" (his131) gene in patients with heparin-induced thrombocytopenia. *J Lab Clin Med* 130:278, 1997.
932. Carlsson LE, Santoso S, Baurichter G, et al: Heparin-induced thrombocytopenia: New insights into the impact of the FcgammaRIIa-R-H131 polymorphism. *Blood* 92:1526, 1998.
933. Williams Y, Lynch S, McCann S, et al: Correlation of platelet Fc gammaRIIA polymorphism in refractory idiopathic (immune) thrombocytopenic purpura. *Br J Haematol* 101:779, 1998.
934. Trikalinos TA, Karassa FB, Ioannidis JP: Meta-analysis of the association between low-affinity Fcgamma receptor gene polymorphisms and hematologic and autoimmune disease. *Blood* 98:1634, 2001.
935. Gruel Y, Pouplard C, Lasne D, et al: The homozygous FcgammaRIIIa-158V genotype is a risk factor for heparin-induced thrombocytopenia in patients with antibodies to heparin-platelet factor 4 complexes. *Blood* 104:2791, 2004.
936. Kannan M, Saxena R, Adiguzel C, et al: An update on the prevalence and characterization of H-PF4 antibodies in Asian-Indian patients. *Semin Thromb Hemost* 35:337, 2009.
937. Diacovo TG, deFougerolles AR, Bainton DF, et al: A functional integrin ligand on the surface of platelets: Intercellular adhesion molecule-2. *J Clin Invest* 94:1243, 1994.
938. Joseph M, Gounni AS, Kusnierz JP, et al: Expression and functions of the high-affinity IgE receptor on human platelets and megakaryocyte precursors. *Eur J Immunol* 27:2212, 1997.
939. Hasegawa S, Pawankar R, Suzuki K, et al: Functional expression of the high affinity receptor for IgE (FcepsilonRI) in human platelets and its intracellular expression in human megakaryocytes. *Blood* 93:2543, 1999.
940. Kasperska-Zajac A, Rogala B: Platelet function in anaphylaxis. *J Investig Allergol Clin Immunol* 16:1, 2006.
941. McMorran BJ, Marshall VM, de GC, et al: Platelets kill intraerythrocytic malarial parasites and mediate survival to infection. *Science* 323:797, 2009.
942. Gupta SK, Pillarisetti K, Ohlstein EH: Platelet agonist F11 receptor is a member of the immunoglobulin superfamily and identical with junctional adhesion molecule (JAM): Regulation of expression in human endothelial cells and macrophages. *IUBMB Life* 50:51, 2000.
943. Naik UP, Naik MU, Eckfeld K, et al: Characterization and chromosomal localization of JAM-1, a platelet receptor for a stimulatory monoclonal antibody. *J Cell Sci* 114:539, 2001.
944. Kornecki E, Walkowiak B, Naik UP, et al: Activation of human platelets by a stimulatory monoclonal antibody. *J Biol Chem* 265:10042, 1990.
945. Sobocka MB, Sobocki T, Banerjee P, et al: Cloning of the human platelet F11 receptor: A cell adhesion molecule member of the immunoglobulin superfamily involved in platelet aggregation. *Blood* 95:2600, 2000.
946. Sobocki T, Sobocka MB, Babinska A, et al: Genomic structure, organization and promoter analysis of the human F11R/F11 receptor/junctional adhesion molecule-1/JAM-A. *Gene* 366:128, 2006.
947. Naik UP, Eckfeld K: Junctional adhesion molecule 1 (JAM-1). *J Biol Regul Homeost Agents* 17:341, 2003.
948. Sugano Y, Takeuchi M, Hirata A, et al: Junctional adhesion molecule-A, JAM-A, is a novel cell-surface marker for long-term repopulating hematopoietic stem cells. *Blood* 111:1167, 2008.
949. Santoso S, Sachs UJ, Kroll H, et al: The junctional adhesion molecule 3 (JAM-3) on human platelets is a counterreceptor for the leukocyte integrin Mac-1. *J Exp Med* 196:679, 2002.
950. Larsen E, Celi A, Gilbert GE, et al: PADGEM protein: A receptor that mediates the interaction of activated platelets with neutrophils and monocytes. *Cell* 59:305, 1989.
951. Haskard DO: Adhesive proteins, in *Haemostasis and Thrombosis*, 3 ed, edited by AL Bloom, CD Forbes, DP Thomas, EGD Tuddenham, p 233. Churchill Livingstone, Edinburgh, Scotland, 1994.
952. Ishiwata N, Takio K, Katayama M, et al: Alternatively spliced isoform of P-selectin is present *in vivo* as a soluble molecule. *J Biol Chem* 269:23708, 1994.
953. Hartwell DW, Mayadas TN, Berger G, et al: Role of P-selectin cytoplasmic domain in granular targeting *in vivo* and in early inflammatory responses. *J Cell Biol* 143:1129, 1998.
954. Hamburger SA, McEver RP: GMP-140 mediates adhesion of stimulated platelets to neutrophils. *Blood* 75:550, 1990.
955. Geng JG, Bevilacqua P, Moore KL, et al: Rapid neutrophil adhesion to activated endothelium mediated by GMP-140. *Nature* 343:757, 1990.
956. Handa K, Nudelman ED, Stroud MR, et al: Selectin GMP-140 (CD62;PADGEM) binds to sialosyl-Le(a) and sialosyl-Le(x), and sulfated glycans modulate this binding. *Biochem Biophys Res Commun* 181:1223, 1991.
957. Polley MJ, Phillips ML, Wayner E, et al: CD62 and endothelial cell-leukocyte adhesion molecule I (ELAM-1) recognize the same carbohydrate ligand, sialyl-Lewis^x. *Proc Natl Acad Sci U S A* 88:6224, 1991.
958. Aruffo A, Kolanus W, Walz G, et al: CD62/P-selectin recognition of myeloid and tumor cell sulfatides. *Cell* 67:35, 1991.
959. Stone JP, Wagner DD: P-selectin mediates adhesion of platelets to neuroblastoma and small cell lung cancer. *J Clin Invest* 92:804, 1993.
960. Sako D, Chang XJ, Barone KM, et al: Expression cloning of a functional glycoprotein ligand for P-selectin. *Cell* 75:1179, 1993.
961. Yang J, Furie BC, Furie B: The biology of P-selectin glycoprotein ligand-1: Its role as a selectin counterreceptor in leukocyte-endothelial and leukocyte-platelet interaction. *Thromb Haemost* 81:1, 1999.
962. McEver RP, Cummings RD: Perspectives series: Cell adhesion in vascular biology. Role of PSGL-1 binding to selectins in leukocyte recruitment. *J Clin Invest* 100:485, 1997.
963. Falati S, Liu Q, Gross P, et al: Accumulation of tissue factor into developing thrombi *in vivo* is dependent upon microparticle P-selectin glycoprotein ligand 1 and platelet P-selectin. *J Exp Med* 197:1585, 2003.
964. Celi A, Pellegrini G, Lorenzet R, et al: P-selectin induces the expression of tissue factor on monocytes. *Proc Natl Acad Sci U S A* 91:8767, 1994.
965. Hrachovinova I, Cambien B, Hafezi-Moghadam A, et al: Interaction of P-selectin and PSGL-1 generates microparticles that correct hemostasis in a mouse model of hemophilia A. *Nat Med* 9:1020, 2003.
966. Ridker PM, Buring JE, Rifai N: Soluble P-selectin and the risk of future cardiovascular events. *Circulation* 103:491, 2001.
967. Mayadas TN, Johnson RC, Rayburn H, et al: Leukocyte rolling and extravasation are severely compromised in P selectin-deficient mice. *Cell* 74:541, 1993.
968. Padilla A, Moake JL, Bernardo A, et al: P-selectin anchors newly released ultralarge von Willebrand factor multimers to the endothelial cell surface. *Blood* 103:2150, 2004.
969. Ludwig RJ, Schon MP, Boehncke WH: P-selectin: A common therapeutic target for cardiovascular disorders, inflammation and tumour metastasis. *Expert Opin Ther Targets* 11:1103, 2007.
970. Polgar J, Matuskova J, Wagner DD: The P-selectin, tissue factor, coagulation triad. *J Thromb Haemost* 3:1590, 2005.
971. Ozaki Y, Suzuki-Inoue K, Inoue O: Novel interactions in platelet biology: CLEC-2/podoplanin and laminin/GPVI. *J Thromb Haemost* 7:191, 2009.
972. Tsuruo T, Fujita N: Platelet aggregation in the formation of tumor metastasis. *Proc Jpn Acad Ser B Phys Biol Sci* 84:189, 2008.

973. Schacht V, Ramirez MI, Hong YK, et al: T1alpha/podoplanin deficiency disrupts normal lymphatic vasculature formation and causes lymphedema. *EMBO J* 22:3546, 2003.
974. Suzuki-Inoue K, Kato Y, Inoue O, et al: Involvement of the snake toxin receptor CLEC-2, in podoplanin-mediated platelet activation, by cancer cells. *J Biol Chem* 282:25993, 2007.
975. Christou CM, Pearce AC, Watson AA, et al: Renal cells activate the platelet receptor CLEC-2 through podoplanin. *Biochem J* 411:133, 2008.
975a. May F, Hagedorn I, Pleines I, et al: CLEC-2 is an essential platelet activating receptor in hemostasis and thrombosis. *Blood* 114:3364, 2009.
976. Hemler ME: Tetraspanin functions and associated microdomains. *Nat Rev Mol Cell Biol* 6:801, 2005.
977. Goschnick MW, Lau LM, Wee JL, et al: Impaired "outside-in" integrin alphaIIbbeta3 signaling and thrombus stability in TSSC6-deficient mice. *Blood* 108:1911, 2006.
978. Protty MB, Watkins NA, Colombo D, et al: Identification of Tspan9 as a novel platelet tetraspanin and the collagen receptor GPVI as a component of tetraspanin microdomains. *Biochem J* 417:391, 2009.
979. Boucheix C, Benoit P, Frachet P, et al: Molecular cloning of the CD9 antigen. A new family of cell surface proteins. *J Biol Chem* 266:117, 1991.
980. Lanza F, Wolf D, Fox CF, et al: CDNA cloning and expression of platelet p24/CD9. Evidence for a new family of multiple membrane-spanning proteins. *J Biol Chem* 266:10638, 1991.
981. Hato T, Ikeda K, Yasukawa M, et al: Exposure of platelet fibrinogen receptors by a monoclonal antibody to CD9 antigen. *Blood* 72:224, 1988.
982. Brisson C, Azorsa DO, Jennings LK, et al: Co-localization of CD9 and GPIIb-IIIa (alpha IIb beta 3 integrin) on activated platelet pseudopods and alpha-granule membranes. *Histochem J* 29:153, 1997.
983. Jennings LK, Fox CF, Kouns WC, et al: The activation of human platelets mediated by anti-human platelet p24/CD9 monoclonal antibodies. *J Biol Chem* 265:3815, 1990.
984. Hato T, Sumida M, Yasukawa M, et al: Induction of platelet Ca2+ influx and mobilization by a monoclonal antibody to CD9 antigen. *Blood* 75:1087, 1990.
985. Worthington RE, Carroll RC, Boucheix C: Platelet activation by CD9 monoclonal antibodies is mediated by the Fc gamma II receptor. *Br J Haematol* 74:216, 1990.
986. Slupsky JR, Seehafer JG, Tang SC, et al: Evidence that monoclonal antibodies against CD9 antigen induce specific association between CD9 and the platelet glycoprotein IIb-IIIa complex. *J Biol Chem* 264:12289, 1989.
987. Nishibori M, Cham B, McNicol A, et al: The protein CD63 is in platelet dense granules, is deficient in a patient with Hermansky-Pudlak syndrome, and appears identical to granulophysin. *J Clin Invest* 91:1775, 1993.
988. Metzelaar MJ, Wijngaard PL, Peters PJ, et al: CD63 antigen. A novel lysosomal membrane glycoprotein, cloned by a screening procedure for intracellular antigens in eukaryotic cells. *J Biol Chem* 266:3239, 1991.
989. Roberts JJ, Rodgers SE, Drury J, et al: Platelet activation induced by a murine monoclonal antibody directed against a novel tetra-span antigen. *Br J Haematol* 89:853, 1995.
990. Fitter S, Tetaz TJ, Berndt MC, et al: Molecular cloning of cDNA encoding a novel platelet-endothelial cell tetra-span antigen, PETA-3. *Blood* 86:1348, 1995.
991. Sincock PM, Mayrhofer G, Ashman LK: Localization of the transmembrane 4 superfamily (TM4SF) member PETA-3 (CD151) in normal human tissues: Comparison with CD9, CD63, and alpha5beta1 integrin. *J Histochem Cytochem* 45:515, 1997.
992. Lau LM, Wee JL, Wright MD, et al: The tetraspanin superfamily member, CD151 regulates outside-in integrin {alpha}IIb{beta}3 signalling and platelet function. *Blood* 104:2368, 2004.
993. Robb L, Tarrant J, Groom J, et al: Molecular characterisation of mouse and human TSSC6: Evidence that TSSC6 is a genuine member of the tetraspanin superfamily and is expressed specifically in haematopoietic organs. *Biochim Biophys Acta* 1522:31, 2001.
994. Polgar J, Clemetson JM, Gengenbacher D, et al: Additional GPI-anchored glycoproteins on human platelets that are absent or deficient in paroxysmal nocturnal haemoglobinuria. *FEBS Lett* 327:49, 1993.
995. Kelton JG, Smith JW, Horsewood P, et al: ABH antigens on human platelets: Expression on the glycosyl phosphatidylinositol-anchored protein CD109. *J Lab Clin Med* 132:142, 1998.
996. Grunewald M, Grunewald A, Schmid A, et al: The platelet function defect of paroxysmal nocturnal haemoglobinuria. *Platelets* 15:145, 2004.
997. Hernandez-Campo PM, Martin-Ayuso M, Almeida J, et al: Comparative analysis of different flow cytometry-based immunophenotypic methods for the analysis of CD59 and CD55 expression on major peripheral blood cell subsets. *Cytometry* 50:191, 2002.
998. Jin JY, Tooze JA, Marsh JC, et al: Glycosylphosphatidyl-inositol (GPI)-linked protein deficiency on the platelets of patients with aplastic anaemia and paroxysmal nocturnal haemoglobinuria: Two distinct patterns correlating with expression on neutrophils. *Br J Haematol* 96:493, 1997.
999. Holada K, Mondoro TH, Muller J, et al: Increased expression of phosphatidylinositol-specific phospholipase C resistant prion proteins on the surface of activated platelets. *Br J Haematol* 103:276, 1998.
1000. Barclay GR, Hope J, Birkett CR, et al: Distribution of cell-associated prion protein in normal adult blood determined by flow cytometry. *Br J Haematol* 107:804, 1999.
1001. Starke R, Cramer E, Harrison P: Expression of cell-associated prion protein on normal human platelets. *Br J Haematol* 110:748, 2000.
1002. MacGregor I, Hope J, Barnard G, et al: Application of a time-resolved fluoroimmunoassay for the analysis of normal prion protein in human blood and its components. *Vox Sang* 77:88, 1999.
1003. Prevost N, Woulfe D, Tanaka T, et al: Interactions between Eph kinases and ephrins provide a mechanism to support platelet aggregation once cell-to-cell contact has occurred. *Proc Natl Acad Sci U S A* 99:9219, 2002.
1004. Prevost N, Woulfe DS, Tognolini M, et al: Signaling by ephrinB1 and Eph kinases in platelets promotes Rap1 activation, platelet adhesion, and aggregation via effector pathways that do not require phosphorylation of ephrinB1. *Blood* 103:1348, 2004.
1005. Prevost N, Woulfe DS, Jiang H, et al: Eph kinases and ephrins support thrombus growth and stability by regulating integrin outside-in signaling in platelets. *Proc Natl Acad Sci U S A* 102:9820, 2005.
1006. Fielder PJ, Hass P, Nagel M, et al: Human platelets as a model for the binding and degradation of thrombopoietin. *Blood* 89:2782, 1997.
1007. dem Borne AE, Folman C, Linthorst GE, et al: Thrombopoietin and its receptor: Structure, function and role in the regulation of platelet production. *Baillieres Clin Haematol* 11:409, 1998.
1008. Kaushansky K: Thrombopoietin: A tool for understanding thrombopoiesis. *J Thromb Haemost* 1:1587, 2003.
1009. Kaushansky K: Historical review: Megakaryopoiesis and thrombopoiesis. *Blood* 111:981, 2008.
1010. Ezumi Y, Takayama H, Okuma M: Thrombopoietin, c-Mpl ligand, induces tyrosine phosphorylation of Tyk2, JAK2, and STAT3, and enhances agonists-induced aggregation in platelets *in vitro*. *FEBS Lett* 374:48, 1995.
1011. Chen J, Herceg-Harjacek L, Groopman JE, et al: Regulation of platelet activation in vitro by the c-Mpl ligand, thrombopoietin. *Blood* 86:4054, 1995.
1012. Kojima H, Hamazaki Y, Nagata Y, et al: Modulation of platelet activation *in vitro* by thrombopoietin. *Thromb Haemost* 74:1541, 1995.
1013. Rodriguez-Linares B, Watson SP: Thrombopoietin potentiates activation of human platelets in association with JAK2 and TYK2 phosphorylation. *Biochem J* 316(Pt 1):93, 1996.
1014. Oda A, Miyakawa Y, Druker BJ, et al: Thrombopoietin primes human platelet aggregation induced by shear stress and by multiple agonists. *Blood* 87:4664, 1996.
1015. Kubota Y, Arai T, Tanaka T, et al: Thrombopoietin modulates platelet activation in vitro through protein-tyrosine phosphorylation. *Stem Cells* 14:439, 1996.
1016. Fox NE, Chen R, Hitchcock I, et al: Compound heterozygous c-Mpl mutations in a child with congenital amegakaryocytic thrombocytopenia: Functional characterization and a review of the literature. *Exp Hematol* 37:495, 2009.
1017. Kilpivaara O, Levine RL: JAK2 and MPL mutations in myeloproliferative neoplasms: Discovery and science. *Leukemia* 22:1813, 2008.
1018. Tandon NN, Lipsky RH, Burgess WH, et al: Isolation and characterization of platelet glycoprotein IV (CD36). *J Biol Chem* 264:7570, 1989.
1019. Legrand C, Pidard D, Beiso P, et al: Interaction of a monoclonal antibody to glycoprotein IV (CD36) with human platelets and its effect on platelet function. *Platelets* 2:99, 1991.
1020. Daviet L, McGregor JL: Vascular biology of CD36: Roles of this new adhesion molecule family in different disease states. *Thromb Haemost* 78:65, 1997.
1021. Febbraio M, Silverstein RL: CD36: Implications in cardiovascular disease. *Int J Biochem Cell Biol* 39:2012, 2007.
1022. Valiyaveettil M, Podrez EA: Platelet hyperreactivity, scavenger receptors and atherothrombosis. *J Thromb Haemost* 7:218, 2009.
1023. Oquendo P, Hundt E, Lawler J, et al: CD36 directly mediates cytoadherence of *Plasmodium falciparum* infected erythrocytes. *Cell* 58:95, 1989.
1024. Huang MM, Bolen JB, Barnwell JW, et al: Membrane glycoprotein IV (CD36) is physically associated with the Fyn, Lyn, and Yes protein-tyrosine kinases in human platelets. *Proc Natl Acad Sci U S A* 88:7844, 1991.
1025. Taketani T, Ito K, Mishima S, et al: Neonatal isoimmune thrombocytopenia caused by type I CD36 deficiency having novel splicing isoforms of the CD36 gene. *Eur J Haematol* 81:70, 2008.
1026. Thorne RF, Meldrum CJ, Harris SJ, et al: CD36 forms covalently associated dimers and multimers in platelets and transfected COS-7 cells. *Biochem Biophys Res Commun* 240:812, 1997.
1027. Thibert V, Bellucci S, Cristofari M, et al: Increased platelet CD36 constitutes a common marker in myeloproliferative disorders. *Br J Haematol* 91:618, 1995.
1028. Aiken JW, Ginsberg MH, Plow EF: Mechanisms for expression of thrombospondin on the platelet surface. *Semin Thromb Hemost* 13:307, 1987.
1029. Yamashita S, Hirano K, Kuwasako T, et al: Physiological and pathological roles of a multi-ligand receptor CD36 in atherogenesis; insights from CD36-deficient patients. *Mol Cell Biochem* 299:19, 2007.
1030. Collot-Teixeira S, Martin J, McDermott-Roe C, et al: CD36 and macrophages in atherosclerosis. *Cardiovasc Res* 75:468, 2007.
1031. Korporaal SJ, Van EM, Adelmeijer J, et al: Platelet activation by oxidized low density lipoprotein is mediated by CD36 and scavenger receptor-A. *Arterioscler Thromb Vasc Biol* 27:2476, 2007.
1032. Podrez EA, Byzova TV, Febbraio M, et al: Platelet CD36 links hyperlipidemia, oxidant stress and a prothrombotic phenotype. *Nat Med* 13:1086, 2007.
1033. Chen K, Febbraio M, Li W, et al: A specific CD36-dependent signaling pathway is required for platelet activation by oxidized low-density lipoprotein. *Circ Res* 102:1512, 2008.

1034. Ghosh A, Li W, Febbraio M, et al: Platelet CD36 mediates interactions with endothelial cell-derived microparticles and contributes to thrombosis in mice. *J Clin Invest* 118:1934, 2008.
1035. Hirano K, Kuwasako T, Nakagawa-Toyama Y, et al: Pathophysiology of human genetic CD36 deficiency. *Trends Cardiovasc Med* 13:136, 2003.
1036. Hajjar DP, Gotto AM: Targeting CD36: Modulating inflammation and atherogenesis. *Curr Atheroscler Rep* 5:155, 2003.
1037. Pravenec M, Kurtz TW: Genetics of Cd36 and the hypertension metabolic syndrome. *Semin Nephrol* 22:148, 2002.
1038. Su X, Abumrad NA: Cellular fatty acid uptake: A pathway under construction. *Trends Endocrinol Metab* 20:72, 2009.
1039. Asch AS, Barnwell J, Silverstein RL, et al: Isolation of the thrombospondin membrane receptor. *J Clin Invest* 79:1054, 1987.
1040. Tandon NN, Kralisz U, Jamieson GA: Identification of glycoprotein IV (CD36) as a primary receptor for platelet-collagen adhesion. *J Biol Chem* 264:7576, 1989.
1041. Diaz-Ricart M, Tandon NN, Gomez-Ortiz G, et al: Antibodies to CD36 (GPIV) inhibit platelet adhesion to subendothelial surfaces under flow conditions. *Arterioscler Thromb Vasc Biol* 16:883, 1996.
1042. Saelman EU, Kehrel B, Hese KM, et al: Platelet adhesion to collagen and endothelial cell matrix under flow conditions is not dependent on platelet glycoprotein IV. *Blood* 83:3240, 1994.
1043. Wun T, Paglieroni T, Field CL, et al: Platelet-erythrocyte adhesion in sickle cell disease. *J Investig Med* 47:121, 1999.
1044. Valiyaveettil M, Kar N, Ashraf MZ, et al: Oxidized high-density lipoprotein inhibits platelet activation and aggregation via scavenger receptor BI. *Blood* 111:1962, 2008.
1045. Choi WS, Jeon OH, Kim HH, et al: MMP-2 regulates human platelet activation by interacting with integrin alphaIIbbeta3. *J Thromb Haemost* 6:517, 2008.
1046. Aukrust P, Damas JK, Solum NO: Soluble CD40 ligand and platelets: Self-perpetuating pathogenic loop in thrombosis and inflammation? *J Am Coll Cardiol* 43:2326, 2004.
1047. Varo N, de Lemos JA, Libby P, et al: Soluble CD40L: Risk prediction after acute coronary syndromes. *Circulation* 108:1049, 2003.
1048. Inwald DP, McDowall A, Peters MJ, et al: CD40 is constitutively expressed on platelets and provides a novel mechanism for platelet activation. *Circ Res* 92:1041, 2003.
1049. Urbich C, Dernbach E, Aicher A, et al: CD40 ligand inhibits endothelial cell migration by increasing production of endothelial reactive oxygen species. *Circulation* 106:981, 2002.
1050. Czapiga M, Kirk AD, Lekstrom-Himes J: Platelets deliver costimulatory signals to antigen-presenting cells: A potential bridge between injury and immune activation. *Exp Hematol* 32:135, 2004.
1051. Elzey BD, Tian J, Jensen RJ, et al: Platelet-mediated modulation of adaptive immunity. A communication link between innate and adaptive immune compartments. *Immunity* 19:9, 2003.
1052. Ahmad R, Menezes J, Knafo L, et al: Activated human platelets express Fas-L and induce apoptosis in Fas-positive tumor cells. *J Leukoc Biol* 69:123, 2001.
1053. Crist SA, Elzey BD, Ludwig AT, et al: Expression of TNF-related apoptosis-inducing ligand (TRAIL) in megakaryocytes and platelets. *Exp Hematol* 32:1073, 2004.
1054. Otterdal K, Smith C, Oie E, et al: Platelet-derived LIGHT induces inflammatory responses in endothelial cells and monocytes. *Blood* 108:928, 2006.
1055. Silverstein RL, Febbraio M: Identification of lysosome-associated membrane protein-2 as an activation-dependent platelet surface glycoprotein. *Blood* 80:1470, 1992.
1056. Peerschke EIB, Ghebrehiwet B: Human blood platelets possess specific binding sites for C1q. *J Immunol* 138:1537, 1987.
1057. Peerschke EI, Ghebrehiwet B: Platelet receptors for the complement component C1q: Implications for hemostasis and thrombosis. *Immunobiology* 199:239, 1998.
1058. Ghebrehiwet B, Lim BL, Kumar R, et al: GC1q-R/p33, a member of a new class of multifunctional and multicompartmental cellular proteins, is involved in inflammation and infection. *Immunol Rev* 180:65, 2001.
1059. Ghebrehiwet B, Lim BL, Peerschke EI, et al: Isolation, cDNA cloning, and overexpression of a 33-kD cell surface glycoprotein that binds to the globular "heads" of C1q. *J Exp Med* 179:1809, 1994.
1060. Herwald H, Dedio J, Kellner R, et al: Isolation and characterization of the kininogen-binding protein p33 from endothelial cells. Identity with the gC1q receptor. *J Biol Chem* 271:13040, 1996.
1061. Nepomuceno RR, Tenner AJ: C1qRP, the C1q receptor that enhances phagocytosis, is detected specifically in human cells of myeloid lineage, endothelial cells, and platelets. *J Immunol* 160:1929, 1998.
1062. Peerschke EI, Reid KB, Ghebrehiwet B: Platelet activation by C1q results in the induction of alpha IIb/beta 3 integrins (GPIIb-IIIa) and the expression of P-selectin and procoagulant activity. *J Exp Med* 178:579, 1993.
1063. Peerschke EI, Ghebrehiwet B: Platelet membrane receptors for the complement component C1q. *Semin Hematol* 31:320, 1994.
1064. Jiang J, Zhang Y, Krainer AR, et al: Crystal structure of human p32, a doughnut-shaped acidic mitochondrial matrix protein. *Proc Natl Acad Sci U S A* 96:3572, 1999.
1065. Metzelaar MJ, Heijnen HF, Sixma JJ, et al: Identification of a 33-Kd protein associated with the alpha-granule membrane (GMP-33) that is expressed on the surface of activated platelets. *Blood* 79:372, 1992.
1066. Damas C, Vink T, Nieuwenhuis HK, et al: The 33-kDa platelet alpha-granule membrane protein (GMP-33) is an N-terminal proteolytic fragment of thrombospondin. *Thromb Haemost* 86:887, 2001.
1067. Rosenstein Y, Park JK, Hahn WC, et al: CD43, a molecule defective in Wiskott-Aldrich syndrome, binds ICAM-1. *Nature* 354:233, 1991.
1068. Beutler B: Inferences, questions and possibilities in toll-like receptor signalling. *Nature* 430:257, 2004.
1068a. Gerold G, Abu Ajaj K, Bienert M, et al: A Toll-like receptor 2-integrin $\beta3$ complex senses bacterial lipopeptides via vitronectin. *Nat Immun* 9:7671, 2008.
1069. Semple JW, Aslam R, Kim M, et al: Platelet-bound lipopolysaccharide enhances Fc receptor-mediated phagocytosis of IgG-opsonized platelets. *Blood* 109:4803, 2007.
1070. Zhang G, Han J, Welch EJ, et al: Lipopolysaccharide stimulates platelet secretion and potentiates platelet aggregation via TLR4/MyD88 and the cGMP-dependent protein kinase pathway. *J Immunol* 182:7997, 2009.
1071. Stahl AL, Svensson M, Morgelin M, et al: Lipopolysaccharide from enterohemorrhagic *Escherichia coli* binds to platelets through TLR4 and CD62 and is detected on circulating platelets in patients with hemolytic uremic syndrome. *Blood* 108:167, 2006.
1072. Cognasse F, Hamzeh-Cognasse H, Lafarge S, et al: Toll-like receptor 4 ligand can differentially modulate the release of cytokines by human platelets. *Br J Haematol* 141:84, 2008.
1073. Scott T, Owens MD: Thrombocytes respond to lipopolysaccharide through Toll-like receptor-4, and MAP kinase and NF-kappaB pathways leading to expression of interleukin-6 and cyclooxygenase-2 with production of prostaglandin E2. *Mol Immunol* 45:1001, 2008.
1074. Clark SR, Ma AC, Tavener SA, et al: Platelet TLR4 activates neutrophil extracellular traps to ensnare bacteria in septic blood. *Nat Med* 13:463, 2007.
1075. Akbiyik F, Ray DM, Gettings KF, et al: Human bone marrow megakaryocytes and platelets express PPARgamma, and PPARgamma agonists blunt platelet release of CD40 ligand and thromboxanes. *Blood* 104:1361, 2004.
1076. Ray DM, Spinelli SL, Pollock SJ, et al: Peroxisome proliferator-activated receptor gamma and retinoid X receptor transcription factors are released from activated human platelets and shed in microparticles. *Thromb Haemost* 99:86, 2008.
1077. Borchert M, Schondorf T, Lubben G, et al: Review of the pleiotropic effects of peroxisome proliferator-activated receptor gamma agonists on platelet function. *Diabetes Technol Ther* 9:410, 2007.
1078. Ali FY, Davidson SJ, Moraes LA, et al: Role of nuclear receptor signaling in platelets: Antithrombotic effects of PPARbeta. *FASEB J* 20:326, 2006.
1079. Santos-Martinez MJ, Medina C, Gilmer JF, et al: Matrix metalloproteinases in platelet function: Coming of age. *J Thromb Haemost* 6:514, 2008.
1080. Trivedi V, Boire A, Tchernychev B, et al: Platelet matrix metalloprotease-1 mediates thrombogenesis by activating PAR1 at a cryptic ligand site. *Cell* 137:332, 2009.
1081. Coller BS: Platelets and thrombolytic therapy. *N Engl J Med* 322:33, 1990.
1082. Coller BS: Augmentation of thrombolysis with antiplatelet drugs. Overview. *Coron Artery Dis* 6:911, 1995.
1083. Korbut R, Gryglewski RJ: Platelets in fibrinolytic system. *J Physiol Pharmacol* 46:409, 1995.
1084. Kolev K, Machovich R: Molecular and cellular modulation of fibrinolysis. *Thromb Haemost* 89:610, 2003.
1085. Maron BA, Loscalzo J: The role of platelets in fibrinolysis, in *Platelets*, 2nd ed, edited by AD Michelson, p 415. Academic Press, San Diego, 2007.
1086. Thorsen S, Brakman P, Astrup T: Influence of platelets on fibrinolysis: A critical review, in *Hematologic Reviews,* 3rd ed, edited by JL Ambrole, p 123. Marcel Dekker, New York, 1972.
1087. Carroll RC, Radcliffe RD, Taylor FB, et al: Plasminogen, plasminogen activator and platelets in the regulation of clot lysis. *J Lab Clin Med* 100:986, 1982.
1088. Miles LA, Plow EF: Binding and activation of plasminogen on the platelet surface. *J Biol Chem* 260:4303, 1985.
1089. Stricker RB, Wong D, Shiu DT, et al: Activation of plasminogen by tissue plasminogen activator on normal and thrombasthenic platelets: Effects on surface proteins and platelet aggregation. *Blood* 68:275, 1986.
1090. Jeanneau C, Sultan Y: Tissue plasminogen activator in human megakaryocytes and platelets: Immunocytochemical localization, immunoblotting and zymographic analysis. *Thrombosis Haemostasis* 19:529, 1988.
1091. Park S, Harker LA, Marzec UM, et al: Demonstration of single chain urokinase-type plasminogen activator on human platelet membrane. *Blood* 73:1421, 1989.
1092. de Haan J, van Oeveren W: Platelets and soluble fibrin promote plasminogen activation causing downregulation of platelet glycoprotein Ib/IX complexes: Protection by aprotinin. *Thromb Res* 92:171, 1998.
1093. Plow EF, Collen D: The presence and release of α_2-antiplasmin from human platelets. *Blood* 58:1069, 1981.
1094. Smariga PE, Maynard JR: Purification of a platelet protein which stimulates fibrinolytic inhibition and tissue factor in human fibroblasts. *J Biol Chem* 257:11960, 1982.
1095. Erickson LA, Ginsberg MH, Loskutoff DJ: Detection and partial characterization of an inhibitor of plasminogen activator in human platelets. *J Clin Invest* 74:1465, 1984.
1096. Kruithof EKO, Tran-Thang C, Bachmann F: Studies on the release of plasminogen activator inhibitor from human platelets. *Thromb Haemost* 55:201, 1986.
1097. Francis CW, Marder VJ: Rapid formation of large molecular weight alpha-polymers in cross-linked fibrin induced by high factor XIII concentrations: Role of platelet factor XIII. *J Clin Invest* 80:1459, 1987.
1098. Fay WP, Eitzman DT, Shapiro AD, et al: Platelets inhibit fibrinolysis *in vitro* by both plasminogen activator inhibitor-1 dependent and independent mechanisms. *Blood* 83:351, 1994.

1099. Cox AD, Devine DV: Factor XIIIa binding to activated platelets is mediated through activation of glycoprotein IIb-IIIa. *Blood* 83:1006, 1994.
1100. Kawasaki T, Dewerchin M, Lijnen HR, et al: Vascular release of plasminogen activator inhibitor-1 impairs fibrinolysis during acute arterial thrombosis in mice. *Blood* 96:153, 2000.
1101. Binder BR, Christ G, Gruber F, et al: Plasminogen activator inhibitor 1: Physiological and pathophysiological roles. *News Physiol Sci* 17:56, 2002.
1102. Jang I-K, Gold HK, Ziskind AA, et al: Differential sensitivity of erythrocyte-rich and platelet-rich arterial thrombi to lysis with recombinant tissue-type plasminogen activator. A possible explanation for resistance to coronary thrombolysis. *Circulation* 79:920, 1989.
1103. Ohlstein EH, Storer B, Fujita T, et al: Tissue-type plasminogen activator and streptokinase induce platelet hyperaggregability in the rabbit. *Thromb Res* 46:575, 1987.
1104. Fitzgerald DJ, Catella F, Roy L, et al: Marked platelet activation *in vivo* after intravenous streptokinase in patients with acute myocardial infarction. *Circulation* 77:142, 1988.
1105. Shebuski RJ: Principles underlying the use of conjunctive agents with plasminogen activators. *Ann N Y Acad Sci* 667:382, 1992.
1106. Rudd MA, George D, Amarante P, et al: Temporal effects of thrombolytic agents on platelet function *in vivo* and their modulation by prostaglandins. *Circ Res* 67:1175, 1990.
1107. Kerins DM, Roy L, FitzGerald GA, et al: Platelet and vascular function during coronary thrombolysis with tissue-type plasminogen activator. *Circulation* 80:1718, 1990.
1108. Fitzgerald DJ, Wright F, FitzGerald GA: Increased thromboxane biosynthesis during coronary thrombolysis: Evidence that platelet activation and thromboxane A_2 modulate the response to tissue-type plasminogen activator *in vivo*. *Circ Res* 65:83, 1989.
1109. Penny WF, Ware JA: Platelet activation and subsequent inhibition by plasmin and recombinant tissue-type plasminogen activator. *Blood* 79:91, 1992.
1110. Niewiarowski S, Senyi AF, Gillies P: Plasmin-induced platelet aggregation and platelet release reaction. *J Clin Invest* 52:1647, 1973.
1111. Schafer AI, Maas AK, Ware JA, et al: Platelet protein phosphorylation, elevation of cytosolic calcium, and inositol phospholipid breakdown in platelet activation induced by plasmin. *J Clin Invest* 78:73, 1986.
1112. Ervin AL, Peerschke EI: Platelet activation by sustained exposure to low-dose plasmin. *Blood Coagul Fibrinolysis* 12:415, 2001.
1113. Ishii-Watabe A, Uchida E, Mizuguchi H, et al: On the mechanism of plasmin-induced platelet aggregation. Implications of the dual role of granule ADP. *Biochem Pharmacol* 59:1345, 2000.
1114. Quinton TM, Kim S, Derian CK, et al: Plasmin-mediated activation of platelets occurs by cleavage of protease-activated receptor 4. *J Biol Chem* 279:18434, 2004.
1115. Eisenberg PR, Sherman LA, Jaffe AS: Paradoxic elevation of fibrinopeptide A after streptokinase: Evidence for continued thrombosis despite intense fibrinolysis. *J Am Coll Cardiol* 10:527, 1987.
1116. Owen J, Friedman KD, Grossman BA, et al: Thrombolytic therapy with tissue plasminogen activator or streptokinase induces transient thrombin activity. *Blood* 72:616, 1988.
1117. Leopold JA, Loscalzo J: Platelet activation by fibrinolytic agents: A potential mechanism for resistance to thrombolysis and reocclusion after successful thrombolysis. *Coron Artery Dis* 6:923, 1995.
1118. Szczeklik A: Thrombin generation in myocardial infarction and hypercholesterolemia: Effects of aspirin. *Thromb Haemost* 74:77, 1995.
1119. Weitz JI, Cruickshank MK, Though D, et al: Human tissue-type plasminogen activator releases fibrinopeptides A and B from fibrinogen. *J Clin Invest* 82:1700, 1988.
1120. Coller BS: Inhibitors of the platelet glycoprotein IIb/IIIa receptor as conjunctive therapy for coronary artery thrombolysis. *Coron Artery Dis* 3:1016, 1992.
1121. Eccleston D, Topol EJ: Inhibitors of platelet glycoprotein IIb/IIIa as augmenters of thrombolysis. *Coron Artery Dis* 6:947, 1995.
1122. O'Donnell CJ, Jonas MA, Hennekens CH: Aspirin augmentation of the efficacy of thrombolysis. *Coron Artery Dis* 6:936, 1995.
1123. Topol EJ: Reperfusion therapy for acute myocardial infarction with fibrinolytic therapy or combination reduced fibrinolytic therapy and platelet glycoprotein IIb/IIIa inhibition: The GUSTO V randomised trial. *Lancet* 357:1905, 2001.
1124. Di MC, Dudek D, Piscione F, et al: Immediate angioplasty versus standard therapy with rescue angioplasty after thrombolysis in the Combined Abciximab REteplase Stent Study in Acute Myocardial Infarction (CARESS-in-AMI): An open, prospective, randomised, multicentre trial. *Lancet* 371:559, 2008.
1125. Ellis SG, Tendera M, de Belder MA, et al: Facilitated PCI in patients with ST-elevation myocardial infarction. *N Engl J Med* 358:2205, 2008.
1126. Lapchak PA, Araujo DM, Song D, et al: The nonpeptide glycoprotein IIb/IIIa platelet receptor antagonist SM-20302 reduces tissue plasminogen activator-induced intracerebral hemorrhage after thromboembolic stroke. *Stroke* 33:147, 2002.
1127. Zhang L, Zhang ZG, Zhang R, et al: Adjuvant treatment with a glycoprotein IIb/IIIa receptor inhibitor increases the therapeutic window for low-dose tissue plasminogen activator administration in a rat model of embolic stroke. *Circulation* 107:2837, 2003.
1128. Adams HP Jr, Effron MB, Torner J, et al: Emergency administration of abciximab for treatment of patients with acute ischemic stroke: Results of an international phase III trial: Abciximab in Emergency Treatment of Stroke Trial (AbESTT-II). *Stroke* 39:87, 2008.
1129. Mandava P, Thiagarajan P, Kent TA: Glycoprotein IIb/IIIa antagonists in acute ischaemic stroke: Current status and future directions. *Drugs* 68:1019, 2008.
1130. Kowalski E, Kopec M, Wegrzynowicz A: Influence of fibrinogen degradation products (FDP) on platelet aggregation, adhesiveness and viscous metamorphosis. *Thromb Diath Haemorrh* 10:406, 1963.
1131. Schafer AL, Adelman B: Plasmin inhibition of platelet function and of arachidonic acid metabolism. *J Clin Invest* 75:456, 1985.
1132. Adelman B, Michelson AD, Loscalzo J, et al: Plasmin effect on platelet glycoprotein Ib-von Willebrand factor interactions. *Blood* 64:32, 1985.
1133. Loscalzo J, Vaughan DE: Tissue plasminogen activator promotes platelet disaggregation in plasma. *J Clin Invest* 79:1749, 1987.
1134. Schafer AL, Zavoico GB, Loscalzo J, et al: Synergistic inhibition of platelet activation by plasmin and prostaglandin I_2. *Blood* 69:1504, 1987.
1135. Adnot S, Ferry N, Nanoune J, et al: Plasmin: A possible physiological modulator of human platelet adenylate cyclase system. *Clin Sci* 72:467, 1987.
1136. Gimple LW, Gold HK, Leinbach RC, et al: Correlation between template bleeding times and spontaneous bleeding during treatment of acute myocardial infarction with recombinant tissue-type plasminogen activator. *Circulation* 80:581, 1989.
1137. Michelson AD, Gore JM, Rybak ME, et al: Effect of *in vivo* infusion of recombinant tissue-type plasminogen activator on platelet glycoprotein Ib. *Thromb Res* 60:421, 1990.
1138. Federici AB, Berkowitz SD, Mannucci PM, et al: Proteolysis of von Willebrand factor in patients undergoing thrombolytic therapy [abstract]. *Circulation* 78(Suppl II):II-120, 1988.
1139. Johnstone MT, Andrews T, Ware JA, et al: Bleeding time prolongation with streptokinase and its reduction with 1-desamino-8-D-arginine vasopressin. *Circulation* 82:2142, 1990.
1140. Kamat SG, Schafer AI: Antiplatelet effects of fibrinolytic agents: A potential contributor to the hemostatic defect after thrombolysis. *Coron Artery Dis* 6:930, 1995.
1141. Coller BS: Binding of abciximab to $\alpha V\beta 3$ and activated $\alpha M\beta 2$ receptors: With a review of platelet-leukocyte interactions. *Thromb Haemost* 82:326, 1999.
1142. Farb A, Sangiorgi G, Carter AJ, et al: Pathology of acute and chronic coronary stenting in humans. *Circulation* 99:44, 1999.
1143. Merhi Y, Provost P, Chauvet P, et al: Selectin blockade reduces neutrophil interaction with platelets at the site of deep arterial injury by angioplasty in pigs. *Arterioscler Thromb Vasc Biol* 19:372, 1999.
1144. Smyth SS, Reis ED, Zhang W, et al: $\beta 3$-Integrin-deficient mice, but not P-selectin-deficient mice, develop intimal hyperplasia after vascular injury: Correlation with leukocyte recruitment to adherent platelets 1 hour after injury. *Circulation* 103:2501, 2001.
1145. Wehner J, Morrell CN, Reynolds T, et al: Antibody and complement in transplant vasculopathy. *Circ Res* 100:191, 2007.
1146. Nishimura S, Manabe I, Nagasaki M, et al: *In vivo* imaging in mice reveals local cell dynamics and inflammation in obese adipose tissue. *J Clin Invest* 118:710, 2008.
1147. Bozza FA, Shah AM, Weyrich AS, et al: Amicus or adversary: Platelets in lung biology, acute injury, and inflammation. *Am J Respir Cell Mol Biol* 40:123, 2009.
1148. von Hundelshausen P, Weber KS, Huo Y, et al: RANTES deposition by platelets triggers monocyte arrest on inflamed and atherosclerotic endothelium. *Circulation* 103:1772, 2001.
1149. Schober A, Manka D, von Hundelshausen P, et al: Deposition of platelet RANTES triggering monocyte recruitment requires P-selectin and is involved in neointima formation after arterial injury. *Circulation* 106:1523, 2002.
1150. Huo Y, Schober A, Forlow SB, et al: Circulating activated platelets exacerbate atherosclerosis in mice deficient in apolipoprotein E. *Nat Med* 9:61, 2003.
1151. Yeo EL, Sheppard JA, Feuerstein IA: Role of P-selectin and leukocyte activation in polymorphonuclear cell adhesion to surface adherent activated platelets under physiologic shear conditions (an injury vessel wall model). *Blood* 83:2498, 1994.
1152. Diacovo TG, Roth SJ, Buccola JM, et al: Neutrophil rolling, arrest, and transmigration across activated, surface-adherent platelets via sequential action of P-selectin and the beta 2-integrin CD11b/CD18. *Blood* 88:146, 1996.
1153. Sheikh S, Nash GB: Continuous activation and deactivation of integrin CD11b/CD18 during *de novo* expression enables rolling neutrophils to immobilize on platelets. *Blood* 87:5040, 1996.
1154. Kirchhofer D, Riederer MA, Baumgartner HR: Specific accumulation of circulating monocytes and polymorphonuclear leukocytes on platelet thrombi in a vascular injury model. *Blood* 89:1270, 1997.
1155. Konstantopoulos K, Neelamegham S, Burns AR, et al: Venous levels of shear support neutrophil-platelet adhesion and neutrophil aggregation in blood via P-selectin and beta2-integrin. *Circulation* 98:873, 1998.
1156. Weber C, Springer TA: Neutrophil accumulation on activated, surface-adherent platelets in flow is mediated by interaction of Mac-1 with fibrinogen bound to alphaIIbbeta3 and stimulated by platelet-activating factor. *J Clin Invest* 100:2085, 1997.
1157. Altieri DC, Plescia J, Plow EF: The structural motif glycine 190-valine 202 of the fibrinogen gamma chain interacts with CD11b/CD18 integrin (alpha M beta 2, Mac-1) and promotes leukocyte adhesion. *J Biol Chem* 268:1847, 1993.
1158. Ugarova TP, Solovjov DA, Zhang L, et al: Identification of a novel recognition sequence for integrin alphaM beta2 within the gamma-chain of fibrinogen. *J Biol Chem* 273:22519, 1998.
1159. Silverstein RL, Asch AS, Nachman RL: Glycoprotein IV mediates thrombospondin-dependent platelet-monocyte and platelet-U937 cell adhesion. *J Clin Invest* 84:546, 1989.

1160. Marcus AJ, Safier LB: Thromboregulation: Multicellular modulation of platelet reactivity in hemostasis and thrombosis. *FASEB J* 7:516, 1993.
1161. Lindemann S, Tolley ND, Dixon DA, et al: Activated platelets mediate inflammatory signaling by regulated interleukin 1beta synthesis. *J Cell Biol* 154:485, 2001.
1162. Alderson MR, Armitage RJ, Tough TW, et al: CD40 expression by human monocytes: Regulation by cytokines and activation of monocytes by the ligand for CD40. *J Exp Med* 178:669, 1993.
1163. Yellin MJ, Brett J, Baum D, et al: Functional interactions of T cells with endothelial cells: The role of CD40L-CD40-mediated signals. *J Exp Med* 182:1857, 1995.
1164. Slupsky JR, Kalbas M, Willuweit A, et al: Activated platelets induce tissue factor expression on human umbilical vein endothelial cells by ligation of CD40. *Thromb Haemost* 80:1008, 1998.
1165. Del PD, Frega G, Savini I, et al: The plasma membrane redox system in human platelet functions and platelet-leukocyte interactions. *Thromb Haemost* 101:284, 2009.
1166. Goel MS, Diamond SL: Neutrophil cathepsin G promotes prothrombinase and fibrin formation under flow conditions by activating fibrinogen-adherent platelets. *J Biol Chem* 278:9458, 2003.
1167. Goel MS, Diamond SL: Neutrophil enhancement of fibrin deposition under flow through platelet-dependent and -independent mechanisms. *Arterioscler Thromb Vasc Biol* 21:2093, 2001.
1168. Pluskota E, Woody NM, Szpak D, et al: Expression, activation, and function of integrin alphaMbeta2 (Mac-1) on neutrophil-derived microparticles. *Blood* 112:2327, 2008.
1169. Andre P, Hartwell D, Hrachovinova I, et al: Pro-coagulant state resulting from high levels of soluble P-selectin in blood. *Proc Natl Acad Sci U S A* 97:13835, 2000.
1170. Ott I, Neumann FJ, Gawaz M, et al: Increased neutrophil-platelet adhesion in patients with unstable angina. *Circulation* 94:1239, 1996.
1171. Mickelson JK, Lakkis NM, Villarreal-Levy G, et al: Leukocyte activation with platelet adhesion after coronary angioplasty: A mechanism for recurrent disease? *J Am Coll Cardiol* 28:345, 1996.
1172. Michelson AD, Barnard MR, Krueger LA, et al: Circulating monocyte-platelet aggregates are a more sensitive marker of *in vivo* platelet activation than platelet surface P-selectin: Studies in baboons, human coronary intervention, and human acute myocardial infarction. *Circulation* 104:1533, 2001.
1173. Lozano ML, Gonzalez-Conejero R, Corral J, et al: Polymorphisms of P-selectin glycoprotein ligand-1 are associated with neutrophil-platelet adhesion and with ischaemic cerebrovascular disease. *Br J Haematol* 115:969, 2001.
1174. Bugert P, Hoffmann MM, Winkelmann BR, et al: The variable number of tandem repeat polymorphism in the P-selectin glycoprotein ligand-1 gene is not associated with coronary heart disease. *J Mol Med* 81:495, 2003.
1175. Roldan V, Gonzalez-Conejero R, Marin F, et al: Short alleles of P-selectin glycoprotein ligand-1 protect against premature myocardial infarction. *Am Heart J* 148:602, 2004.
1176. Ozben B, Diz-Kucukkaya R, Bilge AK, et al: The association of P-selectin glycoprotein ligand-1 VNTR polymorphisms with coronary stent restenosis. *J Thromb Thrombolysis* 23:181, 2007.
1177. Diz-Kucukkaya R, Inanc M, fshar-Kharghan V, et al: P-selectin glycoprotein ligand-1 VNTR polymorphisms and risk of thrombosis in the antiphospholipid syndrome. *Ann Rheum Dis* 66:1378, 2007.
1178. Tauxe C, Xie X, Joffraud M, et al: P-selectin glycoprotein ligand-1 decameric repeats regulate selectin-dependent rolling under flow conditions. *J Biol Chem* 283:28536, 2008.
1179. Li N: Platelet-lymphocyte cross-talk. *J Leukoc Biol* 83:1069, 2008.
1180. Pawelczyk T: Isozymes delta of phosphoinositide-specific phospholipase C. *Acta Biochim Pol* 46:91, 1999.
1181. Hirata T, Ushikubi F, Kakizuka A, et al: Two thromboxane A2 receptor isoforms in human platelets. Opposite coupling to adenylyl cyclase with different sensitivity to Arg60 to Leu mutation. *J Clin Invest* 97:949, 1996.
1182. Murphy CT, Westwick J: Selective inhibition of protein kinase C. Effect on platelet-activating-factor-induced platelet functional responses. *Biochem J* 283:159, 1992.
1183. Kunapuli SP: Funcional characterization of platelet ADP. *Platelets* 9:343, 1998.
1184. Cattaneo M: The platelet P2 receptors, in *Platelets*, 2nd ed, edited by AD Michelson, p 201. Academic Press, San Diego, 2007.
1185. Murugappa S, Kunapuli SP: The role of ADP receptors in platelet function. *Front Biosci* 11:1977, 2006.
1186. Hollopeter G, Jantzen HM, Vincent D, et al: Identification of the platelet ADP receptor targeted by antithrombotic drugs. *Nature* 409:202, 2001.
1187. Conley PB, Delaney SM: Scientific and therapeutic insights into the role of the platelet P2Y12 receptor in thrombosis. *Curr Opin Hematol* 10:333, 2003.
1188. Dorsam RT, Kunapuli SP: Central role of the P2Y12 receptor in platelet activation. *J Clin Invest* 113:340, 2004.
1189. Aleil B, Ravanat C, Cazenave JP, et al: Flow cytometric analysis of intraplatelet VASP phosphorylation for the detection of clopidogrel resistance in patients with ischemic cardiovascular diseases. *J Thromb Haemost* 3:85, 2005.
1190. Jin J, Daniel JL, Kunapuli SP: Molecular basis for ADP-induced platelet activation. II. The P2Y1 receptor mediates ADP-induced intracellular calcium mobilization and shape change in platelets. *J Biol Chem* 273:2030, 1998.
1191. Mills DC, Puri R, Hu CJ, et al: Clopidogrel inhibits the binding of ADP analogues to the receptor mediating inhibition of platelet adenylate cyclase. *Arterioscler Thromb* 12:430, 1992.
1192. Andre P, Delaney SM, LaRocca T, et al: P2Y12 regulates platelet adhesion/activation, thrombus growth, and thrombus stability in injured arteries. *J Clin Invest* 112:398, 2003.
1193. Foster CJ, Prosser DM, Agans JM, et al: Molecular identification and characterization of the platelet ADP receptor targeted by thienopyridine antithrombotic drugs. *J Clin Invest* 107:1591, 2001.
1194. Fontana P, Dupont A, Gandrille S, et al: Adenosine diphosphate-induced platelet aggregation is associated with P2Y12 gene sequence variations in healthy subjects. *Circulation* 108:989, 2003.
1195. Staritz P, Kurz K, Stoll M, et al: Platelet reactivity and clopidogrel resistance are associated with the H2 haplotype of the P2Y(12)-ADP receptor gene. *Int J Cardiol* 133:341, 2009.
1196. Henderson DJ, Elliot DG, Smith GM, et al: Cloning and characterisation of a bovine P2Y receptor. *Biochem Biophys Res Commun* 212:648, 1995.
1197. Fabre JE, Nguyen M, Latour A, et al: Decreased platelet aggregation, increased bleeding time and resistance to thromboembolism in $P2Y_1$-deficient mice. *Nat Med* 5:1199, 1999.
1198. Leon C, Hechler B, Freund M, et al: Defective platelet aggregation and increased resistance to thrombosis in purinergic P2Y(1) receptor-null mice. *J Clin Invest* 104:1731, 1999.
1199. Offermanns S, Toombs CF, Hu YH, et al: Defective platelet activation in G alpha(q)-deficient mice. *Nature* 389:183, 1997.
1200. MacKenzie AB, Mahaut-Smith MP, Sage SO: Activation of receptor-operated cation channels via P2X1 not P2T purinoceptors in human platelets. *J Biol Chem* 271:2879, 1996.
1201. Valera S, Hussy N, Evans RJ, et al: A new class of ligand-gated ion channel defined by P2x receptor for extracellular ATP. *Nature* 371:516, 1994.
1202. Oury C, Toth-Zsamboki E, Vermylen J, et al: Does the P(2X1del) variant lacking 17 amino acids in its extracellular domain represent a relevant functional ion channel in platelets? *Blood* 99:2275, 2002.
1203. Vial C, Pitt SJ, Roberts J, et al: Lack of evidence for functional ADP-activated human P2X1 receptors supports a role for ATP during hemostasis and thrombosis. *Blood* 102:3646, 2003.
1204. Oury C, Toth-Zsamboki E, Vermylen J, et al: P2X(1)-mediated activation of extracellular signal-regulated kinase 2 contributes to platelet secretion and aggregation induced by collagen. *Blood* 100:2499, 2002.
1205. Vial C, Rolf MG, Mahaut-Smith MP, et al: A study of P2X1 receptor function in murine megakaryocytes and human platelets reveals synergy with P2Y receptors. *Br J Pharmacol* 135:363, 2002.
1206. Hechler B, Lenain N, Marchese P, et al: A role of the fast ATP-gated P2X1 cation channel in thrombosis of small arteries *in vivo*. *J Exp Med* 198:661, 2003.
1207. Oury C, Kuijpers MJ, Toth-Zsamboki E, et al: Overexpression of the platelet P2X1 ion channel in transgenic mice generates a novel prothrombotic phenotype. *Blood* 101:3969, 2003.
1208. Greco NJ, Tonon G, Chen W, et al: Novel structurally altered P(2X1) receptor is preferentially activated by adenosine diphosphate in platelets and megakaryocytic cells. *Blood* 98:100, 2001.
1209. Raju NC, Eikelboom JW, Hirsh J: Platelet ADP-receptor antagonists for cardiovascular disease: Past, present and future. *Nat Clin Pract Cardiovasc Med* 5:766, 2008.
1210. Gayle RB3, Maliszewski CR, Gimpel SD, et al: Inhibition of platelet function by recombinant soluble ecto-ADPase/CD39. *J Clin Invest* 101:1851, 1998.
1211. Banga HS, Simons ER, Brass LF, et al: Activation of phospholipases A and C in human platelets exposed to epinephrine: Role of glycoproteins IIb/IIIa and dual role of epinephrine. *Proc Natl Acad Sci U S A* 83:9197, 1986.
1212. Shattil SJ, Budzynski A, Scrutton MC: Epinephrine induces platelet fibrinogen receptor expression, fibrinogen binding, and aggregation in whole blood in the absence of other excitatory agonists. *Blood* 73:150, 1989.
1213. Lanza F, Beretz A, Stierle A, et al: Epinephrine potentiates human platelet activation but is not an aggregating agent. *Am J Physiol* 255:1276, 1988.
1214. Regan JW, Nakata H, DeMarinis RM, et al: Purification and characterization of the human platelet alpha 2- adrenergic receptor. *J Biol Chem* 261:3894, 1986.
1215. Kobilka BK, Matsui H, Kobilka TS, et al: Cloning, sequencing, and expression of the gene coding for the human platelet alpha 2-adrenergic receptor. *Science* 238:650, 1987.
1216. Yang J, Wu J, Kowalska MA, et al: Loss of signaling through the G protein, Gz, results in abnormal platelet activation and altered responses to psychoactive drugs. *Proc Natl Acad Sci U S A* 97:9984, 2000.
1217. Homcy CJ, Graham RM: Molecular characterization of adrenergic receptors. *Circ Res* 56:635, 1985.
1218. Yang J, Wu J, Jiang H, et al: Signaling through Gi family members in platelets. Redundancy and specificity in the regulation of adenylyl cyclase and other effectors. *J Biol Chem* 277:46035, 2002.
1219. Haslam RJ, Davidson MM, Fox JE, et al: Cyclic nucleotides in platelet function. *Thromb Haemost* 40:232, 1978.
1220. Salzman EW, Ware JA: Ionized calcium as an intracellular messenger in blood platelets. *Prog Hemost Thromb* 9:177, 1989.
1221. Patel YM, Patel K, Rahman S, et al: Evidence for a role for Galphai1 in mediating weak agonist-induced platelet aggregation in human platelets: Reduced Galphai1 expression and defective Gi signaling in the platelets of a patient with a chronic bleeding disorder. *Blood* 101:4828, 2003.

1222. Freeman K, Farrow S, Schmaier A, et al: Genetic polymorphism of the alpha 2-adrenergic receptor is associated with increased platelet aggregation, baroreceptor sensitivity, and salt excretion in normotensive humans. *Am J Hypertens* 8:863, 1995.
1223. Small KM, Forbes SL, Brown KM, et al: An asn to lys polymorphism in the third intracellular loop of the human alpha 2A-adrenergic receptor imparts enhanced agonist-promoted Gi coupling. *J Biol Chem* 275:38518, 2000.
1224. von KR, Dimsdale JE: Effects of sympathetic activation by adrenergic infusions on hemostasis *in vivo*. *Eur J Haematol* 65:357, 2000.
1225. Folts JD, Rowe GG: Epinephrine potentiation of *in vivo* stimuli reverses aspirin inhibition of platelet thrombus formation in stenosed canine coronary arteries. *Thromb Res* 50:507, 1988.
1226. Bertha BG, Folts JD: Inhibition of epinephrine-exacerbated coronary thrombus formation by prostacyclin in the dog. *J Lab Clin Med* 103:204, 1984.
1227. Sibbing D, von BO, Schomig A, et al: Platelet function in clopidogrel-treated patients with acute coronary syndrome. *Blood Coagul Fibrinolysis* 18:335, 2007.
1228. Marcus A: Platelet eicosanoid metabolism, in *Hemostasis and Thrombosis; Basic Principles and Clinical Practice*, 2nd ed, edited by RW Colman, J Hirsch, VJ Marder, EW Salzman, p 676. JB Lippincott, Philadelphia, 1987.
1229. Puri RN: Phospholipase A2: Its role in ADP- and thrombin-induced platelet activation mechanisms. *Int J Biochem Cell Biol* 30:1107, 1998.
1230. Wong DA, Kita Y, Uozumi N, et al: Discrete role for cytosolic phospholipase A(2)alpha in platelets: Studies using single and double mutant mice of cytosolic and group IIA secretory phospholipase A(2). *J Exp Med* 196:349, 2002.
1231. Adler DH, Cogan JD, Phillips JA, et al: Inherited human cPLA(2alpha)deficiency is associated with impaired eicosanoid biosynthesis, small intestinal ulceration, and platelet dysfunction. *J Clin Invest* 118:2121, 2008.
1232. Prevost N, Mitsios JV, Kato H, et al: Group IVA cytosolic phospholipase A2 (cPLA2alpha) and integrin alphaIIbbeta3 reinforce each other's functions during alphaIIbbeta3 signaling in platelets. *Blood* 113:447, 2009.
1233. Crofford LJ: COX-1 and COX-2 tissue expression: Implications and predictions. *J Rheumatol* 24:15, 1997.
1234. Warner TD, Mitchell JA: Cyclooxygenases: New forms, new inhibitors, and lessons from the clinic. *FASEB J* 18:790, 2004.
1235. Dubois RN, Abramson SB, Crofford L, et al: Cyclooxygenase in biology and disease. *FASEB J* 12:1063, 1998.
1236. Smith JB, Willis AL: Aspirin selectively inhibits prostaglandin production in human platelets. *Nat New Biol* 231:235, 1971.
1237. Svensson J, Hamberg M, Samuelsson B: On the formation and effects of thromboxane A2 in human platelets. *Acta Physiol Scand* 98:285, 1976.
1238. Weber AA, Zimmermann KC, Meyer-Kirchrath J, et al: Cyclooxygenase-2 in human platelets as a possible factor in aspirin resistance. *Lancet* 353:900, 1999.
1239. Rocca B, Secchiero P, Ciabattoni G, et al: Cyclooxygenase-2 expression is induced during human megakaryopoiesis and characterizes newly formed platelets. *Proc Natl Acad Sci U S A* 99:7634, 2002.
1240. Funk CD, FitzGerald GA: COX-2 inhibitors and cardiovascular risk. *J Cardiovasc Pharmacol* 50:470, 2007.
1241. Parent JL, Labrecque P, Orsini MJ, et al: Internalization of the TXA2 receptor alpha and beta isoforms. Role of the differentially spliced COOH terminus in agonist-promoted receptor internalization. *J Biol Chem* 274:8941, 1999.
1242. Habib A, FitzGerald GA, Maclouf J: Phosphorylation of the thromboxane receptor alpha, the predominant isoform expressed in human platelets. *J Biol Chem* 274:2645, 1999.
1243. Komiotis D, Wencel-Drake JD, Dieter JP, et al: Labeling of human platelet plasma membrane thromboxane A2/prostaglandin H2 receptors using SQB, a novel biotinylated receptor probe. *Biochem Pharmacol* 52:763, 1996.
1244. Kim SO, Lim CT, Lam SC, et al: Purification of the human blood platelet thromboxane A2/prostaglandin H2 receptor protein. *Biochem Pharmacol* 43:313, 1992.
1245. Ushikubi F, Nakajima M, Hirata M, et al: Purification of the thromboxane A2/prostaglandin H2 receptor from human blood platelets. *J Biol Chem* 264:16496, 1989.
1246. Takahara K, Murray R, FitzGerald GA, et al: The response to thromboxane A2 analogues in human platelets. Discrimination of two binding sites linked to distinct effector systems. *J Biol Chem* 265:6836, 1990.
1247. Thomas DW, Mannon RB, Mannon PJ, et al: Coagulation defects and altered hemodynamic responses in mice lacking receptors for thromboxane A2. *J Clin Invest* 102:1994, 1998.
1248. Gabbeta J, Yang X, Kowalska MA, et al: Platelet signal transduction defect with Galpha subunit dysfunction and diminished Galphaq in a patient with abnormal platelet responses. *Proc Natl Acad Sci U S A* 94:8750, 1997.
1249. Djellas Y, Manganello JM, Antonakis K, et al: Identification of Galpha13 as one of the G-proteins that couple to human platelet thromboxane A2 receptors. *J Biol Chem* 274:14325, 1999.
1250. Allan CJ, Higashiura K, Martin M, et al: Characterization of the cloned HEL cell thromboxane A2 receptor: Evidence that the affinity state can be altered by G alpha 13 and G alpha q. *J Pharmacol Exp Ther* 277:1132, 1996.
1251. Nakahata N, Miyamoto A, Ohkubo S, et al: Gq/11 communicates with thromboxane A2 receptors in human astrocytoma cells, rabbit astrocytes and human platelets. *Res Commun Mol Pathol Pharmacol* 87:243, 1995.
1252. Ushikubi F, Nakamura K, Narumiya S: Functional reconstitution of platelet thromboxane A2 receptors with Gq and Gi2 in phospholipid vesicles. *Mol Pharmacol* 46:808, 1994.
1253. Paul BZ, Jin J, Kunapuli SP: Molecular mechanism of thromboxane A(2)-induced platelet aggregation. Essential role for p2t(ac) and alpha(2a) receptors. *J Biol Chem* 274:29108, 1999.
1254. Klages B, Brandt U, Simon MI, et al: Activation of G12/G13 results in shape change and Rho/Rho-kinase-mediated myosin light chain phosphorylation in mouse platelets. *J Cell Biol* 144:745, 1999.
1255. Nieswandt B, Schulte V, Zywietz A, et al: Costimulation of Gi- and G12/G13-mediated signaling pathways induces integrin alpha IIbbeta 3 activation in platelets. *J Biol Chem* 277:39493, 2002.
1256. Dorsam RT, Kim S, Jin J, et al: Coordinated signaling through both G12/13 and G(i) pathways is sufficient to activate GPIIb/IIIa in human platelets. *J Biol Chem* 277:47588, 2002.
1257. Pulcinelli FM, Ashby B, Gazzaniga PP, et al: Protein kinase C activation is not a key step in ADP-mediated exposure of fibrinogen receptors on human platelets. *FEBS Lett* 364:87, 1995.
1258. Knezevic I, Dieter JP, Le Breton GC: Mechanism of inositol 1,4,5-trisphosphate-induced aggregation in saponin-permeabilized platelets. *J Pharmacol Exp Ther* 260:947, 1992.
1259. Nugteren DH: Arachidonate lipoxygenase in blood platelets. *Biochim Biophys Acta* 380:299, 1975.
1260. Johnson EN, Brass LF, Funk CD: Increased platelet sensitivity to ADP in mice lacking platelet-type 12-lipoxygenase. *Proc Natl Acad Sci U S A* 95:3100, 1998.
1261. Coffey MJ, Jarvis GE, Gibbins JM, et al: Platelet 12-lipoxygenase activation via glycoprotein VI: Involvement of multiple signaling pathways in agonist control of H(P)ETE synthesis. *Circ Res* 94:1598, 2004.
1262. Dasari VR, Jin J, Kunapuli SP: Distribution of leukotriene B4 receptors in human hematopoietic cells. *Immunopharmacology* 48:157, 2000.
1263. Maclouf JA, Murphy RC: Transcellular metabolism of neutrophil-derived leukotriene A4 by human platelets. A potential cellular source of leukotriene C4. *J Biol Chem* 263:174, 1988.
1264. Maugeri N, Evangelista V, Celardo A, et al: Polymorphonuclear leukocyte-platelet interaction: Role of P-selectin in thromboxane B2 and leukotriene C4 cooperative synthesis. *Thromb Haemost* 72:450, 1994.
1265. Levy BD, Bertram S, Tai HH, et al: Agonist-induced lipoxin A4 generation: Detection by a novel lipoxin A4-ELISA. *Lipids* 28:1047, 1993.
1266. Ofosu FA, Liu L, Freedman J: Control mechanisms in thrombin generation. *Semin Thromb Hemost* 22:303, 1996.
1267. Phillips DR: Thrombin interaction with human platelets. Potentiation of thrombin-induced aggregation and release by inactivated thrombin. *Thromb Diath Haemorrh* 32:207, 1974.
1268. Hung DT, Vu TK, Wheaton VI, et al: Cloned platelet thrombin receptor is necessary for thrombin-induced platelet activation. *J Clin Invest* 89:1350, 1992.
1269. Vu TK, Hung DT, Wheaton VI, et al: Molecular cloning of a functional thrombin receptor reveals a novel proteolytic mechanism of receptor activation. *Cell* 64:1057, 1991.
1270. Bahou W: Thrombin receptors, in *Platelets*, 2nd ed, edited by AD Michelson, p 179. Academic Press, San Diego, 2007.
1271. Furman MI, Liu L, Benoit SE, et al: The cleaved peptide of the thrombin receptor is a strong platelet agonist. *Proc Natl Acad Sci U S A* 95:3082, 1998.
1272. Ishihara H, Zeng D, Connolly AJ, et al: Antibodies to protease-activated receptor 3 inhibit activation of mouse platelets by thrombin. *Blood* 91:4152, 1998.
1273. Kahn ML, Zheng YW, Huang W, et al: A dual thrombin receptor system for platelet activation. *Nature* 394:690, 1998.
1274. Kahn ML, Nakanishi-Matsui M, Shapiro MJ, et al: Protease-activated receptors 1 and 4 mediate activation of human platelets by thrombin. *J Clin Invest* 103:879, 1999.
1275. Andrade-Gordon P, Maryanoff BE, Derian CK, et al: Design, synthesis, and biological characterization of a peptide-mimetic antagonist for a tethered-ligand receptor. *Proc Natl Acad Sci U S A* 96:12257, 1999.
1276. Shapiro MJ, Weiss EJ, Faruqi TR, et al: Protease-activated receptors 1 and 4 are shut off with distinct kinetics after activation by thrombin. *J Biol Chem* 275:25216, 2000.
1277. Covic L, Gresser AL, Kuliopulos A: Biphasic kinetics of activation and signaling for PAR1 and PAR4 thrombin receptors in platelets. *Biochemistry* 39:5458, 2000.
1278. Sambrano GR, Weiss EJ, Zheng YW, et al: Role of thrombin signalling in platelets in haemostasis and thrombosis. *Nature* 413:74, 2001.
1279. Nakanishi-Matsui M, Zheng YW, Sulciner DJ, et al: PAR3 is a cofactor for PAR4 activation by thrombin. *Nature* 404:609, 2000.
1280. Weiss EJ, Hamilton JR, Lease KE, et al: Protection against thrombosis in mice lacking PAR3. *Blood* 100:3240, 2002.
1281. Becker RC, Moliterno DJ, Jennings LK, et al: Safety and tolerability of SCH 530348 in patients undergoing non-urgent percutaneous coronary intervention: A randomised, double-blind, placebo-controlled phase II study. *Lancet* 373:919, 2009.
1282. Hoxie JA, Ahuja M, Belmonte E, et al: Internalization and recycling of activated thrombin receptors. *J Biol Chem* 268:13756, 1993.
1283. Trejo J, Coughlin SR: The cytoplasmic tails of protease-activated receptor-1 and substance P receptor specify sorting to lysosomes versus recycling. *J Biol Chem* 274:2216, 1999.
1284. Gibbins JM: Tweaking the gain on platelet regulation: The tachykinin connection. *Atherosclerosis* 206:1, 2009.
1285. Graham GJ, Stevens JM, Page NM, et al: Tachykinins regulate the function of platelets. *Blood* 104:1058, 2004.

1286. Gleissner CA, von HP, Ley K: Platelet chemokines in vascular disease. *Arterioscler Thromb Vasc Biol* 28:1920, 2008.
1287. McIntyre TM, Zimmerman GA, Prescott SM: Biologically active oxidized phospholipids. *J Biol Chem* 274:25189, 1999.
1288. Honda Z, Nakamura M, Miki I, et al: Cloning by functional expression of platelet-activating factor receptor from guinea-pig lung. *Nature* 349:342, 1991.
1289. Nakamura M, Honda Z, Izumi T, et al: Molecular cloning and expression of platelet-activating factor receptor from human leukocytes. *J Biol Chem* 266:20400, 1991.
1290. Carlson SA, Chatterjee TK, Fisher RA: The third intracellular domain of the platelet-activating factor receptor is a critical determinant in receptor coupling to phosphoinositide phospholipase C-activating G proteins. Studies using intracellular domain minigenes and receptor chimeras. *J Biol Chem* 271:23146, 1996.
1291. Chao W, Liu H, Hanahan DJ, et al: Protein tyrosine phosphorylation and regulation of the receptor for platelet-activating factor in rat Kupffer cells. Effect of sodium vanadate. *Biochem J* 288:777, 1992.
1292. Stafforini DM: Biology of platelet-activating factor acetylhydrolase (PAF-AH, lipoprotein associated phospholipase A2). *Cardiovasc Drugs Ther* 23:73, 2009.
1293. Korporaal SJ, Van EM, Adelmeijer J, et al: Platelet activation by oxidized low density lipoprotein is mediated by CD36 and scavenger receptor-A. *Arterioscler Thromb Vasc Biol* 27:2476, 2007.
1294. Eitzman DT, Westrick RJ, Xu Z, et al: Hyperlipidemia promotes thrombosis after injury to atherosclerotic vessels in apolipoprotein E-deficient mice. *Arterioscler Thromb Vasc Biol* 20:1831, 2000.
1295. Sano T, Baker D, Virag T, et al: Multiple mechanisms linked to platelet activation result in lysophosphatidic acid and sphingosine 1-phosphate generation in blood. *J Biol Chem* 277:21197, 2002.
1296. Smyth SS, Cheng HY, Miriyala S, et al: Roles of lysophosphatidic acid in cardiovascular physiology and disease. *Biochim Biophys Acta* 1781:563, 2008.
1297. Umezu-Goto M, Kishi Y, Taira A, et al: Autotaxin has lysophospholipase D activity leading to tumor cell growth and motility by lysophosphatidic acid production. *J Cell Biol* 158:227, 2002.
1298. Siess W, Zangl KJ, Essler M, et al: Lysophosphatidic acid mediates the rapid activation of platelets and endothelial cells by mildly oxidized low density lipoprotein and accumulates in human atherosclerotic lesions. *Proc Natl Acad Sci U S A* 96:6931, 1999.
1299. Retzer M, Essler M: Lysophosphatidic acid-induced platelet shape change proceeds via Rho/Rho kinase-mediated myosin light-chain and moesin phosphorylation. *Cell Signal* 12:645, 2000.
1300. Haseruck N, Erl W, Pandey D, et al: The plaque lipid lysophosphatidic acid stimulates platelet activation and platelet-monocyte aggregate formation in whole blood: Involvement of P2Y1 and P2Y12 receptors. *Blood* 103:2585, 2004.
1301. Olorundare OE, Peyruchaud O, Albrecht RM, et al: Assembly of a fibronectin matrix by adherent platelets stimulated by lysophosphatidic acid and other agonists. *Blood* 98:117, 2001.
1302. Maschberger P, Bauer M, Baumann-Siemons J, et al: Mildly oxidized low density lipoprotein rapidly stimulates via activation of the lysophosphatidic acid receptor Src family and Syk tyrosine kinases and Ca2+ influx in human platelets. *J Biol Chem* 275:19159, 2000.
1303. Siess W: Athero- and thrombogenic actions of lysophosphatidic acid and sphingosine-1-phosphate. *Biochim Biophys Acta* 1582:204, 2002.
1304. Motohashi K, Shibata S, Ozaki Y, et al: Identification of lysophospholipid receptors in human platelets: The relation of two agonists, lysophosphatidic acid and sphingosine 1-phosphate. *FEBS Lett* 468:189, 2000.
1305. Siess W, Tigyi G: Thrombogenic and atherogenic activities of lysophosphatidic acid. *J Cell Biochem* 92:1086, 2004.
1306. Yatomi Y, Ruan F, Hakomori S, et al: Sphingosine-1-phosphate: A platelet-activating sphingolipid released from agonist-stimulated human platelets. *Blood* 86:193, 1995.
1307. Nugent D, Xu Y: Sphingosine-1-phosphate: Characterization of its inhibition of platelet aggregation. *Platelets* 11:226, 2000.
1308. Hoyer D, Clarke DE, Fozard JR, et al: International Union of Pharmacology classification of receptors for 5-hydroxytryptamine (serotonin). *Pharmacol Rev* 46:157, 1994.
1309. De Clerck F, Xhonneux B, Leysen J, et al: Evidence for functional 5-HT2 receptor sites on human blood platelets. *Biochem Pharmacol* 33:2807, 1984.
1310. Cook EH, Jr, Fletcher KE, Wainwright M, et al: Primary structure of the human platelet serotonin 5-HT2A receptor: Identify with frontal cortex serotonin 5-HT2A receptor. *J Neurochem* 63:465, 1994.
1311. Roth BL, Willins DL, Kristiansen K, et al: 5-Hydroxytryptamine2-family receptors (5-hydroxytryptamine2A, 5-hydroxytryptamine2B, 5-hydroxytryptamine2C): Where structure meets function. *Pharmacol Ther* 79:231, 1998.
1312. Allen JA, Yadav PN, Roth BL: Insights into the regulation of 5-HT2A serotonin receptors by scaffolding proteins and kinases. *Neuropharmacology* 55:961, 2008.
1313. Leysen JE, Eens A, Gommeren W, et al: Identification of nonserotonergic [3H]ketanserin binding sites associated with nerve terminals in rat brain and with platelets; relation with release of biogenic amine metabolites induced by ketans. *J Pharmacol Exp Ther* 244:310, 1988.
1314. Ozaki N, Manji H, Lubierman V, et al: A naturally occurring amino acid substitution of the human serotonin 5- HT2A receptor influences amplitude and timing of intracellular calcium mobilization. *J Neurochem* 68:2186, 1997.
1315. Shimizu M, Kanazawa K, Matsuda Y, et al: Serotonin-2A receptor gene polymorphisms are associated with serotonin-induced platelet aggregation. *Thromb Res* 112:137, 2003.
1316. Arora RC, Meltzer HY: Serotonin2 receptor binding in blood platelets of schizophrenic patients. *Psychiatry Res* 47:111, 1993.
1317. Coccaro EF, Kavoussi RJ, Sheline YI, et al: Impulsive aggression in personality disorder correlates with platelet 5-HT2A receptor binding. *Neuropsychopharmacology* 16:211, 1997.
1318. Pandey GN: Altered serotonin function in suicide. Evidence from platelet and neuroendocrine studies. *Ann N Y Acad Sci* 836:182, 1997.
1319. Wolfe BE, Metzger E, Jimerson DC: Research update on serotonin function in bulimia nervosa and anorexia nervosa. *Psychopharmacol Bull* 33:345, 1997.
1320. Tomiyoshi R, Kamei K, Muraoka S, et al: Serotonin-induced platelet intracellular Ca2+ responses in untreated depressed patients and imipramine responders in remission. *Biol Psychiatry* 45:1042, 1999.
1321. Cho R, Kapur S, Du L, et al: Relationship between central and peripheral serotonin 5-HT2A receptors: A positron emission tomography study in healthy individuals. *Neurosci Lett* 261:139, 1999.
1322. Schins A, Honig A, Crijns H, et al: Increased coronary events in depressed cardiovascular patients: 5-HT2A receptor as missing link? *Psychosom Med* 65:729, 2003.
1323. de Chaffoy dC, Leysen JE, De Clerck F, et al: Evidence that phospholipid turnover is the signal transducing system coupled to serotonin-S2 receptor sites. *J Biol Chem* 260:7603, 1985.
1324. Erne P, Pletscher A: Rapid intracellular release of calcium in human platelets by stimulation of 5-HT2-receptors. *Br J Pharmacol* 84:545, 1985.
1325. Li N, Wallen NH, Ladjevardi M, et al: Effects of serotonin on platelet activation in whole blood. *Blood Coagul Fibrinolysis* 8:517, 1997.
1326. Houston DS, Shepherd JT, Vanhoutte PM: Aggregating human platelets cause direct contraction and endothelium- dependent relaxation of isolated canine coronary arteries. Role of serotonin, thromboxane A2, and adenine nucleotides. *J Clin Invest* 78:539, 1986.
1327. Golino P, Ashton J, Glas-Grewaalt P, et al: Mediation or reocclusion by thromboxane A2 and serotonin after thrombolysis with tissue-type plasminogen activator in a canine preparation of coronary thrombosis. *Circulation* 77:678, 1988.
1328. Alberio LJ, Clemetson KJ: All platelets are not equal: COAT platelets. *Curr Hematol Rep* 3:338, 2004.
1329. Dale GL, Friese P, Batar P, et al: Stimulated platelets use serotonin to enhance their retention of procoagulant proteins on the cell surface. *Nature* 415:175, 2002.
1330. Walther DJ, Peter JU, Winter S, et al: Serotonylation of small GTPases is a signal transduction pathway that triggers platelet alpha-granule release. *Cell* 115:851, 2003.
1331. Carneiro AM, Cook EH, Murphy DL, et al: Interactions between integrin alphaIIbbeta3 and the serotonin transporter regulate serotonin transport and platelet aggregation in mice and humans. *J Clin Invest* 118:1544, 2008.
1332. McCloskey DJ, Postolache TT, Vittone BJ, et al: Selective serotonin reuptake inhibitors: Measurement of effect on platelet function. *Transl Res* 151:168, 2008.
1333. Haslam RJ, Rosson GM: Aggregation of human blood platelets by vasopressin. *Am J Physiol* 223:958, 1972.
1334. Pollock WK, MacIntyre DE: Desensitization and antagonism of vasopressin-induced phosphoinositide metabolism and elevation of cytosolic free calcium concentration in human platelets. *Biochem J* 234:67, 1986.
1335. Thomas ME, Osmani AH, Scrutton MC: Some properties of the human platelet vasopressin receptor. *Thromb Res* 32:557, 1983.
1336. Thibonnier M, Roberts JM: Characterization of human platelet vasopressin receptors. *J Clin Invest* 76:1857, 1985.
1337. Siess W, Stifel M, Binder H, et al: Activation of V1-receptors by vasopressin stimulates inositol phospholipid hydrolysis and arachidonate metabolism in human platelets. *Biochem J* 233:83, 1986.
1338. Thibonnier M, Goraya T, Berti-Mattera L: G protein coupling of human platelet V1 vascular vasopressin receptors. *Am J Physiol* 264:C1336, 1993.
1339. Berrettini WH, Post RM, Worthington EK, et al: Human platelet vasopressin receptors. *Life Sci* 30:425, 1982.
1340. Siess W: Molecular mechanisms of platelet activation. *Physiol Rev* 69:58, 1989.
1341. Wun T, Paglieroni T, Lachant NA: Physiologic concentrations of arginine vasopressin activate human platelets *in vitro*. *Br J Haematol* 92:968, 1996.
1342. Serradeil-Le Gal C, Wagnon J, Valette G, et al: Nonpeptide vasopressin receptor antagonists: Development of selective and orally active V1a, V2 and V1b receptor ligands. *Prog Brain Res* 139:197, 2002.
1343. Gunnet JW, Wines P, Xiang M, et al: Pharmacological characterization of RWJ-676070, a dual vasopressin V(1A)/V(2) receptor antagonist. *Eur J Pharmacol* 590:333, 2008.
1344. Crabos M, Bertschin S, Buhler FR, et al: Identification of AT1 receptors on human platelets and decreased angiotensin II binding in hypertension. *J Hypertens Suppl* 11 Suppl 5:S230, 1993.
1345. Lopez-Farre A, Sanchez dM, Monton M, et al: Angiotensin II AT(1) receptor antagonists and platelet activation. *Nephrol Dial Transplant* 16 Suppl 1:45, 2001.
1346. Jagroop IA, Mikhailidis DP: Angiotensin II can induce and potentiate shape change in human platelets: Effect of losartan. *J Hum Hypertens* 14:581, 2000.
1347. Larsson PT, Schwieler JH, Wallen NH: Platelet activation during angiotensin II infusion in healthy volunteers. *Blood Coagul Fibrinolysis* 11:61, 2000.
1348. Li P, Fukuhara M, Diz DI, et al: Novel angiotensin II AT(1) receptor antagonist irbesartan prevents thromboxane A(2)-induced vasoconstriction in canine coronary arteries and human platelet aggregation. *J Pharmacol Exp Ther* 292:238, 2000.

1349. Monton M, Jimenez A, Nunez A, et al: Comparative effects of angiotensin II AT-1-type receptor antagonists *in vitro* on human platelet activation. *J Cardiovasc Pharmacol* 35:906, 2000.
1350. Kalinowski L, Matys T, Chabielska E, et al: Angiotensin II AT1 receptor antagonists inhibit platelet adhesion and aggregation by nitric oxide release. *Hypertension* 40:521, 2002.
1351. Jimenez AM, Monton M, Garcia R, et al: Inhibition of platelet activation in stroke-prone spontaneously hypertensive rats: Comparison of losartan, candesartan, and valsartan. *J Cardiovasc Pharmacol* 37:406, 2001.
1352. Owens P, Kelly L, Nallen R, et al: Comparison of antihypertensive and metabolic effects of losartan and losartan in combination with hydrochlorothiazide—A randomized controlled trial. *J Hypertens* 18:339, 2000.
1353. Schieffer B, Bunte C, Witte J, et al: Comparative effects of AT1-antagonism and angiotensin-converting enzyme inhibition on markers of inflammation and platelet aggregation in patients with coronary artery disease. *J Am Coll Cardiol* 44:362, 2004.
1354. Yamada K, Hirayama T, Hasegawa Y: Antiplatelet effect of losartan and telmisartan in patients with ischemic stroke. *J Stroke Cerebrovasc Dis* 16:225, 2007.
1355. Serebruany VL, Pokov AN, Malinin AI, et al: Valsartan inhibits platelet activity at different doses in mild to moderate hypertensives: Valsartan Inhibits Platelets (VIP) trial. *Am Heart J* 151:92, 2006.
1356. Chung J, Gao AG, Frazier WA: Thrombospondin acts via integrin-associated protein to activate the platelet integrin alphaIIbbeta3. *J Biol Chem* 272:14740, 1997.
1357. Dorahy DJ, Thorne RF, Fecondo JV, et al: Stimulation of platelet activation and aggregation by a carboxyl-terminal peptide from thrombospondin binding to the integrin-associated protein receptor. *J Biol Chem* 272:1323, 1997.
1358. Lindberg FP, Gresham HD, Schwarz E, et al: Molecular cloning of integrin-associated protein: An immunoglobulin family member with multiple membrane-spanning domains implicated in alpha v beta 3-dependent ligand binding. *J Cell Biol* 123:485, 1993.
1359. Wang XQ, Frazier WA: The thrombospondin receptor CD47 (IAP) modulates and associates with alpha2 beta1 integrin in vascular smooth muscle cells. *Mol Biol Cell* 9:865, 1998.
1360. Frazier WA, Gao AG, Dimitry J, et al: The thrombospondin receptor integrin-associated protein (CD47) functionally couples to heterotrimeric Gi. *J Biol Chem* 274:8554, 1999.
1361. Isenberg JS, Romeo MJ, Yu C, et al: Thrombospondin-1 stimulates platelet aggregation by blocking the antithrombotic activity of nitric oxide/cGMP signaling. *Blood* 111:613, 2008.
1362. Lagadec P, Dejoux O, Ticchioni M, et al: Involvement of a CD47-dependent pathway in platelet adhesion on inflamed vascular endothelium under flow. *Blood* 101:4836, 2003.
1363. Huang MM, Bolen JB, Barnwell JW, et al: Membrane glycoprotein IV (CD36) is physically associated with the Fyn, Lyn, and Yes protein-tyrosine kinases in human platelets. *Proc Natl Acad Sci U S A* 88:7844, 1991.
1364. Pimanda JE, Annis DS, Raftery M, et al: The von Willebrand factor-reducing activity of thrombospondin-1 is located in the calcium-binding/C-terminal sequence and requires a free thiol at position 974. *Blood* 100:2832, 2002.
1365. Pimanda JE, Ganderton T, Maekawa A, et al: Role of thrombospondin-1 in control of von Willebrand factor multimer size in mice. *J Biol Chem* 279:21439, 2004.
1366. van Zanten GH, de Graaf S, Slootweg PJ, et al: Increased platelet deposition on atherosclerotic coronary arteries. *J Clin Invest* 93:615, 1994.
1367. van der Rest M, Garrone R: Collagen family of proteins. *FASEB J* 5:2814, 1991.
1368. Ruggeri ZM, Mendolicchio GL: Adhesion mechanisms in platelet function. *Circ Res* 100:1673, 2007.
1369. Ichinohe T, Takayama H, Ezumi Y, et al: Collagen-stimulated activation of Syk but not c-Src is severely compromised in human platelets lacking membrane glycoprotein VI. *J Biol Chem* 272:63, 1997.
1370. Ishibashi T, Ichinohe T, Sugiyama T, et al: Functional significance of platelet membrane glycoprotein p62 (GP VI), a putative collagen receptor. *Int J Hematol* 62:107, 1995.
1371. Kehrel B, Wierwille S, Clemetson KJ, et al: Glycoprotein VI is a major collagen receptor for platelet activation: It recognizes the platelet-activating quaternary structure of collagen, whereas CD36, glycoprotein IIb/IIIa, and von Willebrand factor do not. *Blood* 91:491, 1998.
1372. Poole A, Gibbins JM, Turner M, et al: The Fc receptor gamma-chain and the tyrosine kinase Syk are essential for activation of mouse platelets by collagen. *EMBO J* 16:2333, 1997.
1373. Clemetson KJ, Clemetson JM: Platelet receptors, in *Platelets*, 2nd ed, edited by AD Michelson, p 117. Academic Press, San Diego, 2007.
1374. Stout JG, Basse F, Luhm RA, et al: Scott syndrome erythrocytes contain a membrane protein capable of mediating Ca2+-dependent transbilayer migration of membrane phospholipids. *J Clin Invest* 99:2232, 1997.
1375. Horii K, Kahn ML, Herr AB: Structural basis for platelet collagen responses by the immune-type receptor glycoprotein VI. *Blood* 108:936, 2006.
1376. Chiang TM: Collagen-platelet interaction: Platelet non-integrin receptors. *Histol Histopathol* 14:579, 1999.
1377. Keely PJ, Parise LV: The alpha2beta1 integrin is a necessary co-receptor for collagen-induced activation of Syk and the subsequent phosphorylation of phospholipase Cgamma2 in platelets. *J Biol Chem* 271:26668, 1996.
1378. Sugiyama T, Okuma M, Ushikubi F, et al: A novel platelet aggregating factor found in a patient with defective collagen-induced platelet aggregation and autoimmune thrombocytopenia. *Blood* 69:1712, 1987.
1379. Briddon SJ, Watson SP: Evidence for the involvement of p59fyn and p53/56lyn in collagen receptor signalling in human platelets. *Biochem J* 338:203, 1999.
1380. Fujii C, Yanagi S, Sada K, et al: Involvement of protein-tyrosine kinase p72syk in collagen-induced signal transduction in platelets. *Eur J Biochem* 226:243, 1994.
1381. Shattil SJ, Ginsberg MH, Brugge JS: Adhesive signaling in platelets. *Curr Opin Cell Biol* 6:695, 1994.
1382. Soriano P, Montgomery C, Geske R, et al: Targeted disruption of the c-src proto-oncogene leads to osteopetrosis in mice. *Cell* 64:693, 1991.
1383. Daniel JL, Dangelmaier C, Smith JB: Evidence for a role for tyrosine phosphorylation of phospholipase Cg2 in collagen-induced platelet cytosolic calcium mobilization. *Biochem J* 302:617, 1994.
1384. Quek LS, Bolen J, Watson SP: A role for Bruton's tyrosine kinase (Btk) in platelet activation by collagen. *Curr Biol* 8:1137, 1998.
1385. Jung SM, Moroi M: Platelet collagen receptor integrin alpha2beta1 activation involves differential participation of ADP-receptor subtypes P2Y1 and P2Y12 but not intracellular calcium change. *Eur J Biochem* 268:3513, 2001.
1386. Wang Z, Leisner TM, Parise LV: Platelet alpha2beta1 integrin activation: Contribution of ligand internalization and the alpha2-cytoplasmic domain. *Blood* 102:1307, 2003.
1387. Bertoni A, Tadokoro S, Eto K, et al: Relationships between Rap1b, affinity modulation of integrin alpha IIbbeta 3, and the actin cytoskeleton. *J Biol Chem* 277:25715, 2002.
1388. Larson MK, Chen H, Kahn ML, et al: Identification of P2Y12-dependent and -independent mechanisms of glycoprotein VI-mediated Rap1 activation in platelets. *Blood* 101:1409, 2003.
1389. Auger JM, Best D, Snell DC, et al: C-Cbl negatively regulates platelet activation by glycoprotein VI. *J Thromb Haemost* 1:2419, 2003.
1390. Locke D, Liu C, Peng X, et al: Fc Rgamma -independent signaling by the platelet collagen receptor glycoprotein VI. *J Biol Chem* 278:15441, 2003.
1391. Inoue O, Suzuki-Inoue K, Dean WL, et al: Integrin alpha2beta1 mediates outside-in regulation of platelet spreading on collagen through activation of Src kinases and PLCgamma2. *J Cell Biol* 160:769, 2003.
1392. Chen H, Kahn ML: Reciprocal signaling by integrin and nonintegrin receptors during collagen activation of platelets. *Mol Cell Biol* 23:4764, 2003.
1393. Galt SW, Lindemann S, Allen L, et al: Outside-in signals delivered by matrix metalloproteinase-1 regulate platelet function. *Circ Res* 90:1093, 2002.
1394. Best D, Senis YA, Jarvis GE, et al: GPVI levels in platelets: Relationship to platelet function at high shear. *Blood* 102:2811, 2003.
1395. Chen H, Locke D, Liu Y, et al: The platelet receptor GPVI mediates both adhesion and signaling responses to collagen in a receptor density-dependent fashion. *J Biol Chem* 277:3011, 2002.
1396. Furihata K, Clemetson KJ, Deguchi H, et al: Variation in human platelet glycoprotein VI content modulates glycoprotein VI-specific prothrombinase activity. *Arterioscler Thromb Vasc Biol* 21:1857, 2001.
1397. Suzuki H, Murasaki K, Kodama K, et al: Intracellular localization of glycoprotein VI in human platelets and its surface expression upon activation. *Br J Haematol* 121:904, 2003.
1398. Nakamura T, Jamieson GA, Okuma M, et al: Platelet adhesion to type I collagen fibrils: Role of GPVI in divalent cation-dependent and -independent adhesion and thromboxane A2 generation. *J Biol Chem* 273:4338, 1998.
1399. Matsuno K, az-Ricart M, Montgomery RR, et al: Inhibition of platelet adhesion to collagen by monoclonal anti-CD36 antibodies. *Br J Haematol* 92:960, 1996.
1400. Daniel JL, Dangelmaier C, Strouse R, et al: Collagen induces normal signal transduction in platelets deficient in CD36 (platelet glycoprotein IV). *Thromb Haemost* 71:353, 1994.
1401. az-Ricart M, Tandon NN, Carretero M, et al: Platelets lacking functional CD36 (glycoprotein IV) show reduced adhesion to collagen in flowing whole blood. *Blood* 82:491, 1993.
1402. Smith JB, Selak MA, Dangelmaier C, et al: Cytosolic calcium as a second messenger for collagen-induced platelet responses. *Biochem J* 288:925, 1992.
1403. Greenwalt DE, Tandon NN: Platelet shape change and Ca2+ mobilization induced by collagen, but not thrombin or ADP, are inhibited by phenylarsine oxide. *Br J Haematol* 88:830, 1994.
1404. Chow TW, Hellums JD, Moake JL, et al: Shear stress-induced von Willebrand factor binding to platelet glycoprotein Ib initiates calcium influx associated with aggregation. *Blood* 80:113, 1992.
1405. Gu M, Xi X, Englund GD, et al: Analysis of the roles of 14-3-3 in the platelet glycoprotein Ib-IX-mediated activation of integrin alpha(IIb)beta(3) using a reconstituted mammalian cell expression model. *J Cell Biol* 147:1085, 1999.
1406. Zaffran Y, Meyer SC, Negrescu E, et al: Signaling across the platelet adhesion receptor glycoprotein Ib-IX induces alpha IIbbeta 3 activation both in platelets and a transfected Chinese hamster ovary cell system. *J Biol Chem* 275:16779, 2000.
1407. Kasirer-Friede A, Cozzi MR, Mazzucato M, et al: Signaling through GP Ib-IX-V activates {alpha}IIb{beta}3 independently of other receptors. *Blood* 103:3403, 2004.
1408. Marshall SJ, Senis YA, Auger JM, et al: GPIb-dependent platelet activation is dependent on Src kinases but not MAP kinase or cGMP-dependent kinase. *Blood* 103:2601, 2004.
1409. Mangin P, Yuan Y, Goncalves I, et al: Signaling role for phospholipase C gamma 2 in platelet glycoprotein Ib alpha calcium flux and cytoskeletal reorganization. Involvement of a pathway distinct from FcR gamma chain and Fc gamma RIIA. *J Biol Chem* 278:32880, 2003.

1410. Li Z, Xi X, Gu M, et al: A stimulatory role for cGMP-dependent protein kinase in platelet activation. *Cell* 112:77, 2003.
1411. Andrews RK, Munday AD, Mitchell CA, et al: Interaction of calmodulin with the cytoplasmic domain of the platelet membrane glycoprotein Ib-IX-V complex. *Blood* 98:681, 2001.
1412. Gu M, Du X: A novel ligand-binding site in the zeta-form 14-3-3 protein recognizing the platelet glycoprotein Ibalpha and distinct from the c-Raf-binding site. *J Biol Chem* 273:33465, 1998.
1413. Du X, Harris SJ, Tetaz TJ, et al: Association of a phospholipase A2 (14-3-3 protein) with the platelet glycoprotein Ib-IX complex. *J Biol Chem* 269:18287, 1994.
1414. Kasirer-Friede A, Ware J, Leng L, et al: Lateral clustering of platelet GP Ib-IX complexes leads to up-regulation of the adhesive function of integrin alpha IIbbeta 3. *J Biol Chem* 277:11949, 2002.
1415. Fox JE, Berndt MC: Cyclic AMP-dependent phosphorylation of glycoprotein Ib inhibits collagen-induced polymerization of actin in platelets. *J Biol Chem* 264:9520, 1989.
1416. Phillips DR, Agin PP: Thrombin-induced alterations in the surface structure of the human platelet plasma membrane. *Ser Haematol* 6:292, 1973.
1417. Ramakrishnan V, Reeves PS, DeGuzman F, et al: Increased thrombin responsiveness in platelets from mice lacking glycoprotein V. *Proc Natl Acad Sci U S A* 96:13336, 1999.
1418. Ni H, Ramakrishnan V, Ruggeri ZM, et al: Increased thrombogenesis and embolus formation in mice lacking glycoprotein V. *Blood* 98:368, 2001.
1419. Rink TJ: Cytosolic calcium in platelet activation. *Experientia* 44:97, 1988.
1420. Kovacs T, Felfoldi F, Papp B, et al: All three splice variants of the human sarco/endoplasmic reticulum Ca2+-ATPase 3 gene are translated to proteins: A study of their co-expression in platelets and lymphoid cells. *Biochem J* 358:559, 2001.
1421. Hassock SR, Zhu MX, Trost C, et al: Expression and role of TRPC proteins in human platelets: Evidence that TRPC6 forms the store-independent calcium entry channel. *Blood* 100:2801, 2002.
1422. Roberts DE, McNicol A, Bose R: Mechanism of collagen activation in human platelets. *J Biol Chem* 279:19421, 2004.
1423. Jones GD, Gear AR: Subsecond calcium dynamics in ADP- and thrombin-stimulated platelets: A continuous-flow approach using indo-1. *Blood* 71:1539, 1988.
1424. Rybak ME, Renzulli LA: Effect of calcium channel blockers on platelet GPIIb-IIIa as a calcium channel in liposomes: Comparison with effects on the intact platelet. *Thromb Haemost* 67:131, 1992.
1425. Dessen A, Tang J, Schmidt H, et al: Crystal structure of human cytosolic phospholipase A2 reveals a novel topology and catalytic mechanism. *Cell* 97:349, 1999.
1426. Khan WA, Blobe G, Halpern A, et al: Selective regulation of protein kinase C isoenzymes by oleic acid in human platelets. *J Biol Chem* 268:5063, 1993.
1427. Scholey JM, Taylor KA, Kendrick-Jones J: Regulation of non-muscle myosin assembly by calmodulin-dependent light chain kinase. *Nature* 287:233, 1980.
1428. Naik MU, Naik UP: Calcium-and integrin-binding protein regulates focal adhesion kinase activity during platelet spreading on immobilized fibrinogen. *Blood* 102:3629, 2003.
1429. Barry WT, Boudignon-Proudhon C, Shock DD, et al: Molecular basis of CIB binding to the integrin alpha IIb cytoplasmic domain. *J Biol Chem* 277:28877, 2002.
1430. Zhang J, Zhang J, Shattil SJ, et al: Phosphoinositide 3-kinase gamma and p85/phosphoinositide 3-kinase in platelets. Relative activation by thrombin receptor or beta-phorbol myristate acetate and roles in promoting the ligand-binding function of alphaIIbbeta3 integrin. *J Biol Chem* 271:6265, 1996.
1431. Rittenhouse SE: Phosphoinositide 3-kinase activation and platelet function. *Blood* 88:4401, 1996.
1432. Hartwig JH, Kung S, Kovacsovics T, et al: D3 phosphoinositides and outside-in integrin signaling by glycoprotein IIb-IIIa mediate platelet actin assembly and filopodial extension induced by phorbol 12-myristate 13-acetate. *J Biol Chem* 271:32986, 1996.
1433. Kucera GL, Rittenhouse SE: Human platelets form 3-phosphorylated phosphoinositides in response to alpha-thrombin, U46619, or GTP gamma S. *J Biol Chem* 265:5345, 1990.
1434. Banfic H, Downes CP, Rittenhouse SE: Biphasic activation of PKBalpha/Akt in platelets. Evidence for stimulation both by phosphatidylinositol 3,4-bisphosphate, produced via a novel pathway, and by phosphatidylinositol 3,4,5-trisphosphate. *J Biol Chem* 273:11630, 1998.
1435. Gibbins JM, Briddon S, Shutes A, et al: The p85 subunit of phosphatidylinositol 3-kinase associates with the Fc receptor gamma-chain and linker for activator of T cells (LAT) in platelets stimulated by collagen and convulxin. *J Biol Chem* 273:34437, 1998.
1436. Watanabe N, Nakajima H, Suzuki H, et al: Functional phenotype of phosphoinositide 3-kinase p85alpha-null platelets characterized by an impaired response to GP VI stimulation. *Blood* 102:541, 2003.
1437. Gratacap MP, Payrastre B, Viala C, et al: Phosphatidylinositol 3,4,5-trisphosphate-dependent stimulation of phospholipase C-gamma2 is an early key event in FcgammaRIIA-mediated activation of human platelets. *J Biol Chem* 273:24314, 1998.
1438. Canobbio I, Stefanini L, Cipolla L, et al: Genetic evidence for a predominant role of PI3K{beta} catalytic activity in platelets. *Blood* 114:2193, 2009.
1439. Hirsch E, Bosco O, Tropel P, et al: Resistance to thromboembolism in PI3Kgamma-deficient mice. *FASEB J* 15:2019, 2001.
1440. Leevers SJ, Vanhaesebroeck B, Waterfield MD: Signalling through phosphoinositide 3-kinases: The lipids take centre stage. *Curr Opin Cell Biol* 11:219, 1999.
1441. Bae YS, Cantley LG, Chen CS, et al: Activation of phospholipase C-gamma by phosphatidylinositol 3,4,5- trisphosphate. *J Biol Chem* 273:4465, 1998.
1442. Salim K, Bottomley MJ, Querfurth E, et al: Distinct specificity in the recognition of phosphoinositides by the pleckstrin homology domains of dynamin and Bruton's tyrosine kinase. *EMBO J* 15:6241, 1996.
1443. Li Z, Wahl MI, Eguinoa A, et al: Phosphatidylinositol 3-kinase-gamma activates Bruton's tyrosine kinase in concert with Src family kinases. *Proc Natl Acad Sci U S A* 94:13820, 1997.
1444. Alessi DR, James SR, Downes CP, et al: Characterization of a 3-phosphoinositide-dependent protein kinase which phosphorylates and activates protein kinase Balpha. *Curr Biol* 7:261, 1997.
1445. Stokoe D, Stephens LR, Copeland T, et al: Dual role of phosphatidylinositol-3,4,5-trisphosphate in the activation of protein kinase B. *Science* 277:567, 1997.
1446. Kroner C, Eybrechts K, Akkerman JW: Dual regulation of platelet protein kinase B. *J Biol Chem* 275:27790, 2000.
1447. Li D, August S, Woulfe DS: GSK3beta is a negative regulator of platelet function and thrombosis. *Blood* 111:3522, 2008.
1448. Stojanovic A, Marjanovic JA, Brovkovych VM, et al: A phosphoinositide 3-kinase-AKT-nitric oxide-cGMP signaling pathway in stimulating platelet secretion and aggregation. *J Biol Chem* 281:16333, 2006.
1449. Zhang W, Colman RW: Thrombin regulates intracellular cyclic AMP concentration in human platelets through phosphorylation/activation of phosphodiesterase 3A. *Blood* 110:1475, 2007.
1450. Woulfe D, Jiang H, Morgans A, et al: Defects in secretion, aggregation, and thrombus formation in platelets from mice lacking Akt2. *J Clin Invest* 113:441, 2004.
1451. Chen J, De S, Damron D, et al: Impaired platelet response to thrombin and collagen in AKT-1 deficient mice. *Blood* 104:1703, 2004.
1452. Woulfe D, Jiang H, Morgans A, et al: Defects in secretion, aggregation, and thrombus formation in platelets from mice lacking Akt2. *J Clin Invest* 113:441, 2004.
1453. Karniguian A, Zahraoui A, Tavitian A: Identification of small GTP-binding rab proteins in human platelets: Thrombin-induced phosphorylation of rab3B, rab6, and rab8 proteins. *Proc Natl Acad Sci U S A* 90:7647, 1993.
1454. Richards-Smith B, Novak EK, Jang EK, et al: Analyses of proteins involved in vesicular trafficking in platelets of mouse models of Hermansky Pudlak syndrome. *Mol Genet Metab* 68:14, 1999.
1455. Wilson SM, Yip R, Swing DA, et al: A mutation in Rab27a causes the vesicle transport defects observed in ashen mice. *Proc Natl Acad Sci U S A* 97:7933, 2000.
1456. Bao X, Faris AE, Jang EK, et al: Molecular cloning, bacterial expression and properties of Rab31 and Rab32. *Eur J Biochem* 269:259, 2002.
1457. Choi W, Karim ZA, Whiteheart SW: Arf6 plays an early role in platelet activation by collagen and convulxin. *Blood* 107:3145, 2006.
1458. Hall A: Rho GTPases and the actin cytoskeleton. *Science* 279:509, 1998.
1459. Bishop AL, Hall A: Rho GTPases and their effector proteins. *Biochem J* 348 Pt 2:241, 2000.
1460. Polakis PG, Snyderman R, Evans T: Characterization of G25K, a GTP-binding protein containing a novel putative nucleotide binding domain. *Biochem Biophys Res Commun* 160:25, 1989.
1461. Polakis PG, Weber RF, Nevins B, et al: Identification of the ral and rac1 gene products, low molecular mass GTP-binding proteins from human platelets. *J Biol Chem* 264:16383, 1989.
1462. Schoenwaelder SM, Hughan SC, Boniface K, et al: RhoA sustains integrin alpha IIbbeta 3 adhesion contacts under high shear. *J Biol Chem* 277:14738, 2002.
1463. Soulet C, Gendreau S, Missy K, et al: Characterisation of Rac activation in thrombin- and collagen-stimulated human blood platelets. *FEBS Lett* 507:253, 2001.
1464. Vidal C, Geny B, Melle J, et al: Cdc42/Rac1-dependent activation of the p21-activated kinase (PAK) regulates human platelet lamellipodia spreading: Implication of the cortical-actin binding protein cortactin. *Blood* 100:4462, 2002.
1465. Soulet C, Hechler B, Gratacap MP, et al: A differential role of the platelet ADP receptors P2Y1 and P2Y12 in Rac activation. *J Thromb Haemost* 3:2296, 2005.
1466. Moers A, Wettschureck N, Offermanns S: G13-mediated signaling as a potential target for antiplatelet drugs. *Drug News Perspect* 17:493, 2004.
1467. Azim AC, Barkalow K, Chou J, et al: Activation of the small GTPases, rac and cdc42, after ligation of the platelet PAR-1 receptor. *Blood* 95:959, 2000.
1468. Shock DD, He K, Wencel-Drake JD, et al: Ras activation in platelets after stimulation of the thrombin receptor, thromboxane A2 receptor or protein kinase C. *Biochem J* 321(Pt 2):525, 1997.
1469. Omerovic J, Hammond DE, Clague MJ, et al: Ras isoform abundance and signalling in human cancer cell lines. *Oncogene* 27:2754, 2008.
1470. Omerovic J, Laude AJ, Prior IA: Ras proteins: Paradigms for compartmentalised and isoform-specific signalling. *Cell Mol Life Sci* 64:2575, 2007.
1471. Tulasne D, Bori T, Watson SP: Regulation of RAS in human platelets. Evidence that activation of RAS is not sufficient to lead to ERK1–2 phosphorylation. *Eur J Biochem* 269:1511, 2002.
1472. Bauer M, Retzer M, Wilde JI, et al: Dichotomous regulation of myosin phosphorylation and shape change by Rho-kinase and calcium in intact human platelets. *Blood* 94:1665, 1999.
1473. Nemoto Y, Namba T, Teru-uchi T, et al: A rho gene product in human blood platelets. I. Identification of the platelet substrate for botulinum C3 ADP-ribosyltransferase as rhoA protein. *J Biol Chem* 267:20916, 1992.

1474. Morii N, Teru-uchi T, Tominaga T, et al: A rho gene product in human blood platelets. II. Effects of the ADP-ribosylation by botulinum C3 ADP-ribosyltransferase on platelet aggregation. *J Biol Chem* 267:20921, 1992.
1475. Leng L, Kashiwagi H, Ren XD, et al: RhoA and the function of platelet integrin alphaIIbbeta3. *Blood* 91:4206, 1998.
1476. Klages B, Brandt U, Simon MI, et al: Activation of G12/G13 results in shape change and Rho/Rho-kinase-mediated myosin light chain phosphorylation in mouse platelets. *J Cell Biol* 144:745, 1999.
1477. Schwartz M: Rho signalling at a glance. *J Cell Sci* 117:5457, 2004.
1478. McCarty OJ, Larson MK, Auger JM, et al: Rac1 is essential for platelet lamellipodia formation and aggregate stability under flow. *J Biol Chem* 280:39474, 2005.
1479. Akbar H, Kim J, Funk K, et al: Genetic and pharmacologic evidence that Rac1 GTPase is involved in regulation of platelet secretion and aggregation. *J Thromb Haemost* 5:1747, 2007.
1480. Pleines I, Elvers M, Strehl A, et al: Rac1 is essential for phospholipase C-gamma2 activation in platelets. *Pflugers Arch* 457:1173, 2009.
1481. Falet H, Hoffmeister KM, Neujahr R, et al: Normal Arp2/3 complex activation in platelets lacking WASP. *Blood* 100:2113, 2002.
1482. Pula G, Poole AW: Critical roles for the actin cytoskeleton and cdc42 in regulating platelet integrin alpha2beta1. *Platelets* 19:199, 2008.
1483. Kooistra MR, Dube N, Bos JL: Rap1: A key regulator in cell-cell junction formation. *J Cell Sci* 120:17, 2007.
1484. Franke B, Akkerman JW, Bos JL: Rapid Ca2+-mediated activation of Rap1 in human platelets. *EMBO J* 16:252, 1997.
1485. Greco F, Sinigaglia F, Balduini C, et al: Activation of the small GTPase Rap2B in agonist-stimulated human platelets. *J Thromb Haemost* 2:2223, 2004.
1486. Chrzanowska-Wodnicka M, Smyth SS, Schoenwaelder SM, et al: Rap1b is required for normal platelet function and hemostasis in mice. *J Clin Invest* 115:680, 2005.
1487. Eto K, Murphy R, Kerrigan SW, et al: Megakaryocytes derived from embryonic stem cells implicate CalDAG-GEFI in integrin signaling. *Proc Natl Acad Sci U S A* 99:12819, 2002.
1488. Crittenden JR, Bergmeier W, Zhang Y, et al: CalDAG-GEFI integrates signaling for platelet aggregation and thrombus formation. *Nat Med* 10:982, 2004.
1489. Cifuni SM, Wagner DD, Bergmeier W: CalDAG-GEFI and protein kinase C represent alternative pathways leading to activation of integrin alphaIIbbeta3 in platelets. *Blood* 112:1696, 2008.
1490. Watanabe N, Bodin L, Pandey M, et al: Mechanisms and consequences of agonist-induced talin recruitment to platelet integrin alphaIIbbeta3. *J Cell Biol* 181:1211, 2008.
1491. Cullen PJ, Lockyer PJ: Integration of calcium and Ras signalling. *Nat Rev Mol Cell Biol* 3:339, 2002.
1492. Bodemann BO, White MA: Ral GTPases and cancer: Linchpin support of the tumorigenic platform. *Nat Rev Cancer* 8:133, 2008.
1493. Mark BL, Jilkina O, Bhullar RP: Association of Ral GTP-binding protein with human platelet dense granules. *Biochem Biophys Res Commun* 225:40, 1996.
1494. Wolthuis RM, Franke B, van Triest M, et al: Activation of the small GTPase Ral in platelets. *Mol Cell Biol* 18:2486, 1998.
1495. Kawato M, Shirakawa R, Kondo H, et al: Regulation of platelet dense granule secretion by the Ral GTPase-exocyst pathway. *J Biol Chem* 283:166, 2008.
1496. Zerial M, McBride H: Rab proteins as membrane organizers. *Nat Rev Mol Cell Biol* 2:107, 2001.
1497. Kuchay SM, Chishti AH: Calpain-mediated regulation of platelet signaling pathways. *Curr Opin Hematol* 14:249, 2007.
1498. Lai KC, Flaumenhaft R: SNARE protein degradation upon platelet activation: Calpain cleaves SNAP-23. *J Cell Physiol* 194:206, 2003.
1499. Kuchay SM, Kim N, Grunz EA, et al: Double knockouts reveal that protein tyrosine phosphatase 1B is a physiological target of calpain-1 in platelets. *Mol Cell Biol* 27:6038, 2007.
1500. Vinogradova O, Vaynberg J, Kong X, et al: Membrane-mediated structural transitions at the cytoplasmic face during integrin activation. *Proc Natl Acad Sci U S A* 101:4094, 2004.
1501. Martel V, Racaud-Sultan C, Dupe S, et al: Conformation, localization, and integrin binding of talin depend on its interaction with phosphoinositides. *J Biol Chem* 276:21217, 2001.
1502. Di Paolo G, Pellegrini L, Letinic K, et al: Recruitment and regulation of phosphatidylinositol phosphate kinase type 1 gamma by the FERM domain of talin. *Nature* 420:85, 2002.
1503. Ling K, Doughman RL, Firestone AJ, et al: Type I gamma phosphatidylinositol phosphate kinase targets and regulates focal adhesions. *Nature* 420:89, 2002.
1504. Calderwood DA, Yan B, de Pereda JM, et al: The phosphotyrosine binding-like domain of talin activates integrins. *J Biol Chem* 277:21749, 2002.
1505. Garcia-Alvarez B, de Pereda JM, Calderwood DA, et al: Structural determinants of integrin recognition by talin. *Mol Cell* 11:49, 2003.
1506. Wegener KL, Campbell ID: Transmembrane and cytoplasmic domains in integrin activation and protein-protein interactions [review]. *Mol Membr Biol* 25:376, 2008.
1507. Ling K, Doughman RL, Iyer VV, et al: Tyrosine phosphorylation of type Igamma phosphatidylinositol phosphate kinase by Src regulates an integrin-talin switch. *J Cell Biol* 163:1339, 2003.
1508. Xing B, Jedsadayanmata A, Lam SC: Localization of an integrin binding site to the C terminus of talin. *J Biol Chem* 276:44373, 2001.
1509. Montanez E, Ussar S, Schifferer M, et al: Kindlin-2 controls bidirectional signaling of integrins. *Genes Dev* 22:1325, 2008.
1510. Ma YQ, Qin J, Wu C, et al: Kindlin-2 (Mig-2): A co-activator of beta3 integrins. *J Cell Biol* 181:439, 2008.
1511. Moser M, Nieswandt B, Ussar S, et al: Kindlin-3 is essential for integrin activation and platelet aggregation. *Nat Med* 14:325, 2008.
1512. Kuijpers TW, van de Vijver E, Weterman MA, et al: LAD-1/variant syndrome is caused by mutations in FERMT3. *Blood* 113:3740, 2008.
1513. Mory A, Feigelson SW, Yarali N, et al: Kindlin-3: A new gene involved in the pathogenesis of LAD-III. *Blood* 112:2591, 2008.
1514. Svensson L, Howarth K, McDowall A, et al: Leukocyte adhesion deficiency-III is caused by mutations in KINDLIN3 affecting integrin activation. *Nat Med* 15:306, 2009.
1515. Malinin NL, Zhang L, Choi J, et al: A point mutation in KINDLIN3 ablates activation of three integrin subfamilies in humans. *Nat Med* 15:313, 2009.
1516. Harburger DS, Bouaouina M, Calderwood DA: Kindlin-1 and -2 directly bind the C-terminal region of beta integrin cytoplasmic tails and exert integrin-specific activation effects. *J Biol Chem* 284:11485, 2009.
1517. Li R, Babu CR, Lear JD, et al: Oligomerization of the integrin alphaIIbbeta3: Roles of the transmembrane and cytoplasmic domains. *Proc Natl Acad Sci U S A* 98:12462, 2001.
1518. Arias-Salgado EG, Lizano S, Sarkar S, et al: Src kinase activation by direct interaction with the integrin beta cytoplasmic domain. *Proc Natl Acad Sci U S A* 100:13298, 2003.
1519. Obergfell A, Eto K, Mocsai A, et al: Coordinate interactions of Csk, Src, and Syk kinases with [alpha]IIb[beta]3 initiate integrin signaling to the cytoskeleton. *J Cell Biol* 157:265, 2002.
1520. Newman DK: The Y's that bind: Negative regulators of Src family kinase activity in platelets. *J Thromb Haemost* 7:195, 2009.
1521. Woodside DG, Obergfell A, Leng L, et al: Activation of Syk protein tyrosine kinase through interaction with integrin beta cytoplasmic domains. *Curr Biol* 11:1799, 2001.
1522. Woodside DG, Obergfell A, Talapatra A, et al: The N-terminal SH2 domains of Syk and ZAP-70 mediate phosphotyrosine-independent binding to integrin beta cytoplasmic domains. *J Biol Chem* 277:39401, 2002.
1523. De Virgilio M, Kiosses WB, Shattil SJ: Proximal, selective, and dynamic interactions between integrin {alpha}IIb{beta}3 and protein tyrosine kinases in living cells. *J Cell Biol* 165:305, 2004.
1524. Patil S, Newman DK, Newman PJ. PECAM-1 serves as an inhibitory receptor that modulates platelet responses to collagen [abstract]. *Blood* 96:446a, 2009.
1525. Falati S, Patil S, Gross PL, et al: Platelet PECAM-1 inhibits thrombus formation in vivo. *Blood* 107:535, 2006.
1526. Newman PJ, Newman DK: Signal transduction pathways mediated by PECAM-1: New roles for an old molecule in platelet and vascular cell biology. *Arterioscler Thromb Vasc Biol* 23:953, 2003.
1527. Wong C, Liu Y, Yip J, et al: CEACAM1 negatively regulates platelet-collagen interactions and thrombus growth *in vitro* and *in vivo*. *Blood* 113:1818, 2009.
1528. Newland SA, Macaulay IC, Floto AR, et al: The novel inhibitory receptor G6B is expressed on the surface of platelets and attenuates platelet function *in vitro*. *Blood* 109:4806, 2007.
1529. Mori J, Pearce AC, Spalton JC, et al: G6b-B inhibits constitutive and agonist-induced signaling by glycoprotein VI and CLEC-2. *J Biol Chem* 283:35419, 2008.
1530. Kumar G, Wang S, Gupta S, et al: The membrane immunoglobulin receptor utilizes a Shc/Grb2/hSOS complex for activation of the mitogen-activated protein kinase cascade in a B-cell line. *Biochem J* 307:215, 1995.
1531. Miranti CK, Leng L, Maschberger P, et al: Identification of a novel integrin signaling pathway involving the kinase Syk and the guanine nucleotide exchange factor Vav1. *Curr Biol* 8:1289, 1998.
1532. Majerus PW: Arachidonate metabolism in vascular disorders. *J Clin Invest* 72:1521, 1983.
1533. Moncada S, Whittle BJ: Biological actions of prostacyclin and its pharmacological use in platelet studies. *Adv Exp Med Biol* 192:337, 1985.
1534. Marcus AJ: The role of lipids in platelet function: With particular reference to the arachidonic acid pathway. *J Lipid Res* 19:793, 1978.
1535. Katsuyama M, Sugimoto Y, Namba T, et al: Cloning and expression of a cDNA for the human prostacyclin receptor. *FEBS Lett* 344:74, 1994.
1536. Kunapuli SP, Fen MG, Bastepe M, et al: Cloning and expression of a prostaglandin E receptor EP3 subtype from human erythroleukaemia cells. *Biochem J* 298(Pt 2):263, 1994.
1537. Hung SH, Zhang W, Pixley RA, et al: New insights from the structure-function analysis of the catalytic region of human platelet phosphodiesterase 3A: A role for the unique 44-amino acid insert. *J Biol Chem* 281:29236, 2006.
1538. Feijge MA, Ansink K, Vanschoonbeek K, et al: Control of platelet activation by cyclic AMP turnover and cyclic nucleotide phosphodiesterase type-3. *Biochem Pharmacol* 67:1559, 2004.
1539. Sun B, Li H, Shakur Y, et al: Role of phosphodiesterase type 3A and 3B in regulating platelet and cardiac function using subtype-selective knockout mice. *Cell Signal* 19:1765, 2007.
1540. Chapman TM, Goa KL: Cilostazol: A review of its use in intermittent claudication. *Am J Cardiovasc Drugs* 3:117, 2003.

1541. Manganello JM, Huang JS, Kozasa T, et al: Protein kinase A-mediated phosphorylation of the Galpha13 switch I region alters the Galphabetagamma13-G protein-coupled receptor complex and inhibits Rho activation. *J Biol Chem* 278:124, 2003.
1542. Bodnar RJ, Xi X, Li Z, et al: Regulation of glycoprotein Ib-IX-von Willebrand factor interaction by cAMP-dependent protein kinase-mediated phosphorylation at Ser 166 of glycoprotein Ib(beta). *J Biol Chem* 277:47080, 2002.
1543. Cavallini L, Coassin M, Borean A, et al: Prostacyclin and sodium nitroprusside inhibit the activity of the platelet inositol 1,4,5-trisphosphate receptor and promote its phosphorylation. *J Biol Chem* 271:5545, 1996.
1544. Nishimura T, Yamamoto T, Komuro Y, et al: Antiplatelet functions of a stable prostacyclin analog, SM-10906 are exerted by its inhibitory effect on inositol 1,4,5-trisphosphate production and cytosolic Ca2++ increase in rat platelets stimulated by thrombin. *Thromb Res* 79:307, 1995.
1545. Cook SJ, McCormick F: Inhibition by cAMP of Ras-dependent activation of Raf. *Science* 262:1069, 1993.
1546. Dumaz N, Marais R: Protein kinase A blocks Raf-1 activity by stimulating 14-3-3 binding and blocking Raf-1 interaction with Ras. *J Biol Chem* 278:29819, 2003.
1547. Fischer TH, Collins JH, Gatling MN, et al: The localization of the cAMP-dependent protein kinase phosphorylation site in the platelet rat protein, rap 1B. *FEBS Lett* 2832:173, 1991.
1548. Siess W, Grunberg B: Phosphorylation of rap1B by protein kinase A is not involved in platelet inhibition by cyclic AMP. *Cell Signal* 5:209, 1993.
1549. Lou L, Urbani J, Ribeiro-Neto F, et al: CAMP inhibition of Akt is mediated by activated and phosphorylated Rap1b. *J Biol Chem* 277:32799, 2002.
1550. Fabre JE, Nguyen M, Athirakul K, et al: Activation of the murine EP3 receptor for PGE2 inhibits cAMP production and promotes platelet aggregation. *J Clin Invest* 107:603, 2001.
1551. Shio H, Ramwell P: Effect of prostaglandin E2 and aspirin on the secondary aggregation of human platelets. *Nat New Biol* 236:45, 1972.
1552. Gross S, Tilly P, Hentsch D, et al: Vascular wall-produced prostaglandin E2 exacerbates arterial thrombosis and atherothrombosis through platelet EP3 receptors. *J Exp Med* 204:311, 2007.
1553. Luscher TF, Diederich D, Siebenmann R, et al: Difference between endothelium-dependent relaxation in arterial and in venous coronary bypass grafts. *N Engl J Med* 319:462, 1988.
1554. Goretski J, Hollocher TC: Trapping of nitric oxide produced during denitrification by extracellular hemoglobin. *J Biol Chem* 263:2316, 1988.
1555. Loscalzo J, Welch G: Nitric oxide and its role in the cardiovascular system. *Prog Cardiovasc Dis* 38:87, 1995.
1556. Mellion BT, Ignarro LJ, Ohlstein EH, et al: Evidence for the inhibitory role of guanosine 3′, 5′-monophosphate in ADP-induced human platelet aggregation in the presence of nitric oxide and related vasodilators. *Blood* 57:946, 1981.
1557. Radomski MW, Palmer RM, Moncada S: Modulation of platelet aggregation by an L-arginine-nitric oxide pathway. *Trends Pharmacol Sci* 12:87, 1991.
1558. Wang GR, Zhu Y, Halushka PV, et al: Mechanism of platelet inhibition by nitric oxide: *In vivo* phosphorylation of thromboxane receptor by cyclic GMP-dependent protein kinase. *Proc Natl Acad Sci U S A* 95:4888, 1998.
1559. Massberg S, Sausbier M, Klatt P, et al: Increased adhesion and aggregation of platelets lacking cyclic guanosine 3′,5′-monophosphate kinase I. *J Exp Med* 189:1255, 1999.
1560. Aszodi A, Pfeifer A, Ahmad M, et al: The vasodilator-stimulated phosphoprotein (VASP) is involved in cGMP- and cAMP-mediated inhibition of agonist-induced platelet aggregation, but is dispensable for smooth muscle function. *EMBO J* 18:37, 1999.
1561. Butt E, Abel K, Krieger M, et al: CAMP- and cGMP-dependent protein kinase phosphorylation sites of the focal adhesion vasodilator-stimulated phosphoprotein (VASP) *in vitro* and in intact human platelets. *J Biol Chem* 269:14509, 1994.
1562. Hauser W, Knobeloch KP, Eigenthaler M, et al: Megakaryocyte hyperplasia and enhanced agonist-induced platelet activation in vasodilator-stimulated phosphoprotein knockout mice. *Proc Natl Acad Sci U S A* 96:8120, 1999.
1563. Massberg S, Gruner S, Konrad I, et al: Enhanced *in vivo* platelet adhesion in vasodilator-stimulated phosphoprotein (VASP)-deficient mice. *Blood* 103:136, 2004.
1564. Maurice DH, Haslam RJ: Molecular basis of the synergistic inhibition of platelet function by nitrovasodilators and activators of adenylate cyclase: Inhibition of cyclic AMP breakdown by cyclic GMP. *Mol Pharmacol* 37:671, 1990.
1565. Kaczmarek E, Koziak K, Sevigny J, et al: Identification and characterization of CD39/vascular ATP diphosphohydrolase. *J Biol Chem* 271:33116, 1996.
1566. Atkinson B, Dwyer K, Enjyoji K, et al: Ecto-nucleotidases of the CD39/NTPDase family modulate platelet activation and thrombus formation: Potential as therapeutic targets. *Blood Cells Mol Dis* 36:217, 2006.
1567. Le F, Townsend-Nicholson A, Baker E, et al: Characterization and chromosomal localization of the human A2a adenosine receptor gene: ADORA2A. *Biochem Biophys Res Commun* 223:461, 1996.
1568. Pulte D, Olson KE, Broekman MJ, et al: CD39 activity correlates with stage and inhibits platelet reactivity in chronic lymphocytic leukemia. *J Transl Med* 5:23, 2007.
1569. White JG: Platelet ultrastructure, in *Hemostasis and Thrombosis*, 3rd ed, edited by AL Bloom, CD Forbes, PT Duncan, EGD Tuddenham, p 49. Churchill Livingstone, Edinburgh, 1994.
1570. Li R, Babu CR, Valentine K, et al: Characterization of the monomeric form of the transmembrane and cytoplasmic domains of the integrin beta 3 subunit by NMR spectroscopy. *Biochemistry* 41:15618, 2002.
1571. Smyth SS, Woulfe DS, Weitz JI, et al: G-protein-coupled receptors as signaling targets for antiplatelet therapy. *Arterioscler Thromb Vasc Biol* 29:449, 2009.
1572. Andrews RK, Gardiner EE, Shen Y, et al: Glycoprotein Ib-IX-V. *Int J Biochem Cell Biol* 35:1170, 2003.
1573. Coller BS: Disorders of platelets, in *Disorders of Hemostasis*, edited by OD Ratnoff, CD Forbes, p 73. Grune & Stratton, Orlando, FL, 1984.
1574. Holmsen H, Weiss HJ: Secretable storage pools in platelets. *Annu Rev Med* 30:119, 1979.
1575. Pollard TD: Actin. *Curr Opin Cell Biol* 2:33, 1990.
1576. Vandekerckhove J: Actin-binding proteins. *Curr Opin Cell Biol* 2:41, 1990.
1577. Weeds AG, Gooch J, Pope B, et al: Preparation and characterization of pig plasma and platelet gelsolins. *Eur J Biochem* 161:69, 1986.
1578. Smillie LB: Structure and function of tropomyosins from muscle and non-muscle. *Trends Biochem Sci* 4:151, 1981.
1579. Vandekerckhove J: Structural principles of actin-binding proteins. *Curr Opin Cell Biol* 1:15, 1989.
1580. Lind SE, Stossel TP: The microfilament network of the platelet. *Prog Hemost Thromb* 6:63, 1982.
1581. Chen M, Stracher A: In situ phosphorylation of platelet actin-binding protein by cAMP-dependent protein kinase stabilizes it against proteolysis by calpain. *J Biol Chem* 264:14282, 1989.
1582. Beckerle MC, Miller DE, Bertagnolli ME, et al: Activation-dependent redistribution of the adhesion plaque protein, talin, in intact human platelets. *J Cell Biol* 109:3333, 1989.
1583. O'Halloran T, Beckerle MC, Burridge K: Identification of talin as a major cytoplasmic protein implicated in platelet activation. *Nature* 317:449, 1985.
1584. Koteliansky VE, Gneushev GN, Glukhova MA, et al: Identification and isolation of vinculin from platelets. *FEBS Lett* 165:26, 1984.
1585. Langer B, Gonnella PA, Nachmias VT: α-actinin and vinculin in normal and thrombasthenic platelets. *Blood* 63:606, 1984.
1586. Lucas RC, Rosenberg S, Shafiq S, et al: The isolation and characterization of a cytoskeleton and a contractile apparatus from platelets, in *Protides of Biological Fluids*, edited by H Peeters, p 465. Pergamon Press, New York, 1975.
1587. Wang L-L, Bryan J: Isolation of calcium-dependent platelet proteins that interact with actin. *Cell* 25:637, 1981.
1588. Hathaway DR, Adelstein RS: Human platelet myosin light chain kinase requires the calcium binding protein calmodulin for activity. *Proc Natl Acad Sci U S A* 76:1653, 1979.
1589. Wolff DJ, Brostrom CO: Properties and functions of the calcium-dependent regulator protein. *Adv Cyclic Nucleotide Res* 11:27, 1979.
1590. Daniel JL: Platelet contractile proteins, in *Hemostasis and Thrombosis: Basic Principles and Clinical Practice*, 3rd ed, edited by RW Colman, J Hirsh, VJ Marder, EW Salzman, p 557. Philadelphia, JB Lippincott, Philadelphia, 1993.

CHAPTER 115

MOLECULAR BIOLOGY AND BIOCHEMISTRY OF THE COAGULATION FACTORS AND PATHWAYS OF HEMOSTASIS

Dougald M. Monroe III, Maureane Hoffman, and Harold R. Roberts

SUMMARY

Blood coagulation is a very delicately balanced system. When it functions as it should, the blood is maintained in a fluid state in the vasculature, yet rapidly clots to seal an injury. When hemostatic functions fail, hemorrhage or thromboembolic phenomena result. This chapter addresses molecular and biochemical features of the proteins of the coagulation system, and how they interact with cells and with one another to provide hemostasis in the living organism. We have grouped the coagulation factors as (1) the vitamin-K-dependent zymogens (prothrombin, and factors VII, IX, X, and protein C); (2) the soluble cofactors (protein S, factor V, factor VIII, and von Willebrand factor); (3) factor XI and the other "contact" factors; (4) cell-associated cofactors (tissue factor and thrombomodulin); (5) fibrinogen; (6) factor XIII and TAFI; and (7) the plasma coagulation protease inhibitors. Table 115–1 shows the major features of the coagulation factors addressed in this chapter. A model of the coagulation pathway is presented that is based on current understanding of cell-cell and cell-protein interactions that regulate hemostasis. This scheme emphasizes the importance of cellular localization and plasma protease inhibitors in confining the coagulation reactions to a specific site of vascular injury.

Acronyms and abbreviations that appear in this chapter include: ADAMTS, a disintegrin and metalloproteinase with thrombospondin motifs; APC, activated protein C; aPTT, activated partial thromboplastin time; AT, antithrombin; BiP, immunoglobulin-binding protein; CYP2C9, cytochrome P450 complex that metabolizes warfarin; C/EB, CCAAT/enhancer binding protein; EGF, epidermal growth factor; EPCR, endothelial cell protein C receptor; ERGIC, endoplasmic reticulum-Golgi intermediate compartment; GLA, γ-carboxyglutamic acid; HC II, heparin cofactor II; HK, high-molecular-weight kininogen; HNF, hepatic nuclear factor; IL, interleukin; LMAN1, mannose-binding lectin-1 gene product; MCFD2, multiple coagulation deficiency protein 2; MZF, myeloid-enriched transcription factor; NF-κB, nuclear factor kappa-light-chain-enhancer of activated B cells; PAR, proteolytically activated receptor; PK, prekallikrein; PS, phosphatidylserine; RFLP, restriction fragment length polymorphism; SCR, short consensus repeat; Serpin, serine protease inhibitor; TAFI, thrombin-activatable fibrinolytic inhibitor; TF, tissue factor; TFPI, tissue factor pathway inhibitor; TM, thrombomodulin; VKORC1, vitamin K epoxide reductase complex 1; VWF, von Willebrand factor; ZPI, protein Z-dependent protease inhibitor.

MOLECULAR BIOLOGY, BIOCHEMISTRY, AND LIFE SPAN OF THE COAGULATION FACTORS

VITAMIN K-DEPENDENT ZYMOGENS (PROTHROMBIN AND FACTORS VII, IX, X, AND PROTEIN C)

Common Structural and Functional Features

The vitamin K-dependent coagulation zymogens are precursors of serine proteases that must be proteolytically activated to express their enzymatic activity. They all share a similar protein domain structure (Fig. 115–1). Each of the mature vitamin K-dependent coagulation zymogen proteins has an amino-terminal γ-carboxy glutamic acid (GLA) domain with 9 to 12 GLA residues. This is followed by a hydrophobic region. All except prothrombin have two epidermal growth factor (EGF)-like domains, and all have a serine protease domain in their carboxy-terminal region. Prothrombin has two kringle domains instead of EGF-like domains. Specific functions are associated, at least in part, with specific domains.

In addition to the functional modules found in the mature protein, each vitamin K-dependent factor is synthesized with an amino-terminal signal sequence directing it to the endoplasmic reticulum, followed by a 19- to 25-amino-acid propeptide that is recognized by the γ-glutamyl carboxylase that catalyzes carboxylation of glutamic acid residues in the amino-terminal portion of the molecule. Following translocation into the endoplasmic reticulum, the signal sequence is removed by a microsomal signal peptidase. The propeptide is cleaved following carboxylation before the mature protein is secreted.

Not only are the proteins homologous, but their gene structures also are highly similar. The coding regions of the vitamin K-dependent factors are quite similar in size. However, the intron lengths vary substantially and account for the differences in the overall size of the genes (20 kb for prothrombin, 13 kb for factor VII, 33 kb for factor IX, 25 kb for factor X, and 10 kb for protein C). Although the complementary DNA (cDNA) of all of the vitamin K-dependent factors has been sequenced, the noncoding regions have only been characterized to varying degrees of detail. The vitamin K-dependent coagulation zymogens are synthesized primarily by the liver and thus they all have regulatory elements that direct liver-specific expression. The regulatory elements vary however among the proteins.

In factors VII, IX, and X and proteins C and Z, the introns are located in identical positions in the genes,[1–3] suggesting that these enzymes evolved by duplication of a common ancestral precursor gene. The regions of the molecules that constitute "functional" domains tend to be encoded in their entirety by a single exon, that is, the signal peptide by one exon, the propeptide and GLA region by the next exon, and so forth. This "modular" design suggests how "exon shuffling" could splice together intact functional units of different proteins to give rise to new proteins with novel properties.

The GLA domain that is characteristic of the vitamin K-dependent factors mediates interaction of the protein with lipid membranes. The GLA domain is named for the modified amino acids found in the first 42 residues of the mature protein. GLA residues are produced by the posttranslational modification of glutamic acid residues carried out by a specific γ-glutamyl carboxylase[4] in the endoplasmic reticulum (Fig. 115–2). This carboxylase requires oxygen, carbon dioxide, and the reduced form of vitamin K for its action. For each glutamyl residue that is carboxylated, one molecule of reduced vitamin K is converted to the epoxide form. The propeptide sequence is required for γ-carboxylation to take place, and is highly conserved among the vitamin K-dependent factors. Amino acids at positions −18, −17, −16, −15, and −10 are critical to recognition by the carboxylase.[5,6] Mutations of the carboxylase can lead to low levels of all of the GLA-containing factors.[7]

TABLE 115–1 Characteristics of Coagulation Proteins

	Protein	Concentration	Plasma Half-Life (hours)	Chromosome
ZYMOGENS				
GLA[a]	Prothrombin (factor II)	100–150 mcg/mL	60–70	11p11-q12
	Factor VII	0.5 mcg/mL	3–6	13q34
	Factor IX	4–5 mcg/mL	18–24	Xq27.1-q27.2
	Factor X	8–10 mcg/mL	30–40	13q34
	Protein C	4–5 mcg/mL	6	2q13-q14
non-GLA	Factor XI	5 mcg/mL	52	4q32-q35
	Factor XII	30 mcg/mL	60 hours	5q33
	Prekallikrein	50 mcg/mL	35	4q35
	Factor XIII-A chain[b,c]	10 mcg/mL	240	6p24-p25
	Factor XIII-B chain[b]	22 mcg/mL		1q31-q32.1
	Thrombin activatable fibrinolysis inhibitor	6 mcg/mL		13q14
COFACTORS				
Soluble	Factor V[c]	5–10 mcg/mL	12	1q21-q25
	Factor VIII	0.1–0.2 mcg/mL	8–12	Xq28
	VWF	10 mcg/mL	12	12p13.2
	Protein S	25 mcg/mL[d]	42	3p11.1-q11.2
	Protein Z	2–3 mcg/mL	60	13q34
	High-molecular-weight kininogen	70 mcg/mL	150	3q26
Cellular	Tissue factor	–	–	1p21-p22
	thrombomodulin	–	–	20p12-cen
STRUCTURAL PROTEIN	Fibrinogen	2000–4000 mcg/mL	72–120	
	$A\alpha$ chain			4q23-q32
	$B\beta$ chain			4q23-q32
	γ Chain			4q23-q32
INHIBITORS	Antithrombin	150–400 mcg/mL	72	1q23-q25
	Tissue factor pathway inhibitor	0.1 mcg/mL	8	2q31-q32.1
	Protein Z-dependent protease inhibitor	1–1.6 mcg/mL	[e]	14q32

[a] γ-Carboxyglutamic acid.

[b] All of the factor XIII-A chain is in complex with factor XIII-B chain; only half of factor XIII-B chain is in complex with factor XIII-A chain, the rest is free in plasma.

[c] Platelets carry significant amounts of factor XIIIa (roughly half of the total factor XIII activity) and factor V (20% of circulating factor V).

[d] Approximately 60% of the protein S is in complex with C4b binding protein.

[e] Protein Z-dependent protease inhibitor circulates in complex with protein Z.

Although the γ-glutamyl carboxylase is directly responsible for modification of the vitamin K-dependent factors, a separate enzyme complex, the vitamin K epoxide reductase, is required to convert the epoxide form of vitamin K back to the reduced form. Warfarin inhibits the activity of the vitamin K epoxide reductase and prevents recycling of vitamin K back to the reduced form. The effect of warfarin is, therefore, to inhibit γ-glutamyl carboxylation, resulting in the presence of a heterogeneous population of undercarboxylated forms of the GLA-containing factors in the circulation. These undercarboxylated forms have reduced activity. Because warfarin blocks the reductase (rather than blocking the carboxylase) and prevents recycling of vitamin K, the effects of warfarin poisoning can be (temporarily) reversed by administration of vitamin K. The gene for the epoxide reductase has been sequenced.[8] Mutations in this gene have been linked both to warfarin resistance and to a combined deficiency of the vitamin K-dependent clotting factors (type 2).[9,10]

Genetic variants in the vitamin K epoxide reductase complex 1 (VKORC1), as well as in the cytochrome P450 complex that metabolizes warfarin (CYP2C9), are associated with the dose of warfarin required to achieve therapeutic anticoagulation.[11] Interestingly, polymorphisms in the γ-glutamyl carboxylase do not seem to contribute to individual differences in warfarin sensitivity.[12] There are large variations in the effective warfarin dose among patients, and significant clinical consequences when the degree of anticoagulation is either insufficient or excessive. Thus, individualization of warfarin dosing appears to be one of the most promising clinical applications of pharmacogenetics.

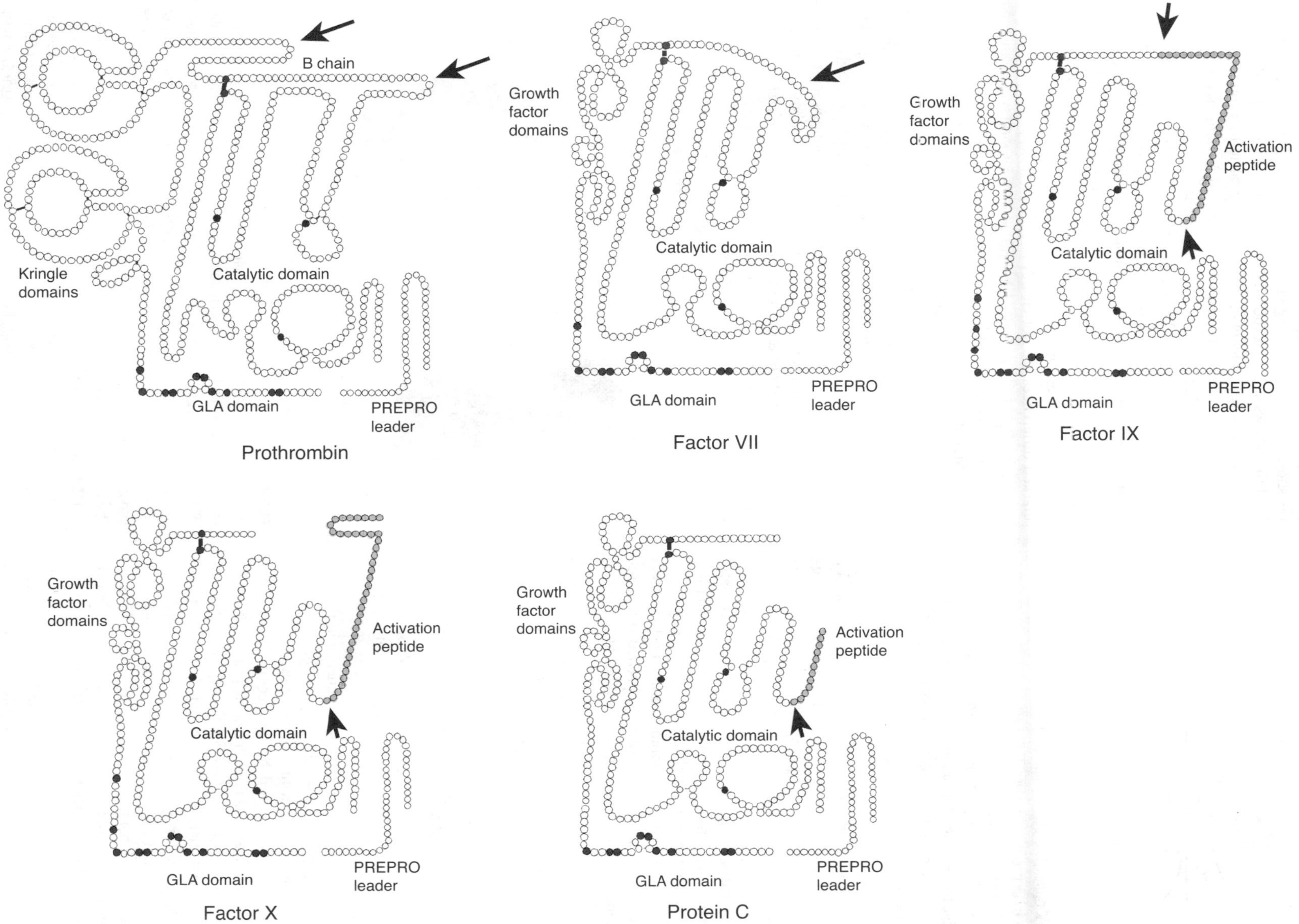

FIGURE 115–1. Comparison of the GLA containing zymogens. The figure shows basic structural elements of the GLA-containing zymogens. Each *circle* is an amino acid. The prepro leader sequence contains the signal peptide, as well as elements that direct carboxylation of glutamyl residues. Cleavage of the leader sequence is indicated by showing a slight separation from the mature protein. All have a GLA domain with the GLA residues indicated by filled *blue circles*. Prothrombin has a finger loop followed by two Kringle domains. Factors VII, IX, X, and protein C have epidermal growth factor-like domains. Prothrombin, factor VII, and factor IX circulate as single-chain molecules. Factor X and protein C circulate as two chains that are disulfide linked. All have a catalytic domain that is homologous between the GLA-containing zymogens. The active site His, Asp, and Ser residues are indicated by the *black circles* in the catalytic domain. Cleavages that convert the zymogen to an active enzyme are indicated by the *arrows*. In factor IX, factor X, and protein C, the released activation peptide is indicated by the *yellow circles*. After cleavage, all of the molecules are two-chain disulfide-linked molecules. The disulfide connecting the catalytic domain with the rest of the molecule is shown by the heavy bond. All catalytic domains but that of prothrombin remain attached to the GLA domain following activation.

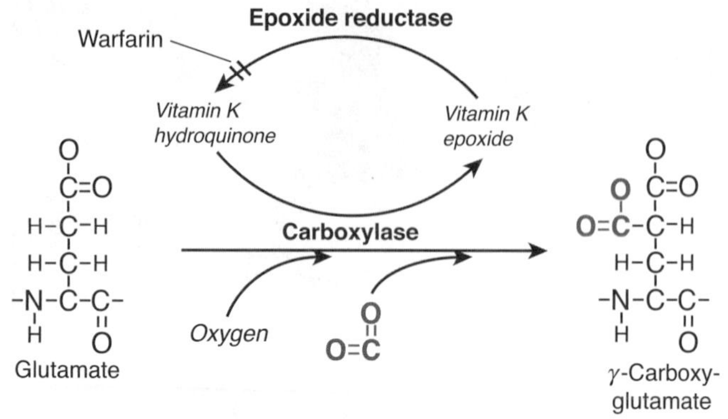

FIGURE 115–2. Vitamin K carboxylase activity. Glutamyl residues are converted to γ-carboxy glutamyl residues by a specific carboxylase. This reaction requires oxygen, carbon dioxide (shown in green), and reduced vitamin K in the form of a hydroquinone. Carbon dioxide is incorporated onto the γ carbon, providing a second carboxylate group on that residue. In the process of this reaction, reduced vitamin K is converted to an epoxide. Reduced vitamin K is recycled by a specific epoxide reductase, a reaction that can be blocked by warfarin.

The calcium-bound form of the GLA domain is responsible for mediating association with phospholipid membranes. Lipids with negatively charged head groups, primarily phosphatidylserine (PS), are required for this binding. Even in the absence of the appropriate protein cofactor, binding to phospholipids increases the proteolytic activity of GLA-containing proteases. PS is required for activity on synthetic phospholipid membranes. The role of PS in mediating coagulation reactions on cellular membranes, such as platelets, is more complex. PS is not normally exposed on the outer membrane leaflet of cells in contact with flowing blood. Further, activation of cells (particularly platelets) is often accompanied by exposure of PS on the outer leaflet of cell membranes. Because this activation enhances the ability to support coagulation reactions, it has often been assumed that exposure of PS on the outer surface of cells is sufficient to account for the ability of a cell to support coagulation reactions. However, other studies show that the level of coagulant activity on cells does not directly correlate with the amount of PS exposure. This result is in direct contrast to studies with phospholipid membranes in which the level of coagulant activity is directly related to the amount of PS expressed. From these studies, it can be concluded that PS exposure is necessary for cells to support coagulation reactions, but that other features, such as cell receptors and/or binding proteins, are also necessary.[13]

There is very high homology in the amino acid sequence in the first 42 residues of GLA-containing proteins. This implies that the three-dimensional structure of the GLA-domain is highly conserved and that few specific interactions are determined by this region. It was once thought that the binding of GLA-containing proteins to phospholipids was mediated by calcium ion "bridging" between the negatively charged GLA residues and negatively charged phospholipid. This mechanism provided a good explanation for why both calcium and negatively charged phospholipid were required for binding. It is currently believed, however, that binding of GLA-containing factors to lipid surfaces is mediated by membrane insertion of hydrophobic residues in the first 10 amino acids of the GLA domain. Calcium is essential for this to occur because calcium binding to some of the GLA residues induces a dramatic conformational change that exposes the hydrophobic amino acid residues in a contiguous patch. This hydrophobic patch is located at the tip of a structural feature that sticks out from the surface of the GLA-containing protease like the keel of a ship. This conformation allows insertion of the "keel" into a phospholipid membrane.[14,15] A computer modeling study suggests a refinement of this hypothesis.[16] This model suggests that the "keel" is inserted more deeply into the membrane than previously thought. The hydrophobic tip is buried in the membrane, but (as shown in Fig. 115–3) the keel is inserted in the membrane up to a level that allows surface-exposed GLA-residues to interact with PS molecules in the outer leaflet of the membrane by calcium bridging. In addition, lysine and arginine residues in the GLA-domain can interact directly with PS headgroups in the membrane.

The striking degree of homology among the GLA domains of the vitamin K-dependent clotting factors suggest that the affinity of the calcium–GLA complexes for phospholipids would also be very similar. However, this turns out not to be the case. Factor IX and factor X bind much more strongly to phosphatidylcholine/phosphatidylserine-containing vesicles than does factor VII.[17] The reasons for these marked differences are not clear, but may be related to differences in presence of positively charged amino acids in the GLA-domain that might interact directly with PS.

The first EGF domain of the vitamin K-dependent proteins has a calcium ion binding site that does not involve GLA residues, but does involve a β-hydroxy aspartic acid. This conserved aspartic acid residue is modified posttranslationally by a β-hydroxylase about which little is known. Binding of calcium to this EGF-1 site appears to be important for activity and probably serves to orient the GLA domain relative to the rest of the molecule. The EGF-1 and EGF-2 domains serve, at least in part, to space the serine protease domain above the lipid membrane surface. Factor VIIa interaction with its cofactor, tissue factor, is mediated at least in part, by direct interaction between tissue factor and both EGF domains of factor VIIa, as shown in Figure 115–4.

All of the GLA-containing zymogens undergo activation by cleavage of at least one peptide bond (see Fig. 115–1). Activation is indicated by

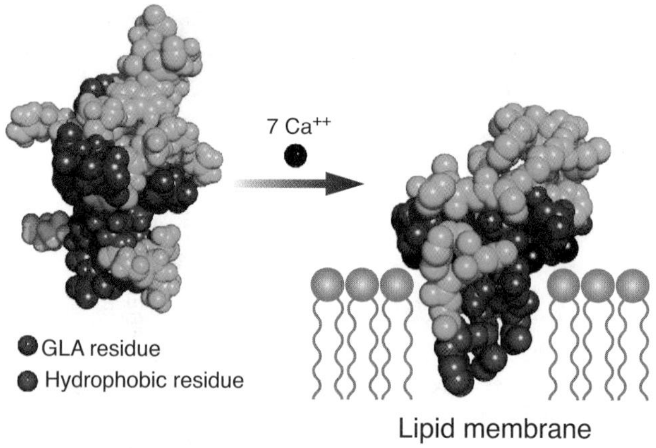

FIGURE 115–3. Calcium ion binding to the GLA domain alters the conformation of the GLA domain. The figure shows molecular models of the GLA domain of prothrombin. The calcium bound form is taken from the x-ray crystal structure of prothrombin (PDB structure 2PF2).[14] The noncalcium form is modeled from the nuclear magnetic resonance structure of factor X (PDB structure 1WHE).[15] Each *circle* shows the position of an amino acid. GLA residues are colored red. Hydrophobic residues believed to be important in membrane insertion are shown in dark blue (residues 6, 7, and 9). In the absence of calcium, the negatively charged GLA residues are exposed to the solution and the hydrophobic residues are buried. Calcium ion binding to the GLA residues provides sufficient energy to alter the overall conformation of the GLA domain and expose the hydrophobic residues (residues 6, 7, and 9). In this view, only 3 of the 7 bound calcium ions can be seen. Insertion of the hydrophobic residues into a membrane is illustrated schematically. Modeling suggests that the GLA domain inserts into the membrane to a level where the calcium ions can interact with negatively charged phospholipid head groups.[16] Molecular models were made with the program PyMol.

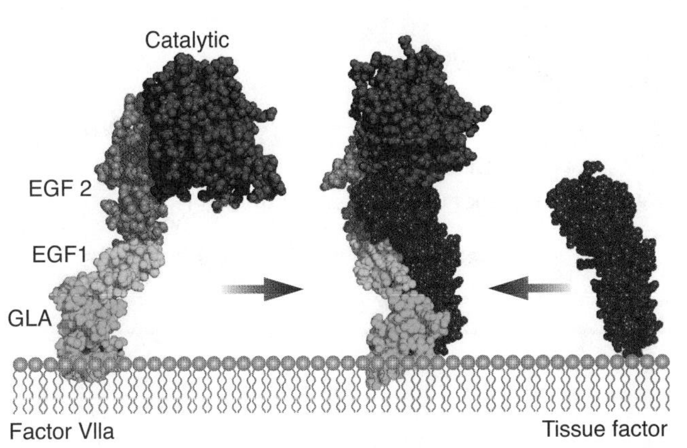

FIGURE 115–4. Complex of factor VIIa and tissue factor. The crystal structure of tissue factor (PDB structure 2HFT)[21] and the tissue factor complex (PDB structure 1DAN)[22] are shown along with a model of the free structure of factor VIIa (constructed from PDB structures 1QHK, 1WHF, 1RFN,[23] and 1DAN). The structure of the transmembrane domain of tissue factor has not been elucidated, so only the extracellular domain is shown. The GLA domain, EGF domains, and catalytic domain of factor VIIa are indicated. Calcium ions are shown in black. Binding to tissue factor alters the overall structure of factor VIIa. The crystal structure of the complex shows multiple close contacts between tissue factor and multiple domains of factor VIIa. Molecular models were made with the program PyMol.

appending the letter "a" to the name of the factor, except for protein C which is often abbreviated APC. The cleavage that leads to activation generates a new amino terminal that folds back and interacts with specific residues in the serine protease domain. This interaction changes the conformation of the protein such that the active site residues (His, Ser, Asp) are aligned and the protease activity of the factor is expressed.

The serine protease domains of all the GLA-containing proteases show a high homology to each other and to chymotrypsin and trypsin; all have trypsin-like activity, with an almost absolute specificity for cleaving at the carboxy terminal of arginyl residues. However, unlike trypsin which shows little specificity beyond cleaving after an arginyl or lysyl residue, the activated coagulation factors have extended substrate specificity pockets, such that only a small number of amino acid sequences are recognized by each activated factor. Despite the high degree of homology between the protease domains of protein C, prothrombin, and factors VII, IX and X, each of these factors has a highly specific function in coagulation that is mediated by surface loops that are not highly homologous.

The activated forms of factors VII, IX, and X each associate with a specific cofactor. Tissue factor (TF) is the cofactor for factor VIIa; factor VIIIa is the cofactor for factor IXa; and factor Va is the cofactor for factor Xa. The factors and cofactors associate on cell membranes to form proteolytically active complexes. Thrombin does not require a cofactor for its coagulant activity. However, upon association with the cofactor thrombomodulin (TM), its specificity is changed from coagulant (clotting fibrinogen) to anticoagulant (cleaving and activating protein C). Although each of the proteases has some activity in the absence of its cofactor, association with cofactor dramatically enhances its activity. This is illustrated in Table 115–2, which shows the enhancement of factor IXa activity by calcium, activated platelets, and the factor VIII cofactor.[18,19] Thus, the physiologic coagulant activity of factors VIIa, IXa, and Xa is only expressed as a part of a complete procoagulant complex (Table 115–3). The complexes are sometimes named for their physiologic substrate: the factor IXa/VIIIa complex is termed the "tenase" or "intrinsic tenase" complex; the factor VIIa/tissue factor complex the "extrinsic tenase" complex; and the factor Xa/Va complex the "prothrombinase" complex. The cofactors enhance proteolytic activity by two basic mechanisms: (1) they have binding sites for both substrate and enzyme and bring the two into close proximity, and (2) they associate with the protease and induce a conformational change that enhances enzymatic activity. The structure of the factor VIIa/TF complex has been determined by x-ray crystallography.[20] Figure 115–4[21–23] illustrates the projected change in conformation of the factor VIIa molecule when it binds to its cofactor, tissue factor. The factor IXa/VIIIa and Xa/Va complexes have not been crystallized, but it is likely that generally similar conformational changes occur during formation of these complexes.

TABLE 115–2. Cofactor Enhancement of Factor IXa Activity

Conditions	Relative Rate[b]
IXa/Ca^{2+}	1
IXa/Ca^{2+}/platelets[a]	150[18]
IXa/Ca^{2+}/VIIIa	250[19]
IXa/Ca^{2+}/platelet[a]/VIIIa	9,000,000[18]

[a]Platelets were activated with thrombin.

[b]Rates are given as k_{cat}/K_m.

PROTHROMBIN (FACTOR II)

Protein Structure

Like the other vitamin K-dependent zymogens, plasma prothrombin is primarily synthesized in the liver. It circulates as a single-chain zymogen of Mr ~72,000 and has a plasma half-life of about 60 hours. Figure 115–5 is a schematic representation. It has 10 GLA residues. Instead of the EGF region present in most vitamin K-dependent zymogens, prothrombin has two kringle domains. Kringle domains are structures held together by three disulfide bonds that schematically resemble a Danish pastry called a "kringle." The primary function of kringle structures appears to be to bind other proteins such as activators, substrates, cofactors, or receptors.[24]

TABLE 115–3. Protease/Cofactor Complexes

Enzyme	Cofactor	Substrate	Cellular Location
Factor VIIa	Tissue factor	Factor X Factor IX	Many cells[a]
Factor IXa	Factor VIIIa	Factor X	Platelets
Factor Xa	Factor Va	Prothrombin	Platelets[b]
Thrombin	Thrombomodulin	Protein C	Endothelium
Activated protein C	Protein S	Factor Va Factor VIIIa	Endothelium

[a]TF is constitutively expressed on many extravascular cells (e.g., stromal cells, epithelial cells, astrocytes) and is induced by inflammatory mediators in many other cells (e.g., monocytes, endothelial cells).

[b]Many other cells have low levels of factor Xa/factor Va activity.

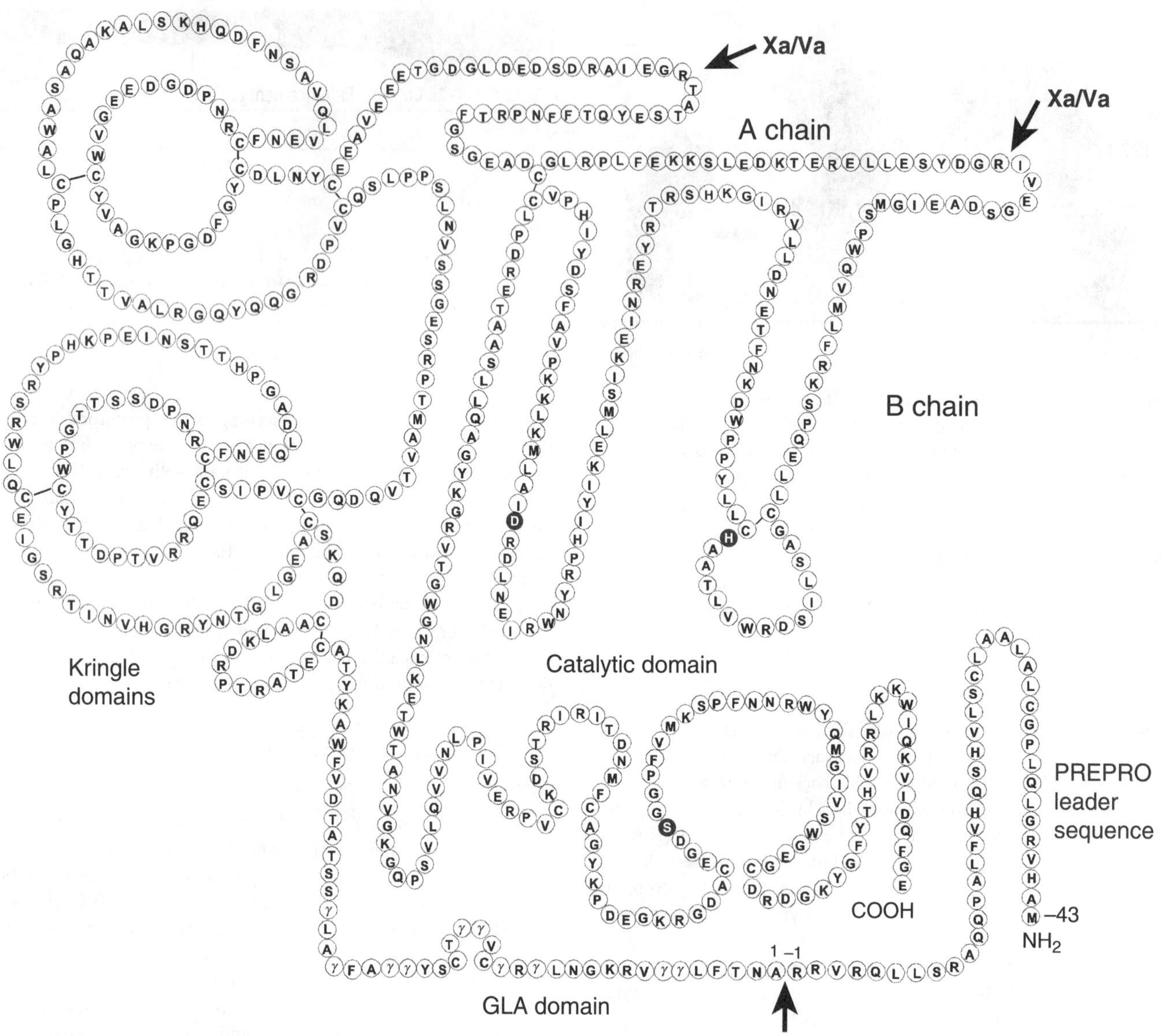

FIGURE 115–5. Domains of prothrombin. Each amino acid in prothrombin is shown. GLA residues are indicated by γ. The cleavage site to remove the prepro leader sequence is indicated by an *arrow*. The active sites His, Asp, and Ser are shown by *blue circles*. Cleavage sites for factor Xa/factor Va are shown by *arrows*. Cleavage removes the GLA domain and kringles, leaving thrombin composed of a small A chain disulfide linked to the catalytic domain (B chain; the disulfide link is indicated by the heavy bond).

Molecular Biology The human prothrombin gene has been localized to chromosome 11, near the centromere.[25] It has been completely sequenced and is composed of 14 exons separated by 13 introns (Fig. 115–6). The 5′ flanking region of the prothrombin gene contains the promoter region and two or more *cis*-acting enhancer sequences. *Cis*-acting sequences are portions of the DNA that act as promoters, enhancers, or silencers. Unlike many other promoters, the promoter region of the prothrombin gene does not contain a TATA box. It has multiple potential sites of transcription initiation extending from 3 to 38 base pairs (bp) upstream from the initial methionine. The site at −31 is the most likely start site. The region between −887 and −875 is likely to be a binding site for hepatic nuclear factor 1 (HNF-1), a DNA-binding protein that plays a role in the liver-specific expression of a number of genes.[26] HNF-1 is an example of a *trans*-acting factor, which is a molecule that binds to a DNA sequence and affects expression of the associated gene. An additional site in the prothrombin promoter region with non–tissue-specific enhancer activity lies just upstream to the HNF-1 site.

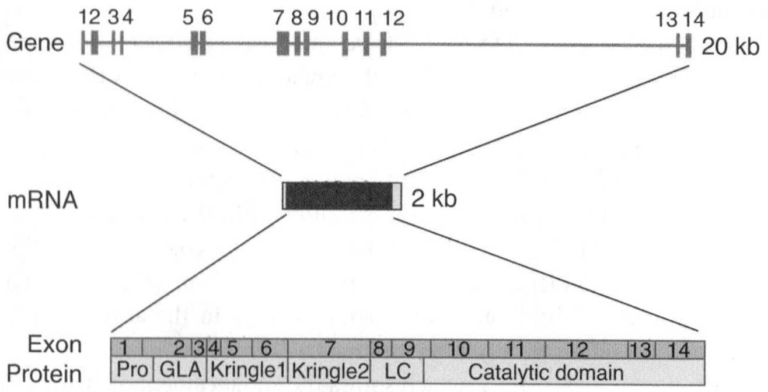

FIGURE 115–6. Relationship of gene structure to protein structure in prothrombin. The exons, introns, messenger ribonucleic acid (mRNA), and protein structure are as indicated. Promoter elements upstream from exon 1 are not shown but are discussed in the text. The mRNA is 2 Kb with small 5′ and 3′ untranslated regions (shown in light blue). In the protein, Pro indicates the prepro leader sequence; GLA indicates the GLA domain. Kringles 1 and 2 are shown. *LC* indicates the light chain, also called the A chain.

One unusual feature of the prothrombin gene is the presence of many repetitive sequences in its 5′ flanking region.[27] Approximately 41 percent of the gene and upstream sequence consists of Alu repeats. The function of these repetitive sequences, if any, is not known.

Several polymorphisms of the prothrombin gene have been described and one of these is now recognized to have important functional consequences. This G-to-A transition in the 3′ untranslated region (20210 G→A) of the prothrombin gene is associated with higher-than-normal levels of plasma prothrombin.[28] Increased prothrombin levels are associated with an increased risk of venous thromboembolism (see Chap. 131).

Knockout of the prothrombin gene in a mouse model results in intrauterine and neonatal lethality.[29]

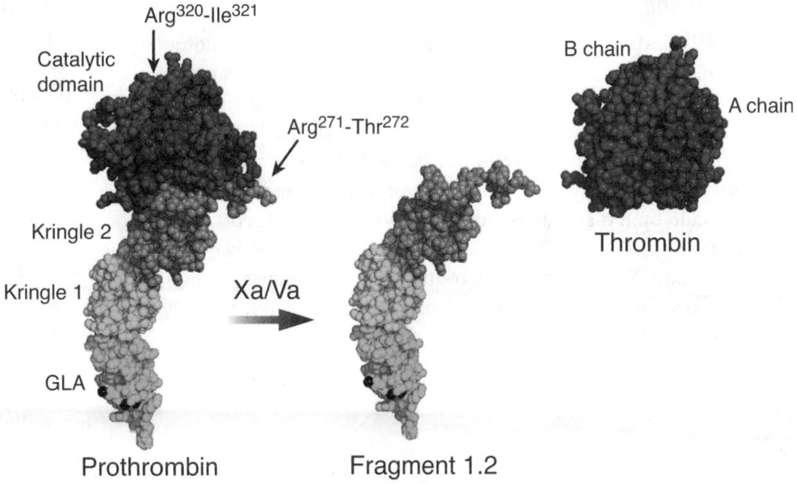

FIGURE 115–7. Activation of prothrombin. A model of prothrombin constructed from four crystal structures (PDB structures 2PF2, 1HAG, 1A0H, and 1HAI) is shown.[14,30–32] The GLA domain, both kringle domains, and the catalytic domain are shown. Calcium ions are shown in black. Cleavage by factor Xa/factor Va releases thrombin (with small A chain and catalytically active B chains) from the rest of the molecule, fragment 1.2. Molecular models were made with the program PyMol.

Activation and Activity

Prothrombin is cleaved by the factor Xa/Va prothrombinase complex in two places (Arg 271 and Arg 320), as shown in Figure 115–7.[14,30–32] The catalytic domain (thrombin), Mr 36,600, is released from the remainder of the molecule (prothrombin fragment 1.2). Because one molecule of prothrombin fragment 1.2 is released for each molecule of thrombin, assays for fragment 1.2 reflect the level of prothrombin activation.

Thrombin cleaves a number of biologically important substrates. It removes fibrinopeptides A and B from fibrinogen to form fibrin monomers, which then spontaneously polymerize to form a fibrin clot (see Chap. 126). The anion-binding exosite spans residues 387 to 398 and is involved in binding to fibrinogen, thrombomodulin, hirudin, heparin cofactor II (HC II), and the proteolytically activated thrombin receptors. Interestingly, this region of thrombin is identical in human, bovine, rat, and mouse.[33] In addition to directly clotting fibrinogen, thrombin has a procoagulant effect by participating in positive feedback loops by activating platelets and coagulation factors V, VIII, XI, and XIII.

Thrombin is a potent platelet activator through at least two types of receptors. These include the G-protein-linked proteolytically activated receptors, PAR-1 and PAR-4, as well as platelet glycoprotein Ibα (see Chap. 114).

Another function of thrombin is to activate a procarboxypeptidase B-like enzyme to its active state, a reaction enhanced by thrombomodulin. The active carboxypeptidase inhibits plasmin-mediated fibrinolysis by removing C-terminal lysine residues from fibrin, which facilitate plasminogen binding, from partially degraded fibrin. Thus, the carboxypeptidase has been termed *thrombin-activatable fibrinolysis inhibitor* (TAFI).[34,35]

In addition to its procoagulant activity, thrombin has an anticoagulant function. Thus, thrombin binds to the cofactor thrombomodulin on endothelial cells, allowing it to activate protein C which inactivates factors Va and VIIIa (see Chap. 116).[36,37] Thrombin also has growth factor and cytokine-like activities that may play a role in atherosclerosis, wound healing, and inflammation.[38]

The primary plasma inhibitor of thrombin in coagulation is antithrombin (AT). HC II also inhibits thrombin, and may serve as an extravascular thrombin inhibitor that regulates the growth factor and cytokine-like activities of thrombin.[38]

FACTOR VII

Protein Structure

Factor VII circulates as a single-chain zymogen of Mr 50,000. It has the shortest half-life of the procoagulant factors, approximately 3 to 6 hours (see Table 115–1), and has 10 GLA residues.

Molecular Biology

The human factor VII gene is located on chromosome 13, very close to the gene for factor X. The gene consists of eight exons and seven introns, with an overall size of about 13 kb, and an organization similar to the other vitamin K-dependent factors (Fig. 115–8).[1,2]

The major transcription start site in the factor VII gene is at −51. Three other minor start sites have been described.[39] A hormone-responsive element and binding sites for the *trans*-acting factors HNF-4 and Sp-1 are located between −233 and −58 in the promoter region of the factor VII gene.

In contrast to the intrauterine lethality observed in TF-deficient mice, embryos deficient in factor VII developed normally, without evidence of hemorrhage. However, factor VII-deficient newborns sometimes succumb to intraabdominal or intracranial hemorrhage.[40]

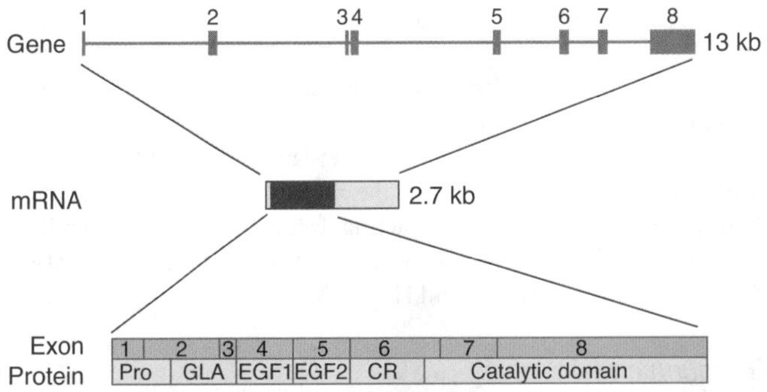

FIGURE 115–8. Relationship of gene structure to protein structure in factor VII. The exons, introns, messenger ribonucleic acid (mRNA), and protein structure are as indicated. Promoter elements upstream from exon 1 are not shown but are discussed in the text. The mRNA is 2.7 kb with a small 5′ untranslated region and a relatively large 3′ untranslated region (light blue). In the protein, Pro indicates the prepro leader sequence; GLA indicates the GLA domain; EGF indicates the epidermal growth factor-like domains; and CR indicates the connecting region. The site of proteolytic activation is in this region.

Activation and Activity

Factor VII binds to tissue factor with a kDa in the subnanomolar range. Once bound to its cofactor, factor VII can be activated by a number of different proteases that cleave between Arg152 and Ile153. The physiologic activator of factor VII is thought to be factor Xa, although significant autoactivation by factor VIIa can occur.[41] Unlike prothrombin, the catalytic domain of factor VII is linked to the rest of the molecule by a disulfide bond, so no portion is cleaved from the protein (see Fig. 115–1). The factor VIIa/TF complex activates both factors IX and X. It is inhibited by tissue factor pathway inhibitor (TFPI) in complex with factor Xa. It is also inhibited by AT, but only in the presence of heparin.

FACTOR IX

Protein Structure

Factor IX is synthesized in hepatocytes and circulates as a single-chain zymogen of Mr ~57,000 with a plasma half-life of 18 to 24 hours. It has 12 GLA residues. Only approximately 40 percent of factor IX molecules are hydroxylated at aspartic acid 64 in the EGF-1 domain. All the other GLA-containing zymogens have complete hydroxylation of the homologous residues (Fig. 115–9). Factor IX contains N- and O-linked carbohydrate moieties found mostly in the activation peptide. In the mature molecule, the tyrosine residue at position 155 is sulfated, whereas the serine residue at position 158 is phosphorylated. Factor IX, unlike other vitamin K-dependent factors, has been shown to bind effectively to collagen IV *in vitro*.[42] The molecule appears to bind to collagen IV *in vivo*, which may account for the observation that when factor IX is infused into hemophilia B patients, recovery is only 50 percent of that expected (see Chap. 124).[43] The physiologic relevance of this observation remains to be precisely determined, but studies suggest that factor IX mutants lacking collagen IV binding exhibit a greater recovery but may be associated with a mild bleeding tendency.[44,44a]

Molecular Biology

The gene for factor IX is located on the tip of the long arm of the X chromosome at position Xq27.1-q27.2.[45] Therefore, deficiency of factor IX (hemophilia B) is sex linked. The gene contains eight exons, seven introns, and a long 1.4 kb 3′-untranslated region, for an overall size of 33 kb (Fig. 115–10).

Eight polymorphisms have been described within or flanking the factor IX gene. These polymorphisms can be useful for antenatal diagnosis and carrier detection of hemophilia B by restriction fragment length polymorphism (RFLP) analysis.[46]

The promoter activity of the 5′ untranslated region of the factor IX gene resides 274 bp upstream of the major transcription start site.[47] Binding sites for several *trans*-acting factors have been identified, including sites for CCAAT/enhancer binding protein (C/EBP),[48] D-site binding protein,[49] HNF-4,[50] and HNF-1.[51]

Activation and Activity

Factor IX can be activated either by factor XIa or by the factor VIIa/TF complex. Full activation requires cleavage of two bonds (Arg 145 and Arg 180) releasing an activation peptide of Mr ~10,000 (see Fig. 115–9). This results in an Mr 17,000 light chain connected to an Mr 30,000 heavy chain that contains the active sites Asp, His, and Ser.

In complex with its cofactor, factor VIIIa, on a phospholipid membrane surface, factor IXa activates factor X. Physiologically this activity is primarily expressed on the surface of activated platelets, and there is preliminary evidence suggesting that platelets express a receptor/binding protein for factor IXa that promotes assembly of the factor IXa/VIIIa complex.[52]

The primary plasma inhibitor of factor IXa appears to be AT. Inhibition of factor IXa by AT is slow compared to AT inhibition of thrombin. However, it is enhanced in the presence of heparin.

FACTOR X

Protein Structure

Factor X circulates as a 2-chain, disulfide-linked zymogen of Mr 59,000 (see Fig. 115–1) with a plasma half life of approximately 34 to 40 hours. A 3-amino-acid sequence between the light and heavy chains (Arg140-Lys141-Arg142) is cleaved from the protein during intracellular processing. The resulting light chain Mr is ~17,000 and the heavy chain Mr is ~40,000. The light chain contains the GLA domain, with its 11 GLA residues, and the two EGF domains. The heavy chain contains the 52-amino-acid activation peptide and the catalytic domain. Like all other vitamin K-dependent factors, it is synthesized in the liver.

Molecular Biology

The gene for human factor X is on chromosome 13q34-qter[53] in close proximity to the factor VII gene. It is composed of eight exons and seven introns,[1] with a size of ~25 kb (Fig. 115–11). The 3′ untranslated region is unusually short, with only 10 base pairs. A number of potentially useful polymorphisms have been identified.[54]

The factor X promoter region has been sequenced and characterized. It lacks a typical TATA box, but contains a CCAAT sequence at −120 to −116. Factor X appears to have multiple start sites of transcription.[55] This finding is consistent with multiple start sites reported for other promoters lacking a TATA box. Like the factor IX gene, a binding site for HNF-4 has been identified.[56] However, unlike the factor IX gene, there does not appear to be a binding site for C/EBP.

Complete deficiency of FX induced by targeted gene disruption in a mouse model often resulted in embryonic lethality. Most of the deficient mice that survived to term succumbed to hemorrhage within 5 days after birth.[57]

Activation and Activity

Factor X can be activated to fully active factor Xaα by factor VIIa/TF or factor IXa/VIIIa by cleavage at the Arg 194–Ile 195 bond in the heavy chain. Further autocatalytic cleavage near the carboxy terminus of the heavy chain releases a 19-amino-acid peptide to yield "β-factor Xa" which is also enzymatically active.

Factor Xa in complex with factor Va on a phospholipid membrane surface activates prothrombin to thrombin by cleaving two peptide bonds. Factor Xa may also play a physiologic role in activation of factors VII,[58] VIII,[59] and V.[60] Although any membrane surface that expresses anionic phospholipid can support prothrombinase complex assembly, the activated platelet surface is especially well suited for this purpose. Prothrombinase assembly on platelets is not strictly a function of phospholipid composition, but is likely coordinated by one or more specific binding proteins.[61]

Like thrombin, factor X has biologic activities not directly related to coagulation. It is reported to have mitogenic activity for smooth muscle cells.[62] Factor Xa also possesses receptor-mediated proinflammatory activities.[63] The primary plasma inhibitor of factor Xa is the serine protease inhibitor (Serpin) AT. The inhibition of factor Xa by AT is accelerated by heparin. Tissue factor pathway inhibitor (TFPI) is also a potent inhibitor of factor Xa, as shown in Table 115–4.

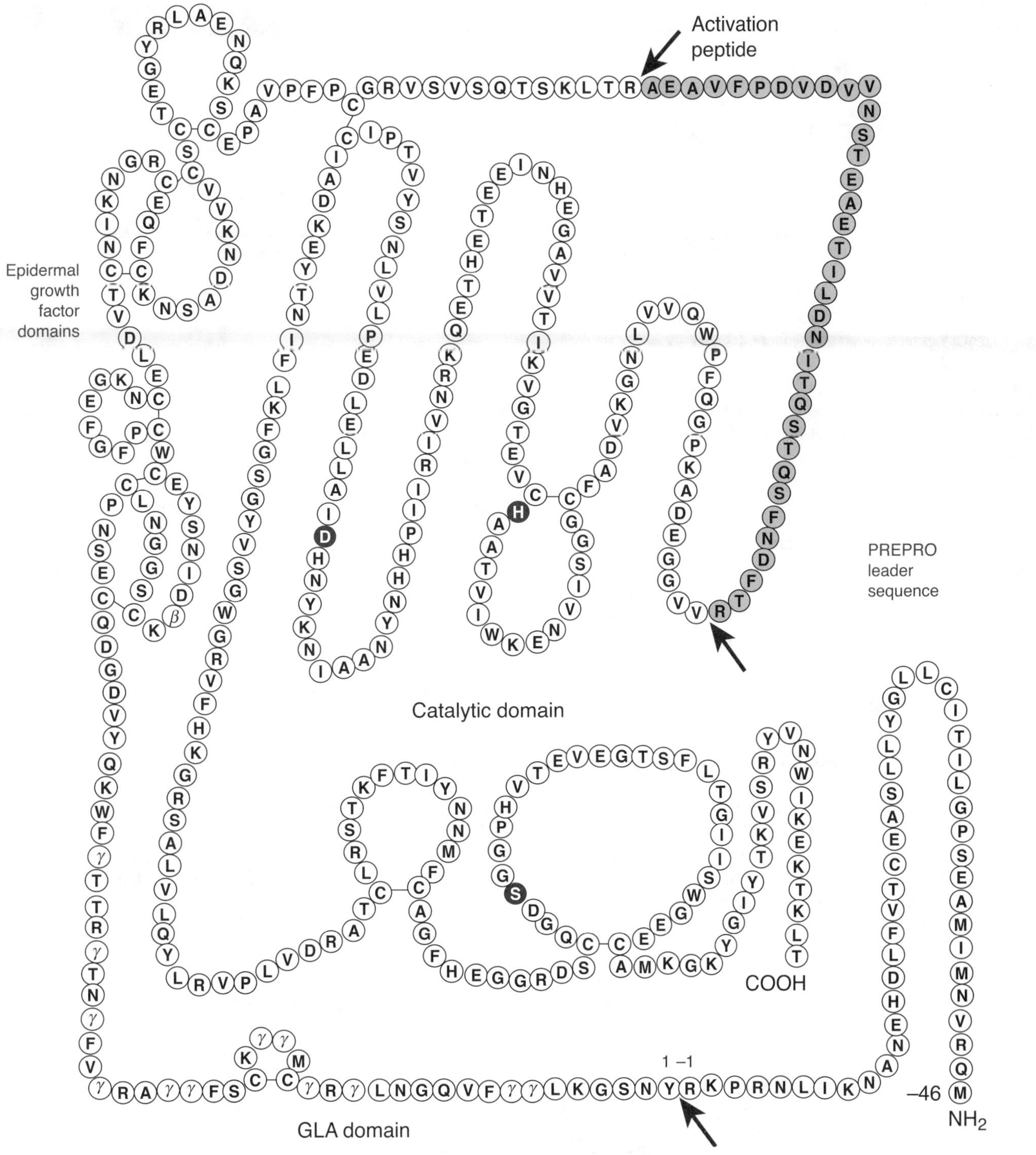

FIGURE 115–9. Domains of factor IX. Each amino acid in factor IX is shown. GLA residues are indicated by γ. The cleavage site to remove the prepro leader sequence is indicated by an *arrow*. The active site His, Asp, and Ser are shown by blue circles. Cleavage sites for factor XIa and factor VIIa/tissue factor are shown by *arrows* leading to removal of the activation peptide (shown in yellow).

PROTEIN C

Protein Structure

Protein C, unlike the other vitamin K-dependent zymogens, is not a procoagulant, but controls coagulation, when activated, by inactivating factors Va and VIIIa (see Chap. 116). It circulates as a two-chain disulfide-linked zymogen with nine GLA residues (see Fig. 115–1). It has an Mr of 59,000 and a short plasma half-life of approximately 6 hours.

Molecular Biology

The gene for human protein C is on chromosome 2q13–14.[64] It was originally described as being composed of eight exons with a size of

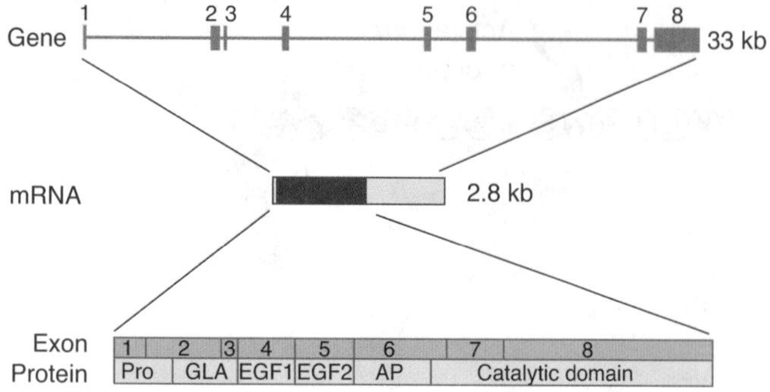

FIGURE 115–10. Relationship of gene structure to protein structure in factor IX. The exons, introns, messenger ribonucleic acid (mRNA), and protein structure are as indicated. Promoter elements upstream from exon 1 are not shown but are discussed in the text. The mRNA is 2.8 kb with a small 5′ untranslated region and a relatively large 3′ untranslated region (light blue). In the protein, Pro indicates the prepro leader sequence; GLA indicates the GLA domain; EGF indicates the epidermal growth factor like domains; and AP indicates the activation peptide that is released after cleavage of two bonds.

TABLE 115–4. Characterization of TFPI and AT Inhibition of Coagulation Factors

		Time to 50% Inhibition[a] (min)	
Inhibitor	Protease	– Heparin	+ Heparin
Antithrombin	Thrombin	1.5	<0.1
	Factor Xa	4	<0.1
	Factor IXa	60	0.6
Tissue factor pathway inhibitor	Factor Xa	0.3	<0.1

[a]Time to 50% inhibition in plasma. *In vivo*, natural glycosaminoglycan molecules on endothelium and other cells accelerate the rate of inhibition.

~10 kb.[65] Other workers have described it as having nine exons and eight introns,[66] with the first exon corresponding to the 5′-noncoding region (Fig. 115–12). Thus, the first exon is transcribed from the gene into messenger ribonucleic acid (mRNA), but is not translated into protein. The gene structure is very similar to the other vitamin K-dependent factors, with especially close homology to factor IX.

Activation and Activity

Protein C is activated by thrombin in complex with the cell-surface cofactor thrombomodulin. A single cleavage at Arg169-Leu170 releases a 12-amino-acid activation peptide leading to APC with a molecular weight of 56,000. Activation of protein C is modulated in part by the endothelial cell protein C receptor (EPCR).[67] EPCR concentrates protein C on the endothelial cell membrane, thereby enhancing the activation of protein C by the thrombin–thrombomodulin complex.[68] The EPCR is preferentially expressed by the endothelium of larger vessels.

APC, in complex with its cofactor protein S, proteolytically inactivates factors Va and VIIIa. Data suggest that inactivation of these factors is much more likely to occur on endothelial cells than on platelet surfaces.[69] Thus, APC primarily acts to prevent thrombin generation on intact endothelial cells that might lead to thrombosis. It has also been reported that factor V can act as a cofactor for the inactivation of factors Va and VIIIa by APC.[70] The primary inhibitor of APC is the serpin protein C inhibitor, also known as plasminogen activator inhibitor-3 (PAI-3) and SERPINA5.[71]

In addition to its antithrombotic effects, APC has a variety of antiinflammatory activities (see Chap. 116). It suppresses inflammatory cytokine production in animal models of sepsis, inhibits leukocyte adhesion and chemotaxis, reduces endothelial cell apoptosis, helps maintain endothelial cell barrier function, and minimizes hypotension associated with severe sepsis.[72] Most of these functions require binding to EPCR and cleavage of proteolytically activated receptor (PAR)-1. Although the antiinflammatory functions of APC require proteolytic activity, they are not mediated by its inhibitory effects on thrombin generation.[73] Overall the protein C system has important roles in controlling inappropriate or excessive activity of both the coagulation and inflammatory responses.

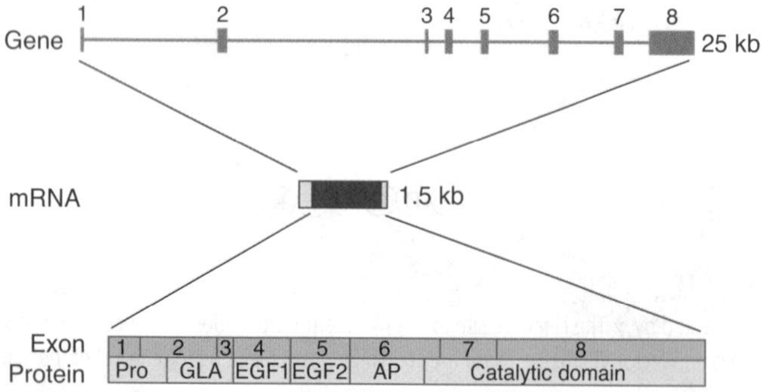

FIGURE 115–11. Relationship of gene structure to protein structure in factor X. The exons, introns, messenger ribonucleic acid (mRNA), and protein structure are as indicated. Promoter elements upstream from exon 1 are not shown but are discussed in the text. The mRNA is 1.5 Kb with a relatively large 5′ untranslated region and a small 3′ untranslated region. In the protein, Pro indicates the prepro leader sequence; GLA indicates the GLA domain; EGF indicates the epidermal growth factor-like domains; and AP indicates the activation peptide. Before secretion, cleavage in this domain processes factor X to the two-chain zymogen that circulates. A second cleavage releases the activation peptide and generates factor Xa activity.

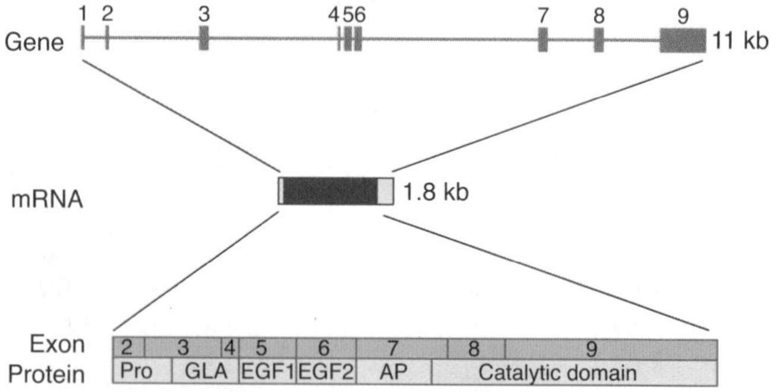

FIGURE 115–12. Relationship of gene structure to protein structure in protein C. The exons, introns, messenger ribonucleic acid (mRNA), and protein structure are as indicated. The mRNA is 1.8 kb with a small 5′ untranslated region coded for by exon 1 and a relatively small 3′ untranslated region (light blue). In the protein, Pro indicates the prepro leader sequence; GLA indicates the GLA domain; EGF indicates the epidermal growth factor-like domains; and AP indicates the activation peptide. Before secretion, cleavage in this domain processes protein C to the two-chain zymogen that circulates. A second cleavage releases the very small activation peptide and generates activated protein C.

SOLUBLE COFACTORS (PROTEIN S, FACTOR V, FACTOR VIII, AND VON WILLEBRAND FACTOR)

PROTEIN S

Protein Structure

Protein S is a single-chain plasma glycoprotein of Mr ~75,000 with a plasma half-life of approximately 42 hours. It is dependent on vitamin K for its synthesis and contains 11 GLA residues in the amino-terminal region. Its structure is quite different from the GLA-containing zymogens (Fig. 115–13). Protein S is organized into a GLA domain, a thrombin-sensitive finger region, four EGF domains, and a region with homology to glucocorticoid-binding proteins. Unlike the other vitamin K-dependent factors, it does not contain a serine protease domain and so does not have the potential to catalyze reactions. Each EGF domain contains a modified amino acid, either β-hydroxyaspartic acid or β-hydroxyasparagine. Protein S circulates both in the free form (~40% of the total amount) and in a form bound to the complement regulatory protein C4b-binding protein. The glucocorticoid hormone-binding globulin-like region of protein S is involved in binding to the β subunit of C4b-binding protein. Like the GLA-containing zymogens, protein S is synthesized with a signal peptide that directs it to the endoplasmic reticulum, and a propeptide that binds to the γ-glutamyl carboxylase. The signal sequence and propeptide are removed before the mature protein is secreted.

Protein S is synthesized primarily by hepatocytes,[74] as well as by endothelial cells,[75] megakaryocytes,[76] Leydig cells,[77] and osteoblasts.[78]

Molecular Biology

The human protein S gene is on chromosome 3, spanning the centromere from p11.1 to q11.2. It is more than 80 kb in length and contains 15 exons and 14 introns (see Fig. 115–13).[79] Exons 1 to 8 encode protein domains that are homologous to the GLA-containing zymogens. The intron–exon structure is typical of the members of this family. Exons 9 to 15 encode protein segments homologous to glucocorticoid hormone-binding globulin. There is also a pseudogene of protein S located on the same chromosome. It is approximately 55 kb in size and contains coding sequences for regions corresponding to amino acids 46 to 635 of protein S.

Activity

Protein S serves as a cofactor for the cleavage and inactivation of factors Va and VIIIa by APC. In contrast to factors V and VIII, it does not require proteolytic activation for its cofactor activity. Until recently, it had been thought that protein S can only serve as a cofactor for APC when in the free form, rather than when bound to C4b-binding protein. However, reevaluation of the data suggests that C4b-binding protein-bound protein S does, indeed, express APC-cofactor activity.[80]

Protein S alone also has a low level of anticoagulant activity by virtue of its ability to compete with factor Xa for binding to factor Va[81] and this activity is not reduced by binding to C4b-binding protein.[82] In addition, data show that protein S can act to enhance the effectiveness of TFPI in inhibiting the factor VIIa/TF complex.[83]

FACTOR V

Protein Structure

Factors V and VIII are homologous in their gene structures, amino acid sequences, and protein domain structures. They have similar mechanisms of intracellular processing in the endoplasmic reticulum (ER) and Golgi apparatus and defects in these mechanisms can result in combined deficiency of factors V and VIII. The mannose-binding lectin-1 gene product LMAN1 (also called endoplasmic reticulum-Golgi intermediate compartment [ERGIC]-53) is a protein found in the intermediate compartment of the Golgi apparatus that facilitates secretion of both factor V and factor VIII.[84] Mutations in the LMAN1 gene lead to a hereditary deficiency of both factors V and VIII[85] which accounts for about two-thirds of the cases of combined deficiency (see Chap. 125). Analysis of patients without defects in LMAN1 suggests that mutations of a second protein, MCFD2 (multiple coagulation deficiency protein 2), also account for a number of the cases of combined factors V and VIII deficiency.[86] The gene product of MCFD2 is an Mr 16,000 protein localized to the ERGIC through a direct, calcium-dependent interaction with LMAN1. The MCFD2–LMAN1 complex appears to form a specific cargo receptor for the ER-to-Golgi transport of selected proteins, including both factors V and VIII.

Factor V is a large glycoprotein of Mr ~330,000 and has a plasma half-life of approximately 12 hours, with some reports of a half-life of up to 36 hours.[87] It has the following domain organization: A1-A2-B-A3-C1-C2 (Fig. 115–14). The three A domains have significant homology to the copper-binding plasma protein ceruloplasmin. The C domains have some homology to fat globule proteins. The C2 domain of factor V mediates binding to lipid membranes.[88] The A and C domains of factor V are approximately 40 percent identical to the homologous regions in

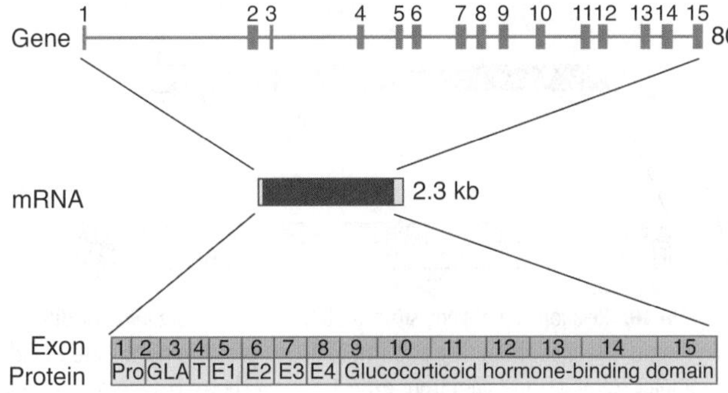

FIGURE 115–13. Relationship of gene structure to protein structure in protein S. The exons, introns, messenger ribonucleic acid (mRNA), and protein structure are as indicated. The mRNA is 2.3 kb with a small 5′ and 3′ untranslated region (light blue). In the protein, Pro indicates the prepro leader sequence; GLA indicates the GLA domain; T indicates the thrombin-sensitive finger region; and E indicates the epidermal growth factor-like domains.

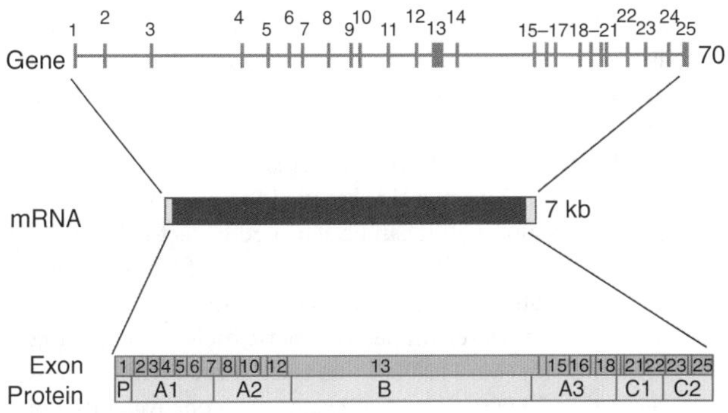

FIGURE 115–14. Relationship of gene structure to protein structure in factor V. The exons, introns, messenger ribonucleic acid (mRNA), and protein structure are as indicated. The mRNA is 7 kb with some 5′ and 3′ untranslated sequences (light blue). In the protein, P indicates the propeptide leader sequence. The A domains have homology to ceruloplasmin. The C domains have homology to fat globule proteins. The B domain is released on activation and has no significant homology to any other identified protein.

factor VIII. In contrast, the B domains show little homology between the two proteins and are not known to be homologous to any other proteins. In factor V, unlike factor VIII, sequences in the B domain appear to be important in promoting its activation by thrombin. The acidic regions of factor V have a high proportion of Asp and Glu residues. These regions are thought to be important in promoting activation, possibly by providing a site of interaction with the anion binding exosite of thrombin.

Factor V shows five potential sites for tyrosine sulfation at residues 696, 698, 1494, 1510, and 1565. Sulfation of factor V also plays a role in factor V activity by enhancing activation by thrombin and by promoting maximal factor Xa activation of prothrombin.[89] Factor V contains both N- and O-linked carbohydrate moieties, most of which are clustered in the B domain.

Molecular Biology

The gene for factor V is located on chromosome 1q21 to q25. It is located very close to the genes for the selectin family of leukocyte adhesion molecules. The factor V gene spans approximately 70 kb and consists of 25 exons (see Fig. 115–14). The gene structure is very similar to that of the factor VIII gene, with exon–intron boundaries occurring at exactly the same location in 21 of 24 cases.[90] The mechanisms governing factor V gene transcription and translation are not clear.

Activation and Activity

Factor V circulates in plasma as a single-chain molecule. As much as 20 percent of the circulating factor V pool is found in platelet α granules, where it is localized by uptake from the plasma.[91] Platelet factor V appears to be sufficient for hemostatic function, at least in mice.[92] Interestingly, the origin of factor V in mouse platelets is different from human. Mouse platelet factor V is synthesized in megakaryocytes and packaged into the α granules before platelet release from the marrow.[92,93] This very clear difference between mouse and human platelets should serve to remind us that one should not assume, without validation, that any animal model reproduces human biology and pathophysiology.

Platelet factor V is heterogeneous because of cleavages in the B domain by calpain and other platelet proteases. These cleavages produce a partially activated form of platelet factor V. Activated platelet factor V is also more resistant to inactivation by activated protein C.[69,94] In platelets, but not in plasma, factor V is complexed to a large multimeric protein called *multimerin*.[95] Multimerin has a massive repeating structure, with some of the multimers having molecular weights of several million. Multimerin has structural features that suggest it may mediate adhesive interactions. Although multimerin interactions with factor V are functionally similar to von Willebrand factor (VWF) interactions with factor VIII, multimerin and VWF share no structural homology.

Full factor V cofactor activity is achieved only after cleavage at several bonds (Fig. 115–15). Factor V is believed to be primarily activated by thrombin *in vivo*, although it can be activated by factor Xa as well,[60] and factor Xa appears to be the preferred activator of factor V released from platelet α granules.[94] Thrombin cleaves factor V at Arg 709 and Arg 1545 to produce a two-chain heterodimeric molecule consisting of an A1-A2 heavy chain (Mr 110,000) that is associated with an A3-C1-C2 light chain (Mr 73,000). The two chains are noncovalently linked through metal ions (probably calcium). APC catalyzes inactivation of factor Va by proteolysis of Arg 306 and Arg 506, resulting in dissociation of the cleaved A2 fragments[87] (Fig. 115–15). A common Arg 506 Gln mutation in factor V leads to resistance to inactivation by APC (factor V Leiden) and is associated with an increased risk of venous thromboembolism (see Chap. 131).[96] Disruption of the factor V gene in mice leads to the death of approximately half of the homozygous factor V-deficient embryos dying at embryonic days 9 to 10. The remaining factor V-deficient embryos survive to term, but die from massive bleeding within 2 hours of birth.[97]

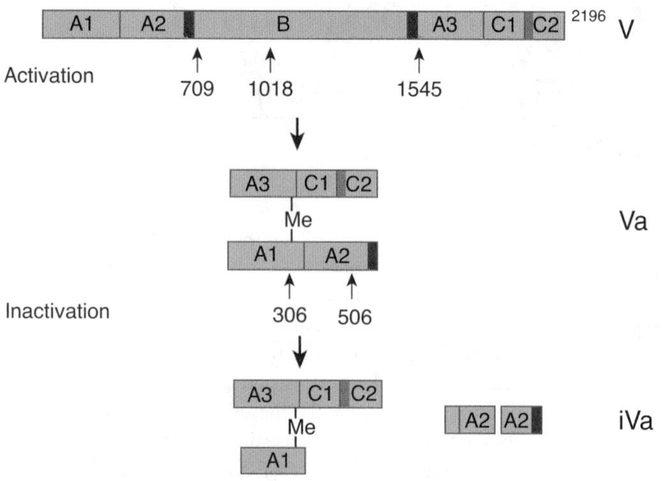

FIGURE 115–15. Activation and inactivation of factor V. For full cofactor activity, factor V requires cleavage by thrombin or factor Xa. The acidic domains, shown in dark blue, are believed to bind to the anion binding exosite in thrombin and enhance thrombin activation of factor V. Cleavage of residue 1018 enhances cleavage at residue 1545. Heavy and light chains are held together by noncovalent interactions mediated by metal ions (Me). Membrane binding is mediated through a site in the C2 domain (shown in gold). Cleavage at residues 306 and 506 inactivates factor V by releasing two A2 fragments (iVa).

FACTOR VIII

Protein Structure

The domain organization of the factor VIII protein is A1-A2-B-A3-C1-C2, like that of factor V (Fig. 115–16). In factor VIII, the B domain does not appear to play a significant role in stability or activation. B-domainless

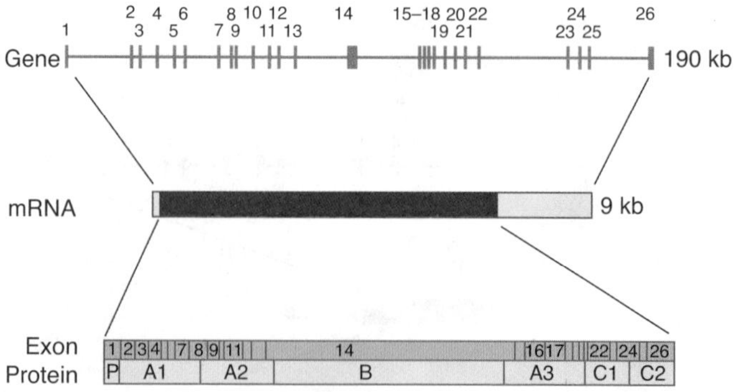

FIGURE 115–16. Relationship of gene structure to protein structure in factor VIII. The exons, introns, messenger ribonucleic acid (mRNA), and protein structure are as indicated. Promoter elements upstream from exon 1 are not shown but are discussed in the text. The mRNA is 9 kb with some 5′ untranslated sequence and a large 3′ untranslated region (light blue). In the protein, P indicates the propeptide leader sequence. The A domains have homology to ceruloplasmin. The C domains have homology to fat globule proteins. The B domain is released on activation and has no significant homology to any other identified protein.

factor VIII has been used successfully as a therapeutic agent in patients with classic hemophilia.

Factor VIII is synthesized in the liver,[98] although not in hepatocytes. Hepatic endothelial cells appear to be a major site of synthesis.[99] This conclusion is supported by the effects of transplantation in hemophilia A (factor VIII deficiency). Hemophilia A has been cured by liver transplantation in human and canine subjects.[100] However, spleen transplantation was not curative in a dog model.[101] Transplantation of isolated hepatocytes did not correct hemophilia A in a mouse model, but transplantation of a cellular fraction enriched in liver endothelial cells did.[102]

Factor VIII is secreted into the plasma as a heterogeneous collection of partially cleaved forms resulting from different cleavages in the B domain. Factor VIII circulates in a noncovalent complex with VWF. The normal half-life of factor VIII is 8 to 12 hours when associated with VWF. The half-life is markedly reduced in the absence of VWF, accounting for the reduced factor VIII levels observed in many patients with a deficiency of VWF.

Factor VIII is not secreted very efficiently from the cell. In addition to LMAN1 and MCDF2, several molecular chaperone proteins have been identified that appear to play a role in regulating transit of the large factor VIII protein through secretory and/or degradative pathways. Calnexin and calreticulin are chaperone proteins that preferentially interact with glycoproteins containing monoglucosylated N-linked oligosaccharides. These proteins bind to the heavily glycosylated B-domain of factor VIII and enhance both its intracellular degradation and secretion.[103] Factor V associates with calreticulin, but not calnexin. Factor VIII, but not factor V, also interacts through its A1-domain with another chaperone protein, immunoglobulin-binding protein (BiP). Association with BiP appears to enhance the stability of factor VIII, but also retards its secretion.[104]

Factor VIII has six tyrosine residues that are modified by sulfation (residues 346, 718, 719, 723, 1664, and 1680). Sulfation of these residues is required for optimal activation by thrombin, maximal activity in complex with factor IXa, and maximal affinity of factor VIIIa for VWF.

The acidic regions of factor VIII appear to promote activation by interacting with the anion-binding exosite of thrombin. In addition, the site for factor VIII binding to VWF is in the acidic domain in the light chain of factor VIII.[105]

Molecular Biology

The factor VIII gene is on the X chromosome at q28. Deficiency of factor VIII results in classic sex-linked hemophilia A. The factor VIII gene contains 26 exons (see Fig. 115–16), one more than factor V. Exon 5 of factor V corresponds to exons 5 and 6 of the factor VIII gene.[106] The gene for factor VIII is much larger than that for factor V, spanning approximately 190 kb. This is largely because six of the introns in the factor VIII gene are much larger than the corresponding introns in the factor V gene. The mRNA for factor VIII is also much larger than that for factor V because of a 1.8-kb 3′-untranslated region in the factor VIII message.

Activation and Activity

Factor VIII is activated by thrombin or factor Xa by cleavages at arginyl residues 372, 740, and 1689 (Fig. 115–17). This produces a heterotrimeric molecule consisting of A1 and A2 domains noncovalently linked with an A3-C1-C2 light chain through calcium ions. Activation also results in the release of factor VIIIa from VWF. The factor VIIIa molecule is thermodynamically unstable and dissociation of the A2 domain results in the spontaneous loss of activity. Factor VIIIa is also inactivated by thrombin or APC through additional cleavages at arginyl residues 336 and 562 (Fig. 115–17).

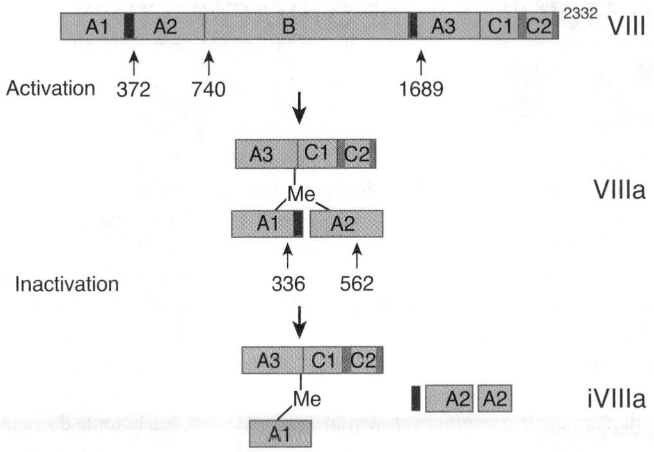

FIGURE 115–17. Activation and inactivation of factor VIII. For full cofactor activity, factor VIII requires cleavage by thrombin or factor Xa. The acidic domains, shown in dark blue, are believed to bind to the anion binding exosite in thrombin and enhance thrombin activation of factor VIII. The acidic domain in the A3 domain mediates VWF binding. The chains of factor VIIIa are held together by noncovalent interactions mediated by metal ions (Me). Factor VIIIa is thermodynamically unstable because the A2 domain can spontaneously dissociate from the complex. Membrane binding is mediated through sites in the C2 domain (shown in gold). Cleavages at residues 336 and 562 inactivate factor VIIIa, releasing the A2 fragments (iVIIIa).

VON WILLEBRAND FACTOR

Chapter 127 discusses the structure, molecular biology, and activities of VWF in greater detail.

Protein Structure and Activity

VWF is a large multimeric glycoprotein that serves as a carrier for factor VIII and is required for normal platelet adhesion to components of the vessel wall. It is synthesized as a prepropolypeptide with a 22-amino-acid signal sequence, a 741-amino-acid precursor polypeptide called VWF antigen II, and the mature VWF polypeptide chain.[107] The mature VWF protein contains three A domains, three B domains, two C domains, and four D domains. The A domains are structurally homologous to a family of proteins involved in extracellular matrix or cell-adhesive functions.[108] Factor VIII binds to the amino-terminal region of VWF, within the first 272 amino acids of the mature protein subunit.[109]

In the ER, the pro-VWF monomers form disulfide-stabilized dimers. The dimers move to the Golgi apparatus where they assemble into high-molecular-weight multimers, which are also held together by disulfide bonds. The propeptide is essential for multimerization to occur. It is usually removed before secretion of the mature VWF multimers. After secretion from its cells of origin, endothelial cells, VWF is further cleaved by a metalloprotease named ADAMTS13 (a disintegrin and metalloproteinase with thrombospondin domain 13).[110] The circulating VWF multimers range in size from Mr ~500,000 to larger than 20,000,000.[111] The higher-molecular-weight multimers are most effective in promoting platelet adhesion. However, all multimers can bind factor VIII and enhance its stability. The plasma half-life of VWF is approximately 12 hours.

Molecular Biology

The VWF gene is located on chromosome 12 and spans approximately 180 kb. It contains 52 exons.[112] VWF is synthesized only in endothelial cells and megakaryocytes.

FACTOR XI AND THE CONTACT FACTORS

■ FACTOR XI

Protein Structure

Factor XI, along with factor XII, high-molecular-weight kininogen (HK) and prekallikrein (PK) are sometimes referred to as the *contact factors*. Factor XI is a zymogen precursor of a serine protease. Factor XI circulates in complex with the nonenzymatic cofactor, HK.

Factor XI is synthesized in the liver and has a plasma mean half-life of approximately 52 hours. Although synthesized as a single chain, it circulates as a homodimer held together by a disulfide bond through Cys321 residues.[113] Each monomer has a Mr ~80,000, including approximately 5 percent carbohydrate and contains four repeats of a structural motif called an *apple domain*, as shown in Figure 115–18. Each apple domain contains 90 or 91 amino acids held together by 3 disulfide bonds. Specific functions have been assigned to the different apple domains within factor XI,[114–117] including sites for binding to HK, prothrombin, platelets, factor IX, thrombin, and factor XIIa.

Molecular Biology

The human factor XI gene is 23 kb in length and is localized to chromosome 4q32–35.[118] It consists of 15 exons and 14 introns (Fig. 115–19).[119] The gene lacks canonical CAAT and TATA boxes, which may account for the multiple transcription initiation sites that have been identified. Exon 1 encodes a 5′ untranslated region that is transcribed into mRNA, but not translated into protein. The signal peptide is encoded in exon 2. Each of the four apple domains is encoded in two exons. The light chain is encoded in five exons, with an organization similar to the homologous proteins PK, tissue plasminogen activator, urokinase, and factor XII. An HNF-4α binding site required for liver-specific expression is located between −375 and −363 bp.[120]

Activation and Activity

Factor XI can be activated by more than one mechanism *in vitro*. *In vitro*, factor XI can be activated by factor XIIa. In the fluid phase and on charged surfaces thrombin can activate factor XI even in the absence of the other contact factors.[121,122] Factor XI can also be activated by

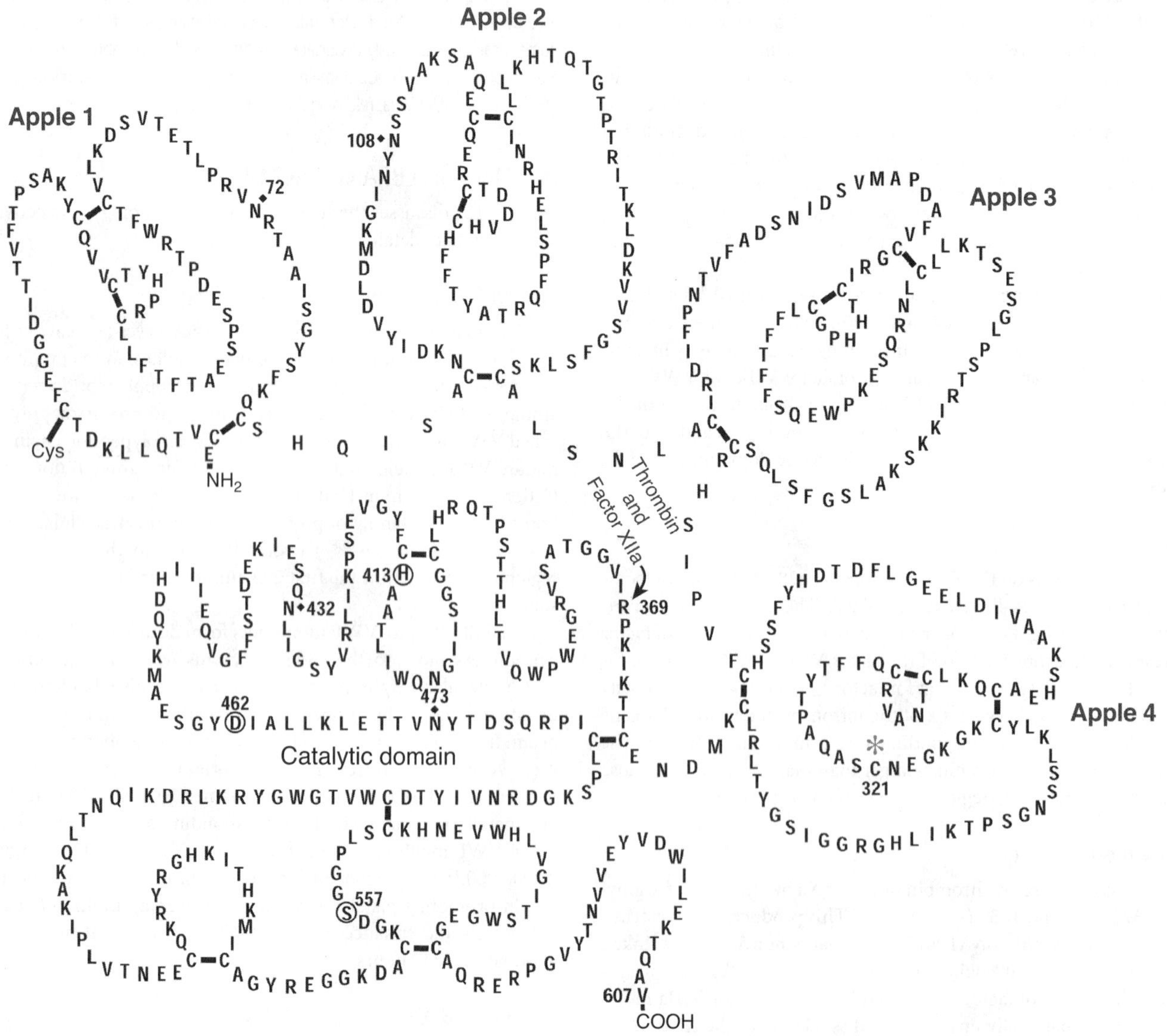

FIGURE 115–18. Domains of factor XI. Factor XI circulates as a dimer. The amino acids of one monomer are shown. The disulfide bond that links the factor XI homodimers is indicated by the asterisk at the Cys 321 residue in the fourth apple domain. The apple domains (A1–A4) are named for their appearance in this type of schematic. A free Cys in the Apple 1 domain is indicated. The active site His, Asp, and Ser residues are *circled*. The cleavage site for thrombin and factor XIIa is shown by the *arrow*.

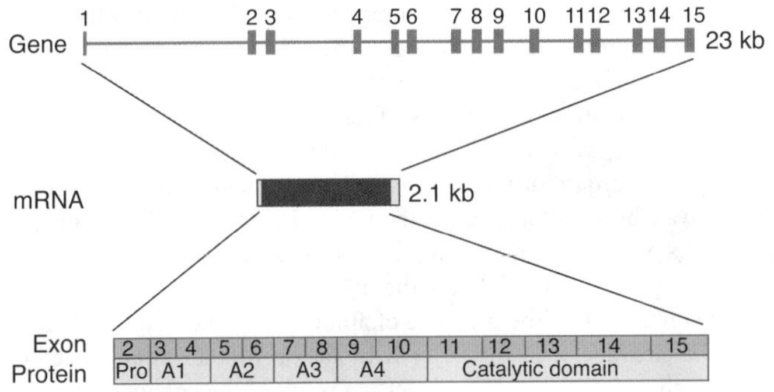

FIGURE 115–19. Relationship of gene structure to protein structure in factor XI. The exons, introns, messenger ribonucleic acid (mRNA), and protein structure are as indicated. The mRNA is 2.1 kb with a small 5′ and 3′ untranslated region (light blue). In the protein, Pro indicates the prepro leader sequence; A indicates apple domains.

thrombin on the surface of activated platelets, and this pathway is the most likely mechanism of activation during hemostasis *in vivo*.[123] At least in a mouse model, factor XI may play a more significant role in thrombosis than in hemostasis.[124]

As discussed below in the section "A Cell-Based Model of Coagulation," factor XI serves as a "booster" mechanism, enhancing platelet surface thrombin generation. Knockout of the factor XI gene in mice does not result in intrauterine death.[125] However, deficiencies of factor XI in humans can lead to a bleeding tendency,[126] although it is not as severe as in hemophilia A or B. This reflects the significant role of factor XI in hemostasis, in contrast to the other contact factors (see below).

Activation of factor XI by either factor XIIa or thrombin is caused by cleavage of the Arg369–Ile370 bond in the factor XI subunits. This yields two active sites in each factor XIa dimer. Each subunit has a heavy chain containing the apple domains and a light chain containing the catalytic domain (see Fig. 115–18). Both the heavy and light chains interact with the substrate, factor IX.[127] Factor XIa activation of factor IX is calcium dependent, but does not require any other cofactor. Factor XIa binds with high affinity to activated platelets and can activate factor IX with the same efficiency as unbound factor XIa.[128] Binding to activated platelets could serve to localize factor XIa to the site of clot formation, as well as protect it from plasma protease inhibitors.

Factor XIa is susceptible to inhibition by several plasma protease inhibitors that circulate in high concentrations. The Serpin protease nexin 1 has the highest affinity for factor XIa, followed by C1-esterase inhibitor, antithrombin, α_1-protease inhibitor, and α_2-plasmin inhibitor.[129] Platelets also contain a tight-binding Kunitz-type inhibitor of factor XIa, protease nexin 2.[130]

FACTOR XII, PREKALLIKEIN, AND HIGH-MOLECULAR-WEIGHT KININOGEN

Protein Structure

Factor XII and PK are zymogen precursors of proteases. PK has four apple domains, and is highly homologous to factor XI. Factor XII is homologous to plasminogen activators. HK is a nonenzymatic cofactor that circulates in complex with Factor XI and with PK. In addition to its nonenzymatic role in contact activation, HK acts as a thiol protease inhibitor and as an antiadhesive protein. HK is cleaved at two sites by kallikrein to release the bioactive nonapeptide bradykinin, a potent vasodilator. Table 115–1 shows the plasma levels, plasma half-lives, and chromosomal locations of factor XII, PK, and HK.[131] All three proteins are synthesized in the liver.

Molecular Biology

The gene for factor XII is located on chromosome 5q33-qter and spans approximately 12 kb. It contains 14 exons. The intron–exon structure of the gene is similar to the plasminogen activator family of serine proteases. Portions of the gene are homologous to domains found in fibronectin and tissue-type plasminogen activator. The gene for PK is located on chromosome 4q35, close to the factor XI gene. It spans 30 kb and has 15 exons with 14 introns and is homologous to the factor XI gene.[132] The gene for HK is located on chromosome 3 and contains 11 exons and spans 27 kb. HK and low-molecular-weight kininogen are produced from the same gene by alternative splicing. Both proteins serve as precursors to bradykinin, but low-molecular-weight kininogen has no interaction with the coagulation proteins.

Activation and Activity

Factor XII, HK, and PK are responsible for the contact activation of blood coagulation as seen in the activated partial thromboplastin time test (aPTT). In this clinical laboratory test, plasma is mixed with a reagent such as glass, kaolin, celite, or ellagic acid that provides a negatively charged surface. Contact activation involves both protein–protein and protein–surface interactions that lead to the activation of factor XII. Factor XIIa activates factor XI, which then activates factor IX. In spite of the fact that factor XII, HK, and PK are required for a normal aPTT, they do not appear to be required for normal hemostasis. Individuals who are deficient in any of these factors do not have a bleeding tendency, even after significant trauma or surgery. However, factor XII, HK, and PK, along with complement factor C1q, do participate in inflammatory responses that involve the blood clotting system, fibrinolysis, and generation of kinins.[133,134] Targeted deletion of factor XII in a mouse model does not impair hemostasis,[135] but does result in reduced generation of inflammatory mediators. Factor XII deficiency is associated with an increased tendency toward thrombosis in animal models,[136,137] and perhaps in patients.[138,139] Thus, activation of the contact factors likely plays a much greater role in thrombosis than hemostasis. The available data suggest that the contact system may normally function on the surface of endothelial cells. PK and factor XI, through its binding to HK, assemble on a multiprotein receptor complex on endothelial cells.[140] PK is activated to kallikrein by a membrane-expressed carboxypeptidase, releasing bradykinin in the process. Kallikrein activates factor XII, which, in turn, initiates fibrinolysis by activating urokinase. Thus, activation of the contact system *in vivo* on cell surfaces is mechanistically quite different from activation on a charged surface in the aPTT. The kallikrein/kinin system has been hypothesized to serve *in vivo* as a physiologic counterbalance to the renin–angiotensin system by lowering blood pressure and preventing thrombosis.[141]

CELL-ASSOCIATED COFACTORS

TISSUE FACTOR

Protein Structure

TF is the cellular receptor and cofactor for factor VII and VIIa (see Fig. 115–4). TF is composed of 263 amino acids, and consists of a 219-amino-acid extracellular domain, a 23-residue transmembrane portion, and a 21-residue intracytoplasmic domain (Fig. 115–20).[142] A cysteine in the intracytoplasmic domain is linked to a palmityl fatty acid, which downregulates phosphorylation of the cytoplasmic domain.[143] Although many of the coagulation factors share a high degree of homology, the structure of TF is unique. It is the only one of the procoagulant proteins that is an integral membrane protein, and it is homologous to the type 2

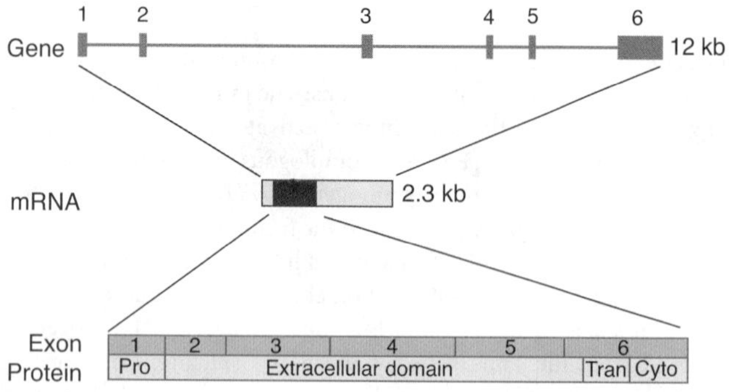

FIGURE 115–20. Relationship of gene structure to protein structure in tissue factor. The exons, introns, messenger ribonucleic acid (mRNA), and protein structure are as indicated. The mRNA is 2.3 kb with 5′ untranslated region and a large 3′ untranslated region (light blue). Pro indicates the prepro leader sequence; Tran indicates the transmembrane region; Cyto indicates the cytoplasmic domain.

cytokine receptors.[144] This family includes the receptors for interleukin-10 and interferons α, β, and γ. The extracellular domain of TF complexed with factor VIIa has been crystallized, and the extracellular domain has been found to fold in a manner typical of the cytokine receptor homology unit (see Fig. 115–4).[22,145] These structural features suggest that TF may be a multifunctional protein with both signal transducing and procoagulant functions.

Molecular Biology

The human TF gene is located on chromosome 1p21-p22.[146] The DNA sequence of the TF gene has been determined and consists of 6 exons and 5 introns that span approximately 12 kb.[147] The first exon codes for the signal peptide, whereas the second through fifth encode the extracellular domain. The sixth exon codes for the transmembrane and cytoplasmic domains, as well as a relatively long 3′ untranslated region. An alternatively spliced form of TF that lacks the membrane-anchoring domain has been described in humans and mice.[148,149] It is reported to be present in the blood and to possess cofactor activity, but its role in hemostasis or thrombosis remains to be clarified.

The initiation site for transcription of the TF gene is well defined, and the region with promoter activity is from −383 to −121 bp relative to the start site.[150] The promoter contains a serum response element with a putative binding site for Sp-1, and a lipopolysaccharide responsive element with AP-1 and nuclear factor κB (NF-κB)-like sites.

TF is expressed constitutively on many extravascular tissues. Although it is not normally expressed by cells in contact with flowing blood, TF expression can be induced on blood monocytes by bacterial products, inflammatory cytokines, and engagement of P-selectin glycoprotein ligand-1 on monocytes.[151–154] Small amounts of TF protein have been reported to be present in platelets, but the physiologic and/or pathophysiologic roles of this phenomenon are not yet clear.[155]

Activation and Activity

The factor VIIa/TF complex is thought to be the major physiologic initiator of blood coagulation. TF is normally expressed on pericytes surrounding blood vessels and by epidermal, stromal, and glial cells.[156,157] It has also been shown that monocytes, which normally have no TF activity, can express TF when exposed to vessel media or collagen.[158] The process of coagulation is initiated when an injury ruptures a vessel and allows blood to come in to contact with extravascular TF. It is often said that release of blood from the vessel allows factor VII to bind to extravascular TF and initiate coagulation. However, it is very likely that TF around vessels in most sites already has bound factor VIIa in the absence of injury.[159] An injury allows the extravascular factor VIIa/TF complexes to come into contact with platelets, and initiate large-scale thrombin generation on platelet surfaces.

The binding of factor VIIa to TF enhances its proteolytic activity almost three orders of magnitude.[160,161] The factor VIIa/TF complex can activate both factor IX and factor X.[162] However, unlike binding of factor IXa or Xa to their cofactors, binding of factor VIIa to TF does not strictly require calcium,[163] and the affinity of the interaction is only slightly enhanced by the presence of anionic phospholipid.[164,165] However, the cleavage of factor IX or X by factor VIIa/TF is enhanced by anionic phospholipid.[165] This effect is a result of the enhanced binding of the substrate, rather than of any effect of the phospholipid on the catalytic efficiency of the VIIa/TF complex.

The affinity of factor VIIa binding for TF on cells is very high (20–80 pM). Binding of factor VIIa to TF that is reconstituted into synthetic phospholipid vesicles always results in enhanced factor VIIa proteolytic activity. However, binding of factor VIIa to cellular sources of TF does not always correlate with enhanced enzymatic activity. This suggests that cells can regulate the cofactor activity of TF in a manner that is not reproduced by synthetic phospholipid vesicles.

TF does not require proteolytic activation to express its activity. However, it appears that TF can occur in a latent or "encrypted" form[166,167]; that is, TF detected as antigen on the cell surface may not express detectable clotting activity. It has been hypothesized that the TF could form dimers that block access to the substrate binding site on TF. Dimerized ("encrypted") TF could still bind factor VII, but would be inactive because it could not bind either factor IX or X. The physiologic regulators that control TF encryption are not clear and it remains to be determined whether this is an important regulatory mechanism *in vivo*.

In addition to its role as a cofactor in coagulation, tissue factor is thought to play important roles in cell signaling. This signaling can occur both through proteolytic activity of factor VIIa bound to tissue factor[168] and through the formation of a VIIa/TF/Xa complex.[169] This cell signaling has been suggested to play important roles in the cell migration needed for wound healing, inflammation, and vasculogenesis. The importance of this signaling in vasculogenesis is suggested by the observation that mice in which the tissue factor gene has been knocked out die during embryonic development partly as a result of disorganization of the yolk sac vasculature.[170]

THROMBOMODULIN

Protein Structure

Thrombomodulin is a transmembrane protein of Mr of 78,000.[171] It is the cellular cofactor for thrombin.[172] TM has a leader sequence followed by lectin-like domains homologous to the asialoglycoprotein receptor (Fig. 115–21).[173] However, TM has no known lectin-like activity. Following the lectin-like domain are six EGF-like domains, the fourth, fifth, and sixth of which are responsible for both thrombin-binding and protein-C activating activities (Fig. 115–21).[174] A serine- and threonine-rich region follows the EGF domains and is the site of O-linked glycosylation. A chondroitin sulfate moiety, which enhances TM anticoagulant activity, is attached to Ser492 in this region.[175] The 23-amino-acid transmembrane domain follows the serine and threonine-rich region, followed by a short cytoplasmic tail.

Molecular Biology

The human TM gene is located on chromosome 20p12-cen[176] and spans approximately 3.5 kb. It consists of a single exon (see Fig. 115–21). Intronless genes are uncommon and include rhodopsin, angiogenin,

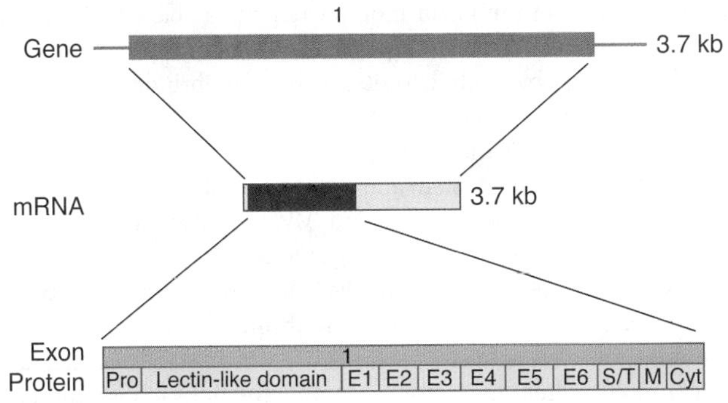

FIGURE 115–21. Relationship of gene structure to protein structure in thrombomodulin. The thrombomodulin gene has no introns. It covers 3.7 kb on chromosome 20 (p12-centromere). The messenger ribonucleic acid (mRNA) is the same size, with a small 5′ untranslated region and a large 3′ untranslated region (light blue). In the protein, Pro indicates the prepro leader sequence; E indicates epidermal growth factor-like domains; S/T indicates a serine, threonine-rich region; M indicates the transmembrane region; and Cyt indicates the cytoplasmic domain.

mitochondrial genes, interferons α- and β-adrenergic receptors. The functional significance of the lack of introns is not known.

Activation and Activity

Thrombin can cleave a number of substrates without a cofactor, such as fibrinogen, factors V and VIII, and the protease-activated thrombin receptors. However, binding to the cofactor TM localizes thrombin to endothelial cell surfaces and induces a conformational change such that its ability to activate protein C is enhanced 1000- to 2000-fold. Thrombin bound to TM no longer activates platelets, nor does it cleave fibrinogen or activate factor V or factor VIII.[177] Thus, TM changes the activity of thrombin from procoagulant to anticoagulant. TM also enhances the ability of thrombin to activate TAFI.[34]

TM is expressed on the surface of vascular endothelial cells. In conjunction with EPCR, TM appears to play a major role in preventing thrombosis from occurring on intact endothelium in the microcirculation.[178] In mice, knocking out either TM or EPCR creates an embryonically lethal phenotype correlated with increased placental fibrin deposition.[179,180] TM has also been detected in mesothelial cells,[181] mononuclear phagocytes,[182] squamous epithelium,[183] megakaryocytes, and malignant cells,[36,184] where its function is unknown. The level of TM expression differs among endothelial cells from different sites.[185] Endothelial TM and TF expression are regulated by inflammatory cytokines in a reciprocal fashion. Thus, thrombosis may be favored at sites of inflammation by a concurrent elevation of endothelial TF and depression of endothelial TM.

Protein C inhibitor is an effective inhibitor of the thrombin/TM complex.[186]

FIBRINOGEN

Protein Structure

Fibrinogen, when converted to fibrin, forms the structural meshwork that consolidates an initial platelet plug into a solid hemostatic clot. The physiologic importance of fibrinogen is underscored by the bleeding diathesis associated with afibrinogenemia[187,188] and some dysfibrinogenemias[189] (see Chap. 126). Other dysfibrinogenemias are associated with thromboembolic disease.[188,190] Although afibrinogenemia is associated with a bleeding tendency, it is usually not as severe as classical hemophilia. This is possibly explained by findings in mice demonstrating that fibronectin can accumulate in platelets and assume the adhesive functions of fibrinogen to a limited extent.[191]

Fibrinogen is a dimeric glycoprotein whose dominant form has an Mr of 340,000. It is found in plasma and in platelet α granules. Each of the two subunits contains three disulfide-linked polypeptide chains[192] that are referred to as the Aα (Mr 66,500), Bβ (Mr 52,000), and γ (Mr 46,500) chains. Fibrinopeptides A and B are released from the amino termini of the Aα and Bβ chains by thrombin cleavage of the Argl6-Glyl7 and Argl4-Glyl5 bonds, respectively.[193] The central globular domain of fibrinogen is called the E-domain. It includes the disulfide-linked amino-termini of all six polypeptide chains referred to as the N-terminal disulfide knot.[194] The E domain is linked by helical, coiled-coil domains to the carboxy-terminal globular domains of the three chains, designated the D domains. A trinodular model of fibrinogen structure has been established from the crystal structure of fibrinogen (Fig. 115–22).[195] N-linked glycosylation occurs at Asn364 of the Bβ chain and Asn52 of the γ chain.

Because human fibrinogen is subject to modification at a number of different sites both during and after biosynthesis, the fibrinogen present in the circulation is a heterogeneous mixture of molecules. These normal variants are caused by alternative splicing, modification of certain amino acids by sulfation, phosphorylation, and hydroxylation, different degrees of glycosylation, and proteolysis. It has been estimated that the number of nonidentical fibrinogen molecules that can be produced by these mechanisms is in excess of 1 million.[196] Some of these variations may have significant functional consequences. For example, the level of one variant of fibrinogen with an alternatively spliced γ chain (fibrinogen-γ) is associated with a decreased risk of venous thrombosis,[197,198] but an increased risk of myocardial infarction.[199]

In normal individuals, the plasma half-life of fibrinogen is 3 to 5 days,[200] with only a small proportion of the catabolism caused by consumption. Plasma fibrinogen is synthesized in the liver. Fibrinogen is an acute-phase reactant and its synthesis can be increased up to 20-fold with a strong inflammatory stimulus.[201,202] Interleukin-6 (IL-6) is an important mediator of increased fibrinogen synthesis during an acute-phase response,[203] and IL-6 secretion can be upregulated by fibrin(ogen)-degradation products.

Molecular Biology

The genes for the three chains of fibrinogen are found within a 50-kb length of DNA on chromosome 4 at q23-q32[204] (Fig. 115–23). The genes for all three chains have been sequenced. The genomic sequences show a high degree of homology, suggesting they were derived through

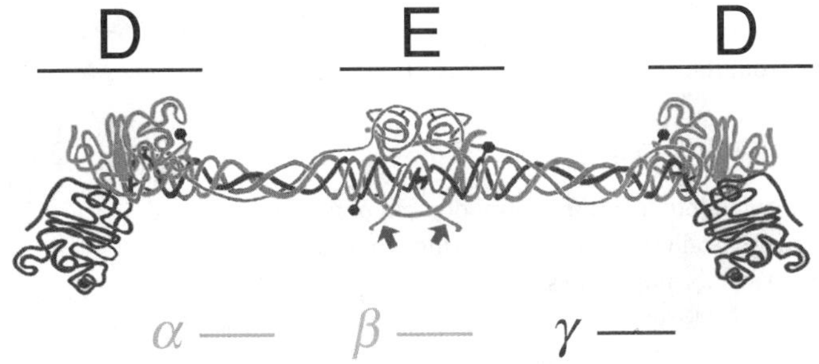

FIGURE 115–22. Structure of fibrinogen. Fibrinogen is a dimer. Each dimer consists of three chains: Aα shown in light blue, Bβ shown in pink, and γ shown in dark blue. The disulfides that link the two dimers are in the central E domain. The D domains consist primarily of the carboxy-terminal regions of the Bβ and γ chains. The helical region connecting the two domains consists of all three chains intertwined. *(From HC Côté, ST Lord, KP Pratt,[195a] with permission.)*

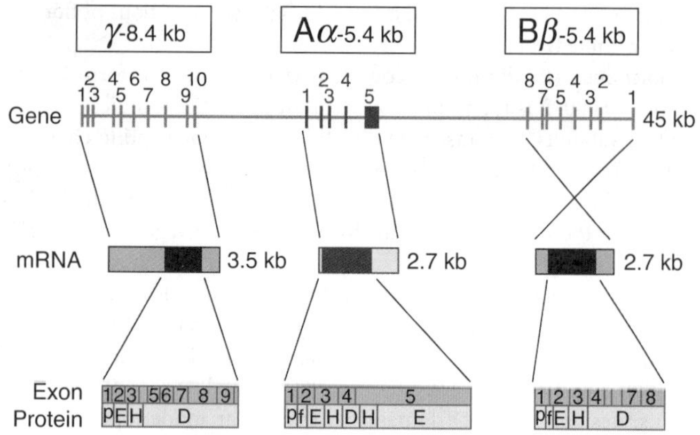

FIGURE 115–23. Relationship of gene structure to protein structure in fibrinogen. The exons, introns, messenger ribonucleic acid (mRNA), and protein structure for the three chains of fibrinogen are shown. The Bβ chain is translated in the opposite direction from the Aα and γ chains. Lighter colors in the mRNA indicate 5′ and 3′ untranslated regions. In the proteins, P designates the prepro leader sequence; f designates fibrinopeptide (A in Aα and B in Bβ); E designates residues in the E domain; H designates residues in the helical connecting region; and D designates residues in the D domain.

duplication of a common ancestral gene.[205,206] The homology extends to sites upstream of the gene, suggesting that common regulatory elements may reside in these areas, thus helping to coordinate synthesis of the three chains.[207]

Studies of tissue-specific expression and acute-phase regulation of the mRNA of the fibrinogen chains have revealed some surprises. The expression of the γ chain is regulated by ubiquitous factors such as SP1, whereas transcription of the Aα and Bβ genes requires the liver-specific factor HNF-1.[208] The Bβ-chain promoter contains an IL-6–responsive element[209] that appears to be present in the upstream sequences of the other chains as well. Because of the differences in the promoter regions of the genes for the three chains, the tissue distribution differs. The highest levels of mRNA for all three chains are found in the liver. However, γ-chain transcripts have been found in a number of organs that lack transcripts of the other chains. mRNA for Aα and Bβ has been found in the kidney, consistent with the presence of HNF-1 in kidney.[210]

Because of the presence of fibrinogen in the α granules of platelets, it was initially assumed that megakaryocytes synthesized fibrinogen. However, although some γ-chain transcripts are present in marrow precursors, it appears that most of the fibrinogen found within platelets is taken up from the plasma by endocytosis (see Chap. 114).[211,212]

Activation and Activity

Thrombin binds to the central domain of fibrinogen[213] and proteolytically releases two fibrinopeptides A (Aα 1–16) and two fibrinopeptides B (Bβ 1–14) from each fibrinogen molecule. Release of the fibrinopeptides exposes binding sites in the E domain that have complementary sites in the D domains of other fibrin monomers.[214,215] These complementary binding sites lead to the initial formation of two-stranded protofibrils with a half-staggered overlap configuration (Fig. 115–24). Protofibrils then aggregate into thick fibers consisting of 14 to 22 protofibrils that branch into a meshwork of interconnected thick fibers.[216] The half-staggered overlap of the fibrin monomers gives a characteristic cross-banded pattern on electron micrographs.[217] Calcium appears to enhance lateral fiber growth by binding to sites on human fibrinogen.[218,219]

During fibrin monomer polymerization, other plasma proteins also bind to the surface of the developing meshwork. These include elements of the fibrinolytic system and a variety of adhesive proteins, such as fibronectin, thrombospondin, and VWF. These surface proteins influence the generation, cross-linking, and lysis of fibrin. Fibrin(ogen) also has specific integrin-binding sites that are essential for platelet binding (see Chaps. 114 and 126). The thrombin that initiates fibrin polymerization also activates factor XIII, which stabilizes the fibrin polymer by cross-linking. Factor XIIIa also crosslinks other bound proteins, for example, plasminogen activator-1, vitronectin, fibronectin, and α_2-antiplasmin, to the fibrin network.

Once formed, the fibrin mesh can be degraded by the fibrinolytic system. Plasmin cleaves fibrin and fibrinogen in an ordered sequence at arginyl and lysyl bonds, giving rise to a series of soluble degradation products.[220] The plasmin digestion of fibrinogen initially cleaves the Aα polar appendage and the Bβ 1–42 fragment, generating fragment X (Mr 250,000), which can still form a clot, albeit slowly. Further action of plasmin releases a D fragment (Mr 100,000) from fragment X to form fragment Y (Mr 150,000). Fragment Y is further cleaved to form another fragment D and a fragment E (Mr 50,000). Similar fragments are generated during plasmin digestion of cross-linked fibrin, with two exceptions: (1) the Bβ 15–42 is released from the des 1–14 Bβ chain of fibrin, and (2) D-dimer and other covalently cross-linked degradation products are cleaved from the cross-linked fibrin polymer. Monoclonal antibodies recognizing the fibrin D-dimer fragments can help to discriminate fibrin-degradation products from fibrinogen-degradation products.[221] Although the large X fragment can still polymerize into a weak clot,[222] the smaller Y and D fragments inhibit normal fibrin monomer polymerization.[223] The inhibition of polymerization can prolong the thrombin time and lead to spuriously low values of fibrinogen when measured by thrombin-dependent clotting assays.

In addition to its obvious procoagulant role in stabilizing the initial platelet hemostatic plug, fibrin can also act as an important inhibitor of thrombin generation. Fibrin functions as "antithrombin I" by sequestering thrombin in the developing fibrin clot, and also by reducing the catalytic activity of fibrin-bound thrombin.[224]

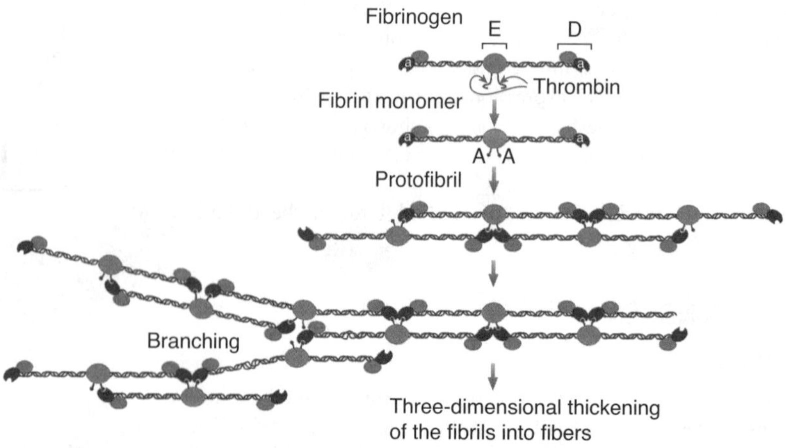

FIGURE 115–24. Cleavage of fibrinogen and polymerization of fibrin. The structure of fibrinogen is indicated schematically. Cleavage sites for fibrinopeptide A by thrombin are shown. Cleavage of the B peptide is not shown in this figure. Release of fibrinopeptide A exposes binding sites in the E domain that match complementary sites in the D domain. Fibrin monomers polymerize by half-staggered overlaps. Polymerization can also lead to branched structures. *(From HC Côté, ST Lord, KP Pratt,[195a] with permission.)*

FACTOR XIII

Protein Structure

Factor XIII is a 320,000 Mr glycoprotein composed of A and B subunits with a plasma half-life of approximately 10 days. It is a protransglutaminase that is activated by thrombin in the presence of calcium.[225] The A chain contains the cysteine active site, whereas the B chain is not enzymatically active and functions as a carrier protein. The cDNA and protein sequences of both subunits have been determined.[226–228]

The factor XIII A chain is a unique member of the transglutaminase family, which is composed of calcium- and thiol-dependent enzymes found in all human tissues and fluids. Factor XIIIa crosslinks proteins between the γ-carbon of glutamine in one protein and the ε amino group of lysine in the other. The A chain contains 731 amino acids with a Mr of ~83,000 (Fig. 115–25).

The factor XIII B chain is homologous to complement regulatory proteins. It is synthesized as a chain of 661 amino acids starting with a signal peptide. The mature B chain comprises 641 amino acids,[228] with a Mr of ~76,500, including 8.5 percent carbohydrate. The B chain contains 10 short consensus repeat (SCR) units (also called GP-1 or Sushi domains; Fig. 115–26). Each SCR contains 60 to 70 amino acids, containing 4 conserved cysteine residues with a characteristic pattern of disulfide bonds.[229] In plasma, the B subunit is found in molar excess over the A component. So all circulating A subunit is bound to B subunit. The B subunit can also be found free in circulation.

In addition to plasma, factor XIII also is present in platelets, monocytes, and monocyte-derived macrophages. The plasma factor is a heterotetramer consisting of paired A and B subunits (A2B2). In platelet and other cells, factor XIII exists as an A2 dimer and lacks the B domain. Monocytes/macrophages can synthesize factor XIII,[230] and the factor XIII found in platelets is probably synthesized by megakaryocytes.[231] Cells of marrow origin seem to be the primary site for the synthesis of subunit A in plasma factor XIII, but hepatocytes might also contribute.[225] The B subunit of plasma factor XIII is synthesized in the liver.

Molecular Biology

The factor XIII A chain gene has been localized to chromosome 6 p24-p25.[232] It contains 15 exons and 14 introns and is larger than 160 kb in size (see Fig. 115–25).[227] The fibrin-binding domain is encoded by exons 2 to 12. The active site, with its reactive thiol at Cys314, is present in exon 7. Although the structure of the factor XIII A-chain gene is quite similar to that of other transglutaminases, it has unique regulatory

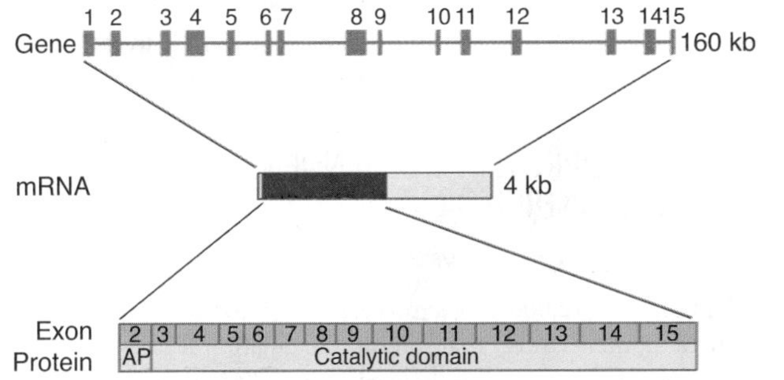

FIGURE 115–25. Relationship of gene structure to protein structure in the factor XIII A chain. The exons, messenger ribonucleic acid (mRNA), and protein structure for the factor XIII A chain are shown (taken from the National Center for Biotechnology Information submission Gene ID 2162, F13A1). The mRNA is 4 kb with some 5′ untranslated sequence coded in exon 1 and a large 3′ untranslated region (light blue). In the protein, AP indicates the activation peptide.

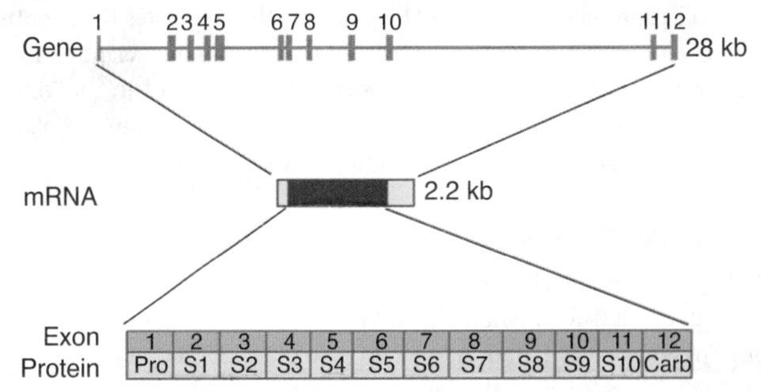

FIGURE 115–26. Relationship of gene structure to protein structure in the factor XIII B chain. The exons, introns, messenger ribonucleic acid (mRNA), and protein structure are as indicated. The mRNA is 2.2 kb with small 3′ and 5′ untranslated noncoding regions (light blue). In the protein, Pro indicates the propeptide; S indicates sushi (SCR) domains. The carboxy-terminal region is indicated by carb.

mechanisms. Transcription is regulated by a myeloid-enriched transcription factor (MZF-1–like protein) and two ubiquitous transcription factors (NF-1 and SP-1).[233] The myeloid-enriched factor GATA-1 acts as an enhancer, as does Ets-1. The transcription initiation site for the A-chain is 76 bp upstream from the first intron–exon boundary.[233]

The factor XIII B chain has been localized to chromosome 1q31-q32.1. It has 12 exons separated by 11 introns and is about 28 kb in size (see Fig. 115–26).[226] Each SCR is encoded by a single exon. The regulation of the factor XIII B-chain expression is poorly understood. A total of 30 potential start sites are located upstream of the initial methionine.

Activation and Activity

Plasma factor XIII circulates in association with its substrate, fibrinogen. The key step in the activation of plasma factor XIII is thrombin cleavage of the Arg37-Gly38 bond in the A chain to release a Mr 4500 activation peptide. This leads to dissociation of the A and B subunits and exposure of the active site on the free A subunits. Cellular factor XIII in platelets becomes activated through a nonproteolytic process. When intracytoplasmic Ca^{2+} is elevated during platelet activation, the zymogen, in the absence of the B-chain, assumes an active configuration.[225] The main physiologic function of plasma factor XIIIa is to crosslink the α and γ chains of fibrin to stabilize the fibrin plug.[234] In the absence of factor XIII a clot forms, but is inadequate for hemostasis. Additional protein substrates of factor XIIIa include components of the clotting and fibrinolytic system, as well as multiple adhesive and contractile proteins. Factor XIIIa also protects fibrin from fibrinolysis by crosslinking it to α_2-antiplasmin.[235] Plasma factor XIII is also involved in wound healing and tissue repair, and is essential to maintaining pregnancy.

THROMBIN-ACTIVATABLE FIBRINOLYSIS INHIBITOR

Protein Structure

TAFI is the zymogen precursor to a zinc-bound metalloprotease, and has been called carboxypeptidase B, R, and U in the literature. It has an Mr of 60,000 with 20 percent of that mass a result of carbohydrate attached to 4 sites within the first 92 amino acids. In sequence alignments with other members of the carboxypeptidase A family, active site residues (Glu 271 and Arg 125), and zinc-binding residues (His 67, Glu 70, and His 196) in TAFI are conserved.

Molecular Biology

The gene for TAFI has been localized to 13q14. The gene contains 11 exons with 10 introns and spans 48 kb.[236] TAFI is synthesized in the liver.

The TAFI promoter has a C/EBP binding site that regulates liver synthesis.[237] The promoter lacks a consensus TATA box and transcription is initiated from multiple sites. Plasma concentration of TAFI in individuals can vary from 4 to 15 mcg/mL with a strong correlation between plasma levels and polymorphisms in the promoter and 3′ region.[238]

Activation and Activity

TAFI is activated by cleavage by plasmin or thrombin, a reaction that is accelerated 1000-fold when thrombin is bound to thrombomodulin. Both enzymes cleave after Arg-92 to give a Mr 37,000 activated form (TAFIa) with release of the large activation peptide. TAFIa catalyzes removal of carboxy-terminal lysine and arginine residues from fibrin and fibrin cleavage products. These residues are important for binding and activation of plasminogen. Removal of these residues by TAFIa reduces clot catalyzed formation of plasmin resulting in decreased clot lysis. TAFIa may also have an antiinflammatory role as it can efficiently cleave bradykinin. A polymorphism in TAFI is associated with lower blood pressure in individuals homozygous for this polymorphism.[239]

Inhibitors of TAFIa have not been identified, however the molecule is thermodynamically unstable with a half-life at 37°C (98.6°F) of less than 15 minutes.[240]

INHIBITORS

There are many protease inhibitors in plasma, but the two most specifically involved in inhibition of coagulation factors are TFPI and AT (see Table 115–4). The protein Z/protein Z-dependent protease inhibitor (ZPI) system is also emerging as a potentially important regulator of the coagulation system.[241]

Chapter 116 discusses coagulation inhibitors in detail.

TISSUE FACTOR PATHWAY INHIBITOR

Protein Structure and Activity

TFPI is a single-chain polypeptide with a Mr of 34,000 to 40,000, depending upon the degree of proteolysis of the carboxy-terminal region. TFPI contains three Kunitz-type protease inhibitor domains. The second Kunitz domain binds and inhibits factor Xa; this is required for the first Kunitz domain to bind and inhibit the factor VIIa/TF complex. The function of the third Kunitz domain is not clear, but it may be involved in binding to glycosaminoglycans. Thus, TFPI is unique among the coagulation protease inhibitors in two respects. First, it has inhibitory sites for both factor Xa and for the factor VIIa/TF complex. Second, TFPI cannot inhibit the factor VIIa/TF complex unless it has also bound factor Xa.[242,243]

The primary site of plasma TFPI synthesis is endothelial cells.[244] Most circulating TFPI is bound to lipoproteins. A second pool of TFPI is bound to heparan sulfates on the surface of endothelial cells. Administration of heparin releases the endothelial cell bound TFPI and raises the plasma level severalfold.[245] A third pool is an alternatively spliced form of TFPI (TFPI-β) that is anchored to endothelial cells via a glycosyl phosphatidylinositol linkage.[246]

TFPI is only present in the plasma at about 2.5 nM, compared to AT at about 2 μM. However, its rate of reaction with factor Xa in plasma is similar to that of AT. Therefore, TFPI contributes significantly to the inhibition of factor Xa *in vivo*.

Molecular Biology

The gene for human TFPI is located on chromosome 2q31-q32.1 and has 9 exons that span 70 kb. The first two exons code for a 5′ untranslated region, and coding begins at exon 3. No TATA box is present in the promoter region of the TFPI gene. DNA sequences that are consistent with binding sites for the transcription factors GATA-2, AP-1, and NF-1 are present in the 5′ untranslated region of the TFPI gene. It is thought that GATA-2 binding is necessary for constitutive expression of TFPI by endothelial cells.[244]

TFPI is synthesized in two alternatively spliced forms, α and β. TFPI-β lacks the third Kunitz domain and instead has a unique carboxy-terminal. TFPI-α is the predominant form in circulation. Although a significant fraction of TFPI-β is linked to the endothelial cells via a glycosyl phosphatidylinositol anchor,[246] it is also found in plasma and has inhibitory activity similar to that of TFPI-α.[247]

ANTITHROMBIN

Protein Structure and Activity

AT is a member of the large family of serine protease inhibitors (serpins) and in the systematic nomenclature is SERPINC1. These inhibitors act as "suicide" substrates for their target proteases through a surface-exposed structure termed a *reactive site loop*. An amino acid sequence in the reactive site loop of AT is cleaved by the target protease to form a 1:1 covalent complex that blocks the active site of the protease. AT is an important physiologic inhibitor of the blood coagulation proteases, as its deficiency leads to a significantly increased risk of thrombosis. The primary proteases targeted by AT are thrombin, factor Xa, and factor IXa.[248–250] Inhibition of these proteases is accelerated by heparin. Factor VIIa is resistant to inhibition by AT unless it is complexed to TF in the presence of heparin or cell surface glycosaminoglycans.[251,252]

Heparin and related molecules accelerate inhibition of proteases by AT by two distinct mechanisms, as illustrated in Figure 115–27. As shown in the middle panel, binding of a specific pentasaccharide sequence in a heparin molecule results in a conformational change in the AT molecule that increases the accessibility of the reactive site loop to a target protease. This results in an increased rate of inhibition of proteases by AT. In addition, as shown in the right panel of the figure, a larger heparin molecule can bind to both AT and a target protease. This serves to align the two molecules and facilitates their interaction, again increasing the rate of inhibition of the protease by AT.

The protease–serpin complex is cleared from the circulation by receptor-mediated endocytosis in the liver.[253]

Molecular Biology

The gene for AT is on the long arm of chromosome 1. The gene has seven exons and spans about 13.5 kb. Little is known about transcriptional regulation of AT. The region from −89 to −68 has been implicated in the binding of transcription factors from rat liver,[254] but the specific transcription factors involved are not clear.

PROTEIN Z/PROTEIN Z-DEPENDENT PROTEASE INHIBITOR

Protein Structure and Activity

The ZPI is a Mr 72,000 serine protease inhibitor (SERPINA10 in the systematic nomenclature) that inhibits coagulation factors XIa and Xa. Its inhibition of factor Xa is enhanced over 1000-fold in the presence of a vitamin K-dependent plasma protein, protein Z.[255] Protein Z is a plasma glycoprotein of Mr 62,000. Like the other GLA-containing proteins, it consists of a GLA domain, hydrophobic region, and two EGF domains. However, instead of a catalytic domain, the carboxy-terminal region of protein Z contains a domain that, while homologous to the catalytic domain of the other GLA containing proteins, lacks the His

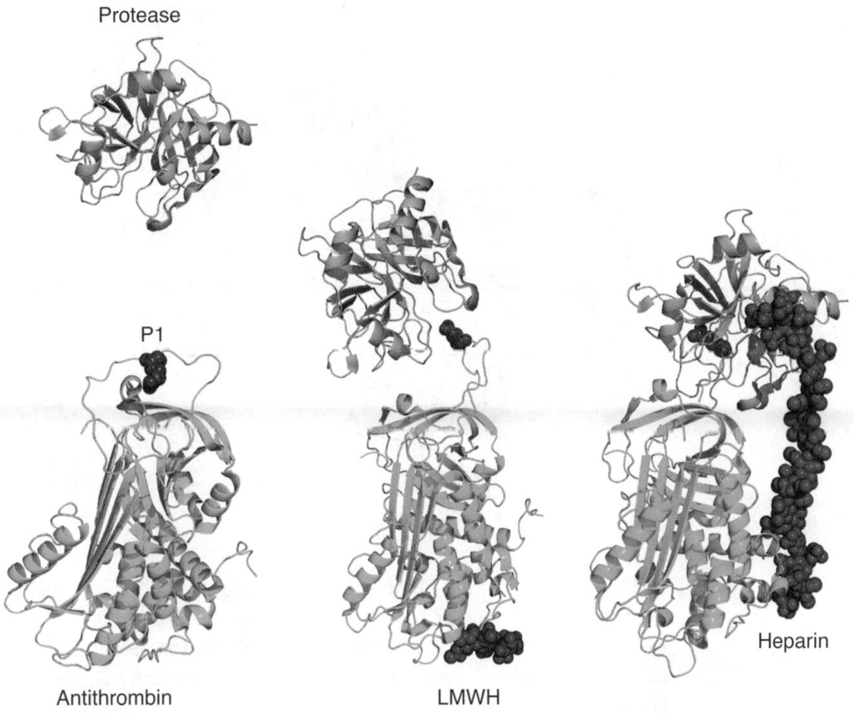

FIGURE 115–27. Effect of glycosaminoglycans on antithrombin inhibition. *Left panel:* Protease (cyan) and antithrombin (green) structures are shown as cartoons. The red spheres show the location in the reactive loop of the P1 residue that binds to the target protease (thrombin). *Middle panel:* Binding of a specific pentasaccharide sequence (blue) to antithrombin alters the flexibility of the reactive loop and increases exposure of the P1 residue, enhancing the rate of interaction with the target protease (allosteric effect). *Right panel:* If a heparin molecule (blue) is sufficiently long, the target protease (thrombin) can bind to heparin in a proper orientation to also bind the P1 residue of antithrombin (template effect). Models were created in the program PyMol (www.pymol.org) from PDB structures 1T1F, 2GD4, and 1TB6.

and Ser residues characteristic of the catalytic triad of trypsin-like serine proteases. Thus, protein Z has no protease activity. In normal plasma, which has a molar excess of ZPI over protein Z, all protein Z circulates in complex with ZPI.[256]

The physiologic role of protein Z/ZPI in the coagulation system is not yet clear. Deficiency of protein Z in a mouse model does not lead to thrombosis, but dramatically worsens the thrombotic tendency of mice who simultaneously express the factor V Leiden genotype, a known risk factor for thrombosis.[257]

Molecular Biology

The chromosomal location of the gene for ZPI is not known. The gene for protein Z is on the long arm of chromosome 13 (q34) in close proximity to the genes for factor X and factor VII.[3] The gene spans 14 kb and consists of 9 exons and 8 introns. The intron/exon boundaries are identical to the other GLA-containing coagulation proteins. There is an alternative exon that codes for a unique peptide of 22 amino acids in the preproleader sequence. The gene is transcribed into a 1.6 kb mRNA.

PATHWAYS OF HEMOSTASIS

Early Models of Coagulation

In the 1960s, two groups proposed a model of coagulation that envisaged a sequential series of steps in which activation of one clotting factor led to the activation of another, finally leading to a burst of thrombin generation.[258,259] Each clotting factor was thought to exist as a proenzyme that could be converted to an active enzyme.

The original cascade models were subsequently modified to include the observation that some procoagulants were cofactors and did not possess enzymatic activity. In addition the clotting sequences were divided into so-called extrinsic and intrinsic systems, as shown in Figure 115–28. As can be seen, the extrinsic system consisted of factor VIIa and tissue factor, the latter being viewed as extrinsic to the circulating blood. The factors in the intrinsic system were all viewed as being intravascular. Both pathways could activate factor X, which, in complex with its cofactor Va, could convert prothrombin to thrombin. Although these earlier concepts of coagulation were extremely valuable, investigators recognized that the intrinsic and extrinsic systems could not operate independently of one another and that all the clotting factors were somehow interrelated. Only in this way could hemostasis *in vivo* be explained.

REVISION OF THE COAGULATION MODELS

Key observations made by several groups have led to a revision of earlier models of coagulation. A major observation was that a complex of factor VIIa/TF activated not only factor X but also factor IX.[162] Furthermore, it was observed that thrombin could directly activate factor XI.[121,122] Together with other important observations, this led to the conclusion that the major initiating event in hemostasis *in vivo* was the formation of a factor VIIa/TF complex at the site of injury.[260–262] This led to the belief that factor VIII and IX deficiency, which resulted in hemophilia A and B, respectively, were in fact, abnormalities of the VIIa/TF pathway, even though factors IX and VIII were considered components of the intrinsic system. It was also recognized that *in vivo* coagulation was regulated by control mechanisms, one of which was the localization of the coagulation reactions to cell surfaces. In addition, earlier and more recent observations emphasized the importance of plasma inhibitors of each step of the coagulation process. These include TFPI, which inhibits the factor VIIa/TF/Xa complex,[243,263] proteins C and S, which inactivate factors Va and VIIIa,[178,264,265] and AT, which inhibits thrombin and other coagulation proteases.[266]

A CELL-BASED MODEL OF COAGULATION

The Role of the TF-bearing Cell

The goal of hemostasis it to produce a fibrin clot to seal a site of injury or rupture in the blood vessel wall. This process is initiated when TF-bearing cells are exposed to blood at a site of injury. TF is anchored to cells via a transmembrane domain and acts as a receptor for plasma factor VII. Once bound to TF, zymogen factor VII is rapidly converted to factor VIIa through mechanisms incompletely understood, but which may involve factor Xa and autoactivation. TF is expressed around vessels and in the epithelium, where it has been described as forming a "hemostatic envelope." The TF around vessels has likely already bound factor VII(a), even in the absence of an injury.[159] The factor VIIa/TF complex catalyzes two very important reactions: (1) activation of factor X to factor Xa and (2) activation of factor IX to IXa. The factor Xa and

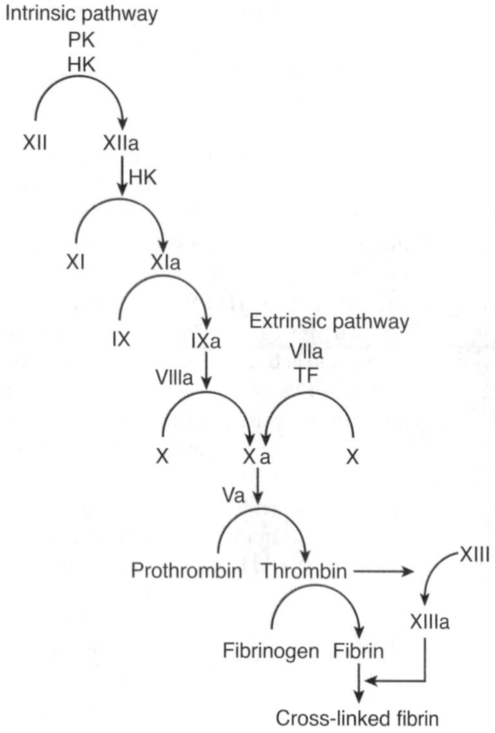

FIGURE 115–28. Cascade model of coagulation. This model shows successive activation of coagulation factors proceeding from the top of the schematic to thrombin generation and fibrin formation at the bottom of the schematic. The intrinsic and extrinsic pathways are as indicated.

IXa formed on the TF-bearing cells have very distinct and separate functions in initiating the process of blood coagulation.[13] When a vessel is injured, the blood delivers platelets to the site of injury. They bind to extravascular matrix components to produce the primary hemostatic plug and become partially activated in the process. The platelets are thereby localized in close proximity to active factor VIIa/TF complexes.

The factor Xa formed on the TF-bearing cell interacts with factor Va released from the activated platelets to form prothrombinase complexes sufficient to generate a small amount of thrombin in the vicinity of the TF cells (Fig. 115–29). Although this amount of thrombin may not be sufficient to clot fibrinogen, it is sufficient to initiate events that "prime" the clotting system for a subsequent burst of thrombin generation. Experiments using a cell-based model have shown that minute amounts of thrombin are formed in the milieu of TF-bearing cells exposed to plasma concentrations of procoagulants, even in the absence of platelets. The small amounts of factor Va required for prothrombinase assembly on the TF-bearing cells are likely provided by release from platelets, or activated by factor Xa[60] or noncoagulation proteases elaborated by the cells.[267] The small amounts of thrombin generated on the TF-bearing cells are capable of accomplishing the following: (1) activating platelets; (2) activating factor V; (3) activating factor VIII and dissociating factor VIII from VWF; and (4) activating factor XI (Fig. 115–30).[123,268] The activity of the factor Xa formed by the factor VIIa/TF complex is restricted to the TF-bearing cell. Factor Xa that diffuses off the cell surface is rapidly inhibited by TFPI or AT.

Unlike factor Xa, the primary site of activity of the factor IXa formed by factor VIIa/TF is on activated platelets in close proximity to the TF-bearing cell. Factor IXa can diffuse to adjacent cell surfaces because it is not inhibited by TFPI and is inhibited much more slowly by AT than is factor Xa (see Table 115–4).

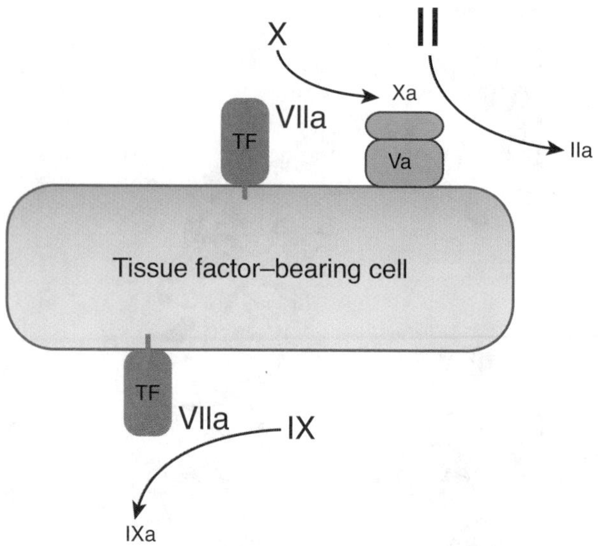

FIGURE 115–29. The role of TF-bearing cells: initiation. Factor VIIa bound to tissue factor can activate both factor X and factor IX. Factors Xa and IXa activated by factor VIIa/TF play distinct roles in coagulation. Factor Xa is assembled into a prothrombinase complex on the surface of the tissue factor-bearing cell. This generates a small amount of thrombin.

In addition to the pool of extravascular, cell-anchored TF, many reports now document the presence of TF antigen and active TF protein in the circulating blood. This tissue factor can be found either associated with so-called microparticles[269] or as an alternatively spliced form that has no membrane association. The microparticles are membrane vesicles that can be shed from many cell types, particularly in the setting of inflammation or during apoptosis. Their presence in the blood has been reported in association with a wide range of inflammatory and prothrombotic states, including atherosclerotic vascular disease, severe infections and malignancy. Less information is available

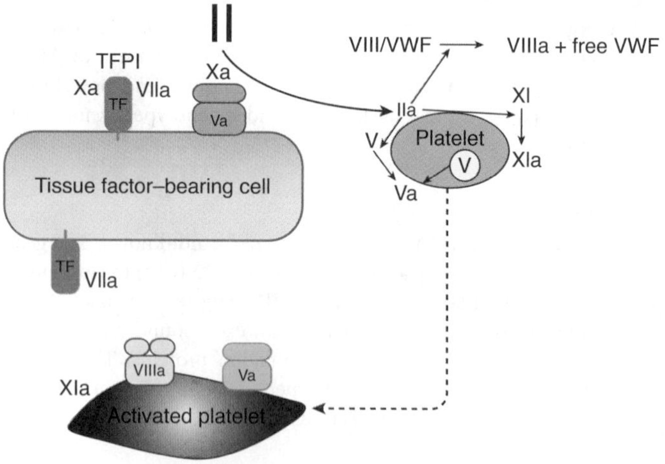

FIGURE 115–30. The role of thrombin generated by TF-bearing cells: Amplification. After the initial generation of factor Xa on tissue factor-bearing cells, subsequent factor Xa generation is shut down when TFPI reacts with factor Xa to inactivate the factor VIIa/TF complex. The small amount of thrombin generated on the tissue factor bearing cell (see Fig. 115–28) plays a critical role in priming platelets for subsequent coagulation steps. This thrombin activates platelets, releases factor V from α granules, activates factor V, activates factor VIII releasing it from VWF, and activates factor XI.

about the alternatively spliced form. However, it is not clear that the alternatively spliced form of tissue factor can effectively promote factor Xa and thrombin generation.[270]

Tissue factor mRNA has also been reported to be present and transcribed in platelets after they are strongly activated.[271] The time course of these events appears to be too slow to play a role in normal hemostasis, but could play a role in thrombosis or inflammation and wound healing following injury.

There are data showing that thrombi formed in flowing blood accumulate significant amounts of tissue factor as they develop.[158] This tissue factor accumulation is very different than what is seen in wounds where the only detectable tissue factor is present at the periphery of the hemostatic clot where it contacts the injured tissue.[272] In animal models of thrombosis induced by stasis, microparticles containing tissue factor enhanced thrombus formation in a dose-dependent fashion.[273] A study in a mouse model suggested that tissue factor in microparticles contributes to thrombus formation *in vivo*.[274] However, another study in mice, using a different model of thrombosis, suggested that circulating tissue factor did not contribute significantly to thrombus formation.[275]

Thus, based on the available data, it can be provisionally concluded that circulating tissue factor is present at a low level in normal individuals and higher levels in some disease states. The circulating tissue factor likely contributes to thrombosis in some settings, but is less likely to play a significant role in normal hemostasis.

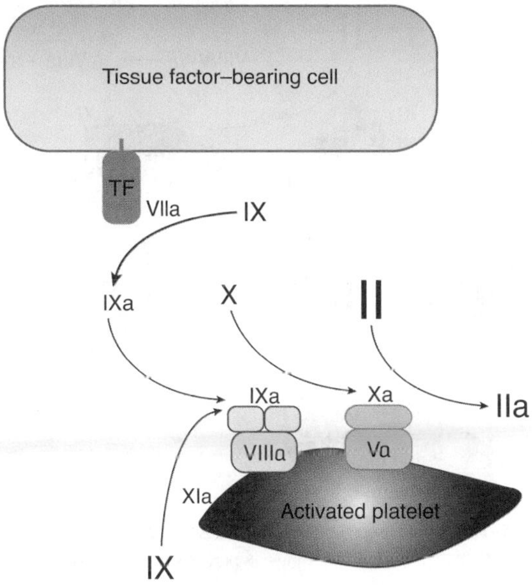

FIGURE 115–31. The role of platelets: propagation. Factor IXa, generated on tissue factor-bearing cells, is only slowly inhibited by plasma inhibitors and so can make its way to the primed platelet surface where it binds to factor VIIIa. This factor IXa activates factor X on the platelet surface. This factor Xa complexes to factor Va and activates prothrombin leading to the burst of thrombin generation responsible for cleaving fibrinogen. Additional factor IXa is supplied by factor XIa on the platelet surface.

The Role of Activated Platelets

Platelets also play a major role in localizing clotting reactions to the site of injury, as they adhere and aggregate at the same sites where TF is exposed. Platelet localization and activation are mediated by VWF, thrombin, platelet receptors, and vessel wall components such as collagen (see Chap. 114).[276]

Once platelets are activated, the cofactors Va and VIIIa are rapidly localized to the platelet membrane surface (see Fig. 115–30). Cofactor binding is mediated in part by the exposure of phosphatidyl serine on the platelet membrane, a process resulting from a flip-flop mechanism whereby phosphatidyl serine on the inner leaflet of the membrane bilayer flips to the outside.[277] In addition, it appears that the cofactors bind to platelet surface before the binding of the respective enzymes.[278]

The factor IXa formed by the factor VIIa/TF complex binds to the surface of activated platelets (Fig. 115–31). Specific receptors on the activated platelets bind factor IXa and promote formation of active factor IXa/VIIIa complexes.[279,280] Once the platelet "tenase" complex is assembled, factor X is recruited from the plasma and is activated to factor Xa on the platelet surface. Factor Xa then associates with factor Va on the surface to generate a burst of thrombin sufficient to clot fibrinogen and form a hemostatic plug (Fig. 115–31). Factor XIII, activated by thrombin, crosslinks fibrin and stabilizes the hemostatic plug, rendering it impermeable. Thrombin also activates TAFI which helps to stabilize the fibrin clot.

Thrombin can directly activate factor XI.[121,122,280a] This reaction is enhanced when factor XI and thrombin bind to platelet surfaces,[123,128,281] thus bypassing the need for factor XIIa in hemostasis. The platelet-bound factor XIa can then activate more factor IX to IXa. Thus, it appears that factor XI activation enhances the platelet tenase activity and serves as a "booster" mechanism to enhance thrombin generation. The enhanced thrombin generation resulting from the effect of factor XIa probably ensures activation of TAFI.[282]

The role of factor XI in hemostasis has been a point of major interest, as even severe factor XI deficiency does not result in a hemorrhagic tendency comparable to that seen in severe factor VIII or IX deficiency. This observation can be explained if factor XI is viewed as an "enhancer" or "booster" of thrombin generation. In factor VIII and IX deficiency, the individual has a markedly decreased ability to generate factor Xa on the platelet surface. Thus, one would expect that patients with a severe deficiency of either factor VIII or factor IX would generate insufficient thrombin for hemostasis as the tenase and hence prothrombinase activity would be markedly reduced. In contrast, patients with factor XI deficiency would always possess some baseline tenase activity. Such patients only lack the ability to "boost" platelet surface factor X activation by producing extra factor IXa.

Our knowledge of the platelet contribution to thrombin generation has been expanded. There is evidence that there is more than one population of activated platelets, one of which has been referred to as COAT (collagen and thrombin stimulated) platelets.[283] These platelets have enhanced thrombin-generating ability as a result of enhanced binding of both tenase and prothrombinase complexes.[284,285] The *in vivo* relevance of these findings is not clear.

Even though each step of the model has been depicted as an isolated set of reactions including initiation, amplification, and propagation, they should be viewed as an overlapping continuum of events, as illustrated in Figure 115–32.

The Role of Endothelial Cells

Once a fibrin/platelet clot is formed over an area of injury, the clotting process must be terminated to avoid thrombotic occlusion in adjacent normal areas of the vasculature. If the coagulation mechanism were not controlled, clotting could occur throughout the entire vascular tree after even a modest procoagulant stimulus.

Endothelial cells play a major role in confining the coagulation reactions to a site of injury and preventing clot extension to areas where an intact endothelium is present (see Chap. 116). Endothelial cells have two major types of anticoagulant/antithrombotic activities, as illustrated in Figure 115–33. The protein C/S/TM system is activated in response to thrombin generation.[69] Some of the thrombin formed during the coagulation process can diffuse away or be swept downstream

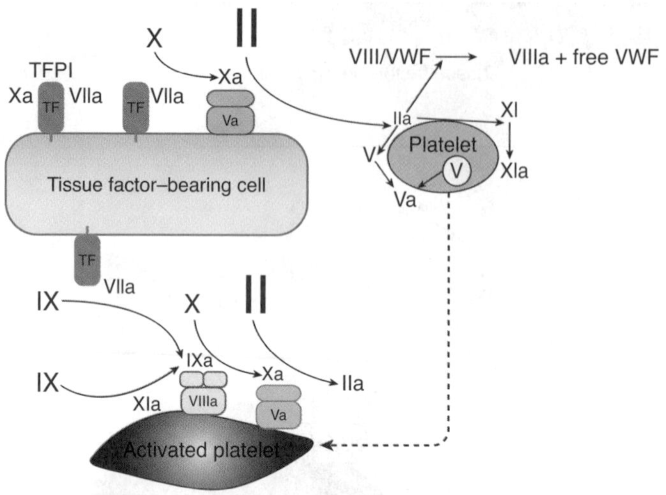

FIGURE 115–32. A cell-based model of hemostasis. The sequence of events, Initiation, Amplification, and Propagation, shown in previous figures are summarized here.

from a site of injury. When thrombin reaches an intact endothelial cell, it binds to TM on the endothelial surface. The thrombin/TM complex, in conjunction with the EPCR, then activates protein C, which binds to its cofactor protein S and inactivates any factor Va or VIIIa that finds its way to the adjacent endothelial cell membrane. This prevents the generation of additional thrombin in the vasculature. The endothelial cell also possesses other anticoagulant features. The protease inhibitors AT and TFPI are always present bound to heparan sulfates expressed on the endothelial surface where they can inactivate proteases near an intact endothelium.[286] Glycosyl phosphatidylinositol (GPI)-anchored TFPI-β may also play a role in controlling intravascular thrombin generation. Endothelial cells also inhibit platelet activation by releasing the inhibitors prostacyclin (PGI_2) and nitric oxide (NO), as well as degrading ADP by their membrane ecto-ADPase, CD39.[287]

Role of Plasma Protease Inhibitors

Like cell-based coagulation, circulating protease inhibitors are also critical in localizing the coagulation reactions to specific cell surfaces by directly inhibiting proteases that escape into the fluid phase. Not only are the plasma protease inhibitors key players in confining a clot to the proper location, they also impose a threshold effect on the coagulation process.[288] Thus, in the presence of inhibitors, coagulation does not proceed unless procoagulant factors are generated in sufficient amounts to overcome the effects of inhibitors. If the triggering event is insufficiently strong, the system returns to baseline rather than continuing through the coagulation process. Under pathologic conditions the trigger for clotting may be so strong as to overwhelm the control mechanisms, leading to disseminated intravascular coagulation or thrombosis (see Chaps. 116 and 130).

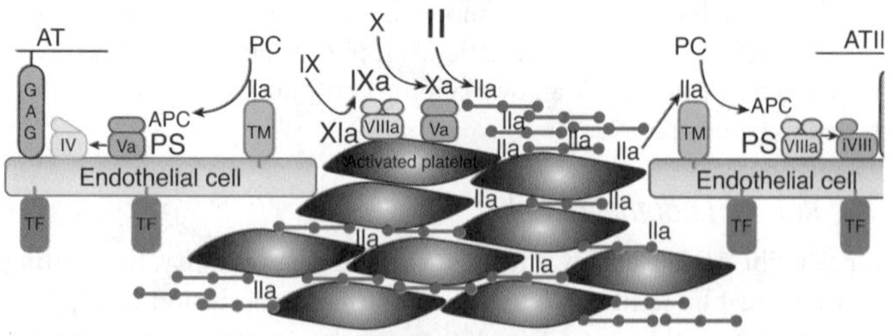

FIGURE 115–33. The role of endothelial cells. Activated coagulation proteins generated on platelets localized to the site of an injury need to be confined to the site of injury. Activated coagulation factors that move to an endothelial cell surface are rapidly inhibited by AT associated with glycosaminoglycans (GAG) on the endothelial surface. Furthermore, thrombin that reaches the endothelial cell surface binds to thrombomodulin (TM). Once bound, thrombin can no longer cleave fibrinogen. Instead this thrombin activates protein C, leading to the formation of APC/PS complexes on the endothelial cell surface. APC/PS on the endothelial cell surface inactivates procoagulant factors VIIIa (VIIIi) and Va (Vi, not shown).

ROLE OF FIBRINOLYSIS

Once a hemostatic clot has been formed, some provision must be made for its eventual removal as wound healing takes place. Dissolution of clots is accomplished by the fibrinolytic system, as discussed in detail in Chap. 136. In addition, small clots formed inappropriately within the vasculature can sometimes be removed by fibrinolysis.

The Concept of Basal Coagulation and Anticoagulation

The coagulation process only proceeds when enough thrombin is generated on or near the TF-bearing cell to trigger activation of platelets and cofactors. One wonders, however, if minute hemostatic plugs are not constantly formed throughout the body to maintain the integrity of the vascular tree. A low level of coagulation factor activation probably occurs at all times.[289] It was shown more than 30 years ago that fibrinopeptides are continuously cleaved from fibrinogen at low levels in normal individuals.[290] It has also been shown that there are low levels of circulating factor VIIa, as well as low levels of the activation peptides from factors IX and X in the blood of normal individuals.[291–293] This has been called *basal* coagulation or *idling*. Some have speculated that circulating TF drives this idling process.[294] The authors of this chapter favor the explanation that basal activation of coagulation factors results from minor injuries that occur during normal daily activities, and as the coagulation factors percolate through the extravascular spaces.[159]

This basal coagulation must be balanced by basal activity of the anticoagulation and fibrinolytic systems. This is evidenced by the presence of low levels of the protein C activation peptide and tissue plasminogen activator activity in normal individuals.[295]

Blood Coagulation as a Part of the Host Defense Mechanism

The process of hemostasis is only one part of the overall host response to injury. Although different parts of the host response are presented as if they were truly separate processes, in fact, coagulation, fibrinolysis, inflammation, the immune response, and wound healing are interrelated parts of the overall response to injury. This close interaction is reflected in the close structural relationships between many proteins of the coagulation and immune/inflammatory systems. For example, tissue factor is structurally analogous to type 2 cytokine receptors.[296] Furthermore, a number of coagulation proteins have multiple diverse activities in the host response to injury. Thrombin not only acts as a procoagulant to clot fibrinogen, but also as a growth factor and cytokine that promotes monocyte, fibroblast, and endothelial cell influx and proliferation in an area of recent injury. By generating thrombin, the coagulation process not only stops bleeding in the short-term, but also sets the stage for removal of damaged tissue and wound healing in the long-term.[38] Platelets also have multiple roles in the response to injury. They release growth factors and cytokines upon activation, some of which play key roles in wound healing and atherosclerosis. Factor Xa, TF, and fibrinogen fragments similarly seem to have roles as inflammatory mediators and cell growth regulators. The contact factors (factor XII, PK, and HK) also may play a role as a bridge between the coagulation reactions and other host defense mechanisms. The roles of the coagulation system in the host response to injury are emphasized by the finding that wound healing is impaired in hemophilia.[297] No doubt the list of multifunctional molecules will grow as understanding of the blood clotting mechanism increases.

REFERENCES

1. Leytus S, Foster D, Kurachi K, Davie E: Gene for human factor X, a blood coagulation factor whose gene organization is essentially identical to that of factor IX and protein C. *Biochemistry* 25:5098, 1986.
2. Yoshitake S, Schach BG, Forter DC, et al: Nucleotide sequence of the gene for human factor IX (antihemophilic factor B). *Biochemistry* 24:3736, 1985.
3. Fujimaki K, Yamazaki T, Taniwaki M, Ichinose A: The gene for human protein Z is localized to chromosome 13 at band q34 and is coded by eight regular exons and one alternative exon. *Biochemistry* 37:6838, 1998.
4. Wu SM, Cheung WF, Frazier D, Stafford DW: Cloning and expression of the cDNA for human gamma-glutamyl carboxylase. *Science* 254:1634, 1991.
5. Jorgensen M, Cantor A, Furie B, et al: Recognition site directing vitamin K-dependent gamma-carboxylation residues on the propeptide of factor IX. *Cell* 48:185, 1987.
6. Huber P, Schmitz T, Griffin J, et al: Identification of amino acids in the gamma-carboxylation recognition site on the propeptide of prothrombin. *J Biol Chem* 265:12467, 1990.
7. Brenner B, Sánchez-Vega B, Wu SM, et al: A missense mutation in gamma-glutamyl carboxylase gene causes combined deficiency of all vitamin K-dependent blood coagulation factors. *Blood* 92:4554, 1998.
8. Li T, Chang CY, Jin DY, et al: Identification of the gene for vitamin K epoxide reductase. *Nature* 427:541, 2004.
9. Oldenburg J, von Brederlow B, Fregin A, et al: Congenital deficiency of vitamin K dependent coagulation factors in two families presents as a genetic defect of the vitamin K-epoxide-reductase-complex. *Thromb Haemost* 84:937, 2000.
10. Rost S, Fregin A, Ivaskevicius V, et al: Mutations in VKORC1 cause warfarin resistance and multiple coagulation factor deficiency type 2. *Nature* 427:537, 2004.
11. Kamali F: Genetic influences on the response to warfarin. *Curr Opin Hematol* 13:357, 2006.
12. Cooper GM, Johnson JA, Langaee TY, et al: KA genome-wide scan for common genetic variants with a large influence on warfarin maintenance dose. *Blood* 112:1022, 2008.
13. Monroe DM, Hoffman M, Roberts HR: Platelets and thrombin generation. *Arterioscler Thromb Vasc Biol* 22:1381, 2002.
14. Soriano-Garcia M, Padmanabhan K, de Vos AM, Tulinsky A: The Ca^{2+} ion and membrane binding structure of the Gla domain of Ca-prothrombin fragment 1. *Biochemistry* 31:2554, 1992.
15. Sunnerhagen M, Forsen S, Hoffren AM, et al: Structure of the Ca(2+)-free Gla domain sheds light on membrane binding of blood coagulation proteins. *Nat Struct Biol* 2:504, 1995.
16. Ohkubo YZ, Tajkhorshid E: Distinct structural and adhesive roles of Ca2+ in membrane binding of blood coagulation factors. *Structure* 16:72, 2008.
17. Nelsestuen G, Kisiel W, RG DS: Interaction of vitamin K-dependent proteins with membranes. *Biochemistry* 12:2134, 1978.
18. Rawal-Sheikh R, Ahmad SS, Ashby B, Walsh PN: Kinetics of coagulation factor X activation by platelet-bound factor IXa. *Biochemistry* 29:2606, 1990.
19. Gilbert GE, Arena AA: Partial activation of the factor VIIIa-factor IXa enzyme complex by dihexanoic phosphatidylserine at submicellar concentrations. *Biochemistry* 36:10768, 1997.
20. Kirchhofer D, Guha A, Nemerson Y, et al: Activation of blood coagulation factor VIIa with cleaved tissue factor extracellular domain and crystallization of the active complex. *Proteins* 22:419, 1995.
21. Muller Y, Ultsch M, de Vos A: The crystal structure of the extracellular domain of tissue factor refined to 1.7 Å resolution. *J Mol Biol* 256:144, 1996.
22. Banner DW, D'Arcy A, Chene C, et al: The crystal structure of the complex of blood coagulation factor VIIa with human soluble tissue factor. *Nature* 380:41, 1996.
23. Brandstetter H, Bauer M, Huber R, et al: X-ray structure of clotting factor IXa: Active site and module structure related to Xase activity and hemophilia B. *Proc Natl Acad Sci U S A* 92:9796, 1995.
24. Patthy L, Trexler M, Vali Z, et al: Kringles: Modules specialized for protein binding. Homology of the gelatin-binding region of fibronectin with the kringle structure of proteases. *FEBS Lett* 171:131, 1984.
25. Royle N, Irwin D, Koschinsky ML, et al: Human genes encoding prothrombin and ceruloplasmin map to 11p11-q12 and 3q21-q24, respectively. *Somat Cell Mol Genet.* 13:285, 1987.
26. Chow B-C, Ting V, Tufaro F, MacGillivray R: Characterization of a novel liver-specific enhancer in the human prothrombin gene. *J Biol Chem* 266:18927, 1991.
27. Degen S: The prothrombin gene and its liver-specific expression. *Semin Thromb Hemost* 18:230, 1992.
28. Poort S, Rosendaal F, Bertina R: A common genetic variant in the 3′-untranslated region of the prothrombin gene is associated with elevated plasma prothrombin levels and an increase in venous thrombosis. *Blood* 88:3698, 1996.
29. Sun WY, Witte DP, Degen JL, et al: Prothrombin deficiency results in embryonic and neonatal lethality in mice. *Proc Natl Acad Sci U S A* 95:7597, 1998.
30. Bode W, Mayr I, Baumann U, et al: The refined 1.9 Å crystal structure of human alpha-thrombin: Interaction with D-Phe-Pro-Arg chloromethylketone and significance of the Try-Pro-Pro-Trp insertion segment. *EMBO J* 8:3467, 1989.
31. Martin PD, Malkowski MG, Box J, et al: New insights into the regulation of the blood clotting cascade derived from the X-ray crystal structure of bovine meizothrombin des F1 in complex with PPACK. *Structure* 5:1681, 1997.
32. Vijayalakshmi J, Padmanabhan KP, Mann KG, Tulinsky A: The isomorphous structures of prethrombin2, hirugen-, and PPACK-thrombin: Changes accompanying activation and exosite binding to thrombin. *Protein Sci* 3:2254, 1994.
33. Banefield D, MacGillivray R: Partial characterization of vertebrate prothrombin cDNAs: Amplification and sequence analysis of the B chain of thrombin from nine different species. *Proc Natl Acad Sci U S A* 89:2779, 1992.
34. Nesheim M: Fibrinolysis and the plasma carboxypeptidase. *Curr Opin Hematol* 5:309, 1998.
35. Boffa MB, Nesheim ME, Koschinsky ML: Thrombin activatable fibrinolysis inhibitor (TAFI): Molecular genetics of an emerging potential risk factor for thrombotic disorders. *Curr Drug Targets Cardiovasc Haematol Disord* 1:59, 2001.
36. Dittman W, Nelson S: Thrombomodulin, in *Molecular Basis of Thrombosis and Hemostasis*, edited by KA High, HR Roberts, p 425. Marcel Dekker, New York, 1995.
37. Esmon CT: The protein C pathway. *Chest* 124:26S, 2003
38. Church FC, Hoffman MR: Heparin cofactor II and thrombin: Heparin-binding proteins linking hemostasis and inflammation. *Trends Cardiovasc Med* 4:140, 1994.
39. Pollak E, Hung H, Godin W, et al: Functional characterization of the human factor VII 5′-flanking region. *J Biol Chem* 271:1738, 1996.
40. Rosen ED, Chan JC, Idusogie E, et al: Mice lacking factor VII develop normally but suffer fatal perinatal bleeding. *Nature* 390:290, 1997.
41. Hedner U, Kisiel W: Use of human factor VIIa in the treatment of two hemophilia A patients with high-titer inhibitors. *J Clin Invest* 71:1836, 1983.
42. Wolberg AS, Stafford DW, Erie DA: Human factor IX binds to specific sites on the collagenous domain of collagen IV. *J Biol Chem* 272:16717, 1997.
43. Cheung WF, van den Born J, Kuhn K, et al: Identification of the endothelial cell binding site for factor IX. *Proc Natl Acad Sci U S A* 93:11068, 1996.
44. Gui T, Lin HF, Jin DY, et al: Circulating and binding characteristics of wild-type factor IX and certain Gla domain mutants *in vivo*. *Blood* 100:153, 2002.
44a. Gui T, Reheman A, Ni H, et al: Abnormal hemostasis in a knock-in mouse carrying a variant of Factor IX with impaired binding to collagen type IV. *J Thromb Haemost* 2009:epub ahead of press.
45. Camerino G, Grzeschik K, Jaye M, et al: Regional localization on the human X chromosome and polymorphism of the coagulation factor IX gene (hemophilia B locus). *Proc Natl Acad Sci U S A* 81:498, 1984.
46. Winship P, Rees D, Alkan M: Detection of polymorphisms at cytosine phosphoguanidine dinucleotides and diagnosis of haemophilia B carriers. *Lancet* 1:631, 1989.
47. High K, Roberts H: Factor IX, in *Molecular Basis of Thrombosis and Hemostasis*, edited by KA High, HR Roberts, p 215. Marcel Dekker, New York, 1995.
48. Landschulz W, Johnson P, McKnight S: Homologous recognition of a promoter domain common to the MSV LTR and the HSV tk gene. *Cell* 44:565, 1986.
49. Mueller C, Maire P, Schibler U: DBP, a liver-enriched transcriptional activator, is expressed late in ontogeny and its tissue specificity is determined posttranslationally. *Cell* 61:279, 1990.
50. Sladek F, Zhong W, Lai E, Darnell JJ: Liver-enriched transcription factor NHF-4 is a novel member of the steroid hormone receptor superfamily. *Genes Dev* 4:2353, 1990.
51. Paonessa G, Gounari F, Frank R, Cortese R: Purification of a NF1-like DNA-binding protein from rat liver and cloning of the corresponding cDNA. *EMBO J* 7:3115, 1988.
52. London FS, Walsh PN: Activation dependent appearance of a platelet protein that recognizes coagulation factor IXa. *Circulation* 86:I465, 1992.
53. Scambler P, Williamson R: The structural gene for human coagulation factor X is located on chromosome 13q34. *Cytogenet Cell Genet* 39:231, 1985.
54. Watzke H, High K: Factor X, in *Molecular Basis of Thrombosis and Hemostasis*, edited by KA High, HR Roberts, p 239. Marcel Dekker, New York, 1995.
55. Huang M, Hung H, Stanfield-Oakley S, High K: Characterization of the human coagulation factor X promoter. *J Biol Chem* 267:15440, 1992.
56. Hung H, High K: Liver-enriched transcription factor HNF-4 and ubiquitous factor NF-Y are critical for expression of blood coagulation factor X. *J Biol Chem* 271:2323, 1996.
57. Dewerchin M, Liang Z, Moons L, et al: Blood coagulation factor X deficiency causes partial embryonic lethality and fatal neonatal bleeding in mice. *Thromb Haemost* 83:185, 2000.
58. Rao L, Rapaport SI: Activation of factor VII bound to tissue factor: A key early step in the tissue factor pathway of blood coagulation. *Proc Natl Acad Sci U S A* 85:6687, 1988.
59. Neuenschwander PF, Jesty J: Thrombin-activated and factor Xa-activated human factor VIII: Differences in cofactor activity and decay rate. *Arch Biochem Biophys* 296:426, 1992.
60. Monkovic DD, Tracy PB: Activation of human factor V by factor Xa and thrombin. *Biochemistry* 29:1118, 1990.
61. Bouchard BA, Catcher CS, Thrash BR, et al: Effector cell protease receptor-1, a platelet activation-dependent membrane protein, regulates prothrombinase-catalyzed thrombin generation. *J Biol Chem* 272:9244, 1997.
62. Gasic GP, Arenas CP, Gasic TB, Gasic GJ: Coagulation factors X, Xa, and protein S as potent mitogens of cultured aortic smooth muscle cells. *Proc Natl Acad Sci U S A* 89:2317, 1992.

63. Altieri DC, Edgington TS: Identification of effector cell protease receptor-1. A leukocyte-distributed receptor for the serine protease factor Xa. *J Immunol* 145:246, 1990.
64. Patrucchini P, Aiello V, Palazzi P, et al: Sublocalization of the human protein C gene on chromosome 2q13-q14. *Hum Genet* 81:191, 1989.
65. Foster D, Yoshitake S, Davie E: The nucleotide sequence for the gene for human protein C. *Proc Natl Acad Sci U S A* 82:4673, 1985.
66. Plutzky J, Hoskins J, Long G, Crabtree G: Evolution and organization of the human protein C gene. *Proc Natl Acad Sci U S A* 83:546, 1986.
67. Esmon CT: Inflammation and thrombosis. *J Thromb Haemost* 1:1343, 2003.
68. Stearns-Kurosawa DJ, Kurosawa S, Mollica JS, et al: The endothelial cell protein C receptor augments protein C activation by the thrombin-thrombomodulin complex. *Proc Natl Acad Sci U S A* 93:10212, 1996.
69. Oliver JA, Monroe DM, Church FC, et al: Activated protein C cleaves factor Va more efficiently on endothelium than on platelet surfaces. *Blood* 100:539, 2002.
70. Shen L, Dahlbäck B: Factor V and protein S as synergistic cofactors to activated protein C in degradation of factor VIIIa. *J Biol Chem* 269:18735, 1994.
71. Cooper S, Church F: PCI: Protein C inhibitor? *Adv Exp Med Biol* 425:45, 1997.
72. Esmon CT: Inflammation and the activated protein C anticoagulant pathway. *Semin Thromb Hemost* 32 Suppl 1:49, 2006.
73. Kerschen EJ, Fernandez JA, Cooley BC, et al: Endotoxemia and sepsis mortality reduction by non-anticoagulant activated protein C. *J Exp Med* 204:2439, 2007.
74. Fair D, Marlar R: Biosynthesis and secretion of factor VII, protein C, protein S and the protein inhibitor from a human hepatoma cell line. *Blood* 6:64, 1986.
75. Fair D, Marlar R, Levin E: Human endothelial cells synthesize protein S. *Blood* 67:1168, 1986.
76. Ogura M, Tanabe N, Nishioka J, et al: Biosynthesis and secretion of functional protein S by a human megakaryoblastic cell line. *Blood* 70:301, 1987.
77. Dahlback B: Protein S and C4b-binding protein: Components involved in the regulation of the protein C anticoagulant system. *Thromb Haemost* 66:49, 1991.
78. Maillard C, Berruyer M, Serre C, et al: Protein S, a vitamin K-dependent protein, is a bone matrix component synthesized and secreted by osteoblasts. *Endocrinology* 130:1599, 1992.
79. Edenbrandt C-M, Lundvall A, Wydro R, Stenflo J: Molecular analysis of the gene for vitamin K-dependent protein S and its pseudogene: Cloning and partial characterization. *Biochemistry* 29:7861, 1990.
80. Castoldi E, Hackeng TM: Regulation of coagulation by protein S. *Curr Opin Hematol* 15:529, 2008.
81. Hackeng T, van't Veer C, Meijers J, Bouma B: Human protein S inhibits prothrombinase complex activity on endothelial cells and platelets via direct interactions with factors Va and Xa. *J Biol Chem* 269:21051, 1994.
82. Rezende SM, Simmonds RE, Lane DA: Coagulation, inflammation, and apoptosis: Different roles for protein S and the protein S-C4b binding protein complex. *Blood* 103:1192, 2004.
83. Hackeng TM, Sere KM, Tans G, Rosing J: Protein S stimulates inhibition of the tissue factor pathway by tissue factor pathway inhibitor. *Proc Natl Acad Sci U S A* 103:3106, 2006.
84. Moussalli M, Pipe SW, Hauri HP, et al: Mannose-dependent endoplasmic reticulum (ER)-Golgi intermediate compartment-53-mediated ER to Golgi trafficking of coagulation factors V and VIII. *J Biol Chem* 274:32539, 1999.
85. Nichols W, Seligsohn U, Zivelin A, et al: Mutations in the ER-Golgi intermediate compartment protein ERGIC-53 cause combined deficiency of coagulation factors V and VIII. *Cell* 93:61, 1998.
86. Zhang B, Ginsburg D: Familial multiple coagulation factor deficiencies: New biological insights from rare genetic bleeding disorders. *J Thromb Haemost* 2:1564, 2004.
87. Ortel T, Keller F, Kane W: Factor V, in *Molecular Basis of Thrombosis and Hemostasis*, edited by KA High, HR Roberts, p 19. Marcel Dekker, New York, 1995.
88. Ortel TL, Quinn-Allen MA, Keller FG, et al: Localization of functionally important epitopes within the second C-type domain of coagulation factor V using recombinant chimeras. *J Biol Chem* 269:15898, 1994.
89. Pittman DD, Tomkinson KN, Michnick D, et al: Posttranslational sulfation of factor V is required for efficient thrombin cleavage and activation and for full procoagulant activity. *Biochemistry* 33:6592, 1994.
90. Cripe L, Moore K, Kane W: Structure of the gene for human factor V. *Biochemistry* 31:3777, 1992.
91. Gould WR, Simioni P, Silveira JR, et al: Megakaryocytes endocytose and subsequently modify human factor V in vivo to form the entire pool of a unique platelet-derived cofactor. *J Thromb Haemost* 3:450, 2005.
92. Sun H, Yang TL, Yang A, et al: The murine platelet and plasma factor V pools are biosynthetically distinct and sufficient for minimal hemostasis. *Blood* 102:2856, 2003.
93. Yang TL, Pipe SW, Yang A, Ginsburg D: Biosynthetic origin and functional significance of murine platelet factor V. *Blood* 102:2851, 2003.
94. Gould WR, Silveira JR, Tracy PB: Unique in vivo modifications of coagulation factor V produce a physically and functionally distinct platelet-derived cofactor: Characterization of purified platelet-derived factor V/Va. *J Biol Chem* 279:2383, 2004.
95. Hayward C: Multimerin: A bench-to-bedside chronology of a unique platelet and endothelial cell protein—From discovery to function to abnormalities in disease. *Clin Invest Med* 20:176, 1997.
96. Bertina RM, Koeleman BP, Koster T, et al: Mutation in blood coagulation factor V associated with resistance to activated protein C. *Nature* 369:64, 1994.
97. Cui J, O'Shea KS, Purkayastha A, et al: Fatal haemorrhage and incomplete block to embryogenesis in mice lacking coagulation factor V. *Nature* 384:66, 1996.
98. Shaw E, Giddings JC, Peake IR, Bloom AL: Synthesis of procoagulant factor VIII, factor VIII related antigen and other coagulation factors by the isolated perfused rat liver. *Br J Haematol* 41:585, 1979.
99. Hellman L, Smedsrod B, Sandberg H, Pettersson U: Secretion of coagulant factor VIII activity and antigen by in vitro cultivated rat liver sinusoidal endothelial cells. *Br J Haematol* 73:348, 1989.
100. Bontempo FA, Lewis JH, Gorenc TJ, et al: Liver transplantation in hemophilia A. *Blood* 69:1721, 1987.
101. Marchioro TL, Hougie C, Ragde H, et al: Hemophilia: Role of organ homografts. *Science* 163:188, 1969.
102. Kumaran V, Benten D, Follenzi A, et al: Transplantation of endothelial cells corrects the phenotype in hemophilia A mice. *J Thromb Haemost* 3:2022, 2005.
103. Pipe S, Morris J, Shah J, Kaufman R: Differential interaction of coagulation factor VIII and factor V with protein chaperones calnexin and calreticulin. *J Biol Chem* 273:8537, 1998.
104. Swaroop M, Moussalli M, Pipe S, Kaufman R: Mutagenesis of a potential immunoglobulin-binding protein-binding site enhances secretion of coagulation factor VIII. *J Biol Chem* 272:24121, 1997.
105. Lollar P, Hill-Eubanks E, Parker C: Association of the FVIII light chain with von Willebrand factor. *J Biol Chem* 263:10451, 1988.
106. Gitschier J, Wood W, Goralka T, et al: Characterization of the human factor VIII gene. *Nature* 312:326, 1984.
107. Bonthron D, Handin R, Kaufman R, et al: Structure of pre-pro-von Willebrand factor and its expression in heterologous cells. *Nature* 324:270, 1986.
108. Colombatti A, Bonaldo P: The superfamily of proteins with von Willebrand factor type A-domains: One theme common to components of extracellular matrix, hemostasis, cellular adhesion, and defense mechanisms. *Blood* 77:2305, 1991.
109. Foster P, Fulcher C, Marti T, et al: A major factor VIII binding domain resides within the amino-terminal 272 amino acid residues of von Willebrand factor. *J Biol Chem* 262:8443, 1987.
110. Dong JF, Moake JL, Nolasco L, et al: ADAMTS-13 rapidly cleaves newly secreted ultralarge von Willebrand factor multimers on the endothelial surface under flowing conditions. *Blood* 100:4033, 2002.
111. Zimmerman T, Roberts J, Edgington T: Factor VIII-related antigen: Multiple molecular forms in human plasma. *Proc Natl Acad Sci U S A* 72:5121, 1975.
112. Mancuso D, Tuley E, Westfield L, et al: Structure of the gene for human von Willebrand factor. *J Biol Chem* 264:19514, 1989.
113. Fujikawa K, Chung DW: Factor XI, in *Molecular Basis of Thrombosis and Hemostasis*, edited by KA High, HR Roberts, p 257. Marcel Dekker, New York, 1995.
114. Baglia FA, Seaman FS, Walsh PN: The Apple 1 and Apple 4 domains of factor XI act synergistically to. *Blood* 85:2078, 1995.
115. Baglia FA, Jameson BA, Walsh PN: Identification and characterization of a binding site for platelets in the Apple 3 domain of coagulation factor XI. *J Biol Chem* 270:6734, 1995.
116. Baglia FA, Jameson BA, Walsh PN: Identification and characterization of a binding site for factor XIIa in the Apple 4 domain of coagulation factor XI. *J Biol Chem* 268:3838, 1993.
117. Baglia FA, Walsh PN: A binding site for thrombin in the apple 1 domain of factor XI. *J Biol Chem* 271:3652, 1996.
118. Kato A, Asaki R, Davie E, Aoki N: Factor XI gene (F11) is located on the distal end of the long arm of chromosome 4. *Cytogenet Cell Genet* 52:77, 1989.
119. Asakai R, Davie E, Chung D: Organization of the gene for human factor XI. *Biochemistry* 26:7221, 1987.
120. Tarumi T, Kravtsov DV, Zhao M, et al: Cloning and characterization of the human factor XI gene promoter: Transcription factor hepatocyte nuclear factor 4alpha (HNF-4alpha) is required for hepatocyte-specific expression of factor XI. *J Biol Chem* 277:18510, 2002.
121. Gailani D, Broze Jr. GJ: Factor XI activation in a revised model of blood coagulation. *Science* 253:909, 1991.
122. Naito K, Fujikawa K: Activation of human blood coagulation factor XI independent of factor XII. Factor XI is activated by thrombin and factor XIa in the presence of negatively charged surfaces. *J Biol Chem* 266:7353, 1991.
123. Oliver J, Monroe D, Roberts H, Hoffman M: Thrombin activates factor XI on activated platelets in the absence of factor XII. *Arterioscler Thromb Vasc Biol* 19:170, 1999.
124. Rosen ED, Gailani D, Castellino FJ: FXI is essential for thrombus formation following FeCl3-induced injury of the carotid artery in the mouse. *Thromb Haemost* 87:774, 2002.
125. Gailani D, Lasky NM, Broze GJ Jr: A murine model of factor XI deficiency. *Blood Coagul Fibrinolysis* 8:134, 1997.
126. Ragni MV, Sinha D, Seaman F, et al: Comparison of bleeding tendency, factor XI coagulant activity, and factor XI antigen in 25 factor XI-deficient kindreds. *Blood* 65:719, 1985.
127. Sinha D, Seaman FS, Walsh PN: Role of calcium ions and the heavy chain of factor XIa in the activation of human coagulation factor IX. *Biochemistry* 26:3768, 1987.
128. Sinha D, Seaman FS, Koshy A, et al: Blood coagulation factor XIa binds specifically to a site on activated human platelets distinct from that for factor XI. *J Clin Invest* 73:1550, 1984.
129. Knauer DJ, Majumdar D, Fong PC, Knauer MF: SERPIN regulation of factor XIa. The novel observation that protease nexin 1 in the presence of heparin is a more potent inhibitor of factor XIa than C1 inhibitor. *J Biol Chem* 275:37340, 2000.

130. Cronlund AL, Walsh PN: A low molecular weight platelet inhibitor of factor XIa: Purification, characterization, and possible role in blood coagulation. *Biochemistry* 31:1685, 1992.
131. Saito H, Kojima T: Factor XII, prekallikrein and high-molecular-weight kininogen, in *Molecular Basis of Thrombosis and Hemostasis*, edited by KA High, HR Roberts, p 269. Marcel Dekker, New York, 1995.
132. Yu H, Anderson PJ, Freedman BI, et al: Genomic structure of the human plasma prekallikrein gene, identification of allelic variants, and analysis in end-stage renal disease. *Genomics* 69:225, 2000.
133. Colman RW: Biologic activities of the contact factors in vivo—potentiation of hypotension, inflammation, and fibrinolysis, and inhibition of cell adhesion, angiogenesis and thrombosis. *Thromb Haemost* 82:1568, 1999.
134. Schmaier AH: The plasma kallikrein-kinin system counterbalances the renin-angiotensin system. *J Clin Invest* 109:1007, 2002.
135. Pauer HU, Renne T, Hemmerlein B, et al: Targeted deletion of murine coagulation factor XII gene—A model for contact phase activation *in vivo*. *Thromb Haemost* 92:503, 2004.
136. Renne T, Gailani D: Role of Factor XII in hemostasis and thrombosis: Clinical implications. *Expert Rev Cardiovasc Ther* 5:733, 2007.
137. Kleinschnitz C, Stoll G, Bendszus M, et al: Targeting coagulation factor XII provides protection from pathological thrombosis in cerebral ischemia without interfering with hemostasis. *J Exp Med* 203:513, 2006.
138. Castaman G, Ruggeri M, Tosetto A, et al: Thrombosis in patients with heterozygous and homozygous factor XII deficiency is not explained by the associated presence of factor V Leiden. *Thromb Haemost* 76:275, 1996.
139. Dyerberg J, Stoffersen E: Recurrent thrombosis in a patient with factor XII deficiency. *Acta Haematol* 63:278, 1980.
140. Mahdi F, Madar ZS, Figueroa CD, Schmaier AH: Factor XII interacts with the multiprotein assembly of urokinase plasminogen activator receptor, gC1qR, and cytokeratin 1 on endothelial cell membranes. *Blood* 99:3585, 2002.
141. Shariat-Madar Z, Mahdi F, Schmaier AH: Assembly and activation of the plasma kallikrein/kinin system: A new interpretation. *Int Immunopharmacol* 2:1841, 2002.
142. Morrissey JH, Fakhrai H, Edgington TS: Molecular cloning of the cDNA for tissue factor, the cellular receptor for the initiation of the coagulation protease cascade. *Cell* 50:129, 1987.
143. Dorfleutner A, Ruf W: Regulation of tissue factor cytoplasmic domain phosphorylation by palmitoylation. *Blood* 102:3998, 2003.
144. Martin D, Boys C, Ruf W: Tissue factor: Molecular recognition and cofactor function. *FASEB J* 9:852, 1995.
145. Minazzo AS, Darlington RC, Ross JB: Loop dynamics of the extracellular domain of human tissue factor and activation of factor VIIa. *Biophys J* 96:681, 2009.
146. Kao F-T, Hartz J, Horton R, et al: Regional assignment of human tissue factor gene (F3) to chromosome 1p21–22. *Somat Cell Mol Genet* 14:407, 1988.
147. Mackman N, Morrissey JH, Fowler B, Edgington TS: Complete sequence of the human tissue factor gene, a highly regulated cellular receptor that initiates the coagulation protease cascade. *Biochemistry* 28:1755, 1989.
148. Bogdanov VY, Balasubramanian V, Hathcock J, et al: Alternatively spliced human tissue factor: A circulating, soluble, thrombogenic protein. *Nat Med* 9:458, 2003.
149. Bogdanov VY, Kirk RI, Miller C, et al: Identification and characterization of murine alternatively spliced tissue factor. *J Thromb Haemost* 4:158, 2006.
150. Mackman N, Fowler B, Edgington TS, Morrissey JH: Functional analysis of the human tissue factor promoter and induction by serum. *Proc Natl Acad Sci U S A* 87:2254, 1990.
151. Gregory SA, Morrissey JH, Edgington TS: Regulation of tissue factor gene expression in the monocyte procoagulant response to endotoxin. *Mol Cell Biol* 9:2752, 1989.
152. Schecter AD, Rollins BJ, Zhang YJ, et al: Tissue factor is induced by monocyte chemoattractant protein-1 in human aortic smooth muscle and THP-1 cells. *J Biol Chem* 272:28568, 1997.
153. Conway EM, Bach R, Rosenberg RD, Konigsberg WH: Tumor necrosis factor enhances expression of tissue factor mRNA in endothelial cells. *Thromb Res* 53:231, 1989.
154. Hoffman M, Cooper S: Thrombin enhances monocyte secretion of tumor necrosis factor and Interleukin-1 beta by two distinct mechanisms. *Blood Cells Mol Dis* 21:156, 1995.
155. Key NS: Platelet tissue factor: How did it get there and is it important? *Semin Hematol* 45: S16, 2008.
156. Drake TA, Morrissey JH, Edgington TS: Selective cellular expression of tissue factor in human tissues. Implications for disorders of hemostasis and thrombosis. *Am J Pathol* 134:1087, 1989.
157. Eddleston M, de la Torre J, Oldstone M, et al: Astrocytes are the primary source of tissue factor in the murine central nervous system. A role for astrocytes in cerebral hemostasis. *J Clin Invest* 92:349, 1993.
158. Giesen PLA, Rauch U, Bohrmann B, et al: Blood-borne tissue factor: Another view of thrombosis. *Proc Natl Acad Sci U S A* 96:2311, 1999.
159. Hoffman M, Colina CM, McDonald AG, et al: Tissue factor around dermal vessels has bound factor VII in the absence of injury. *J Thromb Haemost* 5:1403, 2007.
160. Shigematsu Y, Miyata T, Higashi S: Expression of human soluble tissue factor in yeast and enzymatic properties of its complex with factor VIIa. *J Biol Chem* 267:21329, 1992.
161. Lawson JH, Butenas S, Mann KG: The evaluation of complex-dependent alterations in human factor VIIa. *J Biol Chem* 267:4834, 1992.
162. Østerud B, Rapaport SI: Activation of factor IX by the reaction product of tissue factor and factor VII: Additional pathway for initiating blood coagulation. *Proc Natl Acad Sci U S A* 74:5260, 1977.
163. Neuenschwander PF, Morrissey JH: Roles of the membrane-interactive regions of factor VIIa-tissue factor. *J Biol Chem* 269:8007, 1994.
164. Neuenschwander PF, Morrissey JH: Deletion of the membrane anchoring region of tissue factor abolishes autoactivation of factor VII but not cofactor function. Analysis of a mutant with a selective deficiency in activity. *J Biol Chem* 267:14477, 1992.
165. Krishnaswamy S, Field KA, Edgington TS, et al: Role of the membrane surface in the activation of human coagulation factor X. *J Biol Chem* 267:26110, 1992.
166. Bach R, Moldow C: Mechanism of tissue factor activation on HL-60 cells. *Blood* 89:3270, 1997.
167. Bach R, Rifkin DB: Expression of tissue factor procoagulant activity: Regulation by cytosolic calcium. *Proc Natl Acad Sci U S A* 87:6995, 1990.
168. Versteeg HH, Sorensen BB, Slofstra SH, et al: VIIa/tissue factor interaction results in a tissue factor cytoplasmic domain-independent activation of protein synthesis, p70, and p90 S6 kinase phosphorylation. *J Biol Chem* 277:27065, 2002.
169. Riewald M, Ruf W: Mechanistic coupling of protease signaling and initiation of coagulation by tissue factor. *Proc Natl Acad Sci U S A* 98:7742, 2001.
170. Mackman N: Role of tissue factor in hemostasis, thrombosis, and vascular development. *Arterioscler Thromb Vasc Biol* 24:1015, 2004.
171. Wen D, Dittman W, Ye R, et al: Human thrombomodulin: Complete cDNA sequence and chromosome localization of the gene. *Biochemistry* 26:4350, 1987.
172. Esmon N, Owen W, Esmon C: Isolation of a membrane-bound cofactor for thrombin-catalyzed activation of protein C. *J Biol Chem* 257:859, 1982.
173. Patthy L: Detecting distant homologies of mosaic proteins: Analysis of thrombomodulin, thrombospondin, complement components C9, C8 alpha, C8 beta, vitronectin and plasma cell membrane glycoprotein PC-1. *J Mol Biol* 202:689, 1988.
174. Stearns D, Kurosawa S, Esmon C: Microthrombomodulin. Residues 310–486 from the epidermal growth factor homology domain of rabbit thrombomodulin will accelerate protein C activation. *J Biol Chem* 264:3352, 1989.
175. Parkinson J, Vlahos C, Yan S, Bang N: Recombinant human thrombomodulin: Regulation of cofactor activity and anticoagulant function by a glycosaminoglycan side chain. *Biochem J* 283:151, 1992.
176. Espinosa R, Sadler J, LeBeau M: Regional localization of the human thrombomodulin gene to 20p12-cen. *Genomics* 5:649, 1989.
177. Esmon C, Esmon N, Hams K: Complex formation between thrombin and thrombomodulin inhibits both thrombin-catalyzed fibrin formation and factor V activation. *J Biol Chem* 257:7944, 1982.
178. Cadroy Y, Diquelou A, Dupouy D, et al: The thrombomodulin/protein C/protein S anticoagulant pathway modulates the thrombogenic properties of the normal resting and stimulated endothelium. *Arterioscler Thromb Vasc Biol* 17:520, 1997.
179. Healy AM, Rayburn HB, Rosenberg RD, Weiler H: Absence of the blood-clotting regulator thrombomodulin causes embryonic lethality in mice before development of a functional cardiovascular system. *Proc Natl Acad Sci U S A* 92:850, 1995.
180. Gu JM, Crawley JT, Ferrell G, et al: Disruption of the endothelial cell protein C receptor gene in mice causes placental thrombosis and early embryonic lethality. *J Biol Chem* 277:43335, 2002.
181. Verhagen HJ, Heijnen-Snyder GJ, Pronk A, et al: Thrombomodulin activity on mesothelial cells: Perspectives for mesothelial cells as an alternative for endothelial cells for cell seeding on vascular grafts. *Br J Haematol* 95:542, 1996.
182. McCachren SS, Diggs J, Weinberg JB, Dittman WA: Thrombomodulin expression by human blood monocytes and by human synovial tissue lining macrophages. *Blood* 78:3128, 1991.
183. Raife TJ, Demetroulis EM, Lentz SR: Regulation of thrombomodulin expression by all-trans retinoic acid and tumor necrosis factor-alpha: Differential responses in keratinocytes and endothelial cells. *Blood* 88:2043, 1996.
184. Ishii H, Nakana M, Tsubouchi J, et al: Distribution of thrombomodulin in human tissues and characterization of thrombomodulin in plasma. *Nippon Ketsueki Gakkai Zasshi* 51:1218, 1998.
185. Dichek D, Quertermous T: Variability in mRNA levels in HUVECs of different lineage and time in culture. *In Vitro Cell Dev Biol* 25:289, 1989.
186. Rezaie A, Cooper S, Church F, Esmon C: Protein C inhibitor is a potent inhibitor of the thrombin-thrombomodulin complex. *J Biol Chem* 270:25336, 1995.
187. Neerman-Arbez M: The molecular basis of inherited afibrinogenaemia. *Thromb Haemost* 86:154, 2001.
188. Hanss M, Biot F: A database for human fibrinogen variants. *Ann N Y Acad Sci* 936:89, 2001.
189. Carrell N, McDonagh J. Functional defects in abnormal fibrinogens, in *Fibrinogen: Structural Variants and Interaction*, edited by A Henschen, B Hesse, J McDonagh, T Saldeen, p 155. Walter DeGruyter, Berlin, 1985.
190. Egeberg O: Inherited fibrinogen abnormality causing thrombophilia. *Thromb Diath Haemorrh* 17:176, 1967.
191. Ni H, Papalia JM, Degen JL, Wagner DD: Control of thrombus embolization and fibronectin internalization by integrin alpha IIb beta 3 engagement of the fibrinogen gamma chain. *Blood* 102:3609, 2003.
192. Gardlund B, Hessel B, Marguerie G, et al: Primary structure of human fibrinogen. Characterization of disulfide-containing cyanogen-bromide fragments. *Eur J Biochem* 77:595, 1977.

193. Blomback B: Studies on the action of thrombotic enzymes on bovine fibrinogen as measured by N-terminal analysis. *Ark Kemi* 12:321, 1958.
194. Blomback B, Blomback M, Henschen A, et al: N-terminal disulfide knot of human fibrinogen. *Nature* 218:130, 1968.
195. Doolittle RF: Determining the crystal structure of fibrinogen. *J Thromb Haemost* 2:683, 2004.
195a. Côté HC, Lord ST, Pratt KP: gamma-Chain dysfibrinogenemias: Molecular structure-function relationships of naturally occurring mutations in the gamma chain of human fibrinogen. *Blood* 92:2195, 1998.
196. Henschen AH: Human fibrinogen—Structural variants and functional sites. *Thromb Haemost* 70:42, 1993.
197. Mosesson MW, Cooley BC, Hernandez I, et al: Thrombosis risk modification in transgenic mice containing the human fibrinogen thrombin-binding gamma′ chain sequence. *J Thromb Haemost* 7:102, 2009.
198. Uitte de Willige S, de Visser MC, Houwing-Duistermaat JJ, et al: Genetic variation in the fibrinogen gamma gene increases the risk for deep venous thrombosis by reducing plasma fibrinogen gamma′ levels. *Blood* 106:4176, 2005.
199. Mannila MN, Lovely RS, Kazmierczak SC, et al: Elevated plasma fibrinogen gamma′ concentration is associated with myocardial infarction: Effects of variation in fibrinogen genes and environmental factors. *J Thromb Haemost* 5:766, 2007.
200. Collen D, Tytgat C, Claeys H: Metabolism and distribution of fibrinogen I. Fibrinogen turnover in physiological conditions in humans. *Br J Haematol* 22:681, 1972.
201. Reeve K, Franks J: Fibrinogen synthesis, distribution and degradation. *Semin Thromb Hemost* 1:129, 1974.
202. Fuller G, Otto J, Woloski B: The effects of hepatocyte-stimulating factor on fibrinogen biosynthesis in hepatocyte monolayers. *J Cell Biol* 101:1481, 1985.
203. Huber P, Laurent M, Dalmon J: Human beta-fibrinogen gene expression. Upstream sequences involved in its tissue specific expression and its dexamethasone and interleukin-6 stimulation. *J Biol Chem* 265:5695, 1990.
204. Chung D, Harris I, Davie E: Nucleotide sequences of the three genes coding for human fibrinogen, in *Advances in Experimental Medicine and Biology*, edited by C Liu, S Chien S, p 39. Plenum, New York, 1990.
205. Doolittle R, Watt KW, Cottrell BA, et al: The amino acid sequence of the alpha-chain of human fibrinogen. *Nature* 280:464, 1979.
206. Kant I, Fornace A, Saxe D: Evolution and organization of the fibrinogen locus on chromosome 4: Gene duplication accompanied by transposition and inversion. *Proc Natl Acad Sci U S A* 82:2344, 1985.
207. Morgan J, Courtois G, Fourel G: Spl, a CAAT binding factor and the adenovirus major late promoter transcription factor interact with functional regions of the gamma-fibrinogen promoter. *Mol Cell Biol* 8:2628, 1988.
208. Courtois G, Morgan J, Campbell L, et al: Interaction of a liver-specific nuclear factor with the fibrinogen and a1 antitrypsin promoters. *Science* 238:688, 1987.
209. Dalmon J, Laurent M, Courtois G: The human b fibrinogen promoter contains a HAF-1 dependent IL-6 responsive element. *Mol Cell Biol* 13:1183, 1993.
210. Haidaris P, Courtney M: Molecular biology and regulation of the fibrinogen gene: Tissue-specific and ubiquitous expression of fibrinogen gamma-chain mRNA. *Blood Coagul Fibrinolysis* 1:433, 1990.
211. Handagama PJ, Shuman MA, Bainton DF: *In vivo* defibrination results in markedly decreased amounts of fibrinogen in rat megakaryocytes and platelets. *Am J Pathol* 137:1393, 1990.
212. Louache F, Debili N, Cramer E, et al: Fibrinogen is not synthesized by human megakaryocytes. *Blood* 77:311, 1991.
213. Vali Z, Scheraga H: Localization of the binding site on fibrin for the secondary binding site of thrombin. *Biochemistry* 27:1956, 1988.
214. Olexa S, Budzynaski A: Evidence for four different polymerization sites involved in human fibrin formation. *Proc Natl Acad Sci U S A* 77:1374, 1980.
215. Kaczmarek E, McDonagh J: Thrombin binding to the A alpha-, B beta-, and gamma-chains of fibrinogen and to their remnants contained in fragment E. *J Biol Chem* 263:13896, 1988.
216. Weisel I, Phillips G, Cohen C: The structure of fibrinogen and fibrin: II. Architecture of the fibrin clot. *Ann N Y Acad Sci* 408:367, 1983.
217. Hantgan R, Fowler R, Erickson H, Hermans J: Fibrin assembly: A comparison of electron microscopic and light scattering results. *Thromb Haemost* 44:119, 1980.
218. Dang C, Shin C, Bell W: Fibrinogen sialic acid residues are low affinity calcium-binding sites that influence fibrin assembly. *J Biol Chem* 264:1989, 1989.
219. Nieuwenhuizen W, van Ruijven-Vermneer J, Nooijen W: Recalculation of calcium-binding properties of human and rat fibrin(ogen) and their degradation products. *Thromb Res* 22:653, 1981.
220. Marder V, Budzynski A: Degradation products of fibrinogen and crosslinked fibrin: Projected clinical applications. *Thromb Diath Haemorrh* 32:49, 1974.
221. Elms M, Bunce I, Bundesen P, et al: Measurement of cross-linked fibrin degradation products: An immunoassay using monoclonal antibodies. *Thromb Haemost* 50:591, 1983.
222. Hermans J, McDonagh J: Fibrin: Structure and interactions. *Semin Thromb Hemost* 8:11, 1982.
223. Williams J, Hantgan R, Hermanns J, McDonagh J: Characterization of the inhibition of fibrin assembly by fibrinogen fragment D. *Biochemistry* 197:661, 1981.
224. Mosesson MW: Update on antithrombin I (fibrin). *Thromb Haemost* 98:105, 2007.
225. Lai T-S, Greenberg C: Factor XIII, in *Molecular Basis of Thrombosis and Hemostasis*, edited by KA High, HR Roberts, p 287. Marcel Dekker, New York, 1995.
226. Bottenus R, Ichinose A, Davie E: Nucleotide sequence of the gene for the b subunit of human factor XIII. *Biochemistry* 29:11195, 1990.
227. Ichinose A, Davie E: Characterization of the gene for the a subunit of human factor XIII (plasma transglutaminase) a blood coagulation factor. *Proc Natl Acad Sci U S A* 85:5829, 1988.
228. Ichinose A: Amino acid sequence of the b subunit of human factor XIII, a protein composed of 109 repetitive segments. *Biochemistry* 25:4633, 1986.
229. Ichinose A, Bottenus R, Davie E: Structure of transglutaminase. *J Biol Chem* 265:13411, 1990.
230. Henricksson P, Becker S, McDonagh J: Identification of intracellular factor XIII in human monocytes and macrophages. *J Clin Invest* 76:528, 1985.
231. McDonagh J, McDonagh R, Deleage J, Wagner R: Factor XIII in human plasma and platelets. *J Clin Invest* 48:940, 1969.
232. Weisberg L, Shiu D, Greenberg C, et al: Localization of the gene for coagulation factor XIII a-chain to chromosome 6 and identification of sites of synthesis. *J Clin Invest* 79:649, 1987.
233. Kida M, Souri M, Yamamoto M, et al: Transcriptional regulation of cell type-specific expression of the TATA-less A subunit gene for human coagulation factor XIII. *J Biol Chem* 274:6138, 1999.
234. Lewis KB, Teller DC, Fry J, et al: Crosslinking kinetics of the human transglutaminase, factor XIII[A2], acting on fibrin gels and gamma-chain peptides. *Biochemistry* 36:995, 1997.
235. Sakata Y, Aoki N: Cross-linking of alpha 2-plasmin inhibitor to fibrin by fibrin-stabilizing factor. *J Clin Invest* 65:290, 1980.
236. Boffa MB, Reid TS, Joo E, et al: Characterization of the gene encoding human TAFI (thrombin-activatable fibrinolysis inhibitor; plasma procarboxypeptidase B). *Biochemistry* 38:6547, 1999.
237. Boffa MB, Hamill JD, Bastajian N, et al: A role for CCAAT/enhancer-binding protein in hepatic expression of thrombin-activatable fibrinolysis inhibitor. *J Biol Chem* 277:25329, 2002.
238. Henry M, Aubert H, Morange PE, et al: Identification of polymorphisms in the promoter and the 3′ region of the TAFI gene: Evidence that plasma TAFI antigen levels are strongly genetically controlled. *Blood* 97:2053, 2001.
239. Koschinsky ML, Boffa MB, Nesheim ME, et al: Association of a single nucleotide polymorphism in CPB2 encoding the thrombin-activatable fibrinolysis inhibitor (TAF1) with blood pressure. *Clin Genet* 60:345, 2001.
240. Schneider M, Boffa M, Stewart R, et al: Two naturally occurring variants of TAFI (Thr-325 and Ile-325) differ substantially with respect to thermal stability and antifibrinolytic activity of the enzyme. *J Biol Chem* 277:1021, 2002.
241. Broze GJ Jr: Protein Z-dependent regulation of coagulation. *Thromb Haemost* 86:8, 2001.
242. Broze GJ Jr, Warren LA, Novotny WF, et al: The lipoprotein-associated coagulation inhibitor that inhibits the factor VII-tissue factor complex also inhibits factor Xa: Insight into its possible mechanism of action. *Blood* 71:335, 1988.
243. Warn-Cramer B, Rao L, Maki S, Rapaport SI: Modifications of extrinsic pathway inhibitor (EPI) and factor Xa that affect their ability to interact and to inhibit factor VIIa/tissue factor: Evidence for a two-step model of inhibition. *Thromb Haemost* 60:453, 1988.
244. Ameri A, Kuppuswamy M, Basu S, Bajaj S: Expression of tissue factor pathway inhibitor by cultured endothelial cells in response to inflammatory mediators. *Blood* 79:3219, 1992.
245. Sandset P, Abildgaard U, Larsen M: Heparin induces release of extrinsic coagulation pathway inhibitor (EPI). *Thromb Res* 50:803, 1988.
246. Zhang J, Piro O, Lu L, Broze GJ Jr: Glycosyl phosphatidylinositol anchorage of tissue factor pathway inhibitor. *Circulation* 108:623, 2003.
247. Chang J-Y, Monroe DM, Oliver JA, Roberts HR: TFPIbeta, a second product from the mouse tissue factor pathway inhibitor (TFPI) gene. *Thromb Haemost* 81:45, 1999.
248. Griffith MJ: Measurement of the heparin enhanced-antithrombin III/thrombin reaction rate in the presence of synthetic substrates. *Thromb Res* 25:245, 1982.
249. Fuchs HE, Trapp HG, Griffith MJ, et al: Regulation of Factor IXa *in vitro* in human and mouse plasma and *in vivo* in the mouse. *J Clin Invest* 73:1696, 1984.
250. Sheffield W, Wu Y, Blajchman M: Antithrombin: Structure and function, in *Molecular Basis of Thrombosis and Hemostasis*, edited by KA High, HR Roberts, p 355. Marcel Dekker, New York, 1995.
251. Hamamoto T, Kisiel W: The effect of cell surface glycosaminoglycans (GAGs) on the inactivation of factor VIIa—Tissue factor activity by antithrombin III. *Int J Hematol* 68:67, 1998.
252. Rao LV, Rapaport SI, Hoang AD: Binding of factor VIIa to tissue factor permits rapid antithrombin III/heparin inhibition of factor VIIa. *Blood* 81:2600, 1993.
253. Pizzo S: Serpin receptor 1: A hepatic receptor that mediates the clearance of antithrombin II protease complexes. *Am J Med* 87:10S, 1989.
254. Ochoa A, Brunel F, Mendelson D, et al: Different liver nuclear proteins bind to similar DNA sequences in the 5′ flanking regions of three hepatic genes. *Nucleic Acids Res* 17:116, 1989.
255. Han X, Fiehler R, Broze GJ Jr: Isolation of a protein Z-dependent plasma protease inhibitor. *Proc Natl Acad Sci U S A* 95:9250, 1998.
256. Tabatabai A, Fiehler R, Broze GJ Jr: Protein Z circulates in plasma in a complex with protein Z-dependent protease inhibitor. *Thromb Haemost* 85:655, 2001.
257. Yin ZF, Huang ZF, Cui J, et al: Prothrombotic phenotype of protein Z deficiency. *Proc Natl Acad Sci U S A* 97:6734, 2000.

258. MacFarlane RG: An enzyme cascade in the blood clotting mechanism, and its function as a biological amplifier. *Nature* 202:498, 1964.
259. Davie EW, Ratnoff OD: Waterfall sequence for intrinsic blood clotting. *Science* 145:1310, 1964.
260. Nemerson Y, Esnouf MP: Activation of a proteolytic system by a membrane lipoprotein: Mechanism of action of tissue factor. *Proc Natl Acad Sci U S A* 70:310, 1973.
261. Nemerson Y: The tissue factor pathway of blood coagulation. *Semin Hematol* 29:170, 1992.
262. Repke D, Gemmell CH, Guha A, et al: Hemophilia as a defect of the tissue factor pathway of blood coagulation: Effect of factors VIII and IX on factor X activation in a continuous-flow reactor. *Proc Natl Acad Sci U S A* 87:7623, 1990.
263. Broze GJ Jr, Girard TJ, Novotny WF: Regulation of coagulation by a multivalent Kunitz-type inhibitor. *Biochemistry* 29:7539, 1990.
264. Hockin MF, Kalafatis M, Shatos M, Mann KG: Protein C activation and factor Va inactivation on human umbilical vein endothelial cells. *Arterioscler Thromb Vasc Biol* 17:2765, 1997.
265. Fay PJ, Smudzin TM, Walker FJ: Activated protein C-catalyzed inactivation of human factor VIII and VIIIa. *J Biol Chem* 266:20139, 1991.
266. Pieters J, Willems G, Hemker HC, Lindhout T: Inhibition of factor IXa and factor Xa by antithrombin III/heparin during factor X activation. *J Biol Chem* 263:15313, 1988.
267. Allen DH, Tracy PB: Human coagulation factor V is activated to the functional cofactor by elastase and cathepsin G expressed at the monocyte surface. *J Biol Chem* 270:1408, 1995.
268. Monroe DM, Hoffman M, Roberts HR: Transmission of a procoagulant signal from tissue factor-bearing cells to platelets. *Blood Coagul Fibrinolysis* 7:459, 1996.
269. Eilertsen KE, Osterud B: Tissue factor: (Patho)physiology and cellular biology. *Blood Coagul Fibrinolysis* 15:521, 2004.
270. Censarek P, Bobbe A, Grandoch M, et al: Alternatively spliced human tissue factor (asHTF) is not pro-coagulant. *Thromb Haemost* 97:11, 2007.
271. Schwertz H, Tolley ND, Foulks JM, et al: Signal-dependent splicing of tissue factor pre-mRNA modulates the thrombogenicity of human platelets. *J Exp Med* 203:2433, 2006.
272. Hoffman M, Whinna HC, Monroe DM: Circulating tissue factor accumulates in thrombi, but not in hemostatic plugs. *J Thromb Haemost* 4:2092, 2006.
273. Biro E, Sturk-Maquelin KN, Vogel GM, et al: Human cell-derived microparticles promote thrombus formation *in vivo* in a tissue factor-dependent manner. *J Thromb Haemost* 1:2561, 2003.
274. Chou J, Mackman N, Merrill-Skoloff G, et al: Hematopoietic cell-derived microparticle tissue factor contributes to fibrin formation during thrombus propagation. *Blood* 104:3190, 2004.
275. Day SM, Reeve JL, Pedersen B, et al: Macrovascular thrombosis is driven by tissue factor derived primarily from the blood vessel wall. *Blood* 105:192, 2005.
276. Falati S, Gross P, Merrill-Skoloff G, et al: Real-time *in vivo* imaging of platelets, tissue factor and fibrin during arterial thrombus formation in the mouse. *Nat Med* 8:1175, 2002.
277. Williamson P, Bevers EM, Smeets EF, et al: Continuous analysis of the mechanism of activated transbilayer lipid movement in platelets. *Biochemistry* 34:10448, 1995.
278. Monroe DM, Roberts HR, Hoffman M: Platelet procoagulant complex assembly in a tissue factor-initiated system. *Br J Haematol* 88:364, 1994.
279. Ahmad SS, Rawala-Sheikh R, Walsh PN: Platelet receptor occupancy with factor IXa promotes factor X activation. *J Biol Chem* 264:20012, 1989.
280. Ahmad SS, Rawala-Sheikh R, Ashby B, Walsh PN: Platelet receptor-mediated factor X activation by factor IX. High-affinity factor IXa receptors induced by factor VIII are deficient on platelets in Scott syndrome. *J Clin Invest* 84:824, 1998.
280a. Kravtsov DV, Matafonov A, Tucker EI: Factor XI contributes to thrombin generation in the absence of factor XII. *Blood* 114:452, 2009.
281. Baglia FA, Walsh PN: Prothrombin is a cofactor for the binding of factor XI to the platelet surface and for platelet-mediated factor XI activation by thrombin. *Biochemistry* 37:2271, 1998.
282. von dem Borne PA, Bajzar L, Meijers JC, et al: Thrombin-mediated activation of factor XI results in a thrombin-activatable fibrinolysis inhibitor-dependent inhibition of fibrinolysis. *J Clin Invest* 99:2323, 1997.
283. Alberio L, Safa O, Clemetson KJ, et al: Surface expression and functional characterization of alpha-granule factor V in human platelets: Effects of ionophore A23187, thrombin, collagen, and convulxin. *Blood* 95:1694, 2000.
284. Dale GL, Friese P, Batar P, et al: Stimulated platelets use serotonin to enhance their retention of procoagulant proteins on the cell surface. *Nature* 415:175, 2002.
285. Kempton CL, Hoffman M, Roberts HR, Monroe DM: Platelet heterogeneity: Variation in coagulation complexes on platelet subpopulations. *Arterioscler Thromb Vasc Biol* 25:861, 2005.
286. de Agostini A, Watkins S, Slayter H, et al: Localization of the anticoagulantly active heparan sulphate proteoglycans in vascular endothelium: Antithrombin binding on cultured endothelial cells and perfused rat aorta. *J Cell Biol* 111:1293, 1990.
287. Marcus AJ, Broekman MJ, Drosopoulos JHF, et al: The endothelial cell ecto-ADPase responsible for inhibition of platelet function is CD39. *J Clin Invest* 99:1351, 1997.
288. Jesty J, Beltrami E, Willems G: Mathematical analysis of a proteolytic positive-feedback loop: Dependence of lag time and enzyme yields on the initial conditions and kinetic parameters. *Biochemistry* 32:6266, 1993.
289. Brakman P, Albrechtsen OK, Astrup T: A comparative study of coagulation and fibrinolysis in blood from normal men and women. *Br J Haematol* 12:74, 1966.
290. Nossel H, Yudelman I, Canfield Rea: Measurement of fibrinopeptide A in human blood. *J Clin Invest* 54:43, 1974.
291. Bauer KA, Kass BL, ten Cate H, et al: Factor IX is activated *in vivo* by the tissue factor mechanism. *Blood* 76:731, 1990.
292. Bauer KA, Kass BL, ten Cate H, et al: Detection of factor X activation in humans. *Blood* 74:2007, 1989.
293. Morrissey JH: Tissue factor modulation of factor VIIa activity: Use in measuring trace levels of factor VIIa in plasma. *Thromb Haemost* 74:185, 1995.
294. Jesty J, Beltrami E: Positive feedbacks of coagulation: Their role in threshold regulation. *Arterioscler Thromb Vasc Biol* 25:2463, 2005.
295. Conard J, Bauer KA, Gruber A, et al: Normalization of markers of coagulation activation with a purified protein C concentrate in adults with homozygous protein C deficiency. *Blood* 82:1159, 1993.
296. Harlos K, Martin DM, O'Brien DP, et al: Crystal structure of the extracellular region of human tissue factor. *Nature* 370:662, 1994.
297. Hoffman M, Harger A, Lenkowski A, et al: Cutaneous wound healing is impaired in hemophilia B. *Blood* 108:3053, 2006.

CHAPTER 116

CONTROL OF COAGULATION REACTIONS

John H. Griffin

SUMMARY

The blood coagulation system, like a powerful idling engine, is always active and generating thrombin at very low levels and is poised for explosive thrombin generation. Positive feedback activation of factors V, VIII, XI, and VII imparts special threshold properties to blood coagulation, making the coagulant response nonlinearly responsive to stimuli. Overt blood coagulation represents a threshold system with apparent all-or-none responses to various levels of stimuli, and an ensemble of opposing reactions determines the ultimate upregulation and downregulation of thrombin generation both locally and systemically. Cellular and humoral anticoagulant mechanisms synergize with plasma coagulation inhibitors to prevent massive thrombin generation in the absence of a substantial procoagulant stimulus. This chapter highlights mechanisms that inhibit blood coagulation, with an emphasis on defects of plasma proteins that cause hereditary thrombophilias. Major thrombophilic defects involve the anticoagulant protein C pathway comprising multiple cofactors or effectors that besides protein C include thrombomodulin, endothelial protein C receptor, protein S, high-density lipoprotein, and factor V. Activated protein C exerts multiple protective homeostatic actions, including proteolytic inactivation of factors Va and VIIIa, as well as direct cell-signaling activities involving protease activated receptor-1, endothelial cell protein C receptor, and apolipoprotein E receptor 2. The factor V Leiden variant causes hereditary activated protein C resistance by impairing the ability of the protein C pathway to inhibit coagulation because it cannot properly cleave factor Va Leiden. Plasma protease inhibitors are also key to block coagulation. Antithrombin inhibits thrombin and factors Xa, IXa, XIa, and XIIa, in reactions stimulated by physiologic heparan sulfate or pharmacologic heparins. Tissue factor pathway inhibitor neutralizes the extrinsic coagulation pathway factors VIIa and Xa. Other plasma protease inhibitors can also neutralize various coagulation proteases.

Control of coagulation reactions is essential for normal hemostasis. As part of the tangled web of host defense systems that respond to vascular injury, the blood coagulation factors (see Chap. 115) act in concert with the endothelium and blood cells, especially platelets, to generate a protective fibrin-platelet clot, forming a hemostatic plug. Pathologic thrombosis occurs when the protective clot is extended beyond its beneficial size, when a clot occurs inappropriately at sites of vascular disease, or when a clot embolizes to other sites in the circulatory bed. For normal hemostasis, both procoagulant and anticoagulant factors must interact with the vascular components and cell surfaces, including the vessel wall (see Chap. 117) and platelets (see Chap. 114). Moreover, the action of the fibrinolytic system must be integrated with coagulation reactions for timely formation and dissolution of blood clots (see Chap. 136). This chapter on control of coagulation highlights the major physiologic mechanisms for downregulation of blood coagulation reactions and the plasma proteins that inhibit blood coagulation, with an emphasis on those mechanisms whose defects are clinically significant based on insights gleaned from consideration of the hereditary thrombophilias (see Chap. 131). Chap. 115 provides a complete description of blood coagulation factors and hemostatic pathways.

Acronyms and abbreviations that appear in this chapter include: APC, activated protein C; apoER2, apolipoprotein E receptor 2; EPCR, endothelial cell protein C receptor; GLA, γ-carboxyglutamic acid; HDL, high-density lipoprotein; NMDA, *N*-methyl-D-aspartate; PAR-1, protease activated receptor-1; serpin, serine protease inhibitor; SHBG, sex-hormone-binding globulin-like; TFPI, tissue factor pathway inhibitor; ZPI, protein Z-dependent protease inhibitor.

BLOOD COAGULATION PATHWAYS AND THE PROTEIN C PATHWAYS

Although decades have elapsed since the elaboration of the cascade model[1,2] for blood coagulation (see Fig. 115–28), the basic outline of sequential conversions of protease zymogens to active serine proteases is still useful, albeit with important modifications, to represent blood coagulation reactions. The major conceptual advances for procoagulant pathways in the past two decades emphasize both positive and negative feedback reactions affecting thrombin generation as depicted in Figure 116–1.

In positive feedback reactions, procoagulant thrombin activates platelets and factors V, VIII, and XI (see Chap. 115).[3–7] Small amounts of thrombin can be generated by trace amounts of tissue factor via the extrinsic pathway. Subsequently, thrombin can activate factors XI, VIII, and V, thereby stimulating each of the steps in the intrinsic pathway and thus amplifying thrombin generation (see Fig. 116–1).

In negative feedback reactions, anticoagulant activated protein C (APC) that is generated on endothelial cell surfaces[8,9] (Fig. 116–2) downregulates coagulation (see Figs. 116–1 and 116–3). Furthermore, APC can exert direct cytoprotective effects on cells via reactions that involve certain receptors, including endothelial protein C receptor (EPCR) and protease activated receptor-1 (PAR-1) (Fig. 116–4),[9] and possibly apolipoprotein E receptor 2 (apoER2). APC's cytoprotective effects include antiinflammatory and antiapoptotic activities, as well as alterations of gene expression profiles and stabilization of endothelial barriers (see "Activated Protein C Activities" below). Because inflammation, apoptosis, and vascular barrier breakdown contribute significantly to reactions that promote thrombin generation, such direct cytoprotective effects of APC on cells indirectly downregulate thrombin generation.[9]

For APC generation by the protein C cellular pathway, binding of thrombin to thrombomodulin converts the bound thrombin from a procoagulant enzyme to an anticoagulant enzyme that converts the protein C zymogen to an anticoagulant serine protease, APC (see Figs. 116–1 and 116–2). This surface-dependent reaction is enhanced by the EPCR that binds protein C.[8,10,11] With the aid of its nonenzymatic cofactor, protein S, as well as other potential lipid and protein cofactors, APC inactivates factors Va and VIIIa by highly selective proteolysis, yielding inactive (i) cofactors, that is, factors V_i and VIII_i (see Fig. 116–3 and Figs. 115–15 and 115–17). Protein S also can directly inhibit factors VIIIa, Xa, and Va.[12–15] Thus, APC and protein S inhibit multiple steps in the intrinsic coagulation pathway.

At each step in the coagulation pathways, each clotting protease can be inhibited by one or more plasma protease inhibitors in reactions stimulated by negatively charged glycosaminoglycans such as heparan sulfate or heparin (see "Inhibition of Coagulation Proteases by Protease Inhibitors" below).[16] Given the highly nonlinear nature of the coagulation pathways with both positive and negative feedback reactions,

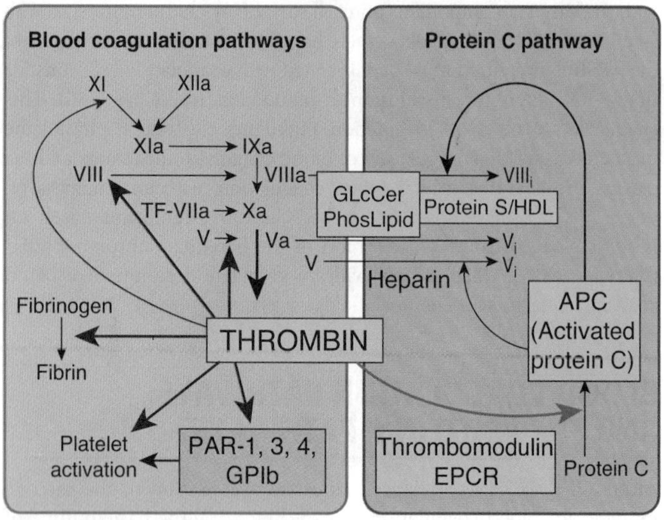

FIGURE 116–1. Blood coagulation pathways and protein C anticoagulant pathway. Thrombin can be either a procoagulant (*left*) or an anticoagulant (*right*) depending on cofactors and surfaces. Coagulant thrombin clots fibrinogen and activates platelets and factors V, VIII, XI, and XIII. Conversion of zymogen protein C to the active protease, APC, by thrombomodulin-bound thrombin is enhanced by endothelial protein C receptor (EPCR). APC with its nonenzymatic cofactor, protein S, inactivates factors Va and VIIIa by highly selective proteolysis (e.g., at Arg506 and Arg306 in factor Va), yielding inactivated (i) factors V_i and VIII_i. This anticoagulant action may be enhanced by phospholipid (PL) surfaces on platelets, endothelial cells, or their microparticles. High-density lipoprotein (HDL) can also provide protein S-dependent anticoagulant APC-cofactor activity. Similarly, neutral glycosphingolipids such as glucosylceramide can enhance APC anticoagulant activity. *(Adapted with permission from Griffin JH.[8])*

synergy between the protein C pathway and plasma protease inhibitors is important for regulating thrombin generation.

There is continuous activation of coagulation factors at a basal physiologic low level. Plasma from all normal subjects contains circulating active enzymes, factor VIIa,[17] and APC,[18] as well as various polypeptide fragments generated by the action of clotting proteases, namely fibrinopeptides,[19,20] prothrombin fragment 1+2,[21] and activation peptides for factors IX and X.[22,23] The presence of multiple clotting factors that require positive feedback activation (e.g., factors V, VIII, XI, and VII) imparts special threshold properties to the blood coagulation pathways, making the coagulant response nonlinearly responsive to stimuli. Theoretical analysis of blood coagulation as a threshold system suggests there can be an all-or-none response to various levels of stimulation, depending on the ensemble of activating and inhibitory reactions that defines upregulation and downregulation of thrombin generation.[24,25] The coagulation system is active, but idling, and is poised for extensive and explosive generation of thrombin. Because of synergy among various cellular and humoral anticoagulant mechanisms that establish a threshold system, the presence of multiple coagulation inhibitors with complementary modes of action prevents massive thrombin generation in the absence of a substantial procoagulant stimulus.

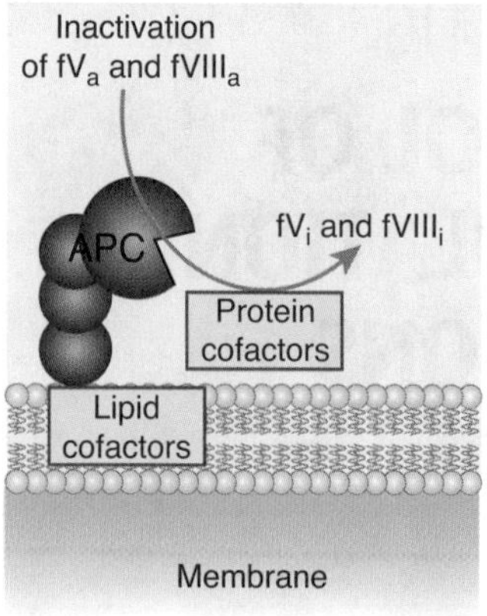

FIGURE 116–3. Activated protein C (APC) exerts its anticoagulant activity by proteolytic inactivation of factors Va and VIIIa on membrane surfaces containing phospholipids that are derived from cells, lipoproteins, or cellular microparticles. A variety of lipid and protein cofactors (see Fig. 116–1 legend and text) accelerate the inactivation of factors Va and VIIIa to yield the irreversibly inactivated factors Vi and VIIIi. *(Adapted with permission from Mosnier LO, Zlokovic BV, Griffin JH.[9])*

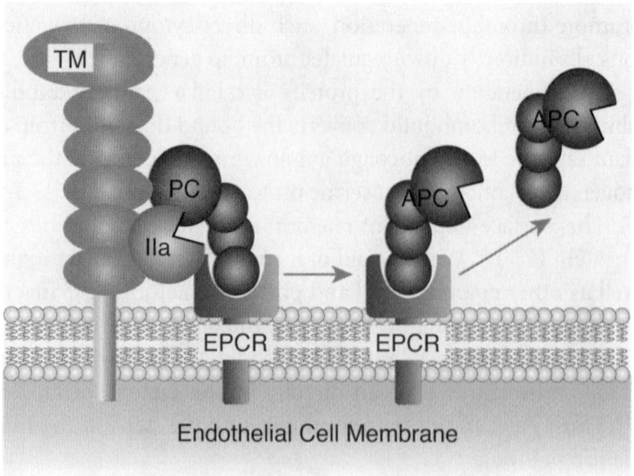

FIGURE 116–2. Protein C activation on endothelial cell surface. On an endothelial surface, activated protein C (APC) generation follows binding of protein C (PC) to endothelial protein C receptor (EPCR) where PC is activated by limited proteolysis by the thrombin:thrombomodulin complex (IIa:TM). This action of thrombin liberates a dodecapeptide (residues 158–169) from protein C to generate the multifunctional protease APC. *(Adapted with permission from Mosnier LO, Zlokovic BV, Griffin JH.[9])*

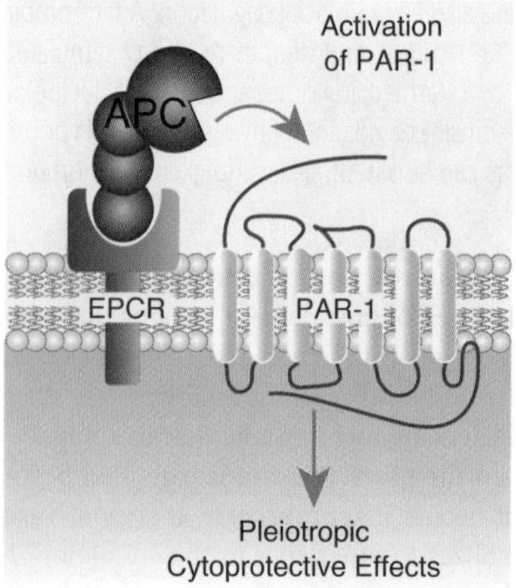

FIGURE 116–4. Paradigm for activated protein C (APC)'s initiation of cell signaling and multiple cytoprotective effects. Direct effects of APC on cells are initiated by activation of the G-protein-coupled receptor, protease activated receptor-1 (PAR-1), by endothelial protein C receptor (EPCR)-bound APC. The γ-carboxyglutamic acid (GLA) domain of APC binds to EPCR to help position APC's protease domain for efficient cleavage of the extracellular N-terminal tail of PAR-1, which results in G-protein-coupled receptor activation and subsequent antiinflammatory and antiapoptotic effects, alterations of gene expression profiles, and stabilization of endothelial junctions. *(Adapted with permission from Mosnier LO, Zlokovic BV, Griffin JH.[9])*

HEREDITARY DEFICIENCIES ASSOCIATED WITH THROMBOTIC DISEASE

Evidence for the physiologic importance of specific factors for controlling coagulation reactions comes from clinical observations and animal model studies. Major identified genetic risk factors for venous thrombosis involve protein structural defects in factor V, protein C, protein S, and antithrombin (see Chap. 131). There are also gene regulatory defects associated with thrombotic disease such as the nt G20210A polymorphism in the prothrombin gene that causes elevated levels of prothrombin and the defects in protein C gene regulatory elements that decrease the expression of protein C. Deficiencies of thrombomodulin might also be associated with increased risk of arterial thrombosis. Association of hereditary abnormalities of EPCR with increased risks of thrombosis has been suggested, but this remains somewhat controversial.

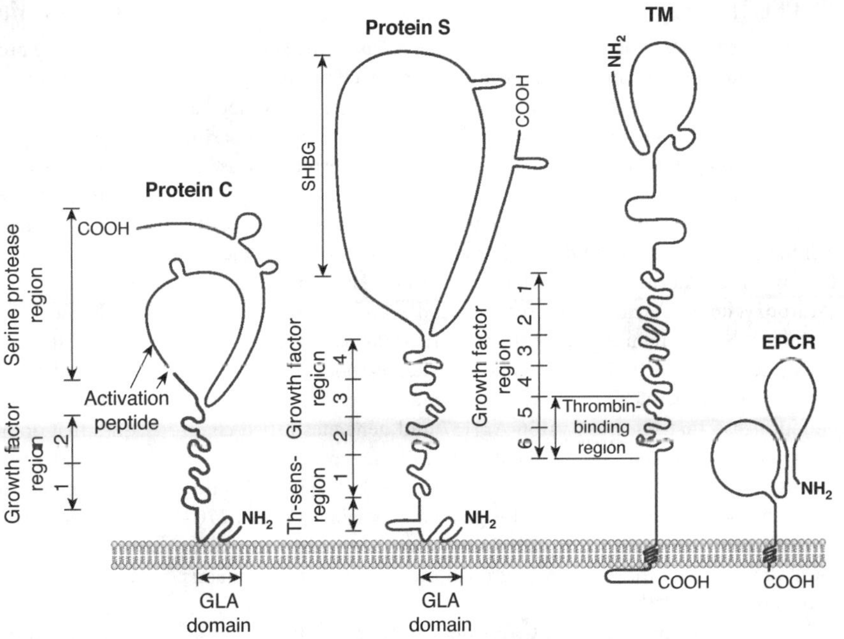

FIGURE 116–5. Membrane-bound protein C, protein S, thrombomodulin$_{TM}$, and endothelial cell protein C receptor (EPCR). Each protein is a multidomain protein that extends above the surface of cell membranes, and different domains mediate different functions of each protein. Proteins C and S can bind reversibly to phospholipid membranes through their NH_2-terminal γ-carboxyglutamic acid (GLA) domains which contain 9 or 11 GLA residues that bind four to six Ca^{2+} ions. TM and EPCR are integral membrane proteins that are embedded in cell membranes by a single hydrophobic transmembrane sequence. *(Adapted with permission from Esmon CT.[91])*

PROTEIN C PATHWAY COMPONENTS

Figure 116–5 provides schematic representations of the structures of protein C, protein S, thrombomodulin, and EPCR. These proteins contain multiple domains, each of which may mediate different molecular functions. Values for the molecular weight, normal plasma concentration, chromosomal location, and gene structures of these factors are given in Tables 115–1 and 116–1. Factors Va and VIIIa, as substrates of APC, are also participants in the reactions of the anticoagulant protein C pathway. Moreover, factor V, but not factor V Leiden, appears to act as an APC cofactor for the inactivation of factor VIIIa (see "Factor V as Activated Protein C Cofactor" below).[26,27]

TABLE 116–1. Characteristics of Blood Coagulation Regulatory Molecules

	Molecular Weight (kDa)	Plasma Concentration (mcg/mL)	Half-Life (h)	Chromosome	Gene (kb)	Exon (N)	Function
Protein C	62	4	6	2q13–14	11	9	Anticoagulant protease
Protein S	75	26	42	3p11.1–11.2	80	15	APC-cofactor and coagulation inhibitor
Thrombomodulin	60–105	0.020	ND	20p11.2–cen	3.7	1	Receptor for thrombin/protein C
Endothelial protein C receptor (EPCR)	46	0.098	ND	20q11.2	6	4	Receptor for protein C/APC
Protease activated receptor-1 (PAR-1)	68	NA	NA	5q13	27	2	G-protein-coupled receptor
Antithrombin	58	150	70	1q23–25	14	7	Protease inhibitor
Tissue factor pathway inhibitor (TFPI)	34	0.1	ND	2q31–32.1	85	9	Protease inhibitor
Heparin cofactor II	66	70	60	22q11	16	5	Protease inhibitor
Protein Z	70	1.7	60	13q34		9	Plasma protein
Protein Z-dependent protease inhibitor (ZPI)	72	1.5		14q32.13		5	Protease inhibitor

NA, not applicable; ND, not determined.

PROTEIN C

In 1976, Stenflo designated a bovine plasma vitamin K-dependent protein that eluted in the third peak (peak C) from an anion exchange column as bovine "protein C."[28] Protein C, actually previously described as the anticoagulant factor autoprothrombin II-A,[29] is a plasma serine protease zymogen that can be converted to an active serine protease by the action of thrombin.

Protein C is synthesized in the liver as a polypeptide precursor of 461 residues, with a prepropeptide of 42 amino acids that contains the signal for carboxylation of Glu residues by a carboxylase that forms nine γ-carboxyglutamic acid (GLA) residues and secretion of the mature protein.[30–32] The mature glycoprotein of Mr 62,000 contains 419 residues (see Figs. 115–1 and 116–5) and *N*-linked carbohydrate, and the majority of the secreted protein C molecules are cleaved by a furin-like endoprotease that releases Lys156-Arg157 and generates a two-chain zymogen that circulates in plasma at 70 nM (4 mcg/mL).[33] The heavy and light chains of plasma protein C are covalently linked by a disulfide bond that keeps the serine protease globular domain (residues 170–419) covalently tethered to the N-terminal string of three domains, the GLA domain and the epidermal growth factor (EGF)-like domains EGF1 and EGF2.[30–34]

The GLA domain of protein C (residues 1–42) and APC is important for a number of functions, including binding to phospholipid-containing membranes (see Fig. 115–3), thrombomodulin, and EPCR; thus, incomplete carboxylation impairs the functional anticoagulant activity of APC.[35–38] The two EGF modules in the light chain may contribute to interactions of APC with protein S and of protein C with thrombomodulin.

The serine protease domain of protein C is homologous to other trypsin-like proteases, and three-dimensional modeling[39] and X-ray crystallographic structures[34] reflect the structural similarity of APC to members of the serine protease family of which chymotrypsin is the prototype. APC's trypsin-like protease domain exerts its anticoagulant activity by highly specific interactions with factors Va and VIIIa followed by cleavage at only two Arg-containing peptide bonds in factors Va and VIIIa (see "Factors Va and VIIIa as Substrates for Activated Protein C" below). These stereo-specific interactions involve both the APC enzymatic active site region and a number of APC residues that are termed *exosites* because they are not located in the immediate vicinity of APC's enzymatic active site. Such APC exosites are essential for specific recognition of the macromolecular substrates, factors Va and VIIIa as well as recognition of cellular APC receptors.[40–49]

Protein C and Activated Protein C Therapy

Purified plasma protein C concentrate (Ceprotin) is FDA-approved for treating protein C-deficient patients.[50–52] Recombinant APC (Xigris) reduces all-cause 28-day mortality in severe sepsis adult patients and is FDA-approved for this indication.[53] The successful therapy of adult severe sepsis using APC followed preclinical antithrombotic and sepsis studies in baboons.[54,55] Various preclinical studies suggest APC therapy may be useful in multiple settings,[9,56,57] including ischemic stroke,[58] wound healing,[57] and islet transplantation for diabetes.[59] Animal injury model studies have also shed light on *in vivo* mechanisms for APC beneficial effects, which can appear to be independent of APC's anticoagulant actions (see "Activated Protein C Direct Cellular Effects Activities" below).

Protein C Gene

The protein C gene, comprising nine exons and eight introns, is located on chromosome 2q14–21 and spans 11 kb (see Fig. 115–12 and Table 116–1).[60–63] The protein C gene is homologous to the genes for factors VII, IX, and X (see Chap. 115).

Protein C Mutations

Hereditary protein C deficiency associated with thrombosis is caused by numerous mutations (see protein C mutation databases[64,65]). Based on three-dimensional structures of the protein C, the structural basis for hereditary protein C defects has been rationalized.[39,66,67] Most mutations that cause type I protein C deficiency, characterized by parallel reductions in activity and antigen, involve amino acid residues that form the hydrophobic cores of the two folded globulin-like domains that are characteristic of serine proteases. These mutations destabilize either the process or the product of protein folding, and they result in unstable molecules that are poorly secreted and/or exhibit a very short circulatory half-life. In contrast, most mutations that cause type II defects (reduced anticoagulant or enzymatic activity but normal antigen levels), that is, circulating dysfunctional molecules, involve polar surface residues that do not affect polypeptide folding or thermodynamic stability; these polar residues presumably are involved in protein–protein interactions important for expression of anticoagulant activity.

Severe protein C deficiency as a consequence of homozygous knockout of the mouse protein C gene showed a similar phenotype as severe human protein C deficiency (Chap. 131), with perinatal consumptive coagulopathy in the brain and liver and either death or massive thrombosis that occurred either intrauterine or shortly after birth.[68]

PROTEIN S

Plasma "protein S" which was named in honor of Seattle, the city of its discovery, is a vitamin K-dependent glycoprotein[69,70] that is synthesized by hepatocytes, neuroblastoma cells, kidney cells, testis, megakaryocytes, and endothelial cells, and is also found in platelet α-granules.[71]

Protein S is synthesized as a precursor protein of 676 amino acids, which gives rise to a mature secreted single-chain glycoprotein of 635 residues with three *N*-linked carbohydrate side chains (see Figs. 115–13 and 116–5).[72–74] Eleven GLA residues in the N-terminal region of mature protein S contribute to Ca^{2+}-mediated binding of the protein to phospholipid membranes. The thrombin-sensitive region, residues 47 to 72, follows the GLA-domain (see Fig. 116–5).

The C-terminal region of protein S, residues 270 to 635, the sex-hormone-binding globulin-like (SHBG) region contains binding sites for C4b-binding protein (see "Activated Protein C–Independent Anticoagulant Activity of Protein S" below)[75] and for factor V as well as factor Va.[76,77] Protein S, like the homologous gas6, also binds to receptor tyrosine kinases, for example, Axl, and initiates cell signaling, and the SHBG region binds the receptor.[78] Thus, for the expression of its multiple activities, different domains of protein S exhibit a number of different binding sites for different proteins.

Protein S Gene

The protein S gene, comprising 15 exons and 14 introns, is located on chromosome 3p11.1–11.2 and spans 80 kb (see Fig. 115–13 and Table 116–1).[62,79–81] The protein S gene has limited homology with other genes for vitamin K–dependent factors in the GLA and EGF domains and notable homology of the region coding for residues 240 to 635 with genes of the SHBG family. Humans contain a protein S pseudogene that contains several stop codons and is not translated and that is located very near the normal protein S gene on chromosome 3.

Protein S Mutations

The molecular basis for hereditary protein S deficiency associated with venous thrombosis (see Chap. 131) is linked to more than 100 different mutations.[82] A protein S polymorphism that is strongly linked to risk for venous thrombosis in Japanese subjects, is known as protein S Tokushima. It involves K155E, which ablates APC-cofactor activity.[83,84] But the K155E apparently is not present in whites, thus mirroring the presence of factor V Leiden and prothrombin G20210A that are risk factors in whites but not in the Japanese population.[85] Another single nucleotide polymorphism present in approximately 1 percent of whites is S460P, which is designated protein S Heerlen; it results in absence of *N*-linked carbohydrate on Asn458 but has no accepted significant functional consequence.[86]

THROMBOMODULIN

Thrombomodulin was discovered as an endothelial cell surface receptor that binds protein C and thrombin, thereby accelerating protein C activation.[87,88] Binding of thrombin to thrombomodulin converts thrombin from a procoagulant enzyme to an anticoagulant enzyme because thrombomodulin-bound thrombin loses its normal ability to clot fibrinogen or activate platelets.[89,90] Thrombomodulin is a multidomain transmembrane protein comprising an N-terminal lectin-like domain, six EGF domains, a Ser/Thr-rich region, a single membrane-spanning sequence, and an intracellular C-terminal tail (see Fig. 116–5).[7–9,87–93] EGF domains 4, 5, and 6 are essential for activation of protein C, with the latter two domains binding thrombin and the first domain binding protein C. The mature protein has 557 amino acid residues and variable amounts of *N*- and *O*-linked carbohydrate modifications that cause variability in molecular size. Glycosaminoglycans, notably chondroitin sulfate, covalently attached to the Ser/Thr-rich region, contribute to the functional properties of thrombomodulin by enhancing either protein C activation by thrombin or by accelerating neutralization of thrombin by protease inhibitors. Modulation of the substrate specificity of thrombin by thrombomodulin involves conformational changes in thrombin caused by binding of thrombomodulin.

Low levels of soluble thrombomodulin circulate in plasma, presumably as a result of limited proteolysis of the protein near its transmembrane cell surface anchor. The functional significance of circulating thrombomodulin is unknown, although variations in its plasma level arise in different clinical conditions.

Thrombomodulin Gene

The thrombomodulin gene, which lacks introns, is located on chromosome 20p12 and spans 3.7 kb (see Figs. 115–21 and 116–5 and Table 116–1).[92,95] Deletion of the thrombomodulin gene in mice is embryonically lethal.[96] Downregulation of thrombomodulin gene expression is promoted by a variety of inflammatory agents, including endotoxin, interleukin-1, and tumor necrosis factor-α, whereas its expression is upregulated by retinoic acid.[7–9,97,98] Generally, thrombomodulin is a key member among the counterbalancing factors that contribute to inflammation, thrombin generation and coagulation in the endothelium.

Thrombomodulin Mutations

Thrombomodulin mutations are well documented in atypical hemolytic uremic syndrome patients,[99] and they may also be associated with an increased risk of arterial thrombosis and myocardial infarction. In contrast, there is less supportive data for association with risk for venous thrombosis (see Chap. 131).[100–104] Atypical hemolytic uremic syndrome is strongly linked to excessive complement activation, and thrombomodulin's lectin-like domain inhibits complement activation.[105] Furthermore, besides promoting protein C activation by thrombin, thrombomodulin also supports activation of the carboxypeptidase, also known as thrombin-activatable fibrinolysis inhibitor, that is a potent inactivator of activated complement component, C5a.[106]

ENDOTHELIAL PROTEIN C RECEPTOR

EPCR binds both protein C and APC with similar affinities through their GLA domains and mediates multiple activities of this zymogen and activated protease.[10,11,38,97,107–117] The mature EPCR glycoprotein contains 221 amino acid residues and *N*-linked carbohydrate, giving an Mr of 46,000. EPCR is an integral membrane protein that is homologous to CD1/major histocompatibility complex class I molecules. The N-terminus is part of an extracellular domain which is connected to a single transmembrane sequence that is followed by a short Arg-Arg-Cys-COOH cytoplasmic tail (see Fig. 116–5). The cytoplasmic tail can be palmitoylated, and this modification may help localize EPCR to certain lipid rafts or caveolae. In blood vessels, EPCR is mainly located on the surface of large vessels, in contrast to the predominant localization of thrombomodulin in the microcirculation. EPCR on endothelial surfaces enhances by fivefold the rate of activation of protein C by thrombin:thrombomodulin, as depicted in Figure 116–2. The three-dimensional structure of EPCR determined by X-ray crystallography or inferred by molecular modeling established that the overall folding of the protein is as expected, and various studies identified the binding site for the protein C GLA domain.[117,118]

Soluble EPCR is found in normal human plasma at 100 ng/mL; in purified reaction mixtures, soluble EPCR at relatively high levels inhibits the anticoagulant action of APC against factor Va but not the reaction of APC with protease inhibitors.[11,97,108,119] Levels of soluble EPCR are increased in patients with disseminated intravascular coagulation and patients with systemic lupus erythematosus, and EPCR increases are not correlated with alterations in circulating thrombomodulin levels.[120] Because soluble EPCR binds protein C and APC with an affinity similar to the membrane-bound molecule, it has been speculated that EPCR binds the protein C and the APC GLA domains without thermodynamically significant contributions from membrane phospholipids, a speculation seemingly confirmed by the EPCR crystallographic structure, although the crystal structure revealed an unexpected phospholipid bound in a groove on the surface of EPCR.[117]

APC exerts multiple cytoprotective activities that are completely independent of its anticoagulant activity (see "Activated Protein C Direct Cellular Activities" below).[9,56,57,97] EPCR modulates the activities of APC by inhibiting its anticoagulant actions that target factors Va and VIIIa (see Fig. 115–3) and promoting its cleavage of PAR-1 (see Fig. 116–4) and cytoprotective actions, which may also potentially involve APC binding to apoER2.[121] The physiologic requirement for EPCR is established by the embryonic lethality caused by knockout of the murine EPCR gene.[122]

Endothelial Protein C Receptor Gene

The EPCR gene, comprising four exons and three introns, is located on human chromosome 20q11.2 and spans 6 kb (see Table 116–1).[123]

PROTEASE ACTIVATED RECEPTOR-1

PAR-1, discovered as a high-affinity human platelet receptor for thrombin,[124] is the prototype of a four-member subfamily of G-protein-coupled receptors that share an unusual mechanism of activation, namely activation by proteases.[124–130] Each PAR contains seven transmembrane helical domains and an extracellular N-terminal tail that is cleaved by a activating protease such that the newly generated amino-terminus is a tethered ligand that triggers activation of the coupled G-protein. Human platelets employ PAR-1 and PAR-3 for activation by thrombin whereas, curiously, murine platelets require PAR-3 and PAR-4, but not PAR-1, for thrombin's normal effects. PAR-1 is activated by various plasma proteases and is generally required for APC's cytoprotective activities (see "Cellular Receptors for Physiologic Effects of Activated Protein C on Cells" below).[9,56,57]

Protease Activated Receptor-1 Gene

The PAR-1 gene contains only two introns, is located on chromosome 5q13, and spans 25 kb (see Table 116–1).[125] Much is known about many factors that can either upregulate or downregulate the PAR-1 gene.[124–130]

ACTIVATION OF PROTEIN C

Protein C is activated from zymogen to active protease as a result of cleavage by thrombin at the Arg169-Leu170 peptide bond in a reaction that is accelerated by thrombomodulin and EPCR (see Fig. 116–2 and "Thrombomodulin" above).[7,9,88,91,97] Thrombin infusions into animals generate anticoagulant activity because of APC.[131,132] Interestingly, thrombin infusion into hyperlipidemic monkeys with atherosclerosis generates less APC and causes a poorer *ex vivo* response to APC compared with normolipidemic control monkeys,[133] showing that hyperlipidemia and vascular disease can affect protein C activation.

Ischemia causes protein C activation *in vivo*. A brief occlusion of the left anterior descending coronary artery in pigs results in APC generation.[134] During cerebral ischemia in humans undergoing routine endarterectomy, APC increases in the venous cerebral blood.[135] Protein C is significantly activated during cardiopulmonary bypass, mainly during the minutes immediately after aortic unclamping in the ischemic vascular beds.[136] Streptokinase therapy for acute myocardial infarction increases circulating APC.[137]

Circulating APC concentration in normal human subjects is highly correlated with circulating levels of protein C zymogen.[138] Based on protein C infusion studies in protein C-deficient subjects, the level of circulating APC is strongly determined by the concentration of protein C.[139] EPCR appears to be required for normal protein C activation in response to thrombin infusions in experimental animals.[140] EPCR and thrombomodulin must be in close proximity on cell surfaces (see Fig. 116–2), although this has yet to be experimentally demonstrated.

Thrombomodulin and EPCR appear to differ markedly in their relative distribution densities on blood vessels as the former is abundantly present in the small blood vessels but less so in large vessels, whereas the latter is more abundant in large vessels than in small vessels.[96,97] Thrombomodulin levels vary markedly in different tissues,[141] with significant consequences for a variable tendency for fibrin deposition in different organs.[91,142,143] In contrast to an initial report that thrombomodulin is absent in brain,[144] low levels are expressed in brain,[145] and brain-specific activation of protein C in humans occurs during carotid occlusion.[135]

Proteolytic cleavage and activation of protein C can also be effected by meizothrombin, plasmin, or factor Xa.[146–149] On the surface of cultured endothelial cells, negatively charged sulfated polysaccharides in the presence of phospholipid vesicles containing phosphatidylethanolamine can enhance the rate of protein C activation by factor Xa to approach the protein C activation rate of thrombin:thrombomodulin.[149] No data yet indicate whether protein C activation by meizothrombin, plasmin, or factor Xa is either physiologically or pharmacologically relevant.

Protein C activation is stimulated by platelet factor 4. Both *in vitro* and *in vivo* data imply that platelet factor 4 may play a physiologic role in enhancing APC generation and protecting against septic shock.[150–153]

ACTIVATED PROTEIN C ACTIVITIES

The clinical phenotype of severe protein C deficiency in neonatal purpura fulminans implies that APC exerts multiple physiologically essential activities, including potent anticoagulant and antiinflammatory actions (see Chap. 131). Recent advances establish that APC's antiinflammatory actions are but one manifestation of its ability to interact directly with cell receptors to provide multiple cytoprotective activities.[9,56,57] These two distinct types of activities of APC, intravascular anticoagulant activity and initiation of cell signaling, are mediated by different sets of molecular interactions, and both types of activities are clinically relevant.

ACTIVATED PROTEIN C ANTICOAGULANT ACTIVITY

Mechanisms for APC's direct anticoagulant activity involve factors V and VIII, the two homologous coagulation cofactors that circulate as inactive molecules and that are converted to active cofactors by limited proteolysis (see Chap. 115 and Figs. 115–15 and 115–17). APC circulates at 40 picomolars in normal humans, and there is an inverse correlation between fibrinopeptide A, the product that is cleaved from fibrinogen by thrombin, and APC levels in healthy nonsmoking adults, suggesting APC is a significant regulator of basal thrombin activity.[18,154]

Factors V and VIII are synthesized as large single-chain precursor coagulation cofactors of Mr 330,000, consisting of three homologous A domains (A1, A2, and A3) and two homologous C domains (C1 and C2) with a very large intervening, generally nonhomologous domain, designated the *B domain*, that connects the A2 and A3 domains (see Chap. 115). In factors V/Va and VIII/VIIIa, the A domains form heterotrimeric structures like ceruloplasmin, while the C domains form head-to-tail heterodimeric structures; activation of the inactive precursor forms of these two cofactors involves limited proteolysis.[27,155–163] Factor V involves cleavages at Arg709, Arg1018, and Arg1545 by thrombin, factor Xa, or other proteases. Cleavage at Arg1545 is the key step for generating factor Va activity because this proteolysis releases the B domain that blocks binding of factor Xa to factor Va.[160–163] The various forms of factor Va (see Fig. 115–15) are composed of two polypeptide chains, one bearing the A1-A2 domains and the other bearing the A3-C1-C2 domains. Although generally similar to factor V activation, factor VIII activation (see Fig. 115–17) involves formation of a heterotrimer of polypeptide chains containing the A1 domain, the A2 domain, and the A3-C1-C2 domains, respectively. In contrast to heterodimeric factor Va, heterotrimeric factor VIIIa is intrinsically unstable as a consequence of spontaneous dissociation of the A2 domain.[164]

Factors Va and VIIIa as Substrates for Activated Protein C

Irreversible proteolytic inactivation of factors Va and VIIIa by APC can be accomplished by proteolysis at Arg506 and Arg306 in factor Va and Arg562 and Arg362 in factor VIIIa (see Figs. 115–15 and 115–17).[27,165–168] Currently, the most common identifiable venous thrombosis risk factor involves a mutation of Arg506 to Gln in factor V that results in APC resistance (see Chap. 131). The complexities of APC-dependent inactivation of factor Va and VIIIa are compounded by the number of different molecular forms of Va and VIIIa that can be generated by limited proteolysis by a variety of proteases and by their differing susceptibilities to APC and to the different APC cofactors.

Activated Protein C Resistance

APC resistance is defined as an abnormally reduced anticoagulant response of a plasma sample to APC (see Chap. 131) and can be caused by many potential abnormalities in the protein C anticoagulant pathway. Such abnormalities could include defective APC cofactors, defective APC substrates, or other molecules that interfere with the normal functioning of the protein C anticoagulant pathway (e.g., autoantibodies against APC, APC cofactors, or APC substrates).

A report of familial venous thrombosis associated with APC resistance without any identifiable defect in four Swedish families[169] led to an intensive search for a genetic explanation that was soon found to involve replacement of G by A at nucleotide 1691 in exon 10 of the factor V gene which causes the amino acid replacement of Arg506 by Gln.[170–172] This factor V variant, like the prothrombin variant nt G20210A, arose in a single white founder some 18,000 to 29,000 years ago,[173,174] and is known as *Gln506-factor V* or *factor V Leiden*. This mutation is currently a common, but not the only, cause of APC resistance (see Chap. 131).

The molecular mechanism for APC resistance of Gln506-factor V is based on the fact that the variant molecule is inactivated 10 times slower than normal Arg506-factor Va.[27,172,175–179] The variant factor Va exhibits only a partial resistance to APC because cleavage at Arg306 in factor Va also occurs, causing complete loss of factor Va activity. This finding helps explain why APC resistance due to Gln506-factor V is a rather mild risk factor for venous thrombosis and why a combination of genetic risk factors or a combination of a genetic and acquired risk factors for venous thrombosis is found in a significant fraction of symptomatic patients (see Chap. 131). Another possibility to help explain the mild risk of venous thrombosis associated with Gln506-factor V is that factor Va may be inactivated *in vivo* by proteases other than APC that cleave at sites other than residue Arg506.

A factor V haplotype, designated R2, is also associated with mild APC resistance, although it appears that the R2 haplotype may only be a risk factor when present along with a Gln506-factor V allele.[180,181]

Plasma and recombinant factor V can exist in two biochemically distinct forms, designated *factor V1* and *factor V2* that differ in *N*-linked carbohydrate on Asn2181, near the phospholipid binding region of the C2 domain as factor V2 has none.[182–185] Because the *N*-linked carbohydrate appears to decrease the apparent affinity of factor V1 or Va1 for phospholipid, it reduces the specific clotting activity and susceptibility to APC. Normal plasma contains a mixture of factors V1 and V2. Removal of the carbohydrate attached to factor V increases the rate of inactivation of factor Va by APC, although the clinical significance of this phenomenon is unknown.[186]

APC resistance with no identifiable genetic or acquired abnormalities is well described in patients with venous and arterial thrombosis and should be therefore examined in patients with a suspected thrombophilia. Further studies are needed to identify the causes of APC resistance in such patients.[187–191] One major challenge involves defining the normal range for the clotting assays that are actually used to characterize APC resistance and the multiple plasma analytes or nonplasma assay components that are present in the assays. For example, activated partial thromboplastin time-based assays are not equivalently sensitive as are dilute tissue-factor-based assays to plasma high-density lipoprotein (HDL) levels or oral contraceptive use.[192,193] Plasma variables, such as elevated prothrombin levels,[194,195] may affect the response to APC by inhibiting APC anticoagulant actions. Endogenous thrombin potential assays involving dilute tissue factor as the procoagulant initiator provide additional tools for defining and characterizing APC resistance and extend the tools for shedding light on the gray area of APC resistance that is not linked to currently known factors.

Functional Variability in Forms of Cleaved Factors Va and VIIIa

Proteolytic activation of factors Va and VIIIa can generate different forms of each active cofactor that differ in specific activity. For example, factor VIIIa generated by factor Xa has lower specific activity and longer half-life than that generated by thrombin,[163,196] and factor Va generated by cleavage only at Arg709 and Arg1018 (without cleavage at Arg1545) has a lower specific activity than that generated after cleavage at Arg1545.[160–162,197] Factor Va can be cleaved at Arg1765, and this could generate forms of factor Va with differing specific activities.[163] Factor VIIa–tissue factor complexes can cleave factor V at novel sites to produce a form of factor V that can be destroyed by APC without the requirement for full activation of the cofactor precursor.[198]

ACTIVATED PROTEIN C ANTICOAGULANT COFACTORS

APC anticoagulant activity is enhanced by a number of factors that may be termed *APC anticoagulant cofactors*; these include Ca^{2+} ions; certain, but not all, phospholipids; protein S; factor V; certain glycosphingolipids; and HDL.

Phospholipids as Activated Protein C Cofactors

Certain phospholipids, such as phosphatidylserine, phosphatidylethanolamine, and cardiolipin, enhance the anticoagulant activity of APC. In addition, phosphatidylethanolamine and cardiolipin stimulate the APC pathway anticoagulant activities much more than they stimulate the procoagulant pathway activities.[199–202]

Protein S as Activated Protein C Cofactor

Protein S structure–activity relationships are informed by much biochemical work and the large number of mutations.[82,203] Protein S, as an anticoagulant APC cofactor, forms a 1:1 complex with APC and enhances by 10- to 20-fold the rate of APC's cleavage at Arg306 in factor Va but not the Arg506 cleavage.[176–179,204] Part of the mechanism for this activity of protein S may be related to its ability to bring the active site of APC closer to the plane of the phospholipid membrane on which the APC–protein S complex is located when the complex is formed.[205,206] Protein S also facilitates the action of APC against factor VIIIa.[207,208] Protein S enhances APC's action, in part at least, by ablating the ability of factor Xa to protect factor Va from APC.[209] The GLA domain, thrombin-sensitive region, and EGF1 and EGF2 domains of protein S are implicated in binding APC for expression of anticoagulant activity by the APC–protein S complex.[203,210–212] Cleavage of the thrombin-sensitive region by thrombin abolishes normal binding of protein S to phospholipid and its normal APC-cofactor anticoagulant activity.[212–215]

Factor V as Activated Protein C Cofactor

Factor V apparently can have anticoagulant as well as procoagulant properties because it enhances the anticoagulant action of APC against factor VIIIa in a reaction in which protein S acts synergistically with factor V.[26,27,216,217] Cleavage at Arg1545, which optimizes factor Va procoagulant activity, ablates the molecule's anticoagulant cofactor activity. However, when factor V is cleaved at Arg506 by APC, its APC cofactor activity is increased 10-fold. This suggests that Gln506-factor V has two potential prothrombotic defects, namely, resistance of the variant factor Va to APC inactivation and resistance of the variant factor V to activation of its APC cofactor function.[26,27,217]

High-Density Lipoprotein as Activated Protein C Cofactor

HDL enhances the anticoagulant activity of APC both in plasma and in purified reaction mixtures, and this APC cofactor activity requires protein S and involves, at least in part, stimulation of APC's cleavage at Arg306 in factor Va.[192] In animal models, HDL inhibits the disseminated intravascular coagulation induced by endotoxin infusion in baboons and ferric chloride-induced arterial thrombosis in rats.[218,219] HDL is heterogeneous in both protein and lipid composition, and the components responsible for this activity have not been identified, although large HDL, but not small HDL, possesses APC anticoagulant cofactor activity.[220] HDL can exert antithrombotic activity via multiple potential mechanisms.[221] Venous thrombosis in males and in subjects experiencing venous thrombosis recurrence are associated with a pattern of dyslipoproteinemia and low HDL, consistent with the hypothesis that deficiency of large HDL is a risk factor for venous thrombosis.[222,223]

Glycosphingolipids as Activated Protein C Cofactors

Although both procoagulant and anticoagulant reactions are markedly enhanced by the presence of negatively charged phospholipid surfaces *in vitro*, certain lipoproteins, for example, HDL,[192] and certain lipids, for example, glycosphingolipids and sphingosine,[220,224–227] selectively enhance anticoagulant reactions in plasma. Plasma glucosylceramide (GlcCer) deficiency is a biomarker and may be a potential risk factor for venous thrombosis.[224] Sphingosine and several of its common analogues are potent inhibitors of thrombin generation in plasma and on cell surfaces because they inhibit interactions between factors Va and Xa.[227] Further studies are needed to characterize the anticoagulant or procoagulant properties of minor abundance plasma and their significance for clinical thrombotic events.

ACTIVATED PROTEIN C DIRECT CELLULAR ACTIVITIES

As noted in Chap. 115, control of coagulation reactions does not occur in the absence of an integrated host defense system that involves a tangled web of biologic processes involving multiple overlapping and integrated pathways. Reactions of the innate and acquired immune system including inflammatory processes, blood coagulation reactions, fibrinolysis, and thrombotic processes are intertwined *in vivo* via multiple molecular and cellular mechanisms.[7–9,91,97,98,221,228,229] In addition to its anticoagulant activity, APC acts directly on cells to cause multiple cytoprotective effects including (1) alteration of gene expression profiles, (2) antiinflammatory activities, (3) antiapoptotic activity, and (4) protection of endothelial barrier function.[9,56,57,230–235]

Apoptosis and thrombin generation may be reciprocally interrelated. Circulating cell-derived microparticles carrying procoagulant tissue factor and adhesive molecules can promote thrombin formation that might be either hemostatic or pathogenic for thrombosis.[236–245] Many such microparticles arise from apoptosis and can promote thrombin generation.[236–249] Hence, because APC inhibits endothelial and circulating blood cell apoptosis,[9,56,57,230,232,233] APC can indirectly decrease thrombin generation and reduce thrombogenesis *in vivo*. APC also can suppress tissue factor expression on stimulated monocytes.[121,250] Thus, there are multiple mechanisms for APC's cell-signaling effects to exert antithrombotic activity.

Although APC infusion shows benefits in numerous animal injury models systems, the most studied and most informative clinical experience is in treating severe sepsis in adults, and the most informative animal studies are in sepsis models and in neuroprotection experiments.[9,56,57]

Activated Protein C and Sepsis

Strong evidence for the physiologic significance of the APC's direct effects on cells come from clinical research and animal model studies. In the PROWESS (Recombinant Human Activated Protein C Worldwide Evaluation in Severe Sepsis) trial, recombinant human APC reduced all-cause 28-day relative mortality by 19 percent in patients with severe sepsis.[53] However, two other potent anticoagulants, namely antithrombin and recombinant tissue factor pathway inhibitor (TFPI), failed to do so in similar large, multicenter phase III studies.[251,252] A reasonable inference is that APC's direct effects on cells involving antiinflammatory and antiapoptotic activities are invoked to help explain the success of APC in reducing mortality in severe sepsis. Protein engineering has permitted the molecular dissection of APC's anticoagulant activity from its cytoprotective activities[9,45–49] and led to proof of principle that APC's cell-signaling activity is both necessary and most likely sufficient for reducing lethality in murine septic shock models.[47,253,254] Notably, recombinant APC mutants that lack anticoagulant activity but retain cell signaling are able to reduce lethality caused by intermediate or high-dose endotoxin, simple bacteremia, or polymicrobial insult caused by cecal puncture and ligation.[47,253–255] Such APC mutants[45–49] might provide APC's cytoprotective actions without a notable risk for serious bleeding that complicated sepsis therapy using wild-type APC.[53]

Activated Protein C Neuroprotective Effects

Neuroprotective effects of APC have been convincingly demonstrated in rodent ischemic stroke models and *N*-methyl-D-aspartate (NMDA) excitotoxic injury models.[58,233,256–264] Interestingly, besides direct cytoprotection *in vitro* and *in vivo* for brain endothelium against ischemic injury, APC directly protects neurons against NMDA-induced excitotoxic injury both *in vivo* and *in vitro*. APC mutants with reduced anticoagulant activity were as neuroprotective as wild-type APC, and certain cellular receptors were required for APC's neuroprotection, strongly implying that neuroprotection by APC involves its actions directly on the endothelium and on neurons. Remarkably, in the ischemic penumbra in a murine stroke model, APC caused neovascularization and neurogenesis.[262]

Cellular Receptors for Physiologic Effects of Activated Protein C on Cells

Receptors that bind APC on the cell surface and that mediate signal initiation have been identified and characterized, although the current paradigm (see Fig. 115–4) is incomplete.[9,56,57,121] The ability of exogenously administered APC to alter the gene expression profile of cultured endothelial cells, to stabilize endothelial barriers, to reduce lethality caused by endotoxin in murine sepsis models, to prevent apoptosis of stressed endothelial cells, and to provide neuroprotection all require EPCR and PAR-1 (see Fig. 115–4).[9,45–49,231–235,253–255,258–260,262,263,266] Curiously, the cytoprotective effects of APC on neurons that are subjected to NMDA-induced excitotoxicity requires PAR-3 in addition to PAR-1.[259] In baboons, EPCR is required for APC-dependent reduction of mortality in *Escherichia coli*–induced sepsis.[140] ApoER2 is a newly identified receptor for APC high-affinity binding and signal initiation that may expand and help clarify the paradigm for APC's cell signaling.[121]

Although few details are known about intracellular mechanisms for APC's multiple cytoprotective actions, some mechanistic details have become clear. These effects involve extensive alterations in gene expression profiles in a manner suggestive of antiinflammatory alterations of nuclear factor-κB–dependent pathways, increases in intracellular Ca^{2+} ion flux, phosphorylation of intracellular effectors (MAPK [mitogen-activated protein kinase], ERK1/2 [extracellular signal-regulated kinase 1/2], Src, PI3K [phosphoinositol 3 kinase], Akt, RhoA, Rac1, Dab1, etc.), and major shifts in levels of proapoptotic and antiapoptotic factors.[9,56,57,97,230,231,233–235,258–266] Notably, APC downregulates the key regulatory transcription factor, p53, in stressed cells and reduces upregulation of the proapoptotic Bax while blunting downregulation of the antiapoptotic factor, Bcl-2, among others.[233,258] Thus, evidence from *in vivo* and *in vitro* studies strongly supports the scheme for APC direct effects on cells involving EPCR and PAR-1, as depicted in the scheme of Figure 115–4. Other receptors are recognized to play key roles for APC's beneficial signaling effects, including S1P1, a receptor for sphingosine-1-phosphate. ApoER2 can initiate Dab1-dependent activation of the PI3K-Akt cell-survival pathway,[121] which may ultimately help explain some aspects of APC's cytoprotection.

Although most studies demonstrating the cell-signaling activities of APC have focused on pharmacologic APC, several reports of murine injury models demonstrate the physiologic importance of cell signaling by endogenous APC,[254,267–269] implying that defects in APC's endogenous cytoprotective actions might have as yet undocumented pathophysiologic relevance. Future investigations on APC cellular receptors and on intracellular mechanisms involved in the protein C cellular pathway will likely provide novel clinical insights with diagnostic and therapeutic potential.

INHIBITION OF ACTIVATED PROTEIN C

Blood contains circulating APC in a well-defined normal concentration range that contributes to antithrombotic surveillance mechanisms and possibly to homeostatic cell signaling.[18,137,139] Circulating APC levels are determined by the balance between countervailing mechanisms for APC generation and for APC inhibition and clearance. APC generation is influenced by protein C zymogen levels; endogenous thrombin generation; and the availability of thrombomodulin and EPCR. Clearance of circulating APC is based on inhibition of APC by protease inhibitors and clearance of APC:inhibitor complexes.[270–279] The major plasma inhibitors of APC include α_1-antitrypsin, protein C inhibitor, and α_2-macroglobulin.

ACTIVATED PROTEIN C–INDEPENDENT ANTICOAGULANT ACTIVITY OF PROTEIN S

Because hereditary protein S deficiency[280,281] is strongly linked to increased venous thrombosis risk (see Chap. 131), protein S is a significant anticoagulant factor.[82,203] In addition to its anticoagulant cofactor activity for APC, protein S can also inhibit coagulation reactions independently of APC. Several plausible mechanisms have been described for protein S's anticoagulant activity independent of APC. First, protein S can bind directly to procoagulant factors Xa and Va and thereby inhibit directly the activity of the prothrombinase complex.[12–15] It is possible that ternary complexes of protein S–factor Va–factor Xa might be formed.[83] The thrombin-sensitive region and the EGF3 domains of protein S (see Fig. 116–5) likely bind factor Xa, contributing to APC-independent anticoagulant activity.[282,283] Second, protein S can also bind factor VIIIa and inhibit activation of factor X by factor IXa–factor VIIIa complexes.[284–286] Third, protein S binds TFPI and enhances its ability to inhibit factor Xa.[287–289] Zn^{2+} ions might play a key role for APC-independent protein S activity.[290] It is not easy to decipher the relative importance of each of these three mechanisms for APC-independent anticoagulant activities of protein S or to establish their physiologic relevance.

The activities of protein S can be strongly influenced by C4b-binding protein, a plasma protein that enhances inactivation of the complement cascade by binding to C4b and promoting its proteolytic inactivation by the protease, factor I. C4b-binding protein reversibly binds protein S with high affinity,[291–293] and formation of this complex affects some of the anticoagulant activities of protein S.[82,203,204,281,294–296] When factor Va is targeted by APC, the anticoagulant cofactor activity of protein S is substantially neutralized by binding to C4b-binding protein for one but not both cleavages at Arg306 and Arg506 in the substrate. However, the association of C4b-binding protein with protein S does not ablate its ability to serve as an APC cofactor when the substrate is factor VIIIa or its ability to inhibit the prothrombinase complex independent of APC. This latter observation is explained by the ability of C4b-binding protein to block binding of protein S to factor Va but apparently not to factor Xa.

Because of the influence of C4b-binding protein on protein S activities and plasma levels, interpretation of clinical assays for protein S requires evaluation of free and bound protein S as plasma contains approximately 240 nM protein S–C4b-binding protein complexes and 120 nM free protein S.[292] C4b-binding protein is a heteropolymer containing six or seven α chains that are disulfide linked to a single β chain that binds protein S.[297–299] Residues 30 to 45 of the β chain bind with high affinity to the C-terminal SHBG domain of protein S.[75,300,301] During an acute phase reaction, the level of the C4b-binding protein α chain, but not the β chain, is increased, so that the acute phase change in total C4b-binding protein does not alter the level of free and bound protein S.[302]

Another potential mechanism for the antithrombotic actions protein S is based on its APC-independent direct interactions with cells that might contribute to its antithrombotic actions. Protein S promotes clearance of apoptotic cells,[78,82,203,303–306] and this antiapoptotic activity of protein S might contribute to its antithrombotic activity, as discussed above for the indirect antithrombotic activity of APC. Protein S has direct effects on cells by activating one or more transmembrane receptor tyrosine kinases.[78,203,304] Protein S is a potent neuroprotectant as it can protect brain endothelium against ischemic injury in murine stroke models and can protect neurons against NMDA-induced excitotoxic injury, presumably acting via transmembrane receptor tyrosine kinases.[307]

INHIBITION OF COAGULATION PROTEASES BY PROTEASE INHIBITORS

Antithrombin, initially designated *antithrombin III*, is clinically the best known inhibitor of clotting factor proteases. Antithrombin can neutralize all coagulation proteases in reactions that are enhanced by heparin and related glycosaminoglycans (see Chap. 115).[16] However, antithrombin does not inhibit the anticoagulant protease APC. TFPI can neutralize factors VIIa and Xa, proteases of the extrinsic coagulation pathway.[6,288,289,308–310] In addition, other plasma protease inhibitors such as α_1-antitrypsin, heparin cofactor II, protein C inhibitor, α_2-macroglobulin, or protein Z-dependent protease inhibitor, can neutralize various coagulation proteases, although the ultimate clinical significance of these reactions is less-well defined than the clinical relevance of antithrombin for thrombophilia (see Chap. 131). Antithrombin is key for anticoagulant therapy based on the heparin-stimulated inhibition of thrombin and factor Xa.

ANTITHROMBIN AND HEPARINS

Antithrombin is synthesized in the liver and is present in plasma at 150 mcg/mL, and it is a typical member of the serine protease inhibitor (SERPIN) superfamily and is denoted as SERPINC1.[311–313] Based on X-ray crystallographic studies,[314–318] pictures of serpin–protease complexes in various reaction states have emerged and the mechanism for the effects of heparin on the reaction of thrombin with antithrombin is reasonably clear.

The neutralization of proteases by antithrombin is a result of a stable enzyme–antithrombin complex that is formed by a molecular mechanism characteristic of inhibitory serpins.[311–319] Following binding of a protease to a "reactive site" loop in a serpin, a single peptide bond in the serpin is cleaved with formation of an acyl-enzyme intermediate via the active site Ser residue. This metastable enzyme–serpin complex can either break apart because of deacylation, or it can form a more stable covalent enzyme–serpin complex. To break apart the enzyme–serpin covalent complex, deacylation liberates the cleaved product and regenerates the active site Ser residue of the protease. However, serpins have an ability to undergo major conformational changes following cleavage at the reactive site residue that can distort that protease's active site region and lock the enzyme into the protease–serpin complex in which both the serpin and the protease are essentially deformed.[16,311–319] The dominant structural feature of native serpins is a large five-stranded β-sheet that defines the structure of an ellipsoidal protein. Following cleavage at the reactive residue in the reactive center loop by a protease, this extended loop is able to partially or completely insert itself into the five-stranded β-sheet, forming a very stable six-stranded β-sheet. If this insertion reaction proceeds before deacylation occurs, then the protease remains covalently attached to the reactive center P1 residue through the protease's active site Ser residue, and a stable covalent protease–inhibitor complex with each protein in an altered conformation, is formed.[317]

Heparin enhancement of the rate of reaction between antithrombin and thrombin or other clotting factors is caused by two distinct effects of heparin, one involving conformational effects on antithrombin and the other involving "approximation" effects on both antithrombin and thrombin.[16,318–324] For the first effect, a particular pentasaccharide sequence within heparin binds antithrombin and potently causes a conformational change that converts antithrombin from its native state of moderate reactivity to a conformation with relatively high reactivity. This pentasaccharide contains a specific sulfated sequence of glucosamine and iduronic acid residues,[16,318–324] and when it is present in a large heparin molecule, in low-molecular-weight heparin, or in a synthetic pentasaccharide, it alters antithrombin conformation and greatly accelerates the reaction of antithrombin, especially with factor Xa. Synthetic pentasaccharides, such as fondaparinux, that are analogues of the naturally occurring sequence are often termed to be indirect factor Xa inhibitors and have significant clinical utility. For the second mechanistic effect, namely the approximation effect, unfractionated heparin or low-molecular-weight heparins simultaneously bind to antithrombin and the target protease to promote frequent and geometrically productive encounters between protease and inhibitor, thus increasing the reaction rate. Heparan sulfates to some extent can also act in this manner.

The mature antithrombin polypeptide chain contains 432 amino acid residues after cleavage of a propeptide from a 464-amino-acid-residue precursor.[325] It has four sites for *N*-linked carbohydrate attachment, one of which (Asn135) is variably glycosylated, giving rise to a β-isoform that has higher affinity for heparin.[326,327] Heparin binding to antithrombin is mediated by a number of positively charged Arg and Lys residues in the N-terminal region of the molecule, including Lys11, Arg13 and Asn45, Arg46, Arg47, Glu113, Lys114, and Lys125 and Arg129, whereas the reactive center loop containing the scissile peptide bond at Arg393-Ser394 is near the C-terminus.[318]

ANTITHROMBIN GENE

The antithrombin gene comprising seven exons and six introns spans 13.4 kb and is located on chromosome 1q23–25 (see Table 116–1).[328–330]

ANTITHROMBIN MUTATIONS

Hereditary deficiencies of antithrombin are risk factors for venous thrombosis (see Chap. 131). More than 100 different antithrombin mutations are associated with thrombosis. An extensive database of mutations is published and is available through the courtesy of Lane and colleagues[331] at http://www1.imperial.ac.uk/medicine/about/divisions/is/haemo/coag/antithrombin/.

Mutations that cause antithrombin deficiency are scattered throughout the gene. Molecular defects can be classified as type I, characterized by parallel decreases in antigen and activity, or type II, characterized by circulating dysfunctional molecules such that plasma has decreased functional activity but normal or near-normal antigen levels. Type II defects are further classified based on whether the dysfunction involves only reactive center defects that can be tested in the absence of heparin, only heparin-binding defects that can be tested only in the presence of heparin, or both of these defects (pleiotropic effects). Reactive center defects carry the largest risk of thrombosis, whereas heparin-binding defects are associated with less risk of venous thrombosis (see Chap. 131). For example, an unusual variant, designated antithrombin London, was described in which the reactive center Arg residue was missing while the molecule had high affinity for heparin, and this mutation was associated with an early onset of thrombotic symptoms.[332]

TISSUE FACTOR PATHWAY INHIBITOR

TFPI, also known as *lipoprotein-associated coagulation inhibitor* or *extrinsic pathway inhibitor*, has a predicted mature protein sequence of 276 residues and an Mr of 34,000, although posttranslational modifications yield a protein with an Mr of 43,000; TFPI is a complex protein.[6,288,289,308–310,333–340] Full-length mature TFPI contains an acidic N-terminal sequence, three homologous but distinct Kunitz-type protease inhibitor domains, and a C-terminal positively charged basic amino acid sequence. Although present

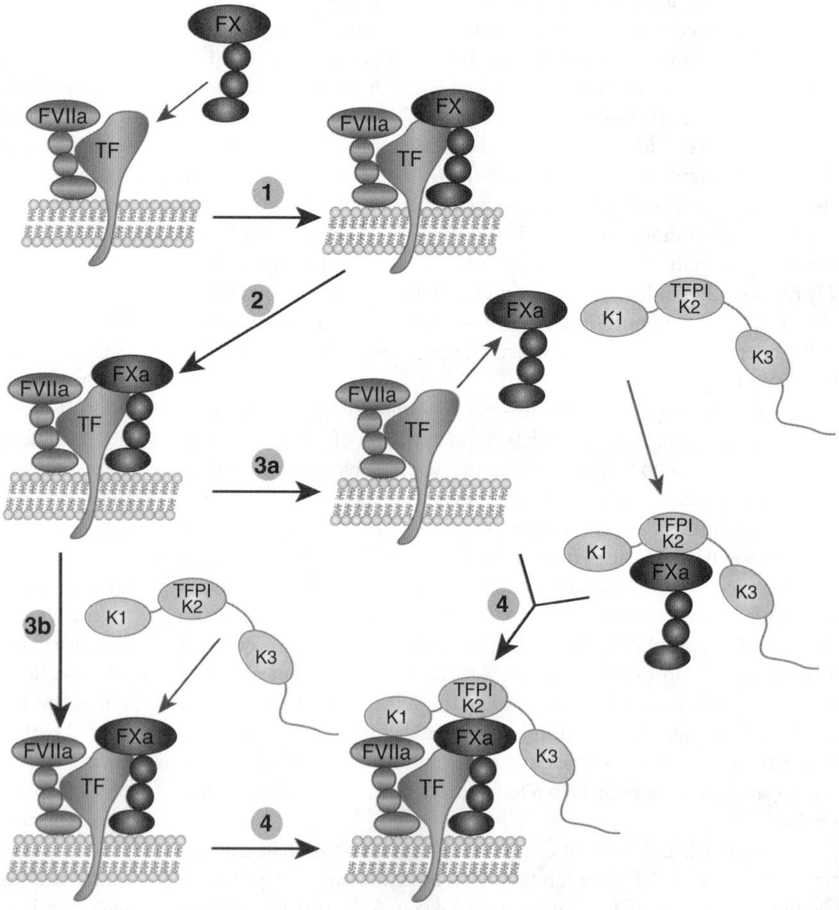

FIGURE 116–6. Inhibition of factors VIIa and Xa by tissue factor pathway inhibitor (TFPI). Free TFPI is a multivalent protease inhibitor containing three Kunitz-type protease inhibitor domains. Factor VIIa complexes with and is inhibited by the Kunitz-1 (K1) domain of TFPI, whereas factor Xa complexes with and is inhibited by the Kunitz-2 (K2) domain. The most productive inhibitory complex is thought to consist of TFPI complexed with both proteases and tissue factor (TF). This scheme represents pathways of formation of such a quaternary complex. Factor X binds to membrane-bound tissue factor–factor VIIa (*step 1*) and is subsequently activated (*step 2*). Then factor Xa can dissociate (*step 3a*) and react with TFPI in solution or on another surface and subsequently this TFPI–Xa complex can combine with tissue factor–factor VIIa to form the quaternary complex (*step 4*). Alternatively, factor Xa that remains bound to tissue factor–factor VIIa (*step 3b*) combines with TFPI (*alternative step 4*) to yield the surface-bound quaternary complex. *(Adapted with permission from Crawley JT, Lane DA.[289])*

at only 2.5 nM in normal plasma, TFPI is a significant inhibitor of the extrinsic coagulation pathway that can function synergistically with the protein C pathway and antithrombin to suppress thrombin generation. TFPI is synthesized by endothelial cells and smooth muscle cells.[6,288,289] More than half of TFPI in plasma is associated with lipoproteins, especially low-density lipoprotein, and a substantial amount of TFPI is released when heparin is infused.[340] There are multiple forms of TFPI in blood and on the endothelium, not only because of its association with lipoproteins but also because there are two alternatively spliced forms of TFPI designated TFPIα and TFPIβ.[333,334] TFPIα is the full-length protein, whereas TFPIβ contains an unrelated sequence that replaces the third Kunitz-type domain and the C-terminus. Each form of TFPI, especially TFPIβ, can be covalently modified by addition of phosphatidylinositol that localizes the TFPI to cell membranes. The interaction of TFPI with lipoproteins greatly reduces the measurable anticoagulant activity, and when TFPI is bound to cells, lipoprotein (a) inhibits activity.[6,288,289] The C-terminus and the third Kunitz-type domain of TFPIα are required for normal binding to the endothelial surface. No protease has yet been identified as the target of the third Kunitz-type protease inhibitor domain.

TFPI neutralizes factors Xa and VIIa by somewhat complicated mechanisms.[6,288,289] Two distinct viewpoints have been advanced. In both mechanisms, Kunitz domains reversibly bind with high affinity to factors VIIa and Xa. In one mechanism, initially the second Kunitz-type inhibitor domain of TFPI reacts with and inhibits the active site of factor Xa. Subsequently, this binary complex reacts with factor VIIa in the tissue factor–VIIa complex to form a quaternary protein complex on a membrane with both proteases neutralized. In an alternative proposed scheme (Fig. 116–6), TFPI first reacts with factor VIIa in a tissue factor–factor VIIa complex that has generated factor Xa, and thereafter rapidly reacts with factor Xa before it can dissociate from the ternary tissue factor–factor VIIa–factor Xa complex. Possibly each proposal is valid. Some argue that because some kinetic studies showed that TFPI requires factor Xa for kinetically favorable reactions with factor VIIa, TFPI does not shut off the initiation of the extrinsic pathway by tissue factor until some significant though small amount of factor Xa is generated, in which case TFPI provides negative feedback inhibition of the generation of factor Xa by the factor VIIa–tissue factor complex. An additional property of TFPI involves its inhibition of factor Xa in the absence of factor VIIa, and this reaction is accelerated by protein S.[287–289]

Animal model studies show that TFPI functions physiologically as an inhibitor of coagulation as mice carrying complete deficiency of TFPI in gene knockout studies do not survive beyond the neonatal period and die of hemorrhage with signs of fibrin formation, suggestive of consumptive coagulopathy.[342]

TFPI GENE

The sequence of TFPI was established from cloning of its complementary DNA. The gene contains 9 exons, spans 85 kb, and is located on chromosome 2q31–32.1 (see Table 116–1).[343,344]

TFPI MUTATIONS

Hereditary abnormalities of *TFPI* were suggested to be associated with a modestly increased risk of venous thrombosis although TFPI assays and the modest reported relative risk limit clinical implications and utility at this point[289] (see Chap. 131).

OTHER PROTEASE INHIBITORS

HEPARIN COFACTOR II

Heparin cofactor II, a serpin whose inhibitory activity is enhanced by dermatan sulfate, inhibits thrombin *in vivo* and *in vitro* by an approximation mechanism.[345] A few data are reported linking heparin cofactor II deficiency to venous thrombosis, but no significant clinical relevance has been established[346]; curiously, a severe heparin cofactor II deficiency was reported in an asymptomatic subject.[347]

PROTEIN Z–DEPENDENT PROTEASE INHIBITOR

Protein Z–dependent protease inhibitor (ZPI) is a plasma serpin that inhibits factors Xa, XIa, and IXa.[348–351] Protein Z stimulates factor Xa inhibition but not factor XIa inhibition by ZPI. Protein Z is a vitamin K–dependent protein that contains a GLA domain, two EGF-like domains, and a protease-like domain.[352] However, the protease-like domain lacks any protease activity because it has mutations at two of the three active site triad residues. The major hypothesis for stimulation of inhibition of factor Xa by protein Z is based on a structural model in which three proteins assemble on a phospholipid membrane via the two GLA domains (Fig. 116–7).[352] In this putative ternary complex, the protease-like domain and the second EGF-like domain of protein Z bind ZPI in an alignment that facilitates reaction of factor Xa with the reactive center loop of ZPI.

In plasma, ZPI is in slight protein molar excess over protein Z with which it can noncovalently associate, and it has been speculated but not proven that almost all plasma protein Z is associated with ZPI.[353–358] If the ZPI is a physiologic coagulation inhibitor, the deficiency of either protein Z or ZPI might be associated with thrombosis. Knocking out the protein Z gene in a mouse does not produce a remarkable phenotype unless protein Z deficiency coexists with factor V Leiden in the mouse, in which case the mouse exhibits a hypercoagulable, prothrombotic

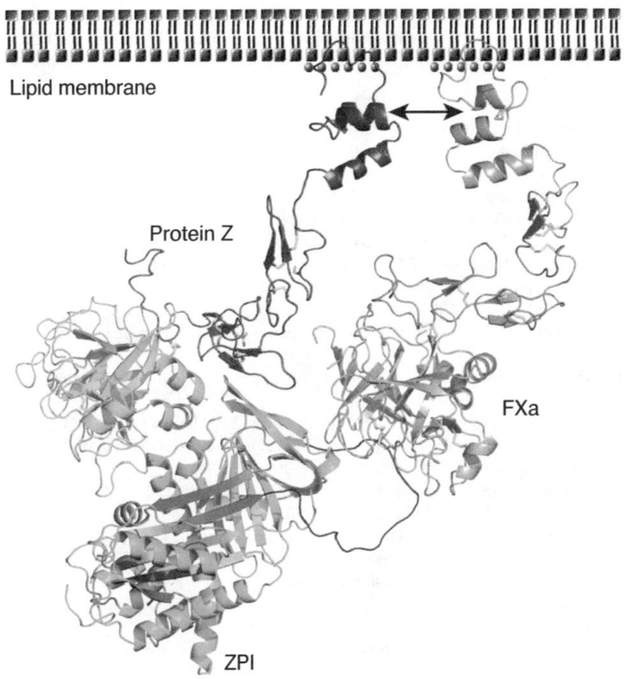

FIGURE 116–7. Mechanism for protein Z–dependent protease inhibitor (ZPI) inhibition of factor Xa mediated by protein Z. This scheme depicts a model of the ternary complex of protein Z/ZPI/factor Xa on the phospholipid membrane surface. ZPI is colored in *green* with its reactive center loop in *red*. The protease-like domain of protein Z (*cyan*) binds ZPI (*green*) and orients the reactive center loop (*red*) to target the active site of the factor Xa protease domain (*gray*). The GLA domains of protein Z and factor Xa mediate binding to the lipid membrane. The N-terminal domains (GLA, epidermal growth factor [EGF] 1, and EGF2) of protein Z are in *brown*. *(Adapted with permission from Wei Z, Yan Y, Carrell RW, Zhou A.[352])*

state.[354] This murine observation is mirrored by a clinical report that subnormal levels of protein Z are associated with venous thrombosis in subjects who are heterozygous for factor V Leiden.[355] Some associations between venous thrombosis and defects in protein Z or ZPI have been reported but not uniformly confirmed.[353,355–358] An association with peripheral arterial disease has appeared.[359] Overall, no convincing pattern between thrombosis and defects in protein Z or ZPI has yet been firmly established.

OTHER MINOR PROTEASE INHIBITORS

Thrombin in plasma can be inhibited not only by antithrombin but also by α_2-macroglobulin, an acute-phase reactant. No association between defects in bleeding or thrombosis is associated with this inhibitor. In purified reaction mixtures, protein C inhibitor also efficiently neutralizes thrombin in the presence of thrombomodulin,[360] although no studies show that this is a physiologic reaction or that it is associated with thrombosis.

REFERENCES

1. MacFarlane RG: An enzyme cascade in the blood clotting mechanism and its function as a biological amplifier. *Nature* 202:498, 1964.
2. Davie EW, Ratnoff OD: Waterfall sequence for intrinsic blood clotting. *Science* 145:1310, 1964.
3. Davie EW, Fujikawa K, Kisiel W: The coagulation cascade: Initiation, maintenance, and regulation. *Biochemistry* 30:10363, 1991.
4. Furie B, Furie BC: Mechanisms of thrombus formation. *N Engl J Med* 359:938, 2008.
5. Lammle B, Griffin JH: Formation of the fibrin clot: The balance of procoagulant and inhibitory factors. *Clin Haematol* 14:281, 1985.
6. Broze GJ Jr: Tissue factor pathway inhibitor and the revised theory of coagulation. *Annu Rev Med* 46:103, 1995.
7. Van de Wouwer M, Collen D, Conway EM: Thrombomodulin-protein C-EPCR system integrated to regulate coagulation and inflammation. *Arterioscler Thromb Vasc Biol* 24:1, 2004.
8. Griffin JH: The thrombin paradox. *Nature* 378:337, 1995.
9. Mosnier LO, Zlokovic BV, Griffin JH: The protein C cellular pathway. *Blood* 109:3161, 2007.
10. Fukudome K, Esmon CT: Identification, cloning, and regulation of a novel endothelial cell protein C/activated protein C receptor. *J Biol Chem* 269:26486, 1994.
11. Esmon CT: Structure and functions of the endothelial cell protein C receptor. *Crit Care Med* 32(5 Suppl):S298, 2004.
12. Mitchell CA, Kelemen SM, Salem HH: The anticoagulant properties of a modified form of protein S. *Thromb Haemost* 60:298, 1988.
13. Heeb MJ, Mesters RM, Tans G, et al: Binding of protein S to factor Va associated with inhibition of prothrombinase that is independent of activated protein C. *J Biol Chem* 268:2872, 1993.
14. Heeb MJ, Rosing J, Bakker HM, et al: Protein S binds to and inhibits factor Xa. *Proc Natl Acad Sci U S A* 91:2728, 1994.
15. Hackeng TM, van't Veer C, Meijers JCM, Bouma BN: Human protein S inhibits prothrombinase complex activity on endothelial cells and platelets via direct interactions with factors Va and Xa. *J Biol Chem* 269:21051, 1994.
16. Huntington JA: Mechanisms of glycosaminoglycan activation of the serpins in hemostasis. *J Thromb Haemost* 1:1535, 2003.
17. Morrissey JH, Macik BG, Neuenschwander PF, Comp PC: Quantitation of activated factor VII levels in plasma using a tissue factor mutant selectively deficient in promoting factor VII activation. *Blood* 81:734, 1993.
18. Gruber A, Griffin JH: Direct detection of activated protein C in blood from human subjects. *Blood* 79:2340, 1992.
19. Nossel HL, Yudelman I, Canfield RE, et al: Measurement of fibrinopeptide A in human blood. *J Clin Invest* 54:43, 1974.
20. Nossel HL: Radioimmunoassay of fibrinopeptides in relation to intravascular coagulation and thrombosis. *N Engl J Med* 295:428, 1976.
21. Bauer KA, Rosenberg RD: The pathophysiology of the prethrombotic state in humans: Insights gained from studies using markers of hemostatic system activation. *Blood* 70:343, 1987.
22. Bauer KA, Kass BL, ten Cate H, et al: Detection of factor X activation in humans. *Blood* 74:2007, 1989.
23. Bauer KA, Kass BL, ten Cate H, et al: Factor IX is activated *in vivo* by the tissue factor mechanism. *Blood* 76:731, 1990.
24. Jesty J, Beltrami E, Willems G: Mathematical analysis of a proteolytic positive-feedback loop: Dependence of lag time and enzyme yields on the initial conditions and kinetic parameters. *Biochemistry* 32:6266, 1993.
25. Beltrami E, Jesty J: Mathematical analysis of activation thresholds in enzyme-catalyzed positive feedbacks: Application to the feedbacks of blood coagulation. *Proc Natl Acad Sci U S A* 92:8744, 1995.
26. Shen L, Dahlbäck B: Factor V and protein S as synergistic cofactors to activated protein C in degradation of factor VIIIa. *J Biol Chem* 269:18735, 1994.
27. Nicolaes, GA, Dahlback, B: Factor V and thrombotic disease: Description of a Janus-faced protein. *Arterioscler Thromb Vasc Biol* 22:530, 2002.
28. Stenflo JA: A new vitamin K-dependent protein: Purification from bovine plasma and preliminary characterization. *J Biol Chem* 251:355, 1976.
29. Seegers WH, Novoa E, Henry RL, Hassouna HI: Relationship of "new" vitamin K–dependent protein C and "old" autoprothrombin II-A. *Thromb Res* 8:543, 1976.
30. Kisiel W: Human plasma protein C. Isolation, characterization and mechanism of activation by α-thrombin. *J Clin Invest* 64:761, 1979.
31. Foster D, Davie EW: Characterization of a cDNA coding for human protein C. *Proc Natl Acad Sci U S A* 81:4766, 1984.
32. Beckman RJ, Schmidt RJ, Santerre RF, et al: The structure and evolution of a 461 amino acid human protein C precursor and its messenger RNA, based upon the DNA sequence of cloned human liver cDNA's. *Nucleic Acids Res* 13:5233, 1985.
33. Griffin JH, Evatt B, Zimmerman TS, et al: Deficiency of protein C in congenital thrombotic disease. *J Clin Invest* 68:1370, 1981.
34. Mather T, Oganessyan V, Hof P, et al: The 2.8 Å crystal structure of Gla-domainless activated protein C. *EMBO J* 15:6822, 1996.
35. Kurosawa S, Galvin JB, Esmon NL, Esmon CT: Proteolytic formation and properties of functional domains of thrombomodulin. *J Biol Chem* 262:2206, 1987.
36. Jhingan A, Zhang L, Christiansen WT, Castellino FJ: The activities of recombinant gamma-carboxyglutamic-acid-deficient mutants of activated human protein C toward human coagulation factor Va and factor VIII in purified systems and in plasma. *Biochemistry* 33:1869, 1994.
37. Zhang L, Castellino FJ: The binding energy of human coagulation protein C to acidic phospholipid vesicles contains a major contribution from leucine 5 in the gamma-carboxyglutamic acid domain. *J Biol Chem* 269:3590, 1994.
38. Regan LM, Mollica JS, Rezaie AR, Esmon CT: The interaction between the endothelial cell protein C receptor and protein C is dictated by the gamma-carboxyglutamic acid domain of protein C. *J Biol Chem* 272:26279, 1997.
39. Greengard JS, Fisher CL, Villoutreix B, Griffin JH: Structural basis for type I and type II deficiencies of antithrombotic plasma protein C: Patterns revealed by three-dimensional molecular modeling of mutations of the protease domain. *Proteins* 18:367, 1994.
40. Gale AJ, Heeb MJ, Griffin JH: The autolysis loop of activated protein C interacts with factor Va and differentiates between the Arg506 and Arg306 cleavage sites. *Blood* 96:585, 2000.
41. Friedrich U, Nicolaes GA, Villoutreix BO, Dahlback B: Secondary substrate-binding exosite in the serine protease domain of activated protein C important for cleavage at Arg-506 but not at Arg- 306 in factor Va. *J Biol Chem* 276:23105, 2001.
42. Rezaie AR: Exosite-dependent regulation of the protein C anticoagulant pathway. *Trends Cardiovasc Med* 13:8, 2003.
43. Gale AJ, Griffin JH: Characterization of a thrombomodulin binding site on protein C and its comparison to an activated protein C binding site for factor Va. *Proteins* 54:433, 2004.
44. Gale AJ, Tsavaler A, Griffin JH: Molecular characterization of an extended binding site for coagulation factor Va in the positive exosite of activated protein C. *J Biol Chem* 277:28836, 2002.
45. Mosnier LO, Gale AJ, Yegneswaran S, Griffin JH: Activated protein C variants with normal cytoprotective but reduced anticoagulant activity. *Blood* 104:1740, 2004.
46. Mosnier LO, Yang XV, Griffin JH: Activated protein C mutant with minimal anticoagulant activity, normal cytoprotective activity, and preservation of thrombin activatable fibrinolysis inhibitor-dependent cytoprotective functions. *J Biol Chem* 282:33022, 2007.
47. Mosnier LO, Zampolli A, Kerschen EJ, et al: Hyperantithrombotic, noncytoprotective Glu149Ala-activated protein C mutant. *Blood* 113:5970, 2009.
48. Bae JS, Yang L, Manithody C, Rezaie AR: Engineering a disulfide bond to stabilize the calcium-binding loop of activated protein C eliminates its anticoagulant but not its protective signaling properties. *J Biol Chem* 282:9251, 2007.
49. Yang L, Bae JS, Manithody C, Rezaie AR: Identification of a specific exosite on activated protein C for interaction with protease-activated receptor 1. *J Biol Chem* 282:25493, 2007.
50. Dreyfus M, Magny JF, Bridey F, et al: Treatment of homozygous protein C deficiency and neonatal purpura fulminans with a purified protein C concentrate. *N Engl J Med* 325:1565, 1991.
51. Rivard GE, David M, Farrell C, Schwarz HP: Treatment of purpura fulminans in meningococcemia with protein C concentrate. *J Pediatr* 126:646, 1995.
52. Tcheng WY, Dovat S, Gurel Z et al: Severe congenital protein C deficiency: Description of a new mutation and prophylactic protein C therapy and *in vivo* pharmacokinetics. *J Pediatr Hematol Oncol* 30:166, 2008.
53. Bernard GR, Vincent JL, Laterre PF, et al: Efficacy and safety of recombinant human activated protein C for severe sepsis. *N Engl J Med* 344:699, 2001.
54. Gruber A, Griffin JH, Harker LA, Hanson SR: Inhibition of platelet-dependent thrombus formation by human activated protein C in a primate model. *Blood* 73:639, 1989.
55. Taylor FB, Chang A, Esmon CT, et al: Protein C prevents the coagulopathic and lethal effects of *Escherichia coli* infusion in the baboon. *J Clin Invest* 79:918, 1987.

56. Toltl LJ, Swystun LL, Pepler L, Liaw PC: Protective effects of activated protein C in sepsis. *Thromb Haemost* 100:582, 2008.
57. Jackson C, Whitmont K, Tritton S et al: New therapeutic applications for the anticoagulant, activated protein C. *Expert Opin Biol Ther* 8:1109, 2008.
58. Griffin JH, Fernandez JA, Liu D et al: Activated protein C and ischemic stroke. *Crit Care Med* 32:S247, 2004.
59. Contreras JL, Eckstein C, Smyth CA, et al: Activated protein C preserves functional islet mass after intraportal transplantation: A novel link between endothelial cell activation, thrombosis, inflammation, and islet cell death. *Diabetes* 53:2804, 2004.
60. Foster DC, Yoshitake S, Davie EW: The nucleotide sequence of the gene for human protein C. *Proc Natl Acad Sci U S A* 82:4673, 1985.
61. Rocchi M, Roncuzzi L, Santamaria R, et al: Mapping through somatic cell hybrids and cDNA probes of protein C to chromosome 2, factor X to chromosome 13, and alpha 1-acid glycoprotein to chromosome 9. *Hum Genet* 74:30, 1986.
62. Long GL, Marshall A, Gardner JC, Naylor SL: Genes for human vitamin K–dependent plasma proteins C and S are located on chromosomes 2 and 3, respectively. *Somat Cell Mol Genet* 140:93, 1988.
63. Patracchini P, Aiello V, Palazzi P, et al: Sublocalization of the human protein C gene on chromosome 2q13-q14. *Hum Genet* 81:191, 1989.
64. D'Ursi P, Marino F, Caprera A, et al: ProCMD: A database and 3D web resource for protein C mutants. *BMC Bioinformatics* 8(Suppl 1):S11, 2007.
65. Saunders RE, Perkins SJ: CoagMDB: A database analysis of missense mutations within four conserved domains in five vitamin K-dependent coagulation serine proteases using a text-mining tool. *Hum Mutat* 29:333, 2008.
66. Greengard JS, Griffin JH, Fisher CL: Possible structural implications of 20 mutations in the protein C protease domain. *Thromb Haemost* 72:869, 1994.
67. Rovida E, Merati G, D'Ursi P, et al: Identification and computationally-based structural interpretation of naturally occurring variants of human protein C. *Hum Mutat* 28:345, 2007.
68. Jalbert LR, Rosen ED, Moons L, et al: Inactivation of the gene for anticoagulant protein C causes lethal perinatal consumptive coagulopathy in mice. *J Clin Invest* 102:1481, 1998.
69. DiScipio RG, Hermodson MA, Yates SG, Davie EW: A comparison of human prothrombin, factor IX (Christmas factor), factor X (Stuart factor), and protein S. *Biochemistry* 16:698, 1977.
70. DiScipio RG, Davie EW: Characterization of protein S, a gamma-carboxyglutamic acid containing protein from bovine and human plasma. *Biochemistry* 18:899, 1979.
71. Schwarz HP, Heeb MJ, Wencel-Drake JD, Griffin JH: Identification and characterization of protein S in human platelets. *Blood* 66:1452, 1985.
72. Lundwall A, Dackowski W, Cohen E, et al: Isolation and sequence of the cDNA for human protein S, a regulator of blood coagulation. *Proc Natl Acad Sci U S A* 83:6716, 1986.
73. Ploos van Amstel HK, van der Zanden L, Reitsma PH, Bertina RM: Human protein S cDNA encodes Phe-16 and Tyr 222 in consensus sequences for the post-translational processing. *FEBS Lett* 222:186, 1987.
74. Hoskins J, Norman DK, Beckmann RJ, Long GL: Cloning and characterization of human liver cDNA encoding a protein S precursor. *Proc Natl Acad Sci U S A* 84:349, 1987.
75. Fernández JA, Heeb MJ, Griffin JH: Identification of residues 413–433 of plasma protein S as essential for binding to C4b-binding protein. *J Biol Chem* 268:16788, 1993.
76. Heeb MJ, Kojima Y, Tans G, et al: C-terminal residues 621–635 of protein S are essential for binding to factor Va. *J Biol Chem* 274:36187, 1999.
77. Nyberg P, Dahlback B, Garcia DF: The SHBG-like region of protein S is crucial for factor V–dependent APC-cofactor function. *FEBS Lett* 433:28, 1998.
78. Hafizi S, Dahlback B: Gas6 and protein S. *FEBS J* 273:5231, 2006.
79. Ploos van Amstel JK, Van der Zanden AL, Bakker E, et al: Two genes homologous with human protein S cDNA are located on chromosome 3. *Thromb Haemost* 58:982, 1987.
80. Watkins PC, Eddy R, Fukushima Y, et al: The gene for protein S maps near the centromere of human chromosome 3. *Blood* 71:238, 1988.
81. Schmidel DK, Tatro AV, Phelps LG, et al: Organization of the human protein S gene. *Biochemistry* 29:7845, 1990.
82. de Frutos P, Fuentes-Prior P, Hurtado B, Sala N: Molecular basis of protein S deficiency. *Thromb Haemost* 98:543, 2007.
83. Hayashi T, Nishioka J, Suzuki K: Molecular mechanism of the dysfunction of protein S (Tokushima) (Lys155ÆGlu) for the regulation of the blood coagulation system. *Biochim Biophys Acta* 1272:159, 1995.
84. Kimura R, Honda S, Kawasaki T, et al. Protein S-K196E mutation as a genetic risk factor for deep vein thrombosis in Japanese subjects. *Blood* 107:1737, 2006.
85. Pecheniuk NM, Elias DJ, Xu X, Griffin JH: Failure to validate association of gene polymorphisms in EPCR, PAR-1, FSAP and protein S Tokushima with venous thromboembolism among Californians of European ancestry. *Thromb Haemost* 99:453, 2008.
86. Bertina RM, Ploos van Amstel HK, van Wijngaarden A, et al: Heerlen polymorphism of protein S, an immunologic polymorphism due to dimorphism of residue 460. *Blood* 76:538, 1990.
87. Esmon CT, Owen WG: Identification of an endothelial cell cofactor for thrombin-catalyzed activation of protein C. *Proc Natl Acad Sci U S A* 78:2249, 1981.
88. Esmon CT, Owen WG: The discovery of thrombomodulin. *J Thromb Haemost* 2:209, 2004.
89. Esmon CT, Esmon NL, Harris KW: Complex formation between thrombin and thrombomodulin inhibits both thrombin-catalyzed fibrin formation and factor V activation. *J Biol Chem* 257:7944, 1982.
90. Esmon NL, Carroll RC, Esmon CT: Thrombomodulin blocks the ability of thrombin to activate platelets. *J Biol Chem* 258:12238, 1983.
91. Esmon CT: The roles of protein C and thrombomodulin in the regulation of blood coagulation. *J Biol Chem* 264:4743, 1989.
92. Jackman RW, Beeler DL, Fritze L, et al: Human thrombomodulin gene is intron depleted: Nucleic acid sequences of the cDNA and gene predict protein structure and suggest sites of regulatory control. *Proc Natl Acad Sci U S A* 84:6425, 1987.
93. Sadler JE, Lentz SR, Sheehan JP, et al: Structure-function relationships of the thrombin-thrombomodulin interaction. *Haemostasis* 23(Suppl 1):183, 1993.
94. Shirai T, Shiojiri S, Ito H, et al: Gene structure of human thrombomodulin, a cofactor for thrombin-catalyzed activation of protein C. *J Biochem* 103:281, 1988.
95. Esmon CT: Cell mediated events that control blood coagulation and vascular injury. *Annu Rev Cell Biol* 9:1, 1993.
96. Healy AM, Rayburn HB, Rosenberg RD, Weiler H: Absence of the blood-clotting regulator thrombomodulin causes embryonic lethality in mice before development of a functional cardiovascular system. *Proc Natl Acad Sci U S A* 92:850, 1995.
97. Esmon CT: Inflammation and the activated protein C anticoagulant pathway. *Semin Thromb Hemost* 32(Suppl 1):49, 2006.
98. Schouten M, Wiersinga, Levi M, van der Poll T: Inflammation, endothelium, and coagulation in sepsis. *J Leukoc Biol* 83:536, 2008.
99. Delvaeye M, Noris M, De Vriese A, et al: Thrombomodulin mutations in atypical hemolytic-uremic syndrome. *N Engl J Med* 361:345, 2009.
100. Norlund L, Holm J, Zoller B, Ohlin AK: A common thrombomodulin amino acid dimorphism is associated with myocardial infarction. *Thromb Haemost* 77:248, 1997.
101. Ireland H, Kunz G, Kyriakoulis K, et al: Thrombomodulin gene mutations associated with myocardial infarction. *Circulation* 96:15, 1997.
102. Doggen CJ, Kunz G, Rosendaal FR, et al: A mutation in the thrombomodulin gene, 127G to A coding for Ala25Thr, and the risk of myocardial infarction in men. *Thromb Haemost* 80:743, 1998.
103. Wu KK: Soluble thrombomodulin and coronary heart disease. *Curr Opin Lipidol* 14:373, 2003.
104. Ohlin AK, Marlar RA: Thrombomodulin gene defects in families with thromboembolic disease—A report on four families. *Thromb Haemost* 81:338, 1999.
105. Van de Wouwer M, Plaisance S, De Vriese A, et al. The lectin-like domain of thrombomodulin interferes with complement activation and protects against arthritis. *J Thromb Haemost* 4:1813, 2006.
106. Myles T, Nishimura T, Yun TH, et al: Thrombin activatable fibrinolysis inhibitor: A potential regulator of vascular inflammation. *J Biol Chem* 278:51059, 2003.
107. Fukudome K, Esmon CT: Molecular cloning and expression of murine and bovine endothelial cell protein C–activated protein C receptor (EPCR). The structural and functional conservation in human, bovine, and murine EPCR. *J Biol Chem* 270:5571, 1995.
108. Regan LM, Stearns-Kurosawa DJ, Kurosawa S, et al: The endothelial cell protein C receptor. Inhibition of activated protein C anticoagulant function without modulation of reaction with proteinase inhibitors. *J Biol Chem* 271:17499, 1996.
109. Fukudome K, Kurosawa S, Stearns-Kurosawa DJ, et al: The endothelial cell protein C receptor. Cell surface expression and direct ligand binding by the soluble receptor. *J Biol Chem* 271:17491, 1996.
110. Stearns-Kurosawa DJ, Kurosawa S, Mollica JS, et al: The endothelial cell protein C receptor augments protein C activation by the thrombin–thrombomodulin complex. *Proc Natl Acad Sci U S A* 93:10212, 1996.
111. Laszik Z, Mitro A, Taylor FB Jr, et al: Human protein C receptor is present primarily on endothelium of large blood vessels: Implications for the control of the protein C pathway. *Circulation* 96:3633, 1997.
112. Xu J, Esmon NL, Esmon CT: Reconstitution of the human endothelial cell protein C receptor with thrombomodulin in phosphatidylcholine vesicles enhances protein C activation. *J Biol Chem* 274:6704, 1999.
113. Fukudome K, Ye X, Tsuneyoshi N, et al: Activation mechanism of anticoagulant protein C in large blood vessels involving the endothelial cell protein C receptor. *J Exp Med* 187:1029, 1998.
114. Liang Z, Rosen ED, Castellino FJ: Nucleotide structure and characterization of the murine gene encoding the endothelial cell protein C receptor. *Thromb Haemost* 81:585, 1999.
115. Ye X, Fukudome K, Tsuneyoshi N, et al: The endothelial cell protein C receptor (EPCR) functions as a primary receptor for protein C activation on endothelial cells in arteries, veins, and capillaries. *Biochem Biophys Res Commun* 259:671, 1999.
116. Simmonds RE, Lane DA: Structural and functional implications of the intron/exon organization of the human endothelial cell protein C–activated protein C receptor (EPCR) gene: Comparison with the structure of CD1/major histocompatibility complex alpha1 and alpha2 domains. *Blood* 94:632, 1999.
117. Oganesyan V, Oganesyan N, Terzyan S, et al: The crystal structure of the endothelial protein C receptor and a bound phospholipid. *J Biol Chem* 277:24851, 2002.
118. Villoutreix BO, Blom AM, Dahlback B: Structural prediction and analysis of endothelial cell protein C–activated protein C receptor. *Protein Eng* 12:833, 1999.
119. Kurosawa S, Stearns-Kurosawa DJ, Hidari N, Esmon CT: Identification of functional endothelial protein C receptor in human plasma. *J Clin Invest* 100:411, 1997.
120. Kurosawa S, Stearns-Kurosawa DJ, Carson CW, et al: Plasma levels of endothelial cell protein C receptor are elevated in patients with sepsis and systemic lupus erythematosus: Lack of correlation with thrombomodulin suggests involvement of different pathological processes [letter]. *Blood* 91:725, 1998.
121. Yang XV, Banerjee Y, Fernández JA et al: Activated protein C ligation of ApoER2 (LRP8) causes Dab1-dependent signaling in U937 cells. *Proc Natl Acad Sci U S A* 106:274, 2009.

122. Gu JM, Crawley JT, Ferrell G et al: Disruption of the endothelial cell protein C receptor gene in mice causes placental thrombosis and early embryonic lethality. *J Biol Chem* 277:43335, 2002.
123. Hayashi T, Nakamura H, Okada A, et al: Organization and chromosomal localization of the human endothelial protein C receptor gene. *Gene* 238:367, 1999.
124. Vu TK, Hung DT, Wheaton VI, Coughlin SR: Molecular cloning of a functional thrombin receptor reveals a novel proteolytic mechanism of receptor activation. *Cell* 64:1057, 1991.
125. Kahn ML, Nakanishi-Matsui M, Shapiro MJ, et al: Protease-activated receptors 1 and 4 mediate activation of human platelets by thrombin. *J Clin Invest* 103:879, 1999.
126. Coughlin SR: Thrombin signaling and protease-activated receptors. *Nature* 407:258, 2000.
127. Macfarlane SR, Seatter MJ, Kanke T, et al: Proteinase-activated receptors. *Pharmacol Rev* 53:245, 2001.
128. Steinhoff M, Buddenkotte J, Shpacovitch V, et al: Proteinase-activated receptors: Transducers of proteinase-mediated signaling in inflammation and immune response. *Endocr Rev* 26:1, 2005.
129. Leger AJ, Covic L, Kuliopulos A: Protease-activated receptors in cardiovascular diseases. *Circulation* 114:1070, 2006.
130. Traynelis SF, Trejo J. Protease-activated receptor signaling: New roles and regulatory mechanisms. *Curr Opin Hematol* 14:230, 2007.
131. Comp PC, Jacocks RM, Ferrell GL, Esmon CT: Activation of protein C *in vivo*. *J Clin Invest* 70:127, 1982.
132. Hanson SR, Griffin JH, Harker LA, et al: Antithrombotic effects of thrombin-induced activation of endogenous protein C in primates. *J Clin Invest* 92:2003, 1993.
133. Lentz SR, Fernandez JA, Griffin JH, et al: Impaired anticoagulant response to infusion of thrombin in atherosclerotic monkeys associated with acquired defects in the protein C system. *Arterioscler Thromb Vasc Biol* 19:1744, 1999.
134. Snow TR, Deal MT, Dickey DT, Esmon CT: Protein C activation following coronary artery occlusion in the in situ porcine heart. *Circulation* 84:293, 1991.
135. Macko RF, Killewich LA, Fernandez JA, et al: Brain-specific protein C activation during carotid artery occlusion in humans. *Stroke* 30:542, 1999.
136. Petaja J, Pesonen E, Fernandez JA, et al: Cardiopulmonary bypass and activation of antithrombotic plasma protein C. *J Thorac Cardiovasc Surg* 118:422, 1999.
137. Gruber A, Pal A, Kiss RG, et al: Generation of activated protein C during thrombolysis. *Lancet* 342:1275, 1993.
138. Macko RF, Ameriso SF, Gruber A, et al: Impairments of the protein C system and fibrinolysis in infection-associated stroke. *Stroke* 27:2005, 1996.
139. Conard J, Bauer KA, Gruber A, et al: Normalization of markers of coagulation activation with a purified protein C concentrate in adults with homozygous protein C deficiency. *Blood* 82:1159, 1993.
140. Taylor FB Jr, Peer GT, Lockhart MS, et al: Endothelial cell protein C receptor plays an important role in protein C activation *in vivo*. *Blood* 97:1685, 2001.
141. Bajaj MS, Kuppuswamy MN, Manepalli AN, Bajaj SP: Transcriptional expression of tissue factor pathway inhibitor, thrombomodulin and von Willebrand factor in normal human tissues. *Thromb Haemost* 82:1047, 1999.
142. Christie PD, Edelberg JM, Picard MH, et al: A murine model of myocardial microvascular thrombosis. *J Clin Invest* 104:533, 1999.
143. Healy AM, Rayburn HB, Rosenberg RD, Weiler H: Absence of the blood-clotting regulator thrombomodulin causes embryonic lethality in mice before development of a functional cardiovascular system. *Proc Natl Acad Sci U S A* 92:850, 1995.
144. Ishii H, Salem HH, Bell CE, et al: Thrombomodulin, an endothelial anticoagulant protein, is absent from the human brain. *Blood* 67:362, 1986.
145. Wong VL, Hofman FM, Ishii H, Fisher M: Regional distribution of thrombomodulin in human brain. *Brain Res* 556:1, 1991.
146. Hackeng TM, Tans G, Koppelman SJ, et al: Protein C activation on endothelial cells by prothrombin activation products generated *in situ*: Meizothrombin is a better protein C activator than α-thrombin. *Biochem J* 319:399, 1996.
147. Varadi K, Philapitsch A, Santa T, Schwarz HP: Activation and inactivation of human protein C by plasmin. *Thromb Haemost* 71:615, 1994.
148. Haley PE, Doyle MF, Mann KG: The activation of bovine protein C by factor Xa. *J Biol Chem* 264:16303, 1989.
149. Rezaie AR: Rapid activation of protein C by factor Xa and thrombin in the presence of polyanionic compounds. *Blood* 91:4572, 1998.
150. Slungaard A, Key NS: Platelet factor 4 stimulates thrombomodulin protein C-activating cofactor activity. A structure-function analysis. *J Biol Chem* 269:25549, 1994.
151. Dudek AZ, Pennell CA, Decker TD, et al: Platelet factor 4 binds to glycanated forms of thrombomodulin and to protein C. A potential mechanism for enhancing generation of activated protein C. *J Biol Chem* 272:31785, 1997.
152. Slungaard A, Fernandez JA, Griffin JH, et al: Platelet factor 4 enhances generation of activated protein C *in vitro* and *in vivo*. *Blood* 102:146, 2003.
153. Kowalska MA, Mahmud SA, Lambert MP, et al: Endogenous platelet factor 4 stimulates activated protein C generation *in vivo* and improves survival after thrombin or lipopolysaccharide challenge. *Blood* 110:1903, 2007.
154. Fernandez JA, Petaja J, Gruber A, Griffin JH: Activated protein C correlates inversely with thrombin levels in resting healthy individuals. *Am J Hematol* 56:29, 1997.
155. Villoutreix BO, Dahlback B: Structural investigation of the A domains of human blood coagulation factor V by molecular modeling. *Protein Sci* 7:1317, 1998.
156. Pellequer JL, Gale AJ, Griffin JH, Getzoff ED: Homology modeling of factor Va, a cofactor of the prothrombinase complex. *Protein Sci* 7:159, 1998.
157. Pellequer JL, Gale AJ, Griffin JH, Getzoff ED: Homology models of the C domains of blood coagulation factors V and VIII: A proposed membrane binding mode for FV and FVIII C2 domains. *Blood Cells Mol Dis* 24:448, 1998.
158. Autin L, Steen M, Dahlbäck B, Villoutreix BO: Proposed structural models of the prothrombinase (FXa-FVa) complex. *Proteins* 63:440, 2006.
159. Adams TE, Hockin MF, Mann KG, Everse SJ: The crystal structure of activated protein C-inactivated bovine factor Va: Implications for cofactor function. *Proc Natl Acad Sci U S A* 101:8918, 2004.
160. Camire RM, Kalafatis M, Tracy PB: Proteolysis of factor V by cathepsin G and elastase indicates that cleavage at Arg1545 optimizes cofactor function by facilitating factor Xa binding. *Biochemistry* 37:11896, 1998.
161. Steen M, Dahlback B: Thrombin-mediated proteolysis of factor V resulting in gradual B-domain release and exposure of the factor Xa-binding site. *J Biol Chem* 277:38424, 2002.
162. Toso R, Camire RM: Removal of B-domain sequences from factor V rather than specific proteolysis underlies the mechanism by which cofactor function is realized. *J Biol Chem* 279:21643, 2004.
163. Thorelli E, Kaufman RJ, Dahlbäck B: Cleavage requirements for activation of factor V by factor Xa. *Eur J Biochem* 247:12, 1997.
164. Fay PJ: Regulation of factor VIIIa in the intrinsic factor Xase. *Thromb Haemost* 82:193, 1999.
165. Marlar RA, Kleiss AJ, Griffin JH: Mechanism of action of human activated protein C, a thrombin-dependent anticoagulant enzyme. *Blood* 59:1067, 1982.
166. Suzuki K, Stenflo JA, Dahlbäck B, Teodorsson B: Inactivation of human coagulation factor V by activated protein C. *J Biol Chem* 258:1914, 1983.
167. Fulcher CA, Gardiner JE, Griffin JH, Zimmerman TS: Proteolytic inactivation of activated human factor VIII procoagulant protein by activated protein C and its analogy to factor V. *Blood* 63:486, 1984.
168. Kalafatis M, Rand MD, Mann KG: The mechanism of inactivation of human factor V and human factor Va by activated protein C. *J Biol Chem* 269:31869, 1994.
169. Dahlbäck B, Carlsson M, Svensson PJ: Familial thrombophilia due to a previously unrecognized mechanism characterized by poor anticoagulant response to activated protein C: Prediction of a cofactor to activated protein C. *Proc Natl Acad Sci U S A* 90:1004, 1993.
170. Bertina RM, Koeleman BPC, Koster T, et al: Mutation in blood coagulation factor V associated with resistance to activated protein C. *Nature* 369:64, 1994.
171. Greengard JS, Sun X, Xu X, et al: Activated protein C resistance caused by Arg506Gln mutation in factor Va. *Lancet* 343:1361, 1994.
172. Sun X, Evatt B, Griffin JH: Blood coagulation factor Va abnormality associated with resistance to activated protein C in venous thrombophilia. *Blood* 83:3120, 1994.
173. Zivelin A, Griffin JH, Xi X, et al: A single genetic origin for a common Caucasian risk factor for venous thrombosis. *Blood* 89:397, 1997.
174. Zivelin A, Mor-Cohen R, Kovalsky V, et al: Prothrombin 20210G>A is an ancestral prothrombotic mutation that occurred in whites approximately 24,000 years ago. *Blood* 107:4666, 2006.
175. Heeb MJ, Kojima Y, Greengard J, Griffin JH: Activated protein C resistance: Molecular mechanisms based on studies using purified Gln506-factor V. *Blood* 85:3405, 1995.
176. Kalafatis M, Bertina RM, Rand MD, Mann KG: Characterization of the molecular defect in factor VR506Q. *J Biol Chem* 270:4053, 1995.
177. Rosing J, Hoekema L, Nicolaes GA, et al: Effects of protein S and factor Xa on peptide bond cleavages during inactivation of factor Va and factor VaR506Q by activated protein C. *J Biol Chem* 270:27852, 1995.
178. Gale AJ, Xu X, Pellequer JL, et al: Interdomain engineered disulfide bond permitting elucidation of mechanisms of inactivation of coagulation factor Va by activated protein C. *Protein Sci* 11:2091, 2002.
179. Maurissen LF, Thomassen MC, Nicolaes GA, et al: Re-evaluation of the role of the protein S-C4b binding protein complex in activated protein C-catalyzed factor Va-inactivation. *Blood* 111:3034, 2008.
180. Bernardi F, Faioni EM, Castoldi E, et al: A factor V genetic component differing from factor V R506Q contributes to the activated protein C resistance phenotype. *Blood* 90:1552, 1997.
181. Faioni EM, Franchi F, Bucciarelli P, et al: Coinheritance of the HR2 haplotype in the factor V gene confers an increased risk of venous thromboembolism to carriers of factor V R506Q (factor V Leiden). *Blood* 94:3062, 1999.
182. Rosing J, Bakker H, Thomassen MC, et al: Characterization of two forms of human factor Va with different cofactor activities. *J Biol Chem* 268:21130, 1993.
183. Hoekema L, Nicolaes GA, Hemker HC, et al: Human factor Va1 and factor Va2: Properties in the procoagulant and anticoagulant pathways. *Biochemistry* 36:3331, 1997.
184. Kim SW, Ortel TL, Quinn-Allen MA, et al: Partial glycosylation at asparagine-2181 of the second C-type domain of human factor V modulates assembly of the prothrombinase complex. *Biochemistry* 38:11448, 1999.
185. Nicolaes GA, Villoutreix BO, Dahlbäck B: Partial glycosylation of Asn2181 in human factor V as a cause of molecular and functional heterogeneity. Modulation of glycosylation efficiency by mutagenesis of the consensus sequence for N-linked glycosylation. *Biochemistry* 38:13584, 1999.
186. Fernández JA, Hackeng TM, Kojima K, Griffin JH: The carbohydrate moiety of factor V modulates inactivation by activated protein C. *Blood* 89:4348, 1997.
187. Fisher M, Fernández JA, Ameriso SF, et al: Activated protein C resistance in ischemic stroke not due to factor V arginine506Æglutamine mutation. *Stroke* 27:1163, 1996.

188. Van der Bom JG, Bots ML, Haverkate F, et al: Reduced response to activated protein C is associated with increased risk for cerebrovascular disease. *Ann Intern Med* 125:265, 1996.
189. De Visser MC, Rosendaal FR, Bertina RM: A reduced sensitivity for activated protein C in the absence of factor V Leiden increases the risk of venous thrombosis. *Blood* 93:1271, 1999.
190. Rodeghiero F, Tosetto A: Activated protein C resistance and factor V Leiden mutation are independent risk factors for venous thromboembolism. *Ann Intern Med* 130:643, 1999.
191. Kiechl S, Muigg A, Santer P, et al: Poor response to activated protein C as a prominent risk predictor of advanced atherosclerosis and arterial disease. *Circulation* 99:614, 1999.
192. Griffin JH, Kojima K, Banka CL, et al: High-density lipoprotein enhancement of anticoagulant activities of plasma protein S and activated protein C. *J Clin Invest* 103:219, 1999.
193. Curvers J, Thomassen MC, Nicolaes GA, et al: Acquired APC resistance and oral contraceptives: Differences between two functional tests. *Br J Haematol* 105:88, 1999.
194. Smirnov MD, Safa O, Esmon NL, Esmon CT: Inhibition of activated protein C anticoagulant activity by prothrombin. *Blood* 94:3839, 1999.
195. Brugge JM, Tans G, Rosing J, Castoldi E: Protein S levels modulate the activated protein C resistance phenotype induced by elevated prothrombin levels. *Thromb Haemost* 95:236, 2006.
196. Neuenschwander P, Jesty J: A comparison of phospholipid and platelets in the activation of human factor VIII by thrombin and factor Xa, and in the activation of factor X. *Blood* 72:1761, 1988.
197. Keller FG, Ortel TL, Quinn-Allen MA, Kane WH: Thrombin-catalyzed activation of recombinant human factor V. *Biochemistry* 34:4118, 1995.
198. Safa O, Morrissey JH, Esmon CT, Esmon NL: Factor VIIa/tissue factor generates a form of factor V with unchanged specific activity, resistance to activation by thrombin, and increased sensitivity to activated protein C. *Biochemistry* 38:1829, 1999.
199. Bakker HM, Tans G, Jannssen-Claessen T, et al: The effect of phospholipids, calcium ions and protein S on rate constants of human factor Va inactivation by activated human protein C. *Eur J Biochem* 208:171, 1992.
200. Smirnov MD, Esmon C: Phosphatidylethanolamine incorporation into vesicles selectively enhances factor Va inactivation by activated protein C. *J Biol Chem* 269:816, 1994.
201. Smirnov MD, Triplett DT, Comp PC, et al: On the role of phosphatidylethanolamine in the inhibition of activated protein C activity by antiphospholipid antibodies. *J Clin Invest* 95:309, 1995.
202. Fernández JA, Kojima K, Hackeng TM, Griffin JH: Cardiolipin, a protein C pathway cofactor: Implications for anticardiolipin antibody syndrome. *Thromb Haemost* 73(6):1392, 1995.
203. Rezende SM, Simmonds RE, Lane DA: Coagulation, inflammation, and apoptosis: Different roles for protein S and the protein S-C4b binding protein complex. *Blood* 103:1192, 2004.
204. Nishioka J, Suzuki K: Inhibition of cofactor activity of protein S by a complex of protein S and C4b-binding protein: Evidence for inactive ternary complex formation between protein S, C4b-binding protein, and activated protein C. *J Biol Chem* 265:9072, 1990.
205. Yegneswaran S, Wood GM, Esmon CT, Johnson AE: Protein S alters the active site location of activated protein C above the membrane surface. A fluorescence resonance energy transfer study of topography. *J Biol Chem* 272:25013, 1997.
206. Yegneswaran S, Smirnov MD, Safa O, et al: Relocating the active site of activated protein C eliminates the need for its protein S cofactor. A fluorescence resonance energy transfer study. *J Biol Chem* 274:5462, 1999.
207. Gardiner JE, McGann MA, Berridge CW, et al: Protein S as a cofactor for activated protein C in plasma and in the inactivation of purified factor VIII:C. *Circulation* 70:205a, 1984.
208. Koedam JA, Meijers JCM, Sixma JJ, Bouma BN: Inactivation of human factor VIII by activated protein C. Cofactor activity of protein S and protective effect of von Willebrand factor. *J Clin Invest* 82:1236, 1988.
209. Solymoss S, Tucker MM, Tracy PB: Kinetics of inactivation of membrane-bound factor Va by activated protein C: Protein S modulates factor Xa protection. *J Biol Chem* 263:14884, 1988.
210. Dahlback B, Hildebrand B, Malm J: Characterization of functionally important domains in human vitamin K-dependent protein S using monoclonal antibodies. *J Biol Chem* 265:8127, 1990.
211. Saller F, Villoutreix BO, Amelot A et al: The gamma-carboxyglutamic acid domain of anticoagulant protein S is involved in activated protein C cofactor activity, independently of phospholipid binding. *Blood* 105:122, 2005.
212. Saller F, Kaabache T, Aiach M, et al: The protein S thrombin-sensitive region modulates phospholipid binding and the gamma-carboxyglutamic acid-rich (Gla) domain conformation in a non-specific manner. *J Thromb Haemost* 4:704, 2006.
213. Suzuki K, Nishioka J, Hashimoto S: Regulation of activated protein C by thrombin-modified protein S. *J Biochem* 94:699, 1983.
214. Walker FJ: Regulation of vitamin K-dependent protein S: Inactivation by thrombin. *J Biol Chem* 259:10335, 1984.
215. Dahlbäck B, Lundwall A, Stenflo JA: Localization of thrombin cleavage sites in the amino-terminal region of bovine protein S. *J Biol Chem* 261:5111, 1986.
216. Váradi K, Rosing J, Tans G, et al: Factor V enhances the cofactor function of protein S in the APC-mediated inactivation of factor VIII: Influence of the factor VR506Q mutation. *Thromb Haemost* 76:208, 1996.
217. Thorelli E, Kaufman RJ, Dahlback B: Cleavage of factor V at Arg 506 by activated protein C and the expression of anticoagulant activity of factor V. *Blood* 93:2552, 1999.
218. Pajkrt D, Lerch PG, van der Poll T, et al: Differential effects of reconstituted high-density lipoprotein on coagulation, fibrinolysis and platelet activation during human endotoxemia. *Thromb Haemost* 77:303, 1997.
219. Li D, Weng S, Yang B, et al: Inhibition of arterial thrombus formation by ApoA1 Milano. *Arterioscler Thromb Vasc Biol* 19:378, 1999.
220. Griffin JH, Fernandez JA, Deguchi H: Plasma lipoproteins, hemostasis and thrombosis. *Thromb Haemost* 86:386, 2001.
221. Mineo C, Deguchi H, Griffin JH, Shaul PW. Endothelial and antithrombotic actions of HDL. *Circ Res* 98:1352, 2006.
222. Deguchi H, Pecheniuk NM, Elias DJ, et al: High density lipoprotein deficiency and dyslipoproteinemia associated with venous thrombosis in males. *Circulation* 112:893, 2005.
223. Eichinger S, Pecheniuk NM, Hron G et al: High-density lipoprotein and the risk of recurrent venous thromboembolism. *Circulation* 115:1609, 2007.
224. Deguchi H, Fernandez JA, Pabinger I, et al: Plasma glucosylceramide deficiency as potential risk factor for venous thrombosis and modulator of anticoagulant protein C pathway. *Blood* 97:1907, 2001.
225. Deguchi H, Fernandez JA, Griffin JH: Neutral glycosphingolipid-dependent inactivation of coagulation factor Va by activated protein C and protein S. *J Biol Chem* 277:8861, 2002.
226. Yegneswaran S, Deguchi H, Griffin JH: Glucosylceramide, a neutral glycosphingolipid anticoagulant cofactor, enhances the interaction of human- and bovine-activated protein C with negatively charged phospholipid vesicles. *J Biol Chem* 278:14614, 2003.
227. Deguchi H, Yegneswaran S, Griffin JH: Sphingolipids as bioactive regulators of thrombin generation. *J Biol Chem* 279:12036, 2004.
228. Esmon CT: Interactions between the innate immune and blood coagulation systems. *Trends Immunol* 25:536, 2004.
229. Levi M, van der Poll T, Buller HR: Bidirectional relation between inflammation and coagulation. *Circulation* 109:2698, 2004.
230. Joyce DE, Gelbert L, Ciaccia A, et al: Gene expression profile of antithrombotic protein C defines new mechanisms modulating inflammation and apoptosis. *J Biol Chem* 276:11199, 2001.
231. Riewald M, Petrovan RJ, Donner A, et al: Activation of endothelial cell protease activated receptor 1 by the protein C pathway. *Science* 296:1880, 2002.
232. Mosnier LO, Griffin JH: Inhibition of staurosporine-induced apoptosis of endothelial cells by activated protein C requires protease activated receptor-1 and endothelial cell protein C receptor. *Biochem J* 373:65, 2003.
233. Cheng T, Liu D, Griffin JH, et al: Activated protein C blocks p53-mediated apoptosis in ischemic human brain endothelium and is neuroprotective. *Nat Med* 9:338, 2003.
234. Feistritzer C, Riewald M: Endothelial barrier protection by activated protein C through PAR1-dependent sphingosine 1-phosphate receptor-1 crossactivation. *Blood* 105:3178, 2005.
235. Finigan JH, Dudek SM, Singleton PA et al: Activated protein C mediates novel lung endothelial barrier enhancement: Role of sphingosine 1-phosphate receptor transactivation. *J Biol Chem* 280:17286, 2005.
236. Giesen PL, Rauch U, Bohrmann B, et al: Blood-borne tissue factor: Another view of thrombosis. *Proc Natl Acad Sci U S A* 96:2311, 1999.
237. Nieuwland R, Berckmans RJ, McGregor S, et al: Cellular origin and procoagulant properties of microparticles in meningococcal sepsis. *Blood* 95:930, 2000.
238. Berckmans RJ, Neiuwland R, Boing AN, et al: Cell-derived microparticles circulate in healthy humans and support low grade thrombin generation. *Thromb Haemost* 85:639, 2001.
239. Shet AS, Aras O, Gupta KMJH, et al: Sickle blood contains tissue factor positive microparticles derived from endothelial cells and monocytes. *Blood* 102:2678, 2003.
240. Freyssinet JM: Cellular microparticles: What are they bad or good for? *J Thromb Haemost* 1:1655, 2003.
241. Chou J, Mackman N, Merrill-Skoloff G, et al: Hematopoietic cell-derived microparticle tissue factor contributes to fibrin formation during thrombus propagation. *Blood* 104:3190, 2004.
242. Morel O, Toti F, Hugel B et al: Procoagulant microparticles: Disrupting the vascular homeostasis equation? *Arterioscler Thromb Vasc Biol* 26:2594, 2006.
243. Mackman N, Tilley RE, Key NS: Role of the extrinsic pathway of blood coagulation in hemostasis and thrombosis. *Arterioscler Thromb Vasc Biol* 27:1687, 2007.
244. George FD: Microparticles in vascular diseases. *Thromb Res* 122(Suppl 1):S55, 2008.
245. Nomura S, Ozaki Y, Ikeda Y: Function and role of microparticles in various clinical settings. *Thromb Res* 123:8, 2008.
246. Casciola-Rosen L, Rosen A, Petri M, Schlissel M: Surface blebs on apoptotic cells are sites of enhanced procoagulant activity: Implications for coagulation events and antigenic spread in systemic lupus erythematosus. *Proc Natl Acad Sci U S A* 93:1624, 1996.
247. Bombeli T, Karsan A, Tait JF, Harlan JM: Apoptotic vascular endothelial cells become procoagulant. *Blood* 89:2429, 1997.
248. Wang J, Weiss I, Svoboda K, Kwaan HC: Thrombogenic role of cells undergoing apoptosis. *Br J Haematol* 115:382, 2001.
249. Diamant M, Tushuizen ME, Sturk A, Nieuwland R. Cellular microparticles: New players in the field of vascular disease? *Eur J Clin Invest* 34:392, 2004.
250. Shu F, Kobayashi H, Fukudome K, et al: Activated protein C suppresses tissue factor expression on U937 cells in the endothelial protein C receptor-dependent manner. *FEBS Lett* 477:208, 2000.

251. Warren BL, Eid A, Singer P, et al: For the KyberSept trail study group. High-dose antithrombin III in severe sepsis: A randomized controlled trial. *JAMA* 286:1869, 2001.
252. Abraham E, Reinhart K, Opal S, et al: For the OPTIMIST trial study group. Efficacy and safety of tifacogin (recombinant tissue factor pathway inhibitor) in severe sepsis: A randomized controlled trail. *JAMA* 290:238, 2003.
253. Kerschen EJ, Fernandez JA, Cooley BC et al: Endotoxemia and sepsis mortality reduction by non-anticoagulant activated protein C. *J Exp Med* 204:2439, 2007.
254. Niessen F, Furlan-Freguia C, Fernandez JA et al: Endogenous EPCR/aPC-PAR1 signaling prevents inflammation-induced vascular leakage and lethality. *Blood* 113:2859, 2009.
255. Schuepbach RA, Feistritzer C, Fernández JA, et al: Protection of vascular barrier integrity by activated protein C in murine models depends on protease-activated receptor-1. *Thromb Haemost* 101:724, 2009.
256. Shibata M, Kumar SR, Amar A, et al: Anti-inflammatory, antithrombotic, and neuroprotective effects of activated protein C in a murine model of focal ischemic stroke. *Circulation* 103:1799, 2001.
257. Fernández JA, Xu X, Liu D, et al: Recombinant murine-activated protein C is neuroprotective in a murine ischemic stroke model. *Blood Cells Mol Dis* 30:271, 2003.
258. Liu D, Cheng T, Guo H, et al: Tissue plasminogen activator neurovascular toxicity is controlled by activated protein C. *Nat Med* 10:1379, 2004.
259. Guo H, Liu D, Gelbard H, et al: Activated protein C prevents neuronal apoptosis via protease activated receptors 1 and 3. *Neuron* 41:563, 2004.
260. Domotor E, Benzakour O, Griffin JH, et al: Activated protein C alters cytosolic calcium flux in human brain endothelium via binding to endothelial protein C receptor and activation of protease activated receptor-1. *Blood* 101:4797, 2003.
261. Zlokovic BV, Zhang C, Liu D, et al: Functional recovery after embolic stroke in rodents by activated protein C. *Ann Neurol* 58:474, 2005.
262. Cheng T, Petraglia AL, Li Z, et al: Activated protein C inhibits tissue plasminogen activator-induced brain hemorrhage. *Nat Med* 12:1278, 2006.
263. Thiyagarajan M, Fernández JA, Lane SM, et al: Activated protein C promotes neovascularization and neurogenesis in postischemic brain via protease-activated receptor 1. *J Neurosci* 28:12788, 2008.
264. Guo H, Singh I, Wang Y, et al: Neuroprotective activities of activated protein C mutant with reduced anticoagulant activity. *Eur J Neurosci* 29:1119, 2009.
265. Guo H, Wang Y, Singh I, et al: Species-dependent neuroprotection by activated protein C mutants with reduced anticoagulant activity. *J Neurochem* 109:116, 2009.
266. Riewald M, Ruf W: Protease-activated receptor-1 signaling by activated protein C in cytokine-perturbed endothelial cells is distinct from thrombin signaling. *J Biol Chem* 280:19808, 2005.
267. Chesebro BB, Rahn P, Carles M, et al: Increase in activated protein c mediates acute traumatic coagulopathy in mice. *Shock* 32:659, 2009.
268. Finigan JH, Boueiz A, Wilkinson E, et al: Activated protein C protects against ventilator-induced pulmonary capillary leak. *Am J Physiol Lung Cell Mol Physiol* 296:L1002, 2009.
269. Xu J, Ji Y, Zhang X, et al: Endogenous activated protein C signaling is critical to protection of mice from lipopolysaccharide-induced septic shock. *J Thromb Haemost* 7:851, 2009.
270. Heeb MJ, Gruber A, Griffin JH: Identification of divalent metal ion–dependent inhibition of activated protein C by α_2-macroglobulin and α_2-antiplasmin in blood and comparisons to inhibition of factor Xa, thrombin, and plasmin. *J Biol Chem* 226:17606, 1991.
271. Okajima K, Koga S, Kaji M, et al: Effect of protein C and activated protein C on coagulation and fibrinolysis in normal human subjects. *Thromb Haemost* 63:48, 1990.
272. Heeb MJ, Griffin JH: Physiologic inhibition of human activated protein C by α_1-antitrypsin. *J Biol Chem* 263:11613, 1988.
273. Heeb MJ, España F, Geiger M, et al: Immunological identity of heparin-dependent plasma and urinary protein C inhibitor and plasminogen activator inhibitor-3. *J Biol Chem* 262:15813, 1987.
274. Heeb MJ, España F, Griffin JH: Inhibition and complexation of activated protein C by two major inhibitors in plasma. *Blood* 73:446, 1989.
275. España F, Vicente V, Tabernero D, et al: Determination of plasma protein C inhibitor and of two activated protein C-inhibitor complexes in normals and in patients with intravascular coagulation and thrombotic disease. *Thromb Res* 59:593, 1990.
276. España F, Gilabert J, Aznar J, et al: Complexes of activated protein C with α_1-antitrypsin in normal pregnancy and in severe preeclampsia. *Am J Obstet Gynecol* 164:1310, 1991.
277. Scully MF, Toh CH, Hoogendoorn H, et al: Activation of protein C and its distribution between its inhibitors, protein C inhibitor, α_1-antitrypsin and α_2-macroglobulin, in patients with disseminated intravascular coagulation. *Thromb Haemost* 69:448, 1993.
278. Strandberg K, Astermark J, Björgell O, et al: Complexes between activated protein C and protein C inhibitor measured with a new method: Comparison of performance with other markers of hypercoagulability in the diagnosis of deep vein thrombosis. *Thromb Haemost* 86:1400, 2001.
279. Bhiladvala P, Strandberg K, Stenflo J, Holm J: Early identification of acute myocardial infarction by activated protein C–protein C inhibitor complex. *Thromb Res* 118:213, 2006.
280. Schwarz HP, Fischer M, Hopmeier P, et al: Plasma protein S deficiency in familial thrombotic disease. *Blood* 646:1297, 1984.
281. Comp PC, Nixon RR, Cooper MR, Esmon CT: Familial protein S deficiency is associated with recurrent thrombosis. *J Clin Invest* 74:2082, 1984.
282. Stenberg Y, Muranyi A, Steen C, et al: EGF-like module pair 3–4 in vitamin K–dependent protein S: Modulation of calcium affinity of module 4 by module 3 and interaction with factor X. *J Mol Biol* 293:653, 1999.
283. Yegneswaran S, Hackeng T, Johnson AE, Griffin JH: Phospholipid-dependent protein S interaction with factor Xa mediated through the thrombin-sensitive region of protein S. *Thromb Haemost* 82:428, 1999.
284. Van't Veer C, Hackeng TM, Biesbroeck D, et al: Increased prothrombin activation in protein S-deficient plasma under flow conditions on endothelial cell matrix: An independent anticoagulant function of protein S in plasma. *Blood* 85:1815, 1995.
285. Koppelman SJ, Hackeng TM, Sixma JJ, Bouma BN: Inhibition of the intrinsic factor X activating complex by protein S: Evidence for a specific binding of protein S to factor VIII. *Blood* 86:1062, 1995.
286. Koppelman SJ, van't Veer C, Sixma JJ, Bouma BN: Synergistic inhibition of the intrinsic factor X activation by protein S and C4b-binding protein. *Blood* 86:2653, 1995.
287. Hackeng TM, Sere KM, Tans G, Rosing J: Protein S stimulates inhibition of the tissue factor pathway by tissue factor pathway inhibitor. *Proc Natl Acad Sci U S A* 103:3106, 2006.
288. Hackeng TM, Rosing J: Protein S as cofactor for TFPI. *Arterioscler Thromb Vasc Biol* 29:2015, 2009.
289. Crawley JT, Lane DA: The haemostatic role of tissue factor pathway inhibitor. *Arterioscler Thromb Vasc Biol* 28:233, 2008.
290. Heeb MJ, Prashun D, Griffin JH, Bouma BN: Plasma protein S contains zinc essential for efficient activated protein C-independent anticoagulant activity and binding to factor Xa, but not for efficient binding to tissue factor pathway inhibitor. *FASEB J* 23:2244, 2009.
291. Dahlbäck B: Purification of human C4b-binding protein and formation of its complex with vitamin K-dependent protein S. *Biochem J* 209:847, 1983.
292. Griffin JH, Gruber A, Fernández JA: Reevaluation of total, free and bound protein S and C4b-binding protein levels in plasma anticoagulated with citrate or hirudin. *Blood* 79:32003, 1992.
293. Schwarz HP, Muntean W, Watzke H, et al: Low total protein S antigen but high protein S activity due to decreased C4b-binding protein in neonates. *Blood* 71:562, 1988.
294. Dahlbäck B: Inhibition of the protein Ca cofactor function of human and bovine protein S by C4b-binding protein. *J Biol Chem* 261:12022, 1986.
295. Maurissen LF, Thomassen MC, Nicolaes GA, et al: Re-evaluation of the role of the protein S-C4b binding protein complex in activated protein C-catalyzed factor Va-inactivation. *Blood* 111:3034, 2008.
296. van de Poel RH, Meijers JC, Bouma BN: C4b-binding protein inhibits the factor V-dependent but not the factor V-independent cofactor activity of protein S in the activated protein C-mediated inactivation of factor VIIIa. *Thromb Haemost* 85:761, 2001.
297. Hillarp A, Dahlbäck B: Novel subunit in C4b-binding protein required for protein S binding. *J Biol Chem* 263:12759, 1988.
298. Hillarp A, Hessing M, Dahlbäck B: Protein S binding in relation to the subunit composition of human C4b-binding protein. *FEBS Lett* 259:53, 1989.
299. Hillarp A, Dahlbäck B: Cloning of cDNA coding for the beta chain of human complement component C4b-binding protein: Sequence homology with the alpha chain. *Proc Natl Acad Sci U S A* 87:1183, 1990.
300. Fernández JA, Griffin JH: A protein S binding site on C4b-binding protein involves β chain residues 31–45. *J Biol Chem* 269:2535, 1994.
301. Fernández JA, Griffin JH, Chang GTG, et al: Involvement of amino acid residues 423–429 of human protein S in binding to C4b-binding protein. *Blood Cells Mol Dis* 24:101, 1998.
302. García de Frutos P, Alim RI, et al: Differential regulation of α and β chains of C4b-binding protein during acute-phase response resulting in stable plasma levels of free anticoagulant protein S. *Blood* 84:815, 1994.
303. Anderson HA, Maylock CA, Williams JA, et al: Serum-derived protein S binds to phosphatidylserine and stimulates the phagocytosis of apoptotic cells. *Nat Immunol* 4:87, 2003.
304. Prasad D, Rothlin CV, Burrola P, et al: TAM receptor function in the retinal pigment epithelium. *Mol Cell Neurosci* 33:96, 2006.
305. Uehara H, Shacter E: Auto-oxidation and oligomerization of protein S on the apoptotic cell surface is required for Mer tyrosine kinase-mediated phagocytosis of apoptotic cells. *J Immunol* 180:2522, 2008.
306. McColl A, Bournazos S, Franz S, et al: Glucocorticoids induce protein S-dependent phagocytosis of apoptotic neutrophils by human macrophages. *J Immunol* 183:2167, 2009.
307. Liu D, Guo H, Griffin JH, et al: Protein S confers neuronal protection during ischemic/hypoxic injury in mice. *Circulation* 107:1791, 2003.
308. Wun TC, Kretzmer KK, Girard TJ, et al: Cloning and characterization of a cDNA coding for the lipoprotein-associated coagulation inhibitor shows that it consists of three tandem Kunitz-type inhibitory domains. *J Biol Chem* 263:6001, 1988.
309. Bajaj MS, Birktoft JJ, Steer SA, Bajaj SP: Structure and biology of tissue factor pathway inhibitor. *Thromb Haemost* 86:959, 2001.
310. Rao LV, Rapaport SI: Studies of a mechanism inhibiting the initiation of the extrinsic pathway of coagulation. *Blood* 69:645, 1987.
311. Gettins PG: Serpin structure, mechanism, and function. *Chem Rev* 102:4751, 2002.
312. Whisstock JC, Bottomley SP: Molecular gymnastics: Serpin structure, folding and misfolding. *Curr Opin Struct Biol* 16:761, 2006.
313. Rau JC, Beaulieu LM, Huntington JA, Church FC: Serpins in thrombosis, hemostasis and fibrinolysis. *J Thromb Haemost* 5(Suppl 1):102, 2007.
314. Schreuder HA, de Boer B, Dijkema R, et al: The intact and cleaved human antithrombin III complex as a model for serpin-proteinase interactions. *Nat Struct Biol* 1:48, 1994.
315. Whisstock J, Skinner R, Lesk AM: An atlas of serpin conformations. *Trends Biochem Sci* 23:63, 1998.

316. Skinner R, Abrahams JP, Whisstock JC, et al: The 2.6 Å structure of antithrombin indicates a conformational change at the heparin binding site. *J Mol Biol* 266:601, 1997.
317. Huntington JA, Read RJ, Carrell RW: Structure of a serpin-protease complex shows inhibition by deformation. *Nature* 407:923, 2000.
318. Li W, Johnson DJ, Esmon CT, Huntington JA: Structure of the antithrombin-thrombin-heparin ternary complex reveals the antithrombotic mechanism of heparin. *Nat Struct Mol Biol* 11:857, 2004.
319. Huber R, Carrell RW: Implications of the three-dimensional structure of α_1-antitrypsin for structure and function of serpins. *Biochemistry* 28:8951, 1989.
320. Rosenberg RD, Rosenberg JS: Natural anticoagulant mechanisms. *J Clin Invest* 74:1, 1984.
321. Olson ST, Bjork I, Sheffer R, et al: Role of the antithrombin-binding pentasaccharide in heparin acceleration of antithrombin-proteinase reactions. Resolution of the antithrombin conformational change contribution to heparin rate enhancement. *J Biol Chem* 267:12528, 1992.
322. Choay J, Petitou M, Lormeau JC, et al: Structure-activity relationship in heparin: A synthetic pentasaccharide with high affinity for antithrombin III and eliciting high anti-factor Xa activity. *Biochem Biophys Res Commun* 116:492, 1983.
323. Bourin MC, Lindahl U: Glycosaminoglycans and the regulation of blood coagulation. *Biochem J* 289:313, 1993.
324. Hirsh J, O'Donnell M, Eikelboom JW: Beyond unfractionated heparin and warfarin: Current and future advances. *Circulation* 1165:552, 2007.
325. Olds RJ, Lane DA, Chowdhury V, et al: Complete nucleotide sequence of the antithrombin gene: Evidence for homologous recombination causing thrombophilia. *Biochemistry* 32:4216, 1993.
326. Picard V, Ersdal-Badju E, Bock SC: Partial glycosylation of antithrombin III asparagine-135 is caused by the serine in the third position of its N-glycosylation consensus sequence and is responsible for production of the beta-antithrombin III isoform with enhanced heparin affinity. *Biochemistry* 34:8433, 1995.
327. Turko IV, Fan B, Gettins PG: Carbohydrate isoforms of antithrombin variant N135Q with different heparin affinities. *FEBS Lett* 335:9, 1993.
328. Bock SC, Harris JF, Balazs I, Trent JM: Assignment of the human antithrombin III structural gene to chromosome 1q23–25. *Cytogenet Cell Genet* 39:67, 1985.
329. Chandra T, Stackhouse R, Kidd VJ, Woo SL: Isolation and sequence characterization of a cDNA clone of human antithrombin III. *Proc Natl Acad Sci U S A* 80:1845, 1983.
330. Prochownik EV, Markham AF, Orkin SH: Isolation of a cDNA clone for human antithrombin III. *J Biol Chem* 258:8389, 1983.
331. Lane DA, Bayston T, Olds RJ, et al: Antithrombin mutation database: 2nd (1997) update. For the Plasma Coagulation Inhibitors Subcommittee of the Scientific and Standardization Committee of the International Society on Thrombosis and Haemostasis. *Thromb Haemost* 77:197, 1997.
332. Raja SM, Chhablani N, Swanson R, et al: Deletion of P1 arginine in a novel antithrombin variant (antithrombin London) abolishes inhibitory activity but enhances heparin affinity and is associated with early onset thrombosis. *J Biol Chem* 278:13688, 2003.
333. Chang JY, Monroe DM, Oliver JA, Roberts HR: TFPIbeta, a second product from the mouse tissue factor pathway inhibitor (TFPI) gene. *Thromb Haemost* 81:45, 1999.
334. Zhang J, Piro O, Lu L, Broze GJ: Glycosyl phosphatidylinositol anchorage of tissue factor pathway inhibitor. *Circulation* 108:623, 2003.
335. Caplice NM, Panetta C, Peterson TE, et al: Lipoprotein (a) binds and inactivates tissue factor pathway inhibitor: A novel link between lipoproteins and thrombosis. Blood 98:2980, 2001.
336. Piro O, Broze GJ Jr: Role for the Kunitz-3 domain of tissue factor pathway inhibitor-alpha in cell surface binding. *Circulation* 110:3567, 2004.
337. Piro O, Broze GJ Jr: Comparison of cell-surface TFPIappha and beta. *J Thromb Haemost* 3:2677, 2005.
338. Kato H: Regulation of functions of vascular wall cells by tissue factor pathway inhibitor: Basic and clinical aspects. *Arterioscler Thromb Vasc Biol* 22:539, 2002.
339. Girard TJ, Warren LA, Novotny WF, et al: Functional significance of the Kunitz-type inhibitory domains of lipoprotein-associated coagulation inhibitor. *Nature* 338:518, 1989.
340. Lesnik P, Vonica A, Guerin M, et al: Anticoagulant activity of tissue factor pathway inhibitor in human plasma is preferentially associated with dense subspecies of LDL and HDL and with Lp(a). *Arterioscler Thromb* 13:1066, 1993.
341. Sandset PM, Abildgaard U, Larsen ML: Heparin induces release of extrinsic coagulation pathway inhibitor (EPI). *Thromb Res* 50:803, 1988.
342. Huang ZF, Broze G Jr: Consequences of tissue factor pathway inhibitor gene-disruption in mice. *Thromb Haemost* 78:699, 1997.
343. Van der Logt CP, Reitsma PH, Bertina RM: Intron-exon organization of the human gene coding for the lipoprotein-associated coagulation inhibitor: The factor Xa dependent inhibitor of the extrinsic pathway of coagulation. Biochemistry 30:1571, 1991.
344. Girard TJ, Eddy R, Wesselschmidt RL, et al: Structure of the human lipoprotein-associated coagulation inhibitor gene. Intron/exon gene organization and localization of the gene to chromosome 2. *J Biol Chem* 266:5036, 1991.
345. Tollefsen DM, Majerus DW, Blank MK: Heparin cofactor II. Purification and properties of a heparin-dependent inhibitor of thrombin in human plasma. *J Biol Chem* 257:2162, 1982.
346. Bertina RM, van der Linden IK, Engesser L, et al: Hereditary heparin cofactor II deficiency and the risk of development of thrombosis. *Thromb Haemost* 57:196, 1987.
347. Corral J, Aznar J, Gonzalez-Conejero R, et al: Homozygous deficiency of heparin cofactor II: Relevance of P17 glutamate residue in serpins, relationship with conformational diseases, and role in thrombosis. *Circulation* 110:1303, 2004.
348. Broze GJ: Protein Z dependent regulation of coagulation. *Thromb Haemost* 86:813, 2001.
349. Han X, Huang Z-F, Fiehler R, Broze GJ: The protein Z-dependent protease inhibitor is a serpin. *Biochemistry* 38:11073, 1999.
350. Han X, Fiehler R, Broze GJ: Characterization of the protein Z-dependent protease inhibitor. *Blood* 99:3049, 2000.
351. Heeb MJ, Cabral KM, Ruan L: Down-regulation of factor IXa in the factor Xase complex by protein Z-dependent protease inhibitor. *J Biol Chem* 280:33819, 2005.
352. Wei Z, Yan Y, Carrell RW, Zhou A: Crystal structure of protein Z-dependent inhibitor complex shows how protein Z functions as a cofactor in the membrane inhibition of factor X. *Blood* 114:3662, 2009.
353. Corral J, González-Conejero R, Hernández-Espinosa D, Vicente V: Protein Z/Z-dependent protease inhibitor (PZ/ZPI) anticoagulant system and thrombosis. *Br J Haematol* 137:99, 2007.
354. Yin Z-F, Huang Z-F, Cui J, et al: Prothrombotic phenotype of protein Z deficiency. *Proc Natl Acad Sci U S A* 97:6734, 2000.
355. Kemkes-Matthes B, Nees M, Kuhnel G, et al: Protein Z influences the prothrombotic phenotype in factor V Leiden patients. *Thromb Res* 106:183, 2002.
356. Water N, Tan T, Ashton F, et al: Mutations within the protein Z-dependent protease inhibitor gene are associated with venous thromboembolic disease: A new form of thrombophilia. *Br J Haematol* 127:190, 2004.
357. Vasse M: Protein Z, a protein seeking a pathology. *Thromb Haemost* 100:548, 2008.
358. Dentali F, Gianni M, Lussana F, et al: Polymorphisms of the Z protein protease inhibitor and risk of venous thromboembolism: A meta-analysis. *Br J Haematol* 143:284, 2008.
359. Sofi F, Cesari F, Tu Y, et al: Protein Z-dependent protease inhibitor and protein Z in peripheral arterial disease patients. *J Thromb Haemost* 7:731, 2009.
360. Rezaie AR, Cooper ST, Church FC, Esmon CT: Protein C inhibitor is a potent inhibitor of the thrombin-thrombomodulin complex. *J Biol Chem* 270:25336, 1995.

CHAPTER 117

VASCULAR FUNCTION IN HEMOSTASIS

Katherine A. Hajjar, Aaron J. Marcus, and William A. Muller

SUMMARY

Blood vessels and their constitutive endothelium play a critical role in the maintenance of vascular fluidity, the arrest of hemorrhage (hemostasis), prevention of occlusive vascular phenomena (thrombosis), and regulation of the inflammatory process. The endothelium extends to all recesses of the body and maintains an intimate association with flowing blood and blood cells. However, endothelial cell morphologies, gene-expression profiles, and functions vary among different vascular beds. In straight arterial segments, but not at branch points or curvatures of the arteries or veins, for example, endothelial cells align themselves in parallel to the direction of blood flow. Similarly, endothelial cells in post capillary venules are primarily responsible for mediating adhesion and transmigration of leukocytes, whereas arteriolar endothelium is important for regulation of vasomotor tone. Recent proteomic approaches, moreover, have revealed that endothelial cells have the unique capacity to express and elaborate thromboregulatory molecules which can be classified according to their chronological appearance. Early thromboregulators appear prior to thrombin formation and late thromboregulators arrive after thrombin has formed. This chapter reviews some of the mechanisms that impart thromboresistance to the vascular wall, and discusses their implication for blood vessel health and disease.

THE ENDOTHELIUM

The endothelium represents a dynamic interface between flowing blood and the vessel wall, and produces a variety of factors that regulate blood fluidity (Fig. 117–1). Endothelial cells are subject to unique shear stress, to soluble factors in the blood, to signals emanating from the large variety of cells in the circulation, and to cell–cell interactions in the vascular wall, all of which create region-specific phenotypes.[1] In addition to modulating vascular permeability and fragility, the endothelium regulates the fluid state of blood by displaying thromboresistance and profibrinolytic potential. All of the above activities serve to maintain patency of all the lumens in the circulation (Fig. 117–1).[2]

Acronyms and abbreviations that appear in this chapter include: ADAMTS, a disintegrin and metalloproteinase with thrombospondin repeats; ADP, adenosine diphosphate; APC, activated protein C; Apo(a), apolipoprotein(a); ApoE, apolipoprotein E; CD, cluster of differentiation; CD39/ENTPD1, ectonucleotidase triphosphate diphosphohydrolase 1; COX, cyclooxygenase; DDAVP, desmopressin acetate; EPCR, endothelial cell protein C receptor; ET-1, endothelin-1; GP, glycoprotein; HC, homocysteine; ICAM, intercellular adhesion molecule; IFN, interferon; IL, interleukin; JAM, junctional adhesion molecule; LFA, lymphocyte function-associated antigen; Lp(a), lipoprotein(a); Mac-1, macrophage-1; MAdCAM-1, mucosal addressin cell adhesion molecule-1; MHC, major histocompatibility complex; NK, natural killer; NO, nitric oxide; NOS, nitric oxide synthase; p11, protein p11, the annexin A2 binding partner; PAF, platelet-activating factor; PAI-1, plasminogen activator inhibitor-1; PECAM, platelet/endothelial cell adhesion molecule; PGI_2, prostaglandin I_2; PSGL-1, P-selectin glycoprotein ligand-1; TAFI, thrombin-activatable fibrinolysis inhibitor; TF, tissue factor; TM, thrombomodulin; TNF-α, tumor necrosis factor-α; t-PA, tissue-type plasminogen activator; u-PA, urokinase plasminogen activator; uPAR, urokinase receptor; VCAM, vascular cell adhesion molecule; VLA-1, very-late antigen-1; VWF, von Willebrand factor.

ENDOTHELIAL CELL HETEROGENEITY

The heterogeneity of endothelial cells is mediated by two mechanisms.[3] The first involves biochemical and biomechanical signals within the extracellular environment that trigger posttranscriptional and/or posttranslational changes in these cells. Both the net signal input and the endothelial cell output (cellular phenotype) vary across the vascular tree. Second, certain site-specific properties of the endothelium are genetically programmed and, therefore, independent of the extracellular milieu. Although explanations for the existence of endothelial cell heterogeneity are still somewhat speculative, phenotypic variability serves at least two important purposes: (1) It allows endothelial cells to meet the specific needs of the surrounding tissue. For example, the tight junctions of the blood–brain barrier protect neurons from fluctuations in composition of the blood supply. In contrast, the fenestrated discontinuous endothelium of hepatic sinusoids allows for ready access of nutrient-rich portal venous blood for the metabolic systems in hepatocytes. (2) It provides endothelial cells with site-specific mechanisms for thriving within many different microenvironments. For example, endothelial cells in the inner medulla of the kidney must survive the profoundly hypoxic and hyperosmolar local environment. One can assume that these cells made adaptations that differ significantly from those of the endothelial cells in the oxygen-rich environment of the pulmonary capillary bed.

Because of the necessity for a rapid response to sudden environmental perturbation, translational control mechanisms probably play a significant role in regulating endothelial cell phenotype and function, and regulate up to 10 percent of genes expressed in these cells.[4] Compared to transcriptional control pathways, translational control provides a much more rapid mechanism for responses to environmental cues. Because of their close association with both flowing blood and solid tissues, endothelial cells are subject to a broad spectrum of agonistic and inhibitory external signals that frequently require rapid functional and phenotypic responses. Such stimuli are associated with sepsis, inflammation, ischemia-reperfusion injury, and direct mechanical trauma induced clinically by stents, balloon catheters, and graft procedures.

ENDOTHELIAL CELL PRODUCTION OF THROMBOREGULATORY MOLECULES

Thromboregulatory compounds control platelet and vascular reactivity during the early stages of thrombus formation (Table 117–1).[5] They include eicosanoids, nitric oxide, endothelin, and the CD39/ecto-nucleoside triphosphate diphosphohydrolase 1 (CD39/ENTPD1). The endothelial cell eicosanoids are hydrocarbon compounds derived from essential fatty acids in the diet. The most important endothelial eicosanoid is prostacyclin (PGI_2), which blocks platelet reactivity, induces vascular relaxation, and stimulates cytokine production.[6] Nitric oxide is a naturally occurring gas released from vascular endothelial cells in response to binding of vasodilators to endothelial cell membrane receptors. It is therefore a short-lived vasodilator and inhibitor of platelet reactivity. By activating guanylate cyclase, the resulting increase in cyclic guanosine monophosphate inhibits platelet function and induces vascular relaxation.[7,8] Endothelin is a short polypeptide that regulates vascular tone by binding to a G-protein-coupled receptor on

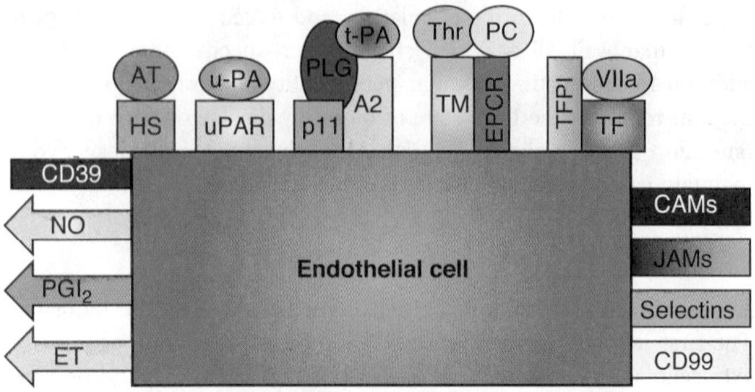

FIGURE 117–1. Schematic depiction of endothelial cell thromboregulatory molecules. Products that are secreted and exert their effects in the fluid phase are represented by *arrows*. Cell surface-associated molecules are shown as *rectangles*. Thromboregulators that modulate platelet activation, recruitment, and blood vessel contractility are shown on the *left*. Agents that regulate components of the coagulation cascade and/or fibrinolytic system are located at the *top*. Inflammatory molecules whose expression or activity is directed by inflammatory mediators are shown at the *right*. A2, annexin A2; AT, antithrombin; CAMs, cellular adhesion molecules; CD39/ENTPD1, ectonucleoside triphosphate diphosphohydrolase 1; EPCR, endothelial cell protein C receptor; ET, endothelin; HS, heparan sulfate; JAMs, junctional adhesion molecules; NO, nitric oxide; PC, protein C; PGI_2, prostacyclin; PLG, plasminogen; TF, tissue factor; TFPI, tissue factor pathway inhibitor; TM, thrombomodulin; t-PA, tissue-type plasminogen activator; u-PA, urokinase plasminogen activator; uPAR, u-PA receptor; VIIa, factor VIIa. These components are discussed further in the text.

smooth muscle cells. Endothelial cell CD39/ENTPD1 is a membrane-associated apyrase which metabolizes adenosine diphosphate (ADP) in the primary platelet releasate. This prevents further platelet activation and recruitment, and has considerable therapeutic potential.[9,10]

Late thromboregulators act either to prevent excessive thrombin generation or to promote lysis of intravascular thrombi (Table 117–2). Antithrombin, a natural anticoagulant, acts as an inhibitor of thrombin and factor Xa in the circulation. Endothelial cell heparan proteoglycans act as cofactors for antithrombin. The tissue factor pathway inhibitor inhibits the complex between factor VIIa and tissue factor. The thrombomodulin/endothelial cell protein C receptor (EPCR)/protein C system in the vascular wall is involved in regulation of hemostasis through a direct anticoagulant effect on thrombin (see Chap. 116). Cellular signals resulting from thrombin-mediated activation of protein C and the interaction of activated protein C with the EPCR are linked to the inflammatory process. The fibrinolytic system is intimately involved with the vascular endothelium because endothelial cells not only synthesize and secrete components of the fibrinolytic system, but also regulate formation of plasmin from its precursor, plasminogen, through the expression of receptors. Impairment of fibrinolytic synthetic and assembly systems probably plays a central role in the etiology of occlusive vascular disease.[11]

In the setting of inflammation, pathologic alterations in the thromboregulatory balance are evidenced by increased expression of tissue factor and modulation of the thrombomodulin/EPCR/protein C system. In addition, endothelial cell adhesion molecules constitute a special class of glycoproteins which mediate physical interactions between endothelial cells and leukocytes. Such glycoproteins include members of two molecular families, the cell adhesion molecules (MAdCAM-1 [mucosal addressin cell adhesion molecule-1], ICAM-1 [intercellular adhesion molecule-1], VCAM-1 [vascular cell adhesion molecule-1], and PECAM-1 [platelet endothelial adhesion molecule-1]) and the selectins (P and E). In concert, these molecules create a dynamic interface that modulates multiple interactions between the endothelium and various classes of circulating leukocytes.[12]

Thromboregulation defines a process or group of processes by which hematologic cells in the circulation and cells of the vessel wall interact in order to facilitate or inhibit thrombus formation.[13,14] Thromboregulation is accomplished through cell proximity or contact. The process can be cell-associated or involve compounds which have been released into the aqueous phase during agonist exposure. Thromboregulatory systems are an intricate homeostatic component which can prevent or reverse platelet accumulation, coagulation factor activation, and fibrin formation. In this manner blood fluidity is maintained.[15]

The physiologic defense systems that render endothelial surfaces and blood cells antithrombotic can be overwhelmed by excessive shear stress, increased turbulence, injury, inflammation, and severe atherosclerosis.[16] These events may transform the endothelial cells into a prothrombotic and antifibrinolytic phenotype.[17] This transformation is accompanied by upregulation of leukocyte and endothelial cell adhesion molecules, increased expression of tissue factor, and accumulation of monocytes/macrophages in the vessel wall.[18] These events commonly occur at the site of fissured or fractured atherosclerotic plaques in the coronary and cerebrovascular circulation.[18]

The above events are closely associated with activity of the early thromboregulatory systems—the eicosanoids such as PGI_2, nitric oxide (NO), and the CD39/ENTPD1 systems. Because these systems reach peak activity very early in the hemostatic/thrombotic cascade, they represent important new targets for therapeutic intervention. Figures 117–2 through 117–4 depict the sequence of events beginning with platelet activation, coagulation, thrombosis, and atherogenesis. These involve interactions between platelets, leukocytes, and endothelial cells. These cascades highlight the molecular mechanisms and inflammatory pathways used by platelets to initiate and accelerate atherothrombosis.[18,19]

TABLE 117–1. Early Pro- and Antithrombotic Thromboregulators Associated with Human Endothelial Cells

Class	Type	Site of Action	Aspirin Sensitivity	Mode of Action
Eicosanoids	PGI_2, PGD_2	Fluid phase autacoid	Sensitive	Elevation of platelet cAMP
Nitrovasodilators	EDRF/NO	Fluid phase autacoid	Insensitive	Elevation of platelet cGMP
Ecto-nucleotidases	CD39/ENTPD1	Endothelial cell surface	Insensitive	Enzymatic removal of secreted ADP
Thromboxane	TXA_2	Fluid phase vasoconstrictor	Sensitive	Lowers platelet cAMP and platelet agonist
Endothelins	ET-1, ET-2	Fluid phase vasoconstrictor	Insensitive	Direct vasoconstrictor peptide

ADP, adenosine diphosphate; cAMP, cyclic adenosine monophosphate; cGMP, cyclic guanosine monophosphate; EDRF, endothelium-derived relaxing factor; ET, endothelin; NO, nitric oxide; PGD_2, prostaglandin D_2; PGI_2, prostacyclin; TXA_2, thromboxane A_2.

TABLE 117–2. Chronology of Endothelial Cell Thromboregulators

Early thromboregulators
Nitric oxide (NO)
Eicosanoids (prostacyclin and prostaglandin D_2)
Endothelial cell CD39/ENTPDase1
Endothelin
Late thromboregulators
Endothelin
Antithrombin
Endothelial cell/heparin proteoglycans
Tissue factor pathway inhibitor
Thrombomodulin-protein C-protein S pathway
Fibrinolytic system (plasminogen activators, inhibitors, and receptors)
Inflammatory thromboregulators
Thrombomodulin-protein C-protein S pathway
Cellular adhesion molecules
Selectins

Another aspect of thromboregulation concerns the endothelial cell–platelet axis, which prevents extravasation of erythrocytes and other hematologic cells at inter-endothelial junctions in the absence of physical or immunologic trauma.[1] Functional and physical contacts between platelets and endothelial cells are of critical importance for the maintenance of vascular integrity and cell permeability.[20] Proangiogenic cytokines and growth factors, stored in platelet granules and released upon platelet activation, bind to specific receptors on the surface of endothelial cells.[1] This results in intracellular signaling, which serves to stabilize a vascular–endothelium intercellular–adhesion protein complex between endothelial cells. Importantly, during thrombocytopenia, the adjacent intercellular junctions disassemble, resulting in extravasation of erythrocytes and other circulating cells into the surrounding tissue, and this extravasation results in petechiae, which, if uncontrolled, evolve into purpura and then ecchymosis.[1] These signaling pathways may vary in tissue-specific vascular beds to satisfy the needs of that particular tissue. This information indicates that platelets actually serve as a "biochemical reservoir" that stabilizes the endothelium and may also lead to new therapeutic approaches for thrombocytopenia.

THE EICOSANOID PATHWAY

Eicosanoids are a group of biologically active substances derived from the essential fatty acid, arachidonate, which must be obtained from the diet. Oxygenation and further enzymatic transformation of arachidonic acid gives rise to eicosanoids (formerly classified as prostaglandins) and hydroxy acids, such as the leukotrienes. Eicosanoids are autacoids, a group of transient, physiologically active endogenous substances acting on the immediate environment of the cell to promote or inhibit its functions. Intermediates of the arachidonic acid pathway from different cells can interact with each other and produce new products with new biologic activities.[21] The main basic and clinical issue is whether these short-lived autacoids can have a longer life span than a classical autacoid, which is a few seconds, or whether they are released constantly at baseline.

In 1975, Hamberg, Svensson, and Samuelsson discovered a new eicosanoid, thromboxane, which is derived from arachidonic acid in activated platelets. This was the second vasoconstrictor released from activated platelets in addition to serotonin.[22] Moreover, thromboxane promoted platelet aggregation, operative via release of ADP from platelet-dense granules. While attempting to study thromboxane from arterial tissue, Moncada and associates identified a substance that acted as a transient autacoid that displayed vasodilation and inhibition of platelet aggregation contrasting with the effect of thromboxane.[23] The new autacoid was initially named PGX,[23] but later designated PGI_2 or prostacyclin.[24] Similarly to thromboxane, its biologic half-life was in the vicinity of 10 to 20 seconds, and its synthesis was inhibitable by acetyl salicylic acid (aspirin).[24]

BIOSYNTHESIS OF PROSTACYCLIN IN ENDOTHELIAL CELLS

Prostacyclin is the most important eicosanoid produced by endothelial cells. A wide range of stimuli, including hormones, biochemicals, or physical forces in the form of shear stress, elicit its release. Kinetic studies have revealed two patterns of prostacyclin production: (1) rapid release, independent of new cyclooxygenase (COX) messenger RNA (mRNA) or protein synthesis, and (2) slower production reflecting increased COX-2 expression. As will be described, the mechanisms of these two patterns of stimulation are distinct and separate.

In the case of rapid stimulation of PGI_2 production, as induced by thrombin, histamine, bradykinin, and ionophore, the response plateaus at 10 minutes. These agonists activate phospholipase C which generates inositol trisphosphate and diacylglycerol. The released inositol trisphosphate induces an elevation of intracellular calcium, which translocates phospholipase A to the outer portion of the nuclear envelope and endoplasmic reticulum. Phospholipase A then couples functionally to COX-1, which is localized on the luminal membrane. Prostacyclin synthase colocalizes with COX-1 in endothelial cells. Activated cytosol phospholipase

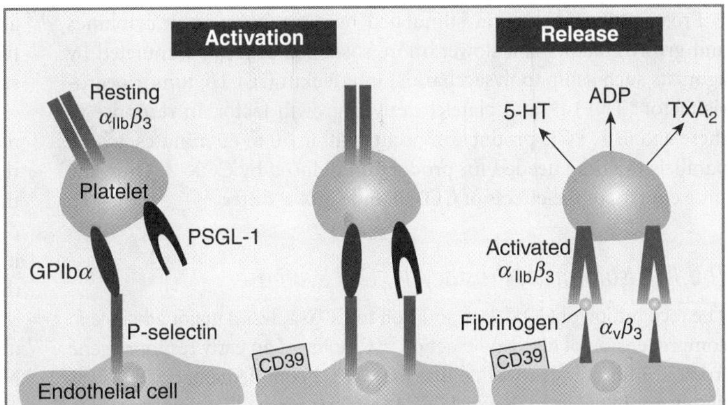

FIGURE 117–2. Following injury or severance of the vessel wall, platelets adhere to the damaged surface of the endothelial cell. Concomitant with adhesion, platelets and endothelial cells become activated. P-selectin is expressed on the endothelial cell surface. Platelet surface receptors GP1bα (glycoprotein 1bα) and PSGL-1 (P-selectin glycoprotein ligand-1) interact with endothelial P-selectin, thereby mediating platelet rolling. Firm adhesion is mediated by the β_3 integrins. In parallel with these intercellular events, platelet activation and release occur. The enzyme CD39 on the endothelial surface serves to control for excessive quantities of adenosine diphosphate (ADP) in the releasate by further metabolizing it. 5-HT, 5-hydroxytryptamine; TXA_2, thromboxane A_2. *(Adapted from Gawaz M, Langer H, May AE,[18] with permission.)*

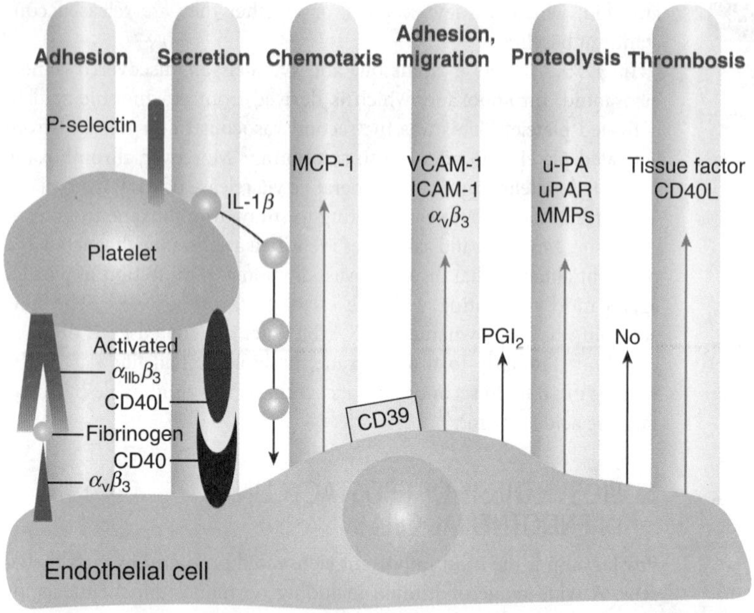

FIGURE 117–3. Adherent activated platelets induce an inflammatory response in endothelial cells. Platelet adhesion involving $\alpha_{IIb}\beta_3$ induces exposure of P-selectin (CD62P) and release of platelet CD40L and interleukin (IL)-1β, which then stimulate endothelial cells to respond with an inflammatory reaction that supports prothrombotic and proatherogenic alterations in the endothelium. IL-8 and MCP-1 (monocyte chemoattractant protein-1) are the principal chemoattractants for neutrophils and monocytes. The thromboregulator, CD39/ENTPD1, is substrate-activated and metabolizes released platelet ADP, thereby exerting an inhibitory effect on platelet activation and recruitment. ICAM, intercellular adhesion molecule; MMP, matrix metalloproteinase; NO, nitric oxide; PGI_2, prostacyclin; u-PA, urokinase plasminogen activator; uPAR, u-PA receptor; VCAM, vascular cell adhesion molecule. *(Adapted from Gawaz M, Langer H, May AE,[18] with permission.)*

A_2 catalyzes the release of arachidonic acid from membrane phospholipids, and the free arachidonate interacts with COX-1 and is converted to the endoperoxide prostaglandin H_2. The prostacyclin synthase converts prostaglandin H_2 to prostacyclin. The half-life of COX-1 is approximately 10 minutes, whereupon it autoinactivates.

Prostacyclin production stimulated by proinflammatory cytokines and growth factors is a slower, more sustained process, stimulated by agonists such as lipopolysaccharide, interleukin (IL)-1β, tumor necrosis factor (TNF)-α, and platelet-derived growth factor. In response to these agonists, PGI_2 production occurs within 30 to 60 minutes, which parallels the time needed for production induced by COX-2. Thus, the time courses of the effects of COX-1 and COX-2 differ.[25]

The Two Isoforms of Prostacyclin G/H Synthase

The recognition of COX-2, in addition to COX-1, was a major advance in comprehension of eicosanoid action.[26] Cloning of an early response gene from 3T3 fibroblasts revealed that the COX-2 complementary DNA was highly homologous to that of COX-1.[27,28] This meant that there were two different forms of COX, COX-1 (constitutive) and COX-2 (inducible), the latter of which was produced as an intermediate-early gene in monocytes, neutrophils, and endothelial cells.[26,29,30] COX-2 is inducible in endothelial cells by prothrombotic, inflammatory, or mitogenic stimuli, and in neutrophils by inflammatory stimuli.[31,32]

Within a specific species, there is approximately 60 percent homology between deduced amino acid sequences of COX-1 and COX-2. COX-1 contains 576 residues as compared to 587 for COX-2. The C-terminal sequence of 18 amino acids in COX-2 is absent in COX-1. Therefore, antibodies directed at this C-terminal sequence can identify COX-2 in a tissue by immunoblotting. The catalytic activity of both COX enzymes are similar and all amino acids critical for COX-1 activity are conserved in COX-2. The active site in COX-1 is slightly larger than that of COX-2, a fact that has impacted on the design of COX inhibitors. COX-2 contains mannose, and an *N*-glycosylation site within the 18-amino-acid C-terminal sequence. An *N*-glycosylation site at Asn410 is required for COX-1 to fold into its active conformation.

The gene for COX-1 is located on chromosome 9 and spans 22 kb of genomic DNA, whereas the gene for COX-2 is located on chromosome 1 and spans 8 kb of DNA. Transcription of COX-2 proceeds via several signaling mechanisms initiated by cMAP/protein kinase A, protein kinase C, tyrosine kinases, and pathways activated by growth factors, endotoxin, and cytokines.[29,33–35] The discoveries of COX-1 and COX-2 led to new concepts concerning the structure and function of COX-induced autacoids.[36]

Prostacyclin as an Autacoid

Prostacyclin is released from activated endothelial cells by a broad range of agonists. Prostacyclin also plays a critical role in the maintenance of vascular integrity by promoting thromboresistance and inhibiting inflammatory responses in the vasculature. Production of PGI_2 is dynamically regulated to meet the challenges arising from frequent prothrombotic and proinflammatory insults.[25] The molecule has a half-life of 3 minutes, whereupon it undergoes chemical hydrolysis to 6-keto-$PGF_{1\alpha}$. This is in keeping with its classification as an autacoid. It acts on platelets by increasing cyclic adenosine monophosphate levels in a paracrine manner.[37] Platelets have a specific prostacyclin receptor known as the I type prostaglandin receptor. This is a seven-transmembrane G-coupled receptor that couples with adenylyl cyclase. The latter binds to and activates protein kinase A, which results in inhibition of platelet activation and recruitment.[38] Physical or chemical perturbation of endothelial cells results in enhanced PGI_2 production. The action of prostacyclin increases the concentration of cyclic adenosine monophosphate in the platelet resulting in abolition of platelet shape change, inhibition of platelet secretion and recruitment, and impaired binding of von Willebrand factor and fibrinogen to the platelet surface. PGI_2 also inhibits platelet adhesion to subendothelium, especially at high shear rates.[39]

The discovery of prostacyclin revealed that the vascular endothelium has a protective effect on blood fluidity. It also meant that prostacyclin released from endothelial cells could counteract the effect of excessive thromboxane production. In addition, it was appreciated that intermediates in the synthesis of prostacyclin from arachidonic acid could also interact with other cells and tissues. Thus, prostacyclin could be synthesized from platelet-derived endoperoxides by cultured human endothelial cells.[40] Because of a low threshold for toxicity (hypotension and diarrhea), prostacyclin has had a rather narrow therapeutic window. Nevertheless, it was one of the major substances contributing to our concepts of thromboregulation.[5,41]

NITRIC OXIDE

In vascular endothelial cells, nitric oxide synthase (NOS) catalyzes formation of NO from L-arginine, in the presence of NADPH and oxygen.[42] The L-arginine is subsequently converted to citrulline and nitric oxide. The endothelial cell isoform of NO synthase (eNOS or the NOS3 gene product) functions constitutively, and is further activated by receptor-agonists that elevate intracellular calcium. Major stimuli include

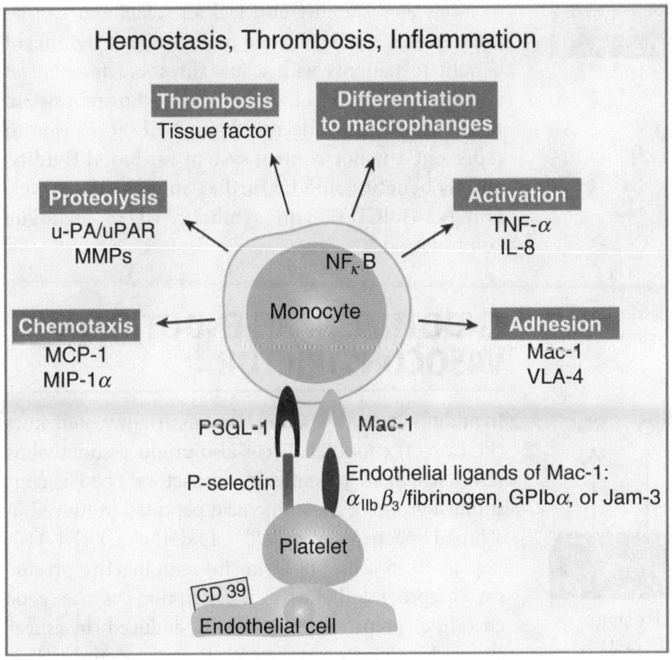

FIGURE 117–4. Adherent/activated platelets recruit and promote an NF-κB inflammatory response in monocytes. The platelets mainly interact with monocyte PSGL-1 (P-selectin glycoprotein ligand-1) with monocytic PSGL-1 via P-selectin and with monocyte Mac-1 ($\alpha_M\beta_2$) via $\alpha_{IIb}\beta_3$ (and fibrinogen bridging) or GP1bα (glycoprotein 1bα). Through this mechanism platelets initiate monocyte secretion of chemokines, cytokines, and procoagulant tissue factor. These serve to upregulate and activate adhesion receptors and proteases. In parallel, they induce monocyte differentiation into macrophages. Therefore, platelet–monocyte interactions provide a prothrombotic and atherogenic milieu at the vascular wall, which can eventually support plaque formation. CD39/ENTPD1 serves to modify excessive platelet recruitment via conversion of AMP to adenosine by 5′-nucleotidase. IL, interleukin; JAM, junctional adhesion molecule; MCP, monocyte chemoattractant protein; MIP, macrophage inflammatory protein; MMP, matrix metalloproteinase; NF-κB, nuclear factor-κB; TNF, tumor necrosis factor; u-PA, urokinase plasminogen activator; uPAR, u-PA receptor; VLA, very-late antigen. *(Adapted from Gawaz M, Langer H, May AE,[18] with permission.)*

ADP, thrombin, bradykinin, and shear stress.[39] Shear forces induce transcriptional activation of the eNOS gene because its promoter contains a shear response consensus sequence (GAGACC).[39] The NO that forms activates guanylate cyclase, thereby generating cyclic guanosine monophosphate. NO becomes oxidized to nitrite and then to nitrate, which is measurable in blood samples. NO in the circulation is rapidly inactivated by erythrocytes.[8,43,44] Its half-life is 5 to 10 minutes. NO has a vasodilatory effect on the pulmonary vasculature, and, in patients with congestive heart failure, its inhalation decreases pulmonary hypertension and increases pulmonary ventilation.[7,8,43–50] Acetylcholine released by activated nerve terminals in the vessel wall activate the endothelial cell to produce and release NO. This NO effect also explains the action of nitroglycerin, an NO donor that has been used for more than a 100 years to treat patients with angina resulting from coronary artery disease.[50]

Production of NO by endothelial cells is impaired in the presence of the thiol-containing amino acid, homocysteine. Cynomolgus monkeys with diet-induced hyperhomocysteinemia (11 μM) demonstrated reduced blood flow in the lower extremity and an impaired response to endothelial cell-dependent vasodilators.[47] Similarly, production of NO by endothelial cells *in vitro* is significantly inhibited in the presence of homocysteine, possibly by a mechanism involving impairment of the enzyme glutathione peroxidase.[48,49]

STRUCTURE AND BIOCHEMICAL PROPERTIES OF NITRIC OXIDE SYNTHASE

There are two isoforms of NOS: (1) the constitutive form, synthesized and regulated by Ca^{2+} and calmodulin, and (2) the cytokine-inducible, posttranscriptionally regulated form.[43] Both constitutive and inducible forms are mainly cytosolic, although a membrane-bound constitutive NOS isoform containing a myristoylation consensus sequence has been isolated from bovine aortic endothelial cells.[43] Endothelial NOS is M_r 144,000 and shares 57 percent amino acid sequence identity with neuronal NOS. The cofactor (6R-tetrahydro-L-biopterin, H_4B) participates in inducible and constitutive NOS isoform reactions. It is thought that H_4B stabilizes the enzyme in a manner allowing for maximum activity of the NOS subunit to which the pterin binds.[7,8,43,50]

BLOCKADE OF PLATELET AGGREGATION AND SECRETION BY NITRIC OXIDE

Platelet activation and recruitment in response to agonists, such as ADP, collagen, epinephrine, and thrombin, are blocked by NO. Blockade also occurs *in vivo* via formation of NO from endothelium.[7] Importantly, the inhibitory action of NO is not affected by aspirin either *in vivo* or *ex vivo*. Consequently, NO production is not a result of participation of endothelial cell eicosanoids.

In addition to the constitutive isoform of NOS (eNOS, the NOS3 gene product), endothelial cells stimulated by agonists such as cytokines will express the inducible form of NOS, iNOS, which is the NOS2 gene product. Through this mechanism, NO can further inhibit platelet reactivity and reduce basal vessel tone by inducing relaxation of vascular smooth muscle. The biochemical basis for the reaction is that NO binds to the heme prosthetic group of guanylyl cyclase. The inhibitory effect of NO on platelet activation can be monitored by measuring surface expression of P-selectin. The property of NO to inhibit mobilization of intracellular platelet calcium results in reduction of the conformational changes in platelet membrane $\alpha_{IIb}\beta_3$—an absolute requirement for fibrinogen binding and subsequent platelet aggregation. There is a broad spectrum of other effects of NO including inhibition of leukocyte adhesion to endothelial cell surfaces, inhibition of smooth muscle migration, and reduction of smooth muscle cell proliferation. These phenomena suggest that secretion of NO into the microenvironment is a major component of the response of the vasculature to injury.[39]

INHIBITION OF PLATELET ACTIVATION AND RECRUITMENT BY CD39/ENTPD1

In addition to the platelet inhibition by PGI_2 and NO, endothelial cells inhibit platelet function via the action of endothelial cell CD39/ENTPD1, an ecto-apyrase with adenosine diphosphatase and adenosine triphosphatase activities. The gene symbol for this compound is *ENTPD1*—ecto-nucleoside triphosphate diphosphohydrolase 1.[51] CD39 is localized mainly in endothelial cells and leukocytes. In endothelial cells, CD39 is located on the cell surface with the major portion of the molecule facing the vessel lumen. This is where the enzyme activity actually resides.[9,10,52] The enzyme has both N- and C-terminal transmembrane regions with small cytosolic portions anchoring the molecule.[53] In addition to CD39, CD73 (5′-nucleotidase) is present on vascular cells and converts the adenosine monophosphate generated from CD39 metabolism to adenosine (Fig. 117–5). In contrast to all other known platelet inhibitors, CD39 acting in concert with CD73 can

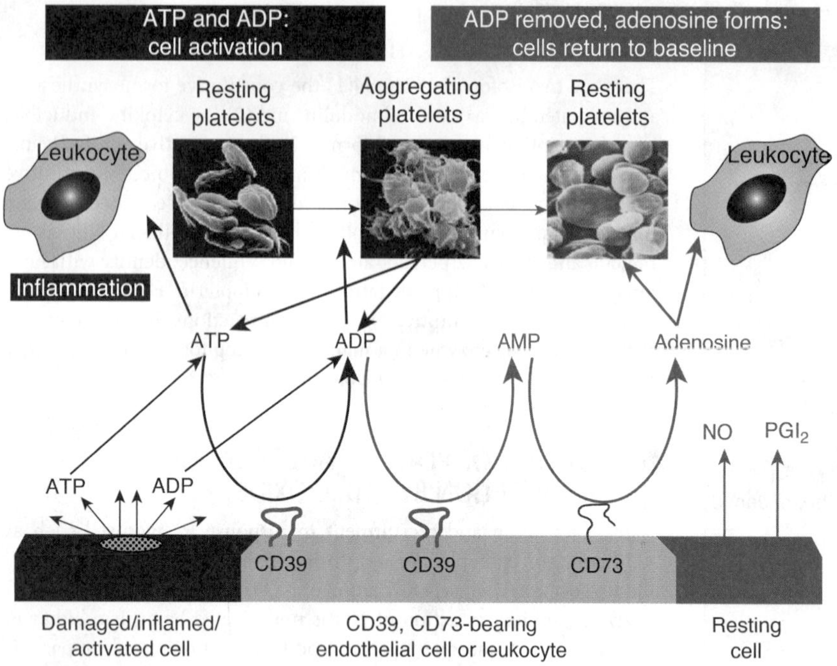

FIGURE 117–5. Biochemical transition and amplification of released platelet ADP as the major control system for hemostasis: ADP → AMP → adenosine. In parallel, perturbation of endothelial cells as a consequence of vascular injury initiates the process of thromboregulation. This includes release of newly synthesized prostacyclin as well as nitric oxide, both of which inhibit platelet reactivity in the fluid phase. The apyrase CD39 is the cell-associated inhibitory thromboregulator. CD39 is substrate-activated and in concert with CD39, CD73 brings the reaction to completion with the formation of adenosine.[321,322] The overall theme of this sequence of biochemical interactions is reminiscent of the enzyme cascade/waterfall of blood coagulation which functions as a biochemical amplifier. The early metabolic deletion of ADP from the system may also serve as a biologic safeguard to avoid excessive platelet accumulation, which would result in thrombosis.[18,19,321,322] ADP, adenosine diphosphate; AMP, adenosine monophosphate; ATP, adenosine triphosphate; NO, nitric oxide; PGI_2, prostacyclin.

convert the local environment from a prothrombotic ADP/ATP-rich entity to an antithrombotic adenosine-rich environment.[15] This phenomenon was quite evident from observations that platelets became unresponsive to all agonists when in motion and in proximity to endothelial cells even when eicosanoid and NO production were blocked.[41] It is of importance to emphasize that CD39 and CD73 do not exert their action on the platelet per se but act in series to metabolize ATP and ADP secreted from activated platelets to adenosine monophosphate and hence to adenosine.[10,54]

Most platelet agonists initiate secretion of dense granule contents within 15 to 20 seconds. The enhanced metabolism of ATP and ADP by therapeutically administered soluble CD39 (solCD39) also reduces secondary autoamplification and recruitment and consequently thrombus formation.[6,24,55] Because CD39 and CD73 are probably acting together, they theoretically will elevate levels of endogenous adenosine and increase the threshold for platelet activation in the local microenvironment. SolCD39 administration *in vivo* ameliorates the extent of stroke and reverses excessive platelet reactivity in a murine model, even if administered 3 hours following stroke induction. This is not associated with bleeding complications as observed with currently available therapeutic modalities.[56] It can be inferred that solCD39 does not interfere with the major signaling pathways which promote hemostasis. Therapeutic benefit of solCD39 has also been demonstrated in animal models of cardiac ischemia,[57] in the development of atherosclerosis,[58] regulation of leukocyte proinflammatory activity,[59] inhibition of metastasis,[60] and in transplantation.[61]

Therapy with solCD39 can abrogate thrombosis without inducing hemorrhage such as seen with existing antiplatelet therapies.[62] Because of its *in vivo* stability and lack of toxicity, it can be inferred that solCD39 could probably be of significant benefit to patients with a low threshold for platelet activation (as in diabetes) or to those who are resistant to existing therapeutic paradigms.[6] CD39 appears to represent a major control system for blood fluidity, and its benefit could be further enhanced by developing a solCD39 and synthetic CD73 analogue combination.[63]

ENDOTHELIN: AN ENDOTHELIAL VASOCONSTRICTOR

In addition to synthesizing two important vasodilators (PGI_2, NO) endothelial cells also produce endothelins (ETs), which are potent vasoconstrictors. The ETs constitute a group of 21-amino acid peptides, produced in a broad spectrum of cells.[64,65] Endothelin-1 (ET-1) is not stored in cells, but forms from an inactive precursor, preproendothelin-1. Transcription of the gene encoding preproendothelin-1 is induced by shear stress, hypoxia, or ischemia. Preproendothelin-1 is cleaved by an ET-1 converting enzyme, thereby forming the active peptide. ET-1, released from the activated endothelial cell binds to a G-protein-coupled receptor in smooth muscle. The binding process induces an increase in cytosolic calcium concentration, resulting in smooth muscle contraction. When concentrations of other thromboregulators such as NO are decreased, the action of ET-1 may be amplified and result in greater vasoconstriction.[64,65]

Release of ET-1 has been reported in the hepatorenal syndrome, a form of renal failure occurring in patients with severe liver disease. This disorder is characterized by intense and prolonged renal vasoconstriction. The hypoxia, oxidant injury, and endotoxemia, characteristic of end-stage liver disease, are probably agonists for endothelin production. The renal vasoconstriction has been attributed to activation of the sympathetic and renin-angiotensin systems in the kidney.[50,64,65] ET receptor antagonists may have therapeutic potential in hepatorenal syndrome, persistent pulmonary artery hypertension of the newborn, shunt-related pulmonary hypertension in patients with congenital heart disease, and possibly portal hypertension.[42,66–69]

THE PROTEIN C PATHWAY

The protein C pathway[70] plays a critical role in the prevention of thrombosis and is an integral part of the host inflammatory response as described in detail in Chap. 116. This pathway is initiated on the endothelial cell surface when thrombin combines with the endothelial receptor protein thrombomodulin (TM). Although thrombin is capable of slowly activating protein C, this reaction is markedly inhibited in the presence of physiologic concentrations of calcium ions. Once thrombin is bound to TM, the rate of protein C activation is dramatically enhanced[71] and is dependent on the presence of calcium. The detailed biochemistry of this activation reaction has been reviewed elsewhere.[72,73] Another protein found predominantly in large vessels, the EPCR, can bind protein C and further augment its activation by the thrombin–TM complex.[74] Presumably, the activated protein C (APC) can dissociate from EPCR and interact with protein S on either the endothelial cell or other membrane surface to exert its anticoagulant function. The function of APC can be found in detail in Chap. 116.

By far, the best known function of TM is its role in protein C activation. When thrombin is bound to TM, it is no longer able to clot fibrinogen, activate platelets, activate factors V and VIII,[79] or interact with the protease-activated receptors.[80,81] Instead, thrombin bound to TM acts as a direct anticoagulant.

TM also promotes the activation of a plasma procarboxypeptidase B by thrombin. This carboxypeptidase, also referred to as *thrombin-activatable fibrinolysis inhibitor* (TAFI),[82] or carboxypeptidase R, causes partial inhibition of fibrin degradation by plasmin, presumably by removing carboxy-terminal lysine residues from fibrin, thereby decreasing the binding of fibrin to certain forms of plasminogen and plasmin (see Chap. 136). However, TAFI has functions outside its antifibrinolytic role. TAFI is the major enzyme responsible for the removal of a C terminal arginine from C5a,[83–85] leading to its inactivation. C5a is a potent anaphylotoxin generated during complement activation and other vasoactive substances are most likely also inactivated by this enzyme by a similar mechanism.

TM also accelerates the proteolytic inactivation of prourokinase (also called single-chain urokinase-type plasminogen activator) by thrombin,[86,87] which may affect both fibrinolysis and tissue remodeling.[88] Despite these antifibrinolytic affects of TM, many *in vivo* experiments have demonstrated that soluble TM infusion results in a net antithrombotic and/or antiinflammatory effect.[89]

Independent of its effect on hemostasis, TM is essential to normal fetal development. When the TM gene is deleted by homologous recombination in mice, embryos die on day 8.5, prior to the development of a functional cardiovascular system,[90] implying that TM has functions in addition to its anticoagulant and fibrinolytic properties. TM,[91] in addition to EPCR,[92] is highly expressed on the giant trophoblast cells of the placenta. If TM expression is maintained on these cells, the TM null embryos survive[93,94] past this blockade point.

EPCR[95] is a 220-amino-acid type 1 transmembrane protein.[96–98] EPCR has two extracellular domains that show structural homology with the α and β domains of major histocompatibility complex (MHC) class 1 molecules, most notably the CD1d family. Because there are 3 Cys residues in the extracellular domain, the possibility of crosslinking with another protein exists. The cytoplasmic domain of human EPCR is only three amino acids long—Arg-Arg-Cys. The terminal Cys can be acylated with palmitate and this may have functional consequences.[99] Both protein C and APC bind to EPCR with similar affinity, about 30 nM.[95] Binding requires the presence of calcium and is tightened by the presence of magnesium ions. In addition, a soluble form of EPCR found normally in plasma[100] is also capable of binding both protein C and APC with equivalent affinity.

EPCR augments protein C activation by the thrombin–TM complex *in vitro* and *in vivo*, primarily through decreasing the K_m for protein C.[74,101,102] Just as thrombin changes its function from procoagulant to anticoagulant when it binds to TM, it appears that APC bound to EPCR undergoes a similar switch from anticoagulant to antiinflammatory molecule.[103,104] APC protects against septic shock,[75] a function that requires its interaction with EPCR.[105] Deletion of the *EPCR* gene by homologous recombination leads to early embryonic lethality around day 9.5,[106] at which time EPCR is highly expressed in the giant trophoblasts of the placenta, but not in the embryo itself.[92] In contrast to TM knockout animals,[107] the placentas of EPCR knockout embryos show significant fibrin deposition at the fetal maternal interface.

VASCULAR FIBRINOLYSIS

Plasmin, the major clot-dissolving protease in humans, is formed upon the cleavage of a single peptide bond within the zymogen plasminogen (see Chap. 136). This tightly regulated reaction is strongly influenced by cells of the blood vessel wall, including endothelial cells, smooth muscles cells, and macrophages, which express plasminogen activators, plasminogen activator inhibitors, and fibrinolytic receptors. Here we consider the interplay between the cells of the vascular wall and the fibrinolytic system in the maintenance of blood vessel patency. In addition, we review how vascular cells employ the fibrinolytic system to execute the remodeling response to blood vessel injury.

ENDOTHELIAL CELL PRODUCTION OF FIBRINOLYTIC PROTEINS

Plasmin generation is a property of blood vessels. In 1958, Todd demonstrated that fibrinolytic activity in human tissues is focally distributed, relating consistently to blood vessels, especially veins and venous sinusoids, and, to a lesser extent, arteries.[108] This activity was localized primarily to the wall of the blood vessel and depended upon an intact endothelium.[109] We now know that plasminogen activator activity may also be associated with certain extravascular cells.[110]

Although endothelial cells cultured from multiple sources (umbilical vein, umbilical artery, pulmonary artery, and vena cava) synthesize tissue plasminogen activator (t-PA), and although the endothelium appears to be the principal source of t-PA in blood,[111] t-PA expression *in vivo* appears to be highly restricted to smaller vessels in specific anatomic locations. This pattern of expression likely reflects the heterogeneity of endothelial cells as they respond to a myriad of cues specific to a given tissue.[112] In the baboon, for example, neither t-PA antigen nor t-PA mRNA were detected in femoral artery or vein, carotid artery, or aorta, whereas positive signals were readily apparent in precapillary arterioles, postcapillary venules, and the vasa vasorum, ranging in diameter from 7 to 30 μm.[113] In the mouse lung, similarly, bronchial blood vessels displayed endothelial cell-associated t-PA antigen while pulmonary blood vessels were uniformly negative.[114] Expression of t-PA at branch points of pulmonary blood vessels may reflect stimulation by laminar shear stress.[115] In addition, peripheral sympathetic neurons localized at the walls of small arteries may represent a significant source of circulating t-PA.[116]

Although *in vitro* studies suggest that t-PA expression in cultured endothelial cells is regulated by a wide array of factors, only a few of these have been confirmed *in vivo*. Thrombin,[117] histamine,[118,119] oxygen radicals,[120] phorbol myristate acetate,[121] DDAVP (1-deamino-8-D-arginine vasopressin),[122] and butyric acid liberated from dibutyryl cyclic adenosine monophosphate[123] all increase t-PA mRNA in the cultured endothelial cell. Both thrombin and histamine appear to act via a receptor-mediated activation of the protein kinase C pathway.[111] Laminar shear stress stimulates both t-PA secretion[124] and steady-state mRNA levels.[125] Hyperosmotic stress and repetitive stretch also enhance t-PA expression.[126,127] In addition, differentiating agents, such as retinoids[128,129] and butyrate,[123] stimulate transcription of t-PA in endothelial cells *in vitro*.

In vivo, the circulating half-life of t-PA is approximately 5 minutes. Infusion of DDAVP, bradykinin, platelet-activating factor (PAF), endothelin, or thrombin is associated with an acute release of t-PA, and a burst of fibrinolytic activity can be detected within minutes.[111] In the mouse lung, exposure to hyperoxia leads to 4.5-fold upregulation of t-PA mRNA in small vessel endothelial cells.[114] In humans, infusion of TNF into patients with malignancy is associated with an increase in t-PA,[130] while treatment of cultured endothelial cells with TNF either has no effect or decreases t-PA production.[131] Deficient release of t-PA in response to venous occlusion in humans has been associated with deep venous thrombotic vascular disease,[132] as well as atrophie blanche and other cutaneous vasculitides.[133]

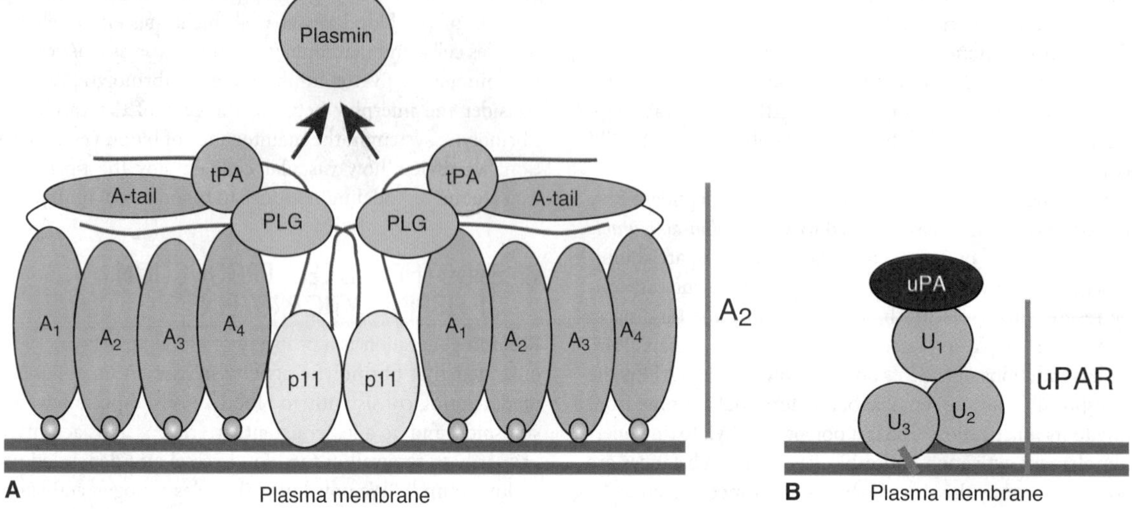

FIGURE 117–6. Two-dimensional representation of the structure of principal endothelial cell fibrinolytic receptors. **A.** Annexin A2 consists of a hydrophilic amino terminal tail domain (A-Tail, ~3 kDa), and a membrane-oriented carboxyl-terminal core domain (~33 kDa).[323,324] The tail domain contains residues required for t-PA binding. The core domain is composed of four homologous annexin repeats (A_1, A_2, A_3, and A_4), each consisting of five α-helical regions that contribute to calcium-dependent phospholipid binding sites. Repeat A_2 appears to be most important for the interaction of annexin A2 with the endothelial cell surface. Plasminogen (PLG) binding requires lysine residue 307 within helix C of repeat 4. (Adapted with permission from Gerke V, Creutz CE, Moss SE.[325]) **B.** uPAR is a 55–60-kDa glycosylphosphatidylinositol-linked protein that consists of three disulfide-linked domains (U_1, U_2, U_3).[326] Domain 1 contains sequences required for u-PA binding, while domains 2 and 3 mediate the receptor's interaction with matrix proteins such as vitronectin. Domain 3 contains its membrane anchor. t-PA, tissue-type plasminogen activator; u-PA, urokinase plasminogen activator; uPAR, u-PA receptor.

In vivo, urokinase plasminogen activator (u-PA) is not a product of resting endothelium,[134] but is produced primarily by renal tubular epithelium.[135] Expression of u-PA mRNA in endothelium, however, is strongly stimulated during wound repair and physiologic angiogenesis within ovarian follicles, corpus luteum, and maternal decidua.[136] Endothelial cells passaged in culture do synthesize u-PA,[137] and expression of its mRNA is stimulated by tumor necrosis factor by 5- to 30-fold.[138] Small increases in u-PA have also been observed *in vitro* in response to IL-1 and lipopolysaccharide.[139–141]

The association of u-PA with the blood vessel wall appears to reflect its association with the u-PA receptor, uPAR (Fig. 117–6). In the adult mouse, uPAR mRNA is not normally detected by *in situ* hybridization in the endothelium of either large or small blood vessels.[142] However, upon stimulation with endotoxin, expression is detected in endothelium lining aorta, arteries, veins, and capillaries of a variety of organs including heart, kidney, brain, and liver,[142] whereas the same stimulus leads to a dramatic decrease in expression in the renal tubules.[135] Indeed, uPAR may fulfill a variety of nonproteolytic functions ranging from directed cell migration, to cellular adhesion, differentiation, and proliferation.[143]

Plasminogen activator inhibitor (PAI-1) is likely to function as a major regulator of plasmin generation in the vicinity of the endothelial cell. *In vitro*, PAI-1 appears to be associated mainly with the substratum of cultured human umbilical vein endothelial cells, rather than the external face of the plasma membrane.[144,145] Thrombin, IL-1, transforming growth factor-β, tumor necrosis factor, and endotoxin all induce dramatic increases in steady-state PAI-1 message levels.[117,139,140,146] In addition, the low-density lipoprotein-like particle, lipoprotein(a), which contains an apoprotein homologous to plasminogen, also induces a two- to fourfold increase in PAI-1 mRNA without affecting mRNA for t-PA.[147] Heparin-binding growth factor 1 (endothelial cell growth factor) is recognized as a downregulator of PAI-1 mRNA production by cultured endothelial cells; this agent has no effect on t-PA.[148] These studies suggest that *in vitro* synthesis and secretion of PAI-1 by the endothelial cell may be regulated independently of t-PA.

Elevated levels of circulating PAI-1 have been linked epidemiologically to risk for myocardial infarction.[132] Although quiescent endothelial cells express little or no PAI-1 *in vivo*, the liver being the major source of plasma PAI-1, endothelial expression of PAI-1 is detected near neovascular sprouts that also express u-PA during decidual neovascularization in the ovary.[136] In addition, inflammatory cytokines are powerful stimuli for induction of PAI-1 in a variety of tissues including liver. In both rats and humans with active malignancy, injection of TNF results in a striking increase of plasma concentrations of PAI-1.[111,130]

In contrast, the endothelial cell coreceptor for t-PA and plasminogen, the annexin A2/p11 complex (see Fig. 117–6), appears to be expressed constitutively *in vivo* in association with blood vessels in a wide variety of tissues. In the adult chicken, endothelial cells of vessels in the dermis, lung, renal glomeruli, pancreas, liver, and meninges stain intensely positive by immunohistology.[149] Blood vessels of the developing mouse brain are also strongly cross-reactive,[150] and in rats[151] and humans,[152] vascular endothelial cells are positive for annexin A2 in most tissues studied so far.

The evidence that annexin A2 plays a role in maintaining vascular patency includes the findings (1) that individuals with acute promyelocytic leukemia who overexpress annexin A2 usually present with a hemorrhagic disorder associated with fibrinolysis,[153] (2) that systemic injection of annexin A2 can diminish thrombotic vascular occlusion following vascular injury,[154] and (3) that annexin A2-deficient mice display fibrin deposition on microvessels and impaired clearance of arterial thrombi following vascular injury.[155] Expression of annexin A2 in neuronal-like PC12 cells is transcriptionally upregulated upon stimulation with nerve growth factor, suggesting the potential for regulation by receptor tyrosine kinases.[156] In addition, the *in vitro* transition of human monocyte to macrophage is associated with a severalfold increase in annexin A2 protein and steady-state mRNA expression, and an even more dramatic (8–10-fold) increase in cell surface expression.[157] These data suggest that annexin A2 is subject to regulation in a variety of cell types found both within and outside of the vasculature.

NONFIBRINOLYTIC VASCULAR FUNCTIONS OF PLASMIN

Plasmin has been shown to inactivate bovine factor Va *in vitro* by cleaving both the heavy and light chains of this Mr 168,000 protein.[158] This lipid-dependent inactivation results in a series of plasmin-specific cleavages that are distinct from those produced by activated protein C.[159] The inactivation of human factor V by plasmin may be preceded by transient generation of procoagulant fragments that are subsequently degraded to inactive form.[160] Plasmin can also inactivate factor VIIIa, another coagulant cofactor that is structurally homologous to factor Va.[161] Factor X is subject to a well-defined pattern of cleavage events, some of the products of which may stimulate t-PA–dependent plasminogen activation.[162]

The effects of plasmin on *in vitro* platelet function are complex. Platelet $\alpha_{IIb}\beta_3$ and glycoprotein Ib, the cell surface receptors for fibrinogen and von Willebrand factor, respectively, are both plasmin substrates.[163,164] Thus, plasmin formation in the vicinity of a hemostatic plug could lead to impaired adhesion and poor aggregation in response to agonists. Plasmin generation has been shown to be associated with both platelet activation[165,166] and platelet inhibition[167] or disaggregation.[168] The ultimate effect of plasmin appears to depend upon the incubation conditions, particularly the dose and duration of plasmin treatment. These findings are of potential significance in view of reports that plasminogen can interact with platelets in a manner that is enhanced upon thrombin-mediated conversion of platelet fibrinogen to fibrin.[169] *In vivo*, prolonged bleeding times were found in patients 90 minutes after t-PA infusion for thrombolysis, suggesting early impairment of platelet function upon plasmin generation.[170] However, there is also evidence that platelets may play a role in thrombotic reocclusion following successful thrombolytic therapy.[171]

FIBRINOLYTIC FUNCTION IN VASCULAR INJURY

A number of transgenic mouse models of vascular disease have begun to elucidate the complex role of the fibrinolytic system in atherosclerotic vascular disease (Table 117–3).[172,173] In mice, the general effects of plasminogen deficiency include runting, fibrin deposition in intra- and extravascular locations, and premature death.[174,175] In addition, the mice display impaired healing of cutaneous wounds,[176] a response that appears to depend largely on the fibrinolytic action of plasmin as loss of fibrinogen eliminates these defects.[177] Based on these results, one might expect to see increased plaque formation as a result of accumulation in atherosclerosis-prone mice with plasminogen deficiency (Fig. 117–7). Indeed, mice doubly deficient in plasminogen and apolipoprotein E (ApoE) showed an increased predisposition to atherosclerosis compared to animals deficient in ApoE alone.[178] Mice with ApoE deficiency combined with deficiency of either u-PA or t-PA showed the same predilection for early fatty streaks and advanced plaques as was observed in mice with isolated ApoE deficiency, suggesting that complete elimination of plasmin generating activity is required to exacerbate the proatherogenic state.[179] Mice doubly deficient in ApoE and PAI-1 exhibited no change in early plaque size at the aortic root,[180,181] decreased early plaque size at the carotid bifurcation,[180,181] but increased advanced plaque size with accelerated deposition of matrix.[182] Thus, rather than promote cellular invasion during initial plaque formation, the role of plasmin in degrading fibrin and other matrix constituents in the early lesion may supersede its ability to promote cellular invasion later on.

Once the atherosclerotic plaque is established, plasmin may affect its evolution by mediating invasion of leukocytes.[183] In the peritoneal cavity, recruitment of inflammatory cells is profoundly influenced by the presence or absence of plasminogen.[184] In transplantation-associated arteriosclerosis, the extent of disease is significantly reduced in plasminogen-deficient mice, reflecting, at least in part, reduced influx of macrophages, with an associated reduction in medial necrosis, fragmentation of elastic laminae, and remodeling of the adventitia.[185]

TABLE 117–3. The Fibrinolytic System in Cardiovascular Disease—Transgenic Mouse Models

Genotype	Result	Reference
Atherogenesis:		
$PLG^{-/-}$ $ApoE^{-/-}$	Increased atherogenesis	178
$t\text{-}PA^{-/-}$ $ApoE^{-/-}$	Unchanged atherogenesis	179
$u\text{-}PA^{-/-}$ $ApoE^{-/-}$	Unchanged atherogenesis	179
$PAI\text{-}1^{-/-}$ $ApoE^{-/-}$	Decrease in early plaque size; increase in advanced plaque size	180–182
Transplant arteriosclerosis:		
$PLG^{-/-}$	Reduced leukocyte invasion in transplantation model; reduced extent of disease	185
Coronary ligation:		
$u\text{-}PA^{-/-}$	Protection from ventricular rupture; but poor revascularization and late death from heart failure	186
$t\text{-}PA^{-/-}$	No protection	186
$uPAR^{-/-}$	No protection	186
Aortic aneurysm:		
$u\text{-}PA^{-/-}$ $ApoE^{-/-}$	Protected	179
$t\text{-}PA^{-/-}$ $ApoE^{-/-}$	Not protected	179
Early oxidative injury:		
$PAI\text{-}1^{-/-}$	Attenuated thrombotic occlusion (Rose Bengal)	194
$PAI\text{-}1^{-/-}$	Attenuated thrombotic occlusion ($FeCl_3$)	195
$u\text{-}PA^{-/-}$	Increased thrombosis ($FeCl_3$)	196
$t\text{-}PA^{-/-}$	Increased thrombosis ($FeCl_3$)	196
$A2^{-/-}$	Increased thrombosis ($FeCl_3$)	155
Restenosis with prominent thrombosis:		
$PAI\text{-}1^{-/-}$	No neointima (Cu cuff)	199
$PAI\text{-}1^{-/-}$	Reduced neointima (ligation)	317
	Reduced neointima ($FeCl_3$)	317
$PAI\text{-}1^{-/-}$ $ApoE^{-/-}$	Reduced neointima ($FeCl_3$)	198
Restenosis without prominent thrombosis:		
$PLG^{-/-}$	Reduced neointima (electrical)	187, 188
$t\text{-}PA^{-/-}$	No change (electrical or mechanical)	187, 189
$u\text{-}PA^{-/-}$	Reduced neointima (electrical or mechanical)	187, 189
$u\text{-}PA^{-/-}$ $t\text{-}PA^{-/-}$	Reduced neointima (electrical or mechanical)	187, 189
$uPAR^{-/-}$	No change (electrical)	190
$PAI\text{-}1^{-/-}$	Increased neointima (ligation)	318
$PAI\text{-}1^{-/-}$	Increased neointima (electrical or mechanical)	191

ApoE, apolipoprotein E; PAI-1, plasminogen-activator inhibitor-1; PLG, plasminogen; t-PA, tissue-type plasminogen activator; u-PA, urokinase plasminogen activator; uPAR, u-PA receptor.

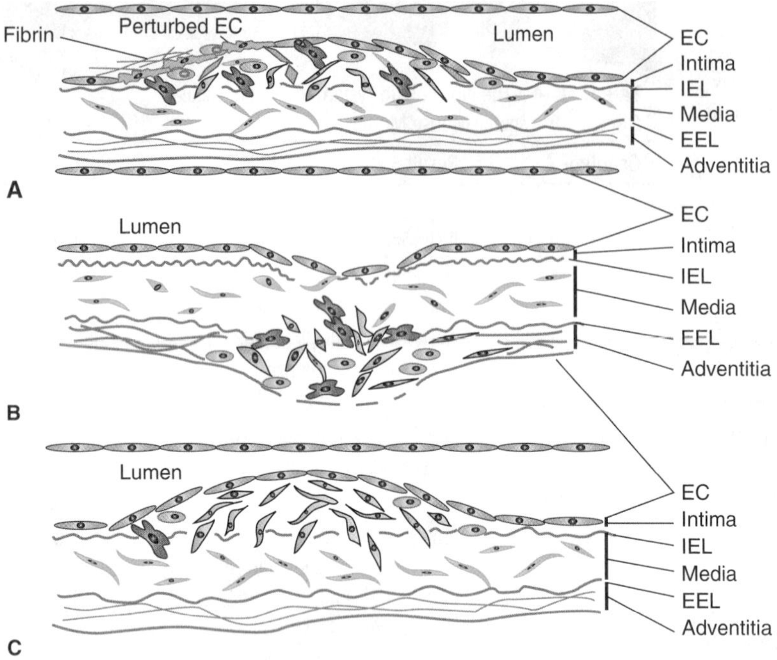

FIGURE 117–7. Schematic representation of the suggested role of the fibrinolytic system in vascular disease. **A.** Plaque formation. Atheromatous plaque is thought to form in response to endothelial cell (orange) injury or perturbation. Following the initial injury, perturbed endothelial cells may fail to clear fibrin on the blood vessel surface, and may also promote adhesion and invasion of leukocytes (blue). In addition, smooth muscle cells arising in the tunica media invade the developing plaque within the intima (green). Endothelial cells may utilize cell surface receptors for focal activation of plasmin to maintain a thromboresistant vascular surface. Leukocytes, macrophages, and smooth muscle cells may use plasmin to migrate into the evolving plaque (cells in brown, blue, and yellow). **B.** Aneurysm. Fragmentation and dissolution of the elastic laminae of the arterial wall may occur upon matrix metalloproteinase activation via plasmin-dependent pathways, possibly mediated by smooth muscle cells. Cells migrating outward toward the adventitial surface of the vessel induce further matrix degradation, and the potential for rupture. **C.** Restenosis. In response to vascular injury, smooth muscle cells proliferate and, together with leukocytes, invade the subendothelial space establishing a thickened neointima that compromises vascular patency. In all three scenarios, cell migration is thought to require plasmin activity, possibly in association with cell surfaces. EC, endothelial cell; EEL, external elastic lamina; IEL, internal elastic lamina.

During aneurysm formation, the fibrinolytic system seems to be central (see Fig. 117–7). In a model of aortic disease, u-PA, but not t-PA, deficiency was associated with reduced medial destruction and reduced activation of downstream plasmin-dependent matrix metalloproteinases.[179] Similarly, u-PA– but not t-PA–deficient mice were protected from cardiac rupture secondary to ventricular aneurysm. In this study, temporary administration of PAI-1 or the general matrix metalloproteinase inhibitor, TIMP-1, completely protected wild-type mice from aortic rupture.[186]

Vascular remodeling may occur following acute arterial injury induced by interventions for vascular compromise, leading to a secondary phase of blood vessel narrowing known as restenosis (see Fig. 117–7). This process reflects leukocyte invasion, proliferation and migration of smooth muscle cells, deposition of extracellular matrix, and reendothelialization, and may require plasmin activity at several stages. Electrical and mechanical injury studies in gene-targeted mice indicate that neointima formation, an initial step in restenosis, requires intact expression of plasminogen and u-PA, but not t-PA.[187–189] Loss of uPAR has no effect on neointima formation,[190] whereas loss of PAI-1 is associated with increased neointimal stenosis.[191] In these injury models, which do not induce severe thrombosis, it is thought that vascular occlusion, and hence migration of smooth muscle cells and leukocytes, is impaired when fibrinolytic potential is attenuated.[192] Consistent with this hypothesis is the observation that stenosis in vein segments grafted to the arterial circulation did not require the presence of background plasminogen, suggesting that plasmin proteolysis may be most important in neointima formation in settings where structural barriers impede cellular invasion.[193]

In the ferric chloride, Rose Bengal, and copper cuff models, on the other hand, thrombosis is observed within minutes following arterial injury. In these systems, deficiency of PAI-1 is associated with later and less-extensive thrombotic occlusion of the injured artery,[194,195] whereas loss of u-PA or loss of annexin A2 is associated with more rapid and more significant thrombotic occlusion.[155,196] At the same time, the absence of PAI-1 led to reduced vascular stenosis, regardless of whether ApoE was absent[197,198] or present.[199] In balloon-injured rat carotid arteries, finally, transduction of a PAI-1–expressing gene led to increased restenosis of the vessel, again suggesting that clearance of the initial thrombus may have long-term effects on vessel patency and neointima formation.[200] In these models, the predominant effect of the fibrinolytic system may be to clear the initial thrombus, which may provide a provisional scaffolding for later restenosis.

The fibrinolytic system also the modulates growth factor activity. Circulating levels of transforming growth factor-β are reduced in individuals with atherosclerosis, possibly reflecting impaired activation by plasmin.[201] *In vitro*, u-PA–mediated plasmin activity appears to generate active transforming growth factor-β, which is antiapoptotic for smooth muscle cells.[202] Furthermore, the *in vitro* mitogenic and chemotactic effects of basic fibroblast growth factor and platelet-derived growth factor depend upon u-PA and t-PA, respectively.[203]

FIBRINOLYTIC ASSEMBLY AND VASCULAR DISEASE

Both plasminogen and plasminogen activators can assemble on cell surface receptors in a manner that enhances the potential for plasmin activation (Chap. 136). The major endothelial cell fibrinolytic receptors are uPAR and the annexin A2/p11 complex (see Fig. 117–6). Both have significant roles in vascular homeostasis in gene-targeted mice.

Lipoprotein(a)

Lipoprotein(a) [Lp(a)] is a low-density lipoprotein-like particle that is an independent risk factor for atherosclerosis.[204–207] Lp(a) contains, in addition to apolipoprotein B-100, a disulfide-linked moiety called apolipoprotein(a) [apo(a)]. Apo(a) shares a remarkable degree of homology with plasminogen,[208] including multiple tandem repeats of domains similar to kringle four, a single region resembling kringle five, and a pseudoprotease segment.[209] Furthermore, plasminogen and apo(a) are genetically linked on chromosome 6 and may have arisen from a common ancestral gene.[210]

Although Lp(a) levels are only transiently responsive to diet,[211,212] plasma levels appear to be subject to mendelian inheritance.[213–215] Plasma Lp(a) concentrations seem to correlate inversely with the ratio of kringle IV to kringle V encoding domains within the apo(a) gene,[216,217] such that larger apo(a) gene products are associated with lower plasma concentrations of apo(a). In addition, Lp(a) appears to represent an acute phase reactant in the postsurgical and postmyocardial infarction setting,[214] and in patients with cancer,[215] suggesting a role for soluble inflammatory mediators in regulating its synthesis or assembly. Apo(a) possesses a high-affinity lysine binding site within kringle 4, which closely resembles kringle 1 of plasminogen with its lysine-binding amino acid tetrad consisting of anionic Asp-55 and Asp-57 plus cationic Arg-34 and Arg-71.[218] Kringle 37 of the originally cloned apo(a) resembles plasminogen kringle 4 of plasminogen which possesses three of the four lysine-binding amino acids (Asp-55, Asp-57, and Arg-71).[219] *In vivo*, Lp(a) colocalizes histologically with fibrin in atheromatous tissue.[220]

When apo(a) is overexpressed in transgenic mice,[221] cell-associated plasmin activity is reduced such that the animals are resistant to t-PA thrombolysis.[222] There are three potential mechanisms to explain the prothrombotic, proatherogenic effect of Lp(a). First, both Lp(a) and apo(a) inhibit Lys-plasminogen binding to endothelial cells (ID_{50} = 36-fold excess).[223] Lp(a) binds to annexin A2 *in vitro*,[224] and can inhibit 95 percent of plasminogen activation by t-PA at the endothelial cell surface. The estimated dissociation constants for apo(a) and plasminogen with respect to the endothelial cell surface are comparable, suggesting that receptor occupancy *in vivo* is largely determined by the ambient level of Lp(a), as plasminogen concentrations do not appear to change significantly.[225–227] Furthermore, anti-Lp(a) cross-reactive material can be detected within atherosclerotic lesions.[223] Second, endothelial cell exposure to Lp(a) *in vitro* is associated with increased levels of PAI-1 that were not found with low-density lipoprotein or plasminogen,[147] but have been reported for very-low-density lipoprotein.[228] Third, Lp(a) may act as a competitive inhibitor of t-PA in the presence of fibrinogen,[229] or as a noncompetitive inhibitor of the fibrin-dependent enhancement of t-PA induced plasmin generation.[230]

When Lp(a) was overexpressed in mice receiving a high-fat diet, atherosclerotic lesions containing both lipid and anti-apo(a) cross-reactive material were observed.[231] Deposition of both lipid and apo(a) was reduced in mice expressing apo(a) in which lysine-binding sites had been mutated.[232] These data indicate that lysine-binding sites of apo(a) play a role in its atherogenicity *in vivo*, possibly by competing with plasminogen for cell surface receptors.

Homocysteine

Homocysteine is a thiol-containing amino acid that accumulates in nutritional deficiencies of vitamin B_6, vitamin B_{12}, or folic acid, or in inherited abnormalities of cystathionine β-synthase, methylene tetrahydrofolate reductase, or methionine synthase.[233] A meta-analysis of 27 studies including approximately 4000 patients showed homocysteine to be an independent risk factor for atherosclerosis of coronary, cerebral, and peripheral arteries.[234] Of 10 subsequent prospective studies, 8 demonstrated an increased risk of coronary heart disease, venous thromboembolism, cardiovascular complications, and death.[235] *In vitro*, homocysteine-treated endothelial cells bind approximately 50 percent less t-PA than untreated cells, and activate approximately 50 percent less plasminogen.[236] Mass spectrometry studies indicate that homocysteine directly disables the t-PA–binding domain of annexin A2 by forming a covalent adduction product with cysteine 9 within the tail domain of purified annexin A2.[237] Homocysteine treatment of annexin A2, further, inhibits its ability to bind t-PA with half-maximal effect observed at approximately 11 μM, a value close to the upper limit of normal for homocysteine in plasma (14 μM). This was confirmed in vivo in mice with diet-induced hyperhomocysteinemia, where A2 was shown to be derivatized by HC, leading to loss of fibrinolytic activity and angiogenic potential.[327] Thus, inhibition of t-PA–annexin A2 assembly on the endothelial cell may contribute to the prothrombotic, proatherogenic effect of homocysteine.

Antiphospholipid Syndrome

Antiphospholipid syndrome is an autoimmune disorder characterized by thrombosis, recurrent pregnancy loss, and persistently positive antiphospholipid antibodies.[238,239] The latter can include lupus anticoagulant, anticardiolipin antibodies, or antibodies directed against β_2-glycoprotein I. Compared to patients with lupus erythematosus, nonimmune thrombosis, or healthy controls, a relatively high proportion of patients with antiphospholipid syndrome have antibodies directed against annexin A2 (22.6% vs. 6.3%, 1.4%, and 0%, respectively), suggesting a pathogenic role for this protein in the disorder. Such antibodies can induce a prothrombotic endothelial cell phenotype by inhibiting t-PA–dependent cell surface plasmin generation, and inducing expression of procoagulant molecules, such as tissue factor.[240] These adverse signaling events may require crosslinking of β_2-glycoprotein I bound to closely associated cell surface annexin A2,[241,242] and a myeloid differentiation protein 88 (MyD88) and nuclear factor-κB–dependent pathway.[243] Additional evidence shows that annexin A2 is required for the pathogenic effects of antiphospholipid antibodies *in vivo*.[244]

ROLE OF ADHESION MOLECULES

A proinflammatory environment is also prothrombotic. Endothelial cells express molecules that regulate binding of leukocytes to their surface during inflammation. These interactions have both direct and indirect roles in hemostasis and thrombosis, as many of the cytokines and bioactive molecules that promote the inflammatory response also trigger the former. Moreover, the inflammatory response itself results in expression of adhesion molecules and mediators that secondarily promote hemostasis. These processes are not limited to the surfaces of endothelium. Membrane microparticles derived from platelets, leukocytes, and perhaps endothelium provide circulating sources of tissue factor, proinflammatory lipids, and other molecules that have the potential to regulate thrombosis and inflammation at a distance from the primary site.[245–248]

MOLECULAR CHANGES IN AN INFLAMMATORY MILIEU

Immediate Changes

Histamine produced locally at the site of inflammation by degranulation of resident tissue mast cells stimulates the overlying endothelial cells to express P-selectin on their surfaces. This change occurs within minutes and is caused by the rapid fusion of Weibel-Palade bodies, with the plasma membrane bringing P-selectin to the surface. Along with P-selectin expression, fusion of the Weibel-Palade bodies also results in the release of von Willebrand Factor (VWF) into the local environment. In addition to its ability to induce release of platelet α granules and expression of P-selectin on the surface of platelets, thrombin can also trigger the release of P-selectin on the endothelial cell surface at sites of inflammation.

P-selectin serves as a receptor for P-selectin glycoprotein ligand 1 (PSGL-1), L-selectin, and probably other unidentified ligands on leukocytes. PSGL-1 is a specific sialomucin containing sialylated, fucosylated *O*-linked oligosaccharides, as well as an unusual sulfated tyrosine residue motif.[249] Dimerization of PSGL-1 may be required for optimal recognition of P-selectin.[250] Adhesive interactions between P-selectin and its ligands result in the tethering of passing leukocytes to, and rolling on, the surface of the endothelial cell—the first step in leukocyte emigration. L-selectin, another member of the selectin family of adhesion molecules, is constitutively expressed on the surfaces of most leukocytes. It binds to sialylated, fucosylated glycoprotein ligands

TABLE 117–4. Common Leukocyte–Endothelial Cell Adhesion Molecule Pairs in Inflammation

Leukocyte Molecule	CD and Integrin Nomenclature	Leukocytes Expressing*	Action	Endothelial Counter Ligand	CD Number
L-selectin	CD62L	PMN, Mo, T, B, NK	Tethering, rolling	MAdCAM-1†	Pending
				GP105–120	CD34
PSGL-1	CD162	PMN, Mo, T, B, NK	Tethering, rolling	P-selectin	CD62P
Sialyl Lewis^X ESL-1, CLA‡	CD15s	PMN, Mo, T, B, NK	Tethering, rolling	E-selectin	CD62E
LFA-1	CD11a/CD18 ($\alpha_L\beta_2$)	PMN, Mo, T, B, NK	Tight adhesion	ICAM-1	CD54
				ICAM-2	CD102
				ICAM-3	CD50
			Adhesion, diapedesis	JAM-A	Pending
Mac-1	CD11b/CD18	PMN, Mo, NK	Tight adhesion	ICAM-1	CD54
VLA-4	CD49d/CD29	Mo, B, Eo§ > NK, T	Tight adhesion¶ Rolling	VCAM-1	CD106
PECAM-1	CD31	PMN, Mo, NK Subsets of T	Diapedesis	PECAM-1	CD31
CD99	CD99	All leukocytes to varying degrees	Diapedesis	CD99	CD99
JAM-C?	Pending	T	Diapedesis	JAM-C?	Pending

GP, glycoprotein; ICAM, intercellular adhesion molecule; JAM, junctional adhesion molecule; PECAM, platelet endothelial adhesion molecule; VCAM, vascular cell adhesion molecule.

*B, B lymphocytes; Eo, eosinophils; Mo, monocytes; NK, natural killer cells; PMN, neutrophils; T, T lymphocytes.

†MAdCAM-1 (mucosal addressin cell-adhesion molecule) and CD34 have been shown to be important for homing of T cells to lymph nodes via high endothelial venules. The protein structures bearing the L-selectin ligands, including CD15s, at sites of inflammation have not been identified.

‡ESL-1 (E-selectin ligand), a protein with homology to fibroblast growth factor receptor, has been identified in mice. CLA (cutaneous lymphocyte antigen), a molecule on the surface of skin-homing T cells related to PSGL-1, directs them to skin via E-selectin expressed on dermal venules.

§Expression of very-late antigen (VLA)-4 on granulocytes is limited to eosinophils and basophils. Adult human neutrophils do not express it under normal circumstances.

¶Although VLA-4/VCAM-1 interactions are generally thought to be important for tight adhesion of leukocytes to endothelium, there are reports[319,320] that leukocytes can use VLA-4 to roll on endothelial VCAM-1, as well.

expressed by endothelial cells in response to inflammation, as well as to CD34 constitutively expressed by cells of the high endothelial venules.

The low affinity reversible adhesions of leukocytes to the endothelium at the site of inflammation result in their rolling along the luminal surface. This stage serves to slow down the movement of leukocytes and bring them into contact with a variety of chemical mediators that trigger the next stage of leukocyte emigration—tight adhesion to the endothelial surface. These mediators include surface bound chemokines,[251] new adhesion molecules expressed by the endothelium in response to inflammatory cytokines,[252] PAF,[253] soluble chemokines,[254] and ligands that crosslink leukocyte CD31.[255–257] The variety of chemical signals that can trigger tight adhesion is large (reviewed in reference 258), and may vary according to the nature of the inflammatory stimulus, the tissue involved, and the chronology of the response. However, they all seem to work by stimulating the activation of leukocyte integrin adhesion molecules by so-called inside-out signaling. This process involves a conformational change and/or clustering of the two chains of these heterodimeric surface molecules such that the affinity or avidity, respectively, for their ligands on the surfaces of endothelial cells is increased.[259] The ligands identified are members of a third family of adhesion molecules, the immunoglobulin gene superfamily.[258] While immunoglobulin gene superfamily members have not been shown to undergo conformational change, there is evidence that the active form of ICAM-1 is dimerized.[260,261]

Table 117–4 lists some of the more common leukocyte/endothelial cell adhesion molecule pairs participating in the inflammatory response. It is interesting to note that the mucosal addressin MAdCAM-1, a unique molecule expressed by endothelial cells of high endothelial venules of mesenteric lymph nodes and Peyer patches, has structural features of both a mucin and an immunoglobulin superfamily molecule. It can bind both L-selectin and the leukocyte integrin $\alpha_4\beta_7$, expressed by a subset of memory T cells. It is believed to interact with L-selectin through its mucin (carbohydrate) domain and with $\alpha_4\beta_7$ through its immunoglobulin domains. However, identified protein ligands for L-selectin (MAdCAM-1 and CD34) have been demonstrated to bind to L-selectin only in the context of lymphocyte homing. Their role in leukocyte rolling and adhesion in postcapillary venules during an inflammatory response has not been demonstrated.

PAF is made and secreted acutely by leukocytes and mast cells at the site of inflammation. In addition, PAF is rapidly made and expressed on the surfaces of stimulated endothelial cells. PAF (1-alkyl-2-acetyl-*sn*-glycero-3-phosphocholine) is produced enzymatically from phosphatidyl choline in the plasma membrane. Although its role as an activator of neutrophils in this environment has been established,[253] it appears to be a relatively weak agonist of platelet activation in this location.

Examination of the rolling phenomenon *in vivo* by intravital microscopy shows that leukocytes may roll on other leukocytes that are already tightly adherent. These interactions, which are promoted through L-selectin and PSGL-1 on the leukocytes amplify the inflammatory process.[262,263]

Adherent leukocytes migrate to nearby interendothelial junctions by repeated cycles of adhesion in the front and disadhesion in the rear.[258,264] At the junction, additional distinct molecular interactions between leukocytes and endothelial cells regulate transendothelial migration for the vast majority of neutrophils, monocytes, and natural killer (NK) cells. For a more complete review of transendothelial migration, a synopsis of the molecules involved, and an explanation of the nomenclature of the junctional adhesion molecule (JAM) family, readers are referred to recent reviews.[265–267] Platelet/endothelial cell adhesion molecule-1 (PECAM/CD31) on the leukocyte contacts the same molecule concentrated at the endothelial junctions in a homophilic manner.[268–270] The relevant signal(s) transduced by this interaction have not been worked out. However, a transient rise in the intracellular calcium ion content of the endothelial cell cytoplasm accompanies transmigration, and is required for the process to proceed.[271] Blocking the function of either leukocyte PECAM or endothelial cell PECAM arrests the leukocyte poised over the junction, tightly adherent to the apical side of the endothelial cell,[270,272,273] a phenotype very similar to that seen when the rise in endothelial cell intracellular calcium was blocked by the intracellular chelator, bis(2-amino-5-methylphenoxy)ethane-*N,N,N',N'*-tetraacetic acid tetraacetoxymethyl ester (MAPTAM).[271]

Anti-PECAM reagents never block diapedesis completely; therefore, PECAM-independent pathways of transendothelial migration must exist. The leukocyte integrins $\alpha_4\beta_1$ (very-late antigen [VLA]-4) and $\alpha_L\beta_2/\alpha_M\beta_2$ (lymphocyte function-associated antigen [LFA]-1/macrophage [Mac]-1) and their endothelial counterreceptors VCAM-1 and ICAM-1, have been implicated in transmigration.[258] In addition, interaction of leukocyte LFA-1 with JAM-A on endothelial cells has been implicated in leukocyte recruitment.[274] Similarly, antibodies against JAM-C blocked migration of lymphocytes across endothelial cell monolayers, implicating its role in lymphocyte migration.[275] In addition, under certain specialized conditions, there appear to be pathways across the endothelial cell that bypass the intercellular junction.[276,277]

CD99, a GP expressed on the surfaces of leukocytes, platelets, and erythrocytes, and concentrated at the endothelial cell borders, controls a step in diapedesis distal to the step controlled by PECAM,[278] interfering with homophilic interaction between leukocyte CD99 and endothelial cell CD99-arrested monocytes midway through the process of diapedesis. Their leading edges were below the endothelial cell monolayer, while their trailing uropods remained on the apical surface of the endothelial cell. These data have been verified *in vivo*.[279,280]

At the onset of most acute inflammatory responses, vascular permeability transiently increases as a result of histamine release. The endothelial junctions are soon reestablished, and the junctions are closed to the leukocytes that arrive at the scene over the next hour. During diapedesis—the passage of leukocytes across the endothelium—leukocytes migrate in ameboid fashion across the junction between tightly apposed endothelial cells. Studies performed both *in vivo* and *in vitro* indicate that, during diapedesis, leukocytes penetrate the vessel wall without breaching the vascular permeability barrier.[271,281] This prevents exposure of subendothelial collagen and VWF deposits to circulating platelets. Although PECAM-1 has no known role in binding platelets to endothelial cells, PECAM-1 has been hypothesized to maintain the tight apposition of endothelial cells and leukocytes during diapedesis.[270]

Acute Changes

In addition to the stimulation of immediate responses by endothelial cells, cytokines and inflammatory mediators released at the site of inflammation activate the surrounding endothelial cells to initiate new genetic programs. *De novo* synthesis of mRNA and protein leads to the establishment of an inflammatory phenotype within several hours of exposure to adequate levels of the mediator. These changes induce a procoagulant and proadhesive phenotype in the endothelial cell.

Stimulated by inflammatory cytokines like TNF-α or IL-1, vascular endothelial cells express several important cell adhesion molecules on their surface. E-selectin expression is induced within hours of cytokine stimulation. Expression peaks at 4 to 6 hours *in vitro*; however, *in vivo* in the presence of interferon (IFN)-γ, expression is maintained over several days.[282,283] E-selectin mediates rolling of leukocytes bearing sialylated, fucosylated carbohydrate receptors similar to sialylated Lewis X antigen. This molecule is important for the slow rolling seen in some vascular beds.[284] P-selectin expression on the endothelial cell surface stimulated by thrombin or histamine is transient, but expression can be prolonged by IL-3,[285] IL-4, or oncostatin M stimulation[286] of human endothelium, and by TNF-α stimulation of murine, but not human endothelium.[287,288] Expression often lasts for hours to days. This prolonged expression requires *de novo* message and protein synthesis.

In general, expression of the immunoglobulin superfamily members ICAM-1 and VCAM-1 is induced by the same stimuli that induce E-selectin. Some specializations exist, at least *in vitro*. For example, IL-4 induces VCAM-1 but not E-selectin or ICAM-1 in microvascular endothelial cells.[289,290] These molecules serve as counterreceptors for the leukocyte integrins in the tight adhesion step, as discussed above.

Chronic Changes

Prolonged stimulation of endothelial cells with interferon-γ leads to expression of MHC class II molecules (human leukocyte antigen [HLA]-DR and -DQ) on their surfaces. This takes several days *in vitro*. In human tissues such as skin and gut, class II is commonly seen even in the absence of overt inflammation, and is thought to be caused by chronic exposure of these sites to subclinical inflammation and antigenic stimulation. Cytokines can also induce the expression of CD40 ligand on endothelial cells. The significance of class II expression on endothelial cells is as follows. When costimulatory molecules such as CD40, ICAM-1, or LFA-3 are induced by inflammatory stimuli, the endothelial cell becomes capable (at least *in vitro*) of acting as an antigen presenting cell that can stimulate CD4+ memory T cells. Although this process may not be a major threat in the normal host, this mechanism may stimulate graft rejection by the host when the endothelium belongs to an organ graft with foreign MHC class II.[291–293]

In contrast to these changes, the expression of the adhesion molecule ICAM-2 does not change in response to inflammatory mediators. PECAM-1 shows a unique expression pattern in response to IFN-γ *in vitro*[294] and *in vivo*.[295] The distribution, but not absolute amount of PECAM, on the surface changes as the molecule is no longer concentrated at intercellular borders, but becomes expressed diffusely over the surface of the cell. *In vitro* chronic exposure of human umbilical vein endothelial cells to a combination of IFN-γ and TNF-α at relatively high doses leads to a decrease in total PECAM-1 expression.[296] Such a cytokine milieu could exist *in vivo*, but a similar phenotype has not been described to date.

Adhesion Molecules in a Thrombotic Milieu

In addition to the adhesive interactions germane to thrombosis and hemostasis, such an environment exposes leukocytes to ligands that promote their adhesion and recruitment to the vessel wall. For example, *in vitro* thrombin induces E-selectin expression and IL-8 secretion by human umbilical vein endothelial cells.[297] These changes are classically induced by inflammatory cytokines such as IL-1 and TNF-α.

TABLE 117–5. Dual Roles of Inflammatory Mediators in Thrombosis and Hemostasis

Mediator	Role in Inflammation	Role in Thrombosis or Hemostasis
Histamine, thrombin	P-selectin expression induced on vascular endothelium	Degranulation of Weibel-Palade bodies; extrusion of VWF
Platelet activating factor	Activation of leukocyte integrins	Activation of platelets
Expression of P-selectin glycoprotein ligand 1 (PSGL-1)	Adhesion of leukocytes to endothelial P-selectin	Adhesion of platelets to adherent leukocytes via P-selectin bidirectionally
Adherent platelets	Leukocyte rolling on platelet P-selectin; tight adhesion to platelet membrane component	Thrombosis
Fibrinogen	Adhesion of leukocytes to fibrinogen via CD11b/CD18	Bridging of platelets to VWF and matrix via α_{IIb}/β_{III}
Thrombin	Induction of E-selectin expression and IL-8 secretion by endothelial cells	Fibrinogen formation and platelet aggregation
Leukocyte Integrin CD11b/CD18	Adhesion of leukocytes to endothelium; phagocytosis CD11b/CD18	Binding and activation of factor X, adhesion of platelets via GPIbα; adhesion of platelets via JAM-C

IL, interleukin; JAM, junctional adhesion molecule; VWF, von Willebrand factor.

Table 117–5 lists some mediators that could have dual roles in inflammation and hemostasis/thrombosis.

Leukocyte–Platelet and Endothelial Cell–Platelet Interactions

Activated platelets bind to circulating lymphocytes in a P-selectin-dependent manner. This interaction can facilitate rolling on the endothelium[298] and can allow homing of lymphocytes to peripheral lymph nodes in the absence of L-selectin, because P-selectin on the adherent platelets will interact with the peripheral lymph node addressin.[299] *In vitro,* neutrophils are capable of rolling on immobilized platelets via PSGL-1 on the leukocyte interacting with degranulated P-selectin on the platelet membranes.[300] Moreover, $\alpha_M\beta_2$ (CD11b/CD18)-dependent arrest and tight adhesion of neutrophils to bound platelets following P-selectin–dependent rolling has been described.[300,301] The endothelial ligand for this is not known. ICAM-2 has been found on the surface of activated platelets, but it is not a ligand for $\alpha_M\beta_2$. In fact, antibodies against neither ICAM-2 nor its neutrophil receptor α_L (CD11) blocked this adhesion.[301,302] On the other hand, neutrophil $\alpha_M\beta_2$ reportedly binds to fibrinogen, which may be present on the surfaces of activated platelets bound to $\alpha_{IIb}\beta_3$. Two additional platelet surface molecules, GPIbα and JAM-C, have been demonstrated as ligands for leukocyte CD11b/CD18. GPIbα is part of the GP1b-IX-V complex, the platelet VWF receptor,[303,304] and JAM-C was originally described as a component of epithelial and endothelial cell tight junctions.

Platelets can interact with activated endothelial cells. Platelets express PSGL-1 and can use this expression to interact with P-selectin on the surfaces of activated endothelial cells.[305] Activated platelets can also bind to endothelial cell via fibrinogen, fibrin, or VWF, forming a molecular bridge between platelet $\alpha_{IIb}\beta_3$ and endothelial cell $\alpha_v\beta_3$ and ICAM-1.

Levels of VWF are elevated under inflammatory conditions. Ultralarge VWF molecules are stored in Weibel-Palade bodies and released upon endothelial cell activation. Ultralarge VWF is normally cleaved by endothelial cell surface proteases, notably the metalloprotease ADAMTS13 (a disintegrin and metalloprotease with thrombospondin repeats 13). Ultralarge VWF multimers have been found in blood of patients with thrombotic thrombocytopenic purpura.[306] Most patients with thrombotic thrombocytopenic purpura have a congenital or acquired deficiency or reduced activity of ADAMTS-13 (a disintegrin and metalloproteinase with thrombospondin domain 13) (see Chap. 133).[307] Data in mice indicate that ADAMTS-13 plays a homeostatic role in dampening inflammation.[308] ADAMTS-13–deficient mice showed platelet-dependent rolling on venules in the absence of overt inflammation, slower rolling, and higher levels of leukocyte extravasation in models of inflammation. The studies provided evidence that platelets bound to ultralarge VWF on the endothelium of ADAMTS-13–deficient mice supported slower leukocyte rolling on the platelet-coated endothelium.[308]

Leukocyte-Endothelial Cell Matrix Interactions That Promote Coagulation

The same proinflammatory stimuli that stimulate *de novo* expression of E-selectin and VCAM-1, and augment expression of ICAM-1 for the recruitment of leukocytes, may stimulate synthesis and expression of tissue factor (TF) by endothelial cells.[309] Furthermore, interaction of monocytes with endothelium stimulates production of TF on monocytes. Adhesion of monocytic cell lines to cytokine-activated endothelial cells in culture leads to rapidly increased procoagulant activity because of induction of TF. This effect is partially blocked by a monoclonal antibody directed against E-selectin on endothelium and is mimicked by crosslinking Lewis X on the monocyte cell lines.[310] A similar increase in TF gene expression can be induced by crosslinking α_4- or β_1-integrin chains, the components of VLA-4 on monocytic cell lines.[311]

A study of prolonged interaction of blood monocytes with human endothelial cells showed that, within a few hours of transendothelial migration, monocytes in the collagen matrix expressed functional TF on their surfaces.[312] Furthermore, over the next several days, approximately half of these monocytes had differentiated into immature dendritic cells, and, bearing even higher levels of TF, migrated back across the intact endothelial cell monolayer in the abluminal-to-luminal direction. TF on the surface of monocytes was involved in this migration, as it could be blocked by soluble fragments of TF. The same TF fragments blocked adhesion of endothelial cells to TF *in vitro.* Therefore, TF expressed by the emigrating dendritic cells was hypothesized to be directly involved in a adhesive step of this process and in any procoagulant role it may play.[312]

Leukocytes bound to P-selectin exposed on the surfaces of platelets on adherent thrombi promote the conversion of fibrinogen to fibrin.[313] The leukocyte integrin CD11b/CD18 has been shown to bind fibrinogen.[314] The same integrin has a conformational form that binds coagulation factor X.[315] Monocytic cells are capable of activating the bound factor X to Xa when activated,[316] defining a pathway for activation of factor X that is independent of TF.

REFERENCES

1. Nachman RL, Rafii S: Platelets, petechiae, and preservation of the vascular wall. *N Engl J Med* 359:1261, 2008.
2. Furie B, Furie BC: Mechanisms of thrombus formation. *N Engl J Med* 359:938, 2008.

3. Aird WC: The endothelium in health and disease, in *Endothelial Biomedicine*, edited by WC Aird, p 1111. Cambridge University Press, Cambridge, 2007.
4. Brant-Zawadzki PB, Schmid DI, Jiang H, et al: Translational control in endothelial cells. *J Vasc Surg* 45 Suppl A:A8, 2007.
5. Marcus AJ, Safier LB, Hajjar KA, et al: Inhibition of platelet function by an aspirin-insensitive endothelial cell ADPase. Thromboregulation by endothelial cells. *J Clin Invest* 88:1690, 1991.
6. Marcus AJ, Broekman MJ, Drosopoulos JH, et al: Role of CD39 (NTPDase-1) in thromboregulation, cerebroprotection, and cardioprotection. *Semin Thromb Hemost* 31:234, 2005.
7. Broekman MJ, Eiroa AM, Marcus AJ: Inhibition of human platelet reactivity by endothelium-derived relaxing factor from human umbilical vein endothelial cells in suspension. Blockade of aggregation and secretion by an aspirin-insensitive mechanism. *Blood* 78:1033, 1991.
8. Moncada S, Higgs EA: Molecular mechanisms and therapeutic strategies related to nitric oxide. *FASEB J* 9:1319, 1995.
9. Kaczmarek E, Koziak K, Sevigny J, et al: Identification and characterization of CD39 vascular ATP diphosphohydrolase. *J Biol Chem* 271:33116, 1996.
10. Marcus AJ, Broekman MJ, Drosopoulos JHF, et al: The endothelial cell ecto-ADPase responsible for inhibition of platelet function is CD39. *J Clin Invest* 99:1351, 1997.
11. Dahlback B: Advances in understanding pathogenic mechanisms of thrombophilic disorders. *Blood* 112:19, 2008.
12. Esmon CT: Inflammation and the activated protein C anticoagulant pathway. *Semin Thromb Hemost* 32 Suppl 1:49, 2006.
13. Marcus AJ, Safier LB: Thromboregulation: Multicellular modulation of platelet reactivity in hemostasis and thrombosis. *FASEB J* 7:516, 1993.
14. Pulte D, Olson KE, Broekman MJ, et al: CD39 activity correlates with stage and inhibits platelet recovery in chronic lymphocytic leukemia. *J Transl Med* 5:23, 2007.
15. Hyman MC, Ptrovic-Djergovic D, Visovatti SH, et al: Self-regulation of inflammatory cell trafficking in mice by the leukocyte surface apyrase CD39. *J Clin Invest* 119:1136, 2009.
16. Ross R: Atherosclerosis: An inflammatory disease. *N Engl J Med* 340:115, 1999.
17. Garlanda C, Dejana E: Heterogeneity of endothelial cells: Specific markers. *Arterioscler Thromb Vasc Biol* 17:1193, 1997.
18. Gawaz M, Langer H, May AE: Platelets in inflammation and atherogenesis. *J Clin Invest* 115:3378, 2005.
19. May AE, Langer H, Seizer P, et al: Platelet-leukocyte interactions in inflammation and atherothrombosis. *Semin Thromb Hemost* 33:123, 2007.
20. Brass LF, Zhu L, Stalker TJ: Novel therapeutic targets at the platelet vascular interface. *Arterioscler Thromb Vasc Biol* 28:s43, 2008.
21. Marcus AJ: Transcellular metabolism of eicosanoids. *Prog Hemost Thromb* 8:127, 1986.
22. Hamberg M, Svensson J, Samuelsson B: Thromboxanes: A new group of biologically active compounds derived from prostaglandin endoperoxides. *Proc Natl Acad Sci U S A* 72:2994, 1975.
23. Moncada S, Gryglewski R, Bunting S, et al: An enzyme isolated from arteries transforms prostaglandin endoperoxides to an unstable substance that inhibits platelet aggregation. *Nature* 263:663, 1976.
24. Woulfe D, Yang J, Brass L: ADP and platelets: The end of the beginning. *J Clin Invest* 107:1503, 2001.
25. Wu KK: Endothelial eicosanoids, in *Endothelial Biomedicine*, edited by WC Aird, p 1004. Cambridge University Press, Cambridge, 2009.
26. McAdam BF, Catella-Lawson F, Mardini IA, et al: Systemic biosynthesis of prostacyclin by cyclooxygenase (COX)-2: The human pharmacology of a selective inhibitor of COX-2. *Proc Natl Acad Sci U S A* 96:272, 1999.
27. Herschman HR: Prostaglandin synthase 2. *Biochim Biophys Acta* 1299:125, 1996.
28. Maclouf J, Folco G, Patrono C: Eicosanoids and iso-eicosanoids: Constitutive, inducible and transcellular biosynthesis in vascular disease. *Thromb Haemost* 79:691, 1998.
29. Smith WL, DeWitt DL: Prostaglandin endoperoxide H synthases-1 and -2. *Adv Immunol* 62:167, 1996.
30. Xie WL, Chipman JG, Robertson DL, et al: Expression of a mitogen-responsive gene encoding prostaglandin synthase is regulated by mRNA splicing. *Proc Natl Acad Sci U S A* 88:2692, 1991.
31. Kurumbail RG, Stevens Am, Gierse JK, et al: Structural basis for selective inhibition of cyclooxygenase-2 by anti-inflammatory agents [published erratum appears in *Nature* 385:555, 1997]. *Nature* 384:644, 1996.
32. Pouliot M, Gilbert C, Borgeat P, et al: Expression and activity of prostaglandin endoperoxide synthase-2 in agonist-activated human neutrophils. *FASEB J* 12:1109, 1998.
33. DeWitt DL, Smith WL: Cloning of sheep and mouse prostaglandin endoperoxide synthases. *Methods Enzymol* 187:469, 1990.
34. Dubois RN, Abramson SB, Crofford L, et al: Cyclooxygenase in biology and disease. *FASEB J* 12:1063, 1998.
35. Lipsky LPE, Abramson SB, Crofford L, et al: The classification of cyclooxygenase inhibitors. *J Rheumatol* 25:2298, 1998.
36. Marnett LJ: The COXIB experience: A look in the rear-view mirror. *Annu Rev Pharmacol Toxicol* 49:265, 2008.
37. Moncada S, Vane JR: Pharmacology and endogenous roles of prostaglandin endoperoxides, thromboxane A2, and prostacyclin. *Pharmacol Rev* 30:293, 1978.
38. Narumiya S, FitzGerald GA: Genetic and pharmacologic analysis prostanoid receptor function. *J Clin Invest* 108:25, 2001.
39. Cines DB, Pollak ES, Buck CA, et al: Endothelial cells in physiology and in the pathophysiology of vascular disorders. *Blood* 91:3527, 1998.
40. Marcus AJ, Weksler BB, Jaffe EA, et al: Synthesis of prostacyclin from platelet-derived endoperoxides by cultured human endothelial cells. *J Clin Invest* 66:979, 1980.
41. Marcus AJ, Broekman MJ, Drosopoulos JH, et al: Heterologous cell-cell interactions: Thromboregulation, cerebroprotection and cardioprotection by CD39 (NTPDase-1). *J Thromb Haemost* 1:2497, 2003.
42. Pepine CJ: Impact of nitric oxide on cardiovascular medicine: Untapped potential utility. *Am J Med* 122:S10-S15, 2009.
43. Marletta MA: Nitric oxide synthase structure and mechanism. *J Biol Chem* 268:12231, 1993.
44. Moncada S, Palmer RMJ, Higgs EA: Nitric oxide: Physiology, pathophysiology, and pharmacology. *Pharmacol Rev* 43:109, 1991.
45. Furchgott RF, Zawadzki JV: The obligatory role of endothelial cells in the relaxation of arterial smooth muscle by acetylcholine. *Nature* 288:373, 1980.
46. Matsumoto A, Momomura S, Sugiura S, et al: Effect of inhaled nitric oxide on gas exchange in patients with congestive heart failure. *Ann Intern Med* 130:40, 1999.
47. Lentz SR, Sobey CG, Piegers DJ, et al: Vascular dysfunction in monkeys with diet-induced hyperhomocyst(e)inemia. *J Clin Invest* 98:24, 1996.
48. Stamler JS, Osborne JA, Jaraki O, et al: Adverse vascular effects of homocysteine are modulated by endothelium-derived relaxing factor and related oxides of nitrogen. *J Clin Invest* 91:308, 1993.
49. Upchurch GR Jr, Welch GN, Fabian AJ, et al: Homocyst(e)ine decrease bioavailable nitric oxide by a mechanism involving glutathione peroxidase. *J Biol Chem* 272:17012, 1997.
50. Voetsch B, Loscalzo J: Genetic determinants of arterial thrombosis. *Arterioscler Thromb Vasc Biol* 24:216, 2004.
51. Robson SC, Sevigny J, Zimmermann H: The E-NTPDase family of ectonucleotidases: Structure function relationships and pathophysiological significance. *Purinergic Signal* 2:409, 2006.
52. Gayle RB, Maliszewski CR, Gimpel SD, et al: Inhibition of platelet function by recombinant soluble ecto-ADPase/CD39. *J Clin Invest* 101:1851, 1998.
53. Handa M, Guidotti G: Purification and cloning of a soluble ATP-diphosphohydrolase (apyrase) from potato tubers (*Solanum tuberosum*). *Biochem Biophys Res Commun* 218:916, 1996.
54. Colgan S, Eltzschig H, Eckle T, et al: Physiological roles for ecto-5'-nucleotidase (CD73). *Purinergic Signal* 2:351, 2006.
55. Atkinson BT, Jarvis GE, Watson SP: Activation of GPVI by collagen is regulated by alpha2beta1 and secondary mediators. *J Thromb Haemost* 1:1278, 2003.
56. Pinsky DJ, Broekman MJ, Peschon JJ, et al: Elucidation of the thromboregulatory role of CD39/ectoapyrase in the ischemic brain. *J Clin Invest* 109:1031, 2002.
57. Marcus AJ, Broekman MJ, Drosopoulos JHF, et al: Metabolic control of excessive extracellular nucleotide accumulation by CD39/ectonucleotidase-1: Implications for ischemic vascular diseases. *J Pharmacol Exp Ther* 305:9, 2003.
58. Koziak K, Bojakowska M, Robson SC, et al: Overexpression of CD39/nucleoside triphosphate diphosphohydrolase-1 decreases smooth muscle cell proliferation and prevents neointima formation after angioplasty. *J Thromb Haemost* 6:1191, 2008.
59. Deaglio S, Dwyer KM, Gao W, et al: Adenosine generation catalyzed by CD39 and CD73 expressed on regulatory T cells mediates immune suppression. *J Exp Med* 204:1257, 2007.
60. Uluckan O, Eagleton MC, Floyd DH, et al: APT102, a novel ADPase, cooperates with aspirin to disrupt bone metastasis in mice. *J Cell Biochem* 104:1311, 2008.
61. Dwyer KM, Robson SC, Nandurkar HH, et al: Thromboregulatory manifestations in human CD39 transgenic mice and the implications for thrombotic disease and transplantation. *J Clin Invest* 113:1440, 2004.
62. Serebrauny VL, Malinin AI, Ferguson JJ, et al: Bleeding risks of combination vs. single antiplatelet therapy: A meta-analysis of 18 randomized trials comprising 129,314 patients. *Fundam Clin Pharmacol* 22:315, 2008.
63. Fung CY, Marcus AJ, Broekman MJ, et al: P2X1 receptor inhibition and soluble CD39 administration as novel approaches to widen the cardiovascular therapeutic window. *Trends Cardiovasc Med* 19:1, 2009.
64. Moore K, Wendon J, Frazer M, et al: Plasma endothelin immunoreactivity in liver disease and the hepatorenal syndrome. *N Engl J Med* 327:1774, 1992.
65. Rubanyi GM, Polokoff MA: Endothelins: Molecular biology, biochemistry, pharmacology, physiology, and pathophysiology. *Pharmacol Rev* 46:325, 1994.
66. Fine N, Dias B, Shoemaker G, et al: Endothelin receptor antagonist therapy in congenital heart disease with shunt-associated pulmonary arterial hypertension: A qualitative systematic review. *Can J Cardiol* 25:e63, 2009.
67. Konduri GG, Kim UO: Advances in the diagnosis and management of persistent pulmonary hypertension of the newborn. *Pediatr Clin North Am* 56:579, 2009.
68. Pitts KR: Endothelin receptor antagonism in portal hypertension. *Expert Opin Investig Drugs* 18:135, 2009.
69. Steiner MK, Preston IR: Optimizing endothelin receptor antagonism use in the management of pulmonary arterial hypertension. *Vasc Health Risk Manag* 4:943, 2008.
70. Hajjar KA, Esmon NL, Marcus AJ, et al: Vascular function in hemostasis, in *Williams Hematology*, 7th ed, edited by MA Lichtman, E Beutler, TJ Kipps, U Seligsohn, K Kaushansky, JT Prchal, p 1715. McGraw-Hill, New York, 2006.

71. Esmon CT, Owen WG: Identification of an endothelial cell cofactor for thrombin-catalyzed activation of protein C. *Proc Natl Acad Sci U S A* 78:2249, 1981.
72. Esmon CT: Anticoagulant properties of vascular cells: Thrombomodulin and protein C activation pathway, in *Vascular Control of Hemostasis*, edited by VWM Van Hinsbergh, p 9. Harwood Academic, Newark, New Jersey, 1996.
73. Esmon CT: Regulation of blood coagulation. *Biochim Biophys Acta* 1477:349, 2000.
74. Stearns-Kurosawa DJ, Kurosawa S, Mollica JS, et al: The endothelial cell protein C receptor augments protein C activation by the thrombin-thrombomodulin complex. *Proc Natl Acad Sci U S A* 93:10212, 1996.
75. Esmon CT: Protein C pathway in sepsis. *Ann Med* 34:598, 2002.
76. Esmon CT: Inflammation and thrombosis. *J Thromb Haemost* 1:1343, 2003.
77. Esmon CT: The protein C pathway. *Chest* 124:26S, 2003.
78. Esmon CT: Protein C, protein S, and thrombomodulin, in *Hemostasis and Thrombosis: Basic Principles and Clinical Practice*, 5th ed, edited by RW Colman, J Hirsh, VJ Marder, AW Clowes, JN George, p 249. Lippincott Williams & Wilkins, Philadelphia, 2005.
79. Esmon CT: The roles of protein C and thrombomodulin in the regulation of blood coagulation. *J Biol Chem* 264:4743, 1989.
80. Grinnell BW, Berg DT: Surface thrombomodulin modulates thrombin receptor responses on vascular smooth muscle cells. *Am J Physiol* 270:H603, 1996.
81. Lafay M, Laguna R, Le Bonniec BF, et al: Thrombomodulin modulates the mitogenic response to thrombin of human umbilical vein endothelial cells. *Thromb Haemost* 79:848, 1998.
82. Bajzar L, Manuel R, Nesheim M: Purification and characterization of TAFI, a thrombin activatable fibrinolysis inhibitor. *J Biol Chem* 270:14477, 1995.
83. Campbell W, Okada N, Okada H: Carboxypeptidase R is an inactivator of complement-derived inflammatory peptides and an inhibitor of fibrinolysis. *Immunol Rev* 180:162, 2001.
84. Campbell WD, Lazoura E, Okada N, et al: Inactivation of C3a and C5a octapeptides by carboxypeptidase R and carboxypeptidase N. *Microbiol Immunol* 46:131, 2002.
85. Ikeguchi H, Fujita Y, Kato T, et al: Effects of human soluble thrombomodulin on experimental glomerulonephritis. *Kidney Int* 61:490, 2002.
86. de Munk GAW, Groeneveld E, Rijken DC: Acceleration of the thrombin inactivation of single chain urokinase-type plasminogen activator (pro-urokinase) by thrombomodulin. *J Clin Invest* 88:1680, 1991.
87. Molinari A, Giogetti C, Lansen J, et al: Thrombomodulin is a cofactor for thrombin degradation of recombinant single-chain urokinase plasminogen activator in vitro and in a perfused rabbit heart model. *Thromb Haemost* 67:226, 1992.
88. Preissner KT, May AE, Wohn KD, et al: Molecular crosstalk between adhesion receptors and proteolytic cascades in vascular remodeling. *Thromb Haemost* 78:88, 1997.
89. Esmon CT: Anticoagulant protein C/thrombomodulin pathway, in *The Metabolic and Molecular Bases of Inherited Disease*, edited by CR Scriver, AL Beaudet, WS Sly, D Valle, p 4327. McGraw-Hill, New York, 1999.
90. Healy AM, Rayburn HB, Rosenberg RD, et al: Absence of the blood-clotting regulator thrombomodulin causes embryonic lethality in mice before development of a functional cardiovascular system. *Proc Natl Acad Sci U S A* 92:850, 1995.
91. Weiler-Guettler H, Aird WC, Rayburn H, et al: Developmentally regulated gene expression of thrombomodulin in postimplantation mouse embryos. *Development* 122:2271, 1996.
92. Crawley JTB, Gu AM, Ferrell G, et al: Distribution of endothelial cell protein C/activated protein C receptor (EPCR) during mouse embryo development. *Thromb Haemost* 88:259, 2002.
93. Isermann B, Hendrickson SB, Hutley K, et al: Tissue-restricted expression of thrombomodulin in the placenta rescues thrombomodulin-deficient mice from early lethality and reveals a secondary developmental block. *Development* 128:827, 2001.
94. Isermann B, Hendrickson SB, Zogg M, et al: Endothelium-specific loss of murine thrombomodulin disrupts the protein C anticoagulant pathway and causes juvenile-onset thrombosis. *J Clin Invest* 108:537, 2001.
95. Fukodome K, Esmon CT: Identification, cloning, and regulation of a novel endothelial cell protein C/activated protein C receptor. *J Biol Chem* 269:26486, 1994.
96. Esmon CT, Gu J, Xu J, et al: Regulation and functions of the protein C anticoagulant pathway. *Haematologica* 84:363, 1999.
97. Esmon CT, Xu J, Gu J, et al: Endothelial protein C receptor. *Thromb Haemost* 82:251, 1999.
98. Esmon CT: The endothelial cell protein C receptor. *Curr Opin Hematol* 13:382, 2006.
99. Xu J, Liaw PCY, Esmon CT: A novel transmembrane domain of the endothelial cell protein C receptor (EPCR) dictates receptor localization of sphingolipid-cholesterol rich regions on plasma membrane while EPCR palmitoylation modulates intracellular trafficking patterns. *Suppl Thromb Haemost* 1999:695a, 1999.
100. Kurosawa S, Stearns-Kurosawa DJ, Hidari N, et al: Identification of functional endothelial protein C receptor in human plasma. *J Clin Invest* 100:411, 1997.
101. Fukudome K, Ye X, Tsuneyoshi N, et al: Activation mechanism of anticoagulant protein C in large blood vessels involving the endothelial cell protein C receptor. *J Exp Med* 187:1029, 1998.
102. Taylor FB Jr, Peer GT, Lockhart MS, et al: Endothelial cell protein C receptor plays an important role in protein C activation *in vivo*. *Blood* 97:1685, 2001.
103. Esmon CT, Taylor FB, Snow TR: Inflammation and coagulation: Linked processes potentially regulated through a common pathway mediated by protein C. *Thromb Haemost* 66:160, 1991.
104. Esmon CT, Schwarz HP: An update on clinical and basic aspects of the protein C anticoagulant pathway. *Trends Cardiovasc Med* 5:141, 1995.
105. Taylor FB, Stearns-Kurosawa DJ, Kurasawa S, et al: The endothelial cell protein C receptor aids in host defense against *Escherichia coli* sepsis. *Blood* 95:1680, 2000.
106. Gu JM, Crawley JTB, Ferrell G, et al: Disruption of the endothelial cell protein C receptor gene in mice causes placental thrombosis and early embryonic lethality. *J Biol Chem* 277:43335, 2002.
107. Weiler H, Isermann B: Thrombomodulin. *J Thromb Haemost* 1:1515, 2003.
108. Todd AS: Fibrinolysis autographs. *Nature* 181:495, 1958.
109. Todd AS: Localization of fibrinolytic activity in tissues. *Br Med Bull* 20:210, 1964.
110. Pandolfi M: Histochemistry of tissue plasminogen activator. *Thromb Diath Haemorrh* 34:661, 1975.
111. Van Hinsbergh VWM, Kooistra T, Emeis JJ, et al: Regulation of plasminogen activator production by endothelial cells: Role in fibrinolysis and local proteolysis. *Int J Radiat Biol* 60:261, 1991.
112. Augustin HG, Kozian DH, Johnson RC: Differentiation of endothelial cells: Analysis of the constitutive and activated endothelial cell phenotypes. *Bioessays* 16:901, 1994.
113. Levin EG, del Zoppo GJ: Localization of tissue plasminogen activator in the endothelium of a limited number of vessels. *Am J Pathol* 144:855, 1994.
114. Levin EG, Santell L, Osborn KG: The expression of endothelial tissue plasminogen activator *in vivo*: A function defined by vessel size and anatomic location. *J Cell Sci* 110:139, 1997.
115. Levin EG, Osborn KG, Schleuning WD: Vessel-specific gene expression in the lung: Tissue plasminogen activator is limited to bronchial arteries and pulmonary vessels of discrete size. *Chest* 114:68S, 1998.
116. O'Rourke J, Jiang X, Hao Z, et al: Distribution of sympathetic tissue plasminogen activator (tPA) to a distant microvasculature. *J Neurosci* 79:727, 2005.
117. Dichek D, Quertermous T: Thrombin regulation of mRNA levels of tissue plasminogen activator inhibitor-1 in cultured human umbilical vein endothelial cells. *Blood* 74:222, 1989.
118. Hanss M, Collen D: Secretion of tissue-type plasminogen activator and plasminogen activator inhibitor by cultured human endothelial cells: Modulation by thrombin, endotoxin, and histamine. *J Lab Clin Med* 109:97, 1987.
119. Levin EG, Santell L: Stimulation and desensitization of tissue plasminogen activator release from human endothelial cells. *J Biol Chem* 263:9360, 1988.
120. Shatos MA, Doherty JM, Orfeo T, et al: Modulation of the fibrinolytic response of cultured human vascular endothelium by extracellularly generated oxygen radicals. *J Biol Chem* 267:597, 1992.
121. Levin EG, Marotti KR, Santell L: Protein kinase C and the stimulation of tissue plasminogen activator release from human endothelial cells. *J Biol Chem* 264:16030, 1989.
122. Cugno M, Uziel L, Fabrizi I, et al: Fibrinolytic response in normal subjects to venous occlusion and DDAVP infusion. *Thromb Res* 56:625, 1989.
123. Kooistra T, Van den Berg J, Tons A, et al: Butyrate stimulates tissue type plasminogen activator synthesis in cultured human endothelial cells. *Biochem J* 247:605, 1987.
124. Diamond SL, Eskin SG, McIntire LV: Fluid flow stimulates tissue plasminogen activator secretion by cultured human endothelial cells. *Science* 243:1483, 1989.
125. Diamond SL, Sharefkin JB, Dieffenbach C, et al: Tissue plasminogen activator messenger RNA levels increase in cultured human endothelial cells exposed to laminar shear stress. *J Cell Physiol* 143:364, 1990.
126. Levin EG, Santell L, Saljooque F: Hyperosmotic stress stimulates tissue plasminogen activator expression by a PKC-dependent pathway. *Am J Physiol* 265:C387-C396, 1993.
127. Iba T, Shin T, Sonoda T, et al: Stimulation of endothelial secretion of tissue-type plasminogen activator by repetitive stretch. *J Surg Res* 50:457, 1991.
128. Thompson EA, Nelles L, Collen D: Effect of retinoic acid on the synthesis of tissue-type plasminogen activator and plasminogen activator inhibitor 1 in human endothelial cells. *Eur J Biochem* 201:627, 1991.
129. Bulens F, Ibanez-Tallon I, Van Acker P, et al: Retinoic acid induction of human tissue-type plasminogen activator gene expression via a direct repeat element (DR5) located at – 7 kilobases. *J Biol Chem* 270:7167, 1995.
130. Van Hinsbergh VWM, Bauer KA, Kooistra T, et al: Progress of fibrinolysis during tumor necrosis factor infusions in humans. Concomitant increase in tissue-type plasminogen activator, plasminogen activator inhibitor type-1, and fibrin(ogen) degradation products. *Blood* 76:2284, 1990.
131. Schleef RR, Bevilacqua MP, Sawdey M, et al: Cytokine activation of vascular endothelium: Effects on tissue-type plasminogen activator and type 1 plasminogen activator inhibitor. *J Biol Chem* 263:5797, 1988.
132. Hamsten A, Wiman B, De Faire U, et al: Increased plasma levels of a rapid inhibitor of tissue plasminogen activator in young survivors of myocardial infarction. *N Engl J Med* 313:1557, 1985.
133. Pizzo SV, Murray JC, Gonias SL: Atrophie blanche: A disorder associated with defective release of tissue plasminogen activator. *Arch Pathol Lab Med* 110:517, 1986.
134. Kristensen P, Larson LI, Nielsen LS, et al: Human endothelial cells contain one type of plasminogen activator. *FEBS Lett* 168:33, 1984.
135. Yamamoto K, Loskutoff DJ: Fibrin deposition in tissues from endotoxin-treated mice correlates with decreases in the expression of urokinase-type but not tissue-type plasminogen activator. *J Clin Invest* 97:2440, 1996.
136. Bacharach E, Itin A, Keshet E: In vivo patterns of expression of urokinase and its inhibitor PAI-1 suggest a concerted role in regulating physiological angiogenesis. *Proc Natl Acad Sci U S A* 89:10686, 1992.

137. Booyse FM, Scheinbuks J, Radek J, et al: Immunological identification and comparison of plasminogen activator forms in cultured normal human endothelial cells and smooth muscle cells. *Thromb Res* 24:495, 1981.
138. Van Hinsbergh VWM, Van den Berg EA, Fiers W, et al: Tumor necrosis factor induces the production of urokinase-type plasminogen activator by human endothelial cells. *Blood* 75:1991, 1990.
139. Sawdey M, Podor TJ, Loskutoff DJ: Regulation of type-1 plasminogen activator inhibitor gene expression in cultured bovine aortic endothelial cells. *J Biol Chem* 264:10396, 1989.
140. Van den Berg EA, Sprengers ED, Jaye M, et al: Regulation of plasminogen activator inhibitor-1 mRNA in human endothelial cells. *Thromb Haemost* 60:63, 1988.
141. Ellis V, Scully MF, Kakkar VV: Plasminogen activation by single-chain urokinase in functional isolation. *J Biol Chem* 262:14998, 1987.
142. Almus-Jacobs F, Varki N, Sawdey MS, et al: Endotoxin stimulates expression of the murine urokinase receptor gene *in vivo*. *Am J Pathol* 147:688, 1995.
143. Blasi F, Carmeliet P: UPAR: A versatile signalling orchestrator. *Nat Rev Mol Cell Biol* 3:932, 2002.
144. Schleef RR, Podor TJ, Dunne E, et al: The majority of type 1 plasminogen activator inhibitor associated with cultured human endothelial cells is located under the cells and is accessible to solution-phase tissue-type plasminogen activator. *J Cell Biol* 110:155, 1990.
145. Levin EG, Santell L: Association of a plasminogen activator inhibitor (PAI-1) with the growth substratum and membrane of human endothelial cells. *J Cell Biol* 105:2543, 1987.
146. Medina R, Socher SH, Han JH, et al: Interleukin-1, endotoxin, or tumor necrosis factor/cachectin enhance the level of plasminogen activator inhibitor messenger RNA in bovine aortic endothelial cells. *Thromb Res* 54:41, 1989.
147. Etingin OR, Hajjar DP, Hajjar KA, et al: Lipoprotein(a) regulates plasminogen activator inhibitor-1 expression in endothelial cells. *J Biol Chem* 266:2459, 1990.
148. Konkle B, Ginsburg D: The addition of endothelial cell growth factor and heparin to human endothelial cell cultures decrease plasminogen activator. *J Clin Invest* 82:579, 1988.
149. Greenberg ME, Brackenbury R, Edelman GM: Changes in the distribution of the 34-kdalton tyrosine kinase substrate during differentiation and maturation of chicken tissues. *J Cell Biol* 98:473, 1984.
150. Hamre KM, Chepenik KP, Goldowitz D: The annexins: Specific markers of midline structures and sensory neurons in the developing murine central nervous system. *J Comp Neurol* 352:421, 1995.
151. Gould KL, Cooper JA, Hunter T: The 46,000-dalton tyrosine kinase substrate is widespread, whereas the 36,000-dalton substrate is only expressed at high levels in certain rodent tissues. *J Cell Biol* 98:487, 1984.
152. Dreier R, Schmid KW, Gerke V, et al: Differential expression of annexins I, II, and IV in human tissues: An immunohistochemical study. *Histochem Cell Biol* 110:137, 1998.
153. Menell JS, Cesarman GM, Jacovina AT, et al: Annexin II and bleeding in acute promyelocytic leukemia. *N Engl J Med* 340:994, 1999.
154. Ishii H, Yoshida M, Hiraoka M, et al: Recombinant annexin II modulates impaired fibrinolytic activity in vitro and in rat carotid artery. *Circ Res* 89:1240, 2001.
155. Ling Q, Jacovina AT, Deora AB, et al: Annexin II is a key regulator of fibrin homeostasis and neoangiogenesis . *J Clin Invest* 113:38, 2004.
156. Jacovina AT, Zhong F, Khazanova E, et al: Neuritogenesis and the nerve growth factor-induced differentiation of PC-12 cells requires annexin II-mediated plasmin generation. *J Biol Chem* 276:49350, 2001.
157. Brownstein C, Deora AB, Jacovina AT, et al: Annexin II mediates plasminogen-dependent matrix invasion by human monocytes: Enhanced expression by macrophages. *Blood* 103:317, 2004.
158. Omar MN, Mann KG: Inactivation of Factor Va by plasmin. *J Biol Chem* 262:9750, 1987.
159. Esmon CT: The regulation of natural anticoagulant pathways. *Science* 235:1348, 1987.
160. Lee CD, Mann KG: Activation/inactivation of human factor V by plasmin. *Blood* 73:185, 1989.
161. McKee PA, Anderson JC, Switzer ME: Molecular structural studies of human factor VIII. *Ann N Y Acad Sci* 240:8, 1975.
162. Moser TL, Stack MS, Asplin I, et al: Angiostatin binds ATP synthase on the surface of human endothelial cells. *Proc Natl Acad Sci U S A* 96:2811, 1999.
163. Stricker RB, Wong D, Shiu DT, et al: Activation of plasminogen by tissue plasminogen activator on normal and thrombasthenic platelets: Effects on surface proteins and platelet aggregation. *Blood* 68:275, 1986.
164. Adelman B, Michelson AD, Greenberg J, et al: Proteolysis of platelet glycoprotein by plasmin is facilitated by plasmin lysine-binding regions. *Blood* 68:1280, 1986.
165. Schafer AI, Adelman B: Plasmin inhibition of platelet function and of arachidonate metabolism. *J Clin Invest* 75:456, 1985.
166. Puri RN, Zhou FX, Colman RF, et al: Plasmin-induced platelet aggregation is accompanied by cleavage of aggregin and indirectly mediated by calpain. *Am J Physiol* 259:C862-C868, 1990.
167. Schafer AI, Maas AK, Ware JA, et al: Platelet protein phosphorylation, elevation of cytosolic calcium, and inositol phospholipid breakdown in platelet activation induced by plasmin. *J Clin Invest* 78:73, 1986.
168. Loscalzo J, Vaughan DE: Tissue plasminogen activator promotes platelet disaggregation. *J Clin Invest* 79:1749, 1986.
169. Miles LA, Ginsberg MA, White JG, et al: Plasminogen interacts with platelets through two distinct mechanisms. *J Clin Invest* 77:2001, 1986.
170. Gimple LW, Gold HK, Leinbach RC, et al: Correlation between template bleeding times and spontaneous bleeding during treatment of acute myocardial infarction with recombinant issue type plasminogen activator. *Circulation* 80:581, 1989.
171. Coller BS: Platelets and thrombolytic therapy. *N Engl J Med* 322:33, 1990.
172. Fay WP, Garg N, Sunkar M: Vascular function of the plasminogen activation system. *Arterioscler Thromb Vasc Biol* 27:1231, 2007.
173. Libby P, Aikawa M, Jain MK: Vascular endothelium and atherosclerosis. *Handb Exp Pharmacol* 176 Part 2:285, 2006.
174. Ploplis VA, Carmeliet P, Vazirzadeh S, et al: Effects of disruption of the plasminogen gene on thrombosis, growth, and health in mice. *Circulation* 92:2585, 1995.
175. Bugge TH, Flick MJ, Daugherty CC, et al: Plasminogen deficiency causes severe thrombosis but is compatible with development and reproduction. *Genes Dev* 9:794, 1995.
176. Romer J, Bugge TH, Pyke C, et al: Impaired wound healing in mice with a disrupted plasminogen gene. *Nat Med* 2:287, 1996.
177. Bugge TH, Kombrinck KW, Flick MJ, et al: Loss of fibrinogen rescues mice from the pleiotropic effects of plasminogen deficiency. *Cell* 87:709, 1996.
178. Xiao Q, Danton MJS, Witte DP, et al: Plasminogen deficiency accelerates vessel wall disease in mice predisposed to atherosclerosis. *Proc Natl Acad Sci U S A* 94:10335, 1997.
179. Carmeliet P, Moons L, Lijnen R, et al: Urokinase-generated plasmin activates matrix metalloproteinases during aneurysm formation. *Nat Genet* 17:439, 1997.
180. Eitzman DT, Westrick RJ, Xu Z, et al: Plasminogen activator inhibitor-1 deficiency protects against atherosclerosis progression in the mouse carotid artery. *Blood* 96:4212, 2000.
181. Sjoland H, Eitzman DT, Gordon D, et al: Atherosclerosis progression in LDL receptor-deficient and apolipoprotein E-deficient mice is independent of genetic alterations in plasminogen activator inhibitor-1. *Arterioscler Thromb Vasc Biol* 20:846, 1999.
182. Luttun A, Lupu F, Storkebaum E, et al: Lack of plasminogen activator inhibitor-1 promotes growth and abnormal remodeling of advanced atherosclerotic plaque in apolipoprotein E-deficient mice. *Arterioscler Thromb Vasc Biol* 22:499, 2002.
183. Plow EF, Ploplis VA, Busuttil S, et al: A role of plasminogen in atherosclerosis and restenosis models in mice. *Thromb Haemost* 82 Suppl:4, 1999.
184. Ploplis VA, French EL, Carmeliet P, et al: Plasminogen deficiency differentially affects recruitment of inflammatory cell populations in mice. *Blood* 91:2005, 1998.
185. Moons L, Wi C, Ploplis V, et al: Reduced transplant arteriosclerosis in plasminogen-deficient mice. *J Clin Invest* 102:1788, 1998.
186. Heymans S, Luttun A, Nuyens D, et al: Inhibition of plasminogen activators or matrix metalloproteinases prevents cardiac rupture but impairs therapeutic angiogenesis and causes cardiac failure. *Nat Med* 5:1135, 2003.
187. Lijnen HR, Van Hoef B, Lupu F, et al: Function of the plasminogen/plasmin and matrix metalloproteinase systems after vascular injury in mice with targeted inactivation of fibrinolytic system genes. *Arterioscler Thromb Vasc Biol* 18:1035, 1998.
188. Carmeliet P, Moons L, Ploplis VA, et al: Impaired arterial neointima formation in mice with disruption of the plasminogen gene. *J Clin Invest* 99:200, 1997.
189. Carmeliet P, Moons L, Herbert JM, et al: Urokinase but not tissue plasminogen activator mediates arterial neointima formation in mice. *Circ Res* 81:829, 1997.
190. Carmeliet P, Moons L, Dewerchin M, et al: Receptor-independent role of urokinase-type plasminogen activator in pericellular plasmin and matrix metalloproteinase proteolysis during vascular wound healing in mice. *J Cell Biol* 140:233, 1998.
191. Carmeliet P, Moons L, Lijnen R, et al: Inhibitory role of plasminogen activator inhibitor-1 in arterial wound healing and neointima formation. *Circulation* 96:3180, 1997.
192. Konstantinides S, Schafer K, Loskutoff DJ: Do PAI-1 and vitronectin promote or inhibit neointima formation? *Arterioscler Thromb Vasc Biol* 22:1943, 2002.
193. Shi C, Patel A, Zhang D, et al: Plasminogen is not required for neointima formation in a mouse model of vein graft stenosis. *Circ Res* 84:883, 1999.
194. Eitzman DT, Westrick RJ, Nabel EG, et al: Plasminogen activator inhibitor-1 and vitronectin promote vascular thrombosis in mice. *Blood* 95:577, 2000.
195. Konstantinides S, Schafer K, Thinnes T, et al: Plasminogen activator inhibitor-1 and its cofactor vitronectin stabilize arterial thrombi following vascular injury in mice. *Circulation* 103:576, 2001.
196. Schafer K, Konstantinides S, Riedel C, et al: Different mechanisms of increased luminal stenosis after arterial injury in mice deficient for urokinase- or tissue-type plasminogen activator. *Circulation* 106:1847, 2002.
197. Schafer K, Muller K, Hecker A, et al: Enhanced thrombosis in atherosclerosis-prone mice is associated with increased arterial expression of plasminogen activator. *Arterioscler Thromb Vasc Biol* 23:2097, 2003.
198. Zhu Y, Farrehi PM, Fay WP: Plasminogen activator inhibitor type 1 enhances neointima formation after oxidative vascular injury in atherosclerosis-prone mice. *Circulation* 103:3105, 2001.
199. Ploplis VA, Cornelissen I, Sandoval-Cooper MJ, et al: Remodeling of the vessel wall after copper-induced injury is highly attenuated in mice with a total deficiency of plasminogen activator inhibitor-1. *Am J Pathol* 158:107, 2001.
200. DeYoung MB, Tom C, Dichek DA: Plasminogen activator inhibitor type 1 increases neointima formation in balloon-injured rat carotid arteries. *Circulation* 104:1972, 2001.
201. Grainger DJ, Kemp PR, Metcalfe JC, et al: The serum concentration of active transforming growth factor-β is severely depressed in advanced atherosclerosis. *Nat Med* 1:74, 1995.

202. Herbert JM, Carmeliet P: Involvement of u-PA in the anti-apoptotic activity of TGF-beta for vascular smooth muscle cells. *FEBS Lett* 413:401, 1997.
203. Herbert JM, Lamarche I, Carmeliet P: Urokinase and tissue-type plasminogen activator are required for the mitogenic and chemotactic effects of bovine fibroblast growth factor and platelet-derived growth factor-BB for vascular smooth muscle cells. *J Biol Chem* 272:23585, 1997.
204. Scanu AM, Fless GM: Lipoprotein(a) heterogeneity and biologic relevance. *J Clin Invest* 85:1709, 1990.
205. Utermann G: The mysteries of lipoprotein(a). *Science* 246:904, 1989.
206. Loscalzo J: Lipoprotein(a), a unique risk factor for atherothrombotic disease. *Arteriosclerosis* 10:672, 1990.
207. Hajjar KA, Nachman RL: The role of lipoprotein(a) in atherogenesis and thrombosis. *Annu Rev Med* 47:423, 1996.
208. Bauer PI, Machovich R, Buki KG, et al: Interaction of plasmin with endothelial cells. *Biochem J* 218:119, 1984.
209. McLean JW, Tomlinson JE, Kuang WJ, et al: CDNA sequence of human apolipoprotein(a) is homologous to plasminogen. *Nature* 330:132, 1987.
210. Weitkamp LR, Guttormsen SA, Schultz JS: Linkage between the loci for the Lp(a) lipoprotein (Lp) and plasminogen (PLG). *Hum Genet* 79:80, 1988.
211. Neven L, Khalil A, Pfaffinger D, et al: Rhesus monkey model of familial hypercholesterolemia: Relation between plasma Lp(a) levels, apo(a) isoforms and LDL-receptor function. *J Lipid Res* 31:633, 1990.
212. Pfaffinger D, Schuelke J, Kim C, et al: Relationship between apo(a) isoforms and Lp(a) density in subjects with different apo(a) phenotype: A study before and after a fatty meal. *J Lipid Res* 32:679, 1991.
213. Utermann G, Menzel HJ, Kraft HG, et al: Lp(a) glycoprotein phenotypes. *J Clin Invest* 80:458, 1987.
214. Maeda S, Abe A, Seishima M, et al: Transient changes of serum lipoprotein(a) as an acute phase protein. *Atherosclerosis* 78:145, 1989.
215. Wright LC, Sullivan DR, Muller M, et al: Elevated apolipoprotein(a) levels in cancer patients. *Int J Cancer* 43:241, 1989.
216. Gavish D, Azrolan N, Breslow JL: Fish oil reduces plasma Lp(a) levels and affects post-prandial association of apo(a) with triglyceride rich lipoproteins. *J Clin Invest* 84:2021, 1989.
217. Koschinsky ML, Beisiegel U, Henne-Bruns D, et al: Apolipoprotein(a) size heterogeneity is related to variable number of repeat sequences in its mRNA. *Biochemistry* 29:640, 1990.
218. Lerch PG, Rickli EE, Lergier W, et al: Localization of individual lysine-binding regions in human plasminogen and investigations on their complex-forming properties. *Eur J Biochem* 107:7, 1980.
219. Armstrong VW, Harrach B, Robenek H, et al: Heterogeneity of human lipoprotein Lp(a): Cytochemical and biochemical studies on the interaction of two Lp(a) species with the LDL receptor. *J Lipid Res* 31:429, 1990.
220. Wolf K, Rith M, Niendorf A, et al: Thrombosis: Cellular elements of the vasculature. *Circulation* 80:522, 1989.
221. Grainger DJ, Kemp PR, Liu AC, et al: Activation of transforming growth factor-beta is inhibited in transgenic apolipoprotein(a) mice. *Nature* 370:460, 1994.
222. Palabrica TM, Liu AC, Aronovitz MJ, et al: Antifibrinolytic activity of apolipoprotein(a) *in vivo*: Human apolipoprotein(a) transgenic mice are resistant to tissue plasminogen activator-mediated thrombolysis. *Nat Med* 1:256, 1995.
223. Petros AM, Ramesh V, Llinas M: NMR studies of aliphatic ligand binding to human plasminogen kringle 4. *Biochemistry* 28:1368, 1989.
224. Hajjar KA: The endothelial cell tissue plasminogen activator receptor: Specific interaction with plasminogen. *J Biol Chem* 266:21962, 1991.
225. Hajjar KA, Gavish D, Breslow J, et al: Lipoprotein(a) modulation of endothelial cell surface fibrinolysis and its potential role in atherosclerosis. *Nature* 339:303, 1989.
226. Gonzales-Gronow M, Edelberg JM, Pizzo SV: Further characterization of the cellular plasminogen binding site: Evidence that plasminogen 2 and lipoprotein a compete for the same site. *Biochemistry* 28:2374, 1989.
227. Miles LA, Fless GM, Levin EG, et al: A potential basis for the thrombotic risks associated with lipoprotein(a). *Nature* 339:301, 1989.
228. Stiko-Rahm A, Wiman B, Hamsten A, et al: Secretion of plasminogen activator inhibitor-1 from cultured human umbilical vein endothelial cells is induced by very low density lipoprotein. *Arteriosclerosis* 10:1067, 1990.
229. Edelberg JM, Gonzalez-Gronow M, Pizzo SV: Lipoprotein(a) inhibition of plasminogen activation by tissue-type plasminogen activator. *Thromb Res* 57:155, 1990.
230. Loscalzo J, Weinfeld M, Fless G, et al: Lipoprotein(a), fibrin binding, and plasminogen activation. *Arteriosclerosis* 10:240, 1990.
231. Lawn RM, Wade DP, Hammer RE, et al: Atherogenesis in transgenic mice expressing human apolipoprotein(a). *Nature* 360:670, 1992.
232. Boonmark NW, Lou XJ, Schwartz K, et al: Modification of apolipoprotein(a) lysine binding site reduces atherosclerosis in transgenic mice. *J Clin Invest* 100:558, 1997.
233. Kraus JP: Molecular basis of phenotype expression in homocystinuria. *J Inherit Metab Dis* 17:383, 1994.
234. Boushey CJ, Beresford SAA, Omenn GS, et al: A quantitative assessment of plasma homocysteine as a risk factor for vascular disease. *JAMA* 274:1049, 1995.
235. Refsum H, Ueland PM, Nygard O, et al: Homocysteine and cardiovascular disease. *Annu Rev Med* 49:31, 1998.
236. Hajjar KA: Homocysteine-induced modulation of tissue plasminogen activator binding to its endothelial cell membrane receptor. *J Clin Invest* 91:2873, 1993.
237. Hajjar KA, Mauri L, Jacovina AT, et al: Tissue plasminogen activator binding to the annexin II tail domain: Direct modulation by homocysteine. *J Biol Chem* 273:9987, 1998.
238. Miyakis S, Lockshin MD, Atsumi T, et al: International consensus statement on an update of the classification criteria for definite antiphospholipid syndrome (APS). *J Thromb Haemost* 4:295, 2006.
239. Cockrell.E., Espinola RG, McCrae KR: Annexin A2: Biology and relevance to the antiphospholipid syndrome. *Lupus* 17:943, 2008.
240. Cesarman-Maus G, Rios-Luna NP, Deora AB, et al: Autoantibodies against the fibrinolytic receptor, annexin 2, in antiphospholipid syndrome. *Blood* 107:4375, 2006.
241. Ma K, Simantov R, Zhang JC, et al: High affinity binding of beta 2-glycoprotein I to human enodhtelial cells is mediated by annexin II. *J Biol Chem* 275:15541, 2000.
242. Zhang J, McCrae KR: Annexin A2 mediates endothelial cell activation by antiphospholipid/anti-{beta}2-glycoprotein I antibodies. *Blood* 105:1964, 2005.
243. Raschi E, Testoni C, Bosisio D, et al: Role of the My88 transduction signaling pathway in endothelial activation by antiphospholipid antibodies. *Blood* 101:3295, 2003.
244. Romay-Penabad Z, Montiel-Manzano MG, Shilagard T, et al: Annexin A2 is involved in antiphospholipid antibody-mediated pathogenic effects in vitro and in vivo. *Blood* 114:3074, 2009.
245. Ardoin SP, Shanahan JC, Pisetsky DS: The role of microparticles in inflammation and thrombosis. *Scand J Immunol* 66:159, 2007.
246. George FD: Microparticles in vascular diseases. *Thromb Res* 122:S55, 2008.
247. Lechner D, Weltermann A: Circulating tissue factor-exposing microparticles. *Thromb Res* 122:S47-S54, 2008.
248. Peerschke EI, Yin W, Ghebrehiwet B: Platelet mediated complement activation. *Adv Exp Med Biol* 632:81, 2008.
249. Wilkins PP, Moore KL, McEver RP, et al: Tyrosine sulfation of P-selectin glycoprotein ligand-1 is required for high affinity binding to P-selectin. *J Biol Chem* 270:22677, 1995.
250. Snapp KR, Craig R, Herron M, et al: Dimerization of P-selectin glycoprotein ligand-1 (PSGL-1) required for optimal recognition of P-selectin. *J Cell Biol* 142:263, 1998.
251. Tanaka Y, Adams Dh, Hubscher S, et al: T-cell adhesion induced by proteoglycan-immobilized cytokine MIP-1 beta. *Nature* 361:79, 1993.
252. Lo SK, Lee S, Ramos RA, et al: Endothelial-leukocyte adhesion molecule 1 stimulates the adhesive activity of leukocyte integrin CD3 [CD11B/CD18, Mac-1, alpha m beta 2] on human neutrophils. *J Exp Med* 173:1493, 1991.
253. Lorant DE, Patel KD, McIntyre TM, et al: Coexpression of GMP-140 and PAF by endothelium stimulated by histamine or thrombin: A juxtacrine system for adhesion and activation of neutrophils. *J Cell Biol* 115:223, 1991.
254. Huber AR, Kunkel SL, Todd RF, et al: Regulation of transendothelial neutrophil migration by endogenous interleukin-8. *Science* 254:99, 1991.
255. Tanaka Y, Albelda SM, Horgan KJ, et al: CD31 expressed on distinctive T cell subsets is a preferential amplifier of beta 1 integrin-mediated adhesion. *J Exp Med* 176:245, 1992.
256. Piali L, Albelda SM, Baldwin HS, et al: Murine platelet endothelial cell adhesion molecule (PECAM-1/CD31) modulates beta2 integrins on lymphokine-activated killer cells. *Eur J Immunol* 23:2464, 1993.
257. Berman ME, Muller WA: Ligation of platelet/endothelial cell adhesion molecule 1 (PECAM-1/CD31) on monocytes and neutrophils increases binding capacity of leukocyte CR3 (CD11b/CD18). *J Immunol* 154:299, 1995.
258. Carlos TM, Harlan JM: Leukocyte-endothelial cell adhesion molecules. *Blood* 84:2068, 1994.
259. Hynes RO: Integrins: Versatility, modulation, and signalling in cell adhesion. *Cell* 69:11, 1992.
260. Miller J, Knorr R, Ferrone M, et al: Intercellular adhesion molecule-1 dimerization and its consequences for adhesion mediated by lymphocyte function associated molecule-1. *J Exp Med* 182:1231, 1995.
261. Reilly PL, Woska RJR, Jeanfavre DD, et al: The native structure of intercellular adhesion molecule-1(ICAM-1) is a dimer. Correlation with binding to LFA-1. *J Immunol* 155:529, 1995.
262. Bargatze RF, Kurk S, Butcher EC, et al: Neutrophils roll on adherent neutrophils bound to cytokine-induced endothelial cells via L-selectin on the rolling cells. *J Exp Med* 180:1785, 1994.
263. Walcheck B, Moore KL, McEver RP, et al: Neutrophil-neutrophil interactions under hydrodynamic shear stress involve L-selectin and PSGL-1. *J Clin Invest* 98:1081, 1996.
264. Muller WA: Migration of leukocytes across the vascular intima. Molecules and mechanisms. *Trends Cardiovasc Med* 5:15, 1995.
265. Muller WA: Leukocyte-endothelial cell interactions in leukocyte transmigration and the inflammatory response. *Trends Immunol* 24:326, 2003.
266. Ley K, Laudanna C, Cybulsky MI, et al: Getting to the site of inflammation: The leukocyte adhesion cascade updated. *Nat Rev Immunol* 218:178, 2007.
267. Vestweber D: Adhesion and signaling molecules controlling the transmigration of leukocytes through endothelium. *Immunol Rev* 218:178, 2007.
268. Muller WA, Ratti CM, McDonnell SL, et al: A human endothelial cell-restricted, externally disposed plasmalemmal protein enriched in intercellular junctions. *J Exp Med* 170:399, 1989.
269. Newman PJ, Berndt MC, Gorski J, et al: PECAM-1 [CD31] cloning and relation to adhesion molecules of the immunoglobulin gene superfamily. *Science* 247:1219, 1990.

270. Muller WA, Weigl SA, Deng X, et al: PECAM-1 is required for transendothelial migration of leukocytes. *J Exp Med* 178:449, 1993.
271. Huang AJ, Manning JE, Bandak TM, et al: Endothelial cell cytosolic free calcium regulates neutrophil migration across monolayers of endothelial cells. *J Cell Biol* 120:1371, 1993.
272. Liao F, Huynh HK, Eiroa A, et al: Migration of monocytes across endothelium and passage through extracellular matrix involve separate molecular domains of PECAM-1. *J Exp Med* 182:1337, 1995.
273. Liao F, Ali J, Greene T, et al: Soluble domain 1 of platelet-endothelial cell adhesion molecule (PECAM) is sufficient to block transendothelial migration in vitro and in vivo. *J Exp Med* 185:1349, 1997.
274. Ostermann G, Weber KSC, Zernecke A, et al: JAM-1 is a ligand for the b2 integrin LFA-1 involved in transendothelial migration of leukocytes. *Nat Immunol* 3:151, 2002.
275. Johnson-Leger C, Aurrand-Lions M, Beltraminelli N, et al: Junctional adhesion molecule-2 (JAM-2) promotes lymphocyte transendothelial migration. *Blood* 100:2479, 2002.
276. Feng D, Nagy JA, Pyne K, et al: Neutrophils emigrate from venules by a transendothelial cell pathway in response to fMLP. *J Exp Med* 187:903, 1999.
277. Carman CV, Springer TA: Trans-cellular migration: Cell-cell contacts get intimate. *Curr Opin Cell Biol* 20:533, 2008.
278. Schenkel AR, Mamdouh Z, Chen X, et al: CD99 plays a major role in the migration of monocytes through endothelial junctions. *Nat Immunol* 3:2479, 2002.
279. Bixel MG, Petri B, Khandoga AG, et al: A CD99-related antigen on endothelial cells mediates neutrophil, but not lymphocyte extravasation *in vivo*. *Blood* 109:5327, 2009.
280. Dufour EM, Deroche A, Bae Y, et al: CD99 is essential for leukocyte diapedesis in vivo. *Cell Commun Adhes* 15:351, 2008.
281. Marchesi VT, Florey HW: Electron micrographic observations on the emigration of leukocytes. *Q J Exp Physiol Cogn Med Sci* 45:343, 1960.
282. Leeuwenberg JFM, Von Asmuth EJ, Jeunhomme TM, et al: IFN-gamma regulates the expression of the adhesion molecule ELAM-1 and IL-6 production by human endothelial cells *in vitro*. *J Immunol* 145:2110, 1990.
283. Strindall J, Lundblad A, Pahlsson P: Interferon-gamma enhancement of E-selectin expression on endothelial cells is inhibited by monensin. *Scand J Immunol* 46:338, 1997.
284. Ley K, Arbones ML, Bosse R, et al: Sequential contribution of L- and P-selectin to leukocyte rolling *in vivo*. *J Exp Med* 181:669, 1995.
285. Khew-Goodall Y, Butcher E, Litwin MS, et al: Chronic expression of P-selectin on endothelial cells stimulated by the T-cell cytokine, interleukin-3. *Blood* 87:1432, 1999.
286. Yao L, Pan J, Setiadi H, et al: Interleukin-4 or oncostatin M induces a prolonged increase in P-selectin mRNA and protein in human endothelial cells. *J Exp Med* 184:81, 1996.
287. Jung U, Ley K: Regulation of E-selectin, P-selectin, and intercellular adhesion molecule-1 expression in mouse cremaster vasculature. *Microcirculation* 4:311, 1997.
288. Pan J, Xia L, Yao L, et al: Tumor necrosis factor-alpha- or lipopolysaccharide-induced expression of the murine P-selectin gene in endothelial cells involves novel kappaB sites and a variant activating transcription factor/cAMP response element. *J Biol Chem* 273:10067, 1998.
289. Masinovsky B, Urdal D, Gallatin WM: IL-4 acts synergistically with IL-1 beta to promote lymphocyte adhesion to microvascular endothelium by induction of vascular cell adhesion molecule-1. *J Immunol* 145:2886, 1990.
290. Blease K, Seybold J, Adcock IM, et al: Interleukin-4 and lipopolysaccharide synergize to induce vascular adhesion molecule-1 expression in human lung microvascular endothelial cells. *Am J Respir Cell Mol Biol* 18:620, 1998.
291. Pober JS, Collins T, Gimbrone M, et al: Inducible expression of class II major histocompatibility complex antigens and the immunogenicity of vascular endothelium. *Transplantation* 41:141, 1986.
292. Savage COS, Hughes CCW, McIntyre BW, et al: Human CD4+ cells proliferate to HLA-DR+ allogeneic vascular endothelium. Identification of accessory interactions. *Transplantation* 56:128, 1993.
293. Pober JS, Orosz CG, Rose ML, et al: Can graft endothelial cells initiate a host anti-graft immune response? *Transplantation* 61:343, 1996.
294. Romer LH, McLean NV, Horng-Chin Y, et al: IFN-gamma and TNF-alpha induce redistribution of PECAM-1 [CD31] on human endothelial cells. *J Immunol* 154:6582, 1995.
295. Tang Q, Hendricks RL: Interferon gamma regulates platelet endothelial cell adhesion molecule-1 expression and neutrophil infiltration into herpes simplex virus-infected mouse corneas. *J Exp Med* 184:1435, 1996.
296. Rival Y, Del Maschio A, Rabiet MJ, et al: Inhibition of platelet endothelial cell adhesion molecule-1 synthesis and leukocyte transmigration in endothelial cells by the combined action of TNFα and IFNγ. *J Immunol* 157:1233, 1996.
297. Kaplanski G, Fabrigoule M, Boulay V, et al: Thrombin induces endothelial type II activation in vitro: IL-1- and TNF-alpha-independent IL-8 secretion and E-selectin expression. *J Immunol* 158:5435, 1997.
298. Diacovo TG, Puri KD, Warnock RA, et al: Platelet-mediated lymphocyte delivery to high endothelial venules. *Science* 273:252, 1996.
299. Diacovo TG, Catalina MD, Siegelman MH, et al: Circulating activated platelets reconstitute lymphocyte homing and immunity in L-selectin-deficient mice. *J Exp Med* 187:197, 1998.
300. Buttrum SM, Hatton R, Nash GB: Selectin-mediated rolling of neutrophils on immobilized platelets. *Blood* 82:1165, 1993.
301. Diacovo TG, Roth SJ, Buccola JM, et al: Neutrophil rolling, arrest, and transmigration across activated, surface-adherent platelets via sequential action of P-selectin and the beta 2-integrin CD11b/CD18. *Blood* 88:146, 1996.
302. Diacovo TG, de Fougerolles AR, Bainton DF, et al: A functional integrin ligand on the surface of platelets: Intercellular adhesion molecule-2. *J Clin Invest* 94:1243, 1994.
303. Simon DI, Chen Z, Xu H, et al: Platelet glycoprotein Iba is a counterreceptor for the leukocyte integrin Mac-1 (CD11b/CD18). *J Exp Med* 192:193, 2000.
304. Santoso S, Sachs UJ, Kroll H, et al: The junctional adhesion molecule 3 (JAM-3) on human platelets is a counterreceptor for the leukocyte integrin Mac-1. *J Exp Med* 196:679, 2002.
305. Frenette PS, Denis CV, Weiss L, et al: P-selectin glycoprotein ligand 1 (PSGL-) is expressed on platelets and can mediate platelet-endothelial interactions *in vivo*. *J Exp Med* 191:1413, 2000.
306. Moake JL, Rudy.C.K., Troll JH, et al: Unusually large plasma factor VIII:von Willebrand factor multimers in chronic relapsing thrombotic thrombocytopenic purpura. *N Engl J Med* 307:1432, 1982.
307. Zheng XL, Sadler JE: Pathogenesis of thrombotic microangiopathies. *Annu Rev Pathol* 3:249, 2008.
308. Chauhan AK, Kisucka J, Brill A, et al: ADAMTS13: A new link between thrombosis and inflammation. *J Exp Med* 205:2065, 2008.
309. Altieri DC: Cogulation assembly on leukocytes in transmembrane signaling and cell adhesion. *Blood* 81:569, 1993.
310. Lo SK, Cheung A, Zheng Q, et al: Induction of tissue factor in monocytes by adhesion to endothelial cells. *J Immunol* 154:4768, 1995.
311. Fan ST, Mackman N, Cui MZ, et al: Integrin regulation of an inflammatory effector gene: Direct induction of the tissue factor promoter by engagement of β_1 or α_4 integrin chains. *J Immunol* 154:3266, 1995.
312. Randolph GJ, Luther T, Albrecht S, et al: Role of tissue factor adhesion of mononuclear phagocytes to and trafficking through endothelium. *Blood* 92:4167, 1998.
313. Palabrica T, Lobb R, Furie BC, et al: Leukocyte accumulation promoting fibrin deposition is mediated *in vivo* by P-selectin on adherent platelets. *Nature* 359:848, 1992.
314. Wright SD, Weitz JI, Huang AJ, et al: Complement receptor type [CR3, CD11b/CD18] of human polymorphonuclear leukocytes recognizes fibrinogen. *Proc Natl Acad Sci U S A* 85:7734, 1988.
315. Altieri DC, Morrisey JH, Edgington TS: Adhesive receptor Mac-1 coordinates the activation of factor X on stimulated cells of monocytic and myeloid differentiation: An alternative initiation of the coagulation protease cascade. *Proc Natl Acad Sci U S A* 85:7462, 1988.
316. Altieri DC, Edgington TS: The saturable high affinity association of factor X to ADP-stimulated monocytes defines a novel function of the Mac-1 receptor. *J Biol Chem* 263:7007, 1988.
317. Peng L, Bhatia N, Parker AC, et al: Endogenous vitronectin and plasminogen activator inhibitor-1 promote neointima formation in murine carotid arteries. *Arterioscler Thromb Vasc Biol* 22:934, 2002.
318. de Waard V, Armitage RJ, Carmeliet P, et al: Plasminogen activator inhibitor-1 and vitronectin protect against stenosis in a murine carotid ligation model. *Arterioscler Thromb Vasc Biol* 22:1978, 2002.
319. Alon R, Fassner PD, Carr MW, et al: The integrin VLA-4 supports tethering and rolling on VCAM-1. *J Cell Biol* 128:1243, 1995.
320. Berlin CBRF, Campbell JJ, Von Andrian UH, et al: Alpha 4 integrins mediate lymphocyte attachment and rolling under physiologic flow. *Cell* 80:413, 1995.
321. Davie EW, Ratnoff OD: Waterfall sequence for intrinsic blood clotting. *Science* 145:1310, 1964.
322. MacFarlane RG: An enzyme cascade in the blood clotting mechanism, and its function as a biochemical amplifier. *Nature* 202:498, 1964.
323. Huber R, Berendes R, Burger A, et al: Crystal and molecular structure of human annexin V after refinement: Implications for structure, membrane binding and ion channel formation of the annexin family of proteins. *J Mol Biol* 223:683, 1992.
324. Huang K-S, Wallner BP, Mattaliano RJ, et al: Two human 35 kd inhibitors of phospholipase A2 are related to substrates of pp60 v-src and of the epidermal growth factor receptor/kinase. *Cell* 46:191, 1986.
325. Gerke V, Creutz CE, Moss SE: Annexins: Linking Ca++ signalling to membrane dynamics. *Nat Rev Mol Cell Biol* 6:449, 2005.
326. Blasi F, Conese M, Moller LB, et al: The urokinase receptor: Structure, regulation and inhibitor-mediated internalization. *Fibrinolysis* 8:182, 1994.
327. Jacovina AT, Deora AB, Ling Q, et al: Homocysteine inhibits neoangiogenesis through blockade of annexin A2-dependent angiogenesis. *J Clin Invest* 119:3385, 2009.

CHAPTER 118

CLASSIFICATION, CLINICAL MANIFESTATIONS, AND EVALUATION OF DISORDERS OF HEMOSTASIS

Uri Seligsohn and Kenneth Kaushansky

SUMMARY

Evaluation of a hemostatic disorder is commonly initiated when (1) a patient or referring physician suspects a bleeding tendency, (2) a bleeding tendency is discovered in one or more family members, (3) an abnormal coagulation assay result is obtained from an individual as part of a routine examination, (4) an abnormal assay result is obtained from a patient during preparation for surgery, or (5) a patient has unexplained diffuse bleeding during or after surgery or following trauma. Evaluation of a possible hemostatic disorder in each of these scenarios is a stepwise process that requires knowledge of the various classes of hemostatic disorders commonly found under the particular circumstances. The patient's history, the results of physical examination, and an initial set of hemostatic tests usually enable a tentative diagnosis. However, more specific tests are commonly necessary to make a definitive diagnosis. This chapter reviews the necessary steps.

CLASSIFICATION OF HEMOSTATIC DISORDERS

Hemostatic disorders can conveniently be classified as either hereditary or acquired (Table 118–1). Alternatively, hemostatic disorders can be classified according to the mechanism of the defect. Of the acquired disorders, the thrombocytopenias are the most frequently encountered entities. Thrombocytopenias can result from reduced production of platelets, excessive destruction caused by antibodies or other consumptive processes, or pooling of platelets in the spleen, as in hypersplenism (see Chap. 119); however, if hypersplenism is the sole cause of a hemostatic disorder, it is rarely severe enough to cause pathologic bleeding.

BLEEDING HISTORY

The bleeding history is a crucial element in the evaluation of a patient with a hemorrhagic disorder. The bleeding history helps define the subsequent diagnostic approach and the likelihood of future bleeding. Eliciting and interpreting all of the relevant information requires a systematic and methodical approach. The following points are worth considering.

1. Patients vary in their responses to hemorrhagic symptoms. Some patients ignore significant symptoms, whereas other patients are highly sensitive to even minor symptoms. When asked in standardized questionnaires, many normal, healthy people indicate they have excessive bleeding or bruising.[1,2] Therefore, some experts believe the question "Do you bruise easily?" is virtually worthless. Women more likely respond that they have excessive bleeding or bruising than do men.
2. Patients with severe hemorrhagic disorders invariably have very abnormal bleeding histories, for example, severe hemophilia A or hemophilia B, type 3 von Willebrand disease, and Glanzmann thrombasthenia.
3. The diagnostic value of any specific symptom varies in the different disorders. Therefore, recognizing typical patterns of bleeding is important (Table 118–2). Unprovoked hemarthroses and muscle hemorrhages suggest one of the hemophilias, whereas mucocutaneous bleeding (epistaxis, gingival bleeding, menorrhagia) are more characteristic of patients with qualitative platelet disorders, thrombocytopenia, or von Willebrand disease.
4. Assessing the extent of hemorrhage against the background of any trauma or provocation that may have elicited the hemorrhage is important. If a patient has never had a significant hemostatic challenge, such as tooth extraction, surgery, trauma, or childbirth, the lack of a significant bleeding history is much less valuable in excluding a mild hemorrhagic disorder. For example, a significant percentage of patients with mild von Willebrand disease or mild forms of hemophilia may have negative bleeding histories,[1] even though they may be at considerable risk for excessive bleeding after surgery or other interventions. Thus, these diagnoses must be considered even in elderly patients if their first severe hemostatic challenge occurs at that age.
5. Obtaining objective confirmation of the subjective information conveyed in the bleeding history is valuable. Objective data include (a) previous hospital or physician visits for bleeding symptoms, (b) results of previous laboratory evaluations, (c) previous transfusions of blood products for bleeding episodes, and (d) a history of anemia and/or previous treatment with iron.
6. Although self-administered questionnaires may provide useful background information, they cannot substitute for a dialogue between the physician and the patient. Thus, history taking in general, but especially in the often subtle histories related to hemostatic disorders, is an intellectually active process involving data collection, hypothesis development, new question formulation, additional data gathering, and new hypothesis development. However, this procedure has its limitations even when it is carefully pursued.[3,4]
7. A medication history is a crucial component of the bleeding history, with particular attention to nonprescription drugs, such as aspirin and nonsteroidal antiinflammatory agents, which may affect bleeding symptoms. A medication history is especially important in patients with thrombocytopenia, because drug-induced thrombocytopenia is common (see Chap. 119 and Table 118–1). Medication also may affect hemostasis through deleterious effects on the liver or kidney functions. The increased use of herbal and alternative medicines poses particular problems, because patients may not readily share information about what they are taking, and the dose they are taking of any particular active ingredient may be difficult to determine. *Ginkgo biloba* and ginseng are the most commonly used herbals that can cause platelet dysfunction and induce bleeding.[5] Other dietary supplements can display similar effects.[5,6]

Acronyms and abbreviations that appear in this chapter include: aPTT, activated partial thromboplastin time; BT, bleeding time; DIC, disseminated intravascular coagulation; ELISA, enzyme-linked immunosorbent assay; PT, prothrombin time; RCF, ristocetin cofactor.

TABLE 118–1. Classification of Disorders of Hemostasis

Major Types	Disorders	Examples
Acquired	Thrombocytopenias	Autoimmune and alloimmune, drug-induced, hypersplenism, hypoplastic (primary, myelosuppressive therapy, myelophthisic marrow infiltration), disseminated intravascular coagulation (DIC), thrombotic thrombocytopenic purpura, hemolytic-uremic syndrome (see Chaps. 119, 130, and 133)
	Liver diseases	Cirrhosis, acute hepatic failure, liver transplantation (see Chap. 129), thrombopoietin deficiency
	Renal failure	
	Vitamin K deficiency	Malabsorption syndrome, hemorrhagic disease of the newborn, prolonged antibiotic therapy, malnutrition, prolonged biliary obstruction
	Hematologic disorders	Acute leukemias (particularly promyelocytic), myelodysplasias, monoclonal gammopathies, essential thrombocythemia (see Chaps. 87–89 and 108)
	Acquired antibodies against coagulation factors	Neutralizing antibodies against factors V, VIII, and XIII, accelerated clearance of antibody-factor complexes, e.g., acquired von Willebrand disease, hypoprothrombinemia associated with antiphospholipid antibodies (see Chaps. 127, 128, and 132)
	DIC	Acute (sepsis, malignancies, trauma, obstetric complications) and chronic (malignancies, giant hemangiomas, retained products of conception) (see Chap. 130)
	Drugs	Antiplatelet agents, anticoagulants, antithrombins, and thrombolytic, hepatotoxic, and nephrotoxic agents (see Chaps. 23, 134–136)
	Vascular	Nonpalpable purpura ("senile," solar, and factitious purpura), use of corticosteroids, vitamin C deficiency, child abuse, thromboembolic, purpura fulminans; palpable-purpura (Henoch-Schönlein, vasculitis, dysproteinemias; see Chap. 123), amyloidosis
Inherited	Deficiencies of coagulation factors	Hemophilia A (factor VIII deficiency), hemophilia B (factor IX deficiency), deficiencies of fibrinogen factors II, V, VII, X, XI, and XIII and von Willebrand disease (see Chaps. 124–127)
	Platelet disorders	Glanzmann thrombasthenia, Bernard-Soulier syndrome, platelet granule disorders (see Chap. 121)
	Fibrinolytic disorders	α_2-Antiplasmin deficiency, plasminogen activator inhibitor-1 deficiency (see Chap. 136)
	Vascular	Hemorrhagic telangiectasias (see Chap. 123)
	Connective tissue disorders	Ehlers-Danlos syndrome (see Chap. 123)

8. A nutrition history should be obtained to assess the likelihood of (a) vitamin K deficiency, especially if the patient also is taking broad-spectrum antibiotics, (b) vitamin C deficiency, especially if the patient has skin bleeding consistent with scurvy (perifollicular purpura), and (c) general malnutrition and/or malabsorption.
9. Several tissues have an increased local fibrinolytic activity. Such tissues include the urinary tract, endometrium, and mucous membranes of the nose and oral cavity. These sites are particularly likely to have prolonged oozing of blood after trauma in patients with hemostatic abnormalities. Excessive bleeding following tooth extraction is one of the most common manifestations.
10. Bleeding isolated to a single organ or system (e.g., hematuria, hematemesis, melena, hemoptysis) is less likely to result from a hemostatic abnormality than from a local cause such as neoplasm, ulcer, or angiodysplasia. Thus, careful anatomic evaluation of the involved organ or system should be performed.
11. Bleeding may result from blood vessel disorders such as hereditary hemorrhagic telangiectasias, Cushing disease, scurvy, or Ehlers-Danlos syndrome. Many primary dermatologic disorders also have a purpuric or hemorrhagic component and must also be considered in the differential diagnosis (see Chap. 123).
12. A family history is particularly important when hereditary disorders are considered. Patients usually will not spontaneously offer a history of consanguinity, so specific inquiry should be made about this possibility. A diagram of the patient's genealogic tree, extending back at least two generations, should be included to document consideration of genetic disorders. A sex-linked pattern of inheritance is consistent with hemophilia A or B (see Chap. 124). An autosomal dominant pattern is characteristic of most forms of von Willebrand disease (see Chap. 127). An autosomal recessive pattern is typical for all other coagulation factor deficiencies (see Chap. 125), inherited platelet disorders (see Chap. 121), and the rare, severe, type 3 von Willebrand disease. Population genetic information may be helpful; for example, the higher prevalence of factor XI deficiency in Ashkenazi Jews (see Chap. 125).
13. The history should include information on diseases and organs that may affect hemostasis, such as cirrhosis, renal insufficiency, myeloproliferative disorders (e.g., essential thrombocythemia), acute leukemia, myelodysplasia, systemic lupus erythematosus, and Gaucher disease (see Table 118–1).

CLINICAL MANIFESTATIONS

Individual hemorrhagic symptoms often require detailed analysis before the significance of the symptoms and the resulting diagnosis or therapy can be determined. Some of the more common symptoms are discussed below, and Table 118–2 summarizes clinical manifestations that are typical for specific hemostatic disorders.

TABLE 118–2. Clinical Manifestations Typically Associated with Specific Hemostatic Disorders

Clinical Manifestations	Hemostatic Disorders
Mucocutaneous bleeding	Thrombocytopenias, platelet dysfunction, von Willebrand disease
Cephalhematomas in newborns, hemarthroses, hematuria, and intramuscular, intracerebral, and retroperitoneal hemorrhages	Severe hemophilias A and B, severe deficiencies of factor VII, X, or XIII, severe type 3 von Willebrand disease, afibrinogenemia
Injury-related bleeding and mild spontaneous bleeding	Mild and moderate hemophilias A and B, severe factor XI deficiency, moderate deficiencies of fibrinogen and factors II, V, VII, or X, combined factors V and VIII deficiency, α_2-antiplasmin deficiency
Bleeding from stump of umbilical cord and habitual abortions	Afibrinogenemia, hypofibrinogenemia, dysfibrinogenemia, factor XIII deficiency
Impaired wound healing	Factor XIII deficiency
Facial purpura in newborns	Glanzmann thrombasthenia, severe thrombocytopenia
Recurrent severe epistaxis and chronic iron deficiency anemia	Hereditary hemorrhagic telangiectasias

1. Epistaxis is one of the most common symptoms of platelet disorders and von Willebrand disease. It also is the most common symptom of hereditary hemorrhagic telangiectasia. In the latter condition, epistaxis almost always becomes more severe with advancing age. Epistaxis is not uncommon in normal children, but it usually resolves before puberty. Dry air heating systems can provoke epistaxis even in otherwise normal individuals. Bleeding confined to a single nostril more likely results from a local vascular problem than a systemic coagulopathy.
2. Gingival hemorrhage is very common in patients with both qualitative and quantitative platelet abnormalities and von Willebrand disease. Occasional gum bleeding occurs in normal individuals, especially if they use a hard bristle tooth brush and dental hygiene procedures. Thus, establishing whether the bleeding is excessive may be difficult. Frequent gingival hemorrhage can occur in individuals with normal hemostasis if they have gingivitis.
3. Oral mucous membrane bleeding in the form of blood blisters is a common manifestation of severe thrombocytopenia. Such bleeding usually has a predilection for sites where teeth can traumatize the inner surface of the cheek.
4. Skin hemorrhage in the form of petechiae and ecchymoses are common manifestations of hemostatic disorders. However, skin hemorrhage also is common among individuals without hemostatic disorders. Excessive bruising is more common in women than men. Moreover, women frequently note that the severity of their bruising varies with the phase of their menstrual cycle, although the most severe phase of the cycle may differ in different women. Features that help establish the severity of skin hemorrhage include the size of the bruises, the frequency of bruising, whether the bruises occur spontaneously or only with trauma, and the appearance of bruises on regions of the body that usually are not traumatized, such as the trunk and back. The color of the bruise may yield information. Red bruises on the extensor surfaces of the arms and hands indicate loss of supporting tissues, as occurs in Cushing syndrome, glucocorticoid therapy, senile purpura, and damage from chronic sun exposure. Jet-black bruises may be caused by warfarin-induced skin necrosis and similar disorders. Easy bruising can also occur in patients with Ehlers-Danlos syndrome manifested by distensible skin or extraordinary ligament laxness, and in patients with hyperflexibility of the thumb.[8]
5. Tooth extractions are common hemostatic challenges and may be helpful in defining the risk of bleeding. Molar extractions are greater hemostatic challenges than extractions of other teeth. Objective data regarding excessive bleeding based on the need for blood products or the need to pack or suture the extraction site are valuable.
6. Excessive bleeding in response to razor nicks is common in patients with platelet disorders or von Willebrand disease.
7. Hemoptysis almost never is the presenting symptom of a bleeding disorder and is rare even in patients with serious bleeding disorders. However, blood-tinged sputum in association with upper respiratory tract infections may be more common in patients with hemostatic disorders.
8. Hematemesis, like hemoptysis, almost never is the presenting symptom of a hemostatic disorder. However, a hemostatic disorder may lead to hematemesis because of an anatomic abnormality in the upper gastrointestinal tract. Some hemostatic disorders more likely result in hematemesis because of a combination of effects, such as liver disease with deficient synthesis of coagulation proteins and with esophageal varices and aspirin ingestion with gastritis.
9. Hematuria is rarely the presenting symptom of a hemostatic disorder except for the hemophilias. However, hemostatic disorders can exacerbate hematuria caused by other disorders, including simple urinary tract infections.
10. Rectal bleeding in individuals with normal hemostasis most often results from hemorrhoids. However, von Willebrand disease and platelet disorders may contribute to repeated episodes of rectal bleeding when associated with a number of different underlying causes, including diverticuli, hemorrhoids, or angiodysplasia. Melena is also only rarely the presenting symptom of a hemorrhagic disorder. However, repeated episodes of melena may occur in patients with hemorrhagic disorders.
11. Menorrhagia is common in women with platelet disorders and von Willebrand disease. In general, menstrual bleeding is considered excessive if the patient indicates she has heavy flow for more than 3 days or total flow for more than 7 days. However, an objective distinction between menorrhagia (loss of more than 80 mL blood per period) and normal blood loss can only be made by a visual assessment technique using pictorial charts of towels or tampons.[7]
12. Postpartum hemorrhage. Childbirth poses a considerable hemostatic challenge. Consequently, patients with bleeding disorders commonly manifest excessive bleeding during or after labor necessitating blood transfusion.
13. Habitual spontaneous abortions raise the possibility that the patient has a quantitative or qualitative abnormality of fibrinogen (see Chap. 126), factor XIII deficiency (see Chap. 125), or the antiphospholipid syndrome (see Chap. 132).
14. Hemarthroses are the hallmark abnormality in the hemophiliac; they are rare in other disorders except in severe factor VII deficiency and type 3 von Willebrand disease (see Chaps. 125 and 127). Because discoloration of the skin overlying the joint with hemarthroses does not occur, patients may not recognize that their symptoms (pain, swelling, and limitation of motion) are caused by bleeding into their joints.

15. Excessive hemorrhage associated with surgical procedures is common in patients with hemorrhagic disorders. Procedures involving tissues with increased local fibrinolytic activity like urinary tract, nose, tonsils and oral cavity are particularly prone to bleed.
16. Excessive bleeding following circumcision is common in males with severe hemostatic disorders such as hemophilia A, hemophilia B, or Glanzmann thromboasthenia, and often is the patient's first symptom.
17. Bleeding from the umbilical stump is characteristic of factor XIII deficiency (see Chap. 125) and afibrinogenemia (see Chap. 126).

PHYSICAL EXAMINATION

Physical examination is essential for identifying signs of bleeding or their sequelae and for signs of a possible underlying disorder that can cause the hemostatic derangement (see Table 118–1). Careful examination of the skin is essential for detecting petechiae and ecchymoses. These signs may be prominent on the legs, where the hydrostatic pressure is greatest, or around the hair follicles in vitamin C deficiency.

Telangiectasias may range from pinpoint erythematous dots that blanch with pressure to classic cherry angiomata ranging in size up to several centimeters. Many normal individuals develop increasing numbers of telangiectasias with aging. Patients with hereditary hemorrhagic telangiectasia have more florid lesions that characteristically affect the vermilion border of the lips and the tongue (including the underside of the tongue), but not all patients have these classic features. Thus, a systematic search of the integument is necessary. Spider telangiectasias found in patients with chronic liver disease have a more splotchy and serpiginous appearance than the telangiectasias associated with hereditary hemorrhagic telangiectasia. In addition, the telangiectasias tend to be concentrated on the shoulders, chest, and face.

Chap. 123 details the differential diagnosis of nonpalpable purpuras and palpable purpuras. Hematomas, ecchymoses, and protracted oozing should be sought at venipuncture sites, injection sites, and arterial and venous catheter insertion sites. Joint deformities and limited joint mobility are suggestive of severe hemophilia A or B, severe deficiency of factor VII, or type 3 von Willebrand disease (see Chaps. 124, 125, and 127). Hyperelasticity of the skin and hyperextensibility of joints are typical of Ehlers-Danlos syndrome, and hyperextensibility of only the thumb probably is a variant.[8]

EVALUATION BASED ON BLEEDING HISTORY, PHYSICAL EXAMINATION, AND BASIC LABORATORY TESTS

The patient's history and results of physical examination provide important information on the likelihood of the patient having a hemostatic defect and the possible cause of the defect, if one is present. However, performing an initial set of widely available and inexpensive tests, including prothrombin time (PT), activated partial thromboplastin time (aPTT), and platelet count, is important for the following reasons: (1) The patient's history sometimes is unreliable; (2) the patient may have a mild hemostatic abnormality that has not manifested itself for lack of hemostatic challenge; (3) the patient may have developed an acquired hemostatic defect that has remained asymptomatic; and (4) the tests may reveal more than one abnormality.[9]

Figure 118–1 shows a series of algorithms that integrate the patient's bleeding history and the results of the initial hemostatic tests. A prolonged aPTT as a sole abnormality can be caused by a deficiency of factor VIII, IX, XI, or XII or by an inhibitor, which can be either factor specific, such as an antibody against factor VIII, or factor nonspecific, such as the presence of heparin or a lupus anticoagulant (Fig. 118–1A). A prolonged PT as the sole finding can indicate a factor VII deficiency or the presence of an inhibitor (Fig. 118–1B). Abnormalities of both PT and aPTT may indicate a deficiency of fibrinogen, prothrombin, factor V or factor X, an inhibitor to one of these factors, or a combined deficiency of coagulation factors (Fig. 118–1C).

To distinguish between a deficiency state and the presence of an inhibitor, repeating the abnormal test, the PT and/or aPTT, using a 1:1 mixture of the patient's plasma and normal plasma is useful. If the mixture normalizes the prolonged PT or aPTT, a deficiency state is likely as most coagulation tests are calibrated to produce a normal result if each of the relevant factor levels are 50 percent of normal or greater. If the mixture still yields a significantly prolonged PT or aPTT, an inhibitor probably is present. Some inhibitors, such as antibodies to factor VIII, require time to inhibit the factor VIII activity in the assay, whereas other inhibitors, such as lupus anticoagulant or heparin, do not. Consequently, incubating the mixture for 1 or 2 hours at 37°C (98.6°F) before performing the coagulation assay is desirable.

When the results of none of the initial tests (PT, aPTT, and platelet count) is abnormal and the patient exhibits bleeding manifestations, the template bleeding time (BT), ristocetin cofactor (RCF) activity, and examination of the blood film can be helpful for distinguishing among various candidate hemostatic abnormalities. Although the BT can be useful in diagnosis, an experienced technician is a requisite for proper interpretation because the test is highly operator dependent. Figure 118–2 shows an algorithm that includes these secondary tests. Patients with type 1 and type 2 von Willebrand disease often have normal findings on initial laboratory tests because factor VIII levels are sufficiently high (>30 U/dL) for a normal aPTT result (see Chap. 127). Examination of the blood film is helpful for distinguishing between Bernard-Soulier syndrome and von Willebrand disease because giant platelets are characteristic of the former (see Chap. 121). Distinguishing mild-type von Willebrand disease from normal is difficult because of the broad distribution of von Willebrand factor level partly related to ABO blood types. In fact, some investigators have questioned whether patients with von Willebrand factor levels as low as 35 percent should be labeled as having von Willebrand disease.[10] The likelihood of having von Willebrand disease is a function of bleeding score, the von Willebrand factor level and the number of first degree family members with reduced von Willebrand factor levels.[11]

The ristocetin-induced platelet aggregation test is useful for distinguishing type 2B and platelet-type von Willebrand disease from the other types of von Willebrand disease. In type 2B and platelet-type von Willebrand disease, an enhanced response to low concentrations of ristocetin is observed, whereas in the other types of von Willebrand disease, a decreased response is found. Total absence of platelet aggregates in a blood film prepared from nonanticoagulated blood and absent clot retraction are characteristic of Glanzmann thrombasthenia (see Chap. 121).

Another simple test that may be useful for distinguishing among hemostatic disorders is the thrombin time (i.e., time for plasma to clot after adding thrombin). The thrombin time is prolonged in (1) afibrinogenemia, hypofibrinogenemia, and dysfibrinogenemias (see Chap. 126), (2) the presence of heparin, (3) disseminated intravascular coagulation (DIC) causing increased levels of fibrin(ogen) degradation products, which inhibit fibrin monomer polymerization (see Fig. 118–1D and Chap. 130), and (4) patients with amyloidosis and an immunoglobulin inhibitor of thrombin.[12]

PREOPERATIVE ASSESSMENT OF HEMOSTASIS

Because surgical procedures are a great challenge to the hemostatic system, careful assessment of the risk of bleeding in every patient is important.

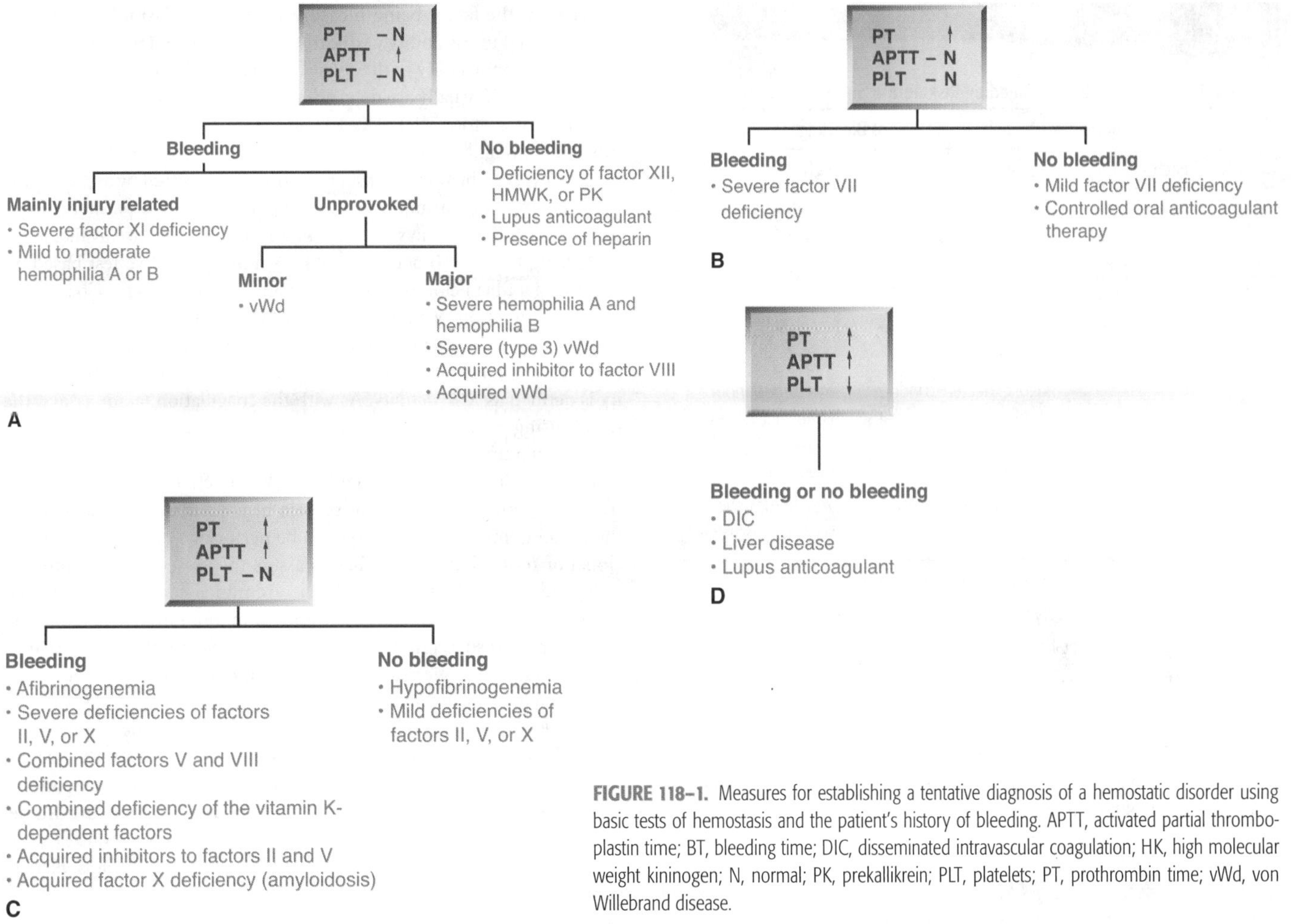

FIGURE 118–1. Measures for establishing a tentative diagnosis of a hemostatic disorder using basic tests of hemostasis and the patient's history of bleeding. APTT, activated partial thromboplastin time; BT, bleeding time; DIC, disseminated intravascular coagulation; HK, high molecular weight kininogen; N, normal; PK, prekallikrein; PLT, platelets; PT, prothrombin time; vWd, von Willebrand disease.

The risk assessment is based on the bleeding history, physical examination, the underlying disorder if any, the type and site of surgery that is planned and the results of basic hemostatic tests (PT, aPTT, platelet count). Several studies have indicated that unselected coagulation tests have no significant predictive value of perioperative bleeding, and that patients with a negative bleeding history do not require routine coagulation screening.[13] However, this conclusion does not take into account that patients with mild to moderate bleeding disorders who can bleed excessively following surgery may have a negative bleeding history because they have not been challenged, obtaining a good bleeding history is an expertise that is not shared by all physicians, and if bleeding occurs during or after surgery for whatever reason, the basic tests performed preoperatively are an essential reference for determining the cause of bleeding.

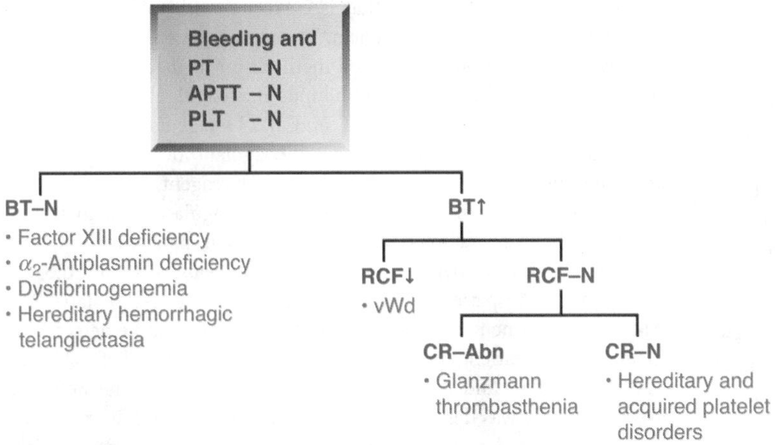

FIGURE 118–2. Tentative diagnoses in patients with bleeding manifestations and normal primary hemostatic tests using secondary tests. Abn, abnormal; APTT, activated partial thromboplastin time; BT, bleeding time; CR, clot retraction; N, normal; PK, prekallikrein; PLT, platelets; PT, prothrombin time; RCF, ristocetin cofactor activity; vWd, von Willebrand disease.

Table 118–3 lists low-risk and high-risk conditions. A critical analysis of each potential cause of bleeding should be undertaken for the high-risk conditions. In addition to the extent of the surgical trauma, the magnitude of the fibrinolytic activity at the surgical site must be considered. For example, prostatectomy carries considerable risk of prolonged bleeding because of the presence of high fibrinolytic activity in the urine. Some surgical procedures can be anticipated to cause hemostatic abnormalities, such as operations in which extracorporeal circulation is used (because the extracorporeal circuits and/or the anticoagulation cause platelet dysfunction) and operations on patients with extensive malignancies or brain injury, which can give rise to DIC. Finally, the ability to institute local hemostatic measures should be considered. Thus, liver, lung, and kidney biopsies, although considered minor procedures, have a significant

TABLE 118–3. Evaluation of Bleeding Risk during Surgery

	Risk of Bleeding	
Assessed Factor	Low	High
Bleeding history	Negative	Positive*
Underlying conditions that compromise hemostasis (see Table 118–1)	Absent	Present
Initial hemostatic tests	Normal	Abnormal
Type of surgery	Minor	Major
	Not expected to induce a hemostatic defect at a site without local fibrinolysis	Expected to induce a hemostatic defect† at a site with local fibrinolysis‡
	Local hemostatic measures effective	Local hemostatic measures ineffective§

*Spontaneous bleeding episodes or injury-related hemorrhage.

†Open heart surgery or brain surgery.

‡Prostatectomy, tonsillectomy, oral or nasal surgery.

§Liver, lung, or kidney biopsy.

risk of bleeding because local measures, such as direct pressure, cannot be used to control bleeding.

SPECIFIC ASSAYS FOR ESTABLISHING THE DIAGNOSIS

A tentative diagnosis can be made by following the stepwise process of evaluation outlined in Figures 118–1 and 118–2. However, further testing usually is required to establish a definitive diagnosis.

THROMBOCYTOPENIAS

When the laboratory reports an abnormally low platelet count, looking at the blood film to exclude pseudothrombocytopenia as a result of anticoagulant-induced platelet clumping is essential.[14] Examination of the blood film also can reveal the presence of giant platelets, as in some inherited thrombocytopenias; giant platelets and Döhle bodies in leukocytes, as in May-Hegglin and other MYH9 platelet syndromes; moderately enlarged platelets, as in immune thrombocytopenia or other conditions associated with shortened platelet survival; small platelets, as in Wiskott-Aldrich syndrome; schistocytes and burr cells, as in the hemolytic uremic syndrome and thrombotic thrombocytopenic purpura, and occasionally in DIC; rouleaux formation, as in monoclonal gammopathies; macrocytosis and/or hypersegmentation, as in vitamin B_{12} or folic acid deficiency; and abnormal white blood cells, as in leukemias and myeloproliferative disorders. Chapter 119 further discusses the evaluation and differential diagnosis of the thrombocytopenias.

FACTOR DEFICIENCIES

Coagulation factors usually are assayed by measuring their clotting activity. The most common assays analyze the ability of dilutions of the patient's plasma to correct the clotting time of a plasma known to be deficient in the factor being measured (substrate plasma). The results are compared to the ability of dilutions of a normal reference plasma to correct the abnormality in the substrate plasma. The activities of factors II, V, VII, and X usually are determined in PT-based assays, whereas the activities of factors VIII, IX, XI, and XII, prekallikrein, and high-molecular-weight kininogen are measured in aPTT-based assays. The plasma level of fibrinogen most commonly is measured by assessing the time required for thrombin to clot the patient's diluted plasma (Clauss method).[15] Several assays of transglutaminase activity are available for measuring factor XIII activity,[16] but a simple qualitative test based on dissolving a fibrin clot in 5 M urea usually is sufficient (see Chap. 125). The RCF function of von Willebrand factor can be measured by the ability of the patient's plasma to support the agglutination of a suspension of formaldehyde-fixed normal platelets by ristocetin.[17] This activity is defined as *RCF activity*. As with the coagulation factor assays, the results using patient plasma are compared to the results obtained with a normal reference plasma.

To determine whether a coagulation factor activity deficiency results from a quantitative decrease in protein or a qualitative abnormality in the protein, immunologic assays can be performed using specific polyclonal or monoclonal antibodies to assess the presence of the protein, independent of its function. Electroimmunoassays, enzyme-linked immunosorbent assays (ELISAs), and immunoradiometric assays all have been used successfully. Crossed immunoelectrophoresis measures both the immunologic reactivity and the mobility of the protein in an electric field; thus, it can detect protein abnormalities that affect electrophoretic migration. The abnormalities include the presence of antibody–antigen complexes that migrate differently from the protein itself, such as antiprothrombin–prothrombin complexes in patients with systemic lupus erythematosus or antiphospholipid syndrome. Diagnosis of the specific type of von Willebrand disease requires additional tests of the multimeric structure of plasma and, perhaps, platelet von Willebrand factor.

INHIBITORS TO COAGULATION FACTORS

If an inhibitor is suspected as a result of a prolonged PT or aPTT performed on a 1:1 mixture of the patient's plasma and normal plasma, further studies can help define the nature of the inhibitor and its titer. Among inhibitors that do not require incubation (i.e., immediate-type), perhaps the most common cause is the presence of heparin in the sample. This cause can be verified by finding a prolonged thrombin time on a test of the patient's plasma that is corrected with toluidine blue or other agents that neutralize heparin. The lupus anticoagulant also does not require incubation, and several methods for its detection are available (see Chap. 132). However, with lupus anticoagulant, the PT usually is less prolonged than is the aPTT, and aPTT reagents have markedly different sensitivity to lupus-type anticoagulant depending on the amount of phosphatidyl serine present in each reagent.

Immunoglobulin inhibitors to specific coagulation factors may develop either after factor replacement therapy in patients with inherited deficiencies of coagulation factors (see Chaps. 124 and 125) or spontaneously in patients without factor deficiencies (see Chap. 128). Antibodies that neutralize factor activity frequently can be detected by incubating the patient's plasma with normal plasma, usually for 2 hours at 37°C (98.6°F), and then assaying the specific factor. The Bethesda assay originally was designed to quantify factor VIII inhibitors but can be modified to detect other inhibitors of coagulation factors[18] (see Chap. 124). Some inhibitors do not directly neutralize clotting activity; instead they reduce factor levels by forming complexes with coagulation factors, which then are rapidly cleared from the circulation. Such plasmas do not produce prolonged clotting times when mixed 1:1 with normal plasma and thus may be confused with inherited deficiency states. More elaborate assays are required to identify this type of inhibitor, which may, for example, produce severe deficiency of prothrombin in some patients with the antiphospholipid syndrome (see Chap. 132) and deficiency of von Willebrand factor in some acquired forms of von Willebrand disease (see Chap. 127).[19]

PLATELET FUNCTION DISORDERS

A prolonged BT suggests a platelet function disorder (inherited or acquired) or von Willebrand disease. Use of the RCF activity assay, platelet aggregation, and/or clot retraction are useful for assessing whether the patient has von Willebrand disease or a platelet function disorder (see Fig. 118–2). Chapter 121 contains a flow diagram of the steps required to diagnose the different qualitative disorders of platelet function. Additional platelet function assays and glycoprotein analysis may be required to establish the diagnosis.

REFERENCES

1. Miller CH, Graham JB, Goldin LR, Elston RC: Genetics of classic von Willebrand's disease: II. Optimal assignment of the heterozygous genotype (diagnosis) by discriminant analysis. *Blood* 54:137, 1979.
2. Wahlberg T, Blomback M, Hall P, Axelsson G: Application of indicators, predictors and diagnostic indices in coagulation disorders: I. Evaluation of a self-administered questionnaire with binary questions. *Methods Inf Med* 19:194, 1980.
3. Eikenboom JCJ, Rosendaal FR, Briet E: Value of the patient interview: All but consensus among haemostasis experts. *Haemostasis* 22:221, 1992.
4. Sramek A, Eikenboom JC, Briet E, et al: Usefulness of patient interview in bleeding disorders. *Arch Intern Med* 155:1409, 1995.
5. Dinehart SM, Henry L: Dietary supplements: Altered coagulation and effects on bruising. *Dermatol Surg* 31:819, 2005.
6. Basila D, Yuan C-S: Effects of dietary supplements on coagulation and platelet function. *Thromb Res* 117:49, 2005.
7. Janssen CAH, Scholten PC, Heintz APM: A simple visual assessment technique to discriminate between menorrhagia and normal menstrual blood loss. *Obstet Gynecol* 85:977, 1995.
8. Kaplinsky C, Kenet G, Seligsohn U, Rechavi G: Association between hyperflexibility of the thumb and an unexplained bleeding tendency: Is it a rule of thumb? *Br J Haematol* 101:260, 1998.
9. Rapaport SI: Preoperative hemostatic evaluation: Which tests, if any? *Blood* 61:229, 1983.
10. Sadler JE: Von Willebrand disease type 1: A diagnosis in search of a disease. *Blood* 101:2089, 2003.
11. Tosetto A, Castaman G, Rodeghiero F: Evidence-based diagnosis of type 1 von Willebrand disease: a Bayes theorem approach. *Blood* 111:3998, 2008.
12. Gastineau DA, Gertz MA, Daniels TM, et al: Inhibitor of the thrombin time in systemic amyloidosis: A common coagulation abnormality. *Blood* 77:2637, 1991.
13. Chee YL, Crawford JC, Watson HG, Greaves M: Guidelines on the assessment of bleeding risk prior to surgery or invasive procedures. *Br J Haematol* 140:496, 2008.
14. Payne BA, Pierre RV: Pseudothrombocytopenia: A laboratory artifact with potentially serious consequences. *Mayo Clin Proc* 59:123, 1984.
15. Clauss A: Gerinnungsphysiologische schnell methodes zur des fibrinogens. *Acta Haematol* 17:327, 1957.
16. Fickenscher K, Aab A, Stuber W: A photometric assay for blood coagulation factor XIII. *Thromb Haemost* 65:535, 1991.
17. McFarlane DE, Stibbe J, Kirby EP, et al: A method for assaying von Willebrand factor (ristocetin cofactor). *Thromb Diath Haemorrh* 34:306, 1975.
18. Kasper CK, Aledort L, Aronson D, et al: Proceedings: A more uniform measurement of factor VIII inhibitors. *Thromb Diath Haemorrh* 34:612, 1975.
19. Inbal A, Bank I, Zivelin A, et al: Acquired von Willebrand disease in a patient with angiodysplasia resulting from immune-mediated clearance of von Willebrand factor. *Br J Haematol* 96:179, 1997.

CHAPTER 119
THROMBOCYTOPENIA

Reyhan Diz-Küçükkaya, Junmei Chen,
Amy Geddis, and José A. López

SUMMARY

Thrombocytopenia is one of the most frequent causes for hematologic consultation in the practice of medicine, and potentially one of the most life-threatening. Although the normal platelet count in humans ($150–400 \times 10^9$/L) far exceeds the minimal level required to avoid pathologic hemorrhage ($<50 \times 10^9$/L), a number of medical conditions cause either increased destruction or reduced production of platelets, increasing the risk of pathologic bleeding. This chapter discusses an approach to the diagnosis of thrombocytopenia, grouping various causes by mechanism of action, and describing our current understanding of pathogenesis, treatment, and prognostication. In the vast majority of patients, a cause for thrombocytopenia can be identified, and effective therapy instituted.

PLATELET KINETICS

Platelet kinetic studies have been performed to determine the pathophysiologic mechanisms in various thrombocytopenic states, particularly in complicated clinical situations. For instance, the thrombocytopenia seen in patients with HIV infection can result from many factors, including platelet destruction (because of an autoimmune mechanism or drug toxicity) or decreased platelet production because of direct megakaryocyte infection by the virus, or by marrow-based malignancy or opportunistic infection.

Platelet kinetic studies are performed using autologous platelets, which are labeled *ex vivo* with radioactive isotopes and then infused back into the patient. The radioisotope indium-111 (^{111}In) oxine is most commonly used because it binds platelets very efficiently, which allows kinetic studies even in subjects with very low platelet counts.[1–3] Platelet recovery, platelet survival, and platelet turnover are calculated based on the radioactivity of blood samples drawn from the patient during the several days following injection of the radiolabeled platelets. Platelet recovery is determined by the percentage of radiolabeled platelets detected in blood 1 hour after the injection. It takes approximately 10 to 12 minutes for the platelets to pass through a normal spleen; nearly one-third of reinfused platelets are sequestered during the first hour before reaching equilibrium with the circulating platelets.[4] The normal value of initial platelet recovery is between 50 and 70 percent. The initial platelet recovery is high in patients who have undergone splenectomy and low in patients with immune thrombocytopenic purpura (ITP) or hypersplenism.[4–6]

The mean platelet life span is generally calculated in reference to a standard curve generated using radioactivity measurements taken over time in normal controls.[2] Under normal conditions, human platelets have a mean life span in the circulation of between 7 and 10 days.[7,8] Patients with thrombocytopenia because of platelet destruction have a markedly decreased platelet survival.[9,10] Patients with thrombocytopenia because of marrow failure have mildly decreased platelet survival because the body's fixed daily consumption of platelets accounts for a progressively larger fraction of the reduced total daily production.[11] Platelet turnover is a measure of the net effect of platelet production and platelet destruction under steady-state conditions.[10] Several studies using ^{111}In oxine have established that, under normal conditions, platelet turnover in humans ranges from 40 to 50 $\times$ 10^9/L per day.[10] Although a high platelet turnover is expected in patients with ITP, platelet production measured as turnover is not always increased in this disorder.[10] Low production may result from binding of the antibodies to megakaryocytes that inhibit their development or lead to their destruction, causing an inappropriate marrow response to the degree of thrombocytopenia.[12]

The number of platelets entering the circulation to maintain the platelet count defines platelet production rate. This rate is calculated from mean platelet life span, platelet count, blood volume, and the initial platelet recovery. The normal rate of platelet production varies from 160×10^9 to 280×10^9 per day.

Platelet kinetic studies also usually measure hepatic and splenic platelet uptake, estimated by the radioactivity from these organs detected by a gamma camera connected to a computerized data collection system. Images are taken during the first hour after injection and followed for 5 to 7 days. In normal subjects, platelet uptake by the liver and spleen usually is constant for 5 days. Thus, increased sequestration beyond this time is suggestive of increased platelet destruction. Patients with ITP and increased splenic sequestration respond better to splenectomy than do patients with liver sequestration only or with combined liver and splenic uptake.[13] The scan is useful for determining spleen size and other sites of platelet sequestration, such as an accessory spleen or congenital hemangiomas, which also are associated with thrombocytopenia.

SPURIOUS THROMBOCYTOPENIA (PSEUDOTHROMBOCYTOPENIA)

Spurious thrombocytopenia, also called *pseudothrombocytopenia*, is a relatively uncommon phenomenon caused by *ex vivo* agglutination of platelets. As a result of platelet clumping, platelet counts reported by automated counters may be much lower than the actual count in the blood because these devices cannot differentiate platelet clumps from individual cells. The incidence of pseudothrombocytopenia reported

Abbreviations and acronyms that appear in this chapter include: ADAMTS, a disintegrin and metalloproteinase with thrombospondin repeats; ALL, acute lymphocytic leukemia; APLA, antiphospholipid antibody; APS, antiphospholipid antibody syndrome; CAMT, congenital amegakaryocytic thrombocytopenia; CTP, cyclic thrombocytopenia; DIC, disseminated intravascular coagulation; EDTA, ethylenediaminetetraacetic acid; Flt, fms-like tyrosine kinase; FOG, friend of GATA1; FPS/AML, familial platelet syndrome with predisposition to acute myelogenous leukemia; GP, glycoprotein; HAART, highly active antiretroviral therapy; HELLP, hemolysis, elevated liver enzymes, and low platelet count; HIT, heparin-induced thrombocytopenia; HLA, human leukocyte antigen; HPA, human platelet antigen; HSC, hematopoietic stem cell; HUS, hemolytic uremic syndrome; Ig, immunoglobulin; IL, interleukin; ITP, immune thrombocytopenic purpura; IVIg, intravenous immunoglobulin; KMS, Kasabach-Merritt syndrome; MACA, modified antigen-capture enzyme-linked immunoadsorbent assay; MDS, myelodysplastic syndrome; NAIT, neonatal alloimmune thrombocytopenia; NICU, neonatal intensive care unit; NMMHC, nonmuscle myosin heavy chain; PAICA, platelet-associated IgG characterization assay; PAIgG, platelet-associated immunoglobulin G; RAEB, refractory anemia with excess blasts; SLE, systemic lupus erythematosus; TAR, thrombocytopenia with absent radii; TPO, thrombopoietin; TTP, thrombotic thrombocytopenic purpura; VEGF, vascular endothelial growth factor; VWF, von Willebrand factor; WAS, Wiskott-Aldrich syndrome; WASP, WAS protein.

TABLE 119–1. Classification of Thrombocytopenia

Pseudothrombocytopenia	Parvovirus (see Chap. 35)
Platelet agglutination	Cytomegalovirus (see Chap. 35)
Platelet satellitism	Others
Antiphospholipid antibodies	Radiotherapy and chemotherapy (see Chap. 20)
GpIIa-IIIa antagonists	Folic acid and vitamin B_{12} deficiency (see Chap. 41)
Giant platelets	Paroxysmal nocturnal hemoglobinuria (see Chap. 40)
Miscellaneous associations	Acquired aplastic anemia (see Chap. 34)
Impaired platelet production	Myelodysplastic syndromes (see Chap. 88)
Congenital	Acquired pure megakaryocytic thrombocytopenia
Autosomal dominant	Accelerated platelet destruction
MYH9-related	Immune-mediated thrombocytopenia
May-Hegglin anomaly	Autoimmune thrombocytopenic purpura
Fechtner syndrome	Idiopathic
Epstein syndrome	Secondary (infections, pregnancy-related, lymphoproliferative disorders, collagen vascular diseases)
Sebastian syndrome	
Mediterranean macrothrombocytopenia	Alloimmune thrombocytopenia
Familial platelet syndrome with predisposition to acute myelogenous leukemia	Neonatal thrombocytopenia
Thrombocytopenia with linkage to chromosome 10	Posttransfusion purpura
Paris-Trousseau syndrome	Nonimmune thrombocytopenia
Thrombocytopenia with radial synostosis	Thrombotic microangiopathies
Autosomal recessive	Thrombotic thrombocytopenic purpura and hemolytic uremic syndrome
Congenital amegakaryocytic thrombocytopenia	Disseminated intravascular coagulopathy
Thrombocytopenia with absent radius (TAR) syndrome	Kasabach-Merritt syndrome
Bernard-Soulier syndrome (see Chap. 121)	Platelet destruction by artificial surfaces
Gray platelet syndrome (see Chap. 121)	Hemophagocytosis
X-linked thrombocytopenias	Abnormal platelet distribution or pooling
Wiskott-Aldrich syndrome	Splenomegaly (see Chap. 55)
X-linked thrombocytopenia	Hypersplenism (see Chap. 55)
X-linked thrombocytopenia with dyserythrocytosis	Hypothermia
Acquired	Massive transfusion
Marrow infiltration (see Chap. 44)	Drug-induced thrombocytopenia
Infectious disease	Heparin-induced thrombocytopenia (see Chap. 133)
HIV (see Chap. 83)	Other drug-induced thrombocytopenias

in different studies ranges from 0.09 to 0.21 percent, which accounts for 15 to 30 percent of all cases of isolated thrombocytopenia.[14–21] Pseudothrombocytopenia has been reported in association with the use of ethylenediaminetetraacetic acid (EDTA) as an anticoagulant, with platelet cold agglutinins,[22] and with multiple myeloma.[23] A very interesting recent report demonstrates pseudothrombocytopenia caused by platelet phagocytosis *ex vivo* in the presence of EDTA anticoagulant.[24] An example of *ex vivo* platelet clumping is shown in Chap. 1, Figure 1–6H, accompanied by platelet–neutrophil satellitism (see "Platelet Satellitism" below). Table 119–1 outlines the classification of thrombocytopenia.

ANTIBODY-INDUCED PLATELET AGGLUTINATION

Platelet agglutination *ex vivo* can be induced by antiplatelet antibodies or by activation of the platelets during collection. The responsible antibodies do not appear to be associated with a pathologic process, as they are found in normal individuals. One hypothesis put forth to explain their presence is that the antibodies are responsible for clearing aged and damaged platelets. Most antibodies implicated in pseudothrombocytopenia recognize platelet membrane glycoproteins that are modified or exposed when calcium is chelated. Typically, the artifact is most prominent in the presence of EDTA, but other anticoagulants, such as sodium citrate, sodium oxalate, acid citrate dextrose, and heparin, also can cause platelet clumping. The antibodies usually are of the immunoglobulin (Ig) G type; IgM and IgA antibodies also have been described.[25–27] Most antibodies react at room temperature; thus, the reaction can be prevented when the blood sample is kept at 37°C. In 20 percent of cases, the antibodies, usually of the IgM type, are reactive at both 22°C and 37°C.[26] Clumping usually is evident within 60 minutes after the blood is drawn, but may require incubations of 2 to 3 hours. Agglutination can be reproduced by incubating plasma from patients with pseudothrombocytopenia with blood from normal individuals in the presence of EDTA.

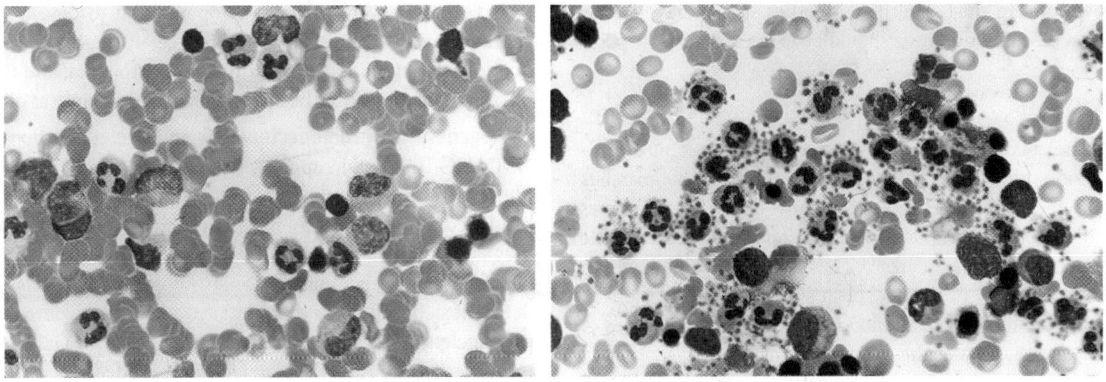

FIGURE 119–1. Platelet satellitism. **A.** Direct (non-anticoagulated) marrow film. No platelet satellitism. **B.** A concentrated marrow film anticoagulated with Na_2EDTA from same specimen as in **(A)**. Note platelets are adherent to the mature neutrophil surface (satellitism) in the presence of Na_2EDTA. The neutrophil precursors do not have surface features that interact with platelets, apparently a feature only present after the final steps in maturation. *(Used with permission from* Lichtman's Atlas of Hematology, *www.accessmedicine.com.)*

In most cases, the antibodies are directed against glycoprotein (GP) IIb/IIIa (GPIIb/IIIa), a conclusion supported by the observation that platelets from patients with Glanzmann thrombasthenia, who lack the GPIIb/IIIa complex, fail to agglutinate in the presence of patient sera.[28–31] Moreover, pretreatment of fresh blood with anti–GPIIb/IIIa dramatically reduces EDTA-induced platelet agglutination.[32] The responsible epitope normally is cryptic and located in the GPIIb subunit. Low temperature and calcium chelation combine to change the conformation of GPIIb/IIIa and expose the epitope.[29]

PLATELET SATELLITISM

Antibodies directed against GPIIb/IIIa may react simultaneously with the leukocyte Fcγreceptor III (FcγRIII) and attach the platelets to neutrophils and monocytes, inducing a phenomenon known as *platelet leukocyte satellitism*,[28] another form of pseudothrombocytopenia (Fig. 119–1). These antibodies fail to produce satellitism in the presence of platelets from patients with type I Glanzmann thrombasthenia or in the presence of neutrophils from patients with congenital absence of FcγRIII.[28] Typically, the platelets form a rosette around the periphery of leukocytes. Neutrophils are most frequently involved, but the phenomenon also is occasionally observed with monocytes.[33,34] These antibodies also are naturally occurring, and their presence does not clearly correlate with any specific clinical situation, disease, or drug. As with the antibodies that induce only platelet clumping, exposure of a cryptic antigen on EDTA-treated platelets and leukocytes may trigger this phenomenon.

ANTIPHOSPHOLIPID ANTIBODIES

Some antiplatelet antibodies from patients with pseudothrombocytopenia cross-react with negatively charged phospholipids and may exhibit anticardiolipin activity.[26] The sera of these patients lose their ability to clump platelets when adsorbed onto either cardiolipin or activated normal platelets, supporting the hypothesis that antibody subpopulations directed against negatively charged phospholipids can bind to antigens modified by EDTA on the platelet membrane. Another possibility is that the antigens in this case are negatively charged phospholipids on the surface of platelets.

GLYCOPROTEIN IIB/IIIA ANTAGONISTS

Thrombocytopenia has been described in patients suffering from acute coronary syndromes treated with the GPIIb/IIIa antagonist abciximab and other GPIIb/IIIa antagonists.[35–37] Abciximab is associated with both pseudothrombocytopenia and true thrombocytopenia. The mechanism for platelet clumping with abciximab is unknown, and the drug itself likely is not crosslinking the platelets because it is monovalent. More likely, other agglutinins bind GPIIb/IIIa at new epitopes induced by the combination of abciximab binding and calcium chelation. True abciximab-induced thrombocytopenia occurs in approximately 0.3 to 1 percent of patients treated with the drug.[38] The mechanism is incompletely understood, but likely includes formation or reaction of preformed antibodies to a neoepitope expressed after binding of abciximab to GPIIb/IIIa (ligand-induced binding sites) or abciximab-induced platelet activation with subsequent platelet sequestration from the circulation. In some abciximab-treated patients, high antibody titers are detected in the plasma.

The incidence of pseudothrombocytopenia and thrombocytopenia related to abciximab was determined in four large placebo-controlled trials:[36] c7E3 Fab Antiplatelet Therapy in Unstable Refractory Angina (CAPTURE), Evaluation of 7E3 for the Prevention of Ischemic Complications (EPIC), Evaluation of Percutaneous Transluminal Coronary Angioplasty to Improve Long-term Outcome of c7E3 GPIIb/IIIa Receptor Blockade (EPILOG), and Evaluation of Platelet IIb/IIIa Inhibitor for Stenting (EPISTENT). In these studies, pseudothrombocytopenia accounted for more than one-third of low platelet counts in patients undergoing coronary interventions and treated with abciximab. These studies demonstrated that pseudothrombocytopenia is a benign laboratory condition not associated with increased bleeding, stroke, transfusion requirements, or the need for repeat revascularization.

MISCELLANEOUS ASSOCIATIONS

Some studies suggest that platelet agglutinins occur more frequently in hospitalized patients and in association with medical conditions such as autoimmune diseases, malignancy, liver disease, and sepsis.[21,39–42] However, others found no association with any particular pathology or with use of specific drugs.[26]

One study showed that antibodies from patients with pseudothrombocytopenia can induce agglutination of donor platelets in the presence of EDTA. This agglutination was prevented by warming the donor platelets to 37°C or by pretreating the platelets with aspirin, prostaglandin E_1, apyrase, and monoclonal antibodies against GPIIb/IIIa that block the binding site for fibrinogen and the von Willebrand factor (VWF) or RGD peptide, which binds the site on GPIIb/IIIa that recognizes cytoadhesive proteins.[29] Whether the same reaction occurs *in vivo* is not known, but in that case the antibodies should have a slow reactivity, or else a bleeding diathesis should be expected.

DIAGNOSIS

An automated platelet count must be confirmed by microscopic examination of the blood film. Automated cell counters identify platelets merely based on their small volumes, generally defined as volumes between 2 and 20 fl. Because the platelet clumps tend to exceed 20 fl, the clumps may be counted as leukocytes.[14] Thus, pseudothrombocytopenia may be accompanied by pseudoleukocytosis.[1,8,17,20] The greater the delay in processing of anticoagulated blood, the greater is the degree of platelet clumping and the greater the potential for artifact.[17]

Platelet clumping can be prevented by collecting the sample in EDTA and maintaining its temperature at 37°C. Even with these measures, however, clumping still will be present in approximately 20 percent of cases.[26] Another alternative is use of sodium citrate, which chelates calcium more weakly than does EDTA but still causes platelet clumping in approximately 10 to 20 percent of cases with EDTA-induced clumping. In some patients, an accurate platelet count can be obtained only by sampling blood directly into ammonium oxalate and manually counting the platelets using a Bruker chamber.[26]

IMPLICATIONS

Platelet agglutinins are not associated with bleeding or thrombosis, so they appear to have no clinical implications. Transplacental transmission has been documented, but the pseudothrombocytopenia induced by these antibodies in the neonate resolves spontaneously.[43] No complications have been reported when platelet agglutinins are discovered during pregnancy.[43,44] Transfusion of blood products from patients with pseudothrombocytopenia produces an acceptable corrected count increment in the recipient, again supporting its benign nature.[19] Thus, the clinical importance of pseudothrombocytopenia concerns conditions with which it is confused rather than any pathology associated with the condition. It is important that this syndrome be recognized promptly to avoid unnecessary diagnostic tests and treatment.

THROMBOCYTOPENIA RESULTING FROM IMPAIRED PLATELET PRODUCTION

CONGENITAL THROMBOCYTOPENIA RESULTING FROM IMPAIRED PLATELET PRODUCTION

MYH9-*Related Thrombocytopenia Syndromes*

Genetics May-Hegglin anomaly, Fechtner syndrome, Sebastian syndrome, and Epstein syndrome are autosomal dominant macrothrombocytopenias with mutations in the *MYH9* gene,[45–49] located on chromosome 22q12–13. This gene encodes nonmuscle myosin heavy chain (NMMHC)-IIA, which is expressed in platelets, kidney, leukocytes, and the cochlea.[50–54] Breeding of genetically engineered mice deficient in *MYH9* failed to yield homozygous animals, strongly arguing for a critical developmental role for the gene.[55] In all cells in which the gene product is expressed, except platelets and leukocytes, other NMMHC isoforms (IIB and IIC) are also expressed, and these can compensate functionally for the defective IIA isoform, restricting the most profound manifestations of NMMHC-IIA deficiency to platelets and leukocytes.[56] Several studies demonstrate that mutations affecting the motor domain at the N-terminus of NMMHC-IIA cause a more severe phenotype than those affecting the tail domain at the C-terminus of the protein. Those individuals with motor domain mutations tended to have more severe thrombocytopenia and to develop nephritis and deafness at an earlier age (before age 40 years).[57] Those with tail domain mutations have milder thrombocytopenia, and the hearing and renal impairments may be subclinical or occur only at older ages.

Pathogenesis of Thrombocytopenia and Platelet Functional Defects The NMMHC-IIA protein appears to be an important cytoskeletal contractile protein in hematopoietic cells.[52] One mutation in the *MYH9* gene produced a highly unstable protein with abnormal organization of the megakaryocyte cytoskeleton.[58] The defect in platelet number is likely a defect in platelet maturation from proplatelets, as when *MYH9*-deficient stem cells were differentiated to megakaryocytes they produced proplatelets normally.[59] Unexpectedly, when *MYH9* was introduced into these cells, the proplatelet number decreased, suggesting that NMMHC-IIA is actually a negative regulator of thrombopoiesis. Megakaryocyte/platelet–specific knockout of *MYH9* produced mice with markedly prolonged bleeding times and platelets defective in thrombus growth and organization.[60] Interestingly, platelet aggregation in response to almost all agonists was near normal but clot retraction was defective. Near-normal aggregation also has been demonstrated with platelets from patients,[61] with the exception that the shape change reaction was absent.

Clinical Findings Affected patients have the triad of thrombocytopenia, macrothrombocytes, and Döhle body-like inclusions in the leukocytes (Fig. 119–2), except for those with Epstein syndrome, which lacks the latter, and various degrees of high-tone sensorineural deafness, nephritis, and cataracts.[46] Hematuria and proteinuria are manifestations of the glomerulonephritic lesions present in a proportion of patients. Selective high-tone hearing loss and cataracts also develop in varying proportions of patients. Patients may have a history of mild bleeding, but they may be completely asymptomatic and discovered incidentally. Conversely, patients may have a bleeding tendency despite a seemingly adequate platelet count and normal standard platelet function test results. Expression of GPIb/IX/V on the surface of platelets from May-Hegglin anomaly is reduced and could account for this finding.[50]

One hallmark feature of *MYH9*-related disorders is revealed on the blood film, where neutrophilic inclusions that appear blue with Wright-Giemsa stain are noted. The inclusions correspond to cytoplasmic aggregates of NMMHC-IIA, which are readily detected by immunocytochemistry (see Fig. 119–2).[62–65]

Treatment Patients with *MYH9*-related disorders may be misdiagnosed with ITP and subjected to inappropriate treatment with glucocorticoids, intravenous immunoglobulin (IVIg), or splenectomy. Thus, the patient and the patient's relatives should be educated to avoid potentially dangerous treatments for presumed ITP. Treatment of *MYH9*-related disorders generally is supportive, with platelet transfusions given only in specific instances, such as uncontrolled bleeding, prior to major surgery, and with a complicated delivery. 1-Deamino-8-D-arginine vasopressin (DDAVP) is recommended before surgical procedures (0.3 mcg/kg) and 24 hours after surgery, combined with tranexamic acid.[56] Caution should be exercised when using these measures, as the platelet defect does not protect the patients from postsurgical venous thrombosis, and thromboprophylaxis should be considered when the risk is high.[66,67] It has been suggested that because of the large platelets found in the disorder, it is important to treat anemia, as a normal complement of red cells is necessary for optimal platelet–endothelial interactions.[56] To prevent renal disease, blockade of the renin–angiotensin system may delay the onset of proteinuria and renal impairment.[68]

Mediterranean Macrothrombocytopenia

Mediterranean macrothrombocytopenia is a mild congenital thrombocytopenia with an autosomal dominant pattern of inheritance.[69] The

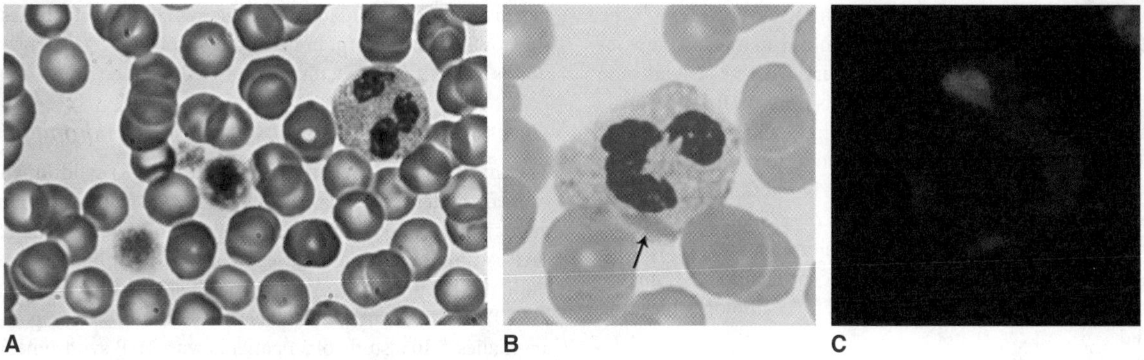

FIGURE 119–2. *MYH9* abnormality. **A.** Blood film. May-Hegglin anomaly. Macrothrombocytes, thrombocytopenia, and light blue cytoplasmic inclusions in neutrophils. Note two giant platelets approximately the diameter of red cells. The neutrophil has a large gray-blue inclusion in the cytoplasm at the 9 o'clock position. **B.** Blood film. Neutrophil of an individual with a mutation (E1841K) in exon 38 of the *MYH9* gene. This mutation results in macrothrombocytopenia and Döhle-body–like inclusions in neutrophils (*arrow*). **C.** Blood film. Immunofluorescent analysis with antibodies to the A heavy-chain of nonmuscle myosin in the neutrophils of the same patient as in (**B**). The fluorescent body in the neutrophil indicates that the inclusion contains precipitated nonmuscle myosin heavy chains, characteristic of this family of disorders. *(Used with permission from* Lichtman's Atlas of Hematology, *www.accessmedicine.com. Images **B** and **C** kindly were provided for the* Atlas *by Dr. Shinji Kunishima, the Japanese Red Cross Aichi Blood Center, Nagoya, Japan.)*

condition initially was described in a group of 145 apparently healthy subjects from Italy and the Balkan Peninsula.[69] Because the undefined macrothrombocytopenia was not present in controls from northern Europe, it was named *Mediterranean macrothrombocytopenia*. Many of the patients shared clinical and molecular features with the heterozygous Bernard-Soulier syndrome phenotype.[70] Linkage analyses revealed a heterozygous Ala156Val missense substitution in the *GPIbα* gene (also known as the *Bolzano mutation*), which is also present in patients with Bernard-Soulier syndrome. Patients with true autosomal hereditary thrombocytopenia without the mutation have a normal content of platelet glycoproteins, whereas the content is abnormal in those with the mutation, similar to that found in Bernard-Soulier syndrome heterozygotes.[70] The clinical manifestations of Mediterranean macrothrombocytopenia are variable, with the severity of bleeding related to both platelet number and function.

A related syndrome with concomitant stomatocytosis and hemolysis (Mediterranean stomatocytosis/macrothrombocytopenia) and autosomal recessive transmission is caused by mutations in the genes *ABCG5* and *ABCG8*, encoding two subunits of a ABC cassette sterol transporter expressed in the gut.[71] This disorder is a variant of phytosterolemia (sitosterolemia), a syndrome caused by unrestricted cholesterol and plant sterol absorption in the gut. In addition to hemolysis, all of the patients also had defective ristocetin-induced platelet aggregation, an indication that the abnormal sterol content of the platelets somehow interferes with the function of the GPIb/IX/V complex. This also suggests that the large platelets reflect abnormal GPIb/IX/V function in megakaryocytes.

Familial Platelet Syndrome with Predisposition to Acute Myelogenous Leukemia

Pathogenesis Familial platelet syndrome with predisposition to acute myelogenous leukemia (FPS/AML) is a rare autosomal dominant condition characterized by qualitative and quantitative platelet defects resulting in pathologic bleeding and predisposition to the development of AML.[72] Genetic analysis of several pedigrees linked the causative defect to a mutation in the transcription factor Runx-1 (also known as AML1 and CBFA2).[73] Runx-1 binds to transcriptional complexes and regulates many genes important in hematopoiesis. Mutations of *Runx*-1 are commonly involved in the pathogenesis of sporadic leukemias and myelodysplastic syndromes (MDSs), stressing the importance of this transcription factor in normal hematopoiesis.[74] Genetic studies performed in animals engineered to have altered expression of *Runx*-1 and in humans affected with FPS/AML suggest that a deficiency of the full-length Runx-1 leads to an expanded population of undifferentiated hematopoietic stem cells (HSCs).[75] In animal models, at least one functional copy of Runx-1 is required to affect definitive embryonic hematopoiesis. In contrast, patients with point mutations in one allele are predisposed to develop AML in adult life.[73,75] The reason for the thrombocytopenia seen in this disorder is unknown, but the explanation may lie in the interaction of Runx-1 with the megakaryocytic transcription factors GATA-1 and Fli-1 (see Chap. 113).[76,77]

Clinical Features The degree of thrombocytopenia in FPS/AML is mild to moderate. Platelets are of normal size and morphology but may have functional defects that lead to a prolonged bleeding time and clinical bleeding. The marrow may show decreased levels of megakaryocytic progenitor cells.

Autosomal Dominant Thrombocytopenia with Linkage to Human Chromosome 10

This autosomal dominant thrombocytopenia has a genetic defect localized to 10p11–12 on the short arm of chromosome 10.[78,79] In one large kindred with the disorder, a missense mutation was identified within the gene *FLJ14813*a,[80] which encodes a putative tyrosine kinase of unknown function. Pedigree studies show that the thrombocytopenia segregates with incomplete differentiation of megakaryocytes. Megakaryocyte precursors from affected individuals produce low numbers of polyploid cells *in vitro*, with delayed nuclear and cytoplasmic differentiation when analyzed by electron microscopy.[78] Thus, the newly identified kinase (possibly a tyrosine kinase) seems to be involved in megakaryocyte endomitosis and terminal maturation. Affected family members have lifelong moderate thrombocytopenia, with a risk of bleeding proportionate to the degree of thrombocytopenia, but without any association with hematopoietic malignancy or progression to aplastic anemia.[78]

Paris-Trousseau Syndrome

Paris-Trousseau syndrome and its variant Jacobsen syndrome are congenital dysmorphology syndromes in which affected individuals manifest trigonocephaly, facial dysmorphism, heart defects, and mental retardation.[81] Both disorders result from deletion of the long arm of chromosome 11 at 11q23, a region that includes the *FLI1* gene,[82] the product of which is a transcription factor involved in megakaryopoiesis.[9,83] The dominant inheritance pattern of Paris-Trousseau syndrome despite the presence of one normal allele seems to result from monoallelic expression of *FLI1* only during a brief window in megakaryocyte differentiation.[83,84] All affected patients have mild to moderate thrombocytopenia and dysfunctional platelets.[81] The blood film shows a subpopulation of platelets containing giant α granules.[82] Marrow examination reveals two distinct subpopulations of megakaryocytes with expansion of immature megakaryocytic progenitors, dysmegakaryopoiesis, and many micromegakaryocytes.[83] Pathologic bleeding usually is mild.

Thrombocytopenia with Radial-Ulnar Synostosis

Clinical Features Patients with amegakaryocytic thrombocytopenia with radioulnar synostosis present at birth with severe normocytic thrombocytopenia with absent marrow megakaryocytes, proximal radioulnar synostosis, and other skeletal anomalies such as clinodactyly and shallow acetabulae.[85] Bleeding complications are proportional to the degree of thrombocytopenia. Subsequent development of hypoplastic anemia and pancytopenia occurred in several individuals, suggesting that the defect is not limited to megakaryocytic progenitors.

Pathogenesis Genetic analysis of patients with thrombocytopenia and radioulnar synostosis revealed a mutation in *HoxA11*.[86] The Hox family of genes is characterized by a conserved DNA-binding domain, termed the *homeobox*, a region that helps direct their transcriptional activity. These genes are known primarily for their role in embryonic development and cell fate determination. Studies have shown that members of Hox clusters A and B are expressed in HSCs. By manipulating the levels of HoxB4 and HoxA9 in mice, several investigators have shown that these genes are important in maintaining adequate numbers of HSCs.[87] Although defects in *HoxA10* and *HoxA11* result in forearm defects and expression of each gene has been detected in HSCs, only *HoxA10* has been shown to be expressed in megakaryocytes.[88] Mice that are genetically null for *HoxA11* have forearm defects and impaired fertility, but no description of hematopoiesis in these mice has been reported. Thus, how elimination of HoxA11 function alters thrombopoiesis in humans is not clear, but the associated development of aplastic anemia suggests that the defect is at the level of the HSC.

Congenital Amegakaryocytic Thrombocytopenia

Congenital amegakaryocytic thrombocytopenia (CAMT) is a rare disease that in most cases presents with severe thrombocytopenia without physical abnormalities at birth. Bleeding complications usually are substantial because of the severe thrombocytopenia present in these children. The disorder progresses to aplastic anemia before age 3 to 5 years in most patients. CAMT results from mutations in the thrombopoietin (TPO) receptor c-Mpl, rendering it deficient (type I CAMT) or of reduced function (type II CAMT).[89,90] The first patient in whom the pathogenesis of the disorder was identified displayed compound heterozygosity for two mutations in the *c-MPL* gene, both of which encoded truncated c-Mpl receptor polypeptides lacking all domains essential for intracellular signals.[91] Sequence analysis in eight patients with CAMT uncovered nonsense or missense mutations in all of them.[92]

Mutations of the TPO receptor are associated with greatly reduced megakaryopoiesis, which correlates with the decreased number of megakaryocyte precursors seen in the marrow at birth. TPO affects megakaryocytes but also multipotent hematopoietic stem and progenitor cells.[93–95] The gradual loss of CD34+ cells and hematopoietic progenitor cells in the blood and marrow of CAMT patients with increasing age, eventuating in marrow failure, establishes the critical role for TPO and c-Mpl in human HSC biology.[96] Marrow transplantation is the only curative therapy for CAMT.

Thrombocytopenia with Absent Radius Syndrome

The thrombocytopenia and absent radii (TAR) syndrome is a rare disease, first identified[97] in 1959, that occurs with an approximate frequency of 1 in 500,000 to 1,000,000 births. The inheritance pattern of TAR is unknown. The disease is characterized by the absence of both radii in the presence of both thumbs and thrombocytopenia (Fig. 119–3).[98] The disorder is associated with a broad range of congenital anomalies.[98] In a study of 34 patients with TAR syndrome, all cases had documented thrombocytopenia and bilateral radial aplasia, 47 percent had lower-limb anomalies, 47 percent had intolerance to cow's milk, 23 percent had renal anomalies, and 15 percent had cardiac anomalies,[99] results consistent with previous reports.[100]

The thrombocytopenia in TAR syndrome usually is moderate, with platelet counts of approximately 50×10^9/L. Although occasionally more severe early in life, the platelet count in patients with TAR tend to improve with age. Thus, given a strong clinical suspicion, the diagnosis should not be excluded based on one isolated normal count. The etiology of the thrombocytopenia is unknown, but most authors agree the defect directly involves the megakaryocytes and causes an early arrest in megakaryopoiesis.[101] Serum TPO levels are normal,[102] and marrow cellularity is normal or increased. Megakaryocytes are low in number, or absent, or appear immature.

Affected patients can be managed with platelet transfusions and supportive treatment. Treatment usually is required only at early ages when the thrombocytopenia is more severe. Death is most commonly caused by bleeding in very young patients. In a review of 77 patients, only 1 death related to thrombocytopenia occurred after age 14 months.[100]

Wiskott-Aldrich Syndrome

Definition, Genetics, and Pathogenesis Wiskott-Aldrich syndrome (WAS) is a rare X-linked immunodeficiency disorder characterized by microthrombocytopenia, eczema, recurrent infections, T-cell deficiency, and increased risk for autoimmune and lymphoproliferative disorders (see Chap. 82).[103,104] The syndrome is caused by mutations of the *WASP* gene located on the short arm of the X chromosome (Xp11.22).[105–107] The product of this gene, the WAS protein (WASP), is expressed in hematopoietic cells. WASP regulates actin polymerization and coordinates reorganization of the actin cytoskeleton and signal transduction pathways that occur during cell movement and cell–cell interaction.[108] Microthrombocytopenia is the most consistent feature of WASP-associated disease, but the mechanism of reduced production and abnormal size remains incompletely understood. Mutant WASP is uniformly absent in platelets, even in the mildest patient phenotypes, suggesting a direct role of WASP deficiency in producing thrombocytopenia.[109] In some patients, destruction of platelets is increased as they may experience a significant rise in platelet count after splenectomy.[110] Because of a compromise in the cytoskeleton, a selective physical restriction to transmigration of larger platelets through the splenic vasculature leads to destruction of larger platelets in the spleen with resulting microthrombocytopenia.[111] Some studies have suggested a defect of platelet production, but the mechanism remains unclear.

Clinical Findings Clinically, the genetic defect produces cellular and humoral immunodeficiency, high susceptibility to autoimmune diseases, and increased risk for developing hematologic malignancies. This is the classic presentation, but the disease has a broad clinical spectrum that tends to correlate with the location and nature of the causative mutation.[108,111] More than 300 mutations have been described, and the

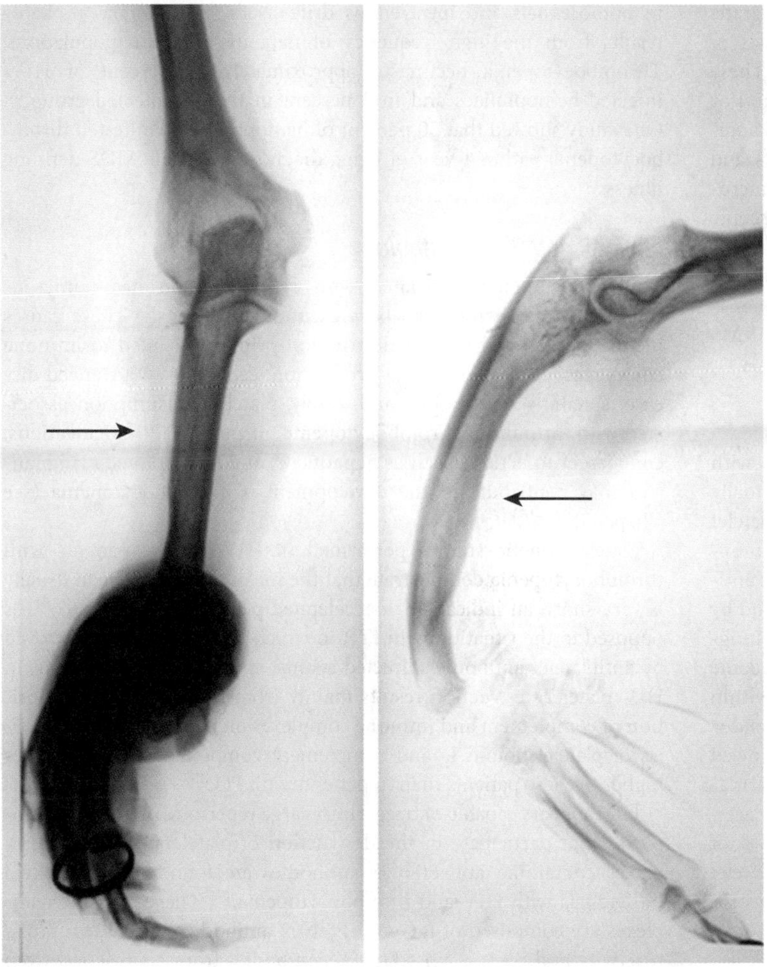

FIGURE 119–3. Thrombocytopenia with absent radii (TAR syndrome). Radiograph of right forearm. A 48-year-old woman with repeated platelet counts in the range of 85–100 × 10^9/L. Bleeding time was 11 minutes. No laboratory evidence of von Willebrand disease. Marrow examination was normal. Both forearms were short and bowed with angulated wrists and normal hands. No family history of forearm deformity. **A.** Anterior-posterior film of right arm. **B.** Lateral film of right arm. Absence of radius and bowed, hypertrophied ulna (*arrows*). Angulation deformity at wrist. *(Used with permission from* Lichtman's Atlas of Hematology, *www.accessmedicine.com. Kindly provided for the* Atlas *by Timothy J. Woodlock, Unity Health Systems, Rochester, NY.)*

clinical picture varies from mild microthrombocytopenia alone (also called *X-linked thrombocytopenia*) to the full-blown syndrome.[112,113]

Treatment HSC transplantation is the treatment of choice for patients with severe WAS. It corrects both thrombocytopenia and immunodeficiency and should always be considered, even in patients with milder phenotypes, because of the risk of developing hematologic malignancies.[114,115] Supportive treatment during acute bleeding and disease complications consists of platelet transfusions, antibiotics, and systemic glucocorticoids when eczema is severe. Patients with mild phenotypes and severe thrombocytopenia may respond to splenectomy, but the risk of infection in these already immunocompromised patients may outweigh the benefit. Some patients may have a rise in platelet count in response to prednisolone or methylprednisolone pulse therapy, but the response is only transient. The thrombocytopenia is not mediated by the humoral immune system, as platelet autoantibodies are absent and patients do not respond to IVIg therapy. Gene therapy, with retrovirus-mediated transfer of the *WASP* gene, is under active investigation and shows promise in experimental animals.[116–118]

X-linked Thrombocytopenia with Dyserythropoiesis

A family of X-linked disorders of thrombocytopenia associated with dyserythropoiesis and thalassemia has been described.[119] GATA-1 (named after the core nucleotide binding sequence guanine-adenine-thymidine-adenine) is a transcription factor containing two zinc fingers: the carboxyl-terminal finger supports DNA binding and the amino-terminal finger stabilizes its binding to DNA and interacts with the cofactor friend of GATA-1 (FOG-1). In several families, mutation in the amino-terminal finger is associated with macrothrombocytopenia and variable abnormalities in the erythroid lineage, whereas in other families, mutations in the amino-terminal finger that disrupt the interaction of GATA-1 with FOG-1 lead to macrothrombocytopenia with dyserythropoietic anemia or β-thalassemia.[120] Although GATA-1 was first recognized for its vital role in erythropoiesis, GATA-1 and FOG-1 subsequently were shown to be critical for megakaryopoiesis,[121,122] as the GATA-1 consensus motif is found in the 5′ flanking regions of almost all characterized erythroid and megakaryocyte specific genes.[123] Although GATA-1 null mice die in embryogenesis of severe anemia, a megakaryocyte-specific deletion of the transcription factor allows sufficient erythropoiesis for survival, revealing the role of the transcription factor in megakaryopoiesis. These mice demonstrate hyperproliferation of immature low ploidy megakaryocyte progenitor cells associated with abnormal maturation and reduced expression of platelet specific genes.[124] Chapter 113 discusses the role of GATA-1 and FOG in megakaryopoiesis.

Fanconi Anemia

Patients with Fanconi anemia occasionally present with predominant thrombocytopenia, but the coexistent anemia and dysmorphogenesis usually make the diagnosis obvious. Chapter 34 discusses the disorder in greater detail.

THROMBOCYTOPENIA RESULTING FROM PLATELET TRAPPING

■ KASABACH-MERRITT SYNDROME

Definition

Kasabach-Merritt syndrome (KMS) is defined as profound thrombocytopenia related to platelet trapping within a vascular tumor, either a Kaposi-like hemangioendothelioma or a tufted angioma.[125–128] The syndrome presents predominantly during infancy, but several adult cases have been reported.[129] These vascular tumors should be differentiated from vascular malformations such as classic benign hemangiomas. Benign hemangiomas usually are superficial, multiple, not associated with severe thrombocytopenia or disseminated intravascular coagulopathy (DIC; see Chap. 130), and usually disappear during childhood. On the other hand, Kaposi-like hemangioendothelioma and tufted angioma are low-grade malignant vascular tumors associated with high morbidity and mortality.

Histopathology

Vascular tumors usually are solitary, may reach 20 cm in diameter, and may be superficial or invade internal organs and the retroperitoneum.[130–132] Superficial tumors can be recognized by the local red to purple discoloration of the skin.

The histologic types more frequently associated with KMS are Kaposi-like hemangioendothelioma and tufted angiomas or angioblastomas.[125,126,133,134]

Kaposi-like hemangioendothelioma is a locally aggressive, low-grade malignant tumor characterized by infiltrating sheets or lobules of poorly formed vascular channels and aberrant lymphatic vessels. These tumors are composed predominantly of plump, round, oval, and/or spindled endothelial cells with hemosiderin deposits.[125] A tufted angioma is a lesion characterized by the presence of vascular tufts and aggregates of round dilated capillaries, lymphangiomatosis, microthrombi, and hemosiderin deposits.[125,126,135,136] Electron microscopic examination shows abnormal endothelial cells with prominent cytoplasmic projections and wide intercellular gaps, fibrin deposition, and platelet aggregates within the vessels.[126] The histology of the tumor is useful for differentiating the vascular tumors associated with KMS from benign capillary hemangiomas.[137]

Clinical Findings

Thrombocytopenia in KMS usually is severe and associated with DIC.[138] Contributing factors include "platelet trapping" by abnormally proliferating endothelium within the hemangioma[139,140] and platelet consumption associated with DIC. Platelet trapping has been demonstrated by immunohistochemical staining of the tumors with anti-CD61 antibodies (a marker of platelets and megakaryocytes)[141] and by nuclear studies using ^{51}Cr-labeled platelets[142] and ^{111}In platelet scintigraphy to monitor response to therapy.[143,144] How platelets become trapped is not clear. Initial physical entrapment of the platelets within twisted abnormal vessels may favor their adhesion to abnormal endothelium, which may lead to platelet activation and aggregation followed by activation of the coagulation cascade, fibrin deposition, and formation of microthrombi. Excessive flow and shear rates generated by arteriovenous shunting within the tumor further increase the level of platelet activation. Continuous thrombus formation leads to platelet consumption and activation of the fibrinolytic cascade. Severe thrombocytopenia and DIC result.

Treatment and Course

The mainstay of treatment is eradication of the tumor. Several specific therapeutic modalities have been proposed, but none has been established as consistently effective.[145] Among the therapies are high-dose glucocorticoids,[145] interferon-α,[145,146] vincristine,[147] cyclophosphamide,[148] combination chemotherapy,[149] and radiation.[150–152] For severe cases, interventions such as arterial embolization[153,154] surgical resection,[155,156] and pneumatic compression can be attempted.

The mortality rate for advanced KMS is approximately 12 percent; the rate is higher when associated with retroperitoneal or intraabdominal tumors. Patients die of complications resulting from DIC, low platelet count, and infections secondary to immunosuppression.

ACQUIRED THROMBOCYTOPENIA RESULTING FROM IMPAIRED PLATELET PRODUCTION

THROMBOCYTOPENIA ASSOCIATED WITH HIV INFECTION

Prevalence

Thrombocytopenia is common in patients infected with HIV, with the prevalence of thrombocytopenia, depending on the subpopulation of patients studied (see Chap. 83).[157] Among HIV-infected drug users, the prevalence is approximately 36.9 percent, compared to 8.7 percent in drug users without HIV infection.[158] In homosexual men, the prevalence is approximately 16 percent in the HIV-infected group and 3 percent in the HIV-negative group.[158] The high prevalence of thrombocytopenia in homosexuals and intravenous drug users without HIV probably results from the high frequency of hepatitis in these populations. Thrombocytopenia occurs in approximately 19 percent of HIV-infected hemophiliacs and in 3 percent in the noninfected group.[159] One study showed that 50 percent of hemophiliacs manifested thrombocytopenia within 1 year of being diagnosed with an AIDS-defining illness.[159]

Etiology and Physiopathology

Thrombocytopenia associated with HIV infection has numerous causes, many of which can be present simultaneously. These causes include accelerated platelet destruction primarily related to immune complexes, decreased platelet production, especially in advanced disease, splenic sequestration, and, rarely, platelet consumption associated with thrombotic thrombocytopenic purpura (TTP). Medications, concurrent infections such as hepatitis C, and hematologic malignancies may contribute to the development of thrombocytopenia (see Chap. 83).[160–163]

Platelet kinetic studies performed in HIV-positive patients with thrombocytopenia demonstrate that the mean platelet life span usually is very short, an indication of accelerated platelet destruction.[10,164] As opposed to the situation with ITP, in which the platelets are destroyed by antiplatelet antibodies directed against specific platelet antigens, in HIV platelet destruction results mainly from the nonspecific deposition of complement and immune complexes on platelets.[165,166] The levels of platelet-bound Ig and complement components are four times higher in these patients than in patients with ITP.[167–170]

HIV appears capable of triggering a large repertoire of immune complexes that participate in the destruction of platelets. Immune complexes containing anti-F(ab′)2 antibodies are found in homosexual individuals with HIV and thrombocytopenia.[171] These immune complexes are composed of IgG anti-F(ab′)2 antibodies that have a broad reactivity and react against F(ab′)2 antibodies from control and from HIV-infected patients. Part of the immune complex bound to platelets has been proposed to correspond to IgG anti-F(ab′)2 antibodies.[171]

Antibodies against CD4 and the CD4 receptor gp120 have been found in HIV-positive patients with and without thrombocytopenia.[172] Studies with affinity-purified anti-CD4 and anti-gp120 have shown that the antibodies are capable of forming complexes through their specificity-determining regions.[172–174] These immune complexes can bind platelets and have been postulated to play a role in the thrombocytopenia associated with HIV.

High-affinity antibodies against platelet GPIIIa have been eluted from the platelets of thrombocytopenic patients infected with HIV.[175] These antibodies react against a specific region on the molecule located between amino acids 49 and 66. That these antibodies are physiologically relevant is supported by *in vivo* studies showing that administration of the antibodies systemically produces significant thrombocytopenia, an effect that can be prevented by coadministration of an albumin conjugate of $GPIIIa_{49-66}$.[175] The presence of this immunodominant epitope appears unique to thrombocytopenia associated with HIV infection and may reflect cross-reactivity with antibodies directed against particular HIV antigens. Several studies suggest cross-reactivity of antibodies directed against viral antigens gp120 and p24 with platelet glycoproteins.[176–181]

Antiidiotype antibodies directed against anti-$GPIIIa_{49-66}$ can be detected in HIV patients, whether or not they are thrombocytopenic.[182] In the plasma, these antibodies (which usually are of the IgM type) are found as part of immune complexes. They are capable of blocking the destruction of platelets induced by anti-$GPIIIa_{49-66}$. The levels of the antiidiotype antibodies appear to be inversely related to the degree of platelet destruction. Thus, the levels are higher in HIV patients without thrombocytopenia than in patients with thrombocytopenia.

One study proposed that the mechanism of platelet destruction by anti-GPIIIa$_{49-66}$ is independent of complement.[183] Anti-GPIIIa$_{49-66}$ antibodies were shown to induce platelet fragmentation through the generation of reactive oxygen species such as H_2O_2 through the reduced nicotinamide adenine dinucleotide phosphate (NADPH) oxidase pathway. These findings where observed *in vitro* using inhibitors of reactive oxygen species and *in vivo* using p47phox-deficient mice lacking NADPH oxidase.[183,184]

Circulating immune complexes containing the head domain of talin (talin-H) associated with thrombocytopenia in HIV have been described.[185] Talin-H is a cleavage product of talin that can be generated by calpain when platelets become activated or by HIV-1 protease. Antitalin antibodies have been detected in the serum of HIV patients with thrombocytopenia but not in controls subjects with ITP. These antibodies are highly mutated, suggesting an antigen-driven, affinity-matured response that may result from exposure of immunodominant epitopes on talin-H. The role of these antibodies in producing thrombocytopenia is unknown. The fact that they are directed against a cytoskeletal antigen argues against a causative role.

In addition to increased platelet destruction, reduced platelet production appears to play a role in the thrombocytopenia observed in HIV patients.[164,186,187] A direct effect of viral infection on platelet production is suggested by the observation that platelet production increases when patients are treated with zidovudine, an antiretroviral drug.[188] Infected patients with thrombocytopenia also have increased levels of TPO, again supporting the notion of ineffective platelet production in the origin of HIV-associated thrombocytopenia.[189,190] The defect appears to lie at the level of megakaryopoiesis, as decreased levels of megakaryocyte progenitors in marrow have been observed.[186,191]

How HIV decreases megakaryopoiesis is not known. The response to antiretroviral therapy suggests that the virus infects megakaryocytes or their precursors in the marrow. HIV-1 entry into cells requires sequential interaction of the viral envelope glycoprotein gp120 with CD4 and a coreceptor on the host cell plasma membrane, either C-C chemokine receptor-5 (CCR5) or CXC chemokine receptor-4 (CXCR4).[192] All of these receptors are expressed by megakaryocytes.[193,194] CD4, the receptor for HIV-1 on T cells, has been detected by flow cytometry in approximately 25 percent of human megakaryocytes at a density comparable to that of CD4+ T cells.[195] Anti-CD4 antibodies inhibit HIV infection of megakaryocytic cell lines *in vitro*.[196]

One study determined the biologic characteristics of HIV-1 in the marrow of HIV-1–infected patients and identified distinct amino acids in the third hypervariable loop (V3) of HIV-1 envelope glycoprotein gp120 that distinguish patients with thrombocytopenia from those without thrombocytopenia.[197] This study suggests that a particular strain of HIV-1 may be causally related to the development of thrombocytopenia, either by infection of megakaryocytes or their precursors or by infection of cells of the marrow microenvironment.[197,198]

Defective modulation of hematopoiesis by HIV-infected T lymphocytes can explain impairment of megakaryopoiesis. T cells from infected patients reduce the growth *in vitro* of colony-forming units for granulocytes, erythrocytes, monocytes/macrophages, and megakaryocytes.[199] A significant increase in the growth of these colonies in marrow from HIV-infected patients was observed when the cultures were depleted of T cells. Growth inhibition recurred upon readministration of the T cells. This effect was dependent on the ratio of T4 to T8 cells.[199]

Patients with HIV are at higher risk for developing thrombotic microangiopathies.[200,201] A cohort study from New York found that one-third of patients diagnosed with TTP also were infected with HIV. The incidence of TTP was much greater in the HIV-infected patients than in the general patient population, suggesting a causal association. The causative role for HIV is also supported by the observation that the incidence of TTP associated with HIV has decreased since the advent of highly active antiretroviral therapy (HAART).[202] The relationship of HIV-associated TTP with diminished activity of the VWF-cleaving protease a disintegrin and metalloproteinase with thrombospondin repeats (ADAMTS) 13 is inconsistent, with some patients displaying low activity and inhibitors, and others not.[203–205] It has been suggested that HIV infection itself may trigger TTP in susceptible individuals,[205] a suggestion bolstered by the observation that VWF plasma levels increase with progression of HIV infection, being highest in those with full-blown AIDS.[206] In other cases, the clinical syndrome of HIV infection may overlap the clinical features of TTP, for example, in those with disseminated Kaposi sarcoma.[205]

Clinical Course

Thrombocytopenic patients with HIV rarely experience clinically important bleeding (except, of course, those with hemophilia). The platelet counts rarely dip below 50×10^9/L, and the thrombocytopenia often spontaneously resolves.[159,207–210] Thrombocytopenia in the early stages often is discovered through routine blood testing.[209] In the late stages of the disease, decreased platelet production may become more apparent, and marrow aspiration may be required to rule out infiltrative processes, although such processes are not routinely seen. One study examining the marrow in 42 patients with HIV infection found trilineage dysplasia, increased plasma cells and eosinophils, increased megakaryocytes, increased iron, and reticulin fibrosis.[211] Granulomata were found in two cases. Another study that reviewed marrow biopsies from 85 patients with HIV infection, at different stages, found increased cellularity in 72.9 percent, dysmyelopoiesis in 78.8 percent, plasma cell hyperplasia in 97.7 percent, lymphoid infiltration in 27 percent, and histiocytosis with or without granulomata in 11.7 percent.[212] In patients with end-stage AIDS, 28.2 percent had marrow hypoplasia. Opportunistic infections were seen occasionally, with agents such as *Mycobacterium avium*, *Cryptococcus neoformans*, *Toxoplasma gondii*, and *Leishmania donovani*. Malignancies were found in seven cases, including three cases of lymphoma.[212]

Treatment

Antiretroviral therapy is generally the first-line and most effective therapy for the thrombocytopenia associated with HIV infection.[209,213] Although improvements in platelet counts were previously achieved with zidovudine,[214–216] current combination antiretroviral regimens likely are more effective in increasing platelet counts as they are for enhancing CD4 cell counts and reducing HIV viral loads.[217] One retrospective study compared patients with severe thrombocytopenia treated with zidovudine to those treated with HAART. After 6 months, HAART more frequently resulted in complete and sustained recovery of platelet counts.[218] Responses were achieved even in those with zidovudine-resistant thrombocytopenia.

Management of patients with severe and symptomatic thrombocytopenia is similar to the management of patients with severe ITP. A retrospective study analyzed the response to prednisone, splenectomy, and other therapeutic modalities in 208 cases.[219] As in ITP, patients initially were treated with prednisone for 1 month; refractory or relapsed patients underwent splenectomy and/or other therapeutic modalities. An initial complete response with prednisone was seen in 38.8 percent of patients, a sustained remission that lasted for more than 6 months was observed in 18.7 percent, but only a few patients remained in remission. Splenectomy was performed in 63 patients, of whom 47 had an initial response, 41 had sustained remission, and 12 experienced sustained partial remission. Spontaneous remissions were observed in eight of 87 untreated cases. The patients who underwent splenectomy were more likely to experience a sustained complete remission. Similarly, another study of 185 HIV-infected patients showed an increase in the mean platelet count from 18×10^9/L to 223×10^9/L in those patients who underwent splenectomy, with a sustained response in 82 percent.[220] Neither AIDS progression rate nor AIDS-free survival was influenced by splenectomy. Thus, as in ITP, splenectomy is an effective therapy and appears to have no adverse effect on the progression of HIV disease.[221,222]

Other treatment modalities, such as IVIg[223,224] anti-D,[225] megakaryocyte growth factor,[226] and interferon-α,[227] have been used and reportedly were successful in particular cases. TPO-mimetic agents such as eltrombopag and romiplostim may also be effective.[228]

For HIV-associated thrombotic microangiopathy, plasma exchange may be insufficient and should always be accompanied by potent antiretroviral therapy.[203] It has also been argued that plasma exchange may have no role in this syndrome in the absence of severely depressed ADAMTS-13 activity or a detectable inhibitor.[203]

CHEMOTHERAPY AND RADIATION THERAPY

The hematopoietic system appears to promptly recover after doses of chemotherapy and radiotherapy. However, heavily treated patients have a reduced tolerance to additional therapy, showing lower nadirs of blood counts, particularly platelets.[229] Depressed marrow function has been demonstrated up to 5 years following treatment. Hypoplastic syndromes or MDSs have been observed at late intervals. During the recovery phase, severe thrombocytopenia requires prompt attention. The current American Society of Clinical Oncology recommendations for platelet transfusions include prophylactic platelet transfusions when the platelet concentration is less than 10×10^9/L (grade 4 toxicity), when the platelet concentration is less than 20×10^9/L in patients with necrotic tumors (e.g., colorectal or bladder tumors), or when performance status is decreased.[230] Several completed trials evaluated optimal dosing of platelets for patients with hypoproliferative thrombocytopenia, and whether such patients can be treated as effectively with therapeutic platelet transfusions (given only for significant bleeding) as with prophylactic transfusions (given when a specific platelet-count trigger is reached).[231] Thus far, no consensus has been reached as to whether the trigger platelet count can be lowered or what is the optimal platelet dose to be given.

Patients given multiple platelet transfusions may become refractory and show inadequate increments in the posttransfusion platelet counts. A platelet count increment less than 7×10^9/L 1 hour posttransfusion or less than 20×10^9/L 20 hours posttransfusion should raise the possibility of platelet refractoriness.[232] A true refractory state is encountered in less than half of patients treated for hematologic malignancies and results from alloimmunization against human leukocyte antigens (HLA) on leukocytes in the transfused platelets. Other potential causes of poor platelet count increments following transfusion include fever, infections, bleeding, autoantibodies, and splenomegaly. Several strategies have been proposed in an effort to minimize the risks of allogeneic platelet transfusions, including routine transfusion of leukocyte-poor platelets[233] and transfusion of autologous cryopreserved platelets obtained with recombinant human TPO or with TPO mimetics.[234] A patient with thrombocytopenia refractory to platelet transfusion can be treated with HLA-compatible platelets or large quantities of platelet concentrates.[233]

Administration of growth factors, such as interleukin (IL)-1, IL-4, IL-6, IL-3,[235–237] or IL-11,[238–244] have been used to manage thrombocytopenia by stimulating uncommitted progenitors. Several studies have shown that administration of recombinant human (rh) TPO after chemotherapy reduces the degree and duration of thrombocytopenia[245–252]; however, additional studies are needed to validate the benefit of this drug in the treatment of myelosuppressive forms of thrombocytopenia.

NUTRITIONAL DEFICIENCIES AND ALCOHOL-INDUCED THROMBOCYTOPENIA

Mild thrombocytopenia occurs in approximately 20 percent of patients with megaloblastic anemia resulting from vitamin B_{12} deficiency in the United States.[253] The frequency may be higher in patients with folic acid deficiency because of the high frequency of concomitant alcohol abuse (see Chap. 41). One large study of 139 patients examined the rates of cytopenias associated with megaloblastic anemia in India.[254] In this study, 76 percent had isolated vitamin B_{12} deficiency, 7 percent had isolated folate deficiency, 9 percent had a combined deficiency, and 8 percent had normal vitamin levels. All by definition were anemic, and 80 percent had thrombocytopenia with mild to moderate depression of the platelet count. In more than half of those with thrombocytopenia, neutropenia was also present. The authors suggested that the cytopenias tended to progress from isolated anemia, to anemia plus thrombocytopenia, to pancytopenia, with the degree of cytopenia related to the severity of vitamin deficiency. Occasionally, thrombocytopenia is severe in the megaloblastic anemias and, when accompanied by fever, hepatomegaly, and splenomegaly, the presenting features may suggest acute leukemia. In these syndromes the primary mechanism of thrombocytopenia is ineffective platelet production[255]; marrow megakaryocyte number usually is normal or increased. Abnormalities of megakaryocyte morphology are much less distinctive than the characteristic erythroid and myeloid defects, but larger size and dispersed nuclear segments, rather than polyploid single nuclei, may be seen.[256]

Thrombocytopenia may be seen in association with vitamin B_{12} deficiency when the latter results from autoantibodies against parietal cells or intrinsic factor and is associated with immune thrombocytopenia.[257,258] Various other autoimmune disorders can coexist with pernicious anemia, including autoimmune vitiligo and autoimmune thyroiditis.[259]

Abnormalities of platelet function are sometimes seen associated with vitamin B_{12} deficiency.[260,261] Diminished platelet aggregation and reduced release of adenosine diphosphate and adenosine triphosphate from granular stores in response to different agonists have been reported, and vitamin deficiency has been suggested to induce an acquired storage pool disease (see Chap. 41).[261]

Thrombocytopenia has been reported in association with iron deficiency, although thrombocytosis is a much more common association (see Chap. 42). One study described thrombocytopenia in six iron-deficient children ranging in age from 14 months to 17 years, with the platelet counts ranging from 11 to 102×10^9/L. In all patients, platelet counts returned to normal with iron repletion. Another study reported the case of a multiparous woman who presented with a platelet count of 9×10^9/L, menorrhagia, and severe anemia because of iron deficiency. The marrow revealed no evidence of an underlying hematologic abnormality, and all findings resolved with repletion of iron stores.[262] These reports illustrate the extent to which severe iron deficiency can diminish the platelet count.

Thrombocytopenia in alcoholic patients almost always results from liver cirrhosis with relative TPO deficiency (the liver is the primary origin of circulating TPO levels), congestive splenomegaly, and/or from folic acid deficiency. In some patients, thrombocytopenia results primarily from direct marrow suppression by alcohol of platelet production.[263–267] Suppression of platelet production sufficient to produce thrombocytopenia requires consumption of large quantities of ethanol over several days.[263] However, one study of guinea pigs allowed to ingest ethanol *ad libitum* showed that, although blood ethanol never reached measurable levels, the average platelet count declined 16 percent in the 4 weeks of study.[265] The platelets of the ethanol-imbibing guinea pigs were smaller than those of the control animals.

Thrombocytopenia induced by alcohol ingestion is accompanied by a decreased number of marrow megakaryocytes. Vacuolated proerythroblasts and granulocyte precursors are sometimes seen, as are multinuclear erythroblasts and megaloblasts.[266] Vacuolization of the periphery of mature megakaryocytes has been reported.[264] Thrombocytopenia usually resolves in 5 to 21 days with cessation of ethanol ingestion, sometimes with a transient rebound thrombocytosis.

PAROXYSMAL NOCTURNAL HEMOGLOBINURIA

Thrombocytopenia in patients with paroxysmal nocturnal hemoglobinuria primarily results from marrow failure (see Chap. 40). Decreased platelet production has been shown by kinetic studies using autologous radiolabeled platelets[268] and by *in vitro* studies using CD34+ cells from paroxysmal nocturnal hemoglobinuria patients.[269,270] These cells demonstrate decreased proliferation and differentiation of megakaryocyte progenitors, as is seen in aplastic anemia, suggesting a defect at the stem cell level.[270] Thrombocytopenia also may be explained by platelet consumption associated with ongoing thrombosis. The molecular bases of thrombophilia in these patients are unknown. Several mechanisms have been proposed, including excessive generation of platelet microvesicles released from complement-injured and -activated platelets,[271,272] increased prothrombinase activity on C5b-C9–injured platelets,[273] increased tissue factor expression by complement-injured CD55- and CD59-deficient monocytes and macrophages,[274] resistance to fibrinolytic stimuli because of detachment of the glycosylphosphatidylinositol-anchored urokinase plasminogen activator receptor from monocytes and neutrophils,[275,276] and elevated microparticles from damaged endothelium.[277]

MYELODYSPLASTIC SYNDROMES

Myelodysplastic syndromes are clonal myeloid disorders characterized by blood cytopenias in combination with a hypercellular marrow that often exhibit dysplastic changes in any of the three hematopoietic lineages (see Chap. 88).[278–280] Thrombocytopenia is present in approximately 50 percent of patients and usually occurs in conjunction with other cytopenias. Isolated thrombocytopenia at initial presentation occurs in less than 5 percent of cases.[281] Thrombocytopenia is seen more frequently in patients with oligoblastic myelogenous leukemia (refractory anemia with excess blasts [RAEB]) than in those with clonal cytopenias (refractory anemia and refractory anemia with ringed sideroblasts; see Chap. 88).[282] Moreover, platelets from patients with MDS often display functional abnormalities (see Chaps. 88 and 132) and, when present, usually augment the thrombocytopenia-related bleeding disorder.

The presence of micromegakaryocytes or micromononuclear megakaryocytes in marrow from MDS patients indicates altered megakaryopoiesis. Normal megakaryocytes have a diameter of 25 to 35 μm and a peak ploidy of 16N, whereas micromegakaryocytes have a diameter less than 20 μm and a peak ploidy of 4N or 8N.[283–288] The relationship between these morphologic changes and the pathophysiology of abnormal megakaryopoiesis in MDS is unknown.

Maturation of megakaryocytes is arrested in MDS, as suggested by immunohistochemistry studies showing an increased number of megakaryocytic precursors in the marrow of affected patients.[286] Besides the maturational arrest, as measured by enumeration of denuded megakaryocytic nuclei, an increased rate of apoptosis has been detected in all subtypes of MDS.[289] Immunohistochemistry studies of the marrow biopsies from patients with MDS suggest that the mechanism of programmed cell death of megakaryocytes is independent of activated caspase 3 or cathepsin D.[290] Abnormal megakaryopoiesis seems to be worse and clinically more significant in the high-risk group of patients with MDS, such as those with RAEB.[282,291] Abnormal proliferation and differentiation of megakaryocytes have been observed *in vitro*, during evaluation of the number and growth of megakaryocyte colony-forming units of mononuclear cells in marrow from patients with MDS.[292,293] Although the TPO receptor is present on megakaryocytes of patients with MDS, *in vitro* administration of TPO overcomes the underlying maturation defect in only a subset of patient cells.[294] These findings suggest that the defective response may result from either a dysfunctional receptor or an abnormality in the downstream signaling pathway rather than from diminished expression of the receptor itself.[295] In accordance with this hypothesis, some studies have shown TPO induction of blast cell proliferation in marrow from patients with RAEB and the condition previously termed RAEB-T.[296–298] Many ongoing studies aim to identify the molecular bases of the hematopoietic insufficiency and the leukemic progression in patients with the MDSs.[281] Until this goal is achieved, supportive therapy in addition to chemotherapy and marrow transplantation remain the mainstays of therapy.

APLASTIC ANEMIA

Aplastic anemia is a pancytopenia that results from failure of marrow hematopoiesis (see Chap. 34). However, some patients with MDS or amegakaryocytic thrombocytopenia present with low platelet counts and then progress to pancytopenia and aplastic anemia.[299–301] In aplastic anemia, blood testing reveals markedly decreased cell counts, reticulocytopenia, and lack of circulating blasts.

A considerable amount of data support the hypothesis that aplastic anemia results from an autoimmune attack directed against HSC.[302–304] Activated T-helper type 1 T cells that produce interferon-α, tumor necrosis factor, and IL-2 are responsible for suppression of the hematopoietic cell compartment. This cytotoxic activation leads to a Fas-mediated cell-cycle arrest and death of CD34+ cells. The majority of cases are idiopathic; however, idiosyncratic reactions to some drugs, chemicals, and viruses have been implicated in the etiology (see Chap. 34).

The development of alloantibodies to platelets is a major problem in the supportive management of thrombocytopenia in patients with severe aplastic anemia. Leukocyte-reduced platelets are helpful in preventing alloimmunization. Cyclosporine has been used to modulate alloimmunization in these patients. Platelet counts greater than 10×10^9/L should be adequate to prevent catastrophic bleeding, except in the case of breeches in vascular integrity or surgical challenge. Experimental treatment with rhIL-11 (Neumega) and with rhTPO reportedly is effective for treatment of thrombocytopenia in some patients with aplastic anemia.[305,306]

ACQUIRED PURE AMEGAKARYOCYTIC THROMBOCYTOPENIA

Thrombocytopenia attributable to pure aplasia or hypoplasia of megakaryocytes is rare.[307] More common are instances in which amegakaryocytic thrombocytopenia is seen preceding the development of full-blown myelodysplastic syndromes or aplastic anemia and is associated with subtle abnormalities of other lineages, such as macrocytosis and dyserythropoiesis.[308–312] Most commonly the disorder is caused by autoimmune suppression of megakaryocyte development, either idiopathic,[313] associated with autoimmune disorders such as systemic lupus erythematosus[314] and eosinophilic fasciitis, or associated with infections such as hepatitis C.[301] Antibodies against TPO[315] have been described to cause the disorder, as have antibodies against the TPO receptor.[316] Patients may achieve durable remission with therapies designed to blunt the autoimmune response, such as cyclosporine or antithymocyte globulin (ATG).[317]

CYCLIC THROMBOCYTOPENIA

Cyclic thrombocytopenia (CTP) is a rare acquired disorder characterized by a periodic decrease in the platelet count, sometimes followed by rebound thrombocytosis without therapy ($> 500 \times 10^9/L$).[318] Each cycle typically spans a period of 3 to 6 weeks, and women are more often affected than men. The platelet counts may fluctuate across a wide range. In reported cases, the median nadir and peak platelet counts were $10 \times 10^9/L$ (range: $1–90 \times 10^9/L$) and $330 \times 10^9/L$ (range: $72–2300 \times 10^9/L$), respectively.[319] Rebound thrombocytosis is an important and distinctive feature for CTP. Although some cases are reported as associated with myeloproliferative diseases, most CTP cases are idiopathic.[320,321] The pathophysiology is unclear and a number of potential mechanisms have been proposed, including autoimmune platelet destruction, megakaryocytic hypoplasia/aplasia, infections, and hormonal disturbances. Although most premenopausal female CTP patients studied have had low platelet counts during their menstrual periods, hysterectomy and bilateral salpingo-oophorectomy has not been shown to affect the course of the platelet fluctuations.[319]

The clinical presentation of CTP is similar to that of ITP. The bleeding tendency ranges from asymptomatic, to easy bruising, gingival bleeding, recurrent epistaxis, menorrhagia, and hematuria; to more serious bleeding, including gastrointestinal or central nervous system hemorrhage.[319] CTP is rarely considered as a differential diagnosis of thrombocytopenia, so patients are usually diagnosed and treated as having ITP. CTP is a rare disorder, but in patients with ITP who have not responded to therapies such as glucocorticoids, splenectomy, and IVIg, and who have rebound thrombocytosis, this diagnosis should be considered. Responses have been reported to hormone therapy and to cyclosporine. In female patients, oral contraceptives may be useful to prolong the menstrual cycle and cover low-platelet-count days. Antifibrinolytic drugs such as epsilon aminocaproic acid or tranexamic acid may also be useful to decrease bleeding symptoms.

THROMBOCYTOPENIA RESULTING FROM ACCELERATED PLATELET DESTRUCTION

IMMUNE (IDIOPATHIC) THROMBOCYTOPENIC PURPURA IN ADULTS

Definition and Classification

Immune (autoimmune, idiopathic) thrombocytopenic purpura is a common acquired autoimmune disorder defined by a low platelet count secondary to accelerated platelet destruction or impaired thrombopoiesis by antiplatelet antibodies. The diagnosis of ITP requires decreased platelets on the blood film and the exclusion of other causes of thrombocytopenia. Normal or increased numbers of marrow megakaryocytes are found in the majority of patients.[322] ITP can be classified based on the absence or presence of other diseases (primary or secondary), patient age (adult or childhood ITP), and duration of thrombocytopenia (acute or chronic). Antibody-mediated platelet destruction may develop in several infectious diseases, lymphoproliferative diseases, and autoimmune diseases, and in association with drug therapy (Table 119–2).

TABLE 119–2. Causes of Immune-Mediated Thrombocytopenia

1. Primary
   A. Idiopathic autoimmune thrombocytopenic purpura
2. Secondary
   A. Autoimmune diseases: systemic lupus erythematosus, antiphospholipid syndrome, autoimmune hepatitis, autoimmune thyroiditis
   B. Lymphoproliferative disorders: chronic lymphocytic leukemia, Hodgkin lymphoma, large granular lymphocytic leukemia
   C. Infections: HIV, hepatitis C, *Helicobacter pylori*
   D. Myelodysplastic syndrome
   E. Agammaglobulinemia, hypogammaglobulinemia, immunoglobulin A deficiency
   F. Drugs: quinidine, gold, heparin, penicillin, procainamide, α-methyldopa, sulfamethoxazole

The presentation and management of ITP are different in adults and children. Childhood ITP typically is acute in onset. Boys and girls are equally affected, and the condition often develops after a viral infection or vaccination. Although thrombocytopenia may be severe, it usually resolves spontaneously, within a few weeks up to 6 months.[323] A general approach to thrombocytopenia in pediatric patients is provided below (see "An Approach to Thrombocytopenia in Children"). In contrast to childhood ITP, adult ITP generally is a chronic disease of insidious onset, is predominant in women, and rarely resolves spontaneously (Table 119–3).

Incidence

ITP is relatively common, but demographic studies have yielded a wide range of incidence rates largely because of differences in the age and gender distribution of the populations studied and differences in cutoff platelet counts used to define the syndrome. In one detailed study, the reported annual incidence of ITP was 5.5 per 100,000 persons when defined by a platelet count of less than $100 \times 10^9/L$ and 3.2 per 100,000 using a cutoff platelet count less than $50 \times 10^9/L$.[324] The estimated female-to-male ratio was 1.7. The incidence of ITP increases with age, being twofold higher in populations older than age 60 years than in those younger than age 60 years.[324,325]

Pathophysiology

More than 50 years ago, Harrington and colleagues provided the first evidence that ITP could be caused by antiplatelet antibodies. In this pioneering work, normal volunteers (including Harrington himself) were infused with the plasma from patients with ITP, resulting in severe thrombocytopenia in the recipients.[326,327] Subsequently, Shulman and coworkers[328] showed that the thrombocytopenic effect of ITP plasma was dose dependent and associated with globulin fraction. Additional findings suggested that splenic clearance was the major mechanism of thrombocytopenia.[328]

In the early 1970s, two groups showed that platelets from chronic ITP patients had elevated levels of platelet-associated immunoglobulin G (PAIgG).[329,330] Elevated levels of PAIgG later were seen often in nonimmune thrombocytopenic patients.[331,332] In 1982, the first platelet target was identified. Autoantibodies from patients with ITP were shown not to bind to platelets deficient in the GPIIb/IIIa complex (i.e., from patients with Glanzmann thrombasthenia).[333] In the late 1980s, two specific assays for the target antigens were described: the immunobead assay[334] and the monoclonal antibody-specific immobilization of platelet

TABLE 119–3. Clinical Features of Idiopathic Thrombocytopenic Purpura in Children and Adults

	Children	Adults
Occurrence		
Peak age (years)	2–4	15–40
Sex (F:M)	Equal	1.2–1.7
Presentation		
Onset	Acute (most with symptoms <1 week)	Insidious (most with symptoms >2 months)
Symptoms	Purpura (<10% with severe bleeding)	Purpura (typically bleeding not severe)
Platelet count	Most <20,000/μL	Most <20,000/μL
Course		
Spontaneous remission	83%	2%
Chronic disease	24%	43%
Response to splenectomy	71%	66%
Eventual complete recovery	89%	64%
Morbidity and mortality		
Cerebral hemorrhage	<1%	3%
Hemorrhagic death	<1%	4%
Mortality of chronic refractory disease	2%	5%

antigens assay.[335] These assays showed that the majority of antiplatelet antibodies in patients with ITP are directed against GPIIb/IIIa (~80%), and the remainder against the GPIb/IX complex and other platelet glycoproteins such as GPIV and GPIa/IIa.[336,337] Antibodies in some sera recognize several antigens. Most antiplatelet autoantibodies are IgG; the remainder are IgM and IgA. Antibody-coated platelets bind antigen-presenting cells through Fcγ receptors, primarily in the spleen but also in other organs of the mononuclear phagocyte system.[338,339] It has been postulated that platelet destruction also amplifies the immune response. The mechanism involves presentation of platelet antigens by activated antigen-presenting cells, which thereby activate both CD4+ T-cell clones and antigen-specific T-cell clones. These T-cell clones, having different antigen specificities, induce different B-cell clones to produce antibodies against distinct platelet antigens.[337–339]

In the initial studies with PAIgG, antibodies in ITP reportedly were polyclonal.[340] However, later studies showed that at least some ITP patients had clonal B-cell proliferation, as determined by DNA analysis for immunoglobulin heavy- and light-chain rearrangements and by flow cytometry of B cells from blood and spleen for surface Ig light chains.[341,342]

Although in most patients ITP is antibody mediated, the autoantibodies are under the control of T helper cells and their cytokines. Abnormal T-cell responses drive the differentiation of autoreactive B-cell clones and autoantibody secretion. GPIIb/IIIa-reactive CD4+ T cells from patients with ITP promote the production of anti–GPIIb/IIIa antibodies capable of binding normal platelets,[343] and the clones respond to chemically modified GPIIb/IIIa and recombinant GPIIb/IIIa fragments but not to native GPIIb/IIIa. Thus, autoreactive CD4+ T-helper cells in patients with ITP may recognize a modified GPIIb/IIIa molecule (the cryptic epitope theory[27]). Although specific GPIIb/IIIa peptide fragments have been identified that are recognized by autoreactive CD4+ T cells,[338,344,345] the initial event that induces these abnormalities is not clear.

It was suggested that CD8+ cytotoxic T cells might be involved in the pathogenesis of ITP through cell-mediated destruction of platelets, and through suppression of megakaryocyte apoptosis leading to impaired platelet production.[346,347]

Complement activation may also play a role in thrombocytopenia in some patients with ITP. Increased platelet-associated C3, C4, and C9 have been demonstrated on the platelets from patients with ITP.[348,349] *In vitro* studies have shown that, in the presence of antiplatelet antibodies, C3 and C4 can bind platelets and cause their lysis.[350]

The potential role of *Helicobacter pylori* in the pathogenesis of chronic ITP is controversial. Japanese and Italian studies showed that eradication of *H. pylori* with antibiotics resulted in marked platelet count increases in patients with ITP. However, this success was not reproduced in American and European studies.[351] ITP patients treated for *H. pylori* had higher platelet counts than untreated ITP patients, even if the therapy was unsuccessful in eradicating the infection.[352] It has therefore been speculated that the antibiotic therapy, rather than eradication of *H. pylori*, may be the factor improving platelet counts. However, a recent meta-analysis found that the likelihood that *H. pylori* eradication therapy would increase the platelet count was 14.5 times higher in patients with *H. pylori* infection than in uninfected patients,[353] strengthening the case for a causal relationship between infection and thrombocytopenia.

Platelet Production and Destruction

Early studies of platelet survival demonstrated that platelet survival is shortened in ITP patients and returns to normal after splenectomy-induced remission.[354] Platelet transfusion only transiently increases a patient's platelet count, and the transfused platelets also have shortened survival, reflecting the fact that the major problem in ITP is platelet destruction. The antibody-coated platelets are destroyed by tissue macrophages located primarily in the spleen and, to a lesser extent, in the liver and marrow. However, later studies showed that platelet life span was not short enough to account for the observed thrombocytopenia on the basis of destruction alone, suggesting a concomitant defect in platelet production.[12] These studies confirmed the very early observation by Frank, in 1915, of a defect in platelet production,[355] which was later bolstered by the studies of Dameshek and Miller, who described markedly decreased platelet production in both acute and chronic ITP, despite the presence of increased numbers of megakaryocytes in the marrow.[356] These investigators attributed the defective platelet production to "abnormal splenic activity." Potential mechanisms for this observation were provided by later studies that showed that autoantibodies against platelet glycoproteins might interfere with the maturation of megakaryocytes, resulting in reduced platelet production, contributing to the severity of thrombocytopenia in some ITP patients.[357] Antibodies that target the GPIb/IX/V complex may induce thrombocytopenia by decreasing platelet production, as GPIb autoantibodies have been shown to inhibit megakaryopoiesis *in vitro*,[357] and GPIb monoclonal antibodies inhibit proplatelet formation *in vitro*.[358]

The severity of thrombocytopenia in ITP patients reflects the balance between platelet destruction and platelet production. In most cases of ITP, the marrow has a normal or increased number of megakaryocytes.

The compensatory increase in platelet production in ITP is generally associated with large platelets on the blood film and an elevated mean platelet volume on automated cell counters. Large, young platelets have increased granular contents and enhanced function both *in vitro* and *in vivo*,[359–361] likely explaining the observation that the bleeding time is generally less severely affected in patients with ITP, even when severe, than in patients with thrombocytopenia from myelosuppression or aplastic anemia with equivalent platelet levels. Although the mean platelet volume is increased, the ultrastructure of ITP platelets viewed by electron microscopy is similar to that of normal platelets.[362]

The large size and increased function of the platelets in ITP can be largely attributed to the actions of TPO, the major regulator of megakaryopoiesis and thrombopoiesis. TPO is synthesized in greatest quantity in the liver but is found in other organs (kidney, muscle), including the marrow in patients with ITP.[363] This protein hormone enhances megakaryocyte colony formation and increases the size, number, and ploidy of megakaryocytes and platelet production (see Chap. 113).[363–365] TPO is also required to maintain the viability of stem cells.[366] The hepatic production of TPO is not regulated, rather, the concentration of TPO to which megakaryocytes are exposed is determined by the platelet concentration. Platelets, having TPO receptors, remove the hormone from the circulation, at least partially accounting for the inverse relationship between TPO and platelet levels. TPO levels are markedly elevated in patients with thrombocytopenia associated with megakaryocytic hypoplasia, disorders such as aplastic anemia or acute leukemia. The association of TPO levels with ITP is not clear. In most reports, ITP patients have normal or slightly elevated TPO levels whether measured in plasma or serum, but the levels are always lower than the concentrations found in thrombocytopenias resulting from megakaryocytic hypoplasia.[363–365,367,368]

Genetics

ITP has been documented in monozygotic twins[369] and in some families.[370] As with other autoimmune disorders, heredity may contribute to the development of ITP and may affect the response to therapy. HLA class I and class II allele frequencies in patients with ITP have been studied by several investigators, with inconsistent results. Some investigators reported an increased frequency of HLA Aw32, DRw2, and DRB1*0410.[339,371–373] Investigation has focused on genetic differences associated with dysregulation of immune tolerance and humoral immunity, but results have been inconclusive. For example, genetic polymorphisms of cytotoxic T-lymphocyte antigen (CTLA)-4, tumor necrosis factor, and Fcγ receptors IIA and IIIA have been suggested to influence the development of ITP and the response to therapy,[157,373,374] but as yet no strong association has been found.

Clinical Features

ITP usually is a chronic disease in adults. Chronic ITP is traditionally defined as ITP with a platelet count less than 150×10^9/L for more than 6 months without other cause. A significant portion of patients are diagnosed incidentally in routine complete blood counts. Symptoms and signs of ITP depend on the platelet count. Approximately one-third of patients have platelet counts greater than 30×10^9/L at diagnosis and no significant bleeding,[375] although bleeding symptoms are generally seen in patients with counts below this level. Purpura (ecchymoses and petechiae), epistaxis, menorrhagia, and gingival bleeding are common. Hematuria, hemoptysis, and gastrointestinal bleeding are less common. Intracerebral hemorrhage is rare and generally occurs in patients with platelet counts less than 10×10^9/L and usually is associated with trauma or vascular lesions. The incidence of life-threatening complications is highest in patients older than 60 years; however, mortality rates are low in patients with ITP, even in those with severe thrombocytopenia.[375–378]

The purpuric lesions seen in ITP are not palpable, do not blanch with pressure, and often develop on distal regions of the extremities and on skin areas exposed to pressure (e.g., around tight belts and stockings and at tourniquet sites). Hemorrhagic bullae, which may develop in the buccal mucosa, generally reflect acute, severe thrombocytopenia. Bleeding after surgery, trauma, or tooth extraction is common.

Besides the physical findings associated with platelet-type bleeding, the history and physical examination usually are normal. Family history is especially important to discriminate familial thrombocytopenic syndromes from ITP. The spleen usually is not enlarged but may be palpable in some patients, a finding considered to occur with the same incidence as in normal adults.[379] Constitutional symptoms, such as fever, significant weight loss, marked splenomegaly, hepatomegaly, and lymphadenopathy, provide evidence against the possibility that the thrombocytopenia results from ITP and strongly suggest an alternative diagnosis, such as immune platelet destruction associated with a lymphoproliferative disorder.

Laboratory Features

Platelet Counts and Size Thrombocytopenia is defined as a blood platelet count less than 150×10^9/L. The blood film usually demonstrates isolated thrombocytopenia without erythrocyte or leukocyte abnormalities. Platelet anisocytosis is a common finding in ITP. Mean platelet volume and platelet distribution width are increased. Platelets may be abnormally large or abnormally small. The former reflect accelerated platelet production,[380] and the latter platelet microparticles reflect platelet destruction.[381] The observation of giant platelets should trigger consideration of inherited platelet disorders, which often are misdiagnosed as ITP.[382] Bleeding time correlates inversely with platelet count if the count is less than 100×10^9/L, but may be normal in patients with mild or moderate thrombocytopenia.[383] The ultrastructure of ITP platelets viewed by electron microscopy is similar to that of normal platelets.[362]

Other Blood Findings Hemoglobin concentration and hematocrit are generally normal in patients with ITP. The presence of anemia that is not easily explained (e.g., resulting from iron deficiency in bleeding patients or associated with thalassemia minor in endemic areas) requires further investigation. Autoimmune hemolytic anemia with a positive direct antiglobulin (Coombs) test and reticulocytosis may accompany ITP; this association is termed *Evans syndrome*.[384] The latter syndrome can include immune neutropenia.[385] Neither erythrocyte poikilocytosis nor schistocytes should be present. Total leukocyte counts and differential are generally normal. Although atypical lymphocytes and eosinophilia may occur in children with ITP, leukocytosis and leukopenia with immature cells are not consistent with the diagnosis.[385]

Marrow examination, which is not always required to make a diagnosis of ITP in adults, generally reveals normal or increased numbers of megakaryocytes of normal morphology, although a decreased number of megakaryocytes does not rule out ITP.[386] Erythropoiesis and myelopoiesis are normal. The American Society of Hematology guidelines for ITP state that marrow aspiration is unnecessary in the initial evaluation of ITP if the patient is younger than age 60 years, has a typical presentation, has a good response to first-line therapy, and if splenectomy is not being considered.[322] Nevertheless, some hematologists recommend that the marrow be evaluated to rule out leukemia and myelodysplasia, especially in children and those older than age 40 years.[339,385]

Measuring Platelet Antibodies Because ITP is caused by autoantibodies, specific measurement of such antibodies is expected to provide useful diagnostic clues, much as the direct antiglobulin (Coombs) test is used to diagnose autoimmune hemolytic anemia. Various antiplatelet antibody tests have been described, but none is sufficiently sensitive or specific to be of widespread clinical use. Three types of antiplatelet antibody tests have been developed.

Phase 1 assays were developed after the demonstration that infusion of ITP plasma to healthy subjects resulted in platelet destruction.[326] In these, the patient's serum is incubated with control platelets, and platelet-dependent endpoints are measured, such as platelet aggregation or agglutination, granule release, or platelet lysis. Phase 1 tests are neither sensitive nor specific and are of no diagnostic value for ITP.[386,387]

Phase 2 assays measure PAIgG and other antibodies that can bind the platelet plasma membrane. Antibodies found in platelet granules and in the open canalicular system also are detected with these assays. In these assays, total and surface PAIgG can be measured with different methods.[388] PAIgG is increased in patients with ITP but is also found in healthy subjects and in patients with nonimmune thrombocytopenia. Normal platelets contain immunoglobulins in their α-granules, and plasma immunoglobulin levels affect the amount of immunoglobulins in platelets.[389–391] Although the sensitivity of phase 2 assays has been reported to be as high as 91 percent, the specificity is very low. PAIgG assays cannot discriminate immune from nonimmune thrombocytopenia.[332,388,389]

Phase 3 assays measure platelet glycoprotein-specific autoantibodies. Three techniques are most widely used: immunoblotting, immunoprecipitation, and glycoprotein immobilization assays. In the *immunoblot assay*, platelet membrane proteins are separated by electrophoresis, transferred to membranes, and the membranes incubated with the patient's serum. Serum autoantibodies bound to platelet proteins then are detected by radiolabeled or enzyme-conjugated antihuman IgG. Platelet autoantigens are identified based on their electrophoretic migration.[387,392] The sensitivity of the immunoblot assay is low, and nonspecific binding may occur with normal sera.[393] In the *immunoprecipitation assay*, platelet glycoprotein–autoantibody complexes are captured from the serum using Sepharose beads coated with staphylococcal protein A. This technique may be useful for identifying novel platelet antigens, but its sensitivity is low.[387] *Glycoprotein immobilization assays* include five different assays: microtiter well assay, immunobead assay, modified antigen-capture enzyme-linked immunoadsorbent assay (MACA), monoclonal antibody-specific immobilization of platelet antigen (MAIPA), and platelet-associated IgG characterization assay (PAICA). The microtiter well assay is an indirect test, and both sensitivity and specificity are low.[387,394] The immunobead assay, MACA, MAIPA, and PAICA all appear to be more sensitive and specific than the microtiter well assay.[335] PAICA has several advantages because it can detect both surface and intracellular autoantibodies. These tests may be useful for discriminating immune from nonimmune thrombocytopenia and for monitoring response to treatment. Although phase 3 tests are specific, they are not sensitive enough for ITP screening.

Differential Diagnosis

The diagnosis of ITP is based on its clinical manifestations because no laboratory parameters can accurately diagnose the condition. The diagnosis is based on history, physical examination, blood count, and blood film. The American Society of Hematology guidelines recommend no further diagnostic studies for the typical patient. Additional tests, such as lupus anticoagulant, antiplatelet antibody testing, direct antiglobulin test, reticulocyte count, urinalysis, and thyroid function tests, are generally unnecessary but may be appropriate when other patient characteristics call attention to underlying disorders. Bleeding time, platelet survival studies, serum complement, abdominal ultrasonography, computed tomography, and PAIgG assays are unnecessary and inappropriate.[386] Antiphospholipid antibodies (lupus anticoagulant and anticardiolipin antibodies) are seen frequently in patients with ITP.[395] Although some researchers report these autoantibodies have no clinical significance,[219,396] others find an increased risk for thrombosis in ITP patients with antiphospholipid antibodies[397,398] (see "Thrombocytopenia in Patients with Systemic Lupus Erythematosus" and "Thrombocytopenia in Patients with Antiphospholipid Syndrome" below).

Therapy, Course, and Prognosis

What little is known of the natural course of moderate or severe ITP derives from before the glucocorticoid era, and suggests that left untreated, ITP in adults typically is a chronic disease, with infrequent spontaneous remissions, in contrast to ITP in children. Even with glucocorticoid therapy, complete remission usually is not seen. An analysis of 12 series of 1761 adults with ITP reported a complete remission rate of only 25 percent with glucocorticoids and a mortality rate of 5 percent, predominantly because of intracerebral hemorrhage.[376] The risk of hemorrhagic complications is greater in patients older than age 60 years.[324]

ITP may respond to various agents or manipulations, including glucocorticoids, splenectomy, IVIg, anti-(Rh)D, danazol, and antineoplastic drugs such as vincristine and azathioprine. Thus, the patient's symptoms and initial response to therapy should dictate ongoing therapy.

Initial Management

Observation Because most ITP patients are diagnosed incidentally in routine evaluation, signs and symptoms of bleeding are important in determining whether any treatment is required. Patients with no bleeding and consistent platelet counts in excess of 50×10^9/L do not require treatment and can be observed periodically. These patients are at low risk for clinically important bleeding and may safely undergo invasive procedures.[376,377,399] Patients with platelet counts between 30 and 50×10^9/L generally do not experience clinically important bleeding but may manifest easy bruising. They usually do not require treatment. Careful followup is necessary for these patients because the clinical course is difficult to predict. Simple observation is not recommended for patients with platelet counts less than 10×10^9/L, in those with platelet counts between 10 and 50×10^9/L and significant mucosal bleeding, or in those with risk factors for bleeding, such as uncontrolled hypertension, peptic ulcer, or a vigorous lifestyle.[386]

Emergency Treatment of Acute Bleeding Resulting from Severe Thrombocytopenia Fortunately, bleeding symptoms generally are not severe in adult patients with ITP, even with very low platelet counts. However, life-threatening bleeding may occur in patients with platelet counts less than 10×10^9/L. Emergent treatment should be instituted in patients with intracranial or gastrointestinal bleeding, massive hematuria, internal hematoma, or in need of emergent surgical intervention. The presence of extensive purpura or hemorrhagic bullae in mucosal tissues is a harbinger of life-threatening bleeding and warrants therapy. Patients with any of these findings should be hospitalized and monitored closely. High-dose parenteral glucocorticoid therapy (methylprednisolone 1 g/day in divided doses for 1–3 days), IVIg (1 g/kg per day for 2 days), or IVIg and parenteral glucocorticoids in combination are generally recommended for those patients.[322] In most patients, IVIg increases the platelet count within 2 to 3 days.[322,339,376] Although platelet transfusions may not increase the platelet counts because the transfused platelets are destroyed rapidly, they nevertheless may contribute to the formation of platelet plugs at sites of bleeding and improve hemostasis. Platelet transfusion following IVIg infusion may increase the platelet count because IVIg may improve platelet survival.[400] Aminocaproic acid, which inhibits fibrinolysis, can be used to reduce bleeding[400] and is safe except in the presence of hematuria, in which it can cause thrombi of the glomeruli, renal pelves, and ureters. This agent does not affect platelet count or function. Aminocaproic acid usually is administered intravenously (initial dose 0.1 g/kg over 30 minutes, then given either by continuous infusion at 0.5–1 g/h or as an equivalent intermittent dose every 2–4 hours). Aminocaproic acid also can be administered orally in a similar dose in emergency situations because it is absorbed very rapidly from the gastrointestinal tract. Vincristine can be used in combination with glucocorticoid and IVIg treatment in older patients.[339]

Glucocorticoid Therapy Glucocorticoids are recommended as initial treatment for patients with platelet counts less than 20×10^9/L and in patients with platelet counts between 20 and 50×10^9/L and significant bleeding. Oral prednisone 1 to 2 mg/kg per day is generally accepted for initial treatment in patients with ITP. Glucocorticoids increase the platelet count through several mechanisms, including inhibition of phagocytosis of antibody-coated platelets by macrophages, decreasing autoantibody production, and improving marrow platelet production.[401,402] They also appear to reduce capillary leakage. Although no consensus exists regarding the duration of initial therapy, treatment should continue until platelet counts reach a safe range. Patients generally respond to initial prednisone therapy within the first 3 weeks of treatment. In approximately two-thirds of patients, platelet counts increase to greater than 50×10^9/L within 1 week but decrease again when the prednisone dose is tapered.[322,376] Thus, in patients who respond, the recommendation is to continue glucocorticoid therapy 1 mg/kg per day for a total of 3 weeks before initiating the taper.

The glucocorticoid-dosing regimen that achieves the best response of the platelet count in patients with ITP is still under investigation. In addition to the standard 1 to 2 mg/kg per day dose of prednisone, lower doses[403,404] and high doses[405–408] have been investigated, with good results. Methylprednisolone or dexamethasone can be used for high-dose initial therapy by either oral or intravenous route.

The major drawback of glucocorticoid therapy is that the adverse effects may be worse than the disease itself. Facial swelling, weight gain, folliculitis, hyperglycemia, hypertension, cataracts, osteoporosis, opportunistic infections, and behavioral disturbances are common side effects and can be severe.[322,409] A study showed that a short course of treatment with high-dose glucocorticoids (dexamethasone 40 mg/day for 4 consecutive days) as initial therapy for ITP was well tolerated and effective[408] compared to standard-dose therapy. Despite this success, the use of this regimen as first-line therapy has not been validated.

Sustained remissions with glucocorticoids are infrequent, with reported rates ranging from 5 to 30 percent.[322,339] If the patient does not respond to 3 weeks of prednisone therapy, other therapeutic options should be considered.

Splenectomy Splenectomy was first demonstrated by Kaznelson in 1916 to be effective in patients with ITP.[410] Splenectomy is indicated in adult ITP patients whose platelet counts remain less than 10×10^9/L and in patients whose platelet counts remain less than 30×10^9/L and who continue to experience excessive bleeding after 4 to 6 weeks of appropriate medical treatment. Splenectomy also should be considered in patients who have experienced a transient response to primary treatment and have platelet counts less than 30×10^9/L after 3 months or who require continuous glucocorticoid therapy to maintain safe platelet counts.[322,410] At least 2 weeks before splenectomy, patients should be immunized with polyvalent pneumococcal vaccine, *Haemophilus influenzae* type B vaccine, and quadrivalent meningococcal polysaccharide vaccine[411] because they are susceptible to overwhelming sepsis, especially from these bacterial infections. Patients with platelet counts less than 50×10^9/L, and especially less than 30×10^9/L, may require glucocorticoid and/or IVIg therapy before the procedure to reach platelet levels that minimize the risk of surgical bleeding. Platelet transfusions may be required during the perioperative period in severely thrombocytopenic patients.

Two-thirds of patients who undergo splenectomy achieve normal platelet counts.[322,410] In the remaining third of patients, platelet counts recover only partially or transiently, and most of these patients relapse within 6 months of splenectomy. The duration of the disease prior to splenectomy does not affect the results of the procedure. Splenectomy can be performed even years after ITP is diagnosed.[412,413] Both the time required to reach a normal platelet count and the magnitude of platelet recovery are useful predictors of the long-term efficacy of splenectomy. In most cases, platelet counts recover within 10 days. Patients who attain a normal platelet count within 3 days of splenectomy or platelet counts greater than 500×10^9/L by day 10 generally have a good long-term response to splenectomy. Younger patients respond better to splenectomy.

The mortality rate associated with splenectomy is very low (<1%), even in patients with severe thrombocytopenia. The rate increases in older patients and in the presence of coexisting illnesses.[322,414] Postsplenectomy sepsis is a major cause of morbidity and mortality in those patients. Splenectomized patients should be informed to be alert for the symptoms and signs of infection and be prepared for an emergency situation. Any febrile situation should be carefully evaluated, and should be treated with broad spectrum antibiotics. Patients should be revaccinated with quadrivalent *meningococcal* polysaccharide vaccine and polyvalent *pneumococcal* vaccine at 3- to 5-year intervals; vaccination with only one dose of *H. influenzae* type B vaccine is recommended in adults.[415]

Laparoscopic splenectomy, first introduced in 1991, is an alternative to open splenectomy because the spleen is of normal size and vascularity in ITP patients. In experienced hands, laparoscopic splenectomy is cost-effective and safe. Long-term and short-term benefits and complications are similar to those seen with open splenectomy. This procedure is limited by a high frequency of retained splenic tissue, especially in those with an accessory spleen, and increased risk of splenosis.[339,416] Preoperative imaging of accessory splenic tissues by ultrasonography or computed tomography is of limited benefit. A handheld gamma probe may be used for the detection of accessory splenic tissues during laparoscopy.[417] Splenic irradiation or splenic artery embolization can be used in glucocorticoid-resistant ITP patients in whom surgical splenectomy is contraindicated.[322,418] In patients refractory to splenectomy, the presence of accessory splenic tissue should be suspected, particularly if the blood film shows no evidence of splenectomy (i.e., pitting and Howell-Jolly bodies are absent in the erythrocytes; see Chap. 55). Such patients should be screened with sensitive radionuclide or magnetic resonance scans to identify residual splenic tissue.

Intravenous Immunoglobulin IVIg was first shown to be effective in childhood ITP in 1981.[419] IVIg increases the platelet count in more than 75 percent of patients with chronic ITP and normalizes the platelet count in approximately 50 percent of the patients.[322,409] The effect of IVIg is similar whether or not the patient is splenectomized and is transient, generally lasting only 3 to 4 weeks. The patient may become refractory with repeated infusions of IVIg.[420]

Postulated mechanisms for the action of IVIg include blockade of macrophage Fc receptors, which slows clearance of antibody-coated platelets, antiidiotype neutralization of antiplatelet autoantibodies, cytokine modulation, immunomodulation (increased suppressor T-cell function and decreased autoantibody production), complement neutralization, and dendritic cell priming.[409,421,422] The recommended total dose of IVIg is 2 g/kg administered either as 0.4 g/kg per day on 5 consecutive days or as 1 g/kg per day on 2 consecutive days. For maintenance therapy, 0.5 to 1 g/kg as a single dose may be used. Adverse effects of IVIg therapy include headache, backache, nausea, fever, aseptic meningitis, alloimmune hemolysis, hepatitis, renal failure, pulmonary insufficiency, and thrombosis. Anaphylactic reactions may occur in patients with congenital IgA deficiency; therefore, IgA levels should be evaluated before IVIg infusions. The cost of IVIg is considerable, and it is not recommended as initial therapy in adult patients with ITP, except in the setting of life-threatening bleeding.[322]

Anti-(Rh)D Anti-(Rh)D is a polyclonal γ-globulin containing high titers of antibodies against the $Rh_0(D)$ antigen of erythrocytes. It is administered intravenously for treatment of ITP. Anti-(Rh)D binds Rh-positive erythrocytes and leads to their destruction in the spleen. Because splenic Fc receptors are blocked, more antibody-coated platelets survive in the circulation.[423,424] Anti-(Rh)D also can also modulate $Fc\gamma$ receptor expression and regulate the production of various cytokines, including IL-6, IL-10, tumor necrosis factor-α.[425] A positive direct antiglobulin test, a decrease in serum haptoglobin levels, and mild and transient hemolysis occur in all Rh-positive patients after anti-(Rh)D infusion, generally without requiring a blood transfusion,[424] although serious hemolysis can occur. Anti-(Rh)D therapy is not effective in Rh-negative patients, and response rates are very low in splenectomized patients.

A single dose of 50 to 100 mcg/kg is recommended, given by intravenous infusion over 3 to 5 minutes.[225,423,426] Adverse effects of anti-(Rh)D therapy are those seen with both γ-globulin infusion and autoimmune hemolytic anemia; symptoms include headache, asthenia, chills, fever, abdominal pain, diarrhea, vomiting, dizziness, and myalgia. Immediate anaphylactic reactions and both type I (IgE mediated) and type III (immune complex mediated) hypersensitivity reactions can occur.[225,322,423,424,427] Although anti-(Rh)D reportedly increases platelet counts in more than 70 percent of patients who are Rh-positive and not splenectomized[225] and may preclude the need for splenectomy,[427] a randomized, controlled trial comparing anti-(Rh)D with conventional therapy showed no differences in the rates of spontaneous remission or the need for splenectomy.[426]

Treatments for patients refractory to initial therapies. Approximately one-third of patients with ITP do not respond to splenectomy or relapse after a short remission. The therapeutic options for those with moderate to severe thrombocytopenia after splenectomy are many; therapy should be tailored to the individual patient. Bleeding symptoms rather than platelet count should determine whether treatment is required. Patients with platelet counts greater than 30×10^9/L can be followed without therapy because their bleeding risk is very low. The treatment strategy is uncertain for patients with platelet counts less than 30×10^9/L. Observation without therapy may be appropriate if the patient has no signs of bleeding and has no risk factors for bleeding, such as uncontrolled hypertension or peptic ulcer disease. The main goal of therapy in these patients is prevention of bleeding.

Rituximab A chimeric monoclonal antibody against CD20, rituximab binds B cells and causes Fc-mediated lysis, thereby depleting these cells from blood, lymph nodes and marrow. Depletion of autoreactive B cell clones has been shown to be effective in the treatment of autoimmune diseases.[428–432] Rituximab is generally administered at a dose of 375 mg/m^2, as in patients with B-cell lymphoma. Although the optimal dosing and duration of therapy in ITP patients has not been determined, weekly infusion for 4 consecutive weeks has been used in most studies. With initial reports of good results, rituximab has emerged as an effective therapeutic option for refractory ITP patients. Published studies with rituximab, however, have generally not been controlled, have primarily been presented as case reports, and are extremely heterogenous in terms of rituximab dosing and response criteria. A meta-analysis of 19 reviewed studies (313 patients) that evaluated efficacy, and 29 studies (306 patients) that evaluated safety is available. A complete response (platelet counts greater than 150×10^9/L) was observed in 46.3 percent of patients, the overall response rate (platelet counts greater than 50×10^9/L) was 62.5 percent, and partial response (platelet counts between 50 and 150×10^9/L) was 24 percent.[431]

Different patterns of response have been reported in ITP patients treated with rituximab. Although the majority of patients responded within 4 to 6 weeks (early responders), response was delayed until several months in some patients (late responders). It has been suggested that anti-CD20–coated B cells might occupy Fc receptors and save platelets from destruction in early responders, whereas depletion of B cells and reduction of autoantibody production occurs in late responders.[430,432] Approximately one-third of complete rituximab responders remained in remission for more than 1 year, and splenectomy did not affect response rates to rituximab therapy.[430,433]

In a meta-analysis of 306 ITP patients treated with rituximab, adverse reactions were reported as mild-to-moderate in 66 patients (21.6%), life-threatening in 10 (3.7%), and 9 (2.9%) patients died.[431] This mortality rate is higher than expected in ITP patients. More controlled studies with rituximab are expected to identify high-risk patient subgroups, and to increase the efficacy and safety of the drug in refractory ITP patients.

TPO Mimetic Drugs The observations of impaired platelet production from megakaryocytes in patients with ITP, the massive megakaryopoiesis seen in the marrow of mice and humans treated with recombinant thrombopoietin and the unexpectedly normal or only modestly elevated TPO levels in patients with ITP suggested the use of megakaryocyte-stimulation therapy in refractory patients. Early use of two recombinant TPO molecules for the treatment of thrombocytopenia associated with cancer or chemotherapy were limited by the production of autoantibodies that blocked TPO action. Since then, TPO mimetics (TPO mimetic peptides, nonpeptide TPO mimetics, and TPO agonist antibodies) have been developed to stimulate platelet production.[366]

The TPO mimetic peptibody (TPO-receptor-binding peptides fused to an immunoglobulin scaffold) romiplostim (AMG531-Nplate) binds to the TPO-binding site of TPO receptor with high affinity, and induces megakaryocyte proliferation and differentiation. Weekly subcutaneous injection of romiplostim at doses of 1 to 3 mcg/kg produced dose-dependent increases in the platelet count, starting from day 5, with peak platelet levels reached by days 12 to 15.[366,433]

The nonpeptide TPO mimetic eltrombopag (Promacta) is a small molecule that binds to the transmembrane domain of the TPO receptor to also trigger megakaryocyte growth and differentiation, and platelet production. It is used orally at daily doses of 50 or 75 mg. Eltrombopag should be given 2 hours before or after meals because foods may affect its absorption. Divalent cations such as calcium also interfere with absorption of the drug, so it should not be taken with dairy products or antacids. In healthy volunteers, daily doses given for 10 days elevated platelet counts beginning at 8 days and peaking at 16 days.

In earlier trials, 6-week treatment with either eltrombopag or romiplostim were shown to be effective in refractory ITP patients. These drugs increased platelet counts in more than 80 percent of refractory ITP patients regardless of splenectomy status. These drugs are well-tolerated; mild headache is the most common complaint. A rebound thrombocytopenia may occur upon discontinuation of either drug.

Romiplostim was also evaluated for long-term administration in two parallel placebo-controlled trials in both splenectomized and nonsplenectomized patients treated for 24 weeks.[434] Durable platelet responses were achieved by 16 of 42 splenectomized patients and 25 of 41 nonsplenectomized patients given romiplostim, but in only 1 of 42 patients (21 splenectomized and 21 splenectomized) given placebo. The drug was well tolerated. In spite of these successes, however, it is important to recognize the many possible complications that could ensue from long-term administration of these drugs, including increased marrow reticulin or collagen deposition, thrombosis, tumor cell growth, stem cell depletion, and formation of neutralizing antibodies.[366,433]

Vinca Alkaloids Both vincristine and vinblastine transiently increase the platelet count in approximately 70 percent of ITP patients within 5 to 21 days but produce sustained remissions in only 10 percent of treated patients.[322,339,377,435] The recommended dose of vincristine is 1 to 2 mg and of vinblastine is 0.1 mg/kg (maximum: 10 mg), both given by bolus injection at 1-week intervals for a minimum of three courses. It has been proposed that vinca alkaloids bind to platelet microtubules and thereby are transported to the spleen, where they subsequently inhibit the phagocytic functions of splenic macrophages. They may also stimulate megakaryopoiesis. Peripheral neuropathy, neutropenia, jaw pain, alopecia, and constipation are complications of treatment with vinca alkaloids.[435–438]

Cyclophosphamide This alkylating drug can be used orally (50–200 mg/day) or parenterally (1–1.5 g/m^2 IV every 4 weeks) in refractory ITP patients.[439,440] It increases platelet counts in 60 to 80 percent of ITP cases, and 20 to 40 percent of those patients will remain in remission for 2 to 3 years[322] after 2 to 3 months of therapy. Its action in increasing the platelet count involves immunosuppression. The major complications of cyclophosphamide therapy are marrow suppression, hemorrhagic cystitis, infertility, alopecia, and secondary malignancy.

Azathioprine This purine analogue is converted to 6-mercaptopurine following gastrointestinal absorption. It also works through immunosuppression. An azathioprine dose ranging from 50 to 250 mg/day for at least 4 months seems to be necessary before its effectiveness can be evaluated. Azathioprine reportedly produced a sustained normalization of the platelet counts in up to 45 percent of refractory ITP patients.[441] As with other immunosuppressive drugs, major adverse effects are marrow suppression, possible increased risk of secondary malignancy, and teratogenesis.[322,435]

Danazol This synthetic androgen with reduced virilizing effects compared to other androgens has been used for treatment of refractory ITP patients. Given at doses of 400 to 800 mg/day for at least 6 months, reported response rates range from 10 to 80 percent.[322,435] Danazol is postulated to decrease Fc receptor numbers on phagocytic cells by antagonizing the effects of estrogens.[377] Danazol should not be given to pregnant women or patients with liver disease. Common side effects of danazol therapy are weight gain, fluid retention, seborrhea, hirsutism, secondary amenorrhea, vocal changes, acne, hepatic toxicity, headache, lethargy, myalgia, and thrombocytopenia. Because liver dysfunction is common with danazol therapy, liver function should be evaluated monthly.[322,377,435]

Other Therapies Many other therapies, including interferon-α,[442] dapsone,[443] immunoadsorption with staphylococcal protein A,[444] cyclosporine,[445] ascorbic acid,[445] colchicine,[446] and plasmapheresis[447] have been studied for refractory ITP cases, but none has been clearly demonstrated to be effective.

Accessory Therapies Adjunctive therapies include agents designed to reduce bleeding without necessarily affecting the platelet count. For example, aminocaproic acid can be used for excessive menstrual bleeding in young women and may prevent blood loss.

THROMBOCYTOPENIA IN PATIENTS WITH ANTIPHOSPHOLIPID SYNDROME

Antiphospholipid syndrome (APS) is characterized by recurrent arterial and venous thrombosis and well-defined morbidity during pregnancy in the presence of antiphospholipid antibodies (APLAs) (see Chap. 132).[448] APS may affect any system or organ in the body, including the heart, brain, kidney, skin, lung, and placenta. This syndrome predominantly affects females (female-to-male ratio 5:1), especially during the childbearing years.[449] APLAs (lupus anticoagulant; anticardiolipin antibodies; anti-β_2-glycoprotein I antibodies) represent a heterogeneous family of antibodies that react with anionic phospholipids and phospholipid–protein complexes. Despite overwhelming evidence that APLAs are associated with thrombosis, the mechanisms remain uncertain. Many have been proposed, including endothelial cell damage and apoptosis, inhibition of prostacyclin release from endothelial cells, inhibition of the protein C–protein S anticoagulant system, induction of tissue factor, activation of platelets, interference with antithrombin, impairment of fibrinolytic activity, and the effect of APLAs in inhibiting annexin V binding to membrane phospholipids, eliminating the antithrombotic effect of annexin V.[450–453] APS is considered one of the most common causes of acquired thrombophilia.[454,455]

Thrombocytopenia is reported in approximately 20 to 40 percent of patients with APS, usually is mild (70–120 × 10^9/L), and does not require clinical intervention. Severe thrombocytopenia (platelet counts <50 × 10^9/L) may be seen in 5 to 10 percent of patients.[456–458] Although thrombocytopenia was a clinical criterion used to define the syndrome in the initial classification of APS,[459] it was not included in the most recently proposed classification.[460] Because ITP patients who present with APLAs are at increased risk for thrombosis,[397] measurement of APLA, especially lupus anticoagulant, in patients diagnosed with ITP may identify a subgroup at high risk for developing APS.

The pathogenesis of thrombocytopenia in APS is not clear. Potential mechanisms explaining thrombocytopenia in APS patients include APLA-related direct platelet destruction, immune platelet destruction by antibodies against platelet glycoproteins, and platelet aggregation and consumption. Evidence indicates APLAs bind platelet membranes and cause platelet destruction, but the link is not definitive. Some investigators suggest that antibodies against platelet glycoproteins, rather than APLAs, are responsible for thrombocytopenia in patients with APS. Antiglycoprotein antibodies are rare in patients with APS with normal platelet counts.[461,462] Antibodies against the GPIIb/IIIa or GPIb/IX/V complexes are found in approximately 40 percent of thrombocytopenic patients with APS.[463] Such antibodies do not cross-react with antibodies against phospholipids or β_2-glycoprotein I.[464] Immunosuppressive treatment in these patients increases the platelet count and reduces the titers of anti-GP antibodies but not the titers of APLAs.[396] These data suggest that thrombocytopenia is a secondary immune phenomenon that develops concomitantly with APS. Against this conclusion, platelet antigens in thrombocytopenic patients with APS were found to be different from those in ITP and display virtually no reactivity of the antibodies with membrane glycoproteins.[465] CD40 ligand on platelets is another possible antibody target. Anti-CD40 ligand antibodies have been found in patients with APS (13%) and ITP (12%), but not in healthy controls; and it was suggested that these antibodies were associated with the thrombocytopenia.[466] Platelet activation, aggregation, and consumption (APS-associated thrombotic microangiopathy) may also cause thrombocytopenia in patients with APS.[458]

Another issue of clinical importance in evaluating thrombocytopenia associated with APS is the risk for future development of thrombosis. In one study in which APS patients were divided into three groups according to platelet counts as normal, moderately thrombocytopenic (50–100 × 10^9/L), or severely thrombocytopenic (<50 × 10^9/L), the rates of future thrombosis were 40 percent, 32 percent, and 9 percent, respectively.[467] These data show that moderate thrombocytopenia does not prevent thrombosis in patients with APS. Antithrombotic prophylaxis should be considered in these patients.[456,467]

Although thrombocytopenia is a common finding in patients with APS, bleeding complications are rare, even with severe thrombocytopenia. Bleeding in an APS patient with moderate thrombocytopenia should trigger evaluation for the presence of antiprothrombin antibodies[468] and other disorders that may affect hemostasis, such as DIC, liver insufficiency, and uremia. Severe thrombocytopenia may require therapy, with treatment strategies similar to those used for patients with ITP. Glucocorticoids are effective in only 15 percent of patients.[456] IVIg and immunosuppressive drugs such as cyclophosphamide can be used in patients with severe bleeding and "catastrophic" APS. Splenectomy is another option, producing sustained remission in approximately two-thirds of patients.[219,469,470] Preoperative vaccinations should be administered to patients with ITP. Because of their increased risk of thrombosis, patients should be prophylactically anticoagulated in the immediate postoperative period. The anti-CD20 monoclonal antibody rituximab has been used to treat refractory thrombocytopenia in patients with APS, with conflicting results.[471,472] Although there is no consensus on dosing and schedule with rituximab therapy, it is generally administered as in patients with ITP (see ITP therapy in "Therapy, Course, and Prognosis" above).

Cases of thrombocytopenia responding to aspirin,[473,474] warfarin,[475,476] and antimalarial drugs have been reported.[477] Inhibition of platelet activation, aggregation, and platelet consumption have been suggested as helpful in increasing platelet counts in APS patients.

THROMBOCYTOPENIA IN PATIENTS WITH SYSTEMIC LUPUS ERYTHEMATOSUS AND OTHER AUTOIMMUNE CONDITIONS

Systemic lupus erythematosus (SLE) is a complex autoimmune disease that primarily afflicts women of childbearing age. The autoimmune attack in SLE is not organ specific; it may affect any tissue in the body. The diagnostic criteria for SLE are based on a classification system proposed by the American College of Rheumatology. Patients with SLE should fulfill any 4 of 11 criteria.[478,479]

FREQUENCY OF THROMBOCYTOPENIA

Thrombocytopenia is common in patients with SLE, occurring in 20 to 40 percent of patients.[480] Immunologic destruction of platelets is also seen in several other autoimmune conditions, such as polyarteritis nodosa, rheumatoid arthritis and Sjögren syndrome, albeit at much reduced rates than seen in SLE. The causes of thrombocytopenia in SLE are many and include platelet destruction (ITP, DIC, TTP or hemolytic uremic syndrome [TTP-HUS], sepsis), ineffective hematopoiesis (megaloblastic anemia), abnormal platelet pooling (hypersplenism), marrow hypoplasia (from drugs and infections), and dilutional thrombocytopenia related to therapy. Severe thrombocytopenia is relatively rare, seen in 5 percent of patients.[480] Although clinically significant bleeding is uncommon even in patients with severe thrombocytopenia, fatal gastrointestinal, cerebral, and pulmonary bleeding have been reported.

PATHOGENESIS OF THROMBOCYTOPENIA

Among the many potential contributors to thrombocytopenia in SLE patients, destruction of the platelets by autoantibodies is the major mechanism. Antiplatelet antibodies are present in up to 60 percent of SLE patients.[481,482] Although the presence of antiplatelet antibodies is correlated with low platelet counts and increased disease severity,[482] the mechanism of platelet destruction is not clear. Besides the antiplatelet antibodies, antiphospholipid antibodies (see "Thrombocytopenia in Patients with Antiphospholipid Syndrome" above) and circulating immune complexes that bind platelets nonspecifically may accelerate platelet destruction.[483] Specific antiplatelet antibodies, especially those against GPIIb/IIIa, have an important role in the pathogenesis of thrombocytopenia in SLE patients.[462,481,482]

In general, marrow megakaryocytes are normal or increased, and platelet production is not affected in SLE patients with thrombocytopenia. However, decreased numbers of megakaryocytes and even amegakaryocytic thrombocytopenia have been reported.[314,484] High levels of TPO in the serum, and both anti-TPO and anti-TPO receptor antibodies have been found in SLE patients,[485,486] the latter associated with a decrease in marrow megakaryocytes and thrombocytopenia.[486]

Thrombocytopenia in SLE is associated with serious organ pathology, leading to neuropsychiatric disease,[487] renal disease,[488,489] and APS,[490] and is an independent indicator of poor prognosis.[489,491,492] A study of selected SLE families in which at least one affected member was thrombocytopenic reported genetic linkage to loci at chromosomes 11p13 and 1q22–23.[493] Severe lupus phenotype was much more common among patients with thrombocytopenia and their affected family members than in patients from families with no thrombocytopenic patients. Therefore, thrombocytopenia in a family member may herald severe lupus in familial SLE.

TREATMENT OF THROMBOCYTOPENIA

Although thrombocytopenia is a common finding in SLE, treatment strategies for severe thrombocytopenia are not well established. Because SLE ranges in severity from milder forms with easily controlled symptoms and signs to severe forms that may be fatal, the treatment of severe thrombocytopenia should be tailored to the individual patient. Patients with severe thrombocytopenia are generally treated with glucocorticoids as first-line therapy, but sustained remission is infrequent. Because most patients with severe thrombocytopenia also have nephritis and neurologic symptoms for which they receive immunosuppressive therapy either alone or combination with glucocorticoids, immunosuppressive drugs and antimalarials can be used as components of first-line therapy.[494–497] These combined regimens have significant potential for toxicity.

It is well-known that B lymphocytes play an important role in the pathogenesis of SLE. Although lymphopenia is common in patients with active SLE, autoantibody-producing B cells have been shown to be expanded, and B cells were found to be more sensitive to inflammatory cytokines.[498] These data have led to the use of B-cell targeted therapies in SLE. For example, rituximab has been demonstrated to be effective in the treatment of refractory SLE patients, especially those with nephritis and severe thrombocytopenia.[498]

Because of its high cost and transient effect, IVIg is reserved for use in patients with emergent bleeding symptoms.[499,500] If other therapies fail, splenectomy should be considered. Although case reports suggest that—in contrast to other autoimmune disorders—splenectomy increases complications in SLE patients and does not improve thrombocytopenia,[501–503] more comprehensive series indicate that splenectomy yields sustained remission in 61 percent of SLE patients with severe thrombocytopenia.[495]

THROMBOCYTOPENIA DURING PREGNANCY

Evaluation of blood counts of pregnant women has shown that thrombocytopenia is the second most common hematologic problem in pregnancy, after anemia. Table 119–4 lists the major causes of thrombocytopenia in pregnancy (see Chap. 7).

TABLE 119–4. Causes of Thrombocytopenia during Pregnancy

Pseudothrombocytopenia
Gestational thrombocytopenia
Autoimmune thrombocytopenia
Antiphospholipid syndrome and systemic lupus erythematosus
Folate deficiency
Preeclampsia, eclampsia
HELLP (hemolysis, elevated liver function tests, low platelets) syndrome
Thrombotic thrombocytopenic purpura
Disseminated intravascular coagulation
Hypersplenism
Viral infections (HIV, cytomegalovirus, Epstein-Barr virus)
Drug-induced thrombocytopenia
Marrow dysfunction (aplastic anemia, leukemia)
Acute fatty liver
Hereditary disorders (type IIb von Willebrand disease, May-Hegglin anomaly, hereditary macrothrombocytopenia)

Platelet counts tend to decrease during normal pregnancy. Mild thrombocytopenia, with platelet counts ranging from 120 to 150 × 10^9/L, may be present, especially during the third trimester.[504,505] It is important to investigate the cause of thrombocytopenia and exclude the disorders associated with significant morbidity (see Table 119–4). A thorough history, blood pressure measurement, repeated blood count with a fresh sample, and examination of the blood film are the main steps in the diagnosis of pseudothrombocytopenia, leukemia, and microangiopathic disorders such as TTP; microangiopathic hemolysis, elevated liver enzymes, and low platelet counts (HELLP) syndrome; and DIC in pregnant women with thrombocytopenia. Physical examination may be difficult in the third trimester, so an abdominal ultrasound may be required to detect organomegaly.

GESTATIONAL THROMBOCYTOPENIA

Gestational thrombocytopenia is detected in 5 to 7 percent of otherwise healthy pregnant women, accounting for approximately 74 percent of thrombocytopenia cases at term.[390,506,507] Gestational thrombocytopenia is a benign disorder and is not associated with an increased risk of bleeding. It is not associated with decreased platelet counts in the fetus. Platelet counts are generally greater than 70 × 10^9/L[390,504–506] and usually return to normal after delivery. The pathogenesis of gestational thrombocytopenia is unknown. Several mechanisms have been proposed, including hemodilution, a compensated state of subclinical coagulopathy, endothelial cell injury, and immune destruction. Some authors have suggested platelet consumption by the placenta and hormonal depression of megakaryopoiesis as causes of gestational thrombocytopenia, as suggested by the rapid return of platelet count to normal after delivery and by the transient return to normal of platelet count during pregnancy in some cases of essential thrombocythemia.[232,507–509]

Discriminating gestational thrombocytopenia from immune thrombocytopenia can be difficult because ITP is also common in young women, and ITP is often exacerbated by pregnancy. Neither condition can be diagnosed by currently available tests. The diagnosis of ITP is favored if the patient had a previous episode of ITP unassociated with pregnancy or if the thrombocytopenia is severe and associated with bleeding that occurs in the first trimester. In healthy pregnant women, a platelet count greater than 75 × 10^9/L late in pregnancy does not require intensive investigation at that time because bleeding is not likely in the woman or her newborn child.[510]

IMMUNE THROMBOCYTOPENIC PURPURA

ITP is responsible for 4 to 5 percent of all cases of pregnancy-associated thrombocytopenia.[390,507] It generally causes moderate to severe thrombocytopenia in the first trimester. No test for discriminating ITP from gestational thrombocytopenia is available. PAIgG is elevated in patients with ITP and in gestational thrombocytopenia.[511] Diagnosis of ITP in a pregnant woman requires the exclusion of other causes of thrombocytopenia. Given no suspicious clinical or laboratory features, marrow aspiration is considered unnecessary.[505] Diagnosis of ITP is important for the fetus because antiplatelet antibodies decrease the fetal platelet count and may cause bleeding.[506]

According to the American Society of Hematology ITP guidelines, an ITP patient who has platelet counts greater than 50 × 10^9/L should not be discouraged from becoming pregnant, but the patient who has platelet counts less than 10 × 10^9/L after splenectomy should be advised of the high risk to the fetus.[390] ITP may exacerbate during pregnancy, but generally the platelet count returns to the prepregnancy level after delivery.

The approach to treatment of ITP during pregnancy is different from that in nonpregnant women because the potential side effects of the drugs may complicate both fetal development and the course of the pregnancy. Mother and fetus should be managed by close collaboration between a hematologist, an obstetrician, and a neonatologist. Although glucocorticoids are not teratogenic, they may induce gestational diabetes, osteoporosis, hypertension, or psychosis. Fetal side effects are minimal because approximately 90 percent of the glucocorticoid dose is metabolized in the placenta.[505] Cytotoxic drugs, such as vinca alkaloids, azathioprine, and cyclophosphamide, are potentially teratogenic. The rigors of splenectomy may induce preterm labor. IVIg is safe for the fetus but often is associated with maternal side effects. Experience with anti-(Rh)D therapy in pregnant women is limited. Platelet counts and bleeding symptoms are important for management of these patients. If the platelet count is greater than 30 × 10^9/L and the patient has no bleeding symptoms, observation without therapy is appropriate. A pregnant women who has a platelet count less than 10 × 10^9/L in any trimester, a platelet count of 10 to 30 × 10^9/L in the third trimester, or signs of bleeding requires therapy. If the pregnant woman has no life-threatening bleeding symptoms, glucocorticoids are considered for initial therapy. A starting dosage of 1 mg/kg per day and then the minimal dose that will keep platelet counts greater than 50 × 10^9/L are appropriate. If the platelet count is greater than 50 × 10^9/L, vaginal delivery can be performed. If cesarean section or epidural anesthesia is required, the platelet count should be maintained over 80 × 10^9/L.[505] IVIg is indicated in patients who have no response to glucocorticoid treatment, have life-threatening bleeding symptoms, and have platelet count less than 10 × 10^9/L at term. A dosage of 400 mg/kg per day for 5 days or 1 g/kg per day for 2 days can be used. The transient effect and the cost of IVIg therapy should be considered. In patients who have no response to standard glucocorticoid and IVIg therapy and who have bleeding symptoms, a combined therapy with high-dose glucocorticoids (1 g/day) and IVIg (1–2 g/kg per day) may increase platelet counts. Splenectomy can be performed in the second trimester if the patient has not responded to glucocorticoids and IVIg therapy and has a platelet count less than 10 × 10^9/L or has bleeding symptoms. Platelet transfusions may be required in patients who have platelet counts less than 30 × 10^9/L to prevent maternal bleeding during labor.[390,505]

Severe neonatal thrombocytopenia (platelet counts $<20 \times 10^9$/L) occurs in 4 percent of ITP pregnancies and moderate neonatal thrombocytopenia (platelet counts $<50 \times 10^9$/L) in 9 percent.[512] Severe bleeding occurs in less than 1 percent of the babies. Because earlier studies reported that thrombocytopenic neonates have an increased risk for intracranial hemorrhage, some physicians have recommended performing cesarean delivery for all women with ITP to avoid injuries to the fetus during passage through the pelvis.[513] However, because of the rarity of intracerebral hemorrhage, no data prove that cesarean delivery is an effective approach for reducing the occurrence of intracerebral hemorrhage in the thrombocytopenic fetus.[232] Measurement of platelet counts in infants before delivery, such as by percutaneous umbilical cord blood sampling or fetal scalp vein sampling after cervical dilatation, is not recommended routinely because the morbidity and mortality rates of these procedures are high (2%).[512,514,515] Maternal platelet count at delivery does not correlate with the infant's platelet count. In ITP patients who gave birth more than once, however, the first infant's platelet count at birth is an important predictor of severe thrombocytopenia in subsequent pregnancies and may justify further obstetric management.[232,514,516] On the other hand, discordances in degree of thrombocytopenia between dichorionic twins in ITP indicate that fetal factors also are important.[517] Although the risk of neonatal thrombocytopenia is higher in newborns of mothers with ITP, only a small percentage of newborns have severe thrombocytopenia, with the infrequent case of intracranial hemorrhage often associated with other risk factors such as prematurity and alloimmune thrombocytopenia. In a study in which platelet counts were obtained from 6770 pregnant women late in pregnancy and in 6103 of their newborns, severe neonatal thrombocytopenia was found in only one newborn of a thrombocytopenic mother.[510] There are no controlled studies describing the effects of antepartum treatment of the pregnant woman on the fetal platelet count. Treatment with glucocorticoids and IVIg has failed to improve the neonatal platelet count compared to counts obtained prepartum by serial fetal blood sampling.[518] IgG antibodies, especially IgG_4, are transmitted in breast milk. Although ITP reportedly is not a contraindication to breast-feeding,[339] if the neonatal platelet count does not return to normal in the weeks after birth, a trial cessation of breast-feeding should be instituted.[232]

PREECLAMPSIA, ECLAMPSIA, AND HELLP SYNDROME

Preeclampsia, defined by hypertension and proteinuria, complicates 5 to 8 percent of all pregnancies. It usually becomes evident during the second trimester and is a major contributor to maternal and fetal morbidity and mortality (see Chap. 7).[519,520] *Eclampsia* is defined by the occurrence of acute neurologic abnormalities in a preeclamptic woman during the peripartum period.[520–522] Thrombocytopenia is seen in approximately 50 percent of women with preeclampsia, with the severity of thrombocytopenia correlating with the severity of the preeclampsia.[523]

Pathogenesis

Attempts to define the pathogenesis of preeclampsia have engendered numerous theories, to the point that the disorder has been termed *a disease of theories*.[524] One clear aspect of the pathogenesis is the requirement for a placenta, given that the condition can be produced in abdominal pregnancies and molar pregnancies.[525] The disease appears to be initiated by defective invasion of the uterine spiral arteries by placental cytotrophoblasts. During normal implantation, these cells convert from epithelial to endothelial morphology, a process called *pseudovasculogenesis*.[526,527] In preeclampsia, this process is defective, resulting in diminished maternal blood flow to the placenta and placental hypoxia. Through unknown mechanisms, the production of membrane and soluble forms of the vascular endothelial growth factor (VEGF) receptor fms-like tyrosine kinase-1 (Flt1) is increased,[528] with resultant increases of soluble Flt1 (sFlt1) in the amniotic fluid[529] and maternal circulation.[530] sFlt1 is the product of an alternately spliced form of the Flt1 messenger RNA, which lacks the transmembrane and cytoplasmic domains present in the full-length receptor. A large amount of evidence implicates sFlt1 as playing a key role in the pathogenesis of preeclampsia. By binding to VEGF and the related placental growth factor, sFlt1 prevents their favorable effects on vascular endothelium. Its expression in rats produces a syndrome akin to preeclampsia: hypertension and proteinuria associated with glomerular endotheliosis (occlusion of glomerular capillaries by swollen endothelial cells).

Endoglin is another angiogenic receptor expressed on endothelial cells and placental syncytiotrophoblasts, functioning as a co-receptor for the potent angiogenic factor transforming growth factor-β.[531] Expression of its messenger RNA is increased in preeclamptic placenta.[531] The levels of the soluble extracellular domain, produced by proteolysis, are elevated in the blood of preeclamptic patients. In pregnant rats, soluble endoglin works synergistically with sFlt1 to produce vascular damage and a HELLP-like syndrome.[531]

These findings strongly suggest that a tonic level of VEGF-like angiogenic factors is required to maintain the normal function of vascular endothelial cells and that this process is dysregulated during preeclampsia/eclampsia.

The connection between preeclampsia and thrombocytopenia is not clear, although many cases have evidence of activation of blood coagulation detected by elevated levels of fibrin-degradation products and thrombin–antithrombin complexes.[507] Low levels of the VWF-cleaving metalloprotease ADAMTS-13 have also been described,[532] as have elevated levels of VWF, including the hyperadhesive ultralarge forms.[533]

A disorder related to preeclampsia/eclampsia is the HELLP syndrome, seen in the peripartum period and defined by the presence of microangiopathic hemolytic anemia, elevated liver enzymes, and low platelets. This disorder occurs more commonly in white women older than age 25 years and is the most common cause of severe liver disease in pregnancy.[534] Microangiopathic hemolysis results from shearing of the erythrocytes as they pass through arterioles occluded by platelet–fibrin deposits. Adhesion and aggregation of platelets on damaged and activated endothelium presumably accounts for the low platelet count (see Chap. 114). HELLP shares a number of features with TTP, including the presence of microangiopathic hemolysis and thrombocytopenia. Involvement of the central nervous system is a more prominent feature of TTP, whereas HELLP more commonly displays severe liver function abnormalities (see Chaps. 7, 49, and 124).[535] Because the two syndromes can be confused with one other, one study attempted to distinguish the two by measuring the activity of ADAMTS-13, which usually is absent or severely deficient in TTP.[532] The study found that essentially all 17 patients in a cohort with the HELLP syndrome had mild to moderate reductions in the activity of ADAMTS-13 in the plasma, and none was severely deficient.

Delivery of the fetus is the most effective treatment for preeclampsia, eclampsia, and the HELLP syndrome. The nadir of the platelet count and the peak of serum lactate dehydrogenase may occur postpartum, during the first postpartum day in most patients, but as late as 5 to 7 days in some. For patients with severe thrombocytopenia and microangiopathic hemolytic anemia, plasma exchange may be indicated if the fetus cannot be delivered or if improvement does not follow delivery. This treatment is empirically based on the similarity of the clinical picture to that of TTP. Postpartum day 3 often is considered the limit for supportive therapy in anticipation of a spontaneous recovery.[532] If thrombocytopenia and hemolysis (as assessed by serum lactate dehydrogenase levels) continue to worsen beyond this time, intervention with plasma exchange is appropriate for the presumed diagnosis of TTP-HUS (see Chap. 133). At this point, TTP-HUS cannot be distinguished from atypical preeclampsia/eclampsia/HELLP syndrome, for which plasma exchange treatment may be beneficial.[536] Earlier intervention with plasma exchange is indicated for more severe clinical problems, such as neurologic abnormalities or acute, anuric renal failure.

As with TTP-HUS, recurrence of HELLP syndrome in subsequent pregnancies is a concern. In the absence of persistent hypertension between pregnancies, HELLP syndrome is uncommon in subsequent pregnancies (3%), but less-severe complications are more common in subsequent pregnancies (preeclampsia 19% and preterm delivery 21%).[537]

NEONATAL ALLOIMMUNE THROMBOCYTOPENIA

Fetal–neonatal alloimmune thrombocytopenia (NAIT) is caused by the placental transfer of maternal alloantibodies against fetal platelet antigens inherited from the father. NAIT resembles neonatal alloimmune hemolytic anemia (Rh hemolytic disease of the newborn) in many aspects. In both diseases, maternal alloantibodies against fetal blood cell antigens cross the placenta and destroy antigen-positive cells, resulting in significant fetal/neonatal morbidity and mortality. However, unlike neonatal alloimmune hemolytic anemia, which tends to spare the firstborn child, the first child is affected in 40 to 60 percent of NAIT cases.[505] Transplacental transfer of antiplatelet antibodies can occur in babies born from mothers with ITP. Maternal ITP rarely may cause serious thrombocytopenia or bleeding problems in the fetus, including intracranial hemorrhage. In cases of NAIT, thrombocytopenia tends to be more severe and the intracranial hemorrhage rate is higher (10–20%) compared with maternal ITP.[232] In contrast to maternal ITP, in NAIT the maternal platelet count is normal, a key differential diagnostic finding.

Prevalence and Pathogenesis

The estimated frequency of NAIT varies from 1 in 500 to 1 in 2000 livebirths.[232,505,538] Maternal alloantibodies against human platelet antigens (HPAs) are responsible for platelet destruction in NAIT. In whites, the most frequently implicated antigens are HPA-1a or Pl^{A1} (78% of cases) and HPA-5b or Br^{a} (19% of cases).[539] These antigens are rare in Asian populations. HPA-4a (80% of cases) and HPA-3a (15% of cases) are responsible for platelet destruction in most Asian NAIT cases. Besides targeting the HPA system, anti–HLA-2 antibodies have been reported, but whether they are responsible for NAIT is not clear.[538,540,541]

The frequency of NAIT in whites is lower than would be expected given that the incidence of HPA-1a negativity is 2.5 percent. Only 10 percent of HPA-1a–negative mothers exposed to HPA-1a–positive platelets during pregnancy become immunized. HPA alloimmunization is strongly correlated with the presence of specific class II HLA antigens, with increased risk demonstrated in HPA-1a–negative mothers expressing HLA-B8, HLA-DR3, and HLA-DR52a antigens.[505,542,543] The presence of HLA-DRB3*0101 allele in HPA-1a–negative women increases the NAIT risk as much as 140-fold.[543]

NAIT tends to be clinically more severe in cases with alloantibodies against HPA-1a.[232] HPA-1 (Pl^{A}) antigens are expressed on platelet GPIIa. Anti–HPA-1a antibodies have been proposed to impair platelet aggregation, which may explain the severity of bleeding symptoms.[544]

Clinical Features

IgG alloantibodies can cross the placenta as early as week 14 of pregnancy, and passage increases with gestational age.[538] These antibodies bind to fetal platelets and lead to their destruction. In severe cases, intracranial hemorrhage and hydrocephalus may develop and lead to fetal death. The diagnosis is difficult to make in the first fetus affected. An ultrasonography scan may not help unless it detects bleeding or hydrocephalus. Unexplained fetal deaths in the maternal history or fetal hydrocephalus or bleeding in previous pregnancies may alert the physician to the possibility of NAIT. The diagnosis is made by fetal blood sampling.

Usually the diagnosis of NAIT is possible after birth. NAIT should be suspected in a thrombocytopenic neonate with extensive purpura or visceral hemorrhage but no evidence of sepsis, skeletal anomalies, or other systemic diseases that may cause thrombocytopenia, including maternal ITP. Affected babies may have no symptoms (13–59% of cases), or they may have bleeding symptoms (18–65% of cases) and evidence of intracranial hemorrhage (22–23% of cases).[545] In a case series of 88 infants with NAIT resulting from anti–HPA-1a antibodies, 90 percent had purpura, 66 percent had hematomas, 30 percent had gastrointestinal bleeding, and 14 percent had intracerebral hemorrhage. Bleeding may be delayed, as the platelet count usually falls further during the first several days of life. Death or neurologic impairment occurs in up to 25 percent of infants. Platelet counts recover to normal in 1 to 2 weeks.[546]

The diagnosis of NAIT usually can be confirmed by tests for circulating maternal alloantibodies against fetal antigens (usually by MAIPA) or by platelet typing of the parents and neonate by either genotyping or enzyme-linked immunosorbent assay. These tests may fail to yield the diagnosis because private HPA antigens may be responsible for NAIT.[232,505,538]

Management

Postnatal The alternatives in the management of affected neonates are IVIg, glucocorticoids (alone or combined with IVIg), and platelet transfusions. IVIg and/or glucocorticoid therapy may increase platelet counts rapidly, although a substantial increase of platelet counts usually occurs after 24 to 72 hours.[539] In cases with severe bleeding, platelets should be transfused. Transfused platelets should be ABO and (Rh)D compatible and HPA-1a–negative in the majority of cases.[547] Transfusion of washed and irradiated maternal platelets to the affected fetus is an alternative but may not be appropriate for several reasons. Washing of maternal platelets to eliminate maternal alloantibodies and irradiation to prevent graft-versus-host disease may damage the platelets.[232] Repeated platelet transfusions may be required.[505] One alternative in these cases is transfusion of platelets from HPA-1a–negative donors. Platelet counts usually increase rapidly after transfusion.[232,538]

Prenatal The treatment options in high-risk NAIT are maternal weekly IVIg administration with or without glucocorticoids, serial *in utero* platelet transfusions, *in utero* IVIg administration, and early delivery (after 32 weeks of gestation). Maternal IVIg administration at a dosage of 1 g/kg per week with or without glucocorticoids may increase fetal platelet counts,[548] although not all studies support this conclusion.[538,544] Direct administration of IVIg to the fetus also may not consistently raise fetal platelet counts.[549] In patients who do not respond to IVIg and glucocorticoid administration, serial matched platelet transfusions may be used. Matched platelet transfusions will only transiently increase the fetal platelet count because the transfused platelets also are targeted.[505] Serial platelet transfusions may increase the cumulative risk of hemorrhage and procedure-related hemorrhage and fetal loss.[544] In severely thrombocytopenic fetuses, early delivery with cesarean section may help reduce the risk of intracranial hemorrhage.[544]

Current therapeutic alternatives for antenatal management of NAIT are unsatisfactory. Novel therapeutic strategies are under investigation, including vaccines and competitive molecules that competitively bind anti–HPA-1a antibodies.[547]

ABNORMAL PLATELET DISTRIBUTION OR POOLING

SPLENOMEGALY

Splenomegaly may lead to thrombocytopenia by inducing a reversible pooling of up to 90 percent of total body platelets.[550,551] This process can be thought of as an exaggeration of normal splenic pooling, in which approximately one-third of the platelet mass is contained within the spleen at any one time (see Chap. 55). The survival of platelets within the spleen often is normal or may be moderately reduced. Thus, the total blood platelet pool in a patient with splenomegaly could be normal even when the counts measured in venous blood are only 20 percent of normal. In splenomegaly, platelet production usually is normal, as estimated by dividing the total body platelet mass by the platelet life span.[550]

Several lines of evidence support the concept that pooling is the major factor responsible for thrombocytopenia in uncomplicated splenomegaly. First, the fraction of radiolabeled platelets that can be recovered from the circulation after infusion into patients with hypersplenism is small, from 10 to 30 percent, in contrast to 60 to 80 percent in normal subjects and 90 to 100 percent in asplenic patients.[550,552] Second, epinephrine injected intravenously causes an immediate increase in the platelet count in both normal individuals and patients with splenomegaly. The increase in patients with splenomegaly is proportionally greater than the 30 to 40 percent seen in normal individuals.[550,553,554] Epinephrine causes constriction of the splenic artery, with a fivefold decrease in splenic blood flow and passive emptying of the spleen. Third, large quantities of platelets, three to seven times the number present in the circulation, can be flushed from enlarged spleens after surgical removal. Fourth, removal of large numbers of platelets from the circulation through apheresis is followed rapidly by replenishment from the splenic pool, without resultant thrombocytopenia.[551,555]

The finding that thrombocytopenia caused by increased splenic pooling does not stimulate thrombopoiesis is taken as evidence that total blood platelet pool, not the blood platelet concentration, is responsible for regulation of platelet production.

The most common disorder causing thrombocytopenia resulting from splenic pooling is chronic liver disease with portal hypertension and congestive splenomegaly. In patients with cirrhosis and portal hypertension, moderate thrombocytopenia is the rule. However, in such cases the thrombocytopenia often results from both splenic pooling and reduced hepatic production of TPO.

Thrombocytopenia associated with splenomegaly often is of no clinical importance. Signs and symptoms are related to the primary disorder, and bleeding manifestations result primarily from coagulation abnormalities caused by the underlying liver disease. This finding is consistent with the relatively moderate degree of thrombocytopenia, the near-normal total body content of platelets,[550] and the ability to mobilize platelets from the spleen to replenish losses.[555]

Because thrombocytopenia resulting from splenic pooling rarely is of clinical importance, no treatment is indicated. When splenectomy is performed for another reason, however, the platelet count predictably returns to normal and thrombocytosis may even occur.[550] Platelet counts may return to normal in patients following surgical correction of portal hypertension by portosystemic shunting.[556] Platelet transfusions usually are not needed for splenomegaly-associated thrombocytopenia and rarely produce significant increases in platelet count because as much as 90 percent of the transfused platelets will be sequestered in the spleen.

HYPERSPLENISM

Hypersplenism is distinguished from uncomplicated splenomegaly in that pooling is accompanied by increased destruction of platelets, leukocytes, and erythrocytes in association with increased marrow precursors of the deficient lines and correction of the cytopenia by splenectomy.[557–560] The clinical manifestations, laboratory findings, and specific treatment are aimed at the underlying disease (see Chap. 55).[561]

Imaging studies, such as computed tomographic scans, can be useful for defining the size of the spleen and identifying intrasplenic and extrasplenic disease. Magnetic resonance imaging defines blood flow patterns, which is especially useful for detecting portal or splenic vein thromboses. Cell survival studies using radiolabeled platelets or red blood cells may be helpful for identifying hypersequestration when weighing the need for splenectomy. Most patients with splenomegaly require therapy for the underlying disease rather than for thrombocytopenia.

THROMBOCYTOPENIA ASSOCIATED WITH MASSIVE TRANSFUSION

In the era before platelet transfusion, thrombocytopenia often accompanied severe hemorrhage with transfusion of stored blood. In the massively transfused patient, the severity of thrombocytopenia is related to the number of red cell transfusions but does not solely result from dilution of the platelets. Platelet counts may be higher than predicted, possibly by release of platelets from the spleen, or they may be lower than predicted because of consumption in microvascular lesions.[562] Fibrinogen deficiency develops earlier than thrombocytopenia when blood is replaced by red cell concentrates and plasma substitutes.[563] A study of patients requiring massive transfusion, defined as transfusion of 10 or more red cell units within 24 hours, demonstrated that mild thrombocytopenia ($47–100 \times 10^9$/L) occurred in all patients after transfusion of 15 red cell units, and more severe thrombocytopenia ($25–61 \times 10^9$/L) developed after 20 red cell units.[563,564] DIC, triggered by the disease responsible for the blood loss or the hypotension that commonly occurs with massive blood loss, may contribute to the thrombocytopenia (see Chap. 140). Management of the thrombocytopenia depends on its severity and the underlying condition. Massively transfused patients should be treated with fresh-frozen plasma to replace coagulation factors, and with platelets (see Chap. 140).[565] The precise ratio of platelets to red cells has not been determined, but two studies show that massively transfused trauma patients demonstrated improved survival with increased transfusion of platelet concentrates.[566,567]

THROMBOCYTOPENIA RESULTING FROM HYPOTHERMIA

Transient thrombocytopenia occurs during hypothermia, in both animals and humans, when the body temperature falls below 25°C.[568] The degree of thrombocytopenia correlates with the severity of body temperature drop. Thus, thrombocytopenia is less severe in cardiac surgery patients supported by normothermic systemic perfusion (35–37°C) than in those supported by moderately hypothermic systemic perfusion (25–29°C).[569] In this case, the drop in platelet count likely results from splenic and hepatic pooling[570] and from cold activation and clearance of platelets. Cold induces clustering of the GPIb complex and rearrangement of its carbohydrate chains, which then serve as ligands for the macrophage integrin $\alpha_M\beta_2$, which mediates their clearance in hepatic macrophages.[571,572] In hypothermic dogs, radiolabeled platelets are sequestered in the spleen, liver, and other organs; the platelets return to the circulation when normal body temperature is restored.[568,573] The clinical relevance of these observations is illustrated by reports of patients, often elderly, who are hypothermic after periods of unconsciousness in inadequately heated rooms. In one report, a 69-year-old woman had 13 admissions over an 8-year period with repeated hypothermia, 31° to 34°C. On each admission she was thrombocytopenic (platelet count $7–39 \times 10^9$/L).

With no therapy other than rewarming, platelet counts returned to normal in 4 to 10 days.[574] However, a review of 75 patients admitted with hypothermia (body temperatures 26°–35°C) demonstrated that only three patients were thrombocytopenic.[574]

DRUG-INDUCED THROMBOCYTOPENIA

Development of thrombocytopenia after quinine was first described by Vipan in 1865, and since then a large number of drugs have been found to cause thrombocytopenia. Drugs should be considered as potential culprits in any thrombocytopenic patient on medication, taking herbal remedies, or using iodinated radiocontrast solutions.[575] Drug-induced thrombocytopenia generally affects only a small percentage of patients taking a particular drug, and is usually not severe, although it can be fatal. Genetic or environmental factors both influence susceptibility to drugs. Discontinuation of causative drug(s) is the main treatment strategy; glucocorticoids may be used in some patients.

Drugs may cause thrombocytopenia by different mechanisms. Dose-dependent myelosuppression and immune destruction of the platelets are two well-known causes. One of the most severe and life-threatening immune thrombocytopenias is heparin-induced thrombocytopenia (HIT), an immune-mediated disorder caused by antibodies that recognize a neoepitope in platelet factor 4 that is exposed when platelet factor 4 binds heparin. The result is activation of platelets and the coagulation cascade and, ultimately, thrombosis. HIT affects up to 5 percent of patients exposed to heparin (see Chap. 133). This section discusses drugs, other than heparins, that cause isolated thrombocytopenia by immune platelet destruction; Chap. 34 discusses drug-induced aplastic anemia with thrombocytopenia.

Etiology

Reviews of drug-induced thrombocytopenia often contain such extensive lists of implicated drugs, many of which are commonly used, that they are not helpful for decisions regarding which therapy to interrupt first. To address the issue of which drugs most likely cause thrombocytopenia, a systematic review of all published case reports defined levels of evidence to document the causal relation between the drug and thrombocytopenia.[576] This review distinguished drugs with definite or probable causal relationships from those for which the evidence was weaker.[576] Table 119–5 lists the drugs for which there is definite evidence of a causal role in producing thrombocytopenia (which includes recurrent thrombocytopenia with rechallenge in the same patient) and drugs for which the causal relation to thrombocytopenia has been validated by at least two reports with probable evidence (thus meeting all of the criteria for definite evidence except for the lack of rechallenge). Quinidine is by far the most commonly cited drug. Other commonly cited drugs are similar to drugs documented in a

TABLE 119–5. Drugs Causing Thrombocytopenia

Cases: 1			
Adefovir dipivoxil (1, 0)	Diflunisal (0, 1)	Isotretinoin (0, 1)	Penicillin (0, 1)
Alatrofloxacin (0, 1)	Digitoxin (0, 1)	Itraconazole (0, 1)	Pentoxifylline (1, 0)
Albendazole (0, 1)	Diltiazem (0, 1)	Lithium (1, 0)	Piperazine (0, 1)
Alprenolol (1, 0)	Doxepin (0, 1)	Lopinavir/ritonavir (1, 0)	Primidone (0, 1)
Amlodipine (0, 1)	Eflornithine (1, 0)	Losartan (0, 1)	Pyrazinamide (0, 1)
Anakinra (0, 1)	Ezetimibe (0, 1)	Mebhydroline (0, 1)	Recombinant hepatitis B vaccine (0, 1)
Apalcillin (0, 1)	Famotidine (0, 1)	Meloxicam (0, 1)	Rifampicin (1, 0)
Aspirin (0, 1)	Felbamate (0, 1)	Meprobamate (0, 1)	Rituximab (1, 0)
Atorvastatin (1, 0)	Fenoprofen (0, 1)	Mesalamine (1, 0)	Rofecoxib (0, 1)
Bismuth (0, 1)	Feprazone (0, 1)	Methazolamide (0, 1)	Rosiglitazone (0, 1)
Butoconazole (0, 1)	Finasteride (0, 1)	Mexiletine (0, 1)	Sodium stibogluconate (0, 1)
Cefamandole (0, 1)	Formestane (0, 1)	Minoxidil (1, 0)	Sulfadiazine (0, 1)
Cephalothin (1, 0)	G-csf (filgrastim) (0, 1)	Mirtazapine (0, 1)	Sulfamethoxazole (0, 1)
Chlorpheniramine (0, 1)	Haloperidol (1, 0)	Morphine (0, 1)	Sulfathiazole (1, 0)
Chlorpromazine (1, 0)	Inamrinone (1, 0)	Naphazoline (1, 0)	Suramin (0, 1)
Ciprofloxacin (0, 1)	Indomethacin (0, 1)	Nimesulide (0, 1)	Teicoplanin (1, 0)
Clarithromycin (0, 1)	Infliximab (0, 1)	Nitroglycerin (1, 0)	Thiothixene (1, 0)
Clopidogrel (0, 1)	Influenza vaccine (0, 1)	Novobiocin (1, 0)	Tiagabine (0, 1)
Deferoxamine (1, 0)	Interferon 2b (0, 1)	Octreotide (1, 0)	Tolmetin (1, 0)
Desipramine (0, 1)	Iocetamic acid (0, 1)	Oxcarbazepine (0, 1)	Tranilast (0, 1)
Diazepam (1, 0)	Iopamidol (0, 1)	Oxytetracycline (0, 1)	
Diazoxide (1, 0)	Iron dextran (0, 1)	Penicillamine (0, 1)	
Diethylstilbestrol (1, 0)	Isoniazid (1, 0)		
Cases: 2–4			
Acetazolamide (1, 2)	Etretinate (0, 2)	Naproxen (0, 4)	Sulindac (0, 2)
Aminoglutethimide (2, 1)	Fluconazole (0, 2)	Oxaliplatin (0, 2)	Sulfamethoxypyridazine (0, 3)
Aminosalicylic acid (2, 1)	Glibenclamide (0, 2)	Oxprenolol (2, 1)	Sulfasalazine (1, 2)
Amphotericin b (2, 1)	Ibuprofen (0, 2)	Oxyphenbutazone (0, 2)	Tamoxifen (2, 1)
Ampicillin (0, 2)	Indinavir (3, 0)	Phenytoin (0, 3)	Terbinafine (0, 2)
Captopril (0, 2)	Interferon (0, 4)	Piperacillin (1, 1)	Ticlopidine (0, 3)
Chlordiazepoxide (0, 2)	Iopanoic acid (1, 1)	Roxifiban (0, 2)	Trastuzumab (0, 2)
Chlorothiazide (1, 3)	Levamisole (2, 0)	Simvastatin (0, 2)	Vancomycin (3, 0)
Digoxin (3, 0)	Meclofenamate (2, 0)	Sulfapyridine (0, 2)	
Ethambutol (1, 1)	Methicillin (2, 0)		
Cases: 5–10			
Abciximab c7e3 Fab (1, 6)	Danazol (3, 4)	Hydrochlorothiazide (0, 5)	Procainamide (0, 7)
Amiodarone (2, 0)	Diatrizoate meglumine/diatrizoate sodium (3, 2)	Interferon alpha (1, 6)	Ranitidine (0, 5)
Acetaminophen (3, 4)	Diclofenac (2, 3)	Lotrafiban (0, 5)	Rifampin (5, 5)
Carbamazepine (0, 10)	Efalizumab (Raptiva) (0, 6)	Methyldopa (3, 3)	Sulfisoxazole (1, 4)
Chlorpropamide (0, 5)	Eptifibatide (0, 7)	Nalidixic acid (1, 5)	Tirofiban (1, 6)
Cimetidine (1, 5)			
Cases: >10			
Gold (0, 11)	Quinidine (26, 32)	Quinine (14, 9)	Sulfamethoxazole (3, 12)

Table of drugs that cause thrombocytopenia supported by one or more patient case reports with level I (definite) or level II (probable) clinical evidence. The table is broken down by the total number of single case reports with the individual number of level I cases and level II reports denoted in parentheses, respectively. The full list of articles reviewed, the methodology for establishing levels of evidence, and a complete updated database are available at www.ouhsc.edu/platelets/.

SOURCE: Adapted from data obtained at www.ouhsc.edu/platelets/ditp.html, with permission of J. George.

TABLE 119–6. Mechanisms Underlying Drug-Induced Immune Thrombocytopenia

Classification	Mechanism	Incidence	Example
Hapten-dependent antibody	Hapten links covalently to membrane protein and induces drug-specific immune response	Very rare	Penicillin, possibly some cephalosporin antibiotics
Quinine-type drug	Drug induces antibody that binds to membrane protein in presence of soluble drug	26 cases per 1 million users of quinine per week, probably fewer cases with other drugs	Quinine, sulfonamide antibiotics, nonsteroidal anti-inflammatory drugs
Fiban-type drug	Drug reacts with glycoprotein IIb/IIIa to induce a conformational change (neoepitope) recognized by antibody (not yet confirmed)	0.2–0.5%	Tirofiban, eptifibatide
Drug-specific antibody	Antibody recognizes murine component of chimeric Fab fragment specific for platelet membrane glycoprotein IIIa	0.5–1.0% after first exposure, 10–14% after seconds exposure	Abciximab
Autoantibody	Drug induces antibody that reacts with autologous platelets in absence of drug	1.0% with gold, very rare with procainamide and other drugs	Gold salts, procainamide
Immune complex	Drug binds to platelet factor 4, producing immune complex for which antibody is specific; immune complex activates platelets through Fc receptors	3–6% among patients treated with unfractionated heparin for 7 days, rare with low-molecular-weight heparin	Heparins

SOURCE: From Aster RH, Bougie DW[575] with permission of the Massachusetts Medical Society. Copyright © 2007 Massachusetts Medical Society. All rights reserved.

case-control study.[577] A remarkable observation from the systematic review was how many case reports did not provide sufficient clinical information to allow a determination of even a probable causal relation.[390]

Pathogenesis

Thrombocytopenia is usually assumed to result from immune platelet destruction by drug-dependent antibodies.[575] Most of these antibodies bind the platelets only in the presence of the offending drugs. Drugs may trigger different immune mechanisms, as depicted in Table 119–6.

Drugs may bind covalently to membrane proteins, and may induce hapten-dependent antibodies in patients receiving penicillin and cephalosporin. In quinine-induced thrombocytopenia, antibodies bind to membrane proteins only in the presence of soluble drug. In patients receiving tirofiban or eptifibatide, the drug binds to GPIIb/IIIa ($\alpha_{IIb}\beta_3$ integrin), creating a conformation-dependent neoepitope, and inducing antibody production. Gold salts and procainamide, however, may induce true autoantibodies, with those induced by gold being unique in targeting platelet glycoprotein V.[578] These antibodies can bind and destroy platelets in the absence of the drug. In HIT, heparin–platelet factor 4 complexes induce autoantibodies.

Initial experimental observations suggested that drug–antibody complexes bind to platelets via the platelet Fcγ receptor. This mechanism is confirmed for HIT (see below in this section), but for other drugs, the drug-dependent antibodies appear to bind to platelets via their Fab regions.[579]

The target antigens are the major platelet surface glycoproteins (GPIb/IX/V and GPIIb/IIIa). Different drugs may provoke drug-dependent antibodies that preferentially react with one of these glycoproteins, or drug-dependent antibodies from a single patient may react with multiple epitopes on both glycoproteins. For example, a study of sera from 15 patients with quinine-induced thrombocytopenia demonstrated that, in the presence of quinine, the antibodies bound to two distinct domains on GPIb/IX, one on GPIbα and one on GPIX. Some patients had only one of the antibodies; some had both.[580] The same domains on GPIb/IX also appear to be the antigenic targets for quinidine- and ranitidine-dependent antiplatelet antibodies.[580,581] Definition of the specific epitope involved in patient reactions with drug-dependent antibodies may not only elucidate the mechanism of drug-induced thrombocytopenia but also identify polymorphisms in GPIb/IX that cause sensitivity in producing drug-dependent antiplatelet antibodies. Sulfonamides, quinidine, and quinine are frequent causes of drug-induced thrombocytopenia. Studies of sera from 15 patients with thrombocytopenia caused by sulfamethoxazole or sulfisoxazole demonstrated that the antigenic epitope was part of GPIIb/IIIa.[582] Some antibodies from patients with quinidine- and quinine-dependent antiplatelet antibodies also react with GPIIb/IIIa.[583]

In addition to specificity for discrete epitopes on platelet surface glycoproteins, drug-dependent antibodies are highly specific for the structure of the drug. For example, no cross-reactivity occurs between quinidine and quinine-dependent antibodies or between sulfamethoxazole and sulfisoxazole-dependent antibodies, even though both pairs of drugs have similar structures. Therefore, the neoantigens produced by drug binding to platelets create discrete epitopes that are sensitive to minor changes in drug structure.

The implications of this mechanism for platelet destruction are apparent. A patient with prior sensitivity to the drug has preformed antibodies that immediately react with the altered platelets upon repeat drug exposure, as demonstrated. An exception to this situation is the immediate acute thrombocytopenia that may occur with initial administration of antithrombotic agents that bind platelet GPIIb/IIIa,[38,584] especially abciximab. Abciximab is a humanized monoclonal antibody fragment that lacks the Fc domain, so thrombocytopenia is not caused by phagocytosis of the platelets by macrophages. Patients experiencing thrombocytopenia after receiving GPIIb/IIIa inhibitors have been postulated to have preformed antibodies to epitopes exposed on GPIIb/IIIa by drug binding. These could be the same antibodies that cause *in vitro* EDTA-dependent platelet agglutination and pseudothrombocytopenia (see "Pseudothrombopenia" above).[29,585,586]

DIAGNOSIS

The diagnosis of drug-induced thrombocytopenia can be made only by recovery from thrombocytopenia upon discontinuation of the drug and can be confirmed if thrombocytopenia recurs with rechallenge by the drug. Prompt recovery within 5 to 7 days is predictable.[576] Gold-induced thrombocytopenia is an exception because gold salts are retained for a long time within the body and thrombocytopenia can persist for months, becoming indistinguishable from ITP.[587] Rechallenge with a suspected drug is dangerous, because severe thrombocytopenia can develop rapidly with even very small doses. However, when any one of multiple drugs is involved and all are important for management, it may be appropriate to reintroduce them individually, followed by several days of close observation. In general, the smallest possible dose of the drug should be administered. The administration should be performed under direct supervision, with platelets available for bleeding should it occur. If rechallenge leads to thrombocytopenia, the patient should be advised to wear a Medic Alert bracelet. For common drugs, especially those that can be purchased without a prescription, it may be safer to supervise a rechallenge and unequivocally document risk rather than risk future unintentional use.

Laboratory assays can detect drug-dependent antibodies, and positive results can support a clinical diagnosis. However, the laboratory role remains largely investigational because results are not promptly available when a clinical decision must be made about discontinuing a drug. Furthermore, no laboratory test has been validated by continuing a suspected drug with no adverse effects following a negative laboratory test.

Drug-dependent antibodies can be detected by flow cytometric techniques,[582] MAIPA,[588] and solid-phase red cell adherence assays.[589] Strongly positive tests are apparent, but distinction of positive from negative tests is arbitrary and not yet clinically validated. Positive tests for heparin-dependent antibodies have been reported in patients without thrombocytopenia,[590–593] and patients with clinical evidence for drug-induced thrombocytopenia may have negative tests using multiple techniques.[582,594]

CLINICAL AND LABORATORY FEATURES

In patients with newly discovered thrombocytopenia, all medications should be identified. Not only prescription medications but also nonprescription drugs, such as products with acetaminophen,[576] and drinks that may include quinine ("tonic water") must be documented.[595,596]

Drug-induced thrombocytopenia typically produces profoundly low platelet counts. Among the 247 patient case reports with evidence for a definite or probable causal relation of the drug to thrombocytopenia, 23 patients (9%) had major bleeding, including two patients who died of bleeding,[576] and 68 patients (28%) had overt but minor bleeding; 96 patients (39%) had only purpura or trivial bleeding, and the remainder had no bleeding.[576] The time from beginning the drug to the initial occurrence of thrombocytopenia varies from 1 day to 3 years, but the median time is only 14 days. With rechallenge, acute thrombocytopenia may occur within minutes but almost always within 3 days.[576] Patients may have other signs and symptoms of drug sensitivity, such as nausea and vomiting, rash, fever, and abnormal liver function tests.[597] Laboratory data may demonstrate leukopenia, indicating multiple cell targets of the drug-dependent antibodies.[597] Patients who have systemic adverse reactions manifesting TTP-HUS are described in Chap. 133.

Treatment

Withdrawal of the offending drug is the most important therapeutic measure. Prednisone is commonly given because the distinction from ITP almost never is initially clear; however, it does not appear to influence recovery.[597] In patients with major bleeding, emergent treatment should be the same as for ITP: platelet transfusions, high doses of parenteral methylprednisolone, and possibly IVIg.[390]

AN APPROACH TO THROMBOCYTOPENIA IN CHILDREN

In many situations the diagnosis and management of thrombocytopenia in children and adults is similar, but special discussion of thrombocytopenia in the newborn and pediatric ITP is warranted.

NEONATAL THROMBOCYTOPENIA

Although relatively rare in well babies, thrombocytopenia is a common problem in the neonatal intensive care unit (NICU). As many as 25 to 30 percent of infants in the NICU will be affected by thrombocytopenia at some point in their hospitalization.[598,599] The approach to thrombocytopenia in the neonate is somewhat different than in older children and adults, given the unique differential diagnosis in this population.

Platelet counts increase toward adult levels throughout gestation, and a recent study indicates that the lower reference range for platelets in an infant who is less than 32 weeks gestation may extend as low as 104×10^9/L and reach 123×10^9/L in term infants.[600] In addition, neonatal megakaryocytes tend to be smaller and of lower ploidy than those of adults, resulting in a limited ability of the newborn to increase platelet production and compensate for enhanced platelet consumption.[601] These factors combine to explain the susceptibility of neonates to thrombocytopenia, especially when adult normal ranges of 150 to 450 $\times 10^9$/L are used. Severe thrombocytopenia in the newborn period is defined as a platelet count less than 50×10^9/L. The differential diagnosis of thrombocytopenia in the newborn period is driven by the initial assessment of whether the child is sick or well. In addition, the timing of the onset of thrombocytopenia (before or after 72 hours of life) is useful in discriminating between potential causes.

In sick infants, thrombocytopenia is most often attributable to the underlying disorder.[598,599] Etiologies of thrombocytopenia that presents before 72 hours of life include birth asphyxia and chronic placental insufficiency (pregnancy-induced hypertension, intrauterine growth retardation), and less commonly congenital infection with TORCH organisms (i.e., toxoplasmosis, other including HIV, rubella, cytomegalovirus and herpes simplex virus), sepsis, or thrombosis (especially renal vein thrombosis). When thrombocytopenia occurs later, sepsis and necrotizing enterocolitis are leading causes. Treatment is supportive, with platelet transfusions if needed, as well as treatment directed to the underlying diagnosis.

When thrombocytopenia is diagnosed in a well-appearing newborn, the differential includes both immune and nonimmune causes. Immune thrombocytopenia in the newborn is a result of passive transfer of maternal auto- or alloantibodies across the placenta. An important question to ask is whether the mother has a normal platelet count. If the mother has immune thrombocytopenia, then platelet autoantibodies reacting to a common platelet antigen present both in the mother and the child may lead to thrombocytopenia in approximately 10 percent of births.[602] Neonatal autoimmune thrombocytopenia is generally mild to moderate but may be severe with rare intracranial hemorrhage (1% or less); platelet counts usually recover within 1 to 3 weeks. In children with platelets less than 30×10^9/L or other bleeding risks necessitating intervention, treatment may include IVIg, platelet transfusion, or, occasionally, glucocorticoids. Although at risk, the severity of neonatal autoimmune thrombocytopenia is not expected to increase with subsequent pregnancies.

If the mother's platelets are normal, alloimmune thrombocytopenia should be considered. NAIT, analogous to hemolytic disease of the newborn, is a consequence of the development of maternal alloantibodies to human platelet antigens present in the father and infant but absent in the mother. Neonatal alloimmune thrombocytopenia is discussed at length above (see "Neonatal Alloimmune Thrombocytopenia" above).

Nonimmune platelet destruction is another potential cause of thrombocytopenia in clinically well infants. Although cutaneous hemangiomas are obvious, vascular malformations that involve the deep tissues or internal organs such as the liver may not be apparent on physical examination and can be an occult cause of thrombocytopenia. Such lesions often enlarge following birth and throughout the first year of life. Consumption of red cells, platelets, and clotting factors is discussed above (see "Kasabach-Merritt Syndrome" above). Other rare but important causes of nonimmune platelet destruction include congenital thrombotic thrombocytopenic purpura as a consequence of lack of ADAMTS-13[603,604] and von Willebrand disease type IIB.[605] Thrombocytopenia will respond to replacement of ADAMTS-13 by plasma transfusion in congenital TTP, whereas bleeding in von Willebrand disease type IIB is best managed with plasma derived factor VIII–von Willebrand factor complex and antithrombolytics if mucous membrane bleeding is present.

For those infants with persistent thrombocytopenia of unclear etiology, congenital thrombocytopenia should be considered. Although the list of potential inherited defects is long,[606–608] only a subset is likely to result in significant thrombocytopenia in the newborn period. In addition, inheritance pattern and associated congenital abnormalities may help to clarify the diagnosis. CAMT presents at birth with severe thrombocytopenia in an otherwise well and nondysmorphic child.[609] It is caused by autosomal recessive inheritance of mutations in the thrombopoietin receptor c-Mpl. Children with CAMT may be initially presumed to have NAIT, but thrombocytopenia in CAMT does not resolve in the first few weeks of life. Evaluation of the marrow will show a paucity of megakaryocytes; platelets are normal in size and granularity. In some cases, if the marrow is done very early, megakaryocytes may be only minimally decreased and a subsequent marrow is needed to clarify the diagnosis.[610,611] Although CAMT is a disorder of thrombocytopenia, nearly all children will go on to develop pancytopenia and aplastic anemia by age 10 years.[612] The diagnosis of CAMT can be confirmed by genetic analysis of c-Mpl. Whereas platelets in CAMT are morphologically normal, the findings of microthrombocytopenia in a boy should raise suspicion for the X-linked WAS. Although the full syndrome includes eczema and immune defects, mutations that only partially impair the WAS protein may exhibit isolated thrombocytopenia.[613]

Other congenital thrombocytopenias have associated morphologic abnormalities that facilitate their diagnosis. For example, radial defects and thrombocytopenia are linked in TAR and amegakaryocytic thrombocytopenia with radioulnar synostosis syndromes.[614–615] Although absent radii are clinically apparent, radioulnar synostosis may be more subtle and therefore forearm radiographs are useful in evaluation of the infant with thrombocytopenia of unknown etiology. Although platelet counts in TAR tend to improve over the first year of life, children with amegakaryocytic thrombocytopenia with radioulnar synostosis syndrome may progress rapidly to marrow failure. Paris Trousseau syndrome is also associated with significant thrombocytopenia in the newborn period[616]; these children usually have neurologic and cardiac abnormalities, and platelets may be notable for the presence of giant α granules. The diagnosis of Paris Trousseau syndrome is confirmed by detection of terminal deletion of chromosome 11q23 by cytogenetics or fluorescence *in situ* hybridization.

Transfusion parameters are difficult to establish in the neonatal period and practices vary.[617] More importantly, the risk of clinically important bleeding is affected by factors other than the platelet count including gestational age, the mode of delivery and concomitant illnesses. Preterm infants, especially those younger than 32 weeks' gestation or who weigh less than 1500 g and are in the first week of life, are at increased risk of intracranial hemorrhage because of the immaturity of the germinal matrix.[618] Prolonged labor, breech presentation, or use of instrumental or vacuum extraction may be associated with increased bleeding.[619,620] DIC as a consequence of sepsis, necrotizing enterocolitis, or KMS may lead to additional clotting factor deficiencies that exacerbate the bleeding risk from thrombocytopenia. Consequently, the bleeding risk cannot be determined only by the platelet count but must incorporate an assessment of the overall status of the child. One practical guideline suggests that within the first week of life, prophylactic transfusions should be given to keep the platelet count above 50,000/μL, and thereafter can be safely withheld in a nonbleeding infant until platelets are less than 30×10^9/L.[598,599] Transfusion to keep platelets greater than 50 to 100×10^9/L is typically recommended if significant bleeding (intracranial, gastrointestinal) is present. It is important to bear in mind the potential detrimental effects of transfusion. Several studies show that platelet transfusions are associated with an adverse outcome in infants in the NICU.[621–623] Although transfusions may be a marker associated with more severe underlying illness, they should be limited to children with true bleeding risk.

IMMUNE THROMBOCYTOPENIC PURPURA

Although the basic principles are similar, the approach to ITP is somewhat different in young children than in adolescents and adults because of age-related differences in inciting factors, differential diagnosis, clinical course of thrombocytopenia, risks for bleeding, the consequences of empiric therapy, and the side effects of treatment.

ITP in young children may occur as a polyclonal immune response to an external exposure, such as infection, an aberrant immune response because of an innate immune deficiency, or dysregulation.[624] In adolescents the mechanism may be more like that in adults.[625] In approximately two-thirds of cases, ITP in children occurs within 6 weeks of a recent viral illness or, less often, live virus vaccination.[626] Measles, rubella, varicella, influenza, Epstein-Barr, and human immunodeficiency viruses have all been specifically implicated; however, myriad viral syndromes in children go undiagnosed. Although poorly understood, the mechanism may involve molecular mimicry with antibodies formed against viral targets cross-reacting to platelet antigens.[626–628] Alternatively, antiidiotype antibodies produced during viral infection have been proposed to react with platelet antigens, perhaps explaining the lag between viral infection and the onset of thrombocytopenia.[629] The relationship between vaccination and ITP is of particular importance in pediatrics. The incidence of clinically significant thrombocytopenia ($<50 \times 10^9$/L) is estimated to be between 1:30,000 and 1:40,000 MMR (measles, mumps, rubella) vaccinations, although the majority of cases resolved within 1 month.[630–633] Vaccination does not cause relapse of thrombocytopenia in children with a history of non–vaccine-associated ITP[630,631,633,634] but may be associated with a higher risk of recurrence in children whose ITP had onset within 6 weeks of prior vaccination.[635–637] In this situation, measurement of measles and rubella titers may be useful: If protective immunity is present, booster immunizations can be withheld.[638] Importantly, the risk of thrombocytopenia following vaccination is much lower than that following the natural infection, and therefore if protective immunity is not present then the risks and benefits of vaccination must be weighed, taking into consideration the individual patient and the prevalence of disease in the community. As in adults, ITP in children is a clinical diagnosis and rests on the finding of isolated thrombocytopenia in an otherwise well-appearing child without evidence of another cause for thrombocytopenia. Anemia, neutropenia, atypical findings on the blood film, lymphadenopathy, splenomegaly, bony pain, or fevers should raise suspicion for an alternate diagnosis such as aplastic anemia or leukemia, in which event a marrow examination is indicated.[625,639] In young children, an important diagnosis to be distinguished from ITP is acute lymphoblastic leukemia (ALL). ALL can be exquisitely sensitive to glucocorticoids, and empiric treatment of thrombocytopenia with these agents for a presumed diagnosis of ITP can obscure and delay the diagnosis of ALL. In addition, treatment with glucocorticoids prior to the diagnosis of ALL is considered an adverse risk factor in most protocols.[640] A Pediatric Oncology Group study of 2000 children with leukemia, however, found that isolated thrombocytopenia is rare as a presenting finding in leukemia[641] and therefore a marrow examination is not required in children who meet criteria for a clinical diagnosis of ITP. However, most pediatric hematologists recommend a marrow examination prior to initiation of glucocorticoids, particularly at initial diagnosis or if being used for refractory disease.[642,643] Another rare but important diagnosis to exclude is one of the inherited or congenital thrombocytopenia syndromes. It is not uncommon for evaluation of the child to lead to the diagnosis of an inherited disorder affecting adult family members. Thrombocytopenia discovered prior to 1 year of age; subacute presentation of thrombocytopenia; unusually large, small, or hypogranular platelets; associated congenital abnormalities or a family history of thrombocytopenia should lead to consideration of a genetic cause for thrombocytopenia. These children can be spared what would be ineffective treatment for ITP.

Bleeding in children with ITP is most common at initial diagnosis. Most children with ITP present acutely with platelet counts below 20×10^9/L and many are below 10×10^9/L. Of children with ITP, 2.9 percent have severe hemorrhage at the time of diagnosis.[644] The risk of bleeding is greatest in those children whose platelet count is less than 10×10^9/L.[645] The incidence of intracranial hemorrhage in pediatric ITP is very low (0.1–1%).[646,647] Although platelet counts can be made to increase with treatment, it is unclear whether therapy prevents severe bleeding. Of those children with platelet counts less than 20×10^9/L, only 0.6 percent have severe bleeding within 28 days of diagnosis and bleeding in this group is not influenced by treatment.[644] Other age-related factors influence bleeding risk and decision making in individual patients. Toddlers with ITP are often very active, prone to falling, and difficult to confine to quiet play, whereas some teens may not accept restrictions on participation in contact or other high-risk sports.

Although severe at presentation, thrombocytopenia in pediatric ITP tends to be self-limited, and with or without therapy, with platelet counts improving within 6 weeks to 6 months of diagnosis in the majority of children.[649–651] In general, it is not thought that treatment significantly influences the course of ITP, although a recent report suggests that IVIg may speed resolution of thrombocytopenia,[652] and in adults, anti-CD20 is associated with a sustained alteration of the T-cell compartment and potentially the autoimmune response.[653] Traditionally, ITP has been defined as chronic when thrombocytopenia lasts beyond 6 months from diagnosis. However, data from the Intercontinental Childhood ITP Study Group indicate that a 25 percent of children with persistent thrombocytopenia at 6 months from diagnosis will remit within 1 year[654] and therefore continued thrombocytopenia beyond 6 months does not indicate that the disease will be lifelong. The frequency of spontaneous remission, sometimes years from diagnosis, complicates management decisions.

The management of pediatric ITP remains controversial and there are no randomized studies to effectively guide treatment decisions. Given the high rate of eventual remission, lack of evidence that treatment prevents severe bleeding or shortens the disease course, side effects, and expense of available therapeutic agents, some pediatric hematologists believe that it is appropriate to observe nonbleeding children regardless of platelet count without pharmacotherapy if they are able to have close followup; others advocate treatment at platelet counts less than 10 to 20×10^9/L to minimize the small but nevertheless important risk of severe bleeding.[642,643,655–658] To facilitate clinical studies, scoring systems have been devised to more consistently quantify bleeding symptomatology, including petechiae and bruising, epistaxis, and oral bleeding.[659,660] Individual risk factors and quality-of-life assessments contribute to decision making regarding treatment.[661] The goal of therapy in newly diagnosed children is to prevent bleeding while waiting for the disease to spontaneously remit. First-line treatments include IVIg and anti-(Rh)D; glucocorticoids are also effective but may be avoided as an initial intervention to preclude the need for a marrow biopsy or because of concerns regarding side effects of chronic use. Higher-dose, pulse glucocorticoid regimens may be associated with fewer long-term side effects.[662,663] Although there is also controversy on this point, because of the risk of postsplenectomy sepsis most pediatric hematologists would defer splenectomy until ITP has persisted more than 1 year and until the child is at least 5 years old, unless there is an emergent need to increase platelet counts quickly because of severe bleeding.[643,664,665] Prior to splenectomy, patients should be immunized against pneumococcus and meningococcus. Anti-CD20 has emerged as a potential splenectomy-sparing approach, although studies indicate that, as in adults, only approximately 30 percent of children will have a long-term response to this medication[666] and its effects on the developing immune system are unknown. The role of newer thrombopoietin receptor agonists in the management of pediatric ITP is not yet defined.

Thus, when considering the diagnosis and management of thrombocytopenia, children are not small adults. Fortunately, even severe thrombocytopenia in the newborn period or in childhood ITP often resolves, but it is important to establish the correct diagnosis and criteria for intervention in order to prevent serious bleeding while avoiding unnecessary treatments.

REFERENCES

1. Recommended methods for radioisotope platelet survival studies: By the panel on Diagnostic Application of Radioisotopes in Hematology, International Committee for Standardization in Hematology. *Blood* 50:1137, 1977.
2. Recommended method for indium-111 platelet survival studies. International Committee for Standardization in Hematology. Panel on Diagnostic Applications of Radionuclides. *J Nucl Med* 29:564, 1988.
3. Heyns AP, Badenhorst PN, Wessels P, et al: Indium-111-labelled human platelets: A method for use in severe thrombocytopenia. *Thromb Haemost* 52:226, 1984.
4. Brubaker DB, Marcus C, Holmes E: Intravascular and total body platelet equilibrium in healthy volunteers and in thrombocytopenic patients transfused with single donor platelets. *Am J Hematol* 58:165, 1998.
5. Heyns AD, Lotter MG, Badenhorst PN, et al: Kinetics and fate of (111)Indium-oxine labelled blood platelets in asplenic subjects. *Thromb Haemost* 44:100, 1980.
6. Aster RH: Pooling of platelets in the spleen: Role in the pathogenesis of "hypersplenic" thrombocytopenia. *J Clin Invest* 45:645, 1966.
7. Hill-Zobel RL, McCandless B, Kang SA, et al: Organ distribution and fate of human platelets: Studies of asplenic and splenomegalic patients. *Am J Hematol* 23:231, 1986.
8. Heyns AD, Lotter MG, Badenhorst PN, et al: Kinetics, distribution and sites of destruction of 111indium-labelled human platelets. *Br J Haematol* 44:269, 1980.
9. Heyns AD, Lotter MG, Badenhorst PN, et al: Kinetics and sites of destruction of 111Indium-oxine-labeled platelets in idiopathic thrombocytopenic purpura: A quantitative study. *Am J Hematol* 12:167, 1982.
10. Leissinger CA: Platelet kinetics in immune thrombocytopenic purpura and human immunodeficiency virus thrombocytopenia. *Curr Opin Hematol* 8:299, 2001.
11. Hanson SR, Slichter SJ: Platelet kinetics in patients with bone marrow hypoplasia: Evidence for a fixed platelet requirement. *Blood* 66:1105, 1985.
12. Ballem PJ, Segal GM, Stratton JR, et al: Mechanisms of thrombocytopenia in chronic autoimmune thrombocytopenic purpura. Evidence of both impaired platelet production and increased platelet clearance. *J Clin Invest* 80:33, 1987.
13. Lamy T, Moisan A, Dauriac C, et al: Splenectomy in idiopathic thrombocytopenic purpura: Its correlation with the sequestration of autologous indium-111-labeled platelets. *J Nucl Med* 34:182, 1993.
14. Yoneyama A, Nakahara K: [EDTA-dependent pseudothrombocytopenia—differentiation from true thrombocytopenia]. *Nippon Rinsho* 61:569, 2003.

15. Garcia Suarez J, Merino JL, Rodriguez M, et al: [Pseudothrombocytopenia: Incidence, causes and methods of detection]. *Sangre (Barc)* 36:197, 1991.
16. Payne BA, Pierre RV: Pseudothrombocytopenia: A laboratory artifact with potentially serious consequences. *Mayo Clin Proc* 59:123, 1984.
17. Savage RA: Pseudoleukocytosis due to EDTA-induced platelet clumping. *Am J Clin Pathol* 81:317, 1984.
18. Vicari A, Banfi G, Bonini PA: EDTA-dependent pseudothrombocytopaenia: A 12-month epidemiological study. *Scand J Clin Lab Invest* 48:537, 1988.
19. Sweeney JD, Holme S, Heaton WA, et al: Pseudothrombocytopenia in plateletpheresis donors. *Transfusion* 35:46, 1995.
20. Bartels PC, Schoorl M, Lombarts AJ: Screening for EDTA-dependent deviations in platelet counts and abnormalities in platelet distribution histograms in pseudothrombocytopenia. *Scand J Clin Lab Invest* 57:629, 1997.
21. Bragnani G, Bianconcini G, Brogna R, Zoli G: [Pseudothrombocytopenia: Clinical comment on 37 cases]. *Minerva Med* 92:13, 2001.
22. Kurata Y, Hayashi S, Jouzaki K, et al: [Four cases of pseudothrombocytopenia due to platelet cold agglutinins]. *Rinsho Ketsueki* 47:781, 2006.
23. Reed BW, Go RS: Pseudothrombocytopenia associated with multiple myeloma. *Mayo Clin Proc* 81:869, 2006.
24. Campbell V, Fosbury E, Bain BJ: Platelet phagocytosis as a cause of pseudothrombocytopenia. *Am J Hematol* 84:362, 2009.
25. Onder O, Weinstein A, Hoyer LW: Pseudothrombocytopenia caused by platelet agglutinins that are reactive in blood anticoagulated with chelating agents. *Blood* 56:177, 1980.
26. Bizzaro N: EDTA-dependent pseudothrombocytopenia: A clinical and epidemiological study of 112 cases, with 10-year follow-up. *Am J Hematol* 50:103, 1995.
27. Hoyt RH, Durie BG: Pseudothrombocytopenia induced by a monoclonal IgM kappa platelet agglutinin. *Am J Hematol* 31:50, 1989.
28. Bizzaro N, Goldschmeding R, dem Borne AE: Platelet satellitism is Fc gamma RIII (CD16) receptor-mediated. *Am J Clin Pathol* 103:740, 1995.
29. Casonato A, Bertomoro A, Pontara E, et al: EDTA dependent pseudothrombocytopenia caused by antibodies against the cytoadhesive receptor of platelet GPIIB-IIIA. *J Clin Pathol* 47:625, 1994.
30. Nomura S, Nagata H, Oda K, et al: Effects of EDTA on the membrane glycoproteins IIb-IIIa complex—Analysis using flow cytometry. *Thromb Res* 47:47, 1987.
31. Schrezenmeier H, Muller H, Gunsilius E, et al: Anticoagulant-induced pseudothrombocytopenia and pseudoleucocytosis. *Thromb Haemost* 73:506, 1995.
32. Ryo R, Sugano W, Goto M, et al: Platelet release reaction during EDTA-induced platelet agglutinations and inhibition of EDTA-induced platelet agglutination by anti-glycoprotein IIb/IIIa complex monoclonal antibody. *Thromb Res* 74:265, 1994.
33. Cohen AM, Lewinski UH, Klein B, Djaldetti M: Satellitism of platelets to monocytes. *Acta Haematol* 64:61, 1980.
34. Djaldetti M, Fishman P: Satellitism of platelets to monocytes in a patient with hypogammaglobulinaemia. *Scand J Haematol* 21:305, 1978.
35. Schell DA, Ganti AK, Levitt R, Potti A: Thrombocytopenia associated with c7E3 Fab (abciximab). *Ann Hematol* 81:76, 2002.
36. Sane DC, Damaraju LV, Topol EJ, et al: Occurrence and clinical significance of pseudothrombocytopenia during abciximab therapy. *J Am Coll Cardiol* 36:75, 2000.
37. Pinton P: [Abciximab-induced thrombopenia during treatment of acute coronary syndromes by angioplasty]. *Ann Cardiol Angeiol (Paris)* 47:351, 1998.
38. Berkowitz SD, Sane DC, Sigmon KN, et al: Occurrence and clinical significance of thrombocytopenia in a population undergoing high-risk percutaneous coronary revascularization. Evaluation of c7E3 for the Prevention of Ischemic Complications (EPIC) Study Group. *J Am Coll Cardiol* 32:311, 1998.
39. Berkman N, Michaeli Y, Or R, Eldor A: EDTA-dependent pseudothrombocytopenia: A clinical study of 18 patients and a review of the literature. *Am J Hematol* 36:195, 1991.
40. Mori M, Kudo H, Yoshitake S, et al: Transient EDTA-dependent pseudothrombocytopenia in a patient with sepsis. *Intensive Care Med* 26:218, 2000.
41. Bizzaro N, Fiorin F: Coexistence of erythrocyte agglutination and EDTA-dependent platelet clumping in a patient with thymoma and plasmocytoma. *Arch Pathol Lab Med* 123:159, 1999.
42. Matarazzo M, Conturso V, Di Martino M, et al: EDTA-dependent pseudothrombocytopenia in a case of liver cirrhosis. *Panminerva Med* 42:155, 2000.
43. Chiurazzi F, Villa MR, Rotoli B: Transplacental transmission of EDTA-dependent pseudothrombocytopenia. *Haematologica* 84:664, 1999.
44. Solanki DL, Blackburn BC: Spurious thrombocytopenia during pregnancy. *Obstet Gynecol* 65:14S, 1985.
45. Kelley MJ, Jawien W, Ortel TL, Korczak JF: Mutation of MYH9, encoding non-muscle myosin heavy chain A, in May-Hegglin anomaly. *Nat Genet* 26:106, 2000.
46. Seri M, Pecci A, Di Bari F, et al: MYH9-related disease: May-Hegglin anomaly, Sebastian syndrome, Fechtner syndrome, and Epstein syndrome are not distinct entities but represent a variable expression of a single illness. *Medicine (Baltimore)* 82:203, 2003.
47. Heath KE, Campos-Barros A, Toren A, et al: Nonmuscle myosin heavy chain IIA mutations define a spectrum of autosomal dominant macrothrombocytopenias: May-Hegglin anomaly and Fechtner, Sebastian, Epstein, and Alport-like syndromes. *Am J Hum Genet* 69:1033, 2001.
48. Balduini CL, Iolascon A, Savoia A: Inherited thrombocytopenias: From genes to therapy. *Haematologica* 87:860, 2002.
49. Shao XR, Li JZ, Ma J, et al: [Clinical and molecular-biological study of a May-Hegglin anomaly family]. *Zhonghua Xue Ye Xue Za Zhi* 25:548, 2004.
50. Di Pumpo M, Noris P, Pecci A, et al: Defective expression of GPIb/IX/V complex in platelets from patients with May-Hegglin anomaly and Sebastian syndrome. *Haematologica* 87:943, 2002.
51. Ghiggeri GM, Caridi G, Magrini U, et al: Genetics, clinical and pathological features of glomerulonephritis associated with mutations of nonmuscle myosin IIA (Fechtner syndrome). *Am J Kidney Dis* 41:95, 2003.
52. Toothaker LE, Gonzalez DA, Tung N, et al: Cellular myosin heavy chain in human leukocytes: Isolation of 5' cDNA clones, characterization of the protein, chromosomal localization, and upregulation during myeloid differentiation. *Blood* 78:1826, 1991.
53. D'Apolito M, Guarnieri V, Boncristiano M, et al: Cloning of the murine non-muscle myosin heavy chain IIA gene ortholog of human MYH9 responsible for May-Hegglin, Sebastian, Fechtner, and Epstein syndromes. *Gene* 286:215, 2002.
54. Arrondel C, Vodovar N, Knebelmann B, et al: Expression of the nonmuscle myosin heavy chain IIA in the human kidney and screening for MYH9 mutations in Epstein and Fechtner syndromes. *J Am Soc Nephrol* 13:65, 2002.
55. Matsushita T, Hayashi H, Kunishima S, et al: Targeted disruption of mouse ortholog of the human MYH9 responsible for macrothrombocytopenia with different organ involvement: Hematological, nephrological, and otological studies of heterozygous KO mice. *Biochem Biophys Res Commun* 325:1163, 2004.
56. Althaus K, Greinacher A: MYH9-related platelet disorders. *Semin Thromb Hemost* 35:189, 2009.
57. Pecci A, Panza E, Pujol-Moix N, et al: Position of nonmuscle myosin heavy chain IIA (NMMHC-IIA) mutations predicts the natural history of MYH9-related disease. *Hum Mutat* 29:409, 2008.
58. Deutsch S, Rideau A, Bochaton-Piallat ML, et al: Asp1424Asn MYH9 mutation results in an unstable protein responsible for the phenotypes in May-Hegglin anomaly/Fechtner syndrome. *Blood* 102:529, 2003.
59. Chen Z, Naveiras O, Balduini A, et al: The May-Hegglin anomaly gene MYH9 is a negative regulator of platelet biogenesis modulated by the Rho-ROCK pathway. *Blood* 110:171, 2007.
60. Leon C, Eckly A, Hechler B, et al: Megakaryocyte-restricted MYH9 inactivation dramatically affects hemostasis while preserving platelet aggregation and secretion. *Blood* 110:3183, 2007.
61. Canobbio I, Noris P, Pecci A, et al: Altered cytoskeleton organization in platelets from patients with MYH9-related disease. *J Thromb Haemost* 3:1026, 2005.
62. Pujol-Moix N, Kelley MJ, Hernandez A, et al: Ultrastructural analysis of granulocyte inclusions in genetically confirmed MYH9-related disorders. *Haematologica* 89:330, 2004.
63. Kunishima S: [May-Hegglin anomaly—From genome research to clinical laboratory]. *Rinsho Byori* 51:898, 2003.
64. Kunishima S, Matsushita T, Kojima T, et al: Immunofluorescence analysis of neutrophil nonmuscle myosin heavy chain-A in MYH9 disorders: Association of subcellular localization with MYH9 mutations. *Lab Invest* 83:115, 2003.
65. Pecci A, Noris P, Invernizzi R, et al: Immunocytochemistry for the heavy chain of the non-muscle myosin IIA as a diagnostic tool for MYH9-related disorders. *Br J Haematol* 117:164, 2002.
66. Heller PG, Pecci A, Glembotsky AC, et al: Unexplained recurrent venous thrombosis in a patient with MYH9-related disease. *Platelets* 17:274, 2006.
67. Selleng K, Lubenow LE, Greinacher A, Warkentin TE: Perioperative management of MYH9 hereditary macrothrombocytopenia (Fechtner syndrome). *Eur J Haematol* 79:263, 2007.
68. Pecci A, Granata A, Fiore CE, Balduini CL: Renin-angiotensin system blockade is effective in reducing proteinuria of patients with progressive nephropathy caused by MYH9 mutations (Fechtner-Epstein syndrome). *Nephrol Dial Transplant* 23:2690, 2008.
69. Behrens WE: Mediterranean macrothrombocytopenia. *Blood* 46:199, 1975.
70. Savoia A, Balduini CL, Savino M, et al: Autosomal dominant macrothrombocytopenia in Italy is most frequently a type of heterozygous Bernard-Soulier syndrome. *Blood* 97:1330, 2001.
71. Rees DC, Iolascon A, Carella M, et al: Stomatocytic haemolysis and macrothrombocytopenia (Mediterranean stomatocytosis/macrothrombocytopenia) is the haematological presentation of phytosterolaemia. *Br J Haematol* 130:297, 2005.
72. Minelli A, Maserati E, Rossi G, et al: Familial platelet disorder with propensity to acute myelogenous leukemia: Genetic heterogeneity and progression to leukemia via acquisition of clonal chromosome anomalies. *Genes Chromosomes Cancer* 40:165, 2004.
73. Song WJ, Sullivan MG, Legare RD, et al: Haploinsufficiency of CBFA2 causes familial thrombocytopenia with propensity to develop acute myelogenous leukaemia. *Nat Genet* 23:166, 1999.
74. Okuda T, van Deursen J, Hiebert SW, et al: AML1, the target of multiple chromosomal translocations in human leukemia, is essential for normal fetal liver hematopoiesis. *Cell* 84:321, 1996.
75. Michaud J, Wu F, Osato M, et al: *In vitro* analyses of known and novel RUNX1/AML1 mutations in dominant familial platelet disorder with predisposition to acute myelogenous leukemia: Implications for mechanisms of pathogenesis. *Blood* 99:1364, 2002.
76. Elagib KE, Racke FK, Mogass M, et al: RUNX1 and GATA-1 coexpression and cooperation in megakaryocytic differentiation. *Blood* 101:4333, 2003.

77. Geddis AE, Kaushansky K: Inherited thrombocytopenias: Toward a molecular understanding of disorders of platelet production. *Curr Opin Pediatr* 16:15, 2004.
78. Drachman JG, Jarvik GP, Mehaffey MG: Autosomal dominant thrombocytopenia: Incomplete megakaryocyte differentiation and linkage to human chromosome 10. *Blood* 96:118, 2000.
79. Savoia A, Del Vecchio M, Totaro A, et al: An autosomal dominant thrombocytopenia gene maps to chromosomal region 10p. *Am J Hum Genet* 65:1401, 1999.
80. Gandhi MJ, Cummings CL, Drachman JG: FLJ14813 missense mutation: A candidate for autosomal dominant thrombocytopenia on human chromosome 10. *Hum Hered* 55:66, 2003.
81. Grossfeld PD, Mattina T, Lai Z, et al: The 11q terminal deletion disorder: A prospective study of 110 cases. *Am J Med Genet* 129A:51, 2004.
82. Favier R, Jondeau K, Boutard P, et al: Paris-Trousseau syndrome: Clinical, hematological, molecular data of ten new cases. *Thromb Haemost* 90:893, 2003.
83. Raslova H, Komura E, Le Couedic JP, et al: FLI1 monoallelic expression combined with its hemizygous loss underlies Paris-Trousseau/Jacobsen thrombopenia. *J Clin Invest* 114:77, 2004.
84. Shivdasani RA: Lonely in Paris: When one gene copy isn't enough. *J Clin Invest* 114:17, 2004.
85. Thompson AA, Woodruff K, Feig SA, et al: Congenital thrombocytopenia and radio-ulnar synostosis: A new familial syndrome. *Br J Haematol* 113:866, 2001.
86. Thompson AA, Nguyen LT: Amegakaryocytic thrombocytopenia and radio-ulnar synostosis are associated with HOXA11 mutation. *Nat Genet* 26:397, 2000.
87. Sauvageau G, Iscove NN, Humphries RK: *In vitro* and *in vivo* expansion of hematopoietic stem cells. *Oncogene* 23:7223, 2004.
88. Thorsteinsdottir U, Sauvageau G, Hough MR, et al: Overexpression of HOXA10 in murine hematopoietic cells perturbs both myeloid and lymphoid differentiation and leads to acute myeloid leukemia. *Mol Cell Biol* 17:495, 1997.
89. van den Oudenrijn S, de Haas M, dem Borne AE: Screening for c-mpl mutations in patients with congenital amegakaryocytic thrombocytopenia identifies a polymorphism. *Blood* 97:3675, 2001.
90. Tonelli R, Scardovi AL, Pession A, et al: Compound heterozygosity for two different amino-acid substitution mutations in the thrombopoietin receptor (c-mpl gene) in congenital amegakaryocytic thrombocytopenia (CAMT). *Hum Genet* 107:225, 2000.
91. Ihara K, Ishii E, Eguchi M, et al: Identification of mutations in the c-mpl gene in congenital amegakaryocytic thrombocytopenia. *Proc Natl Acad Sci U S A* 96:3132, 1999.
92. Ballmaier M, Germeshausen M, Schulze H, et al: c-mpl mutations are the cause of congenital amegakaryocytic thrombocytopenia. *Blood* 97:139, 2001.
93. Germeshausen M, Schulze H, Gaudig A, et al: [Congenital amegakaryocytic thrombocytopenia (CAMT)—A defect of the thrombopoietin receptor c-Mpl]. *Klin Padiatr* 213:155, 2001.
94. Germeshausen M, Ballmaier M, Welte K: Implications of mutations in hematopoietic growth factor receptor genes in congenital cytopenias. *Ann N Y Acad Sci* 938:305; discussion 320, 2001.
95. van den Oudenrijn S, Bruin M, Folman CC, et al: Mutations in the thrombopoietin receptor, Mpl, in children with congenital amegakaryocytic thrombocytopenia. *Br J Haematol* 110:441, 2000.
96. Ballmaier M, Germeshausen M, Krukemeier S, Welte K: Thrombopoietin is essential for the maintenance of normal hematopoiesis in humans: Development of aplastic anemia in patients with congenital amegakaryocytic thrombocytopenia. *Ann N Y Acad Sci* 996:17, 2003.
97. Shaw S: Congenital hypoplastic thrombocytopenia with skeletal deformities in siblings. *Blood* 14:374, 1959.
98. Hall JG: Thrombocytopenia and absent radius (TAR) syndrome. *J Med Genet* 24:79, 1987.
99. Greenhalgh KL, Howell RT, Bottani A, et al: Thrombocytopenia-absent radius syndrome: A clinical genetic study. *J Med Genet* 39:876, 2002.
100. Hedberg VA, Lipton JM: Thrombocytopenia with absent radii. A review of 100 cases. *Am J Pediatr Hematol Oncol* 10:51, 1988.
101. Letestu R, Vitrat N, Masse A, et al: Existence of a differentiation blockage at the stage of a megakaryocyte precursor in the thrombocytopenia and absent radii (TAR) syndrome. *Blood* 95:1633, 2000.
102. Ballmaier M, Schulze H, Strauss G, et al: Thrombopoietin in patients with congenital thrombocytopenia and absent radii: Elevated serum levels, normal receptor expression, but defective reactivity to thrombopoietin. *Blood* 90:612, 1997.
103. Ochs HD: The Wiskott-Aldrich syndrome. *Clin Rev Allergy Immunol* 20:61, 2001.
104. Rengan R, Ochs HD: Molecular biology of the Wiskott-Aldrich syndrome. *Rev Immunogenet* 2:243, 2000.
105. Derry JM, Kerns JA, Weinberg KI, et al: WASP gene mutations in Wiskott-Aldrich syndrome and X-linked thrombocytopenia. *Hum Mol Genet* 4:1127, 1995.
106. Derry JM, Ochs HD, Francke U: Isolation of a novel gene mutated in Wiskott-Aldrich syndrome. *Cell* 78:635, 1994.
107. Villa A, Notarangelo L, Macchi P, et al: X-linked thrombocytopenia and Wiskott-Aldrich syndrome are allelic diseases with mutations in the WASP gene. *Nat Genet* 9:414, 1995.
108. Imai K, Nonoyama S, Ochs HD: WASP (Wiskott-Aldrich syndrome protein) gene mutations and phenotype. *Curr Opin Allergy Clin Immunol* 3:427, 2003.
109. Burns S, Cory GO, Vainchenker W, Thrasher AJ: Mechanisms of WASp-mediated haematological and immunological disease. *Blood* 104:3454, 2004.
110. Notarangelo LD, Mazza C, Giliani S, et al: Missense mutations of the WASP gene cause intermittent X-linked thrombocytopenia. *Blood* 99:2268, 2002.
111. Zhu Q, Watanabe C, Liu T, et al: Wiskott-Aldrich syndrome/X-linked thrombocytopenia: WASP gene mutations, protein expression, and phenotype. *Blood* 90:2680, 1997.
112. Shcherbina A, Rosen FS, Remold-O'Donnell E: WASP levels in platelets and lymphocytes of Wiskott-Aldrich syndrome patients correlate with cell dysfunction. *J Immunol* 163:6314, 1999.
113. Lum LG, Tubergen DG, Corash L, Blaese RM: Splenectomy in the management of the thrombocytopenia of the Wiskott-Aldrich syndrome. *N Engl J Med* 302:892, 1980.
114. Filipovich AH, Stone JV, Tomany SC, et al: Impact of donor type on outcome of bone marrow transplantation for Wiskott-Aldrich syndrome: Collaborative study of the International Bone Marrow Transplant Registry and the National Marrow Donor Program. *Blood* 97:1598, 2001.
115. Drachman JG: Inherited thrombocytopenia: When a low platelet count does not mean ITP. *Blood* 103:390, 2004.
116. Strom TS, Gabbard W, Kelly PF, Cunningham JM, Nienhuis AW: Functional correction of T cells derived from patients with the Wiskott-Aldrich syndrome (WAS) by transduction with an oncoretroviral vector encoding the WAS protein. *Gene Ther* 10:803, 2003.
117. Wada T, Jagadeesh GJ, Nelson DL, Candotti F: Retrovirus-mediated WASP gene transfer corrects Wiskott-Aldrich syndrome T-cell dysfunction. *Hum Gene Ther* 13:1039, 2002.
118. Klein C, Nguyen D, Liu CH, et al: Gene therapy for Wiskott-Aldrich syndrome: Rescue of T-cell signaling and amelioration of colitis upon transplantation of retrovirally transduced hematopoietic stem cells in mice. *Blood* 101:2159, 2003.
119. Freson K, Devriendt K, Matthijs G, et al: Platelet characteristics in patients with X-linked macrothrombocytopenia because of a novel GATA1 mutation. *Blood* 98:85, 2001.
120. Mehaffey MG, Newton AL, Gandhi MJ, et al: X-linked thrombocytopenia caused by a novel mutation of GATA-1. *Blood* 98:2681, 2001.
121. Shivdasani RA, Fujiwara Y, McDevitt MA, Orkin SH: A lineage-selective knockout establishes the critical role of transcription factor GATA-1 in megakaryocyte growth and platelet development. *EMBO J* 16:3965, 1997.
122. Tsang AP, Fujiwara Y, Hom DB, Orkin SH: Failure of megakaryopoiesis and arrested erythropoiesis in mice lacking the GATA-1 transcriptional cofactor FOG. *Genes Dev* 12:1176, 1998.
123. Orkin SH: GATA-binding transcription factors in hematopoietic cells. *Blood* 80:575, 1992.
124. Vyas P, Ault K, Jackson CW, et al: Consequences of GATA-1 deficiency in megakaryocytes and platelets. *Blood* 93:2867, 1999.
125. Enjolras O, Wassef M, Mazoyer E, et al: Infants with Kasabach-Merritt syndrome do not have "true" hemangiomas. *J Pediatr* 130:631, 1997.
126. Sarkar M, Mulliken JB, Kozakewich HP, et al: Thrombocytopenic coagulopathy (Kasabach-Merritt phenomenon) is associated with Kaposiform hemangioendothelioma and not with common infantile hemangioma. *Plast Reconstr Surg* 100:1377, 1997.
127. Vin-Christian K, McCalmont TH, Frieden IJ: Kaposiform hemangioendothelioma. An aggressive, locally invasive vascular tumor that can mimic hemangioma of infancy. *Arch Dermatol* 133:1573, 1997.
128. Hall GW: Kasabach-Merritt syndrome: Pathogenesis and management. *Br J Haematol* 112:851, 2001.
129. Cooper JG, Edwards SL, Holmes JD: Kaposiform haemangioendothelioma: Case report and review of the literature. *Br J Plast Surg* 55:163, 2002.
130. Hoeger PH, Helmke K, Winkler K: Chronic consumption coagulopathy due to an occult splenic haemangioma: Kasabach-Merritt syndrome. *Eur J Pediatr* 154:365, 1995.
131. Brasanac D, Janic D, Boricic I, et al: Retroperitoneal kaposiform hemangioendothelioma with tufted angioma-like features in an infant with Kasabach-Merritt syndrome. *Pathol Int* 53:627, 2003.
132. Mukhtar IA, Letts M: Hemangioma of the radius associated with Kasabach-Merritt syndrome: Case report and literature review. *J Pediatr Orthop* 24:87, 2004.
133. Fukunaga M, Ushigome S, Ishikawa E: Kaposiform haemangioendothelioma associated with Kasabach-Merritt syndrome. *Histopathology* 28:281, 1996.
134. Alvarez-Mendoza A, Lourdes TS, Ridaura-Sanz C, Ruiz-Maldonado R: Histopathology of vascular lesions found in Kasabach-Merritt syndrome: Review based on 13 cases. *Pediatr Dev Pathol* 3:556, 2000.
135. Jones EW, Orkin M: Tufted angioma (angioblastoma). A benign progressive angioma, not to be confused with Kaposi's sarcoma or low-grade angiosarcoma. *J Am Acad Dermatol* 20:214, 1989.
136. Wong SN, Tay YK: Tufted angioma: A report of five cases. *Pediatr Dermatol* 19:388, 2002.
137. Mueller BU, Mulliken JB: The infant with a vascular tumor. *Semin Perinatol* 23:332, 1999.
138. Mazoyer E, Enjolras O, Laurian C, et al: Coagulation abnormalities associated with extensive venous malformations of the limbs: Differentiation from Kasabach-Merritt syndrome. *Clin Lab Haematol* 24:243, 2002.
139. Lyons LL, North PE, Mac-Moune LF, et al: Kaposiform hemangioendothelioma: A study of 33 cases emphasizing its pathologic, immunophenotypic, and biologic uniqueness from juvenile hemangioma. *Am J Surg Pathol* 28:559, 2004.
140. Gilon E, Ramot B, Sheba C: Multiple hemangiomata associated with thrombocytopenia: Remarks on the pathogenesis of the thrombocytopenia in this syndrome. *Blood* 14:74, 1959.

141. Seo SK, Suh JC, Na GY, et al: Kasabach-Merritt syndrome: Identification of platelet trapping in a tufted angioma by immunohistochemistry technique using monoclonal antibody to CD61. *Pediatr Dermatol* 16:392, 1999.
142. Brizel HE, Raccuglia G: Giant hemangioma with thrombocytopenia. Radioisotopic demonstration of platelet sequestration. *Blood* 26:751, 1965.
143. Shulkin BL, Argenta LC, Cho KJ, Castle VP: Kasabach-Merritt syndrome: Treatment with epsilon-aminocaproic acid and assessment by indium 111 platelet scintigraphy. *J Pediatr* 117:746, 1990.
144. Warrell RP Jr, Kempin SJ, Benua RS, et al: Intratumoral consumption of indium-111 labeled platelets in a patient with hemangiomatosis and intravascular coagulation (Kasabach-Merritt syndrome). *Cancer* 52:2256, 1983.
145. Wananukul S, Nuchprayoon I, Seksarn P: Treatment of Kasabach-Merritt syndrome: A stepwise regimen of prednisolone, dipyridamole, and interferon. *Int J Dermatol* 42:741, 2003.
146. MacArthur CJ, Senders CW, Katz J: The use of interferon alfa-2a for life-threatening hemangiomas. *Arch Otolaryngol Head Neck Surg* 121:690, 1995.
147. Haisley-Royster C, Enjolras O, Frieden IJ, et al: Kasabach-Merritt phenomenon: A retrospective study of treatment with vincristine. *J Pediatr Hematol Oncol* 24:459, 2002.
148. Blei F, Karp N, Rofsky N, et al: Successful multimodal therapy for kaposiform hemangioendothelioma complicated by Kasabach-Merritt phenomenon: Case report and review of the literature. *Pediatr Hematol Oncol* 15:295, 1998.
149. Hu B, Lachman R, Phillips J, et al: Kasabach-Merritt syndrome-associated kaposiform hemangioendothelioma successfully treated with cyclophosphamide, vincristine, and actinomycin D. *J Pediatr Hematol Oncol* 20:567, 1998.
150. Frevel T, Rabe H, Uckert F, Harms E: Giant cavernous haemangioma with Kasabach-Merritt syndrome: A case report and review. *Eur J Pediatr* 161:243, 2002.
151. Atahan IL, Cengiz M, Ozyar E, Gurkaynak M: Radiotherapy in the management of Kasabach-Merritt syndrome: A case report. *Pediatr Hematol Oncol* 18:471, 2001.
152. Ogino I, Torikai K, Kobayasi S, et al: Radiation therapy for life- or function-threatening infant hemangioma. *Radiology* 218:834, 2001.
153. Billio A, Pescosta N, Rosanelli C, et al: Treatment of Kasabach-Merritt syndrome by embolisation of a giant liver hemangioma. *Am J Hematol* 66:140, 2001.
154. Hosono S, Ohno T, Kimoto H, et al: Successful transcutaneous arterial embolization of a giant hemangioma associated with high-output cardiac failure and Kasabach-Merritt syndrome in a neonate: A case report. *J Perinat Med* 27:399, 1999.
155. Zukerberg LR, Nickoloff BJ, Weiss SW: Kaposiform hemangioendothelioma of infancy and childhood. An aggressive neoplasm associated with Kasabach-Merritt syndrome and lymphangiomatosis. *Am J Surg Pathol* 17:321, 1993.
156. George M, Singhal V, Sharma V, Nopper AJ: Successful surgical excision of a complex vascular lesion in an infant with Kasabach-Merritt syndrome. *Pediatr Dermatol* 19:340, 2002.
157. Pavkovic M, Georgievski B, Cevreska L, et al: CTLA-4 exon 1 polymorphism in patients with autoimmune blood disorders. *Am J Hematol* 72:147, 2003.
158. Mientjes GH, van Ameijden EJ, Mulder JW, et al: Prevalence of thrombocytopenia in HIV-infected and non-HIV infected drug users and homosexual men. *Br J Haematol* 82:615, 1992.
159. Ehmann WC, Rabkin CS, Eyster ME, Goedert JJ: Thrombocytopenia in HIV-infected and uninfected hemophiliacs. Multicenter Hemophilia Cohort study. *Am J Hematol* 54:296, 1997.
160. Ciernik IF, Cone RW, Fehr J, Weber R: Impaired liver function and retroviral activity are risk factors contributing to HIV-associated thrombocytopenia. Swiss HIV Cohort Study. *AIDS* 13:1913, 1999.
161. Dominguez A, Gamallo G, Garcia R, et al: Pathophysiology of HIV related thrombocytopenia: An analysis of 41 patients. *J Clin Pathol* 47:999, 1994.
162. Louache F, Vainchenker W: Thrombocytopenia in HIV infection. *Curr Opin Hematol* 1:369, 1994.
163. Brook MG, Ayles H, Harrison C, et al: Diagnostic utility of bone marrow sampling in HIV positive patients. *Genitourin Med* 73:117, 1997.
164. Van W, V, Kotze HF, Heyns AP: Kinetics of indium-111-labelled platelets in HIV-infected patients with and without associated thrombocytopaenia. *Eur J Haematol* 62:332, 1999.
165. Kamiyama M, Arkel YS, Chen K, Shido K: Inhibition of platelet GPIIb/IIIa binding to fibrinogen by serum factors: Studies of circulating immune complexes and platelet antibodies in patients with hemophilia, immune thrombocytopenic purpura, human immunodeficiency virus-related immune thrombocytopenic purpura, and systemic lupus erythematosus. *J Lab Clin Med* 117:209, 1991.
166. Karpatkin S, Nardi MA, Hymes KB: Sequestration of anti-platelet GPIIIa antibody in rheumatoid factor immune complexes of human immunodeficiency virus 1 thrombocytopenic patients. *Proc Natl Acad Sci U S A* 92:2263, 1995.
167. Karpatkin S, Nardi M, Lennette ET, et al: Anti-human immunodeficiency virus type 1 antibody complexes on platelets of seropositive thrombocytopenic homosexuals and narcotic addicts. *Proc Natl Acad Sci U S A* 85:9763, 1988.
168. Fabris F, Cordiano I, Casonato A, et al: "Anti-platelet antibodies" in HIV infected haemophiliacs. *Folia Haematol Int Mag Klin Morphol Blutforsch* 117:709, 1990.
169. Bettaieb A, Oksenhendler E, Fromont P, et al: Immunochemical analysis of platelet autoantibodies in HIV-related thrombocytopenic purpura: A study of 68 patients. *Br J Haematol* 73:241, 1989.
170. Quadri MI, Lee CA, Goodall AH, et al: Antibodies to platelet glycoproteins in haemophiliacs infected with HIV. *Clin Lab Haematol* 14:109, 1992.
171. Yu JR, Lennette ET, Karpatkin S: Anti-F(ab')2 antibodies in thrombocytopenic patients at risk for acquired immunodeficiency syndrome. *J Clin Invest* 77:1756, 1986.
172. Karpatkin S, Nardi MA, Kouri YH: Internal-image anti-idiotype HIV-1GP120 antibody in human immunodeficiency virus 1 (HIV-1)-seropositive individuals with thrombocytopenia. *Proc Natl Acad Sci U S A* 89:1487, 1992.
173. Karpatkin S, Nardi M: Autoimmune anti-HIV-1GP120 antibody with antiidiotype-like activity in sera and immune complexes of HIV-1-related immunologic thrombocytopenia. *J Clin Invest* 89:356, 1992.
174. Karpatkin S, Nardi MA, Liu LX, et al: Production of a human anti-CD4 monoclonal antibody with antiidiotype to anti-HIV type 1 glycoprotein 120. *AIDS Res Hum Retroviruses* 11:509, 1995.
175. Nardi MA, Liu LX, Karpatkin S: GPIIIa-(49–66) is a major pathophysiologically relevant antigenic determinant for anti-platelet GPIIIa of HIV-1-related immunologic thrombocytopenia. *Proc Natl Acad Sci U S A* 94:7589, 1997.
176. Chia WK, Blanchette V, Mody M, et al: Characterization of HIV-1-specific antibodies and HIV-1-crossreactive antibodies to platelets in HIV-1-infected haemophiliac patients. *Br J Haematol* 103:1014, 1998.
177. Gonzalez-Conejero R, Rivera J, Rosillo MC, et al: Association of autoantibodies against platelet glycoproteins Ib/IX and IIb/IIIa, and platelet-reactive anti-HIV antibodies in thrombocytopenic narcotic addicts. *Br J Haematol* 93:464, 1996.
178. Samuel H, Nardi M, Karpatkin M, et al: Differentiation of autoimmune thrombocytopenia from thrombocytopenia associated with immune complex disease: Systemic lupus erythematosus, hepatitis-cirrhosis, and HIV-1 infection by platelet and serum immunological measurements. *Br J Haematol* 105:1086, 1999.
179. Bettaieb A, Oksenhendler E, Duedari N, Bierling P: Cross-reactive antibodies between HIV-GP120 and platelet GPIIIa (CD61) in HIV-related immune thrombocytopenic purpura. *Clin Exp Immunol* 103:19, 1996.
180. Bettaieb A, Fromont P, Louache F, et al: Presence of cross-reactive antibody between human immunodeficiency virus (HIV) and platelet glycoproteins in HIV-related immune thrombocytopenic purpura. *Blood* 80:162, 1992.
181. Hohmann AW, Booth K, Peters V, et al: Common epitope on HIV p24 and human platelets. *Lancet* 342:1274, 1993.
182. Nardi M, Karpatkin S: Antiidiotype antibody against platelet anti-GPIIIa contributes to the regulation of thrombocytopenia in HIV-1-ITP patients. *J Exp Med* 191:2093, 2000.
183. Nardi M, Feinmark SJ, Hu L, et al: Complement-independent Ab-induced peroxide lysis of platelets requires 12-lipoxygenase and a platelet NADPH oxidase pathway. *J Clin Invest* 113:973, 2004.
184. Nardi M, Tomlinson S, Greco MA, Karpatkin S: Complement-independent, peroxide-induced antibody lysis of platelets in HIV-1-related immune thrombocytopenia. *Cell* 106:551, 2001.
185. Koefoed K, Ditzel HJ: Identification of talin head domain as an immunodominant epitope of the antiplatelet antibody response in patients with HIV-1-associated thrombocytopenia. *Blood* 104:4054, 2004.
186. Cole JL, Marzec UM, Gunthel CJ, et al: Ineffective platelet production in thrombocytopenic human immunodeficiency virus-infected patients. *Blood* 91:3239, 1998.
187. Chelucci C, Federico M, Guerriero R, et al: Productive human immunodeficiency virus-1 infection of purified megakaryocytic progenitors/precursors and maturing megakaryocytes. *Blood* 91:1225, 1998.
188. Ballem PJ, Belzberg A, Devine DV, et al: Kinetic studies of the mechanism of thrombocytopenia in patients with human immunodeficiency virus infection. *N Engl J Med* 327:1779, 1992.
189. Espanol I, Muniz-Diaz E, Margall N, et al: Serum thrombopoietin levels in thrombocytopenic and non-thrombocytopenic patients with human immunodeficiency virus (HIV-1) infection. *Eur J Haematol* 63:245, 1999.
190. Young G, Loechelt BJ, Rakusan TA, et al: Thrombopoietin levels in HIV-associated thrombocytopenia in children. *J Pediatr* 133:765, 1998.
191. Zauli G, Catani L, Gibellini D, et al: Impaired survival of bone marrow GPIIb/IIa+ megakaryocytic cells as an additional pathogenetic mechanism of HIV-1-related thrombocytopenia. *Br J Haematol* 92:711, 1996.
192. Sato T, Sekine H, Kakuda H, et al: HIV infection of megakaryocytic cell lines. *Leuk Lymphoma* 36:397, 2000.
193. Kowalska MA, Ratajczak J, Hoxie J, et al: Megakaryocyte precursors, megakaryocytes and platelets express the HIV co-receptor CXCR4 on their surface: Determination of response to stromal-derived factor-1 by megakaryocytes and platelets. *Br J Haematol* 104:220, 1999.
194. Riviere C, Subra F, Cohen-Solal K, et al: Phenotypic and functional evidence for the expression of CXCR4 receptor during megakaryocytopoiesis. *Blood* 93:1511, 1999.
195. Basch RS, Kouri YH, Karpatkin S: Expression of CD4 by human megakaryocytes. *Proc Natl Acad Sci U S A* 87:8085, 1990.
196. Kouri YH, Borkowsky W, Nardi M, et al: Human megakaryocytes have a CD4 molecule capable of binding human immunodeficiency virus-1. *Blood* 81:2664, 1993.
197. Voulgaropoulou F, Tan B, Soares M, et al: Distinct human immunodeficiency virus strains in the bone marrow are associated with the development of thrombocytopenia. *J Virol* 73:3497, 1999.
198. Voulgaropoulou F, Pontow SE, Ratner L: Productive infection of CD34+-cell-derived megakaryocytes by X4 and R5 HIV-1 isolates. *Virology* 269:78, 2000.
199. Stella CC, Ganser A, Hoelzer D: Defective *in vitro* growth of the hemopoietic progenitor cells in the acquired immunodeficiency syndrome. *J Clin Invest* 80:286, 1987.
200. Ahmed S, Sadiq A, Siddiqui AK, et al: Thrombotic thrombocytopenic purpura: A rare cause of thrombocytopenia in HIV-infected hemophiliacs. *Ann Hematol* 83:253, 2004.

201. Sutor GC, Schmidt RE, Albrecht H: Thrombotic microangiopathies and HIV infection: Report of two typical cases, features of HUS and TTP, and review of the literature. *Infection* 27:12, 1999.
202. Gervasoni C, Ridolfo AL, Vaccarezza M, et al: Thrombotic microangiopathy in patients with acquired immunodeficiency syndrome before and during the era of introduction of highly active antiretroviral therapy. *Clin Infect Dis* 35:1534, 2002.
203. Brecher ME, Hay SN, Park YA: Is it HIV TTP or HIV-associated thrombotic microangiopathy? *J Clin Apher* 23:186, 2008.
204. Gunther K, Garizio D, Nesara P: ADAMTS13 activity and the presence of acquired inhibitors in human immunodeficiency virus-related thrombotic thrombocytopenic purpura. *Transfusion* 47:1710, 2007.
205. Benjamin M, Terrell DR, Vesely SK, et al: Frequency and significance of HIV infection among patients diagnosed with thrombotic thrombocytopenic purpura. *Clin Infect Dis* 48:1129, 2009.
206. Aukrust P, Bjornsen S, Lunden B, et al: Persistently elevated levels of von Willebrand factor antigen in HIV infection. Downregulation during highly active antiretroviral therapy. *Thromb Haemost* 84:183, 2000.
207. Peltier JY, Lambin P, Doinel C, et al: Frequency and prognostic importance of thrombocytopenia in symptom-free HIV-infected individuals: A 5-year prospective study. *AIDS* 5:381, 1991.
208. Glatt AE, Anand A: Thrombocytopenia in patients infected with human immunodeficiency virus: Treatment update. *Clin Infect Dis* 21:415, 1995.
209. Scaradavou A: HIV-related thrombocytopenia. *Blood Rev* 16:73, 2002.
210. Mannucci PM, Gringeri A: [HIV-related thrombocytopenias]. *Ann Ital Med Int* 15:20, 2000.
211. Sitalakshmi S, Srikrishna A, Damodar P: Haematological changes in HIV infection. *Indian J Pathol Microbiol* 46:180, 2003.
212. Diebold J, Tabbara W, Marche C, et al: [Bone marrow changes at several stages of HIV infection, studied on bone marrow biopsies in 85 patients]. *Arch Anat Cytol Pathol* 39:137, 1991.
213. Ananworanich J, Phanuphak N, Nuesch R, et al: Recurring thrombocytopenia associated with structured treatment interruption in patients with human immunodeficiency virus infection. *Clin Infect Dis* 37:723, 2003.
214. Ballem PJ, Belzberg A, Devine D, et al: Pathophysiology of thrombocytopenia associated with HIV infection in homosexual men. A preliminary report. *Blut* 59:111, 1989.
215. Panzer S, Stain C, Benda H, Mannhalter C: Effects of 3-azidothymidine on platelet counts, indium-111-labelled platelet kinetics, and antiplatelet antibodies. *Vox Sang* 57:120, 1989.
216. Zidovudine for the treatment of thrombocytopenia associated with human immunodeficiency virus (HIV). A prospective study. The Swiss Group for Clinical Studies on the Acquired Immunodeficiency Syndrome (AIDS). *Ann Intern Med* 109:718, 1988.
217. Aboulafia DM, Bundow D, Waide S, et al: Initial observations on the efficacy of highly active antiretroviral therapy in the treatment of HIV-associated autoimmune thrombocytopenia. *Am J Med Sci* 320:117, 2000.
218. Carbonara S, Fiorentino G, Serio G, et al: Response of severe HIV-associated thrombocytopenia to highly active antiretroviral therapy including protease inhibitors. *J Infect* 42:251, 2001.
219. Stasi R, Stipa E, Masi M, et al: Long-term observation of 208 adults with chronic idiopathic thrombocytopenic purpura. *Am J Med* 98:436, 1995.
220. Oksenhendler E, Bierling P, Chevret S, et al: Splenectomy is safe and effective in human immunodeficiency virus-related immune thrombocytopenia. *Blood* 82:29, 1993.
221. Marroni M, Gresele P: Detrimental effects of high-dose dexamethasone in severe, refractory, HIV-related thrombocytopenia. *Ann Pharmacother* 34:1139, 2000.
222. Brown SA, Majumdar G, Harrington C, et al: Effect of splenectomy on HIV-related thrombocytopenia and progression of HIV infection in patients with severe haemophilia. *Blood Coagul Fibrinolysis* 5:393, 1994.
223. Majluf-Cruz A, Luna-Castanos G, Huitron S, Nieto-Cisneros L: Usefulness of a low-dose intravenous immunoglobulin regimen for the treatment of thrombocytopenia associated with AIDS. *Am J Hematol* 59:127, 1998.
224. Jahnke L, Applebaum S, Sherman LA, et al: An evaluation of intravenous immunoglobulin in the treatment of human immunodeficiency virus-associated thrombocytopenia. *Transfusion* 34:759, 1994.
225. Scaradavou A, Woo B, Woloski BM, et al: Intravenous anti-D treatment of immune thrombocytopenic purpura: Experience in 272 patients. *Blood* 89:2689, 1997.
226. Harker LA, Marzec UM, Novembre F, et al: Treatment of thrombocytopenia in chimpanzees infected with human immunodeficiency virus by pegylated recombinant human megakaryocyte growth and development factor. *Blood* 91:4427, 1998.
227. Marroni M, Gresele P, Landonio G, et al: Interferon-alpha is effective in the treatment of HIV-1-related, severe, zidovudine-resistant thrombocytopenia. A prospective, placebo-controlled, double-blind trial. *Ann Intern Med* 121:423, 1994.
228. Stasi R: Therapeutic strategies for hepatitis- and other infection-related immune thrombocytopenias. *Semin Hematol* 46:S15, 2009.
229. Neben S, Hellman S, Montgomery M, et al: Hematopoietic stem cell deficit of transplanted bone marrow previously exposed to cytotoxic agents. *Exp Hematol* 21:156, 1993.
230. Schiffer CA, Anderson KC, Bennett CL, et al: Platelet transfusion for patients with cancer: Clinical practice guidelines of the American Society of Clinical Oncology. *J Clin Oncol* 19:1519, 2001.
231. Blajchman MA, Slichter SJ, Heddle NM, Murphy MF: New strategies for the optimal use of platelet transfusions. *Hematology Am Soc Hematol Educ Program* 198, 2008.
232. Bishop JF, Matthews JP, Yuen K, et al: The definition of refractoriness to platelet transfusions. *Transfus Med* 2:35, 1992.
233. Helleberg C, Taaning EB, Johnsen HE: [Transfusion-refractory thrombocytopenia during chemotherapy: Pathogenesis, frequency and treatment]. *Ugeskr Laeger* 157:5082, 1995.
234. Vadhan-Raj S, Kavanagh JJ, Freedman RS, et al: Safety and efficacy of transfusions of autologous cryopreserved platelets derived from recombinant human thrombopoietin to support chemotherapy-associated severe thrombocytopenia: A randomised cross-over study. *Lancet* 359:2145, 2002.
235. Leonardi V, Danova M, Fincato G, Palmeri S: Interleukin 3 in the treatment of chemotherapy induced thrombocytopenia. *Oncol Rep* 5:1459, 1998.
236. Farber L, Haus U, Fuchsel G, et al: Treatment of prolonged chemotherapy induced severe thrombocytopenia with recombinant human interleukin-3—A report on four cases. *Anticancer Drugs* 8:288, 1997.
237. Meden H, Fock M, Kuhn W: Effect of recombinant human interleukin-3 (rhIL-3) on persisting chemotherapy-induced thrombocytopenia. *Anticancer Drugs* 5:483, 1994.
238. Chu DT, Xu BH, Song ST, et al: [Recombinant human interleukin-11 in the prevention of chemotherapy-induced thrombocytopenia]. *Zhonghua Zhong Liu Za Zhi* 25:272, 2003.
239. Sun XF, Guan ZZ, Huang H, et al: [Clinical study of rhIL-11 for prevention and treatment of chemotherapy-induced thrombocytopenia]. *Ai Zheng* 21:892, 2002.
240. Chu DT, Xu BH, Song ST, et al: [Recombinant Human Interleukin 11 (Mega) Promotes Thrombopoiesis in Cancer Patients with Chemotherapy-Induced Myelosuppression]. *Zhongguo Shi Yan Xue Ye Xue Za Zhi* 9:314, 2001.
241. Smith JW: Tolerability and side-effect profile of rhIL-11. *Oncology (Williston Park)* 14:41, 2000.
242. Kaye JA: FDA licensure of NEUMEGA to prevent severe chemotherapy-induced thrombocytopenia. *Stem Cells* 16 Suppl 2:207, 1998.
243. Tepler I, Elias L, Smith JW, et al: A randomized placebo-controlled trial of recombinant human interleukin-11 in cancer patients with severe thrombocytopenia due to chemotherapy. *Blood* 87:3607, 1996.
244. Kaye JA: Clinical development of recombinant human interleukin-11 to treat chemotherapy-induced thrombocytopenia. *Curr Opin Hematol* 3:209, 1996.
245. Nichol JL, Hokom MM, Hornkohl A, et al: Megakaryocyte growth and development factor. Analyses of in vitro effects on human megakaryopoiesis and endogenous serum levels during chemotherapy-induced thrombocytopenia. *J Clin Invest* 95:2973, 1995.
246. Bai CM, Xu GX, Zhao YQ, et al: [A multi-center clinical trial of recombinant human thrombopoietin in the treatment of chemotherapy-induced thrombocytopenia in patients with solid tumor]. *Zhongguo Yi Xue Ke Xue Yuan Xue Bao* 26:437, 2004.
247. Bai CM, Zou XY, Zhao YQ, et al: [The clinical study of recombinant human thrombopoietin in the treatment of chemotherapy-induced severe thrombocytopenia]. *Zhonghua Yi Xue Za Zhi* 84:397, 2004.
248. Vadhan-Raj S, Patel S, Bueso-Ramos C, et al: Importance of predosing of recombinant human thrombopoietin to reduce chemotherapy-induced early thrombocytopenia. *J Clin Oncol* 21:3158, 2003.
249. Vadhan-Raj S: Clinical experience with recombinant human thrombopoietin in chemotherapy-induced thrombocytopenia. *Semin Hematol* 37:28, 2000.
250. Nash RA, Kurzrock R, DiPersio J, et al: A phase I trial of recombinant human thrombopoietin in patients with delayed platelet recovery after hematopoietic stem cell transplantation. *Biol Blood Marrow Transplant* 6:25, 2000.
251. Shinjo K, Takeshita A, Nakamura S, et al: Serum thrombopoietin levels in patients correlate inversely with platelet counts during chemotherapy-induced thrombocytopenia. *Leukemia* 12:295, 1998.
252. Heits F, Katschinski DM, Wilmsen U, et al: Serum thrombopoietin and interleukin 6 concentrations in tumour patients and response to chemotherapy-induced thrombocytopenia. *Eur J Haematol* 59:53, 1997.
253. Stabler SP, Allen RH, Savage DG, Lindenbaum J: Clinical spectrum and diagnosis of cobalamin deficiency. *Blood* 76:871, 1990.
254. Sarode R, Garewal G, Marwaha N, et al: Pancytopenia in nutritional megaloblastic anaemia. A study from north-west India. *Trop Geogr Med* 41:331, 1989.
255. Slichter SJ, Harker LA: Thrombocytopenia: Mechanisms and management of defects in platelet production. *Clin Haematol* 7:523, 1978.
256. Epstein RD: Cells of the megakaryocytic series in pernicious anemia: In particular, the effect of specific therapy. *Am J Pathol* 25:239, 1949.
257. Rabinowitz AP, Sacks Y, Carmel R: Autoimmune cytopenias in pernicious anemia: A report of four cases and review of the literature. *Eur J Haematol* 44:18, 1990.
258. Junca J, Flores A, Granada ML, et al: The relationship between idiopathic thrombocytopenic purpura and pernicious anaemia. *Br J Haematol* 111:513, 2000.
259. Dittmar M, Kahaly GJ: Polyglandular autoimmune syndromes: Immunogenetics and long-term follow-up. *J Clin Endocrinol Metab* 88:2983, 2003.
260. Ingeberg S, Stoffersen E: Platelet dysfunction in patients with vitamin B12 deficiency. *Acta Haematol* 61:75, 1979.
261. Terade H, Niikura H, Mori H, et al: [Megaloblastic anemia and platelet function—A qualitative platelet defect in pernicious anemia]. *Rinsho Ketsueki* 31:254, 1990.
262. Berger M, Brass LF: Severe thrombocytopenia in iron deficiency anemia. *Am J Hematol* 24:425, 1987.
263. Sullivan LW, Adams WH, Liu YK: Induction of thrombocytopenia by thrombopheresis in man: Patterns of recovery in normal subjects during ethanol ingestion and abstinence. *Blood* 49:197, 1977.
264. Latvala J, Parkkila S, Niemela O: Excess alcohol consumption is common in patients with cytopenia: Studies in blood and bone marrow cells. *Alcohol Clin Exp Res* 28:619, 2004.

265. Smith CM, Tobin JD Jr, Burris SM, White JG: Alcohol consumption in the guinea pig is associated with reduced megakaryocyte deformability and platelet size. *J Lab Clin Med* 120:699, 1992.
266. Michot F, Gut J: Alcohol-induced bone marrow damage. A bone marrow study in alcohol-dependent individuals. *Acta Haematol* 78:252, 1987.
267. Wolber EM, Jelkmann W: Thrombopoietin: The novel hepatic hormone. *News Physiol Sci* 17:6, 2002.
268. Louwes H, Vellenga E, de Wolf JT: Abnormal platelet adhesion on abdominal vessels in asymptomatic patients with paroxysmal nocturnal hemoglobinuria. *Ann Hematol* 80:573, 2001.
269. Elebute MO, Rizzo S, Tooze JA, et al: Evaluation of the haemopoietic reservoir in de novo haemolytic paroxysmal nocturnal haemoglobinuria. *Br J Haematol* 123:552, 2003.
270. Nishimura J, Ware RE, Burnette A, et al: The hematopoietic defect in PNH is not due to defective stroma, but is due to defective progenitor cells. *Blood Cells Mol Dis* 29:159, 2002.
271. Hugel B, Socie G, Vu T, et al: Elevated levels of circulating procoagulant microparticles in patients with paroxysmal nocturnal hemoglobinuria and aplastic anemia. *Blood* 93:3451, 1999.
272. Gralnick HR, Vail M, McKeown LP, et al: Activated platelets in paroxysmal nocturnal haemoglobinuria. *Br J Haematol* 91:697, 1995.
273. Wiedmer T, Hall SE, Ortel TL, et al: Complement-induced vesiculation and exposure of membrane prothrombinase sites in platelets of paroxysmal nocturnal hemoglobinuria. *Blood* 82:1192, 1993.
274. Liebman HA, Feinstein DI: Thrombosis in patients with paroxysmal nocturnal hemoglobinuria is associated with markedly elevated plasma levels of leukocyte-derived tissue factor. *Thromb Res* 111:235, 2003.
275. Ninomiya H, Hasegawa Y, Nagasawa T, Abe T: Excess soluble urokinase-type plasminogen activator receptor in the plasma of patients with paroxysmal nocturnal hemoglobinuria inhibits cell-associated fibrinolytic activity. *Int J Hematol* 65:285, 1997.
276. Grunewald M, Siegemund A, Grunewald A, et al: Plasmatic coagulation and fibrinolytic system alterations in PNH: Relation to clone size. *Blood Coagul Fibrinolysis* 14:685, 2003.
277. Simak J, Holada K, Risitano AM, et al: Elevated circulating endothelial membrane microparticles in paroxysmal nocturnal haemoglobinuria. *Br J Haematol* 125:804, 2004.
278. Williams JL: The myelodysplastic syndromes and myeloproliferative disorders. *Clin Lab Sci* 17:223, 2004.
279. Lawrence LW: Refractory anemia and the myelodysplastic syndromes. *Clin Lab Sci* 17:178, 2004.
280. Bain B: The WHO classification of the myelodysplastic syndromes. *Exp Oncol* 26:166, 2004.
281. Hofmann WK, Kalina U, Koschmieder S, et al: Defective megakaryocytic development in myelodysplastic syndromes. *Leuk Lymphoma* 38:13, 2000.
282. Hofmann WK, Ottmann OG, Ganser A, Hoelzer D: Myelodysplastic syndromes: Clinical features. *Semin Hematol* 33:177, 1996.
283. Kobayashi Y, Takahashi Y, Chikayama S, et al: Comparison of the DNA content of megakaryocytes identified immunologically with that identified morphologically. *Histochem Cell Biol* 108:115, 1997.
284. Kobayashi Y, Uoshima N, Kimura S, et al: Relationship between morphological classification of the degree of maturation and the ploidy of micromegakaryocytes in myelodysplastic syndrome patients. *Int J Hematol* 61:117, 1995.
285. Ohshima K, Kikuchi M, Takeshita M: A megakaryocyte analysis of the bone marrow in patients with myelodysplastic syndrome, myeloproliferative disorder and allied disorders. *J Pathol* 177:181, 1995.
286. Thiele J, Quitmann H, Wagner S, Fischer R: Dysmegakaryopoiesis in myelodysplastic syndromes (MDS): An immunomorphometric study of bone marrow trephine biopsy specimens. *J Clin Pathol* 44:300, 1991.
287. Mori H, Niikura H, Terada H, Fujita K: [Morphological analysis of the megakaryocytes in myelodysplastic syndrome]. *Rinsho Byori* 38:1347, 1990.
288. Thiele J, Titius BR, Kopsidis C, Fischer R: Atypical micromegakaryocytes, promegakaryoblasts and megakaryoblasts: A critical evaluation by immunohistochemistry, cytochemistry and morphometry of bone marrow trephines in chronic myeloid leukemia and myelodysplastic syndromes. *Virchows Arch B Cell Pathol Incl Mol Pathol* 62:275, 1992.
289. Hatfill SJ, Fester ED, Steytler JG: Apoptotic megakaryocyte dysplasia in the myelodysplastic syndromes. *Hematol Pathol* 6:87, 1992.
290. Houwerzijl EJ, Blom NR, van der Want JJ, et al: Increased peripheral platelet destruction and caspase-3-independent programmed cell death of bone marrow megakaryocytes in myelodysplastic patients. *Blood* 105:3472, 2005.
291. Hofmann WK, Kalina U, Wagner S, et al: Characterization of defective megakaryocytic development in patients with myelodysplastic syndromes. *Exp Hematol* 27:395, 1999.
292. Wang W, Matsuo T, Yoshida S, et al: Colony-forming unit-megakaryocyte (CFR-meg) numbers and serum thrombopoietin concentrations in thrombocytopenic disorders: An inverse correlation in myelodysplastic syndromes. *Leukemia* 14:1751, 2000.
293. Dan K, An E, Futaki M, et al: Megakaryocyte, erythroid and granulocyte-macrophage colony formation in myelodysplastic syndromes. *Acta Haematol* 89:113, 1993.
294. Adams JA, Liu Yin JA, Brereton ML, et al: The in vitro effect of pegylated recombinant human megakaryocyte growth and development factor (PEG rHuMGDF) on megakaryopoiesis in normal subjects and patients with myelodysplasia and acute myeloid leukaemia. *Br J Haematol* 99:139, 1997.
295. Kalina U, Hofmann WK, Koschmieder S, et al: Alteration of c-mpl–mediated signal transduction in CD34(+) cells from patients with myelodysplastic syndromes. *Exp Hematol* 28:1158, 2000.
296. Luo SS, Ogata K, Yokose N, Kato T, Dan K: Effect of thrombopoietin on proliferation of blasts from patients with myelodysplastic syndromes. *Stem Cells* 18:112, 2000.
297. Fontenay-Roupie M, Dupont JM, Picard F, et al: Analysis of megakaryocyte growth and development factor (thrombopoietin) effects on blast cell and megakaryocyte growth in myelodysplasia. *Leuk Res* 22:527, 1998.
298. Hashimoto S, Toba K, Fuse I, et al: Thrombopoietin activates the growth of megakaryoblasts in patients with chronic myeloproliferative disorders and myelodysplastic syndrome. *Eur J Haematol* 64:225, 2000.
299. Nishikawa M: [Thrombocytopenia due to deficient platelet production]. *Nippon Rinsho* 61:575, 2003.
300. King JA, Elkhalifa MY, Latour LF: Rapid progression of acquired amegakaryocytic thrombocytopenia to aplastic anemia. *South Med J* 90:91, 1997.
301. Slater LM, Katz J, Walter B, Armentrout SA: Aplastic anemia occurring as amegakaryocytic thrombocytopenia with and without an inhibitor of granulopoiesis. *Am J Hematol* 18:251, 1985.
302. Kondo Y, Molldrem JJ: Immune-induced cytopenia: Bone marrow failure syndrome. *Curr Hematol Rep* 3:178, 2004.
303. Maciejewski JP, Risitano A, Kook H, et al: Immune pathophysiology of aplastic anemia. *Int J Hematol* 76 Suppl 1:207, 2002.
304. Nakao S: Immune mechanism of aplastic anemia. *Int J Hematol* 66:127, 1997.
305. Kurzrock R, Cortes J, Thomas DA, et al: Pilot study of low-dose interleukin-11 in patients with bone marrow failure. *J Clin Oncol* 19:4165, 2001.
306. Wang WX, Gong CL: [Clinical report on treatment of thrombocytopenia with rhIL-11 (Mega) in 10 chronic aplastic anemia patients]. *Zhongguo Shi Yan Xue Ye Xue Za Zhi* 10:375, 2002.
307. Hoffman R: Acquired pure amegakaryocytic thrombocytopenic purpura. *Semin Hematol* 28:303, 1991.
308. Antonijevic N, Terzic T, Jovanovic V, et al: [Acquired amegakaryocytic thrombocytopenia: Three case reports and a literature review]. *Med Pregl* 57:292, 2004.
309. Dewulf G, Gouin I, Pautas E, et al: [Myelodisplasic syndromes diagnosed in a geriatric hospital: Morphological profile in 100 patients]. *Ann Biol Clin (Paris)* 62:197, 2004.
310. Rochant H: [Myelodysplastic syndromes: Unusual and mild forms]. *Pathol Biol (Paris)* 45:579, 1997.
311. Kini J, Khadilkar UN, Dayal JP: A study of the haematologic spectrum of myelodysplastic syndrome. *Indian J Pathol Microbiol* 44:9, 2001.
312. Nand S, Godwin JE: Hypoplastic myelodysplastic syndrome. *Cancer* 62:958, 1988.
313. Zafar T, Yasin F, Anwar M, Saleem M: Acquired amegakaryocytic thrombocytopenic purpura (AATP): A hospital based study. *J Pak Med Assoc* 49:114, 1999.
314. Nagasawa T, Sakurai T, Kashiwagi H, Abe T: Cell-mediated amegakaryocytic thrombocytopenia associated with systemic lupus erythematosus. *Blood* 67:479, 1986.
315. Shiozaki H, Miyawaki S, Kuwaki T, et al: Autoantibodies neutralizing thrombopoietin in a patient with amegakaryocytic thrombocytopenic purpura. *Blood* 95:2187, 2000.
316. Katsumata Y, Suzuki T, Kuwana M, et al: Anti–c-Mpl (thrombopoietin receptor) autoantibody-induced amegakaryocytic thrombocytopenia in a patient with systemic sclerosis. *Arthritis Rheum* 48:1647, 2003.
317. Leach JW, Hussein KK, George JN: Acquired pure megakaryocytic aplasia report of two cases with long-term responses to antithymocyte globulin and cyclosporine. *Am J Hematol* 62:115, 1999.
318. Balduini CL, Stella CC, Rosti V, et al: Acquired cyclic thrombocytopenia-thrombocytosis with periodic defect of platelet function. *Br J Haematol* 85:718, 1993.
319. Go RS: Idiopathic cyclic thrombocytopenia. *Blood Rev* 19:53, 2005.
320. Steensma DP, Harrison CN, Tefferi A: Hydroxyurea-associated platelet count oscillations in polycythemia vera: A report of four new cases and a review. *Leuk Lymphoma* 42:1243, 2001.
321. Abe Y, Hirase N, Muta K, et al: Adult onset cyclic hematopoiesis in a patient with myelodysplastic syndrome. *Int J Hematol* 71:40, 2000.
322. George JN, Woolf SH, Raskob GE: Idiopathic thrombocytopenic purpura: A guideline for diagnosis and management of children and adults. American Society of Hematology. *Ann Med* 30:38, 1998.
323. Lusher JM, Iyer R: Idiopathic thrombocytopenic purpura in children. *Semin Thromb Hemost* 3:175, 1977.
324. Frederiksen H, Schmidt K: The incidence of idiopathic thrombocytopenic purpura in adults increases with age. *Blood* 94:909, 1999.
325. Neylon AJ, Saunders PW, Howard MR, et al: Clinically significant newly presenting autoimmune thrombocytopenic purpura in adults: A prospective study of a population-based cohort of 245 patients. *Br J Haematol* 122:966, 2003.
326. Harrington WJ, Minnich V, Hollingsworth JW, Moore CV: Demonstration of a thrombocytopenic factor in the blood of patients with thrombocytopenic purpura. *J Lab Clin Med* 38:1, 1951.
327. Altman LK: Black and blue at the flick of a feather, in *Who Goes First?*, p 273. Random House, New York, 1987.
328. Shulman NR, Weinrach RS, Libre EP, Andrews HL: The role of the reticuloendothelial system in the pathogenesis of idiopathic thrombocytopenic purpura. *Trans Assoc Am Physicians* 78:374, 1965.
329. McMillan R, Smith RS, Longmire RL, et al: Immunoglobulins associated with human platelets. *Blood* 37:316, 1971.

330. Dixon R, Rosse W, Ebbert L: Quantitative determination of antibody in idiopathic thrombocytopenic purpura. Correlation of serum and platelet-bound antibody with clinical response. *N Engl J Med* 292:230, 1975.
331. Mueller-Eckhardt C, Mueller-Eckhardt G, Kayser W, et al: Platelet associated IgG, platelet survival, and platelet sequestration in thrombocytopenic states. *Br J Haematol* 52:49, 1982.
332. Kelton JG, Powers PJ, Carter CJ: A prospective study of the usefulness of the measurement of platelet-associated IgG for the diagnosis of idiopathic thrombocytopenic purpura. *Blood* 60:1050, 1982.
333. van Leeuwen EF, van der Ven JT, Engelfriet CP, dem Borne AE: Specificity of autoantibodies in autoimmune thrombocytopenia. *Blood* 59:23, 1982.
334. McMillan R, Tani P, Millard F, et al: Platelet-associated and plasma anti-glycoprotein autoantibodies in chronic ITP. *Blood* 70:1040, 1987.
335. Kiefel V, Santoso S, Weisheit M, Mueller-Eckhardt C: Monoclonal antibody-specific immobilization of platelet antigens (MAIPA): A new tool for the identification of platelet-reactive antibodies. *Blood* 70:1722, 1987.
336. Kiefel V, Santoso S, Kaufmann E, Mueller-Eckhardt C: Autoantibodies against platelet glycoprotein Ib/IX: A frequent finding in autoimmune thrombocytopenic purpura. *Br J Haematol* 79:256, 1991.
337. He R, Reid DM, Jones CE, Shulman NR: Spectrum of Ig classes, specificities, and titers of serum antiglycoproteins in chronic idiopathic thrombocytopenic purpura. *Blood* 83:1024, 1994.
338. McMillan R: Autoantibodies and autoantigens in chronic immune thrombocytopenic purpura. *Semin Hematol* 37:239, 2000.
339. Cines DB, Blanchette VS: Immune thrombocytopenic purpura. *N Engl J Med* 346:995, 2002.
340. Hymes K, Schur PH, Karpatkin S: Heavy-chain subclass of round antiplatelet IgG in autoimmune thrombocytopenic purpura. *Blood* 56:84, 1980.
341. van der HD, de Jong D, Limpens J, et al: Clonal B-cell populations in patients with idiopathic thrombocytopenic purpura. *Blood* 76:2321, 1990.
342. McMillan R, Lopez-Dee J, Bowditch R: Clonal restriction of platelet-associated anti-GPIIb/IIIa autoantibodies in patients with chronic ITP. *Thromb Haemost* 85:821, 2001.
343. Kuwana M, Kaburaki J, Ikeda Y: Autoreactive T cells to platelet GPIIb-IIIa in immune thrombocytopenic purpura. Role in production of anti-platelet autoantibody. *J Clin Invest* 102:1393, 1998.
344. Kuwana M, Kaburaki J, Kitasato H, et al: Immunodominant epitopes on glycoprotein IIb-IIIa recognized by autoreactive T cells in patients with immune thrombocytopenic purpura. *Blood* 98:130, 2001.
345. Semple JW: Pathogenic T-cell responses in patients with autoimmune thrombocytopenic purpura. *J Pediatr Hematol Oncol* 25 Suppl 1:S11, 2003.
346. Zhang F, Chu X, Wang L, et al: Cell-mediated lysis of autologous platelets in chronic idiopathic thrombocytopenic purpura. *Eur J Haematol* 76:427, 2006.
347. Li S, Wang L, Zhao C, et al: CD8+ T cells suppress autologous megakaryocyte apoptosis in idiopathic thrombocytopenic purpura. *Br J Haematol* 139:605, 2007.
348. Hauch TW, Rosse WF: Platelet-bound complement (C3) in immune thrombocytopenia. *Blood* 50:1129, 1977.
349. Kurata Y, Curd JG, Tamerius JD, McMillan R: Platelet-associated complement in chronic ITP. *Br J Haematol* 60:723, 1985.
350. Tsubakio T, Tani P, Curd JG, McMillan R: Complement activation in vitro by antiplatelet antibodies in chronic immune thrombocytopenic purpura. *Br J Haematol* 63:293, 1986.
351. Jackson S, Beck PL, Pineo GF, Poon MC: Helicobacter pylori eradication: Novel therapy for immune thrombocytopenic purpura? A review of the literature. *Am J Hematol* 78:142, 2005.
352. Franchini M, Cruciani M, Mengoli C, et al: Effect of Helicobacter pylori eradication on platelet count in idiopathic thrombocytopenic purpura: A systematic review and meta-analysis. *J Antimicrob Chemother* 60:237, 2007.
353. Arnold DM, Bernotas A, Nazi I, et al: Platelet count response to *H. pylori* treatment in patients with immune thrombocytopenic purpura with and without *H. pylori* infection: A systematic review. *Haematologica* 94:850, 2009.
354. Aster RH, Keene WR: Sites of platelet destruction in idiopathic thrombocytopenic purpura. *Br J Haematol* 16:61, 1969.
355. Frank E: Die essentielle Thrombopenie (Konstitutionelle Purpura-Pseudoha¨mophilie), I: Klinisches Bild. *Berl Klin Wochenschr* 52:454, 1915.
356. Dameshek W, Miller EB: The megakaryocytes in idiopathic thrombocytopenic purpura, a form of hypersplenism. *Blood* 1:27, 1946.
357. Chang M, Nakagawa PA, Williams SA, et al: Immune thrombocytopenic purpura (ITP) plasma and purified ITP monoclonal autoantibodies inhibit megakaryocytopoiesis in vitro. *Blood* 102:887, 2003.
358. Takahashi R, Sekine N, Nakatake T: Influence of monoclonal antiplatelet glycoprotein antibodies on *in vitro* human megakaryocyte colony formation and proplatelet formation. *Blood* 93:1951, 1999.
359. Bessman JD: The relation of megakaryocyte ploidy to platelet volume. *Am J Hematol* 16:161, 1984.
360. Thompson CB, Jakubowski JA: The pathophysiology and clinical relevance of platelet heterogeneity. *Blood* 72:1, 1988.
361. Saxon BR, Mody M, Blanchette VS, Freedman J: Reticulated platelet counts in the assessment of thrombocytopenic disorders. *Acta Paediatr Suppl* 424:65, 1998.
362. Hughes M, Webert K, Kelton JG: The use of electron microscopy in the investigation of the ultrastructural morphology of immune thrombocytopenic purpura platelets. *Semin Hematol* 37:222, 2000.
363. Kaushansky K: Thrombopoietin: The primary regulator of megakaryocyte and platelet production. *Thromb Haemost* 74:521, 1995.
364. Chang M, Qian JX, Lee SM, et al: Tissue uptake of circulating thrombopoietin is increased in immune-mediated compared with irradiated thrombocytopenic mice. *Blood* 93:2515, 1999.
365. Kosugi S, Kurata Y, Tomiyama Y, et al: Circulating thrombopoietin level in chronic immune thrombocytopenic purpura. *Br J Haematol* 93:704, 1996.
366. Kuter DJ: Thrombopoietin and thrombopoietin mimetics in the treatment of thrombocytopenia. *Annu Rev Med* 60:193, 2009.
367. Porcelijn L, Folman CC, Bossers B, et al: The diagnostic value of thrombopoietin level measurements in thrombocytopenia. *Thromb Haemost* 79:1101, 1998.
368. Gouin-Thibault I, Cassinat B, Chomienne C, et al: Is the thrombopoietin assay useful for differential diagnosis of thrombocytopenia? Analysis of a cohort of 160 patients with thrombocytopenia and defined platelet life span. *Clin Chem* 47:1660, 2001.
369. Laster AJ, Conley CL, Kickler TS, et al: Chronic immune thrombocytopenic purpura in monozygotic twins: Genetic factors predisposing to ITP. *N Engl J Med* 307:1495, 1982.
370. Bizzaro N: Familial association of autoimmune thrombocytopenia and hyperthyroidism. *Am J Hematol* 39:294, 1992.
371. Karpatkin S, Fotino M, Winchester R: Hereditary autoimmune thrombocytopenic purpura: An immunologic and genetic study. *Ann Intern Med* 94:781, 1981.
372. Stanworth SJ, Turner DM, Brown J, et al: Major histocompatibility complex susceptibility genes and immune thrombocytopenic purpura in Caucasian adults. *Hematology* 7:119, 2002.
373. Evers KG, Thouet R, Haase W, Kruger J: HLA frequencies and haplotypes in children with idiopathic thrombocytopenic purpura (ITP). *Eur J Pediatr* 129:267, 1978.
374. Foster CB, Zhu S, Erichsen HC, et al: Polymorphisms in inflammatory cytokines and Fcgamma receptors in childhood chronic immune thrombocytopenic purpura: A pilot study. *Br J Haematol* 113:596, 2001.
375. Cortelazzo S, Finazzi G, Buelli M, et al: High risk of severe bleeding in aged patients with chronic idiopathic thrombocytopenic purpura. *Blood* 77:31, 1991.
376. George JN, el Harake MA, Raskob GE: Chronic idiopathic thrombocytopenic purpura. *N Engl J Med* 331:1207, 1994.
377. McMillan R: Therapy for adults with refractory chronic immune thrombocytopenic purpura. *Ann Intern Med* 126:307, 1997.
378. Schattner E, Bussel J: Mortality in immune thrombocytopenic purpura: Report of seven cases and consideration of prognostic indicators. *Am J Hematol* 46:120, 1994.
379. McIntyre OR, Ebaugh FG Jr: Palpable spleens in college freshmen. *Ann Intern Med* 66:301, 1967.
380. Burstein SA, Downs T, Friese P, et al: Thrombocytopoiesis in normal and sublethally irradiated dogs: Response to human interleukin-6. *Blood* 80:420, 1992.
381. Khan I, Zucker-Franklin D, Karpatkin S: Microthrombocytosis and platelet fragmentation associated with idiopathic/autoimmune thrombocytopenic purpura. *Br J Haematol* 31:449, 1975.
382. Lopez JA, Andrews RK, Afshar-Kharghan V, Berndt MC: Bernard-Soulier syndrome. *Blood* 91:4397, 1998.
383. Rodgers RP, Levin J: A critical reappraisal of the bleeding time. *Semin Thromb Hemost* 16:1, 1990.
384. Evans RS, Takahashi K, Duane RT, et al: Primary thrombocytopenic purpura and acquired hemolytic anemia; evidence for a common etiology. *AMA Arch Intern Med* 87:48, 1951.
385. Vesely S, Buchanan GR, Cohen A, et al: Self-reported diagnostic and management strategies in childhood idiopathic thrombocytopenic purpura: Results of a survey of practicing pediatric hematology/oncology specialists. *J Pediatr Hematol Oncol* 22:55, 2000.
386. George JN, Raskob GE: Idiopathic thrombocytopenic purpura: Diagnosis and management. *Am J Med Sci* 316:87, 1998.
387. Chong BH, Keng TB: Advances in the diagnosis of idiopathic thrombocytopenic purpura. *Semin Hematol* 37:249, 2000.
388. Kelton JG, Murphy WG, Lucarelli A, et al: A prospective comparison of four techniques for measuring platelet-associated IgG. *Br J Haematol* 71:97, 1989.
389. George JN, Saucerman S, Levine SP, et al: Immunoglobulin G is a platelet alpha granule-secreted protein. *J Clin Invest* 76:2020, 1985.
390. George JN, Saucerman S: Platelet IgG, IgA, IgM, and albumin: Correlation of platelet and plasma concentrations in normal subjects and in patients with ITP or dysproteinemia. *Blood* 72:362, 1988.
391. Kelton JG, Denomme G: The quantitation of platelet-associated IgG on cohorts of platelets separated from healthy individuals by buoyant density centrifugation. *Blood* 60:136, 1982.
392. Beardsley DS, Spiegel JE, Jacobs MM, et al: Platelet membrane glycoprotein IIIa contains target antigens that bind anti-platelet antibodies in immune thrombocytopenias. *J Clin Invest* 74:1701, 1984.
393. Reid DM, Jones CE, Vostal JG, Shulman NR: Western blot identification of platelet proteins that bind normal serum immunoglobulins. Characteristics of a 95-Kd reactive protein. *Blood* 75:2194, 1990.
394. Nomura S, Yanabu M, Soga T, et al: Analysis of idiopathic thrombocytopenic purpura patients with antiglycoprotein IIb/IIIa or Ib autoantibodies. *Acta Haematol* 86:25, 1991.
395. Harris EN, Gharavi AE, Hegde U, et al: Anticardiolipin antibodies in autoimmune thrombocytopenic purpura. *Br J Haematol* 59:231, 1985.
396. Stasi R, Stipa E, Masi M, et al: Prevalence and clinical significance of elevated antiphospholipid antibodies in patients with idiopathic thrombocytopenic purpura. *Blood* 84:4203, 1994.

397. Diz-Kucukkaya R, Hacihanefioglu A, Yenerel M, et al: Antiphospholipid antibodies and antiphospholipid syndrome in patients presenting with immune thrombocytopenic purpura: A prospective cohort study. *Blood* 98:1760, 2001.
398. Funauchi M, Hamada K, Enomoto H, et al: Characteristics of the clinical findings in patients with idiopathic thrombocytopenic purpura who are positive for anti-phospholipid antibodies. *Intern Med* 36:882, 1997.
399. Lacey JV, Penner JA: Management of idiopathic thrombocytopenic purpura in the adult. *Semin Thromb Hemost* 3:160, 1977.
400. Baumann MA, Menitove JE, Aster RH, Anderson T: Urgent treatment of idiopathic thrombocytopenic purpura with single-dose gammaglobulin infusion followed by platelet transfusion. *Ann Intern Med* 104:808, 1986.
401. Gernsheimer T, Stratton J, Ballem PJ, Slichter SJ: Mechanisms of response to treatment in autoimmune thrombocytopenic purpura. *N Engl J Med* 320:974, 1989.
402. Bussel JB: Fc receptor blockade and immune thrombocytopenic purpura. *Semin Hematol* 37:261, 2000.
403. Mazzucconi MG, Francesconi M, Fidani P, et al: Treatment of idiopathic thrombocytopenic purpura (ITP): Results of a multicentric protocol. *Haematologica* 70:329, 1985.
404. Bellucci S, Charpak Y, Chastang C, Tobelem G: Low doses v conventional doses of corticoids in immune thrombocytopenic purpura (ITP): Results of a randomized clinical trial in 160 children, 223 adults. *Blood* 71:1165, 1988.
405. Ozsoylu S, Irken G, Karabent A: High-dose intravenous methylprednisolone for acute childhood idiopathic thrombocytopenic purpura. *Eur J Haematol* 42:431, 1989.
406. Ozsoylu S, Sayli TR, Ozturk G: Oral megadose methylprednisolone versus intravenous immunoglobulin for acute childhood idiopathic thrombocytopenic purpura. *Pediatr Hematol Oncol* 10:317, 1993.
407. Albayrak D, Islek I, Kalayci AG, Gurses N: Acute immune thrombocytopenic purpura: A comparative study of very high oral doses of methylprednisolone and intravenously administered immune globulin. *J Pediatr* 125:1004, 1994.
408. Cheng Y, Wong RS, Soo YO, et al: Initial treatment of immune thrombocytopenic purpura with high-dose dexamethasone. *N Engl J Med* 349:831, 2003.
409. George JN, Vesely SK: Immune thrombocytopenic purpura—Let the treatment fit the patient. *N Engl J Med* 349:903, 2003.
410. Bell WR Jr: Long-term outcome of splenectomy for idiopathic thrombocytopenic purpura. *Semin Hematol* 37:22, 2000.
411. Atkinson WL, Pickering LK, Schwartz B, et al: General recommendations on immunization. Recommendations of the Advisory Committee on Immunization Practices (ACIP) and the American Academy of Family Physicians (AAFP). *MMWR Recomm Rep* 51:1, 2002.
412. Najean Y, Rain JD, Billotey C: The site of destruction of autologous 111In-labelled platelets and the efficiency of splenectomy in children and adults with idiopathic thrombocytopenic purpura: A study of 578 patients with 268 splenectomies. *Br J Haematol* 97:547, 1997.
413. Pizzuto J, Ambriz R: Therapeutic experience on 934 adults with idiopathic thrombocytopenic purpura: Multicentric Trial of the Cooperative Latin American group on Hemostasis and Thrombosis. *Blood* 64:1179, 1984.
414. Lortan JE: Management of asplenic patients. *Br J Haematol* 84:566, 1993.
415. Melles DC, de MS: Prevention of infections in hyposplenic and asplenic patients: An update. *Neth J Med* 62:45, 2004.
416. Marcaccio MJ: Laparoscopic splenectomy in chronic idiopathic thrombocytopenic purpura. *Semin Hematol* 37:267, 2000.
417. Barbaros U, Dinccag A, Erbil Y, et al: Handheld gamma probe used to detect accessory spleens during initial laparoscopic splenectomies. *Surg Endosc* 21:115, 2007.
418. Callis M, Palacios C, Lopez A, et al: Splenic irradiation as management of ITP. *Br J Haematol* 105:843, 1999.
419. Imbach P, Barandun S, d'Apuzzo V, et al: High-dose intravenous gammaglobulin for idiopathic thrombocytopenic purpura in childhood. *Lancet* 1:1228, 1981.
420. Bussel JB, Pham LC, Aledort L, Nachman R: Maintenance treatment of adults with chronic refractory immune thrombocytopenic purpura using repeated intravenous infusions of gammaglobulin. *Blood* 72:121, 1988.
421. Berchtold P, Dale GL, Tani P, McMillan R: Inhibition of autoantibody binding to platelet glycoprotein IIb/IIIa by anti-idiotypic antibodies in intravenous gammaglobulin. *Blood* 74:2414, 1989.
422. Ramamurthi A, Lewis R: Design of a novel apparatus to study nitric oxide (NO) inhibition of platelet adhesion. *Ann Biomed Eng* 26:1036, 1998.
423. Hong F, Ruiz R, Price H, et al: Safety profile of WinRho anti-D. *Semin Hematol* 35:9, 1998.
424. Ware RE, Zimmerman SA: Anti-D: Mechanisms of action. *Semin Hematol* 35:14, 1998.
425. Crow AR, Lazarus AH: The mechanisms of action of intravenous immunoglobulin and polyclonal anti-D immunoglobulin in the amelioration of immune thrombocytopenic purpura: What do we really know? *Transfus Med Rev* 22:103, 2008.
426. George JN, Raskob GE, Vesely SK, et al: Initial management of immune thrombocytopenic purpura in adults: A randomized controlled trial comparing intermittent anti-D with routine care. *Am J Hematol* 74:161, 2003.
427. Waintraub SE, Brody JI: Use of anti-D in immune thrombocytopenic purpura as a means to prevent splenectomy: Case reports from two University Hospital Medical Centers. *Semin Hematol* 37:45, 2000.
428. Stasi R, Pagano A, Stipa E, Amadori S: Rituximab chimeric anti-CD20 monoclonal antibody treatment for adults with chronic idiopathic thrombocytopenic purpura. *Blood* 98:952, 2001.
429. Narang M, Penner JA, Williams D: Refractory autoimmune thrombocytopenic purpura: Responses to treatment with a recombinant antibody to lymphocyte membrane antigen CD20 (rituximab). *Am J Hematol* 74:263, 2003.
430. Cooper N, Stasi R, Cunningham-Rundles S, et al: The efficacy and safety of B-cell depletion with anti-CD20 monoclonal antibody in adults with chronic immune thrombocytopenic purpura. *Br J Haematol* 125:232, 2004.
431. Arnold DM, Dentali F, Crowther MA, et al: Systematic review: Efficacy and safety of rituximab for adults with idiopathic thrombocytopenic purpura. *Ann Intern Med* 146:25, 2007.
432. Garvey B: Rituximab in the treatment of autoimmune haematological disorders. *Br J Haematol* 141:149, 2008.
433. Psaila B, Bussel JB: Refractory immune thrombocytopenic purpura: Current strategies for investigation and management. *Br J Haematol* 143:16, 2008.
434. Kuter DJ, Bussel JB, Lyons RM, et al: Efficacy of romiplostim in patients with chronic immune thrombocytopenic purpura: A double-blind randomised controlled trial. *Lancet* 371:395, 2008.
435. Blanchette V, Freedman J, Garvey B: Management of chronic immune thrombocytopenic purpura in children and adults. *Semin Hematol* 35:36, 1998.
436. Ahn YS, Byrnes JJ, Harrington WJ, et al: The treatment of idiopathic thrombocytopenia with vinblastine-loaded platelets. *N Engl J Med* 298:1101, 1978.
437. Jackson CW, Edwards CC: Evidence that stimulation of megakaryocytopoiesis by low dose vincristine results from an effect on platelets. *Br J Haematol* 36:97, 1977.
438. Tangun Y, Atamer T: More on vincristine in treatment of ITP. *N Engl J Med* 297:894, 1977.
439. Verlin M, Laros RK Jr, Penner JA: Treatment of refractory thrombocytopenic purpura with cyclophosphamine. *Am J Hematol* 1:97, 1976.
440. Reiner A, Gernsheimer T, Slichter SJ: Pulse cyclophosphamide therapy for refractory autoimmune thrombocytopenic purpura. *Blood* 85:351, 1995.
441. Quiquandon I, Fenaux P, Caulier MT, et al: Re-evaluation of the role of azathioprine in the treatment of adult chronic idiopathic thrombocytopenic purpura: A report on 53 cases. *Br J Haematol* 74:223, 1990.
442. Sekreta CM, Baker DE: Interferon alfa therapy in adults with chronic idiopathic thrombocytopenic purpura. *Ann Pharmacother* 30:1176, 1996.
443. Godeau B, Durand JM, Roudot-Thoraval F, et al: Dapsone for chronic autoimmune thrombocytopenic purpura: A report of 66 cases. *Br J Haematol* 97:336, 1997.
444. Snyder HW Jr, Cochran SK, Balint JP, Jr., et al: Experience with protein A-immunoadsorption in treatment-resistant adult immune thrombocytopenic purpura. *Blood* 79:2237, 1992.
445. Emilia G, Messora C, Longo G, Bertesi M: Long-term salvage treatment by cyclosporin in refractory autoimmune haematological disorders. *Br J Haematol* 93:341, 1996.
446. Strother SV, Zuckerman KS, LoBuglio AF: Colchicine therapy for refractory idiopathic thrombocytopenic purpura. *Arch Intern Med* 144:2198, 1984.
447. Bussel JB, Saal S, Gordon B: Combined plasma exchange and intravenous gammaglobulin in the treatment of patients with refractory immune thrombocytopenic purpura. *Transfusion* 28:38, 1988.
448. Miyakis S, Lockshin MD, Atsumi T, et al: International consensus statement on an update of the classification criteria for definite antiphospholipid syndrome (APS). *J Thromb Haemost* 4:295, 2006.
449. Cervera R, Piette JC, Font J, et al: Antiphospholipid syndrome: Clinical and immunologic manifestations and patterns of disease expression in a cohort of 1,000 patients. *Arthritis Rheum* 46:1019, 2002.
450. Oosting JD, Derksen RH, Bobbink IW, et al: Antiphospholipid antibodies directed against a combination of phospholipids with prothrombin, protein C, or protein S: An explanation for their pathogenic mechanism? *Blood* 81:2618, 1993.
451. D'Cruz D, Hughes G: Antibodies, thrombosis and the endothelium. *Br J Rheumatol* 33:2, 1994.
452. Santoro SA: Antiphospholipid antibodies and thrombotic predisposition: Underlying pathogenetic mechanisms. *Blood* 83:2389, 1994.
453. Rand JH, Wu XX: Antibody-mediated interference with annexins in the antiphospholipid syndrome. *Thromb Res* 114:383, 2004.
454. Asherson RA, Khamashta MA, Ordi-Ros J, et al: The "primary" antiphospholipid syndrome: Major clinical and serological features. *Medicine (Baltimore)* 68:366, 1989.
455. Alarcon-Segovia D, Deleze M, Oria CV, et al: Antiphospholipid antibodies and the antiphospholipid syndrome in systemic lupus erythematosus. A prospective analysis of 500 consecutive patients. *Medicine (Baltimore)* 68:353, 1989.
456. Galli M, Finazzi G, Barbui T: Thrombocytopenia in the antiphospholipid syndrome. *Br J Haematol* 93:1, 1996.
457. Cuadrado MJ, Mujic F, Munoz E, Khamashta MA, Hughes GR: Thrombocytopenia in the antiphospholipid syndrome. *Ann Rheum Dis* 56:194, 1997.
458. Uthman I, Godeau B, Taher A, Khamashta M: The hematologic manifestations of the antiphospholipid syndrome. *Blood Rev* 22:187, 2008.
459. Harris EN: Antiphospholipid antibodies. *Br J Haematol* 74:1, 1990.
460. Wilson WA, Gharavi AE, Koike T, et al: International consensus statement on preliminary classification criteria for definite antiphospholipid syndrome: Report of an international workshop. *Arthritis Rheum* 42:1309, 1999.
461. Godeau B, Piette JC, Fromont P, et al: Specific antiplatelet glycoprotein autoantibodies are associated with the thrombocytopenia of primary antiphospholipid syndrome. *Br J Haematol* 98:873, 1997.
462. Macchi L, Rispal P, Clofent-Sanchez G, et al: Anti-platelet antibodies in patients with systemic lupus erythematosus and the primary antiphospholipid antibody syndrome: Their relationship with the observed thrombocytopenia. *Br J Haematol* 98:336, 1997.
463. Galli M, Daldossi M, Barbui T: Anti-glycoprotein Ib/IX and IIb/IIIa antibodies in patients with antiphospholipid antibodies. *Thromb Haemost* 71:571, 1994.
464. Lipp E, von Felten A, Sax H, et al: Antibodies against platelet glycoproteins and antiphospholipid antibodies in autoimmune thrombocytopenia. *Eur J Haematol* 60:283, 1998.

465. Fabris F, Steffan A, Cordiano I, et al: Specific antiplatelet autoantibodies in patients with antiphospholipid antibodies and thrombocytopenia. *Eur J Haematol* 53:232, 1994.
466. Nakamura M, Tanaka Y, Satoh T, et al: Autoantibody to CD40 ligand in systemic lupus erythematosus: Association with thrombocytopenia but not thromboembolism. *Rheumatology (Oxford)* 45:150, 2006.
467. Thrombosis and thrombocytopenia in antiphospholipid syndrome (idiopathic and secondary to SLE): First report from the Italian Registry. Italian Registry of Antiphospholipid Antibodies (IR-APA). *Haematologica* 78:313, 1993.
468. Bernini JC, Buchanan GR, Ashcraft J: Hypoprothrombinemia and severe hemorrhage associated with a lupus anticoagulant. *J Pediatr* 123:937, 1993.
469. Font J, Jimenez S, Cervera R, et al: Splenectomy for refractory Evans' syndrome associated with antiphospholipid antibodies: Report of two cases. *Ann Rheum Dis* 59:920, 2000.
470. Hakim AJ, Machin SJ, Isenberg DA: Autoimmune thrombocytopenia in primary antiphospholipid syndrome and systemic lupus erythematosus: The response to splenectomy. *Semin Arthritis Rheum* 28:20, 1998.
471. Ames PR, Tommasino C, Fossati G, et al: Limited effect of rituximab on thrombocytopaenia and anticardiolipin antibodies in a patient with primary antiphospholipid syndrome. *Ann Hematol* 86:227, 2007.
472. Ahn ER, Lander G, Bidot CJ, Jy W, Ahn YS: Long-term remission from life-threatening hypercoagulable state associated with lupus anticoagulant (LA) following rituximab therapy. *Am J Hematol* 78:127, 2005.
473. Alarcon-Segovia D, Sanchez-Guerrero J: Correction of thrombocytopenia with small dose aspirin in the primary antiphospholipid syndrome. *J Rheumatol* 16:1359, 1989.
474. Alliot C, Messouak D, Albert F, Barrios M: Correction of thrombocytopenia with aspirin in the primary antiphospholipid syndrome. *Am J Hematol* 68:215, 2001.
475. Wisbey HL, Klestov AC: Thrombocytopenia corrected by warfarin in antiphospholipid syndrome. *J Rheumatol* 23:769, 1996.
476. Ames PR, Orefice G, Brancaccio V: Reversal of thrombocytopenia following oral anticoagulation in two patients with primary antiphospholipid syndrome. *Lupus* 4:491, 1995.
477. Suarez IM, Diaz RA, Aguayo Canela D, Pujol de la Llave E: Correction of severe thrombocytopenia with chloroquine in the primary antiphospholipid syndrome. *Lupus* 5:81, 1996.
478. Tan EM, Cohen AS, Fries JF, et al: The 1982 revised criteria for the classification of systemic lupus erythematosus. *Arthritis Rheum* 25:1271, 1982.
479. Hochberg MC: Updating the American College of Rheumatology revised criteria for the classification of systemic lupus erythematosus. *Arthritis Rheum* 40:1725, 1997.
480. Rabinowitz Y, Dameshek W: Systemic lupus erythematosus after "idiopathic" thrombocytopenic purpura: A review. *Ann Intern Med* 52:1, 1960.
481. Michel M, Lee K, Piette JC, et al: Platelet autoantibodies and lupus-associated thrombocytopenia. *Br J Haematol* 119:354, 2002.
482. Pujol M, Ribera A, Vilardell M, et al: High prevalence of platelet autoantibodies in patients with systemic lupus erythematosus. *Br J Haematol* 89:137, 1995.
483. McMillan R: Immune thrombocytopenia. *Clin Haematol* 12:69, 1983.
484. Griner PF, Hoyer LW: Amegakaryocytic thrombocytopenia in systemic lupus erythematosus. *Arch Intern Med* 125:328, 1970.
485. Fureder W, Firbas U, Nichol JL, et al: Serum thrombopoietin levels and anti-thrombopoietin antibodies in systemic lupus erythematosus. *Lupus* 11:221, 2002.
486. Kuwana M, Okazaki Y, Kajihara M, et al: Autoantibody to c-Mpl (thrombopoietin receptor) in systemic lupus erythematosus: Relationship to thrombocytopenia with megakaryocytic hypoplasia. *Arthritis Rheum* 46:2148, 2002.
487. Feinglass EJ, Arnett FC, Dorsch CA, et al: Neuropsychiatric manifestations of systemic lupus erythematosus: Diagnosis, clinical spectrum, and relationship to other features of the disease. *Medicine (Baltimore)* 55:323, 1976.
488. Miller MH, Urowitz MB, Gladman DD: The significance of thrombocytopenia in systemic lupus erythematosus. *Arthritis Rheum* 26:1181, 1983.
489. Mok CC, Lee KW, Ho CT, et al: A prospective study of survival and prognostic indicators of systemic lupus erythematosus in a southern Chinese population. *Rheumatology (Oxford)* 39:399, 2000.
490. Drenkard C, Villa AR, Alarcon-Segovia D, Perez-Vazquez ME: Influence of the antiphospholipid syndrome in the survival of patients with systemic lupus erythematosus. *J Rheumatol* 21:1067, 1994.
491. Reveille JD, Bartolucci A, Alarcon GS: Prognosis in systemic lupus erythematosus. Negative impact of increasing age at onset, black race, and thrombocytopenia, as well as causes of death. *Arthritis Rheum* 33:37, 1990.
492. Abu-Shakra M, Urowitz MB, Gladman DD, Gough J: Mortality studies in systemic lupus erythematosus. Results from a single center. II. Predictor variables for mortality. *J Rheumatol* 22:1265, 1995.
493. Scofield RH, Bruner GR, Kelly JA, et al: Thrombocytopenia identifies a severe familial phenotype of systemic lupus erythematosus and reveals genetic linkages at 1q22 and 11p13. *Blood* 101:992, 2003.
494. Boumpas DT, Austin HA, III, Fessler BJ, et al: Systemic lupus erythematosus: Emerging concepts. Part 1: Renal, neuropsychiatric, cardiovascular, pulmonary, and hematologic disease. *Ann Intern Med* 122:940, 1995.
495. Arnal C, Piette JC, Leone J, et al: Treatment of severe immune thrombocytopenia associated with systemic lupus erythematosus: 59 cases. *J Rheumatol* 29:75, 2002.
496. Boumpas DT, Barez S, Klippel JH, Balow JE: Intermittent cyclophosphamide for the treatment of autoimmune thrombocytopenia in systemic lupus erythematosus. *Ann Intern Med* 112:674, 1990.
497. Roach BA, Hutchinson GJ: Treatment of refractory, systemic lupus erythematosus-associated thrombocytopenia with intermittent low-dose intravenous cyclophosphamide. *Arthritis Rheum* 36:682, 1993.
498. Ding C, Foote S, Jones G: B-cell–targeted therapy for systemic lupus erythematosus: An update. *BioDrugs* 22:239, 2008.
499. Maier WP, Gordon DS, Howard RF, et al: Intravenous immunoglobulin therapy in systemic lupus erythematosus-associated thrombocytopenia. *Arthritis Rheum* 33:1233, 1990.
500. Cohen MG, Li EK: Limited effects of intravenous IgG in treating systemic lupus erythematosus—associated thrombocytopenia. *Arthritis Rheum* 34:787, 1991.
501. Hall S, McCormick JL Jr, Greipp PR, et al: Splenectomy does not cure the thrombocytopenia of systemic lupus erythematosus. *Ann Intern Med* 102:325, 1985.
502. Rivero SJ, Alger M, Alarcon-Segovia D: Splenectomy for hemocytopenia in systemic lupus erythematosus. A controlled appraisal. *Arch Intern Med* 139:773, 1979.
503. Alarcon-Segovia D: Splenectomy has a limited role in the management of lupus with thrombocytopenia. *J Rheumatol* 29:1, 2002.
504. Burrows RF, Kelton JG: Incidentally detected thrombocytopenia in healthy mothers and their infants. *N Engl J Med* 319:142, 1988.
505. Letsky EA, Greaves M: Guidelines on the investigation and management of thrombocytopenia in pregnancy and neonatal alloimmune thrombocytopenia. Maternal and Neonatal Haemostasis Working Party of the Haemostasis and Thrombosis Task Force of the British Society for Haematology. *Br J Haematol* 95:21, 1996.
506. Burrows RF, Kelton JG: Fetal thrombocytopenia and its relation to maternal thrombocytopenia. *N Engl J Med* 329:1463, 1993.
507. McCrae KR, Samuels P, Schreiber AD: Pregnancy-associated thrombocytopenia: Pathogenesis and management. *Blood* 80:2697, 1992.
508. Shehata N, Burrows R, Kelton JG: Gestational thrombocytopenia. *Clin Obstet Gynecol* 42:327, 1999.
509. Kaplan C, Forestier F, Dreyfus M, et al: Maternal thrombocytopenia during pregnancy: Diagnosis and etiology. *Semin Thromb Hemost* 21:85, 1995.
510. Boehlen F, Hohlfeld P, Extermann P, et al: Platelet count at term pregnancy: A reappraisal of the threshold. *Obstet Gynecol* 95:29, 2000.
511. Lescale KB, Eddleman KA, Cines DB, et al: Antiplatelet antibody testing in thrombocytopenic pregnant women. *Am J Obstet Gynecol* 174:1014, 1996.
512. Gill KK, Kelton JG: Management of idiopathic thrombocytopenic purpura in pregnancy. *Semin Hematol* 37:275, 2000.
513. al Mofada SM, Osman ME, Kides E, et al: Risk of thrombocytopenia in the infants of mothers with idiopathic thrombocytopenia. *Am J Perinatol* 11:423, 1994.
514. Webert KE, Mittal R, Sigouin C, et al: A retrospective 11-year analysis of obstetric patients with idiopathic thrombocytopenic purpura. *Blood* 102:4306, 2003.
515. Stamilio DM, Macones GA: Selection of delivery method in pregnancies complicated by autoimmune thrombocytopenia: A decision analysis. *Obstet Gynecol* 94:41, 1999.
516. Christiaens GC, Nieuwenhuis HK, Bussel JB: Comparison of platelet counts in first and second newborns of mothers with immune thrombocytopenic purpura. *Obstet Gynecol* 90:546, 1997.
517. Moise KJ Jr, Cotton DB: Discordant fetal platelet counts in a twin gestation complicated by idiopathic thrombocytopenic purpura. *Am J Obstet Gynecol* 156:1141, 1987.
518. Kaplan C, Daffos F, Forestier F, et al: Fetal platelet counts in thrombocytopenic pregnancy. *Lancet* 336:979, 1990.
519. Silver RM, Branch DW, Scott JR: Maternal thrombocytopenia in pregnancy: Time for a reassessment. *Am J Obstet Gynecol* 173:479, 1995.
520. Mushambi MC, Halligan AW, Williamson K: Recent developments in the pathophysiology and management of pre-eclampsia. *Br J Anaesth* 76:133, 1996.
521. Leitch CR, Cameron AD, Walker JJ: The changing pattern of eclampsia over a 60-year period. *Br J Obstet Gynaecol* 104:917, 1997.
522. Thomas SV: Neurological aspects of eclampsia. *J Neurol Sci* 155:37, 1998.
523. McCrae KR: Thrombocytopenia in pregnancy: Differential diagnosis, pathogenesis, and management. *Blood Rev* 17:7, 2003.
524. Schlembach D: Pre-eclampsia—Still a disease of theories. *Fukushima J Med Sci* 49:69, 2003.
525. Brittain PC, Bayliss P: Partial hydatidiform molar pregnancy presenting with severe preeclampsia prior to twenty weeks gestation: A case report and review of the literature. *Mil Med* 160:42, 1995.
526. Luttun A, Carmeliet P: Soluble VEGF receptor Flt1: The elusive preeclampsia factor discovered? *J Clin Invest* 111:600, 2003.
527. Torry DS, Hinrichs M, Torry RJ: Determinants of placental vascularity. *Am J Reprod Immunol* 51:257, 2004.
528. Maynard SE, Min JY, Merchan J, et al: Excess placental soluble fms-like tyrosine kinase 1 (sFlt1) may contribute to endothelial dysfunction, hypertension, and proteinuria in preeclampsia. *J Clin Invest* 111:649, 2003.
529. Vuorela P, Helske S, Hornig C, et al: Amniotic fluid—Soluble vascular endothelial growth factor receptor-1 in preeclampsia. *Obstet Gynecol* 95:353, 2000.
530. Zhou Y, McMaster M, Woo K, et al: Vascular endothelial growth factor ligands and receptors that regulate human cytotrophoblast survival are dysregulated in severe preeclampsia and hemolysis, elevated liver enzymes, and low platelets syndrome. *Am J Pathol* 160:1405, 2002.
531. Venkatesha S, Toporsian M, Lam C, et al: Soluble endoglin contributes to the pathogenesis of preeclampsia. *Nat Med* 12:642, 2006.
532. Lattuada A, Rossi E, Calzarossa C, et al: Mild to moderate reduction of a von Willebrand factor cleaving protease (ADAMTS-13) in pregnant women with HELLP microangiopathic syndrome. *Haematologica* 88:1029, 2003.

533. Hulstein JJ, van Runnard Heimel PJ, Franx A, et al: Acute activation of the endothelium results in increased levels of active von Willebrand factor in hemolysis, elevated liver enzymes and low platelets (HELLP) syndrome. *J Thromb Haemost* 4:2569, 2006.
534. Tank PD, Nadanwar YS, Mayadeo NM: Outcome of pregnancy with severe liver disease. *Int J Gynaecol Obstet* 76:27, 2002.
535. Egerman RS, Sibai BM: HELLP syndrome. *Clin Obstet Gynecol* 42:381, 1999.
536. Martin JN Jr, Files JC, Blake PG, et al: Postpartum plasma exchange for atypical preeclampsia-eclampsia as HELLP (hemolysis, elevated liver enzymes, and low platelets) syndrome. *Am J Obstet Gynecol* 172:1107, 1995.
537. Sibai BM, Ramadan MK, Chari RS, Friedman SA: Pregnancies complicated by HELLP syndrome (hemolysis, elevated liver enzymes, and low platelets): Subsequent pregnancy outcome and long-term prognosis. *Am J Obstet Gynecol* 172:125, 1995.
538. Kaplan C: Alloimmune thrombocytopenia of the fetus and the newborn. *Blood Rev* 16:69, 2002.
539. Mueller-Eckhardt C, Kiefel V, Grubert A, et al: 348 cases of suspected neonatal alloimmune thrombocytopenia. *Lancet* 1:363, 1989.
540. Grainger JD, Morrell G, Yates J, Deleacy D: Neonatal alloimmune thrombocytopenia with significant HLA antibodies. *Arch Dis Child Fetal Neonatal Ed* 86:F200, 2002.
541. Chow MP, Sun KJ, Yung CH, et al: Neonatal alloimmune thrombocytopenia due to HLA-A2 antibody. *Acta Haematol* 87:153, 1992.
542. Davoren A, McParland P, Crowley J, et al: Antenatal screening for human platelet antigen-1a: Results of a prospective study at a large maternity hospital in Ireland. *BJOG* 110:492, 2003.
543. Williamson LM, Hackett G, Rennie J, et al: The natural history of fetomaternal alloimmunization to the platelet-specific antigen HPA-1a (PlA1, Zwa) as determined by antenatal screening. *Blood* 92:2280, 1998.
544. Jolly MC, Letsky EA, Fisk NM: The management of fetal alloimmune thrombocytopenia. *Prenat Diagn* 22:96, 2002.
545. Murphy MF, Hambley H, Nicolaides K, Waters AH: Severe fetomaternal alloimmune thrombocytopenia presenting with fetal hydrocephalus. *Prenat Diagn* 16:1152, 1996.
546. Kaplan C, Murphy MF, Kroll H, Waters AH: Feto-maternal alloimmune thrombocytopenia: Antenatal therapy with IVIgG and steroids—More questions than answers. European Working Group on FMAIT. *Br J Haematol* 100:62, 1998.
547. Ouwehand WH, Smith G, Ranasinghe E: Management of severe alloimmune thrombocytopenia in the newborn. *Arch Dis Child Fetal Neonatal Ed* 82:F173, 2000.
548. Porcelijn L, Kanhai HH: Fetal thrombocytopenia. *Curr Opin Obstet Gynecol* 10:117, 1998.
549. Weiner E, Zosmer N, Bajoria R, et al: Direct fetal administration of immunoglobulins: Another disappointing therapy in alloimmune thrombocytopenia. *Fetal Diagn Ther* 9:159, 1994.
550. Aster RH: Platelet sequestration studies in man. *Br J Haematol* 22:259, 1972.
551. Wadenvik H, Denfors I, Kutti J: Splenic blood flow and intrasplenic platelet kinetics in relation to spleen volume. *Br J Haematol* 67:181, 1987.
552. Savage B, McFadden PR, Hanson SR, Harker LA: The relation of platelet density to platelet age: Survival of low- and high-density 111indium-labeled platelets in baboons. *Blood* 68:386, 1986.
553. Wadenvik H, Kutti J: The effect of an adrenaline infusion on the splenic blood flow and intrasplenic platelet kinetics. *Br J Haematol* 67:187, 1987.
554. Vilen L, Freden K, Kutti J: Presence of a non-splenic platelet pool in man. *Scand J Haematol* 24:137, 1980.
555. Heyns AD, Badenhorst PN, Lotter MG, Pieters H, Wessels P: Kinetics and mobilization from the spleen of indium-111-labeled platelets during platelet apheresis. *Transfusion* 25:215, 1985.
556. Lawrence SP, Lezotte DC, Durham JD, et al: Course of thrombocytopenia of chronic liver disease after transjugular intrahepatic portosystemic shunts (TIPS). A retrospective analysis. *Dig Dis Sci* 40:1575, 1995.
557. Peck-Radosavljevic M: Hypersplenism. *Eur J Gastroenterol Hepatol* 13:317, 2001.
558. Eichner ER: Splenic function: Normal, too much and too little. *Am J Med* 66:311, 1979.
559. Jacob HS: Hypersplenism: Mechanisms and management. *Br J Haematol* 27:1, 1974.
560. Cooney DP, Smith BA: The pathophysiology of hypersplenic thrombocytopenia. *Arch Intern Med* 121:332, 1968.
561. McCormick PA, Murphy KM: Splenomegaly, hypersplenism and coagulation abnormalities in liver disease. *Baillieres Best Pract Res Clin Gastroenterol* 14:1009, 2000.
562. Reed RL, Ciavarella D, Heimbach DM, et al: Prophylactic platelet administration during massive transfusion. A prospective, randomized, double-blind clinical study. *Ann Surg* 203:40, 1986.
563. Hiippala ST, Myllyla GJ, Vahtera EM: Hemostatic factors and replacement of major blood loss with plasma-poor red cell concentrates. *Anesth Analg* 81:360, 1995.
564. Leslie SD, Toy PT: Laboratory hemostatic abnormalities in massively transfused patients given red blood cells and crystalloid. *Am J Clin Pathol* 96:770, 1991.
565. Hardy JF, de MP, Samama CM: The coagulopathy of massive transfusion. *Vox Sang* 89:123, 2005.
566. Cosgriff N, Moore EE, Sauaia A, et al: Predicting life-threatening coagulopathy in the massively transfused trauma patient: Hypothermia and acidoses revisited. *J Trauma* 42:857, 1997.
567. Cinat ME, Wallace WC, Nastanski F, et al: Improved survival following massive transfusion in patients who have undergone trauma. *Arch Surg* 134:964, 1999.
568. Villalobos TJ, Adelson E, Riley PA Jr, Crosby WH: A cause of the thrombocytopenia and leukopenia that occur in dogs during deep hypothermia. *J Clin Invest* 37:1, 1958.
569. Yau TM, Carson S, Weisel RD, et al: The effect of warm heart surgery on postoperative bleeding. *J Thorac Cardiovasc Surg* 103:1155, 1992.
570. Pina-Cabral JM, Ribeiro-da-Silva A, Almeida-Dias A: Platelet sequestration during hypothermia in dogs treated with sulphinpyrazone and ticlopidine—Reversibility accelerated after intra-abdominal rewarming. *Thromb Haemost* 54:838, 1985.
571. Hoffmeister KM, Felbinger TW, Falet H, et al: The clearance mechanism of chilled blood platelets. *Cell* 112:87, 2003.
572. Hoffmeister KM, Josefsson EC, Isaac NA, et al: Glycosylation restores survival of chilled blood platelets. *Science* 301:1531, 2003.
573. Reddick RL, Poole BL, Penick GD: Thrombocytopenia of hibernation. Mechanism of induction and recovery. *Lab Invest* 28:270, 1973.
574. Chan KM, Beard K: A patient with recurrent hypothermia associated with thrombocytopenia. *Postgrad Med J* 69:227, 1993.
575. Aster RH, Bougie DW: Drug-induced immune thrombocytopenia. *N Engl J Med* 357:580, 2007.
576. George JN, Raskob GE, Shah SR, et al: Drug-induced thrombocytopenia: A systematic review of published case reports. *Ann Intern Med* 129:886, 1998.
577. Kaufman DW, Kelly JP, Johannes CB, et al: Acute thrombocytopenic purpura in relation to the use of drugs. *Blood* 82:2714, 1993.
578. Garner SF, Campbell K, Metcalfe P, et al: Glycoprotein V: The predominant target antigen in gold-induced autoimmune thrombocytopenia. *Blood* 100:344, 2002.
579. Christie DJ, Mullen PC, Aster RH: Fab-mediated binding of drug-dependent antibodies to platelets in quinidine- and quinine-induced thrombocytopenia. *J Clin Invest* 75:310, 1985.
580. Lopez JA, Li CQ, Weisman S, Chambers M: The glycoprotein Ib-IX complex-specific monoclonal antibody SZ1 binds to a conformation-sensitive epitope on glycoprotein IX: Implications for the target antigen of quinine/quinidine-dependent autoantibodies. *Blood* 85:1254, 1995.
581. Chong BH, Du X, Berndt MC, et al: Characterization of the binding domains on platelet glycoproteins Ib-IX and IIb/IIIa complexes for the quinine/quinidine-dependent antibodies. *Blood* 77:2190, 1991.
582. Curtis BR, McFarland JG, Wu GG, et al: Antibodies in sulfonamide-induced immune thrombocytopenia recognize calcium-dependent epitopes on the glycoprotein IIb/IIIa complex. *Blood* 84:176, 1994.
583. Visentin GP, Newman PJ, Aster RH: Characteristics of quinine- and quinidine-induced antibodies specific for platelet glycoproteins IIb and IIIa. *Blood* 77:2668, 1991.
584. Berkowitz SD, Harrington RA, Rund MM, Tcheng JE: Acute profound thrombocytopenia after C7E3 Fab (abciximab) therapy. *Circulation* 95:809, 1997.
585. Fiorin F, Steffan A, Pradella P, et al: IgG platelet antibodies in EDTA-dependent pseudothrombocytopenia bind to platelet membrane glycoprotein IIb. *Am J Clin Pathol* 110:178, 1998.
586. Cancio LC, Cohen DJ: Heparin-induced thrombocytopenia and thrombosis. *J Am Coll Surg* 186:76, 1998.
587. Coblyn JS, Weinblatt M, Holdsworth D, Glass D: Gold-induced thrombocytopenia. A clinical and immunogenetic study of twenty-three patients. *Ann Intern Med* 95:178, 1981.
588. Nieminen U, Kekomaki R: Quinidine-induced thrombocytopenic purpura: Clinical presentation in relation to drug-dependent and drug-independent platelet antibodies. *Br J Haematol* 80:77, 1992.
589. Leach MF, Cooper LK, AuBuchon JP: Detection of drug-dependent, platelet-reactive antibodies by solid-phase red cell adherence assays. *Br J Haematol* 97:755, 1997.
590. Visentin GP, Malik M, Cyganiak KA, Aster RH: Patients treated with unfractionated heparin during open heart surgery are at high risk to form antibodies reactive with heparin:platelet factor 4 complexes. *J Lab Clin Med* 128:376, 1996.
591. Boon DM, van Vliet HH, Zietse R, Kappers-Klunne MC: The presence of antibodies against a PF4-heparin complex in patients on haemodialysis. *Thromb Haemost* 76:480, 1996.
592. Kappers-Klunne MC, Boon DM, Hop WC, et al: Heparin-induced thrombocytopenia and thrombosis: A prospective analysis of the incidence in patients with heart and cerebrovascular diseases. *Br J Haematol* 96:442, 1997.
593. Bauer TL, Arepally G, Konkle BA, et al: Prevalence of heparin-associated antibodies without thrombosis in patients undergoing cardiopulmonary bypass surgery. *Circulation* 95:1242, 1997.
594. Gentilini G, Curtis BR, Aster RH: An antibody from a patient with ranitidine-induced thrombocytopenia recognizes a site on glycoprotein IX that is a favored target for drug-induced antibodies. *Blood* 92:2359, 1998.
595. Belkin GA: Cocktail purpura. An unusual case of quinine sensitivity. *Ann Intern Med* 66:583, 1967.
596. Siroty RR: Purpura on the rocks—With a twist. *JAMA* 235:2521, 1976.
597. Pedersen-Bjergaard U, Andersen M, Hansen PB: Drug-induced thrombocytopenia: Clinical data on 309 cases and the effect of corticosteroid therapy. *Eur J Clin Pharmacol* 52:183, 1997.
598. Roberts I, Murray NA: Neonatal thrombocytopenia. *Semin Fetal Neonatal Med* 13:256, 2008.
599. Bussel JB, Sola-Visner M: Current approaches to the evaluation and management of the fetus and neonate with immune thrombocytopenia. *Semin Perinatol* 33:35, 2009.
600. Wiedmeier SE, Henry E, Sola-Visner MC, Christensen RD: Platelet reference ranges for neonates, defined using data from over 47,000 patients in a multihospital healthcare system. *J Perinatol* 29:130, 2009.
601. Sola-Visner M, Sallmon H, Brown R: New insights into the mechanisms of nonimmune thrombocytopenia in neonates. *Semin Perinatol* 33:43, 2009.
602. Bussel JB: Immune thrombocytopenia in pregnancy: Autoimmune and alloimmune. *J Reprod Immunol* 37:35, 1997.

603. Schiff DE, Roberts WD, Willert J, Tsai HM: Thrombocytopenia and severe hyperbilirubinemia in the neonatal period secondary to congenital thrombotic thrombocytopenic purpura and ADAMTS13 deficiency. *J Pediatr Hematol Oncol* 26:535, 2004.
604. Levy GG, Nichols WC, Lian EC, et al: Mutations in a member of the ADAMTS gene family cause thrombotic thrombocytopenic purpura. *Nature* 413:488, 2001.
605. Donner M, Kristoffersson AC, Lenk H, et al: Type IIB von Willebrand's disease: Gene mutations and clinical presentation in nine families from Denmark, Germany and Sweden. *Br J Haematol* 82:58, 1992.
606. Noris P, Pecci A, Di Bari F, et al: Application of a diagnostic algorithm for inherited thrombocytopenias to 46 consecutive patients. *Haematologica* 89:1219, 2004.
607. Balduini CL, Savoia A: Inherited thrombocytopenias: Molecular mechanisms. *Semin Thromb Hemost* 30:513, 2004.
608. Geddis AE, Kaushansky K: Inherited thrombocytopenias: Toward a molecular understanding of disorders of platelet production. *Curr Opin Pediatr* 16:15, 2004.
609. Geddis AE: Congenital amegakaryocytic thrombocytopenia and thrombocytopenia with absent radii. *Hematol Oncol Clin North Am* 23:321, 2009.
610. Fox NE, Chen R, Hitchcock I, et al: Compound heterozygous c-Mpl mutations in a child with congenital amegakaryocytic thrombocytopenia: Functional characterization and a review of the literature. *Exp Hematol* 37:495, 2009.
611. Rose MJ, Nicol KK, Skeens MA, et al: Congenital amegakaryocytic thrombocytopenia: The diagnostic importance of combining pathology with molecular genetics. *Pediatr Blood Cancer* 50:1263, 2008.
612. King S, Germeshausen M, Strauss G, et al: Congenital amegakaryocytic thrombocytopenia: A retrospective clinical analysis of 20 patients. *Br J Haematol* 131:636, 2005.
613. Ochs HD: Mutations of the Wiskott-Aldrich syndrome protein affect protein expression and dictate the clinical phenotypes. *Immunol Res* 44:84, 2009.
614. Greenhalgh KL, Howell RT, Bottani A, et al: Thrombocytopenia-absent radius syndrome: A clinical genetic study. *J Med Genet* 39:876, 2002.
615. Thompson AA, Nguyen LT: Amegakaryocytic thrombocytopenia and radio-ulnar synostosis are associated with HOXA11 mutation. *Nat Genet* 26:397, 2000.
616. Grossfeld PD, Mattina T, Lai Z, et al: The 11q terminal deletion disorder: A prospective study of 110 cases. *Am J Med Genet A* 129:51, 2004.
617. Josephson CD, Su LL, Christensen RD, et al: Platelet transfusion practices among neonatologists in the United States and Canada: Results of a survey. *Pediatrics* 123:278, 2009.
618. Volpe JJ: Intracranial hemorrhage: Germinal matrix-intraventricular hemorrhage, in *Neurology of the Newborn*, 4th ed, p 428. WB Saunders, Philadelphia, 2001.
619. Towner D, Castro MA, Eby-Wilkens E, Gilbert WM: Effect of mode of delivery in nulliparous women on neonatal intracranial injury. *N Engl J Med* 341:1709, 1999.
620. Gardella C, Taylor M, Benedetti T, et al: The effect of sequential use of vacuum and forceps for assisted vaginal delivery on neonatal and maternal outcomes. *Am J Obstet Gynecol* 185:896, 2001.
621. Garcia MG, Duenas E, Sola MC, et al: Epidemiologic and outcome studies of patients who received platelet transfusions in the neonatal intensive care unit. *J Perinatol* 21:415, 2001.
622. Baer VL, Lambert DK, Henry E, et al: Do platelet transfusions in the NICU adversely affect survival? Analysis of 1600 thrombocytopenic neonates in a multihospital healthcare system. *J Perinatol* 27:790, 2007.
623. Kenton AB, Hegemier S, Smith EO, et al: Platelet transfusions in infants with necrotizing enterocolitis do not lower mortality but may increase morbidity. *J Perinatol* 25:173, 2005.
624. Nugent DJ: Controversies in the treatment of pediatric immune thrombocytopenias. *Blood Rev* 16:15, 2002.
625. Blanchette V, Carcao M: Approach to the investigation and management of immune thrombocytopenic purpura in children. *Semin Hematol* 37:299, 2000.
626. Rand ML, Wright JF: Virus-associated idiopathic thrombocytopenic purpura. *Transfus Sci* 19:253, 1998.
627. Winiarski J: Antibodies to platelet membrane glycoprotein antigens in three cases of infectious mononucleosis-induced thrombocytopenic purpura. *Eur J Haematol* 43:29, 1989.
628. Taub JW, Warrier I, Holtkamp C, et al: Characterization of autoantibodies against the platelet glycoprotein antigens IIb/IIIa in childhood idiopathic thrombocytopenia purpura. *Am J Hematol* 48:104, 1995.
629. Karpatkin S, Nardi MA, Kouri YH: Internal-image anti-idiotype HIV-1GP120 antibody in human immunodeficiency virus 1 (HIV-1)-seropositive individuals with thrombocytopenia. *Proc Natl Acad Sci U S A* 89:1487, 1992.
630. Rajantie J, Zeller B, Treutiger I, Rosthoj S: Vaccination associated thrombocytopenic purpura in children. *Vaccine* 25:1838, 2007.
631. Miller E, Waight P, Farrington CP, et al: Idiopathic thrombocytopenic purpura and MMR vaccine. *Arch Dis Child* 84:227, 2001.
632. Nieminen U, Peltola H, Syrjala MT, et al: Acute thrombocytopenic purpura following measles, mumps and rubella vaccination. A report on 23 patients. *Acta Paediatr* 82:267, 1993.
633. France EK, Glanz J, Xu S, et al: Risk of immune thrombocytopenic purpura after measles-mumps-rubella immunization in children. *Pediatrics* 121:E687, 2008.
634. Stowe J, Kafatos G, Andrews N, Miller E: Idiopathic thrombocytopenic purpura and the second dose of MMR. *Arch Dis Child* 93:182, 2008.
635. Kelton JG: Vaccination-Associated relapse of immune thrombocytopenia. *JAMA* 245:369, 1981.
636. Vlacha V, Forman EN, Miron D, Peter G: Recurrent thrombocytopenic purpura after repeated measles-mumps-rubella vaccination. *Pediatrics* 97:738, 1996.
637. Drachtman RA, Murphy S, Ettinger LJ: Exacerbation of chronic idiopathic thrombocytopenic purpura following measles-mumps-rubella immunization. *Arch Pediatr Adolesc Med* 148:326, 1994.
638. Bibby AC, Farrell A, Cummins M, Erlewyn-Lajeunesse M: Is MMR immunisation safe in chronic Idiopathic thrombocytopenic purpura? *Arch Dis Child* 93:354, 2008.
639. Geddis AE, Balduini CL: Diagnosis of immune thrombocytopenic purpura in children. *Curr Opin Hematol* 14:520, 2007.
640. Revesz T, Kardos G, Kajtar P, Schuler D: The adverse effect of prolonged prednisolone pretreatment in children with acute lymphoblastic leukemia. *Cancer* 55:1637, 1985.
641. Dubansky AS, Boyett JM, Falletta J, et al: Isolated thrombocytopenia in children with acute lymphoblastic leukemia: A rare event in a Pediatric Oncology Group Study. *Pediatrics* 84:1068, 1989.
642. Vesely S, Buchanan GR, Cohen A, et al: Self-reported diagnostic and management strategies in childhood idiopathic thrombocytopenic purpura: Results of a survey of practicing pediatric hematology/oncology specialists. *J Pediatr Hematol Oncol* 22:55, 2000.
643. George JN, Woolf SH, Raskob GE, et al: Idiopathic thrombocytopenic purpura: A practice guideline developed by explicit methods for the American Society of Hematology. *Blood* 88:3, 1996.
644. Neunert CE, Buchanan GR, Imbach P, et al: Severe hemorrhage in children with newly diagnosed immune thrombocytopenic purpura. *Blood* 112:4003, 2008.
645. Bolton-Maggs PH, Moon I: Assessment of UK practice for management of acute childhood idiopathic thrombocytopenic purpura against published guidelines. *Lancet* 350:620, 1997.
646. Medeiros D, Buchanan GR: Current controversies in the management of idiopathic thrombocytopenic purpura during childhood. *Pediatr Clin North Am* 43:757, 1996.
647. Butros LJ, Bussel JB: Intracranial hemorrhage in immune thrombocytopenic purpura: A retrospective analysis. *J Pediatr Hematol Oncol* 25:660, 2003.
648. Kuhne T, Buchanan GR, Zimmerman S, et al: A prospective comparative study of 2540 infants and children with newly diagnosed idiopathic thrombocytopenic purpura (ITP) from the Intercontinental Childhood ITP Study Group. *J Pediatr* 143:605, 2003.
649. Buchanan GR, Holtkamp CA: Prednisone therapy for children with newly diagnosed idiopathic thrombocytopenic purpura. A randomized clinical trial. *Am J Pediatr Hematol Oncol* 6:355, 1984.
650. Lusher JM, Emami A, Ravindranath Y, Warrier AI: Idiopathic thrombocytopenic purpura in children. The case for management without corticosteroids. *Am J Pediatr Hematol Oncol* 6:149, 1984.
651. Kuhne T, Imbach P, Bolton-Maggs PH, et al: Newly diagnosed idiopathic thrombocytopenic purpura in childhood: An observational study. *Lancet* 358:2122, 2001.
652. Tamminga R, Berchtold W, Bruin M, et al: Possible lower rate of chronic ITP after IVIG for acute childhood ITP an analysis from registry I of the Intercontinental Cooperative ITP Study Group (ICIS). *Br J Haematol* 146:180, 2009.
653. Stasi R, Del Poeta G, Stipa E, et al: Response to B-cell depleting therapy with rituximab reverts the abnormalities of T-cell subsets in patients with idiopathic thrombocytopenic purpura. *Blood* 110:2924, 2007.
654. Imbach P, Kuhne T, Muller D, et al: Childhood ITP: 12 months follow-up data from the prospective registry I of the Intercontinental Childhood ITP Study Group (ICIS). *Pediatr Blood Cancer* 46:351, 2006.
655. Dickerhoff R, von Ruecker A: The clinical course of immune thrombocytopenic purpura in children who did not receive intravenous immunoglobulins or sustained prednisone treatment. *J Pediatr* 137:629, 2000.
656. George JN: Initial management of immune thrombocytopenic purpura in children: Is supportive counseling without therapeutic intervention sufficient? *J Pediatr* 137:598, 2000.
657. Tarantino MD, Bolton-Maggs PH: Update on the management of immune thrombocytopenic purpura in children. *Curr Opin Hematol* 14:526, 2007.
658. Nugent DJ: Immune thrombocytopenic purpura: Why treat? *J Pediatr* 134:3, 1999.
659. Page LK, Psaila B, Provan D, et al: The immune thrombocytopenic purpura (ITP) bleeding score: Assessment of bleeding in patients with ITP. *Br J Haematol* 138:245, 2007.
660. Edslev PW, Rosthoj S, Treutiger I, et al: A clinical score predicting a brief and uneventful course of newly diagnosed idiopathic thrombocytopenic purpura in children. *Br J Haematol* 138:513, 2007.
661. Bolton-Maggs P, Tarantino MD, Buchanan GR, et al: The child with immune thrombocytopenic purpura: Is pharmacotherapy or watchful waiting the best initial management? A panel discussion from the 2002 meeting of the American Society of Pediatric Hematology/Oncology. *J Pediatr Hematol Oncol* 26:146, 2004.
662. Carcao MD, Zipursky A, Butchart S, et al: Short-course oral prednisone therapy in children presenting with acute immune thrombocytopenic purpura (ITP). *Acta Paediatr Suppl* 424:71, 1998.
663. Yetgin S, Yenicesu IC, Ersoy F: The effects of megadose methylprednisolone therapy on the immune system in childhood immune thrombocytopenia. *Pediatr Hematol Oncol* 22:401, 2005.
664. Eden OB, Lilleyman JS: Guidelines for management of idiopathic thrombocytopenic purpura. The British Paediatric Haematology Group. *Arch Dis Child* 67:1056, 1992.
665. Neunert CE, Bright BC, Buchanan GR: Severe chronic refractory immune thrombocytopenic purpura during childhood: A survey of physician management. *Pediatr Blood Cancer* 51:513, 2008.
666. Mueller BU, Bennett CM, Feldman HA, et al: One year follow-up of children and adolescents with chronic immune thrombocytopenic purpura (ITP) treated with rituximab. *Pediatr Blood Cancer* 52:259, 2009.

CHAPTER 120
REACTIVE THROMBOCYTOSIS

Kenneth Kaushansky

SUMMARY

The three major pathophysiologic causes of thrombocytosis are (1) clonal, including essential (or primary) thrombocythemia and other myeloproliferative disorders; (2) familial, including rare cases of nonclonal myeloproliferation resulting from thrombopoietin and thrombopoietin receptor mutations; and (3) reactive, in which thrombocytosis occurs secondary to a variety of acute and chronic clinical conditions.

The upper limit of the normal platelet count in most clinical laboratories is between 350,000/μL (350 × 10^9/L) and 450,000/μL (450 × 10^9/L). In a sample of 10,000 healthy individuals 18 to 65 years of age, 1 percent had platelet counts greater than 400,000/μL. Only in 8 these 99 individuals was thrombocytosis confirmed 6 months to 1 year later.[1] Nevertheless, it is clear that thrombocytosis is a feature of several important disorders, including cancer, and that even a high normal platelet count is associated with morbidity and mortality. In a longitudinal study of healthy Norwegian men, a platelet count in the top quartile of the normal range was associated with a twofold increase in cardiovascular mortality over a 12-year followup.[2] Whether the platelet count per se, or an underlying inflammatory condition resulting in both thrombocytosis and accelerated atherogenesis is responsible for these observations is not certain. The causes of thrombocytosis in which the platelet count exceeds the upper limit can be broadly categorized as (1) reactive, or secondary; (2) clonal, including essential thrombocythemia and other myeloproliferative disorders; and (3) familial (see Table 87–1). This chapter focuses on the causes and molecular mechanisms that underlie reactive, or secondary, thrombocytosis. Clonal and familial thrombocytosis are discussed in detail in Chap. 87.

NORMAL THROMBOPOIESIS

The regulation of platelet production is discussed extensively in Chap. 113, but a brief discussion here will serve to provide the appropriate background for discussion of reactive thrombocytosis. Thrombopoietin (TPO), the ligand for the megakaryocytic growth factor receptor c-mpl, is the major humoral regulator of megakaryocyte survival, growth, and development, although, curiously, it does not stimulate the final step in thrombopoiesis, platelet release from megakaryocyte proplatelet processes. Although TPO supports the entire continuum of megakaryocyte development from stem cell to mature megakaryocyte,[3] other cytokines including interleukin [IL]-6,[4] IL-3,[5,6] IL-11,[7] leukemia inhibitory factor (LIF),[8,9] fibroblast growth factor (FGF)-4,[10] stromal cell-derived factor (SDF)-1,[10,11] interferon (IFN)-γ,[12] and granulocyte-macrophage colony-stimulating factor (GM-CSF)[13] also affect thrombopoiesis, both *in vitro* and *in vivo*. Many of these cytokines act in synergy with other cytokines, including TPO.[11,12,14]

Acronyms and abbreviations that appear in this chapter include: EPO, erythropoietin; ESA, erythropoiesis-stimulating agent; FGF, fibroblast growth factor; GM-CSF, granulocyte-macrophage colony-stimulating factor; IFN, interferon; IL, interleukin; LIF, leukemia inhibitory factor; SCF, stem cell factor; SDF, stromal cell-derived factor; STAT, signal transducer and activator of transcription; TPO, thrombopoietin.

The regulation of thrombopoiesis occurs primarily by humoral mechanisms, with the levels of TPO inversely related to platelet counts.[15,16] In contrast, other cytokines shown to affect megakaryopoiesis *in vitro* do not vary with platelet levels.[17] Despite these important insights, the regulation of TPO blood levels is complex, and incompletely understood. The liver produces approximately half of all the hormone that circulates, based on platelet production in liver specific knockout mice.[18] However, platelet levels do not affect hepatic TPO production; instead, platelets themselves have an important role in regulating plasma levels, as their receptors for TPO (c-mpl) remove it from plasma.[19] Thus, as the platelet count drops, increased free plasma TPO levels stimulate megakaryopoiesis; conversely, as the platelet count rises, depletion of free plasma TPO decreases platelet production. This modulatory mechanism results in the steady-state level of platelet production. However, marrow stromal cells also produce TPO,[20,21] and are responsive to platelet products which serve to down-modulate expression of the hormone.[22]

ENHANCED THROMBOPOIESIS IN PATHOLOGIC STATES

THROMBOCYTOSIS IN INFLAMMATORY CONDITIONS

Inflammation is the most common cause of secondary thrombocytosis. In a one survey, thrombocytosis was believed secondary to one or more inflammatory conditions in nearly 80 percent of all patients with an elevated platelet count. Table 120–1 lists the clinical conditions associated with reactive thrombocytosis. The most common diagnoses in such patients are inflammatory bowel disease and rheumatoid arthritis,[23] although most conditions in which the erythrocyte sedimentation rate or C-reactive protein is elevated have been reported to cause secondary thrombocytosis. Although several cytokines and lymphokines are elevated in the blood of such patients, the most compelling evidence suggests that IL-6 and IFN-γ are responsible for the thrombocytosis seen in patients with inflammation.

Interleukin-6

IL-6 was cloned by several groups of investigators using a number of distinct assays, including antiviral activity, myeloma cell growth, hepatocyte growth, and immunoglobulin secretion.[24] The recombinant protein was later found to affect megakaryocyte growth and differentiation, both *in vitro* and *in vivo*.[4,25,26] The IL-6 gene is present on the short arm of human chromosome 7, and encodes a 26-kDa polypeptide produced in almost all tissues from T cells, fibroblasts, macrophages, and stromal cells, and is a key regulator of the inflammatory response.[27]

IL-6 production is dependent on the presence of IL-1 and tumor necrosis factor (TNF)-α, cytokines produced by lymphocytes and monocytes in response to phagocytosis of microorganisms, the binding of immune complexes, and several other innate immune stimuli. IL-6 production is regulated primarily by transcriptional enhancement; regulatory elements responsible for IL-6 promoter activation include nuclear factor-κB (NF-κB), adapter protein (AP)-1, CCAAT/enhancer binding protein (C/EBP) α and C/EBPβ.

Although not critical for steady-state thrombopoiesis, as the combined genetic elimination of *c-mpl* and the signaling component of the IL-6 receptor (gp130) produces no more severe thrombocytopenia than

TABLE 120–1. Major Causes of Thrombocytosis

Reactive (secondary) thrombocytosis

A. Transient reactive processes
   1. Acute blood loss
   2. Recovery ("rebound") from thrombocytopenia
   3. Acute infection, inflammation
   4. Response to exercise

B. Sustained processes
   1. Iron deficiency
   2. Postsplenectomy, asplenic states
   3. Malignancies
   4. Chronic inflammatory and infectious diseases (inflammatory bowel disease, rheumatoid arteritis, tuberculosis, chronic pneumonitis)
   5. Response to drugs (vincristine, epinephrine, all-*trans*-retinoic acid, some antibiotics, cytokines and growth factors)
   6. Hemolytic anemia

elimination of *c-mpl* alone,[29] IL-6 contributes to inflammatory thrombopoiesis, primarily by stimulating the hepatic production of TPO.[30] Most studies report that patients with inflammation display an increased level of TPO,[31,32] but TPO is not the only cytokine responsible for this effect,[33] especially when corrected for the thrombocytosis which would normally act to reduce levels of the hormone. Stimulation of hepatocytes with IL-6 results in enhanced production of thrombopoietin messenger ribonucleic acid (mRNA) and protein.[34,35]

INTERFERON-γ

A second inflammatory cytokine that contributes to inflammatory thrombopoiesis is IFN-γ. The interferons are proteins first defined by their ability to induce an antiviral state in mammalian cells. Biochemical fractionation revealed three classes of interferons, IFN-α, a family of 17 distinct but highly homologous molecules; IFN-β, a single molecule more distantly related to the various isoforms of IFN-α; and IFN-γ, a unique molecule that shares functional properties but not structure with the others. IFN-γ exerts the most profound hematologic effects of the three classes of protein, including direct suppression of erythroid colony-forming cell growth and the activation of macrophages to secrete a number of inflammatory cytokines; several comprehensive reviews on IFN-γ have been published.[36,37]

IFN-γ is produced by activated T lymphocytes and natural killer (NK) cells in response to T-cell antigen cross-linking and in response to stimulation by the inflammatory mediators TNF-α, IL-12, and IL-15.[38] Prominent hematologic effects include activation of macrophages to assume an inflammatory phenotype (e.g., secretion of TNF-α and enhanced tumor cell killing), upregulation of major histocompatibility complex (MHC) class I and class II molecules enhancing antigen recognition responses,[37] and inhibition of proliferative responses in stem cells and erythroid progenitors.[39,40] These latter effects accounts for the association of IFN-γ and aplastic anemia[41] are discussed more fully in Chap. 34. However, in stark contrast to the inhibitory effects of IFN-γ on erythropoiesis, the cytokine stimulates megakaryocyte growth and differentiation.[42,43] This is likely related to its stimulation of signal transducer and activator of transcription (STAT)-1 in megakaryocytes, as transgenic expression of the transcription factor mimics the effect of the cytokine, and corrects the thrombocytopenia seen in a genetic model system.[44] These findings argue that IFN-γ also contributes to the thrombocytosis seen in inflammatory states in humans.

THROMBOCYTOSIS CAUSED BY IRON DEFICIENCY

Although most patients with inflammation-related thrombocytosis display increased production of the hormone, TPO levels in patients with iron deficiency and thrombocytosis are not elevated.[45] In contrast, erythropoietin (EPO) levels are elevated in patients with iron-deficiency anemia, and are thought by some to be the responsible for the thrombocytosis seen in iron deficiency, at least in part. Consistent with this hypothesis, administration of EPO to animals and humans leads to a modest increase in the platelet count.[46] Although some have suggested that this is a result of cross reactivity of EPO on the TPO receptor,[47] direct EPO and TPO receptor binding studies refute this hypothesis.[48] Rather, megakaryocytic progenitors display EPO receptors, and their binding of the hormone leads to many of the same intracellular biochemical signals as induced by TPO (see Chap. 14).

However, several lines of evidence indicate that pathophysiologic mechanisms other than anemia must be responsible, at least in part, for the thrombocytosis seen in patients with iron deficiency. For example, many patients with iron-deficiency anemia do not have thrombocytosis.[45] Moreover, EPO levels are elevated in nearly all types of anemia, but iron deficiency is the only type of anemia that is regularly associated with thrombocytosis, other than the anemia of chronic inflammation, in which the inflammatory state that causes the anemia by modulation of hepcidin levels (see Chap. 37) also causes thrombocytosis (as discussed in "Thrombocytosis in Inflammatory Conditions" above). Thus, although several lines of evidence suggest that enhanced levels of EPO as a consequence of the anemia associated with iron deficiency contribute to this form of reactive thrombocytosis, elevated EPO levels cannot completely account for it.

THERAPEUTIC ERYTHROPOIETIN AND ENHANCED CARDIOVASCULAR MORTALITY

Several reports have linked the use of large doses of EPO or other erythropoiesis-stimulating agents (ESA) to enhanced cardiovascular mortality,[49] and in patients with renal insufficiency, to progression to dialysis in patients with renal insufficiency,[50] although not all studies concur with these landmark results.[51] Although also discussed in Chap. 16, this finding is presented here because evidence is accumulating that the rapid expansion of erythropoiesis induced by pharmacologic levels of EPO often induces functional iron deficiency. If so, because iron deficiency leads to thrombocytosis, the excessive cardiovascular morbidity and mortality associated with the administration of EPO and ESAs to patients is hypothesized to be secondary to the thrombocytosis. Consistent with this view is that even a high normal platelet count was found associated with enhanced cardiovascular morbidity and mortality in a longitudinal study of healthy Norwegian men.[2] In support of this hypothesis is the finding that patients with renal insufficiency on high therapeutic doses of erythropoietin (>20,000 U/week) and hemoglobin (Hgb) values in excess of 13 g/dL are more likely to develop functional iron deficiency and thrombocytosis, and those individuals in whom the platelet count exceeds 300,000/μL display a statistically significantly higher 3-year mortality rate.[52] An alternate explanation is that EPO directly increases thrombopoiesis independently of iron deficiency and/or enhances the vascular reactivity of platelets. This hypothesis is based on the finding that megakaryocytes and platelets bear EPO receptors,[53] and that TPO, which stimulates very similar signaling pathways as EPO in receptor-bearing cells (see Chap. 14), primes platelets to enhanced aggregation responses to classic platelet agonists.[54] Still other researchers have hypothesized that an alternate form of the EPO receptor, composed of the classic EPO receptor and the β subunit of the GM-CSF, IL-3, and IL-5 receptors is displayed on vascular endothelial cells,[55] and in that site could mediate enhanced vascular events. Thus, given the widespread use of ESAs in patients with anemia caused by cancer, kidney failure, myelodysplastic syndromes, and many other conditions, verifying these hypotheses or disproving them and establishing new ones appears to be important and a field ripe for new discovery.

CLINICAL FEATURES OF REACTIVE THROMBOCYTOSIS

The clinical features of secondary thrombocytosis are almost always a result of the underlying disorder provoking the reaction, usually an inflammatory condition or iron-deficiency anemia. It is also highly unusual for the thrombocytosis per se to provoke any untoward symptoms. Although pathologic thrombosis is a major feature of primary thrombocythemia (see Chap. 87), it is virtually absent in reactive thrombocytosis, unless provoked by other features of the underlying condition (e.g., vasculitis) or completely unrelated conditions in the patient (e.g., atherosclerotic disease). Whether this is because patients with reactive thrombocytosis do not have as high platelet counts, on average, as patients with primary thrombocythemia[56]; or because they have smaller mean platelet volumes[56]; or are a result of the activated signaling characteristic of the platelets or other blood cells in patients with myeloproliferative diseases, or because of the presence of a mutant JAK2 kinase,[57] or a constitutively active TPO receptor,[58] is uncertain at this time. Nevertheless, because vascular complications of reactive thrombocytosis are so unlikely to be a consequence of the elevated platelet count, treatment of the thrombocytosis per se is not recommended in reactive thrombocytosis except in very unusual circumstances.

REFERENCES

1. Ruggeri M, Tosetto A, Frezzato M, Rodeghiero F: The rate of progression to polycythemia vera or essential thrombocythemia in patients with erythrocytosis or thrombocytosis. *Ann Intern Med* 139:470, 2003.
2. Thaulow E, Erikssen J, Sandvik L, et al: Blood platelet count and function are related to total and cardiovascular death in apparently healthy men. *Circulation* 84:613, 1991.
3. Kaushansky K: The molecular mechanisms that control thrombopoiesis. *J Clin Invest* 115:3339, 2005.
4. Williams N, De Giorgio T, Banu N, et al: Recombinant interleukin 6 stimulates immature megakaryocytes. *Exp Hematol* 18:69, 1990.
5. Yonemura Y, Kawakita M, Masuda T, et al: Synergistic effects of interleukin 3 and interleukin 11 on murine megakaryopoiesis in serum-free culture. *Exp Hematol* 20:1011, 1992.
6. Carrington PA, Hill RJ, Stenberg PE, et al: Multiple in vivo effects of interleukin 3 and interleukin 6 on mouse megakaryocytopoiesis. *Blood* 77:34, 1991.
7. Schlerman FJ, Bree AG, Kaviani MD, et al: Thrombopoietic activity of recombinant human interleukin 11 in normal and myelosuppressed nonhuman primates. *Stem Cells* 14:517, 1996.
8. Debili N, Massé J-M, Katz A, et al: Effects of the recombinant hematopoietic growth factors interleukin-3, interleukin-6, stem cell factor, and leukemia inhibitory factor on the megakaryocytic differentiation of CD34+ cells. *Blood* 82:84, 1993.
9. Farese A, Myers LA, MacVittie TJ: Therapeutic efficacy of recombinant leukemia inhibitory factor in a primate model of radiation-induced marrow aplasia. *Blood* 84: 3675, 1994.
10. Avecilla ST, Hattori K, Heissig B, et al: Chemokine-mediated interaction of hematopoietic progenitors with the bone marrow vascular niche is required for thrombopoiesis. *Nat Med* 10:64, 2004.
11. Hodohara K, Fujii N, Yamamoto N, Kaushansky K: Stromal cell derived factor 1 acts synergistically with thrombopoietin to enhance the development of megakaryocytic progenitor cells. *Blood* 95:769, 2000.
12. Tsuji-Takayama K, Tahata H, Izumi N, et al: IFN-gamma in combination with IL-3 accelerates platelet recovery in mice with 5-fluorouracil-induced marrow aplasia. *J Interferon Cytokine Res* 16:447, 1996.
13. Kaushansky K, O'Hara PJ, Berkner K, et al: Genomic cloning, characterization, and multilineage expression of human granulocyte-macrophage colony-stimulating factor. *Proc Natl Acad Sci U S A* 83:3101, 1986.
14. Broudy VC, Lin NL, Kaushansky K: Thrombopoietin (c-mpl ligand) acts synergistically with erythropoietin, stem cell factor, and IL-11 to enhance murine megakaryocyte colony growth and increases megakaryocyte ploidy in vitro. *Blood* 85:1719, 1995.
15. Kuter DJ, Rosenberg RD: The reciprocal relationship of thrombopoietin (c-Mpl Ligand) to changes in the platelet mass during busulfan-induced thrombocytopenia in the rabbit. *Blood* 85:2720, 1995.
16. Kuter DJ: The physiology of platelet production. *Stem Cells* 14(Suppl 1):88, 1996.
17. Cockrell EM, Gorman J, Hord JD, et al: Endogenous interleukin-11 (IL-11) levels in newly diagnosed children with acquired severe aplastic anemia (SAA). *Cytokine* 28:55, 2004.
18. Qian S, Fu F, Li W, et al: Primary role of the liver in thrombopoietin production shown by tissue-specific knockout. *Blood* 92:2189, 1998.
19. Fielder PJ, Hass P, Nagel M, et al: Human platelets as a model for the binding and degradation of thrombopoietin. *Blood* 89: 2782, 1997.
20. McCarty JM, Sprugel KH, Fox NE, et al: Murine thrombopoietin mRNA levels are modulated by platelet count. *Blood* 86:3668, 1995.
21. Sungaran R, Markovic B, Chong BH: Localization and regulation of thrombopoietin mRNA expression in human kidney, liver, bone marrow and spleen using in situ hybridization. *Blood* 89:101, 1997.
22. McIntosh B, Kaushansky K: Marrow stromal production of thrombopoietin is regulated by transcriptional mechanisms in response to platelet products. *Exp Hematol* 36:799, 2008.
23. Griesshammer M, Bangerter M, Sauer T, et al: Aetiology and clinical significance of thrombocytosis: analysis of 732 patients with an elevated platelet count. *J Intern Med* 245:295, 1999.
24. Kishimoto T: The biology of interleukin-6. *Blood* 74:1, 1989.
25. Asano S, Okano A, Ozawa K, et al: In vivo effects of recombinant human interleukin 6 in primates: Stimulated production of platelets. *Blood* 75:1602, 1990.
26. Ishibashi T, Kimura H, Shikama Y, et al: Interleukin-6 is a potent thrombopoietic factor in vivo in mice. *Blood* 74:1241, 1989.
27. Naka T, Nishimoto N, Kishimoto T: The paradigm of IL-6: from basic science to medicine. *Arthritis Res* 4(Suppl 3):S233, 2002.
28. Sehgal PB: Regulation of IL6 gene expression. *Res Immunol* 143:724, 1992.
29. Gainsford T, Nandurkar H, Metcalf D, et al: The residual megakaryocyte and platelet production in c-Mpl-deficient mice is not dependent on the actions of interleukin-6, interleukin-11, or leukemia inhibitory factor. *Blood* 95: 528, 2000.
30. Wolber EM, Fandrey J, Frackowski U, Jelkmann W: Hepatic thrombopoietin mRNA is increased in acute inflammation. *Thromb Haemost* 86:1421, 2001.
31. Heits F, Stahl M, Ludwig D, et al: Elevated serum thrombopoietin and interleukin-6 concentrations in thrombocytosis associated with inflammatory bowel disease. *J Interferon Cytokine Res* 19:757, 1999.
32. Ishiguro A, Suzuki Y, Mito M, et al: Elevation of serum thrombopoietin precedes thrombocytosis in acute infections. *Br J Haematol* 116:612, 2002.
33. Ceresa IF, Noris P, Ambaglio C, et al: Thrombopoietin is not uniquely responsible for thrombocytosis in inflammatory disorders. *Platelets* 18:579, 2007.
34. Wolber EM, Jelkmann W: Interleukin-6 increases thrombopoietin production in human hepatoma cells HepG2 and Hep3B. *J Interferon Cytokine Res* 20:499, 2000.
35. Kaser A, Brandacher G, Steurer W, et al: Interleukin-6 stimulates thrombopoiesis through thrombopoietin: Role in inflammatory thrombocytosis. *Blood* 98:2720, 2001.
36. Theofilopoulos AN, Baccala R, Beutler B, Kono DH: Type I interferons (alpha/beta) in immunity and autoimmunity. *Annu Rev Immunol* 23:307, 2005.
37. Young HA, Bream JH: IFN-gamma: Recent advances in understanding regulation of expression, biological functions, and clinical applications. *Curr Top Microbiol Immunol* 316:97, 2007.
38. Schoenborn JR, Wilson CB: Regulation of interferon-gamma during innate and adaptive immune responses. *Adv Immunol* 96:41, 2007.
39. Choi I, Muta K, Wickrema A, et al: Interferon gamma delays apoptosis of mature erythroid progenitor cells in the absence of erythropoietin. *Blood* 95:3742, 2000.
40. Yu JM, Emmons RV, Hanazono Y, et al: Expression of interferon-gamma by stromal cells inhibits murine long-term repopulating hematopoietic stem cell activity. *Exp Hematol* 27:895, 1999.
41. Young NS, Scheinberg P, Calado RT: Aplastic anemia. *Curr Opin Hematol* 15:162, 2008.
42. Tsuji-Takayama K, Tahata H, Harashima A, et al: Interferon-gamma enhances megakaryocyte colony-stimulating activity in murine bone marrow cells. *J Interferon Cytokine Res* 16:701, 1996.
43. Griffin CG, Grant BW: Effects of recombinant interferons on human megakaryocyte growth. *Exp Hematol* 18:1013, 1990.
44. Huang Z, Richmond TD, Muntean AG, et al: STAT1 promotes megakaryopoiesis downstream of GATA-1 in mice. *J Clin Invest* 117:3890, 2007.

45. Akan H, Güven N, Aydogdu I, et al: Thrombopoietic cytokines in patients with iron deficiency anemia with or without thrombocytosis. *Acta Haematol* 103:152, 2000.
46. Loo M, Beguin Y: The effect of recombinant human erythropoietin on platelet counts is strongly modulated by the adequacy of iron supply. *Blood* 93:3286, 1999.
47. Bilic E, Bilic E: Amino acid sequence homology of thrombopoietin and erythropoietin may explain thrombocytosis in children with iron deficiency anemia. *J Pediatr Hematol Oncol* 25:675, 2003.
48. Geddis AE, Kaushansky K: Cross reactivity between erythropoietin and thrombopoietin at the level of Mpl does not account for the thrombocytosis seen in iron deficiency. *J Pediatr Hematol Oncol* 25:919, 2003.
49. Singh AK, Szczech L, Tang KL, et al: Correction of anemia with epoetin alfa in chronic kidney disease. *N Engl J Med* 355:2085, 2006.
50. Drüeke TB, Locatelli F, Clyne N, et al: Normalization of hemoglobin level in patients with chronic kidney disease and anemia. *N Engl J Med* 355:2071, 2006.
51. Rossert J, Levin A, Roger SD, et al: Effect of early correction of anemia on the progression of CKD. *Am J Kidney Dis* 47:738, 2006.
52. Streja E, Kovesdy CP, Greenland S, et al: Erythropoietin, iron depletion, and relative thrombocytosis: A possible explanation for hemoglobin-survival paradox in hemodialysis. *Am J Kidney Dis* 52:727, 2008.
53. Geddis AE, Fox NE, Hitchcock, I: Erythropoietin stimulates thrombopoiesis in the absence of c-Mpl signaling. *Blood* 112(Suppl 1): 2451, 2008.
54. Rodríguez-Liñares B, Watson SP: Thrombopoietin potentiates activation of human platelets in association with JAK2 and TYK2 phosphorylation. *Biochem J* 316:93, 1996.
55. Brines M, Grasso G, Fiordaliso F, et al: Erythropoietin mediates tissue protection through an erythropoietin and common beta-subunit heteroreceptor. *Proc Natl Acad Sci U S A* 101:14907, 2004.
56. Osselaer JC, Jamart J, Scheiff JM: Platelet distribution width for differential diagnosis of thrombocytosis. *Clin Chem* 43:1072, 1997.
57. Kaushansky K: On the molecular origins of the chronic myeloproliferative disorders: It all makes sense. *Blood* 105:4187, 2005.
58. Pikman Y, Lee BH, Mercher T, et al: MPLW515L is a novel somatic activating mutation in myelofibrosis with myeloid metaplasia. *PLoS Med* 3:e270, 2006.

CHAPTER 121

HEREDITARY QUALITATIVE PLATELET DISORDERS

Barry S. Coller, Deborah L. French, and A. Koneti Rao

SUMMARY

Abnormalities of platelet function manifest themselves primarily as excessive hemorrhage at mucocutaneous sites, with ecchymoses, petechiae, epistaxis, gingival hemorrhage, and menorrhagia most common. Both quantitative and qualitative platelet abnormalities can produce these symptoms, so it is necessary to exclude thrombocytopenia (see Chap. 119) by performing a platelet count. A prolonged bleeding time in a patient with a normal platelet count is indicative of a qualitative platelet abnormality, von Willebrand disease (see Chap. 127), or afibrinogenemia (see Chap. 126). Chap. 122 discusses acquired qualitative platelet abnormalities, and this chapter discusses the hereditary qualitative platelet abnormalities.

The hereditary qualitative platelet disorders can be classified according to the major locus of the defect (Table 121–1; Fig. 121–1). Thus, abnormalities of platelet glycoproteins, platelet granules, and signal transduction and secretion can all result in hemorrhagic diatheses and prolonged bleeding times. Glanzmann thrombasthenia results from abnormalities in one of two integrin subunits, either α_{IIb} (glycoprotein [GP] IIb) or β_3 (GPIIIa), resulting in loss or dysfunction of the $\alpha_{IIb}\beta_3$ (GPIIb/IIIa) receptor. This results in a profound defect in platelet aggregation and secondary defects in platelet adhesion and platelet coagulant activity. Loss of the platelet GPIb/IX/V complex because of abnormalities in GPIbα, GPIbβ, or GPIX results in the Bernard-Soulier syndrome, which is characterized by giant platelets and modest thrombocytopenia. The major defect is in platelet adhesion because of a decrease in platelet interactions with von Willebrand factor, but abnormalities in $\alpha_{IIb}\beta_3$ activation and thrombin-induced aggregation are also present. A gain of function defect in GPIbα (platelet-type [pseudo-] von Willebrand disease) can also produce a hemorrhagic disorder via depletion of high-molecular-weight von Willebrand multimers. Inherited defects in agonist receptors or proteins involved in signal transduction may also produce hemorrhagic symptoms. Abnormalities of platelet coagulant activity, that is, the ability of platelets to facilitate thrombin generation (see Chap. 114), can also lead to a hemorrhagic diathesis, but this platelet defect is unique in not usually producing mucocutaneous hemorrhage or a prolonged bleeding time.

Acronyms and abbreviations that appear in this chapter include: ADP, adenosine diphosphate; ATP, adenosine triphosphate; BLOC, biogenesis of lysosome-related organelles complex; cAMP, cyclic adenosine monophosphate; EDTA, ethylenediaminetetraacetic acid; HLA, human leukocyte antigen; HPS, Hermansky-Pudlak syndrome; Ig, immunoglobulin; LAD, leukocyte adhesion deficiency; MIDAS, metal ion-dependent adhesion site; PAR, protease-activated receptor; PKC; protein kinase C; PLC, phospholipase C; rFVIIa, recombinant factor VIIa.

ABNORMALITIES OF GLYCOPROTEIN ADHESION RECEPTORS

$\alpha_{IIb}\beta_3$ (GLYCOPROTEIN IIb/IIIa; CD41/CD61): GLANZMANN THROMBASTHENIA

Definition and History

Glanzmann thrombasthenia is an inherited hemorrhagic disorder characterized by a severe reduction in, or absence of, platelet aggregation in response to multiple physiologic agonists because of qualitative or quantitative abnormalities of platelet glycoprotein α_{IIb} (GPIIb; CD41) and/or β_3 (GPIIIa, CD61).[1–4]

In 1918, Eduard Glanzmann, a Swiss pediatrician, described a group of patients with hemorrhagic symptoms and a defect in platelet function, namely the ability to retract clots ("weak" platelets or thrombasthenia).[5] Subsequent studies demonstrated that thrombasthenic patients have prolonged bleeding times and that platelets from thrombasthenic patients fail to aggregate in response to physiologic agonists such as adenosine diphosphate (ADP), epinephrine, collagen, and thrombin,[6–9] and have markedly reduced[6,8–10] levels of platelet fibrinogen. In the mid-1970s, Nurden and Caen[11] and Phillips and colleagues[12] discovered that thrombasthenic platelets are deficient in both α_{IIb} and β_3. Later studies demonstrated that α_{IIb} and β_3 form a calcium-dependent complex in the platelet membrane that functions as a receptor for fibrinogen and other adhesive glycoproteins.[13–16] Cloning and sequencing of the complementary DNAs for α_{IIb}[17] and β_3[18] identified them as separate protein subunits that are members of the integrin receptor superfamily[19] and permitted the molecular biologic characterization of patients with the disorder. Identification of the DNA defects in selected patients has provided information on the structure-function relationships of the $\alpha_{IIb}\beta_3$ receptor and permitted DNA-based carrier detection and prenatal diagnosis (see database of Glanzmann patients and their molecular biologic defects at http://med.mssm.edu/glanzmanndb).

Etiology and Pathogenesis

Glanzmann thrombasthenia is a rare disorder characterized by autosomal recessive inheritance with a worldwide distribution. In regions where consanguineous matings are common, groups of patients with the disorder have been identified, and in several populations founder mutations have been identified by analyzing polymorphisms in the DNA surrounding the affected mutation. These include 42 patients from South India; 39 patients from the Iraqi-Jewish population in Israel; 46 Arab patients from Israel, Jordan, and Saudi Arabia; 30 patients from Italy; and a smaller number of patients from 3 Gypsy families.[10,20–27] Perhaps the highest frequency of a Glanzmann thrombasthenia mutation is found in the Iraqi-Jewish population where the most common mutation causing Glanzmann thrombasthenia was found in 6 of 700 individuals in that population.[27]

The platelet $\alpha_{IIb}\beta_3$ receptor is required for platelet aggregation induced by all of the agonists thought to operate *in vivo* (ADP, epinephrine, thrombin, collagen, thromboxane A_2; see Chap. 114).[13–16] Consequently, abnormalities in the receptor result in a failure of platelet plug formation at sites of vascular injury, leading to excessive bleeding and bruising.

The $\alpha_{IIb}\beta_3$ receptor is also responsible for the uptake of fibrinogen from plasma into platelet α granules,[28–31] hence, patients with Glanzmann thrombasthenia have markedly reduced levels of platelet fibrinogen.[6,8,9,32,33] Clot retraction requires platelets with intact $\alpha_{IIb}\beta_3$ receptors,[34–36] presumably to make contact with fibrin, and thus, patients with Glanzmann thrombasthenia usually have abnormal clot retraction.[6]

TABLE 121–1. Inherited Disorders of Platelet Function

I. Abnormalities of Glycoprotein Adhesion Receptors
  A. $\alpha_{IIb}\beta_3$ (Glycoprotein IIb/IIIa; CD41/CD61): Glanzmann thrombasthenia
  B. Glycoproteins Ib (CD42b,c)/IX(CD42a)/V: Bernard-Soulier syndrome
  C. Glycoprotein GPIbα (CD42b): platelet-type (pseudo-) von Willebrand disease
  D. $\alpha_2\beta_1$ (Glycoprotein Ia/IIa; very-late antigen [VLA]-2; CD49b/CD29)
  E. CD36 (Glycoprotein IV)
  F. Glycoprotein VI
II. Abnormalities of Platelet Granules
  A. δ-Storage pool deficiency
  B. Gray platelet syndrome (α-storage pool deficiency)
  C. α,δ-Storage pool deficiency
  D. Quebec platelet disorder
III. Abnormalities of Platelet Coagulant Activity (Scott syndrome)
IV. Abnormalities of Platelet Signaling and Secretion
  A. Defects in platelet agonist receptors or agonist-specific signal transduction (thromboxane A_2 receptor defect, adenosine diphosphate [ADP] receptor defects [$P2Y_{12}$, $P2Y_1$, $P2X_1$], epinephrine receptor defect, platelet-activating factor receptor defect)
  B. Defects in guanosine triphosphate (GTP)-binding proteins (Gαq deficiency, Gαs hyperfunction and genetic variation in extralarge Gαs, Gαi1 deficiency)
  C. Phospholipase C (PLC)-β_2 deficiency and defects in PLC activation
  D. Defects in protein phosphorylation: protein kinase C (PKC)-θ deficiency
  E. Defects in arachidonic acid metabolism and thromboxane production (phospholipase A_2 deficiency, cyclooxygenase [prostaglandin H_2 synthase] deficiency, thromboxane synthase deficiency)
V. Abnormalities of a Cytoskeletal Structural Protein: β_1 Tubulin
VI. Abnormalities in Cytoskeletal Linking Proteins
  A. Wiskott-Aldrich syndrome protein (WASP)
  B. Kindlin-3: Leukocyte adhesion defect-III (LAD-III); LAD-1 variant, integrin activation deficiency disease defect (IADD)
VII. Abnormalities of Ttranscription Factors Leading to Functional Defects
  A. RUNX1 (familial platelet dysfunction with predisposition to acute myelogenous leukemia)
  B. GATA-1
  C. FLI1 (dimorphic dysmorphic platelets with giant α granules and thrombocytopenia; Paris-Trousseau/Jacobsen syndrome)

Defects in either α_{IIb} or β_3 result in the same functional defect because both subunits are required for receptor function (see Chap. 114). Biosynthetic studies indicate that α_{IIb} and β_3 form a complex soon after protein synthesis in the rough endoplasmic reticulum[37–39]; subsequent posttranslational processing[40] and transport to the platelet membrane require that the complex be intact (Fig. 121–2).[41,42] Complex formation protects each of the glycoproteins from proteolytic digestion,[37–40] so if either α_{IIb} or β_3 is absent or unable to form a normal complex, the other subunit will be rapidly degraded. Thus, a deficiency in either glycoprotein produces a deficiency in both. Because complex formation and vesicular transport are also required for proteolytic processing of pro-α_{IIb} into its constituent $\alpha_{IIb}\alpha$ and $\alpha_{IIb}\beta$ subunits,[40] if complex formation and/or vesicular transport does not occur normally, the very small amount of residual α_{IIb} will be pro-α_{IIb}, not mature α_{IIb}.[43] Pro-α_{IIb} has been reported to bind to the membrane-bound endoplasmic reticulum chaperone calnexin, providing a potential mechanism for assessing whether the protein has undergone proper folding (calnexin cycle) and perhaps explaining how the receptor adopts a bent configuration.[44,45]

β_3 (Glycoprotein [GP] IIIa) can also combine with the α_V-integrin (CD51) subunit to form the $\alpha_V\beta_3$ "vitronectin receptor" (see Fig. 121–2 and Chap. 114).[18,46,47] Despite its common name, this receptor can bind many of the same adhesive glycoproteins as $\alpha_{IIb}\beta_3$, although there are some differences in ligand preference and binding sequences.[47–51] A small number of $\alpha_V\beta_3$ receptors are present on platelets (50–100 per platelet)[50,52,53]; osteoclasts, endothelial cells, macrophages, vascular smooth muscle, and uterine cells, among others, also have $\alpha_V\beta_3$ receptors.[54–56] In general, Glanzmann thrombasthenia patients with defects in β_3 also are deficient in $\alpha_V\beta_3$, whereas patients with defects in α_{IIb} have either normal or increased numbers of platelet $\alpha_V\beta_3$ receptors.[50,53,55,57–59] One exception to this rule is a patient with a defect in β_3 (H280P) that interferes with $\alpha_{IIb}\beta_3$ biogenesis to a much greater extent than $\alpha_V\beta_3$ biogenesis.[60] At present, there is no evidence that patients who lack $\alpha_V\beta_3$ receptors in addition to lacking $\alpha_{IIb}\beta_3$ receptors have a more severe hemorrhagic diathesis or suffer from any other abnormalities, perhaps because alternative receptors containing α_V associated with other β subunits can substitute for $\alpha_V\beta_3$.[53] Upregulation of $\alpha_2\beta_1$ on osteoclasts of Iraqi-Jewish patients with Glanzmann thrombasthenia has been reported as a potential compensatory mechanism to explain the lack of bone changes despite the deficiency in osteoclast $\alpha_V\beta_3$.

The molecular biologic abnormalities in more than 100 patients with Glanzmann thrombasthenia have been identified[60a] and they are listed in an Internet database that is updated continuously[61] (http://med.mssm.edu/glanzmanndb). Figure 121–3 contains information on mutations of particular interest. Of note, many of the patients with identified mutations are compound heterozygotes rather than homozygotes, indicating that a sizable number of silent carriers are present in the population. Where consanguinity is common, the disorder is more likely to be caused by a homozygous mutation arising in a founder, but even under these circumstances, more than one mutation may be present. Thus, in the Iraqi-Jewish population, in which consanguinity has been present from 586 BCE to the present, two separate mutations have been identified in more than one family.[27] Most of the missense mutations result in decreased expression of $\alpha_{IIb}\beta_3$ on the surface of platelets. This probably reflects the stringent structural requirements for proper folding and complex formation.

Mutations in $\alpha_{IIb}\beta_3$ Within the Metal Ion-Dependent Adhesion Site of β_3 (GPIIIa) and the Interface with the α_{IIb} (GPIIb) β-Propeller A metal coordination site or metal ion-dependent adhesion site (MIDAS) domain,[62] which is highly conserved in six integrin receptor α-chain subunits and required for ligand-binding,[63] is also present in the βA (or I-like) domain of the β_3 subunit.[64,65] Mutagenesis and molecular modeling experiments suggested that a highly conserved D*x*S*x*S amino acid sequence[66] motif plus additional coordinating residues are brought together in the three-dimensional structure of the β_3 subunit to form a cation-binding sphere of the MIDAS domain,[62] and this was confirmed by the crystal structures of $\alpha_V\beta_3$ and later $\alpha_{IIb}\beta_3$ (see Figs. 114–3 and 121–3).[67,68] Thus, the β_3 MIDAS is composed of Asp^{119}, Ser^{121}, Ser^{123}, Glu^{220}, and Asp^{251}. A region originally termed the ligand-associated metal-binding site (LIMBS) in $\alpha_V\beta_3$,[69] but now termed the synergy metal-binding site (SyMBS) in $\alpha_{IIb}\beta_3$,[65] binds a Ca^{2+} ion and is required for binding of ligands to the MIDAS. It is composed of atoms from D158, N215, D217, P219, and E220. β_3 Residues 214 and 216 are in close proximity with both the SyMBS residues and the interface with

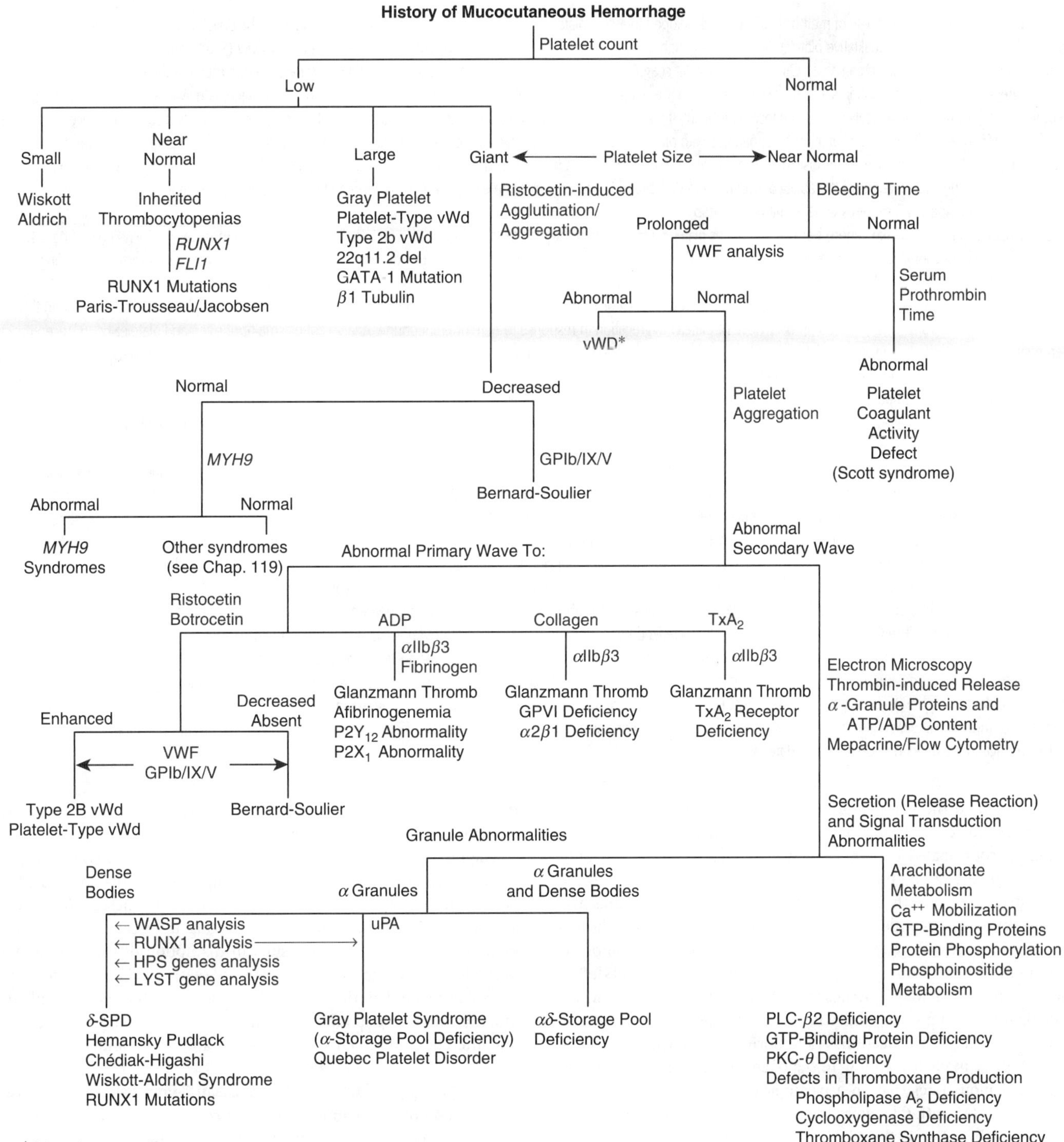

*Other than type 2b

FIGURE 121–1. Evaluation of patients for inherited abnormalities in platelet number or function. A reduced platelet count occurs in patients with purely quantitative platelet disorders (inherited or acquired) as well as in patients who have inherited qualitative platelet disorders associated with thrombocytopenia. Platelet size (determined from the blood film and/or the mean platelet volume) helps to separate the inherited quantitative platelet syndromes from the acquired thrombocytopenias and the inherited combined quantitative and qualitative thrombocytopenias (see Chap. 119). Very small platelets are characteristic of the Wiskott-Aldrich syndrome. The Paris-Trousseau/Jacobsen syndrome is a rare inherited thrombocytopenia with giant α granules in only a fraction of circulating platelets and deletion of chromosome 11q23.3–24 affecting the transcription factor *FLI1*. Transcription factor RUNX-1 mutations are associated with familial thrombocytopenia, abnormal platelet function, and a predisposition to leukemia. Large platelets that lack purple granules are observed in the gray platelet syndrome (α-storage pool deficiency), but one needs to be certain that the stain is working properly. Confirmation of the diagnosis of gray platelet syndrome is obtained with biochemical analysis of α-granule contents. Patients with platelet-type (pseudo-) von Willebrand disease (VWD) and type 2b VWD have moderate thrombocytopenia and large platelets. Studies of glycoprotein (GP) Ib function and biochemistry described below establish the diagnosis. Patients who are hemizygous for GPIbβ because of deletion of 22q11.2, those with mutations in transcription factor *GATA-1* or β_1 tubulin (R318W), and some patients who are heterozygous for defects in GPIb/IX associated with Bernard-Soulier syndrome have variable thrombocytopenia and large platelets. The platelets in Bernard-Soulier syndrome itself are truly giant; the diagnosis is confirmed with biochemical and functional analyses of the GPIb/IX/V complex. (*continued*)

FIGURE 121–1. (*continued*) A variety of methods have been developed to assess platelet function and new instrumentation continues to be developed.[564,799–805] The bleeding time is prolonged in most patients with qualitative platelet disorders (although to various extents) except in the disorder of platelet coagulant activity (Scott syndrome), where the serum prothrombin time is the preferred screening assay. Other tests of platelet coagulant activity, microvesiculation, and phospholipid transfer are used to establish the diagnosis.
Platelet aggregation can separate patients into those with defects in the primary wave of platelet aggregation (dependent on either fibrinogen, von Willebrand factor, their respective receptors, or agonist receptors for collagen or adenosine diphosphate [ADP]) and those with defects in the secondary wave of aggregation. Enhanced ristocetin-induced platelet aggregation at low doses of ristocetin is characteristic of patients with platelet-type VWD (who have a defect in the GPIb receptor that facilitates von Willebrand factor binding) and patients with type 2b VWD (who have an intrinsic defect in von Willebrand factor; see Chap. 127). These two diseases can be separated by analyzing the binding of the patient's von Willebrand factor to normal platelets, or the ability of purified von Willebrand factor, cryoprecipitate or asialo-von Willebrand factor to aggregate patient platelets; confirmation of the diagnosis of platelet-type VWD requires genetic analysis of GPIb.

Neither ristocetin nor the snake venom botrocetin induces platelet aggregation if the plasma lacks functional von Willebrand factor, as in most cases of VWD (see Chap. 127), or if the platelets lack functional GPIb/IX complexes, as in Bernard-Soulier syndrome. The defect in VWD, but not Bernard-Soulier syndrome, can be corrected by adding normal plasma or purified von Willebrand factor. Direct analysis of von Willebrand factor and the platelet GPIb/IX complex[805a] are used to confirm the diagnosis.

Patients whose plasma lacks fibrinogen (afibrinogenemia; see Chap. 126) or whose platelets cannot bind fibrinogen because of abnormal $\alpha_{IIb}\beta_3$ receptors (Glanzmann thrombasthenia; Glanzmann Thromb) will have no primary wave of platelet aggregation in response to ADP or epinephrine. Analysis of plasma fibrinogen and platelet $\alpha_{IIb}\beta_3$ receptors can differentiate between these two groups. Isolated defects in the primary response to collagen have been observed in patients with abnormalities in platelet $\alpha_2\beta_1$ (GPIa/IIa) or GPVI. Platelet glycoprotein analysis can separate these from each other. Because antibodies to GPVI can result in receptor depletion from circulating platelets, a search for an antibody to GPVI should be undertaken in patients with reduced levels of platelet GPVI. Other isolated defects in one or more of the ADP receptor or the thromboxane A_2 (TXA_2) receptor will result in decreased platelet aggregation in response to ADP or the thromboxane analogue U46619, respectively; isolated defects in the receptor for epinephrine will lead to a defect in primary aggregation in response to this agonist.

A heterogeneous group of platelet defects can result in an abnormal secondary wave of platelet aggregation in response to ADP and epinephrine, and diminished responses to low doses of collagen and thrombin. They can be broadly separated into granule defects and defects in the platelet secretion or release reaction. Operationally, these two groups can be separated on the basis of their release of dense granule contents in response to high doses of thrombin. Thrombin activation can overcome most or all of the release reaction abnormalities, so platelets from patients with these disorders will release normal amounts of granule contents; in contrast, patients with reduced granule contents have abnormal release responses even when using high doses of thrombin. α-Granule contents and dense body contents can be measured immunologically and biochemically; electron microscopy can confirm the diagnosis of granule defects. Analysis of the genes or proteins implicated in the different granule defect abnormalities (Wiskott-Aldrich syndrome [WASP], Hermansky-Pudlak syndrome [HPS], Chédiak-Higashi syndrome [*LYST*], Paris-Trousseau/Jacobson syndrome [*FLI1*], and inherited platelet disorder with predisposition to leukemia [*RUNX1*]) can establish the diagnosis. The Quebec platelet disorder is characterized by increased urokinase plasminogen activator (uPA) in α granules and degradation of several α-granule proteins. The diagnosis can be established by immunoblot analysis or analysis of uPA activity. Secretion abnormalities arise due to defects in mechanisms that regulate the release of granule contents, and include abnormalities at the level of guanosine triphosphate (GTP)-binding proteins that link surface receptors to intracellular enzymes, phospholipase C activation, and protein phosphorylation (protein kinase C [PKC]-θ). They also arise from defects in thromboxane A_2 synthesis because of deficiencies of phospholipase A_2 (PLA_2), cyclooxygenase, or thromboxane synthase. Specific studies on signal transduction mechanisms, phosphoinositide metabolism, Ca^{2+} mobilization, protein phosphorylation, and thromboxane production are needed to define these defects.

α_{IIb}. Adjacent to the MIDAS domain is a metal ion site termed the ADMIDAS (adjacent to metal ion-dependent adhesion site), in which calcium is coordinated by Ser^{123}, Asp^{126}, Asp^{127}, and Met^{335} in unliganded $\alpha_V\beta_3$ and $\alpha_{IIb}\beta_3$, but Asp^{251} substitutes for Met^{335} in the ligand bound structures of both $\alpha_V\beta_3$ and $\alpha_{IIb}\beta_3$. The crystal structures also demonstrated that peptide ligands containing the RGD cell adhesion sequence interact with $\alpha_{IIb}\beta_3$ and $\alpha_V\beta_3$ in part by coordination of the metal ion in the MIDAS by the aspartic acid in the RGD peptide.[69,70] The low-molecular-weight drugs eptifibatide and tirofiban, which block ligand binding to α_{IIb}, have negatively charged regions that also interact with the MIDAS cation.[68] The fibrinogen γ-chain C-terminal dodecapeptide mediates binding to $\alpha_{IIb}\beta_3$ and a crystal structure of the complex demonstrates that an aspartic acid carboxyl oxygen coordinates the MIDAS cation whereas the carboxy-terminal valine interacts with the nearby cation in the ADMIDAS.[68,70] A number of mutations in patients with Glanzmann thrombasthenia have been identified within the cation-binding sphere of the MIDAS domain (see Fig. 121–3). Two mutations D119Y (Cam variant)[71] and D119N (patient NR),[72] are located within the conserved DxSxS amino acid motif and produce severe abnormalities of ligand binding to $\alpha_{IIb}\beta_3$, but do not affect $\alpha_{IIb}\beta_3$ surface expression. Mutations at residues R214 and R216 result in abnormal $\alpha_{IIb}\beta_3$ receptors that cannot bind ligand and are very sensitive to dissociation by calcium chelation, perhaps because they are at the α_{IIb}–β_3 interface.[20,73–75] Disrupting the SyMBS with a D217V mutation also leads to Glanzmann thrombasthenia despite the expression of normal amounts of $\alpha_{IIb}\beta_3$.[76] Further support for the importance of the MIDAS domain, SyMBS, and adjacent residues comes from studies in which the mutations D119N, R214W, D217N, E220Q, and E220K were introduced into Chinese hamster ovary (CHO) cells *in vitro* and shown to result in functional abnormalities.[77]

The interface between the α_{IIb} β-propeller β_3 also involves, in part, the interaction between β_3 R261, contained in a four-amino-acid 3_{10} helix, with a number of hydrophobic residues in the α_{IIb} β-propeller arranged as inner and outer rings, making up a cage.[67] A β_3 L262Y mutation, adjacent to R261 results in disruption of the helix and an unstable $\alpha_{IIb}\beta_3$ complex that is expressed on the surface of platelets but is unable to bind fibrinogen.[78] The platelets of the patient with this mutation were able to bind fibrin and support clot retraction, suggesting different requirements for fibrinogen and fibrin binding.

Mutations in $\alpha_{IIb}\beta_3$ Within the GPIIb (α-Chain) β-Propeller Sequence Based on their homology to another integrin α subunit, the amino-terminal 450 amino acids of α_{IIb} and the homologous region in α_V, which contain the minimal ligand-binding sequence,[79] were predicted to fold into seven repeat (blade) β-propellers, containing four cation-binding sites,[80] and this prediction was confirmed by the crystal structures of both α_V and α_{IIb}.[67,68] The upper surface of the propeller interacts with the β_3 subunit β-A (or I-like) domain to form the head of the $\alpha_{IIb}\beta_3$ complex which is the site of ligand binding. Each repeat (blade) contains four β strands that are connected by loops. The four calcium binding sites in α_{IIb}, which are in β-hairpin structures, are located in loops on the undersurface of the propeller. Ligand binding in α_{IIb} has been localized to a hydrophobic (F160, Y190, F231) and negatively charged (D224) pocket that lies adjacent to the MIDAS domain in β_3, and is composed of contributions from the loops that link blade 2 to blade 3 (residues 144–171), β strand 2 to β strand 3 in blade 3 (residues

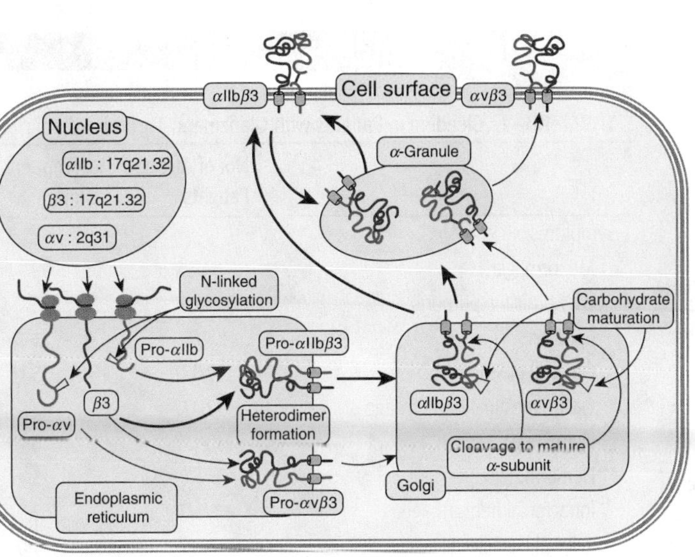

FIGURE 121–2. Biogenesis of integrin receptors $\alpha_{IIb}\beta_3$ and $\alpha_V\beta_3$. The nuclear genes for α_{IIb} (chromosome localization 17q21.32; gene designation *ITGA2B*; 30 exons), α_V (2q31; *ITGAV*; 30 exons), and β_3 (17q21.32; *ITGB3*; 14 exons) are transcribed into messenger RNA and translated by ribosomes attached to the membranes of the endoplasmic reticulum (ER). The proteins undergo initial glycosylation and form the $\alpha_{IIb}\beta_3$ and $\alpha_V\beta_3$ heterodimers in the ER. It is presumed that many more $\alpha_{IIb}\beta_3$ complexes form than $\alpha_V\beta_3$ complexes because the final copy number of platelet $\alpha_{IIb}\beta_3$ receptors is approximately 100,000 whereas it is only 50–100 for $\alpha_V\beta_3$. This is shown schematically by the differences in the width of the *arrows* depicting $\alpha_{IIb}\beta_3$ versus $\alpha_V\beta_3$ complex formation. The heteroduplexes are transported to the Golgi where the carbohydrate chains undergo modification to their mature structures and both α_{IIb} and α_V undergo proteolytic cleavage within a disulfide-bonded loop, resulting in two-chain forms of the receptor subunits. Mature $\alpha_{IIb}\beta_3$ receptors are transported to α-granule membranes, where they undergo cycling to and from the plasma membrane. This process results in the internalization of fibrinogen and perhaps other plasma proteins. $\alpha_{IIb}\beta_3$ may be transported directly to the plasma membrane. Of the total of approximately 100,000 $\alpha_{IIb}\beta_3$ receptors, approximately two-thirds are on the surface at any given time and the remaining one-third can be brought to the surface by platelet activation. The distribution of $\alpha_V\beta_3$ between the plasma membrane and α granules, and the potential cycling of $\alpha_V\beta_3$ receptors between α granules and the plasma membrane have not be defined. *(Courtesy of Dr. W. Beau Mitchell, New York Blood Center, New York, NY.)*

186–193), and blade 3 to blade 4 (residues 223–236). α_{IIb} contains a unique "cap" subdomain made up of four insertions in β propeller loops (residues 72–88, 111–126, 147–166, 200–217) that plays a ligand binding role similar to that of the I domains present in some integrin receptors.[68]

Glanzmann thrombasthenia missense mutations located within the α_{IIb} β-propeller (see Fig. 121–3) primarily affect transport of the $\alpha_{IIb}\beta_3$ complex to the cell surface,[59,81–84] but several missense mutations and an insertion result in functionally defective receptors. Thus, Y143H affects soluble ligand binding but not adhesion or clot retraction,[85] and P145A, which has been identified in several kindreds,[20,86] and P145L, prevent ligand binding. A two-amino-acid insertion at residues 161 and 162, as well as a T176I missense mutation, also affect ligand binding.[87–89] A L183P mutation, which is near to, but not in the loop containing Y190, affects both receptor expression and function.[90]

Mutations in $\alpha_{IIb}\beta_3$ That Affect Receptor Activation Several β_3 missense mutations (C560R, V193M) result in the receptor adopting a high-affinity ligand binding state, which is paradoxical as it results in a bleeding diathesis.[91,92] A β_3 S527F mutation in the third I-EGF domain was also associated with a constitutively active receptor, presumably because it prevents the receptor from assuming a bent, inactive conformation.[93] The cytoplasmic domain of β_3 plays a functional role in integrin activation and the regulation of ligand binding.[94–96] Two Glanzmann thrombasthenia mutations have been identified in this region. One is an R724X nonsense mutation (patient RM)[97] that results in the deletion of the carboxy-terminal 39 residues of β_3 and the other is a β_3 S752P missense mutation (patient P or Paris I).[94,96,98] This latter patient is unusual in that he had a generally mild history of excessive hemorrhage, but he did have a prolonged bleeding time and his platelets did not aggregate in response to ADP. These mutations do not severely affect surface expression of platelet $\alpha_{IIb}\beta_3$ complexes, but both mutant receptors are unresponsive to agonist stimulation. Mammalian cell expression studies of these mutations show normal adhesion to immobilized fibrinogen, but abnormal cell spreading. Cells expressing the S752P mutant receptors have reduced focal adhesion plaque formation and cells expressing the R724X mutant receptors have undetectable tyrosine phosphorylation of focal adhesion kinase, $pp125^{FAK}$. These mutations provide evidence for the role of the β_3 cytoplasmic tail in inside-out signaling (i.e., platelet signals that lead to $\alpha_{IIb}\beta_3$ adopting a high-affinity ligand-binding conformation) and outside-in signaling (i.e., signaling to the interior of the platelet as a result of $\alpha_{IIb}\beta_3$ binding ligand; see Figs. 114–3 and 114–4).

Clinical Features

The clinical manifestations of a total of 232 patients with Glanzmann thrombasthenia have been the subject of two reviews, and Table 121–2 summarizes data from 177 of these patients.[10,21] Menorrhagia occurs in nearly all patients, especially at the time of menarche. Purpura can be present immediately after birth but often is not dramatic. Petechiae of the face and subconjunctival hemorrhage associated with crying may be the first symptoms in neonates and babies. Epistaxis is a common symptom and can be life threatening.[10,21,99] It usually abates in adulthood. Gingival bleeding can be a chronic source of blood (and iron) loss, especially if the teeth are not kept in good repair.[100] Gastrointestinal bleeding was present in 12 percent of patients in one review,[10] but was present in 49 percent of patients in another review.[21] Gastrointestinal bleeding is usually intermittent, and it is often difficult to identify the bleeding site. Patients with Glanzmann thrombasthenia and vascular abnormalities of the gastrointestinal tract such as hereditary hemorrhagic telangiectasias or angiodysplasia can present severe challenges since bleeding may be recurrent and difficult to control.

Hemarthroses are very rare, and spontaneous ones even rarer, distinguishing Glanzmann thrombasthenia from the hemophilias. Having Glanzmann thrombasthenia undoubtedly increases the risk of excessive bleeding when there is trauma to the central nervous system, but it is remarkable that spontaneous central nervous system bleeding is so rare.[10,21]

Patients with Glanzmann thrombasthenia do not appear to bleed excessively during pregnancy, but immediate postpartum hemorrhage is very common unless platelet transfusions are administered.[10] Delayed postpartum hemorrhage can also be severe; it may be less likely to occur in patients delivered by cesarean section.[10] Hypopituitarism after delivery associated with excessive bleeding (Sheehan syndrome) has been reported in a patient with Glanzmann thrombasthenia.[101] Surgical procedures, including oral surgery, are usually complicated by excessive bleeding unless prophylactic platelet transfusions are administered.[10,21,102]

The hemorrhagic diathesis in Glanzmann thrombasthenia is notable for its variability and the lack of correlation between the biochemical platelet abnormalities and clinical severity.[10] Even within groups of patients such as the Iraqi Jews, most of whom share the same genetic abnormality and have very similar platelet function and biochemical

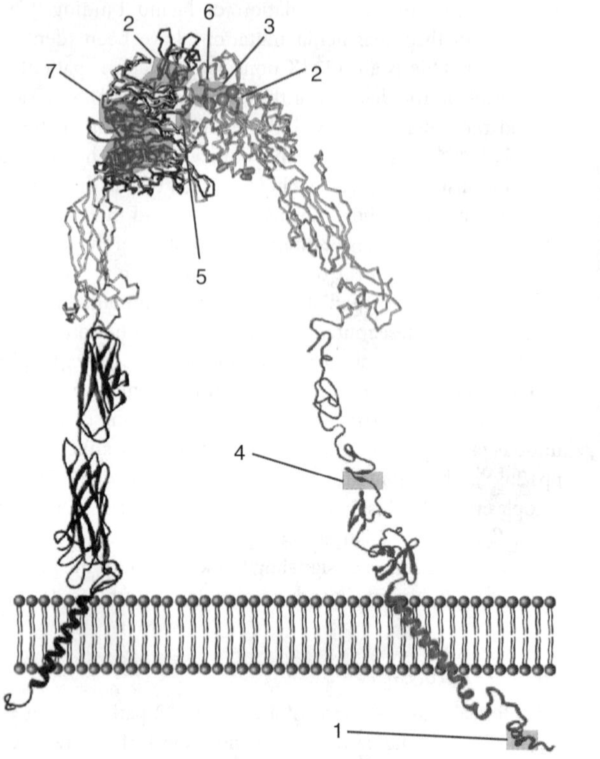

FIGURE 121–3. Diagram of $\alpha_{IIb}\beta_3$ structure and identification of select mutations causing Glanzmann thrombasthenia. The website http://med.mssm.edu/glanzmanndb contains a full listing of reported Glanzmann thrombasthenia mutations. Details of the structure of $\alpha_{IIb}\beta_3$ are given in Figures 114–3 and 114–13. The $\alpha_{IIb}\beta_3$ structure depicted is a composite of data obtained from the headpiece of $\alpha_{IIb}\beta_3$,[68] the extracellular domains of $\alpha_V\beta_3$,[67] and the transmembrane and intracellular domains.[806] Among the missense mutations identified are ones that (1) interfere with inside-out and outside-in signaling (β_3 S752P)[98]; (2) interfere with ligand binding to either the metal ion-dependent adhesion site (MIDAS) in β_3 (β_3 D119Y and D119N) or the α_{IIb} component of the ligand binding site (Y143H, P145L/A, insert R160/T161)[71,85,86,88,94]; (3) result in receptors that are sensitive to dissociation by divalent cation chelation (R214W, R214Q, R216Q)[73–75]; (4) result in a constitutively active receptor (β_3 C560R); (5) alter the interface between α_{IIb} and β_3 and disrupt ligand binding (β_3 L262Y)[78]; (6) result in a β_3 protein that can complex more effectively with α_V than α_{IIb} (S162L, R216Q, H280P)[60]; or (7) alter the α_{IIb} propeller structure and prevent normal $\alpha_{IIb}\beta_3$ complex formation, processing, and/or transport.[59,82–84,807] *(Adapted with permission from Qin J, Vinogradova O, Plow EF,[808] Xiao T, Takagi J, Coller BS, et al,[68] and Xiong JP, Stehle T, Zhang R, et al.[69])*

TABLE 121–2. Bleeding in Patients with Glanzmann Thrombasthenia

	No. of Affected Patients	Frequency (%)
Symptoms		
Menorrhagia	54/55	98
Easy bruising, purpura	152/177	86
Epistaxis	129/177	73
Gingival bleeding	97/177	55
Gastrointestinal hemorrhage	22/177	12
Hematuria	10/177	6
Hemarthrosis	5/177	3
Intracranial hemorrhage	3/177	2
Visceral hematoma	1/177	1
Severity		
Requirement for red cell transfusions		
Patients from literature*	32/48	67
Paris patients	54/64	84

*Data are from 177 patients reviewed by George et al[10] of whom 113 were from the literature and 64 were studied in Paris.

SOURCE: Reproduced with permission from Coller BS.[809]

profiles, there is a wide spectrum of clinical severity.[21,27] Moreover, the severity of bleeding symptoms can vary significantly during the lifetime of individual patients. Thus, factors other than the platelet defect itself play important roles in determining the risk of bleeding.

Arterial thrombosis appears to be very rare among patients with Glanzmann thrombasthenia as judged by a lack of reported cases, but venous thrombosis and pulmonary emboli have been reported in several patients, one of whom also had factor V Leiden.[102a–d] Glanzmann thrombasthenia does not appear to protect against the development of atherosclerosis as judged by the carotid artery intima-to-media ratio.[102e] Carriers of Glanzmann thrombasthenia are usually asymptomatic and generally have normal results in platelet function tests,[10,21] although a prolonged bleeding time has been reported in at least one heterozygote.[103]

Laboratory Features

Table 121–3 provides characteristic laboratory data in patients with Glanzmann thrombasthenia. Patients have normal platelet counts and morphology, prolonged bleeding times, decreased or absent clot retraction, and abnormal platelet aggregation responses to physiologic stimuli. Platelets of patients with Glanzmann thrombasthenia have a normal (or near-normal) initial slope of high-dose ristocetin-induced aggregation, reflecting the normal levels of plasma von Willebrand factor and the normal platelet GPIb/IX content; at lower doses of ristocetin, however, where GPIb/IX-mediated activation of $\alpha_{IIb}\beta_3$ (see Chap. 114) normally contributes to the aggregation response, patient's have decreased second-wave aggregation.[104] The interesting cyclical aggregation observed at high doses of ristocetin[105] probably reflects a complex interaction between ristocetin-induced binding of von Willebrand factor to GPIb/IX and inhibition of this interaction by released ADP and collagen.[106] Glanzmann thrombasthenia platelets undergo normal shape change in response to ADP and thrombin, demonstrating their ability to undergo metabolic and cytoskeletal changes in response to these agents. Similarly, high doses of thrombin and collagen produce normal release of dense body and α-granule contents[6,8,107]; the release reaction abnormalities observed with lower doses of these agents reflect the lack of augmentation of the release reaction normally produced by platelet aggregation.[6,104,108–110]

Platelets in whole blood or platelet-rich plasma adhere to glass because fibrinogen first becomes deposited on the glass and the platelets then adhere to the immobilized fibrinogen.[111,112] Platelets from patients with Glanzmann thrombasthenia fail to adhere to glass,[6,8,111] and this forms the basis of their abnormality in the glass bead retention assay.[113] Platelet coagulant activity has been variably reported as normal or abnormal,[6–9,114–116] probably as a result of variations in the assays used to assess this activity or individual patient differences. A defect in platelet microparticle formation and support of thrombin generation has been identified in some patients,[115–118] but not all patients appear to share this abnormality.[119] $\alpha_{IIb}\beta_3$ and $\alpha_V\beta_3$ have been shown to bind prothrombin, probably accounting for some of the abnormalities identified.[120,121]

In flow chamber studies, thrombasthenic platelets adhere normally to deendothelialized blood vessels at low and intermediate shear rates, but do not spread normally or form platelet thrombi.[122–124] A defect in

TABLE 121–3. Laboratory Features of Glanzmann Thrombasthenia

I. Platelet Count: Normal
II. Bleeding Time: Markedly Prolonged
III. Tests of platelet function
 A. Platelet aggregation
  1. Epinephrine—no observable response
  2. Adenosine diphosphate (ADP) and thrombin—shape change, but no aggregation
  3. Collagen—shape change followed by variable increase in light transmission due most likely to progressive adhesion to collagen fibers (pseudoaggregation)
  4. Ristocetin—normal initial slope of aggregation; at low doses, inhibition of second wave; at high doses, cyclical aggregation–disaggregation
 B. Aperture closure time (PFA-100): Prolonged
 C. Clot retraction: Absent or reduced
 D. Platelet release reaction: Decreased with epinephrine and low dose ADP, thrombin and collagen; normal with high dose thrombin and collagen
 E. Interaction with glass (platelet retention test): Absent or reduced
 F. Platelet coagulant activity: Variably abnormal
 G. Microparticle formation: Variably abnormal
 H. *Ex vivo* interaction with deendothelialized blood vessels in flow chambers: Marked abnormality in platelet thrombus formation and defective platelet spreading. Decreased platelet adhesion at high shear rates
IV. Tests of $\alpha_{IIb}\beta_3$ and $\alpha_V\beta_3$ Receptors: Number and Functional Integrity
 A. $\alpha_{IIb}\beta_3$ content: Reduced or absent, except in variants
 B. $\alpha_V\beta_3$ content: Reduced or absent in patients with β_3 defects; normal or increased in patients with α_{IIb} defects
 C. Platelet binding of fibrinogen and other adhesive glycoproteins to $\alpha_{IIb}\beta_3$: Reduced or absent
 D. Platelet fibrinogen content: Markedly reduced, except in some variants
V. Platelet Coagulant Activity: Normal or Reduced

adhesion occurs at higher shear rates. A paradoxical increase in fibrin formation on these surfaces has been observed with thrombasthenic platelets, but the explanation for this phenomenon remains unknown.[125] In contrast to normal blood, blood from nearly all patients with Glanzmann thrombasthenia fails to occlude a 150-μm aperture in collagen-coated membranes under high sheer, either in the presence of ADP or epinephrine (PFA-100).[126,127]

Platelet $\alpha_{IIb}\beta_3$ and $\alpha_V\beta_3$ can be quantitated by any one of several techniques, including, monoclonal antibody binding (using flow cytometry or radiolabeled binding), immunoblotting, and surface-labeling followed by sodium dodecylsulfate polyacrylamide gel electrophoresis (SDS-PAGE). Based on the results of such studies, patients with Glanzmann thrombasthenia have been subcategorized by $\alpha_{IIb}\beta_3$ content into those with less than 5 percent of normal $\alpha_{IIb}\beta_3$ (type I), 5 to 20 percent (type II), or 50 percent or more (variants).[10,128] In one review of 64 patients, 78 percent were type I, 14 percent were type II, and 8 percent were variants.[10] The subtyping of Glanzmann thrombasthenia into type I, type II, and variants predated the identification of $\alpha_{IIb}\beta_3$ abnormalities as the cause of Glanzmann thrombasthenia and was based on functional data. With current methods of more precise laboratory analysis and the recognition of the diverse clinical and functional abnormalities present in Glanzmann thrombasthenia, this categorization provides only limited information.

Measuring $\alpha_V\beta_3$ content is technically more demanding than measuring $\alpha_{IIb}\beta_3$ because there are so few $\alpha_V\beta_3$ receptors per platelet.[53] The $\alpha_V\beta_3$ level is very useful, however, in making a preliminary assessment of whether the patient has a defect in α_{IIb} or β_3, since, in general, patients who lack $\alpha_V\beta_3$ receptors have a defect in β_3 rather than α_{IIb}.[129] A β_3 missense mutation (H280P) that differentially affected $\alpha_{IIb}\beta_3$ more than $\alpha_V\beta_3$ has, however, been described.[60]

Fibrinogen binding studies assess the function of the $\alpha_{IIb}\beta_3$ complex.[13,14] The method used for early studies was to add radiolabeled fibrinogen to platelets suspended in buffer (prepared either by washing or gel-filtration) and then measure the binding of radioactivity when the platelets were stimulated with ADP[13,14] or a similar agonist. Fibrinogen can also be labeled with a fluorescent molecule and then flow cytometry can be used to measure fibrinogen binding. These techniques are most useful in detecting qualitative abnormalities of $\alpha_{IIb}\beta_3$ in patients with variant Glanzmann thrombasthenia. The binding of a monoclonal antibody (PAC1) to platelets gives similar information because the antibody only binds to the activated form of $\alpha_{IIb}\beta_3$.[130]

Carriers of Glanzmann thrombasthenia have essentially normal platelet function.[22] Their platelets, however, only contain approximately 60 percent of the normal number of $\alpha_{IIb}\beta_3$ receptors; the overlap in values between normals and carriers, however, doesn't permit for unequivocal diagnosis of carriers by this technique.[131] Carrier detection is most accurately performed by DNA analysis when the defect is known, and advances in polymerase chain reaction technology allows this to be performed even with DNA obtained from cells in random urine samples.[132]

Platelet fibrinogen is reduced to approximately 10 percent of normal in patients with marked reductions in $\alpha_{IIb}\beta_3$,[6,9,32,33] but is variably reduced in patients with significant amounts of $\alpha_{IIb}\beta_3$.[128,133,134] Its presence may provide insights into the nature of the functional defect.

Differential Diagnosis

A history of mucocutaneous hemorrhage, as opposed to hemarthroses and muscle hemorrhage, helps to differentiate disorders of platelet function (including von Willebrand disease and afibrinogenemia) from the hemophilias and related disorders. The symptoms of qualitative platelet function disorders and thrombocytopenia are essentially identical, so their differentiation depends on laboratory studies, most importantly the platelet count. Similarly, the symptoms of von Willebrand disease, afibrinogenemia, and the different qualitative platelet disorders are often indistinguishable, and again laboratory tests are required to make the definitive diagnosis. Hereditary disorders, such as Glanzmann thrombasthenia, are usually present at birth or have their onset in early childhood. Thus, the history can be helpful in distinguishing inherited from acquired abnormalities. Figure 121–1 is a flow diagram that depicts a logical series of steps one may take in evaluating patients with mucocutaneous hemorrhage.

Autoantibodies to $\alpha_{IIb}\beta_3$ may produce the phenotype of Glanzmann disease and many of the characteristic laboratory abnormalities.[135–143] Mixing studies using patient plasma and normal platelets should identify these acquired autoimmune disorders.

Therapy, Course, and Prognosis

Therapy involves both preventive measures and treatment of specific bleeding episodes. Dental hygiene is especially important in minimizing gingival hemorrhage.[100] Antiplatelet agents should be avoided. Iron and folate may be needed in patients with sufficient ongoing hemorrhage to cause anemia and iron depletion. Hepatitis B vaccine should be administered early in life, using a small-gauge needle and with prolonged direct pressure to the injection site to prevent excessive bleeding.

Antifibrinolytic agents are useful in patients with gingival bleeding or who are undergoing tooth extractions. Either epsilon aminocaproic acid (40 mg/kg given orally four times daily)[10] or tranexamic acid (0.5–1.0 g given orally three or four times daily)[144,145] have been recommended based on studies in patients with hemophilia A or B; tranexamic acid usually produces fewer gastrointestinal side effects than epsilon aminocaproic acid. These agents are contraindicated if disseminated intravascular coagulation is present. A tranexamic acid mouthwash (10 mL of a 5% solution used four times daily) is effective in controlling gum bleeding in patients treated with oral anticoagulants and in patients with hemophilia,[146] and one of the authors (BC) has found this helpful in Glanzmann thrombasthenia.

Antifibrinolytic agents and desmopressin may also be effective in controlling menstrual bleeding in patients with relatively mild hemorrhagic symptoms.[147,147a] Desmopressin (DDAVP; see Chap. 127) usually does not normalize the bleeding time in patients with Glanzmann thrombasthenia,[10,148] but exceptions have been reported.[149] Anecdotal reports suggest that it may improve hemostasis, even without normalizing the bleeding time.[149,150] Nonsteroidal antiinflammatory drugs, which are commonly prescribed to reduce menstrual bleeding,[150a] should be avoided because of their antiplatelet effects.[147a] In those with more severe menorrhagia, hormonal therapy to suppress menses should be considered, although the long-term consequences of such therapy needs to be considered. Menorrhagia is often most severe at the time of menarche and can result in the need for emergency hysterectomy,[147a,151] and thus patients should be counseled to seek medical attention immediately at the time of menarche. Guidelines for the medical and, if necessary, surgical management of patients with menorrhagia and inherited bleeding disorders provide a framework for a stepwise and individualized approach.[147a,152]

Topical agents can also help arrest bleeding in Glanzmann thrombasthenia patients. Gelfoam (a form of resolvable, oxidized, regenerated cellulose) soaked in either tranexamic acid[153] or topical thrombin may be effective.[154] Fibrin sealants prepared from a source of fibrinogen and a source of thrombin (exogenous or from the patient's own plasma), with or without antifibrinolytic agents or other components[154] have been used successfully in patients with Glanzmann thrombasthenia, and in one study eliminated the need for platelet transfusion at the time of tooth extractions.[155,156] At the time of writing, human thrombin (prepared from plasma and recombinant) and bovine thrombin are available, as is a method for using the patient's own plasma as a source of thrombin.[154] Bovine thrombin has induced antibody formation to itself and contaminating factors V and XI; at least some antibodies to factor V have cross-reacted with human factor V and caused serious hemorrhage.[157–159] Immunoglobulin (Ig) E-mediated anaphylaxis has also been reported with bovine topical thrombin.[160,161] Human thrombin products have variable risks of infection and allergic reactions to thrombin and/or products used in their manufacture.[154] A microfibrillar collagen hemostatic agent of bovine origin has been used to secure hemostasis in bleeding normal individuals. However, antibodies to bovine (and rabbit) tissue factor have been identified in some patients treated with this hemostatic agent, but these did not cross-react with human tissue factor nor did they induce a hemorrhagic diathesis.[162] Polyethylene glycol polymers have also been used to achieve hemostasis.[154] For dental procedures, custom splints of soft acrylic or celluloid help prevent excessive hemorrhage.[156,163]

Control of epistaxis can be particularly difficult.[99,164] When topical measures fail to control bleeding, platelet transfusions or recombinant factor VIIa (rFVIIa; see below) should be considered. Nosebleeds occur primarily along the anterior nasal septum at Kiesselbach area, which receives its blood supply from terminal branches that originate from both the internal and external carotid arteries.[164] Posterior nosebleeds can occur either along the septum or the lateral nasal wall, both of which are supplied by branches of the sphenopalatine artery, which originates from the external carotid artery. The efficacy of moisturizing creams in preventing epistaxis is controversial. Recommendations for treating nosebleeds from the American Academy of Otolaryngology–Head and Neck Surgery can be reviewed at www.entnet.org/healthinformation/nosebleeds.cfm/.

The preferred self-administered home therapy for anterior hemorrhage consists of pinching the outer aspect of the nose by compressing the nasal ala against the septum for 15 minutes to tamponade the septal vessels.[164] If this fails to control the bleeding, topical application by medical personnel of anesthetics such as lidocaine in combination with a vasoconstrictor such as phenylephrine or oxymetazoline is commonly effective in stopping the bleeding. For hemorrhage that does not respond, cauterization with silver nitrate can be effective, being careful to only cauterize one side of the septum at a time to avoid septal perforation. Electrical cautery sometimes is effective when chemical cauterization fails. If bleeding persists from Kiesselbach area despite these interventions, anterior packing with one of a variety of materials for 1 to 3 days can be tried, with especial care when removing the packing. Alternatively, a variety of absorbable or degradable materials that do not require removal and contain prohemostatic agents, including microfibrillar collagen and thrombin, may be used.[154] They generally cause less discomfort and may be associated with less rebleeding, although they are more expensive. For refractory anterior septal bleeding, external ligation of the anterior and posterior ethmoidal arteries using cauterization or clips is recommended.

For posterior bleeding, transpalatal injection of lidocaine and epinephrine around (but not in) the sphenopalatine artery may be effective. If this does not control the bleeding, posterior packing with an inflatable balloon or Foley catheter should be considered. Antibiotic prophylaxis is commonly employed to prevent the rare toxic shock syndrome. If all of the above measures fail, percutaneous embolization or surgical ligation of the sphenopalatine artery can be considered for treatment of posterior nosebleeds, with the latter producing fewer side effects than the former when performed endoscopically.

Postpartum hemorrhage in patients without a bleeding diathesis may be controlled by administration of rFVIIa.[165–169] A Glanzmann thrombasthenia patient with postpartum hemorrhage refractory to platelet transfusion had a rapid response to rFVIIa.[170]

Erythropoietin was reported to improve the bleeding time and glass bead column platelet retention in one patient with Glanzmann thrombasthenia, even without producing a significant increase in hemoglobin concentration.[149] A positive effect of erythropoietin on platelet function, independent of an effect on hemoglobin, has also been reported in uremia.[171–173]

Transfusion of platelets (see Chap. 141) is the most time tested therapy for serious bleeding in Glanzmann thrombasthenia and as prophylaxis prior to surgery or other major hemostatic stresses. Successful control of bleeding episodes in Glanzmann thrombasthenia has also been achieved with the nonblood product rFVIIa, and so the choice between platelet transfusion and rFVIIa will depend on a number of factors, including the nature of the bleeding, previous responses to each therapy, concomitant illnesses, and cost.[165] Judging the effect of transfusion on hemostasis prior to a procedure may be difficult because a platelet count increment may be difficult to establish above a normal baseline level and the bleeding time has major limitations with regard to reproducibility and requires considerable operator skill. A shortening of the closure time of the aperture of a collagen-coated membrane in the presence of ADP or epinephrine (PFA-100) has been recommended to monitor therapy,[174,175] and thus it may be possible to use one or more of the other tests of platelet function that are now available, some of which can be conducted at the bedside.[176]

Because patients may need transfusions throughout their lifetimes, hepatitis B vaccine should be administered at the time of diagnosis and all transfusions of both platelets and packed red blood cells should be given with leukocyte depletion filters to decrease the risk of alloimmunization[177] and cytomegalovirus transmission.[178] Febrile transfusion reactions can be diminished by leukocyte depletion at the time of blood collection.[179,180] Even in patients who are refractory to platelets, leukocyte depletion filters may improve the recovery of transfused platelets in the circulation.[181]

It is reasonable to use only human leukocyte antigen (HLA)-matched platelets, even early in the patient's course, to minimize the risk of alloimmunization.[182] It is preferable to match ABO blood group status in platelet transfusions because it may improve the platelet response and it will decrease the risk of a hemolytic transfusion reactions, which have been reported on rare occasions when transfusing type O platelets into type A individuals.[183] The use of platelets prepared by apheresis of a single individual compared with pooling of platelets concentrates obtained from whole blood donations will decrease the number of donor exposures, but may increase the possibility of a severe lung injury reaction since more plasma (~200 mL) is transfused from a single individual with this product than with pooled donor platelets (~40–60 mL per unit). The use of family members' platelets may be convenient, but if consideration is given to hematopoietic stem cell transplantation from a family member, it may be advisable to avoid donations from family members. Blood from family members should be irradiated to prevent transfusion-related graft-versus-host disease. Similarly, if transplantation is considered, and the patient has not already developed cytomegalovirus infection, it may be desirable to select blood from donors who do not have evidence of cytomegalovirus infection and/or use leukodepletion. Whenever possible, females of childbearing potential who are Rh-negative should be given Rh-negative platelets. If Rh-positive platelets must be given, it is perhaps preferable to use platelets prepared by apheresis, because they may have less erythrocyte contamination, but it is not clear that this translates into decreased immunization.[183] Rh-negative women of child-bearing potential who receive Rh-positive platelets should also receive anti-D therapy to neutralize the Rh antigen.[184]

Platelet alloimmunization poses several different problems in patients with Glanzmann thrombasthenia, depending upon the antigen involved. In addition to antibodies directed at platelet proteins other than $\alpha_{IIb}\beta_3$, such as HLA determinants, patients can make several different types of antibodies to α_{IIb} and/or β_3. These include antibodies to (1) the well-recognized polymorphic alloantigens on α_{IIb} and β_3[185,186] (see Chap. 138); (2) other regions of $\alpha_{IIb}\beta_3$ that are not involved in ligand binding; and (3) the ligand-binding regions of $\alpha_{IIb}\beta_3$. Because the platelets from most patients with Glanzmann thrombasthenia lack $\alpha_{IIb}\beta_3$ and thus the $\alpha_{IIb}\beta_3$ alloantigens, antibodies against these determinants, as well as against other nonligand-binding domains of $\alpha_{IIb}\beta_3$, could theoretically be produced either as a result of transfusions or pregnancy. Such antibodies could result in refractoriness to platelet transfusions, a predisposition to developing posttransfusion purpura, or a predisposition to having children with neonatal isoimmune thrombocytopenia (see Chap. 119).[185] In one report, platelets from Pl^{A2} (HPA1b/b) donors were found to be less reactive with serum from a multiply transfused patient with Glanzmann thrombasthenia than platelets containing the Pl^{A1} alloantigen, and platelets from the Pl^{A2} donors produced good platelet increments when transfused into the patient.[186] One possible case of neonatal thrombocytopenia in a Glanzmann patient has been reported, but an autoantibody could not be excluded.[187]

The development of antibodies that inhibit $\alpha_{IIb}\beta_3$ function has the potential to make further platelet transfusions ineffectual, even if the platelets circulate. Several such cases have been reported.[10,187–191] The antibodies produced by the patients induce a thrombasthenic defect in normal platelets. If patients with antibodies to $\alpha_{IIb}\beta_3$ that block ligand binding have severe hemorrhage, it is reasonable to use rFVIIa (see below) and/or to try to mechanically remove the offending plasma antibodies, but the efficacy of the latter treatment is not defined, and at best it provides only short-term benefit.[191–193] It is notable, however, that at least one patient has been reported to have had an inhibiting antibody for more than 15 years without significant hemorrhage.[10,194]

Allogeneic hematopoietic stem cell transplantation has been reported in several patients with Glanzmann thrombasthenia. The first was a 5-year-old male who had several severe gastrointestinal hemorrhages.[195] His bleeding diathesis was cured and he was alive and well, but with mild graft-versus-host disease, 16 years after the transplant.[196] The second patient, who required multiple hospital admissions to control bleeding, but who only received a platelet transfusion once, was transplanted at age 2.5 years from an HLA-identical sibling who was heterozygous for Glanzmann thrombasthenia.[197] She was well 19 months after the transplant. The third patient was transplanted at age 5 years with marrow from a sibling and did well.[198] The fourth patient, the sister of the first patient, was age 16 years at the time of transplantation and also had an uneventful course.[196] Success has also been reported using an unrelated donor[199] and reduced intensity conditioning regimens (three patients),[200] and in a recipient with antiplatelet antibodies, including antibodies to $\alpha_{IIb}\beta_3$.[199,201] Nonmyeloablative marrow transplantation has been performed successfully in a dog model of Glanzmann thrombasthenia.[202] *In utero* transplantation at 16 weeks of gestation of fetal liver cells from a 16-week fetus led to platelet alloantigen chimerism 3 weeks later (at the time of pregnancy termination), supporting the potential of such therapy for treating fetuses with Glanzmann thrombasthenia.[203]

Treatment of patients with Glanzmann thrombasthenia with rFVIIa has produced considerable, but not universal, success, but rare thromboembolic complications have been reported in association with rFVIIa therapy.[170,174,204–209] The mechanism of action is still under investigation, but current evidence suggests that a pharmacologic dose (90 mcg/kg) results in a peak plasma concentration of approximately 20 nM, which can then (1) bind to platelets via an interaction with platelet-associated tissue factor, negatively charged phospholipids, and/or GPIbα,[210,211] (2) enhance thrombin generation,[212] leading to both platelet activation and fibrin formation, and (3) enhance platelet adhesion and aggregation, even in the absence of $\alpha_{IIb}\beta_3$ or the presence of $\alpha_{IIb}\beta_3$ antagonists.[210,213,214] Several of these phenomena can occur even in the absence of tissue factor.[206,207] The optimal dose and duration of therapy remains uncertain, although doses above 80 mcg/kg and intervals between doses of less than 2.5 hours correlated with improved outcomes.[205] Thus, the justification for rFVIIa is strongest for patients who have failed to respond to platelet transfusions, who are known to have antibodies that are associated with refractoriness to platelet transfusions, or who have antibodies to $\alpha_{IIb}\beta_3$ that inhibit platelet function.[214]

Progress has been made in gene therapy approaches to correcting the genetic defect in Glanzmann thrombasthenia in megakaryocytes.[215,216] Several animal models are available, including α_{IIb}- and β_3-null mouse models,[217] and two dog models involving mutations in α_{IIb}.[218,219] Thus, as methods of hematopoietic stem cell transplantation and gene transfer therapy improve, it will be important to reassess the risk-to-benefit ratios of these therapies for individual patients with Glanzmann thrombasthenia.

Although Glanzmann thrombasthenia is a severe disease, the prognosis for survival is generally good. In one series, 2 of 64 patients died of hemorrhage, and in another series, 3 of 43 patients died of hemorrhage.[10,21] A nationwide survey in Japan identified 98 Glanzmann thrombasthenia patients in 1976 and 192 in 1991.[220] The mortality rate decreased substantially during this time interval.

GLYCOPROTEIN Ib (CD42b,c)/IX (CD42a)/V: BERNARD-SOULIER SYNDROME

Definition and History

Bernard-Soulier syndrome is an inherited disorder of the platelet GPIb/IX/V complex characterized by thrombocytopenia, giant platelets, and a failure of the platelets to bind GPIb ligands, most importantly, von Willebrand factor and thrombin.[221,222]

In 1948, Bernard and Soulier described two children from a consanguineous family who had a severe bleeding disorder characterized by mucocutaneous hemorrhage.[223,224] Evaluation of the patients' blood revealed variable thrombocytopenia and giant platelets. Beginning in the early 1970s, Bernard-Soulier syndrome platelets were shown to have a functional defect in von Willebrand factor-dependent platelet adhesion and agglutination.[225–227] In 1975, Nurden and Caen identified an abnormality in platelet GPIb as the cause of the functional defect.[228] Later studies confirmed the defect in von Willebrand factor-GPIb interactions[229–231] and identified additional defects in platelet GPV and GPIX.[232,233] Subsequent studies have identified additional ligands for the GPIb/IX complex, including thrombin,[234] P-selectin,[235] leukocyte integrin $\alpha_M\beta_2$,[236] high-molecular-weight kininogen,[237] thrombospondin-1,[238] and coagulation factors XI[239] and XII[240] (see Chap. 114), but the precise contributions of these interactions to the disorder are not well defined. Defects in GPIbα, GPIbβ, and GPIX, but not GPV have been identified in Bernard-Soulier syndrome. Mouse models of Bernard-Soulier syndrome have been produced by gene targeting of GPIbα[241] and GPIbβ,[242] and like humans, mice deficient in GPV do not demonstrate the typical features of human Bernard-Soulier syndrome.[243,244]

Etiology and Pathogenesis

Epidemiology This rare disease, with a prevalence estimated as less than 1 in 1,000,000, has been reported from countries around the world.[20,221,224,232,245–335] Consanguinity is common in the families with affected children[224] because the disorder is usually inherited as an autosomal recessive trait and because spontaneous mutations appear infrequently. However, autosomal dominant forms of the disease have been reported.[268,328] Moreover, some forms of autosomal dominant macrothrombocytopenia may result from heterozygous inheritance of select Bernard-Soulier syndrome mutations.[328]

Causes of Hemorrhage Six different features of Bernard-Soulier syndrome may contribute to the hemorrhagic diathesis: thrombocytopenia, abnormal platelet interactions with von Willebrand factor, abnormal platelet interactions with thrombin, abnormal platelet coagulant activity, abnormal platelet interactions with P-selectin, and abnormal platelet interactions with leukocyte integrin $\alpha_M\beta_2$.

The pathophysiology of the thrombocytopenia is uncertain. Early studies suggested a marked shortening of platelet survival, presumably due to the decrease in platelet surface charge resulting from the GPIb defect.[336,337] Later studies using ^{111}In-oxine to label platelets reported more modest or no shortening of platelet survival, indicating that ineffective thrombopoiesis and/or decreased thrombopoiesis may contribute to the thrombocytopenia.[338,339] Morphologic abnormalities have been identified in Bernard-Soulier syndrome megakaryocytes and these may contribute to abnormal platelet production.[340] Based on observations in other giant platelet syndromes (see Chap. 119), the large size of Bernard-Soulier platelets would tend to diminish the adverse hemostatic effects of the thrombocytopenia because the platelet mass is better preserved. With only rare exceptions,[341] however, the bleeding diathesis with Bernard-Soulier syndrome is more severe than expected from the thrombocytopenia, reinforcing the conclusion that a qualitative platelet defect is also present.[194,224]

The platelet GPIb/IX complex functions as a receptor for von Willebrand factor (see Chaps. 114 and 127).[221,342,343] This interaction is crucial in the adhesion of platelets to subendothelial surfaces, especially under high shear conditions, where von Willebrand factor acts as a bridge between the subendothelial matrix and the platelet.[123,124] The relative roles of subendothelial von Willebrand factor, plasma von Willebrand factor, and platelet von Willebrand factor have not been completely defined, but they probably all contribute to platelet adhesion.[343] The interaction of von Willebrand factor with GPIb/IX initiates activation of $\alpha_{IIb}\beta_3$,[344] which can also bind to von Willebrand factor, but at a different site on the molecule. The interaction of GPIb/IX with von Willebrand factor also directly contributes to platelet–platelet interactions.[345,346]

GPIb/IX-von Willebrand factor interactions can also occur in platelet suspensions at high shear rates; this can lead to platelet activation, with subsequent aggregation mediated by $\alpha_{IIb}\beta_3$.[343,347–349] Whether sustained shear rates *in vivo* ever reach the levels required to initiate von Willebrand factor binding, however, is not established.

The platelets of patients with Bernard Soulier syndrome have a decreased response to platelet activation by thrombin, especially at limiting concentrations of thrombin.[350–353] Bernard-Soulier platelets are deficient in two different proteins that interact with thrombin, namely GPIbα, which binds thrombin,[234] and GPV, which is a thrombin substrate (see Chap. 114). The precise nature of the interactions of thrombin with GPIbα and its biologic consequences are still unclear, but binding of thrombin to GPIbα can initiate signaling within the platelet, perhaps directly through GPIbα crosslinking or indirectly by augmenting activation of other thrombin receptors (protease-activated receptors [PARs] 1 and 4) or other thrombin-dependent events at the platelet surface.[234] Paradoxically, mice deficient in GPV actually have increased sensitivity to thrombin activation and variably increased thrombus formation, perhaps because GPV limits access of thrombin to GPIb.[244,354,355] Because thrombin is one of the major physiologic activators of platelets, the loss of thrombin binding to GPIbα may contribute to the hemorrhagic diathesis.

Bernard-Soulier platelets appear defective in supporting thrombin generation as judged by the serum prothrombin time,[356] a test performed with whole blood, but in other tests of platelet coagulant activity, Bernard-Soulier platelets support coagulation as well as, or better than, normal platelets.[114,357] Defects in collagen-induced coagulant activity and the association of factors V, VIII, and XI with Bernard-Soulier platelets have been described,[357] but their significance is unclear. Similarly, GPIb/IX has been identified as a binding site for other proteins involved in coagulation, including high-molecular-weight kininogen and factor XII, but the contributions of these interactions to the coagulant abnormality are also uncertain.[237,239,240] Abnormal membrane lipids have also been reported.[358] Binding of von Willebrand factor to GPIb/IX has been implicated in fibrin-dependent, but not fibrin-independent, augmentation of platelet coagulant activity and thus fibrin-dependent coagulant activity is likely to be abnormal in Bernard-Soulier syndrome.[116] This finding may partially explain the variability in findings between the serum prothrombin time and some of the other assays since fibrin only forms in the serum prothrombin time.

The mechanism(s) producing the giant platelets in Bernard-Soulier syndrome has not been identified, but because giant platelets are found in Bernard-Soulier syndrome variants in which GPIb/IX is present, but unable to bind ligand, it has been postulated that the abnormality is a result of the inability of GPIb/IX to bind an unknown marrow ligand.[221] It cannot be because of an inability to bind von Willebrand factor with only rare exceptions,[221a] as patients lacking von Willebrand factor do not have large platelets. Moreover, in a mouse model of Bernard-Soulier syndrome, restoring a receptor with the GPIb transmembrane and cytoplasmic domains, but not the ligand binding domain, partially corrected both the thrombocytopenia and large platelet size.[359] A defect in GPIb/IX-mediated signaling has also been proposed to cause the large platelets as a deficiency of phospholipase C has been described in Bernard-Soulier syndrome.[221,360] A mechanical alteration in the plasma membrane of Bernard-Soulier platelets has been identified by micropipette experiments, showing the plasma membrane to be more deformable than normal.[361] Megakaryocytes in Bernard-Soulier syndrome have increased ploidy and volume, as well as alterations in the membrane demarcation system, granules, and microtubules.[339,340] Both the increased size and deformability may reflect the loss of the normal interaction of GPIb/IX with the cytoskeleton via actin-binding protein (filamin-1; see Chap. 114).

Bernard-Soulier platelets are deficient not only in GPIbα, GPIbβ, and GPIX, which are known to be associated as a complex, but also in GPV (see Chap. 114).[221,233,362] It is of considerable interest that all of these proteins share highly conserved leucine-rich regions (see Chap. 114).[221,342,343] One possible explanation for the loss of surface expression of all the proteins is that they need to form a complex during biosynthesis in order to get transported to the surface[343]; evidence supports the need for GPIbα, GPIbβ, and GPIX to all be present for optimal surface expression,[363] but data from mice deficient in GPV indicate that this glycoprotein is not required for surface expression of the GPIb/IX complex.[354] GPV may, however, improve the efficiency of expression of the other members of the complex.[364] Moreover, data from the Bernard-Soulier mouse expressing a chimeric GPIbα molecule in which the leucine-rich repeat domain was replaced with the external domain of another receptor indicate that complex formation does not require the GPIbα leucine-rich domain.[359]

At the molecular level, the platelets from different patients with Bernard-Soulier syndrome are heterogeneous, with many having no detectable GPIb and others having variable amounts, up to 50 percent of normal.[221,255,257,262,264,360,365,366] There also is variability in the degree of concordance in the reduction of GPIb and the other deficient proteins.[270,367]

Molecular Biologic Defects The molecular biologic basis of Bernard-Soulier syndrome has been determined in a number of patients and an online registry of defects is available at www.bernardsoulier.org/.[368] As of this writing, 23 mutations have been described in GPIbα, 16 in GPIbβ, and 11 in GPIX. Defects have been identified in GPIbα, GPIbβ, and GPIX, but not in GPV. Many of the defects affect the leucine-rich repeats or the conserved flanking sequences, supporting the importance of these structural elements in the biogenesis and surface expression of the GPIb/IX/V complex (see Figs. 114–15, 114–16, and 121–4). Three patients have been described who are homozygous for a deletion in the last two bases of codon 492 of GPIbα, resulting in a frameshift that alters the membrane spanning region and results in premature termination, and another patient has been described who is heterozygous for this deletion and a missense mutation of GPIbα.[283,285,286,310] These defects appear to result in a poorly anchored GPIbα with GPIbα antigen present in plasma. Haplotype analysis indicated that the three identical mutations in Caucasians may have derived from a common founder. GPIbβ mutations have affected the promoter region (133) at a binding site for the GATA-1 transcription factor,[369] the signal peptide,[324] and the transmembrane and intracellular domains.[319] A homozygous Y88C defect in GPIbβ has been reported to cause Bernard-Soulier syndrome in two Japanese families and heterozygotes with this mutation have a giant platelet syndrome.[286,299] Similarly, a patient heterozygous for a GPIbβ R17C mutation also had a giant platelet syndrome.[302] An N45S mutation in GPIX, affecting leucine-rich repeat 1, has been reported in at least 12 different white patients, including 4 patients from a large Swiss family with variable clinical manifestations[292,303,335,369a] and 1 Turkish patient.[370]

Bernard-Soulier syndrome has been reported in several patients in association with hemizygous deletion of GPIbβ and several neighboring genes on chromosome 22q11.2, the DiGeorge/velocardiofacial syndrome.[278,311–314,371] Hemizygous mutations in the remaining GPIbβ allele

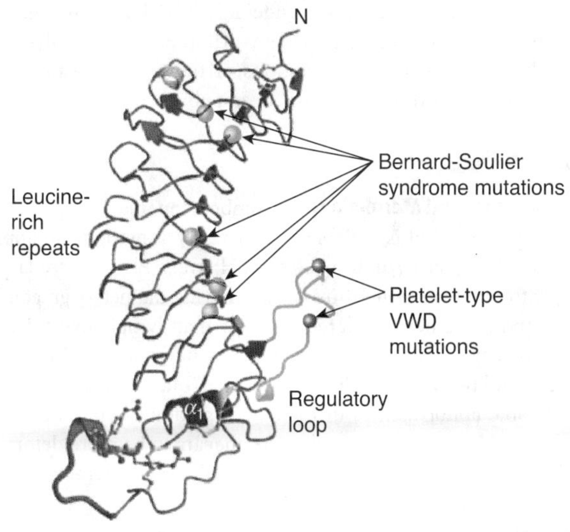

FIGURE 121–4. Localization of select missense mutations causing platelet-type von Willebrand disease and Bernard-Soulier syndrome in the GPIbα N-terminal domain. Ribbon diagram of the topology of GPIbα N-terminal domain viewed from the side. The regulatory loop is colored *green* with activating platelet-type von Willebrand disease (VWD) mutations G233V and M239V indicated as *blue balls*. Five Bernard-Soulier syndrome mutations, which cause loss of von Willebrand factor binding, are shown as *yellow balls*. L57F and C65R localize to leucine-rich repeat (LRR) 2 with L129P, A156V, and L179del localized to the LRR5, LRR6, and LRR7 β-strands respectively. The molecular structure of the sulfated tyrosine residues 276, 278, and 279 are shown. *(Adapted with permission from Uff S, Clemetson JM, Harrison T, et al.[439])*

have included P96S and P29L.[312,313] In other studies of patients with the 22q11.2 deletion syndrome, modest reductions in platelet count and increases in platelet volume, as well as reduced platelet agglutination to ristocetin and decreased platelet GPIb/IX expression have been variably reported, consistent with hemizygosity for GPIbβ.[289,372–375]

Several variants of Bernard-Soulier syndrome have been described. An autosomal dominant form has been ascribed to a heterozygous mutation in the second leucine-rich repeat (L57F).[268] The affected patients have moderate bleeding symptoms, moderate thrombocytopenia, and giant platelets. The residual GPIb is unusually susceptible to proteolysis. The "Bolzano" defect, which has been described in two patients, involves the sixth leucine-rich repeat of GPIbα (A156V). This mutation results in a GPIbα molecule that cannot bind von Willebrand factor, but can bind thrombin. In one patient, the Bolzano defect was homozygous, and the patient had nearly normal levels of GPIb/IX/V complex.[263] In the other, it coexisted with a 12-amino-acid deletion and an amino acid substitution (Q181K); GPIbα platelet expression was markedly reduced in this patient.[293] A Japanese patient heterozygous for two mutations in GPIbβ, one of which produced an additional Cys at amino acid 88, had a mild bleeding disorder, significant amounts of functional platelet GPIb/IX/V complex, and very large platelets; of note, the patient did not have thrombocytopenia. A defect in GPIbβ crosslinking to GPIbα was proposed as the cause of the abnormality.[286]

Clinical Features

Epistaxis is the most common symptom of Bernard-Soulier syndrome (70%); also common are ecchymoses (58%), menometrorrhagia (44%), gingival hemorrhage (42%), and gastrointestinal bleeding (22%).[224] The combination of Bernard Soulier syndrome with angiodysplasia can result in particularly severe recurrent hemorrhage.[376–378] Hemorrhagic symptoms that occur with lower frequency include posttraumatic bleeding (13%), hematuria (7%), cerebral hemorrhage (4%), and retinal hemorrhage (2%). There is considerable variability in symptoms among patients,[194] even among patients within a single family.[221,379] A review that includes brief descriptions of the clinical features of 55 patients, reported through 1998, has been published.[221]

Laboratory Features

Platelet Number and Morphology Thrombocytopenia is present in nearly all patients, but is variable in its severity, ranging from approximately 20,000 platelets/μL to near-normal levels. Platelets are large on smear, with more than one-third usually having diameters greater than 3.5 μm, and some being as large or larger than lymphocytes. By electron microscopy, platelets display only minor variations in vesicular structures and the open canalicular system,[224] but megakaryocytes have more notable abnormalities in their demarcation membranes.[340] The membrane of Bernard-Soulier platelets appears to be more deformable than normal,[361] perhaps because GPIb ordinarily interacts with the platelet cytoskeleton (see Chap. 114).[380]

Bleeding Time and Platelet Aggregation Studies The bleeding time is almost always prolonged but the degree of prolongation is variable. Closure times of the apertures of collagen-coated membranes are markedly prolonged in the presence of ADP or epinephrine (PFA-100).[126]

The hallmark findings in the Bernard-Soulier syndrome are the failure of platelets to aggregate in response to ristocetin[226] or botrocetin,[229,381] agents that require von Willebrand factor–GPIb interactions. In von Willebrand disease, but not Bernard-Soulier syndrome, this defect can be corrected by adding normal plasma (or von Willebrand factor).

Although the large size of the platelets in Bernard-Soulier syndrome and the thrombocytopenia make it technically difficult to perform platelet aggregation studies, in general, aggregation induced by ADP, epinephrine, or collagen is either normal or enhanced.[227,266,382] The aggregation response to thrombin is usually dose-dependent, being essentially normal in response to high doses of thrombin[351] but characterized by a prolonged lag phase and diminished aggregation in response to low doses of thrombin.[350,383]

Platelet Coagulant Activity The coagulant activity of Bernard-Soulier platelets has been variably reported as reduced, normal, or increased.[114,356,357] The variable presence of fibrin in the different assays used to assess platelet coagulant activity may account for these inconsistent results as GPIb–von Willebrand factor interactions enhance platelet coagulant activity when fibrin is present, but not when it is absent.[116]

Platelet–Thrombin Interactions Both GPIb and the seven-transmembrane domains PAR-1 and PAR-4 receptors are required for maximal response to thrombin.[234,383] Two different crystal structures of the interactions between thrombin and GPIbα have been reported; in one, two molecules of thrombin bind to each GPIbα molecule, raising the possibility that free thrombin or thrombin adherent to fibrinogen can cluster GPIb/IX/V complexes.[234,384,385] GPV, which is missing from the platelet surface in Bernard-Soulier syndrome, is cleaved by thrombin, but the cleavage is neither necessary nor sufficient for thrombin-induced platelet activation.[386,387] In fact, platelets of mice lacking GPV have increased responsiveness to thrombin, perhaps because GPV ordinarily limits access of thrombin to GPIbα or inhibits GPIbα crosslinking.[354,355]

***Ex Vivo* Interaction with Subendothelial Surfaces** Bernard-Soulier platelets demonstrate defective adhesion to subendothelial surfaces, especially at shear rates greater than 650 s[1].[123,124,225,388] The results are similar to those in patients with von Willebrand disease.

Shear-Induced Platelet Aggregation Unlike normal platelets, Bernard-Soulier platelets are not aggregated by high shear rates.[347,348] The initial interaction in this process appears to be binding of von Willebrand factor to GPIb,[343] with subsequent activation of $\alpha_{IIb}\beta_3$, perhaps through signaling via the protein 14-3-3ζ associated with the cytoplasmic domain of GPIbα,[349,389] Fcγreceptor IIA, GPVI, and/or the Fc receptor γchain (see Chap. 114).[390–392] Pathologic shear stress has been reported to increase binding of α-actin to GPIb/IX as part of the signaling process.[392–394]

Differential Diagnosis

This is discussed in the differential diagnosis of Glanzmann thrombasthenia above. Acquired Bernard-Soulier syndrome has been reported as a consequence of autoantibodies,[395–399] as part of a juvenile myelodysplastic syndrome,[400,401] and in association with acute myelogenous leukemia.[394,401]

Therapy, Course, and Prognosis

The therapy of Bernard-Soulier syndrome is essentially identical to that for Glanzmann thrombasthenia (see "$\alpha_{IIb}\beta_3$ (Glycoprotein IIb/IIIa; CD41/CD61): Glanzmann Thrombasthenia" above). Splenectomy has been performed when the diagnosis of immune thrombocytopenia was mistakenly made, but this usually does not normalize the platelet count or improve the bleeding diathesis.[293] Oral contraceptives can control menorrhagia.[402] Octreotide has been reported to be beneficial for treating bleeding from gastric angiodysplasia lesions.[378] Desmopressin (DDAVP) has been variably effective in decreasing the bleeding time.[150,254,256,266,281,288,403–406] Platelet transfusions are effective when needed but carry a risk of alloimmunization, including the production of antibodies to the functional region of GPIb.[407,408] Factor VIIa infusion has been reported in several patients and may be beneficial, but the proper indications, dose, and duration are uncertain.[409–414] Patients have had successful pregnancies and deliveries, but serious delayed bleeding can occur, and emergency hysterectomy has been required to control the hemorrhage.[246,249,259,269,290,408,412,415–417] Neonatal thrombocytopenia presumed to be caused by maternal alloimmunization has been reported.[408,418] Two sisters with serious bleeding episodes who developed antibodies to the GPIb/IX/V complex and refractoriness to platelet transfusions underwent successful hematopoietic stem cell transplantation from an HLA-identical sibling and another patient was successfully transplanted from an HLA-matched sibling.[419,420] Allogeneic hematopoietic stem cell transplantation has also been performed successfully.[420] Proof of principle for the development of gene therapy has been achieved by targeting GPIbα to human megakaryocytes and formation of a complex with GPIbβ and GPIX.[422]

As with Glanzmann thrombasthenia, the prognosis of patients with Bernard-Soulier syndrome has improved as platelet transfusion support has become more readily available and other supportive measures have become more effective.

GPIbα (CD42b): PLATELET-TYPE (PSEUDO-) VON WILLEBRAND DISEASE

Definition and History

A heterogeneous group of patients has been described with mild to moderate bleeding symptoms, variably enlarged platelets, variable thrombocytopenia, and diminished plasma high-molecular-weight von Willebrand factor multimers. The fundamental defect in these patients is thought to be an enhanced interaction between an abnormal platelet GPIb/IX receptor and normal plasma von Willebrand factor.[423–433] Because these patients have some of the hallmarks of von Willebrand disease, but the defect is in platelet GPIb/IX, it has been termed both *pseudo-von Willebrand disease* and *platelet-type von Willebrand disease.*

Etiology and Pathogenesis

A qualitative abnormality in GPIb is thought to be responsible for this disorder, with ongoing *in vivo* binding of high-molecular-weight von

Willebrand multimers to platelets causing depletion of the plasma high-molecular-weight multimers. In addition, the binding of the von Willebrand factor to platelets may lead to shortened platelet survival, perhaps accounting for the variable thrombocytopenia. Inheritance appears to be autosomal dominant.

Abnormalities in the Mr of GPIb were identified in two families,[428] but these may have resulted from a now-recognized polymorphism in GPIb (see Chaps. 114 and 138) rather than being related to the functional disorder. Heterozygous point mutations in the GPIbα DNA (G233V, G233S, M239V) have been found in several different families.[429,434–438] These mutations are in a β-hairpin loop in the carboxy-terminal flanking sequence of the leucine-rich repeats, a region implicated in ligand binding (see Fig. 121–4).[221,343,439,440] Molecular modeling suggests that the M239V substitution produces a significant conformational change in the molecule,[441] and this was confirmed by crystallographic analysis.[442] A mouse model of the GPIbα G233V mutation recapitulated many of the human manifestations of the human disease but had an unexpected increase in bone mass.[443] Recombinant GPIbα fragments containing the G233V and M239V mutations demonstrated enhanced interactions with von Willebrand factor in several different systems, including ones under shear stress.[444,445] An increase in platelet GPIb/IX expression has also been reported.[429,432] An in-frame 27-base pair deletion in the macroglycopeptide region of GPIbα has also been reported to cause platelet-type von Willebrand disease, indicating that this region many also control affinity for von Willebrand factor.[430]

Clinical Features

Patients have variable thrombocytopenia and mild to moderate mucocutaneous hemorrhage. Pregnancy may exacerbate the thrombocytopenia.[429]

Laboratory Features and Differential Diagnosis

The bleeding time is often, but not invariably, prolonged. Mild thrombocytopenia and somewhat enlarged platelets are present in some, but not all, patients. Plasma von Willebrand factor levels are variably reduced, with a disproportionate reduction in plasma high-molecular-weight multimers. Platelet von Willebrand factor multimers are normal.

The most characteristic laboratory finding in platelet-type von Willebrand disease is enhanced platelet aggregation in response to low concentrations of ristocetin[423–427,429,438] or botrocetin.[446] This same abnormality is present in patients with type 2b von Willebrand disease, as is selective depletion of plasma high-molecular-weight von Willebrand factor multimers (see Chap. 127). In platelet-type von Willebrand disease, however, the defect is in platelet GPIbα, whereas in type 2b von Willebrand disease, the defect is in the von Willebrand factor molecule. Several assays can help differentiate between these abnormalities:[425,447–449] (1) normal von Willebrand factor (purified or in cryoprecipitate) will aggregate platelets from patients with platelet-type von Willebrand disease, but not platelets from patients with type 2b von Willebrand disease; (2) isolated platelets from patients with platelet-type von Willebrand disease will bind normal von Willebrand factor at lower concentrations of ristocetin than will normal platelets or platelets from patients with type 2b von Willebrand disease; (3) plasma von Willebrand factor from patients with type 2b von Willebrand disease will bind to normal platelets at lower-than-normal concentrations of ristocetin, whereas higher-than-normal concentrations of ristocetin are required to get the plasma von Willebrand factor from patients with platelet-type von Willebrand factor to bind to normal platelets[448]; and (4) von Willebrand factor lacking sialic acid residues (asialo-von Willebrand factor) will agglutinate platelets from patients with platelet-type von Willebrand disease in the presence of ethylenediaminetetraacetic acid (EDTA).[450] A number of patients with platelet-type von Willebrand disease were originally diagnosed as having type 2b von Willebrand disease, leading to the conclusion that platelet-type von Willebrand disease may be under diagnosed.[429,431]

Therapy, Course, and Prognosis

Because normal von Willebrand factor (especially the high-molecular-weight forms) can bind excessively to the platelets of patients with platelet-type von Willebrand disease and potentially lead to rapid platelet clearance from the circulation, increasing the von Willebrand factor level by any means (desmopressin infusion or von Willebrand replacement with cryoprecipitate or von Willebrand factor concentrates) poses a potential risk of inducing thrombocytopenia.[447,451] It may be possible to estimate this risk by assessing whether the patient's platelets aggregate *ex vivo* in response to von Willebrand factor (as in cryoprecipitate).[424] Low-dose cryoprecipitate has successfully supported hemostasis, without inducing thrombocytopenia in patients at risk of having thrombocytopenia.[426,451,452] Currently, cryoprecipitate is generally less favored for von Willebrand factor replacement therapy than plasma-derived concentrates such as Humate-P, which is approved in the United States for the therapy of von Willebrand disease, because the latter are treated to reduce the risk of viral infection. Consideration should also be given to platelet transfusion in appropriate circumstances. Factor VIIa infusion may be beneficial, but this therapy is experimental; it has the theoretical advantage of avoiding excessive interactions between von Willebrand factor and the abnormal GPIbα receptor.[409,453]

$\alpha_2\beta_1$ (GLYCOPROTEIN Ia/IIa; VLA-2; CD49B/CD29)

$\alpha_2\beta_1$ (GPIa/IIa) can mediate platelet adhesion to collagen and platelet activation under certain conditions (see Chap. 114). Nieuwenhuis and coworkers[454,455] reported a female patient with excessive posttraumatic bruising and menorrhagia but no epistaxis, gum bleeding, or excessive bleeding after tonsillectomy or appendectomy, whose platelets selectively failed to aggregate or undergo shape change in response to collagen. The bleeding time was markedly prolonged, and the patient's platelets failed to adhere and spread normally on subendothelial surfaces. The patient's platelets only contained approximately 15 to 25 percent of the normal amount of GPIa,[454,456] and a reduction in GPIIa was also apparent.[454] It is difficult to draw conclusions about the physiologic role of GPIa/IIa in platelet function from this patient because her GPIa/IIa deficiency was incomplete, her bleeding symptoms were mild and variable, and some of the platelet function abnormalities (e.g., abnormal platelet-collagen interactions in the presence of the divalent chelating agent EDTA) are difficult to ascribe to the deficiency in GPIa/IIa.[454,457]

Another patient with GPIa deficiency has been described.[458] She had a history of mucocutaneous and postoperative bleeding. Her bleeding time was prolonged and platelet aggregation in response to collagen was selectively reduced, but not absent. In addition to her GPIa defect, she also had little or no intact thrombospondin, and exogenous thrombospondin corrected the defect in platelet aggregation. The patient's hemorrhagic symptoms and platelet defects disappeared when she entered menopause.

CD36 (GPIV)

CD36 (GPIV) is a highly, but variably expressed platelet glycoprotein that is present on many cell types and documented to participate in long-chain fatty acid transport (see Chap. 114). Approximately 3 percent of Japanese, 2 percent of African Americans, and 0.3 percent of whites in the United States have platelets that lack CD36 (GPIV).[459,460] Although CD36 (GPIV) has been implicated in platelet interactions with collagen and thrombospondin,[461,462,462a] as well as in platelet-monocyte interactions,[463] individuals lacking CD36 (GPIV) do not have a hemorrhagic diathesis. Platelets from these patients can bind thrombospondin via alternative receptors[464] and there is controversy as to whether they have even a mild defect in adhesion to collagen.[465,466] CD36 (GPIV) has been implicated as a receptor for oxidized low-density lipoprotein (LDL), and the binding of very-low-density lipoprotein to CD36 (GPIV) has been reported to enhance collagen-induced platelet aggregation and thromboxane production.[467] Data from animal models suggest that CD36 expression may play an important role in mediating enhanced platelet reactivity in response to oxidized LDL and a prothrombotic state.[468–470]

Two forms of CD36 (GPIV) deficiency have been described in Japan: type I in which both platelets and monocytes are deficient, and type II in which only platelets are deficient.[471–473] A C478T mutation leading to a P90S substitution and abnormal posttranslational modification is a common abnormality contributing to both type I and type II deficiencies. In the type I form, patients are homozygous for the abnormality, whereas in type II deficiency, patients are doubly heterozygous for the P90S abnormality and an unidentified platelet-specific expression defect.[471,474,475] Other abnormalities that have been associated with type I deficiency include a dinucleotide deletion (539–540) in exon 5, a 161 bp deletion (331–491) corresponding to loss of exon 4, a nucleotide insertion at position 1159 in codon 317 leading to a frameshift and premature stop, and splice site mutations.[476–478] CD36 deficiency is very rare in Caucasians, but was found in 2.4 percent of 250 African Americans.[478a] Other mutations have been identified in other populations.

CD36 (GPIV) deficiency can result in refractoriness to platelet transfusions due to isoimmunization and has been implicated in posttransfusion purpura (see Chap. 119)[479] as well as thrombocytopenia caused by the passive transfer of anti-CD36 antibodies.[479a] CD36 (GPIV) has also been implicated in monocyte binding of oxidized LDL and atherosclerosis, especially in diabetes, and myocardial uptake of long-chain fatty acids.[480–482] The abnormality in myocardial long-chain fatty acid uptake in individuals with type I CD36 (GPIV) deficiency can be documented by nuclear medicine studies and there may be an association with hypertrophic cardiomyopathy.[480,483] CD36 (GPIV) has been implicated in the adherence of *Plasmodium falciparum* to erythrocytes and different CD36 (GPIV) mutations in African and Asian populations have been reported to either predispose to, or protect from, cerebral *falciparum* malaria.[484–487] CD36 (GPIV)-mediated platelet clumping of *P. falciparum*-infected erythrocytes has been associated with malaria severity.[488]

GLYCOPROTEIN VI

GPVI can mediate platelet adhesion to collagen and is important in collagen-induced signal transduction (see Chap. 114). Twelve patients with mild to moderate bleeding disorders and variable deficiencies of platelet GPVI or signaling have been described; one had concomitant gray platelet syndrome (α-granule deficiency) and is discussed with that disorder.[489–497,497a] The others had selective abnormalities in platelet-collagen interactions. Platelet GPVI deficiency associated with an autoantibody to GPVI has been described in several patients, one of whom also had systemic lupus erythematosus and another of whom had coexisting antibodies to $\alpha_{IIb}\beta_3$.[498–501] Antibody to GPVI may be detectable in eluates prepared from patient platelets even when it is not detectable in patient plasma.[501] Acquired forms of GPVI-specific signal transduction have also been described in association with myelodysplasia and chronic lymphocytic leukemia.[495] Studies in mice and primates demonstrated that antibodies to GPVI can result in loss of GPVI from the platelet surface through either proteolytic shedding or a cyclic adenosine monophosphate (cAMP)-mediated internalization mechanism, even though the platelets continue to circulate.[494,502] Thus, it is likely that the deficiency of GPVI most commonly results from the presence of autoantibodies.[500] It is unclear whether the patients reported earlier as having GPVI deficiency might also have had an immune basis for their GPVI deficiency. The exception is a patient with a lifelong history of "mild" mucocutaneous, posttraumatic, and post-surgery bleeding with a marked deficiency of platelet membrane GPVI due to both a 16 base out of frame deletion and an S175N missense mutation. The patient's platelets failed to respond to collagen, convulxin, or collagen-related peptide. Of note, FcRγ expression was normal.

ABNORMALITIES OF PLATELET GRANULES

A heterogeneous group of disorders involving platelet granules has been described. They are broadly categorized into defects affecting dense granules (also termed dense bodies; δ-storage pool deficiency), α granules (α-storage pool deficiency, or gray platelet syndrome), or both dense granules and α granules ($\alpha\delta$-storage pool deficiency).

δ-STORAGE POOL DEFICIENCY

Definition and History

Based on the original description of Weiss and associates in 1969,[503] and subsequent studies by other investigators,[504–507] δ-storage pool deficiency is a heterogeneous disorder characterized by a bleeding tendency, abnormalities in the second wave of platelet aggregation, and variable deficiencies of the contents of platelet dense granules.

Etiology and Pathogenesis

δ-Storage pool deficiency can be a primary, inherited platelet disorder or a component of a multisystem (syndromic) disorder, such as the Hermansky-Pudlak syndrome (HPS)[507–512] (variable oculocutaneous albinism, excessive accumulation of ceroid-like material in lysosomes, in monocyte-macrophage cells in marrow and other tissues, variable pulmonary fibrosis and inflammatory bowel disease, and a hemorrhagic diathesis), the Chédiak-Higashi syndrome[513–516] (partial oculocutaneous albinism, giant lysosomal granules, and frequent pyogenic infections), and the Wiskott-Aldrich syndrome (see "Abnormalities of Cytoskeleton Linking Protein" below and Chap. 82). Other diseases are associated with δ-storage pool deficiency (Ehlers-Danlos syndrome, osteogenesis imperfecta, thrombocytopenia with absent radii), but the relationship is less well established.[505] The mode of inheritance is not well defined, but an autosomal dominant pattern for the primary form has been identified in some patients.[517] The inheritance of the forms associated with multisystem disorders follows the autosomal recessive and X-linked patterns characteristic of those disorders.

The etiology of primary human δ-storage pool deficiency is unknown, but based on data from animal models, it is most likely caused by a defect intrinsic to hematopoietic precursors. Studies in patients with the syndromic variants indicate that defects in biogenesis of lysosome-related organelles (which includes melanosomes and dense granules) form the basis of the disorders.[507,518] In δ-storage pool deficiency associated with HPS, there may be a total failure of δ-granule formation as judged by electron microscopy of platelets and megakaryocytes[519] and the absence of CD63 (granulophysin; ME491; lysosome integral membrane protein [LIMP]-1; lysosome-associated membrane protein [LAMP]-3), a lysosomal and dense granule membrane protein of Mr 40,000 that is also found in melanosomes.[507,509,520,521] (A periodically updated review of the clinical findings in HPS is available online at www.ncbi.nlm.nih.gov/bookshelf/br.fcgi?book=gene&part=hps.)

The defect in melanosomes accounts for the oculocutaneous albinism and the defect in membrane trafficking is the probable cause of the accumulation of ceroid lipofuscin, a lipid-protein complex; granulomatous colitis and pulmonary fibrosis (which commonly proves fatal in the fourth to sixth decades) are variably manifest. Abnormalities of eight genes have been implicated in causing eight different subtypes of HPS (Fig. 121–5). Ultrastructural studies in patients with a variety of types of HPS indicate

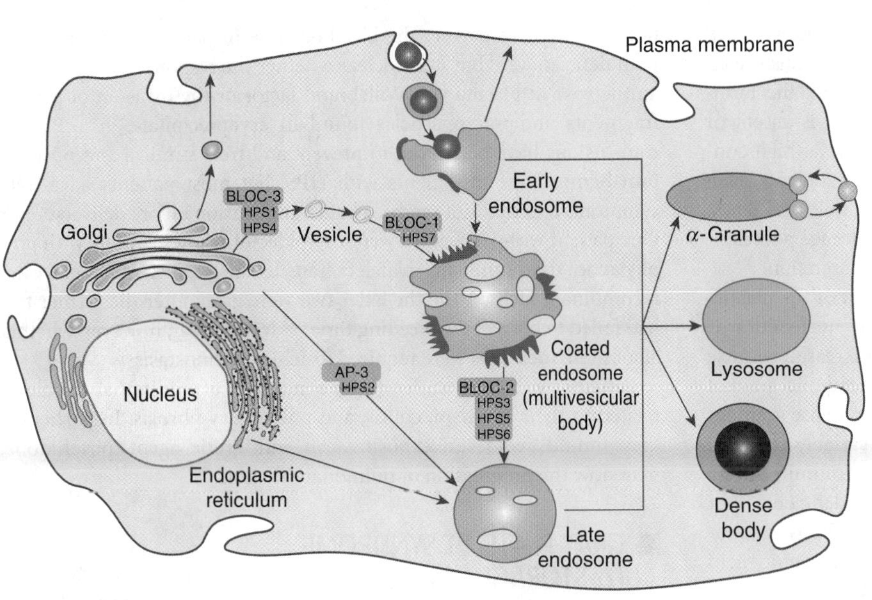

FIGURE 121–5. Hypothetical model of platelet granule formation and location of defects resulting in Hermansky-Pudlak syndrome (HPS). Early endosomes derive from invaginations from the plasma membrane whereas membrane-bound structures from the Golgi and endoplasmic reticulum contribute to the production of coated endosomes and late endosomes. Three multiprotein complexes termed biogenesis of lysosome related organelles complexes (BLOCs) are involved in the transport and interconversion of the different endosomal species. The gene products of HPS-1 and -4 are involved in BLOC-3, whereas those of HPS-3, -5, and -6 are involved in BLOC-2, and those of HPS-7 and HPS-8 contribute to BLOC-1. HPS-2 is caused by mutations in adaptor complex-3 (AP-3). It has not yet been determined which endosomal species contribute to α granules, lysosomes, and dense granules. α Granules are in dynamic exchange with the plasma membrane, selectively taking up fibrinogen via $\alpha_{IIb}\beta_3$ receptors. *(Adapted with permission from Marjan Huizing and William Gahl, National Human Genome Research Institute, National Institutes of Health.)*

that α granules and other organelles (other than dense bodies) are unaffected.[522] The HPS gene products operate in distinct complexes called BLOC (biogenesis of lysosome-related organelles complexes). HPS is unusually common in patients from northwest Puerto Rico, affecting 1 in 1800 individuals; linkage analysis of patients from this area led to the identification of the abnormal gene in these patients (*HPS1*). The gene encodes a 700-amino-acid protein that, along with HPS4, comprises BLOC-3.[509] The mutation in the Puerto Rican kindreds is a 16-bp duplication in exon 15; other mutations of the same gene have been identified in patients from other ethnic groups.[509,523] Mutations in the β3A subunit of the heterotetrameric complex, adaptor protein-3 (AP-3), a group of proteins that facilitates the formation of vesicles of lysosomal lineage from membranes of the *trans*-Golgi network or late endosomes, also have been identified in patients with HPS type 2; HPS-2 patients (eight in the world) have granulocyte colony-stimulating factor-responsive neutropenia and childhood infections.[524,525]

Defects in the *HPS3* gene cause a relatively mild form of HPS and pulmonary involvement is usually minimal.[526] *HPS4* encodes a protein that interacts with the *HPS1* protein in the BLOC-3 complex.[527–530] Patients with mutations in this gene tend to have severe disease, and like patients with defects in *HPS1*, pulmonary involvement is common. The gene products of HPS-5 and *HPS6* interact with the *HPS3* gene product to form BLOC-2,[531,532] As with HPS3 patients, they are spared the complication of pulmonary fibrosis. Improper trafficking of melanocyte-specific proteins, including tyrosinase, was found in the melanosomes of patients with HPS-5.[533] The protein implicated in HPS-7 (*DTNBP1*) is a component of BLOC-1; only a single patient has been reported.[534] Similarly, one family has been reported with mutations in the BLOC-1 protein, HPS8 (BLOS3).[535] A patient with a oculocutaneous albinism type 1, partial δ-storage pool deficiency with aberrant dense granules, recurrent rhabdomyolysis, and a bleeding diathesis but normal known HPS genes has been reported.[536]

In other forms of δ-storage pool disease, data obtained with uranaffin, a dye that specifically stains amine-containing granules, indicate that dense granule membranes are formed but are not properly filled.[505,537,538] The defects in the different substances contained in dense granules are also heterogeneous, with some patients able to secrete significant amounts of calcium and pyrophosphate even when adenine nucleotide secretion is nearly completely absent.[505]

Chédiak-Higashi syndrome results from mutation of the *LYST* gene. The gene encodes a protein of estimated molecular mass of 429 kDa, predicted from domain analysis to participate in vesicle transport and interact with microtubules; an *HPS1*-like region is also present.[539]

The heterogeneity of human δ-storage pool deficiency is matched by a similar heterogeneity among animal models of these disorders. Thus, more than 20 separate inherited mouse defects have been reported to include dense granule deficiencies[507,521,540–544]; of these, pale ear (*ep*) is linked to the mouse equivalent of human HPS-1, pearl (*pe*) to the mouse equivalent of human HPS-2 (mutation in the β3A subunit of AP-3 complex), cocoa is like human HPS-3, light ear (*le*) is like human HPS-4, ruby-eye-2 (*ru2*) is like human HPS-5, ruby-eye (*ru*) is like human HPS-6, sandy (*sdy*) is like human HPS-7, and reduced pigment (rp) is like human HPS-8.[532,541,545,546] Another mouse mutation (the pallid mutation) has been genetically linked to protein 4.2.[540] The beige mouse and rat serve as models for Chédiak-Higashi syndrome.[539,547] Several of these animal disorders are also characterized by abnormalities in lysosomes, pigment, and inner ear function.[540,541]

Clinical Features

Patients with δ-storage pool deficiency as part of the HPS may have severe, or even lethal, hemorrhage.[509,548,549] For all other forms of the disorder, the bleeding tendency is mild to moderate.[505]

Mucocutaneous hemorrhage is most common, with excessive bruising and epistaxis as well as increased bleeding after delivery, tooth extractions, and surgical procedures. The bleeding symptoms can be considerably more severe, however, if patients are taking aspirin or other antiplatelet agents.[504,505] The 15 percent of HPS patients with granulomatous colitis experience gastrointestinal bleeding worse than expected as a consequence of inflammatory bowel disease alone.

Laboratory Features

The bleeding time is usually prolonged, and there may be some correlation between the severity of dense granule deficiency and the bleeding time prolongation[550]; however, patients with δ-storage pool deficiency may have normal bleeding times. In one report, patients with δ-storage pool deficiency had normal aperture closure times (PFA-100) utilizing collagen/ADP and only a minority had prolonged closure times with collagen/epinephrine (PFA-100); the sensitivity was similar to that of the bleeding time.[551] In another report, 13 of 19 patients had abnormal closure times, but the closure times did not correlate with bleeding symptoms.[549]

Platelet aggregation abnormalities are characteristic. ADP and epinephrine induce normal primary waves of aggregation, but the secondary waves are variably abnormal, with the defects ranging from minor to major. The abnormal platelet response is more easily discernible at low collagen concentrations than at high concentrations.[505] Secretion of ATP from platelets can be measured by luminescence simultaneously with platelet aggregation using a specially designed instrument, the lumi-aggregometer.[552,553] ATP release in response to activation is absent or decreased in δ-storage pool deficiency patients. Thrombin at high concentrations causes maximal release of platelet dense body contents, even in patients with secretion abnormalities unrelated to granule deficiency, and, therefore, this reagent may distinguish between δ-storage pool deficiency (diminished release) and abnormalities of platelet secretion.

More sophisticated tests can define further the extent of the platelet abnormality. The total platelet content of adenine nucleotides is reduced, and the ratio of total platelet ATP to ADP is increased because it more closely reflects the ratio in the cytoplasmic, "metabolic" pool of adenine nucleotides (~8:1) than in the "storage" pool in dense granules (~2:3; see Chap. 114).[505,550,554] Platelet serotonin is variably reduced, with the lowest levels found in patients with HPS.[555] Serotonin can be taken up by platelets of patients with δ-storage pool deficiency, but because it cannot be stored in dense granules, it is rapidly catabolized.[555] Abnormalities in platelet secretion and arachidonic acid metabolism have been identified, but are quite variable, and it is not clear whether they result from the aggregation abnormalities.[505,556–558] Reduced levels of plasma and platelet von Willebrand factor activity in association with a decrease in plasma high-molecular-weight multimers and an increase in low-molecular-weight multimers has been reported in HPS.[559,560] Combined δ-storage pool diseases in HPS and reduced von Willebrand factor activity may result in more severe bleeding,[559] but in one study no association between bleeding and von Willebrand factor levels could be identified.[560]

The decrease or absence of platelet dense granules can be confirmed by electron microscopy, using either whole mounts[561,562] or thin sections of platelets fixed in the presence of calcium,[519] although it requires expertise to interpret the results.[563,564] Some patients have abnormal granules.[538,565,566] Uranaffin and osmium may help to identify dense granules.[537,567] The fluorescent amine mepacrine can be used to quantify dense granules by fluorescent microscopy or by flow cytometry.[568,569] Immunoblot analysis of skin fibroblasts in HPS extracts may identify the protein responsible for the defect.[570] Platelet thrombus formation on subendothelial surfaces is decreased in δ-storage pool deficiency, and a hematocrit-related defect in platelet adhesion has also been noted.[124]

Differential Diagnosis

See "Differential Diagnosis" for Glanzmann thrombasthenia above.

Therapy, Course, and Prognosis

The general principles of patient management are similar to those described for Glanzmann thrombasthenia. Patients should be specifically instructed to avoid aspirin and other antiplatelet agents. Short courses of glucocorticoids before surgery may reduce the operative risk,[505,571] but the effectiveness of this therapy is not clear. Although desmopressin did not shorten the bleeding time at all in three patients with δ-storage pool deficiency in the only reported double-blind placebo-controlled trial,[572] it has been reported to shorten or normalize the bleeding time in some patients.[148,573–577] It is possible, however, that it improves hemostasis even though it does not normalize the bleeding. In one patient with HPS, desmopressin did not prevent excessive hemorrhage after one caesarian section, but did prevent excessive hemorrhage after another.[578] Delivery needs to be carefully coordinated in pregnant HPS patients because severe postpartum hemorrhage has been reported both in the bleeding disorder and in the concomitant pulmonary disease, which might affect the choice of anesthesia.[579] Cryoprecipitate has been reported to correct the bleeding time in patients with δ-storage pool deficiency,[580] but it is unclear whether the response was a result of an increase in plasma von Willebrand factor or the infusion of platelet fragments and microparticles found in cryoprecipitate.[581,582] Platelet transfusions have been used to prevent and treat surgical and postpartum hemorrhage in patients with HPS, but most patients have mild symptoms and may not require platelet transfusion before delivery.[578,583] One patient with HPS underwent thyroidectomy uneventfully with prophylactic desmopressin, platelet transfusion, tranexamic acid, and recombinant factor VIIa; the latter two were given after the former two had failed to correct the bleeding time.[584] It is unclear, however, whether all of these measures were required to achieve hemostasis.

Patients with HPS suffer from a number of additional problems related to their albinism, colitis, and pulmonary fibrosis. In particular, they should avoid sun exposure. An antifibrotic agent, pirfenidone, may slow the progression of pulmonary fibrosis.[584]

GRAY PLATELET SYNDROME (α-STORAGE POOL DEFICIENCY)

Definition and History

Raccuglia[585] reported the first patient with gray platelet syndrome, an 11-year-old female with a lifelong bleeding tendency, in 1971. Since then a number of additional patients with isolated abnormalities in platelet α granules have been reported,[491,586–607] including one patient with Goldenhar syndrome,[586] one patient with Marfan syndrome,[598] and one patient with concomitant TREM (triggering receptors express on myeloid cells)-like transcript-1 (TLT-1), P-selectin, and GPVI deficiency.[491,606] The inheritance is not certain, but because many parents are normal and more than one sibling may be affected, at least some cases are probably a result of recessive inheritance.[600,603–605] A Japanese family with 24 affected members has also been reported,[608] but these patients were atypical in having only an approximately 50 percent reduction in platelet factor 4 and only a partial loss of platelet granularity; they also had apparently coincidental reductions in von Willebrand factor.

Etiology and Pathogenesis

Studies using antibodies to the α-granule membrane protein P-selectin (CD62P) and other α-granule membrane proteins indicate that gray platelets contain α-granule membranes, but the membranes form abnormal vesicular structures rather than α granules.[609,610] The P-selectin (CD62P) molecules join the plasma membrane when platelets are stimulated with thrombin, indicating that the membranes are able to fuse with the plasma membrane. Antibodies specific for proteins contained in α granules, such as fibrinogen and von Willebrand factor, identify small and misshapen α granules in gray platelets, further supporting a defect in packaging, as does the observation that the von Willebrand factor lacks high-molecular-weight multimers.[603,611] Plasma levels of the α-granule proteins β-thromboglobulin and platelet factor 4 are normal or increased, indicating that the defect is not in the synthesis of α-granule proteins.[586] One study of the megakaryocytes in patients with the gray platelet syndrome identified von Willebrand factor, platelet-derived growth factor, and platelet factor 4 in early megakaryocytes, but a failure of the proteins to be retained in α granules as the megakaryocytes matured.[362] In another study, megakaryocytes were observed to have increased P-selectin staining, decreased von Willebrand staining, and extensive neutrophil emperipolesis (the passage of blood cells through megakaryocytes), perhaps as a result of neutrophil interactions with P-selectin.[603] It is postulated that the emperipolesis of neutrophils results in megakaryocyte leakage of platelet-derived growth factor from platelet α granules, and this may be responsible for the mild reticulin fibrosis that has been observed in some patients[589,591,599,612,613]; marrow fibrosis is associated with splenomegaly and evidence of extramedullary hematopoiesis.[599,603] The fibrosis does not, however, appear to be progressive. An association with pulmonary fibrosis also is reported,[596] raising the possibility of leakage of growth factors from megakaryocytes in the lung, but this remains speculative. In one family with three affected siblings, neutrophils were gray on blood film and electron microscopy confirmed decreased numbers of secondary granules.[602]

The primary defect responsible for abnormal granule formation has not been identified, but it could involve membrane production, protein targeting, granule formation, proteolysis or protein retention.[606] The evidence for constant recycling of α granules to and from the plasma membrane adds additional loci where defects may result in abnormalities in α granules.[614] An X-linked form of the gray platelet syndrome has been described in association with a *GATA-1* mutation,[615] and giant α granules have been reported in association with mutations in *FLI1* (Paris-Trousseau/Jacobson syndrome). These disorders are discussed in "Transcription Factor Mutations and Associated Platelet Dysfunction" below.

The pathophysiology of the thrombocytopenia is uncertain, but reports of increased marrow megakaryocytes, shortened platelet survival, and elevated levels of plasma glycocalicin (a fragment of GPIbα) relative to the platelet count, suggest that decreased platelet survival and/or ineffective thrombopoiesis contribute.[590,603,616]

Clinical Features

Hemorrhagic manifestations are usually mild in the gray platelet syndrome, but severe bleeding has been noted in a patient with head trauma.[592]

Laboratory Features

Platelets appear as larger-than-normal, pale, ghostlike, oval forms on blood films (Fig. 121–6). Often they can be extremely difficult to identify. Thrombocytopenia is common and can be moderately severe, with the count dropping below 50,000/μL. Platelet aggregation abnormalities are present, but the reported abnormalities vary considerably. ADP- and epinephrine-induced aggregation is normal or nearly normal. Collagen- and thrombin-induced aggregation tend to be more abnormal, but this is an inconsistent finding; concomitant GPVI deficiency has been reported in one patient and if the association is more widespread, it may explain the variable abnormalities in collagen-induced aggregation.[491,593,597,617] The abnormal thrombin-induced aggregation was studied further in one patient; abnormal platelet aggregation in response to thrombin receptor-activating peptide and normal numbers of thrombin PAR-1 receptors were found.[597] Additional abnormalities in phosphoinositide metabolism, protein phosphorylation, calcium mobilization, platelet factor Va, and platelet secretion have been described.[618–620] Thus, it is unclear whether the α-granule protein deficiency, the defects in signal transduction, or both are responsible for the platelet aggregation abnormalities. The failure of α-granule proteins to fully correct the aggregation defects suggests that the signal transduction defects may be significant.[593]

Gray platelets are deficient in α-granule contents, including fibrinogen, von Willebrand factor, thrombospondin, platelet factor 4, β-thromboglobulin, and platelet-derived growth factor; these can be analyzed by immunologic assays or polyacrylamide gel electrophoresis. Platelet IgG and albumin are less severely affected. Electron microscopy confirms a selective absence of α granules, with normal numbers of dense granules.[519,591,611]

Differential Diagnosis

See "Differential Diagnosis" for Glanzmann thrombasthenia above. Degranulated platelets are sometimes observed in myelodysplastic and myeloproliferative disorders, but the clinical setting should provide enough information to establish the diagnosis. Some normal individuals' platelets degranulate *in vitro* when anticoagulated with EDTA and thus can appear gray on smear.[621]

Therapy, Course, and Prognosis

The general measures for treating this disorder are similar to those for Glanzmann thrombasthenia. Desmopressin produces inconsistent correction of the bleeding time,[590,622] but hemostasis after a tooth extraction was acceptable after desmopressin treatment in one patient, even without correction of the bleeding time.[590] Antifibrinolytic therapy may also be beneficial.[592] Platelet transfusions are rarely needed but should be given for serious hemorrhage.

Thrombocytopenia can contribute to the hemostatic defect. Glucocorticoid therapy may or may not increase the platelet count but usually does not result in a normal count.[585,590] The mechanism for this effect is unknown, but it raises the possibility that an immune mechanism may contribute to the thrombocytopenia in some patients. Splenectomy resulted in normalization of the platelet count in two patients soon after the surgery,[585,599] but in one of them the count slowly decreased thereafter.[586]

$\alpha\delta$-STORAGE POOL DEFICIENCY

This rare disorder is characterized by moderate to severe defects in both α and δ granules, with heterogeneous expression in the few patients in whom it has been reported.[505,517] One severely affected patient also had decreased platelet P-selectin (CD62P), a point of distinction from other patients with the disorder and patients with gray platelet syndrome.[623] Clinical and laboratory features are similar to those of δ-storage pool deficiency. In general, the defect in dense granules is more severe than the defect in α granules. Decreased α_2-adrenergic receptors[624] and increased platelet CD36 (GPIV)[625] have been reported in isolated cases, as has an association with hematologic malignancy.[626]

QUEBEC PLATELET DISORDER

Originally described as factor V Quebec, the early description of this autosomal dominant disorder included severe bleeding after trauma, mild thrombocytopenia, decreased functional platelet factor V, and normal plasma factor V.[627–629] The bleeding time is abnormal, as is epinephrine-induced platelet aggregation. Subsequent studies demonstrated that the platelets of these patients had markedly reduced levels of multimerin and thrombospondin (see Chap. 114), and both reduced levels and proteolysis of a number of α-granule proteins, including factor V, fibrinogen, von Willebrand factor, fibronectin, and osteonectin.[630] Platelet factor 4 and β-thromboglobulin, which are also α-granule proteins, did not, however, show evidence of proteolysis. The defect in these patients' platelets appears to be excessive plasmin generation as a result of increased expression of urokinase-type plasminogen activator; increased megakaryocyte expression of the urokinase-type plasminogen activator gene because of an abnormality in a *cis* regulatory element may be the primary abnormality.[631,632] The amount of plasminogen available for conversion to plasmin may affect the severity of the disorder.[633,634] The diagnosis can be established by analysis of platelet urokinase-type plasminogen activator or the identification of degraded α-granule proteins by immunoblot analysis. Treatment with fibrinolytic inhibitors appears to be effective in controlling bleeding, even without factor V replacement therapy.[635] Because the platelet factor V abnormality is prominent, this defect may also be classified as a defect in platelet coagulant activity (see "Abnormalities of Platelet Coagulant Activity (Scott Syndrome)" below).[629]

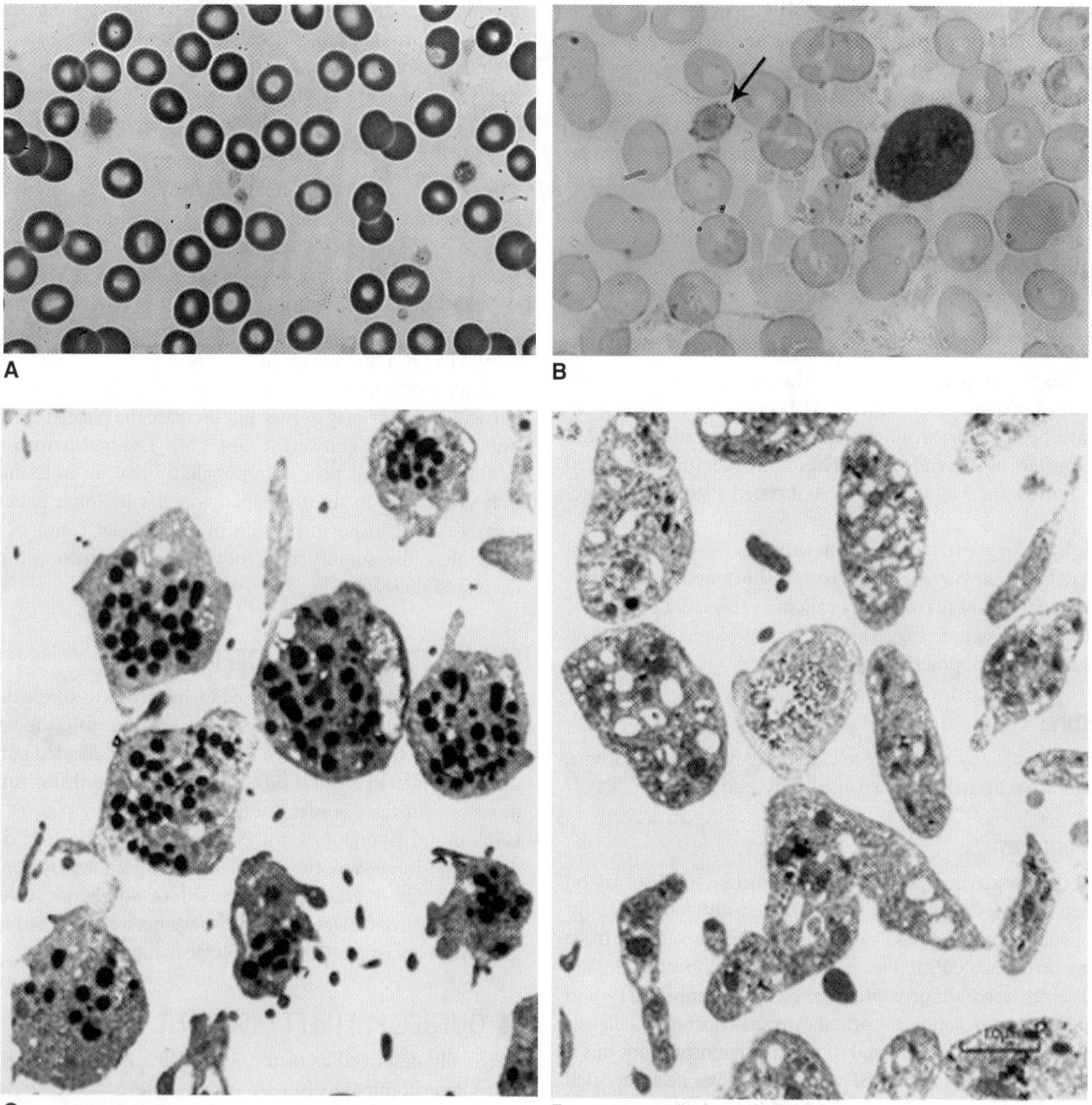

FIGURE 121–6. Gray platelet syndrome (α-granule deficiency). **A.** Blood film. Note gray-staining of many, but not all, platelets with loss of internal granular structure. Two are megathrombocytes, one platelet being very large, almost the size of a red cell (giant platelet). **B.** Blood film. Treated with periodic acid-Schiff (PAS) stain for carbohydrate. Note large "gray platelet" stained with PAS (*arrow*) and typical PAS staining of neutrophil cytoplasm. **C.** Transmission electron microscopy of normal human platelets with abundant electron-dense α granules. **D.** Transmission electron microscopy of platelets from a patient with gray platelet syndrome. Note profound reduction in electron-dense α granules. *(Used with permission from* Lichtman's Atlas of Hematology, *www.accessmedicine.com.)*

ABNORMALITIES OF PLATELET COAGULANT ACTIVITY (SCOTT SYNDROME)

DEFINITION AND HISTORY

Activated platelets play an essential role in providing the membrane surface on which specific blood coagulation reactions occur leading to thrombin generation.[629] Patients whose platelets fail to facilitate thrombin generation are defined as having defects in platelet coagulant activity (PCA; (see Chap. 114). Only a few patients have been described with isolated defects in PCA and normal aggregation and secretion responses.[629,636–643] In general, defects in PCA secondary to abnormalities in platelet aggregation are more common and noted in disorders such as storage pool deficiency and thrombasthenia (see "Abnormalities of Platelet Granules" and "$\alpha_{IIb}\beta_3$ (Glycoprotein IIb/IIIa; CD41/CD61): Glanzmann Thrombasthenia" above).[644] Patients with isolated abnormalities in PCA are referred to as having the Scott syndrome after the first patient described in 1979 by Weiss and associates.[629,636,638–640]

ETIOLOGY AND PATHOGENESIS

The primary functional abnormality in the Scott syndrome is the impaired ability of platelets to promote coagulation reactions, whereas the primary anatomic abnormality is a defect in microvesiculation in response to several different stimuli.[637,645] In resting platelet plasma membranes, phospholipids are asymmetrically distributed, with the aminophospholipids phosphatidylserine (PS) and phosphatidylethanolamine concentrated in the inner membrane leaflet while phosphatidylcholine and sphingomyelin are concentrated in the outer leaflet of the membrane. On cell activation, there is translocation of these lipids, with

PS moving to the outer leaflet. This process is regulated by several membrane proteins that can transport lipid. These include a "flippase" (aminophospholipid translocase), which promotes inward-directed transport of lipids, a "floppase" that regulates outward-directed transport, and a "scramblase" that promotes mixing of the lipids between the two layers.[641] Activation-induced surface expression of PS is essential for platelets to accelerate coagulation, in particular, to enhance the assembly and catalytic activity of the Xase complex leading to the activation of factor X to Xa and of the prothrombinase complex that converts prothrombin to thrombin (see Chap. 115). Platelets in the Scott syndrome have a defect in the translocation of PS to the platelet outer membrane leaflet, which results in decreased binding of factors Va-Xa and VIIIa-IXa[645–648] and impaired blood coagulation. The defects are not confined to platelets, and erythrocytes and lymphocytes demonstrate similar defects in both microvesicle formation and coagulant activity.[641,642,649] Complementation studies using the patient Scott's lymphocytes and a myeloma cell line suggested that the patient's cells lack a functional gene product.[650] Two other patients with sporadic defects in platelet coagulant activity have been described, and in both cases, the most significant abnormality was in collagen plus thrombin-induced prothrombinase activity in the absence of added factor Va. In one of these patients, this may have been because of a defect in α-granule factor V distinct from the abnormality found in the Quebec platelet syndrome (see "Quebec Platelet Syndrome" above).[639] In a French family with Scott syndrome[638] the propositus' platelets were found to have a defect in protein tyrosine phosphorylation, suggesting a defect in signal transduction.[640]

In the few studies reported to date the inheritance pattern in the Scott syndrome seems to be autosomal recessive.[629,638] The specific protein and genetic mechanisms in the Scott syndrome remain to be defined. The phospholipids and scramblase levels have been normal in the patients studied.[651,652] A heterozygous missense mutation was reported in one patient in the gene *ABCA1*, which codes for an ATP-binding cassette transporter protein implicated in PS translocation.[653] This patient was postulated to have an additional defect(s) as the messenger RNA (mRNA) levels of both the mutant and normal allele were reduced.

Apart from the above patients with the Scott syndrome, four patients from three unrelated families have been reported to have abnormal PCA, a bleeding disorder, impaired serum prothrombin consumption, and reduced microparticle formation.[654] However, in contrast to the Scott syndrome, the prothrombinase activity was normal.

CLINICAL FEATURES

Platelet coagulant defects differ from other platelet function disorders in that the hemorrhagic manifestations are not primarily mucocutaneous. For example, the patient Scott [636,637] did not have easy bruising or excessive bleeding after superficial cuts. She did, however, have variably severe bleeding after tooth extractions, menorrhagia, severe postpartum hemorrhage requiring transfusions and hysterectomy, and a spontaneous pelvic hematoma. Bleeding after surgery was present in the two sporadic cases, but epistaxis and easy bruising were only present in one of the two patients.[639] In the French family, the 71-year-old female propositus had epistaxis, trauma-related hematomas, bleeding after tooth extractions, and severe postpartum hemorrhage.[638] Her two older sisters died from hemorrhage during childbirth.

LABORATORY FEATURES

The bleeding time is usually normal.[637–639] The serum prothrombin time, which reflects the completeness of clotting of whole blood as reflected in consumption of prothrombin, is consistently abnormal and serves as a convenient screening assay.[636,638,639] More specific assays of "platelet factor 3," the phenomenologic designation of all of the platelet's contributions to accelerating clot formation, are also abnormal.[644]

Patients with the Scott syndrome have normal platelet aggregation and secretion in response to the usually used agonists. The patient Scott[645,647,648,651,652] also had normal platelet phospholipid content, normal to enhanced platelet adhesion to subendothelium with diminished thrombus formation, severely impaired fibrin formation on subendothelium, diminished factor Va binding to platelets and platelet microparticles, and diminished platelet acceleration of both factor X activation and prothrombin activation. Abnormalities in exposure of negatively charged phospholipids and shedding of microparticles, measured by any one of several techniques, including the binding of annexin V to the surface of platelets and microparticles, have been consistent findings in all of the patients described.[638–642]

DIFFERENTIAL DIAGNOSIS

The normal bleeding time, abnormal serum prothrombin time, and in several of the reported cases, the lack of the characteristic mucocutaneous pattern of bleeding, distinguish platelet coagulant defects from the other qualitative platelet disorders. See "Differential Diagnosis" for Glanzmann thrombasthenia above.

THERAPY, COURSE, AND PROGNOSIS

Platelet or whole blood transfusions have been effective as prophylaxis and as therapy for bleeding episodes.[636–639] Prothrombin complex concentrates, which may contain activated coagulation species that can bypass some of the activation steps, were effective in the patient Scott.[505] These preparations may, however, induce thrombosis and so this needs to be considered seriously in deciding whether to administer them.

ABNORMALITIES OF PLATELET SIGNALING AND SECRETION

A sizable percentage of patients with variably severe mucocutaneous bleeding manifestations, mostly mild, have defects in platelet aggregation and secretion. In most of these patients, the underlying platelet abnormality(ies) is(are) unknown. The most common pattern is blunted platelet aggregation with absence of the second wave of aggregation on exposure to ADP, epinephrine, or collagen, and decreased release of dense granule contents. Such patients have been lumped together, more out of convenience than because of an understanding of the mechanism, under the rubric of primary secretion defects, activation defects, or signal transduction defects.[655,656] Platelet activation is a complex phenomenon involving agonist binding to receptors; signal transduction through G-protein coupled receptors and other types of receptors; phosphoinositol metabolism resulting in calcium mobilization and phosphorylation of target proteins; arachidonic acid metabolism leading to thromboxane A_2 production; activation of the $\alpha_{IIb}\beta_3$ receptor; and release of granule contents (see Chap. 114). Defects involving any of these processes can result in impaired platelet function.[505,657]

DEFECTS IN PLATELET AGONIST RECEPTORS OR AGONIST-SPECIFIC SIGNAL TRANSDUCTION

Thromboxane A_2 Receptor Defect

Platelets contain two different isoforms of the thromboxane A_2 receptor that can activate phospholipase C (PLC), but which differ in their effects on adenylyl cyclase with one stimulating and the other inhibiting this enzyme.[658] A mutation in the thromboxane A_2 receptor (R601L) has been described as causing an inherited bleeding disorder in several unrelated families from Japan.[659,660] In these patients, the abnormal aggregation responses are not restricted to thromboxane A_2 and extend to several agonists, including ADP. The mutation is in the first cytoplasmic loop of the receptor and studies with a recombinant mutated receptor indicate a defect in signal initiation rather than ligand binding. Of note, the mutation appears to inhibit PLC activation of both isoforms and impairs adenylyl cyclase stimulation by one of the isoforms; it does not, however, affect the inhibition of adenylyl cyclase produced by the other isoform. Both dominant and recessive inheritance patterns have been reported; the homozygotes had more severe abnormalities in PLC activation. Nonetheless, the abnormal aggregation responses in heterozygous family members suggest a dominant negative effect of the mutation; the inhibition may be mediated by a mechanism independent of PLC.[660]

ADP Receptor Defects ($P2Y_{12}$, $P2Y_1$, and $P2X_1$)

Multiple receptors ($P2Y_{12}$, $P2Y_1$, and $P2X_1$) mediate ADP interaction with platelets (see Chap. 114).[661,662] $P2Y_1$ receptors induce PLC activation, intracellular Ca^{2+} mobilization, and shape change, whereas $P2Y_{12}$ receptors mediate inhibition of cAMP formation by adenylyl cyclase. ADP-induced platelet aggregation requires activation of both $P2Y_1$ and $P2Y_{12}$ receptors. $P2X_1$ receptors function as an ATP- and ADP-gated cation channels (see Chap. 114). Several patients have been described with $P2Y_{12}$ receptor abnormalities, characterized by blunted ADP-induced platelet aggregation responses, impaired suppression of prostaglandin E_1 (PGE_1)-induced elevations in cAMP, and normal ADP-stimulated shape change.[663–667,667a] Patients symptoms range in severity, with some demonstrating moderately severe hemorrhage in association with surgery and trauma.[668,669] Bleeding time prolongation has been described.[669] Because released ADP potentiates the responses to other agonists, such as collagen and thromboxane A_2, platelet aggregation in response to these agonists are also abnormal in these patients. Platelet binding of ADP or the ADP analogous 2-methylthio-ADP (2MeS-ADP)[663–665,667] was decreased in all but one of these patients.[669] Decreased platelet 2MeS-ADP binding has also been reported in other patients with impaired aggregation and secretion in response to several agonists, including ADP.[670]

The genetic defects have been defined in some of these patients. In several patients, homozygous deletions, or a hemizygous deletion in association with haploinsufficiency,[667a] have been demonstrated in the $P2Y_{12}$ gene, resulting in premature termination and a lack of $P2Y_{12}$ protein.[663,667a,671,672] A homozygous missense mutation in the translation initiation codon was described in another patient,[665] and another patient was reported to have a two nucleotide deletion (at amino acid 240) in one $P2Y_{12}$ gene allele, resulting in a frameshift and a premature stop codon.[664,673] Although this last patient had one $P2Y_{12}$ allele with a normal coding region, the patient's platelets lacked $P2Y_{12}$ receptors, suggesting repression of the normal allele or an unrelated abnormality in its transcriptional regulation. In contrast, platelets from the patient's daughter had an intermediate number of ADP-binding sites, a normal platelet response to ADP, and one frameshifted allele and one normal allele, suggesting that the mutant allele does not act in a dominant negative manner.[664] Studies in yet another patient with abnormal ADP-induced aggregation revealed a compound heterozygous state with one allele containing an R256N substitution, and the other allele containing an R265W substitution.[669] The former mutation was in the sixth transmembrane domain and the latter was in the third extracellular loop of the receptor. Platelet binding of 2MeS-ADP was normal. In expression studies in CHO cells, neither mutation affected the translocation of the $P2Y_{12}$ receptor to the cell surface, but ADP-induced inhibition of adenylyl cyclase was partially reduced, indicating that the mutant receptors were functionally abnormal. In screening 92 patients with type 1 von Willebrand disease, a heterozygous mutation in the second extracellular loop of $P2Y_{12}$ was identified in one patient and several of the family members of this patient.[666] This mutation was associated with decreased 2MeS-ADP binding and modest defects in ADP-induced platelet aggregation. Thus, it is possible that the added platelet defect contributed to the bleeding. Another heterozygous mutation, P258T, in the third extracellular loop has been described in association with a bleeding diathesis.[674]

A defect in the $P2X_1$ purinergic receptor has been described in a 6-year-old patient with a history of petechiae, ecchymoses, and severe epistaxis requiring tranexamic acid treatment and platelet transfusion.[675] The patient had isolated impairment of ADP-induced platelet aggregation and was heterozygous for a deletion of a single leucine in a stretch of 4 leucine residues (351–354) in the second transmembrane domain of $P2X_1$. The mutant protein apparently caused a dominant negative effect on $P2X_1$-mediated calcium channel activity.

A preliminary report of one patient with a defect in the $P2Y_1$ platelet receptor, which is coupled to PLC and mediates ADP induced calcium mobilization (see Chap. 114), described impaired platelet aggregation in response to ADP and other agonists.[676]

Epinephrine Receptor Defects

Abnormalities of α-adrenergic receptors or α-adrenergic–specific signal transduction have been described in several patients,[655,656,677–680] but the relationship to bleeding manifestations remains unclear, particularly because responses to epinephrine are blunted even in some otherwise normal individuals.

Platelet-Activating Factor Receptor Defect

A defect in the platelet-activating factor receptor or platelet-activating factor-specific signal transduction has been reported.[681]

DEFECTS IN GUANOSINE TRIPHOSPHATE-BINDING PROTEINS

Guanosine triphosphate-binding proteins are a heterotrimeric class of proteins (consisting of α, β, and γ subunits) that link surface receptors and intracellular enzymes (see Chap. 114). Abnormalities involving $G\alpha q$, $G\alpha i1$, and $G\alpha s$ subclass proteins have been described in human platelets.

$G\alpha q$ Deficiency

$G\alpha q$ plays a major role in mediating platelet responses to activation of G-protein-coupled receptors. One patient has been described with $G\alpha q$ deficiency in association with a mild bleeding disorder, abnormal platelet aggregation and secretion in response to a number of agonists, and diminished guanosine triphosphatase activity (a reflection of $G\alpha$-subunit dysfunction) in response to platelet activation.[682] The binding of ^{35}S-$GT\gamma S$ to a preparation of the patient's platelet membranes was diminished, and this was associated with a selective decrease in platelet membrane $G\alpha q$, with normal levels of $G\alpha i2$, $G\alpha 12$, $G\alpha 13$, and $G\alpha z$. The downstream events from $G\alpha q$, including Ca^{2+} mobilization, release of arachidonic acid from phospholipids upon platelet activation, and activation of $\alpha_{IIb}\beta_3$ receptors, were impaired. The $G\alpha q$ coding sequence in this patient was normal, but $G\alpha q$ mRNA levels were decreased in platelets, suggesting a potential defect in transcriptional regulation of the gene. This abnormality appeared to be selective for platelets as the patient's neutrophils had normal $G\alpha q$ protein and normal function.[683] Similar impairment in platelet function has been noted in $G\alpha q$-deficient mice.[684]

$G\alpha s$ Hyperfunction and Genetic Variation in Extra Large $G\alpha s$

$G\alpha s$ activation increases platelet cAMP levels and inhibits platelet aggregation and secretion. Two unrelated families have been described with inducible hyperactivity of Gαs.[685] These patients had a bleeding diathesis, prolonged bleeding times, variable mental retardation, and mild skeletal malformations. Platelet aggregation responses to physiologic agonists were normal, but the platelets showed increased sensitivity to inhibition by agents (PGE_1, prostacyclin [PGI_2]) that elevate cAMP levels. The platelet Gαs protein level was increased in these patients. The Gαs gene (*GNAS1*) has multiple alternative promoters and exons, including those associated with extra-large Gαs (XLαs). XLαs is imprinted and thus normally only expressed from the paternal allele. A heterozygous 36-bp insertion and a 2-bp substitution were identified in exon 1 of the paternal XLαs gene in these patients. Because XLαs is not activated by the usual platelet Gαs-coupled receptors, the mechanisms leading to increased cAMP levels and enhanced expression of Gαs protein remains unclear. Of note, 2.2 percent of control subjects also had the same polymorphism, but only those individuals inheriting it from their father had inducible Gαs hyperfunction and increased platelet Gαs protein.

Platelet Gαs deficiency has also been described in a patient with pseudohypoparathyroidism Ib (PHPIb) in association with disturbed imprinting and altered methylation in the *GNAS1* gene cluster that encompasses the four *GNAS1* splice variants, including the Gαs subunit.[686] The Gαs coding sequence was normal. As expected from the deficiency in Gαs protein, there was decreased platelet cAMP formation upon activation of receptors linked to Gαs. The authors did not indicate whether the patient had a bleeding diathesis.

Gαi1 Deficiency

Platelet Gαi1 deficiency has been reported in association with a bleeding disorder and abnormalities in $\alpha_{IIb}\beta_3$ activation, platelet aggregation, and dense granule secretion upon activation with one or more agonists.[687] In keeping with the known function of Gαi inhibiting both the activation of adenylyl cyclase and the subsequent increases in cAMP levels, the patient's platelets did not demonstrate inhibition of forskolin-stimulated cAMP levels on exposure to ADP, thrombin, or epinephrine. In contrast, Gαq-mediated Ca^{2+} mobilization and pleckstrin phosphorylation were normal in response to ADP, thrombin, and collagen. Platelet Gαi1 protein was decreased by 75 percent, whereas other members of the Gαi family (Gαi2, Gαi3, Gαiz) and Gαq were normal. These studies underscore the physiologic role of Gαi1 in human platelet responses.

PLC-β_2 DEFICIENCY AND DEFECTS IN PHOSPHOLIPASE C ACTIVATION

Several investigators have described patients with relatively mild bleeding diatheses and impaired platelet aggregation and dense granule secretion, despite normal granule stores and the ability to synthesize thromboxane A_2.[672,688–690] An early event after stimulating several platelet G-protein-coupled receptors is activation of PLC-β leading to formation of the intracellular mediators IP_3 (inositol 1,4,5-trisphosphate) and diacylglycerol (see Chap. 114); the former is responsible for Ca^{2+} mobilization and the latter for protein kinase C (PKC)-induced protein phosphorylation. Defects in one or more of these responses have been documented in several patients. In one study of eight patients with abnormal platelet aggregation and secretion in response to several different receptor-mediated agonists, Ca^{2+} mobilization and/or pleckstrin phosphorylation was abnormal in seven patients, suggesting that the impaired secretion and aggregation resulted from upstream abnormalities in early signaling events.[690] In fact, specific defects at the level of PLC-β_2,[691,692] Gαq,[682] and PKC-θ[693] were identified in these eight patients. In another study, eight patients were described who had decreased initial rates and extents of platelet aggregation in response to ADP, epinephrine, and U44069[688]; subsequent studies demonstrated impaired phosphatidylinositol hydrolysis, phosphatidic acid formation, and pleckstrin phosphorylation in one patient.[694,695]

In two related patients described with PLC-β_2 deficiency, platelet aggregation and secretion were impaired in association with impaired IP_3 and diacylglycerol formation, calcium mobilization, and pleckstrin phosphorylation following activation with ADP, collagen, platelet-activating factor, or thrombin, indicating a defect in PLC activation.[691] Human platelets contain at least seven PLC isozymes and a selective decrease was observed in only the PLC-β_2 isozyme.[692] The decreased platelet PLC-β_2 protein levels were associated with a normal gene coding sequence but with diminished PLC-β_2 mRNA levels in platelets, but not neutrophils, suggesting a hematopoietic lineage-specific defect in PLC-β_2 gene regulation.[696] Additional studies in this patient documented a 13-bp deletion in the 5 promoter region of PLC-β_2 gene, providing evidence for defective transcriptional regulation.[697] These studies support the importance of PLC-β_2 in hemostasis. Defects in phosphatidylinositol metabolism and protein phosphorylation have been described in other such patients, although the primary protein abnormalities were not defined.[694,695,698–701]

DEFECTS IN PROTEIN PHOSPHORYLATION: PKC-θ DEFICIENCY

PKC isozymes, a family of serine and threonine specific protein kinases, phosphorylate a wide array of proteins involved in signal transduction. PKC enzymes regulate several aspects of platelet function, including activation of $\alpha_{IIb}\beta_3$ receptors, platelet aggregation and secretion, and platelet production (see Chap. 114). Deficiency of a human platelet PKC isozyme (PKC-θ) has been described in a patient with lifelong mucocutaneous bleeding manifestations, mild thrombocytopenia, and markedly abnormal platelet aggregation (including primary wave) and dense granule secretion in response to multiple agonists.[693,702] Agonist-induced phosphorylation of pleckstrin and myosin light chain were diminished in the patient's platelets. This subject had a heterozygous mutation in a transcription factor, core-binding factor A2 (CBFA2, also called *RUNX1* or *AML1*), which has been linked to a familial platelet function defect, thrombocytopenia, and predisposition to acute leukemia (see "Transcription Factor Mutations and Associated Platelet Dysfunction" below).[693,703] Expression profiling of platelets from this patient revealed downregulation of several genes, including myosin light chain (*MYL9*) and 12-lipoxygenase (*ALOX12*),[704] indicating that these genes may be transcriptional targets of *RUNX1*.

DEFECTS IN ARACHIDONIC ACID METABOLISM AND THROMBOXANE PRODUCTION

Defects in Arachidonic Acid Release from Phospholipids and Phospholipase A_2 Deficiency

Release of free arachidonic acid from phospholipids, mediated by phospholipase A_2, (PLA_2) is the initial and rate-limiting step in thromboxane synthesis upon platelet activation (see Fig. 114–11). Several patients have been described with abnormalities in the release of arachidonic acid.[698,705–707] Their platelets aggregated normally in response to arachidonic acid but not to ADP, epinephrine, and/or collagen. In one of these patients, this defect was related to an upstream abnormality in Gαq (see "Defects in Guanosine Triphosphate-Binding Proteins" above).[682] Another patient had the HPS with δ-storage pool deficiency and abnormal PLA_2 activity.[705] An inherited deficiency in cytosolic PLA_2, the principal enzyme that regulates the release of arachidonic acid, has been reported in a patient with recurrent small intestinal ulceration, markedly decreased eicosanoid synthesis (including in thromboxane, 12-hydroxyeicosatetraenoic acid, and leukotriene B_4) and platelet dysfunction (see Fig. 114–11).[707] This patient had two heterozygous single-base-pair mutations in the PLA_2 coding region, leading to S111P and R485H substitutions.

Cyclooxygenase (Prostaglandin H_2 Synthase-1) Deficiency

Deficient platelet cyclooxygenase (prostaglandin H_2 synthase-1) activity leading to impaired platelet function has been identified in a number of patients.[708–715] Platelets from such patients cannot make thromboxane from arachidonic acid but can make it from cyclic endoperoxides. If cyclooxygenase activity is also deficient in endothelial cells, prostacyclin production will also be impaired. The clinical manifestations of patients with cyclooxygenase deficiency are, therefore, of interest, as they presumably reflect the competing influences of thromboxane A_2 and prostacyclin. One patient with both platelet and vessel-wall deficiency had a mild bleeding disorder.[710] Although some patients have had decreased platelet cyclooxygenase protein, others have had evidence of a dysfunctional molecule.[714,715]

Thromboxane Synthase Deficiency

Presumed platelet thromboxane synthase deficiencies have been identified in two families based on the failure of cyclic endoperoxides to be converted into thromboxane A_2.[716,717] An otherwise mild bleeding disorder associated with one life-threatening hemorrhage and a variably prolonged bleeding time was found in one patient.[717]

ABNORMALITIES OF A CYTOSKELETAL STRUCTURAL PROTEIN: β_1-TUBULIN

Megakaryocytes and platelets express primarily and selectively the β_1 isoform of tubulin. Mice deficient in β_1-tubulin have moderate thrombocytopenia and abnormally spherocytic platelets (see Chap. 114). In 2005, a heterozygous β_1-tubulin Q43P polymorphism was identified in a group of patients with a recessive form of macrothrombocytopenia; the polymorphism could not account fully for the macrothrombocytopenia because of the difference in inheritance and its presence in approximately 11 percent of the normal population.[718] Individuals heterozygous for the polymorphism had normal platelet counts, relatively high mean platelet volume values, abnormally rounded platelets with abnormal marginal bands of microtubules, and mild abnormalities of platelet aggregation, secretion, and adhesion to collagen. In one study, the Q43P polymorphism was associated with decreased risk of cardiovascular disease in men,[718] but in another, there was no association with myocardial infarction.[719] One study found the polymorphism associated with decreased collagen-induced platelet aggregation and increased risk of intracerebral hemorrhage in men.[720]

Subsequently, two patients with macrothrombocytopenia from a single kindred were reported to be heterozygous for a R318W β_1-tubulin mutation.[721] The mutation is strategically located at the α–β tubulin interface. Of note, the Q43P polymorphism and an R207H substitution were also found in this family, but neither was judged to be responsible for the macrothrombocytopenia.

ABNORMALITIES OF CYTOSKELETAL LINKING PROTEINS

WISKOTT-ALDRICH SYNDROME PROTEIN

Definition and History

The Wiskott-Aldrich syndrome, which affects 4 of every 1 million males worldwide, is an X chromosome-linked inherited disorder characterized by small platelets, thrombocytopenia, recurrent infections, and eczema, although only a minority of patients have all of the classic manifestations.[722–724] In addition, a variety of immunologic abnormalities affecting T-lymphocyte function, immunoglobulin levels, cellular immunity, and responsiveness to polysaccharide antigens are commonly present.[725,726] The immune defects are probably responsible for an increase in autoimmune phenomena and lymphoreticular malignancies associated with the disorder. Death from infection, hemorrhage, or malignancy is common before adulthood.

Etiology and Pathogenesis

The Wiskott-Aldrich syndrome protein (WASP) has been cloned and its amino acid sequence deduced from the complementary DNA. The protein contains a unique Wiskott homology domain, which is also present in a number of other genes that convey signals from the surface of cells to the actin cytoskeleton. A number of other domains interact with a large number of other proteins.[725,727] WASP is found in all hematopoietic stem cell-derived lineages. It is likely that signals from G-protein-coupled receptors can initiate actin bundling via WASP. Most, but not all patients with Wiskott-Aldrich syndrome have mutations in the WASP protein[723] and so other genes may be involved. Moreover, some patients with X-linked thrombocytopenia without the other associated features of Wiskott-Aldrich syndrome have been found to have mutations in WASP.[728] Of note, an apparently X-linked severe congenital neutropenia was found in a family with a constitutively activating mutation in WASP.[729] An international database of WASP mutations[730] was compiled through 2004 and can be accessed at http://homepage.mac.com/kohsukeimai/wasp/WASPbase.html.

A defect in the surface glycoprotein sialophorin (CD43, gp115, leukosialin) has also been described in Wiskott-Aldrich syndrome,[731] but its significance is uncertain. Deficiencies in platelet GPIb have also been described in some patients with the Wiskott-Aldrich syndrome,[731,732] but this is not an invariant finding.[733,734] Deficiencies in platelet integrin α_2 have also been recorded in some, but not all, patients.[731] Similarly, decreases in platelet $\alpha_{IIb}\beta_3$ and GPIV have been reported based on flow cytometry studies even after normalizing for platelet size.[734]

The mechanism(s) underlying the thrombocytopenia and small platelet size in Wiskott-Aldrich syndrome remains uncertain despite extensive investigation. Inconsistent data have been reported on shortened platelet survival, and in those studies in which shortened survival has been observed, it is unclear whether the defect was selective for patient platelets compared to normal platelets.[735–739] Marrow megakaryocyte numbers have been reported to be normal in most, but not all patients[735,738,740,741]; similarly, *ex vivo* defects in megakaryopoiesis and/or proplatelet formation have been described in some, but not all, studies.[742–745] Moreover, both decreased and increased levels of immature platelets (thiazole orange-positive; "reticulated") have been reported in Wiskott-Aldrich patients.[734,746] Splenectomy consistently improves the platelet count,[747,748] but recurrent severe thrombocytopenia and hemorrhage can occur, often on an autoimmune basis.[725,741,749]

A specific connection between Wiskott-Aldrich syndrome and immune thrombocytopenia has been proposed and an increase in other autoimmune diseases is found in Wiskott-Aldrich syndrome.[750] Thus, immune mechanisms may contribute to the thrombocytopenia in some patients[734,738,751–753] and the patients' other abnormalities in platelet production and removal may make them particularly susceptible to even low-level immune-mediated premature removal.[750] Moreover, based on data from the murine model, opsonized Wiskott-Aldrich platelets may be especially susceptible to clearance because of increased *ex vivo* phagocytosis.[754] This observation has also been proposed to explain why intravenous immunoglobulin G usually fails to increase the platelet count in patients with Wiskott-Aldrich syndrome, as the abnormality(ies) leading to enhanced phagocytosis may limit the effectiveness of intravenous immunoglobulin G. It is also possible that enhanced phagocytosis of Wiskott-Aldrich platelets contributes to the development of immune thrombocytopenia.[750]

The cause of the small size of the platelets is unknown. Although it is likely related in part to an abnormality in the connection between the membrane and the cytoskeleton caused by the defect in the WASP, it is less clear whether this becomes manifest before and/or after platelets enter the circulation. Intrinsic cytoskeletal defects in Wiskott-Aldrich platelets may also result in a greater propensity to develop microparticles, which may contribute to both the small size and the documented increase in plasma microparticles.[755]

Variant forms of Wiskott-Aldrich syndrome characterized by thrombocytopenia and X chromosome-linked inheritance (XLT) have been reported,[728,756] some of which are associated with mutations of WASP.[728,740,757] The WASP mutations in XLT are primarily in the N-terminal region of the molecule, which is the region that links WASP to $\alpha_{IIb}\beta_3$ via calcium and integrin binding protein.[757] Platelets from patients with XLT have been reported to have reduced adhesion to fibrinogen and have a defect in $\alpha_{IIb}\beta_3$ activation.[757]

Platelets from most patients with Wiskott-Aldrich syndrome have qualitative as well as quantitative abnormalities. Most common is a deficiency in the storage pool of adenine nucleotides, producing a reduced positive feedback mechanism during platelet activation and aggregation.[735,737,756] Abnormalities in platelet energy metabolism have also been described.[737,758]

Platelet aggregation in Wiskott-Aldrich syndrome has been reported to be reduced, normal, or enhanced.[755,757,759,760] These studies are confounded by the low platelet count. Despite the role of the WASP protein in cytoskeletal reorganization, shape change and actin polymerization are normal in Wiskott-Aldrich platelets.[760–762] Similarly, although WASP undergoes tyrosine phosphorylation in response to collagen and collagen-related peptide, aggregation in response to the latter has been reported to be normal.[760,763] Although it is not possible to reconcile all of the reported findings, the subcellular localization of WASP and its association with $\alpha_{IIb}\beta_3$ may be functionally important. Thus, although in nucleated cells WASP is predominantly a cytosolic protein that becomes activated when it is recruited to the membrane, in platelets, approximately 25 percent of WASP in unactivated platelets is associated with the membrane skeleton. WASP undergoes transient phosphorylation, redistribution, and cleavage by calpain (or a similar enzyme) with platelet activation; all of these changes require $\alpha_{IIb}\beta_3$ outside-in signaling. WASP has been shown to bind to calcium and integrin binding protein when platelets are activated, and the latter protein is known to bind the cytoplasmic domain of α_{IIb}. Inhibiting the interaction between WASP and calcium and integrin binding protein inhibits inside-out signaling of $\alpha_{IIb}\beta_3$ and fibrinogen binding. Because cytoskeletal traction has been implicated in activation of $\alpha_{IIb}\beta_3$,[65] the loss of WASP binding to α_{IIb} via calcium and integrin binding protein may contribute to the reduced ability to activate $\alpha_{IIb}\beta_3$.

Clinical Features

Hemorrhage, recurrent infections, eczema, and lymphoreticular malignancies dominate the clinical picture. Autoimmune diseases, including arthritis, vasculitis, autoimmune hemolytic anemia, and immune thrombocytopenia, may complicate the disorders.[749] There is enormous variability in disease severity, and this even extends to variability within individual kindreds.[725] Correlations between WASP gene mutations and clinical manifestations are inexact, but patients whose cells express full-length protein may have better immunologic function.[725,730]

Laboratory Features

The platelet count is variably reduced, with 44 percent of patients in a large study having platelet counts ≤20,000/μL at the time of diagnosis, and the platelet volume is significantly reduced in nearly all patients.[722,741] Lymphopenia and eosinophilia are present in a minority of patients. The bleeding time is usually prolonged to a greater extent than would be expected from the platelet count, but when the reduced platelet mass is considered, the bleeding time prolongation may not be inappropriate. Platelet aggregation and release of dense body contents are variably abnormal. Platelet ultrastructural abnormalities have been reported, but on balance it appears that platelet morphology is essentially normal.[519]

Results of immunologic evaluations vary significantly, but some patients have decreased numbers of CD8+ T cells.[722] Serum levels of IgG are usually normal, whereas serum levels of IgM are usually depressed and serum levels of IgA and IgE are usually elevated.[741] Variable deficiencies in immune response to antigenic challenge, especially polysaccharide antigens, are common.[741]

Flow cytometry may be used to assess quantitative abnormalities of WASP in blood mononuclear cells and may be useful in carrier detection under certain circumstances.[764,765] X-inactivation in some carriers of Wiskott-Aldrich syndrome is nonrandom, however, and thus caution is required in interpreting such studies.[766]

Therapy, Course, and Prognosis

Splenectomy usually, but not invariably, improves the thrombocytopenia and usually partially corrects the defect in platelet size, at least temporarily.[722,747,748] It may also improve platelet function. Thus, splenectomy should be considered in patients with excessive hemorrhage. Opportunistic infections present serious problems.[725,741,747] There is an increased risk of overwhelming bacterial sepsis after splenectomy, but this can be reduced by the use of pneumococcal, meningococcal, and *Haemophilus influenzae* vaccines, as well as prophylactic antibiotics and intravenous immunoglobulin. Patients with Wiskott-Aldrich syndrome tend to have hypercatabolism of IgG and thus may require both a higher dose and more frequent dosing of IgG.[741] If platelet transfusion is required to stop hemorrhage, the platelets should be irradiated to prevent transfusion-related graft-versus-host disease. It is preferable to obtain platelets from donors who are free of cytomegalovirus.

Hematopoietic reconstitution with stem cells from blood, cord blood or marrow can cure the disorder.[725,748] Because the prognosis is otherwise very poor, intervening before the onset of significant immunodeficiency has been recommended when a histocompatible donor is available.[725,748] Transplantation from matched unrelated donors can be successful in young patients, but the success rate declines after 5 to 6 years of age.[741]

KINDLIN-3 (LEUKOCYTE ADHESION DEFECT-III; LAD-1 VARIANT; INTEGRIN ACTIVATION DEFICIENCY DISEASE)

Definition and History/Etiology and Pathogenesis

A syndrome with the features of both mild leukocyte adhesion deficiency type 1 and Glanzmann thrombasthenia was first described in 1997[767] and termed leukocyte adhesion deficiency (LAD)-1 variant or LAD-III. Since then, more than 10 families have been reported, with several from Turkey.[768–771] The etiology is a deficiency or defect in the cytoskeletal linking protein kindlin-3 (*FERMTS3*). Kindlin3 is a protein expressed exclusively in hematopoietic cells with homology to talin that also binds to the cytoplasmic domain of the integrin β_3 subunit of the $\alpha_{IIb}\beta_3$ receptor (see Chap. 114). It has been implicated in the inside-out activation of $\alpha_{IIb}\beta_3$ in mice.[772] It also participates in the function of leukocyte integrins, which accounts for the defects in immunity. It may also affect red blood cell structure. Defects in *CALDAGGEF1*, an exchange factor important in integrin activation, have also been reported to cause LAD-III, but it is unclear if these are disease causing.[768,773]

Clinical Features

The disorder is characterized by a variable predisposition to infections and inflammation without pus formation, poor wound healing, delayed umbilical cord stump detachment, and variable osteopetrosis. Intracerebral hemorrhage at birth or soon thereafter has been reported in several of the patients, as well as relatively severe mucosal and gastrointestinal bleeding. Thus, the bleeding diathesis is more severe than is found in patients with Glanzmann thrombasthenia. The need for red blood cell transfusions in infancy has been reported in several patients because of blood loss from mucosal surfaces and perhaps red blood cell abnormalities.

Laboratory Features

Leukocytosis, as is found in other LAD syndromes, is a constant finding. Normal platelet counts are the usual finding, but thrombocytopenia has been reported. Platelet aggregation studies demonstrate defects similar to those observed in Glanzmann thrombasthenia.

Therapy, Course, and Prognosis

Hematopoietic stem cell transplantation has been successful in restoring normal hematopoietic function in patients with life threatening hemorrhagic and infectious complications of the disease.

TRANSCRIPTION FACTOR MUTATIONS AND ASSOCIATED PLATELET DYSFUNCTION

Transcription factors regulate the expression of proteins in platelets and megakaryocytes and play an important role in megakaryopoiesis and platelet production. Several reports have demonstrated impaired platelet function in patients with mutations in specific transcription factors, and these have been associated with congenital thrombocytopenia.

■ *RUNX1* (FAMILIAL PLATELET DISORDER WITH PREDISPOSITION TO ACUTE MYELOGENOUS LEUKEMIA)

An association between inherited platelet abnormalities and a predisposition to acute myelogenous leukemia has been reported in several different families in which the thrombocytopenia and abnormal platelet aggregation responses antedated the leukemia and were linked to inherited mutations or a deletion in the gene *RUNX1* (*AML1, CBFA2*).[693,774–785] This gene is involved in the sporadic mutations and the t(8;21), t(3;21), and t(12;21) translocations found in more than 10 percent of patients with acute myelogenous leukemia.[775,786,787] The platelet defect and the predisposition to leukemia with *RUNX1* mutations is inherited as an autosomal dominant trait and individuals generally have mild thrombocytopenia from birth and a bleeding disorder that is disproportionate to the degree of thrombocytopenia. Prior to developing the leukemia, the marrow may be normal or demonstrate mild morphologic abnormalities in megakaryocytes or changes consistent with myelodysplasia. The overall frequency of leukemia is 35 percent with a median age of onset of 33 years.[785] In a study of 10 families with a history of more than one first-degree relative with myeloid dysplasia and/or acute myeloid leukemia, germ-line *RUNX1* mutations were identified in 5 families.[785] Of note, some of the individuals harboring the mutations had normal platelet counts and function. The authors also reported relatively poor outcomes from hematopoietic stem cell transplantation from family members, and suggested screening potential family donors for the mutation.

Most of the mutations of *RUNX1* affected the Runt domain.[781,784] An exception, involving the transactivating domain (Y260X), was identified in a family with only very mild thrombocytopenia and defects in platelet α granules and α_2-adrenergic receptors in addition to defects in dense granules.[781] A partial α-granule abnormality was identified in another patient with this syndrome.[774] Another patient with a splice-site mutation leading to a frameshift and premature termination in the Runt domain was found to have abnormal $\alpha_{IIb}\beta_3$ activation, decreased platelet myosin light chain and pleckstrin phosphorylation, and a selective decrease in platelet protein kinase C-θ; the patient also had diminished PF4, platelet albumin, and IgG, suggesting an α granule abnormality, but normal levels of the α-granule proteins fibrinogen and β-thromboglobulin.[693,702] It is possible that this disorder more generally affects both dense granules and α granules. Expression profiling of platelets from this last patient revealed downregulation of several genes, including *MYL9* (myosin light chain), *ALOX12* (12-lipoxygenase), and *PF4* (platelet factor 4), suggesting that these genes may be regulated by *RUNX1*.[704] *ALOX12*, *PKC-θ*, and *MYL9* have been shown to be direct transcriptional targets of *RUNX1*.[788–790] Patients with *RUNX1* haplodeficiency have been shown to have impaired megakaryopoiesis[782] and decreased platelet thrombopoietin receptors (Mpl).[791]

GATA-1

GATA-1 is a major transcription factor that regulates both erythropoiesis and megakaryopoiesis. *GATA-1* mutations have been associated with an X-linked syndrome consisting of dyserythropoiesis, anemia, thrombocytopenia, and large platelets[792]; selectively impaired responses to collagen and ristocetin related to abnormalities in GPIbβ;[793,794] diminished levels of platelet Gαs protein and mRNA[793]; and a form of gray platelet syndrome (R216N).[615] Some of the *GATA-1* mutations affect the site at which the transcription factor interacts with another megakaryocytic cotranscription factor, friend of GATA (FOG).

■ *FLI1* (DIMORPHIC DYSMORPHIC PLATELETS WITH GIANT α-GRANULES AND THROMBOCYTOPENIA [PARIS-TROUSSEAU/JACOBSEN SYNDROME])

The Paris-Trousseau syndrome, a variant of Jacobsen syndrome, is a rare autosomal dominant disorder[795–798] characterized by mental retardation, congenital thrombocytopenia, giant α granules in a subpopulation of circulating platelets, and marrow dysmegakaryopoiesis in association with deletion of the distal part of either the maternally or paternally derived chromosome 11 (11q23.3–24). Although platelet survival is normal, there is dramatic expansion of marrow megakaryocytes as a result of an arrest in megakaryocyte development. Among the genes deleted is the transcription factor *FLI1*, which plays an important role in megakaryocyte development. Remarkably, during a period in early megakaryocyte development, only one of the two *FLI1* alleles appears to be expressed in any single megakaryocyte precursor, thus accounting for both the inheritance pattern and the dimorphic platelet population in which there are both normal platelets and platelets that have dysmorphic giant α granules.[797,798] It also can explain the expansion of dysmorphic megakaryocytes in the marrow. It is not clear, however, whether this gene defect is also responsible for the abnormalities in α granules and mental function.

REFERENCES

1. Nurden P, Nurden AT: Congenital disorders associated with platelet dysfunctions. *Thromb Haemost* 99:253, 2008.

2. Nurden AT: Glanzmann thrombasthenia. *Orphanet J Rare Dis* 1:10, 2006.
3. Simon D, Kunicki T, Nugent D: Platelet function defects. *Haemophilia* 14:1240, 2008.
4. Salles II, Feys HB, Iserbyt BF, et al: Inherited traits affecting platelet function. *Blood Rev* 22:155, 2008.
5. Glanzmann E: Hereditäre hämmorhagische Thrombasthenie. *Ein Beitrag zur Pathologie der Blutplättchen Jahrbuch fur Kinderheilkunde und physiche Erziehung* 88:113, 1918.
6. Caen JP, Castaldi PA, Leclerc JC, et al: Congenital bleeding disorders with long bleeding time and normal platelet count. I. Glanzmann's thrombasthenia. *Am J Med* 41:4, 1966.
7. Hardisty RM, Dormandy KM, Hutton RA: Thrombasthenia: Studies on three cases. *Br J Haematol* 10:371, 1964.
8. Zucker MB, Pert JH, Hilgartner MW: Platelet function in a patient with thrombasthenia. *Blood* 28:524, 1966.
9. Weiss HJ, Kochwa S: Studies of platelet function and proteins in 3 patients with Glanzmann's thrombasthenia. *J Lab Clin Med* 71:153, 1968.
10. George JN, Caen JP, Nurden AT: Glanzmann's thrombasthenia: The spectrum of clinical disease. *Blood* 75:1383, 1990.
11. Nurden AT, Caen JP: An abnormal platelet glycoprotein pattern in three cases of Glanzmann's thrombasthenia. *Br J Haematol* 28:253, 1974.
12. Phillips DR, Jenkins CS, Luscher EF, et al: Molecular differences of exposed surface proteins on thrombasthenic platelet plasma membranes. *Nature* 257:599, 1975.
13. Peerschke EI: The platelet fibrinogen receptor. *Semin Hematol* 22:241, 1985.
14. Bennett JS: The platelet-fibrinogen interaction, in *Platelet Membrane Glycoproteins*, edited by JN George, AT Nurden, DR Phillips, p 193. Plenum, New York, 1985.
15. Phillips DR, Charo IF, Parise LV, et al: The platelet membrane glycoprotein IIb-IIIa complex. *Blood* 71:831, 1988.
16. Plow EF, Ginsberg MH: Cellular adhesion: GPIIb-IIIa as a prototypic adhesion receptor. *Prog Hemost Thromb* 9:117, 1989.
17. Poncz M, Eisman R, Heidenreich R, et al: Structure of the platelet membrane glycoprotein IIb. Homology to the alpha subunits of the vitronectin and fibronectin membrane receptors. *J Biol Chem* 262:8476, 1987.
18. Fitzgerald LA, Steiner B, Rall SC Jr, et al: Protein sequence of endothelial glycoprotein IIIa derived from a cDNA clone. Identity with platelet glycoprotein IIIa and similarity to "integrin." *J Biol Chem* 262:3936, 1987.
19. Hynes RO: Integrins: Bidirectional, allosteric signaling machines. *Cell* 110:673, 2002.
20. D'Andrea G, Colaizzo D, Vecchione G, et al: Glanzmann's thrombasthenia: Identification of 19 new mutations in 30 patients. *Thromb Haemost* 87:1034, 2002.
21. Seligsohn U, Peretz H, Newman PJ, et al: Glanzmann thrombasthenia in Israel: Clinical, biochemical and molecular genetic characterization, in *Genetic Diversity Among Jews*, edited by B Bonné-Tamir, A Adam, p 275. Oxford University Press, New York, 1992.
22. Reichert N, Seligsohn U, Ramot B: Clinical and genetic studies of Glanzmann's thrombasthenia in Israel. *Thromb Diath Haemorrh* 34:806, 1975.
23. Awidi AS: Increased incidence of Glanzmann's thrombasthenia in Jordan as compared with Scandinavia. *Scand J Haematol* 30:218, 1983.
24. Khanduri U, Pulimood R, Sudarsanam A, et al: Glanzmann's thrombasthenia. A review and report of 42 cases from South India. *Thromb Haemost* 46:717, 1981.
25. Ahmed MA, Al Sohaibani MO, Al Mohaya SA, et al: Inherited bleeding disorders in the Eastern Province of Saudi Arabia. *Acta Haematol* 79:202, 1988.
26. Awidi AS: Rare inherited bleeding disorders secondary to coagulation factors in Jordan: A nine-year study. *Acta Haematol* 88:11, 1992.
27. Rosenberg N, Yatuv R, Orion Y, et al: Glanzmann thrombasthenia caused by an 11.2-kb deletion in the glycoprotein IIIa (beta3) is a second mutation in Iraqi Jews that stemmed from a distinct founder. *Blood* 89:3654, 1997.
28. Handagama PJ, Shuman MA, Bainton DF: Incorporation of intravenously injected albumin, immunoglobulin G, and fibrinogen in guinea pig megakaryocyte granules. *J Clin Invest* 84:73, 1989.
29. Harrison P, Wilbourn BR, Debili N, et al: Uptake of plasma fibrinogen into the alpha granules of human megakaryocytes and platelets. *J Clin Invest* 84:1320, 1989.
30. Handagama P, Rappolee DA, Werb Z, et al: Platelet alpha-granule fibrinogen, albumin, and immunoglobulin G are not synthesized by rat and mouse megakaryocytes. *J Clin Invest* 86:1364, 1990.
31. Harrison P: Platelet α-granular fibrinogen. *Platelets* 3:1, 1992.
32. Coller BS, Seligsohn U, West SM, et al: Platelet fibrinogen and vitronectin in Glanzmann thrombasthenia: Evidence consistent with specific roles for glycoprotein IIb/IIIA and $\alpha V\beta 3$ integrins in platelet protein trafficking. *Blood* 78:2603, 1991.
33. Disdier M, Legrand C, Bouillot C, et al: Quantitation of platelet fibrinogen and thrombospondin in Glanzmann's thrombasthenia by electroimmunoassay. *Thromb Res* 53:521, 1989.
34. Degos L, Dautigny A, Brouet JC, et al: A molecular defect in thrombasthenic platelets. *J Clin Invest* 56:236, 1975.
35. Cohen I, Gerrard JM, White JG: Ultrastructure of clots during isometric contraction. *J Cell Biol* 91:775, 1982.
36. Gartner TK, Ogilvie ML: Peptides and monoclonal antibodies which bind to platelet glycoproteins IIb and/or IIIa inhibit clot retraction. *Thromb Res* 49:43, 1988.
37. Duperray A, Troesch A, Berthier R, et al: Biosynthesis and assembly of platelet GPIIb-IIIa in human megakaryocytes: Evidence that assembly between pro-GPIIb and GPIIIa is a prerequisite for expression of the complex on the cell surface. *Blood* 74:1603, 1989.
38. Bodary SC, Napier MA, McLean JW: Expression of recombinant platelet glycoprotein IIbIIIa results in a functional fibrinogen-binding complex. *J Biol Chem* 264:18859, 1989.
39. O'Toole TE, Loftus JC, Plow EF, et al: Efficient surface expression of platelet GPIIb-IIIa requires both subunits. *Blood* 74:14, 1989.
40. Kolodziej MA, Vilaire G, Gonder D, et al: Study of the endoproteolytic cleavage of platelet glycoprotein IIb using oligonucleotide-mediated mutagenesis. *J Biol Chem* 266:23499, 1991.
41. Bennett JS: The molecular biology of platelet membrane proteins. *Semin Hematol* 27:186, 1990.
42. Kieffer N, Phillips DR: Platelet membrane glycoproteins: Functions in cellular interactions. *Annu Rev Cell Biol* 6:329, 1990.
43. Seligsohn U, Coller BS, Zivelin A, et al: Immunoblot analysis of platelet GPIIb in patients with Glanzmann thrombasthenia in Israel. *Br J Haematol* 72:415, 1989.
44. Mitchell WB, Li J, French DL, et al: AlphaIIbbeta3 biogenesis is controlled by engagement of alphaIIb in the calnexin cycle via the N15-linked glycan. *Blood* 107:2713, 2006.
45. Mitchell WB, Li J, Murcia M, et al: Mapping early conformational changes in alphaIIb and beta3 during biogenesis reveals a potential mechanism for alphaIIbbeta3 adopting its bent conformation. *Blood* 109:3725, 2007.
46. Zimrin AB, Eisman R, Vilaire G, et al: Structure of platelet glycoprotein IIIa. A common subunit for two different membrane receptors. *J Clin Invest* 81:1470, 1988.
47. Cheresh DA: Human endothelial cells synthesize and express an Arg-Gly-Asp-directed adhesion receptor involved in attachment to fibrinogen and von Willebrand factor. *Proc Natl Acad Sci U S A* 84:6471, 1987.
48. Smith JW, Cheresh DA: The Arg-Gly-Asp binding domain of the vitronectin receptor. *J Biol Chem* 263:18726, 1988.
49. Cheresh DA, Berliner SA, Vicente V, et al: Recognition of distinct adhesive sites on fibrinogen by related integrins on platelets and endothelial cells. *Cell* 58:945, 1989.
50. Lawler J, Hynes RO: An integrin receptor on normal and thrombasthenic platelets which binds thrombospondin. *Blood* 74:2022, 1989.
51. Yokoyama K, Zhang XP, Medved L, et al: Specific binding of integrin alpha v beta 3 to the fibrinogen gamma and alpha E chain C-terminal domains. *Biochemistry* 38:5872, 1999.
52. Lam SC, Plow EF, D'Souza SE, et al: Isolation and characterization of a platelet membrane protein related to the vitronectin receptor. *J Biol Chem* 264:3742, 1989.
53. Coller BS, Cheresh DA, Asch E, et al: Platelet vitronectin receptor expression differentiates Iraqi-Jewish from Arab Patients with Glanzmann thrombasthenia in Israel. *Blood* 77:75, 1991.
54. Beckstead JH, Stenberg PE, McEver RP, et al: Immunohistochemical localization of membrane and alpha-granule proteins in human megakaryocytes: Application to plastic-embedded bone marrow biopsy specimens. *Blood* 67:285, 1986.
55. Krissansen GW, Elliott MJ, Lucas CM, et al: Identification of a novel integrin beta subunit expressed on cultured monocytes (macrophages). *J Biol Chem* 265:823, 1990.
56. Byzova TV, Rabbani R, D'Souza SE, et al: Role of integrin alpha(v)beta3 in vascular biology. *Thromb Haemost* 80:726, 1998.
57. Newman PJ, Seligsohn U, Lyman S, et al: The molecular genetic basis of Glanzmann thrombasthenia in the Iraqi-Jewish and Arab populations in Israel. *Proc Natl Acad Sci U S A* 88:3160, 1991.
58. Burk CD, Newman PJ, Lyman S, et al: A deletion in the gene for glycoprotein IIb associated with Glanzmann's thrombasthenia. *J Clin Invest* 87:270, 1991.
59. Poncz M, Rifat S, Coller BS, et al: Glanzmann thrombasthenia secondary to a Gly273Asp mutation adjacent to the first calcium-binding domain of platelet glycoprotein IIb. *J Clin Invest* 93:172, 1994.
60. Tadokoro S, Tomiyama Y, Honda S, et al: Missense mutations in the beta(3) subunit have a different impact on the expression and function between alpha(IIb)beta(3) and alpha(v)beta(3). *Blood* 99:931, 2002.
60a. Nurden AT, Fiore M, Pillois X, Nurden P: Genetic testing in the diagnostic evaluation of inherited platelet disorders. *Semin Thromb Hemost* 35:204, 2009.
61. French DL, Coller BS: Hematologically important mutations: Glanzmann thrombasthenia. *Blood Cells Mol Dis* 23:39, 1997.
62. Lee JO, Rieu P, Arnaout MA, et al: Crystal structure of the A domain from the alpha subunit of integrin CR3 (CD11b/CD18). *Cell* 80:631, 1995.
63. Michishita M, Videm V, Arnaout MA: A novel divalent cation-binding site in the A domain of the beta 2 integrin CR3 (CD11b/CD18) is essential for ligand binding. *Cell* 72:857, 1993.
64. Collins Tozer EC, Liddington RC, Sutcliffe MJ, et al: Ligand binding to integrin $\alpha IIb\beta 3$ is dependent on a MIDAS-like domain in the beta3 subunit. *J Biol Chem* 271:21978, 1996.
65. Zhu J, Luo BH, Xiao T, et al: Structure of a complete integrin ectodomain in a physiologic resting state and activation and deactivation by applied forces. *Mol Cell* 32:849, 2008.
66. Bajt ML, Loftus JC: Mutation of a ligand binding domain of beta 3 integrin. Integral role of oxygenated residues in alpha IIb beta 3 (GPIIb-IIIa) receptor function. *J Biol Chem* 269:20913, 1994.
67. Xiong JP, Stehle T, Diefenbach B, et al: Crystal structure of the extracellular segment of integrin alphaVbeta3. *Science* 294:339, 2001.
68. Xiao T, Takagi J, Coller BS, et al: Structural basis for allostery in integrins and binding to fibrinogen-mimetic therapeutics. *Nature* 432:59, 2004.

69. Xiong JP, Stehle T, Zhang R, et al: Crystal structure of the extracellular segment of integrin alpha Vbeta3 in complex with an Arg-Gly-Asp ligand. *Science* 296:151, 2002.
70. Springer TA, Zhu J, Xiao T: Structural basis for distinctive recognition of fibrinogen gammaC peptide by the platelet integrin alphaIIbbeta3. *J Cell Biol* 182:791, 2008.
71. Loftus JC, O'Toole TE, Plow EF, et al: A β3 integrin mutation abolishes ligand binding and alters divalent cation-dependent conformation. *Science* 249:915, 1990.
72. Ward CM, Chao YL, Kato GJ, et al: Substitution of Asn, but not Tyr, for ASP119 of the β3 integrin subunit preserves fibrin binding and clot retraction. *Blood* 90:26a, 1997.
73. Fournier DJ, Kabral A, Castaldi PA, et al: A variant of Glanzmann's thrombasthenia characterized by abnormal glycoprotein IIb/IIIa complex formation. *Thromb Haemost* 62:977, 1989.
74. Newman PJ, Weyerbusch-Bottum S, Visentin GP, et al: Type II Glanzmann thrombasthenia due to a destabilizing amino acid substitution in platelet membrane glycoprotein IIIa. *Thromb Haemost* 69:1017, 1993.
75. Lanza F, Stierle A, Fournier D, et al: A new variant of Glanzmann's thrombasthenia (Strasbourg I). Platelets with functionally defective glycoprotein IIb-IIIa complexes and a glycoprotein IIIa Arg214Trp mutation. *J Clin Invest* 89:1995, 1992.
76. D'Andrea G, Bafunno V, Del VL, et al: A beta3 Asp217Val substitution in a patient with variant Glanzmann Thrombasthenia severely affects integrin alphaIIBbeta3 functions. *Blood Coagul Fibrinolysis* 19:657, 2008.
77. Baker EK, Tozer EC, Pfaff M, et al: A genetic analysis of integrin function: Glanzmann thrombasthenia in vitro. *Proc Natl Acad Sci U S A* 94:1973, 1997.
78. Ward CM, Kestin AS, Newman PJ: A Leu262Pro mutation in the integrin beta(3) subunit results in an alpha(IIb)-beta(3) complex that binds fibrin but not fibrinogen. *Blood* 96:161, 2000.
79. Loftus JC, Halloran CE, Ginsberg MH, et al: The amino-terminal one-third of alpha IIb defines the ligand recognition specificity of integrin alpha IIb beta 3. *J Biol Chem* 271:2033, 1996.
80. Springer TA: Folding of the N-terminal, ligand-binding region of integrin α-subunits into a β-propeller domain. *Proc Natl Acad Sci U S A* 94:65, 1997.
81. Ruan J, Peyruchaud O, Alberio L, et al: Double heterozygosity of the GPIIb gene in a Swiss patient with Glanzmann's thrombasthenia. *Br J Haematol* 102:918, 1998.
82. Wilcox DA, Paddock CM, Lyman S, et al: Glanzmann thrombasthenia resulting from a single amino acid substitution between the second and third calcium-binding domains of GPIIb. Role of the GPIIb amino terminus in integrin subunit association. *J Clin Invest* 95:1553, 1995.
83. Wilcox DA, Wautier JL, Pidard D, et al: A single amino acid substitution flanking the fourth calcium binding domain of alpha IIb prevents maturation of the alpha IIb beta 3 integrin complex. *J Biol Chem* 269:4450, 1994.
84. Basani RB, Vilaire G, Shattil SJ, et al: Glanzmann thrombasthenia due to a two amino acid deletion in the fourth calcium-binding domain of alpha IIb: Demonstration of the importance of calcium-binding domains in the conformation of alpha IIb beta 3. *Blood* 88:167, 1996.
85. Kiyoi T, Tomiyama Y, Honda S, et al: A naturally occurring Tyr143His alpha IIb mutation abolishes alpha IIb beta 3 function for soluble ligands but retains its ability for mediating cell adhesion and clot retraction: Comparison with other mutations causing ligand-binding defects. *Blood* 101:3485, 2003.
86. Basani RB, French DL, Vilaire G, et al: A naturally-occurring mutation near the amino terminus of αIIb defines a new region involved in ligand binding to αIIbβ3. *Blood* 95:180, 2000.
87. Westrup D, Santoso S, Becker-Hagendorff K, et al: Transfection of GPIIbIIe176/IIIa (Frankfurt I) in mammalian cells. *Thromb Haemost* 77:671, 1997.
88. Honda S, Tomiyama Y, Shiraga M, et al: A two-amino acid insertion in the Cys146-Cys167 loop of the αIIb subunit is associated with a variant of Glanzmann thrombasthenia. *J Clin Invest* 102:1183, 1998.
89. Kirchmaier CM, Westrup D, Becker-Hagendorff K, et al: A new variant of Glanzmann thrombasthenia (Frankfurt I). *Thromb Haemost* 73:1058, 1995.
90. Grimaldi CM, Chen F, Wu C, et al: Glycoprotein IIb Leu214Pro mutation produces Glanzmann thrombasthenia with both quantitative and qualitative abnormalities in GPIIb/IIIa. *Blood* 91:1562, 1998.
91. Fullard J, Murphy R, O'Neill S, et al: A Val193Met mutation in GPIIIa results in a GPIIb/IIIa receptor with a constitutively high affinity for a small ligand. *Br J Haematol* 115:131, 2001.
92. Ruiz C, Liu CY, Sun QH, et al: A point mutation in the cysteine-rich domain of glycoprotein (GP) IIIa results in the expression of a GPIIb-IIIa (alphaIIbbeta3) integrin receptor locked in a high-affinity state and a Glanzmann thrombasthenia-like phenotype. *Blood* 98:2432, 2001.
93. Vanhoorelbeke K, De Meyer SF, Pareyn I, et al: The novel S527F mutation in the integrin beta3 chain induces a high affinity alphaIIbbeta3 receptor by hindering adoption of the bent conformation. *J Biol Chem* 284:14914, 2009.
94. Chen Y-P, Djaffar I, Pidard E: Ser752Pro mutation in the cytoplasmic domain of integrin β3 subunit and defective activation of platelet integrin αIIbβ3 (glycoprotein IIb-IIIa) in a variant of Glanzmann thrombasthenia. *Proc Natl Acad Sci U S A* 89:10169, 1992.
95. Ylanne J, Chen Y, O'Toole TE, et al: Distinct functions of integrin alpha and beta subunit cytoplasmic domains in cell spreading and formation of focal adhesions. *J Cell Biol* 122:223, 1993.
96. Ylanne J, Huuskonen J, O'Toole TE, et al: Mutation of the cytoplasmic domain of the integrin beta 3 subunit. Differential effects on cell spreading, recruitment to adhesion plaques, endocytosis, and phagocytosis. *J Biol Chem* 270:9550, 1995.
97. Wang R, Shattil SJ, Ambruso DR, et al: Truncation of the cytoplasmic domain of β3 in a variant form of Glanzmann thrombasthenia abrogates signaling through the integrin αIIbβ3 complex. *J Clin Invest* 100:2393, 1997.
98. Chen YP, O'Toole TE, Ylanne J, et al: A point mutation in the integrin beta 3 cytoplasmic domain (S752P) impairs bidirectional signaling through alpha IIb beta 3 (platelet glycoprotein IIb-IIIa). *Blood* 84:1857, 1994.
99. Guarisco JL, Cheney ML, Ohene-Frempong K, et al: Limited septoplasty as treatment for recurrent epistaxis in a child with Glanzmann's thrombasthenia. *Laryngoscope* 97:336, 1987.
100. Ranjith A, Nandakumar K: Glanzmann thrombasthenia: A rare hematological disorder with oral manifestations: A case report. *J Contemp Dent Pract* 9:107, 2008.
101. Bayraktaroglu T, Colak N, Nalcaci M, et al: Sheehan's syndrome associated with Glanzmann's thrombasthenia: Case report and literature review. *Exp Clin Endocrinol Diabetes* 116:549, 2008.
102. Seligsohn U, Rososhansky S: A Glanzmann's thrombasthenia cluster among Iraqi Jews in Israel. *Thromb Haemost* 52:230, 1984.
102a. Gruel Y, Pacouret G, Bellucci S, Caen J: Severe proximal deep vein thrombosis in a Glanzmann thrombasthenia variant successfully treated with a low molecular weight heparin. *Blood* 90:888, 1997.
102b. Ten Cate H, Brandjes DP, Smits PH, van Mourik JA: The role of platelets in venous thrombosis: A patient with Glanzmann's thrombasthenia and a factor V Leiden mutation suffering from deep vein thrombosis. *J Thromb Haemost* 1:394, 2003.
102c. Phillips R, Richards M: Venous thrombosis in Glanzmann's thrombasthenia. *Haemophilia* 13:758, 2007.
102d. Seretny M, Senadheera N, Miller E, et al: Pulmonary embolus in Glanzmann's thrombasthenia treated with warfarin. *Haemophilia* 14:1128, 2008.
102e. Shpilberg O, Rabi I, Schiller K, et al: Patients with Glanzmann thrombasthenia lacking platelet glycoprotein alpha(IIb)beta(3) (GPIIb/IIIa) and alpha(v)beta(3) receptors are not protected from atherosclerosis. *Circulation* 105:1044, 2002.
103. Ruan J, Schmugge M, Clemetson KJ, et al: Homozygous Cys542Arg substitution in GPIIIa in a Swiss patient with type I Glanzmann's thrombasthenia. *Br J Haematol* 105:523, 1999.
104. Coller BS, Peerschke EI, Scudder LE, et al: A murine monoclonal antibody that completely blocks the binding of fibrinogen to platelets produces a thrombasthenic-like state in normal platelets and binds to glycoproteins IIb and/or IIIa. *J Clin Invest* 72:325, 1983.
105. Chediak J, Telfer MC, Vander LB, et al: Cycles of agglutination-disagglutination induced by ristocetin in thrombasthenic platelets. *Br J Haematol* 43:113, 1979.
106. Grant RA, Zucker MB, McPherson J: ADP-induced inhibition of von Willebrand factor-mediated platelet agglutination. *Am J Physiol* 230:1406, 1976.
107. Malmsten C, Kindahl H, Samuelsson B, et al: Thromboxane synthesis and the platelet release reaction in Bernard- Soulier syndrome, thrombasthenia Glanzmann and Hermansky-Pudlak syndrome. *Br J Haematol* 35:511, 1977.
108. Charo IF, Feinman RD, Detwiler TC: Interrelations of platelet aggregation and secretion. *J Clin Invest* 60:866, 1977.
109. Heptinstall S, Taylor PM: The effects of citrate and extracellular calcium ions on the platelet release reaction induced by adenosine diphosphate and collagen. *Thromb Haemost* 42:778, 1979.
110. Caen JP, Cronberg S, Levy-Toledano S, et al: New data on Glanzmann's thrombasthenia. *Proc Soc Exp Biol Med* 136:1082, 1971.
111. Zucker MB, Vroman L: Platelet adhesion induced by fibrinogen adsorbed onto glass. *Proc Soc Exp Biol Med* 131:318, 1969.
112. Stanford MF, Munoz PC, Vroman L: Platelets adhere where flow has left fibrinogen on glass. *Ann N Y Acad Sci* 416:504, 1983.
113. Zucker MB, McPherson J: Reactions of platelets near surfaces *in vitro*: Lessons from the platelet retention test. *Ann N Y Acad Sci* 283:128, 1977.
114. Bevers EM, Comfurius P, Nieuwenhuis HK, et al: Platelet prothrombin converting activity in hereditary disorders of platelet function. *Br J Haematol* 63:335, 1986.
115. Reverter JC, Beguin S, Kessels H, et al: Inhibition of platelet-mediated, tissue factor-induced thrombin generation by the mouse/human chimeric 7E3 antibody. Potential implications for the effect of c7E3 Fab treatment on acute thrombosis and "clinical restenosis." *J Clin Invest* 98:863, 1996.
116. Beguin S, Kumar R, Keularts I, et al: Fibrin-dependent platelet procoagulant activity requires GPIb receptors and von Willebrand factor. *Blood* 93:564, 1999.
117. Gemmell CH, Sefton MV, Yeo EL: Platelet-derived microparticle formation involves glycoprotein IIb- IIIa. Inhibition by RGDS and a Glanzmann's thrombasthenia defect. *J Biol Chem* 268:14586, 1993.
118. Nomura S, Komiyama Y, Matsuura E, et al: Participation of $\alpha_{IIb}\beta_3$ in platelet microparticle generation by collagen plus thrombin. *Haemostasis* 26:31, 1996.
119. Nomura S, Komiyama Y, Murakami T, et al: Flow cytometric analysis of surface membrane proteins on activated platelets and platelet-derived microparticles from healthy and thrombasthenic individuals. *Int J Hematol* 58:203, 1993.
120. Byzova TV, Plow EF: Networking in the hemostatic system. Integrin alphaiibbeta3 binds prothrombin and influences its activation. *J Biol Chem* 272:27183, 1997.
121. Byzova TV, Plow EF: Activation of alphaVbeta3 on vascular cells controls recognition of prothrombin. *J Cell Biol* 143:2081, 1998.
122. Tschopp TB, Weiss HJ, Baumgartner HR: Interaction of thrombasthenic platelets with subendothelium: Normal adhesion, absent aggregation. *Experientia* 31:113, 1975.
123. Sakariassen KS, Nievelstein PFEM, Coller BS, et al: The role of platelet membrane glycoproteins Ib and IIb-IIIa in platelet adherence to human artery subendothelium. *Br J Haematol* 63:681, 1986.

124. Weiss HJ, Turitto VT, Baumgartner HR: Platelet adhesion and thrombus formation on subendothelium in platelets deficient in glycoproteins IIb-IIIa, Ib, and storage granules. *Blood* 67:322, 1986.
125. Weiss HJ, Turitto VT, Baumgartner HR: The role of shear rate and platelets in promoting fibrin formation on rabbit subendothelium: Studies utilizing patients with quantitative and qualitative platelet defects. *J Clin Invest* 78:1072, 1986.
126. Harrison P, Robinson M, Liesner R, et al: The PFA-100: A potential rapid screening tool for the assessment of platelet dysfunction. *Clin Lab Haematol* 24:225, 2002.
127. Buyukasik Y, Karakus S, Goker H, et al: Rational use of the PFA-100 device for screening of platelet function disorders and von Willebrand disease. *Blood Coagul Fibrinolysis* 13:349, 2002.
128. Lee H, Nurden AT, Thomaidis A, et al: Relationship between fibrinogen binding and platelet glycoprotein deficiencies in Glanzmann's thrombasthenia type I and type II. *Br J Haematol* 48:47, 1981.
129. Coller BS, Seligsohn U, Peretz H, et al: Glanzmann thrombasthenia: New insights from an historical perspective. *Semin Hematol* 31:301, 1994.
130. Shattil SJ, Hoxie JA, Cunningham M, et al: Changes in the platelet membrane glycoprotein IIb/IIIa complex during platelet activation. *J Biol Chem* 260:11107, 1985.
131. Coller BS, Seligsohn U, Zivelin A, et al: Immunologic and biochemical characterization of homozygous and heterozygous Glanzmann's thrombasthenia in Iraqi-Jewish and Arab populations of Israel: Comparison of techniques for carrier detection. *Br J Haematol* 62:723, 1986.
132. Peretz H, Seligsohn U, Zwang E, et al: Detection of the Glanzmann's thrombasthenia mutations in Arab and Iraqi-Jewish patients by polymerase chain reaction and restriction analysis of blood or urine samples. *Thromb Haemost* 66:500, 1991.
133. Karpatkin M, Howard L, Karpatkin S: Studies of the origin of platelet-associated fibrinogen. *J Lab Clin Med* 104:223, 1984.
134. Grimaldi CM, Chen F, Scudder LE, et al: A Cys374Tyr homozygous mutation of platelet glycoprotein IIIa (beta 3) in a Chinese patient with Glanzmann's thrombasthenia. *Blood* 88:1666, 1996.
135. Diminno G, Coraggio F, Cerbone AM, et al: A myeloma paraprotein with specificity for platelet glycoprotein IIIa in a patient with a fatal bleeding disorder. *J Clin Invest* 77:157, 1986.
136. Niessner H, Clemetson KJ, Panzer S, et al: Acquired thrombasthenia due to GPIIb/IIIa-specific platelet autoantibodies. *Blood* 68:571, 1986.
137. Kubota T, Tanoue K, Murohashi I, et al: Autoantibody against platelet glycoprotein IIb/IIIa in a patient with non-Hodgkin's lymphoma. *Thromb Res* 53:379, 1989.
138. Malik U, Dutcher JP, Oleksowicz L: Acquired Glanzmann's thrombasthenia associated with Hodgkin's lymphoma: A case report and review of the literature. *Cancer* 82:1764, 1998.
139. Macchi L, Nurden P, Marit G, et al: Autoimmune thrombocytopenic purpura (AITP) and acquired thrombasthenia due to autoantibodies to GP IIb-IIIa in a patient with an unusual platelet membrane glycoprotein composition. *Am J Hematol* 57:164, 1998.
140. Thomas RV, Bessos H, Turner ML, et al: The successful use of plasma exchange and immunosuppression in the management of acquired Glanzmann's thrombasthenia. *Br J Haematol* 119:878, 2002.
141. Dinakaran S, Edwards MP, Hampton KK: Acquired Glanzmann's thrombasthenia causing prolonged bleeding following phacoemulsification. *Br J Ophthalmol* 87:1189, 2003.
142. Rawal A, Sarode R, Curtis BR, et al: Acquired Glanzmann's thrombasthenia as part of multiple-autoantibody syndrome in a pediatric heart transplant patient. *J Pediatr* 144:672, 2004.
143. Granel B, Swiader L, Veit V, et al: [Pseudo-Glanzmann thrombasthenia in the course of autoimmune thrombocytopenic purpura]. *Rev Med Interne* 19:823, 1998.
144. Ratnoff OD: Some therapeutic agents influencing hemostasis, in *Hemostasis and Thrombosis: Basic Principles and Clinical Practice*, 2nd ed, edited by RW Colman, J Hirsh, VJ Marder, EW Salzman, p 1026. Lippincott, Philadelphia, 1987.
145. Berliner S, Horowitz I, Martinowitz U, et al: Dental surgery in patients with severe factor XI deficiency without plasma replacement. *Blood Coagul Fibrinolysis* 3:465, 1992.
146. Sindet-Pedersen S, Ramstrom G, Bernvil S, et al: Hemostatic effect of tranexamic acid mouthwash in anticoagulant-treated patients undergoing oral surgery. *N Engl J Med* 320:840, 1989.
147. Rodeghiero F: Management of menorrhagia in women with inherited bleeding disorders: General principles and use of desmopressin. *Haemophilia* 14(Suppl 1):21, 2008.
147a. Rodeghiero F: Management of menorrhagia in women with inherited bleeding disorders: General principles and use of desmopressin. *Haemophilia* 14(Suppl 1):21, 2008.
148. Mannucci PM: Desmopressin (DDAVP) for treatment of disorders of hemostasis. *Prog Hemost Thromb* 8:19, 1986.
149. Lethagen S, Karlsson MK: Erythropoietin and desmopressin obviated transfusion in a thromboasthenic Jehovah's witness undergoing scoliosis surgery. *Thromb Haemost* 2:11, 1996.
150. DiMichele DM, Hathaway WE: Use of DDAVP in inherited and acquired platelet dysfunction. *Am J Hematol* 33:39, 1990.
150a. Lethaby A, Augood C, Duckitt K: Nonsteroidal anti-inflammatory drugs for heavy menstrual bleeding. *Cochrane Database Syst Rev* 2:CD000400, 2000.
151. Markovitch O, Ellis M, Holzinger M, et al: Severe juvenile vaginal bleeding due to Glanzmann's thrombasthenia: Case report and review of the literature. *Am J Hematol* 57:225, 1998.
152. Demers C, Derzko C, David M, et al: Gynaecological and obstetric management of women with inherited bleeding disorders. *Int J Gynaecol Obstet* 95:75, 2006.
153. Tengborn L, Petruson B: A patient with Glanzmann thrombasthenia and epistaxis successfully teated with recombinant factor VIIa. *Thromb Haemost* 75:981, 1996.
154. Spotnitz WD, Burks S: Hemostats, sealants, and adhesives: Components of the surgical toolbox. *Transfusion* 48:1502, 2008.
155. Rakocz M, Lavie G, Martinowitz U: Glanzmann's thrombasthenia: The use of autologous fibrin glue in tooth extractions. *ASDC J Dent Child* 62:129, 1995.
156. Chuansumrit A, Suwannuraks M, Sri-Udomporn N, et al: Recombinant activated factor VII combined with local measures in preventing bleeding from invasive dental procedures in patients with Glanzmann thrombasthenia. *Blood Coagul Fibrinolysis* 14:187, 2003.
157. Cmolik BL, Spero JA, Magovern GJ, et al: Redo cardiac surgery: Late bleeding complications from topical thrombin-induced factor V deficiency. *J Thorac Cardiovasc Surg* 105:222, 1993.
158. Banninger H, Hardegger T, Tobler A, et al: Fibrin glue in surgery: Frequent development of inhibitors of bovine thrombin and human factor V. *Br J Haematol* 85:528, 1993.
159. Streiff MB, Ness PM: Acquired FV inhibitors: A needless iatrogenic complication of bovine thrombin exposure. *Transfusion* 42:18, 2002.
160. Tadokoro K, Ohtoshi T, Takafuji S, et al: Topical thrombin-induced IgE-mediated anaphylaxis: RAST analysis and skin test studies. *J Allergy Clin Immunol* 88:620, 1991.
161. Wai Y, Tsui V, Peng Z, et al: Anaphylaxis from topical bovine thrombin (Thrombostat) during haemodialysis and evaluation of sensitization among a dialysis population. *Clin Exp Allergy* 33:1730, 2003.
162. Tsuda H, Higashi S, Iwanaga S, et al: Development of antitissue factor antibodies in patients after liver surgery. *Blood* 82:96, 1993.
163. Jasmin JR, Dupont D, Velin P: Multiple dental extractions in a child with Glanzmann's thrombasthenia: Report of case. *ASDC J Dent Child* 54:208, 1987.
164. Schlosser RJ: Clinical practice. Epistaxis. *N Engl J Med* 360:784, 2009.
165. Hedner U: Factor VIIa and its potential therapeutic use in bleeding-associated pathologies. *Thromb Haemost* 100:557, 2008.
166. Searle E, Pavord S, Alfirevic Z: Recombinant factor VIIa and other pro-haemostatic therapies in primary postpartum haemorrhage. *Best Pract Res Clin Obstet Gynaecol* 22:1075, 2008.
167. Nicklin J, Perrin L, Crandon A, et al: Re: Guidelines for the use of recombinant activated factor VII in massive obstetric haemorrhage. *Aust N Z J Obstet Gynaecol* 48:447, 2008.
168. Mechsner S, Baessler K, Brunne B, et al: Using recombinant activated factor VII, B-Lynch compression, and reversible embolization of the uterine arteries for treatment of severe conservatively intractable postpartum hemorrhage: New method for management of massive hemorrhage in cases of placenta increta. *Fertil Steril* 90:2012, 2008.
169. Franchini M, Franchi M, Bergamini V, et al: A critical review on the use of recombinant factor VIIa in life-threatening obstetric postpartum hemorrhage. *Semin Thromb Hemost* 34:104, 2008.
170. Sugihara S, Katsutani S, Hyodo H, et al: [Postpartum hemorrhage successfully treated with recombinant factor VIIa in Glanzmann thromboasthenia]. *Rinsho Ketsueki* 49:46, 2008.
171. Cases A, Escolar G, Reverter JC, et al: Recombinant human erythropoietin treatment improves platelet function in uremic patients. *Kidney Int* 42:668, 1992.
172. Tsao CJ, Kao RH, Cheng TY, et al: The effect of recombinant human erythropoietin on hemostatic status in chronic uremic patients. *Int J Hematol* 55:197, 1992.
173. Borawski J, Rydzewski A, Pawlak K, et al: Long-term effects of erythropoietin on platelet serotonin storage and platelet aggregation in hemodialysis patients with reference to ketanserin treatment. *Thromb Res* 90:171, 1998.
174. Bell JA, Savidge GF: Glanzmann's thrombasthenia proposed optimal management during surgery and delivery. *Clin Appl Thromb Hemost* 9:167, 2003.
175. Smith JW, Steinhubl SR, Lincoff AM, et al: Rapid platelet-function assay (RPFA): An automated and quantitative cartridge-based method. *Circulation* 99:620, 1999.
176. Gurbel PA, Becker RC, Mann KG, et al: Platelet function monitoring in patients with coronary artery disease. *J Am Coll Cardiol* 50:1822, 2007.
177. Leukocyte reduction and ultraviolet B irradiation of platelets to prevent alloimmunization and refractoriness to platelet transfusions. The Trial to Reduce Alloimmunization to Platelets Study Group. *N Engl J Med* 337:1861, 1997.
178. Bowden RA, Slichter SJ, Sayers M, et al: A comparison of filtered leukocyte-reduced and cytomegalovirus (CMV) seronegative blood products for the prevention of transfusion-associated CMV infection after marrow transplant. *Blood* 86:3598, 1995.
179. Heddle NM, Klama L, Meyer R, et al: A randomized controlled trial comparing plasma removal with white cell reduction to prevent reactions to platelets. *Transfusion* 39:231, 1999.
180. Heddle NM, Klama L, Singer J, et al: The role of the plasma from platelet concentrates in transfusion reactions. *N Engl J Med* 331:625, 1994.
181. Saarinen UM, Kekomaki R, Siimes MA, et al: Effective prophylaxis against platelet refractoriness in multitransfused patients by use of leukocyte-free blood components. *Blood* 75:512, 1990.
182. Slichter SJ: Platelet transfusions a constantly evolving therapy. *Thromb Haemost* 66:178, 1991.
183. Lozano M, Cid J: The clinical implications of platelet transfusions associated with ABO or Rh(D) incompatibility. *Transfus Med Rev* 17:57, 2003.
184. Anderson B, Shad AT, Gootenberg JE, et al: Successful prevention of post-transfusion Rh alloimmunization by intravenous Rho (D) immune globulin (WinRho SD). *Am J Hematol* 60:245, 1999.

185. Newman PJ, McFarland JG, Aster RH: The alloimmune thrombocytopenias, in *Thrombosis and Hemorrhage*, edited by J Loscalzo, AI Schafer, p 531. Blackwell Scientific, Boston, 1994.
186. Conte R, Cirillo D, Ricci F, et al: Platelet transfusion in a patient affected by Glanzmann's thrombasthenia with antibodies against GPIIb-IIIa. *Haematologica* 82:73, 1997.
187. Jallu V, Pico M, Chevaleyre J, et al: Characterization of an antibody to the integrin beta 3 subunit (GP IIIa) from a patient with neonatal thrombocytopenia and an inherited deficiency of GP IIb-IIIa complexes in platelets (Glanzmann's thrombasthenia). *Hum Antibodies Hybridomas* 3:93, 1992.
188. Levy-Toledano S, Tobelem G, Legrand C, et al: Acquired IgG antibody occurring in a thrombasthenic patient: Its effect on human platelet function. *Blood* 51:1065, 1978.
189. Rosa JP, Kieffer N, Didry D, et al: The human platelet membrane glycoprotein complex GP IIb-IIIa expresses antigenic sites not exposed on the dissociated glycoproteins. *Blood* 64:1246, 1984.
190. Coller BS, Peerschke EI, Seligsohn U, et al: Studies on the binding of an alloimmune and two murine monoclonal antibodies to the platelet glycoprotein IIb-IIIa complex receptor. *J Lab Clin Med* 107:384, 1986.
191. Martin I, Kriaa F, Proulle V, et al: Protein A Sepharose immunoadsorption can restore the efficacy of platelet concentrates in patients with Glanzmann's thrombasthenia and anti-glycoprotein IIb-IIIa antibodies. *Br J Haematol* 119:991, 2002.
192. Ito K, Yoshida H, Hatoyama H, et al: Antibody removal therapy used successfully at delivery of a pregnant patient with Glanzmann's thrombasthenia and multiple antiplatelet antibodies. *Vox Sang* 61:40, 1991.
193. Kriaa F, Laurian Y, Hiesse C, et al: Five years' experience at one centre with protein A immunoadsorption in patients with deleterious allo/autoantibodies (anti-HLA antibodies, autoimmune bleeding disorders) and post-transplant patients relapsing with focal glomerular sclerosis. *Nephrol Dial Transplant* 10 Suppl 6:108, 1995.
194. George JN, Nurden AT: Inherited disorders of the platelet membrane: Glanzmann's thrombasthenia and Bernard-Soulier syndrome., in *Hemostasis and Thrombosis: Basic Principles and Clinical Practice*, edited by RW Colman, J Hirsh, VJ Marder, EW Salzman, p 726. Lippincott, Philadelphia, 1987.
195. Bellucci S, Devergie A, Gluckman E, et al: Complete correction of Glanzmann's thrombasthenia by allogeneic bone marrow transplantation. *Br J Haematol* 59:635, 1985.
196. Bellucci S, Damaj G, Boval B, et al: Bone marrow transplantation in severe Glanzmann's thrombasthenia with antiplatelet alloimmunization. *Bone Marrow Transplant* 25:327, 2000.
197. Johnson A, Goodall AH, Downie CJ, et al: Bone marrow transplantation for Glanzmann's thrombasthenia. *Bone Marrow Transplant* 14:147, 1994.
198. McColl MD, Gibson BE: Sibling allogeneic bone marrow transplantation in a patient with type I Glanzmann's thrombasthenia. *Br J Haematol* 99:58, 1997.
199. Flood VH, Johnson FL, Boshkov LK, et al: Sustained engraftment post bone marrow transplant despite anti-platelet antibodies in Glanzmann thrombasthenia. *Pediatr Blood Cancer* 45:971, 2005.
200. Connor P, Khair K, Liesner R, et al: Stem cell transplantation for children with Glanzmann thrombasthenia. *Br J Haematol* 140:568, 2008.
201. Ishaqi MK, El-Hayek M, Gassas A, et al: Allogeneic stem cell transplantation for Glanzmann thrombasthenia. *Pediatr Blood Cancer* 52:682, 2009.
202. Niemeyer GP, Boudreaux MK, Goodman-Martin SA, et al: Correction of a large animal model of type I Glanzmann's thrombasthenia by nonmyeloablative bone marrow transplantation. *Exp Hematol* 31:1357, 2003.
203. Chen F, Xie Q, Jian Z, et al: Chimera formation of platelet GP II b Bak a/b by intrauterine transplantation of fetal liver stem cells. *Chin Med J (Engl)* 114:676, 2001.
204. d'Oiron R, Menart C, Trzeciak MC, et al: Use of recombinant factor VIIa in 3 patients with inherited type I Glanzmann's thrombasthenia undergoing invasive procedures. *Thromb Haemost* 83:644, 2000.
205. Poon MC, d'Oiron R, von Depka M, et al: Prophylactic and therapeutic recombinant factor VIIa administration to patients with Glanzmann's thrombasthenia: Results of an international survey. *J Thromb Haemost* 2:1096, 2004.
206. Lisman T, Adelmeijer J, Heijnen HF, et al: Recombinant factor VIIa restores aggregation of alphaIIbbeta3-deficient platelets via tissue factor-independent fibrin generation. *Blood* 103:1720, 2004.
207. Lisman T, Moschatsis S, Adelmeijer J, et al: Recombinant factor VIIa enhances deposition of platelets with congenital or acquired alpha IIb beta 3 deficiency to endothelial cell matrix and collagen under conditions of flow via tissue factor-independent thrombin generation. *Blood* 101:1864, 2003.
208. Poon MC: The evidence for the use of recombinant human activated factor VII in the treatment of bleeding patients with quantitative and qualitative platelet disorders. *Transfus Med Rev* 21:223, 2007.
209. Poon MC: Clinical use of recombinant human activated factor VII (rFVIIa) in the prevention and treatment of bleeding episodes in patients with Glanzmann's thrombasthenia. *Vasc Health Risk Manag* 3:655, 2007.
210. Hers I, Mumford A: Understanding the therapeutic action of recombinant factor VIIa in platelet disorders. *Platelets* 19:571, 2008.
211. Weeterings C, de Groot PG, Adelmeijer J, et al: The glycoprotein Ib-IX-V complex contributes to tissue factor-independent thrombin generation by recombinant factor VIIa on the activated platelet surface. *Blood* 112:3227, 2008.
212. Galan AM, Tonda R, Pino M, et al: Increased local procoagulant action: A mechanism contributing to the favorable hemostatic effect of recombinant FVIIa in PLT disorders. *Transfusion* 43:885, 2003.
213. Lisman T, Adelmeijer J, Cauwenberghs S, et al: Recombinant factor VIIa enhances platelet adhesion and activation under flow conditions at normal and reduced platelet count. *J Thromb Haemost* 3:742, 2005.
214. Croom KF, McCormack PL: Recombinant factor VIIa (eptacog alfa): A review of its use in congenital hemophilia with inhibitors, acquired hemophilia, and other congenital bleeding disorders. *BioDrugs* 22:121, 2008.
215. Wilcox DA, Olsen JC, Ishizawa L, et al: Integrin alphaIIb promoter-targeted expression of gene products in megakaryocytes derived from retrovirus-transduced human hematopoietic cells. *Proc Natl Acad Sci U S A* 96:9654, 1999.
216. Wilcox DA, White GC: Gene therapy for platelet disorders, in *Platelets*, edited by AD Michelson, p 927. Academic Press, San Diego, 2000.
217. Hodivala-Dilke KM, Tsakiris DA, Rayburn H, et al: Beta3-integrin-deficient mice are a model for Glanzmann thrombasthenia showing placental defects and reduced survival. *J Clin Invest* 103:229, 1999.
218. Boudreaux MK, Lipscomb DL: Clinical, biochemical, and molecular aspects of Glanzmann's thrombasthenia in humans and dogs. *Vet Pathol* 38:249, 2001.
219. Niemeyer GP, Boudreaux MK, Goodman-Martin SA, et al: Correction of a large animal model of type I Glanzmann's thrombasthenia by nonmyeloablative bone marrow transplantation. *Exp Hematol* 31:1357, 2003.
220. Yasunaga K, Nomura S: Statistical analysis of Glanzmann's thrombasthenia in Japan. *Acta Haematol* 89:165, 1993.
221. Lopez JA, Andrews RK, Afshar-Kharghan V, et al: Bernard-Soulier syndrome. *Blood* 91:4397, 1998.
221a. Nurden P, Nurden AT, La Marca S, et al: Platelet morphological changes in 2 patients with von Willebrand disease type 3 caused by large homozygous deletions of the von Willebrand factor gene. *Haematologica* 94:1627, 2009.
222. Lopez JA, Berndt MC: The GPIb-IX-V complex, in *Platelets*, edited by AD Michelson, p 85. Academic Press, San Diego, 2002.
223. Bernard J, Soulier J-P: Sur une nouvelle variete de dystrophie thrombocytaire-hemorragipare congenitale. *Sem Hop* 24:3217, 1948.
224. Bernard J: History of congenital hemorrhagic thrombocytopathic dystrophy. *Blood Cells* 9:179, 1983.
225. Weiss HJ, Tschopp TB, Baumgartner HR, et al: Decreased adhesion of giant (Bernard-Soulier) platelets to subendothelium. Further implications on the role of the von Willebrand factor in hemostasis. *Am J Med* 57:920, 1974.
226. Howard MA, Hutton RA, Hardisty RM: Hereditary giant platelet syndrome: A disorder of a new aspect of platelet function. *Br Med J* 2:586, 1973.
227. Bithell TC, Parekh SJ, Strong RR: Platelet-function studies in the Bernard-Soulier syndrome. *Ann N Y Acad Sci* 201:145, 1972.
228. Nurden AT, Caen JP: Specific roles for platelet surface glycoproteins in platelet function. *Nature* 255:720, 1975.
229. Howard MA, Perkin J, Salem HH, et al: The agglutination of human platelets by botrocetin: Evidence that botrocetin and ristocetin act at different sites on the factor VIII molecule and platelet membrane. *Br J Haematol* 57:25, 1984.
230. Moake JL, Olson JD, Troll JH, et al: Binding of radioiodinated human von Willebrand factor to Bernard- Soulier, thrombasthenic and von Willebrand's disease platelets. *Thromb Res* 19:21, 1980.
231. Zucker MB, Kim SJ, McPherson J, et al: Binding of factor VIII to platelets in the presence of ristocetin. *Br J Haematol* 35:535, 1977.
232. Berndt MC, Gregory C, Chong BH, et al: Additional glycoprotein defects in Bernard-Soulier's syndrome: Confirmation of genetic basis by parental analysis. *Blood* 62:800, 1983.
233. Clemetson KJ, McGregor JL, James E, et al: Characterization of the platelet membrane glycoprotein abnormalities in Bernard-Soulier syndrome and comparison with normal by surface-labeling techniques and high-resolution two-dimensional gel electrophoresis. *J Clin Invest* 70:304, 1982.
234. Vanhoorelbeke K, Ulrichts H, Romijn RA, et al: The GPIbalpha-thrombin interaction: Far from crystal clear. *Trends Mol Med* 10:33, 2004.
235. Romo GM, Dong JF, Schade AJ, et al: The glycoprotein Ib-IX-V complex is a platelet counterreceptor for P-selectin. *J Exp Med* 190:803, 1999.
236. Simon DI, Chen Z, Xu H, et al: Platelet glycoprotein Ibα is a counterreceptor for the leukocyte integrin Mac-1 (CD11b/CD18). *J Exp Med* 192:193, 2000.
237. Bradford HN, Dela Cadena RA, Kunapuli SP, et al: Human kininogens regulate thrombin binding to platelets through the glycoprotein Ib-IX-V complex. *Blood* 90:1508, 1997.
238. Jurk K, Clemetson KJ, de Groot PG, et al: Thrombospondin-1 mediates platelet adhesion at high shear via glycoprotein Ib (GPIb): An alternative/backup mechanism to von Willebrand factor. *FASEB J* 17:1490, 2003.
239. Baglia FA, Badellino KO, Li CQ, et al: Factor XI binding to the platelet glycoprotein Ib-IX-V complex promotes factor XI activation by thrombin. *J Biol Chem* 277:1662, 2002.
240. Bradford HN, Pixley RA, Colman RW: Human factor XII binding to the glycoprotein Ib-IX-V complex inhibits thrombin-induced platelet aggregation. *J Biol Chem* 275:22756, 2000.
241. Ware J, Russell S, Ruggeri ZM: Generation and rescue of a murine model of platelet dysfunction: The Bernard-Soulier syndrome. *Proc Natl Acad Sci U S A* 97:2803, 2000.
242. Kato K, Martinez C, Russell S, et al: Genetic deletion of mouse platelet glycoprotein Ibbeta produces a Bernard-Soulier phenotype with increased alpha-granule size. *Blood* 104:2339, 2004.

243. Ramakrishnan V, Reeves PS, DeGuzman F, et al: Increased thrombin responsiveness in platelets from mice lacking glycoprotein V. *Proc Natl Acad Sci U S A* 96:13336, 1999.
244. Nonne C, Hechler B, Cazenave JP, et al: Reassessment of *in vivo* thrombus formation in glycoprotein V deficient mice backcrossed on a C57Bl/6 strain. *J Thromb Haemost* 6:210, 2008.
245. McGill M, Jamieson GA, Drouin J, et al: Morphometric analysis of platelets in Bernard-Soulier syndrome: Size and configuration in patients and carriers. *Thromb Haemost* 52:37, 1984.
246. Michalas S, Malamitsi-Puchner A, Tsevrenis H: Pregnancy and delivery in Bernard-Soulier syndrome. *Acta Obstet Gynecol Scand* 63:185, 1984.
247. Suhasini G, Nanivadekar SA, Sawant PD, et al: Bernard-Soulier syndrome presenting as recurrent exsanguinating haematemesis. *Indian J Gastroenterol* 5:137, 1986.
248. Heslop HE, Hickton CM, Laird E, et al: Twin pregnancy and parturition in a patient with the Bernard Soulier syndrome. *Scand J Haematol* 37:71, 1986.
249. De Marco L, Fabris F, Casonato A, et al: Bernard-Soulier syndrome: Diagnosis by an ELISA method using monoclonal antibodies in 2 new unrelated patients. *Acta Haematol* 75:203, 1986.
250. Sheffer R, Ilan Y, Eldor A: [Bernard-Soulier syndrome]. *Harefuah* 111:119, 1986.
251. Ingerslev J, Stenbjerg S, Taaning E: A case of Bernard-Soulier syndrome: Study of platelet glycoprotein Ib in a kindred. *Eur J Haematol* 39:182, 1987.
252. Oki Y, Yoshioka K, Konishi M, et al: [A case of Bernard-Soulier syndrome]. *Nippon Naika Gakkai Zasshi* 76:1414, 1987.
253. de Moerloose P, Vogel JJ, Clemetson KJ, et al: [Bernard-Soulier syndrome in a Swiss family]. *Schweiz Med Wochenschr* 117:1817, 1987.
254. Cuthbert RJ, Watson HH, Handa SI, et al: DDAVP shortens the bleeding time in Bernard-Soulier syndrome. *Thromb Res* 49:649, 1988.
255. Drouin J, McGregor JL, Parmentier S, et al: Residual amounts of glycoprotein Ib concomitant with near-absence of glycoprotein IX in platelets of Bernard-Soulier patients. *Blood* 72:1086, 1988.
256. Mant MJ: DDAVP in Bernard-Soulier syndrome. *Thromb Res* 52:77, 1988.
257. Stevens MC, Blanchette VS, Freedman MH, et al: A variant form of Bernard-Soulier syndrome: Mild haemostatic defect associated with partial platelet GPIb deficiency. *Clin Lab Haematol* 10:443, 1988.
258. Shimamoto Y, Kaneoka H, Matsuzaki M, et al: [Genetic markers and thrombin reaction in a family of Bernard-Soulier syndrome]. *Nippon Ketsueki Gakkai Zasshi* 52:1155, 1989.
259. Peaceman AM, Katz AR, Laville M: Bernard-Soulier syndrome complicating pregnancy: A case report. *Obstet Gynecol* 73:457, 1989.
260. Nichols WL, Kaese SE, Gastineau DA, et al: Bernard-Soulier syndrome: Whole blood diagnostic assays of platelets. *Mayo Clin Proc* 64:522, 1989.
261. Ware J, Russell SR, Vicente V, et al: Nonsense mutation in the glycoprotein Ib alpha coding sequence associated with Bernard-Soulier syndrome. *Proc Natl Acad Sci U S A* 87:2026, 1990.
262. Finch CN, Miller JL, Lyle VA, et al: Evidence that an abnormality in the glycoprotein Ib alpha gene is not the cause of abnormal platelet function in a family with classic Bernard-Soulier disease. *Blood* 75:2357, 1990.
263. De Marco L, Mazzucato M, Fabris F, et al: Variant Bernard-Soulier syndrome type Bolzano. A congenital bleeding disorder due to a structural and functional abnormality of the platelet glycoprotein Ib-IX complex. *J Clin Invest* 86:25, 1990.
264. Poulsen LO, Taaning E: Variation in surface platelet glycoprotein Ib expression in Bernard- Soulier syndrome. *Haemostasis* 20:155, 1990.
265. Ware J, Russell SR, Vicente V, et al: Nonsense mutation in the glycoprotein Ib alpha coding sequence associated with Bernard-Soulier syndrome. *Proc Natl Acad Sci U S A* 87:2026, 1990.
266. Waldenstrom E, Holmberg L, Axelsson U, et al: Bernard-Soulier syndrome in two Swedish families: Effect of DDAVP on bleeding time. *Eur J Haematol* 46:182, 1991.
267. Humphries JE, Yirinec BA, Hess CE: Atherosclerosis and unstable angina in Bernard-Soulier syndrome. *Am J Clin Pathol* 97:652, 1992.
268. Miller JL, Lyle VA, Cunningham D: Mutation of leucine-57 to phenylalanine in a platelet glycoprotein Ib alpha leucine tandem repeat occurring in patients with an autosomal dominant variant of Bernard-Soulier disease. *Blood* 79:439, 1992.
269. Avila MA, Jacyntho C, Santos ML, et al: [Bernard-Soulier syndrome and pregnancy: A case report]. *J Gynecol Obstet Biol Reprod (Paris)* 21:73, 1992.
270. Wright SD, Michaelides K, Johnson DJ, et al: Double heterozygosity for mutations in the platelet glycoprotein IX gene in three siblings with Bernard-Soulier syndrome. *Blood* 81:2339, 1993.
271. Ware J, Russell SR, Marchese P, et al: Point mutation in a leucine-rich repeat of platelet glycoprotein Ibalpha in the Bernard-Soulier syndrome. *J Clin Invest* 92:1213, 1993.
272. Simsek S, Admiraal LG, Modderman PW, et al: Identification of a homozygous single base pair deletion in the gene coding for the human platelet glycoprotein Ibalpha causing Bernard-Soulier syndrome. *Thromb Haemost* 72:444, 1994.
273. Simsek S, Noris P, Lozano M, et al: Cys209Ser mutation in the platelet membrane glycoprotein Ibalpha gene is associated with Bernard Soulier syndrome. *Br J Haematol* 88:839, 1994.
274. Kunishima S, Miura H, Fukutani H, et al: Bernard-Soulier syndrome Kagoshima: Ser 444-Stop mutation of glycoprotein (GP) Ibalpha resulting in circulating truncated GPIbalpha and surface expression of GPIbbeta and GPIX. *Blood* 84:3356, 1994.
275. Li C, Martin SE, Roth GJ: The genetic defect in two well-studied cases of Bernard-Soulier syndrome: A point mutation in the fifth leucine-rich repeat of platelet glycoprotein Ibα. *Blood* 86:3805, 1995.
276. De La Salle C, Baas M-J, Lanza F, et al: A three-base deletion removing a leucine residue in a leucine-rich repeat of platelet glycoprotein Ibalpha associated with a variant of Bernard-Soulier syndrome (Nancy I). *Br J Haematol* 89:386, 1995.
277. Noda M, Fujimura K, Takafuta T, et al: Heterogenous expression of glycoprotein Ib, IX and V in platelets from two patients with Bernard-Soulier syndrome caused by different genetic abnormalities. *Thromb Haemost* 74:1411, 1995.
278. Budarf ML, Konkle BA, Ludlow LB, et al: Identification of a patient with Bernard-Soulier syndrome and a deletion in the DiGeorge/Velo-cardio-facial chromosomal region in 22q11.2. *Hum Mol Genet* 4:763, 1995.
279. Ludlow LB, Schick BP, Budarf ML, et al: Identification of a mutation in a GATA binding site of the platelet glycoprotein Ibbeta promoter resulting in the Bernard-Soulier syndrome. *J Biol Chem* 271:22076, 1996.
280. Li C, Pasquale DN, Roth GJ: Bernard-Soulier syndrome with severe bleeding: Absent platelet glycoprotein Ib alpha due to a homozygous one-base deletion. *Thromb Haemost* 76:670, 1996.
281. Martinez-Murillo C, Quintana-Gonzalez S, Ambriz-Fernandez R, et al: [Utility of desmopressin in 4 cases of thrombocytopathies associated with giant platelets]. *Rev Invest Clin* 49:281, 1997.
282. Kanaji T, Okamura T, Kuroiwa M, et al: Molecular and genetic analysis of two patients with Bernard-Soulier syndrome: Identification of new mutations in glycoprotein Ibalpha gene. *Thromb Haemost* 77:1055, 1997.
283. Kenny D, Newman PJ, Morateck PA, et al: A dinucleotide deletion results in defective membrane anchoring and circulating soluble glycoprotein Ibalpha in a novel form of Bernard-Soulier syndrome. *Blood* 90:2626, 1997.
284. Afshar-Kharghan V, Lopez JA: Bernard-Soulier syndrome caused by a dinucleotide deletion and reading frameshift in the region encoding the glycoprotein Ibalpha transmembrane domain. *Blood* 90:2634, 1997.
285. Holmberg L, Karpman D, Nilsson I, et al: Bernard-Soulier syndrome Karlstad: Trp 498-Stop mutation resulting in a truncated glycoprotein Ibalpha that contains part of the transmembrane domain. *Br J Haematol* 98:57, 1997.
286. Kunishima S, Lopez JA, Kobayashi S, et al: Missense mutations of the glycoprotein (GP) Ib beta gene impairing the GPIb alpha/beta disulfide linkage in a family with giant platelet disorder. *Blood* 89:2404, 1997.
287. Noris P, Simsek S, Stibbe J, et al: A phenylalanine-55 to serine amino-acid substitution in the human glycoprotein IX leucine-rich repeat is associated with Bernard-Soulier syndrome. *Br J Haematol* 97:312, 1997.
288. Noris P, Arbustini E, Spedini P, et al: A new variant of Bernard-Soulier syndrome characterized by dysfunctional glycoprotein (GP) Ib and severely reduced amounts of GPIX and GPV. *Br J Haematol* 103:1004, 1998.
289. Van Geet C, Devriendt K, Eyskens B, et al: Velocardiofacial syndrome patients with a heterozygous chromosome 22q11 deletion have giant platelets. *Pediatr Res* 44:607, 1998.
290. Khalil A, Seoud M, Tannous R, et al: Bernard-Soulier syndrome in pregnancy: Case report and review of the literature. *Clin Lab Haematol* 20:125, 1998.
291. Kenny D, Morateck PA, Gill JC, et al: The critical interaction of glycoprotein (GP) Ibβ with GPIX-a genetic cause of Bernard-Soulier syndrome. *Blood* 93:2968, 1999.
292. Koskela S, Javela K, Jouppila J, et al: Variant Bernard-Soulier syndrome due to homozygous Asn45Ser mutation in the platelet glycoprotein (GP) IX in seven patients of five unrelated Finnish families. *Eur J Haematol* 62:256, 1999.
293. Margaglione M, D'Andrea G, Grandone E, et al: Compound heterozygosity (554–589 del, C515-T transition) in the platelet glycoprotein Ib alpha gene in a patient with a severe bleeding tendency. *Thromb Haemost* 81:486, 1999.
294. Sachs UJ, Kroll H, Matzdorff AC, et al: Bernard-Soulier syndrome due to the homozygous Asn-45Ser mutation in GPIX: An unexpected, frequent finding in Germany. *Br J Haematol* 123:127, 2003.
295. Watanabe R, Ishibashi T, Saitoh Y, et al: Bernard-Soulier syndrome with a homozygous 13 base pair deletion in the signal peptide-coding region of the platelet glycoprotein Ib(beta) gene. *Blood Coagul Fibrinolysis* 14:387, 2003.
296. Strassel C, Pasquet JM, Alessi MC, et al: A novel missense mutation shows that GPIbbeta has a dual role in controlling the processing and stability of the platelet GPIb-IX adhesion receptor. *Biochemistry* 42:4452, 2003.
297. Kunishima S, Matsushita T, Ito T, et al: Novel nonsense mutation in the platelet glycoprotein Ibbeta gene associated with Bernard-Soulier syndrome. *Am J Hematol* 71:279, 2002.
298. Lanza F, De La SC, Baas MJ, et al: A Leu7Pro mutation in the signal peptide of platelet glycoprotein (GP)IX in a case of Bernard-Soulier syndrome abolishes surface expression of the GPIb-V-IX complex. *Br J Haematol* 118:260, 2002.
299. Kurokawa Y, Ishida F, Kamijo T, et al: A missense mutation (Tyr88 to Cys) in the platelet membrane glycoprotein Ibbeta gene affects GPIb/IX complex expression—Bernard-Soulier syndrome in the homozygous form and giant platelets in the heterozygous form. *Thromb Haemost* 86:1249, 2001.
300. Gonzalez-Manchon C, Larrucea S, Pastor AL, et al: Compound heterozygosity of the GPIbalpha gene associated with Bernard-Soulier syndrome. *Thromb Haemost* 86:1385, 2001.
301. Wang Z, Shi J, Han Y: [A novel point mutation in the transmembrane domain of platelet glycoprotein IX gene identified in a Bernard-Soulier syndrome patient]. *Zhonghua Xue Ye Xue Za Zhi* 22:464, 2001.
302. Kunishima S, Naoe T, Kamiya T, et al: Novel heterozygous missense mutation in the platelet glycoprotein Ib beta gene associated with isolated giant platelet disorder. *Am J Hematol* 68:249, 2001.

303. Vanhoorelbeke K, Schlammadinger A, Delville JP, et al: Occurrence of the Asn45Ser mutation in the GPIX gene in a Belgian patient with Bernard Soulier syndrome. *Platelets* 12:114, 2001.
304. Rivera CE, Villagra J, Riordan M, et al: Identification of a new mutation in platelet glycoprotein IX (GPIX) in a patient with Bernard-Soulier syndrome. *Br J Haematol* 112:105, 2001.
305. Afshar-Kharghan V, Craig FE, Lopez JA: Bernard-Soulier syndrome in a patient doubly heterozygous for two frameshift mutations in the glycoprotein ib alpha gene. *Br J Haematol* 110:919, 2000.
306. Antonucci JV, Martin ES, Hulick PJ, et al: Bernard-Soulier syndrome: Common ancestry in two African American families with the GP Ib alpha Leu129Pro mutation. *Am J Hematol* 65:141, 2000.
307. Kunishima S, Tomiyama Y, Honda S, et al: Homozygous Pro74-->Arg mutation in the platelet glycoprotein Ibbeta gene associated with Bernard-Soulier syndrome. *Thromb Haemost* 84:112, 2000.
308. Moran N, Morateck PA, Deering A, et al: Surface expression of glycoprotein ib alpha is dependent on glycoprotein ib beta: Evidence from a novel mutation causing Bernard-Soulier syndrome. *Blood* 96:532, 2000.
309. Kunishima S, Tomiyama Y, Honda S, et al: Cys97Tyr mutation in the glycoprotein IX gene associated with Bernard-Soulier syndrome. *Br J Haematol* 107:539, 1999.
310. Koskela S, Partanen J, Salmi TT, et al: Molecular characterization of two mutations in platelet glycoprotein (GP) Ibalpha in two Finnish Bernard-Soulier syndrome families. *Eur J Haematol* 62:160, 1999.
311. Lascone MR, Sacchelli M, Vittorini S, et al: Complex conotruncal heart defect, severe bleeding disorder and 22q11 deletion: A new case of Bernard-Soulier syndrome and of 22q11 deletion syndrome? *Ital Heart J* 2:475, 2001.
312. Tang J, Stern-Nezer S, Liu PC, et al: Mutation in the leucine-rich repeat C-flanking region of platelet glycoprotein Ibbeta impairs assembly of von Willebrand factor receptor. *Thromb Haemost* 92:75, 2004.
313. Hillmann A, Nurden A, Nurden P, et al: A novel hemizygous Bernard-Soulier Syndrome (BSS) mutation in the amino terminal domain of glycoprotein (GP)Ibbeta—Platelet characterization and transfection studies. *Thromb Haemost* 88:1026, 2002.
314. Nakagawa M, Okuno M, Okamoto N, et al: Bernard-Soulier syndrome associated with 22q11.2 microdeletion. *Am J Med Genet* 99:286, 2001.
315. Bowers MJ, Orr NJ, Dempsey S, et al: Molecular genetics and transfusion management in a child with Bernard Soulier syndrome. *Blood Coagul Fibrinolysis* 17:409, 2006.
316. Kunishima S, Yamada T, Hamaguchi M, et al: Bernard-Soulier syndrome due to GPIX W127X mutation in Japan is frequently misdiagnosed as idiopathic thrombocytopenic purpura. *Int J Hematol* 83:366, 2006.
317. Prabu P, Parapia LA: Bernard-Soulier syndrome in pregnancy. *Clin Lab Haematol* 28:198, 2006.
318. Kunishima S, Imai T, Hamaguchi M, et al: Novel heterozygous missense mutation in the second leucine rich repeat of GPIbalpha affects GPIb/IX/V expression and results in macrothrombocytopenia in a patient initially misdiagnosed with idiopathic thrombocytopenic purpura. *Eur J Haematol* 76:348, 2006.
319. Strassel C, David T, Eckly A, et al: Synthesis of GPIb beta with novel transmembrane and cytoplasmic sequences in a Bernard-Soulier patient resulting in GPIb-defective signaling in CHO cells. *J Thromb Haemost* 4:217, 2006.
320. Picu M, Kahwash S, Crumbacher J, et al: An 8-year-old girl with thrombocytopenia. Bernard-Soulier syndrome variant. *Arch Pathol Lab Med* 129:e214, 2005.
321. Liang HP, Morel-Kopp MC, Clemetson JM, et al: A common ancestral glycoprotein (GP) 9 1828A>G (Asn45Ser) gene mutation occurring in European families from Australia and Northern Europe with Bernard-Soulier Syndrome (BSS). *Thromb Haemost* 94:599, 2005.
322. Drouin J, Carson NL, Laneuville O: Compound heterozygosity for a novel nine-nucleotide deletion and the Asn45Ser missense mutation in the glycoprotein IX gene in a patient with Bernard-Soulier syndrome. *Am J Hematol* 78:41, 2005.
323. Wang Z, Zhao X, Duan W, et al: A novel mutation in the transmembrane region of glycoprotein IX associated with Bernard-Soulier syndrome. *Thromb Haemost* 92:606, 2004.
324. Strassel C, Alessi MC, Juhan-Vague I, et al: A 13 base pair deletion in the GPIbbeta gene in a second unrelated Bernard-Soulier family due to slipped mispairing between direct repeats. *J Thromb Haemost* 2:1663, 2004.
325. Hadjkacem B, Elleuch H, Trigui R, et al: The same genetic defect in three Tunisian families with Bernard Soulier syndrome: A probable founder Stop mutation in GPIbbeta. *Ann Hematol* 2009 (Epub ahead of print).
326. Imai C, Kunishima S, Takachi T, et al: A novel homozygous 8-base pair deletion mutation in the glycoprotein Ibalpha gene in a patient with Bernard-Soulier syndrome. *Blood Coagul Fibrinolysis* 20:470, 2009.
327. Hadjkacem B, Elleuch H, Gargouri J, et al: Bernard-Soulier syndrome: Novel nonsense mutation in GPIbbeta gene affecting GPIb-IX complex expression. *Ann Hematol* 88:465, 2009.
328. Vettore S, Scandellari R, Moro S, et al: Novel point mutation in a leucine-rich repeat of the GPIbalpha chain of the platelet von Willebrand factor receptor, GPIb/IX/V, resulting in an inherited dominant form of Bernard-Soulier syndrome affecting two unrelated families: The N41H variant. *Haematologica* 93:1743, 2008.
329. Vettore S, Scandellari R, Scapin M, et al: A case of Bernard-Soulier Syndrome due to a homozygous four bases deletion (TGAG) of GPIbalpha gene: Lack of GPIbalpha but absence of bleeding. *Platelets* 19:388, 2008.
330. Dagistan N, Kunishima S: First Turkish case of Bernard-Soulier syndrome associated with GPIX N45S. *Acta Haematol* 118:146, 2007.
331. Afrasiabi A, Lecchi A, Artoni A, et al: Genetic characterization of patients with Bernard-Soulier syndrome and their relatives from Southern Iran. *Platelets* 18:409, 2007.
332. Knofler R, Olivieri M, Weickardt S, et al: [First results of the THROMKID study: A quality project for the registration of children und adolescents with hereditary platelet function defects in Germany, Austria, and Switzerland]. *Hamostaseologie* 27:48, 2007.
333. Rosenberg N, Lalezari S, Landau M, et al: Trp207Gly in platelet glycoprotein Ibalpha is a novel mutation that disrupts the connection between the leucine-rich repeat domain and the disulfide loop structure and causes Bernard-Soulier syndrome. *J Thromb Haemost* 5:378, 2007.
334. Kunishima S, Sako M, Yamazaki T, et al: Molecular genetic analysis of a variant Bernard-Soulier syndrome due to compound heterozygosity for two novel glycoprotein Ibbeta mutations. *Eur J Haematol* 77:501, 2006.
335. Zieger B, Jenny A, Tsakiris DA, et al: A large Swiss family with Bernard-Soulier syndrome—Correlation phenotype and genotype. *Hamostaseologie* 29:161, 2009.
336. Grottum KA, Solum NO: Congenital thrombocytopenia with giant platelets: A defect in the platelet membrane. *Br J Haematol* 16:277, 1969.
337. Greenberg JP, Packham MA, Guccione MA, et al: Survival of rabbit-platelets treated in vitro with chymotrypsin, plasmin, trypsin, and neuraminidase. *Blood* 53:916, 1979.
338. Heyns Ad, Badenhorst PN, Wessels P, et al: Kinetics, *in vivo* redistribution and sites of sequestration of indium-111-labelled platelets in giant platelet syndromes. *Br J Haematol* 60:323, 1985.
339. Tomer A, Scharf RE, McMillan R, et al: Bernard-Soulier syndrome: Quantitative characterization of megakaryocytes and platelets by flow cytometric and platelet kinetic measurements. *Eur J Haematol* 52:193, 1994.
340. Nurden P, Nurden A: Giant platelets, megakaryocytes and the expression of glycoprotein Ib- IX complexes. *C R Acad Sci III* 319:717, 1996.
341. Vettore S, Scandellari R, Scapin M, et al: A case of Bernard-Soulier Syndrome due to a homozygous four bases deletion (TGAG) of GPIbalpha gene: Lack of GPIbalpha but absence of bleeding. *Platelets* 19:388, 2008.
342. Ruggeri Z: The platelet glycoprotein Ib-IX complex. *Prog Hemost Thromb* 10:35, 1991.
343. Roth GJ: Developing relationships: Arterial platelet adhesion, glycoprotein Ib, and leucine-rich glycoproteins. *Blood* 77:5, 1991.
344. Yap CL, Hughan SC, Cranmer SL, et al: Synergistic adhesive interactions and signaling mechanisms operating between platelet glycoprotein Ib/IX and integrin alpha IIbbeta 3. Studies in human platelets ans transfected Chinese hamster ovary cells. *J Biol Chem* 275:41377, 2000.
345. Wu YP, Vink T, Schiphorst M, et al: Platelet thrombus formation on collagen at high shear rates is mediated by von Willebrand factor-glycoprotein Ib interaction and inhibited by von Willebrand factor-glycoprotein IIb/IIIa interaction. *Arterioscler Thromb Vasc Biol* 20:1661, 2000.
346. Kulkarni S, Dopheide SM, Yap CL, et al: A revised model of platelet aggregation. *J Clin Invest* 105:783, 2000.
347. Ikeda Y, Handa M, Kawano K, et al: The role of von Willebrand factor and fibrinogen in platelet aggregation under varying shear stress. *J Clin Invest* 87:1234, 1991.
348. Peterson DM, Stathopoulos NA, Giorgio TD, et al: Shear-induced platelet aggregation requires von Willebrand factor and platelet membrane glycoproteins Ib and IIb-IIIa. *Blood* 69:625, 1987.
349. Ruggeri ZM: Mechanisms of shear-induced platelet adhesion and aggregation. *Thromb Haemost* 70:119, 1993.
350. Jamieson GA, Okumura T: Reduced thrombin binding and aggregation in Bernard-Soulier platelets. *J Clin Invest* 61:861, 1978.
351. Nurden AT, George JN, Phillips DR: Human platelet membrane glycoproteins, in *Biochemistry of the Platelet*, edited by M Shuman, DR Phillips, p 159. Academic Press, New York, 1986.
352. Jandrot-Perrus M, Rendu F, Caen JP, et al: The common pathway for alpha- and gamma-thrombin-induced platelet activation is independent of GPIb: A study of Bernard-Soulier platelets. *Br J Haematol* 75:385, 1990.
353. De Marco L, Mazzucato M, Masotti A, et al: Function of glycoprotein Ib alpha in platelet activation induced by alpha-thrombin. *J Biol Chem* 266:23776, 1991.
354. Ramakrishnan V, Reeves PS, DeGuzman F, et al: Increased thrombin responsiveness in platelets from mice lacking glycoprotein V. *Proc Natl Acad Sci U S A* 96:13336, 1999.
355. Ni H, Ramakrishnan V, Ruggeri ZM, et al: Increased thrombogenesis and embolus formation in mice lacking glycoprotein V. *Blood* 98:368, 2001.
356. Caen J, Bellucci S: The defective prothrombin consumption in Bernard-Soulier syndrome. Hypotheses from 1948 to 1982. *Blood Cells* 9:389, 1983.
357. Walsh PN, Mills DC, Pareti FI, et al: Hereditary giant platelet syndrome. Absence of collagen-induced coagulant activity and deficiency of factor-XI binding to platelets. *Br J Haematol* 29:639, 1975.
358. Perret B, Levy-Toledano S, Plataivd M: Abnormal phospholipid organization in Bernard-Soulier platelets. *Thromb Res* 31:529, 1983.
359. Kanaji T, Russell S, Ware J: Amelioration of the macrothrombocytopenia associated with the murine Bernard-Soulier syndrome. *Blood* 100:2102, 2002.
360. McNicol A, Drouin J, Clemetson KJ, et al: Phospholipase C activity in platelets from Bernard-Soulier syndrome patients. *Arterioscler Thromb* 13:1567, 1993.
361. White JG, Burris SM, Hasegawa D, et al: Micropipette aspiration of human blood platelets: A defect in Bernard-Soulier's syndrome. *Blood* 63:1249, 1984.

362. Nurden AT: Congenital abnormalities of platelet membrane glycoproteins, in *Platelet Immunobiology, Molecular and Clinical Aspects*, edited by TJ Kunicki, JN George, p 95. Lippincott, Philadelphia, 1989.
363. Lopez JA, Leung B, Reynolds CC, et al: Efficient plasma membrane expression of a functional platelet glycoprotein Ib-IX complex requires the presence of its three subunits. *J Biol Chem* 267:12851, 1992.
364. Li CQ, Dong JF, Lanza F, et al: Expression of platelet glycoprotein (GP) V in heterologous cells and evidence for its association with GP Ib alpha in forming a GP Ib-IX-V complex on the cell surface. *J Biol Chem* 270:16302, 1995.
365. Nurden AT, Didry-Dupies V, Rosa JP: Molecular defects of platelets in Bernard Soulier Syndrome. *Blood Cells* 9:333, 1983.
366. Nurden AT: Inherited abnormalities of platelets. *Thromb Haemost* 82:468, 1999.
367. Nurden AT, Jallu V, Hourdille P: GP Ib and Bernard-Soulier platelets. *Blood* 73:2225, 1989.
368. Nurden AT, Nurden P: Inherited disorders of platelet function, in *Platelets*, edited by AD Michelson, p 1029. Academic Press, San Diego, 2007.
369. Ludlow LB, Schick BP, Budarf ML, et al: Identification of a mutation in a GATA binding site of the platelet glycoprotein Ibbeta promoter resulting in the Bernard-Soulier syndrome. *J Biol Chem* 271:22076, 1996.
369a. Zieger B, Jenny A, Tsakiris DA, et al: A large Swiss family with Bernard-Soulier syndrome—Correlation phenotype and genotype. *Haostaseologie* 29:161, 2009.
370. Dagistan N, Kunishima S: First Turkish case of Bernard-Soulier syndrome associated with GPIX N45S. *Acta Haematol* 118:146, 2007.
371. Liang HP, Morel-Kopp MC, Curtin J, et al: Heterozygous loss of platelet glycoprotein (GP) Ib-V-IX variably affects platelet function in velocardiofacial syndrome (VCFS) patients. *Thromb Haemost* 98:1298, 2007.
372. Lawrence S, McDonald-McGinn DM, Zackai E, et al: Thrombocytopenia in patients with chromosome 22q11.2 deletion syndrome. *J Pediatr* 143:277, 2003.
373. Kato T, Kosaka K, Kimura M, et al: Thrombocytopenia in patients with 22q11.2 deletion syndrome and its association with glycoprotein Ib-beta. *Genet Med* 5:113, 2003.
374. Latger-Cannard V, Bensoussan D, Gregoire MJ, et al: Frequency of thrombocytopenia and large platelets correlates neither with conotruncal cardiac anomalies nor immunological features in the chromosome 22q11.2 deletion syndrome. *Eur J Pediatr* 163:327, 2004.
375. Ryan AK, Goodship JA, Wilson DI, et al: Spectrum of clinical features associated with interstitial chromosome 22q11 deletions: A European collaborative study. *J Med Genet* 34:798, 1997.
376. Yuksel O, Koklu S, Ucar E, et al: Severe recurrent gastrointestinal bleeding due to angiodysplasia in a Bernard-Soulier patient: An onerous medical concomitance. *Dig Dis Sci* 49:885, 2004.
377. Okita R, Hihara J, Konishi K, et al: Intractable gastrointestinal bleeding from angiodysplasia in a patient of Bernard-Soulier syndrome—Report of a case. *Hiroshima J Med Sci* 54:113, 2005.
378. Kaya Z, Gursel T, Dalgic B, et al: Gastric angiodysplasia in a child with Bernard-Soulier syndrome: Efficacy of octreotide in long-term management. *Pediatr Hematol Oncol* 22:223, 2005.
379. George JN, Reimann TA, Moake JL, et al: Bernard-Soulier disease: A study of four patients and their parents. *Br J Haematol* 48:459, 1981.
380. Fox JEB: Linkage of a membrane skeleton to integral membrane glycoproteins in human platelets. Identification of one of the glycoproteins as glycoprotein Ib. *J Clin Invest* 76:1673, 1985.
381. Eaton LA Jr, Read MS, Brinkhous KM: Glycoprotein Ib bioassays. Activity levels in Bernard-Soulier syndrome and in stored blood bank platelets. *Arch Pathol Lab Med* 115:488, 1991.
382. Evensen SA, Solum NO, Grottum KA, et al: Familial bleeding disorder with a moderate thrombocytopenia and giant blood platelets. *Scand J Haematol* 13:203, 1974.
383. Greco NJ, Tandon NN, Jones GD, et al: Contributions of glycoprotein Ib and the seven transmembrane domain receptor to increases in platelet cytoplasmic [Ca^{2+}] induced by α-thrombin. *Biochemistry* 35:906, 1996.
384. Celikel R, McClintock RA, Roberts JR, et al: Modulation of alpha-thrombin function by distinct interactions with platelet glycoprotein Ibalpha. *Science* 301:218, 2003.
385. Dumas JJ, Kumar R, Seehra J, et al: Crystal structure of the GpIbalpha-thrombin complex essential for platelet aggregation. *Science* 301:222, 2003.
386. McGowan EB, Ding A, Detwiler TC: Correlation of thrombin-induced glycoprotein V hydrolysis and platelet activation. *J Biol Chem* 258:11243, 1983.
387. Bienz D, Schnippering W, Clemetson KJ: Glycoprotein V is not the thrombin activation receptor on human blood platelets. *Blood* 68:720, 1986.
388. Caen JP, Nurden AT, Jeanneau C, et al: Bernard-Soulier syndrome: A new platelet glycoprotein abnormality. Its relationship with platelet adhesion to subendothelium and with the factor VIII von Willebrand protein. *J Lab Clin Med* 87:586, 1976.
389. Andrews RK, Harris SJ, McNally T, et al: Binding of purified 14–3-3 zeta signaling protein to discrete amino acid sequences within the cytoplasmic domain of the platelet membrane glycoprotein Ib-IX-V complex. *Biochemistry* 37:638, 1998.
390. Sullam PM, Hyun WC, Szollosi J, et al: Physical proximity and functional interplay of the glycoprotein Ib-IX-V complex and the Fc receptor FcgammaRIIA on the platelet plasma membrane. *J Biol Chem* 273:5331, 1998.
391. Falati S, Edmead CE, Poole AW: Glycoprotein Ib-V-IX, a receptor for von Willebrand factor, couples physically and functionally to the Fc receptor γ-chain, Fyn, and Lyn to activate human platelets. *Blood* 94:1648, 1999.
392. Arthur JF, Gardiner EE, Matzaris M, et al: Glycoprotein VI is associated with GPIb-IX-V on the membrane of resting and activated platelets. *Thromb Haemost* 93:716, 2005.
393. Feng S, Resendiz JC, Christodoulides N, et al: Pathological shear stress stimulates the tyrosine phosphorylation of alpha-actinin associated with the glycoprotein Ib-IX complex. *Biochemistry* 41:1100, 2002.
394. Aziz KA: An acquired form of Bernard Soulier syndrome associated with acute myeloid leukemia. *Saudi Med J* 26:1095, 2005.
395. Stricker RB, Wong D, Saks SR, et al: Acquired Bernard-Soulier syndrome. Evidence for the role of a 210,000-molecular weight protein in the interaction of platelets with von Willebrand factor. *J Clin Invest* 76:1274, 1985.
396. Deckmyn H, Vanhoorelbeke K, Peerlinck K: Inhibitory and activating human antiplatelet antibodies. *Baillieres Clin Haematol* 11:343, 1998.
397. Devine DV, Currie MS, Rosse WF, et al: Pseudo-Bernard-Soulier syndrome: Thrombocytopenia caused by autoantibody to platelet glycoprotein Ib. *Blood* 70:428, 1987.
398. Varon D, Gitel SN, Varon N, et al: Immune Bernard Soulier-like syndrome associated with anti-glycoprotein- IX antibody. *Am J Hematol* 41:67, 1992.
399. Beales IL: An acquired-pseudo Bernard Soulier syndrome occurring with autoimmune chronic active hepatitis and anti-cardiolipin antibody. *Postgrad Med J* 70:305, 1994.
400. Berndt MC, Kabral A, Grimsley P, et al: An acquired Bernard-Soulier-like platelet defect associated with juvenile myelodysplastic syndrome. *Br J Haematol* 68:97, 1988.
401. Hicsonmez G, Gumruk F, Cetin M, et al: Bernard-Soulier-like functional platelet defect in myelodysplastic syndrome and in acute myeloblastic leukemia associated with trilineage myelodysplasia. *Turk J Pediatr* 37:425, 1995.
402. Sharma JB, Buckshee K, Sharma S: Puberty menorrhagia due to Bernard Soulier syndrome and its successful treatment by "Ovral" hormonal tablets. *Aust N Z J Obstet Gynaecol* 31:369, 1991.
403. Greinacher A, Potzsch B, Kiefel V, et al: Evidence that DDAVP transiently improves hemostasis in Bernard-Soulier syndrome independent of von Willebrand-factor. *Ann Hematol* 67:149, 1993.
404. Kemahli S, Canatan D, Uysal Z, et al: DDAVP shortens bleeding time in Bernard-Soulier syndrome. *Thromb Haemost* 71:675, 1994.
405. Greinacher A, Potzsch B, Kiefel V, et al: Evidence that DDAVP transiently improves hemostasis in Bernard-Soulier syndrome independent of von Willebrand-factor. *Ann Hematol* 67:149, 1993.
406. Saade G, Homsi R, Seoud M: Bernard-Soulier syndrome in pregnancy; a report of four pregnancies in one patient, and review of the literature. *Eur J Obstet Gynecol Reprod Biol* 40:149, 1991.
407. Degos L, Tobelem G, Lethielleux P, et al: Molecular defect in platelets from patients with Bernard-Soulier syndrome. *Blood* 50:899, 1977.
408. Peng TC, Kickler TS, Bell WR, et al: Obstetric complications in a patient with Bernard-Soulier syndrome. *Am J Obstet Gynecol* 165:425, 1991.
409. Poon M-C: Factor VIIa, in *Platelets*, 2nd ed, edited by AD Michelson, p 867. Academic Press, San Diego, 2007.
410. Peters M, Heijboer H: Treatment of a patient with Bernard-Soulier syndrome and recurrent nosebleeds with recombinant factor VIIa. *Thromb Haemost* 80:352, 1998.
411. Tonda R, Galan AM, Pino M, et al: Hemostatic effect of activated recombinant factor VIIa in Bernard-Soulier syndrome: Studies in an *in vitro* model. *Transfusion* 44:1790, 2004.
412. Kriplani A, Singh BM, Sowbernika R, et al: Successful pregnancy outcome in Bernard-Soulier syndrome. *J Obstet Gynaecol Res* 31:52, 2005.
413. Hacihanefioglu A, Tarkun P, Gonullu E: Use of recombinant factor VIIa in the management and prophylaxis of bleeding episodes in two patients with Bernard-Soulier syndrome. *Thromb Res* 120:455, 2007.
414. Ozelo MC, Svirin P, Larina L: Use of recombinant factor VIIa in the management of severe bleeding episodes in patients with Bernard-Soulier syndrome. *Ann Hematol* 84:816, 2005.
415. Prabu P, Parapia LA: Bernard-Soulier syndrome in pregnancy. *Clin Lab Haematol* 28:198, 2006.
416. Rahimi G, Rellecke S, Mallmann P, et al: Course of pregnancy and birth in a patient with Bernard-Soulier syndrome—A case report. *J Perinat Med* 33:264, 2005.
417. Kriplani A, Singh BM, Sowbernika R, et al: Successful pregnancy outcome in Bernard-Soulier syndrome. *J Obstet Gynaecol Res* 31:52, 2005.
418. Uotila J, Tammela O, Makipernaa A: Fetomaternal platelet immunization associated with maternal Bernard-Soulier syndrome. *Am J Perinatol* 25:219, 2008.
419. Locatelli F, Rossi G, Balduini C: Hematopoietic stem-cell transplantation for the Bernard-Soulier syndrome. *Ann Intern Med* 138:79, 2003.
420. Rieger C, Rank A, Fiegl M, et al: Allogeneic stem cell transplantation as a new treatment option for patients with severe Bernard-Soulier Syndrome. *Thromb Haemost* 95:190, 2006.
421. Rieger C, Rank A, Fiegl M, et al: Allogeneic stem cell transplantation as a new treatment option for patients with severe Bernard-Soulier Syndrome. *Thromb Haemost* 95:190, 2006.
422. Shi Q, Wilcox DA, Morateck PA, et al: Targeting platelet GPIbalpha transgene expression to human megakaryocytes and forming a complete complex with endogenous GPIbbeta and GPIX. *J Thromb Haemost* 2:1989, 2004.
423. Takahashi H: Studies on the pathophysiology and treatment of von Willebrand's disease. IV. Mechanism of increased ristocetin-induced platelet aggregation in von Willebrand's disease. *Thromb Res* 19:857, 1980.
424. Krizek DM, Rick ME, Williams SB, et al: Cryoprecipitate transfusion in variant von Willebrand's disease and thrombocytopenia. *Ann Intern Med* 98:484, 1983.

425. Weiss HJ, Meyer D, Rabinowitz R, et al: Pseudo-von Willebrand's disease. An intrinsic platelet defect with aggregation by unmodified human factor VIII/von Willebrand factor and enhanced adsorption of its high-molecular-weight multimers. *N Engl J Med* 306:326, 1982.
426. Miller JL, Castella A: Platelet-type von Willebrand's disease: Characterization of a new bleeding disorder. *Blood* 60:790, 1982.
427. Gralnick HR, Williams SB, Shafer BC, et al: Factor VIII/von Willebrand factor binding to von Willebrand's disease platelets. *Blood* 60:328, 1982.
428. Takahashi H, Handa M, Watanabe K, et al: Further characterization of platelet-type von Willebrand's disease in Japan. *Blood* 64:1254, 1984.
429. Nurden P, Lanza F, Bonnafous-Faurie C, et al: A second report of platelet-type von Willebrand disease with a Gly233Ser mutation in the GPIBA gene. *Thromb Haemost* 97:319, 2007.
430. Othman M, Notley C, Lavender FL, et al: Identification and functional characterization of a novel 27-bp deletion in the macroglycopeptide-coding region of the GPIBA gene resulting in platelet-type von Willebrand disease. *Blood* 105:4330, 2005.
431. Enayat MS, Guilliatt AM, Lester W, et al: Distinguishing between type 2B and pseudo-von Willebrand disease and its clinical importance. *Br J Haematol* 133:664, 2006.
432. Bryckaert MC, Pietu G, Ruan C, et al: Abnormality of glycoprotein Ib in two cases of "pseudo"-von Willebrand's disease. *J Lab Clin Med* 106:393, 1985.
433. Ozelo MC, Svirin P, Larina L: Use of recombinant factor VIIa in the management of severe bleeding episodes in patients with Bernard-Soulier syndrome. *Ann Hematol* 84:816, 2005.
434. Miller JL, Cunningham D, Lyle VA, et al: Mutation in the gene encoding the alpha chain of platelet glycoprotein Ib in platelet-type von Willebrand disease. *Proc Natl Acad Sci U S A* 88:4761, 1991.
435. Russell SD, Roth GJ: Pseudo-von Willebrand disease: A mutation in the platelet glycoprotein Ib alpha gene associated with a hyperactive surface receptor. *Blood* 81:1787, 1993.
436. Takahashi H, Murata M, Moriki T, et al: Substitution of Val for Met at residue 239 of platelet glycoprotein Ib alpha in Japanese patients with platelet-type von Willebrand disease. *Blood* 85:727, 1995.
437. Kunishima S, Heaton DC, Naoe T, et al: De novo mutation of the platelet glycoprotein Ib alpha gene in a patient with pseudo-von Willebrand disease. *Blood Coagul Fibrinolysis* 8:311, 1997.
438. Matsubara Y, Murata M, Sugita K, et al: Identification of a novel point mutation in platelet glycoprotein Ibalpha, Gly to Ser at residue 233, in a Japanese family with platelet-type von Willebrand disease. *J Thromb Haemost* 1:2198, 2003.
439. Uff S, Clemetson JM, Harrison T, et al: Crystal structure of the platelet glycoprotein Ib(alpha) N-terminal domain reveals an unmasking mechanism for receptor activation. *J Biol Chem* 277:35657, 2002.
440. Huizinga EG, Tsuji S, Romijn RA, et al: Structures of glycoprotein Ibalpha and its complex with von Willebrand factor A1 domain. *Science* 297:1176, 2002.
441. Pincus MR, Carty RP, Miller JL: Structural implications of the substitution of Val for Met at residue 239 in the alpha chain of human platelet glycoprotein Ib. *J Protein Chem* 13:629, 1994.
442. Dumas JJ, Kumar R, McDonagh T, et al: Crystal structure of the wild-type von Willebrand factor A1-glycoprotein Ibalpha complex reveals conformation differences with a complex bearing von Willebrand disease mutations. *J Biol Chem* 279:23327, 2004.
443. Suva LJ, Hartman E, Dilley JD, et al: Platelet dysfunction and a high bone mass phenotype in a murine model of platelet-type von Willebrand disease. *Am J Pathol* 172:430, 2008.
444. Doggett TA, Girdhar G, Lawshe A, et al: Alterations in the intrinsic properties of the GPIbalpha-VWF tether bond define the kinetics of the platelet-type von Willebrand disease mutation, Gly233Val. *Blood* 102:152, 2003.
445. Tait AS, Cranmer SL, Jackson SP, et al: Phenotype changes resulting in high-affinity binding of von Willebrand factor to recombinant glycoprotein Ib-IX: Analysis of the platelet-type von Willebrand disease mutations. *Blood* 98:1812, 2001.
446. Takahashi H, Nagayama R, Hattori A, et al: Botrocetin- and polybrene-induced platelet aggregation in platelet-type von Willebrand disease. *Am J Hematol* 18:179, 1985.
447. Miller JL, Kupinski JM, Castella A, et al: Von Willebrand factor binds to platelets and induces aggregation in platelet-type but not type IIB von Willebrand disease. *J Clin Invest* 72:1532, 1983.
448. Scott JP, Montgomery RR: The rapid differentiation of type IIb von Willebrand's disease from platelet-type (pseudo-) von Willebrand's disease by the "neutral" monoclonal antibody binding assay. *Am J Clin Pathol* 96:723, 1991.
449. Miller JL: Sorting out heightened interactions between platelets and von Willebrand factor. "IIB or not IIB?" is becoming an increasingly answerable question in the molecular era. *Am J Clin Pathol* 96:681, 1991.
450. Miller JL, Ruggeri ZM, Lyle VA: Unique interactions of asialo von Willebrand factor with platelets in platelet-type von Willebrand disease. *Blood* 70:1804, 1987.
451. Takahashi H: Replacement therapy in platelet-type von Willebrand disease. *Am J Hematol* 18:351, 1985.
452. Miller JL: Platelet-type von Willebrand's disease. *Clin Lab Med* 4:319, 1984.
453. Fressinaud E, Signaud-Fiks M, Le Boterff C, Piot B. Use of recombinant factor VIIa (NovoSeven) for dental extraction in a patient affected by platelet-type (pseudo-) von Willebrand disease. *Haemophilia* 4:299, 1998.
454. Nieuwenhuis HK, Akkerman JWN, Houdijk WPM, et al: Human blood platelets showing no response to collagen fail to express surface glycoprotein Ia. *Nature* 318:470, 1985.
455. Nieuwenhuis HK, Sakariassen KS, Houdijk WPM, et al: Deficiency of platelet membrane glycoprotein Ia associated with a decreased platelet adhesion to subendothelium: A defect in platelet spreading. *Blood* 68:692, 1986.
456. Beer JH, Nieuwenhuis HK, Sixma JJ, Coller BS: Deficiency of antibody 6F1 binding to the platelets of a patient with an isolated defect in platelet-collagen interaction. *Circulation* 78(Suppl):II-308, 1988.
457. Coller BS, Beer JH, Scudder LE, et al: Collagen-platelet interactions: Evidence for a direct interaction of collagen with platelet GPIa/IIa and an indirect interaction with platelet GPIIb/IIa mediated by adhesive proteins. *Blood* 74:182, 1989.
458. Kehrel B, Balleisen L, Kokott R, et al: Deficiency of intact thrombospondin and membrane glycoprotein Ia in platelets with defective collagen-induced aggregation and spontaneous loss of disorder. *Blood* 71:1074, 1988.
459. Yamamoto N, Ikeda H, Tandon NN, et al: A platelet membrane glycoprotein (GP) deficiency in healthy blood donors: Nak[a]-platelets lack detectable GPIV (CD36). *Blood* 76:1698, 1990.
460. Curtis BR, Aster RH: Incidence of the Nak(a)-negative platelet phenotype in African Americans is similar to that of Asians. *Transfusion* 36:331, 1996.
461. Asch AS, Barnwell J, Silverstein RL, et al: Isolation of the thrombospondin membrane receptor. *J Clin Invest* 79:1054, 1987.
462. Tandon NN, Kralisz U, Jamieson GA: Identification of glycoprotein IV (CD36) as a primary receptor for platelet-collagen adhesion. *J Biol Chem* 264:7576, 1989.
462a. Matsuno K, Diaz-Ricart M, Montgomery RR, et al: Inhibition of platelet adhesion to collagen by monoclonal anti-CD36 antibodies. *Br J Haematol* 92:960, 1996.
463. Silverstein RL, Asch AS, Nachman RL: Glycoprotein IV mediates thrombospondin-dependent platelet-monocyte and platelet-U937 cell adhesion. *J Clin Invest* 84:546, 1989.
464. Kehrel B, Kronenberg A, Schwippert B, et al: Thrombospondin binds normally to glycoprotein IIIb deficient platelets. *Biochem Biophys Res Commun* 179:985, 1991.
465. Tandon NN, Ockenhouse CF, Greco NJ, et al: Adhesive functions of platelets lacking glycoprotein IV (CD36). *Blood* 78:2809, 1991.
466. Saelman EU, Kehrel B, Hese KM, et al: Platelet adhesion to collagen and endothelial cell matrix under flow conditions is not dependent on platelet glycoprotein IV. *Blood* 83:3240, 1994.
467. Englyst NA, Taube JM, Aitman TJ, et al: A novel role for CD36 in VLDL-enhanced platelet activation. *Diabetes* 52:1248, 2003.
468. Korporaal SJ, Van EM, Adelmeijer J, et al: Platelet activation by oxidized low density lipoprotein is mediated by CD36 and scavenger receptor-A. *Arterioscler Thromb Vasc Biol* 27:2476, 2007.
469. Podrez EA, Byzova TV, Febbraio M, et al: Platelet CD36 links hyperlipidemia, oxidant stress and a prothrombotic phenotype. *Nat Med* 13:1086, 2007.
470. Chen K, Febbraio M, Li W, et al: A specific CD36-dependent signaling pathway is required for platelet activation by oxidized low-density lipoprotein. *Circ Res* 102:1512, 2008.
471. Kashiwagi H, Tomiyama Y, Honda S, et al: Molecular basis of CD36 deficiency. Evidence that a 478CT substitution (proline90serine) in CD36 cDNA accounts for CD36 deficiency. *J Clin Invest* 95:1040, 1995.
472. Hirano K, Kuwasako T, Nakagawa-Toyama Y, et al: Pathophysiology of human genetic CD36 deficiency. *Trends Cardiovasc Med* 13:136, 2003.
473. Febbraio M, Silverstein RL: CD36: Implications in cardiovascular disease. *Int J Biochem Cell Biol* 39:2012, 2007.
474. Kashiwagi H, Tomiyama Y, Kosugi S, et al: Family studies of type II CD36 deficient subjects: Linkage of a CD36 allele to a platelet-specific mRNA expression defect(s) causing type II CD36 deficiency. *Thromb Haemost* 74:758, 1995.
475. Ikeda H: Platelet membrane protein CD36. *Hokkaido Igaku Zasshi* 74:99, 1999.
476. Kashiwagi H, Tomiyama Y, Kosugi S, et al: Identification of molecular defects in a subject with type I CD36 deficiency. *Blood* 83:3545, 1994.
477. Kashiwagi H, Tomiyama Y, Nozaki S, et al: A single nucleotide insertion in codon 317 of the CD36 gene leads to CD36 deficiency. *Arterioscler Thromb Vasc Biol* 16:1026, 1996.
478. Hanawa H, Watanabe K, Nakamura T, et al: Identification of cryptic splice site, exon skipping, and novel point mutations in type I CD36 deficiency. *J Med Genet* 39:286, 2002.
478a. Curtis BR, Aster RH: Incidence of the Nak(a)-negative platelet phenotype in African Americans is similar to that of Asians. *Transfusion* 36:331, 1996.
479. Bierling P, Godeau B, Fromont P, et al: Posttransfusion purpura-like syndrome associated with CD36 (Naka) isoimmunization. *Transfusion* 35:777, 1995.
479a. Morishita K, Wakamoto S, Miyazaki T: Life-threatening adverse reaction followed by thrombocytopenia after passive transfusion of fresh frozen plasma containing anti-CD36 (Nak) isoantibody. *Transfusion* 45:803, 2005.
480. Nozaki S, Tanaka T, Yamashita S, et al: CD36 mediates long-chain fatty acid transport in human myocardium: Complete myocardial accumulation defect of radiolabeled long-chain fatty acid analog in subjects with CD36 deficiency. *Mol Cell Biochem* 192:129, 1999.
481. Griffin E, Re A, Hamel N, et al: A link between diabetes and atherosclerosis: Glucose regulates expression of CD36 at the level of translation. *Nat Med* 7:840, 2001.
482. Coburn CT, Knapp FF Jr, Febbraio M, et al: Defective uptake and utilization of long chain fatty acids in muscle and adipose tissues of CD36 knockout mice. *J Biol Chem* 275:32523, 2000.
483. Okamoto F, Tanaka T, Sohmiya K, et al: CD36 abnormality and impaired myocardial long-chain fatty acid uptake in patients with hypertrophic cardiomyopathy. *Jpn Circ J* 62:499, 1998.

484. Aitman TJ, Cooper LD, Norsworthy PJ, et al: Malaria susceptibility and CD36 mutation. *Nature* 405:1015, 2000.
485. Omi K, Ohashi J, Patarapotikul J, et al: CD36 polymorphism is associated with protection from cerebral malaria. *Am J Hum Genet* 72:364, 2003.
486. Pain A, Urban BC, Kai O, et al: A non-sense mutation in CD36 gene is associated with protection from severe malaria. *Lancet* 357:1502, 2001.
487. Oquendo P, Hundt E, Lawler J, et al: CD36 directly mediates cytoadherence of Plasmodium falciparum parasitized erythrocytes. *Cell* 58:95, 1989.
488. Pain A, Ferguson DJ, Kai O, et al: Platelet-mediated clumping of Plasmodium falciparum-infected erythrocytes is a common adhesive phenotype and is associated with severe malaria. *Proc Natl Acad Sci U S A* 98:1805, 2001.
489. Moroi M, Jung SM, Okuma M, et al: A patient with platelets deficient in glycoprotein VI that lack both collagen-induced aggregation and adhesion. *J Clin Invest* 84:1440, 1989.
490. Ryo R, Yoshida A, Sugano W, et al: Deficiency of P62, a putative collagen receptor, in platelets from a patient with defective collagen-induced platelet aggregation. *Am J Hematol* 39:25, 1992.
491. Nurden P, Jandrot-Perrus M, Combrie R, et al: Severe deficiency of glycoprotein VI in a patient with gray platelet syndrome. *Blood* 104:107, 2004.
492. Arai M, Yamamoto N, Moroi M, et al: Platelets with 10% of the normal amount of glycoprotein VI have an impaired response to collagen that results in a mild bleeding tendency. *Br J Haematol* 89:124, 1995.
493. Arthur JF, Dunkley S, Andrews RK: Platelet glycoprotein VI-related clinical defects. *Br J Haematol* 139:363, 2007.
494. Chu XX, Hou M: [Advances in the studies of platelet glycoprotein VI (GPVI): Review]. *Zhongguo Shi Yan Xue Ye Xue Za Zhi* 14:1040, 2006.
495. Bellucci S, Huisse MG, Boval B, et al: Defective collagen-induced platelet activation in two patients with malignant haemopathies is related to a defect in the GPVI-coupled signalling pathway. *Thromb Haemost* 93:130, 2005.
496. Kojima H, Moroi M, Jung SM, et al: Characterization of a patient with glycoprotein (GP) VI deficiency possessing neither anti-GPVI autoantibody nor genetic aberration. *J Thromb Haemost* 4:2433, 2006.
497. Dunkley S, Arthur JF, Evans S, et al: A familial platelet function disorder associated with abnormal signalling through the glycoprotein VI pathway. *Br J Haematol* 137:569, 2007.
497a. Hermans C, Wittervrongel C, Thys C, et al: A compound heterozygous mutation in glycoprotein VI in a patient with a bleeding disorder. *J Thromb Haemostas* 7:1356, 2009.
498. Sugiyama T, Okuma M, Ushikubi F, et al: A novel platelet aggregating factor found in a patient with defective collagen-induced platelet aggregation and autoimmune thrombocytopenia. *Blood* 69:1712, 1987.
499. Takahashi H, Moroi M: Antibody against platelet membrane glycoprotein VI in a patient with systemic lupus erythematosus. *Am J Hematol* 67:262, 2001.
500. Boylan B, Chen H, Rathore V, et al: Anti-GPVI-associated ITP: An acquired platelet disorder caused by autoantibody-mediated clearance of the GPVI/FcR{gamma}-chain complex from the human platelet surface. *Blood* 104:1350, 2004.
501. Akiyama M, Kashiwagi H, Todo K, et al: Presence of platelet-associated anti-GPVI autoantibodies and restoration of GPVI expression in patients with GPVI deficiency. *J Thromb Haemost* 7:1373, 2009.
502. Nieswandt B, Schulte V, Bergmeier W, et al: Long-term antithrombotic protection by *in vivo* depletion of platelet glycoprotein VI in mice. *J Exp Med* 193:459, 2001.
503. Weiss HJ, Chervenick PA, Zalusky R, et al: A familial defect in platelet function associated with impaired release of adenosine diphosphate. *N Engl J Med* 281:1264, 1969.
504. Nieuwenhuis HK, Akkerman JW, Sixma JJ: Patients with a prolonged bleeding time and normal aggregation tests may have storage pool deficiency: Studies on one hundred six patients. *Blood* 70:620, 1987.
505. Weiss HJ: Inherited disorders of platelet granules and signal transduction, in *Hemostasis and Thrombosis: Basic Principles and Clinical Practice*, 3rd ed, edited by RW Colman, J Hirsh, VJ Marder, M Samama, p 673. Lippincott, Philadelphia, 1993.
506. Rao SV, O'Grady K, Pieper KS, et al: A comparison of the clinical impact of bleeding measured by two different classifications among patients with acute coronary syndromes. *J Am Coll Cardiol* 47:809, 2006.
507. Huizing M, Helip-Wooley A, Westbroek W, et al: Disorders of lysosome-related organelle biogenesis: Clinical and molecular genetics. *Annu Rev Genomics Hum Genet* 9:359, 2008.
508. Hermansky F, Pudlak P: Albinism associated with hemorrhagic diathesis and unusual pigmented reticular cells in the bone marrow: Report of two cases with histochemical studies. *Blood* 14:162, 1959.
509. Gahl WA, Brantly M, Kaiser-Kupfer MI, et al: Genetic defects and clinical characteristics of patients with a form of oculocutaneous albinism (Hermansky-Pudlak syndrome). *N Engl J Med* 338:1258, 1998.
510. Wei ML: Hermansky-Pudlak syndrome: A disease of protein trafficking and organelle function. *Pigment Cell Res* 19:19, 2006.
511. Di Pietro SM, Dell'Angelica EC: The cell biology of Hermansky-Pudlak syndrome: Recent advances. *Traffic* 6:525, 2005.
512. Gunay-Aygun M, Huizing M, Gahl WA: Molecular defects that affect platelet dense granules. *Semin Thromb Hemost* 30:537, 2004.
513. Buchanan GR, Handin RI: Platelet function in the Chédiak-Higashi syndrome. *Blood* 47:941, 1976.
514. Costa JL, Fauci AS, Wolff SM: A platelet abnormality in the Chédiak-Higashi syndrome of man. *Blood* 48:517, 1976.
515. Boxer GJ, Holmsen H, Robkin L, et al: Abnormal platelet function in Chédiak-Higashi syndrome. *Br J Haematol* 35:521, 1977.
516. Apitz-Castro R, Cruz MR, Ledezma E, et al: The storage pool deficiency in platelets from humans with the Chédiak-Higashi syndrome: Study of six patients. *Br J Haematol* 59:471, 1985.
517. Weiss HJ, Witte LD, Kaplan KL, et al: Heterogeneity in storage pool deficiency: Studies on granule-bound substances in 18 patients including variants deficient in alpha-granules, platelet factor 4, beta-thromboglobulin, and platelet-derived growth factor. *Blood* 54:1296, 1979.
518. Bonifacino JS: Insights into the biogenesis of lysosome-related organelles from the study of the Hermansky-Pudlak syndrome. *Ann N Y Acad Sci* 1038:103, 2004.
519. White JG: Inherited abnormalities of the platelet membrane and secretory granules. *Hum Pathol* 18:123, 1987.
520. Nishibori M, Cham B, McNicol A, et al: The protein CD63 is in platelet dense granules, is deficient in a patient with Hermansky-Pudlak syndrome, and appears identical to granulophysin. *J Clin Invest* 91:1775, 1993.
521. Huizing M, Boissy RE, Gahl WA: Hermansky-Pudlak syndrome: Vesicle formation from yeast to man. *Pigment Cell Res* 15:405, 2002.
522. Huizing M, Parkes JM, Helip-Wooley A, et al: Platelet alpha granules in BLOC-2 and BLOC-3 subtypes of Hermansky-Pudlak syndrome. *Platelets* 18:150, 2007.
523. Hermos CR, Huizing M, Kaiser-Kupfer MI, et al: Hermansky-Pudlak syndrome type 1: Gene organization, novel mutations, and clinical-molecular review of non-Puerto Rican cases. *Hum Mutat* 20:482, 2002.
524. Dell'Angelica EC, Shotelersuk V, Aguilar RC, et al: Altered trafficking of lysosomal proteins in Hermansky-Pudlak syndrome due to mutations in the beta 3A subunit of the AP-3 adaptor. *Mol Cell* 3:11, 1999.
525. Shotelersuk V, Dell'Angelica EC, Hartnell L, et al: A new variant of Hermansky-Pudlak syndrome due to mutations in a gene responsible for vesicle formation. *Am J Med* 108:423, 2000.
526. Huizing M, Anikster Y, Fitzpatrick DL, et al: Hermansky-Pudlak syndrome type 3 in Ashkenazi Jews and other non-Puerto Rican patients with hypopigmentation and platelet storage-pool deficiency. *Am J Hum Genet* 69:1022, 2001.
527. Nazarian R, Falcon-Perez JM, Dell'Angelica EC: Biogenesis of lysosome-related organelles complex 3 (BLOC-3): A complex containing the Hermansky-Pudlak syndrome (HPS) proteins HPS1 and HPS4. *Proc Natl Acad Sci U S A* 100:8770, 2003.
528. Martina JA, Moriyama K, Bonifacino JS: BLOC-3, a protein complex containing the Hermansky-Pudlak syndrome gene products HPS1 and HPS4. *J Biol Chem* 278:29376, 2003.
529. Suzuki T, Li W, Zhang Q, et al: Hermansky-Pudlak syndrome is caused by mutations in HPS4, the human homolog of the mouse light-ear gene. *Nat Genet* 30:321, 2002.
530. Anderson PD, Huizing M, Claassen DA, et al: Hermansky-Pudlak syndrome type 4 (HPS-4): Clinical and molecular characteristics. *Hum Genet* 113:10, 2003.
531. Huizing M, Helip-Wooley A, Dorward H, et al: Hermansky-Pudlak syndrome: A model for abnormal vesicle formation and trafficking. *Pigment Cell Res* 16:584, 2003.
532. Zhang Q, Zhao B, Li W, et al: Ru2 and Ru encode mouse orthologs of the genes mutated in human Hermansky-Pudlak syndrome types 5 and 6. *Nat Genet* 33:145, 2003.
533. Helip-Wooley A, Westbroek W, Dorward HM, et al: Improper trafficking of melanocyte-specific proteins in Hermansky-Pudlak syndrome type-5. *J Invest Dermatol* 127:1471, 2007.
534. Li W, Zhang Q, Oiso N, et al: Hermansky-Pudlak syndrome type 7 (HPS-7) results from mutant dysbindin, a member of the biogenesis of lysosome-related organelles complex 1 (BLOC-1). *Nat Genet* 35:84, 2003.
535. Morgan NV, Pasha S, Johnson CA, et al: A germline mutation in BLOC1S3/reduced pigmentation causes a novel variant of Hermansky-Pudlak syndrome (HPS8). *Am J Hum Genet* 78:160, 2006.
536. Contopoulos-Ioannidis D, Evangeliou A, ter LH, et al: Recurrent rhabdomyolysis in a patient with oculocutaneous albinism type 1 and platelet storage-pool deficiency. *Am J Med Genet A* 146A:3100, 2008.
537. Payne CM: A qualitative ultrastructural evaluation of the cell organelle specificity of the uranaffin reaction to normal human platelets. *Am J Clin Pathol* 31:62, 1984.
538. Weiss HJ, Lages B, Vicic W, et al: Heterogeneous abnormalities of platelet dense granule ultrastructure in 20 patients with congenital storage pool deficiency. *Br J Haematol* 83:282, 1993.
539. Huizing M, Anikster Y, Gahl WA: Hermansky-Pudlak syndrome and Chédiak-Higashi syndrome: Disorders of vesicle formation and trafficking. *Thromb Haemost* 86:233, 2001.
540. White RA, Peters LL, Adkison LR, et al: The murine pallid mutation is a platelet storage pool disease associated with the protein 4.2 (pallidin) gene. *Nat Genet* 2:80, 1992.
541. Swank RT, Novak EK, McGarry MP, et al: Mouse models of Hermansky Pudlak syndrome: A review. *Pigment Cell Res* 11:60, 1998.
542. Shotelersuk V, Gahl WA: Hermansky-Pudlak syndrome: Models for intracellular vesicle formation. *Mol Genet Metab* 65:85, 1998.
543. Novak EK, Gautam R, Reddington M, et al: The regulation of platelet-dense granules by Rab27a in the ashen mouse, a model of Hermansky-Pudlak and Griscelli syndromes, is granule-specific and dependent on genetic background. *Blood* 100:128, 2002.
544. Suzuki T, Oiso N, Gautam R, et al: The mouse organellar biogenesis mutant buff results from a mutation in Vps33a, a homologue of yeast vps33 and *Drosophila* carnation. *Proc Natl Acad Sci U S A* 100:1146, 2003.

545. Zhen L, Jiang S, Feng L, et al: Abnormal expression and subcellular distribution of subunit proteins of the AP-3 adaptor complex lead to platelet storage pool deficiency in the pearl mouse. *Blood* 94:146, 1999.
546. Gautam R, Chintala S, Li W, et al: The Hermansky-Pudlak syndrome 3 (cocoa) protein is a component of the biogenesis of lysosome-related organelles complex-2 (BLOC-2). *J Biol Chem* 279:12935, 2004.
547. Spritz RA: Genetic defects in Chédiak-Higashi syndrome and the beige mouse. *J Clin Immunol* 18:97, 1998.
548. Hardisty RM, Mills DC, Ketsa-Ard K: The platelet defect associated with albinism. *Br J Haematol* 23:679, 1972.
549. Harrison C, Khair K, Baxter B, et al: Hermansky-Pudlak syndrome: Infrequent bleeding and first report of Turkish and Pakistani kindreds. *Arch Dis Child* 86:297, 2002.
550. Akkerman JW, Nieuwenhuis HK, Mommersteeg-Leautaud ME, et al: ATP-ADP compartmentation in storage pool deficient platelets: Correlation between granule-bound ADP and the bleeding time. *Br J Haematol* 55:135, 1983.
551. Cattaneo M, Lecchi A, Agati B, et al: Evaluation of platelet function with the PFA-100 system in patients with congenital defects of platelet secretion. *Thromb Res* 96:213, 1999.
552. White MM, Foust JT, Mauer AM, et al: Assessment of lumiaggregometry for research and clinical laboratories. *Thromb Haemost* 67:572, 1992.
553. Cattaneo M: Light transmission aggregometry and ATP release for the diagnostic assessment of platelet function. *Semin Thromb Hemost* 35:158, 2009.
554. Pareti FI, Day HJ, Mills DC: Nucleotide and serotonin metabolism in platelets with defective secondary aggregation. *Blood* 44:789, 1974.
555. Weiss HJ, Tschopp TB, Rogers J, et al: Studies of platelet 5-hydroxytryptamine (serotonin) in storage pool disease and albinism. *J Clin Invest* 54:421, 1974.
556. Willis AL, Weiss HJ: A congenital defect in platelet prostaglandin production associated with impaired hemostasis in storage pool disease. *Prostaglandins* 4:783, 1973.
557. Holmsen H, Setkowsky CA, Lages B, et al: Content and thrombin-induced release of acid hydrolases in gel-filtered platelets from patients with storage pool disease. *Blood* 46:131, 1975.
558. Weiss HJ, Lages B: Platelet malondialdehyde production and aggregation responses induced by arachidonate, prostaglandin-G2, collagen, and epinephrine in 12 patients with storage pool deficiency. *Blood* 58:27, 1981.
559. Witkop CJ Jr, Bowie EJ, Krumwiede MD, et al: Synergistic effect of storage pool deficient platelets and low plasma von Willebrand factor on the severity of the hemorrhagic diathesis in Hermansky-Pudlak syndrome. *Am J Hematol* 44:256, 1993.
560. McKeown LP, Hansmann KE, Wilson O, et al: Platelet von Willebrand factor in Hermansky-Pudlak syndrome. *Am J Hematol* 59:115, 1998.
561. Israels SJ, McNicol A, Robertson C, et al: Platelet storage pool deficiency: Diagnosis in patients with prolonged bleeding times and normal platelet aggregation. *Br J Haematol* 75:118, 1990.
562. Witkop CJ, Krumwiede M, Sedano H, et al: Reliability of absent platelet dense bodies as a diagnostic criterion for Hermansky-Pudlak syndrome. *Am J Hematol* 26:305, 1987.
563. White JG: Electron opaque structures in human platelets: Which are or are not dense bodies? *Platelets* 19:455, 2008.
564. Hayward CP, Moffat KA, Spitzer E, et al: Results of an external proficiency testing exercise on platelet dense-granule deficiency testing by whole mount electron microscopy. *Am J Clin Pathol* 131:671, 2009.
565. White JG, Witkop CJ: Studies of platelets in a variant of the Hermansky-Pudlak syndrome. *Am J Pathol* 63:319, 1971.
566. Weiss HJ, Ames RP: Ultrastructural findings in storage-pool disease and aspirin-like defects in platelets. *Am J Pathol* 71:447, 1973.
567. Richards JG, DaPrada M: Uranaffin reaction: A new cytochemical technique for the localization of adenine nucleotides in organelles storing biogenic amines. *J Histochem Cytochem* 25:1322, 1977.
568. Lorez HP, Richards JG, Da Prada M, et al: Storage pool disease: Comparative fluorescence microscopical, cytochemical and biochemical studies on amine-storing organelles of human blood platelets. *Br J Haematol* 43:297, 1979.
569. Gordon N, Thom J, Cole C, et al: Rapid detection of hereditary and acquired platelet storage pool deficiency by flow cytometry. *Br J Haematol* 89:117, 1995.
570. Nazarian R, Huizing M, Helip-Wooley A, et al: An immunoblotting assay to facilitate the molecular diagnosis of Hermansky-Pudlak syndrome. *Mol Genet Metab* 93:134, 2008.
571. Mielke CH Jr, Levine PH, Zucker S: Preoperative prednisone therapy in platelet function disorders. *Thromb Res* 21:655, 1981.
572. Rao AK, Ghosh S, Sun L, et al: Mechanisms of platelet dysfunction and response to DDAVP in patients with congenital platelet function defects. A double-blind placebo-controlled trial. *Thromb Haemost* 74:1071, 1995.
573. Kobrinsky NL, Israels ED, Gerrard JM, et al: Shortening of bleeding time by 1-deamino-8-D-arginine vasopressin in various bleeding disorders. *Lancet* 1:1145, 1984.
574. Nieuwenhuis HK, Sixma JJ: 1-Desamino-8-D-arginine vasopressin (desmopressin) shortens the bleeding time in storage pool deficiency. *Ann Intern Med* 108:65, 1988.
575. Wijermans PW, van Dorp DB: Hermansky-Pudlak syndrome: Correction of bleeding time by 1-desamino-8D-arginine vasopressin. *Am J Hematol* 30:154, 1989.
576. van Dorp DB, Wijermans PW, Meire F, et al: The Hermansky-Pudlak syndrome. Variable reaction to 1-desamino-8D-arginine vasopressin for correction of the bleeding time. *Ophthalmic Paediatr Genet* 11:237, 1990.
577. Castaman G, Rodeghiero F: Consistency of responses to separate desmopressin infusion in patients with storage pool disease and isolated prolonged bleeding time. *Thromb Res* 69:407, 1993.
578. Zatik J, Poka R, Borsos A, et al: Variable response of Hermansky-Pudlak syndrome to prophylactic administration of 1-desamino 8D-arginine in subsequent pregnancies. *Eur J Obstet Gynecol Reprod Biol* 104:165, 2002.
579. Spencer J, Rosengren S: Hermansky-Pudlak syndrome in pregnancy. *Am J Perinatol* 26:617, 2009.
580. Gerritsen SW, Akkerman JW, Sixma JJ: Correction of the bleeding time in patients with storage pool deficiency by infusion of cryoprecipitate. *Br J Haematol* 40:153, 1978.
581. Coller BS, Hirschman RJ, Gralnick HR: Studies of the factor VIII/von Willebrand factor antigen on human platelets. *Thromb Res* 6:469, 1975.
582. George JN, Pickett EB, Heinz R: Platelet membrane microparticles in blood bank fresh frozen plasma and cryoprecipitate. *Blood* 68:307, 1986.
583. Wax JR, Rosengren S, Spector E, et al: DNA diagnosis and management of Hermansky-Pudlak syndrome in pregnancy. *Am J Perinatol* 18:159, 2001.
584. Pozo Pozo AI, Jimenez-Yuste V, Villar A, et al: Successful thyroidectomy in a patient with Hermansky-Pudlak syndrome treated with recombinant activated factor VII and platelet concentrates. *Blood Coagul Fibrinolysis* 13:551, 2002.
585. Raccuglia G: Gray platelet syndrome. A variety of qualitative platelet disorder. *Am J Med* 51:818, 1971.
586. Gerrard JM, Phillips DR, Rao GH, et al: Biochemical studies of two patients with the gray platelet syndrome. Selective deficiency of platelet alpha granules. *J Clin Invest* 66:102, 1980.
587. Levy-Toledano S, Caen JP, Breton-Gorius J, et al: Gray platelet syndrome: Alpha-granule deficiency. Its influence on platelet function. *J Lab Clin Med* 98:831, 1981.
588. Nurden AT, Kunicki TJ, Dupuis D, et al: Specific protein and glycoprotein deficiencies in platelets isolated from two patients with the gray platelet syndrome. *Blood* 59:709, 1982.
589. Coller BS, Hultin MB, Nurden AT. Isolated alpha-granule deficiency (gray platelet syndrome) with slight increase in bone marrow reticulin and possible glycoprotein and/or protease defect. *Thromb Haemost* 50:211, 1983.
590. Kohler M, Hellstern P, Morgenstern E, et al: Gray platelet syndrome: Selective alpha-granule deficiency and thrombocytopenia due to increased platelet turnover. *Blut* 50:331, 1985.
591. Berndt MC, Castaldi PA, Gordon S, et al: Morphological and biochemical confirmation of gray platelet syndrome in two siblings. *Aust N Z J Med* 13:387, 1983.
592. Gootenberg JE, Buchanan GR, Holtkamp CA, et al: Severe hemorrhage in a patient with gray platelet syndrome. *J Pediatr* 109:1017, 1986.
593. Srivastava PC, Powling MJ, Nokes TJ, et al: Grey platelet syndrome: Studies on platelet alpha-granules, lysosomes and defective response to thrombin. *Br J Haematol* 65:441, 1987.
594. Berrebi A, Klepfish A, Varon D, et al: Gray platelet syndrome in the elderly. *Am J Hematol* 28:270, 1988.
595. Wills EJ: Gray platelet syndrome. *Ultrastruct Pathol* 13:451, 1989.
596. Facon T, Goudemand J, Caron C, et al: Simultaneous occurrence of grey platelet syndrome and idiopathic pulmonary fibrosis: A role for abnormal megakaryocytes in the pathogenesis of pulmonary fibrosis? *Br J Haematol* 74:542, 1990.
597. Lages B, Sussman II, Levine SP, et al: Platelet alpha granule deficiency associated with decreased P-selectin and selective impairment of thrombin-induced activation in a new patient with gray platelet syndrome (alpha-storage pool deficiency). *J Lab Clin Med* 129:364, 1997.
598. Martinez-Murillo C, Payns BE, Arzate HG, et al: Gray-platelet syndrome associated with Marfan disease in a Mexican family. *Sangre (Barc)* 39:287, 1994.
599. Jantunen E, Hanninen A, Naukkarinen A, et al: Gray platelet syndrome with splenomegaly and signs of extramedullary hematopoiesis: A case report with review of the literature. *Am J Hematol* 46:218, 1994.
600. Alkhairy KS: The gray platelet syndrome of four members of a Palestinian Arab family. *Emirates Medical Journal* 13:137, 1995.
601. Lutz P, Roth-Pougheon A, Wiesel ML, et al: [Gray platelet syndrome]. *Arch Fr Pediatr* 49:637, 1992.
602. Drouin A, Favier R, Masse JM, et al: Newly recognized cellular abnormalities in the gray platelet syndrome. *Blood* 98:1382, 2001.
603. Falik-Zaccai TC, Anikster Y, Rivera CE, et al: A new genetic isolate of gray platelet syndrome (GPS): Clinical, cellular, and hematologic characteristics. *Mol Genet Metab* 74:303, 2001.
604. Elliott MA, White JG, Charlesworth JE, et al: Gray platelet syndrome (GPS) in a Native American female. *Thromb Haemost* 508:(Suppl S), 1999.
605. Laskey AL, Tobias JD: Anesthetic complications of the gray platelet syndrome. *Can J Anaesth* 47:1224, 2000.
606. Nurden AT, Nurden P, Bermejo E, et al: Phenotypic heterogeneity in the Gray platelet syndrome extends to the expression of TREM family member, TLT-1. *Thromb Haemost* 100:45, 2008.
607. Nurden AT, Nurden P: The gray platelet syndrome: Clinical spectrum of the disease. *Blood Rev* 21:21, 2007.
608. Mori K, Suzuki S, Sugai K: Electron microscopic and functional studies on platelets in gray platelet syndrome. *Tohoku J Exp Med* 143:261, 1984.
609. Berger G, Masse JM, Cramer EM: Alpha-granule membrane mirrors the platelet plasma membrane and contains the glycoproteins Ib, IX, and V. *Blood* 87:1385, 1996.

610. Rosa JP, George JN, Bainton DF, et al: Gray platelet syndrome. Demonstration of alpha granule membranes that can fuse with the cell surface. *J Clin Invest* 80:1138, 1987.
611. Cramer EM, Vainchenker W, Vinci G, et al: Gray platelet syndrome: Immunoelectron microscopic localization of fibrinogen and von Willebrand factor in platelets and megakaryocytes. *Blood* 66:1309, 1985.
612. Caen JP, Deschamps JF, Bodevin E, et al: Megakaryocytes and myelofibrosis in gray platelet syndrome. *Nouv Rev Fr Hematol* 29:109, 1987.
613. Schmitt A, Jouault H, Guichard J, et al: Pathologic interaction between megakaryocytes and polymorphonuclear leukocytes in myelofibrosis. *Blood* 96:1342, 2000.
614. Wencel-Drake JD: Plasma membrane GPIIb/IIIa. Evidence for a cycling receptor pool. *Am J Clin Pathol* 136:61, 1990.
615. Tubman VN, Levine JE, Campagna DR, et al: X-linked gray platelet syndrome due to a GATA1 Arg216Gln mutation. *Blood* 109:3297, 2007.
616. Steinberg MH, Kelton JG, Coller BS: Plasma glycocalicin: An aid in the classification of thrombocytopenic disorders. *N Engl J Med* 317:1037, 1987.
617. Greenberg-Sepersky SM, Simons ER, White JG: Studies of platelets from patients with the grey platelet syndrome. *Br J Haematol* 59:603, 1985.
618. Rendu F, Marche P, Hovig T, et al: Abnormal phosphoinositide metabolism and protein phosphorylation in platelets from a patient with the grey platelet syndrome. *Br J Haematol* 67:199, 1987.
619. Baruch D, Lindhout T, Dupuy E, et al: Thrombin-induced platelet factor Va formation in patients with a gray platelet syndrome. *Thromb Haemost* 58:768, 1987.
620. Enouf J, Lebret M, Bredoux R, et al: Abnormal calcium transport into microsomes of grey platelet syndrome. *Br J Haematol* 65:437, 1987.
621. Cockbill SR, Burmester HB, Heptinstall S: Pseudo grey platelet syndrome—Grey platelets due to degranulation in blood collected into EDTA. *Eur J Haematol* 41:326, 1988.
622. Pfueller SL, Howard MA, White JG, et al: Shortening of bleeding time by 1-deamino-8-arginine vasopressin (DDAVP) in the absence of platelet von Willebrand factor in Gray platelet syndrome. *Thromb Haemost* 58:1060, 1987.
623. Lages B, Shattil SJ, Bainton DF, et al: Decreased content and surface expression of alpha-granule membrane protein GMP-140 in one of two types of platelet alpha delta storage pool deficiency. *J Clin Invest* 87:919, 1991.
624. Weiss HJ, Lages B: The response of platelets to epinephrine in storage pool deficiency—Evidence pertaining to the role of adenosine diphosphate in mediating primary and secondary aggregation. *Blood* 72:1717, 1988.
625. Jamieson GA, Okumara T, Fishback B, et al: Platelet membrane glycoproteins in thrombasthenia, Bernard-Soulier syndrome, and storage pool disease. *J Lab Clin Med* 93:652, 1979.
626. Gerrard JM, McNicol A: Platelet storage pool deficiency, leukemia, and myelodysplastic syndromes. *Leuk Lymphoma* 8:277, 1992.
627. Tracy PB, Giles AR, Mann KG, et al: Factor V (Quebec): A bleeding diathesis associated with a qualitative platelet Factor V deficiency. *J Clin Invest* 74:1221, 1984.
628. Janeway CM, Rivard GE, Tracy PB, et al: Factor V Quebec revisited. *Blood* 87:3571, 1996.
629. Weiss HJ: Impaired platelet procoagulant mechanisms in patients with bleeding disorders. *Semin Thromb Hemost* 35:233, 2009.
630. Hayward CP, Rivard GE, Kane WH, et al: An autosomal dominant, qualitative platelet disorder associated with multimerin deficiency, abnormalities in platelet factor V, thrombospondin, von Willebrand factor, and fibrinogen and an epinephrine aggregation defect. *Blood* 87:4967, 1996.
631. Veljkovic DK, Rivard GE, Diamandis M, et al: Increased expression of urokinase plasminogen activator in Quebec platelet disorder is linked to megakaryocyte differentiation. *Blood* 113:1535, 2009.
632. Diamandis M, Paterson AD, Rommens JM, et al: Quebec platelet disorder is linked to the urokinase plasminogen activator gene (PLAU) and increases expression of the linked allele in megakaryocytes. *Blood* 113:1543, 2009.
633. Kahr WH, Zheng S, Sheth PM, et al: Platelets from patients with the Quebec platelet disorder contain and secrete abnormal amounts of urokinase-type plasminogen activator. *Blood* 98:257, 2001.
634. Sheth PM, Kahr WH, Haq MA, et al: Intracellular activation of the fibrinolytic cascade in the Quebec platelet disorder. *Thromb Haemost* 90:293, 2003.
635. McKay H, Derome F, Haq MA, et al: Bleeding Risks Associated with Inheritance of the Quebec Platelet Disorder. *Blood* 104:159, 2004.
636. Weiss HJ, Vicic WJ, Lages BA, et al: Isolated deficiency of platelet procoagulant activity. *Am J Med* 67:206, 1979.
637. Weiss HJ: Scott syndrome—A disorder of platelet coagulant activity. *Semin Hematol* 31:312, 1994.
638. Toti F, Satta N, Fressinaud E, et al: Scott syndrome, characterized by impaired transmembrane migration of procoagulant phosphatidylserine and hemorrhagic complications, is an inherited disorder. *Blood* 87:1409, 1996.
639. Weiss HJ, Lages B: Platelet prothrombinase activity and intracellular calcium responses in patients with storage pool deficiency, glycoprotein IIb-IIIa deficiency, or impaired platelet coagulant activity—A comparison with Scott syndrome. *Blood* 89:1599, 1997.
640. Dachary-Prigent J, Pasquet JM, Fressinaud E, et al: Aminophospholipid exposure, microvesiculation and abnormal protein tyrosine phosphorylation in the platelets of a patient with Scott syndrome: A study using physiologic agonists and local anaesthetics. *Br J Haematol* 99:959, 1997.
641. Zwaal RF, Comfurius P, Bevers EM: Scott syndrome, a bleeding disorder caused by defective scrambling of membrane phospholipids. *Biochim Biophys Acta* 1636:119, 2004.
642. Munnix IC, Harmsma M, Giddings JC, et al: Store-mediated calcium entry in the regulation of phosphatidylserine exposure in blood cells from Scott patients. *Thromb Haemost* 89:687, 2003.
643. Solum NO: Procoagulant expression in platelets and defects leading to clinical disorders. *Arterioscler Thromb Vasc Biol* 19:2841, 1999.
644. Weiss HJ: Platelet aggregation, adhesion and adenosine diphosphate release in thrombopathia (platelet factor 3 deficiency). A comparison with Glanzmann's thrombasthenia and von Willebrand's disease. *Am J Med* 43:570, 1967.
645. Sims PJ, Wiedmer T, Esmon CT, et al: Assembly of the platelet prothrombinase complex is linked to vesiculation on the platelet plasma membrane. Studies in Scott syndrome: An isolated defect in platelet procoagulant activity. *J Biol Chem* 264:137, 1989.
646. Miletich JP, Kane WH, Hofmann SL, et al: Deficiency of factor Xa-factor Va binding sites on the platelets of a patient with a bleeding disorder. *Blood* 54:1015, 1979.
647. Rosing J, Bevers EM, Comfurius P, et al: Impaired factor X and prothrombin activation associated with decreased phospholipid exposure in platelets from a patient with a bleeding disorder. *Blood* 65:1557, 1985.
648. Ahmad SS, Rawala-Sheikh R, Ashby B, et al: Platelet receptor-mediated factor X activation by factor IXa. High- affinity factor IXa receptors induced by factor VIII are deficient on platelets in Scott syndrome. *J Clin Invest* 84:824, 1989.
649. Bevers EM, Wiedmer T, Comfurius P, et al: Defective Ca(2+)-induced microvesiculation and deficient expression of procoagulant activity in erythrocytes from a patient with a bleeding disorder: A study of the red blood cells of Scott syndrome. *Blood* 79:380, 1992.
650. Kojima H, Newton-Nash D, Weiss HJ, et al: Production and characterization of transformed B-lymphocytes expressing the membrane defect of Scott syndrome. *J Clin Invest* 94:2237, 1994.
651. Zhou Q, Sims PJ, Wiedmer T: Expression of proteins controlling transbilayer movement of plasma membrane phospholipids in the B lymphocytes from a patient with Scott syndrome. *Blood* 92:1707, 1998.
652. Stout JG, Basse F, Luhm RA, et al: Scott syndrome erythrocytes contain a membrane protein capable of mediating Ca2+-dependent transbilayer migration of membrane phospholipids. *J Clin Invest* 99:2232, 1997.
653. Albrecht C, McVey JH, Elliott JI, et al: A novel missense mutation in ABCA1 results in altered protein trafficking and reduced phosphatidylserine translocation in a patient with Scott syndrome. *Blood* 106:542, 2005.
654. Castaman G, Yu-Feng L, Battistin E, et al: Characterization of a novel bleeding disorder with isolated prolonged bleeding time and deficiency of platelet microvesicle generation. *Br J Haematol* 96:458, 1997.
655. Rao AK: Hereditary disorders of platelet secretion and signal transduction, in *Hemostasis and Thrombosis: Basic Principles and Clinical Practice*, 5th ed, edited by RW Colman, VJ Marder, AW Clowes, JN George, SZ Goldhaber, p 961. Lippincott Williams & Wilkins, Philadelphia, 2006.
656. Rao AK, Jalagadugula G, Sun L: Inherited defects in platelet signaling mechanisms. *Semin Thromb Hemost* 30:525, 2004.
657. Rao AK: Inherited defects in platelet signaling mechanisms. *J Thromb Haemost* 1:671, 2003.
658. Hirata T, Ushikubi F, Kakizuka A, et al: Two thromboxane A2 receptor isoforms in human platelets. Opposite coupling to adenylyl cyclase with different sensitivity to Arg60 to Leu mutation. *J Clin Invest* 97:949, 1996.
659. Hirata T, Kakizuka A, Ushikubi F, et al: Arg60 to Leu mutation of the human thromboxane A2 receptor in a dominantly inherited bleeding disorder. *J Clin Invest* 94:1662, 1994.
660. Higuchi W, Fuse I, Hattori A, et al: Mutations of the platelet thromboxane A2 (TXA2) receptor in patients characterized by the absence of TXA2-induced platelet aggregation despite normal TXA2 binding activity. *Thromb Haemost* 82:1528, 1999.
661. Cattaneo M: The platelet P2 receptors, in *Platelets*, 2nd ed, edited by AD Michelson, p 201. Academic Press, San Diego, 2007.
662. Gachet C: P2 receptors, platelet function and pharmacological implications. *Thromb Haemost* 99:466, 2008.
663. Cattaneo M, Lecchi A, Randi AM, et al: Identification of a new congenital defect of platelet function characterized by severe impairment of platelet responses to adenosine diphosphate. *Blood* 80:2787, 1992.
664. Nurden P, Savi P, Heilmann E, et al: An inherited bleeding disorder linked to a defective interaction between ADP and its receptor on platelets. Its influence on glycoprotein IIb-IIIa complex function. *J Clin Invest* 95:1612, 1995.
665. Shiraga M, Miyata S, Kato H, et al: Impaired platelet function in a patient with P2Y12 deficiency caused by a mutation in the translation initiation codon. *J Thromb Haemost* 3:2315, 2005.
666. Daly ME, Dawood BB, Lester WA, et al: Identification and characterization of a novel P2Y 12 variant in a patient diagnosed with type 1 von Willebrand disease in the European MCMDM-1VWD study. *Blood* 113:4110, 2009.
667. Cattaneo M, Lecchi A, Lombardi R, et al: Platelets from a patient heterozygous for the defect of P2CYC receptors for ADP have a secretion defect despite normal thromboxane A2 production and normal granule stores: Further evidence that some cases of platelet 'primary secretion defect' are heterozygous for a defect of P2CYC receptors. *Arterioscler Thromb Vasc Biol* 20:E101, 2000.
667a. Fontana G, Ware J, Cattaneo M: Haploinsufficiency of the platelet *P2Y12* gene in a family with congenital bleeding diathesis. *Haematologica* 94:581, 2009.

668. Nurden P, Savi P, Heilmann E, et al: An inherited bleeding disorder linked to a defective interaction between ADP and its receptor on platelets. Its influence on glycoprotein IIb-IIIa complex function. *J Clin Invest* 95:1612, 1995.
669. Cattaneo M, Zighetti ML, Lombardi R, et al: Molecular bases of defective signal transduction in the platelet P2Y12 receptor of a patient with congenital bleeding. *Proc Natl Acad Sci U S A* 100:1978, 2003.
670. Cattaneo M, Lombardi R, Zighetti ML, et al: Deficiency of (33)P-2MeS-ADP binding sites on platelets with secretion defect, normal granule stores and normal thromboxane A2 production. *Thromb Haemost* 77:986, 1997.
671. Cattaneo M, Lecchi A, Lombardi R, et al: Platelets from a patient heterozygous for the defect of P2(CYC) receptors for ADP have a secretion defect despite normal thromboxane A(2) production and normal granule stores: Further evidence that some cases of platelet 'Primary secretion Defect' are heterozygous for a defect of P2(CYC) receptors. *Arterioscler Thromb Vasc Biol* 20:E101, 2000.
672. Cattaneo M: Inherited platelet-based bleeding disorders. *J Thromb Haemost* 1:1628, 2003.
673. Hollopeter G, Jantzen HM, Vincent D, et al: Identification of the platelet ADP receptor targeted by antithrombotic drugs. *Nature* 409:202, 2001.
674. Remijn JA, Ijsseldijk MJ, Strunk AL, et al: Novel molecular defect in the platelet ADP receptor P2Y12 of a patient with haemorrhagic diathesis. *Clin Chem Lab Med* 45:187, 2007.
675. Oury C, Toth-Zsamboki E, Van Geet C, et al: A natural dominant negative P2X1 receptor due to deletion of a single amino acid residue. *J Biol Chem* 275:22611, 2000.
676. Oury C, Lenaerts T, Peerlinck K, Vermylen J. Congential deficiency of the phospholipase C coupled platelet P2Y1 receptor leads to a mild bleeding disorder. *Thromb Haemost* 82:20, 1999.
677. Rao AK: Congenital disorders of platelet function: Disorders of signal transduction and secretion. *Am J Med Sci* 316:69, 1998.
678. Scrutton MC, Clare KA, Hutton RA, et al: Depressed responsiveness to adrenaline in platelets from apparently normal human donors: A familial trait. *Br J Haematol* 49:303, 1981.
679. Tamponi G, Pannocchia A, Arduino C, et al: Congenital deficiency of alpha-2-adrenoceptors on human platelets: Description of two cases. *Thromb Haemost* 58:1012, 1987.
680. Rao AK, Willis J, Kowalska MA, et al: Differential requirements for platelet aggregation and inhibition of adenylate cyclase by epinephrine. Studies of a familial platelet alpha 2-adrenergic receptor defect. *Blood* 71:494, 1988.
681. Pelczar-Wissner CJ, McDonald EG, Sussman II: Absence of platelet activating factor (PAF) mediated platelet aggregation: A new platelet defect. *Am J Hematol* 16:419, 1984.
682. Gabbeta J, Yang X, Kowalska MA, et al: Platelet signal transduction defect with Galpha subunit dysfunction and diminished Galphaq in a patient with abnormal platelet responses. *Proc Natl Acad Sci U S A* 94:8750, 1997.
683. Gabbeta J, Vaidyula VR, Dhanasekaran DN, et al: Human platelet Gaq deficiency is associated with decreased Gaq gene expression in platelets but not neutrophils. *Thromb Haemost* 87:129, 2002.
684. Offermanns S, Toombs CF, Hu YH, et al: Defective platelet activation in G alpha(q)-deficient mice. *Nature* 389:183, 1997.
685. Freson K, Hoylaerts MF, Jaeken J, et al: Genetic variation of the extra-large stimulatory G protein alpha-subunit leads to Gs hyperfunction in platelets and is a risk factor for bleeding. *Thromb Haemost* 86:733, 2001.
686. Freson K, Thys C, Wittevrongel C, et al: Pseudohypoparathyroidism type Ib with disturbed imprinting in the GNAS1 cluster and Gsalpha deficiency in platelets. *Hum Mol Genet* 11:2741, 2002.
687. Patel YM, Patel K, Rahman S, et al: Evidence for a role for Galphai1 in mediating weak agonist-induced platelet aggregation in human platelets: Reduced Galphai1 expression and defective Gi signaling in the platelets of a patient with a chronic bleeding disorder. *Blood* 101:4828, 2003.
688. Lages B, Weiss HJ: Heterogeneous defects of platelet secretion and responses to weak agonists in patients with bleeding disorders. *Br J Haematol* 68:53, 1988.
689. Koike K, Rao AK, Holmsen H, et al: Platelet secretion defect in patients with the attention deficit disorder and easy bruising. *Blood* 63:427, 1984.
690. Yang X, Sun L, Gabbeta J, et al: Platelet activation with combination of ionophore A23187 and a direct protein kinase C activator induces normal secretion in patients with impaired receptor mediated secretion and abnormal signal transduction. *Thromb Res* 88:317, 1997.
691. Yang X, Sun L, Ghosh S, et al: Human platelet signaling defect characterized by impaired production of inositol-1,4,5-triphosphate and phosphatidic acid and diminished Pleckstrin phosphorylation: Evidence for defective phospholipase C activation. *Blood* 88:1676, 1996.
692. Lee SB, Rao AK, Lee KH, et al: Decreased expression of phospholipase C-beta 2 isozyme in human platelets with impaired function. *Blood* 88:1684, 1996.
693. Sun L, Mao G, Rao AK: Association of CBFA2 mutation with decreased platelet PKC-theta and impaired receptor-mediated activation of GPIIb-IIIa and pleckstrin phosphorylation: Proteins regulated by CBFA2 play a role in GPIIb-IIIa activation. *Blood* 103:948, 2004.
694. Lages B, Weiss HJ: Impairment of phosphatidylinositol metabolism in a patient with a bleeding disorder associated with defects of initial platelet responses. *Thromb Haemost* 59:175, 1988.
695. Speiser-Ellerton S, Weiss HJ: Studies on platelet protein phosphorylation in patients with impaired responses to platelet agonists. *J Lab Clin Med* 115:104, 1990.
696. Mao GF, Vaidyula VR, Kunapuli SP, et al: Lineage-specific defect in gene expression in human platelet phospholipase C-beta2 deficiency. *Blood* 99:905, 2002.
697. Mao GF, Kunapuli SP, Rao AK: NF-κB regulates platelet PLC-β2 expression studies in human platelet PLC-β2 deficiency. *Thromb Haemost* 5(Suppl 2):22, 2007.
698. Holmsen H, Walsh PN, Koike K, et al: Familial bleeding disorder associated with deficiencies in platelet signal processing and glycoproteins. *Br J Haematol* 67:335, 1987.
699. Cartwright J, Hampton KK, Macneil S, et al: A haemorrhagic platelet disorder associated with altered stimulus-response coupling and abnormal membrane phospholipid composition. *Br J Haematol* 88:129, 1994.
700. Fuse I, Mito M, Hattori A, et al: Defective signal transduction induced by thromboxane A2 in a patient with a mild bleeding disorder: Impaired phospholipase C activation despite normal phospholipase A2 activation. *Blood* 81:994, 1993.
701. Mitsui T: Defective signal transduction through the thromboxane A2 receptor in a patient with a mild bleeding disorder. Deficiency of the inositol 1,4,5-triphosphate formation despite normal G-protein activation. *Thromb Haemost* 77:991, 1997.
702. Gabbeta J, Yang X, Sun L, et al: Abnormal inside-out signal transduction-dependent activation of glycoprotein IIb-IIIa in a patient with impaired pleckstrin phosphorylation. *Blood* 87:1368, 1996.
703. Song WJ, Sullivan MG, Legare RD, et al: Haploinsufficiency of CBFA2 causes familial thrombocytopenia with propensity to develop acute myelogenous leukaemia. *Nat Genet* 23:166, 1999.
704. Sun L, Gorospe JR, Hoffman EP, et al: Decreased platelet expression of myosin regulatory light chain polypeptide (MYL9) and other genes with platelet dysfunction and CBFA2/RUNX1 mutation: Insights from platelet expression profiling. *J Thromb Haemost* 5:146, 2007.
705. Rendu F, Breton-Gorius J, Trugnan G, et al: Studies on a new variant of the Hermansky-Pudlak syndrome: Qualitative, ultrastructural, and functional abnormalities of the platelet-dense bodies associated with a phospholipase A defect. *Am J Hematol* 4:387, 1978.
706. Rao AK, Koike K, Willis J, et al: Platelet secretion defect associated with impaired liberation of arachidonic acid and normal myosin light chain phosphorylation. *Blood* 64:914, 1984.
707. Adler DH, Cogan JD, Phillips JA, et al: Inherited human cPLA(2alpha)deficiency is associated with impaired eicosanoid biosynthesis, small intestinal ulceration, and platelet dysfunction. *J Clin Invest* 118:2121, 2008.
708. Malmsten C, Hamberg M, Svensson J, et al: Physiological role of an endoperoxide in human platelets: Hemostatic defect due to platelet cyclo-oxygenase deficiency. *Proc Natl Acad Sci U S A* 72:1446, 1975.
709. Lagarde M, Byron PA, Vargaftig BB, et al: Impairment of platelet thromboxane A2 generation and of the platelet release reaction in two patients with congenital deficiency of platelet cyclo-oxygenase. *Br J Haematol* 38:251, 1978.
710. Pareti FI, Mannucci PM, D'Angelo A, et al: Congenital deficiency of thromboxane and prostacyclin. *Lancet* 1:898, 1980.
711. Rak K, Boda Z: Haemostatic balance in congenital deficiency of platelet cyclo-oxygenase. *Lancet* 2:44, 1980.
712. Horellou MH, Lecompte T, Lecrubier C, et al: Familial and constitutional bleeding disorder due to platelet cyclo- oxygenase deficiency. *Am J Hematol* 14:1, 1983.
713. Rao AK, Koike K, Day HJ, et al: Bleeding disorder associated with albumin-dependent partial deficiency in platelet thromboxane production. Effect of albumin on arachidonate metabolism in platelets. *Am J Clin Pathol* 83:687, 1985.
714. Roth GJ, Machuga R: Radioimmune assay of human platelet prostaglandin synthetase. *J Lab Clin Med* 99:187, 1982.
715. Matijevic-Aleksic N, McPhedran P, Wu KK: Bleeding disorder due to platelet prostaglandin H synthase-1 (PGHS-1) deficiency. *Br J Haematol* 92:212, 1996.
716. Defreyn G, Machin SJ, Carreras LO, et al: Familial bleeding tendency with partial platelet thromboxane synthetase deficiency: Reorientation of cyclic endoperoxide metabolism. *Br J Haematol* 49:29, 1981.
717. Mestel F, Oetliker O, Beck E, et al: Severe bleeding associated with defective thromboxane synthetase. *Lancet* 1:157, 1980.
718. Freson K, De Vos R, Wittevrognel C, et al: The β1-tubulin Q43P functional polymorphism reduces the risk of cardiovascular disease in men by modulating platelet function and structure. *Blood* 106:2356, 2005.
719. Navarro-Nunez L, Roldan V, Lozano ML, et al: TUBB1 Q43P polymorphism does not protect against acute coronary syndrome and premature myocardial infarction. *Thromb Haemost* 100:1211, 2008.
720. Navarro-Nunez L, Lozano ML, Rivera J, et al: The association of the beta1-tubulin Q43P polymorphism with intracerebral hemorrhage in men. *Haematologica* 92:513, 2007.
721. Kunishima S, Kobayashi R, Itoh TJ, et al: Mutation of the beta1-tubulin gene associated with congenital macrothrombocytopenia affecting microtubule assembly. *Blood* 113:458, 2009.
722. Sullivan KE, Mullen CA, Blaese RM, et al: A multiinstitutional survey of the Wiskott-Aldrich syndrome. *J Pediatr* 125:876, 1994.
723. Notarangelo LD, Miao CH, Ochs HD: Wiskott-Aldrich syndrome. *Curr Opin Hematol* 15:30, 2008.
724. Imai K, Morio T, Zhu Y, et al: Clinical course of patients with WASP gene mutations. *Blood* 103:456, 2004.
725. Sullivan KE: Recent advances in our understanding of Wiskott-Aldrich syndrome. *Curr Opin Hematol* 6:8, 1999.

726. Ochs HD: The Wiskott-Aldrich syndrome. *Semin Hematol* 35:332, 1998.
727. Notarangelo LD, Miao CH, Ochs HD: Wiskott-Aldrich syndrome. *Curr Opin Hematol* 15:30, 2008.
728. Thompson LJ, Lalloz MR, Layton DM: Unique and recurrent WAS gene mutations in Wiskott-Aldrich syndrome and X-linked thrombocytopenia. *Blood Cells Mol Dis* 25:218, 1999.
729. Devriendt K, Kim AS, Mathijs G, et al: Constitutively activating mutation in WASP causes X-linked severe congenital neutropenia. *Nat Genet* 27:313, 2001.
730. Zhu Q, Watanabe C, Liu T, et al: Wiskott-Aldrich syndrome/X-linked thrombocytopenia: WASP gene mutations, protein expression, and phenotype. *Blood* 90:2680, 1997.
731. Parkman R, Remold-O'Donnell E, Kenney DM, et al: Surface protein abnormalities in lymphocytes and platelets from patients with Wiskott-Aldrich syndrome. *Lancet* 2:1387, 1981.
732. Higgins EA, Siminovitch KA, Zhuang DL, et al: Aberrant O-linked oligosaccharide biosynthesis in lymphocytes and platelets from patients with the Wiskott-Aldrich syndrome. *J Biol Chem* 266:6280, 1991.
733. Pidard D, Didry D, Le Deist F, et al: Analysis of the membrane glycoproteins of platelets in the Wiskott- Aldrich syndrome. *Br J Haematol* 69:529, 1988.
734. Semple JW, Siminovitch KA, Mody M, et al: Flow cytometric analysis of platelets from children with the Wiskott-Aldrich syndrome reveals defects in platelet development, activation and structure. *Br J Haematol* 97:747, 1997.
735. Grottum KA, Hovig T, Holmsen H, et al: Wiskott-Aldrich syndrome: Qualitative platelet defects and short platelet survival. *Br J Haematol* 17:373, 1969.
736. Murphy S, Oski FA, Naiman JL, et al: Platelet size and kinetics in hereditary and acquired thrombocytopenia. *N Engl J Med* 286:499, 1972.
737. Baldini MG: Nature of the platelet defect in the Wiskott-Aldrich syndrome. *Ann N Y Acad Sci* 201:437, 1972.
738. Ochs HD, Slichter SJ, Harker LA, et al: The Wiskott-Aldrich syndrome: Studies of lymphocytes, granulocytes, and platelets. *Blood* 55:243, 1980.
739. Pearson HA, Shulman NR, Oski FA, et al: Platelet survival in Wiskott-Aldrich syndrome. *J Pediatr* 68:754, 1966.
740. Villa A, Notarangelo L, Macchi P, et al: X-linked thrombocytopenia and Wiskott-Aldrich syndrome are allelic diseases with mutations in the WASP gene. *Nat Genet* 9:414, 1995.
741. Ochs HD: The Wiskott-Aldrich syndrome. *Springer Semin Immunopathol* 19:435, 1998.
742. Kajiwara M, Nonoyama S, Eguchi M, et al: WASP is involved in proliferation and differentiation of human haemopoietic progenitors in vitro. *Br J Haematol* 107:254, 1999.
743. Haddad E, Cramer E, Riviere C, et al: The thrombocytopenia of Wiskott Aldrich syndrome is not related to a defect in proplatelet formation. *Blood* 94:509, 1999.
744. Luthi JN, Gandhi MJ, Drachman JG: X-linked thrombocytopenia caused by a mutation in the Wiskott-Aldrich syndrome (WAS) gene that disrupts interaction with the WAS protein (WASP)-interacting protein (WIP). *Exp Hematol* 31:150, 2003.
745. Schulze H, Korpal M, Hurov J, et al: Characterization of the megakaryocyte demarcation membrane system and its role in thrombopoiesis. *Blood* 107:3868, 2006.
746. Matzdorff A, Kemkes-Matthes B, Pralle H: Microparticles and reticulated platelets in Wiskott-Aldrich syndrome patients. *Br J Haematol* 109:673, 2000.
747. Litzman J, Jones A, Hann I, et al: Intravenous immunoglobulin, splenectomy, and antibiotic prophylaxis in Wiskott-Aldrich syndrome. *Arch Dis Child* 75:436, 1996.
748. Mullen CA, Anderson KD, Blaese RM: Splenectomy and/or bone marrow transplantation in the management of the Wiskott-Aldrich syndrome: Long-term follow-up of 62 cases. *Blood* 82:2961, 1993.
749. Akman IO, Ostrov BE, Neudorf S: Autoimmune manifestations of the Wiskott-Aldrich syndrome. *Semin Arthritis Rheum* 27:218, 1998.
750. Strom TS: The thrombocytopenia of WAS: A familial form of ITP? *Immunol Res* 44:42, 2009.
751. Corash L, Shafer B, Blaese RM: Platelet-associated immunoglobulin, platelet size, and the effect of splenectomy in the Wiskott-Aldrich syndrome. *Blood* 65:1439, 1985.
752. Kanegane H, Nomura K, Miyawaki T, et al: X-linked thrombocytopenia identified by flow cytometric demonstration of defective Wiskott-Aldrich syndrome protein in lymphocytes. *Blood* 95:1110, 2000.
753. Litzman J, Jones A, Hann I, et al: Intravenous immunoglobulin, splenectomy, and antibiotic prophylaxis in Wiskott-Aldrich syndrome. *Arch Dis Child* 75:436, 1996.
754. Prislovsky A, Marathe B, Hosni A, et al: Rapid platelet turnover in WASP() mice correlates with increased *ex vivo* phagocytosis of opsonized WASP() platelets. *Exp Hematol* 36:609, 2008.
755. Shcherbina A, Rosen FS, Remold-O'Donnell E: Pathological events in platelets of Wiskott-Aldrich syndrome patients. *Br J Haematol* 106:875, 1999.
756. Stormorken H, Hellum B, Egeland T, et al: X-linked thrombocytopenia and thrombocytopathia: Attenuated Wiskott-Aldrich syndrome. Functional and morphological studies of platelets and lymphocytes. *Thromb Haemost* 65:300, 1991.
757. Tsuboi S, Nonoyama S, Ochs HD: Wiskott-Aldrich syndrome protein is involved in alphaIIb beta3-mediated cell adhesion. *EMBO Rep* 7:506, 2006.
758. Verhoeven AJ, van Oostrum IE, van Haarlem H, et al: Impaired energy metabolism in platelets from patients with Wiskott-Aldrich syndrome. *Thromb Haemost* 61:10, 1989.
759. Marone G, Albini F, di ML, et al: The Wiskott-Aldrich syndrome: Studies of platelets, basophils and polymorphonuclear leucocytes. *Br J Haematol* 62:737, 1986.
760. Gross BS, Wilde JI, Quek L, et al: Regulation and function of WASp in platelets by the collagen receptor, glycoprotein VI. *Blood* 94:4166, 1999.
761. Rengan R, Ochs HD, Sweet LI, et al: Actin cytoskeletal function is spared, but apoptosis is increased, in WAS patient hematopoietic cells. *Blood* 95:1283, 2000.
762. Falet H, Hoffmeister KM, Neujahr R, et al: Normal Arp2/3 complex activation in platelets lacking WASp. *Blood* 100:2113, 2002.
763. Oda A, Ochs HD, Druker BJ, et al: Collagen induces tyrosine phosphorylation of Wiskott-Aldrich syndrome protein in human platelets. *Blood* 92:1852, 1998.
764. Yamada M, Ariga T, Kawamura N, et al: Determination of carrier status for the Wiskott-Aldrich syndrome by flow cytometric analysis of Wiskott-Aldrich syndrome protein expression in peripheral blood mononuclear cells. *J Immunol* 165:1119, 2000.
765. Yamada M, Ohtsu M, Kobayashi I, et al: Flow cytometric analysis of Wiskott-Aldrich syndrome (WAS) protein in lymphocytes from WAS patients and their familial carriers. *Blood* 93:756, 1999.
766. Wengler G, Gorlin JB, Williamson JM, et al: Nonrandom inactivation of the X chromosome in early lineage hematopoietic cells in carriers of Wiskott-Aldrich syndrome. *Blood* 85:2471, 1995.
767. Kuijpers TW, Van Lier RA, Hamann D, et al: Leukocyte adhesion deficiency type 1 (LAD-1)/variant. A novel immunodeficiency syndrome characterized by dysfunctional beta2 integrins. *J Clin Invest* 100:1725, 1997.
768. Kuijpers TW, van de Vijver E, Weterman MA, et al: LAD-1/variant syndrome is caused by mutations in FERMT3. *Blood* 113:4740, 2009.
769. Mory A, Feigelson SW, Yarali N, et al: Kindlin-3: A new gene involved in the pathogenesis of LAD-III. *Blood* 112:2591, 2008.
770. Svensson L, Howarth K, McDowall A, et al: Leukocyte adhesion deficiency-III is caused by mutations in KINDLIN3 affecting integrin activation. *Nat Med* 15:306, 2009.
771. Malinin NL, Zhang L, Choi J, et al: A point mutation in KINDLIN3 ablates activation of three integrin subfamilies in humans. *Nat Med* 15:313, 2009.
772. Moser M, Nieswandt B, Ussar S, et al: Kindlin-3 is essential for integrin activation and platelet aggregation. *Nat Med* 14:325, 2008.
773. Pasvolsky R, Feigelson SW, Kilic SS, et al: A LAD-III syndrome is associated with defective expression of the Rap-1 activator CalDAG-GEFI in lymphocytes, neutrophils, and platelets. *J Exp Med* 204:1571, 2007.
774. Gerrard JM, Israels ED, Bishop AJ, et al: Inherited platelet-storage pool deficiency associated with a high incidence of acute myeloid leukaemia. *Br J Haematol* 79:246, 1991.
775. Ganly P, Walker LC, Morris CM: Familial mutations of the transcription factor RUNX1 (AML1, CBFA2) predispose to acute myeloid leukemia. *Leuk Lymphoma* 45:1, 2004.
776. Dowton SB, Beardsley D, Jamison D, et al: Studies of a familial platelet disorder. *Blood* 65:557, 1985.
777. Ho CY, Otterud B, Legare RD, et al: Linkage of a familial platelet disorder with a propensity to develop myeloid malignancies to human chromosome 21q22.1–22.2. *Blood* 87:5218, 1996.
778. Arepally G, Rebbeck TR, Song W, et al: Evidence for genetic homogeneity in a familial platelet disorder with predisposition to acute myelogenous leukemia (FPD/AML). *Blood* 92:2600, 1998.
779. Song WJ, Sullivan MG, Legare RD, et al: Haploinsufficiency of CBFA2 causes familial thrombocytopenia with propensity to develop acute myelogenous leukaemia. *Nat Genet* 23:166, 1999.
780. Buijs A, Poddighe P, van Wijk R, et al: A novel CBFA2 single-nucleotide mutation in familial platelet disorder with propensity to develop myeloid malignancies. *Blood* 98:2856, 2001.
781. Michaud J, Wu F, Osato M, et al: In vitro analyses of known and novel RUNX1/AML1 mutations in dominant familial platelet disorder with predisposition to acute myelogenous leukemia: Implications for mechanisms of pathogenesis. *Blood* 99:1364, 2002.
782. Walker LC, Stevens J, Campbell H, et al: A novel inherited mutation of the transcription factor RUNX1 causes thrombocytopenia and may predispose to acute myeloid leukaemia. *Br J Haematol* 117:878, 2002.
783. Minelli A, Maserati E, Rossi G, et al: Familial platelet disorder with propensity to acute myelogenous leukemia: Genetic heterogeneity and progression to leukemia via acquisition of clonal chromosome anomalies. *Genes Chromosomes Cancer* 40:165, 2004.
784. Matheny CJ, Speck ME, Cushing PR, et al: Disease mutations in RUNX1 and RUNX2 create nonfunctional, dominant-negative, or hypomorphic alleles. *EMBO J* 26:1163, 2007.
785. Owen CJ, Toze CL, Koochin A, et al: Five new pedigrees with inherited RUNX1 mutations causing familial platelet disorder with propensity to myeloid malignancy. *Blood* 112:4639, 2008.
786. Taketani T, Taki T, Takita J, et al: AML1/RUNX1 mutations are infrequent, but related to AML-M0, acquired trisomy 21, and leukemic transformation in pediatric hematologic malignancies. *Genes Chromosomes Cancer* 38:1, 2003.
787. Asou N: The role of a Runt domain transcription factor AML1/RUNX1 in leukemogenesis and its clinical implications. *Crit Rev Oncol Hematol* 45:129, 2003.
788. Jalagadugula GS, Kaur G, Mao G, et al: RUNX1/CBFA2 regulates myosin light chain9 (MYL9) in megakaryocytic cells: Decreased MYL9 expression in human RUNX1 haplodeficiency. *Blood* 112:645A, 2008.
789. Jalagadugula GS, Kaur G, Mao G, et al: Platelet/megakaryocyte PKC-θ, is a transcriptional target of RUNX1/CBFA2: Studies in human RUNX1 haplodeficiency. *Blood* 112:649A, 2008.
790. Kaur G, Jalagadugula G, Rao AK: CBFA2/RUNX1 regulates human platelet 12-lipoxygenase: Studies in runx1 haplodeficiency. *Blood* 118:1066A, 2007.

791. Heller PG, Glembotsky AC, Gandhi MJ, et al: Low Mpl receptor expression in a pedigree with familial platelet disorder with predisposition to acute myelogenous leukemia and a novel AML1 mutation. *Blood* 105:4664, 2005.
792. Geddis AE, Kaushansky K: Inherited thrombocytopenias: Toward a molecular understanding of disorders of platelet production. *Curr Opin Pediatr* 16:15, 2004.
793. Freson K, Devriendt K, Matthijs G, et al: Platelet characteristics in patients with X-linked macrothrombocytopenia because of a novel GATA1 mutation. *Blood* 98:85, 2001.
794. Hughan SC, Senis Y, Best D, et al: Selective impairment of platelet activation to collagen in the absence of GATA1. *Blood* 105:4369, 2005.
795. Breton-Gorius J, Favier R, Guichard J, et al: A new congenital dysmegakaryopoietic thrombocytopenia (Paris-Trousseau) associated with giant platelet alpha-granules and chromosome 11 deletion at 11q23. *Blood* 85:1805, 1995.
796. Favier R, Jondeau K, Boutard P, et al: Paris-Trousseau syndrome: Clinical, hematological, molecular data of ten new cases. *Thromb Haemost* 90:893, 2003.
797. Raslova H, Komura E, Le Couedic JP, et al: FLI1 monoallelic expression combined with its hemizygous loss underlies Paris-Trousseau/Jacobsen thrombopenia. *J Clin Invest* 114:77, 2004.
798. Shivdasani RA: Lonely in Paris: When one gene copy isn't enough. *J Clin Invest* 114:17, 2004.
799. Cattaneo M, Hayward CP, Moffat KA, et al: Results of a worldwide survey on the assessment of platelet function by light transmission aggregometry: A report from the platelet physiology subcommittee of the scientific and standardization committee of the International Society on Thrombosis and Haemostasis. *J Thromb Haemost* 7:1029, 2009.
800. Hayward CP, Pai M, Liu Y, et al: Diagnostic utility of light transmission platelet aggregometry: Results from a prospective study of individuals referred for bleeding disorder assessments. *J Thromb Haemost* 7:676, 2009.
801. Hayward CP, Moffat KA, Pai M, et al: An evaluation of methods for determining reference intervals for light transmission platelet aggregation tests on samples with normal or reduced platelet counts. *Thromb Haemost* 100:134, 2008.
802. Moffat KA, Ledford-Kraemer MR, Nichols WL, et al: Variability in clinical laboratory practice in testing for disorders of platelet function: Results of two surveys of the North American Specialized Coagulation Laboratory Association. *Thromb Haemost* 93:549, 2005.
803. Zhou L, Schmaier AH: Platelet aggregation testing in platelet-rich plasma: Description of procedures with the aim to develop standards in the field. *Am J Clin Pathol* 123:172, 2005.
804. Gurbel PA, Becker RC, Mann KG, et al: Platelet function monitoring in patients with coronary artery disease. *J Am Coll Cardiol* 50:1822, 2007.
805. Michelson AD: Methods for the measurement of platelet function. *Am J Cardiol* 103:20A, 2009.
805a. Miller JL: Glycoprotein analysis for the diagnostic evaluation of platelet disorders. *Semin Thromb Hemost* 35:224, 2009.
806. Vinogradova O, Velyvis A, Velyviene A, et al: A Structural mechanism of integrin alpha(IIb)beta(3) "inside-out" activation as regulated by its cytoplasmic face. *Cell* 110:587, 2002.
807. Mitchell WB, Li JH, Singh F, et al: Two novel mutations in the alpha IIb calcium-binding domains identify hydrophobic regions essential for alpha IIbbeta 3 biogenesis. *Blood* 101:2268, 2003.
808. Qin J, Vinogradova O, Plow EF: Integrin bidirectional signaling: A molecular view. *PLoS Biol* 2:726, 2004.
809. Coller BS: Inherited disorders of platelet function, in *Hemostasis and Thrombosis*, edited by AL Bloom, p 721. Churchill Livingstone, Edinburgh, Scotland, 1994.

CHAPTER 122
ACQUIRED QUALITATIVE PLATELET DISORDERS

Charles S. Abrams, Sanford J. Shattil, and Joel S. Bennett

SUMMARY

Acquired qualitative platelet disorders are frequent causes of abnormal platelet function *in vitro* and prolonged bleeding times, and occasionally of mild bleeding diatheses. However, their clinical importance increases in the presence of thrombocytopenia or additional disorders of hemostasis. Acquired disorders of platelet function can be conveniently classified into those that result from drugs, hematologic diseases, and systemic disorders. Drugs are the most frequent cause of acquired qualitative platelet dysfunction. Aspirin is the most notable drug in this regard because of its frequent use, its irreversible effect on platelet prostaglandin synthesis, and its documented effect on hemostatic competency, although this effect is minimal in normal individuals. Other nonsteroidal antiinflammatory drugs reversibly inhibit platelet prostaglandin synthesis and usually have little effect on hemostasis. The antiplatelet effect of a number of drugs has proven useful in preventing arterial thrombosis, but as would be anticipated, excessive bleeding can be a complication of their use. In addition to aspirin, these drugs include the thienopyridines ticlopidine, clopidogrel, and prasugrel that primarily antagonize adenosine diphosphate (ADP)-stimulated platelet aggregation and drugs that specifically inhibit the platelet integrin $\alpha_{IIb}\beta_3$ (glycoprotein IIb/IIIa) receptor. Other drugs used to treat thrombosis, such as heparin and fibrinolytic agents, can also impair platelet function *in vitro* and *ex vivo*, but the clinical significance of these observations is uncertain. High doses of the β-lactam antibiotics can impair platelet function *in vitro* and prolong the bleeding time, whereas clinically significant bleeding is unusual in the absence of a coexisting hemostatic defect. Similarly, a number of miscellaneous drugs, including a variety of psychotropic, chemotherapeutic, and anesthetic agents, as well as a number of foods and food additives affect platelet function *in vitro*, but these effects do not appear to be of clinical significance. Hematologic diseases associated with abnormal platelet function include processes in which platelets may be intrinsically abnormal, such as the myelodysplastic syndromes and myeloproliferative disorders, acute myelogenous leukemias, and very rarely, chronic lymphocytic leukemia; dysproteinemias in which abnormal plasma proteins can bind to and impair platelet function; and acquired forms of von Willebrand disease. Of the systemic diseases, renal failure is most prominently associated with abnormal platelet function because of retention of platelet inhibitory compounds in the plasma. Platelet function may also be abnormal in the presence of antiplatelet antibodies, following cardiopulmonary bypass, and in association with liver disease or disseminated intravascular coagulation.

Acronyms and abbreviations that appear in this chapter include: ADP, adenosine diphosphate; cAMP, cyclin adenosine monophosphate; cGMP, cyclic guanosine monophosphate; COX, cyclooxygenase; DDAVP, desmopressin or 1-desamino-8-D-arginine vasopressin; GP, glycoprotein; Ig, immunoglobulin; ITP, idiopathic thrombocytopenic purpura; NO, nitric oxide; PG, prostaglandin; SLE, systemic lupus erythematosus; t-PA, tissue-type plasminogen activator; VWF, von Willebrand factor.

Platelet function may be adversely affected by drugs and by hematologic and nonhematologic disorders. Because the use of aspirin and other nonsteroidal antiinflammatory agents is pervasive in current medical practice, acquired platelet dysfunction is much more frequent than inherited platelet dysfunction. Acquired disorders of platelet function can be classified according to the underlying clinical conditions with which they are associated (Table 122–1).

It is important to have a balanced view of the clinical significance of acquired disorders of platelet function. On the one hand, their severity is usually mild. On the other hand, there are important exceptions to this rule, particularly when platelet dysfunction is associated with other hemostatic defects. If the patient does not present with a history of bleeding, it may be difficult to predict the risk of future bleeding. This is not surprising as even patients with thrombocytopenia may experience little or no spontaneous bleeding until their platelet count is less than 10,000/μL. Furthermore, clinical assessment of these disorders is made problematic by difficulties in standardization and interpretation of laboratory tests of platelet function, including the bleeding time and platelet aggregometry. These tests are more useful in diagnosing platelet dysfunction than in predicting the risk of bleeding.[1,2]

DRUGS THAT AFFECT PLATELET FUNCTION

Drugs represent the most common cause of platelet dysfunction (Table 122–2).[3] For example, in an analysis of 72 hospitalized patients with a prolonged bleeding time, 54 percent were receiving large doses of antibiotics known to prolong the bleeding time, and 10 percent were taking aspirin or other nonsteroidal antiinflammatory drugs.[4] Some drugs can prolong the bleeding time and either cause or exacerbate a bleeding diathesis. Other drugs may prolong the bleeding time but not cause bleeding, whereas many only affect platelet function *ex vivo* or when added to platelets *in vitro*.

ASPIRIN AND OTHER NONSTEROIDAL ANTIINFLAMMATORY DRUGS

Aspirin

Aspirin irreversibly inactivates the enzyme cyclooxygenase (COX), also known as prostaglandin endoperoxide H synthase, by acetylating a serine residue at position 529.[5] Two isoforms of cyclooxygenase have been identified (COX-1 and COX-2),[6] as well as a splice variant of COX-1, called COX-1b (or COX-3), whose functional significance is uncertain.[7] COX-1 is constitutively expressed by many tissues, including platelets, the gastric mucosa, and endothelial cells (see Chap. 135).[6] COX-2 is undetectable in most tissues, but its synthesis is rapidly induced in cells such as endothelial cells, fibroblasts, and monocytes by growth factors, cytokines, endotoxin, and hormones.[6] Platelets and endothelial cells express both COX-1 and COX-2,[8] although COX-2 expression is not thought to be important for platelet function.[9] In the cardiovascular system, COX products regulate complex interactions between platelets and the vessel wall. The platelet product, thromboxane A_2, produces vasoconstriction, and is an agonist for platelet aggregation and secretion.[5] Thus, inactivation of COX-1 by aspirin prevents platelet synthesis of thromboxane A_2, thereby inhibiting platelet responses that depend on this substance. Accordingly, platelet responses to adenosine diphosphate (ADP), epinephrine, arachidonic acid, and low doses of collagen and thrombin are affected, but there is almost no effect on the responses to higher doses of collagen or thrombin.[10,11] On the other hand, the endothelial cell prostaglandin (PG) product, PGI_2, produces smooth muscle cell relaxation and vasodilation

TABLE 122–1. Acquired Qualitative Platelet Disorders

Drugs that affect platelet function
Thienopyridines (ticlopidine, clopidogrel, and prasugrel)
$\alpha_{IIb}\beta_3$ receptor antagonists
Drugs that increase platelet cyclic adenosine monophosphate
Antibiotics
Anticoagulants and fibrinolytic agents
Cardiovascular drugs
Volume expanders
Psychotropic agents and anesthetics
Antineoplastic drugs
Foods and food additives
Hematologic disorders associated with abnormal platelet function
Chronic myeloproliferative disorders
Leukemias and myelodysplastic syndromes
Dysproteinemias
Acquired von Willebrand disease
Systemic disorders associated with abnormal platelet function
Uremia
Antiplatelet antibodies
Cardiopulmonary bypass
Liver disease
Disseminated intravascular coagulation

and by increasing the platelet content of cyclic adenosine monophosphate (cAMP), decreases overall platelet reactivity.[12]

Platelet prostaglandin synthesis in an adult is nearly completely inhibited by a single 100-mg dose of aspirin or by 30 mg taken daily for 7 to 10 days.[5] Although small doses of aspirin irreversibly inhibit platelet and endothelial cell COX,[13] they have no lasting effect on prostaglandin synthesis by endothelial cells because of the ability of endothelial cells to synthesize additional COX unaffected by aspirin.[14,15] *In vitro* studies also suggest that the presence of erythrocytes contributes to agonist-stimulated platelet reactivity,[16] an effect that can be inhibited by aspirin at doses greater than those required to inhibit platelet COX-1.[17] A meta-analysis of clinical trials indicates that aspirin doses varying from 50 to 1500 mg daily are equally efficacious in preventing adverse cardiovascular and cerebrovascular events.[18] This has led many to suggest that the lowest effective doses should be prescribed to minimize gastrointestinal toxicity. Nonetheless, even low doses of aspirin can be associated with gastrointestinal hemorrhage.[19–21]

Aspirin is one of the few drugs that prolongs the bleeding time in humans and appears to do so by blocking aggregation rather than adhesion. In normal individuals, the effect on the bleeding time is slight (generally no more than 1.2 to 2.0 times the preaspirin bleeding time),[22,23] observed in both males and females, and requires that almost all the cyclooxygenase in the circulating platelets be inhibited.[22] The sensitivity of the bleeding time to aspirin is dependent on such technical variables as the direction of the incision on the forearm and the degree of hydrostatic pressure applied to the arm.[24] The bleeding time may remain prolonged for 1 to 4 days after the aspirin has been discontinued and platelet aggregation tests may remain abnormal for up to a week until affected platelets are replaced.[25]

TABLE 122–2. Drugs That Affect Platelet Function

Nonsteroidal antiinflammatory drugs
Aspirin, ibuprofen, sulindac, naproxen, meclofenamic acid, mefenamic acid, diflunisal, piroxicam, tolmetin, zomepirac, sulfinpyrazone, indomethacin, phenylbutazone, celecoxib
Thienopyridines
Ticlopidine, clopidogrel, and prasugrel
$\alpha_{IIb}\beta_3$ antagonists
Abciximab, tirofiban, eptifibatide
Drugs that affect platelet cyclic adenosine monophosphate levels or function
Prostacyclin, iloprost, dipyridamole, cilostazol,
Antibiotics
Penicillins
Penicillin G, carbenicillin, ticarcillin, methicillin, ampicillin, piperacillin, azlocillin mezlocillin, sulbenicillin, temocillin
Cephalosporins
Cephalothin, moxalactam, cefoxitin, cefotaxime, cefazolin
Nitrofurantoin
Miconazole
Anticoagulants, fibrinolytic agents, and antifibrinolytic agents
Heparin
Streptokinase, tissue-type plasminogen activator, urokinase
ε-Aminocaproic acid
Cardiovascular drugs
Nitroglycerin, isosorbide dinitrate, propranolol, nitroprusside, nifedipine, verapamil, diltiazem, quinidine
Volume expanders
Dextran, hydroxyethyl starch
Psychotropic drugs and anesthetics
Psychotropic drugs
Imipramine, amitriptyline, nortriptyline, chlorpromazine, promethazine, fluphenazine, trifluoperazine, haloperidol
Anesthetics
Local
Dibucaine, tetracaine, Cyclaine, butacaine, Nupercaine, procaine, cocaine
General
Halothane
Oncologic drugs
Mithramycin, daunorubicin, BCNU (carmustine)
Miscellaneous drugs
Ketanserin
Antihistamines
Diphenhydramine, chlorpheniramine, mepyramine
Radiographic contrast agent
Iopamidol, iothalamate, ioxaglate, meglumine diatrizoate, sodium diatrizoate
Foods and food additives
ω-3 Fatty acids, ethanol, Chinese black tree fungus, onion extract ajoene, cumin, turmeric

The significance of aspirin ingestion on the hemostatic competency of normal individuals appears to be minimal. Nevertheless, patients chronically taking aspirin report a significant increase in bruising, epistaxis, and gastrointestinal blood loss.[26] The latter appears to be a direct effect of the drug on the gastric mucosa.[27,28] Furthermore, there is an increase in the incidence of hemorrhagic stroke when aspirin is used in the primary and secondary prevention of vascular disease, as well as an increase in major gastrointestinal and other extracranial bleeding.[29] Aspirin may also increase bleeding in the mother and the neonate during parturition.[30] In addition, some, but not all, studies show that aspirin taken preoperatively increases the amount of blood loss following cardiothoracic surgery.[31,32] On the other hand, a retrospective analysis has documented the safety of performing epidural and spinal anesthesia in patients who had ingested aspirin.[33] Although aspirin may increase the amount of blood loss following general surgery,[34] the significance of aspirin ingestion in this setting has never been tested in a prospective, randomized, double-blind study with objective endpoints. Many surgeons ask their patients to avoid aspirin, particularly prior to cardiothoracic, plastic, or neurosurgical procedures, in which the limits of tolerable bleeding are narrow.[35] Aspirin causes a marked prolongation of the bleeding time and precipitates hemorrhage in individuals with preexistent hemostatic defects such as von Willebrand disease, hemophilia A, warfarin ingestion, uremia, or disorders of platelet function.[36–38] Although ingestion of ethanol has no direct effect on the bleeding time, it can potentiate the effect of aspirin.[39,40] Infusion of DDAVP has been effective in correcting a prolonged bleeding time because of aspirin.[41,42]

Traditional Nonsteroidal Antiinflammatory Drugs

Unlike aspirin, nonsteroidal antiinflammatory drugs (NSAIDs) such as ibuprofen, naproxen, diclofenac, sulindac, piroxicam, indomethacin, and sulfinpyrazone reversibly inhibit COX enzymes.[43,44] Furthermore, although these drugs may cause a transient prolongation of the bleeding time when given in therapeutic doses, this is usually not clinically significant.[45–47] As evidence of the modest effect of NSAIDs on platelet function, ibuprofen has been given safely to patients with hemophilia A.[48,49] However, care must be taken when ibuprofen is given to patients with hemophilia and HIV infection who are receiving zidovudine, as increased bleeding has been reported in this circumstance.[50] Furthermore, because ibuprofen, and probably other NSAIDs, binds to COX and blocks its acetylation by aspirin,[44] coadministration of NSAIDs may impair the irreversible effects of aspirin on platelets. For this reason, patients who require both medications should ingest aspirin at least 2 hours prior to the ingestion of other NSAIDs.

Cyclooxygenase-2 Inhibitors

COX-1 is present in the gastric mucosa where its products protect the integrity of the gastric lining cells. In inflammatory cells, COX-2 products such as prostaglandin E_2 and PGI_2 elicit an increased sense of pain and perpetuate the inflammatory process.[12] Thus, the cyclooxygenase inhibitors, designed to be relatively more specific for COX-2 versus COX-1, were intended to reduce pain and inflammation with less gastric side-effects than traditional NSAIDs.[12,51] However, clinical trials revealed that administration of cyclooxygenase inhibitors was associated with cardiovascular toxicity (myocardial infarction, stroke, edema, exacerbation of hypertension), partly as a result of the inhibition of PGI_2 synthesis.[12,52–54] On the basis of these results, rofecoxib and valdecoxib were withdrawn from the market (valdecoxib was also associated with cases of Stevens-Johnson syndrome) and a black box warning regarding serious cardiovascular events was added to prescribing information for celecoxib, the only cyclooxygenase inhibitor now available in the United States.[53] Clinical evidence through 2008 suggests there is no excess cardiovascular risk from daily doses of celecoxib of 200 mg or less.[54] Because traditional NSAIDs also inhibit COX-2 and several clinical trials have suggested excess cardiovascular events with the use of some of these agents,[53,55] a warning has also been added to their prescribing information. If indicated, analgesics such as acetaminophen, sodium or choline salicylate and narcotics may be substituted for aspirin and NSAIDs for treating musculoskeletal pain.[53] A recent report suggests that acetaminophen can selectively inhibit COX-2,[56] but the clinical significance of this observation has not been determined.

THIENOPYRIDINES

The thienopyridines ticlopidine and clopidogrel have been used as antithrombotic agents in arterial diseases (see Chap. 135). They are more effective than aspirin in the secondary prevention of cerebrovascular and cardiovascular events.[57–63]

Ticlopidine and clopidogrel differ from aspirin in the mechanism of their antiplatelet activity and in their toxicity profile. Both thienopyridines are prodrugs that depend on metabolites to competitively inhibit the platelet P2Y12 ADP receptor.[64–72] Ticlopidine at 250 mg by mouth twice a day or clopidogrel at 75 mg once per day have been shown to inhibit platelet aggregation *ex vivo* and to prolong the bleeding time in humans. The degree of prolongation of the bleeding time is equivalent to or greater than that of aspirin and the effect of thienopyridines and aspirin appears additive.[62,73] Effects of ticlopidine and clopidogrel on platelet aggregation and the bleeding time may be seen within 24 to 48 hours of the first dose, but are not maximal for 4 to 6 days. A loading dose of 300 mg of clopidogrel followed by a daily dose of 75 mg per day shortens the time required for the maximal antiplatelet effect.[74] The presence of the common polymorphism of cytochrome P450, termed *CYP2C19*, results in lower levels of the active metabolite in patients. This effect can lead to decreased inhibition of platelet function, and elevated risk for major adverse cardiovascular events.[75–77] The effects of these drugs may persist for 4 to 10 days after they have been discontinued, either because of their extended half-life after multiple dosing or because of an irreversible effect on platelets.[64]

Ticlopidine administration is associated with potentially serious hematologic complications, including neutropenia ($<1200/\mu L$ in 2.4% of individuals),[64,78,79] and less commonly, aplastic anemia and thrombocytopenia.[80,81] In addition, at least 1 in 5000 patients treated with ticlopidine develop thrombotic thrombocytopenic purpura.[82–84] Results from a large clinical trial suggest that hematologic complications may be less common with clopidogrel.[57] One study suggested that clopidogrel may also be rarely associated with thrombotic thrombocytopenic purpura (1 in 270,000 patients),[85] although this rate is close to the incidence of this disease in the general population. Because of their toxicity profiles, the use of ticlopidine has been replaced by clopidogrel in the United States.

Because aspirin and clopidogrel inhibit platelets by different mechanisms, their antithrombotic effects ought to be additive. In theory, this could be beneficial in the treatment of diseases associated with platelet activation such as ischemic heart disease, peripheral vascular disease, and ischemic strokes.[59,61,62,86,87] This theory was tested in the CURE (Clopidogrel in Unstable Angina to Prevent Recurrent Ischemic Events) trial that analyzed the outcome of 12,562 patients with acute coronary syndrome.[62] In this study, the addition of clopidogrel to aspirin decreased the combined incidence of cardiovascular deaths, myocardial infarctions, and strokes from 11.4 percent to 9.3 percent. The benefit of double therapy was partially offset by an increase in severe bleeding from 2.7 percent to 3.7 percent.

The findings of the CURE trial spawned a new series of trials investigating whether double platelet blockade was better than single antiplatelet therapy in a variety of patients at risk for arterial thrombi. Additional studies of patients who had myocardial infarctions or angioplasty appeared to confirm a modest benefit to double platelet blockade that outweighed the associated bleeding risk. However, in the MATCH (Management of Atherothrombosis with Clopidogrel in High-Risk Patients with Recent Transient Ischemic Attack or Ischemic Stroke) study, the bleeding complications of patients who received dual antiplatelet therapy for the prevention of strokes offset any benefit.[88,89]

The CHARISMA (Clopidogrel for High Atherothrombotic Risk and Ischemic Stabilization, Management and Avoidance) study was designed to determine whether long-term treatment with both clopidogrel and aspirin was better than aspirin alone in a broad population at risk for cardiovascular events.[90] As found in the other trials, any benefit for double antiplatelet therapy was at best modest. In total, there were 94 fewer ischemic events in patients treated with both clopidogrel and aspirin, but at the expense of 93 more moderate or severe bleeding events. Except in special circumstances such as angioplasty, it appears that the added benefit of double antiplatelet therapy for most patients is small, and at times dangerous.

Prasugrel is another thienopyridine prodrug that was approved by an advisory panel to the FDA in the United States, and is approved in Europe. Like clopidogrel and ticlopidine, prasugrel is metabolized by cytochrome P450 into a P2Y12 antagonist. In contrast to the older thienopyridines, prasugrel is efficiently converted into its active metabolite.[91] Consequently, a 60-mg loading dose of prasugrel produces much more rapid and consistent inhibition of platelet activation than clopidogrel or ticlopidine.[92–94] The available evidence suggests that prasugrel has a more potent and consistent inhibition of platelet function than clopidogrel.[95]

Prasugrel was compared with clopidogrel in 13,608 patients with acute coronary syndrome scheduled for percutaneous coronary intervention in the Triton-TIMI 38 (Trial to Assess Improvement in Therapeutic Outcomes by Optimizing Platelet Inhibition with Prasugrel—Thrombolysis in Myocardial Infarction) trial. Patients who received prasugrel had a 9.9 percent incidence of ischemic events compared to the 12.1 percent incidence in patients who received clopidogrel.[96] However, major bleeding was also increased in patients receiving prasugrel (2.4%) compared to clopidogrel (1.8%). These data indicate that at the recommended doses, prasugrel is more effective than clopidogrel at preventing ischemic events in patients with acute coronary syndrome, but it is also associated with slightly more major bleeding events. It is notable that several more antagonists of the P2Y12 receptor currently in development are not members of the thienopyridine family. These agents include cangrelor[97] and ticagrelor.[98]

$\alpha_{IIB}\beta_3$ RECEPTOR ANTAGONISTS

Drugs that specifically impair the function of integrin $\alpha_{IIb}\beta_3$ (glycoprotein [GP] IIb/IIIa) have been developed for short-term use as antithrombotic agents in the setting of ischemic coronary artery disease.[99–101] Abciximab, eptifibatide, and tirofiban are three FDA-approved $\alpha_{IIb}\beta_3$ inhibitors that are structurally dissimilar, but all rapidly impair platelet aggregation. Abciximab is a human-murine chimeric Fab fragment, eptifibatide is a cyclic heptapeptide, and tirofiban is a nonpeptide mimetic. Because inherited $\alpha_{IIb}\beta_3$ abnormalities result in the bleeding disorder Glanzmann thrombasthenia,[102,103] it is not surprising that these drugs can predispose patients to bleeding. In EPIC (Evaluation of 7E3 for the Prevention of Ischemic Complications), a clinical trial of the efficacy of abciximab in patients undergoing percutaneous coronary angioplasty, 14 percent of patients given abciximab experienced major bleeding compared to 7 percent of patients given placebo.[104] However, the patients were also given aspirin and heparin. When the heparin dose was decreased in the subsequent EPILOG (Evaluation in PTCA to Improve Long-term Outcome with Abciximab GP IIb/IIIa Blockade) trial, the incidence of major bleeding in patients receiving abciximab decreased to 2.0 percent compared to 3.1 percent in the control group that received heparin and aspirin alone.[105] Nonetheless, in both EPIC and EPILOG, minor bleeding was significantly more frequent in patients given abciximab and standard dose heparin compared to patients given standard dose heparin alone, attesting to the ability of an $\alpha_{IIb}\beta_3$ antagonist to impair normal hemostasis. In the PRISM-PLUS (Platelet Receptor Inhibition in Ischemic Syndrome Management in Patients Limited by Unstable Signs and Symptoms) trial of tirofiban, and the PURSUIT (Platelet Glycoprotein IIb/IIIa in Unstable Angina: Receptor Suppression Using Integrilin Therapy) trial of eptifibatide, major and minor bleeding were slightly more frequent in patients receiving the study drug compared to controls.[106,107] Similarly, patients receiving the oral $\alpha_{IIb}\beta_3$ inhibitors xemilofiban and sibrafiban for 30 and 28 days, respectively, frequently experienced mucocutaneous bleeding similar to that experienced by patients with Glanzmann thrombasthenia.[108,109] Although the short-term use of $\alpha_{IIb}\beta_3$ antagonists is often beneficial in patients with acute coronary syndrome or following percutaneous coronary intervention, paradoxically the long-term use is associated with an increase in mortality.[110] The cause of this paradoxical effect is not clear, but has been attributed by some to the antagonists causing a conformational change in $\alpha_{IIb}\beta_3$ that induces it to stimulate platelet activation.[111]

The risk of bleeding in patients undergoing percutaneous coronary intervention given $\alpha_{IIb}\beta_3$ antagonists can be minimized by using heparin on a weight basis (such as 70 U/kg as in EPILOG),[105] by avoiding treatment of patients who are receiving warfarin at therapeutic doses, by early vascular sheath removal, and by meticulous care of vascular puncture sites.[112] Platelet transfusions appear to rapidly reverse the defect in platelet function in patients receiving abciximab, primarily by decreasing the overall extent of $\alpha_{IIb}\beta_3$ blockade. The ability of platelet transfusion to reverse the effects of the other $\alpha_{IIb}\beta_3$ antagonists is less clear, but these drugs have short half-lives if renal and hepatic function are normal. When bleeding requiring intervention does occur, platelet transfusion should be considered to try to decrease the concentration of platelet-bound drug.

Thrombocytopenia occurring within 24 hours of initiating therapy has been observed in small numbers of patients following the administration of all types of $\alpha_{IIb}\beta_3$ antagonists.[106,107,109,112,113] In the EPIC trial, the incidence of platelet counts less than 100,000/μL and less than 50,000/μL in patients receiving abciximab for the first time was 3.9 percent and 0.9 percent, respectively.[113] The incidence of profound thrombocytopenia after administration of abciximab has been confirmed in subsequent publications.[104,105,114,115] Thrombocytopenia has also been reported in patients receiving eptifibatide, tirofiban, as well as a variety of small molecule RGD- and non–RGD-based $\alpha_{IIb}\beta_3$ inhibitors. The incidence of thrombocytopenia has varied from 0 to 13 percent in several studies, depending on the specific inhibitor studied.[106,107,109,113,116–119] The mechanism responsible for the decrease in platelet count is uncertain, but it may be related to the presence of preexisting anti-$\alpha_{IIb}\beta_3$ antibodies that recognize epitopes (so-called ligand-induced binding sites) on $\alpha_{IIb}\beta_3$ that are exposed upon binding of the $\alpha_{IIb}\beta_3$ antagonist, or in the case of abciximab, to murine sequences incorporated into the therapeutic Fab fragment.[120] It is unknown whether prescreening patients for preexisting antibodies, and avoiding use of these drugs in antibody-positive individuals, will reduce the incidence of severe thrombocytopenia.[121] The thrombocytopenia usually reverses readily when the drug is stopped, but it may also be reversed by platelet transfusion if clinically indicated.[112] Thrombocytopenia in patients receiving $\alpha_{IIb}\beta_3$ antagonists must be differentiated from pseudothrombopenia caused by drug-induced platelet clumping, from heparin-induced thrombocytopenia in patients receiving heparin concurrently, and from other causes of thrombocytopenia, depending on the clinical circumstances.[122,123] It is particularly important to identify thrombocytopenia early, as $\alpha_{IIb}\beta_3$ antagonists are administered as long infusions, and the drug should be stopped as soon as true thrombocytopenia is confirmed. In most cases of profound thrombocytopenia, a platelet count obtained 2 to 4 hours after initiating therapy will provide evidence of a significant decrease in platelet count, although cases of delayed thrombocytopenia have been observed after abciximab.[120]

DRUGS THAT AFFECT PLATELET CYCLIC NUCLEOTIDE LEVELS OR FUNCTION

The pyrimidopyrimidine derivative dipyridamole inhibits cyclic nucleotide phosphodiesterase, resulting in the intracellular accumulation of cAMP. Dipyridamole may also inhibit the breakdown of cyclic guanosine monophosphate (cGMP), resulting in the potentiation of a nitric oxide effect.[124] Although dipyridamole inhibits platelet function *in vitro*, its clinical utility is controversial.[125,126] One early meta-analysis failed to demonstrate a benefit for the addition of dipyridamole to aspirin therapy.[127] However, many of the older dipyridamole trials used formulations with limited bioavailability.[128] In a meta-analysis of five major studies, aspirin plus dipyridamole was found to be superior to aspirin alone (relative risk: 0.77) in preventing stroke and other cardiovascular events in patients with minor stroke and transient ischemic attacks.[129] Subset analysis to dissect out the role of different formulations of dipyridamole indicated that the clinical advantage resides with the extended release form of the drug; the study was insufficiently powered to determine whether the clinical advantage extended to other formulations of dipyridamole.

Intravenous infusions of PGE_1, prostacyclin, or stable analogues of prostacyclin stimulate platelet adenylyl cyclase, causing an increase in platelet cAMP levels and a decrease in platelet responsiveness.[130–132] These agents cause a transient prolongation of the bleeding time and inhibit platelet shape change, aggregation, and secretion. However, their clinical utility is limited by their short half-life and side effects that include peripheral vasodilation.[130,133] Cilostazol, a phosphodiesterase III inhibitor, has been approved in the United States for the treatment of peripheral vascular disease,[134] and may have utility in the prevention of cardiac stent occlusion.[135] Nitric oxide and organic nitrates such as nitroglycerin inhibit platelet function *in vitro*, probably by activating guanylyl cyclase, thereby increasing cGMP.[136] Their effect on *in vivo* platelet function is uncertain. High concentrations of caffeine and theophylline also inhibit platelet phosphodiesterases *in vitro*.

ANTIBIOTICS

The various penicillins contain a β-lactam ring and a unique side chain. Most penicillins cause a dose-dependent prolongation of the bleeding time in normal volunteers.[137] Because they reduce platelet aggregation and secretion, as well as ristocetin-induced platelet agglutination, they may affect both platelet adhesion and platelet activation. Tests of platelet aggregation are abnormal in at least 50 to 75 percent of individuals receiving large doses (at least several grams per day) of carbenicillin, penicillin G, ticarcillin, ampicillin, nafcillin, and azlocillin, and in 25 to 50 percent of patients taking piperacillin, azlocillin, or mezlocillin.[137–139] Differences in the antiplatelet effects of these antibiotics probably relate to differences in blood levels and drug potency. Their effect on platelets is maximal after 1 to 3 days of administration, and may remain for several days after the antibiotic has been stopped, suggesting that the effect of these antibiotics on platelets *in vivo* is irreversible.

Penicillins may impair the interaction of agonists and von Willebrand factor (VWF) with the platelet membrane.[140] Indeed, when many penicillins are incubated with washed platelets, albeit at concentrations higher than those attained *in vivo*, they inhibit the interaction of VWF and agonists, such as ADP and epinephrine, with their platelet receptors.[141] The relative *in vitro* antiplatelet potency of the penicillins correlates well with their lipid solubility and with the inhibitory potency of the isolated side chains.[142] Moreover, the inhibitory effect of penicillin G on platelet function *in vitro* is potentiated by the presence of probenecid.[143] When platelet function was tested after intravenous administration of penicillin, oxacillin, or mezlocillin for 3 to 17 days to patients or normal volunteers, irreversible inhibition of agonist-induced aggregation was noted, along with a 40 percent reduction in low-affinity thromboxane A_2 receptors.[144] Thus, penicillins probably inhibit platelet function by binding to one or more membrane components necessary for adhesive interactions with the vessel wall or for stimulus-response coupling.

Although clinically significant bleeding is associated with the use of carbenicillin, penicillin G, ticarcillin, and nafcillin, it is far less common than prolongation of the bleeding time.[137,145] Patients with coexisting hemostatic defects (e.g., thrombocytopenia, vitamin K deficiency, uremia) may be particularly prone to this complication. On the other hand, high doses of penicillin G did not increase gastrointestinal blood loss in a thrombocytopenic rabbit model.[146] In the authors' experience, bleeding caused by antibiotic-induced platelet dysfunction is uncommon and unpredictable. Because β-lactam–induced platelet dysfunction resolves with time following cessation of the drug, this class of drugs should only be considered as a cause of bleeding in the appropriate clinical setting. A similar pattern of platelet dysfunction has been reported with some cephalosporins or related antibiotics but not with others.[137,147,148] Broad-spectrum antibiotics can also cause a bleeding diathesis attributable to the killing of gut flora and resulting vitamin K deficiency. Nitrofurantoin, a structurally unrelated antibiotic, may cause a mild prolongation of the bleeding time and impair platelet aggregation when blood levels of the drug are higher than 20 μM.[149] Miconazole, an antifungal agent, inhibits human and rabbit platelet cyclooxygenase *in vitro* and rabbit platelet cyclooxygenase after intravenous infusion.[150]

ANTICOAGULANTS, FIBRINOLYTIC AGENTS, ANTIFIBRINOLYTIC AGENTS

Heparin predisposes patients to bleeding primarily through its anticoagulant effect, but it may also affect platelet function. For example, a bolus injection of heparin (100 U/kg) can cause a significant prolongation of the bleeding time in normal subjects and in patients prior to cardiopulmonary bypass, suggesting that therapeutic doses of heparin may impair platelet function.[151] Heparin likely impairs platelet function by inhibiting the generation and action of thrombin, a potent platelet agonist. Paradoxically, heparin can also enhance platelet aggregation induced by other platelet agonists.[152] However, the clinical significance of this *in vitro* effect is unclear. Heparin binds to a single class of high affinity binding sites on resting platelets, and to an additional class of lower-affinity binding sites on fully activated platelets.[153] High heparin doses have also been found to impair VWF-dependent platelet function, possibly by binding to the heparin-binding domain of VWF.[154] The contributions of these effects on platelet function to the bleeding complications of heparin therapy are uncertain.

Bleeding during fibrinolytic therapy is predominantly a result of the combined effects of structural lesions in blood vessels and the fibrin(ogen)olytic activity of the agent used. However, pharmacologic doses of streptokinase, urokinase, and tissue-type plasminogen activator (t-PA) can affect platelet function.[155] High concentrations of plasmin *ex vivo* cause platelet aggregation.[156] Moreover, marked increases in the urinary excretion of the thromboxane A_2 metabolite 2,3-dinor-thromboxane B_2 have been detected in patients receiving streptokinase or t-PA for coronary thrombolysis, suggesting that *in vivo* platelet activation had occurred during infusion of the drug.[157,158] Nevertheless, several *in vitro* studies indicate that plasmin generation has an inhibitory effect on platelet function. First, very high levels of fibrin(ogen) degradation products, coupled with very low levels of fibrinogen, may impair platelet aggregation.[159] Second, plasminogen can bind to platelets[160] and after its conversion to plasmin, it can enzymatically degrade platelet GPIb, impairing the interaction of platelets with VWF.[161,162] Third, plasmin can inhibit platelet arachidonic acid metabolism.[163] Fourth, t-PA promotes the disaggregation of platelet aggregates, presumably by inducing lysis of the fibrinogen that mediates aggregate formation.[164] Finally, after initial activation, platelets incubated with plasmin and recombinant t-PA *in vitro* become refractory to activation by other agonists.[165] Whether any of these *in vitro* and *ex vivo* observations apply to the *in vivo* situation and are clinically significant remains to be determined.[166] The antifibrinolytic drug, ε-aminocaproic acid, can increase the bleeding time when administered for several days at doses ≥24 g/day.[167]

CARDIOVASCULAR DRUGS

Administration of nitroprusside (which increases platelet cGMP),[168–172] nitroglycerine,[173] and propranolol[174,175] can decrease platelet aggregation and secretion *ex vivo*. Nitroprusside can increase the bleeding time twofold when administered at infusion rates of 6 to 8 mcg/kg per minute.[168,176] Inhalation of nitric oxide, advocated for the treatment of pulmonary hypertension and the adult respiratory distress syndrome, can impair agonist-induced platelet aggregation *ex vivo*, although effects on the bleeding time have been variable.[177–179] The clinical significance of these observations is unclear. "Calcium channel blockers," such as verapamil, nifedipine, and diltiazem inhibit platelet aggregation when added at very high concentrations to washed platelets.[180] This effect is seen primarily with epinephrine-induced aggregation and does not appear to be related to calcium channel blockade. For example, verapamil can act as an α_2-adrenergic receptor antagonist at concentrations that inhibit platelet function.[181] At therapeutic doses, calcium channel blockers do not prolong the bleeding time, although one agent, nisoldipine, has been reported to inhibit agonist-induced calcium transients and platelet aggregation after 10 days of oral administration.[182] At high concentrations, the antiarrhythmic drug quinidine has been reported to cause a mild prolongation of the bleeding time and can potentiate the effect of aspirin.[183]

VOLUME EXPANDERS

Dextran is a neutral polysaccharide that is heterogeneous in molecular size. Two preparations with average molecular weights of 40,000 and 70,000 are in clinical use. Although dextran infusions may prolong the bleeding time in normal subjects and in patients with von Willebrand disease, this has not been observed in most of the normal subjects.[184–186] Infused dextran adsorbs to the platelet surface and can impair platelet aggregation, secretion, and procoagulant activity. The maximal effect of dextran may require several hours, suggesting that larger molecules with a slower rate of clearance are responsible.[184] Curiously, the drug has no effect when added to platelet-rich plasma.[184] Dextran infusion produces a modest reduction in plasma VWF antigen levels and ristocetin cofactor activity.[185] Despite these effects on primary hemostasis and the use of dextran in the operative setting as a volume expander or for antithrombotic prophylaxis, prospective studies indicate that dextran is not associated with significant postoperative bleeding, unless it is administered together with low-dose heparin.[187,188] Hydroxyethyl starch, another volume expander, while generally safe, may prolong the bleeding time and predispose patients to hemorrhage, particularly if it is administered in doses exceeding 20 mL/kg of a 6 percent solution. Lower doses of hydroxyethyl starch may contribute to bleeding if administered simultaneously with low-dose heparin, or if given to patients with a preexistent hemostatic defect, or after major cardiothoracic surgery.[189–192] Different hydroxyethyl starch preparations vary in the average number of hydroxymethyl groups per glucose unit, and this may affect both intravascular survival and effects on hemostasis.[193,194]

PSYCHOTROPIC DRUGS, ANESTHETICS, AND COCAINE

Platelets from patients taking antidepressants or phenothiazines may exhibit impaired aggregation responses, but this is not associated with bleeding.[195,196] The effect on aggregation has been attributed to inhibition of intracellular signaling molecules such as protein kinase C.[197] Selective serotonin reuptake inhibitors such as paroxetine decrease serotonin storage within platelets.[198] Fluoxetine does not appear to impair platelet aggregation *in vitro* and has only rarely been associated with clinical bleeding.[199,200] General anesthesia with halothane or propofol may cause a slight prolongation of the bleeding time, most likely because of an effect on calcium signaling, but this has no adverse effect on surgical hemostasis.[201,202] In addition to an association with thrombocytopenia, cocaine is reported to either inhibit platelet function[203,204] or to induce platelet activation.[205] It has been suggested that heroin decreases platelet nitric oxide production.[206] The clinical relevance of these observations is unknown.

ANTINEOPLASTIC AND OTHER HEMATOLOGIC DRUGS

Administration of mithramycin to a total dose of 6 to 21 mg is associated with mucocutaneous bleeding, an increase in the bleeding time, and decreased platelet aggregation.[207] An *ex vivo* defect in platelet secretion and secondary aggregation has been reported in patients with solid tumors within 48 hours of receiving infusions of autologous marrow and high-dose chemotherapy consisting of cisplatin, cyclophosphamide, and either BCNU (carmustine) or melphelan.[208] Both daunorubicin and BCNU can inhibit platelet aggregation and secretion when added to platelet-rich plasma, but as single agents they have not been shown to cause clinically significant platelet dysfunction.[209–211] Administration of recombinant forms of thrombopoietin to thrombocytopenic patients with cancer results in the production of normally functioning platelets.[212,213] The broad-spectrum protein tyrosine kinase inhibitor dasatinib impairs collagen-induced platelet activation *in vitro* and increases tail bleeding times in mice, perhaps explaining some bleeding episodes in patients with chronic myelogenous leukemia who have been treated with the drug.[214]

MISCELLANEOUS AGENTS

The immunosuppressive drug cyclosporine A has been reported to enhance ADP-stimulated platelet aggregation *in vitro*.[215–217] It is unclear whether this contributes to the thrombotic thrombocytopenic purpura syndrome associated with this drug. Antihistamines,[218] the serotonin antagonist ketanserin,[219] and some radiographic contrast agents[220,221] can impair platelet aggregation responses *ex vivo* by unknown mechanisms.

FOODS AND FOOD ADDITIVES

Certain foods and food additives can effect platelet function. For example, a diet rich in fish oils containing ω-3 fatty acids (eicosapentaenoic acid; docosahexaenoic acid) causes a slight prolongation of the bleeding time.[222] These fatty acids act by reducing the platelet content of arachidonic acid and by competing with arachidonic acid for cyclooxygenase.[223,224] Easy bruising noted after eating Chinese food has been attributed to an antiplatelet effect of the black tree fungus.[225] A component of extract of onion can inhibit platelet arachidonic acid metabolism.[226] Ajoene, a component of garlic, is an inhibitor of fibrinogen binding and platelet aggregation.[227,228] Extracts of two commonly used spices, cumin and turmeric, inhibit platelet aggregation and eicosanoid biosynthesis.[229]

HEMATOLOGIC DISORDERS ASSOCIATED WITH ABNORMAL PLATELET FUNCTION

CHRONIC MYELOPROLIFERATIVE DISORDERS

Definition and History

Bleeding and thrombosis are significant causes of morbidity and mortality in the chronic myeloproliferative disorders, particularly in essential thrombocythemia, polycythemia vera, and primary myelofibrosis.[230–232] Most of the information about platelets, bleeding and thrombosis in the myeloproliferative disorders comes from studies of essential thrombocythemia and polycythemia vera.

Etiology and Pathogenesis

Several factors contribute to the hemostatic abnormalities in the myeloproliferative disorders: (1) Increased whole-blood viscosity in polycythemia vera: The engorgement of blood vessels associated with polycythemia is a risk factor for thrombosis and bleeding, particularly in postoperative situations.[233–235] (2) Intrinsic defects in platelet function: A number of intrinsic platelet function defects have been reported in the myeloproliferative disorders. However, the bleeding time, a poor predictor of clinical bleeding in general, is prolonged in only a minority of patients and bleeding can occur in individuals with normal bleeding times.[236,237] (3) Elevated platelet counts: The contribution of an elevated platelet count, by itself, to the risk of hemorrhage and thrombosis in myeloproliferative disorders is controversial.[238,239] A number of retrospective studies indicate that the risk of abnormal hemostasis cannot be confidently predicted from the degree of thrombocytosis.[236] On the other hand, acquired von Willebrand disease, which represents one potential cause of bleeding in the chronic myeloproliferative disorders, is most frequently associated with extreme elevations of the platelet count (e.g., $\geq 1000–1500 \times 10^9/L$)[240–242]; in some, the VWF abnormality can be corrected transiently by infusion of desmopressin (DDAVP),[243,244] whereas in others they can be partially or completely corrected by cytoreductive therapy.[242,245,246] (4) Leukocyte and/or endothelial dysfunction might contribute to the thrombotic phenotype in some individuals with polycythemia vera[247,248] or essential thrombocythemia,[249–251] perhaps through leukocyte–platelet and leukocyte–endothelial cell interactions.[241,252,253] (5) The increased red cell mass displaces platelets from the periphery of the blood cell column, reducing their interaction with endothelial cells, reducing their hemostatic function, indirectly.

Under the light or electron microscope, platelets in these disorders may be larger or smaller than normal, may be abnormally shaped, and may exhibit a reduction in the number of storage granules.[254] In essential thrombocythemia, platelet survival may be modestly reduced.[255] A number of functional and biochemical abnormalities have been described in platelets from patients with myeloproliferative disorders. The most frequently encountered functional abnormality is a decrease in platelet aggregation and secretion in response to epinephrine, ADP or collagen.[236] The defect in epinephrine-induced aggregation often includes absence of the primary wave of aggregation, which is unusual in other conditions. This is not simply the result of an elevated platelet count, because it is not encountered in reactive thrombocytosis.[232,256] Thus, loss of platelet responsiveness to epinephrine may help to support the presence of a myeloproliferative disorder in otherwise ambiguous cases.

Reduced platelet aggregation and secretion in myeloproliferative disorders is associated with one or more of the following: decreased agonist-induced release of arachidonic acid from membrane phospholipids[257,258]; reduced conversion of arachidonic acid to prostaglandin endoperoxides or lipoxygenase products[259]; reduced platelet responsiveness to thromboxane A_2[260]; deficiency of dense or α granules[261,262]; deficiency of integrin $\alpha_2\beta_1$, resulting in variable changes in platelet responsiveness to collagen,[263] and decreased numbers of α_2-adrenergic receptors associated with reduced or absent platelet responses to epinephrine.[264,265] On the other hand, spontaneous platelet aggregation in a patient with essential thrombocythemia and thrombosis has been reported,[266] as has increased thromboxane biosynthesis by platelets from patients with essential thrombocythemia[267] or polycythemia vera.[268] Reduction in platelet procoagulant activity has been reported in some patients with myeloproliferative disorders and thrombocytosis,[269] as have specific platelet membrane abnormalities, including decreased expression and activation of $\alpha_{IIb}\beta_3$,[270] decreased amounts of the GPIb/V/IX complex, resulting in an acquired form of Bernard-Soulier syndrome[271]; decreased numbers of receptors for PGD_2[272]; increased numbers of FcγRIIa receptors[273]; an increase in GPIV (CD36) with[243,274] or without[275] a corresponding decrease in GPIb; and impaired expression of thrombopoietin (c-Mpl) receptors in polycythemia vera[276] and essential thrombocythemia.[277]

Several features of these *in vitro* platelet functional defects require emphasis relative to the clinical setting. First, none are unique to a particular myeloproliferative disorder. Second, their relative frequencies have varied widely in reported series. Third, none has been predictive of bleeding or thrombosis. Fourth, although the chronic myeloproliferative disorders comprise several distinct clinicopathologic entities, they represent clonal abnormalities of hematopoiesis. Therefore, megakaryocytes and their platelet progeny may acquire genetic, biochemical and structural abnormalities as they develop from a clone of abnormal progenitors. An example of this is acquisition of activating mutations in JAK2 (e.g., V617F or exon 12)[278–282] or c-Mpl (W515L/K)[283,284] in polycythemia vera, essential thrombocythemia or primary myelofibrosis. Although it is biologically plausible that activating mutations in these leukocyte and platelet proteins might influence hemostatic mechanisms, including the activation state of platelets,[285–287] the precise impact of their presence or allele burden on human platelet function remains to be fully assessed, as does their impact on thrombotic risk.[241,288] For example, some studies have concluded that the presence of the JAK2 (V617F) mutation or a high JAK2 (V617F) allele burden[289,290] may confer increased thrombotic risk in essential thrombocythemia, whereas others have failed to show such an association.[291,292] It may be useful in future studies to focus on the JAK2 (V617F) allele burden in platelets and granulocytes separately.[292,293]

Clinical and Laboratory Features

Bleeding occurs in a significant number of patients with myeloproliferative disorders and contributes to mortality in up to 10 percent of these patients. Thrombosis also occurs in one-third of cases, contributing to mortality in 15 to 40 percent of these cases.[237,241] Most symptomatic patients experience either bleeding or thrombosis; however, some develop both complications during the course of their disease. Bleeding usually involves the skin or mucous membranes, but may also occur after surgery or trauma. Thrombosis can involve arteries or veins, and may occur in unusual locations such as abdominal wall vessels or the hepatic, portal, and mesenteric circulations.[294–297] Indeed, full-blown or latent myeloproliferative disorders account for a substantial proportion of patients with the Budd-Chiari syndrome or portal vein thrombosis.[294,298–300] Individuals with essential thrombocythemia may experience ischemia and necrosis of the fingers and toes as a consequence of digital artery thrombosis, microvascular occlusion in the coronary circulation, and transient neurologic symptoms caused by cerebrovascular occlusion.[301] A syndrome of redness and burning pain in the extremities, termed erythromelalgia, is associated with essential thrombocythemia and polycythemia vera and is thought to be caused, in part, by arteriolar platelet thrombi, although it may also have vasculopathic and neuropathic components.[302,303] It has been difficult to predict the risk of bleeding or thrombosis in an asymptomatic patient,[238] but an increase in leukocyte count[249–251] or the number of reticulated platelets in patients with thrombocytosis, thought to reflect an increase in platelet turnover, has been associated with an increased risk for thrombosis.[304] Vascular complications are also more likely to occur in patients older than age 60 years and in patients with other risk factors for vascular disease.[305–308]

Therapy

Therapy should be considered for the symptomatic patient, for patients older than 60 years of age, and for individuals about to undergo surgery. Readers are referred to published expert recommendations for a summary of the treatment of essential thrombocythemia and polycythemia vera, with particular relevance to risk factors for hemostasis and thrombosis.[241,306,308,309] Treatment includes correction of polycythemia and maintenance of a normal red cell mass, which may be approximated by a hematocrit less than 45 percent in males and less than 42 percent in females,[310] as well as treatment of the underlying disorder.[237,241,311–313] Platelet count reduction to less than 400,000/μL in patients with thrombocytosis, either by plateletpheresis or cytoreductive agents, generally has been considered to be the target value associated with clinical improvement.[237,307,314]

Effective cytoreductive agents include the ribonuclease reductase inhibitor hydroxyurea,[315] interferon-α, and anagrelide.[306,314,316,317] In a prospective, randomized trial of 114 "high-risk" individuals with essential thrombocythemia who were either older than 60 years of age or had a previous history of thrombosis, hydroxyurea significantly reduced the incidence of new thrombosis from 24 percent to 3.6 percent.[315] Anagrelide, an imidazoquinazolin derivative, is thought to decrease platelet counts by specifically impairing megakaryocyte maturation.[318] Anagrelide has essentially no effect on red and white cells counts and is not known to be leukemogenic. Nevertheless, 10 to 20 percent of patients experience neurologic, gastrointestinal, and cardiac side effects, in particular fluid retention, often necessitating discontinuation of the drug.[317,319,320] When hydroxyurea and anagrelide were compared head-to-head in a randomized trial of 809 patients with essential thrombocythemia, subjects in the anagrelide group showed an increased rate of arterial thrombosis, major bleeding, and transformation to myelofibrosis relative to the group treated with hydroxyurea. However, the anagrelide group showed a relative decreased rate of venous thrombosis.[321] Progression to myelofibrosis despite treatment with anagrelide also was observed in a phase II study.[322] During an episode of acute bleeding in chronic myeloproliferative disorders, DDAVP infusion may temporarily improved hemostasis if the patient has an acquired storage pool defect or acquired von Willebrand disease.[244,262]

Low-dose aspirin (80–325 mg/day) may be useful in patients with essential thrombocythemia and thrombosis, particularly in those with erythromelalgia or with digital or cerebrovascular ischemia.[241,303,313,323,324] However, the evidence to date remains largely anecdotal, and aspirin can exacerbate a bleeding tendency in patients with myeloproliferative disorders.[306,325] In a double-blind, placebo-controlled study of 518 patients with polycythemia vera who were judged to have no contraindications to daily low-dose (100-mg) aspirin, the subjects in the aspirin arm exhibited a reduced risk of nonfatal arterial and venous cardiovascular endpoints. Although aspirin was well-tolerated, there was no effect of aspirin on overall and cardiovascular mortality.[326] As has been noted,[310] this study population was heavily pretreated to normalize the platelet count, although some individuals may have had residual elevations in red cell mass. Consequently, aspirin's safety and efficacy as documented in this study may not be relevant to all patients with polycythemia vera.

Essential thrombocythemia or polycythemia vera in pregnancy poses special challenges because of an apparent increased risk of unsuccessful pregnancy, thrombotic or bleeding complications, and potential teratogenicity of hydroxyurea.[327] In essential thrombocythemia, the risk of first trimester miscarriages may be higher among women with the *JAK2* (V617F) mutation.[328] A risk-stratified approach to management in pregnancy has been proposed in which high risk is defined as either previous major bleeding or thrombotic episodes, previous pregnancy complications, or a platelet count greater than 1500×10^9/L.[329] Low-risk individuals are recommended to be maintained at a hematocrit of less than 45 percent and to receive aspirin, 100 mg/day during pregnancy and subcutaneous low-molecular-weight heparin, 4000 U/day for 6 weeks after delivery. Interferon-α can be considered in place of aspirin if there has been previous major bleeding or if platelets are greater than 1500×10^9/L. In addition, high-risk patients are recommended to receive low-molecular-weight heparin throughout pregnancy.

LEUKEMIAS AND MYELODYSPLASTIC SYNDROMES

Clinical and Laboratory Features

The most frequent cause of bleeding in these disorders is thrombocytopenia. However, abnormal platelet function *in vitro* has been described in acute myelogenous leukemia, especially if the diagnosis of acute leukemia was preceded by a myelodysplastic syndrome, and in some patients the platelet dysfunction may be clinically significant. In acute myelogenous leukemia and its variants, platelets may be larger than normal, abnormally shaped, and exhibit a marked variation in the number of granules. There may be decreased aggregation and serotonin release in response to ADP, epinephrine, or collagen, decreased surface P-selectin expression in response to platelet activation through the PAR1 thrombin receptor, and decreased platelet procoagulant activity. The functional abnormalities may be a result of either acquired storage pool deficiency or a defect in the process of platelet activation through one or more signaling pathways.[330–334] These defects are intrinsic to the platelet and probably relate to the fact that the megakaryocytes from which platelets are derived have originated from a leukemic stem cell. In addition, drugs used to treat acute leukemias may affect platelet function, at least *in vitro*. Bleeding in the acute leukemias usually responds to platelet transfusions and to treatment of the underlying disease. Similar *in vitro* platelet abnormalities may be seen in the myelodysplastic syndromes, sometimes accompanied by clinical bleeding out of proportion to that expected for the degree of thrombocytopenia.[330,335–338] In these syndromes, platelets may be less uniformly affected; perhaps because there is a residual population of normal platelets admixed with those from the malignant clone.

Reduced platelet aggregation has been reported in children with acute lymphocytic leukemia.[331] Unless the leukemia is biphenotypic, it is difficult to ascribe the platelet defect to the leukemic process itself. Platelets are normal in children with lymphoblastic leukemia in complete remission.[339] A single case has been reported of a patient with acute B-lymphoblastic leukemia and thrombocytopenia whose severe bleeding was attributed, in part, to acquired Glanzmann thrombasthenia associated with anti-$\alpha_{IIb}\beta_3$ antibodies.[340] Hairy-cell leukemia is a lymphoproliferative disease in which platelet dysfunction may rarely complicate the clinical picture. Bleeding is responsible for death in 8 percent of patients, but it is usually caused by thrombocytopenia rather than platelet dysfunction.[341] Some patients may exhibit storage pool deficiency or a defect in the process of platelet activation, and these abnormalities have been reported to disappear following splenectomy.[342] However, this conclusion should be interpreted with caution because splenectomy usually corrects the thrombocytopenia as well. Acquired von Willebrand disease has been reported in association with hairy-cell leukemia.[343]

DYSPROTEINEMIAS

Definition and History

Platelet dysfunction is observed in approximately one-third of patients with immunoglobulin (Ig) A myeloma or Waldenström macroglobulinemia, 15 percent of patients with IgG myeloma, and occasionally in patients with essential monoclonal gammopathy.[344] In addition to platelet dysfunction, other causes of bleeding should be considered in these patients, including the hyperviscosity syndrome,[345] thrombocytopenia, complications of amyloidosis (such as amyloid angiopathy[346] or acquired factor X deficiency[347,348]), and, rarely, a circulating heparin-like anticoagulant[349–351] or systemic fibrino(gen)lysis.[352,353] The myeloma protein may also affect *in vitro* coagulation tests, but not *in vivo* hemostasis, by interfering with fibrin polymerization and with the function of other coagulation proteins.

Etiology and Pathogenesis

The bleeding time may be prolonged in patients with dysproteinemias, even in the absence of clinical bleeding. The platelet defect is caused by the monoclonal protein. It has been suggested that some monoclonal immunoglobulins interact with the platelet surface to interfere nonspecifically with platelet adhesion or stimulus-response coupling. This concept is supported by the observations that platelet dysfunction is more common when the concentration of the paraprotein in plasma or on the platelet membrane is very high[354]; that platelet aggregation, secretion, clot retraction, and platelet procoagulant activity may all be affected; and that normal platelets can acquire these defects when incubated with the purified monoclonal immunoglobulin.[355]

In some cases, specific interactions of the monoclonal protein with platelets or components of the extracellular matrix have been described. One IgA myeloma protein inhibited the ability of a suspension of aortic connective tissue to aggregate normal platelets.[356] The bleeding time and bleeding diathesis of the patient from whom this myeloma protein was obtained were corrected by removal of the protein by plasmapheresis. In another patient with IgD myeloma, immunoglobulin dimers bound to the A1 domain of VWF and inhibited shear-induced platelet aggregation.[357] In still another patient, an IgG myeloma protein bound specifically to the platelet integrin β_3 subunit. Both the intact immunoglobulin and its $F(ab')_2$ fragment inhibited the binding of fibrinogen to activated platelets, thus inducing a thrombasthenic-like state.[358] Several patients with myeloma, essential monoclonal gammopathy, or chronic lymphocytic leukemia have been reported to have an acquired form of von Willebrand disease in which the plasma level of VWF is reduced and/or the high-molecular-weight multimers of VWF are lacking.[359–363]

Therapy

When clinically significant platelet dysfunction occurs in a patient with a dysproteinemia, cytoreductive therapy should be considered as a means to reduce the production and plasma level of the monoclonal immunoglobulin.[344] Plasmapheresis can also control bleeding by reducing the level of the abnormal protein and can be lifesaving during acute bleeding episodes.[364,365] Cryoprecipitate, DDAVP, and/or plasmapheresis may be transiently effective in patients with acquired von Willebrand disease.[360,361,366,367] However, high-dose intravenous immunoglobulin appears to be particularly effective in individuals with essential IgG monoclonal gammopathy and acquired von Willebrand disease, although intermittent infusions may be necessary at approximately 3-week intervals.[362,363,368,369] The reported experience with rituximab for acquired von Willebrand disease is extremely limited, but so far disappointing.[370]

ACQUIRED VON WILLEBRAND DISEASE

Acquired von Willebrand disease is a relatively rare disorder that typically occurs in the setting of an autoimmune or clonal hematologic disease (see Chap. 127).[371–374] The latter includes myeloma,[361,366] Waldenström macroglobulinemia,[375] essential monoclonal gammopathy,[363] low-grade non-Hodgkin lymphoma,[376,377] chronic lymphocytic leukemia,[378] and chronic myeloproliferative disorders, particularly in association with very high platelet counts.[242] In many hematologic disorders, a specific anti-VWF antibody is present,[361,366,379] whereas in autoimmune disorders, anti-VWF antibodies are part of a generalized autoimmune response.[380] When acquired von Willebrand disease occurs in other clinical situations such as cancer (e.g., Wilms tumor), hypothyroidism, or aortic stenosis, it may result from the nonspecific direct absorption of VWF onto tumor cells, shear-induced adsorption onto platelets,[246,343,381–383] or decreased VWF production.[384,385]

Mucocutaneous bleeding and a prolonged bleeding time should raise the suspicion of acquired von Willebrand disease in patients without a prior personal or family history of bleeding. This is especially important in patients with known autoimmune disease or lymphoproliferative or myeloproliferative disorders.[246] Diagnostic evaluation includes measurements of factor VIII coagulant activity, VWF antigen, ristocetin cofactor activity, and VWF multimer analysis.[386] The presence of an *in vitro* inhibitor may, or may not, be detected, depending on whether the antibody binds to VWF and neutralizes its function or merely leads to accelerated VWF clearance by the reticuloendothelial system.[246] Given the uncommon frequency of this disease, reports of patient management have been retrospective and largely anecdotal, and treatment should be reserved for patients with active bleeding or those who are likely to bleed if left untreated. Treatment has included glucocorticoids in patients with lupus,[373,374] and infusions of DDAVP,[361,378,380] VWF-containing factor VIII concentrates,[387] recombinant factor VIIa,[388] or high-dose intravenous immunoglobulin.[372,389,390] The latter is particularly efficacious in patients when acquired von Willebrand disease is associated with a lymphoproliferative disorder or, as discussed above (see "Dysproteinemia" above), with an essential IgG monoclonal gammopathy. Intravenous immunoglobulin likely acts by delaying VWF clearance via reticuloendothelial cell blockade, although other mechanisms have been postulated.[302,362,363,368,369,391,392] Treatment of the underlying disease can be effective in some situations[393] (e.g., hypothyroidism[394,395]; aortic stenosis and other high-shear vascular abnormalities[396,397]; and extreme thrombocytosis[242,245,246,398]).

SYSTEMIC DISORDERS ASSOCIATED WITH ABNORMAL PLATELET FUNCTION

UREMIA

Definition and History

In the predialysis era, hemorrhage occurred in approximately 50 percent of uremic patients and was a cause of death in approximately 30 percent.[399,400] With the advent of dialysis, the frequency of spontaneous hemorrhage in patients with renal failure has decreased.[400] Experience with percutaneous renal biopsy in several thousand patients with renal disease supports the notion that the hemostatic defect in patients with renal disease is usually mild. Although the incidence of small perirenal hematomas following biopsy may be as high as 85 percent when patients are examined by computerized tomography, gross hematuria is observed in only 5 to 10 percent of cases and is usually transient.[401,402] Severe bleeding following biopsy requiring surgical intervention is even less common and usually can be attributed to factors other than a uremic hemostatic defect, such as needle lacerations of the kidney or spleen, anomalous vessels, heparin anticoagulation, or the presence of amyloid in the kidney.

Etiology and Pathogenesis

The hemostatic defect in uremia has been attributed to defects in platelet function and appears to be multifactorial.[400,401–406] One prominent factor is renal failure-associated anemia.[407] A lowered hematocrit *ex vivo* induces a defect in platelet adhesion that can be corrected by increasing the hematocrit to ≥30 percent.[404] In uremic patients, successful treatment of anemia with red blood cell transfusion or recombinant human erythropoietin results in partial or complete correction of prolonged bleeding times when the hematocrit is increased to 27 to 32 percent.[403,408–412] Moreover, the effect of anemia on primary hemostasis is not unique to uremia. In normal individuals, the bleeding time correlates with the hematocrit, and bleeding times can be prolonged in patients with severe anemia of any etiology.[407] Red cells may have a beneficial effect on hemostasis both because they displace platelets to the periphery of the column of circulating blood[413] and they may enhance platelet reactivity.[16]

Correction of anemia does not always return the bleeding time to normal, thus other factors must also be present.[403] Ristocetin-induced platelet aggregation, an *in vitro* surrogate for VWF binding to the platelet GPIb/IX/V complex, may be decreased in uremia. However, plasma VWF concentrations are normal or elevated in renal failure[414] and qualitative VWF abnormalities have not been uniformly observed.[405,415] Mixing studies using uremic platelets and normal plasma, and vice versa, do not demonstrate consistent quantitative or qualitative abnormalities in GPIb/IX/V.[405,415,416] Nonetheless, uremic plasma can inhibit the adhesion of normal platelets to deendothelialized human umbilical artery segments, whereas uremic platelets adhere normally in the presence of normal plasma.[405] Because the defective adhesion appears independent of VWF, an unidentified component of uremic plasma may be responsible for the adhesion defect.[405] Uremic platelets also exhibit markedly reduced spreading on the subendothelium of rabbit vessels, a defect attributed to impaired VWF binding to platelet $\alpha_{IIb}\beta_3$.[417] Because VWF binding to $\alpha_{IIb}\beta_3$ requires platelet stimulation, this observation suggests a uremia-induced defect in platelet signal transduction.

There are a number of reports describing defective agonist-induced platelet activation in uremic patients, including reduced fibrinogen binding, aggregation, and secretion. These abnormalities may be retained after platelets are separated from uremic plasma, and in some cases, uremic plasma imparts the defect to normal platelets.[418] Furthermore, the ability of activated platelets to express procoagulant activity is also reduced in uremia.[419] These functional defects likely result from uremia-induced abnormalities in platelet biochemistry, including reduced agonist-induced increases in cytoplasmic free calcium,[420] reduced release of arachidonic acid from platelet phospholipids,[399] and reduced conversion of released arachidonic acid to prostaglandin endoperoxides and thromboxane A_2.[421–424] In addition, decreased platelet dense-granule ADP and serotonin have been observed,[425] as has an increased level of cAMP.[426] Because ADP and serotonin are platelet agonists and cAMP is an inhibitor of platelet function, these abnormalities could contribute to a platelet activation defect.

A number of dialyzable and nondialyzable substances are reported to be responsible for platelet function defects in uremia. *Ex vivo* platelet aggregation can be inhibited by small dialyzable substances, such as guanidinosuccinic acid and phenolic acids, as well as by poorly characterized "middle molecules" at concentrations found in uremic plasma.[427,428] Venous and arterial segments from uremic patients are reported to produce more PGI_2 than segments from normal individuals, an abnormality not corrected by dialysis.[429] Altered nitric oxide (NO) metabolism has been observed in uremia. In a uremic rat model, prolonged bleeding times and defective platelet adhesion were normalized by an inhibitor of NO formation,[430] suggesting that increased NO synthesis by endothelial cells or platelets is at least partially responsible for defective platelet function in uremia.[431] Why renal failure would increase NO synthesis is not entirely clear, although exposing endothelial cells to guanidinosuccinic acid can mimic the effects of NO, suggesting that retained guanidinosuccinic acid may be the relevant substrate.[432] Uremia has been reported to upregulate the y^+L system for L-arginine transport into platelets, enabling platelets to maintain or enhance NO synthesis, even in the face of low circulating L-arginine concentrations.[433,434] On the other hand, some substances found in high concentrations in uremic plasma, such as urea and parathyroid hormone, appear to play no role in platelet dysfunction.

Concurrent medications and thrombocytopenia must always be considered when a patient with renal failure exhibits a bleeding tendency. Aspirin can prolong the bleeding time inordinately in uremia. Unlike aspirin's effect on COX, this effect is transient and correlates with blood levels of aspirin.[36,37] Bleeding may be potentiated by the administration of heparin during hemodialysis; in this situation, the use of an ethylene-vinyl alcohol copolymer hollow fiber dialyzer or intermittent saline infusion and high blood flow rates may eliminate the need for heparin.[435] β-Lactam antibiotics that prolong the bleeding time may have a greater effect in uremic patients and increase the occurrence of bleeding.[436]

Mild thrombocytopenia has been reported in chronic renal failure, particularly in patients on dialysis,[437] as a result of diminished marrow production and decreased platelet survival.[438] Serum thrombopoietin levels in hemodialysis patients are increased,[437,439] perhaps reflecting a decrease in megakaryocyte mass. But when platelet counts are less than $100 \times 10^5/\mu L$, it is necessary to consider whether a systemic disease or medication, such as multiple myeloma, systemic vasculitis, hemolytic uremic syndrome, eclampsia, renal allograft rejection, or heparin, could be responsible.

Clinical and Laboratory Features

Despite dialysis, abnormal platelet function in uremia remains a clinical issue because it may contribute to bleeding following surgery or trauma or in conjunction with anatomic lesions of the gastrointestinal tract.[421,435] The bleeding time has often been used as an indication of hemorrhagic risk in uremia, but critical reviews of the literature indicate that it is inappropriate to use it for this purpose.[440,441]

Therapy

Abnormal platelet aggregation and a prolonged bleeding time are common in uremic patients, but by themselves, are not indications for therapeutic intervention. The frequency of excessive bleeding after biopsies or other surgical procedures in uremic patients who have not received specific treatment is not known, but may be uncommon. Thus, if bleeding does complicate a procedure, a thorough search for causes of bleeding other than uremia should be initiated without assuming that uremia is the etiology. However, when therapy for a uremic bleeding diathesis is necessary, the uremic platelet defect can usually be successfully treated.

There are several therapeutic maneuvers that can either partially or completely correct an abnormal bleeding time in uremic patients and anecdotal observations indicate that they may also improve hemostasis. Because prospective studies comparing various treatment regimens have not been performed, the choice of therapy should be based on the severity of the bleeding, the anticipated severity of the hemostatic stress imposed by surgery or trauma, the predicted duration of the therapeutic effect, and the risks of therapy.

The mainstay of therapy is dialysis. Intensive dialysis can correct the bleeding time and bleeding diathesis in many patients, but is only partially effective in others.[442] Peritoneal dialysis and hemodialysis are equally effective.[442,443] If a patient undergoing dialysis bleeds, it may be worthwhile to increase the intensity of the dialysis.

In uremic individuals, increasing the hematocrit by transfusion or treatment with recombinant human erythropoietin to 27 to 32 percent is associated with correction of the bleeding time and a suggestion of diminished clinical bleeding.[403,408–411] A number of reports suggest that erythropoietin has an effect on platelets independent of an increase in hematocrit,[412] perhaps the result of an increase in the number of young platelets in the circulation.[444]

DDAVP, a vasopressin analogue whose pressor effects are substantially less than its antidiuretic effects, and causes the release of VWF from tissue stores, has been reported to shorten the bleeding time in 50 to 75 percent of patients with uremia. In many cases, surgery has been carried out safely after administration of this drug, although no controlled trial has been performed.[445] DDAVP is usually administered intravenously in a dose of 0.3 mcg/kg over 15 to 30 minutes (maximum dose 20 mcg) but it is also effective at this dose when given subcutaneously.[445] Alternatively, the drug can be given intranasally.[446] Improvement in the bleeding time is seen within 30 to 60 minutes of administration, lasts for approximately 4 hours, and roughly correlates with the rise in the plasma levels of VWF and the appearance in the circulation of high-molecular-weight VWF multimers.[445] In some patients, the drug has been given repeatedly at 12- to 24-hour intervals, although tachyphylaxis often occurs.[447]

Side effects of DDAVP have been mild and uncommon and have included a 10 to 15 percent decrease in mean arterial pressure, a 20 to 30 percent increase in pulse rate, facial flushing, water retention, and hyponatremia, rarely leading to seizures. Seizures are most common after repeated administration and when fluids are given freely.[445] Water retention and hyponatremia have not been observed in patients whose kidneys cannot respond to the hormone. Several uremic and nonuremic individuals with atherosclerosis have been reported to develop stroke or myocardial infarction after DDAVP administration, although such complications appear to be rare.[448,449] If dialysis is not effective, DDAVP is the treatment of choice for uremic bleeding, particularly if only a short-term benefit is required.[445]

Conjugated estrogens at a dose of 0.6 mg/kg intravenously for 5 days have also been reported to shorten the bleeding time in most, but not all, uremic individuals, both in uncontrolled studies and in randomized, double-blind studies.[450–453] They may also be useful in some patients with uremia who bleed from gastrointestinal telangiectasia.[454] No changes in the plasma levels or multimer distribution of VWF have been noted with this treatment, and it has been postulated that the active component in conjugated estrogens, 17β-estradiol, acts through an estrogen receptor mechanism.[455] Uncontrolled studies suggest that infusions of cryoprecipitate can shorten the bleeding time in uremic patients and ameliorate bleeding,[456] but other studies report inconsistent results.[457]

ANTIPLATELET ANTIBODIES

Definition and History

Antibody binding to platelets in several pathologic conditions, including immune thrombocytopenic purpura (ITP), system lupus erythematosus (SLE), and platelet alloimmunization, can produce thrombocytopenia caused by decreased platelet survival. Less commonly, bleeding times may be shorter than expected for the degree of thrombocytopenia, suggesting enhanced platelet function.[458] On occasion, however, platelet function is impaired. Although a platelet count above 30,000 to 40,000/μL is generally regarded as "safe,"[459] this cannot always be assumed in patients with immune thrombocytopenia.

Etiology and Pathogenesis

The mechanism by which autoantibodies or alloantibodies impair platelet function is often not apparent, but antibody binding to specific platelet glycoproteins could be responsible. Most antiplatelet antibodies are directed at $\alpha_{IIb}\beta_3$, but antibodies directed against GPIb/IX/V, $\alpha_2\beta_1$, and GPIV have been detected as well.[460,461] In most instances, the functional consequences of antibody binding are obscured by the presence of thrombocytopenia. However, in several patients with normal platelet counts and autoantibodies against $\alpha_{IIb}\beta_3$, there was absent platelet aggregation and a bleeding diathesis reminiscent of Glanzmann thrombasthenia.[462–465] Similarly, two IgG autoantibodies against GPIb were reported to selectively inhibit ristocetin-induced platelet aggregation,[466,467] as were two autoantibodies against $\alpha_2\beta_1$ that impaired collagen-induced platelet aggregation.[468,469] Finally, a patient with ITP has been identified whose anti-GPVI autoantibody produced GPVI shedding from the platelet surface and platelets that were unresponsive to collagen stimulation.[470]

Besides interfering with platelet function, some autoantibodies can activate platelets and induce aggregation and secretion. *In vitro*, antibodies can activate platelets through immune complex binding to platelet Fc receptors, by depositing sublytic quantities of the membrane attack complex of complement (C5b-9) on the cell surface,[471] or by binding to a specific membrane antigen.[472] The prototypic example of this phenomenon is heparin-induced thrombocytopenia in which antibodies bound to neoepitopes exposed on the platelet factor 4 molecule by heparin binding activate platelets by binding to platelet Fc receptors (see Chap. 133).[473]

Clinical Laboratory Features and Therapy

Platelet dysfunction should be suspected in any patient with ITP or SLE who has mucocutaneous bleeding with a platelet count that is not ordinarily associated with bleeding (e.g., ≥30–40,000/μL). In such cases, the bleeding time may be longer than expected for the platelet count. The clinical spectrum of autoimmune platelet dysfunction may also include some individuals, usually women, with "easy bruising" and a normal platelet count. These patients may have ITP with "compensated thrombocytolysis," as a substantial proportion of these patients have circulating antiplatelet antibodies and megathrombocytes.[474]

Patients with antiplatelet antibodies may exhibit defective platelet function *in vitro*, even if they do not manifest a prolonged bleeding time or excessive bleeding. These abnormalities include impaired platelet aggregation to ADP, epinephrine, or collagen,[475–478] as well as impaired adhesion to the subendothelial matrix.[479] The most frequently reported abnormalities are absence of platelet aggregation in response to low concentrations of collagen, and absence of the second wave of aggregation in response to ADP or epinephrine. This pattern is identical to that seen in individuals with congenital storage pool disease. In fact, both ITP and SLE may be associated with an acquired form of storage pool disease manifested by a reduced platelet content of dense and α-granule components.[480,481] In one report, platelets in ITP also exhibited an activation defect manifested by impaired conversion of arachidonic acid to thromboxane A_2.[482] Because antibody-mediated platelet dysfunction and bleeding almost always occur in the setting of immune thrombocytopenia, therapeutic efforts should be directed to the treatment of these disorders.

CARDIOPULMONARY BYPASS

Definition and History

Circulating blood through an extracorporeal bypass circuit during cardiac surgery induces a variety of hemostatic defects. The most significant of these are thrombocytopenia, platelet dysfunction, and hyperfibrinolysis.[483–485] At their extreme, these defects can result in substantial postoperative bleeding that may last hours to days after bypass. Approximately 5 percent of patients experience excessive postoperative bleeding after extracorporeal bypass; roughly half of the bleeding is a result of surgical causes; much of the remainder is a result of qualitative platelet defects and hyperfibrinolysis.

Etiology and Pathogenesis

Thrombocytopenia is a consistent feature of bypass surgery.[151,484] Typically, platelet counts decrease to 50 percent of presurgical levels by 25 minutes after the initiation of bypass, but thrombocytopenia can occur within 5 minutes and may persist for as long as several days.[483,485,486] The major factor responsible for thrombocytopenia is hemodilution from priming the pump with colloid or crystalloid solutions, but it is often more profound than can be accounted for by hemodilution alone.[485–487] Platelet adhesion to artificial surfaces in the circuit has been demonstrated by scanning electron micrographs.[488] The mechanism of this interaction is uncertain, but it may be a result of the deposition of fibrinogen onto the bypass circuit and platelet adhesion mediated by $\alpha_{IIb}\beta_3$.[489] Less common causes of thrombocytopenia during bypass are disseminated intravascular coagulation, sequestration of damaged platelets in the liver, and heparin-induced thrombocytopenia.[490]

Qualitative platelet defects induced by the bypass circuit[484,491] are manifested as prolonged bleeding times, abnormal *ex vivo* platelet aggregation, decreased ristocetin-induced platelet agglutination, deficiency of platelet α and granules, release of soluble CD40 ligand, and the generation of platelet microparticles.[483,485,486,492–495] The severity of these abnormalities correlates with the duration of extracorporeal bypass[496] and they generally resolve within 2 to 24 hours.[484]

The bypass-induced defects in platelet function are likely caused by platelet activation and fragmentation,[494,497] hypothermia, contact with fibrinogen-coated synthetic surfaces, contact with the blood–air interface, cardiotomy suction, and exposure to thrombin, plasmin, ADP, or complement.[489,498–501] Drugs such as heparin, protamine, $\alpha_{IIb}\beta_3$ antagonists, and aspirin, as well as the production of fibrin degradation products, can also impair platelet function.[151,502–504] Controversy exists about the significance of these defects *in vivo*. Some investigators suggest that the entire qualitative platelet defect is a result of the use of heparin during bypass surgery, and its inhibitory effect on thrombin activity[502]; however, this would not account for the bleeding diathesis that can exist hours after reversal of heparin.

Hyperfibrinolysis may also contribute to the bleeding diathesis associated with cardiopulmonary bypass.[505,506] This is likely caused by thrombus formation in the pericardial cavity followed by local and subsequently systemic, fibrinolysis.[505] The relevance of hyperfibrinolysis to post-bypass bleeding is bolstered by the efficacy of antifibrinolytic therapy in minimizing cardiopulmonary bypass surgery blood loss.

Therapy

A preoperative evaluation of cardiac surgical candidates should include a history of bleeding in either the patient or family members. Some authors recommend a screening prothrombin time, partial prothrombin time, and bleeding time even in individuals with no history of bleeding.[507] However, the validity of this approach is controversial.[508] Regardless, prophylactic transfusion of allogeneic blood components is not indicated.[484,509,510] Studies of the preoperative use of recombinant human erythropoietin in anemic patients, or erythropoietin plus autologous blood donation in nonanemic patients suggest that these approaches are reasonable.[511–513] Cell savers are now often used during bypass surgery, and the collected washed autologous red blood cells are reinfused after completion of the cardiopulmonary bypass. In addition, blood collected from chest tube drainage has been reinfused to minimize allogeneic transfusions.[514] The safety of transfusing large quantities of blood by this technique has not fully been established.[515]

A number of maneuvers have been taken to reduce the hemostatic abnormalities associated with cardiac surgery. These include coating the artificial surfaces of cardiopulmonary bypass devices with heparin[516–520] using centrifugal rather than roller pumps,[521] use of a number of pharmacologic agents,[522] and performing coronary artery surgery without bypass.[523,524] Off-pump coronary artery bypass surgery appears to preserve platelet function, but concerns have been raised about adverse thromboembolic events after surgery because of the concurrence of normal platelet function, late thrombin generation, and reduced fibrinolysis.[525–527] Several pharmacologic maneuvers have been tried to assist in the management of postoperative bleeding. Postoperative patients with a prolonged bleeding time and excessive blood loss may respond to DDAVP, as evidenced by a shortening of the bleeding time. However, results of trials using this agent have been contradictory, some studies showing a reduced blood loss and others showing no benefit.[528,529] Based on the assumption that platelet activation during bypass surgery could be a major cause of postoperative platelet dysfunction, infusion of platelet activation inhibitors, such as PGE_1, prostacyclin, or stable prostacyclin analogues, have been carried out in animal models and in humans. By increasing platelet cAMP and reducing platelet responsiveness, these agents prevent bypass-induced thrombocytopenia and platelet dysfunction. However, randomized trials using prostacyclin and its analogue, iloprost, have not shown a clear overall benefit, in part because of significant toxicity, including hypotension.[130,133] Recombinant factor VIIa has been used empirically and successfully to treat uncontrolled postoperative bleeding.[530,531] Primarily on the basis of the cardiovascular complications encountered by patients in two randomized studies of the use of parecoxib/valdecoxib to treat pain after cardiac surgery, the use of cyclooxygenase inhibitors and of traditional NSAIDs is contraindicated in this setting.[532,533]

Inhibiting fibrinolysis using ε-aminocaproic acid or tranexamic acid during cardiopulmonary bypass can reduce mediastinal blood loss and transfusion requirements.[522] Although aprotinin (Trasylol), a broad-spectrum protease inhibitor, was also used for this purpose, observational studies,[534–536] as well as a blinded clinical trial,[537] revealed that its use is associated with serious end-organ damage and a higher mortality than the use of ε-aminocaproic acid or no antifibrinolytic agent.

The most important determinant of blood loss following cardiopulmonary surgery is the surgical procedure itself. If excessive nonsurgical postoperative bleeding occurs, one should verify that the patient is no longer hypothermic and that heparin has been fully reversed. At this point, the administration of pharmacologic agents, along with judicious transfusions of platelets, cryoprecipitate, fresh-frozen plasma and red blood cells, is appropriate.

MISCELLANEOUS DISORDERS

Chronic liver disease of various etiologies has been reported to cause a prolonged bleeding time and reduced platelet aggregation and procoagulant activity (see Chap. 129).[538–540] The prolonged bleeding time in such patients may respond to infusion of DDAVP.[541] However, the existence of a platelet function defect specific to liver disease was placed in doubt by a study of 60 patients with cirrhosis in whom aggregation studies and bleeding times were compatible with the degree of thrombocytopenia.[542] The etiology of the bleeding diathesis associated with fulminant or end-stage liver disease is multifactorial and includes decreased coagulation factor production, fibrinolysis, dysfibrinogenemia, thrombocytopenia as a consequence of hypersplenism and thrombopoietin deficiency,[543,544] and, occasionally, disseminated intravascular coagulation.[540] Thus, the prolonged bleeding time reported in some patients with severe liver disease may be a result of multiple factors, including thrombocytopenia, hypofibrinogenemia, and anemia, none of which imply an intrinsic defect in platelet function.[545]

Patients with disseminated intravascular coagulation may exhibit reduced platelet aggregation and acquired storage pool deficiency.[546,547] These result from platelet activation *in vivo* by thrombin or other agonists. Alternatively, elevated levels of fibrin(ogen) degradation products and low fibrinogen levels that accompany disseminated intravascular coagulation may also contribute to the platelet defect. Although purified low-molecular-weight fibrinogen degradation products can impair platelet aggregation, this effect requires concentrations of degradation products unlikely to occur *in vivo*.[548] Moreover, it is difficult to assess the significance of platelet dysfunction in most patients with disseminated intravascular coagulation because of the simultaneous presence of thrombocytopenia and other hemostatic defects.

Decreased platelet aggregation and secretion in response to ADP and epinephrine has been reported in Bartter syndrome, a group of rare inherited disorders characterized by severe restrictions of salt reabsorption by thick ascending limb of Henle, perhaps caused by excessive prostaglandin E_2 synthesis.[549–552] However, reviews of Bartter syndrome make no mention of hemostatic problems[550] so that the clinical significance of the platelet aggregation abnormalities is doubtful.

There are isolated reports of a slight prolongation of the bleeding time and/or *ex vivo* platelet function defects in a number of other clinical conditions. These include nonthrombocytopenic purpura with eosinophilia,[553–555] atopic asthma and hay fever,[556] acute respiratory failure,[557] and Wilms tumor elaborating hyaluronic acid.[558] The clinical significance of these associations is not clear.

REFERENCES

1. Rodgers RP, Levin J: A critical reappraisal of the bleeding time. *Semin Thromb Hemost* 16:1, 1990.
2. Carr ME Jr: *In vitro* assessment of platelet function. *Transfus Med Rev* 11:106, 1997.
3. George J, Shattil S: The clinical importance of acquired abnormalities of platelet function. *N Engl J Med* 324:27, 1991.
4. Wisloff F, Godal H: Prolonged bleeding time with adequate platelet count in hospital patients. *Scand J Haematol* 27:45, 1981.
5. Patrono C: Aspirin as an antiplatelet drug. *N Engl J Med* 330:1287, 1994.
6. Smith WL, DeWitt DL, Garavito RM: Cyclooxygenases: Structural, cellular, and molecular biology. *Annu Rev Biochem* 69:145, 2000.
7. Kis B, Snipes JA, Busija DW: Acetaminophen and the cyclooxygenase-3 puzzle: Sorting out facts, fictions, and uncertainties. *J Pharmacol Exp Ther* 315:1, 2005.
8. Smith W, Garavito R, DeWitt D: Prostaglandin endoperoxide H synthases (cyclooxygenases)-1 and -2. *Biol Chem* 271:33157, 1996.
9. Riondino S, Trifirò E, Principessa L, et al: Lack of biological relevance of platelet cyclooxygenase-2 dependent thromboxane A2 production. *Thromb Res* 122:359, 2008.
10. Weiss H, Aledort L: Impaired platelet/connective tissue reaction in man after aspirin ingestion. *Lancet* 2:495, 1967.
11. O'Brien JR: Effect of salicylates on human platelets. *Lancet* 1:1431, 1968.
12. Grosser T, Fries S, FitzGerald GA: Biological basis for the cardiovascular consequences of COX-2 inhibition: Therapeutic challenges and opportunities. *J Clin Invest* 116:4, 2006.
13. Kyrle PA, Eichler HG, Jager U, Lechner K: Inhibition of prostacyclin and thromboxane A2 generation by low-dose aspirin at the site of plug formation in man *in vivo*. *Circulation* 75:1025, 1987.
14. Clarke RJ, Mayo G, Price P, FitzGerald GA: Suppression of thromboxane A2 but not of systemic prostacyclin by controlled-release aspirin. *N Engl J Med* 325:1137, 1991.
15. Jaffe EA, Weksler BB: Recovery of endothelial cell prostacyclin production after inhibition by low doses of aspirin. *J Clin Invest* 63:532, 1979.
16. Marcus AJ, Safier LB: Thromboregulation: Multicellular modulation of platelet reactivity in hemostasis and thrombosis. *FASEB J* 7:516, 1993.
17. Rich JB: The efficacy and safety of aprotinin use in cardiac surgery. *Ann Thorac Surg* 66:S6, 1998.
18. Johnson ES, Lanes SF, Wentworth CE 3rd, et al: A metaregression analysis of the dose-response effect of aspirin on stroke. *Arch Intern Med* 159:1248, 1999.
19. A comparison of two doses of aspirin (30 mg vs. 283 mg a day) in patients after a transient ischemic attack or minor ischemic stroke. The Dutch TIA Trial Study Group. *N Engl J Med* 325:1261, 1991.
20. Derry S, Loke YK: Risk of gastrointestinal haemorrhage with long term use of aspirin: Meta-analysis. *BMJ* 321:1183, 2000.
21. Campbell CL, Smyth S, Montalescot G, Steinhubl SR: Aspirin dose for the prevention of cardiovascular disease: A systematic review. *JAMA* 297:2018, 2007.
22. Kallmann R, Nieuwenhuis HK, de Groot PG, et al: Effects of low doses of aspirin, 10 mg and 30 mg daily, on bleeding time, thromboxane production and 6-keto-PGF1a excretion in healthy subjects. *Thromb Res* 45:355, 1987.
23. Nakajima H, Takami H, Yamagata K, et al: Aspirin effects on colonic mucosal bleeding. *Dis Colon Rectum* 40:1484, 1997.
24. Mielke CH Jr: Aspirin prolongation of the template bleeding time: Influence of venostasis and direction of incision. *Blood* 60:1139, 1982.
25. Hirsh J, Salzman EW, Harker L, et al: Aspirin and other platelet active drugs. Relationship among dose, effectiveness, and side effects. *Chest* 95:12S,1989.
26. Final report on the aspirin component of the ongoing physicians' health study. Steering Committee of the Physicians' Health Study Research Group. *N Engl J Med* 321:129, 1989.
27. Page IH: Salicylate damage to the gastric mucosal barrier. *N Engl J Med* 276:1307, 1967.
28. Leonards JR, Levy G: The role of dosage form in aspirin-induced gastrointestinal bleeding. *Clin Pharmacol Ther* 8:400, 1967.
29. Baigent C, Blackwell L, Collins R, et al: Aspirin in the primary and secondary prevention of vascular disease: Collaborative meta-analysis of individual participant data from randomised trials. *Lancet* 373:1849, 2009.
30. Stuart MJ, Gross SJ, Elrad H, Graeber JE: Effects of acetylsalicylic-acid ingestion on maternal and neonatal hemostasis. *N Engl J Med* 307:909, 1982.
31. Ferraris VA, Ferraris SP, Lough FC, Berry WR: Preoperative aspirin ingestion increases operative blood loss after coronary artery bypass grafting. *Ann Thorac Surg* 45:71, 1988.
32. Sethi GK, Copeland JG, Goldman S, et al: Implications of preoperative administration of aspirin in patients undergoing coronary artery bypass grafting. Department of Veterans Affairs Cooperative Study on Antiplatelet Therapy. *J Am Coll Cardiol* 15:15, 1990.
33. Horlocker TT, Wedel DJ, Offord KP: Does preoperative antiplatelet therapy increase the risk of hemorrhagic complications associated with regional anesthesia? *Anesth Analg* 70:631, 1990.
34. Kitchen L, Erichson RB, Sideropoulos H: Effect of drug-induced platelet dysfunction on surgical bleeding. *Am J Surg* 143:215, 1982.
35. Kennedy BM: Aspirin and surgery—A review. *Ir Med J* 77:363, 1984.
36. Livio M, Benigni A, Vigano G, et al: Moderate doses of aspirin and risk of bleeding in renal failure. *Lancet* 1:414, 1986.
37. Gaspari F, Vigano G, Orisio S, et al: Aspirin prolongs bleeding time in uremia by a mechanism distinct from platelet cyclooxygenase inhibition. *J Clin Invest* 79:1788, 1987.
38. Chesebro JH, Fuster V, Elveback LR, et al: Trial of combined warfarin plus dipyridamole or aspirin therapy in prosthetic heart valve replacement: Danger of aspirin compared with dipyridamole. *Am J Cardiol* 51:1537, 1983.
39. Deykin D, Janson P, McMahon L: Ethanol potentiation of aspirin-induced prolongation of the bleeding time. *N Engl J Med* 306:852, 1982.
40. Rosove MH, Hocking WG, Harwig SS, Perloff JK: Studies of beta-thromboglobulin, platelet factor 4, and fibrinopeptide A in erythrocytosis due to cyanotic congenital heart disease. *Thromb Res* 29:225, 1983.
41. Kobrinsky NL, Israels ED, Gerrard JM, et al: Shortening of bleeding time by 1-deamino-8-D-arginine vasopressin in various bleeding disorders. *Lancet* 1:1145, 1984.
42. Lethagen S, Rugarn P: The effect of DDAVP and placebo on platelet function and prolonged bleeding time induced by oral acetyl salicylic acid intake in healthy volunteers. *Thromb Haemost* 67:185, 1992.
43. Simon LS, Mills JA: Drug therapy: Nonsteroidal antiinflammatory drugs (first of two parts). *N Engl J Med* 302:1179, 1980.
44. Catella-Lawson F, Reilly MP, Kapoor SC, et al: Cyclooxygenase inhibitors and the antiplatelet effects of aspirin. *N Engl J Med* 345:1809, 2001.
45. Buchanan GR, Martin V, Levine PH, et al: The effects of "anti-platelet" drugs on bleeding time and platelet aggregation in normal human subjects. *Am J Clin Pathol* 68:355, 1977.

46. Nadell J, Bruno J, Varady J, Segre EJ: Effect of naproxen and of aspirin on bleeding time and platelet aggregation. *J Clin Pharmacol* 14:176, 1974.
47. Mielke CH Jr, Kahn SB, Muschek LD, et al: Effects of zomepirac on hemostasis in healthy adults and on platelet function *in vitro*. *J Clin Pharmacol* 20:409, 1980.
48. Thomas P, Hepburn B, Kim HC, Saidi P: Nonsteroidal anti-inflammatory drugs in the treatment of hemophilic arthropathy. *Am J Hematol* 12:131, 1982.
49. McIntyre BA, Philp RB, Inwood MJ: Effect of ibuprofen on platelet function in normal subjects and hemophiliac patients. *Clin Pharmacol Ther* 24:616, 1978.
50. Ragni MV, Miller BJ, Whalen R, Ptachcinski R: Bleeding tendency, platelet function, and pharmacokinetics of ibuprofen and zidovudine in HIV(+) hemophilic men. *Am J Hematol* 40:176, 1992.
51. FitzGerald GA, Patrono C: The coxibs, selective inhibitors of cyclooxygenase-2. *N Engl J Med* 345:433, 2001.
52. Kearney PM, Baigent C, Godwin J, et al: Do selective cyclo-oxygenase-2 inhibitors and traditional non-steroidal anti-inflammatory drugs increase the risk of atherothrombosis? Meta-analysis of randomised trials. *BMJ* 332:1302, 2006.
53. Antman EM, Bennett JS, Daugherty A, et al: Use of nonsteroidal antiinflammatory drugs: An update for clinicians: A scientific statement from the American Heart Association. *Circulation* 115:1634, 2007.
54. Solomon SD, Wittes J, Finn PV, et al: Cardiovascular risk of celecoxib in 6 randomized placebo-controlled trials: The cross trial safety analysis. *Circulation* 117:2104, 2008.
55. McGettigan P, Henry D: Cardiovascular risk and inhibition of cyclooxygenase: A systematic review of the observational studies of selective and nonselective inhibitors of cyclooxygenase 2. *JAMA* 296:1633, 2006.
56. Hinz B, Cheremina O, Brune K: Acetaminophen (paracetamol) is a selective cyclooxygenase-2 inhibitor in man. *FASEB J* 22:383, 2008.
57. A randomised, blinded, trial of clopidogrel versus aspirin in patients at risk of ischaemic events (CAPRIE). CAPRIE Steering Committee. *Lancet* 348:1329, 1996.
58. Rupprecht HJ, Darius H, Borkowski U, et al: Comparison of antiplatelet effects of aspirin, ticlopidine, or their combination after stent implantation. *Circulation* 97:1046, 1998.
59. Leon MB, Baim DS, Popma JJ, et al: A clinical trial comparing three antithrombotic-drug regimens after coronary-artery stenting. Stent Anticoagulation Restenosis Study Investigators. *N Engl J Med* 339:1665, 1998.
60. Sharis PJ, Cannon CP, Loscalzo J: The antiplatelet effects of ticlopidine and clopidogrel. *Ann Intern Med* 129:394, 1998.
61. Schomig A, Neumann FJ, Kastrati A, et al: A randomized comparison of antiplatelet and anticoagulant therapy after the placement of coronary-artery stents. *N Engl J Med* 334:1084, 1996.
62. Yusuf S, Zhao F, Mehta SR, et al: Effects of clopidogrel in addition to aspirin in patients with acute coronary syndromes without ST-segment elevation. *N Engl J Med* 345:494, 2001.
63. Bhatt DL, Chew DP, Hirsch AT, et al: Superiority of clopidogrel versus aspirin in patients with prior cardiac surgery. *Circulation* 103:363, 2001.
64. McTavish D, Faulds D, Goa KL: Ticlopidine. An updated review of its pharmacology and therapeutic use in platelet-dependent disorders. *Drugs* 40:238, 1990.
65. Hardisty RM, Powling MJ, Nokes TJ: The action of ticlopidine on human platelets. Studies on aggregation, secretion, calcium mobilization and membrane glycoproteins. *Thromb Haemost* 64:150, 1990.
66. Humbert M, Nurden P, Bihour C, et al: Ultrastructural studies of platelet aggregates from human subjects receiving clopidogrel and from a patient with an inherited defect of an ADP-dependent pathway of platelet activation. *Arterioscler Thromb Vasc Biol* 16:1532, 1996.
67. Hechler B, Eckly A, Ohlmann P, et al: The P2Y1 receptor, necessary but not sufficient to support full ADP-induced platelet aggregation, is not the target of the drug clopidogrel. *Br J Haematol* 103:858, 1998.
68. Geiger J, Honig-Liedl P, Schanzenbacher P, Walter U: Ligand specificity and ticlopidine effects distinguish three human platelet ADP receptors. *Eur J Pharmacol* 351:235, 1998.
69. Geiger J, Brich J, Honig-Liedl P, et al: Specific impairment of human platelet P2Y(AC) ADP receptor-mediated signaling by the antiplatelet drug clopidogrel. *Arterioscler Thromb Vasc Biol* 19:2007, 1999.
70. Savi P, Laplace MC, Maffrand JP, Herbert JM: Binding of [3H]-2-methylthio ADP to rat platelets—Effect of clopidogrel and ticlopidine. *J Pharmacol Exp Ther* 269:772, 1994.
71. Daniel JL, Dangelmaier C, Jin J, et al: Molecular basis for ADP-induced platelet activation. I. Evidence for three distinct ADP receptors on human platelets. *J Biol Chem* 273:2024, 1998.
72. Jantzen HM, Gousset L, Bhaskar V, et al: Evidence for two distinct G-protein-coupled ADP receptors mediating platelet activation. *Thromb Haemost* 81:111, 1999.
73. De Caterina R, Sicari R, Bernini W, et al: Benefit/risk profile of combined antiplatelet therapy with ticlopidine and aspirin. *Thromb Haemost* 65:504, 1991.
74. Helft G, Osende JI, Worthley SG, et al: Acute antithrombotic effect of a front-loaded regimen of clopidogrel in patients with atherosclerosis on aspirin. *Arterioscler Thromb Vasc Biol* 20:2316, 2000.
75. Collet JP, Hulot JS, Pena A, et al: Cytochrome P450 2C19 polymorphism in young patients treated with clopidogrel after myocardial infarction: A cohort study. *Lancet* 373:309, 2009.
76. Simon T, Verstuyft C, Mary-Krause M, et al: Genetic determinants of response to clopidogrel and cardiovascular events. *N Engl J Med* 360:363, 2009.
77. Mega JL, Close SL, Wiviott SD, et al: Cytochrome p-450 polymorphisms and response to clopidogrel. *N Engl J Med* 360:354, 2009.
78. Hass WK, Easton JD, Adams HP Jr, et al: A randomized trial comparing ticlopidine hydrochloride with aspirin for the prevention of stroke in high-risk patients. Ticlopidine Aspirin Stroke Study Group. *N Engl J Med* 321:501, 1989.
79. Gent M, Blakely JA, Easton JD, et al: The Canadian American Ticlopidine Study (CATS) in thromboembolic stroke. *Lancet* 1:1215, 1989.
80. Mataix R, Ojeda E, Perez MC, Jimenez S: Ticlopidine and severe aplastic anaemia. *Br J Haematol* 80:125, 1992.
81. Garnier G, Taillan B, Pesce A, et al: Ticlopidine and severe aplastic anaemia. *Br J Haematol* 81:459, 1992.
82. Bennett CL, Weinberg PD, Rozenberg-Ben-Dror K, et al: Thrombotic thrombocytopenic purpura associated with ticlopidine. A review of 60 cases. *Ann Intern Med* 128:541, 1998.
83. Steinhubl SR, Tan WA, Foody JM, Topol EJ: Incidence and clinical course of thrombotic thrombocytopenic purpura due to ticlopidine following coronary stenting. EPISTENT Investigators. Evaluation of Platelet IIb/IIIa Inhibitor for Stenting. *JAMA* 281:806, 1999.
84. Chen DK, Kim JS, Sutton DM: Thrombotic thrombocytopenic purpura associated with ticlopidine use: A report of 3 cases and review of the literature. *Arch Intern Med* 159:311, 1999.
85. Bennett CL, Connors JM, Carwile JM, et al: Thrombotic thrombocytopenic purpura associated with clopidogrel. *N Engl J Med* 342:1773, 2000.
86. Bossavy JP, Thalamas C, Sagnard L, et al: A double-blind randomized comparison of combined aspirin and ticlopidine therapy versus aspirin or ticlopidine alone on experimental arterial thrombogenesis in humans. *Blood* 92:1518, 1998.
87. Steinhubl SR, Berger PB, Mann JT 3rd, et al: Early and sustained dual oral antiplatelet therapy following percutaneous coronary intervention: A randomized controlled trial. *JAMA* 288:2411, 2002.
88. Diener HC, Bogousslavsky J, Brass LM, et al: Aspirin and clopidogrel compared with clopidogrel alone after recent ischaemic stroke or transient ischaemic attack in high-risk patients (MATCH): Randomised, double-blind, placebo-controlled trial. *Lancet* 364:331, 2004.
89. Rothwell PM: Lessons from MATCH for future randomised trials in secondary prevention of stroke. *Lancet* 364:305, 2004.
90. Bhatt DL, Fox KA, Hacke W, et al: Clopidogrel and aspirin versus aspirin alone for the prevention of atherothrombotic events. *N Engl J Med* 354:1706, 2006.
91. Sugidachi A, Ogawa T, Kurihara A, et al: The greater *in vivo* antiplatelet effects of prasugrel as compared to clopidogrel reflect more efficient generation of its active metabolite with similar antiplatelet activity to that of clopidogrel's active metabolite. *J Thromb Haemost* 5:1545, 2007.
92. Jernberg T, Payne CD, Winters KJ, et al: Prasugrel achieves greater inhibition of platelet aggregation and a lower rate of non-responders compared with clopidogrel in aspirin-treated patients with stable coronary artery disease. *Eur Heart J* 27:1166, 2006.
93. Brandt JT, Payne CD, Wiviott SD, et al: A comparison of prasugrel and clopidogrel loading doses on platelet function: Magnitude of platelet inhibition is related to active metabolite formation. *Am Heart J* 153:66 e9, 2007.
94. Wiviott SD, Trenk D, Frelinger AL, et al: Prasugrel compared with high loading- and maintenance-dose clopidogrel in patients with planned percutaneous coronary intervention: The Prasugrel in Comparison to Clopidogrel for Inhibition of Platelet Activation and Aggregation—Thrombolysis in Myocardial Infarction 44 trial. *Circulation* 116:2923, 2007.
95. Michelson AD, Frelinger AL 3rd, Braunwald E, et al: Pharmacodynamic assessment of platelet inhibition by prasugrel vs. clopidogrel in the TRITON-TIMI 38 trial. *Eur Heart J* 30:1753, 2009.
96. Wiviott SD, Braunwald E, McCabe CH, et al: Prasugrel versus clopidogrel in patients with acute coronary syndromes. *N Engl J Med* 357:2001, 2007.
97. Greenbaum AB, Grines CL, Bittl JA, et al: Initial experience with an intravenous P2Y12 platelet receptor antagonist in patients undergoing percutaneous coronary intervention: Results from a 2-part, phase II, multicenter, randomized, placebo- and active-controlled trial. *Am Heart J* 151:689.e1, 2006.
98. Storey RF, Husted S, Harrington RA, et al: Inhibition of platelet aggregation by AZD6140, a reversible oral P2Y12 receptor antagonist, compared with clopidogrel in patients with acute coronary syndromes. *J Am Coll Cardiol* 50:1852, 2007.
99. Lefkovits J, Plow EF, Topol EJ: Platelet glycoprotein IIb/IIIa receptors in cardiovascular medicine. *N Engl J Med* 332:1553, 1995.
100. Nurden AT, Poujol C, Durrieu-Jais C, Nurden P: Platelet glycoprotein IIb/IIIa inhibitors: Basic and clinical aspects. *Arterioscler Thromb Vasc Biol* 19:2835, 1999.
101. Bennett JS, Mousa S: Platelet function inhibitors in the year 2000. *Thromb Haemost* 85:395, 2001.
102. French DL, Seligsohn U: Platelet glycoprotein IIb/IIIa receptors and Glanzmann's thrombasthenia. *Arterioscler Thromb Vasc Biol* 20:607, 2000.
103. Nurden AT: Inherited abnormalities of platelets. *Thromb Haemost* 82:468, 1999.
104. Use of a monoclonal antibody directed against the platelet glycoprotein IIb/IIIa receptor in high-risk coronary angioplasty. The EPIC Investigation. *N Engl J Med* 330:956, 1994.
105. Platelet glycoprotein IIb/IIIa receptor blockade and low-dose heparin during percutaneous coronary revascularization. The EPILOG Investigators. *N Engl J Med* 336:1689, 1997.
106. Inhibition of the platelet glycoprotein IIb/IIIa receptor with tirofiban in unstable angina and non-Q-wave myocardial infarction. Platelet Receptor Inhibition in

Ischemic Syndrome Management in Patients Limited by Unstable Signs and Symptoms (PRISM-PLUS) Study Investigators. *N Engl J Med* 338:1488, 1998.

107. Inhibition of platelet glycoprotein IIb/IIIa with eptifibatide in patients with acute coronary syndromes. The PURSUIT Trial Investigators. Platelet Glycoprotein IIb/IIIa in Unstable Angina: Receptor Suppression Using Integrilin Therapy. *N Engl J Med* 339:436, 1998.
108. Simpfendorfer C, Kottke-Marchant K, Lowrie M, et al: First chronic platelet glycoprotein IIb/IIIa integrin blockade. A randomized, placebo-controlled pilot study of xemilofiban in unstable angina with percutaneous coronary interventions. *Circulation* 96:76, 1997.
109. Cannon CP, McCabe CH, Borzak S, et al: Randomized trial of an oral platelet glycoprotein IIb/IIIa antagonist, sibrafiban, in patients after an acute coronary syndrome: Results of the TIMI 12 trial. Thrombolysis in Myocardial Infarction. *Circulation* 97:340, 1998.
110. Chew DP, Bhatt DL, Sapp S, Topol EJ: Increased mortality with oral platelet glycoprotein IIb/IIIa antagonists: A meta-analysis of phase III multicenter randomized trials. *Circulation* 103:201, 2001.
111. Bassler N, Loeffler C, Mangin P, et al: A mechanistic model for paradoxical platelet activation by ligand-mimetic alphaIIb beta3 (GPIIb/IIIa) antagonists. *Arterioscler Thromb Vasc Biol* 27:e9, 2007.
112. Ferguson JJ, Kereiakes DJ, Adgey AA, et al: Safe use of platelet GP IIb/IIIa inhibitors. *Eur Heart J* 19 Suppl D:D40, 1998.
113. Berkowitz SD, Sane DC, Sigmon KN, et al: Occurrence and clinical significance of thrombocytopenia in a population undergoing high-risk percutaneous coronary revascularization. Evaluation of c7E3 for the Prevention of Ischemic Complications (EPIC) Study Group. *J Am Coll Cardiol* 32:311, 1998.
114. Randomised placebo-controlled trial of abciximab before and during coronary intervention in refractory unstable angina: The CAPTURE Study. *Lancet* 349:1429, 1997.
115. Jubelirer SJ, Koenig BA, Bates MC: Acute profound thrombocytopenia following C7E3 Fab (abciximab) therapy: Case reports, review of the literature and implications for therapy. *Am J Hematol* 61:205, 1999.
116. Giugliano RP, McCabe CH, Sequeira RF, et al: First report of an intravenous and oral glycoprotein IIb/IIIa inhibitor (RPR 109891) in patients with recent acute coronary syndromes: Results of the TIMI 15A and 15B trials. *Am Heart J* 140:81, 2000.
117. Comparison of sibrafiban with aspirin for prevention of cardiovascular events after acute coronary syndromes: A randomised trial. The SYMPHONY Investigators. Sibrafiban versus Aspirin to Yield Maximum Protection from Ischemic Heart Events Post-acute Coronary Syndromes. *Lancet* 355:337, 2000.
118. Hongo RH, Brent BN: Association of eptifibatide and acute profound thrombocytopenia. *Am J Cardiol* 88:428, 2001.
119. McClure MW, Berkowitz SD, Sparapani R, et al: Clinical significance of thrombocytopenia during a non-ST-elevation acute coronary syndrome. The platelet glycoprotein IIb/IIIa in unstable angina: Receptor suppression using integrilin therapy (PURSUIT) trial experience. *Circulation* 99:2892, 1999.
120. Aster RH: Immune thrombocytopenia caused by glycoprotein IIb/IIIa inhibitors. *Chest* 127(2 Suppl):535, 2005.
121. Brassard JA, Curtis BR, Cooper RA, et al: Acute thrombocytopenia in patients treated with the oral glycoprotein IIb/IIIa inhibitors xemilofiban and orbofiban: Evidence for an immune etiology. *Thromb Haemost* 88:892, 2002.
122. Christopoulos CG, Machin SJ: A new type of pseudothrombocytopenia: EDTA-mediated agglutination of platelets bearing Fab fragments of a chimaeric antibody. *Br J Haematol* 87:650, 1994.
123. Sane DC, Damaraju LV, Topol EJ, et al: Occurrence and clinical significance of pseudothrombocytopenia during abciximab therapy. *J Am Coll Cardiol* 36:75, 2000.
124. Ivy DD, Kinsella JP, Ziegler JW, Abman SH: Dipyridamole attenuates rebound pulmonary hypertension after inhaled nitric oxide withdrawal in postoperative congenital heart disease. *J Thorac Cardiovasc Surg* 115:875, 1998.
125. Gresele P, Arnout J, Deckmyn H, Vermylen J: Mechanism of the antiplatelet action of dipyridamole in whole blood: Modulation of adenosine concentration and activity. *Thromb Haemost* 55:12, 1986.
126. FitzGerald GA: Dipyridamole. *N Engl J Med* 316:1247, 1987.
127. Antithrombotic Trialists' Collaboration: Collaborative meta-analysis of randomised trials of antiplatelet therapy for prevention of death, myocardial infarction, and stroke in high risk patients. *BMJ* 324:71, 2002.
128. Reilly M, FitzGerald GA: Gathering intelligence on antiplatelet drugs: The view from 30,000 feet. When combined with other information overviews lead to conviction. *BMJ* 324:59, 2002.
129. Verro P, Gorelick PB, Nguyen D. Aspirin plus dipyridamole versus aspirin for prevention of vascular events after stroke or TIA: A meta-analysis. Stroke 39:1358, 2008.
130. Walker ID, Davidson JF, Faichney A, Wheately DJ, Davidson KG: A double-blind study of prostacyclin in cardiopulmonary bypass surgery. *Br J Haematol* 49:415, 1981.
131. Huddleston CB, Wareing TH, Clanton JA, Bender HW Jr: Amelioration of the deleterious effects of platelets activated during cardiopulmonary bypass: Comparison of a thromboxane synthetase inhibitor and a prostacyclin analogue. *J Thorac Cardiovasc Surg* 89:190, 1985.
132. Fisher CA, Kappa JR, Sinha AK, et al: Comparison of equimolar concentrations of iloprost, prostacyclin, and prostaglandin E_1 on human platelet function. *J Lab Clin Med* 109:184, 1987.
133. Fish KJ, Sarnquist FH, van Steennis C, et al: A prospective, randomized study of the effects of prostacyclin on platelets and blood loss during coronary bypass operations. *J Thorac Cardiovasc Surg* 91:436, 1986.
134. Sorkin EM, Markham A: Cilostazol. *Drugs Aging* 14:63, 1999.
135. Biondi-Zoccai GG, Lotrionte M, Anselmino M, et al: Systematic review and meta-analysis of randomized clinical trials appraising the impact of cilostazol after percutaneous coronary intervention. *Am Heart J* 155:1081, 2008.
136. Loscalzo J, Welch G: Nitric oxide and its role in the cardiovascular system. *Prog Cardiovasc Dis* 38:87, 1995.
137. Sattler FR, Weitekamp MR, Ballard JO: Potential for bleeding with the new beta-lactam antibiotics. *Ann Intern Med* 105:924, 1986.
138. Pillgram-Larsen J, Wisloff F, Jorgensen JJ, Godal HC, Semb G: Effect of high-dose ampicillin and cloxacillin on bleeding time and bleeding in open-heart surgery. *Scand J Thorac Cardiovasc Surg* 19:45, 1985.
139. Fass RJ, Copelan EA, Brandt JT, Moeschberger ML, Ashton JJ: Platelet-mediated bleeding caused by broad-spectrum penicillins. *J Infect Dis* 155:1242, 1987.
140. Cazenave JP, Packham MA, Guccione MA, Mustard JF: Effects of penicillin G on platelet aggregation, release, and adherence to collagen. *Proc Soc Exp Biol Med* 142:159, 1973.
141. Shattil SJ, Bennett JS, McDonough M, Turnbull J: Carbenicillin and penicillin G inhibit platelet function *in vitro* by impairing the interaction of agonists with the platelet surface. *J Clin Invest* 65:329, 1980.
142. Fletcher C, Pearson C, Choi SC, et al: *In vitro* comparison of antiplatelet effects of beta-lactam penicillins. *J Lab Clin Med* 108:217, 1986.
143. Packham MA, Rand ML, Perry DW, et al: Probenecid inhibits platelet responses to aggregating agents *in vitro* and has a synergistic inhibitory effect with penicillin G. *Thromb Haemost* 76:239, 1996.
144. Burroughs SF, Johnson GJ: Beta-lactam antibiotic-induced platelet dysfunction: Evidence for irreversible inhibition of platelet activation *in vitro* and *in vivo* after prolonged exposure to penicillin. *Blood* 75:1473, 1990.
145. Sattler FR, Weitekamp MR, Sayegh A, Ballard JO: Impaired hemostasis caused by beta-lactam antibiotics. *Am J Surg* 155:30, 1988.
146. Giles AR, Greenwood P, Tinlin S: A platelet release defect induced by aspirin or penicillin G does not increase gastrointestinal blood loss in thrombocytopenic rabbits. *Br J Haematol* 57:17, 1984.
147. Andrassy K, Koderisch J, Trenk D, et al: Hemostasis in patients with normal and impaired renal function under treatment with cefodizime. *Infection* 15:348, 1987.
148. Brown RB, Klar J, Lemeshow S, et al: Enhanced bleeding with cefoxitin or moxalactam. Statistical analysis within a defined population of 1493 patients. *Arch Intern Med* 146:2159, 1986.
149. Rossi EC, Levin NW: Inhibition of primary ADP-induced platelet aggregation in normal subjects after administration of nitrofurantoin (Furadantin). *J Clin Invest* 52:2457, 1973.
150. Ishikawa S, Manabe S, Wada O: Miconazole inhibition of platelet aggregation by inhibiting cyclooxygenase. *Biochem Pharmacol* 35:1787, 1986.
151. Khuri SF, Valeri CR, Loscalzo J, et al: Heparin causes platelet dysfunction and induces fibrinolysis before cardiopulmonary bypass [see comments]. *Ann Thorac Surg* 60:1008, 1995.
152. Salzman EW, Rosenberg RD, Smith MH, et al: Effect of heparin and heparin fractions on platelet aggregation. *J Clin Invest* 65:64, 1980.
153. Horne MK 3rd, Chao ES: Heparin binding to resting and activated platelets. *Blood* 74:238, 1989.
154. Sobel M, McNeill PM, Carlson PL, et al: Heparin inhibition of von Willebrand factor-dependent platelet function *in vitro* and *in vivo*. *J Clin Invest* 87:1787, 1991.
155. Coller BS: Platelets and thrombolytic therapy. *N Engl J Med* 322:33, 1990.
156. Niewiarowski S, Senyi AF, Gillies P: Plasmin-induced platelet aggregation and platelet release reaction. Effects on hemostasis. *J Clin Invest* 52:1647, 1973.
157. Fitzgerald DJ, Catella F, Roy L, FitzGerald GA: Marked platelet activation *in vivo* after intravenous streptokinase in patients with acute myocardial infarction. *Circulation* 77:142, 1988.
158. Kerins DM, Roy L, FitzGerald GA, Fitzgerald DJ: Platelet and vascular function during coronary thrombolysis with tissue-type plasminogen activator. *Circulation* 80:1718, 1989.
159. Thorsen LI, Brosstad F, Gogstad G, et al: Competitions between fibrinogen with its degradation products for interactions with the platelet-fibrinogen receptor. *Thromb Res* 44:611, 1986.
160. Miles LA, Ginsberg MH, White JG, Plow EF: Plasminogen interacts with human platelets through two distinct mechanisms. *J Clin Invest* 77:2001, 1986.
161. Adelman B, Michelson AD, Loscalzo J, et al: Plasmin effect on platelet glycoprotein Ib-von Willebrand factor interactions. *Blood* 65:32, 1985.
162. Stricker RB, Wong D, Shiu DT, et al: Activation of plasminogen by tissue plasminogen activator on normal and thrombasthenic platelets: Effects on surface proteins and platelet aggregation. *Blood* 68:275, 1986.
163. Schafer AI, Adelman B: Plasmin inhibition of platelet function and of arachidonic acid metabolism. *J Clin Invest* 75:456, 1985.
164. Loscalzo J, Vaughan DE: Tissue plasminogen activator promotes platelet disaggregation in plasma. *J Clin Invest* 79:1749, 1987.
165. Penny WF, Ware JA: Platelet activation and subsequent inhibition by plasmin and recombinant tissue-type plasminogen activator. *Blood* 79:91, 1992.
166. Winters KJ, Eisenberg PR, Jaffe AS, Santoro SA: Dependence of plasmin-mediated degradation of platelet adhesive receptors on temperature and Ca2+. *Blood* 76:1546, 1990.
167. Green D, Ts'ao CH, Cerullo L, et al: Clinical and laboratory investigation of the effects of epsilon-aminocaproic acid on hemostasis. *J Lab Clin Med* 105:321, 1985.

168. Hines R, Barash PG: Infusion of sodium nitroprusside induces platelet dysfunction *in vitro*. *Anesthesiology* 70:611, 1989.
169. Kroll MH, Schafer AI: Biochemical mechanisms of platelet activation. *Blood* 74:1181, 1989.
170. Anfossi G, Russo I, Massucco P, et al: Studies on inhibition of human platelet function by sodium nitroprusside. Kinetic evaluation of the effect on aggregation and cyclic nucleotide content. *Thromb Res* 102:319, 2001.
171. Bozzo J, Hernandez MR, Galan AM, et al: Antiplatelet effects of sodium nitroprusside in flowing human blood: Studies under normoxic and hypoxic conditions. *Thromb Res* 97:217, 2000.
172. Jang EK, Azzam JE, Dickinson NT, et al: Roles for both cyclic GMP and cyclic AMP in the inhibition of collagen-induced platelet aggregation by nitroprusside. *Br J Haematol* 117:664, 2002.
173. Schafer AI, Alexander RW, Handin RI: Inhibition of platelet function by organic nitrate vasodilators. *Blood* 55:649, 1980.
174. Weksler BB, Gillick M, Pink J: Effect of propranolol on platelet function. *Blood* 49:185, 1977.
175. Leon R, Tiarks CY, Pechet L: Some observations on the *in vivo* effect of propranolol on platelet aggregation and release. *Am J Hematol* 5:117, 1978.
176. Hines R: Preservation of platelet function during trimethaphan infusion. *Anesthesiology* 72:834, 1990.
177. Hogman M, Frostell C, Arnberg H, Hedenstierna G: Bleeding time prolongation and NO inhalation. *Lancet* 341:1664, 1993.
178. Samama CM, Diaby M, Fellahi JL, et al: Inhibition of platelet aggregation by inhaled nitric oxide in patients with acute respiratory distress syndrome. *Anesthesiology* 83:56, 1995.
179. Gries A, Bode C, Peter K, et al: Inhaled nitric oxide inhibits human platelet aggregation, P-selectin expression, and fibrinogen binding *in vitro* and *in vivo*. *Circulation* 97:1481, 1998.
180. Ring ME, Corrigan JJ Jr, Fenster PE: Effects of oral diltiazem on platelet function: Alone and in combination with "low dose" aspirin. *Thromb Res* 44:391, 1986.
181. Barnathan ES, Addonizio VP, Shattil SJ: Interaction of verapamil with human platelet alpha-adrenergic receptors. *Am J Physiol* 242:H19, 1982.
182. Fujinishi A, Takahara K, Ohba C, et al: Effects of nisoldipine on cytosolic calcium, platelet aggregation, and coagulation/fibrinolysis in patients with coronary artery disease. *Angiology* 48:515, 1997.
183. Lawson D, Mehta J, Mehta P, et al: Cumulative effects of quinidine and aspirin on bleeding time and platelet α_2-adrenoceptors: Potential mechanism of bleeding diathesis in patients receiving this combination. *J Lab Clin Med* 108:581, 1986.
184. Weiss HJ: The effect of clinical dextran on platelet aggregation, adhesion, and ADP release in man: *In vivo* and *in vitro* studies. *J Lab Clin Med* 69:37, 1967.
185. Aberg M, Hedner U, Bergentz SE: Effect of dextran 70 on factor VIII and platelet function in von Willebrand's disease. *Thromb Res* 12:629, 1978.
186. Mishler JMt: Synthetic plasma volume expanders—Their pharmacology, safety and clinical efficacy. *Clin Haematol* 13:75, 1984.
187. Kelton JG, Hirsh J: Bleeding associated with antithrombotic therapy. *Semin Hematol* 17:259, 1980.
188. Korttila K, Lauritsalo K, Sarmo A, et al: Suitability of plasma expanders in patients receiving low-dose heparin for prevention of venous thrombosis after surgery. *Acta Anaesthesiol Scand* 27:104, 1983.
189. Cope JT, Banks D, Mauney MC, et al: Intraoperative hetastarch infusion impairs hemostasis after cardiac operations. *Ann Thorac Surg* 63:78, 1997.
190. Ruttmann TG, James MF, Aronson I: *In vivo* investigation into the effects of haemodilution with hydroxyethyl starch (200/0.5) and normal saline on coagulation. *Br J Anaesth* 80:612, 1998.
191. Roberts JS, Bratton SL: Colloid volume expanders. Problems, pitfalls and possibilities. *Drugs* 55:621, 1998.
192. Avorn J, Patel M, Levin R, Winkelmayer WC: Hetastarch and bleeding complications after coronary artery surgery. *Chest* 124:1437, 2003.
193. Treib J, Haass A, Pindur G: Coagulation disorders caused by hydroxyethyl starch. *Thromb Haemost* 78:974, 1997.
194. Scharbert G, Deusch E, Kress HG, et al: Inhibition of platelet function by hydroxyethyl starch solutions in chronic pain patients undergoing peridural anesthesia. *Anesth Analg* 99:823, 2004.
195. Svehla C, Spankova H, Mlejnkova M: The effect of tricyclic antidepressive drugs on adrenaline and adenosine diphosphate induced platelet aggregation. *J Pharm Pharmacol* 18:616, 1966.
196. Warlow C, Ogston D, Douglas AS: Platelet function after the administration of chlorpromazine to human subjects. *Haemostasis* 5:21, 1976.
197. Morishita S, Aoki S, Watanabe S: Different effect of desipramine on protein kinase C in platelets between bipolar and major depressive disorders. *Psychiatry Clin Neurosci* 53:11, 1999.
198. Hergovich N, Aigner M, Eichler HG, et al: Paroxetine decreases platelet serotonin storage and platelet function in human beings. *Clin Pharmacol Ther* 68:435, 2000.
199. Alderman CP, Seshadri P, Ben-Tovim DI: Effects of serotonin reuptake inhibitors on hemostasis. *Ann Pharmacother* 30:1232, 1996.
200. Pai VB, Kelly MW: Bruising associated with the use of fluoxetine. *Ann Pharmacother* 30:786, 1996.
201. Corbin F, Blaise G, Sauve R: Differential effect of halothane and forskolin on platelet cytosolic Ca2+ mobilization and aggregation. *Anesthesiology* 89:401, 1998.
202. Aoki H, Mizobe T, Nozuchi S, Hiramatsu N: *In vivo* and *in vitro* studies of the inhibitory effect of propofol on human platelet aggregation. *Anesthesiology* 88:362, 1998.
203. Heesch CM, Negus BH, Steiner M, et al: Effects of *in vivo* cocaine administration on human platelet aggregation. *Am J Cardiol* 78:237, 1996.
204. Jennings LK, White MM, Sauer CM, et al: Cocaine-induced platelet defects. *Stroke* 24:1352, 1993.
205. Togna G, Graziani M, Sorrentino C, Caprino L: Prostanoid production in the presence of platelet activation in hypoxic cocaine-treated rats. *Haemostasis* 26:311, 1996.
206. Batista A, Macedo T, Tavares P, et al: Nitric oxide production and nitric oxide synthase expression in platelets from heroin abusers before and after ultrarapid detoxification. *Ann N Y Acad Sci* 965:479, 2002.
207. Ahr DJ, Scialla SJ, Kimbali DB Jr: Acquired platelet dysfunction following mithramycin therapy. *Cancer* 41:448, 1978.
208. Panella TJ, Peters W, White JG, et al: Platelets acquire a secretion defect after high-dose chemotherapy. *Cancer* 65:1711, 1990.
209. Pogliani EM, Fantasia R, Lambertenghi-Deliliers G, Cofrancesco E: Daunorubicin and platelet function. *Thromb Haemost* 45:38, 1981.
210. McKenna R, Ahmad T, Ts'ao CH, Frischer H: Glutathione reductase deficiency and platelet dysfunction induced by 1,3-bis(2-chloroethyl)-1-nitrosourea. *J Lab Clin Med* 102:102, 1983.
211. Karolak L, Chandra A, Khan W, et al: High-dose chemotherapy-induced platelet defect: Inhibition of platelet signal transduction pathways. *Mol Pharmacol* 43:37, 1993.
212. O'Malley CJ, Rasko JE, Basser RL, et al: Administration of pegylated recombinant human megakaryocyte growth and development factor to humans stimulates the production of functional platelets that show no evidence of *in vivo* activation. *Blood* 88:3288, 1996.
213. Vadhan-Raj S, Murray LJ, Bueso-Ramos C, et al: Stimulation of megakaryocyte and platelet production by a single dose of recombinant human thrombopoietin in patients with cancer. *Ann Intern Med* 126:673, 1997.
214. Gratacap M-P, Martin V, Valera M-C, et al: The new tyrosine-kinase inhibitor and anticancer drug dasatinib reversibly affects platelet activation *in vitro* and *in vivo*. *Blood* 114:1884, 2009.
215. Vanrenterghem Y, Roels L, Lerut T, et al: Thromboembolic complications and haemostatic changes in cyclosporin-treated cadaveric kidney allograft recipients. *Lancet* 1:999, 1985.
216. Cohen H, Neild GH, Patel R, et al: Evidence for chronic platelet hyperaggregability and *in vivo* activation in cyclosporin-treated renal allograft recipients. *Thromb Res* 49:91, 1988.
217. Grace AA, Barradas MA, Mikhailidis DP, et al: Cyclosporine A enhances platelet aggregation. *Kidney Int* 32:889, 1987.
218. Thomson C, Forbes CD, Prentice CR: A comparison of the effects of antihistamines on platelet function. *Thromb Diath Haemorrh* 30:547, 1973.
219. Platelet function during long-term treatment with ketanserin of claudicating patients with peripheral atherosclerosis. A multi-center, double-blind, placebo-controlled trial. The PACK Trial Group. *Thromb Res* 55:13, 1989.
220. Parvez Z, Moncada R, Fareed J, Messmore HL: Antiplatelet action of intravascular contrast media. Implications in diagnostic procedures. *Invest Radiol* 19:208, 1984.
221. Rao AK, Rao VM, Willis J, et al: Inhibition of platelet function by contrast media: Iopamidol and ioxaglate versus iothalamate. Work in progress. *Radiology* 156:311, 1985.
222. Goodnight SH Jr, Harris WS, Connor WE: The effects of dietary omega 3 fatty acids on platelet composition and function in man: A prospective, controlled study. *Blood* 58:880, 1981.
223. Moncada S, Higgs EA: Arachidonate metabolism in blood cells and the vessel wall. *Clin Haematol* 15:273, 1986.
224. Leaf A, Weber PC: Cardiovascular effects of n-3 fatty acids. *N Engl J Med* 318:549, 1988.
225. Hammerschmidt DE: Szechwan purpura. *N Engl J Med* 302:1191, 1980.
226. Srivastava KC: Onion exerts antiaggregatory effects by altering arachidonic acid metabolism in platelets. *Prostaglandins Leukot Med* 24:43, 1986.
227. Apitz-Castro R, Ledezma E, Escalante J, Jain MK: The molecular basis of the antiplatelet action of ajoene: Direct interaction with the fibrinogen receptor. *Biochem Biophys Res Commun* 141:145, 1986.
228. Apitz-Castro R, Escalante J, Vargas R, Jain MK: Ajoene, the antiplatelet principle of garlic, synergistically potentiates the antiaggregatory action of prostacyclin, forskolin, indomethacin and dipyridamole on human platelets. *Thromb Res* 42:303, 1986.
229. Srivastava KC: Extracts from two frequently consumed spices—cumin (*Cuminum cyminum*) and turmeric (*Curcuma longa*)—inhibit platelet aggregation and alter eicosanoid biosynthesis in human blood platelets. *Prostaglandins Leukot Essent Fatty Acids* 37:57, 1989.
230. Pearson TC: The risk of thrombosis in essential thrombocythemia and polycythemia vera. *Semin Oncol* 29:16, 2002.
231. Kessler CM: Propensity for hemorrhage and thrombosis in chronic myeloproliferative disorders. *Semin Hematol* 41:10, 2004.
232. Schafer AI: Thrombocytosis. *N Engl J Med* 350:1211, 2004.
233. Wasserman LR, Gilbert HS: The treatment of polycythemia vera. *Med Clin North Am* 50:1501, 1966.
234. Murphy S: Polycythemia vera. *Dis Mon* 38:153, 1992.
235. Ruggeri M, Rodeghiero F, Tosetto A, et al: Postsurgery outcomes in patients with polycythemia vera and essential thrombocythemia: A retrospective survey. *Blood* 111:666, 2008.

236. Schafer AI: Essential thrombocythemia. *Prog Hemost Thromb* 10:69, 1990.
237. Elliott MA, Tefferi A: Pathogenesis and management of bleeding in essential thrombocythemia and polycythemia vera. *Curr Hematol Rep* 3:344, 2004.
238. Kessler CM, Klein HG, Havlik RJ: Uncontrolled thrombocytosis in chronic myeloproliferative disorders. *Br J Haematol* 50:157, 1982.
239. McIntyre KJ, Hoagland HC, Silverstein MN, Petitt RM: Essential thrombocythemia in young adults. *Mayo Clin Proc* 66:149, 1991.
240. Michiels JJ, Berneman Z, Schroyens W, et al: The paradox of platelet activation and impaired function: Platelet-von Willebrand factor interactions, and the etiology of thrombotic and hemorrhagic manifestations in essential thrombocythemia and polycythemia vera. *Semin Thromb Hemost* 32:589, 2006.
241. Finazzi G, Barbui T: Evidence and expertise in the management of polycythemia vera and essential thrombocythemia. *Leukemia* 22:1494, 2008.
242. Budde U, Schaefer G, Mueller N, et al: Acquired von Willebrand's disease in the myeloproliferative syndrome. *Blood* 64:981, 1984.
243. Eche N, Sie P, Caranobe C, et al: Platelets in myeloproliferative disorders. III: Glycoprotein profile in relation to platelet function and platelet density. *Scand J Haematol* 26:123, 1981.
244. Mohri H, Ohkubo T: Acquired von Willebrand's syndrome due to an inhibitor of IgG specific for von Willebrand's factor in polycythemia rubra vera. *Acta Haematol* 78:258, 1987.
245. van Genderen PJ, Prins FJ, Lucas IS, et al: Decreased half-life time of plasma von Willebrand factor collagen binding activity in essential thrombocythaemia: Normalization after cytoreduction of the increased platelet count. *Br J Haematol* 99:832, 1997.
246. Tefferi A, Nichols WL: Acquired von Willebrand disease: Concise review of occurrence, diagnosis, pathogenesis, and treatment. *Am J Med* 103:536, 1997.
247. Landolfi R, Di Gennaro L, Barbui T, et al: Leukocytosis as a major thrombotic risk factor in patients with polycythemia vera. *Blood* 109:2446, 2007.
248. Gangat N, Strand J, Li CY, et al: Leucocytosis in polycythaemia vera predicts both inferior survival and leukaemic transformation. *Br J Haematol* 138:354, 2007.
249. Carobbio A, Finazzi G, Guerini V, et al: Leukocytosis is a risk factor for thrombosis in essential thrombocythemia: Interaction with treatment, standard risk factors, and Jak2 mutation status. *Blood* 109:2310, 2007.
250. Carobbio A, Finazzi G, Antonioli E, et al: Thrombocytosis and leukocytosis interaction in vascular complications of essential thrombocythemia. *Blood* 112:3135, 2008.
251. Carobbio A, Antonioli E, Guglielmelli P, et al: Leukocytosis and risk stratification assessment in essential thrombocythemia. *J Clin Oncol* 26:2732, 2008.
252. Villmow T, Kemkes-Matthes B, Matzdorff AC: Markers of platelet activation and platelet-leukocyte interaction in patients with myeloproliferative syndromes. *Thromb Res* 108:139, 2002.
253. Falanga A, Marchetti M, Vignoli A, et al: Leukocyte-platelet interaction in patients with essential thrombocythemia and polycythemia vera. *Exp Hematol* 33:523, 2005.
254. Maldonado JE, Pintado T, Pierre RV: Dysplastic platelets and circulating megakaryocytes in chronic myeloproliferative diseases. I. The platelets: Ultrastructure and peroxidase reaction. *Blood* 43:797, 1974.
255. Bautista AP, Buckler PW, Towler HM, et al: Measurement of platelet life-span in normal subjects and patients with myeloproliferative disease with indium oxine labelled platelets. *Br J Haematol* 58:679, 1984.
256. Ginsberg AD: Platelet function in patients with high platelet counts. *Ann Intern Med*82, 1975.
257. Jubelirer SJ, Russel F, Vaillancourt R, Deykin D: Platelet arachidonic acid metabolism and platelet function in ten patients with chronic myelogenous leukemia. *Blood* 56:728, 1980.
258. Pareti FI, Gugliotta L, Mannucci L, et al: Biochemical and metabolic aspects of platelet dysfunction in chronic myeloproliferative disorders. *Thromb Haemost* 47:84, 1982.
259. Schafer AI: Deficiency of platelet lipoxygenase activity in myeloproliferative disorders. *N Engl J Med* 306:381, 1982.
260. Ushikubi F, Okuma M, Kanaji K, et al: Hemorrhagic thrombocytopathy with platelet thromboxane A2 receptor abnormality: Defective signal transduction with normal binding activity. *Thromb Haemost* 57:158, 1987.
261. Malpass TW, Savage B, Hanson SR, et al: Correlation between prolonged bleeding time and depletion of platelet dense granule ADP in patients with myelodysplastic and myeloproliferative disorders. *J Lab Clin Med* 103:894, 1984.
262. Mohri H: Acquired von Willebrand disease and storage pool disease in chronic myelocytic leukemia. *Am J Hematol* 22:391, 1986.
263. Handa M, Watanabe K, Kawai Y, et al: Platelet unresponsiveness to collagen: Involvement of glycoprotein Ia-IIa (alpha 2 beta 1 integrin) deficiency associated with a myeloproliferative disorder. *Thromb Haemost* 73:521, 1995.
264. Kaywin P, McDonough M, Insel PA, Shattil SJ: Platelet function in essential thrombocythemia: Decreased epinephrine responsiveness associated with a deficiency of platelet alpha-adrenergic receptors. *N Engl J Med* 299:505, 1978.
265. Swart SS, Pearson D, Wood JK, Barnett DB: Functional significance of the platelet alpha2-adrenoceptor: Studies in patients with myeloproliferative disorders. *Thromb Res* 33:531, 1984.
266. Nurden P, Bihour C, Smith M, et al: Platelet activation and thrombosis: Studies in a patient with essential thrombocythemia. *Am J Hematol* 51:79, 1996.
267. Rocca B, Ciabattoni G, Tartaglione R, et al: Increased thromboxane biosynthesis in essential thrombocythemia. *Thromb Haemost* 74:1225, 1995.
268. Landolfi R, Ciabattoni G, Patrignani P, et al: Increased thromboxane biosynthesis in patients with polycythemia vera: Evidence for aspirin-suppressible platelet activation *in vivo*. *Blood* 80:1965, 1992.
269. Walsh PN, Murphy S, Barry WE: The role of platelets in the pathogenesis of thrombosis and hemorrhage in patients with thrombocytosis. *Thromb Haemost* 38:1085, 1977.
270. Kaplan R, Gabbeta J, Sun L, et al: Combined defect in membrane expression and activation of platelet GPIIb-IIIa complex without primary sequence abnormalities in myeloproliferative disease. *Br J Haematol* 111:954, 2000.
271. Berndt MC, Kabral A, Grimsley P, et al: An acquired Bernard-Soulier-like platelet defect associated with juvenile myelodysplastic syndrome. *Br J Haematol* 68:97, 1988.
272. Cooper B, Schafer AI, Puchalsky D, Handin RI: Platelet resistance to prostaglandin D2 in patients with myeloproliferative disorders. *Blood* 52:618, 1978.
273. Moore A, Nachman RL: Platelet Fc receptor. Increased expression in myeloproliferative disease. *J Clin Invest* 67:1064, 1981.
274. Bolin RB, Okumura T, Jamieson GA: Changes in distribution of platelet membrane glycoproteins in patients with myeloproliferative disorders. *Am J Hematol* 3:63, 1977.
275. Thibert V, Bellucci S, Cristofari M, et al: Increased platelet CD36 constitutes a common marker in myeloproliferative disorders. *Br J Haematol* 91:618, 1995.
276. Moliterno AR, Hankins WD, Spivak JL: Impaired expression of the thrombopoietin receptor by platelets from patients with polycythemia vera. *N Engl J Med* 338:572, 1998.
277. Li J, Xia Y, Kuter DJ: The platelet thrombopoietin receptor number and function are markedly decreased in patients with essential thrombocythaemia. *Br J Haematol* 111:943, 2000.
278. Baxter EJ, Scott LM, Campbell PJ, et al: Acquired mutation of the tyrosine kinase JAK2 in human myeloproliferative disorders. *Lancet* 365:1054, 2005.
279. Levine RL, Wadleigh M, Cools J, et al: Activating mutation in the tyrosine kinase JAK2 in polycythemia vera, essential thrombocythemia, and myeloid metaplasia with myelofibrosis. *Cancer Cell* 7:387, 2005.
280. James C, Ugo V, Le Couedic JP, et al: A unique clonal JAK2 mutation leading to constitutive signalling causes polycythaemia vera. *Nature* 434:1144, 2005.
281. Kralovics R, Passamonti F, Buser AS, et al: A gain-of-function mutation of JAK2 in myeloproliferative disorders. *N Engl J Med* 352:1779, 2005.
282. Scott LM, Tong W, Levine RL, et al: JAK2 exon 12 mutations in polycythemia vera and idiopathic erythrocytosis. *N Engl J Med* 356:459, 2007.
283. Pardanani AD, Levine RL, Lasho T, et al: MPL515 mutations in myeloproliferative and other myeloid disorders: A study of 1182 patients. *Blood* 108:3472, 2006.
284. Schnittger S, Bacher U, Haferlach C, et al: Characterization of 35 new cases with four different MPLW515 mutations and essential thrombocytosis or primary myelofibrosis. *Haematologica* 94:141, 2009.
285. Arellano-Rodrigo E, Alvarez-Larran A, Reverter JC, et al: Increased platelet and leukocyte activation as contributing mechanisms for thrombosis in essential thrombocythemia and correlation with the JAK2 mutational status. *Haematologica* 91:169, 2006.
286. Falanga A, Marchetti M, Vignoli A, et al: V617F JAK-2 mutation in patients with essential thrombocythemia: Relation to platelet, granulocyte, and plasma hemostatic and inflammatory molecules. *Exp Hematol* 35:702, 2007.
287. Robertson B, Urquhart C, Ford I, et al: Platelet and coagulation activation markers in myeloproliferative diseases: Relationships with JAK2 V6I7 F status, clonality, and antiphospholipid antibodies. *J Thromb Haemost* 5:1679, 2007.
288. Vannucchi AM, Antonioli E, Guglielmelli P, et al: Clinical correlates of JAK2V617F presence or allele burden in myeloproliferative neoplasms: A critical reappraisal. *Leukemia* 22:1299, 2008.
289. Campbell PJ, Scott LM, Buck G, et al: Definition of subtypes of essential thrombocythaemia and relation to polycythaemia vera based on JAK2 V617F mutation status: A prospective study. *Lancet* 366:1945, 2005.
290. Finazzi G, Rambaldi A, Guerini V, et al: Risk of thrombosis in patients with essential thrombocythemia and polycythemia vera according to JAK2 V617F mutation status. *Haematologica* 92:135, 2007.
291. Tefferi A, Strand JJ, Lasho TL, et al: Bone marrow JAK2V617F allele burden and clinical correlates in polycythemia vera. *Leukemia* 21:2074, 2007.
292. Pemmaraju N, Moliterno AR, Williams DM, et al: The quantitative JAK2 V617F neutrophil allele burden does not correlate with thrombotic risk in essential thrombocytosis. *Leukemia* 21:2210, 2007.
293. Bellosillo B, Martinez-Aviles L, Gimeno E, et al: A higher JAK2 V617F-mutated clone is observed in platelets than in granulocytes from essential thrombocythemia patients, but not in patients with polycythemia vera and primary myelofibrosis. *Leukemia* 21:1331, 2007.
294. Mitchell MC, Boitnott JK, Kaufman S, et al: Budd-Chiari syndrome: Etiology, diagnosis and management. *Medicine (Baltimore)* 61:199, 1982.
295. Murphy S: Thrombocytosis and thrombocythaemia. *Clin Haematol* 12:89, 1983.
296. Schafer AI: Bleeding and thrombosis in the myeloproliferative disorders. *Blood* 64:1, 1984.
297. Gangat N, Wolanskyj AP, Tefferi A: Abdominal vein thrombosis in essential thrombocythemia: Prevalence, clinical correlates, and prognostic implications. *Eur J Haematol* 77:327, 2006.
298. Valla D, Casadevall N, Huisse MG, et al: Etiology of portal vein thrombosis in adults. A prospective evaluation of primary myeloproliferative disorders. *Gastroenterology* 94:1063, 1988.

299. Hoekstra J, Janssen HL: Vascular liver disorders (II): Portal vein thrombosis. *Neth J Med* 67:46, 2009.
300. Hoekstra J, Janssen HL: Vascular liver disorders (I): Diagnosis, treatment and prognosis of Budd-Chiari syndrome. *Neth J Med* 66:334, 2008.
301. Singh AK, Wetherley-Mein G: Microvascular occlusive lesions in primary thrombocythaemia. *Br J Haematol* 36:553, 1977.
302. van Genderen PJ, Terpstra W, Michiels JJ, et al: High-dose intravenous immunoglobulin delays clearance of von Willebrand factor in acquired von Willebrand disease. *Thromb Haemost* 73:891, 1995.
303. Michiels JJ, Berneman ZN, Schroyens W, Van Vliet HH: Pathophysiology and treatment of platelet-mediated microvascular disturbances, major thrombosis and bleeding complications in essential thrombocythaemia and polycythaemia vera. *Platelets* 15:67, 2004.
304. Rinder HM, Schuster JE, Rinder CS, et al: Correlation of thrombosis with increased platelet turnover in thrombocytosis. *Blood* 91:1288, 1998.
305. Besses C, Cervantes F, Pereira A, et al: Major vascular complications in essential thrombocythemia: A study of the predictive factors in a series of 148 patients. *Leukemia* 13:150, 1999.
306. Barbui T, Barosi G, Grossi A, et al: Practice guidelines for the therapy of essential thrombocythemia. A statement from the Italian Society of Hematology, the Italian Society of Experimental Hematology and the Italian Group for Bone Marrow Transplantation. *Haematologica* 89:215, 2004.
307. De Stefano V, Za T, Rossi E, et al: Recurrent thrombosis in patients with polycythemia vera and essential thrombocythemia: Incidence, risk factors, and effect of treatments. *Haematologica* 93:372, 2008.
308. Tefferi A: Essential thrombocythemia, polycythemia vera, and myelofibrosis: Current management and the prospect of targeted therapy. *Am J Hematol* 83:491, 2008.
309. Schafer AI: Molecular basis of the diagnosis and treatment of polycythemia vera and essential thrombocythemia. *Blood* 107:4214, 2006.
310. Spivak J: Daily aspirin—Only half the answer. *N Engl J Med* 350:99, 2004.
311. Kaplan ME, Mack K, Goldberg JD, et al: Long-term management of polycythemia vera with hydroxyurea: A progress report. *Semin Hematol* 23:167, 1986.
312. Gilbert HS: Modern treatment strategies in polycythemia vera. *Semin Hematol* 40:26, 2003.
313. Finazzi G, Barbui T: How I treat patients with polycythemia vera. *Blood* 109:5104, 2007.
314. Barbui T, Finazzi G: Treatment indications and choice of a platelet-lowering agent in essential thrombocythemia. *Curr Hematol Rep* 2:248, 2003.
315. Cortelazzo S, Finazzi G, Ruggeri M, et al: Hydroxyurea for patients with essential thrombocythemia and a high risk of thrombosis. *N Engl J Med* 332:1132, 1995.
316. Pescatore SL, Lindley C: Anagrelide: A novel agent for the treatment of myeloproliferative disorders. *Expert Opin Pharmacother* 1:537, 2000.
317. Emadi A, Spivak JL: Anagrelide: 20 years later. *Expert Rev Anticancer Ther* 9:37, 2009.
318. Solberg LA Jr, Tefferi A, Oles KJ, et al: The effects of anagrelide on human megakaryocytopoiesis. *Br J Haematol* 99:174, 1997.
319. Fruchtman SM, Petitt RM, Gilbert HS, et al: Anagrelide: Analysis of long-term efficacy, safety and leukemogenic potential in myeloproliferative disorders. *Leuk Res* 29:481, 2005.
320. Wagstaff AJ, Keating GM: Anagrelide: A review of its use in the management of essential thrombocythaemia. *Drugs* 66:111, 2006.
321. Harrison CN, Campbell PJ, Buck G, et al: Hydroxyurea compared with anagrelide in high-risk essential thrombocythemia. *N Engl J Med* 353:33, 2005.
322. Hultdin M, Sundstrom G, Wahlin A, et al: Progression of bone marrow fibrosis in patients with essential thrombocythemia and polycythemia vera during anagrelide treatment. *Med Oncol* 24:63, 2007.
323. Michiels JJ, Abels J, Steketee J, et al: Erythromelalgia caused by platelet-mediated arteriolar inflammation and thrombosis in thrombocythemia. *Ann Intern Med* 102:466, 1985.
324. Michiels JJ, Berneman Z, Schroyens W, et al: Platelet-mediated erythromelalgic, cerebral, ocular and coronary microvascular ischemic and thrombotic manifestations in patients with essential thrombocythemia and polycythemia vera: A distinct aspirin-responsive and coumadin-resistant arterial thrombophilia. *Platelets* 17:528, 2006.
325. Van Genderen PJJ, Mulder PGH, Waleboer M, et al: Prevention and treatment of thrombotic complications in essential thrombocythaemia: Efficacy and safety of aspirin. *Br J Haematol* 97:179, 1997.
326. Landolfi R, Marchioli R, Kutti J, et al: Efficacy and safety of low-dose aspirin in polycythemia vera. *N Engl J Med* 350:114, 2004.
327. Gangat N, Wolanskyj AP, Schwager S, Tefferi A: Predictors of pregnancy outcome in essential thrombocythemia: A single institution study of 63 pregnancies. *Eur J Haematol* 82:350, 2009.
328. Passamonti F, Randi ML, Rumi E, et al: Increased risk of pregnancy complications in patients with essential thrombocythemia carrying the JAK2 (617V>F) mutation. *Blood* 110:485, 2007.
329. Barbui T, Finazzi G: Myeloproliferative disease in pregnancy and other management issues. *Hematology Am Soc Hematol Educ Program* 246, 2006.
330. Sultan Y, Caen JP: Platelet dysfunction in preleukemic states and in various types of leukemia. *Ann N Y Acad Sci* 201:300, 1972.
331. Cowan DH, Haut MJ: Platelet function in acute leukemia. *J Lab Clin Med* 79:893, 1972.
332. Cowan DH, Graham RC Jr, Baunach D: The platelet defect in leukemia. Platelet ultrastructure, adenine nucleotide metabolism, and the release reaction. *J Clin Invest* 56:188, 1975.
333. Foss B, Bruserud O: Platelet functions and clinical effects in acute myelogenous leukemia. *Thromb Haemost* 99:27, 2008.
334. Leinoe EB, Hoffmann MH, Kjaersgaard E, et al: Prediction of haemorrhage in the early stage of acute myeloid leukaemia by flow cytometric analysis of platelet function. *Br J Haematol* 128:526, 2005.
335. Meschengieser S, Blanco A, Maugeri N, et al: Platelet function and intraplatelet von Willebrand factor antigen and fibrinogen in myelodysplastic syndromes. *Thromb Res* 46:601, 1987.
336. Zeidman A, Sokolover N, Fradin Z, et al: Platelet function and its clinical significance in the myelodysplastic syndromes. *Hematol J* 5:234, 2004.
337. Bellucci S, Huisse MG, Boval B, et al: Defective collagen-induced platelet activation in two patients with malignant haemopathies is related to a defect in the GPVI-coupled signalling pathway. *Thromb Haemost* 93:130, 2005.
338. Girtovitis FI, Ntaios G, Papadopoulos A, et al: Defective platelet aggregation in myelodysplastic syndromes. *Acta Haematol* 118:117, 2007.
339. Pui CH, Jackson CW, Chesney C: Normal platelet function after therapy for acute lymphocytic leukemia. *Arch Intern Med* 143:73, 1983.
340. Andre JM, Galambrun C, Trzeciak MC, et al: Acquired Glanzmann's thrombasthenia associated with acute lymphoblastic leukemia. *J Pediatr Hematol Oncol* 27:554, 2005.
341. Westbrook CA, Golde DW: Clinical problems in hairy cell leukemia: Diagnosis and management. *Semin Oncol* 11:514, 1984.
342. Rosove MH, Naeim F, Harwig S, Zighelboim J: Severe platelet dysfunction in hairy cell leukemia with improvement after splenectomy. *Blood* 55:903, 1980.
343. Roussi JH, Houbouyan LL, Alterescu R, et al: Acquired Von Willebrand's syndrome associated with hairy cell leukaemia. *Br J Haematol* 46:503, 1980.
344. Lackner H: Hemostatic abnormalities associated with dysproteinemias. *Semin Hematol* 10:125, 1973.
345. Perkins HA, MacKenzie MR, Fudenberg HH: Hemostatic defects in dysproteinemias. *Blood* 35:695, 1970.
346. Rapoport M, Yona R, Kaufman S, et al: Unusual bleeding manifestations of amyloidosis in patients with multiple myeloma. *Clin Lab Haematol* 16:349, 1994.
347. Furie B, Greene E, Furie BC: Syndrome of acquired factor X deficiency and systemic amyloidosis *in vivo* studies of the metabolic fate of factor X. *N Engl J Med* 297:81, 1977.
348. McPherson RA, Onstad JW, Ugoretz RJ, Wolf PL: Coagulopathy in amyloidosis: Combined deficiency of factors IX and X. *Am J Hematol* 3:225, 1977.
349. Palmer RN, Rick ME, Rick PD, et al: Circulating heparan sulfate anticoagulant in a patient with a fatal bleeding disorder. *N Engl J Med* 310:1696, 1984.
350. Chapman GS, George CB, Danley DL: Heparin-like anticoagulant associated with plasma cell myeloma. *Am J Clin Pathol* 83:764, 1985.
351. Torjemane L, Guermazi S, Ladeb S, et al: Heparin-like anticoagulant associated with multiple myeloma and neutralized with protamine sulfate. *Blood Coagul Fibrinolysis* 18:279, 2007.
352. Liebman H, Chinowsky M, Valdin J, et al: Increased fibrinolysis and amyloidosis. *Arch Intern Med* 143:678, 1983.
353. Meyer K, Williams EC: Fibrinolysis and acquired alpha-2 plasmin inhibitor deficiency in amyloidosis. *Am J Med* 79:394, 1985.
354. McGrath KM, Stuart JJ, Richards F 2nd: Correlation between serum IgG, platelet membrane IgG, and platelet function in hypergammaglobulinaemic states. *Br J Haematol* 42:585, 1979.
355. Kasturi J, Saraya AK: Platelet functions in dysproteinaemia. *Acta Haematol* 59:104, 1978.
356. Vigliano EM, Horowitz HI: Bleeding syndrome in a patient with IgA myeloma: Interaction of protein and connective tissue. *Blood* 29:823, 1967.
357. Shinagawa A, Kojima H, Berndt MC, et al: Characterization of a myeloma patient with a life-threatening hemorrhagic diathesis: Presence of a lambda dimer protein inhibiting shear-induced platelet aggregation by binding to the A1 domain of von Willebrand factor. *Thromb Haemost* 93:889, 2005.
358. DiMinno G, Coraggio F, Cerbone AM, et al: A myeloma paraprotein with specificity for platelet glycoprotein IIIa in a patient with a fatal bleeding disorder. *J Clin Invest* 77:157, 1986.
359. Mannucci PM, Lombardi R, Bader R, et al: Studies of the pathophysiology of acquired von Willebrand's disease in seven patients with lymphoproliferative disorders or benign monoclonal gammopathies. *Blood* 64:614, 1984.
360. Takahashi H, Nagayama R, Tanabe Y, et al: DDAVP in acquired von Willebrand syndrome associated with multiple myeloma. *Am J Hematol* 22:421, 1986.
361. Mohri H, Noguchi T, Kodama F, et al: Acquired von Willebrand disease due to inhibitor of human myeloma protein specific for von Willebrand factor. *Am J Clin Pathol* 87:663, 1987.
362. Lamboley V, Zabraniecki L, Sie P, et al: Myeloma and monoclonal gammopathy of uncertain significance associated with acquired von Willebrand's syndrome. Seven new cases with a literature review. *Joint Bone Spine* 69:62, 2002.
363. Federici AB: Acquired von Willebrand syndrome: Is it an extremely rare disorder or do we see only the tip of the iceberg? *J Thromb Haemost* 6:565, 2008.
364. Wallace MR, Simon SR, Ershler WB, Burns SL: Hemorrhagic diathesis in multiple myeloma. *Acta Haematol* 72:340, 1984.
365. Hyman BT, Westrick MA: Multiple myeloma with polyneuropathy and coagulopathy. A case report of the polyneuropathy, organomegaly, endocrinopathy, M-protein, and skin change (POEMS) syndrome. *Arch Intern Med* 146:993, 1986.

366. Bovill EG, Ershler WB, Golden EA, et al: A human myeloma-produced monoclonal protein directed against the active subpopulation of von Willebrand factor. *Am J Clin Pathol* 85:115, 1986.
367. Silberstein LE, Abrahm J, Shattil SJ: The efficacy of intensive plasma exchange in acquired von Willebrand's disease. *Transfusion* 27:234, 1987.
368. Federici AB, Stabile F, Castaman G, et al: Treatment of acquired von Willebrand syndrome in patients with monoclonal gammopathy of uncertain significance: Comparison of three different therapeutic approaches. *Blood* 92:2707, 1998.
369. Federici AB: Use of intravenous immunoglobulin in patients with acquired von Willebrand syndrome. *Hum Immunol* 66:422, 2005.
370. Mazoyer E, Fain O, Dhote R, Laurian Y: Is rituximab effective in acquired von Willebrand syndrome? *Br J Haematol* 144:967, 2009.
371. Michiels JJ, Budde U, van der Planken M, et al: Acquired von Willebrand syndromes: Clinical features, aetiology, pathophysiology, classification and management. *Best Pract Res Clin Haematol* 14:401, 2001.
372. Kumar S, Pruthi RK, Nichols WL: Acquired von Willebrand disease. *Mayo Clin Proc* 77:181, 2002.
373. Michiels JJ, Berneman Z, Gadisseur A, et al: Immune-mediated etiology of acquired von Willebrand syndrome in systemic lupus erythematosus and in benign monoclonal gammopathy: Therapeutic implications. *Semin Thromb Hemost* 32:577, 2006.
374. Hong S, Lee J, Chi H, et al: Systemic lupus erythematosus complicated by acquired von Willebrand's syndrome. *Lupus* 17:846, 2008.
375. Mazurier C, Parquet-Gernez A, Descamps J, et al: Acquired von Willebrand's syndrome in the course of Waldenström's disease. *Thromb Haemost* 44:115, 1980.
376. Handin RI, Martin V, Moloney WC: Antibody-induced von Willebrand's disease: A newly defined inhibitor syndrome. *Blood* 48:393, 1976.
377. Van Genderen PJJ, Vink T, Michiels JJ, et al: Acquired von Willebrand disease caused by an autoantibody selectively inhibiting the binding of von Willebrand factor to collagen. *Blood* 84:3378, 1994.
378. Goudemand J, Samor B, Caron C, et al: Acquired type II von Willebrand's disease: Demonstration of a complexed inhibitor of the von Willebrand factor-platelet interaction and response to treatment. *Br J Haematol* 68:227, 1988.
379. Mohri H, Hisanaga S, Mishima A, et al: Autoantibody inhibits binding of von Willebrand factor to glycoprotein Ib and collagen in multiple myeloma: Recognition sites present on the A1 loop and A3 domains of von Willebrand factor. *Blood Coagul Fibrinolysis* 9:91, 1998.
380. Igarashi N, Miura M, Kato E, et al: Acquired von Willebrand's syndrome with lupus-like serology. *Am J Pediatr Hematol Oncol* 11:32, 1989.
381. Scott JP, Montgomery RR, Tubergen DG, Hays T: Acquired von Willebrand's disease in association with Wilm's tumor: Regression following treatment. *Blood* 58:665, 1981.
382. Rao KP, Kizer J, Jones TJ, et al: Acquired von Willebrand's syndrome associated with an extranodal pulmonary lymphoma. *Arch Pathol Lab Med* 112:47, 1988.
383. Baxter PA, Nuchtern JG, Guillerman RP, et al: Acquired von Willebrand syndrome and Wilms tumor: Not always benign. *Pediatr Blood Cancer* 52:392, 2009.
384. Levesque H, Borg JY, Cailleux N, et al: Acquired von Willebrand's syndrome associated with decrease of plasminogen activator and its inhibitor during hypothyroidism. *Eur J Med* 2:287, 1993.
385. Aylesworth CA, Smallridge RC, Rick ME, Alving BM: Acquired von Willebrand's disease: A rare manifestation of postpartum thyroiditis. *Am J Hematol* 50:217, 1995.
386. Tiede A, Priesack J, Werwitzke S, et al: Diagnostic workup of patients with acquired von Willebrand syndrome: A retrospective single-centre cohort study. *J Thromb Haemost* 6:569, 2008.
387. Joist JH, Cowan JF, Zimmerman TS: Acquired von Willebrand's disease. Evidence for a quantitative and qualitative factor VIII disorder. *N Engl J Med* 298:988, 1978.
388. Sucker C, Scharf RE, Zotz RB: Use of recombinant factor VIIa in inherited and acquired von Willebrand disease. *Clin Appl Thromb Hemost* 15:27, 2009.
389. Macik BG, Gabriel DA, White GC 2nd, et al: The use of high-dose intravenous gamma-globulin in acquired von Willebrand syndrome. *Arch Pathol Lab Med* 112:143, 1988.
390. White LA, Chisholm M: Gastro-intestinal bleeding in acquired von Willebrand's disease: Efficacy of high-dose immuno-globulin where substitution treatments failed. *Br J Haematol* 84:332, 1993.
391. Rinder MR, Richard RE, Rinder HM: Acquired von Willebrand's disease: A concise review. *Am J Hematol* 54:139, 1997.
392. Van Genderen PJ, Papatsonis DN, Michiels JJ, et al: High-dose intravenous gamma-globulin therapy for acquired von Willebrand disease. *Postgrad Med J* 70:916, 1994.
393. Franchini M, Lippi G: Recent acquisitions in acquired and congenital von Willebrand disorders. *Clin Chim Acta* 377:62, 2007.
394. Oliveira MC, Kramer CK, Marroni CP, et al: Acquired factor VIII and von Willebrand factor (aFVIII-VWF) deficiency and hypothyroidism in a case with hypopituitarism. *Clin Appl Thromb Hemost* 16:107, 2010.
395. Manfredi E, van Zaane B, Gerdes VE, et al: Hypothyroidism and acquired von Willebrand's syndrome: A systematic review. *Haemophilia* 14:423, 2008.
396. Yoshida K, Tobe S, Kawata M: Acquired von Willebrand disease type IIA in patients with aortic valve stenosis. *Ann Thorac Surg* 81:1114, 2006.
397. Shimizu M, Masai H, Miwa Y: Occult gastrointestinal bleeding due to acquired von Willebrand syndrome in a patient with hypertrophic obstructive cardiomyopathy. *Intern Med* 46:481, 2007.
398. Budde U, Scharf RE, Franke P, et al: Elevated platelet count as a cause of abnormal von Willebrand factor multimer distribution in plasma. *Blood* 82:1749, 1993.
399. Rao AK: Uraemic platelets. *Lancet* 1:913, 1986.
400. Boccardo P, Remuzzi G, Galbusera M: Platelet dysfunction in renal failure. *Semin Thromb Hemost* 30:579, 2004.
401. Rosenbaum R, Hoffstein PE, Stanley RJ, Klahr S: Use of computerized tomography to diagnose complications of percutaneous renal biopsy. *Kidney Int* 14:87, 1978.
402. Diaz-Buxo JA, Donadio JVJ: Complications of percutaneous renal biopsy: An analysis of 1000 consecutive biopsies. *Clin Nephrol* 4:223, 1975.
403. Weigert AL, Schafer AI: Uremic bleeding: Pathogenesis and therapy. *Am J Med Sci* 316:94, 1998.
404. Castillo R, Lozano T, Escolar G, et al: Defective platelet adhesion on vessel subendothelium in uremic patients. *Blood* 68:337, 1986.
405. Zwaginga JJ, Ijsseldijk MJW, Beeser-Visser N, et al: High von Willebrand factor concentration compensates a relative adhesion defect in uremic blood. *Blood* 75:1498, 1990.
406. Zwaginga JJ, Ijsseldijk I, de Groot PG, et al: Defects in platelet adhesion and aggregate formation in uremic bleeding disorder can be attributed to factors in plasma. *Arterioscler Thromb* 11:733, 1991.
407. Valeri CR, Cassidy G, Pivacek LE, et al: Anemia-induced increase in the bleeding time: Implications for treatment of nonsurgical blood loss. *Transfusion* 41:977, 2001.
408. Livio M, Gotti E, Marchesi D, et al: Uraemic bleeding: Role of anaemia and beneficial effect of red cell transfusions. *Lancet* 2:1013, 1982.
409. Fernandez F, Goudable C, Sie P, et al: Low haematocrit and prolonged bleeding time in uraemic patients: Effect of red cell transfusions. *Br J Haematol* 59:139, 1985.
410. Moia M, Mannucci PM, Vizzotto L, et al: Improvement in the haemostatic defect of uraemia after treatment with recombinant human erythropoietin. *Lancet* 2:1227, 1987.
411. Vigano G, Benigni A, Mendogni D, et al: Recombinant human erythropoietin to correct uremic bleeding. *Am J Kidney Dis* 18:44, 1991.
412. Tang WW, Stead RA, Goodkin DA: Effects of epoetin alfa on hemostasis in chronic renal failure. *Am J Nephrol* 18:263, 1998.
413. Turrito VT, Weiss HJ: Red blood cells: Their dual role in thrombus formation. *Science* 207:541, 1980.
414. Casonato A, Pontara E, Vertolli UP, et al: Plasma and platelet von Willebrand factor abnormalities in patients with uremia: Lack of correlation with uremic bleeding. *Clin Appl Thromb Hemost* 7:81, 2001.
415. Sloand EM, Sloand JA, Prodouz K, et al: Reduction of platelet glycoprotein Ib in uremia. *Br J Haematol* 77:375, 1991.
416. Gralnick HR, McKeown LP, Williams SB, et al: Plasma and platelet von Willebrand factor defects in uremia. *Am J Med* 85:806, 1988.
417. Escolar G, Cases A, Bastida E, et al: Uremic platelets have a functional defect affecting the interaction of von Willebrand factor with glycoprotein IIb-IIIa. *Blood* 76:1336, 1990.
418. Di Minno G, Cerbone A, Usberti M, et al: Platelet dysfunction in uremia. II. Correction by arachidonic acid of the impaired exposure of fibrinogen receptors by adenosine diphosphate or collagen. *J Lab Clin Med* 108:246, 1986.
419. Rabiner SF, Hrodek O: Platelet factor 3 in normal subjects and patients with renal failure. *J Clin Invest* 47:901, 1968.
420. Ware JA, Clark BA, Smith M, Salzman EW: Abnormalities of cytoplasmic Ca^{2+} in platelets from patients with uremia. *Blood* 73:172, 1989.
421. Mannucci PM, Remuzzi G, Pusineri F, et al: Deamino-8-arginine vasopressin shortens the bleeding time in uremia. *N Engl J Med* 308:8, 1983.
422. Winter M, Frampton G, Bennett A, et al: Synthesis of thromboxane B_2 in uraemia and the effects of dialysis. *Thromb Res* 30:265, 1983.
423. Bloom A, Greaves M, Preston FE, Brown CB: Evidence against a platelet cyclooxygenase defect in uraemic subjects on chronic haemodialysis. *Br J Haematol* 62:143, 1986.
424. Remuzzi G, Benigni A, Dodesini P, et al: Reduced platelet thromboxane formation in uremia: Evidence for a functional cyclooxygenase defect. *J Clin Invest* 71:762, 1983.
425. Eknoyan G, Brown CH: Biochemical abnormalities of platelets in renal failure. Evidence for decreased platelet serotonin, adenosine diphosphate and Mg-dependent adenosine triphosphatase. *Am J Nephrol* 1:17, 1981.
426. Vlachoyannis J, Schoeppe W: Adenylate cyclase activity and cAMP content of human platelets in uraemia. *Eur J Clin Invest* 12:379, 1982.
427. Bazilinski N, Shaykh M, Dunea G, et al: Inhibition of platelet function by uremic middle molecules. *Nephron* 40:423, 1985.
428. Remuzzi G, Livio M, Marchiaro G, et al: Bleeding in renal failure: Altered platelet function in chronic uraemia only partially corrected by haemodialysis. *Nephron* 22:347, 1978.
429. Livio M, Benigni A, Remuzzi G: Coagulation abnormalities in uremia. *Semin Nephrol* 5:82, 1985.
430. Remuzzi G, Perico N, Zoja C, et al: Role of endothelium-derived nitric oxide in the bleeding tendency of uremia. *J Clin Invest* 86:1768, 1990.
431. Aiello S, Noris M, Todeschini M, et al: Renal and systemic nitric oxide synthesis in rats with renal mass reduction. *Kidney Int* 52:171, 1997.
432. Noris M, Remuzzi G: Uremic bleeding: Closing the circle after 30 years of controversies? *Blood* 94:2569, 1999.
433. Mendes Ribeiro AC, Brunini TM, Ellory JC, Mann GE: Abnormalities in L-arginine transport and nitric oxide biosynthesis in chronic renal and heart failure. *Cardiovasc Res* 49:697, 2001.
434. Brunini TM, Yaqoob MM, Novaes Malagris LE, et al: Increased nitric oxide synthesis in uraemic platelets is dependent on L-arginine transport via system y(+)L. *Pflugers Arch* 445:547, 2003.

435. Remuzzi G: Bleeding disorders in uremia: Pathophysiology and treatment. *Adv Nephrol Necker Hosp* 18:171, 1989.
436. Andrassy K, Ritz E: Uremia as a cause of bleeding. *Am J Nephrol* 5:313, 1985.
437. Ando M, Iwamoto Y, Suda A, et al: New insights into the thrombopoietic status of patients on dialysis through the evaluation of megakaryocytopoiesis in bone marrow and of endogenous thrombopoietin levels. *Blood* 97:915, 2001.
438. George CRP, Slichter SJ, Quadracci LJ: A kinetic evaluation of hemostasis in renal disease. *N Engl J Med* 291:1111, 1974.
439. Linthorst GE, Folman CC, van Olden RW, von dem Borne AE: Plasma thrombopoietin levels in patients with chronic renal failure. *Hematol J* 3:38, 2002.
440. Lind SE: The bleeding time does not predict surgical bleeding. *Blood* 77:2547, 1991.
441. Peterson P, Hayes TE, Arkin CF, et al: The preoperative bleeding time test lacks clinical benefit. *Arch Surg* 133:134, 1998.
442. Stewart JH, Castaldi PA: Uraemic bleeding: A reversible platelet defect corrected by dialysis. *Q J Med* 36:409, 1967.
443. Lindsay RM, Friesen M, Koens F, et al: Platelet function in patients on long term peritoneal dialysis. *Clin Nephrol* 6:335, 1976.
444. Tassies D, Reventer JC, Cases A, et al: Effect of recombinant human erythropoietin treatment on circulating reticulated platelets in uremic patients: Association with early improvement in platelet function. *Am J Hematol* 59:105, 1998.
445. Mannucci PM: Desmopressin: A non-transfusional form of treatment for congenital and acquired bleeding disorders. *Blood* 72:1449, 1988.
446. Rose EH, Aledort LM: Nasal spray desmopressin (DDAVP) for mild hemophilia A and von Willebrand disease. *Ann Intern Med* 114:563, 1991.
447. Canavese C, Salomone M, Pacitti A, et al: Reduced response of uraemic bleeding time to repeated doses of desmopressin. *Lancet* 1:867, 1985.
448. Byrnes JJ, Larcada A, Moake JL: Thrombosis following desmopressin for uremic bleeding. *Am J Hematol* 28:63, 1988.
449. Mannucci PM: Desmopressin and thrombosis. *Lancet* 2:675, 1989.
450. Liu YK, Kosfeld RE, Marcum SG: Treatment of uremic bleeding with conjugated estrogen. *Lancet* 2:887, 1984.
451. Livio M, Mannucci PM, Vigano G, et al: Conjugated estrogens for the management of bleeding associated with renal failure. *N Engl J Med* 315:731, 1986.
452. Vigano G, Gaspari F, Locatelli M, et al: Dose-effect and pharmacokinetics of estrogens given to correct bleeding time in uremia. *Kidney Int* 34:853, 1988.
453. Heistinger M, Stockenhuber F, Schneider B, et al: Effect of conjugated estrogens on platelet function and prostacyclin generation in CRF. *Kidney Int* 38:1181, 1990.
454. Bronner MH, Pate MD, Cunningham JT: Estrogen-progesterone therapy for bleeding of gastrointestinal telangiectasias in chronic renal failure. *Ann Intern Med* 105:371, 1986.
455. Vigano G, Zoja C, Corna D, et al: 17β-estradiol is the most active component of the conjugated estrogen mixture active on uremic bleeding by a receptor mechanism. *Mol Pharmacol* 252:344, 1990.
456. Janson PA, Jubelirer SJ, Weinstein MS, Deykin D: Treatment of bleeding tendency in uremia with cryoprecipitate. *N Engl J Med* 303:1318, 1980.
457. Triulzi DJ, Blumber N: Variability in response to cryoprecipitate treatment for hemostatic defects in uremia. *Yale J Biol Med* 63:1, 1990.
458. Thompson AR, Harker LA: Approach to bleeding disorders, in *Manual of Hemostasis and Thrombosis*, 3rd ed, edited by AR Thompson, LA Harker, p 57 FA Davis, Philadelphia, 1983.
459. George JN, Woolf SH, Raskob GE, et al: Idiopathic thrombocytopenic purpura: A practice guideline developed by explicit methods for the American Society of Hematology. *Blood* 88:3, 1996.
460. George JN, El-Harake MA, Raskob GE: Chronic idiopathic thrombocytopenic purpura. *N Engl J Med* 331:1207, 1994.
461. McMillan R: Antiplatelet antibodies in chronic adult immune thrombocytopenic purpura: Assays and epitopes. *J Pediatr Hematol Oncol* 25 Suppl 1:S57, 2003.
462. Meyer M, Kirchmaier CM, Schirmer A, et al: Acquired disorder of platelet function associated with autoantibodies against membrane glycoprotein IIb-IIIa complex-1. Glycoprotein analysis. *Thromb Haemost* 65:491, 1991.
463. Balduini CL, Grignani G, Sinigaglia F, et al: Severe platelet dysfunction in a patient with autoantibodies against membrane glycoproteins IIb-IIIa. *Haemostasis* 7:98, 1987.
464. Balduini CL, Bertolino G, Noris P, et al: Defect of platelet aggregation and adhesion induced by autoantibodies against platelet glycoprotein IIIa. *Thromb Haemost* 68:208, 1992.
465. Fuse I, Higuchi W, Narita M, et al: Overproduction of antiplatelet antibody against glycoprotein IIb after splenectomy in a patient with Evans syndrome resulting in acquired thrombasthenia [see comments]. *Acta Haematol* 99:83, 1998.
466. Stricker RB, Wong D, Saks SR, et al: Acquired Bernard-Soulier syndrome: Evidence for the role of a 210,000-molecular weight protein in the interaction of platelets with von Willebrand factor. *J Clin Invest* 76:1274, 1985.
467. Devine DV, Currie MS, Rosse WF, Greenberg CS: Pseudo-Bernard-Soulier syndrome: Thrombocytopenia caused by autoantibody to platelet glycoprotein Ib. *Blood* 70:428, 1987.
468. Deckmyn H, Zhang J, Van Houtte E, Vermylen J: Production and nucleotide sequence of an inhibitory human IgM autoantibody directed against platelet glycoprotein Ia/IIa. *Blood* 84:1968, 1994.
469. Dromigny A, Triadou P, Lesavre P, et al: Lack of platelet response to collagen associated with autoantibodies against glycoprotein (GP) Ia/IIa and Ib/IX leading to the discovery of SLE. *Hematol Cell Ther* 38:355, 1996.
470. Boylan B, Chen H, Rathore V, et al: Anti-GPVI-associated ITP: An acquired platelet disorder caused by autoantibody-mediated clearance of the GPVI/FcRgamma-chain complex from the human platelet surface. *Blood* 104:1350, 2004.
471. Wiedmer T, Ando B, Sims PJ: Complement C5b-9-stimulated platelet secretion is associated with a calcium-initiated activation of cellular protein kinases. *J Biol Chem* 262:13674, 1987.
472. Sugiyama T, Okuma M, Ushikubi F, et al: A novel platelet aggregating factor found in a patient with defective collagen-induced platelet aggregation and autoimmune thrombocytopenia. *Blood* 69:1712, 1987.
473. Warkentin TE: Heparin-induced thrombocytopenia: Pathogenesis and management. *Br J Haematol* 121:535, 2003.
474. Lackner H, Karpatkin S: On the "easy bruising" syndrome with normal platelet count: A study of 75 patients. *Ann Intern Med* 83:190, 1975.
475. Clancy R, Jenkins E, Firkin B: Qualitative platelet abnormalities in idiopathic thrombocytopenic purpura. *N Engl J Med* 286:622, 1972.
476. Heyns DA, Fraser J, Retief FP: Platelet aggregation in chronic idiopathic thrombocytopenic purpura. *J Clin Pathol* 31:1239, 1978.
477. Regan MG, Lackner H, Karpatkin S: Platelet function and coagulation profile in lupus erythematosus. *Am J Med* 81:462, 1974.
478. Dorsch CA, Meyerhoff J: Mechanisms of abnormal platelet aggregation in systemic lupus erythematosus. *Arthritis Rheum* 25:966, 1982.
479. Nieuwenhuis HK, Zwaginga JJ, Sixma JJ: Analysis of patients with a prolonged bleeding time. *Thromb Haemost* 58:527, 1987.
480. Weiss HJ, Rosove MH, Lages BA, Kaplan KL: Acquired storage pool deficiency with increased platelet-associated IgG. *Am J Med* 69:711, 1980.
481. Meyerhoff J, Dorsch CA: Decreased platelet serotonin levels in systemic lupus erythematosus. *Arthritis Rheum* 24:1495, 1981.
482. Stuart MJ, Kelton JG, Allen JB: Abnormal platelet function and arachidonate metabolism in chronic idiopathic thrombocytopenic purpura. *Blood* 58:326, 1981.
483. Harker LA, Malpass TW, Branson HE, et al: Mechanism of abnormal bleeding in patients undergoing cardiopulmonary bypass: Acquired transient platelet dysfunction associated with selective alpha-granule release. *Blood* 56:824, 1980.
484. Woodman RC, Harker LA: Bleeding complications associated with cardiopulmonary bypass. *Blood* 76:1680, 1990.
485. Mammen EF, Koets MH, Washington BC, et al: Hemostasis changes during cardiopulmonary bypass surgery. *Semin Thromb Hemost* 11:281, 1985.
486. Khuri SF, Wolfe JA, Josa M, et al: Hematologic changes during and after cardiopulmonary bypass and their relationship to the bleeding time and nonsurgical blood loss. *J Thorac Cardiovasc Surg* 104:94, 1992.
487. Martin JF, Daniel TD, Trowbridge EA: Acute and chronic changes in platelet volume and count after cardiopulmonary bypass induced thrombocytopenia in man. *Thromb Haemost* 57:55, 1987.
488. Chandler AB, Hutson MS: Platelet plug formation in an extracorporeal unit. *Am J Clin Pathol* 64:101, 1975.
489. Lindon JN, McManama, Kushner L: Does the conformation of adsorbed fibrinogen dictate platelet interactions with artificial surfaces? *Blood* 68:355, 1986.
490. Singer RL, Mannion JD, Bauer TL, et al: Complications from heparin-induced thrombocytopenia in patients undergoing cardiopulmonary bypass. *Chest* 104:1436, 1993.
491. Bick RL: Hemostasis defects associated with cardiac surgery, prosthetic devices, and other extracorporeal circuits. *N Engl J Med* 22:1446, 1986.
492. McKenna R, Bachmann F, Whittaker B, et al: The hemostatic mechanism after open heart surgery. II. Frequency of abnormal platelet functions during and after extracorporeal circulation. *J Thorac Cardiovasc Surg* 70:298, 1975.
493. Beurling-Harbury C, Galvan CA: Acquired decrease in platelet secretory ADP associated with increased post-operative bleeding in post-cardiopulmonary bypass patients and in patients with severe valvular heart disease. *Blood* 52:13, 1978.
494. Abrams CS, Ellison N, Budzynski AZ, Shattil S: Direct detection of activated platelets and platelet-derived microparticles in humans. *Blood* 75:128, 1990.
495. Nannizzi-Alaimo L, Rubenstein MH, Alves VL, et al: Cardiopulmonary bypass induces release of soluble CD40 ligand. *Circulation* 105:2849, 2002.
496. Wahba A, Rothe G, Lodes H, et al: The influence of the duration of cardiopulmonary bypass on coagulation, fibrinolysis and platelet function. *Thorac Cardiovasc Surg* 49:153, 2001.
497. George JN, Pickett EB, Saucerman S, et al: Platelet surface glycoproteins. Studies on resting and activated platelets and platelet membrane microparticles in normal subjects, and observations in patients during adult respiratory distress syndrome and cardiac surgery. *J Clin Invest* 78:340, 1986.
498. Bachmann F, McKenna R, Cole ER, Najafi H: The hemostatic mechanism after open heart surgery. I. Studies on plasma coagulation factors and fibrinolysis in 512 patients after extracorporeal circulation. *J Thorac Cardiovasc Surg* 70:76, 1975.
499. Gluszko P, Ricinski B, Musial J, et al: Fibrinogen receptors in platelet adhesion to surfaces of extracorporeal circuit. *Am J Physiol* 252:H615, 1987.
500. van den Dengen JJAM, Karliczek GF, Brenken W, et al: Clinical study of blood trauma during perfusion with membrane and bubble oxygenators. *Thorac Cardiovasc Surg* 83:108, 1982.
501. Edmunds LH Jr, Colman RW: Thrombin during cardiopulmonary bypass. *Ann Thorac Surg* 82:2315, 2006.
502. Kestin AS, Valeri CR, Khuri SF, et al: The platelet function defect of cardiopulmonary bypass. *Blood* 82:107, 1993.

503. Weksler BB, Pett SB, Alonso D, et al: Differential inhibition of aspirin of vascular prostaglandin synthesis in atherosclerotic patients. *N Engl J Med* 308:800, 1983.
504. Levy JH: Pharmacologic preservation of the hemostatic system during cardiac surgery. *Ann Thorac Surg* 72:S1814, 2001.
505. Tabuchi N, de Haan J, Boonstra PW, van Oeveren W: Activation of fibrinolysis in the pericardial cavity during cardiopulmonary bypass. *J Thorac Cardiovasc Surg* 106:828, 1993.
506. Hunt BJ, Parratt RN, Segal HC, et al: Activation of coagulation and fibrinolysis during cardiothoracic operations. *Ann Thorac Surg* 65:712, 1998.
507. Rapaport SI: Preoperative hemostatic evaluation: Which tests, if any? *Blood* 61:229, 1983.
508. Magovern JA, Sakert T, Benckart DH, et al: A model for predicting transfusion after coronary artery bypass grafting [see comments]. *Ann Thorac Surg* 61:27, 1996.
509. Simon TA, Akl BF, Murphy W: Controlled trial of routine administration of platelet concentrates in cardiopulmonary bypass surgery. *Ann Thorac Surg* 37:359, 1987.
510. Wasser MNJM, Houbiers JGA, D'Amaro J, et al: The effect of fresh versus stored blood on post-operative bleeding after coronary bypass surgery: A prospective randomized study. *Br J Haematol* 72:81, 1989.
511. Sowade O, Warnke H, Scigalla P, et al: Avoidance of allogeneic blood transfusions by treatment with epoetin beta (recombinant human erythropoietin) in patients undergoing open- heart surgery. *Blood* 89:411, 1997.
512. Shimpo H, Mizumoto T, Onoda K, et al: Erythropoietin in pediatric cardiac surgery: Clinical efficacy and effective dose. *Chest* 111:1565, 1997.
513. Schmoeckel M, Nollert G, Mempel M, et al: Effects of recombinant human erythropoietin on autologous blood donation before open heart surgery. *Thorac Cardiovasc Surg* 41:364, 1993.
514. Axford TC, Dearani JA, Ragno G, et al: Safety and therapeutic effectiveness of reinfused shed blood after open heart surgery [see comments]. *Ann Thorac Surg* 57:615, 1994.
515. Griffith LD, Billman GF, Daily PO, Lane TA: Apparent coagulopathy caused by infusion of shed mediastinal blood and its prevention by washing of the infusate [see comments]. *Ann Thorac Surg* 47:400, 1989.
516. Hsu LC: Heparin-coated cardiopulmonary bypass circuits: Current status. *Perfusion* 16:417, 2001.
517. Spijker HT, Graaff R, Boonstra PW, et al: On the influence of flow conditions and wettability on blood material interactions. *Biomaterials* 24:4717, 2003.
518. Lappegard KT, Fung M, Bergseth G, et al: Effect of complement inhibition and heparin coating on artificial surface-induced leukocyte and platelet activation. *Ann Thorac Surg* 77:932, 2004.
519. Weerwind PW, Caberg NE, Reutelingsperger CP, et al: Exposure of procoagulant phospholipids on the surface of platelets in patients undergoing cardiopulmonary bypass using non-coated and heparin-coated extracorporeal circuits. *Int J Artif Organs* 25:770, 2002.
520. Johnell M, Elgue G, Larsson R, et al: Coagulation, fibrinolysis, and cell activation in patients and shed mediastinal blood during coronary artery bypass grafting with a new heparin-coated surface. *J Thorac Cardiovasc Surg* 124:321, 2002.
521. Linneweber J, Chow TW, Kawamura M, et al: *In vitro* comparison of blood pump induced platelet microaggregates between a centrifugal and roller pump during cardiopulmonary bypass. *Int J Artif Organs* 25:549, 2002.
522. Despotis GJ, Avidan MS, Hogue CW Jr: Mechanisms and attenuation of hemostatic activation during extracorporeal circulation. *Ann Thorac Surg* 72:S1821, 2001.
523. Nuttall GA, Erchul DT, Haight TJ, et al: A comparison of bleeding and transfusion in patients who undergo coronary artery bypass grafting via sternotomy with and without cardiopulmonary bypass. *J Cardiothorac Vasc Anesth* 17:447, 2003.
524. Lo B, Fijnheer R, Castigliego D, et al: Activation of hemostasis after coronary artery bypass grafting with or without cardiopulmonary bypass. *Anesth Analg* 99:634, 2004.
525. Mariani MA, Gu YJ, Boonstra PW, et al: Procoagulant activity after off-pump coronary operation: Is the current anticoagulation adequate? *Ann Thorac Surg* 67:1370, 1999.
526. Paparella D, Galeone A, Venneri MT, et al: Activation of the coagulation system during coronary artery bypass grafting: Comparison between on-pump and off-pump techniques. *J Thorac Cardiovasc Surg* 131:290, 2006.
527. Vallely MP, Bannon PG, Bayfield MS, et al: Quantitative and temporal differences in coagulation, fibrinolysis and platelet activation after on-pump and off-pump coronary artery bypass surgery. *Heart Lung Circ* 18:123, 2009.
528. Hackmann T, Gascoyne R, Naiman SC, et al: A trial of desmopressin to reduce blood loss in uncomplicated cardiac surgery. *N Engl J Med* 321:1437, 1989.
529. Seear MD, Wadsworth LD, Rogers PC, et al: The effect of desmopressin acetate (DDAVP) on postoperative blood loss after cardiac operations in children [see comments]. *J Thorac Cardiovasc Surg* 98:217, 1989.
530. Pychynska-Pokorska M, Moll JJ, Krajewski W, Jarosik P: The use of recombinant coagulation factor VIIa in uncontrolled postoperative bleeding in children undergoing cardiac surgery with cardiopulmonary bypass. *Pediatr Crit Care Med* 5:246, 2004.
531. Herbertson M: Recombinant activated factor VII in cardiac surgery. *Blood Coagul Fibrinolysis* 15 Suppl 1:S31, 2004.
532. Ott E, Nussmeier NA, Duke PC, et al: Efficacy and safety of the cyclooxygenase 2 inhibitors parecoxib and valdecoxib in patients undergoing coronary artery bypass surgery. *J Thorac Cardiovasc Surg* 125:1481, 2003.
533. Nussmeier NA, Whelton AA, Brown MT, et al: Complications of the COX-2 inhibitors parecoxib and valdecoxib after cardiac surgery. *N Engl J Med* 352:1081, 2005.
534. Mangano DT, Tudor IC, Dietzel C: The risk associated with aprotinin in cardiac surgery. *N Engl J Med* 354:353, 2006.
535. Schneeweiss S, Seeger JD, Landon J, Walker AM: Aprotinin during coronary-artery bypass grafting and risk of death. *N Engl J Med* 358:771, 2008.
536. Shaw AD, Stafford-Smith M, White WD, et al: The effect of aprotinin on outcome after coronary-artery bypass grafting. *N Engl J Med* 358:784, 2008.
537. Fergusson DA, Hebert PC, Mazer CD, et al: A comparison of aprotinin and lysine analogues in high-risk cardiac surgery. *N Engl J Med* 358:2319, 2008.
538. Krauss JS, Jonah MH: Platelet dysfunction (thrombocytopathy) in extra-hepatic biliary obstruction. *South Med J* 75:506, 1982.
539. Hillbom M, Muuronen A, Neiman J: Liver disease and platelet function in alcoholics. *Br Med J* 295:581, 1987.
540. Amitrano L, Guardascione MA, Brancaccio V, Balzano A: Coagulation disorders in liver disease. *Semin Liver Dis* 22:83, 2002.
541. Mannucci PM, Vicente V, Vianello L, et al: Controlled trial of desmopressin in liver cirrhosis and other conditions associated with a prolonged bleeding time. *Blood* 67:1148, 1986.
542. Stein SF, Harker LA: Kinetic and functional studies of platelets, fibrinogen, and plasminogen in patients with hepatic cirrhosis. *J Lab Clin Med* 99:217, 1982.
543. Peck-Radosavljevic M, Wichlas M, Zacherl J, et al: Thrombopoietin induces rapid resolution of thrombocytopenia after orthotopic liver transplantation through increased platelet production. *Blood* 95:795, 2000.
544. Giannini E, Botta F, Borro P, et al: Relationship between thrombopoietin serum levels and liver function in patients with chronic liver disease related to hepatitis C virus infection. *Am J Gastroenterol* 98:2516, 2003.
545. Violi F, Leo R, Vezza E, et al: Bleeding time in patients with cirrhosis: Relation with degree of liver failure and clotting abnormalities. C.A.L.C. Group. Coagulation Abnormalities in Cirrhosis Study Group. *J Hepatol* 20:531, 1994.
546. Pareti FI, Capitanio A, Mannucci L: Acquired storage pool disease in platelets during disseminated intravascular coagulation. *Blood* 48:511, 1976.
547. Pareti FI, Capitanio A, Mannucci L, et al: Acquired dysfunction due to the circulation of "exhausted" platelets. *Am J Med* 69:235, 1980.
548. Solum NO, Rigollot C, Budzynski A, Marder VJ: A quantitative evaluation of the inhibition of platelet aggregation by low molecular weight degradation products of fibrinogen. *Br J Haematol* 24:619, 1973.
549. Stoff JS, Stemerman M, Steer M, et al: A defect in platelet aggregation in Bartter's syndrome. *Am J Med* 68:171, 1980.
550. van Wersch J, Rodriques Pereira R: Platelet aggregation in six families with Bartter's syndrome. *Clin Chim Acta* 130:363, 1983.
551. Nusing RM, Reinalter SC, Peters M, et al: Pathogenetic role of cyclooxygenase-2 in hyperprostaglandin E syndrome/antenatal Bartter syndrome: Therapeutic use of the cyclooxygenase-2 inhibitor nimesulide. *Clin Pharmacol Ther* 70:384, 2001.
552. Hebert SC: Bartter syndrome. *Curr Opin Nephrol Hypertens* 12:527, 2003.
553. Lim SH, Tan CE, Agasthian T, Chew LS: Acquired platelet dysfunction with eosinophilia: Review of seven adult cases. *J Clin Pathol* 42:950, 1989.
554. Poon MC, Ng SC, Coppes MJ: Acquired platelet dysfunction with eosinophilia in white children. *J Pediatr* 126:959, 1995.
555. Laosombat V, Wongchanchailert M, Sattayasevana B, et al: Acquired platelet dysfunction with eosinophilia in children in the south of Thailand. *Platelets* 12:5, 2001.
556. Szczeklik A, Milner PC, Birch J, et al: Prolonged bleeding time, reduced platelet aggregation, altered PAF-acether sensitivity and increased platelet mass are a trait of asthma and hay fever. *Thromb Haemost* 56:283, 1986.
557. Carvalho AC, Quinn DA, DeMarinis SM, et al: Platelet function in acute respiratory failure. *Am J Hematol* 25:377, 1987.
558. Bracey AW, Wu AH, Aceves J, et al: Platelet dysfunction associated with Wilms tumor and hyaluronic acid. *Am J Hematol* 24:247, 1987.

CHAPTER 123
THE VASCULAR PURPURAS

Doru T. Alexandrescu and Richard L. Gallo

SUMMARY

Purpura, the clinical manifestation of red blood cell extravasation into mucosa or skin, results from various conditions, including rheumatologic, infectious, dermatologic, traumatic, and hematologic disorders. This chapter does not address purpura resulting from quantitative or functional deficiencies of platelets or coagulation factors; these causes are discussed in other chapters. The differential diagnosis of the disparate causes of nonthrombocytopenic purpura is best approached by stratifying purpura into three types of lesions: (1) palpable or retiform and noninflammatory, such as hyperglobulinemic purpura of Waldenström; (2) palpable or nonpalpable but inflammatory, such as Henoch-Schönlein purpura; and (3) nonpalpable and noninflammatory, such as senile purpura. By accounting for palpability, presence of inflammation, size, and shape, the differential diagnosis of a particular lesion can be significantly reduced.

DEFINITION AND DIAGNOSTIC APPROACH

Purpura, from the Latin for purple, refers to visible hemorrhage into mucous membranes or skin, which corresponds to extravasation of red blood cells around dermal small vessels and chronic hemosiderin deposition.[1] Purpuric lesions, by definition, do not blanch completely upon compression, as opposed to erythema. Blanching is commonly tested by compression of skin lesions with a glass slide, referred to as diascopy (Fig. 123–1). Certain conditions give rise to lesions that mimic purpura with incomplete blanching upon diascopy, but are not purpura because no hemorrhage has occurred. Examples include disorders that impede on the red cell flow, such as tortuous veins.[1]

Assessing lesion palpability is the first step in evaluating purpuric lesions (Fig. 123–2). The causes for palpability are varied and include fibrin deposition, localized edema, significant cellular infiltration, and subcutaneous extravasation of red blood cells.

Inspecting the lesion for inflammatory changes is the next step in evaluating purpuric lesions. The presence of pain, erythema, and palpation for warmth and localized swelling are signs of inflammation and suggest a vasculitis or immune complex disorder.

The shape of a purpuric lesion, either round or retiform (branching), is important in assessing the lesion. In the absence of accompanying inflammation, retiform purpuric lesions suggest small vessel occlusion. A retiform, inflammatory purpuric lesion supports the diagnosis of vasculitis as a result of immunoglobulin (Ig) complex formation.[2] Small, focal areas of hemorrhage are referred to as *petechiae* (≤4 mm). Larger lesions are referred to as *intermediate* or *mid-size purpura* (>4 mm, <1 cm) or *ecchymosis* (≥1 cm).[3]

Purpuric lesions frequently appear purple; however, they can take on a variety of colors, according to age of the lesion and the hemoglobin saturation of the extravasated blood. Ecchymosis usually starts as blue or purple, evolves to a greenish brown, and ultimately changes with variable speed to yellow as hemoglobin degrades to bilirubin.[4] These examples of hemorrhage into the dermis must be distinguished from telangiectasia, which are vascular anomalies that blanch with pressure (see Fig. 123–1). Tables 123–1 through 123–3 classify the etiologies for purpura discussed in this chapter.

Acronyms and abbreviations that appear in this chapter include: ANCA, antineutrophil cytoplasmic antibody; APS, antiphospholipid syndrome; CREST, calcinosis, Raynaud phenomenon, esophageal motor dysfunction, sclerodactyly, and telangiectasia; CSS, Churg-Strauss syndrome; DIC, disseminated intravascular coagulation; HCV, hepatitis C virus; HP, hypergammaglobulinemic purpura; HSP, Henoch-Schönlein purpura; MELAS, mitochondrial encephalopathy, lactic acidosis, stroke-like; SLE, systemic lupus erythematosus; WG, Wegener granulomatosis.

PALPABLE OR RETIFORM, NONINFLAMMATORY PURPURIC LESIONS (Table 123–1)

DYSPROTEINEMIAS

Cryoglobulinemia

Cryoglobulinemia refers to the presence in plasma of cold-insoluble immunoglobulins,[5] and is a secondary finding associated with several disease states. Cryoglobulins are commonly present in low concentrations, therefore approximately 90 percent of patients are asymptomatic or have minimal symptoms.[6] Symptoms occur when the abnormal protein precipitates at the temperatures present in superficial venules in the skin and acral parts of the body. Cryoglobulinemia syndromes are divided into three main types based on the Ig composition of the precipitate. Type I cryoglobulinemia results from the accumulation of monoclonal IgG, IgM, or IgA. It is most commonly seen in association with lymphoproliferative disorders, such as myeloma, Waldenström macroglobulinemia, or lymphoma. Type II, or mixed cryoglobulinemia involves formation of complexes composed of polyclonal IgG with monoclonal Igs, typically IgM with anti-IgG specificity. Exposure to exogenous antigens appears to cause polyclonal Ig production, with activity against bacteria, viruses, and fungi. Mixed cryoglobulinemia is commonly seen secondary to hepatitis C virus (HCV) infection,[7] other causes including HIV, collagen vascular disorders, and hematologic neoplasias.[8,9] In mixed cryoglobulinemia secondary to HCV infection, the presence of active cutaneous vasculitis correlates with increased levels of the B-cell-attracting chemokine 1 (CXCL 13).[10] It manifests with petechiae of the legs, palpable purpura, and necrotic skin ulcerations. First-line treatment of HCV-associated mixed cryoglobulinemia includes use of interferon-α, often with adjunct glucocorticoids or plasmapheresis.[11] Direct treatment of the HCV infection with ribavirin and interferon therapy ameliorates this associated lymphoproliferative disorder.[12] Deposition of immune complexes on vessel walls leads to tissue damage in the vasculature, nerves, joints, and skin leading to the hallmark findings of mixed cryoglobulinemia: weakness, arthralgia, and purpura. This purpura often is palpable and is accompanied by areas of hemorrhagic necrosis (Fig. 123–3) and occasionally follicular pustular purpura. Other cutaneous manifestations include lower extremity ulcerations, urticaria, Raynaud phenomena, and subungual purpura (Fig. 123–4). Type III cryoglobulinemia associates polyclonal IgG and IgM complexes, also resulting in symptoms of mixed cryoglobulinemia.[6] It is associated with a variety of infections, systemic lupus erythematous (SLE), and poststreptococcal glomerulonephritis.

Waldenström Hyperglobulinemic Purpura

A polyclonal increase of immunoglobulins, most commonly IgG_1, appears to be responsible for the varied cutaneous findings seen in this

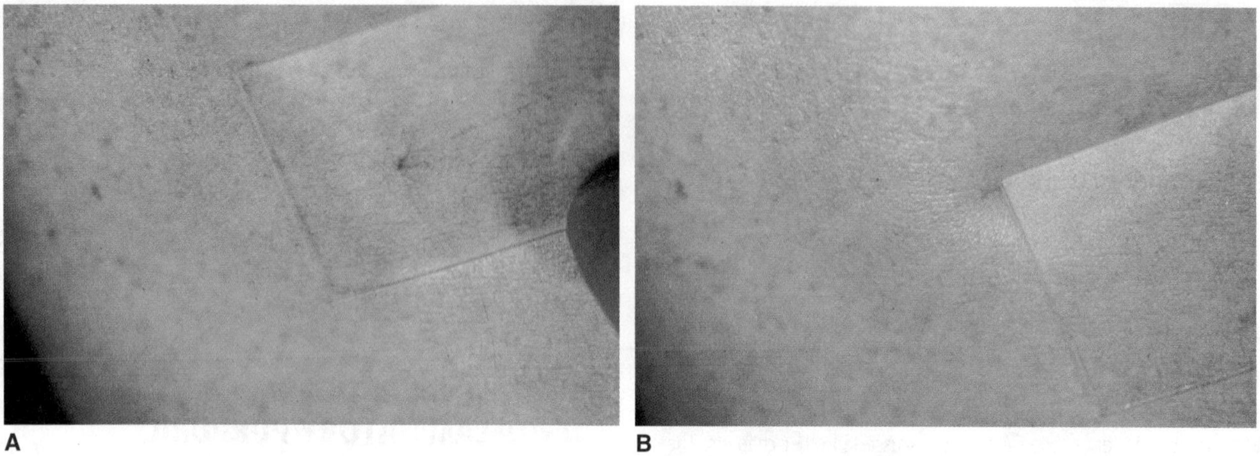

FIGURE 123–1. **A.** Spider telangiectasia. **B.** Blanching of spider telangiectasia. Note that spider telangiectasia blanches with diascopy.

hypergammaglobulinemic purpura (HP). Waldenström first described a hyperproteinemic syndrome characterized by hypergammaglobulinemia, recurrent purpura, elevated erythrocyte sedimentation rate, and anemia.[13] Most commonly seen in young women, this syndrome has been associated with a large number of autoimmune disorders, including SLE, rheumatoid arthritis, Sjögren syndrome, hepatitis C, polymyositis, sarcoidosis, and multiple sclerosis. Discrete to confluent collections of lower limb petechiae are its most common skin findings (Fig. 123–5), but lesions can occur in various body locations.[14] Although lesions are usually self-limited and resolve in 7 to 10 days, recurrence of purpura is common and is associated with exposure to cold temperatures or increases in hydrostatic pressure, such as with the use of tight stockings or prolonged standing.[15] Clinical manifestations consist of palpable purpura or diminutive macular erythematous lesions occurring on the lower legs. A reticulate purpura pattern has been described.[16] Development of edema and arthralgia has also been described.[17]

Common histologic findings include perivascular infiltrates, hemorrhage, vascular necrosis, and leukocytoclastic vasculitis. In addition to the polyclonal increase in either IgA, IgM, or IgG, serology may reveal cryoglobulinemia, rheumatoid factor, or antinuclear antibodies.[18] Imbalances in IgG subclass expression, usually because of a decrease in IgG_2, appear to be associated with recurrent infections.[17] Development of antilymphocyte antibodies results in lymphopenia. Anti-Ro/SSA antibodies occur in up to 78 percent of HP patients, suggesting that screening for anti-Ro/SSA should be considered in cases suspicious for Waldenström.[19]

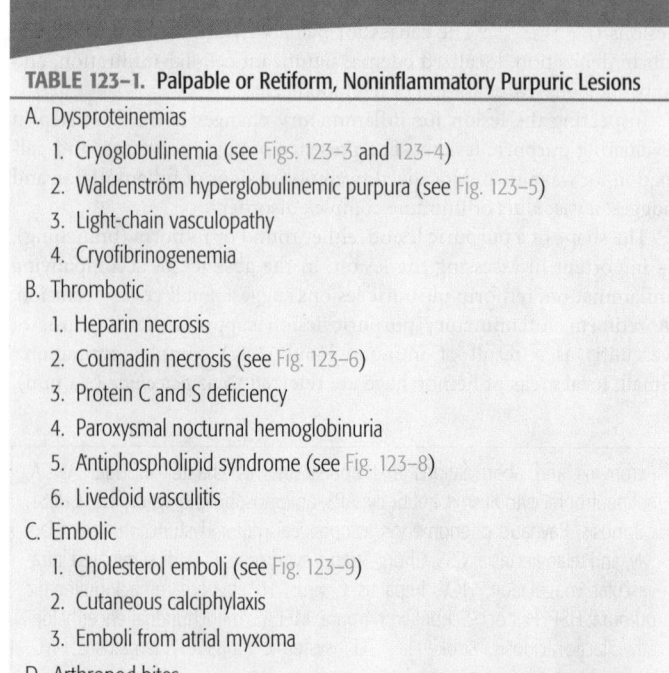

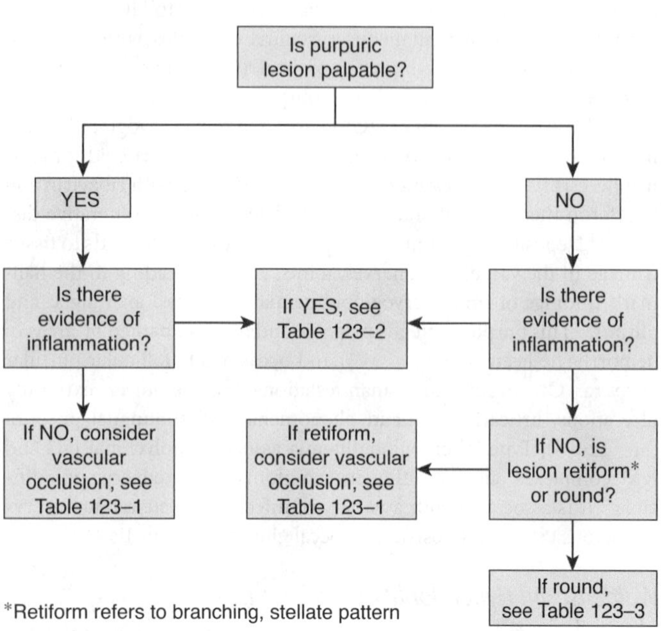

FIGURE 123–2. Bedside approach to purpuric lesion diagnosis.

Light-Chain Vasculopathy

Precipitates of Ig light chains that form crystalline deposits in the skin cause hemorrhagic palpable purpura. A nonamyloid monoclonal light chain of predominant κ type is involved in two-thirds of the cases.[20] An 82-year-old man and a 34-year-old woman were found by direct immunofluorescence to have crystalline deposits containing monoclonal λ

TABLE 123–1. Palpable or Retiform, Noninflammatory Purpuric Lesions

A. Dysproteinemias
1. Cryoglobulinemia (see Figs. 123–3 and 123–4)
2. Waldenström hyperglobulinemic purpura (see Fig. 123–5)
3. Light-chain vasculopathy
4. Cryofibrinogenemia

B. Thrombotic
1. Heparin necrosis
2. Coumadin necrosis (see Fig. 123–6)
3. Protein C and S deficiency
4. Paroxysmal nocturnal hemoglobinuria
5. Antiphospholipid syndrome (see Fig. 123–8)
6. Livedoid vasculitis

C. Embolic
1. Cholesterol emboli (see Fig. 123–9)
2. Cutaneous calciphylaxis
3. Emboli from atrial myxoma

D. Arthropod bites

TABLE 123–2. Palpable and Nonpalpable Inflammatory Purpuric Lesions

A.	Pyoderma gangrenosum (see Fig. 123–7)
B.	Sweet syndrome (see Fig. 123–10)
C.	Behçet disease
D.	Serum sickness (Fig. 123–11)
E.	Henoch-Schönlein purpura (see Fig. 123–12)
F.	Infections
G.	Erythema multiforme (see Fig. 123–20)
H.	Cutaneous polyarteritis nodosum (see Fig. 123–21)
I.	Paraneoplastic vasculitis
J.	Drug-induced vasculitis
K.	ANCA-associated vasculitides
	1. Wegener granulomatosis (see Fig. 123–23)
	2. Churg-Strauss
	3. Microscopic angiitis

light chains in their skin and multiple tissues.[21] Both patients subacutely developed ischemic necrosis and rapidly progressive renal failure. Although clinical presentation suggested a systemic vasculitis, no histologic signs of inflammation were seen. Light-chain vasculopathy with cutaneous findings has also been described in a 37-year-old man with multiple myeloma. Intravascular deposition of crystals containing IgG and λ light chains were found on immunohistochemical analysis and manifested with gangrene of the feet and intestinal perforation.[22]

Cryofibrinogenemia

First described by Korst and Kratochvil in 1955, cryofibrinogenemia is a form of serum dysproteinemia characterized by formation of an abnormal cold-precipitable fibrinogen. Cutaneous manifestations include

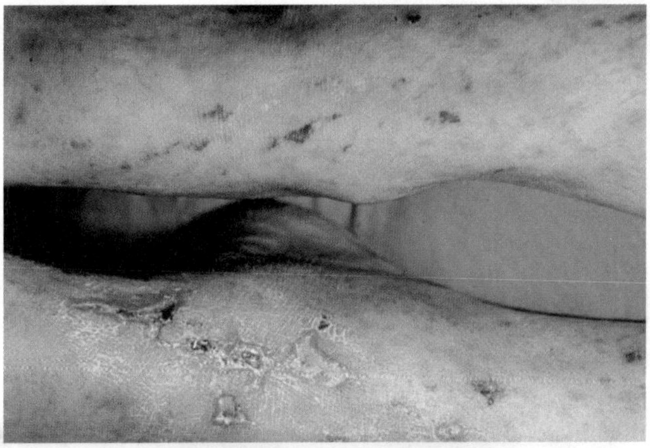

FIGURE 123–3. Cryoglobulinemia: peripheral purpura.

cyanosis, erythema, Raynaud phenomenon, and palpable purpura of the nose, ears, and distal extremities.[23] Tissue ischemia and gangrene may result. Pathogenesis of cryofibrinogenemia may involve an inhibition of normal fibrinolysis produced by a high plasma level of α_1-antitripsin and α_2-macroglobulin proteases.[24] Cryofibrinogenemia is commonly secondary to thromboembolic disorders, metastatic malignancies, infections, and collagen vascular disease.[25] Treatment modalities include avoidance of cold, plasmapheresis, fibrinolytics, and Stanozolol, a fibrinolytic anabolic glucocorticoid, or immunosuppression with glucocorticoids or cytotoxic agents.

THROMBOTIC

Heparin Necrosis

Cutaneous reactions to heparin administration vary greatly from a type I urticarial rash to purpuric plaques with cutaneous ulceration or necrosis.[26] The syndrome occurs after both subcutaneous and intravenous administration of heparin, but recently it was described after dalteparin.[27] A delayed-type hypersensitivity reaction to the medication is involved. Skin lesions appear within 1 to 2 weeks after treatment initiation and include necrotic purpuric lesions.[28] Development of cutaneous lesions is closely related to heparin-induced thrombocytopenia, which involves anti-FP4 antibody-mediated platelet aggregation with development of thrombosis and microvascular occlusion.[27] However, most patients do not develop thrombocytopenia. A platelet count

TABLE 123–3. Nonpalpable, Noninflammatory, Round Purpuric Lesions

A.	Increased transmural pressure gradient
B.	Drug reactions
C.	Coagulation disorders
D.	Decreased vessel integrity without trauma
	1. Senile purpura
	2. Excess glucocorticoid (Cushing syndrome, glucocorticoid treatment)
	3. Scurvy–vitamin C deficiency (see Fig. 123–25)
	4. Systemic amyloidosis
	5. Connective tissue disorders (Ehlers-Danlos syndrome, pseudoxanthoma elasticum)
	6. Mitochondrial encephalomyopathy with lactic acidosis and stroke-like syndrome (MELAS)
E.	Trauma
F.	Waldenström hypergammaglobulinemic purpura (see Table 123–1 and Fig. 123–5)
G.	Schamberg disease (progressive pigmentary dermatosis; see Fig. 123–26)

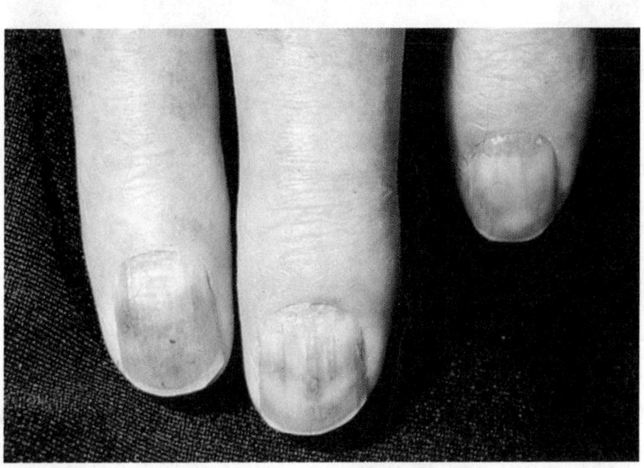

FIGURE 123–4. Cryoglobulinemia: subungual purpura.

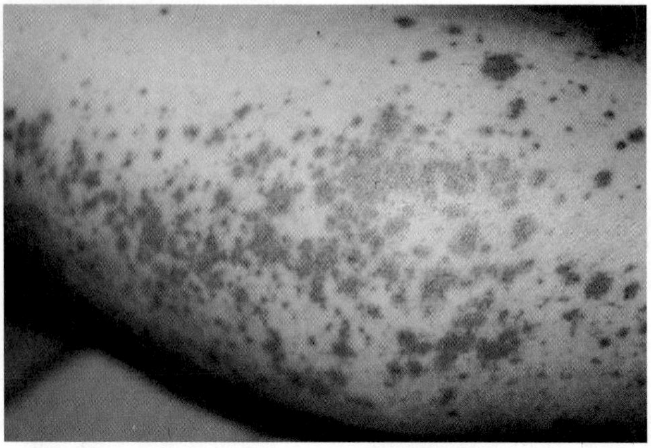

FIGURE 123–5. Waldenström hyperglobulinemic purpura. Note discrete and coalescing petechiae on lower limb.

should be considered in patients developing a skin reaction following initiation of heparin.

Coumadin Necrosis

The development of painful erythematous plaques and nodules is a potential complication of Coumadin therapy (Fig. 123–6). These lesions can rapidly become hemorrhagic and necrotic, leading to large areas of infarct with black eschar formation and subsequent skin sloughing. Purpura, vesicular, maculopapular, or urticarial eruptions can be encountered.[1] More common in perimenopausal obese women, Coumadin-induced necrosis has a prevalence between 0.01 and 0.1 percent and presents typically 3 to 10 days after initiation of anticoagulant treatment for intravascular thrombosis.[29,30] Late-onset Coumadin necrosis has been reported in a patient who developed palpable purpura with rapid progression to hemorrhagic bullae 56 days after initiation of Coumadin treatment.[31] However, an atypical presentation can ensure several years later, such as the one described in a patient with protein S deficiency.[32] Although Coumadin necrosis tends to develop in areas of greatest fat deposition, such as breasts, thighs, and buttocks, acral areas, including penis, fingers, and toes, can also be involved.[33] Coumadin necrosis results from the rapid decrease of vitamin K-dependent coagulation factors, such as proteins C and S. Microvascular occlusion of small dermal and subcutaneous vessels by fibrin deposits is seen on histologic analysis, but true vasculitis is infrequent.[29] Treatment involves prompt cessation of Coumadin and occasionally surgical debridement. Methicillin-resistant *Staphylococcus aureus* infection of areas involved with Coumadin necrosis leading to fatal septic shock has been described.[31] Because patients with protein C or S deficiency are at increased susceptibility to Coumadin necrosis, heparin should always be administered prior to initiation of Coumadin.[34]

Proteins C and S Deficiencies

Clinical manifestations of proteins C and S deficiencies include venous thromboembolism, warfarin-induced skin necrosis, and neonatal purpura fulminans. Congenital and acquired deficiencies in these proteins can lead to palpable necrotic purpura and ecchymosis.[35,36] Erythematous purpuric lesions associated with homozygous protein C deficiency can develop within hours of birth and can rapidly progress to hemorrhagic necrosis (see Chap. 131).[37] Acquired deficiencies of protein C are associated with autoantibodies to protein C, antibiotics administration, septic shock, HIV, and liver disease.[38] Acquired protein S deficiency may occur after varicella infection, when it is associated with the generation of antiprotein S immunoglobulins.[39] Treatment involves prompt cessation of warfarin, along with administration of heparin and vitamin K. Protein repletion with fresh-frozen plasma is effective as initial treatment for protein C or S deficiency to help clear both cutaneous lesions and venous occlusion, while lifelong Coumadin treatment is used for recurrence prevention.[34] Retreatment with warfarin for patients with prior skin necrosis can be employed in selected cases under a steady-state degree of anticoagulation provided by administration of protein C concentrate or fresh-frozen plasma.[40]

Paroxysmal Nocturnal Hemoglobinuria

Paroxysmal nocturnal hemoglobinuria (see Chap. 40) is a hematopoietic clonal disorder resulting in defective production of cell surface-binding proteins.[41] Cutaneous manifestations are secondary to a hypercoagulable state and include palpable purpura, petechiae, ecchymosis, leg ulcers, plaques, necrosis, and hemorrhagic bullae.[42] Parvovirus B19 may play an etiologic role in the development of cutaneous necrosis.[43] An association with pyoderma gangrenosum (Fig. 123–7)[44] and

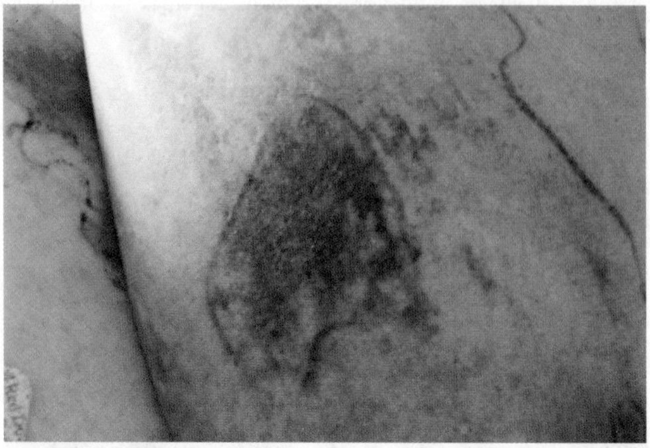

FIGURE 123–6. Coumadin necrosis. Develops in acral areas and areas of fat deposition such as buttocks or breast. Typically, lesions develop 3 to 10 days after initiation of anticoagulant treatment and are caused by rapid clearing of protein C. The lesions are characterized microscopically by small-vessel thrombosis.

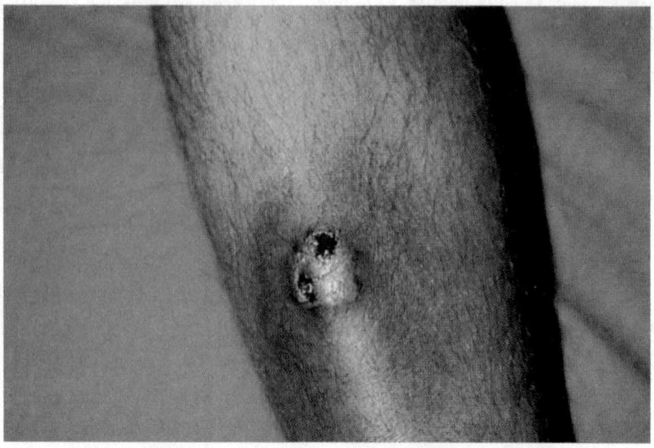

FIGURE 123–7. Pyoderma gangrenosum. A large number of systemic diseases are associated with pyoderma gangrenosum, including inflammatory bowel diseases, hematologic and solid malignancies, and rheumatologic disorders. Microscopically, the lesions are characterized by central necrotizing, neutrophilic infiltration, and a surrounding perivascular and intramural lymphocytic infiltration.

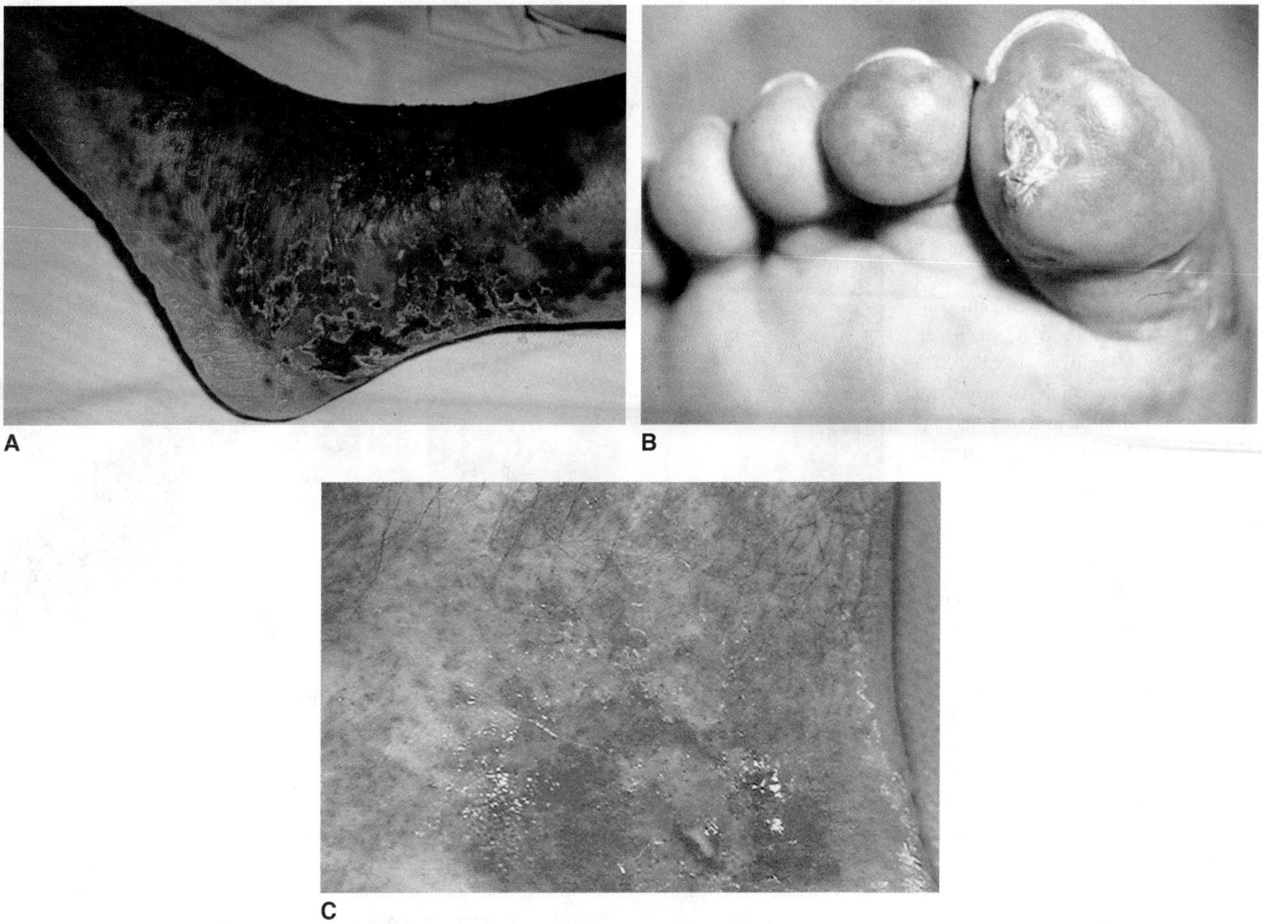

FIGURE 123–8. A. Antiphospholipid antibody syndrome. A number of skin lesions can be seen, including ecchymosis, livedo reticularis and racemosa, leg ulcerations, bullae, splinter hemorrhages, superficial venous thrombosis, atrophie blanche, and, as shown here, extensive necrosis. **B.** Anticardiolipin antibody. **C.** Lupus anticoagulant.

occurrence of purpura fulminans[45] have been described. Histology reveals formation of microvascular fibrin thrombi.[42]

Antiphospholipid Syndrome

Antiphospholipid syndrome (APS) is a disease characterized by hypercoagulability associated with the presence of antibodies against phospholipids, such as anticardiolipin and lupus anticoagulant (see Chap. 132).[46] Approximately 40 percent of patients with APS present with cutaneous lesions secondary to both large-vessel and microvascular thrombosis.[47] Skin manifestations include ecchymosis, livedo reticularis and racemosa, leg ulcerations, bullae, splinter hemorrhages, livedoid vasculopathy, superficial venous thrombosis, atrophie blanche, and extensive necrosis (Fig. 123–8).[47,48] Presence of livedo reticularis is frequently the presenting symptom of APS, most commonly when the syndrome is secondary to SLE, and its presence commonly presages arterial events.[49] Development of acute bullous purpura has been described.[50] Treatment includes anticoagulant and antiplatelet agents with immunosuppressant administration for associated thrombocytopenia. Prevention of thromboembolic events with aspirin is yet of uncertain value.[51]

Livedoid Vasculitis

First described by Bard and Winkelmann in 1967, livedoid vasculitis (segmental hyalinizing vasculitis) is a chronic recurrent thrombo-occlusive disorder characterized by the initial development of erythematous purpuric lesions with telangiectasis and peripheral petechiae, and lower-extremity ulcerations. Subsequent healing leads to atrophie blanche, a term that refers to the appearance of ivory-white stellate scars commonly surrounded by hyperpigmented areas and telangiectasia. These lesions appear to be caused by small-vessel fibrin thrombi in the middle and lower dermis as a result of a procoagulant tendency.[52] Although most commonly arising without associated cause, livedoid vasculitis is associated with polyarteritis nodosa, APS, and SLE.[53,54] Although not consistently beneficial, common therapies include discontinuation of oral contraceptives, anticoagulation and antiplatelet medications, glucocorticoids, and dapsone. Ketanserin, an S_2 serotoninergic receptor blocker, psoralen plus UV-A therapy, and intravenous immunoglobulins also have been used successfully.[55]

■ EMBOLIC

Cholesterol Crystal Emboli

Also known as atheroemboli, cholesterol crystal emboli are responsible for a syndrome characterized by lower extremity pain and livedo reticularis with preservation of peripheral pulses. Other common cutaneous findings include gangrene, purpura, ulcerations, cyanosis, and nodules (Fig. 123–9).[56] Clinical symptoms include fever, myalgia, and altered mental status. Laboratory features include an elevated erythrocyte sedimentation rate, eosinophilia, and acute renal failure. Onset of symptoms varies from immediate after physical dislodgement of plaque, up to months later when caused by anticoagulant therapy.[1] A blue toe syndrome is, in fact, rare, and most atheroemboli are clinically silent.[57] Cholesterol crystal emboli usually dislodge from atherosclerotic lesions in the descending aorta. This explains the propensity for lower-extremity findings during intravascular procedures or initiation of thrombolytic or anticoagulant therapy.[56] Histologic evaluation can offer a definitive diagnosis with findings of birefringent cholesterol crystals within blood vessel lumen in the absence of vasculitis.[58] No effective treatment is in use. Nevertheless, supportive care with proper hydration and dialysis may lessen the potential for end-organ damage.

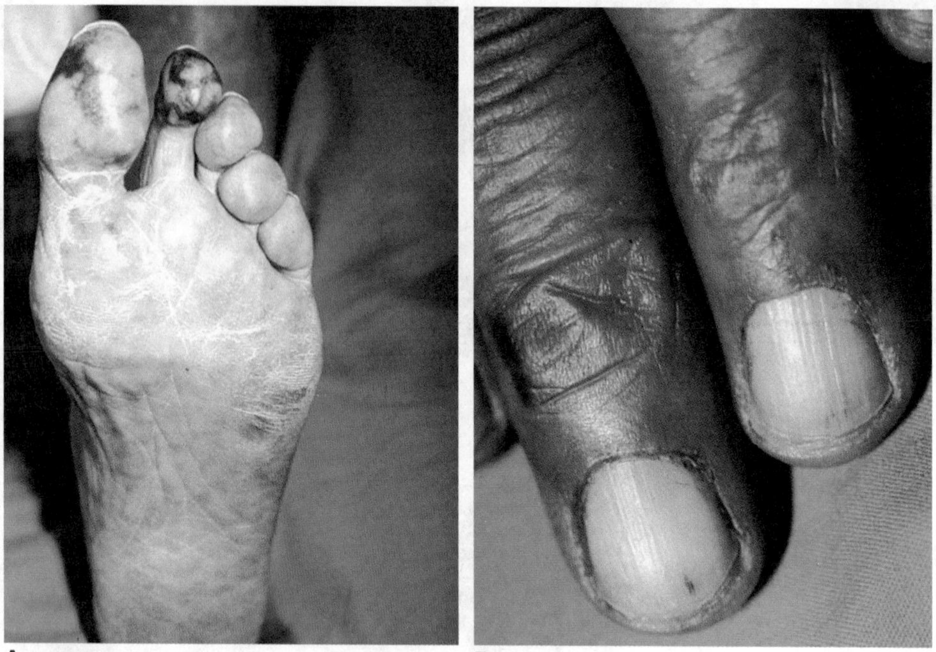

FIGURE 123–9. A. Cholesterol emboli. **B.** Rupture of an atherosclerotic plaque can result in showers of microemboli that lodge in distal arterioles, causing splinter hemorrhages.

Cutaneous Calciphylaxis

Calciphylaxis (calcific uremic arteriolopathy)[59] is a thrombo-occlusive disorder involving formation of cutaneous, subcutaneous, and vascular calcifications. It is most commonly seen in patients with end-stage renal disease, classically caused by the development of secondary hyperparathyroidism.[60] Approximately 4 percent of hemodialysis-dependent patients suffer from calciphylaxis, with less than 50 percent survival at 5 years after diagnosis.[61] Other etiologies include primary hyperparathyroidism, malignancy, alcoholic liver disease, and collagen tissue disorders.[62] Cutaneous lesions present initially as reddish-purple plaques, evolving to tender, gangrenous ulcers or reticular hemorrhagic necrosis. Treatment involves a combination of medical and surgical interventions, such as parathyroidectomy, renal transplantation, wound debridement, and amputation.[61]

Emboli from Atrial Myxoma

Acral purpuric lesions secondary to emboli arise from left atrial myxomas or right atrial clots through paradoxical embolization.[63] These purpuric lesions include palpable purpura, livedo reticularis, erythematous macules and papules, cyanosis, petechiae, splinter hemorrhages, ulcerations, and cutaneous necrosis. Cyanosis, livedo reticularis, and lower extremity ulcerations can also be seen.[64]

ARTHROPOD BITES

Purpuric lesions are not uncommon after arthropod bites. Bites from bed bugs, *Cimex lectularius*, can give rise to localized purpuric macules or papules, while bites from kissing bugs, *Reduviidae*, often manifest as urticaria with hemorrhagic bulla.[65] Cutaneous findings after envenomation from a brown recluse spider, *Loxosceles reclusa*, include purpuric necrosis with surrounding erythema evolving to ulcer formation.

PALPABLE AND NONPALPABLE, INFLAMMATORY PURPURIC LESIONS (Table 123–2)

PYODERMA GANGRENOSUM

Pyoderma gangrenosum is an idiopathic skin eruption characterized by early follicular erythematous papules and pustules or tender, fluctuant nodules with surrounding erythema that spread peripherally and ulcerate, surrounded by a violaceous rim (see Fig. 123–7).[66] In 50 percent of cases of pyoderma gengrenosum, there is an associated disorder, such as inflammatory bowel disorders (classically ulcerative colitis), arthritis, hematologic disorders, and solid tumors.[67] All four main clinical variants (ulcerative, pustular, bullous, and vegetative) share the histopathologic finding of a sterile abscess with central necrotizing, neutrophilic infiltration, and a surrounding perivascular and intramural lymphocytic infiltration. First-line treatment involves wound care and immunosuppressants, such as glucocorticoids, cyclosporine, dapsone, azathioprine, and infliximab.[68]

SWEET SYNDROME

Also referred to as acute, febrile neutrophilic dermatosis, Sweet syndrome is characterized by the acute manifestation of painful erythematous and violaceous papules, nodules, and plaques accompanied by fever and elevated neutrophil count (Fig. 123–10).[69] These papules,

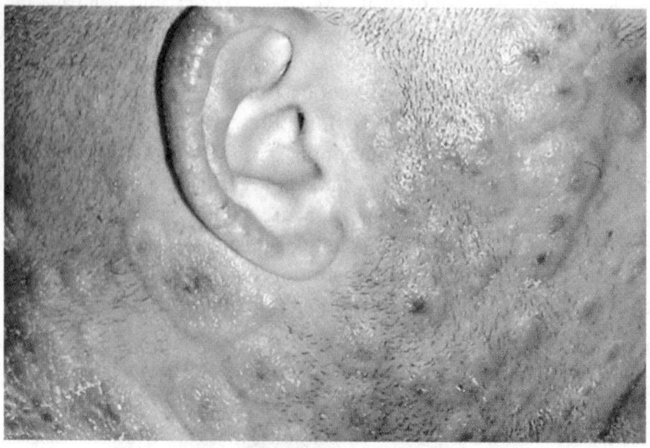

FIGURE 123–10. Sweet syndrome. The lesions are characterized by nonvasculitic neutrophilic infiltration, commonly on the face.

which most commonly appear on face, neck, and upper extremities, present a central yellowish discoloration and tend to coalesce, forming well-circumscribed, irregularly bordered plaques. Other organs can be involved, including the central nervous system, kidneys, lungs, and bones.[70] Classically more prominent in middle-aged women, this syndrome associates a complex cytokine dysregulation. Other manifestations include respiratory and urinary infections and autoimmune disorders (including rheumatoid arthritis, SLE, inflammatory bowel disease). Histologic analysis shows a distinct nonvasculitic neutrophilic infiltrate in the superficial dermis with dermal edema. Although systemic glucocorticoid treatment is the standard treatment, clofazimine, dapsone, colchicines, indomethacin, and cyclosporine have also been used successfully.[71]

BEHÇET DISEASE

Besides its classification as a neutrophilic dermatosis, Behçet disease is also an inflammatory disorder that affects multiple organ systems. Clinical features are chronic and relapsing cutaneous manifestations, such as palpable purpura, infiltrative erythema, and papulopustular lesions, as well as oral mucosal and genital ulcers, arthralgias, and gastrointestinal and central nervous system involvement.[72] Genetic studies show an association between Behçet disease and human leukocyte antigen B51.[73] Histologic features include leukocytoclastic or lymphocytic vasculitis, hence its previous classification as a vasculitis. Antitumor necrosis factor (anti-TNF)-α directed therapies (infliximab, etanercept), interferon-α, immunosuppressive and immunomodulatory agents such as thalidomide, intravenous immunoglobulin, dapsone, and stem cell transplantation are utilized in Behçet disease.[74,75]

SERUM SICKNESS

Serum sickness refers to the systemic manifestation of immune complex formation and deposition. Cutaneous lesions such as urticarial and morbilliform eruptions predominate, though palpable purpura and erythema multiforme are also often seen. Serum sickness associated with infection or medical therapy can result in specific characteristic lesions. The use of antithymocyte globulin for marrow failure, for instance, results in 75 percent of patients developing serpiginous bands of erythema and purpura on the sides of their hands and feet (Fig. 123–11).[76] These characteristic lesions consistently appear 1 to 2 days prior to the onset of systemic symptoms of serum sickness, which include fever and malaise. Analysis of biopsies by direct immunofluorescence reveals deposition of IgM, IgE, IgA, and C3. This deposition appears to activate neutrophils leading to release of lysosomal enzymes and, in turn, dermal vasculitis.[77]

HENOCH-SCHÖNLEIN PURPURA

Henoch-Schönlein purpura (HSP), a predominantly pediatric vasculitic syndrome characterized by the acute onset of abdominal pain and lower extremity eruption of diffuse urticarial plaques and palpable purpura, was first described in 1801 by Dr. William Heberden.[78] HSP predominantly affects patients 2 to 20 years of age, 90 percent of patients being younger than 10 years old.[79] Several environmental triggers precede HSP onset, such as viral (upper respiratory infections, hepatitis B virus, HCV, parvovirus B19, and HIV) and bacterial (*Streptococcus spp.*, *S. aureus*, and *Salmonella spp.*) infections in children. Adult disease is precipitated by medications (nonsteroidal antiinflammatory drugs [NSAIDs], angiotensin-converting enzyme inhibitors, and antibiotics), food allergies, vaccinations, and insect bites.[80] The pathogenesis of HSP leukocytoclastic vasculitis is complex and, appears to involve IgA_1 immune complex and complement deposition on vessel walls. Elevated values of thrombomodulin, tissue plasminogen activator, and plasminogen activator inhibitor-1 appear to correlate with endothelial injury and fibrinolytic activity in the acute phase of HSP.[81]

Cutaneous eruptions often begin acutely as urticarial papules and plaques evolving to petechiae, ecchymoses, and palpable and nonpalpable purpura over the lower extremities and buttocks (Fig. 123–12). Palpable purpura is a universal finding, being present in one series in 98.6 percent of patients.[82] Clinically, lesions may take the form of retiform or patterned purpura, presence of a retiform edge of various inflammatory lesions, or skin necrosis.[83] Other common manifestations include localized subcutaneous edema, nephritis, arthritis, and abdominal pain.

In spite of its chronic relapsing pattern, the long-term evolution is benign in the majority of patients.[82] The self-limited course of HSP may be contributed by an enhanced apoptosis of immune cells, which

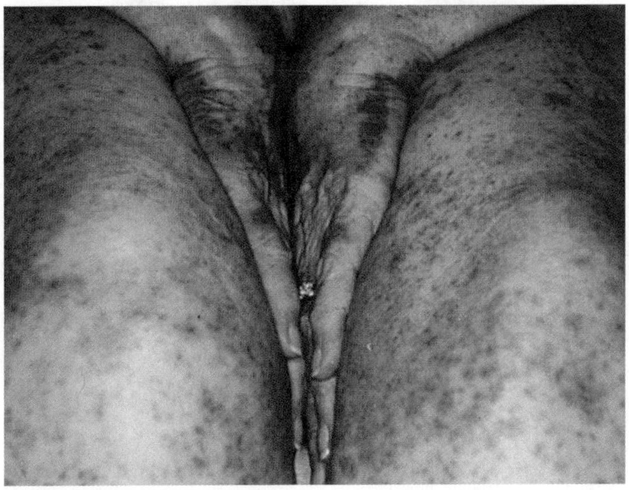

FIGURE 123–11. Serum sickness caused by antithymocyte globulin. The lesions consist of immunoglobulins and neutrophils.

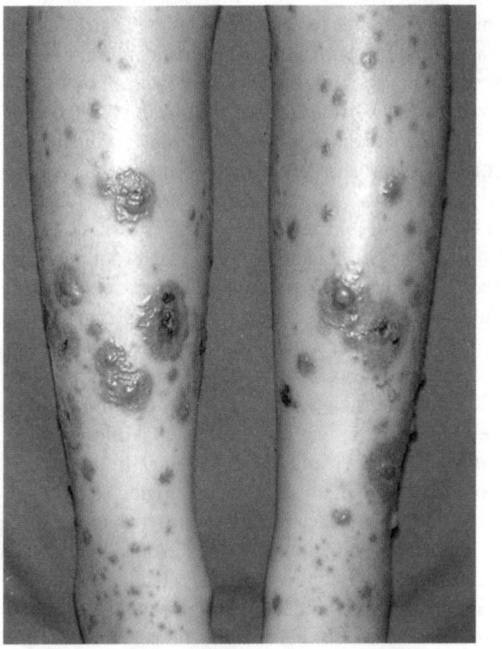

FIGURE 123–12. Henoch-Schönlein purpura. Urticarial papules and plaques can evolve into palpable purpura. The lesions are characterized by leukocytoclastic vasculitis.

diminishes the severity of the acute inflammatory response.[84] Consequently, treatment is generally supportive. Immunosuppressive drugs, including glucocorticoids, are typically reserved for cases with renal involvement.[78] Persistent purpura, severe abdominal symptoms, and diminished plasma coagulation factor XIII activity are predictive of renal involvement, requiring initiation of glucocorticoids.[85]

INFECTIONS

Careful analysis of skin lesions associated with an infection can provide important hints toward identifying the responsible pathogen. Purpura is one such lesion arising through a variety of pathophysiologic mechanisms associated with infection: (1) direct invasion of vessels with subsequent vascular occlusion, (2) septic emboli, (3) vascular effects of toxins, and (4) immune complex formation.[86] Although the morphology of these purpuric lesions may be nonspecific, many pathogens lead to characteristic findings.

Bacterial

Gram-positive and Gram-negative infections give rise to a large array of purpuric patterns depending on organism virulence and patient immune status. Skin lesions range from simple macules and papules to bullae, ulcers, and necrosis. Purpura fulminans, a hemorrhagic infarction syndrome consisting of fever, disseminated intravascular coagulation (DIC), acral purpura, and hypotension may manifest in the setting of bacterial sepsis with encapsulated organisms (*Streptococcus pneumoniae*, group A and B *β*-hemolytic streptococci, *S. aureus, Neisseria meningitidis*, and *Haemophilus influenzae*; see Chap. 130).[87]

Most commonly seen in immunocompromised hosts, purpura fulminans can also be produced by bacterial pathogens in immunocompetent hosts.[88] The syndrome was associated with asplenism and functional hyposplenism.[89] Although most affected individuals are younger than the age of 10 years, adults can also be affected.[90] Retiform purpuric lesions result from fibrin-induced microvascular occlusion, and commonly have a rapid evolution toward necrosis and eschar formation. Adult patients with purpura fulminans as a result of meningococcemia have significantly depressed antithrombin III and proteins C and S levels, which may explain this tendency toward fibrin deposition and development of cutaneous ischemic lesions, such as symmetrical peripheral gangrene.[91] Similarly characteristic in immunocompromised patients, ecthyma gangrenosum is seen with Gram-negative sepsis caused by *Pseudomonas aeruginosa, Klebsiella spp.*, or *Escherichia coli* (Fig. 123–13). Cutaneous lesions begin as acral erythematous or purpuric macules that evolve into erythematous plaques with surrounding purpura. Rapid progression to hemorrhagic vesicles or bullae surrounded by a halo of normal skin with an erythematous rim occurs in 24 to 48 hours. The vesicles and bullae can then rupture, leaving an ulcer with a necrotic center. Facial purpura and livedo reticularis may be seen during fulminant pneumococcal infection in asplenic patients.[92] Postinfectious purpura fulminans may occur after infections with streptococci, varicella zoster,[39] and was associated with anti-protein S antibodies.

In children, more than 20 percent of cases admitted to the hospital with petechiae and fever had invasive bacterial infections (*N. meningitidis, H. influenzae type B*, and *S. pneumoniae)*. In fact, approximately 7 percent of cases are diagnosed with meningiococcemia.[93] Sepsis secondary to *N. meningitidis* can also produce a characteristic pattern of purpuric lesions. Erythematous papules can quickly progress to numerous petechiae combined with violaceous reticular purpuric lesions.[94] A retiform aspect can be seen during progression of the infection to purpura fulminans. Although their pathogenesis is unclear, the finding of petechiae on a patient with symptoms and signs of bacterial meningitis is predictive of meningococcal meningitis.[95]

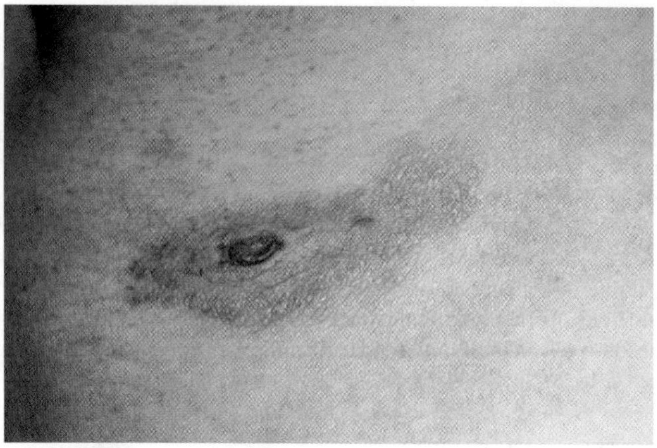

FIGURE 123–13. Ecthyma gangrenosum. Associated with Gram-negative sepsis, disseminated fungal infection, or other serious infectious diseases, these hemorrhagic bullae evolve from erythematosus plaques, both of which are shown here.

Borrelia burgdorferi infection gives rise to erythema migrans, the characteristic lesion of Lyme disease. The lesion is classically a nonpruritic erythematous expanding plaque, occasionally including a central hemorrhagic bullae (Fig. 123–14). Other reported cutaneous findings associated with this infection include papular urticaria, Henoch-Schönlein–like purpura, and morphea.[96]

Viral

Purpuric lesions can also be a manifestation of a viral infection. For example, the adenovirus and enterovirus family of viruses have been associated with the development of fever and petechiae in children.[97] Similarly, parvovirus B19 can produce a syndrome of petechiae or purpuric papules progressing to confluent purpuric papules or plaques in a sharply demarcated glove-and-sock distribution.[98] In addition to the cutaneous findings, the "gloves-and-socks syndrome" is characterized by fever and occasionally leukopenia.[99] Purpura in the axilla and chest also has been described during parvovirus B19 infection (Fig. 123–15).[100] Histopathologic analysis of these purpuric lesions show an evolution from superficial perivascular lymphocytic infiltrate to a dermatitis accompanied by necrotic keratinocytes and hemorrhage.[101] Other viruses known to cause purpuric lesions are measles and *Hantavirus*. The later causes a syndrome of hemorrhagic fever and renal

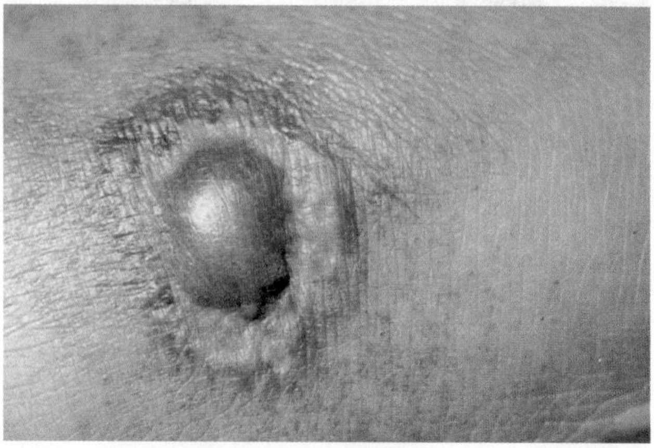

FIGURE 123–14. Lyme disease. Erythema migrans with a central hemorrhagic bulla is the characteristic lesion.

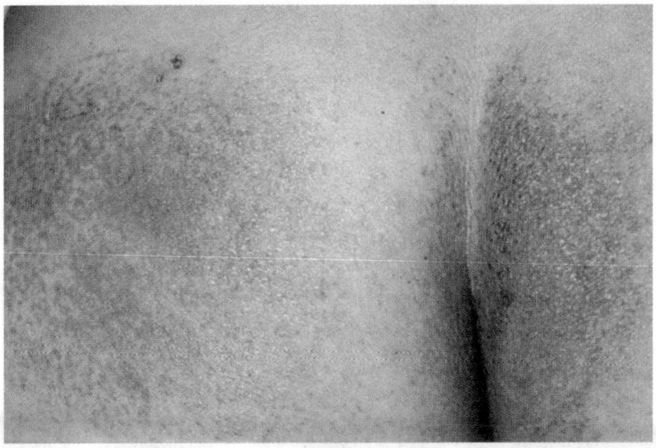

FIGURE 123–15. Parvovirus B19 erythema and petechiae. The classic slapped-cheek rash on the face can appear on other areas of the body, sometimes punctuated with petechiae of unclear etiology.

failure accompanied by headache, vomiting, and cutaneous and mucosal petechiae and ecchymosis.[102]

Fungal

Fungal infections in the immunocompromised population are a growing medical issue, given the increasing number of patients receiving immunosuppressants for organ transplantation or malignancy. Disseminated or locally invasive infections can give rise to petechiae and hemorrhagic necrosis. Common fungal pathogens in disseminated disease includes *Candida* (Fig. 123–16), *Aspergillus* (Fig. 123–17), *Histoplasma*, and *Fusarium*.[103] Disseminated candidiasis can manifest as ecthyma gangrenosum in immunocompromised patients, suggesting that pursuing a skin biopsy should be considered.[104] Cutaneous aspergillosis can occur in immunocompetent individuals, and manifest as eruptive maculopapules, necrotizing plaques, or subcutaneous granuloma.[105]

Parasitic

Immunocompromised patients are at risk of developing purpuric lesions secondary to parasitic infections, such as *Pneumocystis carinii*. Disseminated strongyloidiasis is characterized by larva currens, a serpiginous urticarial eruption caused by the migration of filiform larvae through the dermis.[106] Other cutaneous lesions include generalized

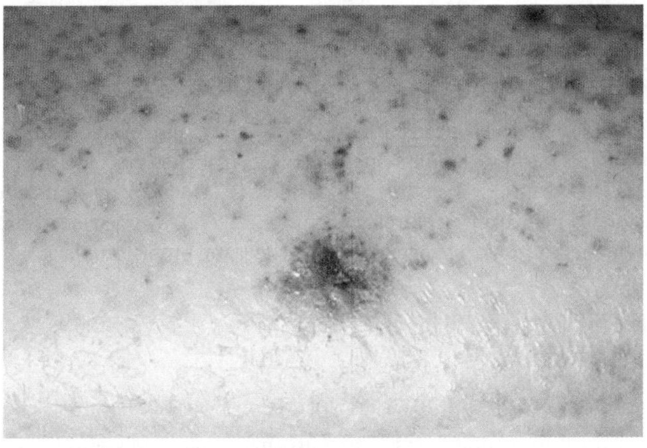

FIGURE 123–16. Disseminated candidiasis. Purpuric nodules in a patient with acute myelogenous leukemia. Ecthyma gangrenosum can also occur in this disease.

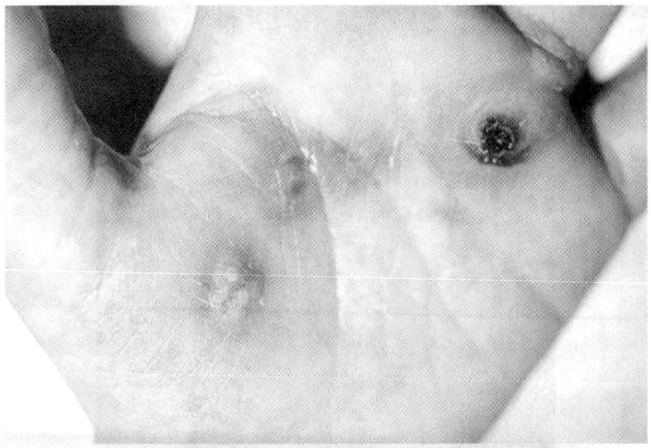

FIGURE 123–17. Aspergillosis: primary cutaneous inoculation from contaminated armboard.

petechiae and widespread reticular purpura of the arms, legs, and abdomen (Fig. 123–18), with a characteristic *thumbprint* periumbilical distribution.[107]

Rickettsial

Infections caused by *Rickettsia* species can also lead to purpuric lesions as a result of their direct invasion of endothelial cell cytoplasm and nuclei. This is followed by medial and intimal necrosis with subsequent thrombosis and hemorrhage.[86] Cutaneous lesions in Rocky Mountain spotted fever range from petechiae to acral purpuric lesions and hemorrhagic necrosis (Fig. 123–19). Maculopapular and vesicular rashes along with lower extremity eschars produced by *Rickettsia africae* may also occur in travelers to sub-Saharan Africa.[108]

ERYTHEMA MULTIFORME

Erythema multiforme (EM) is a cutaneous disorder characterized by the development of crops of well-demarcated, erythematous target lesions with central clearing,[109] most commonly representing a hypersensitivity reaction triggered by infection or drug exposure (Fig. 123–20). The severity of this disorder ranges from mild (EM minor), to severe (EM major or Stevens-Johnson syndrome). EM has been reported to be triggered by a number of viruses (most commonly herpes simplex, but also adenovirus, cytomegalovirus, and HIV),[110,111] and medications (sulfonamides, penicillins, bupropion, phenylbutazone,

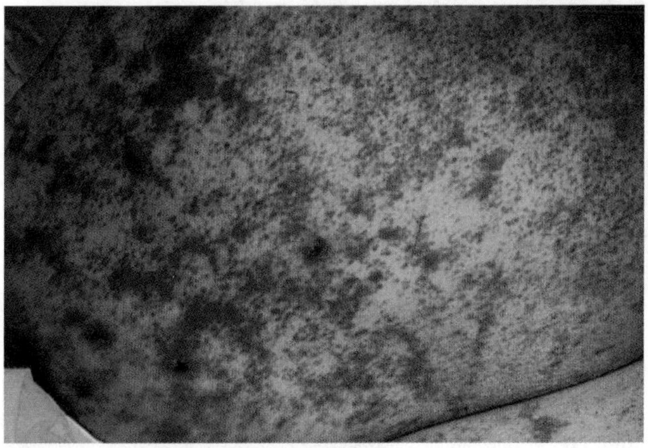

FIGURE 123–18. Disseminated strongyloidiasis.

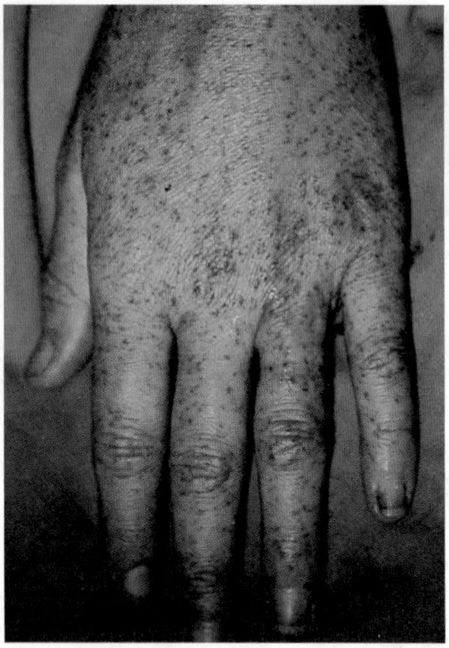

FIGURE 123–19. Rocky Mountain spotted fever. This rickettsial disorder can present with petechiae on the dorsum of the hand.

phenytoin, NSAIDs, adalimumab).[112] A cellular allergic reaction coupled with impaired histamine metabolism because of a decrease in histamine-*N*-methyltransferase activity may be causative.[113] Treatment for mild cases is supportive, while glucocorticoid use is often warranted in severe cases.

CUTANEOUS POLYARTERITIS NODOSA

Classic polyarteritis nodosa represents a systemic small- and medium-size vessel vasculitis most commonly involving the skin, heart, liver, and kidneys. A relatively benign cutaneous form exists that lacks significant systemic involvement[114] and consistently involves the deep dermis and panniculus.[115] Lesions develop as tender erythematous nodules[116] with occasional retiform purpura and livedo reticularis localized to the upper and lower extremities, but the trunk, neck, and face can also be involved (Fig. 123–21). The duration of lesions varies

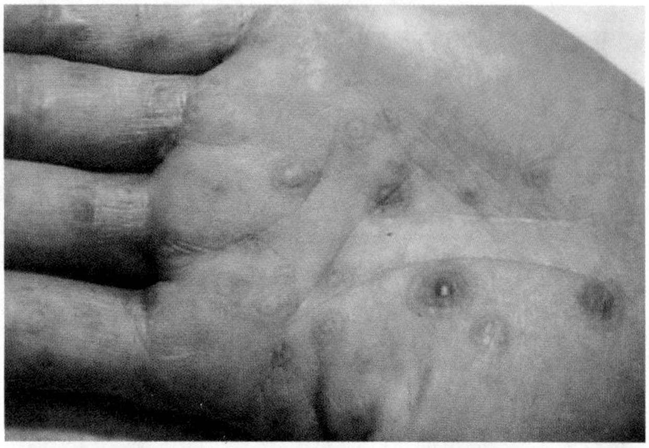

FIGURE 123–20. Erythema multiforme. This hypersensitivity reaction, usually to one of various drugs, characteristically presents with targetoid lesions.

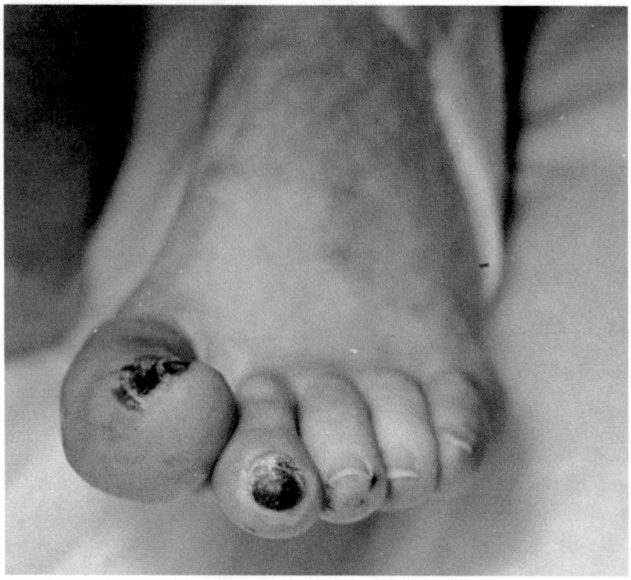

FIGURE 123–21. Polyarteritis nodosa. Acral purpura accompanying tender erythematous nodules.

from days to a few months.[115] Histologic analysis of involved skin shows deep dermal artery necrosis with infiltration of neutrophils and eosinophils, and fibrin deposition. Treatment typically involves the use of NSAIDs and glucocorticoids, alone or in combination. Some cases of cutaneous polyarteritis nodosum are reported to have progressed on long-term followup.[117] Thus, close monitoring of patients diagnosed with an apparently benign, cutaneous form of disease is warranted.[118]

PARANEOPLASTIC VASCULITIS

Most common vasculitis associated with neoplasia are cutaneous leukocytoclastic vasculitis, paraneoplastic vasculitis, and Henoch-Schönlein purpura.[119,120] Paraneoplastic vasculitis is most commonly associated with hematologic neoplasia,[121] and is commonly a result of paraproteinemia.[122] However, an association with carcinomas of the lung, colon, breast, and cervix has been observed.[123,124] Solid tumors predominate in certain types of paraneoplastic vasculitis, such as the Henoch-Schönlein purpura.[125] Cutaneous manifestations include petechiae, urticaria, and palpable purpura, and are often intensely pruritic. In hematologic disorders, these lesions often precede the development of malignancy by an average of 10 months.[126] Histologic examination shows necrotizing leukocytoclastic vasculitis with neutrophilic infiltration.

DRUG-INDUCED VASCULITIS

A long list of drugs are reported to cause a vasculitis resulting in erythematous purpuric lesions. One-fifth of all cutaneous vasculitis are produced by drugs,[122] including allopurinol, cefaclor, colony-stimulating factors, D-penicillamine, furosemide (Fig. 123–22), hydralazine, isotretinoin, methotrexate, phenytoin, minocycline, and propylthiouracil.[127]

ANTINEUTROPHIL CYTOPLASMIC ANTIBODY-ASSOCIATED VASCULITIS

Wegener Granulomatosis

This small to medium vessel vasculitis most commonly affects upper and lower respiratory tracts and kidneys and is strongly associated with the development of circulating antineutrophil cytoplasmic antibodies

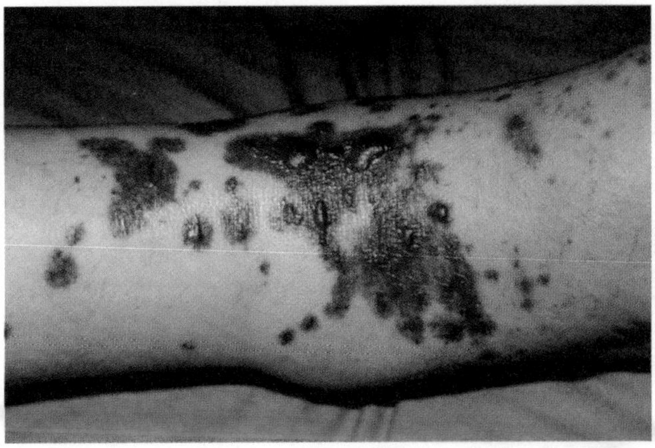

FIGURE 123-22. Leukocytoclastic vasculitis secondary to furosemide.

(ANCA).[128] Skin involvement has been reported in 35 to 50 percent of cases.[129] Although variable, cutaneous eruptions include a combination of palpable purpura, oral ulcers, and erythematous cutaneous and subcutaneous nodules (Fig. 123-23).[130] Necrotizing vasculitis, palisading granulomas, and granulomatous vasculitis are characteristic histologic findings.[131]

Churg-Strauss Syndrome

Churg-Strauss syndrome (CSS) is characterized by granulomatous inflammation in the lungs associated with asthma and eosinophilia.[132] Cutaneous findings such as ulcers, papules, palpable purpura, cutaneous nodules, and infarcts of fingers and toes are encountered in 50 to 80 percent of cases.[130] CSS limited to the skin was described.[133] Eosinophilia accompanies elevated IgE levels and a positive perinuclear ANCA. Granulomatous inflammation and necrotizing vasculitis of small- to medium-size blood vessels are present histologically.[131]

Microscopic Angiitis

This is a predominantly small-vessel vasculitis that carries a strong association with perinuclear ANCA. It differs from other small-vessel vasculitides, like cryoglobulinemic vasculitis and HSP, in its absence or paucity of immune complex involvement. Skin involvement is seen in 40 to 70 percent of patients, and consists of purpura, livedo, papules, urticaria, nodules, and ulcerations.[116,130] Histologic assessment shows necrotizing vasculitis of small vessels.

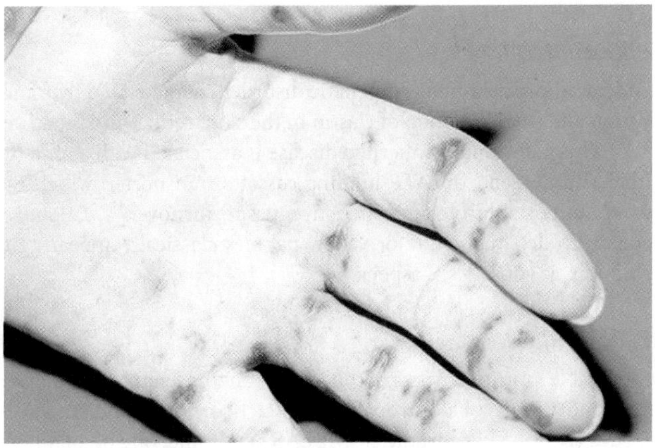

FIGURE 123-23. Wegener granulomatosis.

Treatment of ANCA-positive vasculitis includes an induction phase consisting of glucocorticoids alone for good prognosis CSS and microscopic polyangiitis, or a combination of the former with cyclophosphamide for Wegener granulomatosis. Maintenance treatment with azathioprine or other immunosuppressive drugs (mycophenolate, methotrexate) reduces relapses. Biologic therapies such as B-cell depletion with rituximab or TNF-α antagonists emerge as effective modalities for refractory disease.[130,134–136]

NONPALPABLE, NONINFLAMMATORY, ROUND PURPURIC LESIONS (Table 123-3)

INCREASED TRANSMURAL PRESSURE GRADIENT

Acute increases in vascular transmural pressure gradients lead to extravasation of red blood cells resulting in nonpalpable, noninflammatory petechial and larger purpuric lesions. Examples include postictal purpura,[137] weightlifting,[138] postemesis facial purpura,[139] prolonged Valsalva, and childbirth. Acute decreases in extravascular negative pressure, referred to as suction purpura from gas mask, kissing, or cupping, can also increase this gradient, resulting in well-circumscribed lesions in the shape of the causative device.[140] The development of petechiae in mountain climbers has also been described, presumably caused by significantly reduced atmospheric pressures at high elevations.[141] Lower-extremity venous incompetence, predominantly at the medial ankle, can result in macules or patches of yellowish-brown purpura.

THROBOCYTOPENIAS

Disseminated Intravascular Coagulation

DIC is defined as widespread, amplified and uncontrolled intravascular coagulation with a range of causes including sepsis, trauma, and malignancy.[142] Petechiae and purpuric plaques result from thrombocytopenia, and are common manifestations of DIC (see Chap. 130).

Idiopathic Thrombocytopenia Purpura

Idiopathic thrombocytopenia purpura is an acquired disease characterized by autoantibody-mediated platelet destruction commonly resulting in purpuric lesions of the skin and mucosa as well as other sites of abnormal bleeding.[143]

Thrombotic Thrombocytopenia Purpura

Thrombotic thrombocytopenia purpura is characterized by nonimmune platelet consumption, organ damage, and microvascular hemolysis, and appears to be associated with a deficiency in the von Willebrand factor cleaving protease, ADAMTS-13 (a disintegrin and metalloproteinase with thrombospondin domain 13; see Chap. 133).[144] Petechiae and purpuric plaques are common.

DRUG REACTIONS

A large number of medications are reported to result in vasculitic and nonvasculitic purpuric eruptions.[145] Nevertheless, *any* drug on the medication list of a patient with a purpuric lesion (within 2 weeks of starting a new drug or a few days if prior sensitization is suspected) may be involved.[146]

COAGULATION DISORDERS

A large number of disorders manifest with increased bruising including, but not limited to, anticoagulant use, vitamin K deficiency, and poor hepatic function (see Chap. 118).

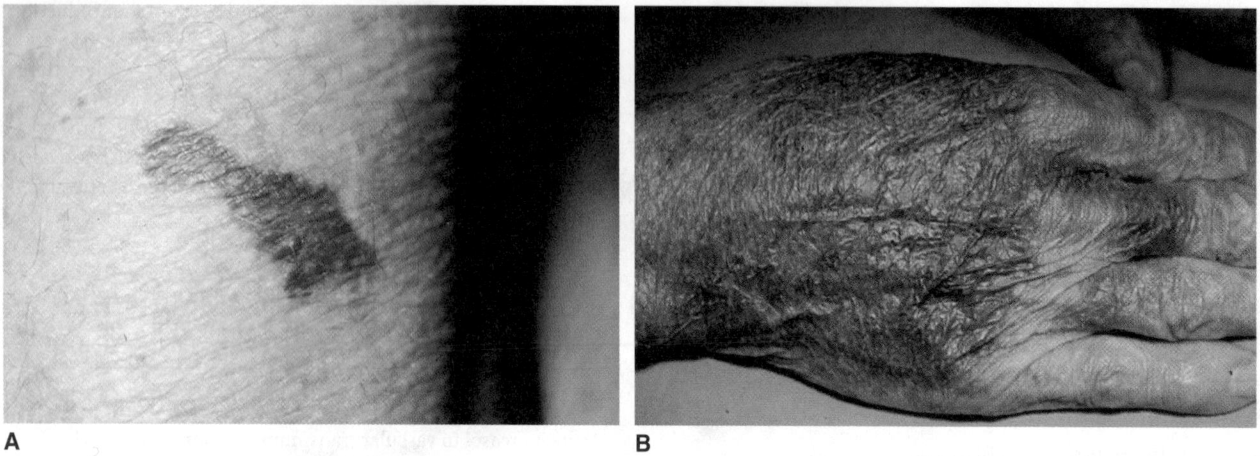

FIGURE 123–24. Senile purpura. Note accompanying skin atrophy.

DECREASED VESSEL INTEGRITY WITHOUT TRAUMA

Senile Purpura

Synonymous with actinic purpura, senile purpura refers to the easy bruising seen in the aged and sun-damaged skin, commonly appearing on the dorsal aspect of the hands and forearms (Fig. 123–24). One proposed etiology is the degeneration of skin extracellular matrix components leaving dermal capillaries unsupported and vulnerable to shearing injuries,[147] but zinc deficiency has also been suspected.[148]

Excess Glucocorticoid

The presence of excess endogenous (Cushing syndrome) or exogenous glucocorticoid use can result in dermal thinning and vessel fragility. Consequently, bright red, nonpalpable purpuric lesions tend to arise after slight or even undetected trauma and manifest in a linear or geometric pattern.[149]

Scurvy–Vitamin C Deficiency

Vitamin C (ascorbic acid) deficiency occurs because of reduced dietary intake or absorption. A consequent disruption in normal collagen production results in blood vessel fragility leading to petechiae, perifollicular hemorrhage, and larger purpuric plaques, most commonly on the lower extremities (Fig. 123–25).[150] Cutaneous features can also include follicular hyperkeratotic papules, poor wound healing, and bent or corkscrew-shaped body hairs.[151] Scurvy is usually a clinical diagnosis. Vitamin C supplementation is initiated after a thorough investigation of all factors leading to malnutrition.

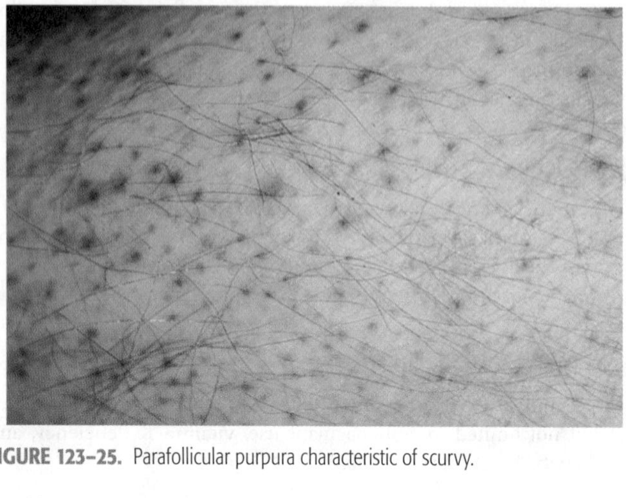

FIGURE 123–25. Parafollicular purpura characteristic of scurvy.

Systemic Amyloidosis

Systemic amyloidosis is characterized by a clonal proliferation of plasma cells with consequent immunoglobulin light-chain deposition in vital organs. Microscopic 8 to 10 nm protofilaments aggregate to form fibrils.[152] It can present as a primary disorder or secondarily to multiple myeloma (see Chaps. 109 and 110). Characteristic features are periorbital "pinch purpura," "raccoon eyes," and macroglosia.[153]

Waxy, purpuric cutaneous and mucocutaneous lesions manifest when light-chain aggregates deposit in dermal blood vessels. Although rare, palmodigital purpura has been reported as the sole cutaneous finding in a case of myeloma-associated systemic amyloidosis.[154] A distinct localized form, primary cutaneous amyloidosis, is caused by local dermal infiltration of plasma cells.[155]

CONNECTIVE TISSUE DISORDERS

Ehlers-Danlos Syndrome

A rare autosomal dominant syndrome, Ehlers-Danlos syndrome is a consequence of a mutation in collagen synthesis leading to loss of skin elasticity, delayed wound healing, easy bruising, joint hypermobility, and systemic organ tissue fragility.[156] Cutaneous findings include thin skin and a tendency to develop nonpalpable purpuric lesions.[157]

Pseudoxanthoma Elasticum

Pseudoxanthoma elasticum is genetic disorder characterized by mineralization and fragmentation of elastin in the skin, retina, and blood vessels.[158] This autosomally inherited disease is associated with a mutation in the ABCC6 gene, an ATP-binding cassette transporter, which may play an important role in connective tissue turnover.[159] Cutaneous lesions include small white or yellow papules classically appearing on the neck in a "gooseflesh" aspect.[160]

MELAS Syndrome

Nonpalpable purpuric lesions can occur on the palms and soles in *m*itochondrial *e*ncephalomyopathy with *l*actic *a*cidosis and *s*troke-like episodes (MELAS) syndrome.[161] MELAS syndrome, one of a family of mitochondrial encephalomyopathies, has been associated with a muta-

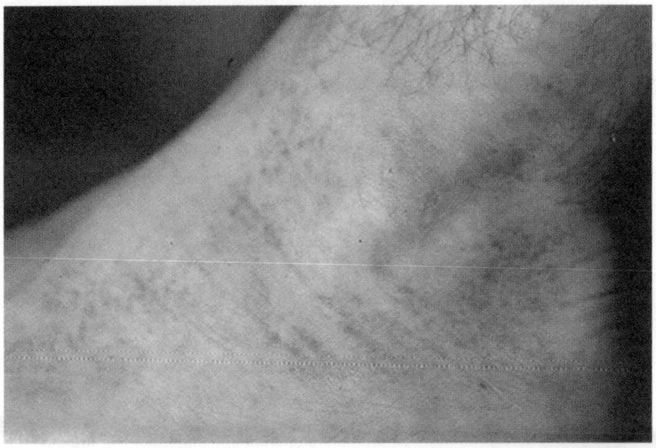

FIGURE 123–26. Schamberg disease. Note characteristic "cayenne pepper" petechiae.

tion in a mitochondrial transfer RNA.[162] Skin manifestations can also include hypertrichosis, ichthyosis, and vitiligo.[163]

TRAUMA

Focal ecchymosis and other purpuric lesions can manifest as a result of trauma. Characteristic patterns of purpuric lesions are commonly used in forensic science. Traumatic asphyxia, for instance, is characterized by cervicofacial cyanosis and swelling, petechiae, and subconjunctival hemorrhage.[164] Factitious purpura, often related to deliberate suction purpura, should be considered in the differential for purpura.[165] Other physical causes of purpura consist of physical remedies, such as spooning (Quat Sha) or coin rubbing (Cao Gio). Exercise-induced purpura results in purpuric, erythematous, or urticarial lesions distributed on the lower legs.[166]

SCHAMBERG DISEASE

Also referred to as progressive pigmentary purpura, Schamberg disease is characterized by the development of "cayenne pepper" petechiae on a background of hyperpigmented brown or orange oval patches often seen in tibial regions bilaterally as a chronic eruption (Fig. 123–26).[167] Histologic analysis reveals capillaritis with a perivascular infiltrate of dendritic cells suggesting that this disease may involve a cell-mediated immune response. Extravasated red blood cells and hemosiderin-laden macrophages are also commonly seen.

REFERENCES

1. Carlson JA, Chen KR: Cutaneous pseudovasculitis. *Am J Dermatopathol* 29:44, 2007.
2. Piette WW: The differential diagnosis of purpura from a morphologic perspective. *Adv Dermatol* 9:3, discussion 24, 1994.
3. Piette WW: Hematologic diseases, in *Fitzpatrick's Dermatology in General Medicine*, 6th ed, edited by IM Freedburg, AZ Eisen, K Wolff, KF Austen, LA Goldsmith, SI Katz, p 1523. McGraw-Hill, New York, 2003.
4. Stephenson T: Ageing of bruising in children. *J R Soc Med* 90:312, 1997.
5. Winfield JB: Cryoglobulinemia. *Hum Pathol* 14:350, 1983.
6. Galossi A, Guarisco R, Bellis L, Puoti C: Extrahepatic manifestations of chronic HCV infection. *J Gastrointestin Liver Dis* 16:65, 2007.
7. Agnello V, Romain PL: Mixed cryoglobulinemia secondary to hepatitis C virus infection. *Rheum Dis Clin North Am* 22:1, 1996.
8. Braun GS, Horster S, Wagner KS, et al: Cryoglobulinaemic vasculitis: Classification and clinical and therapeutic aspects. *Postgrad Med J* 83:87, 2007.
9. Sansonno D, Dammacco F: Hepatitis C virus, cryoglobulinaemia, and vasculitis: Immune complex relations. *Lancet Infect Dis* 5:227, 2005.
10. Sansonno D, Tucci FA, Troiani L, et al: Increased serum levels of the chemokine CXCL13 and up-regulation of its gene expression are distinctive features of HCV-related cryoglobulinemia and correlate with active cutaneous vasculitis. *Blood* 112:1620, 2008.
11. Dispenzieri A: Symptomatic cryoglobulinemia. *Curr Treat Options Oncol* 1:105, 2000.
12. Casato M, Mecucci C, Agnello V, et al: Regression of lymphoproliferative disorder after treatment for hepatitis C virus infection in a patient with partial trisomy 3, Bcl-2 overexpression, and type II cryoglobulinemia. *Blood* 99:2259, 2002.
13. Waldenström J: Clinical methods for determination of hyperproteinemia and their practical value for diagnosis. *Nord Med* 20:2288, 1943.
14. Finder KA, McCollough ML, Dixon SL, et al: Hypergammaglobulinemic purpura of Waldenstrom. *J Am Acad Dermatol* 23:669, 1990.
15. Malaviya AN, Kaushik P, Budhiraja S, et al: Hypergammaglobulinemic purpura of Waldenström: Report of 3 cases with a short review. *Clin Exp Rheumatol* 18:518, 2000.
16. Tan E, Ng SK, Tan SH, Wong GC: Hypergammaglobulinaemic purpura presenting as reticulate purpura. *Clin Exp Dermatol* 24:469, 1999.
17. Al-Mayouf SM, Ghonaium A, Bahabri S: Hypergammaglobulinaemic purpura associated with IgG subclass imbalance and recurrent infection. *Clin Rheumatol* 19:499, 2000.
18. Oosterkamp HM, van der Pijl H, Derksen J, et al: Arthritis and hypergammaglobulinemic purpura in hypersensitivity pneumonitis. *Am J Med* 100:478, 1996.
19. Miyagawa S, Fukumoto T, Kanauchi M, et al: Hypergammaglobulinaemic purpura of Waldenstrom and Ro/SSA autoantibodies. *Br J Dermatol* 134:919, 1996.
20. Pozzi C, D'Amico M, Fogazzi GB, et al: Light chain deposition disease with renal involvement: Clinical characteristics and prognostic factors. *Am J Kidney Dis* 42:1154, 2003.
21. Stone GC, Wall BA, Oppliger IR, et al: A vasculopathy with deposition of lambda light chain crystals. *Ann Intern Med* 110:275, 1989.
22. Usuda H, Emura I, Naito M: Crystal globulin-induced vasculopathy accompanying ischemic intestinal lesions of a patient with myeloma. *Pathol Int* 46:165, 1996.
23. Sankarasubbaiyan S, Scott G, Holley JL: Cryofibrinogenemia: An addition to the differential diagnosis of calciphylaxis in end-stage renal disease. *Am J Kidney Dis* 32:494, 1998.
24. Amdo TD, Welker JA. An approach to the diagnosis and treatment of cryofibrinogenemia. *Am J Med* 116:332, 2004.
25. Blain H, Cacoub P, Musset L, et al: Cryofibrinogenaemia: A study of 49 patients. *Clin Exp Immunol* 120:253, 2000.
26. Wutschert R, Piletta P, Bounameaux H: Adverse skin reactions to low molecular weight heparins: Frequency, management and prevention. *Drug Saf* 20:515, 1999.
27. Moore A, Lau E, Yang C, et al: Dalteparin-induced skin necrosis in a patient with metastatic lung adenocarcinoma. *Am J Clin Oncol* 30:329, 2007.
28. Chong BH: Heparin-induced thrombocytopenia. *J Thromb Haemost* 1:1471, 2003.
29. Chan YC, Valenti D, Mansfield AO, Stansby G: Warfarin induced skin necrosis. *Br J Surg* 87:266, 2000.
30. Harenberg J, Hoffmann U, Huhle G, et al: Cutaneous reactions to anticoagulants. Recognition and management. *Am J Clin Dermatol* 2:69, 2001.
31. Scarff CE, Baker C, Hill P, Foley P: Late-onset warfarin necrosis. *Australas J Dermatol* 43:202, 2002.
32. Ward CT, Chavalitanonda N: Atypical warfarin-induced skin necrosis. *Pharmacotherapy* 26:1175, 2006.
33. Stone MS, Rosen T: Acral purpura: An unusual sign of coumarin necrosis. *J Am Acad Dermatol* 14:797, 1986.
34. Segel GB, Francis CA: Anticoagulant proteins in childhood venous and arterial thrombosis: A review. *Blood Cells Mol Dis* 26:540, 2000.
35. Marlar RA, Neumann A: Neonatal purpura fulminans due to homozygous protein C or protein S deficiencies. *Semin Thromb Hemost* 16:299,1990.
36. Kemahli S, Alhenc-Gelas M, Gandrille S, et al: Homozygous protein C deficiency with a double variant His 202 to Tyr and Ala 346 to Thr. *Blood Coagul Fibrinolysis* 9:351, 1998.
37. Ezer U, Misirlioglu ED, Colba V, et al: Neonatal purpura fulminans due to homozygous protein C deficiency. *Pediatr Hematol Oncol* 18:453, 2001.
38. Gruber A, Blasko G, Sas G: Functional deficiency of protein C and skin necrosis in multiple myeloma. *Thromb Res* 42:579, 1986.
39. van Ommen CH, van Wijnen M, de Groot FG, et al: Postvaricella purpura fulminans caused by acquired protein s deficiency resulting from antiprotein s antibodies: Search for the epitopes. *J Pediatr Hematol Oncol* 24:413, 2002.
40. De Stefano V, Mastrangelo S, Schwarz HP, et al: Replacement therapy with a purified protein C concentrate during initiation of oral anticoagulation in severe protein C congenital deficiency. *Thromb Haemost* 70:247, 1993.
41. Hillman RS, Ault, KA: The dysplastic and sideroblastic anemias, in *Hematology in Clinical Practice*, 2nd ed, edited by J Morgan, P Hanley, p 151. McGraw-Hill, New York, 1998.
42. White JM, Watson K, Arya R, Du Vivier AW: Haemorrhagic bullae in a case of paroxysmal nocturnal haemoglobinuria. *Clin Exp Dermatol* 28:504, 2003.
43. Cholez C, Schmutz JL, Hulin C, et al: Cutaneous necrosis during paroxysmal nocturnal haemoglobinuria: Role of parvovirus B19? *J Eur Acad Dermatol Venereol* 19:381, 2005.
44. Goulden V, Bond L, Highet AS: Pyoderma gangrenosum associated with paroxysmal nocturnal haemoglobinuria. *Clin Exp Dermatol* 19:271, 1994.
45. Watt SG, Winhoven S, Hay CR, Lucas GS: Purpura fulminans in paroxysmal nocturnal haemoglobinuria. *Br J Haematol* 137:271, 2007.

46. Blume JE, Miller CC: Antiphospholipid syndrome: A review and update for the dermatologist. *Cutis* 78:409, 2006.
47. DiFrancesco LM, Burkart P, Hoehn JG: A cutaneous manifestation of antiphospholipid antibody syndrome. *Ann Plast Surg* 51:517, 2003.
48. Weinstein S, Piette W: Cutaneous manifestations of antiphospholipid antibody syndrome. *Hematol Oncol Clin North Am* 22:67, 2008.
49. Uthman IW, Khamashta MA: Livedo racemosa: A striking dermatological sign for the antiphospholipid syndrome. *J Rheumatol* 33:2379, 2006.
50. Martin L, Armingaud P, Georgescu V, et al: Acute bullous purpura associated with hyperhomocysteinemia and antiphospholipid antibodies. *J Am Acad Dermatol* 49:S161, 2003.
51. Hereng T, Lambert M, Hachulla E, et al: Influence of aspirin on the clinical outcomes of 103 anti-phospholipid antibodies-positive patients. *Lupus* 17:11, 2008.
52. Hairston BR, Davis MD, Pittelkow MR, Ahmed I. Livedoid vasculopathy: Further evidence for procoagulant pathogenesis. *Arch Dermatol* 142:1413, 2006.
53. Mimouni D, Ng PP, Rencic A, et al: Cutaneous polyarteritis nodosa in patients presenting with atrophie blanche. *Br J Dermatol* 148:789, 2003.
54. Acland KM, Darvay A, Wakelin SH, Russell-Jones R: Livedoid vasculitis: A manifestation of the antiphospholipid syndrome? *Br J Dermatol* 140:131, 1999.
55. Ravat FE, Evans AV, Russell-Jones R: Response of livedoid vasculitis to intravenous immunoglobulin. *Br J Dermatol* 147:166, 2002.
56. Donohue KG, Saap L, Falanga V: Cholesterol crystal embolization: An atherosclerotic disease with frequent and varied cutaneous manifestations. *J Eur Acad Dermatol Venereol* 17:504, 2003.
57. Jucgla A, Moreso F, Muniesa C, et al: Cholesterol embolism: Still an unrecognized entity with a high mortality rate. *J Am Acad Dermatol* 55:786, 2006.
58. Meyrier A: Cholesterol crystal embolism: Diagnosis and treatment. *Kidney Int* 69:1308, 2006.
59. Floege J: When man turns to stone: Extraosseous calcification in uremic patients. *Kidney Int* 65:2447, 2004.
60. Parker RW, Mouton CP, Young DW, Espino DV: Early recognition and treatment of calciphylaxis. *South Med J* 96:53, 2003.
61. Trent JT, Kirsner RS: Calciphylaxis: Diagnosis and treatment. *Adv Skin Wound Care* 14:309, 2001.
62. Nigwekar SU, Wolf M, Sterns RH, Hix JK: Calciphylaxis from nonuremic causes: A systematic review. *Clin J Am Soc Nephrol* 3:1139, 2008.
63. Alexandrescu DT, Wiernik PH: Cutaneous manifestations of a catheter-related thrombus. *Arch Dermatol* 141:1049, 2005.
64. García-F-Villalta MJ, Sanz-Sánchez T, Aragüés M, et al: Cutaneous embolization of cardiac myxoma. *Br J Dermatol* 147:379, 2002.
65. Zhu YI, Stiller MJ: Arthropods and skin diseases. *Int J Dermatol* 41:533, 2002.
66. Shankar S, Sterling JC, Rytina E: Pustular pyoderma gangrenosum. *Clin Exp Dermatol* 28:600, 2003.
67. Crowson AN, Mihm MC Jr, Magro C: Pyoderma gangrenosum: A review. *J Cutan Pathol* 30:97, 2003.
68. Gettler S, Rothe M, Grin C, Grant-Kels J: Optimal treatment of pyoderma gangrenosum. *Am J Clin Dermatol* 4:597, 2003.
69. Cohen PR, Kurzrock R: Sweet's syndrome: A neutrophilic dermatosis classically associated with acute onset and fever. *Clin Dermatol* 18:265, 2000.
70. Nobeyama Y, Kamide R: Sweet's syndrome with neurologic manifestation: Case report and literature review. *Int J Dermatol* 42:438, 2003.
71. Cohen PR, Kurzrock R: Sweet's syndrome: A review of current treatment options. *Am J Clin Dermatol* 3:117, 2002.
72. Chen KR, Kawahara Y, Miyakawa S, Nishikawa T: Cutaneous vasculitis in Behçet disease: A clinical and histopathologic study of 20 patients. *J Am Acad Dermatol* 36:689, 1997.
73. Yurdakul S, Hamuryudan V, Yazici H: Behçet syndrome. *Curr Opin Rheumatol* 16:38, 2004.
74. Olivieri I, Latanza L, Siringo S, et al: Successful treatment of severe Behçet's disease with infliximab in an Italian Olympic athlete. *J Rheumatol* 35:930, 2008.
75. Curigliano V, Giovinale M, Fonnesu C, et al: Efficacy of etanercept in the treatment of a patient with Behçet's disease. *Clin Rheumatol* 27:933, 2008.
76. Bielory L, Gascon P, Lawley TJ, et al: Human serum sickness: A prospective analysis of 35 patients treated with equine anti-thymocyte globulin for bone marrow failure. *Medicine (Baltimore)* 67:40, 1988.
77. Jegasothy BV: Immune complexes in the reactive inflammatory vascular dermatoses. *Dermatol Clin* 3:185, 1985.
78. Ballinger S: Henoch-Schönlein purpura. *Curr Opin Rheumatol* 15:591, 2003.
79. Saulsbury FT: Henoch-Schönlein purpura. *Curr Opin Rheumatol* 13:35, 2001.
80. Eftychiou C, Samarkos M, Golfinopoulou S, et al: Henoch-Schönlein purpura associated with methicillin-resistant *Staphylococcus aureus* infection. *Am J Med* 119:85, 2006.
81. Besbas N, Saatci U, Ruacan S, et al: The role of cytokines in Henoch-Schönlein purpura. *Scand J Rheumatol* 26:456, 1997.
82. Fretzayas A, Sionti I, Moustaki M, et al: Henoch-Schönlein purpura: A long-term prospective study in Greek children. *J Clin Rheumatol* 14:324, 2008.
83. Carlson JA, Chen KR: Cutaneous vasculitis update: Small vessel neutrophilic vasculitis syndromes. *Am J Dermatopathol* 28:486, 2006.
84. Ozaltin F, Besbas N, Uckan D, et al: The role of apoptosis in childhood Henoch-Schönlein purpura. *Clin Rheumatol* 22:265, 2003.
85. Kaku Y, Nohara K, Honda S: Renal involvement in Henoch-Schönlein purpura: A multivariate analysis of prognostic factors. *Kidney Int* 53: 1755, 1998.
86. Kingston ME, Mackey D: Skin clues in the diagnosis of life-threatening infections. *Rev Infect Dis* 8:1, 1986.
87. Childers BJ, Cobanov B: Acute infectious purpura fulminans: A 15-year retrospective review of 28 consecutive cases. *Am Surg* 69:86, 2003.
88. Cnota JF, Barton LL, Rhee KH: Purpura fulminans associated with *Streptococcus pneumoniae* infection in a child. *Pediatr Emerg Care* 15:187, 1999.
89. Ward KM, Celebi JT, Gmyrek R, Grossman ME: Acute infectious purpura fulminans associated with asplenism or hyposplenism. *J Am Acad Dermatol* 47:493, 2002.
90. Betrosian AP, Berlet T, Agarwal B: Purpura fulminans in sepsis. *Am J Med Sci* 332:339, 2006.
91. Rintala E, Kauppila M, Seppala OP, et al: Protein C substitution in sepsis-associated purpura fulminans. *Crit Care Med* 28:2373, 2000.
92. Rusonis PA, Robinson HN, Lamberg SI: Livedo reticularis and purpura: Presenting features in fulminant pneumococcal septicemia in an asplenic patient. *J Am Acad Dermatol* 15:1120, 1986.
93. Baker RC, Seguin JH, Leslie N, et al: Fever and petechiae in children. *Pediatrics* 84:1051, 1989.
94. Baselga E, Drolet BA, Esterly NB: Purpura in infants and children. *J Am Acad Dermatol* 37:673, quiz 706, 1997.
95. Mancebo J, Domingo P, Blanch L, et al: The predictive value of petechiae in adults with bacterial meningitis. *JAMA* 256:2820, 1986.
96. Berger BW: Dermatologic manifestations of Lyme disease. *Rev Infect Dis* 11(Suppl 6):S1475, 1989.
97. Nielsen HE, Andersen EA, Andersen J, et al: Diagnostic assessment of haemorrhagic rash and fever. *Arch Dis Child* 85:160, 2001.
98. McNeely M, Friedman J, Pope E: Generalized petechial eruption induced by parvovirus B19 infection. *J Am Acad Dermatol* 52:S109, 2005.
99. Perez-Ferriols A, Martinez-Aparicio A, Aliaga-Boniche A: Papular-purpuric "gloves and socks" syndrome caused by measles virus. *J Am Acad Dermatol* 30:291, 1994.
100. Shiraishi H, Umetsu K, Yamamoto H, et al: Human parvovirus (HPV/B19) infection with purpura. *Microbiol Immunol* 33:369, 1989.
101. Smith SB, Libow LF, Elston DM, et al: Gloves and socks syndrome: Early and late histopathologic features. *J Am Acad Dermatol* 47:749, 2002.
102. Bruno P, Hassell LH, Brown J, et al: The protean manifestations of hemorrhagic fever with renal syndrome. A retrospective review of 26 cases from Korea. *Ann Intern Med* 113:385, 1990.
103. Helm TN, Longworth DL, Hall GS, et al: Case report and review of resolved fusariosis. *J Am Acad Dermatol* 23:393, 1990.
104. Fine JD, Miller JA, Harrist TJ, Haynes HA: Cutaneous lesions in disseminated candidiasis mimicking ecthyma gangrenosum. *Am J Med* 70: 1133, 1981.
105. Galimberti R, Kowalczuk A, Hidalgo Parra I, et al: Cutaneous aspergillosis: A report of six cases. *Br J Dermatol* 139:522, 1998.
106. von Kuster LC, Genta RM: Cutaneous manifestations of strongyloidiasis. *Arch Dermatol* 124:1826, 1988.
107. Ly MN, Bethel SL, Usmani AS, et al: Cutaneous Strongyloides stercoralis infection: An unusual presentation. *J Am Acad Dermatol* 49:S157, 2003.
108. Jensenius M, Fournier PE, Kelly P, et al: African tick bite fever. *Lancet Infect Dis* 3:557, 2003.
109. Lamoreux MR, Sternbach MR, Hsu WT: Erythema multiforme. *Am Fam Physician* 74:1883, 2006.
110. Ng PP, Sun YJ, Tan HH, Tan SH: Detection of herpes simplex virus genomic DNA in various subsets of erythema multiforme by polymerase chain reaction. *Dermatology* 207:349, 2003.
111. Schechner AJ, Pinson AG: Acute human immunodeficiency virus infection presenting with erythema multiforme. *Am J Emerg Med* 22:330, 2004.
112. Yang YH, Tsai MJ, Tsau YK, et al: Clinical observations of erythema multiforme in children. *Acta Paediatr Taiwan* 40:107, 1999.
113. Imamura S, Horio T, Yanase K, et al: Erythema multiforme: Pathomechanism of papular erythema and target lesion. *J Dermatol* 19:524, 1992.
114. Siberry GK, Cohen BA, Johnson B: Cutaneous polyarteritis nodosa. Reports of two cases in children and review of the literature. *Arch Dermatol* 130:884, 1994.
115. Díaz-Pérez JL, De Lagrán ZM, Díaz-Ramón JL, Winkelmann RK: Cutaneous polyarteritis nodosa. *Semin Cutan Med Surg* 26:77, 2007.
116. Kluger N, Pagnoux C, Guillevin L, et al: Comparison of cutaneous manifestations in systemic polyarteritis nodosa and microscopic polyangiitis. *Br J Dermatol* 159:615, 2008.
117. Minkowitz G, Smoller BR, McNutt NS: Benign cutaneous polyarteritis nodosa. Relationship to systemic polyarteritis nodosa and to hepatitis B infection. *Arch Dermatol* 127:1520, 1991.
118. Chen KR: Cutaneous polyarteritis nodosa: A clinical and histopathological study of 20 cases. *J Dermatol* 16:429, 1989.
119. Diez-Porres L, Rios-Blanco JJ, Robles-Marhuenda A, et al: ANCA-associated vasculitis as paraneoplastic syndrome with colon cancer: A case report. *Lupus* 14:632, 2005.
120. Solans-Laqué R, Bosch-Gil JA, Pérez-Bocanegra C, et al: Mitochondrial encephalopathy, lactic acidosis, and strokelike episodes: Basic concepts, clinical phenotype, and therapeutic management of MELAS syndrome. *Ann N Y Acad Sci* 1142:133, 2008.
121. Farrell AM, Stern SC, El-Ghariani K, et al: Splenic lymphoma with villous lymphocytes presenting as leucocytoclastic vasculitis. *Clin Exp Dermatol* 24:19, 1999.

122. Carlson JA, Ng BT, Chen KR: Cutaneous vasculitis update: Diagnostic criteria, classification, epidemiology, etiology, pathogenesis, evaluation and prognosis. *Am J Dermatopathol* 27:504, 2005.
123. Ponge T, Boutoille D, Moreau A, et al: Systemic vasculitis in a patient with small-cell neuroendocrine bronchial cancer. *Eur Respir J* 12:1228, 1998.
124. Nakajima H, Ikeda M, Yamamoto Y, Kodama H: Large annular purpura and paraneoplastic purpura in a patient with Sjögren's syndrome and cervical cancer. *J Dermatol* 27:40, 2000.
125. El Tal AK, Tannous Z: Cutaneous vascular disorders associated with internal malignancy. *Dermatol Clin* 26:45, 2008.
126. Greer JM, Longley S, Edwards NL, et al: Vasculitis associated with malignancy. Experience with 13 patients and literature review. *Medicine (Baltimore)* 67:220, 1988.
127. Wiik A: Drug-induced vasculitis. *Curr Opin Rheumatol* 20:35, 2008.
128. Seo P, Stone JH: The antineutrophil cytoplasmic antibody-associated vasculitides. *Am J Med* 117:39, 2004.
129. Daoud MS, Gibson LE, DeRemee RA, et al: Cutaneous Wegener's granulomatosis: Clinical, histopathologic, and immunopathologic features of thirty patients. *J Am Acad Dermatol* 31:605, 1994.
130. Puéchal X: Antineutrophil cytoplasmic antibody-associated vasculitides. *Joint Bone Spine* 74:427, 2007.
131. Csernok E, Gross WL: Primary vasculitides and vasculitis confined to skin: Clinical features and new pathogenic aspects. *Arch Dermatol Res* 292:427, 2000.
132. Keogh KA, Specks U: Churg-Strauss syndrome. *Semin Respir Crit Care Med* 27:148, 2006.
133. Khan NA, Shenoy PK, McClymont L, Palmer TJ: Exophthalmos and facial swelling: A case of limited Churg-Strauss syndrome. *J Laryngol Otol* 110:578, 1996.
134. Seo P, Specks U, Keogh KA: Efficacy of rituximab in limited Wegener's granulomatosis with refractory granulomatous manifestations. *J Rheumatol* 35:2017, 2008.
135. Sánchez-Cano D, Callejas-Rubio JL, Ortego-Centeno N: Effect of rituximab on refractory Wegener granulomatosis with predominant granulomatous disease. *J Clin Rheumatol* 14:92, 2008.
136. Josselin L, Mahr A, Cohen P, et al: Cholesterol embolism: Still an unrecognized entity with a high mortality rate. *J Am Acad Dermatol* 55:786, 2006.
137. Reis JJ, Kaplan PW: Postictal hemifacial purpura. *Seizure* 7:337, 1998.
138. Pierson JC, Suh PS: Powerlifter's purpura: A Valsalva-associated phenomenon. *Cutis* 70:93, 2002.
139. Alcalay J, Ingber A, Sandbank M: Mask phenomenon: Postemesis facial purpura. *Cutis* 38:28, 1986.
140. Metzker A, Merlob P: Suction purpura. *Arch Dermatol* 128:822, 1992.
141. Forster PJ: Microvascular fragility at high altitude. *Br Med J (Clin Res Ed)* 296:1004, 1988.
142. Toh CH, Dennis M: Disseminated intravascular coagulation: Old disease, new hope. *BMJ* 327:974, 2003.
143. Beardsley DS: Pathophysiology of immune thrombocytopenic purpura. *Blood Rev* 16:13, 2002.
144. Tsai HM: Advances in the pathogenesis, diagnosis, and treatment of thrombotic thrombocytopenic purpura. *J Am Soc Nephrol* 14:1072, 2003.
145. Bruinsma W: The file of side effects to the skin: A guide to drug eruptions. *Semin Dermatol* 8:141, 1989.
146. Stern, RS, Shear, NH: Cutaneous reactions to drugs and biological modifiers, in *Cutaneous Medicine and Surgery*, vol 1, edited by KA Arndt, PE LeBoit, JK Robinson, BU Wintroub, p 412. WB Saunders, Philadelphia, 1996.
147. Feinstein RJ, Halprin KM, Penneys NS, et al: Senile purpura. *Arch Dermatol* 108:229, 1973.
148. Haboubi NY, Haboubi NA, Gyde OH, et al: Zinc deficiency in senile purpura. *J Clin Pathol* 38:1189, 1985.
149. Del Rosso J, Friedlander SF. Corticosteroids: Options in the era of steroid-sparing therapy. *J Am Acad Dermatol* 53:S50, 2005.
150. Nguyen RT, Cowley DM, Muir JB: Scurvy: A cutaneous clinical diagnosis. *Australas J Dermatol* 44:48, 2003.
151. Olmedo JM, Yiannias JA, Windgassen EB, Gornet MK: Scurvy: A disease almost forgotten. *Int J Dermatol* 45:909, 2006.
152. Goldsbury C, Green J: Time-lapse atomic force microscopy in the characterization of amyloid-like fibril assembly and oligomeric intermediates. *Methods Mol Biol* 299:103, 2005.
153. Eder L, Bitterman H: Image in clinical medicine. Amyloid purpura. *N Engl J Med* 356:2406, 2007.
154. Vella FS, Simone B, Antonaci S: Palmodigital purpura as the only skin abnormality in myeloma-associated systemic amyloidosis. *Br J Haematol* 120:917, 2003.
155. Breathnach SM: Amyloid and amyloidosis. *J Am Acad Dermatol* 18:1, 1988.
156. Fernandes NF, Schwartz RA: A "hyperextensive" review of Ehlers-Danlos syndrome. *Cutis* 82:242, 2008.
157. Germain DP: Clinical and genetic features of vascular Ehlers-Danlos syndrome. *Ann Vasc Surg* 16:391, 2002.
158. Bercovitch L, Terry P: Pseudoxanthoma elasticum 2004. *J Am Acad Dermatol* 51:S13, 2004.
159. Hu X, Plomp AS, Van Soest S, et al: Pseudoxanthoma elasticum: A clinical, histopathological, and molecular update. *Surv Ophthalmol* 48:424, 2003.
160. Laube S, Moss C: Pseudoxanthoma elasticum. *Arch Dis Child* 90:754, 2005.
161. Horiguchi Y, Fujii T, Imamura S: Purpuric cutaneous manifestations in mitochondrial encephalomyopathy. *J Dermatol* 18:295, 1991.
162. Kubota Y, Ishii T, Sugihara H, et al: Skin manifestations of a patient with mitochondrial encephalomyopathy with lactic acidosis and strokelike episodes (MELAS syndrome). *J Am Acad Dermatol* 41:469, 1999.
163. Sproule DM, Kaufmann P: Mitochondrial encephalopathy, lactic acidosis, and strokelike episodes: Basic concepts, clinical phenotype, and therapeutic management of MELAS syndrome. *Ann N Y Acad Sci* 1142:133, 2008.
164. Kondo T, Betz P, Eisenmenger W: Retrospective study on skin reddenings and petechiae in the eyelids and the conjunctivae in forensic physical examinations. *Int J Legal Med* 110:204, 1997.
165. Urkin J, Katz M: Suction purpura. *Isr Med Assoc J* 2:711, 2000.
166. Ramelet AA: Exercise-induced purpura. *Dermatology* 208:293, 2004.
167. Tristani-Firouzi P, Meadows KP, Vanderhooft S: Pigmented purpuric eruptions of childhood: A series of cases and review of literature. *Pediatr Dermatol* 18:299, 2001.

CHAPTER 124
HEMOPHILIA A AND HEMOPHILIA B

Harold R. Roberts, Nigel S. Key, and Miguel A. Escobar

SUMMARY

Hemophilia A and B are the only two bleeding disorders inherited in a sex-linked pattern. The gene for both disorders is on the long arm of the X-chromosome. Both hemophilias appear as severe, moderate, or mild hemorrhagic diseases each being clinically indistinguishable, at least in individual patients. In the severe form, both hemophilia A and B are characterized by multiple bleeding episodes into joints and other tissues leading to chronic crippling hemarthropathy unless treated early or prophylactically with factor VIII or IX concentrates, respectively. Even though phenotypically similar, both diseases are genetically heterogeneous with more than 1000 mutations leading to dysfunctional factor VIII or IX molecules that do not support normal thrombin generation nor adequate fibrin clot formation.

Despite similarities in hemorrhagic symptoms, there are major differences between hemophilia A and B. Hemophilia A is more common and is caused by defects in the factor VIII gene, a large 186-kb gene with 26 exons. A common mutation results from inversion and crossing over of intron 22 during meiosis, resulting in homologous recombination between an a_1 gene within intron 22 and extragenic homologous sequences 5′ to intron 22. This leads to severe hemophilia, and these patients are prone to developing antibody inhibitors that neutralize factor VIII coagulant function. Approximately 20 percent of severely affected hemophilia A patients develop inhibitors, whereas only 3 percent or fewer of severely affected hemophilia B patients develop inhibitors against factor IX.

About one-third of the mutations in hemophilia A and B arise *de novo* at CpG "hotspots." These mutations are apt to occur in the germ cells of a maternal grandfather whose daughters will be carriers and whose grandsons will have a 50 percent chance of having hemophilia. Replacement therapy is available for both hemophilia A and B patients. Safe, effective, and highly purified factor VIII and IX concentrates derived from plasma or made by recombinant technology are available for prophylactic therapy to prevent bleeding episodes or prompt treatment of hemorrhagic events. Prophylaxis is the treatment of choice and can prevent disabling joint disease and other hemorrhagic events such that patients can expect a relatively normal life span provided that adequate replacement therapy is available. For patients with inhibitors, factor VIIa and factor VIII inhibitor bypassing activity can be used to "by-pass" the factor VIII or factor IX deficiency. Both disorders are good candidates for gene therapy that may eventually lead to their cure.

Abbreviations and acronyms that appear in this chapter include: AAV, adeno-associated virus; aPTT, activated partial thromboplastin time; BT, bleeding time; BU, Bethesda unit; cDNA, complementary deoxyribonucleic acid; CGA, cytosine, guanine, adenine; CJD, Creutzfeldt-Jakob disease; COX, cyclooxygenase; CRM, cross-reacting material; CT, computerized tomography; DDAVP, 1-desamino-8-D-arginine vasopressin, desmopressin; DVT, deep vein thrombosis; EACA, ε-aminocaproic acid; FEIBA, factor VIII inhibitor bypassing activity; GLA, γ-carboxyglutamic acid; Ig, immunoglobulin; PT, prothrombin time; PTC, plasma thromboplastin component (factor IX); RFLP, restriction fragment length polymorphism; TCT, thrombin clotting time; TF, tissue factor; VNTR, variable number of tandem repeats; VWD, von Willebrand disease; VWF, von Willebrand factor.

HEMOPHILIA A (CLASSIC HEMOPHILIA, FACTOR VIII DEFICIENCY)

DEFINITION AND HISTORY

Hemophilia A is an X-linked hereditary disorder caused by defective synthesis of factor VIII. Hemophilia A is less common than von Willebrand disease (see Chap. 127), but it is more common than other inherited clotting factor abnormalities. The estimated incidence of hemophilia A is 1 in every 5000 to 7000 live male births. It occurs in all ethnic groups in all parts of the world.[1]

Sex-linked hemophilia was recognized at least as early as the second century, when a rabbi correctly deduced that sons of hemophilic carriers were at risk for bleeding following circumcision.[2] In the 19th century, several authors noted the sex-linked inheritance pattern of the disease and ascribed the hemorrhagic episodes to delayed blood coagulation. Morawitz[3] developed the classic theory of blood coagulation, which recognized two major reactions: (1) conversion of prothrombin to thrombin by a tissue substance that Morawitz termed *thrombokinase*, and (2) conversion of fibrinogen to fibrin by thrombin. In 1911, Addis[4] demonstrated that thrombin formed more slowly in hemophilic blood than in normal blood and that the defect could be corrected by small amounts of normal plasma. However, he incorrectly theorized that hemophilia resulted from prothrombin deficiency. As protein purification techniques improved throughout the 1930s and 1940s, thrombokinase was resolved into several distinct components. Brinkhous[5] demonstrated that the prothrombin content of hemophilic plasma was normal and that the basic defect in hemophilia was the delayed conversion of prothrombin to thrombin. The defect could be corrected by a fraction of normal plasma containing the antihemophilic factor, later named *factor VIII*. In 1947, Pavlovsky[6] observed that when blood from one patient with hemophilia was transfused into another patient with a similar clinical phenotype, the prolonged clotting time in the recipient was corrected. At the time, Pavlovsky did not recognize that he was dealing with two different types of hemophilia. This fact was recognized by Aggeler and coworkers[7] in 1952, when they described a patient deficient in "plasma thromboplastin component" (PTC), a blood clotting factor different from factor VIII. A deficiency of "plasma thromboplastin component," later termed factor IX, was identified as the cause of hemophilia B. A month later, Biggs and colleagues described a similar patient whose surname was Christmas, thus the synonym "Christmas disease."[8] Hemophilia A and B are the only two hereditary clotting factor defects inherited in a sex-linked pattern and they are clinically indistinguishable, although recent data suggest that on the whole, hemophilia B may be less severe than hemophilia A.[8a] However, in an individual patient, the disorders cannot be distinguished without a specific assay for factor VIII or IX.

In 1964, a proposal to organize the growing number of coagulation factors into a cascade or waterfall mechanism was put forth by Davie and Ratnoff and by Macfarlane.[9,10] In this scheme, each zymogen clotting factor was sequentially activated to a protease that subsequently activated the next zymogen until thrombin ultimately was produced. In this scheme, factors VIII and IX were considered to be proenzymes. Later, however, factor VIII, when activated by thrombin, was shown not to be a proenzyme but rather an essential cofactor for factor IXa. The waterfall hypothesis has been modified so that the primary role of the tissue factor–factor VII complex in the initiation of coagulation is emphasized (see Chap. 115).[11]

ETIOLOGY AND PATHOGENESIS

Hemophilia A is a heterogeneous disorder resulting from defects in the factor VIII gene that leads to absent or reduced circulating levels of functional factor VIII. The reduced activity can result from a decreased

Hemophilic male
X^hY

Normal female	X	XX^h (Carrier female)	XY (Normal male)
	X	XX^h (Carrier female)	XY (Normal male)

Normal male
XY

Carrier female	X^h	XX^h (Carrier female)	X^hY (Hemophilic male)
	X	XX (Normal female)	XY (Normal male)

FIGURE 124–1. Inheritance pattern of hemophilia A. All daughters of a hemophilic male are carriers of hemophilia, whereas all sons are normal. Daughters of carriers have a 50% chance of being a carrier, whereas sons of carriers have a 50% chance of having hemophilia. (X, normal; X^h, abnormal X chromosome with the hemophilic gene; X^hY, hemophilic male; XX, normal female; XX^h, carrier female; XY, normal male; Y, normal.)

amount of factor VIII protein, the presence of a functionally abnormal protein, or a combination of both. For factor VIII to be an effective cofactor for factor IXa, it must first be activated by thrombin, a reaction that results in the formation of a heterotrimer composed of the A_1, A_2, A_3, C_1, and C_2 domains of factor VIII in a complex with calcium (see Chap. 115).[12] Activated factor VIII (factor VIIIa) and activated factor IX (factor IXa) associate on the surface of activated platelets, forming a functional factor X-activating complex ("tenase" or "Xase").[13] In the presence of factor VIIIa, the rate of factor X activation by factor IXa is dramatically enhanced. That hemophilia A and hemophilia B have similar clinical manifestations is not surprising, because both factor VIIIa and factor IXa are required to form the Xase complex. The lack of either activated factor leads to a similar lack of platelet surface Xase activity with subsequent decreased thrombin generation. In patients with hemophilia, clot formation is delayed because of the decreased thrombin generation. The clot that is formed is friable, easily dislodged, and highly susceptible to fibrinolysis, all of which lead to excessive bleeding and poor wound healing.[14]

GENETICS

Hemophilia A results when mutations occur in the factor VIII gene located on the long arm of the X-chromosome (X-q28). The disease occurs almost exclusively in males. Figure 124–1 shows the inheritance pattern of hemophilia A and hemophilia B. All the sons of affected hemophilic males are normal, whereas all the daughters are obligatory carriers of the factor VIII defect. Sons of carriers have a 50 percent chance of being affected, whereas daughters of carriers have a 50 percent chance of being carriers themselves.

The factor VIII gene is very large, approximately 186 kb, with approximately 9 kb of exons. The gene contains 26 exons and 25 intervening sequences or introns.[15] The size and complexity of the gene make it difficult to routinely sequence the gene to detect specific mutations resulting in hemophilia. Nevertheless, the factor VIII gene has been cloned and sequenced, and numerous specific mutations have been described.[15,16] As of 2008, more than 1000 specific mutations in the factor VIII gene resulting in classic hemophilia have been described.[16]

Hemophilia A can result from multiple alterations in the factor VIII gene. These include gene rearrangements; missense mutations, in which a single base substitution leads to an amino acid change in the molecule; nonsense mutations, which result in a stop codon; abnormal splicing of the gene; deletions of all or portions of the gene; and insertions of genetic elements.[17] The genetic defects leading to hemophilia have been reviewed.[16] Table 124–1 presents a summary of the different mutations.[16]

One of the most common mutations, accounting for 40 to 50 percent of patients, is a unique "combined gene inversion and crossing over" that disrupts the factor VIII gene.[18,19] Figures 124–2 and 124–3 schematically depict the factor VIII gene and the mechanism of the "inversion–crossing over" mechanism as initially described by Gitschier.[20] Within intron 22 are two other genes: (1) $F8A(a_1)$, which is transcribed

TABLE 124–1. Summary of Different Mutations Reported for Hemophilia A

	Point Mutations			Deletions		
Exon	Missense	Nonsense (Stop)	Splicing	Small	Large	Insertions
1	15	2	4	2	na	1
2	10	1	5	8	na	4
3	25	0	6	5	na	0
4	35	7	4	1	na	1
5	13	1	10	4	na	1
6	11	2	6	4	na	2
7	38	5	4	8	na	1
8	27	6	1	8	na	1
9	27	3	5	7	na	3
10	10	3	3	5	na	0
11	36	1	4	2	na	1
12	20	5	4	2	na	1
13	32	3	2	7	na	3
14	43	52	6	77	na	39
15	19	2	3	4	na	0
16	26	7	2	7	na	0
17	28	3	2	6	na	5
18	34	5	1	5	na	4
19	16	1	8	4	na	4
20	8	1	0	2	na	2
21	9	5	1	0	na	1
22	19	5	4	3	na	1
23	30	1	4	7	na	0
24	13	5	4	3	na	2
25	13	2	2	7	na	3
26	26	3	0	9	na	0
TOTAL	583	131	95	197	135	80

SOURCE: Information received from HAMSTeRS website, with permission. Available at: http://europium.csc.mrc.ac.uk.

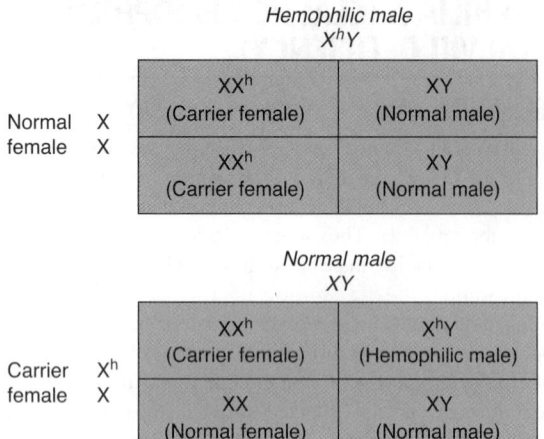

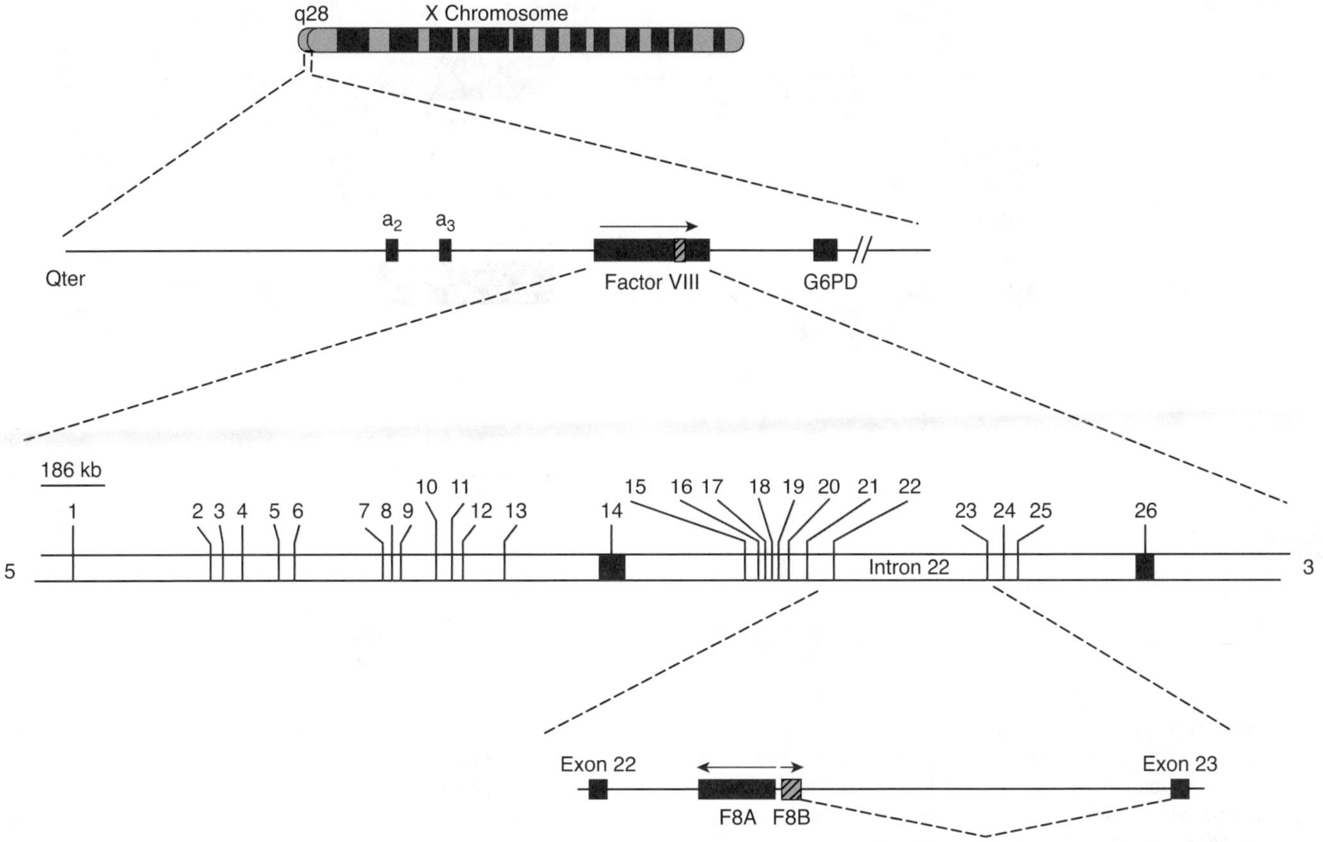

FIGURE 124–2. Schematic of the factor VIII gene. The factor VIII gene is located at q28 on the long arm of the X chromosome. The region of the factor VIII gene is enlarged on the *second line*. Note that two genes, designated a_2 and a_3, are 5′ to the factor VIII gene. The *hatched area* indicated on the factor VIII gene corresponds to intron 22 shown on the *third line*. Within intron 22 (*fourth line*) are two nested genes, one designated *F8A*, which is transcribed in a direction opposite to that of the whole factor VIII gene and is homologous to the a_2 and a_3 genes shown on *line 2*. *(From Kazazian HK, Tuddenham EGD, Antonorakis SE: Hemophilia A: Deficiency of coagulation factor VIII, in* Metabolic and Molecular Basis of Inherited Diseases, *8th ed, vol 4, edited by CR Scriver, AL Beaudet, WS Sly, D Valle, B Childs, KW Kinzler, B Vogelstein, p 4367. McGraw-Hill, New York, 1995, with permission.)*

in the 5′ direction, and (2) *F8B*, which is transcribed in the 3′ direction of the factor VIII gene. The hatched boxes in Figure 124–3 show two other extragenic homologous sequences (a_2,a_3) 5′ to the *F8A* gene that lies within intron 22 (a_1). The presence of extragenic *F8A* sequences 5′ to the *F8A* gene within intron 22 is central to the inversion and translocation of part of the factor VIII gene from exon 1 to exon 22. The mechanism is homologous recombination between the *F8A* sequence that lies within intron 22 and one of the homologous extragenic sequences of the *F8A* gene 5′ to the factor VIII gene. During meiosis, crossing over of homologous sequences occurs between the *F8A* gene lying within intron 22 and one of the extragenic homologous *F8A* sequences 5′ to intron 22. Thus, the transcription of the complete factor VIII sequence is interrupted (Fig. 124–3). Figure 124–3 shows a common inversion and crossing over but homologous recombinations can occur with either of the extragenic genes. Occasionally, there are duplications of a_2 or a_3 genes 5′ to the intron 22 a_1 gene such that there are four possible types of inversion.[21] The "inversion–crossing over" mutations result in severe hemophilia, and approximately 50 percent of these patients are susceptible to developing antibody inhibitors that neutralize factor VIII coagulant function.

Of the different insertions in the factor VIII gene that have been reported, a few are LINE (L_1) elements that are transposon sequences; that is, sequences that have been inserted frequently throughout the genome.[22] Most of these insertions result in severe hemophilia.

In many cases of hemophilia, there is no family history of the disease, and at least 30 percent of the cases of hemophilia are a result of spontaneous (*de novo*) mutations. Most of these occur at CpG dinucleotides in the factor VIII gene.[22] *De novo* occurrences of hemophilia usually result from a mutation in the gamete of a normal male; for example, a mutation in the germ cell of a maternal grandfather will give rise to the hemophilia gene in his daughters such that his grandsons may have hemophilia.[17] Because the restriction fragment enzyme *Taq*I recognizes the sequence TCGA, CpG mutations at this site can be directly detected by loss of a *Taq*I cleavage site. Codons for the amino acid arginine (CGA) are frequently affected by mutations at CG doublets. A C→T transition often results in a stop codon (Fig. 124–4). A stop codon results in synthesis of a truncated factor VIII molecule and usually is associated with severe hemophilia. However, as shown in the figure, a G→A transition results in a missense mutation, which often leads to a dysfunctional factor VIII molecule that may be associated with mild, moderate, or severe hemophilia. Some missense mutations result in the production of normal or near-normal amounts of factor VIII antigen, while the coagulant activity may be dramatically or only slightly reduced. Many other single-base substitutions have been described, resulting in hemophilia of varying degrees of severity.

Large deletions in the factor VIII gene almost always are associated with severe hemophilia. On the other hand, a small deletion that does not change the reading frame of the gene may result in milder disease. Patients with large deletions who have no detectable factor VIII antigen are more susceptible to the development of antifactor VIII antibodies, although antibodies clearly also occur in patients without deletions.[15,22]

Hemophilia A in females is extremely rare, although an affected female offspring from a hemophilic father and carrier mother have been reported. Hemophilia A may occur in females with X chromosomal

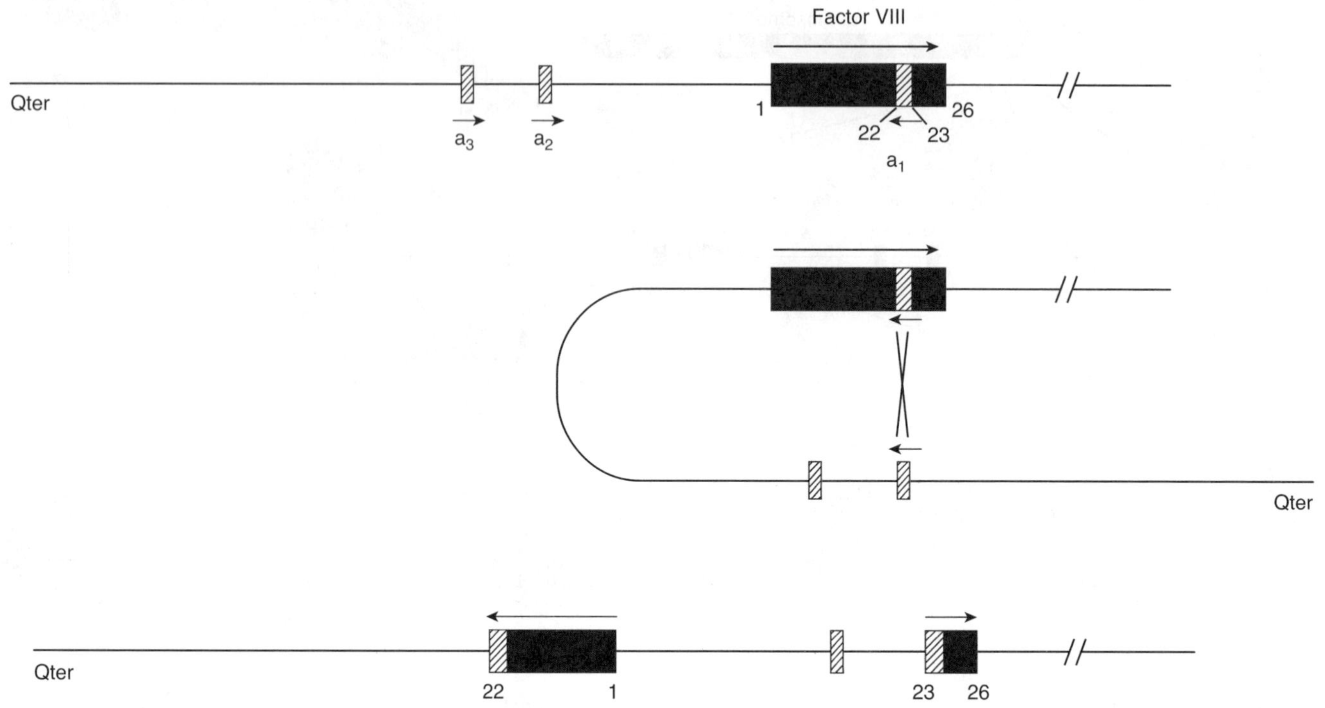

FIGURE 124–3. Schematic of inversion and crossing over at intron 22. Inversion and crossing-over of the a_3 gene with its homologous sequence a_1 nested within intron 22 are shown. *Middle panel:* When crossing over of the a_1 gene nested within intron 22 and the a_3 gene extragenic to factor VIII occurs, a portion of the factor VIII gene is transcribed in a reverse manner from exon 1 through exon 22. Homologous recombination with the extragenic a_2 gene is also possible. In some individuals there are two a_2 or a_3 extragenic sequences giving rise to four possible types of the "inversion–crossing over" mechanism. *(From Antonarakis SE, Kazazian HH, Tuddenham EG: Molecular etiology of factor VIII deficiency in hemophilia A.* Hum Mutat *5:1, 1995, with permission.)*

abnormalities such as Turner syndrome, X chromosomal mosaicism, and other X chromosomal defects.[22,23] If the normal X chromosome is inactivated disproportionately ("imbalanced X inactivation") in a carrier female, factor VIII levels may be sufficiently low to cause bleeding manifestations. Usually these manifestations are mild, but they may be serious during surgical procedures or following significant trauma.

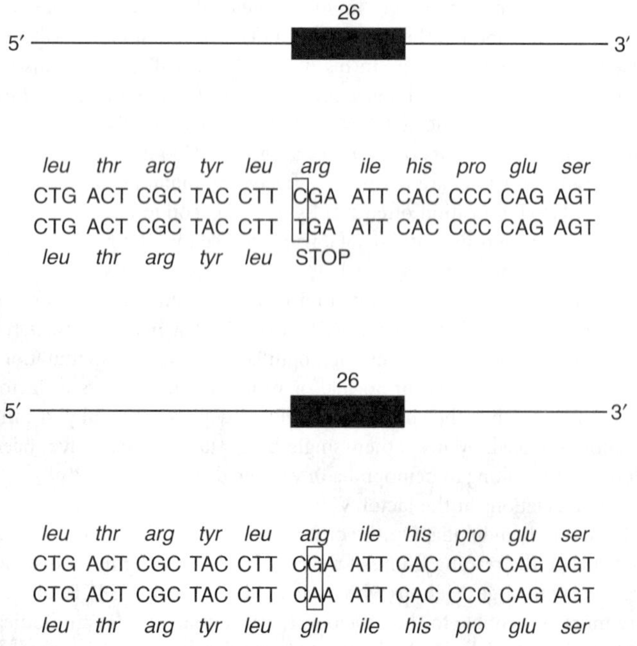

FIGURE 124–4. Examples of mutations and CG doublets. The *red box* denotes exon 26. A C→T transition results in a stop codon (TGA), whereas a G→A transition results in substitution of a glutamine for an arginine residue.

PRENATAL DIAGNOSIS AND CARRIER DETECTION

A careful and complete family history is important for carrier detection.[24] All daughters of a hemophilic father are obligatory carriers of the hemophilic defect. If a known carrier has a daughter, that daughter has a 50 percent chance of being a carrier.

Carrier detection is important when a daughter of a known carrier or a female offspring of a hemophilic patient wishes to become pregnant. At times, the history of hemophilia in the family is in a distant blood relative, and the gene for hemophilia may skip several generations (Fig. 124–5). Although the current standard for identifying carrier status is genotyping, an older method for testing for the carrier state required measurement of factor VIII coagulant activity and the von Willebrand factor (VWF) antigen level. The ratio of VWF to factor VIII is higher in carrier females than in noncarriers; thus, determining the ratio adds to test sensitivity. Carriers generally have 50 percent or less of the normal factor VIII level. When these data are added to the family history, the probability of whether a woman is a carrier can be calculated.[24] However, the physician or genetic counselor must carefully explain to the subjects being tested that the test results carry a significant error rate, and accurate determination of the carrier state using the ratio of VWF to factor VIII cannot be guaranteed.

Carriers who harbor the intron 22 inversion can be identified using the Southern blot technique.[24] Where the capability exists, analysis of the complete coding region can be performed using gradient gel electrophoresis and single-stranded conformation polymorphism technology or by restriction fragment length polymorphism (RFLP) analysis.[25]

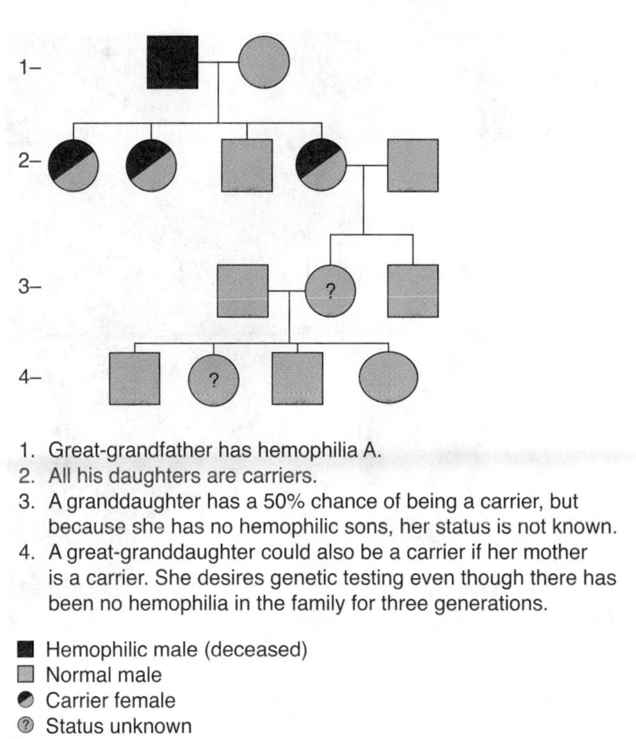

1–
2–
3–
4–
?
?
1. Great-grandfather has hemophilia A.
2. All his daughters are carriers.
3. A granddaughter has a 50% chance of being a carrier, but because she has no hemophilic sons, her status is not known.
4. A great-granddaughter could also be a carrier if her mother is a carrier. She desires genetic testing even though there has been no hemophilia in the family for three generations.
Hemophilic male (deceased)
Normal male
Carrier female
Status unknown

FIGURE 124–5. Example of a hemophilic kindred "skipping" generations. Carriers and potential carriers are identified. Note that the deceased male hemophiliac has carrier daughters but in subsequent generations, no hemophilic males are born. Nevertheless, the females in generations 3 and 4 could be carriers. DNA sequencing for carrier detection is now available.

Use of markers for RFLP is simpler than direct sequencing of the coding region of the factor VIII gene, but use of the RFLP technique requires that the pedigree analyses include at least one hemophilic male whose mother is heterozygous for one or more RFLP markers. Figure 124–6 shows an example of RFLP analysis.[25–28] The polymorphic markers include the variable number of tandem repeats (VNTR) in introns 13 and 22 and *BclI* and *XbaI* restriction sites. The female III-2 has the same polymorphic marker in intron 13 and the same *XbaI* restriction site as her hemophilic brother, carrier mother, and hemophilic grandfather. Therefore, female III-2 is a carrier. In contrast, the female III-1 inherited markers that are not linked with hemophilia.

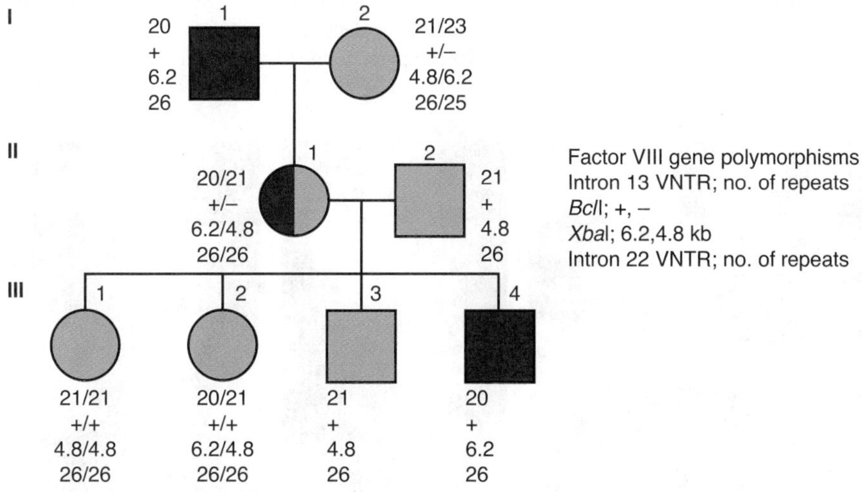

FIGURE 124–6. Use of RFLP and variable number of tandem repeats (VNTR) for carrier diagnosis of hemophilia. The carrier female (II-1) is informative for polymorphisms at intron 13 and the *XbaI* site but not informative for markers on *BclI* or intron 22. III-2 is a carrier of the hemophilic trait with markers similar to the hemophilic grandfather (I-1) and hemophilic brother (III-4). BclI and XbaI are sites cleaved by VNTR restriction endonucleases. *(From Goodeve AC, Peake IR: Diagnosis of hemophilia A and B carriers and prenatal diagnosis, in* Haemophilia, *edited by CD Forbes, L Aledort, R Madhok, p 63. Chapman & Hall, London, 1997, with permission.)*

Prenatal diagnosis of hemophilia now can be performed almost routinely.[27] If a carrier female has a fetus that can be identified as a female by chromosomal analysis of cells obtained by amniocentesis (at approximately 16 weeks of gestation) or by chorionic villus sampling at week 10 of gestation, little concern exists regarding whether the female fetus is a carrier because carriers usually have no bleeding tendency. If the fetus is a male, sufficient cells can be obtained to perform DNA analysis using the methods described above. The decision on whether to carry an affected male fetus to term should be decided by the parents after they are appropriately counseled and provided with all the necessary genetic, clinical, and therapeutic information about hemophilia.

CLINICAL FEATURES

Hemophilia A is characterized by excessive bleeding into various tissues of the body, including soft-tissue hematomas and hemarthroses that lead to severe crippling hemarthropathy. Recurrent hemarthroses are characteristic of the disease. The disease has been broadly classified as mild, moderate, and severe, although overlap exists between these categories. Table 124–2 shows a classification based on the severity of clinical manifestations. A range of plasma factor VIII concentrations in percentages of normal and in units per milliliter is given for each category. Some patients with factor VIII levels compatible with severe hemophilia may exhibit milder symptoms because of the coinheritance of the factor V Leiden mutation (R506Q) with the hemophilic gene.[29,30] Severely affected patients (<1% factor VIII) frequently experience "spontaneous" bleeding without known trauma other than that associated with the usual day-to-day activities. Without effective treatment, recurrent hemarthroses, resulting in chronic hemophilic arthropathy, occur by young adulthood and are highly characteristic of the severe form of the disorder. Severely affected patients are subject to serious hemorrhages that may dissect through tissue planes, ultimately leading to compromise of vital organs. However, bleeding episodes are intermittent, and some patients do not bleed for weeks or months. Except for intracranial bleeding, sudden death because of hemorrhage is rare.

Moderately affected patients with hemophilia may have occasional hematomas. Hemarthroses, usually, associated with a known trauma may occur as well. These patients have greater than 1 but less than 5 percent of normal factor VIII activity.

Mildly affected patients with hemophilia who have factor VIII levels of 6 to 30 percent have infrequent bleeding episodes. The disease may go undiagnosed and be discovered only because of excessive hemorrhage postoperatively, following trauma, or after the toss and tumble of contact sports.

Most carriers have approximately 50 percent factor VIII activity and experience no bleeding symptoms, even with surgical procedures. Carriers with factor VIII levels less than 50 percent, as a result of imbalanced X chromosome inactivation, may experience excessive bleeding after trauma (e.g., childbirth or surgery). Therefore, measurement of factor VIII level is recommended in all carriers.

TABLE 124–2. Clinical Classification of Hemophilia

Classification	Factor VIII Level	Clinical Features
Severe	≤1% of normal (≤0.01 U/mL)	1. Spontaneous hemorrhage from early infancy 2. Frequent spontaneous hemarthroses and other hemorrhages, requiring clotting factor replacement
Moderate	1–5% of normal (0.01–0.05 U/mL)	1. Hemorrhage secondary to trauma or surgery 2. Occasional spontaneous hemarthroses
Mild	6–30% of normal (0.06–0.30 U/mL)	1. Hemorrhage secondary to trauma or surgery 2. Rare spontaneous hemorrhage

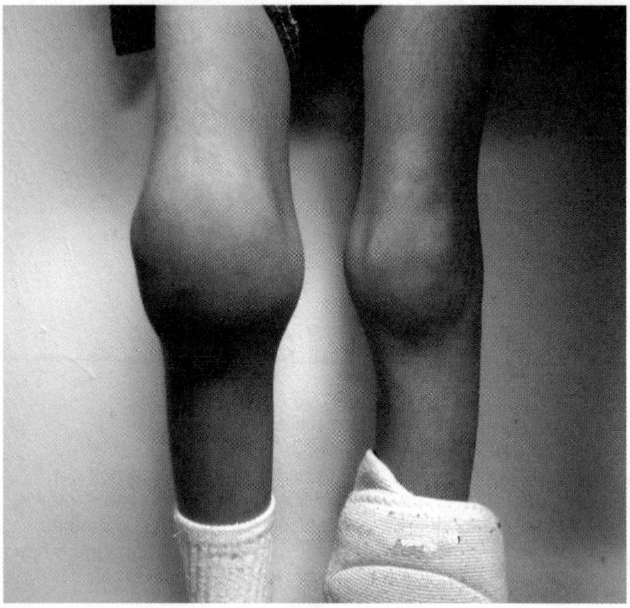

FIGURE 124–7. Hemophilic arthropathy. The chronic effects of repeated hemorrhage into the knee of a severely affected hemophilic patient are seen. Note swelling and deformity with atrophy of muscle tissue.

Hemarthroses

Bleeding into joints accounts for approximately 75 percent of bleeding episodes in severely affected patients with hemophilia A.[31,32] The normal synovium has few cells, but numerous capillaries beneath the synovial layer can be damaged by the mechanical trauma associated with daily use of joints. The joints most frequently involved, in decreasing order of frequency are knees, elbows, ankles, shoulders, wrists, and hips. Hinge joints are much more likely to be involved than are ball-and-socket joints. Hemarthroses usually occur when an affected child begins to walk.

Hemarthroses are heralded by an aura of mild discomfort that, over a period of minutes to hours, becomes progressively painful. The joint usually swells, becomes warm, and exhibits limited motion. Occasionally, the patient experiences a mild fever. Significant and sustained fever, however, suggests an infected joint. When joint bleeding does not respond to replacement therapy, one should suspect an inhibitor of factor VIII or an infected joint. Bleeding into the knee joint is more easily detected by physical findings than is bleeding into either the elbow or shoulder. When bleeding stops, the blood resorbs, and the symptoms gradually subside over a period of several days. If hemarthroses are treated early and the joint is not chronically involved, pain usually subsides in 6 to 8 hours and disappears in 12 to 24 hours. However, repeated hemorrhage into the joints eventually results in extensive destruction of articular cartilage, synovial hyperplasia, and other reactive changes in the adjacent bone and tissues. Iron deposits from residual blood is a major factor in the pathogenesis of hemophilic arthropathy.[32] Acute bleeding into a chronically affected joint may be difficult to distinguish from the pain of degenerative arthritis.

A major complication of repeated hemarthroses is joint deformity complicated by muscle atrophy and soft-tissue contractures (Fig. 124–7). Figure 124–8 shows the various radiologic stages of progressive destruction of joint cartilage and adjacent bone. Osteoporosis and cystic areas in the subchondral bone may develop, and progressive loss of joint space occurs. Figure 124–9 shows a magnetic resonance image (MRI) of a normal knee and Figures 124–10 and 124–11 depict bleeding into a hemophilic knee and ankle, which can be compared to the MRI of the normal knee.

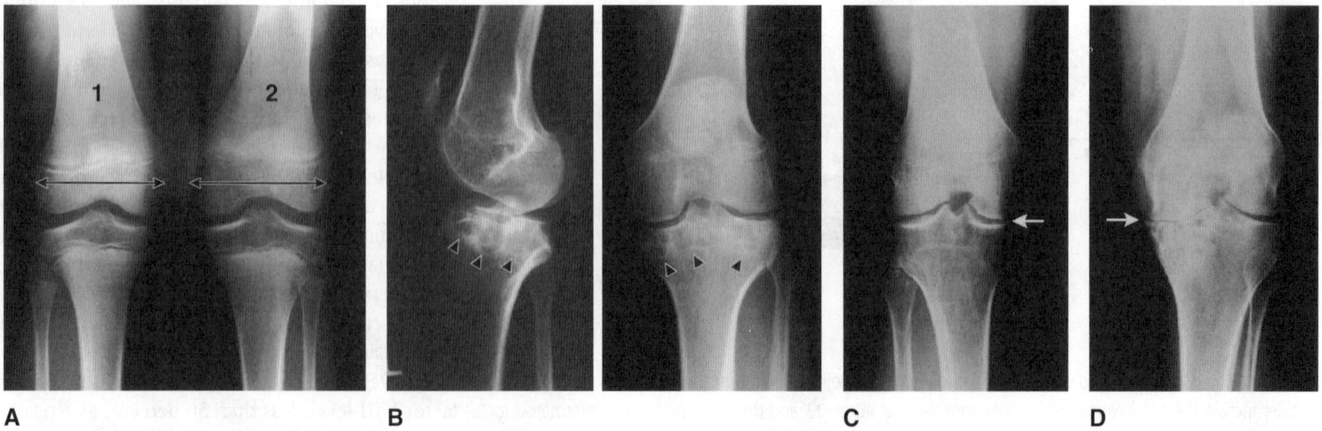

FIGURE 124–8. Various radiologic stages of hemophilic arthropathy. Stages 0 (normal joint) and 1 (fluid in the joint) are not shown. **A.** Stage 2. Some osteoporosis and epiphyseal overgrowth are present in knee 2. Epiphysis is wider in knee 2 than in knee 1 (*arrows*). **B.** Stage 3. Subchondral bone cysts (*arrowheads*). Joint spaces exhibit irregularities. **C.** Stage 4. Prominent bone cysts with marked narrowing of joint space (*arrow*). **D.** Stage 5. Obliteration of joint space with epiphyseal overgrowth (*arrow*).

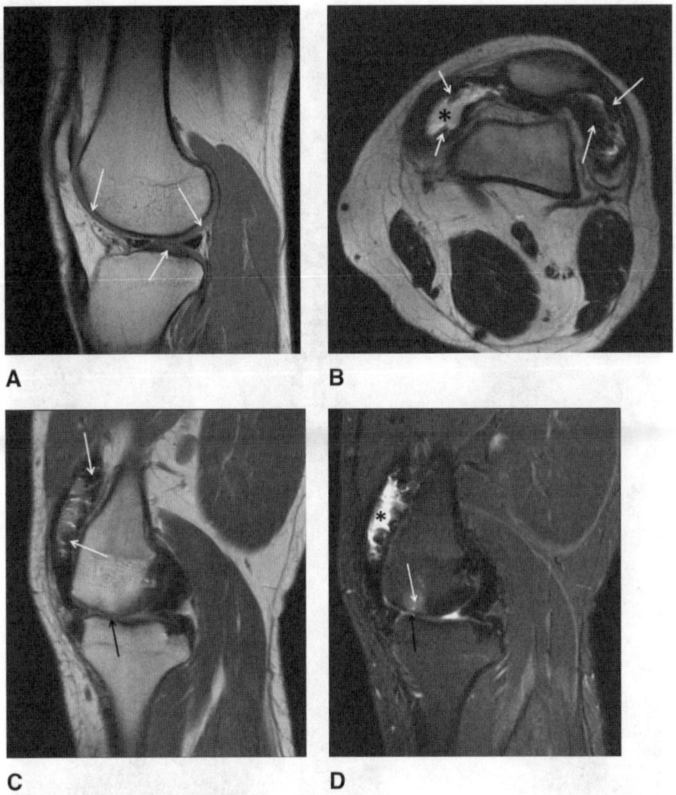

FIGURE 124–9. MRI of normal and hemophilic knees. **A.** MRI of normal knee. **B.** A transverse T2-weighted spin-echo image of the knee shows an effusion (*) and multiple foci of hemosiderin deposition (*arrows*) along the synovium lining the suprapatellar bursa. **C.** A sagittal T2-weighted spin-echo image of the knee shows dark foci of synovial hemosiderin deposition (*white arrows*) accompanied by narrowing of the femorotibial joint (*black arrow*). **D.** A sagittal STIR (short tau inversion recovery) image of the knee (in the same patient as *B*) demonstrates an effusion in the suprapatellar bursa (*asterisks*). The irregular, lumpy surface of the bursa represents thickened, hemosiderin-laden synovium. Femorotibial joint narrowing (*black arrow*) is associated with edema in the subchondral bone of the femoral condyle (*white arrow*). *(MRI images were obtained and interpreted by Dr. Jordan Renner, University of North Carolina.)*

Repeated bleeding into a joint results in synovial hypertrophy and inflammation. The synovium is thickened and folded, leading to limited joint motion. The result is a tendency for repeated hemorrhages leading to a so-called target joint.[31] The joints most often involved are the knees, ankles, and elbows, which become chronically swollen. Chronic synovitis may persist for months or years unless the condition is adequately treated.

Infection of hemophilic joints is not common but must be suspected in all patients with fever, leukocytosis, or other systemic manifestations. Rapid diagnosis is mandatory, because infection of such joints leads to rapid loss of joint architecture and function. A painful and swollen joint may require aspiration, which should be performed by experienced personnel using meticulous aseptic techniques and appropriate factor replacement therapy prior to aspiration.

Hematomas

Soft-tissue hematomas are also characteristic of hemophilia A. Hemorrhage into subcutaneous connective tissues or into muscles may occur with or without a known trauma. Hematomas, once formed, may stabilize and slowly resorb. However, in moderately and severely affected patients, hematomas have a tendency to enlarge progressively and to dissect in all directions, unless appropriately treated. Rarely, retroperitoneal hematomas, after beginning in the iliopsoas muscle, can dissect superiorly through the diaphragm, into the chest, and sometimes even into the soft tissues of the neck, compromising the airway. A retroperitoneal hematoma is more likely to compromise renal function by causing ureteral obstruction. Figure 124–11 shows the computed tomography (CT) scan of a patient with a retroperitoneal hemorrhage. Other hematomas expand locally and may compress adjacent organs, blood vessels, and nerves. A rare, and often fatal, complication of an abdominal hematoma is perforation and drainage into the colon. Subcutaneous hematomas may dissect into muscle. Pharyngeal and retropharyngeal hematomas, sometimes complicating simple colds, may enlarge and obstruct the airway. Hemorrhage in or around the airway is a potentially life-threatening situation that requires prompt administration of factor VIII.

Hemorrhages occur into muscle in the following order of frequency: calf, thigh, buttocks, and forearm. Recurrent hematomas often lead to muscle contractures, nerve palsies, and muscle atrophy. Bleeding into

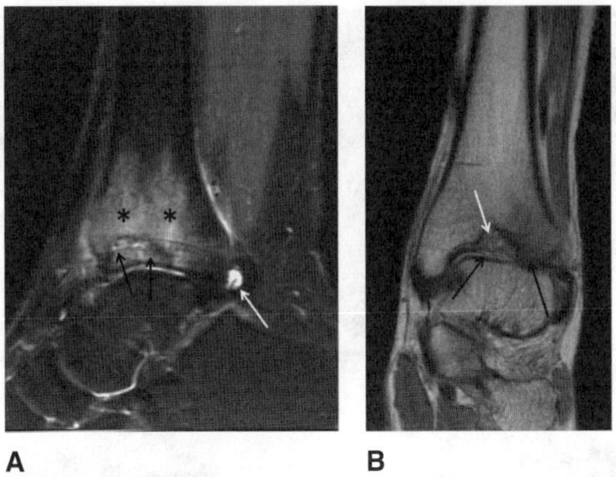

FIGURE 124–10. **A.** A sagittal STIR (short tau inversion recovery) image of an ankle shows an effusion (*white arrow*). Edema in the distal tibia (*asterisks*) surrounds a debris-filled defect in the subchondral bone of the distal tibia (*black arrows*). **B.** A coronal proton density of the ankle in the same patient as in *A* shows the defect in the subchondral bone of the distal tibia (*white arrow*). Mild narrowing of the tibiotalar joint (*black arrows*) is more apparent laterally.

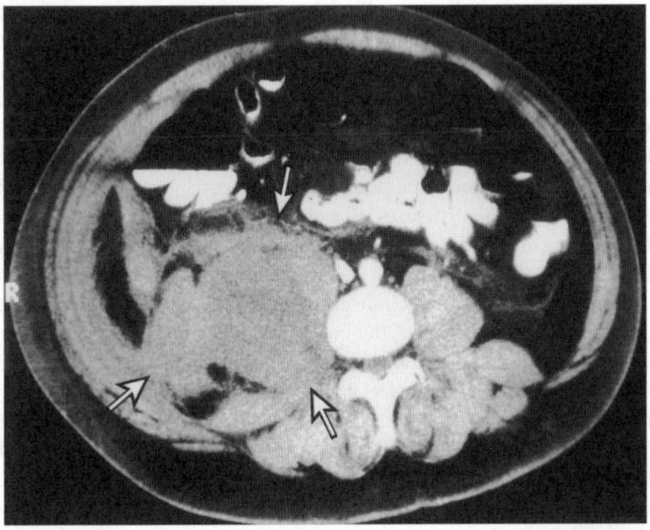

FIGURE 124–11. Computed tomography scan of a retroperitoneal hematoma in a patient with severe hemophilia A. Extent of the hematoma is indicated by the *arrows*.

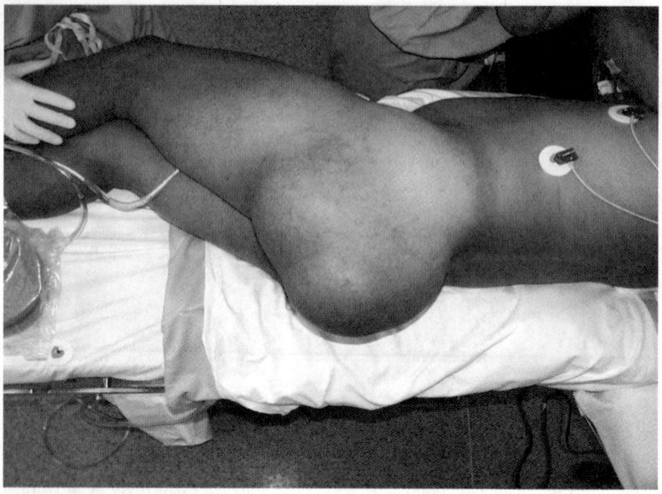

FIGURE 124–12. Photograph of a pseudotumor of the gluteal region.

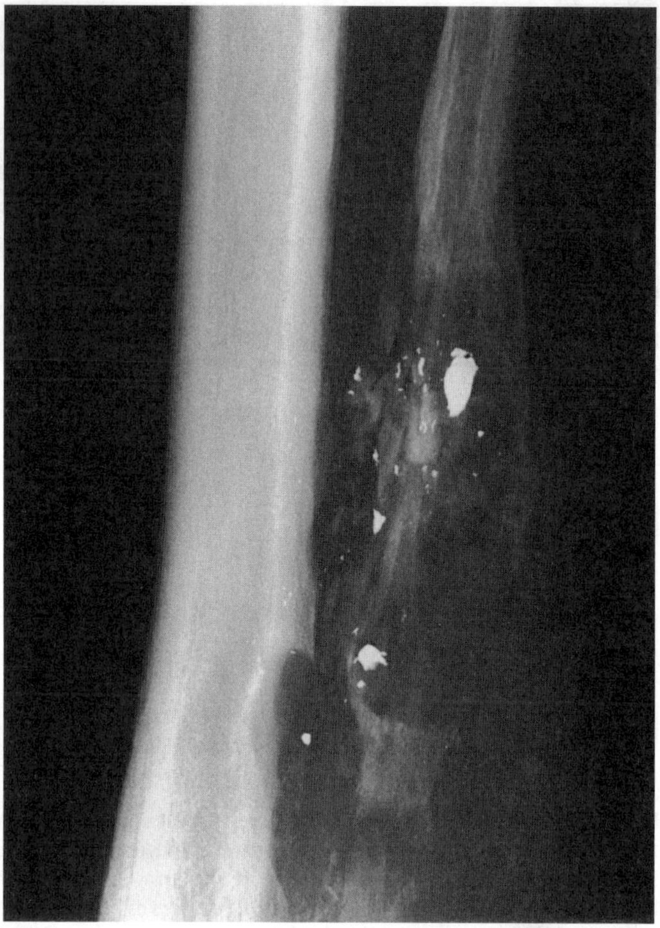

FIGURE 124–13. Pseudotumor of the fibula in a severely affected hemophilic. Note the virtual destruction of the bone with cysts and calcifications. The tibia also is involved.

the tongue or frenulum is particularly frequent in young children and usually is caused by trauma.

Bleeding into fascia and muscle can result in so-called compartment syndrome. This results when hemorrhage in a confined space compresses the arterial vasculature resulting in ischemic muscle injury. Compartment syndrome tends to occur in the distal part of the extremities, particularly in the flexor muscles, and requires urgent fasciotomy under cover of clotting factor replacement therapy. Bleeding into the myocardium or erect penis is very unusual, raising the interesting question as to why these tissues seem to be protected from hemorrhage.

Pseudotumors (Blood Cysts)

Pseudotumors are blood cysts that occur in soft tissues or bone. They are rare but dangerous complications of hemophilia (Figs. 124–12 and 124–13).[33] They are classified into three types. One type is a simple cyst that is confined by tendinous attachments within the fascial envelope of a muscle. The second type initially develops as a simple cyst in soft tissues such as a tendon, but it interferes with the vascular supply to the adjacent bone and periosteum, resulting in cyst formation and resorption of bone. The third type is thought to result from subperiosteal bleeding that separates the periosteum from the bony cortex (Fig. 124–13). Most pseudotumors are not associated with pain unless rapid growth or nerve compression occurs. As the volume of the cyst increases, the cyst compresses and destroys the adjacent muscle, nerve, and/or bone. Pseudotumors usually contain either serosanguineous fluid or a viscous brownish material surrounded by a fibrous membrane. The pseudotumors have a tendency to expand over several years and eventually become multiloculated. Some reach enormous size and involve so many structures that make them inoperable. Erosion through surrounding tissues and penetration into viscera or through the skin can occur, usually as a late event. Sinus tracts from the pseudotumor predispose to infection and septicemia. Pseudotumors often develop in the lower half of the body, usually in the thigh, buttock, or pelvis, but they can occur anywhere, including the temporal bone. The small bones of the hands or feet are most frequently affected in younger patients. CT or MRI are useful for diagnosis. Needle biopsies of pseudotumors should be avoided because of the risk of infection and hemorrhage. A reliable treatment is operative removal of the entire mass because the pseudotumor likely will reform if it is not completely removed. Radiotherapy of a pseudotumor has been reported to be successful and may be of value in hemophiliacs with inhibitors when surgery is not possible.[34]

Hematuria

Many severely affected patients with hemophilia experience episodes of hematuria. The urine may be brown or red, depending upon the rate of bleeding. Most bleeding arises from the renal pelvis, usually from one kidney but occasionally from both. Appropriate studies to exclude a structural lesion in the kidneys should be performed.

Neurologic Complications

Intracranial bleeding is one of the most dangerous hemorrhagic events in hemophilic patients.[35] Currently, bleeding into the brain is the leading cause of death in hemophilic patients. Hemorrhage into the central nervous system may be "spontaneous" but usually follows trauma, which may be trivial. Symptoms often occur soon after trauma, but sometimes they are delayed. For example, symptoms of a subdural hematoma may be delayed for days or several weeks. Hemorrhage into the brain parenchyma or a subdural or epidural hematoma should always be suspected in hemophilic patients with unusual headaches (Fig. 124–14). When intracranial bleeding is suspected, the patient should be treated immediately with factor VIII and diagnostic procedures, such as CT scans or MRI studies, should be delayed until after treatment is initiated. Although lumbar puncture has been performed safely in severe hemophilic patients without replacement therapy, replacing factor VIII to a level of approximately 50 percent of normal prior to the procedure is safer.

Hemorrhage into the spinal canal is an uncommon neurologic complication in hemophilia but can result in paraplegia. Bleeding may

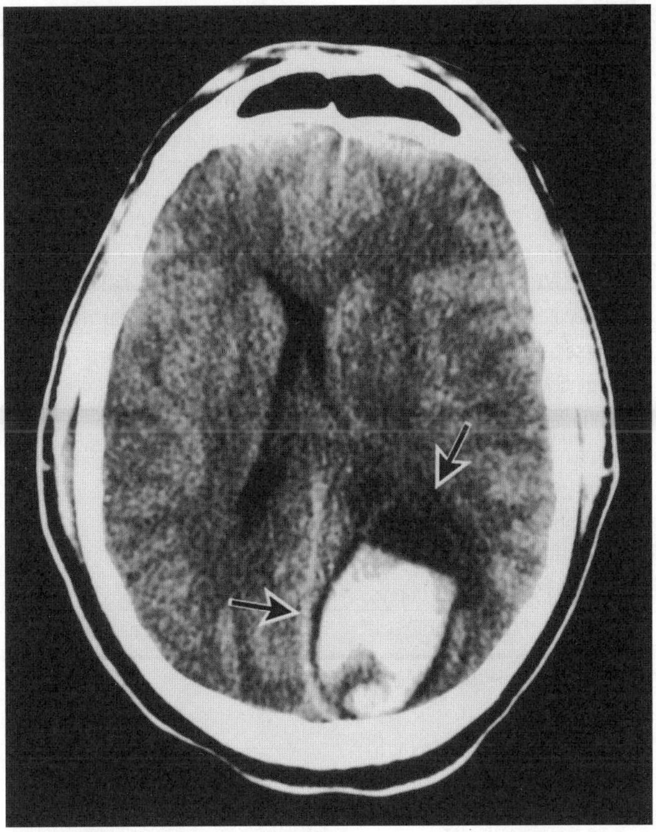

FIGURE 124–14. CT scan of an intracerebral hematoma in a severely affected hemophilic. The lesion is indicated by the *arrows*. Note compression of the ventricles.

occur within the spinal cord itself, but epidural bleeding compressing the cord is more common.[36]

Peripheral nerve compression is a frequent complication of muscle hematomas, particularly in the extremities. Compression of the femoral nerve by a hematoma in the iliopsoas muscle can result in sensory loss over the lateral and anterior thigh, weakness and atrophy of the quadriceps, and loss of the patellar reflex. The ulnar nerve is the next most frequently involved peripheral nerve. Bleeding may occur in any muscle and may compress local neural blood supply. This situation can be followed by permanent neuromuscular defects and multiple contractures.

Mucous Membrane Hemorrhage

Mucous membrane bleeding is common in hemophilia. Epistaxis and hemoptysis, often resulting from allergic reactions or trauma, can be associated with local structural lesions involving the upper and/or lower respiratory tract. Treatment of epistaxis by cautery or nasal packing sometimes is followed by recurrent bleeding because of sloughing of the cauterized area or dislodging of a poorly formed clot when the packing is removed. Peptic ulcer disease has been found to be more frequent in the adult hemophilia A population than in the general male population.[37] Ingestion of antiinflammatory drugs for relief of pain of hemophilic arthropathy is a frequent cause of upper gastrointestinal hemorrhage, and a history of ingestion of aspirin and other antiinflammatory drugs should be specifically addressed when assessing the etiology of such bleeding.[38]

Dental and Surgical Bleeding

Hemophilic patients are treated preoperatively and postoperatively to prevent bleeding. Mildly or sometimes moderately affected patients may go unrecognized until surgery results in excessive bleeding at the surgical site. Bleeding may be delayed for several hours or, occasionally, for several days. Surgery in such patients is characterized by delayed wound healing because of poor clot formation.[14] Prolonged bleeding and subsequent infection of the wound hematoma may further complicate healing. Appropriate factor VIII replacement therapy, sometimes supplemented by antifibrinolytic agents, can prevent intraoperative and postoperative hemorrhages.

Dental extraction is the most frequent surgical procedure performed on hemophilic patients. Loss of deciduous teeth seldom causes excessive bleeding, but extraction of permanent teeth may result in excessive hemorrhage that can persist intermittently for several days to weeks unless appropriate treatment is administered. In the untreated patient with severe hemophilia, life-threatening, dissecting pharyngeal and/or sublingual hematomas may result from dental procedures or from administration of regional block anesthesia.

LABORATORY FEATURES

Patients with severe hemophilia A have a prolonged activated partial thromboplastin time (aPTT). The prothrombin time (PT), thrombin clotting time (TCT), and bleeding time (BT) are normal, although some investigators have reported minor increases in the BT. Different combinations of aPTT reagents and instrumentation exhibit varying sensitivities to factor VIII levels. In mild hemophilia, the aPTT may be only slightly prolonged or at the upper limit of normal, especially if factor VIII activity is 20 percent or greater of normal. The aPTT is corrected when hemophilic plasma is mixed with an equal volume of normal plasma. If the hemophilic plasma contains an anti-factor VIII inhibitor antibody, the aPTT on a similar mixture is prolonged, but incubation of the mixture for 1 or 2 hours at 37°C (98.6°F) is required to detect the prolongation. A definitive diagnosis of hemophilia A should be based on a specific assay for factor VIII activity.

Functional factor VIII coagulant activity is measured by one-stage clotting assays based on the aPTT.[39] Chromogenic assays for factor VIII activity also are used widely, but do not always agree with one-stage assays.[39] Although infrequently measured in practice, factor VIII antigen is measured by immunologic assays, which detect normal and most abnormal factor VIII molecules. If the factor VIII antigen level is normal but the clotting activity is reduced, the patient has a dysfunctional factor VIII molecule. Such patients have antigen-positive hemophilia, also referred to as cross-reacting material (CRM)-positive.[40] Patients in whom both the factor VIII antigen level and activity are nearly undetectable are CRM-negative.

Factor VIII activity is expressed as percent of normal or as units per milliliter of plasma. By definition, 1 U of factor VIII equals the amount of factor VIII in 1 mL of pooled fresh, normal, human plasma. Also by definition, 1 U of factor VIII per milliliter is 100 percent of normal.

DIFFERENTIAL DIAGNOSIS

von Willebrand disease (VWD) sometimes is confused with hemophilia A. The basic defect in VWD is reduced activity of VWF, which acts as a carrier of factor VIII *in vivo* (see Chap. 127). Thus, in VWD, factor VIII levels are reduced, although considerable variability exists. Although factor VIII is synthesized normally in patients with VWD, the half-life of factor VIII is markedly shortened because the VWF "carrier" molecule is decreased or absent. Other abnormalities in VWD that distinguish VWD from hemophilia A are prolonged BT, decreased VWF antigen level, and decreased VWF activity, often measured using the ristocetin cofactor activity assay. In type III VWD, factor VIII levels may be very low (<5% of normal), making it difficult to distinguish from classical hemophilia. A long BT and lack of a sex-linked pattern of inheritance in the family will help in the differential diagnosis.

Another variant of VWD that is particularly difficult to distinguish from hemophilia A is VWD-Normandy, in which VWF multimers are normal but factor VIII levels are low.[41,42] Several mutations causing VWD-Normandy have been described, but all of them result in decreased binding of factor VIII to VWF.[43] The result is shortening of the intravascular survival of factor VIII and thus reduced factor VIII activity. The Normandy variant of VWD should be suspected in patients with mild hemophilia A who do not exhibit a sex-linked recessive inheritance pattern.[42]

Hemophilia A must be distinguished from other hereditary blood clotting factor deficiencies that exhibit a prolonged aPTT, including deficiencies of factors IX, XI, and XII, prekallikrein, and high-molecular-weight kininogen. Only deficiencies of factors VIII and IX cause chronic crippling hemarthroses with a family history suggestive of an X-linked bleeding disorder. Only specific assays can distinguish hemophilia A from factor IX deficiency (hemophilia B). Factor XI deficiency occurs in males and females and is a milder hemorrhagic disorder compared to severe hemophilia A or B. Factor XI deficiency can be confused with mild hemophilia A or B on screening laboratory tests, but specific assays distinguish them. Deficiencies of factor XII, prekallikrein, and high-molecular-weight kininogen can be distinguished from hemophilia because they are not associated with bleeding. Mild hemophilia A, with factor VIII levels of approximately 10 to 20 percent of normal, must be distinguished from combined deficiency of factors V and VIII.[44,45] Both the PT and aPTT are moderately prolonged in the combined disorder.[45]

TABLE 124–3. Currently Available Factor VIII Products[a]

	Origin	Viral Inactivation
Intermediate purity		
Humate P[b]	Plasma	Pasteurization[c]
High purity		
Koate DVI[b]	Plasma	Solvent-detergent[d], heat treated[i]
Alphanate[b]	Plasma	Solvent-detergent, heat treated[i]
Ultrapure[e]		
Hemofil M	Plasma	Solvent-detergent[d]
Monoclate P	Plasma	Pasteurization[c]
Recombinant		
Advate[h]	CHO cells[f]	Solvent-detergent[d]
Recombinate[e]	CHO cells[f]	
Kogenate FS[e]	BHK cells[g]	Solvent-detergent
Helixate FS[e]	BHK cells[g]	Solvent-detergent
Xyntha[h]	CHO cells[f]	Solvent-detergent, nanofiltration

[a]Additional concentrates are available in Europe.
[b]Contains VWF.
[c]Pasteurization at 60°C (140°F) for 10 h.
[d]Solvent-detergent: tri-n-butyl phosphate (TNBP) + polysorbate 80.
[e]Human albumin added; insignificant VWF.
[f]Chinese hamster ovarian cells.
[g]Baby hamster kidney cells.
[h]Not exposed to human or animal protein during manufacture.
[i]Heat treated at 80°C (176°F) for 72 h.

THERAPY

General

General principles applicable to therapy for hemophilia A include avoidance of aspirin, nonsteroidal antiinflammatory drugs, and other agents that interfere with platelet aggregation. Acetaminophen or relatively specific cyclooxygenase (COX)-2 inhibitors such as celecoxib have been recommended, but these drugs can be harmful when taken in excessive doses or for prolonged periods. Patients should be advised of the numerous over-the-counter analgesics that contain aspirin or other antiplatelet agents. Addictive narcotic agents should be used with great caution and only when clearly indicated, because drug dependency can be a major problem for patients with hemophilia. In general, intramuscular injections should be avoided unless the patient receives adequate replacement therapy. In the absence of prophylactic therapy, patients with hemophilia A must be treated as early as possible to avoid bleeding complications. Surgical procedures in hemophilic patients should be scheduled early in the week to avoid "weekend crises." Ample supplies of factor VIII should be available in the blood bank or pharmacy to ensure rapid access to treatment when needed. All hemophilic patients should have access to home treatment and periodic examinations at a comprehensive hemophilia diagnostic and treatment center. Prophylactic therapy is recommended in all severely affected patients, and it should be initiated before the onset of recurrent hemarthroses (primary prophylaxis) or as directed. Secondary prophylaxis (daily therapy) for an established "target" joint may be necessary.

Factor VIII Replacement Therapy

Hemorrhagic episodes in patients with hemophilia A can be managed by replacing factor VIII. Several products are available for use in raising factor VIII to hemostatic levels (see Fig. 124–3). Fresh-frozen plasma and cryoprecipitate both contain factor VIII and once were the only products available for treatment. A disadvantage of plasma is that large volumes must be infused to achieve and maintain even minimal factor VIII levels. The highest factor VIII level that can be achieved with plasma is approximately 20 percent of normal, which is not always attainable or sufficient for hemostasis. Cryoprecipitate, containing approximately 80 U of factor VIII in 10 mL of solution, can be used to attain normal factor VIII levels, but individual bags of cryoprecipitate must be pooled; the factor VIII dose can only be estimated; and the product must be stored frozen. Several commercial lyophilized factor VIII concentrates, using cryoprecipitate of pooled normal human plasmas as starting material (2000–20,000 donors), are available and do not have the disadvantages of plasma and cryoprecipitate (Table 124–3). Factor VIII concentrates have been sterilized by heating in solution, by superheating to 80°C (176°F) after lyophilization, and by exposure to organic solvent-detergents that inactivate lipid-enveloped viruses, including HIV and hepatitis B and C viruses, but do not inactivate parvovirus or hepatitis A.[46,47] Parvovirus infection does not occur frequently in hemophilia A patients because parvovirus is transmitted by cellular elements of the blood. Nevertheless, seroconversion to B19 parvovirus has been observed in patients receiving plasma-derived concentrates undergoing solvent-detergent extraction or pasteurization.

Some of these products contain significant amounts of VWF (see Table 124–3). Plasma-derived factor VIII concentrates prepared by monoclonal antibody techniques, and subjected to viral inactivation techniques, are highly purified and, barring breakdown in manufacturing procedures, are considered to be safe in terms of transmission of viral diseases.

Factor VIII produced by recombinant DNA techniques is available, safe, and effective (see Table 124–3). There are new "third-generation" factor VIII products, Advate and Xyntha, that are manufactured without exposure to animal or human protein. These products were developed because of fear of transmission of new-variant Creutzfeldt-Jakob disease (CJD) disease by blood products.[48–51] This concern was accelerated by reports of possible transmission of CJD to a hemophilic patient who received a plasma-derived factor VIII concentrate, which contained plasma from one donor who had new-variant CJD. Although the patient did not have clinical evidence of CJD, postmortem examination revealed prions in the patient's spleen.[49] Although all factor VIII products, both recombinant and plasma-derived, are currently safe and effective, some physicians and patients prefer products that are not exposed to human or animal proteins during the manufacturing process. There are continuing reports of the emergence of potentially pathogenic viruses that infect humans.[52] These viruses have a viremic phase and could contaminate the blood supply, but whether they are inactivated by present technology is unknown. For fear of a repeat of an "AIDS-like" crisis by contamination of the blood supply with transmissible infectious agents not inactivated by current technology, constant vigilance to insure a safe blood supply is warranted.

The dose of factor VIII can be determined as follows. If 1 U of factor VIII per milliliter of plasma is considered 100 percent of normal, the dose required to raise the level to a given value depends upon the patient's plasma volume (approximately 5% of body weight in kilograms) and the level to which factor VIII is to be raised. Thus, the plasma volume of a 70-kg adult is approximately equivalent to 3500 mL ($5\% \times 70$ kg = 3.5 kg = 3500 g, approximately equivalent to 3500 mL). To achieve normal factor VIII levels of 1 U/mL (100%), 3500 U of factor VIII should be given. This scenario assumes a 100 percent recovery of the administered dose. Recovery has approached 100 percent in studies, but depends upon the method of assay and the factor VIII standard used for comparison.[53] After the initial dose of factor VIII, further doses of factor VIII are based on a half-life of 8 to 12 hours. Thus, after a loading dose of 3500 U of factor VIII, a dose of 1750 U could be given in 12 hours. However, for practical purposes, the dose of factor VIII is based on the knowledge that 1 U of factor VIII per kilogram of body weight raises the circulating factor VIII level approximately 0.02 U/mL. Thus, to raise the factor VIII level to 100 percent, that is, 1 U/mL, the dose of factor VIII required is approximately 50 U per kilogram of body weight, assuming the patient's baseline factor VIII level is less than 1 percent of normal. The site and severity of hemorrhage determine the frequency and dose of factor VIII to be infused.

Table 124–4 summarizes the recommended doses of factor VIII for various types of hemorrhage.[53] These doses are not based on rigorous randomized studies, and recommendations vary among hemophilia centers. Given the high cost of factor VIII, some physicians prefer the lower doses.

Factor VIII can be given as a constant infusion to hospitalized patients. Following a loading dose to raise factor VIII to the desired level, 150 to 200 U of factor VIII per hour can be infused. Factor VIII levels can be conveniently monitored in blood obtained from veins other than the vein into which factor VIII was infused intravenously.[54] In selected patients, factor VIII can be given outside the hospital in a continuous infusion using pump devices.[55]

DDAVP (Desmopressin)

During the 1970s, 1-desamino-8-D-arginine vasopressin (DDAVP; desmopressin) was found to cause a transient increase in factor VIII in normal subjects and in patients with mild to moderate hemophilia. After a dose of DDAVP (0.3 mcg per kilogram body weight), given intravenously or subcutaneously, factor VIII levels increase two- to threefold above baseline in most, but not all, mildly or moderately affected hemophilia A patients. Patients with severe hemophilia A do not respond to DDAVP.[56] A concentrated intranasal spray of DDAVP also can be used (150 mcg in each nostril for adults and 150 mcg in one nostril for children weighing less than 50 kg). The degree of response to the drug should always be determined in patients before a bleeding episode, because occasionally mildly or moderately affected patients do not respond. The peak response to DDAVP usually occurs 30 to 60 minutes after dosing. In patients with mild or moderate hemophilia A and in carriers whose baseline factor VIII levels are less than 0.5 U/mL, DDAVP may be used in lieu of blood products. The mechanism by which DDAVP increases factor VIII is unknown.

Repeated administration of DDAVP results in a diminished response to the agent (tachyphylaxis). In many patients, the response to the second

TABLE 124–4. Doses of Factor VIII for Treatment of Hemorrhage*

Site of Hemorrhage	Desired Factor VIII Level (% of normal)	Factor VIII Dose† (U/kg body weight)	Frequency of Dose‡ (every no. of hours)	Duration (days)
Hemarthroses	30–50	~25	12–24	1–2
Superficial intramuscular hematoma	30–50	~25	12–24	1–2
Gastrointestinal tract	~50	~25	12	7–10
Epistaxis	30–50	~25	12	Until resolved
Oral mucosa	30–50	~25	12	Until resolved
Hematuria	30–100	~25–50	12	Until resolved
Central nervous system	50–100	50	12	At least 7–10 days
Retropharyngeal	50–100	50	12	At least 7–10 days
Retroperitoneal	50–100	50	12	At least 7–10 days

*Mild or moderately affected patients may respond to 1-deamino-8-D-arginine vasopressin (DDAVP), which should be used in lieu of blood or blood products whenever possible.

†Factor VIII may be administered in a continuous infusion if the patient is hospitalized. After initial bolus, approximately 150 U of factor VIII per hour usually are sufficient in an average-size adult. Doses are given every 12 to 24 hours.

‡The frequency of dosing and duration of therapy can be adjusted, depending on the severity and duration of the patient's bleeding episode.

DDAVP dose averages 30 percent less than the response to the first dose, and the response rate may be even less after additional doses.[57] DDAVP is a potent antidiuretic. As a result, hyponatremia has been reported in some patients whose water intake exceeds approximately 1 L per 24 hours after dosing. There is no convincing evidence to indicate that DDAVP administration is associated with thrombosis in hemophilic patients.

Antifibrinolytic Agents

Antifibrinolytic agents, such as ε-aminocaproic acid (EACA) and tranexamic acid, have been used to enhance hemostasis in patients with hemophilia A.[58,59] Fibrinolytic inhibitors may be given as adjunctive therapy for bleeding from mucous membranes and are particularly valuable as adjunctive therapy for dental procedures. The usual oral dose of tranexamic acid for adults is 1 g four times per day. EACA can be given as a loading dose of 4 to 5 g followed by 1 g/h by continuous IV infusion in adults. Another regimen of EACA is 4 g every 4 to 6 hours orally for 2 to 8 days, depending upon the severity of the bleeding episode. Antifibrinolytic therapy is contraindicated in the presence of hematuria because clots resistant to lysis may obstruct the ureters.

Fibrin Glue

Fibrin glue, otherwise known as fibrin tissue adhesive, has been used as adjunctive therapy to factor VIII in hemophilic patients.[60] Briefly, fibrin glue contains fibrinogen, thrombin, and factor XIII. Fibrinolytic inhibitors are added to some commercial products. The fibrinogen–factor XIII mixture is placed on the injury site and clotted with a human thrombin solution containing calcium. As a result, the fibrin clot is crosslinked and anchored to tissue. It is especially useful for hemostasis in patients undergoing dental surgery who receive a preextraction bolus of factor VIII followed by application of fibrin glue to the tooth socket. Fibrin glue also has been used as adjunctive therapy to factor VIII following orthopedic procedures and circumcision. It is very valuable for controlling bleeding when applied to the bed of a surgical wound following removal of large pseudotumors. Some hemophilia centers prepare their own "homemade" fibrin glue using cryoprecipitate as a source of fibrinogen and factor XIII. In some cases, bovine thrombin preparations are used for clotting the fibrinogen solution. Bovine thrombin can result in complications because it is contaminated with small amounts of bovine factor V. As a result, human antibodies to bovine factor V and bovine thrombin may develop in patients receiving such products. These antibodies may cross-react with human factor V and/or human thrombin, resulting in a transient but sometimes severe hemorrhagic disorder.[61]

Treatment of Minor or Moderate Hemorrhage

On occasion, superficial cuts and abrasions are managed with local measures, that is, application of pressure sometimes suffices to control bleeding, although oozing may continue intermittently for several hours. Topical thrombin is of little value in this type of bleeding. In general, cautery should be avoided because bleeding may restart when the cauterized area sloughs.

When replacement therapy for epistaxis is needed, the factor VIII level should be raised to approximately 30 to 50 percent of normal. For treatment of hematuria, patients should be instructed to drink large quantities of fluids. If hematuria is mild, uncomplicated, and painless, factor VIII replacement may not be necessary unless the hematuria persists. Gross or protracted hematuria requires replacement therapy. In these patients, factor VIII levels of at least 50 percent of normal or higher are needed, probably because urine is rich in urokinase that rapidly lyses clots.

Hemophilic patients requiring endoscopic procedures first should be treated with factor VIII to raise levels to at least 0.5 U/mL before the procedure. Only one dose may be necessary if endoscopy is uncomplicated. In cases of severe abrasions or perforations following endoscopy, factor VIII replacement should be continued until healing of the lesion is complete. For expanding soft-tissue hematomas, factor VIII therapy should be started immediately and maintained until the hematoma begins to resolve. With effective therapy, the patient usually experiences rapid relief from pain. For treatment of acute hemarthroses, prompt administration of factor VIII decreases the occurrence of extensive degenerative joint changes, deformity, and muscle wasting. For chronic synovitis and for bleeding into "target" joints, daily administration of factor VIII to raise levels to 100 percent of normal for 6 to 8 weeks ("secondary prophylaxis") is usually indicated.

Treatment of Major Nonsurgical Hemorrhages

Any hemorrhage in a patient with hemophilia A may become major, but the following hemorrhages are common and frequently life-threatening: retropharyngeal, retroperitoneal, and central nervous system bleeding, whether subdural, subarachnoid, or into the brain parenchyma.[62]

For treatment of retropharyngeal bleeding, particularly that associated with a sensation of tightness in the throat, pain in the neck, dysphagia, or difficulty breathing, patients should receive factor VIII immediately in doses sufficient to raise factor VIII levels to normal (1.0 U/mL). Near-normal levels should be maintained until bleeding ceases and the hematoma begins to resolve. For retroperitoneal hemorrhage, early treatment is required, and therapy should be continued for 7 to 10 days; otherwise, bleeding may recur upon resumption of activity.

Immediate administration of factor VIII, sufficient to raise the level to normal, should be started upon the first sign of an intracranial hemorrhage or following a history of head trauma. Even *asymptomatic* patients with a history of head trauma should receive at least one dose of factor VIII as a prophylactic measure, and this dose should be given before diagnostic procedures such as a CT scan. Treatment of a known intracranial hemorrhage should be maintained for a minimum of 7 to 10 days, and the circulating factor VIII level should be kept normal throughout this period. Prolonged secondary prophylaxis is often indicated following an intracerebral hemorrhage, particularly in patients with HIV disease, who seem to have a high recurrence rate. Evacuation of subdural hematomas and surgical removal of hematomas involving the brain parenchyma can be performed, depending upon location. Despite aggressive replacement therapy, however, mortality from central nervous system bleeding is high.

Replacement of Factor VIII for Surgical Procedures

For major surgical procedures, factor VIII should be raised to normal levels before operation and maintained for 7 to 10 days or until healing is complete. Treatment can be started a few hours before surgery and continued intraoperatively using a continuous infusion protocol. Postoperatively, factor VIII levels should be monitored at least one or two times per day to ensure that adequate levels are maintained. Because factor VIII may be "consumed" during surgery, factor VIII levels should be monitored intraoperatively and doses of factor VIII higher than normal may be required. Bone and joint surgery may require longer periods of factor VIII coverage. Replacement of knee, hip, and elbow joints is now possible, and several weeks of replacement therapy may be needed.[63]

Home Therapy

Home therapy using available factor VIII concentrates was introduced in the United States in 1977 and was a major advance in the treatment of all forms of hemophilia.[64,65] Current practice for home therapy is to treat patients at home using a regular prophylactic regimen. Patients, age 6 years and older, can be taught to treat themselves with factor VIII in the correct dose for an appropriate length of time. The training of patients and their families for home therapy is best accomplished in a regional comprehensive hemophilia diagnostic and treatment center or an affiliate of one of these centers. Patients are given an adequate supply of factor concentrates and the paraphernalia required for intravenous administration. Prompt treatment of hemarthroses and hematomas made possible by home therapy has markedly improved the morbidity and mortality associated with hemophilia. In addition, the quality of life of hemophilia A patients has improved dramatically.[65,66]

Prophylactic Therapy

The advent of stable and safe factor VIII concentrates has made prophylactic therapy for hemophilia A in severely affected patients feasible. Such therapy is now the treatment of choice for all severely affected hemophilia patients (unfortunately, such treatment is not available or affordable for all patients). Administration of 25 to 40 U of factor VIII per kilogram of body weight every other day markedly decreases the frequency of hemophilic arthropathy and other long-term effects of hemorrhagic episodes.[66–68] For prophylactic therapy to be successful in young children, patients should be selected for their reliability in managing central venous catheter devices.[69,70] Analysis of the economic impact of prophylactic therapy, weighing the benefits against the high costs of factor VIII concentrates, suggests the clinical benefit of prophylaxis is warranted, as evidenced by significant improvement in the clinical condition of patients and improvement in the quality of life.[68,71]

Liver Transplantation and Gene Therapy

Normal livers have been transplanted successfully into patients with hemophilia, with resulting cure of the hemophilic condition.[72,73] The procedure is performed not only to cure hemophilia but also for therapy for chronic hepatitis that afflicts many older hemophilic patients.

Gene replacement therapy for classic hemophilia offers an ideal theoretical approach for prophylactic therapy or even for a final cure of the disorder. Gene therapy trials in human hemophilic patients have included *ex vivo* transduction of human fibroblasts with a plasmid containing the factor VIII gene and subsequent implantation of the transduced cells into patients. Infusion of a retroviral vector containing the complementary deoxyribonucleic acid (cDNA) for B domainless factor VIII has also been tried.[74,75] Although no serious side effects were observed in either trial, in both trials the expression level of factor VIII was low (approximately 1% of normal) and persisted for only a few months to 1 year. Despite these disappointing early results, however, gene therapy still holds promise for cure of hemophilia. Factor VIII is a difficult protein to express because of its large size and because it must transit the endoplasmic reticulum–Golgi apparatus, which requires chaperone proteins for proper protein folding and other posttranslational modifications.[76,77] Molecular manipulations of factor VIII such that the protein is easier to express should make gene therapy with factor VIII more feasible in the future. Large and small animal models of hemophilia A exist and can be used to test new approaches to gene therapy.[78,79] Development of better viral and nonviral vectors is possible and promises to improve chances for future successful gene transfer in hemophilic patients.[80]

COURSE AND PROGNOSIS

After the advent of factor VIII concentrates in the 1960s, the morbidity and mortality from bleeding in hemophilia were significantly reduced, and by the late 1970s the life expectancy of hemophilia A patients began to approach that of normal individuals. However, use of replacement therapy has not been without significant complications. Prior to 1985, common and serious adverse side effects of treatment included chronic liver disease resulting from hepatitis B and C and, from about 1978, infection with HIV.[81] Factor VIII concentrates were prepared from many thousands of donors, making contamination of factor VIII concentrates highly likely. With the introduction of heat- or solvent-detergent-treated concentrates in 1985, contamination of blood products with these viruses has been eliminated for all practical purposes. However, AIDS became a leading cause of death in older patients with hemophilia.[81] Chronic liver disease in hemophilia A patients resulting from transfusion-related hepatitis B and C may be accelerated by HIV infection and by the associated hepatotoxicity of antiviral drug therapy.[82] Fortunately, patients treated prophylactically after 1985 can expect almost normal life spans free of the complications of hepatitis, AIDS, and other currently recognized bloodborne viral diseases. However, the development of inhibitor antibodies against factor VIII has been, and continues to be, one of the more serious complications of replacement therapy.

Factor VIII Inhibitors

Other than the transmission of viral diseases by factor VIII infusions, the main complication of hemophilia A replacement therapy is the development of specific inhibitor antibodies that neutralize factor VIII.[83] Current debate centers around the true frequency of anti-factor VIII inhibitors in severe hemophilia A patients. However, analysis reveals the frequency of inhibitors in a large group of patients was approximately 40 percent in patients with large deletions, and approximately 35 percent in patients with nonsense mutations.[84] When the whole population of severe hemophilia A patients is included, the overall incidence of inhibitor formation appears to be approximately 20 percent over a long followup period. Frequent testing for inhibitors in previously untreated patients receiving newer highly purified factor VIII products from plasma or by recombinant technology revealed the frequent occurrence of transient inhibitors to factor VIII, many of which were of low titer and did not necessitate cessation of treatment with the same product. Although still controversial, some believe that the risk of inhibitors does not appear to be higher with the use of highly purified products than the risk reported in earlier studies using products of intermediate purity that contain VWF.[85–90] Some physicians believe that VWF is immunomodulatory so that products containing VWF are less likely to induce inhibitors than highly purified products. One outbreak of inhibitors appeared to be related to an intermediate-purity plasma-derived factor VIII concentrate. Fortunately, inhibitors disappeared from affected patients when use of the product was stopped.[91]

Table 124–5 lists the factors related to development of inhibitors. They arise most frequently in severely affected patients, following treatment at an early age. Many have gross gene rearrangements or the intron 22 inversion abnormality of the factor VIII gene.

Factor VIII inhibitors are antibodies (almost always alloantibodies, although some mild hemophilic patients develop autoantibodies against the factor), most often of the immunoglobulin (Ig)-G class and frequently restricted to the IgG_4 subclass.[83] Antibodies against the A_2 and C domains of factor VIII are most common. These antibodies interfere with the interactions of factor VIII with other hemostatic components.[83,92]

Early diagnosis of factor VIII inhibitors is essential. Although the presence of an inhibitor can be suspected on clinical grounds, as when a patient does not respond to conventional doses of factor VIII, laboratory diagnosis is required for confirmation. Factor VIII inhibitors are time and temperature dependent. The prolonged aPTT of the plasma of a patient without an inhibitor is corrected when mixed 1:1 with normal plasma even after incubation at 37°C (98.6°F) for 1 to 2 hours. In

TABLE 124–5. Risk Factors for Development of Anti-Factor VIII Antibodies in Hemophilia A Patients

Disease severity: 80% of hemophilia A patients with inhibitors have <1% factor VIII activity

Early exposure to factor VIII concentrates: majority of high-titer inhibitors develop after <90 days of exposure to factor VIII

Genetic factors

1. Family history of inhibitor development
2. Negative correlation with human leukocyte antigen (HLA) Cw5 antigen
3. Molecular defects: inversion and crossing over defect in intron 22, gene deletions, and nonsense point mutations resulting in patients without factor VIII antigen

Method of purification of factor VIII concentrate

SOURCE: Roberts HR: Inhibitors and their management, in *Haemophilia & Other Bleeding Disorders*, edited by C Rizza, G Lowe, p 371. WB Saunders, New York, 1997, with permission.

contrast, the aPTT of a 1:1 mixture of plasma from a patient with an inhibitor and normal plasma is significantly prolonged after incubation at 37°C (98.6°F) for 1 to 2 hours. Specific diagnosis rests upon demonstrating that an appropriate dilution of the patient's plasma, when added to normal plasma, specifically neutralizes factor VIII and not other blood clotting factors that influence the aPTT (i.e., factors IX, XI, XII, prekallikrein, high-molecular-weight kininogen). The demonstration that the inhibitor is specific for factor VIII distinguishes it from inhibitors of other clotting factors, for example, the lupus anticoagulant, and nonspecific inhibitors. A common assay used for inhibitor detection and quantification is the Bethesda assay.[93] In the Bethesda assay, the patient's plasma is diluted such that, when the plasma is mixed with an equal volume of normal pooled human plasma and incubated for 2 hours at 37° C (98.6°F), the factor VIII activity in the mixture is decreased by 50 percent. A modification of the Bethesda assay is the Nijmegen assay, in which the pH of the sample over the 2-hour incubation period is maintained at 7.4.[94]

Several approaches to treatment of factor VIII inhibitors are available (Table 124–6). Use of these treatments requires knowledge of whether the patient with an inhibitor is a "high" or "low" responder and whether the bleeding episode requiring treatment is minor or major.[83]

High-Responder Patients Approximately 60 percent of patients who have inhibitors are high responders. High responders are defined as patients whose inhibitor titer is higher than 5 Bethesda units (BU) at baseline or whose initial inhibitor titer is less than 5 BU but rises to greater than 10 BU after administration of factor VIII. Thus, high responders who are not treated with factor VIII for long periods may have a sustained high level of inhibitor, or they may have a very low to undetectable level of inhibitor until they are challenged with factor VIII.

Major bleeding episodes in a high-responder patient whose initial inhibitor titer is less than 5 BU can be treated with human factor VIII concentrate (see Table 124–6). When the initial titer is low, sufficient factor VIII can be administered in high doses to neutralize the inhibitor and attain adequate factor VIII levels for hemostasis. Although factor VIII inhibitor bypassing agents can be used (see below), they are not as reliable as factor VIII in achieving hemostasis, and their effect cannot be adequately monitored with specific laboratory tests. If human factor VIII is used, a loading dose of 10,000 to 15,000 U may be required, followed by up to 1000 U of factor VIII per hour, depending upon the factor VIII level. One can expect an anamnestic response approximately 5 days after administration of factor VIII.

In high-responder patients whose initial inhibitor titer is less than 5 BU and who experience a minor bleeding episode, the agent of choice is a factor VIII inhibitor bypassing agent. Recombinant factor VIIa in doses of 90 to 120 mcg per kilogram of body weight or higher every 2 to 3 hours is safe and effective in most hemorrhagic episodes.[95] The dosing frequency is based on a factor VIIa plasma half-life of approximately 2 to 3 hours. The mechanisms of action of factor VIIa have been investigated using *in vitro* techniques. After coagulation is initiated by the tissue factor/factor VIIa pathway, factor VIIa at recommended doses is hypothesized to activate factor X on the surface of activated platelets, even in the absence of additional tissue factor activity.[94] Factor Xa then can associate with factor Va and convert prothrombin to thrombin. Because activated platelets are localized to the site of vessel injury, thrombin generation by factor VIIa is localized to the site of bleeding. This process may account for the reported safety of factor VIIa.[96] If this agent is not available, activated or inactivated prothrombin complex concentrates may be used. Factor VIII inhibitor bypassing activity (FEIBA), a plasma-derived agent, has been used successfully to treat many bleeding episodes and is both safe and effective.[97]

High-responder patients whose initial inhibitor titer is greater than 5 BU usually do not respond to even very high doses of human factor VIII. Thus, recombinant factor VIIa or FEIBA should be used.[97] If these agents are not available, unactivated prothrombin complex concentrates or exchange transfusion can be considered (see Table 124–6).

Low-Responder Patients Low-responder patients are arbitrarily defined as patients whose inhibitor titer is less than 5 BU even after a challenge with factor VIII. For major bleeding episodes, high doses of human factor VIII can be used as recommended above. For minor bleeds, recombinant factor VIIa, FEIBA, or prothrombin complex concentrates

TABLE 124–6. Treatment of Inhibitors in Hemophilia A Patients

Type of Patient	Initial Titer	Minor Hemorrhage*	Major Hemorrhage*
High responder	<5 BU	Recombinant factor VIIa; FEIBA; prothrombin complex concentrates	Human factor VIII†; recombinant factor VIIa; FEIBA; prothrombin complex concentrates
High responder	>5 BU	Recombinant factor VIIa; FEIBA; prothrombin complex concentrates	Recombinant factor VIIa; FEIBA; plasma exchange
Low responder	<5 BU	Recombinant factor VIIa; FEIBA; prothrombin complex concentrates	High-dose human factor VIII; recombinant factor VIIa; FEIBA

BU, Bethesda unit; FEIBA, factor VIII inhibitor bypassing activity.

*Choice of agents for treatment of major and minor hemorrhage are listed. Some physicians will choose the first product listed as the agent of choice, but the choice varies among physicians.

†High dose of factor VIII may overcome an initial low-titer inhibitor, although an anamnestic response can be expected in high responders

SOURCE: Roberts HR: Inhibitors and their management, in *Haemophilia & Other Bleeding Disorders*, edited by C Rizza, G Lowe, p 376. WB Saunders, New York, 1997, with permission.

(activated or unactivated) are recommended because some "low" responders may convert to high responders when they are challenged repeatedly with factor VIII.

Nonactivated or activated prothrombin complex concentrates contain variable amounts of activated factors, including factors VIIa, IXa, and Xa. The activated products have higher concentrations of activated factors than do unactivated products. FEIBA contains a complex of prothrombin and factor Xa that can bind to membrane surfaces and enhance thrombin generation in the absence of factors VIII or IX.[96,97]

Surgery in Inhibitor Patients The question of whether major surgery can be performed in patients with hemophilia A and B with inhibitors arises now that joint replacement is possible. Knee and hip replacements have been carried out successfully in patients with inhibitor antibodies using factor VIIa.[98] Basically, the patient is given a loading dose of factor VIIa followed by bolus doses of factor VIIa and use of fibrin sealant and antifibrinolytic therapy until healing is complete. FEIBA has also been successfully used in surgery in hemophilic patients with inhibitors.[99]

Immunosuppression Removal of the antibody by plasmapheresis, adsorption of the antibody on an affinity column during plasma exchange, and administration of intravenous γ-globulin have been used in patients with an inhibitor. The Malmö protocol uses nearly all of these approaches in combination, including extracorporeal adsorption of antibody to a Sepharose A column, administration of cyclophosphamide, daily administration of factor VIII, and intravenous γ-globulin.[100]

The most promising approach to eradication of an inhibitor is use of immune tolerance regimens. The basis of this approach is administration of daily doses of factor VIII until the inhibitor titer is undetectable.[101] Low-dose and high-dose regimens have been described (Table 124–7). Factor VIII inhibitor bypassing agents are used for acute bleeds that occur during immune tolerance induction.

Other approaches to treatment of factor VIII inhibitors include immunosuppressive drugs, like cyclosporine and rituximab.[101–103] However, these drugs, although occasionally successful, seem to be more effective in patients with acquired hemophilia resulting from autoantibodies against factor VIII.

Infectious Complications

Hepatitis Almost all multitransfused patients with hemophilia treated before 1985 were infected with one or more viruses that caused hepatitis. Although many infected patients did not suffer acute symptoms, at least 50 percent developed chronic persistent or chronic active hepatitis that led to cirrhosis. Hepatitis C and B viruses are commonly associated with chronic liver disease. Many adult hemophilic patients treated with concentrates before 1985 have antibodies to hepatitis B surface antigen, and some of them have circulating hepatitis B surface antigen. The antigen-positive adult patients frequently have a superimposed infection with the delta agent, leading to severe active hepatitis and cirrhosis and an increased risk of hepatocellular carcinoma.[104–106] Therapy with recombinant interferon-α and ribavirin can reduce viral load and improve survival of affected patients.[107] All patients with hemophilia should be vaccinated against hepatitis A and hepatitis B.

TABLE 124–7. Examples of Tolerance Protocols for Hemophilia A Inhibitor Patients

Immune Tolerance Protocols	Dose	Initial Response
High-dose regimen	100 U/kg factor VIII two times per day until antibody reaches 1 BU/mL, then 150 U/kg factor VIII per day until factor VIII half-life is normal	In 16 of 21 patients, titer fell to <1 BU/mL
Low-dose regimen	50 U/kg factor VIII per day	9 of 12 patients responded
Netherlands protocol	25 U/kg factor VIII per day	11 of 18 patients responded

SOURCE: Roberts HR: Inhibitors and their management, in *Haemophilia & Other Bleeding Disorders*, edited by C Rizza, G Lowe, p 376. WB Saunders, New York, 1997, with permission.

Human Immunodeficiency Virus Many of the older, severely affected hemophilia A patients who were treated before 1985 have antibodies to HIV, indicating infection with the virus. The incidence of HIV antibodies in mildly affected patients is much lower and correlates with treatment with factor VIII concentrates before viral inactivation procedures were used. In one study, 14 percent of patients treated only with cryoprecipitate from 1979 to 1985 were infected with HIV, whereas 88 percent of patients treated with factor VIII concentrates became infected.[108] Screening of donor populations and new techniques for preparing factor VIII concentrates since 1985 have eliminated the risk of HIV transmission.

Risk of Viral Disease Transmission by New Factor VIII Products All available factor VIII concentrates, both plasma-derived and recombinant products, are considered safe and effective with almost no risk of transmitting currently known viral diseases. However, occasional exceptions have been observed. For example, solvent-detergent extraction does not inactivate viruses without lipid envelopes, including the hepatitis A virus and parvovirus. As a result, outbreaks of hepatitis A have been reported in patients receiving some solvent-detergent–treated products. These outbreaks of viral diseases usually are related to breakdowns during the manufacturing process.

Prions Prions are infectious particles consisting of proteinaceous material devoid of a nucleic acid genome.[109] They are thought to be variant forms of a normal protein with an altered conformation. The "infectious" nature of prions may result from their ability to bind to other proteins and induce similar conformational changes in them such that new "infectious" particles can be generated. Prions are responsible for several neurodegenerative disorders, including CJD in humans, scrapie in sheep, and spongiform encephalopathy in cows. Prions are resistant to most currently available viral inactivation techniques. Removal of prion particles using iodine column chromatography has been claimed.[110] Although prion diseases generally are transmitted by ingestion of infected neural tissues, a new variant of CJD appears to occur in people who have eaten beef from cows infected with a form of prion causing bovine spongiform encephalopathy. This form of CJD has been reported mainly in the United Kingdom and in certain other European countries and has been related to the bovine disease.[111] For example, prions have been found in tonsillar tissue of patients with new-variant CJD, heightening concern about whether prions of this type might be transmitted by blood products.[112] One case of a hemophilic patient suspected of being infected with new-variant CJD following transfusion of a blood product from a donor later found to be infected has been reported.[113] This patient had no symptoms of CJD, but the agent was found in the spleen at autopsy. Conclusive data about possible prion infection of hemophilic patients are lacking, so continued vigilance is necessary. For this reason, certain plasma products prepared from blood of donors in the United Kingdom have been withdrawn until more data are available.

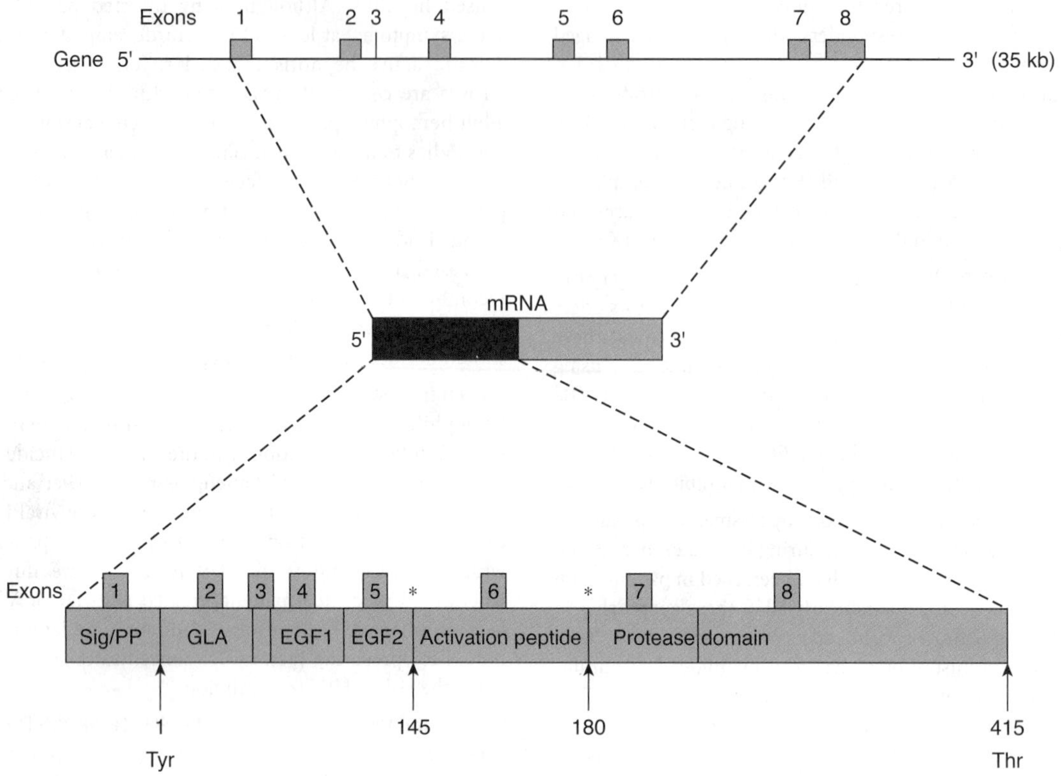

FIGURE 124–15. Schematic of the factor IX gene, the messenger RNA, and the protein. Exons are depicted by the tan boxes. The light 3′ portion of the mRNA is untranslated. The diagram of the protein shows the domains and the exons that encode each portion of the protein. The cleavage sites of factor XIa or factor VIIa–tissue factor complex are indicated by *asterisks*.

HEMOPHILIA B (FACTOR IX DEFICIENCY, CHRISTMAS FACTOR DEFICIENCY)

ETIOLOGY AND PATHOGENESIS

Hemophilia B occurs in 1 of every 25,000 to 30,000 live male births. As with hemophilia A, hemophilia B is found in all ethnic groups and has no geographic predilection.

Factor IX is a vitamin K-dependent, single-chain glycoprotein consisting of 415 amino acids. It is activated by the factor VIIa–tissue factor complex, or factor XIa, forming the active enzyme factor IXa (see Chap. 115). Once activated, factor IXa activates factor X in the presence of factor VIIIa, phospholipid (activated platelets), and calcium. Factor VIIIa is a necessary cofactor for activity of factor IXa. Therefore, deficiency of either factor IX or VIII leads to a similar lack of factor X-activating activity on the platelet surface. Factor Xa converts prothrombin to thrombin in the presence of factor Va, activated platelets, and calcium. Thus, deficiency of factor IX results in delayed conversion of prothrombin to thrombin, which is the cause of the bleeding tendency. Hemophilia B can result from either the absence or the dysfunction of factor IX molecules. Clinical severity of hemophilia B is roughly correlated with factor IX functional activity.

GENETICS AND MOLECULAR BIOLOGY

The factor IX gene is located on the long arm of the X chromosome. It is approximately 33 kb long, which is much smaller than the gene for factor VIII.[114] Because it is less complex, the factor IX gene has been studied in greater detail than the factor VIII gene. Figure 124–15 is a schematic of the gene and the protein product. The protein consists of a signal peptide that targets the protein for secretion from the hepatocyte to the circulation. The propeptide is necessary for posttranslational modification of 12 amino-terminal glutamic acid residues by an intracellular vitamin K-dependent carboxylase. The propeptide is cleaved from the mature protein before it enters the circulation. The amino-terminus of factor IX contains 12 γ-carboxyglutamic acid (GLA) residues necessary for calcium-dependent lipid binding. The activation peptide is cleaved from the zymogen form of factor IX by either factor VIIa/tissue factor or factor XIa, resulting in the two-chain active enzyme, factor IXaβ. The catalytic triad (histidine 221, aspartic acid 229, serine 365) resides on the heavy chain (see Chap. 115).[114]

There are more than 1000 distinct mutations or deletions in the factor IX gene reported in the factor IX database, including more than 900 distinct amino acid substitutions and numerous complete gene deletions.[115,116] More than 30 percent of factor IX mutations occur at CpG dinucleotides. These mutations often involve critical arginine residues that result in a dysfunctional molecule.[116–119] Many mutations have been reported in more than one kindred, and some of these mutations derive from the same "founder."[120] As predicted by genetic theory of X chromosome-linked recessive disorders, approximately one-third of mutations resulting in hemophilia B arise *de novo*.

Mutations in regulatory regions of the factor IX gene have been identified. Particularly interesting examples are mutations in the 5′ promoter region that lead to the hemophilia B Leyden phenotype (Table 124–8).[121] This disorder is characterized by very low levels of factor IX antigen and activity at birth and during early childhood. The factor IX levels gradually rise to 60 percent of normal or greater following puberty, apparently in response to endogenous androgen synthesis. Several different mutations in the promoter region of the factor IX gene

TABLE 124–8. Mutations in the Promoter Region of the Factor IX GENE

Nucleotide Substitution	Nucleotide Change	Factor IX Percent Activity	Factor IX Percent Antigen	Comments
−21	T→G	<1–70	–	Disruption of HNF-4 binding site; factor IX activity increases after puberty
−20	T→A	<1–60	<1–60	Factor IX activity increases after puberty
−20	T→C	9	–	Factor IX activity increases after puberty
−6	G→A	13–70	–	Factor IX activity increases after puberty
−5	A→T	3	–	Factor IX activity increases after puberty
6	T→A	<2–20	–	Factor IX activity increases after puberty
8	T→C	1–2	–	C/EBP binding site: factor IX clotting activity increases after puberty
13	A→G	<1–60	<1–60	C/EBP binding site: factor IX clotting activity increases after puberty
13	delete 1	<1–60	<1–60	C/EBP binding site: factor IX clotting activity increases after puberty

SOURCE: Roberts HR: Molecular biology of hemophilia B. *Thromb Haemost* 70:3, 1993, with permission.

disrupt binding of transcription factors, resulting in reduced transcription of the factor IX gene.[121–123] The hormonal changes occurring at puberty apparently can overcome the transcription defect and maintain hemostatically adequate levels of factor IX.

Hemophilia Bm, a unique form of hemophilia B, is characterized by a deficiency of factor IX clotting activity and a prolonged ox brain PT. The original hemophilia Bm patient with a prolonged ox brain PT had the surname Martin, which led to the term *hemophilia Bm*.[124] A number of missense mutations affecting amino acid residues at positions 180, 181, and 182 of the protein and several residues close to the active site region have been identified in patients with the characteristic findings of hemophilia Bm. These mutations result in a factor IX molecule that exhibits abnormal interaction with ox brain tissue factor.[124] Ox brain TF is currently not used in the United States. However, using recombinant TF for the PT, the hemophilia Bm variants may exhibit a slightly prolonged PT, for example, 13 to 14 seconds.

Hemophilia B inheritance is similar to that of hemophilia A. All daughters of affected males are obligatory carriers, whereas all sons are normal. Female carriers may have factor IX levels ranging from less than 10 to 100 percent of normal, but the mean level is approximately 50 percent of normal. Carriers of hemophilia B usually are asymptomatic, except in cases of extreme X chromosome inactivation, X mosaicism, Turner syndrome, or testicular feminization.[125] When the level of factor IX activity is less than 25 percent of normal, abnormal bleeding may occur, especially after trauma.

Carrier Detection and Prenatal Diagnosis

Carrier detection and genetic screening are possible through use of DNA probes to directly identify known mutations. As with factor VIII, mutations at CpG nucleotide pairs disrupt TaqI cleavage sites and therefore can be directly detected by restriction endonuclease mapping. More commonly, RFLP analysis is used. Prenatal diagnosis has been reliably accomplished by RFLP analysis of DNA obtained by chorionic villus sampling as early as 8 to 10 weeks after conception.[126] This procedure also can be performed on fetal cells obtained by amniocentesis and is more accurate than fetal blood sampling for factor IX activity and factor IX antigen. Direct sequencing of the factor IX gene can be used for carrier detection but is not available in most clinical laboratories.

CLINICAL FEATURES

Bleeding episodes in patients with hemophilia B are clinically indistinguishable to episodes in patients with hemophilia A, although as stated elsewhere, the hemophilia B population as a whole seem to have fewer and less severe complications as severely affected hemophilia A patients[8a] (see "Clinical Features" under "Hemophilia A" above). When patients are inadequately treated, repeated hemarthroses leading to chronic, crippling hemarthropathy occur. Hematoma formation with dissection into surrounding tissues is possible. Hematuria, bleeding from mucous membranes, and other bleeding manifestations are as described in the section on hemophilia A. The physical, psychological, vocational, and social aspects of the disease are similar to those encountered with hemophilia A. Classification of hemophilia B is based on clinical severity and roughly correlates with the level of factor IX coagulant activity. Severe disease usually is associated with factor IX levels of less than 1 percent of normal; moderate disease is associated with factor IX levels of 1 to 5 percent; and mild disease is associated with factor IX levels ranging from 5 to 40 percent of normal.

The occurrence of factor IX inhibitor antibodies is much less common in hemophilia B patients than in hemophilia A patients. Only approximately 3 percent of severely affected patients develop inhibitors.

LABORATORY FEATURES

The screening tests used in the diagnosis of hemophilia A also are used in the diagnosis of hemophilia B. In most cases of hemophilia B, PT is normal and aPTT is prolonged. However, specific assay of factor IX coagulant activity is required for definitive diagnosis. The most commonly used test is a one-stage clotting assay based on aPTT. Determination of factor IX antigen levels is valuable in further classifying the disorder. PTs usually are normal in hemophilia B, but occasionally they are prolonged, especially when ox brain thromboplastin is the source of tissue factor (hemophilia Bm). Because most PT reagents contain rabbit brain or human tissue factor, the PTs recorded for patients with hemophilia Bm usually are normal, but are occasionally prolonged by one or two seconds. In all forms of hemophilia B, the bleeding time usually is normal.

DIFFERENTIAL DIAGNOSIS

Hemophilia B must be distinguished from hemophilia A. Both forms are inherited as X-linked recessive disorders, and both have almost identical hemorrhagic and clinical manifestations. The only method for differentiating hemophilia B from hemophilia A is performing specific assays for factors VIII and IX on the patient's plasma.

Inherited and acquired deficiencies of other vitamin K-dependent factors, liver disease, and warfarin overdose must be distinguished from hemophilia B. In these cases, not only factor IX but all other vitamin K-dependent clotting factors, including prothrombin, factor VII, and factor X, are decreased. Acquired antibodies specific for factor IX occur in nonhemophilic patients but are very rare.

THERAPY

Factor IX Replacement

The basic treatment of hemophilia B is replacement of factor IX. Several products are available for use (Table 124–9). The older factor IX-containing products often are referred to as prothrombin complex concentrates. These products, which are prepared from large pools of human plasma (several thousand donors), contain not only factor IX but also prothrombin, factors VII and X, and proteins C and S. In addition, the products may contain small amounts of activated factors, such as factors VIIa, IXa, and Xa. Some of these products are associated with thromboembolic events, presumably resulting from contamination with the activated components. Deep venous thrombosis and disseminated intravascular coagulation have been reported in some patients who receive large doses of prothrombin complex concentrates, but these complications seem to occur less frequently with currently available purified factor IX products than with earlier preparations. Prothrombin complex concentrates are not the best choice for replacement therapy in hemophilia B, even though they are much less expensive than the highly purified factor IX concentrates. When prothrombin complex concentrates are used for replacement therapy, factor IX levels greater than 50 percent of normal should not be exceeded in order to minimize the risk of thrombosis. Use of these products in factor IX-deficient patients with liver dysfunction may be hazardous because the activated factors contaminating these preparations may not be cleared efficiently by a diseased liver, and thrombosis might be induced.

Table 124–9 lists the highly purified factor IX products. Some products are prepared from human plasma; one product (BeneFIX) is produced by recombinant DNA technology. Although all available factor IX concentrates are considered safe and effective, the recombinant product undergoes a final viral inactivation step. In addition, the recombinant product is not exposed to human albumin or bovine serum during preparation. Thus, even the theoretical risk of transmission of prion diseases is averted with this preparation. Some clinicians consider the recombinant product to be the agent of choice, although it has a major drawback in that the intravascular recovery of factor IX generally is lower than the recovery of highly purified factor IX product prepared from plasma.[127] The recombinant factor IX product is not thought to be thrombogenic. Special new factor IX products are currently being developed by several pharmaceutical companies so one can expect the number of available factor IX products to increase in the near future.

Dosing of Factor IX

The dose calculations for all factor IX products are different from those used in hemophilia A because intravascular recovery of factor IX is only approximately 50 percent, and the recovery is even lower with the recombinant product. The reason for this finding is unclear, but factor IX binding to elements on the vessel wall has been proposed. In fact, factor IX binds specifically to collagen type IV, a component of the vessel wall.[128] The dose of factor IX can be estimated by assuming that 1 U of factor IX per kilogram body weight increases circulating factor IX by 1 percent of normal or 0.01 U/mL.[129] Thus, to achieve 100 percent of normal (using only highly purified factor IX products) in a severely affected patient, 100 U of factor IX per kilogram body weight should be given as a bolus, followed by half this amount every 12 to 18 hours. Dosing should be monitored by assays of factor IX before and after bolus administration. Factor IX also can be administered as a constant infusion in hospitalized patients after the bolus administration. The dose of factor IX to be infused per hour can be estimated based on a factor IX half-life of 18 to 24 hours. Thus, in a 60-kg adult who receives highly purified factor IX, 6000 U of the factor should raise the factor IX level to approximately 100 percent of normal. Over the next 12 to 18 hours, the level decreases by approximately 50 percent. Thus, the patient needs approximately 3000 U of factor IX during that period or 250 U of factor IX per hour as an infusion.[129] These calculations are only estimates of average responses, so factor IX dosing should be monitored by factor IX assays and the dose adjusted appropriately. Prophylactic therapy for hemophilia B also can be attempted in individuals selected in the same manner as that described for hemophilia A patients. The prophylactic dose of factor IX is 25 to 40 U/kg of body weight two times per week.

Although currently available factor IX concentrates are safe in terms of transmission of HIV and hepatitis B and C viruses, patients treated prior to 1985 may have been infected with these agents.

TABLE 124–9. Currently Available Factor IX Products*

	Origin	Viral Inactivation
Intermediate purity (prothrombin complex concentrates)		
Profilnine SD	Plasma	Solvent-detergent
Bebulin VH	Plasma	Vapor heating
High purity		
Mononine	Plasma	Ultra filtration; chemical
AlphaNine	Plasma	Solvent-detergent; virus filtered
Recombinant		
BeneFIX	CHO cells	Nanofiltration

*Additional factor IX concentrates are available in Europe.

COURSE AND PROGNOSIS

Unless treated properly, severe hemophilia B is fraught with the same complications of recurrent hemorrhages as hemophilia A. Thus, hemarthroses and chronic hemophilic arthropathy are common in inadequately treated patients. In addition to joint deformities, chronic active hepatitis and chronic persistent hepatitis are common in patients treated before 1985. Approximately 50 percent of older and severely affected patients now are HIV-positive. Patients treated after 1985 are not likely to have contracted HIV and can expect to have a relatively normal life span.

Patients with severe hemophilia B may develop inhibitory antibodies against factor IX, making treatment very difficult.[130,131] Approximately 3 percent of patients with severe hemophilia B develop specific inhibitor antibodies, frequently restricted in immunoglobulin composition to the IgG_4 subclass and κ light chains.[131] Most inhibitors can be detected when the aPTT of a mixture of normal plasma and the patient's plasma is prolonged. In contrast to the inhibitors in hemophilia A patients, inhibitor antibodies against factor IX are not time and temperature dependent; thus, incubating the mixtures for 2 hours at 37°C (98.6°F) usually is unnecessary. Inhibitors to factor IX can be quantitated by modifying the Bethesda method for detecting factor VIII inhibitors. Many patients with inhibitors have mutations that result in the absence of circulating factor IX antigen, most commonly because of deletions and nonsense mutations.

TREATMENT OF PATIENTS WITH FACTOR IX INHIBITOR ANTIBODIES

When the inhibitor titer is less than 5 BU/mL, the factor IX inhibitor possibly can be neutralized using large doses of highly purified factor IX concentrates. However, when the inhibitor titer is greater than 5 BU/mL, acute bleeding in patients should be treated with the same agents used to bypass factor VIII inhibitors (see Table 124–6). Recombinant factor VIIa in doses of 90 to 120 mcg per kilogram body weight administered intravenously every 2 to 3 hours can be used. Alternatively, FEIBA or nonactivated prothrombin complex concentrates can be used (see Table 124–6).

Induction of immune tolerance can be attempted in hemophilia B patients using daily infusions of purified factor IX preparations. However, significant adverse reactions, including anaphylaxis and nephrotic syndrome, have been reported in severely affected patients.[132] Of the reported cases, many patients were younger than age 12 years and suffered from severe hemophilia B as a result of large deletions of the factor IX gene. The nephrotic syndrome may be transient and remit upon cessation of factor IX replacement. The pathogenesis of the nephrotic syndrome is not known. Patients with hemophilia B and factor IX antibodies who experience anaphylaxis with factor IX infusions should be treated with factor VIIa concentrates because both unactivated prothrombin complex concentrates and FEIBA contain factor IX.[132]

GENE THERAPY FOR HEMOPHILIA B

Long-term correction of hemophilia B has been achieved in animal models.[133] Transduction of muscle cells by an adeno-associated virus (AAV) vector containing a factor IX construct resulted in phenotypic correction of the clotting defect in hemophilia B dogs for more than 17 months.[133] Likewise, transduction of hepatocytes with an AAV vector containing factor IX DNA reportedly corrected the hemophilia defect in hemophilia B mice and dogs for approximately 7 and 8 months, respectively. Sustained factor IX levels up to 25 percent of normal were obtained in one study in mice,[134] whereas levels exceeding 100 percent were achieved in another study.[135] The results in animals are encouraging and suggest that corrections of the hemophilic defect using gene transfer technology in humans are possible. Clinical trials of gene transfer therapy for hemophilia B in humans are not in progress, but investigations in animals continue.[125] Recent studies in hemophilia A and B dogs reveal that the insertion of the factor VIIa gene into the liver results in long-term expression of factor VIIa with the result that bleeding in these dogs is virtually eliminated.[136] In earlier experiments, it was shown that long-term expression of factor VIIa in hemophilia B mice also could correct the bleeding defect and was safe at low doses, but when expressed in high doses, death occurred as a result of pulmonary and cardiac thrombi.[137] Although gene transfer trials for hemophilic patients currently are suspended, ongoing studies of new vectors and in animal models of hemophilia are encouraging.

SPECIAL PROBLEMS ASSOCIATED WITH HEMOPHILIA A AND B

Unusual problems are occasionally encountered in both hemophilias A and B. Some of these are discussed at www.isth-forum.org, and some are summarized in a brief publication.[138] For example, scuba diving can be dangerous in severely affected hemophiliacs and should be avoided. Hemophilic patients requiring laser treatment for visual problems may not require replacement therapy provided that a surgical incision is not required during such therapy. Carriers of either hemophilia A or B may have bleeding problems during delivery and will require replacement therapy. Carriers whose fetuses have hemophilia may require cesarean section if vaginal delivery is found to be difficult. Forceps and mechanical devices should be avoided during delivery of infants who are hemophilic. Some patients with hemophilia may also have another familial bleeding disorder, such as VWD.

Hemophilic patients requiring valve replacement should receive a biologic rather than a mechanical valve when possible. Obviously valve replacement can only be carried out following replacement therapy for major surgery.

The deficiency of either factor VIII or IX seems to provide some protection against thrombosis.[139] However, myocardial infarction has been reported in hemophilic patients even without treatment.[139] Deep venous thrombosis (DVT) has also been reported following replacement therapy in both hemophilias A and B. Acute DVT can be treated with heparin for 7 to 10 days as long as the patient receives replacement therapy. Thereafter, anticoagulation is not recommended. Thromboembolic episodes in hemophilia B are much less common since the advent of highly purified factor IX products.

Hemophilia patients who have atrial fibrillation should undergo cardioversion when possible. If cardioversion is not successful, some physicians recommend treatment with aspirin but coumarin therapy is not recommended even in patients with mild disease.[140]

REFERENCES

1. Brinkhous KM: A short history of hemophilia, with some comments on the word "hemophilia," in *Handbook of Hemophilia*, edited by KM Brinkhous, HC Hemker, p 3. Elsevier, New York, 1975.
2. Katznelson JL: Hemophilia, with special reference to the Talmud. *Harofe Haivri Heb Med J* 1:165, 1958.
3. Morawitz P: Die Chemie der Blutgerinnung. *Ergeb Physiol* 4:307, 1905.
4. Addis T: The pathogenesis of hereditary haemophilia. *J Pathol Bacteriol* 15:427, 1911.
5. Brinkhous KM: A study of the clotting defect in hemophilia. The delayed formation of thrombin. *Am J Med Sci* 198:509, 1939.
6. Pavlovsky A: Contribution to the pathogenesis of hemophilia. *Blood* 2:185, 1947.
7. Aggeler PM, White SG, Glendenning MB: Plasma thromboplastin component (PTC) deficiency: A new disease resembling hemophilia. *Proc Soc Exp Biol Med* 79:692, 1952.
8. Biggs R, Douglas AS, Macfarlane AG, et al: Christmas disease: A condition previously mistaken for hemophilia. *Br Med J* 2:1378, 1952.

8a. Tagariello G, Lorio A, Santagustino E, et al: Comparison of the rates of joint arthroplasty in patients with severe factor VIII and IX deficiency: An index of different clinical severity of the 2 coagulation disorders. *Blood* 114:779, 2009.

9. Davie EW, Ratnoff OD: Waterfall sequence for intrinsic blood clotting. *Science* 145:1310, 1964.
10. Macfarlane RG: An enzyme cascade in the blood clotting mechanism, and its function as a biological amplifier. *Nature* 202:498, 1964.
11. Broze GR Jr: Tissue factor pathway inhibitor and the revised theory of coagulation. *Annu Rev Med* 46:103, 1995.
12. Fay PJ: Reconstitution of human factor VIII from isolated subunits. *Arch Biochem Biophys* 262:525, 1988.
13. Roberts HR: Contributions to the evolution of knowledge about hereditary hemorrhagic disorders. *Cell Mol Life Sci* 64:517, 2007.
14. Hoffman M, Hargen A, Lewkowski A, et al: Cutaneous wound healing is impaired in hemophilia B. *Blood* 108:3053, 2006.
15. Tuddenham EGD: Factor VIII, in *Molecular Basis of Thrombosis and Hemostasis*, edited by KA High, HR Roberts, p 167. Marcel Dekker, New York, 1995.
16. Hemophilia A mutation, structure, test and resource site (HAMSTeRS). Available at: http://europium.csc.mrc.ac.uk.
17. Tuddenham EGD, Cooper DN, Gitschier J, et al: Haemophilia A: Database of nucleotide substitutions, deletions, insertions and rearrangements of the factor VIII gene. *Nucleic Acids Res* 22:4851, 1996.
18. Lakich D, Kazazian HH, Antonarakis SE, Gitschier J: Inversions disrupting the factor VIII gene are a common cause of severe hemophilia A. *Nat Genet* 5:236, 1993.
19. Higuchi M, Kazazian HH Jr, Kasch L, et al: Molecular characterization of severe hemophilia A suggests that about half the mutations are not within the coding regions and splice junctions of the factor VIII gene. *Proc Natl Acad Sci U S A* 88:7405, 1991.
20. Gitschier J, Kogan S, Diamond C, Levinson B: Genetic basis of hemophilia A. *Thromb Haemost* 66:37, 1991.
21. Bagnall RD, Waseem N, Green PM, Giannelli F: Recurrent inversion breaking intron 1 of the factor VIII gene is a frequent cause of severe hemophilia A. *Blood* 99:168, 2002.
22. Antonarakis SE, Youssoufian H, Kazazian H: Molecular genetics of hemophilia in man (factor VIII deficiency). *Mol Biol Med* 4:81, 1987.
23. Mori PG, Pasino M, Vadala CR, et al: Haemophilia "A" in a 46Xi(Xq) female. *Br J Haematol* 43:143, 1979.

24. Green PP, Mannucci PM, Briet E, et al: Carrier detection in hemophilia A: A cooperative international study. *Blood* 67:1560, 1986.
25. Peake IR, Lillicrap DP, Boulyjenkov V, et al: Report of a joint WHO/WFH meeting on control of haemophilia: Carrier detection and prenatal diagnosis. *Blood Coagul Fibrinolysis* 4:313, 1993.
26. Ljung RC: Prenatal diagnosis of haemophilia. *Haemophilia* 5:84, 1999.
27. Goodeve AC, Peake IR: Diagnosis of hemophilia A and B carriers and prenatal diagnosis, in *Haemophilia*, edited by CD Forbes, L Aledort, R Madhok, p 63. Chapman & Hall, London, 1997.
28. Poon MC, Hoar DI, Low S, et al: Hemophilia A carrier detection by restriction fragment length polymorphism analysis and discriminant analysis based on ELISA of factor VIII and vWf. *J Lab Clin Med* 119:751, 1992.
29. Nichols WC, Amano K, Cacheris PM, et al: Moderation of hemophilia A phenotype by the factor V R506Q mutation. *Blood* 88:1183, 1996.
30. Arbini AA, Mannucci PM, Bauer K: Low prevalence of the factor V Leiden mutation among "severe" hemophiliacs with a "milder" bleeding diathesis. *Thromb Haemost* 74:1255, 1995.
31. Gilbert MS: Musculoskeletal complications of haemophilia: The joint. *Haemophilia* 6:34, 2000.
32. Jansen NA, Rosendaal G, Lafeber FP: Understanding haemophilic arthropathy: An exploration of current issues. *Br J Haematol* 143:632, 2008.
33. Gilbert MS: The hemophilic pseudotumor. *Prog Clin Biol Res* 324:257, 1990.
34. Subasi M, Direr A, Kapukaya A, et al: Successful treatment of hemophilic pseudotumor by radiotherapy. *Ann Plast Surg* 59:338, 2007.
35. Hanley JP, Ludlam CA: Central and peripheral nervous system bleeding, in *Hemophilia*, edited by CD Forbes, L Aledort, R Madhok, p 87. Chapman & Hall, London, 1997.
36. Kulkarni R, Lusher J: Intracranial and intracranial hemorrhages in newborns with hemophilia: A review of the literature. *J Pediatr Hematol Oncol* 21:254, 1999.
37. Schulman S, Rehnberg AS, Hein M, et al: *Helicobacter pylori* causes gastrointestinal hemorrhage in patients with congenital disorders. *Thromb Haemost* 89:741, 2003.
38. Griffin PH, Chopra S: Spontaneous intramural gastric hematoma: A unique presentation for hemophilia. *Am J Gastroenterol* 80:430, 1985.
39. Cinotti S, Longo G, Messori A, et al: Reproducibility of one-stage, two-stage and chromogenic assays of factor VIII activity: A multi-center study. *Thromb Res* 61:385, 1991.
40. Hoyer LW, Breckenridge RT: Immunologic studies of antihemophilic factor (AHF, factor VIII): Cross-reacting material in a genetic variant of hemophilia A. *Blood* 32:962, 1968.
41. Morales-de la Vega A, Reyes-Maldonado E, Martinez-Murillo E, Quintano-Gonzalez S: Type 2N von Willebrand disease (Normandy). *Rev Med Inst Mex Seguro Soc* 46:55, 2008.
42. Tully EA, Gaucher C, Jorieux S, et al: Expression of von Willebrand factor "Normandy." An autosomal mutation that mimics hemophilia A. *Proc Natl Acad Sci U S A* 88:6377, 1991.
43. Jorieux S, Tuley EA, Gaucher C, et al: The mutation Arg (53)→Trp causes von Willebrand disease Normandy by abolishing binding to factor VIII. Studies with recombinant von Willebrand factor. *Blood* 79:563, 1992.
44. Seligsohn U, Zwang E, Zivelin A: Combined factor V and factor VIII deficiency among non-Ashkenazi Jews. *N Engl J Med* 307:1191, 1982.
45. Ginsberg D: Identifying novel genetic determinants of hemostatic balance. *J Thromb Haemost* 8:1561, 2005.
46. Santagostino E, Mannucci PM, Gringeri A, et al: Transmission of parvovirus B19 by coagulation factor concentrates exposed to 100 degrees C of heat after lyophilization. *Transfusion* 37:517, 1997.
47. Robertson BH, Alter MJ, Bell BP, et al: Hepatitis A virus sequence detected in clotting factor concentrates associated with disease transmission. *Biologicals* 26:95, 1998.
48. Llewelyn CA, Hewitt PE, Knight RS, et al: Possible transmission of variant Creutzfeldt-Jakob disease by blood transfusion. *Lancet* 363:411, 2004.
49. World Federation of Hemophilia website. Available at: www.wfh.org.
50. International Society on Thrombosis and Haemostasis website. Available at: www.med.unc.edu/isth/welcome.
51. Turner ML, Ludlam CA: An update on the assessment and management of the risk of transmission of variant Creutzfeldt-Jakob disease by blood and plasma products. *Br J Haematol* 144:14, 2009.
52. Ludlam CA, Powderly WG, Bozzette S, et al: Clinical perspectives of emerging pathogens in bleeding disorders. *Lancet* 367:252, 2006.
53. Escobar MA: Treatment on demand—*In vivo* dose finding studies. *Haemophilia* 9:360, 2003.
54. McMillan CW, Webster WP, Roberts HR, Blythe WB: Continuous intravenous infusion of factor VIII in classic hemophilia. *Br J Haematol* 18:659, 1972.
55. Schulman S: Continuous infusion. *Haemophilia* 9:368, 2003.
56. Rodeghiero F, Castaman G, Di Bona E, Ruggeri M: Consistency of responses to repeated DDAVP infusions in patients with von Willebrand's disease and hemophilia A. *Blood* 74:1997, 1989.
57. Mannucci PM, Bettega D, Cattaneo M: Patterns of development of tachyphylaxis in patients with haemophilia and von Willebrand disease after repeated doses of desmopressin (DDAVP). *Br J Haematol* 82:87, 1992.
58. Porte RJ, Leebeek FW: Pharmacological strategies to decrease transfusion requirements in patients undergoing surgery. *Drugs* 62:2193, 2002.
59. Ghosh K, Shetty S, Jijina F, Mohanty D: Role of epsilon amino caproic acid in the management of haemophilic patients with inhibitors. *Haemophilia* 10:58, 2004.
60. Martinowitz U, Saltz R: Fibrin sealant. *Curr Opin Hematol* 3:395, 1996.
61. Ortel TL, Charles LA, Keller FG, et al: Topical thrombin and acquired coagulation factor inhibitors: Clinical spectrum and laboratory diagnosis. *Am J Hematol* 45:128, 1994.
62. Revel-Vilk S, Golomb MR, Achonu C, et al: Effect of intracranial bleeds on the health and quality of life of boys with hemophilia. *J Pediatr* 144: 490, 2004.
63. Rodriguez-Merchan EC: Orthopaedic surgery in persons with haemophilia. *Thromb Haemost* 89:34, 2003.
64. Rabiner SF, Telfer MC: Home transfusion for patients with hemophilia A. *N Engl J Med* 283:1011, 1977.
65. Teitel JM, Barnard D, Israels S, et al: Home management of haemophilia. *Haemophilia* 10:118, 2004.
66. Manco-Johnson MJ, Riske B, Kasper CK: Advances in care of children with hemophilia. *Semin Thromb Hemost* 29:585, 2003.
67. Nilsson IM, Berntorp E, Lofqvist T, Pettersson H: Twenty-five years' experience of prophylactic treatment in severe haemophilia A and B. *J Intern Med* 232:25, 1992.
68. Manco-Johnson MJ, Abshire TC, Shapiro AD et al: Prophylaxis versus episodic treatment to prevent joint disease in boys with severe hemophilia. *N Engl J Med* 357:535, 2007.
69. Price VE, Carcao M, Connolly B, et al: A prospective, longitudinal study of central venous catheter-related deep venous thrombosis in boys with hemophilia. *J Thromb Haemost* 2:737, 2004.
70. Lofqvist T, Nilsson IM, Berntorp E, Pettersson H: Haemophilia prophylaxis in young patients—A long-term follow-up. *J Intern Med* 241:395, 1997.
71. Globe DR, Curtis RG, Koerper MA: Utilization of care in haemophilia: A resource-based method for cost analysis from the Haemophilia Utilization Group Study (HUGS). *Haemophilia* 10(Suppl 1):63, 2004.
72. Bontempo FA, Lewis JH, Gorenc TJ, et al: Liver transplantation in hemophilia A. *Blood* 69:1721, 1987.
73. Wilde J, Teixeira P, Bramhall SR, et al: Liver transplantation in haemophilia. *Br J Haematol* 117:952, 2002.
74. Roth DA, Tawa NE Jr, O'Brien JM, et al: Nonviral transfer of the gene encoding coagulation factor VIII in patients with severe hemophilia A. *N Engl J Med* 344:1735, 2001.
75. Powell JS, Ragni MV, White GC 2nd, et al: Phase 1 trial of FVIII gene transfer for severe hemophilia A using a retroviral construct administered by peripheral intravenous infusion. *Blood* 102:2038, 2003.
76. Pipe SW: Coagulation factors with improved properties for hemophilia gene therapy. *Semin Thromb Hemost* 30:227, 2004.
77. Kaufman RJ: Good things come in small packages for hemophilia. *J Thromb Haemost* 1:2472, 2003.
78. Wilcox DA, Shi Q, Nurden P, et al: Induction of megakaryocytes to synthesize and store a releasable pool of human factor VIII. *J Thromb Haemost* 1:274, 2003.
79. Miao HZ, Sirachainan N, Palmer L, et al: Bioengineering of coagulation factor VIII for improved secretion. *Blood* 103:3412, 2004.
80. Pierce GF, Lillicrap D, Pipe SW, Vandendriessche T: Gene therapy, bioengineered clotting factors and novel technologies for hemophilia treatment. *J Thromb Haemost* 5:901, 2007.
81. Levetow LB, Sox HCJ, Stoto MA: *HIV and the Blood Supply: An Analysis of Crisis Decision Making, Institute of Medicine*, p 1. National Academy Press, Washington, DC, 1994.
82. Santagostino E, De Filippi F, Rumi MG, et al: Sustained suppression of hepatitis C virus by high doses of interferon and ribavirin in adult hemophilic patients. *Transfusion* 44:790, 2004.
83. Lollar P: Pathogenic antibodies to coagulation factors: I. Factor VIII and factor IX. *J Thromb Haemost* 2:1082, 2004.
84. Goodeve A: The incidence of inhibitor development according to specific mutations—And treatment? *Blood Coagul Fibrinolysis* 14(Suppl 1):17, 2003.
85. Lusher JM: Is the incidence and prevalence of inhibitors greater with recombinant products? No. *J Thromb Haemost* 2:863, 2004.
86. Aledort L: Is the incidence and prevalence of inhibitors greater with recombinant products? Yes. *J Thromb Haemost* 2:861, 2004.
87. Hoots WK, Lusher J: High-titer inhibitor development in hemophilia A: Lack of product specificity. *J Thromb Haemost* 2:358, 2004.
88. Gouw SC, van der Bom JG, Auerswald G, et al: Recombinant versus plasma-derived factor VIII products and the development of inhibitors in previously untreated patients with severe hemophilia A: The CANAL cohort study. *Blood* 109:4693, 2007.
89. ter Avest PC, Fischer K, Mancuso ME, et al: Risk stratification for inhibitor development at first treatment for severe hemophilia A: A tool for clinical practice. *J Thromb Haemost* 6:2048, 2008.
90. Gouw SC, van den Berg HM, le Cessie S, van der Bom JG: Treatment characteristics and the risk of inhibitor development: a multicenter cohort study among previously untreated patients with severe hemophilia A. *Blood* 109:4648, 2007.
91. Peerlinck K, Arnout J, Gilles JH, et al: A higher than expected incidence of factor VIII inhibitors in multitransfused haemophilia A patients treated with an intermittent purity pasteurized factor VIII concentrate. *Thromb Haemost* 69:115, 1993.
92. Parker ET, Healey JF, Barrow RT, et al: Reduction of the inhibitory antibody response to human factor VIII in hemophilia A mice by mutagenesis of the A2 domain B cell epitope. *Blood* 104:704, 2004.
93. Kasper CK: Laboratory tests for factor VIII inhibitors, their variation, significance and interpretation. *Blood Coagul Fibrinolysis* 2:S7, 1991.

94. Verbruggen B, Novakova I, Wessels H, et al: The Nijmegen modification of the Bethesda assay for factor VIII:C inhibitors: Improved specificity and reliability and specificity. *Thromb Haemost* 73:247, 1995.
95. Roberts HR: The use of agents that by-pass factor VIII inhibitors in patients with hemophilia. *Vox Sang* 77(Suppl 1):38, 1999.
96. Monroe DM, Roberts HR: Mechanism of action of high-dose factor VIIa: Points of agreement and disagreement. *Arterioscler Thromb Vasc Biol* 23:8, 2003.
97. Varadi K, Negrier C, Berntorp E, et al: Monitoring the bioavailability of FEIBA with a thrombin generation assay. *J Thromb Haemost* 1:2374, 2003.
98. Tjønnfjord GE: Surgery in patients with hemophilia and inhibitors: A review of the Norwegian experience with FEIBA. *Semin Hematol* 43(2 Suppl 4):S18, 2006.
99. Toomey JR, Blackburn MN, Storer BL, et al: Comparing the antithrombotic efficacy of a humanized anti-factor IX(a) monoclonal antibody (SB 249417) to the low-molecular-weight heparin enoxaparin in a rat model of arterial thrombosis. *Thromb Res* 100:73, 2000.
100. Makris M: Systematic review of the management of patients with haemophilia A and inhibitors. *Blood Coagul Fibrinolysis* 15(Suppl 1):S25, 2004.
101. Brackmann HH, Effenberger W, Heiss L, et al: Immune tolerance induction: A role for recombinant activated factor VII (rVIIa)? *Eur J Haematol* 63:18, 1998.
102. Kempton CL, White CG II: How we treat a patient with a factor VIII inhibitor. *Blood* 113:11, 2009.
103. White CG II, Kempton CL, Grimsley A, et al: Cellular immune responses in hemophilia: why do inhibitors develop in some but not all hemophiliacs. *J Thromb Haemost* 3:1676, 2005.
104. Lemon SM, Becherer PR, Wang JG, et al: Hepatitis delta infection among multiply-transfused hemophiliacs. *Prog Clin Biol Res* 364:351, 1991.
105. Rosina F, Saracco G, Rizzetto M: Risk of post-transfusion infection with the hepatitis delta virus. A multicenter study. *N Engl J Med* 312:1488, 1985.
106. Gerritzen A, Brackmann H, Van Loo B, et al: Chronic delta hepatitis in haemophiliacs. *J Med Virol* 34:188, 1991.
107. Gotto J, Dusheiko GM: Hepatitis C and treatment with pegylated interferon and ribavirin. *Int J Biochem Cell Biol* 36:1874, 2004.
108. Gjerset GF, Clements MJ, Counts RB, et al: Treatment type and amount influenced human immunodeficiency virus seroprevalence of patients with congenital bleeding disorders. *Blood* 78:1623, 1991.
109. Prusiner SB: Molecular biology of prion diseases. *Science* 252:1515, 1991.
110. Shanbrom E, Owens W: Cascade iodination: a novel method to enhance the safety and efficacy of therapeutic proteins. *J Thromb Haemost* 2:836, 2004.
111. Lee CA, Ironside JW, Bell JE, et al: Retrospective neuropathological review of prion disease in U.K. haemophilic patients. *Thromb Haemost* 80:909, 1998.
112. Farrugia A: Risk of variant Creutzfeldt-Jakob disease from factor concentrates: Current perspectives. *Haemophilia* 8:350, 2002.
113. Report put on the World Federation of Hemophilia website. Available at: www.wfh.org.
114. Kurachi K, Davie EW: Isolation and characterization of a cDNA coding for factor IX. *Proc Natl Acad Sci U S A* 79:6461, 1982.
115. Noyes CM, Griffith MJ, Roberts HR, Lundblad RL: Identification of the molecular defect in factor IX Chapel Hill: Substitution of a histidine for an arginine at position 145. *Proc Natl Acad Sci U S A* 80:4200, 1983.
116. http://www.kcl.ac.uk/ip/petergreen/intro.html
117. Monroe DM, McCord DM, Huang MN, et al: Functional consequences of an arginine 180 to glutamine mutation in factor IX Hilo. *Blood* 73:1540, 1989.
118. Bertina RM, van der Linden IK, Mannucci PM, et al: Mutations in hemophilia Bm occur at the Arg180-Val activation site or in the catalytic domain of factor IX. *J Biol Chem* 265:10876, 1990.
119. Bottema CD, Ketterling RP, Ii S, et al: Missense mutations and evolutionary conservation of amino acids: Evidence that many of the amino acids in factor IX function as "spacer" elements. *Am J Hum Genet* 49:820, 1991.
120. Ketterling RP, Bottema CD, Phillips JA III, Sommer SS: Evidence that descendants of three founders constitute about 25% of hemophilia B in the United States. *Genomics* 10:1093, 1991.
121. Briet E, Bertina RM, van Tilburg NH, Veltkamp JJ: Hemophilia B Leyden: A sex-linked hereditary disorder that improves after puberty. *N Engl J Med* 306:788, 1982.
122. Crossley M, Ludwig M, Stowell KM, et al: Recovery from hemophilia B Leyden: An androgen-responsive element in the factor IX promoter. *Science* 257:377, 1992.
123. Reijnen MJ, Sladek FM, Bertina RM, Reitsma PH: Disruption of a binding site for hepatocyte nuclear factor 4 results in hemophilia B Leyden. *Proc Natl Acad Sci U S A* 89:6300, 1992.
124. Hamaguchi N, Roberts H, Stafford DW: Mutations in the catalytic region of factor IX that are related to the subclass hemophilia Bm. *Biochemistry* 32:6324, 1993.
125. Lusher JM, McMillan CW: Severe factor VIII and factor IX deficiency in females. *Am J Med* 65:637, 1978.
126. McGraw RA, Davis LM, Lundblad RL, et al: Structure and function of factor IX: Defects in haemophilia B. *Clin Haematol* 14:359, 1985.
127. White GC, Bebe A, Nielsen B: Recombinant factor IX. *Thromb Haemost* 78:261, 1997.
128. Wolberg AS, Stafford DW, Erie DA: Human factor IX binds to specific sites on the collagenous domain of collagen IV. *J Biol Chem* 272:16717, 1997.
129. Kim HC, McMillan CW, White GC, et al: Purified factor IX using monoclonal immunoaffinity technique: Clinical trials in hemophilia B and comparison to prothrombin complex concentrates. *Blood* 79:568, 1992.
130. Briet E, Reisner HM, Roberts HR: Inhibitors in Christmas disease, in *Factor VIII Inhibitors*, edited by LW Hoyer, p 408. Alan R. Liss, New York, 1984.
131. High KA: Factor IX: Molecular structure, epitopes, and mutations associated with inhibitor formation, in *Inhibitors to Coagulation Factors*, edited by LM Aledort, LW Hoyer, JM Lusher, HM Reisner, CG White, p 79. Plenum, New York, 1995.
132. Warrier I, Ewenstein BM, Koerper MA, et al: Factor IX inhibitors and anaphylaxis in hemophilia B. *J Pediatr Hematol Oncol* 19:23, 1997.
133. Herzog RW, Yang EY, Couto LB, et al: Long term correction of hemophilia B by gene transfer of blood coagulation factor IX mediated by adeno-associated viral vector. *Nat Med* 5:56, 1999.
134. Arruda VR, Schuettrumpf J, Herzog RW, et al: Safety and efficacy of factor IX gene transfer to skeletal muscle in murine and canine hemophilia B models by adeno-associated viral vector serotype 1. *Blood* 103:85, 2004.
135. Kaiser J: Gene therapy: Side effects sideline hemophilia trial. *Science* 304:1423, 2004.
136. Margaritis P, Roy E, Aljamali MN, Downey HD, et al: Successful treatment of canine hemophilia by continuous expression of canine FVIIa. *Blood* 113:3682, 2009.
137. Aljamali MN, Margaritis P, Schlachterman A, et al: Long-term expression of murine activated factor VII is safe, but elevated levels cause premature mortality. *J Clin Invest* 118:1825–34, 2008.
138. Roberts HR, Carrizosa D, Ma A (eds): *Haemophilia and Haemostasis: A Case-based Approach to Management*. Blackwell, Oxford, 2007.
139. Girolami A, Ruzzon E, Fabris F, et al: Myocardial infarction and other arterial occlusions in hemophilia A patients. A cardiological evaluation of all 42 cases reported in the literature. *Acta Haemotol* 116:120, 2006.
140. Brand B: Anticoagulation for atrial fibrillation in a haemophiliac, in *Haemophilia and Haemostasis: A Case-based Approach to Management*, edited by HR Roberts, D Carrizosa, A Ma, p. 43. Blackwell, Oxford, 2007.

CHAPTER 125

INHERITED DEFICIENCIES OF COAGULATION FACTORS II, V, VII, X, XI, AND XIII AND COMBINED DEFICIENCIES OF FACTORS V AND VIII AND OF THE VITAMIN K-DEPENDENT FACTORS

Uri Seligsohn, Ariella Zivelin, and Ophira Salomon

SUMMARY

Bleeding tendencies caused by inherited deficiencies of one or more coagulation factors are rare disorders distributed worldwide. Homozygotes or compound heterozygotes for the mutant genes responsible for these defects exhibit bleeding manifestations that are of variable severity and usually related to the extent of the decreased activity of the particular coagulation factor. Heterozygotes for the various deficiencies rarely display a bleeding tendency. Numerous mutations have been identified in genes encoding coagulation factors II, V, VII, X, XI, and XIII. For some factors, such as factors II, VII, and X, mutations giving rise to dysfunctional proteins predominate, whereas for other factors, such as factors V, XI, and XIII, true protein deficiencies usually are found. Combined deficiency of factors V and VIII, inherited as an autosomal recessive trait, results from mutations in genes encoding two proteins that transport factors V and VIII out of the endoplasmic reticulum to the Golgi compartment. The very rare combined deficiency of the vitamin K-dependent coagulation factors can be caused by mutations in the gene encoding for a carboxylase that γ-carboxylates glutamic acid residues in these proteins or in the gene encoding vitamin K epoxide reductase. Treatment of patients with the various coagulation factor deficiencies may be necessary during spontaneous bleeding episodes, during and after surgical procedures, and for prevention of intracranial hemorrhage. In most deficiency states, plasma replacement has been used, but specific concentrates of all the vitamin K-dependent factors and of factors VII, XI, and XIII are available.

Acronyms and abbreviations that appear in this chapter include: aPTT, activated partial thromboplastin time; CRM, cross-reacting material; DIC, disseminated intravascular coagulation; ELISA, enzyme-linked immunosorbent assay; ERGIC, endoplasmic reticulum-Golgi intermediate compartment; GGCX, γ-glutamyl carboxylase; Gla, γ-carboxyglutamic acid; HK, high-molecular-weight kininogen; LMAN1, mannose-binding lectin; MCFD, multiple combined-factor deficiency; MRP, multidrug resistance protein; PAR, protease-activated receptor; PK, prekallikrein; PT, prothrombin time; TAFI, thrombin-activatable fibrinolysis inhibitor; VKDFD, vitamin K-dependent factors deficiency; VKORC1, vitamin K epoxide reductase complex.

Inherited deficiencies of the coagulation factors other than factor VIII (hemophilia A), factor IX (hemophilia B) are rare bleeding disorders that have been described in most populations. Their relative frequency varies among populations partly as a result of high frequencies of specific mutant genes in inbred populations. Several population surveys indicate that common among these bleeding disorders are factors XI and VII deficiency, less common disorders are factors V and X deficiency and afibrinogenemia, and the rarest disorders are factor II (prothrombin) deficiency, combined factor V and VIII deficiency, factor XIII deficiency, and deficiency of all the vitamin K-dependent factors (Table 125–1). The severity of bleeding manifestations in affected patients who are homozygotes or compound heterozygotes for a mutant gene is variable and usually related to the extent of the deficiency. Some patients have only mild bruising or display excessive bleeding only following trauma. Other patients, usually with less than 1 percent of normal factor VII, XIII, or X activity, can exhibit intracranial hemorrhages and hemarthroses similar to patients with severe hemophilias A and B. Heterozygotes for the coagulation factor deficiencies usually do not manifest a bleeding tendency, and if they do, an additional hemostatic disorder should be sought.

The study of these disorders has significantly advanced the understanding of the pathophysiology of blood coagulation mechanisms (see Chap. 115). Following characterization of the genes encoding for the coagulation factors, a host of mutations causing the various deficiencies have been identified (Table 125–2). This chapter reviews the clinical, biochemical, and genetic aspects of the inherited deficiencies of coagulation factors that cause bleeding tendencies other than the hemophilias (see Chap. 124), von Willebrand disease (see Chap. 127), and inherited fibrinogen disorders (see Chap. 126). Published mutations causing the coagulation factor deficiencies reviewed in this chapter and their characteristics have been compiled and placed as supplementary material of this chapter, and on the International Society of Thrombosis and Hemostasis website (www.isth.org) under databases. This list is updated periodically.

FACTOR II DEFICIENCY

DEFINITION

Inherited factor II (prothrombin) deficiency is one of the rarest coagulation factor deficiencies. It presents in two forms: type I, true deficiency (hypoprothrombinemia), and type II, in which dysfunctional prothrombin is produced (dysprothrombinemia). These autosomal recessive disorders are genetically heterogeneous, and characterized by a mild to moderate bleeding tendency. Both types of prothrombin deficiency impair the generation or function of thrombin, the central enzyme of the blood coagulation system.

BIOCHEMISTRY AND MOLECULAR FEATURES

Prothrombin, Mr approximately 72,000, is structurally homologous with other members of the vitamin K-dependent proteins, factors VII, IX, and X, proteins C, S, and Z, and bone γ-carboxyglutamic acid (Gla) protein. Prothrombin is synthesized in the liver as a prepropeptide of 622 amino acids. Its plasma concentration is 100 to 150 mcg/mL and its half-life is 60 to 70 hours (see Chap. 115). Prothrombin is composed of the following domains: a prepropeptide domain (residues –43 to –1), a Gla domain (residues 1–37), kringle 1 domain (F1; residues 38–155), kringle 2 domain (F2; residues 156–271), and catalytic domain (residues 272–579).[1–3] The prepropeptide domain is responsible for protein processing, targeting, and carboxylation, and it is removed prior to secretion from the cell. The Gla domain constitutes the amino-terminus of the mature

TABLE 125–1. Relative Prevalence of Rare Bleeding Disorders*

Deficiency	WFH Survey (2002)†		Six National Registries (2007)†		UK Data (Oct. 2008)‡		Survey of 64 Centers (Aug. 2008)†	
	N	%	N	%	N	%	N	%
Factor XI	2446	35.3	1947	39.4	1762	59.5	770	23.5
Factor VII	1689	24.4	1050	21.3	580	19.6	927	28.3
Afibrinogenemia	644	9.3	496	10.0	203	6.9	241	7.4
Factor X	597	8.6	446	9.0	190	6.4	339	10.4
Factor V	769	11.1	415	8.4	129	4.4	233	7.1
Factor XIII	434	6.3	282	5.7	60	2.0	211	6.5
Factor V/Factor VIII	188	2.7	203	4.1	25	0.8	495	15.1
Factor II	167	2.4	101	2.0	13	0.4	55	1.7
Total	6934	100.1	4940	99.9	2962	100.0	3271	100.0

*Patients with partial deficiency were included.

†Data courtesy of Professor Flora Peyvandi, Milan, Italy.

‡Data courtesy of Professor Paula Bolton-Maggs, Manchester, UK.

prothrombin molecule and contains the 10 glutamic acid residues that are posttranslationally modified through action of vitamin K-dependent carboxylase to Gla. As a result of this modification, prothrombin acquires the capacity to bind calcium and membranes containing acidic phospholipids. The kringle domain contains two extensively folded, disulfide-bonded "kringle" motifs, the functions of which are not fully understood (see Chap. 115).[4] They are present in diverse proteins and are thought to mediate protein–protein interactions. For example, the second kringle mediates interaction of prothrombin with activated factor V (factor Va).[5] The catalytic domain contains the enzyme's active site, which is responsible for fibrinogen cleavage. The residues characteristic for the serine protease family, His363, Asp419, and Ser525, constitute a charge relay system responsible for bond cleavage. The crystal structure of prothrombin has not been determined, but the crystal structure of human α-thrombin complexed with *D-Phe-Pro-Arg chloromethylketone* (an inhibitor that is a transition state analogue covalently bound to the enzyme) has been determined.[6]

The prothrombin gene is located on chromosome 11 near the centromere.[7] It is 20 kb long and consists of 14 exons separated by 13 introns. Comparison of the organization of the prothrombin gene shows homology with the organization of other vitamin K-dependent serine protease genes, with the highest degree of homology in the part encoding the Gla domain. An unusual feature of the prothrombin gene is the presence of 41 copies of Alu-repetitive sequences in the upstream and intervening sequences.[8,9] The function, if any, of these sequences is unknown.

Prothrombin plays a central role in coagulation, functioning in both tissue factor and contact activation pathways. Prothrombin is converted to its proteolytically active form thrombin by the prothrombinase

TABLE 125–2. Mutations Causing Rare Bleeding Disorders

Deficiency	Gene	Total Number	Promoter	Missense	Nonsense	Splicing	Insertion/ Deletion	Gross Deletion
Prothrombin	*F2*	49		38	3	2	5	1
Factor V	*F5*	72		24	10	9	28	1
Factor VII	*F7*	180*	11	115	13	19	19	3
Factor X	*F10*	95		74	1	9	9	2
Factor XI	*F11*	152	1	99	21	16	12	3
Factor XIII	*F13A1*	99	1	45	7	15	28	3
Factor XIII	*F13B1*	4		1		1	2	
Combined factors V and VIII	*LMAN1*	32		2	7	7	16	
Combined factors V and VIII	*MCFD2*	15		5	1	3	5	1
Vitamin K-dependent factors	*GGCX*	8		6		2		
Vitamin K-dependent factors	*VKORC1*	1		1				

*Forty-one additional mutations were reported but not included because no information about the patients was disclosed.[66,98]

complex consisting of activated factor X (factor Xa), factor Va, and phospholipid surface of platelets and other cells (see Chap. 115). Two forms of thrombin are generated: meizothrombin if prothrombin is cleaved at residue 320, and α-thrombin if cleavage occurs first at residue 271, removing prothrombin fragment 1.2, and subsequently cleaved at residue 320. The α-thrombin A-chain (residues 272–320) formed by factor Xa cleavage is encoded by exons 8 and 9. The B-chain (residues 321–579) containing the catalytic site and regulatory elements is encoded by exons 9 to 14.

Thrombin is a multifunctional serine protease. In addition to converting fibrinogen to fibrin (see Chap. 126), thrombin also activates (1) platelets by cleavage of the protease-activated receptor (PAR)-1 and PAR-4, initiating signals leading to adhesion and aggregation; (2) factors V, VIII, and XI, yielding factors Va, VIIIa, and XIa, which promote the generation of additional thrombin; (3) factor XIII, which leads to crosslinking of fibrin; (4) plasminogen, converting it to plasmin and thereby activating the fibrinolytic system; (5) thrombin-activatable fibrinolysis inhibitor (TAFI), which leads to fibrinolysis inhibition; and (6) protein C after binding to thrombomodulin in the presence of endothelial protein C receptor (see Chap. 116). Thrombin also stimulates wound healing through its action as a growth factor and its proangiogenic activity.[10]

GENETICS

Abnormalities of prothrombin are inherited in an autosomal recessive manner. Among individuals with type I deficiency, heterozygotes exhibit prothrombin levels that are approximately 50 percent of normal, whereas homozygotes display levels that typically are less than 10 percent of normal. Prothrombin activity and antigen levels are reduced concordantly in these patients, who are designated as cross-reacting material (CRM) negative (CRM^-). Heterozygotes for type II deficiency exhibit a prothrombin activity level approximately 50 percent of normal, with antigen levels that are normal or nearly normal. Homozygotes for type II deficiency display a prothrombin activity level 1 to 20 percent of normal, with antigen levels that are either normal (CRM^+) or partially reduced (CRM^{red}). Compound heterozygotes with one type I deficiency allele and one type II deficiency allele have been reported. They typically have a prothrombin activity level between 1 and 20 percent, with antigen levels between 13 and 50 percent of normal. Undetectable plasma prothrombin probably is incompatible with life, as inferred from the embryonic and neonatal lethality of prothrombin knockout mice.[11]

Forty-nine mutations that cause prothrombin deficiency have been identified, of which 38 are missense, 3 nonsense, 6 deletions/insertions, and 2 splicing mutations (see Table 125–2). Type II deficiency (dysprothrombinemias) results from missense mutations that are located throughout the gene. However, many mutations are in the catalytic domain, imparting dysfunction of thrombin (Arg418Trp [Tokushima, Molise], Met337Thr [Himi I], Arg388His [Himi II], Arg382His, Arg382Cys [Quick I, Corpus Christi], Gly558Val [Quick II], Glu466Ala [Salakta, Frankfurt], Arg517Gln [Greenville], Gly548Ala [Perija], Lys556Thr [Scranton]).[12–21] Other mutations give rise to abnormally slow activation of prothrombin (Arg271Cys [Barcelona, Madrid, Obihirio], Arg271His [Padual, Dhahran], Arg320His [San Antonio], Arg457Gln [Puerto Rico I]).[22–25] Only 10 mutations were identified in patients with type I deficiency, of which 5 were present in homozygotes. Two mutations clustered in distinct populations suggest common ancestry: prothrombin Puerto Rico I reported in several unrelated families from Puerto Rico,[25] and prothrombin Perija, which is found in 35 percent of Yukba Indians living in a small village in Venezuela.[26,27]

A number of polymorphisms have been identified in the prothrombin gene. One of these polymorphisms, a G>A change at nucleotide 20210 in the 3′ untranslated region of the prothrombin gene, is associated with increased plasma levels of prothrombin and an increased tendency to venous thrombosis (see Chap. 131).[28,29]

CLINICAL MANIFESTATIONS

Inherited types I and II deficiencies are characterized by mild to moderate mucocutaneous and soft-tissue bleeding that usually correlates with the degree of functional prothrombin deficiency. With prothrombin levels of approximately 1 percent of normal, bleeding may occur spontaneously or following trauma. Surgical bleeding may be significant. Menorrhagia, epistaxis, gingival bleeding, easy bruising, and subcutaneous hematomas may occur. Hemarthrosis has been observed, but is less frequent than in the hemophilias. In patients with prothrombin activities 2 to 5 percent of normal, bleeding is variable. Some individuals bleed following minimal trauma, whereas others are asymptomatic. Patients with prothrombin activity 5 to 50 percent of normal usually bleed only following major trauma and surgery, or they do not bleed at all.

DIFFERENTIAL DIAGNOSIS

The activated partial thromboplastin time (aPTT) and prothrombin time (PT) are variably prolonged in inherited hypoprothrombinemia and dysprothrombinemia. The diagnosis of all prothrombin abnormalities is established by demonstrating decreased functional levels of prothrombin. Determination of both functional and antigenic levels of prothrombin distinguishes among CRM^-, CRM^+ and CRM^{red} prothrombin deficiencies.

Acquired prothrombin deficiency occurs in patients with liver disease, in patients on oral anticoagulant therapy, and, rarely, in patients who develop nonneutralizing antibodies against prothrombin that remove prothrombin from the circulation and cause a significant bleeding tendency. Such antibodies to prothrombin have been described in patients with lupus anticoagulant (the hypoprothrombinemia–lupus anticoagulant syndrome), malignant lymphoma, or in patients with no underlying disorder (see Chap. 132). A family study is helpful in establishing the diagnosis of an inherited deficiency.

Prothrombin can be activated by enzymes of several snake venoms, and the pattern of activation can provide clues to the nature of the prothrombin abnormality. Activation of prothrombin by *Taipan* viper venom and by *Pseudonaja textilis* venom is independent of factor V. Thus, normal Taipan viper venom or *P. textilis* venom times with an abnormal classic one-stage assay for prothrombin implies a defect in the region of prothrombin that binds factor V. *Echis carinatus* venom activates prothrombin in the absence of factor V, phospholipid, and calcium and therefore can be used with other prothrombin activators to test the requirement for each of these components.

Plasma prothrombin immunoelectrophoresis is useful for the diagnosis of dysprothrombinemias. Prolonged aPTT and PT with a normal thrombin time are seen in inherited factor V and factor X deficiency, acquired conditions such as vitamin K deficiency, therapeutic or surreptitious use of warfarin, liver disease, and lupus anticoagulants. These various disorders are readily distinguished by taking the patient's history and performing additional factor assays (see Chap. 118).

THERAPY

Replacement therapy in patients with inherited prothrombin deficiency consists of administration of prothrombin complex concentrates containing coagulation factors II, VII, IX, and X. These concentrates are heated or treated with solvent–detergent, processes that remove HIV, hepatitis B, hepatitis C, and other viruses, but which do not remove parvovirus B19 or hepatitis A virus[30–32]; the latter viruses can be effectively removed by dry heat and nanofiltration.[33] However, transmission of other possible bloodborne agents, such as prions causing Creutzfeldt-Jakob disease and its new variant, have not been totally eliminated. Thus, these concentrates are not without risk. In addition to the zymogen forms of factors II, VII, IX, and X, prothrombin complex concentrates contain small amounts of activated forms of some of these factors. As a result, their administration may cause venous thromboembolism, myocardial infarction, or stroke.[34] Because the risk of thrombosis appears to increase with the dose, repeated administration of small doses probably is safer.

Fresh-frozen plasma is effective but confers a very low but measurable risk of HIV and hepatitis B and C virus transmission. Solvent–detergent-treated fresh-frozen plasma has been developed, providing increased safety. However, because solvent–detergent-treated fresh-frozen plasma is prepared from large pools of plasma, it may increase the risk of transmitting agents that are not destroyed by solvent–detergent treatment. Volume overload is a limiting factor, which should be reckoned with when plasma is used.

In many cases, the decision is not what to use for treatment but whether treatment is needed. Bruises and mild superficial bleeding generally do not require replacement therapy. Because the half-life of prothrombin is 60 to 70 hours, in many cases a single treatment is sufficient for prevention of surgical bleeding or to arrest spontaneous bleeding.

FACTOR VII DEFICIENCY

DEFINITION AND HISTORY

Hereditary deficiency of factor VII, first described by Alexander and colleagues[35] in 1951, is a rare autosomal recessive disorder that has been observed in most populations. Among the rare clotting factor deficiencies described in this chapter, the relative frequency of factor VII deficiency is high (see Table 125–1).[36,37] The disorder is symptomatic mainly in homozygotes or compound heterozygotes, and the symptoms vary greatly from mild to severe. A presumptive diagnosis can be easily made because, except for very rare cases of factor X deficiency only affecting the tissue factor pathway of coagulation, factor VII deficiency is the only coagulation disorder that produces a prolonged PT and a normal aPTT (see Chap. 118).

BIOCHEMISTRY AND MOLECULAR FEATURES

Human factor VII is a single-chain glycoprotein (Mr ~50,000) that is secreted from the liver parenchymal cells as a zymogen. The mature protein consists of 406 amino acids organized in three main domains: a Gla domain at the N-terminus containing 10 Gla residues, an epidermal growth factor domain in the center, and a serine protease domain at the C-terminus.[38] Vitamin K is required for formation of the Gla residues that bind calcium ions and permit interactions with phospholipid membranes. The factor VII gene spans approximately 12.8 kb[39] and is located on chromosome 13q34,[40,41] 2.8 kb upstream from the factor X gene.[42] The gene contains a pre-pro leader sequence and eight exons that encode the mature protein. Promoter and silencer elements of the 5′ flanking region have been characterized.[43,44] Factor VII zymogen circulates in blood at an extremely low concentration (~500 ng/mL)[45] and has the shortest half-life of all coagulation factors (5 hours).[46]

Factor VII is converted to activated factor VII (factor VIIa) by cleavage of an Arg152-Ile153 bond, resulting in a two-chain molecule held together by a disulfide bond. The cleavage can be caused by factor Xa,[47] factor IXa,[48] factor XIIa,[48,49] thrombin,[47] and factor VIIa in the presence of tissue factor in an autoactivation reaction.[50] Binding of factor VII to tissue factor strikingly enhances these reactions.[51–55]

Factor VIIa can be detected in plasma by a sensitive assay using a recombinant soluble form of tissue factor.[56] The mean concentration of plasma factor VIIa is 3.6 ng/mL in normal individuals, which is 0.76 percent of the total factor VII mass in plasma.[56] The half-life of factor VIIa is relatively long (~2.5 hours)[57] compared to other activated coagulation factors. Factor IXa, which activates factor VII,[48] probably is responsible for the basal levels of plasma factor VIIa in normal individuals, but its origin is unknown. This supposition is supported by the observation that patients with severe hemophilia B, unlike patients with severe hemophilia A, have a very low concentration of circulating factor VIIa.[58,59] Moreover, hemophilia B patients acquire normal levels of factor VIIa within a few hours of purified factor IX infusion.[60]

The initial generation of thrombin that heralds blood coagulation occurs when blood is exposed to tissue factor present in the subendothelium, in tissues, on the surface of stimulated monocytes or microparticles (see Chap. 115). The exposed tissue factor forms a complex with circulating factor VIIa, which activates factor X, and factor Xa converts prothrombin to thrombin in the presence of factor Va, derived probably from activated platelets, negatively charged phospholipids, and calcium ions. The factor VIIa–tissue factor complex also activates factor IX.[61] Once factor VIII is activated by the initial amounts of generated thrombin, factor IXa in the presence of factor VIIIa, negatively charged phospholipids, and calcium ions activates factor X at a rate 50-fold higher than the rate of factor X activation by factor VIIa–tissue factor complex.[62]

When factor VII is completely lacking, as in knockout mice, fatal hemorrhage occurs perinatally.[63] Mice lacking tissue factor die during the embryonal phase because of abnormalities in the vascular wall,[64] whereas transgenic mice, rescued by incorporation of approximately 1 percent human tissue factor activity, develop normally and exhibit normal hemostasis.[65]

GENETICS

Factor VII deficiency is inherited as an autosomal recessive trait. The disorder manifests in homozygotes or compound heterozygotes, some of whom are also homozygotes for polymorphisms associated with reduced factor VII levels.[53,66,67]

The heterogeneity of factor VII deficiency was apparent in 1971, when 2 of 4 patients studied were found to have dysfunctional factor VII demonstrable by the presence of antibody-neutralizing material.[68] Later studies confirmed these observations and classified subjects with factor VII deficiency into CRM^-, CRM^+ (having normal levels of factor VII antigen), and CRM^{red} having reduced amounts of factor VII antigen.[69,70] The latter two categories predominated.[70] Further heterogeneity was exhibited by variable reactivities of plasma from individuals with factor VII deficiency to bovine, rabbit, and human tissue factor.[70] Following the characterization of the factor VII gene, the heterogeneity of factor VII deficiency was confirmed. At the time of this writing, more than 180 mutations have been reported (see Table 125–2). The mutations are distributed throughout the gene, and most are missense mutations. Eleven single-base substitutions are in the promoter region; four disrupt binding to transcriptional factors such as the hepatocyte nuclear factor-4 and SP1.[71–74] Two homozygotes bearing such mutations exhibited a very severe bleeding tendency.[71,72] Four mutations (Phe24del, Asn57Asp, Arg79Gln, and Gln100Arg) affect binding to tissue factor.[75–79] The Arg152Gln mutation located at the cleavage site prevents activation of the factor VII zymogen,[77] and other mutations at the catalytic domain impair factor VIIa activity on its substrates.

Most mutations causing factor VII deficiency have been observed in individual patients. However, one missense mutation (Ala244Val) was detected in 102 (84 percent) of 121 independent mutant alleles discerned in 88 unrelated patients in Israel.[75] Most subjects were of Iranian and Moroccan-Jewish origin and shared an identical haplotype, consistent with a founder effect. In the general Iranian-Jewish and Moroccan-Jewish populations, the prevalences of the Ala244Val allele are 0.023 and 0.025, respectively.[67]

The Dubin-Johnson syndrome caused by mutations in the multidrug resistance protein-2 (MRP2) is associated with factor VII deficiency in Iranian and Moroccan Jews.[80] This association reflects the high consanguinity rates, the relatively high prevalence of the Ala244Val mutation in both populations, a high prevalence of an MRP2 Ile1173Phe mutation in Iranian Jews, and a high prevalence of the MRP2 Arg1150His mutation in Moroccan Jews.[81]

Several additional clusters of patients with a specific mutation were reported: (1) Ala294Val, with or without a deletion of nt C at position 11128, prevails in patients from Poland and Germany but also was identified in other Europeans.[66,82,83] All subjects bearing Ala294Val have an identical haplotype, suggesting common ancestry.[82] (2) Twelve unrelated families from Norway carry Gln100Arg.[77] (3) IVS75G>A was detected in six unrelated patients from the Lazio region in Italy. All bear the same haplotype, suggesting a founder effect.[84] (4) Gly331Ser was identified in 10 Italian and 4 German patients on one haplotype.[85] The widely distributed and common Arg304Gln mutation probably is a recurrent mutation.[86]

Three polymorphisms in the factor VII gene are associated with reduced plasma levels of factor VII. The first polymorphism, an Arg353Gln substitution, results in impaired secretion of factor VII from cells[87] and gives rise to a 20 to 25 percent decrease in plasma factor VII level in heterozygotes and a 40 to 50 percent decrease in homozygotes.[88,89] The allele frequency of the Arg353Gln polymorphism varies significantly in different populations.[90–93] The second polymorphism associated with a diminished factor VII level is a decanucleotide insertion upstream from the 5′ end of the gene at –323, which confers a 33 percent decrease in the promoter activity.[44] The relative effects of this polymorphism and the Arg353Gln polymorphism on factor VII level are difficult to assess because linkage disequilibrium exists between these markers.[89] A third polymorphism associated with factor VII level is a hypervariable region 4 polymorphism (HVR4) in intron 7.[94] The variable number of tandem repeats (5 to 8 copies of 37 bp) apparently influences the splicing efficiency. The effect of the variable repeats on factor VII level is less conspicuous than the decanucleotide insertion at the promoter region and the Arg353Gln polymorphism.

All homozygotes for the Ala244Val mutation also are homozygotes for the Arg353Gln polymorphism.[67,75] In coexpression studies performed in COS-1 and BHK cells, the two gene alterations have an additive effect in reducing secretion of factor VII.[75,95]

CLINICAL FEATURES

Bleeding manifestations occur in homozygotes and in compound heterozygotes for factor VII deficiency. Heterozygotes who have partial factor VII deficiency may present with mild bleeding manifestations, for example, epistaxis, menorrhagia, and easy bruising.[37,96] A recent survey of 499 heterozygotes revealed that 19 percent had bleeding manifestations.[66] Patients who have factor VII activity less than 1 percent of normal, frequently present with a disease that is indistinguishable from severe hemophilias A or B. Such patients are afflicted by hemarthroses leading to severe arthropathy[46,66,97] and can present with life-threatening intracerebral hemorrhage.[46,98] Patients with slightly higher levels of factor VII can also manifest such severe bleeding episodes, but this finding seems to be exceptional because most patients with factor VII activity of 5 percent of normal or more have a much milder disease, characterized by epistaxis, gingival bleeding, menorrhagia, and easy bruising. Dental extractions, tonsillectomy, and surgical procedures involving the urogenital tracts frequently are accompanied by bleeding when no prior therapy is instituted.[46] In contrast, surgical procedures such as laparotomy, herniorrhaphy, appendectomy, and hysterectomy have been uneventful.[46] This apparent discrepancy can be explained by different extents of local fibrinolysis exhibited by the respective traumatized tissues. Factor VII levels rise during pregnancy in healthy females,[99] but do not change in homozygous patients with the deficiency.[100] Nevertheless, postpartum hemorrhage has not been observed in patients with factor VII deficiency, except for a few instances.[46,100] Inhibitors to factor VII have been rarely described in patients with inherited factor VII deficiency.[101]

Venous and arterial thromboses have been described in several patients. A survey of 514 cases with severe or partial factor VII deficiency recorded 7 patients with venous thrombosis and 1 patient with arterial thrombosis.[102] In 6 of the 8 patients, the thrombotic event occurred after surgery or labor. These data suggest severe factor VII deficiency confers no protection against thrombosis.

LABORATORY FEATURES

A normal aPTT and a prolonged PT in a patient with a lifelong history of a mild or severe bleeding tendency is consistent with the diagnosis of factor VII deficiency (see Chap. 118). Only in very rare cases of inherited factor X in which the tissue factor pathway of coagulation is impaired and the intrinsic pathway is intact, a prolonged PT and normal aPTT are discernible (see "Factor X Deficiency" below). The prolonged PT in inherited factor VII deficiency can be corrected by normal serum (containing factor VII) but not by barium sulfate-absorbed plasma (devoid of factor VII). Determining the diagnosis depends on a specific assay of factor VII activity using known factor VII-deficient plasma. Factor VII antigen can be measured by a commercial enzyme-linked immunosorbent assay (ELISA). Factor VIIa can be measured by a clotting assay using soluble tissue factor, which is insensitive to native factor VII,[56] or by an ELISA using an antibody that exhibits 3000-fold greater reactivity with factor VIIa than with factor VII.[103] Heterozygous carriers have reduced mean levels of factor VII activity, but the range of activity overlaps with normal values. Factor VII activity also can be decreased when the subject being studied has vitamin K deficiency, which occurs frequently. Detection of heterozygotes can be facilitated by concomitant measurements of factor VII activity and antigen levels following administration of vitamin K. Because many factor VII deficiency states are CRM^+ or CRM^{red},[69,70] findings of reduced factor VII activity and significantly higher factor VII antigen level are consistent with heterozygosity. A more definitive approach is identifying the mutant gene in the involved family and tracking it among family members.

DIFFERENTIAL DIAGNOSIS

The common causes of acquired factor VII deficiency must be excluded before diagnosing inherited factor VII deficiency. These causes include liver disease, vitamin K deficiency, use of warfarin or related anticoagulants, and, rarely, a lupus anticoagulant with severely deficient factor VII associated with severe bleeding.[104] Very rare hereditary defects that must be distinguished from factor VII deficiency are the combined deficiency of all vitamin K-dependent factors (see "Combined Deficiency of the Vitamin K-Dependent Coagulation Factors" below), combined deficiency of factors VII and X,[105] and combined deficiency of factors VII and factor V, factor VIII, factor X, or factor XI.[106]

THERAPY

Replacement therapy is unnecessary for minor bleeding episodes. Local hemostasis for skin lacerations and administration of an antifibrinolytic agent for menorrhagia, epistaxis, and gingival hemorrhage usually are sufficient to arrest bleeding. Replacement therapy is essential in patients who present with severe hemorrhage, such as hemarthrosis or intracerebral bleeding. When surgery is required, the following issues should be considered: (1) the site of surgery, as dental extractions, tonsillectomy, nose surgery, and urologic interventions likely are associated with bleeding because of local fibrinolysis; (2) history of bleeding, as patients who have experienced hemarthroses, intracerebral hemorrhage, or other severe bleeding episodes have a much higher risk of bleeding than those who have not had such symptoms; (3) basic level of factor VII, as patients with very low activities (<3% of normal) more likely will bleed; (4) trough factor VII level 20 to 25 percent of normal probably is sufficient even when extensive trauma is present[46,107]; (5) volume overload should be expected if plasma is used as the replacement material; (6) short half-life of factor VII (~5 hours)[46]; and (7) safety of the blood component to be used.

Prothrombin complex concentrates containing activated clotting factors[57] can be used, but they confer a risk of thrombosis.[107] Specific factor VII concentrates have been used successfully in series of patients.[108] The dose during surgery usually ranges between 8 and 40 U/kg given at 4- to 6-hour intervals. Another option is use of recombinant factor VIIa, which has been successful in managing patients with hemarthroses and during surgery.[109,110] During surgery, recombinant factor VIIa doses of 20 to 25 mcg/kg were used at intervals of 2 to 3 hours. In children and in females during pregnancy, the half-life of factor VIIa is even shorter than the usual 2.5 hours, so treating such patients is a challenge. When plasma is used for major surgery, a loading dose of 15 mL/kg should be administered, followed by 4 mL/kg every 6 hours for 7 to 10 days. Diuretics or even plasmapheresis may be necessary because of volume overload.[111]

FACTOR X DEFICIENCY

Factor X deficiency, a moderate to severe bleeding tendency, is an autosomal recessive disorder first reported by Telfer and colleagues[112] and Hougie and colleagues.[113]

BIOCHEMISTRY AND MOLECULAR FEATURES

The gene encoding factor X is located on chromosome 13q34-qter, adjacent to the gene encoding factor VII.[114,115] The gene spans approximately 25 kb and is composed of 8 exons.[116] The factor X gene shows significant homology with the genes of other vitamin K-dependent serine proteases, which suggests all of these multidomain genes evolved from a common ancestral gene.[117]

The protein encoded by the factor X gene is 488 amino acids long. A 23-amino-acid signal peptide is located at the N-terminus. The Gla domain forms the N-terminus of the mature protein and contains 11 Gla residues that are responsible for calcium and phospholipid binding.[118] Adjacent to the Gla domain is a short aromatic amino acid stack of predominantly hydrophobic amino acids, followed by the epidermal growth factor domain, which contains two epidermal growth factor motifs that are believed to mediate protein–protein interactions. The heavily glycosylated 52-amino-acid activation peptide of factor X separates the epidermal growth factor domain from the C-terminal catalytic domain. Factor X zymogen is synthesized in the liver, its plasma concentration is 8 to 10 mcg/mL and its half-life is 30 to 40 hours (see Chap. 115).

Factor X undergoes proteolytic processing in the endoplasmic reticulum so that circulating factor X is a two-chain, disulfide-linked protein consisting of a 17-kDa light chain composed of the Gla and epidermal growth factor domains and a 40-kDa heavy chain composed of the activation and catalytic domains.[119] Factor X can be activated by a complex of negatively charged phospholipids, factor IXa, and factor VIIIa, or by membrane-bound factor VIIa–tissue factor complex.[120] Factor X also can be activated by a component of Russell viper venom[121] and by trypsin. In each case, activation of factor X is accomplished by proteolytic cleavage and subsequent removal of the activation peptide. Factor Xa, in turn, activates prothrombin to thrombin in a reaction that requires negatively charged phospholipids, calcium ions, and factor Va.

GENETICS

Factor X deficiency is inherited in an autosomal recessive manner. Heterozygotes have factor X levels that are approximately 50 percent of normal and are generally asymptomatic. The genetic defects causing a deficiency of factor X are classified according to functional and immunologic analysis as CRM^+, CRM^-, and CRM^{red}.

The currently described 95 mutations that cause factor X deficiency include large deletions, small frameshift deletions, nonsense mutation, and missense mutations. The deletions result in impaired protein synthesis or in synthesis of unstable or dysfunctional proteins. CRM^+ or CRM^{red} variants may affect factor X function in several ways.[122] Activation through the tissue factor pathway may be affected when the mutations are located for example in the Gla domain, as in Glu7Gly (St. Louis II), or Glu19Ala.[122–124] Activation through factor IXa is affected by, for example, Thr318Met (Roma).[122,125] Activation of factor X through Russell viper venom is almost intact in the Pro343Ser (Friuli) mutation,[126] whereas its activation through the intrinsic and tissue factor pathways is only 5 to 9 percent of normal. Missense mutations also may affect synthesis or secretion, thus producing CRM^- phenotypes, as with the mutation identified in Mr. Stuart, one of the first two patients described with factor X deficiency (Val298Met).[127] An interesting cluster of unrelated families with a Phe31Ser mutation was described in Algeria and haplotype analysis was consistent with a founder effect.[128]

CLINICAL MANIFESTATIONS

The clinical manifestations of factor X deficiency are related to the functional levels of factor X. Individuals with severe factor X deficiency and functional factor X levels less than 1 percent of normal bleed spontaneously and following trauma. Bleeding occurs primarily into joints and soft tissues, from the umbilical cord and mucous membranes.[129] Menorrhagia may be especially problematic in women. More unusual bleedings are intracerebral hemorrhage, intramural intestinal bleeding (which can produce symptoms like those of an acute abdomen), urinary tract bleeding, and soft tissue bleeding with development of hemorrhagic pseudocysts or pseudotumors. In an analysis of 102 patients from Europe and Latin America, three mutations were associated with intracerebral hemorrhage (Gly380Arg, IVS7–1G>A, and Tyr163delAT) and Gly(−20)Arg mutation was associated with severe hemarthrosis.[129] In individuals homozygous for moderate or mild deficiencies of factor X and in heterozygotes, bleeding is less common, usually occurring only after trauma or during or after surgery. Such patients may experience easy bruising as the only clinical manifestation.

DIFFERENTIAL DIAGNOSIS

The diagnosis of factor X deficiency is suggested in most cases by assays demonstrating prolonged PT, aPTT, and Russell viper venom time, which is based on the activation of factor X by the venom. However, patients harboring mutations that cause a defect only in the tissue factor pathway will only display a prolonged PT and their aPTT will be normal. Other patients who carry mutations that only affect the intrinsic activity of FX, will exhibit a normal PT and prolonged aPTT.[122] The definitive diagnosis of factor X deficiency depends on demonstrating an isolated deficiency of factor X by a specific factor X assay.

Prolonged PT and aPTT and a normal thrombin time can be observed in patients with prothrombin deficiency, factor V deficiency, multiple factor deficiencies, vitamin K deficiency, liver disease, and lupus anticoagulant. These disorders are distinguished from factor X deficiency by measuring the levels of factor X and other specific factors, including factors II, V, VII, and IX (see Chap. 118). Combined deficiencies of FX with FVII or FVIII are extremely rare.[130]

Inherited factor X deficiency must be differentiated from various acquired causes of isolated factor X deficiency, such as systemic amyloidosis.[131,132] Factor X deficiency that sometimes occurs in this disorder can result from (1) selective binding of factor X to the amyloid fibrils, which can be erroneously attributed to the presence of an inhibitor when exogenously infused factor X is rapidly removed from the circulation, and (2) presence of abnormal factor X molecules with reduced activity versus antigen level. Amyloidosis associated with factor X deficiency resulting from both causes is generally of the primary type. Acquired isolated factor X deficiency with severe bleeding manifestations occurs rarely because of the formation of specific antibodies with no underlying autoimmune disorder.[133]

THERAPY

Therapy for inherited factor X deficiency usually is administration of heated and solvent–detergent-treated prothrombin complex concentrates containing factor X, in addition to factors II, VII, and IX. Use of these concentrates carries a low risk of transmission of bloodborne viruses. However, a risk of thrombosis, including venous thromboembolism, diffuse intravascular coagulation, and myocardial infarction,[34] which is thought to be dose dependent, exists. As a result, administration of doses greater than 2000 U is not recommended. If a larger dose is needed, divided doses are recommended.

For soft tissue, mucous membrane, and joint hemorrhages, the aim of treatment should be maintaining a factor X level that is at least 30 percent of normal. For more serious hemorrhages, a factor X level that is 50 to 100 percent of normal should be the goal. The biologic half-life of factor X is 30 to 40 hours.[134,135] Based on this, if continued treatment is needed, prothrombin complex concentrates should be administrated every 24 hours until hemostasis is achieved. In patients with particularly severe bleeding manifestations, prophylactic therapy with regular infusion of prothrombin complex concentrate is used.[136] Fresh-frozen plasma also can be used to treat patients with factor X deficiency. The issue of volume overload with plasma and the relative merits of using solvent–detergent-treated plasma are discussed above for therapy of prothrombin deficiency.

COMBINED DEFICIENCY OF VITAMIN K-DEPENDENT COAGULATION FACTORS

In 1966, McMillan and Roberts reported the first case of vitamin K-dependent coagulation factors deficiency (VKDFD).[137] This autosomal recessive disorder is the most infrequent inherited bleeding tendency, and so far has been described in 26 unrelated families.[138,139] There are two types of the disorder: VKDFD1 which is caused by mutations in the γ-glutamyl carboxylase gene (*GGCX*), and VKDFD2 which is caused by a mutation in the vitamin K 2,3-epoxide reductase (VKORC1) gene (*VKORC1*).

BIOCHEMISTRY AND MOLECULAR FEATURES

For their full function, vitamin K-dependent proteins—for example, factors II, VII, IX and X, proteins C, S, and Z and osteocalcin—must undergo γ-carboxylation of glutamic acid residues located at their N-terminal regions. This reaction is driven by GGCX that uses oxygen and reduced vitamin K (vitamin KH2) to introduce carbon dioxide into glutamic acid residues after binding of the enzyme to an 18-amino-acid propeptide that is conserved in all vitamin K-dependent proteins. The γ-carboxylation is coupled with the conversion of vitamin KH2 to vitamin K 2,3-epoxide. The Gla residues of coagulation factors II, VII, IX, and X and the natural inhibitors, proteins C and S, enable calcium-dependent interactions between these proteins and phospholipid membranes. VKORC1, the target enzyme for inhibition by warfarin, reduces vitamin K 2,3-epoxide to vitamin KH2, thereby replenishing this essential cofactor of γ-carboxylation. Both GGCX and VKORC1 are located in the endoplasmic reticulum. The *GGCX* gene spans 13 kb, contains 15 exons, and is located on chromosome 2p12. The protein comprises 758 residues (Mr ~94,000) and was crystallized.[140] The *VKORC1* gene spans 5.2 kb comprising 3 exons and is located on chromosome 16p12.[141–143] The protein consists of 163 residues (Mr ~18,000) and exhibits a three-transmembrane topology.[144,145] Formation of a complex between VKORC1 and protein disulfide isomerase is responsible for the reduction of vitamin K 2,3-epoxide.[146]

GENETICS

In 8 of 19 families of unrelated probands, consanguinity was reported.[138] In the remaining families described, this information was not disclosed.

The molecular genetic bases for VKDFD1 have been established in 10 unrelated probands, of whom 7 were homozygotes and 3 were compound heterozygotes (see database at www.isth.org). So far, only one mutation in *VKORC1* gene, an Arg98Trp substitution, has been found to cause VKDFD2. This mutation was detected in three unrelated probands of Lebanese, German, and Italian origins.[141,147,148] For VKDFD1, eight mutations in the *GGCX* gene have been identified: Leu394Arg, Trp501Ser, Arg485Pro, His404Pro, Trp157Arg, Thr591Lys, IVS2–1 G>T, and IVS-1 del nt. 1056–1069.[139,149–154] In several additional families with other mutations in the *GGCX* gene, pseudoxanthoma elasticum-like phenotype was described.[155]

CLINICAL MANIFESTATIONS

The clinical manifestations of VKDFD1 and VKDFD2 are similar. The severity of the bleeding tendency varies substantially and roughly correlates with the extent of the deficiency of the coagulation factors. Symptoms that have been observed are easy bruising, bleeding from the umbilical stump, menorrhagia, hematuria, gastrointestinal bleeding, and intracerebral hemorrhage presenting shortly after birth. In three families, the affected patients had skeletal abnormalities resembling warfarin embryopathy, which probably stemmed from impaired carboxylation of osteocalcin or matrix Gla protein.[138]

DIAGNOSIS AND DIFFERENTIAL DIAGNOSIS

Both PT and aPTT are prolonged in patients with VKDFD1 and VKDFD2 but not in heterozygous carriers. The activities of all circulating vitamin K-dependent proteins usually range between 20 and 40 U/dL, whereas their antigen levels are normal or slightly reduced. VKDFD1 can be distinguished from VKDFD2 by measuring the plasma level of vitamin K 2,3-epoxide; in the former, vitamin K 2,3-epoxide will be low or undetectable, whereas in the latter, the level will be high. VKDFD1 and VKDFD2 must be distinguished from acquired causes for deficiencies of factors II, VII, IX, and X, that is, liver disease, vitamin K deficiency, or use of warfarin. The definitive diagnosis of VKDFD1 or VKDFD2 can be made at the present time by identifying the responsible mutation in the *VKORC1* and *GGCX* genes.

THERAPY

Large doses of vitamin K correct at least partially the reduced levels of the vitamin K-dependent factors resulting in amelioration and prevention of bleeding manifestations.[138] During acute bleeding episodes, fresh-frozen plasma or prothrombin complex concentrates can be used.

FACTOR V DEFICIENCY

DEFINITION AND HISTORY

Hereditary factor V deficiency was initially termed parahemophilia.[156] It is among the less common inherited bleeding disorders and manifests in homozygotes or compound heterozygotes as a moderate bleeding tendency.

BIOCHEMISTRY AND MOLECULAR GENETIC FEATURES

Human plasma factor V is a high-molecular-weight (Mr ~330,000) single-chain glycoprotein that consists of 2196 amino acids.[157] Analysis of the approximately 7-kb factor V complementary DNA (cDNA) showed that the protein is organized according to the following domain structure: A_1-A_2-B-A_3-C_1-C_2. The A- and C-domains have approximately 40 percent homology with analogous domains in factor VIII. The large B-domain shows no homology with the corresponding B-domain of factor VIII. The gene contains 25 exons and was mapped to chromosome 1q21–25.[158] Factor V is converted to its activated form following several proteolytic cleavages by thrombin[159] or factor Xa.[160] These cleavages remove the B-domain and yield factor Va, which consists of a heavy chain (A_1-A_2 domains) associated by Ca^{2+} with a light chain (A_3-C_1-C_2 domains). The light chain contains the binding sites for membrane phospholipids, prothrombin, and activated protein C; both light and heavy chains probably are necessary for factor Xa binding.

Assembly of factors Va and Xa on the phospholipid membrane of platelets in the presence of calcium ions forms the prothrombinase complex, which catalyzes the conversion of prothrombin to thrombin. Exclusion of factor Va from the prothrombinase complex reduces the rate of thrombin generation by four orders of magnitude.[161]

Factor V is synthesized by the liver.[162] Its plasma concentration is approximately 7 mcg/mL,[163] and its half-life is 12 to 15 hours.[164] Approximately 20 percent of factor V in whole blood is localized in the α granules of platelets, where it is complexed with an extremely large protein multimerin.[165] Megakaryocyte endocytosis of plasma-derived factor V accounts for the platelet factor V pool.[166] Following absorption, factor V undergoes partial proteolysis forming a partially activated factor V cofactor.[167] The release from platelets upon their activation at injury sites exerts a powerful hemostatic effect.[166]

Factor Va is inactivated by activated protein C through limited proteolysis at Arg506, Arg306, and Arg679 in the presence of protein S, calcium ions, and either platelet or endothelial cell membrane phospholipids.[168] Partial protection from this cleavage is provided by factor Xa when bound to factor Va on the surface of platelets.[169] Partial resistance to inactivation by activated protein C occurs when the cleavage sites Arg306 or Arg506 are mutated (see Chaps. 116 and 131). The procofactor, factor V, accelerates the inactivation of factor VIIIa by activated protein C in the presence of protein S (see Chap. 116).

Factor V deficiency is inherited as an autosomal recessive trait. Heterozygotes, whose plasma factor V activity ranges between 25 and 60 percent of normal, usually are asymptomatic, although an American registry recorded mild bleeding in 50 percent of the cases.[37]

Assays of factor V antigen indicate that most homozygotes and compound heterozygotes have a true deficiency rather than a dysfunctional protein. A total of 72 distinct mutations have been identified, of which 24 are missense, 28 are small insertions/deletions, 10 are nonsense, 9 are splice site mutations, and 1 is a deletion of the whole gene (see Table 125–2). Most mutations cause truncations and are localized throughout the gene. Several mutations have interesting features. One, a Tyr1702Cys transition, was identified in eight unrelated families, of whom six were Italian. The frequency of this mutant allele in Italy is 0.002.[170] Another mutation, an Ala221Val (New Brunswick) alteration, characterized in the homozygous state by activity and antigen levels of 29 and 39 percent of normal, respectively displays decreased stability of the expressed protein.[171] Additional mutations exhibit decreased secretion of the protein from producing cells.[172,173] Remarkably, the Gln773ter and Arg1133ter mutations and a 4-bp deletion mutation, all present in exon 13 and predicted to result in partial truncation of the B-domain and complete truncation of the A3-, C1-, and C2-domains, cause no bleeding or only a mild bleeding tendency in affected patients having factor V antigen and activity levels 1 percent of normal.[174–176] This finding contrasts with the phenotype of factor V knockout mice, which have defective embryonic development and early hemorrhagic death.[177]

Subjects who are compound heterozygotes for factor V Arg506Gln (factor V Leiden) and for a factor V null allele have normal hemostasis (despite reduced factor V clotting activity). However, because they phenotypically resemble homozygotes for activated protein C resistance, these patients may present with thrombosis (see Chap. 131).[178]

Among several polymorphisms detected in the factor V gene, His1299Arg in exon 13 is particularly interesting because it is associated with a reduced plasma factor V level and mild activated protein C resistance.[179] His1299Arg co-segregates with several other polymorphisms encoding several amino acid changes, together named R2 haplotype. In two heterozygotes for factor V Arg506Gln mutation (factor V Leiden) who presented with venous thrombosis, reduced factor V activity resulting from the His1299Arg polymorphism harbored by the non-Leiden chromosome, imparted a pseudohomozygous phenotype for activated protein C resistance.[180] Additional polymorphisms or mutations in the factor V gene have been observed to increase the risk of venous thrombosis (see Chap. 131).[181]

Factor V Quebec initially was described as an autosomal dominant disorder with severe bleeding manifestations.[182] Affected patients had platelet factor V activity 2 to 4 percent of normal, slightly reduced platelet factor V antigen, moderately decreased plasma factor V activity, and mild thrombocytopenia. The inactive platelet factor V in these patients is caused by proteolysis of several platelet α-granule proteins, including fibrinogen, von Willebrand factor, thrombospondin, and factor V complexed with multimerin.[183] Thus, factor V Quebec, described in two unrelated families, is a deficiency of platelet factor V activity caused by a generalized platelet defect.

CLINICAL MANIFESTATIONS

Homozygous or compound heterozygous patients whose factor V level ranges from less than 1 to 10 percent of normal exhibit a lifelong bleeding tendency. Common manifestations include ecchymoses, epistaxis, gingival bleeding, hemorrhage following minor lacerations, and menorrhagia.[36,37,184] Postpartum hemorrhage occurs in more than 50 percent of pregnancies in patients with severe factor V deficiency.[185] Bleeding from other sites is less common, but instances of hemarthroses unrelated to trauma and intracerebral hemorrhage have been reported.[36] Trauma, dental extractions, and surgery confer a high risk of excessive bleeding.

A low concentration of tissue factor pathway inhibitor, observed in patients with severe factor V deficiency, was proposed to ameliorate the bleeding tendency.[186] Venous and arterial thromboses have been described in patients with factor V levels ranging between 2 and 14 percent of normal.[187] These observations indicate that factor V deficiency, like deficiencies of other coagulation factors, does not provide protection against thrombosis. Factor V deficiency deprives activated protein C of one of its essential substrates, thereby downregulating the inhibitory function of the protein C system. As discussed in "Biochemistry and Molecular Genetic Features" above, this situation is highlighted in patients with thrombosis who are compound heterozygotes for a factor V deficiency allele and an allele bearing the factor V Leiden mutation.

Only two patients with hereditary factor V deficiency who developed an inhibitor after receiving plasma transfusions were reported.[188,189] The inhibitor disappeared in one patient, but a low titer of the inhibitor persisted in the other patient.[189]

DIFFERENTIAL DIAGNOSIS

Hereditary factor V deficiency must be distinguished from hereditary combined deficiency of factors V and VIII, acquired factor V deficiency associated with severe liver dysfunction or disseminated intravascular coagulation (DIC). In both factor V deficiency and combined deficiency of factors V and VIII, PT and aPTT are prolonged, inheritance is autosomal recessive, and bleeding manifestations are similar, making an assay of factor VIII essential for distinguishing between these entities (see Chap. 118). The clinical manifestations of severe liver disease or DIC are sufficient to allow easy distinction between acquired and inherited factor V deficiency. Rare instances of an acquired factor V inhibitor as a result of exposure to bovine thrombin preparations and drugs, or because of an unknown cause, should also be taken into account (see Chap. 128).[190]

THERAPY

Patients with epistaxis and gingival bleeding may respond to tranexamic acid (1 g qid), and local hemostatic measures may suffice for minor lacerations. If these measures fail, severe spontaneous bleeding occurs, or surgery is performed, fresh-frozen plasma replacement should be given. The following factors should be considered when planning plasma replacement therapy: (1) half-life of factor V is approximately 12 to 15 hours; (2) a factor V level of 25 percent of normal usually is adequate even for major surgery[191,192]; (3) surgical procedures at sites having high local fibrinolytic activity such as the urogenital tract, oral cavity, and nose, likely will result in excessive bleeding, and late bleeding may occur; and (4) postpartum hemorrhage is common.[185] Infusion of a loading dose of 20 mL/kg of fresh-frozen plasma followed by 5 to 10 mL/kg every 12 hours for 7 days usually is adequate to ensure hemostasis during and after surgery. To prevent postpartum hemorrhage, the same regimen can be used but for a shorter period of time.

COMBINED DEFICIENCY OF FACTORS V AND VIII

DEFINITION AND HISTORY

Combined deficiency of factors V and VIII, first described in 1954,[193] is a rare moderate bleeding disorder that is transmitted as an autosomal recessive trait.[194] Affected homozygotes have plasma levels of factors V and VIII ranging from 5 to 30 percent of normal.[195] The disorder results from a deficiency of either mannose-binding lectin (LMAN1), also called endoplasmic reticulum–Golgi intermediate compartment protein (ERGIC)-53, or multiple combined-factor deficiency protein (MCFD2), which form a specific calcium-dependent cargo receptor complex for the endoplasmic reticulum to Golgi transport of factors V and VIII.[196–198] The disorder has been detected in many populations, but a relatively high frequency occurs among Tunisian and Middle Eastern Jews residing in Israel[194] and among Iranians.[199]

BIOCHEMISTRY AND MOLECULAR GENETIC FEATURES

Factors V and VIII are essential coagulation factors that circulate in plasma as precursors. Upon limited proteolysis by thrombin or factor Xa and in concert with negatively charged phospholipid surfaces, factors VIIIa and Va exhibit profound cofactor activities for activation of factor X by factor IXa and for activation of prothrombin by factor Xa, respectively. Inactivation of factors Va and VIIIa is accomplished by activated protein C in the presence of protein S and phospholipids through several proteolytic cleavages at distinct sites (see Chap. 116). Factors V and VIII have similar domain organizations with partial homology (see "Factor V Deficiency" above and Chap. 115).

The pathogenesis of combined deficiency of factors V and VIII puzzled investigators for more than 40 years. The enigma was resolved by the finding that the disease stems from a deficiency of either one of two interacting proteins, LMAN1 and MCFD2, which play a role in the intracellular transport of factors V and VIII.[196,197] LMAN1 is a type-1 transmembrane protein and MCFD2 is an EF-hand domain soluble luminal protein. Together they form a stable calcium-dependent complex that sorts and transports factors V and VIII from the endoplasmic reticulum to the Golgi in COPII-coated vesicles. Homozygosity mapping and positional cloning in nine unrelated Jewish families demonstrated that the LMAN1 gene (*LMAN1*) was localized on the long arm of chromosome 18.[196,200,201] Using a similar approach in other families with the combined factors V and VIII deficiency identified the MCFD2 gene (*MCFD2*) encoding on the short arm of chromosome 2.[197] Thirty-two mutations identified in *LMAN1* predicted either a truncated protein product or no protein at all, and one mutation, a Cys475Arg substitution, disrupts a disulfide bond which is required for oligomerization.[202] In contrast, of the 15 mutations identified in the *MCFD2*, 5 are missense and 10 are null mutations. Missense mutations are located at the EF-2 domains giving rise to defective binding to LMAN1.[202]

A distinct founder haplotype was found in patients belonging to six unrelated families of Tunisian-Jewish origin bearing a donor splice site mutation in intron 9 of *LMAN1*.[200,202] All six families originated from an ancient Jewish community that has resided on the island of Djerba for more than 2 millennia. A survey of this community, which presently lives in Israel, disclosed that the mutation is prevalent at an allele frequency of 0.0107.[203] Another founder effect for a G insertion in exon 1 of *LMAN1* was observed in eight unrelated Jewish families of Middle Eastern origin.[200,202] An M1T mutation in *LMAN1* has been detected in several unrelated Italian families likely implying another founder effect.[202] Although deficiencies of either LMAN1 or MCFD2 proteins give rise to indistinguishable clinical manifestations, the mean levels of factor V and factor VIII are significantly lower in patients harboring an MCFD2 mutation.[202] This finding may imply that MCFD2 plays a more important role in transporting factors V and VIII. Because all patients with the combined deficiency have residual plasma levels of factor V and VIII ranging from 5 to 30 percent of normal, alternative mechanisms of intracellular transport of factors V and VIII probably exist.

CLINICAL MANIFESTATIONS

Homozygous patients exhibit spontaneous and posttraumatic bleeding. Menorrhagia, epistaxis, easy bruising, and gingival hemorrhage are common observations.[195,199] Hemarthrosis, unrelated to trauma, was described in approximately 20 percent of cases.[195,199] Hematuria, gastrointestinal hemorrhage, and spontaneous intracranial hemorrhage are less common.[199] Dental extractions and surgical procedures almost always are accompanied by excessive bleeding when the missing factors are not replaced. Interestingly, bleeding was noted in only 1 of 6 Jewish infants patients who underwent circumcision on day 8 of life.[194] In contrast, Muslim patients bled excessively following circumcision performed at age 5 to 7 years.[199] Postpartum hemorrhage was noted in 13 of 17 women.[195,199]

Heterozygotes exhibit slight but significantly reduced mean levels of factors V and VIII.[194] In a literature survey of 161 heterozygotes, 22 reported having significant bleeding manifestations.[204] However, no correlation between the factor V or factor VIII levels and bleeding tendency was noted.[195,204]

DIFFERENTIAL DIAGNOSIS

Coincidental association between hemophilia A and factor V deficiency is estimated to be extremely rare.[205] The association has been reported in only 5 families.[206–210] The following features that help distinguish between this association and the combined deficiency: (1) Consanguinity frequently is present in parents of patients with combined deficiency of factors V and VIII. (2) Independent segregation of factor V and factor VIII deficiency can be observed among immediate relatives of patients with the coincidental association. (3) Concordant reductions in levels of factors V and VIII more likely occur in patients afflicted by the combined deficiency. Hereditary factor V deficiency can be confused with combined deficiency of factors V and VIII because the two entities are inherited as autosomal recessive traits, have similar manifestations, and are characterized by prolonged PT and aPTT. Consequently, assays of factors V and VIII are essential for making the distinction (see Chap. 118).

THERAPY

An antifibrinolytic agent such as tranexamic acid or ε-aminocaproic acid can be helpful in patients exhibiting menorrhagia, epistaxis, or gingival bleeding. Patients with severe bleeding episodes or patients undergoing surgical procedures, including dental extractions, should receive fresh-frozen plasma as replacement for factor V and cryoprecipitate or factor VIII concentrate as a source of factor VIII. Desmopressin can be used to increase factor VIII level,[195] but this treatment sometimes fails.[211] As with other clotting factor deficiencies, replacement therapy in patients undergoing major surgery should be maintained for at least 7 days after the operation. Hemostatically safe levels of factor V and VIII have not been established, but given the significant bleeding experienced by patients with factor V and VIII levels up to 30 percent of normal, a reasonable aim is trough factor levels greater than 50 percent of normal during and after surgery. Volume overload can be a serious problem but can be circumvented by plasma exchange and concomitant use of a factor VIII concentrate.[211]

FACTOR XI DEFICIENCY

DEFINITION AND HISTORY

Factor XI deficiency initially was described as a "new hemophilia" in two sisters and their maternal uncle by Rosenthal and colleagues[212] in 1953. The deficiency was erroneously thought to be transmitted as an autosomal dominant disorder with variable expressivity. Later studies clearly established that, in most cases, the mode of transmission of factor XI deficiency is autosomal recessive.[213,214] The disorder is exhibited in homozygotes or compound heterozygotes as a mild to moderate bleeding tendency that is mainly injury related. Affected subjects have been described in most populations but in Jews, particularly of Ashkenazi origin, the disorder is common.[214]

Until 1991, factor XI was regarded as one of the "contact" coagulation factors, functioning in the initiation of the intrinsic coagulation system. Numerous studies showed that when blood or plasma is exposed to negatively charged surfaces *in vitro*, a series of reactions involving factor XII, high-molecular-weight kininogen (HK), and prekallikrein (PK) yields α-factor XIIa. α-Factor XIIa then activates factor XI, and factor XIa, in turn, activates factor IX in the presence of calcium ions, leading through additional reactions to thrombin generation. All attempts to ascribe to the contact activation pathway an essential function *in vivo* have been futile because, unlike factor XI deficiency, severe deficiencies of factor XII, HK, and PK have not been associated with a bleeding tendency. Studies in 1991 showed that factor XI can be activated by thrombin,[215,216] thereby bypassing the contact reactions. This finding and new observations on the involvement of factor XI in the intrinsic coagulation system (see Chap. 115) and in the fibrinolytic system (see "Biochemistry and Molecular Features" below) explain why factor XI is important for hemostasis, whereas factor XII, HK, and PK probably are not.

BIOCHEMISTRY AND MOLECULAR FEATURES

Factor XI is a glycoprotein that consists of two identical 80-kDa polypeptide chains linked by a disulfide bond.[217] Each subunit contains 607 amino acids with a serine protease domain at the C-terminus and four tandem repeats of 90 or 91 amino acids, designated "apple domains," at the N-terminus. The described crystal structure of factor XI dimer[218] defined the interface of the monomers in apple 4 domains in which three residues—Leu284, Ile290, and Tyr329—are essential for noncovalent binding between the monomers. This binding enables the formation of a disulfide bond between Cys321 residues in the fourth apple domain of each monomer.[219,220] In blood, factor XI is complexed noncovalently with HK through binding primarily to the apple 2 domain and secondarily to other apple domains.[221] The normal plasma concentration of factor XI is 5 mcg/mL. The 23-kb gene encoding for factor XI consists of 15 exons and 14 introns[222] and is located on chromosome 4q34–35.[223]

Activation of factor XI involves cleavage of an Arg369-Ile370 bond, yielding a heavy chain containing the four apple domains linked by a disulfide bond to a light chain that contains the catalytic domain.[217] Each activated molecule thus contains two catalytic sites. Factor XI adhered to negatively charged surfaces by HK can be activated by α-factor XIIa[224] or through autoactivation by factor XIa,[216] but whether these reactions are important for hemostasis is questionable. The major activator of factor XI *in vivo* is thrombin.[215,216] Factor XI binds through its apple 3 domain to lipid rafts on platelets containing glycoprotein Ib–IX–V complex. This glycoprotein complex also binds thrombin; thus, both substrate and enzyme are colocalized at the same site.[225] Optimal binding of factor XI to these membrane rafts requires HK and Zn^{2+} or prothrombin and Ca^{2+} (see Chap. 115). Factor XI activation also can occur on the fibrin surface after a clot forms.[226] Factor XIa, once generated, activates factor IX by limited proteolysis of two peptide bonds in the presence of calcium ions.[227] Factor IXa then activates factor X in the presence of factor VIIIa, negatively charged phospholipids, and calcium ions. Thus, additional thrombin is generated through thrombin-mediated activation of factor XI.

The presence of factor XI contributes to the activation of procarboxypeptidase B by thrombin. When procarboxypeptidase B, also termed TAFI, is activated, it removes terminal lysine residues from fibrin, which impairs binding of certain forms of plasminogen to fibrin and disrupts tissue plasminogen activator-induced plasmin generation in the blood clot.[228] Thus, activated TAFI is a strong inhibitor of fibrinolysis. Large amounts of thrombin are necessary for TAFI activation, but the reaction is substantially augmented when thrombin is bound to thrombomodulin.[229] It follows that impaired generation of thrombin, for example, in inherited deficiency of factor VIII, IX, or XI, not only delays clot formation but also enhances premature lysis of clots.[230] Activation of factor XI by thrombin, particularly within the blood clot, is essential for adequate TAFI activation and protection of the clot from lysis.[230–232] These data fit well with clinical observations in factor XI-deficient patients who are particularly susceptible to bleeding following injury at sites exhibiting local fibrinolytic activity[233] and with the effective prevention of such episodes by antifibrinolytic agents (see "Therapy" below).[234]

Factor XI is synthesized by the liver. The case of acquired factor XI deficiency as a result of liver transplantation from a donor who, in retrospect, had the deficiency has been reported.[235]

Factor XI deficiency as a result of a dysfunctional protein is rare. In a study of 125 patients of various ethnic origins, none had discordant levels of factor XI activity and antigen.[236] Only several patients with deficiency of factor XI activity and seemingly normal antigen levels have been described.[237–240] (See also database at www.isth.org.)

GENETICS

Inheritance

In most cases, factor XI deficiency is inherited as an autosomal recessive trait characterized by plasma factor XI levels less than 15 percent of normal in homozygotes and compound heterozygotes.[213,214,233] In heterozygotes, factor XI levels frequently range between 25 and 70 percent of normal, but can be higher.[214,241] Exceptional cases of patients in whom dominantly transmitted heterozygosity is associated with a significant bleeding tendency and factor XI levels of approximately 10 to 20 percent of normal (see "Mutations" below) have been described.

Mutations

Three mutations, designated type I, II, and III, were first described in six Ashkenazi-Jewish patients with severe factor XI deficiency.[242] The type I mutation is a G>A change at the splice site of the last intron of the gene. The type II mutation is a G>T change in exon 5 at Glu117 leading to a stop codon –TAA. The type III mutation is a T>C change in exon 9 that results in a substitution of Phe283 by Leu in the fourth apple domain of the protein. A fourth mutation designated type IV, later identified in another Ashkenazi-Jewish patient, consists of a 14-bp deletion at the exon 14–intron N junction.[243] Of the four mutations, the predominant mutations in Jewish persons are types II and III. Altogether, 152 mutations have been reported in non-Jewish and Jewish patients of various origins (see Table 125–2). These comprise 99 missense and 21 nonsense mutations, with the remaining being deletions, insertions (including the whole gene) and splice site mutations. Expression of several missense mutations revealed impaired factor XI secretion from transfected cells.[244–246]

The homodimeric structure of factor XI implies that for certain mutations in heterozygotes, the mutant allele imparts a dominant negative effect by impairing secretion of wild-type mutant heterodimers. Cotransfection experiments with Gly400Val or Trp569Ser yielded decreased secretion of wild-type factor XI by 50 percent.[247] The heterozygotes for these mutations manifest a significant bleeding tendency and a factor XI level as low as 10 percent of normal.

The Gly555Glu mutation located two amino acids before the active serine yields a dysfunctional protein that is normally activated by factor XIIa or thrombin, but its activated form fails to activate factor IX and is resistant to inhibition by antithrombin.[238]

Ethnic Distribution and Prevalence

Most patients with factor XI deficiency are Jewish.[213,214,233,241] Several instances of vertical transmission of severe factor XI deficiency in Ashkenazi-Jewish families (consistent with pseudodominance) suggested that the mutant gene frequency in this segment of Jewish individuals is very high. The high frequency was indeed found in two surveys of this population performed in Israel.[214,248]

Types II and III are the predominant mutations causing factor XI deficiency in Jewish persons.[233,249] Of 590 mutant alleles in 295 unrelated patients with severe deficiency, 577 (97.8%) were either type II (306 alleles) or type III (271 alleles). Screening of the general Ashkenazi-Jewish population for these mutations disclosed allele frequencies of 0.0217 for type II mutation and 0.0254 for type III mutation.[250] Hence, the estimated frequency of subjects with severe factor XI deficiency in Ashkenazi Jews is 1:450 and of heterozygotes for either type of mutation is 1:11. These data indicate factor XI deficiency is the most frequent hereditary disorder in this population. Interestingly, the type II mutation was observed in Iraqi Jews with a similar allele frequency of 0.0167,[250] but in Palestinian Arabs and in Sephardic and other Middle Eastern Jews at frequencies of 0.0065 and 0.0027, respectively.[251] In sharp contrast, the type III mutation was not detected among 1343 Jewish persons of non-Ashkenazi origin or in 313 Palestinian Arabs.[251] A recent study indicated that both type II and type III mutations are prevalent in the Italian population, although at a much lower rate.[252]

A second cluster of patients with factor XI deficiency was observed in Basques living in southwestern France in whom the predominant mutation is a Cys38Arg substitution.[246] The frequency of this mutant allele in the general Basque population is 0.005. A third cluster of factor XI-deficient patients was reported in whites residing in or originating from the United Kingdom.[253] The mutation, a Cys128stop nonsense alteration, is predicted to produce a truncated protein and has an estimated allele frequency of 0.01 in the general British white population.

Founder Effects

Haplotype analysis based on examination of factor XI gene polymorphisms disclosed distinct founder effects for type II and type III mutations.[251] In view of the similar prevalences of the type II mutation in Iraqi Jews and Ashkenazi Jews, the presence of the type II mutation in Palestinian Arabs and Sephardic Jews, and the historical information about the divergence of these populations 2000 to 2500 years ago, the type II mutation seems to have occurred in ancient times. Type III mutation, which is confined to Ashkenazi Jews, probably stems from a founder who lived in more recent times. There is reported evidence to support these hypotheses.[254] Haplotype analyses have suggested founder effects for the Cys38Arg mutation in Basques and for the Cys128stop mutation in British whites.[246,253]

CLINICAL FEATURES

Bleeding Manifestations in Homozygotes and Compound Heterozygotes

Most bleeding manifestations in homozygotes and compound heterozygotes are injury related. Excessive bleeding can occur at the time of injury or begin several hours or days following trauma. Some patients with severe factor XI deficiency may not bleed at all following trauma.[213] In other patients, the bleeding tendency varies depending upon the hemostatic challenge and the variable sites of injury.[233,241,255] Surgical procedures involving tissues with high fibrinolytic activity (urinary tract, tonsils, nose, tooth sockets) frequently are associated with excessive bleeding in patients with severe factor XI deficiency, irrespective of the genotype.[233,256] A significantly lower frequency of bleeding complications follows surgical interventions at sites without excessive local fibrinolysis, such as appendicectomy, cholecystectomy, circumcision, and orthopedic surgery.[256] Site-related bleeding tendency now can be understood in light of the demonstrated function of factor XI in preventing clot lysis (see "Biochemistry and Molecular Features" above).

Spontaneous bleeding manifestations such as menorrhagia, gingival bleeding, ecchymoses, and epistaxis occur in patients with severe factor XI deficiency but are uncommon.[255] Postpartum hemorrhage occurs in only 24 percent of affected women.[257]

Bleeding Manifestations in Heterozygotes

Whether heterozygotes exhibit a bleeding tendency (except for those bearing mutations causing a dominant negative effect) is controversial. In one extensive study, heterozygotes had almost no bleeding complications following a variety of surgical procedures, including operations at sites with enhanced local fibrinolysis.[213] In another study, all heterozygotes who underwent urologic surgery did well except for one patient whose factor XI level was 25 percent of normal.[248] Other studies identified a bleeding tendency, particularly following injury, in 33 percent,[241] 48 percent,[255] and 20 percent[258] of heterozygotes. Variable definitions of what constitutes a bleeding tendency[259] can only partially explain this discrepancy. A more likely explanation for the variable manifestations in heterozygotes is the coexistence of additional hemostatic abnormalities in patients who do bleed. Thus, heterozygotes who were defined as bleeders tended to have lower levels of factor VIII and von Willebrand factor, and to have blood group O, which is associated with reduced von Willebrand factor levels. Moreover, in another study, most heterozygotes who presented with a bleeding tendency also had a platelet function abnormality.[260] A study that assessed the risk of bleeding in patients from 45 families showed that the odds ratio for bleeding was 13.0 in homozygotes and compound heterozygotes, but was only 2.6 in heterozygotes.[258] It can be concluded that heterozygotes for factor XI deficiency may display a small risk of bleeding but that this risk is significantly lower than the risk of bleeding exhibited by homozygotes and compound heterozygotes.

Thrombosis

Although factor XI plays an essential role in promoting blood coagulation and prevention of fibrinolysis, severe factor XI deficiency does not confer protection against myocardial infarction. Of 96 unrelated patients who were older than age 35 years and who had severe factor XI deficiency, 16 had a myocardial infarction.[261] In contrast, severe factor XI deficiency was shown to confer protection against ischemic stroke.[262] This remarkable difference probably relates to variable undefined characteristics of the cerebral and myocardial vascular beds. Venous thromboembolism was described in two reports,[253,263] but whether this finding suggests no protection against venous thrombosis remains to be determined. Thrombotic events have been described in patients with severe factor XI deficiency following infusion of factor XI concentrates (see "Therapy" below).

Association of Factor XI Deficiency with Other Disorders

Factor XI deficiency has been described in patients with Gaucher disease. In view of the independent segregation of the two disorders,[264] the coincidental occurrence of Gaucher disease and hereditary factor XI deficiency appears to stem from the high frequency of the respective mutant genes in the Ashkenazi-Jewish population. Patients with Noonan syndrome display factor XI deficiency as well as several other abnormalities in coagulation factors and platelet function for which no explanation has been provided.[265] A variety of other inherited disorders of hemostasis have been described in association with factor XI deficiency, including von Willebrand disease,[266,267] factor VIII deficiency,[241,268,269] and factor VII deficiency.[270] Because of the high prevalence of factor XI deficiency in Jewish persons, these associations are expected to occur in this population.

Acquired Inhibitors

Inhibitors that neutralize factor XI activity have been described in patients with severe hereditary factor XI deficiency who received plasma replacement therapy. Of 118 Israeli patients examined, 7 had an inhibitor to factor XI.[271] All the patients belonged to a subgroup of 21 patients who were homozygotes for the Glu117stop mutation and had received plasma prior to development of the inhibitor. Of six additional patients who received plasma or factor XI concentrate and had an inhibitor, five had the same genotype and one was homozygous for another null mutation, Gln88stop.[239] Thus, approximately one-third of patients who are homozygous for a null mutation can be expected to develop an inhibitor following blood component therapy.

An interesting patient harboring homozygosity for the Glu117stop mutation and Rh negativity developed an inhibitor antibody against factor XI following anti-D therapy during pregnancy.[272] This patient had not received plasma derivatives before. The development of the inhibitor was attributed to the presence of small amounts of factor XI in anti-D immunoglobulin (Ig) preparations.[272] Inhibitors that were characterized are of the IgG type recognizing different epitopes of factor XI and giving rise to impaired binding to HK, abrogation of activation by thrombin and factor XIIa, and diminished activation of factor IX. Spontaneous bleeding manifestations usually do not occur following the development of an inhibitor to factor XI. However, in one patient whose antibody titer was extremely high, spontaneous bleeding did occur.[273] Securing hemostasis during and after surgery in such cases is a great challenge (see "Therapy" below).

■ LABORATORY FEATURES

Patients with factor XI deficiency have a prolonged aPTT and normal PT (see Chap. 118). All homozygotes and compound heterozygotes have aPTTs that are longer than 2 standard deviations above the normal mean.[274] However, aPTT values in heterozygotes substantially overlap the normal range.[233,274] Consequently, screening of patients for a hemostatic abnormality prior to surgery (which is recommended for Jewish patients because of the high prevalence of factor XI deficiency) identifies all patients with a severe factor XI deficiency. The diagnosis is established by an aPTT-based assay using factor XI-deficient plasma.[213] Factor XI antigen also can be measured by ELISA.[238] For known mutations, analysis by polymerase chain reaction and restriction enzyme digestion, or by multiplex real-time polymerase chain reaction can identify the patient's genotype.[233,252] Mean factor XI levels are 1.2 percent of normal in type II homozygotes, 3.3 percent of normal in compound heterozygotes for the type II and type III mutations, and 9.7 percent of normal in type III homozygotes.[233] Although one study reported heterozygotes for the type II mutation have a significantly lower mean factor XI level than heterozygotes for the type III mutation,[233] another study found similar values in patients bearing the two genotypes.[249]

■ THERAPY

Patients with Severe Deficiency

Patients with severe factor XI deficiency who must undergo a surgical procedure should be carefully evaluated and meticulously prepared for the operation. A negative history of excessive bleeding following previous procedures does not preclude an increased bleeding tendency. Other hemostatic abnormalities and the presence of an inhibitor to factor XI should be excluded. Aspirin or other antiplatelet agents should not be given during the week prior to surgery.

When choosing the treatment modality and the intensity of treatment, the following issues should be considered: (1) patient's age and history of cardiovascular disease, as use of plasma may create volume overload and use of a factor XI concentrate can induce thrombosis; (2) presence of an inhibitor to factor XI, as plasma or factor XI concentrate cannot be used in such patients; (3) use of an antifibrinolytic agent should be considered in patients undergoing operation at a site with high local fibrinolytic activity, as in oral or lower urinary tract surgery; (4) PT and platelet count should be tested; (5) safety, as transmission of infectious agents and allergic reactions are more common following plasma transfusions compared to factor XI concentrate; however, concentrates can induce thrombosis; (6) half-life of factor XI, as a mean half-life of 52 hours was recorded following infusions of a factor XI concentrate[275] and 45 hours following plasma transfusion.[276]

Patients undergoing dental extractions do not require replacement therapy. Tranexamic acid administration (1 g qid) starting 12 hours before surgery until 7 days after surgery effectively prevents bleeding.[234] ε-Aminocaproic acid (5–6 g qid) given similarly is expected to achieve the same results. For major surgery or surgery at sites with increased fibrinolytic activity, fresh-frozen plasma should be transfused for approximately 10 days, targeting trough factor XI levels 45 percent of normal.[277] For surgery at tissues not displaying high levels of local fibrinolysis, fresh-frozen plasma can be transfused for approximately 5 days, targeting trough factor XI levels 30 percent of normal. Following prostatectomy and bladder operations, continuous flushing of the bladder with saline containing tranexamic acid 0.5 to 1 g/L can be helpful for hemostasis. For nose surgery or tonsillectomy, apart from replacement therapy, tranexamic acid or ε-aminocaproic acid given as for dental extraction should be considered. No plasma replacement therapy is necessary during or after labor unless excessive bleeding occurs.[257]

Two viral-inactivated factor XI concentrates have been used for treatment of patients with factor XI deficiency.[275,278,279] However, infusions of the two concentrates result in laboratory signs of DIC.[280,281] Pulmonary embolism and arterial thrombosis, including fatal cases, have been reported in patients receiving the concentrates,[282,283] albeit mostly in elderly patients who had preexisting cardiovascular disease and were given a dose greater than 30 U/kg. Consequently, these concentrates must be used with great caution.

Patients with Partial Factor XI Deficiency

Heterozygotes with a negative history of a bleeding tendency who do not exhibit any other hemostatic abnormality and whose plasma factor XI level is more than 40 percent of normal probably do not require treatment while undergoing surgery.[248] However, if a positive bleeding history is elicited in such patients, a detailed investigation of the hemostatic system should be performed. If another abnormality is found, adequate measures should be taken to correct that abnormality, in addition to replacement therapy for 5 days targeting trough factor XI levels 45 percent of normal.

Patients with Inhibitor Antibodies to Factor XI

Most reported patients have not exhibited aggravation of bleeding tendency following development of an inhibitor. Consequently, when such patients undergo dental extraction, use of tranexamic acid and fibrin glue may be sufficient,[284] but limited evidence supporting this contention is available. Activated prothrombin complex[273,285] and recombinant factor VIIa[286] have been used successfully for major surgical procedures, and an *in vitro* study revealed that abnormal thrombin generation in the plasma of patients with an inhibitor was corrected by adding moderate amounts of recombinant factor VIIa.[271,287] A recent study showed that the use of a one-time low dose of recombinant factor VIIa (15–30 mcg/kg) given at the end of surgery and tranexamic acid 1 g four times daily from 2 hours before surgery until 7 days after surgery secured normal hemostasis in three patients with an inhibitor.[288]

FACTOR XIII DEFICIENCY

DEFINITION AND HISTORY

Factor XIII (fibrin-stabilizing factor) is a plasma transglutaminase that crosslinks γ-glutamyl–ε-lysine residues of fibrinogen chains, thereby stabilizing the fibrin clot. Severe deficiency of factor XIII, first described by Duckert and colleagues[289] in 1960, causes a moderate to severe hemorrhagic disorder, recurrent abortions, and impaired wound healing in some patients.

BIOCHEMISTRY AND MOLECULAR FEATURES

Plasma factor XIII is an Mr 340,000 heterotetramer composed of two catalytic A-subunits and two carrier B-subunits linked by noncovalent bonds. The average concentration of the A_2B_2 tetramer in plasma is approximately 22 mcg/mL, and its half-life is 9 to 14 days.[290] The A-subunit (Mr ~82,000) contains an activation peptide, the catalytic site of factor XIII, and a calcium binding site.[291] It is structurally homologous with the α chain of tissue transglutaminase,[292] the α chain of keratinocyte transglutaminase,[293] and band 4.2 of erythrocytes,[294] although the latter lacks transglutaminase activity. The first 37 amino acids of the N-terminus of the factor XIII A-subunit constitute an activation peptide that is removed by thrombin cleavage of an Arg37-Gly38 bond in the presence of calcium ions.[295] An active site sulfhydryl residue, which is characteristic for this class of enzymes, is located at Cys314. Two calcium-binding domains, which have weak homology with the canonical EF calcium-binding hands of calmodulin, flank the active site cysteine.

The three-dimensional structure of factor XIII A-subunit determined by x-ray crystallography disclosed the A-subunit is divided into four sequential domains: β-sandwich (Glu43-Phe184), catalytic core (Asn185-Arg515), and two barrel domains (Ser516-Thr628, Ile629-Arg727).[296] The catalytic triad Cys314-His373-Asp396 is very similar to the Cys-His-Asp triad of papain-like cysteine proteases.

The two B-subunits of factor XIII function as carrier proteins for the A-subunits,[297,298] stabilizing them in the circulation and regulating the calcium-dependent activation of factor XIII. The B-subunit of Mr 76,500, is composed of 10 homologous consensus or "sushi" repeats, each consisting of approximately 60 amino acids.[299]

The gene for the factor XIII A-subunit is located on chromosome 6p24-p25.[300,301] It spans more than 170 kb and is composed of 15 exons.[302] The B-subunit gene is located on chromosome 1q31-q32.1.[303] Interestingly, a number of other genes encoding for proteins with "sushi" repeats also are located on chromosome 1. The gene for the B-subunit spans 28 kb and is composed of 12 exons.[299]

Factor XIII A-subunit is synthesized in megakaryocytes and is packed into newly formed platelets.[304] Monocytes and tissue macrophages/histiocytes in the placenta, uterus, and liver also produce A-subunits.[290,305] Because factor XIII-A subunit lacks a signal sequence, it cannot be released by the classic secretory pathway through the Golgi. Conceivably, factor XIII A-subunit is released into the circulation from cells as a consequence of cell injury.[302] The B-subunit is synthesized in the liver.[306,307] Assembly of the A- and B-subunits probably occurs in the circulation.

Factor XIII circulates in plasma as an inactive tetramer (A_2B_2). Cleavage of the Arg37-Gly38 peptide bond of the A-subunit by thrombin releases a 4500-kDa activation peptide that is required for activation of the tetramer.[308] Thereafter, calcium ions induce dissociation of the A- and B-subunits. In the absence of inhibitory B-subunits, the active site sulfhydryl residue of the A-subunit is exposed and proteolytically activated (activated factor XIII [factor XIIIa]).[290] Fibrin polymer is an important cofactor for generation of factor XIIIa.[309]

Factor XIIIa catalyzes the formation of peptide bonds between adjacent molecules of fibrin monomer, thus imparting chemical and mechanical stability to a clot. The peptide bond that is formed consists of an amide bond between the γ-carbonyl group of glutamine and the ε-amino group of lysine. In fibrin, this amide bond is located between Aα-chain sequences and between γ-chain sequences.[309,310] Factor XIIIa also crosslinks α_2-antiplasmin to the α-chain of fibrin,[311] thereby increasing the resistance of fibrin to plasmin degradation, and crosslinks fibronectin to the α-chain of fibrin,[312] thereby affecting the mechanical properties of the clot and increasing cell adhesion. A number of other proteins also are substrates for factor XIIIa, including factor V, plasminogen activator inhibitor-2, collagen, thrombospondin, von Willebrand factor, vinculin, vitronectin, actin, myosin, and lipoprotein(a), but the physiologic significance of these reactions is less clear.[290]

GENETICS

Inherited factor XIII deficiency is transmitted in an autosomal recessive fashion. Parents of affected individuals typically are asymptomatic, and consanguinity is common. Deficiency of the factor XIII A-subunit is the predominant abnormality and occurs at a frequency of approximately 1 in 2 to 3 million.[313] A higher prevalence was described in the Finnish, Swiss, and Palestinian Arab populations.[314–316] At the time of this writing, 99 mutations causing factor XIII A-subunit deficiency have been reported, of which 1 is in the promoter region, 45 are missense mutations, 7 are nonsense mutations, 15 are splice-site mutations, 28 are small deletions/insertions, and 3 are gross deletions (see Table 125–2). For two mutations, a splice-site IVS5–1G>A prevalent in European populations, and Arg660Pro in Palestinian Arabs, haplotype analyses were consistent with founder effects, respectively.[316,317] It is likely that the Arg661stop mutation in Finnish patients and the Arg77Cys mutation in Swiss patients are also a result of founder effects, although both are at CpG dinucleotides and therefore can be considered recurrent mutations.[314,315,317] Another mutation, Ser295Arg, was identified in six Pakistani families and may also stem from a common founder but this remains to be established.[318]

Six common nonsynonymous polymorphisms have been identified in the A-subunit gene.[319] One is a common G>T alteration resulting in Val34Leu substitution that affects factor XIII function.[309] Some but not all studies found the Leu34 allele was protective against myocardial infarction and venous thrombosis.[309]

Four mutations causing deficiency of B-subunits have been described. One is a missense mutation (Cys430Phe); the remaining are small deletions/insertions.[320]

CLINICAL MANIFESTATIONS

Factor XIII deficiency causes formation of blood clots that are unstable and susceptible to fibrinolytic degradation by plasmin. As a result, affected individuals have an increased tendency to bleed. Factor XIII A-subunit knockout mice manifest bleeding into the thoracic cavity, peritoneum, and subcutis.[321] In humans, bleeding from the umbilical stump during the first few days of life is common, and intracranial hemorrhage is observed more frequently than in other inherited bleeding disorders. This finding forms the basis for recommending prophylaxis against intracranial hemorrhage by regular replacement therapy. Ecchymoses, muscle hematomas, prolonged bleeding following trauma and hemarthroses also are characteristic.[317,322]

Delayed wound healing occurs in approximately 15 percent of patients deficient in factor XIII. The exact mechanism by which factor XIII, or its activated form, exerts its beneficial effect on wound healing is unknown. A proangiogenic effect of factor XIIIa was described and thus it is conceivable that in the absence of factor XIII, decreased vascularization of wounds results in improper repair.[323]

Habitual abortions are commonly observed in affected patients and in mice deficient in factor XIII A-subunit.[317,324] In affected women, formation of the cytotrophoblastic shell is impaired.[325] Conceivably, factor XIII A-subunit deficiency at the implantation site abrogates fibrin/fibronectin crosslinking, which is essential for attachment of the placenta to the uterus.[326]

Inhibitor antibodies against factor XIII have been described in three patients with severe inherited factor XIII deficiency.[37,317]

DIAGNOSIS

PT and aPTT are normal in factor XIII deficiency (see Chap. 118). Because of increased fibrin breakdown, levels of fibrin degradation products may be increased and result in a minimally prolonged thrombin time. This finding may be the only clue to the diagnosis based on simple coagulation screening tests. Diagnosis of factor XIII deficiency is established by demonstrating increased clot solubility in 5 M urea, dilute monochloroacetic acid, or acetic acid. Factor XIII activity also can be determined quantitatively by a chromogenic assay (Dade-Behring, Germany) or by an incorporation assay (Pentapharm, Switzerland).[315,317] Factor XIII A-subunit antigen can be measured by ELISA.[327]

DIFFERENTIAL DIAGNOSIS

Severe inherited factor XIII deficiency is easily differentiated from other deficiencies of plasma coagulation factors by demonstrating normal results of screening coagulation tests and increased fibrin solubility. The very rare deficiency of α_2-antiplasmin may cause an increased tendency to bleed, also with normal screening tests and increased clot solubility. A specific assay for α_2-antiplasmin is required to distinguish between the two disorders. However, patients with α_2-antiplasmin deficiency appear to have a milder bleeding disorder and do not manifest umbilical cord or intracranial hemorrhages.

A family history and a lifelong history of bleeding help distinguish inherited factor XIII deficiency from acquired inhibitor antibodies against factor XIII-A subunit, an extremely rare entity which can be idiopathic, drug induced or related to systemic lupus erythematosus or lymphoproliferation disorders (see Chap. 128).[328] An autoantibody against factor XIII-B subunit associated with severe bleeding was described in one patient with systemic lupus erythematosus.[329]

THERAPY

Plasma replacement therapy for factor XIII deficiency is highly satisfactory because of the small quantities of factor XIII needed for effective hemostasis and the long half-life of factor XIII (9–14 days).[290] Plasma-derived, virus-inactivated concentrates of factor XIII are available[330] and are the treatment of choice. Recombinant factor XIII-A2 has been tested successfully in a phase 1 study.[331] The recombinant product binds to the endogenous plasma factor XIII-B and displays a half-life of 8.5 days. Fresh-frozen plasma or solvent–detergent-treated plasma can be used when factor XIII concentrates are unavailable. Prophylactic therapy with factor XIII concentrate at a regimen of 10 to 20 U/kg every 5 to 6 weeks is sufficient to secure normal hemostasis.[330,332] During pregnancy, more frequent replacement therapy is needed to prevent fetal loss. On the basis of prophylactic therapy during eight pregnancies in patients with severe factor XIII deficiency and review of the literature it was recommended to administer factor XIII concentrate 250 U/week from early gestation, to increase the weekly dose to 500 U as of the twenty-third week, and to give 1000 U during labor.[333] A one-time infusion of 10 to 20 U/kg is sufficient when impaired wound healing occurs in patients with hereditary factor XIII deficiency.

REFERENCES

1. Walz DA, Hewett-Emmett D, Seegers WH: Amino acid sequence of human prothrombin fragments 1, and 2. *Proc Natl Acad Sci U S A* 74:1969, 1977.
2. Butkowski RJ, Elion J, Downing MR, Mann KG: Primary structure of human prethrombin 2, and alpha-thrombin. *J Biol Chem* 252:4942, 1977.
3. Degen SJ, MacGillivray RT, Davie EW: Characterization of the complementary deoxyribonucleic acid and gene coding for human prothrombin. *Biochemistry* 22:2087, 1983.
4. Degen SJ, Sun WY: The biology of prothrombin. *Crit Rev Eukaryot Gene Expr* 8:203, 1998.
5. Kotkow KJ, Deitcher SR, Furie B, Furie BC: The second kringle domain of prothrombin promotes factor Va-mediated prothrombin activation by prothrombinase. *J Biol Chem* 270:4551, 1995.
6. Bode W, Mayr I, Baumann U, et al: The refined 1.9, A crystal structure of human α-thrombin interaction with D-Phe-Pro-Arg chloromethylketone and significance of the Tyr-Pro-Pro-Trp insertion segment. *EMBO J* 8:3467, 1989.
7. Royle NJ, Irwin DM, Koschnsky ML, et al: Human genes encoding prothrombin and ceruloplasmin map to 11p11-q12, and 3q21–24, respectively. *Somat Cell Mol Genet* 13:285, 1987.
8. Degen SJ, Davie EW: Nucleotide sequence of the gene for human prothrombin. *Biochemistry* 26:6165, 1987.
9. Bancroft JD, Schaefer LA, Degen SJ: Characterization of the Alu-rich 5′-flanking region of the human prothrombin-encoding gene: Identification of a positive *cis*-acting element that regulates liver-specific expression. *Gene* 95:253, 1990.
10. Lane DA, Phillipu H, Huntington JA: Directing thrombin. *Blood* 106:2605, 2005.
11. Sun WY, Witte DP, Degen JL, et al: Prothrombin deficiency results in embryonic and neonatal lethality in mice. *Proc Natl Acad Sci U S A* 95:7597, 1998.
12. Miyata T, Moita T, Inomoto T, et al: Prothrombin Tokushima, a replacement of arginine-418, by tryptophan that impairs the fibrinogen clotting activity of derived thrombin Tokushima. *Biochemistry* 26:1117, 1987.
13. Morishita E, Saito M, Asakura H, et al: Prothrombin Himi: An abnormal prothrombin characterized by a defective thrombin activity. *Thromb Res* 62:697, 1991.
14. Akhavan S, De Cristofaro R, Peyvandi F, et al: Molecular and functional characterization of a natural homozygous Arg67His mutation in the prothrombin gene of a patient with a severe procoagulant defect contrasting with a mild hemorrhagic phenotype. *Blood* 100:1347, 2002.
15. O'Marcaigh AS, Nichols WL, Hassinger NL, et al: Genetic analysis and functional characterization of prothrombins Corpus Christi (Arg382-Cys), Dhahran (Arg271-His), and hypoprothrombinemia. *Blood* 88:2611, 1996.
16. Henriksen RA, Mann KG: Identification of the primary structural defect in the dysthrombin thrombin Quick I: Substitution of cysteine for arginine-382. *Biochemistry* 27:9160, 1988.
17. Henriksen RA, Mann KG: Substitution of valine for glycine-558, in the congenital dysthrombin thrombin Quick II alters primary substrate specificity. *Biochemistry* 28:2078, 1989.
18. Miyata T, Aruga R, Umeyama H, et al: Prothrombin Salakta: Substitution of glutamic acid-466, by alanine reduces the fibrinogen clotting activity and the esterase activity. *Biochemistry* 31:7457, 1992.
19. Henriksen RA, Dunham CK, Miller LD, et al: Prothrombin Greenville, Arg517Gln, identified in an individual heterozygous for dysprothrombinemia. *Blood* 91:2026, 1998.
20. Sekine O, Sugo T, Ebisawa K, et al: Substitution of Gly-548, to Ala in the substrate binding pocket of prothrombin Perija leads to the loss of thrombin proteolytic activity. *Thromb Haemost* 87:282, 2002.
21. Sun WY, Smirnow D, Jenkins ML, Degen SJ: Prothrombin Scranton: Substitution of an amino acid residue involved in the binding of Na^+ (Lys-556, to Thr) leads to dysprothrombinemia. *Thromb Haemost* 85:651, 2001.
22. Diuguid DL, Rabiet MJ, Furie BC, Furie B: Molecular defects of factor IX Chicago-2, (Arg 145His) and prothrombin Madrid (Arg 271Cys): Arginine mutations that preclude zymogen activation. *Blood* 74:193, 1989.
23. James HL, Kim DJ, Zheng DQ, Girolami A: Prothrombin Padua I: Incomplete activation due to an amino acid substitution at a factor Xa cleavage site. *Blood Coagul Fibrinolysis* 5:841, 1994.
24. Sun WY, Burkart MC, Holahan JR, Degen SJ: Prothrombin San Antonio: A single amino acid substitution at a factor Xa activation site (Arg320, to His) results in dysprothrombinemia. *Blood* 95:711, 2000.
25. Lefkowitz JB, Weller A, Nuss R, et al: A common mutation, Arg457Gln, links prothrombin deficiencies in the Puerto Rican population. *J Thromb Haemost* 1:2381, 2003.
26. Ruiz-Saez A, Luengo J, Rodriguez A, et al: Prothrombin Perija: A new congenital dysprothrombinemia in an Indian family. *Thromb Res* 44:587, 1986.
27. Ruiz-Saez A, Bosch N, Echenagucia M, et al: High prevalence of an abnormal prothrombin in an Indian population of Venezuela [abstract]. *Thromb Haemost* 73:1438, 1995.
28. Poort SR, Rosendaal FR, Reitsma PH, Bertina RM: A common genetic variation in the 3′-untranslated region of the prothrombin gene is associated with elevated plasma prothrombin levels and an increase in venous thrombosis. *Blood* 88:3698, 1996.
29. Gehring NH, Frede U, Neu-Yilik G, et al: Increased efficiency of mRNA 3′ end formation: A new genetic mechanism contributing to hereditary thrombophilia. *Nat Genet* 28:389, 2001.
30. Mannucci PM: Outbreak of hepatitis A among Italian patients with haemophilia. *Lancet* 339:819, 1992.
31. Gerritzen A, Schneweis KE, Brackmann HH, et al: Acute hepatitis A in haemophilias. *Lancet* 340:1231, 1992.
32. Ragni MV, Koch WC, Jorda JA: Parvovirus B19, infection in patients with hemophilia. *Transfusion* 36:238, 1996.
33. Jorquera JI: Safety procedures of coagulation factors. *Haemophilia* 13(Suppl 5):41, 2007.
34. Lusher JM: Thrombogenicity associated with factor IX complex concentrates. *Semin Hematol* 28:3, 1991.
35. Alexander B, Goldstein R, Landwehr G, Cook CD: Congenital SPCA deficiency: A hitherto unrecognized coagulation defect with hemorrhage rectified by serum and serum fractions. *J Clin Invest* 30:596, 1951.
36. Peyvandi F, Duga S, Akhavan S, Mannucci PM: Rare coagulation deficiencies. *Haemophilia* 8:308, 2002.
37. Acharya SS, Coughlin A, Dimichele DM: Rare Bleeding Disorder Registry: Deficiencies of factors II V, VII X, XIII, fibrinogen and dysfibrinogenemias. *J Thromb Haemost* 2:248, 2004.
38. Hagen FS, Gray CL, O'Hara P, et al: Characterization of a cDNA coding for human factor VII. *Proc Natl Acad Sci U S A* 83:2412, 1986.
39. O'Hara PJ, Grant FJ, Haldeman BA, et al: Nucleotide sequence of the gene coding for human factor VII, a vitamin K-dependent protein participating in blood coagulation. *Proc Natl Acad Sci U S A* 84:5158, 1987.
40. Ott R, Pfeiffer RA: Evidence that activities of coagulation factors VII and X are linked to chromosome 13, (q34). *Hum Hered* 34:123, 1984.
41. Gilgenkrantz S, Briquel ME, Andre E, et al: Structural genes of coagulation factors VII and X located on 13q34. *Ann Genet* 29:32, 1986.
42. Miao CH, Leytus SP, Chung DW, Davie EW: Liver-specific expression of the gene coding for human factor X, a blood coagulation factor. *J Biol Chem* 267:7395, 1992.
43. Greenberg D, Miao CH, Ho WT, et al: Liver-specific expression of the human factor VII gene. *Proc Natl Acad Sci U S A* 92:12347, 1995.
44. Pollak ES, Hung HL, Godin W, et al: Functional characterization of the human factor VII 5′-flanking region. *J Biol Chem* 271:1738, 1996.
45. Fair DS: Quantitation of factor VII in the plasma of normal and warfarin-treated individuals by radioimmunoassay. *Blood* 62:784, 1983.
46. Marder VJ, Shulman NR: Clinical aspects of congenital factor VII deficiency. *Am J Med* 37:182, 1964.
47. Radcliffe R, Nemerson Y: Activation and control of factor VII by activated factor X and thrombin: Isolation and characterization of a single chain form of factor VII. *J Biol Chem* 250:388, 1975.
48. Seligsohn U, Osterud B, Brown SF, et al: Activation of human factor VII in plasma and in purified systems: Roles of activated factor IX, kallikrein, and activated factor XII. *J Clin Invest* 64:1056, 1979.
49. Radcliffe R, Bagdasarian A, Colman R, Nemerson Y: Activation of bovine factor VII by Hageman factor fragments. *Blood* 50:611, 1977.
50. Nakagaki T, Foster DC, Berkner KL, Kisiel W: Initiation of the extrinsic pathway of blood coagulation: Evidence for the tissue factor dependent autoactivation of human coagulation factor VII. *Biochemistry* 30:10819, 1991.
51. Rapaport SI, Rao LV: The tissue factor pathway: How it has become a "prima ballerina." *Thromb Haemost* 74:7, 1995.
52. Banner DW, D'Arcy A, Chene C, et al: The crystal structure of the complex of blood coagulation factor VIIa with soluble tissue factor. *Nature* 380:41, 1996.
53. Cooper DN, Millar DS, Wacey A, et al: Inherited factor VII deficiency: Molecular genetics and pathophysiology. *Thromb Haemost* 78:151, 1997.
54. Edgington TS, Dickinson CD, Ruf W: The structural basis of function of the TF-VIIa complex in the cellular initiation of coagulation. *Thromb Haemost* 78:401, 1997.
55. Morrissey JH, Neuenschwander PF, Huang Q, et al: Factor VIIa–tissue factor: Functional importance of protein-membrane interactions. *Thromb Haemost* 78:112, 1997.
56. Morrissey JH, Macik BG, Neuenschwander PF, Comp PC: Quantitation of activated factor VII levels in plasma using a tissue factor mutant selectively deficient in promoting factor VII activation. *Blood* 81:734, 1993.
57. Seligsohn U, Kasper CK, Osterud B, Rapaport SI: Activated factor VII: Presence in factor IX concentrates and persistence in the circulation after infusion. *Blood* 53:828, 1979.
58. Miller BC, Hultin MB, Jesty J: Altered factor VII activity in hemophilia. *Blood* 65:845, 1985.
59. Wildgoose P, Nemerson Y, Hansen LL, et al: Measurement of basal levels of factor VIIa in hemophilia A and B patients. *Blood* 80:25, 1992.
60. Eichinger S, Mannucci PM, Tradati F, et al: Determinants of plasma factor VIIa levels in humans. *Blood* 86:3021, 1995.
61. Osterud B, Rapaport SI: Activation of factor IX by the reaction product of tissue factor and factor VII: Additional pathway for initiating blood coagulation. *Proc Natl Acad Sci U S A* 74:5260, 1977.

62. Butenas S, Van't Veer C, Mann KG: Evaluation of the initiation phase of blood coagulation using ultrasensitive assays for serine proteases. *J Biol Chem* 272:21527, 1997.
63. Rosen ED, Chan JC, Idusogie E, et al: Mice lacking factor VII develop normally but suffer fatal perinatal bleeding. *Nature* 390:290, 1997.
64. Carmeliet P, Mackman N, Moons L, et al: Role of tissue factor in embryonic blood vessel development. *Nature* 383:73, 1996.
65. Parry GC, Erlich JH, Carmeliet P, et al: Low levels of tissue factor are compatible with development and hemostasis in mice. *J Clin Invest* 101:560, 1998.
66. Herrmann FH, Wulff K, Auerswald G, et al: Factor VII deficiency: clinical manifestation of 717, subjects from Europe and Latin America with mutations in the factor 7, gene. *Haemophilia* 15:267, 2008.
67. Tamary H, Fromovich Y, Shalmon L, et al: Ala244Val is a common, probably ancient mutation causing factor VII deficiency in Moroccan and Iranian Jews. *Thromb Haemost* 76:283, 1996.
68. Goodnight SH Jr, Feinstein DI, Osterud B, Rapaport SI: Factor VII antibody-neutralizing material in hereditary and acquired factor VII deficiency. *Blood* 38:1, 1971.
69. Mariani G, Mazzucconi MG, Hermans J, et al: Factor VII deficiency: Immunological characterization of genetic variants and detection of carriers. *Br J Haematol* 48:7, 1981.
70. Triplett DA, Brandt JT, Batard MA, et al: Hereditary factor VII deficiency: Heterogeneity defined by combined functional and immuno-chemical analysis. *Blood* 66:1284, 1985.
71. Arbini AA, Pollak ES, Bayleran JK, et al: Severe factor VII deficiency due to a mutation disrupting a hepatocyte nuclear factor 4, binding site in the factor VII promoter. *Blood* 89:176, 1997.
72. Carew JA, Pollak ES, High KA, Bauer KA: Severe factor VII deficiency due to a mutation disrupting an Sp1, binding site in the factor VII promoter. *Blood* 92:1639, 1998.
73. Nagaizumi K, Inaba H, Suzuki T, et al: Two double heterozygous mutations in the F7, gene show different manifestations. *Br J Haematol* 119:1052, 2002.
74. Carew JA, Pollak ES, Lopaciuk S, Bauer KA: A new mutation in the HNF4, binding region of the factor VII promoter in a patient with severe factor VII deficiency. *Blood* 96:4370, 2000.
75. Fromovich-Amit Y, Zivelin A, Rosenberg N, et al: Characterization of mutations causing factor VII deficiency in 61, unrelated Israeli patients. *J Thromb Haemost* 2:1774, 2004.
76. Leonard BJN, Chen Q, Blajchman MA, et al: Factor VII deficiency caused by a structural variant N57D of the first epidermal growth factor domain. *Blood* 91:142, 1998.
77. Chaing S, Clarke B, Sridhara S, et al: Severe factor VII deficiency caused by mutations abolishing the cleavage site for activation and altering binding to tissue factor. *Blood* 83:3524, 1994.
78. Kavlie A, Orning L, Grindflek A, et al: Characterization of a factor VII molecule carrying a mutation in the second epidermal growth factor-like domain. *Thromb Haemost* 79:1136, 1998.
79. Kemball-Cook G, Johnson DJD, Takamiya O, et al: Coagulation factor VII $Gln^{100}Arg$. Amino acid substitution at the epidermal growth factor 2-protease domain interface results in severely reduced tissue factor binding and procoagulant function. *J Biol Chem* 273:8516, 1998.
80. Seligsohn U, Shani M, Ramot B, et al: Dubin-Johnson syndrome in Israel: II. Association with factor VII deficiency. *Q J Med* 39:569, 1970.
81. Mor-Cohen R, Zivelin A, Rosenberg N, et al: Identification and functional analysis of two novel mutations in the multidrug resistance protein 2, gene in Israeli patients with Dubin-Johnson syndrome. *J Biol Chem* 276:36923, 2001.
82. Wulff K, Herrmann FH: Twenty-two novel mutations of the factor VII gene in factor VII deficiency. *Hum Mutat* 15:489, 2000.
83. Giansily-Blaizot M, Aguilar-Martinez P, Biron-Andreani C, et al: Analysis of the genotypes and phenotypes of 37, unrelated patients with inherited factor VII deficiency. *Eur J Hum Genet* 9:105, 2001.
84. Bernardi F, Patracchini P, Gemmati D, et al: Molecular analysis of factor VII deficiency in Italy: A frequent mutation (FVII Lazio) in a repeated intronic region. *Hum Genet* 92:446, 1993.
85. Etro D, Pinotti M, Wulff K, et al: The Gly331Ser mutation in factor VII in Europe and the Middle East. *Haematologica* 88:1434, 2003.
86. Bernardi F, Liney DL, Patracchini P, et al: Molecular defects in CRM+ factor VII deficiencies: Modeling of missense mutations in the catalytic domain of FVII. *Br J Haematol* 86:610, 1994.
87. Hunault M, Arbini AA, Lopaciuk S, et al: The Arg353,Gln polymorphism reduces the level of coagulation factor VII: In vivo and in vitro studies. *Arterioscler Thromb Vasc Biol* 17:2825, 1997.
88. Green F, Kelleher C, Wilkes H, et al: A common genetic polymorphism associated with lower coagulation factor VII levels in healthy individuals. *Arterioscler Thromb* 11:540, 1991.
89. Bernardi F, Marchetti G, Pinotti M, et al: Factor VII gene polymorphisms contribute about one-third of the factor VII level variation in plasma. *Arterioscler Thromb Vasc Biol* 16:72, 1996.
90. Kario K, Narita N, Matsuo T, et al: Genetic determinants of plasma factor VII activity in the Japanese. *Thromb Haemost* 73:617, 1995.
91. Lane A, Cruickshank JK, Mitchell J, et al: Genetic and environmental determinants of factor VII coagulant activity in ethnic groups at differing risk of coronary heart disease. *Atherosclerosis* 94:43, 1992.
92. La Coviello L, Di Castelnuovo A, DeKnijff P, et al: Polymorphisms in the coagulation factor VII gene and the risk of myocardial infarction. *N Engl J Med* 338:79, 1998.
93. Saha N, Liu Y, Hong CK, et al: Association of factor VII genotype with plasma factor VII activity and antigen levels in healthy Indian adults and interaction with triglycerides. *Arterioscler Thromb* 14:1923, 1994.
94. Marchetti G, Gemmati D, Patracchini P, et al: PCR detection of a repeat polymorphism within the F7, gene. *Nucleic Acids Res* 19:4570, 1991.
95. Hunault M, Arbini AA, Carew JA, Bauer KA: Mechanism underlying factor VII deficiency in Jewish populations with the Ala244Val mutation. *Br J Haematol* 105:1101, 1999.
96. Hermann FH, Wulff K, Strey R, et al: Variability of clinical manifestation of factor VII-deficiency in homozygous and heterozygous subjects of the European F7, gene mutation A294V. *Haematologica* 93:1273, 2008.
97. Mariani G, Mazzucconi MG: Factor VII congenital deficiency: Clinical picture and classification of the variants. *Haemostasis* 13:169, 1983.
98. Mariani G, Herrman FH, Dolce A, et al: The International factor VII deficiency study group. Clinical phenotypes and factor VII genotype in congenital factor VII deficiency. *Thromb Haemost* 93:481, 2005.
99. de Moerloose P, Amiral J, Vissac AM, Reber G: Longitudinal study on activated factors XII and VII levels during normal pregnancy. *Br J Haematol* 100:40, 1998.
100. Kulkarni AA, Lee CA, Kadir RA: Pregnancy in women with congenital factor VII deficiency. *Haemophilia* 12:413, 2006.
101. Pruthi RK, Rodriguez V, Allen C, et al: Molecular analysis in a patient with severe factor VII deficiency and an inhibitor: report of a novel mutation (S103G). *Eur J Haematol* 79:354, 2007.
102. Mariani G, Herrmann FH, Schulman S, et al: Thrombosis in inherited factor VII deficiency. *J Thromb Haemost* 1:2153, 2003.
103. Philippou H, Adami A, Amersey RA, et al: A novel specific immunoassay for plasma two-chain factor VIIa: Investigation of FVIIa levels in normal individuals and in patients with acute coronary syndromes. *Blood* 89:767, 1997.
104. Lim S, Zuha R, Burt T, et al: Life-threatening bleeding in a patient with a lupus inhibitor and probable acquired factor VII deficiency. *Blood Coagul Fibrinolysis* 17:867, 2006.
105. Boxus G, Slacmeulder M, Ninane J: Combined hereditary deficiency in factors VII and X revealed by a prolonged partial thromboplastin time. *Arch Pediatr* 4:44, 1997.
106. Girolami A, Ruzzon E, Tezza F, et al: Congenital combined defects of factor VII: A critical review. *Acta Haematol* 117:51, 2007.
107. Cederbaum AI, Blatt PM, Roberts HR: Intravascular coagulation with use of human prothrombin complex concentrates. *Ann Intern Med* 84:683, 1976.
108. Perry DJ: Factor VII deficiency. *Blood Coagul Fibrinolysis* 14(Suppl 1):S47, 2003.
109. Mariani G, Konkle BA, Ingerslev J: Congenital factor VII deficiency: Therapy with recombinant activated factor VII—A critical appraisal. *Haemophilia* 12:19, 2006.
110. Tcheng WY, Donkin J, Konzal S, Wong WY: Recombinant factor VIIa in a patient with severe congenital factor VII deficiency. *Haemophilia* 10:295, 2004.
111. Briet E, Onvlee G: Hip surgery in a patient with severe factor VII deficiency. *Haemostasis* 17:273, 1987.
112. Telfer TP, Denson KW, Wright DW: A "new" coagulation defect. *Br J Haematol* 2:308, 1956.
113. Hougie C, Barrow EM, Graham JB: Stuart clotting defect: I. Segregation of an hereditary hemorrhagic state from the heterogeneous group heretofore called "stable factor" (SPCA, proconvertin, factor VII) deficiency. *J Clin Invest* 36:485, 1957.
114. Scambler PJ, Williamson R: The structural gene for human coagulation factor X is located on chromosome 13q34. *Cytogenet Cell Genet* 39:231, 1985.
115. Royle NJ, Fung MR, McGillivray RT, Hamerton JL: The gene for clotting factor 10, is mapped to 13q32-qter. *Cytogenet Cell Genet* 41:185, 1986.
116. Leytus SP, Foster DC, Kurachi K, Davie EW: Gene for human factor X: A blood coagulation factor whose gene organization is essentially identical with that of factor IX and protein C. *Biochemistry* 25:5098, 1986.
117. Neurath H: Evolution of proteolytic enzymes. *Science* 224:350, 1984.
118. McMullen BA, Fujikawa K, Kisiel W, et al: Complete amino acid sequence of the light chain of human blood coagulation factor X: Evidence for identification of residue 63, as beta-hydroxyaspartic acid. *Biochemistry* 22:2875, 1983.
119. Jackson CM: Characterization of two glycoprotein variants of bovine factor X and demonstration that the factor X zymogen contains two polypeptide chains. *Biochemistry* 11:4873, 1972.
120. Fujikawa K, Coan MH, Legaz ME, Davie EW: The mechanism of activation of bovine factor X (Stuart factor) by intrinsic and extrinsic pathways. *Biochemistry* 13:5290, 1974.
121. Fujikawa K, Legaz ME, Davie EW: Bovine factor X (Stuart factor): Mechanism of activation by protein from Russell's viper venom. *Biochemistry* 11:4892, 1972.
122. Girolami A, Scarparo P, Scandellari R, Allemand E: Congenital factor X deficiencies with a defect only or predominantly in the extrinsic or in the intrinsic system: A critical evaluation. *Am J Hematol* 83:668, 2008.
123. Rudolph AE, Mullane MP, Porche-Sorbet R, et al: Factor X St. Louis II. Identification of a glycine substitution at residue 7, and characterization of the recombinant protein. *J Biol Chem* 271:28601, 1996.
124. Pinotti M, Marchetti G, Baroni M, et al: Reduced activation of the Gla19Ala FX variant via the extrinsic coagulation pathway results in symptomatic CRMred FX deficiency. *Thromb Haemost* 88:236, 2002.
125. De Stefano V, Leone G, Ferrelli R, et al: Factor X Roma: A congenital factor X variant defective at different degrees in the intrinsic and the extrinsic activation. *Br J Haematol* 69:387, 1988.
126. James HL, Girolami A, Fair DS: Molecular defect in coagulation factor X_{Friuli} results from a substitution of serine for proline at position 343. *Blood* 77:317, 1991.

127. Cooper DN, Millar DS, Wacey A, et al: Inherited factor X deficiency: Molecular genetics and pathophysiology. *Thromb Haemost* 78:161, 1997.
128. Akhavan S, Chafa O, Obame FN, et al: Recurrence of a Phe31Ser mutation in the Gla domain of blood coagulation factor X, in unrelated Algerian families: a founder effect? *Eur J Haematol* 78:405, 2007.
129. Herrmann FH, Auerswald G, Ruiz-Saez A, et al: Factor X deficiency: clinical manifestation of 102, subjects from Europe and Latin America with mutations in the factor 10, gene. *Haemophilia* 12:479, 2006.
130. Girolami A, Ruzzon E, Tezza F, et al: Congenital FX deficiency combined with other clotting defects or with other abnormalities: A critical evaluation of the literature. *Haemophilia* 14:323, 2008.
131. Furie B, Voo L, McAdam KP, Furie BC: Mechanism of factor X deficiency in systemic amyloidosis. *N Engl J Med* 304:827, 1981.
132. Fair DS, Edgington TS: Heterogeneity of hereditary and acquired factor X deficiencies by combined immunochemical and functional analyses. *Br J Haematol* 59:235, 1985.
133. Rao LVM, Zivelin A, Iturbe I, Rapaport SI: Antibody-induced acute factor X deficiency: Clinical manifestations and properties of the antibody. *Thromb Haemost* 72:363, 1994.
134. Biggs R, Denson KWE: The fate of prothrombin and factors VIII, IX, and X transfused to patients deficient in these factors. *Br J Haematol* 9:532, 1963.
135. Roberts HR, Lechler E, Webster WP, Penick GD: Survival of transfused factor X in patients with Stuart disease. *Thromb Diath Haemorrh* 18:305, 1965.
136. Auerswald G: Prophylaxis in rare coagulation disorders—Factor X deficiency. *Thromb Res* 118(Suppl 1):S29, 2006.
137. McMillan CW, Roberts HR: Congenital combined deficiency of coagulation factors II, VII, IX and X: Report of a case. *N Engl J Med* 274:1313, 1966.
138. Girolami A, Scandellari R, Scapin M, Vettore S: Congenital bleeding disorders of the vitamin K-dependent clotting factors. *Vitam Horm* 78:281, 2008.
139. Darghouth D, Hallgren KW, Shtofman RL, et al: Compound heterozygosity of novel missense mutations in the gamma-glutamyl-carboxylase gene causes hereditary combined vitamin K-dependent coagulation factor deficiency. *Blood* 108:1925, 2006.
140. Schmidt-Krey I, Haase W, Mutucumarana V, et al: Two-dimensional crystallization of human vitamin K-dependent gamma-glutamyl carboxylase. *J Struct Biol* 157:437, 2007.
141. Rost S, Fregin A, Ivaskevicius V, et al: Mutations in VKORC1, cause warfarin resistance and multiple coagulation factor deficiency type 2. *Nature* 427:537, 2004.
142. Li T, Chang CY, Jin DY, et al: Identification of the gene for vitamin K epoxide reductase. *Nature* 427:541, 2004.
143. Fregin A, Rost S, Wolz W, et al: Homozygosity mapping of a second gene locus for hereditary combined deficiency of vitamin K-dependent clotting factors to the centromeric region of chromosome 16. *Blood* 100:3229, 2002.
144. Chu PH, Huang TY, Williams J, Stafford DW: Purified vitamin K epoxide reductase alone is sufficient for conversion of vitamin K epoxide to vitamin K and vitamin K to vitamin KH2. *Proc Natl Acad Sci U S A* 103:19308, 2006.
145. Garcia AA, Reitsma PH: VKORC1, and the vitamin K cycle. *Vitam Horm* 78:23, 2008.
146. Wallin R, Wajih N, Hutson SM: VKORC1: A warfarin-sensitive enzyme in vitamin K metabolism and biosynthesis of vitamin K-dependent blood coagulation factors. *Vitam Horm* 78:227, 2008.
147. Oldenburg J, von Brederlow B, Fregin A, et al: Congenital deficiency of vitamin K dependent coagulation factors in two families presents as a genetic defect of the vitamin K-epoxide-reductase-complex. *Thromb Haemost* 84:937, 2000.
148. Marchetti G, Caruso P, Lunghi B, et al: Vitamin K-induced modification of coagulation phenotype in VKORC1, homozygous deficiency. *J Thromb Haemost* 6:797, 2008.
149. Brenner B, Sanchez-Vega B, Wu SM, et al: A missense mutation in gamma-glutamyl carboxylase gene causes combined deficiency of all vitamin K-dependent blood coagulation factors. *Blood* 92:4554, 1998.
150. Spronk HM, Farah RA, Buchanan GR, et al: Novel mutation in the gamma-glutamyl carboxylase gene resulting in congenital combined deficiency of all vitamin K-dependent blood coagulation factors. *Blood* 96:3650, 2000.
151. Mousallem M, Spronk HM, Sacy R, et al: Congenital combined deficiencies of all vitamin K-dependent coagulation factors. *Thromb Haemost* 86:1334, 2001.
152. Rost S, Fregin A, Koch D, et al: Compound heterozygous mutations in the gamma-glutamyl carboxylase gene cause combined deficiency of all vitamin K-dependent blood coagulation factors. *Br J Haematol* 126:546, 2004.
153. Soute BA, Jin DY, Spronk HM, et al: Characteristics of recombinant W501S mutated human gamma-glutamyl carboxylase. *J Thromb Haemost* 2:597, 2004, .
154. Rost S, Geisen C, Fregin A, et al: Founder mutation Arg485Pro led to recurrent compound heterozygous GGCX genotypes in two German patients with VKCFD type 1. *Blood Coagul Fibrinolysis* 17:503, 2006.
155. Vanakker OM, Martin L, Gheduzzi D, et al: Pseudoxanthoma elasticum-like phenotype with cutis laxa and multiple coagulation factor deficiency represents a separate genetic entity. *J* Invest *Dermatol* 127:581, 2006.
156. Owren PA: Parahemophilia: Hemorrhagic diathesis due to absence of a previously unknown factor. *Lancet* 1:446, 1947.
157. Mann KG, Kalafatis M: Factor V: A combination of Dr Jekyll and Mr Hyde. *Blood* 101:20, 2003.
158. Wang H, Riddell DC, Guinto ER, et al: Localization of the gene encoding human factor V to chromosome 1q21–25. *Genomics* 2:324, 1988.
159. Suzuki K, Dahlback B, Stenflo J: Thrombin-catalyzed activation of human coagulation factor V. *J Biol Chem* 257:6556, 1982.
160. Foster WB, Nesheim ME, Mann KG: The factor Xa-catalyzed activation of factor V. *J Biol Chem* 258:13970, 1983.
161. Tracy PB, Mann KG: Abnormal formation of the prothrombinase complex: Factor V deficiency and related disorders. *Hum Pathol* 18:162, 1987.
162. Wilson DB, Salem HH, Mruk JS, et al: Biosynthesis of coagulation factor V by human hepatocellular carcinoma cell line. *J Clin Invest* 73:654, 1983.
163. Tracy PB, Eide LL, Bowie EJ, Mann KG: Radioimmunoassay of factor V in human plasma and platelets. *Blood* 60:59, 1982.
164. Seeler RA: Parahemophilia: Factor V deficiency. *Med Clin North Am* 56:119, 1972.
165. Hayward CP, Furmaniak-Kazmierczak E, Cieutat AM, et al: Factor V is complexed with multimerin in resting platelet lysates and colocalizes with multimerin in platelet alpha-granules. *J Biol Chem* 270:19217, 1995.
166. Gould WR, Simioni P, Silveira JR, et al: Megakaryocytes endocytose and subsequently modify human factor V in vivo to form the entire pool of a unique platelet-derived cofactor. *J Thromb Haemost* 3:450, 2005.
167. Gould WR, Silveira JR, Tracy PB: Unique in vivo modifications of coagulation factor V produce a physically and functionally distinct platelet-derived cofactor: Characterization of purified platelet-derived factor V/Va. *J Biol Chem* 279:2383, 2004.
168. Suzuki K, Stenflo J, Dahlback B, et al: Inactivation of human coagulation factor V by activated protein. C. *J Biol Chem* 258:1914, 1983.
169. Nesheim ME, Canfield WM, Kisiel W, et al: Studies of the capacity of factor Xa to protect factor Va from inactivation by activated protein C. *J Biol Chem* 257:1443, 1982.
170. Castoldi E, Lunghi B, Mingozzi F, et al: A missense mutation (Y1702C) in the coagulation factor V gene is a frequent cause of factor V deficiency in the Italian population. *Haematologica* 86:629, 2001.
171. Steen M, Miteva M, Villoutreix BO, et al: Factor V New Brunswick: Ala221Val associated with FV deficiency reproduced in vitro and functionally characterized. *Blood* 102:1316, 2003.
172. Duga S, Montefusco MC, Asselta R, et al: Arg2074Cys missense mutation in the C2, domain of factor V causing moderately severe factor V deficiency: Molecular characterization by expression of the recombinant protein. *Blood* 101:173, 2003.
173. Montefusco MC, Duga S, Asselta R, et al: Clinical and molecular characterization of 6 patients affected by severe deficiency of coagulation factor V: Broadening of the mutational spectrum of factor V gene and in vitro analysis of the newly identified missense mutations. *Blood* 102:3210, 2003.
174. Van Wijk R, Nieuwenhuis K, van den Berg M, et al: Five novel mutations in the gene for human blood coagulation factor V associated with type I factor V deficiency. *Blood* 98:358, 2001.
175. Van Wijk R, Montefusco MC, Duga S, et al: Coexistence of a novel homozygous nonsense mutation in exon 13, of the factor V gene with the homozygous Leiden mutation in two unrelated patients with severe factor V deficiency. *Br J Haematol* 114:871, 2001.
176. Guasch JF, Cannegieter S, Reitsma PH, et al: Severe coagulation factor V deficiency caused by a 4 bp deletion in the factor V gene. *Br J Haematol* 101:32, 1998.
177. Cui J, O'Shea KS, Purkayastha A, et al: Fatal haemorrhage and incomplete block to embryogenesis in mice lacking coagulation factor V. *Nature* 384:66, 1996.
178. Guasch JF, Lensen RP, Bertina RM: Molecular characterization of a type I quantitative factor V deficiency in a thrombosis patient that is "pseudohomozygous" for activated protein C resistance. *Thromb Haemost* 77:252, 1997.
179. Lunghi B, Iacoviello L, Gemmati D, et al: Detection of new polymorphic markers in the factor V gene: Association with factor V levels in plasma. *Thromb Haemost* 75:45, 1996.
180. Castaman G, Lunghi B, Missiaglia E, et al: Phenotypic homozygous activated protein C resistance associated with compound heterozygosity for Arg506Gln (factor V Leiden) and His1299Arg substitutions in factor V. *Br J Haematol* 99:257, 1997.
181. Vos HL: Inherited defects of coagulation Factor V: The thrombotic side. *J Thromb Haemost* 4:35, 2006.
182. Tracy PB, Giles AR, Mann KG, et al: Factor V (Quebec): A bleeding diathesis associated with a qualitative platelet factor V deficiency. *J Clin Invest* 74:1221, 1984.
183. Hayward CP, Cramer EM, Kane WH, et al: Studies of a second family with the Quebec platelet disorder: Evidence that the degradation of the alpha-granule membrane and its soluble contents are not secondary to a defect in targeting proteins to alpha-granules. *Blood* 89:1243, 1997.
184. Asselta R, Tenchini ML, Duga S: Inherited defects of coagulation factor V: The hemorrhagic side. *J Thromb Haemost* 4:26, 2006.
185. Girolami A, Scandellari R, Lombardi AM, et al: Pregnancy and oral contraceptives in factor V deficiency: A study of 22, patients (five homozygotes and 17 heterozygotes) and review of the literature. *Haemophilia* 11:26, 2005.
186. Duckers C, Simioni P, Spiezia L, at al: Low plasma levels of tissue factor pathway inhibitor in patients with congenital factor V deficiency. *Blood* 112:3615, 2008.
187. Girolami A, Ruzzon E, Tezza F: Arterial and venous thrombosis in rare congenital bleeding disorders: A critical review. *Haemophilia* 12:345, 2006.
188. Fratantoni JC, Hilgartner M, Nachman RL: Nature of the defect in congenital factor V deficiency: Study in a patient with an acquired circulating anticoagulant. *Blood* 39:751, 1972.
189. Mazzucconi MG, Solinas S, Chistolini A, et al: Inhibitor to factor V in severe factor V congenital deficiency: A case report. *Nouv Rev Fr Hematol* 27:303, 1985.
190. Wiwanitkit V: Spectrum of bleeding in acquired factor V inhibitor: A summary of 33 cases. *Clin Appl Thromb Hemost* 12:485, 2006.
191. Webster WP, Roberts HR, Penick GD: Hemostasis in factor V deficiency. *Am J Med Sci* 248:194, 1964.
192. Tanis BC, van der Meer FJ, Bloem RM, Vlasveld LT: Successful excision of a pseudotumour in a congenitally factor V deficient patient. *Br J Haematol* 100:380, 1998.

193. Oeri J, Matter M, Isenschmid H, et al: [Congenital factor V deficiency (parahemophilia) with true hemophilia in two brothers]. *Bibl J Paediatr* 58:575, 1954.
194. Seligsohn U, Zivelin A, Zwang E: Combined factor V and factor VIII deficiency among non-Ashkenazi Jews. *N Engl J Med* 307:1191, 1982.
195. Seligsohn U: Combined factor V and factor VIII deficiency, in *Factor VIII: Von Willebrand Factor*, vol 2, edited by J Seghatchian, GT Savidge, p 89. CRC Press, Boca Raton, FL, 1989.
196. Nichols WC, Seligsohn U, Zivelin A, et al: Mutations in the ER-Golgi intermediate compartment protein ERGIC-53, cause combined deficiency of coagulation factors V and VIII. *Cell* 93:61, 1998.
197. Zhang B, Cunningham MA, Nichols WC, et al: Bleeding due to disruption of a cargo-specific ER-to-Golgi transport complex. *Nat Genet* 34:220, 2003.
198. Zhang B, McGee B, Yamaoka JS, et al: Combined deficiency of factor V and factor VIII is due to mutations in either LMAN1, or MCFD2. *Blood* 107:1903, 2006.
199. Peyvandi F, Tuddenham EG, Akhtari AM, et al: Bleeding symptoms in 27 Iranian patients with the combined deficiency of factor V and factor VIII. *Br J Haematol* 100:773, 1998.
200. Nichols WC, Seligsohn U, Zivelin A, et al: Linkage of combined factors V and VIII deficiency to chromosome 18q by homozygosity mapping. *J Clin Invest* 99:596, 1997.
201. Neerman-Arbez M, Antonarakis SE, Blouin JL, et al: The locus for combined factor V-factor VIII deficiency (F5F8D) maps to 18q21, between D18S849, and D18S1103. *Am J Hum Genet* 61:143, 1997.
202. Zhang B, Spreafico M, Zheng C, et al: Genotype-phenotype correlation in combined deficiency of factor V and factor VIII. *Blood* 111:5592, 2008.
203. Segal A, Zivelin A, Rosenberg N, et al: A mutation in LMAN 1, (ERGIC-53) causing combined factor V and factor VIII deficiency is prevalent in Jews originating from the island of Djerba in Tunisia. *Blood Coagul Fibrinolysis* 15:99, 2004.
204. Fischer RR, Giddings JC, Roisenberg I: Hereditary combined deficiency of clotting factors V and VIII with involvement of von Willebrand factor. *Clin Lab Haematol* 10:53, 1988.
205. Soff GA, Levin J, Bell WR: Familial multiple coagulation factor deficiencies: I. Review of the literature: Differentiation of single hereditary disorders associated with multiple factor deficiencies from coincidental concurrence of single factor deficiency states. *Semin Thromb Hemost* 7:112, 1981.
206. Gobbi F: Heredity of combined deficiency of AHG and proaccelerin. *Scand J Haematol* 3:222, 1966.
207. Girolami A, Gastaldi G, Patrassi G, Galletti A: Combined congenital deficiency of factor V and factor VIII: Report of a further case with some considerations on the hereditary transmission of this disorder. *Acta Haematol* 55:234, 1976.
208. Mazzone D, Fichera A, Pratico G, Sciacca F: Combined congenital deficiency of factor V and factor VIII. *Acta Haematol* 68:337, 1982.
209. Bartlett JA, Sweeney JD, Sadowsky D: Exodontia in combined factor V and factor VIII deficiency. *Br J Oral Maxillofac Surg* 43:537, 1985.
210. Tsurumi H, Takahashi T, Moriwaki H, Muto Y: Congenital combined deficiency of factor V and factor VIII with acquired ichthyosis, epidermodysplasia verruciformis, and immunological abnormalities. *Am J Hematol* 40:320, 1992.
211. Sallah AS, Angchaisuksiri P, Roberts HR: Use of plasma exchange in hereditary deficiency of factor V and factor VIII. *Am J Hematol* 52:229, 1996.
212. Rosenthal RL, Dreskin OH, Rosenthal N: A new hemophilia like disease caused by deficiency of a third plasma thromboplastin factor. *Proc Soc Exp Biol Med* 82:171, 1953.
213. Rapaport SI, Proctor RR, Patch NJ, Yettra M: The mode of inheritance of PTA deficiency: Evidence for the existence of major PTA deficiency and minor PTA deficiency. *Blood* 18:149, 1961.
214. Seligsohn U: High gene frequency of factor XI (PTA) deficiency in Ashkenazi-Jews. *Blood* 51:1223, 1978.
215. Gailani D, Broze GJ Jr: Factor XI activation in a revised model of blood coagulation. *Science* 253:909, 1991.
216. Naito K, Fujikawa K: Activation of human blood coagulation factor XI independent of factor XII: Factor XI is activated by thrombin and factor XIa in the presence of negatively charged surfaces. *J Biol Chem* 266:7353, 1991.
217. McMullen BA, Fujikawa K, Davie EW: Location of the disulfide bonds in human coagulation factor XI: The presence of tandem apple domains. *Biochemistry* 30:2056, 1991.
218. Papagrigoriou E, McEwan PA, Walsh PN, Emsley J: Crystal structure of the factor XI zymogen reveals a pathway for transactivation. *Nat Struct Mol Biol* 13:557, 2006.
219. Zucker M, Zivelin A, Landau M, et al: Three residues at the interface of factor XI monomers augment covalent dimerization of factor XI. *J Thromb Haemost* 7:970, 2009.
220. Wu W, Sinha D, Shikov S, et al: Factor XI homodimer structure is essential for normal proteolytic activation by factor XIIa, thrombin, and factor XIa. *J Biol Chem* 283:18655, 2008.
221. Renne T, Gailani D, Meijers JC, Muller-Esterl W: Characterization of the H-kininogen-binding site on factor XI: A comparison of factor XI and plasma prekallikrein. *J Biol Chem* 277:4892, 2002.
222. Asakai R, Davie EW, Chung DW: Organization of the gene for human factor XI. *Biochemistry* 26:7221, 1987.
223. Kato A, Asakai R, Davie EW, Aoki N: Factor XI gene (F11) is located on the distal end of the long arm of human chromosome 4. *Cytogenet Cell Genet* 52:77, 1989.
224. Bouma BN, Griffin JH: Human blood coagulation factor XI: Purification, properties, and mechanism of activation by activated factor XII. *J Biol Chem* 252:6432, 1977.
225. Baglia FA, Shrimpton CN, Lopez JA, Walsh PN: The glycoprotein Ib-IX-V complex mediates localization of factor XI to lipid rafts on the platelet membrane. *J Biol Chem* 278:21744, 2003.
226. Von dem Borne PA, Meijers JC, Bouma BN: Effect of heparin on the activation of factor XI by fibrin-bound thrombin. *Thromb Haemost* 76:347, 1996.
227. Osterud B, Bouma BN, Griffin JH: Human blood coagulation factor IX: Purification, properties, and mechanism of activation by activated factor XI. *J Biol Chem* 253:5946, 1978.
228. Bouma BN, Meijers JC: Thrombin-activatable fibrinolysis inhibitor (TAFI, plasma procarboxypeptidase B, procarboxypeptidase R, procarboxypeptidase U). *J Thromb Haemost* 1:1566, 2003.
229. Bajzar L, Morser J, Nesheim M: TAFI, or plasma procarboxypeptidase B, couples the coagulation and fibrinolytic cascades through the thrombin-thrombomodulin complex. *J Biol Chem* 271:16603, 1996.
230. Broze GJ Jr, Higuchi DA: Coagulation-dependent inhibition of fibrinolysis: Role of carboxypeptidase-U and the premature lysis of clots from hemophilic plasma. *Blood* 88:3815, 1996.
231. Von dem Borne PA, Bajzar L, Meijers JC, et al: Thrombin-mediated activation of factor XI results in a thrombin-activatable fibrinolysis inhibitor-dependent inhibition of fibrinolysis. *J Clin Invest* 99:2323, 1997.
232. Minnema MC, Friederich PW, Levi M, et al: Enhancement of rabbit jugular vein thrombolysis by neutralization of factor XI: In vivo evidence for a role of factor XI as an anti-fibrinolytic factor. *J Clin Invest* 101:10, 1998.
233. Asakai R, Chung DW, Davie EW, Seligsohn U: Factor XI deficiency in Ashkenazi Jews in Israel. *N Engl J Med* 325:153, 1991.
234. Berliner S, Horowitz I, Martinowitz U, et al: Dental surgery in patients with severe factor XI deficiency without plasma replacement. *Blood Coagul Fibrinolysis* 3:465, 1992.
235. Clarkson K, Rosenfeld B, Fair J, et al: Factor XI deficiency acquired by liver transplantation. *Ann Intern Med* 115:877, 1991.
236. Saito H, Ratnoff OD, Bouma BN, Seligsohn U: Failure to detect variant (CRM+) plasma thromboplastin antecedent (factor XI) molecules in hereditary plasma thromboplastin antecedent deficiency: A study of 125 patients of several ethnic backgrounds. *J Lab Clin Med* 106:718, 1985.
237. Mannhalter C, Hellstern P, Deutsch E: Identification of a defective factor XI cross-reacting material in a factor XI-deficient patient. *Blood* 70:31, 1987.
238. Zivelin A, Ogawa T, Bulvik S, et al: Severe Factor XI deficiency caused by a Gly^{555} to Glu mutation (factor XI-Glu555): A cross-reactive material positive variant defective in factor IX activation. *J Thromb Haemost* 2:1782, 2004.
239. Quelin F, Trossaert M, Sigaud M, et al: Molecular basis of severe factor XI deficiency in seven families from the west of France. Seven novel mutations, including an ancient Q88X mutation. *J Thromb Haemost* 2:71, 2004.
240. Martincic D, Zimmerman SA, Ware RE, et al: Identification of mutations and polymorphisms in the factor XI genes of an African-American family by dideoxy fingerprinting. *Blood* 92:3309, 1998.
241. Bolton-Maggs PH, Young Wan-Yin B, McCraw AH, et al: Inheritance and bleeding in factor XI deficiency. *Br J Haematol* 69:521, 1988.
242. Asakai R, Chung DW, Ratnoff OD, Davie EW: Factor XI (plasma thromboplastin antecedent) deficiency in Ashkenazi Jews is a bleeding disorder that can result from three types of point mutations. *Proc Natl Acad Sci U S A* 86:7667, 1989.
243. Peretz H, Zivelin A, Usher S, Seligsohn U: A 14-bp deletion (codon 554, del AAGgtaacagagtg) at exon 14/intron N junction of the coagulation factor XI gene disrupts splicing and causes severe factor XI deficiency. *Hum Mutat* 8:77, 1996.
244. Meijers JC, Davie EW, Chung DW: Expression of human blood coagulation factor XI: Characterization of the defect in factor XI type III deficiency. *Blood* 79:1435, 1992.
245. Pugh RE, McVey JH, Tuddenham EGD, Hancock JF: Six point mutations that cause factor XI deficiency. *Blood* 85:1509, 1995.
246. Zivelin A, Bauduer F, Ducout L, et al: Factor XI deficiency in French Basques is caused predominantly by an ancestral Cys38Arg mutation in the factor XI gene. *Blood* 99:2448, 2002.
247. Kravtsov DV, Wu W, Meijers JC, et al: Dominant factor XI deficiency caused by mutations in the factor XI catalytic domain. *Blood* 104:128, 2004.
248. Sidi A, Seligsohn U, Jonas P, Many M: Factor XI deficiency: Detection and management during urological surgery. *J Urol* 119:528, 1978.
249. Hancock JF, Wieland K, Pugh RE, et al: A molecular genetic study of factor XI deficiency. *Blood* 77:1942, 1991.
250. Shpilberg O, Peretz H, Zivelin A, et al: One of the two common mutations causing factor XI deficiency in Ashkenazi Jews (type II) is also prevalent in Iraqi Jews, who represent the ancient gene pool of Jews. *Blood* 85:429, 1995.
251. Peretz H, Mulai A, Usher S, et al: The two common mutations causing factor XI deficiency in Jews stem from distinct founders: One of ancient Middle Eastern origin and another of more recent European origin. *Blood* 90:2654, 1997.
252. Zadra G, Asselta R, Tenchini ML, et al: Simultaneous genotyping of coagulation factor XI type II and type III mutations by multiplex real-time polymerase chain reaction to determine their prevalence in healthy and factor XI-deficient Italians. *Haematologica* 93:715, 2008.
253. Bolton-Maggs PHB, Peretz H, Butler R, et al: A common ancestral mutation (C128X) occurring in 11 non-Jewish families from the U.K. with factor XI deficiency. *J Thromb Haemost* 2:918, 2004.
254. Goldstein DB, Reich DE, Bradman N, et al: Age estimates of two common mutations causing factor XI deficiency: Recent genetic drift is not necessary for elevated disease incidence among Ashkenazi Jews. *Am J Hum Genet* 64:1071, 1999.

255. Bolton-Maggs PH, Patterson DA, Wensley RT, Tuddenham EG: Definition of the bleeding tendency in factor XI-deficient kindreds: A clinical and laboratory study. *Thromb Haemost* 73:194, 1995.
256. Salomon O, Steinberg DM, Seligsohn U: Variable bleeding manifestations characterize different types of surgery in patients with severe factor XI deficiency enabling parsimonious use of replacement therapy. *Haemophilia* 12:490, 2006.
257. Salomon O, Steinberg DM, Tamarin I, et al: Plasma replacement therapy during labor is not mandatory for women with severe factor XI deficiency. *Blood Coagul Fibrinolysis* 16:37, 2005.
258. Brenner B, Laor A, Lupo H, et al: Bleeding predictors in factor-XI deficient patients. *Blood Coagul Fibrinolysis* 8:511, 1997.
259. Eikenboon JC, Rosendaal FR, Briet E: Value of the patient interview: All but consensus among haemostasis experts. *Haemostasis* 22:221, 1992.
260. Peter MK, Meili EO, Von Felten A: Factor XI deficiency: Do patients with hemorrhagic diathesis also have hemostasis defects? *Schweiz Med Wochenschr* 126:999, 1996.
261. Salomon O, Steinberg DM, Dardik R, et al: Inherited factor XI deficiency confers no protection against acute myocardial infarction. *J Thromb Haemost* 1:658, 2003.
262. Salomon O, Steinberg DM, Koren-Morag N, et al: Reduced incidence of ischemic stroke in patients with severe factor XI deficiency. *Blood* 111:4113, 2008.
263. Brodsky JB, Burgess GE: Pulmonary embolism with factor XI deficiency. *JAMA* 534:1156, 1975.
264. Seligsohn U, Zitman D, Many A, Klibansky C: Coexistence of factor XI (plasma thromboplastin antecedent) deficiency and Gaucher's disease. *Isr J Med Sci* 12:1448, 1976.
265. Singer ST, Hurst D, Addiego JE Jr: Bleeding disorders in Noonan syndrome: Three case reports and review of the literature. *J Pediatr Hematol Oncol* 19:130, 1997.
266. Chediak J, Lambert E, Johnson EI, Telfer MC: Combined severe factor XI deficiency and von Willebrand's disease. *Am J Clin Pathol* 74:108, 1980.
267. Tavori S, Brenner B, Tatarsky I: The effect of combined factor XI deficiency with von Willebrand factor abnormalities on haemorrhagic diathesis. *Thromb Haemost* 63:36, 1990.
268. Lian EC, Deykin D, Harkness DR: Combined deficiencies of factor VIII (AHF) and factor XI (PTA). *Am J Hematol* 1:319, 1976.
269. Berg LP, Varon D, Martinowitz U, et al: Combined factor VIII/factor XI deficiency may cause intra-familial clinical variability in haemophilia A among Ashkenazi Jews. *Blood Coagul Fibrinolysis* 5:59, 1994.
270. Berube C, Ofosu FA, Kelton JG, Blajchman MA: A novel congenital haemostatic defect: Combined factor VII and factor XI deficiency. *Blood Coagul Fibrinolysis* 3:357, 1992.
271. Salomon O, Zivelin A, Livnat T, et al: Prevalence, causes, and characterization of factor XI inhibitors in patients with inherited factor XI deficiency. *Blood* 101:4783, 2003.
272. Zucker M, Zivelin A, Teitel J, Seligsohn U: Induction of an inhibitor antibody to factor XI in a patient with severe inherited factor XI deficiency by Rh immune globulin. *Blood* 111:1306, 2008.
273. Stern DM, Nossel HL, Owen J: Acquired antibody to factor XI in a patient with congenital factor XI deficiency. *J Clin Invest* 69:1270, 1982.
274. Seligsohn U, Modan M: Definition of the population at risk of bleeding due to factor XI deficiency in Ashkenazic Jews and the value of activated partial thromboplastin time in its detection. *Isr J Med Sci* 17:413, 1981.
275. Bolton-Maggs PHB, Wensley RT, Kernoff PBA, et al: Production and therapeutic use of a factor XI concentrate from human plasma. *Thromb Haemost* 67:314, 1992.
276. Inbal A, Epstein O, Blickstein D, et al: Evaluation of solvent/detergent treated plasma in the management of patients with hereditary and acquired coagulation disorders. *Blood Coagul Fibrinolysis* 4:599, 1993.
277. Seligsohn U: Factor XI deficiency. *Thromb Haemost* 70:68, 1993.
278. De Raucourt MH, Aurousseau MH, Denninger MH, et al: Use of a factor XI concentrate in three severe factor XI-deficient patients. *Blood Coagul Fibrinolysis* 6:486, 1995.
279. Aledort LM, Forster A, Maksoud J, Isola L: BPL factor XI concentrate: Clinical experience in the U.S.A. *Haemophilia* 3:59, 1997.
280. Mannucci PM, Bauer KA, Santagostino E, et al: Activation of the coagulation cascade after infusion of a factor XI concentrate in congenitally deficient patients. *Blood* 84:1314, 1994.
281. Richards EM, Makris MM, Cooper P, Preston FE: In vivo coagulation activation following infusion of highly purified factor XI concentrate. *Br J Haematol* 96:293, 1997.
282. Bolton-Maggs PHB, Colvin BT, Satchi G, et al: Thrombogenic potential of factor XI concentrate. *Lancet* 344:748, 1994.
283. Briggs N, Harman C, Dash CH: A decade of experience with factor XI concentrate. *Haemophilia* 2:14, 1996.
284. Rakocz M, Mazar A, Varon D, et al: Dental extractions in patients with bleeding disorders. *Oral Surg Oral Med Oral Pathol* 75:280, 1993.
285. Connelly NR, Brull SJ: Anesthetic management of a patient with factor XI deficiency and factor XI inhibitor undergoing a cesarean section. *Anesth Analg* 76:1365, 1993.
286. Hedner U: Factor VIIa in the treatment of haemophilia. *Blood Coagul Fibrinolysis* 1:307, 1990.
287 Livnat T, Zivelin A, Martinowitz U, et al: Prerequisites for recombinant factor VIIa-induced thrombin generation in plasmas deficient in factors VIII, IX or XI. *J Thromb Haemost* 4:192, 2006.
288. Livnat T, Tamarin I, Mor Y, et al: Recombinant activated factor VII and tranexamic acid are haemostatically effective during major surgery in factor XI-deficient patients with inhibitor antibodies. *Throm Haemost*, 102:487, 2009.
289. Duckert F, Jung E, Sherling DH: An undescribed congenital haemorrhagic diathesis probably due to fibrin stabilizing factor deficiency. *Thromb Diath Haemorrh* 5:179, 1960.
290. Muszbek L, Adany R, Mikkola H: Novel aspects of blood coagulation factor XIII: I. Structure, distribution, activation, and function. *Crit Rev Clin Lab Sci* 33:357, 1996.
291. Chung SI, Lewis MS, Folk JE: Relationships of the catalytic properties of human plasma and platelet transglutaminases (activated blood coagulation factor XIII) to their subunit structures. *J Biol Chem* 249:940, 1974.
292. Gentile V, Saydak M, Chiocca EA, et al: Isolation and characterization of cDNA clones to mouse macrophage and human endothelial cell tissue transglutaminases. *J Biol Chem* 266:478, 1991.
293. Phillips MA, Stewart BE, Qin Q, et al: Primary structure of keratinocyte transglutaminase. *Proc Natl Acad Sci U S A* 87:9333, 1990.
294. Sung LA, Chien S, Chang LS, et al: Molecular cloning of human protein 4.2: A major component of the erythrocyte membrane. *Proc Natl Acad Sci U S A* 87:955, 1990.
295. Lorand L, Graham RM: Transglutaminases: Crosslinking enzymes with pleiotropic functions. *Nat Rev Mol Cell Biol* 4:140, 2003.
296. Yee VC, Pedersen LC, Le Trong I, et al: Three-dimensional structure of a transglutaminase: Human blood coagulation factor XIII. *Proc Natl Acad Sci U S A* 91:7296, 1994.
297. Lorand L, Gray AJ, Brown K, Credo RB, et al: Dissociation of the subunit structure of fibrin stabilizing factor during activation of the zymogen. *Biochem Biophys Res Commun* 56:914, 1974.
298. Mary A, Achyuthan KE, Greenberg CS: B-chains prevent the proteolytic inactivation of the a-chains of plasma factor XIII. *Biochim Biophys Acta* 966:328, 1988.
299. Bottenus RE, Ichinose A, Davie EW: Nucleotide sequence of the gene for the b subunit of human factor XIII. *Biochemistry* 29:11195, 1990.
300. Board PG, Webb GC, McKee J, Ichinose A: Localization of the coagulation factor XIII A subunit gene (F13A) to chromosome bands 6p24-p25. *Cytogenet Cell Genet* 48:25, 1988.
301. Weisberg LJ, Shiu DT, Greenberg CS, et al: Localization of the gene for coagulation factor XIII a-chain to chromosome 6, and identification of sites of synthesis. *J Clin Invest* 79:649, 1987.
302. Ichinose A, Davie EW: Characterization of the gene for the a subunit of human factor XIII (plasma transglutaminase), a blood coagulation factor. *Proc Natl Acad Sci U S A* 85:5829, 1988.
303. Webb GC, Coggan M, Ichinose A, Board PG: Localization of the coagulation factor XIII B subunit gene (F13B) to chromosome bands 1q31–32.1, and restriction fragment length polymorphism at the locus. *Hum Genet* 81:157, 1989.
304. Adany R, Kiss A, Muszbek L: Factor XIII: A marker of mono- and megakaryocytopoiesis. *Br J Haematol* 67:167, 1987.
305. Inbal A, Muszbek L, Lubetsky A, et al: Platelets but not monocytes contribute to the plasma levels of factor XIII subunit A in patients undergoing autologous peripheral blood stem cell transplantation. *Blood Coagul Fibrinolysis* 15:249, 2004.
306. Wolpl A, Lattke H, Board PG, et al: Coagulation factor XIII A and B subunits in bone marrow and liver transplantation. *Transplantation* 43:151, 1987.
307. Nagy JA, Kradin RL, McDonagh J: Biosynthesis of factor XIII A and B subunits. *Adv Exp Med Biol* 231:29, 1988.
308. Takagi T, Doolittle RF: Amino acid sequence studies on factor XIII and the peptide released during its activation by thrombin. *Biochemistry* 13:750, 1974.
309. Ariens RA, Lai TS, Weisel JW, et al: Role of factor XIII in fibrin clot formation and effects of genetic polymorphisms. *Blood* 100:743, 2002.
310. Varadi A, Scheraga HA: Localization of segments essential for polymerization and for calcium binding in the gamma-chain of human fibrinogen. *Biochemistry* 25:519, 1986.
311. Sakata Y, Aoki N: Cross-linking of alpha 2-plasmin inhibitor to fibrin by fibrin-stabilizing factor. *J Clin Invest* 65:290, 1980.
312. Mosher DF, Schad PE, Vann JM: Cross-linking of collagen and fibronectin by factor XIIIa: Localization of participating glutaminyl residues to a tryptic fragment of fibronectin. *J Biol Chem* 255:1181, 1980.
313. Board PG, Losowsky MS, Miloszewski KJ: Factor XIII: Inherited and acquired deficiency. *Blood Rev* 7:229, 1993.
314. Mikkola H, Syrjala M, Rasi V, et al: Deficiency in the A-subunit of coagulation factor XIII: Two novel point mutations demonstrate different effects on transcript level. *Blood* 84:517, 1994.
315. Schroeder V, Durrer D, Meili E, et al: Congenital factor XIII deficiency in Switzerland: from the worldwide first case in 1960, to its molecular characterisation in 2005. *Swiss Med Wkly* 137:272, 2007.
316. Inbal A, Yee VC, Kornbrot N, et al: Factor XIII deficiency due to a Leu660Pro mutation in the factor XIII subunit-a gene in three unrelated Palestinian Arab families. *Thromb Haemost* 77:1062, 1997.
317. Ivaskevicius V, Seitz R, Kohler HP, et al: International registry on factor XIII deficiency: a basis formed mostly on European data. *Thromb Haemost* 97:914, 2007.
318. Aslam S, Standen GR, Khurshid M, Bilwani F: Molecular analysis of six factor XIII-A-deficient families in Southern Pakistan. *Br J Haematol* 109:463, 2000.
319. Cargill M, Altshuler D, Ireland J, et al: Characterization of single-nucleotide polymorphisms in coding regions of human genes. *Nat Genet* 22:231, 1999.
320. Ichinose A: Physiopathology and regulation of factor XIII. *Thromb Haemost* 86:57, 2001.
321. Lauer P, Metzner HJ, Zettlmeissl G, et al: Targeted inactivation of the mouse locus encoding coagulation factor XIII-A: Hemostatic abnormalities in mutant mice and characterization of the coagulation deficit. *Thromb Haemost* 88:967, 2002.
322. Lak M, Peyvandi F, Ali Sharifian A, et al: Pattern of symptoms in 93, Iranian patients with severe factor XIII deficiency. *J Thromb Haemost* 1:1852, 2003.
323. Dardik R, Loscalzo J, Inbal A: Factor XIII (FXIII) and angiogenesis. *J Thromb Haemost* 4:19, 2006.

324. Koseki-Kuno S, Yamakawa M, Dickneite G, Ichinose A: Factor XIII A subunit-deficient mice developed severe uterine bleeding events and subsequent spontaneous miscarriages. *Blood* 102:4410, 2003.
325. Asahina T, Kobayashi T, Okada Y, et al: Maternal blood coagulation factor XIII is associated with the development of cytotrophoblastic shell. *Placenta* 21:388, 2000.
326. Inbal A, Muszbek L: Coagulation factor deficiencies and pregnancy loss. *Semin Thromb Hemost* 29:171, 2003.
327. Katona E, Haramura G, Karpati L, et al: A simple, quick one-step ELISA assay for the determination of complex plasma factor XIII (A2B2). *Thromb Haemost* 83:268, 2000.
328. Nijenhuis AV, van Bergeijk L, Huijgens PC, Zweegman S: Acquired factor XIII deficiency due to an inhibitor: A case report and review of the literature. *Haematologica* 89:ECR14, 2004.
329. Ajzner E, Schlammadinger A, Kerenyi A, et al: Severe bleeding complications caused by an autoantibody against the B subunit of plasma factor XIII; a novel form of acquired factor XIII deficiency. *Blood* 113:723, 2009.
330. Gootenberg JE: Factor concentrates for the treatment of factor XIII deficiency. *Curr Opin Hematol* 5:372, 1998.
331. Lovejoy AE, Reynolds TC, Visich JE, et al: Safety and pharmacokinetics of recombinant factor XIII-A2, administration in patients with congenital factor XIII deficiency. *Blood* 108:57, 2006.
332. Nugent DJ: Prophylaxis in rare coagulation disorders—Factor XIII deficiency. *Thromb Res* 118(Suppl 1):S23, 2006.
333. Asahina T, Kobayashi T, Takeuchi K, Kanayama N: Congenital blood coagulation factor XIII deficiency and successful deliveries: a review of the literature. *Obstet Gynecol Surv* 62:255, 2007.

CHAPTER 126
HEREDITARY FIBRINOGEN ABNORMALITIES

Marguerite Neerman-Arbez and Philippe de Moerloose

SUMMARY

Hereditary fibrinogen abnormalities comprise two classes of plasma fibrinogen defects: (1) type I, afibrinogenemia or hypofibrinogenemia, in which there are low or absent plasma fibrinogen antigen levels (quantitative fibrinogen deficiencies), and (2) type II, dysfibrinogenemia or hypodysfibrinogenemia, in which there are normal or reduced antigen levels associated with disproportionately low functional activity (qualitative fibrinogen deficiencies). In afibrinogenemia, most mutations of the three encoding genes of fibrinogen chains are null mutations. In some cases, missense or truncating nonsense mutations allow synthesis of the corresponding fibrinogen chain, but intracellular fibrinogen assembly and/or secretion are impaired. In certain hypofibrinogenemic cases, the mutant fibrinogen molecules are produced and retained in the rough endoplasmic reticulum of hepatocytes in the form of inclusion bodies, causing endoplasmic reticulum storage disease. Afibrinogenemia is associated with mild to severe bleeding, whereas hypofibrinogenemia is most often asymptomatic. Thromboembolism also occurs either spontaneously or in association with infusions of fibrinogen-rich fractions. Because fibrin is an antithrombin (termed *antithrombin I*), the absence of fibrin in afibrinogenemia can render affected patients vulnerable to thrombosis. Women suffer from recurrent pregnancy loss. Hereditary dysfibrinogenemias are characterized by biosynthesis of a structurally abnormal fibrinogen molecule that exhibits reduced functional properties. Dysfibrinogenemia is commonly associated with bleeding, thrombophilia, and both thrombosis and bleeding, but in many patients it is asymptomatic. Hypodysfibrinogenemia is a subcategory of this disorder. Certain mutations involving the C-terminus of the fibrinogen α chain are associated with amyloidosis, in which an abnormal fragment from the fibrinogen αC domain is deposited in the kidneys. The cause for thrombophilia in type II fibrinogen abnormalities often is uncertain but may involve defective calcium binding, impaired tissue-type plasminogen activator-mediated fibrinolysis, resistance to fibrinolysis, defective fibrin polymerization, or reduced thrombin binding to fibrin.

Several detailed and thoroughly annotated reviews of identified mutations causing inherited fibrinogen disorders have been published[1–5] and a registry for hereditary fibrinogen abnormalities[6] can be accessed at http://www.geht.org/databaseang/fibrinogen/. Fibrinogen plays a major role in hemostasis as the precursor molecule for the insoluble fibrin clot (Fig. 126–1), but in addition participates in numerous other biologic processes such as inflammation, wound healing, and angiogenesis. Fibrinogen binds plasminogen, α_2-antiplasmin, fibronectin, and factor XIII, among other proteins. It also binds to platelets and supports platelet aggregation. After fibrinogen is converted to fibrin by thrombin, it provides nonsubstrate binding sites for thrombin and therefore, fibrinogen is sometimes termed antithrombin I.[7] Fibrinogen also binds to vascular endothelial and other cells, plasma or tissue matrix components such as fibronectin and glycosaminoglycans, and peptide growth factors. Fibrin provides a template for assembly and activation of the fibrinolytic system components and is the major substrate for the enzyme plasmin (see Chap. 136). Both fibrinogen and fibrin serve as substrates for plasma factor XIIIa that catalyzes covalent crosslinking/ligation.

Acronyms and abbreviations that appear in this chapter include: FFP, fresh-frozen plasma; *FGA*, fibrinogen Aα-chain gene; *FGB*, fibrinogen Bβ-chain gene; *FGG*, fibrinogen γ-chain gene; FpA, fibrinopeptide A; FpB, fibrinopeptide B; LMWH, low-molecular-weight heparin; TAFI, thrombin-activatable fibrinolysis inhibitor; t-PA, tissue-type plasminogen activator.

Diseases affecting fibrinogen may be acquired or inherited. Acquired fibrinogen disorders include liver disease, disseminated intravascular coagulation, and primary fibrinolysis, and can be caused by certain drugs. Inherited disorders of fibrinogen are rare and can be subdivided into type I and type II disorders. Type I disorders affect the quantity of fibrinogen in the circulation: hypofibrinogenemia is characterized by fibrinogen levels lower than 1.5 g L^{-1} and afibrinogenemia is characterized by complete or almost complete absence of fibrinogen. Type II disorders affect the quality of circulating fibrinogen: In dysfibrinogenemia, fibrinogen antigen levels are normal, whereas in hypodysfibrinogenemia levels are reduced.

STRUCTURE AND SYNTHESIS

Fibrinogen is a 340-kDa glycoprotein synthesized in hepatocytes[8] that circulates in plasma at a concentration of 1.5 to 3.5 mg/mL (~4–10 μM). Each fibrinogen molecule is approximately 45 nm in length. The core structure consists of two outer D regions[9] (or D domains) and a central E region (or E domain) connected through coiled-coil connectors (Fig. 126–2). The molecule exhibits a twofold axis of symmetry perpendicular to the long axis, consisting of two sets of three polypeptide chains (Aα, Bβ, γ) that are joined in their amino-terminal regions by disulfide bridges to form the E region. The outer D regions contain the globular C terminal domains of the Bβ chain (βC) and γ chain (γC). The βC and γC domains, which are highly conserved in vertebrates, are members of the FreD (fibrinogen-related domain) family of proteins. Unlike the βC and γC domains, the C-terminal domains of the Aα chain (αC) are intrinsically unfolded and flexible and tend to be noncovalently tethered in the vicinity of the central E region (Fig. 126–2).

The three genes encoding fibrinogen Bβ (*FGB*), Aα (*FGA*), and γ (*FGG*), ordered from centromere to telomere, are clustered in a region of approximately 50 kilobases on human chromosome 4.[10] *FGA* and *FGG* are transcribed from the reverse strand, in the opposite direction to *FGB*. Alternative splicing[11] results in two isoforms for the fibrinogen α chain: the common Aα chain, encoded by exons 1 to 5, and an extended Aα-E isoform, encoded by exons 1 to 6 which represents only 1 to 2 percent of transcripts. Alternative splicing for *FGG* also produces two transcripts: the major messenger ribonucleic acid (mRNA) species contains all 10 exons and encodes the common γ chain (or γA), while the minor product (γ') does not splice out intron 9 and the corresponding open reading frame replaces the 4 codons of exon 10 with 20 alternative codons. *FGB* encodes a single 1.9-kb transcript with a 1.5-kb coding sequence. Each gene is separately transcribed and translated to produce nascent polypeptides of 644 amino acids (Aα), 491 amino acids (Bβ), and 437 amino acids (γ).

During translocation of the single chains into the lumen of the endoplasmic reticulum (ER), a signal peptide is cotranslationally cleaved from each chain. The resulting chains have 610 amino acids (Aα), 461 amino acids (Bβ), and 411 amino acids (γ). Assembly proceeds in the ER with the formation of an Aα-γ or Bβ-γ intermediate. The addition of either a Bβ or Aα chain gives rise to a [AαB$\beta\gamma$] half-molecule, which dimerizes to form the functional hexamer.[12] The protein undergoes several posttranslational modifications in the Golgi complex, including maturation of N-linked oligosaccharides, phosphorylation, hydroxylation, and sulfation.[13]

Following assembly, which is completed within minutes, the mature molecule is constitutively secreted into the circulation, where it exhibits a half-life of approximately 4 days.[14] In addition to plasma fibrinogen, blood contains an internalized intracellular fibrinogen pool that is stored within platelet α granules. Both megakaryocytes and platelets are capable of internalizing plasma fibrinogen via the fibrinogen integrin $\alpha_{IIb}\beta_3$ receptor,[15] which binds to a C-terminal platelet recognition sequence that is present on γA chains but is absent from γ' chains. Consequently, internalized platelet fibrinogen molecules contain only γ_A chains.[16]

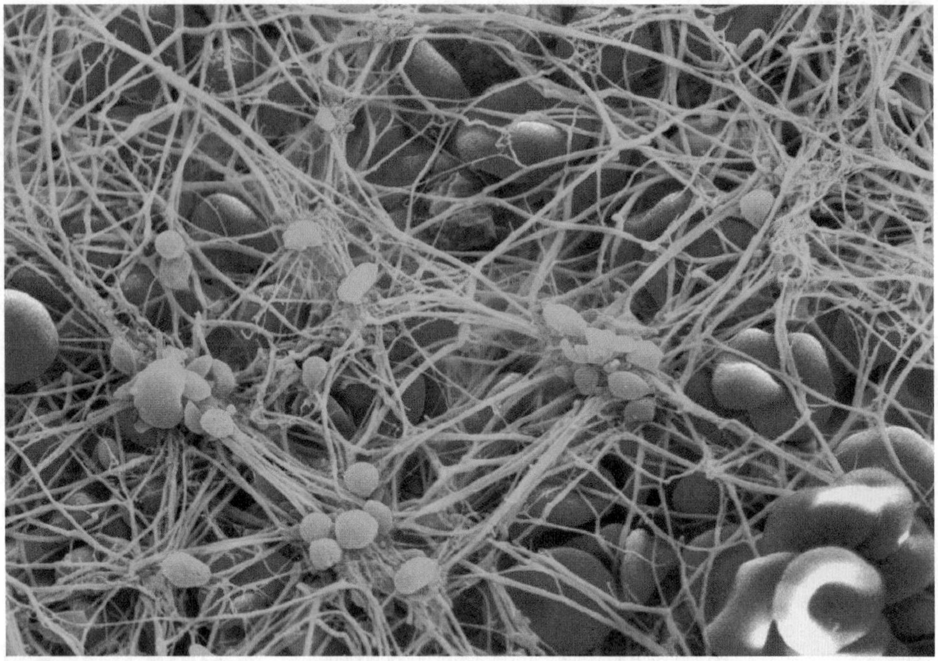

FIGURE 126–1. Colorized scanning electron micrograph of a whole blood clot. The fibrin mesh is shown in green, trapped platelets and erythrocytes are colored violet and red, respectively. *(Used with permission of Yuri Veklich and John W. Weisel, University of Pennsylvania School of Medicine.)*

FIBRINOGEN CONVERSION TO FIBRIN AND NETWORK ASSEMBLY

Conversion of fibrinogen to a fibrin clot[17,18] occurs in three distinct phases: (1) enzymatic cleavage by thrombin to produce fibrin monomers; (2) self-assembly of fibrin units to form an organized polymeric structure; and (3) covalent crosslinking of fibrin by factor XIIIa. In the first phase of conversion to fibrin, cleavage of fibrinogen at AαR35/G36 (R16/G17)* and later Bβ R44/G45 (R14/G15) results in release of fibrinopeptides A (FpA) and B (FpB), respectively, thus exposing "A" knobs and "B" knobs[9] (or E_A and E_B polymerization sites; Fig. 126–3). The "A" knob located at the new amino-terminal end of the fibrin α chain starts with the GPRV amino acid sequence. The "A" knob in fibrin interacts with the constitutive complementary association site known as hole "a" (or site Da) in another molecule to initiate the fibrin assembly process. Hole "a" is encompassed by residues 363–405 (337–379) of the γ-chain.[19]

A knob-a hole interaction results in formation of double-stranded fibrils in which fibrin molecules become aligned in an end-to-middle, staggered overlapping arrangement (see Fig. 126–3).[17,18,20,21] Fibrils subsequently undergo branching by lateral fibril associations ("bilateral branch junctions") in which two fibrils converge to form a four-stranded "bilateral" fibril junction. Progressive lateral associations among fibrils result in larger fibril bundles or fibers. A second type of junction, known as *equilateral branching* (Fig. 126–4), is formed by three fibrils converging to form a three-member junction.[22] Together these two types of branch junctions provide scaffolding for the clot network, the ultimate structure of which is governed by several variables, including salt concentration, pH, and thrombin concentration.[23,24]

FpB release occurs more slowly than FpA release and exposes another polymerization site known as the "B" knob (or E_B) beginning with the amino acid sequence GHRP.[25,26] GHRP interacts with a constitutive "b" hole (or Db site) in the β chain encompassed by residues 427–462 (397–432). FpB cleavage is accelerated by fibrin polymerization, whereas FpA cleavage is independent of fibrin polymerization. B knob-b hole interactions are not required for lateral fibril associations, but they contribute to lateral association by inducing rearrangements in βC that allow βC:βC contacts to occur.[27,28]

The flexible αC domains also participate in fibrin polymerization.[29,30] Fibrin clots made from plasma fibrinogen molecules lacking more than 100 C-terminal residues from the αC domain display prolonged thrombin times, reduced turbidity, and produce thinner fibers, indicating that αC domains participate in lateral fibril associations. In addition, αC domains become dissociated as a result of FpB cleavage. This allows αC domains to participate in noncovalent interactions with other αC domains, thereby promoting lateral fibril associations and fibrin network assembly.

Finally, additional self-associating sites in the D region participate in fibrin assembly. These are the D:D sites and γ_{XL} sites that promote end to end alignment of assembling fibrin units and factor XIIIa crosslinking, respectively.[31,32]

*The recommendation of the Human Genome Variation Society (HGVS) is to number amino acid residues from the initiator Met, with the protein reference sequences representing the primary translation product, not the processed, mature, protein. This is the standard nomenclature used by geneticists. For fibrinogen, however, as for many other secreted proteins such as the coagulation factors, this is not the nomenclature used in earlier publications (historically fibrinogen residues are numbered according to the secreted product lacking the signal peptide). In this text both nomenclatures are used: amino acid residues and substitutions are described first according to HGVS guidelines followed in brackets by the corresponding amino acid in the mature chain lacking the signal peptide. To convert from the HGVS nomenclature to the mature protein nomenclature, subtract 19 for Aα, 30 for Bβ or 26 for γ. A one-letter abbreviation for amino acids is used in this chapter. A, alanine; C, cysteine; D, aspartic acid; E, glutamic acid; F, phenylalanine; G, glycine; H, histidine; I, isoleucine; K, lysine; L, leucine; M, methionine; N, asparagine; P, proline; Q, glutamine; R, arginine; S, serine; T, threonine; V, valine; W, tryptophan; Y, tyrosine.

CROSSLINKING BY FACTOR XIII

The C-terminal region of each fibrinogen or fibrin γ chain contains one crosslinking site for factor XIII or factor XIIIa. Factor XIIIa catalyzes the formation of γ dimers by forming ε-(γ-glutamyl) lysine isopeptide

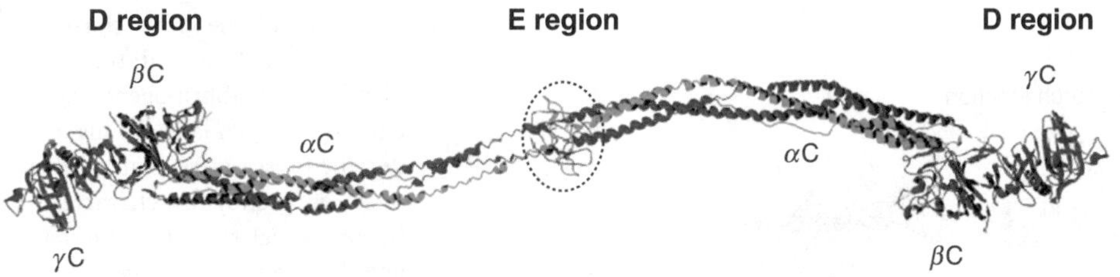

FIGURE 126–2. Ribbon representation of native chicken fibrinogen[28] modified from PDB file 1M1J (www.pdb.org/pdb/). α chains are in green, β chains are in purple, and γ chains are in blue. The globular C-terminal domains of the Bβ and γ chains forming the D regions are shown, as well as the central E region, which contains the N-terminal portions of all three chains. Unlike the βC and γC domains, the C-terminal domains of the Aα chain (αC) are flexible and tend to be noncovalently tethered in the vicinity of the central E region.

bonds.[33] These occur between lysine 432 (406) of one γ chain and glutamine 424 (398) or 425 (399) of another chain. Crosslinking increases the resistance of the clot to deformation. The same process occurs, but at lower rate, between α chains and also between α chains and γ chains. In the presence of factor XIIIa, α_2-antiplasmin becomes covalently bound to the distal α-chains of fibrin or fibrinogen. α_2-Antiplasmin becomes ligated to fibrinogen already prior to the initiation of clotting through the action of factor XIII which may be important for the regulation of *in vivo* fibrinolysis.[33] Fibronectin is also incorporated into the fibrin clot. This occurs by noncovalent interactions between the two proteins through specific binding sites, followed by their covalent crosslinking with factor XIIIa.[34] Fibronectin incorporation appears to affect the adhesion and migration of cells at sites of fibrin deposition, thereby contributing to wound healing and other cell-dependent processes.

CELLULAR AND OTHER BINDING SITES ON FIBRIN(OGEN)

Many sites in fibrinogen and fibrin are involved in interactions with other proteins and cells. For example, neutrophils and monocytes can bind to the fibrin(ogen) D region through their $\alpha_M\beta_2$/Mac-1 integrin receptor.[35] After fibrinopeptide cleavage by thrombin, the β45–72 (15–42) sequence binds heparin and allows endothelial cell binding.[36,37] Exposure of the β45–72 (15–42) sequence also promotes platelet spreading, fibroblast proliferation, endothelial cell spreading, proliferation and capillary tube formation, and release of von Willebrand factor.[36–43] Fibrinogen also contains two integrin-binding sites at Aα114–117 (95–98) (i.e., RGDF) and Aα591–594 (572–575) (i.e., RGDS). Many cellular interactions with fibrinogen and fibrin occur through binding to one or more of these recognition sequences. Crosslinking of αC domains promotes integrin-dependent cell adhesion and signaling. In the case of platelets, RGD sites compete with the fibrinogen γ_A426–437 (400–411) sequence for binding to platelet integrin $\alpha_{IIb}\beta_3$ receptor.

FIBRINOLYSIS

Plasminogen and tissue-type plasminogen activator (t-PA) binding sites in the D regions (i.e., γ337–350) (312–324), and αC domains (i.e., Aα167–179) (148–160), are cryptic in fibrinogen and become exposed during fibrin assembly or during formation of cross-linked fibrinogen fibrils.[44] Two phases can be distinguished in the t-PA induced lysis of a fibrin-clot (see Chap. 136). In the first slow phase, t-PA activates plasminogen on the intact fibrin surface.[45] The generation of C-terminal lysine residues in partially degraded fibrin (by plasmin) in the second phase of clot lysis may result in accumulation of plasminogen at the clot surface and a concomitant increase in lysis rate.[46] Thrombin-activatable fibrinolysis inhibitor (TAFI) removes C-terminal lysine residues, resulting in a strongly reduced binding of plasminogen and in an inhibition of the second phase of clot lysis by a reduction of the activation of plasminogen on the fibrin surface.[47] TAFI, as well as α_2-antiplasmin, lipoprotein(a), and histidine-rich glycoprotein, bind to fibrin and all have an inhibitory effect on fibrinolysis through various mechanisms.

THROMBIN BINDING TO FIBRINOGEN AND FIBRIN

Thrombin binds to its substrate, fibrinogen, through a fibrinogen recognition site in thrombin, referred to as exosite 1.[48] The fibrin clot itself also exhibits significant thrombin-binding potential; this nonsubstrate binding potential of fibrin for thrombin is referred to as antithrombin activity I.[7] This activity is defined by two classes of nonsubstrate thrombin-binding sites in fibrin, one of "low-affinity" in the E-region and the other of "high-affinity" in D regions of fibrin(ogen) molecules containing the variant γ′ chain. Altogether, heterodimeric γA/γ′ and homodimeric molecules γ′/γ′ chains comprise approximately 8 percent

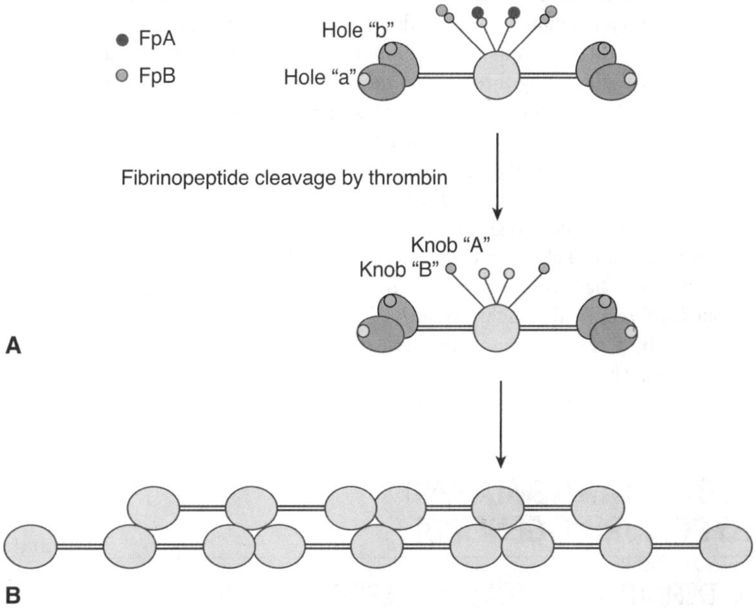

FIGURE 126–3. First steps of fibrinogen conversion to fibrin and fibrin assembly. **A.** Schematic of fibrinogen showing fibrinopeptides A (FpA) and B (FpB), the constitutive "a" and "b" holes in the globular C-terminal domains of the γ chains and β chains, respectively, and the "A" and "B" knobs, which are exposed only after FpA and FpB cleavage by thrombin. Here the globular βC and γC domains are shown separately, βC in purple, γC in blue as in Figure 126–2. **B.** Self-assembly of fibrin units to form an organized polymeric structure. Here, for simplicity, the D regions are represented as a single globular unit.

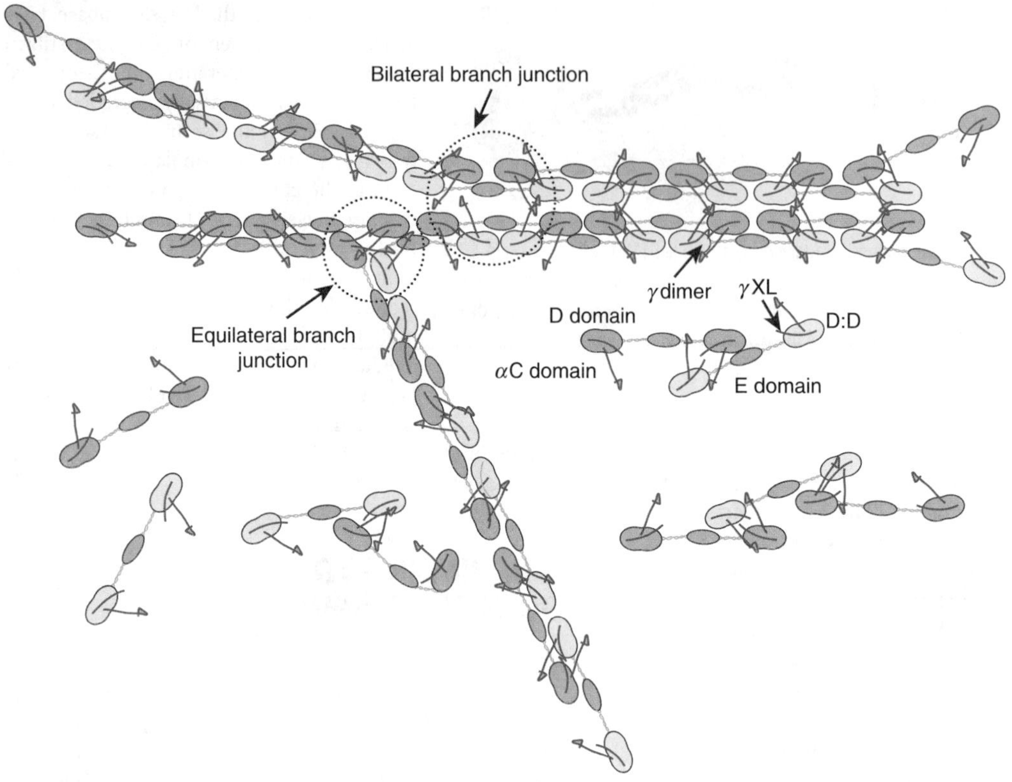

FIGURE 126–4. Fibrin assembly and γ-chain crosslinking.

of the total γ chain population.[11] Low-affinity thrombin-binding activity reflects thrombin exosite 1 binding in the E region of fibrin, whereas high-affinity thrombin binding to γ' chains takes place through exosite 2. The binding affinity of thrombin for γ'-containing fibrin molecules is increased by concomitant fibrin binding to thrombin exosite 1. Antithrombin I (fibrin) is an important inhibitor of thrombin generation that functions by sequestering thrombin in the forming fibrin clot, and also by reducing the catalytic activity of fibrin-bound thrombin. Vascular thrombosis may result from absence of antithrombin I (as in afibrinogenemia; see "Afibrinogenemia and Hypofibrinogenemia" below), reduced plasma γ' chain content,[49] or defective thrombin binding to fibrin as found in certain dysfibrinogenemias (see "Dysfibrinogenemia and Hypodysfibrinogenemia" below). In contrast, an increased susceptibility to arterial thrombosis has been reported when γ'-chain levels are significantly elevated. Moreover, thrombin bound to γ_A/γ'-fibrin is protected from inhibition by antithrombin to a greater extent than thrombin bound to γ_A/γ_A-fibrin. Thus, γ_A/γ'-fibrin serves as a reservoir of active thrombin, which may contribute to the prothrombotic nature of thrombi.[50]

AFIBRINOGENEMIA AND HYPOFIBRINOGENEMIA

DEFINITION, HISTORY, AND EPIDEMIOLOGY

Diseases affecting fibrinogen may be both acquired or inherited. Inherited disorders of fibrinogen are rare and can be subdivided into type I and type II disorders. Type I disorders (afibrinogenemia and hypofibrinogenemia) affect the quantity of fibrinogen in circulation. Type II disorders (dysfibrinogenemia and hypodysfibrinogenemia) affect the quality of circulating fibrinogen. While the first dysfibrinogenemia mutation was identified as early as 1968,[51] even before the genomic sequences of the three fibrinogen genes were determined, the molecular basis of afibrinogenemia was elucidated much later.[52] This disorder, the most severe form of fibrinogen deficiency, is characterized by autosomal recessive inheritance and the complete absence of fibrinogen in plasma.

The disease was originally described in 1920[53] with an estimated prevalence of around 1 in 1,000,000.[54] In populations where consanguineous marriages are common, however, the prevalence of afibrinogenemia, as for other autosomal recessive coagulation disorders, is increased.[55,56] Because hypofibrinogenemia (fibrinogen levels below 1.5 g L^{-1}) is often caused by heterozygosity for a fibrinogen gene mutation, this is much more frequent than afibrinogenemia. If one applies the Hardy Weinberg binomial distribution of alleles in the population to afibrinogenemia, carriers of fibrinogen deficiency causing mutations could be as frequent as 1:500.

ETIOLOGY AND PATHOGENESIS

Since the identification of the first causative mutation for congenital afibrinogenemia in 1999,[52] more than 80 distinct mutations, the majority in *FGA*, have been identified in patients with afibrinogenemia (in homozygosity or in compound heterozygosity) or in hypofibrinogenemia.[5] The mutations that lead to complete fibrinogen deficiency, identified either in afibrinogenemic and/or hypofibrinogenemic individuals, are listed together in Table 126–1.[52–121] Causative mutations can be divided into two main classes: null mutations with no protein production at all and mutations producing abnormal protein chains which are retained inside the cell.

Large Deletions

Four large deletions (>1 kb) have been identified to date (see Table 126–1). A nonconsanguineous Swiss family with two pairs of afibrinogenemic brothers was studied by microsatellite analysis, polymerase chain reaction (PCR) amplification, and Southern blotting.[52] In a first step toward establishing whether or not the disease was linked to the fibrinogen gene cluster on chromosome 4, haplotype data were obtained for five microsatellite markers surrounding this locus. One of these, FGAi3, a (TCTT)n polymorphic marker located in intron 3 of the *FGA* gene, was found to be deleted in all four affected individuals and was hemizygous in the obligate carriers. Analysis of the flanking microsatellite markers revealed that the deletions had occurred on three different ancestral chromosomes, implying that homozygous deletion of at least part of the *FGA* gene was responsible for the congenital afibrinogenemia in this family and that this mutation was either very ancient, or the fibrinogen locus is susceptible to deletion by a common mechanism.

PCR amplification of portions of the three fibrinogen genes revealed that the *FGG* and *FGB* genes were intact in the affected individuals. In contrast, for *FGA*, only exon 1, which encodes the first 18 of the 19 amino acid signal peptides, could be amplified from patient's DNA, thus

TABLE 126–1. Mutations Resulting in Afibrinogenemia and Hypofibrinogenemia*

	Mutation				
cDNA	Nascent	Mature Chain	Etiology/Pathology	Clinical Manifestation	Reference
FGA					
4.1 kb deletion	–	–	Large deletion of exon 1	AFIB	61
−1138C→T	–	–	Promoter mutation, reduces enhancer activity	HYPO	62
c. 3_4insC	F2Lfs	F-17Lfs	Frameshift mutation exon 1	AFIB	63
c. 54+1G→A	–	–	Splice site mutation intron 1	AFIB	82
c. 54+3A→G	–	–	Splice site mutation intron 1	AFIB	63
11 kb deletion	–	–	Large deletion of exons 2–6, recurrent	AFIB	52, 57, 63
c. 94G→T	G32X	G13X	Nonsense mutation exon 2, escapes NMD	AFIB	83
c. 117delT	V40Wfs	V21Wfs	Frameshift mutation exon 2, escapes NMD	AFIB	64, 83
c. 180+2T→C	–	–	Splice-site mutation intron 2	HYPO	5
c. 191G→T	C64F	C45F	Missense mutation exon 3, impairs fibrinogen secretion	HYPO	84
c. 196_197insT	S66Ffs	S47Ffs	Frameshift mutation exon 3	AFIB	82
c. 209T→G	M70R	M51R	Missense mutation exon 3, impairs fibrinogen secretion	AFIB	85
c. 229_231del3ins12	V77insPLMX	V58insPLMX	Deletion insertion in exon 3, premature stop codon	AFIB	61
c. 285T→A	Y95X	Y76X	Nonsense mutation exon 3	AFIB	64
c. 356C→G	S119X	S100X	Nonsense mutation exon 3, escapes NMD	AFIB	83
c. 364+1_+4delGTAA	–	–	Splice-site mutation intron 3, causes exon 3 skipping	AFIB	64, 86
1.2 kb deletion	–	–	Large deletion of exon 4	AFIB	59
c. 385C→T	R129X	R110X	Nonsense mutation exon 4, escapes NMD	AFIB	83
c. 431_432delAA	K144Sfs	K125Sfs	Frameshift mutation exon 4	AFIB	63
c. 448C→T	Q150X	Q131X	Nonsense mutation exon 4	AFIB	87
c. 502C→T	R168X	R149X	Nonsense mutation exon 4, escapes NMD	AFIB	88, 83
c. 510+1G→T	–	–	Splice site mutation intron 4, recurrent, causes cryptic splice site usage	AFIB	63–65
15 kb deletion	–	–	Large deletion of exons 5–6	AFIB	60
c. 541C→T	R181X	R162X	Nonsense mutation exon 5	AFIB	5
c. 563_564insT	L188Ffs	L169Ffs	Frameshift mutation exon 5	AFIB	5
c. 607C→T	Q203X	Q184X	Nonsense mutation exon 5	AFIB	89
c. 609_610insTGA	L204X	L185X	Insertion stop codon exon 5	AFIB	82
c. 635T→G	L212X	L166X	Nonsense mutation exon 5	AFIB	5
c. 711_712insT	K238X	K219X	Frameshift mutation exon 5	AFIB	90
c. 743G→A	W248X	W229X	Nonsense mutation exon 5	AFIB	5
c. 786_789delGAGA	E262Dfs	E243Dfs	Frameshift mutation exon 5, predicted to encode 157 aberrant aa	AFIB	91
c. 835delA	T279Pfs	T260Pfs	Frameshift mutation exon 5, predicted to encode 141 aberrant aa	AFIB	92
c. 885G→A	W295X	W276X	Nonsense mutation exon 5	AFIB	5
c. 934delA	S312Afs	S293Afs	Frameshift mutation exon 5, predicted to encode 108 aberrant aa	AFIB	64
c. 945delT	G316Efs	G297Efs	Frameshift mutation exon 5, predicted to encode 103 aberrant aa	AFIB	64
c. 946G→T	G316X	G297X	Nonsense mutation exon 5	AFIB	63
c. 1001G→A	W334X	W315X	Nonsense mutation exon 5	AFIB	63
c. 1025delG	G342Efs	G323Efs	Frameshift mutation exon 5, predicted to encode 78 aberrant aa	AFIB	5
c. 1037delA	N346Tfs	N327Tfs	Frameshift mutation exon 5, predicted to encode 74 aberrant aa	AFIB	5
c. 1055delC	P352Lfs	P333Lfs	Frameshift mutation exon 5, predicted to encode 68 aberrant aa	AFIB	63

(*continued*)

TABLE 126–1. Mutations Resulting in Afibrinogenemia and Hypofibrinogenemia* (Continued)

	Mutation				
cDNA	Nascent	Mature Chain	Etiology/Pathology	Clinical Manifestation	Reference
FGB					
c. 114+2076→G	–	–	Mutation intron 1, causes inclusion of 50bp cryptic exon	AFIB	93, 94
c. 139C→T	R47X	R17X	Nonsense mutation exon 2	AFIB	66, 71
c. 213T→G	Y71X	Y41X	Nonsense mutation exon 2	HYPO	95
c. 248_249delAGinsT	K83Ifs	K53Ifs	Frameshift mutation exon 2	AFIB	5
c. 264delA	A89Pfs	A59Pfs	Frameshift mutation exon 2	HYPO	96
c. 605T→A	L202N	L172N	"Missense" mutation exon 4, leads to aberrant splicing	AFIB	97
c. 854G→A	R285H	R255H (Merivale)	Missense mutation exon 6	HYPO	98
c. 880A→G	R294G	R264G (Nottingham II)	Missense mutation exon 6	HYPO	99
c. 887G→A	W296X	W266X	Nonsense mutation exon 6	AFIB	61
c. 958+1G→A	–	–	Splice-site mutation intron 6	HYPO	100
c. 958+13C→T	–	–	Splice-site mutation intron 6	AFIB	101
c. 1036G→T	D346Y	D316Y	Missense mutation exon 7	HYPO	102
c. 1148T→G	L383R	L353R	Missense mutation exon 7, impairs fibrinogen secretion	AFIB	70
c. 1244+1G→T	–	–	Splice-site mutation intron 7	AFIB	101
c. 1245–1G→C	–	–	Splice-site mutation intron 7	HYPO	103
c. 1267C→T	Q423X	Q393X	Nonsense mutation exon 8	HYPO	104
c. 1296G→A	W432X	W402X	Nonsense mutation exon 8	HYPO	105
c. 1289G→A	G430D	G400D	Missense mutation exon 8, impairs fibrinogen secretion	AFIB	70
c. 1330G→C	G444S	G414S	Missense mutation exon 8, impairs fibrinogen secretion	AFIB	71
c. 1346delG	G449Vfs	G419Vfs	Frameshift mutation exon 8	AFIB	106
c. 1391G→A	G464D	G434D	Missense mutation exon 8, impairs fibrinogen secretion	AFIB	73
c. 1399T→G	W467G	W437G	Missense mutation exon 8, impairs fibrinogen secretion	AFIB	72
c. 1400G→A	W467X	W437X	Nonsense mutation exon 8, impairs fibrinogen secretion	AFIB	68
c. 1409G→A	W470X	W440X	Nonsense mutation exon 8, impairs fibrinogen secretion	HYPO	67, 69
FGG					
c. 78+5G→A	–	–	Splice-site mutation intron 1	AFIB	108
c. 98delA	N33Tfs	N7Tfs	Frameshift mutation exon 2	AFIB	64
c. 123+1G→A	–	–	Splice-site mutation intron 2	HYPO	109
c. 124–3C→G	–	–	Splice-site mutation intron 2	AFIB	64
c. 307+5G→A	–	–	Splice site mutation intron 3	AFIB	110
c. 400C→T	R134X	R108X	Nonsense mutation split between exons 4 and 5, escapes NMD	AFIB	111
c. 448delC	L150X	L124X	Frameshift mutation exon 5, creates stop codon	AFIB	5
c. 535T→C	C179R	C153R (Matsumoto IV)	Missense mutation exon 6, impairs fibrinogen assembly/secretion	HYPO	74
c. 666+660A→T	–	–	Mutation intron 6, causes inclusion of 75 bp cryptic exon	AFIB	112
c. 667A→T	R223X	R197X	Nonsense mutation exon 7	AFIB	64
c. 677G→T	G226V	G200V (Colombus)	Missense mutation exon 7	HYPO	113
c. 759G→T	W253C	W227C (Bratislava)	Missense mutation exon 7, impairs fibrinogen secretion	HYPO	75
c. 769G→T	E257X	E231X	Nonsense mutation exon 7	AFIB	114
c. 835T→G	W279G	W253G (Darlinghurst, homozygous)	Missense mutation exon 7	HYPO	115
c. 928G→C	G310R	G284R (Brescia)	Missense mutation exon 8, causes hepatic ER storage disease	HYPO	76
c. 944C→T	A315V	A289V (Dorfen)	Missense mutation exon 8	HYPO	116

(*continued*)

TABLE 126–1. Mutations Resulting in Afibrinogenemia and Hypofibrinogenemia* (Continued)

Mutation				Clinical	
cDNA	Nascent	Mature Chain	Etiology/Pathology	Manifestation	Reference
c. 997C→T	H333Y	H307Y (Mannheim II)	Missense mutation exon 8	HYPO	117
c. 1016C→A	S339N	S313N	Missense mutation exon 8	HYPO	118
c. 1100C→T	A367V	A341V (Tolaga Bay)	Missense mutation exon 8	HYPO	119
c. 1112A→G	N371S	N345S (Saint Germain II)	Missense mutation exon 8	HYPO	120
c. 1116_1129+1del	del372–376	del346–350 (Angers)	15 bp deletion including intron 8 donor splice-site, aberrant splicing leads to inframe deletion of 5 aa, causes hepatic ER storage disease	HYPO	80
c. 1190C→T	T397I	T371I	Missense mutation exon 8	HYPO	121
c. 1201C→T	R401W	R375W (Aguadilla)	Missense mutation exon 8, causes hepatic ER storage disease	HYPO	77–79

aa, Amino acids; AFIB, afibrinogenemia; bp, base pairs; del, deletion; fs, frameshift; HYPO, hypofibrinogenemia; ins, insertion; NMD, nonsense-mediated decay.

*Mutations are listed here if the causative nature has been demonstrated by functional analysis or if the type of mutation leaves no doubt that they are indeed responsible for the fibrinogen deficiency. Distinct mutations published in peer-reviewed journals before January 2009 are listed. For recurrent mutations, not all are referenced due to limited space. A complete list is available at www.geht.org/databaseang/fibrinogen/, which also lists variants reported in abstracts and submitted online. Unless specified otherwise, mutations were identified in homozygosity or compound heterozygosity in afibrinogenemia (AFIB) and heterozygosity in hypofibrinogenemia (HYPO).

placing the 5′ deletion breakpoint in *FGA* intron 1. Bam HI Southern blot analysis placed the 3′ deletion breakpoint in the *FGA-FGB* intergenic region, approximately 11 kb downstream. The deletion junction sequences were found to be identical to the base pair in all the affected individuals and in their heterozygous parents.[57] The genetic defect in this family was an apparently recurrent deletion of approximately 11 kb of DNA, which eliminated most of the *FGA* gene resulting in an absence of fibrinogen. These results demonstrated that afibrinogenemia is caused by a defect in fibrinogen synthesis and demonstrated unequivocally that humans, like mice,[58] may be born without any functional fibrinogen.

Three other large deletions in the fibrinogen gene cluster have been identified, all involving part of the *FGA* gene. The first, a deletion of 1.2 kb eliminating the entire *FGA* exon 4, was identified in homozygosity in a Japanese patient.[59] The second, a deletion of 15 kb, with breakpoints situated in *FGA* intron 4 and in the *FGA-FGB* intergenic region, was identified in a Thai patient.[60] Interestingly, although the patient was apparently homozygous for the deletion, this was found to be transmitted only by the heterozygous mother. Nonpaternity was ruled out, and complete maternal uniparental disomy was confirmed for chromosome 4 by analysis of microsatellite markers spanning the entire chromosome. As for the 11-kb deletion identified earlier,[54,57] short direct repeats were found in the vicinity of the deletion breakpoints, indicating nonhomologous recombination as the most likely mechanism causing this deletion. However, in contrast to the 11-kb deletion, recurrence of the 15-kb deletion has not been reported. Finally a 4.1-kb deletion encompassing *FGA* exon 1 was identified in an Italian patient.[61]

Promoter Mutations

To date only one mutation has been identified in a promoter. This was a heterozygous variant −1138C→T upstream of *FGA* identified in heterozygosity in a Japanese patient with hypofibrinogenemia.[62]

Splice-Site Mutations

Thirteen splice-site mutations have been identified so far: five in *FGA*, four in *FGB*, and four in *FGG*. In afibrinogenemic patients of European origin, the most common mutation is a donor splice mutation in intron 4, c.510+1G→T (previously described as IVS4+1 G→T).[5,63,64] Haplotype data suggest that this mutation, like the *FGA* 11-kb deletion, is also recurrent, or a very ancient mutation, because the c.510+1G→T mutation is found on multiple discrete haplotypes. Functional analysis of the mutation in transfected COS cells demonstrated that the c.510+1G→T mutation abolishes the normal donor site and leads to aberrant usage of an alternative downstream donor site and a consequent 4-bp frameshift mutation in the majority of transcripts.[65]

Frameshift Mutations

To date, the total number of frameshift mutations leading to complete fibrinogen deficiency amounts to 17 (12 in *FGA*, 3 in *FGB* and 2 in *FGG*). Frameshift mutations that cause hypodysfibrinogenemia are not included in this number and are discussed separately (see "Dysfibrinogenemia and Hypodysfibrinogenemia" below). *FGA* exon 5 has the largest number of frameshift mutations. Interestingly, seven single base-pair deletions in *FGA* exon 5 (see Table 126–1) result in usage of the same new reading frame. All seven mutations are predicted to encode a long stretch of aberrant amino acids before terminating at the same premature stop codon, 69 to 158 codons downstream. The aberrant amino acid sequence (if the abnormal protein is synthesized and stable, which remains to be determined) may lead to abnormal folding of the Aα chain, thus affecting fibrinogen chain assembly or secretion. Computer-assisted analysis of two of these putative C-terminal sequences (S312Afs and G316Efs) predicted the presence of several α helices in the mutant domains as a result of enrichment in leucine and valine residues.[66] These motifs, which are absent in the wild-type fibrinogen Aα chain, may perturb the assembly and/or secretion of the fibrinogen hexamer molecule; the longer the aberrant polypeptide, the likelier the deleterious effect on fibrinogen synthesis.

Nonsense Mutations

More than 20 nonsense mutations accounting for afibrinogenemia and hypofibrinogenemia have been identified (see Table 126–1). Of the seven nonsense mutations identified in *FGB*, four are located in *FGB* exon 8. In particular, two *FGB* nonsense mutations—W467X (W437X) and W470X (W440X)—are localized very close to the β-chain C-terminus and are expected to cause the synthesis of β chains truncated of only 25 and 22 residues, respectively.[67,68] Expression studies in transfected COS cells performed for both mutations showed that the mutations allowed individual chain synthesis and intracellular assembly of the hexamer but impaired secretion, suggesting that an intact *FGB* C-terminal domain is necessary for fibrinogen secretion into the circulation.[68,69]

Missense Mutations

Null mutations, that is, large deletions, frameshift, early truncating nonsense, and splice-site mutations expectedly account for the majority of afibrinogenemia alleles.[5] Of particular interest are missense mutations leading to complete fibrinogen deficiency. These are clustered in the highly conserved C-terminal globular domains of the Bβ and γ chains (see Table 126–1). Expression studies of transfected cells for five of these in *FGB*, all identified in homozygosity or compound heterozygosity in afibrinogenemic patients, showed that these mutations also allowed individual chain synthesis and intracellular assembly of the hexamer but impaired secretion, suggesting again that an intact *FGB* C-terminal domain is necessary for fibrinogen secretion into the circulation.[70–73]

Further characterization of the *FGB* G444S (G414S) mutant using immunostaining for fibrinogen and visualization by confocal microscopy revealed that the secretion-impaired mutant was retained in the ER proving the existence of an efficient quality control mechanism for fibrinogen secretion.[69]

Ten missense mutations have also been identified in *FGG* in heterozygosity in patients with hypofibrinogenemia. For the majority of these mutations, analysis of patient plasma fibrinogen by mass spectrometry has confirmed absence of the mutant γ chain in the circulation. Others have been studied at the functional level in transfected cells: fibrinogen Matsumoto IV C179R (C153R) was found to impair intracellular hexamer assembly,[74] whereas fibrinogen Bratislava W253C (W227C) was found to impair fibrinogen secretion.[75]

Mutations Causing Hepatic Endoplasmic Reticulum Retention and Hypofibrinogenemia

In the majority of patients with afibrinogenemia or hypofibrinogenemia there is no evidence of intracellular accumulation of the mutant fibrinogen chain. This implies the existence of an efficient degradation pathway for fibrinogen mutants that allow individual chain synthesis and assembly but not secretion. Three mutations, all in *FGG*, are known to cause hypofibrinogenemia accompanied by hepatic storage disease. Two are missense mutations in *FGG*, which cause fibrinogen deficiency in the heterozygous state because of the absence of the mutant γ chain in patient plasma, but also progressive liver disease associated with hepatocellular cytoplasmic inclusions. The fibrinogen Brescia mutation *FGG* G310R (G284R) was the first to be identified in heterozygosity in a patient suffering from liver cirrhosis. The globular inclusions in the liver of the proband corresponded to dilated rough ER cisternae filled with densely packed tubular structures. Intracisternal material selectively and exclusively reacted with antifibrinogen antibodies.[76]

The second case of hypofibrinogenemia associated with hepatic inclusion bodies with fibrinogen aggregates was reported in a young girl heterozygous for a *FGG* R401W (R375W) mutation (fibrinogen Aguadilla).[77] The patient was asymptomatic and only presented chronically elevated liver function test results. The same mutation was identified later in a 61-year-old Swiss man with progressive liver disease.[78] In this patient, a liver biopsy revealed chronic hepatitis complicated by cirrhosis and weakly eosinophilic globular cytoplasmic inclusions within the hepatocytes. Both the propositus and his two sons showed low functional and antigenic fibrinogen concentrations, and all three were heterozygous for the Aguadilla mutation. A liver biopsy performed in the older son demonstrated the same globular cytoplasmic inclusions, but without chronic liver disease. This mutation was also identified in a young boy with liver storage disease and hypofibrinogenemia.[79]

A third mutation was identified in *FGG* (fibrinogen Angers) in a woman with chronic abnormal liver function tests.[80] The propositus and her brother were heterozygous for a 15-bp deletion at the end of *FGG* exon 8, which creates a new *FGG* exon 8–intron 8 junction and donor splice site. Usage of this splice site was predicted to result in an aberrant mRNA with an in-frame deletion of five amino acids: del372–376GVYYQ (del346–350). The production of this abnormal mRNA was confirmed by reverse-transcription polymerase chain reaction (RT-PCR) on a liver biopsy obtained from the patient's brother followed by sequencing. The five amino acids missing in fibrinogen Angers are located in the "a" hole, which is crucial for fibrin polymerization. The molecular mechanism by which the fibrinogen Angers mutation as well as the fibrinogen Brescia and Aguadilla mutations, localized in the five-stranded beta sheet of γC and the "a" hole, respectively, leads to impaired secretion, retention in the ER, and formation of aggregates remains to be determined.[81]

CLINICAL FEATURES

Afibrinogenemia

Bleeding because of afibrinogenemia usually manifests in the neonatal period, with 85 percent of cases presenting umbilical cord bleeding,[55] but a later age of onset is not unusual. Bleeding may occur in the skin, gastrointestinal tract, genitourinary tract, or the central nervous system with intracranial hemorrhage being the major cause of death. Joint bleeding, which is common in patients with severe hemophilia, is infrequent: In a series of 72 patients with severe fibrinogen deficiency, hemarthrosis was observed in 25 percent of cases.[122] There is an intriguing susceptibility of spontaneous rupture of the spleen in afibrinogenemic patients.[121–123]

Menstruating women may experience menometrorrhagia but some have normal menses. First trimester abortion is usual in afibrinogenemic women. The importance of fibrinogen in pregnancy was demonstrated in studies with fibrinogen knockout mice that do not reach term.[58,124] Women may also have antepartum and postpartum hemorrhage. Hemoperitoneum after rupture of the corpus luteum has also been observed.

Paradoxically both arterial and venous thromboembolic complications are observed in afibrinogenemic patients. These complications can occur in the presence of concomitant risk factors such as a coinherited thrombophilic risk factor or after replacement therapy. However, in many patients, no known risk factors are present. Many hypotheses have been put forward to explain this predisposition to thrombosis. One explanation is that even in the absence of fibrinogen platelet aggregation is possible because of the action of von Willebrand factor[125] and, in contrast to patients with severe hemophilia, afibrinogenemic patients are able to generate thrombin, both in the initial phase of limited production and also in the secondary burst of thrombin generation. In some patients, an increase of prothrombin activation fragments or thrombin–antithrombin complexes has been observed, which may reflect enhanced thrombin generation.[126] These abnormal levels can be normalized by fibrinogen infusions.

As previously mentioned, fibrin also acts as antithrombin I by both sequestering and downregulating thrombin activity.[7] Thrombin which is not trapped by the clot is available for platelet activation and smooth muscle cell migration and proliferation, particularly in the arterial vessel wall. Thrombus formation is maintained in fibrinogen-deficient mice, but the thrombus is unstable and has a tendency to embolize.[127] Similarly, the absence of fibrinogen in human plasma results in large but loosely packed thrombi under flow conditions.[128]

Hypofibrinogenemia

Hypofibrinogenemia patients are very often heterozygous carriers of afibrinogenemia mutations. These patients are usually asymptomatic with fibrinogen levels around 1.0 g L^{-1}, levels which are in theory high enough to protect against bleeding and maintaining pregnancy. However they can bleed when exposed to trauma, or if they have a second associated hemostatic abnormality. Hypofibrinogenemic women may also suffer from pregnancy loss.

LABORATORY FEATURES

The clinical diagnosis is established by immunologic measurements of fibrinogen concentration backed by genetic analyses.

Phenotype Analysis

Absence of immunoreactive fibrinogen is essential for the diagnosis of congenital afibrinogenemia. All coagulation tests that depend on the formation of fibrin as the end point—that is, prothrombin time (PT), partial thromboplastin time (PTT), or thrombin time (TT)—are infinitely prolonged. Plasma activity of all other clotting factors is normal. Some abnormalities in platelet functions tests can be observed which can be reversed upon addition of fibrinogen.[129] Because fibrinogen is one of the main determinants of erythrocyte sedimentation, it is not surprising that afibrinogenemic patients have very low erythrocyte sedimentation rates. When skin testing is performed for delayed hypersensitivity, there is no induration because of the lack of fibrin deposition.[130]

Hypofibrinogenemia is defined as a proportional decrease of functional and immunoreactive fibrinogen. Coagulation tests depending on the formation of fibrin are variably prolonged, the most sensitive assay being the TT.

Genotype Analysis

The large number of mutations identified in patients with afibrinogenemia allows the design of an efficient flow-chart for mutation detection in new cases.[131] Two common mutations are found in individuals of European origin, both in *FGA*: the c.510+1G→T intron 4 donor splice-site mutation and the *FGA* 11-kb deletion, both found on multiple haplotypes. In all new patients of European origin, the *FGA* c.510+1G→ T should be the first mutation to be screened. Southern blot or PCR analysis of the *FGA* 11 kb deletion should also be performed, because it is the second most common mutation in patients of European origin and because of the risk of diagnostic error: A nonconsanguineous patient who appears to be homozygous for a mutation in *FGA* exons 2–6 may in reality be a heterozygous carrier of the large 11-kb deletion.[132] Given the high frequency of mutations in *FGA*, the other *FGA* exons (starting with exon 5) should then be studied for mutations before screening *FGB* (starting with exon 8) and *FGG* (starting with exons 7 and 8). The same strategy can also be applied to afibrinogenemic patients of non-European origin for whom recurrent mutations have yet to be identified. If the patient comes from a geographical region or population in which a mutation has already been identified, that mutation should be the first to be screened for. Screening of patients with hypofibrinogenemia can follow the same strategy apart from patients with ER fibrinogen-positive liver inclusions, for which three mutations in *FGG* are known so far to cause hepatic storage disease (see Table 126–1).

Prenatal diagnosis has been performed in a few cases.[68] This is particularly important in families with afibrinogenemia since the prenatal diagnosis of an affected infant allows initiation of treatment immediately after birth before the first bleeding manifestation.

Genotype-Phenotype Correlations: The Importance of Global Assays

Current diagnostic tests are appropriate for establishing the diagnosis but clearly additional tests are required for a more accurate prediction of the clinical phenotype of a patient and consequently the appropriate treatment. Indeed, although in afibrinogenemia all patients have unmeasurable functional fibrinogen, the severity of bleeding is highly variable amongst patients, even amongst those with the same genotype. Similarly, there is no clear relationship between the molecular defect and the risk of thrombosis.

One possible explanation for the observed variability of clinical manifestations is the existence of modifier genes/alleles: some variants may increase the severity of bleeding while others may ameliorate the phenotype. Such modifiers have yet to be identified. However, the common thrombophilias (e.g., factor V Leiden) most certainly play a role in decreasing the severity of bleeding. The existence of modifying genes/polymorphisms is also strongly suspected in the previously discussed cases of hypofibrinogenemia associated with fibrinogen inclusion bodies in hepatocytes. Indeed, all individuals heterozygous for one of the three causative mutations identified in *FGG* have hypofibrinogenemia, but not all have fibrinogen aggregates and associated liver disease.

Global assays such as thromboelastography and thrombin generation test may provide a complementary and in some cases a better evaluation of an individual's hemostatic state.[133] Such global assays could be useful for the design of individual therapeutic strategies as was shown in hemophilia A patients.[134,135]

DIFFERENTIAL DIAGNOSIS

Inherited afibrinogenemia and hypofibrinogenemia have to be distinguished from acquired disorders. These include disseminated intravascular coagulation, primary fibrinolysis, liver disease, and can be caused by certain drugs (e.g., thrombolytic agents and L-asparaginase). In addition, one should be aware that artifactually low levels of fibrinogen can be observed with samples that have clotted as a result of improper collection. In most cases, the clinical context as well as the association with other laboratory abnormalities will allow differentiation of inherited from acquired disorders. Identification of a causative mutation in one of the three fibrinogen genes will confirm the diagnosis.

THERAPY

Available Treatments and Modalities

Replacement therapy is effective in treating bleeding episodes in congenital fibrinogen disorders. Depending on the country of residence, patients receive fresh-frozen plasma (FFP), cryoprecipitate or fibrinogen concentrates.[131] Fibrinogen concentrate preparations include safety steps for inactivation or removal of viruses, which make them safer than cryoprecipitate or FFP. Furthermore, more precise dosing can be accomplished with fibrinogen concentrates because their potency is known, in contrast to FFP or cryoprecipitates.

The conventional treatment is on demand, in which fibrinogen is administered as soon as possible after onset of bleeding. Another approach is primary prophylaxis that includes administration of fibrinogen concentrates from an early age to prevent bleeding and, in the case of pregnancy, to prevent miscarriage. Effective long-term secondary prophylaxis with administration of fibrinogen every 7 to 14 days (particularly after central nervous system bleeds) has been advocated. The frequency and dose of fibrinogen concentrates should be adjusted to maintain a level above 0.5 g L^{-1}.[131]

The United Kingdom guidelines on therapeutic products for coagulation disorders[136] provide recommendations about the best treatment options (dosage, management of bleeding, surgery and pregnancy as well as prophylaxis). According to these guidelines, in case of bleeding fibrinogen levels should be increased to 1.0 g L^{-1} and maintained above this threshold until hemostasis is secured, and above 0.5 g L^{-1} until wound healing is complete. To increase the fibrinogen concentration of 1 g L^{-1}, a dose of approximately 50 mg/kg is required. The doses and duration of treatment also vary depending on the type of injury or operative procedure and on the patient's personal and familial history of bleeding and thrombosis.

Women with congenital afibrinogenemia are able to conceive and embryonic implantation is normal, but the pregnancy usually results in spontaneous abortion at 5 to 8 weeks of gestation unless fibrinogen replacement is given.[137] Maintaining the fibrinogen level above 0.6 g L^{-1} and if possible over 1.0 g L^{-1} is recommended. Lower fibrinogen concentrations (<0.4 g L^{-1}) have proven adequate to maintain pregnancy but not to avoid hemorrhagic complications. Continuous infusion of fibrinogen concentrate should be performed during labor to maintain fibrinogen higher than 1.5 g L^{-1} (ideally greater than 2.0 g L^{-1}).[138] Thromboembolic events can occur, particularly with the use of cryoprecipitates that contain appreciable quantities of factor VIII and von Willebrand factor in addition to fibrinogen.

In addition to fibrinogen substitution, antifibrinolytic agents may be given, particularly to treat mucosal bleeding or to prevent bleeding following procedures such as dental extraction. Fibrin glue is useful to treat superficial wounds or following dental extractions. Oestrogen-progestogen preparations are useful in case of menorrhagia.[136] Oral iron preparations can be given in cases with associated iron-deficiency anemia. Routine vaccination against hepatitis, as well as a regular surveillance for both the disease and treatment-related complications in a comprehensive care setting, is highly recommended.[131]

Complications of Therapy

In many countries only FFP or cryoprecipitate are available, which is problematic because the viral inactivation process is in general not as efficient as it is for fibrinogen concentrates (although emerging non-viral pathogens such as the prion responsible for variant Creutzfeldt-Jacob disease must be considered, even for concentrates). Even if viral inactivation steps are performed, these preparations (particularly FFP) can induce volume overload. There is also a risk of transfusion-related acute lung injury, because of the presence of cytotoxic antibodies in the infused plasma.

Acquired inhibitors to fibrinogen after replacement therapy have been reported in only two cases.[139,140] It is not clear why afibrinogenemic patients do not develop inhibitors more frequently. One explanation for some cases is that minute amounts of fibrinogen, which can only be detected by highly sensitive immunoassays, are present in the circulation.

One of the major complications in afibrinogenemic patients is thrombosis, which can occur spontaneously following blood component therapy. Some clinicians give small doses of heparin or low-molecular-weight heparin (LMWH) during administration of fibrinogen. Before surgery, patients with a thrombotic phenotype should be treated with compression stockings and LMWH. Successful use of lepirudin has been reported for an afibrinogenemic patient who suffered recurrent arterial thrombosis despite treatment with heparin and aspirin.[141] Thromboembolic complications are difficult to manage because both anticoagulants and fibrinogen preparations have to be administered.

New Preparations

The increasing need for fibrinogen preparations in congenital but also in acquired deficiencies has stimulated some companies to improve existing preparations or to develop new ones.[131] A recombinant fibrinogen molecule, purified from the milk of transgenic cows is also under development.

DYSFIBRINOGENEMIA AND HYPODYSFIBRINOGENEMIA

■ DEFINITION, HISTORY, AND EPIDEMIOLOGY

The second class of hereditary fibrinogen abnormalities comprises the type II disorders, that is, dysfibrinogenemia and hypodysfibrinogenemia. Dysfibrinogenemia is defined by the presence of normal levels of functionally abnormal plasma fibrinogen. Hypodysfibrinogenemia is defined by low levels of a dysfunctional protein. As in afibrinogenemia and hypofibrinogenemia, both are heterogeneous disorders caused by many different mutations in the three fibrinogen-encoding genes. Dysfibrinogenemias and hypodysfibrinogenemias are autosomal dominant disorders. Most affected patients are heterozygous for missense mutations in the coding region of one of the three fibrinogen genes. Because the secreted fibrinogen hexamer contains two copies of each of the three fibrinogen chains, and the resulting fibrin network contains multiple copies of the molecule, heterozygosity for one mutant allele is sufficient to impair the structure and function of the fibrin clot (Fig. 126–5).

With a few exceptions, the causative mutation results in impairment of one or more steps of fibrinogen conversion to fibrin and the fibrin assembly process (Table 126–2).[147–207] More than 400 cases have been reported to date, with more than 60 distinct mutations identified in patients with dysfibrinogenemia and hypodysfibrinogenemia (Table 126–2). The described mutants are most often named after the city of origin of the family or the city of the laboratory characterizing the mutation. Most cases are asymptomatic and are only identified as a result of routine coagulation screening. Approximately 25 percent of the patients with dysfibrinogenemia have a history of bleeding, and in approximately 20 percent, a tendency toward thrombosis is observed.[6]

■ ETIOLOGY AND PATHOGENESIS

Dysfibrinogenemic abnormalities usually are reflected in one or more phases of the fibrinogen-fibrin conversion and fibrin assembly process, including (1) impaired release of fibrinopeptides, (2) defects in fibrin polymerization, and (3) defective factor XIIIa-mediated crosslinking. Other significant abnormalities involve related aspects of fibrinogen/fibrin function or metabolism, abnormal tissue deposition, defective assembly of the fibrinolytic system, and abnormal interactions with platelets, endothelial cells, or calcium binding.

Mutations Resulting in Abnormal "A" Knobs or Deficient Fibrinopeptide Release

Fibrinogen Detroit was the first abnormal fibrinogen in which the specific mutation was identified at the protein level.[51] This *FGA* R38S (R19S) mutation is located in the "A" knob (i.e., GPRV) resulting in impaired fibrin polymerization and a bleeding tendency. Other substitutions involving residue R38(R19) have been found to be associated with bleeding in some cases, for example, Munich I, R38N (R19N), and Mannheim I, R38G (R19G), and with thrombosis in other cases, for example, Aarhus and Kumamoto, which are also a result of R38G (R19G). The mechanism for thrombophilia remains unclear, but

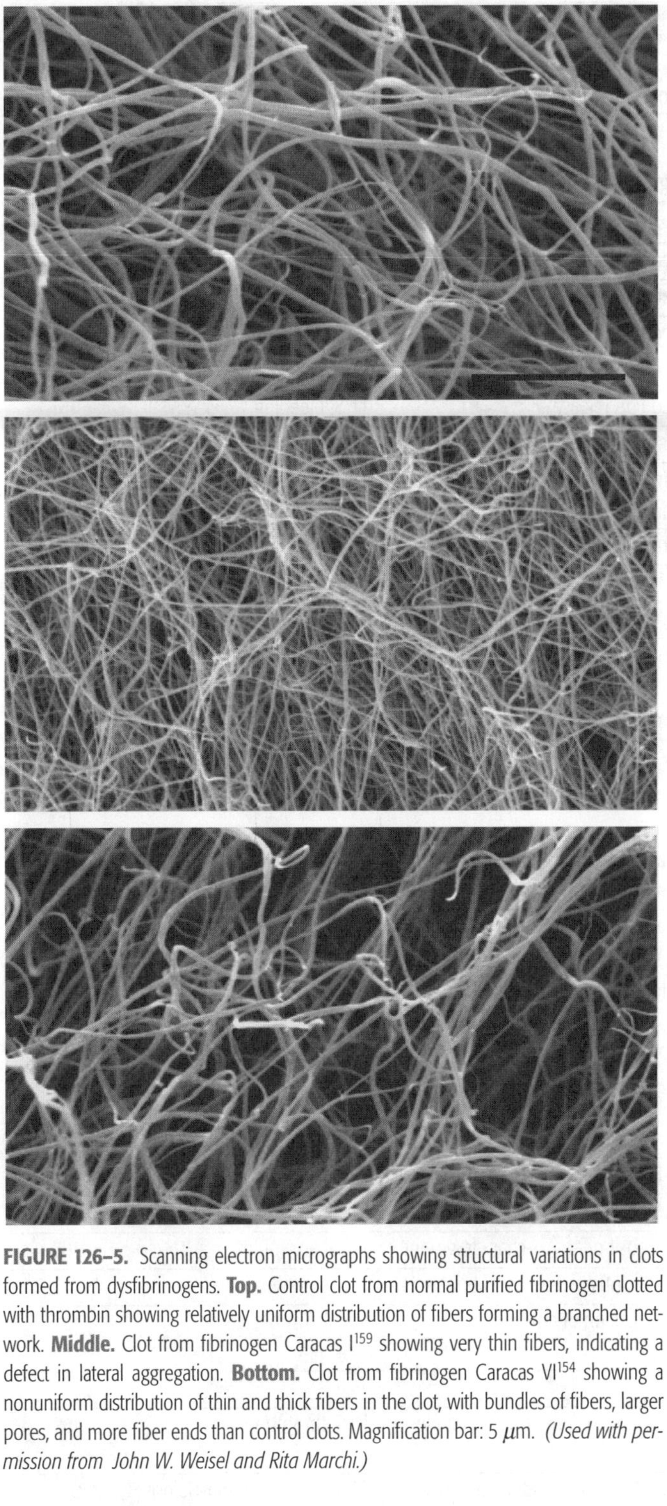

FIGURE 126–5. Scanning electron micrographs showing structural variations in clots formed from dysfibrinogens. **Top.** Control clot from normal purified fibrinogen clotted with thrombin showing relatively uniform distribution of fibers forming a branched network. **Middle.** Clot from fibrinogen Caracas I[159] showing very thin fibers, indicating a defect in lateral aggregation. **Bottom.** Clot from fibrinogen Caracas VI[154] showing a nonuniform distribution of thin and thick fibers in the clot, with bundles of fibers, larger pores, and more fiber ends than control clots. Magnification bar: 5 μm. *(Used with permission from John W. Weisel and Rita Marchi.)*

coexisting risk factors may contribute to the clinical manifestations. Furthermore, the inability of a mutant fibrin to effectively bind and sequester thrombin[7] may play a role in such a clinical presentation. Bleeding that occurs under conditions involving defective fibrinopeptide release or production of a defective A knob is most likely related to the reduced polymerization potential of the mutant fibrins that are produced, with resulting defective clot formation.

Missense mutations at residue *FGA* R35 (R16) which is part of the thrombin cleavage site in the fibrinogen α chain are the most common causative mutations accounting for dysfibrinogenemia, found in approximately 40 percent of cases.[6] The R35 (R16) residue can be mutated to either H (CGT→CAT) or C (CGT→TGT) leading to delayed or absent fibrinopeptide A release, respectively, and subsequent delayed polymerization. A prolonged reptilase time is observed for both variants. Most patients do not have a bleeding tendency. Some patients have been found to be homozygous for these mutations or phenotypically homozygous, due to compound heterozygosity for an R35 (R16) missense mutation and the large 11-kb *FGA* deletion first characterized in afibrinogenemia.[132] In these cases, a mild bleeding tendency is observed.

Missense mutations in *FGB* affecting FpB release have been identified but are much less common than those affecting FpA release (see Table 126–2).

Mutations Leading to Polymerization Defects in the D Region

Sites in the D region important for fibrin polymerization, that is, the "a" hole and D:D sites are affected in many dysfibrinogenemias (see Table 126–2). Mutations affecting the "a" hole in the γ chain are numerous while none specifically involving the "b" hole in the Bβ chain have been described.

The interface for the end-to-end D:D site in the γ chain lies between R301 (R275) and S326 (S300), with T306 (T280) contacting R301 (R275) at the D:D interface.[20] Mutations at the R301 (R275) residue to C (CGT→TGT) or H (CGT→CAT) are the second most common cause of dysfibrinogenemia, accounting for approximately more than 10 percent of fibrinogen variants.[6] Impaired polymerization has been observed for all substitutions at this position. Most of these cases are asymptomatic, but some patients heterozygous for R301C (R275C) have thrombophilia, sometimes in association with an additional thrombotic risk factor such as factor V Leiden.[142]

Mutations Leading to Abnormal Factor XIII Crosslinking

The γ_{XL} self-association site contains the factor XIIIa crosslinking sequence and overlaps the platelet fibrinogen receptor $\alpha_{IIb}\beta_3$ binding site. No mutations specifically involving this region of the molecule have been reported, although markedly impaired to absent factor XIIIa-mediated γ-chain crosslinking has been reported for fibrinogen Paris I.[143]

Mutations Accounting for Hypodysfibrinogenemia

Hypodysfibrinogenemia which is defined by low levels of a dysfunctional protein can be caused by different molecular mechanisms (see Table 126–2). One mechanism is heterozygosity for a single mutation that leads to synthesis of an abnormal fibrinogen chain which is secreted less efficiently than normal fibrinogen, for example, fibrinogen Kyoto IV.[144] Another mechanism is the presence of two different mutations with one mutation responsible for the fibrinogen deficiency (the "hypo phenotype") and one mutation responsible for the abnormal function of the molecule (the "dys phenotype"). For example, in fibrinogen Keokuk,[45] there is compound heterozygosity for the common afibrinogenemia splice-site mutation c.510G→T and a premature truncating nonsense mutation in *FGA* Q347X (Q328X). Another example is fibrinogen Leipzig II in which the common hypofibrinogenemia mutation *FGG* A108G (A82G) and *FGG* G377S (G351S) are located on the same allele.[146] Homozygosity for a single mutation, which allows reduced secretion of a functionally impaired molecule, has been described in fibrinogens Otago[147] and Marburg.[148,149]

■ CLINICAL FEATURES

Patients with inherited dysfibrinogenemia are frequently asymptomatic and are usually discovered incidentally because of abnormal coagulation

TABLE 126–2. Mutations Resulting in Dysfibrinogenemia and Hypodysfibrinogenemia*

Mutation					
cDNA	Nascent	Mature Chain	Etiology/Pathology	Clinical Manifestations†	Reference
FGA					
c. 83T→C	L28P	L9P (Magdeburg I)	Delayed FpA release	DYS, none	150
c. 89A→G	E30G	E11G (Mikata II)	Delayed FpA release	DYS, bleeding	3
c. 103C→T	R35C	R16C (Metz I, Zurich I, etc.)	Delayed FpA release	DYS, none, or bleeding	1, 6
c. 104G→A	R35H	R16H (Bicêtre I, Giessen I, etc.)	Delayed FpA release	DYS, none, or bleeding	1, 6
c. 107G→T	G36V	G17V (Bremen I)	Delayed FpA release	DYS, bleeding	151
c. 110C→T	P37L	P18L (Kyoto II)	Abnormal polymerization	DYS, bleeding	152
c. 112A→G	R38G	R19G (Mannheim I, Aarhus I)	Abnormal polymerization	DYS, bleeding, or thrombophilia	1, 3, 6
c. 114G→C/T	R38S	R19S (Detroit)	Abnormal polymerization	DYS, bleeding	51
?	R38N	R19N (Munich I)	Abnormal polymerization	DYS, bleeding	3
c. 116T→A	V39D	V20D (Canterbury)	Intracellular cleavage by furin	HYPODYS, bleeding	153
c. 295_297del	delN99	delN80 (Caracas IV)	Abnormal polymerization	DYS, bleeding, and thrombophilia	154
c. 480A→C/T	R160S	R141S (Lima, homozygous)	Abnormal polymerization	DYS, none	155
c. 858_859insC	R287Qfs	R268Qfs (Otago, homozygous)	Diminished assembly and secretion	Severe HYPODYS, bleeding	147
c. 1358G→A	S453N	S434N (Caracas II)	Impaired fibrin gelation with thinner fibers	DYS, none	156
c. 1410_1411insT	G471Wfs	G452Wfs (Milano III, homozygous)	Premature Aα-chain truncation	DYS, thrombophilia	157
c. 1438A→T	K480X	K461X (Marburg, homozygous)	Premature Aα-chain truncation	HYPODYS, bleeding, thrombophilia	148, 149
c. 1452delC	S485Pfs	S466Pfs(Wilmington)	Premature Aα-chain truncation	DYS, bleeding	158
c. 1456G→T	E486X	E467X (Caracas I)	Defective lateral aggregation	DYS, bleeding	159
c. 1482-1495del	M495Hfs	M476Hfs (Lincoln)	Premature Aα-chain truncation	DYS, bleeding	160
c. 1541delC	P514Lfs	P495Lfs (Perth)	Thinner clot fibers	DYS, bleeding	161
c. 1554delC	F519Sfs	F500Sfs (San Giovanni Rotundo)	Abnormal polymerization	DYS, None	162
c. 1622delT	V541Afs	V522Afs	Renal deposit of an Aα-chain fragment	Renal amyloidosis	163
c. 1629delG	T544Lfs	T525Lfs	Renal deposit of an Aα-chain fragment	Renal amyloidosis	164
c. 1634A→T	E545V	E526V	Renal deposit of an Aα-chain fragment	Renal amyloidosis	165
c. 1717C→G	R573C	R554C (Dusart)	Abnormal clot structure and fibrinolysis	DYS, thrombophilia	166, 167
c. 1718G→T	R573L	R554L	Renal deposition of an Aα-chain fragment	Renal amyloidosis	168
FGB					
c. 130C→T	R44C	R14C (Ijmuiden)	Large fibrinogen complexes; disulfide-linked albumin	DYS, thrombophilia	169
c. 133G→T	G45C	G15C (Ise, Fukuoka II, Kosai)	Defective lateral association, defective FpB release	DYS, none, or arteriosclerosis	170, 171
? (del exon 2)	del39-102	del9-72 (New York I)	Defective thrombin binding	DYS, thrombophilia	172
c. 220C→T	R74C	R44C (Nijmegen)	Impaired fibrinolysis	DYS, thrombophilia	169, 173
c. 292G→A	A98T	A68T (Naples, homozygous)	Defective thrombin binding	DYS, thrombophilia	174
c. 421_423del	delS141	delS111 (Kyoto IV)	Augmented lateral aggregation	HYPODYS, none	144
c. 1093G→A	A365T	A335T (Pontoise)	Defective polymerization	DYS, none	175

(continued)

TABLE 126–2. Mutations Resulting in Dysfibrinogenemia and Hypodysfibrinogenemia* (Continued)

Mutation					
cDNA	Nascent	Mature Chain	Etiology/Pathology	Clinical Manifestations†	Reference
FGG					
c. 571G→C	G191R	G165R (Milano XII, compound het with AαR16C)	Modified plasmin digestion	DYS, none	176
c. 795G→T	Q265H	Q239H (Vicenza)	Defective polymerization	DYS, bleeding	177
c. 863A→G	Y288C	Y262C (Liberec)	Defective polymerization	DYS, none	178
c. 881G→A	G294E	G268E (Kurashiki)	Impaired D:D interactions	DYS, none	179
c. 901C→T	R301C	R275C (Baltimore IV, Milano IV, Bologna I, Cedar Rapids. . .)	Impaired D:D interactions	DYS, none, or thrombophilia	1, 6, 142
c. 902G→A	R301H	R275H (Barcelona IV, Claro I, Haifa I, Barcelona III. . .)	Impaired D:D interactions	DYS, none, or thrombophilia	1,6
c. 902G→C	R301S	R275S (Kamogawa)	Impaired D:D interactions	DYS, none	180
c. 917A→G	Y306C	Y280C (Banks Peninsula)	Impaired D:D interactions	DYS, bleeding	181
c. 953G→T	G318V	G292V (Baltimore I)	Impaired D:D function?	DYS, bleeding, or thrombophilia	182
c. 1001A→T	N334I	N308I (Baltimore III)	?	DYS, none	183
c. 1002T→G	N334K	N308K (Kyoto I, Bicêtre II, Matsumoto II)	?	DYS, none, bleeding, or thrombophilia	184–186
c. 1007T→C	M336T	M310 T (Asahi I, Frankfurt VII)	?	DYS, bleeding	187
c. 1032A→G	D344G	D318G (Giessen IV)	Defective calcium binding	DYS, bleeding, thrombophilia	188
c. 1031A→T	D344V	D318V (Caen)	Defective calcium binding	DYS, thrombophilia	189
c. 1033_1038del	delN345-D346	delN319-D320 (Vlissingen, Otsu I)	Defective calcium binding	DYS, none or thrombophilia	190, 191
c. 1036_1038del	delD346	delD320 (Des Moines)	Defective calcium binding	HYPODYS, thrombophilia	192
c. 1055G→A	C352Y	C326Y (Suhl)	Defective polymerization	HYPODYS, thrombophilia	193
c. 1057G→A	A353T	A327T (Tokyo V)	Defective fibrin assembly, crosslinking, fibrinolysis, defective calcium binding	HYPODYS, thrombophilia	194
c. 1064A→G	Q355R	Q329R (Nagoya I)	Defective polymerization	DYS, none	195
c. 1066G→T	D356Y	D330Y (Kyoto III)	Defective polymerization	DYS, none	196
c. 1067A→T	D356V	D330V (Milano I)	Defective polymerization	DYS, none	197
c. 1085T→?	M362I	M336I (Hannover VI)	Defective polymerization	HYPODYS, thrombophilia	193
?	N382K	N337K (Bern I‡)	Defective polymerization	DYS, none	198
c. 1100C→A	A367D	A341D (Seoul)	Defective polymerization	HYPODYS, thrombophilia	199
c. 1129+632A→G	376_377ins 15 aa	350_351ins 15 aa (Paris I)	Absent γ-chain crosslinking, defective platelet aggregation	DYS, bleeding	143
c. 1129G→A	G377S	G351S (Leipzig II, with γA82G on the same allele)	Defective polymerization	HYPODYS, bleeding	146
c. 1139A→G	Y380C	Y354C (Homburg VII)	Defective polymerization	HYPODYS, thrombophilia	193
c. 1147G→A	A383T	A357T (Frankfurt I)	Defective platelet aggregation	DYS, bleeding	200
c. 1151C→G	S384C	S358C (Milano VII)	Defective fibrin polymerization	None	201
c. 1161T→A	N387K	N361K (Poissy II)	Impaired FpB release, defective fibrin polymerization	DYS, DIC	202
c. 1168G→C	D390H	D364H (Matsumoto I)	Defective fibrin polymerization	DYS, none	203
c. 1169A→T	D390V	D364V (Melun I)	Defective fibrin polymerization	DYS, thrombophilia	204
c. 1201C→G	R401G	R375G (Osaka V)	Defective calcium binding	DYS, none	205

(continued)

TABLE 126–2. Mutations Resulting in Dysfibrinogenemia and Hypodysfibrinogenemia* (Continued)

Mutation					
cDNA	Nascent	Mature Chain	Etiology/Pathology	Clinical Manifestations†	Reference
c. 1210T→C	S404P	S378P (Philadelphia)	Hypercatabolism	HYPODYS, bleeding	206
c. 1218G→T	K406N	K380N (Kaiserslautern)	Defect normalized with calcium or removal of sialic acid residues	DYS, thrombophilia	207

aa, Amino acids; bp, base pairs; del, deletion; DIC, disseminated intravascular coagulation; DYS, dysfibrinogenemia; fs, frameshift; HYPODYS, hypodysfibrinogenemia; ins, insertion; NMD, nonsense-mediated decay.

*Distinct mutations published in peer-reviewed journals before January 2009 are listed. For recurrent mutations, not all are referenced due to limited space. A complete list is available at www.geht.org/databaseang/fibrinogen/, which also lists variants reported in abstracts and online submissions. Unless specified otherwise, mutations were identified in heterozygosity. If the mutation is not characterized at the DNA level, the change at the complementary DNA level is inferred by the amino acid substitution when possible.

†Although the distinction between dysfibrinogenemia (DYS) and hypodysfibrinogenemia (HYPODYS) is not always clear-cut, most authors consider that normal levels of a dysfunctional protein constitute a dysfibrinogenemia, even if the variant is present at lower levels than the normal chain in plasma.

‡For this variant, the reference sequence from National Center for Biotechnology Information indicates that K is the normal residue.

tests or because a case of dysfibrinogenemia has been previously discovered in the family. However some patients suffer from bleeding, thromboembolic complications, or both (see Table 126–2). A compilation of more than 260 cases of dysfibrinogenemia revealed that 55 percent of the patients had no clinical complications, 25 percent exhibited bleeding, and 20 percent had a tendency to thrombosis, mainly venous.[188] However, when 2376 patients with deep vein thrombosis were screened for thrombophilia, the prevalence of dysfibrinogenemia was very low (0.8%) and hence testing for dysfibrinogenemia in patients with deep vein thrombosis is not recommended.[208] Patients with dysfibrinogenemia associated with hemorrhage bleed most often after trauma, surgery, or during the puerperium. Thrombosis may also occur in the postpartum period. Two mechanisms may explain why thrombosis can occur in patients with dysfibrinogenemia: (1) The abnormal fibrinogen is defective in binding thrombin, which results in elevated levels of thrombin, and (2) the abnormal fibrinogen forms a fibrin clot that is resistant to plasmin degradation. Women with dysfibrinogenemia can also suffer from spontaneous abortions. The problems during and after pregnancy are not necessarily correlated to the fibrinogen concentration.

Some mutations in the Aα chain of fibrinogen are associated with a particular form of hereditary amyloidosis.[209] The E545V (E526V) amino acid substitution is the most common of these mutations. The abnormal fibrinogen fragments form amyloid fibrils and the extracellular deposition of these fibrils leads to renal failure. Chronic renal dialysis is performed for managing renal failure. Renal transplantation should be considered as an alternative to chronic dialysis. However, renal transplantation is not a curative solution because continuous fibrinogen-related amyloid deposition ultimately results in allograft destruction. Combined liver and kidney transplantation prevents further amyloid deposition in the renal allograft and elsewhere but is associated with additional perioperative and subsequent risks.

LABORATORY FEATURES

Phenotype Analysis

Initial screening tests for fibrinogen dysfunction should include fibrinogen concentration, measured functionally and immunochemically, thrombin time, and reptilase (a snake venom which removes only FpA but also triggers fibrin polymerization) time. Dysfibrinogenemia is diagnosed by a discrepancy between clottable and immunoreactive fibrinogen. However, even in specialized laboratories, this diagnosis can be difficult because the sensitivity of the tests depends on the specific mutation, reagents, and techniques. A diagnostic algorithm based on the thrombin time as an initial test has been proposed.[210] However, it has to be noted that some dysfibrinogenemic patients have a normal thrombin time. In classical dysfibrinogenemias, the functional assay of fibrinogen yields low levels compared with the immunologic assays, but levels are sometimes concordant and the functional level may even be normal. The determination of the precise nature of a fibrinogen defect has to be performed in highly specialized laboratories since it involves purification of fibrinogen, measurement of the rate of fibrinopeptide cleavage, analysis of fibrin monomer polymerization, and fibrinolysis.

Genotype Analysis

The gold standard for the diagnosis of dysfibrinogenemia is the characterization of the molecular defect. However, although advances in DNA analysis have made mutation detection easier, it is not always clear whether the identified mutation is the cause of the presenting phenotype. Family studies showing segregation of the mutation with the phenotype, exclusion that the DNA alteration is a common polymorphism in the general population, and structural correlations are necessary for establishing the link between the DNA alteration and the disorder. As previously mentioned, two mutation "hotspots" are of prime interest in screening for dysfibrinogenemia mutations: residue R35 (R16) situated in *FGA* exon 2, and residue R301 (R275) in *FGG* exon 8. Other causative mutations are common in the surrounding residues. Thus, it is recommended to initially screen *FGA* exon 2 and *FGG* exon 8 in cases of dysfibrinogenemia. It should be noted that most individuals heterozygous for these two mutations are asymptomatic.[6,211]

Some mutations are predictive of the clinical phenotype, such as the R573C (R554C) substitution in the Aα chain (e.g., fibrinogens Chapel Hill III, Paris V, and Dusart) that predisposes patients to thrombosis. Impaired fibrinolysis exhibited by this dysfibrinogen appears to be responsible for the thrombotic complications. Other examples associated with thrombosis include dysfibrinogens Barcelona III, Haifa I, or Bergamo II as a result of the common R301H (R275H) mutation in the γ chain and Cedar Rapids I due to R301C (R275C). Interestingly, in fibrinogen Cedar Rapids I, only patients heterozygous for both factor V Leiden and the *FGG* R301C (R275C) substitution were symptomatic, suggesting that this mutation causes thrombosis when associated with another defect. On the other hand, several dysfibrinogenemias, particularly those caused by mutations in the amino-terminal region of the Aα chain, such as fibrinogen Detroit R38S (R19S) and Mannheim I R38G (R19G), are associated with bleeding. These examples illustrate how determining the causative mutation permits, at least in some cases, to predict the clinical manifestations.

DIFFERENTIAL DIAGNOSIS

Inherited dysfibrinogenemia has to be distinguished from acquired dysfibrinogenemia. Liver diseases (e.g., cirrhosis, chronic active liver disease, hepatoma, liver failure) are the main causes of acquired dysfibrinogenemia. L-Asparaginase treatment also may result in the production of abnormal fibrinogen. In addition, there are a few case reports of acquired dysfibrinogenemia secondary to pancreatitis, paraneoplastic syndrome, and renal carcinoma. The acquired dysfibrinogenemias represent a heterogeneous group of disorders with multiple pathogenetic mechanisms, the most clearly defined fibrinogen abnormalities being an increase in carbohydrate content in patients with liver disease. These abnormal fibrinogens are usually characterized by prolonged thrombin and reptilase times, by abnormal fibrin monomer polymerization but with normal fibrinopeptide release. Fibrinogen concentration is variable.

In some cases no underlying disease is found, and to determine whether a fibrinogen abnormality is congenital or acquired may be difficult. The demonstration of the same fibrinogen abnormality in another family member is a strong argument for a congenital disorder. When measured in newborns, fibrinogen levels should be interpreted with caution since neonatal fibrinogen has an altered content of carbohydrate that can mimic dysfibrinogenemia in certain laboratory tests.

Rare cases of circulating autoantibodies to fibrinogen have also been reported. These antibodies can inhibit each of the reactions necessary for normal fibrin formation: fibrinopeptide A or B cleavage, fibrin monomer polymerization, and covalent crosslinking. These autoantibodies may be associated with severe bleeding. Antibodies to fibrinogen have been also detected in patients with systemic lupus erythematosus as well as in patients receiving surgical sealants containing bovine fibrinogen. In the latter cases the antibodies do not cross-react with human fibrinogen. Patients with multiple myeloma may also have abnormal fibrinogen tests but here the mechanism for antibody interference with fibrinogen function is not clear.

THERAPY

Any treatment considered in patients with dysfibrinogenemia should be based on the personal and family history. Indeed, as already discussed, subjects with hereditary dysfibrinogenemias may be asymptomatic throughout their whole life or may suffer from bleeding and/or thrombotic complications. In cases with bleeding, functional levels of fibrinogen should be raised above 1.0 g L^{-1} and maintained above this threshold until hemostasis is secured and above 0.5 g L^{-1} until wound healing is complete. Topical fibrin glue or antifibrinolytic agents may be used for superficial bleeds. In pregnant women with a bleeding phenotype, the recommendations for afibrinogenemia and hypofibrinogenemia can be followed. With a personal or familial history of thrombosis, thromboprophylaxis and antithrombotic treatments may be proposed after a careful analysis of each particular situation. Long-term management strategies for thrombophilic dysfibrinogenemia are the same as the strategies for patients with recurrent thromboembolism and may include long-term anticoagulant therapy.

REFERENCES

1. Mosesson MW: Hereditary fibrinogen abnormalities, in *Williams Hematology,* 7th ed, edited by M Lichtman, E Beutler, TJ Kipps, U Seligsohn, K Kaushansky, J Prchal, p 1909. McGraw-Hill, New York, 2006.
2. Maghzal GJ, Brennan SO, Homer VM, George PM: The molecular mechanisms of congenital hypofibrinogenemia. *Cell Mol Life Sci* 61:1427, 2004.
3. Ebert RF: *Index of Variant Human Fibrinogens.* CRC Press, Boca Raton, 1994.
4. Asselta R, Duga S, Tenchini ML: The molecular basis of quantitative fibrinogen disorders. *J Thromb Haemost* 4:2115, 2006.
5. Neerman-Arbez M, de Moerloose P: Mutations in the fibrinogen gene cluster accounting for congenital afibrinogenemia: An update and report of 10 novel mutations. *Hum Mutat* 28:540, 2006.
6. Hanss M, Biot F: A database for human fibrinogen variants. *Ann N Y Acad Sci* 936:89, 2001.
7. Mosesson MW: Update on antithrombin I (fibrin). *Thromb Haemost* 98:105, 2007.
8. Tennent GA, Brennan SO, Stangou AJ, et al: Human plasma fibrinogen is synthesized in the liver. *Blood* 109:1971, 2007.
9. Medved L, Weisel JW: Recommendations for nomenclature on fibrinogen and fibrin. *J Thromb Haemost* 7:355, 2009.
10. Kant J, Fornace AJ Jr, Saxe D, et al: Organization and evolution of the human fibrinogen locus on chromosome four. *Proc Natl Acad Sci U S A* 82:2344, 1985.
11. de Maat M, Verschuur M: Fibrinogen heterogeneity: Inherited and noninherited. *Curr Opin Hematol* 12:377, 2005.
12. Huang S, Mulvihill ER, Farrell DH, et al: Biosynthesis of human fibrinogen. Subunit interactions and potential intermediates in the assembly. *J Biol Chem* 268:8919, 1993.
13. Henschen-Edman AH: On the identification of beneficial and detrimental molecular forms of fibrinogen. *Haemostasis* 29:179, 1999.
14. Collen D, Tytgat GN, Claeys H, Piessens R: Metabolism and distribution of fibrinogen I. *Br J Haematol* 22:681, 1972.
15. Handagama P, Scarborough RM, Shuman MA, Bainton DF: Endocytosis of fibrinogen into megakaryocytes and platelet α-granules is mediated by $\alpha II_b b_3$ (glycoprotein IIb-IIIa). *Blood* 82:135, 1993.
16. Francis CW, Nachman RL, Marder VJ: Plasma and platelet fibrinogen differ in gamma chain content. *Thromb Haemost* 51:84, 1984.
17. Mosesson MW: The structure and biological features of fibrinogen and fibrin. *Ann N Y Acad Sci* 936:11, 2001.
18. Weisel JW: Fibrinogen and fibrin. *Adv Protein Chem* 70:247, 2005.
19. Shimizu A, Nagel GM, Doolittle RF: Photoaffinity labeling of the primary fibrin polymerization site: Isolation of a CNBr fragment corresponding to γ337–379. *Proc Natl Acad Sci U S A* 89:2888, 1992.
20. Spraggon G, Everse SJ, Doolittle RF: Crystal structures of fragment D from human fibrinogen and its crosslinked counterpart from fibrin. *Nature* 389:455, 1997.
21. Fowler WE, Hantgan RR, Hermans J, et al: Structure of the fibrin protofibril. *Proc Natl Acad Sci U S A* 78:4872, 1981.
22. Mosesson MW, DiOrio JP, Siebenlist KR, et al: Evidence for a second type of fibril branch point in fibrin polymer networks, the trimolecular junction. *Blood* 82:1517, 1993.
23. Lord ST: Fibrinogen and fibrin: Scaffold proteins in hemostasis. *Curr Opin Hematol* 14:236, 2007.
24. Weisel JW: Structure of fibrin: Impact on clot stability. *J Thromb Haemost* 5(Suppl 1):116, 2007.
25. Shainoff JR, Dardik BN: Fibrinopeptide B in fibrin assembly and metabolism: Physiologic significance in delayed release of the peptide. *Ann N Y Acad Sci* 408:254, 1983.
26. Everse SJ, Spraggon G, Veerapandian L, et al: Crystal structure of fragment double-D from human fibrin with two different bound ligands. *Biochemistry* 37:8637, 1998.
27. Medved LV, Litvinovich SV, Ugarova TP, et al: Localization of a fibrin polymerization site complimentary to Gly-His-Arg sequence. *FEBS Lett* 320:239, 1993.
28. Yang Z, Mochalkin I, Doolittle RF: A model of fibrin formation based on crystal structures of fibrinogen and fibrin fragments complexed with synthetic peptides. *Proc Natl Acad Sci U S A* 97:14156, 2000.
29. Weisel JW, Medved LV: The structure and function of the αC domains of fibrinogen. *Ann N Y Acad Sci* 936:312, 2001.
30. Gorkun OV, Veklich YI, Medved LV, et al: Role of the αC domains of fibrin in clot formation. *Biochemistry* 33:6986, 1994.
31. Mosesson MW, Siebenlist KR, Hainfeld JF, Wall JS: The covalent structure of factor XIIIa crosslinked fibrinogen fibrils. *J Struct Biol* 115:88, 1995.
32. Siebenlist KR, Meh D, Mosesson MW: Protransglutaminase (factor XIII) mediated crosslinking of fibrinogen and fibrin. *Thromb Haemost* 86:1221, 2001.
33. Mosesson MW, Siebenlist KR, Hernandez I, et al: Evidence that α2-antiplasmin becomes covalently ligated to plasma fibrinogen in the circulation: A new role for plasma factor XIII in fibrinolysis regulation. *J Thromb Haemost* 6:1565, 2008.
34. Makogonenko E, Ingham KC, Medved L: Interaction of the fibronectin COOH-terminal Fib-2 regions with fibrin: Further characterization and localization of the Fib-2-binding sites. *Biochemistry* 46:5418, 2006.
35. Flick MJ, Du X, Degen JL: Fibrin(ogen)-$\alpha M\beta 2$ interactions regulate leukocyte function and innate immunity *in vivo*. *Exp Biol Med* 229:1105, 2004.
36. Odrljin TM, Shainoff JR, Lawrence SO, Simpson-Haidaris PJ: Thrombin cleavage enhances exposure of a heparin binding domain in the N-terminus of the fibrin β chain. *Blood* 88:2050, 1996.

37. Odrljin TM, Francis CW, Sporn LA, et al: Heparin-binding domain of fibrin mediates its binding to endothelial cells. *Arterioscler Thromb Vasc Biol* 16:1544, 1996.
38. Bach TL, Barsigian C, Yaen CH, Martinez J: Endothelial cell VE-cadherin functions as a receptor for the β15–42 sequence of fibrin. *J Biol Chem* 273:30719, 1998.
39. Hamaguchi M, Bunce LA, Sporn LA, Francis CW: Spreading of platelets on fibrin is mediated by the amino terminus of the β chain including peptide β 15–42. *Blood* 81:2348, 1993.
40. Sporn LA, Bunce LA, Francis CW: Cell proliferation on fibrin: Modulation by fibrinopeptide cleavage. *Blood* 86:1801, 1995.
41. Chalupowicz DG, Chowdhury ZA, Bach TL, et al: Fibrin II induces endothelial cell capillary tube formation. *J Cell Biol* 130:207, 1995.
42. Ribes JA, Bunce LA, Francis CW: Mediation of fibrin-induced release of von Willebrand factor from cultured endothelial cells by the fibrin β chain. *J Clin Invest* 84:435, 1989.
43. Francis CW, Bunce LA, Sporn LA: Endothelial cell responses to fibrin mediated by FPB cleavage and the amino terminus of the β chain. *Blood Cells* 19:291, 1993.
44. Mosesson MW, Siebenlist KR, Voskuilen M, Nieuwenhuizen W: Evaluation of the factors contributing to fibrin-dependent plasminogen activation. *Thromb Haemost* 79:796, 1998.
45. Medved L, Niewenhuizen W: Molecular mechanisms of initiation of fibrinolysis by fibrin. *Thromb Haemost* 89:409, 2003.
46. Rijken DC, Lijnen HR: New insights into the molecular mechanisms of the fibrinolytic system. *J Thromb Haemost* 7:4, 2009.
47. Sakharov DV, Plow EF, Rijken DC: On the mechanism of the antifibrinolytic activity of plasma carboxypeptidase B. *J Biol Chem* 272:14477, 1997.
48. Fenton JW II, Olson TA, Zabinski MP, Wilner GD: Anion-binding exosite of human α-thrombin and fibrin(ogen) recognition. *Biochemistry* 27:7106, 1988
49. Uitte de Willige S, de Visser MC, Houwing-Duistermaat JJ, et al: Genetic variation in the fibrinogen gamma gene increases the risk for deep venous thrombosis by reducing plasma fibrinogen gamma′ levels. *Blood* 106:4176, 2005.
50. Fredenburgh JC, Stafford AR, Leslie BA, Weitz JI: Bivalent binding to to γ_A/γ'- fibrin engages both exosites of thrombin and protects it from inhibition by the antithrombin-heparin complex. *J Biol Chem* 283:2470, 2008.
51. Blomback M, Blomback B, Mammen EF, Prasad AS: Fibrinogen Detroit—A molecular defect in the N-terminal disulphide knot of human fibrinogen? *Nature* 218:134, 1968.
52. Neerman-Arbez M, Honsberger A, Antonarakis SE, Morris MA: Deletion of the fibrinogen alpha-chain gene (FGA) causes congenital afibrinogenemia. *J Clin Invest* 103:215, 1999.
53. Rabe F, Salomon E: Ueber-faserstoffmangel im Blute bei einem Falle von Hämophilie. *Arch Intern Med* 95:2, 1920.
54. Martinez J: Congenital dysfibrinogenemia. *Curr Opin Hematol* 4:357, 1997.
55. Lak M, Keihani M, Elahi F, et al: Bleeding and thrombosis in 55 patients with inherited afibrinogenaemia. *Br J Haematol* 107:204, 1999.
56. Peyvandi F, Mannucci PM: Rare coagulation disorders. *Thromb Haemost* 82:1207, 1999.
57. Neerman-Arbez M, Antonarakis SE, Honsberger A, Morris MA: The 11 kb FGA deletion responsible for congenital afibrinogenaemia is mediated by a short direct repeat in the fibrinogen gene cluster. *Eur J Hum Genet* 7:897, 1999.
58. Suh TT, Holmback K, Jensen NJ, et al: Resolution of spontaneous bleeding events but failure of pregnancy in fibrinogen-deficient mice. *Genes Dev* 9:2020, 1995.
59. Watanabe K, Shibuya A, Ishii E, et al: Identification of simultaneous mutation of fibrinogen alpha chain and protein C genes in a Japanese kindred. *Br J Haematol* 120:101, 2003.
60. Spena S, Duga S, Asselta R, et al: Congenital afibrinogenaemia caused by uniparental isodisomy of chromosome 4 containing a novel 15-kb deletion involving fibrinogen Aα-chain gene. *Eur J Hum Genet* 12:891, 2004.
61. Monaldini L, Asselta R, Duga S, et al: Mutational screening of six afibrinogenemic patients: Identification and characterization of four novel molecular defects. *Thromb Haemost* 97:546, 2007.
62. Okumura N, Terasawa F, Yonekawa O, et al: Hypofibrinogenemia associated with a heterozygous C→T nucleotide substitution at position -1138 BP of the 5′-flanking region of the fibrinogen A alpha-chain gene. *Ann N Y Acad Sci* 936:526, 2001.
63. Neerman-Arbez M, de Moerloose P, Bridel C, et al: Mutations in the fibrinogen A-alpha gene account for the majority of cases of congenital afibrinogenemia. *Blood* 96:149, 2000.
64. Neerman-Arbez M, de Moerloose P, Honsberger A, et al: Molecular analysis of the fibrinogen gene cluster in 16 patients with congenital afibrinogenemia: Novel truncating mutations in the FGA and FGG genes. *Hum Genet* 108:237, 2001.
65. Attanasio C, de Moerloose P, Antonarakis SE, et al: Activation of multiple cryptic donor splice sites by the common congenital afibrinogenemia mutation, FGA IVS4 + 1 G→T. *Blood* 97:1879, 2001.
66. Asselta R, Spena S, Duga S, et al: Analysis of Iranian patients allowed the identification of the first truncating mutation in the fibrinogen Bbeta-chain gene causing afibrinogenemia. *Haematologica* 87:855, 2002.
67. Homer VM, Brennan SO, Ockelford P, George PM: Novel fibrinogen truncation with deletion of Bbeta chain residues 440–461 causes hypofibrinogenaemia. *Thromb Haemost* 88:427, 2002.
68. Neerman-Arbez M, Vu D, Abu-Libdeh B, et al: Prenatal diagnosis for congenital afibrinogenemia caused by a novel nonsense mutation in the FGB gene in a Palestinian family. *Blood* 101:3492, 2003.
69. Vu D, Di Sanza C, Caille D, et al: Quality control of fibrinogen secretion in the molecular pathogenesis of congenital afibrinogenemia. *Hum Mol Genet* 14:3271, 2005.
70. Duga S, Asselta R, Santagostino E, et al: Missense mutations in the human beta fibrinogen gene cause congenital afibrinogenemia by impairing fibrinogen secretion. *Blood* 95:1336, 2000.
71. Vu D, Bolton-Maggs PH, Parr JR, et al : Congenital afibrinogenemia: Identification and expression of a missense mutation in FGB impairing fibrinogen secretion. *Blood* 102:4413, 2003.
72. Spena S, Asselta R, Duga S, et al: Congenital afibrinogenemia: Intracellular retention of fibrinogen due to a novel W437G mutation in the fibrinogen Bbeta-chain gene. *Biochim Biophys Acta* 1639:87, 2003.
73. Monaldini L, Asselta R, Duga S, et al: Fibrinogen Mumbai: Intracellular retention due to a novel G434D mutation in the Bbeta-chain gene. *Haematologica* 91:628, 2006.
74. Terasawa F, Okumura N, Kitano K, et al: Hypofibrinogenemia associated with a heterozygous missense mutation gamma153Cys to Arg (Matsumoto IV): *In vitro* expression demonstrates defective secretion of the variant fibrinogen. *Blood* 94:4122, 1999.
75. Vu D, de Moerloose P, Batorova A, et al: Hypofibrinogenaemia caused by a novel FGG missense mutation (W253C) in the gamma chain globular domain impairing fibrinogen secretion. *J Med Genet* 42:e57, 2005.
76. Brennan SO, Wyatt J, Medicina D, et al: Fibrinogen Brescia: Hepatic endoplasmic reticulum storage and hypofibrinogenemia because of a gamma284 Gly→Arg mutation. *Am J Pathol* 157:189, 2000.
77. Brennan SO, Maghzal G, Shneider BL, et al: Novel fibrinogen gamma375 Arg→Trp mutation (fibrinogen Aguadilla) causes hepatic endoplasmic reticulum storage and hypofibrinogenemia. *Hepatology* 36:652, 2002.
78. Rubbia-Brandt L, Neerman-Arbez M, Rougemont A-L, et al: Fibrinogen gamma 375Arg→Trp mutation (fibrinogen Aguadilla) causes hereditary hypofibrinogenemia, hepatic endoplasmic reticulum storage disease and cirrhosis. *Am J Surg Pathol* 30:906, 2006.
79. Francalanci P, Santorelli FM, Talini I, et al: Severe liver disease in early childhood due to fibrinogen storage and de novo gamma375Arg→Trp gene mutation. *J Pediatr* 148:396–8, 2006.
80. Dib N, Quelin F, Ternisien C, et al: Fibrinogen Angers with a new deletion gamma GVYYQ 346–350 causes hypofibrinogenemia with hepatic storage. *J Thromb Haemost* 5:1999, 2007.
81. Neerman-Arbez M: To aggregate or not to aggregate. *J Thromb Haemost* 5:1997, 2007.
82. Monaldini L, Asselta R, Malcovati M, et al: The DNA-pooling technique allowed for the identification of three novel mutations responsible for afibrinogenemia. *J Thromb Haemost* 3:2591, 2005.
83. Asselta R, Duga S, Spena S, et al: Congenital afibrinogenemia: Mutations leading to premature termination codons in fibrinogen A alpha-chain gene are not associated with the decay of the mutant mRNAs. *Blood* 98:3685, 2001.
84. Platè M, Asselta R, Spena S et al: Congenital hypofibrinogenemia: Characterization of two missense mutations affecting fibrinogen assembly and secretion. *Blood Cells Mol Dis* 41:292, 2008.
85. Platé M, Asselta R, Peyvandi F, et al: Molecular characterization of the first missense mutation in the fibrinogen Aalpha-chain gene identified in a compound heterozygous afibrinogenemic patient. *Biochim Biophys Acta* 1772:781, 2007.
86. Attanasio C, David A, Neerman-Arbez M: Outcome of donor splice site mutations accounting for congenital afibrinogenemia reflects order of intron removal in the fibrinogen alpha gene (FGA). *Blood* 101:1851, 2003.
87. Wu SY, Wang ZY, Dong NZ, et al: Congenital afibrinogenemia associated with a novel nonsense mutation in the FGA gene. *Zhonghua Xue Ye Xue Za Zhi* 26:133, 2005.
88. Fellowes AP, Brennan SO, Holme R, et al: Homozygous truncation of the fibrinogen A alpha chain within the coiled coil causes congenital afibrinogenemia. *Blood* 96:773, 2000.
89. Fang Y, Dai BT, Wang XF et al: Identification of three FGA mutations in two Chinese families with congenital afibrinogenemia. *Haemophilia* 12:615, 2006.
90. Vlietman JJ, Verhage J, Vos HL et al: Congenital afibrinogenaemia in a newborn infant due to a novel mutation in the fibrinogen Aalpha gene. *Br J Haematol* 119:282, 2002.
91. Robert-Ebadi H, de Moerloose P, El Khorassani M, et al: A novel frameshift mutation in FGA accounting for congenital afibrinogenemia predicted to encode an aberrant peptide terminating 158 amino acids downstream. *Blood Coagul Fibrinolysis* 20:385, 2009.
92. Anglès-Cano E, Mathonnet F, Dreyfus M, et al: A case of afibrinogenemia associated with A-alpha chain gene compound heterozygosity (HUMFIBRA c.[4110delA]+[3200+1G→T]) *Blood Coagul Fibrinolysis* 18:73, 2007.
93. Dear A, Daly J, Brennan SO, et al: An intronic mutation within FGB (IVS1+2076 a→g) is associated with afibrinogenemia and recurrent transient ischemic attacks. *J Thromb Haemost* 4:471, 2006.
94. Davis RL, Homer VM, George PM, Brennan SO: A deep intronic mutation in FGB creates a consensus exonic splicing enhancer motif that results in afibrinogenemia caused by aberrant mRNA splicing, which can be corrected in vitro with antisense oligonucleotide treatment. *Hum Mutat* 30:221, 2009.
95. Mimuro J, Hamano A, Tanaka T et al: Hypofibrinogenemia caused by a nonsense mutation in the fibrinogen Bbeta chain gene. *J Thromb Haemost* 1:2356, 2003.
96. Brennan SO, Mosesson MW, Lowen R, et al: Hypofibrinogenaemia resulting from novel single nucleotide deletion at codon Bbeta58 (3404del A) associated with thrombotic stroke in infancy. *Thromb Haemost* 95:738, 2006.
97. Asselta R, Duga S, Spena S, et al: Missense or splicing mutation? The case of a fibrinogen Bbeta-chain mutation causing severe hypofibrinogenemia. *Blood* 103:3051, 2004.

98. Maghzal GJ, Brennan SO, Fellowes AP, et al: Familial hypofibrinogenaemia associated with heterozygous substitution of a conserved arginine residue; Bbeta255 Arg→His (Fibrinogen Merivale). *Biochim Biophys Acta* 1645:146, 2003.
99. Hill MB, Brennan SO, Dear A, et al: Fibrinogen Nottingham II: A novel Bbeta Arg264gly substitution causing hypofibrinogenaemia. *Thromb Haemost* 96:378, 2006.
100. Homer VM, Brennan SO, George PM: Novel fibrinogen Bbeta gene mutation causing hypofibrinogenaemia. *Thromb Haemost* 88:1066, 2002.
101. Spena S, Duga S, Asselta R, et al: Congenital afibrinogenemia: First identification of splicing mutations in the fibrinogen Bbeta-chain gene causing activation of cryptic splice sites. *Blood* 100:4478, 2002.
102. Brennan SO, Wyatt JM, May S, et al: Hypofibrinogenemia due to novel 316 Asp→Tyr substitution in the fibrinogen Bbeta chain. *Thromb Haemost* 85:450, 2001.
103. Horellou MH, Chevreaud C, Mathieux V, et al: Fibrinogen Paris IX: A case of symptomatic hypofibrinogenaemia with Bbeta Y236C and Bbeta IVS7–1G→C mutations. *J Thromb Haemost* 4:1134, 2006.
104. Castaman G, Giacomelli SH, Duga S, Rodeghiero F: Congenital hypofibrinogenemia associated with novel heterozygous fibrinogen Bβ and γ mutations. *Haemophilia* 14:630, 2008.
105. Hanss M, Ffrench P, Vinciguerra C, et al: Four cases of hypofibrinogenemia associated with four novel mutations. *J Thromb Haemost* 3:2347, 2005.
106. Xu X, Wu J, Zhai Z, et al: A novel fibrinogen Bbeta chain frameshift mutation in a patient with severe congenital hypofibrinogenaemia. *Thromb Haemost* 95:931, 2006.
107. Asselta R, Duga S, Simonic T, et al: Afibrinogenemia: First identification of a splicing mutation in the fibrinogen gamma chain gene leading to a major gamma chain truncation. *Blood* 96:2496, 2000.
108. Wyatt J, Brennan SO, May S, George PM: Hypofibrinogenaemia with compound heterozygosity for two gamma chain mutations—Gamma 82 Ala→Gly and an intron two GT→AT splice site mutation. *Thromb Haemost* 84:449, 2000.
109. Margaglione M, Santacroce R, Colaizzo D, et al: A G-to-A mutation in IVS-3 of the human gamma fibrinogen gene causing afibrinogenemia due to abnormal RNA splicing. *Blood* 96:2501, 2000.
110. Neerman-Arbez M, Germanos-Haddad M, Tzanidakis K, et al: Expression and analysis of a split premature termination codon in FGG responsible for congenital afibrinogenemia: Escape from RNA surveillance mechanisms in transfected cells. *Blood* 104:3618, 2004.
111. Spena S, Asselta R, Platè M, et al: Pseudo-exon activation caused by a deep-intronic mutation in the fibrinogen γ-chain gene as a novel mechanism for congenital afibrinogenemia. *Br J Haematol* 139:128, 2007.
112. Davis RL, Mosesson MW, Kerlin BA, et al: Fibrinogen Columbus: A novel gamma Gly200Val mutation causing hypofibrinogenemia in a family with associated thrombophilia. *Haematologica* 92:1151, 2007.
113. Iida H, Ishii E, Nakahara M, et al: A case of congenital afibrinogenemia: Fibrinogen Hakata, a novel nonsense mutation of the fibrinogen gamma-chain gene. *Thromb Haemost* 84:49, 2000.
114. Sheen CR, Low J, Joseph J, et al: Fibrinogen Darlinghurst: Hypofibrinogenaemia caused by a W253G mutation in the gamma chain in a patient with both bleeding and thrombotic complications. *Thromb Haemost* 96:685, 2006.
115. Dear A, Brennan SO, Dempfle CE, et al: Hypofibrinogenaemia associated with a novel heterozygous gamma289 Ala→Val substitution (fibrinogen Dorfen). *Thromb Haemost* 92:1291, 2004.
116. Dear A, Dempfle CE, Brennan SO, et al: Fibrinogen Mannheim II: A novel gamma307 His→Tyr substitution in the gammaD domain causes hypofibrinogenemia. *J Thromb Haemost* 2:2194, 2004.
117. Meyer M, Bergmann F, Brennan SO: Novel fibrinogen mutation (gamma 313 Ser→Asn) associated with hypofibrinogenemia in two unrelated families. *Blood Coagul Fibrinolysis* 17:63, 2006.
118. Davis RL, Brennan SO: Fibrinogen Tologa Bay: A novel gammaAla341Val mutation causing hypofibrinogenemia. *Thromb Haemost* 98:1136, 2007.
119. de Raucourt E, de Mazancourt P, Maghzal GJ, et al: Fibrinogen Saint-Germain II: Hypofibrinogenemia due to heterozygous gamma N345S mutation. *Thromb Haemost* 94:965, 2005.
120. Brennan SO, Wyatt JM, Fellowes AP, et al: Gamma371 Thr→Ile substitution in the fibrinogen gammaD domain causes hypofibrinogenaemia. *Biochim Biophys Acta* 1550:183, 2001.
121. Acharya SS, Coughlin A, DiMichele DM: North American Rare Bleeding Disorder Study Group. Rare Bleeding Disorder Registry: Deficiencies of factors II, V, VII, X, XIII, fibrinogen and dysfibrinogenemias. *J Thromb Haemost* 2:248, 2004.
122. Peyvandi F, Kaufman RJ, Seligsohn U, et al: Rare bleeding disorders. *Haemophilia* 12(Suppl 3):137, 2006.
123. Ehmann WC, al-Mondhiry H. Congenital afibrinogenemia and splenic rupture. *Am J Med* 96:92, 1994.
124. Iwaki T, Sandoval-Cooper MJ, Paiva M, et al: Fibrinogen stabilizes placental-maternal attachment during embryonic development in the mouse. *Am J Pathol* 160:1021, 2002.
125. De Marco L, Girolami A, Zimmerman TS, Ruggeri ZM: Von Willebrand factor interaction with the glycoprotein IIb/IIa complex. Its role in platelet function as demonstrated in patients with congenital afibrinogenemia. *J Clin Invest* 77:1272, 1986.
126. Korte W, Feldges A: Increased prothrombin activation in a patient with congenital afibrinogenemia is reversible by fibrinogen substitution. *Clin Investig* 72:396, 1994.
127. Ni H, Denis CV, Subbarao S, et al: Persistence of platelet thrombus formation in arterioles of mice lacking both von Willebrand factor and fibrinogen. *J Clin Invest* 106:385, 2000.
128. Remjin JA, Wu Y-P, Ijsseldijk W, et al: Absence of fibrinogen in afibrinogenemia results in large but loosely packed thrombi under flow conditions. *Thromb Haemost* 85:736, 2001.
129. Dupuy E, Soria C, Molho P, et al: Embolized ischemic lesions of toes in an afibrinogenemic patient: Possible relevance to in vivo circulating thrombin. *Thromb Res* 102:211, 2001.
130. Colvin RB, Mosesson MW, Dvorak HF: Delayed-type hypersensitivity skin reactions in congenital afibrinogenemia lack fibrin deposition and induration. *J Clin Invest* 63:1302, 1979.
131. de Moerloose P, Neerman-Arbez M: Treatment of congenital fibrinogen disorders. *Expert Opin Biol Ther* 8:979, 2008.
132. Galanakis DK, Neerman-Arbez M, Scheiner T, et al: Homophenotypic A-alpha R16H fibrinogen (Kingsport): Uniquely altered polymerization associated with slower fibrinopeptide A than fibrinopeptide B release. *Blood Coagul Fibrinolysis* 18:731, 2007.
133. Barrowcliffe TW, Cattaneo M, Poda GM, et al: New approaches for measuring coagulation. *Haemophilia* 12(Suppl 3):76, 2006.
134. Goldenberg NA, Hathaway WE, Jacobson L, et al: Influence of factor VIII on overall coagulability and fibrinolytic potential of haemophilic plasma as measured by global assay: Monitoring in haemophilia A. *Haemophilia* 12:805, 2006.
135. Lewis SJ, Stephens E, Florou G, et al: Measurement of global haemostasis in severe haemophilia A following factor VIII infusion. *Br J Haematol* 138:775, 2007.
136. Bolton-Maggs PHB, Perry DJ. Chalmers EA, et al: The rare coagulation disorders—Review with guidelines for management from the United Haemophilia Centre Doctor's Organisation. *Haemophilia* 10:593, 2004.
137. Grech H, Majumdar G, Lawrie AS, Savidge GF: Pregnancy in congenital afibrinogenaemia: Report of a successful case and review of the literature. *Br J Haematol* 78:571, 1991.
138. Kobayashi T, Kanayama N, Tokunaga N, et al: Prenatal and peripartum management of congenital afibrinogenaemia. *Br J Haematol* 109:364, 2000.
139. De Vries A, Rosenberg T, Kochwa S, Boss JH: Precipitating antifibrinogen antibody appearing after fibrinogen infusions in a patient with congenital afibrinogenemia. *Am J Med* 30:486, 1961.
140. Ra'anani P, Levi Y, Varon D, et al: Congenital afibrinogenemia with bleeding, bone cysts and antibodies to fibrinogen. *Harefuah* 121:291, 1991.
141. Schuepbach RA, Meili EO, Schneider E, et al: Lepirudin therapy for thrombotic complications in congenital afibrinogenaemia. *Thromb Haemost* 91:1044, 2004.
142. Siebenlist KR, Mosesson MW, Meh DA, et al: Coexisting dysfibrinogenemia (γR275C) and factor V Leiden deficiency associated with thromboembolic disease (fibrinogen Cedar Rapids). *Blood Coagul Fibrinolysis* 11:293, 2000.
143. Rosenberg JB, Newman PJ, Mosesson MW, et al: Paris I dysfibrinogenemia: A point mutation in intron 8 results in insertion of a 15 amino acid sequence in the fibrinogen gamma-chain. *Thromb Haemost* 69:217, 1993.
144. Okumura N, Terasawa F, Hirota-Kawadobora M et al: A novel variant fibrinogen, deletion of Bbeta111Ser in coiled-coil region, affecting fibrin lateral aggregation. *Clin Chim Acta* 365:160, 2006.
145. Lefebvre P, Velasco PT, Dear A, et al: Severe hypodysfibrinogenemia in compound heterozygotes of the fibrinogen AalphaIVS4 + 1G→T mutation and an AalphaGln328 truncation (fibrinogen Keokuk). *Blood* 103:2571, 2004.
146. Meyer M, Dietzel H, Kaetzel R, et al: Fibrinogen Leipzig II (gamma351Gly→Ser and gamma82Ala→Gly): Hypodysfibrinogenaemia due to two independent amino acid substitutions within the same polypeptide chain. *Thromb Haemost* 98:903, 2007.
147. Ridgway HJ, Brennan SO, Faed JM, George PM: Fibrinogen Otago: A major alpha chain truncation associated with severe hypofibrinogenaemia and recurrent miscarriage. *Br J Haematol* 98:632, 1997.
148. Koopman J, Haverkate F, Grimbergen J, et al: Fibrinogen Marburg: A homozygous case of dysfibrinogenemia, lacking amino acids A alpha 461–610 (Lys 461 AAA→stop TAA). *Blood* 80:1972, 1992.
149. Sugo T, Nakamikawa C, Takebe M, et al: Factor XIIIa cross-linking of the Marburg fibrin: Formation of alpha and gamma-heteromultimers and the alpha-chain-linked albumin gamma complex, and disturbed proto-fibril assembly resulting in acquisition of plasmin resistance relevant to thrombophilia. *Blood* 91:3282, 1998.
150. Meyer M, Kutscher G, Sturzebecher J, et al: Fibrinogen Magdeburg I: A novel variant of human fibrinogen with an amino acid exchange in the fibrinopeptide A (Aalpha 9, Leu→Pro). *Thromb Res* 100:145, 2003.
151. Wada Y, Niwa K, Maekawa H, et al: A new type of congenital dysfibrinogen, fibrinogen Bremen, with an A alpha Gly-17 to Val substitution associated with hemorrhagic diathesis and delayed wound healing. *Thromb Haemost* 70:397, 1993.
152. Yoshida N, Okuma M, Hirata H, et al: Fibrinogen Kyoto II, a new congenitally abnormal molecule, characterized by the replacement of A alpha proline-18 by leucine. *Blood* 78:149, 1991.
153. Brennan SO, Hammonds B, George PM: Aberrant hepatic processing causes removal of activation peptide and primary polymerisation site from fibrinogen Canterbury (A alpha 20 Val→Asp). *J Clin Invest* 96:2854, 1995.
154. Marchi CR, Meyer MH, de Bosch NB, et al: A novel mutation (deletion of Aα-Asn 80) in an abnormal fibrinogen: Fibrinogen Caracas VI. Consequences of disruption of the coiled-coil for the polymerization of fibrin: Peculiar clot structure and diminished stiffness of the clot. *Blood Coagul Fibrinolysis* 15:559, 2004.
155. Maekawa H, Yamazumi K, Muramatsu S, et al: Fibrinogen Lima: A homozygous dysfibrinogen with an A alpha-arginine-141 to serine substitution associated with extra N-glycosylation at A alpha-asparagine-139. Impaired fibrin gel formation but nor-

mal fibrin-facilitated plasminogen activation catalyzed by tissue-type plasminogen activator. *J Clin Invest* 90:67, 1992.
156. Maekawa H, Yamazumi K, Muramatsu S, et al: An Aα Ser 434 to Nglycosylated Asn substitution in a dysfibrinogen, fibrinogen Caracas II, characterized by impaired fibrin gel formation. *J Biol Chem* 266:11575, 1991.
157. Furlan M, Steinmann C, Jungo M, et al: A frameshift mutation in Exon V of the A alpha-chain gene leading to truncated A alpha-chains in the homozygous dysfibrinogen Milano III. *J Biol Chem* 269:33129, 1994.
158. Brennan SO, Mosesson MW, Lowen R, Frantz C: Dysfibrinogenemia (fibrinogen Wilmington) due to a novel Aalpha chain truncation causing decreased plasma expression and impaired fibrin polymerisation. *Thromb Haemost* 96:88, 2006.
159. Marchi R, Meyer M, de Bosch N, et al: Biophysical characterization of fibrinogen Caracas I with an Aalpha-chain truncation at Aalpha-466 Ser: Identification of the mutation and biophysical characterization of properties of clots from plasma and purified fibrinogen. *Blood Coagul Fibrinolysis* 15:285, 2004.
160. Ridgway HJ, Brennan SO, Gibbons S, George PM: Fibrinogen Lincoln: A new truncated alpha chain variant with delayed clotting. *Br J Haematol* 93:177, 1996.
161. Homer VM, Mullin JL, Brennan SO, et al: Novel Aalpha chain truncation (fibrinogen Perth) resulting in low expression and impaired fibrinogen polymerization. *J Thromb Haemost* 1:1245, 2003.
162. Margaglione M, Vecchione G, Santacroce R, et al: A frameshift mutation in the human fibrinogen Aalpha-chain gene (Aalpha(499)Ala frame-shift stop) leading to dysfibrinogen San Giovanni Rotondo. *Thromb Haemost* 86:1483, 2001.
163. Hamidi AL, Liepnieks JJ, Uemichi T, et al: Renal amyloidosis with a frame shift mutation in fibrinogen alpha-chain gene producing a novel amyloid protein. *Blood* 90:4799, 1997.
164. Uemichi T, Liepnieks JJ, Yamada T, et al: A frame shift mutation in the fibrinogen A alpha chain gene in a kindred with renal amyloidosis. *Blood* 87:4197, 1996.
165. Uemichi T, Liepnieks JJ, Benson MD: Hereditary renal amyloidosis with a novel variant fibrinogen. *J Clin Invest* 93:731, 1994.
166. Collet JP, Soria J, Mirshahi M, et al: Dusart syndrome: A new concept of the relationship between fibrin clot architecture and fibrin clot degradability: Hypofibrinolysis related to an abnormal clot structure. *Blood* 82:2462, 1993.
167. Koopman J, Haverkate F, Grimbergen J, et al: Molecular basis for fibrinogen Dusart (A alpha 554 Arg→Cys) and its association with abnormal fibrin polymerization and thrombophilia. *J Clin Invest* 91:1637, 1993.
168. Benson MD, Liepnieks J, Uemichi T, et al: Hereditary renal amyloidosis associated with a mutant fibrinogen alpha-chain. *Nat Genet* 3:252, 1993.
169. Koopman J, Haverkate F, Grimbergen J, et al: Abnormal fibrinogens IJmuiden (B beta Arg14—Cys) and Nijmegen (B beta Arg44—Cys) form disulfide-linked fibrinogen-albumin complexes. *Proc Natl Acad Sci U S A* 89:3478, 1992.
170. Kamura T, Tsuda H, Yae Y, et al: An abnormal fibrinogen Fukuoka II (Gly-B beta 15→Cys) characterized by defective fibrin lateral association and mixed disulfide formation. *J Biol Chem* 270:29392, 1995.
171. Hirota-Kawadobora M, Terasawa F, Yonekawa O, et al: Fibrinogens Kosai and Ogasa: Bbeta15Gly→Cys (GGT→TGT) substitution associated with impairment of fibrinopeptide B release and lateral aggregation. *J Thromb Haemost* 1:275, 2003.
172. Liu CY, Koehn JA, Morgan FJ: Characterization of fibrinogen New York 1. *J Biol Chem* 260:4390, 1985.
173. Engesser L, Koopman J, de Munk G, et al: Fibrinogen Nijmegen: Congenital dysfibrinogenemia associated with impaired t-PA mediated plasminogen activation and decreased binding of t-PA. *Thromb Haemost* 60:113, 1988.
174. Koopman J, Haverkate F, Lord ST, et al: Molecular basis of fibrinogen Naples associated with defective thrombin binding and thrombophilia. Homozygous substitution of B beta 68 Ala→Thr. *J Clin Invest* 90:238, 1992.
175. Kaudewitz H, Henschen A, Soria J, Soria C: Fibrinogen Pontoise—A genetically abnormal fibrinogen with defective fibrin polymerization but normal fibrinopeptide release, in *Fibrinogen, Fibrin Formation and Fibrinolysis*, edited by DA Lane, A Henschen, MK Jasani, p 91. W de Gruyter, Berlin, 1986.
176. Bolliger-Stucki B, Lord ST, Furlan M: Fibrinogen Milano XII: A dysfunctional variant containing 2 amino acid substitutions, Aalpha R16C and gamma G165R. *Blood* 98:351, 2001.
177. Castaman G, Ghiotto R, Duga S, Rodeghiero F: A novel fibrinogen gamma chain mutation (gamma 239 Gln→His) is the cause of dysfibrinogenemia Vicenza. *J Thromb Haemost* 3:600, 2005.
178. Kotlín R, Sobotková A, Suttnar J, et al: A novel fibrinogen variant Liberec: Dysfibrinogenaemia associated with gamma Tyr262Cys substitution. *Eur J Haematol* 81:123, 2008.
179. Niwa K, Takebe M, Sugo T, et al: A γ Gly-268 to Glu substitution is responsible for impaired fibrin assembly in a homozygous dysfibrinogen Kurashiki. *Blood* 87:4686, 1996.
180. Niwa K, Kawata Y, Madoiwa S, et al: Fibrinogen Kamogawa: A new type of gamma Arg-275 to Ser substitution characterized by delayed fibrin gel formation [abstract]. *Thromb Haemost* 73:1229, 1995.
181. Fellowes AP, Brennan SO, Ridgway HJ, et al: Electrospray ionization mass spectrometry identification of fibrinogen Banks Peninsula (gamma280Tyr→Cys): A new variant with defective polymerization. *Br J Haematol* 101:24, 1998.
182. Bantia S, Mane SM, Bell WR, Dang CV: Fibrinogen Baltimore I: Polymerization defect associated with a gamma 292Gly→Val (GGC→GTC) mutation. *Blood* 76:2279, 1990.
183. Bantia S, Bell WR, Dang CV: Polymerization defect of fibrinogen Baltimore III due to a gamma Asn308→Ile mutation. *Blood* 75:1659, 1990.
184. Yoshida N, Terukina S, Okuma M, et al: Characterization of an apparently lower molecular weight gamma-chain variant in fibrinogen Kyoto I. The replacement of gamma-asparagine 308 by lysine which causes accelerated cleavage of fragment D1 by plasmin and the generation of a new plasmin cleavage site. *J Biol Chem* 263:13848, 1988.
185. Grailhe P, Boyer-Neumann C, Haverkate F, et al: The mutation in fibrinogen Bicetre II (gamma Asn308→Lys) does not affect the binding of t-PA and plasminogen to fibrin. *Blood Coagul Fibrinolysis* 4:679, 1993.
186. Okumura N, Furihata K, Terasawa F, et al: Fibrinogen Matsumoto II: Gamma 308 Asn→Lys (AAT→AAG) mutation associated with bleeding tendency. *Br J Haematol* 94:526, 1996.
187. Yamazumi K, Shimura K, Terukina S, et al: A gamma methionine-310 to threonine substitution and consequent N-glycosylation at gamma asparagine-308 identified in a congenital dysfibrinogenemia associated with posttraumatic bleeding, fibrinogen Asahi. *J Clin Invest* 83:1590, 1989.
188. Haverkate F, Samama M: Familial dysfibrinogenemia and thrombophilia. Report on a study of the SSC Subcommittee on Fibrinogen. *Thromb Haemost* 73:151, 1995.
189. Robert-Ebadi H, Le Querrec A, de Moerloose P, et al: A novel Asp344Val substitution in the fibrinogen gamma chain (fibrinogen Caen) causes dysfibrinogenemia associated with thrombosis. *Blood Coagul Fibrinolysis* 19:697, 2008.
190. Koopman J, Haverkate F, Briet E, Lord ST: A congenitally abnormal fibrinogen (Vlissingen) with a 6-base deletion in the gamma-chain gene, causing defective calcium binding and impaired fibrin polymerization. *J Biol Chem* 266:13456, 1991.
191. Terasawa F, Hogan KA, Kani S, et al: Fibrinogen Otsu I: A gamma Asn319,Asp320 deletion dysfibrinogen identified in an asymptomatic pregnant woman. *Thromb Haemost* 90:757, 2003.
192. Brennan SO, Davis RL, Mosesson MW, et al: Congenital hypodysfibrinogenaemia (Fibrinogen Des Moines) due to a gamma320Asp deletion at the Ca2+ binding site. *Thromb Haemost* 98:467, 2007.
193. Meyer M, Franke K, Richter W, et al: New molecular defects in the gamma subdomain of fibrinogen D-domain in four cases of (hypo)dysfibrinogenemia: Fibrinogen variants Hannover VI, Homburg VII, Stuttgart and Suhl. *Thromb Haemost* 89:637, 2003.
194. Hamano A, Mimuro J, Aoshima M, et al: Thrombophilic dysfibrinogen Tokyo V with the amino acid substitution of gammaAla327Thr: Formation of fragile but fibrinolysis-resistant fibrin clots and its relevance to arterial thromboembolism. *Blood* 103:3045, 2004.
195. Miyata T, Furukawa K, Iwanaga S, et al: Fibrinogen Nagoya, a replacement of glutamine-329 by arginine in the gamma-chain that impairs the polymerization of fibrin monomer. *J Biochem* 105:10, 1989.
196. Yoshida N, Terukina S, Okuma M, et al: Characterization of an apparently lower molecular weight gamma-chain variant in fibrinogen Kyoto I. The replacement of gamma-asparagine 308 by lysine which causes accelerated cleavage of fragment D1 by plasmin and the generation of a new plasmin cleavage site. *J Biol Chem* 263:13848, 1988.
197. Reber P, Furlan M, Rupp C, et al: Characterization of fibrinogen Milano I: Amino acid exchange gamma 330 Asp→Val impairs fibrin polymerization. *Blood* 67:1751, 1986.
198. Steinmann C, Reber P, Jungo M, et al: Fibrinogen Bern I: Substitution gamma 337 Asn→Lys is responsible for defective fibrin monomer polymerization. *Blood* 82:2104, 1993.
199. Song KS, Park NJ, Choi JR, et al: Fibrinogen Seoul (FGG Ala341Asp): A novel mutation associated with hypodysfibrinogenemia. *Clin Appl Thromb Hemost* 12:338, 2006.
200. Galanakis DK, Peerschke EIB, Spitzer S, Scharrer I: Fibrinogen Frankfurt I, a γ357 Ala→Thr substitution associated with impaired fibrin polymerization and decreased platelet aggregation support. *Blood* 86(Suppl 1):76a, 1995.
201. Steinmann C, Bogli C, Jungo M, et al: A new substitution, gamma 358 Ser→Cys, in fibrinogen Milano VII causes defective fibrin polymerization. *Blood* 84:1874, 1994.
202. Mathonnet F, Guillon L, Detruit H, et al: Fibrinogen Poissy II (gammaN361K): A novel dysfibrinogenemia associated with defective polymerization and peptide B release. *Blood Coagul Fibrinolysis* 14:293, 2003.
203. Okumura N, Furihata K, Terasawa F, et al: Fibrinogen Matsumoto I: A gamma 364 Asp→His (GAT→CAT) substitution associated with defective fibrin polymerization. *Thromb Haemost* 75:887, 1996.
204. Bentolila S, Samama MM, Conard J, et al: Association of dysfibrinogenemia and thrombosis. Apropos of a family (Fibrinogen Melun) and review of the literature. *Ann Med Interne (Paris)* 146:575, 1995.
205. Yoshida N, Hirata H, Morigami Y, et al: Characterization of an abnormal fibrinogen Osaka V with the replacement of gamma-arginine 375 by glycine. The lack of high affinity calcium binding to D-domains and the lack of protective effect of calcium on fibrinolysis. *J Biol Chem* 267:2753, 1992.
206. Keller MA, Martinez J, Baradet TC, et al: Fibrinogen Philadelphia, a hypodysfibrinogenemia characterized by abnormal polymerization and fibrinogen hypercatabolism due to γS378P mutation. *Blood* 105:3162, 2005.
207. Ridgway HJ, Brennan SO, Loreth RM, George PM: Fibrinogen Kaiserslautern (gamma 380 Lys to Asn): A new glycosylated fibrinogen variant with delayed polymerization. *Br J Haematol* 99:562, 1997.
208. Hayes T: Dysfibrinogenemia and thrombosis. *Arch Pathol Lab Med* 126:1387, 2002.
209. Gillmore JD, Lachmann HJ, Rowczenio D, et al: Diagnosis, pathogenesis, treatment, and prognosis of hereditary fibrinogen A alpha-chain amyloidosis. *J Am Soc Nephrol* 20:444, 2009.
210. Roberts HR, Stinchcombe TE, Gabriel DA: The dysfibrinogenaemias. *Br J Haematol* 114:249, 2001.
211. Hill M, Dolan G: Diagnosis, clinical features and molecular assessment of the dysfibrinogenaemias. *Haemophilia* 14:889, 2008.

CHAPTER 127
VON WILLEBRAND DISEASE

Jill M. Johnsen and David Ginsburg

SUMMARY

von Willebrand factor (VWF) is a central component of hemostasis, serving both as a carrier for factor VIII and as an adhesive link between platelets and the injured blood vessel wall. Abnormalities in VWF function result in von Willebrand disease (VWD), the most common inherited bleeding disorder in humans. The overall prevalence of VWD has been estimated to be as high as 1 percent of the general population, although the prevalence of clinically significant disease is probably closer to 1:1000. VWD is associated with either quantitative deficiency (type 1 and type 3) or qualitative abnormalities of VWF (type 2). The uncommon type 3 variant is the most severe form of VWD and is characterized by very low or undetectable levels of VWF, a severe bleeding diathesis, and a generally autosomal recessive pattern of inheritance. Type 1 VWD, the most common variant, is characterized by VWF that is normal in structure and function but decreased in quantity (in the range of 20–50% of normal). In type 2 VWD, the VWF is abnormal in structure and/or function. Type 2A VWD is associated with selective loss of the largest and most functionally active VWF multimers. Type 2A is further subdivided into group 1, as a result of mutations that interfere with biosynthesis and secretion, and group 2, in which the mutant VWF exhibits an increased sensitivity to proteolysis in plasma. Type 2B VWD is caused by mutations clustered within the VWF A1 domain, in a segment critical for binding to the platelet glycoprotein Ib (GPIb) receptor. These mutations produce a "gain of function" resulting in spontaneous VWF binding to platelets and clearance of the resulting platelet complexes, leading to thrombocytopenia and loss of the most active (large) VWF multimers. Type 2N VWD is characterized by mutations within the factor VIII binding domain of VWF, leading to disproportionately decreased factor VIII and a disorder resembling mild hemophilia A, but with autosomal recessive inheritance. Type 1 VWD can often be effectively managed by treatment with desmopressin (DDAVP), which transiently produces a two- to threefold increase in plasma VWF level. Response to DDAVP is generally poor in type 3 and some type 2 VWD variants. These disorders often require treatment with factor replacement in the form of factor VIII concentrates containing large quantities of intact VWF multimers.

DEFINITION AND HISTORY

In 1926, Eric von Willebrand described a bleeding disorder in 24 of 66 members of a family from the Åland Islands.[1] Both sexes were afflicted, and the bleeding time was prolonged despite normal platelet counts and normal clot retraction. von Willebrand distinguished this condition from the other hemostatic diseases known at the time and recognized its genetic basis, calling the disorder "hereditary pseudohemophilia," but incorrectly characterizing the inheritance as X-linked dominant. von Willebrand's confusion about the inheritance pattern was probably partly the result of the greater recognition of bleeding symptoms in women because of the hemostatic stresses of menstruation and parturition. The proband in the original family, Hjördis, was 5 years old at the time of von Willebrand's initial evaluation and ultimately died at age 13 during her fourth menstrual cycle. Four of Hjördis' sisters died between the ages of 2 and 4 years, and deaths in the family were also noted during childbirth.

An apparently similar disorder was independently reported in the United States by Minot and others in 1928. The original family in the Åland Islands was reexamined by von Willebrand and Jürgens in 1933, leading to the conclusion that the defect in this disorder was caused by an impairment of platelet function. It was not until 1953 that Alexander and Goldstein demonstrated reduced levels of coagulation factor VIII in von Willebrand disease (VWD) patients, along with prolonged bleeding time. This observation was confirmed by others, including studies of the original von Willebrand pedigree by Nilsson and coworkers. In the late 1950s, the latter group demonstrated that a fraction of plasma referred to as "I-O" could correct the factor VIII deficiency and normalize the bleeding time, indicating that the defect in VWD was a result of the deficiency of a plasma factor rather than an intrinsic platelet abnormality. Infusion of fraction I-O promptly increased the factor VIII level in a hemophilic patient, whereas in VWD the factor VIII level rose gradually, peaking at 5 to 8 hours. Fraction I-O prepared from a hemophilia A patient was also shown to correct the defect in VWD, demonstrating that these disorders were caused by deficiencies of distinct plasma factors (reviewed in references 2 and 3).

It was not until 1971 that Zimmerman, Ratnoff, and Powell prepared the first antibodies against what was thought to be a highly purified form of factor VIII.[4] This factor VIII-related antigen was found to be normal in hemophilia A patients but decreased in VWD. This puzzle was finally resolved with the demonstration that von Willebrand factor (VWF) and factor VIII are closely associated, with more than 98 percent of the mass of the complex composed of VWF (see "VWF Biosynthesis" below). Thus, antibodies raised against this complex predominantly recognize VWF. The first direct assay of VWF function was based on the observation that the antibiotic ristocetin induced thrombocytopenia and the demonstration by Howard and Firkin[5] that ristocetin-induced platelet aggregation was absent in some VWD patients. Weiss and coworkers[6] used this observation to develop a quantitative assay for VWF function that remains a mainstay of laboratory evaluation for VWD to this day. In 1973, several groups succeeded in dissociating VWF from factor VIII procoagulant activity.[7,8]

Final proof that VWF and factor VIII are independent proteins encoded by distinct genes came with the complementary DNA (cDNA) cloning of the two molecules in 1984 and 1985.[9–14] These discoveries also marked the beginning of the molecular genetic era for the study of VWF and factor VIII, leading to the identification of gene mutations in many patients with hemophilia and VWD as well as considerable insight into the structure and function of these related proteins.

Table 127–1 summarizes the current nomenclature and terminology for factor VIII and VWF. VWD is a heterogeneous disorder with more than 20 variants described. The previous complex and confusing classification has been consolidated and simplified into 6 distinct types,[15] as summarized in Table 127–2. Type 3 VWD is associated with very low or undetectable levels of VWF and severe bleeding. Type 1 VWD is characterized by concordant reductions in factor VIII activity, VWF antigen, and ristocetin cofactor activity, generally to the range of 20 to 50 percent of normal, in association with a normal VWF multimer distribution. Type 2 VWD is heterogeneous and further divided into

Acronyms and abbreviations that appear in this chapter include: ADAMTS-13, a disintegrin and metalloprotease with thrombospondin type 1 motifs; aPTT, activated partial thromboplastin time; DDAVP, 1-desamino-8-D-arginine vasopressin, or desmopressin; ER, endoplasmic reticulum; GPIb, glycoprotein Ib; HHT, hereditary hemorrhagic telangiectasia; PCR, polymerase chain reaction; RIPA, ristocetin-induced platelet aggregation; t-PA, tissue-type plasminogen activator; VWD, von Willebrand disease; VWF, von Willebrand factor.

TABLE 127–1. VWF and Factor VIII Terminology

Factor VIII	
	Antihemophilic factor, the protein that is reduced in plasma of patients with classic hemophilia A and most VWD and is measured in standard coagulation assays
Factor VIII activity (factor VIII:C)	
	The coagulant property of the factor VIII protein (this term is sometimes used interchangeably with factor VIII)
Factor VIII antigen (VIII:Ag)	
	The antigenic determinant(s) on factor VIII measured by immunoassays, which may employ polyclonal or monoclonal antibodies
von Willebrand factor (VWF)	
	The large multimeric glycoprotein that is necessary for normal platelet adhesion, a normal bleeding time, and stabilizing factor VIII
von Willebrand factor antigen (VWF:Ag)	
	The antigenic determinant(s) on VWF measured by immunoassays, which may employ polyclonal or monoclonal antibodies; *inaccurate designations of historical interest only* include factor VIII-related antigen (VIIIR:Ag), factor VIII antigen, AHF antigen, and AHF-like antigen
Ristocetin cofactor activity (VWF:RCo)	
	The property of VWF that supports ristocetin-induced agglutination of washed or fixed normal platelets
von Willebrand factor collagen-binding activity (VWF:CB)	
	The property of VWF that supports binding to collagen, measured by enzyme-linked immunosorbent assay (ELISA)

four subtypes (2A, 2B, 2M, and 2N). Type 2A VWD results from abnormal VWF proteolysis and is characterized by a disproportionately low level of ristocetin cofactor activity relative to VWF antigen and absence of large and intermediate-sized multimers. Type 2B VWD is also associated with reduced high-molecular-weight VWF multimers, but as the result of an abnormal VWF molecule with increased affinity for platelet GPIb. Functional abnormalities in VWF can also result in defective interactions with platelets, as in type 2M VWD, or decreased factor VIII binding to VWF, designated type 2N VWD and characterized by mild to moderate factor VIII deficiency. Many other subtypes have been reported, including platelet-type (pseudo-) VWD, which is actually an intrinsic platelet disorder caused by mutations in GPIb (see Chap. 121). Finally, acquired forms of VWD also occur, resulting in accelerated loss of circulating VWF.

ETIOLOGY AND PATHOGENESIS

VWF is synthesized exclusively in endothelial cells and megakaryocytes and performs two major functions in hemostasis. First, VWF serves as the initial critical bridge between circulating platelets and the injured blood vessel wall, accounting for the apparent defect in platelet function and prolonged bleeding time observed in VWD patients. The VWF monomer is assembled into higher-order multimers, a structure required for optimal adhesive function. Second, VWF serves as the carrier in plasma for factor VIII, ensuring its stability and localizing it to the initial platelet plug for participation in thrombin generation and fibrin clot formation (see Chap. 115). This tight, noncovalent interaction between VWF and factor VIII accounts for the copurification of these two molecules and the resulting initial confusion as to the origin of hemophilia and VWD. Factor VIII is encoded by the factor VIII gene on the X chromosome (see Chaps. 115 and 124), whereas VWF is encoded by a distinct gene on human chromosome 12.

THE VWF GENE AND cDNA

The VWF cDNA was initially cloned from endothelial cells,[11–14] and the corresponding gene mapped to the short arm of chromosome 12 (12p13.3).[11] The VWF messenger RNA (mRNA) is approximately 9 kb in length, encoding a primary translation product of 2813 amino acid residues with an estimated Mr of 310,000. Comparison of the primary peptide sequence obtained from plasma VWF[16] with the VWF cDNA sequence established the prepropolypeptide nature of VWF.[17] Prepropolypeptide VWF is composed of a 22-amino-acid signal peptide, a 741-amino-acid precursor polypeptide (propeptide) termed *VWF antigen II,* and the mature subunit.[11,17–20] Cleavage of the 741-amino-acid propeptide from the amino terminus produces the mature VWF subunit of 2050 amino acids (Fig. 127–1).

Analysis of the VWF sequence identifies four distinct types of repeated domains: three A domains, three B domains, two C domains, and four D domains.[18,21] The first pair of D domains is arranged in tandem in the VWF propeptide, followed by a partial and full D domain at the N terminus of the mature subunit. The final complete D domain is separated by a segment of more than 600 amino acids containing the triplicated A domains. The repeated domain structure of VWF suggests that the gene may have evolved via a complex series of partial duplications, although exon structure is not highly conserved between homologous domains.

Comparison of the VWF amino acid sequence to other proteins identifies a superfamily of related proteins that all share sequence similarity with the VWF A domains.[22] The common theme among these potentially evolutionarily related genes is a role in extracellular matrix or adhesive function. Consistent with this notion, VWF functional domains for binding to the platelet receptor GPIb and specific ligands within the extracellular matrix have been localized to the VWF A repeats. A potential relationship between the VWF C domains and portions of thrombospondin and procollagen has also been proposed.[23]

The *VWF* gene spans 178 kb and is divided into 52 exons.[24] Exons range in size from 40 bases to 1.4kb (exon 28). The latter exon is unusually large, encoding the entire Al and A2 domains, and containing most of the known type 2A and all of the type 2B VWD mutations. The concentration of these defects within one exon has facilitated the identification of human mutations responsible for these VWD variants (see "Molecular Genetics of VWD" below). A partial, nonfunctional duplication of the *VWF* gene, termed a *pseudogene*, is located on human chromosome 22.[25] The pseudogene duplicates the middle portion of the *VWF* gene, from exons 23 to 34, and includes the intervening sequences. The pseudogene is approximately 97 percent identical in sequence to the authentic VWF gene, indicating that it is of fairly recent evolutionary origin.[26] Gene conversion involving the pseudogene, possibly through recombination with the large homologous exon 28 sequence, has been proposed as a mechanism for introducing mutations into the *VWF* gene.[27–30]

VWF is synthesized exclusively in megakaryocytes and endothelial cells and, as a result, has frequently been used as a specific histochemical marker to identify cells of endothelial cell origin. Although generally assumed to mark all endothelial cells, VWF is expressed at widely varying levels among endothelial cells, depending on the size and location of the associated blood vessel.[31,32] A careful survey in the mouse identified wide differences in the level of VWF mRNA, with 5 to 50 times higher concentrations in the lung and brain, particularly in small vessels, than in comparable vessels in the liver and kidney. In general, the higher levels of VWF mRNA and antigen were found in the

TABLE 127–2. Classification of VWD

Type	Molecular Characteristics	Inheritance	Frequency	Factor VIII Activity	VWF Antigen	Ristocetin Cofactor Activity	RIPA	Plasma VWF Multimer Structure
Type 1	Partial quantitative VWF deficiency	Autosomal dominant, incomplete penetrance	1–30:1000; most common VWD variant (>70% of VWD)	Decreased	Decreased	Decreased	Decreased or normal	Normal distribution (mutant subunits permitted)
Type 3	Severe quantitative reduction or absence of VWF	Autosomal recessive (or codominant)	1–5:1,000,000	Markedly decreased	Very low or absent	Very low or absent	Absent	Usually absent
Type 2A	Qualitative VWF defect; loss of large VWF multimers, decreased VWF-dependent platelet adhesion	Usually autosomal dominant	~10–15% of clinically significant VWD	Decreased to normal	Usually low	Markedly decreased	Decreased	Largest and intermediate multimers absent
Type 2B	Qualitative VWF defect; increased VWF-platelet interaction (GPIb)	Autosomal dominant	Uncommon variant (<5% of clinical VWD)	Decreased to normal	Usually low	Decreased to normal	Increased to low concentrations of ristocetin	Largest multimers reduced/absent
Type 2M	Qualitative VWF defect; decreased VWF-platelet interaction, no loss of large VWF multimers	Usually autosomal dominant	Rare (case reports)	Variably decreased	Variably decreased	Decreased	Variably decreased	Normal and occasionally ultralarge forms
Type 2N	Qualitative VWF defect; decreased VWF-factor VIII binding capacity	Autosomal recessive	Uncommon; heterozygotes may be prevalent in some populations	Decreased	Normal	Normal	Normal	Normal
Platelet-type (pseudo-)	Platelet defect; decreased platelet-VWF interactions	Autosomal dominant	Rare	Decreased to normal	Decreased to normal	Decreased	Increased to low concentrations of ristocetin	Largest multimers absent

GPIb, glycoprotein Ib; RIPA, ristocetin-induced platelet aggregation.

endothelial cells of large vessels rather than in microvasculature, and in venous rather than arterial endothelial cells.[32]

Specific DNA sequences within or near the proximal promoter of the *VWF* gene appear to be required for endothelial-specific gene expression,[33–38] although it is likely that additional important regulatory elements exist outside of this region, some of which may lie at a great distance.[39] VWF is expressed in most, but not all, endothelial cells,[40] and this vascular-bed specific gene expression program is likely a result of the concerted action of multiple regulatory elements. Endothelial *VWF* gene expression also appears to be upregulated by exposure to shear stress. The length of a polymorphic GT repeat in the proximal *VWF* promoter correlates with the magnitude of this response, and several other more distal DNA sequences are predicted to be involved in a shear stress response.[41] However, this GT repeat does not appear to influence circulating VWF levels.[42]

VWF BIOSYNTHESIS

The processing steps involved in the biosynthesis of VWF are similar in megakaryocytes and endothelial cells (reviewed in references 44 and 45). VWF is first synthesized as a large precursor monomer polypeptide, as depicted schematically in Figure 127–1. VWF is unusually rich in cysteine, which accounts for 8.3 percent of its amino acid content. All cysteines in the mature VWF molecule are thought to be involved in disulfide bonds,[46] although these bonds may be exposed in circulating mature VWF by shear stress.[47] Pro-VWF monomers are assembled into dimers through disulfide bonds at both C termini, and only dimers are exported from the endoplasmic reticulum (ER).[46,48,49]

Glycosylation begins in the ER, with 12 potential *N*-linked glycosylation sites present on the mature subunit and 3 on the propeptide. Extensive additional posttranslational modification of VWF occurs in the Golgi apparatus, including the addition of multiple *O*-linked carbohydrate structures, sulfation, and multimerization through the formation of disulfide bonds at the N termini of adjacent dimers. VWF is the only protein known to undergo extensive disulfide bond formation at this late stage, and this unique process appears to be catalyzed by a novel disulfide isomerase activity present within the VWF propeptide.[50] Mutations at either of two specific cysteines within the propeptide that are thought to be critical for disulfide isomerase activity, or a

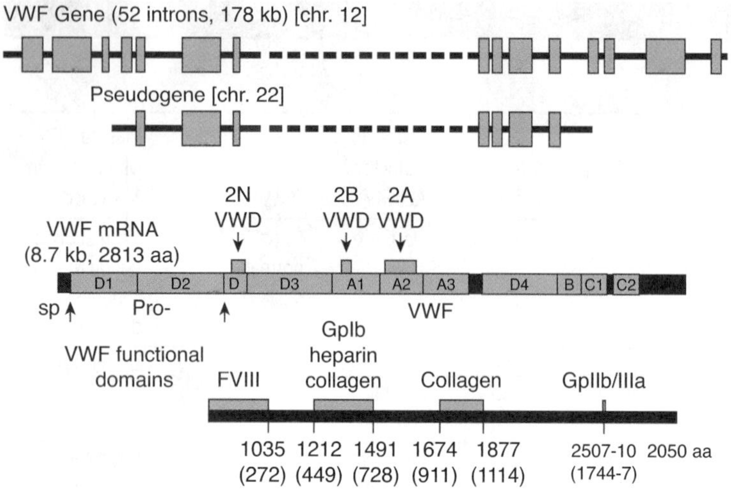

FIGURE 127–1. Schematic of the human VWF gene, mRNA, and protein. The VWF gene and pseudogene are depicted at the top, with *boxes* representing exons and the *solid line* representing introns. The VWF mRNA encoding the full prepro-VWF subunit is depicted in the middle as the *bar* and *lettered boxes*. The locations of signal peptide (*sp*) and propeptide (*Pro*) cleavage sites are indicated by *arrowheads*, and the lettered boxes denote regions of internally repeated sequence. The approximate localizations for known VWF functional domains within the mature VWF subunit are indicated at the bottom. Numbers underneath the domains refer to amino acid residues numbered from the ATG start site; numbers in parentheses indicate the amino acid residue position in the mature VWF subunit. aa, amino acids; chr, chromosome. *(Adapted from Ginsburg D, Bowie EJW[43] with permission.)*

shift in the spacing between them, results in loss of multimer formation.[50] An intermediate species with disulfide bonds between the propeptide and VWF D′D3 domain appears briefly in either the late ER or early Golgi,[51] which may position these domains for subsequent multimerization. The multimerization process appears to require the slightly acidic environment of the distal Golgi.[52] The VWF propeptide self-associates and may also serve to align VWF subunits for multimer assembly.[53] However, the propeptide facilitates multimer assembly even when coexpressed as a separate molecule from the mature VWF monomer.[54,55]

Propeptide cleavage occurs late in VWF synthesis or just prior to secretion. Cleavage occurs adjacent to two basic amino acids, Lys-Arg at positions −2 and −1. An Arg at position −4 is also required for recognition by the intracellular protease responsible for propeptide cleavage.[56] Multimerization and propeptide cleavage are not linked to each other. The multimers secreted by cultured endothelial cells contain both pro-VWF and mature subunits,[57,58] and recombinant VWF with a point mutation inhibiting propeptide cleavage is still assembled into normal multimer structures.[59] Although propeptide cleavage appears to occur primarily intracellularly, cleavage may also occur after secretion.

VWF is secreted from endothelial cells continuously via constitutive and constitutive-like (or basal) pathways and upon stimulation via a classic regulated pathway.[44,60] VWF is stored in tubular structures within the α-granules of platelets and within the Weibel-Palade bodies in endothelial cells[61,62] (reviewed in reference 63). These large VWF structures may be formed by tubular packing of the VWF N-terminal domains within the secretory granules.[64] Weibel-Palade bodies are derived from the Golgi apparatus and are found in most endothelial cells, though the number varies considerably. Although a number of other hemostatic proteins are also stored in the platelet α-granule, the Weibel-Palade body appears to be relatively specific for VWF and its propeptide.[65,66] It has been shown that VWF and factor VIII co-localize in storage granules. Although VWF is not required to traffic factor VIII to platelets,[67] VWF appears to play a role in trafficking factor VIII to Weibel-Palade bodies in endothelial cells.[68,69] Mature Weibel-Palade bodies acquire Rab27a, Rab3D, and CD63 as they move to the periphery of the cell. Rab27a (and possibly Rab3) may anchor Weibel-Palade bodies to cytoskeleton structures, in effect providing a brake on exocytosis.[70] The transmembrane glycoprotein P-selectin is also found in the membranes of both the α-granule and the Weibel-Palade body.[71] The VWF D′D3 domain has been shown *in vitro* to associate with P-selectin and to be necessary for the recruitment of P-selectin to Weibel-Palade bodies.[72] There appears to be heterogeneity within Weibel-Palade body populations both in relative content of VWF and P-selectin and in response to regulated secretion by different stimuli.[73] In addition to VWF and P-selectin, the Weibel-Palade body also contains tissue-type plasminogen activator (t-PA), a thrombolytic secreted protein which also may be released distinctly from VWF,[74] and several other proteins that are known to participate in inflammation or angiogenesis (for a complete list of Weibel-Palade contents see reference 75).

Regulated secretion of VWF from its storage site in the Weibel-Palade body is triggered by a number of secretagogues, including thrombin,[76] fibrin,[77] histamine,[78] the C5b-9 complement complex,[79] and several inflammatory cytokines.[80] Recent *in vitro* data suggests that there may also be suppression of regulated VWF secretion by statins.[81,82] The secretagogue desmopressin acetate (DDAVP), a vasopressin analogue, is used clinically for its capacity to cause a marked release of VWF and factor VIII *in vivo* by acting through type 2 vasopressin receptors to induce secretion from the Weibel-Palade bodies in endothelial cells.[83] Constitutive-like secretion of VWF occurs evenly at the luminal and abluminal surface, while regulated secretion from the Weibel-Palade body is highly polarized in the luminal direction (Fig. 127–2).[60,84] While constitutively secreted multimers are of relatively small size, the multimers stored within the Weibel-Palade body are the largest, most biologically potent form.[66,85] The VWF stored in platelet α-granules is also enriched for large multimers.[86] The N-terminal D domains appear to be required for VWF storage, with deletion of any of the individual domains resulting in constitutive secretion.[87,88] It also appears that cleavage of the VWF propeptide is required for efficient formation of storage granules.[89]

The concentration of VWF in plasma is approximately 10 mcg/mL, with approximately 15 percent of circulating VWF localized to the platelet compartment.[90] Marrow transplants between normal and VWD pigs demonstrate that platelet VWF is derived entirely from synthesis within the marrow and does not contribute to the normal plasma VWF pool.[91–93] These studies also demonstrate that both the plasma and the platelet VWF pools are required for full hemostasis, although the plasma pool appears to be more critical.

Plasma VWF is further processed in the circulation through cleavage by a specific protease, ADAMTS-13 (a disintegrin and metalloprotease with thrombospondin type 1 motifs), resulting in reduction in the size of the largest multimers (reviewed in reference 94). After regulated secretion *in vitro*, ultralarge VWF multimers may anchor to the endothelial cell surface via P-selectin[95,96] resulting in shear stress and VWF cleavage by ADAMTS-13. The major proteolytic cleavage site maps to the peptide bond between Tyr1605 and Met1606 in the VWF A2 domain,[97] and recombinant VWF missing the A2 domain is resistant to proteolysis.[98] VWF carrying a subgroup of type 2A VWD mutations exhibits increased susceptibility to cleavage by this protease,[99] and this is the proposed mechanism for the selective loss of large VWF multimers in this group of patients (see "Molecular Genetics of VWD" below). Increased VWF susceptibility to proteolysis by ADAMTS-13 has also been described in a subset of type 1 VWD patients, but the clinical significance of this is unclear as increased proteolysis appears to only occur under certain conditions.[100,101] Decreased ADAMTS-13 activity, either as a result of congenital deficiency

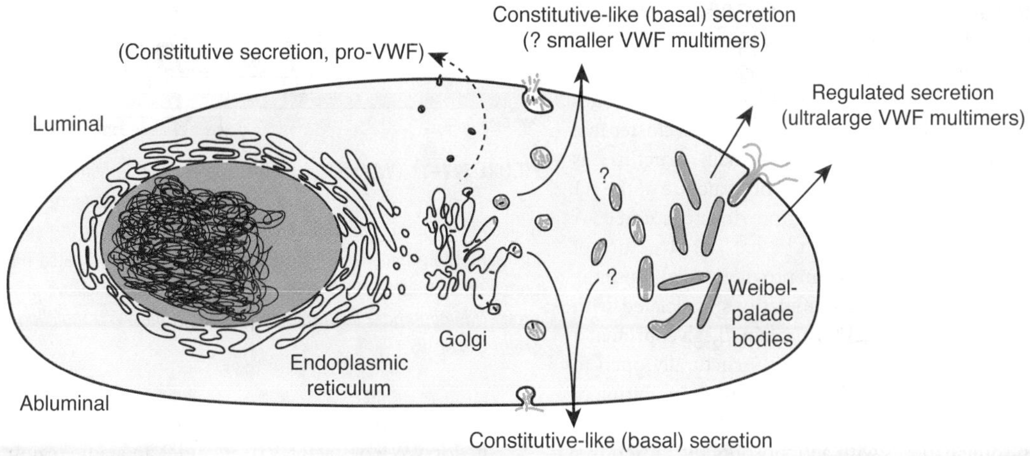

FIGURE 127–2. Schematic of VWF processing and secretion from endothelial cells. VWF dimers are formed in the endoplasmic reticulum, where VWF begins to be glycosylated. VWF dimers are transported to the Golgi, where the VWF undergoes further glycosylation and sulfation. Multimerization begins in the Golgi and continues within the secretory granules (Weibel-Palade bodies). A small amount of immature VWF is released constitutively (i.e., without regulation or storage) from endothelial cells as dimers or very small multimers. VWF is also released continuously from both the luminal and abluminal endothelial cell surfaces by constitutive-like (or basal) secretion. This VWF has been processed in the Golgi and may be transiently stored in an intermediate secretory granule or Weibel-Palade bodies. Mature VWF is packaged and stored as ultralarge multimers in Weibel-Palade bodies. This ultralarge VWF is released from the luminal surface of stimulated endothelial cells by regulated secretion. Once in circulation, VWF multimers undergo proteolysis by ADAMTS-13 (a disintegrin and metalloprotease with thrombospondin type 1 motifs) under moderate to high shear conditions. *(Adapted from Johnsen J, Lopez JA,[102] with permission.)*

or acquired inhibitors, plays a central role in the pathophysiology of thrombotic thrombocytopenic purpura (see Chap. 133).

THE FUNCTION OF VWF

VWF is a large multivalent adhesive protein that plays an important role in platelet attachment to subendothelial surfaces, platelet aggregation at sites of vessel injury, and stabilization of coagulation factor VIII in the circulation. Not only is the interaction of VWF and factor VIII important for the protection of factor VIII from inactivation or degradation, factor VIII bound to VWF may localize to cells and/or sites where it can more readily participate in the promotion of blood coagulation and/or thrombus formation.

VWF is required for the adhesion of platelets to the subendothelium, particularly at moderate to high shear force. VWF performs this bridging function by binding to two platelet receptors, GPIb and integrin αIIbβ_3, as well as to specific ligands within the exposed subendothelium at sites of vascular injury (reviewed in references 102, 103). Binding of VWF to its platelet receptors generally does not occur in the circulation under normal conditions. However, the interaction of VWF with exposed ligands in the vessel wall, combined with high shear stress conditions, facilitates VWF binding to platelet GPIb and subsequent platelet adhesion and activation. Activation of platelets leads to the exposure of the integrin αIIbβ_3 complex, an integrin receptor that can bind to fibrinogen, VWF, and other ligands, to form the platelet-platelet bridges required for thrombus propagation. Platelet adhesion to VWF immobilized at a site of injury appears to be a two-step process, with the initial tethering of the rapidly moving platelet dependent on the VWF/GPIb interaction and subsequent firm adhesion occurring through integrin αIIbβ_3 after platelet activation.[104,105] VWF may also play a role in inflammation by directly interacting with leukocytes,[106] but the clinical significance of this observation is not clear.

VWF Binding to the Vessel Wall

VWF binds to the vessel wall at sites of vascular endothelial injury (reviewed in reference 107). VWF binds to several different types of collagens, including types I through VI. Two distinct binding domains for the fibrillar collagens, types I and III, have been localized to specific segments within the VWF A1 and A3 repeats (see Fig. 127–1),[108,109] and a potential third domain has been identified in the propeptide.[110] Studies of recombinant VWF suggest that the A3 collagen-binding domain may be the most important.[111,112] The physiologic relevance of VWF interactions with fibrillar collagens has been questioned, as VWF still binds to extracellular matrix depleted of these molecules by treatment with collagenase.[113] VWF has also been shown to bind to the nonfibrillar collagen type VI, which is resistant to collagenase[114] and colocalizes with VWF in the subendothelium.[115] Type VI collagen supports the binding of VWF under high shear through cooperative interactions between binding domains within the VWF A1 and A3 repeat.[116] Although VWF binding has also been demonstrated to a number of other potential components of the subendothelium, including glycosaminoglycans[117,118] and sulfatides,[119] the biologic significance of these interactions remains to be demonstrated.

VWF Binding to Platelets

VWF interacts with platelets both to mediate platelet aggregation and platelet localization to sites of vascular injury (reviewed in reference 107). Circulating VWF does not spontaneously interact with platelets, but once bound to an injured vessel wall VWF is subjected to higher shear stresses and a platelet-binding site in the VWF A1 domain is uncovered. VWF interacts with a receptor complex on the surface of platelets composed of the disulfide-linked GPIbα and GPIbβ chains noncovalently associated with GPIX and GpV. The binding site for VWF is within a 293-amino-acid segment at the N-terminus of GPIb and requires sulfation of several key tyrosine residues for optimal binding.[120] The GPIb binding domain within VWF lies within the A1 segment, within the disulfide loop formed between the cysteine residues at 1272 (509) and 1458 (695) (see Fig. 127–1).[121,122] GPIb binding to the A1 domain enhances proteolysis of recombinant VWF fragments by ADAMTS-13 and suggests a feedback mechanism for limiting thrombus propagation *in vivo*.[123] Scanning mutagenesis studies of recombinant VWF characterized a number of amino acid residues within the

VWF A1 domain that are critical for binding to GPIb and for interaction with botrocetin (this section).[124] Several mutations were also identified that increase platelet binding, an effect similar to that of mutations associated with type 2B VWD (see "Molecular Genetics of VWD" below). These natural and synthetic mutations cluster in a small area on the surface of the VWF A1 domain structure, as revealed by x-ray crystallographic studies.[125] The structure of the A1 domain closely resembles that of other previously studied A domains, including the VWF A3 domain.[126–128] The structure of GPIb in complex with the VWF A1 domain provides insight into the structural basis for the gain of function mutations associated with type 2B VWD.[129] The abundant plasma protein β_2-glycoprotein I can bind the VWF A1 domain when VWF is structurally open to GPIbα binding. This may result in biologically relevant inhibition of the VWF-platelet interaction, as inhibitory anti-β_2-glycoprotein I autoantibodies found in some patients with antiphospholipid antibody syndrome are associated with thrombosis (see Chap. 132).[130]

Ristocetin binds to both VWF and platelets, but the mechanism by which it enhances the VWF/GPIb interaction is still poorly understood.[131,132] The snake venom botrocetin appears to induce GPIb binding through a different alteration in the VWF A1 domain and is also used to study this interaction.[128] Heparin binds the VWF A1 domain within the loop formed by the disulfide bond formed between the residues Cys1272 and Cys1458,[133] where it appears to competitively inhibit VWF binding to GPIb[134,135] and enhance VWF proteolysis by ADAMTS-13 *in vitro*.[136] Although it has been suggested that this may account for hemorrhage not predicted by conventional heparin monitoring, the clinical significance of the VWF–heparin interaction is not clear.

The Arg-Gly-Asp-Ser (RGDS) sequence at amino acids 2507–2510 of the mature VWF subunit serves as the binding site within VWF for integrin αIIbβ_3. The latter complex is a member of the integrin family of cell surface receptors. αIIbβ_3 undergoes a conformational change to a high-affinity ligand-binding state following platelet activation and, in addition to VWF, can bind a number of other adhesive proteins, including fibrinogen. Although VWF is present in blood at much lower concentrations than is fibrinogen, evidence suggests that VWF may be a critical ligand. VWF participates in platelet tethering and adhesion to fibrin under flow conditions,[104,105,137] where the C1C2 domains of VWF are required for fibrin binding.[137] An RGD sequence is also present in the VWF propeptide (VWF antigen II), although its functional significance is unknown.

The Interaction of VWF with Factor VIII

The noncovalent interaction between factor VIII and VWF is required for the stability of factor VIII in the circulation, as is evident from the factor VIII levels of less than 10 percent that are observed in most severe VWD patients. Although each VWF subunit appears to carry a binding site for factor VIII, the stoichiometry for the VWF/factor VIII complex found in normal plasma is approximately 1 to 2 factor VIII molecules per 100 VWF monomers.[138] Factor VIII bound to VWF is also protected from proteolytic degradation by activated protein C (reviewed in references 139 and 140). Interestingly, factor VIII also appears to increase the susceptibility of VWF to proteolysis by ADAMTS-13 under shear conditions.[141]

The factor VIII binding domain within VWF has been localized to the first 272 N-terminal amino acids of the mature subunit,[142] with antibody studies suggesting a particularly critical role for amino acids 78–96.[143,144] The mutations identified in patients with type 2N VWD, in which VWF binding to factor VIII is specifically affected (see "Molecular Genetics of VWD" below), are all clustered in this region, including the most common type 2N mutation at Arg854.[145] It is noteworthy that the same amino acid substitution at Arg852 is a common polymorphism that does not affect factor VIII binding.[146] The corresponding binding site for VWF on factor VIII includes an acidic region at the N-terminus of the light chain (residues 1669–1689)[147] and requires sulfation of Tyr1680 for optimal binding.[148] Thrombin cleavage after Arg1689 in factor VIII activates and releases factor VIII from VWF. Thus, VWF may serve to efficiently deliver factor VIII to the sites of clot formation, where it can complex with factor IXa on the platelet surface.

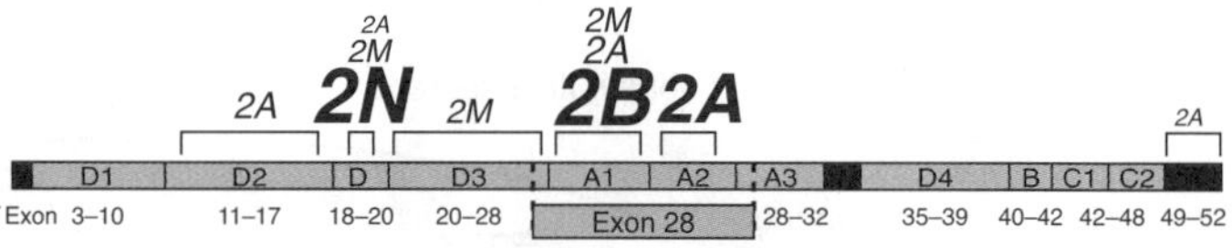

FIGURE 127–3. VWD mutations. The VWF domain locations of all reported mutations associated with type 2A, 2B, 2M, and 2N VWD. Lettering size represents the proportion of total mutations reported within the designated VWF domain for that subtype, with larger letters indicating more mutations. Type 1 and Type 3 VWD associated mutations have been reported throughout the *VWF* gene. Shown below are the relative positions of the *VWF* gene exons. *(Mutation data from reference 149 and the VWD mutation database at www.vwf.group.shef.ac.uk/.)*

MOLECULAR GENETICS OF VWD

VWD is an extremely heterogeneous and complex disorder, with more than 20 distinct subtypes reported (reviewed in references 149 and 150). A large number of mutations within the *VWF* gene have now been identified (Fig. 127–3). Previous definitions of VWD required the presence of a *VWF* gene mutation. However, because of both the genetic complexity of VWD and the practical considerations of *VWF* gene sequencing in most clinical settings, a *VWF* gene mutation is no longer included in the criteria for the diagnosis of VWD.[15] A list is maintained by a consortium of VWD investigators and can be accessed through the Internet at http://www.vwf.group.shef.ac.uk/. These findings form the basis for the simplified classification of VWD that is outlined in Table 127–2 and used throughout this chapter. Types 1 and 3 VWD are defined as pure quantitative deficiencies of VWF that are either partial (type 1) or complete (type 3). Type 2 VWD is characterized by qualitative abnormalities of VWF structure and/or function. The quantity of VWF found in type 2 VWD may be normal, but it is usually mildly to moderately decreased (see Table 127–2).

Type 1 VWD

Type 1 is the most common form, accounting for approximately 70 percent of VWD patients. Type 1 VWD is generally autosomal dominant in inheritance and is associated with coordinate reductions in factor VIII, ristocetin cofactor activity, and VWF antigen with maintenance of the full complement of multimers (Fig. 127–4). Subgroups within type 1 VWD have been proposed based on the relative levels of VWF present in the plasma and platelet pools,[151–154] but this distinction is not generally used in clinical practice.

Type 1 VWF was previously assumed to simply represent the heterozygous form of type 3 VWD. However, the majority of heterozygous carriers of VWF gene deletions, as well as carriers of VWF mRNA expression defects,[25,155–158] are asymptomatic and have normal VWF laboratory values, consistent with an autosomal recessive pattern of inheritance for type 3 VWD. Furthermore, although two large studies of type 1 VWD families identified numerous putative *VWF* mutations, very few were predictive of null alleles.[30,159] Nonetheless, in some families with nonsense or frameshift mutations, heterozygotes with apparent type 1 VWD have been identified, indicating that some, but probably not all (this section), type 1 VWD may be a result of such

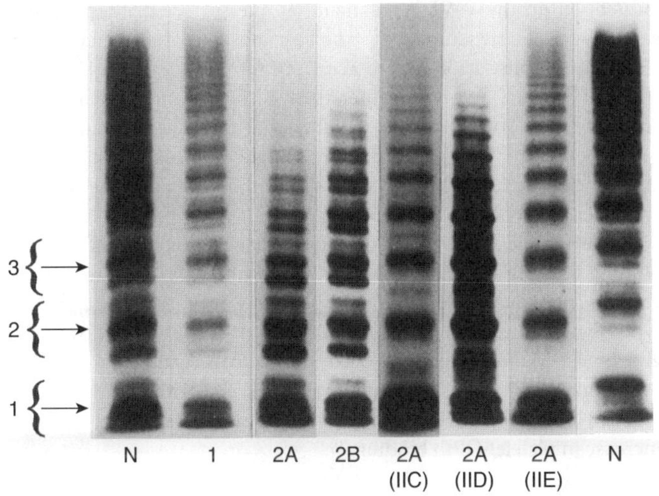

FIGURE 127–4. Agarose gel electrophoresis of plasma VWF. VWF multimers from plasma of patients with various subtypes of VWD are shown. The brackets to the left encompass three individual multimer subunits, including the main band and its associate satellite bands. N indicates normal control lanes. Lanes 5 through 7 are rare variants of type 2A VWD. The former designations for these variants are indicated in parentheses below the lanes (IIC through IIE). *(Adapted from Zimmerman TS, Dent JA, Ruggeri ZM, Nannini LH:* J Clin Invest *77:947, 1986, with permission.)*

defects within the VWF gene (see Fig. 127–3). Mutations that give rise to defective VWF subunits that interfere in a dominant negative way with the normal allele may be particularly likely to cause symptomatic VWD in the heterozygote.[160] Mutations have been identified at several cysteine residues in the VWF D3 domain and in the VWF propeptide of patients with moderately severe type 1 VWD. VWF carrying one of these mutations is retained in the ER, where it is proposed to exert a dominant negative effect on VWF derived from the normal allele via heterodimerization and degradation.[161,162] A subgroup of type 1 VWD patients exhibit variably decreased survival of VWF after DDAVP challenge. Several novel polymorphisms within the *VWF* gene have been associated with the accelerated clearance of VWF from circulation.[163]

To date, most mutation studies and genetic linkage analysis of type 1 VWD have been consistent with defects within the *VWF* gene. Although no single mutation can explain the majority of type 1 VWD, a common *VWF* founder mutation, Tyr1584Cys, has been identified in 14 percent of Canadian type 1 VWD patients, and possibly a similar proportion of patients in Europe.[159,164] This mutation is associated with decreased VWF survival, likely because of increased susceptibility to proteolysis by ADAMTS-13.[165–168] A recent large multicenter Canadian study of 123 type 1 VWD families found candidate *VWF* mutations in 63 percent of families with type 1 VWD, again with Tyr1584Cys being the most common mutation (15%), leaving 37 percent of type 1 VWD index cases in the study without a putative mutation in *VWF*. Cases with *VWF* gene mutations tended to be more severe and highly heritable, while cases without an identifiable *VWF* mutation generally had higher von Willebrand factor antigen (VWF:Ag) levels (>0.30 IU/mL).[30] Another large, multicenter European study of 150 type 1 VWD families found a similar prevalence of candidate *VWF* mutations (70% of index cases) within their cohort. Interestingly, about one-third of cases that were historically diagnosed to have type 1 VWD were found to have abnormal multimers in this study, and of these nearly all (95%) had a putative *VWF* gene mutation and significantly lower VWF:Ag, VWF ristocetin cofactor activity (VWF:RCo), factor VIII:C, and von Willebrand factor collagen-binding activity (VWF:CB) levels. Conversely, index cases with normal multimers had higher laboratory VWF values and fewer identifiable *VWF* mutations (55%), suggesting that the pathogenic mechanism(s) underlying this cohort of "true" type 1 VWD patients is more genetically complex.[159]

Given the complex biosynthesis and processing of VWF, defects at a number of other loci could also be expected to result in quantitative VWF abnormalities (reviewed in reference 160). This concept is supported by families with type 1 VWD in which bleeding histories and low ristocetin cofactor activities do not always cosegregate with genetic markers at the VWF locus,[30,169] whereas one or more genetic factors outside the *VWF* locus may be associated with the variation in bleeding severity observed within VWD pedigrees.[170,171] It is interesting to note that a mouse model for type 1 VWD associated with an up to 20-fold reduction in plasma VWF is a result of an unusual mutation in a glycosyltransferase gene, leading to aberrant posttranslational processing of VWF and accelerated clearance from plasma.[172] A similar mechanism affecting VWF survival, perhaps combined with accelerated proteolysis,[173–175] may explain the observed modifying effect of the ABO blood group glycosyltransferases on plasma VWF survival.[176]

The diagnosis of type 1 VWD can be confounded by the incomplete penetrance of the disease, the wide range of VWF levels in "normals," the inherent difficulties in obtaining reliable bleeding histories, and borderline laboratory results. An alternative strategy has been proposed to classify some patients for whom the diagnosis of VWD is ambiguous as "low VWF," recognizing that these patients may have an increased risk of bleeding without labeling them as type 1 VWD.[177,178] This proposal has yet to be tested in clinical practice.

Type 3 VWD

Patients with type 3 VWD account for 1 to 5 percent of clinically significant VWD, have very low or undetectable levels of plasma and platelet VWF antigen and ristocetin cofactor activity, and generally present early in life with severe bleeding.[179] Factor VIII coagulant activity is markedly reduced but usually detectable at levels of 3 to 10 percent of normal. Type 3 VWD appears to be inherited as an autosomal recessive trait in most families, but parents of affected individuals may have mildly reduced VWF levels and are occasionally given the diagnosis of mild type 1 VWD.

Mutations associated with type 3 VWD have been reported throughout the *VWF* gene (www.vwf.group.shef.ac.uk/). Southern blot analysis has identified gross gene deletion as the molecular mechanism for type 3 VWD in only a small subset of families[25,155,156,180,181]; however, large deletions may confer an increased risk for the development of alloantibodies against VWF.[25,180] A similar correlation has been reported for hemophilia B (see Chap. 124). Comparative analysis of VWF genomic DNA and platelet VWF mRNA has identified nondeletion defects resulting in complete loss of VWF mRNA expression as a molecular mechanism in some patients with type 3 VWD.[157,158] A number of nonsense and frameshift mutations that would be predicted to result in loss of VWF protein expression or in expression of a markedly truncated or disrupted protein have been identified in some type 3 VWD families (see Fig. 127–3).[149,160,182,183] A frameshift mutation in exon 18 appears to be a particularly common cause of type 3 VWD in the Swedish population and is the defect responsible for VWD in the original Åland Island pedigree.[184,185] This mutation results in a stable mRNA encoding a truncated protein that is rapidly degraded in the cell.[186] This mutation also appears to be common among type 3 VWD patients in Germany[187] but not in the United States.[186]

Type 2A VWD

Type 2A is the most common qualitative variant of VWD and is generally associated with autosomal dominant inheritance and selective loss of the large and intermediate VWF multimers from plasma (see Fig. 127–4). A 176-kDa proteolytic fragment present in normal individuals is markedly increased in quantity in many type 2A VWD patients. This fragment is caused by proteolytic cleavage of the peptide bond between Tyr1605 (842) and Met1606 (843).[97,188] Based on this observation, initial DNA sequence analysis in patients centered on VWF exon 28, in the region encoding this segment of the VWF protein, leading to the identification of the first point mutations responsible for VWD.[189] Since that time, a large number of mutations have been identified, accounting for the majority of type 2A VWD patients.[149] Most of these mutations are clustered within a 134-amino-acid segment of the VWF A2 domain (between Gly1505 and Glu1638; see Fig. 127–3), and the most common, Arg1597Trp, appears to account for about one-third of type 2A VWD patients.[149,182,190]

Expression of recombinant VWF containing type 2A VWD mutations has identified two distinct molecular mechanisms for the loss of large VWF multimers characteristic of this disorder.[191] In the first subset, classified as group 1, the type 2A VWD mutation results in a defect in intracellular transport, with retention of mutant VWF in the ER. In the second subset, or group 2, mutant VWF is normally processed and secreted *in vitro*, and thus loss of multimers *in vivo* was presumed to occur as a result of increased susceptibility to proteolysis in plasma[97,191–194] at the same Tyr1605-Met1606 site cleaved by ADAMTS-13.[195,196] The susceptibility of type 2A VWD mutations to proteolysis by ADAMTS-13 *in vitro* supports accelerated proteolysis as a mechanism for the loss of high molecular weight VWF multimers in these patients.[190]

The multimer structure of platelet VWF correlates well with this subclassification. Group 1 patients show loss of large VWF multimers within platelets because of defective synthesis, whereas group 2 patients have normal VWF multimers within the protected environment of the α granule.[191] These observations confirm the earlier subclassification of type 2A VWD based on platelet multimers.[151] Subclassification into group 1 or 2 might be expected to predict response to desmopressin therapy, although this remains to be demonstrated.

In addition to the major class of type 2A VWD described above, a number of rare variants previously classified as types IIC to IIH, type IB, and "platelet discordant" are now included in the new, more general type 2A category. Most of these rare variants were distinguished on the basis of subtle differences in the multimer pattern (see Fig. 127–4; reviewed in reference 150). The IIC variant is usually inherited as an autosomal recessive trait and is associated with loss of large multimers and a prominent dimer band. Several mutations have been identified in the VWF propeptide of these patients,[197,198] presumably interfering with multimer assembly. A mutation at the C terminus of VWF, interfering with dimer formation, was described in a patient with the IID variant.[199] Most of the other reported variants of type 2A VWD are quite rare, often limited to single case reports.

Type 2B VWD

Type 2B VWD is usually inherited as an autosomal dominant disorder and is characterized by thrombocytopenia and loss of large VWF multimers. The plasma VWF in type 2B VWD binds to normal platelets in the presence of lower concentrations of ristocetin than does normal VWF and often binds spontaneously. Accelerated clearance of the resulting complexes between platelets and the large, most adhesive forms of VWF accounts for the thrombocytopenia and the characteristic multimer pattern (see Fig. 127–4).

The peculiar functional abnormality characteristic of type 2B VWD suggested a molecular defect within the GPIb binding domain of VWF. For this reason, initial DNA sequence analysis focused on the corresponding portion of VWF exon 28.[200,201] All of these mutations are located within the VWF A1 domain, at one surface of the described crystallographic structure.[125,129] The four most common mutations are clustered within a 36-amino-acid stretch between Arg1306 and Arg1341 (see Fig. 127–3); together, these account for more than 80 percent of type 2B VWD patients.[182] Functional analysis of mutant recombinant VWF[202–206] confirms that these single-amino-acid substitutions are sufficient to account for increased GPIb binding and the resulting characteristic type 2B VWD phenotype.

Three families have been described that exhibit enhanced VWF binding to GPIb but a normal distribution of VWF multimers. These variants, previously referred to as type I New York, type I Malmö, and type I Sydney, are now all designated as type 2B VWD. Type I New York and type I Malmö have now been shown to be caused by the same mutation, Pro1266Leu. This mutation is located within the cluster of type 2B mutations in the VWF A1 domain and results in a similar increase in platelet GPIb binding.[207]

Type 2N VWD

As described in Chap. 124, hemophilia A results from defects in the factor VIII gene and is inherited in an X-linked recessive manner. Rare families have been reported in which the inheritance of hemophilia appears to be autosomal, based on the occurrence of affected females or direct transmission from an affected father.[208,209] Several cases of an apparent autosomal recessive decrease in factor VIII have been shown to be caused by decreased binding of factor VIII by VWF.[210–212] This disorder has also been referred to as VWD Normandy, after the province of origin of the first patient. DNA sequence analysis has identified a total of 37 mutations associated with this disorder, which are summarized in the ISTH SSC VWF Database (http://www.vwf.group.shef.ac.uk/), all located at the VWF N terminus (see Fig. 127–3). One of these mutations, Arg854Gln, appears to be particularly common and may contribute to variability in the severity of type 1 VWD in some cases.[213]

Type 2M VWD

This category is reserved for rare VWD variants in which a defect in VWF platelet-dependent function leads to significant bleeding but VWF multimer structure is not affected (although some have subtle multimer abnormalities). Most of these variants were previously classified as type I. The variant previously referred to as type B is associated with absent ristocetin cofactor activity but normal platelet binding with other agonists. This variant is caused by a mutation in the A1 domain (Gly1324Ser).[214] Mutations have also been identified in a number of other families with normal VWF multimers and disproportionately decreased ristocetin cofactor activity.[150,215] Several families have been described with a VWD variant (VWD Vicenza) characterized by larger than normal VWF multimers.[216] Genetic linkage analysis indicates that the defect lies within the VWF gene.[217] Although mutations within the VWF gene have been reported to be associated with VWD Vicenza[218] (which is also sometimes classified as type 1 VWD), the underlying molecular mechanism responsible for the VWD Vicenza phenotype remains controversial.[219]

CLINICAL FEATURES

INHERITANCE

Type 1 VWD is the most common form of VWD, with a prevalence that has been estimated to be as high as 1 percent.[221,222] Type 1 VWD is generally transmitted as an autosomal dominant disorder and accounts for approximately 70 percent of clinically significant VWD. However, disease expressivity is variable, and penetrance is incomplete.[160] Laboratory values and clinical symptoms can vary considerably, even within the same individual, and establishing a definite diagnosis of VWD is often difficult. In two large families with type 1 VWD, only 65 percent of individuals with both an affected parent and an affected descendent had significant clinical symptoms.[223] For comparison, 23 percent of the unrelated spouses of the patients, who presumably did not have a bleeding disorder, were judged to have a positive bleeding history.

A number of factors are known to modify VWF levels, including ABO blood group, Secretor blood group, estrogens, thyroid hormone, age, and stress.[224–226] ABO blood group is the best characterized of these factors (reviewed in reference 227). A genomewide linkage screen has confirmed strong linkage between the ABO locus and VWF levels.[228] Mean VWF antigen levels are approximately 75 percent for type O individuals and 123 percent for type AB individuals when compared to a pool of normal donor plasmas. Thus, it may be difficult to differentiate between a low-normal value and mild type 1 VWD in blood group O individuals. The variable expressivity and incomplete penetrance of type 1 VWD has complicated the determination of accurate incidence figures for VWD, with estimates ranging from as high as 1 percent[221,222] to as low as 2 to 10 per 100,000.[229]

In general, the type 2 variants are more uniformly penetrant. Type 2A and type 2B VWD account for the vast majority of patients with qualitative VWF abnormalities. No accurate incidence figures are available for these subtypes, but the type 2 variants are generally felt to comprise 20 to 30 percent of all VWD diagnoses. The type 2 variants are generally autosomal dominant in inheritance, although type 2N and other rare cases of apparent recessive inheritance have been reported.

Estimates of prevalence for severe (type 3) VWD range from 0.5 to 5.3 per 1,000,000 persons.[230–232] Although this variant is frequently defined as autosomal recessive in inheritance, this is not a consistent finding. As described above, one or both parents of a severe VWD patient are frequently clinically asymptomatic and often have entirely normal laboratory test results, but many families have also been reported in which one or both parents appear to be affected with classic type 1 VWD. Thus, in some families, severe VWD may represent the homozygous form of type 1 VWD. In this model, the apparent recessive inheritance in a subset of families could simply be the result of the incomplete penetrance of type 1 VWD. Alternatively, there may be a fundamental difference in the molecular mechanisms responsible for type 1 and type 3 VWD.[160]

Compound heterozygosity (the presence of more than one *VWF* gene mutation) can occur, and the clinical presentation in such cases can depend on the interaction between the different mutant VWF proteins. Compound heterozygosity can impact response to therapy as a result of a complex VWD phenotype and has implications for genetic counseling. If compound heterozygosity is deduced from the family history and/or laboratory studies, or discovered during genetic testing, the most recent update to the VWD nomenclature represents both types separated by a slash (/), such as VWD type 2B/2N.[15]

CLINICAL SYMPTOMS

Mucocutaneous bleeding is the most common symptom in patients with type 1 VWD.[223] It is important to note that more than 20 percent of normal individuals may give a positive bleeding history.[233] Although several bleeding questionnaires have been developed for research purposes, none are diagnostic for VWD. This observation, together with the limited sensitivity and specificity of the currently available laboratory tests (see "Laboratory Features" below), makes the diagnosis of mild VWD quite difficult and probably contributes to the wide range of prevalence figures for type 1 VWD currently in the literature. A recent National Heart, Lung, and Blood Institute Expert Panel has proposed clinical guidelines for evaluating patients to determine whether laboratory testing for VWD or other bleeding disorders is warranted.[234]

Epistaxis occurs in approximately 60 percent of type 1 VWD patients, 40 percent have easy bruising and hematomas, 35 percent have menorrhagia, and 35 percent have gingival bleeding. Gastrointestinal bleeding occurs in approximately 10 percent of patients.[235] An apparent association between hereditary hemorrhagic telangiectasia (HHT) and VWD had been reported in several families. The causative genes in HHT have been identified and are located on chromosomes 9q33–34, and 12q13,[236] distinct from the VWF gene on chromosome 12p13. However, because inheriting VWD is likely to increase the severity of bleeding from HHT, the diagnosis is more likely to be made in patients inheriting both defects.[237] Mucocutaneous bleeding is common after trauma, with approximately 50 percent of patients reporting bleeding after dental extraction, approximately 35 percent after trauma or wounds, 25 percent postpartum, and 20 percent postoperatively. Hemarthroses in patients with moderate disease are extremely rare and are generally only encountered after major trauma. The bleeding symptoms can be quite variable among patients within the same family and even in the same patient over time. An individual may experience postpartum bleeding with one pregnancy but not with others, and clinical symptoms in mildly to moderately affected type 1 individuals often ameliorate by the second or third decade of life. Aside from an infrequent type 3 patient, death from bleeding rarely occurs in VWD.

Patients with type 3 VWD can suffer from severe clinical bleeding and experience hemarthroses and muscle hematomas, as in severe hemophilia A (see Chap. 124). The bleeding time is very prolonged. After infusion of VWF-containing plasma fractions, some of these patients develop anti-VWF antibodies that neutralize VWF. Development of antibodies has been correlated with the presence of gene deletions.[25,180]

Thrombocytopenia is a common feature of type 2B VWD and is not seen in any other form of VWD. Most patients only experience thrombocytopenia at times of increased VWF production or secretion, such as during physical effort, in pregnancy, in newborn infants, postoperatively, or if an infection develops. The platelet count rarely drops sufficiently to contribute to clinical bleeding.[238,239] Infants with type 2B VWD may present with neonatal thrombocytopenia, which could be confused with neonatal sepsis or congenital thrombocytopenia.

Patients who are homozygous or compound heterozygous for type 2N VWD generally have normal levels of VWF antigen and ristocetin cofactor activity and normal VWF platelet adhesive function. However, factor VIII levels are moderately decreased, resulting in a mild to moderate hemophilia-like phenotype.[145] However, in contrast to patients with classic hemophilia A (factor VIII deficiency), these patients do not respond to infusion of purified factor VIII and should be treated with VWF-containing concentrates. Heterozygotes for this disorder may have mildly decreased factor VIII levels but are generally asymptomatic. Although type 2N VWD appears to be considerably less common than classic hemophilia A, it should be considered in the differential diagnosis of factor VIII deficiency, particularly if any features suggest an autosomal pattern of inheritance. Although the factor VIII level rarely drops below 5 percent, at least one type 2N VWD mutation has been associated with factor VIII levels as low as 1 percent, when coinherited with a type 3 VWD allele.[240] The latter observation suggests that a diagnosis of type 2N VWD should also be considered in patients with marked reductions of factor VIII.

Other heritable coagulopathies can coexist with VWF deficiency. An evaluation for other factor deficiencies or platelet disorders should be considered in patients that have a suggestive family history, a bleeding phenotype out of proportion or inconsistent with an expected VWD pattern, or a poor response to therapy. In VWD patients with combination coagulopathies, treatment of both disorders may be necessary to achieve a good clinical result.[241]

LABORATORY FEATURES

In the initial laboratory evaluation of patients suspected by history of having VWD, the following tests are routinely performed: assay of factor VIII activity, VWF:Ag, and VWF:RCo. In a large epidemiologic study, the ristocetin cofactor assay was found to be more sensitive than the VWF:Ag for the diagnosis of type 1 VWD.[242] Other tests that are commonly used include ristocetin-induced platelet aggregation (RIPA), VWF:CB, and VWF multimer analysis. Routine coagulation studies, such as prothrombin time or activated partial-thromboplastin time, are generally not useful in the evaluation of VWD. However, the activated partial thromboplastin time can be prolonged in subjects with VWF deficiency[243] because of the secondary reduction in factor VIII level. As noted above, results of these tests can all be normal in some patients with type 1 VWD. In addition, the wide range of normal and the considerable overlap with the levels observed in type 1 VWD make borderline levels difficult to interpret. A variety of concurrent diseases and drugs may modify the results of individual tests, including aspirin or other nonsteroidal antiinflammatory drugs, which often prolong the bleeding time. Many conditions, such as pregnancy, age, time of the menstrual cycle, hypo- or hyperthyroidism, uremia, recent exercise, liver disease, infection, diabetes, estrogen therapy, myeloproliferative disorders, or malignancy can affect the factor VIII activity, VWF:Ag, and VWF:RCo levels. These values can be regarded as acute-phase reactants, and even minor illnesses can increase the levels in a VWD patient to normal. Appropriate processing of laboratory specimens is also critical as VWF parameters can be artifactually skewed (either high or low) by phlebotomy conditions or specimen handling (reviewed in reference 234). Even controlling for many of these factors, the coefficients of variation of repeated VWF:Ag and VWF:RCo assays in a single person are quite large.[244] For this reason, repeated measurements are usually necessary, and the diagnosis of VWD or its exclusion should not be based on a single set of laboratory values unless they are well below or well above the limits of normal.

FACTOR VIII

Factor VIII levels in VWD patients are generally coordinately decreased along with plasma VWF. Levels in type 3 VWD generally range from 3 to 10 percent. In contrast, the levels in type 1 and the type 2 VWD variants (other than 2N) are variable and usually only mildly or moderately decreased. The factor VIII level in type 2N VWD is more severely decreased, but rarely to less than 5 percent.

VWF ANTIGEN

Plasma VWF:Ag is usually quantitated by electroimmunoassay, radioimmunoassay, or an enzyme-linked immunosorbent assay (ELISA) technique. In type 1 VWD, the VWF:Ag assay usually parallels the ristocetin cofactor activity, but it has lower specificity and sensitivity than the ristocetin cofactor assay. In patients with type 2A VWD, the VWF:Ag is usually low but can be normal.[244]

RISTOCETIN COFACTOR ACTIVITY

The standard measure of VWF activity quantitates the ability of plasma VWF to agglutinate platelets via platelet membrane glycoprotein GPIbα in the presence of ristocetin,[245] also referred to as the ristocetin cofactor assay. Normal platelets washed free of plasma VWF are used either as fresh platelets or after formaldehyde fixation. This assay has been reported to be the most sensitive and specific single test for the detection of VWD.[242] An ELISA has been proposed as an alternative to the standard platelet-based ristocetin cofactor activity assay.[246,247] However, there is high interassay and interlaboratory variability,[248,249] leading to the recommendation by the UK Haemophilia Doctors' Organization VWD Working Party that only platelet-based ristocetin cofactor activity assays be used.[250] Because the ELISA appears to be more sensitive than the platelet-based VWF:RCo assay, an effort to standardize this technique for routine clinical laboratory use has been undertaken.[251] A flow cytometry based VWF:RCo assay has also been developed,[252] but this method remains to be validated in clinical practice. Ristocetin cofactor activity is generally decreased coordinately with VWF:Ag and factor VIII in type 1 VWD patients. In type 2 VWD variants, ristocetin cofactor activity can be disproportionately decreased, as is usually the case in type 2A variants (and sometimes type 2B) because of the greater dependence of the ristocetin-mediated platelet-VWF interaction on the presence of larger VWF multimers, and in type 2M because of decreased VWF-platelet interactions (see Table 127–2). Thus, the VWF:RCo-to-VWF:Ag ratio has been proposed as means to distinguish between type 1 and type 2 VWD, with a ratio of VWF:RCo-to-VWF:Ag <0.7 indicative of a qualitative (type 2) VWF defect.[15] However, in patients with very low VWF:Ag levels, this ratio may not be reliable because of the limits of sensitivity of most VWF:RCo assays.

RISTOCETIN-INDUCED PLATELET AGGLUTINATION

Similar to the ristocetin cofactor assay above, the RIPA assay also measures platelet agglutination caused by ristocetin-mediated VWF binding to platelet membrane glycoprotein GPIbα. In the case of RIPA, ristocetin is added directly to patient platelet-rich plasma. This activity is generally reduced in most VWD patients. Hyperresponsiveness to RIPA results either from a type 2B VWD mutation or an intrinsic defect in the platelet (platelet-type or pseudo-VWD). In these disorders, patient platelet-rich plasma agglutinates spontaneously or at ristocetin concentrations of only 0.2 to 0.7 mg/mL. At these concentrations, normal platelet-rich plasma does not agglutinate. Type 2B and platelet-type VWD can be distinguished by RIPA experiments performed with separated patient platelets or plasma mixed with the corresponding component from a normal individual or paraformaldehyde-fixed platelets.

MULTIMER ANALYSIS

Analysis of plasma VWF multimers is critical for the proper diagnosis and subclassification of VWD (see Fig. 127–4). This is generally accomplished by agarose gel electrophoresis of plasma VWF to separate VWF multimers on the basis of molecular size, with the largest multimers migrating more slowly than the intermediate or smaller multimers. The multimers may be visualized by autoradiography after incubation with ^{125}I-monospecific antihuman VWF antibody or by nonradioactive immunologic techniques. The normal multimeric distribution is an orderly ladder of major protein bands of increasing molecular weight, going from the smallest to the largest VWF multimers (see Fig. 127–4). Each normal multimer has a fine structure consisting of one major component and two to four satellite bands.[253] Type 2B and most of the type 2A variants were initially distinguished from each other on the basis of subtle variations in the satellite band pattern. In a large European multicenter type 1 VWD study, careful analysis of VWF multimers in subjects historically diagnosed as type 1 VWD, including patients diagnosed at experienced centers, found one-third of "type 1" VWD patients had subtly abnormal multimers.[254] Although this previously would have required reclassification of these patients as type 2 VWD, the most recent update on the classification of von Willebrand disease by the ISTH Subcommittee on von Willebrand Factor expanded the category of type 1 VWD to permit subtle VWF multimer abnormalities.[15] The authors of the European type 1 VWD study note that having samples from the index case, affected family members, and unaffected family members on one gel made qualitative defects more readily detectable, and that intermediate-resolution multimer gels were superior to low-resolution multimer gels in detecting abnormalities in this population. Furthermore, the VWF:RCo-to-VWF:Ag ratio was less sensitive than either multimer gel technique in identifying qualitative VWF defects, indicating an important role for VWF multimer analysis in the laboratory evaluation of VWD.[254]

ADDITIONAL LABORATORY TESTS

The bleeding time was previously used as a standard screening test for VWD and other abnormalities of platelet function.[255] However, results can vary considerably with the experience of the operator and a variety of other factors, and its value as a screening test has been questioned. Furthermore, although bleeding time does not prolong with factor VIII deficiency, low factor VIII levels have been shown to correlate with operative bleeding.[256] There is now a general consensus that the bleeding time should not be used for routine patient screening in the preoperative setting.[234,257–259] Although the bleeding time probably also should not be used as a routine screening test for VWD, it may still be of value in selected patients when taken together with the clinical history and the results of other laboratory tests. It may also be useful as a means of monitoring therapy in some settings.

Because of the variable sensitivity and specificity of laboratory testing for VWD, additional select diagnostic studies may be useful in the classification of VWD patients. The VWF:CB measures VWF binding to collagen (type I, type III, type VI, or mixed) by ELISA. Abnormalities in VWF:CB can reflect loss of high-molecular-weight VWF multimers. Assays based on VWF:CB can complement the VWF:RCo in detecting type 2 VWD variants,[260–263] and an abnormal VWF:CB-to-VWF:Ag is suggestive of a qualitative VWF defect.[15] When type 2N VWD is suspected, VWF:factor VIII binding capacity can be measured.[212] Specific assays of factor VIII binding to VWF (VWF:FVIIIB) have been developed and can be used to confirm the diagnosis of type 2N VWD.[264,265] Type 2N carriers do not always exhibit a decrease in VWF:FVIIIB, but a decreased VWF:FVIIIB-to-VWF:Ag ratio may correlate with heterozygosity for a type 2N *VWF* mutation.[266] Although this assay is widely used in European hemostasis laboratories, its availability in the United States is currently limited to a few specialized reference laboratories.

An assay measuring the VWF propeptide (VWFpp) has been developed as a means to detect a subset of VWD patients with decreased VWF survival. Good correlation has been reported between subjects with significantly shortened VWF half-life after DDAVP challenge and an increased VWFpp-to-VWF:Ag ratio.[267] This assay is currently only available in a few reference laboratories or for research purposes. A normal platelet VWF:Ag in the setting of decreased plasma VWF laboratory parameters also suggests an accelerated clearance phenotype such as that seen in VWD type Vicenza,[268] but platelet VWF:Ag testing also is not widely available in clinical laboratories.

A number of other assays for VWF activity have been developed. The PFA-100 system, which measures platelet binding under high shear,[269,270] is controversial in the diagnosis and monitoring of VWD. Although the PFA-100 is usually abnormal in type 2 VWD and in more severe type 1 and type 3 VWD cases, milder type 1 VWD and some type 2 VWD patients can have normal results.[234] Another VWF assay measures binding of an antibody to the GPIb binding site on VWF and has also been proposed as an automated screening test for VWD.[271–274] Additional assays can measure platelet agglutination induced by botrocetin and other snake venom proteins.[275] In the most recent National Heart, Lung, and Blood Institute Expert Panel guidelines, none of these tests are recommended for screening for VWD.[234]

With advances in understanding the molecular genetics of VWD, it is now possible to precisely diagnose and subclassify many variants of VWD on the basis of DNA mutations (reviewed in reference 276). DNA testing, particularly for type 2 VWD mutations, which cluster within specific regions of the cDNA (see Fig. 127–3), can be used to confirm the diagnosis and is available in specialized reference laboratories. The analysis of type 3 and type 1 VWD is more complex, as the currently known mutations account only for a small subset of these patients, except in selected populations.[184]

PRENATAL TESTING

Given the mild clinical phenotype of most patients with the common variants of VWD, prenatal diagnosis for the purpose of deciding on terminating a pregnancy is rarely performed. However, type 3 VWD patients often have a profound bleeding disorder, similar to or more severe than classic hemophilia, and some families may request prenatal diagnosis. In those cases of VWD in which the precise mutation is known, DNA diagnosis can be performed rapidly and accurately by polymerase chain reaction from amniotic fluid or chorionic villus biopsies.[277] In those cases where the mutation is unknown, diagnosis can still be attempted by genetic linkage analysis using the large panel of known polymorphisms within the VWF gene.[278] One of these polymorphisms, a TCTA tetranucleotide repeat of variable length in intron 40, is particularly useful, with more than 100 known polymorphic alleles. Several cases of successful prenatal diagnosis have been reported.[277,279–281] Although all cases of VWD analyzed to date appear to be linked to the VWF gene, the possibility of locus heterogeneity (i.e., a similar phenotype caused by a mutation in a gene other than VWF) should be considered.[160] As with all DNA testing, if prenatal testing is being considered, genetic counseling should be provided before the decision to test is made as well as following the procedure.

DIFFERENTIAL DIAGNOSIS

PLATELET-TYPE (PSEUDO-) VWD

Platelet-type (pseudo-) VWD is a platelet defect that phenotypically mimics VWD (see Chap. 121).[282] The plasma VWD lacks the largest multimers, RIPA is enhanced at low concentrations of ristocetin, and thrombocytopenia of variable degree is often present. Clinically, these patients have primarily mucocutaneous bleeding. Molecular analysis has identified mutations within the GPIbα chain as the molecular basis for pseudo-VWD. These mutations are located within the segment of GPIb that encodes the VWF binding domain and appear to induce the conformational change complementary to that produced in the corresponding fragment of VWF by type 2B VWD mutations.[129,282]

The specialized RIPA test should be performed at low ristocetin concentrations to distinguish type 2B and platelet type VWD from type 2A VWD. Purified plasma VWF or cryoprecipitate causes platelet aggregation when added to platelet-rich plasma from patients with platelet-type VWD, distinguishing this disorder from type 2B VWD. In addition, type 2B VWD plasma transfers the enhanced RIPA to normal platelets, whereas plasma from patients with platelet-type VWD interacts normally with control platelets.

ACQUIRED VWD

Acquired VWD is a relatively rare acquired bleeding disorder that usually presents as a late-onset bleeding diathesis in a patient with no prior bleeding history and a negative family history of bleeding (reviewed in references 283 and 284). Decreased levels of factor VIII, VWF:Ag, and VWF:RCo are common, and VWF multimers can be abnormal. Acquired VWD is usually associated with another underlying disorder and has been reported to occur in patients with myeloproliferative disorders,[285] amyloidosis,[286] benign or malignant B-cell disorders,[287] hypothyroidism,[288] autoimmune disorders,[289] several solid tumors (particularly Wilms tumor),[290] cardiac or vascular defects (notably aortic stenosis),[291] and in association with several drugs, including ciprofloxacin and valproic acid,[292,293] and ventricular assist devices.[294]

A variety of B-cell disorders are associated with the development of anti-VWF autoantibodies. In most cases the acquired VWD appears to be a result of rapid clearance of VWF induced by the circulating inhibitor, although these antibodies may also interfere with VWF function. Hypothyroidism results in decreased VWF synthesis,[288] and, in some cases of malignancy, acquired VWD is thought to be caused by selective adsorption of VWF to the tumor cells. In acquired VWD associated with valvular heart disease, ventricular assist devices, or certain drugs, VWF may be lost by accelerated destruction or proteolysis.[292–294]

Although the VWF multimers in acquired VWD usually exhibit a type 2A pattern with relative depletion of the large multimer forms, acquired VWD can manifest as a wide range of VWD phenotypes.[295,296] Distinguishing acquired VWD from genetic VWD can be difficult, as testing for the associated autoantibodies is generally not available in the clinical setting. The diagnosis often rests on the late onset of the disease, the absence of a family history, and the identification of an associated underlying disorder.

Management of acquired VWD is generally aimed at treating the underlying disorder. VWF levels and bleeding symptoms often improve with successful treatment of hypothyroidism or an associated malignancy. Refractory patients have been treated with glucocorticoids, plasma exchange, intravenous gamma-globulin, DDAVP, and VWF containing factor VIII concentrates.[293,297]

THERAPY, COURSE, AND PROGNOSIS

The mainstays of therapy for VWD are DDAVP, which induces secretion of both VWF and factor VIII, and replacement therapy with VWF-containing plasma concentrates. The choice of treatment in any given patient depends upon the type and severity of VWD, the clinical setting, and the type of hemostatic challenge that must be met. Type 1 patients are most often treated with DDAVP alone, types 2A and 2B with a combination of DDAVP and a VWF-containing factor VIII product, and type 2N and type 3 patients with VWF-containing concentrates.[298] A previous history of trauma or surgery and the success of previous treatment are important parameters to include in assessing the risk of bleeding. Prophylaxis is generally not used except in anticipation of hemostatic challenges, such as dental extractions, and in the most severe Type 3 VWD patients[299,300] who exhibit recurrent hemarthroses or gastrointestinal bleeding (reviewed in reference 301). Although in general there is a correlation between normal hemostasis and correction of the bleeding time and factor VIII activity, this does not occur in all cases. Factor VIII has been found to be the most important determinant of soft-tissue and postoperative hemorrhage, but no laboratory test clearly correlates with mucosal bleeding or response to therapy.[302]

DESMOPRESSIN

Desmopressin (1-desamino-8-D-arginine vasopressin, DDAVP) is an analogue of antidiuretic hormone that acts through type 2 vasopressin receptors to induce secretion of factor VIII and VWF, likely via cyclic adenosine monophosphate-mediated secretion from the Weibel-Palade bodies in endothelial cells.[303] When DDAVP is administered to healthy subjects, it causes sustained increases of factor VIII and ristocetin cofactor activity for approximately 4 hours.[304] DDAVP also releases t-PA, presumably from endothelial cells. Patients with type 1 VWD treated with DDAVP release unusually high-molecular-weight VWF multimers into the circulation for 1 to 3 hours after the infusion.[304,305] Therapy with DDAVP increases the factor VIII activity, VWF:Ag, and VWF:RCo to two to five times the basal level and, in many instances, corrects the bleeding time of type 1 VWD patients.

DDAVP has become a mainstay for the treatment of mild hemophilia and VWD[306] because it is relatively inexpensive, widely available, and avoids the risks of plasma-derived products. Approximately 80 percent of type 1 VWD patients have excellent responses to DDAVP, although this figure may be substantially lower depending on the criteria for diagnosis and response.[307] It is regularly used in the setting of mild to moderate bleeding and for prophylaxis of patients undergoing surgical procedures. DDAVP is administered at a dose of 0.3 mcg/kg continuous intravenous infusion over 30 minutes. DDAVP is also available for subcutaneous injection (at the same 0.3 mcg/kg dose) and in intranasal form (at a fixed dose of 300 mcg for adults and 150 mcg for children), which appears to be similar in efficacy to intravenous administration,[308,309] although the response may be more variable.

The response to DDAVP in any given individual with VWD is generally reproducible and predicts response to future doses. In one study, 22 type 1 VWD patients showed a departure of less than 20 percent from the mean factor VIII peak level calculated from two separate infusions. In addition, the consistency of response in one patient reliably predicted the future response of that patient and other affected family members.[310] In another study of 77 type 1 VWD patients, DDAVP response was associated both with *VWF* mutation and baseline multimeric pattern, although subtle abnormalities in VWF multimers did not preclude a patient response to DDAVP. Interestingly, patients with the same *VWF* mutation did not necessarily exhibit the same degree of responsiveness to DDAVP, implying the influence of other factors in the magnitude of DDAVP effect.[311] For patients requiring repeated infusions of DDAVP, the factor VIII activity and VWF responses may not be of the same magnitude as after the first infusion. Although this decay in response has considerable individual variability, after one infusion of DDAVP per day for 4 days it was found that the responses on days 2 to 4 were reduced approximately 30 percent compared to day 1.[308–310,312]

Consequently, in patients for whom DDAVP is potentially the treatment of choice, a test dose should be given at the planned therapeutic dose and route in advance of the first required course of treatment with measurements of before and after VWF and factor VIII:C levels to ensure an adequate therapeutic response. Sampling additional time points after DDAVP infusion should be considered as a subgroup of type 1 VWD patients that have a significantly shortened half-life of VWF may be more appropriate to treat with VWF replacement therapy in clinical scenarios requiring more durable therapy to maintain hemostasis. For patients with type 1 VWD who are undergoing surgical procedures, DDAVP can be administered 1 hour before surgery and approximately every 12 hours thereafter for up to four doses before loss of clinically significant response. The response of factor VIII and ristocetin cofactor activity should be monitored when DDAVP is administered at frequent intervals. VWF-containing factor VIII concentrates and/or cryoprecipitate should be available for transfusion as backup.

Approximately 20 to 25 percent of patients with VWD do not respond adequately to DDAVP. Type 2 VWD patients are less likely to have a response than type 1 patients,[307,313] and nearly all patients with type 3 VWD cannot respond. The response to DDAVP of patients with type 2A VWD is variable. Although most patients respond only transiently, some patients exhibit complete hemostatic correction after DDAVP infusion.[314,315] It has been hypothesized that the differences in DDAVP efficacy among type 2A patients may correspond to the type of mutation, with better responses predicted in patients with group 2 mutations. A prospective study of the biologic response to DDAVP in well-characterized VWD patients included type 2A VWD patients with both group 1 and group 2 defects. Although patients with group 2 mutations had greater improvements in VWF:RCo and bleeding time than did patients with group 1 defects, neither group could be classified as being responsive.[316]

Common side effects of DDAVP administration are mild cutaneous vasodilation resulting in a feeling of heat, facial flushing, tachycardia, tingling, and headaches. The potential for dilutional hyponatremia, especially in elderly and very young patients, requires appropriate attention to fluid restriction, as it may result in seizures. There are isolated reports of acute arterial thrombosis associated with administration of DDAVP, but the risk appears to be very low when judged against the total number of patients treated. However, DDAVP is contraindicated in patients with unstable coronary artery disease because of increased risk of thrombotic events, such as myocardial infarction.[317] As above, patients receiving DDAVP at closely spaced intervals of less than 24 to 48 hours can develop tachyphylaxis.[312]

Many experts consider DDAVP to be contraindicated in the treatment of type 2B VWD, as the high-molecular-weight VWF released from storage sites has an increased affinity for binding to GPIb and might be expected to induce spontaneous platelet aggregation and worsening thrombocytopenia.[318] However, there are reports of DDAVP used successfully in type 2B VWD patients, with an associated shortening or correction of the bleeding time and variable thrombocytopenia.[319,320] Although type 2N patients can exhibit increased factor VIII:C levels after DDAVP, in some cases the factor VIII:C levels rapidly decline in the absence of stabilizing normal VWF, attenuating clinical efficacy. Type 2M patients generally do not have a satisfactory response to DDAVP.[321,322]

VWF REPLACEMENT THERAPY

It is important to determine the response to DDAVP for each individual in order to avoid the unnecessary use of plasma products. For type 3 VWD patients and other patients unresponsive to DDAVP, the use of selected virus-inactivated, VWF-containing factor VIII concentrates is generally safe and effective.[323] Cryoprecipitate has been successfully used in the past, but since it is not currently treated to inactivate viruses, it is less desirable. Solvent-detergent-treated plasma is available, and cryoprecipitate prepared from such plasma may be an appropriate choice. It is important to note that most standard factor VIII concentrates and all recombinant factor VIII products are not effective in VWD because they lack clinically significant quantities of VWF. Although such products can substantially increase circulating factor VIII:C, the infused factor is short-lived in the circulation in the absence of stabilizing VWF.[324] Only preparations that contain large quantities of VWF with well-preserved multimer structure are suitable for use in VWD patients. Humate-P and Alphanate are both acceptable commercial VWF-containing plasma concentrates that have been evaluated in VWD replacement therapy in clinical studies, although other VWF-containing factor VIII concentrates may also be effective (reviewed in reference 325).

In practice, VWD replacement therapy dosing and timing has been largely empiric. Recent recommendations for therapy have been outlined based upon the degree and nature of hemorrhage.[325,326] The recommended treatment goals are similar to the posttreatment factor VIII:C and VWF activity level goals currently used in clinical practice.[327] The objective is to elevate factor VIII:C and VWF activity until bleeding stops and healing is complete. In general, replacement goals of factor VIII:C and VWF activity should be greater than 50 to 80 percent for major trauma, surgery, or central nervous system hemorrhage, greater than 50 percent factor VIII:C and VWF activity for delivery and in the postpartum period, greater than 30 to 50 percent factor VIII:C and VWF activity for dental extractions and minor surgery, and 20 to 80 percent factor VIII:C and VWF activity for mucous membrane bleeding or menorrhagia. Laboratory monitoring of posttreatment factor VIII:C and VWF levels is important in guiding therapy and avoidance of supratherapeutic replacement doses (>200%), which have been associated with an increased risk of thrombosis.[328,329]

In patients who have concomitant thrombocytopenia associated with or in addition to VWD, it may be necessary to transfuse platelets in addition to factor VIII concentrates. If clinical bleeding continues, additional replacement therapy must be given and searches undertaken for other hemostatic defects.

Type 3 VWD patients receiving multiple transfusions can develop antibodies directed against VWF, and continued replacement with VWF-containing concentrates is contraindicated because of the risk of anaphylaxis.[330,331] A variety of approaches to the management of VWD inhibitors, similar to the treatment of factor VIII inhibitors in hemophilia A (see Chap. 124), have been tried. Immunosuppression, recombinant factor VIII, and recombinant factor VIIa have been reported to be useful in patients with type 3 VWD who have developed anti-VWF antibodies.

THERAPY DURING PREGNANCY

In pregnant patients with type 1 VWD, the factor VIII and ristocetin cofactor activities usually rise above 50 percent. These patients usually do not require any specific therapy at the time of parturition. In contrast, individuals who have 30 percent or less factor VIII or variant forms of VWD are more likely to require prophylactic therapy with DDAVP or plasma products before delivery. Postpartum hemorrhage within the first few days after parturition may be related to the relatively rapid return to pre-pregnancy levels of factor VIII and VWF activities, and postpartum hemorrhage in all forms of VWD may occur as long as 1 month postpartum. Therefore, laboratory monitoring is recommended at term and for 2 weeks postpartum to identify patients at risk for immediate and/or delayed bleeding complications.

NONREPLACEMENT THERAPIES

Estrogens or oral contraceptives have been used empirically in treating menorrhagia. In addition to their effects on the ovaries and uterus, estrogens also tend to increase plasma VWF levels. Patients with VWD frequently normalize their levels of factor VIII, VWF:Ag, and VWF:RCo during pregnancy. The mechanism of action of estrogens may be related in part to the increased production of VWF through a direct effect on endothelial cells.[332]

Fibrinolytic inhibitors, such as ε-aminocaproic acid or tranexamic acid, have been used effectively in some VWD patients. Antifibrinolytics are commonly used alone or in conjunction with DDAVP or a plasma-derived VWF replacement product in patients with mucous membrane bleeding or undergoing dental extraction.[333] Fibrinolytic inhibitors are generally well tolerated, but rarely can cause nausea or diarrhea and are contraindicated in patients with gross hematuria.

Recombinant activated factor VII (rFVIIa, or NovoSeven) has also been successfully used in VWD patients with severe hemorrhage refractory to VWF replacement therapy and in bleeding patients with anti-VWF antibodies (reviewed in reference 334). In the case of minor accessible bleeding, topical drugs such as fibrin sealants or topical bovine thrombin may also be considered when standard VWD therapies fail to provide adequate local hemostasis.[234]

REFERENCES

1. von Willebrand EA: Hereditär Pseudohemofili. *Fin Lakaresallsk Handl* 67:7, 1926.
2. Hoyer LW: Von Willebrand's disease. *Prog Hemost Thromb* 3:231, 1976.
3. Nilsson IM: Von Willebrand's disease—Fifty years old. *Acta Med Scand* 201:497, 1977.
4. Zimmerman TS, Ratnoff OD, Powell AE: Immunologic differentiation of classic hemophilia (Factor VIII deficiency) and von Willebrand disease. *J Clin Invest* 50:244, 1971.
5. Howard MA, Firkin BG: Ristocetin—A new tool in the investigation of platelet aggregation. *Thromb Diath Haemorrh* 76:362, 1971.
6. Weiss HJ, Rogers J, Brand H: Defective ristocetin-induced platelet aggregation in von Willebrand's disease and its correction by Factor VIII. *J Clin Invest* 52:2697, 1973.
7. Weiss HJ, Hoyer LW: Von Willebrand factor: Dissociation from antihemophilic factor procoagulant activity. *Science* 182:1149, 1973.
8. Zimmerman TS, Edgington TS: Factor VIII Coagulant activity and Factor VIII-like antigen: Independent molecular entities. *J Exp Med* 138:1015, 1973.
9. Gitschier J, Wood WI, Goralka TM, et al: Characterization of the human factor VIII gene. *Nature* 312:326, 1984.
10. Toole JJ, Knopf JL, Wozney JM, et al: Molecular cloning of a cDNA encoding human antihaemophilic factor. *Nature* 312:342, 1984.
11. Ginsburg D, Handin RI, Bonthron DT, et al: Human von Willebrand factor (vWF): Isolation of complementary DNA (cDNA) clones and chromosomal localization. *Science* 228:1401, 1985.
12. Lynch DC, Zimmerman TS, Collins CJ, et al: Molecular cloning of cDNA for human von Willebrand factor: Authentication by a new method. *Cell* 41:49, 1985.
13. Sadler JE, Shelton-Inloes BB, Sorace JM, et al: Cloning and characterization of two cDNAs coding for human von Willebrand factor. *Proc Natl Acad Sci U S A* 82:6394, 1985.
14. Verweij CL, de Vries CJM, Distel B, et al: Construction of cDNA coding for human von Willebrand factor using antibody probes for colony-screening and mapping of the chromosomal gene. *Nucleic Acids Res* 13:4699, 1985.
15. Sadler JE, Budde U, Eikenboom JC, et al: Update on the pathophysiology and classification of von Willebrand disease: A report of the Subcommittee on von Willebrand Factor. *J Thromb Haemost* 4:2103, 2006.
16. Titani K, Kumar S, Takio K, et al: Amino acid sequence of human von Willebrand Factor. *Biochemistry* 25:3171, 1986.
17. Fay PJ, Kawai Y, Wagner DD, et al: Propolypeptide of von Willebrand factor circulates in blood and is identical to von Willebrand antigen II. *Science* 232:995, 1986.
18. Bonthron DT, Handin RI, Kaufman RJ, et al: Structure of pre-pro-von Willebrand factor and its expression in heterologous cells. *Nature* 324:270, 1986.
19. Bonthron DT, Orr EC, Mitsock LM, et al: Nucleotide sequence of pre-pro-von Willebrand factor cDNA. *Nucleic Acids Res* 14:7125, 1986.
20. Shelton-Inloes BB, Broze GJ Jr, Miletich JP, Sadler JE: Evolution of human von Willebrand Factor: CDNA sequence polymorphisms, repeated domains, and relationship to von Willebrand antigen II. *Biochem Biophys Res Commun* 144:657, 1987.
21. Shelton-Inloes BB, Titani K, Sadler JE: CDNA sequences for human von Willebrand Factor reveal five types of repeated domains and five possible protein sequence polymorphisms. *Biochemistry* 25:3164, 1986.
22. Colombatti A, Bonaldo P: The superfamily of proteins with von Willebrand factor type A-like domains: One theme common to components of extracellular matrix, hemostasis, cellular adhesion, and defense mechanisms. *Blood* 77:2305, 1991.
23. Hunt LT, Barker WC: Von Willebrand factor shares a distinctive cysteine-rich domain with thrombospondin and procollagen. *Biochem Biophys Res Commun* 144:876, 1987.
24. Mancuso DJ, Tuley EA, Westfield LA, et al: Structure of the gene for human von Willebrand factor. *J Biol Chem* 264:19514, 1989.
25. Shelton-Inloes BB, Chehab FF, Mannucci PM, et al: Gene deletions correlate with the development of alloantibodies in von Willebrand Disease. *J Clin Invest* 79:1459, 1987.
26. Mancuso DJ, Tuley EA, Westfield LA, et al: Human von Willebrand factor gene and pseudogene: Structural analysis and differentiation by polymerase chain reaction. *Biochemistry* 30:253, 1991.
27. Zhang ZP, Blomback M, Nyman D, Anvret M: Mutations of von Willebrand factor gene in families with von Willebrand disease in the Aland Islands. *Proc Natl Acad Sci U S A* 90:7937, 1993.
28. Eikenboom JC, Vink T, Briet E, et al: Multiple substitutions in the von Willebrand factor gene that mimic the pseudogene sequence. *Proc Natl Acad Sci U S A* 91:2221, 1994.
29. Eikenboom JC, Castaman G, Vos HL, et al: Characterization of the genetic defects in recessive type 1 and type 3 von Willebrand disease patients of Italian origin. *Thromb Haemost* 79:709, 1998.
30. James PD, Notley C, Hegadorn C, et al: The mutational spectrum of type 1 von Willebrand disease: Results from a Canadian cohort study. *Blood* 109:145, 2007.
31. Rand JH, Badimon L, Gordon RE, et al: Distribution of von Willebrand factor in porcine intima varies with blood vessel type and location. *Arteriosclerosis* 7:287, 1987.
32. Yamamoto K, de Waard V, Fearns C, Loskutoff DJ: Tissue distribution and regulation of murine von Willebrand factor gene expression *in vivo*. *Blood* 92:2791, 1998.
33. Jahroudi N, Lynch DC: Endothelial-cell-specific regulation of von Willebrand factor gene expression. *Mol Cell Biol* 14:999, 1994.
34. Harvey PJ, Keightley AM, Lam YM, et al: A single nucleotide polymorphism at nucleotide -1793 in the von Willebrand factor (VWF) regulatory region is associated with plasma VWF:Ag levels. *Br J Haematol* 109:349, 2000.
35. Guan J, Guillot PV, Aird WC: Characterization of the mouse von Willebrand factor promoter. *Blood* 94:3405, 1999.
36. Hough C, Cuthbert CD, Notley C, et al: Cell type-specific regulation of von Willebrand factor expression by the E4BP4 transcriptional repressor. *Blood* 105:1531, 2005.
37. Kleinschmidt AM, Nassiri M, Stitt MS, et al: Sequences in intron 51 of the von Willebrand factor gene target promoter activation to a subset of lung endothelial cells in transgenic mice. *J Biol Chem* 283:2741, 2008.
38. Aird WC, Jahroudi N, Weiler-Guettler H, et al: Human von Willebrand factor gene sequences target expression to a subpopulation of endothelial cells in transgenic mice. *Proc Natl Acad Sci U S A* 92:4567, 1995.
39. Bernat JA, Crawford GE, Ogurtsov AY, et al: Distant conserved sequences flanking endothelial-specific promoters contain tissue-specific DNase-hypersensitive sites and over-represented motifs. *Hum Mol Genet* 15:2098, 2006.
40. Pusztaszeri MP, Seelentag W, Bosman FT: Immunohistochemical expression of endothelial markers CD31, CD34, von Willebrand factor, and Fli-1 in normal human tissues. *J Histochem Cytochem* 54:385, 2006.
41. Hough C, Cameron CL, Notley CR, et al: Influence of a GT repeat element on shear stress responsiveness of the VWF gene promoter. *J Thromb Haemost* 6:1183, 2008.
42. Daidone V, Cattini MG, Pontara E, et al: Microsatellite (GT)(n) repeats and SNPs in the von Willebrand factor gene promoter do not influence circulating von Willebrand factor levels under normal conditions. *Thromb Haemost* 101:298, 2009.
43. Ginsburg D, Bowie EJW: Molecular genetics of von Willebrand disease. *Blood* 79:2507, 1992.
44. Wagner DD: Cell biology of von Willebrand factor. *Annu Rev Cell Biol* 6:217, 1990.
45. de Wit TR, van Mourik JA: Biosynthesis, processing and secretion of von Willebrand factor: Biological implications. *Best Pract Res Clin Haematol* 14:241, 2001.
46. Marti T, Rosselet SJ, Titani K, Walsh KA: Identification of disulfide-bridged substructures within human von Willebrand factor. *Biochemistry* 26:8099, 1987.
47. Choi H, Aboulfatova K, Pownall HJ, et al: Shear-induced disulfide bond formation regulates adhesion activity of von Willebrand factor. *J Biol Chem* 282:35604, 2007.
48. Wagner DD, Lawrence SO, Ohlsson-Wilhelm BM, et al: Topology and order of formation of interchain disulfide bonds in von Willebrand factor. *Blood* 69:27, 1987.
49. Voorberg J, Fontijn R, Calafat J, et al: Assembly and routing of von Willebrand factor variants: The requirements for disulfide-linked dimerization reside within the carboxy-terminal 151 amino acids. *J Cell Biol* 113:195, 1991.
50. Mayadas TN, Wagner DD: Vicinal cysteines in the prosequence play a role in von Willebrand factor multimer assembly. *Proc Natl Acad Sci U S A* 89:3531, 1992.
51. Purvis AR, Sadler JE: A covalent oxidoreductase intermediate in propeptide-dependent von Willebrand factor multimerization. *J Biol Chem* 279:49982, 2004.
52. Mayadas TN, Wagner DD: In vitro multimerization of von Willebrand factor is triggered by low pH: Importance of the propolypeptide and free sulfhydryls. *J Biol Chem* 264:13497, 1989.
53. Wagner DD, Fay PJ, Sporn LA, et al: Divergent fates of von Willebrand factor and its propolypeptide (von Willebrand antigen II) after secretion from endothelial cells. *Proc Natl Acad Sci U S A* 84:1955, 1987.
54. Verweij CL, Hart M, Pannekoek H: Expression of variant von Willebrand factor (vWF) cDNA in heterologous cells: Requirement of the pro-polypeptide in vWF multimer formation. *EMBO J* 6:2885, 1987.
55. Wise RJ, Pittman DD, Handin RI, et al: The propeptide of von Willebrand factor independently mediates the assembly of von Willebrand multimers. *Cell* 52:229, 1988.
56. Rehemtulla A and Kaufman RJ: Preferred sequence requirements for cleavage of pro-von Willebrand propeptide-processing enzymes. *Blood* 79:2349, 1992.
57. Wagner DD, Marder VJ: Biosynthesis of von Willebrand protein by human endothelial cells: Processing steps and their intracellular localization. *J Cell Biol* 99:2123, 1984.
58. Lynch DC, Zimmerman TS, Ling EH, Browning PJ: An explanation for minor multimer species in endothelial cell-synthesized von Willebrand factor. *J Clin Invest* 77:2048, 1986.
59. Verweij CL, Hart M, Pannekoek H: Proteolytic cleavage of the precursor of von Willebrand Factor is not essential for multimer formation. *J Biol Chem* 263:7921, 1988.
60. Giblin JP, Hewlett LJ, Hannah MJ: Basal secretion of von Willebrand factor from human endothelial cells. *Blood* 112:957, 2008.
61. Weibel ER, Palade GE: New cytoplasmic components in arterial endothelia. *J Biol Chem* 23:101, 1964.
62. Wagner DD, Olmsted JB, Marder VJ: Immunolocalization of von Willebrand protein in Weibel-Palade bodies of human endothelial cells. *J Cell Biol* 95:355, 1982.
63. Metcalf DJ, Nightingale TD, Zenner HL, et al: Formation and function of Weibel-Palade bodies. *J Cell Sci* 121:19, 2008.

64. Huang RH, Wang Y, Roth R, et al: Assembly of Weibel-Palade body-like tubules from N-terminal domains of von Willebrand factor. *Proc Natl Acad Sci U S A* 105:482, 2008.
65. McCarroll DR, Levin EG, Montgomery RR: Endothelial cell synthesis of von Willebrand antigen II, von Willebrand factor, and von Willebrand factor/von Willebrand antigen II complex. *J Clin Invest* 75:1089, 1985.
66. Ewenstein BM, Warhol MJ, Handin RI, Pober JS: Composition of the von Willebrand factor storage organelle (Weibel-Palade body) isolated from cultured human umbilical vein endothelial cells. *J Cell Biol* 104:1423, 1987.
67. Yarovoi H, Nurden AT, Montgomery RR, et al: Intracellular interaction of von Willebrand factor and factor VIII depends on cellular context: Lessons from platelet-expressed factor VIII. *Blood* 105:4674, 2005.
68. Rosenberg JB, Foster PA, Kaufman RJ, et al: Intracellular trafficking of factor VIII to von Willebrand factor storage granules. *J Clin Invest* 101:613, 1998.
69. van den Biggelaar M, Bierings R, Storm G, et al: Requirements for cellular co-trafficking of factor VIII and von Willebrand factor to Weibel-Palade bodies. *J Thromb Haemost* 5:2235, 2007.
70. Nightingale TD, Pattni K, Hume AN, et al: Rab27a and MyRIP regulate the amount and multimeric state of VWF released from endothelial cells. *Blood* 14:5010, 2009.
71. Bonfanti R, Furie BC, Furie B, Wagner DD: PADGEM (GMP140) is a component of Weibel-Palade bodies of human endothelial cells. *Blood* 73:1109, 1989.
72. Michaux G, Pullen TJ, Haberichter SL, Cutler DF: P-selectin binds to the D′-D3 domains of von Willebrand factor in Weibel-Palade bodies. *Blood* 107:3922, 2006.
73. Cleator JH, Zhu WQ, Vaughan DE, Hamm HE: Differential regulation of endothelial exocytosis of P-selectin and von Willebrand factor by protease-activated receptors and cAMP. *Blood* 107:2736, 2006.
74. Knop M, Aareskjold E, Bode G, Gerke V: Rab3D and annexin A2 play a role in regulated secretion of vWF, but not tPA, from endothelial cells. *EMBO J* 23:2982, 2004.
75. Rondaij MG, Bierings R, Kragt A, et al: Dynamics and plasticity of Weibel-Palade bodies in endothelial cells. *Arterioscler Thromb Vasc Biol* 26:1002, 2006.
76. Levine JD, Harlan JM, Harker LA, et al: Thrombin-mediated release of factor VIII antigen from human umbilical vein endothelial cells in culture. *Blood* 60:531, 1982.
77. Ribes JA, Francis CW, Wagner DD: Fibrin induces release of von Willebrand factor from endothelial cells. *J Clin Invest* 79:117, 1987.
78. Hamilton KK, Sims PJ: Changes in cytosolic Ca^{2+} associated with von Willebrand factor release in human endothelial cells exposed to histamine. Study of microcarrier cell monolayers using the fluorescent probe indo-1. *J Clin Invest* 79:600, 1987.
79. Hattori R, Hamilton KK, McEver RP, Sims PJ: Complement proteins C5b-9 induce secretion of high molecular weight multimers of endothelial von Willebrand factor and translocation of granule membrane protein GMP-140 to the cell surface. *J Biol Chem* 264:9053, 1989.
80. Bernardo A, Ball C, Nolasco L, et al: Effects of inflammatory cytokines on the release and cleavage of the endothelial cell-derived ultralarge von Willebrand factor multimers under flow. *Blood* 104:100, 2004.
81. Fish RJ, Yang H, Viglino C, et al: Fluvastatin inhibits regulated secretion of endothelial cell von Willebrand factor in response to diverse secretagogues. *Biochem J* 405:597, 2007.
82. Yamakuchi M, Greer JJ, Cameron SJ, et al: HMG-CoA reductase inhibitors inhibit endothelial exocytosis and decrease myocardial infarct size. *Circ Res* 96:1185, 2005.
83. Kaufmann JE, Oksche A, Wollheim CB, et al: Vasopressin-induced von Willebrand factor secretion from endothelial cells involves V2 receptors and cAMP. *J Clin Invest* 106:107, 2000.
84. Sporn LA, Marder VJ, Wagner DD: Differing polarity of the constitutive and regulated secretory pathways for von Willebrand factor in endothelial cells. *J Cell Biol* 108:1283, 1989.
85. Sporn LA, Marder VJ, Wagner DD: Inducible secretion of large, biologically potent von Willebrand factor multimers. *Cell* 46:185, 1986.
86. Fernandez MF, Ginsberg MH, Ruggeri ZM, et al: Multimeric structure of platelet factor VIII/von Willebrand factor: The presence of larger multimers and their reassociation with thrombin-stimulated platelets. *Blood* 60:1132, 1982.
87. Wagner DD, Saffaripour S, Bonfanti R, et al: Induction of specific storage organelles by von Willebrand factor propolypeptide. *Cell* 64:403, 1991.
88. Voorberg J, Fontijn R, Calafat J, et al: Biogenesis of Von Willebrand factor-containing organelles in heterologous transfected CV-1 cells. *EMBO J* 12:749, 1993.
89. Journet AM, Saffaripour S, Cramer EM, et al: Von Willebrand factor storage requires intact prosequence cleavage site. *Eur J Cell Biol* 60:31, 1993.
90. Nachman RL, Jaffe EA: Subcellular platelet factor VIII antigen and von Willebrand factor. *J Exp Med* 141:1101, 1975.
91. Bowie EJW, Solberg LA Jr, Fass DN, et al: Transplantation of normal bone marrow into a pig with severe von Willebrand's disease. *J Clin Invest* 78:26, 1986.
92. Nichols TC, Samama CM, Bellinger DA, et al: Function of von Willebrand factor after crossed bone marrow transplantation between normal and von Willebrand disease pigs: Effect on arterial thrombosis in chimeras. *Proc Natl Acad Sci U S A* 92:2455, 1995.
93. André P, Brouland JP, Roussi J, et al: Role of plasma and platelet von Willebrand factor in arterial thrombogenesis and hemostasis in the pig. *Exp Hematol* 26:620, 1998.
94. Bowen DJ and Collins PW: Insights into von Willebrand factor proteolysis: Clinical implications. *Br J Haematol* 133:457, 2006.
95. Padilla A, Moake JL, Bernardo A, et al: P-selectin anchors newly released ultralarge von Willebrand factor multimers to the endothelial cell surface. *Blood* 103:2150, 2004.
96. Lopez JA, Dong JF: Shear stress and the role of high molecular weight von Willebrand factor multimers in thrombus formation. *Blood Coagul Fibrinolysis* 16(Suppl 1):S11, 2005.
97. Dent JA, Berkowitz SD, Ware J, et al: Identification of a cleavage site directing the immunochemical detection of molecular abnormalities in type IIA von Willebrand factor. *Proc Natl Acad Sci U S A* 87:6306, 1990.
98. Lankhof H, Damas C, Schiphorst ME, et al: Von Willebrand factor without the A2 domain is resistant to proteolysis. *Thromb Haemost* 77:1008, 1997.
99. Tsai HM, Sussman II, Ginsburg D, et al: Proteolytic cleavage of recombinant type 2A von Willebrand factor mutants R834W and R834Q: Inhibition by doxycycline and by monoclonal antibody VP-1. *Blood* 89:1954, 1997.
100. Bowen DJ, Collins PW: An amino acid polymorphism in von Willebrand factor correlates with increased susceptibility to proteolysis by ADAMTS13. *Blood* 103:941, 2004.
101. Bowen DJ: Increased susceptibility of von Willebrand factor to proteolysis by ADAMTS13: Should the multimer profile be normal or type 2A? *Blood* 103:3246, 2004.
102. Johnsen J, Lopez JA: VWF secretion: What's in a name? *Blood* 112:926, 2008.
103. Reininger AJ: Function of von Willebrand factor in haemostasis and thrombosis. *Haemophilia* 14 Suppl 5:11, 2008.
104. Savage B, Saldívar E, Ruggeri ZM: Initiation of platelet adhesion by arrest onto fibrinogen or translocation on von Willebrand factor. *Cell* 84:289, 1996.
105. Savage B, Almus-Jacobs F, Ruggeri ZM: Specific synergy of multiple substrate-receptor interactions in platelet thrombus formation under flow. *Cell* 94:657, 1998.
106. Pendu R, Terraube V, Christophe OD, et al: P-selectin glycoprotein ligand 1 and beta2-integrins cooperate in the adhesion of leukocytes to von Willebrand factor. *Blood* 108:3746, 2006.
107. Ruggeri ZM, Ware J, Ginsburg D: von Willebrand factor, in *Thrombosis and Hemorrhage*, 3rd ed, edited by J Loscalzo, AI Schafer, p 246. Lippincott Williams & Wilkins, Philadelphia, 2003.
108. Kalafatis M, Takahashi Y, Girma J-P, Meyer D: Localization of a collagen-interactive domain of human von Willebrand factor between amino acid residues Gly 911 and Glu 1365. *Blood* 70:1577, 1987.
109. Pareti FI, Niiya K, McPherson JM, Ruggeri ZM: Isolation and characterization of two domains of human von Willebrand Factor that interact with fibrillar collagen types I and III. *J Biol Chem* 262:13835, 1987.
110. Takagi J, Sekiya F, Kasahara K, et al: Inhibition of platelet-collagen interaction by propolypeptide of von Willebrand factor. *J Biol Chem* 264:6017, 1989.
111. Cruz MA, Yuan H, Lee JR, et al: Interaction of the von Willebrand factor (vWF) with collagen. Localization of the primary collagen-binding site by analysis of recombinant vWF A domain polypeptides. *J Biol Chem* 270:10822, 1995.
112. Lankhof H, Van Hoeij M, Schiphorst ME, et al: A3 domain is essential for interaction of von Willebrand factor with collagen type III. *Thromb Haemost* 75:950, 1996.
113. Wagner DD, Urban-Pickering M, Marder VJ: Von Willebrand protein binds to extracellular matrices independently of collagen. *Proc Natl Acad Sci U S A* 81:471, 1984.
114. Rand JH, Patel ND, Schwartz E, et al: 150-kD von Willebrand factor binding protein extracted from human vascular subendothelium is Type VI collagen. *J Clin Invest* 88:253, 1991.
115. Rand JH, Wu X-X, Potter BJ, et al: Co-localization of von Willebrand factor and type VI collagen in human vascular subendothelium. *Am J Pathol* 142:843, 1993.
116. Mazzucato M, Spessotto P, Masotti A, et al: Identification of domains responsible for von Willebrand factor type VI collagen interaction mediating platelet adhesion under high flow. *J Biol Chem* 274:3033, 1999.
117. Fretto LJ, Fowler WE, McCaslin DR, et al: Substructure of human von Willebrand factor: Proteolysis by V8 and characterization of two functional domains. *J Biol Chem* 261:15679, 1986.
118. Fujimura Y, Titani K, Holland LZ, et al: A heparin-binding domain of human von Willebrand factor. Characterization and localization to a tryptic fragment extending from amino acid residue Val^{449} to Lys^{728}. *J Biol Chem* 262:1734, 1987.
119. Christophe O, Obert B, Meyer D, Girma J-P: The binding domain of von Willebrand factor to sulfatides is distinct from those interacting with glycoprotein Ib, heparin, collagen and residues between amino acid residues Leu 512 and Lys 673. *Blood* 78:2310, 1991.
120. Marchese P, Murata M, Mazzucato M, et al: Identification of three tyrosine residues of glycoprotein IBα with distinct roles in von Willebrand factor and α-thrombin binding. *J Biol Chem* 270:9571, 1995.
121. Fujimura Y, Titani K, Holland LZ, et al: von Willebrand factor: A reduced and alkylated 52/48-kDa fragment beginning at amino acid residue 449 contains the domain interacting with platelet glycoprotein Ib. *J Biol Chem* 261:381, 1986.
122. Mohri H, Fujimura Y, Shima M, et al: Structure of the von Willebrand factor domain interacting with glycoprotein Ib. *J Biol Chem* 263:17901, 1988.
123. Nishio K, Anderson PJ, Zheng XL, Sadler JE: Binding of platelet glycoprotein Ibalpha to von Willebrand factor domain A1 stimulates the cleavage of the adjacent domain A2 by ADAMTS13. *Proc Natl Acad Sci U S A* 101:10578, 2004.
124. Matsushita T, Sadler JE: Identification of amino acid residues essential for von Willebrand factor binding to platelet glycoprotein Ib. Charged-to-alanine scanning mutagenesis of the A1 domain of human von Willebrand factor. *J Biol Chem* 270:13406, 1995.
125. Emsley J, Cruz M, Handin RI, Liddington R: Crystal structure of the von Willebrand factor A1 domain and implications for the binding of platelet glycoprotein Ib. *J Biol Chem* 273:10396, 1998.

126. Bienkowska J, Cruz M, Atiemo A, et al: The von Willebrand factor A3 domain does not contain a metal ion-dependent adhesion site motif. *J Biol Chem* 272:25162, 1997.
127. Huizinga EG, Van der Plas RM, Kroon J, et al: Crystal structure of the A3 domain of human von Willebrand factor: Implications for collagen binding. *Structure* 5:1147, 1997.
128. Fukuda K, Doggett TA, Bankston LA, et al: Structural basis of von Willebrand factor activation by the snake toxin botrocetin. *Structure* 10:943, 2002.
129. Huizinga EG, Tsuji S, Romijn RA, et al: Structures of glycoprotein Ibalpha and its complex with von Willebrand factor A1 domain. *Science* 297:1176, 2002.
130. Hulstein JJ, Lenting PJ, de Laat B, et al: Beta2-glycoprotein I inhibits von Willebrand factor dependent platelet adhesion and aggregation. *Blood* 110:1483, 2007.
131. Scott JP, Montgomery RR, Retzinger GS: Dimeric ristocetin flocculates proteins, binds to platelets, and mediates von Willebrand factor-dependent agglutination of platelets. *J Biol Chem* 266:8149, 1991.
132. Berndt MC, Du XP, Booth WJ: Ristocetin-dependent reconstitution of binding of von Willebrand factor to purified human platelet membrane glycoprotein Ib-IX complex. *Biochemistry* 27:633, 1988.
133. Adachi T, Matsushita T, Dong Z, et al: Identification of amino acid residues essential for heparin binding by the A1 domain of human von Willebrand factor. *Biochem Biophys Res Commun* 339:1178, 2006.
134. Sobel M, McNeill PM, Carlson PL, et al: Heparin inhibition of von Willebrand factor-dependent platelet function *in vitro* and *in vivo*. *J Clin Invest* 87:1787, 1991.
135. Sobel M, Bird KE, Tyler-Cross R, et al: Heparins designed to specifically inhibit platelet interactions with von Willebrand factor. *Circulation* 93:992, 1996.
136. Nishio K, Anderson PJ, Zheng XL, Sadler JE: Binding of platelet glycoprotein Ibalpha to von Willebrand factor domain A1 stimulates the cleavage of the adjacent domain A2 by ADAMTS13. *Proc Natl Acad Sci U S A* 101:10578, 2004.
137. Keuren JF, Baruch D, Legendre P, et al: Von Willebrand factor C1C2 domain is involved in platelet adhesion to polymerized fibrin at high shear rate. *Blood* 103:1741, 2004.
138. Vlot AJ, Koppelman SJ, Van den Berg MH, et al: The affinity and stoichiometry of binding of human factor VIII to von Willebrand factor. *Blood* 85:3150, 1995.
139. Sadler JE: Biochemistry and genetics of von Willebrand factor. *Annu Rev Biochem* 67:395, 1998.
140. Vlot AJ, Koppelman SJ, Bouma BN, Sixma JJ: Factor VIII and von Willebrand factor. *Thromb Haemost* 79:456, 1998.
141. Cao W, Krishnaswamy S, Camire RM, et al: Factor VIII accelerates proteolytic cleavage of von Willebrand factor by ADAMTS13. *Proc Natl Acad Sci U S A* 105:7416, 2008.
142. Foster PA, Fulcher CA, Marti T, et al: A major factor VIII binding domain resides within the amino-terminal 272 amino acid residues of von Willebrand factor. *J Biol Chem* 262:8443, 1987.
143. Bahou WF, Ginsburg D, Sikkink R, et al: A monoclonal antibody to von Willebrand factor (vWF) inhibits factor VIII binding. Localization of its antigenic determinant to a nonadecapeptide at the amino terminus of the mature vWF polypeptide. *J Clin Invest* 84:56, 1989.
144. Ginsburg D, Bockenstedt PL, Allen EA, et al: Fine mapping of monoclonal antibody epitopes on human von Willebrand factor using a recombinant peptide library. *Thromb Haemost* 67:166, 1992.
145. Mazurier C: Von Willebrand disease masquerading as haemophilia A. *Thromb Haemost* 67:391, 1992.
146. Cacheris PM, Nichols WC, Ginsburg D: Molecular characterization of a unique von Willebrand disease variant. A novel mutation affecting von Willebrand factor/factor VIII interaction. *J Biol Chem* 266:13499, 1991.
147. Lollar P, Hill-Eubanks DC, Parker CG: Association of the factor VIII light chain with von Willebrand factor. *J Biol Chem* 263:10451, 1988.
148. Leyte A, van Schijndel HB, Niehrs C, et al: Sulfation of Tyr^{1680} of human blood coagulation factor VIII is essential for the interaction of factor VIII with von Willebrand factor. *J Biol Chem* 266:740, 1991.
149. Nichols WC and Ginsburg D: von Willebrand disease. *Medicine (Baltimore)* 76:1, 1997.
150. Nichols WC, Cooney KA, Ginsburg D, Ruggeri ZM: von Willebrand disease, in *Thrombosis and Hemorrhage,* 3rd ed, edited by J Loscalzo, AI Schafer, p 539. Lippincott Williams & Wilkins, Philadelphia, 2003.
151. Weiss HJ, Piétu G, Rabinowitz R, et al: Heterogeneous abnormalities in the multimeric structure, antigenic properties, and plasma-platelet content of factor VIII/von Willebrand factor in subtypes of classic (type I) and variant (type IIA) von Willebrand's disease. *J Lab Clin Med* 101:411, 1983.
152. Hoyer LW, Rizza CR, Tuddenham EGD, et al: Von Willebrand factor multimer patterns in von Willebrand's disease. *Br J Haematol* 55:493, 1983.
153. Mannucci PM, Lombardi R, Bader R, et al: Heterogeneity of type I von Willebrand disease: Evidence for a subgroup with an abnormal von Willebrand factor. *Blood* 66:796, 1985.
154. Mannucci PM: Platelet von Willebrand factor in inherited and acquired bleeding disorders. *Proc Natl Acad Sci U S A* 92:2428, 1995.
155. Ngo KY, Glotz VT, Koziol JA, et al: Homozygous and heterozygous deletions of the von Willebrand factor gene in patients and carriers of severe von Willebrand Disease. *Proc Natl Acad Sci U S A* 85:2753, 1988.
156. Peake IR, Liddell MB, Moodie P, et al: Severe type III von Willebrand's disease caused by deletion of Exon 42 of the von Willebrand factor gene: Family studies that identify carriers of the condition and a compound heterozygous individual. *Blood* 75:654, 1990.
157. Nichols WC, Lyons SE, Harrison JS, et al: Severe von Willebrand disease due to a defect at the level of von Willebrand factor mRNA expression: Detection by exonic PCR-restriction fragment length polymorphism analysis. *Proc Natl Acad Sci U S A* 88:3857, 1991.
158. Eikenboom JCJ, Ploos van Amstel HK, Reitsma PH, Briët E: Mutations in severe, type III von Willebrand's disease in the Dutch population: Candidate missense and nonsense mutations associated with reduced levels of von Willebrand factor messenger RNA. *Thromb Haemost* 68:448, 1992.
159. Goodeve A, Eikenboom J, Castaman G, et al: Phenotype and genotype of a cohort of families historically diagnosed with type 1 von Willebrand disease in the European study, Molecular and Clinical Markers for the Diagnosis and Management of Type 1 von Willebrand Disease (MCMDM-1VWD). *Blood* 109:112, 2007.
160. Mohlke KL, Ginsburg D: von Willebrand disease and quantitative deficiency of von Willebrand factor. *J Lab Clin Med* 130:252, 1997.
161. Eikenboom JCJ, Matsushita T, Reitsma PH, et al: Dominant type 1 von Willebrand disease caused by mutated cysteine residues in the D3 domain of von Willebrand factor. *Blood* 88:2433, 1996.
162. Bodo I, Katsumi A, Tuley EA, et al: Type 1 von Willebrand disease mutation Cys1149Arg causes intracellular retention and degradation of heterodimers: A possible general mechanism for dominant mutations of oligomeric proteins. *Blood* 98:2973, 2001.
163. Millar CM, Riddell AF, Brown SA, et al: Survival of von Willebrand factor released following DDAVP in a type 1 von Willebrand disease cohort: Influence of glycosylation, proteolysis and gene mutations. *Thromb Haemost* 99:916, 2008.
164. O'Brien LA, James PD, Othman M, et al: Founder von Willebrand factor haplotype associated with type 1 von Willebrand disease. *Blood* 102:549, 2003.
165. Bowen D: Type 1 von Willebrand disease: A possible novel mechanism. *Blood Coagul Fibrinolysis* 15 Suppl 1:S21, 2004.
166. Bowen DJ, Collins PW, Lester W, et al: The prevalence of the cysteine1584 variant of von Willebrand factor is increased in type 1 von Willebrand disease: Co-segregation with increased susceptibility to ADAMTS13 proteolysis but not clinical phenotype. *Br J Haematol* 128:830, 2005.
167. Davies JA, Collins PW, Hathaway LS, Bowen DJ: von Willebrand factor: Evidence for variable clearance in vivo according to Y/C1584 phenotype and ABO blood group. *J Thromb Haemost* 6:97, 2008.
168. Keeney S, Grundy P, Collins PW, Bowen DJ: C1584 in von Willebrand factor is necessary for enhanced proteolysis by ADAMTS13 *in vitro*. *Haemophilia* 13:405, 2007.
169. Castaman G, Eikenboom JC, Bertina RM, Rodeghiero F: Inconsistency of association between type 1 von Willebrand disease phenotype and genotype in families identified in an epidemiological investigation. *Thromb Haemost* 82:1065, 1999.
170. Kunicki TJ, Federici AB, Salomon DR, et al: An association of candidate gene haplotypes and bleeding severity in von Willebrand disease (VWD) type 1 pedigrees. *Blood* 104:2359, 2004.
171. Kunicki TJ, Baronciani L, Canciani MT, et al: An association of candidate gene haplotypes and bleeding severity in von Willebrand disease type 2A, 2B, and 2M pedigrees. *J Thromb Haemost* 4:137, 2006.
172. Mohlke KL, Purkayastha AA, Westrick RJ, et al: *Mvwf*, a dominant modifier of murine von Willebrand factor, results from altered lineage-specific expression of a glycosyltransferase. *Cell* 96:111, 1999.
173. McKinnon TA, Chion AC, Millington AJ, et al: N-linked glycosylation of VWF modulates its interaction with ADAMTS13. *Blood* 111:3042, 2008.
174. O'Donnell JS, McKinnon TA, Crawley JT, et al: Bombay phenotype is associated with reduced plasma-VWF levels and an increased susceptibility to ADAMTS13 proteolysis. *Blood* 106:1988, 2005.
175. Bowen DJ: An influence of ABO blood group on the rate of proteolysis of von Willebrand factor by ADAMTS13. *J Thromb Haemost* 1:33, 2003.
176. Gallinaro L, Cattini MG, Sztukowska M, et al: A shorter von Willebrand factor survival in O blood group subjects explains how ABO determinants influence plasma von Willebrand factor. *Blood* 111:3540, 2008.
177. Sadler JE: Von Willebrand disease type 1: A diagnosis in search of a disease. *Blood* 101:2089, 2003.
178. Sadler JE: New concepts in von Willebrand disease. *Annu Rev Med* 56:173, 2005.
179. Zimmerman TS, Abildgaard CF, Meyer D: The factor VIII abnormality in severe von Willebrand's disease. *N Engl J Med* 301:1307, 1979.
180. Mancuso DJ, Tuley EA, Castillo R, et al: Characterization of partial gene deletions in type III von Willebrand disease with alloantibody inhibitors. *Thromb Haemost* 72:180, 1994.
181. Xie F, Wang X, Cooper DN, et al: A novel Alu-mediated 61-kb deletion of the von Willebrand factor (VWF) gene whose breakpoints co-locate with putative matrix attachment regions. *Blood Cells Mol Dis* 36:385, 2006.
182. Ginsburg D, Sadler JE: von Willebrand disease: A database of point mutations, insertions, and deletions. *Thromb Haemost* 69:177, 1993.
183. Eikenboom JCJ, Castaman G, Vos HL, et al: Characterization of the genetic defects in recessive type 1 and type 3 von Willebrand disease patients of Italian origin. *Thromb Haemost* 79:709, 1998.
184. Zhang ZP, Falk G, Blombäck M, et al: A single cytosine deletion in exon 18 of the von Willebrand factor gene is the most common mutation in Swedish vWD type III patients. *Hum Mol Genet* 1:767, 1992.

185. Zhang ZP, Blombäck M, Nyman D, Anvret M: Mutations of von Willebrand factor gene in families with von Willebrand disease in the Åland Islands. *Proc Natl Acad Sci U S A* 90:7937, 1993.
186. Mohlke KL, Nichols WC, Rehemtulla A, et al: A common frameshift mutation in von Willebrand factor does not alter mRNA stability but interferes with normal propeptide processing. *Br J Haematol* 95:184, 1996.
187. Schneppenheim R, Krey S, Bergmann F, et al: Genetic heterogeneity of severe von Willebrand disease type III in the German population. *Hum Genet* 94:640, 1994.
188. Berkowitz SD, Dent JA, Roberts J, et al: Epitope mapping of the von Willebrand factor subunit distinguishes fragments present in normal and type IIA von Willebrand Disease from those generated by plasmin. *J Clin Invest* 79:524, 1987.
189. Ginsburg D, Konkle BA, Gill JC, et al: Molecular basis of human von Willebrand disease: Analysis of platelet von Willebrand factor mRNA. *Proc Natl Acad Sci U S A* 86:3723, 1989.
190. Hassenpflug WA, Budde U, Obser T, et al: Impact of mutations in the von Willebrand factor A2 domain on ADAMTS13-dependent proteolysis. *Blood* 107:2339, 2006.
191. Lyons SE, Bruck ME, Bowie EJW, Ginsburg D: Impaired intracellular transport produced by a subset of type IIA von Willebrand disease mutations. *J Biol Chem* 267:4424, 1992.
192. Dent JA, Galbusera M, Ruggeri ZM: Heterogeneity of plasma von Willebrand factor multimers resulting from proteolysis of the constituent subunit. *J Clin Invest* 88:774, 1991.
193. Gralnick HR, Williams SB, McKeown LP, et al: *In vitro* correction of the abnormal multimeric structure of von Willebrand factor in Type IIA von Willebrand's disease. *Proc Natl Acad Sci U S A* 82:5968, 1985.
194. Kunicki TJ, Montgomery RR, Schullek J: Cleavage of human von Willebrand factor by platelet calcium-activated protease. *Blood* 65:352, 1985.
195. Bowen DJ: Increased susceptibility of von Willebrand factor to proteolysis by ADAMTS13: Should the multimer profile be normal or type 2A? *Blood* 103:3246, 2004.
196. Chung DW, Fujikawa K: Processing of von Willebrand Factor by ADAMTS-13. *Biochemistry* 41:11065, 2003.
197. Schneppenheim R, Thomas KB, Krey S, et al: Identification of a candidate missense mutation in a family with von Willebrand disease type IIC. *Hum Genet* 95:681, 1995.
198. Gaucher C, Diéval J, Mazurier C: Characterization of von Willebrand factor gene defects in two unrelated patients with type IIC von Willebrand disease. *Blood* 84:1024, 1994.
199. Schneppenheim R, Brassard J, Krey S, et al: Defective dimerization of von Willebrand factor subunits due to a Cys→Arg mutation in type IID von Willebrand disease. *Proc Natl Acad Sci U S A* 93:3581, 1996.
200. Cooney KA, Nichols WC, Bruck ME, et al: The molecular defect in type IIB von Willebrand disease. Identification of four potential missense mutations within the putative GPIb binding domain. *J Clin Invest* 87:1227, 1991.
201. Ribba AS, Lavergne JM, Bahnak BR, et al: Duplication of a methionine within the glycoprotein Ib binding domain of von Willebrand factor detected by denaturing gradient gel electrophoresis in a patient with type IIB von Willebrand disease. *Blood* 78:1738, 1991.
202. Cooney KA, Ginsburg D: Comparative analysis of type 2B von Willebrand disease mutations: Implications for the mechanism of von Willebrand factor to binding platelets. *Blood* 87:2322, 1996.
203. Cooney KA, Lyons SE, Ginsburg D: Functional analysis of a type IIB von Willebrand disease missense mutation: Increased binding of large von Willebrand factor multimers to platelets. *Proc Natl Acad Sci U S A* 89:2869, 1992.
204. Ware J, Dent JA, Azuma H, et al: Identification of a point mutation in type IIB von Willebrand disease illustrating the regulation of von Willebrand factor affinity for the platelet membrane glycoprotein Ib-IX receptor. *Proc Natl Acad Sci U S A* 88:2946, 1991.
205. Kroner PA, Kluessendorf ML, Scott JP, Montgomery RR: Expressed full-length von Willebrand factor containing missense mutations linked to type IIB von Willebrand disease shows enhanced binding to platelets. *Blood* 79:2048, 1992.
206. Randi AM, Jorieux S, Tuley EA, et al: Recombinant von Willebrand factor Arg578Gln: A type IIB von Willebrand disease mutation affects binding to glycoprotein Ib but not to collagen or heparin. *J Biol Chem* 267:21187, 1992.
207. Holmberg L, Dent JA, Schneppenheim R, et al: Von Willebrand factor mutation enhancing interaction with platelets in patients with normal multimeric structure. *J Clin Invest* 91:2169, 1993.
208. Veltkamp JJ, van Tilburg NH: Autosomal haemophilia: A variant of von Willebrand's disease. *Br J Haematol* 26:141, 1974.
209. Graham JB, Barrow ES, Roberts HR, et al: Dominant inheritance of hemophilia A in three generations of women. *Blood* 46:175, 1975.
210. Mazurier C, Gaucher C, Jorieux S, et al: Evidence for a von Willebrand factor defect in factor VIII binding in three members of a family previously misdiagnosed mild haemophilia A and haemophilia A carriers: Consequences for therapy and genetic counselling. *Br J Haematol* 76:372, 1990.
211. Mazurier C, Diéval J, Jorieux S, et al: A new von Willebrand Factor (vWF) defect in a patient with factor VIII (FVIII) deficiency but with normal levels and multimeric patterns of both plasma and platelet vWF. Characterization of abnormal vWF/FVIII interaction. *Blood* 75:20, 1990.
212. Nishino M, Girma J-P, Rothschild C, et al: New variant of von Willebrand disease with defective binding to factor VIII. *Blood* 74:1591, 1989.
213. Eikenboom JCJ, Reitsma PH, Peerlinck KMJ, Briët E: Recessive inheritance of von Willebrand's disease type I. *Lancet* 341:982, 1993.
214. Rabinowitz I, Tuley EA, Mancuso DJ, et al: von Willebrand disease type B: A missense mutation selectively abolishes ristocetin-induced von Willebrand factor binding to platelet glycoprotein Ib. *Proc Natl Acad Sci U S A* 89:9846, 1992.
215. Meyer D, Fressinaud E, Gaucher C, et al: Gene defects in 150 unrelated French cases with type 2 von Willebrand disease: From the patient to the gene. *Thromb Haemost* 78:451, 1997.
216. Mannucci PM, Lombardi R, Castaman G, et al: von Willebrand disease "Vicenza" with larger-than-normal (supranormal) von Willebrand factor multimers. *Blood* 71:65, 1988.
217. Randi AM, Sacchi E, Castaman GC, et al: The genetic defect of type I von Willebrand disease "Vicenza" is linked to the von Willebrand factor gene. *Thromb Haemost* 69:173, 1993.
218. Casonato A, Pontara E, Sartorello F, et al: Reduced von Willebrand factor survival in type Vicenza von Willebrand disease. *Blood* 99:180, 2002.
219. Castaman G, Rodeghiero F, Mannucci PM: The elusive pathogenesis of von Willebrand disease Vicenza. *Blood* 99:4243, 2002.
220. Berkowitz SD, Ruggeri ZM, Zimmerman TS: von Willebrand disease, in *Coagulation and Bleeding Disorders. The Role of Factor VIII and von Willebrand Factor,* edited by TS Zimmerman, ZM Ruggeri, p 215. Marcel Dekker, New York, 1989.
221. Rodeghiero F, Castaman G, Dini E: Epidemiological investigation of the prevalence of von Willebrand's disease. *Blood* 69:454, 1987.
222. Werner EJ, Broxson EH, Tucker EL, et al: Prevalence of von Willebrand disease in children: A multiethnic study. *J Pediatr* 123:893, 1993.
223. Miller CH, Graham JB, Goldin LR, Elston RC: Genetics of classic von Willebrand's disease. I. Phenotypic variation within families. *Blood* 54:117, 1979.
224. Gill JC, Endres-Brooks J, Bauer PJ, et al: The effect of ABO blood group on the diagnosis of von Willebrand Disease. *Blood* 69:1691, 1987.
225. Orstavik KH, Kornstad L, Reisner H, Berg K: Possible effect of secretor locus on plasma concentration of Factor VIII and von Willebrand factor. *Blood* 73:990, 1989.
226. O'Donnell J, Boulton FE, Manning RA, Laffan MA: Genotype at the secretor blood group locus is a determinant of plasma von Willebrand factor level. *Br J Haematol* 116:350, 2002.
227. Millar CM and Brown SA: Oligosaccharide structures of von Willebrand factor and their potential role in von Willebrand disease. *Blood Rev* 20:83, 2006.
228. Souto JC, Almasy L, Soria JM, et al: Genome-wide linkage analysis of von Willebrand factor plasma levels: Results from the GAIT project. *Thromb Haemost* 89:468, 2003.
229. Sadler JE: Von Willebrand disease type 1: A diagnosis in search of a disease. *Blood* 101:2089, 2003.
230. Weiss HJ, Ball AP, Mannucci PM: Incidence of severe von Willebrand's disease. *N Engl J Med* 307:127, 1982.
231. Berliner SA, Seligsohn U, Zivelin A, et al: A relatively high frequency of severe (type III) von Willebrand's disease in Israel. *Br J Haematol* 62:535, 1986.
232. Mannucci PM, Bloom AL, Larrieu MJ, et al: Atherosclerosis and von Willebrand factor. I. Prevalence of severe von Willebrand's disease in western Europe and Israel. *Br J Haematol* 57:163, 1984.
233. Nosek-Cenkowska B, Cheang MS, Pizzi NJ, et al: Bleeding/bruising symptomatology in children with and without bleeding disorders. *Thromb Haemost* 65:237, 1991.
234. Nichols WL, Hultin MB, James AH, et al: von Willebrand disease (VWD): Evidence-based diagnosis and management guidelines, the National Heart, Lung, and Blood Institute (NHLBI) Expert Panel report (USA). *Haemophilia* 14:171, 2008.
235. Silwer J: von Willebrand's disease in Sweden. *Acta Paediatr Scand Suppl* 238:1, 1973.
236. van den Driesche S, Mummery CL, Westermann CJ: Hereditary hemorrhagic telangiectasia: An update on transforming growth factor beta signaling in vasculogenesis and angiogenesis. *Cardiovasc Res* 58:20, 2003.
237. Iannuzzi MC, Hidaka N, Boehnke ML, et al: Analysis of the relationship of von Willebrand disease (vWD) and hereditary hemorrhagic telangiectasia and identification of a potential type IIA vWD mutation (IIe865 to Thr). *Am J Hum Genet* 48:757, 1991.
238. Rick ME, Williams SB, Sacher RA, McKeown LP: Thrombocytopenia associated with pregnancy in a patient with type IIB von Willebrand's disease. *Blood* 69:786, 1987.
239. Mazurier C, Parquet-Gernez A, Goudemand J, et al: Investigation of a large kindred with type IIB von Willebrand's disease, dominant inheritance and age-dependent thrombocytopenia. *Br J Haematol* 69:499, 1988.
240. Schneppenheim R, Budde U, Krey S, et al: Results of a screening for von Willebrand disease type 2N in patients with suspected haemophilia A or von Willebrand disease type 1. *Thromb Haemost* 76:598, 1996.
241. Asatiani E, Kessler CM: Multiple congenital coagulopathies co-expressed with Von Willebrand's disease: The experience of Hemophilia Region III Treatment Centers over 25 years and review of the literature. *Haemophilia* 13:685, 2007.
242. Rodeghiero F, Castaman G, Tosetto A: Von Willebrand factor antigen is less sensitive than ristocetin cofactor for the diagnosis of Type I von Willebrand disease—Results based on a epidemiological investigation. *Thromb Haemost* 64:349, 1990.
243. Lippi G, Franchini M, Poli G, et al: Is the activated partial thromboplastin time suitable to screen for von Willebrand factor deficiencies? *Blood Coagul Fibrinolysis* 18:361, 2007.
244. Abildgaard CF, Suzuki Z, Harrison J, et al: Serial studies in von Willebrand's disease: Variability versus "variants." *Blood* 56:712, 1980.

245. Weiss HJ, Hoyer LW, Rickles FR, et al: Quantitative assay of a plasma factor deficient in von Willebrand's disease that is necessary for platelet aggregation. *J Clin Invest* 52:2708, 1973.
246. Murdock PJ, Woodhams BJ, Matthews KB, et al: Von Willebrand factor activity detected in a monoclonal antibody-based ELISA: An alternative to the ristocetin cofactor platelet agglutination assay for diagnostic use. *Thromb Haemost* 78:1272, 1997.
247. Federici AB, Canciani MT, Forza I, et al: A sensitive ristocetin co-factor activity assay with recombinant glycoprotein Ibalpha for the diagnosis of patients with low von Willebrand factor levels. *Haematologica* 89:77, 2004.
248. Preston FE: Assays for von Willebrand factor functional activity: A UK NEQAS survey. National External Quality Assessment Scheme. *Thromb Haemost* 80:863, 1998.
249. Favaloro EJ, Henniker A, Facey D, Hertzberg M: Discrimination of von Willebrand's disease (VWD) subtypes: Direct comparison of von Willebrand factor:collagen binding assay (VWF:CBA) with monoclonal antibody (MAB) based VWF-capture systems. *Thromb Haemost* 84:541, 2000.
250. Laffan M, Brown SA, Collins PW, et al: The diagnosis of von Willebrand disease: A guideline from the UK Haemophilia Centre Doctors' Organization. *Haemophilia* 10:199, 2004.
251. Federici AB: Update on the management of von Willebrand disease. *Clin Adv Hematol Oncol* 6:29, 2008.
252. Chen D, Daigh CA, Hendricksen JI, et al: A highly-sensitive plasma von Willebrand factor ristocetin cofactor (VWF:RCo) activity assay by flow cytometry. *J Thromb Haemost* 6:323, 2008.
253. Ruggeri ZM and Zimmerman TS: The complex multimeric composition of Factor VIII/von Willebrand Factor. *Blood* 57:1140, 1981.
254. Budde U, Schneppenheim R, Eikenboom J, et al: Detailed von Willebrand factor multimer analysis in patients with von Willebrand disease in the European study, molecular and clinical markers for the diagnosis and management of type 1 von Willebrand disease (MCMDM-1VWD). *J Thromb Haemost* 6:762, 2008.
255. Harker LA and Slichter SJ: The bleeding time as a screening test for evaluation of platelet function. *N Engl J Med* 287:155, 1972.
256. Mannucci PM: Treatment of von Willebrand's Disease. *N Engl J Med* 351:683, 2004.
257. Lind SE: The bleeding time does not predict surgical bleeding. *Blood* 77:2547, 1991.
258. De Caterina R, Lanza M, Manca G, et al: Bleeding time and bleeding: An analysis of the relationship of the bleeding time test with parameters of surgical bleeding. *Blood* 84:3363, 1994.
259. Peterson P, Hayes TE, Arkin CF, et al: The preoperative bleeding time test lacks clinical benefit: College of American Pathologists' and American Society of Clinical Pathologists' position article. *Arch Surg* 133:134, 1998.
260. Favaloro EJ, Dean M, Grispo L, et al: Von Willebrand's disease: Use of collagen binding assay provides potential improvement to laboratory monitoring of desmopressin (DDAVP) therapy. *Am J Hematol* 45:205, 1994.
261. Riddell AF, Jenkins PV, Nitu-Whalley IC, et al: Use of the collagen-binding assay for von Willebrand factor in the analysis of type 2M von Willebrand disease: A comparison with the ristocetin cofactor assay. *Br J Haematol* 116:187, 2002.
262. Popov J, Zhukov O, Ruden S, et al: Performance and clinical utility of a commercial von Willebrand factor collagen binding assay for laboratory diagnosis of von Willebrand disease. *Clin Chem* 52:1965, 2006.
263. Meiring M, Badenhorst PN, Kelderman M: Performance and utility of a cost-effective collagen-binding assay for the laboratory diagnosis of Von Willebrand disease. *Clin Chem Lab Med* 45:1068, 2007.
264. Mazurier C, Meyer D: Factor VIII binding assay of von Willebrand factor and the diagnosis of type 2N von Willebrand disease—Results of an international survey. On behalf of the Subcommittee on von Willebrand Factor of the Scientific and Standardization Committee of the ISTH. *Thromb Haemost* 76:270, 1996.
265. Zhukov O, Popov J, Ramos R, et al: Measurement of von Willebrand factor-FVIII binding activity in patients with suspected von Willebrand disease type 2N: Application of an ELISA-based assay in a reference laboratory. *Haemophilia* 15:788, 2009.
266. Casonato A, Pontara E, Sartorello F, et al: Identifying carriers of type 2N von Willebrand disease: Procedures and significance. *Clin Appl Thromb Hemost* 13:194, 2007.
267. Haberichter SL, Balistreri M, Christopherson P, et al: Assay of the von Willebrand factor (VWF) propeptide to identify patients with type 1 von Willebrand disease with decreased VWF survival. *Blood* 108:3344, 2006.
268. Casonato A, Pontara E, Sartorello F, et al: Identifying type Vicenza von Willebrand disease. *J Lab Clin Med* 147:96, 2006.
269. Fressinaud E, Veyradier A, Truchaud F, et al: Screening for von Willebrand disease with a new analyzer using high shear stress: A study of 60 cases. *Blood* 91:1325, 1998.
270. Cattaneo M, Federici AB, Lecchi A, et al: Evaluation of the PFA-100 system in the diagnosis and therapeutic monitoring of patients with von Willebrand disease. *Thromb Haemost* 82:35, 1999.
271. De Vleeschauwer A, Devreese K: Comparison of a new automated von Willebrand factor activity assay with an aggregation von Willebrand ristocetin cofactor activity assay for the diagnosis of von Willebrand disease. *Blood Coagul Fibrinolysis* 17:353, 2006.
272. Salem RO, Van Cott EM: A new automated screening assay for the diagnosis of von Willebrand disease. *Am J Clin Pathol* 127:730, 2007.
273. Sucker C, Senft B, Scharf RE, Zotz RB: Determination of von Willebrand factor activity: Evaluation of the HaemosIL assay in comparison with established procedures. *Clin Appl Thromb Hemost* 12:305, 2006.
274. Pinol M, Sales M, Costa M, et al: Evaluation of a new turbidimetric assay for von Willebrand factor activity useful in the general screening of von Willebrand disease. *Haematologica* 92:712, 2007.
275. Fujimura Y, Kawasaki T, Titani K: Snake venom proteins modulating the interaction between von Willebrand factor and platelet glycoprotein Ib. *Thromb Haemost* 76:633, 1996.
276. Pruthi RK: A practical approach to genetic testing for von Willebrand disease. *Mayo Clin Proc* 81:679, 2006.
277. Bignell P, Standen GR, Bowen DJ, et al: Rapid neonatal diagnosis of von Willebrand's disease by use of the polymerase chain reaction. *Lancet* 336:638, 1990.
278. Sadler JE, Ginsburg D: A database of polymorphisms in the von Willebrand factor gene and pseudogene. *Thromb Haemost* 69:185, 1993.
279. Peake IR, Bowen D, Bignell P, et al: Family studies and prenatal diagnosis in severe von Willebrand Disease by polymerase chain reaction amplification of a variable number tandem repeat region of the von Willebrand factor gene. *Blood* 76:555, 1990.
280. Mannhalter C, Kyrle PA, Brenner B, Lechner K: Rapid neonatal diagnosis of Type IIB von Willebrand disease using the polymerase chain reaction. *Blood* 77:2538, 1991.
281. Gupta PK, Kannan M, Saxena R: Carrier detection in severe von Willebrand's disease. *Ann Hematol* 83:625, 2004.
282. Miller JL: Platelet-type von Willebrand disease. *Thromb Haemost* 75:865, 1996.
283. Franchini M, Lippi G: Acquired von Willebrand syndrome: An update. *Am J Hematol* 82:368, 2007.
284. Federici AB: Acquired von Willebrand syndrome: Is it an extremely rare disorder or do we see only the tip of the iceberg? *J Thromb Haemost* 6:565, 2008.
285. Budde U, Schaefer G, Mueller N, et al: Acquired von Willebrand's disease in the myeloproliferative syndrome. *Blood* 64:981, 1984.
286. Kos CA, Ward JE, Malek K, et al: Association of acquired von Willebrand syndrome with AL amyloidosis. *Am J Hematol* 82:363, 2007.
287. Mannucci PM, Lombardi R, Bader R, et al: Studies of the pathophysiology of acquired von Willebrand's disease in seven patients with lymphoproliferative disorders or benign monoclonal gammopathies. *Blood* 64:614, 1984.
288. Rogers JS, Shane SR, Jencks FS: Factor VIII activity and thyroid function. *Ann Intern Med* 97:713, 1982.
289. Viallard JF, Pellegrin JL, Vergnes C, et al: Three cases of acquired von Willebrand disease associated with systemic lupus erythematosus. *Br J Haematol* 105:532, 1999.
290. Scott JP, Montgomery RR, Tubergen DG, and Hays T: Acquired von Willebrand's disease in association with Wilms' tumor: Regression following treatment. *Blood* 58:665, 1981.
291. Warkentin TE, Moore JC, Morgan DG: Aortic stenosis and bleeding gastrointestinal angiodysplasia: Is acquired von Willebrand's disease the link? *Lancet* 340:35, 1992.
292. Castaman G, Lattuada A, Mannucci PM, Rodeghiero F: Characterization of two cases of acquired transitory von Willebrand syndrome with ciprofloxacin: Evidence for heightened proteolysis of von Willebrand factor. *Am J Hematol* 49:83, 1995.
293. Tefferi A, Nichols WL: Acquired von Willebrand disease: Concise review of occurrence, diagnosis, pathogenesis, and treatment. *Am J Med* 103:536, 1997.
294. Geisen U, Heilmann C, Beyersdorf F, et al: Non-surgical bleeding in patients with ventricular assist devices could be explained by acquired von Willebrand disease. *Eur J Cardiothorac Surg* 33:679, 2008.
295. Viallard JF, Pellegrin JL, Vergnes C, et al: Three cases of acquired von Willebrand disease associated with systemic lupus erythematosus. *Br J Haematol* 105:532, 1999.
296. Kumar S, Pruthi RK, Nichols WL: Acquired von Willebrand disease. *Mayo Clin Proc* 77:181, 2002.
297. Sucker C, Michiels JJ, Zotz RB: Causes, etiology and diagnosis of acquired von Willebrand disease: a prospective diagnostic workup to establish the most effective therapeutic strategies. *Acta Haematol* 121:177, 2009.
298. Cohen AJ, Kessler CM, Ewenstein BM: Management of von Willebrand disease: A survey on current clinical practice from the haemophilia centres of North America. *Haemophilia* 7:235, 2001.
299. Sumner M and Williams J: Type 3 von Willebrand disease: Assessment of complications and approaches to treatment—Results of a patient and Hemophilia Treatment Center Survey in the United States. *Haemophilia* 10:360, 2004.
300. Berntorp E, Petrini P: Long-term prophylaxis in von Willebrand disease. *Blood Coagul Fibrinolysis* 16 Suppl 1:S23, 2005.
301. Franchini M, Targher G, Lippi G: Prophylaxis in von Willebrand disease. *Ann Hematol* 86:699, 2007.
302. Mannucci PM: Treatment of von Willebrand's Disease. *N Engl J Med* 351:683, 2004.
303. Kaufmann JE, Oksche A, Wollheim CB, et al: Vasopressin-induced von Willebrand factor secretion from endothelial cells involves V2 receptors and cAMP. *J Clin Invest* 106:107, 2000.
304. Mannucci PM, Ruggeri ZM, Pareti FI, Capitanio A: 1-Deamino-8-D-arginine vasopressin: A new pharmacological approach to the management of haemophilia and von Willebrand's diseases. *Lancet* 1:869, 1977.
305. Ruggeri ZM, Mannucci PM, Lombardi R, et al: Multimeric composition of factor VIII/von Willebrand Factor following administration of DDAVP: Implications for pathophysiology and therapy of von Willebrand's disease subtypes. *Blood* 59:1272, 1982.
306. Mannucci PM: Desmopressin (DDAVP) in the treatment of bleeding disorders: The first 20 years. *Blood* 90:2515, 1997.
307. Federici AB, Mazurier C, Berntorp E, et al: Biologic response to desmopressin in patients with severe type 1 and type 2 von Willebrand disease: Results of a multicenter European study. *Blood* 103:2032, 2004.
308. Lethagen S, Harris AS, Nilsson IM: Intranasal desmopressin (DDAVP) by spray in mild hemophilia A and von Willebrand's disease type I. *Blut* 60:187, 1990.

309. Rose EH, Aledort LM: Nasal spray desmopressin (DDAVP) for mild hemophilia A and von Willebrand disease. *Ann Intern Med* 114:563, 1991.
310. Rodeghiero F, Castaman G, Di Bona E, Ruggeri M: Consistency of responses to repeated DDAVP infusions in patients with von Willebrand's disease and hemophilia A. *Blood* 74:1997, 1989.
311. Castaman G, Lethagen S, Federici AB, et al: Response to desmopressin is influenced by the genotype and phenotype in type 1 von Willebrand disease (VWD): Results from the European Study MCMDM-1VWD. *Blood* 111:3531, 2008.
312. Mannucci PM, Bettega D, Cattaneo M: Patterns of development of tachyphylaxis in patients with haemophilia and von Willebrand disease after repeated doses of desmopressin (DDAVP). *Br J Haematol* 82:87, 1992.
313. Federici AB, Mazurier C, Berntorp E, et al: Biologic response to desmopressin in patients with severe type 1 and type 2 von Willebrand disease: Results of a multicenter European study. *Blood* 103:2032, 2004.
314. de la Fuente B, Kasper CK, Rickles FR, Hoyer LW: Response of patients with mild and moderate hemophilia A and von Willebrand's disease to treatment with desmopressin. *Ann Intern Med* 103:6, 1985.
315. Gralnick HR, Williams SB, McKeown LP, et al: DDAVP in type IIa von Willebrand's disease. *Blood* 67:465, 1986.
316. Federici AB, Mazurier C, Berntorp E, et al: Biologic response to desmopressin in patients with severe type 1 and type 2 von Willebrand disease: Results of a multicenter European study. *Blood* 103:2032, 2004.
317. Mannucci PM: Treatment of von Willebrand's Disease. *N Engl J Med* 351:683, 2004.
318. Holmberg L, Nilsson IM, Borge L, et al: Platelet aggregation induced by 1-desamino-8-D-arginine vasopressin (DDAVP) in Type IIB von Willebrand's disease. *N Engl J Med* 309:816, 1983.
319. Casonato A, Sartori MT, De Marco L, Girolami A: 1-Desamino-8-D-arginine vasopressin (DDAVP) infusion in type IIB von Willebrand's disease: Shortening of bleeding time and induction of a variable pseudothrombocytopenia. *Thromb Haemost* 64:117, 1990.
320. McKeown LP, Connaghan G, Wilson O, et al: 1-Desamino-8-arginine-vasopressin corrects the hemostatic defects in type 2B von Willebrand's disease. *Am J Hematol* 51:158, 1996.
321. Federici AB, Mazurier C, Berntorp E, et al: Biologic response to desmopressin in patients with severe type 1 and type 2 von Willebrand disease: Results of a multicenter European study. *Blood* 103:2032, 2004.
322. Mazurier C, Gaucher C, Jorieux S, et al: Biological effect of desmopressin in eight patients with type 2N ("Normandy") von Willebrand disease. *Br J Haematol* 88:849, 1994.
323. Foster PA: A perspective on the use of FVIII concentrates and cryoprecipitate prophylactically in surgery or therapeutically in severe bleeds in patients with von Willebrand disease unresponsive to DDAVP: Results of an international survey. *Thromb Haemost* 74:1370, 1995.
324. Morfini M, Mannucci PM, Tenconi PM, et al: Pharmacokinetics of monoclonally-purified and recombinant factor VIII in patients with severe von Willebrand disease. *Thromb Haemost* 70:270, 1993.
325. Mannucci PM: Treatment of von Willebrand's disease. *N Engl J Med* 351:683, 2004.
326. Pasi KJ, Collins PW, Keeling DM, et al: Management of von Willebrand disease: A guideline from the UK Haemophilia Centre Doctors' Organization. *Haemophilia* 10:218, 2004.
327. Cohen AJ, Kessler CM, Ewenstein BM: Management of von Willebrand disease: A survey on current clinical practice from the haemophilia centres of North America. *Haemophilia* 7:235, 2001.
328. Makris M, Colvin B, Gupta V, et al: Venous thrombosis following the use of intermediate purity FVIII concentrate to treat patients with von Willebrand's disease. *Thromb Haemost* 88:387, 2002.
329. Mannucci PM, Chediak J, Hanna W, et al: Treatment of von Willebrand disease with a high-purity factor VIII/von Willebrand factor concentrate: A prospective, multicenter study. *Blood* 99:450, 2002.
330. Mannucci PM, Tamaro G, Narchi G, et al: Life-threatening reaction to factor VIII concentrate in a patient with severe von Willebrand disease and alloantibodies to von Willebrand factor. *Eur J Haematol* 39:467, 1987.
331. Bergamaschini L, Mannucci PM, Federici AB, et al: Posttransfusion anaphylactic reactions in a patient with severe von Willebrand disease: Role of complement and alloantibodies to von Willebrand factor. *J Lab Clin Med* 125:348, 1995.
332. Harrison RL, McKee PA: Estrogen stimulates von Willebrand Factor production by cultured endothelial cells. *Blood* 63:657, 1984.
333. Cohen AJ, Kessler CM, Ewenstein BM: Management of von Willebrand disease: A survey on current clinical practice from the haemophilia centres of North America. *Haemophilia* 7:235, 2001.
334. Franchini M, Veneri D, Lippi G: The use of recombinant activated factor VII in congenital and acquired von Willebrand disease. *Blood Coagul Fibrinolysis* 17:615, 2006.

CHAPTER 128
ANTIBODY-MEDIATED COAGULATION FACTOR DEFICIENCIES

Pete Lollar

SUMMARY

Clinically significant autoantibodies to coagulation factors are uncommon, but can produce life-threatening bleeding and death. The most commonly targeted coagulation factor by an autoantibody is factor VIII. Acquired hemophilia A, which results from these antibodies, can either be idiopathic or associated with other autoimmune disorders, malignancy, the postpartum period, and the use of drugs such as penicillin and sulfonamides. Idiopathic autoantibodies occur most often in older persons. Bleeding in acquired hemophilia A is treated with factor VIII bypassing agents. The underlying autoimmune disorder frequently responds to immunosuppressive drugs or to the induction of immune tolerance. Antiprothrombin antibodies found in patients with lupus anticoagulant are often associated with bleeding. Antibodies to factor V can occur as autoantibodies or as cross-reacting antibovine factor V antibodies that develop after exposure to bovine thrombin products that are contaminated with factor V. Pathogenic autoantibodies also have been described that target thrombin, factor IX, factor XI, factor XIII, protein C, protein S, and the endothelial cell protein C receptor.

DEFINITION AND HISTORY

Antibodies directed against coagulation factors can develop as an acquired, autoimmune phenomenon or, as described in Chaps. 124 and 125, in response to replacement therapy in hereditary coagulation factor deficiencies. These "circulating anticoagulants" or "inhibitors" were recognized as early as 1906 as a cause of an acquired bleeding disorder.[1,2] In 1966, factor VIII inhibitors were shown to be antibodies.[3] The key feature that distinguishes antibody-mediated from other acquired coagulation factor deficiencies, such as impaired synthesis (e.g., as a consequence of vitamin K deficiency) or increased consumption (e.g., in disseminated intravascular coagulation), is the ability of the patient's plasma to inhibit the coagulation of normal plasma.

ACQUIRED HEMOPHILIA A

INCIDENCE AND ASSOCIATED DISORDERS

The clinical condition associated with acquired (spontaneous) factor VIII antibodies is called *acquired hemophilia A*. The incidence of autoantibodies to factor VIII is 0.2 to 1 per 1 million persons per year.[4] This disorder is the most common spontaneous antibody-induced bleeding disorder involving a specific coagulation factor. The associated clinical condition is called acquired hemophilia A. Approximately 50 percent of acquired hemophilia A patients have an underlying condition, such as an autoimmune disorder (e.g., rheumatoid arthritis or systemic lupus erythematosus), malignancy, pregnancy, or a history consistent with a drug reaction.[5] The remaining cases, referred to as idiopathic, commonly occur in older patients of either sex.

Acronyms and abbreviations that appear in this chapter include: aPTT, activated partial thromboplastin time; BU, Bethesda unit.

MECHANISMS OF AUTOANTIBODY DEVELOPMENT

In addition to non-self-antigen, antigen products of infection and cellular damage of the host can promote an immune response.[6] These inciting agents include microbial products and host proteins associated with inflammation, such as heat shock proteins.[6] It was proposed that in the absence of these "danger" signals, autoimmunity can be avoided.[7] Additionally, several other mechanisms exist that prevent an immune response to self-antigens, which collectively are known as immunologic tolerance (see Chap. 77). Coagulation frequently occurs at sites of inflammation and injury where "danger" signals presumably are generated. Additionally, nonproteolytic and proteolytic degradation of coagulation proteins potentially could present neoepitopes. Thus, the fact that autoantibodies to coagulation proteins are uncommon is a testimony to the ability of the immune system to discriminate efficiently between infectious non-self from noninfectious self. Essentially, nothing is known about the breakdown of tolerance in patients that develop autoantibodies to coagulation factors.

MOLECULAR PATHOLOGY

Factor VIII inhibitors in hereditary and acquired hemophilia are nearly always polyclonal immunoglobulin (Ig) G antibodies. Although IgG_4 accounts for only 5 percent of the total IgG in normal plasma, it usually is a major, but not the sole, component of the anti-factor VIII antibody population.[8] IgG_4 antibodies do not fix complement, which has been cited as a reason that immune complex disease is not observed in factor VIII inhibitor patients. However, it is more likely that factor VIII simply is not present in sufficient quantity to form enough immune complex deposition to mediate tissue damage.

Factor VIII contains a sequence of domains designated A1-A2-B-ap-A3-C1-C2. During the activation of factor VIII by thrombin, the B and ap domains are released, producing an A1/A2/A3-C1-C2 activated factor VIII heterotrimer.[9] Anti-factor VIII antibodies in both congenital and acquired hemophilia A inhibitor disease are primarily directed to the A2 and C2 domains, suggesting that albeit different immunologic settings, structural features in the factor VIII molecule are an important determinant driving the immune response.[10–12] Epitope spreading from a single "problem" epitope, which has been implicated in some autoantibody phenomena,[13] does not appear to be a property of factor VIII inhibitors because anti-C2 antibodies can occur in the absence of anti-A2 antibodies and *vice versa.*

The only known biologic function of factor VIII is to become proteolytically activated and participate as a cofactor for factor IXa during factor X activation on phospholipid membranes. Theoretically, antibodies could inhibit factor VIII procoagulant function in several ways, including blocking the binding of factor VIIIa to factor IXa, factor X, or phospholipid, or by interfering with the proteolytic activation of factor VIII. Some anti-A2 antibodies map to a region bounded by Arg484 Ile508[14] and inhibit activated factor VIII by blocking its ability to bind factor X.[15] Anti-C2 antibodies bind to the NH_2-terminal half of the C2 domain.[16] Anti-C2 antibodies have been identified that inhibit the binding of activated factor VIII to phospholipid membranes,[17] which is critical for its interaction with the platelet surfaces. However, the C2 domain also apparently contributes to the binding of factor VIII to its activators, thrombin, and factor Xa.[18–20] Consistent with this, anti-C2 inhibitors have been identified that block factor VIII activation.[20,21]

Factor VIII inhibitors also have been identified in approximately 20 percent of normal healthy donors.[22] These inhibitors inhibit factor VIII activity in pooled normal plasma, but not autologous plasma, indicating that they are not autoantibodies, but rather alloantibodies directed against an unidentified polymorphism. Anti-factor VIII IgG also has been identified in all normal plasmas tested by affinity chromatography on immobilized factor VIII.[23] The increased sensitivity of the method is because of its ability to resolve anti-factor VIII antibodies from anti–anti-factor VIII idiotypic antibodies that also are present. Idiotypic regulation has been proposed as a mechanism for controlling autoantibody activity *in vivo*.[24]

CLINICAL FEATURES

Acquired hemophilia A patients usually present with spontaneous bleeding, which often is severe and life- or limb-threatening. These patients are more likely to have a more severe bleeding diathesis than patients with hemophilia A and an inhibitor.[25] Common bleeding sites are soft tissues, skin, and mucous membranes. In contrast to patients with hemophilia A, hemarthroses, intramuscular, and central nervous system bleeding are rare. The reason for these differences is puzzling, especially in light of the fact that the properties of factor VIII inhibitors in the two patient populations are similar. Inhibitors can block factor VIII function in several ways (see "Molecular Pathology" above). Conceivably, unidentified mechanistic differences in inhibitor action account for the difference in clinical severity. Acquired factor VIII inhibitors sometimes resolve spontaneously. However, it is not possible to predict in which subset of patients this will occur.

LABORATORY FEATURES AND DIFFERENTIAL DIAGNOSIS

The new onset of an acquired bleeding disorder should immediately lead to screening tests that include an activated partial thromboplastin time (aPTT), a prothrombin time, and a platelet count. Patients with acquired hemophilia A have a prolonged aPTT caused by decreased or absent factor VIII activity in the intrinsic pathway of blood coagulation. The autoantibody inhibits the factor VIII in the plasma from normal individuals, which forms the basis of a plasma mixing test that is used to screen for inhibitors. The presence of a prolonged aPTT in a 1:1 mixture between patient and normal plasma establishes the diagnosis of a circulating anticoagulant. Specific factor assays then are performed to determine whether a specific coagulation factor inhibitor or a lupus anticoagulant is present. The activity of other intrinsic pathway coagulation factors may be decreased in the presence of high titer factor VIII inhibitors. However, the levels of these factors normalize at increasing dilutions of patient plasma, whereas factor VIII activity remains decreased.

Once the identity of an inhibitor has been established, its titer is determined using the Bethesda assay.[26] Inhibitors frequently take minutes to hours to maximally inhibit factor VIII. Therefore, dilutions of patient's plasma are preincubated with normal plasma for 2 hours at 37°C (98.6°F). The inhibitor titer is defined as the dilution of patient plasma that produces 50 percent inhibition of the factor VIII activity and is expressed as Bethesda units per mL (BU/mL). Inhibitors are classified informally as low titer or high titer when the titers are less than 5 or greater than 5 BU/mL, respectively. The Bethesda assay has been modified by the addition of 0.1 M imidazole, pH 7.4, and by diluting test plasma into factor VIII-deficient plasma during the preincubation phase to prevent assay variation because of pH changes and adsorptive losses of factor VIII.[27] This "Nijmegen" modification of the Bethesda assay has been shown to decrease false-positive low-titer inhibitors.[28]

Factor VIII inhibitors are classified based on the kinetics and extent of inactivation of factor VIII.[29] Type I inhibitors follow second-order kinetics and inactivate factor VIII completely, which would be expected for a simple bimolecular antigen–antibody reaction. Type II inhibitors inactivate factor VIII incompletely and display more complex kinetics of inhibition. Hemophilia A patients with an inhibitor and patients with acquired hemophilia A tend to have type I and type II inhibitors, respectively.[30] However, the borderline between type I and type II inhibitors is not always clear and the distinction is not useful clinically.

TREATMENT

The severe bleeding that often is the presenting feature of this disorder requires urgent action to establish a diagnosis and initiate therapeutic measures. Ideally, this is carried out in a setting where factor VIII inhibitors can be identified and quantitated and where there is subspecialty expertise in the management of bleeding disorders. Treatment of patients with acquired hemophilia A depends on the inhibitor titer.

Factor VIII Concentrates

Although no prospective trials are available, clinical experience indicates that patients with a factor VIII inhibitor titer of less than 5 BU/mL often are treated successfully with sufficient doses of recombinant or plasma-derived factor VIII concentrates to neutralize the inhibitor. Patients with titers between 5 and 10 BU/mL also may respond to factor VIII concentrates, whereas those with titers greater than 10 BU/mL generally do not respond.

Factor VIII Bypassing Agents

Factor VIII bypassing agents, which drive the coagulation mechanism through the extrinsic pathway, are the mainstays of management of patients with a high titer of an inhibitor. Two agents, recombinant activated factor VII (rFVIIa; NovoSeven RT) and plasma-derived anti-inhibitor coagulant complex (AICC; FEIBA VH Immuno, also called activated prothrombin complex concentrate) are commercially available and approved by the U.S. Food and Drug Administration for treatment of acquired hemophilia A. The recommended dose range of rFVIIa for the treatment of patients with acquired hemophilia is 70 to 90 mcg/kg repeated every 2 to 3 hours until hemostasis is achieved. The minimum effective dose in acquired hemophilia has not been determined. Recommended doses of AICC depend on the type of bleeding. In joint hemorrhage, 50 U/kg is recommended at 12-hour intervals, which may be increased to doses of 100 U/kg. Treatment should be continued until clear signs of clinical improvement appear, such as relief of pain, reduction of swelling, or mobilization of the joint. For mucous membrane bleeding, 50 U/kg is recommended at 6-hour intervals under careful monitoring. If hemorrhage does not stop, the dose may be increased to 100 U/kg at 6-hour intervals. For severe soft-tissue bleeding, such as retroperitoneal bleeding, 100 U/kg at 12-hour intervals is recommended. Central nervous system bleeding has been effectively treated with doses of 100 U/kg at 6- to 12-hour intervals. One should not exceed a daily dose of AICC of 200 U/kg.

The response to bypassing agents is variable and does not correlate with the inhibitor titer. A major concern with the use of rFVIIa and AICC is that there is no laboratory method available for predicting response to therapy or monitoring patients on therapy. A retrospective analysis indicates that rFVIIa is effective in 75 percent of bleeding episodes in acquired hemophilia A.[31] Retrospective analysis of the use of AICC indicates that it has similar efficacy.[32] The major serious adverse event associated with bypassing agents is thrombosis. The incidence of thrombosis in patients with acquired hemophilia A treated with bypassing agents is not known. However, it is considered low when used for approved indications at the recommended doses. Escalating doses of either bypassing agent or combination of the two agents should be done with caution, especially in older patients.

Porcine Factor VIII

Factor VIII inhibitors usually cross-react poorly with porcine factor VIII.[33] A commercial plasma-derived porcine factor VIII concentrate was useful in the treatment of factor VIII inhibitor patients for approximately 20 years,[34] but was discontinued in 2004 because of viral contamination of the product. Porcine factor VIII has the advantage of potentially being guided by laboratory monitoring of recovery of factor VIII activity in plasma. However, the development of antiporcine factor VIII antibodies may preclude its long-term use. A phase II clinical trial of a recombinant porcine factor VIII product has been completed in patients with hemophilia A and an inhibitor.[35,36]

Immunosuppressive Therapy

Although acquired inhibitors may remit spontaneously, fatal bleeding may occur up to several months after the initial diagnosis, even in patients who present with mild bleeding. Therefore, immunosuppressive therapy at the time of diagnosis to eradicate the inhibitor is recommended.[37] A variety of immunosuppressive agents have been used, including cyclophosphamide, azathioprine, cyclosporine A, intravenous immunoglobulin, and rituximab. Additionally, plasmapheresis and immunoadsorption of the inhibitory antibody have been used. Finally, immune tolerance induction using human factor VIII has been used successfully. It is difficult to compare these regimens because the rarity of the disease has contributed to the lack of controlled trials. Several recent excellent reviews are available that address this complex subject.[35,36,38]

ANTI-FACTOR V AND ANTITHROMBIN ANTIBODIES

Thrombin and factor V inhibitors are discussed together because of their frequent coexistence in immune responses to commercial products that contain thrombin. Thrombin products have been used widely in surgical and endoscopic procedures. It has been estimated that more than 500,000 patients are treated annually with products containing thrombin.[39] Thrombin is used either alone or as a component of fibrin sealants, which consist of fibrinogen and thrombin preparations that are mixed together at the wound site to form a topical fibrin clot.[40] Factor XIII sometimes is added to cross-link and stabilize the clot.

Fibrin sealants contain thrombin and fibrinogen derived from human plasma, whereas stand-alone thrombin products are prepared from bovine plasma. Both types of products are heavily contaminated with other plasma proteins, including factor V and prothrombin.[41,42] Almost all patients exposed to bovine proteins develop a detectable immune response. In half of these patients antibovine antibodies cross-react with human thrombin, factor V, or prothrombin.[43] Usually, these antibodies cause no clinical manifestation.[44] However, mild to life-threatening hemorrhage can occur, especially if the titer of antihuman factor V antibodies is high. The risk of bleeding is higher in patients who receive bovine thrombin products more than once because of the development of a secondary immune response.

There have been no clinical trials comparing the safety and efficacy of fibrin sealants to stand-alone thrombin products. Because fibrin sealants are composed mainly of human proteins, they may be less immunogenic. However, anti-factor V antibodies have been reported in a patient receiving fibrin sealant.[45] Currently there is no stand-alone human thrombin product. It seems likely that the development of highly purified plasma-derived or recombinant products containing human thrombin in the presence or absence of human fibrinogen would decrease the incidence of antithrombin and anti-factor V antibodies.[42]

Autoantibodies to thrombin are rare.[46] In contrast, approximately half of the 105 cases of inhibitory anti-factor V antibodies reported and reviewed between 1955 and 1997 appeared to be autoantibodies not associated with the exposure to bovine thrombin products.[44] Beta-lactam antibiotics also have been associated with anti-factor V autoantibodies and may partly explain the increased incidence with surgery. In approximately 20 percent of cases of autoantibody formation, no underlying disease was identified. Anti-factor V autoantibodies have been identified rarely in patients with autoimmune diseases, solid tumors, and monoclonal gammopathies. In addition to autoantibody formation, alloantibodies to factor V have developed in patients with severe factor V deficiency in response to replacement therapy with fresh-frozen plasma (see Chap. 125).

Patients with inhibitory antibodies to factor V have prolonged prothrombin and activated partial thromboplastin times, low factor V levels and a normal thrombin time. The diagnosis of a factor V inhibitor is based on the specific loss of factor V coagulant activity when patient and normal plasma are mixed in a coagulation assay. The antibody titer can be defined as in the factor VIII Bethesda assay as the dilution of test plasma that produces 50 percent inhibition of factor V activity.

Not all patients with factor V inhibitors have hemorrhagic manifestations. Factor V inhibitors produce a less serious bleeding disorder than factor VIII inhibitors. The relationship between inhibitor titer and bleeding has not been studied. The reported incidence of bleeding has been higher in patients with autoantibodies to factor V compared to anti-factor V antibodies in patients receiving bovine thrombin. However, this may reflect a bias resulting from the reason the patient sought medical attention.

Factor V contains an A1-A2-B-A3-C1-C2 domain structure that is homologous to factor VIII. Also, like factor VIII, the N-terminal half of the factor V C2 domain contains a phospholipid-binding site[47] that is necessary for normal procoagulant function[48] and is targeted by factor V inhibitors.[49,50]

ANTIPROTHROMBIN ANTIBODIES

Antiprothrombin antibodies are most commonly associated with the antiphospholipid syndrome (see Chap. 132). The antiphospholipid syndrome is caused by lupus anticoagulants, which are defined as antibodies that produce phospholipid-dependent prolongation of *in vitro* coagulation assays. Anionic phospholipids participate as cofactors for the lupus anticoagulant binding to protein antigens, primarily β_2-glycoprotein I[51] and prothrombin.[52] The antibody–antigen complexes compete for the binding of coagulation factors to the phospholipid present in coagulation assays and produce the lupus anticoagulant phenomenon.

The role of prothrombin in the generation of lupus anticoagulant activity initially was suggested from studies of a bleeding patient with severe hypoprothrombinemia.[53] However, in the absence of hypoprothrombinemia, lupus anticoagulants do not produce a bleeding diathesis, and bleeding in patients with lupus anticoagulants is uncommon.[54] In patients with antiprothrombin antibodies and hypoprothrombinemia, precipitating, noninhibitory antibodies are present and prothrombin antigen levels are low, indicating that the hypoprothrombinemia is caused by rapid clearance of antigen–antibody complexes.[55] However, most patients with lupus anticoagulants have demonstrable antiprothrombin antibodies but do not have hypoprothrombinemia.[56] Thus, antibody-mediated hypoprothrombinemia appears to represent a relatively uncommon evolution of the autoimmune response to prothrombin in patients with lupus anticoagulants.

ANTIBODIES TO COMPONENTS OF THE PROTEIN C SYSTEM

An acquired inhibitor to protein C associated with a fatal thrombotic disorder has been reported,[57] but evidently is rare. In contrast, there is a relatively high prevalence of pathogenic anti-protein S antibodies. Inhibitory antibodies to protein S were detected in 5 of 15 patients with acquired protein S deficiency.[58] Anti-protein S antibodies, but not antibodies to cardiolipin, β_2-glycoprotein I, prothrombin, or protein C, appear to be a risk factor for venous thrombosis and can be manifested *in vitro* as activated protein C resistance.[59] Antibodies to endothelial cell protein C receptor have been identified in patients with the antiphospholipid syndrome and were associated with fetal death.[60]

ACQUIRED ANTIBODIES TO OTHER COAGULATION FACTORS

Clinically significant antibodies to coagulation factors other than factor VIII, factor V and prothrombin that produce acquired bleeding disorders are rare. In contrast to acquired hemophilia A, acquired hemophilia B is extremely rare.[61] Patients with antifibrinogen antibodies have been identified in asymptomatic patients and patients with abnormal bleeding.[62,63] Patients with excessive bleeding associated with acquired inhibitors to factor XI,[64] and factor XIII subunits A[65] or B[66] also have been described.

REFERENCES

1. Weil PE: Etude du sang chez les hemophiles. *Bull e Mem Soc Med Hôp Par* 23:101, 1906.
2. Margolius A Jr, Jackson DP, Ratnoff OD: Circulating anticoagulants: A study of 40 cases and a review of the literature. *Medicine (Baltimore)* 40:145, 1961.
3. Bidwell E, Denson KWE, Dike GWR, et al: Antibody nature of the inhibitor to antihemophilic globulin (Factor VIII). *Nature* 210:746, 1966.
4. Cohen AJ, Kessler CM: Acquired inhibitors. *Baillieres Clin Haematol* 9:331, 1996.
5. Green D, Lechner K: A survey of 215 non-hemophilic patients with inhibitors to factor VIII. *Thromb Haemost* 45:2000, 1981.
6. Janeway CA Jr: Approaching the asymptote? Evolution and revolution in immunology. *Cold Spring Harb Symp Quant Biol* 54 Pt 1:1, 1989.
7. Matzinger P: Tolerance, danger, and the extended family. *Annu Rev Immunol* 12:991, 1994.
8. Hoyer LW, Gawryl MS, de la Fuente B: Immunochemical characterization of factor VIII inhibitors, in *Factor VIII Inhibitors*, edited by LW Hoyer, p73. Alan R. Liss, New York, 1984.
9. Lollar P, Parker CG: Subunit structure of thrombin-activated porcine factor VIII. *Biochemistry* 28:666, 1989.
10. Fulcher CA, Mahoney SD, Roberts JR, et al: Localization of human factor FVIII inhibitor epitopes to two polypeptide fragments. *Proc Natl Acad Sci U S A* 82:7728, 1985.
11. Prescott R, Nakai H, Saenko EL, et al: The inhibitory antibody response is more complex in hemophilia A patients than in most nonhemophiliacs with fVIII autoantibodies. *Blood* 89:3663, 1997.
12. Scandella D, Mattingly M, de Graaf S, et al: Localization of epitopes for human factor VIII inhibitor antibodies by immunoblotting and antibody neutralization. *Blood* 74:1618, 1989.
13. James JA, Harley JB: B-cell epitope spreading in autoimmunity. *Immunol Rev* 164:185, 1998.
14. Healey JF, Barrow RT, Tamim HM, et al: Residues Glu2181Val2243 contain a major determinant of the inhibitory epitope in the C2 domain of human factor VIII. *Blood* 92:3701, 1998.
15. Lollar P, Parker ET, Curtis JE, et al: Inhibition of human factor VIIIa by anti-A2 subunit antibodies. *J Clin Invest* 93:2497, 1994.
16. Healey JF, Lubin IM, Nakai H, et al: Residues 484–508 contain a major determinant of the inhibitory epitope in the A2 domain of human factor VIII. *J Biol Chem* 270:14505, 1995.
17. Arai M, Scandella D, Hoyer LW: Molecular basis of factor VIII inhibition by human antibodies—Antibodies that bind to the factor VIII light chain prevent the interaction of factor VIII with phospholipid. *J Clin Invest* 83:1978, 1989.
18. Saenko EL, Shima M, Rajalakshmi KJ, Scandella D: A role for the C2 domain of factor binding to von Willebrand factor. *J Biol Chem* 269:11601, 1994.
19. Nogami K, Shima M, Hosokawa K, et al: Role of factor VIII C2 domain in factor VIII binding to factor Xa. *J Biol Chem* 274:31000, 1999.
20. Nogami K, Shima M, Hosokawa K, et al: Factor VIII C2 domain contains the thrombin-binding site responsible for thrombin-catalyzed cleavage at Arg1689. *J Biol Chem* 275:25774, 2000.
21. Meeks SL, Healey JF, Parker ET, et al: Non-classical anti-C2 domain antibodies are present in patients with factor VIII inhibitors. *Blood* 112:1151, 2008.
22. Algiman M, Dietrich G, Nydegger UE, et al: Natural antibodies to factor VIII (antihemophilic factor) in healthy individuals. *Proc Natl Acad Sci U S A* 89:3795, 1992.
23. Gilles JG, Saint-Remy JM: Healthy subjects produce both anti-factor VIII and specific anti-idiotypic antibodies. *J Clin Invest* 94:1496, 1994.
24. Guilbert B, Dighiero G, Avrameas S: Naturally occurring antibodies against nine common antigens in human sera. I. Detection, isolation and characterization. *J Immunol* 128:2779, 1982.
25. Ludlam CA, Morrison AE, Kessler C: Treatment of acquired hemophilia. *Semin Hematol* 31(2 Suppl 4):16, 1994.
26. Kasper CK, Aledort LM, Counts RB, et al: A more uniform measurement of factor VIII inhibitors. *Thromb Diath Haemorrh* 34:869, 1975.
27. Verbruggen B, Novakova I, Wessels H, et al: The Nijmegen modification of the Bethesda assay for factor VIII: C inhibitors: Improved specificity and reliability. *Thromb Haemost* 73:247, 1995.
28. Giles AR, Verbruggen B, Rivard GE, et al: A detailed comparison of the performance of the standard versus the Nijmegen modification of the Bethesda assay in detecting factor VIII:C inhibitors in the haemophilia A population of Canada. Association of Hemophilia Centre Directors of Canada. Factor VIII/IX Subcommittee of Scientific and Standardization Committee of International Society on Thrombosis and Haemostasis. *Thromb Haemost* 79:872, 1998.
29. Biggs R, Austen DE, Denson KW, et al: The mode of action of antibodies which destroy factor VIII. II. Antibodies which give complex concentration graphs. *Br J Haematol* 23:137, 1972.
30. Hoyer LW, Scandella D: Factor VIII inhibitors: Structure and function in autoantibody and hemophilia A patients. *Semin Hematol* 31:1, 1994.
31. Sumner MJ, Geldziler BD, Pedersen M, Seremetis S: Treatment of acquired haemophilia with recombinant activated FVII: A critical appraisal. *Haemophilia* 13:451, 2007.
32. Sallah S: Treatment of acquired haemophilia with factor eight inhibitor bypassing activity. *Haemophilia* 10:169, 2004.
33. Brettler DB, Forsberg AD, Levine PH, et al: The use of porcine factor VIII concentrate (Hyate:C) in the treatment of patients with inhibitor antibodies to factor VIII. A multicenter US experience. *Arch Intern Med* 149:1381, 1989.
34. Hay CR: Porcine factor VIII: Past, present and future. *Haematologica* 85:21, 2000.
35. Barnett B, Kruse-Jarres R, Leissinger CA: Current management of acquired factor VIII inhibitors. *Curr Opin Hematol* 15:451, 2008.
36. Collins PW: Treatment of acquired hemophilia A. *J Thromb Haemost* 5:893, 2007.
37. Hay CR, Brown S, Collins PW, et al: The diagnosis and management of factor VIII and IX inhibitors: A guideline from the United Kingdom Haemophilia Centre Doctors Organisation. *Br J Haematol* 133:591, 2006.
38. Franchini M, Lippi G: Acquired factor VIII inhibitors. *Blood* 112:250, 2008.
39. Schoenecker JG, Johnson RK, Lesher AP, et al: Exposure of mice to topical bovine thrombin induces systemic autoimmunity. *Am J Pathol* 159:1957, 2001.
40. Ortel TL, Charles LA, Keller FG, et al: Topical thrombin and acquired coagulation factor inhibitors: Clinical spectrum and laboratory diagnosis. *Am J Hematol* 45:128, 1994.
41. Zehnder JL, Leung LL: Development of antibodies to thrombin and factor V with recurrent bleeding in a patient exposed to topical bovine thrombin. *Blood* 76:2011, 1990.
42. Schoenecker JG, Johnson RK, Fields RC, et al: Relative purity of thrombin-based hemostatic agents used in surgery. *J Am Coll Surg* 197:580, 2003.
43. Ortel TL, Mercer MC, Thames EH, et al: Immunologic impact and clinical outcomes after surgical exposure to bovine thrombin. *Ann Surg* 233:88, 2001.
44. Knobl P, Lechner K: Acquired factor V inhibitors. *Baillieres Clin Haematol* 11:305, 1998.
45. Caers J, Reekmans A, Jochmans K, et al: Factor V inhibitor after injection of human thrombin (Tissucol) into a bleeding peptic ulcer. *Endoscopy* 35:542, 2003.
46. Lollar P: Pathogenic antibodies to coagulation factors. II. Fibrinogen, prothrombin, thrombin, factor V, factor XI, factor XII, factor XIII, the protein C system and von Willebrand factor. *J Thromb Haemost* 3:1385, 2005.
47. Macedo-Ribeiro S, Bode W, Huber R, et al: Crystal structures of the membrane-binding C2 domain of human coagulation factor V. *Nature* 402:434, 1999.
48. Ortel TL, Devore-Carter D, Quinn-Allen MA, Kane WH: Deletion analysis of recombinant human factor V. Evidence for a phosphatidylserine binding site in the second C-type domain. *J Biol Chem* 267:4189, 1992.
49. Ortel TL, Moore KD, Quinn-Allen MA, et al: Inhibitory anti-factor V antibodies bind to the factor V C2 domain and are associated with hemorrhagic manifestations. *Blood* 91:4188, 1998.
50. Izumi T, Kim SW, Greist A, et al: Fine mapping of inhibitory anti-factor V antibodies using factor V C2 domain mutants. Identification of two antigenic epitopes involved in phospholipid binding. *Thromb Haemost* 85:1048, 2001.
51. McNeil HP, Simpson RJ, Chesterman CN, Krilis SA: Anti-phospholipid antibodies are directed against a complex antigen that includes a lipid-binding inhibitor of coagulation: Beta 2-glycoprotein I (apolipoprotein H). *Proc Natl Acad Sci U S A* 87:4120, 1990.

52. Fleck RA, Rapaport SI, Rao LV: Anti-prothrombin antibodies and the lupus anticoagulant. *Blood* 72:512, 1988.
53. Loeliger A: Prothrombin as a co-factor of the circulating anticoagulant in systemic lupus erythematosus? *Thromb Diath Haemorrh* 3:273, 1959.
54. Feinstein DI, Rapaport SI: Acquired inhibitors of blood coagulation. *Prog Hemost Thromb* 1:75, 1972.
55. Bajaj SP, Rapaport SI, Fierer DS, et al: A mechanism for the hypoprothrombinemia of the acquired hypoprothrombinemia-lupus anticoagulant syndrome. *Blood* 61:684, 1983.
56. Edson JR, Vogt JM, Hasegawa DK: Abnormal prothrombin crossed-immunoelectrophoresis in patients with lupus inhibitors. *Blood* 64:807, 1984.
57. Mitchell CA, Rowell JA, Hau L, et al: A fatal thrombotic disorder associated with an acquired inhibitor of protein C. *N Engl J Med* 317:1638, 1987.
58. Sorice M, Arcieri P, Griggi T, et al: Inhibition of protein S by autoantibodies in patients with acquired protein S deficiency. *Thromb Haemost* 75:555, 1996.
59. Nojima J, Kuratsune H, Suehisa E, et al: Acquired activated protein C resistance associated with anti-protein S antibody as a strong risk factor for DVT in non-SLE patients. *Thromb Haemost* 88:716, 2002.
60. Hurtado V, Montes R, Gris JC, et al: Autoantibodies against EPCR are found in antiphospholipid syndrome and are a risk factor for fetal death. *Blood* 104:1369, 2004.
61. Boggio LN, Green D: Acquired hemophilia. *Rev Clin Exp Hematol* 5:389, 2001.
62. Nawarawong W, Wyshock E, Meloni FJ, et al: The rate of fibrinopeptide B release modulates the rate of clot formation: A study with an acquired inhibitor to fibrinopeptide B release. *Br J Haematol* 79:296, 1991.
63. Ruiz-Arguelles A: Spontaneous reversal of acquired autoimmune dysfibrinogenemia probably due to an antiidiotypic antibody directed to an interspecies cross-reactive idiotype expressed on antifibrinogen antibodies. *J Clin Invest* 82:958, 1988.
64. Goodrick MJ, Prentice AG, Copplestone JA, et al: Acquired factor XI inhibitor in chronic lymphocytic leukaemia. *J Clin Pathol* 45:352, 1992.
65. Lorand L, Maldonado N, Fradera J, et al: Haemorrhagic syndrome of autoimmune origin with a specific inhibitor against fibrin stabilizing factor (factor XIII). *Br J Haematol* 23:17, 1972.
66. Ajzner E, Schlammadinger A, Kerenyi A, et al: Severe bleeding complications caused by an autoantibody against the B subunit of plasma factor XIII: A novel form of acquired factor XIII deficiency. *Blood* 113:723, 2009.

CHAPTER 129

HEMOSTATIC DYSFUNCTION RELATED TO LIVER DISEASES AND LIVER TRANSPLANTATION

Ton Lisman and Philip G. De Groot

SUMMARY

Chronic or acute liver failure caused by, for example, viral hepatitis, alcohol abuse, or acetaminophen intoxication, results in substantial changes in the hemostatic system. Because the liver is involved in the synthesis of procoagulant and antifibrinolytic proteins, reduced amounts of these proteins are found if the synthetic function of the liver is compromised. Furthermore, a diseased liver has a reduced ability to clear activated hemostatic proteins, activators of fibrinolysis, or protein–inhibitor complexes from the circulation. A reduced platelet count and impaired platelet function are also commonly observed in patients with liver disease. These defects in hemostatic pathways are counteracted by concomitant defects in anticoagulant and profibrinolytic systems. Furthermore, highly elevated levels of von Willebrand factor that may compensate for impaired platelet function are present in patients with liver disease. Prolonged prothrombin time (PT) and activated partial thromboplastin time do not correlate very well with a bleeding tendency because these tests do not measure the reduced activity of the physiologic anticoagulants like protein C, protein S, and antithrombin. More sophisticated tests of hemostasis, such as total thrombin generation tests, can be normal in patients with stable liver disease. Thus, in many patients there is "rebalanced" hemostasis represented by limited bleeding during surgery including liver transplantation and sometimes even by thromboembolic complications. The new concept of rebalanced hemostasis has been translated to a more restricted prophylactic use of blood components in patients undergoing liver transplantation.

The liver plays a central role in hemostasis and thrombosis. Liver parenchymal cells are the site of synthesis of most coagulation factors, the physiologic inhibitors of coagulation, protein C, protein S, and antithrombin, and essential components of the fibrinolytic system, plasminogen, α_2-antiplasmin, and thrombin activatable fibrinolysis inhibitor (TAFI). The liver also regulates hemostasis and fibrinolysis by clearing activated coagulation factors and enzyme-inhibitor complexes from the circulation. Therefore, when liver dysfunction occurs in patients with liver disease, a complicated hemostatic derangement ensues, which can lead to bleeding, thrombosis, or neither bleeding nor thrombosis.

Acronyms and abbreviations that appear in this chapter include: ADAMTS13, a disintegrin-like and metalloprotease with thrombospondin domain 13; aPTT, activated partial thromboplastin time; DDAVP, 1-deamino-8-D-arginine vasopressin; DIC, disseminated intravascular coagulation; FFP, fresh-frozen plasma; HAT, hepatic artery thrombosis; INR, international normalized ratio; ISI, international sensitivity index; MELD, model of end-stage liver disease; PAI-1, plasminogen activator inhibitor 1; PT, prothrombin time; PVT, portal vein thrombosis; TAFI, thrombin-activatable fibrinolysis inhibitor; TFPI, tissue factor pathway inhibitor; t-PA, tissue-type plasminogen activator; VWF, von Willebrand factor.

PATHOGENESIS

PLATELETS

Thrombocytopenia

A mild to moderate thrombocytopenia (platelet counts between 50,000 and 100,000/μL) is frequently observed in patients with liver disease. The main causes for thrombocytopenia are increased platelet sequestration in the spleen because of congestive splenomegaly related to portal hypertension[1,2] and reduced thrombopoietin production by the liver.[3] Alternative mechanisms of thrombocytopenia include a reduced platelet half-life, possibly related to autoantibodies.[4] In patients with alcohol-induced liver disease, defective platelet production also occurs as a result of toxic effects of alcohol and folic acid deficiency on megakaryocytopoiesis.[5] Low-grade disseminated intravascular coagulation (DIC) may result in further platelet consumption, but its presence in patients with liver disease but without other causes, such as sepsis, is controversial.[6]

Platelet Function Defects

Platelet aggregation in response to various agonists is frequently diminished in patients with liver disease. Defective platelet function results from impaired signal transduction, decreased levels of proaggregatory components in the platelet granules (i.e., acquired storage pool deficiency), proteolysis of platelet membrane proteins presumably as a result of excessive plasmin formation, and increased production of the endothelial-derived platelet inhibitors, nitric oxide, and prostacyclin.[7] The presence of abnormal high-density lipoprotein or the presence of bile salts may also impair platelet function, and a reduced hematocrit may contribute to defective platelet–vessel wall interaction. Patients with cholestatic liver disease as a result of primary sclerosing cholangitis or primary biliary cirrhosis exhibit normal or even hyperactive platelets,[8,9] which is possibly related to the systemic inflammatory state in these patients. Platelet adhesion defects were also found under conditions of flow,[10] but were in some studies attributed to thrombocytopenia and a low hematocrit.[11,12] Platelet procoagulant activity measured by a thrombin generation assay using platelet-rich plasma was similar in patients and healthy controls, which casts additional doubt on the extent of the functional defects of platelets in patients with liver disease.[13]

VON WILLEBRAND FACTOR

Profoundly elevated levels of von Willebrand factor (VWF) antigen are frequently observed in patients with liver disease and were suggested to result from endothelial damage possibly mediated by bacterial infection.[14,15] VWF messenger ribonucleic acid (mRNA) and protein expression in the liver itself are substantially increased in cirrhosis,[16] but VWF activity measured by ristocetin or botrocetin-induced agglutination is variable.[12,14,15,17] The high levels of VWF may ameliorate the hemostatic defect caused by thrombocytopenia and platelet function defects.[15] In patients with liver disease the regulation of VWF multimer size and activity can be impaired because of reduced synthesis of VWF-cleaving protease ADAMTS13 (a disintegrin-like and metalloprotease with thrombospondin type 1 repeats) by stellate cells in the liver.[18] However, a reduced multimer size of VWF was found in patients with liver disease, suggesting that other proteases, such as plasmin, elastase, and granzyme B, contribute to VWF proteolysis.[19]

COAGULATION AND ANTICOAGULATION

Procoagulant Factors

The liver is the site of synthesis of most procoagulant proteins. As a result, decreased levels of coagulation factors V, VII, IX, X, and XI and prothrombin are commonly observed in patients with liver failure.[20] In contrast, factor VIII levels are increased which may be related to the elevated level of its carrier protein VWF and to decreased clearance of factor VIII from the circulation by the liver low-density lipoprotein-related receptor.[16] Factor VIII is synthesized primarily in hepatic sinusoidal endothelial cells, whose function is preserved in liver disease.[21]

Qualitative defects in clotting factors can arise as a consequence of hepatic failure. Because of vitamin K deficiency or decreased production of gamma glutamic carboxylase, a proportion of circulating vitamin K–dependent coagulation factors II, VII, IX, and X may be deficient in γ-carboxylated glutamic acid residues giving rise to impaired function of these factors.[22] Notably, increased levels of des-γ-carboxyprothrombin were observed in patients with hepatocellular carcinoma and can be used to distinguish between malignant and nonmalignant liver disease.[23]

Anticoagulant Factors

Levels of anticoagulant protein C, protein S, antithrombin, heparin cofactor II, and α_2-macroglobulin are decreased in patients with liver disease. Because tissue factor pathway inhibitor (TFPI) is mainly synthesized by endothelial cells, normal levels of this protein are present in patients with hepatic failure,[24] although one study found decreased levels.[25]

Dysfibrinogenemia

Fibrinogen levels are in the normal range in patients with chronic liver disease, but may be decreased in patients with decompensated cirrhosis or acute liver failure.[26] A qualitative defect in fibrinogen is frequently found in patients with all types of liver disease. The dysfibrinogen is characterized by an increased content of sialic acid,[27] possibly caused by enhanced levels of glycosyltransferases in hepatocytes.[28] Hypersialization of fibrinogen impairs its polymerization but does not affect the interaction of fibrinogen with platelets.[29]

FIBRINOLYTIC SYSTEM

Synthesis of Proteins Involved in Fibrinolysis

Except for tissue plasminogen activator (t-PA) and plasminogen-activator inhibitor (PAI)-1, all proteins involved in fibrinolysis are synthesized by the liver. Consequently, liver disease leads to decreased plasma levels of plasminogen, α_2-antiplasmin, TAFI, and factor XIII. Plasma levels of t-PA are elevated as a result of increased secretion from endothelial cells and/or reduced clearance by the diseased liver.[30] Plasma levels of PAI-1 also are increased but not to the same extent as t-PA.[31] In patients with acute hepatic failure PAI-1 levels are particularly high.[32]

Hyperfibrinolysis

Accelerated lysis of fibrin clots prepared from plasma of patients with chronic liver disease was described in 1914.[33] Since then, *in vitro* hyperfibrinolysis has been demonstrated by using various clot lysis assays and by measurements of D-dimer, fibrin(ogen) degradation products, and plasmin–antiplasmin complexes.[6,34–37] However, one study found no hyperfibrinolysis in patients with cirrhosis despite decreased levels of TAFI and elevated D-dimer levels.[38]

Hyperfibrinolysis in patients with cirrhosis has been associated with low-grade DIC induced by endotoxemia and was manifested by increased levels of prothrombin fragment 1+2, fibrinopeptide A, D-dimer, thrombin–antithrombin complex, and plasmin–antiplasmin complex.[39,40] However, it has been argued that the increased levels of these markers may result from their decreased clearance by the liver rather than from DIC. This argument was supported by postmortem studies that showed little evidence of fibrin deposition in organs of patients with liver disease (see Chap. 130).[41] Thus, whether or not low-grade DIC contributes to the hemostatic impairment in patients with uncomplicated liver disease is uncertain.

In patients with liver disease who presented with gastrointestinal bleeding or soft-tissue bleeding after trauma, *in vitro* signs of increased fibrinolysis were reported.[35,42] Intriguingly, unlike patients with α_2-antiplasmin or PAI-1 deficiency who have a delayed type of bleeding following trauma,[43,44] patients with liver disease exhibit an immediate type of bleeding diathesis.[45]

In patients with acute liver failure, there is an increased level of PAI-1 which is consistent with a hypofibrinolytic state. In contrast, the finding of an increased level of D-dimers in such patients is consistent with hyperfibrinolysis.[32,38] These conflicting observations make it difficult to discern whether or not hyperfibrinolysis is associated with liver disease.

TABLE 129–1. Alterations in the Hemostatic System in Patients with Liver Disease That Contribute to Bleeding (Left) or Counteract Bleeding (Right)

Changes That Impair Hemostasis	Changes That Promote Hemostasis
Thrombocytopenia	Elevated levels of VWF
Platelet function defects	Decreased levels of ADAMTS-13
Enhanced production of nitric oxide and prostacyclin	Elevated levels of factor VIII
Low levels of factors II, V, VII, IX, X, and XI	Decreased levels of protein C, protein S, antithrombin, α_2-macroglobulin, and heparin cofactor II
Vitamin K deficiency	Low levels of plasminogen
Dysfibrinogenemia	
Low levels of α_2-antiplasmin, factor XIII, and TAFI	
Elevated t-PA levels	

SOURCE: Modified with permission from the European Association for the Study of the Liver from Lisman T, Leebeek FWG, de Groot PG.[118]

THE CONCEPT OF A REBALANCED HEMOSTATIC SYSTEM

Because both procoagulant and anticoagulant proteins decline in patients with liver diseases, it appears that the hemostatic system is rebalanced (Table 129–1).[46–49] This may explain why most patients with liver disease usually do not exhibit severe bleeding manifestations during invasive procedures,[50,51] and why patients are not protected against thrombosis.[52–55] This balance is quite delicate and vulnerable to be tipped toward bleeding or thrombosis depending on the particular trigger that is inflicted.

PITFALLS IN DIAGNOSIS OF HEMOSTATIC DISORDERS IN LIVER DISEASE

Assessment of Platelet Function

The thrombocytopenia in patients with stable cirrhosis is often mild and does not cause spontaneous bleeding or bleeding following minimally invasive procedures. There is little evidence that tests showing platelet dysfunction predict bleeding in patients with cirrhosis. Nevertheless, one study showed that a prolonged bleeding time was associated with a fivefold increase in the risk of bleeding after liver biopsy.[56] Although shortening of the bleeding time was achieved by administration of 1-deamino-8-D-arginine vasopressin (DDAVP),[57] no effect of this drug was observed in patients with bleeding from esophageal varices or on the blood loss in patients undergoing hepatectomy or liver transplantation.[58–60]

Assessment of Coagulation

Screening tests of coagulation, such as the prothrombin time (PT) or activated partial thromboplastin time (aPTT), are frequently prolonged in patients with liver failure. These results have been traditionally interpreted to reflect a hypocoagulable state, but with no impact on the bleeding risk after invasive procedures.[61] The PT and aPTT are sensitive to levels of procoagulant proteins in plasma, but not to the natural anticoagulants, proteins C, protein S, and antithrombin. The use of the more sophisticated test of coagulation, such as total thrombin generation tests, illustrates the limitation of the PT and aPTT assays. In a dilute PT-like assay, total thrombin generation was significantly lower in patients with stable cirrhosis than in controls.[62] Yet, when measured in the presence of thrombomodulin to enable protein C activation, thrombin generation was indistinguishable from controls. These results suggest that thrombin generation *in vivo* can be normal in patients with liver failure, and that a prolonged PT does not indicate a bleeding risk.

A second important problem with coagulation tests in patients with liver disease is the use of the international normalized ratio (INR) in prognostic scores such as the Child-Pugh and model of end-stage liver disease (MELD) presently employed to prioritize patients for liver transplantation. The INR was developed and validated only to monitor anticoagulant therapy with vitamin K antagonists. The interlaboratory variation of the INR in patients with liver disease is substantial, and its use results in significant differences in MELD scores when a single patient sample is tested in different laboratories.[63,64] The main reason for this large interlaboratory variation is the use of different reagents with variable international sensitivity indices (ISI) that have been determined by calibration against plasma samples from patients treated with vitamin K antagonists. Although the use of alternative ISI values obtained by calibration against plasma samples from patients with liver disease was shown to decrease this variability,[65,66] this modification has not as yet been introduced by most centers.

HEMOSTATIC ALTERATIONS DURING LIVER TRANSPLANTATION

During the first stage of liver transplantation, the removal of the diseased liver, no significant worsening of the preoperative hemostatic functions occurs.[67] Following removal of the diseased liver, the anhepatic stage, significant hemostatic changes can occur. Because activated clotting factors are not removed from the circulation, DIC can develop, with consumption of platelets and clotting factors and secondary hyperfibrinolysis.[68] Moreover, primary hyperfibrinolysis also occurs as a result of defective clearance of t-PA.[69,70] The most severe hemostatic changes during liver transplantation occur after reperfusion of the donor liver. Platelets are trapped in the graft, giving rise to an aggravation of thrombocytopenia and causing damage to the graft by induction of endothelial cell apoptosis.[71] Release of tissue factor and t-PA from the reperfused graft results from endothelial damage and causes DIC with secondary fibrinolysis and primary fibrinolysis.[69,72] Moreover, the graft releases heparin-like substances that can inhibit coagulation.[73] In addition, other factors such as hypothermia, metabolic acidosis, and hemodilution adversely affect hemostasis during this phase.

During transplantation, the levels of VWF remain high, the functional properties of VWF improve, and the levels of ADAMTS13 decline, which may partially compensate for the hemostatic dysfunction, but may also increase the risk for postoperative thrombosis.[74,75] The platelets count and hemostatic proteins are at their nadir after reperfusion and rise gradually during the early postoperative period.[76] However, the levels of procoagulant factors rise more rapidly than the levels of anticoagulant factors, which results in a temporary hypercoagulable state.[77] A transiently increased level of PAI-1 immediately after surgery can result in a hypofibrinolytic state that may aggravate the hypercoagulable status.[78]

CLINICAL FEATURES

BLEEDING IN PATIENTS WITH LIVER DISEASE AND DURING LIVER TRANSPLANTATION

Although it is currently debated whether patients with liver disease have a bleeding tendency,[47,79] bleeding does occur and may be related to nonhemostatic factors. The most common bleeding manifestation in patients with liver disease is bleeding from ruptured esophageal varices. This results from local vascular abnormalities and increased splanchnic blood pressure, and not necessarily from deranged hemostasis.[80] Occasionally, impaired hemostasis does cause easy bruising, purpura, epistaxis, gingival bleeding, menorrhagia, gastrointestinal bleeding, and bleeding associated with invasive procedures. Bleeding following liver biopsy is uncommon.[45]

Liver transplantation is a lengthy procedure with extensive surgical wound surfaces including potential transection of collateral veins. In earlier years, liver transplantation was thought to require massive transfusion of blood product to correct the hemostatic dysfunction before, during, and after transplantation.[68] Improved surgical techniques and anesthesiologic care have led to a remarkable reduction of blood loss during liver transplantation. Currently, no blood transfusion is given in up to 50 percent of patients undergoing a liver transplantation, depending on the center.[50]

THROMBOSIS IN PATIENTS WITH LIVER DISEASE AND IN PATIENTS FOLLOWING LIVER TRANSPLANTATION

Venous Thrombosis

Deep vein thromboses and pulmonary emboli can occur in patients with cirrhosis.[52–55] A large nationwide population-based case-control study in Denmark indicated that patients with liver disease have a substantially increased risk for venous thromboembolism compared to controls with an odds ratio of 1.74 (95% confidence interval [CI] 1.54–1.95) for patients with cirrhosis, and an odds ratio of 1.87 (95% CI 1.73–2.03) for patients with other liver diseases.[52] Between 0.5 and 1.8 percent of all hospitalized patients with cirrhosis developed venous thrombosis, but this rate is probably an underestimation because edema and dyspnea, commonly observed in patients with cirrhosis, may mask thromboembolism. Treatment of venous thromboembolism in patients with liver disease is difficult, because the risk of bleeding associated with anticoagulant treatment is greater than in healthy individuals.[54] This again indicates that the balanced hemostatic system in patients with cirrhosis involves a narrow safety margin. Pulmonary emboli and intracardiac thrombosis may occur during liver transplantation, indicating that the hemostatic system may also tip toward thrombus formation during this procedure.[81]

Liver-Related Thrombosis

Patients with liver disease can develop thrombosis in the portal and mesenteric veins. These complications presumably are caused by (1) decreased levels of the natural inhibitors of coagulation, antithrombin, protein C, and protein S; (2) the common inherited thrombophilias such as factor V Leiden, prothrombin G20210A, and homozygous methylenetetrahydrofolate reductase C677T[82]; and (3) decreased blood flow in the splanchnic venous circulation because of portal hypertension. The prevalence of portal vein thrombosis (PVT) in patients with cirrhosis without hepatocellular carcinoma increases with the progression of the disease, being less than 1 percent in patients with compensated cirrhosis, and 8 to 25 percent in liver transplantation candidates.[83,84]

Following liver transplantation, both immediate and delayed thrombotic complications frequently occur.[85] Thrombosis of the hepatic artery occurs in 1.6 to 8.9 percent of patients and may lead to graft failure, requiring retransplantation.[86] Hepatic artery thrombosis (HAT) may occur early after transplantation, but may also occur years after the procedure. Thrombosis of the portal vein or the vena cava are much less common, but these complications also contribute to poorer outcome of transplantation.[87] Although HAT has been considered a surgical complication, recent evidence suggests that excessive coagulation activation also may contribute to HAT.[88] Small studies and case reports have suggested that factor V Leiden may be associated with the occurrence of HAT.[89,90] In patients undergoing liver transplantation for familial amyloidotic polyneuropathy who do not have liver failure, there is a substantially increased risk for HAT, which may be related to the fully competent hemostatic system in these patients.[91]

Hypercoagulation and Progression of Fibrosis

Activation of the coagulation pathways has been suggested to directly contribute to the progression of fibrosis in patients with chronic liver disease for which several mechanism have been proposed.[92] Thrombin was shown to promote fibrogenesis by enhancing stellate cell activation via protease activated receptors[93]; formation of microthrombi within the hepatic parenchyma caused ischemia, parenchymal extinction, and fibrosis[94]; promotion of carbon tetrachloride-induced fibrosis was shown in mice carrying factor V Leiden[95]; anticoagulants slowed down the progression of fibrosis in rodent models[96,97]; hepatitis C-related liver disease in patients with hemophilia was milder compared to hepatitis C progression in patients without hemophilia[98]; and in patients with chronic hepatitis B, heparin or low-molecular-weight heparin was associated with improved serum levels of alanine aminotransferase, hyaluronic acid, and collagen IV, and improved histologic features of fibrosis.[99]

HEMOSTATIC MANAGEMENT

General Considerations

Traditional guidelines have advised not to perform invasive procedures in patients with liver disease when routine hemostatic tests are abnormal unless they are corrected by blood products or pharmacologic prohemostatic agents. In recent years, the rationale for such a prophylactic approach has been questioned because (1) abnormal coagulation tests in patients with liver disease are not necessarily associated with a bleeding risk,[46] (2) normalization of tests is rarely achieved,[100] (3) the adverse effects of blood products are increasingly recognized,[101] and (4) the efficacy of prophylactic treatment has not been proven.[102] Consequently, consensus guidelines do not recommend the use of fresh-frozen plasma transfusion for prophylactic correction of an abnormal PT.[102–104] Another guideline states that the available evidence suggests that patients with liver disease with a PT more than 4 seconds longer than control are unlikely to benefit from fresh-frozen plasma (grade C recommendation, level IV evidence).[103] A novel strategy to improve platelet function in patients with hepatitis C is the administration of a thrombopoietin analogue (Eltrombopag), which has been shown to substantially increase the platelet count in these patients, but has not been approved for patients with cirrhosis by the FDA at the time of this writing.[105] However, because Eltrombopag administration can result in thrombocytosis, a theoretical risk of thrombosis ensues, especially in light of the highly elevated VWF levels in patients with liver disease.[15]

Hemostatic Management during Liver Transplantation

For many years excessive blood loss during liver transplantation has been recognized as an important cause of morbidity and mortality; consequently, transfusion of a combination of blood products has been advocated for correction of the hemostatic derangements.[68,106] Because prophylactic transfusion of blood products is associated with serious side effects,[107,108] many centers have discontinued to attempt to improve hemostatic functions by administration of blood products prior to liver transplantation.[50] Many centers report that liver transplant procedures can be performed without a requirement for transfusion of blood products in a substantial proportion of patients. One study reported that 79 percent of patients could be transplanted without the use of any blood product, provided the patient's central venous pressure was controlled through restriction of volume replacement, and by using intraoperative phlebotomy during the transplantation.[51] Increased experience and improvements in surgical technique, anesthesiologic care, and better graft preservation methods have contributed to a steady decrease in blood transfusion requirements. When uncontrolled bleeding does occur, packed red cells, platelets, and fresh-frozen plasma can be transfused guided by laboratory values or thromboelastography. Hyperfibrinolysis is thought to contribute significantly to impaired hemostasis during the anhepatic and reperfusion phases.[68] Use of synthetic antifibrinolytic agents, such as tranexamic acid (a lysine analogue) and aprotinin (a serine protease inhibitor) have reduced red cell and plasma transfusion.[110,111] These agents also improve hemostasis by modulating vascular tone, preservation of platelet function, and inhibiting inflammation.[112] Notably, however, aprotinin was taken off the market in 2008 because of severe adverse events and mortality in patients undergoing cardiac surgery.[113]

Adverse Effects of Blood Products

Blood transfusions have an immunosuppressive effect and can be associated with transmission of infectious agents, transfusion reactions, pulmonary edema and transfusion-related acute lung injury (see Chaps. 140 and 141).[114] Also, in patients undergoing liver transplantations, there is an increased rate of postoperative infection, morbidity, and mortality with increased use of packed red cells.[50,107,115] Also platelet transfusions are associated with increased mortality after liver transplantation, possibly by an increased risk of acute lung injury.[116]

Anticoagulation

Postoperative use of anticoagulants has been limited in liver transplant recipients as a result of the perceived bleeding risk. However, thrombotic complications do occur, and liver-related thromboses in particular, such as HAT and PVT, are of concern as they often lead to graft loss. A single, uncontrolled retrospective study showed aspirin to substantially reduce the risk of post transplantation HAT.[117] None of the 236 patients followed for a median of 1704 days had bleeding manifestations related to aspirin therapy. Whether or not other anticoagulants will prevent postoperative thrombosis remains to be established.

REFERENCES

1. Aster RH: Pooling of platelets in the spleen: Role in the pathogenesis of "hypersplenic" thrombocytopenia. *J Clin Invest* 45:645, 1966.

2. Schmidt KG, Rasmussen JW, Bekker C, Madsen PE: Kinetics and *in vivo* distribution of 111-In-labelled autologous platelets in chronic hepatic disease: Mechanisms of thrombocytopenia. *Scand J Haematol* 34:39, 1985.
3. Goulis J, Chau TN, Jordan S, et al: Thrombopoietin concentrations are low in patients with cirrhosis and thrombocytopenia and are restored after orthotopic liver transplantation. *Gut* 44:754, 1999.
4. Kajihara M, Kato S, Okazaki Y, et al: A role of autoantibody-mediated platelet destruction in thrombocytopenia in patients with cirrhosis. *Hepatology* 37:1267, 2003.
5. Levine RF, Spivak JL, Meagher RC, Sieber F: Effect of ethanol on thrombopoiesis. *Br J Haematol* 62:345, 1986.
6. Ben Zimran A, Osman E, Hutton RA, Burroughs AK: Disseminated intravascular coagulation in liver cirrhosis: Fact or fiction? *Am J Gastroenterol* 94:2977, 1999.
7. Witters P, Freson K, Verslype C, et al: Review article: Blood platelet number and function in chronic liver disease and cirrhosis. *Aliment Pharmacol Ther* 27:1017, 2008.
8. Pihusch R, Rank A, Gohring P, et al: Platelet function rather than plasmatic coagulation explains hypercoagulable state in cholestatic liver disease. *J Hepatol* 37:548, 2002.
9. Ben Zimran A, Panagou M, Patch D, et al: Hypercoagulability in patients with primary biliary cirrhosis and primary sclerosing cholangitis evaluated by thrombelastography. *J Hepatol* 26:554, 1997.
10. Ordinas A, Escolar G, Cirera I, et al: Existence of a platelet-adhesion defect in patients with cirrhosis independent of hematocrit: Studies under flow conditions. *Hepatology* 24:1137, 1996.
11. Lisman T, Adelmeijer J, de Groot PG, et al: No evidence for an intrinsic platelet defect in patients with liver cirrhosis—Studies under flow conditions. *J Thromb Haemost* 4:2070, 2006.
12. Escolar G, Cases A, Vinas M, et al: Evaluation of acquired platelet dysfunctions in uremic and cirrhotic patients using the platelet function analyzer (PFA-100): Influence of hematocrit elevation. *Haematologica* 84:614, 1999.
13. Tripodi A, Primignani M, Chantarangkul V, et al: Thrombin generation in patients with cirrhosis: The role of platelets. *Hepatology* 44:440, 2006.
14. Ferro D, Quintarelli C, Lattuada A, et al: High plasma levels of von Willebrand factor as a marker of endothelial perturbation in cirrhosis: Relationship to endotoxemia. *Hepatology* 23:1377, 1996.
15. Lisman T, Bongers TN, Adelmeijer J, et al: Elevated levels of von Willebrand Factor in cirrhosis support platelet adhesion despite reduced functional capacity. *Hepatology* 44:53, 2006.
16. Hollestelle MJ, Geertzen HGM, Straatsburg IH, et al: Factor VIII expression in liver disease. *Thromb Haemost* 91:267, 2004.
17. Beer JH, Clerici N, Baillod P, et al: Quantitative and qualitative analysis of platelet GPIb and von Willebrand factor in liver cirrhosis. *Thromb Haemost* 73:601, 1995.
18. Mannucci PM, Canciani MT, Forza I, et al: Changes in health and disease of the metalloprotease that cleaves von Willebrand factor. *Blood* 98:2730, 2001.
19. Federici AB, Berkowitz SD, Lattuada A, Mannucci PM: Degradation of von Willebrand factor in patients with acquired clinical conditions in which there is heightened proteolysis. *Blood* 81:720, 1993.
20. Kerr R, Newsome P, Germain L, et al: Effects of acute liver injury on blood coagulation. *J Thromb Haemost* 1:754, 2003.
21. Hollestelle MJ, Thinnes T, Crain K, et al: Tissue distribution of factor VIII gene expression *in vivo*—A closer look. *Thromb Haemost* 86:855, 2001.
22. Blanchard RA, Furie BC, Jorgensen M, et al: Acquired vitamin K-dependent carboxylation deficiency in liver disease. *N Engl J Med* 305:242, 1981.
23. Marrero JA, Su GL, Wei W, et al: Des-gamma carboxyprothrombin can differentiate hepatocellular carcinoma from nonmalignant chronic liver disease in American patients. *Hepatology* 37:1114, 2003.
24. Bajaj MS, Kuppuswamy MN, Saito H, et al: Cultured normal human hepatocytes do not synthesize lipoprotein-associated coagulation inhibitor: Evidence that endothelium is the principal site of its synthesis. *Proc Natl Acad Sci U S A* 87:8869, 1990.
25. Oksuzoglu G, Simsek H, Haznedaroglu IC, Kirazli S: Tissue factor pathway inhibitor concentrations in cirrhotic patients with and without portal vein thrombosis. *Am J Gastroenterol* 92:303, 1997.
26. de Maat MP, Nieuwenhuizen W, Knot EA, et al: Measuring plasma fibrinogen levels in patients with liver cirrhosis. The occurrence of proteolytic fibrin(ogen) degradation products and their influence on several fibrinogen assays. *Thromb Res* 78:353, 1995.
27. Francis JL, Armstrong DJ: Acquired dysfibrinogenaemia in liver disease. *J Clin Pathol* 35:667, 1982.
28. Martinez J, MacDonald KA, Palascak JE: The role of sialic acid in the dysfibrinogenemia associated with liver disease: Distribution of sialic acid on the constituent chains. *Blood* 61:1196, 1983.
29. Harfenist EJ, Packham MA, Mustard JF: Effects of variant gamma chains and sialic acid content of fibrinogen upon its interactions with ADP-stimulated human and rabbit platelets. *Blood* 64:1163,1984.
30. Leiper K, Croll A, Booth NA, et al: Tissue plasminogen activator, plasminogen activator inhibitors, and activator-inhibitor complex in liver disease. *J Clin Pathol* 47:214, 1994.
31. Leebeek FWG, Kluft C, Knot EAR, et al: A shift in balance between profibrinolytic and antifibrinolytic factors causes enhanced fibrinolysis in cirrhosis. *Gastroenterology* 101:1382, 1991.
32. Pernambuco JR, Langley PG, Hughes RD, et al: Activation of the fibrinolytic system in patients with fulminant liver failure. *Hepatology* 18:1350, 1993.
33. Goodpasture EW: Fibrinolysis in chronic hepatic insufficiency. *Johns Hopkins Hosp Bull* 25:330, 1914.
34. Vukovich T, Teufelsbauer H, Fritzer M, et al: Hemostasis activation in patients with liver cirrhosis. *Thromb Res* 77:271, 1995.
35. Francis RB Jr, Feinstein DI: Clinical significance of accelerated fibrinolysis in liver disease. *Haemostasis* 14:460, 1984.
36. Colucci M, Binetti BM, Branca MG, et al: Deficiency of thrombin activatable fibrinolysis inhibitor in cirrhosis is associated with increased plasma fibrinolysis. *Hepatology* 38:230, 2003.
37. Wilde JT, Kitchen S, Kinsey S, et al: Plasma D-dimer levels and their relationship to serum fibrinogen/fibrin degradation products in hypercoagulable states. *Br J Haematol* 71:65, 1989.
38. Lisman T, Leebeek FW, Mosnier LO, et al: Thrombin-activatable fibrinolysis inhibitor deficiency in cirrhosis is not associated with increased plasma fibrinolysis. *Gastroenterology* 121:131, 2001.
39. Violi F, Ferro D, Basili S, et al: Hyperfibrinolysis resulting from clotting activation in patients with different degrees of cirrhosis. *Hepatology* 17:78, 1993.
40. Violi F, Ferro D, Basili S, et al: Association between low-grade disseminated intravascular coagulation and endotoxemia in patients with liver cirrhosis. *Gastroenterology* 109:531, 1995.
41. Oka K, Tanaka K: Intravascular coagulation in autopsy cases with liver diseases. *Thromb Haemost* 42:564, 1979.
42. Violi F, Ferro D, Basili S, et al: Hyperfibrinolysis increases the risk of gastrointestinal hemorrhage in patients with advanced cirrhosis. *Hepatology* 15:672, 1992.
43. Kluft C, Nieuwenhuis HK, Rijken DC, et al: Alpha 2-Antiplasmin Enschede: Dysfunctional alpha 2-antiplasmin molecule associated with an autosomal recessive hemorrhagic disorder. *J Clin Invest* 80:1391, 1987.
44. Lee MH, Vosburgh E, Anderson K, McDonagh J: Deficiency of plasma plasminogen activator inhibitor 1 results in hyperfibrinolytic bleeding. *Blood* 81:2357, 1993.
45. Piccinino F, Sagnelli E, Pasquale G, Giusti G: Complications following percutaneous liver biopsy. A multicentre retrospective study on 68,276 biopsies. *J Hepatol* 2:165, 1986.
46. Caldwell SH, Hoffman M, Lisman T, et al: Coagulation disorders and hemostasis in liver disease: Pathophysiology and critical assessment of current management. *Hepatology* 44:1039, 2006.
47. Lisman T, Caldwell SH, Leebeek FWG, Porte RJ: Hemostasis in chronic liver disease—Is chronic liver disease associated with a bleeding diathesis? *J Thromb Haemost* 4:2059, 2006.
48. Warnaar N, Lisman T, Porte RJ: The two tales of coagulation in liver transplantation. *Curr Opin Organ Transplant* 13:298, 2008.
49. Tripodi A, Mannucci PM: Abnormalities of hemostasis in chronic liver disease: Reappraisal of their clinical significance and need for clinical and laboratory research. *J Hepatol* 46:727, 2007.
50. de Boer MT, Molenaar IQ, Hendriks HG, et al: Minimizing blood loss in liver transplantation: Progress through research and evolution of techniques. *Dig Surg* 22:265, 2005.
51. Massicotte L, Lenis S, Thibeault L, et al: Effect of low central venous pressure and phlebotomy on blood product transfusion requirements during liver transplantations. *Liver Transpl* 12:117, 2006.
52. Sogaard KK, Horvath-Puho E, Gronbaek H, et al: Risk of venous thromboembolism in patients with liver disease: A nationwide population-based case-control study. *Am J Gastroenterol* 104:96, 2009.
53. Northup PG, McMahon MM, Ruhl AP, et al: Coagulopathy does not fully protect hospitalized cirrhosis patients from peripheral venous thromboembolism. *Am J Gastroenterol* 101:1524, 2006.
54. Garcia-Fuster MJ, Abdilla N, Fabia MJ, et al: [Venous thromboembolism and liver cirrhosis]. *Rev Esp Enferm Dig* 100:259, 2008.
55. Gulley D, Teal E, Suvannasankha A, et al: Deep vein thrombosis and pulmonary embolism in cirrhosis patients. *Dig Dis Sci* 53:3012, 2008.
56. Boberg KM, Brosstad F, Egeland T, et al: Is a prolonged bleeding time associated with an increased risk of hemorrhage after liver biopsy? *Thromb Haemost* 81:378, 1999.
57. Agnelli G, Parise P, Levi M, et al: Effects of desmopressin on hemostasis in patients with liver cirrhosis. *Haemostasis* 25:241, 1995.
58. de Franchis R, Arcidiacono PG, Carpinelli L, et al: Randomized controlled trial of desmopressin plus terlipressin vs. terlipressin alone for the treatment of acute variceal hemorrhage in cirrhotic patients: A multicenter, double-blind study. New Italian Endoscopic Club. *Hepatology* 18:1102, 1993.
59. Wong AY, Irwin MG, Hui TW, et al: Desmopressin does not decrease blood loss and transfusion requirements in patients undergoing hepatectomy. *Can J Anaesth* 50:14, 2003.
60. Pivalizza EG, Warters RD, Gebhard R: Desmopressin before liver transplantation. *Can J Anaesth* 50:748, 2003.
61. Tripodi A, Caldwell SH, Hoffman M, et al: Review article: The prothrombin time test as a measure of bleeding risk and prognosis in liver disease. *Aliment Pharmacol Ther* 26:141, 2007.
62. Tripodi A, Salerno F, Chantarangkul V, et al: Evidence of normal thrombin generation in cirrhosis despite abnormal conventional coagulation tests. *Hepatology* 41:553, 2005.
63. Trotter JF, Brimhall B, Arjal R, Phillips C: Specific laboratory methodologies achieve higher model for endstage liver disease (MELD) scores for patients listed for liver transplantation. *Liver Transpl* 10:995, 2004.

64. Lisman T, van Leeuwen Y, Adelmeijer J, et al: Interlaboratory variability in assessment of the model of end-stage liver disease score. *Liver Int* 28:1344, 2008.
65. Tripodi A, Chantarangkul V, Primignani M, et al: The international normalized ratio calibrated for cirrhosis (INR(liver)) normalizes prothrombin time results for model for end-stage liver disease calculation. *Hepatology* 46:520, 2007.
66. Bellest L, Eschwege V, Poupon R, et al: A modified international normalized ratio as an effective way of prothrombin time standardization in hepatology. *Hepatology* 46:528, 2007.
67. Kang YG, Martin DJ, Marquez J, et al: Intraoperative changes in blood coagulation and thrombelastographic monitoring in liver transplantation. *Anesth Analg* 64:888, 1985.
68. Porte RJ, Knot EAR, Bontempo FA: Hemostasis in liver transplantation. *Gastroenterology* 97:488, 1989.
69. Porte RJ, Bontempo FA, Knot EA, et al: Systemic effects of tissue plasminogen activator-associated fibrinolysis and its relation to thrombin generation in orthotopic liver transplantation. *Transplantation* 47:978, 1989.
70. Bakker CM, Metselaar HJ, Groenland TN, et al: Increased fibrinolysis in orthotopic but not in heterotopic liver transplantation: The role of the anhepatic phase. *Transpl Int* 5:S173, 1992.
71. Sindram D, Porte RJ, Hoffman MR, et al: Platelets induce sinusoidal endothelial cell apoptosis upon reperfusion of the cold ischemic rat liver. *Gastroenterology* 118:183, 2000.
72. Suzumura N, Monden M, Gotoh M, et al: Coagulation disorders during orthotopic liver transplantation: Inhibition of tissue thromboplastin activity by its antibody. *Transplant Proc* 21:2367, 1989.
73. Agarwal S, Senzolo M, Melikian C, et al: The prevalence of a heparin-like effect shown on the thromboelastograph in patients undergoing liver transplantation. *Liver Transpl* 14:855, 2008.
74. Pereboom ITA, Adelmeijer J, van Leeuwen Y, et al: Development of a severe von Willebrand factor/ADAMTS13 dysbalance during orthotopic liver transplantation. *Am J Transpl* 9:1189, 2009.
75. Kobayashi T, Wada H, Usui M, et al: Decreased ADAMTS13 levels in patients after living donor liver transplantation. *Thromb Res* 124:541, 2009.
76. Meijer K, Hendriks HG, de Wolf JT, et al: Recombinant factor VIIa in orthotopic liver transplantation: Influence on parameters of coagulation and fibrinolysis. *Blood Coagul Fibrinolysis* 14:169, 2003.
77. Stahl RL, Duncan A, Hooks MA, et al: A hypercoagulable state follows orthotopic liver transplantation. *Hepatology* 12:553, 1990.
78. Lisman T, Leebeek FWG, Meijer K, et al: Recombinant Factor VIIa improves clot formation but not fibrinolytic potential in patients with cirrhosis and during liver transplantation. *Hepatology* 35:616, 2002.
79. Reverter JC: Abnormal hemostasis tests and bleeding in chronic liver disease: Are they related? Yes. *J Thromb Haemost* 4:717, 2006.
80. Sharara AI, Rockey DC: Gastroesophageal variceal hemorrhage. *N Engl J Med* 345:669, 2001.
81. Warnaar N, Molenaar IQ, Colquhoun SD, et al: Intraoperative pulmonary embolism and intracardiac thrombosis complicating liver transplantation: A systematic review. *J Thromb Haemost* 6:297, 2008.
82. Amitrano L, Brancaccio V, Guardascione MA, et al: Inherited coagulation disorders in cirrhotic patients with portal vein thrombosis. *Hepatology* 31:345, 2000.
83. Okuda K, Ohnishi K, Kimura K, et al: Incidence of portal vein thrombosis in liver cirrhosis. An angiographic study in 708 patients. *Gastroenterology* 89:279, 1985.
84. Francoz C, Belghiti J, Vilgrain V, et al: Splanchnic vein thrombosis in candidates for liver transplantation: Usefulness of screening and anticoagulation. *Gut* 54:691, 2005.
85. Washington K: Update on post-liver transplantation infections, malignancies, and surgical complications. *Adv Anat Pathol* 12:221, 2005.
86. Silva MA, Jambulingam PS, Gunson BK, et al: Hepatic artery thrombosis following orthotopic liver transplantation: A 10-year experience from a single centre in the United Kingdom. *Liver Transpl* 12:146, 2006.
87. Quiroga S, Sebastia MC, Margarit C, et al: Complications of orthotopic liver transplantation: Spectrum of findings with helical CT. *Radiographics* 21:1085, 2001.
88. Lisman T, Porte RJ: Hepatic artery thrombosis after liver transplantation: More than just a surgical complication? *Transpl Int* 22:162, 2009.
89. Hirshfield G, Collier JD, Brown K, et al: Donor factor V Leiden mutation and vascular thrombosis following liver transplantation. *Liver Transpl Surg* 4:58, 1998.
90. Tanyel FC, Ocal T, Balkanci F, et al: The factor V Leiden mutation: A possible contributor to the hepatic artery thrombosis encountered after liver transplantation in a child. *J Pediatr Surg* 35:607, 2000.
91. Bispo M, Marcelino P, Freire A, et al: High incidence of thrombotic complications early after liver transplantation for familial amyloidotic polyneuropathy. *Transpl Int* 22:165, 2009.
92. Calvaruso V, Maimone S, Gatt A, et al: Coagulation and fibrosis in chronic liver disease. *Gut* 57:1722, 2008.
93. Rullier A, Gillibert-Duplantier J, Costet P, et al: Protease-activated receptor 1 knockout reduces experimentally induced liver fibrosis. *Am J Physiol Gastrointest Liver Physiol* 294:G226, 2008.
94. Wanless IR, Wong F, Blendis LM, et al: Hepatic and portal vein thrombosis in cirrhosis: Possible role in development of parenchymal extinction and portal hypertension. *Hepatology* 21:1238, 1995.
95. Anstee QM, Goldin RD, Wright M, et al: Coagulation status modulates murine hepatic fibrogenesis: Implications for the development of novel therapies. *J Thromb Haemost* 6:1336, 2008.
96. Duplantier JG, Dubuisson L, Senant N, et al: A role for thrombin in liver fibrosis. *Gut* 53:1682, 2004.
97. Abe W, Ikejima K, Lang T, et al: Low molecular weight heparin prevents hepatic fibrogenesis caused by carbon tetrachloride in the rat. *J Hepatol* 46:286, 2007.
98. Assy N, Pettigrew N, Lee SS, et al: Are chronic hepatitis C viral infections more benign in patients with hemophilia? *Am J Gastroenterol* 102:1672, 2007.
99. Shi J, Hao JH, Ren WH, Zhu JR: Effects of heparin on liver fibrosis in patients with chronic hepatitis B. *World J Gastroenterol* 9:1611, 2003.
100. Youssef WI, Salazar F, Dasarathy S, et al: Role of fresh frozen plasma infusion in correction of coagulopathy of chronic liver disease: A dual phase study. *Am J Gastroenterol* 98:1391, 2003.
101. Alter HJ, Klein HG: The hazards of blood transfusion in historical perspective. *Blood* 112:2617, 2008.
102. Segal JB, Dzik WH: Paucity of studies to support that abnormal coagulation test results predict bleeding in the setting of invasive procedures: An evidence-based review. *Transfusion* 45:1413, 2005.
103. O'Shaughnessy DF, Atterbury C, Bolton MP, et al: Guidelines for the use of fresh-frozen plasma, cryoprecipitate and cryosupernatant. *Br J Haematol* 126:11, 2004.
104. Ramsey G: Treating coagulopathy in liver disease with plasma transfusions or recombinant factor VIIa: An evidence-based review. *Best Pract Res Clin Haematol* 19:113, 2006.
105. McHutchison JG, Dusheiko G, Shiffman ML, et al: Eltrombopag for thrombocytopenia in patients with cirrhosis associated with hepatitis C. *N Engl J Med* 357:2227, 2007.
106. Ozier Y, Steib A, Ickx B, et al: Haemostatic disorders during liver transplantation. *Eur J Anaesthesiol* 18:208, 2001.
107. de Boer MT, Christensen MC, Asmussen M, et al: The impact of intraoperative transfusion of platelets and red blood cells on survival after liver transplantation. *Anesth Analg* 106:32, 2008.
108. Spiess BD: Risks of transfusion: Outcome focus. *Transfusion* 44:4S, 2004.
109. Coakley M, Reddy K, Mackie I, Mallett S: Transfusion triggers in orthotopic liver transplantation: A comparison of the thromboelastometry analyzer, the thromboelastogram, and conventional coagulation tests. *J Cardiothorac Vasc Anesth* 20:548, 2006.
110. Porte RJ, Molenaar IQ, Begliomini B, et al: Aprotinin and transfusion requirements in orthotopic liver transplantation: A multicentre randomised double-blind study. EMSALT Study Group. *Lancet* 355:1303, 2000.
111. Boylan JF, Klinck JR, Sandler AN, et al: Tranexamic acid reduces blood loss, transfusion requirements, and coagulation factor use in primary orthotopic liver transplantation. *Anesthesiology* 85:1043, 1996.
112. Peters DC, Noble S: Aprotinin: An update of its pharmacology and therapeutic use in open heart surgery and coronary artery bypass surgery. *Drugs* 57:233, 1999.
113. Fergusson DA, Hebert PC, Mazer CD, et al: A comparison of aprotinin and lysine analogues in high-risk cardiac surgery. *N Engl J Med* 358:2319, 2008.
114. Brand A: Immunological aspects of blood transfusions. *Transpl Immunol* 10:183, 2002.
115. Ramos E, Dalmau A, Sabate A, et al: Intraoperative red blood cell transfusion in liver transplantation: Influence on patient outcome, prediction of requirements, and measures to reduce them. *Liver Transpl* 9:1320, 2003.
116. Pereboom IT, de Boer MT, Haagsma EB, et al: Platelet transfusion during liver transplantation is associated with increased postoperative mortality due to acute lung injury. *Anesth Analg* 108:1083, 2009.
117. Vivarelli M, La BG, Cucchetti A, et al: Can antiplatelet prophylaxis reduce the incidence of hepatic artery thrombosis after liver transplantation? *Liver Transpl* 13:651, 2007.
118. Lisman T, Leebeek FWG, de Groot PG: Haemostatic abnormalities in patients with liver disease. *J Hepatol* 37:280, 2002.

CHAPTER 130

DISSEMINATED INTRAVASCULAR COAGULATION

Marcel Levi and Uri Seligsohn

SUMMARY

When procoagulants are produced or introduced into the blood and overcome the anticoagulant mechanisms of coagulation, intravascular thrombin is generated systemically, which can lead to disseminated intravascular coagulation (DIC). The clinical manifestations of intravascular coagulation include (1) multiorgan dysfunction caused by microthrombi; (2) bleeding caused by consumption of platelets, fibrinogen, and other coagulation factors; and (3) secondary fibrinolysis. Exposure of blood to tissue factor is the most common trigger. This event can occur when mononuclear cells and endothelial cells are induced to generate and express tissue factor during the systemic inflammatory response syndrome (e.g., Gram-negative and Gram-positive infections, fungemia, burns, severe trauma), or when contact is established between blood and tissue factor constitutively present on membranes of cells foreign to blood (e.g., malignant, placental, brain, adventitial cells, or traumatized tissues). Laboratory features include thrombocytopenia, reduced levels of fibrinogen and other factors (leading to prolonged partial thromboplastin, prothrombin, and thrombin times), and elevated levels of D-dimer and fibrin(ogen) degradation products. Several underlying disorders affect these hemostatic parameters and can lead to a false-positive diagnosis of DIC (e.g., liver disease-related coagulation abnormalities and thrombocytopenia) or to a false-negative diagnosis (e.g., pregnancy-related high fibrinogen levels). Reexamining these variables every 6 to 8 hours may permit a specific diagnosis. Early detection, vigorous treatment of the underlying disorder, and support of vital functions are essential for survival of affected patients. Blood component therapy is effective in patients who bleed excessively, whereas heparin administration is indicated in a limited number of circumstances. Infusion of recombinant activated protein C, which exerts antiinflammatory and anticoagulant effects, reduces mortality caused by sepsis related intravascular coagulation. Intravascular coagulation and the underlying disorders causing it contribute to a high rate of mortality. The severity of the organ dysfunction and extent of hemostatic failure, as well as increasing patient age, have been associated with a grave prognosis.

Acronyms and abbreviations that appear in this chapter include: APACHE, acute physiology and chronic health evaluation; APC, activated protein C; APL, acute promyelocytic leukemia; aPTT, activated partial thromboplastin time; ARDS, adult respiratory distress syndrome; AT, antithrombin; CAM, cell adhesion molecule; DIC, disseminated intravascular coagulation; EPCR, endothelial protein C receptor; FDP, fibrinogen degradation product; HELLP, hemolysis, elevated liver enzymes, low platelet count; IL, interleukin; LCAD, long-chain acyl-coenzyme A dehydrogenase; LPS, lipopolysaccharide; MP, microparticles; PAI, plasminogen-activator inhibitor; PAR, protease-activated receptor; TAFI, thrombin-activatable fibrinolysis inhibitor; TAT, thrombin–antithrombin; TF, tissue factor; TFPI, tissue factor pathway inhibitor; TM, thrombomodulin; TNF, tumor necrosis factor; t-PA, tissue-type plasminogen activator; VWF, von Willebrand factor.

DEFINITION AND HISTORY

Disseminated intravascular coagulation (DIC) is a clinicopathologic syndrome in which widespread intravascular coagulation occurs as a result of exposure or production of procoagulants insufficiently balanced by natural anticoagulant mechanisms and endogenous fibrinolysis. Perturbation of the endothelium in the microcirculation along with stimulated inflammatory cells and release of inflammatory mediators play a key role in this mechanism. DIC may cause tissue ischemia from occlusive microthrombi, and bleeding from the consumption of platelets and coagulation factors and, in some cases, an excessive fibrinolytic response. DIC complicates a variety of disorders, and the complexity of its pathophysiology has made it the subject of a voluminous literature.[1–7]

In 1834, Dupuy reported that injection of brain material into animals caused widespread clots in blood vessels, thus providing the first description of DIC.[8] In 1865, Trousseau described the tendency to thrombosis, sometimes disseminated, in cachectic patients with malignancies.[9] In 1873, Naunyn showed that disseminated thrombosis could be evoked by intravenous injection of dissolved red cells, and Wooldridge demonstrated that the procoagulant involved was a substance contained in the stroma of the red cells.[10–12]

In 1955 Ratnoff and associates described the hemostatic abnormalities, which we would currently classify as DIC, that occur in women with fetal death or amniotic fluid embolism.[13] The mechanism by which DIC can lead to bleeding was clarified only in 1961, when Lasch and coworkers introduced the concept of consumption coagulopathy, and McKay established that DIC is a pathogenetic feature of a variety of diseases.[1,14] Sizable series of cases were first described in the late 1960s, following the introduction of defined laboratory criteria for DIC.[15] Yet despite the vast experience that has been accumulated, DIC still constitutes a major clinicopathologic and therapeutic challenge.

PATHOLOGY

Diffuse multiorgan bleeding, hemorrhagic necrosis, microthrombi in small blood vessels, and thrombi in medium and large blood vessels are common findings at autopsy, although patients who had unequivocal clinical and laboratory signs of DIC may not have confirming postmortem findings.[16,17] Conversely, some patients in whom clinical and laboratory signs were not consistent with DIC had typical autopsy findings.[18,19] This occasional lack of correlation among clinical, laboratory, and pathologic findings is partly a result of extensive postmortem changes in the blood, for example, excessive fibrinolysis, but remains unexplained in most instances.[17] Organs most frequently involved by diffuse microthrombi are the lungs and kidneys, followed by the brain, heart, liver, spleen, adrenal glands, pancreas, and gut. Specific immunohistologic techniques and ultrastructural analysis have revealed that most thrombi consist of fibrin monomers or polymers in combination with platelets. In addition, involvement of activated mononuclear cells and other signs of inflammatory activation are frequently present.[20] In cases of long-lasting DIC, organization and endothelialization of the microthrombi are often observed. Acute tubular necrosis is more frequent than renal cortical necrosis.[16]

A significant proportion of patients with chronic DIC have nonbacterial thrombotic endocarditis involving mainly the mitral and aortic valves.[19] Moreover, in a retrospective pathologic study, approximately 50 percent of patients with nonbacterial thrombotic endocarditis had DIC.[18] These heart lesions can be a source of arterial embolization, leading to infarction of the brain, kidneys, and myocardium.

PATHOGENESIS

INFLAMMATION AND ENDOTHELIUM IN DIC

Various triggers cause an hemostatic imbalance that gives rise to a procoagulant state (Fig. 130–1). The most important mediators that are responsible for this imbalance are cytokines.[21] There is an extensive crosstalk between coagulation and inflammatory systems, whereby inflammation leads to activation of coagulation, and coagulation stimulates inflammatory activity.[22] These interactions are highlighted in sepsis-induced systemic activation of coagulation and inflammation that lead to specific organ dysfunctions.[23] The endothelium of the capillary bed is the most important interface in which the interaction between inflammation and coagulation takes place. Endothelial cells may be a source of tissue factor and can thereby be involved in the initiation of coagulation activation. All physiologic anticoagulant systems and various adhesion molecules that may modulate both inflammation and coagulation are connected to the endothelium. In sepsis, endothelial glycosaminoglycans present in the glycocalyx are downregulated by proinflammatory cytokines, thereby impairing the functions of antithrombin (AT), tissue factor pathway inhibitor (TFPI), leukocyte adhesion, and leukocyte transmigration. Because the glycocalyx also plays a role in other endothelial functions, including maintenance of the vascular barrier function, nitric oxide-mediated vasodilation, and antioxidant activity, all these processes can be impaired in DIC (see "Role of Oxidative Stress and Vasoactive Molecules" below).[24,25] Moreover, specific disruption of the glycocalyx results in thrombin generation and platelet adhesion within a few minutes.[26,27]

Endothelial perturbation constitutes a *sine qua non* for most patients with DIC. Following injury or infection, the integrity of the endothelium is compromised, mononuclear cells are activated by cytokine and hormonal signals, additional cytokines and surface receptors are upregulated, procoagulant proteins and platelets are activated, the endothelium changes from an anticoagulant to procoagulant surface, and fibrinolysis is impeded. This sequence of events is typical for the so-called *systemic inflammatory response syndrome* and can lead to microvascular thrombosis with ensuing multiorgan dysfunction and eventually to multiorgan failure.

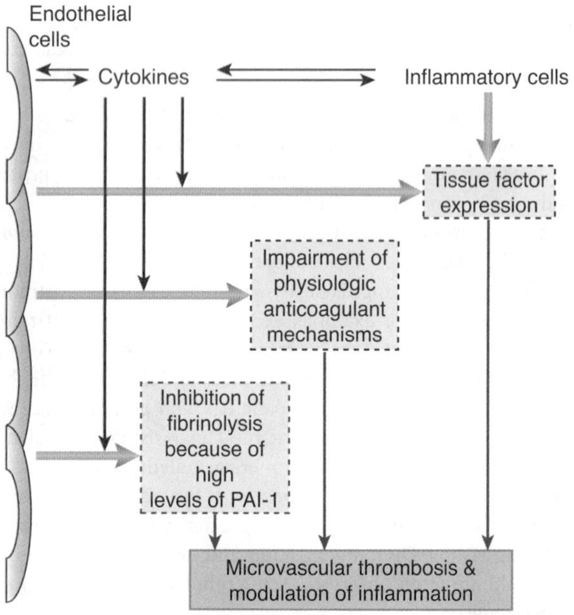

FIGURE 130–1. Schematic presentation of pathogenetic pathways involved in the activation of coagulation in DIC. In DIC, both perturbed endothelial cells and activated mononuclear cells may produce proinflammatory cytokines that mediate coagulation activation. Activation of coagulation is initiated by tissue factor expression on activated mononuclear cells and endothelial cells. In addition, downregulation of physiologic anticoagulant mechanisms and inhibition of fibrinolysis by endothelial cells further promote intravascular fibrin deposition. PAI-1, plasminogen-activator inhibitor type 1.

ROLE OF CYTOKINES AND TISSUE FACTOR

Tissue factor (TF) plays a central role in the initiation of inflammation-induced coagulation in DIC.[28] Blocking TF activity completely inhibits inflammation-induced thrombin generation in experimental models of endotoxemia or bacteremia.[29,30] Most cells constitutively expressing TF are found in tissues not in direct contact with blood, such as the adventitial layer of larger blood vessels. Tissue factor becomes exposed to blood upon disruption of the vascular integrity, or when cells present in the circulation, such as monocytes, are triggered to express tissue factor. The *in vivo* expression of tissue factor is dependent on interleukin (IL)-6 generation; inhibition of IL-6, unlike inhibition of other proinflammatory cytokines, completely abrogates tissue factor-dependent thrombin generation in experimental endotoxemia.[21,31] In severe sepsis, monocytes, stimulated by proinflammatory cytokines, express TF, which leads to systemic activation of coagulation.[32] Even in experimental low-dose endotoxemia in healthy subjects, a 125-fold increase in tissue factor messenger RNA (mRNA) levels in blood monocytes can be detected.[33] A potential alternative source of TF may be endothelial cells, polymorphonuclear cells, and other cell types. It is hypothesized that TF from these sources is shuttled between cells through microparticles derived from activated mononuclear cells.[34] However, it is unlikely that cells other than monocytes synthesize tissue factor in substantial quantities.[32,35]

Tumor necrosis factor-α (TNF-α), and IL-1, also generated during inflammation, impair the physiologic anticoagulant pathways.[31,36,37]

AMPLIFYING ROLE OF THROMBIN AND PLATELETS

The complex of TF–factor VIIa catalyzes the conversion of factor X to Xa, and factor Xa, in turn, forms the prothrombinase complex with factor Va, prothrombin (factor II), and calcium ions, thereby generating thrombin, and converting fibrinogen into fibrin. The TF–factor VIIa complex can also activate factor IX, and factor IXa forms the tenase complex with activated factor VIII and calcium ions, generating additional factor Xa, thereby forming an essential amplification loop of thrombin generation. The assembly of the prothrombinase and tenase complexes are markedly facilitated if a suitable phospholipid surface is available, such as the membrane of activated platelets. In the setting of inflammation-induced activation of coagulation, platelets can be activated directly by endotoxin or by proinflammatory mediators, such as the membrane of platelet-activating factor. Thrombin itself is one of the strongest platelet activators (see Chap. 115).

Activation of platelets may also accelerate fibrin formation by another mechanism. The expression of TF on monocytes is markedly stimulated by the presence of platelets and granulocytes in a P-selectin–dependent reaction.[38] This effect may be the result of nuclear factor kappa B (NF-κB) activation induced by binding of activated platelets to neutrophils and mononuclear cells.[39] This cellular interaction also markedly enhances the production of IL-1β, IL-8, monocyte chemotactic protein (MCP)-1, and TNF-α.[40]

Thrombin generated by the TF pathway amplifies both clotting and inflammation through the following activities: (1) it activates platelets, giving rise to platelet aggregation and augmenting platelet functions in coagulation; (2) it activates factors VIII, V, and XI, yielding further thrombin generation; (3) it activates proinflammatory factors via protease-activated receptors (PARs); (4) it activates factor XIII to factor

XIIIa, which crosslinks fibrin clots; (5) it activates thrombin-activatable fibrinolysis inhibitor (TAFI), making clots resistant to fibrinolysis; and (6) it increases expression of adhesion molecules, such as L-selectin, thereby promoting the inflammatory effects of leukocytes.[41]

Paradoxically, at low concentrations, thrombin exhibits both antiinflammatory and anticoagulant effects because it binds to thrombomodulin and activates protein C to the activated form, which, in turn, downregulates inflammation and serves as an "off switch" for further thrombin generation (see Chap. 116).

ROLE OF COAGULATION PROTEASES IN UPREGULATING INFLAMMATION

Coagulation proteases and protease inhibitors not only interact with coagulation proteins, but also with specific cell receptors to induce signaling pathways. In particular, protease interactions that affect inflammatory processes may be important in critically ill patients. Coagulation of whole blood *in vitro* results in a detectable expression of IL-1β mRNA in blood cells,[42] and thrombin markedly enhances endotoxin-induced IL-1 activity in culture supernatants of guinea pig macrophages.[43] Similarly, clotted blood produces IL-8 *in vitro*.[44]

Factor Xa, thrombin, and fibrin can also activate endothelial cells, eliciting the synthesis of IL-6 and IL-8.[45,46] Coagulation proteases such as thrombin, factor Xa, and factor VIIa–TF complex induce inflammatory upregulation via leukocyte, endothelial cell, and platelet PAR-1, PAR-2, PAR-3, and PAR-4, which are located on leukocytes, endothelial cells, and platelets.[47] PARs have an extracellular domain, seven transmembrane domains, and an intracellular domain that is coupled to specific G-proteins that transmit signaling. PAR-1, PAR-3, and PAR-4 are activated by thrombin through cleavage of a specific amino-terminus bond creating a tethered ligand that activates the receptor. PAR-2 can be cleaved by factor Xa–TF–factor VIIa complex and by other proteases.[48] Activated PARs then lead through mitogen-activated protein kinase and NF-κB signaling pathways to cell motility, shape change, proliferation, endogenous secretagogue release, and apoptosis. The activated protein C (APC)–endothelial protein C receptor complex (see "Role of Natural Anticoagulant Pathways" below) appears to be the "off switch" for PAR activation by the proteases. These counterbalances determine the magnitude of coagulation and inflammatory upregulation by PARs. For example, factor VIIa–TF binding to PAR-2 in the lungs is proinflammatory and appears to play a role in acute respiratory distress syndrome (ARDS), raising the possibility that TFPI might be therapeutic in this circumstance.[49] This finding is consistent with data from animal studies demonstrating that TFPI can protect baboons from an LD100 of *Escherichia coli*, likely by impeding factor VIIa–TF activation of PAR-2 and thereby attenuating release of IL-6 and other proinflammatory agents.

ROLE OF FIBRINOGEN AND FIBRIN

Fibrinogen and fibrin directly influence the production of proinflammatory cytokines and chemokines (including TNF-α, IL-1β, and MCP-1) by mononuclear cells and endothelial cells.[50] Fibrinogen-deficient mice display inhibition of macrophage adhesion and less thrombin-mediated cytokine production *in vivo*. The effects of fibrinogen on mononuclear cells seem to be mediated by toll-like receptor-4, which is also the receptor of endotoxin.

ROLE OF NATURAL ANTICOAGULANT PATHWAYS

Procoagulant activity is regulated by three important anticoagulant pathways: AT, the protein C system, and TFPI. In DIC, the function of all three pathways can be impaired (Fig. 130–2).[51]

The serine protease inhibitor AT is the main inhibitor of thrombin and factor Xa. Without heparin, AT neutralizes coagulation enzymes in a slow, progressive manner.[52] Heparin induces conformational changes in AT that result in at least a 1000-fold enhancement of AT activity. Thus, the clinical efficacy of heparin is attributed to its interaction with AT. Endogenous glycosaminoglycans, such as heparan sulfate, also promote on the vessel wall AT-mediated inhibition of thrombin and other coagulation enzymes. During severe inflammatory responses, AT levels are markedly decreased because of impaired synthesis, degradation by elastase from activated neutrophils, and consumption as a consequence of ongoing thrombin generation.[53] Proinflammatory cytokines also cause reduced synthesis of glycosaminoglycans on the endothelial surface, thereby reducing AT function.[54]

APC appears to play a central role in the pathogenesis of sepsis and associated organ dysfunction.[55] There is ample evidence that decreased function of the protein C pathway contributes to the derangement of coagulation in sepsis.[49,56] The circulating zymogen protein C is activated by thrombin when it is bound to thrombomodulin at the endothelial cell surface.[57] APC acts with its cofactor protein S and degrades the essential cofactors Va and VIIIa, and hence, is an effective anticoagulant. The endothelial protein C receptor (EPCR) accelerates the activation of protein C several-fold, and also serves as a receptor for APC, thereby augmenting APC's anticoagulant and antiinflammatory activities.[58]

In patients with severe inflammation, the protein C pathway malfunctions at virtually all levels. Plasma levels of the zymogen protein C

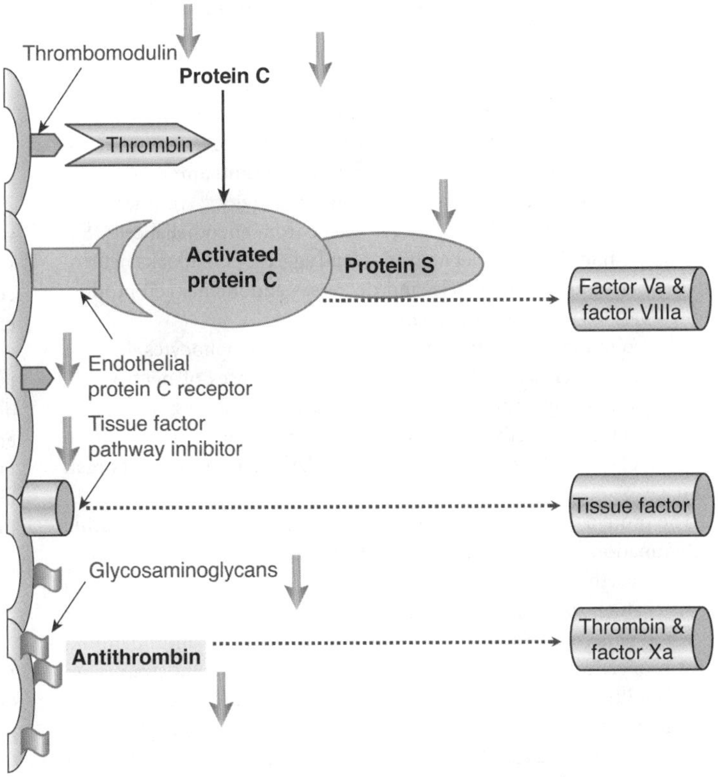

FIGURE 130–2. Schematic of the three important physiologic anticoagulant mechanisms and their point of impact in the coagulation system. In sepsis, these mechanisms are impaired by various mechanisms (*green arrows*). The protein C system is dysfunctional as a result of low levels of zymogen protein C, downregulation of thrombomodulin and the endothelial protein C receptor, and low levels of free protein S because of acute phase-induced high levels of its binding protein (i.e., C4b-binding protein). There is a relative insufficiency of the endothelial cell-associated tissue factor pathway inhibitor. The antithrombin system is defective because of low levels of antithrombin and impaired glycosaminoglycan expression on perturbed endothelial cells.

are decreased because of impaired synthesis, consumption, and degradation by proteolytic enzymes, such as neutrophil elastase.[59–61] Furthermore, a significant downregulation of thrombomodulin, caused by proinflammatory cytokines such as TNF-α and IL-1, results in diminished protein C activation.[62,63] Low levels of free protein S may further compromise the function of the protein C system. In plasma, 60 percent of protein S is complexed with a complement regulatory protein, C4b-binding protein (C4bBP), and exhibits no activity. The remaining protein S in plasma is free and functional. It was suggested that increased plasma levels of C4bBP caused by the acute phase reaction in inflammatory diseases results in a relative protein S deficiency, which further contributes to a procoagulant state during sepsis. Indeed, infusion of C4bBP in combination with a sublethal dose of *E. coli* into baboons resulted in a lethal response with severe organ damage because of DIC.[64]

In sepsis, the EPCR is downregulated, which further impairs the function of the protein C pathway.[65] Sepsis can also cause resistance toward APC because of a substantial increase in factor VIII levels.[66]

A third inhibitory mechanism of thrombin generation involves TFPI, the main inhibitor of the TF–factor VIIa complex and factor Xa. The role of TFPI in the regulation of inflammation-induced coagulation activation is not completely clear. Administration of recombinant TFPI blocks inflammation-induced thrombin generation in humans, and pharmacologic doses of TFPI prevent mortality during systemic infection and inflammation in experimental animals suggesting that TFPI can modulate tissue factor–mediated coagulation.[67,68]

NATURAL ANTICOAGULANTS AND INFLAMMATION

AT possesses antiinflammatory properties, many of which are mediated by its actions in the coagulation cascade.[69] By inhibiting thrombin, AT blunts activation of many inflammatory mediators released by platelets and endothelial cells that recruit and activate leukocytes.[70] At high concentrations, AT also possesses potent antiinflammatory properties that are independent of its anticoagulant activity.[70] Another effect of AT is the induction of prostacyclin release from endothelial cells.[71–73] Prostacyclin inhibits platelet activation and aggregation, blocks neutrophil tethering to blood vessels, and decreases endothelial cell production of various cytokines and chemokines.[74]

AT also interacts directly with leukocytes and lymphocytes. It binds to receptors, such as syndecan-4, on the cell surfaces of neutrophils, monocytes, and lymphocytes, thereby blocking the adhesion of these cells to endothelial cells, their activation and migration. This effect, in turn, ameliorates the severity of capillary leakage and subsequent organ damage.

The protein C system also has an important function in modulating inflammation.[75,76] Blocking the protein C pathway in septic baboons exacerbates the inflammatory response, and in contrast, administration of APC ameliorates the inflammatory activation upon the intravenous infusion of *E. coli*.[77] Support for the notion that APC has antiinflammatory properties comes from *in vitro* observations, demonstrating an APC binding site on monocytes, that may mediate downstream inflammatory processes,[78,79] and from experiments showing that APC can block NF-κB nuclear translocation, which is a prerequisite for increased proinflammatory cytokine levels and adhesion molecules.[80] These *in vitro* findings are supported by *in vivo* studies in mice with targeted disruption of the protein C gene. In these mice with genetic deficiencies of protein C, endotoxemia was associated with a more marked increase in proinflammatory cytokines and other inflammatory responses as compared with wild-type mice.[81,82]

It is likely that the antiinflammatory effects of APC are mediated by the EPCR.[75] Binding of APC to EPCR influences gene expression profiles of cells by inhibiting NF-κB nuclear translocation.[79,80] The EPCR-APC complex itself can translocate from the plasma membrane into the cell nucleus, which may be another mechanism of modulating gene expression, although the relative contribution of this nuclear translocation and cell surface signaling is uncertain.[56] Like APC, EPCR itself may have antiinflammatory properties. Blocking the EPCR with a specific monoclonal antibody aggravates both the coagulation and the inflammatory response to *E. coli* infusion.[65]

Apart from the effect on cytokine levels, APC causes diminished leucocyte chemotaxis and adhesion to the activated endothelium.[83–85] A localized antiinflammatory effect of APC has been demonstrated in the lung.[86] One mechanism for this effect may be inhibition of the expression of platelet-derived growth factor in the lung.[87] Also, APC protects against the disruption of endothelial cell barrier in sepsis.[88–90] APC also inhibits endothelial cell apoptosis by a mechanism that seems to be mediated by binding of APC to EPCR and requires PAR-1.[91,92] Signaling through this pathway can affect Bcl-2 homologue protein, which can inhibit apoptosis, and further suppresses p53, that is a proapoptotic transcription factor.[93,94]

DYSREGULATION OF FIBRINOLYSIS

In experimental models of DIC, fibrinolysis is initially activated but subsequently inhibited, because of an increased release of plasminogen activator inhibitor-I (PAI-1) by endothelial cells.[95] These effects are mediated by TNF-α and IL-1.[96,97] In a study of 69 DIC patients (31 with multiorgan failure), higher levels of tissue-type plasminogen activator (t-PA) antigen and PAI-1 with depressed levels of α_2-antiplasmin were observed in patients with DIC and multiorgan failure compared to DIC patients without multiorgan failure.[98] This finding supports the conclusion that fibrinolysis is an important mechanism in preventing multiorgan failure.

Experiments in mice with targeted disruptions of genes encoding components of the plasminogen–plasmin system confirm that fibrinolysis plays a major role in inflammation. Mice with a deficiency of plasminogen activators have more extensive fibrin deposition in organs when challenged with endotoxin, whereas PAI-1 knockout mice, in contrast to wild-type controls, have no microvascular thrombosis upon endotoxin administration.[99]

TAFI, like PAI-1, may play a role in impeding fibrinolysis and in augmenting formation of microvascular thrombi. Studies in a DIC cohort demonstrated very low levels of TAFI proportionate to thrombin generation in such patients, particularly in those with infection-associated DIC.[100] Hence, TAFI may contribute (along with PAI-1) to microvascular thrombosis-induced ischemia in organs resulting in multiorgan dysfunction.

ROLE OF OXIDATIVE STRESS AND VASOACTIVE MOLECULES

Superoxides and hydroxyl radicals are generated during sepsis and other organ injury states that predispose to DIC. Each is a proinflammatory agent that may lead to recruitment of neutrophils, formation of chemotactic factors, lipid peroxidation, and stimulation of NF-κB, which induces cytokine upregulation.[101] In addition, formation of peroxynitrite by these radicals exacerbates inflammation by (1) deactivating superoxide dismutase, which ordinarily would eliminate these superoxides and other radicals, and (2) exerting damaging effects on deoxyribonucleic acid, nicotinamide adenine dinucleotide, and ATP. For example, evidence indicates that the poor response to pressors in shock-like states associated with DIC may be directly related to their deactivation by superoxides.

Adding further insult, high levels of superoxide impair vascular response to nitrous oxide, thereby creating an imbalance in the signaling to vascular cells. Because of the strategic importance of an intact endothelium for attenuating any microangiopathic process, the most devastating effect of excessive generation of superoxides and associated free radicals may be their role in inducing endothelial apoptosis, which exacerbates capillary leak.[101]

Vasoactive substances play a critical role in the evolution of DIC. The vasodilatory agent nitric oxide (NO) and the vasoconstrictor endothelin have been measured in experimental rat models of DIC induced by both TF infusion and lipopolysaccharide (LPS) infusion.[102] LPS infusion increased both NO and endothelin remarkably, whereas TF infusion increased NO more than did LPS but did not stimulate endothelin significantly. The differential stimuli–response mechanisms may explain why LPS-induced DIC so prominently displays tissue infarction leading to multiorgan dysfunction (e.g., sepsis) compared to DIC that is predominately induced by TF exposure (e.g., head trauma).

■ METABOLIC MODULATION OF COAGULATION IN DIC

Because there is a tight relation between plasma lipoproteins and coagulation, it has been suggested that lipoprotein metabolism modulates coagulation in DIC.[103] *In vitro* experiments showed that plasma large very-low-density lipoprotein, small very-low-density lipoprotein, intermediate-density lipoprotein, and low-density lipoprotein stimulate activation of coagulation by supporting factor VII activation or by stimulating monocytes to express TF.[104] Lipid infusion potentiates in animals endotoxin-induced coagulation activation, as indicated by increased plasma levels of prothrombin fragments 1 and 2, thrombin–antithrombin III complex, and PAI-1.[105] High-density lipoprotein (HDL) exerts opposite effects. Administration of recombinant HDL (rHDL) ameliorates the inflammatory response, inhibits coagulation, and augments fibrinolysis,[106] as reflected by reduced thrombin generation and increased levels of t-PA antigen following administration of endotoxin.

Endogenous lipid levels may have similar effects. Human subjects with low endogenous HDL-cholesterol plasma levels injected with small doses of endotoxin had a more pronounced increase in markers of coagulation activation in comparison with subjects with high endogenous HDL levels.[107] Also, patients heterozygous for familial hypercholesterolemia whose low-density lipoproteins level is increased were more prone to activation of coagulation upon an inflammatory stimulus.[108]

Hyperglycemia and hyperinsulinemia, as seen in type 2 diabetes mellitus and the associated metabolic syndrome, affect hemostasis.[109–111] In these circumstances, there is a marked decrease of endogenous fibrinolysis because of increased upregulation of plasma levels of PAI-1. Also, a modulatory effect of glucose/insulin on coagulation in an inflammatory setting has been described. Inflammation-induced TF gene expression was elevated in the brain, lung, kidney, heart, liver, and adipose tissues of diabetic mice compared with controls. Administration of insulin to lean mice induced enhanced inflammation-driven TF mRNA in the kidney, brain, lung, and adipose tissue.[112] In a hyperglycemic normoinsulinemic study in healthy subjects, there was an increased sensitivity toward endotoxin exhibited by upregulation of TF expression.[113] Strict glucose regulation in critically ill patients improves survival and reduces morbidity that is probably related to a better control of the derangement of coagulation and a faster resolution of coagulation abnormalities.[103]

■ CONSUMPTION OF HEMOSTATIC FACTORS

The widespread generation of thrombin in DIC induces deposition of fibrin, which leads to the consumption of substantial amounts of platelets, fibrinogen, factors V and VIII, protein C, AT, and components of the fibrinolytic system. This situation results in massive depletion of these components that is further aggravated because of their decreased synthesis by the liver, which frequently is affected in DIC. Depending on the magnitude and nature of component depletion, bleeding, enhanced thrombosis, or both can result. Bleeding can be promoted by fibrinolysis-derived fibrin degradation products (FDPs) that exhibit anticoagulant and antiplatelet aggregation effects (see Fig. 130–1). Microangiopathic hemolytic anemia also occurs as a result of blood cells passing through vessels that are partially occluded by thrombi.

CLINICAL FEATURES

Numerous disorders can provoke DIC, but only a few constitute major causes, as can be inferred from retrospective clinical studies (Table 130–1).[114] Infectious diseases and malignant disorders together account for approximately two-thirds of DIC cases in the major series (Table 130–2). Trauma was a major cause of DIC in some series, probably reflecting the specialized nature of the clinical practice in those centers.[115] Clinical manifestations are attributable to DIC, the underlying disease, or both (Table 130–3). Bleeding manifestations were common in all series of DIC cases, but considerable variation existed in the relative frequency of shock and of dysfunction of the liver, kidney, lungs, and central nervous system. These variations probably reflect the different nature of the underlying disorders in the respective series.

■ BLEEDING

Acute DIC frequently is heralded by hemorrhage into the skin at multiple sites.[115] Petechiae, ecchymoses, and oozing from venipunctures, arterial lines, catheters, and injured tissues are common. Bleeding also may occur on mucosal surfaces. Hemorrhage may be life-threatening, with massive bleeding into the gastrointestinal tract, lungs, central nervous system, or orbit. Patients with chronic DIC usually exhibit only minor skin and mucosal bleeding.

TABLE 130–1. Clinical Conditions That May Be Complicated by DIC

Sepsis/severe infection
Trauma
Malignancy
Solid tumors
Acute leukemia
Obstetrical conditions
Amniotic fluid embolism
Abruptio placentae
HELLP syndrome
Vascular abnormalities
Kasabach-Merritt syndrome
Other vascular malformations
Aortic aneurysms
Severe allergic/toxic reactions
Severe immunologic reactions (e.g., transfusion reaction)
Heatstroke

HELLP, hemolysis, elevated liver enzymes, and low platelet count.

TABLE 130–2. Relative Frequency (%) of Major Underlying Diseases in Case Series of Patients with DIC

Study	Number of Patients	Infectious Disease	Trauma and Major Surgery	Malignant Disease	Liver Disease	Obstetric Complications	Miscellaneous Diseases
Minna et al.[347]	60	41	30	2	5	2	20
Siegal et al.[115]	118	40	24	7	4	4	21
Spero et al.[122]	346	26	19	24	8	0	23
Matsuda et al.[348]	503	15	2	61	6	4	12
Kobayash, et al.[139]	345	16	–	55	4	5	20
Larcan et al.[349]	361	15	14	6	3	38	24

TABLE 130–3. Frequency (%) and Type of Organ Dysfunction or Other Clinical Manifestations in Case Series of Patients with DIC

Study	Number of Patients	Bleeding	Thromboembolism	Renal Failure	Liver Failure	Respiratory Failure	CNS Manifestation	Shock	Acral Cyanosis*
Minna et al.[347]	60	87	22	67	NR	78	65	NR	14
Al-Mondhiry et al.[116]	89	76	23	39	NR	NR	11	NR	0
Siegal et al.[115]	118	64	8	25	22	16	2	14	0
Matsuda et al.[348]	47	87	47	40	NR	38	NR	NR	NR
Spero et al.[122]	346	77	NR	NR	NR	NR	NR	NR	NR
Larcan et al.[349]	361	73	11	61	57	37	13	55	13

CNS, central nervous system; NR, not reported.

*Including necrotizing purpura and acral gangrene.

THROMBOSIS AND THROMBOEMBOLISM

Extensive organ dysfunction can result from microvascular thrombi or from venous and/or arterial thromboembolism (Table 130–4). For example, involvement of the skin can cause hemorrhagic bullae, acral necrosis, and gangrene. Thrombosis of major veins and arteries and pulmonary embolism occur but are rare. Cerebral embolism can complicate nonbacterial thrombotic endocarditis in patients with chronic DIC.

SHOCK

Both the diseases underlying DIC and the DIC itself can cause shock. For example, septicemia and excessive blood loss because of trauma or obstetric complications by themselves can cause shock. Whatever the cause of shock, its advent in cases with DIC is a serious adverse event.

RENAL DYSFUNCTION

Renal cortical ischemia induced by microthrombosis of afferent glomerular arterioles and acute tubular necrosis related to hypotension are the major causes of renal dysfunction in DIC. Oliguria, anuria, azotemia, and hematuria were observed in 25 to 67 percent of cases in all series (see Table 130–3).

LIVER DYSFUNCTION

Hepatocellular dysfunction sufficient to cause jaundice has been reported in 20 to 50 percent of patients with DIC.[4,115] Infectious diseases and prolonged hypotension contribute to hepatic dysfunction.

CENTRAL NERVOUS SYSTEM DYSFUNCTION

Microthrombi, macrothrombi, emboli, and hemorrhage in the cerebral vasculature all have been held responsible for the nonspecific neurologic symptoms and signs displayed by patients with DIC.[116] These

TABLE 130–4. Organ Dysfunction Associated with Severe DIC

Organ	Manifestation
Skin	Purpura, bleeding from injury sites, hemorrhagic bullae, focal necrosis, acral gangrene
Cardiovascular	Shock, acidosis, myocardial infarction, cerebrovascular events, thromboembolism in all types and caliber blood vessels
Renal	Acute renal insufficiency (acute tubular necrosis), oliguria, hematuria, renal cortical necrosis
Liver	Hepatic failure, jaundice
Lungs	Adult respiratory distress syndrome, hypoxemia, edema, hemorrhage
Gastrointestinal	Bleeding, mucosal necrosis and ulceration, intestinal ischemia
Central nervous system	Coma, convulsions, focal lesions, bleeding
Adrenals	Adrenal insufficiency (hemorrhagic necrosis)

manifestations include coma, delirium, transient focal neurologic symptoms, and signs of meningeal irritation. Careful exclusion of causes other than DIC is essential.

PULMONARY DYSFUNCTION

Symptoms and signs of respiratory dysfunction in DIC range from transient hypoxemia in mild cases to pulmonary hemorrhage and ARDS in severe cases.[117–119] Pulmonary hemorrhage is heralded by hemoptysis, dyspnea, and chest pain. Physical examination reveals rales, wheezing, and occasionally a pleural friction rub. Chest imaging shows diffuse infiltration resulting from excessive intraalveolar hemorrhage. ARDS is characterized by tachypnea, auscultatory silence, hypoxemia, low lung compliance, normal wedge pressure, and "white lungs" on chest images.[120] It stems from severe damage to the pulmonary vascular endothelium, which permits egress of blood components into the pulmonary interstitium and alveoli. This situation leads to intraalveolar hyaline membrane formation and severe respiratory insufficiency. ARDS can be caused by septic shock, severe trauma, fat embolism, amniotic fluid embolism, and heat stroke, all of which can also incite DIC. Yet only a fraction of patients with ARDS exhibit signs of DIC. When DIC and ARDS are simultaneously triggered, each aggravates the other. Regardless of the mechanism, ARDS is a serious complication in patients with DIC.

MORTALITY

Both DIC and its underlying disorders contribute to the high mortality rate. Mortality correlates independently with the extent of organ dysfunction,[115] the degree of hemostatic failure,[121] and increasing age.[122] Mortality rates in major series of patients with DIC ranged from 31 to 86 percent,[121–124] whether or not heparin was administrated. Of note, there is a clear correlation between the severity of DIC and the mortality rate.[121,123,124] In patients with sepsis, the presence of DIC is one of the strongest predictors of 28-day mortality.[124]

LABORATORY FEATURES AND DIAGNOSIS

No single laboratory test is sensitive or specific enough to allow a definite diagnosis of DIC (Table 130–5). However, some sophisticated laboratory tests, for example, thrombin–antithrombin complex, prothrombin fragment 1.2, are sensitive to ongoing activation of coagulation pathways. Determination of soluble fibrin in plasma is one of the best parameters for detection of ongoing DIC[125–128]; when the concentration is above a defined threshold, a diagnosis of DIC is likely.[129,130] Most of the other parameters show a sensitivity of 90 to 100 percent for the diagnosis of DIC but have a rather low specificity,[131] and a wide discordance among various assays.[132] FDPs may be detected by specific enzyme-linked immunosorbent assays or by latex agglutination assays, allowing rapid and bedside determination.[133] None of the available assays discriminates between degradation products of crosslinked fibrin and fibrinogen, a situation that may cause spuriously high results.[134,135] The specificity of high levels of FDPs is therefore limited and many other conditions, such as trauma, recent surgery, inflammation or venous thromboembolism, are associated with elevated FDPs.

Newly developed tests are aimed at the detection of neoantigens on degraded crosslinked fibrin, one of which detects an epitope related to plasmin-degraded crosslinked γ-chain, associated with D-dimer formation. These tests better differentiate degradation of crosslinked fibrin from fibrinogen or fibrinogen degradation products.[136] D-dimer level is substantially elevated in patients with DIC, but this poorly distinguishes patients with DIC from patients with venous thromboembolism, recent surgery, or inflammatory conditions.[133,137]

TABLE 130–5. Routine Laboratory Value Abnormalities in DIC

Test	Abnormality	Causes Other Than DIC Contributing to Test Result
Platelet count	Decreased	Sepsis, impaired production, major blood loss, hypersplenism
Prothrombin time	Prolonged	Vitamin K deficiency, liver failure, major blood loss
aPTT	Prolonged	Liver failure, heparin treatment, major blood loss
Fibrin degradation products	Elevated	Surgery, trauma, infection, hematoma
Protease inhibitors (e.g., protein C, AT, protein S)	Decreased	Liver failure, capillary leakage

aPTT, activated partial thromboplastin time.

In routine practice, simple laboratory tests in conjunction with clinical considerations are used for establishing the diagnosis of DIC. The simple tests include platelet count, prothrombin time, fibrinogen level, and fibrin-related markers, such as FDP or D-dimer. Caution should be exercised when using these laboratory parameters in the algorithms described below, because an underlying disease by itself can cause an abnormality. For example, impairment of hemostasis and/or thrombocytopenia unrelated to DIC can arise from hepatic disease and from marrow involvement by leukemia. Impaired hemostasis also may occur normally in the neonatal period. Conversely, the elevated levels of some hemostatic components that are normally observed during pregnancy may obscure the presence of DIC. These limitations in laboratory diagnosis of DIC can be overcome by repeated testing, thereby following the dynamics of the process.

A scoring system utilizing the simple laboratory tests has been developed by the subcommittee on DIC of the International Society on Thrombosis and Haemostasis,[138] and Table 130–6 summarizes a five-step diagnostic algorithm to calculate a DIC score. Tentatively, a score of 5 or more is compatible with DIC, whereas a score of less than 5 may be indicative but is *not* affirmative for nonovert DIC. By using receiver-operating characteristics curves, an optimal cut-off for a quantitative D-dimer assay was determined, thereby optimizing sensitivity and the negative predictive value of the system.[131] Prospective studies show that the sensitivity of the DIC score is 93 percent, and the specificity is 98 percent.[123] The severity of DIC according to this scoring system is related to the mortality in patients with sepsis (Fig. 130–3).[124] Linking prognostic determinants from critical care measurement scores such as acute physiology and chronic health evaluation (APACHE-II) to DIC scores is an important means to assess prognosis in critically ill patients. In addition, certain biochemical indicators of organ dysfunction may imply a DIC risk. For example, serial assessment of arterial lactate has proved to be a reliable prognostic indicator of DIC development among patients with the systemic inflammatory response syndrome.[139]

Criteria for less-overt DIC have been more difficult to establish.[138,140] In the algorithm for nonovert DIC, the global coagulation tests are scored as with the overt DIC algorithm; however, when scoring by the algorithm is being serially repeated, improvement in any laboratory test confers a negative score (rather than a zero or neutral score). This

TABLE 130–6. Diagnostic Algorithm for the Diagnosis of Overt DIC*

1. Presence of an underlying disorder known to be associated with DIC (see Table 130–2) ❑
   (no = 0, yes = 2)
2. Score global coagulation test results
   Platelet count *(>100 = 0; <100 = 1; <50= 2)* ❑
   Level of fibrin markers (soluble fibrin monomers/fibrin degradation products) ❑
   (no increase: 0; moderate increase: 2; strong increase: 3)
   Prolonged prothrombin time ❑
   (<3 s.= 0; >3 s. but <6 s.= 1; >6 s = 2)
   Fibrinogen level ❑
   (>1.0 g/L = 0; <1.0 g/L = 1)
3. Calculate score ❑
4. If ≥5: compatible with overt DIC; repeat scoring daily
   If <5: suggestive (not affirmative) for nonovert DIC; repeat next 1–2 days

*According to the Scientific Standardization Committee of the International Society of Thrombosis and Haemostasis.[138]

SOURCE: Reference 138.

"trend" scoring allows longitudinal assessment of the patient's microangiopathy and, when therapy has been instituted, inference on whether the therapy has improved the course of the disease.[121,141] Measurements of several markers for assessing the risk of progression from nonovert to overt DIC and prediction of multiorgan dysfunction are potentially valuable and in the future can be accommodated in the nonovert DIC score. For example, impaired fibrinolysis may play a particularly important role in multiorgan dysfunction resulting from DIC of sepsis.[142] Therefore, assaying PAI-1, plasmin–antiplasmin complexes, or TAFI in septic patients may be important. Another highly sensitive early marker of impending DIC is a monoclonal antibody against activated protein C that identifies a calcium ion-dependent epitope involved in factor Va inactivation.[143] Whether serial measurement of von Willebrand factor-cleaving protease also will identify individuals at risk early in their disease course, or will help differentiate individuals with microangiopathy who are not prone to progress, needs further data.[144,145]

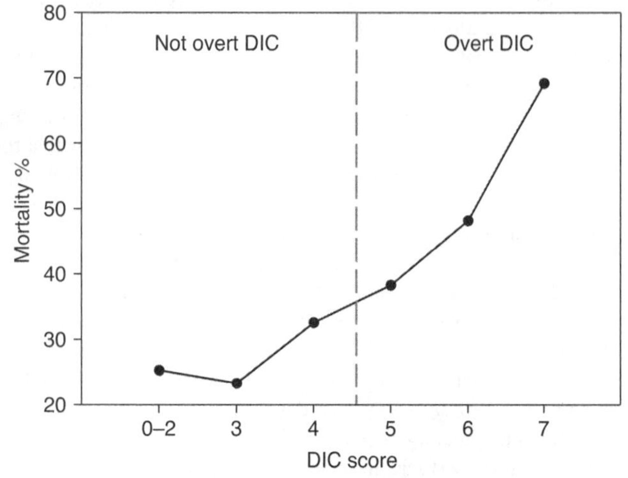

FIGURE 130–3. Number of points on the International Society of Thrombosis and Haemostasis DIC score and 28-day mortality in patients with severe sepsis. Data were derived from the placebo group (n = 840) in the Prowess trial on the efficacy of activated protein C in sepsis.

One new method that has proved highly sensitive and specific for nonovert (impending) DIC is the partial thromboplastin test biphasic waveform analysis.[146,147] This test, which requires specific instrumentation, detects the presence of precipitates of a complex of very-low-density lipoprotein and C-reactive protein that appears very early in DIC. When such complexes first appear in the plasma of individuals with diseases known to predispose to DIC, they confer a greater than 90 percent sensitivity and specificity for subsequent development of DIC and fatal outcome.[148]

SPECIFIC UNDERLYING DISORDERS

INFECTIOUS DISEASES

Bacterial infections are among the most common causes of DIC.[5,149] Certain patients are particularly vulnerable to infection-induced DIC, such as immune-compromised hosts, asplenic patients whose ability to clear bacteria, particularly pneumococci and meningococci, is impaired, and newborns whose coagulation inhibitory systems are immature. Infections are frequently superimposed on trauma and malignancies, which themselves are potential triggers of DIC. In addition, infections can aggravate bleeding and thrombosis by directly inducing thrombocytopenia, hepatic dysfunction, and shock associated with diminished blood flow in the microcirculation.[150] Clinically overt DIC may occur in 30 to 50 percent of patients with Gram-negative sepsis.[151,152] DIC is similarly common in patients with Gram-positive sepsis.[153,154] Extreme examples of sepsis-related DIC are (1) group A streptococcus toxic shock syndrome, characterized by deep tissue infection, vascular collapse, vascular leakage, and multiorgan dysfunction; a streptococcal M protein forms complexes with fibrinogen, and these complexes bind to β_2 integrins of neutrophils leading to their activation[155]; and (2) meningococcemia, a fulminant Gram-negative infection characterized by extensive hemorrhagic necrosis, DIC, and shock. The extent of hemostatic derangement in patients with meningococcemia correlates with prognosis.[156,157] More frequent Gram-negative infections associated with DIC are caused by *Pseudomonas aeruginosa, E. coli,* and *Proteus vulgaris*. Patients affected by such bacteremias may have only laboratory signs of activated coagulation or may present with severe DIC, especially when shock develops.[158,159]

Severe secondary deficiency of a disintegrin-like metalloprotease with thrombospondin type 1 repeats (ADAMTS-13), the von Willebrand cleaving protease, occurs in patients with sepsis-induced DIC and is associated with a high incidence of acute renal failure.[160]

Among the Gram-positive infections, *Staphylococcus aureus* bacteremia can cause DIC accompanied by renal cortical and dermal necrosis. The mechanism by which DIC is elicited may be related to an α-toxin that activates platelets and induces IL-1 secretion by macrophages.[161] *Streptococcus pneumoniae* infection is associated with the Waterhouse-Friderichsen syndrome,[162] particularly in asplenic patients. Initiation of DIC in these conditions is ascribed to the capsular antigen of the bacterium and to antigen–antibody complex formation.[163] Other Gram-positive bacteria that can cause DIC are the anaerobic clostridia. Clostridial bacteremia is a highly lethal disease characterized by septic shock, DIC, renal failure, and hemolytic anemia.[164]

Activation of the coagulation system has also been documented for nonbacterial pathogens, that is, viruses (causing hemorrhagic fevers),[164,165] protozoa (Malaria),[166,167] and fungi.[168] Common viral infections, such as influenza, varicella, rubella, and rubeola, rarely are associated with DIC.[169]

However, purpura fulminans associated with DIC has been reported in patients with infections and either hereditary thrombophilias,[170,171] or acquired antibodies to protein S.[172] Other viral infections can cause "hemorrhagic fevers" characterized by fever, hypotension, bleeding, and renal failure. Laboratory evidence of DIC can accompany Korean, rift valley, and dengue-related hemorrhagic fevers.[173–175] Release of TF from cells in which viruses replicate[28] and increased levels of proinflammatory cytokines have been suggested as mechanisms for initiation of the TF pathway in these conditions.[163]

PURPURA FULMINANS

Purpura fulminans is a severe, often lethal form of DIC in which extensive areas of the skin over the extremities and buttocks undergo hemorrhagic necrosis.[176] The disease affects infants and children predominantly, and occasionally adults.[177,178] Diffuse microthrombi in small blood vessels, necrosis, and occasionally vasculitis are present in biopsies of skin lesions. Onset can be within 2 to 4 weeks of a mild infection such as scarlet fever, varicella, or rubella, or can occur during an acute viral or bacterial infection in patients with acquired or hereditary thrombophilias affecting the protein C inhibitory pathway.[156,177] Homozygous protein C deficiency presents in neonates soon after birth as purpura fulminans, with or without extensive thrombosis.[179,180] Patients affected by purpura fulminans are acutely ill with fever, hypotension, and hemorrhage from multiple sites; they frequently have typical laboratory signs of DIC.[177] Excision of necrotic skin areas and grafting are indispensable at a later stage.

SOLID TUMORS

Trousseau was the first to describe the propensity to thrombosis of patients with cancer and cachexia, and evidence for malignancy-related primary fibrinolysis and/or DIC was provided 75 years ago.[9,181,182]

In 182 patients with malignant disorders, excessive bleeding was recorded in 75 cases, venous thrombosis in 123, migratory thrombophlebitis in 96, arterial thrombosis in 45, and arterial embolism resulting from nonbacterial thrombotic endocarditis in 31.[183] Multifocal hemorrhagic infarctions of the brain, caused by fibrin microemboli and manifested as disorders of consciousness, have been described. Patients with solid tumors and DIC are more prone to thrombosis than to bleeding, whereas patients with leukemia and DIC are more prone to hemorrhage. The incidence of DIC in consecutive patients with solid tumors was 7 percent.[184]

Solid-tumor cells can express different procoagulant molecules including tissue factor, which forms a complex with factor VII(a) to activate factors IX and X, and a cancer procoagulant, a cysteine protease with factor X activating properties.[185,186] In breast cancer, TF is expressed by vascular endothelial cells as well as the tumor cells.[187,188] Tissue factor also appears to be involved in tumor metastasis and angiogenesis.[189–191] Cancer procoagulant is an endopeptidase that can be found in extracts of neoplastic cells but also in the plasma of patients with solid tumors.[192,193] The exact role of cancer procoagulant in the pathogenesis of cancer-related DIC is unclear.

Interactions of P- and L-selectins with mucin from mucinous adenocarcinoma can induce formation of platelet microthrombi and probably constitute a third mechanism of cancer-related thrombosis.[194] Depending on the rate and quantity of exposure or influx of shed vesicles from tumors containing TF, a nonovert or overt DIC develops.[39,195,196] For instance, a patient may be asymptomatic or present with venous thromboembolism if the tumor cells expose or release TF slowly or intermittently and the ensuing utilization of fibrinogen and platelets is compensated by increased production of these components. Conversely, massive thrombosis or severe bleeding may supervene in a patient whose circulation is deluged by TF.[184,186]

Another mechanism by which tumor cells may contribute to the pathogenesis of DIC is by expressing fibrinolytic proteins.[197,198] Despite the ability of many malignant cells to express urokinase-type plasminogen activator and t-PA, most tumors induce a hypofibrinolytic state. Because DIC is commonly characterized by a shutdown of the fibrinolytic system, mostly because of high levels of PAI-1, this may represent an alternative mechanism for the development of DIC in cancer.

Virtually all pathways that contribute to the occurrence of DIC are driven by cytokines. IL-6 has been identified as one of the most important proinflammatory cytokines that is able to induce TF expression on cells.[21,199] Indeed, inhibition of IL-6 results in an inhibition of endotoxin-stimulated activation of coagulation. In contrast, changes in fibrinolysis and microvascular physiologic anticoagulant pathways are mostly dependent on TNF-α.[200–202] Other cytokines that participate in the systemic activation of coagulation are IL-1β and IL-8, whereas anti-inflammatory cytokines, such as IL-10, are able to inhibit DIC.[203–205] Because many types of tumors have the ability to synthesize and release cytokines or to stimulate other cells to activate the cytokine network, it is likely that cytokine-dependent modulation of coagulation and fibrinolysis plays a role in cancer-related DIC.

Patients with solid tumors are vulnerable to risk factors and additional triggers of DIC that can aggravate thromboembolism and bleeding.[182] Risk factors include advanced age, stage of the disease, and use of chemotherapy or antiestrogen therapy.[197] Triggers include septicemia, immobilization, and involvement of the liver by metastases that impede the function of the liver in controlling DIC. Microangiopathic hemolytic anemia frequently is induced by DIC in patients with malignancies and is particularly severe in patients with widespread intravascular metastases of mucin-secreting adenocarcinomas.[206]

LEUKEMIAS

Numerous reports on DIC and fibrinolysis complicating the course of acute leukemias have been published. In 161 consecutive patients who presented with acute myeloid leukemia, DIC was diagnosed in 52 (32%).[207] In acute lymphoblastic leukemia, DIC was diagnosed in 15 to 20 percent.[208] Some reports indicate that the incidence of DIC in acute leukemia patients might further increase during remission induction with chemotherapy.[209] In patients with acute promyelocytic leukemia (APL) DIC is present in more than 90 percent of patients at the time of diagnosis or after initiation of remission induction.[210,211]

The pathogenesis of hemostatic disturbance in APL is related to properties of the malignant cells and their interaction with the host's endothelial cells.[192,208] APL cells express TF and the cancer procoagulant that can initiate coagulation, and they release IL-1β and TNF-α, which downregulate endothelial thrombomodulin, thereby compromising the protein C anticoagulant pathway. APL cells also express increased amounts of annexin II, which mediates augmented conversion of plasminogen to plasmin (see Chap. 136). The overall results of these processes are DIC and hyperfibrinolysis, followed by major bleeding that can lead to death.[212] All-*trans*-retinoic acid, used for induction and maintenance therapy of APL, inhibits *in vitro* and *in vivo* the deleterious effect of APL cells and has led to a reduced frequency of early hemorrhagic death.[192,213]

TRAUMA

When DIC complicates trauma, it usually occurs in severely injured patients. Extensive exposure of TF to the blood circulation and hemorrhagic shock probably are the most immediate triggers of DIC in such instances, although direct proof of this mechanism is lacking. An alternative hypothesis is that cytokines play a pivotal role in the occurrence of DIC in trauma patients. In fact, the changes in cytokine levels are virtually identical in trauma patients and septic patients.[214] The levels of TNF-α, IL-1β, PAI-1, circulating TF, plasma elastase derived from neutrophils, and soluble thrombomodulin all can be elevated in patients with signs of DIC, predicting multiorgan dysfunction (ARDS included) and death.[215,216] Careful monitoring of laboratory signs of DIC, reduced fibrinolytic activity, and perhaps low AT levels also are useful for predicting the outcome of such patients.[217]

DIC can be aggravated in patients with severe trauma who require massive blood replacement because stored blood components are diluted and do not contain sufficient amounts of viable platelets and factors V and VIII. Moreover, in such patients, there is an activation of fibrinolysis that further aggravate bleeding in combination with acidosis, and hypotension.[218–221] Infection commonly occurs in such patients and may contribute to the DIC.

The time interval between trauma and medical intervention correlates with the development and magnitude of DIC. Experience during wars proved that fast evacuation and prompt medical care reduce the risk of DIC.[222–224]

BRAIN INJURY

Brain injury can be associated with DIC, most likely because the injury exposes the abundant TF of brain to blood. Specimens of contused brain, obtained during surgery in patients with head injury and of liver, lungs, kidneys, and pancreas obtained during autopsy, revealed microthrombi in arterioles and venules.[225,226] In adults and children with head injuries, a high rate of mortality occurred when DIC was present.[227] A laboratory DIC score has predictive value for prognosis in patients with head injuries, thereby supplementing the Glasgow coma score.[228] Bleeding in patients with DIC that is related to brain injury can be managed by replacement therapy.

BURNS

Tissue factor exposed to blood at sites of burned tissue, the systemic inflammatory response syndrome induced by the burn, and the common presence of superimposed infections, all can trigger DIC.[229] Bleeding, laboratory tests indicative of DIC, and vascular microthrombi in biopsies of undamaged skin have been described in patients with extensive burns.[230] Kinetic studies with labeled fibrinogen and labeled platelets disclosed that, in addition to systemic consumption of hemostatic factors, significant local consumption occurs in burned areas.[231] Laboratory signs of DIC are associated with organ failure; the extent of protein C and AT deficiencies correlates with a poor outcome.[230] A clinicopathologic study of 139 patients who died during treatment for a severe burn disclosed that 18 percent had cerebral infarctions caused by septic arterial occlusions or DIC and approximately 4 percent had intracranial hemorrhage.[232]

LIVER DISEASES

Very complicated derangements of hemostasis occur in patients with severe liver disease and during liver transplantation (see Chap. 129). Synthesis of most coagulation factors and natural anticoagulants (protein C, protein S, and AT) and of the main components of the fibrinolytic system (plasminogen, TAFI, and α_2-antiplasmin) is reduced. The capacity of the liver to clear the circulation of activated factors IX, X, and XI and of t-PA is decreased. Moreover, thrombocytopenia is common as a result of hypersplenism and decreased production of thrombopoietin by the liver. The similarities between the hemostatic defects observed in patients with liver disease and in patients with DIC are striking and have evoked an ongoing controversy as to whether or not DIC contributes to hemostatic derangements associated with liver disease.[233]

Several laboratory and clinical observations support the hypothesis that DIC accompanies hepatic disorders. They include a shortened half-life of radiolabeled fibrinogen and prolongation of fibrinogen half-life by administration of heparin[234,235]; failure of replacement therapy to significantly increase the levels of hemostatic factors (suggesting continuous consumption); and increased blood levels of D-dimer, thrombin–antithrombin (TAT) complexes, and fibrinopeptide A, all consistent with ongoing thrombin generation.[236–238]

Other observations and considerations argue against the hypothesis that DIC accompanies liver diseases. They include (1) a very low incidence (2.2%) of microthrombosis in the tissues of patients who die of liver disease and (2) causes other than, or inconsistent with, DIC for the deranged findings in liver disease.[237] Examples of alternative explanations include the following: (1) a prolonged thrombin time may result from acquired dysfibrinogenemia[239]; (2) low levels of coagulation factors and inhibitors may result from reduced synthesis[240]; (3) increased FDP levels may be a consequence of primary fibrinogenolysis induced by reduced synthesis of α_2-antiplasmin and PAI-1 and by decreased clearance of t-PA; (4) factor VIII levels are commonly increased rather than decreased[241]; (5) the kinetic data show that the apparently excessive consumption of fibrinogen can be explained by loss of fibrinogen into extravascular spaces[242]; and (6) fibrinogen and plasminogen do not appear to be removed rapidly when labeled endogenously by ^{75}Se-selenomethionine.[243]

A third hypothesis maintains that patients with liver disease usually do not present with DIC but are extremely sensitive to the various triggers of DIC because of their impeded capacity to clear procoagulants and to synthesize essential components of the coagulation, inhibitory, and fibrinolytic systems. Patients with primary or metastatic liver disease who undergo a peritoneovenous shunt operation for severe ascites are more likely to develop DIC than are patients with ascites who undergo the same procedure because of other causes.[244]

What, then, should be the approach to patients with liver disease and bleeding without an apparent local cause? First, possible underlying causes of DIC should be considered and identified, and then a hemostatic profile should be examined at frequent intervals so as to detect any dynamic changes that may be helpful in recognizing DIC. The sensitive assays that reflect thrombin generation (TAT complex and prothrombin fragments 1.2) or concomitant thrombin and plasmin generation (D-dimer), as well as finding a normal or decreased level of factor VIII may help establish the diagnosis of DIC in a patient with liver disease.[245]

HEAT STROKE

In 1841, James Wellstead published his book *Travels to the City of the Caliphs* (currently known as Baghdad) and vividly described that on an extremely hot day in the Persian Gulf the decks of the ship *Liverpool* resembled a slaughterhouse, so numerous were the bleeding patients.[246] This is probably one of the first written reports on the occurrence of DIC in humans who suffer from heatstroke.[229] Heat stroke is a syndrome characterized by a rise in body temperature to higher than 42°C, which follows collapse of the thermoregulatory mechanism. The following predisposing factors have been identified: high environmental temperature, strenuous physical activity, infection, dehydration, and lack of acclimatization.[247,248] Extensive hemorrhage, unclottable blood, and venous engorgement were found as early as 1838 in postmortem examinations of patients who died of heat stroke.[246] Investigations confirm that a severe hemorrhagic diathesis and multiple organ failure often accompany heat stroke.[229,249–251] Diffuse fibrin deposition and hemorrhagic infarctions are found in fatal human cases. DIC associated with profound fibrin(ogen)olysis is evident in patients with heat stroke. The possible triggers of DIC in patients with heat stroke include endothelial cell damage and TF released from heat-damaged tissues.[249]

In a series of 18 critically ill patients from Paris with heat stroke during the 2003 heat wave in Western Europe that caused numerous deaths in France alone,[251] patients had very high levels of IL-6 and IL-8. In addition, there was a striking activation of white blood cells, as demonstrated by β_2-integrin upregulation and increased production of reactive oxygen species. All patients also had evidence of a significant systemic activation of coagulation and DIC was present in approximately 35 percent of patients. There was a marked correlation between the extent of inflammation and coagulation activation and the clinical severity of the heat stroke.

The severity of the syndrome and the stage of its development affect the type and magnitude of hemostatic alterations. Thus, in a study of 56 patients, three groups were discernible: nonbleeders, bleeders without DIC but with slight consumption of hemostatic factors, and bleeders with typical signs of DIC.[252] Prompt cooling and support of vital functions have substantially reduced the high mortality that was commonly observed in early studies.

SNAKE BITES

Several species of snakes belonging to the Viperidae family produce venoms that have a wide range of activities affecting hemostasis. Prominent among these species are the *Vipera, Echis (E. carinatus* or *E. coloratus), Aspis, Crotalus, Bothrops*, and *Agkistrodon*. Venoms of these snakes contain enzymes or peptides that exert the following activities[253–255]: (1) thrombin-like activity, cleaving fibrinopeptide A from the Aα chain of fibrinogen *(Agkistrodon rhodostoma)*; (2) activation of prothrombin even in the absence of calcium ions *(E. carinatus)*; (3) activation of factors X and V (Russell viper venom); (4) fibrinogenolytic activity *(Agkistrodon acutus)*; (5) induction of thrombocytopenia by platelet aggregation; (6) inhibition of platelet aggregation by the low-molecular-weight arginine-glycine-aspartic acid–containing peptides from a variety of snake species; (7) activation of protein C; and (8) activities causing damage to endothelial cells, leading to bleeding, tissue ischemia, and edema. Interestingly, victims of snake bites rarely experience excessive bleeding or thromboembolism, in spite of the serious derangements in hemostatic tests and findings that are sometimes consistent with DIC.[256–258]

The major symptoms and signs related to envenomation are vomiting, diarrhea, apprehension, hypotension, local swelling, ischemia, and necrosis. Consequently, treatment for victims of snake bites consists of immediate immobilization, administration of antivenom and fluids, and other general measures to preserve vital functions. Local incisions, cooling, and application of tourniquet should be avoided.[253]

HEMANGIOMAS

In 1940, Kasabach and Merritt described the association between giant hemangioma and a bleeding tendency occurring mainly in infants. The pathogenesis and management of this syndrome have been reviewed.[259] Studies using radiolabeled fibrinogen and platelets provided evidence that within the hemangioma, consumption of platelets and fibrinogen occurs because of localized intravascular clotting and excessive fibrinogenolysis.[260,261] Conceivably, concomitant local activation of the coagulation pathway and release of large amounts of t-PA by the abnormal endothelium lining the tumor vessels occur. Microangiopathic hemolytic anemia and laboratory signs of DIC and fibrinolysis have been demonstrated in patients with giant hemangiomas.[262] Accelerated growth of these hemangiomas in infants is associated with augmented consumption of hemostatic factors, and can be effectively treated with glucocorticoids. Radiotherapy and interferon-α are also effective, but should only be used in life-threatening circumstances after failure of glucocorticoid therapy because of severe adverse events.[263] Spontaneous mild to moderate bleeding manifestations have been observed, but severe bleeding generally occurs only after surgery or trauma.

Extensive vascular malformation may persist and cause pain, probably resulting from thrombosis, and bleeding following trauma, which is related to the localized or generalized consumption of clotting factors and platelets and hyperfibrinolysis.[264] Graded permanent elastic compression, when possible, and low-molecular-weight heparin constitute the only effective treatment in such cases.

AORTIC ANEURYSM

An association between aortic aneurysm and DIC is well documented.[265,266] In a series of patients with aortic aneurysm, 40 percent had elevated levels of fibrin(ogen) degradation products, but only 4 percent had significant bleeding and laboratory evidence of DIC.[265] Several factors predispose patients with aortic aneurysms to the development of DIC: a large surface area, dissection, and expansion of the aneurysm.[267] Clinical and laboratory signs of DIC should be carefully sought in patients with an aortic aneurysm because bleeding may seriously complicate surgical repair of the aneurysm.[267,268] The initiation of localized and generalized intravascular coagulation can be ascribed to activation of the TF pathway by the abundant amounts of TF present in atherosclerotic plaques.[269] When patients present with significant bleeding or when surgery is planned, hemostatic defects should be sought and corrected by low-molecular-weight heparin.[270] Stent-grafting, which is a common procedure for repair of aortic aneurysms, was complicated by DIC and death in two patients, of whom one had cirrhosis and the other underwent a lengthy procedure.[271] However, a study of 31 such patients failed to detect DIC following stent-grafting of thoracic aneurysms.[272]

TRANSFUSION REACTION

DIC accompanies incompatible blood transfusion, in which massive hemolysis is commonly associated with excessive bleeding with widespread thrombosis in fatal cases (see Chap. 140). The trigger of DIC in these cases cannot be simply ascribed to the release of red cell stroma, as patients with massive oxidative hemolysis because of glucose-6-phosphate dehydrogenase deficiency do not develop DIC.[273] Rather, extensive antigen–antibody reaction appears to cause DIC as a result of release of elastase and TNF-α from neutrophils, and activation of monocytes that release TNF-α express TF and complement, with assembly of the membrane attack complex inflicting damage to endothelial cells.[274,275]

DIC DURING PREGNANCY

Pregnancy predisposes patients to DIC for at least four reasons: (1) pregnancy itself produces a hypercoagulable state, manifested by evidence of low-grade thrombin generation, with elevated levels of fibrin monomer complexes and fibrinopeptide A; (2) during labor, leakage of tissue factor from placental tissue into the maternal circulation causes a hypercoagulable state; (3) pregnancy is associated with reduced fibrinolytic activity because of increased plasma levels of PAI-1; and (4) pregnancy is associated with a decline in the plasma level of protein S. DIC may be difficult to diagnose during pregnancy because of the high initial levels of coagulation factors such as fibrinogen, factor VIII, and factor VII.[276,277] Progressive reductions in these factors, however, can confirm or exclude the diagnosis of DIC in suspected cases. Thrombocytopenia may be particularly helpful in determining whether DIC is present, provided other causes of thrombocytopenia are excluded.[278]

Abruptio Placentae

The dramatic clinical presentation of abruptio placentae was first reported by DeLee in 1901,[279] but the immediate cause of sudden rupture of uterine spiral arteries and detachment of the placenta is still unknown. Placental abruption is a leading cause of perinatal death.[280] Older multiparous women or patients with one of the hypertensive disorders of pregnancy are thought to be at highest risk. The severe hemostatic failure accompanying abruptio placentae is the result of acute DIC emanating from the introduction of large amounts of TF into the blood circulation from the damaged placenta and uterus.[281] Amniotic fluid is able to activate coagulation *in vitro*, and the degree of placental separation correlates with the extent of DIC, suggesting that leakage of thromboplastin-like material from the placental system is responsible for the occurrence of DIC. Abruptio placentae occurs in 0.2 to 0.4 percent of pregnancies,[282] but only 10 percent of these cases are associated with DIC.[278] Different grades of severity are found among those who develop DIC, with only the more severe forms resulting in shock and fetal death. Rapid volume replenishment and evacuation of the uterus is the treatment of choice.[280] Transfusion of cryoprecipitate, fresh-frozen plasma, and platelets should be given when profuse bleeding occurs. However, in the absence of severe bleeding, administration of blood components may not be necessary because depleted coagulation factors increase rapidly following delivery. Heparin or antifibrinolytic agents are not indicated.

Amniotic Fluid Embolism

This rare catastrophic disorder, described by Steiner and Lushbaugh in 1941, occurs only in 1 in 8000 to 1 in 80,000 deliveries.[283] A maternal mortality rate of 86 percent was reported in a 1979 review of 272 cases, but in a later population-based study, the maternal mortality (26.4%) was significantly lower.[284,285] Patients predisposed to amniotic fluid embolism are multiparous women whose pregnancies are postmature with large fetuses and women undergoing a tumultuous labor after pharmacologic or surgical induction. Apparently, amniotic fluid is introduced into the maternal circulation through tears in the chorioamniotic membranes, rupture of the uterus, and injury of uterine veins.[284] The trigger of DIC probably is TF present in amniotic fluid.[286,287] The mechanical obstruction of pulmonary blood vessels by fetal debris, meconium, and other particulate matter in the amniotic fluid enhances local fibrin–platelet thrombus formation and fibrinolysis. The extensive occlusion of the pulmonary arteries and an acute anaphylactoid response reminiscent of severe systemic inflammatory response syndrome provoke sudden dyspnea, cyanosis, acute cor pulmonale, left ventricular dysfunction, shock, and convulsions. These symptoms are followed within minutes to several hours by severe bleeding in 37 percent of patients.[284] Hemorrhage is particularly severe from the atonic uterus, puncture sites, gastrointestinal tract, and other organs. The best prospect for decreasing mortality lies in early termination of parturition in patients at high risk and prevention of hypertonic and tetanic uterine contractions during labor. When the syndrome is recognized, immediate termination of pregnancy under pulmonary and cardiovascular support is essential.

Preeclampsia and Eclampsia

Thrombocytopenia described in early reports of eclampsia and widespread deposition of fibrin in blood vessels observed in fatal cases were interpreted as evidence of DIC triggered by placental TF exposure to the circulation.[1] A critical analysis of the literature concluded that the thrombocytopenia in these patients stems from endothelial injury rather than DIC.[288] However, other investigators provided evidence for significant DIC in preeclampsia and eclampsia.[289,290] Moreover, in a large series of patients, a good correlation was noted between the clinical severity and abnormalities in platelet counts and fibrin(ogen) degradation products.[291] Also consistent with DIC were results of assays of sensitive parameters of thrombin generation and activation of fibrinolysis, such as TAT complexes, D-dimer, and fibrinopeptide Bβ_{1-42}. Despite these observations, administration of heparin to patients with preeclampsia and eclampsia has not resulted in convincing benefits.[292]

HELLP Syndrome

The syndrome of hemolysis (H), elevated liver enzymes (EL), low platelet count (LP), and severe epigastric pain is a complication of pregnancy-induced hypertension.[293] Seventy percent of the cases occur during the third trimester of pregnancy and 30 percent occur during the postpartum period.[294] HELLP syndrome occurs more often in whites, multipara, and women older than 35 years.[292] Liver biopsy findings of fibrin deposition in hepatic blood vessels and laboratory tests consistent with DIC in a significant proportion of patients imply that DIC plays a role in the pathogenesis of the syndrome.[294–296] Hepatic imaging in 33 patients revealed subcapsular hematomas in 13 and intraparenchymal hemorrhage in 6.[297] What actually triggers DIC in these cases is not known but has been related to endothelial dysfunction.[292] Multiple organ dysfunctions manifested by acute renal failure, ascites, pulmonary edema, and severe hemorrhage resulting from DIC may develop, leading to significant maternal and perinatal mortality rates. Management of patients with HELLP syndrome consists of supportive care, careful monitoring, and blood component replacement therapy. With few exceptions, immediate delivery, not necessarily by cesarian section, is indicated. HELLP syndrome tends to recur in subsequent gestations.[298]

Sepsis during Pregnancy

Gram-negative bacteria, group A streptococci, and *Clostridium perfringens* are among the more common causes of sepsis during pregnancy. These infections are frequently associated with fulminant DIC. The pathogens gain entry into the circulation during abortion, via amnionitis that may follow invasive procedures or rupture of membranes, by endometritis developing during labor, and by way of the urinary tract. Approximately 40 percent of bacteremic patients experience shock, which is associated with significant mortality.[299] In addition, a high rate of bleeding and organ dysfunction affects the kidneys, lungs, and central nervous system.

Treatment of all cases of sepsis-related DIC should include antibiotics, support of vital functions, and surgical intervention to remove any local nidus of infection. Abortion or hysterectomy may be considered.

Dead Fetus Syndrome

Several weeks after intrauterine fetal death, approximately one-third of patients may exhibit laboratory signs of DIC, occasionally accompanied by bleeding.[278,300] Apparently, TF from the retained dead fetus or placenta slowly enters the maternal circulation and initiates DIC, which sometimes is accompanied by significant fibrinolysis.[13] This complication currently is rarely observed because labor is induced promptly after the diagnosis of fetal death is made. However, if labor induction is unavoidably delayed, serial blood coagulation tests should be performed.

The entity of fetal death and DIC can occur following the demise of one of multiple gestations. If it occurs at term, therapy is started as discussed. If it occurs prior to fetal maturity, prolonged administration of heparin can be useful. Interestingly, when selective termination of the life of an anomalous fetus is performed in women with multiple pregnancies, hemostatic abnormalities develop in only approximately 3 percent of cases.[301]

Acute Fatty Liver

Acute fatty liver of pregnancy is a rare disorder that occurs during the third trimester of pregnancy.[302] It can lead to hepatic failure, encephalopathy, and death of the mother and fetus.[303–306] In 15 to 20 percent of cases, acute fatty liver of pregnancy is associated with fetal homozygosity or compound heterozygosity for long-chain acyl-coenzyme A dehydrogenase (LCAD) deficiency.[307] Infants born with LCAD deficiency fail to thrive and are prone to liver failure and death. LCAD is one of four enzymes taking part in β-oxidation of fatty acids in mitochondria. When it is deficient, accumulation of medium- and long-chain fatty acid occurs. One predominant mutation (G1528C) accounts for 65 to 90 percent of cases with the deficiency. The precise mechanism by which LCAD deficiency in the fetus causes the severe liver disease in the heterozygous mother is unclear. The acute fatty liver disease of pregnancy is characterized by severe liver dysfunction, renal failure, hypertension, and signs of DIC.[304,308] The typical histologic feature is microvesicular fatty infiltration of the liver. Exceedingly low levels of AT and other laboratory signs of DIC were observed in a series of 28 patients, but no definite clinical benefit from AT concentrate infusion was achieved.[308] The primary therapy for these patients is early delivery and supportive care, which yield a maternal survival of 90 percent and perinatal survival of more than 85 percent.[304,309] Pancreatitis is a potentially lethal complication of acute fatty liver of pregnancy.[310]

NEWBORNS

Newborns have a limited capacity to cope with triggers of DIC for several reasons: (1) their ability to clear soluble fibrin and activated factors is reduced; (2) their fibrinolytic potential is decreased because of a low plasminogen level; and (3) their capacity to synthesize coagulation factors and inhibitors is limited.[311,312] Criteria for diagnosis of DIC in newborns are different from those for diagnosis in adults.[313] Important to consider are the physiologic hemostatic findings common at this age, which include low levels of the vitamin K-dependent factors, reduced AT and protein C levels, and prolonged thrombin time. The laboratory evidence of DIC in the newborn is based on the progressive decline of hemostatic parameters, thrombocytopenia, and reduced levels of fibrinogen, factor V, and factor VIII.[311,314,315]

DIC occurs in sick neonates and particularly in those who are premature. More than one underlying cause usually can be identified in newborns with DIC. The most frequent underlying conditions are sepsis, hyaline membrane disease (respiratory distress syndrome), asphyxia, necrotizing enterocolitis, intravascular hemolysis, abruptio placentae, and eclampsia.[312,316]

Bleeding from multiple sites is the most common manifestation of DIC in newborns, with intracranial hemorrhage being the most life-threatening condition. No clinical manifestations of DIC are apparent in approximately 20 percent of neonates,[314] so a high index of suspicion in patients at risk is essential.

THERAPY

Controlled studies of patients with DIC are difficult to perform in view of the variabilities in DIC triggers, clinical presentations, and grades of severity. Figure 130–4 shows general guidelines for management of patients with DIC, but decisions regarding treatment must be individualized after careful consideration of all clinically important aspects.

TREATMENT OF UNDERLYING DISORDERS AND VITAL SUPPORT

The survival of patients with DIC depends on vigorous treatment of the underlying disorder to alleviate or remove the inciting injurious cause. For sepsis-induced DIC, treatment includes aggressive use of intravenous organism-directed antibiotics and source control (e.g., by surgery or drainage). Other examples of vigorous treatment of underlying conditions are cancer surgery or chemotherapy, uterus evacuation or even hysterectomy in patients with abruptio placentae, resection of aortic aneurysm, and debridement of crushed tissues.

Intensive support of vital functions is required. Volume replacement and correction of hypotension, acidosis, and oxygenation may improve blood flow and oxygen delivery to the microcirculation. Careful monitoring of pulmonary, cardiac, and renal function enables prompt institution of supportive measures, such as use of a respirator for respiratory support, inotropic and vasoactive drugs for improvement of organ perfusion, renal function, and maintenance of electrolyte balance.

BLOOD COMPONENT THERAPY

Treatment of the underlying disease and vital support are necessary but usually insufficient to treat DIC or forestall progression of nonovert DIC to overt DIC. Additional supportive treatment directly aimed at the coagulation system may be required. These interventions include replacing the coagulation factors, natural anticoagulant, fibrinolytic proteins, and platelets that are actively consumed during DIC.[317]

Low levels of platelets and coagulation factors may increase the risk of bleeding. However, plasma or platelet substitution therapy should not be instituted on the basis of laboratory results alone; it is indicated only in patients with active bleeding and in those requiring an invasive procedure or are at risk for bleeding complications.[318,319] The suggestion that administration of blood components might "add fuel to the fire" has never been proven in clinical or experimental studies. The presumed efficacy of treatment with plasma, fibrinogen concentrate, cryoprecipitate, or platelets is not based on randomized controlled trials but appears to be rational therapy in bleeding patients or in patients at risk of bleeding who have a significant depletion of these hemostatic factors.[319] One of the major challenges of infusion of fresh-frozen plasma in these dire circumstances is the propensity of the added volume, which is necessary to correct the coagulation defect, to exacerbate capillary leak. This situation can increase the risk of inducing or worsening pulmonary edema and, by extension, predispose to ARDS, and induce ascites. Coagulation factor concentrates, such as prothrombin complex concentrate, may partially overcome this obstacle, but do not contain essential factors, such as factor V. Moreover, caution is advocated with the use of prothrombin complex concentrates in DIC, because it may worsen the coagulopathy because of traces of activated factors that are present in these concentrates. Specific deficiencies of coagulation factors, such as fibrinogen, may be corrected by administration of purified coagulation factor concentrates.

Platelet transfusion is often required in patients with DIC to prevent bleeding into already ischemic or damaged organs (particularly the central nervous system). The threshold platelet count that should prompt transfusion is patient and disease specific. Cryoprecipitate can be used to rapidly raise the fibrinogen and factor VIII levels, particularly when bleeding is part of the DIC and fibrinogen level is less than 1 g/L. Cryoprecipitate has at least four to five times the mass of fibrinogen per milliliter of infusate compared to fresh-frozen plasma. Fresh-frozen plasma contains fibrinogen in sufficient amounts for treatment of patients with mild to moderate hypofibrinogemia.

Replacement therapy for thrombocytopenia should consist of 5 to 10 units platelet concentrate or single-donor apheresis-derived platelets to raise the platelet count to 20 to 30 × 10^9/L, and in patients who need an invasive procedure, to 50 × 10^9/L.

RESTORATION OF PHYSIOLOGICAL ANTICOAGULANT PATHWAYS

Because the levels of the physiologic anticoagulants are reduced in patients with DIC, restoration of these inhibitors may be a rational approach.[49,320] Based on successful preclinical studies, the use of AT

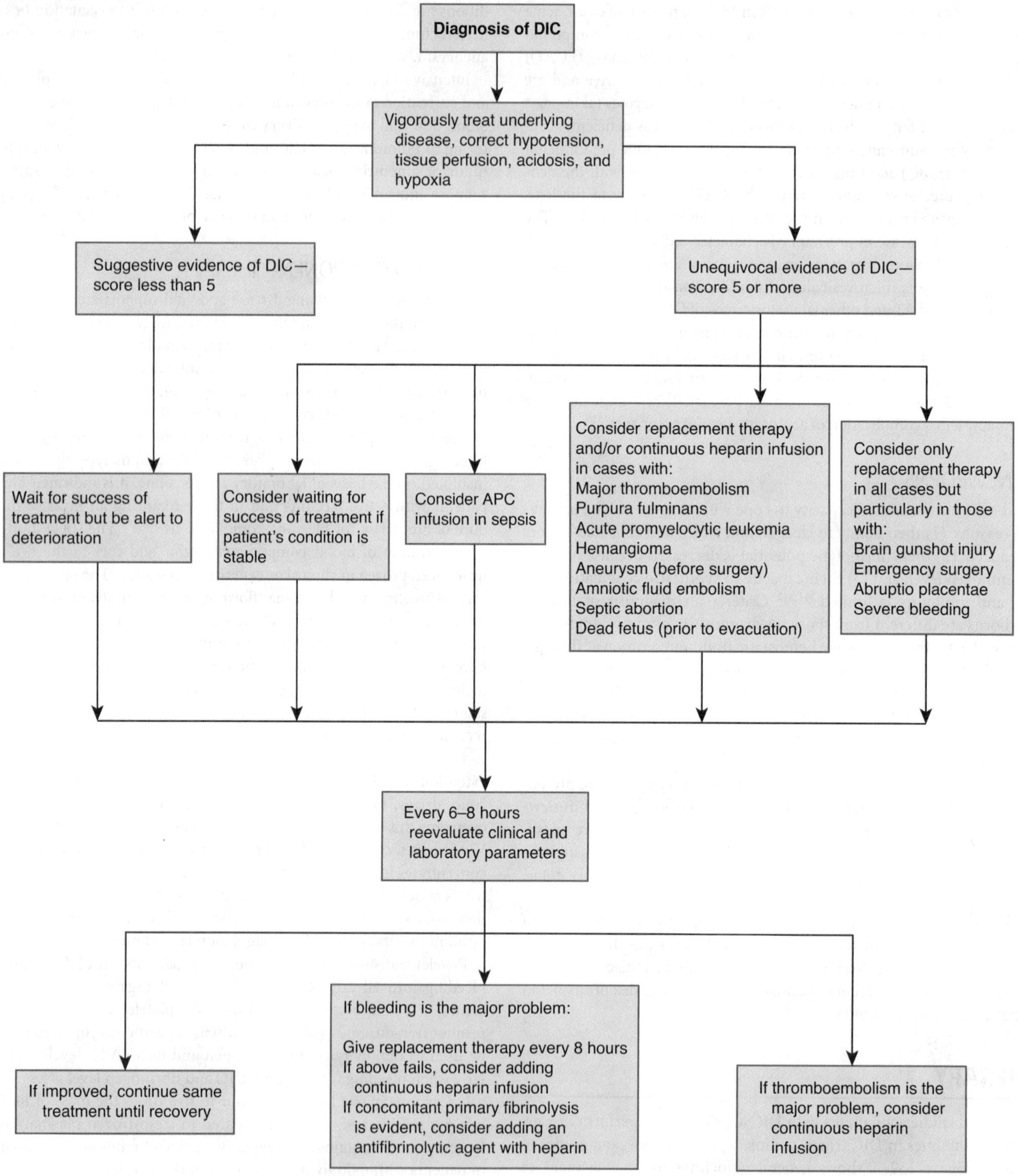

FIGURE 130–4. General guidelines for initial treatment and follow up of patients with DIC. The success of management is related to taking rapid, vigorous measures against the underlying disease, support of vital functions, close clinical observation, thoughtful consideration in each individual patient, availability of 24-hour coagulation laboratory services, and an adequate supply of platelet concentrate, cryoprecipitate, fresh-frozen plasma, and packed red cells for replacement therapy. Heparin, when indicated, should be administered by continuous infusion. The basis and limitations of each of the outlined recommendations are detailed throughout the text. APC, activated protein C.

concentrates and heparin in patients with DIC has been examined mainly in randomized controlled trials, that included patients with sepsis, septic shock, or both. All trials have shown some beneficial effect in terms of improvement of laboratory parameters, shortening of the duration of DIC, or even improvement in organ function.[6,321,322] In several small clinical trials, use of very high doses of AT concentrate showed even a modest reduction in mortality, however, without being statistically significant.[323–325] A large-scale, multicenter, randomized controlled trial also showed no significant reduction in mortality of patients with sepsis.[326] Interestingly, posthoc subgroup analyses of the latter study indicated some benefit in patients who did not receive concomitant heparin, but this observation needs validation. In a small randomized trial in patients with burns and DIC, AT administration decreased mortality, reduced multiple organ failure, and improved coagulation parameters compared to placebo-control patients.[327]

Because a decreased function of the protein C system contributes to the pathogenesis of DIC, therapy by an APC concentrate was predicted to be beneficial.[328] Indeed, a dose-ranging controlled trial using continuous infusion of recombinant human APC disclosed that a dose of 24 mcg/kg per hour was optimal, judged by a decrease of D-dimer level in plasma.[329] A subsequent phase III trial of APC concentrate in patients with sepsis was prematurely stopped because of efficacy in reducing mortality in these patients.[330] All-cause mortality at 28 days after inclusion was 24.7 percent in the APC group versus 30.8 percent in the control group (a 19.4% relative risk reduction). Amelioration of coagulation abnormalities and less organ failure were noted in patients who received the concentrate.[331] Part of the success of therapy could be ascribed to the antiinflammatory effect of APC. Interestingly, patients who manifested "overt DIC" (see "Diagnosis" above) benefited more from the therapy with APC than did patients without overt DIC.[124] The relative risk reduction in mortality of patients with both sepsis and DIC was 38 percent, whereas patients with sepsis and no DIC, only had a risk reduction of 18 percent. This seems to underscore the importance of the coagulation derangement in the pathogenesis of sepsis and implies that the restoration of the protein C pathway in the microvasculature is essential for recovery of patients with sepsis. Recombinant human APC has been licensed in most countries for treatment of patients with severe sepsis involving two or more organ failures.

An extensive analysis of subgroups in the above phase III clinical trial was performed.[332] Administration of recombinant human APC proved to be of benefit in virtually all subgroups defined, including age, type, and site of infection. The efficacy of APC was most prominent in the subgroups of patients with a relatively high disease severity, whereas in patients with a lower disease severity, the drug appeared less effective.

To prospectively analyze this issue, the ADDRESS trial was performed in 2640 patients with sepsis and a relatively low disease severity (defined as a single sepsis-associated organ failure or an APACHE II score below 25).[333] The initial sample size of this trial was 11,400 patients; however, the trial was prematurely stopped after a second interim analysis because of predefined futility rules. The 28-day mortality rates were 18.5 percent in the APC group and 17 percent in the placebo group ($p = 0.34$).[334] Thus, based on the ADDRESS study, treatment with APC seems not to be indicated in patients with sepsis and a relatively low disease severity.

The most frequently encountered adverse effect of APC is bleeding. In the phase III study in patients with severe sepsis, the incidence of major bleeding during the infusion period was 2.4 percent in the APC group as compared with 1 percent in the control group ($p = 0.02$).[330] During the 28-day study period, the incidence of major bleeding was 3.5 percent in the APC group and 2 percent in the placebo group ($p = 0.06$). Gastrointestinal bleeding was the most frequent bleeding manifestation in both groups. Other bleeding manifestations were procedure-related or occurred in patients with a severely deranged coagulation system.[335]

HEPARIN ADMINISTRATION AND OTHER ANTICOAGULANTS

Although the question of heparin therapy in patients with DIC has been studied by several investigators, this therapy remains controversial. Experimental studies have shown that heparin can at least partly inhibit the activation of coagulation in DIC.[336,337] However, a beneficial effect of heparin on clinically important outcome events in patients with DIC has not been demonstrated in controlled clinical trials.[338] Also, the safety of heparin treatment is debatable in DIC patients who are prone to bleeding. A large trial in patients with severe sepsis showed a slight, but nonsignificant benefit, of low-dose heparin on 28-day mortality in patients with severe sepsis.[339]

Notwithstanding these considerations, administration of heparin is beneficial in some categories of chronic DIC, such as metastatic carcinomas, purpura fulminans, and aortic aneurysm (prior to resection). Heparin also is indicated for treating thromboembolic complications in large vessels and before surgery in patients with chronic DIC (see Fig. 130–4). Heparin administration may be helpful in patients with acute DIC when intensive blood component replacement fails to improve excessive bleeding or when thrombosis threatens to cause irreversible tissue injury (e.g., acute cortical necrosis of the kidney or digital gangrene).

Heparin should be used cautiously in all these conditions. In patients with chronic DIC because of metastatic carcinoma or aortic aneurysm, continuous infusion of heparin 500 to 750 U/h without a bolus injection may be sufficient. If no response is obtained within 24 hours, escalating dosages can be used. In hyperacute DIC cases, such as mismatched transfusion, amniotic fluid embolism, septic abortion, and purpura fulminans, intravenous bolus injection of 5000 to 10,000 U heparin may be given simultaneously with replacement therapy with blood products. Some experts would not administer a bolus dose of heparin even under these circumstances. Continuous infusion of 500 to 1000 U/h heparin may be necessary to maintain the benefit until the underlying disease responds to treatment.[339]

Theoretically, the most logical anticoagulant agent to use in DIC is directed against TF activity. Potential agents include recombinant TFPI, inactivated factor VIIa, and recombinant NAPc2, a potent and specific inhibitor of the ternary complex of TF/factor VIIa and factor Xa.[340] Phase II trials of recombinant TFPI in patients with sepsis showed promising results,[341] but a phase III trial did not show an overall survival benefit in patients who were treated with TFPI.[341,342]

Recombinant human soluble thrombomodulin binds to thrombin to form a complex that inactivates thrombin's coagulant activity and activates protein C, and thus, is a potential drug for the treatment of patients with DIC. In a phase III randomized double-blind clinical trial in patients with DIC, administration of the soluble thrombomodulin had a significantly better effect on bleeding manifestations and coagulation parameters than heparin, but the mortality rate at 28 days was similar in the two study groups.[343]

INHIBITORS OF FIBRINOLYSIS

Patients with DIC should not be treated with antifibrinolytic agents such as ε-aminocaproic acid or tranexamic acid because these drugs block fibrinolysis that preserves tissue perfusion in patients with DIC. Use of these agents in patients with DIC has been complicated by severe thrombosis.[344,345]

A different situation prevails in patients with DIC accompanied by primary fibrino(geno)lysis, as in some cases of APL, giant hemangioma, heat stroke, amniotic fluid embolism, some forms of liver disease, and metastatic carcinoma of the prostate. In these conditions, the use of fibrinolytic inhibitors can be considered,[346] provided (1) the patient is bleeding profusely and has not responded to replacement therapy and (2) excessive fibrino(geno)lysis is observed, that is, rapid whole blood clot lysis or a very short euglobulin lysis time. In such circumstances, use of antifibrinolytic agents should be preceded by replacement of depleted blood components and continuous heparin infusion (see Fig. 130–4).

REFERENCES

1. McKay DG: *Disseminated Intravascular Coagulation: an Intermediary Mechanism of Disease*. Hoeber Medical, New York, 1965.
2. Mammen EF: Disseminated intravascular coagulation (DIC). *Clin Lab Sci* 13:239, 2000.
3. Colman RW, Robboy SJ, Minna JD: Disseminated intravascular coagulation: A reappraisal. *Annu Rev Med* 30:359, 1979.
4. Seligsohn U: Disseminated intravascular coagulation, in *Blood: Principles and Practice of Hematology*, edited by RI Handin, SE Lux, TP Stossel, p1289. J.B. Lippincott, Philadelphia, 2000.
5. Levi M, ten Cate H: Disseminated intravascular coagulation. *N Engl J Med* 341:586, 1999.
6. Levi M, ten Cate H, van der Poll T: Disseminated intravascular coagulation: State of the art. *Thromb Haemost* 82:695, 1999.
7. Levi M: Disseminated intravascular coagulation. *Crit Care Med* 29:2191, 2007.
8. Dupuy M: Injections de matière cérébrale dans les veines. *Gaz Med (Paris)* 2:524, 1834.
9. Trousseau A: Phlegmasia alba dolens. *Clin Med Hotel Dieu Paris* 695, 1865.
10. Naunyn C: Untersuchungen uber Blutgerinnung im lebenden tiere and ihre Folgen. *Arch Exp Pathol Pharmacol* 1873.
11. Woolridge LC: Note on the relation of the red cell corpuscles to coagulation. *Practitioner* 187, 1886.
12. Woolridge LC: Ueber intravasculare gerinnungen. *Arch Ant Physiol Abt (Leipzig)* 397, 1886.
13. Ratnoff OD, Pritchard JA, Colopy JE: Hemorraghic states during pregnancy. *N Engl J Med* 253:63,1955.
14. Lasch HG, Heene DL, Huth K, et al: Pathophysiology, clinical manifestations and therapy of consumption-coagulopathy ("Verbrauchskoagulopathie"). *Am J Cardiol* 20:381, 1967.
15. Merskey C, Johnson AJ, Kleiner GJ, et al: The defibrination syndrome: Clinical features and laboratory diagnosis. *Br J Haematol* 13:528, 1967.
16. Robboy SJ, Major MC, Colman RW, et al: Pathology of disseminated intravascular coagulation (DIC). Analysis of 26 cases. *Hum Pathol* 3:327, 1972.
17. Wilde JT, Roberts KM, Greaves M, et al: Association between necropsy evidence of disseminated intravascular coagulation and coagulation variables before death in patients in intensive care units. *J Clin Pathol* 41:138, 1988.
18. Kim HS, Suzuki M, Lie JT, et al: Clinically unsuspected disseminated intravascular coagulation (DIC): An autopsy survey. *Am J Clin Pathol* 66:31, 1976.
19. Watanabe T, Imamura T, Nakagaki K, et al: Disseminated intravascular coagulation in autopsy cases. Its incidence and clinicopathologic significance. *Pathol Res Pract* 165:311, 1979.
20. Shimamura K, Oka K, Nakazawa M, et al: Distribution patterns of microthrombi in disseminated intravascular coagulation. *Arch Pathol Lab Med* 107:543, 1983.
21. Levi M, van der Poll T, ten Cate H, et al: The cytokine-mediated imbalance between coagulant and anticoagulant mechanisms in sepsis and endotoxaemia. *Eur J Clin Invest* 27:3, 1997.
22. Levi M, van der Poll T, Buller HR: The bidirectional relationship between coagulation and inflammation. *Circulation* 109:2698, 2004.
23. Aird WC: Vascular bed-specific hemostasis: Role of endothelium in sepsis pathogenesis. *Crit Care Med* 29:S28, 2001.
24. Weinbaum S, Zhang X, Han Y, et al: Mechanotransduction and flow across the endothelial glycocalyx. *Proc Natl Acad Sci U S A* 100:7988, 2003.
25. Maczewski M, Duda M, Pawlak W, et al: Endothelial protection from reperfusion injury by ischemic preconditioning and diazoxide involves a SOD-like anti-O_2-mechanism. *J Physiol Pharmacol* 55:537, 2004.
26. Vink H, Constantinescu AA, Spaan JA: Oxidized lipoproteins degrade the endothelial surface layer: Implications for platelet-endothelial cell adhesion. *Circulation* 101:1500, 2000.
27. Nieuwdorp M, van Haeften TW, Gouverneur MC, et al: Loss of endothelial glycocalyx during acute hyperglycemia coincides with endothelial dysfunction and coagulation activation *in vivo*. *Diabetes* 55:480, 2006.
28. Levi M, van der Poll T, ten Cate H: Tissue factor in infection and severe inflammation. *Semin Thromb Hemost* 32:33, 2006.
29. Taylor FBJ, Chang A, Ruf W, et al: Lethal *E. coli* septic shock is prevented by blocking tissue factor with monoclonal antibody. *Circ Shock* 33:127, 1991.
30. Levi M, ten Cate H, Bauer KA, et al: Inhibition of endotoxin-induced activation of coagulation and fibrinolysis by pentoxifylline or by a monoclonal anti-tissue factor antibody in chimpanzees. *J Clin Invest* 93:114, 1994.
31. van der Poll T, Levi M, Hack CE, et al: Elimination of interleukin 6 attenuates coagulation activation in experimental endotoxemia in chimpanzees. *J Exp Med* 179:1253, 1994.
32. Osterud B, Rao LV, Olsen JO: Induction of tissue factor expression in whole blood—lack of evidence for the presence of tissue factor expression on granulocytes. *Thromb Haemost* 83:861, 2000.
33. Franco RF, de Jonge E, Dekkers PE, et al: The *in vivo* kinetics of tissue factor messenger RNA expression during human endotoxemia: Relationship with activation of coagulation. *Blood* 96:554, 2000.
34. Rauch U, Bonderman D, Bohrmann B, et al: Transfer of tissue factor from leukocytes to platelets is mediated by CD15 and tissue factor. *Blood* 96:170, 2000.
35. Osterud B, Bjorklid E: Sources of tissue factor. *Semin Thromb Hemost* 32:11, 2006.
36. van Deventer SJ, Buller HR, ten Cate JW, et al: Experimental endotoxemia in humans: Analysis of cytokine release and coagulation, fibrinolytic, and complement pathways. *Blood* 76:2520, 1990.
37. Boermeester MA, van Leeuwen P, Coyle SM, et al: Interleukin-1 blockade attenuates mediator release and dysregulation of the hemostatic mechanism during human sepsis. *Arch Surg* 130:739, 1995.
38. Osterud B: Tissue factor expression by monocytes: Regulation and pathophysiological roles. *Blood Coagul Fibrinolysis* 9 Suppl 1:S9, 1998.
39. Furie B, Furie BC: Role of platelet P-selectin and microparticle PSGL-1 in thrombus formation. *Trends Mol Med* 10:171, 2004.
40. Neumann FJ, Marx N, Gawaz M, et al: Induction of cytokine expression in leukocytes by binding of thrombin-stimulated platelets. *Circulation* 95:2387, 1997.
41. Esmon CT: Protein C anticoagulant pathway and its role in controlling microvascular thrombosis and inflammation. *Crit Care Med* 29:S48, 2001.
42. Mileno MD, Margolis NH, Clark BD, et al: Coagulation of whole blood stimulates interleukin-1 beta gene expression. *J Infect Dis* 172:308, 1995.
43. Jones A, Geczy CL: Thrombin and factor Xa enhance the production of interleukin-1. *Immunology* 71:236, 1990.
44. Johnson K, Choi Y, DeGroot E, et al: Potential mechanisms for a proinflammatory vascular cytokine response to coagulation activation. *J Immunol* 160:5130, 1998.
45. Sower LE, Froelich CJ, Carney DH, et al: Thrombin induces IL-6 production in fibroblasts and epithelial cells. Evidence for the involvement of the seven-transmembrane domain (STD) receptor for alpha-thrombin. *J Immunol* 155:895, 1995.
46. van der Poll T, de Jonge E, Levi M: Regulatory role of cytokines in disseminated intravascular coagulation. *Semin Thromb Hemost* 27:639, 2001.
47. Coughlin SR: Thrombin signalling and protease-activated receptors. *Nature* 407:258, 2000.
48. Versteeg HH, Peppelenbosch MP, Spek CA: The pleiotropic effects of tissue factor: A possible role for factor VIIa-induced intracellular signalling? *Thromb Haemost* 86:1353, 2001.
49. Levi M, de Jonge E, van der Poll T: Rationale for restoration of physiological anticoagulant pathways in patients with sepsis and disseminated intravascular coagulation. *Crit Care Med* 29:S90, 2001.
50. Szaba FM, Smiley ST: Roles for thrombin and fibrin(ogen) in cytokine/chemokine production and macrophage adhesion *in vivo*. *Blood* 99:1053, 2002.
51. Levi M, van der Poll T: The role of natural anticoagulants in the pathogenesis and management of systemic activation of coagulation and inflammation in critically ill patients. *Semin Thromb Hemost* 34:459, 2008.
52. Levi M: Antithrombin in sepsis revisited. *Crit Care* 9:624, 2005.
53. Levi M, van der Poll T: Two-way interactions between inflammation and coagulation. *Trends Cardiovasc Med* 15:254, 2005.
54. Kobayashi M, Shimada K, Ozawa T: Human recombinant interleukin-1 beta- and tumor necrosis factor alpha-mediated suppression of heparin-like compounds on cultured porcine aortic endothelial cells. *J Cell Physiol* 144:383, 1990.
55. Levi M, van der Poll T: Recombinant human activated protein C: Current insights into its mechanism of action. *Crit Care* 11 Suppl 5:S3, 2007.
56. Esmon CT: Role of coagulation inhibitors in inflammation. *Thromb Haemost* 86:51, 2001.
57. Esmon CT: The regulation of natural anticoagulant pathways. *Science* 235:1348, 1987.
58. Esmon CT: The endothelial cell protein C receptor. *Thromb Haemost* 83:639, 2000.
59. Mesters RM, Helterbrand J, Utterback BG, et al: Prognostic value of protein C concentrations in neutropenic patients at high risk of severe septic complications. *Crit Care Med* 28:2209, 2000.
60. Vary TC, Kimball SR: Regulation of hepatic protein synthesis in chronic inflammation and sepsis. *Am J Physiol* 262:C445, 1992.
61. Eckle I, Seitz R, Egbring R, et al: Protein C degradation *in vitro* by neutrophil elastase. *Biol Chem Hoppe Seyler* 372:1007, 1991.
62. Nawroth PP, Stern DM: Modulation of endothelial cell hemostatic properties by tumor necrosis factor. *J Exp Med* 163:740, 1986.
63. Faust SN, Levin M, Harrison OB, et al: Dysfunction of endothelial protein C activation in severe meningococcal sepsis. *N Engl J Med* 345:408, 2001.
64. Taylor FBJ, Dahlback B, Chang AC, et al: Role of free protein S and C4b binding protein in regulating the coagulant response to *Escherichia coli*. *Blood* 86:2642, 1995.
65. Taylor FBJ, Stearns-Kurosawa DJ, Kurosawa S, et al: The endothelial cell protein C receptor aids in host defense against *Escherichia coli* sepsis. *Blood* 95:1680, 2000.
66. De Pont AC, Bakhtiari K, Hutten BA, et al: Endotoxaemia induces resistance to activated protein C in healthy humans. *Br J Haematol* 134:213, 2006.
67. de Jonge E, Dekkers PE, Creasey AA, et al: Tissue factor pathway inhibitor (TFPI) dose-dependently inhibits coagulation activation without influencing the fibrinolytic and cytokine response during human endotoxemia. *Blood* 95:1124, 2000.
68. Creasey AA, Chang AC, Feigen L, et al: Tissue factor pathway inhibitor reduces mortality from *Escherichia coli* septic shock. *J Clin Invest* 91:2850, 1993.
69. Roemisch J, Gray E, Hoffmann JN, et al: Antithrombin: A new look at the actions of a serine protease inhibitor. *Blood Coagul Fibrinolysis* 13:657, 2002.
70. Opal SM: Interactions between coagulation and inflammation. *Scand J Infect Dis* 35:545, 2003.
71. Harada N, Okajima K, Kushimoto S, et al: Antithrombin reduces ischemia/reperfusion injury of rat liver by increasing the hepatic level of prostacyclin. *Blood* 93:157, 1999.
72. Horie S, Ishii H, Kazama M: Heparin-like glycosaminoglycan is a receptor for antithrombin III-dependent but not for thrombin-dependent prostacyclin production in human endothelial cells. *Thromb Res* 59:895, 1990.
73. Mizutani A, Okajima K, Uchiba M, et al: Antithrombin reduces ischemia/reperfusion-induced renal injury in rats by inhibiting leukocyte activation through promotion of prostacyclin production. *Blood* 101:3029, 2003.

74. Uchiba M, Okajima K, Murakami K: Effects of various doses of antithrombin III on endotoxin-induced endothelial cell injury and coagulation abnormalities in rats. *Thromb Res* 89:233, 1998.
75. Esmon CT: New mechanisms for vascular control of inflammation mediated by natural anticoagulant proteins. *J Exp Med* 196:561, 2002.
76. Okajima K: Regulation of inflammatory responses by natural anticoagulants. *Immunol Rev* 184:258, 2001.
77. Taylor FBJ, Chang A, Esmon CT, et al: Protein C prevents the coagulopathic and lethal effects of *Escherichia coli* infusion in the baboon. *J Clin Invest* 79:918, 1987.
78. Hancock WW, Tsuchida A, Hau H, et al: The anticoagulants protein C and protein S display potent antiinflammatory and immunosuppressive effects relevant to transplant biology and therapy. *Transplant Proc* 24:2302, 1992.
79. Hancock WW, Grey ST, Hau L, et al: Binding of activated protein C to a specific receptor on human mononuclear phagocytes inhibits intracellular calcium signaling and monocyte-dependent proliferative responses. *Transplantation* 60:1525, 1995.
80. White B, Schmidt M, Murphy C, et al: Activated protein C inhibits lipopolysaccharide-induced nuclear translocation of nuclear factor kappaB (NF-kappaB) and tumour necrosis factor alpha (TNF-alpha) production in the THP-1 monocytic cell line. *Br J Haematol* 110:130, 2000.
81. Levi M, Dorffler-Melly J, Reitsma PH, et al: Aggravation of endotoxin-induced disseminated intravascular coagulation and cytokine activation in heterozygous protein C deficient mice. *Blood* 101:4823, 2003.
82. Lay AJ, Donahue D, Tsai MJ, et al: Acute inflammation is exacerbated in mice genetically predisposed to a severe protein C deficiency. *Blood* 109:1984, 2007.
83. Feistritzer C, Sturn DH, Kaneider NC, et al: Endothelial protein C receptor-dependent inhibition of human eosinophil chemotaxis by protein C. *J Allergy Clin Immunol* 112:375, 2003.
84. Sturn DH, Kaneider NC, Feistritzer C, et al: Expression and function of the endothelial protein C receptor in human neutrophils. *Blood* 102:1499, 2003.
85. Hoffmann JN, Vollmar B, Laschke MW, et al: Microhemodynamic and cellular mechanisms of activated protein C action during endotoxemia. *Crit Care Med* 32:1011, 2004.
86. Nick JA, Coldren CD, Geraci MW, et al: Recombinant human activated protein C reduces human endotoxin-induced pulmonary inflammation via inhibition of neutrophil chemotaxis. *Blood* 104:3878, 2004.
87. Shimizu S, Gabazza EC, Taguchi O, et al: Activated protein C inhibits the expression of platelet-derived growth factor in the lung. *Am J Respir Crit Care Med* 167:1416, 2003.
88. Zeng W, Matter WF, Yan SB, et al: Effect of drotrecogin alfa (activated) on human endothelial cell permeability and Rho kinase signaling. *Crit Care Med* 32:S302, 2004.
89. Feistritzer C, Riewald M: Endothelial barrier protection by activated protein C through PAR1-dependent sphingosine 1-phosphate receptor-1 cross activation. *Blood* 105:3178, 2005.
90. Finigan JH, Dudek SM, Singleton PA, et al: Activated protein C mediates novel lung endothelial barrier enhancement: Role of sphingosine 1-phosphate receptor transactivation. *J Biol Chem* 280:17286, 2005.
91. Cheng T, Liu D, Griffin JH, et al: Activated protein C blocks p53-mediated apoptosis in ischemic human brain endothelium and is neuroprotective. *Nat Med* 9:338, 2003.
92. Riewald M, Petrovan RJ, Donner A, et al: Activation of endothelial cell protease activated receptor 1 by the protein C pathway. *Science* 296:1880, 2002.
93. Mosnier LO, Griffin JH: Inhibition of staurosporine-induced apoptosis of endothelial cells by activated protein C requires protease activated receptor-1 and endothelial cell protein C receptor. *Biochem J* 373:65, 2003.
94. Mosnier LO, Zlokovic BV, Griffin JH: The cytoprotective protein C pathway. *Blood* 109:3161, 2007.
95. Biemond BJ, Levi M, ten Cate H, et al: Plasminogen activator and plasminogen activator inhibitor I release during experimental endotoxaemia in chimpanzees: Effect of interventions in the cytokine and coagulation cascades. *Clin Sci* 88:587, 1995.
96. Schleef RR, Bevilacqua MP, Sawdey M, et al: Cytokine activation of vascular endothelium. Effects on tissue-type plasminogen activator and type 1 plasminogen activator inhibitor. *J Biol Chem* 263:5797, 1988.
97. van HV, Kooistra T, van den Berg EA, et al: Tumor necrosis factor increases the production of plasminogen activator inhibitor in human endothelial cells *in vitro* and in rats *in vivo*. *Blood* 72:1467, 1988.
98. Asakura H, Ontachi Y, Mizutani T: An enhanced fibrinolysis prevents the development of multiple organ failure in disseminated intravascular coagulation in spite of much activation of blood coagulation. *Crit Care Med* 29:1164, 2001.
99. Yamamoto K, Loskutoff DJ: Fibrin deposition in tissues from endotoxin-treated mice correlates with decreases in the expression of urokinase-type but not tissue-type plasminogen activator. *J Clin Invest* 97:2440, 1996.
100. Nesheim M, Wang W, Boffa M, et al: Thrombin, thrombomodulin and TAFI in the molecular link between coagulation and fibrinolysis. *Thromb Haemost* 78:386, 1997.
101. Salvemini D, Cuzzocrea S: Oxidative stress in septic shock and disseminated intravascular coagulation. *Free Radic Biol Med* 33:1173, 2002.
102. Asakura H, Okudaira M, Yoshida T: Induction of vasoactive substances differs in LPS-induced and TF-induced DIC models in rats. *Thromb Haemost* 88:663, 2002.
103. Levi M, Nieuwdorp M, van der Poll T, et al: Metabolic modulation of inflammation-induced activation of coagulation. *Semin Thromb Hemost* 34:26, 2008.
104. Kjalke M, Silveira A, Hamsten A, et al: Plasma lipoproteins enhance tissue factor-independent factor VII activation. *Arterioscler Thromb Vasc Biol* 20:1835, 2000.
105. van der Poll T, Coyle SM, Levi M, et al: Fat emulsion infusion potentiates coagulation activation during human endotoxemia. *Thromb Haemost* 75:83, 1996.
106. Pajkrt D, Lerch PG, van der Poll T, et al: Differential effects of reconstituted high-density lipoprotein on coagulation, fibrinolysis and platelet activation during human endotoxemia. *Thromb Haemost* 77:303, 1997.
107. Birjmohun RS, van Leuven SI, Levels JH, et al: High-density lipoprotein attenuates inflammation and coagulation response on endotoxin challenge in humans. *Arterioscler Thromb Vasc Biol* 27:1153, 2007.
108. Bisoendial RJ, Kastelein JJ, Peters SL, et al: Effects of CRP infusion on endothelial function and coagulation in normocholesterolemic and hypercholesterolemic subjects. *J Lipid Res* 48:952, 2007.
109. Grant PJ: Diabetes mellitus as a prothrombotic condition. *J Intern Med* 262:157, 2007.
110. Juhan-Vague I, Roul C, Alessi MC, et al: Increased plasminogen activator inhibitor activity in non insulin dependent diabetic patients—Relationship with plasma insulin. *Thromb Haemost* 61:370, 1989.
111. Mansfield MW, Stickland MH, Grant PJ: PAI-1 concentrations in first-degree relatives of patients with non-insulin-dependent diabetes: Metabolic and genetic associations. *Thromb Haemost* 77:357, 1997.
112. Samad F, Pandey M, Loskutoff DJ: Regulation of tissue factor gene expression in obesity. *Blood* 98:3353, 2001.
113. Stegenga ME, van der Crabben SN, Levi M, et al: Hyperglycemia enhances coagulation and reduces neutrophil degranulation, whereas hyperinsulinemia inhibits fibrinolysis during human endotoxemia. *Blood* 112:82, 2008.
114. Levi M: Current understanding of disseminated intravascular coagulation. *Br J Haematol* 124:567, 2004.
115. Siegal T, Seligsohn U, Aghai E, et al: Clinical and laboratory aspects of disseminated intravascular coagulation (DIC): A study of 118 cases. *Thromb Haemost* 39:122, 1978.
116. Al-Mondhiry H: Disseminated intravascular coagulation: Experience in a major cancer center. *Thromb Diath Haemorrh* 34:181, 1975.
117. Hofstra JJ, Haitsma JJ, Juffermans NP, et al: Role of broncho-alveolar hemostasis in the pathogenesis of acute lung injury. *Semin Thromb Hemost* 34:475, 2008.
118. Rinaldo JE, Rogers RM: Adult respiratory distress syndrome [editorial]. *N Engl J Med* 315:578, 1986.
119. Katsumura Y, Ohtsubo K: Incidence of pulmonary thromboembolism, infarction and hemorrhage in disseminated intravascular coagulation. *Thorax* 50:160, 1995.
120. Kollef MH, Schuster DP: The acute respiratory distress syndrome. *N Engl J Med* 332:27, 1995.
121. Dhainaut JF, Shorr AF, Macias WL, et al: Dynamic evolution of coagulopathy in the first day of severe sepsis: Relationship with mortality and organ failure. *Crit Care Med* 33:341, 2005.
122. Spero JA, Lewis JH, Hasiba U: Disseminated intravascular coagulation. Findings in 346 patients. *Thromb Haemost* 43:28, 1980.
123. Bakhtiari K, Meijers JC, de Jonge E, et al: Prospective validation of the international society of thrombosis and haemostasis scoring system for disseminated intravascular coagulation. *Crit Care Med* 32:2416, 2004.
124. Dhainaut JF, Yan SB, Joyce DE, et al: Treatment effects of drotrecogin alfa (activated) in patients with severe sepsis with or without overt disseminated intravascular coagulation. *J Thromb Haemost* 2:1924, 2004.
125. Dempfle CE, Pfitzner SA, Dollman M, et al: Comparison of immunological and functional assays for measurement of soluble fibrin. *Thromb Haemost* 74:673, 1995.
126. Bredbacka S, Blomback M, Wiman B, et al: Laboratory methods for detecting disseminated intravascular coagulation (DIC): New aspects. *Acta Anaesthesiol Scand* 37:125, 1993.
127. Bredbacka S, Blomback M, Wiman B: Soluble fibrin: A predictor for the development and outcome of multiple organ failure. *Am J Hematol* 46:289, 1994.
128. McCarron BI, Marder VJ, Kanouse JJ, et al: A soluble fibrin standard: Comparable dose-response with immunologic and functional assays. *Thromb Haemost* 82:145, 1999.
129. Shorr AF, Thomas SJ, Alkins SA, et al: D-dimer correlates with proinflammatory cytokine levels and outcomes in critically ill patients. *Chest* 121:1262, 2002.
130. Dempfle CE: The use of soluble fibrin in evaluating the acute and chronic hypercoagulable state. *Thromb Haemost* 82:673, 1999.
131. Horan JT, Francis CW: Fibrin degradation products, fibrin monomer and soluble fibrin in disseminated intravascular coagulation. *Semin Thromb Hemost* 27:657, 2001.
132. McCarron BI, Marder VJ, Francis CW: Reactivity of soluble fibrin assays with plasmic degradation products of fibrin and in patients receiving fibrinolytic therapy. *Thromb Haemost* 82:1722, 1999.
133. Carr JM, McKinney M, McDonagh J: Diagnosis of disseminated intravascular coagulation. Role of D-dimer. *Am J Clin Pathol* 91:280, 1989.
134. Boisclair MD, Ireland H, Lane DA: Assessment of hypercoagulable states by measurement of activation fragments and peptides. *Blood Rev* 4:25, 1990.
135. Prisco D, Paniccia R, Bonechi F, et al: Evaluation of new methods for the selective measurement of fibrin and fibrinogen degradation products. *Thromb Res* 56:547, 1989.
136. Shorr AF, Trotta RF, Alkins SA, et al: D-dimer assay predicts mortality in critically ill patients without disseminated intravascular coagulation or venous thromboembolic disease. *Intensive Care Med* 25:207, 1999.
137. Greenberg CS, Devine DV, McCrae KM: Measurement of plasma fibrin D-dimer levels with the use of a monoclonal antibody coupled to latex beads. *Am J Clin Pathol* 87:94, 1987.
138. Taylor FBJ, Toh CH, Hoots WK, et al: Towards definition, clinical and laboratory criteria, and a scoring system for disseminated intravascular coagulation. *Thromb Haemost* 86:1327, 2001.
139. Kobayashi S, Gando S, Morimoto Y: Serial measurement of arterial lactate concentrations as a prognostic indicator in relation to the incidence of disseminated intra-

vascular coagulation in patients with systemic inflammatory response syndrome. *Surg Today* 31:853, 2001.
140. Wada H, Gabazza EC, Asakura H, et al: Comparison of diagnostic criteria for disseminated intravascular coagulation (DIC): Diagnostic criteria of the International Society of Thrombosis and Hemostasis and of the Japanese Ministry of Health and Welfare for overt DIC: *Am J Hematol* 74:17, 2003.
141. Kinasewitz GT, Zein JG, Lee GL, et al: Prognostic value of a simple evolving DIC score in patients with severe sepsis. *Crit Care Med* 33:2214, 2005.
142. Levi M, van der Poll T, de Jonge E, et al: Relative insufficiency of fibrinolysis in disseminated intravascular coagulation. *Sepsis* 3:103, 2000.
143. Liaw PC, Ferrell G, Esmon CT. A monoclonal antibody against activated protein C allows rapid detection of activated protein C in plasma and reveals a calcium ion dependent epitope involved in factor Va inactivation. *J Thromb Haemost* 1:662, 2003.
144. Moore JC, Hayward CP, Warkentin TE, et al: Decreased von Willebrand factor protease activity associated with thrombocytopenic disorders. *Blood* 98:1842, 2001.
145. Levi M, Lowenberg EC: Thrombocytopenia in critically ill patients. *Semin Thromb Hemost* 34:417, 2008.
146. Toh CH, Samis J, Downey C, et al: Biphasic transmittance waveform in the APTT coagulation assay is due to the formation of a Ca(++)-dependent complex of C-reactive protein with very-low-density lipoprotein and is a novel marker of impending disseminated intravascular coagulation. *Blood* 100:2522, 2002.
147. Toh CH: Transmittance waveform of routine coagulation tests is a sensitive and specific method for diagnosing non-overt disseminated intravascular coagulation. *Blood Rev* 16 Suppl 1:S11, 2002.
148. Toh CH, Hoots WK: The scoring system of the Scientific and Standardisation Committee on Disseminated Intravascular Coagulation of the International Society on Thrombosis and Haemostasis: A 5-year overview. *J Thromb Haemost* 5:604, 2007.
149. Bone RC: Modulators of coagulation. A critical appraisal of their role in sepsis. *Arch Intern Med* 152:1381, 1992.
150. Keller TT, Mairuhu AT, de Kruif MD, et al: Infections and endothelial cells. *Cardiovasc Res* 60:40, 2003.
151. Gando S, Nanzaki S, Sasaki S, et al: Activation of the extrinsic coagulation pathway in patients with severe sepsis and septic shock. *Crit Care Med* 26:2005, 1998.
152. Wiersinga WJ, Meijers JC, Levi M, et al: Activation of coagulation with concurrent impairment of anticoagulant mechanisms correlates with a poor outcome in severe melioidosis. *J Thromb Haemost* 6:32, 2008.
153. Bone RC: Gram-positive organisms and sepsis. *Arch Intern Med* 154:26, 1994.
154. Levi M, van der Poll T: Coagulation in sepsis: All bugs bite equally. *Crit Care* 8:99, 2004.
155. Herwald H, Cramer H, Morgelin M. M-protein, a classical bacterial virulence determinant forms complexes with fibrinogen that induce vascular leakage. *Cell* 116:367, 2004.
156. Fijnvandraat K, Derkx B, Peters M, et al: Coagulation activation and tissue necrosis in meningococcal septic shock: Severely reduced protein C levels predict a high mortality. *Thromb Haemost* 73:15, 1995.
157. Hazelzet JA, Risseeuw-Appel IM, Kornelisse RF, et al: Age-related differences in outcome and severity of DIC in children with septic shock and purpura. *Thromb Haemost* 76:932, 1996.
158. Levi M, Opal SM: Coagulation abnormalities in critically ill patients. *Crit Care* 10:222, 2006.
159. Levi M: Hemostasis and thrombosis in critically ill patients. *Semin Thromb Hemost* 34:415, 2008.
160. Ono T, Mimuro J, Madoiwa S, et al: Severe secondary deficiency of von Willebrand factor-cleaving protease (ADAMTS13) in patients with sepsis-induced disseminated intravascular coagulation: Its correlation with development of renal failure. *Blood* 107:528, 2006.
161. Bhakdi S, Muhly M, Mannhardt U: Staphylococcal alpha toxin promotes blood coagulation via attack on human platelets. *J Exp Med* 168:527, 1988.
162. Ratnoff OD, Nebehay WG: Multiple coagulative defects in a patient with the Waterhouse-Friderichsen syndrome. *Ann Intern Med* 56:627, 1962.
163. van Gorp E, Suharti C, ten Cate H, et al: Review: Infectious diseases and coagulation disorders. *J Infect Dis* 180:176, 1999.
164. Levi M, Keller TT, van Gorp E, et al: Infection and inflammation and the coagulation system. *Cardiovasc Res* 60:26, 2003.
165. Heller MV, Marta RF, Sturk A, et al: Early markers of blood coagulation and fibrinolysis activation in Argentine hemorrhagic fever. *Thromb Haemost* 73:368, 1995.
166. Clemens R, Pramoolsinsap C, Lorenz R, et al: Activation of the coagulation cascade in severe falciparum malaria through the intrinsic pathway. *Br J Haematol* 87:100, 1994.
167. Mohanty D, Ghosh K, Nandwani SK, et al: Fibrinolysis, inhibitors of blood coagulation, and monocyte derived coagulant activity in acute malaria. *Am J Hematol* 54:23, 1997.
168. Fera G, Semeraro N, De MV, et al: Disseminated intravascular coagulation associated with disseminated cryptococcosis in a patient with acquired immunodeficiency syndrome. *Infection* 21:171, 1993.
169. Cosgriff TM: Viruses and haemostasis. *Rev Infect Dis* 11:672, 1989.
170. Inbal A, Kenet G, Zivelin A, et al: Purpura fulminans induced by disseminated intravascular coagulation following infection in 2 unrelated children with double heterozygosity for factor V Leiden and protein S deficiency. *Thromb Haemost* 77:1086, 1997.
171. Hofstra JJ, Schouten M, Levi M: Thrombophilia and outcome in severe infection and sepsis. *Semin Thromb Hemost* 33:604, 2007.
172. Levin M, Eley BS, Louis J: Postinfectious purpura fulminans caused by an autoantibody directed against protein S. *J Pediatr* 127:355, 1995.
173. Bhamarapravati N: Hemostatic defects in dengue hemorrhagic fever. *Rev Infect Dis* 11 Suppl 4:S826, 1989.
174. Suvatte V: Dengue hemorrhagic fever: Hematological abnormalities and pathogenesis. *J Med Assoc Thai* 61 Suppl 3:53, 1978.
175. Linder M, Muller-Berghaus G, Lasch HG, et al: Virus infection and blood coagulation. *Thromb Diath Haemorrh* 23:1, 1970.
176. Carpenter CT, Kaiser AB: Purpura fulminans in pneumococcal sepsis: Case report and review. *Scand J Infect Dis* 29:479, 1997.
177. Gerson WT, Dickerman JD, Bovill EG, et al: Severe acquired protein C deficiency in purpura fulminans associated with disseminated intravascular coagulation: Treatment with protein C concentrate. *Pediatrics* 91:418, 1993.
178. Tishler M, Abramov AL, Seligsohn U, et al: Purpura fulminans in an adult. *Isr J Med Sci* 22:820, 1986.
179. Bramson HE, Katz J, Marble R, et al: Inherited protein C deficiency and a coumarin responsive chronic relapsing purpura fulminans in a newborn infant. *Lancet* 2:1156, 1983.
180. Seligsohn U, Berger A, Abend M: Homozygous protein C deficiency manifested by massive venous thrombosis in the newborn. *N Engl J Med* 310:559, 1984.
181. Goad KE, Gralnick HR: Coagulation disorders in cancer. *Hematol Oncol Clin North Am* 10:457, 1996.
182. Levi M: Cancer and DIC: *Haemostasis* 31 Suppl 1:47, 2001.
183. Sack GH Jr, Levin J, Bell WR: Trousseau's syndrome and other manifestations of chronic disseminated coagulopathy in patients with neoplasms: Clinical, pathophysiologic, and therapeutic features. *Medicine (Baltimore)* 56:1, 1977.
184. Sallah S, Wan JY, Nguyen NP, et al: Disseminated intravascular coagulation in solid tumors: Clinical and pathological study. *Thromb Haemost* 86:828, 2001.
185. Donati MB: Cancer and thrombosis: From Phlegmasia alba dolens to transgenic mice. *Thromb Haemost* 74:278, 1995.
186. Levi M: Cancer and thrombosis. *Clin Adv Hematol Oncol* 1:668, 2003.
187. Contrino J, Hair G, Kreutzer DL, et al: *In situ* detection of tissue factor in vascular endothelial cells: Correlation with the malignant phenotype of human breast disease. *Nature Medicine (Baltimore)* 2:209, 1996.
188. Rickles FR, Brenner B: Tissue factor and cancer. *Semin Thromb Hemost* 34:143, 2008.
189. Bromberg ME, Konigsberg WH, Madison JF, et al: Tissue factor promotes melanoma metastasis by a pathway independent of blood coagulation. *Proc Natl Acad Sci U S A* 92:8205, 1995.
190. Zhang Y, Deng Y, Luther T, et al: Tissue factor controls the balance of angiogenic and antiangiogenic properties of tumor cells in mice. *J Clin Invest* 94:1320, 1994.
191. Nadir Y, Vlodavsky I, Brenner B: Heparanase, tissue factor, and cancer. *Semin Thromb Hemost* 34:187, 2008.
192. Falanga A, Consonni R, Marchetti M, et al: Cancer procoagulant and tissue factor are differently modulated by all-trans-retinoic acid in acute promyelocytic leukemia cells. *Blood* 92:143, 1998.
193. Levi M: Disseminated intravascular coagulation in cancer patients. *Best Pract Res Clin Haematol* 22:129, 2009.
194. Wahrenbrock M, Borsig L, Le Duc M: Selectin-mucin interactions as a probable molecular explanation for the association of Trousseau syndrome with mucinous adenocarcinoma. *J Clin Invest* 112:853, 2003.
195. Dvorak HF, Quay SC, Orenstein NS: Tumor shedding and coagulation. *Science* 212:923, 1981.
196. Zwicker JI: Tissue factor-bearing microparticles and cancer. *Semin Thromb Hemost* 34:195, 2008.
197. Nijziel MR, van OR, Hillen HF, et al: From Trousseau to angiogenesis: The link between the haemostatic system and cancer. *Neth J Med* 64:403, 2006.
198. Rickles FR, Falanga A: Molecular basis for the relationship between thrombosis and cancer. *Thromb Res* 102:V215, 2001.
199. Stouthard JM, Levi M, Hack CE, et al: Interleukin-6 stimulates coagulation, not fibrinolysis, in humans. *Thromb Haemost* 76:738, 1996.
200. van der Poll T, Coyle SM, Levi M, et al: Effect of a recombinant dimeric tumor necrosis factor receptor on inflammatory responses to intravenous endotoxin in normal humans. *Blood* 89:3727, 1997.
201. van der Poll T, Levi M, ten Cate H, et al: The role of tumor necrosis factor in systemic inflammatory responses in primate endotoxemia. *Prog Clin Biol Res* 388:425, 1994.
202. van der Poll T, Levi M, van Deventer SJ, et al: Differential effects of anti-tumor necrosis factor monoclonal antibodies on systemic inflammatory responses in experimental endotoxemia in chimpanzees. *Blood* 83:446, 1994.
203. Sewnath ME, Olszyna DP, Birjmohun R, et al: IL-10-deficient mice demonstrate multiple organ failure and increased mortality during *Escherichia coli* peritonitis despite an accelerated bacterial clearance. *J Immunol* 166:6323, 2001.
204. van der Poll T, Jansen J, Levi M, et al: Interleukin 10 release during endotoxaemia in chimpanzees: Role of platelet-activating factor and interleukin 6. *Scand J Immunol* 43:122, 1996.
205. van der Poll T, Jansen PM, Montegut WJ, et al: Effects of IL-10 on systemic inflammatory responses during sublethal primate endotoxemia. *J Immunol* 158:1971, 1997.
206. Seligsohn U, Weber H, Yoran C: Microangiopathic hemolytic anemia and defibrination syndrome in metastatic carcinoma of the stomach. *Isr J Med Sci* 4:69, 1968.
207. Uchiumi H, Matsushima T, Yamane A, et al: Prevalence and clinical characteristics of acute myeloid leukemia associated with disseminated intravascular coagulation. *Int J Hematol* 86:137, 2007.
208. Barbui T, Falanga A: Disseminated intravascular coagulation in acute leukemia. *Semin Thromb Hemost* 27:593, 2001.

209. Sarris AH, Kempin S, Berman E, et al: High incidence of disseminated intravascular coagulation during remission induction of adult patients with acute lymphoblastic leukemia. *Blood* 79:1305, 1992.
210. Avvisati G, ten Cate JW, Sturk A, et al: Acquired alpha-2-antiplasmin deficiency in acute promyelocytic leukaemia. *Br J Haematol* 70:43, 1988.
211. Falanga A: Mechanisms of hypercoagulation in malignancy and during chemotherapy. *Haemostasis* 28 Suppl 3:50, 1998.
212. Stein E, McMahon B, Kwaan H, et al: The coagulopathy of acute promyelocytic leukaemia revisited. *Best Pract Res Clin Haematol* 22:153, 2009.
213. Barbui T, Finazzi G, Falanga A: The impact of all-*trans*-retinoic acid on the coagulopathy of acute promyelocytic leukemia. *Blood* 91:3093, 1998.
214. Gando S, Nakanishi Y, Tedo I: Cytokines and plasminogen activator inhibitor-1 in posttrauma disseminated intravascular coagulation: Relationship to multiple organ dysfunction syndrome. *Crit Care Med* 23:1835, 1995.
215. Gando S: Disseminated intravascular coagulation in trauma patients. *Semin Thromb Hemost* 27:585, 2001.
216. Gando S: Tissue factor in trauma and organ dysfunction. *Semin Thromb Hemost* 32:48, 2006.
217. Owings JT, Gosselin RC, Anderson JT, et al: Practical utility of the D-dimer assay for excluding thromboembolism in severely injured trauma patients. *J Trauma* 51:425, 2001.
218. Attar S, Boyd D, Layne E, et al: Alterations in coagulation and fibrinolytic mechanisms in acute trauma. *J Trauma* 9:939, 1969.
219. Cosgriff N, Moore EE, Sauaia A, et al: Predicting life-threatening coagulopathy in the massively transfused trauma patient: Hypothermia and acidoses revisited. *J Trauma* 42:857, 1997.
220. Hess JR, Holcomb JB: Transfusion practice in military trauma. *Transfus Med* 18:143, 2008.
221. Armand R, Hess JR: Treating coagulopathy in trauma patients. *Transfus Med Rev* 17:223, 2003.
222. Simmons RL, Collins JA, Heisterkamp CA, et al: Coagulation disorders in combat casualties. I: Acute changes after wounding. II: Effects of massive transfusion. 3. Post-resuscitative changes. *Ann Surg* 169:455, 1969.
223. Gomez R, Murray CK, Hospenthal DR, et al: Causes of mortality by autopsy findings of combat casualties and civilian patients admitted to a burn unit. *J Am Coll Surg* 208:348, 2009.
224. Niles SE, McLaughlin DF, Perkins JG, et al: Increased mortality associated with the early coagulopathy of trauma in combat casualties. *J Trauma* 64:1459, 2008.
225. Kaufman HH, Hui KS, Mattson JC, et al: Clinicopathological correlations of disseminated intravascular coagulation in patients with head injury. *Neurosurgery* 15:34, 1984.
226. Stein SC, Chen XH, Sinson GP, et al: Intravascular coagulation: A major secondary insult in nonfatal traumatic brain injury. *J Neurosurg* 97:1373, 2002.
227. Olson JD, Kaufman HH, Moake J, et al: The incidence and significance of hemostatic abnormalities in patients with head injuries. *Neurosurgery* 24:825, 1989.
228. Selladurai BM, Vickneswaran M, Duraisamy S, et al: Coagulopathy in acute head injury—A study of its role as a prognostic indicator. *Br J Neurosurg* 11:398, 1997.
229. Levi M: Burning issues surrounding inflammation and coagulation in heatstroke. *Crit Care Med* 36:2455, 2008.
230. Garcia-Avello A, Lorente JA, Cesar-Perez J, et al: Degree of hypercoagulability and hyperfibrinolysis is related to organ failure and prognosis after burn trauma. *Thromb Res* 89:59, 1998.
231. Simon TL, Curreri PW, Harker LA: Kinetic characterization of hemostasis in thermal injury. *J Lab Clin Med* 89:702, 1977.
232. Winkelman MD, Galloway PG: Central nervous system complications of thermal burns. A postmortem study of 139 patients. *Medicine (Baltimore)* 71:271, 1992.
233. Carr ME Jr: Disseminated intravascular coagulation: Pathogenesis, diagnosis, and therapy. *J Emerg Med* 5:311, 1987.
234. Tytgat GN, Collen D, Verstraete M: Metabolism of fibrinogen in cirrhosis of the liver. *J Clin Invest* 50:169, 1971.
235. Coleman M, Finlayson N, Bettigole RE, et al: Fibrinogen survival in cirrhosis: Improvement by "low dose" heparin. *Ann Intern Med* 83:79, 1975.
236. Coccheri S, Mannucci PM, Palareti G, et al: Significance of plasma fibrinopeptide A and high molecular weight fibrinogen in patients with liver cirrhosis. *Br J Haematol* 52:503, 1982.
237. Oka K, Tanaka K: Intravascular coagulation in autopsy cases with liver diseases. *Thromb Haemost* 42:564, 1979.
238. Paramo JA, Rifon J, Fernandez J, et al: Thrombin activation and increased fibrinolysis in patients with chronic liver disease. *Blood Coagul Fibrinolysis* 2:227, 1991.
239. Palascak JE, Martinez J: Dysfibrinogenemia associated with liver disease. *J Clin Invest* 60:89, 1977.
240. Ben-Ari Z, Osman E, Hutton RA, et al: Disseminated intravascular coagulation in liver cirrhosis: Fact or fiction? [See comments.] *Am J Gastroenterol* 94:2977, 1999.
241. Hollestelle MJ, Geertzen HG, Straatsburg IH, et al: Factor VIII expression in liver disease. *Thromb Haemost* 91:267, 2004.
242. Straub PW: Diffuse intravascular coagulation in liver disease? *Semin Thromb Hemost* 4:29, 1977.
243. Canoso RT, Hutton RA, Deykin D: The hemostatic defect of chronic liver disease. Kinetic studies using ^{75}Se-selenomethionine. *Gastroenterology* 76:540, 1979.
244. Tempero MA, Davis RB, Reed E, et al: Thrombocytopenia and laboratory evidence of disseminated intravascular coagulation after shunts for ascites in malignant disease. *Cancer* 55:2718, 1985.
245. Bakker CM, Knot EA, Stibbe J, et al: Disseminated intravascular coagulation in liver cirrhosis. *J Hepatol* 15:330, 1992.
246. Wakefield EG, Hall WW: Heat injuries: A preparatory study for experimental heatstroke. *JAMA* 89:92, 1927.
247. Chao TC, Sinniah R, Pakiam JE: Acute heat stroke deaths. *Pathology* 13:145, 1981.
248. Bouchama A, Knochel JP: Heat stroke. *N Engl J Med* 346:1978, 2002.
249. Bouchama A, Hammami MM, Haq A, et al: Evidence for endothelial cell activation/injury in heatstroke. *Crit Care Med* 24:1173, 1996.
250. Gauss P, Meyer KA: Heat stroke: Report of one hundred and fifty-eight cases from Cook County Hospital, Chicago. *Am J Med Sci* 154:554, 1917.
251. Huisse MG, Pease S, Hurtado-Nedelec M, et al: Leucocyte activation: The link between inflammation and coagulation during heatstroke. A study of patients during the 2003 heat wave in Paris. *Crit Care Med* 36:2288, 2008.
252. Mustafa KY, Omer O, Khogali M, et al: Blood coagulation and fibrinolysis in heat stroke. *Br J Haematol* 61:517, 1985.
253. Seegers WH, Ouyang C: Snake venoms and blood coagulation, in *Snake Venoms*, edited by L Chen-Yuan L, p 684. Springer Verlag, Berlin, 1979.
254. Huang TF, Holt JC, Lukasiewicz H, et al: Trigramin. A low molecular weight peptide inhibiting fibrinogen interaction with platelet receptors expressed on glycoprotein IIb-IIIa complex. *J Biol Chem* 262:16157, 1987.
255. Klein JD, Walker FJ: Purification of a protein C activator from the venom of the southern copperhead snake (*Agkistrodon contortrix contortrix*). *Biochemistry* 25:4175, 1986.
256. Weiss HJ, Phillips LL, Hopewell WS, et al: Heparin therapy in a patient bitten by a saw-scaled viper (*Echis carinatus*), a snake whose venom activates prothrombin. *Am J Med* 54:653, 1973.
257. Schulchynska-Castel H, Dvilansky A, Keynan A: *Echis colorata* bites: Clinical evaluation of 42 patients. A retrospective study. *Isr J Med Sci* 22:880, 1986.
258. Fainaru M, Eisenberg S, Manny N, et al: The natural course of defibrination syndrome caused by *Echis colorata* venom in man. *Thromb Diath Haemorrh* 31:420, 1974.
259. Hall GW: Kasabach-Merritt syndrome: Pathogenesis and management. *Br J Haematol* 112:851, 2001.
260. Straub PW, Kessler S, Schreiber A, et al: Chronic intravascular coagulation in Kasabach-Merritt syndrome. Preferential accumulation of fibrinogen ^{131}I in a giant hemangioma. *Arch Intern Med* 129:475, 1972.
261. Warrell RPJ, Kempin SJ, Benua RS, et al: Intratumoral consumption of indium-111 labeled platelets in a patient with hemangiomatosis and intravascular coagulation (Kasabach-Merritt syndrome). *Cancer* 52:2256, 1983.
262. Propp RP, Scharfman WB: Hemangioma-thrombocytopenia syndrome associated with microangiopathic hemolytic anemia. *Blood* 28:623, 1966.
263. Hesselmann S, Micke O, Marquardt T, et al: Case report: Kasabach-Merritt syndrome: A review of the therapeutic options and case report of successful treatment with radiotherapy and interferon alpha. *Br J Radiol* 75:180, 2002.
264. Mazoyer E, Enjolras O, Laurian C, et al: Coagulation abnormalities associated with extensive venous malformations of the limbs: Differentiation from Kasabach-Merritt syndrome. *Clin Lab Haematol* 24:243, 2002.
265. Fisher DF Jr, Yawn DH, Crawford ES: Preoperative disseminated intravascular coagulation associated with aortic aneurysms. A prospective study of 76 cases. *Arch Surg* 118:1252, 1983.
266. Bieger R, Vreeken J, Stibbe J, et al: Arterial aneurysm as a cause of consumption coagulopathy. *N Engl J Med* 285:152, 1971.
267. ten Cate JW, Timmers H, Becker AE: Coagulopathy in ruptured or dissecting aortic aneurysms. *Am J Med* 59:171, 1975.
268. Mulcare RJ, Royster TS, Phillips LL: Intravascular coagulation in surgical procedures on the abdominal aorta. *Surg Gynecol Obstet* 143:730, 1976.
269. Wilcox JN, Smith KM, Schwartz SM, et al: Localization of tissue factor in the normal vessel wall and in the atherosclerotic plaque. *Proc Natl Acad Sci U S A* 86:2839, 1989.
270. Cummins D, Segal H, Hunt BJ, et al: Chronic disseminated intravascular coagulation after surgery for abdominal aortic aneurysm: Clinical and haemostatic response to dalteparin. *Br J Haematol* 113:658, 2001.
271. Cross KS, Bouchier-Hayes D, Leahy AL: Consumptive coagulopathy following endovascular stent repair of abdominal aortic aneurysm. *Eur J Vasc Endovasc Surg* 19:94, 2000.
272. Shimazaki T, Ishimaru S, Kawaguchi S, et al: Blood coagulation and fibrinolytic response after endovascular stent grafting of thoracic aorta. *J Vasc Surg* 37:1213, 2003.
273. Mannucci PM, Lobina GF, Caocci L, et al: Effect on blood coagulation of massive intravascular haemolysis. *Blood* 33:207, 1969.
274. Butler J, Parker D, Pillai R, et al: Systemic release of neutrophil elastase and tumour necrosis factor alpha following ABO incompatible blood transfusion. *Br J Haematol* 79:525, 1991.
275. Hamilton KK, Hattori R, Esmon CT, et al: Complement proteins C5b-9 induce vesiculation of the endothelial plasma membrane and expose catalytic surface for assembly of the prothrombinase enzyme complex. *J Biol Chem* 265:3809, 1990.
276. Weiner CP: The obstetric patient and disseminated intravascular coagulation. *Clin Perinatol* 13:705, 1986.
277. Bonnar J: Massive obstetric haemorrhage. *Best Pract Res Clin Obstet Gynaecol* 14:1, 2000.
278. Letsky EA: Disseminated intravascular coagulation. *Best Pract Res Clin Obstet Gynaecol* 15:623, 2001.
279. DeLee JB: Acase of fatal hemorrhagic diathesis with premature detachment of the placenta. *Am J Obstet Gynecol* 44:785, 1901.
280. Eskes TK: Abruptio placentae. A "classic" dedicated to Elizabeth Ramsey. *Eur J Obstet Gynecol Reprod Biol* 75:63, 1997.

281. Kuczynski J, Uszynski W, Zekanowska E, et al: Tissue factor (TF) and tissue factor pathway inhibitor (TFPI) in the placenta and myometrium. *Eur J Obstet Gynecol Reprod Biol* 105:15, 2002.
282. Pritchard JA, Brekken AL: Clinical and laboratory studies on severe abruptio placentae. *Am J Obstet Gynecol* 97:681, 1967.
283. Steiner PE, Lushbaugh CC: Maternal pulmonary embolism by amniotic fluid as a cause of obstetric shock and unexpected deaths in obstetrics. *JAMA* 117:1245, 1941.
284. Morgan M: Amniotic fluid embolism. *Anaesthesia* 34:20, 1979.
285. Gilbert WM, Danielsen B: Amniotic fluid embolism: Decreased mortality in a population-based study. *Obstet Gynecol* 93:973, 1999.
286. Uszynski M, Zekanowska E, Uszynski W, et al: Tissue factor (TF) and tissue factor pathway inhibitor (TFPI) in amniotic fluid and blood plasma: Implications for the mechanism of amniotic fluid embolism. *Eur J Obstet Gynecol Reprod Biol* 95:163, 2001.
287. Boer K, den Hartog I, Meijers JC, et al: Tissue factor-dependent blood coagulation is enhanced following delivery irrespective of the mode of delivery. *J Thromb Haemost* 5:2415, 2007.
288. Gibson B, Hunter D, Neame PB, et al: Thrombocytopenia in preeclampsia and eclampsia. *Semin Thromb Hemost* 8:234, 1982.
289. O'Riordan MN, Higgins JR: Haemostasis in normal and abnormal pregnancy. *Best Pract Res Clin Obstet Gynaecol* 17:385, 2003.
290. Levi M: Disseminated intravascular coagulation (DIC) in pregnancy and the peripartum period. *Thromb Res* 123 Suppl 2:S63, 2009.
291. Giles C: Intravascular coagulation in gestational hypertension and pre-eclampsia: The value of haematological screening tests. *Clin Lab Haematol* 4:351, 1982.
292. Norwitz ER, Hsu CD, Repke JT: Acute complications of preeclampsia. *Clin Obstet Gynecol* 45:308, 2002.
293. Weinstein L: Syndrome of hemolysis, elevated liver enzymes, and low platelet count: A severe consequence of hypertension in pregnancy. *Am J Obstet Gynecol* 142:159, 1982.
294. Sibai BM, Ramadan MK, Usta I, et al: Maternal morbidity and mortality in 442 pregnancies with hemolysis, elevated liver enzymes, and low platelets (HELLP syndrome). *Am J Obstet Gynecol* 169:1000, 1993.
295. Aarnoudse JG, Houthoff HJ, Weits J, et al: A syndrome of liver damage and intravascular coagulation in the last trimester of normotensive pregnancy. A clinical and histopathological study. *Br J Obstet Gynaecol* 93:145, 1986.
296. Audibert F, Friedman SA, Frangieh AY, et al: Clinical utility of strict diagnostic criteria for the HELLP (hemolysis, elevated liver enzymes, and low platelets) syndrome. *Am J Obstet Gynecol* 175:460, 1996.
297. Barton JR, Sibai BM: Hepatic imaging in HELLP syndrome (hemolysis, elevated liver enzymes and low platelet count. *Am J Obstet Gynecol* 174:1820, 1996.
298. Sullivan CA, Magann EF, Perry KG Jr, et al: The recurrence risk of the syndrome of hemolysis, elevated liver enzymes, and low platelets (HELLP) in subsequent gestations. *Am J Obstet Gynecol* 171:940, 1994.
299. Lee W, Clark SL, Cotton DB, et al: Septic shock during pregnancy. *Am J Obstet Gynecol* 159:410, 1988.
300. Romero R, Copel JA, Hobbins JC: Intrauterine fetal demise and hemostatic failure: The fetal death syndrome. *Clin Obstet Gynecol* 28:24, 1985.
301. Berkowitz RL, Stone JL, Eddleman KA: One hundred consecutive cases of selective termination of an abnormal fetus in a multifetal gestation. *Obstet Gynecol* 90:606, 1997.
302. Hay JE: Liver disease in pregnancy. *Hepatology* 47:1067, 2008.
303. Bacq Y, Riely CA: Acute fatty liver of pregnancy: The hepatologist's view. *Gastroenterologist* 1:257, 1993.
304. Usta IM, Barton JR, Amon EA, et al: Acute fatty liver of pregnancy: An experience in the diagnosis and management of fourteen cases. *Am J Obstet Gynecol* 171:1342, 1994.
305. Pereira SP, O'Donohue J, Wendon J, et al: Maternal and perinatal outcome in severe pregnancy-related liver disease. *Hepatology* 26:1258, 1997.
306. Rahman TM, Wendon J: Severe hepatic dysfunction in pregnancy. *Q J Med* 95:343, 2002.
307. Ibdah JA, Yang Z, Bennett MJ: Liver disease in pregnancy and fetal fatty acid oxidation defects. *Mol Genet Metab* 71:182, 2000.
308. Castro MA, Goodwin TM, Shaw KJ, et al: Disseminated intravascular coagulation and antithrombin III depression in acute fatty liver of pregnancy. *Am J Obstet Gynecol* 174:211, 1996.
309. Watson WJ, Seeds JW: Acute fatty liver of pregnancy. *Obstet Gynecol Surv* 45:585, 1990.
310. Moldenhauer JS, O'brien JM, Barton JR, et al: Acute fatty liver of pregnancy associated with pancreatitis: A life-threatening complication. *Am J Obstet Gynecol* 190:502, 2004.
311. Hathaway WE, Mull MM, Pechet GS: Disseminated intravascular coagulation in the newborn. *Pediatrics* 43:233, 1969.
312. Corrigan JJ Jr: Activation of coagulation and disseminated intravascular coagulation in the newborn. *Am J Pediatr Hematol Oncol* 1:245, 1979.
313. Williams MD, Chalmers EA, Gibson BE: The investigation and management of neonatal haemostasis and thrombosis. *Br J Haematol* 119:295, 2002.
314. Buchanan GR: Coagulation disorders in the neonate. *Pediatr Clin North Am* 33:203, 1986.
315. Stanworth SJ, Bennett C: How to tackle bleeding and thrombosis in the newborn. *Early Hum Dev* 84:507, 2008.
316. Corrigan JJ, Ray WL, May N: Changes in the blood coagulation system associated with septicemia. *N Engl J Med* 279:851, 1968.
317. Levi M, de Jonge E, van der Poll T: New treatment strategies for disseminated intravascular coagulation based on current understanding of the pathophysiology. *Ann Med* 36:41, 2004.
318. Alving BM, Spivak JL, DeLoughery TG: Consultative hematology: Hemostasis and transfusion issues in surgery and critical care medicine, in *The American Society of Hematology Education Program Book*, edited by JR McArthur, GP Schechter, SL Schrier, p 320. *American Society of Hematology,* 1998.
319. de Jonge E, Levi M, Stoutenbeek CP, et al: Current drug treatment strategies for disseminated intravascular coagulation. *Drugs* 55:767, 1998.
320. de Jonge E, van der Poll T, Kesecioglu J, et al: Anticoagulant factor concentrates in disseminated intravascular coagulation: Rationale for use and clinical experience. *Semin Thromb Hemost* 27:667, 2001.
321. Abraham E: Coagulation abnormalities in acute lung injury and sepsis. *Am J Respir Cell Mol Biol* 22:401, 2000.
322. Levi M, Schouten M, van der Poll T: Sepsis, coagulation, and antithrombin: Old lessons and new insights. *Semin Thromb Hemost* 34:742, 2008.
323. Fourrier F, Chopin C, Huart JJ, et al: Double-blind, placebo-controlled trial of antithrombin III concentrates in septic shock with disseminated intravascular coagulation. *Chest* 104:882, 1993.
324. Eisele B, Lamy M, Thijs LG, et al: Antithrombin III in patients with severe sepsis. A randomized, placebo-controlled, double-blind multicenter trial plus a meta-analysis on all randomized, placebo-controlled, double-blind trials with antithrombin III in severe sepsis. *Intensive Care Med* 24:663, 1998.
325. Baudo F, Caimi TM, de CF, et al: Antithrombin III (ATIII) replacement therapy in patients with sepsis and/or postsurgical complications: A controlled double-blind, randomized, multicenter study. *Intensive Care Med* 24:336, 1998.
326. Warren BL, Eid A, Singer P, et al: Caring for the critically ill patient. High-dose antithrombin III in severe sepsis: A randomized controlled trial. *JAMA* 286:1869, 2001.
327. Lavrentieva A, Kontakiotis T, Bitzani M, et al: The efficacy of antithrombin administration in the acute phase of burn injury. *Thromb Haemost* 100:286, 2008.
328. Levi M: Activated protein C in sepsis: A critical review. *Curr Opin Hematol* 15:481, 2008.
329. Bernard GR, Ely EW, Wright TJ, et al: Safety and dose relationship of recombinant human activated protein C for coagulopathy in severe sepsis. *Crit Care Med* 29:2051, 2001.
330. Bernard GR, Vincent JL, Laterre PF, et al: Efficacy and safety of recombinant human activated protein C for severe sepsis. *N Engl J Med* 344:699, 2001.
331. Vincent JL, Angus DC, Artigas A, et al: Effects of drotrecogin alfa (activated) on organ dysfunction in the PROWESS trial. *Crit Care Med* 31:834, 2003.
332. Ely EW, Laterre PF, Angus DC, et al: Drotrecogin alfa (activated) administration across clinically important subgroups of patients with severe sepsis. *Crit Care Med* 31:12, 2003.
333. Abraham E, Laterre PF, Garg R, et al: Drotrecogin alfa (activated) for adults with severe sepsis and a low risk of death. *N Engl J Med* 353:1332, 2005.
334. Laterre PF: Clinical trials in severe sepsis with drotrecogin alfa (activated). *Crit Care* 11 Suppl 5:S5, 2007.
335. Levy M, Levi M, Williams MD, et al: Comprehensive safety analysis of concomitant drotrecogin alfa (activated) and prophylactic heparin use in patients with severe sepsis. *Intensive Care Med* 35:1196, 2009.
336. du Toit H, Coetzee AR, Chalton DO: Heparin treatment in thrombin-induced disseminated intravascular coagulation in the baboon. *Crit Care Med* 19:1195, 1991.
337. Pernerstorfer T, Hollenstein U, Hansen JB, et al: Lepirudin blunts endotoxin-induced coagulation activation. *Blood* 95:1729, 2000.
338. Feinstein DI: Diagnosis and management of disseminated intravascular coagulation: The role of heparin therapy. *Blood* 60:284, 1982.
339. Levi M, Levy M, Williams MD, et al: Prophylactic heparin in patients with severe sepsis treated with drotrecogin alfa (activated). *Am J Respir Crit Care Med* 176:483, 2007.
340. Vlasuk GP, Bergum PW, Bradbury AE, et al: Clinical evaluation of rNAPc2, an inhibitor of the fVIIa/tissue factor coagulation complex. *Am J Cardiol* 80:66S, 1997.
341. Abraham E, Reinhart K, Svoboda P, et al: Assessment of the safety of recombinant tissue factor pathway inhibitor in patients with severe sepsis: A multicenter, randomized, placebo-controlled, single-blind, dose escalation study. *Crit Care Med* 29:2081, 2001.
342. Abraham E, Reinhart K, Opal S, et al: Efficacy and safety of tifacogin (recombinant tissue factor pathway inhibitor) in severe sepsis: A randomized controlled trial. *JAMA* 290:238, 2003.
343. Saito H, Maruyama I, Shimazaki S, et al: Efficacy and safety of recombinant human soluble thrombomodulin (ART-123) in disseminated intravascular coagulation: Results of a phase III, randomized, double-blind clinical trial. *J Thromb Haemost* 5:31, 2007.
344. Gralnick HR, Greipp P: Thrombosis with epsilon aminocaproic acid therapy. *Am J Clin Pathol* 56:151, 1971.
345. Naeye RL: Thrombotic state after a hemorrhagic diathesis, a possible complication of therapy with epsilon-aminocaproic acid. *Blood* 19:694, 1962.
346. Mannucci PM, Levi M: Prevention and treatment of major blood loss. *N Engl J Med* 356:2301, 2007.
347. Minna JD, Robboy SJ, Colman RW: *Disseminated Intravascular Coagulation in Man.* Charles C Thomas, Springfield, IL, 1974.
348. Matsuda M, Aoki N: Statistics on underlying and causative diseases of DIC in Japan, in *Disseminated Intravascular Coagulation*, edited by T Abe, M Yamanake, p 15. Karger, Basel, 1983.
349. Larcan A, Lambert H, Gerard A: *Consumption Coagulopathies.* Masson, New York, 1987.

CHAPTER 131
HEREDITARY THROMBOPHILIA

Uri Seligsohn and Aaron Lubetsky

SUMMARY

Venous thromboembolism is a multicausal disease involving one or more genetic defects in conjunction with acquired risk factors such as trauma, immobility, malignancy, inflammation, pregnancy, oral contraceptive use, and autoimmune disease. *Thrombophilia* is defined as a genetically determined increased likelihood of thrombosis. The two most common hereditary defects in whites (found in a substantial proportion of patients presenting with venous thrombosis) include activated protein C resistance caused by replacement of Arg506 by Gln in the factor V gene (factor V Leiden) and a prothrombin single-nucleotide polymorphism (G20210A) that causes elevated plasma prothrombin levels. Also common are hyperhomocysteinemia and increased plasma levels of factor VIII that can result from identified and unidentified genetic defects or from acquired conditions. Less common genetic abnormalities include deficiencies of the anticoagulant proteins, protein C, protein S, and antithrombin. The majority of these thrombophilic defects either enhance procoagulant reactions or hamper anticoagulant mechanisms, thus causing a prothrombotic state resulting from hypercoagulability of the blood. Venous thrombosis or thromboembolism are the most common manifestations of thrombophilia, although a minority of patients, particularly those with other vascular risk factors, also develop arterial thrombosis. Less usual presentations include visceral or cerebral vein thrombosis, second- or third-trimester pregnancy loss, and severe preeclampsia. Laboratory assays are widely available to identify most thrombophilias. Knowledge of these disorders can affect patient management, including the duration of anticoagulant treatment, the use of prophylactic antithrombotic agents, and counseling patients regarding the relative risks of pregnancy and use of oral contraceptives or hormone replacement.

DEFINITION AND HISTORY

Hereditary thrombophilia hereinafter termed *thrombophilia* is defined as a genetically determined increased risk of venous thrombosis or thromboembolism (VTE). Table 131–1 lists the major genetic defects associated with VTE and the acquired predisposing risk factors. Increasing age and interaction among inherited thrombophilias coupled with the effects of acquired predisposing factors are the common causes of VTE (Fig. 131–1).

The first description of thrombophilia caused by a hereditary deficiency of an anticoagulant protein was by Egeberg[1] in 1965. Members of the family described in the report suffered from recurrent venous thrombosis, and the disorder was inherited in an autosomal dominant manner. The plasma of affected family members had reduced levels of antithrombin III, an inhibitor to thrombin, which at present is termed *antithrombin*. Another thrombophilia, hereditary dysfibrinogenemia, was described by Beck and coworkers[2] in the same year. In 1976, Stenflo and coworkers[3] purified and characterized an anticoagulant factor from bovine plasma that was designated protein C because it was present in the third peak on a chromatogram. Subsequently, the first patients with heterozygous protein C deficiency (~50% of normal plasma level) and venous thrombosis in young adults were described by Griffin and colleagues.[4] Three years later, protein S deficiency was reported in several families with thrombosis by Schwarz and coworkers[5] and Comp and coworkers.[6,7] Initial searches for deficiencies of antithrombin, protein C, and protein S in patients with idiopathic venous thrombosis were disappointing because only 5 to 20 percent of such patients had one of these inherited disorders.[8] This situation changed dramatically in 1993 when Dahlback and coworkers reported that venous thrombosis often is associated with hereditary resistance to activated protein C (APC).[9,10] In 1994, three laboratories reported that the underlying genetic defect for most patients with APC resistance (APCR) involved the factor V mutation of Arg506 to Gln, a defect now referred to as factor V Leiden.[11–13] At about the same time, mild to moderate hyperhomocysteinemia was recognized as a risk factor for venous thrombosis,[14] although a predisposition to arterial vascular disease because of elevated homocysteine levels had been known since 1969.[15] In 1996, a single nucleotide polymorphism in the 3′-untranslated region of the prothrombin gene (G20210A) was identified and linked to familial venous thromboembolism by Poort and colleagues.[16] Subsequently, elevated levels of factor VIII were defined as another risk factor for venous thrombosis that is clustered in families, but to date no causal genetic factor has been discerned.[17–19]

Specific thrombophilic risk factors can be identified in approximately 70 percent of patients presenting with an unprovoked first or recurrent episode of venous thromboembolism.[20,21] Patients with VTE may have more than one hereditary thrombophilia[22] associated with acquired abnormalities, such as antiphospholipid antibodies, malignancy, myeloproliferative diseases (see Table 131–1). Thrombophilias confer a modestly increased risk of arterial thrombosis particularly in patients younger than age 55 years and in patients with other cardiovascular risk factor.[23–27]

Acronyms and abbreviations that appear in this chapter include: APC, activated protein C; APCR, activated protein C resistance; aPTT, activated partial thromboplastin time; EPCR, endothelial protein C receptor; IUGR, intrauterine growth restriction; MTHFR, methylenetetrahydrofolate reductase; OR, odds ratio; PAI, plasminogen-activator inhibitor; PCI, protein C inhibitor; PCR, polymerase chain reaction; QTL, quantitative trait loci; sFlt1, soluble fms-like tyrosine kinase 1; TAFI, thrombin-activatable fibrinolysis inhibitor; TFPI, tissue factor pathway inhibitor; VEGF, vascular endothelial growth factor; VTE, venous thrombosis or thromboembolism.

PATHOGENESIS

Thrombosis often is associated with defects in normal, physiologic hemostatic mechanisms that are essential to avoid bleeding. Pathogenesis of thrombosis, according to Virchow's classic triad, involves abnormalities in the vessel wall, blood flow (i.e., stasis), and/or changes in the blood components. Risk of VTE is amplified by both the number and the nature of risk factors present in a given subject, whether genetic or acquired (see Fig. 131–1). Identification of defects in specific blood components, especially plasma factors, thus far has provided most of the molecular insights into the pathogenesis of thrombophilia.

Figure 131–2 presents the major mechanisms of the normal control of coagulation and inherited thrombophilias (see also Chap. 116). Control of coagulation is achieved by the protein C pathway and antithrombin. In the protein C pathway, thrombin bound to thrombomodulin activates protein C, which, in turn, inactivates activated factors V and VIII in the presence of protein S and nonactivated factor V, thereby downregulating the generation of thrombin. The neutralization of thrombin is achieved by antithrombin bound to heparan sulfate located on endothelial cells. In

TABLE 131–1. Thrombophilias and Predisposing Risk Factors for Venous Thromboembolism

Thrombophilias	Acquired Predisposing Risk Factors for Venous Thrombosis
Common	
Factor V Leiden	Increasing age
Prothrombin G20210A	Surgery or trauma
Increased factor VIII level*	Prolonged immobilization
Homozygous C677T polymorphism in methylenetetrahydrofolate reductase†	Obesity
	Smoking
	Arteriosclerotic cardiovascular disease
Rare	Malignant neoplasms
Protein C deficiency	Long flights
Protein S deficiency	Myeloproliferative diseases
Antithrombin deficiency	Superficial vein thrombosis
Very rare	Previous venous thrombosis
Dysfibrinogenemia	Pregnancy and puerperium
Homozygous homocystinuria	Use of female hormones
	Antiphospholipid antibodies
	Hyperhomocysteinemia
	Activated protein C resistance unrelated to factor V Leiden
	Varicose veins

*Heritability is inferred. No gene alteration has been discerned.

†A questionable thrombophilia that can be associated with hyperhomocysteinemia in patients with deficiencies of folic acid or vitamin B_{12}.

the inherited thrombophilias, a deficiency of antithrombin, protein C, or protein S, aberrant activity of factor V, or increased activity of prothrombin results in decreased neutralization of thrombin or increased generation of thrombin. Indeed, asymptomatic carriers of thrombophilias harbor markers of thrombin generation such as increased levels of thrombin–antithrombin complexes, or prothrombin fragments 1 and 2.[28,29] The two most commonly identifiable genetic defects contributing to thrombophilia involve plasma factors, namely, APC-resistant factor V Leiden and elevated prothrombin levels caused by the prothrombin G20210A polymorphism.

Elevated factor VIII levels are associated with increased risk of VTE and of its recurrence. Although the genetic causes are unknown for elevated levels of other clotting factors (XI and IX), such elevations mildly amplify the risk. Such markers of hypercoagulability are each estimated to be 30 to 60 percent heritable,[30–33] where the term *heritability* indicates the relative contributions of heredity versus contributions of environment. Overall, these coagulation factor abnormalities cause an imbalance between the procoagulant and anticoagulant forces in blood with potential mechanistic contributions to thrombosis. Other plasma protein defects contribute to decreased fibrinolytic potential that is caused by either defective molecules, for example, dysfibrinogenemia, dysplasminogenemia or abnormal levels of normal molecules (e.g., thrombin-activatable fibrinolysis inhibitor [TAFI]; see Chaps. 126 and 136).

Males are at greater risk of recurrent VTE for reasons that presently are unclear.[34] Male gender is well known as a risk factor for arterial atherothrombosis, and, intriguingly, atherosclerosis is associated with VTE.[35]

Tissue factor-bearing microparticles in blood play essential roles in experimental thrombogenesis in animal models,[36] and cellular microparticles appear to provide novel mechanisms for cell–cell signaling and communication. This finding suggests that genetically determined cellular processes that regulate the life cycle of prothrombotic (or antithrombotic) microparticles derived from the endothelium and/or bloodborne cells, such as leukocytes or platelets, eventually can be identified as significant thrombophilic factors.

Inflammation contributes to thrombogenesis through various mechanisms, some of which may prove to be genetic and eventually identified as significant thrombophilic factors.[37,38] However, cohort studies failed to establish inflammatory markers, such as C-reactive protein, and several interleukins as risk factors of VTE.[39,40]

EPIDEMIOLOGY

The prevalences of factor V Leiden and prothrombin G20210A vary substantially in human populations. Factor V Leiden and prothrombin G20210A are exceedingly rare in Africans and Orientals, whereas the mean prevalence of heterozygotes in healthy whites is 4.8 and 2.7 percent, respectively (Table 131–2).[41] A particularly high prevalence of heterozygous factor V Leiden (11–14%) was reported in southern Sweden and in Arabs[22,42] and an increased prevalence of prothrombin G20210A was found in southern Europe.[43] Founder effects were demonstrated for both

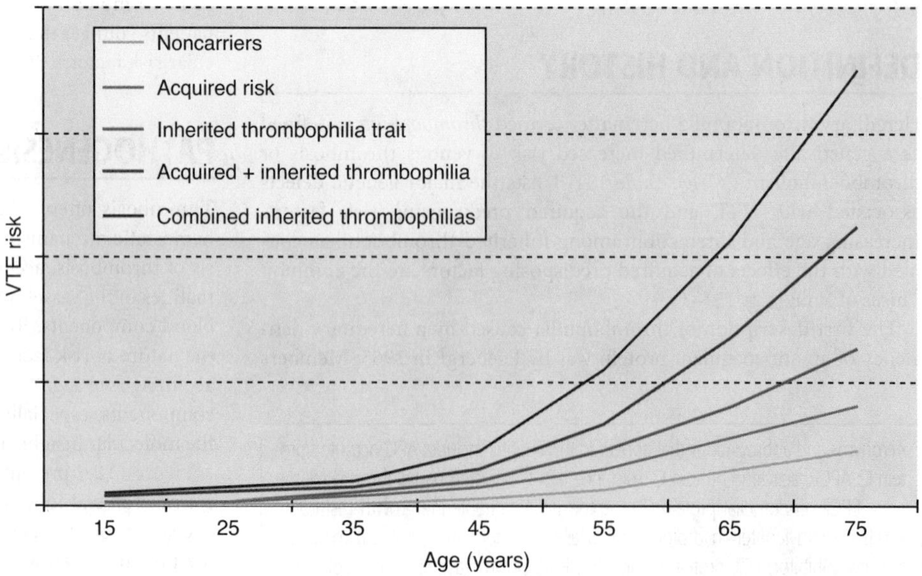

FIGURE 131–1. A paradigm of the occurrence of VTE in the normal population as it relates to increasing age and an increased burden of inherited and/or acquired risk factors. Note the profound effect of age in all risk categories and the younger age at which the risk of VTE occurs in the inherited and acquired thrombophilia.

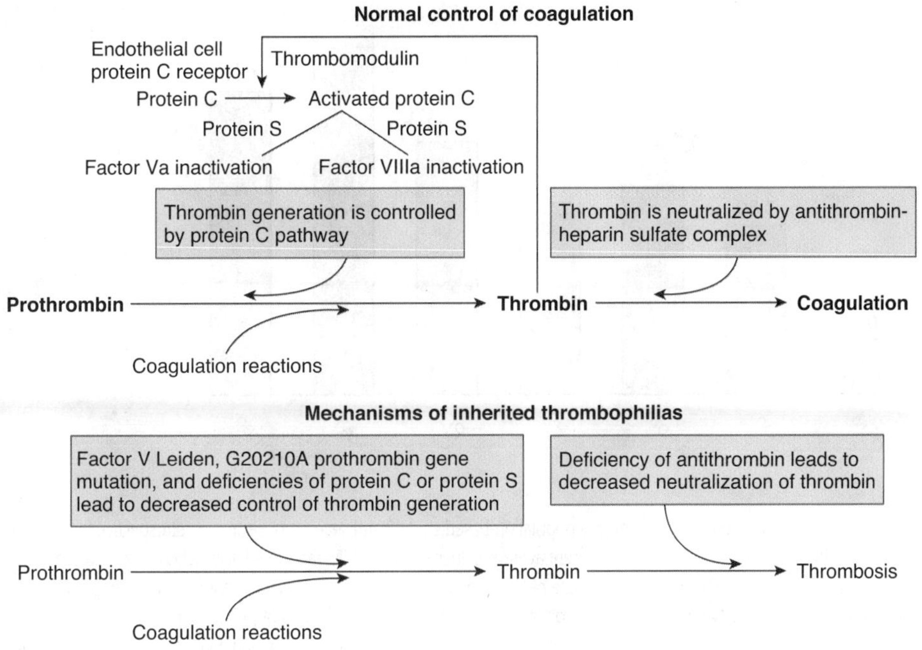

FIGURE 131–2. Major mechanisms involved in the normal control of coagulation and inherited thrombophilias. *(Reproduced with permission from Seligsohn U, Lubetsky A.[41])*

factor V Leiden and prothrombin G20210A, suggesting that they occurred after the evolutionary separation of non-Africans from Africans and after the divergence of whites and Orientals. Analyses based on linkage disequilibria between these mutations and specific markers yielded age estimates of approximately 24,000 years for prothrombin G20210A and approximately 21,000 years for factor V Leiden.[44] The relatively high prevalence of factor V Leiden in whites has been attributed to potential evolutionary advantages, such as decreased bleeding during labor[45] and menstruation,[46] and amelioration of bleeding in acquired and inherited bleeding tendencies.[47,48]

The frequency of thrombophilias is significantly higher in unselected patients with unprovoked VTE than in healthy subjects (see Table 131–2).[41,49] A further twofold increase in the frequency of thrombophilia is demonstrable in selected patients with VTE who are likely, on clinical grounds, to have thrombophilia. The absolute risk of VTE conferred by the thrombophilias has been assessed in a population-based study and in seven longitudinal studies of asymptomatic carriers or noncarriers of thrombophilias who were immediate relatives of probands with VTE.[50–58] These studies showed that the risk of VTE in noncarriers was similar to the risk in the general population, that is, approximately 1 per 1000 patient years. In carriers of factor V Leiden, prothrombin G20210A, or deficiencies of protein C, protein S or antithrombin, the risk was increased. Heterozygosities for factor V Leiden and prothrombin G20210A exerted the lowest risk, and antithrombin deficiency conferred the highest risk (Fig. 131–3). VTE occurred in carriers of thrombophilia at a younger age (35–45 years) than in noncarriers (>60 years). In both carriers and noncarriers, VTE was provoked by environmental risks in approximately 50 percent.

Because factor V Leiden and prothrombin G20210A are relatively common, their coinheritance[59] or inheritance with deficiencies of protein C, protein S, or antithrombin[60–63] is not rare.

TABLE 131–2. Frequency of Thrombophilias in Healthy Subjects and Unselected and Selected Patients with Venous Thrombosis

	Healthy Subjects		Unselected Patients		Selected Patients	
Thrombophilia	No.	Percent Affected	No.	Percent Affected	No.	Percent Affected
Factor V Leiden	16,150*	4.8	1142	18.8	162	40
	2192†	0.05				
Prothrombin G20210A	11,932*	2.7	2884	7.1	551	16
	1811†	0.06				
Protein C deficiency	15,070	0.2–0.4	2008	3.7	767	4.8
Protein S deficiency	3788	0.16–0.21	2008	2.3	649	4.3
Antithrombin deficiency	9669	0.02	2008	1.9	649	4.3

*Whites.

†Africans and Orientals.

Adapted with permission from Seligsohn U, Lubetsky A.[41]

MAJOR HEREDITARY DEFECTS

FACTOR V LEIDEN

Biochemistry and Molecular Features

Any abnormality of a protein C pathway component that interferes with the expression of APC activity can cause APCR, for example, antibodies against protein C pathway components.[64,65] Although the causes in many cases of acquired APCR are unknown, the majority (>90%) of hereditary APCR subjects have the same genetic abnormality, factor V Leiden with a G1691A alteration causing an Arg506Gln substitution. The molecular mechanism for APCR in such probands involves partial resistance of Gln506-factor Va to proteolytic inactivation by APC,[11,66,67] with kinetic studies showing that the Gln506 variant is inactivated 10 times slower than normal Arg506-factor Va.[68,69] Explanation for only a partial resistance to APC derives from the fact that cleavage of factor Va by APC at Arg306 also occurs, causing complete loss of factor Va activity, although this cleavage is slower than that at the Arg506 site.[67,69] This finding helps explain why APCR resulting from Gln506-factor V is a rather mild risk factor for venous thrombosis (see Fig. 131–3) and why a combination of genetic risk factors or a combination of a genetic risk factor and acquired risk factors for VTE is found in a significant fraction of symptomatic patients (see Fig. 131–1).

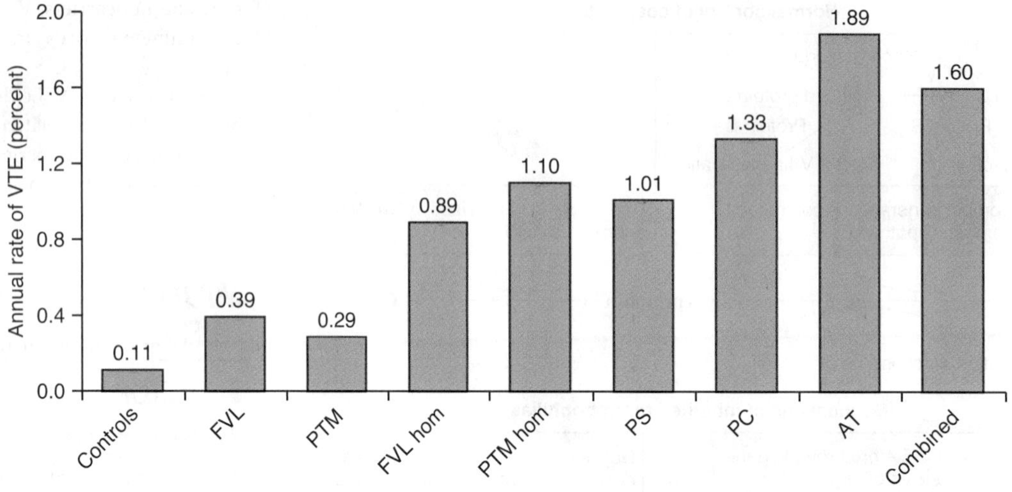

FIGURE 131–3. The absolute risks conferred by the inherited thrombophilias. Data were extracted from a population-based study[50] and seven prospective or retrospective family studies of relatives of probands with venous thrombosis (VTE) and a defined thrombophilia.[51–58] The bars represent average values of annual VTE rates in relatives who harbor the proband's thrombophilia compared to the rates in relatives who do not harbor the thrombophilia. The lowest annual rate of VTE is observed in heterozygotes for factor V Leiden and prothrombin G20210A. A substantially increased annual rate is observed in patients with homozygosity for factor V Leiden or prothrombin G20210A, deficiencies of protein S, protein C, or antithrombin, and patients with combined thrombophilias. AT, antithrombin deficiency; combined, more than one thrombophilia; FVL, heterozygous factor V Leiden; FVL hom, homozygous factor V Leiden; PS, protein S deficiency; PC, protein C deficiency; PTM, heterozygous prothrombin mutation (G20210A); PTM hom, homozygous prothrombin mutation (G20210A).

Additional molecular defects contribute to thrombosis in patients with factor V Leiden. In purified clotting factor reaction mixtures, factor V enhances inactivation of factor VIIIa by APC in the presence of protein S,[70] and APC-resistant subjects carrying factor V Leiden reportedly are defective in this APC cofactor activity.[71,72] This cofactor activity also is impaired in patients with VTE who are pseudohomozygous for an Ile359Thr mutation in factor V with a null allele factor V-Glu119Stop.[73] APCR caused by rare factor V mutations that replace Arg306 by Thr[74] or Gly[75] has been reported, although the relationship to relative risks of VTE has not been established.[76] The reason why these mutated proteins may not confer a risk of thrombosis probably is related to their preserved cofactor activity toward cleavage of factor VIIIa by APC.[77] A factor V haplotype, designated R2, has been associated with mild APCR and was shown to exert reduced factor V cofactor activity in APC mediated factor VIIIa inactivation.[78,79] The molecular mechanisms and thrombotic risks associated with the R2 factor V haplotype remain to be defined.

APC is a normal component of blood that contributes to antithrombotic surveillance mechanisms and prevents thrombosis (see Chap. 116).[80] Normal subjects have a mean APC concentration of 2.3 ng/mL (38 pM) in the circulation,[81] and the *in vivo* half-life of APC in normal adult human subjects and in freshly drawn whole blood is approximately 22 minutes.[82,83] Thus, the protein C pathway undergoes continuous activation *in vivo*. In normal subjects, an inverse relationship exists between levels of circulating APC and thrombin.[84] One report suggests circulating APC deficiency is associated with VTE.[85] APC levels are increased when thrombin is acutely generated, as occurs during disseminated intravascular coagulation, ischemia, or surgical procedures.

Because circulating APC has such a long half-life, it provides systemic anticoagulation to down-regulate thrombin generation and to limit extension of hemostatic plugs. Hence, genetic or acquired defects that impair the response to APC are understandably prothrombotic. Elevated plasma levels of prothrombin fragment F1+2 and thrombin–antithrombin complexes are found in many subjects heterozygous or homozygous for Gln506-factor V,[28,29,86] presumably reflecting impairment of the expression of APC's anticoagulant activity.

Clinical Features

Deep and superficial venous thromboses are the most common manifestations of this disorder, whereas primary pulmonary embolism is less frequent than in subjects with deficiencies in antithrombin, protein C, or protein S.[87–91] In patients with postthrombotic and nonpostthrombotic venous leg ulcers, 38 and 16 percent, respectively, had factor V Leiden.[92,93] Cerebral, hepatic, portal, and upper-extremity venous thromboses have been reported in patients with factor V Leiden.[94–98] In about half of patients with factor V Leiden who present with VTE, the event is unprovoked, and in the second half the event is provoked, with 20 percent occurring after surgery and 30 percent in women who are pregnant or take oral contraceptives.[99] Pregnancy loss during the second and third trimester of pregnancy occurs at an increased rate in women with factor V Leiden (see "Hereditary Thrombophilias during Pregnancy and Puerperium" below).

Because factor V Leiden is so common among known thrombophilic factors, it accounts for the largest proportion of patients presenting with a first VTE (20–25%).[100] The relative risk of deep and superficial vein thrombosis in patients heterozygous for factor V Leiden is increased by four- to eightfold[101–103] and fourfold, respectively,[104] although lower risks have been reported in a population-based study.[50] The risk of idiopathic VTE for men increases with age, from a relative risk of 1.2 at age 40 to 50 years to 6 for those age 70 years and older.[101] Case-control studies indicate that homozygotes for factor V Leiden have an odds ratio (OR) for VTE of 50 to 100,[105] but longitudinal studies of family members of probands carrying factor V Leiden yielded an OR of 9.0.[52,53,106] Despite the increased thrombotic risk, the presence of factor V Leiden does not increase overall mortality.[107–110] In a study of 129 homozygotes for factor V Leiden, environmental risk factors were present in 81 percent of women and 29 percent of men during their first thrombotic episode.[111]

Laboratory Assays

Coagulation assays and DNA-based assays are available for the identification of patients with APCR. Plasma-based coagulation tests depend on the relative prolongation of the activated partial thromboplastin time (aPTT) caused by the addition of purified APC. Individuals with resistance to APC have less prolongation of the aPTT than normal. Although an aPTT assay using patient's plasma originally was used, many current assays use factor V-deficient plasma,[66] which makes the test informative for most patients with lupus anticoagulant, pregnant patients, patients with inflammatory states, and patients on oral anticoagulants. The test is sensitive and specific compared with the genetic test for factor V Leiden.[112] An abnormally low APCR is associated with VTE, in both the presence and absence of the factor V Leiden mutation[113,114] and with ischemic stroke.[115,116] Thus, there is clinically relevant information obtained from the classic aPTT-based APCR test using patient's plasma that is not obtained using factor V-deficient substrate plasma. Tissue factor-based APCR assays can provide additional information about plasma components that differentially modulate the protein C pathway,[117–119] such as "anticoagulant" high-density lipoprotein or glucosylceramide, and possibly as yet unidentified factors that are altered by oral contraceptive usage. The presence of platelets or platelet microparticles in plasma tested for APCR using aPTT assays,[120–122] and autoantibodies against APC,[65] can reduce the anticoagulant response to APC, indicating the need to carefully prepare plasma prior to testing.

Many DNA-based assays for the factor V Leiden are available. Genomic DNA is isolated, amplified by polymerase chain reaction (PCR), subjected to restriction fragment length polymorphism analysis, and analyzed for G or A at nucleotide 1691.[11] Plasma coagulation tests are often used for screening patients, followed by confirmation of positive results with the DNA assay. Only DNA tests clearly distinguish factor V Leiden heterozygosity from homozygosity. "Pseudohomozygotes" who are heterozygous for factor V Leiden and for a dysfunctional factor V allele have very low APC resistance ratios in the plasma test but are heterozygous by the DNA assay for factor V Leiden.[123]

PROTHROMBIN G20210A SUBSTITUTION

Biochemistry and Molecular Features

Replacement of G by A at nt 20210 in the 3′-untranslated region of the prothrombin gene augments translation and stability of prothrombin messenger ribonucleic acid (mRNA).[124] This process results in increased synthesis and secretion of prothrombin by the liver. The elevated level of plasma prothrombin with a mean of 132 percent of normal in heterozygotes[16] may contribute directly to increased thrombotic risk by causing increased thrombin generation[125] or decreased fibrinolytic activity because of enhanced activation of TAFI.[126] Another mechanism for prothrombotic action might derive from the ability of prothrombin to inhibit APC's inactivation of factor Va.[127]

Clinical Features

The prothrombin gene mutation is found largely in white populations.[44] In contrast to factor V Leiden, the frequency of the mutation seems to increase from northern Europe to southern Europe, that is, only 1.7 percent of the population in northern Europe has the abnormality compared with 3 to 5 percent in southern Europe and the Middle East.[43,128] The prothrombin gene mutation is associated with venous thrombosis in all age groups.[129] When sequential patients presenting with a first VTE are analyzed, 4 to 8 percent have the mutation, and the relative risk of thrombosis in subjects with prothrombin 20210A is increased approximately 2-fold to 5.5-fold.[16,20,51,130–135] For patients with superficial vein thrombosis, an OR of 4.3 (95% confidence interval [CI] 1.5–12.6) was reported.[104]

As in other forms of hereditary thrombophilia, the prothrombin gene mutation has been found in patients with thrombosis in unusual sites, particularly hepatic, portal, and cerebral sinus vein thrombosis.[95,136–141] For example, in a study of 40 patients with cerebral vein thrombosis, 20 percent had the gene defect (OR 10.2). Many of these thromboses were in young women taking oral contraceptives, which raises the likelihood of thrombosis even higher.[138] Notably, a large proportion of a group of young women with acute unexplained spinal cord infarction had the mutation.[142] All were taking oral contraceptives, and most were smokers.

Individuals who are homozygous for the prothrombin gene mutation display substantial heterogeneity in thrombotic manifestations, with 40 percent remaining asymptomatic.[143]

Laboratory Features

Identification of the mutation in the 3′-untranslated region of the prothrombin gene requires DNA analysis following PCR amplification of the pertinent region.[16] Although prothrombin levels are elevated, assay of prothrombin activity or prothrombin antigen usually is not sufficiently sensitive or specific for the presence of the mutation or as a more effective predictor of thrombosis.[144–146] Interestingly, an A19911G polymorphism in the prothrombin gene also is associated with mildly increased prothrombin level and risk of VTE.[147]

HYPERHOMOCYSTEINEMIA

Biochemistry and Molecular Features

Homocysteine is an intermediate in the metabolism of the sulfur-containing amino acids methionine and cysteine and participates in several metabolic pathways. Remethylation of homocysteine to generate methionine requires the vitamin B_{12}-dependent enzyme methionine synthase and 5-methyltetrahydrofolate, which are part of a metabolic pathway that recycles tetrahydrofolate and 5-methyltetrahydrofolate and involves the enzyme methylenetetrahydrofolate reductase (MTHFR). For synthesis of cysteine from homocysteine, a transsulfuration pathway first involves condensation of homocysteine with serine to generate cystathionine by the vitamin B_6-dependent enzyme cystathionine β-synthase, then deamination and cleavage of cystathionine to yield cysteine and α-ketobutyrate, which are accomplished by the vitamin B_6-dependent enzyme cystathioninase.

A plasma homocysteine level above the normal range defines hyperhomocysteinemia.[148] Severe hyperhomocysteinemia (plasma levels >100 μmol/L), also identifiable as homocystinuria, occurs in approximately 1 in 200,000 to 300,000 individuals in the general population and is transmitted as an autosomal recessive trait. The most common causes for homocystinuria are mutations in cystathionine β-synthase. Rarely, other mutations in 5,10-MTHFR, or methionine synthase give rise to homocystinuria. Such severe abnormalities are associated with neurologic abnormalities, mental retardation, ectopia lentis, premature cardiovascular disease, stroke, venous thrombosis, and arterial thrombosis.[148] The most common genetic cause of mild hyperhomocysteinemia involves an MTHFR gene polymorphism, ntC677T, which causes a conservative replacement of Ala222 by Val that results in a variant enzyme with reduced specific activity and increased thermolability. Homozygosity for TT at nt677 occurs in 10 to 20 percent of healthy whites and 10 percent of Orientals, but is rare in Africans.[149] The MTHFR C677T polymorphism can be associated with mild hyperhomocysteinemia, particularly when plasma folate level is low.[150] A second polymorphism, ntA1298C, also can be associated with mild hyperhomocysteinemia. Suboptimal levels of folate or vitamin B_6 or B_{12} can contribute to acquired mild to moderate hyperhomocysteinemia by providing inadequate cofactor levels to support the enzymes that regulate homocysteine metabolism. Other causes for hyperhomocysteinemia are renal failure, hypothyroidism, smoking, excessive coffee consumption, inflammatory bowel disease, psoriasis, and rheumatoid arthritis.[151]

The exact mechanisms by which hyperhomocysteinemia causes increased risk of thrombosis have not been defined. Deleterious effects on the endothelium, enhanced smooth muscle proliferation, induction of tissue factor by monocytes, reduced cleavage of factor Va by APC, suppression of heparan sulfate synthesis, and downregulation of thrombomodulin all have been described, but these effects were mainly based on *in vitro* studies that used homocysteine concentrations that exceeded the highest pathologic levels observed in homocystinuria.[151]

Clinical Features

Retrospective case-control studies have shown an association between hyperhomocysteinemia and VTE. Meta-analyses of these studies estimated similar pooled ORs of 2.5 (95% CI 1.8–3.5) and 3.0 (95% CI 2.1–4.2), respectively.[152–154] In a non–population-based prospective study and a large population-based cohort study, significant associations between increased homocysteine level and idiopathic venous thrombosis were found in men,[155] but not in women.[156] Cerebral vein thrombosis has been associated with hyperhomocysteinemia. In a large case control study involving 121 patients and 242 controls, the estimated risk conferred by hyperhomocysteinemia was represented by an OR of 19.5 (95% CI 5.7–67.3).[157]

Conflicting results have been reported regarding a possible association between homozygous MTHFR C677T and VTE. A meta-analysis of 53 studies comprising 8364 cases with venous thrombosis and 12,468 controls revealed a borderline degree of risk with pooled OR 1.2 (95% CI 1.08–1.32).[154] In the multiple environmental and genetic assessment of risk factors for VTE (MEGA study) involving 4,375 cases and 4856 controls, MTHFR C677TT was not associated with a risk of VTE (OR 0.99 [95% CI 0.81–1.08]).[158]

Laboratory Features

Plasma homocysteine concentrations can be measured by high-pressure liquid chromatography or immunoassay. Both fasting levels and levels after methionine loading have been used to assess hyperhomocysteinemia.[159,160] Although the methionine loading test may detect additional subjects with hyperhomocysteinemia,[161] relatively few centers have used the test because of practical difficulties involved.[151] Blood samples for homocysteine levels should be obtained in the fasting state, kept cold, and centrifuged immediately. Individual measurements reflect average homocysteine concentrations over time (e.g., 4 weeks) reasonably well.[162] Serum homocysteine levels are higher than plasma levels, and male values are higher than female values.[163]

The MTHFR C677T substitution creates a cleavage site for HinfI; thus, its detection is possible by PCR to amplify a flanking sequence and digestion by the restriction enzyme.[164] Many laboratories have discontinued testing this parameter because it is probably not a risk factor for VTE.

Mutations causing homozygous homocystinuria have mainly been identified in the cystathionine β-synthase gene with more than 130 mutations described.[165] Of these mutations, the T833C and G919A polymorphisms are prevalent and can be detected by relatively simple methods.[165,166] However, detection of these mutations is rarely needed because heterozygotes do not manifest hyperhomocysteinemia.

PROTEIN C DEFICIENCY

Biochemistry and Molecular Features

Protein C is one of the vitamin K-dependent proteins that is synthesized in the liver and circulates in plasma as a serine protease zymogen. Protein C is activated by limited proteolysis by thrombin bound to thrombomodulin, with additional acceleration by an endothelial protein C receptor (EPCR) (see Chap. 116).[167,168] APC is a potent anticoagulant enzyme that downregulates the blood coagulation pathways by proteolytic and irreversible inactivation of factors Va and VIIIa with protein S serving as a cofactor in these reactions (see Fig. 131–2). Thus, decreased levels of protein C zymogen may impair the natural inhibition of thrombin generation and contribute to hypercoagulability. APC also displays a cytoprotective effect, including antiinflammatory and anti-apoptotic actions and stabilization of endothelial barriers.[169] These protective direct effects of APC on endothelial cells require EPCR and protease activated receptor 1 (see Chap. 116).[170] These distinct functions of APC are underscored by an engineered recombinant APC variant which exhibits cytoprotection with less than 10 percent anticoagulant activity and decreases mortality of mice with endotoxemia and sepsis.[171] The APC cellular pathway likely helps explain the success of APC in reducing mortality in patients with severe sepsis,[172] whereas antithrombin and tissue factor pathway inhibitor (TFPI), two other natural plasma anticoagulants, failed to do so.[173,174]

More than 150 mutations in the protein C gene have been identified (see www.itb.cnr.it/procmd). A CC/GG genotype for 2 polymorphisms in the promoter region of the protein C gene are associated with decreased protein C levels and an increased risk of VTE.[175]

Clinical Features

Heterozygous protein C deficiency occurs in 0.2 to 0.4 percent of normal individuals[176,177] and is found in approximately 4 to 5 percent of consecutive outpatients with objectively confirmed deep venous thrombosis.[178] Deficiency of protein C is linked to thrombosis (OR 6.5–8).[178,179] Heterozygotes for protein C deficiency have a normal survival.[180]

Variability in clinical expression is a hallmark of the disorder. Subjects identified by screening large numbers of normal individuals (e.g., blood donors) in most instances have neither a personal nor a family history of thromboembolism.[176,177] The discrepancy in thrombosis rates between these surveys and studies of families who have striking thrombotic symptoms can be explained in part by the coinheritance of factor V Leiden or other thrombophilic loci.[181,182]

Deep and superficial venous thromboses are the most common clinical presentations of protein C deficiency.[183–186] By age 45 years, up to 50 percent of heterozygous subjects in clinically affected families will have venous thromboembolism, and half of the episodes will be spontaneous.[187] Protein C deficiency has been linked to unusual sites of venous thrombosis, including the cerebral and mesenteric veins.[183,188]

Homozygous protein C deficiency with protein C levels of less than 1 percent of normal causes neonatal purpura fulminans and massive thrombosis in affected infants.[189,190] In a similar reaction, "warfarin skin necrosis" (large areas of thrombotic skin necrosis) appears over central areas of the body (breast, abdomen, genitalia) in subjects with heterozygous protein C deficiency given warfarin (Fig. 131–4).[191] In such patients, the vitamin K antagonist rapidly induces a fall in protein C activity from approximately 50 percent of normal to very low levels because of the short half-life of protein C (approximately 8 hours).[192,193] Because the half-lives of prothrombin, factor IX, and factor X are much longer, a transient hypercoagulable state may arise at the onset of vitamin K antagonist therapy.[193]

Laboratory Features

Most laboratories screen for protein C deficiency with a protein C activity assay that uses a highly specific snake venom protease to activate protein C.[194,195] Protein C activity is best assessed with an assay that uses a coagulation rather than a chromogenic end point to identify the greatest number of patients with protein C deficiency.[196] Immunoassays are used to distinguish type I defects (reduced antigen and

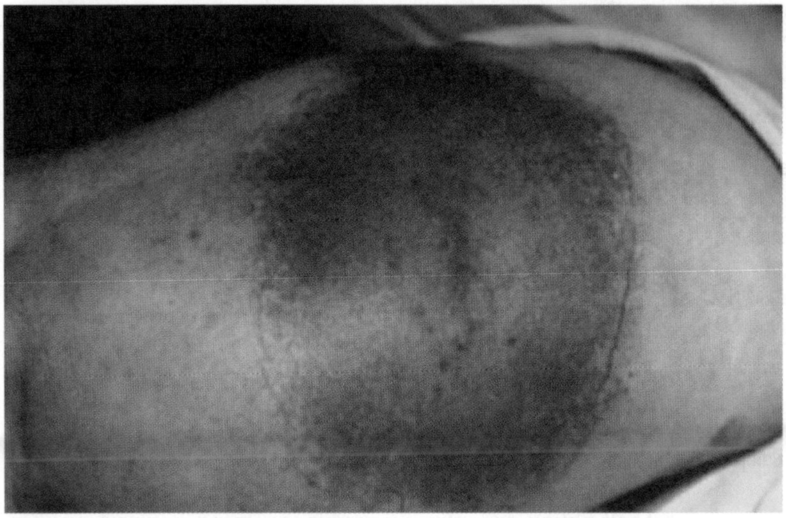

FIGURE 131–4. Warfarin-induced skin necrosis in left flank. *(Used with permission from* Lichtman's Atlas of Hematology, *www.accessmedicine.com.)*

activity) from type II disorders (normal antigen, reduced activity).[197] Protein C gene promotor polymorphisms influence plasma concentrations of the protein,[175,198] and liver disease or use of oral contraceptives can lower or raise protein C levels, respectively (Table 131–3).[199] Consequently, protein C levels of less than 55 percent of normal (in the absence of oral anticoagulant therapy, vitamin K deficiency, or overt liver disease) suggest protein C deficiency, but levels from 55 to 70 percent must be considered borderline, and repeated testing or family studies should be undertaken.[196] Use of DNA-based assays to identify patients with hereditary protein C deficiency is impractical because of the numerous mutations that have been described.

The diagnosis of hereditary protein C deficiency in patients receiving warfarin is particularly difficult. Protein C antigen levels can be compared with antigen levels for other vitamin K-dependent clotting factors, but only if careful control ranges are established for the ratios of protein C to two other vitamin K-dependent factors.[4,200] In most situations, a waiting period of at least 2 weeks after discontinuation of anticoagulant therapy is necessary for a reliable diagnosis. Warfarin should not be restarted before laboratory results are available so as to reduce the possibility of warfarin-induced skin necrosis in patients who are later found to have protein C deficiency. In cases of neonatal purpura fulminans, testing of parents can be useful.

PROTEIN S DEFICIENCY

Biochemistry and Molecular Features

Protein S is one of the vitamin K-dependent coagulation proteins but differs from them by not containing a serine protease domain. It enhances the anticoagulant activity of APC; hence, currently available functional assays of protein S measure APC cofactor activity using protein S-depleted plasma as substrate. Protein S is principally synthesized in the liver, but other organs may be important sites for its synthesis, including the endothelium, kidney, testes, and brain (see Chap. 116). Protein S reversibly associates with the plasma complement factor C4b-binding protein (C4BP), previously known as proline-rich lipoprotein. In normal plasma, approximately 60 percent of protein S is bound to C4BP and 40 percent is free. Importantly, only the free form of protein S functions as a cofactor for APC. Because protein S is a cofactor for APC, decreased levels of free protein S may impair the down-regulation of thrombin generation and contribute to hyper-coagulability (see Fig. 131–2). Protein S also exhibits anticoagulant activity that is independent of APC; it inhibits tissue factor activity by promoting the interaction between tissue factor pathway inhibitor and factor Xa.[201]

Three types of protein S deficiency have been characterized. Type I protein S deficiency is defined as parallel reductions in both antigen and anticoagulant activity levels in plasma. Type II deficiency, which is associated with circulating dysfunctional molecules, involves normal plasma levels of free protein S antigen but low levels of anticoagulant activity. Type III deficiency involves low free protein S level while total protein S antigen usually is in the low to normal range. More than 200 mutations causing protein S deficiency have been described (see *Protein S Deficiency: A Database of Mutations* at www.isth.org).

Clinical Features

In several studies, approximately 2 to 3 percent of unselected outpatients presenting with VTE had low levels of protein S (see Table 131–2).[202,203] In the healthy Japanese population, the prevalence of protein S deficiency is substantially higher than in whites, and hence the prevalence of the deficiency among Japanese patients with VTE is 12.7 percent.[204] A higher prevalence of protein S deficiency is seen in white patients younger than age 50 years and in patients with a personal or family history of VTE. The OR for thrombosis in patients with free protein S deficiency has been variably reported as 1.6,[178] 2.4,[202] and 11.5.[205] Deep venous thrombosis and pulmonary embolism are the most common forms of VTE associated with protein S deficiency, although superficial vein thrombophlebitis and thrombosis in unusual sites also occur.[183–185] As in other forms of thrombophilia, approximately 50 percent of thromboses are unprovoked.[184] Neonatal purpura fulminans has been reported in two patients with homozygous or compound heterozygous protein S deficiency having very low levels of protein S.[206–208] Warfarin-induced skin necrosis has been reported in association with protein S deficiency.[209]

Analysis of four prospective studies showed that the incidence of VTE in asymptomatic protein S-deficient relatives of symptomatic probands was 0.7 to 2.2 percent per year. About half of these events occurred during well-known risk periods, but incidence rates were decreased by prophylactic use of oral anticoagulants.[210]

Laboratory Features

Laboratory assays of plasma protein S must be chosen and interpreted with care because the protein circulates both free and bound to C4BP. Moreover, normal ranges are different for males and females, depend on age, and can be reduced in a variety of conditions (see below). Free protein S antigen and APC cofactor anticoagulant activity are better parameters than total protein S antigen in screening for hereditary protein S deficiency.[178,211] Free protein S antigen can be assayed using monoclonal antibodies specific for free protein S.[212,213] Protein S activity assays may be affected by coexisting APCR, although the second-generation assays in which factor V-deficient plasma is used as substrate have improved specificity.[214–216] Assessment of total and free protein S plus protein S activity should allow classification of patients with protein S defects into type I, II, or III. Type I and type III deficiencies may be phenotypic variants of the same disease given the finding that, within families, different individuals carrying the same DNA mutation in the protein S gene can present with laboratory findings indicating either type I or type III deficiency.[211] Type II deficiency, that is, normal free protein S antigen with reduced protein S activity, is uncommon,[196] so screening patients with free protein S antigen levels is clinically reasonable. In normal subjects, an excellent correlation is seen between free protein S antigen and

TABLE 131–3. Acquired Conditions That Can Yield Abnormal Test Results of Thrombophilia

Tests*	Acquired Conditions That Can Cause Abnormal Test Results
APCR (decreased ratio)	Pregnancy, use of oral contraceptives, stroke, presence of lupus anticoagulant,† increased factor VIII levels,† autoantibodies against activated protein C, use of oral anticoagulants†
Factor V Leiden	–
Prothrombin G20210A	–
Hyperhomocysteinemia	Deficiencies of folate, vitamin B_{12}, or vitamin B_6, old age, renal failure, excessive consumption of coffee, smoking
Increased factor VIII levels	Pregnancy, use of oral contraceptives, exercise, stress, older age, acute phase response, liver disease, hyperthyroidism
Presence of lupus anticoagulant	Systemic lupus erythematosus, antiphospholipid syndrome, autoimmune disease, liver disease, hyperthyroidism, healthy subjects
Increased titer of anticardiolipin antibody	Same as lupus anticoagulant, infectious diseases
Decreased level of protein C	Liver disease, use of oral anticoagulants, vitamin K deficiency, childhood, disseminated intravascular coagulation, presence of autoantibodies against protein C
Decreased level of free protein S	Liver disease, use of oral anticoagulants, vitamin K deficiency, pregnancy, use of oral contraceptives, nephrotic syndrome, childhood, presence of autoantibodies against protein S, disseminated intravascular coagulation
Decreased level of antithrombin	Use of heparin, thrombosis, disseminated intravascular coagulation, liver disease, nephrotic syndrome
Increased level of factor IX	–
Increased level of factor XI	–
Homozygous MTHFR C677T	–
Dysfibrinogenemia	Neonates, liver disease

*Tests are listed in a decreasing order of priority.

†Normal ratios are expected when activated protein C resistance (APCR) is measured in samples diluted with factor V-depleted plasma.

anticoagulant activity. The lower limit of the normal range for free protein S is lower in females than in males (55% vs. 65%).[217] Protein S is remarkably sensitive to hormonal status in females.

The high frequency of acquired protein S deficiency makes identification of hereditary defects more difficult. Oral contraceptives and hormone replacement therapy decrease plasma protein S levels. Reduced levels of free protein S are regularly found during pregnancy (e.g., as low as 20–30% of normal),[218,219] in patients who are taking oral anticoagulants, and in patients with disseminated intravascular coagulation, liver disease, nephrotic syndrome, inflammatory conditions, and acute thromboembolism (see Table 131–3).[220–223] Protein S deficiency can occur in concert with the lupus anticoagulant[224,225] and as a result of autoantibodies to protein S following varicella or other infections in children.[226,227] Thus, these acquired conditions leading to low protein S levels should be excluded and tests repeated before making a diagnosis of hereditary thrombophilia. Family studies may be useful. Diagnosis of hereditary protein S deficiency using DNA techniques is not favored unless the defect has previously been established in the family because numerous different mutations in the protein S gene cause protein S deficiency.

ANTITHROMBIN DEFICIENCY

Biochemistry and Molecular Features

Antithrombin is a plasma protease inhibitor that neutralizes thrombin and factors Xa, IXa, and XIa by irreversibly forming 1:1 complexes in reactions accelerated by heparin or by heparan sulfate on endothelial surfaces (see Chap. 116). Therefore, defects in antithrombin compromise the normal inhibition of the coagulation pathways and cause a hypercoagulable state (see Fig. 131–2). Antithrombin deficiency is classified into two major categories. Type I antithrombin deficiency is defined by low levels of both antigen and activity assayed in the absence or presence of heparin. Type II deficiency is defined by the presence of normal levels of antigen with defects that affect either the inhibitor's active center, which complexes with the target enzyme's active site, or the inhibitor's heparin binding site, which mediates heparin-dependent acceleration of antithrombin activity. Type II antithrombin deficiency is further subdivided into type IIa with mutations affecting the reactive site, type IIb involving mutations in the heparin-binding site, and type IIc that includes a pleiotropic group of mutations. A database of more than 150 mutations in the antithrombin gene is available (www1.imperial.ac.uk/medicine/about/divisions/is/haemo/coag/antithrombin). Severe deficiency of antithrombin (<5% of normal) is rare, involves defects in heparin-dependent enhancement of antithrombin (type IIb), and is associated with severe venous and arterial thrombosis.[228–231] Type I antithrombin deficiency is found in 1:5000 of normal individuals in Scotland, whereas type II defects, mostly observed in asymptomatic individuals, are more common and are found in 1:625 of people screened.[232]

Clinical Features

Antithrombin deficiency is found in approximately 1 to 2 percent of consecutive unselected patients younger than age 70 years with a first objectively documented VTE.[100] The frequency is higher in selected patients with VTE (see Table 131–2). The OR for thrombosis in patients with antithrombin deficiency is approximately 20, which is notably greater than in subjects heterozygous for factor V Leiden.[178,233] No evidence indicates differences in clinical severity between patients with heterozygous type I defects and those with type II mutations involving the thrombin binding site. Mortality rates are not increased in these patients.[234,235] Patients with type II mutations of the heparin binding site have few, if any, thrombotic episodes, although homozygous mutations affecting the heparin binding site are associated with thromboembolism.[236,237]

Venous thrombosis of the lower extremities, which occurs at an early age and peaks in the second decade of life, is the most common symptom in antithrombin deficiency.[236] Superficial venous thrombosis appears to be somewhat less common than in protein C or protein S deficiency or in APCR.[183,184] Thromboses in unusual sites, such as the mesenteric, hepatic, or cerebral veins, have been reported.[183,184,238] Almost 70 percent of patients present with the first thrombotic event before age 35 years and 85 percent before age 50 years.[236] Patients with severe antithrombin deficiency, that is, activity levels less than 5 percent, are rare, most likely because the profound deficiency state causes fetal loss *in utero*. A few infants with homozygous defects involving the heparin-binding region of the molecule have survived, but most have suffered severe venous and arterial thrombosis.[237] No patients homozygous for reactive center defects have been identified, leading to the speculation that complete deficiency of antithrombin in humans is incompatible with life. Complete antithrombin deficiency in knockout mice results in death of the embryo.[239]

Resistance to the anticoagulant effects of heparin has been observed in some patients with antithrombin deficiency. Both acute thrombosis and several days of heparin therapy can decrease antithrombin levels, occasionally to as low as 50 percent of normal, which may lead to an erroneous diagnosis of hereditary antithrombin deficiency.[240,241] Other acquired conditions leading to low levels of antithrombin are common and include liver disease, disseminated intravascular coagulation, nephrotic syndrome, chemotherapy with asparaginase, and preeclampsia (see Table 131–3).[242–246]

Laboratory Features

Antithrombin activity assays that use a chromogenic substrate are widely available.[247] Most laboratories now use factor Xa or bovine thrombin in their antithrombin assays to avoid the inhibitory effects of heparin cofactor II on human thrombin. The normal range for plasma antithrombin levels in healthy subjects is narrow (e.g., 84–116%).[248] Antithrombin antigen measurements are used to help distinguish type I from type II defects. Crossed immunoelectrophoresis using an antithrombin antibody in the presence and absence of heparin can help identify defects in the heparin binding portion of the molecule.

In general, patients with type I deficiency and many of those with type II disorders involving the thrombin-binding site have antithrombin activity levels of 40 to 60 percent. Levels of 60 to 80 percent can be caused by other type II defects, but frequently result from acquired antithrombin deficiency (see Table 131–3). If these confounding conditions are present, measurement of antithrombin level should be repeated and family studies performed if possible.

ELEVATED FACTOR VIII LEVELS

Biochemistry and Molecular Features

Increased factor VIII levels are commonly observed in association with increasing age and body mass index, pregnancy, surgery, chronic inflammation, liver disease, hyperthyroidism, diabetes mellitus, and exercise (see Table 131–3).[249] The ABO blood group system exerts a substantial effect on factor VIII level and von Willebrand factor level, with non-O subjects having significantly higher levels than subjects with blood group O.[250] The mechanisms by which these conditions cause elevated factor VIII levels have not been elucidated, but augmented synthesis of factor VIII or downregulation of low-density lipoprotein-related receptor protein, the liver protein that clears factor VIII from the circulation,[251] is possible. In the Leiden population-based case-control study on VTE, increased factor VIII activity and antigen levels were defined as risk factors independent of all other causes of thrombophilia.[17,249] This observation was confirmed by other studies,[252,253] and the elevated factor VIII levels in patients with VTE were found to persist over time.[249] Clustering of increased factor VIII levels in families of patients with VTE suggests heritability,[18,19] but no gene alteration has been described. How elevated factor VIII levels increase the risk of thrombosis is unknown. The suggestion that increased factor VIII levels enhance thrombin generation[249] has been disputed.[254] It is possible that elevated levels of factor VIII increase the risk of VTE by diminishing the anticoagulant effect of APC, thereby causing acquired APC resistance.[249]

Clinical Features

The clinical presentation of patients with VTE and elevated factor VIII levels does not differ from that of patients with other thrombophilias. The relative risk of VTE is correlated with the extent of increase in factor VIII level. Thus, subjects with factor VIII levels of 100 to 125 percent of normal have an OR of 2.3 (95% CI 1.3–3.8) and those with factor VIII levels of 150 percent of normal or higher have an OR of 4.8 (95% CI 2.3–10).[17] Interestingly, the prevalence of increased factor VIII levels (>150% of normal) in healthy controls of the Leiden study was 10 percent versus 25 percent in patients with a first event of VTE. This finding suggests that increased factor VIII level is one of the most frequent risk factors of VTE.

Laboratory Features

Factor VIII activity is measured by a one-stage assay using factor VIII-depleted plasma and normal reference plasma. Assaying factor VIII antigen is not necessary because factor VIII antigen level correlates well with factor VIII activity, provided plasma is carefully separated and stored at −70°C (−94°F). Factor VIII should not be assayed close to the time of the thrombotic event or when an acute phase reaction is predicted. An assay in more than one blood sample is advisable.

HIGH LEVELS OF OTHER COAGULATION FACTORS

Increased levels of other factors have been associated with an increased risk for VTE.[255] The Leiden population-based case control study revealed that in patients with factor IX levels greater than 129 percent of normal (90th percentile in controls), the OR for VTE was 2.3 (95% CI 1.6–3.5).[256] Adjustments for confounding factors and other hereditary thrombophilias showed that increased factor IX level was an independent risk factor. A "dose–response" relationship also was demonstrated, such that the higher the level, the higher the risk. The thrombotic risk was more pronounced in women than in men and was particularly high in premenopausal women not using oral contraceptives (OR 12.4; 95% CI 3.3–47.2) and in postmenopausal women (OR 6.2; 95% CI 2.4–15.9).

Similar observations were made regarding elevated levels of factor XI in the Leiden study.[257] The adjusted OR for VTE in patients with factor XI levels above the 90th percentile (121% of normal) compared to those who had factor XI levels at or below the 90th percentile was 2.2 (95% CI 1.5–3.2). Stratification of subjects according to factor XI levels disclosed an increase in the relative risk of thrombosis concordant with increasing factor XI levels.

Elevated levels of fibrinogen have been demonstrated to confer a risk of VTE in the Leiden study.[258] However, reanalysis of the data and adjustments for all possible confounding factors disclosed that the estimated risk was small and confined to subjects older than age 45 years.[259]

Regarding possible effects of elevated levels of other coagulation factors (e.g., factors II, V, X, XII), no convincing evidence has been provided.[255]

HEREDITARY THROMBOTIC DYSFIBRINOGENEMIA

Dysfibrinogenemias are defined as qualitative defects in the fibrinogen molecule resulting from mutations in one of the genes encoding for one of the three polypeptide chains (see Chap. 126). The hereditary dysfibrinogenemias represent a heterogeneous group of abnormalities that are asymptomatic in 55 percent of cases. They cause thrombosis with or without bleeding in 20 percent of patients or a bleeding tendency in 25 percent of patients.[260]

Biochemistry and Molecular Features

The mechanisms by which dysfibrinogenemia can cause VTE are not clear. One suggestion is that defective binding of thrombin to an abnormal fibrinogen gives rise to increased plasma thrombin concentrations, which eventually results in thrombosis, and another suggestion is that docking of tissue plasminogen activator on the abnormal fibrinogen is impaired, thereby leading to diminished fibrinolysis and thrombosis.

Also, abnormal fibrin polymerization leading to thrombosis was suggested as one of the mechanisms.[261] Numerous mutations causing structural defects in fibrinogen have been reported, most of which are point mutations that give rise to single amino acid substitutions. The mode of transmission of dysfibrinogenemias is autosomal dominant.

Clinical Features

When VTE is manifested in patients with hereditary dysfibrinogenemias it usually occurs at a young age (27–32 years).[262] When a large number of patients presenting with venous thromboembolism were screened, dysfibrinogenemia was found in only 0.8 percent.[262] An occasional patient has both thrombosis and bleeding (usually postpartum hemorrhage). An increased rate of pregnancy-associated thrombosis, spontaneous abortions, and stillbirth have been described.

Laboratory Features

Prolongation of a dilute thrombin time and/or reptilase time because of delayed fibrin polymerization is common in patients with dysfibrinogenemia, as is a disparity between measurement of immunoreactive and clottable fibrinogen. More sophisticated testing often demonstrates abnormal fibrinogen structure or resistance of fibrin to fibrinolysis. A search for mutations in one of the three genes encoding for fibrinogen is only performed in specialized laboratories.

HEREDITARY DEFECTS IN THE FIBRINOLYTIC SYSTEM

Associations between mutations or polymorphisms in the genes encoding for plasminogen and plasminogen-activator inhibitor (PAI)-1 and VTE are not firmly established.[263–266] Both types of plasminogen deficiency, hypoplasminogenemia (type I) and dysplasminogenemia (type II), have been described in patients with VTE (particularly in Japan), but other studies failed to determine that isolated plasminogen deficiency is a risk factor for VTE.[265] Severe plasminogen deficiency with levels of 5 to 6 percent of normal is a rare entity that is manifested by a pseudomembranous disease affecting mucous membranes, for example, the eyes (ligneous conjunctivitis), but surprisingly not by VTE.[267] Mild to moderate plasminogen deficiency was observed in 28 of 9611 blood donors (1:385) in Scotland.[268] Further analysis of 19 of these subjects and family members (20 with hypoplasminogenemia and 4 with dysplasminogenemia) disclosed that only 1 subject who had venous thrombosis also was heterozygous for prothrombin G20210A.[265]

Increased levels of PAI-1, assumed to cause hypofibrinolysis, have been related to a 4G/5G insertion/deletion at nucleotide −675 of the gene promoter. Homozygotes for the 4G allele have 25 percent higher levels of PAI-1 than homozygotes for the 5G allele.[264] Several studies suggested that the 4G genotype was associated with an increased risk of VTE, but a prospective population-based study of 308 subjects with VTE and 640 controls failed to demonstrate a significant association.[266] Another study that focused on potential factors affecting recurrence of VTE failed to show an association between levels of PAI-1, tissue plasminogen activator, or euglobulin clot lysis time with recurrence.[269]

TAFI is activated by thrombin mostly after blood clots are formed and activated TAFI suppresses fibrinolysis by removing carboxy-terminal lysine residues from fibrin polymers that otherwise promote the binding of tissue plasminogen activator and plasminogen to fibrin.

Increased levels of TAFI (above the 90th percentile in controls, i.e., >122 U/dL) were associated with an increased risk of venous thrombosis (OR 1.7; 95% CI 1.1–2.5) in the Leiden study,[270] but another study of family members of probands with thrombophilia failed to demonstrate an increased absolute risk of VTE in subject with increased TAFI levels.[271] Recurrent venous thrombosis has been associated with increased TAFI level.

Protein C inhibitor (PCI) is another protein that exhibits an antifibrinolytic effect by inhibiting tissue plasminogen activator and urokinase, albeit exerting (1) a profibrinolytic effect (inhibition of TAFI activation by thrombin–thrombomodulin complex); (2) an anticoagulant effect (inhibition of thrombin, factor Xa, and factor XIa); and (3) a procoagulant effect (inhibition of APC).[272]

In the Leiden study, PCI levels above the 95th percentile of controls (136% of normal) were associated with an increased relative risk of VTE with an OR of 1.6 (95% CI 0.9–2.8) compared to PCI levels below the 95th percentile.[273]

OTHER POTENTIAL THROMBOPHILIC DISORDERS

Thrombomodulin is an endothelial receptor that binds thrombin with very high affinity and promotes protein C activation.[167,274] Several mutations in the thrombomodulin gene have been discovered in families with thrombosis.[275–277] The gene alterations are scattered throughout the thrombomodulin gene, and some are associated with variable levels of soluble thrombomodulin in plasma,[276] reduced expression, and impaired function.[278] None of the mutations has been shown to be firmly associated with VTE. A population-based study demonstrated no difference in plasma levels of soluble thrombomodulin in patients with VTE and controls.[279]

EPCR is an endothelial transmembrane protein that promotes interaction between protein C and the thrombin–thrombomodulin complex (see Chap. 116). Changes in the endothelial EPCR have been suggested as being associated with an increased risk of VTE. A soluble form of EPCR lacking the transmembrane and intracellular domains is present in plasma of normal individuals over a broad range of concentrations (70–200 ng/mL), and the plasma level is strongly influenced by EPCR haplotype.[280–283] Soluble EPCR inhibits APC activity and fails to augment activation of protein C by thrombin–thrombomodulin complex. Hence, high levels of soluble EPCR have been suggested to promote thrombosis. Elevated concentrations of soluble EPCR have been observed in approximately 18 percent of healthy individuals bearing a relatively common haplotype.[281,283] In a study of 338 patients with VTE compared to controls, an H3 haplotype constituted a risk factor with ORs of 2.5 (95% CI 1.4–4.5) in men, but only 1.3 (95% CI 0.8–2.2) in women.[281] However, another study of a similar size did not confirm these findings.[282] Another gene alteration, a 23-bp insertion into exon 3 of the EPCR gene, has been suggested to confer a risk of VTE,[284,285] but another study failed to confirm this finding.[286]

Low levels of TFPI have also been implicated in the Leiden and other studies to constitute a weak risk factor of VTE.[287,288] Measuring plasma levels of TFPI poses several challenges. Circulating TFPI represents only 10 to 15 percent of the total TFPI in the intravascular space because most is bound to the endothelium. In plasma, some TFPI is lipoprotein associated, and this association can reduce TFPI functional activity.[289,290] Several polymorphisms in the TFPI gene have been described, but no firm association with venous thrombosis has been discerned. "TFPI resistance," presumably resulting from impaired inhibition of factors VIIa and Xa, reportedly was more prevalent in patients with venous thrombosis who had no other defects than in controls.[291,292] Tests of "TFPI resistance," such as APCR, measure the anticoagulant response of a test plasma to exogenously added TFPI in a prothrombin time performed with diluted tissue factor. Further studies are needed to confirm this finding and clarify the mechanism involved.

NEW METHODS FOR THROMBOPHILIA DISCOVERY

Discovery of thrombophilia risk factors is an important challenge for future genetic studies. Because of the strong evidence for a high degree of heredity in VTE and in causative hypercoagulability factors,[32,293–296] one would posit the existence of a significant number of common, mild genetic risk factors for VTE yet to be discovered. The goal of much future effort will be identifying common genetic risk factors for VTE and quantitating the amount of risk that such factors carry with the related goal of assessing gene–gene and gene–environment interactions (see "Interactions between Different Thrombophilias and between Thrombophilia and Environmental Factors" below).

Methods for future discovery of thrombophilias will draw heavily on the human genome, which will initially provide the necessary platform from which to proceed to discover genotypes underlying VTE.[297] Studies will use both the candidate gene approach in which suspected genes are studied in great detail[298] and the quantitative trait loci (QTL) approach[299,300] in which traits or phenotypes are linked to sites within the genome without an *a priori* prejudice for genetic locus. In the Genetic Analysis of Idiopathic Thrombosis project and in other studies using the QTL methodology, investigators have started to provide remarkable information about potential genetic influences on various plasma risk factors (e.g., protein C and protein S levels, APCR ratios, levels of various clotting factors) that affect venous thrombosis.[181,293,299–304]

INTERACTIONS BETWEEN DIFFERENT THROMBOPHILIAS AND BETWEEN THROMBOPHILIA AND ENVIRONMENTAL FACTORS

Gene–gene interactions or gene–environmental interactions play a profound role in the pathogenesis of venous thromboembolism (see Fig. 131–1). Multiple hereditary thrombophilic defects, or gene–gene interactions, are found in up to 15 percent of patients presenting with VTE.[20] Factor V Leiden has been reported in combination with protein C deficiency,[60,184,305] protein S deficiency,[61,62] antithrombin deficiency,[63] prothrombin 20210A mutation,[306–310] hyperhomocysteinemia,[155,311,312] and increased factor VIII and TAFI levels.[313,314] Except for one large study that failed to demonstrate an interaction of factor V Leiden and hyperhomocysteinemia or MTHFR-TT genotype,[315] all studies demonstrated that these combined defects were associated with an increased risk for VTE and/or its recurrence. Increased risks of thrombosis have been described in subjects with prothrombin G20210A and protein S deficiency[316] or hyperhomocysteinemia.[317] A pooled analysis of 8 case-control studies that included 2310 patients with VTE and 3204 controls showed that the OR for venous thrombosis in heterozygotes for both factor V Leiden and prothrombin G20210A was 20 (95% CI 11.1–36.1).[318] In another study based on retrospective analysis of 400 relatives of 226 probands with factor V Leiden and venous thrombosis, the estimated annual incidence rate of venous thrombosis was 4.8 percent in subjects heterozygous for both factor V Leiden and inherited deficiency of protein C or protein S.[319] In families with combined defects, thromboses occurred not only more frequently in carriers of two thrombophilias but also at an earlier age.[58,60–63,316]

Apart from the strong gene–gene interactions, gene–environment interactions are frequent and impart an augmented increased risk for thrombosis. Oral contraceptives and hormone replacement therapy substantially enhance the risk of VTE in women with factor V Leiden and other thrombophilias. Of women who develop VTE during pregnancy, 28 to 46 percent will carry the factor V mutation.[20,320–322] During pregnancy and puerperium, heterozygotes for factor V Leiden have a 3-fold increase in the relative risk of VTE and a 3.9-fold increased risk of its recurrence compared to women who are not carriers.[322] Several studies have examined the risks of thromboembolism in women with factor V Leiden using third-generation oral contraceptives. A highly significant increase of 30- to 80-fold in the OR for thrombosis was noted, with an absolute increase in risk from 0.8 to 28.5 per 10,000 women per year.[323,324] Even higher risks are seen in women homozygous for factor V Leiden mutation.[325] Among users of oral contraceptives, a 16-fold increased risk was observed in carriers of prothrombin G20210A compared to a 6-fold increased risk in noncarriers.[326] Carriers of prothrombin G20210A also have an excessive risk for cerebral vein thrombosis while using oral contraceptives (OR 149; 95% CI 31–711).[327] Deficiencies of antithrombin, protein C, and protein S also interact with the use of oral contraceptives and synergistically increase the risk of venous thrombosis[328] that occurs in many women within 6 months of starting the pills.[329] The joint effect of increased factor VIII levels (≥150% of normal) and use of oral contraceptives gave an OR of 10.3 (95% CI 3.7–28.9), which was indicative of an additive effect.[330]

Similar synergistic effects have been observed in women receiving hormone replacement therapy who are carriers of factor V Leiden or prothrombin G20210A.[331] Possible interactions between other thrombophilias and hormone replacement therapy have not been sufficiently explored.

Interesting interactions were described between hypofibrinolysis measured by clot lysis time and use of contraceptives, immobilization, and factor V Leiden, but not with prothrombin G20210A.[332]

ARTERIAL THROMBOSIS AND THROMBOPHILIAS

A moderate association between coronary artery disease and factor V Leiden or prothrombin G20210A was established. From a meta-analysis of 191 studies involving 66,155 cases with coronary artery disease and 91,307 controls, data on factor V Leiden and prothrombin G20210A were extracted for at least 5000 cases and 5000 controls. The per-allele relative risks for coronary artery disease of factor V Leiden and prothrombin G20210A were 1.17 (95% CI 1.08–1.28) and 1.31 (95% CI 1.12–1.52), respectively.[23] Coronary artery thrombosis has been notably associated with the factor V Leiden mutation in young women[27] and men[24] who also display other vascular risk factors. Hereditary deficiency of protein C or protein S also confers an increased risk of arterial thromboembolism.[26] In a family cohort study of 552 family members of probands with or without deficiencies of protein C, protein S, or antithrombin, the annual incidence of arterial thromboembolism was 0.34 percent (95% CI 0.23–0.49) in deficient subjects versus 0.17 percent (95% CI 0.09–0.28) in nondeficient subjects. Among subjects who were younger than age 55 years, the risks were 4.7-fold (95% CI 1.5–14.2) higher than in subjects older than age 55 years. Interestingly, antithrombin deficiency did not increase the risk.

Regarding the association between atherothrombosis and hyperhomocysteinemia, numerous retrospective case control studies have found a significant association with hyperhomocysteinemia after adjustment for confounding factors. For an increment of 5 μmol/L homocysteine in plasma, the ORs for coronary heart disease, cerebrovascular disease, and peripheral vascular disease were 1.6, 1.5, and 6.8, respectively.[333] Meta-analysis of 30 prospective or retrospective studies involving more than 5000 cases with ischemic heart disease and more than 1100 cases with stroke showed that a decrease of approximately 3 μmol/L in homocysteine level was associated with an 11 percent lower risk of ischemic heart disease and a 19 percent lower risk of stroke.[334] Also, an association, albeit modest, is observed between homozygosity for MTHFR C677T and cardiovascular disease. Meta-analysis of 40 case-control studies involving more than 11,000 patients with coronary heart disease and more than 12,000 controls yielded an OR of 1.16 (95% CI 1.05–1.28), and in the presence of a low folate status, an OR of 1.44 (95% CI 1.12–1.83).[335] Similar results were obtained in another meta-analysis that included patients with cerebrovascular and peripheral vascular diseases.[336] No increased risk was demonstrated in pooled data from North American study groups compared to European study groups. This difference was attributed to the lower intake of vitamin supplements and higher homocysteine levels for Europeans.[335]

Statistically significant associations with ischemic stroke were identified for factor V Leiden (OR 1.33; 95% CI 1.12–1.58), prothrombin G20210A (OR 1.44; 95% CI 1.11–1.86), and MTHFR C677T homozygosity (OR 1.24; 95% CI 1.08–1.42).[337] Among 860 patients with ischemic stroke, half of those who harbored factor V Leiden had multiple silent brain infarctions, whereas among age- and sex-matched controls these findings were infrequent.[338] The risk of ischemic stroke in young women harboring factor V Leiden or MTHFR C677TT was substantially accentuated in those who used contraceptives.[339]

An increased prevalence of thrombophilias and hyperhomocysteinemia was also found in patients with peripheral vascular disease.[340,341]

Taken together, it appears that thrombophilias confer a modest risk of arterial thromboses, which is highlighted particularly in relatively young individuals who smoke, use contraceptives, or are obese.

RECURRENT VENOUS THROMBOEMBOLISM IN THROMBOPHILIAS

All patients with venous thrombosis, whether or not they have a thrombophilia, are prone to recurrent thromboses for many years after the first incident. Recurrence is fatal in approximately 5 percent of patients,[342] and is associated with the postthrombotic syndrome in one-third of patients.[343]

The effect of inherited and acquired thrombophilias on recurrent VTE has been assessed in retrospective and prospective cohort studies. Table 131–4 shows that there are three categories of risk factors associated with recurrent VTE: patient-related risks, risks emanating from the nature of the thrombotic event, and variable risks related to the type of thrombophilia. Also shown in Table 131–4 are factors or conditions that decrease the chances of recurrent VTE. Regarding the thrombophilias, recurrent VTE is more common in patients with a deficiency of antithrombin, protein C, or protein S.[355–357] High risks were also observed in patients with double heterozygosity for factor V Leiden and prothrombin G20210A,[370] and for factor V Leiden heterozygosity associated with MTHFR C677T homozygosity (see Fig. 131–5).[371]

Hyperhomocysteinemia exerts an increased risk for recurrent venous thrombosis. In one study of 185 patients with a history of recurrent venous thrombosis, 46 (25%) had homocysteine concentrations above the 90th percentile. The adjusted OR (taking into account age, gender, and menopausal status) was 2.0 (95% CI 1.5–2.7).[372] In another study, the relative risk for recurrent venous thrombosis in patients with homocysteine levels above the 95th percentile was 2.7 (95% CI 1.3–5.8) compared to patients with homocysteine concentration below the 95th percentile. At 24-month followup, 19.2 percent of patients with hyperhomocysteinemia had developed a recurrent episode, compared to 6.3 percent of patients with the lower levels of homocysteine.[373] A less strong association between hyperhomocysteinemia and recurrence was observed in a population-based prospective study.[374]

Increased levels of factor VIII have been associated with an increased risk for recurrent venous thrombosis.[362] The likelihood of recurrence at 24-month followup was 37 percent in patients with factor VIII levels above the 90th percentile compared to 5 percent in patients with lower levels. A similar observation was made by the same authors regarding increased factor IX levels. When both factor VIII and factor IX levels were elevated, the relative risk of recurrence was 6.6-fold.[363] Various combinations of elevated levels of factors VIII, IX, and XI, and TAFI have been implicated in increasing the recurrence rate.[363,375] Whether or not factor V Leiden or prothrombin G20210A heterozygosities constitute risk factors for recurrent VTE has been disputed because of conflicting data. Nevertheless, two meta-analyses indicated that the ORs for recurrent VTE in factor Leiden heterozygotes were 1.39 and 1.41, respectively, and for prothrombin G20210A, 1.20 and 1.72, respectively.[359,360] Homozygotes for factor V Leiden have a significantly higher risk of recurrent VTE than heterozygotes (see Fig. 131–5).[358,359]

TABLE 131–4. Risks of Recurrent VTE

Increased Risks	Decreased Risks
Patient-Related Risks	
Male sex[344]	Female sex[344]
Increased age[345]	
Obesity[346]	
Persistence of provocation*[347,348]	Provocation was abolished[347,348]
Related to Thrombotic Event	
Proximal deep vein thrombosis[349]	Distal deep vein thrombosis
Pulmonary emboli[350]	Event occurred after surgery[364]
Unprovoked event[349]	Event occurred during pregnancy‡[365]
Residual thrombosis in ultrasound Doppler[351]	
Postthrombotic syndrome[352]	Event occurred while on female hormones‡[366]
Short duration of anticoagulant therapy[345]	
Increased D-dimer level after discontinuation of anticoagulants[353]	Use of compression stockings?[367]
	Related to anticoagulant treatment:
	Prolonged therapy[345]
	Intensity of anticoagulation[368]
	Adequacy/quality of anticoagulation[369]
Thrombophilia	
Presence of antiphospholipid antibodies[354]	
Deficiencies of antithrombin, protein C or protein S[355–357]	
Homozygous factor V Leiden[358]	
Heterozygous factor V Leiden†[359,360]	
Heterozygous prothrombin G20210A†[359,360]	
Combined inherited thrombophilias[357]	
Increased level of homocysteine[361]	
Increased level of factor VIII[362]	
Increased level of factor IX[363]	

*For example, cancer, immobility.
†Weak risk, if at all.
‡Risk is not decreased if a similar provocation is inflicted.

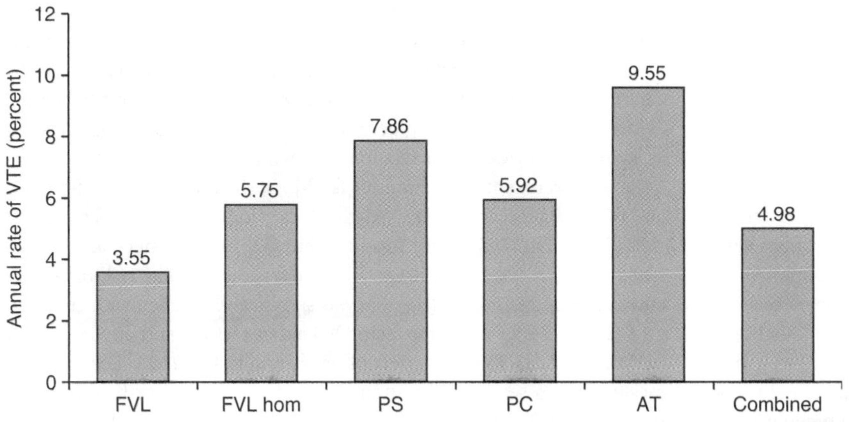

FIGURE 131–5. Annual rates of recurrent VTE in patients with inherited thrombophilias. Data were extracted from family studies as in Figure 131–3.[361–366] The bars represent average values. AT, antithrombin deficiency; combined, more than one thrombophilia; FVL, heterozygous factor V Leiden; FVL Hom, homozygous factor V Leiden; PS, protein S deficiency; PC, protein C deficiency.

HEREDITARY THROMBOPHILIAS DURING PREGNANCY AND PUERPERIUM

Hereditary thrombophilias have been associated with maternal VTE and with major complications of pregnancy, such as placental abruption, preeclampsia, early and late fetal loss, and intrauterine growth restriction (IUGR), all possibly related to compromised blood flow and thrombosis in the maternal–placental–fetal blood circulation.[376] Most studies that found an association of thrombophilia and these complications of pregnancy were case-control studies involving inherent methodologic problems, such as selection bias, relatively small numbers of cases, variable definitions of outcome events, and heterogeneity of controls. Series of prospective cohort studies, that usually yield more reliable results than case-control studies, casted doubt on some of the earlier described associations. The evidence for an association of pregnancy complications with thrombophilias is still robust for VTE and stillbirth, but for other complications of pregnancy, the evidence is only suggestive (severe preeclampsia), controversial (early fetal loss), and probably negative (preeclampsia, placental abruption, and IUGR).

VENOUS THROMBOEMBOLISM

Although VTE only occurs in approximately 1:1000 pregnancies, a rate which is 5 to 10 times higher than in nonpregnant women, pulmonary embolism is the major cause of maternal death.

Pregnancy can be regarded as an acquired temporary thrombophilic state. During gestation, factor VIII and fibrinogen levels increase, protein S levels decrease, fibrinolysis diminishes (because of increased PAI-1 and PAI-2 levels), and acquired APCR occurs. During pregnancy, venous flow in the lower limbs declines because of the enlarging uterus, while at the same time venous flow in the ovarian veins increases markedly. Most thrombotic episodes occur soon after childbirth (57%) or during the third trimester of pregnancy.[377] During pregnancy, thrombosis mainly affects the left iliofemoral vein (~80% of pregnancy-related venous thromboses), probably because of compression by the right iliac and ovarian arteries.

Approximately 50 percent of women with VTE detected during pregnancy or puerperium have an underlying hereditary thrombophilia in addition to the acquired risks.[378] The risk of VTE during pregnancy depends largely on the type of thrombophilia found. Several prospective and retrospective family studies found that VTE occurred in up to 25 percent of patients with antithrombin deficiency compared to 6.5 to 9.5 percent of patients with either protein S or protein C deficiency.[379–382] Regarding the risk conferred by factor V Leiden, a meta-analysis, yielded a rate of 2.1 percent for factor V Leiden carriers and four family studies found an average rate of 9.7 percent for factor V Leiden homozygotes.[383–387] A single retrospective family cohort study disclosed a 2.8 percent risk for carriers of the prothrombin G20210A mutation.[54] Compound heterozygotes for factor V Leiden and prothrombin G20210A carried a risk of approximately 4 percent.[387] Additional risks of VTE, such as a previous thrombotic event, familial history of VTE, obesity, age older than 35 years, cesarean section, varicose veins, and prolonged immobility, augment the VTE risk exerted by the thrombophilias.[378]

PLACENTAL ABRUPTION

The cause of placental abruption, a life-threatening condition for both mother and fetus, is unknown. Predisposing factors include pregnancy-induced hypertension, advanced age, great parity, chorioamnionitis, smoking, and previous abruption. In two prospective large-scale studies and a registry linkage study, the risk rate of abruption was 0.69 percent for factor V Leiden carriers, compared to 0.52 percent in noncarriers with a pooled OR of 1.43 (95% CI 0.75–2.72) (Table 131–5).[388–390]

INTRAUTERINE GROWTH RESTRICTION

IUGR is a significant cause of neonatal and maternal morbidity. It is usually defined as birth weight lower than the 10th percentile, but some

TABLE 131–5. Rates of IUGR, Preeclampsia, and Placental Abruption in Factor V Leiden Carriers and Noncarriers

	IUGR		Preeclampsia		Placental Abruption	
	Cases/No.	OR (95% CI)	Cases/No.	OR (95% CI)	Cases/No.	OR (95% CI)
Noncarriers	989/19,158 (5.2%)	1.09 (0.82–1.44)	476/15,918 (3.0%)	1.16 (0.77–1.74)	42/6961 (0.6%)	0.82 (0.20–3.41)
Carriers	54/963 (5.6%)		25/783 (3.2%)		2/404 (0.5%)	

IUGR, intrauterine growth restriction.

SOURCE: Data extracted from Murphy RP, Donoghue C, Nallen RJ, et al,[388] Lindqvist PG, Svensson PJ, Marsaal K, et al,[389] Clark P, Walker ID, Govan L, et al,[396] Dudding T, Heron J, Thakkinstian A, et al,[397] and Dizon-Townson D, Miller C, Sibai B, et al.[398]

studies refer to IUGR as birth weight below 5th percentile. A meta-analysis of mainly case-control studies[391] suggested that IUGR is associated with factor V Leiden, prothrombin G20210A, and homozygous MTHFR C677T.[376,392–395] However, different definitions of IUGR, different study methodologies, heterogeneity between studies, and suspected publication bias cast doubt on these results. In 5 large-scale prospective studies that included almost 20,000 pregnancies, the rate of IUGR was 5.6 percent among carriers of factor V Leiden compared to 5.2 percent among non carriers (see Table 131–5).[388,389,396–398] These and other studies have clearly established that IUGR is not associated with thrombophilia (an OR of 1.15 [CI 95% 0.95–1.39] for carriers of factor V Leiden).[397]

Multiple infarcts, thromboses of blood vessels, and perivillous fibrin deposition found in the placentas of thrombophilic women who had IUGR, preeclampsia, and abruption were suggested to constitute the link between thrombophilia and these adverse complications of pregnancy.[399] However, two other studies failed to find higher frequencies of pathologic findings in thrombophilic women with IUGR.[400,401] Also, ultrasound-guided measurements of blood flow parameters in the maternal-placental-fetal unit revealed no significant differences between women with or without thrombophilia.[402] Collectively, these data also indicate that there is not a significant association between IUGR and thrombophilias.

PREECLAMPSIA

Preeclampsia complicates 2 to 8 percent of pregnancies and is a major cause of maternal morbidity, prematurity, and neonatal death.[403] In preeclampsia, impaired trophoblastic implantation and diminished placental perfusion occur, leading to placental production of components that are released into the maternal circulation and cause widespread endothelial dysfunction. This process results in secretion of vasopressors with ensuing hypertension, activation of the coagulation system, reduced organ perfusion, increased vascular permeability, proteinuria, and edema.[404] One such component, a soluble fms-like tyrosine kinase 1 (sFlt1), is produced in excessive amounts by preeclamptic placents.[405] This factor is a splice variant of the vascular endothelial growth factor (VEGF) receptor that acts as a potent antagonist of VEGF. Increased plasma concentrations of sFlt1 and decreased concentrations of VEGF were found in women with preeclampsia, and administration of sFlt1 to pregnant rats induced hypertension, proteinuria, and glomerular endotheliosis, the hallmarks of preeclampsia.[405] What causes the increased synthesis of sFlt1 and whether other factors play a role in the pathogenesis of preeclampsia are unknown.

Thrombophilias have been implicated as possible causes or enhancers of preeclampsia. A systematic review of mostly case-control studies disclosed significant associations between preeclampsia and deficiencies of antithrombin, protein C, and protein S, and milder effects of heterozygous factor V Leiden, heterozygous prothrombin G20210A, homozygous MTHFR C677T, and hyperhomocysteinemia.[406] However, several large prospective studies have demonstrated no significant increase in the risk for preeclampsia in patients with factor V Leiden (see Table 131–5).[388,389,396–398] These studies indicated that the rate of preeclampsia was 3.2 percent among factor V Leiden carriers, compared to 3.0 percent in controls, yielding an OR of 1.16 (CI 95% 0.77–1.74). Hence, preeclampsia does not appear to be associated with thrombophilia. Nevertheless, carriership of factor V Leiden and homozygosity for MTHFR C677T are associated with severe preeclampsia.[390,407]

FETAL LOSS

Recurrent habitual abortions (three or more consecutive fetal losses) occur in 1 to 2 percent of women.[408] An early study showed that in patients with deficiencies of antithrombin, protein C, or protein S, the relative risk of habitual abortions was increased (OR 2.0; 95% CI 1.2–3.3).[409] The association between fetal loss and thrombophilia was examined by an extensive meta-analysis of 79 mainly case-control studies.[406] There are very few cohort studies addressing this issue, and hence the evidence for the relationship between fetal loss and thrombophilia is not as solid as the evidence for relationships with other pregnancy complications. For recurrent first trimester fetal loss, the meta-analysis disclosed an OR of 1.91 (95% CI 1.01–3.61) for factor V Leiden carriers, an OR of 2.70 (95% CI 1.37–5.34) for prothrombin G20210A carriers, and a nonsignificant OR for MTHFR C677T homozygotes.[406] The risk of nonrecurrent second trimester fetal loss was significantly higher, with an OR of 4.12 (95% CI 1.93–8.81) for factor V Leiden carriers and an OR of 8.60 (95% CI 2.18–33.95) for carriers of prothrombin G20210A. For third trimester fetal losses, a significant association was found for heterozygosities of factor V Leiden and prothrombin G20210A and for protein S deficiency. Data for other thrombophilias are scarce.

Stillbirth

Third-trimester fetal death is rare in developed countries and is associated with pregnancy-induced hypertension, diabetes mellitus, hydrops fetalis, uterine infections, and congenital anomalies. In many cases, the cause of stillbirth remains unexplained. Several case-control studies show that in such unexplained cases, the prevalence of thrombophilias is significantly increased[410–414] and that thrombosis and infarcts in the placenta are commonly observed.[411,412] The prevalence of thrombophilias in cases was 16 to 43 percent in cases, compared to 4 to 15 percent in controls.[411–413] Protein S deficiency and factor V Leiden predominated in the studies of unexplained stillbirth, with pooled ORs of 16.2 (95% CI 5.0–52) and 6.1 (95% CI 2.8–13.2), respectively.[414]

Prothrombin G20210A is significantly associated with stillbirth, yielding ORs of 2.3 (95% CI 1.3–4) and 3.3 (95% CI 1.1–10.3) in two studies.[411,413] Recurrent late fetal death also occurs more frequently in thrombophilic women.[415]

THROMBOPHILIA IN CHILDREN

VTE is rare in children. Its annual incidence in the general population is 0.07 to 0.14 per 10,000 children, 5.3 per 10,000 hospitalized children, and 24 per 10,000 neonates admitted to intensive care units.[416] VTE in children is usually secondary to a venous or arterial catheter, sepsis, cancer, and congenital heart disease, and occurs mostly at less than 1 year of age and during adolescence. A meta-analysis of 50 case-control studies or case series/registries disclosed that like in adults, deficiencies of antithrombin, protein C, protein S, factor V Leiden, prothrombin G20210A, or combined thrombophilias were significant risk factors, although more than 70 percent of the patients had at least one concomitant clinical risk factor.[416] The greatest risk was exerted by antithrombin deficiency with OR of 9.44 (95% CI 3.34–26.66) and the lowest risk was conferred by prothrombin G20210A with an OR of 2.64 (95% CI 1.6–4.4).

The proportion of children who develop recurrent VTE is 3 percent in neonates, 8 percent in older children, and 21 percent in children with unprovoked VTE.[416] The inherited thrombophilias (except for factor V Leiden), and increased levels of factor VIII are significant risk factors for recurrent VTE in children.[417,418]

Increased prevalence of inherited and acquired thrombophilias have been observed in children with cerebral sinus vein thrombosis,[419,420] and perinatal or early childhood ischemic stroke.[421,422] These entities are very rare, and thus no sizable case-control studies are available for assessing their association with thrombophilias. This issue is further complicated because each of the entities is associated with many other underlying disorders. Notwithstanding these limitations, for cerebral sinus vein thrombosis, an international collaborative study of 396 patients indicated that heterozygosity for prothrombin G20210A, but not for factor V Leiden, exerted a hazard ratio of 4.3 (95% CI 1.1–16.2; p=0.034).[423] Another international collaborative study is under way to determine the role of thrombophilias in perinatal and early childhood stroke.[422]

DIAGNOSIS

In unselected patients with VTE, testing for the more frequent thrombophilias (factor V Leiden, prothrombin G20210A, deficiency of protein C, protein S, or antithrombin, increased factor VIII levels) is expected to yield at least one thrombophilia in 30 percent (or more) of cases.[22] In selected patients, this proportion is 70 percent or even higher.[20] Table 131–3 lists in a decreasing order of priority the abnormal parameters that can be searched for. Tests for lupus anticoagulant, anticardiolipin, anti-β_2-glycoprotein I, and homocysteine concentration should be performed because of their relatively high frequency and known interaction with inherited thrombophilias. It should be borne in mind that acquired conditions can produce abnormal test results that may lead to an erroneous diagnosis of a thrombophilia (see Table 131–3).

A major reason for performing an extensive search for thrombophilia is that the finding(s) might influence therapy and prophylaxis. For example, finding one of the more severe thrombophilias (deficiency of protein C, protein S, or antithrombin, and antiphospholipid antibodies) or combined thrombophilias would entail prolonged anticoagulant therapy, and examination of immediate relatives for identification of the abnormal parameter(s) found in the proband. For affected relatives who are asymptomatic, strict prophylactic measures should be taken because of the relatively high absolute risk of VTE involved (see Fig. 131–3),[51] and for those relatives who have had VTE, anticoagulant therapy should be resumed because of the great risk of recurrent VTE (see Fig. 131–5).

Who should be tested and which tests should be performed are debatable issues. Addressing these issues can be facilitated by evaluating the following questions: (1) What is the likelihood a given patient will be affected? (2) Which are the tests that are predicted to yield abnormal results more frequently? (3) What is the likelihood of recurrence if a given thrombophilia is found? (4) What is the cost? (5) Will abnormal results induce anxiety in a given patient and family? (6) Will abnormal results affect health insurance? and (7) Will the finding of a mild thrombophilia such as heterozygosity for factor V Leiden or prothrombin G20210A alter the health behavior of the patient or family members? Patients should be involved in these considerations and in the decision on whether or not testing for thrombophilia should be performed.

Based in part on published recommendations (levels 1 and 2),[424,425] reviews of other experts,[426,427] and the experience of the authors of this chapter as reviewed elsewhere,[41] the patients who meet one of the following criteria should be tested for all thrombophilias included in Table 131–3: (1) unprovoked VTE; (2) recurrent thrombotic events; (3) provoked VTE in patients younger than age 50 years; (4) VTE provoked by pregnancy, oral contraceptives, or hormone replacement therapy; (5) a family history of VTE; (6) cerebral or visceral vein thrombosis; (7) three or more consecutive unexplained fetal losses during the first trimester of gestation, one or more fetal losses during the second or third trimester, or one or more stillbirths.

Testing for thrombophilia is not necessary for patients who had distal vein thrombosis following trauma or surgery because such patients have a very low recurrence rate (1.5% per year).[428] Similarly, patients whose event was associated with active cancer or an intravascular device should not be tested.

The optimal time for performing tests in most patients is 6 months after the thrombotic event, when the decision as to whether or not treatment should be continued must be made. The results of examinations performed earlier can be misleading, because thrombosis itself can cause low antithrombin levels and elevated levels of factor VIII. At 6 months, while the patient is still undergoing oral anticoagulant therapy, all tests can be performed except for proteins C and S levels, which are decreased because of oral anticoagulant therapy. The patients can then be switched to treatment with low-molecular-weight heparin for 2 weeks and subsequently tested for protein C activity and the level of free protein S antigen. Upon completion of the evaluation and assessment of the risks of thrombosis recurrence and bleeding, a decision can be made regarding discontinuation of treatment or its extension (see "Therapy" below).

In patients who are younger than age 50 years and who had arterial thrombosis with no atherosclerotic risk factors or evidence for atherosclerosis, the following tests should be performed: lupus anticoagulant, anticardiolipin, β_2-glycoprotein I, protein C, protein S, and antithrombin.

THERAPY

Patients with a known thrombophilia who present with VTE should be treated with a standard regimen of heparin overlapped with warfarin until an international normalized ratio of 2.0 to 3.0 is obtained on 2 consecutive days (see Chap. 134). This regimen is sufficient for the prevention of skin necrosis, which may occur during the initiation of warfarin therapy in patients with a protein C deficiency. The chief goal of therapy is to prevent recurrent VTE, because it is fatal in 5 percent of cases,[342] it increases the risk of venous insufficiency,[343] and it imposes prolonged anticoagulant therapy, which carries a significant risk of bleeding. Warfarin therapy reduces the risk of recurrence by 90 to 95 percent, but the annual risk of fatal hemorrhage is 0.25 percent.[429] Consequently, the benefits and hazards associated with prolonging the duration of therapy should be carefully evaluated and discussed with each patient, taking into account the patient's preference and the clinical and laboratory risk factors that might increase the risk of recurrent VTE or hemorrhage. Comprehensive, evidence-based guidelines for therapy cannot yet be formulated, but several reviews have provided reasonable approaches to treatment that are based partly on evidence and partly on expert views.[41,430–434]

During the initiation of therapy, patients are classified according to their likelihood of developing a recurrent event (see Table 131–4). Patients with the lowest likelihood are those who present with distal vein thrombosis after surgery or trauma. Such patients are treated for 3 months by anticoagulants, and no tests for thrombophilia are performed because of a very low recurrence rate (see "Diagnosis" above). All other patients are treated with warfarin for 6 months,[41,432–435] after which they are examined for the presence of thrombophilia (as outlined in "Diagnosis" above) and assessed for risks of recurrence and hemorrhage. Based on this assessment, treatment is discontinued, continued for 6 to 18 more months, or continued indefinitely. Table 131–6 summarizes possible indications for therapy extension or indefinite therapy.

All patients with venous thrombosis of the legs should wear fitted compression stockings for at least 2 years. This measure reduces the incidence of the postthrombotic syndrome by 50 percent.[436] Pregnant patients with thrombophilia who develop VTE should be treated similarly to pregnant women without a thrombophilia. Detailed guidelines are available.[437–439] The preferable anticoagulant is low-molecular-weight heparin, which carries a much smaller risk than heparin for heparin-induced thrombocytopenia, osteoporosis, or bleeding. Warfarin should be avoided because of embryopathy that can occur between 6 and 12 weeks of gestation and because of central nervous

TABLE 131–6. Possible Indications for Extension of Anticoagulant Therapy Beyond 6 Months in Patients with Thrombophilia

Length of Extension	Indication
6–18 months*	Elevated factor VIII level
	Increased level of D-dimer†
	Active cancer
	Severe venous insufficiency
	Iliofemoral venous thrombosis
	Residual thrombosis detected by ultrasound Doppler
	Persistence of inciting cause‡
Indefinite	Life-threatening event
	Cerebral vein thrombosis§
	Visceral vein thrombosis
	Recurrent event
	Deficiencies of antithrombin, protein C, or protein S
	Combined thrombophilias
	Presence of antiphospholipid antibodies

*An extension should be carefully evaluated and probably not applied in patients with a great risk of bleeding, for example, age >70 years, history of hemorrhagic stroke or gastrointestinal bleeding, renal failure, or poorly controlled anticoagulant therapy.

†In samples taken 3 to 4 weeks after cessation of anticoagulation therapy.

‡Examples include immobilization, absolute necessity for female hormone, estrogen modulation therapy.

§The length of therapy is disputed.

system abnormalities that can be observed during all trimesters.[438,439] The dose of low-molecular-weight heparin used throughout pregnancy depends on the patient's weight at the beginning of pregnancy.[437] No monitoring by measurements of anti-factor X levels is necessary unless renal failure is present. Heparin treatment should be given throughout pregnancy and for 6 weeks following delivery, and should not last less than 6 months (see Chap. 134).

Specific therapies are available for some thrombophilic disorders. Antithrombin concentrates, including a recombinant preparation, can be administered for surgery, major trauma, and at the time of delivery in patients with antithrombin deficiency.[440–443] Protein C and APC concentrates are available and can be useful in infants or children with homozygous protein C deficiency or in heterozygous subjects during surgery or other major stresses.[444–446]

PROPHYLAXIS

For thrombophilic patients who had VTE, prophylactic measures should be part of their therapy from its initiation. Measures include weight loss (if necessary), avoiding immobility, and discontinuation of female hormone therapy and smoking (if relevant). Following diagnosis of a thrombophilia, the patient must be educated regarding thrombophilias, future risks of thrombosis (during surgery, air travel, pregnancy, trauma), risk of bleeding during anticoagulant therapy, familial implications, and need for prophylactic therapy during high-risk situations. Followup is advisable for reiteration of prophylactic measures and for updating the patient about new tests and therapy. If gross varicose veins are present, surgery should be considered under appropriate prophylaxis with heparin.

Low-molecular-weight heparin should be given at prophylactic doses prior to surgery, during periods of immobilization, and possibly prior to air travel that will last longer than 4 hours. Use of an antithrombin concentrate should be considered during surgery and delivery in patients with antithrombin deficiency.

Prophylactic oral anticoagulant therapy usually is not warranted in subjects who have not suffered a thrombotic event but who are found to have thrombophilia because of family testing or some other reason. In this instance, the risk of hemorrhage because of warfarin outweighs the risk of thrombosis. However, during exposure to risk periods, use of prophylactic anticoagulant therapy has been suggested to decrease the occurrence of venous thrombosis.[447]

Women who had VTE while receiving hormonal therapy or during pregnancy have a higher risk of recurrence during pregnancy and should receive prophylactic therapy by low-molecular-weight heparin throughout pregnancy and for 6 weeks postpartum. Pregnant women in whom the prior VTE was unprovoked and unrelated to pregnancy or female hormones, or who were found to harbor a thrombophilia, should be treated similarly. Pregnant women without prior VTE who have either protein C, protein S, or antithrombin deficiency should also be considered for such treatment because of the high rate of VTE and fetal loss during pregnancies.[379,448] Patients without a prior VTE who are carriers of factor V Leiden or prothrombin G20210A combined with other risk factors, for example, age >35 years and obesity, should also be considered to receive low-molecular-weight heparin therapy from the third trimester until 6 weeks after delivery. In patients with thrombophilia who had an adverse outcome of pregnancy, such as IUGR, less than three consecutive fetal losses during the first trimester, preeclampsia, and placental abruption, therapy with low-molecular-weight heparin treatment is not supported by firm evidence. Until results of controlled studies will be available, it seems reasonable to use low-molecular-weight heparin prophylaxis throughout pregnancy and 6 weeks postpartum in women with thrombophilia who had three or more consecutive unexplained fetal losses during the first trimester, late pregnancy fetal loss, stillbirth, or severe preeclampsia.

REFERENCES

1. Egeberg O: Inherited antithrombin deficiency causing thrombophilia. *Thromb Diath Haemorrh* 13:516, 1963.
2. Beck EA, Charache P, Jackson DP: A new inherited coagulation disorder caused by an abnormal fibrinogen ("fibrinogen Baltimore"). *Nature* 208:143, 1965.
3. Stenflo J, Fernlund P, Egan W, Roepstorff P: Vitamin K-dependent modifications of glutamic acid residues in prothrombin. *Proc Natl Acad Sci U S A* 71:2730, 1974.
4. Griffin JH, Evatt B, Zimmerman TS, Kleiss AJ: Deficiency of protein C in congenital thrombotic disease. *J Clin Invest* 68:1370, 1981.
5. Schwarz HP, Fischer M, Hopmeier P, et al: Plasma protein S deficiency in familial thrombotic disease. *Blood* 64:1297, 1984.
6. Comp PC, Nixon RR, Cooper MR, Esmon CT: Familial protein S deficiency is associated with recurrent thrombosis. *J Clin Invest* 74:2082, 1984.
7. Comp PC, Esmon CT: Recurrent venous thromboembolism in patients with a partial deficiency of protein S. *N Engl J Med* 311:1525, 1984.
8. Koeleman BP, Reitsma PH, Bertina RM: Familial thrombophilia: A complex genetic disorder. *Semin Hematol* 34:256, 1997.
9. Dahlback B, Carlsson M, Svensson PJ: Familial thrombophilia due to a previously unrecognized mechanism characterized by poor anticoagulant response to activated protein C: Prediction of a cofactor to activated protein C. *Proc Natl Acad Sci U S A* 90:1004, 1993.
10. Svensson PJ, Dahlbäck B: Resistance to activated protein C as a basis for venous thrombosis. *N Engl J Med* 330:517, 1994.
11. Bertina RM, Koeleman BPC, Koster T, et al: Mutation in blood coagulation factor V associated with resistance to activated protein C. *Nature* 369:64, 1994.
12. Greengard JS, Sun X, Xu X, et al: Activated protein C resistance caused by Arg506Gln mutation in factor Va. *Lancet* 343:1361, 1994.
13. Voorberg J, Roelse J, Koopman R, et al: Association of idiopathic venous thromboembolism with single point-mutation at Arg506 of factor V. *Lancet* 343:1535, 1994.

14. Bienvenu T, Ankri A, Chadefaux B, et al: Elevated total plasma homocysteine, a risk factor for thrombosis. Relation to coagulation and fibrinolytic parameters. *Thromb Res* 70:123, 1993.
15. McCully KS: Vascular pathology of homocystinemia: Implications for the pathogenesis of arteriosclerosis. *Am J Pathol* 56:111, 1969.
16. Poort SR, Rosendaal FR, Reitsma PH, Bertina RM: A common genetic variation in the 3′-untranslated region of the prothrombin gene is associated with elevated plasma prothrombin levels and an increase in venous thrombosis. *Blood* 88:3698, 1996.
17. Koster T, Blann AD, Briët E, et al: Role of clotting factor VIII in effect of von Willebrand factor on occurrence of deep-vein thrombosis. *Lancet* 345:152, 1995.
18. Kamphuisen PW, Lensen R, Houwing-Duistermatt JJ, et al: Heritability of elevated factor VIII antigen levels in factor V Leiden families with thrombophilia. *Br J Haematol* 109:519, 2000.
19. Schambeck CM, Hinney K, Haubitz I, et al: Familial clustering of high factor VIII levels in patients with venous thromboembolism. *Arterioscler Thromb Vasc Biol* 21:289, 2001.
20. Salomon O, Steinberg DM, Zivelin A, et al: Single and combined prothrombotic factors in patients with idiopathic venous thromboembolism—Prevalence and risk assessment. *Arterioscler Thromb Vasc Biol* 19:511, 1999.
21. Bertina RM: Genetic approach to thrombophilia. *Thromb Haemost* 86:92, 2001.
22. Seligsohn U, Zivelin A: Thrombophilia as a multigenic disorder. *Thromb Haemost* 78:297, 1997.
23. Ye Z, Liu EH, Higgins JP, et al: Seven haemostatic gene polymorphisms in coronary disease: Meta-analysis of 66,155 cases and 91,307 controls. *Lancet* 367:651, 2006.
24. Inbal A, Freimark D, Modan B, et al: Synergistic effects of prothrombotic polymorphisms and atherogenic factors on the risk of myocardial infarction in young males. *Blood* 93:2186, 1999.
25. Martinelli N, Trabetti E, Pinotti M, et al: Combined effect of hemostatic gene polymorphisms and the risk of myocardial infarction in patients with advanced coronary atherosclerosis. *PLoS ONE* 3:e1523, 2008.
26. Mahmoodi BK, Brouwer JL, Veeger NJ, van der Meer J: Hereditary deficiency of protein C or protein S confers increased risk of arterial thromboembolic events at a young age: Results from a large family cohort study. *Circulation* 118:1659, 2008.
27. Rosendaal FR, Siscovick DS, Schwartz SM, et al: Factor V Leiden (resistance to activated protein C) increases the risk of myocardial infarction in young women. *Blood* 89:2817, 1997.
28. Zoller B, Holm J, Svensson P, Dahlback B: Elevated levels of prothrombin activation fragment 1 + 2 in plasma from patients with heterozygous Arg506 to Gln mutation in the factor V gene (APC-resistance) and/or inherited protein S deficiency. *Thromb Haemost* 75:270, 1996.
29. Simioni P, Scarano L, Gavasso S, et al: Prothrombin fragment 1+2 and thrombin-antithrombin complex levels in patients with inherited APC resistance due to factor V Leiden mutation. *Br J Haematol* 92:435, 1996.
30. Souto JC, Almasy L, Borrell M, et al: Genetic susceptibility to thrombosis and its relationship to physiological risk factors: The GAIT study. Genetic Analysis of Idiopathic Thrombophilia. *Am J Hum Genet* 67:1452, 2000.
31. Ariens RA, De Lange M, Snieder H, et al: Activation markers of coagulation and fibrinolysis in twins: Heritability of the prethrombotic state. *Lancet* 359:667, 2002.
32. Heit JA, Phelps MA, Ward SA, et al: Familial segregation of venous thromboembolism. *J Thromb Haemost* 2:731, 2004.
33. Brinsuk M, Tank J, Luft FC: Heritability of venous function in humans. *Arterioscler Thromb Vasc Biol* 24:207, 2004.
34. Kyrle PA, Minar L, Bialonczyk C, et al: The risk of recurrent venous thromboembolism in men and women. *N Engl J Med* 350:2558, 2004.
35. Prandoni P, Bilora F, Marchen A, et al: An association between atherosclerosis and venous thrombosis. *N Engl J Med* 348:1435, 2003.
36. Chou J, Mackman N, Merrill-Skoloff G, et al: Hematopoietic cell-derived microparticle tissue factor contributes to fibrin formation during thrombus propagation. *Blood* 104:3190, 2004.
37. Esmon CT: Coagulation and inflammation. *J Endotoxin Res* 9:192, 2003.
38. Levi M, Van der Poll T, Buller HR: Bidirectional relation between inflammation and coagulation. *Circulation* 109:2698, 2004.
39. Fox EA, Kahn SR: The relationship between inflammation and venous thrombosis. A systematic review of clinical studies. *Thromb Haemost* 94:362, 2005.
40. Christiansen SC, Naess IA, Cannegieter SC, et al: Inflammatory cytokines as risk factors for a first venous thrombosis: A prospective population-based study. *PLoS Med* 3:e334, 2006.
41. Seligsohn U, Lubetsky A: Genetic susceptibility to venous thrombosis. *N Engl J Med* 344:1222, 2001.
42. Prochazka M, Happach C, Marsal K, et al: Factor V Leiden in pregnancies complicated by placental abruption. *Br J Obstet Gynaecol* 110:462, 2003.
43. Rosendaal FR, Doggen CJ, Zivelin A, et al: Geographic distribution of the 20210 G to A prothrombin variant. *Thromb Haemost* 79:706, 1998.
44. Zivelin A, Mor-Cohen R, Kovalsky V, et al: Prothrombin 20210G>A is an ancestral prothrombotic mutation that occurred in whites approximately 24,000 years ago. *Blood* 107:4666, 2006.
45. Lindqvist PG, Svensson PJ, Dahlback B, Marsal K: Factor V Q^{506} mutation (activated protein C resistance) associated with reduced intrapartum blood loss: A possible evolutionary selection mechanism. *Thromb Haemost* 79:69, 1998.
46. Lindqvist PG, Zoller B, Dahlback B: Improved hemoglobin status and reduced menstrual blood loss among female carriers of factor V Leiden: An evolutionary advantage? *Thromb Haemost* 86:1122, 2001.
47. Corral J, Iniesta JA, Gonzalez-Conejero R, et al: Polymorphisms of clotting factors modify the risk for primary intracranial hemorrhage. *Blood* 97:2979, 2001.
48. Nichols WC, Amano K, Cacheris PM, et al: Moderation of hemophilia A phenotype by the factor V R506Q mutation. *Blood* 88:1183, 1996.
49. Beauchamp NJ, Dykes AC, Parikh N, et al: The prevalence of, and molecular defects underlying, inherited protein S deficiency in the general population. *Br J Haematol* 125:647, 2004.
50. Juul K, Tybjaerg-Hansen A, Schnohr P, Nordestgaard BG: Factor V Leiden and the risk for venous thromboembolism in the adult Danish population. *Ann Intern Med* 140:330, 2004.
51. Lijfering WM, Brouwer JL, Veeger NJ, et al: Selective testing for thrombophilia in patients with first venous thrombosis. Results from a retrospective family cohort study on absolute thrombotic risk for currently known thrombophilic defects in 2479 relatives. *Blood* 113:5314, 2009.
52. Middeldorp S, Meinardi JR, Koopman MM, et al: A prospective study of asymptomatic carriers of the factor V Leiden mutation to determine the incidence of venous thromboembolism. *Ann Intern Med* 135:322, 2001.
53. Simioni P, Tormene D, Prandoni P, et al: Incidence of venous thromboembolism in asymptomatic family members who are carriers of factor V Leiden: A prospective cohort study. *Blood* 99:1938, 2002.
54. Bank I, Libourel EJ, Middeldorp S, et al: Prothrombin 20210A mutation: A mild risk factor for venous thromboembolism but not for arterial thrombotic disease and pregnancy-related complications in a family study. *Arch Intern Med* 164:1932, 2004.
55. Vossen CY, Conard J, Fontcuberta J, et al: Risk of a first venous thrombotic event in carriers of a familial thrombophilic defect. The European Prospective Cohort on Thrombophilia (EPCOT). *J Thromb Haemost* 3:459, 2005.
56. Couturaud F, Kearon C, Leroyer C, et al: Incidence of venous thromboembolism in first-degree relatives of patients with venous thromboembolism who have factor V Leiden. *Thromb Haemost* 96:744, 2006.
57. Coppens M, van de Poel MH, Bank I, et al: A prospective cohort study on the absolute incidence of venous thromboembolism and arterial cardiovascular disease in asymptomatic carriers of the prothrombin 20210A mutation. *Blood* 108:2604, 2006.
58. Brouwer JL, Veeger NJ, Kluin-Nelemans HC, van der Meer J: The pathogenesis of venous thromboembolism: Evidence for multiple interrelated causes. *Ann Intern Med* 145:807, 2006.
59. De Stefano V, Martinelli I, Mannucci PM, et al: The risk of recurrent deep venous thrombosis among heterozygous carriers of both factor V Leiden and the G20210A prothrombin mutation. *N Engl J Med* 341:801, 1999.
60. Koeleman BPC, Reitsma PH, Allaart CF, Bertina RM: Activated protein C resistance as an additional risk factor for thrombosis in protein C deficient families. *Blood* 84:1031, 1994.
61. Zoller B, Berntsdotter A, Garcia de Frutos P, Dahlback B: Resistance to activated protein C as an additional genetic risk factor in hereditary deficiency of protein S. *Blood* 85:3518, 1995.
62. Koeleman PBC, Van Rumpt D, Hamulyak K, et al: Factor V Leiden: An additional risk factor for thrombosis in protein S deficient families? *Thromb Haemost* 74:580, 1995.
63. van Boven HH, Vandenbroucke JP, Briet E, Rosendaal FR: Gene-gene and gene-environment interactions determine risk of thrombosis in families with inherited antithrombin deficiency. *Blood* 94:2590, 1999.
64. Oosting JD, Derksen RHWM, Bobbink IWG, et al: Antiphospholipid antibodies directed against a combination of phospholipids with prothrombin, protein C, or protein S: An explanation for their pathogenic mechanism? *Blood* 81:2618, 1993.
65. Zivelin A, Gitel S, Griffin JH, et al: Extensive venous and arterial thrombosis associated with an inhibitor to activated protein C. *Blood* 94:895, 1999.
66. Sun X, Evatt B, Griffin JH: Blood coagulation factor Va abnormality associated with resistance to activated protein C in venous thrombophilia. *Blood* 83:3120, 1994.
67. Heeb MJ, Kojima Y, Greengard JS, Griffin JH: Activated protein C resistance: Molecular mechanisms based on studies using purified Gln506-factor V. *Blood* 85:3405, 1995.
68. Rosing J, Hoekema L, Nicolaes GA, et al: Effects of protein S and factor Xa on peptide bond cleavages during inactivation of factor Va and factor VaR506Q by activated protein C. *J Biol Chem* 270:27852, 1995.
69. Gale AJ, Xu X, Pellequer JL, et al: Interdomain engineered disulfide bond permitting elucidation of mechanisms of inactivation of coagulation factor Va by activated protein C. *Protein Sci* 11:2091, 2002.
70. Shen L, Dahlback B: Factor V and protein S as synergistic cofactors to activated protein C in degradation of factor VIIIa. *J Biol Chem* 269:18735, 1994.
71. Dahlback B, Hildebrand B: Inherited resistance to activated protein C is corrected by anticoagulant cofactor activity found to be a property of factor V. *Proc Natl Acad Sci U S A* 91:1396, 1994.
72. Nicolaes GA, Dahlback B: Factor V and thrombotic disease: Description of a Janus-faced protein. *Arterioscler Thromb Vasc Biol* 22:530, 2002.
73. Steen M, Norstrom EA, Tholander A-L, et al: Functional characterization of factor V-Ile359Thr: A novel mutation associated with thrombosis. *Blood* 103:3381, 2004.
74. Williamson D, Brown K, Luddington R, et al: Factor V Cambridge: A new mutation (Arg^{306}→Thr) associated with resistance to activated protein C. *Blood* 91:1140, 1998.
75. Chan WP, Lee CK, Kwong YL, et al: A novel mutation of Arg^{306} of factor V gene in Hong Kong Chinese. *Blood* 91:1135, 1998.

76. Franco RF, Maffei FH, Lourenco D, et al: Factor VArg^{306}→Thr (factor V Cambridge) and factor V Arg^{306}→Gly mutations in venous thrombotic disease. *Br J Haematol* 103:888, 1998.
77. Norstrom E, Thorelli E, Dahlback B: Functional characterization of recombinant FV Hong Kong and FV Cambridge. *Blood* 100:524, 2002.
78. Bernardi F, Faioni EM, Castoldi E, et al: A factor V genetic component differing from factor V R506Q contributes to the activated protein C resistance phenotype. *Blood* 90:1552, 1997.
79. Castoldi E, Brugge JM, Nicolaes GA, et al: Impaired APC cofactor activity of factor V plays a major role in the APC resistance associated with the factor V Leiden (R506Q) and R2 (H1299R) mutations. *Blood* 103:4173, 2004.
80. Griffin JH: Blood coagulation. The thrombin paradox [see news; comment]. *Nature* 378:337, 1995.
81. Gruber A, Griffin JH: Direct detection of activated protein C in blood from human subjects. *Blood* 79:2340, 1992.
82. Okajima K, Koga S, Kaji M, et al: Effect of protein C and activated protein C on coagulation and fibrinolysis in normal human subjects. *Thromb Haemost* 63:48, 1990.
83. Heeb MJ, Gruber A, Griffin JH: Identification of divalent metal ion-dependent inhibition of activated protein C by alpha 2-macroglobulin and alpha 2-antiplasmin in blood and comparisons to inhibition of factor Xa, thrombin, and plasmin. *J Biol Chem* 266:17606, 1991.
84. Fernandez JA, Petaja J, Gruber A, Griffin JH: Activated protein C correlates inversely with thrombin levels in resting healthy individuals. *Am J Hematol* 56:29, 1997.
85. Espana F, Vaya A, Mira Y, et al: Low level of circulating activated protein C is a risk factor for venous thromboembolism. *Thromb Haemost* 86:1368, 2001.
86. Greengard JS, Eichinger S, Griffin JH, Bauer KA: Variability of thrombosis among homozygous siblings with resistance to activated protein C due to an Arg→Gln mutation in the gene for factor V. *N Engl J Med* 331:1559, 1994.
87. Desmarais S, De Moerloose P, Reber G, et al: Resistance to activated protein C in an unselected population of patients with pulmonary embolism. *Lancet* 347:1374, 1996.
88. Turkstra F, Karemaker R, Kuijer PMM, et al: Is the prevalence of the factor V Leiden mutation in patients with pulmonary embolism and deep vein thrombosis really different? *Thromb Haemost* 81:345, 1999.
89. de Moerloose P, Reber G, Perrier A, et al: Prevalence of factor V Leiden and prothrombin G20210A mutations in unselected patients with venous thromboembolism. *Br J Haematol* 110:125, 2000.
90. Milio G, Siragusa S, Mina C, et al: Superficial venous thrombosis: Prevalence of common genetic risk factors and their role on spreading to deep veins. *Thromb Res* 123:194, 2008.
91. Rossi E, Za T, Ciminello A, et al: The risk of symptomatic pulmonary embolism due to proximal deep venous thrombosis differs in patients with different types of inherited thrombophilia. *Thromb Haemost* 99:1030, 2008.
92. Munkvad S, Jorgensen M: Resistance to activated protein C: A common anticoagulant deficiency in patients with venous leg ulceration. *Br J Dermatol* 134:296, 1996.
93. Hafner J, Kuhne A, Schar B, et al: Factor V Leiden mutation in postthrombotic and non-postthrombotic venous ulcers. *Arch Dermatol* 137:599, 2001.
94. Janssen HL, Meinardi JR, Vleggaar FP, et al: Factor V Leiden mutation, prothrombin gene mutation, and deficiencies in coagulation inhibitors associated with Budd-Chiari syndrome and portal vein thrombosis: Results of a case control study. *Blood* 96:2364, 2000.
95. Bombeli T, Basic A, Fehr J: Prevalence of hereditary thrombophilia in patients with thrombosis in different venous systems. *Am J Hematol* 70:126, 2002.
96. Linnemann B, Meister F, Schwonberg J, et al: Hereditary and acquired thrombophilia in patients with upper extremity deep-vein thrombosis. Results from the MAISTHRO registry. *Thromb Haemost* 100:440, 2008.
97. Dentali F, Crowther M, Ageno W: Thrombophilic abnormalities, oral contraceptives, and risk of cerebral vein thrombosis: A meta-analysis. *Blood* 107:2766, 2006.
98. Dentali F, Galli M, Gianni M, Ageno W: Inherited thrombophilic abnormalities and risk of portal vein thrombosis. A meta-analysis. *Thromb Haemost* 99:675, 2008.
99. Middeldorp S, Henkens CMA, Koopman MMW, et al: The incidence of venous thromboembolism in family members of patients with factor V Leiden mutation and venous thrombosis. *Ann Intern Med* 128:15, 1998.
100. Rosendaal FR: Venous thrombosis: A multicausal disease. *Lancet* 353:1167, 1999.
101. Ridker PM, Glynn RJ, Miletich JP, et al: Age-specific incidence rates of venous thromboembolism among heterozygous carriers of factor V Leiden mutation. *Ann Intern Med* 126:528, 1997.
102. Ridker PM, Hennekens CH, Lindpaintner K, et al: Mutation in the gene coding for coagulation factor V and the risk of myocardial infarction, stroke, and venous thrombosis in apparently healthy men. *N Engl J Med* 332:912, 1995.
103. Price DT, Ridker PM: Factor V Leiden mutation and the risks for thromboembolic disease: A clinical perspective. *Ann Intern Med* 127:895, 1997.
104. Martinelli I, Cattaneo M, Taioli E, et al: Genetic risk factors for superficial vein thrombosis. *Thromb Haemost* 82:1215, 1999.
105. Rosendaal FR, Koster T, Vandenbroucke JP, Reitsma PH: High risk of thrombosis in patients homozygous for factor V Leiden (activated protein C resistance). *Blood* 85:1504, 1995.
106. Juul K, Tybjaerg-Hansen A, Steffensen R, et al: Factor V Leiden: The Copenhagen City Heart Study and 2 meta-analyses. *Blood* 100:3, 2002.
107. Mari D, Mannucci PM, Duca F, et al: Mutant factor V (Arg506Gln) in healthy centenarians. *Lancet* 347:1044, 1996.
108. Heijmans BT, Westendorp RGJ, Knook DL, et al: The risk of mortality and the factor V Leiden mutation in a population-based cohort. *Thromb Haemost* 80:607, 1998.
109. Hille ETM, Westendorp RGJ, Vandenbroucke JP, Rosendaal FR: Mortality and causes of death in families with the factor V Leiden mutation (resistance to activated protein C). *Blood* 89:1963, 1997.
110. Rees DC, Liu YT, Cox MJ, et al: Factor V Leiden and thermolabile methylenetetrahydrofolate reductase in extreme old age. *Thromb Haemost* 78:1357, 1997.
111. Ehrenforth S, Nemes L, Mannhalter C, et al: Impact of environmental and hereditary risk factors on the clinical manifestation of thrombophilia in homozygous carriers of factor V:G1691A. *J Thromb Haemost* 2:430, 2004.
112. Tripodi A, Negri B, Bertina RM, Mannucci PM: Screening for the FV: Q506 mutation: Evaluation of thirteen plasma-based methods for their diagnostic efficacy in comparison with DNA analysis. *Thromb Haemost* 77:436, 1997.
113. De Visser MCH, Rosendaal FR, Bertina RM: A reduced sensitivity for activated protein C in the absence of factor V Leiden increases the risk of venous thrombosis. *Blood* 93:1271, 1999.
114. Rodeghiero F, Tosetto A: Activated protein C resistance and factor V Leiden mutation are independent risk factors for venous thromboembolism. *Ann Intern Med* 130:643, 1999.
115. Fisher M, Fernandez JA, Ameriso SF, et al: Activated protein C resistance in ischemic stroke not due to factor V arginine506→glutamine mutation. *Stroke* 27:1163, 1996.
116. Van der Bom JG, Bots ML, Haverkate F, et al: Reduced response to activated protein C is associated with increased risk for cerebrovascular disease. *Ann Intern Med* 125:265, 1996.
117. Le DT, Griffin JH, Greengard JS, et al: Use of a generally applicable tissue factor-dependent factor V assay to detect activated protein C resistant factor Va in patients receiving warfarin and in patients with a lupus anticoagulant. *Blood* 85:1704, 1995.
118. Griffin JH, Kojima K, Banka CL, et al: High-density lipoprotein enhancement of anticoagulant activities of plasma protein S and activated protein C. *J Clin Invest* 103:219, 1999.
119. Deguchi H, Fernandez JA, Pabinger I, et al: Plasma glucosylceramide deficiency as potential risk factor for venous thrombosis and modulator of anticoagulant protein C pathway. *Blood* 97:1907, 2001.
120. Stearns-Kurosawa DJ, Kurosawa S, Mollica JS, et al: The endothelial cell protein C receptor augments protein C activation by the thrombin-thrombomodulin complex. *Proc Natl Acad Sci U S A* 93:10212, 1996.
121. Cooper PC, Abuzenadah A, Preston FE: APC resistance test, a new phenomenon—The role of platelets. *Br J Haematol* 86(Suppl):33, 1999.
122. Shizuka R, Kanda T, Amagai H, Kobayashi I: False-positive activated protein C (APC) sensitivity ratio caused by freezing and by contamination of plasma with platelets. *Thromb Res* 78:189, 1995.
123. Simioni P, Scudeller A, Radossi P, et al: "Pseudo homozygous" activated protein C resistance due to double heterozygous factor V defects (factor V Leiden mutation and type I quantitative factor V defect) associated with thrombosis: Report of two cases belonging to two unrelated kindreds. *Thromb Haemost* 75:422, 1996.
124. Carter AM, Sachchithananthan M, Stasinopoulos S, et al: Prothrombin G20210A is a bifunctional gene polymorphism. *Thromb Haemost* 87:846, 2002.
125. Kyrle PA, Mannhalter C, Beguin S, et al: Clinical studies and thrombin generation in patients homozygous or heterozygous for the G20210A mutation in the prothrombin gene. *Arterioscler Thromb Vasc Biol* 18:1287, 1998.
126. Colucci M, Binetti BM, Tripodi A, et al: Hyperprothrombinemia associated with prothrombin G20210A mutation inhibits plasma fibrinolysis through a TAFI-mediated mechanism. *Blood* 103:2157, 2003.
127. Smirnov MD, Safa O, Esmon NL, Esmon CT: Inhibition of activated protein C anticoagulant activity by prothrombin. *Blood* 94:3839, 1999.
128. Souto JC, Coll I, Llobet D, et al: The prothrombin 20210A allele is the most prevalent genetic risk factor for venous thromboembolism in the Spanish population. *Thromb Haemost* 80:366, 1998.
129. Rosendaal FR, Vos HL, Poort SL, Bertina RM: Prothrombin 20210A variant and age at thrombosis. *Thromb Haemost* 79:444, 1998.
130. Leroyer C, Mercier B, Oger E, et al: Prevalence of 20210 A allele of the prothrombin gene in venous thromboembolism patients. *Thromb Haemost* 80:49, 1998.
131. Arruda VR, Annichino-Bizzacchi JM, Gonçalves MS, Costa FF: Prevalence of the prothrombin gene variant (nt20210A) in venous thrombosis and arterial disease. *Thromb Haemost* 78:1430, 1997.
132. Margaglione M, Brancaccio V, Giuliani N, et al: Increased risk for venous thrombosis in carriers of the prothrombin G→A20210 gene variant. *Ann Intern Med* 129:89, 1998.
133. Hillarp A, Zoller B, Svensson PJ, Dahlback B: The 20210 A allele of the prothrombin gene is a common risk factor among Swedish outpatients with verified deep venous thrombosis. *Thromb Haemost* 78:990, 1997.
134. Cumming AM, Keeney S, Salden A, et al: The prothrombin gene G 20210A variant: Prevalence in a U.K. anticoagulant clinic population. *Br J Haematol* 98:353, 1997.
135. Brown K, Luddington R, Williamson D, et al: The risk of venous thromboembolism associated with a G to A transition at position 20210 in the 3′-untranslated region of the prothrombin gene. *Br J Haematol* 98:907, 1997.
136. De Stefano V, Chiusolo P, Paciaroni K, et al: Hepatic vein thrombosis in a patient with mutant prothrombin 20210A allele. *Thromb Haemost* 80:519, 1998.
137. Darnige L, Jezequel P, Amoura Z, et al: Mesenteric venous thrombosis in two patients heterozygous for the 20210 A allele of the prothrombin gene. *Thromb Haemost* 80:703, 1998.

138. Martinelli I, Sacchi E, Landi G, et al: High risk of cerebral-vein thrombosis in carriers of a prothrombin-gene mutation and in users of oral contraceptives. *N Engl J Med* 338:1793, 1998.
139. Biousse V, Conard J, Brouzes C, et al: Frequency of the 20210 G→A mutation in the 3′-untranslated region of the prothrombin gene in 35 cases of cerebral venous thrombosis. *Stroke* 29:1398, 1998.
140. Chamouard P, Pencreach E, Maloisel F, et al: Frequent factor II G20210A mutation in idiopathic portal vein thrombosis. *Gastroenterology* 116:144, 1999.
141. Reuner KH, Ruf A, Grau A, et al: Prothrombin gene G20210→A transition is a risk factor for cerebral venous thrombosis. *Stroke* 29:1765, 1998.
142. Mercier E, Quere I, Campello C, et al: The 20210A allele of the prothrombin gene is frequent in young women with unexplained spinal cord infarction. *Blood* 92:1840, 1998.
143. Bosler D, Mattson J, Crisan D: Phenotypic Heterogeneity in Patients with Homozygous Prothrombin 20210AA Genotype. A paper from the 2005 William Beaumont Hospital Symposium on Molecular Pathology. *J Mol Diagn* 8:420, 2006.
144. Simioni P, Tormene D, Manfrin D, et al: Prothrombin antigen levels in symptomatic and asymptomatic carriers of the 20210A prothrombin variant. *Br J Haematol* 103:1045, 1998.
145. Makris M, Preston FE, Beauchamp NJ, et al: Co-inheritance of the 20210A allele of the prothrombin gene increases the risk of thrombosis in subjects with familial thrombophilia. *Thromb Haemost* 78:1426, 1997.
146. Ceelie H, Bertina RM, van Hylckama Vlieg A, et al: Polymorphisms in the prothrombin gene and their association with plasma prothrombin levels. *Thromb Haemost* 85:1066, 2001.
147. Chinthammitr Y, Vos HL, Rosendaal FR, Doggen CJ: The association of prothrombin A19911G polymorphism with plasma prothrombin activity and venous thrombosis: Results of the MEGA study, a large population-based case-control study. *J Thromb Haemost* 4:2587, 2006.
148. Mudd SH, Levy Hl, Skovby F: Disorders of transsulfuration, in *The Metabolic and Molecular Bases of Inherited Disease*, 7th ed, edited by CR Scriver, AL Beaudet, WS Sly, D Valle, p 1279. McGraw-Hill, New York, 1995.
149. Rosenberg N, Murata M, Ikeda Y, et al: The frequent 5,10-methylenetetrahydrofolate reductase C677T polymorphism is associated with a common haplotype in whites, Japanese, and Africans. *Am J Hum Genet* 70:758, 2002.
150. Jacques PF, Bostom AG, Williams RR, et al: Relation between folate status, a common mutation in methyltetrahydrofolate reductase, and plasma homocysteine concentrations. *Circulation* 93:7,1996.
151. Key NS, McGlennen RC: Hyperhomocyst(e)inemia and thrombophilia. *Arch Pathol Lab Med* 126:1367, 2002.
152. den Heijer M, Rosendaal FR, Blom HJ, et al: Hyperhomocysteinemia and venous thrombosis: A meta-analysis. *Thromb Haemost* 80:874, 1998.
153. Ray JG: Meta-analysis of hyperhomocysteinemia as a risk factor for venous thromboembolic disease. *Arch Intern Med* 158:2101, 1998.
154. Den Heijer M, Lewington S, Clarke R: Homocysteine, MTHFR and risk of venous thrombosis: A meta-analysis of published epidemiological studies. *J Thromb Haemost* 3:292, 2005.
155. Ridker PM, Hennekens CH, Selhub J, et al: Interrelation of hyperhomocyst(e)inemia, factor V Leiden, and risk of future venous thromboembolism. *Circulation* 95:1777, 1997.
156. Naess IA, Christiansen SC, Romundstad PR, et al: Prospective study of homocysteine and MTHFR 677TT genotype and risk for venous thrombosis in a general population—Results from the HUNT 2 study. *Br J Haematol* 141:529, 2008.
157. Martinelli I, Battaglioli T, Pedotti P, et al: Hyperhomocysteinemia in cerebral vein thrombosis. *Blood* 102:1363, 2003.
158. Bezemer ID, Doggen CJ, Vos HL, Rosendaal FR: No association between the common MTHFR 677C->T polymorphism and venous thrombosis: Results from the MEGA study. *Arch Intern Med* 167:497, 2007.
159. Pfeiffer CM, Huff DL, Smith SJ, et al: Comparison of plasma total homocysteine measurements in 14 laboratories: An international study. *Clin Chem* 45:1261, 1999.
160. Tripodi A, Chantarangkul V, Lombardi R, et al: Multicenter study of homocysteine measurement—Performance characteristics of different methods, influence of1standards on interlaboratory agreement of results. *Thromb Haemost* 85:291, 2001.
161. Bostom AG, Jacques PF, Nadeau MR, et al: Post-methionine load hyperhomocysteinemia in persons with normal fasting total plasma homocysteine: Initial results from the NHLBI Family Heart Study. *Atherosclerosis* 116:147, 1995.
162. Garg UC, Zheng ZJ, Folsom AR, et al: Short-term and long-term variability of plasma homocysteine measurement. *Clin Chem* 43:141, 1997.
163. Jacobsen DW, Gatautis VJ, Green R, et al: Rapid HPLC determination of total homocysteine and other thiols in serum and plasma: Sex differences and correlation with cobalamin and folate concentrations in healthy subjects [see comments]. *Clin Chem* 40:873, 1994.
164. Frosst P, Blom HJ, Milos R, et al: A candidate genetic risk factor for vascular disease: A common mutation in methylenetetrahydrofolate reductase. *Nat Genet* 10:111,1995.
165. Moat SJ, Bao L, Fowler B, et al: The molecular basis of cystathionine beta-synthase (CBS) deficiency in U.K. and U.S. patients with homo-cystinuria. *Hum Mutat* 23:206, 2004.
166. Tsai MY, Hanson NQ, Bignell MK, Schwichtenberg KA: Simultaneous detection and screening of T833C and G919A mutations of the cystathionine beta-synthase gene by single-strand conformational polymorphism. *Clin Biochem* 29:473, 1996.
167. Esmon CT: Role of coagulation inhibitors in inflammation. *Thromb Haemost* 86:51, 2001.
168. Esmon CT: Structure and functions of the endothelial cell protein C receptor. *Crit Care Med* 32:S298, 2004.
169. Mosnier LO, Zlokovic BV, Griffin JH: The cytoprotective protein C pathway. *Blood* 109:3161, 2007.
170. Riewald M, Petrovan RJ, Donner A, et al: Activation of endothelial cell protease activated receptor 1 by the protein C pathway. *Science* 296:1880, 2002.
171. Kerschen EJ, Fernandez JA, Cooley BC, et al: Endotoxemia and sepsis mortality reduction by non-anticoagulant activated protein C. *J Exp Med* 204:2439, 2007.
172. Bernard GR, Vincent JL, Laterre PF, et al: Efficacy and safety of recombinant human activated protein C for severe sepsis. *N Engl J Med* 344:699, 2001.
173. Warren BL, Eid A, Singer P, et al: For the KyberSept trail study group. High-dose antithrombin III in severe sepsis: A randomized controlled trial. *JAMA* 286:1869, 2001.
174. Abraham E, Reinhart K, Opal S, et al: For the OPTIMIST trial study group. Efficacy and safety of tifacogin (recombinant tissue factor pathway inhibitor) in severe sepsis: A randomized controlled trail. *JAMA* 290:238, 2003.
175. Pomp ER, Doggen CJ, Vos HL, et al: Polymorphisms in the protein C gene as risk factor for venous thrombosis. *Thromb Haemost* 101:62, 2009.
176. Miletich J, Sherman L, Broze G: Absence of thrombosis in subjects with heterozygous protein C deficiency. *N Engl J Med* 317:991, 1987.
177. Tait RC, Walker ID, Reitsma PH, et al: Prevalence of protein C deficiency in the healthy population. *Thromb Haemost* 73:87, 1995.
178. Koster T, Rosendaal FR, Briët E, et al: Protein C deficiency in a controlled series of unselected outpatients: An infrequent but clear risk factor for venous thrombosis (Leiden thrombophilia study). *Blood* 85:2756, 1995.
179. Folsom AR, Aleksic N, Wang L, et al: Protein C, antithrombin, and venous thromboembolism incidence a prospective population-based study. *Arterioscler Thromb Vasc Biol* 22:1018, 2002.
180. Allaart CF, Rosendaal FR, Noteboom WMP, et al: Survival in families with hereditary protein C deficiency 1820 to 1993. *BMJ* 311:910, 1995.
181. Hasstedt SJ, Scott BT, Callas PW, et al: Genome scan of venous thrombosis in a pedigree with protein C deficiency. *J Thromb Haemost* 2:868, 2004.
182. Brenner B, Zivelin A, Lanir N, et al: Venous thromboembolism associated with double heterozygosity for R506Q mutation of factor V and for T298M mutation of protein C in a large family of a previously described homozygous protein C-deficient newborn with massive thrombosis. *Blood* 88:877, 1996.
183. Pabinger I, Schneider B: Thrombotic risk in hereditary antithrombin III, protein C, or protein S deficiency—A cooperative, retrospective study. *Arterioscler Thromb Vasc Biol* 16:742, 1996.
184. De Stefano V, Leone G, Mastrangelo S, et al: Clinical manifestations and management of inherited thrombophilia: Retrospective analysis and follow-up after diagnosis of 238 patients with congenital deficiency of antithrombin III, protein C, protein S. *Thromb Haemost* 72:352, 1994.
185. Pabinger I, Kyrle PA, Heistinger M, et al: The risk of thromboembolism in asymptomatic patients with protein C and protein S deficiency: A prospective cohort study. *Thromb Haemost* 71:441, 1994.
186. Van den Belt AGM, Sanson BJ, Simioni P, et al: Recurrence of venous thromboembolism in patients with familial thrombophilia. *Arch Intern Med* 157:2227, 1997.
187. Allaart CF, Poort SR, Rosendaal FR, et al: Increased risk of venous thrombosis in carriers of hereditary protein C deficiency defect. *Lancet* 341:134, 1993.
188. De Bruijn SFTM, Stam J, Koopman MMW, Vandenbroucke JP: Cerebral venous sinus thrombosis study: Case-control study of risk of cerebral sinus thrombosis in oral contraceptive users who are carriers of hereditary prothrombotic conditions. *BMJ* 316:589, 1998.
189. Branson HE, Katz J, Marble R, Griffin JH: Inherited protein C deficiency and coumarin-responsive chronic relapsing purpura fulminans in a newborn infant. *Lancet* 2:1165, 1983.
190. Seligsohn U, Berger A, Abend M, et al: Homozygous protein C deficiency manifested by massive venous thrombosis in the newborn. *N Engl J Med* 310:559, 1984.
191. McGehee WG, Klotz TA, Epstein DJ, Rapaport SI: Coumarin necrosis associated with hereditary protein C deficiency. *Ann Intern Med* 101:59, 1984.
192. Vigano D'A, Comp PC, Esmon CT, D'Angelo A: Relationship between protein C antigen and anticoagulant activity during oral anticoagulation and in selected disease states. *J Clin Invest* 77:416, 1986.
193. Weiss P, Soff GA, Halkin H, Seligsohn U: Decline of proteins C and S and factors II, VII, IX, and X during the initiation of warfarin therapy. *Thromb Res* 45:783, 1987.
194. Miletich JP: Laboratory diagnosis of protein C deficiency. *Semin Thromb Hemost* 16:169, 1990.
195. Francis RBJ, Seyfert U: Rapid amidolytic assay of protein C in whole plasma using an activator from the venom of Agkistrodon contortrix. *Am J Clin Pathol* 87:619, 1987.
196. Aiach M, Borgel D, Gaussem P, et al: Protein C and protein S deficiencies. *Semin Hematol* 34:205, 1997.
197. Berdeaux DH, Abshire TC, Marlar RA: Dysfunctional protein C deficiency (type II). A report of 11 cases in 3 American families and review of the literature. *Am J Clin Pathol* 99:677, 1993.
198. Aiach M, Nicaud V, Alhenc-Gelas M, et al: Complex association of protein C gene promoter polymorphism with circulating protein C levels and thrombotic risk. *Arterioscler Thromb Vasc Biol* 19:1573, 1999.
199. Tait RC, Walker ID, Islam SI, et al: Protein C activity in healthy volunteers—Influence of age, sex, smoking, and oral contraceptives. *Thromb Haemost* 70:281, 1993.

200. Bertina RM, Broekmans AW, Van der Linden IK, Mertens K: Protein C deficiency in a Dutch family with thrombotic disease. *Thromb Haemost* 48:1, 1982.
201. Castoldi E, Hackeng TM: Regulation of coagulation by protein S. *Curr Opin Hematol* 15:529, 2008.
202. Faioni EM, Valsecchi C, Palla A, et al: Free protein S deficiency is a risk factor for venous thrombosis. *Thromb Haemost* 78:1343, 1997.
203. Heijboer H, Brandjes DPM, Büller HR, et al: Deficiencies of coagulation-inhibiting and fibrinolytic proteins in outpatients with deep-vein thrombosis. *N Engl J Med* 323:1512, 1990.
204. Adachi T: Protein S and congenital protein S deficiency: The most frequent congenital thrombophilia in Japanese. *Curr Drug Targets* 6:585, 2005.
205. Simmonds RE, Ireland H, Lane DA, et al: Clarification of the risk for venous thrombosis associated with hereditary protein S deficiency by investigation of a large kindred with a characterized gene defect. *Ann Intern Med* 128:8, 1998.
206. Mahasandana C, Suvatte V, Chuansumrit A, et al: Homozygous protein S deficiency in an infant with purpura fulminans. *J Pediatr* 117:750, 1990.
207. Pegelow CH, Ledford M, Young JN, Zilleruelo G: Severe protein S deficiency in a newborn. *Pediatrics* 89:674, 1992.
208. Pung-Amritt P, Poor SR, Vos HL, et al: Compound heterozygosity for one novel and one recurrent mutation in a Thai patient with severe protein S deficiency. *Thromb Haemost* 81:189, 1999.
209. Grimaudo V, Gueissaz F, Hauert J, et al: Necrosis of skin induced by coumarin in a patient deficient in protein S. *BMJ* 298:233, 1989.
210. Langlois NJ, Wells PS: Risk of venous thromboembolism in relatives of symptomatic probands with thrombophilia: A systematic review. *Thromb Haemost* 90:17, 2003.
211. Zoller B, Garcia de Frutos P, Dahlback B: Evaluation of the relationship between protein S and C4b-binding protein isoforms in hereditary protein S deficiency demonstrating type I and type III deficiencies to be phenotypic variants of the same genetic disease. *Blood* 85:3524, 1995.
212. Wolf M, Boyer-Neumann C, Peynaud-Debayle E, et al: Clinical applications of a direct assay of free protein S antigen using monoclonal antibodies. A study of 59 cases. *Blood Coagul Fibrinolysis* 5:187, 1994.
213. Amiral J, Grosley B, Boyer-Neumann C, et al: New direct assay of free protein S antigen using two distinct monoclonal antibodies specific for the free form. *Blood Coagul Fibrinolysis* 5:179, 1994.
214. Faioni EM, Boyer-Neumann C, Franchi F, et al: Another protein S functional assay is sensitive to resistance to activated protein C. *Thromb Haemost* 72:648, 1994.
215. Brunet D, Barthet MC, Morange PE, et al: Protein S deficiency: Different biological phenotypes according to the assays used. *Thromb Haemost* 79:446, 1998.
216. Wolf M, Boyer-Neumann C, Leroy-Matheron C, et al: Functional assay of protein S in 70 patients with congenital and acquired disorders. *Blood Coagul Fibrinolysis* 2:705, 1991.
217. Gari M, Falkon L, Urrutia T, et al: The influence of low protein S plasma levels in young women, on the definition of normal range. *Thromb Res* 73:149, 1994.
218. Comp PC, Thurnau GR, Welsh J, Esmon CT: Functional and immunologic protein S levels are decreased during pregnancy. *Blood* 68:881, 1986.
219. Malm J, Laurell M, Dahlback B: Changes in the plasma levels of vitamin K-dependent proteins C and S and of C4b-binding protein during pregnancy and oral contraception. *Br J Haematol* 68:437, 1988.
220. Comp PC, Doray D, Patton D, Esmon CT: An abnormal plasma distribution of protein S occurs in functional protein S deficiency. *Blood* 67: 504, 1986.
221. D'Angelo A, Vigano-D'Angelo S, Esmon CT, Comp PC: Acquired deficiencies of protein S. Protein S activity during oral anticoagulation, in liver disease, and in disseminated intravascular coagulation. *J Clin Invest* 81:1445, 1988.
222. Vigano-D'Angelo S, D'Angelo A, Kaufman CE, et al: Protein S deficiency occurs in the nephrotic syndrome. *Ann Intern Med* 107:42, 1987.
223. Aadland E, Odegaard OR, Roseth A, Try K: Free protein S deficiency in patients with chronic inflammatory bowel disease. *Scand J Gastroenterol* 27:957, 1992.
224. Parke AL, Weinstein RE, Bona RD, et al: The thrombotic diathesis associated with the presence of phospholipid antibodies may be due to low levels of free protein S. *Am J Med* 93:49, 1992.
225. Song KS, Park YS, Kim HK: Prevalence of anti-protein S antibodies in patients with systemic lupus erythematosus. *Arthritis Rheum* 43:557, 2000.
226. Levin M, Eley BS, Louis J, et al: Postinfectious purpura fulminans caused by an autoantibody directed against protein S. *J Pediatr* 127:355, 1995.
227. D'Angelo A, Della Valle P, Crippa L, et al: Brief report: Autoimmune protein S deficiency in a boy with severe thromboembolic disease. *N Engl J Med* 328:1753, 1993.
228. Sakuragawa N, Takahashi K, Kondo S, Koide T: Antithrombin III Toyama: A hereditary abnormal antithrombin III of a patient with recurrent thrombophlebitis. *Thromb Res* 31:305, 1983.
229. Fischer AM, Cornu P, Sternberg C, et al: Antithrombin III Alger: A new homozygous AT III variant. *Thromb Haemost* 55:218, 1986.
230. Okajima K, Ueyama H, Hashimoto Y, et al: Homozygous variant of antithrombin III that lacks affinity for heparin, AT III Kumamoto. *Thromb Haemost* 61:20, 1989.
231. Boyer C, Wolf M, Vedrenne J, et al: Homozygous variant of antithrombin III: AT III Fontainebleau. *Thromb Haemost* 56:18, 1986.
232. Tait RC, Walker ID, Perry DJ, et al: Prevalence of antithrombin deficiency in the healthy population. *Br J Haematol* 87:106, 1994.
233. Van Boven HH, Vandenbroucke JP, Briët E, Rosendaal FR: Gene-gene and gene-environment interactions determine risk of thrombosis in families with inherited antithrombin deficiency. *Blood* 94:2590, 1999.
234. Rosendaal FR, Heijboer H, Briet E, et al: Mortality in hereditary anti-thrombin III deficiency—1830 to 1989. *Lancet* 337:260, 1991.
235. Van Boven HH, Olds RJ, Thein S-L, et al: Hereditary antithrombin deficiency: Heterogeneity of the molecular basis and mortality in Dutch families. *Blood* 84:4209, 1994.
236. Hirsh J, Piovella F, Pini M: Congenital antithrombin III deficiency. Incidence and clinical features. *Am J Med* 87(Suppl 3B):34S, 1989.
237. Kuhle S, Lane DA, Jochmanns K, et al: Homozygous antithrombin deficiency type II (99 Leu to Phe mutation) and childhood thromboembolism. *Thromb Haemost* 86:1007, 2001.
238. Nakase H, Kawasaki T, Itani T, et al: Budd-Chiari syndrome and extra-hepatic portal obstruction associated with congenital antithrombin III deficiency. *J Gastroenterol* 36:341, 2001.
239. Ishiguro K, Kojima T, Kadomatsu K, et al: Complete antithrombin deficiency in mice results in embryonic lethality. *J Clin Invest* 106:873, 2000.
240. De Boer AC, van Riel LA, den Ottolander GJ: Measurement of anti-thrombin III, alpha 2-macroglobulin and alpha 1-antitrypsin in patients with deep venous thrombosis and pulmonary embolism. *Thromb Res* 15: 17, 1979.
241. Marciniak E, Gockerman JP: Heparin-induced decrease in circulating antithrombin-III. *Lancet* 2:581, 1977.
242. Von Kaulla E, Von Kaulla KN: Antithrombin 3 and diseases. *Am J Clin Pathol* 48:69, 1967.
243. Damus PS, Wallace GA: Immunologic measurement of antithrombin III-heparin cofactor and alpha2 macroglobulin in disseminated intravascular coagulation and hepatic failure coagulopathy. *Thromb Res* 6:27, 1975.
244. Kauffmann RH, Veltkamp JJ, van Tilburg NH, Van Es LA: Acquired antithrombin III deficiency and thrombosis in the nephrotic syndrome. *Am J Med* 65:607, 1978.
245. Buchanan GR, Holtkamp CA: Reduced antithrombin III levels during L-asparaginase therapy. *Med Pediatr Oncol* 8:7, 1980.
246. Weenink GH, Treffers PE, Vijn P, et al: Antithrombin III levels in preeclampsia correlate with maternal and fetal morbidity. *Am J Obstet Gynecol* 148:1092, 1984.
247. Kottke-Marchant K, Duncan A: Antithrombin deficiency: Issues in laboratory diagnosis. *Arch Pathol Lab Med* 126:1326, 2002.
248. Demers C, Henderson P, Blajchman MA, et al: An antithrombin III assay based on factor Xa inhibition provides a more reliable test to identify congenital antithrombin III deficiency than an assay based on thrombin inhibition. *Thromb Haemost* 69:231, 1993.
249. Kamphuisen PW, Eikenboom JC, Bertina RM: Elevated factor VIII levels and the risk of thrombosis. *Arterioscler Thromb Vasc Biol* 21:731, 2001.
250. Morelli VM, De Visser MC, Vos HL, et al: ABO blood group genotypes and the risk of venous thrombosis: Effect of factor V Leiden. *J Thromb Haemost* 3:183, 2005.
251. Saenko EL, Yakhyaev AV, Mikhailenko I, et al: Role of the low density lipoprotein-related protein receptor in mediation of factor VIII catabolism. *J Biol Chem* 274:37685, 1999.
252. O'Donnell J, Tuddenham EG, Manning R, et al: High prevalence of elevated factor VIII levels in patients referred for thrombophilia screening: Role of increased synthesis and relationship to the acute phase reaction. *Thromb Haemost* 77:825, 1997.
253. Kraaijenhagen RA, In't Anker PS, Koopman MM, et al: High plasma concentration of factor VIIIc is a major risk factor for venous thromboembolism. *Thromb Haemost* 83:5, 2000.
254. Siegemund A, Petros S, Siegemund T, et al: The endogenous thrombin potential and high levels of coagulation factor VIII, factor IX and factor XI. *Blood Coagul Fibrinolysis* 15:241, 2004.
255. Tripodi A: Levels of coagulation factors and venous thromboembolism. *Haematologica* 88:705, 2003.
256. Van Hyleckama Vlieg A, van der Linden IK, Bertina RM, Rosendaal FR: High levels of factor IX increase the risk of venous thrombosis. *Blood* 95:3678, 2000.
257. Meijers JC, Tekelenburg WL, Bouma BN, et al: High levels of coagulation factor XI as a risk factor for venous thrombosis. *N Engl J Med* 342:696, 2000.
258. Kamphuisen PW, Eikenboom JC, Vos HL, et al: Increased levels of factor VIII and fibrinogen in patients with venous thrombosis are not caused by acute phase reactions. *Thromb Haemost* 81:680, 1999.
259. Van Hylckama Vlieg A, Rosendaal FR: High levels of fibrinogen are associated with the risk of deep venous thrombosis mainly in the elderly. *J Thromb Haemost* 1:2677, 2003.
260. Hayes T: Dysfibrinogenemia and thrombosis. *Arch Pathol Lab Med* 126:1387, 2002.
261. Robert-Ebadi H, Le Querrec A, de Moerloose P, et al: A novel Asp344Val substitution in the fibrinogen gamma chain (fibrinogen Caen) causes dysfibrinogenemia associated with thrombosis. *Blood Coagul Fibrinolysis* 19:697, 2008.
262. Haverkate F, Samama M: Familial dysfibrinogenemia and thrombophilia. Report on a study of the SSC Subcommittee on Fibrinogen. *Thromb Haemost* 73:151, 1995.
263. Prins MH, Hirsh J: A critical review of the evidence supporting a relationship between impaired fibrinolytic activity and venous thromboembolism. *Arch Intern Med* 151:1721, 1991.
264. Francis CW: Plasminogen activator inhibitor-1 levels and polymorphisms. *Arch Pathol Lab Med* 126:1401, 2002.
265. Tefts K, Tait CR, Walker ID, et al: A K19E missense mutation in the plasminogen gene is a common cause of familial hypoplasminogenaemia. *Blood Coagul Fibrinolysis* 14:411, 2003.
266. Folsom AR, Cushman M, Heckbert SR, et al: Prospective study of fibrinolytic markers and venous thromboembolism. *J Clin Epidemiol* 56: 598, 2003.
267. Mehta R, Shapiro AD: Plasminogen deficiency. *Haemophilia* 14:1261, 2008.

268. Tait RC, Walker ID, Conkie JA, et al: Isolated familial plasminogen deficiency may not be a risk factor for thrombosis. *Thromb Haemost* 76: 1004, 1996.
269. Crowther MA, Roberts J, Roberts R, et al: Fibrinolytic variables in patients with recurrent venous thrombosis: A prospective cohort study. *Thromb Haemost* 85:390, 2001.
270. Van Tilburg NH, Rosendaal FR, Bertina RM: Thrombin activatable fibrinolysis inhibitor and the risk for deep vein thrombosis. *Blood* 95: 2855, 2000.
271. Folkeringa N, Coppens M, Veeger NJ, et al: Absolute risk of venous and arterial thromboembolism in thrombophilic families is not increased by high thrombin-activatable fibrinolysis inhibitor (TAFI) levels. *Thromb Haemost* 100:38, 2008.
272. Mosnier LO, Elisen MG, Bouma BN, Meijers JC: Protein C inhibitor regulates the thrombin-thrombomodulin complex in the up- and down-regulation of TAFI activation. *Thromb Haemost* 86:1057, 2001.
273. Meijers JC, Marquart JA, Bertina RM, et al: Protein C inhibitor (plasminogen activator inhibitor-3) and the risk of venous thrombosis. *Br J Haematol* 118:604, 2002.
274. Van de Wouwer M, Collen D, Conway EM: Thrombomodulin-protein C-EPCR system integrated to regulate coagulation and inflammation. *Arterioscler Thromb Vasc Biol* 24:1, 2004.
275. Ohlin AK, Marlar RA: The first mutation identified in the thrombomodulin gene in a 45-year-old man presenting with thromboembolic disease. *Blood* 85:330, 1995.
276. Ohlin AK, Marlar RA: Thrombomodulin gene defects in families with thromboembolic disease—A report on four families. *Thromb Haemost* 81:338, 1999.
277. Ohlin AK, Norlund L, Marlar RA: Thrombomodulin gene variations and thromboembolic disease. *Thromb Haemost* 78:396, 1997.
278. Kunz G, Ohlin AK, Adami A, et al: Naturally occurring mutations in the thrombomodulin gene leading to impaired expression and function. *Blood* 99:3646, 2002.
279. Aleksic N, Folsom AR, Cushman M, et al: Prospective study of the A455V polymorphism in the thrombomodulin gene, plasma thrombomodulin, and incidence of venous thromboembolism: The LITE study. *J Thromb Haemost* 1:88, 2003.
280. Stearns-Kurosawa DJ, Burgin C, Parker D, et al: Bimodal distribution of soluble endothelial protein C receptor levels in healthy populations. *J Thromb Haemost* 1:855, 2003.
281. Saposnik B, Reny JL, Gaussem P, et al: A haplotype of the EPCR gene is associated with increased plasma levels of sEPCR and is a candidate risk factor for thrombosis. *Blood* 103:1311, 2004.
282. Medina P, Navarro S, Estelles A, Espana F: Polymorphisms in the endothelial protein C receptor gene and thrombophilia. *Thromb Haemost* 98:564, 2007.
283. Uitte de Willige S, Van Marion V, Rosendaal FR, et al: Haplotypes of the EPCR gene, plasma sEPCR levels and the risk of deep venous thrombosis. *J Thromb Haemost* 2:1305, 2004.
284. von Depka M, Czwalinna A, Eisert R, et al: Prevalence of a 23 bp insertion in exon 3 of the endothelial cell protein C receptor gene in venous thrombophilia. *Thromb Haemost* 86:1360, 2001.
285. Biguzzi E, Merati G, Liaw PC, et al: A 23bp insertion in the endothelial protein C receptor (EPCR) gene impairs EPCR function. *Thromb Haemost* 86:945, 2001.
286. Poort SR, Vos HL, Rosendaal FR, Bertina RM: The endothelial protein C receptor (EPCR) 23 bp insert mutation and the risk of venous thrombosis. *Thromb Haemost* 88:160, 2002.
287. Dahm A, Van Hylckama Vlieg A, Bendz B, et al: Low levels of tissue factor pathway inhibitor (TFPI) increase the risk of venous thrombosis. *Blood* 101:4387, 2003.
288. Amini-Nekoo A, Futers TS, Moia M, et al: Analysis of the tissue factor pathway inhibitor gene and antigen levels in relation to venous thrombosis. *Br J Haematol* 113:537, 2001.
289. Kato H: Regulation of the function of vascular wall cells by tissue factor pathway inhibitor. Basic and Clinical Aspects. *Arterioscler Thromb Vasc Biol* 22:539, 2002.
290. Caplice NM, Panetta C, Peterson TE, et al: Lipoprotein (a) binds and inactivates tissue factor pathway inhibitor: A novel link between lipoproteins and thrombosis. *Blood* 98:2980, 2001.
291. Tardy-Poncet B, Tardy B, Laporte S, et al: Poor anticoagulant response to tissue factor pathway inhibitor in patients with venous thrombosis. *J Thromb Haemost* 1:507, 2003.
292. Bombeli T, Piccapietra B, Boersma J, Fehr J: Decreased anticoagulant response to tissue factor pathway inhibitor in patients with venous thromboembolism and otherwise no evidence of hereditary or acquired thrombophilia. *Thromb Haemost* 91:80, 2004.
293. Souto JC, Almasy L, Borrell M, et al: Genetic susceptibility to thrombosis and its relationship to physiological risk factors: The GAIT study. Genetic Analysis of Idiopathic Thrombophilia. *Am J Hum Genet* 67:1452, 2000.
294. Ariens RA, De Lange M, Snieder H, et al: Activation markers of coagulation and fibrinolysis in twins: Heritability of the prethrombotic state. *Lancet* 359:667, 2002.
295. Vossen CY, Hasstedt SJ, Rosendaal FR, et al: Heritability of plasma concentrations of clotting factors and measures of a prethrombotic state in a protein C-deficient family. *J Thromb Haemost* 2:242, 2004.
296. Dunn EJ, Ariens RA, De Lange M, et al: Genetics of fibrin clot structure: A twin study. *Blood* 103:1735, 2004.
297. Botstein D, Risch N: Discovering genotypes underlying human phenotypes: Past successes for Mendelian disease, future approaches for complex disease. *Nat Genet* 33(Suppl):228, 2003.
298. Rosendaal PR: Genetic studies in complex disease: The case proassociation studies. *J Thromb Haemost* 1:1679, 2003.
299. Souto JC: Genetic studies in complex disease: The case prolinkage studies. *J Thromb Haemost* 1:1676, 2003.
300. Blangero J, Williams JT, Almasy L: Novel family-based approaches to genetic risk in thrombosis. *J Thromb Haemost* 1:1391, 2003.
301. Soria JM, Almasy L, Souto JC, et al: A new locus on chromosome 18 that influences normal variation in activated protein C resistance phenotype and factor VIII activity and its relation to thrombosis susceptibility. *Blood* 101:163, 2003.
302. Almasy L, Soria JM, Souto JC, et al: A quantitative trait locus influencing free plasma protein S levels on human chromosome 1q results from the genetic analysis of idiopathic thrombophilia (GAIT) project. *Arterioscler Thromb Vasc Biol* 23:508, 2003.
303. Buil A, Soria JM, Souto JC, et al: Protein C levels are regulated by a quantitative trait locus on chromosome 16. Results from the genetic analysis of idiopathic thrombophilia (GAIT) project. *Arterioscler Thromb Vasc Biol* 24:1321, 2004.
304. Berger M, Mattheisen M, Kulle B, et al: High factor VIII levels in venous thromboembolism show linkage to imprinted loci on chromosomes 5 and 11. *Blood* 105:638, 2004.
305. Gandrille S, Greengard JS, Alhenc-Gelas M, et al: Incidence of activated protein C resistance caused by the ARG 506 GLN mutation in factor V in 113 unrelated symptomatic protein C-deficient patients. The French Network on the behalf of INSERM. *Blood* 86:219, 1995.
306. Tosetto A, Rodeghiero F, Martinelli I, et al: Additional genetic risk factors for venous thromboembolism in carriers of the factor V Leiden mutation. *Br J Haematol* 103:871, 1998.
307. Ehrenforth S, Prondsinski MV, Aygören-Pürsün E, et al: Study of the prothrombin gene 20210 GA variant in FV:Q^{506} carriers in relationship to the presence or absence of juvenile venous thromboembolism. *Arterioscler Thromb Vasc Biol* 19:276, 1999.
308. De Stefano V, Martinelli I, Mannucci PM, et al: The risk of recurrent deep venous thrombosis among heterozygous carriers of both factor V Leiden and the G20210A prothrombin mutation. *N Engl J Med* 341:801, 1999.
309. Howard TE, Marusa M, Boisza J, et al: The prothrombin gene 3′-un-translated region mutation is frequently associated with factor V Leiden in thrombophilic patients and shows ethnic-specific variation in allele frequency. *Blood* 91:1092, 1998.
310. Zoller B, Svensson PJ, Dahlback B, Hillarp A: The A20210 allele of the prothrombin gene is frequently associated with the factor V Arg 506 to Gln mutation but not with protein S deficiency in thrombophilic families. *Blood* 91:2210, 1998.
311. Mandel H, Brenner B, Berant M, et al: Coexistence of hereditary homocystinuria and Factor V Leiden—Effect on thrombosis. *N Engl J Med* 334:763, 1996.
312. Keijzer MB, den Heijer M, Blom HJ, et al: Interaction between hyperhomocysteinemia, mutated methylenetetrahydrofolate reductase (MTHFR) and inherited thrombophilic factors in recurrent venous thrombosis. *Thromb Haemost* 88:723, 2002.
313. Lensen R, Bertina RM, Vandenbroucke JP, Rosendaal FR: High factor VIII levels contribute to the thrombotic risk in families with factor V Leiden. *Br J Haematol* 114:380, 2001.
314. Libourel EJ, Bank I, Meinardi JR, et al: Co-segregation of thrombophilic disorders in factor V Leiden carriers: The contributions of factor VIII, factor XI, thrombin activatable fibrinolysis inhibitor and lipoprotein(a) to the absolute risk of venous thromboembolism. *Haematologica* 87: 1068, 2002.
315. Keijzer MB, Borm GF, Blom HJ, et al: No interaction between factor V Leiden and hyperhomocysteinemia or MTHFR 677TT genotype in venous thrombosis. Results of a meta-analysis of published studies and a large case-only study. *Thromb Haemost* 97:32, 2007.
316. Castaman G, Tosetto A, Cappellari A, et al: The A20210 allele in the prothrombin gene enhances the risk of venous thrombosis in carriers of inherited protein S deficiency. *Blood Coagul Fibrinolysis* 11:321, 2000.
317. De Stefano V, Zappacosta B, Persichilli S, et al: Prevalence of mild hyperhomocysteinaemia and association with thrombophilic genotypes (factor V Leiden and prothrombin G20210A) in Italian patients with venous thromboembolic disease. *Br J Haematol* 106:564, 1999.
318. Emmerich J, Rosendaal FR, Cattaneo M, et al: Combined effect of factor V Leiden and prothrombin 20210A on the risk of venous thromboembolism-pooled analysis of 8 case-control studies including 2,310 cases and 3,204 controls. Study Group for Pooled-Analysis in Venous Thromboembolism. *Thromb Haemost* 86:809, 2001.
319. Meinardi JR, Middeldorp S, de Kam PJ, et al: Risk of venous thromboembolism in carriers of factor V Leiden with a concomitant inherited thrombophilic defect: A retrospective analysis. *Blood Coagul Fibrinolysis* 12:713, 2001.
320. Dizon-Townson DS, Nelson LM, Jang H, et al: The incidence of the factor V Leiden mutation in an obstetric population and its relationship to deep vein thrombosis. *Am J Obstet Gynecol* 176:883, 1997.
321. Hallak M, Senderowicz J, Cassel A, et al: Activated protein C resistance (factor V Leiden) associated with thrombosis in pregnancy. *Am J Obstet Gynecol* 176:889, 1997.
322. Bokarewa MI, Bremme K, Blomback M: Arg^{506}-Gln mutation in factor V and risk of thrombosis during pregnancy. *Br J Haematol* 92:473, 1996.
323. Bloemenkamp KWM, Rosendaal FR, Helmerhorst FM, et al: Enhancement by factor V Leiden mutation of risk of deep-vein thrombosis associated with oral contraceptives containing third-generation progestogen. *Lancet* 346:1593, 1995.
324. Vandenbroucke JP, Koster T, Brit E, et al: Increased risk of venous thrombosis in oral-contraceptive users who are carriers of factor V Leiden mutation. *Lancet* 344:1453, 1994.
325. Rintelen C, Mannhalter C, Ireland H, et al: Oral contraceptives enhance the risk of clinical manifestation of venous thrombosis at a young age in females homozygous for factor V Leiden. *Br J Haematol* 93:487, 1996.
326. Martinelli I, Taioli E, Bucciarelli P, et al: Interaction between the G20210A mutation of the prothrombin gene and oral contraceptive use in deep vein thrombosis. *Arterioscler Thromb Vasc Biol* 19:700, 1999.
327. Martinelli I, Sacchi E, Landi G, et al: High risk of cerebral-vein thrombosis in carriers of a prothrombin-gene mutation and in users of oral contraceptives. *N Engl J Med* 338:1793, 1998.

328. Bloemenkamp KW, Helmerhorst FM, Rosendaal FR, Vandenbroucke JP: Thrombophilias and gynaecology. *Best Pract Res Clin Obstet Gynaecol* 17:509, 2003.
329. Bloemenkamp KW, Rosendaal FR, Helmerhorst FM, Vandenbroucke JP: Higher risk of venous thrombosis during early use of oral contraceptives in women with inherited clotting defects. *Arch Intern Med* 160: 49, 2000.
330. Bloemenkamp KW, Helmerhorst FM, Rosendaal FR, Vandenbroucke JP: Venous thrombosis, oral contraceptives and high factor VIII levels. *Thromb Haemost* 82:1024, 1999.
331. Rosendaal FR, Vessey M, Rumley A, et al: Hormonal replacement therapy, prothrombotic mutations and the risk of venous thrombosis. *Br J Haematol* 116:851, 2002.
332. Meltzer ME, Lisman T, Doggen CJ, et al: Synergistic effects of hypofibrinolysis and genetic and acquired risk factors on the risk of a first venous thrombosis. *PLoS Med* 5:e97, 2008.
333. Boushey CJ, Beresford SA, Omenn GS, Motulsky AG: A quantitative assessment of plasma homocysteine as a risk factor for vascular disease. Probable benefits of increasing folic acid intakes. *JAMA* 274:1049, 1995.
334. Homocysteine Studies Collaboration: Homocysteine and risk of ischemic heart disease and stroke: A meta-analysis. *JAMA* 288:2015, 2002.
335. Klerk M, Verhoef P, Clarke R, et al: MTHFR 677C→T polymorphism and risk of coronary heart disease: A meta-analysis. *JAMA* 288:2023, 2002.
336. Kim RJ, Becker RC: Association between factor V Leiden, prothrombin G20210A, and methylenetetrahydrofolate reductase C677T mutations and events of the arterial circulatory system: A meta-analysis of published studies. *Am Heart J* 146:948, 2003.
337. Casas JP, Hingorani AD, Bautista LE, Sharma P: Meta-analysis of genetic studies in ischemic stroke: Thirty-two genes involving approximately 18,000 cases and 58,000 controls. *Arch Neurol* 61:1652, 2004.
338. Haapaniemi E, Helenius J, Jakovljevic D, et al: Ischaemic stroke patients with heterozygous factor V Leiden present with multiple brain infarctions and widespread atherothrombotic disease. *Thromb Haemost* 101:145, 2009.
339. Slooter AJ, Rosendaal FR, Tanis BC, et al: Prothrombotic conditions, oral contraceptives, and the risk of ischemic stroke. *J Thromb Haemost* 3:1213, 2005.
340. de Moerloose P, Boehlen F: Inherited thrombophilia in arterial disease: A selective review. *Semin Hematol* 44:106, 2007.
341. Vig S, Chitolie A, Bevan D, et al: The prevalence of thrombophilia in patients with symptomatic peripheral vascular disease. *Br J Surg* 93:577, 2005.
342. Douketis JD, Kearon C, Bates S, et al: Risk of fatal pulmonary embolism in patients with treated venous thromboembolism. *JAMA* 279:458, 1998.
343. Prandoni P, Lensing AW, Cogo A, et al: The long-term clinical course of acute deep venous thrombosis. *Ann Intern Med* 125:1, 1996.
344. McRae S, Tran H. Schulman S, et al: Effect of patient's sex on risk of recurrent venous thromboembolism: A meta-analysis. *Lancet* 368:371, 2006.
345. Prandoni P, Noventa F, Ghirarduzzi A, et al: The risk of recurrent venous thromboembolism after discontinuing anticoagulation in patients with acute proximal deep vein thrombosis or pulmonary embolism. A prospective cohort study in 1,626 patients. *Haematologica* 92:199, 2007.
346. Eichinger S, Hron G, Bialonczyk C, et al: Overweight, obesity, and the risk of recurrent venous thromboembolism. *Arch Intern Med* 168:1678, 2008.
347. Prandoni P, Lensing AWA, Piccioli A, et al: Recurrent venous thromboembolism and bleeding complications during anticoagulant treatment in patients with cancer and venous thrombosis. *Blood* 100:3484, 2002.
348. Heit JA, Mohr DN, Silverstein MD, et al: Predictors of recurrence after deep vein thrombosis and pulmonary embolism. A population-based cohort study. *Arch Intern Med* 160:761, 2000.
349. Schulman S, Lindmarker P, Holmstrom M, et al: Post-thrombotic syndrome, recurrence, and death 10 years after the first episode of venous thromboembolism treated with warfarin for 6 weeks or 6 months. *J Thromb Haemost* 4:734, 2006.
350. Eichinger S, Weltermann A, Minar E, et al: Symptomatic pulmonary embolism and the risk of recurrent venous thromboembolism. *Arch Intern Med* 164:92, 2004.
351. Siragusa S, Malato A, Anastasio R, et al: Residual vein thrombosis to establish duration of anticoagulation after a first episode of deep vein thrombosis: The Duration of Anticoagulation based on Compression UltraSonography (DACUS) study. *Blood* 112:511, 2008.
352. Stain M, Schonauer V, Minar E, et al: The post-thrombotic syndrome: Risk factors and impact on the course of thrombotic disease. *J Thromb Haemost* 3:2671, 2005.
353. Palareti G, Cosmi B, Legnani C, et al. D-dimer testing to determine the duration of anticoagulation therapy. *N Engl J Med* 355:1780, 2006.
354. Schulman S, Svenungsson E, Granqvist S: Anticardiolipin antibodies predict early recurrence of thromboembolism and death among patients with venous thromboembolism following anticoagulant therapy. Duration of Anticoagulation Study Group. *Am J Med* 104:332, 1998.
355. Brouwer JL, Lijfering WM, Ten Kate MK, et al: High long-term absolute risk of recurrent venous thromboembolism in patients with hereditary deficiencies of protein S, protein C or antithrombin. *Thromb Haemost* 101:93, 2009.
356. De Stefano V, Simioni P, Rossi E, et al: The risk of recurrent venous thromboembolism in patients with inherited deficiency of natural anticoagulants antithrombin, protein C and protein S. *Haematologica* 91:695, 2006.
357. Vossen CY, Walker ID, Svensson P, et al: Recurrence rate after a first venous thrombosis in patients with familial thrombophilia. *Arterioscler Thromb Vasc Biol* 25:1992, 2005.
358. The Procare Group: Is recurrent venous thromboembolism more frequent in homozygous patients for the factor V Leiden mutation than in heterozygous patients? *Blood Coagul Fibrinolysis* 14:523, 2003.
359. Ho WK, Hankey GJ, Quinlan DJ, Eikelboom JW: Risk of recurrent venous thromboembolism in patients with common thrombophilia: A systematic review. *Arch Intern Med* 166:729, 2006.
360. Marchiori A, Mosena L, Prins MH, Prandoni P: The risk of recurrent venous thromboembolism among heterozygous carriers of factor V Leiden or prothrombin G20210A mutation. A systematic review of prospective studies. *Haematologica* 92:1107, 2007.
361. Eichinger S: Homocysteine, vitamin B_6 and the risk of recurrent venous thromboembolism. *Pathophysiol Haemost Thromb* 33:342, 2003.
362. Kyrle PA, Minar E, Hirschl M, et al: High plasma levels of factor VIII and the risk of recurrent venous thromboembolism. *N Engl J Med* 343:457, 2003.
363. Weltermann A, Eichinger S, Bialonczyk C, et al: The risk of recurrent venous thromboembolism among patients with high factor IX levels. *J Thromb Haemost* 1:28, 2003.
364. Baglin T, Luddington R, Brown K, Baglin C: Incidence of recurrent venous thromboembolism in relation to clinical and thrombophilic risk factors: Prospective cohort study. *Lancet* 362:523, 2003.
365. White RH, Chan WS, Zhou H, Ginsberg JS: Recurrent venous thromboembolism after pregnancy-associated versus unprovoked thromboembolism. *Thromb Haemost* 100:246, 2008.
366. Cushman M, Glynn RJ, Goldhaber SZ, et al: Hormonal factors and risk of recurrent venous thrombosis: The prevention of recurrent venous thromboembolism trial. *J Thromb Haemost* 4:2199, 2006.
367. Kakkos SK, Daskalopoulou SS, Daskalopoulos ME, et al: Review on the value of graduated elastic compression stockings after deep vein thrombosis. *Thromb Haemost* 96:441, 2006.
368. Kearon C, Ginsberg JS, Kovacs MJ, et al: Comparison of low-intensity warfarin therapy with conventional-intensity warfarin therapy for long-term prevention of recurrent venous thromboembolism. *N Engl J Med* 349:631, 2003.
369. Veeger NJ, Piersma-Wichers M, Tijssen JG, et al: Individual time within target range in patients treated with vitamin K antagonists: Main determinant of quality of anticoagulation and predictor of clinical outcome. A retrospective study of 2300 consecutive patients with venous thromboembolism. *Br J Haematol* 128:513, 2005.
370. Meinardi JR, Middeldorp S, De Kam PJ, et al: The incidence of recurrent venous thromboembolism in carriers of factor V Leiden is related to concomitant thrombophilic disorders. *Br J Haematol* 116:625, 2002.
371. Keijzer MB, den Heijer M, Blom HJ, et al: Interaction between hyperhomocysteinemia, mutated methylenetetrahydrofolate reductase (MTHFR) and inherited thrombophilic factors in recurrent venous thrombosis. *Thromb Haemost* 88:723, 2002.
372. Den Heijer M, Blom HJ, Gerrits WB, et al: Is hyperhomocysteinaemia a risk factor for recurrent venous thrombosis? *Lancet* 345:882, 1995.
373. Eichinger S, Stumpflen A, Hirschl M, et al: Hyperhomocysteinemia is a risk factor of recurrent venous thromboembolism. *Thromb Haemost* 80:566, 1998.
374. Tsai AW, Cushman M, Tsai MY, et al: Serum homocysteine, thermolabile variant of methylene tetrahydrofolate reductase (MTHFR), and venous thromboembolism: Longitudinal Investigation of Thromboembolism Etiology (LITE). *Am J Hematol* 72:192, 2003.
375. Eichinger S, Schonauer V, Weltermann A, et al: Thrombin-activatable fibrinolysis inhibitor and the risk for recurrent venous thromboembolism. *Blood* 103:3773, 2004.
376. Kupferminc MJ, Eldor A, Steinman N, et al: Increased frequency of genetic thrombophilia in women with complications of pregnancy. *N Engl J Med* 340:9, 1999.
377. Martinelli I, De Stefano V, Taioli E, et al: Inherited thrombophilia and first venous thromboembolism during pregnancy and puerperium. *Thromb Haemost* 87:791, 2002.
378. Greer IA: Inherited thrombophilia and venous thromboembolism. *Best Pract Res Clin Obstet Gynaecol* 17:413, 2003.
379. Folkeringa N, Brouwer JL, Korteweg FJ, et al: High risk of pregnancy-related venous thromboembolism in women with multiple thrombophilic defects. *Br J Haematol* 138:110, 2007.
380. Conard J, Horellou MH, Van Dreden P, et al: Thrombosis and pregnancy in congenital deficiencies in AT III, protein C or protein S: Study of 78 women. *Thromb Haemost* 63:319, 1990.
381. Friederich PW, Sanson BJ, Simioni P, et al: Frequency of pregnancy-related venous thromboembolism in anticoagulant factor-deficient women: Implications for prophylaxis. *Ann Intern Med* 125:955, 1996.
382. De Stefano V, Leone G, Mastrangelo S, et al: Thrombosis during pregnancy and surgery in patients with congenital deficiency of antithrombin III, protein C, protein S. *Thromb Haemost* 71:799, 1994.
383. Biron-Andreani C, Schved JF, Daures JP: Factor V Leiden mutation and pregnancy-related venous thromboembolism: What is the exact risk? Results from a meta-analysis. *Thromb Haemost* 96:14, 2006.
384. Tormene D, Simioni P, Prandoni P, et al: Factor V Leiden mutation and the risk of venous thromboembolism in pregnant women. *Haematologica* 86:1305, 2001.
385. Middeldorp S, Libourel EJ, Hamulyak K, et al: The risk of pregnancy-related venous thromboembolism in women who are homozygous for factor V Leiden. *Br J Haematol* 113:553, 2001.
386. Pabinger I, Nemes L, Rintelen C, et al: Pregnancy-associated risk for venous thromboembolism and pregnancy outcome in women homozygous for factor V Leiden. *Hematol J* 1:37, 2000.
387. Martinelli I, Legnani C, Bucciarelli P, et al: Risk of pregnancy-related venous thrombosis in carriers of severe inherited thrombophilia. *Thromb Haemost* 86:800, 2001.

388. Murphy RP, Donoghue C, Nallen RJ, et al: Prospective evaluation of the risk conferred by factor V Leiden and thermolabile methylenetetrahydrofolate reductase polymorphisms in pregnancy. *Arterioscler Thromb Vasc Biol* 20:266, 2000.
389. Lindqvist PG, Svensson PJ, Marsaal K, et al: Activated protein C resistance (FV:Q506) and pregnancy. *Thromb Haemost* 81:532, 1999.
390. Nurk E, Tell GS, Refsum H, et al: Factor V Leiden, pregnancy complications and adverse outcomes: The Hordaland Homocysteine Study. *QJM* 99:289, 2006.
391. Howley HE, Walker M, Rodger MA: A systematic review of the association between factor V Leiden or prothrombin gene variant and intrauterine growth restriction. *Am J Obstet Gynecol* 192:694, 2005.
392. Kupferminc MJ, Many A, Bar-Am A, et al: Mid-trimester severe intrauterine growth restriction is associated with a high prevalence of thrombophilia. *Br J Obstet Gynaecol* 109:1373, 2002.
393. Martinelli P, Grandone E, Colaizzo D, et al: Familial thrombophilia and the occurrence of fetal growth restriction. *Haematologica* 86:428, 2001.
394. Grandone E, Margaglione M, Colaizzo D, et al: Lower birth-weight in neonates of mothers carrying factor V G1691A and factor II A(20210) mutations. *Haematologica* 87:177, 2002.
395. Kupferminc MJ, Peri H, Zwang E, et al: High prevalence of the prothrombin gene mutation in women with intrauterine growth retardation, abruption placentae, and second trimester loss. *Acta Obstet Gynecol Scand* 79:963, 2000.
396. Clark P, Walker ID, Govan L, et al: The GOAL study: A prospective examination of the impact of factor V Leiden and ABO(H) blood groups on haemorrhagic and thrombotic pregnancy outcomes. *Br J Haematol* 140:236, 2008.
397. Dudding T, Heron J, Thakkinstian A, et al: Factor V Leiden is associated with pre-eclampsia but not with fetal growth restriction: A genetic association study and meta-analysis. *J Thromb Haemost* 6:1869, 2008.
398. Dizon-Townson D, Miller C, Sibai B, et al: The relationship of the factor V Leiden mutation and pregnancy outcomes for mother and fetus. *Obstet Gynecol* 106:517, 2005.
399. Kupferminc MJ, Eldor A: Inherited thrombophilia and gestational vascular complications. *Semin Thromb Hemost* 29:185, 2003.
400. Mousa HA, Alfirevicl Z: Do Placental lesions reflect thrombophilia state in women with adverse pregnancy outcome? *Hum Reprod* 15:1830, 2000.
401. Sikkema JM, Franx A, Bruinse HW, et al: Placental pathology in early onset pre-eclampsia and intra-uterine growth restriction in women with and without thrombophilia. *Placenta* 23:337, 2002.
402. Salomon O, Seligsohn U, Steinberg DM, et al: The common prothrombotic factors in nulliparous women do not compromise blood flow in the feto-maternal circulation and are not associated with preeclampsia or intrauterine growth restriction. *Am J Obstet Gynecol* 191:2002, 2004.
403. Duley L: Pre-eclampsia and the hypertensive disorders of pregnancy. *Br Med Bull* 67:161, 2003.
404. Roberts JM, Lain KY: Recent insights into the pathogenesis of preeclampsia. *Placenta* 23:359, 2002.
405. Maynard SE, Min JY, Merchan J, et al: Excess placental soluble fms-like tyrosine kinase 1 (sFlt1) may contribute to endothelial dysfunction, hypertension, and proteinuria in preeclampsia. *J Clin Invest* 111:649, 2003.
406. Robertson L, Wu O, Langhorne P, et al: Thrombophilia in pregnancy: A systematic review. *Br J Haematol* 132:171, 2006.
407. Morrison ER, Miedzybrodzka ZH, Campbell DM, et al: Prothrombotic genotypes are not associated with pre-eclampsia and gestational hyper-tension: Results from a large population-based study and systematic review. *Thromb Haemost* 87:779, 2002.
408. Hatasaka HH: Recurrent miscarriage: Epidemiologic factors, definitions, and incidence. *Clin Obstet Gynecol* 37:625, 1994.
409. Sanson BJ, Friederich PW, Simioni P, et al: The risk of abortion and stillbirth in antithrombin-, protein C-, and protein S-deficient women. *Thromb Haemost* 75:387, 1996.
410. Preston FE, Rosendaal FR, Walker ID, et al: Increased fetal loss in women with heritable thrombophilia. *Lancet* 348:913, 1996.
411. Gris JC, Quere I, Monpeyroux F, et al: Case-control study of the frequency of thrombophilic disorders in couples with late fetal loss and no thrombotic antecedent the Nimes Obstetricians and Haematologists Study5 (NOHA5). *Thromb Haemost* 81:891, 1999.
412. Martinelli I, Taioli E, Cetin I, et al: Mutations in coagulation factors in women with unexplained late fetal loss. *N Engl J Med* 343:1015, 2000.
413. Many A, Elad R, Yaron Y, et al: Third-trimester unexplained intrauterine fetal death is associated with inherited thrombophilia. *Obstet Gynecol* 99:684, 2002.
414. Alfirevic Z, Roberts D, Matlew V: How strong is the association between maternal thrombophilia and adverse pregnancy outcome? A systematic review. *Eur J Obstet Gynecol Reprod Biol* 101:6, 2002.
415. Martinelli I, Taioli E, Cetin I, Mannucci PM: Recurrent late fetal death in women with and without thrombophilia. *Thromb Haemost* 87:358, 2002.
416. Young G, Albisetti M, Bonduel M, et al: Impact of inherited thrombophilia on venous thromboembolism in children: A systematic review and meta-analysis of observational studies. *Circulation* 118:1373, 2008.
417. Young G, Becker S, During C, et al: Influence of the factor II G20210A variant or the factor V G1691A mutation on symptomatic recurrent venous thromboembolism in children: An international multicenter cohort study. *J Thromb Haemost* 7:72, 2009.
418. Goldenberg NA, Knapp-Clevenger R, Manco-Johnson MJ: Elevated plasma factor VIII and D-dimer levels as predictors of poor outcomes of thrombosis in children. *N Engl J Med* 351:1081, 2004.
419. deVeber G, Andrew M, Adams C, et al: Cerebral sinovenous thrombosis in children. *N Engl J Med* 345:417, 2001.
420. Heller C, Heinecke A, Junker R, et al: Cerebral venous thrombosis in children: A multifactorial origin. *Circulation* 108:1362, 2003.
421. Simchen MJ, Goldstein G, Lubetsky A, et al: Factor V Leiden and antiphospholipid antibodies in either mothers or infants increase the risk for perinatal arterial ischemic stroke. *Stroke* 40:65, 2009.
422. Mackay MT, Monagle P: Perinatal and early childhood stroke and thrombophilia. *Pathology* 40:116, 2008.
423. Kenet G, Kirkham F, Niederstadt T, et al: Risk factors for recurrent venous thromboembolism in the European collaborative paediatric database on cerebral venous thrombosis: A multicentre cohort study. *Lancet Neurol* 6:595, 2007.
424. Press RD, Bauer KA, Kujovich JL, Heit JA: Clinical utility of factor V Leiden (R506Q) testing for the diagnosis and management of thromboembolic disorders. *Arch Pathol Lab Med* 126:1304, 2002.
425. Van Cott EM, Laposata M, Prins MH: Laboratory evaluation of hyper-coagulability with venous or arterial thrombosis. *Arch Pathol Lab Med* 126:1281, 2002.
426. Tripodi A, Mannucci PM: Laboratory investigation of thrombophilia. *Clin Chem* 47:1597, 2001.
427. Bauer KA: The thrombophilias: Well-defined risk factors with uncertain therapeutic implications. *Ann Intern Med* 135:367, 2001.
428. Schulman S: Duration of anticoagulants in acute or recurrent venous thromboembolism. *Curr Opin Pulm Med* 6:321, 2000.
429. Hirsh J, Kearon C, Ginsberg J: Duration of anticoagulant therapy after first episode of venous thrombosis in patients with inherited thrombophilia. *Arch Intern Med* 157:2174, 1997.
430. Kearon C, Crowther M, Hirsh J: Management of patients with hereditary hypercoagulable disorders. *Annu Rev Med* 51:169, 2000.
431. Bauer KA: Management of thrombophilia. *J Thromb Haemost* 1:1429, 2003.
432. Kearon C, Kahn SR, Agnelli G, et al: Antithrombotic therapy for venous thromboembolic disease: American College of Chest Physicians Evidence-Based Clinical Practice Guidelines (8th edition). *Chest* 133(6 Suppl):454S, 2008.
433. Kearon C: Long-term management of patients after venous thromboembolism. *Circulation* 110(9 Suppl 1):I-100, 2004.
434. Bates SM, Ginsberg JS: Clinical practice. Treatment of deep-vein thrombosis. *N Engl J Med* 351:268, 2004.
435. Schulman S, Rhedin AS, Lindmarker P, et al: A comparison of six weeks with six months of oral anticoagulant therapy after a first episode of venous thromboembolism. Duration of Anticoagulation Trial Study Group. *N Engl J Med* 332:1661, 1995.
436. Brandjes DP, Buller HR, Heijboer H: Randomized trial of effect of compression stockings in patients with symptomatic proximal-vein thrombosis. *Lancet* 349:759, 1997.
437. Marik PE, Plante LA: Venous thromboembolic disease and pregnancy. *N Engl J Med* 359:2025, 2008.
438. Ginsberg JS, Bates SM: Management of venous thromboembolism during pregnancy. *J Thromb Haemost* 1:1435, 2003.
439. Bowles L, Cohen H: Inherited thrombophilias and anticoagulation in pregnancy. *Best Pract Res Clin Obstet Gynaecol* 17:471, 2003.
440. Lechner K, Kyrle PA: Antithrombin III concentrates—Are they clinically useful? *Thromb Haemost* 73:340, 1995.
441. Bucur SZ, Levy JH, Despotis GJ, et al: Uses of antithrombin III concentrate in congenital and acquired deficiency states. *Transfusion* 38: 481, 1998.
442. Menache D, O'Malley JP, Schorr JB, et al: Evaluation of the safety, recovery, half-life, and clinical efficacy of antithrombin III (human) in patients with hereditary antithrombin III deficiency. *Blood* 75:33, 1990.
443. Konkle BA, Bauer KA, Weinstein R: Use of recombinant human anti-thrombin in patients with congenital antithrombin deficiency undergoing surgical procedures. *Transfusion* 43:390, 2003.
444. Vukovich T, Auberger K, Weil J, et al: Replacement therapy for a homozygous protein C deficiency-state using a concentrate of human protein C and S. *Br J Haematol* 70:435, 1988.
445. Manco-Johnson M, Nuss R: Protein C concentrate prevents peripartum thrombosis. *Am J Hematol* 40:69, 1992.
446. Gerson WT, Dickerman JD, Bovill EG, Golden E: Severe acquired protein C deficiency in purpura fulminans associated with disseminated intravascular coagulation: Treatment with protein C concentrate. *Pediatrics* 91:418, 1993.
447. Sanson BJ, Simioni P, Tormene D, et al: The incidence of venous thromboembolism in asymptomatic carriers of a deficiency of antithrombin, protein C, or protein S: A prospective cohort study. *Blood* 94:3702, 1999.
448. Folkeringa N, Brouwer JL, Korteweg FJ, et al: Reduction of high fetal loss rate by anticoagulant treatment during pregnancy in antithrombin, protein C or protein S deficient women. *Br J Haematol* 136:656, 2007.

CHAPTER 132
THE ANTIPHOSPHOLIPID SYNDROME

Jacob H. Rand

SUMMARY

The antiphospholipid (aPL) syndrome (APS) is an acquired thrombophilic disorder in which patients have vascular thrombosis and/or pregnancy complications attributable to placental insufficiency, accompanied by laboratory evidence for the presence of antiphospholipid antibodies in blood. The disorder is referred to as *primary APS* when it occurs in the absence of systemic lupus erythematosus (SLE), and *secondary APS* in its presence. Although the most frequently affected vessels are the deep veins of the lower extremities, any portion of the circulatory tree can be affected. Abnormalities that have been reported in association with the syndrome include virtually all other autoimmune disorders, immune thrombocytopenia, acquired platelet function abnormalities, hypoprothrombinemia, acquired inhibitors of coagulation factors, livedo reticularis, heart valve abnormalities, atherosclerosis, pulmonary hypertension, migraine, and sensorineural hearing loss. Rare patients have a catastrophic form of APS (CAPS) in which there is disseminated thrombosis in large- and small-vessel thrombi, often after a triggering event such as infection or surgery, and often with multiorgan ischemia and infarction.

The main antigenic targets for thrombogenic aPL antibodies are not phospholipids. Rather, they are epitopes on phospholipid-binding proteins, the most important of which appears to be β_2-glycoprotein I (β_2GPI). The syndrome is identified by persistent abnormalities of laboratory tests for antibodies against these phospholipid–protein cofactor complexes, detected by immunoassays and by coagulation assays that, paradoxically, report the inhibition of phospholipid-dependent coagulation reactions. Several conditions, including syphilis, Lyme disease, hepatitis C, alcoholic liver disease, HIV infection, and multiple sclerosis, are associated with increased levels of aPL antibodies that are generally not thrombogenic and are directed against anionic phospholipids themselves rather than the protein cofactors. Long-term warfarin anticoagulant therapy is the usual treatment for thrombosis in patients with APS, although there is some controversy regarding treatment of patients with stroke. Patients with recurrent spontaneous pregnancy losses and APS generally are treated with aspirin and heparin during their pregnancies for prophylaxis against deep vein thrombosis during the postpartum period. CAPS patients have a high mortality and often require additional therapy with anticoagulants, plasmapheresis, and immunosuppressive agents. Patients without clinical manifestations of APS or SLE, should generally not undergo diagnostic screening and, if tested and found to be positive, should not be committed to antithrombotic therapy for the laboratory abnormalities alone. Where anticoagulant therapy is indicated, care should be taken to confirm that prothrombin time and international normalized ratio determinations for monitoring oral anticoagulant therapy reflect true reductions in the levels of the vitamin K-dependent coagulation proteins and are not artifactually altered by a lupus anticoagulant.

Acronyms and abbreviations that appear in this chapter include: aCL, anticardiolipin; APASS, Antiphospholipid Antibodies and Stroke Study; APC, activated protein C; aPL, antiphospholipid; APS, antiphospholipid syndrome; aPTT, activated partial thromboplastin time; ARDS, acute respiratory distress syndrome; AVWS, acquired von Willebrand syndrome; BFP syphilis test, biologic false-positive serologic test for syphilis; β_2GPI, β_2-glycoprotein I; CAPS, catastrophic APS; CMV, cytomegalovirus; dRVVT, dilute Russell viper venom time; EBV, Epstein-Barr virus; ELISA, enzyme-linked immunosorbent assay; HCQ, hydroxychloroquine; ICAM, intercellular adhesion molecule; Ig, immunoglobulin; IL, interleukin; LA, lupus anticoagulant; LDL, low-density lipoprotein; LMWH, low-molecular-weight heparin; mAb, monoclonal antibody; MAPK, mitogen-activated protein kinase; RVV, Russell viper venom; SCR, short consensus repeat; SLE, systemic lupus erythematosus; TM, thrombomodulin; t-PA, tissue-type plasminogen activator; UFH, unfractionated heparin; VCAM, vascular cell adhesion molecule; VWF, von Willebrand factor.

DEFINITION AND HISTORY

The antiphospholipid (aPL) antibody syndrome (APS) is a disorder in which vascular thrombosis or pregnancy complications attributable to placental insufficiency occur in patients with laboratory evidence for antibodies directed against proteins that bind to phospholipids. The syndrome was first proposed to be a distinct entity, "the anticardiolipin (aCL) syndrome," in 1985[1] and soon was renamed APS.[2] While precise data are not available, the syndrome is thought to affect approximately 10 percent of patients with venous thrombosis,[3,4] and approximately 20 percent of women with three unexplained fetal losses before 12 weeks of gestation, or at least one intrauterine fetal death after 12 weeks of gestation.[5]

The term "aPL antibodies" refers to several different assays that do not correlate well with each other; Table 132–1 is a glossary of some frequently used terms. "aPL" can refer to (1) antibodies that recognize protein-phospholipid complexes as in cofactor-dependent anticardiolipin assays, (2) antibodies that recognize the proteins directly as in anti-$\beta_2$glycoprotein I assays (anti-β_2GPI), (3) antibodies that recognize phospholipid directly as in syphilis, and (4) an abnormal coagulation test in several assays that report inhibition of phospholipid-dependent coagulation reactions, collectively as termed lupus anticoagulant (LA) tests.

A brief review of the history of APS will help explain the confusing terminology (Table 132–2); the reader is referred to references 6 to 8 for more detailed accounts. The recognition of this syndrome came about through two diagnostic paths: the progressive development of improved immunoassays and the development of diagnostic coagulation tests. Moore and Mohr's report of the "biologic false-positive" serologic tests for syphilis (BFP syphilis test) in 1952,[9] a test that became associated with systemic lupus erythematosus (SLE),[10] in retrospect, was the first description of aPL autoantibodies. The introduction, at nearly the same time, of the activated partial thromboplastin time (aPTT), which used cephalin, a phospholipid extract of animal brains, as the "partial thromboplastin" (distinct from the "complete thromboplastin," tissue factor and phospholipid)[11] led to the recognition of a unique type of anticoagulant in patients with SLE, that was frequently associated with BFP syphilis tests.[12] Because of its initial association with SLE this phenomenon was misnamed LA.[13] It became recognized that this anticoagulant was not associated with bleeding problems *in vivo* unless another hemostatic defect was present,[6] and also that it was associated with recurrent pregnancy losses[14,15] and with thrombotic and embolic manifestations.[16] The development, in 1983, of the aCL antibody assay that detected antibodies against the anionic phospholipid, cardiolipin (diphosphatidylglycerol), the primary antigen in the syphilis test reagent,[17] was the advance that led to the identification of a new syndrome. Within a few years, it became recognized that these antibodies were actually directed against proteins that bound to the phospholipid, primarily β_2GPI, and generally did not bind cardiolipin directly (see "Pathogenesis" below). This information became important in helping to unravel the mechanisms for APS and in advancing diagnostic testing toward the goal of distinguishing between

TABLE 132–1. Antiphospholipid Terminologies

Anticardiolipin antibodies: Antibodies that recognize cardiolipin–also known as diphosphatidyl glycerol. Cardiolipin, an extract of cardiac intracellular membranes–mainly mitochondria–is the key antigen in the serologic tests for syphilis.

Antidomain specific antibodies: aPL antibodies that recognize specific epitopes on cofactors, e.g., domain I of β_2-glycoprotein I (β_2GPI).

Antiphosphatidyl serine antibodies: aPL antibodies that recognize phosphatidyl serine, the major anionic phospholipid in cytoplasmic membranes.

Antiphospholipid (aPL) antibodies: Antibodies that recognize phospholipids, proteins that bind to phospholipids, complexes of proteins and phospholipids, or inhibit phospholipid-dependent coagulation reactions (see lupus anticoagulant [LA])

aPL cofactors: Proteins, recognized by aPL, that bind to phospholipid, mainly β_2GPI, but includes prothrombin, proteins C and S, and annexins.

APS: The antiphospholipid syndrome: Patients with criteria for clinical manifestations detailed in Table 132–2 who have at least one persistent positive aPL antibody test that is confirmed ≥12 weeks after initial testing. The syndrome is referred to as "primary APS" in the absence of systemic lupus erythematosus (SLE), and "secondary APS" in its presence.

CAPS (Catastrophic APS): A form of APS that is manifest by disseminated thrombosis often microvascular, and frequently by multiorgan failure. CAPS is associated with a high mortality.

Cofactor-dependent aPL antibodies: aPL antibodies that do not bind to phospholipids unless cofactors, such as β_2GPI, are present.

Cofactor-independent aPL antibodies: aPL antibodies that bind phospholipids directly. Antitreponemal antibodies are the paradigm for this.

High-avidity aPL antibodies: Antibodies that bind to phospholipid in the presence of chaotropic agents or high salt concentrations.

LA (Lupus Anticoagulants): aPL antibodies that interfere with phospholipid-dependent coagulation reactions *in vitro*.

TABLE 132–2. Development of aPL Assays: Historical Summary

Immunoassay Path	Coagulation Path
1950s: Syphilis testing	1950s: Partial thromboplastin time (PTT) inhibitor
	1970s: Lupus anticoagulant (LA)
1980s: aPL antibody enzyme-linked immunosorbent assay (ELISA; e.g., anticardiolipin immunoassays)	
	1980s: Recognition that LAs are inhibitors of phospholipid-dependent coagulation reactions
1990s: Anti-cofactor ELISA (anti-β_2GPI, antiprothrombin, etc.)	
2005: Demonstration that antibodies against domain I of β_2GPI are associated with increased risk of thrombosis	2004: Demonstration that resistance to the anticoagulant effect of annexin A5 correlates with thrombosis in APS
Goal: Immunoassays for epitope-specific antibodies that correlate with pathogenic mechanisms of APS and accurately identify high-risk patients	Goal: Functional coagulation assays that correlate with prothrombotic mechanisms and accurately identify high-risk patients

the syndrome and incidental false-positive tests. Table 132–3 states recent consensus investigational criteria for diagnosing APS.[18]

Most patients with elevated aPL antibodies do not have APS; Table 132–4 provides a classification of aPL antibody-positive patients. Elevated aPL antibody levels can occur in patients with a variety of infections that induce formation of antibodies recognizing anionic phospholipids directly, patients taking medications such as chlorpromazine or procainamide, and even in normal healthy individuals. Testing of patients who do not have clinical manifestations or SLE for aPL antibodies may increase the risk of inappropriate diagnostic and treatment decisions.

ETIOLOGY AND PATHOGENESIS

ETIOLOGY

As with most autoimmune conditions, the etiology of APS is not understood. It has been demonstrated that normal healthy individuals without APS have memory B cells that produce aPL antibodies; in a study of patients with infectious mononucleosis, 10 to 60 percent of immunoglobulin (Ig) M aCL-producing cells expressed CD27, the marker of memory B cells.[19] The affinity of aPL antibodies becomes increased by the inclusion of amino acids lysine, arginine, and asparagine within the complementarity determining regions of the heavy and light chains.[20]

Although antibodies against anionic phospholipid moieties arise during the course of infections such as syphilis and Lyme disease, those are distinct from antibodies generated by patients with the syndrome because they generally recognize phospholipid epitopes directly (also referred to as "cofactor independent") and are not associated with the clinical manifestations of the syndrome. There are intriguing hints for molecular mimicry mechanisms for APS. aPL antibodies have been reported in patients who, after varicella infection developed thrombosis,[8,21,22] and in patients with hepatitis C.[23,24] aPL antibodies were reported in a patient with cytomegalovirus (CMV) infection, mesenteric and femoropopliteal thrombosis.[25,26] β_2GPI cofactor-dependent antibodies against cardiolipin, phosphatidyl serine, and phosphatidyl ethanolamine have been identified in sera from patients with parvovirus B19.[27] A high proportion of HIV-1 patients have antiphospholipid antibodies; more than 40 percent in one study, of which 18 percent had aCL and 30 percent had anti-β_2GPI (mostly of the IgA isotype).[28] However, these did not correlate with clinical manifestations of APS. A link has been proposed between the cardiac valvular disease in acute rheumatic fever and the presence of aPL antibodies.[29] aCL antibodies having β_2GPI dependence and LA activity have been generated in rabbits immunized with lipid A and lipoteichoic acid, suggesting that some bacteria can contribute to the production of pathogenic aPL antibodies.[30] It has also been proposed that cellular apoptosis, with the resulting exposure of anionic phospholipids on cell surfaces, triggers the generation of aPL antibodies.[31–33] Molecular mimicry between β_2GPI-related synthetic peptides and structures within bacteria, viruses, and tetanus toxoid[34] have been demonstrated in an experimental model for APS.[35] Mice immunized with a CMV-derived peptide developed aPL antibodies and thrombosis, and showed evidence for endothelial cell activation.[36]

Reports of familial clustering of raised aPL antibody levels[37] indicate that genetic susceptibility can play a role in their development. In one study of 84 APS patients, more than 35 percent had at least one relative, and more than 20 percent had two or more relatives, with evidence of at least one clinical feature of APS, such as thrombosis or recurrent fetal loss.[38]

TABLE 132–3. Sydney Investigational Criteria for Diagnosis of APS

Clinical

Vascular thrombosis (one or more episodes of arterial, venous, or small vessel thrombosis). For histopathologic diagnosis, there should not be evidence of inflammation in the vessel wall.

Pregnancy morbidities attributable to placental insufficiency, including: Three or more otherwise unexplained recurrent spontaneous miscarriages, before 10 weeks of gestation. Also, one or more fetal losses after the 10th week of gestation, stillbirth, episode of preeclampsia, preterm labor, placental abruption, intrauterine growth restriction or oligohydramnios that are otherwise unexplained.

Laboratory

aCL or anti-β_2GPI IgG and/or IgM antibody present in medium or high titer on two or more occasions, at least 12 weeks apart, measured by standard ELISAs.

Lupus anticoagulant in plasma, on two or more occasions, at least 12 weeks apart detected according to the guidelines of the International Society of Thrombosis and Hemostasis Scientific Standardization Committee on Lupus Anticoagulants and Phospholipid-Dependent Antibodies.

"Definite APS" is considered to be present if at least one of the clinical criteria and one of the laboratory criteria are met.

aCL, anticardiolipin; aPL, antiphospholipid; β_2GPI, β_2-glycoprotein I; ELISA, enzyme-linked immunosorbent assay; Ig, immunoglobulin.

SOURCE: Adapted from Miyakis S, Lockshin MD, Atsumi T, et al.[18]

TABLE 132–4. Classification of Patients with aPL Antibodies

aPL Antibodies Usually Not Associated with Thrombosis

aPL antibodies associated with infections: The paradigm for infection-associated aPL is syphilis. However, this has been reported with a variety of other infections including, but not limited to Lyme disease, streptococcal infection, cytomegalovirus (CMV), Epstein-Barr virus (EBV), HIV, and varicella.

aPL antibodies associated with drugs: for example, chlorpromazine, procainamide.

aPL antibodies associated with other clinical conditions: Multiple sclerosis. Migraine symptoms with aPL is controversial, with clinicians viewing the two as coincidental, whereas others view it as a thrombotic manifestation that warrants anticoagulation.

aPL antibodies present in otherwise normal healthy people: These may occur spontaneously, may be associated with genetic factors or subclinical infections, and may vary with seasons, being more prevalent in winter than in summer.

Thrombogenic aPL Antibodies

APS: Patients with the autoimmune aPL disorder. This group constitutes a minority of patients with aPL antibodies. The condition may occur in the absence of SLE (*primary APS*) or in SLE patients (*secondary APS*). These are generally cofactor-dependent.

Catastrophic APS: Relatively rare, but associated with a high mortality.

Pre-APS: Patients with APS antibodies who are thought to be at high risk for thrombosis but who have not yet had a documented event. Until testing methods improve, these patients can only be diagnosed retrospectively.

PATHOGENESIS

Experimental Evidence That aPL Antibodies Are Pathogenic

Experimental animal models of APS indicate that aPL antibodies play a causal role in the development of thrombosis and pregnancy loss. Mice immunized against β_2GPI developed aPL antibodies and pregnancy wastage.[39] Exposure to aPL antibodies caused fetal wastage in mice, a process that involved complement C3 activation.[40] Monoclonal human aPL antibodies promoted thrombosis in experimental vascular injury models in mice[41] and hamsters.[42]

Antigenic Specificities

Antibodies against phospholipid that arise during the immunologic response to syphilis and other infections (with the notable exception of leprosy[43]) recognize anionic phospholipid epitopes directly,[44] whereas pathogenic aPL antibodies recognize phospholipid-binding proteins, primarily β_2GPI.[45,46]

β_2GPI (also named apolipoprotein H), a member of the complement control protein or short consensus repeat superfamily,[47] is a highly glycosylated single-chain plasma protein composed of 326 amino acids, with a molecular weight of approximately 50 kDa (Fig. 132–1A). β_2GPI has five short consensus repeat (SCR) stretches of approximately 60 residues[45] (also referred to as complement control protein [CCP] repeats). Epitopic specificities for individual domains may have pathogenic and prognostic significance (see "Immunoassays" below).[48–50] The protein inserts into phospholipid bilayers through a hydrophobic and cationic region located near the carboxy-terminus of SCR domain V (Fig. 132–1B), and then agglomerates into clusters on phospholipid membranes.[51]

Although the *in vivo* biologic function(s) of the protein has (have) not been established, several interesting properties have been demonstrated. The molecule binds to apoptotic cells,[52] and may play a role in their phagocytosis and clearance.[53] β_2GPI binds to oxidized low-density lipoprotein (LDL) and may play a role in its clearance.[54] β_2GPI reduces platelet adhesion to collagen in flow chambers by interfering with the platelet–von Willebrand factor interaction by binding to its A2 domain, thereby interfering with its binding to the platelet glycoprotein Ib (GpIb) complex.[55] β_2GPI may also promote fibrinolysis as a cofactor for tissue-type plasminogen activator (t-PA) via its SCR domain V, which increases fibrinolytic activity.[56] The protein may have a further effect on fibrinolysis by binding to endothelial cells via annexin A2, a protein that also serves as a receptor for plasminogen and t-PA.[57] However, homozygous β_2GPI-null mice have not been demonstrated to display a disease phenotype.[58] Thrombin generation was also reported to be defective in these animals, but the reason for the defect is unknown and there was no link to increased bleeding. The protein may play a role early in the reproductive process, as fewer than expected numbers of homozygous β_2GPI-null offspring are born from heterozygous parents,[58] however, placental pathology has not been reported.

Other antigenic targets identified for aPL include prothrombin, coagulation factor V, protein C, protein S, annexin A2, annexin A5, high- and low-molecular-weight kininogens, and factors VII/VIIa.[59–61] Antibodies of some APS patients cross-react with heparin and inhibit the formation of antithrombin–thrombin complexes.[62]

Proposed Pathogenic Mechanisms

Table 132–5 summarizes several of the current hypotheses for pathogenic mechanisms in APS. The mechanisms of the human APS disease have resisted elucidation, mainly for two reasons: (1) The phenotypes of vascular thrombosis and pregnancy morbidity are not unique to APS, so it is difficult to ascertain whether the candidate mechanism is playing a causal role or is incidental. (2) Antibodies isolated from APS patients recognize a multiplicity of antigenic determinants,[63] that can have a broad range of effects, so it is difficult to determine which specificities and effects are responsible for disease manifestations in humans.

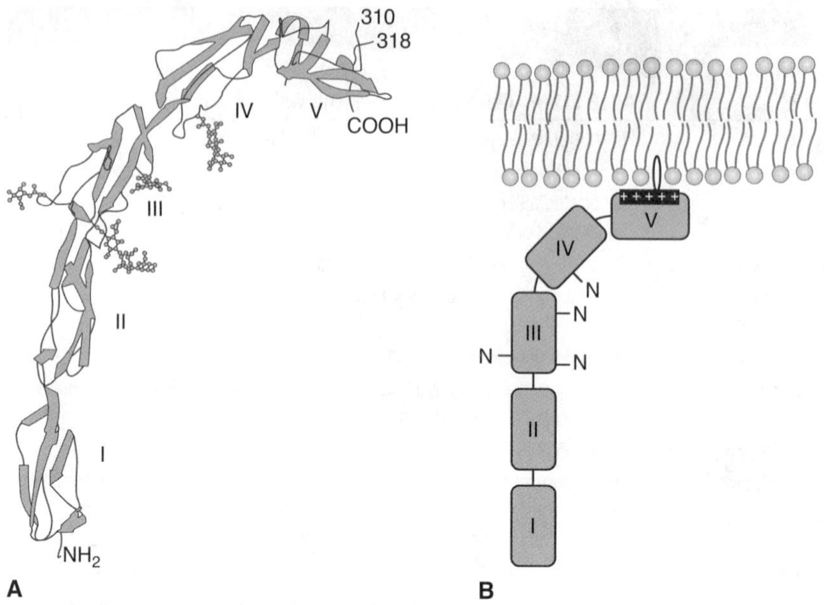

FIGURE 132–1. Structure of human blood plasma β_2-glycoprotein I (β_2GPI).[285] Ribbon **(A)** and domain **(B)** models of β_2GPI based on crystal structure. The protein is composed of an extended chain of five short consensus repeat domains, with a fifth domain having a structure that deviates from the standard fold of the other four and contains the putative phospholipid-binding site. The overall configuration of the molecule is analogous to a J-shaped fishhook with a barb, consisting of the phospholipid binding site near the carboxyterminus of domain V. The portion of Ser311 to Lys317 forms a hydrophobic loop that inserts into the lipid bilayer and positions Trp316 at the interface region between the acyl chains and the phosphate head groups of the lipids, thereby anchoring the β_2GPI in the membrane.[285] Antibodies that recognize epitopes on domain I after the protein binds to phospholipid are particularly associated with thrombosis and pregnancy losses, and correlate with resistance to annexin A5 anticoagulant activity. β-strands are shown in red and helices in light blue. *(Figures reprinted with permission from Bouma B, de Groot PG, van den Elsen JM, et al.[285])*

Disruption of the Annexin A5 Anticoagulant Shield Annexin A5 (previously known as annexin V, placental anticoagulant protein-I, vascular anticoagulant-α and several other names) is a potent anticoagulant protein with high affinity for phospholipid membranes that contain anionic phospholipids, specifically phosphatidyl serine.[64] Annexin A5 forms two-dimensional crystals over the phospholipid bilayers that shield them from binding coagulation factors.[65] It is likely that annexin A5 plays a thrombomodulatory role on the surfaces of cells lining the placental and systemic vasculatures. It is highly expressed on the apical membranes of placental syncytiotrophoblasts, the location where maternal blood interfaces with fetal cells.[66] Pregnant mice treated with antiannexin A5 antibodies developed placental necrosis, fibrosis, and pregnancy loss.[67] Dissociation of annexin A5 from the surface of human placental trophoblasts and human umbilical vein endothelial cells accelerates the coagulation of plasma exposed to those cells.[68] Annexin A5 binds to the surfaces of endothelial cells and inhibits thrombin formation.[69]

aPL antibody-antigen complexes disrupt the crystallization of annexin A5 and displace the protein from phospholipid membrane surfaces (Fig. 132–2).[70–73] In contrast to the LA phenomenon, aPL antibodies accelerate coagulation in reaction systems that include annexin A5.[70,74–77] IgG fractions from APS patients reduce the quantity of annexin A5 on cultured placental trophoblasts[68,78] and endothelial cells[68,79] and accelerate the coagulation of plasma exposed to these cells.[68] This effect of aPL antibodies on annexin A5 binding has been correlated with IgG antibodies that recognize a specific epitope—domain I of β_2GPI in patients with APS who have thrombosis[49] and spontaneous pregnancy losses.[50] Figure 132–3 shows a model for this mechanism.[49]

Interference with Annexin A2 and with Fibrinolysis Several mechanisms have been identified by which aPL antibodies can interfere with fibrinolysis. β_2GPI is a cofactor for t-PA–mediated activation of plasminogen, and aPL antibodies against β_2GPI interfere with its binding to t-PA, thereby downregulating plasminogen activation.[56] APS patients also have increased titers of antibodies against annexin A2, an endothelial surface receptor for t-PA and plasminogen.[80] The blocking of annexin A2 by aPL antibodies impedes plasmin generation in a t-PA-dependent generation assay, and inhibits cell surface plasmin generation on human umbilical vein endothelial cells.[81] Annexin A2 also serves as a receptor for β_2GPI,[57] and anti-β_2GPI antibodies may stimulate expression of tissue factor on endothelial cells.[81] Finally, fibrinolysis may also be impaired by autoantibodies directed against the catalytic site of plasmin or t-PA,[82,83] by an increased level of plasminogen activator inhibitor-1,[84] and by inhibition of autoactivation of factor XII with ensuing reductions of kallikrein and urokinase.[85]

Other Effects on Vascular Endothelial Cells aPL antibodies can bind, injure, and activate cultured vascular endothelial cells.[86–89] Cultured endothelial cells incubated with aPL antibodies with specificity for cell surface β_2GPI express increased levels of cell adhesion molecules,[90] via binding to cell surface β_2GPI.[91] These effects may be mediated by toll-like receptor-4 of the innate immunity system,[92] with downstream signalling that involves TRAF6 (tumor necrosis factor receptor-associated factor 6) and MyD88 (myeloid differentiation factor 88).[93] Increased expression of tissue factor is mediated

TABLE 132–5. Proposed Pathogenic Mechanisms for APS

I. Interference with Endogenous Antithrombotic Mechanisms
   A. Disruption of annexin A5 shield
   B. Interference with protein C and S systems
      1. Acquired resistance to activated protein C
      2. Acquired protein S deficiency
      3. Antibodies to endothelial protein C receptor
   C. Antibodies against tissue factor pathway inhibitor
   D. Interference with fibrinolysis by:
      1. Antibodies to tissue-type plasminogen activator (t-PA)
      2. Antibodies against annexin A2
      3. Interference with β_2GPI complexation with t-PA
      4. Increased level of plasminogen activator inhibitor-1
   E. Interference with β_2GPI dampening of von Willebrand factor (VWF)-mediated platelet adhesion
II. aPL Antibody-Mediated Prothrombotic/Proadhesive Cell Signaling
   A. Induction of endothelial surface proadhesive molecules
   B. Induction of tissue factor expression on monocytes and endothelial cells
   C. Activation of platelets
   D. Complement-mediated injury and signaling

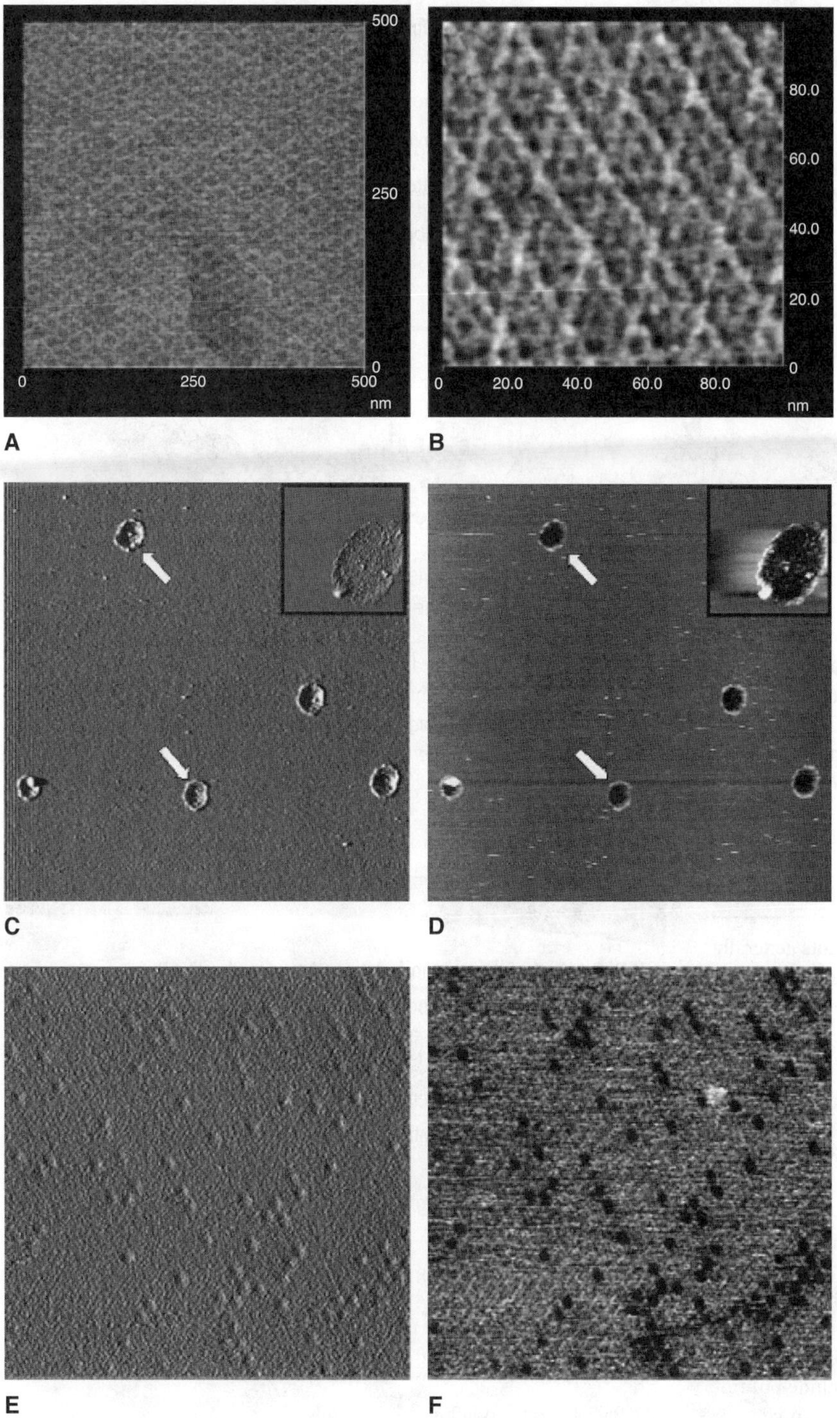

FIGURE 132–2. Atomic force microscopy images showing crystal structure of annexin A5 and the effects of aPL IgG monoclonal antibody on annexin A5 crystallization.[71] **A, B.** Annexin A5 two-dimensional crystalline lattice formed over phospholipid bilayer at low (A) and higher (B) magnifications, showing the ordered arrays of annexin A5 crystal. **C–F.** Effect of a monoclonal aPL antibody (mAb IS3) on an annexin A5 crystal lattice that was preformed over phospholipid bilayer. C and E are amplitude images, D and F are corresponding height images. Addition of the aPL monoclonal antibody (mAb) and the cofactor, β_2GPI, to the fluid over the annexin A5 crystal lattice, resulted in the development of circular craters (*arrows* in C and D) in the crystal lattice that expose underlying anionic phospholipid. A representative crater is shown at higher magnification in the insets. At higher resolution (E, F), more vacancy defects (*small, round, dark holes*) in the crystalline lattice are apparent. These defects, with exposed phospholipid, accelerate phospholipid-dependent coagulation enzyme reactions. Amplitude images (C, E) processed with a 1× convolution and height images (D, F) processed by "zero order flatten." Magnifications 10 μm × 10 mm scan (C, D); 500 nm × 500 nm (E, F). *(Reprinted with permission from Rand JH, Wu XX, Quinn AS, et al.[71])*

by p38 mitogen-activated protein kinase (MAPK).[94] aPL antibodies including species that bind to apoptotic endothelial cells, can promote thrombosis by reducing the clearance of these cells and by increasing phagocytosis by Fc-mediated macrophages.[95]

Complement-Mediated Injury There is evidence that complement activation may play a role in APS. The IgG$_2$ subtype of aPL most closely correlates with thrombosis.[96] Blockade of complement activation using a C3 convertase inhibitor or genetic deletion of C3 protected mice from pregnancy complications induced by aPL antibodies.[97–99] These effects involve the aPL-stimulated expression of tissue factor by myeloid cells,[100] and to involve proteinase-activated G-protein-coupled receptor (PAR)-2 signaling,[101] indicating that complement activation can be pathogenic via both direct injury and downstream signalling.

Induction of Tissue Factor Activity in Leukocytes aPL antibodies can promote tissue factor expression by leukocytes.[100,102–104]

Interference with Components of the Protein C Activation Pathway The protein C pathway (see Chap. 116) is initiated by thrombin binding to thrombomodulin (TM), which activates protein bound to the endothelial protein C receptor (EPCR). Activated protein C (APC), together with free protein S, then proteolyses coagulation factors Va and VIIIa. APC also modulates signalling events by interfering with PAR-1 signalling.[105,106] aPL antibodies can interfere with the activation of protein C by TM–thrombin and with the activity of APC, as well as protect factors Va and VIIIa from proteolysis by APC.[59] APC resistance has been described in APS plasmas[107] and has been correlated with anti-β_2GPI domain I antibodies,[108] a risk factor for thrombosis. The presence of antibodies against EPCR in APS patients was proposed to be a risk factor for fetal death.[109]

Effects of Antiphospholipid Antibodies on Platelets aPL antibodies can stimulate platelet aggregation,[110] an effect that might be promoted via signalling through apolipoprotein E receptor 2 (apoER2) receptors; the β_2GPI binding site for ApoER2 on platelets was localized to its domain V.[111] As described above (see "Antigenic Specificities"), β_2GPI also has a dampening effect on platelet adhesion by interfering with the platelet–von Willebrand factor interaction, and consequently aPL antibodies, by interfering with this dampening, can increase platelet adhesion in flow systems.[55]

Other Prothrombotic Mechanisms APS patients have autoantibodies against tissue factor pathway inhibitor.[112] Some aPL antibodies cross-react with heparin and heparinoid molecules, which are highly polyanionic, and hence, inhibit their contribution to antithrombin activity.[62] aPL antibodies show cross-reactivity against oxidized LDL[113] and are associated with an increased risk of atherosclerosis.[114] Antibodies against β_2GPI-oxidized LDL complexes have been proposed to be atherogenic by reducing their clearance.[115]

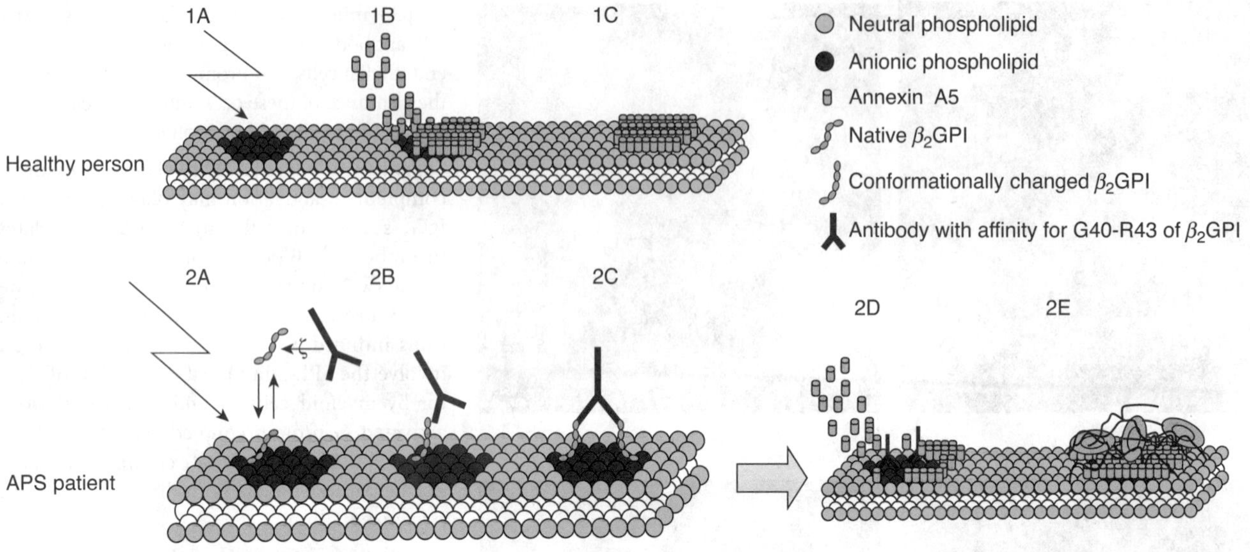

FIGURE 132–3. Proposed mechanism for thrombosis in APS: The antidomain I IgG-mediated disruption of annexin A5 on cell surfaces.[49] In the absence of APS, anionic phospholipids become exposed on cell surfaces, e.g., endothelial cells after injury (*1A*). Annexin A5 assembles over the damaged areas of endothelium and thereby inhibits coagulation which is dependent on anionic phospholipids (*1B* and *1C*). Any β_2GPI that binds to these surfaces would be competed off by the higher affinity annexin A5. In contrast, when damage to endothelial cells occurs in an APS patient with antibodies against epitope G40-R43 on domain I, the following reactions take place: β_2GPI binds to the anionic phospholipids with a rather low affinity (*2A*); the exposure of G40-R43 epitope leads to antibody binding and immune complex formation that dimerizes the β_2GPI molecules (*2B* and *2C*); the immune complexed β_2GPI, which has a high avidity for anionic phospholipids competes with annexin A5 for binding to anionic phospholipid (*2D*); the ordered crystallization of annexin A5 is disrupted thereby causing excessive clotting (*2E*). *(Reprinted with permission from de Laat B, Wu XX, van Lummel M, et al.[49])*

CLINICAL FEATURES

Table 132–6 summarizes the clinical features of APS. Patients generally present with thrombotic manifestations, that is, evidence for vasoocclusion or end-organ ischemia or infarction, and/or pregnancy losses and complications attributable to placental insufficiency. The usual age at presentation with thrombosis is approximately 35 to 45 years.[116] Except for patients with SLE, men and women are equally susceptible to thrombotic manifestations.[116] No differences have been observed between the arterial and venous distributions of thromboses of primary and secondary APS patients.[117]

SYSTEMIC VASCULAR THROMBOSIS

Patients can present with spontaneous venous and/or arterial thrombosis or embolism, involving any site; however, the deep veins of the lower extremities are most common, occurring in about half of patients affected.[118,119] Other sites of venous thrombotic events include pulmonary embolism, thoracic veins (superior vena cava, subclavian vein, or jugular vein), and abdominal or pelvic veins.[119] Approximately one-fourth of patients present with arterial thromboses; the remainder present with concurrent arterial and venous thrombosis.[119] Patients may also present with stroke, cerebral venous thrombosis, upper-extremity venous thrombosis,[118] myocardial infarction, adrenal infarction, acalculous gallbladder infarction, aortic thrombosis with renal infarction,[120] and mesenteric artery thrombosis.[121]

Thrombosis may occur spontaneously or in the presence of some other risk factor such as estrogen replacement therapy, oral contraceptives,[117,122] vascular stasis, surgery, or trauma. Women are at particularly high risk for venous thrombosis during pregnancy and in the postpartum period.[117] Some APS patients with venous thrombosis have concurrent genetic thrombophilic conditions such as the factor

TABLE 132–6. Clinical Manifestations Associated with APS

Venous and arterial thromboembolism*
Pregnancy complications attributable to placental insufficiency, including spontaneous pregnancy losses as detailed in Table 132–3, intrauterine growth restriction, preeclampsia, preterm labor, and placental abruption*
Infertility is not associated with APS
Thrombocytopenia
Thrombotic and embolic stroke*
Cerebral vein thrombosis*
Livedo reticularis, necrotizing skin vasculitis
Coronary artery disease
Valvular heart disease
Kidney disease
Pulmonary hypertension
Acute respiratory distress syndrome
Atherosclerosis and peripheral artery disease
Retinal disease
Adrenal failure, hemorrhagic adrenal infarction*
Budd-Chiari syndrome, mesenteric and portal vein obstructions, hepatic infarction, esophageal necrosis, gastric and colonic ulceration, gallbladder necrosis*
Sensorineural hearing loss
Catastrophic antiphospholipid syndrome with thrombotic microangiopathy*

*Manifestations that qualify as consensus criteria for diagnosis of APS.[18]

V-Leiden.[123–126] A history of a thromboembolic event is probably the most significant risk factor for recurrent thromboembolism in APS; its frequency reached approximately 30 percent in patients followed for 4 years after the first episode of venous thromboembolism.[127] The risk of recurrence correlates with the titer of antibodies,[127,128] and with the presence of LA. In addition, it appears that the presence of anti-β_2GPI domain I antibodies significantly increase the risk of thrombosis, compared to patients who have antibodies that are not domain I dependent and LA that are not domain I dependent.[48]

SYSTEMIC LUPUS ERYTHEMATOSUS AND OTHER AUTOIMMUNE CONDITIONS

APS patients frequently present with other autoimmune conditions. A significant proportion of SLE patients have elevated aPL antibodies, with estimates ranging between 12 to 30 percent for anticardiolipin antibodies and 15 to 34 percent for LA antibodies.[129] APS has been associated with many other autoimmune conditions including, but not limited to, rheumatoid arthritis,[130] Sjögren syndrome,[131] myasthenia gravis,[132] Budd-Chiari syndrome in the setting of SLE,[133] Graves disease,[134] autoimmune hemolytic anemia, progressive systemic sclerosis,[135] Evans syndrome,[136] Takayasu arteritis,[137] and polyarteritis nodosa.[138]

STROKE AND OTHER NEUROLOGIC CONDITIONS

Prospective analysis for the presence of aPL antibodies in stroke patients in the Antiphospholipid Antibody Stroke Study (APASS) demonstrated that elevated levels of aCL antibodies are associated with increased risk for developing stroke but not with subsequent thromboembolic events.[139] Patients who tested positive for both aCL and LA tended to have more subsequent thromboocclusive events than patients who tested negative for both (31.7% vs. 24.0%, $p = 0.07$).[140] Elevated antibodies against β_2GPI and LA, but not aCL and antiphosphatidyl serine, were the most significant risk factors for stroke.[141]

APS should be suspected in young patients with transient ischemic attacks or stroke, particularly when the more typical risk factors for cerebrovascular disease are absent.[142] Most APS patients with stroke have arterial thromboembolic occlusive events that are clinically indistinguishable from the more common arteriosclerotic strokes. Cerebral venous thrombosis is less common in APS patients and presents at a younger age and is more extensive than in non-APS patients with the disorder.[143] In one series of 40 cases of cerebral venous thrombosis, three patients (8%) had elevated aPL antibody levels.[144] Superior sagittal sinus thrombosis has been reported with primary APS.[145]

There is controversy about whether migraines in patients with aPL antibodies should be regarded as thromboocclusive events.[146] Other neurologic abnormalities associated with aPL antibodies include seizures, chorea, Guillain-Barré syndrome, transient global amnesia, dementia, diabetic peripheral neuropathy, and orthostatic hypotension.[147] Recurrent acute transverse myelopathy has been described with APS.[148–152] However, in one study of 315 SLE patients, including 10 with a history of transverse myelopathy, that disorder was not associated with aPL antibodies.[153] Multiple sclerosis patients have a high incidence of elevated aCL antibody levels (in one series, 9% had IgG antibodies and 44% had IgM antibodies)[154]; however, no clinical distinctions were found between aPL-positive and aPL-negative patients and the antibodies do not appear to be associated with thrombosis. Patients with psychotic disorders have an increased prevalence of LA and aCL antibodies, even in the absence of treatment with antipsychotic drugs.[155]

CATASTROPHIC ANTIPHOSPHOLIPID SYNDROME

The catastrophic APS (CAPS), a relatively infrequent but devastating presentation of APS, is characterized by severe widespread vascular occlusions.[156] Diagnostic criteria for CAPS include evidence of involvement of at least three organs, systems, and/or tissues, development of manifestations simultaneously or in less than 1 week, histopathologic confirmation of small-vessel occlusion, and laboratory confirmation of the presence of aPL.[157] Patients present with evidence for severe multiorgan ischemia/infarction, often with concurrent disseminated microvascular thrombosis. Patients with CAPS can present with massive venous thromboembolism, respiratory failure, stroke, abnormal liver function, renal impairment, adrenal insufficiency, and areas of cutaneous infarction. Respiratory failure usually results from acute respiratory distress syndrome (ARDS) and diffuse alveolar hemorrhage. Laboratory evidence for disseminated intravascular coagulation is frequently present. Although most patients are females, often presenting in their late thirties, CAPS can present at any age. Precipitating factors of CAPS include infections, drugs (sulfur-containing diuretics, captopril, and oral contraceptives), surgical procedures, and cessation of prior anticoagulant therapy. Patients usually present with a rapid course of multiple-organ dysfunction leading to failure. Most patients manifest evidence of microangiopathy mainly affecting small vessels of the kidneys, lungs, brain, heart, and liver. Only a minority of patients experience large-vessel occlusions. Improved treatment has reduced mortality from approximately 50 to approximately 20 percent.[156] Relapse is rare in survivors. The only identified predictive factor for adverse outcome is underlying SLE.[158] An international registry named "Registry of the European Forum on Antiphospholipid Antibodies for Patients with CAPS" has been established (www.med.ub.es/MIMMUN/FORUM/CAPS.HTM) and has accumulated almost 300 patients with CAPS at the time of this writing.

PREGNANCY LOSSES, OBSTETRIC COMPLICATIONS, AND INFERTILITY

At this time, aPL screening of asymptomatic obstetrical patients is not warranted because of the high frequency of false positive tests; most studies have estimated the prevalence of aPL antibodies among general obstetric populations to be approximately 5 percent or less and most of these aPL-positive patients are not clinically affected.[159]

Among obstetric patients with recurrent fetal losses, approximately 16 to 38 percent have aPL antibodies. In approximately half of patients, the pregnancy losses occur in the first trimester. Other patients present with later losses, most in the second trimester, but some even later, including stillbirth. Pregnancy complications attributable to APS include three or more recurrent spontaneous first trimester miscarriages, one or more fetal losses during the second trimester, stillbirth, episode of preeclampsia, preterm labor, placental abruption, intrauterine growth restriction, and oligohydramnion.[155] Pregnant patients with APS are also more prone to developing deep vein thrombosis during pregnancy or the puerperium. Rarely, pregnant patients develop CAPS.[160,161] The best predictor for pregnancy loss in a patient who tests positive for aPL antibodies is not the degree of laboratory abnormality but whether the patient has a history of previous pregnancy loss, complications, or thrombosis.[128,162]

Histologic abnormalities were found in many, but not all, placentas of aPL patients.[163] Studies of placental pathology in patients with aPL antibodies, but without a prior history of fetal loss, showed that approximately half had evidence of uteroplacental vascular pathology, approximately half had evidence of thrombotic occlusion, and approximately one-third had chronic villitis and/or decidual plasma cell infiltrates.[164,165]

APS does not appear to be a cause of reproductive failure (i.e., infertility); the presence of aPL antibodies has not been shown to affect either the implantation or ongoing pregnancy rates.[166] The Practice Committee of the American Society for Reproductive Medicine stated that the assessment of aPL antibodies is not indicated among couples undergoing *in vitro* fertilization and that anticoagulant therapy is not justified on the basis of existing data.[167]

CUTANEOUS MANIFESTATIONS

The cutaneous manifestations of APS have been reviewed and may comprise the first signs of APS in some patients.[168,169] Livedo reticularis is relatively common, occurring in 24 percent of a series of 1000 aPL patients,[170] and occasionally presents in a necrosing form.[171] Noninflammatory vascular thrombosis is the most frequent histopathologic feature. Necrotizing vasculitis, livedoid vasculitis, thrombophlebitis, cutaneous ulceration and necrosis, erythematous macules, purpura, ecchymoses, painful skin nodules, and subungual splinter hemorrhages, anetoderma (macular atrophy), discoid lupus erythematosus, and cutaneous T-cell lymphoma have all been reported.

CORONARY ARTERY DISEASE

aPL antibodies are associated with increased susceptibility to coronary artery disease,[172] particularly premature atherosclerosis.[173,174] APS should be considered in patients without the more typical risk factors for coronary artery disease and in patients with evidence for thrombotic or embolic coronary artery occlusion who lack angiographic evidence of atherosclerotic disease. aPL antibodies appear to be a risk factor for adverse outcomes following all coronary revascularization procedures,[172] and for restenosis after percutaneous transluminal coronary angioplasty.[175,176] An ultrasound study of carotid arteries provided evidence supporting an association of aPL antibodies with premature atherosclerosis; relatively young primary APS patients (mean age: 37 ± 11 years) had significantly increased intimal medial thickness compared to control non-APS groups.[177]

VALVULAR HEART DISEASE

Approximately 35 percent of patients with primary APS have cardiac valvular abnormalities detected by echocardiography.[178] In one study, approximately 20 percent of cardiac patients with valvular heart disease had evidence for aPL antibodies compared with approximately 10 percent of matched control subjects.[179] Valvulopathy includes leaflet thickening, vegetations, regurgitation, and stenosis.[180] The mitral valve is mainly affected, followed by the aortic valve.[181] In a prospective followup of 89 patients with severe, nonspecific valvular heart disease, thromboembolic events were significantly more frequent in the aPL-positive group than in the aPL-negative group, however, the presence of aPLs was not an independent risk factor for thromboembolic events in a multivariate analysis.[182]

Histologically, APS valvular lesions consist mainly of superficial or intravalvular fibrin deposits in association with variable degrees of vascular proliferation, fibroblast influx, fibrosis, and calcification. These conditions result in valve thickening, fusion, and rigidity, sometimes leading to functional abnormalities.[183] Deposits of immunoglobulins, including aCL antibodies, and of complement components are commonly found in the affected valves.[184]

PERIPHERAL VASCULAR DISEASE

Approximately one-third of patients with peripheral arterial disease undergoing bypass grafting procedures had elevated aPL antibody levels (mostly aCL antibodies).[185] Intraarterial thromboembolic events are common at presentation of these patients and may complicate surgical management. However, these patients did not have an increased risk for reocclusion, a finding that was attributable to the use of anticoagulant therapy.

PULMONARY MANIFESTATIONS

Patients with APS may present with in situ thrombosis in pulmonary vessels. aPL antibodies have been described in patients with pulmonary hypertension.[186] In one prospective trial of 38 consecutive patients with precapillary pulmonary hypertension, approximately 30 percent had aPL antibodies with various phospholipid specificities.[187] An interinstitutional study of 687 patients with chronic thromboembolic pulmonary hypertension reported that aPL antibodies were a significant risk factor.[188] The majority of patients with CAPS (see "Catastrophic APS" above) have dyspnea, and most of these individuals have ARDS.[189]

ABDOMINAL MANIFESTATIONS

The liver is the most frequently affected abdominal organ because of occlusion of hepatic vessels, including those supplying the biliary tree.[190] aPL antibody levels frequently are elevated in patients with chronic liver disease of various causes. In one prospective study of patients with liver disease, approximately half of patients with alcoholic liver disease and one-third of patients with chronic hepatitis C virus had elevated aPL antibody levels. The frequency was even higher in patients with more severe cirrhosis.[191] A review reported that approximately 20 percent of patients with chronic hepatitis B and hepatitis C had aPL antibodies, most of which were cofactor independent.[192] Some patients with hepatitis C present with true autoimmune aPL antibodies, the most common features reported being intraabdominal thrombosis and myocardial infarction.[193]

Gastrointestinal manifestations of APS also include esophageal necrosis with perforation, intestinal ischemia and infarction, pancreatitis, and colonic ulceration. Primary biliary cirrhosis,[194] acute acalculous cholecystitis with gallbladder necrosis,[195,196] and giant gastric ulceration have been associated with aPL antibody syndrome.[197] APS has been reported in patients with mesenteric inflammatory venoocclusive disease[198] and in patients with mesenteric and portal venous obstruction.[199]

THROMBOCYTOPENIA

Approximately 20 to 40 percent of patients with APS have varying degrees of thrombocytopenia. The decrease in platelet count usually is mild or moderate and rarely is significant enough to cause bleeding complications or affect anticoagulant therapy.[200,201] The thrombocytopenia appears to be a mild form of immune thrombocytopenic purpura, rather than reflecting direct thrombocytopenic effects of aPL antibodies. The majority of patients with APS and thrombocytopenia have antibodies against $\alpha IIb\beta_3$ integrin and/or glycoprotein Ib-IX complex.[202] Conversely, aPL antibodies and antibodies against platelet membrane glycoprotein were present simultaneously in approximately 70 percent of patients with immune-mediated thrombocytopenia.[203] Patients presenting with immune thrombocytopenic purpura frequently have elevated aPL antibodies, and these patients are more prone to thrombosis.[204] Thrombocytopenia itself is not protective against thrombosis in these patients. In a prospective cohort study, 5-year thrombosis-free survival of aPL-positive and aPL-negative immune thrombocytopenic purpura patients were 39 percent and 98 percent, respectively.[205]

BLEEDING

The presence of a concurrent coagulopathy needs to be considered when patients with APS exhibit a bleeding tendency (Table 132–7). Acquired hypoprothrombinemia with severe bleeding has been reported.[206,207]

TABLE 132–7. Causes of Bleeding in APS
Hypoprothrombinemia
Thrombocytopenia
Acquired platelet function abnormality
Acquired inhibitor to specific coagulation factor, e.g., factor VIII
Acquired von Willebrand syndrome

This diagnosis may be missed when coagulation abnormalities are attributed only to the LA effect, so a specific assay for prothrombin should be performed when the prothrombin time is prolonged. Other causes of bleeding in APS include acquired thrombocytopathies, thrombocytopenia (see "Thrombocytopenia," above), acquired inhibitors against specific coagulation factors, such as factor VIII, and the acquired von Willebrand syndrome (AVWS). It is important to note that the mechanism for AVWS in autoimmunity has not been established, and that, contrary to expectation, this deficiency of von Willebrand factor is not usually associated with a demonstrable inhibitor.[208]

RETINAL ABNORMALITIES

The diagnosis of aPL antibody retinopathy should be suspected in patients with diffuse retinal vasoocclusion, particularly when characterized by involvement of arteries and veins, neovascularization at presentation, and symptoms of systemic rheumatologic disease.[209] aPL antibodies were present in 5 to 33 percent of patients with retinal vein occlusion.[210,211] Cilioretinal artery occlusion,[212] optic neuropathy,[213] and severe vasoocclusive retinopathy[214] have been described with APS.

KIDNEY DISEASES

APS may affect the renal system. Patients may present with renal artery stenosis and/or thrombosis, renal infarction, renal vein thrombosis, and glomerulonephritis that is distinct from vasoocclusive disease.[170,215] An entity named "APS nephropathy" has been described, which consists of a vasoocclusive disease of small-size intrarenal vessels.[216] This nephropathy features fibrous intimal hyperplasia, focal cortical atrophy, and thrombotic microangiopathy. A review of 29 consecutive renal biopsies from patients with primary APS, performed at two institutions over 22 years, described 20 cases of APS nephropathy and 9 cases with other distinct pathologic features.[215] These features included membranous nephropathy, minimal change disease/focal segmental glomerulonephritis, mesangial C3 nephropathy, and pauci-immune crescentic glomerulonephritis.

ANTIPHOSPHOLIPID SYNDROME AND AIDS

Although patients with HIV-1 infection frequently have elevated aPL antibody levels, they do not often have thrombotic manifestations. A review indicated that approximately 50 percent of HIV-1 patients have aPL antibodies, most of which are not cofactor dependent.[192] HIV-infected patients with manifestations of APS also presented with avascular bone and cutaneous necrosis.[193]

ANTIPHOSPHOLIPID SYNDROME IN CHILDREN

APS has become increasingly recognized in children,[217] in whom diverse clinical features are common as in adults. A European registry has been reported.[218] Review of the initial 121 cases indicated that although the thrombotic manifestations were similar to adults with APS, there was a significant and interesting difference between children with primary APS and the secondary APS who had other autoimmune disease. The patients with primary APS were younger and had a higher frequency of arterial thrombotic events, whereas secondary APS patients were older and had a higher frequency of venous thrombotic events associated with hematologic and skin manifestations. CAPS has been reported in children, but is rare.[219,220]

OTHER MANIFESTATIONS

Acute adrenal failure secondary to bilateral infarction of the adrenal glands has been reported as the first manifestation of primary APS.[221] Adrenal hemorrhage has been reported.[222] aPL antibodies have been associated with marrow necrosis.[223] Sudden acute sensorineural hearing loss in patients with SLE or lupus-like syndromes has been described as a manifestation of APS.[224]

LABORATORY FEATURES

Diagnosis of APS requires the demonstration of antibodies against phospholipids and/or relevant protein cofactors (Table 132–8). The current tests for APS recommended by the most recent consensus on investigational criteria[18] and the Scientific Standardization Committee of the International Society of Thrombosis and Hemostasis are aCL, anti-β_2GPI (IgG and IgM) and LA.[225] The laboratory diagnosis of APS frequently is problematic, with limitations that have been detailed.[226] aCL IgG and IgM assays are the most sensitive, but the least specific. Anti-β_2GPI IgG and IgM assays are more specific but less sensitive. LA assays, of which the dilute Russell viper venom time (dRVVT) is the most common, generally tend to be the least sensitive but the most specific. The current recommended tests are less than ideal because they

TABLE 132–8. Diagnostic Tests for APS
Immunoassays
Anticardiolipin antibodies*
Anti-β_2GPI antibodies*
Serologic test for syphilis ("biologic false positive")
Antiphosphatidyl serine antibodies
Antiprothrombin antibodies
Coagulation Tests†
Dilute Russell viper venom time with mixing incubations and neutralization with excess phospholipid
aPTT with mixing incubation and neutralization with excess phospholipids
aPL-sensitive and insensitive reagents and platelet neutralization procedure
Kaolin clotting time
Tissue thromboplastin inhibition test ("dilute prothrombin time")
Hexagonal phase array test
Textarin/ecarin test

aPTT, activated partial thromboplastin time; β_2GPI, β_2-glycoprotein I.

*Recommended by ISTH SSC Subcommittee on Lupus Anticoagulants and Antiphospholipid Antibodies.[225]

†The committee recommended that two coagulation assays be performed if LA or APS are suspected, preferably the dilute Russell viper venom time (dRVVT) and aPTT.

are empirically derived phenomenologic tests and do not yet measure antibodies directed against disease specific epitopes or functional parameters that correlate with disease mechanisms. Criteria have nevertheless been developed to identify patients with the "definite" autoimmune APS (see Table 132–3).[18] Because no single test is sufficient for diagnosing the disorder, a panel of tests, including antibodies against cardiolipin, and β_2GPI, and coagulation tests for LA should be performed when APS is suspected.[225] Positive results have to be obtained on 2 or more occasions at least 12 weeks apart.

IMMUNOASSAYS

Anticardiolipin Antibody Assays

Most patients with APS are identified by elevated levels of aCL antibodies, a test with high sensitivity but poor specificity. The prevalence of positive tests in the asymptomatic healthy population has generally ranged from approximately 3 to 10 percent. In a prospective study of 2132 consecutive Spanish patients with venous thromboembolism, 4.1 percent had elevated levels of aCL antibodies (i.e., about the same prevalence as in the asymptomatic healthy population),[227] but in a group of healthy young women, the prevalence of elevated levels of aCL was 18.2 percent.[224] Many individuals have antibody levels that are elevated in response to infections that are not associated with thrombotic complications. Patients with syphilis, Lyme disease, and other infections may be misdiagnosed with APS based on elevated aCL antibody levels when concurrent stroke or arterial thrombosis is present, so these conditions must always be ruled out in susceptible patients. There is also an interesting seasonal variability, with more normal healthy people having increased aPL antibodies in the winter than in the summer months.[228]

In a systematic literature review, 15 of 28 studies showed significant associations between aCL antibodies and thrombosis.[229] In all cases, a correlation existed between high antibody titers and a high risk of thrombosis. Elevated levels of aCL antibodies, whether high or low titer, were significantly associated with both myocardial infarction and cerebral stroke. Only high-titer aCL antibodies significantly increased the risk of deep vein thrombosis. During a 10-year followup of patients with elevated levels of aCL antibodies, approximately 50 percent of patients who presented with the antibodies but without clinical manifestations of the syndrome subsequently developed the APS.[230] The presence of elevated titers of aCL antibodies 6 months after an episode of venous thromboembolism is a predictor for increased risk of recurrence and of death.[127] Women with aCL IgM antibodies, or with an aCL IgG antibody titer less than 20 IgG-binding units, and no LA do not appear to be at risk for APS.[231] In contrast, women with an aCL IgG titer greater than 20 binding units or a positive LA were more likely to develop complications.[231] With respect to pregnancy losses, a meta-analysis of 25 studies on antiphospholipid antibodies in women with recurrent fetal losses showed a significant correlation with increased aCL IgG, and particularly with the LA.[229]

With respect to stroke, elevated levels of aCL antibodies of IgG or IgM isotype were reported to be significant risk factors.[232] aPL antibodies also are an independent risk factor for stroke in young women.[233]

Approximately 20 percent of patients taking procainamide have moderate to high levels of aCL antibodies.[234] In these patients, the antibodies are associated with anti-β_2GPI specificity. There have been case reports of associated thrombosis.[235] Treatment with chlorpromazine is frequently associated with the development of aCL antibodies, and although these antibodies were reported to rarely be associated with thrombosis,[236] this point may require further investigation as it has been reported that the drug alone is associated with increased idiopathic venous thromboembolism.[237]

Antiphosphatidyl Serine Antibody Assay

Tests for antibodies against phosphatidyl serine are hypothesized to be more relevant than antibodies against cardiolipin, because the latter are present in intracellular membranes, whereas phosphatidyl serine is exposed on syncytialized cells, on apoptotic cells, and on activated platelets. Antibodies against phosphatidyl serine are reported to correlate more specifically with APS than aCL antibodies, particularly in arterial thrombosis.[238,239] However, antiphosphatidyl serine antibody tests are not accepted as an international consensus criterion.[225]

Anti-β_2 Glycoprotein I Antibody Assays

β_2GPI is believed to be the major protein cofactor for aPL antibodies. Enzyme-linked immunosorbent assays (ELISAs) for anti-β_2GPI antibodies are considered to be more specific but less sensitive to APS than to aCL assays.[240] In a systematic literature review, 34 of 60 studies showed significant associations between anti-β_2GPI antibodies and thrombosis.[229] None of the studies were prospective. Of the 10 studies that included multivariate analysis, only two confirmed that anti-β_2GPI IgG antibodies were independent risk factors for venous thrombosis. Anti-β_2GPI antibodies were more often associated with venous than arterial thrombosis. Anti-β_2GPI IgA antibodies were significantly associated with thrombosis.

Although these antibodies usually are present in conjunction with abnormal aCL and antiphosphatidyl serine antibodies, some patients with APS present solely with antibodies to β_2GPI.[241,242] Despite their higher specificity for APS (98%), β_2GPI antibodies alone cannot be relied upon for the diagnosis because of their low sensitivity (40–50%).[243,244] Also, interlaboratory variability is a significant problem with anti-β_2GPI antibody assays.[245]

Epitope-specific anti-β_2GPI antibodies, not yet in general use, may offer a better predictive value for diagnosis and prognosis of APS. A recent analysis of 198 samples from patients with a variety of autoimmune conditions revealed that the 52 patients with anti-β_2GPI IgG antibodies could be divided into those that recognize domain I alone and those with reactivity for all domains[48]; the former were positive for LA and were associated with an increased risk for thrombosis. As mentioned earlier, positivity for this assay has been correlated with positivity for a functional coagulation assay that measures resistance to annexin A5 anticoagulant activity.[49]

Antiprothrombin Antibody Assay

Prothrombin is considered the second major cofactor for aPL antibodies. In a systematic literature review, 17 of 46 studies showed significant associations between antiprothrombin antibodies and thrombosis.[229] Of the eight studies that included multivariate analysis, two confirmed that antiprothrombin antibodies were independent risk factors for thrombosis, and three other studies showed that antiprothrombin antibodies added to the risk borne by LA or aCL antibodies.

Assays for Antibodies against Other Phospholipids

Some investigators have advocated testing for antibodies against a panel of phospholipids other than cardiolipin,[246–249] but others have disagreed.[250] The current consensus holds that no benefit has been demonstrated for these panels.[225]

COAGULATION TESTS

Lupus Anticoagulants

One of the most intriguing aspects of APS is the LA phenomenon.[251,252] The various LA tests all report the inhibition of phospholipid-dependent blood coagulation reactions,[6] but by different detection methods.

These include modifications of the aPTT test with LA-sensitive and LA-insensitive reagents, the kaolin clotting time, the dRVVT, the tissue thromboplastin inhibition time, the hexagonal phase array test, and the platelet neutralization procedure.

The results of LA tests can be so variable that even specialized laboratories will disagree as to the results of LA tests. For example, three surveys in the United Kingdom have shown that although most laboratories agreed on identification of plasmas containing strong positive LA activity, they frequently have disagreed about samples with a weak LA activity.[250]

Despite these limitations, the presence of a positive LA appears to be the strongest predictive diagnostic test for future thrombosis. In a meta-analysis of the risk for aPL-associated venous thromboembolism in individuals with aPL antibodies without an underlying autoimmune disease or previous thrombosis, the mean odds ratios were 1.6 for aCL antibodies, 3.2 for high titers of aCL, and 11.0 for LA.[253] In a systematic literature review, 12 of 12 studies showed significant associations between LA and thrombosis, with odds ratios from 5.7 to 9.4.[229] LA increased the risks of arterial and venous events to the same extent. In APASS, positivity for both LA and aCL, but not for aCL alone, predicted a higher risk of recurrent thromboocclusive events in patients with first ischemic stroke.[135]

In patients with SLE as well, the presence of LA activity is more predictive and more specific for the occurrence of thrombosis or pregnancy loss than aCL assays.[254] This was also found in a meta-analysis of women without autoimmune conditions who had recurrent pregnancy losses.[255]

Dilute Russell Viper Venom Time

dRVVT is considered to be one of the most sensitive of the LA tests. The assay uses Russell viper venom (RVV) in a system containing limiting quantities of diluted rabbit brain phospholipid. RVV directly activates coagulation factor X, leading to formation of fibrin clot. LA prolongs dRVVT by interfering with assembly of the prothrombinase complex; however, the prolongation is reversed by adding excess phospholipid to the reaction (sometimes referred to a "confirmatory test"). To ensure that prolongation of the clotting time is not a result of a factor deficiency, the procedure includes mixture of patient and control plasmas. Anticoagulant therapy with heparin, warfarin, or direct thrombin inhibitors can yield falsely abnormal test results.

Activated Partial Thromboplastin Time Tests

Prolongation of the aPTT detects some LAs, and prolonged aPTTs in otherwise healthy individuals are most frequently caused by LAs.[256] The various commercial aPTT reagents vary widely with regard to sensitivity to LA, so it is important to know the characteristics of the particular reagent(s) that is(are) being utilized. When the aPTT of a particular plasma sample is prolonged and not correctable by immediate mixture with normal plasma, the presence of an LA should be suspected, especially if the patient does not have bleeding symptoms. The LA needs to be differentiated from inhibitors of specific coagulation factors and from anticoagulants such as heparin. Besides specific assays to exclude the latter two possibilities, the clinician should check whether the aPTT normalizes when an LA-insensitive aPTT reagent is used or when the assay is performed using frozen washed platelets as the source of phospholipid, a procedure referred to as the platelet neutralization procedure. The effects of incubation with normal plasma may be helpful in differentiating LAs from coagulation factor inhibitors. aPTTs performed on mixtures of normal plasma and plasma containing a factor VIII inhibitor usually show no prolongation immediately after mixing but marked prolongation following incubation for 1 to 2 hours at 37°C, whereas LA-containing plasmas usually prolong the aPTT immediately after mixing with normal plasma and show no further prolongation with incubation. The clinician should be aware that both types of anticoagulants, LA and specific coagulation factor inhibitors, may coexist in rare patients and yield confusing laboratory results. Specific coagulation factor inhibitor assays and using an aPTT reagent that is insensitive to LA are helpful for clarifying most of these cases. LAs may result in artifactual decreases in contact activation pathway coagulation factor assays, because these assays are based on aPTT. Consequently, these patients are sometimes misdiagnosed as having multiple coagulation factor deficiencies. This problem can be handled by repeating the coagulation factor assays following dilution of the plasma samples; this usually results in complete or partial normalization of coagulation factor levels with progressive dilution. The use of an aPTT reagent that is insensitive to LA for specific factor assays is another way to solve this problem.

Other Methods for Detecting LA

The kaolin clotting time (KCT) depends on the ability of aPL antibodies to block the coagulant activity of trace amounts of phospholipid present in centrifuged plasma. Some authors maintain that the kaolin clotting time–LA test reflects dependence on prothrombin as a cofactor and is less likely to be associated with thrombosis than the dRVVT, which appears to be more dependent on β_2GPI.[257,258]

The tissue thromboplastin inhibition test (TTIT; also known as the dilute prothrombin time [dPT]) is essentially a prothrombin time assay done with diluted tissue factor–phospholipid complex. It can be performed with standard or recombinant tissue factor.[259,260] The results are expressed as a ratio of the patient-to-control clotting times.

The hexagonal phase array test is based on the idea that aPL antibodies can recognize phosphatidyl ethanolamine in the hexagonal phase array configuration but not in the lamellar phase. Therefore incubation of plasma with the hexagonal phase phosphatidyl ethanolamine should absorb the LA antibodies, if present, and therefore normalize an aPTT that was prolonged because of LA.

The textarin/ecarin test depends on the difference in phospholipid dependence of coagulation mechanisms triggered by two snake venoms: textarin, which activates prothrombin via a phospholipid-dependent pathway, and ecarin, which activates prothrombin directly without phospholipid.[260]

Annexin A5 Resistance Assay

In addition to the various LA tests, there is a coagulation test that reports on a thrombogenic mechanism—resistance to annexin A5 anticoagulant activity.[72] This assay has been correlated with an immunoassay for IgG antibodies against domain I of β_2GPI.[49] Figure 132–4 illustrates the principle for this assay. The assay has two stages: a first, in which a tissue factor-phospholipid suspension is exposed to test plasma, and a second, in which the washed suspension is used to coagulate pooled normal plasma in the presence and absence of annexin A5. Patients with annexin A5 resistance show a less-than-expected annexin A5 anticoagulant effect, reported as a reduction in the annexin A5 anticoagulant ratio. In contrast to the LA effect, this assay measures and reports a procoagulant effect for the antibodies.[70] (*Disclosure:* The author is inventor of this assay, U.S. Patents #6284475 and #7252959.)

DIFFERENTIAL DIAGNOSIS

Chaps. 134 and 135 address the general subject of vascular occlusion and its differential diagnosis. When vascular occlusion occurs in the setting of a known autoimmune disorder such as SLE, the possibility of a vasculitis, rather than a thrombotic condition, should be considered.

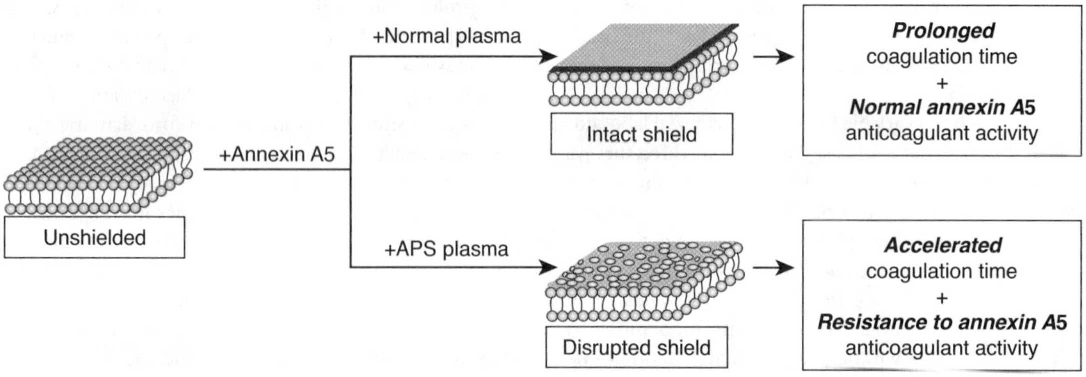

FIGURE 132–4. Principle of annexin A5 resistance assays.[286] This is a two-stage assay to measure annexin A5 anticoagulant activity and is based on the fact that phospholipid bilayers, unshielded by annexin A5, expose thrombogenic phospholipids that accelerate coagulation reactions by serving as scaffolds for the assembly of coagulation enzyme cofactor substrate complexes. In the presence of normal patient plasma, added in the first stage, that lacks interfering aPL antibodies (*top portion*), annexin A5 forms two-dimensional crystals over the bilayer that block the binding coagulation proteins. This prolongs the coagulation time of pooled normal plasma added to the bilayers in the second stage of the test, a result expressed as "normal annexin A5 anticoagulant activity." In contrast, addition of APS plasma containing interfering aPL antibodies will disrupt the binding and assembly of annexin A5 crystals on the phospholipid bilayers. This exposes phospholipids that bind coagulation proteins and accelerates the coagulation time of the pooled normal plasma added to the bilayers in the second stage. The result is expressed as reduced annexin A5 anticoagulant activity, or "annexin A5 resistance." *(Figure designed with assistance of Ethan Rand, 2009.)*

Patients with CAPS may, at first, appear to have other multisystem vasoocclusive disorders, such as thrombotic thrombocytopenic purpura or disseminated vasculitis, and may also manifest laboratory findings of disseminated intravascular coagulation.

The differential diagnosis of a prolonged aPTT includes hereditary and acquired coagulation factor deficiencies, inhibitors to coagulation proteins (e.g., acquired hemophilia A, see Chap. 128), and the presence, or use, of anticoagulants. The diagnosis of LA is substantiated through plasma mixing studies and specific factor assays. A positive immunoassay for aPL—that is, anticardiolipin and/or anti-β_2GPI antibodies—helps confirm the diagnosis.

When an elevated level aPL antibody level is detected, the clinician must exclude the possibility of an infectious etiology for the antibodies; these occur frequently in syphilis, Lyme disease, HIV-1, and hepatitis C. Occasional patients may have artifactually elevated antibodies from increased polyclonal immunoglobulin levels.[261] In such cases, diagnosis is aided by specific tests for suspected infection, quantitative measurement of serum immunoglobulins, and subtraction of background controls using uncoated microtiter wells. Antipsychotic or other medications should be excluded as causative agents.

THERAPY, COURSE, AND PROGNOSIS

There is general agreement that APS patients with recurrent spontaneous thrombosis require long-term, and perhaps lifelong, anticoagulant therapy and APS patients with recurrent spontaneous pregnancy losses require antithrombotic therapy for most of the gestational period. There are differences of opinion among experts regarding the approaches to treatment of patients with a single thrombotic event, patients with a history of thrombotic events in the distant past (>5 years), patients with stroke, and patients with thrombotic events that were associated with a provocative factor such as trauma, surgery, stasis, pregnancy, and estrogens.

THROMBOSIS

The accumulated evidence from randomized controlled trials indicates that patients with APS and thrombosis should be treated with warfarin for the long-term, and maintained at a therapeutic international normalized ratio (INR) of 2.0 to 3.0.[262] Patients with arterial thrombosis may require a higher anticoagulant intensity as a retrospective study showed that a higher intensity (INR >3.0) was necessary for preventing recurrences in this group of patients, but this issue is controversial.[263] Two other studies reported no benefit for high-intensity warfarin but the number of patients with arterial thrombosis was not high.[261,262] The issue of appropriate antithrombotic treatment of aPL-associated stroke is even more controversial (see below). One major study concluded that there was no benefit for warfarin anticoagulation compared to aspirin therapy.[140]

For patients treated acutely with intravenous unfractionated heparin, care must be taken to determine whether the patient has a preexisting LA that can interfere with aPTT monitoring of heparin levels. This problem can be circumvented by using an LA-insensitive aPTT reagent or be avoided by treatment, where appropriate, with a low-molecular-weight heparin (LMWH).

A high titer of aCL antibodies (>30 U/mL) is not sufficient to justify prophylactic anticoagulation therapy in otherwise healthy asymptomatic patients.[264] The same conclusion can be applied to patients with LAs who have not experienced thrombotic or embolic events. Anticoagulant therapy can be considered for occasional asymptomatic patients, such as those with convincing family histories for thromboembolic complications of APS who themselves manifest significant laboratory abnormalities, patients with SLE who have significant aPL laboratory abnormalities, and patients who have other reasons for being at increased risk for thrombosis (e.g., severe valvular heart disease).[182] A study showed no benefit for treating asymptomatic aPL-positive patients with aspirin.[265]

An important practical consequence of the LA effect is that prothrombin time and INR results can be artifactually elevated in some patients with APS and LAs treated with warfarin anticoagulant therapy.[266] A multicenter study reported that all but one of the commercial thromboplastins in use at nine centers provided acceptable INR values for APS patients with LA.[267] New thromboplastins should be checked for their responsiveness to LA prior to their use in monitoring oral anticoagulant treatment in patients with APS.

Fibrinolytic treatment has been reported for patients with primary APS and extensive thrombosis of the common femoral and iliac veins extending to the lower vena cava,[268] acute ischemic stroke,[269] and acute myocardial infarction.[270]

The antimalarial drug hydroxychloroquine has been associated with reduced risk of thrombosis in patients with APS[271–273] and SLE.[273–275] The potential effectiveness of this treatment has been supported by an animal model for aPL thrombosis[276] and by a recent report that hydroxychloroquine directly disrupts aPL IgG–β_2GPI complexes,[277] and also reverses the aPL antibody-mediated disruption of annexin A5 binding.[278] However, the drug has not been tested in randomized controlled trials of APS patients.

Conventional anticoagulant therapy is usually not sufficient for treatment of CAPS; these patients require aggressive treatment because of the high mortality.[156] Treatment modalities may include anticoagulation, immunosuppressive therapy in the form of high-dose glucocorticoids, intravenous immunoglobulin, cyclophosphamide, azathioprine, or rituximab. Plasmapheresis may be a helpful adjunct. Some patients benefit from fibrinolytic agents and prostacyclin.[157]

PREGNANCY COMPLICATIONS

A systematic review of treatments given to maintain pregnancy in women with prior miscarriages and APS concluded that combined unfractionated heparin and aspirin may reduce pregnancy loss by 54 percent compared to aspirin alone.[279] Three trials of aspirin alone showed no significant reduction in pregnancy loss[279]; intravenous immunoglobulin, whether in combination with or without unfractionated heparin and aspirin, was associated with an increased risk of pregnancy loss or premature birth when compared to unfractionated heparin or LMWH combined with aspirin.

Taking together the available data, women with a history of three or more spontaneous pregnancy losses and evidence of aPL antibodies should be treated with a combination of low-dose aspirin (75–81 mg/day) and prophylactic doses of unfractionated heparin (i.e., 5000 U every 12 hours subcutaneously). Treatment should be started as soon as pregnancy is documented and continued until delivery so as to reduce the rate of late complications.[280,281] In especially high-risk situations, induction of early delivery may be necessary. Unfractionated heparin at the prophylactic dosage of 5000 U q12h subcutaneously should be started approximately 4 to 6 hours after delivery, if significant bleeding has ceased, and continued at least until the patient is fully ambulatory. Many physicians recommend to continue prophylactic therapy for 6 weeks after delivery even if the patients have not experienced thrombosis. For patients who experienced thromboembolism, prophylaxis by heparin or oral anticoagulant therapy is warranted for at least 6 weeks after delivery.

Although treatment with LMWH has become widely used for recurrent fetal loss as a replacement for prophylactic dose unfractionated heparin, a prospective randomized controlled trial has questioned the benefit of LMWH treatment versus aspirin therapy. In the LMWH/aspirin group 35/47 (77.8%) had a livebirth, and in the aspirin group 34/43 (79.1%) had a livebirth ($p = 0.7$).[282]

The presence of aPL antibodies is not an indication for treatment in pregnant women without a history of spontaneous pregnancy losses, other attributable pregnancy complications, thrombosis, or SLE. Therefore, the inclusion of aPL tests in prenatal testing panels should be discouraged.

Although prednisone was reported to possibly improve the outcome of pregnancy in women with APS, those benefits are associated with significant toxicity.[283] Glucocorticoids or intravenous IgG should be considered only for patients who are refractory to anticoagulant therapy, who have a severe immune thrombocytopenia or a significant contraindication to heparin therapy. Treatment with the combination of prednisone and heparin is associated with an increased risk of osteopenia and vertebral fractures.[284]

REFERENCES

1. Hughes GR: The anticardiolipin syndrome. *Clin Exp Rheumatol* 3:285, 1985.
2. Harris EN, Hughes GRV, Gharavi AE: The antiphospholipid antibody syndrome. *J Rheumatol* Suppl 13:210, 1987.
3. Simioni P, Prandoni P, Zanon E, et al: Deep venous thrombosis and lupus anticoagulant. A case-control study. *Thromb Haemost* 76:187, 1996.
4. Ginsberg JS, Wells PS, Brill Edwards P, et al: Antiphospholipid antibodies and venous thromboembolism. *Blood* 86:3685, 1995.
5. Out HJ, Bruinse HW, Christiaens GC, et al: Prevalence of antiphospholipid antibodies in patients with fetal loss. *Ann Rheum Dis* 50:553, 1991.
6. Shapiro SS, Thiagarajan P: Lupus anticoagulants. *Prog Hemost Thromb* 6:263, 1982.
7. Shapiro SS: Lupus anticoagulants and anticardiolipin antibodies: Personal reminiscences, a little history, and some random thoughts. *J Thromb Haemost* 3:831, 2005.
8. Asherson RA: The primary, secondary, catastrophic, and seronegative variants of the antiphospholipid syndrome: A personal history long in the making. *Semin Thromb Hemost* 34:227, 2008.
9. Moore JE, Mohr CF: Biologically false positive serological tests for syphilis: Type, incidence, and cause. *J Am Med Assoc* 150:467, 1952.
10. Moore JE, Lutz WB: Natural history of systemic lupus erythematosus: Approach to its study through chronic biologic false positive reactors. *J Chronic Dis* 1:297, 1955.
11. Bell WN, Alton HG: A brain extract as a substitute for platelet suspensions in the thromboplastin generation test. *Nature* 174:880, 1955.
12. Conley CL, Hartmann RC: A hemorrhagic disorder caused by circulating anticoagulant in patients with disseminated lupus erythematosus. *J Clin Invest* 31:621, 1952.
13. Feinstein DI, Rapaport SI: Acquired inhibitors of blood coagulation, in *Progress in Hemostasis and Thrombosis*, edited by TH Spaet, p 75. Grune & Stratton, New York, 1972.
14. Beaumont JL: Acquired hemorrhagic syndrome caused by a circulating anticoagulant; inhibition of the thromboplastic function of the blood platelets; description of a specific test. *Sang* 25:1, 1954.
15. Nilsson IM, Astedt B, Hedner U, et al: Intrauterine death and circulating anticoagulant ("antithromboplastin"). *Acta Med Scand* 197:153, 1975.
16. Bowie WEJ, Thompson JH, Pascuzzi CA, et al: Thrombosis in systemic erythematosus despite circulating anticoagulants. *J Clin Invest* 62:416, 1963.
17. Harris EN, Gharavi AE, Boey ML, et al: Anticardiolipin antibodies: Detection by radioimmunoassay and association with thrombosis in systemic lupus erythematosus. *Lancet* 2:1211, 1983.
18. Miyakis S, Lockshin MD, Atsumi T, et al: International consensus statement on an update of the classification criteria for definite antiphospholipid syndrome (APS). *J Thromb Haemost* 4:295, 2006.
19. Lieby P, Soley A, Knapp AM, et al: Memory B cells producing somatically mutated antiphospholipid antibodies are present in healthy individuals. *Blood* 102:2459, 2003.
20. Giles I, Lambrianides A, Rahman A: Examining the non-linear relationship between monoclonal antiphospholipid antibody sequence, structure and function. *Lupus* 17:895, 2008.
21. Barcat D, Constans J, Seigneur M, et al: Deep venous thrombosis in an adult with varicella. *Rev Med Interne* 19:509, 1998.
22. Peyton BD, Cutler BS, Stewart FM: Spontaneous tibial artery thrombosis associated with varicella pneumonia and free protein S deficiency. *J Vasc Surg* 27:563, 1998.
23. Prieto J, Yuste JR, Beloqui O, et al: Anticardiolipin antibodies in chronic hepatitis C: Implication of hepatitis C virus as the cause of the antiphospholipid syndrome [see comments]. *Hepatology* 23:199, 1996.
24. Cojocaru IM, Cojocaru M, Iacob SA: High prevalence of anticardiolipin antibodies in patients with asymptomatic hepatitis C virus infection associated acute ischemic stroke. *Rom J Intern Med* 43:89, 2005.
25. Labarca JA, Rabaggliati RM, Radrigan FJ, et al: Antiphospholipid syndrome associated with cytomegalovirus infection: Case report and review. *Clin Infect Dis* 24:197, 1997.
26. Delbos V, Abgueguen P, Chennebault JM, et al: Acute cytomegalovirus infection and venous thrombosis: Role of antiphospholipid antibodies. *J Infect* 54:e47-e50, 2007.
27. Loizou S, Cazabon JK, Walport MJ, et al: Similarities of specificity and cofactor dependence in serum antiphospholipid antibodies from patients with human parvovirus B19 infection and from those with systemic lupus erythematosus. *Arthritis Rheum* 40:103, 1997.
28. Galrao L, Brites C, Atta ML, et al: Antiphospholipid antibodies in HIV-positive patients. *Clin Rheumatol* 26:1825, 2007.
29. Blank M, ron-Maor A, Shoenfeld Y: From rheumatic fever to Libman-Sacks endocarditis: Is there any possible pathogenetic link? *Lupus* 14:697, 2005.
30. Gotoh M, Matsuda J: Induction of anticardiolipin antibody and/or lupus anticoagulant in rabbits by immunization with lipoteichoic acid, lipopolysaccharide and lipid A. *Lupus* 5:593, 1996.
31. Eschwege V, Freyssinet JM: The possible contribution of cell apoptosis and necrosis to the generation of phospholipid-binding antibodies. *Ann Med Interne (Paris)* 147(Suppl 1):33, 1996.
32. Price BE, Rauch J, Shia MA, et al: Anti-phospholipid autoantibodies bind to apoptotic, but not viable, thymocytes in a beta 2-glycoprotein I-dependent manner. *J Immunol* 157:2201, 1996.
33. Pittoni V, Isenberg D: Apoptosis and antiphospholipid antibodies. *Semin Arthritis Rheum* 28:163, 1998.
34. Inic-Kanada A, Stojanovic M, Zivkovic I, et al: Murine monoclonal antibody 26 raised against tetanus toxoid cross-reacts with beta2-glycoprotein I: Its characteristics and role in molecular mimicry. *Am J Reprod Immunol* 61:39, 2009.

35. Blank M, Asherson RA, Cervera R, et al: Antiphospholipid syndrome infectious origin. *J Clin Immunol* 24:12, 2004.
36. Gharavi AE, Pierangeli SS, Espinola RG, et al: Antiphospholipid antibodies induced in mice by immunization with a cytomegalovirus-derived peptide cause thrombosis and activation of endothelial cells *in vivo*. *Arthritis Rheum* 46:545, 2002.
37. Hellan M, Kuhnel E, Speiser W, et al: Familial lupus anticoagulant: A case report and review of the literature. *Blood Coagul Fibrinolysis* 9:195, 1998.
38. Weber M, Hayem G, DeBandt M, et al: The family history of patients with primary or secondary antiphospholipid syndrome (APS). *Lupus* 9:258, 2000.
39. Garcia CO, Kanbour-Shakir A, Tang H, et al: Induction of experimental antiphospholipid antibody syndrome in PL/J mice following immunization with beta 2 GPI. *Am J Reprod Immunol* 37:118, 1997.
40. Holers VM, Girardi G, Mo L, et al: Complement C3 activation is required for antiphospholipid antibody-induced fetal loss. *J Exp Med* 195:211, 2002.
41. Pierangeli SS, Liu X, Espinola R, et al: Functional analyses of patient-derived IgG monoclonal anticardiolipin antibodies using *in vivo* thrombosis and *in vivo* microcirculation models. *Thromb Haemost* 84:388, 2000.
42. Jankowski M, Vreys I, Wittevrongel C, et al: Thrombogenicity of beta 2-glycoprotein I-dependent antiphospholipid antibodies in a photochemically induced thrombosis model in the hamster. *Blood* 101:157, 2003.
43. Loizou S, Singh S, Wypkema E, et al: Anticardiolipin, anti-beta(2)-glycoprotein I and antiprothrombin antibodies in black South African patients with infectious disease. *Ann Rheum Dis* 62:1106, 2003.
44. Roubey RA, Pratt CW, Buyon JP, et al: Lupus anticoagulant activity of autoimmune antiphospholipid antibodies is dependent upon beta 2-glycoprotein I. *J Clin Invest* 90:1100, 1992.
45. Galli M, Comfurius P, Maassen C, et al: Anticardiolipin antibodies (ACA) directed not to cardiolipin but to a plasma protein cofactor. *Lancet* 335:1544, 1990.
46. McNeil HP, Simpson RJ, Chesterman CN, et al: Anti-phospholipid antibodies are directed against a complex antigen that includes a lipid-binding inhibitor of coagulation: Beta 2-glycoprotein I (apolipoprotein H). *Proc Natl Acad Sci U S A* 87:4120, 1990.
47. Goldsmith GH, Pierangeli SS, Branch DW, et al: Inhibition of prothrombin activation by antiphospholipid antibodies and beta 2-glycoprotein 1. *Br J Haematol* 87:548, 1994.
48. de Laat HB, Derksen RH, Urbanus RT, et al: IgG antibodies that recognize epitope Gly40-Arg43 in domain I of beta 2-glycoprotein I cause LAC, and their presence correlates strongly with thrombosis. *Blood* 105:1540, 2005.
49. de Laat B, Wu XX, van Lummel M, et al: Correlation between antiphospholipid antibodies that recognize domain I of beta2-glycoprotein I and a reduction in the anticoagulant activity of annexin A5. *Blood* 109:1490, 2007.
50. Hunt BJ, Wu XX, de Laat B, et al: Association of anti-β_2GPI domain I IgG and resistance to annexin A5 with obstetrical antiphospholipid syndrome: Evidence for a specific mechanism in a patient subset. *Blood* 2009 [in press].
51. Gamsjaeger R, Johs A, Gries A, et al: Membrane binding of beta2-glycoprotein I can be described by a two-state reaction model: An atomic force microscopy and surface plasmon resonance study. *Biochem J* 389:665, 2005.
52. Balasubramanian K, Maiti SN, Schroit AJ: Recruitment of beta-2-glycoprotein 1 to cell surfaces in extrinsic and intrinsic apoptosis. *Apoptosis* 10:439, 2005.
53. Maiti SN, Balasubramanian K, Ramoth JA, et al: Beta-2-glycoprotein 1-dependent macrophage uptake of apoptotic cells. Binding to lipoprotein receptor-related protein receptor family members. *J Biol Chem* 283:3761, 2008.
54. Matsuura E, Kobayashi K, Matsunami Y, et al: The immunology of atherothrombosis in the antiphospholipid syndrome: Antigen presentation and lipid intracellular accumulation. *Autoimmun Rev* 8:500, 2009.
55. Hulstein JJ, Lenting PJ, de LB, et al: Beta2-glycoprotein I inhibits von Willebrand factor dependent platelet adhesion and aggregation. *Blood* 110:1483, 2007.
56. Bu C, Gao L, Xie W, et al: Beta2-glycoprotein i is a cofactor for tissue plasminogen activator-mediated plasminogen activation. *Arthritis Rheum* 60:559, 2009.
57. Ma K, Simantov R, Zhang JC, et al: High affinity binding of beta 2-glycoprotein I to human endothelial cells is mediated by annexin II. *J Biol Chem* 275:15541, 2000.
58. Sheng Y, Reddel SW, Herzog H, et al: Impaired thrombin generation in beta 2-glycoprotein I null mice. *J Biol Chem* 276:13817, 2001.
59. de-Groot PG, Horbach DA, Derksen RH: Protein C and other cofactors involved in the binding of antiphospholipid antibodies: Relation to the pathogenesis of thrombosis. *Lupus* 5:488, 1996.
60. Atsumi T, Khamashta MA, Amengual O, et al: Binding of anticardiolipin antibodies to protein C via beta2-glycoprotein I (beta2-GPI): A possible mechanism in the inhibitory effect of antiphospholipid antibodies on the protein C system. *Clin Exp Immunol* 112:325, 1998.
61. Bidot CJ, Jy W, Horstman LL, et al: Factor VII/VIIa: A new antigen in the anti-phospholipid antibody syndrome. *Br J Haematol* 120:618, 2003.
62. Shibata S, Harpel PC, Gharavi A, et al: Autoantibodies to heparin from patients with antiphospholipid antibody syndrome inhibit formation of antithrombin III-thrombin complexes. *Blood* 83:2532, 1994.
63. Lieby P, Soley A, Levallois H, et al: The clonal analysis of anticardiolipin antibodies in a single patient with primary antiphospholipid syndrome reveals an extreme antibody heterogeneity. *Blood* 97:3820, 2001.
64. Andree HAM, Hermens WT, Hemker HC, et al: Displacement of factor Va by annexin V, in *Phospholipid Binding and Anticoagulant Action of Annexin V*, edited by HAM Andree, p 73. Universitaire Pers Maastricht, Maastricht, The Netherlands, 1992.
65. Reviakine I, Bergsma-Schutter W, Brisson A: Growth of protein 2-D crystals on supported planar lipid bilayers imaged *in situ* by AFM. *J Struct Biol* 121:356, 1998.
66. Krikun G, Lockwood CJ, Wu XX, et al: The expression of the placental anticoagulant protein, annexin V, by villous trophoblasts: Immunolocalization and in vitro regulation. *Placenta* 15:601, 1994.
67. Wang X, Campos B, Kaetzel MA, et al: Annexin V is critical in the maintenance of murine placental integrity. *Am J Obstet Gynecol* 180:1008, 1999.
68. Rand JH, Wu XX, Andree HA, et al: Pregnancy loss in the antiphospholipid-antibody syndrome—A possible thrombogenic mechanism. *N Engl J Med* 337:154, 1997.
69. van Heerde WL, Poort S, van 't Veer C, et al: Binding of recombinant annexin V to endothelial cells: Effect of annexin V binding on endothelial-cell-mediated thrombin formation. *Biochem J* 302:305, 1994.
70. Rand JH, Wu XX, Andree HAM, et al: Antiphospholipid antibodies accelerate plasma coagulation by inhibiting annexin-V binding to phospholipids: A "lupus procoagulant" phenomenon. *Blood* 92:1652, 1998.
71. Rand JH, Wu XX, Quinn AS, et al: Human monoclonal antiphospholipid antibodies disrupt the annexin A5 anticoagulant crystal shield on phospholipid bilayers: Evidence from atomic force microscopy and functional assay. *Am J Pathol* 163:1193, 2003.
72. Rand JH, Wu XX, Lapinski R, et al: Detection of antibody-mediated reduction of annexin A5 anticoagulant activity in plasmas of patients with the antiphospholipid syndrome. *Blood* 104:2783, 2004.
73. Wu XX, Pierangeli SS, Rand JH: Resistance to annexin A5 binding and anticoagulant activity in plasmas from patients with the antiphospholipid syndrome but not with syphilis. *J Thromb Haemost* 4:271, 2006.
74. Hanly JG, Smith SA: Anti-beta2-glycoprotein I (GPI) autoantibodies, annexin V binding and the anti-phospholipid syndrome. *Clin Exp Immunol* 120:537, 2000.
75. Tomer A: Antiphospholipid antibody syndrome: Rapid, sensitive, and specific flow cytometric assay for determination of anti-platelet phospholipid autoantibodies. *J Lab Clin Med* 139:147, 2002.
76. Tomer A, Bar-Lev S, Fleisher S, et al: Antiphospholipid antibody syndrome: The flow cytometric annexin A5 competition assay as a diagnostic tool. *Br J Haematol* 139:113, 2007.
77. Gaspersic N, Ambrozic A, Bozic B, et al: Annexin A5 binding to giant phospholipid vesicles is differentially affected by anti-beta2-glycoprotein I and anti-annexin A5 antibodies. *Rheumatology* 46:81, 2007.
78. Rand JH, Wu XX, Guller S, et al: Reduction of annexin-V (placental anticoagulant protein-I) on placental villi of women with antiphospholipid antibodies and recurrent spontaneous abortion. *Am J Obstet Gynecol* 171:1566, 1994.
79. Cederholm A, Svenungsson E, Jensen-Urstad K, et al: Decreased binding of annexin v to endothelial cells: A potential mechanism in atherothrombosis of patients with systemic lupus erythematosus. *Arterioscler Thromb Vasc Biol* 25:198, 2005.
80. Cesarman-Maus G, Rios-Luna NP, Deora AB, et al: Autoantibodies against the fibrinolytic receptor, annexin 2, in antiphospholipid syndrome. *Blood* 107:4375, 2006.
81. Cockrell E, Espinola RG, McCrae KR: Annexin A2: Biology and relevance to the antiphospholipid syndrome. *Lupus* 17:943, 2008.
82. Chen PP, Yang CD, Ede K, et al: Some antiphospholipid antibodies bind to hemostasis and fibrinolysis proteases and promote thrombosis. *Lupus* 17:916, 2008.
83. Cugno M, Cabibbe M, Galli M, et al: Antibodies to tissue-type plasminogen activator (tPA) in patients with antiphospholipid syndrome: Evidence of interaction between the antibodies and the catalytic domain of tPA in 2 patients. *Blood* 103:2121, 2004.
84. Ames PR, Tommasino C, Iannaccone L, et al: Coagulation activation and fibrinolytic imbalance in subjects with idiopathic antiphospholipid antibodies—A crucial role for acquired free protein S deficiency. *Thromb Haemost* 76:190, 1996.
85. Schousboe I, Rasmussen MS: Synchronized inhibition of the phospholipid mediated autoactivation of factor XII in plasma by beta 2-glycoprotein I and anti-beta 2-glycoprotein I. *Thromb Haemost* 73:798, 1995.
86. Dueymes M, Levy Y, Ziporen L, et al: Do some antiphospholipid antibodies target endothelial cells? *Ann Med Interne (Paris)* 147(Suppl 1):22, 1996.
87. Del-Papa N, Raschi E, Catelli L, et al: Endothelial cells as a target for antiphospholipid antibodies: Role of anti-beta 2 glycoprotein I antibodies. *Am J Reprod Immunol* 38:212, 1997.
88. Matsuda J, Gotoh M, Gohchi K, et al: Anti-endothelial cell antibodies to the endothelial hybridoma cell line (EAhy926) in systemic lupus erythematosus patients with antiphospholipid antibodies. *Br J Haematol* 97:227, 1997.
89. Navarro M, Cervera R, Teixido M, et al: Antibodies to endothelial cells and to beta 2-glycoprotein I in the antiphospholipid syndrome: Prevalence and isotype distribution. *Br J Rheumatol* 35:523, 1996.
90. Simantov R, Lo SK, Gharavi A, et al: Antiphospholipid antibodies activate vascular endothelial cells. *Lupus* 5:440, 1996.
91. Meroni PL, Papa ND, Beltrami B, et al: Modulation of endothelial cell function by antiphospholipid antibodies. *Lupus* 5:448, 1996.
92. Raschi E, Borghi MO, Grossi C, et al: Toll-like receptors: Another player in the pathogenesis of the anti-phospholipid syndrome. *Lupus* 17:937, 2008.
93. Raschi E, Testoni C, Bosisio D, et al: Role of the MyD88 transduction signaling pathway in endothelial activation by antiphospholipid antibodies. *Blood* 101:3495, 2003.
94. Vega-Ostertag ME, Ferrara DE, Romay-Penabad Z, et al: Role of p38 mitogen-activated protein kinase in antiphospholipid antibody-mediated thrombosis and endothelial cell activation. *J Thromb Haemost* 5:1828, 2007.

95. Graham A, Ford I, Morrison R, et al: Anti-endothelial antibodies interfere in apoptotic cell clearance and promote thrombosis in patients with antiphospholipid syndrome. *J Immunol* 182:1756, 2009.
96. Sammaritano LR: Significance of aPL IgG subclasses. *Lupus* 5:436, 1996.
97. Salmon JE, Girardi G, Holers VM: Complement activation as a mediator of antiphospholipid antibody induced pregnancy loss and thrombosis. *Ann Rheum Dis* 61(Suppl 2):ii46, 2002.
98. Salmon JE, Girardi G: The role of complement in the antiphospholipid syndrome. *Curr Dir Autoimmun* 7:133, 2004.
99. Girardi G, Redecha P, Salmon JE: Heparin prevents antiphospholipid antibody-induced fetal loss by inhibiting complement activation. *Nat Med* 10:1222, 2004.
100. Redecha P, Tilley R, Tencati M, et al: Tissue factor: A link between C5a and neutrophil activation in antiphospholipid antibody induced fetal injury. *Blood* 110:2423, 2007.
101. Redecha P, Franzke CW, Ruf W, et al: Neutrophil activation by the tissue factor/Factor VIIa/PAR2 axis mediates fetal death in a mouse model of antiphospholipid syndrome. *J Clin Invest* 118:3453, 2008.
102. Zhou H, Wolberg AS, Roubey RA: Characterization of monocyte tissue factor activity induced by IgG antiphospholipid antibodies and inhibition by dilazep. *Blood* 104:2353, 2004.
103. Roubey RA: New approaches to prevention of thrombosis in the antiphospholipid syndrome: Hopes, trials, and tribulations. *Arthritis Rheum* 48:3004, 2003.
104. Martini F, Farsi A, Gori AM, et al: Antiphospholipid antibodies (aPL) increase the potential monocyte procoagulant activity in patients with systemic lupus erythematosus. *Lupus* 5:206, 1996.
105. Riewald M, Ruf W: Protease-activated receptor-1 signaling by activated protein C in cytokine-perturbed endothelial cells is distinct from thrombin signaling. *J Biol Chem* 280:19808, 2005.
106. Niessen F, Furlan-Freguia C, Fernandez JA, et al: Endogenous EPCR/aPC-PAR1 signaling prevents inflammation-induced vascular leakage and lethality. *Blood* 2009.
107. Nojima J, Kuratsune H, Suehisa E, et al: Acquired activated protein C resistance associated with IgG antibodies against beta2-glycoprotein I and prothrombin as a strong risk factor for venous thromboembolism. *Clin Chem* 51:545, 2005.
108. de LB, Eckmann CM, van SM, et al: Correlation between the potency of a beta2-glycoprotein I-dependent lupus anticoagulant and the level of resistance to activated protein C. *Blood Coagul Fibrinolysis* 19:757, 2008.
109. Hurtado V, Montes R, Gris JC, et al: Autoantibodies against EPCR are found in antiphospholipid syndrome and are a risk factor for fetal death. *Blood* 104:1369, 2004.
110. Lin YL, Wang CT: Activation of human platelets by the rabbit anticardiolipin antibodies. *Blood* 80:3135, 1992.
111. van Lummel M, Pennings MT, Derksen RH, et al: The binding site in {beta}2-glycoprotein I for ApoER2 on platelets is located in domain V. *J Biol Chem* 280:36729, 2005.
112. Forastiero RR, Martinuzzo ME, Broze GJ: High titers of autoantibodies to tissue factor pathway inhibitor are associated with the antiphospholipid syndrome. *J Thromb Haemost* 1:718, 2003.
113. Witztum JL, Horkko S: The role of oxidized LDL in atherogenesis: Immunological response and anti-phospholipid antibodies. *Ann N Y Acad Sci* 811:88, 1997.
114. Vaarala O: Antiphospholipid antibodies and atherosclerosis. *Lupus* 5:442, 1996.
115. Lopez LR, Kobayashi K, Matsunami Y, et al: Immunogenic oxidized low-density lipoprotein/beta2-glycoprotein I complexes in the diagnostic management of atherosclerosis. *Clin Rev Allergy Immunol* 37:12, 2009.
116. Stone JH, Amend WJ, Criswell LA: Outcome of renal transplantation in systemic lupus erythematosus. *Semin Arthritis Rheum* 27:17, 1997.
117. Krnic BS, O'Connor CR, Looney SW, et al: A retrospective review of 61 patients with antiphospholipid syndrome. Analysis of factors influencing recurrent thrombosis. *Arch Intern Med* 157:2101, 1997.
118. Martinelli I, Cattaneo M, Panzeri D, et al: Risk factors for deep venous thrombosis of the upper extremities. *Ann Intern Med* 126:707, 1997.
119. Provenzale JM, Ortel TL, Allen NB: Systemic thrombosis in patients with antiphospholipid antibodies: Lesion distribution and imaging findings. *AJR Am J Roentgenol* 170:285, 1998.
120. Poux JM, Boudet R, Lacroix P, et al: Renal infarction and thrombosis of the infrarenal aorta in a 35-year-old man with primary antiphospholipid syndrome. *Am J Kidney Dis* 27:721, 1996.
121. Kojima E, Naito K, Iwai M, et al: Antiphospholipid syndrome complicated by thrombosis of the superior mesenteric artery, co-existence of smooth muscle hyperplasia. *Intern Med* 36:528, 1997.
122. Girolami A, Zanon E, Zanardi S, et al: Thromboembolic disease developing during oral contraceptive therapy in young females with antiphospholipid antibodies. *Blood Coagul Fibrinolysis* 7:497, 1996.
123. Montaruli B, Borchiellini A, Tamponi G, et al: Factor V Arg506→Gln mutation in patients with antiphospholipid antibodies. *Lupus* 5:303, 1996.
124. Simantov R, Lo SK, Salmon JE, et al: Factor V Leiden increases the risk of thrombosis in patients with antiphospholipid antibodies. *Thromb Res* 84:361, 1996.
125. Schutt M, Kluter H, Hagedorn GM, et al: Familial coexistence of primary antiphospholipid syndrome and factor V Leiden. *Lupus* 7:176, 1998.
126. Brenner B, Vulfsons SL, Lanir N, et al: Coexistence of familial antiphospholipid syndrome and factor V Leiden: Impact on thrombotic diathesis. *Br J Haematol* 94:166, 1996.
127. Schulman S, Svenungsson E, Granqvist S: Anticardiolipin antibodies predict early recurrence of thromboembolism and death among patients with venous thromboembolism following anticoagulant therapy. Duration of Anticoagulation Study Group. *Am J Med* 104:332, 1998.
128. Finazzi G, Brancaccio V, Moia M, et al: Natural history and risk factors for thrombosis in 360 patients with antiphospholipid antibodies: A four-year prospective study from the Italian Registry. *Am J Med* 100:530, 1996.
129. Gezer S: Antiphospholipid syndrome. *Dis Mon* 49:696, 2003.
130. Gladd DA, Olech E: Antiphospholipid antibodies in rheumatoid arthritis: Identifying the dominoes. *Curr Rheumatol Rep* 11:43, 2009.
131. Fauchais AL, Lambert M, Launay D, et al: Antiphospholipid antibodies in primary Sjogren's syndrome: Prevalence and clinical significance in a series of 74 patients. *Lupus* 13:245, 2004.
132. Shoenfeld Y, Lorber M, Yucel T, et al: Primary antiphospholipid syndrome emerging following thymectomy for myasthenia gravis: Additional evidence for the kaleidoscope of autoimmunity [see comments]. *Lupus* 6:474, 1997.
133. Yun YY, Yoh KA, Yang HI, et al: A case of Budd-Chiari syndrome with high antiphospholipid antibody in a patient with systemic lupus erythematosus. *Korean J Intern Med* 11:82, 1996.
134. Hofbauer LC, Spitzweg C, Heufelder AE: Graves' disease associated with the primary antiphospholipid syndrome. *J Rheumatol* 23:1435, 1996.
135. Chun WH, Bang D, Lee SK: Antiphospholipid syndrome associated with progressive systemic sclerosis. *J Dermatol* 23:347, 1996.
136. Frolow M, Jankowski M, Swadzba J, et al: Evan's syndrome with antiphospholipid-protein antibodies. *Pol Merkur Lekarski* 1:344, 1996.
137. Yokoi K, Hosoi E, Akaike M, et al: Takayasu's arteritis associated with antiphospholipid antibodies. Report of two cases. *Angiology* 47:315, 1996.
138. Dasgupta B, Almond MK, Tanqueray A: Polyarteritis nodosa and the antiphospholipid syndrome. *Br J Rheumatol* 36:1210, 1997.
139. Anticardiolipin antibodies and the risk of recurrent thrombo-occlusive events and death. The Antiphospholipid Antibodies and Stroke Study Group (APASS). *Neurology* 48:91, 1997.
140. Levine SR, Brey RL, Tilley BC, et al: Antiphospholipid antibodies and subsequent thrombo-occlusive events in patients with ischemic stroke. *JAMA* 291:576, 2004.
141. Amory CF, Levine SR, Brey RL, et al: Persistent antibodies to beta2glycoprotein-I predict shorter time to subsequent thrombo-occlusive events or death after ischemic stroke. *Stroke* 40:E148, 2009.
142. Weingarten K, Filippi C, Barbut D, et al: The neuroimaging features of the cardiolipin antibody syndrome. *Clin Imaging* 21:6, 1997.
143. Carhuapoma JR, Mitsias P, Levine SR: Cerebral venous thrombosis and anticardiolipin antibodies. *Stroke* 28:2363, 1997.
144. Deschiens MA, Conard J, Horellou MH, et al: Coagulation studies, factor V Leiden, and anticardiolipin antibodies in 40 cases of cerebral venous thrombosis. *Stroke* 27:1724, 1996.
145. Nagai S, Horie Y, Akai T, et al: Superior sagittal sinus thrombosis associated with primary antiphospholipid syndrome—Case report. *Neurol Med Chir (Tokyo)* 38:34, 1998.
146. Tanasescu R, Nicolau A, Caraiola S, et al: Antiphospholipid antibodies and migraine: A retrospective study of 428 patients with inflammatory connective tissue diseases. *Rom J Intern Med* 45:355, 2007.
147. Brey RL, Escalante A: Neurological manifestations of antiphospholipid antibody syndrome. *Lupus* 7(Suppl 2):S67, 1998.
148. Matsushita T, Kanda F, Yamada H, et al: Recurrent acute transverse myelopathy: An 83-year-old man with antiphospholipid syndrome. *Rinsho Shinkeigaku* 37:987, 1997.
149. Ruiz AG, Guzman RJ, Flores FJ, et al: Refractory hiccough heralding transverse myelitis in the primary antiphospholipid syndrome. *Lupus* 7:49, 1998.
150. Takamura Y, Morimoto S, Tanooka A, et al: Transverse myelitis in a patient with primary antiphospholipid syndrome—A case report. *No To Shinkei* 48:851, 1996.
151. Campi A, Filippi M, Comi G, et al: Recurrent acute transverse myelopathy associated with anticardiolipin antibodies. *AJNR Am J Neuroradiol* 19:781, 1998.
152. Smyth AE, Bruce IN, McMillan SA, et al: Transverse myelitis: A complication of systemic lupus erythematosus that is associated with the antiphospholipid syndrome. *Ulster Med J* 65:91, 1996.
153. Mok CC, Lau CS, Chan EY, et al: Acute transverse myelopathy in systemic lupus erythematosus: Clinical presentation, treatment, and outcome. *J Rheumatol* 25:467, 1998.
154. Sugiyama Y, Yamamoto T: Characterization of serum anti-phospholipid antibodies in patients with multiple sclerosis. *Tohoku J Exp Med* 178:203, 1996.
155. Schwartz M, Rochas M, Weller B, et al: High association of anticardiolipin antibodies with psychosis. *J Clin Psychiatry* 59:20, 1998.
156. Espinosa G, Bucciarelli S, Asherson RA, et al: Morbidity and mortality in the catastrophic antiphospholipid syndrome: Pathophysiology, causes of death, and prognostic factors. *Semin Thromb Hemost* 34:290, 2008.
157. Erkan D, Cervera R, Asherson RA: Catastrophic antiphospholipid syndrome: Where do we stand? *Arthritis Rheum* 48:3320, 2003.
158. Bucciarelli S, Espinosa G, Cervera R, et al: Mortality in the catastrophic antiphospholipid syndrome: Causes of death and prognostic factors in a series of 250 patients. *Arthritis Rheum* 54:2568, 2006.
159. Lockshin MD: Pregnancy loss and antiphospholipid antibodies. *Lupus* 7(Suppl 2):S86, 1998.
160. Ornstein MH, Rand JH: An association between refractory HELLP syndrome and antiphospholipid antibodies during pregnancy; a report of 2 cases. *J Rheumatol* 21:1360, 1994.
161. Neuwelt CM, Daikh DI, Linfoot JA, et al: Catastrophic antiphospholipid syndrome: Response to repeated plasmapheresis over three years. *Arthritis Rheum* 40:1534, 1997.

162. Ramsey-Goldman R, Kutzer JE, Kuller LH, et al: Pregnancy outcome and anti-cardiolipin antibody in women with systemic lupus erythematosus. *Am J Epidemiol* 138:1057, 1993.
163. Locatelli A, Patane L, Ghidini A, et al: Pathology findings in preterm placentas of women with autoantibodies: A case-control study. *J Matern Fetal Neonatal Med* 11:339, 2002.
164. Salafia CM, Cowchock FS: Placental pathology and antiphospholipid antibodies: A descriptive study. *Am J Perinatol* 14:435, 1997.
165. Salafia CM, Parke AL: Placental pathology in systemic lupus erythematosus and phospholipid antibody syndrome. *Rheum Dis Clin North Am* 23:85, 1997.
166. Backos M, Rai R, Regan L: Antiphospholipid antibodies and infertility. *Hum Fertil (Camb)* 5:30, 2002.
167. Practice Committee of American Society for Reproductive Medicine: Anti-phospholipid antibodies do not affect IVF success. *Fertil Steril* 90(5 Suppl):S172, 2008.
168. Kriseman YL, Nash JW, Hsu S: Criteria for the diagnosis of antiphospholipid syndrome in patients presenting with dermatologic symptoms. *J Am Acad Dermatol* 57:112, 2007.
169. Gibson GE, Su WP, Pittelkow MR: Antiphospholipid syndrome and the skin. *J Am Acad Dermatol* 36:970, 1997.
170. Asherson RA, Cervera R: The antiphospholipid syndrome: Multiple faces beyond the classical presentation. *Autoimmun Rev* 2:140, 2003.
171. Aronoff DM, Callen JP: Necrosing livedo reticularis in a patient with recurrent pulmonary hemorrhage. *J Am Acad Dermatol* 37:300, 1997.
172. Greco TP, Conti-Kelly AM, Matsuura E, et al: Antiphospholipid antibodies in patients with coronary artery disease: New cardiac risk factors? *Ann N Y Acad Sci* 1108:466, 2007.
173. Vaarala O: Antiphospholipid antibodies and myocardial infarction. *Lupus* 7(Suppl 2):S132, 1998.
174. Sherer Y, Shoenfeld Y: Antiphospholipid antibodies: Are they pro-atherogenic or an epiphenomenon of atherosclerosis? *Immunobiology* 207:13, 2003.
175. Ludia C, Domenico P, Monia C, et al: Antiphospholipid antibodies: A new risk factor for restenosis after percutaneous transluminal coronary angioplasty? *Autoimmunity* 27:141, 1998.
176. Chambers-JD J, Haire HD, Deligonul U: Multiple early percutaneous transluminal coronary angioplasty failures related to lupus anticoagulant. *Am Heart J* 132:189, 1996.
177. Ames PR, Antinolfi I, Scenna G, et al: Atherosclerosis in thrombotic primary antiphospholipid syndrome. *J Thromb Haemost* 7:537, 2009.
178. Niaz A, Butany J: Antiphospholipid antibody syndrome with involvement of a bioprosthetic heart valve. *Can J Cardiol* 14:951, 1998.
179. Bouillanne O, Millaire A, de Groote P, et al: Prevalence and clinical significance of antiphospholipid antibodies in heart valve disease: A case-control study. *Am Heart J* 132:790, 1996.
180. Nesher G, Ilany J, Rosenmann D, et al: Valvular dysfunction in antiphospholipid syndrome: Prevalence, clinical features, and treatment. *Semin Arthritis Rheum* 27:27, 1997.
181. Hojnik M, George J, Ziporen L, et al: Heart valve involvement (Libman-Sacks endocarditis) in the antiphospholipid syndrome. *Circulation* 93:1579, 1996.
182. Bulckaen HG, Puisieux FL, Bulckaen ED, et al: Antiphospholipid antibodies and the risk of thromboembolic events in valvular heart disease. *Mayo Clin Proc* 78:294, 2003.
183. Garcia TR, Amigo MC, de-la-Rosa A, et al: Valvular heart disease in primary antiphospholipid syndrome (PAPS): Clinical and morphological findings. *Lupus* 5:56, 1996.
184. Ziporen L, Goldberg I, Arad M, et al: Libman-Sacks endocarditis in the antiphospholipid syndrome: Immunopathologic findings in deformed heart valves. *Lupus* 5:196, 1996.
185. Lee RW, Taylor-LM J, Landry GJ, et al: Prospective comparison of infrainguinal bypass grafting in patients with and without antiphospholipid antibodies. *J Vasc Surg* 24:524, 1996.
186. Porres-Aguilar M, Pena-Ruiz MA, Burgos JD, et al: Chronic thromboembolic pulmonary hypertension as an uncommon presentation of primary antiphospholipid syndrome. *J Natl Med Assoc* 100:734, 2008.
187. Karmochkine M, Cacoub P, Dorent R, et al: High prevalence of antiphospholipid antibodies in precapillary pulmonary hypertension. *J Rheumatol* 23:286, 1996.
188. Bonderman D, Wilkens H, Wakounig S, et al: Risk factors for chronic thromboembolic pulmonary hypertension. *Eur Respir J* 33:325, 2009.
189. Asherson RA: The catastrophic antiphospholipid syndrome, 1998. A review of the clinical features, possible pathogenesis and treatment. *Lupus* 7(Suppl 2):S55, 1998.
190. Uthman I, Khamashta M: The abdominal manifestations of the antiphospholipid syndrome. *Rheumatology (Oxford)* 46:1641, 2007.
191. Biron C, Andreani H, Blanc P, et al: Prevalence of antiphospholipid antibodies in patients with chronic liver disease related to alcohol or hepatitis C virus: Correlation with liver injury. *J Lab Clin Med* 131:243, 1998.
192. Sene D, Piette JC, Cacoub P: Antiphospholipid antibodies, antiphospholipid syndrome and infections. *Autoimmun Rev* 7:272, 2008.
193. Ramos-Casals M, Cervera R, Lagrutta M, et al: Clinical features related to antiphospholipid syndrome in patients with chronic viral infections (hepatitis C virus/HIV infection): Description of 82 cases. *Clin Infect Dis* 38:1009, 2004.
194. Hoffman M, Burke M, Fried M, et al: Primary biliary cirrhosis associated with antiphospholipid syndrome. *Isr J Med Sci* 33:681, 1997.
195. Date K, Shirai Y, Hatakeyama K: Antiphospholipid antibody syndrome presenting as acute acalculous cholecystitis. *Am J Gastroenterol* 92:2127, 1997.
196. Dessailloud R, Papo T, Vaneecloo S, et al: Acalculous ischemic gallbladder necrosis in the catastrophic antiphospholipid syndrome. *Arthritis Rheum* 41:1318, 1998.
197. Kalman DR, Khan A, Romain PL, et al: Giant gastric ulceration associated with antiphospholipid antibody syndrome. *Am J Gastroenterol* 91:1244, 1996.
198. Gul A, Inanc M, Ocal L, et al: Primary antiphospholipid syndrome associated with mesenteric inflammatory veno-occlusive disease. *Clin Rheumatol* 15:207, 1996.
199. Lee HJ, Park JW, Chang JC: Mesenteric and portal venous obstruction associated with primary antiphospholipid antibody syndrome. *J Gastroenterol Hepatol* 12:822, 1997.
200. Galli M, Finazzi G, Barbui T: Thrombocytopenia in the antiphospholipid syndrome. *Br J Haematol* 93:1, 1996.
201. Cuadrado MJ, Mujic F, Munoz E, et al: Thrombocytopenia in the antiphospholipid syndrome. *Ann Rheum Dis* 56:194, 1997.
202. Macchi L, Rispal P, Clofent SG, et al: Anti-platelet antibodies in patients with systemic lupus erythematosus and the primary antiphospholipid antibody syndrome: Their relationship with the observed thrombocytopenia. *Br J Haematol* 98:336, 1997.
203. Lipp E, von-Felten A, Sax H, et al: Antibodies against platelet glycoproteins and antiphospholipid antibodies in autoimmune thrombocytopenia. *Eur J Haematol* 60:283, 1998.
204. Pierrot-Deseilligny DC, Michel M, Khellaf M, et al: Antiphospholipid antibodies in adults with immune thrombocytopenic purpura. *Br J Haematol* 142:638, 2008.
205. Diz-Kucukkaya R, Hacihanefioglu A, Yenerel M, et al: Antiphospholipid antibodies and antiphospholipid syndrome in patients presenting with immune thrombocytopenic purpura: A prospective cohort study. *Blood* 98:1760, 2001.
206. Vivaldi P, Rossetti G, Galli M, et al: Severe bleeding due to acquired hypoprothrombinemia-lupus anticoagulant syndrome. Case report and review of literature. *Haematologica* 82:345, 1997.
207. Hudson N, Duffy CM, Rauch J, et al: Catastrophic haemorrhage in a case of paediatric primary antiphospholipid syndrome and factor II deficiency. *Lupus* 6:68, 1997.
208. Collins P, Budde U, Rand JH, et al: Epidemiology and general guidelines of the management of acquired haemophilia and von Willebrand syndrome. *Haemophilia* 14(Suppl 3):49, 2008.
209. Dunn JP, Noorily SW, Petri M, et al: Antiphospholipid antibodies and retinal vascular disease. *Lupus* 5:313, 1996.
210. Coniglio M, Platania A, Di Nucci GD, et al: Antiphospholipid-protein antibodies are not an uncommon feature in retinal venous occlusions. *Thromb Res* 83:183, 1996.
211. Glacet BA, Bayani N, Chretien P, et al: Antiphospholipid antibodies in retinal vascular occlusions. A prospective study of 75 patients. *Arch Ophthalmol* 112:790, 1994.
212. Dori D, Gelfand YA, Brenner B, et al: Cilioretinal artery occlusion: An ocular complication of primary antiphospholipid syndrome. *Retina* 17:555, 1997.
213. Reino S, Munoz RF, Cervera R, et al: Optic neuropathy in the "primary" antiphospholipid syndrome: Report of a case and review of the literature. *Clin Rheumatol* 16:629, 1997.
214. Au A, O'Day J: Review of severe vaso-occlusive retinopathy in systemic lupus erythematosus and the antiphospholipid syndrome: Associations, visual outcomes, complications and treatment. *Clin Experiment Ophthalmol* 32:87, 2004.
215. Fakhouri F, Noel LH, Zuber J, et al: The expanding spectrum of renal diseases associated with antiphospholipid syndrome. *Am J Kidney Dis* 41:1205, 2003.
216. Nochy D, Daugas E, Droz D, et al: The intrarenal vascular lesions associated with primary antiphospholipid syndrome. *J Am Soc Nephrol* 10:507, 1999.
217. Breda L, Nozzi M, De Sanctis S, et al: Laboratory tests in the diagnosis and follow-up of pediatric rheumatic diseases: An update. *Semin Arthritis Rheum* 2009 [in press].
218. Avcin T, Cimaz R, Silverman ED, et al: Pediatric antiphospholipid syndrome: Clinical and immunologic features of 121 patients in an international registry. *Pediatrics* 122:e1100, 2008.
219. Falcini F, Taccetti G, Ermini M, et al: Catastrophic antiphospholipid antibody syndrome in pediatric systemic lupus erythematosus. *J Rheumatol* 24:389, 1997.
220. Ol'binskaia LI, Poptsov VN, Gofman AM: Hemodynamic changes in patients with myocardial infarct complicated by acute left ventricular failure during combined nitroglycerin and dobutamine therapy. *Kardiologiia* 31:49, 1991.
221. Marie I, Levesque H, Heron F, et al: Acute adrenal failure secondary to bilateral infarction of the adrenal glands as the first manifestation of primary antiphospholipid antibody syndrome. *Ann Rheum Dis* 56:567, 1997.
222. Espinosa G, Santos E, Cervera R, et al: Adrenal involvement in the antiphospholipid syndrome: Clinical and immunologic characteristics of 86 patients. *Medicine (Baltimore)* 82:106, 2003.
223. Paydas S, Kocak R, Zorludemir S, et al: Bone marrow necrosis in antiphospholipid syndrome. *J Clin Pathol* 50:261, 1997.
224. Naarendorp M, Spiera H: Sudden sensorineural hearing loss in patients with systemic lupus erythematosus or lupus-like syndromes and antiphospholipid antibodies. *J Rheumatol* 25:589, 1998.
225. Pengo V, Tripodi A, Reber G, et al: Update of the guidelines for measuring the presence of Lupus anticoagulant. *J Thromb Haemost* 7:1737, 2009.
226. de Groot PG, Derksen RH, de Laat B: Twenty-two years of failure to set up undisputed assays to detect patients with the antiphospholipid syndrome. *Semin Thromb Hemost* 34:347, 2008.
227. Mateo J, Oliver A, Borrell M, et al: Laboratory evaluation and clinical characteristics of 2,132 consecutive unselected patients with venous thromboembolism—Results of the Spanish Multicentric Study on Thrombophilia (EMET-Study). *Thromb Haemost* 77:444, 1997.

228. Luong T-H, Rand JH, Wu XX, et al: Seasonal distribution of antiphospholipid antibodies. *Stroke* 32:1707, 2001.
229. Galli M, Luciani D, Bertolini G, et al: Anti-beta 2-glycoprotein I, antiprothrombin antibodies, and the risk of thrombosis in the antiphospholipid syndrome. *Blood* 102:2717, 2003.
230. Shah NM, Khamashta MA, Atsumi T, et al: Outcome of patients with anticardiolipin antibodies: A 10 year follow-up of 52 patients. *Lupus* 7:3, 1998.
231. Silver RM, Porter TF, van Leeuween I, et al: Anticardiolipin antibodies: Clinical consequences of "low titers." *Obstet Gynecol* 87:494, 1996.
232. Tuhrim S, Rand JH, Wu XX, et al: Elevated anticardiolipin antibody titer is a stroke risk factor in a multiethnic population independent of isotype or degree of positivity. *Stroke* 30:1561, 1999.
233. Brey RL, Stallworth CL, McGlasson DL, et al: Antiphospholipid antibodies and stroke in young women. *Stroke* 33:2396, 2002.
234. Merrill JT, Shen C, Gugnani M, et al: High prevalence of antiphospholipid antibodies in patients taking procainamide. *J Rheumatol* 24:1083, 1997.
235. El-Rayes BF, Edelstein M: Unusual case of antiphospholipid antibody syndrome presenting with extensive cutaneous infarcts in a patient on long-term procainamide therapy. *Am J Hematol* 72:154, 2003.
236. Karmochkine M, Piette JC, Mazoyer E, et al: Antiphospholipid antibodies: Cause of thrombosis or an epiphenomenon? *Presse Med* 24:267, 1995.
237. Zornberg GL, Jick H: Antipsychotic drug use and risk of first-time idiopathic venous thromboembolism: A case-control study. *Lancet* 356:1219, 2000.
238. Lopez LR, Dier KJ, Lopez D, et al: Anti-beta 2-glycoprotein I and antiphosphatidylserine antibodies are predictors of arterial thrombosis in patients with antiphospholipid syndrome. *Am J Clin Pathol* 121:142, 2004.
239. Audrain MA, El-Kouri D, Hamidou MA, et al: Value of autoantibodies to beta(2)-glycoprotein 1 in the diagnosis of antiphospholipid syndrome. *Rheumatology (Oxford)* 41:550, 2002.
240. Amengual O, Atsumi T, Khamashta MA, et al: Specificity of ELISA for antibody to beta 2-glycoprotein I in patients with antiphospholipid syndrome. *Br J Rheumatol* 35:1239, 1996.
241. Alarcon-Segovia D, Mestanza M, Cabiedes J, et al: The antiphospholipid/cofactor syndromes. II. A variant in patients with systemic lupus erythematosus with antibodies to beta 2-glycoprotein I but no antibodies detectable in standard antiphospholipid assays. *J Rheumatol* 24:1545, 1997.
242. Cabral AR, Amigo MC, Cabiedes J, et al: The antiphospholipid/cofactor syndromes: A primary variant with antibodies to beta 2-glycoprotein-I but no antibodies detectable in standard antiphospholipid assays. *Am J Med* 101:472, 1996.
243. Sanmarco M, Soler C, Christides C, et al: Prevalence and clinical significance of IgG isotype anti-beta 2-glycoprotein I antibodies in antiphospholipid syndrome: A comparative study with anticardiolipin antibodies. *J Lab Clin Med* 129:499, 1997.
244. Day HM, Thiagarajan P, Ahn C, et al: Autoantibodies to beta2-glycoprotein I in systemic lupus erythematosus and primary antiphospholipid antibody syndrome: Clinical correlations in comparison with other antiphospholipid antibody tests. *J Rheumatol* 25:667, 1998.
245. Reber G, Schousboe I, Tincani A, et al: Inter-laboratory variability of anti-beta2-glycoprotein I measurement. A collaborative study in the frame of the European Forum on Antiphospholipid Antibodies Standardization Group. *Thromb Haemost* 88:66, 2002.
246. Berard M, Chantome R, Marcelli A, et al: Antiphosphatidylethanolamine antibodies as the only antiphospholipid antibodies. I. Association with thrombosis and vascular cutaneous diseases. *J Rheumatol* 23:1369, 1996.
247. Rauch J, Janoff AS: Antibodies against phospholipids other than cardiolipin: Potential roles for both phospholipid and protein. *Lupus* 5:498, 1996.
248. Yetman DL, Kutteh WH: Antiphospholipid antibody panels and recurrent pregnancy loss: Prevalence of anticardiolipin antibodies compared with other antiphospholipid antibodies. *Fertil Steril* 66:540, 1996.
249. de Maistre E, Gobert B, Bene MC, et al: Comparative assessment of phospholipid-binding antibodies indicates limited overlapping. *J Clin Lab Anal* 10:6, 1996.
250. Branch DW, Silver R, Pierangeli S, et al: Antiphospholipid antibodies other than lupus anticoagulant and anticardiolipin antibodies in women with recurrent pregnancy loss, fertile controls, and antiphospholipid syndrome. *Obstet Gynecol* 89:549, 1997.
251. Shapiro SS: The lupus anticoagulant/antiphospholipid syndrome. *Annu Rev Med* 47:533, 1996.
252. Triplett DA: Lupus anticoagulants/antiphospholipid-protein antibodies: The great imposters. *Lupus* 5:431, 1996.
253. Nojima J, Suehisa E, Akita N, et al: Risk of arterial thrombosis in patients with anticardiolipin antibodies and lupus anticoagulant. *Br J Haematol* 96:447, 1997.
254. Somers E, Magder LS, Petri M: Antiphospholipid antibodies and incidence of venous thrombosis in a cohort of patients with systemic lupus erythematosus. *J Rheumatol* 29:2531, 2002.
255. Opatrny L, David M, Kahn SR, et al: Association between antiphospholipid antibodies and recurrent fetal loss in women without autoimmune disease: A metaanalysis. *J Rheumatol* 33:2214, 2006.
256. Kitchens CS: Prolonged activated partial thromboplastin time of unknown etiology: A prospective study of 100 consecutive cases referred for consultation. *Am J Hematol* 27:38, 1988.
257. Galli M, Barbui T: Prothrombin as cofactor for antiphospholipids. *Lupus* 7(Suppl 2):S37, 1998.
258. Galli M, Finazzi G, Bevers EM, et al: Kaolin clotting time and dilute Russell's viper venom time distinguish between prothrombin-dependent and beta 2-glycoprotein I-dependent antiphospholipid antibodies. *Blood* 86:617, 1995.
259. Liu HW, Wong KL, Lin CK, et al: The reappraisal of dilute tissue thromboplastin inhibition test in the diagnosis of lupus anticoagulant. *Br J Haematol* 72:229, 1989.
260. Forastiero RR, Cerrato GS, Carreras LO: Evaluation of recently described tests for detection of the lupus anticoagulant. *Thromb Haemost* 72:728, 1994.
261. Lenzi R, Rand JH, Spiera H: Anticardiolipin antibodies in pregnant patients with systemic lupus erythematosus. *N Engl J Med* 314:1392, 1986.
262. Lim W, Crowther MA, Eikelboom JW: Management of antiphospholipid antibody syndrome: A systematic review. *JAMA* 295:1050, 2006.
263. Khamashta MA, Cuadrado MJ, Mujic F, et al: The management of thrombosis in the antiphospholipid-antibody syndrome. *N Engl J Med* 332:993, 1995.
264. Urfer C, Pichler WJ, Helbling A: Antiphospholipid antibodies syndrome: Follow-up of patients with a high antiphospholipid antibodies titer. *Schweiz Med Wochenschr* 126:2136, 1996.
265. Erkan D, Harrison MJ, Levy R, et al: Aspirin for primary thrombosis prevention in the antiphospholipid syndrome: A randomized, double-blind, placebo-controlled trial in asymptomatic antiphospholipid antibody-positive individuals. *Arthritis Rheum* 56:2382, 2007.
266. Moll S, Ortel TL: Monitoring warfarin therapy in patients with lupus anticoagulants. *Ann Intern Med* 127:177, 1997.
267. Tripodi A, Chantarangkul V, Clerici M, et al: Laboratory control of oral anticoagulant treatment by the INR system in patients with the antiphospholipid syndrome and lupus anticoagulant. Results of a collaborative study involving nine commercial thromboplastins. *Br J Haematol* 115:672, 2001.
268. Camps GM, Guil M, Sanchez LJ, et al: Fibrinolytic treatment in primary antiphospholipid syndrome. *Lupus* 5:627, 1996.
269. Julkunen H, Hedman C, Kauppi M: Thrombolysis for acute ischemic stroke in the primary antiphospholipid syndrome. *J Rheumatol* 24:181, 1997.
270. Ho YL, Chen MF, Wu CC, et al: Successful treatment of acute myocardial infarction by thrombolytic therapy in a patient with primary antiphospholipid antibody syndrome. *Cardiology* 87:354, 1996.
271. Wallace DJ: The use of chloroquine and hydroxychloroquine for non-infectious conditions other than rheumatoid arthritis or lupus: A critical review. *Lupus* 5(Suppl 1):S59, 1996.
272. Erkan D, Yazici Y, Peterson MG, et al: A cross-sectional study of clinical thrombotic risk factors and preventive treatments in antiphospholipid syndrome. *Rheumatology (Oxford)* 41:924, 2002.
273. Tektonidou MG, Laskari K, Panagiotakos DB, et al: Risk factors for thrombosis and primary thrombosis prevention in patients with systemic lupus erythematosus with or without antiphospholipid antibodies. *Arthritis Rheum* 61:29, 2009.
274. Petri M: Thrombosis and systemic lupus erythematosus: The Hopkins Lupus Cohort perspective. *Scand J Rheumatol* 25:191, 1996.
275. Kaiser R, Cleveland CM, Criswell LA: Risk and protective factors for thrombosis in systemic lupus erythematosus: Results from a large, multi-ethnic cohort. *Ann Rheum Dis* 68:238, 2009.
276. Edwards MH, Pierangeli S, Liu X, et al: Hydroxychloroquine reverses thrombogenic properties of antiphospholipid antibodies in mice. *Circulation* 96:4380, 1997.
277. Rand JH, Wu XX, Quinn AS, et al: Hydroxychloroquine directly reduces the binding of antiphospholipid antibody-beta2-glycoprotein I complexes to phospholipid bilayers. *Blood* 112:1687, 2008.
278. Rand JH, Wu XX, Quinn AS, et al: Hydroxychloroquine reverses a procoagulant mechanism for antiphospholipid syndrome: Evidence for a novel effect for an old antimalarial drug. *Blood* 2009 [in press].
279. Empson M, Lassere M, Craig J, et al: Prevention of recurrent miscarriage for women with antiphospholipid antibody or lupus anticoagulant. *Cochrane Database Syst Rev* 2:CD002859, 2005.
280. Galli M, Barbui T: Antiphospholipid antibodies and pregnancy. *Best Pract Res Clin Haematol* 16:211, 2003.
281. Rai R: Obstetric management of antiphospholipid syndrome. *J Autoimmun* 15:203, 2000.
282. Laskin CA, Spitzer KA, Clark CA, et al: Low molecular weight heparin and aspirin for recurrent pregnancy loss: Results from the randomized, controlled HepASA Trial. *J Rheumatol* 36:279, 2009.
283. Cowchock S, Reece EA: Do low-risk pregnant women with antiphospholipid antibodies need to be treated? Organizing Group of the Antiphospholipid Antibody Treatment Trial. *Am J Obstet Gynecol* 176:1099, 1997.
284. Cowchock S: Treatment of antiphospholipid syndrome in pregnancy. *Lupus* 7(Suppl 2):S95, 1998.
285. Bouma B, de Groot PG, van den Elsen JM, et al: Adhesion mechanism of human beta(2)-glycoprotein I to phospholipids based on its crystal structure. *EMBO J* 18:5166, 1999.
286. Rand JH, Arslan AA, Wu XX, et al: Reduction of circulating Annexin A5 levels and resistance to annexin A5 anticoagulant activity in women with recurrent spontaneous pregnancy losses. *Am J Obstet Gynecol* 194:182, 2006.

CHAPTER 133

ANTIBODY-MEDIATED THROMBOTIC DISORDERS: THROMBOTIC THROMBOCYTOPENIC PURPURA AND HEPARIN-INDUCED THROMBOCYTOPENIA

J. Evan Sadler and Mortimer Poncz

SUMMARY

Idiopathic thrombotic thrombocytopenic purpura (TTP) is associated with microangiopathic hemolytic anemia, thrombocytopenia, and microvascular thrombosis that results in variable injury of the central nervous system, kidney, and other organs. Most cases of TTP are caused by autoantibodies to ADAMTS13, a metalloprotease that cleaves von Willebrand factor (VWF) and inhibits VWF-dependent platelet aggregation. TTP is usually fatal if untreated. Most patients respond to plasma exchange, although many have relapsing disease. Clinically similar thrombotic microangiopathy can occur with normal ADAMTS13 levels. Secondary thrombotic microangiopathy occurs in association with metastatic cancer, infections, organ transplantation, and certain drugs. Secondary thrombotic microangiopathy has a lower likelihood of responding to plasma exchange and a lower survival rate.

Heparin-induced thrombocytopenia (HIT) is a significant complication of treatment with heparin, especially unfractionated high-molecular-weight heparin. It is associated with mild to moderate thrombocytopenia, although the main concern is the high frequency of both arterial and venous thrombotic complications. HIT is an immune complex-based disorder involving heparin/platelet factor 4 (PF4) complexes. Immediate cessation of heparin is required, but the risk of subsequent thrombosis remains high. Direct thrombin inhibitors are the present-day treatment of choice to limit thrombotic complications.

Acronyms and abbreviations that appear in this chapter include: ADAMTS, a disintegrin and metalloprotease with thrombospondin type 1 repeats; APS, antiphospholipid syndrome; aPTT, activated partial thromboplastin time; DDAVP, desmopressin, 1-deamino-8-D-arginine-vasopressin; D$^+$HUS, diarrhea-associated hemolytic uremic syndrome; D$^-$HUS, diarrhea-negative hemolytic uremic syndrome; GP, glycoprotein; HELLP, hemolysis, elevated liver enzymes, and low platelet count; HIT, heparin-induced thrombocytopenia; HUS, hemolytic uremic syndrome; Ig, immunoglobulin; LDH, lactate dehydrogenase; MCP, membrane cofactor protein; MTHFR, methylenetetrahydrofolate reductase; PF4, platelet factor 4; PT, prothrombin time; SLE, systemic lupus erythematosus; TTP, thrombotic thrombocytopenic purpura; VWF, von Willebrand factor.

THROMBOTIC THROMBOCYTOPENIC PURPURA

DEFINITION AND HISTORY

Thrombotic microangiopathy refers to a combination of microangiopathic hemolytic anemia, thrombocytopenia, and microvascular thrombosis, regardless of cause or specific tissue involvement. Various kinds of thrombotic microangiopathy differ in pathogenesis and prognosis, but can be difficult to distinguish because their clinical features overlap.

Thrombotic thrombocytopenic purpura (TTP) is a form of thrombotic microangiopathy in which tissue injury can affect any organ but often results in neurologic damage and fever. Renal involvement is common but oliguric renal failure is not. TTP usually is associated with acquired autoantibodies that inhibit a disintegrin and metalloprotease thrombospondin type 1 repeats (ADAMTS)13.

Congenital TTP, or Upshaw-Schulman syndrome, refers to TTP that is caused by inherited deficiency of ADAMTS13.

Hemolytic uremic syndrome (HUS) refers to thrombotic microangiopathy that mainly affects the kidney and usually causes oliguric or anuric renal failure. *Diarrhea-associated* or *typical* HUS (D$^+$HUS) is caused by enteric infection with Shiga toxin-producing Gram-negative bacilli, and usually is associated with a prodrome of diarrhea. *Diarrhea-negative* or *atypical* HUS (D$^-$HUS) is not associated with diarrhea or Shiga toxin-producing organisms and occurs in patients without an obvious predisposing condition.

Secondary thrombotic microangiopathy occurs in patients with predisposing medical conditions such as metastatic cancer, systemic infection, solid-organ or hematopoietic stem cell transplantation, radiation exposure, chemotherapy, certain other drugs, and various other causes of disseminated intravascular coagulation. For these heterogeneous disorders, the most important clinical intervention is correcting the underlying "primary" condition; with a few specific exceptions, ADAMTS13 levels are normal and plasma exchange is ineffective.

Eli Moschcowitz reported the first detailed description of TTP in 1924.[1,2] The patient was a 16-year-old girl with fever, severe anemia, leukocytosis, petechiae, and hemiparesis. Her renal function was not impaired, but the urine contained albumin, hyaline casts, and granular casts. She became comatose and died 2 weeks after her first symptoms. At autopsy, hyaline thrombi were found diffusely in terminal arterioles and capillaries, particularly of the heart and kidney. For many years, patients with similar findings were said to have Moschcowitz's disease. The name *TTP* was proposed in 1947,[3] and widely adopted thereafter.

In 1955, the term *hemolytic uremic syndrome* was proposed for thrombotic microangiopathy occurring in children and associated with acute anuric renal failure, which is uncommon in TTP.[4] HUS was often preceded by a diarrheal illness and, unlike TTP in adults, the prognosis was favorable. Most patients survived and recovered normal renal function with only supportive care.[5]

In 1966, a review of 272 published cases defined the major clinical features of TTP.[6] Most patients were females between the ages of 10 and 39 years. The symptoms and physical findings included a classic pentad of thrombocytopenia, hemolytic anemia with numerous fragmented red cells or schistocytes, neurologic findings, renal damage, and fever. Mortality exceeded 90 percent: the average hospital stay was only 14 days before death, and 80 percent of patients lived fewer than 90 days after the onset of symptoms. However, dramatic recoveries occurred in some cases following splenectomy.

This grim prognosis was recorded before the recognition that blood or plasma infusions improved the outcome of TTP. A few reports, including one from Moschcowitz in 1925,[2] had suggested that blood transfusion sometimes induced dramatic responses.[7] But interest in transfusion therapy increased after 1976, when whole-blood exchange transfusions reportedly induced prompt remissions in 8 of 14 patients.[8] Similar responses were described after plasmapheresis with plasma replacement.[9] One remarkable case report showed that plasmapheresis was effective if the replacement fluid was plasma or cryoprecipitate-depleted plasma, but ineffective if the replacement fluid contained just albumin.[10] Furthermore, simple plasma infusions without plasmapheresis could induce sustained remissions, suggesting that replacement of a missing plasma factor sometimes was sufficient to ameliorate TTP.[10]

A similar congenital disorder first described by Schulman and colleagues[11] and Upshaw[12] is characterized by autosomal recessive inheritance and chronic relapsing thrombotic microangiopathy from infancy. Congenital TTP, or Upshaw-Schulman syndrome, shared many features with TTP in adults, including the consistent response to plasma.[12]

These reports led to the widespread adoption of plasma therapy for TTP, and two studies published in 1991 provided compelling evidence for its efficacy. Plasma infusion was associated with 91 percent survival in 108 patients, an impressive improvement over historical experience.[13] The same year, a prospective randomized comparison of plasma exchange and plasma infusion in 102 patients with TTP was reported.[14] Long-term survival was 78 percent for the plasma exchange group and 63 percent for the plasma infusion group, a significant difference in favor of plasma exchange.

A link between TTP and von Willebrand factor (VWF) was proposed in 1982, based on studies of four patients with chronic relapsing TTP.[15] Their plasma VWF multimers were much larger than those of healthy controls and similar in size to the VWF multimers secreted by endothelial cells. Patients with TTP were proposed to lack a depolymerase activity, perhaps a protease or a reductase, that shortens newly secreted VWF multimers *in vivo* and produces the multimer distribution of normal plasma. The absence of this depolymerase would cause the persistence of "unusually large" VWF, which promotes intravascular platelet aggregation, thrombocytopenia, and microvascular thrombosis. Plasma exchange therapy could provide the missing depolymerase activity, or remove other factors that provoke clinical relapses.

A candidate depolymerase was identified in 1996, when a metalloprotease in plasma was shown to cleave VWF multimers subjected to high fluid shear stress or to mild protein denaturants.[16,17] Soon thereafter, children with congenital TTP were shown to have inherited deficiency of this metalloprotease,[18] and adults with acquired TTP were shown to have autoantibody inhibitors of the enzyme.[19,20] The VWF cleaving protease was purified,[21,22] cloned,[23,24] and named ADAMTS13, a new member of the ADAMTS family of metalloproteases. Simultaneously, the *ADAMTS13* locus was identified by linkage analysis in families affected by congenital TTP and causative ADAMTS13 mutations were characterized.[25]

Clinical studies confirmed the association of severe ADAMTS13 deficiency with congenital and acquired TTP. In contrast, ADAMTS13 deficiency is almost unknown in HUS or secondary thrombotic microangiopathy. Therefore, ADAMTS13 levels correlate with differences in pathophysiology and prognosis.

ETIOLOGY AND PATHOGENESIS

Unregulated VWF-dependent platelet thrombosis appears to be the mechanism underlying congenital TTP and most instances of TTP. Large VWF multimers mediate platelet adhesion at sites of vascular injury by binding to connective tissue and to glycoprotein Ib (GPIb) on the platelet surface (see Chap. 127). The VWF subunit from which multimers are constructed has a modular structure consisting of five types of conserved structural motifs (Fig. 133–1). VWF multimers bind to collagen through domain A3, and to platelet GPIb through domain A1. When platelets bind to VWF under conditions of high fluid shear stress, the VWF multimer is stretched and the Tyr^{1605}-Met^{1606} bond within domain A2 becomes accessible to ADAMTS13 (Fig. 133–2), which cleaves it and thereby may release any adherent platelets. ADAMTS13 deficiency prevents this feedback inhibition and leads to microvascular platelet thrombosis.

TTP usually is caused by polyclonal immunoglobulin (Ig) G autoantibodies that inhibit ADAMTS13 (Fig. 133–3).[19,20] The antibodies usually bind the cysteine-rich or spacer domain, and often bind to the CUB domains and first thrombospondin-1 repeat; they bind less frequently to other thrombospondin-1 repeats, the metalloprotease domain, or the propeptide.[26,27] Noninhibitory IgG and IgM antibodies have been identified, although their significance is unknown.[28]

The composition of the lesions in TTP is consistent with a pathophysiologic role of VWF-dependent platelet thrombosis. Amorphous thrombi and subendothelial hyaline deposits may be found in the small

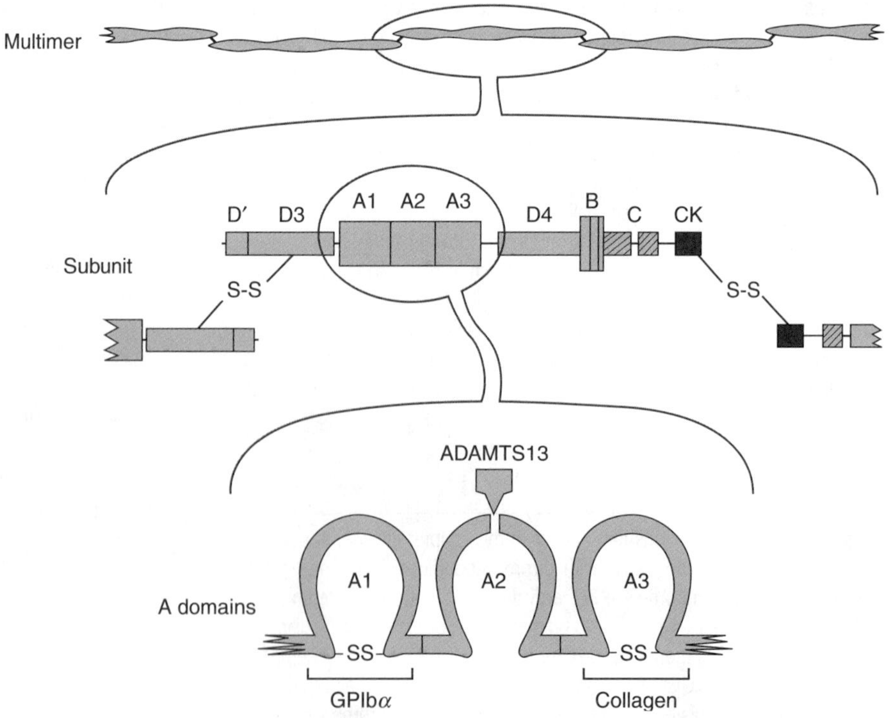

FIGURE 133–1. Structure of von Willebrand factor. Multimeric VWF (*top*) is composed of identical subunits with five kinds of structural motifs, including three A domains, three B domains, two C domains, two complete and one partial D domains, and a cystine knot (CK) domain. Subunits (*middle*) are linked into multimers by disulfide bonds between C-terminal CK domains and N-terminal D3 domains. Domain A1 (*bottom*) binds platelet glycoprotein Ibα (GPIbα), domain A3 binds collagen in extracellular matrix, and domain A2 contains a Tyr-Met bond that is susceptible to cleavage by ADAMTS13.

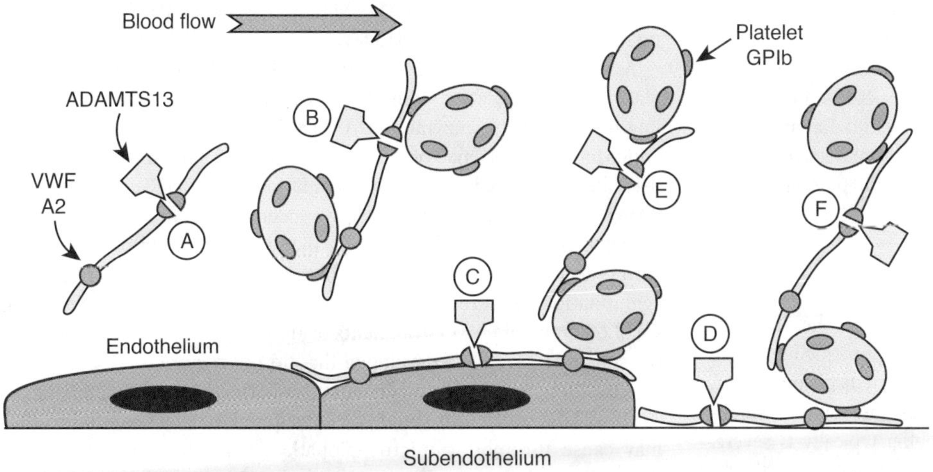

FIGURE 133–2. Regulation of von Willebrand factor (VWF)-dependent platelet thrombosis by ADAMTS13. Endothelial cells secrete VWF as "ultralarge" multimers that enter the circulation (A, B) or adhere to the cell surface (C). VWF also binds to connective tissue at sites of vascular injury (D). Under conditions of high fluid shear stress, platelets may adhere to VWF in solution (B) or on surfaces (C, D) through platelet GPIbα. VWF also can recruit platelets to other adherent platelets (E). ADAMTS13 cleaves the A2 domain of the VWF subunit, severing the multimer. This reaction is slow for VWF in solution (A) but occurs rapidly when platelets adhere to VWF under high fluid shear conditions in suspension (B) or on surfaces (C, D, E, F), presumably as a consequence of conformational changes induced by tensile force on VWF. Failure of this mechanism can cause TTP. *(From Sadler JE,[269] with permission.)*

arterioles and capillaries of any organ, but are particularly common (in order of increasing severity) in the myocardium, pancreas, kidney, adrenal gland, and brain. The liver and lung are relatively spared. The lesions consist mainly of platelets and VWF, with little fibrin and few inflammatory cells. They often include focal endothelial cell proliferation.[29,30] The histologic findings in congenital TTP are similar.[31] In contrast, D$^+$HUS mainly affects the renal cortex, which often shows extensive necrosis. Lesions occur infrequently in the pancreas, brain, adrenal glands, and myocardium. The thrombi of HUS typically involve glomerular capillaries and arterioles and are composed mainly of fibrin with few platelets.[30,32]

Factors other than ADAMTS13 deficiency have been proposed to contribute to TTP, although a causal relationship has not been established. These factors include platelet agglutinating proteins distinct from VWF,[33] antibodies that activate endothelial cells[34] or bind CD36 and activate platelets,[35] and circulating factors causing endothelial cell apoptosis.[36]

Secondary thrombotic microangiopathy is an infrequent complication in many different settings, and the pathophysiology is heterogeneous. Endothelial injury may be a common feature, although the mechanism of injury probably varies and in most cases is not understood. With the exception of some drug-induced TTP, severe ADAMTS13 deficiency is not observed.[37,38] Autopsy studies in a few patients with secondary thrombotic microangiopathy suggest that any microvascular thrombosis tends to be limited to the kidney.[38–40]

EPIDEMIOLOGY

The incidence of TTP in the United States has been estimated at approximately 4.5 per 1 million per year.[41,42] Seasonal or geographical trends have not been observed consistently. TTP is relatively uncommon before age 20 years, with a peak incidence between ages 30 and 50 years.[41,42] Across many reports, the female-to-male ratio averages approximately 2:1, but female preponderance is more pronounced below age 50 years and the ratio approaches equality after age 60 years.[41,42] Other risk factors for TTP include African ancestry[42–44] and obesity.[43,45] Women have a tendency to present during late pregnancy or peripartum (reviewed in references 46 and 47). Congenital TTP[48] and secondary thrombotic microangiopathy[43,44] affect the genders almost equally.

Heritable risk factors probably affect susceptibility to TTP. For example, identical twin sisters developed TTP at ages 23 and 24 years. Both women had autoantibodies against ADAMTS13 and responded completely to plasma exchange, with disappearance of the inhibitors and normalization of ADAMTS13 activity.[49] A low frequency of human leukocyte antigen (HLA)-DR53 was reported in adults with TTP or HUS, suggesting an immunogenetically determined protective effect.[50] A high prevalence of factor V Leiden was reported among patients with TTP who did not have ADAMTS13 deficiency, suggesting that inherited risk factors for venous thrombosis might predispose to thrombotic microangiopathy.[51] However, subsequent studies have not confirmed an association between factor V Leiden and TTP.[52]

CLINICAL FEATURES

The onset of TTP can be dramatically acute or insidious, developing over weeks. Approximately one-third of patients have symptoms of hemolytic anemia.[6,46] Thrombocytopenia typically causes petechiae or purpura; oral, gastrointestinal or genitourinary bleeding is less common but can be severe.

Systemic microvascular thrombosis can affect any organ, and the consequences are variable. Renal involvement is common, but acute renal failure occurs in fewer than 10 percent of cases.[43,44,46] Neurologic findings can be transient or persistent and may include headache, visual disturbances, vertigo, personality change, confusion, lethargy, syncope, coma, seizures, aphasia, hemiparesis, and other focal sensory or motor deficits.[6,46] Many patients have fever. The frequency of neurologic findings or fever has decreased from more than 90 percent to approximately 50 percent over the past 40 years,[6,14,43,44,46] possibly because these features no longer are required for diagnosis of TTP.

The symptoms of TTP sometimes can be quite atypical, either at first presentation or upon relapse. Thrombocytopenia without hemolytic anemia may herald the onset of disease. In rare instances, visual disturbances, pancreatitis, stroke, or other thrombosis may precede overt thrombotic microangiopathy by days to months.[53–56]

Cardiac involvement may cause chest pain, myocardial infarction, congestive heart failure, or arrhythmias.[46,57,58] Direct pulmonary involvement is uncommon but severe acute respiratory distress syndrome may

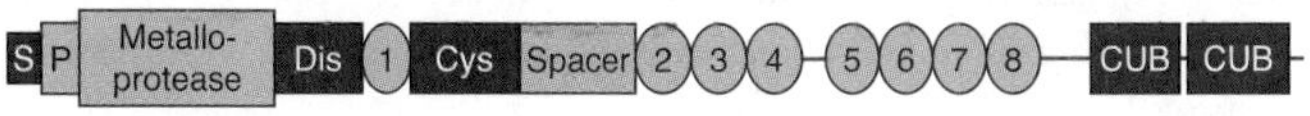

FIGURE 133–3. Structure of ADAMTS13. The ADAMTS13 precursor has a signal peptide (S), a short propeptide (P), a reprolysin-like metalloprotease domain, disintegrin-like domain (Dis), eight thrombospondin type 1 repeats (numbered), characteristic cysteine-rich (Cys) and spacer domains, and two CUB domains (named for motifs in complement C1r and C1s, sea urchin protein UeGF, and bone morphogenetic protein 1). *(Adapted from Zheng X, Chung D, Takayama TK, et al.,[23] with permission.)*

occur,[59] possibly secondary to cardiac failure.[46] Gastrointestinal symptoms are common and can include abdominal pain, nausea, vomiting, and diarrhea.[6,46] Physical examination may suggest acute pancreatitis or mesenteric ischemia. One review reported hepatomegaly and splenomegaly in one-fifth of cases.[6] Infrequent findings include Raynaud phenomenon, arthralgia, myalgia, and retinal hemorrhage or detachment.[6,46]

The clinical features of secondary thrombotic microangiopathy usually are dominated by the underlying condition.

LABORATORY FEATURES

Because the symptoms and signs of TTP are nonspecific, the diagnosis depends on laboratory testing to document microangiopathic hemolytic anemia and thrombocytopenia, without another predisposing cause. Almost all patients have anemia and one-third have hemoglobin values below approximately 6 g/dL.[6,46] Thrombocytopenia typically is severe, and one-half of patients have platelet counts below approximately 20,000/μL.[6,43,44,46,60] Hemolysis is indicated by an elevated reticulocyte count and serum lactate dehydrogenase (LDH) and a decreased serum haptoglobin. The median LDH level is approximately 1200 U/L.[13,14,43,44,60] Direct antiglobulin test (Coombs test) is almost always negative.[13,14,46]

The characteristic morphologic feature of TTP on the blood film is a marked increase in schistocytes. Schistocytes are jagged or irregularly shaped fragments of split red cells with two or more sharply pointed projections, sometimes having the appearance of military helmets (see Chap. 29). Patients with TTP often have markedly increased schistocytes; in a study of six patients, schistocytes comprised a mean of 8.3 percent of all red cells with a range of 1 to 18.4 percent.[61] Spherocytes also may be seen.

Almost all patients have normal values for plasma fibrinogen, prothrombin time (PT), and activated partial thromboplastin time (aPTT),[13,14,46] reflecting a minor role of intravascular coagulation in TTP. Mildly elevated fibrin degradation products have been reported in some patients,[46,62] perhaps as a consequence of fibrin generation triggered by ischemic tissue injury. Evidence of myocardial damage is common, with elevated troponin T levels.[57,58]

Severe congenital ADAMTS13 deficiency (level <5%) is characteristic of congenital TTP. Severe acquired ADAMTS13 deficiency appears to be specific for TTP,[19,20,63,64] although the sensitivity of the association is debated and the frequency of severe ADAMTS13 deficiency in TTP depends on how patients are ascertained. If adult patients with thrombotic microangiopathy are selected with no plausible secondary cause, no diarrheal prodrome, and no features suggestive of HUS (e.g., oliguria, severe hypertension, need for dialysis, serum creatinine >3.5 mg/dL), then at least 80 percent may have undetectable ADAMTS13 activity and the majority will have easily detected autoantibody inhibitors.[19,20,44,65] Among less highly selected patients, severe ADAMTS13 deficiency and inhibitors are less prevalent.[43]

ADAMTS13 levels tend to vary inversely with VWF level.[66] ADAMTS13 levels are normal to moderately decreased in newborns, during pregnancy, and after surgery, and in liver cirrhosis, chronic renal insufficiency, acute inflammatory states, sepsis, and a variety of thrombocytopenic disorders other than TTP.[64,66] Some patients with acute viral hepatitis, severe liver cirrhosis,[67] or venoocclusive disease after stem cell transplantation[68] have had severe ADAMTS13 deficiency (level <5%) at least transiently, which is consistent with the synthesis of ADAMTS13 in liver.[23–25]

Severe sepsis may sometimes cause acquired severe ADAMTS13 deficiency, although the incidence and clinical significance of the finding remain uncertain. One study reported severe ADAMTS13 deficiency (level <5%) in 15 percent (17/109) of patients with sepsis-induced disseminated intravascular coagulation, with a trend toward an association with renal failure.[69] A subsequent study of 40 patients with severe sepsis found no ADAMTS13 levels less than 25 percent and no relationship of ADAMTS13 level to prognosis.[70]

Assays for ADAMTS13 activity usually are performed on citrated plasma; anticoagulation with ethylenediaminetetraacetic acid irreversibly inactivates the enzyme. ADAMTS13 inhibitors can be assayed in anticoagulated plasma or in serum. Several methods have been described that rely on the degradation of VWF multimers by ADAMTS13 in the presence of low concentrations of urea[16] or guanidine hydrochloride.[17] VWF cleavage then is detected indirectly by measuring decreases in VWF-collagen binding or VWF-dependent platelet agglutination, or directly by gel electrophoresis.[71] Rapid assays using small recombinant VWF fragments or fluorogenic synthetic peptides as the substrate have been developed that do not require the use of denaturants; these assays generally have better performance characteristics.[71]

Other laboratory tests should be considered to detect conditions that may cause thrombotic microangiopathy by mechanisms other than ADAMTS13 deficiency. The tests include microbiologic and serologic tests for Shiga toxin-producing organisms, tests for antiphospholipid antibody syndrome, serologies for systemic lupus erythematosus and other autoimmune diseases, and testing suitable for potential causes of secondary thrombotic microangiopathy.

DIFFERENTIAL DIAGNOSIS

The diagnosis of TTP should be entertained for any patient with microangiopathic hemolytic anemia and thrombocytopenia, without evidence for disseminated intravascular coagulation, and without features associated with D^+HUS, such as a prodromal diarrheal illness and acute oliguric or anuric renal failure. These criteria can only be approximate, however, because many diseases associated with secondary thrombotic microangiopathy can produce overlapping clinical and laboratory findings. As a consequence, making a diagnosis of TTP can be a challenge and a wide differential diagnosis often must be considered (Table 133–1).

Schistocytes occur in a variety of conditions besides TTP, although the level seldom enters the 1 to 18 percent range typical of TTP.[61] For example, schistocytes were seen in the blood film of 58 percent of healthy controls, with a mean of 0.05 percent and a range of 0 to 0.27 percent of all red cells.[61] Up to 0.6 percent schistocytes were observed in patients with chronic renal failure, preeclampsia, or properly functioning prosthetic heart valves.[61] Severe hemolysis and marked schistocytosis occur in patients with defective mechanical heart valves. Patients receiving marrow allografts or autografts for a variety of indications had a mean of 0.7 percent schistocytes 6 weeks after transplantation, with a range of 0 to approximately 4 percent schistocytes.[72,73] Approximately 10 percent of patients had at least 1.3 percent schistocytes, placing them at risk for a diagnosis of thrombotic microangiopathy.[73]

Congenital Thrombotic Thrombocytopenic Purpura

Congenital TTP is caused by homozygosity or compound heterozygosity for inactivating mutations in the *ADAMTS13* gene[25] on chromosome 9q34 (reviewed in reference 74). The mutations usually impair the synthesis or secretion of ADAMTS13. Approximately 10 percent of Japanese and Koreans are heterozygous for *ADAMTS13* with the mutation R475S in the cysteine-rich domain. This variant has reduced activity in laboratory assays performed in the presence of urea, but normal activity with other assay designs. ADAMTS13 R475S appears to function satisfactorily *in vivo*, as no association between this mutation and congenital TTP has been observed.[75] As yet no convincing evidence indicates locus heterogeneity in congenital TTP.

The clinical findings in congenital TTP are similar to the findings in TTP, except for age of onset. Most children with congenital ADAMTS13

TABLE 133–1. Classification and Differential Diagnosis of Thrombotic Microangiopathy

Congenital TTP (Upshaw-Schulman Syndrome)
Inherited ADAMTS13 deficiency
TTP
With acquired ADAMTS13 deficiency
Without acquired ADAMTS13 deficiency
Secondary thrombotic microangiopathy
Infections and disseminated intravascular coagulation
Tissue transplant associated
Chemotherapy or radiation injury
Tissue rejection
Graft-versus-host disease
Cancer
Trousseau syndrome
Metastatic carcinoma
Erythroleukemia
Pregnancy associated (preeclampsia, eclampsia, HELLP syndrome)
Autoimmune disorders
Evans syndrome
Systemic lupus erythematosus and other vasculitides
Antiphospholipid syndrome
Drugs (commonly implicated)
Autoimmune with anti–ADAMTS13 antibodies:
Ticlopidine
Clopidogrel (mechanism may be variable)
Autoimmune without anti–ADAMTS13 antibodies
Quinine
Dose-related toxicity
Mitomycin C
Gemcitabine
Cyclosporine
Tacrolimus
Malignant hypertension
Hemolytic uremic syndrome
Diarrhea positive (Infectious, Shiga toxin associated)
Sporadic
Epidemic
Diarrhea negative
Inherited complement regulatory protein deficiencies (factor H, MCP, factor I, factor B, C3, C4BP)

HELLP, hemolysis, elevated liver enzymes, and low platelet count.

deficiency have neonatal jaundice and hemolysis but no evidence of ABO blood group or Rh incompatibility. Approximately half of the children continue to have a chronic relapsing course from infancy. The remaining children usually develop symptoms in their late teens or early twenties. Females may present during their first pregnancy, possibly because VWF levels are increased late in pregnancy. In either case, acute exacerbations often are triggered by infections, otitis media, surgery, or other inflammatory stress.[48,76] Patients may suffer an acute attack after receiving desmopressin (DDAVP), which stimulates the release of VWF from endothelial cell stores; one such patient was receiving a low dose of intranasal desmopressin for enuresis.[77,78] As in acquired TTP, most patients with congenital TTP have some renal involvement with proteinuria, hematuria, or a mildly elevated serum creatinine during acute attacks. Chronic renal failure can occur, usually after a prolonged course of relapsing disease.[76]

Congenital TTP can be treated with periodic infusions of fresh frozen plasma or an equivalent virucidally treated product, if available. The half-life of ADAMTS13 is 2 to 3 days[79] and the level of ADAMTS13 required to avoid symptoms is approximately 5 percent of normal; 5 to 10 mL/kg of plasma every 2 to 3 weeks usually is sufficient to prevent symptoms.[48,76] The frequency of relapses varies considerably among patients, and continuous prophylaxis with plasma may not be necessary in all cases.

Secondary Thrombotic Microangiopathy

Infections and Disseminated Intravascular Coagulation Conditions resulting in disseminated intravascular coagulation sometimes cause microangiopathic changes and thrombocytopenia with little change in blood coagulation tests, which can suggest a diagnosis of TTP. Infections may trigger disease in patients with severe ADAMTS13 deficiency, but more commonly, infections cause secondary thrombotic microangiopathy by other mechanisms (Table 133–2). Secondary thrombotic microangiopathy caused by infections may respond to antimicrobial or antiviral therapy, but generally not to plasma exchange.

Pneumococcal-Related Thrombotic Microangiopathy Thrombotic microangiopathy, often with acute renal failure, is a rare complication of invasive infections with *Streptococcus pneumoniae* in children. A surveillance study in Atlanta, Georgia, identified HUS in 0.6 percent of pneumococcal infections in children younger than 2 years of age.[80] Patients usually have pneumococcal pneumonia or meningitis, with normal plasma fibrinogen and normal or minimally prolonged PT and aPTT. The pathophysiology is thought to involve bacterial neuraminidase, made by *S. pneumoniae* and some other organisms, which removes sialic acid residues from cell surface glycoproteins and exposes Thomsen-Friedenreich antigen (T antigen) that normally is cryptic. T antigen is recognized by naturally occurring antibodies that fix complement, causing hemolysis and damaging the renal microvasculature. Because donor blood usually contains high levels of antibodies against T antigen, red cells and platelets should be washed before transfusion, and plasma should not be used as a replacement fluid. Exchange transfusion has been proposed to stop hemolysis by replacing T-antigen–bearing red blood cells and removing circulating neuraminidase, but the efficacy of this treatment is uncertain.[81]

Tissue Transplants Recipients of solid-organ transplantations can develop thrombotic microangiopathy, often dominated by renal involvement associated with immunosuppression by cyclosporine or tacrolimus.[82] These drugs appear to damage renal endothelial cells directly and can cause neurotoxicity, adding another feature suggestive of TTP.[83] Similarly, hematopoietic stem cell transplantation recipients may develop thrombotic microangiopathy associated with high-dose chemotherapy or radiation, immunosuppressive drugs, graft-versus-host disease, or infections. ADAMTS13 levels are normal,[37,38] and plasma therapy is generally ineffective.[84,85]

Cancer Thrombotic microangiopathy occurs in a small fraction of patients with almost any cancer but most commonly with adenocarcinoma of the pancreas, lung, prostate, stomach, colon, ovary, breast, or unknown primary site (see Chap. 130).[86] In most cases, the cancer is

TABLE 133–2. Some Infectious Agents Associated with Secondary Thrombotic Microangiopathy

	Reference
Bacteria:	
Actinomyces turicensis	270
Campylobacter jejuni	271–273
Enterobacter	274
Escherichia coli (without Shiga toxin)	275
Escherichia coli (with Shiga toxin)	119–121
Group A Streptococci	274
Legionella pneumophila	276, 277
Pseudomonas aeruginosa	274
Salmonella typhi	278
Staphylococcus aureus	274
Shigella dysenteriae	118
Streptococcus pneumoniae	80, 274, 279
Yersinia pseudotuberculosis	280
Ehrlichiosis	281, 282
Brucellosis	283
Fungi:	
Aspergillus fumigatus	274, 284
Blastomyces spp.	274
Candida albicans	274
Candida glabrata	285
Candida krusei	285
Viruses:	
Coxsackie B	286–288
Cytomegalovirus	274
Echovirus	289
Epstein-Barr	290
HIV (usually with a bacterial infectious complication)	60, 274
Herpes simplex (HSV)	292
HSV-6	293
Human T-cell lymphotropic virus (HTLV)-1	294
Influenza	295, 296
Parvovirus B19	297
Dengue	298
Rickettsia:	
Rickettsia rickettsii	274, 299
Mycoplasma:	
Mycoplasma pneumoniae	300, 301

widely metastatic. These cancers also are associated with Trousseau syndrome or paraneoplastic hypercoagulability and thrombosis. Manifestations include arterial thromboembolism, nonbacterial thrombotic endocarditis, venous thrombosis, and hemorrhage.[86] Most patients have variable prolongation of the PT and aPTT and increased fibrin degradation products. These signs of disseminated intravascular coagulation often are intermittent, however,[86] which can suggest a diagnosis of TTP. Clinical studies indicate that the thrombosis of Trousseau syndrome may respond to anticoagulation with heparin but not warfarin,[86] potentially explained by the capacity of heparin (but not warfarin) to inhibit mucin-based platelet-leukocyte interactions. Abundant schistocytes also have been described in acute erythroleukemia.[87] Severe ADAMTS13 deficiency almost never occurs in cancer-associated thrombotic microangiopathy, and plasma exchange is usually ineffective.[43,44,88]

Pregnancy-Associated Thrombotic Microangiopathy The differential diagnosis of thrombotic microangiopathy in pregnancy includes preeclampsia, eclampsia, HELLP (hemolysis, elevated liver enzymes, and low platelet count) syndrome, acute fatty liver of pregnancy, abruptio placenta, amniotic fluid embolism, and retained products of conception (see Chap. 130). In addition, pregnancy can trigger disease in patients with congenital or acquired ADAMTS13 deficiency; in most case series of TTP, between 12 and 31 percent of patients are pregnant women, usually in the third trimester or immediately postpartum.[47] Distinguishing among these various conditions may only be possible by following the course of disease after delivery.

Severe ADAMTS13 deficiency has not been observed in HELLP syndrome and ADAMTS13 assays may help to differentiate it from TTP.[89] Women with congenital ADAMTS13 deficiency or TTP have been carried through pregnancy successfully with plasma therapy.[18,48,90]

Autoimmune Disorders Autoimmune thrombocytopenia may be confused with TTP if other causes of microangiopathic hemolytic anemia are present. Asymptomatic thrombocytopenia also may sometimes be the only finding in TTP, as demonstrated by a previous or subsequent episode of disease. Patients have been described in whom TTP and autoimmune thrombocytopenia appeared to occur simultaneously or sequentially.[91] Evans syndrome (autoimmune hemolytic anemia with autoimmune thrombocytopenia) usually can be distinguished from TTP by a positive Coombs test and the prominence of spherocytes relative to schistocytes in the blood film. Heparin-induced thrombocytopenia (HIT) may sometimes resemble TTP, with thrombocytopenia and disseminated arterial and venous thrombosis (see "Heparin-Induced Thrombocytopenia" below).

Systemic lupus erythematosus (SLE) can cause autoimmune hemolysis and thrombocytopenia, and lupus vasculitis can cause microangiopathic changes, renal insufficiency, and neurologic defects consistent with TTP. Vasculitis associated with other autoimmune disorders can pose a similar diagnostic problem. Although ADAMTS13 deficiency is uncommon among patients with SLE,[92] in rare cases they develop autoimmune ADAMTS13 deficiency and TTP that responds to plasma exchange.[93] Conversely, patients with TTP and autoantibodies against ADAMTS13 may have other markers of autoimmune disease, including antinuclear or anti-DNA antibodies, polyarthritis, discoid lupus, or ulcerative colitis.[94,95] High-titer antinuclear and anti-DNA antibodies, a positive Coombs test, decreased serum complement, and histologic or clinical evidence of active vasculitis suggest a diagnosis of thrombotic microangiopathy secondary to SLE, whereas the absence of these signs plus severe ADAMTS13 deficiency favors a diagnosis of TTP.

Thrombotic microangiopathy can develop in patients with antiphospholipid syndrome (APS), with or without concurrent SLE (see Chap. 132). Among 46 reported cases, the clinical features resembled HUS, catastrophic APS, malignant hypertension, TTP, or HELLP syndrome. One-third of patients presented during pregnancy or in the postpartum period.[96] Mortality was 22 percent; recovery occurred in 34 percent of patients treated with glucocorticoids and 73 percent of patients treated with plasma exchange.[96]

Thrombotic microangiopathy occurs in patients with progressive systemic sclerosis, particularly in association with acute scleroderma renal crisis and malignant hypertension. Treatment with angiotensin-converting enzyme inhibitors is effective; the value of plasma exchange therapy is uncertain.[97]

Drug-Induced Thrombotic Microangiopathy Among the drugs that have been associated with thrombotic microangiopathy (Table 133–3), the antiplatelet drugs ticlopidine and clopidogrel are unusual because they appear to induce autoantibody inhibitors of ADAMTS13, effectively causing TTP. Thrombotic microangiopathy occurs in 200 to 625 per 1 million users of ticlopidine, usually between 2 and 12 weeks after starting therapy.[98] ADAMTS13 levels are undetectable and IgG inhibitors of ADAMTS13 are present in 80 percent of cases.[99] Plasma exchange appears to be effective. The disease usually resolves within 2 weeks of discontinuing the drug and relapses have not been reported. The incidence of TTP with clopidogrel is lower and is estimated to be 10 per 1 million users. TTP usually develops within the first 2 weeks of clopidogrel treatment, is associated with anti-ADAMTS13 antibodies in only 20 percent of cases, and is less responsive to plasma exchange therapy compared to ticlopidine-associated TTP.[99]

Other drugs associated with thrombotic microangiopathy do not cause severe ADAMTS13 deficiency. Comprehensive lists, including single case reports, can be found in Table 133–3 and in several reviews.[100–102] Drugs commonly implicated include selected antineoplastic agents, cyclosporine A, tacrolimus, and quinine.

TABLE 133–3. Drugs and Toxins Associated with Secondary Thrombotic Microangiopathy

	Reference		Reference
Immune-mediated:		Penicillin	332
Quinine	274	Ampicillin	332
Ticlopidine	98, 302	Oxophenarsine	333
Clopidogrel	303, 304	Valacyclovir	334, 335
Antineoplastic agents:		Famciclovir	336
All-*trans* retinoic acid	305	Mefloquine	337
Bleomycin plus cisplatinum	306, 307	Hormones:	
Carmustine	274	Estrogen/progestogen oral contraceptives	338
Chlorozotocin	308	Mestranol, norethindrone	339
Cytosine arabinoside	309	17β-Estradiol transdermal patch	340
Daunorubicin	309	Conjugated estrogens	341
Deoxycoformycin	310	Illicit drugs:	
Estramustine	311	Cocaine	342–344
Gemcitabine	105, 312	Heroin	345
Lomustine (CCNU)	313	Ecstasy	346
Mitomycin C	103, 104	Lipid-lowering agents:	
Tamoxifen (when combined with mitomycin C)	314	Atorvastatin	102
Antiangiogenic agents:		Simvastatin	347
Bevacizumab	315	H_2-receptor antagonists:	
Sunitinib	316	Cimetidine	348
Immunosuppressive and antiinflammatory agents:		Famotidine	348
Cyclosporine	107, 111	Vaccinations:	
Tacrolimus	109, 112	Polio vaccination	349
Penicillamine	317, 318	Measles/mumps/rubella vaccination	350
Muromonab-CD3 (OKT3)	319	Bacillus Calmette-Guerin (intravesicular)	351
Interferon-α	320, 321	Influenza vaccination	352
Interferon-β	322	Miscellaneous:	
Ibuprofen	323	Bee sting	353, 354
Antibiotics:		Bupropion	355
Ciprofloxacin	324	Chlorpropamide	6
Clarithromycin	325	Procainamide	6
Cephalosporin	326	Iodine	6
Piperacillin	327	Carbon monoxide	356
Rifampicin	328	Chloronaphthalene (in varnish)	357
Metronidazole	329, 330	Aminocaproic acid	358
Pentostatin	274	*Echinacea* extract	359
Sulfonamides	331	Quetiapine	360

Mitomycin C is an alkylating agent that is used in a variety of chemotherapy regimens for anal carcinoma and for many adenocarcinomas. It appears to cause dose-dependent nephrotoxicity, with renal failure occurring in approximately 16 percent of patients who receive a cumulative dose of at least 50 mg.[103] About half of the patients with renal toxicity also develop thrombotic microangiopathy, usually 4 to 8 weeks after the latest dose. Mitomycin C-induced thrombotic microangiopathy does not respond to plasma exchange and has a high mortality rate of approximately 70 percent within 4 months of onset.[104]

Gemcitabine is a nucleoside analogue often used for carcinoma of the pancreas, bladder, or lung. Thrombotic microangiopathy with renal failure occurs with an incidence of approximately 0.3 percent.[105] The median time to develop thrombotic microangiopathy is 7 months with a median cumulative dose of 22 g/m^2, although the range of doses is broad and very low doses have been associated with thrombotic microangiopathy.[106] Death or disability usually results from cancer progression or renal failure, not from extrarenal manifestations of thrombotic microangiopathy.

Cyclosporine and tacrolimus are structurally distinct immunosuppressive drugs that indirectly inhibit calcineurin and suppress T-cell activation. Both agents cause dose-dependent nephrotoxicity, neurotoxicity, and thrombotic microangiopathy.[107–109] The renal damage is thought to involve toxic effects on endothelium.[107] Thrombotic microangiopathy can develop during the first few weeks of treatment, and its etiology may be difficult to determine because graft rejection, graft-versus-host disease, or systemic infections can cause similar microangiopathic changes.[107,110] The thrombotic microangiopathy often remits with dose reduction or substitution of other immunosuppressive drugs and may not recur if therapy with cyclosporine or tacrolimus is reinstituted. Plasma exchange has been used as additional therapy but has not been shown to modify the course of disease.[110–112]

Quinine accounts for up to 11 percent of all cases of thrombotic microangiopathy in some series. It has a high risk of chronic renal failure and a high mortality.[100] Most patients are women. Severe thrombotic microangiopathy occurs suddenly within several hours after drug ingestion, with fever, abdominal pain, nausea, vomiting, diarrhea, and oliguric renal failure. Many patients have low fibrinogen, abnormal coagulation test results, abnormal liver function, and leukopenia. Neurologic changes are common and include altered mental status, coma, and seizures.[113–115] ADAMTS13 levels are normal.[102] In a recent series of 17 patients, 14 required dialysis, 8 developed chronic renal failure, and 4 died. Three of the deaths occurred during the initial illness and one occurred during chronic hemodialysis 5 years after a second episode.[114] The mechanism appears to involve a broad range of quinine-dependent antibodies against platelets, endothelium, and other cells.[100] Removal of the antibodies by plasma exchange may be beneficial,[113,114] although recovery without plasma exchange also is common.[115]

Malignant Hypertension Malignant hypertension is associated with microangiopathic hemolytic anemia, thrombocytopenia, neurologic symptoms, and renal insufficiency, and therefore may resemble TTP.[116]

Diarrhea-Associated Hemolytic Uremic Syndrome

The clinical features of TTP and HUS can overlap. D$^+$HUS can occur at any age but affects mainly children younger than 10 years. The disease occurs sporadically and in epidemics, associated with ingestion of foods or other materials contaminated with Shiga toxin-producing bacteria. *Escherichia coli* O157:H7 accounts for at least 80 percent of cases in many series, but D$^+$HUS can be caused by other toxin-bearing *E. coli* serotypes[117] or by *Shigella dysenteriae* type 1.[118] Within 3 days of ingesting the bacteria, patients develop painful diarrhea, without fever, that usually evolves to bloody diarrhea within a few days. From 1 to 20 percent of patients are thought to develop D$^+$HUS during the subsequent 2 weeks, with the acute onset of microangiopathic hemolytic anemia, thrombocytopenia, and renal injury.[119–121] Renal signs may include proteinuria, hematuria, hypertension, and oliguria or anuria. Usually the PT and aPTT are normal or minimally prolonged, plasma fibrinogen is normal or elevated, and fibrin degradation products may be moderately elevated.[122] ADAMTS13 levels are normal in D$^+$HUS.[123,124]

Among 3476 patients with D$^+$HUS, 9 percent died and 3 percent developed end-stage renal failure; these values vary considerably among studies.[125] Central nervous system involvement (seizures, coma, or stroke) occurs in 20 to 40 percent of patients and correlates with a higher risk of death or end-stage renal failure.[117,125] Recurrences after kidney transplantation for D$^+$HUS are very uncommon.

In a study of 268 patients with HUS, 59 percent had prodromal diarrhea plus bacteriologic or serologic evidence of infection by Shiga toxin-producing *E. coli*, 21 percent had only diarrhea, and 10 percent had only positive bacteriologic or serologic studies. All three groups had a similar prognosis: approximately 1 percent died and 73 percent recovered normal renal function. These results emphasize the variability in symptoms and signs among patients with HUS caused by Shiga toxin. In contrast, the 11 percent of patients with neither diarrhea nor documented *E. coli* infection had a significantly worse outcome; 10 percent died and only 34 percent recovered normal renal function.[117]

Several treatments for D$^+$HUS have been evaluated in randomized trials including plasma transfusion, heparin, and glucocorticoids; no intervention has been shown superior to supportive therapy and dialysis, for children or adults.[126] Early intravenous volume expansion seems to reduce the risk of developing HUS.[127] Antibacterial therapy should not be used; several studies suggest antibiotics have no effect or increase the risk of HUS.[128]

Diarrhea-Negative Hemolytic Uremic Syndrome and Inherited Complement Regulatory Defects

Atypical HUS or D$^-$HUS is much less common than D$^+$HUS. At least half of cases appear to be caused by inherited defects in complement regulatory proteins and activating components.[129] These include loss-of-function mutations in factor H, membrane cofactor protein (MCP, CD46), factor I, factor H-related proteins 1 and 3 (CFHR1, CFHR3), and C4 binding protein (C4BP), and gain-of-function mutations in factors B and C3.[130–133] In addition, autoantibodies to factor H have been identified in some patients with atypical HUS, often in association with mutations in CFHR1 and CFHR3.[134] Factor H is a plasma cofactor that promotes the inactivation of complement C3b by the plasma serine protease factor I, and also accelerates the dissociation of factor Bb from the alternative complement convertase C3bBb complex. Factor H and MCP are structurally and functionally similar, but MCP is a transmembrane protein found on the surface of almost all cells. Mutations in these genes impair the regulation of the alternative complement pathway, causing increased endothelial deposition of C3b that attracts phagocytes, promotes membrane attack complex formation, and induces microvascular thrombosis. Some patients have mutations in both factor H alleles or both MCP alleles, but most are heterozygous suggesting that partial deficiency can predispose to disease. The clinical presentation may be sporadic, recessive, or dominant. Many patients develop HUS in childhood, but some have their first episode in adulthood or remain asymptomatic. Occasional patients have long intervals between exacerbations, which may appear to be precipitated by infections, other illness, or pregnancy.

The clinical course correlates with the locus that is mutated. HUS associated with defects in factor H or factor I has responded at least transiently to intensive plasma therapy (20–40 mL/kg once or twice a week by infusion or plasma exchange).[129,135] The disease often recurs in patients with transplanted kidneys, probably because kidney transplantation does not alter the underlying complement defect. Plasma complement proteins are synthesized in the liver, and combined liver–kidney transplantation can be curative.[135,136] In contrast, MCP is membrane-associated and plasma therapy appears to be ineffective; however, disease has not recurred after kidney transplantation, presumably because MCP in the transplanted kidney protects it from complement attack.[135,136]

Two case reports suggest that eculizumab, a monoclonal antibody that blocks the activity of terminal complement component C5, may be useful for treating atypical HUS.[137,138]

THERAPY

Plasma Exchange

The mainstay of therapy for TTP is plasma exchange (Table 133–4), which removes antibody inhibitors of ADAMTS13 and replenishes the enzyme. With the exception of factor H deficiency,[129,135] and possibly APS syndrome[96] and quinine-induced disease,[113,114] no compelling evidence indicates that plasma therapy is effective for thrombotic microangiopathy caused by a mechanism other than ADAMTS13 deficiency. Regardless of mechanism, however, the clinical features are variable and overlapping. Consequently, plasma exchange may sometimes be used to treat apparent HUS or secondary thrombotic microangiopathy, particularly in adults, based on the possibility that such patients may have an atypical presentation of TTP that will respond.

After diagnosing TTP, or determining that the diagnosis is sufficiently likely to justify treatment, plasma exchange therapy should be started immediately. Studies establishing the value of plasma therapy have excluded most forms of secondary thrombotic microangiopathy,[13,14] so the efficacy of plasma exchange has been demonstrated directly only for TTP. The optimal dose of plasma is not known, but a common practice is to perform plasma exchange once daily at a volume of 40 or 60 mL/kg, equivalent to 1 or 1.5 plasma volumes. For refractory disease, the intensity of plasma exchange can be increased to 1 plasma volume twice daily.[139,140] Prompt treatment is essential and if plasma exchange must be delayed more than a few hours, plasma should be given by simple infusion at 20 to 40 mL/kg total dose per day, consistent with the patient's ability to tolerate the fluid load.

The replacement fluid should contain ADAMTS13. Satisfactory results have been obtained with fresh-frozen plasma,[13,14] plasma cryosupernatant,[126,141,142] and various pathogen-inactivated plasma products.[143] The incidence of allergic reactions and transfusion-associated lung injury may be lower with solvent/detergent-treated plasma than with fresh-frozen plasma,[144] but the incidence of thrombosis may be increased with some preparations.[143,145] Cryosupernatant is depleted in the largest VWF multimers but has normal ADAMTS13 levels,[146] which could make cryosupernatant particularly suitable for the treatment of TTP. Nevertheless, small randomized trials suggest that cryosupernatant is not superior to fresh-frozen plasma for the initial treatment of TTP.[141,142] Methylene blue-treated plasma may be less effective than fresh-frozen plasma,[143,147] despite having a similar concentration of ADAMTS13.[143]

Serious catheter-related complications of plasma exchange therapy occur in approximately 26 percent of patients with TTP and include pneumothorax and hemorrhage, cardiac perforation, venous thrombosis, catheter thrombosis, and bacterial or fungal infections.[148,149] Regardless of the platelet count, catheter insertion generally can be performed safely without platelet transfusion.[148,150] Hives or pruritic reactions to fresh-frozen plasma occur in one- to two-thirds of patients but usually can be managed by premedication with antihistamines. High-volume plasma exchange causes metabolic alkalosis and hypocalcemia, and may cause unintentional platelet removal.[151,152] Serious complications attributable to plasma are much less common, occurring in approximately 4 percent of patients, and include bronchospasm, anaphylaxis, hypotension, hypoxia, and serum sickness.[148,149,153]

Plasma exchange should be continued daily until the patient has a complete response, as shown by a platelet count greater than 150,000/μL, LDH within the normal range, and resolution of nonfocal neurologic symptoms.[139,154] The optimal schedule for tapering and discontinuing therapy has not been determined. A typical strategy is to continue plasma exchange until the patient sustained a complete response for a minimum of 2 days, and then reduce the frequency of plasma exchange to every other day (or twice per week) for several days. If the disease remains quiescent, then treatment can be stopped and the patient monitored closely for recurrence.

TABLE 133–4. An Approach to the Treatment and Monitoring of TTP

Treatment:
Glucocorticoids (e.g., prednisone 2 mg/kg per day or equivalent)
Plasma exchange 1.5 volumes per day
Plasma infusion 15–30 mL/kg if plasma exchange will be delayed >12 hours
After the platelet count exceeds 50,000/μL, add aspirin 80 mg/day and routine thromboprophylaxis (e.g., low-molecular-weight heparin)
Continue until complete response for 3 days (platelets >150,000/μL, LDH normal), then decrease plasma exchange to every other day for two more treatments and stop
If response is durable, taper glucocorticoids
Monitoring:
Neurologic status
Hemoglobin and platelet count
Blood film for schistocytes
LDH
Serum electrolytes, calcium, blood urea nitrogen (BUN), creatinine
Electrocardiogram, cardiac enzymes
Common complications:
Cardiac arrhythmias, infarction
Catheter-associated bleeding or thrombosis
Citrate toxicity (hypocalcemia, alkalosis)
Minor allergic reactions to plasma

Glucocorticoids

TTP often is an autoimmune disease and the use of glucocorticoids is logical, although a beneficial effect has not been demonstrated conclusively. Similar results have been reported with[13] and without[14] glucocorticoids. Common practice is to give prednisone or equivalent at a total daily dose of 1 or 2 mg/kg, in one or two doses, for the duration of plasma exchange, followed by tapering. An alternative regimen is methylprednisolone 1 g intravenously daily for 3 days.[154]

Antiplatelet Agents

The use of antiplatelet agents in TTP is controversial. Aspirin and dipyridamole often are combined with plasma exchange but have not been shown conclusively to modify the course of TTP.[14,155] Low-dose aspirin (e.g., 80 mg/day) has been suggested for thromboprophylaxis, once the platelet count exceeds 50,000/μL.[154]

Platelet Transfusion

Transfusion of platelets may sometimes correlate with the acute deterioration and death in TTP, although direct harm is difficult to establish.[13,46,156,157] Consequently, platelet transfusions are relatively contraindicated and should be reserved for the treatment of life-threatening hemorrhage, preferably after plasma exchange treatment has been initiated. Platelets generally need not be given prophylactically before establishing venous access.[148,150] Platelets have been transfused before emergency surgery, immediately after preparation by intensive plasma exchange.[156]

Immunosuppressive Therapy

TTP that is refractory to plasma exchange may respond to immunosuppression. Anecdotal experience suggests that vincristine may be beneficial, although its efficacy is difficult to assess. Dosing schedules have included 2 mg intravenously on day 1 followed by 1 mg on days 4 and 7,[158] or 2 mg intravenously per week for 2 to 14 weeks.[159] However, several newer therapies have emerged with far greater efficacy than vincristine.

Although it can cause secondary thrombotic microangiopathy, cyclosporine has been used to treat TTP and may be effective in refractory disease. Apparent responses, with normalization of ADAMTS13 activity, have been observed with cyclosporine 2 to 3 mg/kg daily in two divided doses as an adjunct to plasma exchange,[160] or without plasma exchange for early recurrences of TTP.[161] Prophylactic cyclosporine therapy continued for 6 months after achieving a response may be associated with a decreased rate of relapse.[162] These results are based on relatively few patients and have not been confirmed in direct comparisons to other treatments.

Rituximab is a monoclonal antibody against CD20, which is expressed on B lymphocytes, and may be preferable to alkylating agents for treating women of childbearing age. Case reports and small case series describe approximately 125 patients with refractory TTP treated with rituximab 375 mg/m^2 weekly for two to eight doses. In most cases, patients had been treated previously for extended periods with plasma exchange, usually with glucocorticoids, and often with multiple other agents.[55,163–166] Approximately 95 percent of patients had complete responses within 1 to 3 weeks of starting treatment, including a normal ADAMTS13 level and disappearance of anti-ADAMTS13 antibodies (if present). Acute reactions to rituximab were controlled by premedication with glucocorticoids, antihistamines, and analgesics. In some settings, rare but serious complications associated with rituximab have included bronchospasm, hypotension, serum sickness, susceptibility to multiple infections, and progressive multifocal leukoencephalopathy.[167,168] Such events have been uncommon for patients with TTP. One patient had transient cardiogenic shock, and another had symptomatic gastrointestinal infection with Strongyloides (reviewed in reference 165).

Relapses have occurred in approximately 10 percent of patients after treatment with rituximab, after intervals of 6 months to 4 years. All but one of these patients had a further prolonged remission after retreatment with rituximab. Some patients have had as many as three relapses at intervals of 1 to 2 years, each responding to retreatment. Rituximab can be removed by plasma exchange, although the efficiency of removal is unknown. Consequently, rituximab should be administered shortly after a session of plasma exchange, and the next plasma exchange should be delayed 1 to several days if the patient's condition will allow.

Other immunosuppressive regimens have included oral or intravenous cyclophosphamide, oral azathioprine (reviewed in reference 169), combination chemotherapy with cyclophosphamide, doxorubicin, vincristine, and prednisone (CHOP),[170] and autologous stem cell transplantation.[171]

Splenectomy

Many reports suggest that splenectomy can result in lasting remissions or reduce the frequency of relapses for some patients with TTP who are refractory to plasma exchange or immunosuppressive therapy, presumably by removing a major site of anti-ADAMTS13 antibody production.[172,173] Laparoscopic splenectomy can be performed safely in most patients regardless of platelet count.[174]

Other Treatments

Extracorporeal protein A immunoadsorption can remove anti-ADAMTS13 IgG, which could increase the intravascular survival of endogenous or transfused ADAMTS13; in practice, the results have been disappointing. The single-use devices available in the United States can remove 550 mg of IgG per treatment, compared to a normal plasma IgG concentration of 8 to 15 g/L. The few reported responses may reflect a coincidental decline of disease activity or the proposed but undocumented changes in antiidiotype antibodies.[175] Higher capacity immunoadsorption methods might be more effective. Prostacyclin analogs[176,177] or high-dose intravenous immunoglobulins[178,179] have been used, without convincing evidence of efficacy.

Supportive Therapy

Daily laboratory monitoring should include complete blood count with platelet count, LDH, electrolytes, blood urea nitrogen, and creatinine. Because of the high incidence of cardiac damage,[46] continuous electrocardiographic monitoring and periodic assessment of cardiac enzymes should be considered. Patients should receive supplemental folic acid and vaccination for hepatitis B.[154] Minor allergic reactions, metabolic alkalosis, and hypocalcemia associated with plasma exchange should be prevented by appropriate adjustments in therapy.

After the platelet count increases to above 50,000/μL, prophylaxis for venous thromboembolism may be instituted with compression stockings, low-molecular-weight heparin,[145] and low-dose aspirin.[154]

COURSE AND PROGNOSIS

The long-term mortality of TTP treated with plasma exchange ranges from 10 to 20 percent. Most deaths occur within a few days after presentation, and almost all occur within the first month.[13,14,44,180–182] The duration of illness is quite variable. Complete response occurs after an average of 9 to 16 days of plasma exchange, and almost all responders are encompassed by a range of 2 to 40 days.[13,14,44,180–182] Renal function abnormalities usually resolve over a similar time course.[60] Within the 2 weeks following a complete response, 25 to 50 percent of patients have an acute exacerbation that requires further treatment with plasma exchange, and some have repeated exacerbations over several months.[180,181]

Relapses, defined as recurrences of disease more than 30 days after a complete response, occur in up to one-third of patients. Most relapses occur during the first year, but have been documented up to 13 years after diagnosis.[44,180–183] Evaluation for relapsing TTP should be considered for any symptom compatible with thrombotic microangiopathy, especially in association with a common trigger of relapse such as infection, surgery, or pregnancy.[55,56] Relapsing patients typically respond to plasma exchange. Relapses in TTP are associated with severe ADAMTS13 deficiency and detectable ADAMTS13 autoantibody inhibitors. Conversely, patients without severe ADAMTS13 deficiency at diagnosis rarely relapse (approximately 9% across several studies; reviewed in reference 165).

Late sequelae of TTP may include long-term deficits in quality of life and cognition in many patients,[184,185] severe persistent neurologic deficits in 5 to 13 percent,[183,186] chronic renal insufficiency in up to 25 percent,[139,186] and dialysis dependent renal failure in 6 to 8 percent of patients.[95,186]

HEPARIN-INDUCED THROMBOCYTOPENIA

DEFINITION AND HISTORY

HIT is a complication of heparin therapy in which the platelet count falls by more than 50 percent or falls to below 150,000/μL in association with heparin therapy. A substantial incidence of arterial and/or venous thromboembolic complications is noted in this disorder.

Although heparin clinical usage as an anticoagulant began in the late 1950s, it was not until the early 1970s that a small percentage of treated patients were noted to develop a complication consisting of thrombocytopenia with paradoxical, life-threatening thromboemboli (for a historical review see reference 187). In the 1980s, it became clear that HIT was a result of IgG antibodies that activated platelets. It was also recognized that HIT could be divided into two types: classic type I disease, which is the focus of this chapter, and type II, which is a benign condition associated with a mild, immediate, and transient drop in platelet count with no immune basis and no increased risk of thrombosis.[188] In the late 1980s and early 1990s, it became clear that HIT antibodies activated both platelets and endothelial cells.[189,190] Further analysis showed that platelet activation involved an immune complex as blocking platelet FcγRIIA inhibited platelet activation by HIT sera *in vitro*.[191] The antigenic immune complex involved heparin bound to the platelet-specific chemokine platelet factor 4 (PF4).[192] Currently, the greatest challenge of this disorder is development of strategies for its prevention and treatment.

EPIDEMIOLOGY

The frequency of HIT in a given hospitalized population depends on the nature of the heparin used, duration of heparin exposure, and clinical setting. Heparin is a negatively charged polysaccharide, enzymatically derived from either bovine or porcine intestines.[193] These products are not homogeneous for either polymer length or sequence. The frequency of HIT in nonsurgical settings is clearly higher in patients treated with unfractionated, high-molecular-weight heparin (1–5%) than in patients treated with low-molecular-weight heparin (0.2–1%).[194–198] Bovine-derived heparin may be associated with a higher incidence of HIT than porcine heparin.[194,199] Newer, synthetic pentasaccharide anticoagulants may have a much lower or no risk of inducing HIT.[200]

No route of unfractionated, high-molecular-weight heparin delivery protects against developing HIT.[196,201] The only recourse to avoid developing HIT is limiting the exposure time,[202] and avoiding heparin flushes thereafter.[203] Heparin-bonded catheters can underlie the development of HIT.[204,205]

The greatest clinical risk factors for developing HIT are the patient's age and the nature of the patient's medical condition. HIT occurs rarely or never in pediatric patients, especially neonates.[206] Patients being treated for medical conditions have a lower risk of developing HIT than do patients who are undergoing surgical procedures. Whether certain subgroups of medical patients, such as hemodialysis patients or pregnant women, have a particularly low incidence of HIT is not clear.[207,208] Among surgical patients, those undergoing coronary artery bypass grafting, orthopedic procedures, or isolated limb perfusion are particularly vulnerable to developing HIT.[197,209,210]

Determination of the incidence of thrombosis in various settings has been hampered by the infrequency of HIT, and the need to carefully document both the diagnosis and the thrombotic complications. Nevertheless, some prospective studies suggest that the incidence of thrombosis is between 35 and 58 percent in patients with documented HIT.[197,211,212] The risk of thromboembolic complications is not altered by discontinuing heparin therapy.[212] Additionally, the ratio of arterial to venous thrombi is high (0.7:1).[212]

ETIOLOGY AND PATHOGENESIS

HIT is an immune complex disorder of heparin therapy involving heparin–PF4 complexes. Such antibodies are not demonstrable in other forms of thrombocytopenia (Fig. 133–4).[213] A murine model involving mice that are transgenic for both human FcγRIIA and human PF4 supports the importance of heparin-PF4 immune complexes in the development of both thrombocytopenia and thrombosis in HIT.[214] Normally, mice lack platelet FcγRIIA. HIT antibodies do not recognize mouse PF4 complexed to heparin. In a murine HIT model, mice were infused with a HIT-like monoclonal antibody termed *KKO*,[215] and then given a course of heparin injections (Fig. 133–5A). Only mice with platelets expressing both FcγRIIA and human PF4 developed thrombocytopenia (Fig. 133–5B) and thrombosis. These studies demonstrate that four components are necessary to induce HIT in a mouse: (1) human PF4 released by platelets, (2) platelet FcγRIIA, (3) heparin infusion, and (4) the presence of an IgG antibody that recognizes PF4–heparin complexes.

The nature of the antigenic heparin–PF4 complex is partially defined. At concentrations reached at injury sites, PF4 exists as a

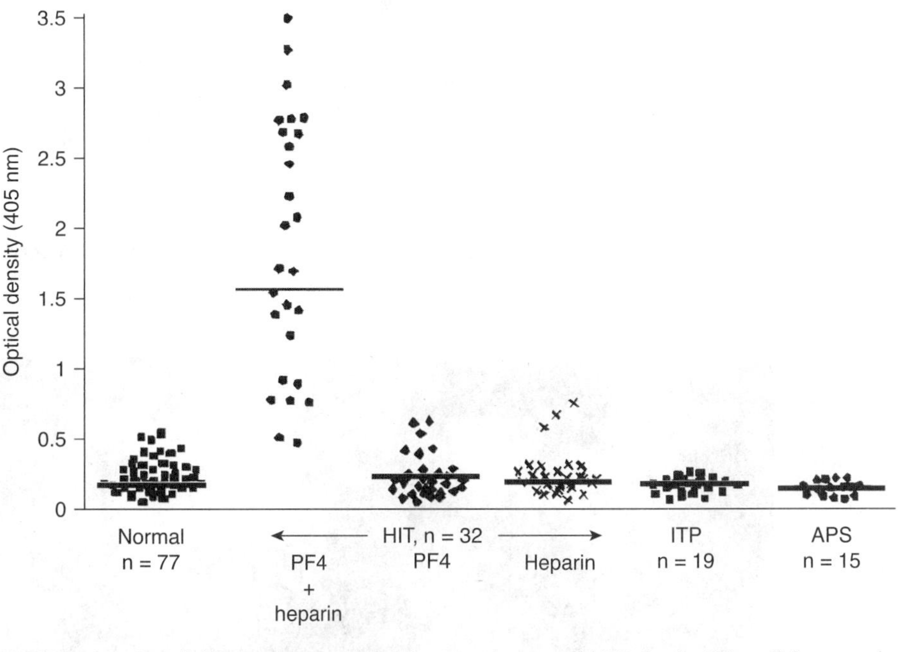

FIGURE 133–4. Heparin/PF4-based enzyme-linked immunosorbent assay (ELISA) showing HIT specificity among the thrombocytopenias. Studies were performed using sera from patients with each of the clinical conditions depicted using the indicated number of samples. All platelets were coated with equimolar amounts of PF4 and unfractionated heparin except as indicated. APS, antiphospholipid syndrome; ITP, immune thrombocytopenic purpura. *(Adapted from Arepally G, Reynolds C, Tomaski A, et al.[213] with permission.)*

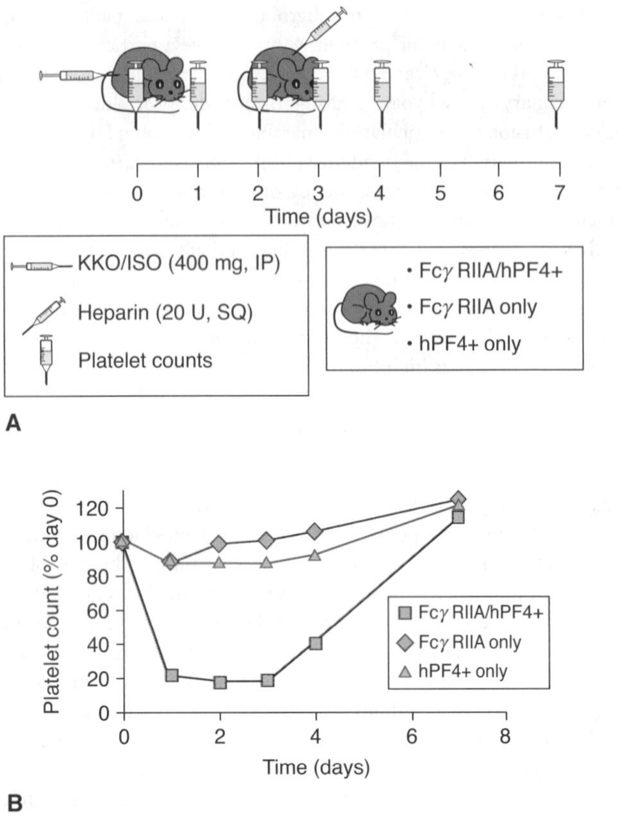

FIGURE 133–5. Murine model of HIT. **A.** Schema of the protocol for HIT mice model. The types of animals studied are shown in the *lower right-hand corner*. FcγRIIA, mice transgenic for the FcγRIIA receptor; hPF4+, mice transgenic for human PF4 expressed in megakaryocytes. On day 0, mice received the HIT-like monoclonal antibody KKO intraperitoneally (IP). On days 1–4, they were injected with heparin. On days 0, 1–4, and 7, blood was drawn. **B.** Platelet counts in each set of transgenic mice at various times in relation to heparin exposure. *(Adapted from Reilly MP, Taylor SM, Hartman NK, et al.[214] with permission.)*

tetramer.[216] Crystal structure analysis shows this tetramer is encircled by a ring of positive charge (Fig. 133–6),[216] and heparin is thought to bind to this region.[217] Two closely spaced HIT antibody recognition domains (Fig. 133–6) [218] are distinct from the heparin-binding domain. About half of patients have antibodies that react with one or the other HIT antigenic domain, and one-third of patients do not have antibodies that react to either domain, suggesting that there are other potential HIT antigenic sites on PF4.

Studies show that tetrameric PF4 and unfractionated heparin must be at an approximately 1:1 molar ratio to display optimal HIT antigenicity.[219,220] At this ratio, an ultralarge complex (>670 kDa) of PF4 and heparin form visible colloidal complexes,[221,222] and these complexes are likely to be the antigenic source in HIT.[221] At higher or lower ratios, PF4 usually forms small and less antigenic PF4-heparin complexes. Low-molecular-weight heparin inefficiently forms ultralarge complexes that may explain the lower incidence of HIT in patients treated with low-molecular-weight heparin. The pentasaccharide fondaparinux does not bind PF4 at all, suggesting that fondaparinux may be useful for the prevention and treatment of HIT.

Other studies in mice that express human PF4 and have the human FcγRIIA receptor on their platelet surface provide insights into why thrombosis is so prevalent in patients with HIT compared to patients with other immune complex disorders.[223] Infusions of the HIT-like monoclonal KKO into these mice cause thrombocytopenia, even without coadministration of heparin. A series of studies *in vitro* and *in vivo* show that the real target in HIT is PF4 complexed to surface GAGs, while the main role of circulating PF4–heparin complexes is to induce increased anti–PF4-heparin levels. At the appropriate molar ratio of PF4:GAG, antigenic complexes form on the cell surface (Fig. 133–7A). Infused heparin actually removes surface bound PF4 (Fig. 133–7B). If the molar ratio of PF4:GAG was initially low, the infused heparin immediately removes surface-bound PF4 and detectable surface antigenicity. If the molar ratio of PF4:GAG was high, removal of excess PF4 by heparin would initially increase surface antigenicity as the ratio approaches 1:1 and then at higher heparin levels, the level of surface antigenicity decreases. Most patients have little surface PF4 and after therapeutic heparinization (Fig. 133–7B), this goes down to even lower levels. The platelets would not bind anti-PF4/heparin antibodies (Fig. 133–8). However, if the patient had high levels of surface PF4 and significant complexes are present after heparinization, then these are patients at risk to have anti-PF4/heparin antibodies bind to their surface (Fig. 133–8). The bound antibodies lead to thrombocytopenia by clearance of the antibody-coated platelets by the reticuloendothelial system. Bound antibodies also lead to activated

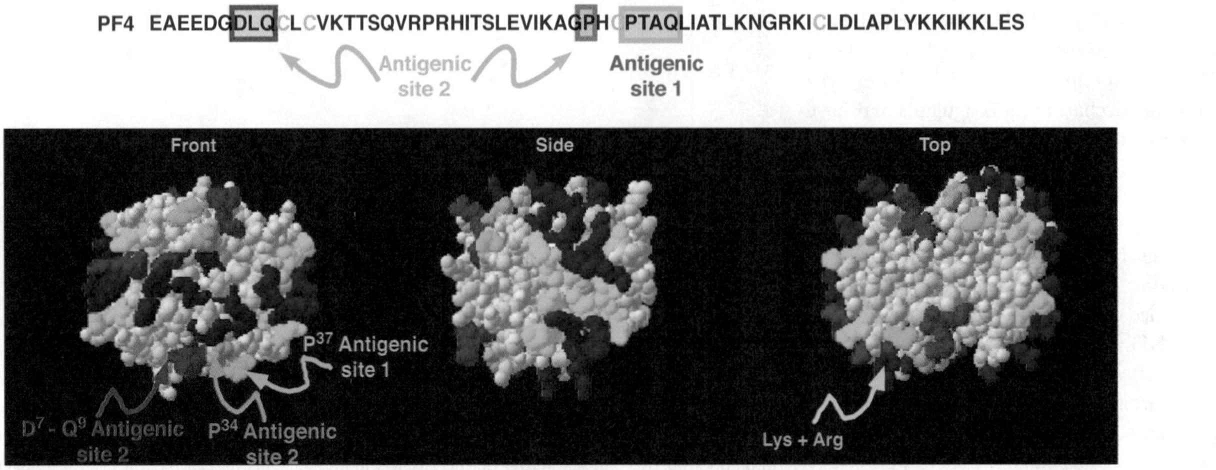

FIGURE 133–6. PF4 tetramer structure. (*Top*) Linear sequence of PF4 and the regions known to contribute to HIT antigenicity when PF4 is complexed to heparin (*boxed*). (*Bottom*) Three views of the PF4 tetramer with the positively charged residues shown in both light and dark blue, and the sites at which HIT neoepitopes are exposed on the PF4 tetramer are indicated. *(Adapted from Li ZQ, Liu W, Park KS, et al.[218] with permission.)*

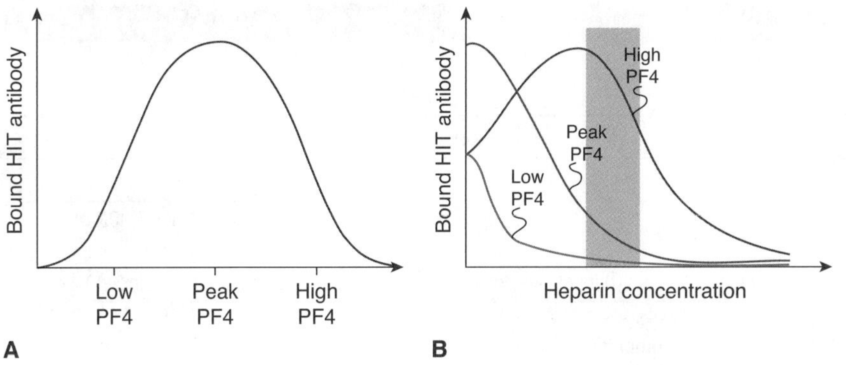

FIGURE 133–7. PF4:GAG complexes in HIT. Schematic models of surface-bound PF4 and HIT antigenicity. **A.** When external PF4 is added to platelets in the absence of added heparin, surface-bound PF4 increases linearly, but surface-bound HIT antigenicity follows a bell-shaped curve. **B.** A similar study was performed at three fixed concentrations of PF4: (1) a level below peak surface HIT antigenicity in (A), (2) at peak, and (3) above peak. In each case, heparin was then added, and surface HIT antigenicity measured. The gray bar represents the therapeutic heparin range. *(Based on data from reference Rauova L, Zhai L, Kowalska MA, et al.[221])*

platelets through the FcγRIIA and the formation of procoagulant platelet microparticles that contribute to the thrombosis.[224]

As part of this activation, HIT antibodies bind to endothelial cells likely via PF4-surface GAG complexes.[190,225] This binding may further increase vascular activation, augmenting local thrombosis. Additionally, HIT antibodies activate monocytes in a PF4-surface GAG-dependent fashion,[226,227] that requires activation through surface FcγRIIA activation[228] with subsequent increased tissue factor expression within hours.

A number of genetic polymorphisms have been examined, but none has shown a clear association with an increased risk of developing HIT or thrombosis. Thus, no association has been shown with known thrombophilic polymorphisms of factor V Leiden, prothrombin G202101A, methylenetetrahydrofolate reductase (MTHFR) C677T, or $\alpha_{IIb}\beta_3$ and $\alpha_2\beta_1$.[229] Studies addressing a functional FcγRIIA R/H131 showed that HIT, with or without thrombosis, occurred equally with either FcγRIIA polymorphism.[230,231] Whether or not patients with HIT have a higher density of FcγRIIA on their platelets is unclear.[232] Whether or not IgG affinity for the heparin-PF4 complex affects the risk of developing thrombosis also is unclear.[230,233]

The model shown in Figure 133–8 suggests that individuals with high platelet PF4 content and platelet activation because of atherosclerosis or other systemic insult associated with high platelet surface-bound PF4, are most likely to develop HIT after heparinization and HIT antibody development. The relationship between baseline platelet PF4 content or surface PF4 levels and the risk of developing HIT has yet to be demonstrated clinically. If such a relationship will be shown, it might offer a method for prescreening patients prior to heparinization for elimination of those who are at increased risk of HIT, and for assessing who among heparinized patients with thrombocytopenia is at risk of developing HIT.

CLINICAL FEATURES

The diagnosis of HIT is difficult to establish in a complicated patient who can have multiple causes for developing thrombocytopenia or thrombosis. A scoring system based on the "4 Ts" was developed to help maintain focus on potentially affected patients.[234] The four Ts are thrombocytopenia, timing of onset of symptoms, thrombosis, and thrombocytopenia from other causes (Table 133–5). Typically, patients develop thrombocytopenia 5 to 10 days after the onset of heparin therapy unless exposure occurred within the preceding 3 months.[234] Bleeding manifestations secondary to the thrombocytopenia, such as petechiae, nosebleeds, and oozing from catheter sites, are not seen in HIT.[197] Symptoms of venous thrombosis include those related to deep vein thrombosis of the lower or upper extremity and pulmonary embolism,[197,235] adrenal infarctions,[236] and cerebral venous thrombosis.[237] Major venous obstruction can lead to limb gangrene.[238] Arterial thrombi in this disease can be striking and

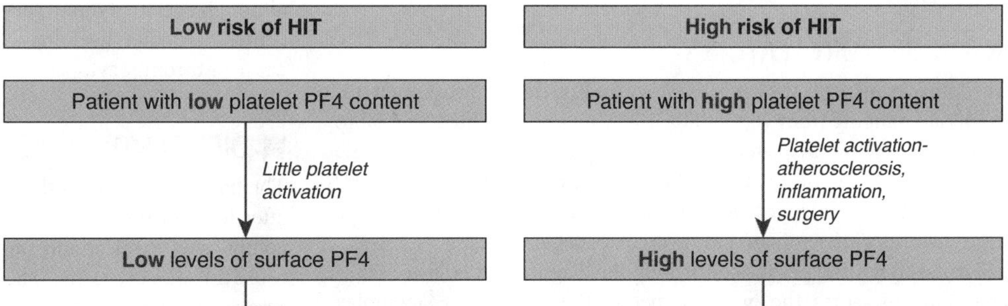

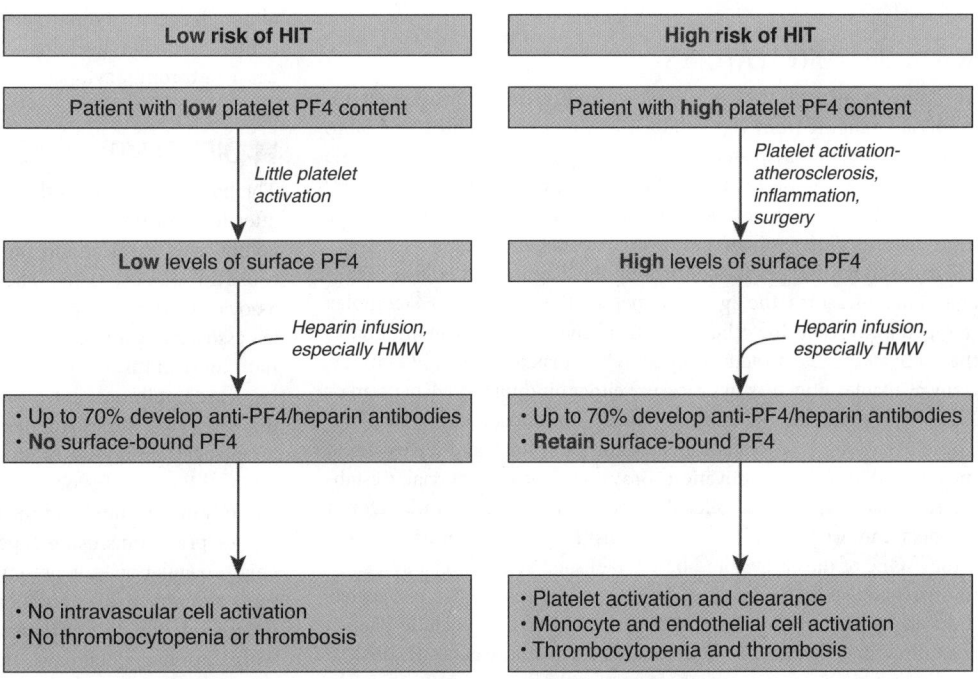

FIGURE 133–8. Model of early events in the etiology of HIT. Schematic of the basis for HIT in heparinized patients relative to surface PF4 levels. Most individuals have little surface PF4 because they either have low platelet stores and/or have little chronic platelet activation (*top left*). A few patients have high platelet PF4 content and chronic platelet activation (*top right*) with high levels of surface-bound PF4. After heparinization, both sets of patients often develop antibodies to PF4-heparin ("HIT antibodies"), although those with higher platelet PF4 release may have a greater antigenic stimulus and perhaps higher frequency of HIT antibodies and/or higher antibody titers. Most heparinized patients with HIT antibodies have no to little surface PF4 and HIT antigenic complexes on their platelets (*middle left*). However, a small percentage of patients retain surface PF4 and target HIT antigenic complexes (*middle right*). Because most patients do not have surface HIT antigenic complexes, they do not develop HIT in spite of the presence of antibodies (*bottom left*). The few patients with retained surface HIT antigenic complexes are at risk of HIT (*bottom right*). HMW, high molecular weight.

TABLE 133–5. The 4 Ts

	Points Per Category		
Clinical Sign	0	1	2
Thrombocytopenia (acute)	Very low nadir (<10 × 103/μL) or <30% fall	Low nadir (10–20 × 103/μL) or 30–50% fall	Moderate nadir (20–100 × 103/μL) or >50% fall
Timing of 1st event (thrombocytopenia or thrombosis)	≤4 days (unless prior heparin exposure in last 3 months)	Within 5–10 days (but not well documented) or ≤1 day (with exposure in last 3 months)	Documented occurrence in 5–10 days or ≤1 day with recent prior exposure
Thrombotic-related event	None	Common thrombi (DVT or line thrombus) or recurrent thrombus; erythematous skin lesion or not suspected thrombus	Major vessel thrombus or skin necrosis or skin lesion at site of heparin infusion
Thrombocytopenia (other causes)	Definite other cause is present	Possible other cause is present	No other strong explanation for thrombocytopenia

A score of 6–8 is high risk for HIT, 4–5 is intermediate risk, and 0–3 is low risk.

SOURCE: Adapted with permission from Warkentin TE.[234]

were the first feature that led to the recognition of HIT as a distinct clinical entity.[187] Other common thrombotic complications include stroke, myocardial infarction, bowel infarction from mesenteric artery thrombosis, and renal infarction.[239,240] Thrombosis of grafts and prosthetic devices has been reported.[238,241] Gangrenous changes in the skin occur at sites of heparin injections,[242] but can occur as well after intravenous heparin administration[243] or after switching to warfarin (Coumadin).[244]

LABORATORY FEATURES

Thrombocytopenia is the key laboratory finding in HIT. Most often it is moderate, ranging from 20 to 100 × 10^9/L, or is represented by a 50 to 70 percent decline in platelet count. Rarely is the thrombocytopenia more severe or absent, as observed in some cases with skin necrosis.[245] Although thrombin generation increases in HIT, patients rarely have decompensated disseminated intravascular coagulation.[246]

Two assay prototypes for confirming the diagnosis of HIT are available. One measures the Ig antibodies to the heparin–PF4 complex (antigen assay), and the other measures heparin-dependent antibodies that activate platelets (activation assay) in plasma or sera. Commercially available antigen assays measure either binding to PF4-heparin or PF4-polyvinylsulfate by enzyme-linked immunosorbent assay.[192,247] These assays are easily established in the laboratory and have a rapid turnaround time. The activation assays are not commercially established because specific platelet donors are needed each time. Donor platelets can vary greatly in their sensitivity to activation by HIT sera.[224] One of the earliest and best-established activation assays, serotonin-release assay,[248] involves ^{14}C-serotonin release from platelets induced by HIT antibodies and heparin. Other tests include platelet activation in a heparin-induced platelet activation assay (HIPA),[249] luminography,[250] and microparticle generation.[224]

In patients with a high clinical risk of having HIT (see Table 133–5), heparin should be stopped and alternative treatment started even before laboratory results are available. A positive antigen test and particularly a progressive increase in the number of platelets over the following days are confirmatory for HIT. A negative antigen test does not rule out HIT and should be repeated after 24 hours while the patient is undergoing alternative anticoagulant therapy. If the repeat assay is negative and platelet count does not increase, alternative diagnoses should be considered. A positive test can be false because many patients who develop anti–PF4-heparin antibodies do not necessarily go on to develop HIT.[202] A recently described cause for such false-positives is the presence of anti-PF4 rather than anti-PF4/heparin antibodies.[251] Such antibodies may occur in patients with lupus or APS, but can be distinguished by continued reactivity even in the presence of excess heparin, which disrupts PF4–heparin complexes. Activation assays take longer to perform and may require sending sera to a reference center. An activation assay will have greater specificity than the antigen assay, although specificity may vary based on the experience of the reference center. Its major usefulness is in *post factum* documentation of the cause of thrombocytopenia.

DIFFERENTIAL DIAGNOSIS

The hallmark of HIT is the onset of thrombocytopenia during or soon after heparin therapy. However, patients who develop HIT often have complicated medical and surgical conditions, many of which can also cause thrombocytopenia. These conditions commonly include disorders associated with increased peripheral destruction of platelets but rarely are associated with decreased platelet production (Table 133–6). A common cause of thrombocytopenia is dilutional thrombocytopenia following cardiopulmonary bypass operations, but this condition slowly improves over time. Another cause is the formation of drug-related, antiplatelet antibodies or the use of anti-$\alpha_{IIb}\beta_3$ drugs such as abciximab.[252] Posttransfusion purpura can begin approximately 1 week after blood transfusion,[253] and the patient often has a history of pregnancies and/or prior transfusion exposures. Sepsis and disseminated intravascular coagulation can present initially with thrombocytopenia as the most prominent manifestation, although often these processes rapidly progress, distinguishing themselves from HIT. TTP and HUS can present with thrombocytopenia as one of the first manifestations. Often, the ensuing clinical course and examination of the blood films distinguish these diseases from HIT. SLE and APS can be confused with HIT because these conditions cause both thrombocytopenia and thrombosis.

THERAPY

Despite greater understanding of the molecular basis of HIT and the availability of a number of new therapeutic agents, management is problematic. Prospective studies of patients with HIT indicate that without treatment, more than 50 percent can develop thrombosis over the ensuing days to weeks.[197,211,212] Current therapies can reduce, but

TABLE 133–6. Alternative Causes of Clinical Conditions Simulating HIT

Thrombocytopenia
Increased destruction
Acute immune thrombocytopenic purpura
Dilutional thrombocytopenia
Posttransfusion purpura
Drug-induced thrombocytopenia
Quinidine, quinine, trimethoprim-sulfamethoxazole, rifampicin, carbamazepine, diclofenac, ibuprofen
Integrin $\alpha_{IIb}\beta_3$ inhibitors: abciximab, tirofiban, eptifibatide
Decreased production
Postsepsis
Chemotherapy
Malignancy
Drug-related
Thrombocytopenia and thrombosis
Consumptive thrombohemorrhagic disorders
Sepsis and disseminated intravascular coagulation
Malignancies
Disseminated intravascular coagulation in pregnancy or after snake bite
TTP
HUS
SLE
Thrombosis alone
Venous stasis
Central catheters
Drugs
Coumadin
Vasculitis
Antiphospholipid syndrome

not eliminate, the risk of this life-threatening complication. For prevention of HIT, many authorities prefer using low-molecular-weight heparin because it confers a lower risk of HIT than high-molecular-weight heparin.[196–198] Thromboprophylaxis with heparin should be limited to the period of high thrombotic risk. Institution of a hospitalwide policy of daily platelet counts in patients receiving heparin therapy may allow early detection of thrombocytopenia and earlier intervention. In addition, elimination of heparin usage in flushes for maintaining patent catheter lines and in impregnation of catheters with heparin decrease the incidence of HIT. Finally, the development of alternative agents to replace heparin therapy, such as synthetic pentasaccharides that do not bind to PF4, may decrease the incidence of HIT. Coumadin should not be used as the sole initial treatment of HIT because of the increased risk of untoward thrombosis.[244] Low-molecular-weight heparin should not replace high-molecular-weight heparin because of cross-reactivity.[253]

Three accepted drugs are used in the treatment of patients with HIT: danaparoid sodium (no longer available in the United States), recombinant hirudin (lepirudin), and argatroban. Danaparoid is a mixture of low-molecular-weight heparanoids consisting of heparan sulfate, dermatan sulfate, and chondroitin sulfate. It has much greater anti-factor Xa activity than anti-factor IIa activity.[254] Danaparoid is an effective anticoagulant[255] that inhibits HIT antibody-induced platelet aggregation *in vitro*.[256] PF4–danaparoid complexes have little cross-reactivity with HIT antibodies.[257] Studies suggest danaparoid use improves platelet count recovery and decreases the incidence of serious thrombosis and death in patients with HIT.[258]

The other two drugs, lepirudin and argatroban, directly inhibit thrombin.[259] Both drugs are given intravenously and have rapid onset of action. Lepirudin binds to two sites on thrombin, the catalytic site and a fibrinogen-binding site, whereas argatroban binds only to the active site. Lepirudin prolongs the aPTT, so this test can be used to monitor effective dosing. Lepirudin is excreted in the urine, and its dosage must be adjusted in patients with renal failure.[260] Lepirudin induces antilepirudin antibodies in approximately half of patients who receive the drug. These antibodies rarely alter biologic activity, but do tend to prolong the drug's half-life, necessitating careful monitoring by aPTT.[261] Argatroban is synthesized from arginine and is rapidly metabolized in the liver.[262] It affects both the aPTT and PT.[263] Use of lepirudin and argatroban is efficacious; the incidence of thrombotic complication is reduced, perhaps by half, and the time to platelet count recovery is shortened. However, bleeding complications can occur.[211,264–266] As with danaparoid, lepirudin or argatroban should be given until patients recover from thrombocytopenia before adding and then switching to a prolonged course of an oral anticoagulant. With argatroban treatment, this switch is slightly more complicated because both argatroban and Coumadin prolong the international normalized ratio.[263]

The synthetic pentasaccharide fondaparinux has been used to treat patients with HIT.[267] Its efficacy relative to the direct thrombin inhibitors needs to be determined. Whether it is completely safe from inducing the HIT state has been questioned.[268]

COURSE AND PROGNOSIS

Unrecognized HIT can lead to life-threatening thrombosis in approximately 50 percent of patients. The percentage of patients with an adverse outcome remains high even if heparin therapy is withdrawn immediately. Intervention with either of the direct thrombin inhibitors or danaparoid significantly reduces the duration of thrombocytopenia, and more importantly, reduces the percent of patients developing thrombosis, with a generally acceptable increased incidence of significant bleeding. The prognosis likely will improve with increasing experience in the care of these patients. Whether alternative treatments based on increased insights into the pathophysiology of HIT will allow more rapid and more effective intervention remains to be seen.

REFERENCES

1. Moschcowitz E: Hyaline thrombosis of the terminal arterioles and capillaries: A hitherto undescribed disease. *Proc N Y Pathol Soc* 24:21, 1924.
2. Moschcowitz E: An acute febrile pleiochromic anemia with hyaline thrombosis of the terminal arterioles and capillaries. *Arch Intern Med* 36:89, 1925.
3. Singer K, Bornstein FP, Wile SA: Thrombotic thrombocytopenic purpura. Hemorrhagic diathesis with generalized platelet thromboses. *Blood* 2:542, 1946.
4. Gasser C, Gautier E, Steck A, et al: Hämolytisch-ürämische Syndrome: Bilaterale Nierenrindennekrosen bei akuten erworbenen hämolytischen Anämien. *Schweiz Med Wochenschr* 85:905, 1955.
5. Kibel MA, Barnard PJ: The haemolytic-uraemic syndrome: A survey in Southern Africa. *S Afr Med J* 42:692, 1968.
6. Amorosi EL, Ultmann JE: Thrombotic thrombocytopenic purpura: Report of 16 cases and review of the literature. *Medicine (Baltimore)* 45:139, 1966.
7. Rubinstein MA, Kagan BM, Macgillviray MH, et al: Unusual remission in a case of thrombotic thrombocytopenic purpura syndrome following fresh blood exchange transfusions. *Ann Intern Med* 51:1409, 1959.
8. Bukowski RM, Hewlett JS, Harris JW, et al: Exchange transfusions in the treatment of thrombotic thrombocytopenic purpura. *Semin Hematol* 13:219, 1976.
9. Bukowski RM, King JW, Hewlett JS: Plasmapheresis in the treatment of thrombotic thrombocytopenic purpura. *Blood* 50:413, 1977.

10. Byrnes JJ, Khurana M: Treatment of thrombotic thrombocytopenic purpura with plasma. *N Engl J Med* 297:1386, 1977.
11. Schulman I, Pierce M, Lukens A, Currimbhoy Z: Studies on thrombopoiesis. I. A factor in normal human plasma required for platelet production; chronic thrombocytopenia due to its deficiency. *Blood* 16:943, 1960.
12. Upshaw JD Jr: Congenital deficiency of a factor in normal plasma that reverses microangiopathic hemolysis and thrombocytopenia. *N Engl J Med* 298:1350, 1978.
13. Bell WR, Braine HG, Ness PM, Kickler TS: Improved survival in thrombotic thrombocytopenic purpura-hemolytic uremic syndrome. Clinical experience in 108 patients. *N Engl J Med* 325:398, 1991.
14. Rock GA, Shumak KH, Buskard NA, et al: Comparison of plasma exchange with plasma infusion in the treatment of thrombotic thrombocytopenic purpura. Canadian Apheresis Study Group. *N Engl J Med* 325:393, 1991.
15. Moake JL, Rudy CK, Troll JH, et al: Unusually large plasma factor VIII:von Willebrand factor multimers in chronic relapsing thrombotic thrombocytopenic purpura. *N Engl J Med* 307:1432, 1982.
16. Furlan M, Robles R, Lämmle B: Partial purification and characterization of a protease from human plasma cleaving von Willebrand factor to fragments produced by *in vivo* proteolysis. *Blood* 87:4223, 1996.
17. Tsai H-M: Physiologic cleavage of von Willebrand factor by a plasma protease is dependent on its conformation and requires calcium ion. *Blood* 87:4235, 1996.
18. Furlan M, Robles R, Solenthaler M, et al: Deficient activity of von Willebrand factor-cleaving protease in chronic relapsing thrombotic thrombocytopenic purpura. *Blood* 89:3097, 1997.
19. Furlan M, Robles R, Galbusera M, et al: von Willebrand factor-cleaving protease in thrombotic thrombocytopenic purpura and the hemolytic-uremic syndrome. *N Engl J Med* 339:1578, 1998.
20. Tsai HM, Lian EC: Antibodies to von Willebrand factor-cleaving protease in acute thrombotic thrombocytopenic purpura. *N Engl J Med* 339:1585, 1998.
21. Fujikawa K, Suzuki H, McMullen B, Chung D: Purification of human von Willebrand factor-cleaving protease and its identification as a new member of the metalloproteinase family. *Blood* 98:1662, 2001.
22. Gerritsen HE, Robles R, Lammle B, Furlan M: Partial amino acid sequence of purified von Willebrand factor-cleaving protease. *Blood* 98:1654, 2001.
23. Zheng X, Chung D, Takayama TK, et al: Structure of von Willebrand factor-cleaving protease (ADAMTS13), a metalloprotease involved in thrombotic thrombocytopenic purpura. *J Biol Chem* 276:41059, 2001.
24. Soejima K, Mimura N, Hirashima M, et al: A novel human metalloprotease synthesized in the liver and secreted into the blood: Possibly, the von Willebrand factor-cleaving protease? *J Biochem* 130:475, 2001.
25. Levy GG, Nichols WC, Lian EC, et al: Mutations in a member of the ADAMTS gene family cause thrombotic thrombocytopenic purpura. *Nature* 413:488, 2001.
26. Klaus C, Plaimauer B, Studt JD, et al: Epitope mapping of ADAMTS13 autoantibodies in acquired thrombotic thrombocytopenic purpura. *Blood* 103:4514, 2004.
27. Luken BM, Turenhout EA, Hulstein JJ, et al: The spacer domain of ADAMTS13 contains a major binding site for antibodies in patients with thrombotic thrombocytopenic purpura. *Thromb Haemost* 93:267, 2005.
28. Scheiflinger F, Knobl P, Trattner B, et al: Nonneutralizing IgM and IgG antibodies to von Willebrand factor-cleaving protease (ADAMTS13) in a patient with thrombotic thrombocytopenic purpura. *Blood* 102:3241, 2003.
29. Asada Y, Sumiyoshi A, Hayashi T, et al: Immunohistochemistry of vascular lesion in thrombotic thrombocytopenic purpura, with special reference to factor VIII related antigen. *Thromb Res* 38:469, 1985.
30. Hosler GA, Cusumano AM, Hutchins GM: Thrombotic thrombocytopenic purpura and hemolytic uremic syndrome are distinct pathologic entities. A review of 56 autopsy cases. *Arch Pathol Lab Med* 127:834, 2003.
31. Wallace DC, Lovric A, Clubb JS, Carseldine DB: Thrombotic thrombocytopenic purpura in four siblings. *Am J Med* 58:724, 1975.
32. Inward CD, Howie AJ, Fitzpatrick MM, et al: Renal histopathology in fatal cases of diarrhoea-associated haemolytic uraemic syndrome. British Association for Paediatric Nephrology. *Pediatr Nephrol* 11:556, 1997.
33. Siddiqui FA, Lian EC: Characterization of platelet agglutinating protein p37 purified from the plasma of a patient with thrombotic thrombocytopenic purpura. *Biochem Mol Biol Int* 30:385, 1993.
34. Praprotnik S, Blank M, Levy Y, et al: Anti-endothelial cell antibodies from patients with thrombotic thrombocytopenic purpura specifically activate small vessel endothelial cells. *Int Immunol* 13:203, 2001.
35. Schultz DR, Arnold PI, Jy W, et al: Anti-CD36 autoantibodies in thrombotic thrombocytopenic purpura and other thrombotic disorders: Identification of an 85 kD form of CD36 as a target antigen. *Br J Haematol* 103:849, 1998.
36. Mitra D, Jaffe EA, Weksler B, et al: Thrombotic thrombocytopenic purpura and sporadic hemolytic-uremic syndrome plasmas induce apoptosis in restricted lineages of human microvascular endothelial cells. *Blood* 89:1224, 1997.
37. van der Plas RM, Schiphorst ME, Huizinga EG, et al: von Willebrand factor proteolysis is deficient in classic, but not in bone marrow transplantation-associated, thrombotic thrombocytopenic purpura. *Blood* 93:3798, 1999.
38. Arai S, Allan C, Streiff M, et al: von Willebrand factor-cleaving protease activity and proteolysis of von Willebrand factor in bone marrow transplant-associated thrombotic microangiopathy. *Hematol J* 2:292, 2001.
39. Iwata H, Kami M, Hori A, et al: An autopsy-based retrospective study of secondary thrombotic thrombocytopenic purpura. *Haematologica* 86:669, 2001.
40. Siami K, Kojouri K, Swisher KK, et al: Thrombotic microangiopathy after allogeneic hematopoietic stem cell transplantation: An autopsy study. *Transplantation* 85:22, 2008.
41. Miller DP, Kaye JA, Shea K, et al: Incidence of thrombotic thrombocytopenic purpura/hemolytic uremic syndrome. *Epidemiology* 15:208, 2004.
42. Terrell DR, Williams LA, Vesely SK, et al: The incidence of thrombotic thrombocytopenic purpura-hemolytic uremic syndrome: All patients, patients, and patients with severe ADAMTS13 deficiency. *J Thromb Haemost* 3:1432, 2005.
43. Vesely SK, George JN, Lammle B, et al: ADAMTS13 activity in thrombotic thrombocytopenic purpura-hemolytic uremic syndrome: Relation to presenting features and clinical outcomes in a prospective cohort of 142 patients. *Blood* 102:60, 2003.
44. Zheng XL, Kaufman RM, Goodnough LT, Sadler JE: Effect of plasma exchange on plasma ADAMTS13 metalloprotease activity, inhibitor level, and clinical outcome in patients with and nonthrombotic thrombocytopenic purpura. *Blood* 103:4043, 2004.
45. Nicol KK, Shelton BJ, Knovich MA, Owen J: Overweight individuals are at increased risk for thrombotic thrombocytopenic purpura. *Am J Hematol* 74:170, 2003.
46. Ridolfi RL, Bell WR: Thrombotic thrombocytopenic purpura. Report of 25 cases and review of the literature. *Medicine (Baltimore)* 60:413, 1981.
47. McMinn JR, George JN: Evaluation of women with clinically suspected thrombotic thrombocytopenic purpura-hemolytic uremic syndrome during pregnancy. *J Clin Apher* 16:202, 2001.
48. Furlan M, Lämmle B: Aetiology and pathogenesis of thrombotic thrombocytopenic purpura and haemolytic uraemic syndrome: The role of von Willebrand factor-cleaving protease. *Best Pract Res Clin Haematol* 14:437, 2001.
49. Studt JD, Hovinga JA, Radonic R, et al: Familial acquired thrombotic thrombocytopenic purpura: ADAMTS13 inhibitory autoantibodies in identical twins. *Blood* 103:4195, 2004.
50. Joseph G, Smith KJ, Hadley TJ, et al: HLA-DR53 protects against thrombotic thrombocytopenic purpura/adult hemolytic uremic syndrome. *Am J Hematol* 47:189, 1994.
51. Raife TJ, Lentz SR, Atkinson BS, et al: Factor V Leiden: A genetic risk factor for thrombotic microangiopathy in patients with normal von Willebrand factor-cleaving protease activity. *Blood* 99:437, 2002.
52. Krieg S, Studt JD, Sulzer I, et al: Is factor V Leiden a risk factor for thrombotic microangiopathies without severe ADAMTS 13 deficiency? *Thromb Haemost* 94:1186, 2005.
53. Piastra M, Curro V, Chiaretti A, et al: Intracranial hemorrhage at the onset of thrombotic thrombocytopenic purpura in an infant: Therapeutic approach and intensive care management. *Pediatr Emerg Care* 17:42, 2001.
54. O'Brien TE, Crum ED: Atypical presentations of thrombotic thrombocytopenic purpura. *Int J Hematol* 76:471, 2002.
55. Tsai H-M, Shulman K: Rituximab induces remission of cerebral ischemia caused by thrombotic thrombocytopenic purpura. *Eur J Haematol* 70:183, 2003.
56. Sarode R: Atypical presentations of thrombotic thrombocytopenic purpura: A review. *J Clin Apher* 24:47, 2009.
57. Hawkins BM, Abu-Fadel M, Vesely SK, George JN: Clinical cardiac involvement in thrombotic thrombocytopenic purpura: A systematic review. *Transfusion* 48:382, 2008.
58. Hughes C, McEwan JR, Longair I, et al: Cardiac involvement in acute thrombotic thrombocytopenic purpura: Association with troponin T and IgG antibodies to ADAMTS 13. *J Thromb Haemost* 7:529, 2009.
59. Chang JC, Aly EM: Acute respiratory distress syndrome as a major clinical manifestation of thrombotic thrombocytopenic purpura. *Am J Med Sci* 321:124, 2001.
60. Thompson CE, Damon LE, Ries CA, Linker CA: Thrombotic microangiopathies in the 1980s: Clinical features, response to treatment, and the impact of the human immunodeficiency virus epidemic. *Blood* 80:1890, 1992.
61. Burns ER, Lou Y, Pathak A: Morphologic diagnosis of thrombotic thrombocytopenic purpura. *Am J Hematol* 75:18, 2004.
62. Takahashi H, Tatewaki W, Nakamura T, et al: Coagulation studies in thrombotic thrombocytopenic purpura, with special reference to von Willebrand factor and protein S. *Am J Hematol* 30:14, 1989.
63. Veyradier A, Obert B, Houllier A, et al: Specific von Willebrand factor-cleaving protease in thrombotic microangiopathies: A study of 111 cases. *Blood* 98:1765, 2001.
64. Bianchi V, Robles R, Alberio L, et al: von Willebrand factor-cleaving protease (ADAMTS13) in thrombocytopenic disorders: A severely deficient activity is specific for thrombotic thrombocytopenic purpura. *Blood* 100:710, 2002.
65. Tsai HM: Is severe deficiency of ADAMTS13 specific for thrombotic thrombocytopenic purpura? Yes. *J Thromb Haemost* 1:625, 2003.
66. Mannucci PM, Canciani MT, Forza I, et al: Changes in health and disease of the metalloprotease that cleaves von Willebrand factor. *Blood* 98:2730, 2001.
67. Uemura M, Fujimura Y, Matsumoto M, et al: Comprehensive analysis of ADAMTS13 in patients with liver cirrhosis. *Thromb Haemost* 99:1019, 2008.
68. Park YD, Yoshioka A, Kawa K, et al: Impaired activity of plasma von Willebrand factor-cleaving protease may predict the occurrence of hepatic veno-occlusive disease after stem cell transplantation. *Bone Marrow Transplant* 29:789, 2002.
69. Ono T, Mimuro J, Madoiwa S, et al: Severe secondary deficiency of von Willebrand factor-cleaving protease (ADAMTS13) in patients with sepsis-induced disseminated intravascular coagulation: Its correlation with development of renal failure. *Blood* 107:528, 2006.

70. Kremer Hovinga JA, Zeerleder S, Kessler P, et al: ADAMTS13, von Willebrand factor and related parameters in severe sepsis and septic shock. *J Thromb Haemost* 5:2284, 2007.
71. Tripodi A, Peyvandi F, Chantarangkul V, et al: Second international collaborative study evaluating performance characteristics of methods measuring the von Willebrand factor cleaving protease (ADAMTS13). *J Thromb Haemost* 6:1534, 2008.
72. Zomas A, Saso R, Powles R, et al: Red cell fragmentation (schistocytosis) after bone marrow transplantation. *Bone Marrow Transplant* 22:777, 1998.
73. Kanamori H, Takaishi Y, Takabayashi M, et al: Clinical significance of fragmented red cells after allogeneic bone marrow transplantation. *Int J Hematol* 77:180, 2003.
74. Zheng XL, Sadler JE: Pathogenesis of thrombotic microangiopathies. *Annu Rev Pathol* 3:249, 2008.
75. Akiyama M, Kokame K, Miyata T: ADAMTS13 P475S polymorphism causes a lowered enzymatic activity and urea lability *in vitro*. *J Thromb Haemost* 6:1830, 2008.
76. Loirat C, Girma JP, Desconclois C, et al: Thrombotic thrombocytopenic purpura related to severe ADAMTS13 deficiency in children. *Pediatr Nephrol* 24:19, 2009.
77. Hara T, Kitano A, Kajiwara T, et al: Factor VIII concentrate-responsive thrombocytopenia, hemolytic anemia, and nephropathy. Evidence that factor VIII:von Willebrand factor is involved in its pathogenesis. *Am J Pediatr Hematol Oncol* 8:324, 1986.
78. Veyradier A, Meyer D, Loirat C: Desmopressin, an unexpected link between nocturnal enuresis and inherited thrombotic thrombocytopenic purpura (Upshaw-Schulman syndrome). *J Thromb Haemost* 4:700, 2006.
79. Furlan M, Robles R, Morselli B, et al: Recovery and half-life of von Willebrand factor-cleaving protease after plasma therapy in patients with thrombotic thrombocytopenic purpura. *Thromb Haemost* 81:8, 1999.
80. Cabrera GR, Fortenberry JD, Warshaw BL, et al: Hemolytic uremic syndrome associated with invasive *Streptococcus pneumoniae* infection. *Pediatrics* 101:699, 1998.
81. Copelovitch L, Kaplan BS: *Streptococcus pneumoniae*–associated hemolytic uremic syndrome. *Pediatr Nephrol* 23:1951, 2008.
82. Singh N, Gayowski T, Marino IR: Hemolytic uremic syndrome in solid-organ transplant recipients. *Transpl Int* 9:68, 1996.
83. Chohan R, Vij R, Adkins D, et al: Long-term outcomes of allogeneic stem cell transplant recipients after calcineurin inhibitor-induced neurotoxicity. *Br J Haematol* 123:110, 2003.
84. Sarode R, McFarland JG, Flomenberg N, et al: Therapeutic plasma exchange does not appear to be effective in the management of thrombotic thrombocytopenic purpura/hemolytic uremic syndrome following bone marrow transplantation. *Bone Marrow Transplant* 16:271, 1995.
85. Ho VT, Cutler C, Carter S, et al: Blood and marrow transplant clinical trials network toxicity committee consensus summary: Thrombotic microangiopathy after hematopoietic stem cell transplantation. *Biol Blood Marrow Transplant* 11:571, 2005.
86. Sack GH Jr, Levin J, Bell WR: Trousseau's syndrome and other manifestations of chronic disseminated coagulopathy in patients with neoplasms: Clinical, pathophysiologic, and therapeutic features. *Medicine (Baltimore)* 56:1, 1977.
87. Domingo-Claros A, Larriba I, Rozman M, et al: Acute erythroid neoplastic proliferations. A biological study based on 62 patients. *Haematologica* 87:148, 2002.
88. Fontana S, Gerritsen HE, Kremer Hovinga J, et al: Microangiopathic haemolytic anaemia in metastasizing malignant tumours is not associated with a severe deficiency of the von Willebrand factor-cleaving protease. *Br J Haematol* 113:100, 2001.
89. Lattuada A, Rossi E, Calzarossa C, et al: Mild to moderate reduction of a von Willebrand factor cleaving protease (ADAMTS13) in pregnant women with HELLP microangiopathic syndrome. *Haematologica* 88:1029, 2003.
90. Scully M, Starke R, Lee R, et al: Successful management of pregnancy in women with a history of thrombotic thrombocytopaenic purpura. *Blood Coagul Fibrinolysis* 17:459, 2006.
91. Baron BW, Martin MS, Sucharetza BS, et al: Four patients with both thrombotic thrombocytopenic purpura and autoimmune thrombocytopenic purpura: The concept of a mixed immune thrombocytopenia syndrome and indications for plasma exchange. *J Clin Apher* 16:179, 2001.
92. Mannucci PM, Vanoli M, Forza I, et al: Von Willebrand factor cleaving protease (ADAMTS13) in 123 patients with connective tissue diseases (systemic lupus erythematosus and systemic sclerosis). *Haematologica* 88:914, 2003.
93. Güngör T, Furlan M, Lämmle B, et al: Acquired deficiency of von Willebrand factor-cleaving protease in a patient suffering from acute systemic lupus erythematosus. *Rheumatology* 40:940, 2001.
94. Ahmed S, Siddiqui AK, Chandrasekaran V: Correlation of thrombotic thrombocytopenic purpura disease activity with von Willebrand factor-cleaving protease level in ulcerative colitis. *Am J Med* 116:786, 2004.
95. Coppo P, Bengoufa D, Veyradier A, et al: Severe ADAMTS13 deficiency in adult thrombotic microangiopathies defines a subset of patients characterized by various autoimmune manifestations, lower platelet count, and mild renal involvement. *Medicine (Baltimore)* 83:233, 2004.
96. Espinosa G, Bucciarelli S, Cervera R, et al: Thrombotic microangiopathic haemolytic anaemia and antiphospholipid antibodies. *Ann Rheum Dis* 63:730, 2004.
97. Steen VD: Scleroderma renal crisis. *Rheum Dis Clin North Am* 29:315, 2003.
98. Bennett CL, Davidson CJ, Raisch DW, et al: Thrombotic thrombocytopenic purpura associated with ticlopidine in the setting of coronary artery stents and stroke prevention. *Arch Intern Med* 159:2524, 1999.
99. Bennett CL, Kim B, Zakarija A, et al: Two mechanistic pathways for thienopyridine-associated thrombotic thrombocytopenic purpura: A report from the SERF-TTP Research Group and the RADAR Project. *J Am Coll Cardiol* 50:1138, 2007.
100. Medina PJ, Sipols JM, George JN: Drug-associated thrombotic thrombocytopenic purpura-hemolytic uremic syndrome. *Curr Opin Hematol* 8:286, 2001.
101. Pisoni R, Ruggenenti P, Remuzzi G: Drug-induced thrombotic microangiopathy: Incidence, prevention and management. *Drug Saf* 24:491, 2001.
102. Dlott JS, Danielson CF, Blue-Hnidy DE, McCarthy LJ: Drug-induced thrombotic thrombocytopenic purpura/hemolytic uremic syndrome: A concise review. *Ther Apher Dial* 8:102, 2004.
103. Valavaara R, Nordman E: Renal complications of mitomycin C therapy with special reference to the total dose. *Cancer* 55:47, 1985.
104. Lesesne JB, Rothschild N, Erickson B, et al: Cancer-associated hemolytic-uremic syndrome: Analysis of 85 cases from a national registry. *J Clin Oncol* 7:781, 1989.
105. Humphreys BD, Sharman JP, Henderson JM, et al: Gemcitabine-associated thrombotic microangiopathy. *Cancer* 100:2664, 2004.
106. Glezerman I, Kris MG, Miller V, et al: Gemcitabine nephrotoxicity and hemolytic uremic syndrome: Report of 29 cases from a single institution. *Clin Nephrol* 71:130, 2009.
107. Remuzzi G, Bertani T: Renal vascular and thrombotic effects of cyclosporine. *Am J Kidney Dis* 13:261, 1989.
108. Bechstein WO: Neurotoxicity of calcineurin inhibitors: Impact and clinical management. *Transpl Int* 13:313, 2000.
109. Scott LJ, McKeage K, Keam SJ, Plosker GL: Tacrolimus: A further update of its use in the management of organ transplantation. *Drugs* 63:1247, 2003.
110. Roy V, Rizvi MA, Vesely SK, George JN: Thrombotic thrombocytopenic purpura-like syndromes following bone marrow transplantation: An analysis of associated conditions and clinical outcomes. *Bone Marrow Transplant* 27:641, 2001.
111. Dzik WH, Georgi BA, Khettry U, Jenkins RL: Cyclosporine-associated thrombotic thrombocytopenic purpura following liver transplantation—Successful treatment with plasma exchange. *Transplantation* 44:570, 1987.
112. Trimarchi HM, Truong LD, Brennan S, et al: FK506-associated thrombotic microangiopathy: Report of two cases and review of the literature. *Transplantation* 67:539, 1999.
113. Gottschall JL, Neahring B, McFarland JG, et al: Quinine-induced immune thrombocytopenia with hemolytic uremic syndrome: Clinical and serological findings in nine patients and review of literature. *Am J Hematol* 47:283, 1994.
114. Kojouri K, Vesely SK, George JN: Quinine-associated thrombotic thrombocytopenic purpura-hemolytic uremic syndrome: Frequency, clinical features, and long-term outcomes. *Ann Intern Med* 135:1047, 2001.
115. Knower MT, Bowton DL, Owen J, Dunagan DP: Quinine-induced disseminated intravascular coagulation: Case report and review of the literature. *Intensive Care Med* 29:1007, 2003.
116. van den Born BJ, van der Hoeven NV, Groot E, et al: Association between thrombotic microangiopathy and reduced ADAMTS13 activity in malignant hypertension. *Hypertension* 51:862, 2008.
117. Gianviti A, Tozzi AE, De Petris L, et al: Risk factors for poor renal prognosis in children with hemolytic uremic syndrome. *Pediatr Nephrol* 18:1229, 2003.
118. Bhimma R, Rollins NC, Coovadia HM, Adhikari M: Post-dysenteric hemolytic uremic syndrome in children during an epidemic of Shigella dysentery in Kwazulu/Natal. *Pediatr Nephrol* 11:560, 1997.
119. Griffin PM, Ostroff SM, Tauxe RV, et al: Illnesses associated with *Escherichia coli* O157:H7 infections. A broad clinical spectrum. *Ann Intern Med* 109:705, 1988.
120. Bell BP, Griffin PM, Lozano P, et al: Predictors of hemolytic uremic syndrome in children during a large outbreak of *Escherichia coli* O157:H7 infections. *Pediatrics* 100:E12, 1997.
121. Havelaar AH, Van Duynhoven YT, Nauta MJ, et al: Disease burden in The Netherlands due to infections with Shiga toxin-producing *Escherichia coli* O157. *Epidemiol Infect* 132:467, 2004.
122. Proesmans W: The role of coagulation and fibrinolysis in the pathogenesis of diarrhea-associated hemolytic uremic syndrome. *Semin Thromb Hemost* 27:201, 2001.
123. Tsai HM, Chandler WL, Sarode R, et al: von Willebrand factor and von Willebrand factor-cleaving metalloprotease activity in *Escherichia coli* O157:H7-associated hemolytic uremic syndrome. *Pediatr Res* 49:653, 2001.
124. Hunt BJ, Lämmle B, Nevard CH, et al: von Willebrand factor-cleaving protease in childhood diarrhoea-associated haemolytic uraemic syndrome. *Thromb Haemost* 85:975, 2001.
125. Garg AX, Suri RS, Barrowman N, et al: Long-term renal prognosis of diarrhea-associated hemolytic uremic syndrome: A systematic review, meta-analysis, and meta-regression. *JAMA* 290:1360, 2003.
126. Michael M, Elliott EJ, Craig JC, et al: Interventions for hemolytic uremic syndrome and thrombotic thrombocytopenic purpura: A systematic review of randomized controlled trials. *Am J Kidney Dis* 53:259, 2009.
127. Ake JA, Jelacic S, Ciol MA, et al: Relative nephroprotection during *Escherichia coli* O157:H7 infections: Association with intravenous volume expansion. *Pediatrics* 115:e673, 2005.
128. Tarr PI, Gordon CA, Chandler WL: Shiga-toxin-producing *Escherichia coli* and haemolytic uraemic syndrome. *Lancet* 365:1073, 2005.
129. Ariceta G, Besbas N, Johnson S, et al: Guideline for the investigation and initial therapy of diarrhea-negative hemolytic uremic syndrome. *Pediatr Nephrol* 24:687, 2009.
130. Zipfel PF, Edey M, Heinen S, et al: Deletion of complement factor H-related genes CFHR1 and CFHR3 is associated with atypical hemolytic uremic syndrome. *PLoS Genet* 3:e41, 2007.
131. Kavanagh D, Richards A, Atkinson JP: Complement regulatory genes and hemolytic uremic syndromes. *Annu Rev Med* 59:61, 2008.

132. Blom AM, Bergstrom F, Edey M, et al: A novel non-synonymous polymorphism (p.Arg240His) in C4b-binding protein is associated with atypical hemolytic uremic syndrome and leads to impaired alternative pathway cofactor activity. *J Immunol* 180:6385, 2008.
133. Fremeaux-Bacchi V, Miller EC, Liszewski MK, et al: Mutations in complement C3 predispose to development of atypical hemolytic uremic syndrome. *Blood* 112:4948, 2008.
134. Jozsi M, Licht C, Strobel S, et al: Factor H autoantibodies in atypical hemolytic uremic syndrome correlate with CFHR1/CFHR3 deficiency. *Blood* 111:1512, 2008.
135. Loirat C, Noris M, Fremeaux-Bacchi V: Complement and the atypical hemolytic uremic syndrome in children. *Pediatr Nephrol* 23:1957, 2008.
136. Saland JM, Ruggenenti P, Remuzzi G: Liver-kidney transplantation to cure atypical hemolytic uremic syndrome. *J Am Soc Nephrol* 20:940, 2009.
137. Gruppo RA, Rother RP: Eculizumab for congenital atypical hemolytic-uremic syndrome. *N Engl J Med* 360:544, 2009.
138. Nurnberger J, Witzke O, Opazo Saez A, et al: Eculizumab for atypical hemolytic-uremic syndrome. *N Engl J Med* 360:542, 2009.
139. George JN: How I treat patients with thrombotic thrombocytopenic purpura-hemolytic uremic syndrome. *Blood* 96:1223, 2000.
140. Nguyen L, Li X, Duvall D, et al: Twice-daily plasma exchange for patients with refractory thrombotic thrombocytopenic purpura: The experience of the Oklahoma Registry, 1989 through 2006. *Transfusion* 48:349, 2008.
141. Zeigler ZR, Shadduck RK, Gryn JF, et al: Cryoprecipitate poor plasma does not improve early response in primary adult thrombotic thrombocytopenic purpura (TTP). *J Clin Apher* 16:19, 2001.
142. Rock G, Anderson D, Clark W, et al: Does cryosupernatant plasma improve outcome in thrombotic thrombocytopenic purpura? No answer yet. *Br J Haematol* 129:79, 2005.
143. Prowse C: Properties of pathogen-inactivated plasma components. *Transfus Med Rev* 23:124, 2009.
144. McCarthy LJ: Evidence-based medicine for apheresis: An ongoing challenge. *Ther Apher Dial* 8:112, 2004.
145. Yarranton H, Cohen H, Pavord SR, et al: Venous thromboembolism associated with the management of acute thrombotic thrombocytopenic purpura. *Br J Haematol* 121:778, 2003.
146. Allford SL, Harrison P, Lawrie AS, et al: von Willebrand factor—Cleaving protease activity in congenital thrombotic thrombocytopenic purpura. *Br J Haematol* 111:1215, 2000.
147. del Rio-Garma J, Alvarez-Larran A, Martinez C, et al: Methylene blue-photoinactivated plasma versus quarantine fresh frozen plasma in thrombotic thrombocytopenic purpura: A multicentric, prospective cohort study. *Br J Haematol* 143:39, 2008.
148. Rizvi MA, Vesely SK, George JN, et al: Complications of plasma exchange in 71 consecutive patients treated for clinically suspected thrombotic thrombocytopenic purpura-hemolytic-uremic syndrome. *Transfusion* 40:896, 2000.
149. Nguyen L, Terrell DR, Duvall D, et al: Complications of plasma exchange in patients treated for thrombotic thrombocytopenic purpura. IV. An additional study of 43 consecutive patients, 2005 to 2008. *Transfusion* 49:392, 2009.
150. Doerfler ME, Kaufman B, Goldenberg AS: Central venous catheter placement in patients with disorders of hemostasis. *Chest* 110:185, 1996.
151. Marques MB, Huang ST: Patients with thrombotic thrombocytopenic purpura commonly develop metabolic alkalosis during therapeutic plasma exchange. *J Clin Apher* 16:120, 2001.
152. Perdue JJ, Chandler LK, Vesely SK, et al: Unintentional platelet removal by plasmapheresis. *J Clin Apher* 16:55, 2001.
153. Reutter JC, Sanders KF, Brecher ME, et al: Incidence of allergic reactions with fresh-frozen plasma or cryo-supernatant plasma in the treatment of thrombotic thrombocytopenic purpura. *J Clin Apher* 16:134, 2001.
154. Allford SL, Hunt BJ, Rose P, Machin SJ: Guidelines on the diagnosis and management of the thrombotic microangiopathic haemolytic anaemias. *Br J Haematol* 120:556, 2003.
155. Bobbio-Pallavicini E, Gugliotta L, Centurioni R, et al: Antiplatelet agents in thrombotic thrombocytopenic purpura (TTP). Results of a randomized multicenter trial by the Italian Cooperative Group for TTP. *Haematologica* 82:429, 1997.
156. Coppo P, Lassoued K, Mariette X, et al: Effectiveness of platelet transfusions after plasma exchange in adult thrombotic thrombocytopenic purpura: A report of two cases. *Am J Hematol* 68:198, 2001.
157. Swisher KK, Terrell DR, Vesely SK, et al: Clinical outcomes after platelet transfusions in patients with thrombotic thrombocytopenic purpura. *Transfusion* 49:873, 2009.
158. Ferrara F, Annunziata M, Pollio F, et al: Vincristine as treatment for recurrent episodes of thrombotic thrombocytopenic purpura. *Ann Hematol* 81:7, 2002.
159. Bobbio-Pallavicini E, Porta C, Centurioni R, et al: Vincristine sulfate for the treatment of thrombotic thrombocytopenic purpura refractory to plasma-exchange. The Italian Cooperative Group for TTP. *Eur J Haematol* 52:222, 1994.
160. Cataland SR, Jin M, Lin S, et al: Cyclosporin and plasma exchange in thrombotic thrombocytopenic purpura: Long-term follow-up with serial analysis of ADAMTS13 activity. *Br J Haematol* 139:486, 2007.
161. Cataland SR, Jin M, Zheng XL, et al: An evaluation of cyclosporine alone for the treatment of early recurrences of thrombotic thrombocytopenic purpura. *J Thromb Haemost* 4:1162, 2006.
162. Cataland SR, Jin M, Lin S, et al: Effect of prophylactic cyclosporine therapy on ADAMTS13 biomarkers in patients with thrombotic thrombocytopenic purpura. *Am J Hematol* 83:911, 2008.
163. Zheng X, Pallera AM, Goodnough LT, et al: Remission of chronic thrombotic thrombocytopenic purpura after treatment with cyclophosphamide and rituximab. *Ann Intern Med* 138:105, 2003.
164. Scully M, Cohen H, Cavenagh J, et al: Remission in acute refractory and relapsing thrombotic thrombocytopenic purpura following rituximab is associated with a reduction in IgG antibodies to ADAMTS13. *Br J Haematol* 136:451, 2007.
165. Sadler JE: von Willebrand factor, ADAMTS13, and thrombotic thrombocytopenic purpura. *Blood* 112:11, 2008.
166. Jasti S, Coyle T, Gentile T, et al: Rituximab as an adjunct to plasma exchange in TTP: A report of 12 cases and review of literature. *J Clin Apher* 23:151, 2008.
167. Kimby E: Tolerability and safety of rituximab (MabThera). *Cancer Treat Rev* 31:456, 2005.
168. Carson KR, Evens AM, Richey EA, et al: Progressive multifocal leukoencephalopathy following rituximab therapy in HIV negative patients: A report of 57 cases from the Research on Adverse Drug Event and Reports (RADAR) project. *Blood* 113:4834, 2009.
169. Allan DS, Kovacs MJ, Clark WF: Frequently relapsing thrombotic thrombocytopenic purpura treated with cytotoxic immunosuppressive therapy. *Haematologica* 86:844, 2001.
170. Spiekermann K, Wormann B, Rumpf KW, Hiddemann W: Combination chemotherapy with CHOP for recurrent thrombotic thrombocytopenic purpura. *Br J Haematol* 97:544, 1997.
171. Passweg JR, Rabusin M, Musso M, et al: Haematopoetic stem cell transplantation for refractory autoimmune cytopenia. *Br J Haematol* 125:749, 2004.
172. Aqui NA, Stein SH, Konkle BA, et al: Role of splenectomy in patients with refractory or relapsed thrombotic thrombocytopenic purpura. *J Clin Apher* 18:51, 2003.
173. Kappers-Klunne MC, Wijermans P, Fijnheer R, et al: Splenectomy for the treatment of thrombotic thrombocytopenic purpura. *Br J Haematol* 130:768, 2005.
174. Katkhouda N, Hurwitz MB, Rivera RT, et al: Laparoscopic splenectomy: Outcome and efficacy in 103 consecutive patients. *Ann Surg* 228:568, 1998.
175. Levy J, Degani N: Correcting immune imbalance: The use of Prosorba column treatment for immune disorders. *Ther Apher Dial* 7:197, 2003.
176. Bobbio-Pallavicini E, Porta C, Tacconi F, et al: Intravenous prostacyclin (as epoprostenol) infusion in thrombotic thrombocytopenic purpura. Four case reports and review of the literature. Italian Cooperative Group for Thrombotic Thrombocytopenic Purpura. *Haematologica* 79:429, 1994.
177. Sagripanti A, Carpi A, Rosaia B, et al: Iloprost in the treatment of thrombotic microangiopathy: Report of thirteen cases. *Biomed Pharmacother* 50:350, 1996.
178. Dervenoulas J, Tsirigotis P, Bollas G, et al: Efficacy of intravenous immunoglobulin in the treatment of thrombotic thrombocytopaenic purpura. A study of 44 cases. *Acta Haematol* 105:204, 2001.
179. Anderson D, Ali K, Blanchette V, et al: Guidelines on the use of intravenous immune globulin for hematologic conditions. *Transfus Med Rev* 21:S9, 2007.
180. Sarode R, Gottschall JL, Aster RH, McFarland JG: Thrombotic thrombocytopenic purpura: Early and late responders. *Am J Hematol* 54:102, 1997.
181. Bandarenko N, Brecher ME: United States Thrombotic Thrombocytopenic Purpura Apheresis Study Group (US TTP ASG): Multicenter survey and retrospective analysis of current efficacy of therapeutic plasma exchange. *J Clin Apher* 13:133, 1998.
182. Lara PN Jr, Coe TL, Zhou H, et al: Improved survival with plasma exchange in patients with thrombotic thrombocytopenic purpura-hemolytic uremic syndrome. *Am J Med* 107:573, 1999.
183. Shumak KH, Rock GA, Nair RC: Late relapses in patients successfully treated for thrombotic thrombocytopenic purpura. Canadian Apheresis Group. *Ann Intern Med* 122:569, 1995.
184. Kennedy AS, Lewis QF, Scott JG: Cognitive deficits after recovery from thrombotic thrombocytopenic purpura. *Transfusion* 49:1092, 2009.
185. Lewis QF, Lanneau MS, Mathias SD, et al: Long-term deficits in health-related quality of life after recovery from thrombotic thrombocytopenic purpura. *Transfusion* 49:118, 2009.
186. Hayward CP, Sutton DM, Carter WH Jr et al: Treatment outcomes in patients with adult thrombotic thrombocytopenic purpura-hemolytic uremic syndrome. *Arch Intern Med* 154:982, 1994.
187. Warkentin TE. History of heparin-induced thrombocytopenia, in *Heparin-Induced Thrombocytopenia,* edited by TE Warkentin, A Greinacher, p 1. Marcel Dekker, New York, 2004.
188. Chong BH, Berndt MC: Heparin-induced thrombocytopenia. *Blut* 58:53, 1989.
189. Fratantoni JC, Pollet R, Gralnick HR: Heparin-induced thrombocytopenia: Confirmation of diagnosis with in vitro methods. *Blood* 45:395, 1975.
190. Cines DB, Tomaski A, Tannenbaum S: Immune endothelial-cell injury in heparin-associated thrombocytopenia. *N Engl J Med* 316:581, 1987.
191. Kelton JG, Sheridan D, Santos A, et al: Heparin-induced thrombocytopenia: Laboratory studies. *Blood* 72:925, 1988.
192. Amiral J, Bridey F, Dreyfus M, et al: Platelet factor 4 complexed to heparin is the target for antibodies generated in heparin-induced thrombocytopenia. *Thromb Haemost* 68:95, 1992.
193. Merton RE, Thomas DP, Havercroft SJ, et al: High and low affinity heparin compared with unfractionated heparin as antithrombotic drugs. *Thromb Haemost* 51:254, 1984.
194. Green D, Martin GJ, Shoichet SH, et al: Thrombocytopenia in a prospective, randomized, double-blind trial of bovine and porcine heparin. *Am J Med Sci* 288:60, 1984.

195. Verma AK, Levine M, Shalansky SJ, et al: Frequency of heparin-induced thrombocytopenia in critical care patients. *Pharmacotherapy* 23:745, 2003.
196. Pouplard C, May MA, Iochmann S, et al: Antibodies to platelet factor 4-heparin after cardiopulmonary bypass in patients anticoagulated with unfractionated heparin or a low-molecular-weight heparin: Clinical implications for heparin-induced thrombocytopenia. *Circulation* 99:2530, 1999.
197. Warkentin TE, Levine MN, Hirsh J, et al: Heparin-induced thrombocytopenia in patients treated with low-molecular-weight heparin or unfractionated heparin. *N Engl J Med* 332:1330, 1995.
198. Lindhoff-Last E, Nakov R, Misselwitz F, et al: Incidence and clinical relevance of heparin-induced antibodies in patients with deep vein thrombosis treated with unfractionated or low-molecular-weight heparin. *Br J Haematol* 118:1137, 2002.
199. Ansell J, Slepchuk N Jr, Kumar R, et al: Heparin induced thrombocytopenia: A prospective study. *Thromb Haemost* 43:61, 1980.
200. D'Amico EA, Villaca PR, Gualandro SF, et al: Successful use of Arixtra in a patient with paroxysmal nocturnal hemoglobinuria, Budd-Chiari syndrome and heparin-induced thrombocytopenia. *J Thromb Haemost* 1:2452, 2003.
201. Girolami B, Prandoni P, Stefani PM, et al: The incidence of heparin-induced thrombocytopenia in hospitalized medical patients treated with subcutaneous unfractionated heparin: A prospective cohort study. *Blood* 101:2955, 2003.
202. Bauer TL, Arepally G, Konkle BA, et al: Prevalence of heparin-associated antibodies without thrombosis in patients undergoing cardiopulmonary bypass surgery. *Circulation* 95:1242, 1997.
203. Doty JR, Alving BM, McDonnell DE, Ondra SL: Heparin-associated thrombocytopenia in the neurosurgical patient. *Neurosurgery* 19:69, 1986.
204. Almeida JI, Liem TK, Silver D: Heparin-bonded grafts induce platelet aggregation in the presence of heparin-associated antiplatelet antibodies. *J Vasc Surg* 27:896, 1998.
205. Laster J, Silver D: Heparin-coated catheters and heparin-induced thrombocytopenia. *J Vasc Surg* 7:667, 1988.
206. Ranze O, Ranze P, Magnani HN, Greinacher A: Heparin-induced thrombocytopenia in paediatric patients—A review of the literature and a new case treated with danaparoid sodium. *Eur J Pediatr* 158 Suppl 3:S130, 1999.
207. O'Shea SI, Sands JJ, Nudo SA, Ortel TL: Frequency of anti-heparin-platelet factor 4 antibodies in hemodialysis patients and correlation with recurrent vascular access thrombosis. *Am J Hematol* 69:72, 2002.
208. Lindhoff-Last E, Bauersachs R: Heparin-induced thrombocytopenia-alternative anticoagulation in pregnancy and lactation. *Semin Thromb Hemost* 28:439, 2002.
209. Warkentin TE, Roberts RS, Hirsh J, Kelton JG: An improved definition of immune heparin-induced thrombocytopenia in postoperative orthopedic patients. *Arch Intern Med* 163:2518, 2003.
210. Masucci IP, Calis KA, Bartlett DL, et al: Thrombocytopenia after isolated limb or hepatic perfusions with melphalan: The risk of heparin-induced thrombocytopenia. *Ann Surg Oncol* 6:476, 1999.
211. Greinacher A, Eichler P, Lubenow N, et al: Heparin-induced thrombocytopenia with thromboembolic complications: Meta-analysis of 2 prospective trials to assess the value of parenteral treatment with lepirudin and its therapeutic aPTT range. *Blood* 96:846, 2000.
212. Wallis DE, Workman DL, Lewis BE, et al: Failure of early heparin cessation as treatment for heparin-induced thrombocytopenia. *Am J Med* 106:629, 1999.
213. Arepally G, Reynolds C, Tomaski A, et al: Comparison of PF4/heparin ELISA assay with the 14C-serotonin release assay in the diagnosis of heparin-induced thrombocytopenia. *Am J Clin Pathol* 104:648, 1995.
214. Reilly MP, Taylor SM, Hartman NK, et al: Heparin-induced thrombocytopenia/thrombosis in a transgenic mouse model requires human platelet factor 4 and platelet activation through FcgammaRIIA. *Blood* 98:2442, 2001.
215. Arepally GM, Kamei S, Park KS, et al: Characterization of a murine monoclonal antibody that mimics heparin-induced thrombocytopenia antibodies. *Blood* 95:1533, 2000.
216. Zhang X, Chen L, Bancroft DP, et al: Crystal structure of recombinant human platelet factor 4. *Biochemistry* 33:8361, 1994.
217. Stuckey JA, St Charles R, Edwards BF: A model of the platelet factor 4 complex with heparin. *Proteins* 14:277, 1992.
218. Li ZQ, Liu W, Park KS, et al: Defining a second epitope for heparin-induced thrombocytopenia/thrombosis antibodies using KKO, a murine HIT-like monoclonal antibody. *Blood* 99:1230, 2002.
219. Greinacher A, Potzsch B, Amiral J, et al: Heparin-associated thrombocytopenia: Isolation of the antibody and characterization of a multimolecular PF4-heparin complex as the major antigen. *Thromb Haemost* 71:247, 1994.
220. Horne MK 3rd, Alkins BR: Platelet binding of IgG from patients with heparin-induced thrombocytopenia. *J Lab Clin Med* 127:435, 1996.
221. Rauova L, Zhai L, Kowalska MA, et al: Role of platelet surface PF4 antigenic complexes in heparin-induced thrombocytopenia pathogenesis: Diagnostic and therapeutic implications. *Blood* 107:2346, 2006.
222. Suvarna S, Espinasse B, Qi R, et al: Determinants of PF4/heparin immunogenicity. *Blood* 110:4253, 2007.
223. Eslin DE, Zhang C, Samuels KJ, et al: Transgenic mice studies demonstrate a role for platelet factor 4 in thrombosis: Dissociation between anticoagulant and antithrombotic effect of heparin. *Blood* 104:3173, 2004.
224. Warkentin TE, Hayward CP, Boshkov LK, et al: Sera from patients with heparin-induced thrombocytopenia generate platelet-derived microparticles with procoagulant activity: An explanation for the thrombotic complications of heparin-induced thrombocytopenia. *Blood* 84:3691, 1994.
225. Visentin GP, Malik M, Cyganiak KA, Aster RH: Patients treated with unfractionated heparin during open heart surgery are at high risk to form antibodies reactive with heparin:platelet factor 4 complexes. *J Lab Clin Med* 128:376, 1996.
226. Pouplard C, Iochmann S, Renard B, et al: Induction of monocyte tissue factor expression by antibodies to heparin-platelet factor 4 complexes developed in heparin-induced thrombocytopenia. *Blood* 97:3300, 2001.
227. Arepally GM, Mayer IM: Antibodies from patients with heparin-induced thrombocytopenia stimulate monocytic cells to express tissue factor and secrete interleukin-8. *Blood* 98:1252, 2001.
228. Ma AD, Arepally G: HIT antibodies and monocyte signaling. *Blood* 100:16a, 2002.
229. Carlsson LE, Lubenow N, Blumentritt C, et al: Platelet receptor and clotting factor polymorphisms as genetic risk factors for thromboembolic complications in heparin-induced thrombocytopenia. *Pharmacogenetics* 13:253, 2003.
230. Arepally G, McKenzie SE, Jiang XM, et al: Fc gamma RIIA H/R 131 polymorphism, subclass-specific IgG anti-heparin/platelet factor 4 antibodies and clinical course in patients with heparin-induced thrombocytopenia and thrombosis. *Blood* 89:370, 1997.
231. Carlsson LE, Santoso S, Baurichter G, et al: Heparin-induced thrombocytopenia: New insights into the impact of the FcgammaRIIa-R-H131 polymorphism. *Blood* 92:1526, 1998.
232. Chong BH, Pilgrim RL, Cooley MA, Chesterman CN: Increased expression of platelet IgG Fc receptors in immune heparin-induced thrombocytopenia. *Blood* 81:988, 1993.
233. Suh JS, Malik MI, Aster RH, Visentin GP: Characterization of the humoral immune response in heparin-induced thrombocytopenia. *Am J Hematol* 54:196, 1997.
234. Warkentin TE: Heparin-induced thrombocytopenia: Pathogenesis and management. *Br J Haematol* 121:535, 2003.
235. Hong AP, Cook DJ, Sigouin CS, Warkentin TE: Central venous catheters and upper-extremity deep-vein thrombosis complicating immune heparin-induced thrombocytopenia. *Blood* 101:3049, 2003.
236. Rowland CH, Woodford PA, De Lisle-Hammond J, Nair B: Heparin-induced thrombocytopenia-thrombosis syndrome and bilateral adrenal haemorrhage after prophylactic heparin use. *Aust N Z J Med* 29:741, 1999.
237. Kyritsis AP, Williams EC, Schutta HS: Cerebral venous thrombosis due to heparin-induced thrombocytopenia. *Stroke* 21:1503, 1990.
238. Towne JB, Bernhard VM, Hussey C, Garancis JC: White clot syndrome. Peripheral vascular complications of heparin therapy. *Arch Surg* 114:372, 1979.
239. Warkentin TE, Kelton JG: A 14-year study of heparin-induced thrombocytopenia. *Am J Med* 101:502, 1996.
240. Nand S, Wong W, Yuen B, et al: Heparin-induced thrombocytopenia with thrombosis: Incidence, analysis of risk factors, and clinical outcomes in 108 consecutive patients treated at a single institution. *Am J Hematol* 56:12, 1997.
241. Lipton ME, Gould D: Case report: Heparin-induced thrombocytopenia—A complication presenting to the vascular radiologist. *Clin Radiol* 45:137, 1992.
242. Wutschert R, Piletta P, Bounameaux H: Adverse skin reactions to low molecular weight heparins: Frequency, management and prevention. *Drug Saf* 20:515, 1999.
243. Warkentin TE: Heparin-induced skin lesions. *Br J Haematol* 92:494, 1996.
244. Srinivasan AF, Rice L, Bartholomew JR, et al: Warfarin-induced skin necrosis and venous limb gangrene in the setting of heparin-induced thrombocytopenia. *Arch Intern Med* 164:66, 2004.
245. Warkentin TE: Heparin-induced thrombocytopenia: IgG-mediated platelet activation, platelet microparticle generation, and altered procoagulant/anticoagulant balance in the pathogenesis of thrombosis and venous limb gangrene complicating heparin-induced thrombocytopenia. *Transfus Med Rev* 10:249, 1996.
246. Betrosian AP, Theodossiades G, Lambroulis G, et al: Heparin-induced thrombocytopenia with pulmonary embolism and disseminated intravascular coagulation associated with low-molecular-weight heparin. *Am J Med Sci* 325:45, 2003.
247. Visentin GP, Ford SE, Scott JP, Aster RH: Antibodies from patients with heparin-induced thrombocytopenia/thrombosis are specific for platelet factor 4 complexed with heparin or bound to endothelial cells. *J Clin Invest* 93:81, 1994.
248. Cines DB, Kaywin P, Bina M, et al: Heparin-associated thrombocytopenia. *N Engl J Med* 303:788, 1980.
249. Greinacher A, Michels I, Kiefel V, Mueller-Eckhardt C: A rapid and sensitive test for diagnosing heparin-associated thrombocytopenia. *Thromb Haemost* 66:734, 1991.
250. Stewart MW, Etches WS, Boshkov LK, Gordon PA: Heparin-induced thrombocytopenia: An improved method of detection based on lumi-aggregometry. *Br J Haematol* 91:173, 1995.
251. Pauzner R, Greinacher A, Selleng K, et al: False positive tests for heparin induced thrombocytopenia in patients with antiphospholipid syndrome and systemic lupus erythematosus. *J Thromb Haemost* 7:1070, 2009.
252. Abrams CS, Cines DB: Thrombocytopenia after treatment with platelet glycoprotein IIb/IIIa inhibitors. *Curr Hematol Rep* 3:143, 2004.
253. Greinacher A, Michels I, Mueller-Eckhardt C: Heparin-associated thrombocytopenia: The antibody is not heparin specific. *Thromb Haemost* 67:545, 1992.
254. Meuleman DG: Orgaran (Org 10172): Its pharmacological profile in experimental models. *Haemostasis* 22:58, 1992.
255. Skoutakis VA: Danaparoid in the prevention of thromboembolic complications. *Ann Pharmacother* 31:876, 1997.
256. Chong BH, Ismail F, Cade J, et al: Heparin-induced thrombocytopenia: Studies with a new low molecular weight heparinoid, Org 10172. *Blood* 73:1592, 1989.

257. Newman PM, Swanson RL, Chong BH: Heparin-induced thrombocytopenia: IgG binding to PF4-heparin complexes in the fluid phase and cross-reactivity with low molecular weight heparin and heparinoid. *Thromb Haemost* 80:292, 1998.
258. Chong BH, Gallus AS, Cade JF, et al: Prospective randomised open-label comparison of danaparoid with dextran 70 in the treatment of heparin-induced thrombocytopaenia with thrombosis: A clinical outcome study. *Thromb Haemost* 86:1170, 2001.
259. Hermann JP, Kutryk MJ, Serruys PW: Clinical trials of direct thrombin inhibitors during invasive procedures. *Thromb Haemost* 78:367, 1997.
260. Vanholder R, Camez A, Veys N, et al: Pharmacokinetics of recombinant hirudin in hemodialyzed end-stage renal failure patients. *Thromb Haemost* 77:650, 1997.
261. Fischer KG, Liebe V, Hudek R, et al: Anti-hirudin antibodies alter pharmacokinetics and pharmacodynamics of recombinant hirudin. *Thromb Haemost* 89:973, 2003.
262. Okamoto S, Hijikata A, Kikumoto R, et al: Potent inhibition of thrombin by the newly synthesized arginine derivative No. 805. The importance of stereo-structure of its hydrophobic carboxamide portion. *Biochem Biophys Res Commun* 101:440, 1981.
263. Hursting MJ, Zehnder JL, Joffrion JL, et al: The international normalized ratio during concurrent warfarin and argatroban anticoagulation: Differential contributions of each agent and effects of the choice of thromboplastin used. *Clin Chem* 45:409, 1999.
264. Lubenow N, Eichler P, Leitz T, Greinacher A: Meta-analysis of three prospective studies of lepirudin in the prevention of thrombosis in patients with heparin-induced thrombocytopenia. *Blood* 100:501a, 2002.
265. Lewis BE, Wallis DE, Berkowitz SD, et al: Argatroban anticoagulant therapy in patients with heparin-induced thrombocytopenia. *Circulation* 103:1838, 2001.
266. Matthai WH, Hursting MJ, Lewis BE: Argatroban use in patients with a history of heparin-induced thrombocytopenia who require acute anticoagulation. *Blood* 98:45a, 2001.
267. Lobo B, Finch C, Howard A, Minhas S: Fondaparinux for the treatment of patients with acute heparin-induced thrombocytopenia. *Thromb Haemost* 99:208, 2008.
268. Alsaleh KA, Al-Nasser SM, Bates SM, et al: Delayed-onset HIT caused by low-molecular-weight heparin manifesting during fondaparinux prophylaxis. *Am J Hematol* 83:876, 2008.
269. Sadler JE: A new name in thrombosis, ADAMTS13. *Proc Natl Acad Sci U S A* 99:11552, 2002.
270. Riegert-Johnson DL, Sandhu N, Rajkumar SV, Patel R: Thrombotic thrombocytopenic purpura associated with a hepatic abscess due to *Actinomyces turicensis*. *Clin Infect Dis* 35:636, 2002.
271. Denneberg T, Friedberg M, Holmberg L, et al: Combined plasmapheresis and hemodialysis treatment for severe hemolytic-uremic syndrome following *Campylobacter* colitis. *Acta Paediatr Scand* 71:243, 1982.
272. Chamovitz BN, Hartstein AI, Alexander SR, et al: *Campylobacter jejuni*-associated hemolytic-uremic syndrome in a mother and daughter. *Pediatrics* 71:253, 1983.
273. Morton AR, Yu R, Waldek S, et al: *Campylobacter* induced thrombotic thrombocytopenic purpura. *Lancet* 2:1133, 1985.
274. George JN, Vesely SK, Terrell DR: The Oklahoma Thrombotic Thrombocytopenic Purpura-Hemolytic Uremic Syndrome (TTP-HUS) Registry: A community perspective of patients with clinically diagnosed TTP-HUS. *Semin Hematol* 41:60, 2004.
275. Coppo P, Adrie C, Azoulay E, et al: Infectious diseases as a trigger in thrombotic microangiopathies in intensive care unit (ICU) patients? *Intensive Care Med* 29:564, 2003.
276. Chang JC, Kathula SK: Various clinical manifestations in patients with thrombotic microangiopathy. *J Investig Med* 50:201, 2002.
277. Riggs SA, Wray NP, Waddell CC, et al: Thrombotic thrombocytopenic purpura complicating Legionnaires' disease. *Arch Intern Med* 142:2275, 1982.
278. Albaqali A, Ghuloom A, Al Arrayed A, et al: Hemolytic uremic syndrome in association with typhoid fever. *Am J Kidney Dis* 41:709, 2003.
279. Brandt J, Wong C, Mihm S, et al: Invasive pneumococcal disease and hemolytic uremic syndrome. *Pediatrics* 110:371, 2002.
280. Prober CG, Tune B, Hoder L: *Yersinia* pseudotuberculosis septicemia. *Am J Dis Child* 133:623, 1979.
281. Marty AM, Dumler JS, Imes G, et al: Ehrlichiosis mimicking thrombotic thrombocytopenic purpura. Case report and pathological correlation. *Hum Pathol* 26:920, 1995.
282. Modi KS, Dahl DC, Berkseth RO, et al: Human granulocytic ehrlichiosis presenting with acute renal failure and mimicking thrombotic thrombocytopenic purpura. A case report and review. *Am J Nephrol* 19:677, 1999.
283. Erdem F, Kiki I, Gundogdu M, Kaya H: Thrombotic thrombocytopenic purpura in a patient with Brucella infection is highly responsive to combined plasma infusion and antimicrobial therapy. *Med Princ Pract* 16:324, 2007.
284. Guidotti TL, Luetzeler J, di Sant' Agnese PA, Escaro DU: Fatal disseminated aspergillosis in a previously well young adult with cystic fibrosis. *Am J Med Sci* 283:157, 1982.
285. Safdar A, van Rhee F, Henslee-Downey JP, et al: *Candida glabrata* and *Candida krusei fungemia* after high-risk allogeneic marrow transplantation: No adverse effect of low-dose fluconazole prophylaxis on incidence and outcome. *Bone Marrow Transplant* 28:873, 2001.
286. Berberich FR, Cuene SA, Chard RL Jr, Hartmann JR: Thrombotic thrombocytopenic purpura. Three cases with platelet and fibrinogen survival studies. *J Pediatr* 84:503, 1974.
287. Glasgow LA, Balduzzi P: Isolation of Coxsackie virus group A, type 4, from a patient with hemolytic-uremic syndrome. *N Engl J Med* 273:754, 1965.
288. Ray CG, Tucker VL, Harris DJ, Cuppage FE, Chin TD: Enteroviruses associated with the hemolytic-uremic syndrome. *Pediatrics* 46:378, 1970.
289. O'Regan S, Robitaille P, Mongeau JG, McLaughlin B: The hemolytic uremic syndrome associated with ECHO 22 infection. *Clin Pediatr (Phila)* 19:125, 1980.
290. Shashaty GG, Atamer MA: Hemolytic uremic syndrome associated with infectious mononucleosis. *Am J Dis Child* 127:720, 1974.
291. Thompson CE, Damon LE, Ries CA, Linker CA: Thrombotic microangiopathies in the 1980s: Clinical features, response to treatment, and the impact of the human immunodeficiency virus epidemic. *Blood* 80:1890, 1992.
292. Myers TJ, Wakem CJ, Ball ED, Tremont SJ: Thrombotic thrombocytopenic purpura: Combined treatment with plasmapheresis and antiplatelet agents. *Ann Intern Med* 92:149, 1980.
293. Matsuda Y, Hara J, Miyoshi H, et al: Thrombotic microangiopathy associated with reactivation of human herpesvirus-6 following high-dose chemotherapy with autologous bone marrow transplantation in young children. *Bone Marrow Transplant* 24:919, 1999.
294. Ucar A, Fernandez HF, Byrnes JJ, et al: Thrombotic microangiopathy and retroviral infections: A 13-year experience. *Am J Hematol* 45:304, 1994.
295. Chan JCM, Eleff MG, Campbell RAA: The hemolytic-uremic syndrome in nonrelated adopted siblings. *J Pediatr* 75:1050, 1969.
296. Wasserstein A, Hill G, Goldfarb S, Goldberg M: Recurrent thrombotic thrombocytopenic purpura after viral infection. Clinical and histologic simulation of chronic glomerulonephritis. *Arch Intern Med* 141:685, 1981.
297. Kok RHJ, Wolfhagen MJHM, Klosters G: A syndrome resembling thrombotic thrombocytopenic purpura associated with human parvovirus B19 infection. *Clin Infect Dis* 32:311, 2001.
298. Wiersinga WJ, Scheepstra CG, Kasanardjo JS, et al: Dengue fever-induced hemolytic uremic syndrome. *Clin Infect Dis* 43:800, 2006.
299. Turner RC, Chaplinski TJ, Adams HG: Rocky Mountain spotted fever presenting as thrombotic thrombocytopenic purpura. *Am J Med* 81:153, 1986.
300. Reynolds PM, Jackson JM, Brine JA, Vivian AB: Thrombotic thrombocytopenic purpura—Remission following splenectomy. Report of a case and review of the literature. *Am J Med* 61:439, 1976.
301. Bar Meir E, Amital H, Levy Y, et al: Mycoplasma-pneumoniae-induced thrombotic thrombocytopenic purpura. *Acta Haematol* 103:112, 2000.
302. Tsai HM, Rice L, Sarode R, et al: Antibody inhibitors to von Willebrand factor metalloproteinase and increased binding of von Willebrand factor to platelets in ticlopidine-associated thrombotic thrombocytopenic purpura. *Ann Intern Med* 132:794, 2000.
303. Zakarija A, Bandarenko N, Pandey DK, et al: Clopidogrel-associated TTP: An update of pharmacovigilance efforts conducted by independent researchers, pharmaceutical suppliers, and the Food and Drug Administration. *Stroke* 35:533, 2004.
304. Bennett CL, Connors JM, Carwile JM, et al: Thrombotic thrombocytopenic purpura associated with clopidogrel. *N Engl J Med* 342:1773, 2000.
305. Fujita H, Takemura S, Hyo R, et al: Pulmonary embolism and thrombotic thrombocytopenic purpura in acute promyelocytic leukemia treated with all-*trans* retinoic acid. *Leuk Lymphoma* 44:1627, 2003.
306. van der Heijden M, Ackland SP, Deveridge S: Haemolytic uraemic syndrome associated with bleomycin, epirubicin and cisplatin chemotherapy—A case report and review of the literature. *Acta Oncol* 37:107, 1998.
307. Palmisano J, Agraharkar M, Kaplan AA: Successful treatment of cisplatin-induced hemolytic uremic syndrome with therapeutic plasma exchange. *Am J Kidney Dis* 32:314, 1998.
308. Kressel BR, Ryan KP, Duong AT, et al: Microangiopathic hemolytic anemia, thrombocytopenia, and renal failure in patients treated for adenocarcinoma. *Cancer* 48:1738, 1981.
309. Byrnes JJ, Baquerizo H, Gonzalez M, Hensely GT: Thrombotic thrombocytopenic purpura subsequent to acute myelogenous leukemia chemotherapy. *Am J Hematol* 21:299, 1986.
310. Sakai C, Takagi T, Wakatsuki S, Matsuzaki O: Hemolytic-uremic syndrome due to deoxycoformycin: A report of the second case. *Intern Med* 34:593, 1995.
311. Tassinari D, Sartori S, Panzini I, et al: Hemolytic-uremic syndrome during therapy with estramustine phosphate for advanced prostatic cancer. *Oncology* 56:112, 1999.
312. Fung MC, Storniolo AM, Nguyen B, et al: A review of hemolytic uremic syndrome in patients treated with gemcitabine therapy. *Cancer* 85:2023, 1999.
313. Laffay DL, Tubbs RR, Valenzuela R, et al: Chronic glomerular microangiopathy and metastatic carcinoma. *Hum Pathol* 10:433, 1979.
314. Montes A, Powles TJ, O'Brien ME, et al: A toxic interaction between mitomycin C and tamoxifen causing the haemolytic uraemic syndrome. *Eur J Cancer* 29A:1854, 1993.
315. Eremina V, Jefferson JA, Kowalewska J, et al: VEGF inhibition and renal thrombotic microangiopathy. *N Engl J Med* 358:1129, 2008.
316. Bollee G, Patey N, Cazajous G, et al: Thrombotic microangiopathy secondary to VEGF pathway inhibition by sunitinib. *Nephrol Dial Transplant* 24:682, 2009.
317. Ahmed F, Sumalnop V, Spain DM, Tobin MS: Thrombohemolytic thrombocytopenic purpura during penicillamine therapy. *Arch Intern Med* 138:1292, 1978.
318. Harrison EE, Hickman JW: Hemolytic anemia and thrombocytopenia associated with penicillamine ingestion. *South Med J* 68:113, 1975.
319. Abramowicz D, Pradier O, Marchant A, et al: Induction of thromboses within renal grafts by high-dose prophylactic OKT3. *Lancet* 339:777, 1992.
320. Ravandi-Kashani F, Cortes J, Talpaz M, Kantarjian HM: Thrombotic microangiopathy associated with interferon therapy for patients with chronic myelogenous leukemia: Coincidence or true side effect? *Cancer* 85:2583, 1999.

321. Al-Zahrani H, Gupta V, Minden MD, et al: Vascular events associated with alpha interferon therapy. *Leuk Lymphoma* 44:471, 2003.
322. Ubara Y, Hara S, Takedatu H, et al: Hemolytic uremic syndrome associated with beta-interferon therapy for chronic hepatitis C. *Nephron* 80:107, 1998.
323. Schoenmaker NJ, Weening JJ, Krediet RT: Ibuprofen-induced HUS. *Clin Nephrol* 68:177, 2007.
324. Allan DS, Thompson CM, Barr RM, et al: Ciprofloxacin-associated hemolytic-uremic syndrome. *Ann Pharmacother* 36:1000, 2002.
325. Alexopoulou A, Dourakis SP, Kaloterakis A: Thrombotic thrombocytopenic purpura in a patient treated with clarithromycin. *Eur J Haematol* 69:191, 2002.
326. Baron BW, van Besien K, Hoffman PC, et al: Thrombotic thrombocytopenic purpura after cephalosporin administration: A possible relationship. *Transfusion* 43:1317, 2003.
327. Yata Y, Miyagiwa M, Inatsuchi S, et al: Thrombotic thrombocytopenia purpura caused by piperacillin successfully treated with plasma infusion. *Ann Hematol* 79:593, 2000.
328. Fahal IH, Williams PS, Clark RE, Bell GM: Thrombotic thrombocytopenic purpura due to rifampicin. *BMJ* 304:882, 1992.
329. Powell HR, Davidson PM, McCredie DA, et al: Haemolytic-uraemic syndrome after treatment with metronidazole. *Med J Aust* 149:222, 1988.
330. Rivkin A: Thrombotic thrombocytopenic purpura induced by metronidazole vaginal gel. *Pharmacotherapy* 27:1058, 2007.
331. Castelman B, McNeely BU: Case records of the Massachusetts General Hospital. Case 1–1968. *N Engl J Med* 278:36, 1968.
332. Parker JC, Barrett DA 2nd: Microangiopathic hemolysis and thrombocytopenia related to penicillin drugs. *Arch Intern Med* 127:474, 1971.
333. Symmers WS: Thrombotic microangiopathy (thrombotic thrombocytopenic purpura) associated with acute haemorrhagic leucoencephalitis and sensitivity to oxophenarsine. *Brain* 79:511, 1956.
334. Bell WR, Chulay JD, Feinberg JE: Manifestations resembling thrombotic microangiopathy in patients with advanced human immunodeficiency virus (HIV) disease in a cytomegalovirus prophylaxis trial (ACTG 204). *Medicine (Baltimore)* 76:369, 1997.
335. Feinberg JE, Hurwitz S, Cooper D, et al: A randomized, double-blind trial of valacyclovir prophylaxis for cytomegalovirus disease in patients with advanced human immunodeficiency virus infection. AIDS Clinical Trials Group Protocol 204/Glaxo Wellcome 123–014 International CMV Prophylaxis Study Group. *J Infect Dis* 177:48, 1998.
336. Ryz K, Klassen J, Gough J, Ahmed SB: Famciclovir and development of thrombotic thrombocytopenic purpura. *Ther Apher Dial* 11:458, 2007.
337. Fiaccadori E, Maggiore U, Rotelli C, et al: Thrombotic-thrombocytopenic purpura following malaria prophylaxis with mefloquine. *J Antimicrob Chemother* 57:160, 2006.
338. Hauglustaine D, Van Damme B, Vanrenterghem Y, Michielsen P: Recurrent hemolytic uremic syndrome during oral contraception. *Clin Nephrol* 15:148, 1981.
339. McShane PM, Bern MM, Schiff I: Thrombotic thrombocytopenic purpura associated with oral contraceptives: A case report. *Am J Obstet Gynecol* 145:762, 1983.
340. Liang R, Wong RW, Cheng IK: Thrombotic thrombocytopenic purpura and 17 beta-estradiol transdermal skin patch. *Am J Hematol* 52:334, 1996.
341. Au WY, Chan KW, Lam CC, Young K: A post-menopausal woman with anuria and uterus bulk: The spectrum of estrogen-induced TTP/HUS. *Am J Hematol* 71:59, 2002.
342. Keung YK, Morgan D, Cobos E: Cocaine-induced microangiopathic hemolytic anemia and thrombocytopenia simulating thrombotic thrombocytopenia purpura. *Ann Hematol* 72:155, 1996.
343. Volcy J, Nzerue CM, Oderinde A, Hewan-Iowe K: Cocaine-induced acute renal failure, hemolysis, and thrombocytopenia mimicking thrombotic thrombocytopenic purpura. *Am J Kidney Dis* 35:E3, 2000.
344. Tumlin JA, Sands JM, Someren A: Hemolytic-uremic syndrome following "crack" cocaine inhalation. *Am J Med Sci* 299:366, 1990.
345. Peces R, Diaz-Corte C, Baltar J, et al: Haemolytic-uraemic syndrome in a heroin addict. *Nephrol Dial Transplant* 13:3197, 1998.
346. Schirren CA, Berghaus TM, Sackmann M: Thrombotic thrombocytopenic purpura after Ecstasy-induced acute liver failure. *Ann Intern Med* 130:163, 1999.
347. McCarthy LJ, Porcu P, Fausel CA, et al: Thrombotic thrombocytopenic purpura and simvastatin. *Lancet* 352:1284, 1998.
348. Kallal SM, Lee M: Thrombotic thrombocytopenic purpura associated with histamine H_2-receptor antagonist therapy. *West J Med* 164:446, 1996.
349. Blecher TE, Raper AB: Early diagnosis of thrombotic microangiopathy by paraffin sections of aspirated bone-marrow. *Arch Dis Child* 42:158, 1967.
350. Karim Y, Masood A: Haemolytic uraemic syndrome following mumps, measles, and rubella vaccination. *Nephrol Dial Transplant* 17:941, 2002.
351. Peyriere H, Klouche K, Beraud JJ, et al: Fatal systemic reaction after multiple doses of intravesical bacillus Calmette-Guerin for polyposis. *Ann Pharmacother* 34:1279, 2000.
352. Brown RC, Blecher TE, French EA, Toghill PJ: Thrombotic thrombocytopenic purpura after influenza vaccination. *Br Med J* 2:303, 1973.
353. Jones MB, Armitage JO, Stone DB: Self-limited TTP-like syndrome after bee sting. *JAMA* 242:2212, 1979.
354. Ashley JR, Otero H, Aboulafia DM: Bee envenomation: A rare cause of thrombotic thrombocytopenic purpura. *South Med J* 96:588, 2003.
355. Mele L, Voso MT, Fianchi L, et al: Thrombotic thrombocytopenic purpura-hemolytic uremic syndrome after bupropion treatment for smoking cessation. *Blood Coagul Fibrinolysis* 14:77, 2003.
356. Stonesifer LD, Bone RC, Hiller FC: Thrombotic thrombocytopenic purpura in carbon monoxide poisoning. Report of a case. *Arch Intern Med* 140:104, 1980.
357. Pilz P: Moschcowitz syndrome with involvement of the central nervous system. Light optical studies on the genesis of hemolytic anemia and vascular changes. *Virchows Arch A Pathol Anat Histol* 366:59, 1975.
358. Mutter WP, Stillman IE, Dahl NK: Thrombotic microangiopathy and renal failure exacerbated by epsilon-aminocaproic acid. *Am J Kidney Dis* 53:346, 2009.
359. Liatsos G, Elefsiniotis I, Todorova R, Moulakakis A: Severe thrombotic thrombocytopenic purpura (TTP) induced or exacerbated by the immunostimulatory herb Echinacea. *Am J Hematol* 81:224, 2006.
360. Huynh M, Chee K, Lau DH: Thrombotic thrombocytopenic purpura associated with quetiapine. *Ann Pharmacother* 39:1346, 2005.

CHAPTER 134
VENOUS THROMBOSIS

Gary E. Raskob, Russell D. Hull, and Graham F. Pineo

SUMMARY

Venous thromboembolism (deep vein thrombosis and/or pulmonary embolism) is a common disorder, which is estimated to affect 900,000 patients each year in the United States. Approximately one-third of these cases are fatal pulmonary emboli, and the remaining two-thirds are nonfatal episodes of symptomatic deep vein thrombosis or pulmonary embolism. The majority of fatal events occur as sudden or abrupt death, underscoring the importance of prevention as the critical strategy for reducing death from pulmonary embolism. Of the estimated 600,000 cases of nonfatal venous thromboembolism each year, approximately 60 percent present clinically as deep vein thrombosis and 40 percent present as pulmonary embolism. Most clinically important pulmonary emboli arise from proximal deep vein thrombosis (thrombosis involving the popliteal, femoral, or iliac veins). Upper extremity deep vein thrombosis also may lead to clinically important pulmonary embolism. The clinical features of deep vein thrombosis and pulmonary embolism are nonspecific. Objective diagnostic testing is required to confirm or exclude the presence of venous thromboembolism. An appropriately validated assay for plasma D-dimer, if available, provides a simple, rapid, and cost-effective first-line exclusion test in patients with low, unlikely, or intermediate clinical probability. Compression ultrasonography of the proximal veins performed at presentation, and if normal, repeated once 5 to 7 days later, can safely exclude clinically important deep vein thrombosis in symptomatic patients. In centers with the expertise, a single comprehensive evaluation of the proximal and calf veins with duplex ultrasonography is sufficient. If capability for combined computed tomographic angiography (CTA) and computed tomographic venography (CTV) exists, it is the preferred approach for most patients with suspected pulmonary embolism because it provides a definitive basis to give or withhold antithrombotic therapy in 90 percent of patients. CTA is not inferior to using ventilation–perfusion lung scanning for excluding the diagnosis of pulmonary embolism when either test is used together with venous ultrasonography of the legs. Anticoagulant therapy is the preferred treatment for most patients with acute venous thromboembolism. Initial treatment with subcutaneous low-molecular-weight heparin or fondaparinux, followed by long-term treatment with an oral vitamin K antagonist such as warfarin sodium, is effective for preventing recurrent venous thromboembolism. Use of low-molecular-weight heparin or fondaparinux enables outpatient therapy and is the preferred initial therapy for most patients. Treatment with low-molecular-weight heparin for at least 6 months is preferred in cancer patients and should be continued if cancer is not resolved. Thrombolytic therapy is indicated for patients with pulmonary embolism who present with cardiovascular collapse and in selected patients who have impaired right ventricular function. Insertion of a vena cava filter is indicated for patients who have an absolute contraindication to anticoagulant therapy or who have recurrent venous thromboembolism despite adequate anticoagulant treatment. Anticoagulant treatment should be continued for at least 3 months in patients with a first episode of venous thromboembolism secondary to a reversible risk factor. Indefinite anticoagulant therapy should be considered for patients with idiopathic venous thromboembolism, certain thrombophilias, or recurrent venous thromboembolism.

Acronyms and abbreviations that appear in this chapter include: aPTT, activated partial thromboplastin time; CT, computed tomography; CTA, computed tomographic angiography; CTV, computed tomographic venography; ELISA, enzyme-linked immunosorbent assay; INR, international normalized ratio; LMW, low molecular weight; MRI, magnetic resonance imaging; PIOPED, Prospective Investigation of Pulmonary Embolism Diagnosis.

DEFINITION AND EPIDEMIOLOGY

Venous thrombosis commonly develops in the deep veins of the leg or the arm or in the superficial veins of these extremities. Superficial venous thrombosis is a relatively benign disorder unless extension into the deep venous system occurs. Thrombosis involving the deep veins of the leg is divided into two prognostic categories: (1) calf vein thrombosis, in which thrombi remain confined to the deep calf veins; and (2) proximal vein thrombosis, in which thrombosis involves the popliteal, femoral, or iliac veins.[1]

Pulmonary emboli originate from thrombi in the deep veins of the leg in 90 percent or more of patients. Other less common sources of pulmonary embolism include the deep pelvic veins, renal veins, inferior vena cava, right side of the heart, and axillary veins. Most clinically important pulmonary emboli arise from proximal deep vein thrombosis of the leg. Upper extremity deep vein thrombosis also may lead to important pulmonary embolism.[2] Deep vein thrombosis and/or pulmonary embolism are referred to collectively as *venous thromboembolism*.

Venous thromboembolism is a common disorder. The estimated annual incidence of clinically evident venous thromboembolism in the United States was 117 per 100,000 population (~250,000 cases per year) through 1998.[3] A more recent modeling suggested that there are more than 900,000 incident or recurrent venous thromboembolism events per year[4] Based on this more recent estimate, approximately one-third of the cases (300,000) are fatal pulmonary embolism, and the remaining two-thirds are nonfatal episodes of deep vein thrombosis or pulmonary embolism. The estimated annual number of deaths from pulmonary embolism in the United States is more than the combined total number of deaths from breast cancer, HIV disease, and motor vehicle crashes.[5] The majority of fatal events occur as sudden or abrupt death, underscoring the importance of prevention as the most critical intervention for reducing death from pulmonary embolism. Of the estimated 600,000 cases of nonfatal venous thromboembolism each year, approximately 60 percent are cases of deep vein thrombosis and 40 percent are episodes of pulmonary embolism. The incidence of venous thromboembolism increases markedly in patients of age 60 years or more. The aging of the population, therefore, has major implications with respect to the expected future burden of disease from venous thromboembolism.

Effective prophylaxis against venous thromboembolism is available for most high-risk patients. Use of prophylaxis is more effective for preventing death and morbidity from venous thromboembolism than is treatment of the established disease. Evidence-based recommendations for prevention of venous thromboembolism are available.[6]

Historically, venous thromboembolism usually occurred in hospitalized patients. The burden of illness from venous thromboembolism has shifted to the community setting such that most patients now present as outpatients to their primary care physician or to the emergency room. The main reason for this shift is the greatly reduced length of hospital stay for most surgical procedures or medical conditions and the discharge of patients from the hospital either before the period of risk of venous thromboembolism has ended or who have subclinical venous thrombi that subsequently evolve and lead to symptomatic deep vein thrombosis or pulmonary embolism. The shift in burden of illness from the hospital to the community setting has led to an emphasis on effective and safe methods for outpatient diagnosis and management.

ETIOLOGY AND PATHOGENESIS

Venous thrombi are composed mainly of fibrin and red blood cells, with variable numbers of platelets and leukocytes. The formation, growth, and breakdown of venous thromboemboli reflect a balance between thrombogenic stimuli and protective mechanisms. The thrombogenic stimuli first identified by Virchow in the 19th century are (1) venous stasis, (2) activation of blood coagulation, and (3) vascular damage. The protective mechanisms are (1) inactivation of activated coagulation factors by circulating inhibitors (e.g., antithrombin bound to heparan sulfate at blood vessel walls and activated protein C), (2) clearance of activated coagulation factors and soluble fibrin polymer complexes by mononuclear phagocytes and the liver, and (3) lysis of fibrin by fibrinolytic enzymes derived from plasma and endothelial cells.

Pulmonary embolism occurs in at least 50 percent of patients with documented proximal vein thrombosis.[1] Many of these emboli are asymptomatic. The clinical importance of pulmonary embolism depends on the size of the embolus and the patient's cardiorespiratory reserve. Usually only part of the thrombus embolizes, and 30 to 70 percent of patients with pulmonary embolism detected by angiography also have identifiable deep vein thrombosis of the legs.[7,8] Deep vein thrombosis and pulmonary embolism are not separate disorders but a continuous syndrome of venous thromboembolism in which the initial clinical presentation may be symptoms of either deep vein thrombosis or pulmonary embolism. Therefore, strategies for diagnosis of venous thromboembolism include both tests for detection of pulmonary embolism (lung scanning, computed tomography [CT], or pulmonary angiography)[8–10] and tests for deep vein thrombosis of the legs (ultrasonography or venography)[11–13] (see "Objective Testing for Pulmonary Embolism" and "Objective Testing for Deep Vein Thrombosis" below).

TABLE 134–1. Risk Factors for Thromboembolism*

Acquired	Hereditary Thrombophilias
Advancing age (age >40 years)	Activated protein C resistance
History of prior thromboembolic event	Prothrombin G20210A
Recent surgery	Antithrombin deficiency
Recent trauma	Protein C deficiency
Prolonged immobilization	Protein S deficiency
Certain forms of cancer	Dysfibrinogenemia
Congestive heart failure	
Recent myocardial infarction	
Paralysis of legs	
Use of female hormones	
Pregnancy or postpartum period	
Varicose veins	
Obesity	
Antiphospholipid antibody syndrome	
Hyperhomocysteinemia	

*See also Chap. 131.

Acquired and inherited risk factors for venous thromboembolism have been identified[14–16] and are shown in Table 134–1 (see also Chap. 131). The risk of thromboembolism increases when more than one predisposing factor is present.

Activated protein C resistance is the most common hereditary abnormality predisposing to venous thromboembolism. The defect results from substitution of glutamine for arginine at residue 506 in the factor V molecule, making factor Va resistant to proteolysis by activated protein C. The gene mutation is commonly designated *factor V Leiden* and follows autosomal dominant inheritance. Patients who are homozygous for the factor V Leiden mutation have a markedly increased risk of thromboembolism and present with clinical thromboembolism at a younger age (median age: 31 years) than those who are heterozygous (median age: 46 years).[14,16] Factor V Leiden is present in approximately 5 percent of the normal white population, 16 percent of patients with a first episode of deep vein thrombosis, and up to 35 percent of patients with idiopathic deep vein thrombosis.[14,16,17] Prothrombin G20210A is another gene mutation that predisposes to venous thromboembolism. It is present in approximately 2 to 3 percent of apparently healthy individuals and in 7 percent of those with deep vein thrombosis.[16] An inherited abnormality cannot be detected in up to 40 to 60 percent of patients with idiopathic deep vein thrombosis, suggesting that as yet undefined gene mutations are present that have an etiologic role (see Chap. 131).

CLINICAL FEATURES

VENOUS THROMBOSIS

The clinical features of venous thrombosis include leg pain, tenderness, and swelling, a palpable cord representing a thrombosed vessel, discoloration, venous distention, prominence of the superficial veins, and cyanosis. The clinical diagnosis of deep vein thrombosis is highly nonspecific because each of the symptoms or signs can be caused by nonthrombotic disorders. The rare exception is the patient with phlegmasia cerulea dolens (occlusion of the whole venous circulation, extreme swelling of the leg, and compromised arterial flow), in whom the diagnosis of massive iliofemoral thrombosis is obvious. This syndrome occurs in less than 1 percent of patients with symptomatic venous thrombosis. In most patients, the symptoms and signs are nonspecific. In 50 to 85 percent of patients, the clinical suspicion of deep vein thrombosis is not confirmed by objective testing.[11–13] Patients with minor symptoms and signs may have extensive deep venous thrombi. Conversely, patients with florid leg pain and swelling, suggesting extensive deep vein thrombosis, may have negative results by objective testing.

Although the clinical diagnosis is nonspecific, prospective studies have established that patients can be categorized as low, moderate, or high probability for deep vein thrombosis using a clinical prediction rule that incorporates signs, symptoms, and risk factors. A systematic review[18] of the studies found that the prevalence of deep vein thrombosis in the low, moderate, and high probability categories was 5 percent (95% confidence interval: 4 to 8%), 17 percent (95% confidence interval: 13 to 23%), and 53 percent (95% confidence interval: 44 to 61%). Thus, the prevalence in the pretest category of "low probability" is not sufficiently low to withhold further diagnostic testing and treatment, and the prevalence in the "high probability" category is not sufficiently high to give anticoagulant therapy without performing further diagnostic testing. The key role for clinical pretest categorization is for use within integrated diagnostic strategies employing measurement of D-dimer and venous imaging.

PULMONARY EMBOLISM

The clinical features of acute pulmonary embolism include the following symptoms and signs that may overlap: (1) transient dyspnea and tachypnea in the absence of other clinical features; (2) pleuritic chest pain, cough, hemoptysis, pleural effusion, and pulmonary infiltrates noted on chest radiogram caused by pulmonary infarction or congestive atelectasis (also known as *ischemic pneumonitis* or *incomplete infarction*); (3) severe dyspnea and tachypnea and right-side heart failure; (4) cardiovascular collapse with hypotension, syncope, and coma (usually associated with massive pulmonary embolism); and (5) several less common and nonspecific clinical presentations, including unexplained tachycardia or arrhythmia, resistant cardiac failure, wheezing, cough, fever, anxiety/apprehension, and confusion. All of these clinical features are nonspecific and can be caused by a variety of cardiorespiratory disorders. Patients can be assigned to categories of pretest probability using implicit clinical judgement, or clinical decision rules such as the Geneva score or approach of Wells.[19,20] However, the prevalences of pulmonary embolism in these categories are not sufficiently low or high to withhold further investigation altogether based on clinical features alone, and the measurement of D-dimer and/or diagnostic imaging is mandatory to exclude or confirm the presence of pulmonary embolism. The assessment of clinical pretest probability is an important first step in integrated diagnostic strategies that employ clinical probability, D-dimer, CT angiography, lung scanning, and objective testing for deep vein thrombosis.[19,20]

LABORATORY FEATURES

Venous thromboembolism is associated with nonspecific laboratory changes that constitute the acute phase response to tissue injury. This response includes elevated levels of fibrinogen and factor VIII, increases in leukocyte and platelet counts, and systemic activation of blood coagulation, fibrin formation, and fibrin breakdown, with increases in plasma concentrations of prothrombin fragment 1.2, fibrinopeptide A, complexes of thrombin–antithrombin, and fibrin degradation products. All of these changes are nonspecific and may occur as a result of surgery, trauma, infection, inflammation, or infarction. None of the reported laboratory changes can be used to predict the development of venous thromboembolism.

The fibrin breakdown fragment D-dimer can be measured by an enzyme-linked immunosorbent assay (ELISA) or by a latex agglutination assay. Some of these assays have a rapid turnaround time and some are quantitative. A negative D-dimer result is useful for excluding the diagnosis in patients with suspected deep vein thrombosis or suspected pulmonary embolism (see "Objective Testing for Pulmonary Embolism" and "Objective Testing for Deep Vein Thrombosis" below).[10,19–21] A positive result is highly nonspecific.

DIFFERENTIAL DIAGNOSIS OF DEEP VEIN THROMBOSIS

The differential diagnosis in patients with clinically suspected deep vein thrombosis includes muscle strain or tear, direct twisting injury to the leg, lymphangitis or lymphatic obstruction, venous reflux, popliteal cyst, cellulitis, leg swelling in a paralyzed limb, and abnormality of the knee joint. An alternate diagnosis frequently is not evident at presentation, so excluding deep vein thrombosis is not possible without objective testing. The cause of symptoms often can be determined by careful followup once deep vein thrombosis has been excluded by objective testing. In approximately 25 percent of patients, however, the cause of pain, tenderness, and swelling remains uncertain even after careful followup.[13]

OBJECTIVE TESTING FOR DEEP VEIN THROMBOSIS

D-DIMER ASSAY

Measurement of plasma D-dimer has been extensively evaluated as an exclusion test in patients with clinically suspected deep vein thrombosis.[21] The different D-dimer assays (ELISA, quantitative rapid ELISA, latex agglutination, and whole blood agglutination) have different sensitivities, specificities, and likelihood ratios for deep vein thrombosis. ELISA and quantitative rapid ELISA have high sensitivity (96%) and negative likelihood ratios of approximately 0.10 for deep vein thrombosis in symptomatic patients. Thus, for excluding deep vein thrombosis in symptomatic patients, a negative D-dimer result by a quantitative rapid ELISA technique is as diagnostically useful as a negative result by duplex ultrasonography.[21] Measurement of D-dimer using an appropriate assay method can be combined with ultrasonograph imaging. If the two tests are negative at presentation, repeat ultrasonograph imaging is unecessary.[22] Use of the D-dimer test for patient care decisions depends on the local availability of an appropriate assay that has high sensitivity and has been validated by clinical outcome studies. Figure 134–1 shows a practical approach for the diagnosis of suspected deep vein thrombosis.

IMAGING TESTS

The objective diagnostic imaging tests that have a role in patients with clinically suspected deep vein thrombosis are ultrasonography and venography. Both of these tests have been validated by properly designed clinical trials, including prospective studies with long-term followup that have established the safety of withholding anticoagulant treatment in patients with negative test results.[11–13,23]

Ultrasonography using vein compression is effective for identifying patients with proximal vein thrombosis. Compression ultrasonography of the proximal veins performed at presentation (and, if normal, repeated once 5 to 7 days later) can safely replace venography in symptomatic patients.[11] In centers with experienced ultrasonography staff, a single comprehensive evaluation of the proximal and calf veins with duplex ultrasonography is sufficient and, if negative, a repeat test is not required.[12] A randomized trial supports the equivalence of a comprehensive whole-leg color-coded Doppler ultrasonography approach to that of an approach using combined D-dimer testing and repeated ultrasonography for the management of suspected deep vein thrombosis.[24]

The positive predictive value of a positive ultrasonographic result isolated to the calf veins may vary among centers based on expertise and thrombosis prevalence. Therefore, the number of repeat ultrasonographic evaluations avoided by evaluating the calf veins may be partially offset by an increased number of patients with positive ultrasonography results confined to the calf, for whom additional diagnostic testing and/or anticoagulant treatment is required. Most patients with a negative ultrasonographic result at presentation require a followup visit to establish the alternate diagnosis and to guide further care, so the return visit for repeat ultrasonography at 5 to 7 days may have added practical value.[11] Venography continues to have a role in selected patients, such as those in whom ultrasonography is unavailable or inconclusive or in whom repeat testing is impractical.

Diagnosis of acute recurrent deep vein thrombosis is particularly challenging because recurrent symptoms such as pain and swelling are common in patients with deep vein thrombosis despite adequate

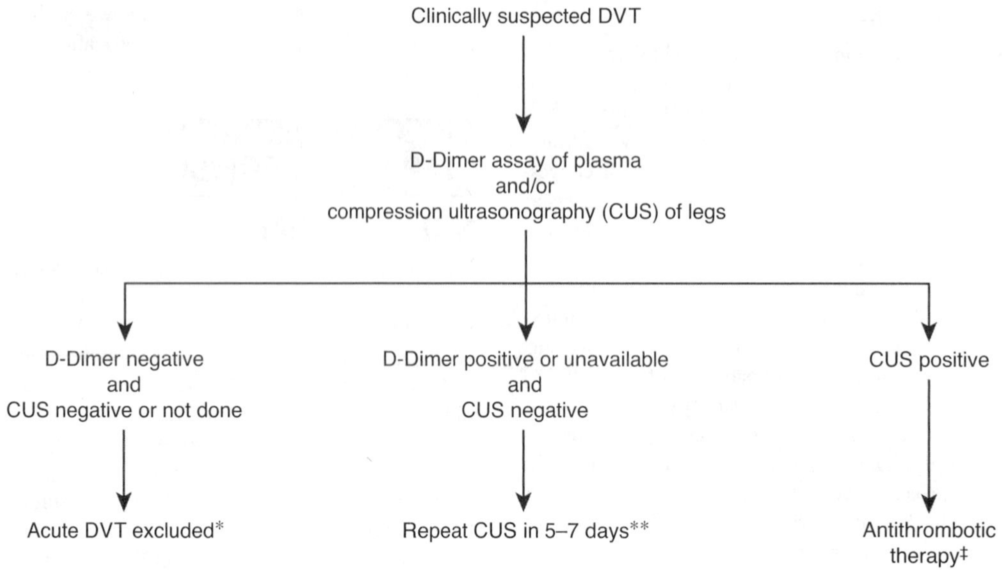

FIGURE 134–1. Diagnosis of patients with suspected first episode of deep vein thrombosis (DVT). *Negative D-dimer can be used to exclude acute DVT, without the need for further diagnostic testing with compression ultrasonography (CUS), if the patient has low, unlikely, moderate, or intermediate clinical probability.[18,21] Ultrasonography should be performed in patients with a high clinical probability. A negative D-dimer can also be used with a negative CUS at presentation to exclude acute DVT without the need for a repeat CUS.[22,24] **CUS is performed with imaging of the common femoral vein in the groin and of the popliteal vein in the popliteal fossa extending distally 10 cm from midpatella. A repeat CUS is required in 5 to 7 days to detect extending calf vein thrombi.[11] In centers with the expertise, a single negative result of full-leg duplex ultrasonography (CUS plus flow evaluation) is sufficient to exclude acute DVT.[12,24] ‡CUS that indicates noncompressibility of deep vein segments is highly predictive of DVT (>95%) and provides an indication for antithrombotic therapy in most patients. If CUS is positive at a single site isolated in the groin, additional testing with venography, computed tomography, or magnetic resonance imaging should be performed because of the potential for false-positive CUS results from disorders producing vein compression in the groin (e.g., tumor mass).

anticoagulant therapy, and because both ultrasonography and venography have limitations for excluding the presence of acute recurrent deep vein thrombosis.[25] Compression ultrasonography may remain abnormal for 1 year in 50 percent of patients, and for even longer in some patients,[26] because of persistent noncompressibility of the vein caused by fibrous organization of the original thrombus. Venography is of limited value for excluding the diagnosis of recurrent deep vein thrombosis because of obliteration or recanalization of the previously affected venous segments or nonfilled venous segments. Thus, measurement of plasma D-dimer may be particularly useful as an exclusion test in patients with suspected acute recurrent deep vein thrombosis. However, use of D-dimer must be evaluated separately in this patient group because many patients with a past history of venous thromboembolism are receiving long-term oral anticoagulant therapy, which has the potential to cause a false-negative D-dimer result. Promising initial results were obtained in one study,[27] but further studies in larger numbers of patients are needed before using a negative D-dimer alone to exclude acute recurrent deep vein thrombosis can be routinely recommended.

DIFFERENTIAL DIAGNOSIS OF PULMONARY EMBOLISM

The differential diagnosis in patients with suspected pulmonary embolism includes cardiopulmonary disorders for each of the modes of presentation (see "Pulmonary Embolism" above). For the presentation of dyspnea and tachypnea, they include atelectasis, pneumonia, pleuritis, pneumothorax, acute pulmonary edema, bronchitis, bronchiolitis, and acute bronchial obstruction. For pulmonary infarction exhibited by pleuritic chest pain or hemoptysis, they include pneumonia, pneumothorax, pericarditis, pulmonary or bronchial neoplasm, bronchiectasis, acute bronchitis, tuberculosis, diaphragmatic inflammation, myositis, muscle strain, and rib fracture. For the clinical presentation of right-side heart failure, they include myocardial infarction, myocarditis, and cardiac tamponade. For cardiovascular collapse, they include myocardial infarction, acute massive hemorrhage, Gram-negative septicemia, cardiac tamponade, and spontaneous pneumothorax.

OBJECTIVE TESTING FOR PULMONARY EMBOLISM

The objective diagnostic imaging tests include CT, computed tomographic angiography (CTA), radionuclide lung scanning, selective pulmonary arteriography, magnetic resonance imaging (MRI), and objective testing for deep vein thrombosis. Measurement of plasma D-dimer is useful as an exclusion test.

D-DIMER ASSAY

The assay for plasma D-dimer is useful as an exclusion test, provided an appropriately validated test is available. A negative result by the rapid quantitative ELISA for D-dimer has a negative likelihood ratio similar to that of a normal perfusion scan.[21] A positive D-dimer result is not useful diagnostically. Several management studies have found that pulmonary embolism can be excluded without performing imaging studies in patients with a low, intermediate, or unlikely clinical probability.[28]

COMPUTED TOMOGRAPHY IMAGING AND ANGIOGRAPHY

Spiral CT imaging has gained an increasingly important role in the diagnosis of pulmonary embolism in recent years and is now the primary imaging test in most centers. Single-detector spiral CT is highly sensitive for large emboli (segmental or larger arteries), but is much less sensitive for emboli in subsegmental pulmonary arteries[10,29]; such emboli may be clinically important in patients with severely impaired cardiorespiratory reserve. Therefore, a negative result by single-detector spiral CT should not be used alone to exclude the diagnosis of pulmonary embolism. A filling defect of a segmental or larger artery on single-detector spiral CT is associated with a high probability (>90%) of pulmonary embolism.[29]

The development of multidetector row CT, together with the use of contrast enhancement, has further improved the utility of CT for the diagnosis of pulmonary embolism.[30–32] Contrast-enhanced CTA has the advantage of providing clear results (positive or negative), with a relatively low rate of nondiagnostic test results, good characterization of nonvascular structures for alternate or associated diagnoses, and the ability to simultaneously evaluate the deep venous system of the legs (computed tomographic venography [CTV]).

The accuracy and clinical utility of multidetector CTA and combined CTA-CTV were evaluated in the recent Prospective Investigation of Pulmonary Embolism Diagnosis (PIOPED) II study.[32] Among 824 patients with a reference diagnosis and a completed CT study, CTA was inconclusive in 51 (6%) because of poor image quality. The sensitivity of CTA was 83 percent and the specificity was 96 percent. CTA-CTV was inconclusive in 87 (11%) of 824 patients because the image quality of either CTA or CTV was poor. Multidetector CTA-CTV had a higher sensitivity (90%) than CTA alone (83%), with similar specificity (~95% for both testing techniques). Positive results on CTA in combination with a high probability or intermediate probability of pulmonary embolism by the clinical assessment, or normal findings on CTA with a low clinical probability had a predictive value (positive or negative) of 92 to 96 percent.[32] Such values are consistent with those generally considered adequate to confirm or rule out the diagnosis of pulmonary embolism. Additional testing is necessary when the clinical probability is discordant with CTA or CTA-CTV imaging results.[32]

RADIONUCLIDE LUNG SCANNING

Radionuclide lung scanning continues to have a role in the diagnosis of suspected pulmonary embolism. A normal perfusion lung scan excludes the diagnosis of clinically important pulmonary embolism.[9,33] A normal perfusion lung scan is found in approximately 10 percent of patients with suspected pulmonary embolism seen at academic health centers or tertiary referral centers. A high-probability lung scan result (i.e., large perfusion defects with ventilation mismatch) has a positive predictive value for pulmonary embolism of 85 percent and provides a diagnostic endpoint to give antithrombotic treatment in most patients.[9,34,35] A high-probability lung scan is found in approximately 10 to 15 percent of symptomatic patients. For patients with a history of pulmonary embolism, careful comparison of the lung scan results to the most recent lung scan is required to ensure the perfusion defects are new. Further diagnostic testing is indicated for patients with a high-probability lung scan who have a "low" pretest clinical suspicion, and in those who are at high risk for major bleeding, to reduce the likelihood of a false-positive diagnosis.

The major limitation of lung scanning is that the results are inconclusive in most patients, even when considered together with the pretest clinical probability.[9] The nondiagnostic lung scan patterns are found in approximately 70 percent of patients with suspected pulmonary embolism.[7,9,35] These lung scan results have historically been called "low-probability" (matching ventilation–perfusion abnormalities or small perfusion defects), "intermediate probability," or indeterminate (because the perfusion defects correspond to an area of abnormality on chest radiograph). Further diagnostic testing is required in most of these patients because, regardless of the pretest clinical suspicion, the posttest probabilities of pulmonary embolism associated with these lung scan results are neither sufficiently high to give antithrombotic treatment nor sufficiently low to withhold therapy. The uncommon exception is the patient with a low clinical suspicion and a so-called low-probability lung scan result. However, even in these patients, objective testing for deep vein thrombosis with ultrasonography and/or measurement of plasma D-dimer is without risk for the patient and may provide added diagnostic value (see "Objective Testing for Deep Vein Thrombosis" below). A randomized trial has established that CTA is not inferior to using ventilation–perfusion lung scanning for excluding the diagnosis of pulmonary embolism when either test is used in an algorithm together with venous ultrasonography of the legs.[36]

MAGNETIC RESONANCE IMAGING

MRI appears to be highly sensitive for pulmonary embolism and is a promising diagnostic approach. However, clinically important interobserver variation exists in the sensitivity for pulmonary embolism, ranging from 70 to 100 percent.[37] Further studies are required to determine the clinical role of MRI in the diagnosis of patients with suspected pulmonary embolism.

PULMONARY ANGIOGRAPHY

Pulmonary angiography using selective catheterization of the pulmonary arteries is a relatively safe technique for patients who do not have pulmonary hypertension or cardiac failure.[9,33] If the expertise is available, pulmonary angiography should be used when other approaches are inconclusive and when definitive knowledge about the presence or absence of pulmonary embolism is required.

OBJECTIVE TESTING FOR DEEP VEIN THROMBOSIS

Objective testing for deep vein thrombosis is useful in patients with suspected pulmonary embolism, particularly those with nondiagnostic lung scan results[23,35] or inconclusive CT results.[38] Detection of proximal vein thrombosis by objective testing provides an indication for anticoagulant treatment, regardless of the presence or absence of pulmonary embolism, and prevents the need for further testing. However, a negative result by objective testing for deep vein thrombosis does not exclude the presence of pulmonary embolism.[7,8]

Currently, the primary role for using ultrasonographic testing of the legs is for those centers which do not have the capability for combined CTA-CTV, or if the results of such imaging are inconclusive. If the patient has adequate cardiorespiratory reserve, then serial ultrasonographic testing for proximal vein thrombosis can be used as an alternative to pulmonary angiography in patients with nondiagnostic lung scan or CT results, and withholding anticoagulant therapy is safe if repeated ultrasonographic testing of the legs is negative.[23,38] The rationale is that the clinical objective in such patients is to prevent recurrent pulmonary embolism, which is unlikely in the absence of proximal vein thrombosis. Selective pulmonary angiography should be done among patients with features suggesting a possible alternate source of embolism to proximal deep vein thrombosis of the leg (e.g., upper-extremity thrombosis, renal vein thrombosis, pelvic vein thrombosis, or right-heart thrombus).

INTEGRATED STRATEGIES FOR DIAGNOSIS OF PULMONARY EMBOLISM

Figure 134–2 summarizes the approach to diagnosis of suspected pulmonary embolism using CTA or CTA-CTV as the primary imaging test. Figure 134–3 summarizes the approach to diagnosis using ventilation–perfusion lung scanning for settings in which CTA capabilities are not available. The specific approach used depends on the local availability of

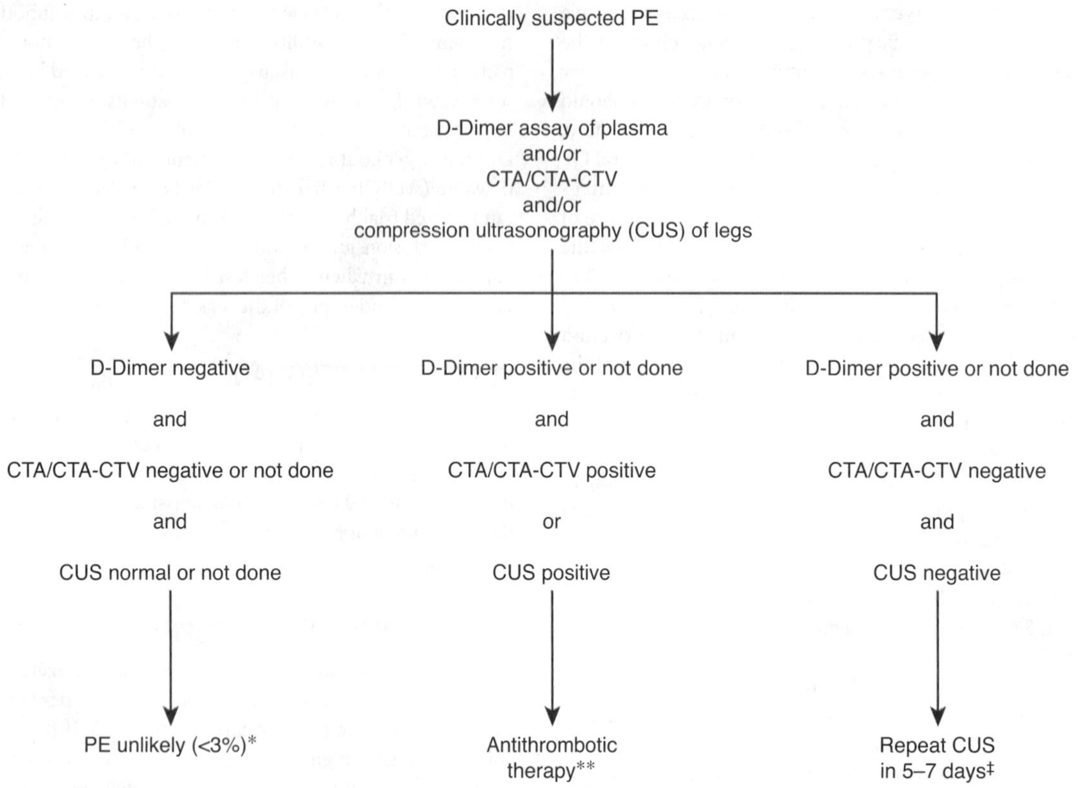

FIGURE 134–2. Integrated strategy for diagnosis of patients with suspected pulmonary embolism (PE) using CTA as the primary imaging test. *Negative D-dimer alone can be used as an exclusion test with high negative predictive value (>96%) in patients with low or moderate probability by the clinical assessment.[21,28] Patients with a high clinical probability should undergo imaging with CTA or combined CTA-CTV. **Positive results on CTA or combined CTA-CTV, in patients with a high or moderate probability of pulmonary embolism by the clinical assessment, have positive predictive value of 90% or more for venous thromboembolism. Similarly, abnormal results by compression ultrasonography (CUS) of the proximal deep veins of the legs have high positive predictive value for proximal vein thrombosis and provide an indication to give antithrombotic therapy. If the patient has a low probability by the clinical assessment, positive results by CTA or CTA-CTV in the main or lobar pulmonary arteries are still highly predictive (97%) for the presence of pulmonary embolism[19]; further testing is recommended for patients with low clinical probability and positive CTA results only of segmental or subsegmental arteries, and the options include pulmonary arteriography or serial CUS. ‡Negative results by CTA or by combined CTA-CTV have high negative predictive value (96%) in patients with low probability by the clinical assessment.[19] For patients with moderate clinical probability, the negative predictive value for combined CTA-CTV is also high (92%), but slightly lower for CTA alone (89%)[19]; in this latter group, and in patients with a high probability by the clinical assessment, serial CUS or pulmonary arteriography are recommended options.

technology, expertise with the different diagnostic techniques, and individual patient circumstances. The pathways in Figures 134–2 and 134–3 incorporate the recommendations of the PIOPED II investigators.[39]

Selective pulmonary arteriography should be done, unless contraindications exist, when other approaches are inconclusive, because the risk of arteriography in properly selected patients is less than the risk of unnecessary anticoagulant therapy.

THERAPY, COURSE, AND PROGNOSIS

■ CLINICAL COURSE OF VENOUS THROMBOEMBOLISM

Proximal Vein Thrombosis

Proximal deep vein thrombosis is a serious and potentially lethal condition. Untreated proximal vein thrombosis is associated with a 10 percent rate of fatal pulmonary embolism. Inadequately treated proximal vein thrombosis results in a 20 to 50 percent risk of recurrent venous thromboembolic events.[40] Prospective studies of patients with clinically suspected deep vein thrombosis or pulmonary embolism indicate that new venous thromboembolic events on followup are rare (≤2%) among patients in whom proximal vein thrombosis is absent by objective testing.[11,22,23,35,38] The aggregate data from diagnostic and treatment studies indicate that the presence of proximal vein thrombosis is the key prognostic marker for recurrent venous thromboembolism.

Distal Vein Thrombosis

Thrombosis that remains confined to the calf veins is associated with low risk (≤1%) of clinically important pulmonary embolism. Extension of thrombosis into the popliteal vein or more proximally occurs in 15 to 25 percent of patients with untreated calf vein thrombosis.[1] Patients with documented calf vein thrombosis should either receive anticoagulant treatment to prevent extension or undergo monitoring for proximal extension using serial ultrasonography.

Postthrombotic Syndrome

The postthrombotic syndrome is a frequent complication of deep vein thrombosis.[41] Patients with the postthrombotic syndrome complain of pain, heaviness, swelling, cramps, and itching or tingling of the affected leg. Ulceration may occur. The symptoms usually are aggravated by standing or walking and improve with rest and elevation of the leg. A prospective study documented a 25 percent incidence of moderate-to-severe postthrombotic symptoms 2 years after the initial diagnosis of proximal vein thrombosis in patients who were treated with initial heparin and oral anticoagulants for 3 months.[42] The study also demon-

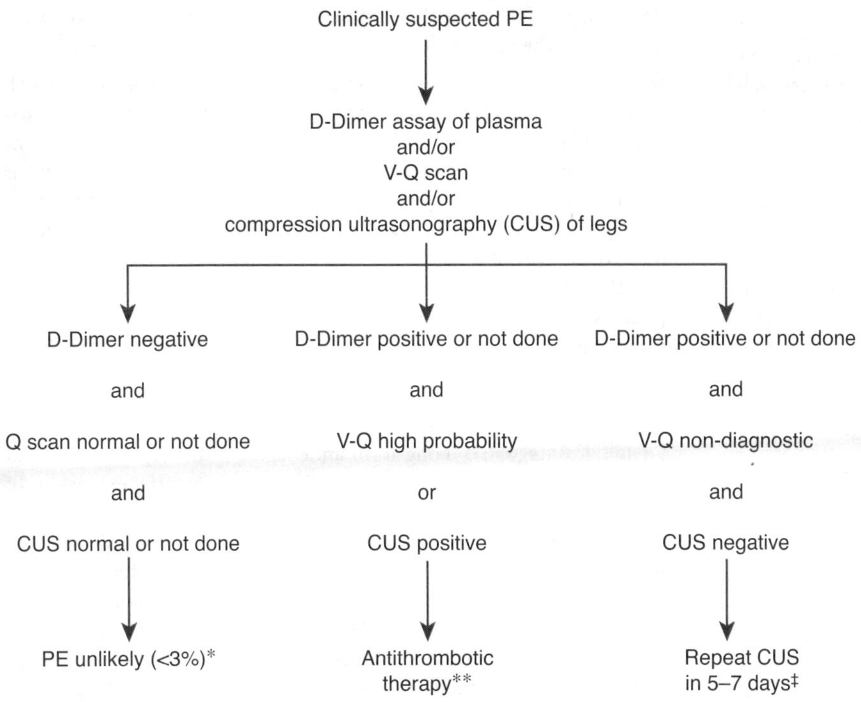

FIGURE 134–3. Integrated strategy for diagnosis of patients with suspected pulmonary embolism (PE) using ventilation (V)–perfusion (Q) lung scanning as the initial imaging test. An appropriately validated assay for plasma D-dimer, if available, provides a simple and rapid first-line exclusion test in patients with low, intermediate, or unlikely clinical probability of pulmonary embolism. The appropriate use of D-dimer can reduce the need for more expensive imaging tests, without compromising patient safety. If a validated D-dimer test is not available, or the patient has high clinical probability for pulmonary embolism, diagnostic imaging should be employed. *Negative D-dimer alone can be used as an exclusion test with high negative predictive value (>96%) in patients with low or moderate probability by the clinical assessment.[21,28] Patients with a high clinical probability should undergo V-Q scanning. A normal Q scan excludes clinically important pulmonary embolism. **A high probability V-Q scan in patients with a high or moderate probability of pulmonary embolism by the clinical assessment has positive predictive value of 85% or more for pulmonary embolism. Abnormal results by compression ultrasonography (CUS) of the proximal deep veins of the legs have high positive predictive value for proximal vein thrombosis and provide an indication to give antithrombotic therapy. Further testing is recommended for patients with a high probability V-Q scan, a low probability by the clinical assessment or a past history of pulmonary embolism, and negative results by CUS, because the positive predictive value is much lower in these patients; the options include CTA or combined CTA-CTV if available, or pulmonary arteriography. ‡Nondiagnostic V-Q lung scan patterns occur in approximately 70% of patients. If CUS is negative, further testing is needed to exclude or confirm the presence of venous thromboembolism. The options include serial CUS, CTA or combined CTA-CTV if available, or pulmonary arteriography. If capability for combined CTA-CTV exists, that is the preferred approach for most patients because it provides a definitive basis to give or withhold antithrombotic therapy in approximately 90 percent of patients. Lung scanning may be indicated as the first-line imaging test in women of reproductive age because the radiation exposure to the breast is significantly less than with CTA.[39]

strated that ipsilateral recurrent venous thrombosis is strongly associated with subsequent development of moderate or severe postthrombotic symptoms. Thus, prevention of ipsilateral recurrent deep vein thrombosis likely reduces the incidence of the postthrombotic syndrome. Application of a properly fitted graded compression stocking, as soon after diagnosis as the patient's symptoms will allow and continued for at least 2 years, is effective in reducing the incidence of postthrombotic symptoms, including moderate-to-severe symptoms.[43]

Chronic Thromboembolic Pulmonary Hypertension

Chronic thromboembolic pulmonary hypertension is a serious complication of pulmonary embolism. Historically, thromboembolic pulmonary hypertension was believed to be relatively rare and to occur only several years after the diagnosis of pulmonary embolism. A prospective cohort study provides important information on the incidence and timing of thromboembolic pulmonary hypertension.[44] The results indicate that thromboembolic pulmonary hypertension is more common and occurs earlier than previously thought. On prospective followup of 223 patients with documented pulmonary embolism, the cumulative incidence of chronic thromboembolic pulmonary hypertension was 3.8 percent at 2 years after diagnosis, despite state-of-the-art treatment for pulmonary embolism. The strongest independent risk factors were a history of pulmonary embolism (odds ratio: 19) and idiopathic pulmonary embolism at presentation (odds ratio: 5.7).[44]

OBJECTIVES AND PRINCIPLES OF ANTITHROMBOTIC TREATMENT

The objectives of treatment in patients with established venous thromboembolism are to (1) prevent death from pulmonary embolism, (2) prevent morbidity from recurrent venous thrombosis or pulmonary embolism, and (3) prevent or minimize the postthrombotic syndrome.

For most patients, the first two objectives are achieved by providing adequate anticoagulant treatment. Thrombolytic therapy is indicated in selected patients with pulmonary embolism (see "Thrombolytic Therapy" below). Use of an inferior vena cava filter is indicated to prevent death from pulmonary embolism in patients in whom anticoagulant treatment is absolutely contraindicated and in other selected patients (see "Anticoagulant Therapy" below). Recommendations for treatment of established venous thromboembolism are linked to the strength of the evidence from clinical trials using the approach for grading evidence of the American College of Chest Physicians guideline committee.[45] Recommendations classified as 1A are supported by evidence from scientifically valid randomized clinical trials (grade A evidence), and the results provide a clear risk-to-benefit conclusion (grade 1). Such recommendations should be implemented for most patients. Grade 2A recommendations also are supported by definitive clinical trial evidence (grade A), but the results indicate a less clear risk-to-benefit conclusion (grade 2); therefore, such recommendations may or may not be appropriate for the individual patient. The remaining grades of recommendation are based on nondefinitive evidence (grade B or C) and are less strong (see Chap. 23).

ANTICOAGULANT THERAPY

Anticoagulant therapy is the treatment of choice for most patients with proximal vein thrombosis or pulmonary embolism (grade 1A). The absolute contraindications to anticoagulant treatment include intracranial bleeding, severe active bleeding, recent brain, eye, or spinal cord surgery, and malignant hypertension. Relative contraindications include recent major surgery, recent cerebrovascular accident, active gastrointestinal tract bleeding, severe hypertension, severe renal or hepatic failure, and severe thrombocytopenia (platelets <50,000/μL).

Heparin and Low-Molecular-Weight Heparin

Patients with proximal deep vein thrombosis require both adequate initial anticoagulant treatment with heparin or low-molecular-weight (LMW) heparin and adequate long-term anticoagulant therapy to prevent recurrent venous thromboembolism.[40,46,47] Adequate anticoagulant treatment reduces the incidence of recurrent venous thromboembolism during the first 3 months after diagnosis from 25 percent to 5 percent or less.[40,46,47]

Initial therapy with continuous intravenous heparin has been the standard approach to treatment of deep vein thrombosis or pulmonary embolism for more than 20 years. During the 1990s, LMW heparin given by subcutaneous injection once or twice daily was evaluated by clinical trials and shown to be as effective and safe as continuous intravenous heparin for the initial treatment of patients with proximal deep vein thrombosis and submassive pulmonary embolism.[45,48] The advantage of LMW heparin is that it does not require anticoagulant monitoring (grade 1A). LMW heparin given subcutaneously once or twice daily is preferred over intravenous unfractionated heparin for the initial treatment of most patients with either deep vein thrombosis or submassive pulmonary embolism (grade 1A).[45] LMW heparin enables outpatient therapy for many patients with uncomplicated proximal vein thrombosis. Intravenous unfractionated heparin remains a useful approach for initial anticoagulant therapy in patients with severe renal failure. Initial treatment with LMW heparin or unfractionated heparin should be continued for at least 5 days (grade 1A). Table 134–2 lists the specific LMW drug regimens that have been effective in the initial treatment of venous thromboembolism.

If unfractionated heparin is used for initial therapy, it is important to achieve an adequate anticoagulant effect, defined as an activated partial thromboplastin time (aPTT) above the lower limit of therapeutic range within the first 24 hours.[49,50] Failure to achieve an adequate aPTT effect early during therapy is associated with a high incidence (25%) of recurrent venous thromboembolism.[49] Two-thirds of the recurrent events occur between 2 and 12 weeks after the initial diagnosis, despite treatment with oral anticoagulants.[50] The clinical trial data indicate that initial management with either unfractionated heparin or LMW heparin is critical to the patient's long-term outcome.[50]

Fondaparinux The synthetic pentasaccharide fondaparinux, which inhibits factor Xa, has been evaluated by large randomized clinical trials.[51,52] These studies indicate fondaparinux is as effective and safe as LMW heparin for treatment of established deep vein thrombosis and as effective and safe as intravenous heparin for treatment of symptomatic submassive pulmonary embolism. Fondaparinux is given subcutaneously once daily at a dose of 7.5 mg for patients weighing between 50 and 100 kg (85% of all patients evaluated in the clinical trials), 5 mg for patients weighing less than 50 kg, and 10 mg for patients weighing more than 100 kg.[51,52]

TABLE 134–2. Regimens of Low-Molecular-Weight Heparin and Fondaparinux for Treatment of Venous Thromboembolism

Drug	Regimen
Enoxaparin	1.0 mg/kg BID*
Dalteparin	200 IU/kg once daily†
Tinzaparin	175 IU/kg once daily‡
Nadroparin	6150 IU BID for 50–70 kg§
Reviparin	4200 IU BID for 46–60 kg¶
Fondaparinux	7.5 mg once daily for 50–100 kg**

*A once-daily regimen of 1.5 mg/kg can be used but probably is less effective in patients with cancer.

†After 1 month, can be followed by 150 IU/kg once daily as an alternative to an oral vitamin K antagonist for long-term treatment.

‡This regimen can also be used for long-term treatment as an alternative to an oral vitamin K antagonist.

§4100 IU BID if patient weighs <50 kg or 9200 IU BID if patient weighs >70 kg.

¶3500 IU BID if patient weighs 35–45 kg or 6300 IU BID if patient weighs >60 kg.

**5 mg once daily if patient weighs <50 kg or 10 mg once daily if patient weighs >100 kg.

Oral Anticoagulants

Vitamin K Antagonists Long-term anticoagulant therapy is required to prevent a high frequency (15–25%) of symptomatic extension of thrombosis and/or recurrent venous thromboembolic events.[40,45,53] Oral anticoagulant treatment using a vitamin K antagonist (e.g., sodium warfarin) currently is the preferred approach for long-term treatment in most patients (grade 1A). Treatment with adjusted doses of unfractionated heparin or LMW heparin is indicated for selected patients in whom vitamin K antagonists are contraindicated (e.g., pregnant women) or impractical, and in patients with concurrent cancer for whom LMW heparin regimens have been shown to be more effective and safer.[45,54,55] Treatment with a vitamin K antagonist is started with initial heparin or LMW heparin therapy and then overlapped for 4 to 5 days (grade 1A).

The preferred intensity of the anticoagulant effect of treatment with a vitamin K antagonist has been established by clinical trials.[45,56–59] The dose of vitamin K antagonist should be adjusted to maintain the international normalized ratio (INR) between 2.0 and 3.0 (grade 1A). High-intensity vitamin K antagonist treatment (INR 3.0–4.0) probably should not be used because it has not improved effectiveness in patients with the antiphospholipid syndrome and recurrent thrombosis[58] and has caused more bleeding.[59] Low-intensity therapy (INR 1.5–1.9) is not recommended routinely because it is less effective than standard-intensity treatment (INR 2.0–3.0) and does not reduce bleeding complications.[57]

New Oral Anticoagulants Several new oral anticoagulants which bind directly to the target coagulation enzyme of either thrombin or factor Xa are currently undergoing evaluation in phase III clinical trials for the treatment of patients with venous thromboembolism (see Chap. 23).[60] The potential advantages of these drugs are: (1) they can be administered orally once or twice daily without the need for anticoagulant monitoring and dose titration, (2) they have fewer clinically relevant drug interactions, and (3) because of a fast onset of anticoagulant action, similar to that of LMW heparin, they have the potential to simplify treatment by replacing the current approach of a parenteral drug (LMW heparin or fondaparinux) followed by an oral vitamin K antagonist with a single drug given for both initial and long-term therapy.

The first such drug to undergo phase III studies was ximelagatran, an oral direct thrombin inhibitor. Ximelagatran was shown to be of similar effectiveness to standard therapy with LMW followed by a vitamin K antagonist,[61] and was also effective for preventing recurrent venous thromboembolism during extended long-term therapy, with a rate of major bleeding similar to placebo.[62] However, the drug was associated with hepatotoxicity.[63] The studies with ximelagatran were nevertheless important conceptually by establishing the feasibility of effectively treating deep vein thrombosis using a single drug given orally without anticoagulant monitoring.

The new oral anticoagulant drugs currently undergoing evaluation in phase III trials for the treatment of deep vein thrombosis are the direct thrombin inhibitor dabigatran, and the direct factor Xa inhibitors rivaroxaban and apixaban.[60] Several other oral direct factor Xa inhibitors are also potential candidates for clinical evaluation for the treatment of deep vein thrombosis.[60]

Long-Acting Pentasaccharides: Idraparinux and Idrabiotaparinux

Idraparinux is a hypermethylated derivative of fondaparinux that inhibits factor Xa indirectly through its action on antithrombin. The very high affinity for antithrombin influences the idraparinux pharmacokinetics, such that the elimination half-life from the plasma of idraparinux is approximately 80 hours.[60] This long elimination half-life enables idraparinux to be given once weekly by subcutaneous injection, instead of once daily as for fondaparinux. Following promising results in a phase II study of patients with deep vein thrombosis,[64] idraparinux 2.5 mg given once weekly was evaluated as an alternative to standard therapy with a heparin and vitamin K antagonist for the treatment of patients with either deep vein thrombosis or pulmonary embolism,[65] and for extended anticoagulant therapy in patients with venous thromboembolism who had completed an initial 6 months of anticoagulant therapy.[66]

In the study of 2904 patients with deep vein thrombosis, the incidence of symptomatic recurrent venous thromboembolism at 3 months was 2.9 percent in the idraparinux group, compared with 3.0 percent for standard therapy, indicating noninferiority of idraparinux.[65] The rates of clinically relevant bleeding during 3 months of treatment were 4.5 percent for idraparinux and 7.0 percent for standard therapy ($p < 0.01$); at 6 months, bleeding rates were similar (8.3% and 8.1% respectively). In the study of 2215 patients with pulmonary embolism, however, the rate of recurrent thromboembolism was 3.4 percent for idraparinux and 1.6% for standard therapy ($p < 0.05$), indicating that idraparinux was less efficacious in this patient group.[65] The difference in efficacy was a result of an excess of fatal and nonfatal recurrent pulmonary emboli within the first 1 to 2 weeks of treatment.

These results establish the concept that patients with deep vein thrombosis can be treated with a single long-acting anticoagulant given once weekly, without anticoagulant monitoring, and achieve similar effectiveness and safety to current standard therapy with LMW heparin overlapped with, and followed by, a vitamin K antagonist, when used for 3 to 6 months of treatment. For patients with pulmonary embolism, either larger doses of idraparinux are needed, or an alternate anticoagulant will need to be given for initial therapy.

In the study of extended anticoagulant therapy, 1215 patients who had received 6 months of anticoagulant therapy were randomly assigned to continue anticoagulant therapy using 2.5 mg idraparinux subcutaneously given once weekly, without anticoagulant monitoring, or to subcutaneous placebo, for a further 6 months.[66] Among the 1215 patients, recurrent venous thromboembolism occurred in 1 percent given idraparinux and in 3.7 percent given placebo ($p < 0.01$). Major bleeding occurred in 11 patients (1.9%) given idraparinux, including three intracranial bleeds, compared with none who received placebo ($p < 0.01$). Thus, idraparinux was effective for preventing recurrent venous thromboembolism, but was associated with an increased risk of major bleeding.[66]

Collectively, the phase III studies with idraparinux suggest that an approach using subcutaneous injection once weekly, without anticoagulant monitoring, is a feasible strategy for long-term anticoagulant therapy of patients with deep vein thrombosis. However, further understanding of the pharmacokinetics of idraparinux, including the time to achieve a steady state and the distribution kinetics of the drug, are needed. The regimen will need to be modified to ensure the drug does not accumulate once a steady state is achieved, and contribute to an increased bleeding incidence. Such studies are in progress with a modified form of idraparinux, known as idrabiotaparinux.

Idrabiotaparinux, formerly known as SSR12517E, is a biotinylated form of idraparinux which exhibits essentially the same pharmacokinetic profile as idraparinux, but which has the advantage that its anticoagulant effect can be rapidly neutralized by the intravenous infusion of avidin.[60] Avidin is a large protein derived from egg white, which binds to the biotin moiety of idrabiotaparinux and the complex is then cleared by the kidneys. Idrabiotaparinux is undergoing phase III evaluation in an equipotency study of patients with deep vein thrombosis, and in patients with pulmonary embolism following an initial course of LMW heparin.

Duration of Anticoagulant Therapy and Recurrent Venous Thromboembolism

The appropriate duration of oral anticoagulant treatment for venous thromboembolism using a vitamin K antagonist has been evaluated by multiple randomized clinical trials.[45,56,67–72] Treatment should be continued for at least 3 months in patients with a first episode of proximal vein thrombosis or pulmonary embolism secondary to a transient (reversible) risk factor (grade 1A). Stopping treatment at 4 to 6 weeks resulted in an increased incidence of recurrent venous thromboembolism during the following 6 to 12 months (absolute risk increase: 8%). In contrast, treatment for 3 to 6 months resulted in a low rate of recurrent venous thromboembolism during the following 1 to 2 years (annual incidence: 3%).

Patients with a first episode of idiopathic (unprovoked) venous thromboembolism should be treated for at least 3 months[45] (grade 1A), and considered for indefinite anticoagulant therapy. This decision should be individualized, taking into consideration the estimated risk of recurrent venous thromboembolism, risk of bleeding, and patient compliance and preference. Indefinite therapy is recommended for patients in whom risk factors for bleeding are absent and in whom good anticoagulant control can be achieved (grade 1A).[45] If indefinite anticoagulant treatment is given, the risk-to-benefit ratio of continuing such treatment should be reassessed at periodic intervals.

A variety of prothrombotic conditions or markers reportedly are associated with an increased risk of recurrent venous thromboembolism. These conditions include deficiencies of the naturally occurring inhibitors of coagulation such as antithrombin, protein C, and protein S; specific gene mutations including factor V Leiden and prothrombin 20210A; elevated levels of coagulation factor VIII; elevated levels of homocysteine; and the presence of antiphospholipid antibodies (see Chap. 131). The presence of residual deep vein thrombosis assessed by compression ultrasonography,[73] elevated levels of plasma D-dimer after discontinuation of anticoagulant treatment,[74] and male gender[75] are associated with an increased incidence of recurrent thromboembolism. However, the available data are limited to subgroup analyses of randomized trials and data from observational studies. No randomized trials have been performed, a priori, in these subgroups of patients with thrombophilic conditions to evaluate the risk-to-benefit ratio of different durations of anticoagulant treatment, so no definitive recommendations can be made.

For patients with a first episode of venous thromboembolism and documented antiphospholipid antibodies or two or more thrombophilic conditions (e.g., combined factor V Leiden and prothrombin 20210A gene mutations), indefinite anticoagulant treatment should be considered. For patients with a first episode of venous thromboembolism who have documented deficiency of antithrombin, protein C, or protein S, or the factor V Leiden or prothrombin 20210A gene mutation, hyperhomocysteinemia, or high factor VIII levels (>90th percentile), the duration of treatment should be individualized after the patients have completed at least 3 months of anticoagulant therapy. Some of these patients also may be candidates for indefinite therapy.

Oral vitamin K antagonist treatment should be given indefinitely for most patients with a second episode of unprovoked venous thromboembolism[45,70] (grade 1A), because stopping treatment at 3 to 6 months in these patients results in a high incidence (21%) of recurrent venous thromboembolism during the following 4 years. The risk of recurrent thromboembolism during 4-year followup was reduced by 87 percent (from 21% to 3%) by continuing anticoagulant treatment; this benefit is partially offset by an increase in the cumulative incidence of major bleeding (from 3% to 9%).[70]

Use of LMW heparin for long-term treatment of venous thromboembolism has been evaluated in clinical trials.[54,55,76] The studies indicate that long-term treatment with subcutaneous LMW heparin for 3 to 6 months is at least as effective as, and in cancer patients is more effective than, an oral vitamin K antagonist adjusted to maintain the INR between 2.0 and 3.0. LMW heparin also was associated with less bleeding complications because of a reduction in minor bleeding. Therefore, patients with venous thromboembolism and concurrent cancer should be treated with LMW heparin for the first 3 to 6 months of long-term treatment (grade 1A).[45] The patients then should receive anticoagulation indefinitely or until the cancer resolves. The regimens of LMW heparin that are established as effective for long-term treatment are dalteparin 200 U/kg once daily for 1 month, followed by 150 U/kg daily thereafter, or tinzaparin 175 U/kg once daily.

Anticoagulant Therapy during Pregnancy

Adjusted-dose subcutaneous heparin is an appropriate long-term anticoagulant regimen for pregnant patients with venous thromboembolism. LMW heparin does not cross the placenta, and initial experience suggests these agents are safe for treatment of venous thromboembolism in pregnant patients.[77,78] With regard to safety advantages, LMW heparin causes less thrombocytopenia and potentially less osteoporosis than unfractionated heparin. An additional advantage is that LMW heparin is effective when given once daily, whereas unfractionated heparin requires twice-daily injection. Large randomized trials comparing the efficacy and safety of LMW heparin with unfractionated heparin in pregnant patients have not been completed. The key uncertainty about use of LMW heparin for treatment of venous thromboembolism during pregnancy is whether the regimens established as effective for initial and long-term therapy in nonpregnant patients, who do not require anticoagulant monitoring, can be generalized to pregnant patients. A study indicates no major change in the peak anti-Xa levels over the course of pregnancy in most patients treated with a once-daily therapeutic LMW heparin regimen (tinzaparin 175 U/kg).[78] Measurement of the anti-Xa level may provide reassurance that major drug accumulation is not occurring. However, the appropriate dose adjustments in response to a decreased anti-Xa level are uncertain. The choice between adjusted-dose unfractionated heparin or LMW heparin therapy during pregnancy is a clinical judgment in the individual patient. The patient should be informed of the pros and cons discussed above and their preference factored into the decision. Evidence-based guidelines for antithrombotic therapy during pregnancy are available.[79]

Side Effects of Anticoagulant Therapy

Bleeding Bleeding is the most common side effect of anticoagulant therapy. Bleeding can be classified as major or minor according to standardized international criteria. *Major bleeding* is defined as clinically overt bleeding resulting in a decline of hemoglobin of at least 2 g/dL, transfusion of at least 2 U of packed red cells, or bleeding that is retroperitoneal or intracranial. The rates of major bleeding in clinical trials of initial therapy with intravenous heparin, LMW heparin, or fondaparinux are 1 to 2 percent.[48,51,52] Patients at increased risk of major bleeding are those who underwent surgery or experienced trauma within the previous 14 days; those with a history of gastrointestinal or intracranial bleeding, peptic ulcer disease, or genitourinary bleeding; and those with miscellaneous conditions predisposing to bleeding, such as thrombocytopenia, liver disease, and multiple invasive lines.

Major bleeding occurs in approximately 2 percent of patients during the first 3 months of oral anticoagulant treatment using a vitamin K antagonist and in 1 to 3 percent per year of treatment thereafter.[80] A meta-analysis suggests the clinical impact of major bleeding during long-term oral vitamin K antagonist treatment is greater than widely appreciated.[80] The estimated case fatality rate for major bleeding is 13 percent, and the rate of intracranial bleeding was 1.15 per 100 patient-years. These risks are important considerations in the decision about extended or indefinite anticoagulant therapy in patients with venous thromboembolism.

Heparin-Induced Thrombocytopenia (see also Chap. 133) Heparin or LMW heparin may cause thrombocytopenia. In large clinical studies of acute venous thromboembolism treatment, thrombocytopenia occurred in less than 1 percent of more than 2000 patients treated with unfractionated heparin or LMW heparin.[49,50] Nevertheless, heparin-induced thrombocytopenia can be a serious complication when accompanied by extension or recurrence of venous thromboembolism or the development of arterial thrombosis. Such complications may precede or coincide with the fall in platelet count and are associated with a high rate of limb loss and a high mortality. Heparin in all forms should be discontinued when the diagnosis of heparin-induced thrombocytopenia is made on clinical grounds, and treatment with an alternative anticoagulant such as danaparoid, bivalirudin, or argatroban should be initiated. Treatment with an oral vitamin K antagonist should be started or resumed once the thrombocytopenia resolves. It is given in low daily doses overlapping for at least 5 days with the alternative anticoagulant that is discontinued once a stable INR is achieved.

Heparin-Induced Osteoporosis Osteoporosis may occur as a result of long-term treatment with heparin or LMW heparin (usually after more than 3 months). The earliest clinical manifestation of heparin-associated osteoporosis usually is nonspecific low back pain primarily involving the vertebrae or the ribs. Patients also may present with spontaneous fractures. Up to one-third of patients treated with long-term heparin may have subclinical reduction in bone density. Whether these patients are predisposed to future fractures is not known. The incidence of symptomatic osteoporosis in clinical trials of LMW heparin treatment for 3 to 6 months was very low and are not increased compared to warfarin treatment. Patients with osteoporosis or fractures often had other risk factors such as bone metastases.

Other Side Effects of Heparin Heparin or LMW heparin may cause elevated liver transaminase levels. These elevations are of unknown clinical significance and usually return to normal after the heparin or LMW heparin is discontinued. Awareness of this biochemical effect is important so as to avoid unnecessary interruption of heparin therapy and unnecessary liver biopsies in patients who may develop elevated transaminase levels during heparin or LMW heparin therapy. Additional rare side effects of heparin include hypersensitivity and skin reactions, such as skin necrosis, alopecia, and hyperkalemia occurring as a result of hypoaldosteronism.

THROMBOLYTIC THERAPY

Thrombolytic therapy is indicated for patients with pulmonary embolism who present with evidence of vascular collapse (hypotension and/

or syncope) and for selected patients with pulmonary embolism who have clinical findings of right ventricular failure or echocardiographic evidence of right ventricular hypokinesia. Thrombolytic therapy provides more rapid lysis of pulmonary emboli and more rapid restoration of right ventricular function and pulmonary perfusion than does anticoagulant treatment.[81] An effective regimen is 100 mg of recombinant tissue plasminogen activator by intravenous infusion over 2 hours (50 mg/h). Heparin then is given by continuous infusion once the thrombin time or aPTT is less than twice the control value.[81] The starting infusion dose is 1000 U/h. Chapters 23 and 136 provide further details of thrombolytic therapy.

The role of thrombolytic therapy in patients with deep vein thrombosis is limited. Thrombolytic therapy may be indicated in patients with acute massive proximal vein thrombosis (phlegmasia cerulea dolens with impending venous gangrene) or in occasional patients with extensive iliofemoral vein thrombosis who have severe symptoms because of venous outflow obstruction. Thrombolytic therapy can be given by systemic infusion or catheter-directed infusion. Whether systemic or catheter-directed thrombolysis reduces the incidence of the postphlebitic syndrome is uncertain. The catheter-directed approach may be associated with a lower risk of major bleeding, particularly intracranial bleeding, than systemic injection, but further clinical trials are required to determine the role of catheter-directed thrombolytic therapy in patients with deep vein thrombosis. The relative benefits and risks of standard anticoagulant therapy versus catheter-directed thrombolysis are currently being evaluated in a large randomized trial, the ATTRACT (*A*cute Venous *T*hrombosis: *T*hrombus *R*emoval with *A*djunctive *C*atheter-Directed *T*hrombolysis) study.

INFERIOR VENA CAVA FILTER

Insertion of an inferior vena cava filter is indicated for patients with acute venous thromboembolism and an absolute contraindication to anticoagulant therapy and for the rare patients who have objectively documented recurrent venous thromboembolism during adequate anticoagulant therapy.

Insertion of a vena cava filter is effective for preventing pulmonary embolism. However, use of a permanent filter results in an increased incidence of recurrent deep vein thrombosis 1 to 2 years after insertion (increase in cumulative incidence at 2 years increases from 12% to 21%).[82] Therefore, if the indication for filter placement is transient, such as a contraindication to anticoagulation due to a temporary high risk of bleeding, a retrievable vena cava filter should be used. A retrievable filter can then be removed in the several weeks to months later, once the filter is no longer required. If a permanent filter is placed, long-term anticoagulant treatment should be given as soon as safely possible to prevent morbidity from recurrent deep vein thrombosis.

REFERENCES

1. Moser KM, Lemoine JR: Is embolic risk conditioned by localization of deep venous thrombosis? *Ann Intern Med* 94:439, 1981.
2. Prandoni P, Polistena P, Bernardi E, et al: Upper-extremity deep vein thrombosis. Risk factors, diagnosis, and complications. *Arch Intern Med* 157:57, 1997.
3. Silverstein MD, Heit JA, Mohr DN, et al: Trends in the incidence of deep vein thrombosis and pulmonary embolism. A 25-year population-based study. *Arch Intern Med* 158:585, 1998.
4. Heit J: The epidemiology of venous thromboembolism in the community. *Arterioscler Thromb Vasc Biol* 28:370, 2008.
5. Kung HC, Hoyert D, Xu J, Murphy S: Deaths: Final data for 2005. National Center for Health Statistics. Centers for Disease Control and Prevention. *Natl Vital Stat Rep* 56:Table 10, 2008.
6. Geerts WH, Bergqvist D, Pineo GF, et al: Prevention of venous thromboembolism: American College of Chest Physicians evidence-based clinical practice guidelines (8th edition). *Chest* 133:381S, 2008.
7. Hull R, Hirsh J, Carter C, et al: Diagnostic value of ventilation-perfusion lung scanning in patients with suspected pulmonary embolism. *Chest* 88:819, 1985.
8. Turkstra F, Kuijer P, van Beck EJ, et al: Diagnostic utility of ultrasonography of leg veins in patients suspected of having pulmonary embolism. *Ann Intern Med* 126:775, 1997.
9. PIOPED Investigators: Value of the ventilation/perfusion scan in acute pulmonary embolism: Results of the Prospective Investigation of Pulmonary Embolism Diagnosis (PIOPED). *JAMA* 263:2753, 1990.
10. Kruip M, Leclercq M, van der Heul C, et al: Diagnostic strategies for excluding pulmonary embolism in clinical outcome studies. A systematic review. *Ann Intern Med* 138:941, 2003.
11. Birdwell BG, Raskob GE, Whitsett TL, et al: The clinical validity of normal compression ultrasonography in outpatients suspected of having deep venous thrombosis. *Ann Intern Med* 128:1, 1998.
12. Stevens S, Elliott CG, Chan K, et al: Withholding anticoagulation after a negative result on Duplex ultrasonography for suspected symptomatic deep venous thrombosis. *Ann Intern Med* 140:985, 2004.
13. Hull R, Hirsh J, Sackett DL, et al: Clinical validity of a negative venogram in patients with clinically suspected venous thrombosis. *Circulation* 64:622, 1981.
14. Rosendaal FR: Risk factors for venous thrombosis: Prevalence, risk and interaction. *Semin Hematol* 34:171, 1997.
15. Heit JA, O'Fallon WM, Peterson TM, et al. Relative impact of risk factors for deep vein thrombosis and pulmonary embolism: A population-based study. *Arch Intern Med* 162:1245, 2002.
16. Bezemer ID, Bare LA, Doggen CJ, et al. Gene variants associated with deep vein thrombosis. *JAMA* 299:1306, 2008.
17. Simioni P, Prandoni P, Lensing AWA, et al: The risk of recurrent venous thromboembolism in patients with an Arg506Gln mutation in the gene for factor V (factor V Leiden). *N Engl J Med* 336:399, 1997.
18. Wells PS, Owen C, Doucette S, et al: Does this patient have deep vein thrombosis? *JAMA* 295:199, 2006.
19. Stein PD, Woodard PK, Weg JG, et al: Diagnostic pathways in acute pulmonary embolism: Recommendations of the PIOPED II Investigators. *Am J Med* 119:1048, 2006.
20. Qaseem A, Snow V, Barry P, et al: Current diagnosis of venous thromboembolism in primary care: A clinical practice guideline from the American Academy of Family Physicians and the American College of Physicians. *Ann Fam Med* 5:57, 2007.
21. Stein P, Hull RD, Patel K, et al: D-dimer for the exclusion of acute venous thrombosis and pulmonary embolism. A systematic review. *Ann Intern Med* 140:589, 2004.
22. Bernardi E, Prandoni P, Lensing AW, et al: D-dimer testing as an adjunct to ultrasonography in patients with clinically suspected deep-vein thrombosis: Prospective cohort study. *BMJ* 317:1037, 1998.
23. Kearon C, Ginsberg J, Hirsh J: The role of venous ultrasonography in the diagnosis of suspected deep vein thrombosis and pulmonary embolism. *Ann Intern Med* 129:1044, 1998.
24. Bernardi E, Camporese G, Buller HR, et al: Serial 2-point ultrasonography plus D-dimer vs whole-leg color-coded Doppler ultrasonography for diagnosing suspected symptomatic deep vein thrombosis: A randomized controlled trial. *JAMA* 300:1653, 2008.
25. Hull RD, Carter CJ, Jay RM, et al: The diagnosis of acute, recurrent deep-vein thrombosis: A diagnostic challenge. *Circulation* 67:901, 1983.
26. Prandoni P, Cogo A, Bernardi E, et al: A simple ultrasound approach for detection of recurrent proximal-vein thrombosis vein diameter. *Circulation* 88:1730, 1993.
27. Rathbun S, Whitsett T, Raskob G: Negative D-dimer to exclude recurrent deep-vein thrombosis in symptomatic patients. *Ann Intern Med* 141:839, 2004.
28. Ten Cate-Hoek AJ, Prins MH: Management studies using a combination of D-dimer test result and clinical probability to rule out venous thromboembolism: A systematic review. *J Thromb Haemost* 3:2465, 2005.
29. Rathbun S, Whitsett T, Raskob G: Sensitivity and specificity of helical computed tomography in the diagnosis of pulmonary embolism: A systematic review. *Ann Intern Med* 132:227, 2000.
30. Patel S, Kazerooni EA, Cascade PN: Pulmonary embolism: Optimization of small pulmonary artery visualization at multi-detector row CT. *Radiology* 227:455, 2003.
31. Perrier A, Roy PM, Sanchez O, et al: Multi-detector row computed tomography in suspected pulmonary embolism. *N Engl J Med* 352:1760, 2005.
32. Stein PD, Fowler SE, Goodman LR, et al: Multi-detector computed tomography for acute pulmonary embolism. *N Engl J Med* 354:2317, 2006.
33. Hull R, Raskob G, Coates G, Panju A: Clinical validity of a normal perfusion lung scan in patients with suspected pulmonary embolism. *Chest* 97:23, 1990.
34. Miniati M, Prediletto A, Fornichi B, et al: Accuracy of clinical assessment in the diagnosis of pulmonary embolism. *Am J Respir Crit Care Med* 159:864, 1999.
35. Hull RD, Raskob GE, Ginsberg JS, et al: A noninvasive strategy for the treatment of patients with suspected pulmonary embolism. *Arch Intern Med* 154:289, 1994.
36. Anderson DR, Kahn SR, Rodger MA, et al: Computed tomographic pulmonary angiography vs ventilation-perfusion lung scanning in patients with suspected pulmonary embolism: A randomized controlled trial. *JAMA* 298:2743, 2007.
37. Meaney JFM, Weg JG, Chenevert TL, et al: Diagnosis of pulmonary embolism with magnetic resonance angiography. *N Engl J Med* 336:1422, 1997.
38. van Strijen M, de Monye W, Schiereck J, et al: Single-detector helical computed tomography as the primary diagnostic test in suspected pulmonary embolism: A

multicenter clinical management study of 510 patients. *Ann Intern Med* 138:307, 2003.
39. Stein PD, Woodward PK, Weg JG, et al. Diagnostic pathways in acute pulmonary embolism: Recommendations of the PIOPED II investigators. *Am J Med* 119:1048, 2006.
40. Hull R, Delmore T, Genton E, et al: Warfarin sodium versus low-dose heparin in the long-term treatment of venous thrombosis. *N Engl J Med* 301:855, 1979.
41. Prandoni P, Kahn S: Post-thrombotic syndrome: Prevalence, prognostication and need for progress. *Br J Haematol* 145:286, 2009.
42. Prandoni P, Lensing AWA, Cogo A, et al: The long-term clinical course of acute deep venous thrombosis. *Ann Intern Med* 125:1, 1996.
43. Prandoni P, Lensing AWA, Prins MH, et al: Below knee elastic compression stockings to prevent the post-thrombotic syndrome: A randomized controlled trial. *Ann Intern Med* 141:249, 2004.
44. Pengo V, Lensing A, Prins M, et al: Incidence of chronic thromboembolic pulmonary hypertension after pulmonary embolism. *N Engl J Med* 350:2257, 2004.
45. Kearon C, Kahn SR, Agnelli G, et al: Antithrombotic therapy for venous thromboembolic disease. American College of Chest Physicians evidence-based clinical practice guidelines (8th edition). *Chest* 133:454S, 2008.
46. Hull R, Raskob G, Hirsh J, et al: Continuous intravenous heparin compared with intermittent subcutaneous heparin in the initial treatment of proximal vein thrombosis. *N Engl J Med* 315:1109, 1986.
47. Brandjes D, Heijboer H, Buller H, et al: Acenocoumarol and heparin compared with acenocoumarol alone in the initial treatment of proximal-vein thrombosis. *N Engl J Med* 327:1485, 1992.
48. Quinlan D, McQuillan A, Eikelboom J: Low-molecular-weight heparin compared with intravenous unfractionated heparin for treatment of pulmonary embolism. *Ann Intern Med* 140:175, 2004.
49. Hull RD, Raskob GE, Brant RF, et al: Relation between the time to achieve the lower limit of the APTT therapeutic range and recurrent venous thromboembolism during heparin treatment for deep vein thrombosis. *Arch Intern Med* 157:2562, 1997.
50. Hull RD, Raskob GE, Brant RF, et al: The importance of initial heparin treatment on long-term clinical outcomes of antithrombotic therapy: The emerging theme of delayed recurrence. *Arch Intern Med* 157:2317, 1997.
51. Buller H, Davidson B, Decousus H, et al: Fondaparinux or enoxaparin for the initial treatment of symptomatic deep venous thrombosis. A randomized trial. *Ann Intern Med* 140:867, 2004.
52. Matisse Investigators: Subcutaneous fondaparinux versus intravenous unfractionated heparin in the initial treatment of pulmonary embolism. *N Engl J Med* 349:1695, 2003.
53. Lagerstedt C, Olsson C, Fagher B, et al: Need for long-term anticoagulant treatment in symptomatic calf-vein thrombosis. *Lancet* 2:515, 1986.
54. Lee A, Levine M, Baker R, et al: Low-molecular-weight heparin versus Coumadin for the prevention of recurrent venous thromboembolism in patients with cancer. *N Engl J Med* 349:146, 2003.
55. Hull R, Pineo G, Brant R, et al: Long-term low-molecular-weight heparin versus usual care in proximal-vein thrombosis patients with cancer. *Am J Med* 119:1062, 2006.
56. Ridker P, Goldhaber S, Danielson E, et al: Long-term low-intensity warfarin therapy for the prevention of recurrent venous thromboembolism. *N Engl J Med* 348:1425, 2003.
57. Kearon C, Ginsberg J, Kovacs M, et al: Comparison of low-intensity warfarin therapy with conventional intensity warfarin therapy for long-term prevention of recurrent venous thromboembolism. *N Engl J Med* 349:631, 2003.
58. Crowther M, Ginsberg J, Julian J, et al: A comparison of two intensities of warfarin for the prevention of recurrent thrombosis in patients with the antiphospholipid antibody syndrome. *N Engl J Med* 349:1133, 2003.
59. Hull R, Hirsh J, Jay R, et al: Different intensities of oral anticoagulant therapy in the treatment of proximal-vein thrombosis. *N Engl J Med* 307:1676, 1982.
60. Weitz J, Hirsh J, Samama M. New antithrombotic drugs: American College of Chest Physicians clinical practice guidelines (8th edition). *Chest* 133:234S, 2008.
61. Fiessinger J, Huisman M, Davidson B, et al: Ximelagatran versus low-molecular-weight heparin and warfarin for the treatment of deep-vein thrombosis. *JAMA* 293:681, 2005.
62. Schulman S, Wahlander K, Lundstrom T, et al: Secondary prevention of venous thromboembolism with the oral direct thrombin inhibitor ximelagatran. The THRIVE III study. *N Engl J Med* 349:1713, 2003.
63. Lee WM, Larrey D, Olsson R, et al: Hepatic findings in long-term clinical trials of ximelagatran. *Drug Saf* 28:351, 2005.
64. Persist Investigators: A novel long-acting synthetic factor Xa inhibitor (SanOrg 34006) to replace warfarin for secondary prevention in deep-vein thrombosis: A phase II evaluation. *J Thromb Haemost* 2:47, 2004.
65. The van Gogh Investigators: Idraparinux versus standard therapy for venous thromboembolic disease. *N Engl J Med* 357:1094, 2007.
66. The van Gogh Investigators: Extended prophylaxis of venous thromboembolism with idraparinux. *N Engl J Med* 357:1105, 2007.
67. Optimum duration of anticoagulation for deep-vein thrombosis and pulmonary embolism. Research Committee of the British Thoracic Society. *Lancet* 340:873, 1992.
68. Schulman S, Rhedin A-S, Lindmarker P, et al: A comparison of six weeks with six months of oral anticoagulant therapy after a first episode of venous thromboembolism. *N Engl J Med* 332:1661, 1995.
69. Levine M, Hirsh J, Gent M, et al: Optimal duration of oral anticoagulant therapy: A randomized trial comparing four weeks with three months of warfarin in patients with proximal deep-vein thrombosis. *Thromb Haemost* 74:606, 1995.
70. Schulman S, Granqvist S, Holmström M, et al: The duration of oral anticoagulant therapy after a second episode of venous thromboembolism. *N Engl J Med* 336:393, 1997.
71. Kearon C, Gent M, Hirsh J, et al: A comparison of three months of anticoagulation with extended anticoagulation for a first-episode of idiopathic venous thromboembolism. *N Engl J Med* 340:901, 1999.
72. Agnelli G, Prandoni P, Santamaria M, et al: Three months versus one year of oral anticoagulant therapy for idiopathic deep-venous thrombosis. *N Engl J Med* 345:165, 2001.
73. Prandoni P, Lensing A, Prins M, et al: Residual venous thrombosis as a predictive factor of recurrent venous thromboembolism. *Ann Intern Med* 137:955, 2002.
74. Palareti G, Cosmi B, Vigano D'Angelo S, et al: D-dimer testing to determine the duration of anticoagulant therapy. *N Engl J Med* 355:1780, 2006.
75. Kyrle P, Minar E, Bialonczyk, et al: The risk of recurrent venous thromboembolism in men and women. *N Engl J Med* 350:2558, 2004.
76. Hull R, Pineo G, Brant R, et al: Self-managed long-term low-molecular-weight heparin therapy: The balance of benefits and harms. *Am J Med* 120:72, 2007.
77. Pettila V, Kaaja R, Leinonen P, et al: Thromboprophylaxis with low molecular weight heparin (dalteparin) in pregnancy. *Thromb Res* 96:275, 1999.
78. Smith M, Norris L, Steer P, et al: Tinzaparin sodium for thrombosis treatment and prevention during pregnancy. *Am J Obstet Gynecol* 190:495, 2004.
79. Bates S, Greer IA, Pabinger I, et al: Venous thromboembolism, thrombophilia, antithrombotic therapy, and pregnancy: American College of Chest Physicians evidence-based clinical practice guidelines (8th edition). *Chest* 133:844S, 2008.
80. Linkins L, Choi P, Douketis J: Clinical impact of bleeding in patients taking oral anticoagulant therapy for venous thromboembolism. A meta-analysis. *Ann Intern Med* 139:893, 2003.
81. Goldhaber SZ, Haire WD, Feldstein ML, et al: Alteplase versus heparin in acute pulmonary embolism: Randomized trial assessing right-ventricular function and pulmonary perfusion. *Lancet* 341:507, 1993.
82. Decousus H, Leizorovicz A, Parent F, et al: A clinical trial of vena caval filters in the prevention of pulmonary embolism in patients with proximal deep-vein thrombosis. *N Engl J Med* 338:409, 1998.

CHAPTER 135

ATHEROTHROMBOSIS: DISEASE INITIATION, PROGRESSION, AND TREATMENT

Emile R. Mohler III and Andrew I. Schafer

SUMMARY

The consequences of atherosclerotic vascular disease are the leading cause of morbidity and mortality in the developed countries of the world and are rapidly approaching that status in the developing world. This chapter reviews the pathologic mechanisms of atherosclerotic disease development and progression, and details the interaction of these processes with the coagulation system. The earliest morphologically visible lesion of arterial atherosclerosis, the fatty streak, already is an advanced metabolic and immunologic locus that manifests as abnormalities of vascular tone, inflammation, cellular growth, and endothelial cell dysfunction. After years to decades, the lesions advance to form plaques that grow and eventually either impinge on the arterial lumen or rupture. Rupture of a vulnerable plaque is a catastrophic event that, through activation of both platelets and the coagulation cascade, triggers thrombosis, which leads to complete occlusion and tissue ischemia. Based on an increased understanding of the pathogenesis and consequences of atheromatous plaque development and progression, medical management of atherothrombotic syndromes has improved and is reviewed for the coronary, cerebrovascular, and peripheral arteries.

ATHEROSCLEROSIS

Atherothrombosis describes a disease process that includes atherosclerosis and thrombosis in the artery. In the 1850s, Virchow[1] described atherosclerosis as an inflammatory and prothrombotic process. Rokitansky, and later Duguid, posited that atherosclerotic lesions are initiated by incorporation of platelet lipids into the vessel wall ("encrustation") following thrombosis. It was subsequently demonstrated that insudation of plasma lipoproteins is responsible for most of the lipid content of the atherosclerotic lesions. In 1913, Anitschkow, in Russia, noted atherosclerosis developing in rabbits fed a relatively high cholesterol diet. Although the involvement of inflammation in atherosclerosis has been known for more than 100 years, the molecular mechanisms of atherosclerotic disease initiation and progression have only become clearer over the past decade.[2]

Acronyms and abbreviations that appear in this chapter include: ACC, American College of Cardiology; ACCP, American College of Chest Physicians; ACS, acute coronary syndrome; AHA, American Heart Association; apo, apolipoprotein; aPTT, activated partial thromboplastin time; CAPRIE, Clopidogrel Versus Aspirin in Patients at Risk of Ischaemic Events; CK, creatine kinase; ECG, electrocardiogram; eNOS, endothelial nitric oxide synthase; HDL, high-density lipoprotein; hsCRP, high-sensitivity C-reactive protein; IFN, interferon; Ig, immunoglobulin; IL, interleukin; LDL, low-density lipoprotein; MCP, monocyte chemoattractant protein; MHC, major histocompatibility complex; MI, myocardial infarction; NO, nitric oxide; NSTEMI, non–ST-segment elevation myocardial infarction; PAD, peripheral arterial disease; PAI, plasminogen-activator inhibitor; PCI, percutaneous coronary intervention; TF, tissue factor; TGF, transforming growth factor; Th, T helper; VCAM, vascular cell adhesion molecule; VLDL, very-low-density lipoprotein.

Lipid accumulation in the arterial intima, a fatty streak (Table 135–1), can occur in adolescents and may progress in paroxysmal fashion to a hemodynamically significant lesion causing arterial insufficiency. Autopsy studies of young soldiers and young trauma victims indicated that occult coronary atherosclerotic plaques are commonly present in healthy individuals in their teens and twenties.[3,4] In addition, intracoronary ultrasonograph studies demonstrated the presence of coronary atherosclerosis in 37 percent of healthy heart donors aged 20 to 29 years, 60 percent of those aged 30 to 39 years, and 85 percent of those older than age 50 years.[5] Several theories have been espoused for this propitious condition. One of these well-recognized theories is the *response to injury hypothesis* whereby the inciting event that predisposes to atherosclerosis is injury to the endothelial lining of the artery. This hypothesis was formulated in animal studies that showed vessel narrowing and intimal thickening after endothelial denudation with angioplasty.[6,7] However, human pathologic studies of early atherosclerotic plaques indicate that endothelium is structurally present but is dysfunctional. The dysfunctional state of endothelium induces abnormalities in vascular tone, inflammation, growth, and thrombosis. Atherosclerotic risk factors contribute to endothelial dysfunction and promote atherosclerosis. This section describes the mechanisms responsible for endothelial dysfunction and the impact of atherosclerotic risk factors.

ATHEROSCLEROTIC RISK FACTORS

Increasing age, male gender, and heredity are the major atherosclerotic cardiovascular disease risk factors that cannot be modified. Abnormal lipids, smoking, hypertension, diabetes mellitus, abdominal obesity, physical inactivity, alcohol, and psychosocial factors are established risk factors that can be modified, accounting for most of the risk of myocardial infarction worldwide in both sexes and at all ages.[8]

In addition to these traditional risk factors, newer risk factors have been recognized in recent years.[9] With the use of highly active antiretroviral therapy (HAART), HIV-infected patients have demonstrated dramatic overall increase in life expectancy. At the same time, HAART-treated HIV patients also have an increased risk of developing premature cardiovascular disease over time. Both HIV viral proteins and the antiretroviral drugs themselves cause endothelial dysfunction. They activate cell signaling cascades, induce oxidative stress, disturb mitochondrial function, alter gene expression, and impair lipid metabolism in vascular cells, macrophages, and adipocytes.[10,11]

Cardiovascular morbidity and mortality is also recognized to be exceedingly high in patients with chronic renal failure.[12] Increased risk of premature atherosclerotic cardiovascular disease in patients on chronic hemodialysis has been known for many years, but recent studies point to an increased risk even at early stages of chronic kidney diseases. Low glomerular filtration rates and/or proteinuria are independently associated with increased rates of cardiovascular disease.[13] Other factors, such as sympathetic overactivity,[14] are likely to contribute to the pathophysiology of cardiac risk in these patients. Among other emerging risk factors is obstructive sleep apnea, in which treatment may improve cardiovascular outcomes.[15]

ENDOTHELIAL DYSFUNCTION

Cardiovascular risk factors and abnormal blood rheology are thought to result in endothelial dysfunction that predisposes the aorta and arteries

TABLE 135–1. Glossary of Terms

Fatty streak	Early accumulation of cholesterol in the intima of an artery
Atherosclerotic lesion	Accumulation of cholesterol, sclerotic tissue, inflammatory cells, smooth muscle cells, and calcium in a lesion that develops in the intima of the artery wall
Vulnerable plaque	Atherosclerotic plaque with high degree of inflammation, vulnerable to rupture or ulceration
Endothelial dysfunction	Abnormal function of endothelial cells lining the lumen of an artery
Foam cells	Lipid-laden macrophages
Scavenger receptors	Cell surface receptors on macrophages that bind and facilitate internalization into the cell of substances such as oxidized low-density lipoprotein and products of apoptotic cells

to atherosclerotic plaque development, sparing the arterioles and capillaries (Fig. 135–1). *Endothelial dysfunction* is a term that encompasses perturbations in the diverse physiologic functions of normal arteries, including regulation of vascular tone, inflammation, growth, and preservation of blood fluidity. Lipid accumulation[16] and endothelial dysfunction are intimately connected and seminal to the initiation and progression of atherosclerosis. Endothelial dysfunction occurs early in the development of plaque and is systemic in nature, afflicting vessels throughout the arterial circulation without gross evidence of atherosclerotic plaque formation. Emerging data indicate that proatherosclerotic genes are upregulated and antiatherosclerotic genes are downregulated in areas of turbulent blood flow, as seen at branch points of arteries,[17] resulting in vascular adhesion molecule expression and recruitment of monocytes.[18] The atherosclerotic plaque initially may expand outward rather than inward into the vessel wall, making some significant lesions difficult to visualize by angiography. The components of the mature atherosclerotic lesion include smooth muscle cells, macrophages, T lymphocytes, and calcification, in addition to accumulation of lipoproteins.[19] Neutrophils and mast cells also are implicated in the atherosclerotic process.[18] Later in the process, increased activity of matrix metalloproteinases in the atherosclerotic cap predisposes to plaque rupture or ulceration, resulting in tissue factor (TF) exposure and platelet adhesion, culminating in thrombus formation.[20] The thrombus may undergo endogenous fibrinolysis with plaque healing or become occlusive and produce organ damage (e.g., myocardial infarction [MI]). In severe lesions, lamellar bone, presumably from endochondral calcification, may appear.[21] The following sections describe in detail the major manifestations of endothelial dysfunction that occur early in the atherosclerotic process.

Abnormal Vascular Tone

The importance of the endothelium in maintaining vascular tone was first recognized when endothelial cells of rabbit aorta were inadvertently removed and resulted in paradoxical vasoconstriction after administration of acetylcholine.[22] The major endothelium-dependent vasodilator normally produced was found to be nitric oxide (NO), a free radical gas with multiple physiologic properties,[23] including inhibition of platelet aggregation and inflammation and stimulation of angiogenesis. Numerous studies indicate that the endothelium does not vasodilate appropriately in the setting of traditional and emerging cardiovascular risk factors. Cardiovascular risk factors (Table 135–2) are thought to reduce NO availability through a variety of mechanisms, including increased oxidative stress, through generation of reactive oxygen species, and in so doing create an environment conducive to development of atherosclerosis.[24] Major sources of reactive oxygen species are nicotinamide adenine dinucleotide phosphate (NADPH) oxidases. The catalytic subunits of the NADPH oxidases are the nicotinamide adenine dinucleotide phosphate oxidase (NOX) proteins and are found in atherosclerotic lesions.[25] A reduction in NO synthesis is thought to occur because of decreased availability of tetrahydrobiopterin, an essential cofactor for synthesis of NO.[26] Administration of sepiapterin, a substrate for tetrahydrobiopterin, improves endothelial dysfunction.[27] Also, recent evidence indicates that the transcription factor p53 and the adaptor protein p66 Shc both play essential roles in impairing endothelium-dependent vascular relaxation.[28] High cholesterol levels are thought to produce oxygen free radicals that may inactivate NO. NO synthases are the enzymes responsible for converting L-arginine to NO (Fig. 135–2). The enzyme may be perturbed by modified low-density lipoprotein (LDL), resulting in decreased NO production. Supplementation of the diet with L-arginine leads to improvement in endothelial-dependent vasodilation.[29] Elevated levels of asymmetric dimethylarginine, an endogenous competitive inhibitor of NO synthase,

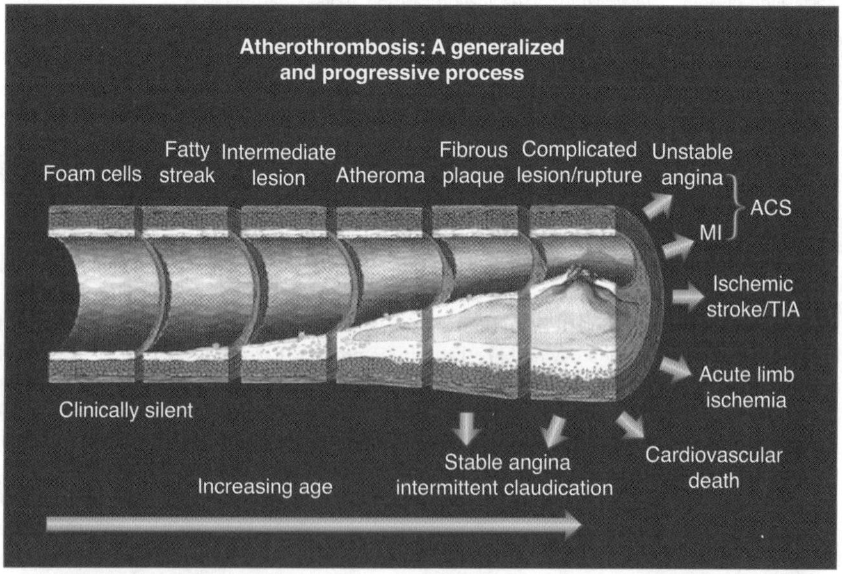

FIGURE 135–1. Schematic showing the life span of the atherosclerotic plaque, beginning with the fatty streak and resulting in a thrombotic event. Cardiovascular risk factors and disturbed blood flow at branch points of vessels are thought to cause endothelial dysfunction that results in atherosclerotic plaque development in the aorta and conduit arteries. Early lipid accumulation in the intimal layer is called the *fatty streak*. A series of stimuli, including lipid peroxidation, are thought to signal adhesion molecule expression on the endothelium, which results in monocyte adhesion and diapedesis into the intimal space. The monocytes develop into macrophages and become sessile with accumulation of lipid (foam cells). Smooth muscle cells, primarily from the media, enter the plaque and participate in cap formation. The plaque accumulates hydroxyapatite mineral and forms calcific deposits. Matrix metalloproteinases also accumulate in the lesion and may predispose to plaque rupture or ulceration resulting in tissue factor exposure and thrombus formation. Risk factor modification favors a more stable plaque, which may have relatively less lipid accumulation and more sclerotic tissue than an unstable plaque. Severe lesions may even develop lamellar bone. ACS, acute coronary syndrome; TIA, transient ischemic attack. *(Adapted with permission from Stary HC.[19])*

TABLE 135–2. Cardiovascular Risk Factors That Cause Impaired Endothelium-Dependent Vasodilatation

Smoking
Dyslipidemia
Hypertension
Diabetes mellitus
Hyperhomocysteinemia

found in patients with hypercholesterolemia and diabetes, also may result in decreased NO availability.[30] Oxidized LDL is thought to increase the elaboration of asymmetric dimethylarginine by endothelial cells and decrease its degradation by the enzyme dimethylarginine dimethylaminohydrolase.[31] Administration of acetylcholine to patients with elevated serum LDL[32] and relatively low high-density lipoprotein (HDL)[33] may result in abnormal vasoconstriction, which can be reversed with nitroglycerin (an endothelium-independent vasodilator).[34] Intravenous infusion of HDL improves endothelial-mediated vasodilation through improved NO availability.[35] The decreased vasodilatory capacity because of dyslipidemia may facilitate the development of coronary ischemia.

Impaired endothelial vasodilation is noted with advanced aging,[36] when the hands are exposed to cold, and during mental stress.[37] The impairment may be mediated by increased production of endothelin, a potent vasoconstrictor.[38] Sex differences are also seen in endothelial function as women in middle age tend to have more endothelial vasodilation than men at all ages.[39] Infection with concomitant inflammation is associated with impaired endothelial vasodilation. For example, repeated infection with *Chlamydia pneumoniae* results in endothelial dysfunction via impaired NO availability.[40] The combination of coronary artery disease and elevated serum levels of high-sensitivity C-reactive protein (hsCRP) is an independent predictor of abnormal endothelial vasoreactivity.[41] External radiation therapy also results in endothelial dysfunction and may explain the increased risk of atherosclerosis in patients receiving mantle irradiation for Hodgkin lymphoma.[42]

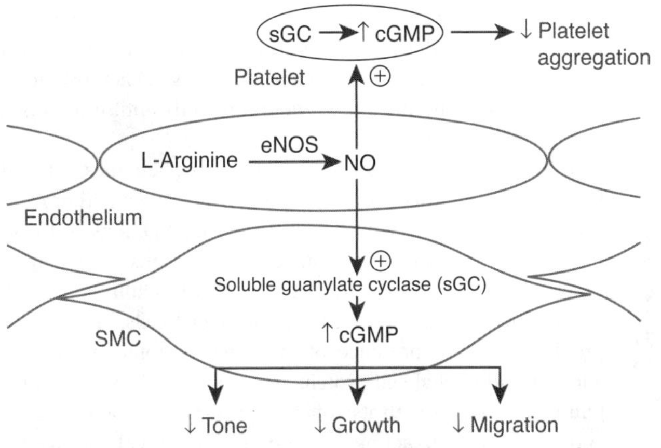

FIGURE 135–2. Vascular tone depends on endothelial production and release of various vasoconstricting and vasodilating substances. The endothelial-derived vasodilators include nitric oxide (NO) and prostacyclin. NO is generated from the amino acid L-arginine by constitutive endothelial NO synthase (eNOS, or NOSIII). The enzyme is stimulated by blood flow across the endothelial surface (shear stress) or by chemical mediators, such as acetylcholine, which stimulate receptors on the endothelial surface. NO diffuses to the underlying smooth muscle cells (SMC), where it stimulates guanylate cyclase to generate cyclic guanosine V monophosphate (cGMP), which causes smooth muscle relaxation and vasodilation. It also diffuses into blood, where it increases intraplatelet cGMP and thereby inhibits platelet adhesion and aggregation.

Endothelial Inflammation

The endothelium does not routinely interact with inflammatory cells but is poised to express adhesion molecules after stimulation with inflammatory mediators. An inflammatory response is thought to begin in the vessel wall after "invasion" of pathogenic lipoproteins.[43] The presence of lipoproteins, especially oxidized LDL, results in expression of adhesion molecules such as vascular cell adhesion molecule (VCAM)-1 on the luminal surface of endothelial cells, leading to adherence of monocytes (Fig. 135–3).[44] Endothelial cell expression of adhesion molecules and recruitment of monocytes can be regarded as endothelial dysfunction because these events may occur in the absence of morphologic changes in the vessel wall. Inflammation may develop without the demonstrable presence of an external microbial pathogen. The complex interactions of inflammation and the endothelium on the initiation and progression of atherosclerosis are reviewed in more detail in "Inflammation and Atherosclerosis" below.

Abnormal Control of Vascular Growth: Smooth Muscle Cells and Extracellular Matrix

Normal endothelium inhibits vascular smooth muscle cell proliferation.[45] The specific function of vascular smooth muscle cells in atherosclerosis is unclear. However, evidence indicates that, in early

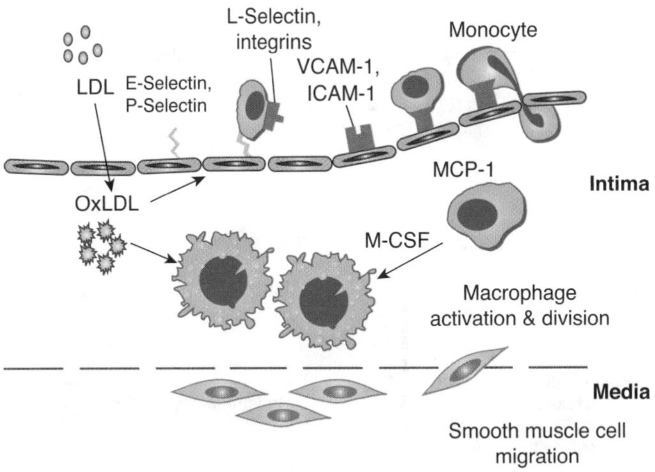

FIGURE 135–3. Atherosclerotic lesion initiation is stimulated by oxidized low-density lipoprotein (OxLDL). Induction of inflammatory gene products in vascular cells is activated by nuclear factor-κB transcription factor, which results in increased expression of cellular adhesion molecules. The adhesion molecules have specific functions for endothelial leukocyte interaction. The selectins tether and trap monocytes and other leukocytes. Vascular cell adhesion molecule-1 (VCAM-1) and intracellular adhesion molecule-1 (ICAM-1) mediate firm attachment of these leukocytes to the endothelial layer. OxLDL also augments expression of monocyte chemoattractant protein-1 (MCP-1) and macrophage colony-stimulating factor (M-CSF). MCP-1 mediates the attraction of monocytes and leukocytes and facilitates diapedesis through the endothelium into the intima. M-CSF is an important cytokine for the transformation of monocytes to macrophage foam cells. Macrophages express scavenger receptors and internalize oxidized LDL during their transformation into foam cells. Smooth muscle cells migrate from the media into the intima and participate in the formation of a fibrous atheroma. *(Adapted with permission from Kinlay S, Selwyn AP, Libby P: Inflammation, the endothelium, and the acute coronary syndromes.* J Cardiovasc Pharmacol *32[Suppl 3]:S62, 1998.)*

atherosclerosis, vascular smooth muscle cells contribute to the development of atheroma through production of proinflammatory mediators such as monocyte chemoattractant protein (MCP)-1 and VCAMs. Although smooth muscle cells primarily play a role in modulating vascular tone, they also are involved in the control of extracellular matrix formation and degradation through matrix modulators such as proteases, protease inhibitors, matrix proteins, and integrins (Fig. 135–4).

The importance of vascular smooth muscle cells in controlling the synthesis of matrix molecules is evident at the clinical level. They provide a thick, fibrous cap that promotes stability and inhibits plaque rupture and ulceration. Factor VII-activating protease, thought to play a role in coagulation and fibrinolysis, is also a potent inhibitor of vascular smooth muscle cell proliferation, and migration *in vitro* and local application of factor VII-activating protease (but not Marburg I variant) in animal models reduces neointima formation.[46] Furthermore, it has been localized to unstable atherosclerotic plaques and may contribute to plaque instability.

Evidence indicates that vascular smooth muscle cells that undergo apoptosis, especially at the shoulder region of the plaque, may create a more unstable cap.[47] Both intact vascular smooth muscle cells and fibroblasts are thought to stabilize plaques through modulation of extracellular calcification and formation of a fibrocalcific plaque.

Vascular smooth muscle cells arise primarily from the medial layer and are considered monoclonal in origin.[48] Evidence also indicates that vascular smooth muscle cells may originate from the adventitia.[49] The rate and timing of smooth muscle cell replication is unclear. It may occur at a constant low rate throughout the development of the atherosclerotic lesion or episodically at a higher rate. Animal studies indicate that new intimal cells may originate from outside the vessel wall from subpopulations of marrow- and non–marrow-derived circulating cells.[50–52] Smooth muscle progenitor cells circulating in blood may contribute to the arterial remodeling that occurs after angioplasty and after bypass graft surgery.[53]

Vascular proliferation and inflammation are linked processes. Inflammation-induced impaired NO bioactivity contributes to vascular smooth muscle proliferation.[2] Overexpression of NO synthase results in reduction of atherosclerotic or restenotic lesion formation in rabbits through both inhibition of vascular smooth muscle cell proliferation and inhibition of adhesion and chemoattractant molecule expression, with subsequent reduction of vascular mononuclear cell infiltration.[54,55] Thus, the vascular smooth muscle cell participates in the atherosclerotic process by affecting lipoprotein retention, modulating inflammation, and controlling plaque stability through formation of the fibrous cap. Several vascular disorders involve vascular smooth muscle proliferation as the primary pathophysiologic mechanism, including in-stent restenosis, transplant vasculopathy, and vein bypass graft failure.[56] The control of smooth muscle proliferation is thought to involve NR4A nuclear receptors that are expressed in atherosclerotic lesion macrophages, smooth muscle cells, and endothelial cells, and are induced by atherogenic stimuli. Inhibition of the transcriptional activity of the NR4A nuclear receptors results in enhanced smooth muscle proliferation.[57] The NR4A nuclear receptors are also expressed in vein segments exposed to arterial pressure and it is postulated that they are responsible for an inhibitory feedback mechanism that occurs in activated vascular cells. Drug-eluting vascular stents that release agents such as sirolimus and paclitaxel interfere with the cell cycle and inhibit restenosis in part via decreased smooth muscle cell proliferation.[58]

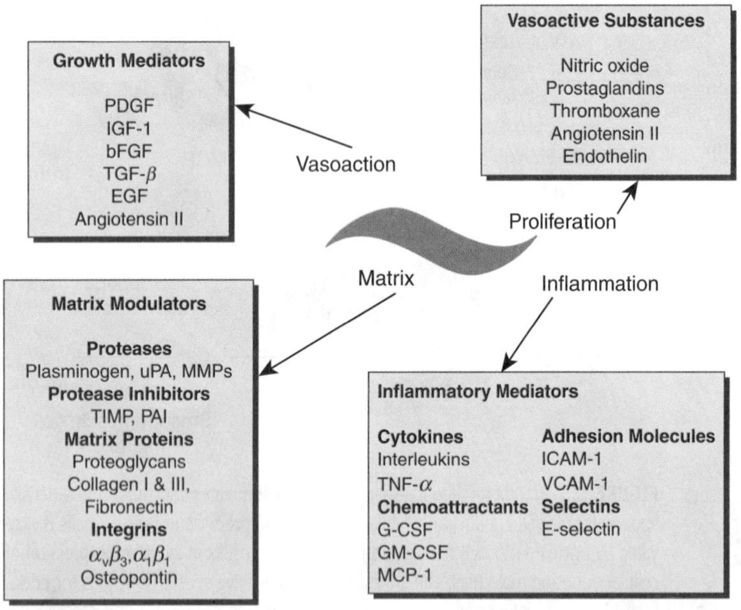

FIGURE 135–4. Vascular smooth muscle cells mediate vascular proliferation, inflammation, matrix composition, and contraction. Many of these mediators have multiple functions. For example, angiotensin is a vasoconstrictor, but it also stimulates proliferation and inflammation. This is only a partial list of mediators secreted by vascular smooth muscle cells. bFGF, basic fibroblast growth factor; EGF, epidermal growth factor; G-CSF, granulocyte colony-stimulating factor; GM-CSF, granulocyte-monocyte colony-stimulating factor; ICAM, intracellular adhesion molecule; IGF, insulin-like growth factor; MCP, monocyte chemoattractant protein; MMPs, matrix metalloproteinases; PAI, plasminogen-activator inhibitor; PDGF, platelet-derived growth factor; TGF-β, transforming growth factor-β; TIMP, tissue inhibitor of metalloproteinases; TNF, tumor necrosis factor; uPA, urokinase-type plasminogen activator; VCAM, vascular cell adhesion molecule. *(Adapted with permission from Dzau VJ, Braun-Dullaeus RC, Sedding DG.[56])*.

Abnormal Endothelial Control of Blood Fluidity

Endothelial cells normally elaborate a number of antithrombotic substances. Some of these substances are released into blood whereas others are properties of the unactivated endothelial cell surface. These antiplatelet, anticoagulant, and profibrinolytic activities of endothelium, some of which also possess vasodilatory properties (e.g., prostacyclin, NO), act in concert to promote blood fluidity under normal circumstances. Acute activation or chronic dysfunction of endothelial cells alters the hemostatic balance, transforming them from predominantly antithrombotic to prothrombotic cells.[59]

To this end, endothelial cells modulate the activities of thrombin in health and disease. In the presence of intact and normally functioning endothelium, the prothrombotic actions of thrombin are quenched and the antithrombotic actions of the enzyme predominate. Thrombin binds to thrombomodulin, an integral membrane protein expressed by endothelial cells, and activates protein C in the presence of endothelial protein C receptor, another endothelial cell protein (see Chap. 116). Activated protein C, in concert with its cofactor, protein S, has anticoagulant and profibrinolytic actions. It degrades by proteolytic digestion factors Va and VIIIa, and inactivates plasminogen-activator inhibitor (PAI)-1. Simultaneously, by binding to thrombomodulin, enzymatically active procoagulant thrombin is removed from the circulation, thereby limiting its availability to catalyze fibrin formation. Endothelial dysfunction causes loss of thrombomodulin activity from the vascular surface. In fact, increased circulating plasma levels of free thrombomodulin represent a marker of endothelial damage. In addition to the role of thrombomodulin in clearance of circulating thrombin, the procoagulant activity of thrombin is normally blocked by endothelial cells through the action of antithrombin, which binds to heparin-like glycosaminoglycans on their luminal surface, thereby catalyzing the inactivation of thrombin by antithrombin. Like thrombomodulin, this thrombin-neutralizing action of endothelial heparan sulfate glycosaminoglycans is lost with endothelial dysfunction.

Endothelial cells do not normally express TF, but they do so upon activation by inflammatory cytokines or exposure to endothelium-activating levels of homocysteine or free thrombin. The procoagulant effects of expression of TF by dysfunctional endothelial cells are potentially compounded by loss of TF pathway inhibitor, which normally is synthesized by endothelial cells.

Normal endothelium is profibrinolytic. It synthesizes and releases tissue-type plasminogen activator; it possesses binding sites for tissue-type plasminogen activator and plasminogen to provide a surface for the concentrated assembly of the fibrinolytic complex and thereby enhance local plasmin generation; and it fails to produce significant amounts of PAI-1. This profibrinolytic state is converted to an antifibrinolytic state in the presence of endothelial dysfunction. In activated or dysfunctional endothelium, PAI-1 gene expression and PAI-1 secretion are induced; simultaneously, the profibrinolytic properties of normal endothelium are lost (see Chap. 136).

The antithrombotic profile of normal endothelium also manifests through the elaboration of several antiplatelet substances. NO is constitutively released into blood by normal endothelial cells and inhibits platelet adhesion and aggregation by stimulating platelet soluble guanylyl cyclase and raising intraplatelet levels of cyclic guanosine monophosphate (see Fig. 135–2).[60] Physiologic flow and shear forces maintain the activity of endothelial (endothelium-derived) nitric oxide synthase (eNOS)[61,62] under normal circumstances. Vascular cell-derived carbon monoxide, a product of heme catabolism by heme oxygenase, may have similar antiplatelet activity.[63] Prostacyclin (prostaglandin I_2) likewise is released basally by normal endothelial cells and inhibits platelet aggregation by inducing platelet adenylyl cyclase and raising intraplatelet levels of cyclic adenosine monophosphate.[64]

NO, carbon monoxide, and prostaglandin I_2 are labile autacoids, acting only in the immediate vicinity of their release into blood from endothelial cells. An endothelial surface ecto-adenosine diphosphatase (CD39) also blocks platelet activity by metabolizing and disposing of platelet aggregatory adenosine diphosphate (ADP).[65] In endothelial dysfunction, these various antiplatelet activities are lost, and endothelial release of von Willebrand factor is increased, which promotes platelet adhesion. In the case of NO, oxidative stress in the microenvironment of endothelial dysfunction actually "uncouples" eNOS activity[62,66] to preferentially generate superoxide over NO. Oxygen-free radicals bind any remaining available NO to produce the toxic product peroxynitrite. Bioactive NO is further reduced in endothelial dysfunction by the presence of asymmetric dimethylarginine, which competes to block eNOS and limit NO production.[61,67]

Progenitor Cells and Atherosclerosis

Endothelial progenitor cells (EPCs) are heterogenous in origin and participate in endothelial cell regeneration and neovascularization of ischemic tissue. The mobilization of EPCs from the marrow is stimulated by hypoxia, cytokines such as vascular endothelial growth factor, hormones such as erythropoietin, and statin drugs, whereas mobilization is inhibited in the diabetic state.[68] The role of EPCs in atherosclerosis is unclear as there are conflicting data.[18] A study in apolipoprotein (apoE)–/– mice showed that there is rapid turnover of endothelial cells in atherosclerosis-prone areas and marrow derived EPCs are recruited to sites of atheroprogression.[69]

INFLAMMATION AND ATHEROSCLEROSIS

Innate Immunity and Atherosclerosis

The endothelial response to injury manifests as a chronic inflammatory response that involves both innate and adaptive immunity.[70] Innate immunity provides the first line of defense for the host and involves several cell types, most importantly macrophages and dendritic cells, which express a limited number of highly conserved sensing molecules such as scavenger receptors and toll-like receptors.[70,71] Microbial infection can be detected by pathogen-associated molecular patterns, which are present in bacteria, viruses, and yeast, but not in mammalian cells, and are recognized by the toll-like receptors.[72] Ligation of a pathogen or other substances containing pathogen-associated molecular patterns (such as lipopolysaccharides, aldehyde-derivatized proteins, mannans, teichoic acids) elicits endocytosis or activation of endothelial cells (e.g., through nuclear factor-κB) that results in an inflammatory response (see Chaps. 17 and 18).[71,73] Proinflammatory cytokines, such as tumor necrosis factor-κB and interleukin (IL)-1, magnify the innate inflammatory response.

Innate defense involves soluble factors, such as complement, which is involved in atherosclerotic lesion formation.[64] hsCRP has been found to be an important and independent predictor for cardiovascular events.[74] Natural antibodies that are generated in the absence of known antigen stimulation, mainly immunoglobulin (Ig) M, provide an immediate response against bacteria and viruses but also may be involved in atherosclerosis. For example, innate B lymphocytes, the so-called B1 cells, express a restricted set of germ-line–encoded antigen receptors that may bind oxidized LDL.

Adaptive Immunity and Atherosclerosis

Compared to innate immunity, adaptive immunity is slower but more precise (see Chap. 77).[70] T cells can be activated by dendritic cells and macrophages, whereas most antigens cannot stimulate B cells without assistance from CD4+ T cells, which recognize the peptide–major histocompatibility complex (MHC) complexes on B cells. By genetic recombination, the number of T-cell and B-cell receptors that can be formed is almost unlimited and far exceed the number of pattern recognition receptors used by the innate immune system. Most CD4+ cells are cytokine-secreting T-helper (Th) cells and express $\alpha\beta$–T-cell receptors, which interact with MHC class II molecules. A smaller number of Th cells express $\gamma\delta$–T-cell receptors, which interact with the nonpolymorphic, nonclassic MHC molecules, CD1, which present certain antigens (particularly lipids and glycolipids). Th cells are classified according to the cytokines they secrete. Th1 cells secrete interferon (IFN)-γ and IL-2 and promote cell-mediated immunity (see Chap. 78). Th2 cells secrete IL-4, IL-5, IL-10, and IL-13 and help B cells produce antibodies. CD8+ T cells are primarily cytotoxic killer cells, although they can secrete cytokines, such as tumor necrosis factor-α, IFN-γ, and lymphotoxin. Some thymus-independent antigens can activate these cells without the help of T cells. Oxidized LDL is considered such an antigen because it expresses multiple copies of oxidation-specific epitopes on a single LDL particle.

Adhesion Molecules and Atherosclerosis

Monocyte recruitment to inflammatory foci initially involves the expression of endothelial cell selectins, which mediate monocyte rolling on the endothelium (see Fig. 135–3). The rolling phenomenon is followed by a firmer attachment to endothelial cells mediated by integrins. Perhaps the most important of these is VCAM-1, which is upregulated in cultured endothelial cells in the presence of oxidized LDL. The appearance of this molecule before the development of grossly visible atherosclerotic lesions supports oxidized LDL as an initial recruiter of macrophages. The finding of reduced atherosclerosis in VCAM-1–deficient mice further supports the important role of macrophages and VCAM-1 in the pathogenesis of atherosclerosis.[75,76] Other adhesion molecules, such as P-selectin and intracellular cell adhesion molecule-1, also may be involved in monocyte adhesion at sites of lesion formation.[77]

Lipoprotein Phospholipase A_2 and Atherosclerosis

Lipoprotein phospholipase A_2 (Lp-PLA_2) is an inflammatory enzyme belonging to the large family of phospholipases that are capable of hydrolyzing the sn-2 ester bond of phospholipids of cell membranes and lipoproteins.[78] This enzyme, produced by macrophages, circulates bound to low-density lipoprotein (LDL) and in the intimal space of the artery can produce oxidized fatty acids and lysophosphatidyl choline. These molecules have a range of potentially atherogenic effects, including chemoattraction of monocytes, increased expression of adhesion molecules, and inhibition of endothelial nitric oxide production.[79] Although originally designated as platelet-activating factor acetylhydrolase because of its ability to degrade platelet-activating factor, the clinical importance of this effect is not thought significant. Numerous epidemiologic studies show that Lp-PLA_2 is a significant biomarker associated with cardiovascular events. The selective inhibition of Lp-PLA_2 with the drug darapladib reduced development of advanced coronary atherosclerosis in diabetic and hypercholesterolemic swine.[80] A phase 2 clinical study of patients with cardiovascular disease showed that sustained inhibition of plasma Lp-PLA_2 activity with background of intensive atorvastatin therapy resulted in reduction in IL-6 and hsCRP after 12 weeks of darapladib 160 mg, suggesting a possible reduction in inflammatory burden.[81]

Immune Cells and Atherosclerosis

Macrophages are essential for the clearance of modified lipoproteins and the efflux of lipoprotein-derived cholesterol to HDL receptors for reverse cholesterol transport, the process by which HDL removes cholesterol from cells. Multiple lines of evidence indicate that macrophages promote lesion initiation and progression. For example, hypercholesterolemic mice become markedly resistant to atherosclerosis if they are bred to macrophage-deficient animals.[82]

The earliest grossly visible sign of atherosclerosis is the fatty streak, which is composed mainly of macrophage foam cells containing relatively large amounts of cholesterol. Foam cells also can derive from smooth muscle cells, as these cells can express scavenger receptors when appropriately activated.[83,84] Formation of the fatty streak is thought to begin with adherence of circulating monocytes to activated endothelial cells at sites in the arterial system prone to atherosclerotic disease, such as at branch points in vessels. Multiple chemoattractant molecules have been identified in these nascent lesions, which recruit monocytes and induce their diapedesis into the subendothelial space where they further differentiate into macrophages.

The chemoattractant MCP-1 facilitates recruitment of monocytes to atherosclerotic lesions, as noted in studies of mouse models of atherosclerosis, such as apolipoprotein E (apoE–/–) or LDL receptor (LDLR–/–)–deficient mice fed a Western-style diet. When these mice are crossed to the model lacking MCP-1 or its receptor CCR-2, lesion development decreases significantly.[85–87]

Macrophages and T cells were once thought to be the only inflammatory cells to significantly promote angiogenesis. More recent data showing that neutrophils are found at sites of plaque rupture or erosion and in thrombus from patients with acute coronary artery syndromes indicate that they also have an important role in atherothrombosis.[18] Mast cells have been found in the adventitia of lesions and in areas of plaque hemorrhage; they have been implicated in macrophage apoptosis, increased vascular permeability, degradation of HDL and reduced cholesterol efflux.[18] Neutrophils and mast cells are recruited to atherosclerotic lesions in response to CXC-chemokine receptor 2 (CXCR2) signals. The mobilization of neutrophils to atherosclerotic lesions is inhibited by CXC-chemokine receptor 4 (CXCR4) and its ligand CXC-chemokine ligand 12 (CXCRL12; also known as SDF 1).

Lipid Peroxidation and Atherosclerosis

Macrophages control the amount of cholesterol loading by downregulating the native LDL receptor. Therefore, knowing how cholesterol is taken up into macrophages is important. Cell culture experiments revealed a "foam cell paradox," in which macrophages engulf only modified lipids. Treatment of native LDL with copper or acetic anhydride (causing acetylation) led to increased LDL uptake through use of the scavenger receptor, leading to the formation of lipid-laden macrophages. These experiments led to the peroxidation theory of atherosclerosis,[84,88] whereby LDL modification is an essential step in the development of foam cells. Although the precise mechanisms responsible for LDL oxidation remain unclear, enzymes including myeloperoxidase, inducible NO synthase, and NADPH oxidases are involved in the process.[88,89] Of note, macrophages express each of these enzymes, which normally are used as antimicrobial reactive oxygen species essential for native immunity.[90] Thus, accumulation of cholesterol in the macrophage occurs via scavenger (not LDL) receptors of oxidized (and not native) LDL.

Scavenger Receptors and Atherosclerosis

Conserved pattern recognition receptors expressed by macrophages include scavenger receptors A and B1 and CD36, all of which internalize oxidized LDL.[91,92] Macrophages express various genes in response to oxidized LDL, including peroxisome proliferator-activated receptor-γ and adenosine triphosphate-binding cassette transporter A1, which profoundly influence macrophage-mediated inflammation and atherosclerotic activity.

Cell culture studies indicate that scavenger receptor A recognizes acetylated LDL but, unlike the LDL receptor, is not downregulated in response to increased cholesterol content and thus likely accounts for foam cell formation.[93] However, no evidence indicates that acetyl LDL is generated *in vivo*, indicating other modifications of LDL, such as oxidation, may be required for foam cell formation.[94,95] Another scavenger receptor presumed to be involved in the atherosclerotic process is CD36, a receptor that avidly binds oxidized LDL.

Circulating IgG and IgM antibodies against products of lipid peroxidation are present in the plasma of animals and humans.[96] These antibodies closely correlate with measures of lipid peroxidation and with atherosclerotic progression and regression in murine models.[97] Immunization of hypercholesterolemic rabbits and mice with products of oxidized LDL, such as malonyldialdehyde LDL or copper-oxidized LDL, inhibits the progression of atherosclerotic lesion formation.[98–101] These experiments have been interpreted to indicate that an immunologic response to oxidized LDL components can alter the atherosclerotic process.

Leukocyte-derived 5-lipoxygenase also contributes to atherosclerosis susceptibility in mice.[102] Animal studies indicate the importance of lipoxygenases in atherosclerosis as disruption of the 12/15-lipoxygenase gene diminishes atherosclerosis in apoE-deficient mice, and overexpression of 15-lipoxygenase in vascular endothelium accelerates early atherosclerosis in LDL receptor-deficient mice.[103,104] This enzyme is under study as a potential target to inhibit the atherosclerotic process.[105]

Accumulation of LDL in the Vascular Wall

Three potential factors lead to accumulation of LDL in the vascular wall: increased permeability of the endothelium, prolonged retention of lipoproteins in the intima, and slow removal of lipoproteins from the vessel wall.[106] Rabbits fed a high-cholesterol diet develop aortic wall lesions at specific lesion-susceptible sites; however, endothelial permeability is not increased at those sites, indicating that LDL is selectively retained in these regions.[107,108] Retention of LDL molecules likely results from their adherence to proteoglycans in the vessel wall.[109] LDL genetically engineered to not bind to proteoglycans is hypothesized to be less atherogenic than native LDL.[16]

Oxidized LDL and its products, oxidized phospholipids and oxysterols, have other properties that make them potentially proatherogenic.[110] These properties include proinflammatory characteristics, such as chemotactic signaling for monocytes, smooth muscle cells, and T lymphocytes (but not for B lymphocytes or neutrophils, neither of which is found in lesions) and increased expression of VCAM-1 on, and stimulation of MCP-1 release from, endothelial cells.[111] Oxidized LDL also may contribute to instability of the atherosclerotic plaque via induction of type 1 metalloproteinase expression and increase in TF activity.[44] For oxidized LDL to be a ligand for the scavenger receptor, extensive degradation of the polyunsaturated fatty acid in the sn-2 position of phospholipids by oxidation is essential.

To test the oxidized LDL hypothesis, several clinical studies have been conducted using antioxidant vitamins, most commonly vitamin E; however, most of the published reports provide negative results.[112,113] At the present time, treatment with vitamin E at doses of 400 to 800 IU daily does not seem adequate to prevent cardiovascular events. However, these studies have been inadequate to prove or disprove the hypothesis; other antioxidant combinations may prove more beneficial.

High-Density Lipoprotein and Atherosclerosis

A low level of HDL cholesterol is a strong predictor of adverse cardiovascular events, presumably because the low level is associated with insufficient reverse cholesterol transport.[114,115] Animal studies using liver-directed gene transfer of human apoA-I resulted in significant promotion of reverse cholesterol transport and regression of preexisting atherosclerotic lesions in LDL receptor-deficient mice.[116,117] However, HDL has additional antiatherogenic properties that may confer protection against atherosclerosis.[118] For example, HDL is protective against oxidation of LDL, at least in part because of paraoxonase, an enzyme physically associated with HDL that degrades organophosphates.[119] Paraoxonase polymorphisms are associated with increased risk of cardiovascular disease, also indicating that oxidized LDL is an important factor in atherosclerotic development.[120]

Research studies currently are evaluating novel ways to increase HDL levels or to use apoA-I variants and mimetics that hopefully will cause regression of atherosclerosis. Cholesteryl ester transfer protein promotes the transfer of cholesteryl esters from antiatherogenic HDLs to proatherogenic apoB-containing lipoproteins, including very-low-density lipoproteins (VLDLs), VLDL remnants, intermediate-density lipoproteins, and LDLs. A deficiency of this molecule results in increased HDL levels and decreased LDL levels, a lipid profile that is antiatherogenic. A large clinical study in humans showed that inhibition of the transfer protein with torcetrapib increased HDL levels but was associated with increased mortality and hypertension.[121] It is supposed that the increase in mortality was a result of an off-target effect of the drug increasing blood pressure and not because of cholesterol ester transfer protein inhibition. Clinical trials evaluating the effect of other inhibitors of cholesteryl ester transfer protein on atherosclerosis and cardiovascular events are underway. Along similar lines, delivery of a mutant form of apoA1 (apoA-1 Milano) resulted in regression of plaque size as measured by intravascular ultrasound in a small phase II clinical trial.[122] Studies evaluating the effect of apoA1 mimetics on atherosclerosis also are underway.[123]

CD40, CD40 Ligand, and Atherosclerosis

Studies indicate that human atherosclerotic lesions express the immune mediator CD40 and its soluble ligand sCD40L. Increasing evidence indicates that the CD40–sCD40L signaling pathway plays a central role in several inflammatory processes, including atherosclerosis and graft rejection following transplantation.[124] Interruption of CD40 signaling in hyperlipidemic mice reduces the size of aortic atherosclerotic lesions and their lipid, macrophage, and T-lymphocyte content.[125] Atorvastatin, lovastatin, pravastatin, and simvastatin reduce IFN-γ–induced CD40 expression in a dose-dependent manner. Activation of atheroma-associated cells with human recombinant sCD40L is reduced when cells are treated with statins. In addition, retrospective *ex vivo* immunostaining of human carotid atherosclerotic lesions of patients treated with simvastatin for more than 3 months revealed less CD40 expression and atheroma-associated cells compared with patients who were not treated with the drug. A reduction in sCD40L is associated with pravastatin or cerivastatin therapy.[126] These findings support the notion that statins have antiinflammatory and cholesterol-lowering effects.

Transforming Growth Factor-β and Atherosclerosis

Transforming growth factor (TGF)-β is a cytokine secreted by macrophages, smooth muscle cells, and the Th3 subset of Th cells that has multiple regulatory functions. TGF-β is speculated to contribute to plaque stabilization because it stimulates collagen synthesis and is fibrogenic. One study found that inhibition of TGF-β signaling by neutralizing antibodies led to a larger plaque size with an unstable phenotype.[127] Further studies are needed to clarify the role of TGF-β in atherosclerotic plaque initiation and growth.

Infection and Atherosclerosis

Several infectious agents have been implicated as pathogens in atherosclerosis.[128] A well-studied infectious pathogen is *C. pneumoniae*. Animals infected with this agent develop atherosclerosis, and patients with cardiovascular disease have higher titers of antibodies against this pathogen. Viruses, such as herpes simplex and cytomegalovirus, also are implicated in human atherosclerotic lesion formation. Poor dental hygiene with associated gingivitis may invoke cellular immune activation and provoke atherosclerosis by cytokines or antibodies.[129] Endogenous proteins, such as heat shock proteins, also are implicated in atherosclerosis. One study showed that progression of carotid disease correlated with antibodies against heat shock proteins 65 and 60.[130]

Splenectomy and Atherosclerosis

The relationship between the immune system and atherosclerosis is complex, as evident from an animal study that showed that splenectomy of cholesterol-fed apoE–/– mice led to significantly increased atherosclerosis.[131] This proatherogenic effect was rescued by transfer of either purified B cells or T cells from the spleens of atherosclerotic apoE–/– donors. A long-term study of soldiers who underwent splenectomy after trauma found the soldiers had a twofold increased incidence of coronary artery disease, providing evidence that the spleen has antiatherogenic activity.[132] Further studies are needed to determine if splenectomy significantly impacts the atherosclerotic process.

Genetics and Myocardial Infarction

Atherosclerotic disease is a complex human trait involving multiple genes and environmental factors. Through the study of linkage analysis of families and sibling pairs as well as candidate genes and genome-wide association studies, the genetic predisposition to MI is starting to be understood.[133] The clinical importance of this knowledge is the potential identification of markers of disease for risk prediction and potential intervention to lower the risk of atherosclerotic-based cardiovascular events.

The use of genome-wide linkage analyses of families or sib-pairs has identified chromosomal loci linked to or genetic variations in the arachidonic 5-lipoxygenase-activating protein gene (ALOX5AP)[134] and leukotriene A_4 hydrolase gene (LTA_4H).[135] The genes are both involved in inflammation-related pathway of leukotriene B_4 production. Interestingly, a small molecule inhibitor of ALOX5AP was shown to reduce leukotriene production and plasma levels of C-reactive protein.

Several association studies of unrelated individuals have identified genetic variations that confer susceptibility to atherosclerotic disease and cardiovascular events. Studies using genome-wide linkage analysis identified four single nucleotide polymorphisms on chromosome 9p21.3 that were associated with MI in white cohorts.[133,136] Other genetic polymorphisms that contribute to increased risk of cardiovascular disease will likely be discovered.

ATHEROSCLEROTIC PLAQUE

Plaque Classification

The American Heart Association classification of atherosclerotic plaques into types I through VIII is based on lesion composition and structure (Fig. 135–5).[19,137] Types I through III atherosclerotic plaques have foam cells organized in a fatty streak, ranging from those not visible on close examination (type I) to those that are apparent on examination (type III). Types I through III lesions are small and clinically silent, whereas types IV through VI lesions may obstruct the lumen and produce a clinical event. Type IV lesions contain a confluent pool of lipid and in most patients do not cause anginal symptoms because of the ability of the artery to remodel outward. Type V lesions contain a fibromuscular cap resulting from replacement of tissue disrupted by accumulated lipid and hematoma or organized thrombotic deposits. Type VI lesions involve thrombosis that may be either mural or obstructive. Of note, a type IV lesion may develop type VI changes without ever passing through a type V change and accumulating significant fibrous tissue. Plaques that are complex and primarily composed of calcium are type VII lesions or, if fibrous tissue predominates, are type VIII lesions.

Vulnerable Plaque and the Vulnerable Patient

The pathologic mechanisms responsible for converting chronic coronary atherosclerosis to an acute coronary event result, in part, from *plaque disruption*, a term that was synonymously used with *plaque rupture*.[138,139] The term *vulnerable plaque* was used by Muller and colleagues[140,141] to describe rupture-prone plaques as the underlying cause of most clinical coronary events. The current definition for "vulnerable plaque" includes all thrombosis-prone plaques and those with a high probability of undergoing rapid progression, thus becoming culprit plaques (Fig. 135–6).[142] Criteria for development of the vulnerable

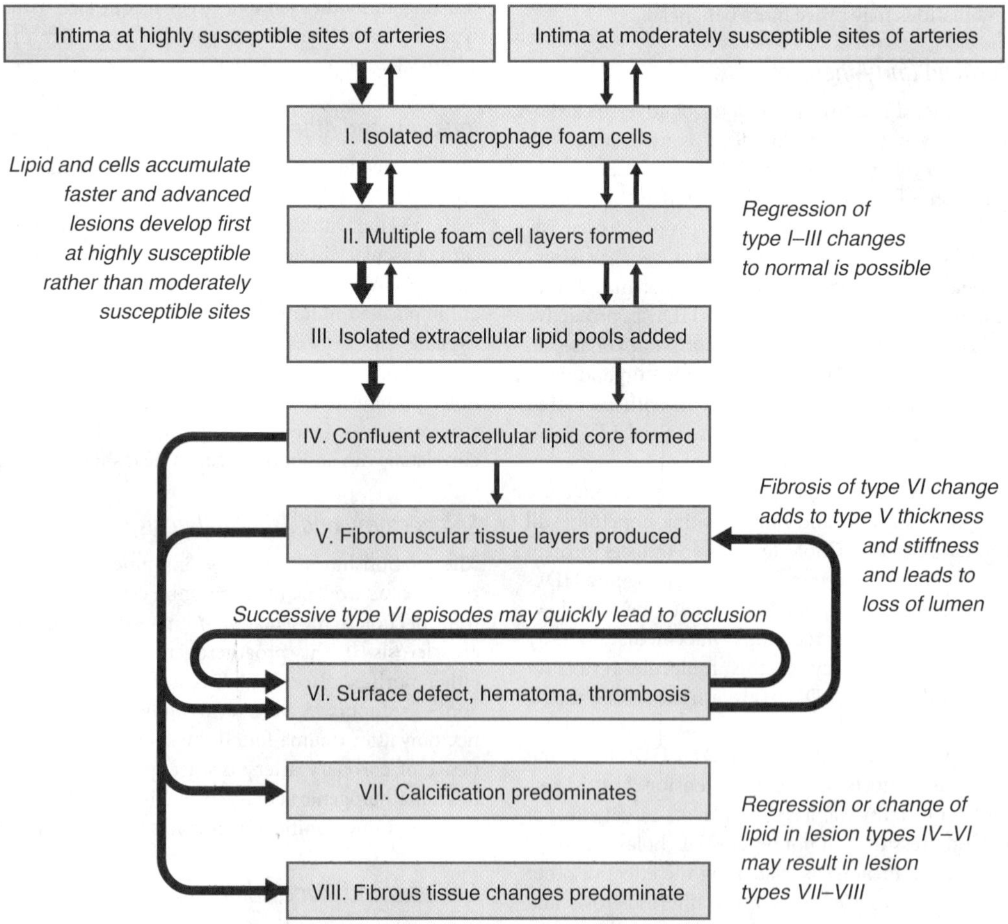

FIGURE 135–5. Flow diagram in *center column* indicates pathways in evolution and progression of human atherosclerotic lesions. *Roman numerals* indicate histologically characteristic types of lesions. The direction of *arrows* indicates sequence in which characteristic morphologies may change. From type I to type IV, changes in lesion morphology occur primarily because of increasing accumulation of lipid. The *loop* between types V and VI illustrates how lesions increase in surfaces. Thrombotic deposits may develop repeatedly over varied time spans in the same location and may be the principal mechanism for gradual occlusion of medium-sized arteries. *(Reproduced with permission from Stary HC.[19])*

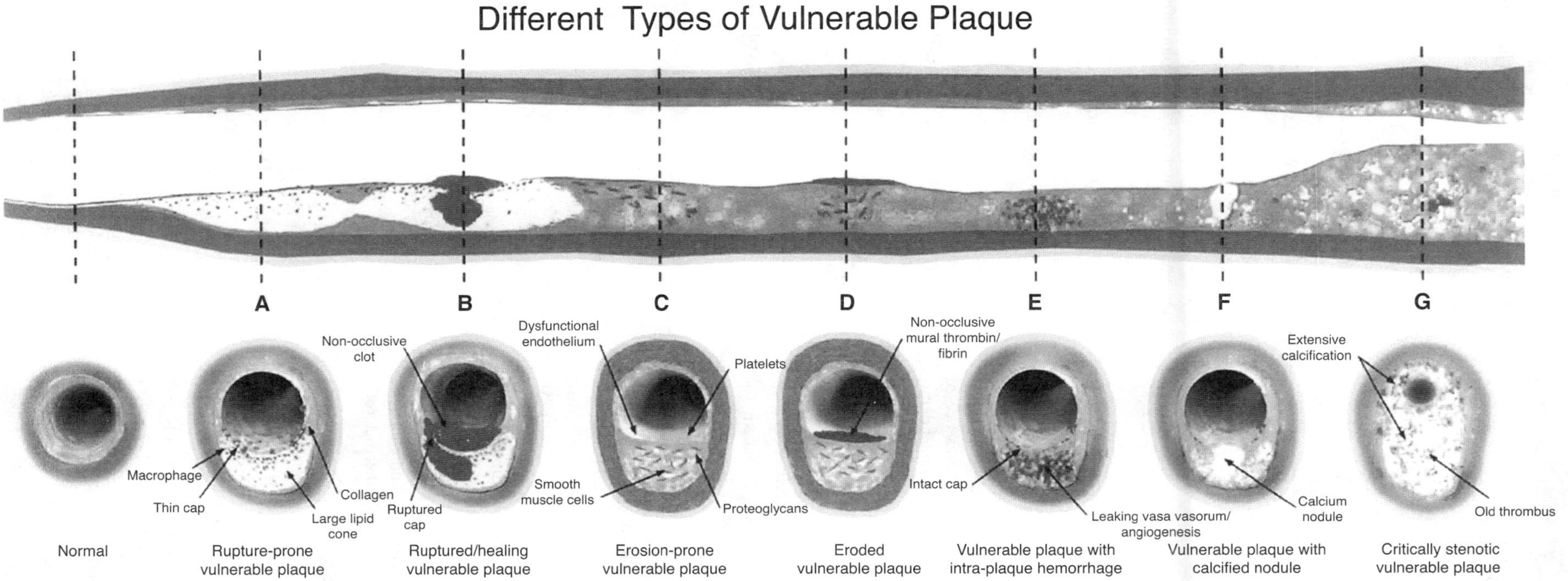

FIGURE 135–6. Different types of vulnerable plaque as underlying cause of acute coronary events and sudden cardiac death. *(A)* Rupture-prone plaque with large lipid core and thin fibrous cap infiltrated by macrophages. *(B)* Ruptured plaque with subocclusive thrombus and early organization. *(C)* Erosion-prone plaque with proteoglycan matrix in a smooth muscle cell-rich plaque. *(D)* Eroded plaque with subocclusive thrombus. *(E)* Intraplaque hemorrhage secondary to leaking vasa vasorum. *(F)* Calcific nodule protruding into the vessel lumen. *(G)* Chronically stenotic plaque with severe calcification, old thrombus, and eccentric lumen. *(Reproduced with permission from Naghavi M, Libby P, Falk E, et al.[142])*

TABLE 135–3. Criteria for Defining the Vulnerable Plaque, Based on the Study of Culprit Plaques

Major criteria
Active inflammation (monocyte/macrophage and sometimes T-cell infiltration)
Thin cap with large lipid core
Endothelial denudation with superficial platelet aggregation
Fissured plaque
Stenosis >90%
Minor criteria
Superficial calcified nodule
Glistening yellow
Intraplaque hemorrhage
Endothelial dysfunction
Outward (positive) remodeling

SOURCE: Naghavi et al,[142] with permission.

plaque have been proposed based on histopathologic study of culprit plaques (Table 135–3).[142] The major criteria involve the presence of active inflammation, a thin cap with large lipid core, endothelial denudation with superficial platelet aggregation, a fissured plaque, and stenosis greater than 90 percent. The minor criteria for a vulnerable plaque include superficial calcified nodule, glistening yellow plaque, intraplaque hemorrhage, endothelial dysfunction, and outward (positive) remodeling. Some studies indicate plaques that are heavily calcified and without a significant lipid core are more stable.[21,143]

An important concept concerning plaque remodeling is that atherosclerotic plaques commonly grow outward (positive remodeling) before a luminal stenosis occurs.[130] Therefore, a contrast dye coronary angiogram may underestimate the plaque burden in the vessel. Arterial thrombosis may result from plaque hemorrhage (majority of events) or occur in an area of endothelial denudation (30–40%) without breach of the intimal space.[144] Thrombosis has also been reported in plaques that have a superficial calcified nodule protruding into the lumen.[144] Most atherosclerotic plaques that underlie a fatal or nonfatal MI are, as shown by angiography, less than 70 percent stenosed.[145] Some patients have more than one vulnerable plaque, which underscores the importance of medical therapy in addition to coronary revascularization.[146] Several technologies are currently being tested to identify the location of the vulnerable plaque.[147] Hopefully these developing technologies will shed more light on the natural history of the vulnerable plaque and afford the ability to conduct studies using local or regional antiatherosclerotic therapy.

Because of the dynamic interaction of atherosclerotic plaque with circulating blood, the term *cardiovascular vulnerable patient* has been proposed to define subjects susceptible to an acute coronary syndrome (ACS) or sudden cardiac death based on atherosclerotic plaque or blood or myocardial vulnerability.[148] The vulnerable (thrombogenic) blood includes serum markers of atherosclerosis and inflammation, such as hsCRP, inflammatory cytokines (e.g., IL-6, sCD40L), and hypercoagulable factors. The blood markers of vulnerability that reflect the hypercoagulable state include those of the fibrinolytic system and platelets (Table 135–4).[148] Patients may have an MI because of a nonfatal or fatal arrhythmia as a result of coronary atherosclerosis or other nonatherosclerotic disease, such as hypertrophic cardiomyopathy or right ventricular dysplasia. Thus, a vulnerable patient should be considered from the standpoint of the combined presence of a vulnerable atherosclerotic plaque, vulnerable blood (prone to thrombosis), and/or vulnerable myocardium (prone to life-threatening arrhythmia).

Arterial Thrombosis

Atherothrombosis refers to the occurrence of thrombosis on atherosclerotic lesions,[149] the typical setting for arterial thrombosis. It represents the acute event that converts chronic atherosclerosis—a silent, asymptomatic, progressive disease—into symptomatic, life-threatening clinical complications, including acute MI, stroke, and critical limb ischemia. The previous section described in detail the current concepts of the consecutive stages of atherosclerotic lesion development.

Thrombosis is not simply the final occlusive event. It also contributes to atherosclerosis lesion development. Intraplaque hemorrhage and *in situ* thrombosis localizes thrombin activity within plaques. Thus, atheroma evolution is not only a proliferative process but also involves thrombosis.[150]

Pathology of Arterial Thrombi

Fundamental pathologic and pathophysiologic distinctions exist between arterial and venous thrombi (Table 135–5). Arterial thrombi usually are occlusive. However, nonocclusive mural thrombi often occur in the lumina of the heart chambers and large arteries, such as the aorta and the iliac and common carotid arteries. Arterial thrombi develop almost invariably upon preexisting abnormal intimal surfaces, which typically are atherosclerotic lesions. Less commonly, arterial thrombosis is superimposed on other forms of vascular disease, such as vasculitis or traumatic injury.[151] Thus, in the high-flow and high-pressure arterial system, thrombi form in response to increased local shear forces and exposure of thrombogenic substances on damaged vascular surfaces. Arterial thrombi, referred to as *white thrombi*, are composed mainly of platelets and relatively little fibrin or red cells. Histopathologic findings and

TABLE 135–4. Blood Hypercoagulability Factors That May Contribute to Patient Vulnerability to Coronary Heart Disease Events

1. Markers of blood hypercoagulability
Decreased anticoagulation factors (e.g., proteins C and S, antithrombin)
Prothrombotic gene polymorphisms (e.g., factor V Leiden, G20210A prothrombin mutation)
Increased coagulation factors (e.g., fibrinogen, factors VII and VIII, von Willebrand factor)
2. Increased platelet activation
(e.g., gene polymorphisms of platelet integrin IIb3, integrin 21, GpIbIX)
3. Decreased endogenous fibrinolysis activity
(e.g., reduced t-PA, increased PAI-1, certain PAI-1 polymorphisms)
4. Other thrombogenic factors
(e.g., anticardiolipin antibodies, thrombocytosis, sickle cell disease, polycythemia, diabetes mellitus, hyperhomocysteinemia, hypercholesterolemia)
5. Increased viscosity
6. Transient hypercoagulability
(e.g., smoking, dehydration, infection, adrenergic surge, cocaine, estrogens, postprandial.)

PAI-1, type 1 plasminogen-activator inhibitor; t-PA, tissue plasminogen activator.

SOURCE: Modified from Naghavi et al.[148]

TABLE 135–5. Pathophysiologic Differences between Arterial and Venous Thrombi

	Arterial Thrombi	Venous Thrombi
Underlying vasculature	Abnormal Atherosclerosis Vasculitis Trauma	Normal
Thrombus pathology	Occlusive or nonocclusive (mural thrombi in large arteries)	Occlusive
	"White thrombus" composed mainly of platelets	"Red thrombus" composed mainly of fibrin, red cells
Pathophysiology	Local shear stress and thrombogenic vascular surface	Stasis and hypercoagulability

imaging and experimental studies have highlighted the important role of leukocytes that are actively recruited into growing, platelet-rich arterial thrombi.[152]

In contrast, venous thrombi almost always are occlusive and may form virtual casts of the vessel in which they arise. Unlike the setting for arterial thrombi, gross vascular damage generally is not found at sites of venous thrombosis. Any ultrastructural abnormalities of adjacent endothelium likely are the consequences rather than the causes of thrombus formation. Therefore, in the low-flow and low-pressure venous system, reduced blood flow (stasis) and systemic activation of the coagulation cascade play the primary pathophysiologic roles. Venous thrombi are composed predominantly of red cells enmeshed in fibrin and contain relatively few platelets; hence, they have been described pathologically as *red thrombi*.

The generalizations described are consistent with the following clinical observations: (1) hereditary hypercoagulable states, characterized by chronic hyperactivity of the coagulation system, are primarily associated with venous rather than arterial thrombosis; and (2) anticoagulants that prevent fibrin formation (e.g., heparin, warfarin) are generally used to prevent venous thrombosis, whereas antiplatelet agents (e.g., aspirin) are more effective in preventing arterial thrombosis. The differences between arterial and venous thrombosis are not, however, absolute because both types of thrombi are composed of different amounts of platelets, fibrin, and leukocytes. In addition, all thrombi continually undergo propagation, organization, embolization, lysis, and rethrombosis, and this dynamic remodeling results in constantly changing compositions.

Site-Specific Arterial Thrombosis

The model of atherothrombosis described has been best characterized in coronary arteries. This pathophysiology may not be entirely applicable to arterial thrombosis at other sites. It cannot be assumed that the local determinants of thrombosis that are operative in the coronary arteries are identical to those encountered in the cerebrovascular and peripheral arterial circulations. Basic regional differences may involve (1) distribution and composition of atherosclerotic lesions, (2) variable local rheology, and (3) underlying vascular cell heterogeneity.

Atherosclerosis is highly localized within the systemic vasculature.[153] Lesion formation particularly affects the carotid artery bifurcation, coronary arteries (especially the left coronary artery bifurcation), abdominal aorta (especially its posterior wall downstream of the renal arteries, but with little disease usually present in the upstream thoracic aorta), and profunda femoral arteries. These lesion-prone sites in the arterial circulation correspond to regions where wall shear stress is very low and may even oscillate between positive and negative directions (i.e., reversal of flow) during the cardiac cycle. A strong correlation exists between local hemodynamic conditions of low shear stress and the development of atherosclerotic plaque formation and intimal thickening.[153–155] However, as arteries become progressively diseased and stenoses develop at these sites, the local hemodynamics change. Stenotic flows are characterized by sharp increases in shear rate that achieve their peak just upstream of the stenosis throat, with development of intensive turbulence downstream of the stenosis. The mechanisms of platelet activation and accumulation that initiate arterial thrombosis at these high-shear sites are described in "Platelet Activation" below.

Striking heterogeneity is seen in the composition of atherothrombotic plaques, even within the same individual. In addition to plaque composition, the basic structural differences between different arteries contribute to differences in thrombogenic substrates that are exposed upon arterial injury. For example, carotid and iliac arteries contain relatively more elastic fibers and proportionately fewer smooth muscle cells than coronary arteries.[156] Furthermore, ACSs typically result from disruption of only modestly stenotic, lipid-rich plaques, whereas disruption-prone, high-risk plaques in the carotid arteries usually are severely stenotic. Thus, a proposed more appropriate term is *high-risk plaque* rather than *vulnerable plaque* (which connotes its composition) to define a disruption-prone or thrombosis-prone plaque in different parts of the circulation.[157]

The pathophysiology of arterial thrombosis at different sites in the circulation may be determined in part by vascular bed-specific heterogeneity of endothelial and smooth muscle cells. Endothelial cell-derived anticoagulant and procoagulant activities are differentially expressed throughout the vascular tree. The heterogeneity of endothelial cells and the vascular bed-specific signaling pathways that control endothelial gene expression have been considered to play an important role in the localization of arterial thrombosis.[158] Heterogeneity of vascular smooth muscle cells likewise exists throughout the arterial tree. They vary in embryonic origin, sources of progenitors, and lineage. With subsequent development, they acquire various phenotypes that can be traced to preferential sites within vessel walls.[159]

Less is known about the pathophysiology of cerebrovascular thrombosis, and even less about peripheral arterial thrombosis, than about coronary artery thrombosis. Future research in these areas should permit the development of more rational antithrombotic strategies in noncoronary artery thrombosis.

Overview of Arterial Thrombotic Process

Arterial thrombosis typically occurs in the presence of underlying atherosclerosis ("atherothrombosis"). Less frequently, however, it may also occur in nonatherosclerotic arteries, such as in the setting of vasculitis.

Atherothrombosis Disruption of an atherosclerotic plaque triggers an explosive cascade of events that results in the formation of a platelet-rich thrombus at the site of arterial injury.[160] Activation of coagulation is determined primarily by local factors (Table 135–6). Focal loss of the antithrombotic and vasodilator properties of endothelium is compounded by plaque rupture or erosion. These events trigger the local activation of platelets and the coagulation system by exposure of blood to previously encrypted thrombogenic substances. The local milieu for thrombus formation is aggravated by focal vasoconstriction, rapidly increased shear forces, and platelet-mediated recruitment of leukocytes. Platelet and coagulation activation are inseparable, reciprocally self-amplifying processes (Fig. 135–7). Activation of platelets generates procoagulant properties on their cell surfaces. Combined with

TABLE 135–6. Local and Systemic Determinants of Arterial Thrombosis

Local factors

1. Loss of antithrombotic and vasodilator properties of endothelium
2. Plaque rupture or erosion
3. Exposure of platelet-activating and procoagulant substances
 Extracellular matrix
 Anionic phospholipids
 Tissue factor
4. Vasoconstriction
5. Increased shear stress
6. Recruitment of leukocytes

Systemic factors

1. Systemic state of activation of platelets and coagulation
 Acquired
 Genetic
2. Adrenergic state
3. Hyperlipidemia
4. Diabetes mellitus

nonplatelet-dependent local activators of the coagulation cascade, platelet activation culminates in the formation of thrombin, which itself is a potent stimulus for further platelet activation. Superimposed on these dominant local determinants of arterial thrombosis, the thrombotic process may be modulated by systemic, circulating factors (Table 135–6). The factors include the systemic state of activation of platelets and coagulation, which may be governed by acquired or genetic factors and by hormonal influences (e.g., adrenergic state).

Arterial thrombi generally are localized to the site of acute vascular injury. They are prevented from extending beyond this site by restoration of hemostatic balance that promotes blood fluidity along adjacent healthy endothelial surfaces. Thrombus propagation may occur, however, through a blood-borne pool of thrombogenic substances that originate at the site of vascular injury and thrombosis. These substances can be in the form of platelet, leukocyte, red cell, endothelial cell, and other cellular microparticles, and circulating active TF derived from leukocytes activated within the thrombus.[161,162] In fact, microparticles constitute the main reservoir of blood-borne TF, the principal initiator of coagulation.

Thrombus persistence within an artery depends on the local balance among prothrombotic, antithrombotic, and fibrinolytic factors. Ulcerated and thrombotic atherosclerotic plaques, particularly in the aorta, tend to persist or recur.[163] Atherosclerotic plaques of the aortic arch have been detected in almost one-third of patients with cryptogenic stroke. Although aortic arch atheroma are more frequent and more severe causes of cryptogenic stroke in individuals older than 55 years of age, patent foramen ovale (and presumably paradoxical embolism) are more strongly associated with cryptogenic stroke in those younger than 55 years of age.[164]

Advances in the development of coronary stents have created a new form of arterial thrombosis. Although drug-eluting stents that deliver sirolimus or paclitaxel have been successful in reducing the problem of restenosis that is caused by smooth muscle cell proliferation and intimal hyperplasia following the coronary intervention, they have actually increased the occurrence of "late stent thrombosis" compared to bare metal stents. This form of arterial thrombosis, which typically occurs after discontinuation of antiplatelet therapy, is probably caused by eluting drugs interfering with endothelialization of the stent surface.[160,165]

Thrombosis in Nonatherosclerotic Arteries Thrombosis may occur in arteries that are affected by vasculitis. As both systemic lupus erythematosus (SLE) and atherosclerosis are immune-driven processes, it is to be expected that some patients with active SLE are more susceptible to accelerated atherosclerosis (and related atherothrombosis) resulting from autoantibody-mediated proatherogenic mechanisms.[166,167] However, in the absence of underlying atherosclerosis, various types of arterial thrombosis can complicate active vasculitis. For example, patients with SLE may have myocardial infarction with angiographically normal coronary arteries. Giant cell arteritis, which characteristically targets the extracranial carotid and vertebral arteries, leads to inflammation and necrosis of the arterial wall and subsequent arterial occlusions in a distribution that is quite different from that of atherosclerosis.[153] Takayasu arteritis has an unusual predilection for the aortic arch and its branches, leading to panarteritis, luminal narrowing, and sometimes thrombotic occlusion. Other types of vasculitis and autoimmune processes that may cause arterial thrombosis include polyarteritis nodosa, Behçet disease, and antiphospholipid antibody syndrome.

Arterial thrombosis in the absence of atherosclerosis is also seen with immune- and nonimmune disorders of platelets and/or the vascular endothelium, such as heparin-induced thrombocytopenia and thrombosis (with arterial thrombosis most commonly occurring in the aorta, iliofemoral arteries, as well as in cerebral and coronary arteries),[168] and in

ACTIVATED PLATELET PROCOAGULANT PROPERTIES

PLATELET ACTIVATORS	COAGULATION ACTIVATORS
↓ Endothelial antiplatelet properties	↓ Endothelial anticoagulant properties
Localized platelet activators: ■ ↑ Shear stress ■ Exposure, binding of platelets to collagen, VWF ■ ↑ Platelet agonists (thrombin, ADP, epinephrine, TXA₂) ■ ↑ Platelet expression of P-selectin, CD40 ligand ■ ↑ Platelet binding to aggregating ligands (fibrinogen, VWF, fibronectin)	Localized coagulation activators: ■ ↑ Tissue factor expression ■ ↑ Phospholipid surface on activated cells and apoptotic cells in lesion, microparticles, plasma lipoproteins ■ Procoagulant effects of oxidized LDL, LDL
Systemic platelet activation	Systemic coagulation activation

THROMBIN

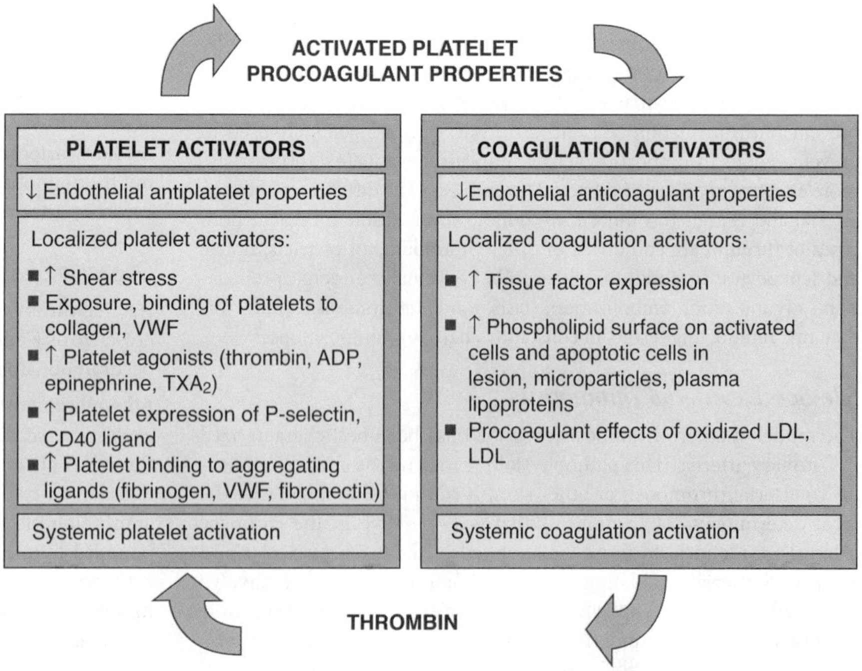

FIGURE 135–7. Atherothrombosis. Reciprocal, mutually amplifying activators of platelets and coagulation occurring on atherosclerotic lesions. ADP, adenosine diphosphate; LDL, low-density lipoprotein; TXA₂, thromboxane A₂; VWF, von Willebrand factor.

the myeloproliferative disorders (e.g., essential thrombocythemia, polycythemia vera).[169,170]

Platelet Activation

Disruption of an advanced atherosclerotic plaque results in abrupt exposure of highly thrombogenic material to flowing blood. This process leads locally to both thrombin generation and platelet activation, which operate simultaneously in a mutually self-amplifying process. Plaque rupture, and the development of new intimal surface irregularities, also suddenly alters local rheologic characteristics, increasing local shear rates. Increased shear stress resulting from sudden changes in degree of stenosis following rupture is compounded by increased focal vasoconstriction induced by thrombin, thromboxane A_2, and other vasoactive substances released in the milieu of acute injury.

In addition to exposure of platelet-activating substances, the high levels of shear stress directly stimulate platelet-rich thrombus formation. Platelets adhere preferentially at the throat of the stenosis, where shear rates are highest. Shear rates in healthy arteries that are subject to thrombosis normally range from approximately 200 s^{-1} (internal carotid arteries) to 500 s^{-1} (left main coronary artery), and up to approximately 1500 s^{-1} at the highest physiologic rates. Pathologic shear rates can rise to 10,000 s^{-1} in stenotic arteries, and with plaque rupture local shear rates can approximate 100,000 s^{-1}.[171,172] Increased shear rate promotes platelet transport, forcing the concentration of platelets outward toward the injured vessel wall to which they can adhere.

At high shear rates (>1000 s^{-1}), platelets must be initially tethered to the vascular surface through a shear-activated interaction between the platelet membrane glycoprotein (GP) Ibα (of the GPIb/IX/V complex) and its adhesive ligand, von Willebrand factor.[173,174] Platelet adhesion also involves collagen binding to platelet collagen receptors (integrin $\alpha_2\beta_1$ and GPVI). Other matrix constituents that become exposed to platelets and serve as adhesive ligands include fibronectin, laminin, fibrinogen, and fibrin. These initial adhesive interactions induce intracellular signaling pathways that activate platelets. High shear stress also activates platelets both directly[175] and by lowering the threshold of platelet activation by chemical agonists to which platelets are exposed in the microenvironment of the arterial thrombus.[176] Thus, following adhesion, platelets are explosively activated by several interacting pathways: (1) intracellular signaling initiated by the adhesion event itself, (2) direct action of locally increased shear stress, and (3) agonists released (e.g., ADP, thromboxane A_2) and generated (e.g., thrombin) at the site of vascular injury.

Finally, the occlusive arterial platelet thrombus is generated by the aggregation of platelets. This process is mediated by several alternative ligands (von Willebrand factor, fibrinogen, fibronectin) that bind to their activated receptors in the platelet integrin $\alpha_{IIb}\beta_3$ complex. Stability of the platelet aggregate is induced by additional ligand–receptor interactions, including CD40L binding to integrin $\alpha_{IIb}\beta_3$.[177] Platelet thrombus stabilization is designed to counteract shear forces that promote not only the formation of arterial thrombi but also their embolization.

The importance of the inflammatory component of arterial thrombosis,[152] which is characterized by complex interactions among leukocytes, endothelial cells, and platelets, is increasingly being recognized. Activated platelets recruit leukocytes to the site of vascular damage, promoting their adhesion to endothelium and their activation on endothelium-bound chemokines.

Tissue Factor and Phospholipids

TF is a cell surface–bound transmembrane protein that normally is not exposed to circulating blood. When expressed, TF initiates coagulation by binding to factor VIIa and activates factors IX and X, thereby triggering the common pathway of coagulation and the formation of thrombin. Strong evidence indicates that TF, particularly the TF expressed on macrophages, is the principal thrombogenic factor in the lipid-rich core of atherosclerotic plaques.[150,178]

Upon rupture of the atherosclerotic plaque, exposure of vascular TF to flowing blood initiates the coagulation cascade. Coagulation reactions are accelerated on the surfaces of activated platelets and on other activated cells in the microenvironment of vascular injury. The surfaces of these activated cells express anionic phospholipids, particularly phosphatidylserine. Apoptotic cells, with which advanced lesions are enriched, likewise translocate phospholipids from the inner to the outer leaflet of the cell membrane.[179] Plasma lipoproteins can provide a phospholipid surface for the assembly of enzymatic complexes of the coagulation cascade; in particular, oxidized LDL, LDL, and VLDL have procoagulant effects.[180,181]

Arterial thrombosis is triggered by the acute exposure of circulating blood to TF and anionic phospholipids, leading to explosive thrombin formation. Thrombin, a potent platelet agonist, further fuels the platelet activation process described in the previous section. These reactions create a self-amplifying process that is tightly localized to the site of vascular injury. The arterial thrombus is further contained to this site by the restoration of normal, antithrombotic endothelium in adjacent areas of the vessel wall.

Systemic Factors

As described above in "Overview of Arterial Thrombotic Process," the pathophysiology of arterial thrombosis is primarily determined by local, "solid-state" factors that operate in concert in the immediate microenvironment of acute vascular injury, typically disruption of an atherosclerotic plaque. However, interindividual differences in systemic, circulating factors can modify individual susceptibility to the focal formation of an arterial thrombus.[182] Systemic determinants of blood thrombogenicity (i.e., hypercoagulability) can enhance the local risk of arterial thrombosis. There is increasing evidence for an association between venous and arterial thrombosis, with several studies now showing that patients with venous thromboembolism (deep vein thrombosis and/or pulmonary embolism) are at increased risk of having coexisting asymptomatic atherosclerosis or subsequent symptomatic atherothrombotic events.[183–186] In addition to certain thrombophilic abnormalities, such as antiphospholipid antibody syndrome, hyperhomocysteinemia, and the myeloproliferative disorders, which are known to predispose individuals to both venous and arterial thromboembolism, some traditional cardiovascular risk factors (e.g., advanced age, obesity, metabolic syndrome, abnormal lipid profiles, immobility, estrogens) also appear to be independent risk factors for venous thromboembolism.[34–36,185–187]

Genetic determinants of the coagulation system may exert modifying effects on susceptibility to arterial thrombosis. The known hypercoagulable states that predispose to venous thrombosis (e.g., factor V Leiden, prothrombin gene mutation, antithrombin, protein C and protein S deficiency) generally are weakly[188] or not at all associated with increased risk of arterial thrombosis. However, decreased mortality from ischemic heart disease has been noted in patients with hemophilia A or B and even in carriers of hemophilia.[189] This finding most likely results from reduced arterial thrombotic tendency in these individuals because early atherogenesis itself does not appear to be significantly affected by the coexistence of hemophilia.[190] Conversely, some epidemiologic studies have correlated elevated levels of fibrinogen and some other coagulation factors with both subclinical atherosclerosis and clinical cardiovascular events,[191,192] although cause-and-effect relationships between elevated levels of hemostatic factors and cardiovascular risk have not been established.

Several lines of evidence suggest that genetic determinants of increased platelet reactivity likewise enhance focal determinants of arterial thrombosis. Animal models of atherosclerosis in pigs and mice with von Willebrand disease suggest that an extremely low or absent von Willebrand factor level exerts a protective effect on the development and distribution of atherosclerotic lesions,[193,194] although these observations are inconclusive. Whether or not von Willebrand disease protects against development of human atherosclerosis remains in dispute.

Platelet membrane glycoproteins are highly polymorphic and can be recognized as alloantigens or autoantigens. Polymorphisms in platelet membrane glycoprotein receptors have been considered to increase platelet reactivity, thereby potentially contributing to susceptibility to arterial thrombosis.[195,196] The first such genetic variation reported involves the HPA-1a/HPA-1b polymorphism, which results in a Leu33Pro substitution in the β_3 subunit of the platelet integrin $\alpha_{IIb}\beta_3$ complex. The 33Pro (HPA-1b) allele was found to be associated with risk of MI in young individuals.[197] Most, but not all, subsequent studies have agreed that the HPA-1b allele represents an inherited risk factor for acute coronary syndromes.[196] Other platelet receptor polymorphisms that have been inconclusively linked to risk of cardiovascular disease include three different polymorphisms of the integrin α_{IIb} (HPA-3), GPIb gene, and a polymorphism of the collagen receptor integrin $\alpha_2\beta_1$. However, as is the case for the soluble hemostatic factors, lack of a clear relationship among genotype, phenotype, and clinical manifestations has failed to establish convincing cause-and-effect relationships for any of these genetic variations.

Although none of these individual hemostatic protein or platelet polymorphisms plays a clear, dominant role in the pathophysiology of arterial thrombosis, future application of platelet genomics may reveal combinations of polymorphisms that, in aggregate, influence disease.[198]

High blood levels of catecholamines likely contribute systemically to localized arterial thrombus formation. Catecholamines may be increased by physical or emotional stress or by cigarette smoking, thereby triggering acute cardiovascular events in these settings. In addition to their vasoactive actions, catecholamines are direct platelet agonists and enhance shear stress-induced platelet activation.[176,199]

Changes in lipid metabolism may exert systemic prothrombotic actions. The thrombogenicity of lipoprotein (a) has been attributed to its structural similarity to plasminogen, leading to reduced plasmin formation and impaired thrombolysis.[163] Elevated LDL cholesterol can contribute to blood hypercoagulability.[200] The prothrombotic state of diabetes involves multiple mechanisms, including platelet hyperreactivity and increased leukocyte procoagulant activity.[163]

ISCHEMIC VASCULAR DISEASE

MYOCARDIAL INFARCTION

MI is a term that reflects necrosis of cardiac myocytes caused by prolonged ischemia. In the past, MI was defined by the combination of two of three characteristics: typical symptoms (i.e., chest discomfort), a rise in serum enzymatic markers derived from myocardial cells, and a typical electrocardiographic pattern involving the development of Q waves. The advent of sensitive and specific serologic biomarkers and precise imaging techniques has led to the development of revised criteria for MI.[202] For example, patients can be diagnosed with a "non-Q wave or non–ST-segment elevation" MI (NSTEMI) if certain criteria are met. The criteria agreed upon by the American College of Cardiology and the European Society of Cardiology for acute, evolving, or recent MI[202] are as follows:

1. Typical rise and gradual fall (troponin) or more rapid rise and fall (creatinine kinase-MB isoform) or biochemical markers of myocardial necrosis with at least one of the following: (A) ischemic symptoms; (B) development of pathologic Q waves on the electrocardiogram (ECG); (C) electrocardiographic changes indicative of ischemia (ST segment elevation or depression); or (D) coronary artery intervention (e.g., coronary angioplasty).
2. Pathologic findings of an acute MI.

The criteria for established MI[202] (i.e., event that occurred in the past) is any one of the following:

1. Development of new pathologic Q waves on serial ECGs. The patient may or may not remember previous symptoms. Biochemical markers of myocardial necrosis may have normalized, depending on the length of time since the infarct developed.
2. Pathologic findings of a healed or healing MI.

Clinical Features of Acute Coronary Syndromes

Stable angina pectoris is ischemic discomfort symptomatology caused by a narrowed coronary artery that does not allow sufficient oxygen delivery to meet the metabolic demands of the myocardium. *Unstable angina* is defined clinically as a change in the pattern of stable angina to more frequent or more severe symptoms, uninterrupted angina symptoms for 20 minutes or more, or the development of angina at rest. The term *acute coronary syndrome* has evolved as a useful description of the spectrum of patients presenting with angina pectoris caused by unstable angina through MI.[203] The underlying pathologic mechanism for the development of ACS is usually a vulnerable atherosclerotic plaque with either plaque rupture or plaque ulceration leading to thrombosis. Unstable angina and non–ST-segment MI are differentiated by pathologic elevation in the levels of cardiac biomarkers that confirm MI.

Angina pectoris can be associated with other symptoms, such as diaphoresis, dizziness, nausea, clamminess, and fatigue. Some patients with ACS present with atypical symptoms rather than chest pain. The presentation may be dyspnea alone, nausea and/or vomiting, palpitations/syncope, or cardiac arrest. Rarely, patients with diabetes mellitus and other patients have a "silent MI" diagnosed incidentally on ECG or cardiac imaging study.

The initial ECG is often not diagnostic in patients with ACS. In one clinical study, the ECG was not diagnostic in 45 percent and was normal in 20 percent of patients who subsequently were shown to have experienced an acute MI.[204,205] ST-segment elevation and Q waves are consistent with STEMI, but other conditions, such as acute pericarditis with early repolarization variant and hypertrophic cardiomyopathy with Q waves, may mimic the ECG manifestations of STEMI.

Laboratory Features of Acute Myocardial Infarction

A variety of serum biomarkers are used to evaluate patients with suspected acute MI. The three most commonly used tests are (1) troponin I and troponin T, (2) creatine kinase (CK) and its isoform CK-MB, and (3) myoglobin. An elevated serum concentration of one or more of the three biomarkers is seen in almost all patients with acute MI. The preferred biomarkers are the troponins because the troponin assays are more specific than the other tests.

Therapy for Acute Coronary Syndromes

Therapy for Acute Myocardial Infarction The initial management of patients with STEMI depends upon prompt recognition and therapy to reduce morbidity and mortality. A carefully coordinated plan of care is essential for optimal results in patients with STEMI, given that multiple therapies usually are initiated simultaneously. The goals of therapy are to reduce ischemic pain, stabilize hemodynamic status, and quickly establish myocardial reperfusion. The American College of Cardiology

(ACC)/American Heart Association (AHA) guidelines for management of patients with acute MI are available at the ACC website.[206]

Antiplatelet Agents Unless contraindicated, all patients with acute MI should be given antiplatelet therapy. The Antiplatelet Trialists' Collaboration indicated a 30 percent reduction in vascular events with an absolute benefit of 38 vascular events prevented per 1000 patients at 1 month with antiplatelet therapy.[206] Aspirin 325 mg/day or an ADP-receptor blocker such as clopidogrel is commonly used. Contraindications to antiplatelet therapy include active bleeding, coagulopathy, and severe, untreated hypertension (a relative contraindication). The combination of dipyridamole and aspirin has not been proven to provide incremental clinical benefit over aspirin alone.

β-Adrenergic Blockade The control of heart rate with β-adrenergic blocker agents has been efficacious in the setting of acute MI or unstable angina.[206,207] According to guidelines, oral β-blocker should be initiated during the first 24 hours of care of STEMI.[206] Intravenous administration of β-blockers should be given only to selected, hemodynamically stable patients according to guidelines.

Management of Chest Pain A cornerstone of ischemic pain management has been intravenous nitroglycerin (beginning at 5–10 mcg/min) in combination with morphine sulfate if necessary. Nitroglycerin also may improve hypertension and symptoms of heart failure, if present. Intravenous nitroglycerin therapy has not been proven to improve mortality and usually is discontinued within 24 to 48 hours of presentation.[203,206] Patients who have taken drugs (e.g., sildenafil) for erectile dysfunction within the preceding 24 hours are at increased risk for vasodilation and hypotension, so caution is advised in these patients when intravenous nitroglycerin is given.

Reperfusion Therapy The overriding goal of treatment of STEMI is restoration of myocardial blood flow and salvage of myocardial tissue. A decision should be made immediately whether the patient will undergo a primary (direct) percutaneous coronary intervention (PCI) or receive a fibrinolytic agent. The currently preferred approach is PCI, but the relative advantages and limitations of each therapy should be considered. The most important factor to consider is whether PCI is immediately available. Several randomized trials indicate enhanced survival with PCI compared to fibrinolysis, with a lower rate of intracranial hemorrhage and recurrent MI.[208–210] Transfer to a center that can provide PCI, if necessary, should be accomplished in less than 2 hours.[210]

Fibrinolytic therapy should be given immediately if PCI cannot be performed promptly.[211] Prior to fibrinolysis, the patient should be initially assessed for possible contraindications, which include active bleeding, history of cerebrovascular disease, intracranial neoplasm, drug allergy, and trauma. A systolic blood pressure greater than 175 torr is a relative contraindication but should not prohibit therapy, especially if the pressure can be rapidly controlled. Many different fibrinolytic regimens with different dosing schemes are available. Streptokinase was the first thrombolytic agent tested but has proved less effective than alteplase.[212] In addition, streptokinase is antigenic and can cause an allergic reaction, particularly with repeat administration. Other thrombolytic agents, such as tenecteplase and reteplase, have reportedly similar results compared to alteplase.[213] Tenecteplase is popular on hospital formularies because of its relatively easy single-bolus administration and reported lower rate of noncerebral bleeding.[214]

Anticoagulation Heparin, both unfractionated and low molecular weight, is commonly used in patients with STEMI. The exact role of heparin therapy with different fibrinolytic agents is evolving. Patients who undergo primary PCI usually are given unfractionated heparin 7500 U subcutaneously twice daily or low-molecular-weight heparin, for example, enoxaparin, 1 mg/kg twice daily unless contraindications are evident. For patients receiving intravenous unfractionated heparin, the recommended dose is an initial 60 to 70 U/kg bolus (maximum 5000 U) followed by 12 to 15 U/kg per hour (maximum 1000 U/h) as continuous infusion with monitoring of the activated partial thromboplastin time (aPTT) measured at 6 hours. The heparin dose is adjusted to maintain an aPTT between 50 and 75 seconds.

Current guidelines recommend maintaining the aPTT at 50 to 75 seconds for short-term use. Heparin should be continued beyond this period only in the case of high risk of systemic or venous thromboembolism.[206,215] Patients can be switched to a subcutaneously administered heparin or converted to oral warfarin during the high-risk period. The anticoagulant drugs unfractionated heparin, enoxaparin, fondaparinux, and bivalirudin are all excreted by the kidneys; consequently, although the first dose is usually safe, longer-term therapy should be guided by assessment of creatinine clearance.[207] The Coumadin-Aspirin Reinfarction Study (CARS) did not show a significant benefit with the combination of low-dose warfarin (1 or 3 mg) and aspirin 80 mg daily compared to aspirin 160 mg daily monotherapy on cardiovascular morbidity in patients who had an MI.[216]

Statins All patients with MI should be started on a 3-hydroxy-3-methylglutaryl-coenzyme A reductase inhibitor (statin) unless the MI was caused by a nonatherosclerotic process such as coronary vasospasm, vasculitis, or embolus. Numerous studies indicate that statins reduce the risk of subsequent MI by approximately 30 to 50 percent.[217] Current evidence suggests that a serum LDL level less than 80 mg/dL with statin treatment is more efficacious in retarding atherosclerotic disease progression than a serum LDL level of 100 mg/dL or above.[218]

Therapy for Unstable Angina Pectoris and Non-ST Elevation Myocardial Infarction The distinction between unstable angina and NSTEMI initially may be difficult because levels of troponins and/or CK-MB may not be elevated until hours after presentation. Similar to STEMI, the initial treatment of unstable angina and NSTEMI includes supplemental oxygen, pain control, and bed rest.[219] Nitrates, given either intravenously or subcutaneously, are the treatment of choice for angina pectoris. Oral β-blockers also are routinely given to patients with unstable angina to relieve symptoms of angina and to reduce the risk of progression to MI.

Treatment of unstable angina and NSTEMI involves administration of an antiplatelet agent and anticoagulation.[219] Fibrinolytic therapy is not beneficial in patients with unstable angina, and its use is associated with unacceptably high bleeding risk. Antiplatelet treatment, most commonly aspirin at a dose of 325 mg daily, was shown in the Antithrombotic Trialists' Collaboration to reduce the combined endpoint of subsequent nonfatal MI, nonfatal stroke, or vascular death (8.0% vs. 13.3%) in patients with non–ST-segment elevation ACS.[220] Clinical trials involving patients with non–ST-segment elevation ACS have demonstrated significantly reduced cardiovascular events and mortality with aspirin administration.[221–223] Some patients do not benefit from aspirin, and this finding has generated an interest as to whether these patients are "aspirin resistant." Nonrandomized studies indicate that aspirin resistance may occur, but because of the limitations of these studies, the definition and prognostic significance of this phenomenon are uncertain.[224–227]

The thienopyridine clopidogrel (75 mg/day) is effective in reducing the risk of MI and mortality in patients with unstable angina.[228,229] The combination of aspirin and clopidogrel has been tested in patients with NSTEMI and unstable angina. The combination of these antiplatelet agents resulted in improved survival and decreased progression to MI.[230] The patients with non–ST-segment elevation ACS who underwent PCI benefited the most from the combination of aspirin and clopidogrel.[231] However, the combination was associated with an increase in major bleeding and reoperation for bleeding in patients who underwent coronary artery bypass grafting (CABG). Therefore, a 5-day, but preferably a 7-day, period off clopidogrel is recommended before CABG.[219,232]

A meta-analysis of randomized clinical trials found that intravenous platelet integrin IIb/IIIa inhibitors substantially benefited patients with non–ST-segment elevation ACS undergoing coronary intervention.[233] The integrin $\alpha_{IIb}\beta_{IIIa}$ receptor antagonist abciximab (ReoPro) is a monoclonal antibody fragment that reduces short-term and long-term clinical events in patients with ACS undergoing angioplasty with or without stent placement.[233–235] Other platelet integrin $\alpha_{IIb}\beta_{IIIa}$ antagonists, such as tirofiban[236,237] and integrilin,[238] also are effective and safe in treating unstable angina when combined with heparin anticoagulation.[239] Current guidelines from an ACC/AHA task force and the American College of Chest Physicians (ACCP) consensus conference recommend administration of an integrin $\alpha_{IIb}\beta_{IIIa}$ inhibitor, in addition to aspirin and heparin, for patients with unstable angina/NSTEMI undergoing planned PCI.[219]

Either intravenous heparin or subcutaneous heparin reduces the rate of MI and death, and relieves anginal pain, when used in combination with an antiplatelet agent.[240] Intravenous heparin usually is given as a 5000-U bolus followed by continuous infusion. Low-molecular-weight heparins can be substituted for unfractionated heparin. Some studies have shown superior efficacy of low-molecular-weight heparins, but other studies have not indicated a significant difference.[219] Direct thrombin inhibitors, such as hirudin and bivalirudin, have been shown to reduce the rate of death, nonfatal MI, and refractory angina compared to heparin.[241,242] The ACCP recommends lepirudin (recombinant hirudin), argatroban, bivalirudin, or danaparoid in patients with a history of heparin-associated thrombocytopenia.[243]

Therapy for Stable Angina Pectoris Patients with stable angina pectoris can be treated with either medical management or revascularization.[244] Limited clinical trial data comparing revascularization, either percutaneous or surgical, to medical therapy are available. The older trials evaluating percutaneous and surgical revascularization were limited by several factors: antiplatelet treatment, angiotensin-converting enzyme inhibitors, and aggressive lipid lowering with statins were not given as background medical therapy of angina. Given these limitations, determining whether revascularization is better than medical management for long-term care of patients with stable angina in modern practice is difficult.

Both PCI and coronary bypass surgery significantly reduce angina. The Coronary Artery Surgery Study (CASS) showed more patients remained symptom-free after CABG compared to medical therapy 5 years after the procedure.[245] At 10 years, however, no significant difference in symptoms was observed. Clinical trials showed significant improvement in angina with PCI compared to medical therapy; however, patients who underwent the former had similar rates of death and MI as those undergoing medical therapy and were less likely to have angina and more likely to have undergone a coronary bypass graft.[244]

Restenosis is a complex process involving inflammation, cellular proliferation, thrombosis, and matrix deposition. Restenosis occurring after PCI may result in flow-limiting luminal narrowing in 20 to 30 percent of therapeutically dilated vessels.[246] Numerous pharmacologic agents, including heparin,[247] have been given in an attempt to reduce the restenosis rate but have met with limited or no success. Intraarterial radiation (brachytherapy) reduces the restenosis rate but is cumbersome to perform because of radiation safety issues. Drug-eluting arterial stents, including the immunosuppressive macrocyclic lactone rapamycin (Sirolimus)[248,249] and the chemotherapeutic agent paclitaxel (Taxol),[250] significantly reduce the rate of restenosis. Because drug-eluting stents were not available at the time of the previous clinical trials, extrapolating the benefits of PCI versus CABG or over medical therapy is difficult. The medical management of patients with stable angina pectoris should include antiplatelet therapy, statin drug treatment, a β-blocker, an angiotensin-converting enzyme inhibitor, and a long-acting nitrate.[244]

PERIPHERAL ARTERIAL DISEASE

Peripheral arterial disease (PAD) is a term that encompasses any arterial disease of the lower extremities, upper extremities, and iliac vessels. It most commonly results from atherosclerosis. Patients who have atherosclerotic disease that compromises blood flow to the extremities may present with exertional pain in a muscle group, called *claudication* (derived from the Latin *claudicare* meaning "to limp"). Claudication is an intermittent but reproducible discomfort of a defined group of muscles that is induced by exercise and relieved with rest.[251] Acute limb ischemia is a relatively rare problem in patients with PAD. In general, it is caused by *in situ* thrombosis or an embolic event from arrhythmias, such as atrial fibrillation, or after manipulation of an artery or aorta with a catheter. Approximately 4 percent of patients with claudication progress to *critical limb ischemia*, which is defined as rest pain and/or foot ulceration that heralds impending tissue loss.

The 5-year mortality rate is estimated to be 30 percent in patients with lower-extremity PAD.[252] Approximately 75 percent of mortality results from a cardiovascular event, such as MI or stroke.[252] The ankle-brachial index is a noninvasive measure of limb vascular pressure in the lower extremities and has been noted in several studies to be predictive of cardiovascular events.[251] However, a decreased index is not just a predictor but is a physical finding that indicates significant atherosclerotic plaque burden is present. Other noninvasive imaging studies for PAD include the combination of segmental pressures and pulse volume recordings,[253] duplex Doppler ultrasound,[253] and magnetic resonance imaging.[254]

Medical therapy for patients with PAD includes risk factor modification, antiplatelet therapy, and treatment of claudication symptoms with exercise rehabilitation and possible pharmacologic agents. The risk factors for development of peripheral atherosclerosis include cigarette smoking, diabetes mellitus, hypertension, and dyslipidemia.[255] Aggressive management of risk factors for PAD is recommended to prevent disease progression.[256] Some emerging risk factors for PAD include hyperhomocysteinemia[257] and elevated fibrinogen levels.[252] Treatment with antiplatelet agents reduces the risk of cardiovascular events, such as MI and stroke, in patients with PAD.[252] The Antithrombotic Trialists' Collaboration evaluated 9214 patients with PAD enrolled in 42 trials and found that use of antiplatelet drugs, such as aspirin 75 to 325 mg/day, resulted in a proportional reduction of 23 percent in serious vascular events.[220] Evaluation of patients with PAD in the Physicians' Health Study found that aspirin 325 mg every other day decreased the need for peripheral artery surgery.[258] However, no difference between the aspirin and placebo groups with regard to development of claudication was observed. Several studies have evaluated the ADP receptor blockers ticlopidine and clopidogrel. Clopidogrel is considered a safer drug of the same class and was evaluated in 19,185 patients in the Clopidogrel Versus Aspirin in Patients at Risk of Ischaemic Events (CAPRIE) study.[229] A dose of clopidogrel 75 mg/day had a modest but significant advantage over aspirin 325 mg/day in preventing stroke, MI, and peripheral vascular disease. Subgroup analysis revealed that the patients with PAD benefited the most with clopidogrel treatment. Antiplatelet therapy should be offered to all patients with PAD unless contraindicated by allergy or comorbidities.[259]

The options for treating claudication symptoms include exercise rehabilitation, pharmacologic agents, and a revascularization procedure. Several studies indicate exercise rehabilitation improves the symptoms of claudication, and a supervised program is better than an unstructured program.[260] Two drugs are approved by the FDA for treatment of claudication symptoms: pentoxifylline, a methylxanthine derivative that may improve abnormal red cell deformability and reduce blood viscosity, and cilostazol, a type III phosphodiesterase inhibitor with antiplatelet and vasodilating properties. Cilostazol is generally considered more effective than pentoxifylline for improving walking distance in patients with claudication.[261] The addition of cilostazol to either aspirin or clopidogrel does not increase the bleeding time or bleeding risk.[262] A revascularization procedure in patients with stable, intermittent claudication generally is reserved for those with severe lifestyle-limiting symptoms or manifestation of critical limb ischemia.

CEREBROVASCULAR DISEASE

The etiology of ischemic stroke is multifactorial and can be categorized into embolic, small-vessel disease, large-vessel disease, and cryptogenic. Carotid artery disease accounts for approximately 30 percent of strokes. Major risk factors for developing carotid artery atherosclerosis are hypertension, diabetes, smoking, and dyslipidemia.[263,264] Emerging risk factors for stroke include hyperhomocysteinemia and an elevated plasma level of lipoprotein (a). An elevated hsCRP level is a risk factor associated with ischemic stroke in both men and women. However, at this time hsCRP is not routinely measured as an additional marker for increased risk of stroke. Similar to coronary and PAD, control of atherosclerotic risk factors is essential in the primary prevention of stroke in patients with evidence of carotid atherosclerosis and for those who have undergone carotid endarterectomy.[112,265]

Carotid endarterectomy is indicated for patients with symptoms and a greater than 50 percent stenosis or for patients who are asymptomatic with a greater than 60 to 70 percent stenosis of the common carotid or internal carotid arteries.[266] Carotid stents with embolic protection appear promising for treatment of carotid atherosclerosis.[267]

Two antiplatelet drug regimens are approved for prevention of stroke: clopidogrel (Plavix) and the combination of aspirin 25 mg and dipyridamole 200 mg daily. Approval of clopidogrel is based on the CAPRIE study, which showed a reduction in the combined endpoint of stroke, MI, and death in patients treated with clopidogrel 75 mg/day compared to those treated with aspirin 325 mg/day.[229] The FDA indication for dipyridamole/aspirin is primarily based on the European Stroke Protection Study 2, which noted a reduction in stroke with the combination of dipyridamole 200 mg and aspirin 25 mg given together (Aggrenox) twice per day.[268] The Prevention Regimen for Effectively Avoiding Second Strokes (PRoFESS) trial was a secondary stroke–prevention trial comparing the combination of aspirin and extended-release dipyridamole (Aggrenox) versus clopidogrel (Plavix) in preventing stroke recurrence after a first event. The difference between the agents was not statistically significant for the primary outcome of recurrent stroke.[269] Fish oil (omega-3 fatty acids) lowers triglycerides and VLDLs and may reduce serum viscosity by lowering fibrinogen. Some studies suggest that fish oil consumption lowers the risk of ischemic stroke. The effect of fish oils on carotid atherosclerosis is unknown.[270]

ATHEROEMBOLISM

Atheromatous embolism refers to the dislodgment into the bloodstream of arterial plaque material, including cholesterol crystals ("cholesterol embolism") from ulcerated vascular plaques. The cholesterol embolization syndrome involves systemic microembolism to the end arteries of almost any circulatory bed. Atheroembolism most characteristically originates from lesions in the abdominal aorta and ileofemoral arteries. Cholesterol emboli that lodge in an arteriole incite an acute inflammatory response, followed by a foreign body reaction, intravascular thrombus formation, endothelial proliferation, and eventually fibrosis. These processes generally result in ischemia that sometimes leads to infarction and necrosis.[271] Mortality rate of clinically diagnosed atheroembolism can be as high as 80 percent, depending on the anatomic location and size of the vascular beds involved.[272]

Patients with atheroembolism, including the cholesterol embolization syndrome, generally have advanced atherosclerosis, often complicated by a history of hypertension, diabetes mellitus, renal failure, or aortic aneurysms. Atherosclerotic plaques can disrupt and embolize spontaneously; however, the clinical syndrome typically is triggered by vascular intervention, including vascular surgery, catheterization, angioplasty, endarterectomy, or angiography.[273] Anticoagulation or thrombolytic therapy may be risk factors with atheroembolism.[272] Clinical presentation depends on the sites of embolization. When these sites involve the distal extremity microcirculation, the "blue toe syndrome" may develop. The syndrome presents with the acute appearance of painful and tender discoloration or mottled blue and patchy appearance of one or more toes that may progress to ulceration and gangrene. Other common cutaneous manifestations are livedo reticularis involving the legs, buttocks, or abdomen, painful nodules, and purpura. Cerebrovascular embolism can cause transient neurologic abnormalities. Cholesterol emboli lodged in retinal arterial bifurcations can be visualized by ophthalmoscopy as bright, refractile, yellow rectangular crystals. Visceral organs most commonly affected by atheroembolism include the kidneys, sometimes causing renal failure, and the gastrointestinal tract, where abdominal pain, ischemic colitis, and bleeding may ensue.

Diagnosis is based on clinical presentation associated with imaging evidence of atherosclerosis of the arterial supply of affected organs.[272] Transient eosinophilia occurs in most cases.[273] Treatment of atheroembolism should include surgical removal or bypass of the source of emboli. No medical treatment modalities have been established to be effective. Anticoagulation or fibrinolytic therapy may increase the risk of further atheroembolism.[274]

REFERENCES

1. Virchow R: *Cellular Pathology: As Based Upon Physiological and Pathological Histology*. Dover, New York, 1863.
2. Ross R: Atherosclerosis—An inflammatory disease. *N Engl J Med* 340:115, 1999.
3. Enos WF, Holmes RH, Beyer J: Coronary disease among United States soldiers killed in action in Korea; preliminary report. *J Am Med Assoc* 152:1090, 1953.
4. Joseph A, Ackerman D, Talley JD, et al: Manifestations of coronary atherosclerosis in young trauma victims—An autopsy study. *J Am Coll Cardiol* 22:459, 1993.
5. Tuzcu EM, Kapadia SR, Tutar E, et al: High prevalence of coronary atherosclerosis in asymptomatic teenagers and young adults: Evidence from intravascular ultrasound. *Circulation* 103:2705, 2001.
6. Ross R, Glomset JA: The pathogenesis of atherosclerosis (first of two parts). *N Engl J Med* 295:369, 1976.
7. Ross R, Glomset JA: The pathogenesis of atherosclerosis (second of two parts). *N Engl J Med* 295:420, 1976.
8. Yusuf S, Hawken S, Ounpuu S, et al: Effect of potentially modifiable risk factors associated with myocardial infarction in 52 countries (the INTERHEART study): Case-control study. *Lancet* 364:937, 2004.
9. Mallika V, Goswami B, Rajappa M: Atherosclerosis pathophysiology and the role of novel risk factors: A clinicobiochemical perspective. *Angiology* 58:513, 2007.
10. Kline ER, Sutliff RL: The roles of HIV-1 proteins and antiretroviral drug therapy in HIV-1-associated endothelial dysfunction. *J Investig Med* 56:752, 2008.
11. Calza L, Manfredi R, Pocaterra D, Chiodo F: Risk of premature atherosclerosis and ischemic heart disease associated with HIV infection and antiretroviral therapy. *J Infect* 57:16, 2008.
12. de Zeeuw D: Renal disease: A common and a silent killer. *Nat Clin Pract Cardiovasc Med* 5 Suppl 1:S27, 2008.
13. Saran AM, DuBose TD Jr: Cardiovascular disease in chronic kidney disease. *Ther Adv Cardiovasc Dis* 2:425, 2008.
14. Vonend O, Rump LC, Ritz E: Sympathetic overactivity—The Cinderella of cardiovascular risk factors in dialysis patients. *Semin Dial* 21:326, 2008.
15. Bradley TD, Floras JS: Obstructive sleep apnoea and its cardiovascular consequences. *Lancet* 373:82, 2009.

16. Skalen K, Gustafsson M, Rydberg EK, et al: Subendothelial retention of atherogenic lipoproteins in early atherosclerosis. *Nature* 417:750, 2002.
17. Passerini AG, Polacek DC, Shi C, et al: Coexisting proinflammatory and antioxidative endothelial transcription profiles in a disturbed flow region of the adult porcine aorta. *Proc Natl Acad Sci U S A* 101:2482, 2004.
18. Weber C, Zernecke A, Libby P: The multifaceted contributions of leukocyte subsets to atherosclerosis: Lessons from mouse models. *Nat Rev Immunol* 8:802, 2008.
19. Stary HC, Chandler AB, Dinsmore RE, et al: A definition of advanced types of atherosclerotic lesions and a histological classification of atherosclerosis. A report from the Committee on Vascular Lesions of the Council on Arteriosclerosis, American Heart Association. *Circulation* 92:1355, 1995.
20. Johnson JL: Matrix metalloproteinases: Influence on smooth muscle cells and atherosclerotic plaque stability. *Expert Rev Cardiovasc Ther* 5:265, 2007.
21. Hunt JL, Fairman R, Mitchell ME, et al: Bone formation in carotid plaques: A clinicopathological study. *Stroke* 33:1214, 2002.
22. Furchgott RF, Zawadzki JV: The obligatory role of endothelial cells in the relaxation of arterial smooth muscle by acetylcholine. *Nature* 288:373, 1980.
23. Furchgott RF: Endothelium-derived relaxing factor: Discovery, early studies, and identification as nitric oxide. *Biosci Rep* 19:235, 1999.
24. Lubos E, Handy DE, Loscalzo J: Role of oxidative stress and nitric oxide in atherothrombosis. *Front Biosci* 13:5323, 2008.
25. Guzik TJ, Chen W, Gongora MC, et al: Calcium-dependent NOX5 nicotinamide adenine dinucleotide phosphate oxidase contributes to vascular oxidative stress in human coronary artery disease. *J Am Coll Cardiol* 52:1803, 2008.
26. Landmesser U, Dikalov S, Price SR, et al: Oxidation of tetrahydrobiopterin leads to uncoupling of endothelial cell nitric oxide synthase in hypertension. *J Clin Invest* 111:1201, 2003.
27. Tiefenbacher CP, Bleeke T, Vahl C, et al: Endothelial dysfunction of coronary resistance arteries is improved by tetrahydrobiopterin in atherosclerosis. *Circulation* 102:2172, 2000.
28. Kim CS, Jung SB, Naqvi A, et al: P53 impairs endothelium-dependent vasomotor function through transcriptional upregulation of p66shc. *Circ Res* 103:1441, 2008.
29. Creager MA, Gallagher SJ, Girerd XJ, et al: L-Arginine improves endothelium-dependent vasodilation in hypercholesterolemic humans. *J Clin Invest* 90:1248, 1992.
30. Boger RH, Bode-Boger SM, Szuba A, et al: Asymmetric dimethylarginine (ADMA): A novel risk factor for endothelial dysfunction: Its role in hypercholesterolemia. *Circulation* 98:1842, 1998.
31. Ito A, Tsao PS, Adimoolam S, et al: Novel mechanism for endothelial dysfunction: Dysregulation of dimethylarginine dimethylaminohydrolase. *Circulation* 99:3092, 1999.
32. Ludmer PL, Selwyn AP, Shook TL, et al: Paradoxical vasoconstriction induced by acetylcholine in atherosclerotic coronary arteries. *N Engl J Med* 315:1046, 1986.
33. Kuhn FE, Mohler ER, Satler LF, et al: Effects of high density lipoprotein on acetylcholine induced coronary vasoreactivity. *Am J Cardiol* 68:1425, 1991.
34. Kuhn FE, Mohler ER, Rackley CE: Cholesterol and lipoproteins: Beyond atherosclerosis. *Clin Cardiol* 15:883, 1992.
35. Spieker LE, Sudano I, Hurlimann D, et al: High-density lipoprotein restores endothelial function in hypercholesterolemic men. *Circulation* 105:1399, 2002.
36. Celermajer DS, Sorensen KE, Spiegelhalter DJ, et al: Aging is associated with endothelial dysfunction in healthy men years before the age-related decline in women. *J Am Coll Cardiol* 24:471, 1994.
37. Ghiadoni L, Donald AE, Cropley M, et al: Mental stress induces transient endothelial dysfunction in humans. *Circulation* 102:2473, 2000.
38. Klemm P, Warner TD, Corder R, Vane JR: Endothelin-1 mediates coronary vasoconstriction caused by exogenous and endogenous cytokines. *J Cardiovasc Pharmacol* 26 Suppl 3:S419, 1995.
39. Mohler ER, III, O'Hare K, Darze ES, et al: Cardiovascular function in normotensive offspring of persons with essential hypertension and black race. *J Clin Hypertens (Greenwich)* 9:506, 2007.
40. Liuba P, Karnani P, Pesonen E, et al: Endothelial dysfunction after repeated *Chlamydia pneumoniae* infection in apolipoprotein E-knockout mice. *Circulation* 102:1039, 2000.
41. Fichtlscherer S, Rosenberger G, Walter DH, et al: Elevated C-reactive protein levels and impaired endothelial vasoreactivity in patients with coronary artery disease. *Circulation* 102:1000, 2000.
42. Beckman JA, Thakore A, Kalinowski BH, et al: Radiation therapy impairs endothelium-dependent vasodilation in humans. *J Am Coll Cardiol* 37:761, 2001.
43. Libby P, Ridker PM, Maseri A: Inflammation and atherosclerosis. *Circulation* 105:1135, 2002.
44. Steinberg D: Atherogenesis in perspective: Hypercholesterolemia and inflammation as partners in crime. *Nat Med* 8:1211, 2002.
45. Ross R, Glomset JA: Atherosclerosis and the arterial smooth muscle cell: Proliferation of smooth muscle is a key event in the genesis of the lesions of atherosclerosis. *Science* 180:1332, 1973.
46. Kanse SM, Parahuleva M, Muhl L, et al: Factor VII-activating protease (FSAP): Vascular functions and role in atherosclerosis. *Thromb Haemost* 99:286, 2008.
47. Fuster V: Lewis A. Conner Memorial Lecture. Mechanisms leading to myocardial infarction: Insights from studies of vascular biology. *Circulation* 90:2126, 1994.
48. Schwartz SM, Murry CE: Proliferation and the monoclonal origins of atherosclerotic lesions. *Annu Rev Med* 49:437, 1998.
49. Scott NA, Cipolla GD, Ross CE, et al: Identification of a potential role for the adventitia in vascular lesion formation after balloon overstretch injury of porcine coronary arteries. *Circulation* 93:2178, 1996.
50. Sata M, Saiura A, Kunisato A, et al: Hematopoietic stem cells differentiate into vascular cells that participate in the pathogenesis of atherosclerosis. *Nat Med* 8:403, 2002.
51. Hillebrands JL, Klatter FA, van den Hurk BM, et al: Origin of neointimal endothelium and alpha-actin-positive smooth muscle cells in transplant arteriosclerosis. *J Clin Invest* 107:1411, 2001.
52. Campbell JH, Han CL, Campbell GR: Neointimal formation by circulating bone marrow cells. *Ann N Y Acad Sci* 947:18, 2001.
53. Simper D, Stalboerger PG, Panetta CJ, et al: Smooth muscle progenitor cells in human blood. *Circulation* 106:1199, 2002.
54. Der Leyen HE, Gibbons GH, Morishita R, et al: Gene therapy inhibiting neointimal vascular lesion: *In vivo* transfer of endothelial cell nitric oxide synthase gene. *Proc Natl Acad Sci U S A* 92:1137, 1995.
55. Qian H, Neplioueva V, Shetty GA, et al: Nitric oxide synthase gene therapy rapidly reduces adhesion molecule expression and inflammatory cell infiltration in carotid arteries of cholesterol-fed rabbits. *Circulation* 99:2979, 1999.
56. Dzau VJ, Braun-Dullaeus RC, Sedding DG: Vascular proliferation and atherosclerosis: New perspectives and therapeutic strategies. *Nat Med* 8:1249, 2002.
57. Bonta PI, Pols TW, de Vries CJ: NR4A nuclear receptors in atherosclerosis and vein-graft disease. *Trends Cardiovasc Med* 17:105, 2007.
58. Lemos PA, Lee CH, Degertekin M, et al: Early outcome after sirolimus-eluting stent implantation in patients with acute coronary syndromes: Insights from the Rapamycin-Eluting Stent Evaluated At Rotterdam Cardiology Hospital (RESEARCH) registry. *J Am Coll Cardiol* 41:2093, 2003.
59. Sagripanti A, Carpi A: Antithrombotic and prothrombotic activities of the vascular endothelium. *Biomed Pharmacother* 54:107, 2000.
60. Feil R, Lohmann SM, de Jonge H, et al: Cyclic GMP-dependent protein kinases and the cardiovascular system: Insights from genetically modified mice. *Circ Res* 93:907, 2003.
61. Gonzalez MA, Selwyn AP: Endothelial function, inflammation, and prognosis in cardiovascular disease. *Am J Med* 115 Suppl 8A:99S, 2003.
62. Anderson TJ: Nitric oxide, atherosclerosis and the clinical relevance of endothelial dysfunction. *Heart Fail Rev* 8:71, 2003.
63. Tulis DA, Durante W, Liu X, et al: Adenovirus-mediated heme oxygenase-1 gene delivery inhibits injury-induced vascular neointima formation. *Circulation* 104:2710, 2001.
64. Sachais BS: Platelet-endothelial interactions in atherosclerosis. *Curr Atheroscler Rep* 3:412, 2001.
65. Marcus AJ, Broekman MJ, Drosopoulos JH, et al: Metabolic control of excessive extracellular nucleotide accumulation by CD39/ecto-nucleotidase-1: Implications for ischemic vascular diseases. *J Pharmacol Exp Ther* 305:9, 2003.
66. Landmesser U, Merten R, Spiekermann S, et al: Vascular extracellular superoxide dismutase activity in patients with coronary artery disease: Relation to endothelium-dependent vasodilation. *Circulation* 101:2264, 2000.
67. Cooke JP: Does ADMA cause endothelial dysfunction? *Arterioscler Thromb Vasc Biol* 20:2032, 2000.
68. Mohler ER 3rd, Shi Y, Moore J, et al: Diabetes reduces bone marrow and circulating porcine endothelial progenitor cells, an effect ameliorated by atorvastatin and independent of cholesterol. *Cytometry A* 75:75, 2009.
69. Foteinos G, Hu Y, Xiao Q, et al: Rapid endothelial turnover in atherosclerosis-prone areas coincides with stem cell repair in apolipoprotein E-deficient mice. *Circulation* 117:1856, 2008.
70. Binder CJ, Chang MK, Shaw PX, et al: Innate and acquired immunity in atherogenesis. *Nat Med* 8:1218, 2002.
71. Medzhitov R: Toll-like receptors and innate immunity. *Nat Rev Immunol* 1:135, 2001.
72. Erridge C: The roles of pathogen-associated molecular patterns in atherosclerosis. *Trends Cardiovasc Med* 18:52, 2008.
73. Medzhitov R, Janeway CA Jr: Decoding the patterns of self and nonself by the innate immune system. *Science* 296:298, 2002.
74. Ridker PM: Clinical application of C-reactive protein for cardiovascular disease detection and prevention. *Circulation* 107:363, 2003.
75. Dansky HM, Barlow CB, Lominska C, et al: Adhesion of monocytes to arterial endothelium and initiation of atherosclerosis are critically dependent on vascular cell adhesion molecule-1 gene dosage. *Arterioscler Thromb Vasc Biol* 21:1662, 2001.
76. Cybulsky MI, Iiyama K, Li H, et al: A major role for VCAM-1, but not ICAM-1, in early atherosclerosis. *J Clin Invest* 107:1255, 2001.
77. Collins RG, Velji R, Guevara NV, et al: P-Selectin or intercellular adhesion molecule (ICAM)-1 deficiency substantially protects against atherosclerosis in apolipoprotein E-deficient mice. *J Exp Med* 191:189, 2000.
78. Zalewski A, Macphee C, Nelson JJ: Lipoprotein-associated phospholipase A2: A potential therapeutic target for atherosclerosis. *Curr Drug Targets Cardiovasc Haematol Disord* 5:527, 2005.
79. Shi Y, Zhang P, Zhang L, et al: Role of lipoprotein-associated phospholipase A(2) in leukocyte activation and inflammatory responses. *Atherosclerosis* 191:54, 2006.
80. Wilensky RL, Shi Y, Mohler ER 3rd, et al: Inhibition of lipoprotein-associated phospholipase A2 reduces complex coronary atherosclerotic plaque development. *Nat Med* 14:1059, 2008.
81. Mohler ER 3rd, Ballantyne CM, Davidson MH, et al: The effect of darapladib on plasma lipoprotein-associated phospholipase A2 activity and cardiovascular biomarkers in patients with stable coronary heart disease or coronary heart disease risk equivalent: The results of a multicenter, randomized, double-blind, placebo-controlled study. *J Am Coll Cardiol* 51:1632, 2008.

82. Smith JD, Trogan E, Ginsberg M, et al: Decreased atherosclerosis in mice deficient in both macrophage colony-stimulating factor (op) and apolipoprotein E. *Proc Natl Acad Sci U S A* 92:8264, 1995.
83. Endemann G, Stanton LW, Madden KS, et al: CD36 is a receptor for oxidized low density lipoprotein. *J Biol Chem* 268:11811, 1993.
84. Steinberg D, Parthasarathy S, Carew TE, et al: Beyond cholesterol: Modifications of low-density lipoprotein that increase its atherogenicity. *N Engl J Med* 320:915, 1989.
85. Boring L, Gosling J, Cleary M, Charo IF: Decreased lesion formation in CCR2−/− mice reveals a role for chemokines in the initiation of atherosclerosis. *Nature* 394:894, 1998.
86. Gu L, Okada Y, Clinton SK, et al: Absence of monocyte chemoattractant protein-1 reduces atherosclerosis in low density lipoprotein receptor-deficient mice. *Mol Cell* 2:275, 1998.
87. Gosling J, Slaymaker S, Gu L, et al: MCP-1 deficiency reduces susceptibility to atherosclerosis in mice that overexpress human apolipoprotein B. *J Clin Invest* 103:773, 1999.
88. Nicholls SJ, Hazen SL: Myeloperoxidase, modified lipoproteins and atherogenesis. *J Lipid Res* 50 Suppl:S346, 2009.
89. Sugiyama S, Okada Y, Sukhova GK, et al: Macrophage myeloperoxidase regulation by granulocyte macrophage colony-stimulating factor in human atherosclerosis and implications in acute coronary syndromes. *Am J Pathol* 158:879, 2001.
90. Babior BM: Phagocytes and oxidative stress. *Am J Med* 109:33, 2000.
91. Suzuki H, Kurihara Y, Takeya M, et al: A role for macrophage scavenger receptors in atherosclerosis and susceptibility to infection. *Nature* 386:292, 1997.
92. Febbraio M, Podrez EA, Smith JD, et al: Targeted disruption of the class B scavenger receptor CD36 protects against atherosclerotic lesion development in mice. *J Clin Invest* 105:1049, 2000.
93. Kodama T, Reddy P, Kishimoto C, Krieger M: Purification and characterization of a bovine acetyl low density lipoprotein receptor. *Proc Natl Acad Sci U S A* 85:9238, 1988.
94. Henriksen T, Mahoney EM, Steinberg D: Enhanced macrophage degradation of low density lipoprotein previously incubated with cultured endothelial cells: Recognition by receptors for acetylated low density lipoproteins. *Proc Natl Acad Sci U S A* 78:6499, 1981.
95. Steinbrecher UP, Parthasarathy S, Leake DS, et al: Modification of low density lipoprotein by endothelial cells involves lipid peroxidation and degradation of low density lipoprotein phospholipids. *Proc Natl Acad Sci U S A* 81:3883, 1984.
96. Shaw PX, Horkko S, Chang MK, et al: Natural antibodies with the T15 idiotype may act in atherosclerosis, apoptotic clearance, and protective immunity. *J Clin Invest* 105:1731, 2000.
97. Tsimikas S, Palinski W, Witztum JL: Circulating autoantibodies to oxidized LDL correlate with arterial accumulation and depletion of oxidized LDL in LDL receptor-deficient mice. *Arterioscler Thromb Vasc Biol* 21:95, 2001.
98. Palinski W, Ord VA, Plump AS, et al: ApoE-deficient mice are a model of lipoprotein oxidation in atherogenesis. Demonstration of oxidation-specific epitopes in lesions and high titers of autoantibodies to malondialdehyde-lysine in serum. *Arterioscler Thromb* 14:605, 1994.
99. Ameli S, Hultgardh-Nilsson A, Regnstrom J, et al: Effect of immunization with homologous LDL and oxidized LDL on early atherosclerosis in hypercholesterolemic rabbits. *Arterioscler Thromb Vasc Biol* 16:1074, 1996.
100. Freigang S, Horkko S, Miller E, et al: Immunization of LDL receptor-deficient mice with homologous malondialdehyde-modified and native LDL reduces progression of atherosclerosis by mechanisms other than induction of high titers of antibodies to oxidative neoepitopes. *Arterioscler Thromb Vasc Biol* 18:1972, 1998.
101. Zhou X, Caligiuri G, Hamsten A, et al: LDL immunization induces T-cell-dependent antibody formation and protection against atherosclerosis. *Arterioscler Thromb Vasc Biol* 21:108, 2001.
102. Mehrabian M, Allayee H, Wong J, et al: Identification of 5-lipoxygenase as a major gene contributing to atherosclerosis susceptibility in mice. *Circ Res* 91:120, 2002.
103. Cyrus T, Witztum JL, Rader DJ, et al: Disruption of the 12/15-lipoxygenase gene diminishes atherosclerosis in apo E-deficient mice. *J Clin Invest* 103:1597, 1999.
104. Harats D, Shaish A, George J, et al: Overexpression of 15-lipoxygenase in vascular endothelium accelerates early atherosclerosis in LDL receptor-deficient mice. *Arterioscler Thromb Vasc Biol* 20:2100, 2000.
105. Whatling C, McPheat W, Herslof M: The potential link between atherosclerosis and the 5-lipoxygenase pathway: Investigational agents with new implications for the cardiovascular field. *Expert Opin Investig Drugs* 16:1879, 2007.
106. Williams KJ, Feig JE, Fisher EA: Cellular and molecular mechanisms for rapid regression of atherosclerosis: From bench top to potentially achievable clinical goal. *Curr Opin Lipidol* 18:443, 2007.
107. Schwenke DC: Comparison of aorta and pulmonary artery: I. Early cholesterol accumulation and relative susceptibility to atheromatous lesions. *Circ Res* 81:338, 1997.
108. Schwenke DC: Comparison of aorta and pulmonary artery: II. LDL transport and metabolism correlate with susceptibility to atherosclerosis. *Circ Res* 81:346, 1997.
109. Camejo G, Hurt-Camejo E, Wiklund O, Bondjers G: Association of apo B lipoproteins with arterial proteoglycans: Pathological significance and molecular basis. *Atherosclerosis* 139:205, 1998.
110. Navab M, Hama SY, Reddy ST, et al: Oxidized lipids as mediators of coronary heart disease. *Curr Opin Lipidol* 13:363, 2002.
111. Rajavashisth TB, Andalibi A, Territo MC, et al: Induction of endothelial cell expression of granulocyte and macrophage colony-stimulating factors by modified low-density lipoproteins. *Nature* 344:254, 1990.
112. MRC/BHF Heart Protection Study of cholesterol lowering with simvastatin in 20,536 high-risk individuals: A randomised placebo-controlled trial. *Lancet* 360:7, 2002.
113. Brown BG, Zhao XQ, Chait A, et al: Simvastatin and niacin, antioxidant vitamins, or the combination for the prevention of coronary disease. *N Engl J Med* 345:1583, 2001.
114. Gordon T, Kannel WB, Castelli WP, Dawber TR: Lipoproteins, cardiovascular disease, and death. The Framingham study. *Arch Intern Med* 141:1128, 1981.
115. Rader DJ, Alexander ET, Weibel GL, et al: Role of reverse cholesterol transport in animals and humans and relationship to atherosclerosis. *J Lipid Res* 50 Suppl:S189, 2009.
116. Tangirala RK, Tsukamoto K, Chun SH, et al: Regression of atherosclerosis induced by liver-directed gene transfer of apolipoprotein A-I in mice. *Circulation* 100:1816, 1999.
117. Zhang Y, Zanotti I, Reilly MP, et al: Overexpression of apolipoprotein A-I promotes reverse transport of cholesterol from macrophages to feces *in vivo*. *Circulation* 108:661, 2003.
118. Mineo C, Deguchi H, Griffin JH, Shaul PW: Endothelial and antithrombotic actions of HDL. *Circ Res* 98:1352, 2006.
119. Shih DM, Gu L, Xia YR, et al: Mice lacking serum paraoxonase are susceptible to organophosphate toxicity and atherosclerosis. *Nature* 394:284, 1998.
120. Mackness MI, Mackness B, Durrington PN, et al: Paraoxonase and coronary heart disease. *Curr Opin Lipidol* 9:319, 1998.
121. Barter PJ, Caulfield M, Eriksson M, et al: Effects of torcetrapib in patients at high risk for coronary events. *N Engl J Med* 357:2109, 2007.
122. Nissen SE, Tsunoda T, Tuzcu EM, et al: Effect of recombinant ApoA-I Milano on coronary atherosclerosis in patients with acute coronary syndromes: A randomized controlled trial. *JAMA* 290:2292, 2003.
123. Van Lenten BJ, Navab M, Anantharamaiah GM, et al: Multiple indications for anti-inflammatory apolipoprotein mimetic peptides. *Curr Opin Investig Drugs* 9:1157, 2008.
124. Rizvi M, Pathak D, Freedman JE, Chakrabarti S: CD40-CD40 ligand interactions in oxidative stress, inflammation and vascular disease. *Trends Mol Med* 14:530, 2008.
125. Mach F, Schonbeck U, Sukhova GK, et al: Reduction of atherosclerosis in mice by inhibition of CD40 signalling. *Nature* 394:200, 1998.
126. Cipollone F, Mezzetti A, Porreca E, et al: Association between enhanced soluble CD40L and prothrombotic state in hypercholesterolemia effects of statin therapy. *Circulation* 106:399, 2002.
127. Mallat Z, Gojova A, Marchiol-Fournigault C, et al: Inhibition of transforming growth factor-beta signaling accelerates atherosclerosis and induces an unstable plaque phenotype in mice. *Circ Res* 89:930, 2001.
128. Gurfinkel E, Lernoud V: The role of infection and immunity in atherosclerosis. *Expert Rev Cardiovasc Ther* 4:131, 2006.
129. Ford PJ, Yamazaki K, Seymour GJ: Cardiovascular and oral disease interactions: What is the evidence? *Prim Dent Care* 14:59, 2007.
130. Mayr M, Kiechl S, Willeit J, et al: Infections, immunity, and atherosclerosis: Associations of antibodies to *Chlamydia pneumoniae, Helicobacter pylori*, and cytomegalovirus with immune reactions to heat-shock protein 60 and carotid or femoral atherosclerosis. *Circulation* 102:833, 2000.
131. Caligiuri G, Nicoletti A, Poirier B, Hansson GK: Protective immunity against atherosclerosis carried by B cells of hypercholesterolemic mice. *J Clin Invest* 109:745, 2002.
132. Robinette CD, Fraumeni JF Jr: Splenectomy and subsequent mortality in veterans of the 1939–45 war. *Lancet* 2:127, 1977.
133. Yamada Y, Ichihara S, Nishida T: Molecular genetics of myocardial infarction. *Genomic Med* 2:7, 2008.
134. Helgadottir A, Manolescu A, Thorleifsson G, et al: The gene encoding 5-lipoxygenase activating protein confers risk of myocardial infarction and stroke. *Nat Genet* 36:233, 2004.
135. Topol EJ, Smith J, Plow EF, Wang QK: Genetic susceptibility to myocardial infarction and coronary artery disease. *Hum Mol Genet* 15 Spec No 2:R117, 2006.
136. Helgadottir A, Thorleifsson G, Manolescu A, et al: A common variant on chromosome 9p21 affects the risk of myocardial infarction. *Science* 316:1491, 2007.
137. Stary HC: Natural history and histological classification of atherosclerotic lesions: An update. *Arterioscler Thromb Vasc Biol* 20:1177, 2000.
138. Falk E: Plaque rupture with severe pre-existing stenosis precipitating coronary thrombosis. Characteristics of coronary atherosclerotic plaques underlying fatal occlusive thrombi. *Br Heart J* 50:127, 1983.
139. Davies MJ, Thomas AC: Plaque fissuring—The cause of acute myocardial infarction, sudden ischaemic death, and crescendo angina. *Br Heart J* 53:363, 1985.
140. Muller JE, Tofler GH, Stone PH: Circadian variation and triggers of onset of acute cardiovascular disease. *Circulation* 79:733, 1989.
141. Muller JE, Abela GS, Nesto RW, Tofler GH: Triggers, acute risk factors and vulnerable plaques: The lexicon of a new frontier. *J Am Coll Cardiol* 23:809, 1994.
142. Naghavi M, Libby P, Falk E, et al: From vulnerable plaque to vulnerable patient: A call for new definitions and risk assessment strategies: Part I. *Circulation* 108:1664, 2003.
143. Beckman JA, Ganz J, Creager MA, et al: Relationship of clinical presentation and calcification of culprit coronary artery stenoses. *Arterioscler Thromb Vasc Biol* 21:1618, 2001.
144. Virmani R, Kolodgie FD, Burke AP, et al: Lessons from sudden coronary death: A comprehensive morphological classification scheme for atherosclerotic lesions. *Arterioscler Thromb Vasc Biol* 20:1262, 2000.
145. Casscells W, Naghavi M, Willerson JT: Vulnerable atherosclerotic plaque: A multifocal disease. *Circulation* 107:2072, 2003.
146. Uchida Y, Nakamura F, Tomaru T, et al: Prediction of acute coronary syndromes by percutaneous coronary angioscopy in patients with stable angina. *Am Heart J* 130:195, 1995.

147. Ambrose JA: In search of the "vulnerable plaque": Can it be localized and will focal regional therapy ever be an option for cardiac prevention? *J Am Coll Cardiol* 51:1539, 2008.
148. Naghavi M, Libby P, Falk E, et al: From vulnerable plaque to vulnerable patient: A call for new definitions and risk assessment strategies: Part II. *Circulation* 108:1772, 2003.
149. Davi G, Patrono C: Platelet activation and atherothrombosis. *N Engl J Med* 357:2482, 2007.
150. Shah PK: Molecular mechanisms of plaque instability. *Curr Opin Lipidol* 18:492, 2007.
151. Frostegard J: Systemic lupus erythematosus and cardiovascular disease. *Lupus* 17:364, 2008.
152. May AE, Langer H, Seizer P, et al: Platelet-leukocyte interactions in inflammation and atherothrombosis. *Semin Thromb Hemost* 33:123, 2007.
153. Aird WC: Vascular bed-specific thrombosis. *J Thromb Haemost* 5 Suppl 1:283, 2007.
154. Chien S: Effects of disturbed flow on endothelial cells. *Ann Biomed Eng* 36:554, 2008.
155. Helderman F, Segers D, de Crom R, et al: Effect of shear stress on vascular inflammation and plaque development. *Curr Opin Lipidol* 18:527, 2007.
156. Badimon JJ, Ortiz AF, Meyer B, et al: Different response to balloon angioplasty of carotid and coronary arteries: Effects on acute platelet deposition and intimal thickening. *Atherosclerosis* 140:307, 1998.
157. Halvorsen B, Otterdal K, Dahl TB, et al: Atherosclerotic plaque stability—What determines the fate of a plaque? *Prog Cardiovasc Dis* 51:183, 2008.
158. Aird WC: Endothelial cell heterogeneity. *Crit Care Med* 31:S221, 2003.
159. Majesky MW: Developmental basis of vascular smooth muscle diversity. *Arterioscler Thromb Vasc Biol* 27:1248, 2007.
160. Mackman N: Triggers, targets and treatments for thrombosis. *Nature* 451:914, 2008.
161. Lechner D, Weltermann A: Circulating tissue factor-exposing microparticles. *Thromb Res* 122 Suppl 1:S47, 2008.
162. George FD: Microparticles in vascular diseases. *Thromb Res* 122 Suppl 1:S55, 2008.
163. Rauch U, Osende JI, Fuster V, et al: Thrombus formation on atherosclerotic plaques: Pathogenesis and clinical consequences. *Ann Intern Med* 134:224, 2001.
164. Molina CA, Santamarina E, and Alvarez-Sabin J: Cryptogenic stroke, aortic arch atheroma and patent foramen ovale. *Cerebrovasc Dis* 24 Suppl 1:84, 2007.
165. Finn AV, Joner M, Nakazawa G, et al: Pathological correlates of late drug-eluting stent thrombosis: Strut coverage as a marker of endothelialization. *Circulation* 115:2435, 2007.
166. Matsuura E, Kobayashi K, Lopez LR: Preventing autoimmune and infection triggered atherosclerosis for an enduring healthful lifestyle. *Autoimmun Rev* 7:214, 2008.
167. Mok CC: Accelerated atherosclerosis, arterial thromboembolism, and preventive strategies in systemic lupus erythematosus. *Scand J Rheumatol* 35:85, 2006.
168. Warkentin TE, Maurer BT, Aster RH: Heparin-induced thrombocytopenia associated with fondaparinux. *N Engl J Med* 356:2653, 2007.
169. Schafer AI: Molecular basis of the diagnosis and treatment of polycythemia vera and essential thrombocythemia. *Blood* 107:4214, 2006.
170. Landolfi R, Di Gennaro L, Falanga A: Thrombosis in myeloproliferative disorders: Pathogenetic facts and speculation. *Leukemia* 22:2020, 2008.
171. Andrews RK, Berndt MC: Platelet adhesion: A game of catch and release. *J Clin Invest* 118:3009, 2008.
172. Wootton DM, Ku DN: Fluid mechanics of vascular systems, diseases, and thrombosis. *Annu Rev Biomed Eng* 1:299, 1999.
173. Ruggeri ZM: Platelets in atherothrombosis. *Nat Med* 8:1227, 2002.
174. Yago T, Lou J, Wu T, et al: Platelet glycoprotein Ibalpha forms catch bonds with human WT vWF but not with type 2B von Willebrand disease vWF. *J Clin Invest* 118:3195, 2008.
175. Kulkarni S, Dopheide SM, Yap CL, et al: A revised model of platelet aggregation. *J Clin Invest* 105:783, 2000.
176. Wagner CT, Kroll MH, Chow TW, et al: Epinephrine and shear stress synergistically induce platelet aggregation via a mechanism that partially bypasses VWF-GP IB interactions. *Biorheology* 33:209, 1996.
177. Andre P, Prasad KS, Denis CV, et al: CD40L stabilizes arterial thrombi by a beta3 integrin-dependent mechanism. *Nat Med* 8:247, 2002.
178. Croce K, Libby P: Intertwining of thrombosis and inflammation in atherosclerosis. *Curr Opin Hematol* 14:55, 2007.
179. Tedgui A, Mallat Z: Apoptosis as a determinant of atherothrombosis. *Thromb Haemost* 86:420, 2001.
180. Shah PK: Inflammation and plaque vulnerability. *Cardiovasc Drugs Ther* 23:31, 2009.
181. Kuge Y, Kume N, Ishino S, et al: Prominent lectin-like oxidized low density lipoprotein (LDL) receptor-1 (LOX-1) expression in atherosclerotic lesions is associated with tissue factor expression and apoptosis in hypercholesterolemic rabbits. *Biol Pharm Bull* 31:1475, 2008.
182. Endler G, Mannhalter C: Polymorphisms in coagulation factor genes and their impact on arterial and venous thrombosis. *Clin Chim Acta* 330:31, 2003.
183. Prandoni P, Bilora F, Marchiori A, et al: An association between atherosclerosis and venous thrombosis. *N Engl J Med* 348:1435, 2003.
184. Sorensen HT, Horvath-Puho E, Pedersen L, et al: Venous thromboembolism and subsequent hospitalisation due to acute arterial cardiovascular events: A 20-year cohort study. *Lancet* 370:1773, 2007.
185. Ageno W, Dentali F: Venous thromboembolism and arterial thromboembolism. Many similarities, far beyond thrombosis per se. *Thromb Haemost* 100:181, 2008.
186. Franchini M, Targher G, Montagnana M, Lippi G: The metabolic syndrome and the risk of arterial and venous thrombosis. *Thromb Res* 122:727, 2008.
187. Lowe GD: Common risk factors for both arterial and venous thrombosis. *Br J Haematol* 140:488, 2008.
188. Ye Z, Liu EH, Higgins JP, et al: Seven haemostatic gene polymorphisms in coronary disease: Meta-analysis of 66,155 cases and 91,307 controls. *Lancet* 367:651, 2006.
189. Tuinenburg A, Mauser-Bunschoten EP, Verhaar MC, et al: Cardiovascular disease in patients with haemophilia. *J Thromb Haemost* 7:247, 2009.
190. Sramek A, Reiber JH, Gerrits WB, Rosendaal FR: Decreased coagulability has no clinically relevant effect on atherogenesis: Observations in individuals with a hereditary bleeding tendency. *Circulation* 104:762, 2001.
191. Haverkate F: Levels of haemostatic factors, arteriosclerosis and cardiovascular disease. *Vascul Pharmacol* 39:109, 2002.
192. Kannel WB: Overview of hemostatic factors involved in atherosclerotic cardiovascular disease. *Lipids* 40:1215, 2005.
193. Badimon L, Badimon JJ, Chesebro JH, Fuster V: Von Willebrand factor and cardiovascular disease. *Thromb Haemost* 70:111, 1993.
194. Methia N, Andre P, Denis CV, et al: Localized reduction of atherosclerosis in von Willebrand factor-deficient mice. *Blood* 98:1424, 2001.
195. Williams MS, Bray PF: Genetics of arterial prothrombotic risk states. *Exp Biol Med (Maywood)* 226:409, 2001.
196. Lekakis J, Bisti S, Tsougos E, et al: Platelet glycoprotein IIb HPA-3 polymorphism and acute coronary syndromes. *Int J Cardiol* 127:46, 2008.
197. Weiss EJ, Bray PF, Tayback M, et al: A polymorphism of a platelet glycoprotein receptor as an inherited risk factor for coronary thrombosis. *N Engl J Med* 334:1090, 1996.
198. Ouwehand WH: Platelet genomics and the risk of atherothrombosis. *J Thromb Haemost* 5 Suppl 1:188, 2007.
199. Birk AV, Leno E, Robertson HD, et al: Interaction between ATP and catecholamines in stimulation of platelet aggregation. *Am J Physiol Heart Circ Physiol* 284:H619, 2003.
200. Rauch U, Osende JI, Chesebro JH, et al: Statins and cardiovascular diseases: The multiple effects of lipid-lowering therapy by statins. *Atherosclerosis* 153:181, 2000.
201. Ikarugi H, Taka T, Nakajima S, et al: Norepinephrine, but not epinephrine, enhances platelet reactivity and coagulation after exercise in humans. *J Appl Physiol* 86:133, 1999.
202. Alpert JS, Thygesen K, Antman E, Bassand JP: Myocardial infarction redefined—A consensus document of The Joint European Society of Cardiology/American College of Cardiology Committee for the redefinition of myocardial infarction. *J Am Coll Cardiol* 36:959, 2000.
203. Braunwald E, Antman EM, Beasley JW, et al: ACC/AHA 2002 guideline update for the management of patients with unstable angina and non-ST-segment elevation myocardial infarction—Summary article: A report of the American College of Cardiology/American Heart Association task force on practice guidelines (Committee on the Management of Patients with Unstable Angina). *J Am Coll Cardiol* 40:1366, 2002.
204. Fesmire FM, Percy RF, Bardoner JB, et al: Usefulness of automated serial 12-lead ECG monitoring during the initial emergency department evaluation of patients with chest pain. *Ann Emerg Med* 31:3, 1998.
205. Pope JH, Ruthazer R, Beshansky JR, et al: Clinical features of emergency department patients presenting with symptoms suggestive of acute cardiac ischemia: A multicenter study. *J Thromb Thrombolysis* 6:63, 1998.
206. Antman EM, Hand M, Armstrong PW, et al: 2007 Focused update of the ACC/AHA 2004 Guidelines for the Management of Patients with ST-Elevation Myocardial Infarction: A report of the American College of Cardiology/American Heart Association Task Force on Practice Guidelines: Developed in collaboration with the Canadian Cardiovascular Society endorsed by the American Academy of Family Physicians: 2007 Writing Group to Review New Evidence and Update the ACC/AHA 2004 Guidelines for the Management of Patients with ST-Elevation Myocardial Infarction, Writing on Behalf of the 2004 Writing Committee. *Circulation* 117:296, 2008.
207. Pollack CV Jr, Antman EM, Hollander JE: 2007 focused update to the ACC/AHA guidelines for the management of patients with ST-segment elevation myocardial infarction: Implications for emergency department practice. *Ann Emerg Med* 52:344, 2008.
208. Grines CL, Browne KF, Marco J, et al: A comparison of immediate angioplasty with thrombolytic therapy for acute myocardial infarction. The Primary Angioplasty in Myocardial Infarction Study Group. *N Engl J Med* 328:673, 1993.
209. Le May MR, Labinaz M, Davies RF, et al: Stenting versus thrombolysis in acute myocardial infarction trial (STAT). *J Am Coll Cardiol* 37:985, 2001.
210. Keeley EC, Grines CL: Primary coronary intervention for acute myocardial infarction. *JAMA* 291:736, 2004.
211. Boersma E, Mercado N, Poldermans D, et al: Acute myocardial infarction. *The Lancet* 361:847, 2003.
212. Califf RM, White HD, Van de WF, et al: One-year results from the Global Utilization of Streptokinase and TPA for Occluded Coronary Arteries (GUSTO-I) trial. GUSTO-I Investigators. *Circulation* 94:1233, 1996.
213. Llevadot J, Giugliano RP, Antman EM: Bolus fibrinolytic therapy in acute myocardial infarction. *JAMA* 286:442, 2001.
214. Brieger DB, Mak KH, White HD, et al: Benefit of early sustained reperfusion in patients with prior myocardial infarction (the GUSTO-I trial). Global Utilization of Streptokinase and TPA for occluded arteries. *Am J Cardiol* 81:282, 1998.
215. Becker RC, Meade TW, Berger PB, et al: The primary and secondary prevention of coronary artery disease: American College of Chest Physicians Evidence-Based Clinical Practice Guidelines (8th edition). *Chest* 133:776S, 2008.
216. Randomised double-blind trial of fixed low-dose warfarin with aspirin after myocardial infarction. Coumadin Aspirin Reinfarction Study (CARS) Investigators. *Lancet* 350:389, 1997.

217. Grundy SM, Cleeman JI, Merz CN, et al: Implications of recent clinical trials for the National Cholesterol Education Program Adult Treatment Panel III Guidelines. *J Am Coll Cardiol* 44:720, 2004.
218. Cannon CP, Braunwald E, McCabe CH, et al: Intensive versus moderate lipid lowering with statins after acute coronary syndromes. *N Engl J Med* 350:1495, 2004.
219. Pollack CV Jr, Braunwald E: 2007 Update to the ACC/AHA guidelines for the management of patients with unstable angina and non-ST-segment elevation myocardial infarction: Implications for emergency department practice. *Ann Emerg Med* 51:591, 2008.
220. Antithrombotic Trialists C: Collaborative meta-analysis of randomised trials of antiplatelet therapy for prevention of death, myocardial infarction, and stroke in high risk patients. *BMJ* 324:71, 2002.
221. Lewis HD Jr, Davis JW, Archibald DG, et al: Protective effects of aspirin against acute myocardial infarction and death in men with unstable angina. Results of a Veterans Administration Cooperative Study. *N Engl J Med* 309:396, 1983.
222. Cairns JA, Gent M, Singer J, et al: Aspirin, sulfinpyrazone, or both in unstable angina. Results of a Canadian multicenter trial. *N Engl J Med* 313:1369, 1985.
223. Boersma E, Harrington RA, Moliterno DJ, et al: Platelet glycoprotein IIb/IIIa inhibitors in acute coronary syndromes: A meta-analysis of all major randomised clinical trials. *Lancet* 359:189, 2002.
224. McKee SA, Sane DC, Deliargyris EN: Aspirin resistance in cardiovascular disease: A review of prevalence, mechanisms, and clinical significance. *Thromb Haemost* 88:711, 2002.
225. Eikelboom JW, Hirsh J, Weitz JI, et al: Aspirin-resistant thromboxane biosynthesis and the risk of myocardial infarction, stroke, or cardiovascular death in patients at high risk for cardiovascular events. *Circulation* 105:1650, 2002.
226. Gum PA, Kottke-Marchant K, Welsh PA, et al: A prospective, blinded determination of the natural history of aspirin resistance among stable patients with cardiovascular disease. *J Am Coll Cardiol* 41:961, 2003.
227. Schafer AI: Genetic and acquired determinants of individual variability of response to antiplatelet drugs. *Circulation* 108:910, 2003.
228. Ryan TJ, Antman EM, Brooks NH, et al: 1999 Update: ACC/AHA guidelines for the management of patients with acute myocardial infarction. A report of the American College of Cardiology/American Heart Association Task Force on Practice Guidelines (Committee on Management of Acute Myocardial Infarction). *J Am Coll Cardiol* 34:890, 1999.
229. Committee CS: A randomised, blinded, trial of clopidogrel versus aspirin in patients at risk of ischaemic events (CAPRIE). *Lancet* 348:1329, 1996.
230. Yusuf S, Zhao F, Mehta SR, et al: Effects of clopidogrel in addition to aspirin in patients with acute coronary syndromes without ST-segment elevation. *N Engl J Med* 345:494, 2001.
231. Mehta SR: Aspirin and clopidogrel in patients with ACS undergoing PCI: CURE and PCI-CURE. *J Invasive Cardiol* 15 Suppl B:17B, 2003.
232. Hongo RH, Ley J, Dick SE, Yee RR: The effect of clopidogrel in combination with aspirin when given before coronary artery bypass grafting. *J Am Coll Cardiol* 40:231, 2002.
233. Antoniucci D, Migliorini A, Parodi G, et al: Abciximab-supported infarct artery stent implantation for acute myocardial infarction and long-term survival. A prospective, multicenter, randomized trial comparing infarct artery stenting plus abciximab with stenting alone. *Circulation* 109:1704, 2004.
234. Antoniucci D, Rodriguez A, Hempel A, et al: A randomized trial comparing primary infarct artery stenting with or without abciximab in acute myocardial infarction. *J Am Coll Cardiol* 42:1879, 2003.
235. Kandzari DE, Hasselblad V, Tcheng JE, et al: Improved clinical outcomes with abciximab therapy in acute myocardial infarction: A systematic overview of randomized clinical trials. *Am Heart J* 147:457, 2004.
236. Topol EJ, Moliterno DJ, Herrmann HC, et al: Comparison of two platelet glycoprotein IIb/IIIa inhibitors, tirofiban and abciximab, for the prevention of ischemic events with percutaneous coronary revascularization. *N Engl J Med* 344:1888, 2001.
237. Servoss SJ, Wan Y, Snapinn SM, et al: Tirofiban therapy for patients with acute coronary syndromes and prior coronary artery bypass grafting in the PRISM-PLUS trial. *Am J Cardiol* 93:843, 2004.
238. Blankenship JC, Sigmon KN, Pieper KS, et al: Effect of eptifibatide on angiographic complications during percutaneous coronary intervention in the IMPACT—(Integrilin to Minimize Platelet Aggregation and Coronary Thrombosis) II Trial. *Am J Cardiol* 88:969, 2001.
239. Nguyen CM, Harrington RA: Glycoprotein IIb/IIIa receptor antagonists: A comparative review of their use in percutaneous coronary intervention. *Am J Cardiovasc Drugs* 3:423, 2003.
240. Braunwald E: Application of current guidelines to the management of unstable angina and non-ST-elevation myocardial infarction. *Circulation* 108: III28, 2003.
241. Direct thrombin inhibitors in acute coronary syndromes: Principal results of a meta-analysis based on individual patients' data. *Lancet* 359:294, 2002.
242. Lincoff AM, Kleiman NS, Kereiakes DJ, et al: Long-term efficacy of bivalirudin and provisional glycoprotein IIb/IIIa blockade vs heparin and planned glycoprotein IIb/IIIa blockade during percutaneous coronary revascularization: REPLACE-2 randomized trial. *JAMA* 292:696, 2004.
243. Warkentin TE, Greinacher A: Heparin-induced thrombocytopenia: Recognition, treatment, and prevention: The Seventh ACCP Conference on Antithrombotic and Thrombolytic Therapy. *Chest* 126: 311S, 2004.
244. Gibbons RJ, Abrams J, Chatterjee K, et al: ACC/AHA 2002 guideline update for the management of patients with chronic stable angina—Summary article: A report of the American College of Cardiology/American Heart Association Task Force on practice guidelines (Committee on the Management of Patients with Chronic Stable Angina). *J Am Coll Cardiol* 41:159, 2003.
245. Kaiser GC, Davis KB, Fisher LD, et al: Survival following coronary artery bypass grafting in patients with severe angina pectoris (CASS). An observational study. *J Thorac Cardiovasc Surg* 89:513, 1985.
246. Mintz GS, Kimura T, Nobuyoshi M, Leon MB: Intravascular ultrasound assessment of the relation between early and late changes in arterial area and neointimal hyperplasia after percutaneous transluminal coronary angioplasty and directional coronary atherectomy. *Am J Cardiol* 83:1518, 1999.
247. Wilensky RL, Tanguay JF, Ito S, et al: Heparin infusion prior to stenting (HIPS) trial: Final results of a prospective, randomized, controlled trial evaluating the effects of local vascular delivery on intimal hyperplasia. *Am Heart J* 139:1061, 2000.
248. Morice MC, Serruys PW, Sousa JE, et al: A randomized comparison of a sirolimus-eluting stent with a standard stent for coronary revascularization. *N Engl J Med* 346:1773, 2002.
249. Moses JW, Leon MB, Popma JJ, et al: Sirolimus-eluting stents versus standard stents in patients with stenosis in a native coronary artery. *N Engl J Med* 349:1315, 2003.
250. Simonton CA, Brodie B, Cheek B, et al: Comparative clinical outcomes of paclitaxel- and sirolimus-eluting stents: Results from a large prospective multicenter registry—STENT Group. *J Am Coll Cardiol* 50:1214, 2007.
251. Mohler ER, III: Peripheral arterial disease: Identification and implications. *Arch Intern Med*163:2306, 2003.
252. Hirsch AT, Haskal ZJ, Hertzer NR, et al: ACC/AHA 2005 practice guidelines for the management of patients with peripheral arterial disease (lower extremity, renal, mesenteric, and abdominal aortic): A collaborative report from the American Association for Vascular Surgery/Society for Vascular Surgery, Society for Cardiovascular Angiography and Interventions, Society for Vascular Medicine and Biology, Society of Interventional Radiology, and the ACC/AHA Task Force on Practice Guidelines (Writing Committee to Develop Guidelines for the Management of Patients with Peripheral Arterial Disease): Endorsed by the American Association of Cardiovascular and Pulmonary Rehabilitation; National Heart, Lung, and Blood Institute; Society for Vascular Nursing; TransAtlantic Inter-Society Consensus; and Vascular Disease Foundation. *Circulation* 113:E463, 2006.
253. Norgren L, Hiatt WR, Dormandy JA, et al: Inter-Society Consensus for the Management of Peripheral Arterial Disease (TASC II). *J Vasc Surg* 45 Suppl S:S5, 2007.
254. Goyen M, Edelman M, Perreault P, et al: MR angiography of aortoiliac occlusive disease: A phase III study of the safety and effectiveness of the blood-pool contrast agent MS-325. *Radiology* 236:825, 2005.
255. Mohler ER, III: Therapy insight: Peripheral arterial disease and diabetes—from pathogenesis to treatment guidelines. *Nat Clin Pract Cardiovasc Med* 4:151, 2007.
256. Mohler ER, Jaff MR: *Peripheral Arterial Disease*. American College of Physicians, Philadelphia, 2008.
257. Malinow MR, Kang SS, Taylor LM, et al: Prevalence of hyperhomocyst(e)inemia in patients with peripheral arterial occlusive disease. *Circulation* 79:1180, 1989.
258. Goldhaber SZ, Manson JE, Stampfer MJ, et al: Low-dose aspirin and subsequent peripheral arterial surgery in the Physicians' Health Study. *Lancet* 340:143, 1992.
259. Mohler E 3rd, and Giri J: Management of peripheral arterial disease patients: Comparing the ACC/AHA and TASC-II guidelines. *Curr Med Res Opin* 24:2509, 2008.
260. Gardner AW, Poehlman ET: Exercise rehabilitation programs for the treatment of claudication pain. A meta-analysis. *JAMA* 274:975, 1995.
261. Reilly MP, Mohler ER, III: Cilostazol: Treatment of intermittent claudication. *Ann Pharmacother* 35:48, 2001.
262. Wilhite DB, Comerota AJ, Schmieder FA, et al: Managing PAD with multiple platelet inhibitors: The effect of combination therapy on bleeding time. *J Vasc Surg* 38:710, 2003.
263. Bogousslavsky J, Regli F, van MG: Risk factors and concomitants of internal carotid artery occlusion or stenosis. A controlled study of 159 cases. *Arch Neurol* 42:864, 1985.
264. Whisnant JP: Modeling of risk factors for ischemic stroke. The Willis Lecture. *Stroke* 28:1840, 1997.
265. Mohler ER, III, Delanty N, Rader DJ, Raps EC: Statins and cerebrovascular disease: Plaque attack to prevent brain attack. *Vasc Med* 4:269, 1999.
266. Rothwell PM, Eliasziw M, Gutnikov SA, et al: Analysis of pooled data from the randomised controlled trials of endarterectomy for symptomatic carotid stenosis. *Lancet* 361:107, 2003.
267. Mohler ER, III: Carotid stenting for atherothrombosis. *Heart* 93:1147, 2007.
268. Diener HC, Cunha L, Forbes C, et al: European Stroke Prevention Study. 2. Dipyridamole and acetylsalicylic acid in the secondary prevention of stroke. *J Neurol Sci* 143:1, 1996.
269. Sacco RL, Diener HC, Yusuf S, et al: Aspirin and extended-release dipyridamole versus clopidogrel for recurrent stroke. *N Engl J Med* 359:1238, 2008.
270. He K, Rimm EB, Merchant A, et al: Fish consumption and risk of stroke in men. *JAMA* 288:3130, 2002.
271. Scolari F, Ravani P, Gaggi R, et al: The challenge of diagnosing atheroembolic renal disease: Clinical features and prognostic factors. *Circulation* 116:298, 2007.
272. Voetsch B, Afshar-Kharghan V, Loscalzo J, Schafer AI: Less common thrombotic and embolic disorders, in *Thrombosis and Hemorrhage*, edited by J Loscalzo, AI Schafer, p 707. Lippincott Williams & Wilkins, Philadelphia, 2003.
273. Bashore TM, Gehrig T: Cholesterol emboli after invasive cardiac procedures. *J Am Coll Cardiol* 42:217, 2003.
274. Applebaum RM, Kronzon I: Evaluation and management of cholesterol embolization and the blue toe syndrome. *Curr Opin Cardiol* 11:533, 1996.

CHAPTER 136
FIBRINOLYSIS AND THROMBOLYSIS

Katherine A. Hajjar and Jia Ruan

SUMMARY

In recent years, an understanding of the molecular mechanisms of fibrinolysis has led to major advances in fibrinolytic and antifibrinolytic therapy. Characterization of the genes for all the major fibrinolytic proteins has revealed the structure and function of the relevant serine proteases, their inhibitors, and their receptors. The development of genetically engineered animals deficient in one or more fibrinolytic protein(s) has revealed both expected and unexpected roles for these proteins in both intravascular and extravascular settings. In addition, genetic analysis of human deficiency syndromes has defined specific mutations that result in human disorders reflective of either fibrinolytic deficiency with thrombosis or fibrinolytic excess with hemorrhage. All of these advances have led to development of more effective and safer protocols for fibrinolytic therapy, and for the rational use of antifibrinolytic agents under certain specific circumstances.

BASIC CONCEPTS OF FIBRINOLYSIS

Fibrin, the insoluble end product of the action of thrombin on fibrinogen, is found in both intravascular and extravascular settings. In response to vascular injury, crosslinked fibrin is deposited in tissues and blood vessels, thus compromising the flow of blood. Once the vessel has healed, the fibrinolytic system is activated, converting fibrin to its soluble degradation products through the action of the serine protease, plasmin (Fig. 136–1A).

Under physiologic conditions, fibrinolysis is precisely regulated by the measured participation of activators, inhibitors, and cofactors.[1] In addition, receptors expressed by endothelial, monocytoid, and myeloid cells provide specialized, protected environments where plasmin can be generated without neutralization by circulating inhibitors (Fig. 136–1B).[2] In addition to soluble circulating factors, endothelial cells, monocytes, macrophages, and myeloid cells participate in all aspects of fibrinolytic regulation. Recent evidence, moreover, indicates that, beyond its more traditional role in fibrin degradation, the fibrinolytic system supports a variety of tissue remodeling mechanisms. This chapter reviews the fundamental features of plasmin generation, considers the major clinical syndromes resulting from abnormalities in fibrinolysis, and discusses approaches to fibrinolytic and antifibrinolytic therapy.

Acronyms and abbreviations that appear in this chapter include: A2, annexin A2; ASK, Australian Streptokinase; ATLANTIS, Alteplase Thrombolysis for Acute Noninterventional Therapy in Ischemic Stroke; cAMP, cyclic adenosine monophosphate; CT, computed tomography; DIC, disseminated intravascular coagulation; EACA, ε-aminocaproic acid; ECASS, European Cooperative Acute Stroke Study; FDA, Food and Drug Administration; HC, homocysteine; IL, interleukin; ISTR, International Stroke Thrombolysis Registry; MAST-E, Multicenter Acute Stroke Trial–Europe; MAST-I, Multicenter Acute Stroke Trial–Italy; MELT, Middle Cerebral Artery Embolism Local Fibrinolytic Intervention Study; MMP, matrix metalloproteinase; Mr, molecular mass; mRNA, messenger ribonucleic acid; NINDS, National Institute of Neurologic Disorders and Stroke; p11, protein p11; PAI, plasminogen-activator inhibitor; PLG, plasminogen; PROACT, Prolyse in Acute Cerebral Thromboembolism; SITS, Safe Implementation of Treatments in Stroke; STILE, Surgery versus Thrombolysis for Ischemia of the Lower Extremity; TAFI, thrombin-activatable fibrinolysis inhibitor; TGF-β, transforming growth factor-β; TOPAS, Thrombolysis or Peripheral Arterial Surgery; t-PA, tissue-type plasminogen activator; u-PA, urokinase plasminogen activator; uPAR, urokinase plasminogen activator receptor.

COMPONENTS OF THE FIBRINOLYTIC SYSTEM

PLASMINOGEN

Synthesized primarily in the liver,[3,4] plasminogen is a Mr ~92,000 single-chain proenzyme that circulates in plasma at a concentration of approximately 1.5 μM (Table 136–1).[5] The plasma half-life of plasminogen in adults is approximately 2 days.[6] Its 791 amino acids are crosslinked by 24 disulfide bridges, 16 of which give rise to 5 homologous triple-loop structures called "kringles" based on the secondary structure resemblance to the Danish pastry of the same name (Fig. 136–2).[7] The first (K1) and fourth (K4) of these 80-amino acid, Mr approximately 10,000 structures impart high- and low-affinity lysine binding, respectively.[8] The lysine-binding domains of plasminogen appear to mediate its specific interactions with fibrin, cell surface receptors, and other proteins including its circulating inhibitor α_2-plasmin inhibitor.[9–13]

Posttranslational modification of plasminogen results in two glycosylation variants (forms 1 and 2) (see Table 136–1).[14–16] *O-linked* oligosaccharide, consisting of sialic acid, galactose, and galactosamine resident on Thr 345, is common to both forms. Only form 2, however, contains *N-linked* oligosaccharide on Asn288 that is comprised of sialic acid, galactose, glucosamine, and mannose. The carbohydrate portion of plasminogen appears to regulate its affinity for cellular receptors, and may also specify its physiologic degradation pathway.

Activation of plasminogen results from cleavage of a single Arg-Val peptide bond at position 560–561,[5] giving rise to the active protease, plasmin (see Table 136–1). Plasmin contains a typical serine protease catalytic triad (His602, Asp645, and Ser740), but exhibits broad substrate specificity when compared to other proteases of this class.[17] The circulating form of plasminogen (PLG), amino-terminal glutamic acid plasminogen (Glu-PLG), is readily converted by limited proteolysis to several modified forms known collectively as Lys-PLG.[18,19] Hydrolysis of the Lys77–Lys78 peptide bond gives rise to a conformationally modified form of the zymogen that more readily binds fibrin, displays two- to threefold higher avidity for cellular receptors, and is activated 10 to 20 times more rapidly than Glu-PLG.[10,20,21] Lys-PLG does not normally circulate in plasma,[20] but has been identified on cell surfaces.[22,23]

Spanning 52.5 kb of DNA on chromosome 6q26-27, the plasminogen gene consists of 19 exons[24,25] and directs expression of a 2.7 kb messenger RNA (mRNA) (see Fig. 136–2).[7] The 5′ upstream region of the plasminogen gene contains two regulatory elements common to genes for acute-phase reactants (CTGGGA) and six interleukin (IL)-6–responsive elements.[25] Plasminogen gene activity, moreover, is stimulated by the acute phase mediator IL-6 both *in vitro* and *in vivo*.[26] The gene is closely linked and structurally related to that of apolipoprotein(a), an apoprotein associated with the highly atherogenic low-density lipoprotein-like particle lipoprotein(a),[27] and more distantly related to other kringle-containing proteins such as tissue plasminogen activator (t-PA), urokinase plasminogen activator (u-PA), macrophage-stimulating protein, and hepatocyte growth factor.[28–32] The latter protein appears to facilitate tissue remodeling and repair following injury.[33]

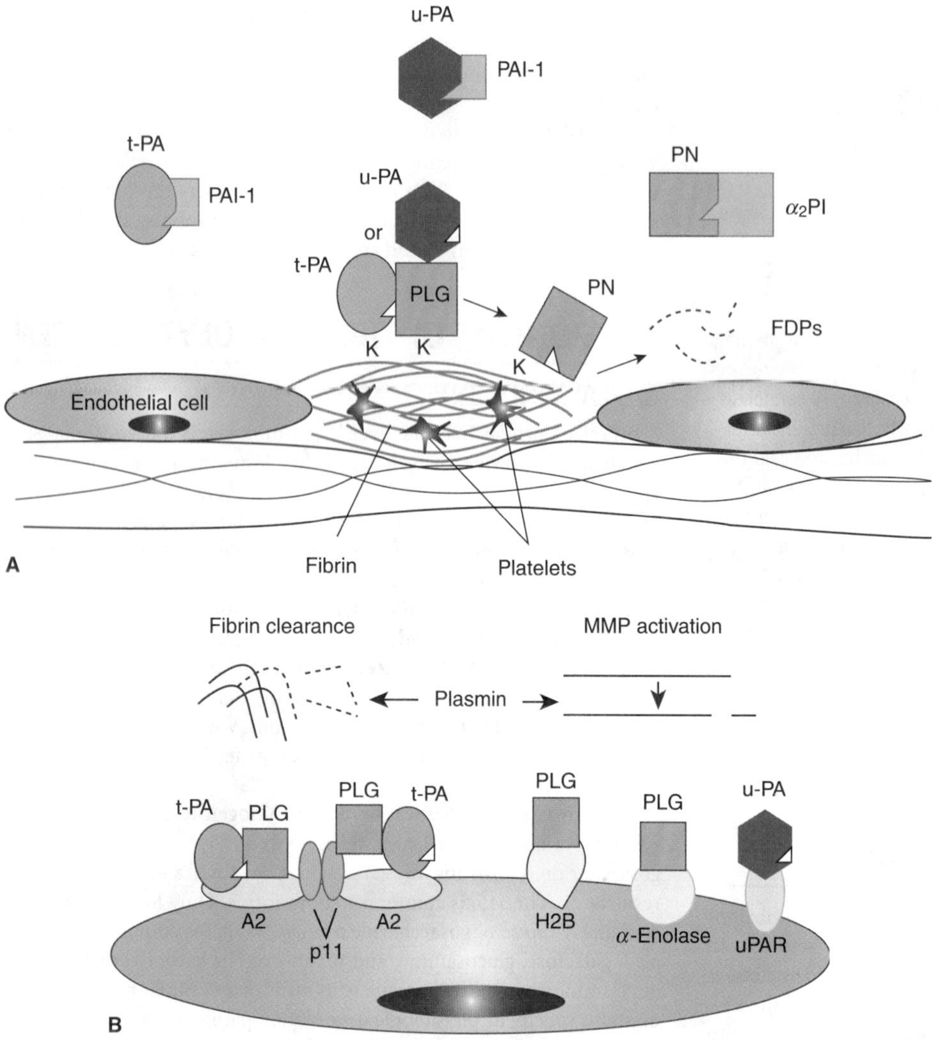

FIGURE 136–1. Overview of the fibrinolytic system. **A.** Fibrin-based plasminogen activation. The zymogen plasminogen (PLG) is converted to the active serine protease, plasmin (PN), through the action of tissue plasminogen activator (t-PA) or urokinase (u-PA). The activity of t-PA is greatly enhanced by its assembly with PLG through lysine residues (K) on a fibrin-containing thrombus. u-PA acts independently of fibrin. Both t-PA and u-PA can be inhibited by plasminogen activator inhibitor-1 (PAI-1), their main physiologic regulator. By binding to fibrin, plasmin is protected from its major inhibitor, α_2-plasmin inhibitor (α_2PI). Bound plasmin degrades crosslinked fibrin, giving rise to soluble fibrin degradation products (FDPs). **B.** Cell surface plasminogen activation. Many cell types express receptors for plasminogen, urokinase, and tissue plasminogen activator. The annexin A2 complex, consisting of annexin A2 (A2) and protein p11 (p11), binds both t-PA and PLG, thereby augmenting the efficiency of plasmin generation on endothelial cells, monocytes, and macrophages. PLG may also bind to other cellular receptors including histone H2B (H2B), and α-enolase on macrophage-like cells. Urokinase binds to the urokinase receptor (uPAR) on monocytes, macrophages, and activated endothelial cells.

The Physiologic Functions of Plasmin(ogen)

The development of the plasminogen-deficient mouse has contributed significantly to our understanding of the physiologic function of the serine protease plasmin. Mice made completely plasminogen deficient through gene targeting undergo normal embryogenesis and development, are fertile, and survive to adulthood (Table 136–2).[34,35] In addition to runting and ligneous conjunctivitis,[36] these animals display a predisposition to thrombosis with spontaneous thrombi appearing in liver, stomach, colon, rectum, lung, and pancreas; fibrin deposition in liver; and ulcerative lesions in the gastrointestinal tract and rectum. These results suggest that plasminogen is not strictly required for normal development, but does play a central role in fibrin homeostasis. In humans, plasminogen deficiency presents most often with ligneous mucositis because of fibrin deposition, and is infrequently a cause of macrovascular thrombosis.

PLASMINOGEN ACTIVATORS

Tissue Plasminogen Activator

One of two major endogenous plasminogen activators, t-PA consists of 527 amino acids comprising a glycoprotein of Mr approximately 72,000 (see Table 136–1).[37] t-PA contains five structural domains including a fibronectin-like "finger," an epidermal growth factor–like domain, two "kringle" structures homologous to those of plasminogen, and a serine protease domain (see Fig. 136–2). Cleavage of the Arg275-Ile276 peptide bond by plasmin converts t-PA to a disulfide-linked, two-chain form.[37] Although single-chain t-PA is less active than two-chain t-PA in the fluid phase, the two forms demonstrate equivalent activity when fibrin-bound.[38]

The two glycosylation forms of t-PA are distinguishable by the presence (type 1) or absence (type 2) of a complex *N-linked* oligosaccharide moiety on Asn184 (see Table 136–1).[39,40] Both types, however, contain high mannose carbohydrate on Asn117, complex oligosaccharide on Asn448, and an *O-linked* α-fucose residue on Thr61.[41] The carbohydrate moieties of t-PA may modulate its functional activity, regulate its binding to cell surface receptors, and specify its degradation pathways.

Located on chromosome 8p12-q11.2, the gene for human t-PA is encoded by fourteen exons spanning a total of 36.6 kb (see Fig. 136–2).[42–44] Although exon 1 encodes a 58-nucleotide mRNA leader sequence, each of the structural domains of t-PA is encoded by 1 or 2 of the remaining 13 exons. This arrangement suggests that the t-PA gene arose by an evolutionary process called "exon shuffling," whereby functionally related genes evolved through rearrangement of exons encoding autonomous domains. Consistent with this hypothesis, deletion of exons encoding the fibronectin-like finger or kringle 2 (but not kringle 1) domains of t-PA results in expression of mutants resistant to the cofactor activity of fibrin, while catalytic activity in the absence of fibrin remains intact.[45]

The proximal promoter of the human t-PA gene contains binding sequences for potentially important transcriptional factors including AP1, NF1, SP1, and AP2,[46,47] as well as a potential cyclic adenosine monophosphate (cAMP)–responsive element.[48] *In vitro*, many agents have been shown to exert small effects on the expression of t-PA mRNA, but relatively few enhance t-PA synthesis without augmenting plasminogen activator inhibitor-I (PAI-1) synthesis as well. Agents that regulate t-PA gene expression independently of PAI-1 include histamine, butyrate, retinoids, arterial levels of shear stress, and dexamethasone.[49–54]

TABLE 136–1. Fibrinolytic Proteins

A. Proteases

Property	Plasminogen	t-PA	u-PA
Molecular mass	92,000	72,000	54,000
Amino acids	791	527	411
Chromosome	6	8	10
Site of synthesis	Liver	Endothelium	Endothelium, kidney
Plasma concentration			
nM	1500	0.075	0.150
mcg/mL	140	0.005	0.008
Plasma half-life	48 h	5 min	8 min
N-glycosylation (%)	2	13	7
Form 1	–	Asn117, Asn184, Asn448	Asn302
Form 2	Asn288	Asn117, –, Asn448	–
O-Glycosylation			
α-Fucose	–	Thr61	Thr18
Complex	Thr345	–	–
Two-chain cleavage site	Arg560-Val561	Arg275-Ile276	Lys158-Ile159
Heavy chain domains			
Finger	No	Yes	No
Growth factor	No	Yes	Yes
Kringles (no.)	5	2	1
Light-chain catalytic triad	His602, Asp645, Ser740	His322, Asp371, Ser478	His204Asp255, Ser356

B. Major Serpin Inhibitors

Property	α_2-PI	PAI-1	PAI-2
Molecular mass	70,000	52,000	60,000 (glycosylated)
			47,000 (nonglycosylated)
Amino acids	452	402	393
Chromosome	18	7	18
Sites of synthesis	Kidney, liver	Endothelium	Placenta
		Monocytes/macrophages	Monocytes/macrophages
		Hepatocytes	Tumor cells
		Adipocytes	
Plasma concentration			
nM	900	0.1–0.4	ND
mcg/mL	50	0.02	ND
Serpin reactive site	Arg364–Met365	Arg346–Met347	Arg358–Thr359
Specificity	Plasmin	u-PA = t-PA	u-PA > t-PA

C. Receptors

Property	uPAR	A2	LRP	Mannose Receptor
Molecular mass	55,000–60,000	36,000	600,000	175,000
Amino acids	313	339	4544	1456
Chromosome	19	15	12	10

(continued)

TABLE 136–1. Fibrinolytic Proteins (Continued)

Property	uPAR	A2	LRP	Mannose Receptor
Source	Endothelial cells	Endothelial cells	Hepatocytes	Macrophages
	Monocytes/macrophages	Monocytes/macrophages	Monocytes/macrophages	
	Fibroblasts	Myeloid cells	Fibroblasts	
	Tumor cells	Smooth muscle cells		
Ligand(s)	u-PA	t-PA, plasminogen	u-PA/PAI-1 u-PA/PAI-2 t-PA/PAI-1 PN/α_2-PI	t-PA

α_2-PI, α_2-plasmin inhibitor; LRP, low-density lipoprotein receptor-like protein; ND, not determined; PAI-1, plasminogen activator inhibitor type 1; PAI-2, plasminogen activator inhibitor type 2; PN, plasmin; t-PA, tissue-type plasminogen activator; u-PA, urokinase plasminogen activator; uPAR, urokinase plasminogen activator receptor.

Forskolin, which increases intracellular cAMP levels, has been reported to decrease synthesis of both t-PA and PAI-1.[47,55]

In the vascular system, t-PA is synthesized and secreted primarily by endothelial cells belonging to a restricted set of blood vessels. In rodents, t-PA expression appears in 7- to 30-μm diameter precapillary arterioles in the lung, postcapillary venules, and vasa vasorum; much less expression is seen in endothelial cells of the femoral artery, femoral vein, carotid artery, or aorta.[56] In the mouse lung, bronchial arteriolar endothelial cells express t-PA antigen, especially at branch points, while pulmonary blood vessels are uniformly negative.[50,57–59] t-PA has also been detected in sympathetic neurons associated with the blood vessel wall.[60] Release of t-PA is governed by a variety of stimuli such as

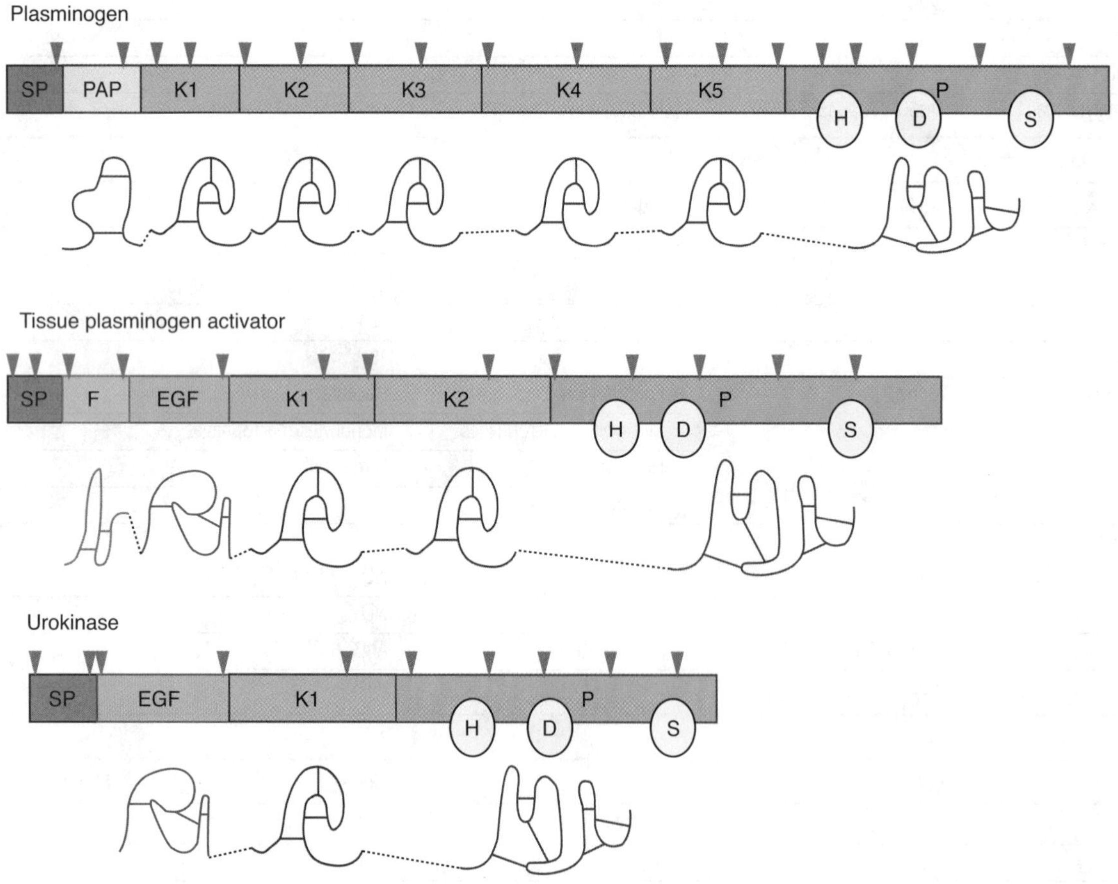

FIGURE 136–2. Structure–function relationships of plasminogen, tissue-type plasminogen activator (t-PA), and urokinase plasminogen activator (u-PA). Alignment of the intron-exon structure of plasminogen, t-PA, and u-PA genes with functional protein domains. Protein domains are labeled signal peptide (SP), preactivation peptide (PAP), "kringle" domains (K), fibronectin-like "finger" (F), epidermal growth factor-like domain (EGF), and protease (P). The position of catalytic triad amino acids histidine (H), aspartic acid (D), and serine (S) are shown within individual protease domains. The positions of individual introns relative to amino acid encoding exons are indicated with inverted triangles.

TABLE 136–2. Genetic Mouse Models Relevant to Fibrinolysis

A. Gene Deletion Models		
Genotype	**Phenotype**	**References**
Plasminogen		
PLG −/−	Spontaneous thrombosis, runting, premature death	34, 469
	Fibrin in liver, lungs, stomach; gastric ulcers	34, 469
	Impaired wound healing; ligneous conjunctivitis	36, 236
	Impaired monocyte recruitment	238
	Impaired neointima formation after electrical injury	239
	Impaired dissemination of *Borrelia burgdorferi*	240
	Reduced excitotoxic neuronal cell death in brain	241
Plasminogen Activators		
t-PA −/−	Reduced lysis of fibrin clot	85
	Increased endotoxin-induced thrombosis	85
u-PA −/−	Occasional fibrin in liver/intestine	85
	Rectal prolapse, ulcers of eyelids, face, ears	85
	Reduced macrophage degradation of fibrin	85
	Increased endotoxin-induced thrombosis	85
u-PA−/− t-PA −/−	Reduced growth, fertility, and life span; cachexia	85
	Fibrin deposits in liver, gonads, lungs	85
	Ulcers in intestine, skin, ears; rectal prolapse	85
	Impaired clot lysis	85
Inhibitors		
PAI-1−/−	Mildly increased lysis of fibrin clot	123
	Resistance to endotoxin-induced thrombosis	470
LRP −/−	Embryonic lethal day 13.5 postconception	199, 200
Receptors		
uPAR −/−	Essentially normal	471
	Reduced macrophage PLG activation *in vitro*	471
	Normal matrix degradation	471
Annexin A2 −/−	Fibrin deposition in microvasculature	195
	Impaired clearance of arterial thrombi	195
	Impaired postnatal neoangiogenesis	195
B. Overexpression Models		
Genotype	**Phenotype**	**Reference**
Apo(a) +/+	Atherosclerotic lesions with high-fat diet	472
	Reduced cell-associated plasmin and activation of TGF-β	473
	Resistance to t-PA–mediated clot lysis	474
Apo(a)ΔLBS +/+	Reduced lipid deposition	475
PAI-1 +++/+++	Venous thrombosis	122
	Tail necrosis, hind foot edema	
u-PA +++/+++	Fatal neonatal hemorrhage	476
	Impaired learning	477

thrombin, histamine, bradykinin, epinephrine, acetylcholine, arginine vasopressin, gonadotropins, exercise, venous occlusion, and shear stress.[49,50,61,62] Its circulating half-life is exceedingly short (~5 minutes). Functionally, t-PA is itself a poor activator of plasminogen. However, in the presence of fibrin, the catalytic efficiency of t-PA–dependent plasmin generation (k_{cat}/K_m) increases by at least two orders of magnitude.[21] This is a result of a dramatic increase in affinity (decreased K_m) between t-PA and its substrate plasminogen in the presence of fibrin. Although it is also expressed by extravascular cells, t-PA appears to represent the major intravascular activator of plasminogen.[17]

Urokinase

The second endogenous plasminogen activator, single-chain u-PA or prourokinase, is a Mr approximately 54,000 glycoprotein consisting of 411 amino acids (see Table 136–1). u-PA possesses an epidermal growth factor-like domain, a single plasminogen-like "kringle," and a classical catalytic triad (His204, Asp255, Ser356) within its serine protease domain (see Fig. 136–2).[63] Cleavage of the Lys158-Ile159 peptide bond by plasmin or kallikrein converts single chain u-PA to a disulfide-linked two-chain derivative.[64] Located on chromosome 10, the human u-PA gene is encoded by 11 exons spanning 6.4 kb, and expressed by activated endothelial cells, macrophages, renal epithelial cells, and some tumor cells.[65,66] Its intron–exon structure is closely related to that of the t-PA gene.

There is circumstantial evidence that u-PA expression may be induced during neoplastic transformation, possibly through a mechanism involving transcription factors AP1 and AP2.[67] Other agents that appear to induce expression of u-PA *in vitro* include hormones, angiogenic growth factors, and cAMP.[54] Inflammatory cytokines such as interleukin-1 and lipopolysaccharide induce only small increments in u-PA expression, although tumor necrosis factor and transforming growth factor (TGF)-β have a more dramatic (5–30-fold) effect.[68–70]

Two-chain u-PA occurs in both high- (Mr 54,000) and low-molecular-weight (Mr 33,000) forms that differ by the presence or absence, respectively, of a 135-residue amino terminal fragment released by plasmin cleavage between Lys135-Lys136.[71,72] Although both forms are capable of activating plasminogen, only the high-molecular-weight form binds to the u-PA receptor. u-PA has much lower affinity for fibrin than t-PA, and is an effective plasminogen activator both in the presence and in the absence of fibrin.[73,74] The extent to which prourokinase possesses intrinsic plasminogen activating capacity is controversial.[75,76]

Accessory Plasminogen Activators and Fibrinolysins

Under certain conditions, proteases traditionally classified within the intrinsic arm of the coagulation cascade have been shown to be capable of activating plasminogen directly. These include kallikrein, factor XIa, and factor XIIa.[77–79] These proteases, however, normally account for no more than 15 percent of total plasmin generating activity in plasma.[80] In addition, the membrane type 1 matrix metalloproteinase (MT1-MMP) appears to exert fibrinolytic activity in the absence of plasminogen, and may explain the unexpectedly mild phenotype observed in plasminogen-deficient mice.[81]

Physiologic Function of the Plasminogen Activators

Although abnormalities of the t-PA release mechanism have been reported in patients with chronic renal disease and hypertension,[82–84] and in a family with an undefined inherited release disorder, no clinical examples of complete deficiency of t-PA or u-PA are available. The most compelling studies of the physiologic functions of t-PA and u-PA come from gene disruption analyses in mice (see Table 136–2).[85] Both u-PA and t-PA null deletion mice exhibit normal fertility and embryonic development. However, u-PA–/– mice developed rectal prolapse, nonhealing ulcerations of the face and eyelids, and occasional fibrin deposition in tissues. Although they show normal lysis rates of pulmonary clots injected via the jugular vein, endotoxin-induced microvascular thrombus formation is significantly enhanced. t-PA–deficient mice display a normal phenotype. However, these animals have a decreased rate of lysis of artificially induced pulmonary thrombi, as well as enhanced thrombus formation in response to injection of endotoxin. Like PLG–/– mice, mice doubly deficient in t-PA and u-PA (t-PA–/–; u-PA–/–) exhibit rectal prolapse, nonhealing ulceration, runting, and cachexia, with extensive fibrin deposition in liver, intestine, gonads, and lung. Not surprisingly, clot lysis is also markedly impaired. These findings demonstrate that t-PA and u-PA are not essential for normal embryologic development, but do play crucial roles in lysis of artificially induced thrombi and in fibrinolytic surveillance in the adult.

INHIBITORS OF FIBRINOLYSIS

Plasmin Inhibitors

The action of plasmin is negatively modulated by a family of serine protease inhibitors, called serpins (see Table 136–1).[86] All serpins share a common mechanism of action by forming an irreversible complex with the active site serine of the target protease following proteolytic cleavage of the inhibitor by the target protease. Within such a complex, both protease and inhibitor lose their activity.

A single-chain glycoprotein of Mr approximately 70,000, α_2-plasmin inhibitor (α_2-PI) is synthesized primarily in the liver, circulates in plasma at relatively high concentrations (~0.9 μM), and has a plasma half-life of 2.4 days (see Table 136–1).[87] This serpin contains approximately 13 percent carbohydrate by mass and consists of 452 amino acids with 2 disulfide bridges.[88] In humans, the gene is located on chromosome 18 and contains 10 exons distributed over 16 kb of DNA.[89] The promoter region of the α_2-PI gene contains a hepatitis B-like enhancer element that directs tissue-specific expression in the liver.[88] α_2-PI is also a constituent of platelet α-granules.[90] Plasmin released into flowing blood or in the vicinity of a platelet-rich thrombus, is immediately neutralized upon forming an irreversible 1:1 stoichiometric, lysine-binding-site-dependent complex with α_2-PI. Interaction with plasmin is accompanied by cleavage of the Arg 364-Met 365 peptide bond, and the resulting covalent complexes are cleared in the liver.

Several additional proteins can act as plasmin inhibitors (see Table 136–1). α_2-Macroglobulin is a Mr 725,000 dimeric protein synthesized by endothelial cells and macrophages, and found in platelet α-granules. This nonserpin inhibits plasmin with approximately 10 percent of the efficiency exhibited by α_2-PI[91] by forming noncovalent complexes with several distinct serine proteases. C_1-esterase inhibitor can also serve as an inhibitor of t-PA in plasma,[92] and the protease nexin may function as a non-circulating cell surface inhibitor of trypsin, thrombin, factor Xa, urokinase, or plasmin, resulting in protease–inhibitor complexes that are endocytosed via a specific nexin receptor.[93,94]

Plasminogen Activator Inhibitors

Plasminogen Activator Inhibitor-1 Of the two major plasminogen activator inhibitors, PAI-1 is the most ubiquitous (see Table 136–1).[95] This Mr approximately 52,000 single-chain, cysteine-less glycoprotein is released by endothelial cells, monocytes, macrophages, hepatocytes, adipocytes, and platelets.[96–98] Release of PAI-1 is stimulated by many cytokines, growth factors, and lipoproteins common to the global inflammatory response.[69,99–101] The PAI-1 gene consists of 9 exons, spanning 12.2 kb on chromosome 7q21.3-q22.[102] The serpin-reactive site is located at Arg 346-Met 347, and activity of this labile serpin is stabilized upon complex formation with vitronectin, a component of plasma and pericellular matrix.[103–105]

Regulation of PAI-1 gene expression is complex.[106,107] The upstream regulatory region of the human PAI-1 gene contains a strong endothelial cell/fibroblast-specific element,[108,109] a glucocorticoid-responsive enhancer,[109] and TGF-β–responsive elements.[110] TGF-β is known to stimulate fos and jun, the two components of the AP1 complex, and an AP1 binding site (GGAGTCA) is located upstream of the PAI-1 cap site.[111] Agents that have been shown to enhance expression of PAI-1 at the message level, the protein level, or both, without affecting t-PA synthesis include the inflammatory cytokines lipopolysaccharide, interleukin-1, tumor necrosis factor-α,[68,69,99,100,112,113] TGF-β and basic fibroblast growth factor,[70,99,110,114] very-low-density lipoprotein and lipoprotein(a),[115,116] angiotensin II,[117] thrombin,[118,119] and phorbol esters.[120] In addition, endothelial cell PAI-1 is downregulated by forskolin[46,55] and by endothelial cell growth factor in the presence of heparin.[121]

PAI-1 is the most important and rapidly acting physiologic inhibitor of both t-PA and u-PA. Transgenic mice that overexpress PAI-1 exhibit thrombotic occlusion of tail veins and swelling of hind limbs within 2 weeks of birth (see Table 136–2).[122] Conversely, Mice deficient in PAI-1 exhibit normal fertility, viability, tissue histology, and development, and show no evidence of hemorrhage.[123] These observations contrast with the moderately severe bleeding disorder observed in a human patient with complete PAI-1 deficiency.[124]

Plasminogen Activator Inhibitor-2 Originally purified from human placenta,[95,125] plasminogen activator inhibitor-2 (PAI-2) is a 393-amino-acid member of the serpin family whose reactive site is the Arg358-Thr359 peptide bond (see Table 136–1).[125] The gene encoding PAI-2 is located on chromosome 18q21-23, spans 16.5 kb, and contains 8 exons.[126] PAI-2 exists as both an Mr 47,000 nonglycosylated intracellular form and an Mr 60,000 glycosylated form secreted by leukocytes and fibrosarcoma cells. Functionally, PAI-2 inhibits both two-chain t-PA and two-chain u-PA with comparable efficiency (second-order rate constants 10^5 $M^{-1}s^{-1}$). However, it is less effective toward single-chain t-PA (second-order rate constant 10^3 $M^{-1}s^{-1}$), and does not inhibit prourokinase.

Significant levels of PAI-2 are found in human plasma primarily during pregnancy. The gene's 5′-untranslated region contains a potent silencer, the PAUSE-1 element, which may be responsible for its low level of expression in nonpregnant individuals.[126,127] The 3′-downstream sequences include the TTATTTAT motif which is acted upon by inflammatory mediators.[128,129] In macrophages *in vitro*, secretion of PAI-2 is enhanced by endotoxin and phorbol esters,[129,130] and dexamethasone decreases PAI-2 expression in HT-1080 cells.[54]

Thrombin-Activatable Fibrinolysis Inhibitor

Thrombin-activatable fibrinolysis inhibitor (TAFI) is a plasma carboxypeptidase with specificity for carboxy-terminal arginine and lysine residues that acts as a potent inhibitor of fibrinolysis.[131] TAFI proteolyses fibrin-associated C-terminal lysine residues on fibrin, thereby eliminating binding sites for plasminogen and t-PA.[132] Identical to the previously cloned carboxypeptidase B[133] and the previously isolated carboxypeptidase U,[134] this single-chain Mr 60,000 polypeptide circulates in plasma at concentrations of about 75 nM, and undergoes limited proteolysis in the presence of thrombin which leads to its activation.[135] The profibrinolytic effect of activated protein C in plasma is a result of its ability to inactivate coagulation factors Va and VIIIa, thereby preventing activation of prothrombin, and inhibiting activation of TAFI.[131] The profibrinolytic effect of activated protein C in an *in vitro* plasma-based system was TAFI-dependent,[136] and, in a system of purified components, TAFI has been shown to downregulate t-PA-induced fibrinolysis half-maximally at a concentration of approximately 1 nM, which is 2 percent of its concentration in plasma.[137] Inhibition of either the intrinsic pathway of coagulation or TAFI activity results in a doubling of endogenous clot lysis in an *in vivo* rabbit jugular vein model of thrombolysis.[138] Although mice globally deficient in TAFI appear to have normal baseline hemostatic parameters,[139] they display increased lysis of plasma clots and reduced fibrin deposition following lung injury, and are protected from injury-induced venous thrombosis.[140,141] In plasma, TAFI may regulate plasminogen binding to both cell surface receptors and to fibrin.[142]

CELLULAR RECEPTORS

Although structurally diverse, cell surface fibrinolytic receptors can be classified into two groups whose integrated actions are likely to be essential for homeostatic control of plasmin activity (see Table 136–1).[2] "Activation" receptors localize and potentiate plasminogen activation while "clearance" receptors eliminate plasmin and plasminogen activators from the blood or focal microenvironments.

Activation Receptors

Plasminogen Receptors Plasminogen receptors are a diverse group of proteins expressed on a wide array of cell types.[2] Proposed receptors, including α-enolase, glycoprotein IIb/IIIa complex, the Heymann nephritis antigen, amphoterin, annexin A2, protein p11, and histone H2B, are expressed on a wide variety of cells, including monocytoid cells, platelets, renal epithelial cells, neuroblastoma cells, endothelial cells, and tumor cells.[143–149] These binding proteins commonly interact with the kringle structures of plasminogen through carboxyl-terminal lysine residues that are either present on the native protein, or generated by limited proteolysis.[143,150] Macrophages express four major plasminogen receptors (H2B, α-enolase, annexin A2, and p11), each of which appears to contribute significantly to plasminogen binding and activation.[150]

Urokinase Plasminogen Activator Receptor The u-PA receptor (uPAR) is expressed on monocytes, macrophages, fibroblasts, endothelial cells, and a wide range of tumor cells (see Table 136–1).[2,151,152] uPAR complementary DNA was cloned and sequenced from a human fibroblast complementary DNA library[153] and encodes a protein of 313 amino acids with a 21-residue signal peptide. The gene consists of 7 exons distributed over 23 kb of genomic DNA, and places this glycoprotein within the Ly-1/elapid venom toxin superfamily of cysteine-rich proteins.[154,155] uPAR is anchored to the plasma membrane through glycosylphosphatidylinositol linkages.[156] u-PA bound to its receptor maintains its activity and susceptibility to the physiologic inhibitor PAI-1.[157] Formation of u-PA–PAI-1 complexes hastens clearance of u-PA by hepatic or monocytoid cells.[157–160]

Although originally thought to function only as a means of localizing plasminogen activation to the cell surface, uPAR now appears to play a central role in cellular signaling and adhesion events.[151,161] uPAR binds the adhesive glycoprotein vitronectin at a site distinct from the u-PA binding domain,[162,163] and u-PA transfected renal epithelial cells acquire enhanced adhesion to vitronectin while they lose their adhesion to fibronectin.[164] uPAR, furthermore, colocalizes with integrins in focal contacts and at the leading edge of migrating cells,[165] and also associates with caveolin, a major component of caveolae, structures abundant in endothelial cells and thought to participate in signaling events.[166–168] In addition, cleaved and soluble forms of uPAR have been detected in the sera of patients with cancer, and these modified forms are thought to regulate the activity of several receptors involved in inflammatory and angiogenic responses.[152] Thus, cell-surface plasmin generation may be linked to cell adhesion, migration, and inflammatory cell recruitment processes via the multifaceted actions of uPAR.

Annexin A2 Annexin A2 is member of the annexin superfamily of calcium-dependent, phospholipid-binding proteins.[169] It is highly conserved, and abundantly expressed on endothelial cells,[170–173] monocyte/macrophages,[174,175] early myeloid cells,[176] developing neuronal cells,[177] and some tumor cells.[178–180] All of the more than 60 annexin family members have in common a conserved membrane-binding C-terminal "core" region and a more variable N-terminal "tail."[181] The human annexin A2 gene consists of 13 exons distributed over 40 kb of genomic DNA on chromosome 15 (15q21).[182]

Annexin A2 is unique among fibrinolytic receptors in that it possesses binding affinity for both plasminogen (Kd 114 nM)[147] and t-PA (Kd 30 nM), but not u-PA.[148] In a fluid-phase system of purified proteins, native human annexin A2 stimulates the catalytic efficiency of t-PA–dependent plasminogen activation by 60-fold.[183] This effect is completely inhibited in the presence of lysine analogues or upon treatment of annexin A2 with carboxypeptidase B, an agent that removes basic carboxyl-terminal amino acids. Although it lacks a classical signal peptide, annexin A2 is constitutively translocated to the endothelial cell surface within 16 hours of its biosynthesis. This translocation event can be stimulated either by thrombin or by heat stress, in a process that requires phosphorylation of annexin A2 at Tyr23, the action of a Src family kinase, and the presence of the annexin A2 binding protein p11 (S100A10).[184]

At the cell surface, annexin A2 in complex with p11 binds phospholipid via core repeat 2, which contains the linear amino acid sequence KGLGT and downstream aspartate residue (Asp161); together these moieties constitute a classical "annexin" motif.[185] The annexin A2 heterotetramer, which consists of two annexin A2 monomers and two protein p11 subunits and constitutes the cell surface form of annexin A2, appears to have even greater stimulatory effects on t-PA–dependent plasmin generation.[172] Interestingly, annexin A2 regulates endogenous levels of protein p11 in the endothelial cell by masking a polyubiquitination site on p11, which otherwise directs p11 to the proteasome where it is rapidly degraded.[186] Plasminogen and t-PA appear to bind to distinct domains. Lys307 appears to be crucial for the effective interaction of plasminogen with annexin A2, and may be revealed upon limited proteolysis of the parent protein.[183] The atherogenic low-density lipoprotein-like particle, lipoprotein(a), competes with plasminogen for binding to annexin A2 *in vitro*,[187] thereby reducing cell surface plasmin generation. t-PA binding to annexin A2 requires a domain consisting of residues 8 to 13 (LCKLSL) within the receptor's amino terminal "tail" domain.[188] This region is a target for homocysteine (HC), a thiol-containing amino acid that accumulates in association with nutritional deficiencies of vitamin B_6, vitamin B_{12}, or folic acid, or in inherited

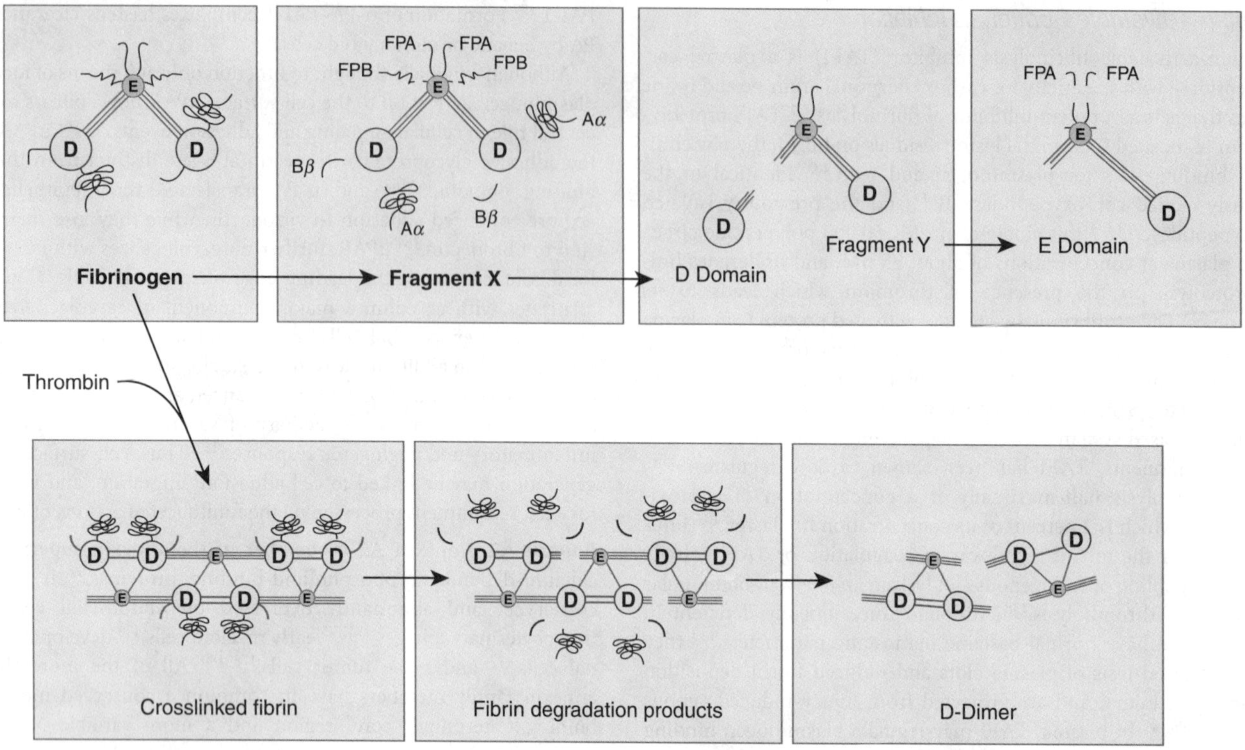

FIGURE 136–3. Degradation of fibrinogen and crosslinked fibrin by plasmin. (*Top panel*) Plasmin initially cleaves the C-terminal regions of the α and β chains within the D domain of fibrinogen, releasing the Aα and Bβ fragments. In addition, a fragment containing fibrinopeptide B (FPB) from the N-terminal region of the β chain is released, giving rise to the intermediate fragment known as "fragment X." Subsequently, plasmin cleaves the three connecting polypeptide chains connecting D and E domains, giving rise to fragments D, E, and Y. (*Bottom panel*) Fibrinogen can also be polymerized by thrombin to form fibrin. When degrading crosslinked fibrin, plasmin initially cleaves the C-terminal region of the α and β chains within the D domain. Subsequently, some of the connecting regions between the D and E domains are severed. Fibrin is ultimately solubilized upon hydrolysis of additional peptide bonds within the central portions of the coiled-coil connectors, giving rise to fibrin degradation products such as D-dimer. *(Reprinted with permission from Hajjar KA.[217])*

abnormalities of cystathionine β-synthase, methylenetetrahydrofolate reductase, or methionine synthase,[189] and is associated with atherothrombotic disease.[189–191] *In vitro*, HC impairs t-PA–dependent plasmin generation at the endothelial cell surface by approximately 50 percent[192] by forming a covalent derivative with Cys9.[188] The half-maximal dose of HC for inhibition of t-PA binding to annexin A2 is approximately 11 μM HC, a value close to the upper limit of normal for HC in plasma (12 μM). This was confirmed *in vivo* in mice with diet-induced hyperhomocysteinemia, where A2 was shown to be derivatized by HC, leading to loss of fibrinolytic activity and angiogenic potential.[478]

Several studies suggest a physiologic role for annexin A2 in fibrin homeostasis. First, blast cells from human patients with acute promyelocytic leukemia overexpress annexin A2 in proportion to their degree of hyperfibrinolytic coagulopathy.[176] Second, in rats, arterial thrombosis can be significantly attenuated by pretreatment with intravenous annexin A2.[193] Third, in humans with antiphospholipid syndrome, the prevalence of high-titer anti-annexin A2 antibodies correlates with a history of severe thrombosis, and anti-annexin A2 antibodies appear to activate endothelial cells and block their profibrinolytic function.[194] Finally, mice with a total deficiency of annexin A2 display impaired clearance of artificial arterial thrombi, fibrin deposition in the microvasculature, and angiogenic defects in a variety of tissues.[195]

Clearance Receptors

Clearance of serpin-enzyme complexes, such as t-PA–PAI-1 and u-PA–PAI-1, occurs mainly in the liver, and is mediated by a large two-chain receptor called the low-density lipoprotein receptor-related protein 1 (LRP1).[196,197] LRP1 binds a large number of serpin-protease complexes and other ligands, indicating a multifunctional role in mammalian physiology. An additional Mr 39,000 "receptor-associated protein" copurifies with LRP1 and appears to regulate the binding and uptake of LRP1 ligands.[198] Interestingly, LRP1 "knockout" embryos undergo developmental arrest by 13.5 days after conception, suggesting that regulation of serine protease activity may be crucial for early embryogenesis.[199,200] Although PAI-1–independent clearance pathways for t-PA have been proposed involving the mannose receptor,[201] or an α-fucose–specific receptor,[202] *in vivo* studies in mice suggest that LRP1 and the mannose receptor play a dominant role in t-PA clearance.[203]

THE FIBRINOLYTIC ACTIONS OF PLASMIN

DEGRADATION OF FIBRINOGEN AND FIBRIN

Fibrinogen

Plasmin releases carboxyl-terminal Aα and N-terminal fibrinopeptide B moieties from fibrinogen (Fig. 136–3; see Chap. 126). This reaction is distinct from the proteolytic cleavage of fibrinogen by thrombin, which releases fibrinopeptide A, exposing the Gly-Pro-Arg tripeptide sequence and allowing fibrinogen to polymerize and form insoluble fibrin.[204] Plasmin cleavage of fibrinogen (Mr 340,000) initially produces carboxyl-terminal fragments from the α chain within the D domain of fibrinogen (Aα fragment).[205–208] Simultaneously, but more slowly, the N-terminal segments of the β chains are cleaved, releasing a peptide containing fibrinopeptide B. The resulting Mr approximately 250,000 molecule is termed *fragment X* and represents a clottable form of fibrinogen. Additional cleavage events may release the Bβ fragment from the β chain's carboxyl-terminus, and, in a series of subsequent reactions, plasmin cleaves the three polypeptide chains that connect the D and E domains giving rise to free D domain (Mr ~100,000) plus the binodular D-E fragment known as fragment Y (Mr ~150,000). Finally, domains D and E are separated from each other, and some of the N-terminal fibrinopeptide A sites on domain E are also modified. Although fragment X can be converted to fibrin by thrombin, the fragments Y, D, and E are all nonclottable, and, in fact, may inhibit polymerization of fibrinogen.[209]

Fibrin

Plasmin degradation of fibrin leads to a distinct set of molecular products.[210] Species similar to fragments Y, D, and E, but lacking fibrinopeptide sites, are released from noncrosslinked fibrin. If fibrin has been extensively crosslinked by factor XIII, however, the resulting D fragments are crosslinked to an E domain fragment. Assay of crosslinked D-dimer fragments is employed clinically to identify disseminated intravascular coagulation-like states associated with excessive plasmin-mediated fibrinolysis (see Chap. 130). Several biologic activities, including inhibition of platelet function,[211] potentiation of the hypotensive effects of bradykinin,[212] chemotaxis,[213] and immune modulation, have been ascribed to fibrin breakdown products.[214]

t-PA–MEDIATED PLASMINOGEN ACTIVATION

With or without fibrin, t-PA-mediated activation of plasminogen follows Michaelis-Menten kinetics.[21] In the absence of fibrin, t-PA is a weak activator of plasminogen. However, in the presence of fibrin, the catalytic efficiency (kcat/K_m) of t-PA–dependent plasminogen activation is enhanced by approximately 500-fold. This is the basis for its specificity as a lytic agent in the treatment of thrombosis. The affinity between t-PA and plasminogen in the absence of fibrin is low (K_m 65 μM), but increases significantly in its presence (K_m 0.16 μM), even though the catalytic rate constant remains essentially unchanged (kcat ~0.05 s^{-1}). When plasmin forms on the fibrin surface, both its lysine-binding sites and its active site are occupied. Thus, it is relatively protected from its physiologic inhibitor, α_2-PI.[215] The interaction of t-PA with fibrin is probably initiated by its "finger" domain. However, once fibrin is modified by plasmin, carboxy-terminal lysine residues are generated, and these become binding sites for "kringle" 2 of t-PA and "kringles" 1 and 4 of plasminogen.[216] Therefore, fibrin accelerates its own destruction by (1) enhancing the catalytic efficiency of plasmin formation by t-PA, (2) protecting plasmin from its physiologic inhibitor, α_2-PI, and (3) providing new binding sites for plasminogen and t-PA once its degradation has begun.

U-PA-MEDIATED PLASMIN GENERATION

For the activation of Glu-plasminogen by u-PA in a fibrin-free system, reported Michaelis constants (K_m) vary from 1.4 to 200 μM, while catalytic rate constants (kcat) range from 0.26 to 1.48 s^{-1}.[217] Interestingly, activation of Glu-plasminogen by two-chain u-PA is increased in the presence of fibrin by about 10-fold even though u-PA does not bind to fibrin.[218] In contrast, single-chain u-PA has considerable fibrin-specificity. This may reflect neutralization by fibrin of components in plasma that impair plasminogen activation.[219] It may also reflect a conformational change in plasminogen upon binding to fibrin.[220] It is important to recognize, however, that the intrinsic plasminogen activating potential of single-chain u-PA is less than 1 percent of that of two-chain u-PA.[217] Two-chain u-PA has been used effectively as a thrombolytic agent for many years.[221]

THE NONFIBRINOLYTIC ACTIONS OF PLASMIN

PLASMIN AS A TISSUE REMODELER

A large number of *in vitro* studies suggest a role for plasmin in tissue remodeling. Basement membrane proteins such as thrombospondin,[222] laminin,[223] fibronectin,[224] and fibrinogen,[225] are readily degraded by plasmin *in vitro*, suggesting possible roles in inflammation,[226] tumor cell invasion,[227] embryogenesis,[228] ovulation,[229] neurodevelopment,[230,231] and prohormone activation.[232–234] Plasmin also activates matrix metalloproteinases (MMPs) 3 and 13 in the mouse, thereby facilitating the degradation of matrix proteins such as the collagens, laminin, fibronectin, vitronectin, elastin, aggrecan, and tenascin C.[235] Conversely, activation of other MMPs apparently proceeds in the absence of plasminogen possibly providing the basis for the mild phenotype observed in plasminogen null homozygote animals.[81]

Roles for plasmin in tissue remodeling and host defense mechanisms are further supported by *in vivo* observations in plasminogen-deficient mice (see Table 136–2). Impaired wound healing is observed in the plasminogen "knockout,"[236] and is reversed upon simultaneous deletion of fibrinogen.[237] Plasminogen-deficient mice also display diminished recruitment of monocytes in response to intraperitoneal thioglycolate,[238] and impaired neointima formation following electrical injury to blood vessels.[239] In studies involving *Borrelia burgdorferi*, the agent of Lyme disease, dissemination of the spirochete within its arthropod vector *Ixodes dammini* is absolutely dependent upon host plasminogen even though the deer tick contains no fibrin.[240] Furthermore, kainate-induced excitotoxicity and attendant neuronal cell dropout in the hippocampus is not observed in plasminogen knockout mice but does occur in fibrinogen-deficient animals.[241] The latter two studies may define new roles for plasmin which appear to be unrelated to degradation of fibrin.

In the lung, the fibrinolytic system mediates lung matrix remodeling, through mechanisms that appear to be independent of fibrin degradation.[242] In mice, deficiency of fibrinogen has no effect on the development of bleomycin-induced pulmonary fibrosis.[243] Mice lacking either PAI-1 or TAFI are protected from lung fibrosis in the same model,[244–246] although inducible expression of u-PA within alveoli abrogates the fibrotic response.[247]

Plasmin may play a role in the activation of growth factors. TGF-β is a Mr 25,000 homodimeric polypeptide that regulates vascular cell responses and epithelial-mesenchymal transformation in development and in tissue fibrosis.[248,249] In culture, cell-associated plasmin appears to convert latent TGF-β to its physiologically relevant active state. Inhibition of wound healing in this system is dependent upon active TGF-β, and activation of this agent can be blocked in the presence of plasmin inhibitors such as aprotinin or α_2-PI. Activation of TGF-β by plasmin may reflect alteration of its tertiary structure upon cleavage of an amino-terminal glycopeptide.[250] Once activated by plasmin, TGF-β can stimulate production of PAI-1, thus impairing further activation of plasminogen.

The role of the fibrinolytic system in vascular remodeling during atherosclerosis appears to be complex.[251] In the evolution of an injury to the endothelial cell lining of blood vessels, deposition of intravascular fibrin and organization of a thrombus occurs.[252] As the injury resolves, fibrin participates in plaque growth and luminal narrowing. Evidence of the importance of fibrinolytic balance in this process is that, in the absence of PAI-1, there is less neointima formation and reduced luminal stenosis, possibly as a result of more rapid resolution of fibrin.[253] In areas of the vasculature where injury is not associated with fibrin deposition, however, absence of PAI-1 may lead to enhanced lesion formation, as cells that invade the developing plaque may require plasmin activity for their directed migration.[254]

FIBRINOLYSIS AND ANGIOGENESIS

Although the fibrinolytic system has generally been assumed to be proangiogenic by virtue of its ability to promote "tunneling" of endothelial cells through fibrin-containing matrices, its effect, in actuality, appears to be context specific.[255,256] PAI-1 deficiency in mice, for example, seems to prevent tumor vascularization in a malignant keratinocyte model.[257] The same mice are also resistant to laser-induced neovascularization of the choroid.[258,259] The paradoxical proangiogenic effect of PAI-1 in some settings may relate to its ability to protect endothelial cells from apoptosis mediated by FasL, which is activated by plasmin.[260]

In the mouse cornea, absence of t-PA, u-PA, or TAFI, had no effect on neovascularization, whereas loss of plasminogen or PAI-1 significantly diminished this response.[261] Within the atherosclerotic plaque, moreover, expression of a truncated form of PAI-1 (rPAI-1_{23}) was antiangiogenic, inhibiting the proliferation of vasa vasorum, and reducing overall plaque area and plaque cholesterol in the descending aorta.[262] Deficiency of annexin A2 is associated with impaired nonmalignant angiogenesis in the retina and cornea.[195]

DISORDERS OF PLASMIN GENERATION

FIBRINOLYTIC DEFICIENCY AND THROMBOSIS

Although partial human plasminogen deficiency was first described in a young man with a history of venous thrombosis and pulmonary embolism,[263] there is currently little evidence that hypoplasminogenemia alone is a significant cause of deep venous thrombosis.[264] In a study of 23 consecutive patients with thrombophilia, the prevalence of plasminogen deficiency was only 1.9 percent.[265] Approximately half of these individuals had other risk factors such as deficiency of antithrombin, protein C, or protein S, or resistance to activated protein C. Among 93 patients with type I plasminogen deficiency, the prevalence of thrombosis was 24 percent, or 9 percent when the propositi were excluded.[266] Two additional epidemiologic studies concluded, moreover, that isolated hypoplasminogenemia is not a risk factor for thrombosis.[267,268]

Although there are no reported cases of complete absence of plasminogen in humans, a large number of plasminogen polymorphisms and dysplasminogenemias have been reported.[264] Congenital plasminogen deficiency has been classified into two types.[264] In type I, the concentration of immunoreactive plasminogen is reduced in parallel with functional activity,[269] whereas in type II (dysplasminogenemia), immunoreactive protein is normal while functional activity is reduced.[270] Patients with type I plasminogen deficiency are most likely to present with ligneous conjunctivitis, which resolves completely upon infusion of lys-plasminogen.[271,272] In a study of a Japanese cohort, approximately 27 percent of individuals with type II deficiency had a clinical history of thrombosis, but it is not clear whether there were other explanations for thrombophilia in these individuals.[273] Acquired plasminogen deficiency may occur in liver disease, sepsis, and Argentine hemorrhagic fever because of decreased synthesis and/or increased catabolism,[274] but associated thrombosis may be a result of abnormalities in other hemostatic factors in these very ill patients.

There are no reported cases of complete t-PA or u-PA deficiency in humans, and no mutations or polymorphisms in these genes have so far been clinically linked to thrombophilia. Defects in plasminogen activator release, as well as increased inhibition of t-PA by PAI-1, have been reported in associated with thrombosis,[275–277] and with chronic renal disease and hypertension.[82,84]

Increased circulating PAI-1 appears to represent an independent risk factor for vascular reocclusion in young survivors of myocardial infarction.[278] In addition, increased levels of PAI-1 have been associated with deep vein thrombosis in patients undergoing hip replacement surgery[279] and in individuals with insulin resistance.[280] Although a 4G versus 5G polymorphism in the PAI-1 promoter has been reported, the 4G form being associated with higher PAI-1 plasma levels, it is not yet established as to whether this allele correlates with elevated thrombotic risk.[281,282] With regard to such studies, one should bear in mind that PAI-1 is itself an acute phase reactant, and thus may not be directly responsible for the observed prothrombotic tendency.[283]

ENHANCED FIBRINOLYSIS AND BLEEDING

Enhanced fibrinolysis caused by congenital or acquired loss of fibrinolytic inhibitor activity may be associated with a bleeding diathesis.[284] Patients with congenital deficiency of α_2-PI may present with a severe hemorrhagic disorder as a result of impaired inactivation of plasmin and premature lysis of the hemostatic plug.[285] Acquired α_2-PI deficiency may be seen in patients with severe liver disease because of decreased synthesis, disseminated intravascular coagulation (DIC) as a consequence of consumption, nephrotic syndrome caused by urinary losses, or during thrombolytic therapy, which induces excessive utilization of the inhibitor.[285] TAFI levels are markedly reduced in liver cirrhosis, correlating with enhanced plasma fibrinolysis, and serving as an independent predictor of mortality.[286]

Patients with acute promyelocytic leukemia demonstrate excessive expression of annexin A2 on their developmentally arrested promyelocytes. Bleeding in this disorder is accompanied by evidence of high levels of plasmin generation and depletion of α_2-PI. Bleeding resolves upon initiation of all-*trans*-retinoic acid therapy, which eliminates expression of promyelocyte annexin A2, probably through a transcriptional mechanism.[176]

Complete loss of PAI-1 expression resulting in hemorrhage in a 9-year-old child was associated with severe hemorrhage in the setting of trauma or surgery.[124] This autosomal recessive trait reflected a frameshift mutation within exon 4 that induced a premature stop codon. This case demonstrates that PAI-1 is a central regulator of fibrinolysis in humans.

DEVELOPMENTAL REGULATION OF THE FIBRINOLYTIC SYSTEM

In the resting, nonstressed state, the plasmin-generating potential in the newborn is significantly less than that of the adult.[287,288] Although the amino acid composition and apparent molecular mass of neonatal plasminogen are indistinguishable from those of the adult protein,[289,290] plasma concentrations of plasminogen in the neonate are approximately 50 to 75 percent of those observed in adults.[289,291,292] Conversely, levels of histidine-rich glycoprotein, a carrier protein that may limit plasminogen's interaction with fibrin, are also reduced by 50 to 80 percent in healthy, term newborns.[293] Neonatal plasminogen is heavily glycosylated, less readily activated by tissue plasminogen activator, and only weakly bound to the endothelial cell surface.[290] Throughout childhood, global plasma fibrinolytic activity and plasmin generation are decreased in comparison to adults, and this relative deficiency may contribute to the high frequency of thrombosis associated with central venous line placement, Kawasaki disease, and Henoch-Schönlein purpura in this age group.[294]

Although t-PA antigen and activity levels are reduced throughout childhood by 50 to 75 percent compared with adult values,[292] stressed infants, such as those with severe congenital heart disease or respiratory distress syndrome, may have t-PA antigen levels that are increased by up to eightfold as a result of the t-PA release response.[295,296] In contrast, the principal plasmin inhibitors undergo only minimal change from birth to adulthood.[291,297–299] Thus, reduced fibrinolytic activity may contribute to the thrombogenic state commonly observed in the newborn,[300] but this predilection may be reversed under conditions of pathophysiologic stress.

FIBRINOLYTIC ACTIVITY DURING PREGNANCY AND PUERPERIUM

Pregnancy is a hypofibrinolytic state.[301–303] Although both plasminogen and fibrinogen levels in plasma increase by 50 to 60 percent in the third trimester, overall fibrinolytic activity, as reflected in euglobulin lysis activity, is reduced, and increased fibrin deposition is suggested by increasing D-dimer levels throughout pregnancy.[304] Between the 20th week of pregnancy and term, PAI-1 levels increase to three times their normal level while PAI-2 levels rise to 25 times their level in early pregnancy.[301] Less dramatic increases in both u-PA and t-PA levels are also observed. Within 1 hour of delivery, however, concentrations of both PAI-1 and PAI-2 begin to decrease, and return to normal within 3 to 5 days.[301] In preeclampsia, the hemostatic and fibrinolytic imbalances seen in pregnancy are further exaggerated.[305] Circulating PAI-1 levels exceed those in normal pregnancy, and fibrin deposition is seen in the glomerular capillaries and spiral arteries of the placenta. Interestingly, levels of PAI-2, a marker of placental function, are reduced during preeclampsia compared with normal pregnancy, and this decrease correlates with intrauterine growth retardation of the fetus. TAFI levels are currently being investigated as an underlying cause of fibrin deposition and occlusion of placental vessels in preeclampsia.[306]

FIBRINOLYTIC THERAPY

The goal of thrombolytic therapy is rapid restoration of flow in an occluded vessel achieved by accelerating fibrinolytic proteolysis of the thrombus.[307] The fibrinolytic system functions physiologically to remove fibrin deposits through the action of plasmin, but this is often too slow to prevent tissue injury following acute vascular occlusion. Because arterial thrombosis immediately renders distal tissue ischemic with rapid onset of dysfunction and necrosis, a critical problem is minimizing time to restoration of flow. Thrombolytic therapy should be viewed as one part of an overall antithrombotic plan that frequently includes anticoagulants, antiplatelet agents and mechanical approaches all designed to rapidly restore flow, prevent reocclusion, and promote healing. Fibrinolytic therapy for acute myocardial infarction (MI) was first attempted in 1958 by Fletcher and colleagues.[308] Since then, advances in biochemistry and pharmacology and the results of numerous clinical trials have led to approval of several therapeutic agents and to the routine use of thrombolysis in common clinical conditions including acute MI, stroke, occlusive peripheral vascular disease, deep vein thrombosis, and pulmonary embolism. This section presents an overview of thrombolytic therapy and reviews approaches to stroke and peripheral vascular disease. Chapter 135 discusses thrombolytic therapy for MI; Chap. 134 discusses therapy for deep vein thrombosis and pulmonary embolism; and Chap. 23 discusses the pharmacology of thrombolytic agents.

PRINCIPLES OF THERAPY

All fibrinolytic drugs are enzymes that accelerate the conversion of plasminogen to plasmin, a serine protease that degrades the insoluble fibrin clot matrix into soluble derivatives. Plasminogen, normally found in plasma at micromolar concentrations, binds specifically to fibrin along with its activators. Physiologically, fibrinolysis is carefully regulated. Small amounts of plasminogen activator present in the blood, or secreted locally by endothelial cells at the site of fibrin deposition, convert fibrin-bound plasminogen to plasmin that then acts locally to slowly dissolve the fibrin deposit, thereby liberating soluble degradation products of fibrin. The biochemical properties of fibrin, plasminogen activators, and inhibitors promote plasmin generation on the fibrin matrix but prevent its activation in the blood. The basic principle of all fibrinolytic therapy, therefore, is administration of pharmacologic amounts of plasminogen activator to achieve a high local concentration at the site of the thrombus and thereby accelerate conversion of plasminogen to plasmin and increase the rate of fibrin dissolution. If large amounts of plasminogen activator overwhelm the natural regulatory systems, plasmin may be formed in the blood resulting in degradation of susceptible proteins, the "lytic state."[309] Additionally, because high concentrations of activator are not limited to the site of thrombosis, fibrin deposits at other sites, including physiologic hemostatic plugs needed at sites of injury, may also dissolve causing local bleeding, often exacerbated by the hypocoagulable state caused by proteolysis of other coagulation factors by plasmin.

Several therapeutic agents are available and approved for thrombolytic use (Table 136–3). Most are produced by recombinant methods, whereas others derive from natural sources and can be antigenic, causing allergic reactions. The degree of "fibrin specificity" also varies; thus, the intensity of action at the site of thrombosis must be compared to proteolysis of plasma proteins. The plasma half-life of most agents is short, ranging from 5 minutes for t-PA to as long as 70 minutes for anistreplase. The method of administration (bolus or continuous infusion) and duration of therapy are determined by the half-life and also by the specific condition being treated.

An important issue for treatment is the use of systemic versus local or regional administration. Systemic therapy is delivered by peripheral vein, offers the advantage of simplicity, and does not require specialized facilities. However, this approach results in relatively greater systemic events, as large dosages must be administered to achieve a sufficiently high concentration at the site of thrombosis. Regional delivery with a catheter placed close to the proximal end of the thrombus can deliver a

TABLE 136–3. Comparison of Plasminogen Activators

Agent (Regimen)	Source (Approved/Available)	Antigenic	Half-Life (min)
Streptokinase (infusion)	Streptococcus (Y/Y)	Yes	20
Urokinase (infusion)	Cell culture; recombinant (Y/N)	No	15
Alteplase (t-PA) (infusion)	Recombinant (Y/Y)	No	5
Anistreplase (bolus)	Streptococcus + plasma product (Y/N)	No	70
Reteplase (double bolus)	Recombinant (Y/Y)	No	15
Saruplase (scu-PA) (infusion)	Recombinant (N/N)	No	5
Staphylokinase (infusion)	Recombinant (N/N)	Yes	
Tenecteplase (bolus)	Recombinant (Y/Y)	No	15

high local concentration with a smaller total dose. This increases the local effect and limits systemic exposure, although a portion of the drug delivered does reach the systemic circulation. For some indications, such as therapy of peripheral vascular disease, the catheter is positioned within the thrombus for direct drug administration and optimum effectiveness.

Fibrinolytic therapy should be viewed as one part of a combined antithrombotic strategy. For best results, thrombolytic therapy is typically given as soon as the patient presents with acute symptoms. This therapy accelerates thrombus dissolution by increasing fibrinolysis, but the overall process of thrombosis is dynamic, with concurrent fibrin formation and platelet deposition. Therefore, the change in thrombus size results from a balance of these processes, and fibrinolytic therapy is often administered in combination with an anticoagulant to block fibrin formation and with an antiplatelet agent to limit continued platelet deposition. Anticoagulant therapy is routinely continued after completion of fibrinolytic therapy to prevent thrombotic reocclusion stimulated by the procoagulant effects of the original lesion and also by prothrombotic effects of fibrinolytic therapy itself. Finally, neither fibrinolytic therapy nor anticoagulant or antiplatelet drugs will alter some local pathologic lesions, such as the atherosclerotic plaque, and mechanical approaches such as percutaneous coronary intervention play a vital role in successful therapy.

Fibrinolytic therapy typically results in proteolytic changes in the blood because plasminogen activation is not limited to the thrombus. These effects are complex and include a reduction in fibrinogen level, increase in fibrinogen degradation products, and decreases in plasminogen and α_2-PI. Screening coagulation tests, including the activated partial thromboplastin time, prothrombin time, and thrombin clotting time, will be prolonged, depending on the intensity of the lytic state. Tests reflecting plasminogen activation such as the euglobulin clot lysis time will be abnormal. Platelet membrane proteins may be degraded, resulting in abnormal platelet function.[310–312] Overall, these effects contribute to a hypocoagulable state that may be beneficial in contributing to vessel patency, but may also cause bleeding complications. The magnitude of the changes depends on both the dose of plasminogen activator administered and its degree of fibrin specificity. Thus, high doses of a nonspecific activator, such as streptokinase, will cause a marked lytic state, whereas a fibrin-specific agent such as reteplase administered as therapy for acute MI infarction will have much less effect. There is limited clinical value to monitoring the hemostatic changes of the lytic state as they are not strongly predictive of either thrombolysis or bleeding complications.[313–316]

The decision to administer fibrinolytic therapy and the choice of agent and regimen depends on careful consideration of risks and benefits for the individual patient (Table 136–4). For patients with acute MI or stroke there is a higher tolerance of bleeding complications, because lytic therapy can be life saving and limit disability. Indeed, in treatment of stroke there is an overall improvement in outcome even though the rate of intracranial hemorrhage is clearly increased. Timing of treatment is critical, with greater benefit achieved with earlier administration. With venous disease, the potential benefits are less. However, fibrinolytic therapy for acute pulmonary embolism with hemodynamic compromise may be life saving. Problems with bleeding become more problematic for treatment of deep vein thrombosis because the benefit of rapid symptomatic relief and possible reduction in long-term complications is less dramatic. The risks of bleeding must be considered in all patients. Local bleeding complications at the site of vascular intervention are frequent, and sites of catheterization must be closely monitored. Major bleeding complications, involving the gastrointestinal tract, retroperitoneum, and especially intracranial hemorrhage, may be life threatening.

TABLE 136–4. Selection of Patients for Thrombolytic Therapy

Treat those most likely to respond and benefit
Acute MI: Within 12 hours of onset; consider percutaneous intervention
Stroke: Ischemic stroke within 4.5 hours of symptom onset
Peripheral arterial obstruction
Acute occlusions
Distal obstruction not correctable by surgery
Deep vein thrombosis
Large proximal thrombi with symptoms for less than 7 days (see Chap. 134)
Pulmonary embolism
Massive or submassive embolism, especially with hemodynamic compromise (see Chap. 134)
Avoid bleeding complications
Major contraindications
Risk of intracranial bleeding
Recent head trauma or central nervous system surgery
History of stroke or subarachnoid bleed
Intracranial metastatic disease
Risk of major bleeding
Active gastrointestinal or genitourinary bleeding
Major surgery or trauma within 7 days
Dissecting aneurysm
Relative contraindications
Remote history of gastrointestinal bleeding
Remote history of genitourinary bleeding
Remote history of peptic ulcer
Other lesion with potential for bleeding
Recent minor surgery or trauma
Severe, uncontrolled hypertension
Coexisting hemostatic abnormalities
Pregnancy

THROMBOLYTIC THERAPY FOR STROKE

Stroke is the third leading cause of death in the United States with an annual incidence of 795,000, including 610,000 new episodes per year.[317] It is also the leading cause of serious disability, and its frequency will increase as the population ages. The incidence has been declining in recent years, and this is most likely related to the control of risk factors. Total numbers are increasing, however, as a consequence of the increasing age of the population. Antithrombotic therapy plays an important role in management, primarily with the use of aspirin in prevention and also anticoagulation for atrial fibrillation (see Chaps. 23 and 135). However, thrombolytic therapy is the only approach currently available to successfully intervene during the acute stage.

Type of Stroke

The appropriate use of thrombolytic therapy for stroke is based on an understanding of its pathogenesis. Ischemic stroke is caused by multiple mechanisms that suddenly block arterial flow in a brain vessel, rendering distal tissue ischemic with immediate dysfunction and leading rapidly to necrosis if blood flow is not restored. The most common underlying cause of ischemic stroke is atherosclerosis that involves large and medium-sized arteries in the neck and cranium. Arterial thrombosis originates in disrupted atherosclerotic plaque and is the most common cause of stroke, but transient ischemic attack and stroke involving small arteries can result from embolization of platelet-fibrin thrombi that form on atherosclerotic vessels in the neck and ascending aorta. Up to 25 percent of strokes result from embolization of thrombi that form in the heart in association with atrial fibrillation, valve dysfunction, artificial valves, and endocardial thrombi. These emboli are typically relatively large and cause serious cortical infarction. A variety of uncommon vascular diseases account for small numbers of stroke, and up to 30 percent have no defined etiology. Therefore, the majority of strokes are caused by thrombi or thromboemboli and are potentially susceptible to thrombolytic therapy.

Pathophysiology of the Lesion

Current approaches to thrombolytic therapy for stroke are based on imaging to define the etiology, results of clinical trials, and the experience with thrombolysis for acute myocardial infarction. Computerized tomography and magnetic resonance imaging can identify ischemic areas quite early and localize areas of hemorrhage. Additionally, arteriography may be useful in some cases and can identify accurately obstructed vessels and follow the course of recanalization during thrombolytic therapy. Clinical studies have generally followed the successful designs used for MI that demonstrated the critical pathologic role of the occluded vessel, the importance of early recanalization in preserving myocardium, the impressive decrease in morbidity and mortality resulting from early reperfusion, and characterized the bleeding risk. The experience with thrombolytic treatment for stroke also highlights important differences from MI. The arterial anatomy of the brain is more complex, the time from onset of ischemia to irreversible necrosis is shorter, the risk and consequences of bleeding are greater, and there is more variability in the thrombo(embolic) occluding lesion. Furthermore, the occlusive platelet-fibrin thrombus that precipitates MI is quite small with a consistent structure. In contrast, the occlusive lesion causing ischemic stroke may be a large in situ thrombus, small platelet-fibrin embolus, or large embolus of varying age and composition originating from the left atrium. Overall, results with thrombolysis for stroke have made a smaller impact than for treatment of myocardial infarction, largely based on these differences.

Early Thrombolytic Studies

The current therapeutic approach began with small studies in the 1980s followed by large multicenter, randomized, controlled trials throughout the 1990s, and is still continuing. Early studies were small, open-labeled, and used streptokinase, urokinase, and t-PA given intravenously or intraarterially to determine the dose, recanalization rate, hemorrhagic potential, and clinical predictors of response.[318–333] The principal findings were that recanalization of occluded vessels could be achieved, recanalization often resulted in clinical improvement, there was a need for treatment very early after presentation, and the rate of intracranial hemorrhage and hemorrhagic transformation within the ischemic area was high. Phase II studies were performed to define the optimum dosage of intravenous t-PA and the time window from symptom onset to treatment as a basis for larger phase III trials. The current approach to thrombolytic therapy for stroke is based on the results of the large clinical trials primarily performed with recombinant t-PA (Table 136–5). The only therapy currently approved for acute stroke by the U.S. Food and Drug Administration (FDA) is intravenous alteplase (recombinant t-PA). Generally, these studies administered intravenous t-PA within 3 hours of symptom onset and demonstrated clinically significant improvements in outcomes.

Tissue Plasminogen Activator Therapy

Treatment within 3 Hours The National Institute of Neurological Disorders and Stroke (NINDS) Study demonstrated the benefit of t-PA most clearly. This was a two-part randomized, double-blind, placebo-controlled study.[334] Part I involved 291 patients and tested whether t-PA had activity as indicated by clinical findings at 24 hours. Part II enrolled 333 patients, and the primary endpoint was clinical outcome at 3 months. All patients were treated within 3 hours of symptom onset with a total dose of 0.9 mg/kg of t-PA. The combined results showed a 30 percent improvement in objectively characterized clinical outcomes at 3 months from a rate of 21 percent to 38 percent of patients with no or minimal disability. This benefit persisted at 12 months and was

TABLE 136–5. Major Fibrinolytic Therapy Trials in Stroke

Study	No. of Patients	Time	Drug	Thrombolytic Dose*†	Main Efficacy Result
NINDS	624	≤3 h	t-PA, IV	0.9 mg/kg	Reduced disability at 3 months
ECASS I	620	≤6 h	t-PA, IV	1.1 mg/kg	No significant difference
ECASS II	800	≤6 h	t-PA, IV	0.9 mg/kg	No significant difference
ECASS III	821	3–4.5 h	t-PA, IV	0.9 mg/kg	Improved outcome at 3 months
ATLANTIS	613	≤6 h‡	t-PA, IV	0.9 mg/kg	No significant difference
SITS-ISTR#	11,865 vs. 664	≤3 vs. 3–4.5 h	t-PA, IV	0.9 mg/kg	No significant difference
ASK	340	≤4 h	SK, IV	1.5 million units	Increased morbidity and mortality
MAST-I	622	≤6 h	SK, IV¶	1.5 million units	Increased mortality
MAST-II	310	≤6 h	SK, IV§	1.5 million units	Increased mortality
PROACT II	180	≤6 h	pro-UK,‖ IA	9 mg	Improved 3-month outcome
MELT	114	≤6 h	u-PA, IA	variableʿ	No significant difference in favorable outcome; significant difference in excellent functional outcome

*All placebo controlled.

†All given over 1 h except PROACT II which was 2 h.

‡547/613 within 3–5 h.

#Observational study without placebo arm.

¶2 × 2 factorial design with acetylsalicylic acid (ASA) 300 mg/day.

§Acetylsalicylic acid (ASA) 100 mg/day.

‖Pro-UK and placebo group also received heparin.

ʿMean doses of u-PA in patients with good and poor outcome were 555,000 IU and 789,000 IU.

observed despite a 10-fold increase in early symptomatic intracranial hemorrhage from 0.6 percent to 6.4 percent. At 3 months, there was no difference in mortality between the groups. This study formed the basis of the approval by the FDA in 1996 of intravenous t-PA for stroke.

Treatment from 3 to 4.5 Hours Early randomized trials of intravenous t-PA did not show a clear benefit for patients treated beyond 3 hours after stroke onset. These trials had treatment time windows up to 6 hours, and included small numbers of patients treated between 3 and 4.5 hours. The European Cooperative Acute Stroke Study (ECASS) had a similar design and included 622 subjects with moderate to severe symptoms who were randomized to placebo or t-PA at a higher dose of 1.1 mg/kg within 6 hours of symptom onset.[335] There was no significant difference between the groups in the primary endpoint of functional status at 90 days, and there was no difference in 30-day mortality. The t-PA group showed some benefits in secondary endpoints such as neurologic recovery at 90 days, shorter hospital stay, and more rapid recovery. The ECASS II included 800 patients randomized to receive either recombinant t-PA (rt-PA) or placebo within 6 hours of symptom onset with stratification for presentation up to 3 hours after symptom onset or between 3 and 6 hours.[336] There was no significant benefit of thrombolytic therapy using the primary endpoint of functional capacity of 90 days. The Alteplase Thrombolysis for Acute Noninterventional Therapy in Ischemic Stroke (ATLANTIS) Study evaluated the safety of rt-PA in a double-blind, placebo-controlled study with administration of drug between 3 and 5 hours after symptom onset.[337] rt-PA was administered in a dose of 0.9 mg/kg over 1 hour. The primary endpoint of excellent neurologic recovery was observed in 32 percent of placebo- and 34 percent of rt-PA–treated patients. There was also no significant difference in secondary functional endpoints. Early symptomatic intracranial hemorrhage occurred in 1.1 percent of control and 7 percent of rt-PA–treated patients. There was a nonsignificant trend toward increased mortality with rt-PA treatment at 90 days (6.9% vs. 11.0%, p = 0.09). A meta-analysis pooling data from 2755 patients who received either alteplase or placebo within 6 hours in the NINDS, ATLANTIS, and ECASS II trials showed that the odds of a favorable 3-month outcome decreased as the interval from stroke onset to the start of alteplase treatment increased. Furthermore, the study alluded to the potential benefit of extending the treatment window to 4.5 hours with a favorable but decreasing odds ratio for alteplase treatment beyond 3 hours.[338]

The benefit of intravenous t-PA for treatment beyond the 3-hour window was established by the ECASS III trial.[339] A total of 821 patients with acute ischemic stroke were randomized to either treatment with intravenous alteplase at 0.9 mg/kg or placebo between 3 and 4.5 hours after the onset of a stroke. The primary endpoint was disability at 90 days assessed by the modified Rankin scale score, and the secondary endpoint was a global outcome analysis of four neurologic and disability scores combined. Safety endpoints included death, symptomatic intracranial hemorrhage, and other serious adverse events. The study results showed that intravenous t-PA treatment initiated at 3 to 4.5 hours after ischemic stroke onset leads to a modest improvement in the 3-month outcome. More patients had a favorable outcome with t-PA than with placebo (52.4% vs. 45.2%; odds ratio: 1.34; 95% confidence interval [CI] 1.02–1.76). Although the incidence of intracranial hemorrhage was higher with t-PA treatment (2.4% vs. 0.2%; p = 0.008), there was no difference in mortality between the two groups.

The observational SITS-ISTR study further lends support for the safety of administering intravenously t-PA between 3 and 4.5 hours after acute ischemic stroke.[340] The study investigators compared outcomes in patients treated between 3 hours and 4.5 hours versus those treated within 3 hours, based on a prospective Internet-based audit known as the Safe Implementation of Treatments in Stroke (SITS) of the International Stroke Thrombolysis Registry (ISTR). Compared to patients treated in under 3 hours (n = 11,865), those treated at 3 to 4.5 hours (n = 664) had similar rates of independence, symptomatic intracranial hemorrhage, and mortality.

Streptokinase Therapy

Streptokinase has been evaluated in three large stroke trials. The Australian Streptokinase (ASK) Study was a double-blind, placebo-controlled trial of 340 patients randomized within 4 hours of symptom onset to receive placebo or 1.5 million units of streptokinase over 1 hour.[341] The early results showed an increase in unfavorable outcomes in streptokinase-treated patients, and the study was prematurely terminated. The death rate at 90 days was significantly higher in patients receiving streptokinase. In the small subgroup of 70 patients who entered the trial within 3 hours of symptom onset, there was evidence of an improved outcome in the streptokinase group. The Multicenter Acute Stroke Trial–Italy (MAST-I) Study examined benefits and risks of streptokinase treatment with or without aspirin in 622 patients with acute ischemic stroke who presented within 6 hours of symptom onset using a 2 × 2 design.[342] Patients received 1.5 million units of streptokinase over 1 hour, and aspirin was given in a dose of 300 mg per day. An interim analysis resulted in early termination because streptokinase treatment was associated with a 2.7-fold increase in fatality at 10 days. This was because of an increased death rate among patients receiving the combination of streptokinase and aspirin. The Multicenter Acute Stroke Trial–Europe (MAST-E) Trial enrolled 310 patients with moderate to severe ischemia in the distribution of the middle cerebral artery that were randomized to receive placebo or 1.5 million units of streptokinase over 1 hour within 6 hours of symptom onset in a double-blind study.[343] The outcome endpoint of mortality or severe disability was not significantly different between the two groups. However, the mortality rate at 10 days was higher in patients who received streptokinase (34.0%) compared with placebo (18.2%, p <0.02) primarily because of hemorrhagic transformation of infarcts.

Intraarterial Thrombolysis

Potential advantages of intraarterial administration include delivery of a higher concentration of an activator delivered proximally or directly into the thrombus using an appropriately placed catheter, more accurate anatomic diagnosis, the ability to observe the course of recanalization, and lower total doses of drug that might reduce intracranial hemorrhage. Problems with this approach include the need for specialized facilities and experienced personnel available at all times to perform arteriography and selective catheterization. These requirements generally result in longer times before the treatment can be delivered, and this is a critical variable in treatment success. Several small open-label trials observed a high rate of recanalization and apparent clinical benefit with intraarterial therapy using urokinase, streptokinase, or t-PA, but hemorrhagic transformation was a frequent problem.[321,325,328,331,344–349] Intraarterial thrombolysis is associated with higher recanalization rates for internal carotid artery, middle cerebral artery stem, and basilar artery occlusions.[350] Intraarterial therapy may have particular value in acute basilar artery occlusion, which has a very high mortality but clinical recovery in up to 50 percent of patients receiving intraarterial thrombolysis.

The Prolyse in Acute Cerebral Thromboembolism (PROACT) and PROACT II Trials evaluated recombinant human prourokinase by catheter-directed intraarterial administration. The PROACT Trial included 26 patients with occlusion in the territory of the middle cerebral artery who received intraarterial prourokinase and heparin and 14 patients treated with heparin alone.[351] A significantly higher recanalization rate was observed with prourokinase treatment with no increase in intracranial hemorrhage. This led to the larger PROACT II Trial, a randomized, placebo-controlled open-label trial that included 180 patients with acute occlusion of the middle cerebral artery who were treated within 6 hours of symptom onset with either heparin alone or 9 mg of intraarterial prourokinase plus heparin.[352] The recanalization rate was significantly higher with prourokinase (66% vs. 18%, $p < 0.001$), and functional improvement at 90 days was also superior. Symptomatic intracranial hemorrhage occurred in 10 percent of patients treated with prourokinase and 2 percent of controls. Although promising, these results did not lead to FDA approval of intraarterial prourokinase for treatment of stroke. Cochrane Reviews of these studies are available.[353,354]

A third study, the Middle Cerebral Artery Embolism Local Fibrinolytic Intervention Trial (MELT) Japan, evaluated 114 patients with middle cerebral artery occlusion of less than 6 hours duration who were randomized to either intraarterial urokinase treatment or placebo.[355] The study was underpowered because of premature study closure. A favorable but not statistically significant outcome at 90 days was more likely with intraarterial urokinase compared with placebo. The proportion of patients with an excellent functional outcome defined by a modified Rankin scale at 90 days was significantly better in the intraarterial urokinase group (42% vs. 23%, $p = 0.045$). Intracerebral hemorrhage within 24 hours of treatment occurred in 9 percent and 2 percent, respectively ($P = 0.206$). This study suggested that intraarterial fibrinolysis has the potential to increase the likelihood of excellent functional outcome in appropriate clinical settings.

Overall, these studies show that treatment of acute stroke with thrombolytic therapy can lead to recanalization of the occluded artery and improvement in clinical outcomes. A critical issue is the time from symptom onset to the start of therapy. Evidence is clear that earlier treatment results in better results. The need for very early treatment is currently the single largest limitation to greater application of thrombolytic therapy for stroke.[356–358] Less than 5 percent of stroke patients currently receive t-PA treatment because treatment is limited to patients presenting within 3 hours of symptom onset and because of the additional contraindication to thrombolytic therapy. The greatest impediment is the delay from the time patients experience symptoms to the time they appear in the emergency room, and focused community educational efforts must be made if this treatment is to have a greater impact. The rate of intracranial hemorrhage is high, principally as a result of hemorrhagic transformation within ischemic tissue. Despite early deaths and increased morbidity in patients affected with intracranial hemorrhage, the overall functional results among stroke patients can be improved. The results are critically dependent on both dose and choice of thrombolytic agent. Clinical studies with intravenous t-PA showed better results, whereas streptokinase was associated with an unacceptably high rate of intracranial hemorrhage. Whether this difference is a result of intrinsic properties of these agents or due to dose and treatment intensity remains controversial.

Thrombolytic therapy for stroke is an area of very active investigation with the primary goal of expanding the proportion of patients who can be successfully treated. Recent randomized studies with recombinant t-PA have provided evidence that intravenous thrombolytic therapy can be safely extended to 4.5 hours after symptom onset in selected patients.[338–340] An additional goal is to reduce intracranial hemorrhage by identifying patients at greatest risk using newer imaging modalities, such as magnetic resonance imaging diffusion/perfusion mismatch to identify reversible ischemia.[359–362] Studies are also evaluating newer agents including reteplase and tenecteplase. The combination of potent antiplatelet therapy using an $\alpha_{IIb}\beta_3$-integrin antagonist with a lower dose of a thrombolytic agent may improve results.[363–368] Other studies are examining the combination of intravenous and intraarterial therapy[369–371] and also the adjunctive use of low-intensity ultrasound to accelerate fibrinolysis.[372–374]

TABLE 136–6. Guidelines for t-PA Therapy in Stroke

Eligibility
Time from symptom onset to therapy ≤3 hours
Results from ECASS III trial suggest treatment within 4.5 h of onset is beneficial
Exclusions
Prior intracranial hemorrhage
Major surgery within 14 days
Gastrointestinal or urinary tract bleeding with 21 days
Arterial puncture in noncompressible site
Recent lumbar puncture
Intracranial surgery, serious head trauma, or prior stroke within 3 months
Minor neurologic deficit
Seizure at time of stroke onset
Clinical findings of subarachnoid hemorrhage
Active bleeding
Persistent systolic blood pressure (BP) >185 and/or diastolic BP >110 or requiring aggressive treatment
Arteriovenous malformation or aneurysm
Evidence of hemorrhage on computed tomography scan
Platelets <100,000/μL
International normalized ratio >1.5 on warfarin
Elevated partial thromboplastin time on heparin
Blood glucose <40 or >400 mg/dL
ECASS III additionally excluded patients >80 years old, patients with a combination of previous stroke and diabetes mellitus, and patients with an National Institutes of Health Stroke Scale score of >25.

Current recommendations limit thrombolytic therapy for stroke to patients presenting within 3 hours of symptom onset.[375–377] The approved therapy is with 0.9 mg/kg (maximum 90 mg) of t-PA administered intravenously with 10 percent as an initial bolus and the remainder infused over 60 minutes. The best results are obtained in patients who meet strict eligibility requirements (Table 136–6). Thrombolytic therapy can be considered for eligible patients within 3 to 4.5 hours of clearly defined symptom onset. Eligible patients should be treated as quickly as possible in general. Patients should be closely monitored for bleeding complications, especially intracranial hemorrhage. Facilities should be available for managing bleeding complications, and careful attention to management of blood pressure and other comorbidities is critical.

THROMBOLYTIC THERAPY FOR PERIPHERAL VASCULAR DISEASE

Most peripheral vascular disease is caused by atherosclerosis which progressively limits flow distally in the legs resulting in clinical presentation with symptoms of claudication, rest pain, and tissue loss in severe cases. Typically, occlusive disease of the leg vessels represent only one aspect of generalized atherosclerosis involving the coronary and cerebral circulation additionally. Treatment seeks to reduce disease progression through amelioration of risk factors and to decrease symptoms by improving flow through exercise, medication, and endovascular or surgical approaches to revascularization. Thrombolysis has very little role in treatment of chronic occlusions.

Acute peripheral arterial occlusion presents with the sudden onset of new, severe leg symptoms or critical acute worsening of chronic ischemia and often involves embolic or acute thrombotic occlusion of leg arteries. The presentation is usually urgent, and the goals of treatment are to preserve limb function through restoration of flow. Anticoagulation is typically administered to prevent thrombus extension, while thrombolytic therapy or surgery can be used to restore perfusion.

The role of thrombolysis in acute peripheral arterial occlusion has evolved from the early application of systemic treatment to the current use of local arterial infusion. Large prospective studies have helped define its role in relation to surgical intervention, and the current approach uses thrombolysis in conjunction with both endovascular and surgical procedures for comprehensive treatment to maximize amputation-free survival. Unique challenges for thrombolytic therapy of peripheral arterial occlusion include the large size of arterial thrombi in comparison with coronary or cranial thrombi and also the variable sites of the occlusion extending from proximal aortoiliac disease to infrapopliteal small vessel occlusion often seen in diabetics. Additionally, patients often have serious vascular comorbidities including hypertension, diabetes, and coronary or cerebrovascular disease that increase risk of bleeding and other operative complications.

Early approaches were with systemic thrombolytic therapy using streptokinase, and the results of small studies demonstrated evidence of reperfusion in approximately 40 percent of patients with greater success in treating occlusions of recent onset. Both embolic and thrombotic occlusions responded, and bleeding complications occurred in up to one-third of all treated patients.[378] Following the report in 1974 by Dotter[379] of successful thrombolysis in peripheral arterial occlusion using locally administered thrombolysis, practice moved progressively to the nearly exclusive use of local intra-arterially administered treatment. Advantages include delivery of a high concentration of drug directly to the site of thrombosis, the ability to follow the course of treatment using the treatment catheter, and identification of local vascular lesions requiring endovascular or surgical treatment after recanalization.

Treatment involves obtaining arterial access from a remote site followed by fluoroscopic guidance of the catheter to the site of the obstruction. A guidewire is extended through the thrombus, and an infusion catheter is advanced to administer drug directly into the thrombus. This is an important determinant of success, which is significantly less if the infusion is administered proximal to, but not within the clot. Therapy is delivered by continuous infusion over a prolonged period of hours to days and requires close monitoring and a large dose of thrombolytic agent. Successful reperfusion occurs in approximately three-quarters of cases overall. Intraarterial t-PA or urokinase is more effective than either intravenous t-PA or intravenous streptokinase.[380]

The relative roles of thrombolysis and surgery were explored in several prospective studies, and demonstrated that thrombolytic therapy is a safe and effective alternative to surgery in certain subsets of patients. Ouriel and associates[381] reported the results of a prospective, randomized trial of 114 patients with limb-threatening ischemia of less than 7 days duration who were assigned to receive either intraarterial urokinase or primary operative intervention. Thrombolytic therapy resulted in a 70 percent recanalization rate, and the frequency of limb salvage was the same in both groups at 1 year. There was, however, a survival advantage in patients receiving primary thrombolytic therapy resulting primarily from a decrease in the occurrence of in-hospital complications. The Surgery versus Thrombolysis for Ischemia of the Lower Extremity (STILE) Trial enrolled 393 patients with nonembolic, native arterial, or graft occlusion of less than 6 months duration who were randomized to undergo the optimal surgical procedure or catheter directed thrombolysis with either t-PA or urokinase.[382] The study was terminated prematurely because of lower ongoing or recurrent ischemia at 30 days in surgically treated patients. Patients with ischemia of longer than 14 days duration did better with surgical revascularization, with significant reductions at 1 year in the rates of major amputation. Some benefit to thrombolysis was observed, however, as patients with symptoms less than 14 days duration who were treated with thrombolysis had a lower amputation rate. More than half of patients receiving thrombolysis had a decrease in the magnitude of the surgical procedure eventually required. There was no difference in results with the use of either t-PA or urokinase.

The Thrombolysis or Peripheral Arterial Surgery (TOPAS) I Study compared recombinant urokinase or surgery for initial therapy of acute lower extremity ischemia of less than 14 days duration in 213 patients who were randomized to one of three doses of urokinase or to surgery for initial therapy.[383] A dose of 4,000 IU/min was selected as the optimum urokinase dose, and this resulted in complete clot lysis in 71 percent of patients with hemorrhagic complications in 2 percent. The 1-year mortality and amputation-free survival were similar in the urokinase and surgery groups. There was a significant reduction in the frequency and magnitude of surgical interventions eventually required in patients randomized to initial thrombolysis. The larger TOPAS II Study included 544 patients with acute arterial obstruction of less than 14 days duration.[384] Patients were randomized to initial therapy with either catheter directed intraarterial recombinant urokinase or to surgery. Recanalization occurred in 80 percent of patients who received urokinase. Amputation-free survival at 1 year was not significantly different between the two groups: 65 percent with urokinase and 70 percent with surgery. Fewer patients in the thrombolysis group required surgical procedures by 6 months. Major hemorrhagic complications were significantly more frequent with urokinase (13%) compared with surgery (6%; $p = 0.005$), with four episodes of intracranial hemorrhage in the urokinase group.

Other studies have investigated modified thrombolytic regimens. Reteplase appears to be equally effective as t-PA or urokinase with comparable recanalization rates, and clinical outcomes and bleeding complications.[385,386] Prourokinase also gave similar overall results to urokinase in a phase II study.[387] Staphylokinase, a highly fibrin-specific plasminogen activator, was given in an open-label trial to 191 patients with peripheral arterial occlusion of less than 120 days duration and resulted in revascularization in 8 percent.[388] Occasional allergic reactions occurred, and severe bleeding complications were comparable to those with other agents. The addition of abciximab, an $\alpha_{IIb}\beta_3$ integrin inhibitor, to urokinase resulted in more rapid clot-like lysis in a randomized study of 70 patients,[389] and good results were also reported with reteplase and abciximab.[390] Intraoperative thrombolysis during thromboembolectomy has been used to improve clearance of distal thromboemboli successfully,[391–394] and mechanical devices have also been used with thrombolysis.[395]

Based on available studies, thrombolysis should be viewed as one part of a combined, comprehensive management approach to peripheral arterial occlusion. Early, accurate angiographic diagnosis is important. With appropriate intrathrombic catheter positioning, recanalization can be achieved in a high percentage of patients. The improved clinical condition and the availability of good angiographic examinations after reperfusion allow a more optimal choice of definitive endovascular or surgical procedures, and surgery can be avoided in some patients. Thrombolysis has particular appeal for patients with serious comorbidities that increase surgical risk and also for lysis of thrombi in small distal vessels that are inaccessible for surgery. Cochrane Reviews of relevant studies are available,[396,397] and an excellent review has been provided from the Working Party on Thrombolysis and Management Limb Ischemia, which provides practical recommendations for management and an overview of dosing regimens for various thrombolytic agents.[398]

In collaboration with vascular medicine, vascular surgery, and interventional radiology societies, the 2005 American College of Cardiology/American Heart Association guidelines on peripheral arterial disease concluded that catheter-based thrombolytic therapy is effective, beneficial, and indicated in patients with acute limb ischemia of less than 14 days duration.[399] Evidence also favors mechanical thromboembolectomy as adjunctive therapy for acute limb ischemia resulting from peripheral arterial occlusion. The 2008 American College of Chest Physicians guideline also suggested long-term anticoagulation with vitamin K antagonist in patients who have undergone embolectomy.[400]

THROMBOLYTIC THERAPY FOR OTHER INDICATIONS

Thrombolytic therapy has been used successfully to treat acute venous and arterial occlusions in a wide variety of sites as reported in small series and case reports. It is difficult to judge the effectiveness based on the available reports, but it is certainly a reasonable choice of therapy for serious acute, symptomatic thrombosis based on a clinical appraisal of bleeding risks and potential benefit. Reports document successful treatment of intra-abdominal thrombosis including Budd-Chiari Syndrome,[401] portal vein thrombosis,[402–404] and mesenteric vein thrombosis.[404–406] Thrombolytic agents are frequently used to open thrombosed central venous catheters that are occluded by a clot.[407–410] Thrombotic occlusion of access devices for hemodialysis represent a major clinical problem, and thrombolysis, often accompanied with mechanical approaches, is often successful in removing the clot.[411–415]

MANAGEMENT OF BLEEDING COMPLICATIONS

Bleeding complications are more frequent with fibrinolytic than with anticoagulant therapy and require rapid diagnosis and management. Two problems contribute to excess bleeding. First, the fibrinolytic effect is not limited to the site of thrombosis but is usually systemic. Therefore, any hemostatic plugs needed to prevent bleeding at sites of vascular injury caused either by catheters needed for treatment or within pathologic lesions in the brain, gastrointestinal tract, or elsewhere are also susceptible to dissolution. Second, fibrinolytic therapy creates a systemic hypocoagulable state to a varying degree dependent on the dose and type of agent administered.

The most serious complication is intracranial hemorrhage which occurs in approximately 1% of patients and is associated with a high mortality and serious disability in survivors. Risk factors for intracranial hemorrhage include prior stroke, serious head trauma, intracranial surgery, tumor, or vascular disease such as aneurysms or arteriovenous malformations and uncontrolled hypertension.[416] These conditions represent strong contraindications to fibrinolytic therapy. The most common bleeding complications are related to invasive vascular procedures such as placement of arterial and venous catheters. Some bleeding at these sites is frequent and should not be a reason for interrupting therapy if it can be managed with local pressure or other simple measures. The problem can be minimized by limiting venous and arterial punctures and by early institution of local measures. Major bleeding may also result from preexisting lesions such as gastrointestinal ulcers or genitourinary lesions. Minor bleeding complications, such as ecchymoses and microscopic hematuria, are frequent and troublesome, but of little clinical consequence.

Before administering thrombolytic therapy, the clinician should be familiar with these bleeding complications and prepared to manage any that develop (Table 136–7).[417] The first step is accurate diagnosis, recognizing that deep bleeding into tissues may appear only as pain and swelling. Intracranial hemorrhage often presents with headache, change in neurologic status and vomiting. These symptoms represent an emergency, and management should include immediate imaging and neurosurgical consultation.

TABLE 136–7. Treatment of Fibrinolytic Bleeding

If intracranial bleeding is suspected, obtain imaging, consult neurosurgery, and correct hemostasis as below.
For major bleeding:
Send diagnostic test: activated partial thromboplastin time (aPTT), platelet count, and fibrinogen.
Attend to local hemostatic problems. Apply pressure if bleeding related to arterial puncture. Proceed with general supportive measures, including intravenous fluid hydration and transfusion of packed red cells if indicated. Proceed with diagnostic evaluation for gastrointestinal or genitourinary tract bleeding.
Correct abnormal hemostasis:
Prevent further fibrinolysis: stop fibrinolytic therapy; consider ε-aminocaproic acid or tranexamic acid.
Replacement therapy to repair hemostasis defect induced by fibrinolytic therapy: give cryoprecipitate 5–10 U and 2 U fresh-frozen plasma; consider platelet transfusion.
Correct other hemostatic defects: stop anticoagulant and antiplatelet agents; consider protamine to reverse heparin.

Treatment of bleeding complications involves measures directed to the local site as well as correction of the systemic hypocoagulable state resulting from proteolysis of plasma proteins and platelets. Initial management includes discontinuation of the fibrinolytic agent, which will be cleared rapidly as most have a short half-life. For serious bleeding, an antifibrinolytic agent such as ε-aminocaproic acid (EACA) can be administered to block fibrinolysis. This is only of value if the fibrinolytic agent remains in the blood, and its appropriate use depends on knowledge of the clearance rate of the agent administered. Replacement therapy to correct the hemostatic defect caused by systemic plasminemia is the next step. Fibrinogen replacement is often needed and can be accomplished by administration of 5 to 10 bags of cryoprecipitate, and fresh-frozen plasma can be used to replace other hemostatic proteins. Replacement treatment should be monitored with repeated coagulation tests. Administration of platelet concentrates may also be useful because fibrinolytic therapy results in platelet dysfunction from proteolysis of surface proteins and because fibrin(ogen) degradation products inhibit platelet function. Additionally, any other anticoagulant and antiplatelet agents should be discontinued. Heparin effect can be reversed by administration of protamine sulfate, and 1-deamino-8-D-arginine vasopressin (DDAVP) may have some value in reversing platelet dysfunction.

ANTIFIBRINOLYTIC THERAPY

PRINCIPLES

The fibrinolytic system functions physiologically to remove fibrin deposits by converting plasminogen to plasmin, which proteolytically degrades and then solubilizes the fibrin matrix. This carefully regulated process is initiated as fibrin is formed but functions slowly, allowing for removal of fibrin after its physiologic need is passed. Pathologic processes that cause abnormal regulation can cause either bleeding or thrombosis, and pharmacologic agents have been developed to inhibit fibrinolysis for treatment of bleeding. They have been used in two different situations. First, excessive systemic fibrinolytic activation can

TABLE 136–8. Principal Uses of Antifibrinolytic Agents

Condition	Comment
Systemic fibrinolysis	
α_2-Plasmin inhibitor or PAI-1 deficiency	Rare inherited disorders
Acute promyelocytic leukemia	Must distinguish fibrinolysis from DIC
Cirrhosis and liver transplantation	Occasional cases of cirrhosis; common in anhepatic phase of liver transplantation
Malignancy	Occasional cases of prostate and other carcinomas
DIC	Must be used with caution; thrombosis can result
Cardiopulmonary bypass	Decreases blood loss and transfusion needs
Fibrinolytic therapy	Can be used in treating bleeding complications
Localized fibrinolysis	
Hemophilia and von Willebrand disease	Decreases bleeding after dental extractions and possibly other procedures
Prostatectomy	Can decrease postoperative bleeding
Kasabach-Merritt syndrome	May shrink hemangioma
Menorrhagia	Often decreases bleeding

cause a hemorrhagic diathesis associated with certain pathologic conditions and also during fibrinolytic therapy. Second, the normal process of fibrinolysis may contribute to local bleeding by prematurely removing needed hemostatic plugs. Inhibition of fibrinolysis can improve hemostasis in both (Table 136–8). Care must be exercised using antifibrinolytic agents to treat bleeding in complicated clinical situations in which thrombosis may also occur, because inhibiting fibrinolysis can worsen thrombosis. For example, in patients with consumption coagulopathies there may be excessive activation of both the coagulation and fibrinolytic systems resulting in clinical manifestations of both bleeding and thrombosis. In this situation, inhibiting fibrinolysis to treat bleeding can precipitate or worsen thrombosis (see Chap. 130).

ANTIFIBRINOLYTIC AGENTS

Two antifibrinolytic agents, EACA and tranexamic acid, are both synthetic lysine analogues. Fibrinolysis is accelerated by binding of plasminogen to lysine residues on fibrin, and these agents inhibit fibrinolysis by competitively blocking this binding.[418–421] Both can be administered orally or intravenously, have rapid absorption after oral administration, and are excreted primarily through the kidneys. Only EACA is approved for use in the United States. Differences in the two agents are primarily in pharmacology. Tranexamic acid is approximately 10-fold more potent than EACA because of its higher binding affinity. Both drugs have a short half-life of 2 to 4 hours and must, therefore, be administered frequently. EACA can be administered intravenously with a loading dose of approximately 100 mg/kg over 30 to 60 minutes followed by a continuous infusion of up to 1 g/h, or the dose can be divided for intermittent administration. For oral treatment, the same loading dose can be administered followed by a maximum dose of 24 g/day in divided doses given every 1 to 6 hours as indicated. The use of tranexamic acid follows similar principles. The intravenous dose is 10 mg/kg followed by 10 mg/kg every 2 to 6 hours as needed. It can also be administered orally in a dose of 25 mg/kg given 3 or 4 times daily. Both EACA and tranexamic acid are generally well tolerated, but patients must be observed for possible thrombotic complications. Additionally, thrombotic ureteral obstruction can occur in patients with upper urinary tract bleeding, and such patients should be treated only after careful consideration. The risks of ureteral obstruction can be decreased by insuring high urine flow. Thrombotic complications can occur in patients with hypercoagulability, and thrombotic events can be precipitated or worsened in patients with DIC. Myonecrosis is a rare complication. Minor complications including rash, abdominal discomfort, nausea, and vomiting are reported.

Aprotinin is a naturally occurring, broad-spectrum proteinase inhibitor derived from bovine lung.[422–424] It has both antiinflammatory and antifibrinolytic properties. Aprotinin was used in the United States for reducing perioperative blood loss and blood transfusions in patients undergoing cardiopulmonary bypass. However, its use has been associated with an increased risk of postoperative renal dysfunction and cardiac and cerebral events.[425,426] Also, several large studies have provided evidence for an increase in both short- and long-term mortality in patients who received aprotinin compared to EACA, tranexamic acid, or placebo. In a retrospective analysis of electronic records from 33,517 aprotinin recipients and 44,682 EACA recipients, the unadjusted risk of death within the first 7 days after coronary artery bypass grafting was 4.5 percent for aprotinin recipients compared to 2.5 percent for EACA recipients. The relative risk of death was significantly increased in the aprotinin group (relative risk: 1.64; 95% CI 1.50–1.78).[427] Another retrospective study on 10,275 consecutive patients undergoing surgical coronary revascularization at Duke University Medical Center found that the mortality risk with aprotinin remained significantly increased at 1 year. Compared with the use of EACA or no antifibrinolytic agents, aprotinin use was also associated with a larger risk-adjusted increase in the serum creatinine level ($p < 0.001$).[428] The prospective Blood Conservation Using Antifibrinolytics in a Randomized Trial (BART) was designed to randomize a total of 3000 patients to either aprotinin, EACA, or tranexamic acid to further assess the safety of aprotinin.[429] The trial was terminated early after enrollment of 2331 patients because of a significantly higher death rate from any cause at 30 days in the aprotinin recipients. Based on results of these studies, aprotinin was removed from U.S. market in May 2008. Access to aprotinin is limited to investigational use only.

CLINICAL USE OF ANTIFIBRINOLYTIC AGENTS

Systemic Fibrinolysis

Excessive systemic fibrinolytic activation can lead to bleeding from premature lysis of hemostatic plugs and also from the hypocoagulable state resulting from the lytic state and, inhibiting fibrinolysis can be useful in treating bleeding complications. Laboratory evaluation can aid in diagnosis and in following the response to treatment. The excessive fibrinolysis is caused by increased levels of plasminogen activator and may result in a shortened euglobulin clot lysis time, decreased levels of plasminogen, α_2-PI, and fibrinogen, and increased levels of plasmin-antiplasmin complexes and fibrinogen degradation products. Screening tests including the prothrombin time and activated partial thromboplastin time may be prolonged. It may be difficult to distinguish between abnormal hemostasis primarily caused by DIC and systemic fibrinolysis. Useful features consistent with primary fibrinolysis include a more prominent decrease in fibrinogen level and increased levels of fibrinogen degradation products, relatively less thrombocytopenia and elevation of D-dimer level (see Chap. 130). Serial measurement of selected tests may be useful in following the course of therapy, as the low fibrinogen and elevated fibrinogen degradation products may normalize.

Rare inherited deficiencies of either α_2-PI or of PAI-1 can cause a life-long bleeding disorder. Inherited deficiency of α_2-PI is an autosomal recessive disorder occurring with homozygous deficiency.[430,431] Individuals with heterozygous deficiency are often asymptomatic but may have a mild bleeding disorder that worsens with age. α_2-Plasmin inhibitor deficiency caused by synthesis of a dysfunctional molecule with a mutation near the reactive site has also been reported and causes a bleeding disorder. Other reports describe an inherited bleeding disorder caused by deficiency of PAI-1 with affected patients having bleeding after surgery or trauma.[432–434] Treatment with antifibrinolytic agents has been effective in these bleeding conditions.

Antifibrinolytic therapy can also be useful in the more common acquired systemic hyperfibrinolytic conditions. Acute promyelocytic leukemia is often associated with a severe bleeding disorder that may have elements of both DIC and systemic fibrinolysis in addition to thrombocytopenia (see Chap. 130). Administration of EACA to inhibit fibrinolysis can be useful.[435–437] However, antifibrinolytic therapy must be used with care in such patients to avoid thrombosis, and treatment may be given in combination with heparin also. The hemostatic abnormality associated with severe liver disease is complex and includes elements of decreased synthesis of coagulation factors and inhibitors, abnormal clearance, thrombocytopenia, abnormal platelet function, and synthesis of abnormal proteins (see Chap. 129). In this setting, fibrinolysis can contribute to bleeding and may occasionally be the primary abnormality.[438–440] During orthotopic liver transplantation, accelerated fibrinolysis often contributes to bleeding, particularly during the anhepatic phase of surgery. Treatment with antifibrinolytic agents can improve bleeding complications and decrease blood loss.[441–444]

Primary fibrinolysis with bleeding may rarely occur with some malignant tumors including prostatic carcinoma[441–450] and also with heat stroke.[451] Fibrinolytic activation routinely occurs as a compensatory mechanism in DIC and may occasionally be prominent, resulting in a short euglobulin lysis time, decreased plasminogen, and other manifestations of fibrinolysis. It is difficult to separate the contribution of excessive fibrinolysis to the development of bleeding complications. The management of DIC is discussed elsewhere (see Chap. 130). It involves treatment of the underlying condition, replacement of coagulation factors, and occasionally the administration of heparin. If fibrinolytic activation is prominent and other measures do not control bleeding, then the use of antifibrinolytic therapy can be helpful. It should be used with caution, however, because inhibiting physiologic fibrinolysis can exacerbate underlying thrombotic events.

The contact system is activated during cardiopulmonary bypass, resulting in alterations in the coagulation, fibrinolytic, and complement systems[452,453] and both postoperative bleeding and the need for large transfusion volumes can be a major problems. Several trials of antifibrinolytic therapy have established that total blood loss and transfusion requirements can be reduced, with EACA and tranexamic acid often used for this purpose.[452–457] Antifibrinolytic therapy can also be useful in treating bleeding associated with some snakebites and following administration of fibrinolytic therapy (see Management of Bleeding Complications, on page 2235).

Excessive bleeding associated with a local lesion in the absence of systemic fibrinolysis may also respond to antifibrinolytic therapy. Bleeding following dental extractions in patients with hemophilia or von Willebrand disease can be reduced.[458–461] The oral mucosa is rich in fibrinolytic activity, and inhibition of normal fibrinolysis prevents premature dissolution of hemostatic thrombi and prevents local bleeding. Fibrinolytic activity is also high in the urinary system and may contribute to excessive bleeding following prostatectomy. Because EACA and tranexamic acid are excreted through the kidneys, their concentration in the urine is high, and antifibrinolytic therapy can inhibit local fibrinolysis and decrease post-prostatectomy bleeding.[462,463] Similarly, endometrial fibrinolysis contributes to menstrual bleeding, and antifibrinolytic therapy can be useful in treating menorrhagia in patients with hemostatic abnormalities or with normal hemostasis in whom other specific therapy is ineffective.[464,465] Antifibrinolytic therapy may also be useful in rare cases of Kasabach-Merritt Syndrome with a symptomatic or expanding hemangioma and consumption coagulopathy. Inhibiting fibrinolysis can result in local thrombosis with shrinkage of the lesion.[466,467] Antifibrinolytic therapy has been used in treating gastrointestinal or genitourinary bleeding in patients with severe thrombocytopenia, ulcerative colitis, hereditary hemorrhagic telangiectasia, traumatic hyphema, following tonsillectomy, and with subarachnoid hemorrhage. Caution is advised in the latter condition, as rebleeding may be decreased with antifibrinolytic therapy but vasospasm and distal ischemia may worsen.[468]

REFERENCES

1. Hajjar KA: The Molecular Basis of Fibrinolysis, in *Nathan and Oski's Hematology of Infancy and Childhood*, 7th ed, edited by SH Orkin, DG Nathan, D Ginsburg, AT Look, DE Fisher, SE Lux, p 1425. Saunders Elsevier, Philadelphia, 2009.
2. Hajjar KA: Cellular receptors in the regulation of plasmin generation. *Thromb Haemost* 74:294, 1995.
3. Raum D, Marcus D, Alper CA, et al: Synthesis of human plasminogen by the liver. *Science* 208:1036, 1980.
4. Bohmfalk J, Fuller G: Plasminogen is synthesized by primary cultures of rat hepatocytes. *Science* 209:408, 1980.
5. Castellino FJ: Biochemistry of human plasminogen. *Semin Thromb Hemost* 10:18, 1984.
6. Collen D, Tytgat G, Claeys H, et al: Metabolism of plasminogen in healthy subjects: Effect of tranexamic acid. *J Clin Invest* 51:1310, 1972.
7. Forsgren M, Raden B, Israelsson M, et al: Molecular cloning and characterization of a full-length cDNA clone for human plasminogen. *FEBS Lett* 213:254, 1987.
8. Miles LA, Dahlberg CM, Plow EF: The cell-binding domains of plasminogen and their function in plasma. *J Biol Chem* 263:11656, 1988.
9. Markus G, De Pasquale JL, Wissler FC: Quantitative determination of the binding of epsilon-aminocaproic acid to native plasminogen. *J Biol Chem* 253:727, 1978.
10. Markus G, Priore RL, Wissler FC: The binding of tranexamic acid to native (glu) and modified (lys) human plasminogen and its effect on conformation. *J Biol Chem* 254:1211, 1979.
11. Hajjar KA, Harpel PC, Jaffe EA, et al: Binding of plasminogen to cultured human endothelial cells. *J Biol Chem* 261:11656, 1986.
12. Miles LA, Plow EF: Cellular regulation of fibrinolysis. *Thromb Haemost* 66:32, 1991.
13. Rakoczi I, Wiman B, Collen D: On the biologic significance of the specific interaction between fibrin, plasminogen, and antiplasmin. *Biochim Biophys Acta* 540:295, 1978.
14. Hayes ML, Castellino FJ: Carbohydrate of the human plasminogen variants. I. Carbohydrate composition, glycopeptide isolation, and characterization. *J Biol Chem* 254:8768, 1979.
15. Hayes ML, Castellino FJ: Carbohydrate composition of the human plasminogen variants. II. Structure of the asparagine-linked oligosaccharide unit. *J Biol Chem* 254:8772, 1979.
16. Hayes ML, Castellino FJ: Carbohydrate of the human plasminogen variants. III. Structure of the O-glycosidically-linked oligosaccharide unit. *J Biol Chem* 254:8777, 1979.
17. Saksela O: Plasminogen activation and regulation of proteolysis. *Biochim Biophys Acta* 823:35, 1985.
18. Wallen P, Wiman B: Characterization of human plasminogen. I. On the relationship between different molecular forms of plasminogen demonstrated in plasma and found in purified preparations. *Biochim Biophys Acta* 221:20, 1970.
19. Wallen P, Wiman B: Characterization of human plasminogen. II. Separation and partial characterization of different molecular forms of human plasminogen. *Biochim Biophys Acta* 157:122, 1972.
20. Holvoet P, Lijnen HR, Collen D: A monoclonal antibody specific for lys-plasminogen. *J Biol Chem* 260:12106, 1985.
21. Hoylaerts M, Rijken DC, Lijnen HR, et al: Kinetics of the activation of plasminogen by human tissue plasminogen activator: Role of fibrin. *J Biol Chem* 257:2912, 1982.
22. Hajjar KA, Nachman RL: Endothelial cell-mediated conversion of glu-plasminogen to lys-plasminogen: Further evidence for assembly of the fibrinolytic system on the endothelial cell surface. *J Clin Invest* 82:1769, 1988.
23. Silverstein RL, Friedlander RJ, Nicholas RL, et al: Binding of lys-plasminogen to monocytes and macrophages. *J Clin Invest* 82:1948, 1988.
24. Murray JC, Buetow KH, Donovan M, et al: Linkage disequilibrium of plasminogen polymorphisms and assignment of the gene to human chromosome 6q26–6q27. *Am J Hum Genet* 40:338, 1987.

25. Petersen TE, Martzen MR, Ichinose A, et al: Characterization of the gene for human plasminogen, a key proenzyme in the fibrinolytic system. *J Biol Chem* 265:6104, 1990.
26. Jenkins GR, Seiffert D, Parmer RJ, et al: Regulation of plasminogen gene expression by interleukin-6. *Blood* 89:2394, 1997.
27. McLean JW, Tomlinson JE, Kuang WJ, et al: CDNA sequence of human apolipoprotein(a) is homologous to plasminogen. *Nature* 330:132, 1987.
28. Nakamura T, Nishizawa T, Hagiya M, et al: Molecular cloning and expression of human hepatocyte growth factor. *Nature* 342:440, 1989.
29. Weissbach L, Treadwell BV: A plasminogen-related gene is expressed in cancer cells. *Biochem Biophys Res Commun* 186:1108, 1992.
30. Yoshimura T, Yuhki N, Wang MH, et al: Cloning, sequencing, and expression of human macrophage stimulating protein (MSP, MST 1) confirms MSP as a member of the family of kringle proteins and locates the MSP gene on chromosome 3. *J Biol Chem* 268:15461, 1993.
31. Byrne CD, Schwartz K, Meer K, et al: The human apolipoprotein(a)/plasminogen gene cluster contains a novel homologue transcribed in liver. *Arterioscler Thromb* 14:534, 1994.
32. Ichinose A: Multiple members of the plasminogen-apolipoprotein(a) gene family associated with thrombosis. *Biochemistry* 31:3113, 1992.
33. Shanmukhappa K, Matte U, Degen JL, et al: Plasmin-mediated proteolysis is required for hepatocyte growth factor activation during liver repair. *J Biol Chem* 284:12917, 2009.
34. Bugge TH, Flick MJ, Daugherty CC, et al: Plasminogen deficiency causes severe thrombosis but is compatible with development and reproduction. *Genes Dev* 9:794, 1995.
35. Carmeliet P, Collen D: Gene targeting and gene transfer studies of the plasminogen/plasmin system: Implications in thrombosis, hemostasis, neointima formation, and atherosclerosis. *FASEB J* 9:934, 1995.
36. Drew AF, Kaufman AH, Kombrinck KW, et al: Ligneous conjunctivitis in plasminogen-deficient mice. *Blood* 91:1616, 1998.
37. Pennica D, Holmes WE, Kohr WJ, et al: Cloning and expression of human tissue-type plasminogen activator cDNA in *E. coli*. *Nature* 301:214, 1983.
38. Tate KM, Higgins DL, Holmes WE, et al: Functional role of proteolytic cleavage at arginine-275 of human tissue plasminogen activator as assessed by site-directed mutagenesis. *Biochemistry* 26:338, 1987.
39. Pohl G, Kenne L, Nilsson B, et al: Isolation and characterization of three different carbohydrate chains from melanoma tissue plasminogen activator. *Eur J Biochem* 170:69, 1987.
40. Spellman MW, Basa LJ, Leonard CK, et al: Carbohydrate structures of tissue plasminogen activator expressed in Chinese hamster ovary cells. *J Biol Chem* 264:14100, 1989.
41. Harris RJ, Leonard CK, Guzzetta AW: Tissue plasminogen activator has an *O*-linked fucose attached to threonine-61 in the epidermal growth factor domain. *Biochemistry* 30:2311, 1991.
42. Ny T, Elgh F, Lund B: Structure of the human tissue-type plasminogen activator gene: Correlation of intron and exon structures to functional and structural domains. *Proc Natl Acad Sci U S A* 81:5355, 1984.
43. Browne MJ, Tyrrell AWR, Chapman CG, et al: Isolation of a human tissue-type plasminogen activator genomic clone and its expression in mouse L cells. *Gene* 33:279, 1985.
44. Degen SJF, Rajput B, Reich E: The human tissue plasminogen activator gene. *J Biol Chem* 261:6872, 1986.
45. Van Zonnefeld A-J, Veerman H, Pannekoek H: Autonomous functions of structural domains on human tissue-type plasminogen activator. *Proc Natl Acad Sci U S A* 83:4670, 1986.
46. Feng P, Ohlsson M, Ny T: The structure of the TATA-less rat tissue-type plasminogen activator gene. *J Biol Chem* 265:2022, 1990.
47. Kooistra T, Bosma PJ, Toet K, et al: Role of protein kinase C and cyclic adenosine monophosphate in the regulation of tissue-type plasminogen activator, plasminogen activator inhibitor-1, and platelet-derived growth factor mRNA levels in human endothelial cells. Possible involvement of proto-oncogenes c-jun and c-fos. *Arterioscler Thromb* 11:1042, 1991.
48. Medcalf RL, Ruegg M, Schleuning WD: A DNA motif related to the cAMP-responsive element and an exon-located activator protein-2 binding site in the human tissue-type plasminogen activator gene promoter cooperate in basal expression and convey activation by phorbol ester and cAMP. *J Biol Chem* 265:14618, 1990.
49. Kooistra T, Van den Berg J, Tons A, et al: Butyrate stimulates tissue type plasminogen activator synthesis in cultured human endothelial cells. *Biochem J* 247:605, 1987.
50. Diamond SL, Eskin SG, McIntire LV: Fluid flow stimulates tissue plasminogen activator secretion by cultured human endothelial cells. *Science* 243:1483, 1989.
51. Hanss M, Collen D: Secretion of tissue-type plasminogen activator and plasminogen activator inhibitor by cultured human endothelial cells: Modulation by thrombin, endotoxin, and histamine. *J Lab Clin Med* 109:97, 1987.
52. Thompson EA, Nelles L, Collen D: Effect of retinoic acid on the synthesis of tissue-type plasminogen activator and plasminogen activator inhibitor 1 in human endothelial cells. *Eur J Biochem* 201:627, 1991.
53. Kooistra T, Opdenberg JP, Toet K, et al: Stimulation of tissue-type plasminogen activator synthesis by retinoids in cultured human endothelial cells and rat tissue *in vivo*. *Thromb Haemost* 65:565, 1991.
54. Medcaf RL, Van den Berg E, Schleuning WD: Glucocorticoid-modulated gene expression of tissue- and urinary-type plasminogen activator and plasminogen activator inhibitor-1 and -2. *J Cell Biol* 106:971, 1988.
55. Santell L, Levin EG: Cyclic AMP potentiates phorbol ester stimulation of tissue plasminogen activator release and inhibits secretion of plasminogen activator inhibitor-1 from human endothelial cells. *J Biol Chem* 263:16802, 1988.
56. Levin EG, del Zoppo GJ: Localization of tissue plasminogen activator in the endothelium of a limited number of vessels. *Am J Pathol* 144:855, 1994.
57. Levin EG, Santell L, Osborn KG: The expression of endothelial tissue plasminogen activator *in vivo*: A function defined by vessel size and anatomic location. *J Cell Sci* 110:139, 1997.
58. Levin EG, Osborn KG, Schleuning WD: Vessel-specific gene expression in the lung: Tissue plasminogen activator is limited to bronchial arteries and pulmonary vessels of discrete size. *Chest* 114:68S, 1998.
59. Diamond SL, Sharefkin JB, Dieffenbach C, et al: Tissue plasminogen activator messenger RNA levels increase in cultured human endothelial cells exposed to laminar shear stress. *J Cell Physiol* 143:364, 1990.
60. O'Rourke J, Jiang X, Hao Z, et al: Distribution of sympathetic tissue plasminogen activator (t-PA) to a distant microvasculature. *J Neurosci* 79:727, 2005.
61. Dichek D, Quertermous T: Thrombin regulation of mRNA levels of tissue plasminogen activator inhibitor-1 in cultured human umbilical vein endothelial cells. *Blood* 74:222, 1989.
62. Levin EG, Marotti KR, Santell L: Protein kinase C and the stimulation of tissue plasminogen activator release from human endothelial cells. *J Biol Chem* 264:16030, 1989.
63. Kasai S, Arimura H, Nishida M, et al: Primary structure of single-chain pro-urokinase. *J Biol Chem* 260:12382, 1985.
64. Gunzler WA, Steffens GJ, Otting F, et al: Structural relationship between high and low molecular mass urokinase. *Hoppe Seylers Z Physiol Chem* 363:133, 1982.
65. Riccio A, Grimaldi G, Verde P, et al: The human urokinase-plasminogen activator gene and its promoter. *Nucleic Acids Res* 13:2759, 1985.
66. Holmes WE, Pennica D, Blaber M, et al: Cloning and expression of the gene for pro-urokinase in *Escherichia coli*. *Biotechnology* 3:923, 1985.
67. Schmitt M, Wilhelm O, Janicke F, et al: Urokinase-type plasminogen activator (u-PA) and its receptor (CD87): A new target in tumor invasion and metastasis. *J Obstet Gynaecol* 21:151, 1995.
68. Van Hinsbergh VWM, Van den Berg EA, Fiers W, et al: Tumor necrosis factor induces the production of urokinase-type plasminogen activator by human endothelial cells. *Blood* 10:1991, 1990.
69. Medina R, Socher SH, Han JH, et al: Interleukin-1, endotoxin, or tumor necrosis factor/cachectin enhance the level of plasminogen activator inhibitor messenger RNA in bovine aortic endothelial cells. *Thromb Res* 54:41, 1989.
70. Gerwin BI, Keski-Oja J, Seddon M, et al: TGF beta 1 modulation of urokinase and PAI-1 expression in human bronchial epithelial cells. *Am J Pathol* 259:262, 1990.
71. Stump DC, Lijnen HR, Collen D: Purification and characterization of a novel low molecular weight form of single-chain urokinase-type plasminogen activator. *J Biol Chem* 261:17120, 1986.
72. Steffens GJ, Gunzler WA, Olting F, et al: The complete amino acid sequence of low molecular mass urokinase from human urine. *Hoppe Seylers Z Physiol Chem* 363:1043, 1982.
73. Lijnen HR, Zamarron C, Blaber M, et al: Activation of plasminogen by pro-urokinase. *J Biol Chem* 261:1253, 1986.
74. Gurewich V, Pannell R, Louie S, et al: Effective and fibrin-specific clot lysis by a zymogen precursor from urokinase (pro-urokinase). A study *in vitro* and in two animal species. *J Clin Invest* 73:1731, 1984.
75. Lijnen HR, Van Hoef B, DeCock F, et al: The mechanism of plasminogen activation and fibrin dissolution by single chain urokinase-type plasminogen activator in a plasma milieu *in vitro*. *Blood* 73:1864, 1989.
76. Petersen LC, Lund LR, Nielsen LS, et al: One-chain urokinase-type plasminogen activator from human sarcoma cells is a precursor with little or no intrinsic activity. *J Biol Chem* 263:11189, 1988.
77. Colman RW: Activation of plasminogen by human plasma kallikrein. *Biochem Biophys Res Commun* 35:273, 1968.
78. Mandle RJ, Kaplan AP: Hageman factor-dependent fibrinolysis: Generation of fibrinolytic activity by the interaction of human activated factor XI and plasminogen. *Blood* 54:850, 1979.
79. Goldsmith GH, Saito H, Ratnoff OD: The activation of plasminogen by Hageman factor (factor XII) and Hageman factor fragments. *J Clin Invest* 62:54, 1978.
80. Ouimet H, Loscalzo J: Fibrinolysis, in *Thrombosis and Hemorrhage*, 1 ed, edited by J Loscalzo, AI Schafer, p 127. Blackwell Scientific, Boston, 1994.
81. Hiraoka N, Allen E, Apel IJ, et al: Matrix metalloproteinases regulate neovascularization by acting as pericellular fibrinolysins. *Cell* 95:365, 1998.
82. Hrafnkelsdottir T, Ottosson P, Gudnason T, et al: Impaired endothelial release of tissue-type plasminogen activator in patients with chronic kidney disease and hypertension. *Hypertension* 44:300, 2004.
83. Patrassi GM, Sartori MT, Viero ML, et al: Venous thrombosis and tissue plasminogen activator release deficiency: A family study. *Blood Coagul Fibrinolysis* 2:231, 1991.
84. Sjogren LS, Doroudi R, Gan L, et al: Elevated intraluminal pressure inhibits vascular tissue plasminogen activator secretion and downregulates its gene expression. *Hypertension* 35:1002, 2000.

85. Carmeliet P, Schoonjans L, Kieckens L, et al: Physiological consequences of loss of plasminogen activator gene function in mice. *Nature* 368:419, 1994.
86. Rau JC, Beaulieu LM, Huntington JA, et al: Serpins in thrombosis, hemostasis and fibrinolysis. *J Thromb Haemost* 5:102, 2007.
87. Aoki N: Genetic abnormalities of the fibrinolytic system. *Semin Thromb Hemost* 10:42, 1984.
88. Holmes WE, Nelles L, Lijnen HR: Primary structure of human alpha2-antiplasmin, a serine protease inhibitor (serpin). *J Biol Chem* 262:1659, 1987.
89. Hirosawa S, Nakamura Y, Miura O, et al: Organization of the human alpha2-antiplasmin inhibitor gene. *Proc Natl Acad Sci U S A* 85:6836, 1988.
90. Plow EF, Collen D: The presence and release of alpha-2-antiplasmin from human platelets. *Blood* 58:1069, 1981.
91. Aoki N, Moroi M, Tachiya K: Effects of alpha-2-plasmin inhibitor on fibrin clot lysis. Its comparison with alpha-2-macroglobulin. *Thromb Haemost* 39:22, 1978.
92. Huisman LG, Van Griensven JM, Kluft C: On the role of C1-inhibitor as inhibitor of tissue-type plasminogen activator in human plasma. *Thromb Haemost* 73:466, 1995.
93. Scott RW, Bergman BL, Bajpai A, et al: Protease nexin: Properties and a modified purification procedure. *J Biol Chem* 260:7029, 1985.
94. Cunningham DD, Van Nostrand WE, Farrell DH, et al: Interactions of serine proteases with cultured fibroblasts. *J Cell Biochem* 32:281, 1986.
95. Sprengers ED, Kluft D: Plasminogen activator inhibitors. *Blood* 69:381, 1987.
96. Ny T, Sawdey M, Lawrence D, et al: Cloning and sequence of a cDNA coding for the human beta-migrating endothelial-cell-type plasminogen activator inhibitor. *Proc Natl Acad Sci U S A* 83:6776, 1986.
97. Kruithof EKO: Plasminogen activator inhibitor type 1: Biochemical, biological, and clinical aspects. *Fibrinolysis* 2:59, 1988.
98. Samad F, Yamamoto K, Loskutoff DJ: Distribution and regulation of plasminogen activator inhibitor-1 in murine adipose tissue *in vivo*. *J Clin Invest* 97:37, 1996.
99. Sawdey M, Podor TJ, Loskutoff DJ: Regulation of type-1 plasminogen activator inhibitor gene expression in cultured bovine aortic endothelial cells. *J Biol Chem* 264:10396, 1989.
100. Van Hinsbergh VWM, Kooistra T, Van den Berg EA, et al: Tumor necrosis factor increases the production of plasminogen activator inhibitor in human endothelial cells *in vitro* and in rats *in vivo*. *Blood* 72:1467, 1988.
101. Van den Berg EA, Sprengers ED, Jaye M, et al: Regulation of plasminogen activator inhibitor-1 mRNA in human endothelial cells. *Thromb Haemost* 60:63, 1988.
102. Loskutoff DJ, Linders M, Keijer J, et al: Structure of the human plasminogen activator inhibitor-1 gene: Non-random distribution of introns. *Biochemistry* 26:3763, 1987.
103. Mottonen J, Strand A, Symersky J, et al: Structural basis of latency in plasminogen activator inhibitor-1. *Nature* 355:270, 1992.
104. Declerck PJ, De Mol M, Alessi MC, et al: Purification and characterization of a plasminogen activator inhibitor-1 binding protein from human plasma. Identification as multimeric form of S protein (vitronectin). *J Biol Chem* 263:15454, 1988.
105. Dupont DM, Madsen JB, Kristensen T, et al: Biochemical properties of plasminogen activator inhibitor-1. *Front Biosci* 14:1337, 2009.
106. Kruithof EK: Regulation of plasminogen activator inhibitor type 1 gene expression by inflammatory mediators and statins. *Thromb Haemost* 100:969, 2008.
107. Nagamine Y: Transcriptional regulation of the plasminogen activator inhibitor type 1 with an emphasis on negative regulation. *Thromb Haemost* 100:1007, 2008.
108. Bosma PJ, Van den Berg EA, Kooistra T, et al: Human plasminogen activator inhibitor-1 gene: Promoter and structural nucleotide sequences. *J Biol Chem* 263:9129, 1988.
109. Van Zonnefeld AJ, Curriden SA, Loskutoff DJ: Type 1 plasminogen activator inhibitor gene: Functional analysis and glucocorticoid regulation of its promoter. *Proc Natl Acad Sci U S A* 85:5525, 1988.
110. Westerhausen DR, Hopkins WE, Billadello JJ: Multiple transforming growth factor beta-inducible elements regulate expression of the plasminogen activator inhibitor type-1 gene in HepG2 cells. *J Biol Chem* 266:1092, 1991.
111. Keeton MR, Curriden SA, Van Zonneveld AJ, et al: Identification of regulatory sequences in the type 1 plasminogen activator inhibitor gene responsive to transforming growth factor. *J Biol Chem* 266:23048, 1991.
112. Emeis JJ, Kooistra T: Interleukin 1 and lipopolysaccharide induce an inhibitor of tissue-type plasminogen activator *in vivo* and in cultured endothelial cells. *J Exp Med* 163:1260, 1986.
113. Schleef RR, Bevilacqua MP, Sawdey M, et al: Cytokine activation of vascular endothelium: Effects on tissue-type plasminogen activator and type 1 plasminogen activator inhibitor. *J Biol Chem* 263:5797, 1988.
114. Craik CS, Rutter WJ, Fletternick R: Splice junctions: Association with variation in protein structure. *Science* 220:1125, 1983.
115. Stiko-Rahm A, Wiman B, Hamsten A, et al: Secretion of plasminogen activator inhibitor-1 from cultured human umbilical vein endothelial cells is induced by very low density lipoprotein. *Arteriosclerosis* 10:1067, 1990.
116. Etingin OR, Hajjar DP, Hajjar KA, et al: Lipoprotein(a) regulates plasminogen activator inhibitor-1 expression in endothelial cells. *J Biol Chem* 266:2459, 1990.
117. Vaughan DE, Shen C, Lazo S: Angiotensin II induces plasminogen activator inhibitor synthesis *in vitro*. *Circulation* 86:I-557, 1992.
118. Gelehrter TD, Scyncer-Laszuk R: Thrombin induction of plasminogen activator-inhibitor synthesis *in vitro*. *J Clin Invest* 77:165, 1986.
119. Van Hinsbergh VWM, Sprengers ED, Kooistra T: Effect of thrombin on the production of plasminogen activators and PA inhibitor-1 by human foreskin microvascular endothelial cells. *Thromb Haemost* 57:148, 1987.
120. Scarpati EM, Sadler JE: Regulation of endothelial cell coagulant properties. Modulation of tissue factor, plasminogen activator inhibitors, and thrombomodulin by phorbol 12-myristate 13-acetate and tumor necrosis factor. *J Biol Chem* 264:20705, 1989.
121. Konkle BA, Kollros PR, Kelly MD: Heparin-binding growth factor-1 modulation of plasminogen activator inhibitor-1 expression. *J Biol Chem* 265:21867, 1990.
122. Erickson LA, Fici GJ, Lund JE, et al: Development of venous occlusions in transgenic mice for the plasminogen activator inhibitor-1 gene. *Nature* 346:74, 1990.
123. Carmeliet P, Kieckens L, Schoonjans L, et al: Plasminogen activator inhibitor-1 gene-deficient mice: I. Generation by homologous recombination and characterization. *J Clin Invest* 92:2746, 1993.
124. Fay WP, Shapiro AD, Shih JL, et al: Complete deficiency of plasminogen activator inhibitor type 1 due to a frame-shift mutation. *N Engl J Med* 327:1729, 1992.
125. Ye RD, Wun T-C, Sadler JE: CDNA cloning and expression in *Escherichia coli* of a plasminogen activator inhibitor from human placenta. *J Biol Chem* 262:3718, 1987.
126. Ye RD, Aherns SM, Le Beau MM, et al: Structure of the gene for human plasminogen activator inhibitor-2. The nearest mammalian homologue of chicken ovalbumin. *J Biol Chem* 264:5495, 1989.
127. Ogbourne SM, Antalis TM: Characterization of PAUSE-1, a powerful silencer in the human plasminogen activator inhibitor type 2 gene promoter. *Nucleic Acids Res* 29:3919, 2001.
128. Antalis TM, Clok MA, Barnes T, et al: Cloning and expression of a cDNA coding for a human monocyte-derived plasminogen activator inhibitor. *Proc Natl Acad Sci U S A* 85:985, 1988.
129. Schleuning WD, Medcalf RL, Hession C, et al: Plasminogen activator inhibitor 2: Regulation of gene transcription during phorbol ester-mediated differentiation of U-937 human histiocytic lymphoma cells. *Mol Cell Biol* 7:4564, 1987.
130. Chapman HA, Stone OL: A fibrinolytic inhibitor of human alveolar macrophages. Induction with endotoxin. *Am Rev Respir Dis* 132:569, 1985.
131. Nesheim M, Wang W, Boffa M, et al: Thrombin, thrombomodulin and TAFI in the molecular link between coagulation and fibrinolysis. *Thromb Haemost* 78:386, 1997.
132. Mosnier LO, Bouma BN: Regulation of fibrinolysis by thrombin activatable fibrinolysis inhibitor, an unstable carboxypeptidase B that unites the pathways of coagulation and fibrinolysis. *Arterioscler Thromb Vasc Biol* 26:2445, 2006.
133. Eaton DL, Malloy BE, Tsai SP, et al: Isolation, molecular cloning, and partial characterization of a novel carboxypeptidase B from plasma. *J Biol Chem* 269:21833, 1991.
134. Wang W, Hendriks DF, Scharpe SS: Carboxypeptidase U, a plasma carboxypeptidase with high affinity for plasminogen. *J Biol Chem* 269:15937, 1994.
135. Bajzar L, Manuel R, Nesheim M: Purification and characterization of TAFI, a thrombin activatable fibrinolysis inhibitor. *J Biol Chem* 270:14477, 1995.
136. Bajzar L, Nesheim ME, Tracy PB: The profibrinolytic effect of activated protein C in clots formed from plasma is TAFI-dependent. *Blood* 88:2093, 1996.
137. Bajzar L, Morser J, Nesheim M: TAFI, or plasma procarboxypeptidase B, couples the coagulation and fibrinolytic cascades through the thrombin-thrombomodulin complex. *J Biol Chem* 271:16603, 1996.
138. Minnema MC, Friederich PW, Levi M, et al: Enhancement of rabbit jugular vein thrombolysis by neutralization of factor XI: *In vivo* evidence for a role of factor XI as an anti-fibrinolytic factor. *J Clin Invest* 101:10, 1998.
139. Nagashima M, Yin ZF, Zhao L, et al: Thrombin-activatable fibrinolysis inhibitor (TAFI) deficiency is compatible with murine life. *J Clin Invest* 109:110, 2002.
140. Wang X, Smith PL, Hsu MY, et al: Deficiency in thrombin-activatable fibrinolysis inhibitor (TAFI) protected mice from ferric chloride-induced vena cava thrombosis. *J Thromb Thrombolysis* 23:41, 2007.
141. Mao SS, Holahan MA, Bailey C, et al: Demonstration of enhanced endogenous fibrinolysis in thrombin activatable fibrinolysis inhibitor-deficient mice. *Blood Coagul Fibrinolysis* 16:407, 2005.
142. Redlitz A, Tan AK, Eaton D, et al: Plasma carboxypeptidases as regulators of the plasminogen system. *J Clin Invest* 96:2534, 1995.
143. Miles LA, Dahlberg CM, Plescia J, et al: Role of cell surface lysines in plasminogen binding to cells: Identification of alpha-enolase as a candidate plasminogen receptor. *Biochemistry* 30:1682, 1991.
144. Miles LA, Ginsberg MA, White JG, et al: Plasminogen interacts with platelets through two distinct mechanisms. *J Clin Invest* 77:2001, 1986.
145. Kanalas JJ, Makker SP: Identification of the rat Heymann nephritis autoantigen (GP330) as a receptor site for plasminogen. *J Biol Chem* 266:10825, 1991.
146. Barnathan ES, Kuo A, Van der Keyl H, et al: Tissue-type plasminogen activator binding to human endothelial cells: Evidence for two distinct binding sites. *J Biol Chem* 263:7792, 1988.
147. Hajjar KA: The endothelial cell tissue plasminogen activator receptor: Specific interaction with plasminogen. *J Biol Chem* 266:21962, 1991.
148. Hajjar KA, Hamel NM: Identification and characterization of human endothelial cell membrane binding sites for tissue plasminogen activator and urokinase. *J Biol Chem* 265:2908, 1990.
149. Herren T, Burke TA, Das R, Plow EF: Identification of histone H2B as a regulated plasminogen receptor. *Biochemistry* 45:9463, 2006.
150. Das R, Burke T, Plow EF: Histone H2B as a functionally important plasminogen receptor on macrophages. *Blood* 110:3763, 2007.
151. D'Alessio S, Blasi F: The urokinase receptor as an entertainer of signal transduction. *Front Biosci* 14:4575, 2009.
152. Montuori N, Ragno P: Multiple activities of a multifaceted receptor: Roles of cleaved and soluble uPAR. *Front Biosci* 14:2492, 2009.

153. Roldan AL, Cubellis MV, Masucci MT, et al: Cloning and expression of the receptor for human urokinase plasminogen activator, a central molecule in cell surface, plasmin-dependent proteolysis. *EMBO J* 9:467, 1990.
154. Casey JR, Petranka JG, Kottra J, et al: The structure of the urokinase-type plasminogen activator receptor gene. *Blood* 84:1151, 1994.
155. Behrendt N, Ronne E, Ploug M, et al: The human receptor for urokinase plasminogen receptor. *J Biol Chem* 265:6453, 1990.
156. Ploug M, Ronne E, Behrendt N, et al: Cellular receptor for urokinase plasminogen activator. Carboxyl-terminal processing and membrane anchoring by glycosylphosphatidylinositol. *J Biol Chem* 266:1926, 1991.
157. Cubellis MV, Andreasson P, Ragno P, et al: Accessibility of receptor-bound urokinase to type-1 plasminogen activator inhibitor. *Proc Natl Acad Sci U S A* 86:4828, 1989.
158. Ellis V, Wun TC, Behrendt N, et al: Inhibition of receptor-bound urokinase by plasminogen activator inhibitor. *J Biol Chem* 265:9904, 1990.
159. Cubellis MV, Wun TC, Blasi F: Receptor-mediated internalization and degradation of urokinase is caused by its specific inhibitor PAI-1. *EMBO J* 9:1079, 1990.
160. Ellis V, Behrendt N, Dano K: Plasminogen activation by receptor-bound urokinase. *J Biol Chem* 266:12752, 1991.
161. Kugler MC, Wei Y, Chapman HA: Urokinase receptor and integrin interactions. *Curr Pharm Des* 9:1565, 2003.
162. Waltz DA, Chapman HA: Reversible cellular adhesion to vitronectin linked to urokinase receptor occupancy. *J Biol Chem* 269:14746, 1994.
163. Wei Y, Waltz DA, Rao N, et al: Identification of the urokinase receptor as an adhesion receptor for vitronectin. *J Biol Chem* 269:32380, 1994.
164. Wei Y, Lukashev M, Simon DI, et al: Regulation of integrin function by the urokinase receptor. *Science* 273:1551, 1996.
165. Xue W, Kindzelskii AL, Todd RF, et al: Physical association of complement receptor type 3 and urokinase-type plasminogen activator in neutrophil membranes. *J Immunol* 152:4630, 1994.
166. Stahl A, Mueller BM: The urokinase-type plasminogen activator receptor, a GPI-linked protein, is localized in caveolae. *J Cell Biol* 129:335, 1995.
167. Anderson RG: Caveolae: Where incoming and outgoing messengers meet. *Proc Natl Acad Sci U S A* 90:10909, 1993.
168. Okamoto T, Schlegel A, Scherer PE, et al: Caveolins, a family of scaffolding proteins for organizing "preassembled signaling complexes" at the plasma membrane. *J Biol Chem* 273:5419, 1998.
169. Gerke V, Creutz CE, Moss SE: Annexins: Linking Ca++ signalling to membrane dynamics. *Nat Rev Mol Cell Biol* 6:449, 2005.
170. Chung CY, Erickson HP: Cell surface annexin II is a high affinity receptor for the alternatively spliced segment of tenascin-C. *J Cell Biol* 126:539, 1994.
171. Wright JF, Kurosky A, Wasi S: An endothelial cell-surface form of annexin II binds human cytomegalovirus. *Biochem Biophys Res Commun* 198:983, 1994.
172. Kassam G, Choi KS, Ghuman J, et al: The role of annexin II tetramer in the activation of plasminogen. *J Biol Chem* 273:4790, 1998.
173. Siever DA, Erickson HP: Extracellular annexin II. *Int J Biochem Cell Biol* 29:1219, 1997.
174. Falcone DJ, Borth W, Faisal Khan KM, et al: Plasminogen-mediated matrix invasion and degradation by macrophages is dependent on surface expression of annexin II. *Blood* 97:777, 2001.
175. Brownstein C, Deora AB, Jacovina AT, et al: Annexin II mediates plasminogen-dependent matrix invasion by human monocytes: Enhanced expression by macrophages. *Blood* 103:317, 2004.
176. Menell JS, Cesarman GM, Jacovina AT, et al: Annexin II and bleeding in acute promyelocytic leukemia. *N Engl J Med* 340:994, 1999.
177. Lee TH, Rhim T, Kim SS: Prothrombin kringle 2 domain has a growth inhibitory activity against basic fibroblast growth factor-stimulated capillary endothelial cells. *J Biol Chem* 273:28805, 1998.
178. Tressler RJ, Updyke TV, Yeatman TJ, et al: Extracellular annexin is associated with divalent cation-dependent tumor cell adhesion of metastatic RAW 117 large-cell lymphoma cells. *J Cell Biochem* 53:265, 1993.
179. Yeatman TJ, Updyke TV, Kaetzel MA, et al: Expression of annexins on the surfaces of non-metastatic human and rodent tumor cells. *Clin Exp Metastasis* 11:37, 1993.
180. Tressler RJ, Nicolson GL: Butanol-extractable and detergent-solubilized cell surface components from murine large cell lymphoma cells associated with adhesion to organ microvessel endothelial cells. *J Cell Biochem* 48:162, 1992.
181. Swairjo MA, Seaton BA: Annexin structure and membrane interactions: A molecular perspective. *Annu Rev Biophys Biomol Struct* 23:193, 1994.
182. Spano F, Raugei G, Palla E, et al: Characterization of the human lipocortin-2-encoding multigene family: Its structure suggests the existence of a short amino acid unit undergoing duplication. *Gene* 95:243, 1990.
183. Cesarman GM, Guevara CA, Hajjar KA: An endothelial cell receptor for plasminogen/tissue plasminogen activator: II. Annexin II-mediated enhancement of t-PA-dependent plasminogen activation. *J Biol Chem* 269:21198, 1994.
184. Deora AB, Kreitzer G, Jacovina AT, et al: An annexin 2 phosphorylation switch mediates its p11-dependent translocation to the cell surface. *J Biol Chem* 279:43411, 2004.
185. Hajjar KA, Guevara CA, Lev E, et al: Interaction of the fibrinolytic receptor, annexin II, with the endothelial cell surface: Essential role of endonexin repeat 2. *J Biol Chem* 271:21652, 1996.
186. He K, Deora AB, Xiong H, et al: Endothelial cell annexin A2 regulates polyubiquitination and degradation of its binding partner, S100A10/p11. *J Biol Chem* 283:19192, 2008.
187. Hajjar KA, Gavish D, Breslow J, et al: Lipoprotein(a) modulation of endothelial cell surface fibrinolysis and its potential role in atherosclerosis. *Nature* 339:303, 1989.
188. Hajjar KA, Mauri L, Jacovina AT, et al: Tissue plasminogen activator binding to the annexin II tail domain: Direct modulation by homocysteine. *J Biol Chem* 273:9987, 1998.
189. Kraus JP: Molecular basis of phenotype expression in homocystinuria. *J Inherit Metab Dis* 17:383, 1994.
190. Boushey CJ, Beresford SAA, Omenn GS, et al: A quantitative assessment of plasma homocysteine as a risk factor for vascular disease. *JAMA* 274:1049, 1995.
191. Refsum H, Ueland PM, Nygard O, et al: Homocysteine and cardiovascular disease. *Annu Rev Med* 49:31, 1998.
192. Hajjar KA: Homocysteine-induced modulation of tissue plasminogen activator binding to its endothelial cell membrane receptor. *J Clin Invest* 91:2873, 1993.
193. Ishii H, Yoshida M, Hiraoka M, et al: Recombinant annexin II modulates impaired fibrinolytic activity *in vitro* and in rat carotid artery. *Circ Res* 89:1240, 2001.
194. Cesarman-Maus G, Rios-Luna NP, Deora AB, et al: Autoantibodies against the fibrinolytic receptor, annexin 2, in antiphospholipid syndrome. *Blood* 107:4375, 2006.
195. Ling Q, Jacovina AT, Deora AB, et al: Annexin II is a key regulator of fibrin homeostasis and neoangiogenesis . *J Clin Invest* 113:38, 2004.
196. Bu G, Warshawsky I, Schwartz AL: Cellular receptors for the plasminogen activators. *Blood* 83:3427, 1994.
197. Lillis AP, Van Duyn LB, Murphy-Ullrich J, et al: LDL receptor-related protein 1: Unique tissue-specific functions revealed by selective gene knockout studies. *Physiol Rev* 88:887, 2008.
198. Herz J, Goldstein JL, Strickland DK, et al: 39 kDa protein modulates binding of ligands to low density lipoprotein receptor-related protein/alpha-2-macroglobulin receptor. *J Biol Chem* 266:21232, 1991.
199. Herz J, Clouthier DE, Hammer RE: LDL receptor-related protein internalizes and degrades u-PA–PAI-1 complexes and is essential for embryo implantation. *Cell* 71:411, 1992.
200. Herz J, Clouthier DE, Hammer RE: Correction: LDL receptor-related protein internalizes and degrades u-PA–PAI-1 complexes and is essential for embryo implantation. *Cell* 73:428, 1993.
201. Otter M, Barrett-Bergshoeff MM, Rijken DC: Binding of tissue type plasminogen activator by the mannose receptor. *J Biol Chem* 266:13931, 1991.
202. Hajjar KA, Reynolds CM: α-Fucose-mediated binding and degradation of tissue plasminogen activator by HepG2 cells. *J Clin Invest* 93:703, 1994.
203. Narita M, Bu G, Herz J, et al: Two receptor systems are involved in the plasma clearance of tissue-type plasminogen activator (t-PA) *in vivo*. *J Clin Invest* 96:1164, 1995.
204. Bailey K, Bettelheim FR, Lorand L, et al: Action of thrombin in the clotting of fibrinogen. *Nature* 167:233, 1951.
205. Doolittle RF: The molecular biology of fibrin, in *The Molecular Basis of Blood Diseases*, 2nd ed, edited by G Stamatoyannopoulos, AW Nienhuis, PW Majerus, H Varmus, p 701. WB Saunders, Philadelphia, 1994.
206. Marder VJ, Budzinski AZ: Data for defining fibrinogen and its plasmic degradation products. *Thromb Diath Haemorrh* 33:199, 1975.
207. Furlan M, Kemp G, Beck EA: Plasmic degradation of fibrinogen. *Biochim Biophys Acta* 400:95, 1975.
208. Gaffney PJ, Dobos P: A structural aspect of human fibrinogen suggested by its plasmin degradation. *FEBS Lett* 15:13, 1971.
209. Latallo ZS, Flether AP, Alkjaersig N, et al: Inhibition of fibrin polymerization by fibrinogen proteolysis products. *Am J Physiol* 202:681, 1962.
210. Pizzo SV, Schwartz ML, Hill RL, et al: The effect of plasmin on the subunit structure of human fibrin. *J Biol Chem* 248:4574, 1973.
211. Culasso DE, Donati MB, DeGaetano G, et al: Inhibition of human platelet aggregation by plasmin digests of human and bovine preparations: Role of contaminating factor VIII-related material. *Blood* 44:169, 1974.
212. Buluk K, Malofiegen M: The pharmacologic properties of fibrinogen degradation products. *Br J Pharmacol* 35:79, 1969.
213. Richardson DL, Pepper DS, Kay AB: Chemotaxis for human monocytes by fibrinogen degradation products. *Br J Haematol* 32:507, 1976.
214. Girmann G, Pees H, Schwarze G, et al: Immunosuppression by micromolecular fibrin-fibrinogen degradation products in cancer. *Nature* 259:399, 1976.
215. Wiman B, Collen D: On the kinetics of the reaction between human antiplasmin and plasmin. *Eur J Biochem* 84:573, 1978.
216. Van Zonnefeld AJ, Veerman H, Pannekoek H: On the interaction of the finger and the kringle-2 domain of tissue-type plasminogen activator with fibrin: Inhibition of kringle-1 binding to fibrin by epsilon-aminocaproic acid. *J Biol Chem* 261:14214, 1986.
217. Hajjar KA: The molecular basis of fibrinolysis, in *Hematology of Infancy and Childhood*, 6th ed, edited by DG Nathan, SH Orkin, D Ginsburg, AT Look, p 1497. WB Saunders, Philadelphia, 2003.
218. Camiolo SM, Thorsen S, Astrup T: Fibrinogenolysis and fibrinolysis with tissue plasminogen activator, urokinase, streptokinase-activated human globulin and plasmin. *Proc Soc Exp Biol Med* 138:277, 1971.
219. Lijnen HR, Zamarron C, Blaber M, et al: Activation of plasminogen by prourokinase: I. Mechanism. *J Biol Chem* 261:1253, 1986.
220. Pannell R, Black J, Gurewich V: Complementary modes of action of tissue-type plasminogen activator and pro-urokinase by which their synergistic effect on clot lysis may be explained. *J Clin Invest* 81:853, 1988.

221. Bell W: Fibrinolytic therapy: Indications and management, in *Hematology: Basic Principles and Practice*, 2nd ed, edited by R Hoffman, EJ Benz, SJ Shattil, B Furie, HJ Cohen, LE Silberstein, p 1814. Churchill Livingstone, New York, 1995.
222. Coligan JE, Slayter HS: Structure of thrombospondin. *J Biol Chem* 259:3944, 1984.
223. Ott U, Odermatt E, Engel J, et al: Protease resistance and conformation of laminin. *Eur J Biochem* 123:63, 1982.
224. Aplin JD, Hughes RC: Complex carbohydrates of the extracellular matrix structures, interactions, and biologic roles. *Biochim Biophys Acta* 694:375, 1982.
225. Marder VJ, Sherry S: Thrombolytic therapy: Current status. *N Engl J Med* 318:1512, 1988.
226. Unkeless JC, Gordon S, Reich E: Secretion of plasminogen activator by stimulated macrophages. *J Exp Med* 139:834, 1974.
227. Ossowski L, Reich E: Antibodies to plasminogen activator inhibit human tumor metastasis. *Cell* 35:611, 1983.
228. Strickland SE, Reich E, Sherman MI: Plasminogen activator in early embryogenesis: Enzyme production by trophoblast and parietal endoderm. *Cell* 9:231, 1976.
229. Strickland SE, Beers WH: Studies on the role of plasmingen activator in ovulation. *J Biol Chem* 254:5694, 1976.
230. Moonen G, Grau-Wagemans MP, Selak I: Plasminogen activator-plasmin system and neuronal migration. *Nature* 298:753, 1982.
231. Pittman RN, Ivins JK, Buettner HM: Neuronal plasminogen activators: Cell surface binding sites and involvement in neurite outgrowth. *J Neurosci* 9:4269, 1989.
232. Virji MA, Vassalli JD, Estensen D, et al: Plasminogen activator of islets of Langerhans: Modulation by glucose and correlation with insulin production. *Proc Natl Acad Sci U S A* 77:875, 1980.
233. Geiger M, Binder BR: Plasminogen activation in diabetes mellitus. *J Biol Chem* 259:2976, 1984.
234. Russell J, Schneider AB, Katzhendler J, et al: Modification of human placental lactogen with plasmin. *J Biol Chem* 254:2296, 1979.
235. Loskutoff DJ, Quigley JP: PAI-1, fibrosis, and the elusive provisional fibrin matrix. *J Clin Invest* 106:1441, 2000.
236. Romer J, Bugge TH, Pyke C, et al: Impaired wound healing in mice with a disrupted plasminogen gene. *Nat Med* 2:287, 1996.
237. Bugge TH, Kombrinck KW, Flick MJ, et al: Loss of fibrinogen rescues mice from the pleiotropic effects of plasminogen deficiency. *Cell* 87:709, 1996.
238. Ploplis VA, French EL, Carmeliet P, et al: Plasminogen deficiency differentially affects recruitment of inflammatory cell populations in mice. *Blood* 91:2005, 1998.
239. Carmeliet P, Moons L, Ploplis VA, et al: Impaired arterial neointima formation in mice with disruption of the plasminogen gene. *J Clin Invest* 99:200, 1997.
240. Coleman JL, Gebbia JA, Piesman J, et al: Plasminogen is required for efficient dissemination of *B. burgdorferi* in ticks and for enhancement of spirochetemia in mice. *Cell* 89:1111, 1997.
241. Chen ZL, Strickland SE: Neuronal death in the hippocampus is promoted by plasmin-catalyzed degradation of laminin. *Cell* 91:917, 1997.
242. Chapman HA: Disorders of lung matrix remodeling. *J Clin Invest* 113:148, 2004.
243. Hattori N, Degen JL, Sisson TH, et al: Bleomycin-induced pulmonary fibrosis in fibrinogen-null mice. *J Clin Invest* 106:1341, 2000.
244. Eitzman DT, McCoy RD, Zheng X, et al: Bleomycin-induced pulmonary fibrosis in transgenic mice that either lack or overexpress the murine plasminogen activator inhibitor-1 gene. *J Clin Invest* 97:232, 1996.
245. Olman MA, Mackman N, Gladson CL, et al: Changes in procoagulant and fibrinolytic gene expression during bleomycin-induced lung injury in the mouse. *J Clin Invest* 96:1621, 1995.
246. Fujimoto H, Gabazza EC, Taguchi O, et al: Thrombin-activatable fibrinolysis inhibitor deficiency attenuates bleomycin-induced lung fibrosis. *Am J Pathol* 168:1086, 2006.
247. Sisson TH, Hanson KE, Subbotina N, et al: Inducible lung-specific urokinase expression reduces fibrosis and mortality after lung injury in mice. *Am J Physiol Lung Cell Mol Physiol* 283:L1023, 2002.
248. Krishnan S, Deora AB, Annes JP, et al: Annexin II-mediated plasmin generation activates TGF-β3 during epithelial-mesenchymal transformation in the developing avian heart. *Dev Biol* 265:140, 2004.
249. Sporn MB, Roberts AB, Wakefield LM, et al: Transforming growth factor-beta: Biological function and chemical structure. *Science* 233:532, 1986.
250. Lyons RM, Gentry LE, Purchio AF, et al: Mechanism of activation of latent recombinant transforming growth factor beta1 by plasmin. *J Cell Biol* 110:1361, 1990.
251. Konstantinides S, Schafer K, Loskutoff DJ: Do PAI-1 and vitronectin promote or inhibit neointima formation? *Arterioscler Thromb Vasc Biol* 22:1943, 2002.
252. Ross R: Atherosclerosis: An inflammatory disease. *N Engl J Med* 340:115, 1999.
253. Konstantinides S, Schafer K, Thinnes T, et al: Plasminogen activator inhibitor-1 and its cofactor vitronectin stabilize arterial thrombi following vascular injury in mice. *Circulation* 103:576, 2001.
254. Peng L, Bhatia N, Parker AC, et al: Endogenous vitronectin and plasminogen activator inhibitor-1 promote neointima formation in murine carotid arteries. *Arterioscler Thromb Vasc Biol* 22:934, 2002.
255. Engelse MA, Hanemaaijer R, Koolwijk P, et al: The fibrinolytic system and matrix metalloproteinases in angiogenesis and tumor progression. *Semin Thromb Hemost* 30:71, 2004.
256. Hajjar KA, Deora AB: New concepts in fibrinolysis and angiogenesis. *Curr Atheroscler Rep* 2:417, 2000.
257. Bajou K, Noel A, Gerard RD, et al: Absence of host plasminogen activator inhibitor 1 prevents cancer invasion and vascularization. *Nat Med* 4:923, 1998.
258. Rakic JM, Lambert V, Munaut C, et al: Mice without u-PA, t-PA, or plasminogen genes are resistant to experimental choroidal neovascularization. *Invest Ophthalmol Vis Sci* 44:1732, 2003.
259. Lambert V, Munaut C, Noel A, et al: Influence of plasminogen activator inhibitor type 1 on choroidal neovascularization. *FASEB J* 15:1021, 2001.
260. Bajou K, Peng H, Laug WE, et al: Plasminogen activator inhibitor-1 protects endothelial cells from FasL-mediated apoptosis. *Cancer Cell* 14:324, 2008.
261. Vogten JM, Reijerkerk A, Meijers JCM, et al: The role of the fibrinolytic system in corneal angiogenesis. *Angiogenesis* 6:311, 2003.
262. Drinane M, Mollmark J, Zagorchev L, et al: The antiangiogenic activity of rPAI-1_{23} inhibits vasa vasorum and growth of atherosclerotic plaque. *Circ Res* 104:337, 2009.
263. Aoki N, Moroi M, Sakata Y, et al: Abnormal plasminogen: A hereditary molecular abnormality found in a patient with recurrent thrombosis. *J Clin Invest* 61:1186, 1978.
264. Schuster V, Hugle B, Tefs K: Plasminogen deficiency. *J Thromb Haemost* 5:2315, 2007.
265. Demarmels Biasiutti F, Sulzer I, Stucki B, et al: Is plasminogen deficiency a thrombotic risk factor? A study on 23 thrombophilic patients and their family members. *Thromb Haemost* 80:167, 1998.
266. Sartori MT, Patrassi GM, Theodoridis P, et al: Heterozygous type I plasminogen deficiency is associated with an increased risk for thrombosis: A statistical analysis of 20 kindreds. *Blood Coagul Fibrinolysis* 5:889, 1994.
267. Shigekiyo T, Uno Y, Tomonari A, et al: Type I congenital plasminogen deficiency is not a risk factor for thrombosis. *Thromb Haemost* 67:189, 1992.
268. Tait RC, Walker ID, Conkie JA, et al: Isolated familial plasminogen deficiency may not be a risk factor for thrombosis. *Thromb Haemost* 76:1004, 1996.
269. Azuma H, Mima N, Shirakawa M, et al: Molecular pathogenesis of type I congenital plasminogen deficiency: Expression of recombinant human mutant plasminogens in mammalian cells. *Blood* 89:183, 1997.
270. Ichinose A, Espling ES, Takamatsu J, et al: Two types of abnormal genes for plasminogen in families with a predisposition for thrombosis. *Proc Natl Acad Sci U S A* 88:115, 1991.
271. Schott D, Dempfle CE, Beck P, et al: Therapy with a purified plasminogen concentrate in an infant with ligneous conjunctivitis and homozygous plasminogen deficiency. *N Engl J Med* 339:1679, 1998.
272. Robbins KC: Dysplasminogenemia. *Prog Cardiovasc Dis* 34:295, 1992.
273. Tsutsumi S, Saito T, Sakata T, et al: Genetic diagnosis of dysplasminogenemia: Detection of an Ala601-Thr mutation in 118 out of 125 families and identification of a new Asp676-Asn mutation. *Thromb Haemost* 76:135, 1996.
274. Lijnen HR, Collen D: Congenital and acquired deficiencies of components of the fibrinolytic system and their relationship to bleeding or thrombosis. *Fibrinolysis* 3:67, 1989.
275. Rakoczi I, Chamone D, Collen D, et al: Prediction of postoperative leg vein thrombosis in gynaecological patients. *Lancet* 1:509, 1978.
276. Nilsson IM, Ljungner H, Tengborn L: Two different mechanisms in patients with venous thrombosis and defective fibrinolysis: Low concentrations of plasminogen activator or increased concentration of plasminogen activator inhibitor. *Br Med J* 290:1453, 1985.
277. Juhan-Vague I, Valadier J, Alessi MC, et al: Deficient t-PA release and elevated PA inhibitor levels in patients with spontaneous or recurrent leg thrombosis. *Thromb Haemost* 57:67, 1987.
278. Hamsten A, Wiman B, De Faire U, et al: Increased plasma levels of a rapid inhibitor of tissue plasminogen activator in young survivors of myocardial infarction. *N Engl J Med* 313:1557, 1985.
279. Paramo JA, Alfaro MJ, Rocha E: Postoperative changes in the plasmatic levels of tissue-type plasminogen activator and its fast-acting inhibitor: Relationship to deep vein thrombosis and influence of prophylaxis. *Thromb Haemost* 54:713, 1985.
280. Juhan-Vague I, Roul C, Alessi MC, et al: Increased plasminogen activator inhibitor activity in non-insulin dependent diabetic patients: Relationship with plasma insulin. *Thromb Haemost* 61:370, 1989.
281. Francis CW: Plasminogen activator inhibitor-1 levels and polymorphisms: Association with venous thromboembolism. *Arch Pathol Lab Med* 126:1401, 2002.
282. Tsantes AE, Nikolopoulos GK, Bagos PG, et al: The effect of the plasminogen activator inhibitor-1 4G/5G polymorphism on the thrombotic risk. *Thromb Res* 122:736, 2008.
283. Juhan-Vague I, Alessi MC, Joly P, et al: Plasma plasminogen activator inhibitor-1 in angina pectoris: Influence of plasma insulin and acute-phase response. *Arteriosclerosis* 9:362, 1989.
284. Stump DC, Taylor FB, Nesheim ME, et al: Pathologic fibrinolysis as a cause of clinical bleeding. *Semin Thromb Hemost* 16:260, 1990.
285. Saito H: Alpha-2-plasmin inhibitor and its deficiency states. *J Lab Clin Med* 112:671, 1988.
286. Gresele P, Binetti BM, Branca G, et al: TAFI deficiency in liver cirrhosis: Relation with plasma fibrinolysis and survival. *Thromb Res* 121:763, 2008.
287. Suarez CR, Walenga J, Mangogna LC, et al: Neonatal and maternal fibrinolysis: Activation at time of birth. *Am J Hematol* 19:365, 1985.
288. Albisetti M: The fibrinolytic system in children. *Semin Thromb Hemost* 29:339, 2009.
289. Summaria L: Comparison of human normal, full-term, fetal and adult plasminogen by physical and clinical analyses. *Haemostasis* 19:266, 1989.

290. Edelberg JM, Enghild JJ, Pizzo SV, et al: Neonatal plasminogen displays altered cell surface binding and activation kinetics: Correlation with increased glycosylation of the protein. *J Clin Invest* 86:107, 1990.
291. Andrew M, Brooker L, Leaker M, et al: Fibrin clot lysis by thrombolytic agents is impaired in newborns due to a low plasminogen concentration. *Thromb Haemost* 68:325, 1992.
292. Corrigan JJ, Sleeth JJ, Jeter MA, et al: Newborn's fibrinolytic mechanism: Components and plasmin generation. *Am J Hematol* 32:273, 1989.
293. Corrigan JJ, Jeter MA: Histidine-rich glycoprotein and plasminogen plasma levels in term and preterm newborns. *Am J Dis Child* 144:825, 1990.
294. Parmar N, Albisetti M, Berry LR, et al: The fibrinolytic system in newborns and children. *Clin Lab* 52:115, 2006.
295. Corrigan JJ, Jeter MA: Tissue-type plasminogen activator, plasminogen activator inhibitor, and histidine-rich glycoprotein in stressed human newborns. *Pediatrics* 89:43, 1992.
296. Brus F, Van Oeveren W, Okkern A, et al: Activation of the plasma clotting, fibrinolytic, and kinin-kallikrein system in preterm infants with severe idiopathic respiratory distress syndrome. *Pediatr Res* 36:647, 1994.
297. Cederholm-Williams SA, Spencer JAD, Wilkerson AR: Plasma levels of selected haemostatic factors in newborn babies. *Thromb Res* 23:555, 1981.
298. Andrew M, Paes B, Milner R, et al: Development of the human coagulation system in the full-term infant. *Blood* 70:165, 1987.
299. Andrew M, Massicotte-Nolan PM, Karpatkin M: Plasma protease inhibitors in premature infants: Influence of gestational age, postnatal age, and health status. *Proc Soc Exp Biol Med* 173:495, 1983.
300. Corrigan JJ: Thrombosis and thromboembolism, in *Hemorrhagic and Thrombotic Disease in Childhood and Adolescence*, edited by JJ Corrigan, p 147. Churchill Livingstone, New York, 1985.
301. Bonnar J, Daly L, Sheppard BL: Changes in the fibrinolytic system during pregnancy. *Semin Thromb Hemost* 16:221, 1990.
302. Brenner B: Haemostatic changes in pregnancy. *Thromb Res* 114:409, 2004.
303. Bremme KA: Haemostatic changes in pregnancy. *Best Pract Res Clin Haematol* 16:153, 2003.
304. Hellgren M: Hemostasis during pregnancy and puerperium. *Haemostasis* 26:244, 1996.
305. Schjetlein R, Haugen G, Wisloff F: Markers of intravascular coagulation and fibrinolysis in preeclampsia: Association with intrauterine growth retardation. *Acta Obstet Gynecol Scand* 76:541, 1997.
306. SantAna Dusse LM, Cooper AJ, Lwaleed BA: Thrombin activatable fibrinolysis inhibitor (TAFI): A role in pre-eclampsia? *Clin Chim Acta* 378:1, 2007.
307. Hajjar KA, Francis CW: Fibrinolysis and thrombolysis, in *Williams Hematology*, 7th ed, edited by MA Lichtman, E Beutler, TJ Kipps, U Seligsohn, K Kaushansky, JT Prchal, p 2089. McGraw-Hill, New York, 2005.
308. Fletcher AP, Alkjaersig N, Smyrniotis FE, et al: The treatment of patients suffering from early myocardial infarction with massive and prolonged streptokinase therapy. *Trans Assoc Am Physicians* 71:287, 1958.
309. Sherry S, Fletcher AP, Alkjaersig N: Fibrinolysis and fibrinolytic activity in man. *Physiol Rev* 39:343, 1959.
310. Adelman B, Michelson AD, Loscalzo J, et al: Plasmin effect on platelet glycoprotein Ib-von Willebrand factor interactions. *Blood* 65:32, 1985.
311. Loscalzo J, Vaughan DE: Tissue plasminogen activator promotes platelet disaggregation in plasma. *J Clin Invest* 79:1749, 1987.
312. Rudd MA, George D, Amarante P, et al: Temporal effects of thrombolytic agents on platelet function *in vivo* and their modulation by prostaglandins. *Circ Res* 67:1175, 1990.
313. The urokinase pulmonary embolism trial. A national cooperative study. *Circulation* 47:1, 1973.
314. Marder VJ: Relevance of changes in blood fibrinolytic and coagulation parameters during thrombolytic therapy. *Am J Med* 83:15, 1987.
315. Rao AK, Pratt C, Berke A, et al: Thrombolysis in Myocardial Infarction (TIMI) Trial—Phase I: Hemorrhagic manifestations and changes in plasma fibrinogen and the fibrinolytic system in patients treated with recombinant tissue plasminogen activator and streptokinase. *J Am Coll Cardiol* 11:1, 1988.
316. Timmis GC, Gangadharan V, Ramos RG, et al: Hemorrhage and the products of fibrinogen digestion after intracoronary administration of streptokinase. *Circulation* 69:1146, 1984.
317. Lloyd-Jones D, Adams R, Carnethon M, et al: Heart disease and stroke statistics—2009 update: A report from the American Heart Association Statistics Committee and Stroke Statistics Subcommittee. *Circulation* 27:480, 2009.
318. Abe T, Kazama M, Naito I, et al: Clinical evaluation for efficacy of tissue culture urokinase (TCUK) on cerebral thrombosis by means of multicenter double blind study. *Blood Vessels* 12:321, 1981.
319. Abe T, Kazama M, Naito I, et al: Clinical effect of urokinase (60,000 units/day) on cerebral infarction comparative study by means of multiple center double blind test. *Blood Vessels* 12:342, 1981.
320. Atarashi J, Otomo E, Araki G, et al: Clinical utility of urokinase in the treatment of acute stage of cerebral thrombosis: Multi-center double-blind study in comparison with placebo. *Clin Eval* 13:659, 1985.
321. del Zoppo GJ, Ferbert A, Otis S, et al: Local intra-arterial fibrinolytic therapy in acute carotid territory stroke. A pilot study. *Stroke* 19:307, 1988.
322. Fletcher AP, Alkjaersig N, Lewis M, et al: A pilot study of urokinase therapy in cerebral infarction. *Stroke* 7:135, 1976.
323. Hacke W, Zeumer H, Ferbert A, et al: Intra-arterial thrombolytic therapy improves outcome in patients with acute vertebrobasilar occlusive disease. *Stroke* 19:1216, 1988.
324. Hanaway J, Torack R, Fletcher AP, et al: Intracranial bleeding associated with urokinase therapy for acute ischemic hemispheral stroke. *Stroke* 7:143, 1976.
325. Matsumoto K, Satoh K: *Topical Intraarterial Urokinase Infusion for Acute Stroke.* Springer-Verlag, Heidelberg, 1991.
326. Meyer JS, Gilroy J, Barnhart MI, et al: Therapeutic thrombolysis in cerebral thromboembolism. Double-blind evaluation of intravenous plasmin therapy in carotid and middle cerebral arterial occlusion. *Neurology* 13:927, 1963.
327. Meyer JS, Gilroy J, Barnhart MI, et al: Anticoagulants plus streptokinase therapy in progressive stroke. *JAMA* 189:373, 1964.
328. Mori E, Tabuchi M, Yoshida T, et al: Intracarotid urokinase with thromboembolic occlusion of the middle cerebral artery. *Stroke* 19:802, 1988.
329. Mori E: *Fibrinolytic Recanalization Therapy in Acute Cerebrovascular Thromboembolism.* Springer-Verlag, Heidelberg, 1991.
330. Otomo E, Araki G, Itoh E, et al: Clinical efficacy of urokinase in the treatment of cerebral thrombosis. *Clin Eval* 13:711, 1985.
331. Theron J, Courtheoux P, Casasco A, et al: Local intraarterial fibrinolysis in the carotid territory. *AJNR Am J Neuroradiol* 10:753, 1989.
332. Zeumer H, Freitag HJ, Grzyska U, et al: Local intra-arterial fibrinolysis in acute vertebrobasilar occlusion. Technical developments and recent results. *Neuroradiology* 31:336, 1989.
333. Zeumer H, Freitag HJ, Zanella F, et al: Local intra-arterial fibrinolytic therapy in patients with stroke: Urokinase versus recombinant tissue plasminogen activator (r-T-PA). *Neuroradiology* 35:159, 1993.
334. Tissue plasminogen activator for acute ischemic stroke. The National Institute of Neurological Disorders and Stroke rt-PA Stroke Study Group. *N Engl J Med* 333:1581, 1995.
335. Hacke W, Kaste M, Fieschi C, et al: Intravenous thrombolysis with recombinant tissue plasminogen activator for acute hemispheric stroke. The European Cooperative Acute Stroke Study (ECASS). *JAMA* 274:1017, 1995.
336. Hacke W, Kaste M, Fieschi C, et al: Randomised double-blind placebo-controlled trial of thrombolytic therapy with intravenous alteplase in acute ischaemic stroke (ECASS II). Second European-Australasian Acute Stroke Study Investigators. *Lancet* 352:1245, 1998.
337. Clark WM, Wissman S, Albers GW, et al: Recombinant tissue-type plasminogen activator (Alteplase) for ischemic stroke 3 to 5 hours after symptom onset. The ATLANTIS Study: A randomized controlled trial. Alteplase Thrombolysis for Acute Noninterventional Therapy in Ischemic Stroke. *JAMA* 282:2019, 1999.
338. Hacke W, Donnan G, Fieschi C, et al: Association of outcome with early stroke treatment: Pooled analysis of ATLANTIS, ECASS, and NINDS rt-PA stroke trials. *Lancet* 363:768, 2004.
339. Hacke W, Kaste M, Bluhmki E, et al: Thrombolysis with alteplase 3 to 4.5 hours after acute ischemic stroke. *N Engl J Med* 359:1317, 2008.
340. Wahlgren N, Ahmed N, Davalos A, et al: Thrombolysis with alteplase 3–4.5 hours after acute ischaemic stroke (SITS-ISTR): An observational study. *Lancet* 372:1303, 2008.
341. Donnan GA, Davis SM, Chambers BR, et al: Streptokinase for acute ischemic stroke with relationship to time of administration: Australian Streptokinase (ASK) Trial Study Group. *JAMA* 276:961, 1996.
342. Randomised controlled trial of streptokinase, aspirin, and combination of both in treatment of acute ischaemic stroke. Multicentre Acute Stroke Trial–Italy (MAST-I) Group. *Lancet* 346:1509, 1995.
343. Thrombolytic therapy with streptokinase in acute ischemic stroke. The Multicenter Acute Stroke Trial–Europe Study Group. *N Engl J Med* 335:145, 1996.
344. Barnwell SL, Clark WM, Nguyen TT, et al: Safety and efficacy of delayed intraarterial urokinase therapy with mechanical clot disruption for thromboembolic stroke. *AJNR Am J Neuroradiol* 15:1817, 1994.
345. Barr JD, Mathis JM, Wildenhain SL, et al: Acute stroke intervention with intraarterial urokinase infusion. *J Vasc Interv Radiol* 5:705, 1994.
346. Casto L, Caverni L, Camerlingo M, et al: Intra-arterial thrombolysis in acute ischaemic stroke: Experience with a superselective catheter embedded in the clot. *J Neurol Neurosurg Psychiatry* 60:667, 1996.
347. Jansen O, von Kummer R, Forsting M, et al: Thrombolytic therapy in acute occlusion of the intracranial internal carotid artery bifurcation. *AJNR Am J Neuroradiol* 16:1977, 1995.
348. Nesbit GM, Clark WM, O'Neill OR, et al: Intracranial intraarterial thrombolysis facilitated by microcatheter navigation through an occluded cervical internal carotid artery. *J Neurosurg* 84:387, 1996.
349. Tarr R, Taylor CL, Selman WR, et al: Good clinical outcome in a patient with a large CT scan hypodensity treated with intra-arterial urokinase after an embolic stroke. *Neurology* 47:1076, 1996.
350. Janjua N, Brisman JL: Endovascular treatment of acute ischaemic stroke. *Lancet Neurol* 6:1086, 2007.
351. del Zoppo GJ, Higashida RT, Furlan AJ, et al: PROACT: A phase II randomized trial of recombinant pro-urokinase by direct arterial delivery in acute middle cerebral artery stroke. PROACT Investigators. Prolyse in Acute Cerebral Thromboembolism. *Stroke* 29:4, 1998.

352. Furlan A, Higashida R, Wechsler L, et al: Intra-arterial prourokinase for acute ischemic stroke. The PROACT II study: A randomized controlled trial. Prolyse in Acute Cerebral Thromboembolism. *JAMA* 282:2003, 1999.
353. Liu M, Wardlaw J: Thrombolysis (different doses, routes of administration and agents) for acute ischaemic stroke. *Cochrane Database Syst Rev* CD000514, 2000.
354. Wardlaw JM, Zoppo G, Yamaguchi T, et al: Thrombolysis for acute ischaemic stroke. *Cochrane Database Syst Rev* CD000213, 2003.
355. Ogawa A, Mori E, Minematsu K, et al: Randomized trial of intraarterial infusion of urokinase within 6 hours of middle cerebral artery stroke: The middle cerebral artery embolism local fibrinolytic intervention trial (MELT) Japan. *Stroke* 38:2633, 2007.
356. Broderick JP: William M. Feinberg Lecture: Stroke therapy in the year 2025: Burden, breakthroughs, and barriers to progress. *Stroke* 35:205, 2004.
357. Kleindorfer D, Khoury J, Alwell K, et al: Eligibility for rt-PA in acute ischemic stroke: A population-based study. *Stroke* 34:281, 2003.
358. Kothari RU, Pancioli A, Liu T, et al: Cincinnati prehospital stroke scale: Reproducibility and validity. *Ann Emerg Med* 33:373, 1999.
359. Albers GW, Thijs VN, Wechsler L, et al: Magnetic resonance imaging profiles predict clinical responses to early reperfusion: The diffusion and perfusion imaging evaluation for understanding stroke evolution (DEFUSE) study. *Ann Neurol* 60:508, 2006.
360. Davis SM, Donnan GA, Parsons MW, et al: Effects of alteplase beyond 3 h after stroke in the Echoplanar Imaging Thrombolytic Evaluation Trial (EPITHET): A placebo-controlled randomised trial. *Lancet Neurol* 7:299, 2008.
361. Furlan A, Eyding D, Albers GW, et al: Dose Escalation of Desmoteplase for Acute Ischemic Stroke (DEDAS): Evidence of safety and efficacy 3 to 9 hours after stroke onset. *Stroke* 37:1227, 2006.
362. Hacke W, Albers G, Al-Rawi Y, et al: The Desmoteplase on Acute Ischemic Stroke Trial (DIAS): A phase II MRI-based 9-hour window acute stroke thrombolysis trial with intravenous desmoteplase. *Stroke* 36:66, 2005.
363. Abciximab in acute ischemic stroke: A randomized, double-blind, placebo-controlled, dose-escalation study. The Abciximab in Ischemic Stroke Investigators. *Stroke* 31:601, 2000.
364. Qureshi AI, Suri MF, Khan J, et al: Abciximab as an adjunct to high-risk carotid or vertebrobasilar angioplasty: Preliminary experience. *Neurosurgery* 46:1316, 2000.
365. Qureshi AI, Ali Z, Suri MF, et al: Intra-arterial third-generation recombinant tissue plasminogen activator (reteplase) for acute ischemic stroke. *Neurosurgery* 49:41, 2001.
366. Seitz RJ, Hamzavi M, Junghans U, et al: Thrombolysis with recombinant tissue plasminogen activator and tirofiban in stroke: Preliminary observations. *Stroke* 34:1932, 2003.
367. Seitz RJ, Meisel S, Moll M, et al: The effect of combined thrombolysis with rt-PA and tirofiban on ischemic brain lesions. *Neurology* 62:2110, 2004.
368. Straub S, Junghans U, Jocanovic V, et al: Systemic thrombolysis with recombinant tissue plasminogen activator and tirofiban in acute middle cerebral artery occlusion. *Stroke* 35:705, 2004.
369. Ernst R, Pancioli A, Tomsick T, et al: Combined intravenous and intra-arterial recombinant tissue plasminogen activator in acute ischemic stroke. *Stroke* 31:2552, 2000.
370. IMS II Trial Investigators: The Interventional Management of Stroke (IMS) II Study. *Stroke* 38:2127, 2007.
371. IMS Study Investigators: Combined intravenous and intra-arterial recanalization for acute ischemic stroke: The Interventional Management of Stroke Study. *Stroke* 35:911, 2004.
372. Alexandrov AV, Demchuk AM, Felberg RA, et al: High rate of complete recanalization and dramatic clinical recovery during t-PA infusion when continuously monitored with 2-MHz transcranial Doppler monitoring. *Stroke* 31:610, 2000.
373. Francis CW: Ultrasound-enhanced thrombolysis. *Echocardiography* 18:239, 2001.
374. Alexandrov AV, Molina CA, Grotta JC, et al: Ultrasound-enhanced systemic thrombolysis for acute ischemic stroke. *N Engl J Med* 351:2170, 2004.
375. Adams HP Jr, Adams RJ, Brott T, et al: Guidelines for the early management of patients with ischemic stroke: A scientific statement from the Stroke Council of the American Stroke Association. *Stroke* 34:1056, 2003.
376. Broderick JP, Hacke W: Treatment of acute ischemic stroke: Part I: Recanalization strategies. *Circulation* 106:1563, 2002.
377. Kaste M, Thomassen L, Grond M, et al: Thrombolysis for acute ischemic stroke: A consensus statement of the 3rd Karolinska Stroke Update, October 30–31, 2000. *Stroke* 32:2717, 2001.
378. Brogden RN, Speight TM, Avery GS: Streptokinase: A review of its clinical pharmacology, mechanism of action and therapeutic uses. *Drugs* 5:357, 1973.
379. Dotter CT, Rosch J, Seaman AJ: Selective clot lysis with low-dose streptokinase. *Radiology* 111:31, 1974.
380. Ouriel K: Current status of thrombolysis for peripheral arterial occlusive disease. *Ann Vasc Surg* 16:797, 2002.
381. Ouriel K, Shortell CK, DeWeese JA, et al: A comparison of thrombolytic therapy with operative revascularization in the initial treatment of acute peripheral arterial ischemia. *J Vasc Surg* 19:1021, 1994.
382. Results of a prospective randomized trial evaluating surgery versus thrombolysis for ischemia of the lower extremity. The STILE trial. *Ann Surg* 220:251, 1994.
383. Ouriel K, Veith FJ, Sasahara AA: Thrombolysis or peripheral arterial surgery: Phase I results. TOPAS Investigators. *J Vasc Surg* 23:64, 1996.
384. Ouriel K, Veith FJ, Sasahara AA: A comparison of recombinant urokinase with vascular surgery as initial treatment for acute arterial occlusion of the legs. Thrombolysis or Peripheral Arterial Surgery (TOPAS) Investigators. *N Engl J Med* 338:1105, 1998.
385. Castaneda F, Swischuk JL, Li R, et al: Declining-dose study of reteplase treatment for lower extremity arterial occlusions. *J Vasc Interv Radiol* 13:1093, 2002.
386. Ouriel K, Katzen B, Mewissen M, et al: Reteplase in the treatment of peripheral arterial and venous occlusions: A pilot study. *J Vasc Interv Radiol* 11:849, 2000.
387. Ouriel K, Kandarpa K, Schuerr DM, et al: Prourokinase versus urokinase for recanalization of peripheral occlusions, safety and efficacy: The PURPOSE trial. *J Vasc Interv Radiol* 10:1083, 1999.
388. Heymans S, Vanderschueren S, Verhaeghe R, et al: Outcome and one year follow-up of intra-arterial staphylokinase in 191 patients with peripheral arterial occlusion. *Thromb Haemost* 83:666, 2000.
389. Duda SH, Tepe G, Luz O, et al: Peripheral artery occlusion: Treatment with abciximab plus urokinase versus with urokinase alone—A randomized pilot trial (the PROMPT Study). Platelet Receptor Antibodies in Order to Manage Peripheral Artery Thrombosis. *Radiology* 221:689, 2001.
390. Drescher P, McGuckin J, Rilling WS, et al: Catheter-directed thrombolytic therapy in peripheral artery occlusions: Combining reteplase and abciximab. *AJR Am J Roentgenol* 180:1385, 2003.
391. Cohen LH, Kaplan M, Bernhard VM: Intraoperative streptokinase. An adjunct to mechanical thrombectomy in the management of acute ischemia. *Arch Surg* 121:708, 1986.
392. Comerota AJ, White JV, Grosh JD: Intraoperative intra-arterial thrombolytic therapy for salvage of limbs in patients with distal arterial thrombosis. *Surg Gynecol Obstet* 169:283, 1989.
393. Parent FN, Bernhard VM, Pabst TS, et al: Fibrinolytic treatment of residual thrombus after catheter embolectomy for severe lower limb ischemia. *J Vasc Surg* 9:153, 1989.
394. Quinones-Baldrich WJ, Zierler RE, Hiatt JC: Intraoperative fibrinolytic therapy: An adjunct to catheter thromboembolectomy. *J Vasc Surg* 2:319, 1985.
395. Vedantham S, Vesely TM, Parti N, et al: Lower extremity venous thrombolysis with adjunctive mechanical thrombectomy. *J Vasc Interv Radiol* 13:1001, 2002.
396. Berridge DC, Kessel D, Robertson I: Surgery versus thrombolysis for acute limb ischaemia: Initial management. *Cochrane Database Syst Rev* CD002784, 2002.
397. Kessel D, Berridge D, Robertson I: Infusion techniques for peripheral arterial thrombolysis. *Cochrane Database Syst Rev* 1:CD000985, 2004.
398. Thrombolysis in the management of lower limb peripheral arterial occlusion—A consensus document. Working Party on Thrombolysis in the Management of Limb Ischemia. *Am J Cardiol* 81:207, 1998.
399. Hirsch AT, Haskal ZJ, Hertzer NR, et al: ACC/AHA 2005 practice guidelines for the management of patients with peripheral arterial disease (lower extremity, renal, mesenteric, and abdominal aortic): A collaborative report. *Circulation* 113:e463, 2006.
400. Sobel M, Verhaeghe R: Antithrombotic therapy for peripheral artery occlusive disease: American College of Chest Physicians Evidence-Based Clinical Practice Guidelines (8th edition). *Chest* 133:815S, 2008.
401. Menon KV, Shah V, Kamath PS: The Budd-Chiari syndrome. *N Engl J Med* 350:578, 2004.
402. Aytekin C, Boyvat F, Kurt A, et al: Catheter-directed thrombolysis with transjugular access in portal vein thrombosis secondary to pancreatitis. *Eur J Radiol* 39:80, 2001.
403. Ciccarelli O, Goffette P, Laterre PF, et al: Transjugular intrahepatic portosystemic shunt approach and local thrombolysis for treatment of early posttransplant portal vein thrombosis. *Transplantation* 72:159, 2001.
404. Tateishi A, Mitsui H, Oki T, et al: Extensive mesenteric vein and portal vein thrombosis successfully treated by thrombolysis and anticoagulation. *J Gastroenterol Hepatol* 16:1429, 2001.
405. Calin GA, Calin S, Ionescu R, et al: Successful local fibrinolytic treatment and balloon angioplasty in superior mesenteric arterial embolism: A case report and literature review. *Hepatogastroenterology* 50:732, 2003.
406. Savassi-Rocha PR, Veloso LF: Treatment of superior mesenteric artery embolism with a fibrinolytic agent: Case report and literature review. *Hepatogastroenterology* 49:1307, 2002.
407. Haire WD, Atkinson JB, Stephens LC, et al: Urokinase versus recombinant tissue plasminogen activator in thrombosed central venous catheters: A double-blinded, randomized trial. *Thromb Haemost* 72:543, 1994.
408. Semba CP, Deitcher SR, Li X, et al: Treatment of occluded central venous catheters with alteplase: Results in 1,064 patients. *J Vasc Interv Radiol* 13:1199, 2002.
409. Shen V, Li X, Murdock M, et al: Recombinant tissue plasminogen activator (alteplase) for restoration of function to occluded central venous catheters in pediatric patients. *J Pediatr Hematol Oncol* 25:38, 2003.
410. Timoney JP, Malkin MG, Leone DM, et al: Safe and cost effective use of alteplase for the clearance of occluded central venous access devices. *J Clin Oncol* 20:1918, 2002.
411. Cooper SG: Original report. Pulse-spray thrombolysis of thrombosed hemodialysis grafts with tissue plasminogen activator. *AJR Am J Roentgenol* 180:1063, 2003.
412. Cynamon J, Pierpont CE: Thrombolysis for the treatment of thrombosed hemodialysis access grafts. *Rev Cardiovasc Med* 3 Suppl 2:84, 2002.
413. Daeihagh P, Jordan J, Chen J, et al: Efficacy of tissue plasminogen activator administration on patency of hemodialysis access catheters. *Am J Kidney Dis* 36:75, 2000.
414. Hilleman DE, Dunlay RW, Packard KA: Reteplase for dysfunctional hemodialysis catheter clearance. *Pharmacotherapy* 23:137, 2003.

415. Shrivastava D, Lundin AP, Dosunmu B, et al: Salvage of clotted jugular vein hemodialysis catheters. *Nephron* 68:77, 1994.
416. Sobel BE: Intracranial bleeding, fibrinolysis, and anticoagulation. Causal connections and clinical implications. *Circulation* 90:2147, 1994.
417. Sane DC, Califf RM, Topol EJ, et al: Bleeding during thrombolytic therapy for acute myocardial infarction: Mechanisms and management. *Ann Intern Med* 111:1010, 1989.
418. Alkjaersig N, Fletcher AP, Sherry S: Xi-Aminocaproic acid: An inhibitor of plasminogen activation. *J Biol Chem* 234:832, 1959.
419. Andersson L, Nilsson IM, Nilehn JE, et al: Experimental and clinical studies on AMCA, the antifibrinolytically active isomer of p-aminomethyl cyclohexane carboxylic acid. *Scand J Haematol* 2:230, 1965.
420. Brockway WJ, Castellino FJ: The mechanism f the inhibition of plasmin by xi-aminocaproic acid. *J Biol Chem* 14:4641, 1971.
421. Alkjaersig N, Fletcher AP, Sherry S. xi-Aminocaproic acid: an inhibitor of plasminogen activation. *J Biol Chem* 234:832, 1959.
422. Huber R, Kukla D, Ruhlmann A, et al: Pancreatic trypsin inhibitor (Kunitz). I. Structure and function. *Cold Spring Harb Symp Quant Biol* 36:141, 1972.
423. Ruhlmann A, Kukla D, Schwager P, et al: Structure of the complex formed by bovine trypsin and bovine pancreatic trypsin inhibitor. Crystal structure determination and stereochemistry of the contact region. *J Mol Biol* 77:417, 1973.
424. Wiman B: On the reaction of plasmin or plasmin-streptokinase complex with aprotinin or alpha 2-antiplasmin. *Thromb Res* 17:143, 1980.
425. Mangano DT, Tudor IC, Dietzel C: The risk associated with aprotinin in cardiac surgery. *N Engl J Med* 354:353, 2006.
426. Mouton R, Finch D, Davis I, et al: Effect of aprotinin on renal dysfunction. *Lancet* 372:1543, 2008.
427. Schneeweiss S, Seeger JD, Landon J, et al: Aprotinin during coronary-artery bypass grafting and risk of death. *N Engl J Med* 358:771, 2008.
428. Shaw AD, Stafford-Smith M, White WD, et al: The effect of aprotinin on outcome after coronary-artery bypass grafting. *N Engl J Med* 358:784, 2008.
429. Fergusson DA, Hebert PC, Mazer CD, et al: A comparison of aprotinin and lysine analogues in high-risk cardiac surgery. *N Engl J Med* 358:2319, 2008.
430. Aoki N, Moro M, Matsuda M, et al: The behavior of alpha-2 plasmin inhibitor in fibrinolytic states. *J Clin Invest* 60:361, 1977.
431. Aoki N, Sakata Y, Matsuda M, et al: Fibrinolytic states in a patient with congenital deficiency of alpha 1-plasmin inhibitor. *Blood* 55:483, 1980.
432. Dieval J, Nguyen G, Gross S, et al: A lifelong bleeding disorder associated with a deficiency of plasminogen activator inhibitor type 1. *Blood* 77:528, 1991.
433. Fay WP, Shapiro AD, Shih JL, et al: Brief report: Complete deficiency of plasminogen-activator inhibitor type 1 due to a frame-shift mutation. *N Engl J Med* 327:1729, 1992.
434. Lee MH, Vosburgh E, Anderson K, et al: Deficiency of plasma plasminogen activator inhibitor 1 results in hyperfibrinolytic bleeding. *Blood* 81:2357, 1993.
435. Avvisati G, Ten Cate JW, Buller HR, et al: Tranexamic acid for control of haemorrhage in acute promyelocytic leukemia. *Lancet* ii:122, 1989.
436. Rodeghiero F, Avvisati G, Castaman G, et al: Early deaths and anti-hemorrhagic treatments in acute promyelocytic leukemia. A GIMEMA retrospective study in 268 consecutive patients. *Blood* 75:2112, 1990.
437. Schwartz BS, Williams EC, Conlan MG, et al: Epsilon-aminocaproic acid in the treatment of patients with acute promyelocytic leukemia and acquired alpha-2-plasmin inhibitor deficiency. *Ann Intern Med* 105:873, 1986.
438. Booth NA, Anderson JA, Bennett B: Plasminogen activators in alcoholic cirrhosis: Demonstration of increased tissue type and urokinase type activator. *J Clin Pathol* 37:772, 1984.
439. Hayashi T, Kamogawa A, Ro S, et al: Plasma from patients with cirrhosis increases tissue plasminogen activator release from vascular endothelial cells *in vitro*. *Liver* 18:186, 1998.
440. Violi F, Basili V, Ferro D, et al: Association between high values of D-dimer and tissue-plasminogen activator activity and first gastrointestinal bleeding in cirrhotic patients. *Thromb Haemost* 76:177, 1996.
441. Boylan JF, Klinck JR, Sandler AN, et al: Tranexamic acid reduces blood loss, transfusion requirements, and coagulation factor use in primary orthotopic liver transplantation. *Anesthesiology* 85:1043, 1996.
442. Kaspar M, Ramsay MA, Nguyen AT, et al: Continuous small-dose tranexamic acid reduces fibrinolysis but not transfusion requirements during orthotopic liver transplantation. *Anesth Analg* 85:281, 1997.
443. Segal HC, Hunt BJ, Cottam S, et al: Fibrinolytic activity during orthotopic liver transplantation with and without aprotinin. *Transplantation* 58:1356, 1994.
444. Soilleux H, Gillon MC, Mirand A, et al: Comparative effects of small and large aprotinin doses on bleeding during orthotopic liver transplantation. *Anesth Analg* 80:349, 1995.
445. Al-Mondhiry H, Manni A, Owen J, et al: Hemostatic effects of hormonal stimulation in patients with metastatic prostate cancer. *Am J Hematol* 28:141, 1988.
446. Bennett B, Croll AM, Robbie LA, et al: Tumour cell u-PA as a cause of fibrinolytic bleeding in metastatic disease. *Br J Haematol* 99:570, 1997.
447. Mannucci PM, Cugno M, Bottasso B, et al: Changes in fibrinolysis in patients with localized tumors. *Eur J Cancer* 26:83, 1990.
448. Meijer K, Smid WM, Geerards S, et al: Hyperfibrinogenolysis in disseminated adenocarcinoma. *Blood Coagul Fibrinolysis* 9:279, 1998.
449. Webber MM, Waghray A: Urokinase-mediated extracellular matrix degradation by human prostatic carcinoma cells and its inhibition by retinoic acid. *Clin Cancer Res* 1:755, 1995.
450. Zacharski LR, Memoli VA, Ornstein DL, et al: Tumor cell procoagulant and urokinase expression in carcinoma of the ovary. *J Natl Cancer Inst* 85:1225, 1993.
451. Bouchama A, Bridey F, Hammami MM, et al: Activation of coagulation and fibrinolysis in heatstroke. *Thromb Haemost* 76:909, 1996.
452. Harker LA: Bleeding after cardiopulmonary bypass. *N Engl J Med* 314:1446, 1986.
453. Williams GD, Bratton SL, Nielsen NJ, et al: Fibrinolysis in pediatric patients undergoing cardiopulmonary bypass. *J Cardiothorac Vasc Anesth* 12:633, 1998.
454. Horrow JC, Hlavacek J, Strong MD, et al: Prophylactic tranexamic acid decreases bleeding after cardiac operations. *J Thorac Cardiovasc Surg* 99:70, 1990.
455. Horrow JC, Van Riper DF, Strong MD, et al: Hemostatic effects of tranexamic acid and desmopressin during cardiac surgery. *Circulation* 84:2063, 1991.
456. Munoz JJ, Birkmeyer NJ, Birkmeyer JD, et al: Is epsilon-aminocaproic acid as effective as aprotinin in reducing bleeding with cardiac surgery? A meta-analysis. *Circulation* 99:81, 1999.
457. Soslau G, Horrow J, Brodsky I: Effect of tranexamic acid on platelet ADP during extracorporeal circulation. *Am J Hematol* 38:113, 1991.
458. Havel M, Grabenwoger F, Schneider J, et al: Aprotinin does not decrease early graft patency after coronary artery bypass grafting despite reducing postoperative bleeding and use of donated blood. *J Thorac Cardiovasc Surg* 107:807, 1994.
459. Laub GW, Riebman JB, Chen C, et al: The impact of aprotinin on coronary artery bypass graft patency. *Chest* 106:1370, 1994.
460. Lemmer JH Jr, Stanford W, Bonney SL, et al: Aprotinin for coronary bypass operations: Efficacy, safety, and influence on early saphenous vein graft patency. A multicenter, randomized, double-blind, placebo-controlled study. *J Thorac Cardiovasc Surg* 107:543, 1994.
461. Sindet-Pedersen S, Stenbjerg S: Effect of local antifibrinolytic treatment with tranexamic acid in hemophiliacs undergoing oral surgery. *J Oral Maxillofac Surg* 44:703, 1986.
462. Blomback M, Johansson G, Johnsson H, et al: Surgery in patients with von Willebrand's disease. *Br J Surg* 76:398, 1989.
463. Hedlund PO: Antifibrinolytic therapy with Cyklokapron in connection with prostatectomy. A double blind study. *Scand J Urol Nephrol* 3:177, 1969.
464. Callender ST, Warner GT, Cope E: Treatment of menorrhagia with tranexamic acid. A double-blind trial. *Br Med J* 4:214, 1970.
465. Ong YL, Hull DR, Mayne EE: Menorrhagia in von Willebrand disease successfully treated with single daily dose tranexamic acid. *Haemophilia* 4:63, 1998.
466. Ortel TL, Onorato JJ, Bedrosian CL, et al: Antifibrinolytic therapy in the management of the Kasabach Merritt syndrome. *Am J Hematol* 29:44, 1988.
467. Stahl RL, Henderson JM, Hooks MA, et al: Therapy of the Kasabach-Merritt syndrome with cryoprecipitate plus intra-arterial thrombin and aminocaproic acid. *Am J Hematol* 36:272, 1991.
468. Roos YB, Vermeulen M, Rinkel GJ, et al: Systematic review of antifibrinolytic treatment in aneurysmal subarachnoid haemorrhage. *J Neurol Neurosurg Psychiatry* 65:942, 1998.
469. Ploplis VA, Carmeliet P, Vazirzadeh S, et al: Effects of disruption of the plasminogen gene on thrombosis, growth, and health in mice. *Circulation* 92:2585, 1995.
470. Carmeliet P, Stassen JM, Schoonjans L, et al: Plasminogen activator inhibitor-1 gene-deficient mice: II. Effects on hemostasis, thrombosis, and thrombolysis. *J Clin Invest* 92:2756, 1993.
471. Dewerchin M, Van Nuffelen A, Wallays G, et al: Generation and characterization of urokinase receptor-deficient mice. *J Clin Invest* 97:870, 1996.
472. Lawn RM, Wade DP, Hammer RE, et al: Atherogenesis in transgenic mice expressing human apolipoprotein(a). *Nature* 360:670, 1992.
473. Grainger DJ, Kemp PR, Liu AC, et al: Activation of transforming growth factor-beta is inhibited in transgenic apolipoprotein(a) mice. *Nature* 370:460, 1994.
474. Palabrica TM, Liu AC, Aronovitz MJ, et al: Antifibrinolytic activity of apolipoprotein(a) *in vivo*: Human apolipoprotein(a) transgenic mice are resistant to tissue plasminogen activator-mediated thrombolysis. *Nat Med* 1:256, 1995.
475. Boonmark NW, Lou XJ, Schwartz K, et al: Modification of apolipoprotein(a) lysine binding site reduces atherosclerosis in transgenic mice. *J Clin Invest* 100:558, 1997.
476. Heckel JL, Sandgren EP, Degen JL, et al: Neonatal bleeding in transgenic mice expressing urokinase-type plasminogen activator. *Cell* 62:447, 1990.
477. Meiri N, Masos T, Rosenblum K, et al: Overexpression of urokinase-type plasminogen activator in transgenic mice is correlated with impaired learning. *Proc Natl Acad Sci U S A* 91:3196, 1994.
478. Jacovina AT, Deora AB, Ling Q, et al: Homocysteine inhibits neoangiogenesis through blockade of annexin A2-dependent angiogenesis. *J Clin Invest* 119:3385, 2009.

PART XIII

Transfusion Medicine

CHAPTER 137

ERYTHROCYTE ANTIGENS AND ANTIBODIES

Marion E. Reid

SUMMARY

Blood group antigens are structures on the outer surface of human red blood cells (RBCs) that can be recognized by the immune system of individuals who lack that particular structure. Identification of RBC antigens and antibodies has been the basis of pretransfusion compatibility testing and the safe transfusion practices used today and also can provide insights into understanding the etiology of hemolytic disease of the fetus and the newborn. Biochemical and molecular studies have led to definition of the biologic functions of molecules expressing blood group antigens. These molecules play a critical role in susceptibility to infection by malarial parasites, some viruses, and bacteria. Alteration of RBC antigen expression is associated with many molecular backgrounds and some play a role in the clinical manifestations of certain diseases. Erythrocytes, far from being inert containers of hemoglobin, are active in a variety of physiologic processes.

DEFINITIONS AND HISTORY

A *blood group system* consists of a group of antigens encoded by alleles at a single gene locus or at gene loci so closely linked that crossing over does not occur or is very rare. An *antigen collection* consists of antigens that are phenotypically, biochemically, or genetically related, but the genes encoding them have not been identified.[1] Placement of a blood group antigen into a system or collection begins with the discovery of an antibody, usually in the serum of a multiparous woman or a multiply transfused recipient, with a unique pattern of reactivity. The antibody can be used to study basic biochemical properties of the corresponding antigen, to enable recognition of the pattern of inheritance of the antigen in families and in populations, to identify red blood cells (RBCs) that lack the antigen, and to search for an antithetical antigen. Identified characteristics, such as prevalence of positive reactions or sensitivity or resistance to specific enzymes, are compared to known systems and collections. A newly recognized antigen is also evaluated using biochemical and molecular genetic methods.

The majority of genes encoding blood group antigens have been cloned and sequenced,[2] and the molecular bases of most blood group antigens have been determined.[3–6] Details on the alleles associated with blood group antigens and phenotypes can be obtained from the following National Center for Biotechnology Information (NCBI) "dbRBC" website: http://www.ncbi.nlm.nih.gov/gv/mhc/xslcgi.cgi?cmd=bgmut/home.

Acronyms and abbreviations that appear in this chapter include: AET, 2-aminoethylisothiouronium bromide; CD, cluster of differentiation; DTT, dithiothreitol; GPA, glycophorin A; GPB, glycophorin B; GPC, glycophorin C; GPD, glycophorin D; GPI, glycosyl phosphatidylinositol; HDFN, hemolytic disease of the fetus and newborn; HEMPAS, hereditary erythroblastic multinuclearity with a positive acidified serum test; Ig, immunoglobulin; ISBT, International Society of Blood Transfusion; LAD, leukocyte adhesion deficiency; 2-ME, 2-mercaptoethanol; PNH, paroxysmal nocturnal hemoglobinuria; RBC, red blood cell.

RBC blood group antigens are inherited carbohydrate or protein structures located on the outside surface of the RBC membrane (Fig. 137–1). Although most of the protein blood group antigens are carried on integral transmembrane proteins (either single-pass type I or type II, or multipass; Fig. 137–1; see Chap. 15), a few are carried on glycosyl phosphatidylinositol (GPI)-linked proteins or adsorbed from plasma. Some carbohydrate antigens are attached to proteins or lipids and some require a combination of a specific portion of protein and carbohydrate. Blood group antigens have revealed that certain transmembrane proteins interact with other transmembrane proteins (e.g., band 3 and glycophorin A [GPA]; Kell and Kx; Rh and RhAG), with lipids (e.g., Rh), or with proteins in the membrane skeleton (e.g., band 3 and ankyrin, glycophorin C [GPC], and protein 4.1 and p55). Many of the proteins carrying blood group antigens reside in the erythrocyte membrane as complexes.[7–10] Many components carrying blood group antigens have been assigned cluster of differentiation (CD) numbers (Table 137–1; see Chap. 15). In human blood grouping, agglutination of RBCs usually serves as the detectable endpoint but it can also be hemolysis.[11] Our ability to detect and identify blood group antigens and antibodies has contributed significantly to current safe blood transfusion practice, reducing death from hemolytic disease of the fetus and newborn (HDFN) from 40 percent to 2 percent and supporting patients receiving chemotherapy or organ transplantation.

The naming of blood group antigens usually does not follow the classic convention wherein dominant traits are given capital letters and recessive traits are designated with lowercase letters. For example, in the ABO blood group system the recessive O phenotype is encoded by a gene designated *O*, whereas in the MNS system the genes *S* and *s* are codominant. To standardize terminology used to describe RBC blood groups, the International Society of Blood Transfusion (ISBT) Committee for Terminology for Red Cell Surface Antigens recommends using the traditional name for an antigen for verbal communication and a numerical system in computer databases (see Blood Group Terminology website at http://ibgrl.blood.co.uk/). The committee has placed blood group antigens into four categories: (1) genetically discrete blood group systems; (2) serologically, biochemically, or genetically related antigens in blood group collections; (3) series of low-incidence antigens; and (4) series of high-incidence antigens. Each system and collection has been given a number and letter designation, and each antigen within the system is numbered sequentially in order of discovery. To date, 30 blood group systems and 6 antigen collections are defined (see Table 137–1).[1,5,6,12–14] Over time, notations devised to describe blood group antigens have changed. A single letter (e.g., A, D, K), a symbol with a superscript (e.g., Fy^a, JK^b, Lu^a), a symbol with a number (e.g., Fy3, Lu4, K12), and three to four letters (e.g., VEL, LAN, FPPT) are all used, sometimes within the same blood group system.

BLOOD GROUP SYSTEMS

Tables 137–1 and 137–2 summarize the characteristics of common blood group antigens. The following sources provide more detail: Issitt and Anstee,[5] Reid and Lomas-Francis,[6,15] Mollison and colleagues,[16] Daniels,[4] and Roback and associates.[11] In the interest of space, reviews or books are referenced in place of original reports.

■ ABO BLOOD GROUP SYSTEM

The ABO blood group system was the first system described and remains the most significant in transfusion medicine. A mismatch of ABO may be fatal, whereas a mismatch of other blood groups initially is harmless. This situation occurs because anti-A and anti-B antibodies

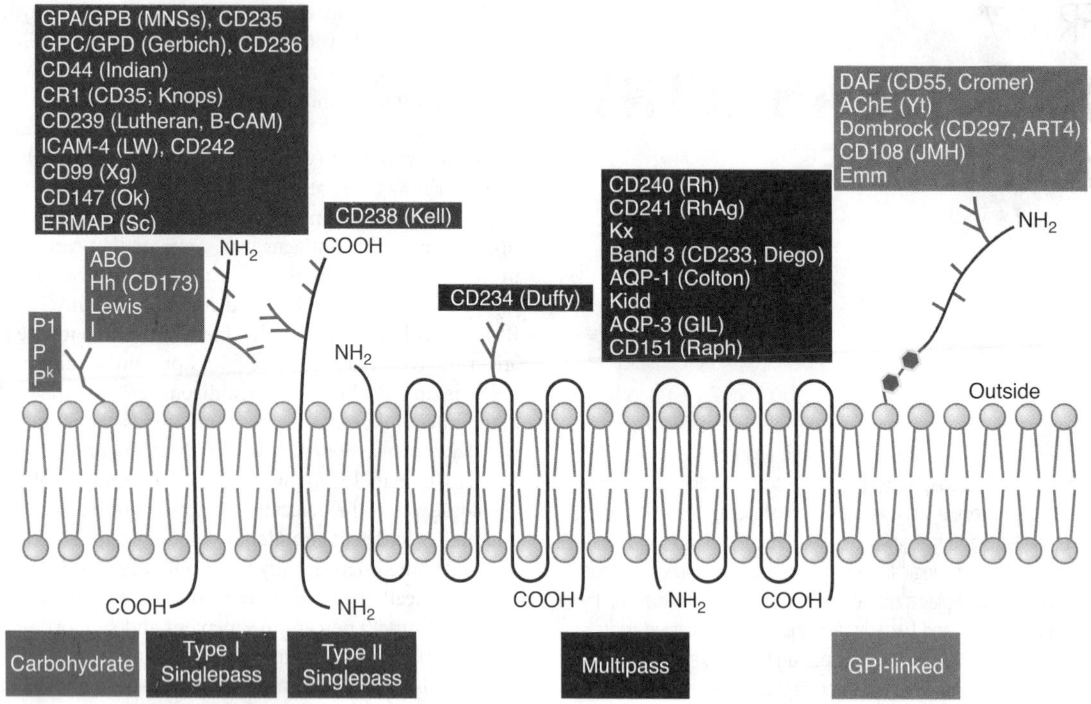

FIGURE 137–1. Membrane structures carrying blood group activity.

usually are present in the blood of adults lacking the corresponding antigen. These antibodies are stimulated by the ubiquitous distribution of the antigen that forms part of the membrane structure of many bacteria, plants, and animals. For this reason, all donor blood for transfusion is tested and labeled with the ABO group. The four main phenotypes are A, B, AB, and O, the latter indicating a lack of A and B antigens. The sugars defining A and B antigens are added to carbohydrate chains carrying the H antigen (fucose), which is "hidden" by the A (GalNAc) or B (Gal) sugar. Thus, group A or B erythrocytes appear to have less H antigen than group O cells. Nonetheless, H is found on all human erythrocytes except those from rare individuals of the O_h (Bombay) phenotype.

Anti-A or anti-B immunoglobulins can cause intravascular hemolysis when ABO-incompatible RBCs are transfused. Because A and B antigens also are expressed on most tissue cells, ABO compatibility is a significant consideration in solid-organ transplantation. However, ABO incompatibility only rarely causes severe HDFN because antibodies directed against A and B antigens are predominantly immunoglobulin (Ig) M, which do not cross the placenta, and A and B antigens are not fully developed on RBCs from a fetus (see Chap. 54).

Although the ABO blood group system has only four phenotypes, more than 200 alleles have been identified by DNA analyses. The *ABO* gene was cloned in 1990 following purification of A transferase.[17,18] A and B transferases have only four amino acid differences in the catalytic domain, two of which (Leu266Met and Gly268Ala) are primarily responsible for substrate specificity.[19] The group O phenotype results from mutations in A and/or B alleles that cause loss of glycosyltransferase activity. The most common group O (O_1) results from a single nucleotide deletion near the 5′ end of the gene that causes a frameshift and early termination with no active enzyme production.[20] The *ABO* gene has seven exons, and A or B subgroups (with only few exceptions) result from a variety of nucleotide changes in exon 7 that cause alterations in the catalytic domain of the glycosyltransferase (reviewed by Chester and Olsson[21]). The rare B(A), A(B), and *cis*-AB phenotypes expressing both A and B antigens result from variant glycosyltransferases that have a combination of A- and B-specific residues.[21] Numerous common and rare *ABO* alleles have been reported, and current information is available on the blood group antigen gene mutation database website: http://www.ncbi.nlm.nih.gov/gv/mhc/xslcgi.cgi?cmd=bgmut/home. In addition to nucleotide changes, recombinations and gene rearrangements can result in hybrids with unexpected activity of the transferase. This situation makes typing of ABO by DNA analysis difficult to interpret.[22] The function of the ABO system is not known, although several disease associations are well established.[23]

■ Rh BLOOD GROUP SYSTEM

The Rh (*not* Rhesus) system is the second most important blood group system in transfusion medicine because antigen-positive RBCs frequently immunize antigen-negative individuals through transfusion and pregnancy.

Inheritance of Rh antigens is determined by a complex of two closely linked genes: one encodes the protein carrying D antigen (RhD); the other encodes the protein carrying C or c and E or e antigens (RhCE). RBCs from Rh-positive people have both RhD and RhCE, whereas Rh-negative RBCs have only RhCE. In the Rh system, eight common antigen combinations or haplotypes are possible: Dce (R_0, Rh_0), DCe (R_1, Rh_1), DcE (R_2, Rh_2), DCE (R_Z, Rh_z), ce (r, rh), Ce (r′, rh′), cE (r″, rh″), and CE (ry, rhy). The letter "d" is commonly used to designate the lack of D, but there is no d antigen or anti-d.

Several nomenclatures can be used to describe Rh genes and antigens. The Fisher-Race nomenclature, which uses CDE terminology, is more commonly used for antigens; the Wiener nomenclature, which uses Rh designations, is favored for haplotypes and gene complexes; and the Rosenfield and Rubinstein nomenclature, which uses numerical designations, was introduced to allow analyses without bias.[24]

The Rh blood group system has 50 antigens (ABO has 4). By far the most important and immunogenic antigen is D (Rh_0 in Weiner terminology, referring to Weiner's discovery that a rhesus monkey injected with human RBCs would produce antibody that agglutinated 85% of white

TABLE 137–1. International Society of Blood Transfusion Defined Blood Group Systems and Antigen Collections with Chromosome and Gene

Conventional Name	ISBT Symbol (No.)	Chromosome Location	ISBT Gene Name (ISGN If Different)	Associated Antigens [Null Phenotype]	Function of RBC Membrane Component (CD No.)	Disease Association
Blood Group Systems						
ABO	ABO (001)	9q34.2	*ABO*	A, B, A, B, A1 [group O]	Glycocalyx	Altered expression in some hematologic disorders
MNS	MNS (002)	4q31.21	*MNS (GYPA, GYPB)*	M, N, S, s, U, He, Mi^a, Vw, M^c, Mur, M^g, Vr, Mt^a St^a, Ri^a, Cl^a, and 29 more [En(a–); U–; M^k M^k]	Binds microbe glycocalyx, complement regulation, chaperone for band 3 (CD235)	Decreased *Plasmodium falciparum* invasion, may be receptor for *Escherichia coli*
P	PI (003)	22q11.2-qter	*P1*	P1	Glycocalyx	
Rh	RH (004)	1p36.11	*RHD, RHCE (RH)*	D, C, E, e, e, f, C^w, C^x, V, G, hr^s, VS, D^w, Rh29, Go^a, hr^B, Rh32, Rh33, and 32 more [Rh$_{null}$]	Possibly transports CO_2 or NH_3 (CD240)	Hemolytic anemia, hereditary stomatocytosis, hematologic malignancies
Lutheran	LU (005)	19q13.2	*LU*	Lu^a, Lu^b, Lu3, Lu4, Lu5, Lu6, Lu7, Lu8, Lu9, Lu11, Lu12, Lu13, and 7 more [recessive Lu(a–b–)]	Binds laminin (CD239)	Increased expressions possibly involved in vasoocclusion in sickle cell disease
Kell	KEL (006)	7q34	*KEL*	K, k, Kp^a, Kp^b, Ku, Js^a, Js^b, and 23 more [K$_0$ or K$_{null}$]	Cleaves big endothelin-3 to ET-3, a potent vasoconstrictor (CD238)	
Lewis	LE (007)	19p13.3	*LE (FUT3)*	Le^a, Le^b, Le^{ab}, Le^{bh}, ALe^b, BLe^b [Le(a–b–)]	Glycocalyx, Le^b is receptor for *Helicobacter pylori*	Increased expression in fucosidosis, Lewis antibodies may be important in graft rejection
Duffy	FY (008)	1q23.2	*FY (DARC)*	Fy^a, Fy^b, Fy3, Fy4, Fy5, Fy6 [Fy(a–b–)]	Chemokine, *Plasmodium vivax* receptor (CD234)	Resistance to *P. vivax* invasion
Kidd	JK (009)	18q12.3	*JK(HUT11, SLC4AI)*	Jk^a, Jk^b, Jk3 [Jk(a–b–)]	Urea transporter	Impaired urea transport, urine concentrating defect
Diego	DI (010)	17q21.31	*DI (SLC4A1; AE1)*	Di^a, Di^b, Wr^a, Wr^b, Wd^a, Rb^a, and 14 more	Anion exchanger (CD233), Band 3 cytoskeletal protein	Southeast Asian ovalocytosis, hereditary spherocytosis, renal tubular acidosis
Yt	YT(O11)	7q22	*Yt (ACHE)*	Yt^a, Yt^b	Acetylcholinesterase	Absent from PNH III RBCs
Xg	XG (012)	Xp22.33	*XG (XG, MIC2)*	Xg^a, CD99	Adhesion molecules (CD99)	
Scianna	SC (013)	1p34.2	*SC (ERMAP)*	Sc1, Sc2, Sc3, Rd [Sc: –1, –2, –3]	Possible adhesion	
Dombrock	DO (014)	12p12.3	*DO (ART4)*	Do^a, Do^b, Gy, Hy, Jo^a [Gy(a–)]	Enzymatic (CD297)	Absent from PNH III RBCs
Colton	CO (015)	7p14	*CO (AQP1)*	Co^a, Co^b, Co3 [Co(a–b–)]	Water transport	Monosomy 7, inability to maximally concentrate urine, congenital dyserythropoietic anemia
Landsteiner-Wiener	LW (016)	19p13.2	*LW (IC AM)*	LW^a, LW^{ab}, LW^b [LW(a–b–)]	Binds CD11/CD18, ligand for integrins (CD242)	Depressed in pregnancy and some malignant diseases
Chido/Rogers	CH/RG (017)	6p21.32	*C4A,C4B*	CH1, CH2, Rgl, and Rg6 more	Complement components	Certain phenotypes have increased susceptibility to certain autoimmune conditions and infections
H	Hh (018)	19q13.33	*H (FUT1)*	H [Bombay, Oh]	Glycocalyx (CD 173)	Decreased in some tumor cells, increased in hematopoietic stress

(continued)

TABLE 137–1. International Society of Blood Transfusion Defined Blood Group Systems and Antigen Collections with Chromosome and Gene (Continued)

Conventional Name	ISBT Symbol (No.)	Chromosome Location	ISBT Gene Name (ISGN If Different)	Associated Antigens [Null Phenotype]	Function of RBC Membrane Component (CD No.)	Disease Association
Kx	XK (019)	Xp21.1	*XK*	Kx [McLeod]	Possible neurotransmitter, function in RBCs not known	Acanthocytosis, muscular dystrophy, hemolytic anemia; McLeod syndrome sometimes associated with CGD, peripheral neuropathy, cardiomyopathy seizures, a late-onset dementia, and behavioral changes
Gerbich	GE (020)	2q14.3	*GE (GYPC)*	Ge2, Ge3, Ge4, Wb, Ls^a, An^a, Dh^a [Leach phenotype]	Membrane attachment; interacts with 4.1R and p55 (CD236)	Hereditary elliptocytosis, hemolytic anemia, decreased 4.1R and p55
Cromer	CROM (021)	1q32.2	*CROM (DAF)*	Cr^a, Tc^a, Tc^b, Tc^c, Dr^a, Es^a, IFC, WES^a, WES^b, UMC, GUTI, SERF, CROV, CRAM [Inab phenotype]	Complement regulation, binds C3b, disassembles C3/C5 convertase (CD55)	Absent from PNH III RBCs, Dr^a is the receptor for uropathogenic *E. coli*
Knops	KN (022)	1q32.2	*KN (CR1)*	Kn^a, Kn^b, McC^a, Sl^a, Yk^a, McC^b, Vil, S13, KCAM [Helgeson phenotype]	Complement regulation, binds C3b and C4b, mediates phagocytosis (CD35)	Antigens depressed in certain autoimmune and malignant conditions
Indian	IN (023)	11p13	*IN (CD44)*	In^a, In$_b$, INFI, INJA	Binds hyaluronic acid, mediates adhesion of leukocytes (CD44)	Depressed in pregnancy, congenital dyserythropoietic anemia
Ok	Ok (024)	19p13.3	*OK (BSB)*	Ok^a	Possible adhesion (CD147)	
Raph	RAPH (025)	11p15.5	*MER2 (CD151)*	MER2 [Raph–]	Adhesion molecule involved in kidney function (CD151)	Renal disease
JMH	JMH (026)	15q24.1	*JMH (SEMA–L)*	JMH, JMHK, JMHL, JMKG, JMKM	Adhesion molecule, function in RBCs not known (CD108)	Absent from PNH III RBCs
I	I (027)	6p24.2	*IGNT*	I [I–; i adult]	Glycocalyx	Congenital cataracts in Asians
GLOB	Globoside (028)	3q26.1	*P (β3GALNT1)*	P [P–]	Glycocalyx	Receptor *E. coli* and parvovirus B19
Gil	GIL (029)	9p13.3	*GIL (AQP3)*	GIL [GIL–]	Glycerol/water/urea transporter	
RhAg	RHAG (030)	6p11.21.1	*RHAG*	Duclos, Os^a, DSLK	Possibly transports CO_2, or NH_3 (CD241)	Hemolytic anemia, hereditary stomatocytosis
Antigen Collections						
Cost	COST (205)	–	–	Cs^a, Cs^b		
Ii	Ii (207)	–	–	i		
Er	ER (208)	–	–	Er^a, Er^b		
(P^k, LKE)	GLOB (209)	–	–	P^k, LKE		
(Lewis-like: Le^c, Le^d)	Unnamed: (210)	–	–	Le^c, Le^d		
Vel	VEL			Vel, ABTI		
Low incidence series	– (700)	–	–	14		
High incidence series	– (901)	–	–	2		

CGD, chronic granulomatous disease; ISGN, International Society for Gene Nomenclature.

SOURCE: Daniels GL, Anstee DJ, Cartron J-P, et al,[13] Issitt PD, Anstee DJ,[5] and Reid ME, Lomas-Francis C.[6,15]

TABLE 137–2. Summary of Common Blood Group Systems or Collections and Their Antigen

Blood Group (Year Reported)	Common Phenotypes	Frequency White/ Black (%)	No. Antigen Copies on Adult RBC × 10^3	Dosage (See Text)	Cord Cell Expression	Biochemistry	Antigen Distribution in Blood, Fluids, and Tissues	Comments
ABO (1901)	A B AB	40/27 11/20 4/4	AB: ~800–1000	A/B: not evident	Weak: ~1/3 adult expression	Carbohydrate on types 1, 2, 3, and 4 precursor chains	RBC, lymphs, plts	Most significant antigens in transfusion and transplantation
H (1948)	O	45/29	H: ~1700	H expression depends on ABO: O>A_2>B>A_2B>A_1>A_1B	Main RBC carrier: bands 3 and 4.5	Attached to lipids in plasma and protein in secretions	Plasma, secretions; broad tissue distribution; most epithelial/endothelial cells	Weak subgroups result from variant transferases
Rh (1940)	R_1 Dce r ce R_2 DcE R_0 Dce r′ Ce r″ cE R_z DCE r^y CE	42/17 37/26 14/11 4/44 2/2 1/0 <1 <1	D on R_2R_2: 15–33 R_1R_1: 14–19 R_0r: 12–20 R_1r: 9–14 c on cc: 70–85 Cc: 37–53 e on ee: 18–24 Ee: 13–14	D: not evident C and c: yes E and e: yes	Normal adult	Multipass, nonglycosylated protein: 30–32 kDa; 417 aa C: serine 103/c: proline 103 E: proline 226/e: alanine 226 Forms "Rh complex" with LW, GPB, and Rh-related glycoprotein (chromosome 6)	Possible cation transport Possible role in RBC membrane integrity	D most significant antigen after A and B Three causes for weak D expression (see text) Nulls: amorphic type and regulator type
Lewis (1946)	Le(a+b–) Le(a–b+) Le(a–b–) Le(a+b+)	22/23 72/55 6/22 Rare	Le^a: ~3	Not evident	Weak: adult expression at age 2 years	Carbohydrate on type 1 precursor chains only Attached to lipids in plasma and protein in secretions	Plasma and secretion antigen; on RBC, lymphs, plts only by adsorption of plasma antigen	Le antigens depend on *Le/Se* interaction; *Le/Se* = Le(a–b+), ABH secretor; *Lel/sese* = Le(a+b–), ABH nonsecretor; *lele* = Le(a–b–), Sese status not apparent Le(a–b+) express some Le^a, do not make anti-Le^a Women test Le(a–b–) during pregnancy
I (1956)	I adult(↑↑I↓i) I_{int} (↑I↓i) i cord (↓I↑i) i adult (↓I↑↑i)	Common Rare Common <1:10,000	I: ~500	Not evident	Strong i; weak I. Adult expressions at age 2 years	Carbohydrate on ABH active chains; lipid on RBC; protein in plasma	Broad tissue distribution; RBCs, plts, lymphs, granules, monos; also in plasma, secretions (e.g., milk, saliva, urine)	I and i expression are inversely proportional but not products of alleles
P1 (1927)	P_1: P^k+P+P_1+	79/94	P1: ~500	Not evident, but inherited variations exist; e.g., P_1 may be normal, strong, or weak	Weak: adult expression by 7 years	Carbohydrate on RBC and plasma glycolipids; not in secretions	RBC, lymphs, plts, monos, fibroblasts, uroepithelial cells	P1-like antigen is associated with pigeon and earthworm protein and parasitic infections

(*continued*)

TABLE 137–2. Summary of Common Blood Group Systems or Collections and Their Antigen (Continued)

Blood Group (Year Reported)	Common Phenotypes	Frequency White/ Black (%)	No. Antigen Copies on Adult RBC × 10^3	Dosage (See Text)	Cord Cell Expression	Biochemistry	Antigen Distribution in Blood, Fluids, and Tissues	Comments
GLOB (1951)	P_2: P^k+P+P_1–	21/6	Globoside: ~15,000					
	p: P^k–P–P_1–	Rare						
	P_1^k:P^k+P–P_1+	Rarer						
	P_2^k: P^k+P–P_1–	Rarest						
MNS	M+N–	28/26	GPA: ~800	Yes	Normal adult	Single-pass sialoglycoprotein type 1	RBCs plus renal capillary epithelial/ endothelium	GPA and GPB carry multiple antigens and many hybrids of GPA–GPB
(M: 1927)	M+N+	50/44	GPB: ~200			GPA: 43 kDa, 131 aa, carries MN		
	M–N+	22/30						
(S: 1947)	S+s–	11/3				GPB: 25 kDa, 72 aa, carries SsU; part of Rh complex		Can have absence of GPA, GPB, or both
	S+s+	44/28						
	S–s+	45/69						
	S–s–U–	0/<1						
Kell(1946)	K–k+	91/98	Kell: 2–6	Yes	Normal adult	Single-pass glycoprotein type II highly folded with S = S bonds: 93	Kell: RBC plus marrow and fetal liver tissue; not on brain, kidney, adult liver	System of high- and low-frequency antigens
(Kp^a/Js^a: 1957)	K+k+	8.8/2				K/k Met 193 Thr	Kx: RBC plus skeletal/ heart muscle, neurologic tissues	Common phenotype: k, Kp^b, Js^b
	K+k–	0.2/rare				Kp^a/Kp^b: Trp 281 Arg		Kell antigen expression depends on both Kell and Xk genes
	Kp(a–b+)	97.7/100				kDa, 732 aa		
	Kp(a+b+)	2.3/rare				Js^a/Js^b: Pro 597 Leu		K_{null} lacks Kell antigens, has Kx
	Kp(a+b–)	Rare/O						Kx_{null} lacks Kx, has poor Kell antigen expression (McLeod phenotype)
	Js(a–b+)	100/80						
	Js(a+b+)	Rare/19						Other causes of poor Kell expression: *cis* Kp^a, Ge-, K_{mod}, autoantibody
	Js(a+b–)	0/1						
Duffy (1950)	Fy(a+b–)	17/9	Fy^a: 6–13	Yes, but not always evident because of *Fy* gene	Normal: adult levels at 12 weeks	Multipass glycoprotein: 35–45 kDa, 338 aa	RBC plus brain, colon, lung, spleen, thyroid, thymus, kidney, endothelium; not in liver or placenta tissue	Fy(a–b–) blacks do not express Fy^b on their RBC, but express it on other tissues and seldom make anti-Fy^b
	Fy(a+b+)	49/1						
	Fy(a–b+)	34/22				Fy^a/Fy^b Gly 42Asp		
	Fy(a–b–)	Rare/68						
Kidd (1951)	Jk(a+b–)	28/57	Jk^a: ~14	Yes	Normal adult	Multipass protein: ~43 kDa, 391 aa 1 potential *N*-glycan Jk^a/Jk^b: Asp284 Asn	RBC specific	Important cause of DHTR
	Jk(a+b+)	49/34						Nulls are unable to fully concentrate urine; dominant inhibitor *In(Jk)* has weak Jk antigen
	Jk(a–b+)	23/9						
	Jk(a–b–)	<1% Polynesians						

Lutheran (1951)	Lu(a+b−) Lu(a+b+) Lu(a−b+) Lu(a−b−)	0.15/− 7.5/0 92.3/− Very rare	Lu^b: 1.5–4	Yes, but family variations exist	Weak: adult level at 15 years	Single-pass glycoprotein type I: 85 kDa, 597 aa 78 kDa 5 Ig superfamily domains: two variable, three constant B-CAM Lu^a/Lu^b: His77Arg	RBC plus brain, heart, kidney, lung, pancreas, placenta, skeletal muscle	System of high- and low-frequency antigens Dominant inhibitor *In(Lu)* and X-linked inhibitor *(XS2)* have weak Lu antigens First known autosomal linkage to *Se*

aa, amino acids; B-CAM, B cell adhesion molecule; DHTR, delayed hemolytic transfusion reactions; GPA, glycophorin A; GPB, glycophorin B; granulos, granulocytes; Ig, immunoglobulin; ISBT, International Society of Blood Transfusion; lymphs, lymphocytes; monos, monocytes; plts, platelets; RBC, red blood cell.

New Yorkers). For most clinical purposes, testing individuals for the D antigen and classifying them as D+ (or Rh-positive), or D– or (Rh-negative) is sufficient. Approximately 85 percent of the white population is Rh-positive, and 15 percent is Rh-negative. Most Rh-negative recipients produce anti-D if they receive Rh-positive blood. Anti-D can cause hemolysis in adults following an Rh-mismatched transfusion and in the newborn (HDFN) if antibodies were made by the mother from a prior transfusion or pregnancy. Thus, donors and recipients are routinely typed and matched for D. The risk of anti-D sensitization by transfusion is essentially eliminated by matching. The risk of anti-D sensitization in pregnancy is minimized by passive immunization of mothers at risk against D.

The antigens C, c, E, and e are less immunogenic and become important in patient care only after the corresponding antibody develops or when the basic Rh haplotype must be determined. The remaining 40+ antigens are other Rh protein epitopes whose corresponding antibodies are seldom encountered. Some are encoded by variant Rh alleles and appear as antithetical antigens to C, c, E, or e, or as related "extra" antigens. Others are referred to as *compound* antigens or *cis* gene products. For example, the protein produced by the gene *ce* encodes c, e, and f (or ce) antigen. Other compound specificities include Ce (rh^{i}), cE, CE, V (ce^{s}), and Ce^{s}. Still other Rh antigens are related to the complex "mosaic" nature of D and e antigens. If immunized, individuals who lack a part of D or e and who make antibody to the portion they lack, can present with a challenging serologic picture. For example, the D+ person who lacks part of the D epitope and makes an antibody to the missing portion appears to make alloanti-D because normal D+ RBCs carry all D epitopes.[25]

Some, but not all, individuals who lack part of the D antigen (partial D) have weak expression of D on their red cells that is detected only by the antiglobulin test. Having a *C* gene in transposition to a *D* gene (e.g., *Dce/Ce* or *DCe/Ce* genotypes) also can weaken expression of D in some individuals. A third type of weak D expression results from inheriting a *D* gene that encodes all epitopes of D, but in less-than-normal quantity.

DNA analyses have revealed the molecular basis underlying antigens and phenotypes in the Rh blood group system. A list of the alleles that have been described to date is available at: http://www.ncbi.nlm.nih.gov/gv/mhc/xslcgi.cgi?cmd=bgmut/home. Rh blood group orthologs are present in nonhuman primates and other species on the evolutionary tree.[26] Rh functions as a CO_2 or an ammonium transporter.

OTHER BLOOD GROUP SYSTEMS

In terms of transfusion and HDFN, the other blood group systems and their antigens become important only when antibody develops. Transfusion service laboratories identify (antibody identification) the specificity and characterize the reactivity of antibodies detected in routine testing (antibody screening). Once this information is known, the blood bank assesses the clinical significance of the antibody and selects the most appropriate blood for transfusion. Tables 137–1 and 137–2 summarize the number of antigens in each blood group system and other relevant information. A detailed description of all the blood group antigens is beyond the scope of this chapter. Because the molecular bases of most blood group antigens and phenotypes are known,[6] DNA analysis can be used to predict the type of transfused patients and to identify the fetus at risk for HDFN.[27]

GENERAL IMMUNOLOGY OF BLOOD GROUP ANTIGENS

An *antigen* is a substance that can evoke an immune response when introduced into an immunocompetent host and react with the antibody produced from that immune response. Its structure and stereochemical fit with its antibody specificity. An antigen can have several *epitopes*, or *antigenic determinants*, each of which is capable of eliciting an antibody response.

The ability of an antigen to stimulate an immune response is called *immunogenicity*, and its ability to react with an antibody is called *antigenicity*. These primary characteristics are affected by antigen size, shape, rigidity, and the number and location of the determinants on the red cell membrane.

IMMUNOGENICITY

Immunogenicity depends on many antigen characteristics, not just the number of antigen sites. Relative immunogenicity is estimated by comparing the actual observed incidence of an antibody to the calculated likelihood of a possible immunizing event. Although numbers vary, researchers agree that after A and B, the D antigen is most immunogenic (approximately 80% of Rh-negative individuals produce anti-D after receiving a single Rh-positive RBC component), followed by K, which stimulates anti-K in approximately 10 percent of cases.[16] The antigens c and E are one-third as immunogenic; Fy^{a} is one-twenty-fifth as potent; and Jk^{a} is one-fiftieth to one-one hundredth times as potent as K.[28] It should be noted that immunogenicity does not always correlate with the hemolytic potential of an antibody specificity; for example, K is more immunogenic than Jk^{a} but anti-Jk^{a} is more likely to cause hemolysis.

ANTIGEN EXPRESSION

NUMBER OF ANTIGEN SITES

The number of antigen sites per RBC has been estimated by measuring the uptake of ^{125}I-labeled antibody or of ferritin-conjugated anti-IgG. Numbers vary widely among blood group systems from a few hundred to over a million (see Table 137–2).

ANTIGEN DEVELOPMENT ON FETAL ERYTHROCYTES

Most RBC antigens can be detected early in fetal development (A, B, and H antigens can be detected at 5–6 weeks' gestation), but not all are fully developed at birth. A, B, H, I, P1, Lu^{a}, Lu^{b}, Yt^{a}, Xg^{a}, Vel, Bg, Knops, and Dombrock antigen expression is considerably weaker on cord RBCs than on RBCs from adults. Le^{a}, sometimes Le^{b}, Ch/Rg, AnWj, and Sd^{a}, are not readily detectable, although 50 percent of cord samples type Le(a+) with more sensitive test methods. Full expression of A, B, H, I, and Lewis antigens usually is present by age 3 years, whereas full expression of P1 and Lutheran antigens may not occur until age 7 years.

VARIATION IN ANTIGEN EXPRESSION

RBCs from individuals who are homozygous for an allele typically have a greater number of antigen sites than do RBCs from individuals who are heterozygous. Consequently, their RBCs can react more strongly with antibody. This difference in expression and antigen–antibody reactivity because of zygosity is known as *dosage*. For example, RBCs from a homozygous *MM* individual carry a double dose of M antigen and react more strongly with anti-M than do RBCs from a *MN* heterozygous individual carrying only a single dose of M. Antithetical antigens C/c, E/e, M/N, S/s, and Jk^{a}/Jk^{b} commonly show dosage effect. Dosage is less obvious with D, K/k, and Lu^{a}/Lu^{b} antigens. It typically is more apparent within a family than between families. Dosage within the Duffy system also may not be serologically obvious because Fy(a+b–) or Fy(a–b+) phenotypes are seen in either homozygous (*Fy^{a}Fy^{a}* or *Fy^{b}Fy^{b}*) or hemizygous (*Fy^{a}Fy* or *Fy^{b}Fy*) individuals.

Some blood group antigens are inherited as closely linked genes or haplotypes. Haplotype pairings and gene interaction (either *cis* or *trans*) also can affect phenotypic expression. For example, the pairing of *C* in *trans* position to *D* can result in weak expression of D (see "Rh Blood Group System" above), whereas *E* in *cis* position with *D* is associated with strong expression of D. Among the common phenotypes, R_2R_2 RBCs carry the strongest expression of D. In the Kell system, *Kp*^{a} is associated with weakened expression of *in cis k* and *Js*^{b}.

Still other antigens are affected by regulator genes.[29] *In(Lu)* is a dominant inhibitor gene (*EKLF*) that suppresses expression of Lutheran, P1, i, and many other antigens.[30] The dominant inhibitor *In(Jk)* suppresses expression of Jk^a and Jk^b antigens.[31] Rare variants of the *RHAG* gene depress or prevent expression of the Rh antigens (see "Rh$_{null}$ Syndrome" below).

BIOCHEMISTRY OF ERYTHROCYTE ANTIGENS

An antibody typically recognizes an epitope consisting of four to five amino acids on linear proteins or one to seven sugars. Alternatively, the antibody-binding site may encompass a more complex three-dimensional structure with branches or folds, and recognition may depend on both amino acids and sugars. Tables 137–2 and 137–3 and Figure 137–1 summarize blood group biochemistry and antigen structure.[4,6,16]

CARBOHYDRATE ANTIGENS

Polysaccharides with blood group activity are made by sequential addition of specific sugars (or sugar derivatives) to specific precursors in specific linkages by specific transferases. Sugars commonly involved are galactose (Gal), *N*-acetyl-D-galactosamine (GalNAc), *N*-acetylglucosamine (GlcNAc), fucose (Fuc), and *N*-acetylneuraminic acid (NeuAc).

ABO, Lewis, and P blood group specificity depends on an immunodominant sugar, usually terminally located, the polysaccharide to which the sugar is attached, and the type of linkage involved. I/i specificity is defined by a series of sugars on the inner portion of ABH saccharide chains. The presence of at least two repeating Gal(β14)GlcNAc(β13)Gal units in a linear structure defines i activity. I activity involves these same sugars in branched form (see Table 137–3). The *I* gene encodes the transferase responsible for branching (β[1–6]glucosaminyltransferase). During the first years of a child's life, linear chains are modified into branched chains, resulting in the appearance of I antigens.[32] The i antigen is reduced on RBCs from fetuses and infants. A rare i phenotype occurs in adults (see "I-Negative Phenotype [i Adult]" below).

Polysaccharide chains are attached to glycoproteins in secretions (on type 2 chains), to glycolipids in plasma (on type 1 chains), and to both on the RBC membrane. Approximately 70 percent of A, B, H, and I antigens on the RBC membrane are carried on glycoproteins, primarily on the anion transporter, but also on the glucose transporter, the Rh glycoprotein, and others. Approximately 10 percent of these antigens are on NeuAc-rich glycoproteins, 5 percent on simple glycolipids, and the remainder on polyglycosylceramide.[16] P, P^k, and P1 antigens are found on glycolipids both on the membrane and in plasma.[33]

Lewis antigens are unique because they occur only on type 1 polysaccharide chains, which are found in plasma and secretions but not made by RBC. Hence, they exist on RBCs only by adsorption of Lewis substance from plasma. The *Le* (or *FUT3)* gene encodes an α(1–4)fucosyltransferase. Whether the resulting antigen is Le^a or Le^b depends on the secretor gene *Se* (or *FUT2*), which encodes an α(1–2)fucosyltransferase.

PROTEIN ANTIGENS

Protein structures that carry blood group antigens can be grouped into three categories: (1) those that make a single pass through the erythrocyte membrane, (2) those that make multiple passes through the membrane, and (3) those that are attached to the membrane through a covalent linkage to lipid (GPI-linked; see Fig. 137–1 and Chap. 15).

Single-pass proteins (type 1) include GPA with M and N antigens, glycophorin B (GPB) with S, s, and U antigens, glycophorins C (GPC) and D (GPD) with Gerbich antigens, and the proteins encoded by Lutheran, LW, Indian, Knops, Xg, Ok, and Scianna genes. These proteins have an extracellular amino-terminus and an intracellular carboxyl-terminus (referred to as *type I*). In contrast, the Kell glycoprotein has an extracellular carboxyl-terminus and an intracellular amino-terminus (referred to as *type II*).

Most proteins that carry blood group antigens and make multiple passes through the erythrocyte membrane have both carboxyl- and amino-terminal ends that are intracellular, are hydrophobic, and have a transport function. Rh, RhAg, Diego, Colton, Kidd, Kx, GIL, and Raph proteins are included in this category. The product of the Duffy gene also is a multipass protein, but it has an extracellular amino-terminus and homology with a family of cytokine receptors.[34]

Lipid-linked proteins have their carboxyl-terminus attached to the lipid GPI and are said to be GPI linked or anchored. Cromer, Yt, Dombrock, and JMH proteins belong to this category. GPI-linked proteins are of special interest to hematologists because defective synthesis of the GPI anchor is responsible for paroxysmal nocturnal hemoglobinuria (PNH).[35] Thus, PNH-III RBCs lack all proteins attached by a GPI anchor, including those carrying blood groups (see Chap. 40).

EFFECT OF ENZYMES AND OTHER CHEMICALS ON ERYTHROCYTE ANTIGENS

Expression of an RBC antigen is determined by its exposure as a result of its position on the cell surface and its biochemical structure. Expression can be modified with treatment of RBCs by enzymes and other chemicals. These reagents are used to help identify complex mixtures of antibodies and to help characterize antibody specificity when identity is not readily apparent.

Proteolytic enzymes, such as ficin, papain, bromelin, trypsin, and α-chymotrypsin, cleave proteins from the erythrocyte membrane at specific amino acids. Enzyme treatment of RBCs cleaves certain protein antigens and allows carbohydrate and other protected protein antigens to react more strongly with their antibody. The reactivity of antibodies to A, B, H, I, P1, Lewis, Rh, and Kidd antigens is enhanced after enzyme treatment of the RBCs, whereas reactivity of antibodies to M, N, Fy^a, Fy^b, and many minor antigens (Xg^a, Ch, Rg, JMH, Indian, Pr, Tn, Ge2, Ge4, and some examples of Yt^a) is reduced or eliminated. S and s are variably affected by enzyme treatment, and Kell and Lutheran antigens are relatively unaffected.[4–6]

Reagents that reduce disulfide bonds, such as 2-mercaptoethanol (2-ME), dithiothreitol (DTT), and 2-aminoethylisothiouronium bromide (AET), denature Kell blood group antigens but enhance Kx. Reducing reagents also denature the minor antigens LW, Scianna, Indian, JMH, and Yt^a and weaken Lutheran, Dombrock, Cromer, Knops, AnWj, and MER2 antigens.[4–6]

Acid treatment of RBCs, which is frequently used to remove IgG from RBCs, can weaken or completely denature antigens in the Kell blood group system. Chloroquine treatment of erythrocytes (also sometimes used to remove IgG from RBCs) at room temperature has little effect on most antigens. However, treatment for 30 minutes at 37°C (98.6°F) can weaken expression of many antigens, including Fy^b, Lu^b, Yt^a, JMH, and those in the Rh, Dombrock, and Knops systems.

GENETICS OF ERYTHROCYTE ANTIGENS

Protein antigens are direct gene products: The gene encodes a protein that expresses one or more antigens. Carbohydrate antigens, made by

TABLE 137–3. Biochemistry of Common Carbohydrate and Antigens on Glycophorin A

Specificity	Structure	Gene for Bolded Determinant
i	**–Gal(β1→4)GlcNAc(β1→3)Gal(β1→4)GLcNAc**(β1→3)Gal–R–	
I	–Gal(β1→4)**GLcNAc(β1→6)** –Gal(β1→4)GlcNAc(β1→3) (both linked to) **Gal(β1→4)GlcNAc**(β1→3)Gal–R	*IGNT*
H	Gal(β1→4 or β1→3)GlcNAc(β1→3)Gal–R | **Fuc(α1→2)**	*H (FUTI)*
A	**GalNAc(α1→3)**Gal(β1→4 or β1→3)GlcNAc(β1→3)Gal–R | Fuc(α1→2)	*A*
B	**Gal(α1→3)**Gal(β1→4 or β1→3)GlcNAc(β1→3)Gal–R | Fuc(α1→2)	*B*
Le^a	Gal(β1→3)GlcNAc(β1→3)Gal–R | **Fuc(α1→4)**	*LE (FUT3)*
Le^b	Gal(β1→3)GlcNAc(β1→3)Gal–R | | **Fuc(α1→2)Fuc(α1→4)**	*SE (FUT2)*
P	Gal(α1→4)Gal(β1→4)Glc-Cer	*Pk**
P	**GalNAc(β1→3)**Gal(α1→4)Gal(β1→4)Glc-Cer	*B3GALNT1*
P_1	**Gal(α1→4)**Gal(β1→4)GlcNAc(β1→3)Gal(α1→4)Gal(β1→4)Glc-Cer	*P1*
M	∇ ∇ ∇ **Ser**–Ser–Thr–Thr–**Gly**–(GPA chain: 131 amino acids)	*GYPA(M)*
N	∇ ∇ ∇ **Leu**–Ser–Thr–Thr–**GluA**–(GPA chain: 131 amino acids)	*GYPA(N)*
S	∇ ∇ ∇ Leu–Ser–Thr–Thr–GluA–**Met29**–(GPA chain: 72 amino acids)	*GPYB(S)*
S	∇ ∇ ∇ Leu–Ser–Thr–Thr–GluA–**Thr29**–(GPA chain: 72 amino acids)	*GPYB(s)*

*Proposed gene.

Immunodominant sugars and amino acids are indicated in bold.

GPA, glycophorin A; GPB, glycophorin B; R, primary glycolipid attachment Glc-Ger, primary glycoprotein attachment GlcNAc-Asp; ∇, –Gal–GalNAc–NeuNAc
|
NeuNac transferase action, are indirect gene products. Most blood group genes are located on autosomes; only two, *Xg* and *XK*, are located on the X chromosome (see Table 137–1 for locations of genes and chromosome).

Most genes that encode blood group antigens have two or more alleles. Individuals who inherit two identical alleles are homozygous and make a double dose of a single gene product, whereas those who inherit two different alleles are heterozygous and make single dose of each of two gene products. Males are hemizygous for the genes located on their single X chromosome and make a single gene product. In contrast, females produce a double dose of the *Xg* and *XK* gene products, as X-chromosome inactivation does not involve Xg^a or Kx antigens.[36]

ALLELES

Alleles encoding blood group antigens commonly arise from single nucleotide changes. For example, *A* and *B* alleles differ by only seven DNA base substitutions, which result in four amino acid substitutions in their respective transferases.[4–6] The common *O* allele is similar to *A* except for a single base deletion at nucleotide 261 that shifts the reading frame during RNA translation. The resulting protein is truncated and has no transferase activity. Another variant *O* allele encodes a transferase identical to that of B except it has arginine instead of alanine at amino acid position 268, which blocks the enzyme activity. A comprehensive listing of blood group alleles is available at the NCBI website: http://www.ncbi.nlm.nih.gov/gv/mhc/xslcgi.cgi?cmd=bgmut/home.

GENE COMPLEXES

Some blood group genes are complexes of several closely linked genes or loci that evolved through duplication of an ancestral gene. The antigens they encode are inherited within families as a haplotype with no or few crossovers. Blood group examples include the Rh system with genes *RHD* and *RHCE*, and the MNS system with genes *GYPA*, *GYPB*, and *GYPE*.

RHD and *RHCE* show remarkable homology between them and with *RHAG*, which encodes the Rh glycoprotein RhAG. *GPYA* and *GPYB* probably arose by duplication of an ancestral *GPYA* gene encoding the N antigen.[37] The most common MNSs complex is Ns, followed by Ms, MS, and NS.

In both Rh and MNS systems, other antigens arose by further nucleotide changes, deletions, or rearrangements within the gene complex. Unequal pairing of *GYPA* and *GYPB* during meiosis, with subsequent recombination, resulted in several hybrids, such as *GYP(A-B)* (called Lepore type, by analogy with a similar hemoglobin hybrid), which encodes a protein with the amino-terminal end of GPA but the carboxyl-terminal end of glycophorin B. Anti–Lepore-type hybrids, *GYP(B-A)* (amino-terminal end of glycophorin B and carboxyl-terminal end of glycophorin A), and other rearrangements (e.g., *GYP[B-A-B]* and *GYP[A-B-A]*) are known. Within the Rh complex, hybrids of *RH(D-CE-D)* and *RH(CE-D-CE)* have been identified. Such hybrids can result in altered antigen expression and new antigens.[4–6]

Kell and Lutheran proteins are single gene products that carry multiple antigens. The most common alleles in humans are $kKp^bJs^bK^{11}$ and $Lu^bLu^6Lu^8Au^a$. Antigens of lower prevalence (K, Kp^a/Kp^c, or Js^a, and Lu^a, Lu9, Lu14, or Au^b) arise from separate nucleotide changes.

SILENT ALLELES

Some blood group alleles are amorphs, or silent; that is, they do not produce a recognizable antigen, although they may encode a product that is simply not detected with standard test methods. As discussed with regard to the ABO system, *A* and *B* genes produce transferases that add GalNAc or Gal, respectively, to the same precursors, but *O* produces no active enzyme. *AB* individuals express both A and B antigen, but *AA* and *AO* individuals express only A, and *BB* and *BO* individuals express only B. Amorphic alleles are recognized only in a homozygous state, and the result is a "null" phenotype. Null phenotypes exist in most blood group systems (see Table 137–1). Group O is the most common, followed by Fy(a–b–) and Le(a–b–) in Africans. Other null phenotypes are rare.

The Fy(a–b–) phenotype is especially interesting. Fy(a–b–) Africans have Fy^b genes that express normal Fy^b glycoprotein on tissue cells but not on RBCs. A nucleotide change that disrupts the GATA-1 binding site for RBC transcription is present in these individuals,[38] which helps explain why many Fy(a–b–) Africans do not make anti-Fy^b despite exposure to antigen-positive RBCs from transfusion.

GENE FREQUENCIES

Gene and phenotype frequencies vary widely with race and geographical boundaries.[6,11,16,39] This information is needed when estimating the availability of compatible blood and the probability of HDFN.

RED CELL ANTIGENS IN HEALTH AND DISEASE

EXPRESSION OF RED CELL ANTIGENS IN OTHER BODY TISSUES AND FLUIDS

Antigens in the Rh and Kidd blood group systems are present only on RBCs and have not been detected on platelets, lymphocytes, or granulocytes or in plasma, other body tissues, or secretions (saliva, milk, amniotic fluid).[4–6,16] MNSs, Lutheran, Kell, and Duffy antigens are found on RBCs and other body tissues (see Table 137–2).

ABH antigens have broad tissue distribution. In embryos, A, B, and H antigens are detectable on all endothelial cells and all epithelial cells except those of the central nervous system. ABH, Lewis, I, and P blood group antigens are in plasma and on platelets and lymphocytes. Granulocytes carry I antigen but no ABH. ABH on platelets and lymphocytes may be acquired at least in part by adsorption from plasma. Lewis antigen is acquired by RBCs by adsorption. Secretions (saliva, milk, sweat, semen, and urine, but not cerebral spinal fluid) contain A, B, H, I, and Lewis antigens but no P or Globoside system antigens. Sd^a antigen is found in most body secretions, with the greatest concentration in urine.[5,16]

ASSOCIATIONS OF RED CELL ANTIGENS WITH DISEASE

ANTIGENS ASSOCIATED WITH POSSIBLE SUSCEPTIBILITY TO DISEASE

Some blood groups are statistically associated with medical conditions or disease (Table 137–4).[4–6,16] For example, blood group A is more common in persons with cancer of the salivary glands, stomach, colon, or ovary and with thrombosis (because of higher levels of coagulation factors VIII, V, and IX). Blood group O is more common in patients with duodenal and gastric ulcers, rheumatoid arthritis, and von Willebrand disease.

Associations with infection arise when microorganisms carry structures homologous with blood group activity. The presence of blood group antibody and/or soluble blood group antigen in secretions may help confer protection. Having anti-B may offer protection against *Salmonella, Shigella, Neisseria gonorrhoeae*, and some *Escherichia coli* infections. An association exists between nonsecretion of ABH antigen and susceptibility to *Candida albicans, Neisseria meningitidis, Streptococcus pneumoniae*, and *Haemophilus influenzae*.[6]

A number of disease associations with globoside have been identified. *Streptococcus suis*, which can cause meningitis and septicemia in

TABLE 137–4. Blood Group Antigens and Antibodies Associated with Disease

Phenotypes Associated with Disease Susceptibility	
Group A	Carcinoma of the salivary glands, stomach, colon, rectum, ovary, uterus, cervix, bladder (T1 and T2 tumors); idiopathic thrombocytopenic purpura, coronary thrombosis, thrombosis (oral contraceptives), pernicious anemia, giardiasis, meningococcal meningitis infections
Group B	*Escherichia coli* urinary tract infection, gonorrhea
Group O	Duodenal and gastric ulcers, rheumatoid arthritis, von Willebrand disease, typhoid, paratyphoid, cholera
ABH nonsecretors	Duodenal ulcers, spondyloarthropathies; increased susceptibility to *Candida albicans, Neisseria meningitidis, Streptococcus pneumoniae, Haemophilus influenzae*
Le(a–b–)	Sjögren syndrome
Group O, Le(a–b+)	*Helicobacter pylori*
Globoside	Parvovirus
Phenotypes Associated with Disease Resistance	
p (PP_1, P^k–)	Pyelonephritogenic infections of *E. coli*
Fy(a–b–)	*Plasmodium vivax, Plasmodium knowlesi*
Tn–, Cad–, En(a–), U–, Ge–	*Plasmodium falciparum*
Diseases Associated with Altered Antigen Expression	
Weakened AB	Leukemia, myelodysplastic syndrome, Hodgkin lymphoma and non-Hodgkin lymphomas, aplastic anemia, bacterial infections
Weakened MN	Bacterial infections, myelodysplastic syndrome, leukemia (Tn, T, Tk activation)
Enhanced i	Thalassemia, sickle cell disease, HEMPAS, Diamond-Blackfan anemia, myeloblastic or sideroblastic erythropoiesis, refractory anemia
Acquired A (Tn)	Myelodysplastic syndrome, acute myelogenous leukemia
Acquired B	Bacterial infections, gastrointestinal lesions or malignancies
Acquired T, Tk	Bacterial infections
Acquired K antigens	*Enterococcus faecium*
Acquired Jk^b antigen	*E. faecium* or *Micrococcus* infection
Absent Cromer, Yt, Dombrock, JMH antigens	Paroxysmal nocturnal hemoglobinuria
Weakened target antigens (Rh, Kell, Kidd, LW)	Autoimmune hemolytic anemia
Weakened I, Rh, S, s, U, Kp^b, Jk^a, Xg^a, or En^a	Stomatocytic hereditary elliptocytosis
Diseases Associated with Null Phenotypes	
Rh_{null} (D–C–E–c–e–)	Hereditary stomatocytosis, mild hemolytic anemia
McLeod phenotype (Kx–)	Hereditary acanthocytosis, mild hemolytic anemia
Ge– (Leach type)	Hereditary elliptocytosis, mild hemolytic anemia
Bombay (Oh)	Leukocyte adhesion deficiency II (some)
I– (i Adult)	Congenital cataracts in Asians (some)
Co(a–b–), Co:–3	Inability to maximally concentrate urine
MER2–	Kidney disease
Diseases Associated with Antibody Production	
Anti-I, -IH, -i, -H, -Pr	Cold agglutinin disease
Anti-"Rh," -"Kell," -U, -Wr^b	Warm autoimmune hemolytic anemia
Anti-I	*Mycoplasma pneumoniae,* chronic lymphocytic leukemia, Hodgkin lymphoma and non-Hodgkin lymphomas
Anti-i	Infectious mononucleosis, reticuloendothelial diseases
Anti-I^T	Hodgkin lymphoma and non-Hodgkin lymphomas
Anti-K	Enterocolitis, bacterial infections (*E. coli* 0125:B15, *Campylobacter jejuni, E. coli)*
Anti-P1	Parasitic infections: hydatid cyst disease, liver flukes
Anti-PP_1P^k	Early spontaneous abortions

(*continued*)

TABLE 137–4. Blood Group Antigens and Antibodies Associated with Disease (Continued)

Anti-P	Paroxysmal cold hemoglobinuria, early spontaneous abortions, lymphoma
Anti-NF	Renal dialysis (formaldehyde exposure)
Anti-Forssman	Neoplastic disorders
Anti-Rx	Virally induced hemolysis
Decreased anti-A or -B	Agammaglobulinemia or hypogammaglobulinemia
"Null" Phenotypes Associated with Biologic Differences but No Disease	
Group O	Lack GalNAc or Gal on terminal Gal
Bombay	Lack Fuc on terminal Gal
Le(a–b–)	Lack Fuc on terminal GlcNAc
M–N– or En(a–)	Lack or have altered GPA
S–s–U–	Lack or have altered GPB
Wr(a–b–)	Lack or have altered GPA
M^k phenotype	Lack GPA and GPB
K_0	Lack Kell glycoprotein
Jk(a–b–)	Lack or have altered Jk protein, reduced ability to concentrate urine
Lu(a–b–)	Lack or have reduced or altered Lu glycoprotein; RBC may show poikilocytosis, potassium loss, increased hemolysis during storage
LW(a–b–)	Lack or have altered LW glycoprotein
Do(a–b–), Gy(a–)	Lack a GPI-linked protein (Do glycoprotein)
Sc:–1,–2,–3	Lack or have altered Sc glycoprotein

HEMPAS, hereditary erythroblastic multinuclearity with positive acidified serum lysis test.

SOURCE: Modified from Issitt PD, Anstee DJ,[5] Daniels G,[4] and Reid ME, Lomas-Francis C.[6,15]

humans, binds exclusively to P^k antigen. A class of toxins secreted by *Shigella dysenteriae, Vibrio cholerae*, and *Vibrio parahaemolyticus* have binding specificity for Gal(α14)-Gal(β14). In addition, globoside is the receptor of human parvovirus B19. Some strains of *E. coli* use the disaccharide receptor Gal(α14)-Galβ on uroepithelial cells to gain entry to the urinary tract receptors associated with P1, P, and P^k antigens.[5,33] People with the rare p phenotype (P_{null}) lack this disaccharide and are not susceptible to acute pyelonephritis from such *E. coli* strains.

PHENOTYPES ASSOCIATED WITH DISEASE RESISTANCE

Erythrocytes lacking Fy^a and Fy^b antigens are not infected by the malarial parasite *Plasmodium vivax* or by the simian malarial parasite *Plasmodium knowlesi*. These parasites attach to the Fy(a–b–) RBC membrane, but penetration does not take place. The Fy6 antigen is the critical receptor for *P. vivax* attachment.[5] *Plasmodium falciparum* attaches to RBC glycophorins and their O-linked oligosaccharides (carrying NeuAc). RBCs with the following phenotypes have a decreased rate of infection: M–N– (GPA-deficient), S–s–U– (GPB-deficient), Ge– (Leach type or GPC/GPD-deficient), and Cad-positive and Tn-positive RBCs (which have abnormal O-linked sugars).

DISEASES ASSOCIATED WITH ALTERED ANTIGEN EXPRESSION

Antigen expression can be altered with inherited or acquired disease. Inherited changes are fixed and consistent; acquired changes can disappear with remission or recovery. In some diseases, antigen expression weakens; in others, antigen expression increases or new antigens appear.

Weakened ABH expression on RBCs has been noted in acute myeloid leukemias and may result from reduced transferase activity.[5,16] Normal antigen expression returns with disease remission. Transient weakened expression of target antigen also occurs in some cases of autoimmune hemolytic anemia. Weak Rh, Kell, and Kidd blood group activity has been reported with concurrent autoantibody.[5,16,40]

Increased expression of i on RBCs is associated with inherited disorders, such as thalassemia, sickle cell disease, Diamond-Blackfan syndrome, and hereditary erythroblastic multinuclearity with a positive acidified serum test (HEMPAS). Increased i expression also is noted with acquired conditions that decrease the red cell maturation time in the marrow, such as myeloblastic or sideroblastic myeloblastic erythropoiesis, refractory anemia, and excessive phlebotomy.[16,23] Expression of the *de novo* antigen Tn is caused by a galactosyltransferase deficiency acquired by somatic mutation in a population of stem cells. The antigen is present on RBCs, platelets, and granulocytes arising from these stem cells. This condition (seen as persistent mixed-field agglutination because of the presence of both normal and abnormal cell clones) causes other RBC changes, such as depressed MN expression, enhanced H, and reduced NeuAc content. Tn antigen exposure is associated with myelodysplastic syndrome and acute myelomonocytic leukemia.[16] Other antigens (T, Tk) occur as a result of infection when microbes produce enzymes that remove some sugars and expose new ones. Group A individuals can appear to acquire a B antigen when bacterial deacetylase removes the acetyl group on GalNAc.[4,16] This phenomenon is associated with severe infection, gastrointestinal lesions, and malignancies.

RBCs may acquire blood group activity when they adsorb material from certain microorganisms. Group B activity has been associated with

E. coli$_{86}$ and *Proteus vulgaris* infection, and K antigen with *Enterococcus faecium*. Acquired Jk^{b}-like activity has been associated with *E. faecium* and *Micrococcus* infections, although the mechanism is not clear.[41]

DISEASES ASSOCIATED WITH ABSENT ANTIGENS OR NULL PHENOTYPES

Rh$_{null}$ Syndrome

The Rh$_{null}$ phenotype is associated with hereditary stomatocytosis, hemolytic anemia (usually mild and well compensated), and a lack of proteins carrying Rh antigens. The Rh protein resides in the RBC membrane, interacts with other membrane proteins and possibly the membrane skeleton, and may help regulate or organize the lipids within the red cell membrane bilayer.[9,10] Hence, it is an important determinant of membrane shape and expression of other antigens. Rh$_{null}$ cells have depressed expression or absence of S, s, U, LW, and Fy5 antigens.

Most Rh$_{null}$ red cells are stomatocytes or occasionally spherocytes and demonstrate increased osmotic fragility, increased potassium permeability, and higher potassium pump activity. They have reduced cation and water content and a relative deficiency of membrane cholesterol. Although these abnormalities are assumed to contribute to shortened *in vivo* survival, Rh$_{null}$ RBCs survive normally in splenectomized patients, suggesting their removal is related more to splenic clearance because of shape rather than some other intrinsic factor.

Two genetic mechanisms account for the Rh$_{null}$ phenotype. Persons with the amorphic type are homozygous for the silent *RHCE* gene on a deleted *RHD* background. Individuals with the more common regulator type of Rh$_{null}$ have normal *RH* genes but an altered (silenced) *RHAG* gene. RhAG is required for expression of Rh antigens. Individuals with the Rh$_{mod}$ phenotype have similar membrane and clinical anomalies associated with Rh$_{null}$ syndrome but demonstrate some Rh antigen expression. The reduced expression of Rh antigens results from the presence of an altered form of RhAG.[24,26,42]

McLeod Phenotype

Numerous males (but no females) with the McLeod phenotype have been identified. These individuals have acanthocytosis, decreased RBC survival, very weak expression of Kell blood group antigens, lack of Kx antigen on RBCs, and a well-compensated hemolytic anemia.[43]

Kx antigen is carried on a 37-kDa protein (XK) encoded by the *XK* gene on the X chromosome, which interacts with the RBC membrane skeleton and helps stabilize the membrane. The absence of Kx is associated with a lipid deficiency in the membrane bilayer that may be critical to the Kell glycoprotein and general RBC discoid shape. RBCs with the McLeod phenotype show a defect in water transport, increased mobility of phosphatidylcholine across the membrane, and increased phosphorylation of protein band 3 and β-spectrin.[43]

After age 40 years, patients with the McLeod phenotype develop a slowly progressive form of muscular dystrophy that is associated with areflexia, choreiform movements, and cardiomegaly, leading to cardiomyopathy. They have elevated levels of serum creatine kinase and carbonic anhydrase III. Some patients with the McLeod phenotype and X-linked chronic granulomatous disease (CGD) have a deletion of both the *XK* and *Phox-91* (see Chap. 66). The McLeod phenotype results from deletions or point mutations on the X chromosome near the *XK* gene at position Xp21[44] (for details, see www.nefo.med.uni-muechen.de/).

Gerbich-Negative Phenotype

The *GYPC* gene on chromosome 2 encodes two proteins: GPC, with antigens Ge3 and Ge4 (the Ge2 portion is "hidden" by the Ge4-bearing terminal end), and its shorter partner GPD, with antigens Ge2 (now exposed) and Ge3. GPC and GPD interact with membrane skeleton proteins 4.1 and p55, which are involved in cell deformability and membrane stability. Gerbich-negative RBCs of the Leach type (Ge:–2, –3, –4) lack both GPC and GPD, have reduced protein 4.1, and elliptocytosis but exhibit normal survival *in vivo*.[6,10]

Bombay (Oh) Phenotype

Rare people lack A, B, and H antigens and have naturally occurring anti-A, -B, and -H in their plasma. Such people are said to have the Bombay (Oh) phenotype. Rare people with the Le(a–b–) Bombay phenotype have a silenced gene that encodes the fucose transporter. As a consequence, all cells lack fucose. Without fucose, neutrophils lack sialyl Le^{X} and thus cannot roll and ingest bacteria. These patients have a high white blood cell count and severe recurrent infections. The condition is called *leukocyte adhesion deficiency II* (LADII) or congenital disorder of glycosylation II.[45,46]

I-negative Phenotype (i Adult)

The gene encoding the I-branching β-1,6-*N*-acetylglucosaminyltransferase *(IGNT)* has three alternative forms of exon 1, with common exons 2 and 3. Mutations in exon 2 or 3 silence *IGNT* and give rise to the form of I-negative phenotype associated with congenital cataracts in Asians.[47,48] Mutations in exon 1C *(IGnTC* or *IGnT3)* silence the gene in RBCs but not in other tissues and lead to the I-negative phenotype (i adult) without cataracts.[49]

Co(a–b–), CO:–3 Phenotype

Antigens of the Colton blood group system are carried on the water transporter (aquaporin). Although an absence of this protein from the RBC membrane was thought to be incompatible with life, in reality these rare individuals have been shown only to be unable to maximally concentrate urine.[50]

MER2 Phenotype

The MER2 antigen in the RAPH blood group system is carried on CD151. Rare individuals who lack CD151 have chronic renal failure and skin ulcers.[51]

Other Null Phenotypes

Patients with null phenotypes can develop RBC antibodies that make it difficult to find compatible blood to avoid the otherwise serious hemolytic transfusion reactions. For example, people with the Bombay phenotype (O$_{h}$ or H$_{null}$) demonstrate no red cell abnormality but make potent hemolytic anti-H as well as anti-A and anti-B. These antibodies are incompatible with all RBCs except those from other persons with the Bombay phenotype. Likewise, p individuals (PP1P^{k}-negative) or P^{k} individuals (P-negative) can make hemolytic antibodies to the antigens they lack. Anti-PP1P^{k} and anti-P also are associated with spontaneous abortions in the first trimester.[16] Women with such antibodies (notably IgG anti-P), even those with a history of spontaneous abortions, have delivered viable infants after plasmapheresis.[52]

Null phenotypes in the MNSs and Lutheran systems are interesting because several types of null phenotypes are known. Within the MNSs blood group system, people may lack GPA (En[a–] or MN-negative), GPB (SsU-negative), or both (M^{k}M^{k} phenotype). The rare Lu(a–b–) phenotype is caused by a dominant inhibitor called *In(Lu)*, by homozygous pairing of the silent allele *Lu*, or by a recessive sex-linked inhibitor *XS2*.[5,16] Only the *LuLu*-type null (recessive Lu[a–b–]) is associated with antibody production because the inhibitor type nulls produce small amounts of Lutheran antigen. *In(Lu)* type, Lu(a–b–) RBCs have low expression of CD44 and have varying degrees of poikilocytosis and acanthocytosis. RBCs of this type tend to hemolyze more quickly during storage, even though they demonstrate normal osmotic fragility.[53] Inactivating nucleotide changes in *EKLF*, which encodes an altered transcription factor, cause this phenotype.[30]

The Jk(a–b–) phenotype is caused by the silent alleles *JkJk* or the dominant inhibitor *In(Jk)*. RBCs having the Jk(a–b–) phenotype resist lysis in 2*M* urea,[54] a solution commonly used in automated platelet counting systems. No significant clinical abnormalities have been identified to date, although Jk(a–b–) individuals have reduced ability to concentrate urine.[55]

The following diagnoses are made easily by simply typing the RBCs with appropriate antisera: Rh syndrome, McLeod syndrome, and LADII.

ANTIERYTHROCYTE ANTIBODIES

IMMUNOLOGY OF RED CELL ANTIBODIES

Blood group antibodies are classified as *alloantibodies* if they react with antigens present on the RBCs of other people and as *autoantibodies* if they are specific for *self-antigens* present on the patient's own RBC. Alloantibodies also can be classified according to their mode of sensitization as *naturally occurring* (no apparent sensitization) or *immune* (following sensitization). Table 137–5 summarizes the common antierythrocyte antibodies.[4,6,15,16]

IMMUNOGLOBULIN CLASSES ASSOCIATED WITH BLOOD GROUP ACTIVITY

Immunoglobulin G

IgG is the predominant antibody made in an immune response and constitutes approximately 80 percent of total serum Ig (see Chap. 77). These antibodies, when specific for RBC antigens, can attach to or lyse transfused antigen-positive RBCs. Receptors on macrophages in the liver and spleen allow the macrophages to remove IgG-coated RBCs from the circulation. IgG blood group antibodies also are capable of fixing complement, although some subclasses do so less efficiently than others: IgG3 > IgG1 > IgG2 > IgG4. How well an IgG antierythrocyte antibody binds complement, depends on the surface density and location of the recognized antigen. This situation occurs because C1q, the initiator of the classic complement cascade, requires binding of at least two IgG molecules to the RBC within a span of 20 to 30 nm to initiate the complement cascade.[16] For example, IgG anti-D rarely binds complement, presumably because most D sites are spaced too far apart.[16] Most IgG blood group antibodies do not agglutinate saline-suspended RBCs, presumably because the IgG molecule is too small to span the distance between RBCs, although some exceptions are known (i.e., potent IgG examples of anti-A, anti-B, anti-M, and anti-K). Some IgG anti-D can directly agglutinate RBCs with the D– – phenotype. Instead, most IgG antibodies sensitize RBCs at 37°C (98.6°F) and are detected with an antiglobulin reagent.[11]

Immunoglobulin M

IgM is a pentamer of five basic units (having μ heavy chains plus a short J, or joining, chain) and makes up only approximately 4 percent of total serum Ig (see Chap. 77). IgM is the first class of Ig produced by the fetus and is the predominant antibody in a primary immune response, but it does not cross the placenta. Because of their pentameric structure, even low-affinity IgM blood group antibodies can agglutinate RBCs and activate complement. Both hemolyzing and agglutinating abilities of IgM molecules are destroyed by reducing reagents, such as 2-ME and DTT. IgM antibodies of low affinity may agglutinate RBCs only at temperatures below 37°C (98.6°F). Such antibodies still may fix complement onto the RBC membrane *in vivo*, at the lower temperatures in the extremities, and activate the complement cascade in the core of the body. Because such IgM antibodies dissociate from RBCs at higher temperatures, their reactivity may be detected in routine antiglobulin tests (using polyspecific antiglobulin) by virtue of the complement components that remain bound to the red cell membrane.[11,16]

Immunoglobulin A

IgA is the primary Ig in body secretions, where it exists predominantly as a dimer with a secretory component (see Chap. 77). IgA does not cross the placenta or fix complement, but aggregated IgA can activate the alternative pathway of complement, and IgA can trigger cell-mediated events. Multimeric IgA antibodies in serum are seen as hemagglutinins in blood bank tests and most often are associated with anti-A or anti-B.

IMMUNOGLOBULIN IN THE FETUS AND NEWBORN

Young fetuses acquire low levels of maternal IgG, probably by diffusion across the placenta. These levels rise significantly between 20 and 33 weeks' gestation as a selective transport system matures and maternal IgG is actively transported across the placenta. Thus, almost all blood group antibodies detected in the fetus and newborn originate from the mother and disappear within the first few months of life.

Actual fetal antibody production begins shortly before birth with low levels of IgM, followed by IgG and IgA several weeks after birth. Anti-A and anti-B usually are readily detected by age 2 to 6 months.

Because of this late immune response in the newborn and because maternal antibody is so predominant at birth, blood bank standards permit abbreviated testing on neonates younger than 4 months.[56] If available, the mother's serum is used (and preferred) for identifying antibodies in a newborn and for cross-matching RBC components.

NATURALLY OCCURRING ANTIBODIES

Naturally Occurring Antibodies in Development

An antibody is said to be *naturally occurring* when it is found in the serum of an individual who has not been exposed to the antigen through transfusion or pregnancy. These antibodies most likely are heteroagglutinins produced in response to substances in the environment that are similar to those on RBC antigens.

Evidence supporting this concept has come from studies on the formation of anti-B in chickens.[57] Chicks raised in a normal environment made anti-B within the first 30 days of life, whereas chicks raised in a germ-free environment did not make anti-B by day 60. Naturally occurring alloanti-A and alloanti-B in humans, also called *isoagglutinins*, can increase in titer following ingestion or inhalation of suitable bacteria.[58]

However, a great many antigens that likely are not present in the environment have been associated with naturally occurring antibodies, so the stimulus for naturally occurring antibodies is not clearly known.

Blood Group Associations and Occurrence of Naturally Occurring Antibodies

Naturally occurring alloantibodies are commonly associated with the carbohydrate antigens of the ABO, Lewis, and P blood group systems. Anti-A and anti-B are expected in people who lack the corresponding antigens, as are antibodies specific for H, $PP1P^k$, or P antigens. Naturally occurring antibodies reactive with A1, Le^a, Le^b, or P1 determinants also are seen frequently. Carbohydrate antigens, especially those with repetitive epitopes, can stimulate B cells to make specific antibody without the aid of helper T cells. Such thymus-independent immune responses typically result in antigen-specific antibodies of the IgM class.

TABLE 137–5. Summary of Antierythrocyte Antibodies

Blood Group	Antibody	Ig Class		Serologic Activity			Activates Complement	Implicated in		Antigen Frequency (%)		Comments
		IgM	IgG	RT	37°C (98.6°F)-AHG	ENZ/DTT		HTR	HDFN	Whites	Blacks	
ABO	A	Most	Some	Most	Most	I/nc	Yes	Yes	Mild	40	27	A/B: very clinically significant, sometimes IgA
	B	Most	Some	Most	Most	I/nc	Yes	Yes	Mild	11	20	
	A1	Most	Rare	Most	Rare	I/nc	Rare	Rare	No	30	–	A1: usually not clinically significant
	H	Most	Rare	Most	Rare	I/nc	Rare	Rare	–	>99.9	–	H: usually weak autoantibody, but strong alloantibody in O_h
Rh	D	Some	Most	Some	Most	I/nc	No	Yes	Sev	85	92	D: most common immune antibody
	C	Few	Most	–	Most	I/nc	No	Yes	Sev	70	33	C: often found with D
	E	Some	Most	S	Most	I/nc	No	Yes	Sev	30	21	E/C: often found together
	c	–	Most	–	Most	I/nc	No	Yes	Sev	80	97	Autoantibodies commonly directed against Rh protein
	e	–	Most	–	Most	I/nc	No	Yes	Mild–sev	98	99	All: clinically significant
	f (ce)	–	M	–	Most	I/nc	No	Yes	Sev	64	–	
	C^w	Some	Most	–	Most	I/nc	No	Yes	Sev	1	–	
	VS/V	–	Most	–	Most	I/nc	No	Yes	Sev	<1	30	
Lewis	Le^a	Most	Rare	Most	Some	I/nc	Yes	Rare	No	22	23	Common in pregnancy
	Le^b	Most	Rare	Most	Some	I/nc	Yes	No	No	72	55	Not clinically significant Le(a–b–) individuals commonly make anti-Le^a
Ii	I	Most	–	Most	Some	I/nc	Yes	Rare	No	>99.9	>99.9	I: common autoantibody, rare significant alloantibody
	i	Most	–	Most	Some	I/nc	Yes	No	Mild	100	100	i: rare autoantibody
P	P1	Most	Rare	Most	Some	I/nc	Few	Rare	No	79	94	P1: usually not clinically significant
GLOB	P	Most	Few	Most	Some	I/nc	Yes	Yes	No–mild	>99.9	>99.9	P: Donath-Landsteiner antibody in PNH
	$PP1P^k$	Most	Few	Most	Some	I/nc	Yes	Yes	Mild–sev	>99.9	>99.9	
MNSs	M	Some	Some	Most	Few	D/nc	No	Rare	(R)	78	70	M: common, usually not clinically significant
	N	Some	Some	Most	Rare	D/nc	No	Rare	(R)	72	74	
	S	Some	Some	Some	Most	V/nc	Some	Yes	Mild	55	31	N: rare, usually not clinically significant
		Few	Most	Few	Most	V/nc	Rare	Yes	Mild–sev	89	97	
	U	–	Most	–	Most	nc/nc	Rare	Yes	Mild–mod	100	99.7	SsU: clinically significant autoantibody specificities reported

Kell	K	Some	Most	Few	Most	nc/D	Rare	Yes	Mild–sev	9	2	K: very common immune antibody
	k	–	Most	Rare	Most	nc/D	No	Yes	Mild–sev	99.9	–	
	Kp^a	–	Most	Rare	Most	nc/D	No	Yes	Mild–mod	2.3	–	
	Kp^b	–	Most	Rare	Most	nc/D	No	Yes	Mild–mod	>99.9	100	Autoantibodies reported
	Js^a	–	Most	Rare	Rare	nc/D	No	Yes	Mild–sev	–	20	
	Js^b	–	Most	–	–	nc/D	No	Yes	Mild–sev	>99.9	99	
Duffy	Fy^a	–	Most	Rare	Most	D/nc	Rare	Yes	Mild–sev	66	10	Fy^a: common immune antibody
	Fy^b	–	Most	Rare	Most	D/nc	Rare	Yes	Mild	83	23	
Kidd	Jk^a	Few	Most	Rare	Most	I/nc	Yes	Yes	Mild–mod	77	92	Jk^a: associated with delayed HTR; hemolytic; disappears quickly from serum
	Jk^b	Few	Most	Rare	Most	I/nc	Yes	Yes	No–mild	72	41	
Lutheran	Lu^a	Some	Few	Most	Few	nc(V)/D	No	No	No–mild	7.7	–	Mild RBC destruction
	Lu^b	Some	Some	Few	Most	nc(V)/D	No	Yes	Mild	99.9	–	
Xg	Xg^a	Some	Most	Rare	Most	D/nc	Some	No	No	64(m)	–	Xg^a: poor immunogen
										89(f)	–	
Yt	Yt^a	–	Most	N	Most	D(V)/D(V)	No	No-mod	No	99.7	–	Yt: some antibody examples clinically significant, others not
	Yt^b	–	Most	N	M	D(V)/D	No	?	No	8	–	
Ch/Rg	Ch	Rare	Most	–	Most	D/nc	No	No	No	96	–	Ch/Rg: associated with C4 complement, clinically insignificant antibodies
	Rg	–	Most	–	Most	D/nc	No	No	No	98	–	
Colton	Co^a	–	Most	Some	Most	nc/nc	No	No	Mild–sev	99.9	–	
	Co^b	–	Most	Some	Most	nc/nc	Rare	No–mod	Mild	10	–	
Cost	Cs^a	–	Most	–	Most	nc/nc	No	No	No	96	98	
Cromer	General group		Most	–	Most	nc/D	No	No–mild	No	>99.9	>99.9	
Diego	Di^a	–	Most	Some	Most	nc/nc	Rare	Yes	Mild–sev	R	–	Di^a: antigen found in South American Indians and Asians
	Di^b	–	Most	N	Most	nc/nc	No	Yes	Mild	100	–	
Dombrock	Do^a	–	Most	N	Most	nc/D(V)	No	Yes	Mild	67	–	Do^a Do^b: poor immunogens
	Do^b	–	Most	N	Most	nc/D(V)	No	Yes	No	83	–	Hy– and Jo(a–): found only in blacks
	Hy	–	Most	–	Most	nc(I)/D(V)	No	Yes	Mild	>99	–	Gy(a–) (Do_{null}) found in eastern Europeans and Japanese
	Gy^a	–	Most	–	Most	nc(I)/D(V)	No	Yes	Mild	>99	–	
	Jo^a	–	Most	–	Most	nc(I)/D(V)	No	No	No	>99	–	
Gerbich	General group		Most	–	Most	D/nc	Yes	No–mod	(+DAT)	>99.9	>99.9	Ge: located on glycophorins C and D
Indian	In^a	–	Most	–	Most	D/D	No	Yes	(+DAT)	<0.1	<0.1	In: located on CD44 adhesion protein
	In^b	–	Most	–	Most	D/D	No	Yes	(+DAT)	99	96	

(*continued*)

TABLE 137–5. Summary of Antierythrocyte Antibodies (Continued)

		Ig Class		Serologic Activity				Implicated in		Antigen Frequency (%)		
Blood Group	Antibody	IgM	IgG	RT	37°C (98.6°F)-AHG	ENZ/DTT	Activates Complement	HTR	HDFN	Whites	Blacks	Comments
Knops	Kn[a]	–	Most	–	Most	D/D/nc	No	No	No	98	99	Knops antigens associated with CR1 (complement) receptor, clinically insignificant antibodies
	McC[a]	–	Most	–	Most	D/D	No	No	No	98	94	
	Yk[a]	–	Most	–	Most	D/D	No	No	No	92	98	
Scianna	Sc1	–	Most	–	Most	nc/D	Yes	No	Mild	>99.9	–	Sc1: some antibodies react in serum but not plasma
	Sc2	–	Most	–	Most	nc/D	No	No	Mild	1	–	
	Sc3	–	Most	–	Most	nc(I)/?	No	No–mild	No	>99.9	–	
JMH	JMH	–	Most	–	Most	D/D	No	No	No	>99.9	>99.9	JMH: carrier protein CDw108

AHG, antiglobulin phase; D, decreased; +DAT, positive direct antiglobulin test result; DTT, dithiothreitol-treated RBC; ENZ, enzyme-treated RBCs; f, female; GPI, glycosyl phosphatidylinositol; HDFN, hemolytic disease of the fetus and newborn; HTR, hemolytic transfusion reactions; I, increased; M, most; m, male; mod, moderate; nc, no significant change using pretreated cells; RT, room temperature; S, some; sev, severe; V, variable.

Within other systems,[16] anti-Sd^a, anti-Vw, and anti-Wr^a are found in up to 2 percent of normal people. Other less common antibody specificities in approximate order of descending occurrence are anti-M, -S, -N, -Ge, -K, -Lu^a, -Di^a, and -Xg^a. Rh antigens are thought to reside only on RBCs, but apparent naturally occurring anti-D has been reported in 0.15 percent of Rh-negative donors and anti-E in more than 0.1 percent of Rh-positive donors when more sensitive enzyme detection methods are used. Examples of naturally occurring anti-C, anti-C^w, and anti-C^x also have been described.

Some naturally occurring antibodies exist as autoagglutinins (anti-H and anti-I). Patients with autoimmune hemolytic anemia can produce many antibodies to low-prevalence antigens with no specific stimulus, in addition to autoantibody.[5,6,16,40]

Characteristics of Naturally Occurring Alloantibodies

Most naturally occurring antibodies are IgM, but some have an IgG component and a few are predominantly IgG. Some anti-A or anti-B may even be of the IgA class. Antibodies that cause direct agglutination of saline-suspended RBCs most commonly are of the IgM class. However, even IgG antibodies may cause agglutination of RBCs when they bind antigens that are present at high density on the RBC membrane, such as the ABO or MN antigens. With the exception of anti-A and anti-B, most common naturally occurring antibodies do not react at body temperature and are considered clinically insignificant. However, if they are found to react at 37°C (98.6°F), providing cross-match–compatible blood for transfusion is prudent.

■ ANTIBODIES GENERATED IN RESPONSE TO IMMUNIZATION: IMMUNE ANTIBODIES

Blood Group Associations and Occurrence of Immune Antibodies

Immune antibodies are produced following exposure to foreign RBC antigens through pregnancy or transfusion. The primary immune response is seen several weeks to several months after the first exposure to antigen. IgM usually is associated with early primary responses, but whether it is always the first antibody class made is unclear. In most individuals, IgG soon predominates. This process is characteristic of a thymus-dependent immune response, where T cells help induce B cells to undergo isotype switching from IgM to IgG.

In a secondary or anamnestic response, antibody concentration starts to increase several days to several weeks following exposure, and IgG may rise to very high levels. Some IgG antibodies remain detectable for decades after a stimulus. Others, especially Kidd antibodies, can disappear after several months and are more commonly associated with delayed hemolytic transfusion reactions.[5,6,16]

Immune antibodies are found more commonly in individuals who have been multiply transfused than in multiparous women. This situation occurs because in pregnancy the immunizing dose of red cells often is too small to elicit a primary response, and the foreign antigens are limited to those of the father.[16]

Anti-D used to be the most common immune antibody, but with the advent of Rh matching of donors and recipients in the late 1940s and use of Rh Ig prophylaxis since the 1970s, its incidence has sharply decreased. Anti-D is present in 0.27 to 0.56 percent of transfusion recipients, 0.10 to 0.20 percent of pregnant women, and 0.16 to 0.25 percent of healthy blood donors.[16]

In contrast, the occurrence of immune antibodies other than anti-D has increased. Specificities other than anti-D have been reported in approximately 0.6 percent of transfusion recipients, 0.14 percent of pregnant women, and 0.19 percent of healthy blood donors. Pooled data from three 5-year periods and approximately 300,000 patients suggest the absolute occurrence of Rh antibodies other than anti-D is 0.22 percent, other than anti-K is 0.19 percent, other than anti-Fy^a is 0.05 percent, and other than anti-Jk^a is 0.04 percent.[16] The rate of alloimmunization in sickle cell anemia was 18.6 percent in one survey, and 55 percent of the immunized patients made more than one antibody. The most common specificities were anti-C, anti-E, and anti-K.[16]

Characteristics of Immune Antibodies

Immune antibodies most often are IgG but may be IgM and sometimes are IgA. Most immune antibodies react at body temperature and are considered clinically significant, except those directed against Bg, Kn^a, McC^a, Sl^a, Yk^a, Cs^a, JMH, and sometimes Yt^a and Lutheran antigens.

CLINICAL SIGNIFICANCE OF ERYTHROCYTE ANTIBODIES

Information about the clinical significance of alloantibodies is available at www.nybloodcenter.org.[59]

■ HEMOLYTIC TRANSFUSION REACTIONS

Clinically significant antibodies are capable of destroying transfused RBCs. The severity of the reaction varies with antigen density and antibody characteristics.

Antibodies commonly associated with intravascular hemolysis include anti-A, anti-B, anti-Jk^a, and anti-Jk^b. ABO incompatibility is the most potent cause of immediate hemolytic reactions because A and B antigens are so strongly expressed on RBCs and the antibodies so efficiently bind complement. Kidd antibodies are associated more often with delayed hemolytic reactions because they typically are difficult to detect and can disappear quickly from the circulation. IgG anti-Jk^a appears to bind complement only when traces of IgM anti-Jk^a are present.[16] Anti-PP1Pk, anti-Vel, and anti-Le^a have been associated with hemolysis, but such examples are rare.

Extravascular hemolysis occurs with IgG_1 and IgG_3 antibodies that react at body temperature, that is, immune antibodies reactive with Rh, Kidd, Kell, Duffy, or Ss antigens. These antibodies make up the bulk of clinically significant antibodies. Antibodies not expected to cause RBC destruction are those that react only at temperatures below 37°C (98.6°F) and IgG antibodies of the IgG_2 or IgG_4 subclass.[16]

■ HEMOLYTIC DISEASE OF THE FETUS AND NEWBORN

HDFN is caused by blood group incompatibility between a sensitized mother and her antigen-positive fetus (see Chap. 54). The antibodies most significant in HDFN are those that cross the placenta (IgG_1 and IgG_3), react at body temperature to cause red cell destruction, and are directed against well-developed RBC antigens. ABO incompatibility most commonly is seen, but ABO HDFN is clinically mild, presumably because the antigens are not fully expressed at birth. Antibodies directed against the D antigen can cause severe HDFN, and fetal health should be carefully monitored when anti-D titers are greater than 1:16. The severity of HDFN is less predictable with other blood group antibodies and can vary from mild to severe. For example, anti-K not only causes red cell hemolysis but also may suppress erythropoiesis.[60]

■ AUTOIMMUNE HEMOLYTIC ANEMIA

Autoimmune hemolytic anemia is caused by the production of "warm-" or "cold-" reactive autoantibodies directed against RBC antigens (see Chap.

53).[40] Production can be triggered by disease, viral infection, or drugs; from breakdown in immune system tolerance to self-antigens; or from exposure to foreign antigens that induce antibodies that cross-react with self-RBC antigens. Autologous specificity is not always obvious because antigen expression can be depressed when autoantibody is present.[40]

Warm autoantibodies react best at 37°C (98.6°F) and are primarily IgG (rarely IgM or IgA). Most are directed against the Rh protein, but Wr^b, Kell, Kidd, and U blood group specificities have been reported.[40]

Cold-reactive autoantibodies are primarily IgM. They react best at temperatures below 25°C (77°F) but can agglutinate RBCs or activate complement at or near 37°C (98.6°F), causing hemolysis or vascular occlusion upon exposure to cold.[16] Patients with cold agglutinin disease often have C3d on their RBCs, which can provide some protection from hemolysis. Most cold-reactive autoantibodies have anti-I activity. Reactivity with i, H, Pr, P, or other antigenic specificities is much less common.

The biphasic cold-reactive IgG antibody associated with paroxysmal cold hemoglobinuria ("Donath-Landsteiner" antibody) typically reacts with the high-prevalence antigen P. It attaches to RBCs in the cold and very efficiently activates complement before it dissociates at warmer temperatures.

DISEASES ASSOCIATED WITH ANTIBODY PRODUCTION

Table 137–4 lists diseases associated with specific antibody production. These antibodies cause autoimmune hemolytic anemia only if the patient carries the corresponding antigen.

TABLE 137–6. Common Causes of ABO Discrepancies

Red cells may appear to have	
Weak or missing antigens	Weak subgroup of A or B antigen
	Excess soluble A or B antigen in plasma
	Disease-associated loss (leukemia)
	ABO nonidentical marrow transplantation
	ABO nonidentical RBC transfusions
Extra antigens	Positive direct antiglobulin test
	Antibody to reagent additive or dye
	Rouleaux or cold agglutinin on cells
	Disease-associated acquisition (polyagglutination)
Serum may appear to have	
Weak or missing antibody	Age related (newborns or the very elderly)
	Disease-associated immunosuppression
	Congenital hypogammaglobulinemia
	ABO nonidentical marrow transplantation
Extra antibody	Alloantibodies (A_1, Le^a, Le^b, P_1, M, N)
	Autoantibodies (I, i, H, Pr, P)
	Rouleaux
	Antibodies to additives in reagent RBCs
	Passive antibody acquisition from transfusion or from passenger lymphocytes in organ transplantation

SEROLOGIC DETECTION OF ERYTHROCYTE ANTIGENS AND ANTIBODIES

ABO

ABO grouping is the single most important test performed in the transfusion service because it is the fundamental basis for determining blood compatibility. ABO grouping is determined by testing RBCs with licensed antisera to identify the A or B antigens they carry (forward, or cell, grouping) and by testing the corresponding serum or plasma with known A and B cells to identify the antibodies present (reverse, or serum, grouping). Positive reactions are seen as hemagglutination or hemolysis, and the results of one test should confirm the results of the other.

If results are discrepant or reactions are weaker than expected, the cause must be investigated before the ABO group can be interpreted with confidence. Discrepancies can be related to RBC anomalies, serum anomalies, or both, and they may be associated with disease.[5,11,16] Table 137–6 lists common causes, excluding clerical and technical error. If the ABO group of a patient cannot be determined, group O blood can be used for transfusion.

Rh

The D type is the next most important test performed for blood compatibility. Individuals whose RBCs type D+ are called *Rh-positive*, and those who type D– are called *Rh-negative*, provided controls are acceptable. Blood donors and pregnant women who type D– using standard typing sera are tested further for weak D expression using more sensitive methods, such as an indirect antiglobulin test. Donors with weak D antigen are considered Rh-positive. Testing for weak D is optional for transfusion recipients.[56]

EXTENDED ANTIGEN PHENOTYPING

Reagent antisera to detect other common antigens (e.g., CcEe, MNSs, Kk, Fy^aFy^b, Jk^aJk^b) are available and used when identification of the red cell phenotype is essential to antibody identification, blood compatibility, determination of zygosity, or paternity or forensic issues. Extended phenotyping is especially important to patients who are at high risk for alloimmunization from chronic blood transfusion, for example, those with sickle cell anemia or thalassemia. Ideally, an extended RBC phenotype of patients who are likely to be chronically transfused should be determined prior to initiation of transfusion therapy. Prediction of a blood group antigen can be made after testing DNA of a patient.[27]

ANTIBODY SCREEN

The antibody screen, or indirect antiglobulin test, detects "atypical" or "unexpected" antibodies in the serum (i.e., other than anti-A and anti-B) using group O reagent red cells that are known to carry various combinations of antigens. The methods used must be able to detect clinically significant antibodies. Typically, serum or plasma and screening cells are incubated at 37°C (98.6°F) with an additive to potentiate antibody-antigen reactions, then an indirect antiglobulin test is performed. Hemagglutination or hemolysis at any point is a positive reaction, indicating the presence of naturally occurring or immune alloantibody or autoantibody. The antibody screen will not detect all atypical antibodies in serum, such as antibodies to low-prevalence antigens not present on screening cells and antibodies that are not apparent at 37°C (98.6°F) and in the antiglobulin phase.

DIRECT ANTIGLOBULIN TEST

The direct antiglobulin test (direct Coombs test) detects antibody or complement bound to RBCs *in vivo*. Red cells are washed free of serum and then mixed with antiglobulin reagents that agglutinate RBCs coated with IgG or the C3 component of complement.

Positive direct antiglobulin test results are associated with the following: (1) transfusion reactions, in which recipient alloantibody coats transfused donor RBCs or transfused donor antibody coats recipient RBCs; (2) HDFN, in which maternal antibody crosses the placenta and coats fetal RBCs; (3) autoimmune hemolytic anemias, in which autoantibody coats the patient's own RBCs; (4) drug or drug–antibody complex interactions with RBCs that sometimes lead to hemolysis; (5) passenger lymphocyte syndrome, in which transient antibody produced by passenger lymphocytes from a transplanted organ coats recipient RBCs; and (6) hypergammaglobulinemia, in which Ig nonspecifically adsorb onto circulating RBCs.

A positive direct antiglobulin test result does not always indicate decreased red cell survival. As many as 10 percent of hospital patients and 0.1 percent of blood donors have a positive direct antiglobulin test result with no clinical indication of hemolysis.[11]

TABLE 137–7. ABO-Rh Compatibility Guidelines

	Antigen on Red Cells	Antibody in Serum	Compatible Blood Groups	
			Donor Red Cells	Donor Plasma
If recipient blood group is				
A	A	Anti-B	A, O	A, AB
B	B	Anti-A	B, O	B, AB
O	O	Anti-A, anti-B	O	O, A, B, AB
AB	A, B	None	AB, A, B, O	AB
Rh-positive	D	None	Rh-positive, Rh-negative	Rh not considered
Rh-negative	–	Anti-D only if immunized	Rh-negative	Rh not considered

NOTE: Whole blood must be identical to recipient's blood group. RBC products must be compatible with recipient's serum. Plasma products should be compatible with recipient's RBCs. Platelet and cryoprecipitate products should be compatible with recipient's RBCs, but any ABO group can be given if compatible units are not available.

COMPATIBILITY TESTING

Compatibility testing refers to a collection of donor and recipient tests that are performed prior to red cell transfusion. The collecting facility tests donors for ABO, Rh, and unexpected antibody. However, transfusing hospitals retest the ABO (and D on Rh-negative units) to verify the accuracy of the blood label.[56] Routine recipient testing includes an ABO, Rh, and antibody screening on a blood sample collected within 3 days of the intended transfusion. Results are checked against historical records to verify ABO, Rh, and antibody status.[56]

If the recipient has a negative antibody screening test result and no history of clinically significant antibodies, a serologic immediate spin cross-match between recipient serum and donor red cells or a "computer cross-match" (wherein computer software compares the ABO test results of both donor and recipient) is required to confirm ABO compatibility.[11]

If clinically significant antibodies are detected in a recipient's serum or previously were identified, red cell components should test negative for the corresponding antigens and be cross-match compatible at 37°C (98.6°F) by the antiglobulin test. The chance of finding compatible units usually reflects the antigen prevalence in the population, that is, 91 percent of units should be compatible with a patient making anti-K because 9 percent of the population is K+. This reasoning will not be valid if the local donor population varies significantly from the general population. When more than one antibody is present, the probability of finding compatible blood is the product of the prevalence (probability) of each independent antigen tested. For example, only 21 percent of units will be compatible for the recipient having both anti-K and anti-Jk^a: (0.91 for K−) × (0.23 for Jk[a−]) = 0.21.

When multiple clinically significant antibodies or antibodies directed against high-prevalence antigens are present, finding compatible RBC components can be extremely difficult. Such antibody producers should be encouraged to give autologous donations prior to their elective blood needs. If the patient is not a candidate for autologous donation, compatible units may be found by testing the patient's siblings or by asking regional blood suppliers to check their rare donor inventories and files. Such procurement requires additional time.

Repeat donor testing and cross-matching are not performed for plasma and platelet components, but the recipient's ABO and Rh phenotypes must be known for appropriate selection of components. Table 137–7 gives general ABO-Rh compatibility guidelines.

ANTIBODY IDENTIFICATION

All unexpected antibodies should be investigated. Those detected in serum or plasma as an ABO discrepancy, a positive antibody screening result, or an incompatible cross-match are identified using a panel of 8 to 16 different group O red cells that have been typed for antigens corresponding to clinically significant antibodies. Serum reactions with these RBCs are compared to their antigen typing to determine specificity.[11] For example, an antibody that reacts with all K+ RBCs but not with K− cells most likely is anti-K.

A control of autologous RBCs and serum is tested concurrently with panel RBCs. Absence of reactivity with autologous cells implies the antibody is an alloantibody, whereas a positive result suggests autoantibody or a positive direct antiglobulin test result. Once antibody specificity is identified, the patient's RBCs are tested for the corresponding antigen. If the alloantibody is anti-K, the cells should type K− Such antigen typing helps to confirm serum findings.

When antibody is detected both on red cells (a positive direct antiglobulin test result) and in serum, only the antibody in serum is identified unless a review of the medical or transfusion history offers evidence that the antibodies might be different. When antibody is detected only on RBCs and *in vivo* hemolysis is suspected, the antibody can be eluted from the patient's RBCs and tested against panel RBCs to identify the specificity.

REFERENCES

1. Lewis M, Anstee DJ, Bird GWG, et al: Blood group terminology 1990. ISBT working party on terminology for red cell surface antigens. *Vox Sang* 58:152, 1990.
2. Lögdberg L, Reid ME, Miller JL: Cloning and genetic characterization of blood group carrier molecules and antigens. *Transfus Med Rev* 16:1, 2002.
3. Cartron JP, Bailly P, Le Van Kim C, et al: Insights into the structure and function of membrane polypeptides carrying blood group antigens. *Vox Sang* 74(Suppl 2):29, 1998.
4. Daniels G: *Human Blood Groups*, 2nd ed. Blackwell Science, Oxford, 2002.
5. Issitt PD, Anstee DJ: *Applied Blood Group Serology*, 4th ed. Montgomery Scientific, Durham, NC, 1998.
6. Reid ME, Lomas-Francis C: *Blood Group Antigen FactsBook*, 2nd ed. Academic Press, San Diego, 2004.
7. Telen MJ: Erythrocyte blood group antigens: Not so simple after all. *Blood* 85:299, 1995.

8. Cartron JP, Colin Y: Structural and functional diversity of blood group antigens. *Transfus Clin Biol* 8:163, 2001.
9. Bruce LJ, Ghosh S, King MJ, et al: Absence of CD47 in protein 4.2-deficient hereditary spherocytosis in man: an interaction between the Rh complex and the band 3 complex. *Blood* 100:1878, 2002.
10. Reid ME, Mohandas N: Red blood cell blood group antigens: Structure and function. *Semin Hematol* 41:93, 2004.
11. Roback JD, Combs MR, Grossman BJ, et al (eds): *Technical Manual*, 16th ed. American Association of Blood Banks, Bethesda, MD, 2008.
12. Daniels GL, Cartron JP, Fletcher A, et al: International Society of Blood Transfusion Committee on terminology for red cell surface antigens: Vancouver report. *Vox Sang* 84:244, 2003.
13. Daniels GL, Anstee DJ, Cartron J-P, et al: Blood group terminology 1995. ISBT working party on terminology for red cell surface antigens. *Vox Sang* 69:265, 1995.
14. Garratty G, Dzik WH, Issitt PD, et al: Terminology for blood group antigens and genes: Historical origins and guidelines in the new millennium. *Transfusion* 40:477, 2000.
15. Reid ME, Lomas-Francis C: *Blood Group Antigens & Antibodies: A Guide to Clinical Relevance & Technical Tips*. Star Bright Books, New York, 2007.
16. Klein HG, Anstee DJ: *Mollison's Blood Transfusion in Clinical Medicine*, 11th ed. Wiley-Blackwell, Oxford, 2006.
17. Clausen H, White T, Takio K, et al: Isolation to homogeneity and partial characterization of a histo-blood group A defined Fuca1—>2Gala1—>3-*N*-acetylglucosaminyltransferase from human lung tissue. *J Biol Chem* 265:1139, 1990.
18. Yamamoto F, Marken J, Tsuji T, et al: Cloning and characterization of DNA complementary to human UDP-GalNAc: Fuca1—>2Gala1—>3GalNAc transferase (histo-blood group A transferase) mRNA. *J Biol Chem* 265:1146, 1990.
19. Yamamoto F, Hakomori S: Sugar-nucleotide donor specificity of histo-blood group A and B transferases is based on amino acid substitutions. *J Biol Chem* 265:19257, 1990.
20. Yamamoto F, Clausen H, White T, et al: Molecular genetic basis of the histo-blood group ABO system. *Nature* 345:229, 1990.
21. Chester MA, Olsson ML: The ABO blood group gene: A locus of considerable genetic diversity. *Transfus Med Rev* 15:177, 2001.
22. Olsson ML, Chester MA: Polymorphism and recombination events at the *ABO* locus: A major challenge for genomic ABO blood grouping strategies. *Transfus Med* 11:295, 2001.
23. Garratty G: Association of blood groups and disease: Do blood group antigens and antibodies have a biological role? *Hist Philos Life Sci* 18:321, 1996.
24. Avent ND, Reid ME: The Rh blood group system: A review. *Blood* 95:375, 2000.
25. Tippett P, Lomas-Francis C, Wallace M: The Rh antigen D: Partial D antigens and associated low incidence antigens. *Vox Sang* 70:123, 1996.
26. Huang C-H, Liu PZ, Cheng JG: Molecular biology and genetics of the Rh blood group system. *Semin Hematol* 37:150, 2000.
27. Reid ME: Applications of DNA-based assays in blood group antigen and antibody identification. *Transfusion* 43:1748, 2003.
28. Giblett ER: A critique of the theoretical hazard of inter *vs.* intra-racial transfusion. *Transfusion* 1:233, 1961.
29. Tippett P: Regulator genes affecting red cell antigens [review]. *Transfus Med Rev* 4:56, 1990.
30. Singleton BK, Burton NM, Green C, et al: Mutations in EKLF/KLF1 form the molecular basis of the rare blood group In(Lu) phenotype. *Blood* 112:2081, 2008.
31. Okubo Y, Yamaguchi H, Nagao N, et al: Heterogeneity of the phenotype Jk(a–b–) found in Japanese. *Transfusion* 26:237, 1986.
32. Hakomori S: Blood group ABH and Ii antigens of human erythrocytes: Chemistry, polymorphism, and their developmental change. *Semin Hematol* 18:39, 1981.
33. Spitalnik PF, Spitalnik SL: The P blood group system: Biochemical, serological, and clinical aspects. *Transfus Med Rev* 9:110, 1995.
34. Pogo AO, Chaudhuri A: The Duffy protein: A malarial and chemokine receptor. *Semin Hematol* 37:122, 2000.
35. Araten DJ, Swirsky D, Karadimitris A, et al: Cytogenetic and morphological abnormalities in paroxysmal nocturnal haemoglobinuria. *Br J Haematol* 115:360, 2001.
36. Tippett P, Ellis NA: The Xg blood group system: A review. *Transfus Med Rev* 12:233, 1998.
37. Cartron J-P, Rahuel C: Human erythrocyte glycophorins: Protein and gene structure analyses. *Transfus Med Rev* 6:63, 1992.
38. Tournamille C, Colin Y, Cartron JP, Le Van Kim C: Disruption of a GATA motif in the *Duffy* gene promoter abolishes erythroid gene expression in Duffy-negative individuals. *Nat Genet* 10:224, 1995.
39. Mourant AE, Kopec AC, Domaniewska-Sobczak K: *Distribution of the Human Blood Groups and Other Polymorphisms*, 2nd ed. Oxford University Press, London, 1976.
40. Petz LD, Garratty G: *Acquired Immune Hemolytic Anemias*, 2nd ed. Churchill Livingstone, New York, 2003.
41. Moulds JM, Moulds JJ: Blood group associations with parasites, bacteria, and viruses. *Transfus Med Rev* 14:302, 2000.
42. Cartron JP: Molecular basis of red cell protein antigen deficiencies. *Vox Sang* 78:7, 2000.
43. Lee S, Russo D, Redman CM: The Kell blood group system: Kell and XK membrane proteins. *Semin Hematol* 37:113, 2000.
44. Danek A, Rubio JP, Rampoldi L, et al: McLeod neuroacanthocytosis: Genotype and phenotype. *Ann Neurol* 50:755, 2001.
45. Luhn K, Wild MK, Eckhardt M, et al: The gene defective in leukocyte adhesion deficiency II encodes a putative GDP-fucose transporter. *Nat Genet* 28:69, 2001.
46. Etzioni A, Tonetti M: Leukocyte adhesion deficiency II-from A to almost Z. *Immunol Rev* 178:138, 2000.
47. Yu L-C, Twu Y-C, Chang C-Y, Lin M: Molecular basis of the adult i phenotype and the gene responsible for the expression of the human blood group I antigen. *Blood* 98:3840, 2001.
48. Inaba N, Hiruma T, Togayachi A, et al: A novel I-branching beta-1,6-*N*-acetylglucosaminyltransferase involved in human blood group I antigen expression. *Blood* 101:2870, 2003.
49. Yu LC, Twu YC, Chou ML, et al: The molecular genetics of the human I locus and molecular background explaining the partial association of the adult i phenotype with congenital cataracts. *Blood* 101:2081, 2003.
50. Agre P, King LS, Yasui M, et al: Aquaporin water channels—From atomic structure to clinical medicine. *J Physiol* 542:3, 2002.
51. Crew VK, Burton N, Kagan A, et al: CD151, the first member of the tetraspanin (TM4) superfamily detected on erythrocytes, is essential for the correct assembly of human basement membranes in kidney and skin. *Blood* 104:2217, 2004.
52. Rock JA, Shirey RS, Braine HG, et al: Plasmapheresis for the treatment of repeated early pregnancy wastage associated with anti-P. *Obstet Gynecol* 66:57S, 1985.
53. Udden MM, Umeda M, Hirano Y, Marcus DM: New abnormalities in the morphology, cell surface receptors, and electrolyte metabolism of In(Lu) erythrocytes. *Blood* 69:52, 1987.
54. Heaton DC, McLoughlin K: Jk(a–b–) red blood cells resist urea lysis. *Transfusion* 22:70, 1982.
55. Sands JM: Molecular mechanisms of urea transport. *J Membr Biol* 191:149, 2003.
56. Standards Committee of American Association of Blood Banks: *Standards for Blood Banks and Transfusion Services*, 24th ed. American Associations of Blood Banks, Bethesda, MD, 2006.
57. Springer GF, Horton RE, Forbes M: Origin of anti-human blood group B agglutinins in white leghorn chicks. *J Exp Med* 110:221, 1959.
58. Springer GF, Horton RE: Blood group isoantibody stimulation in man by feeding blood group-active bacteria. *J Clin Invest* 48:1280, 1969.
59. Reid ME, Øyen R, Marsh WL: Summary of the clinical significance of blood group alloantibodies. *Semin Hematol* 37:197, 2000.
60. Vaughan JI, Warwick R, Letsky E, et al: Erythropoietic suppression in fetal anemia because of Kell alloimmunization. *Am J Obstet Gynecol* 171:247, 1994.

CHAPTER 138
HUMAN LEUKOCYTE AND PLATELET ANTIGENS

Myra Coppage, David Stroncek,
Janice McFarland, and Neil Blumberg

SUMMARY

The human leukocyte antigens (HLAs) are highly polymorphic glycoproteins encoded by the major histocompatibility complex (MHC) on chromosome 6. Their biologic function is presentation of antigenic peptides to T lymphocytes, and there are two major classes: class I (A, B, and C loci) and class II (DR, DQ, and DP loci). Class I antigens are present on almost all nucleated cells, whereas class II antigens are primarily expressed on B cells and other antigen-presenting cells such as dendritic cells, endothelial cells, and monocytes. These antigens play key roles in hematopoietic cell transplantation acceptance/rejection and allosensitization to nonleukoreduced blood transfusions leading to platelet transfusion refractoriness, with lesser, but distinct roles in solid-organ transplantation. Other clinically important lineage-specific white cell antigens include those on neutrophils, which are much less polymorphic and less commonly a cause of clinical problems than the HLA system. Antibody to neutrophil antigens plays a role in autoimmune neutropenia, and reactions such as transfusion-related acute lung injury. Platelets also possess a relatively limited number of polymorphic antigens that are involved in clinical problems such as posttransfusion purpura and platelet transfusion refractoriness, and neonatal problems such as alloimmune thrombocytopenia.

HUMAN LEUKOCYTE ANTIGENS (MAJOR HISTOCOMPATIBILITY COMPLEX)

■ DEFINITION

The human leukocyte antigens (HLAs) are highly polymorphic glycoproteins encoded by a region of genes known as the major histocompatibility complex (MHC) located on chromosome 6p21 and covering a region of about 7.6 Mbp.[1,2] After ABO antigens, HLA antigens are the major barrier to transplantation. Their biologic function is to present antigenic peptides to T lymphocytes. The MHC codes for several groups of antigens. The best understood are the highly polymorphic, classical class I (HLA-A, HLA-B, and HLA-C) and class II (HLA-DR, HLA-DQ, and HLA-DP) antigens. Class I antigens are ubiquitous and present on most nucleated somatic cells. Class II antigens exhibit more restricted distribution, with varying levels of expression on B cells, dendritic cells, monocytes, macrophages, and endothelial cells. However, class II antigens can be induced on many cell types through activation.[3] The nonclassical class Ib antigens HLA-E, HLA-F, and HLA-G, and the more recently described MHC class I chain-related antigens are much less polymorphic, their function less understood, and their tissue expression more limited. In addition the MHC region codes for a number of pseudogenes. This chapter focuses on the classic class I and II molecules because of their importance in transfusion and transplantation.

The two major classes of HLA antigens are homologous. However, there are areas of high variability (polymorphism) that distinguish individual HLA molecules (alleles) and confer antigen specificity. HLA antigens are codominantly expressed so that each individual expresses 2 antigens at each locus (A, B, DR, etc). As of November 2008, 3304 HLA alleles had been characterized.[4] Table 138–1 lists the number of known HLA alleles at each locus.

Acronyms and abbreviations that appear in this chapter include: CDC, complement-dependent cytotoxicity; ELISA, enzyme-linked immunosorbent assay; GP, glycoprotein; GVHD, graft-versus-host disease; HLA, human leukocyte antigens; HNA, human neutrophil antigens; HPA, human platelet antigen; MHC, major histocompatibility complex; NAIT, neonatal alloimmune thrombocytopenia; NMDP, National Marrow Donor Program; PCR, polymerase chain reaction; PRA, panel reactive antibodies; PTP, posttransfusion purpura; SSO, sequence-specific oligonucleotide; SSP, sequence-specific primer; TRALI, transfusion-related acute lung injury; WHO, World Health Organization.

■ GENETICS OF THE MHC

The first sequence map of the MHC encompassed approximately 3.6 Mbp on chromosome 6p21 and was divided into three regions: class I, class II, and class III genes.[2] More recent analysis confirming high linkage disequilibrium and conserved synteny led to the concept of an extended MHC (xMHC), and a new map was produced in 2004.[5] The xMHC occupies about 7.6 Mbp, and is composed of five subregions, which include the classical classes I, II, and III genes. Class II genes are the most centromeric and occupy about 1 Mbp of DNA. The genes are ordered sequentially beginning with HLA-DP genes followed by HLA-DM, TAP, HLA-DQ and lastly the HLA-DR genes. The class III genes occupy space between the class I and class II genes. The class III genes include genes that encode other proteins that participate in immune response such as complement, heat shock proteins, tumor necrosis factor, and other lymphocyte antigens. Telomeric are the class I genes sequentially as MICA, MICB, HLA-B, HLA-C, HLA-E, HLA-A, HLA-F, and HLA-G. Extended class I genes include histone clusters and zinc finger genes. Figure 138–1B is a representative map of the MHC.

■ STRUCTURE AND FUNCTION

Class I Antigens

The HLA-A, -B and -C molecules are transmembrane glycoproteins with an Mr = 56,000.[6] Each is a heterodimer composed of one α heavy chain (Mr = 45,000) noncovalently bound to β_2-microglobulin (Mr = 11,000). The α heavy chain is the polymorphic glycoprotein encoded by the MHC genes. The extracellular region of the α chain consists of three domains (α_1, α_2, α_3) based on folding and disulfide bonding (see Fig. 138–1A). Antigenicity resides in the α_1 and α_2 domains, the areas of highest polymorphism. These two chains form a platform composed of a single β-pleated sheet "floor" topped by two α helices with a cleft or groove between them. The structure is supported by the third, α_3, domain of the heavy chain in conjunction with β_2-microglobulin, which stabilizes the molecule on the cell surface. Class I HLA molecules present peptide fragments from endogenously derived proteins (e.g., viral infection, intracellular bacteria, or transformation) to CD8+ T cells. The highly polymorphic groove permits presentation of highly variable peptides of nine amino acids average length. Class I HLA-A, -B, and -C antigens are found in most nucleated somatic cells.[7] Platelets express HLA-A antigens, but lack some HLA-B and most HLA-C antigens.[8]

Class II Antigens

The class II antigens are also transmembrane glycoproteins formed by two noncovalently bound chains.[11] Both the α heavy chain (Mr = 34,000) and the light β chain (Mr = 29,000) are encoded in the MHC

TABLE 138–1. Number of Known Alleles for Each HLA Locus as of November 2008

HLA Class I						
Gene	A	B	C	E	F	G
Alleles	697	1109	381	9	21	36
HLA Class II						
Gene	DRA	DRB	DQA	DQB	DPA	DPB
Alleles	3	690	34	95	27	131
Non-HLA						
Gene	MICA	MICB	TAP1	TAP2		
Alleles	65	30	7	4		

SOURCE: Adapted and simplified from Robinson J, Waller MJ, Parham P, et al,[4] with permission.

region. Class II molecules, like class I, consist of an extracellular hydrophilic NH_2– terminal region, a hydrophobic transmembrane region, and an intracellular COOH– terminus region. Unlike class I antigens, the extracellular regions of each chain contain only two domains. The two domains of the α chain are designated α_1 and α_2, and the two domains of the β-chain are called β_1 and β_2. The α chain of HLA-DR is constant for all HLA-DR molecules, whereas the β chain is polymorphic and determines specificity of the molecule. Both α and β chains of HLA-DQ and -DP are polymorphic, although the β chain is more so than the α chain. In all class II antigens the β_1 domain represents the most polymorphic region. The structure of HLA-DR is essentially similar to the structure of class I molecules. Class II antigens present peptides from exogenous sources, such as bacterial pathogens, to CD4+ cells. The binding groove is more open than that of class I, and peptides of longer length (11–18 amino acids) are accommodated.[12,13] Class II antigens have a more restricted tissue distribution, being found primarily on B lymphocytes and other antigen-presenting cells such as dendritic cells, monocytes, and macrophages. They may also be expressed on activated endothelial cells and T lymphocytes.[11]

The extraordinarily polymorphic nature of HLA has probably evolved because of the need to present a very large array of different antigenic peptides in host defense. Antigen processing and presentation is a tightly regulated process, especially among the professional antigen-presenting cells such as dendritic cells. A number of alternative mechanisms have been demonstrated *in vitro*, such as cross-presentation, whereby dendritic cells transfer antigen derived from endocytic sources to the class I pathway, but are poorly understood.[14] One promising area of research is the ability of HLA molecules to present antigenic peptides derived from tumors. Such peptides could arise via point mutation, or reactivation of a normally silent gene that produces a peptide that can bind to HLA and induce a T-cell immune response. Several such peptides (MAGE antigens) have been identified for melanoma.[15]

NOMENCLATURE

Distinguishing polymorphic variations among HLA antigens is clinically important in stem cell transplantation. Terminology used to describe accepted HLA alleles or antigens is standardized by the World Health Organization (WHO), Nomenclature Committee for Factors of the HLA System, which issues biannual reports and monthly updates.[4] In addition, an HLA dictionary defining HLA antigens, their assigned nomenclature, and serological equivalents is published periodically.[4a] The nomenclature committee approved major changes to the system that take effect in April 2010 (SG Marsh, oral communication, November 2009). The revisions are designed to accommodate the unexpected number of new sequenced alleles. Under this system, colons are used as delimiters to separate fields. The first field signifies the allele family that often corresponds to the serological antigen. The second field denotes the alleles, assigned in order of determination. The third field is used for

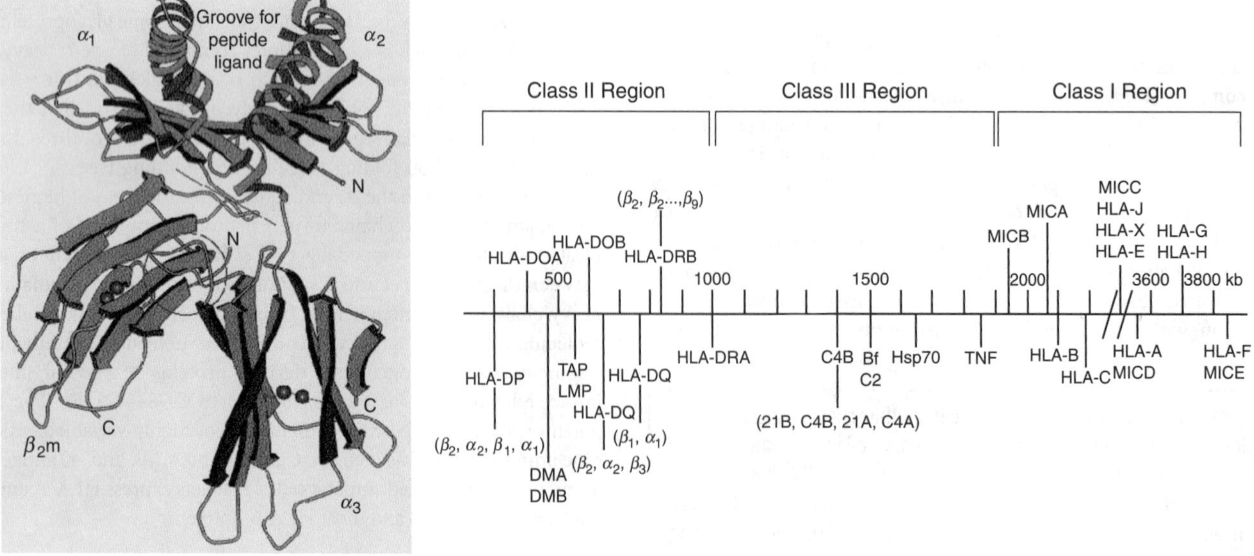

A B

FIGURE 138–1. A. Schematic of the HLA-A2 molecule. The peptide groove is formed by the α helices and β-pleated sheet floor. The groove holds processed peptide antigen. The peptide and the polymorphic α helices interact with the T-cell receptor. *(Reproduced from Bjorkman PJ, Saper MA, Samraoui B, et al[9] with permission.)* **B.** Representative diagram of the genes of the MHC on chromosome 6. *(Adapted and simplified from Campbell RD, Trowsdale J[10] with permission.)*

defining synonymous nucleotide substitutions. The last field defines alleles that differ by sequence polymorphisms in introns or in the 5′ or 3′ untranslated regions that flank the exons and introns. In addition, there are suffixes that are used to describe expression status. Null alleles (not expressed) are identified by the suffix "N." Low surface expression is represented by "L." Secreted molecules not present at the surface are assigned "S."

■ INHERITANCE OF MHC ANTIGENS

The genes of the MHC demonstrate more polymorphism than any other genetic system; that is, many alleles exist for each locus. Each individual, however, has one allele for each locus per chromosome, and therefore, encodes two HLA antigens per locus. The identification of each HLA antigen of an individual is called a *phenotype.* Because HLA genes are closely linked, recombination within the MHC is rare (≤1%), and a complete set of HLA genes usually is inherited from each parent as a unit. The genes inherited from each parent are referred to as a *haplotype.* Maternal and paternal haplotypes can be identified through family studies. Identification of both haplotypes of an individual provides the *genotype.* Family studies consist of typing for the HLA-A, HLA-B, HLA-C, HLA-DR, and HLA-DQ antigens to identify haplotypes and to rule out genetic recombination within the MHC. Because HLA genes are inherited together on a single chromosome, four combinations of maternal and paternal haplotypes are possible provided no recombination occurs (Fig. 138–2).

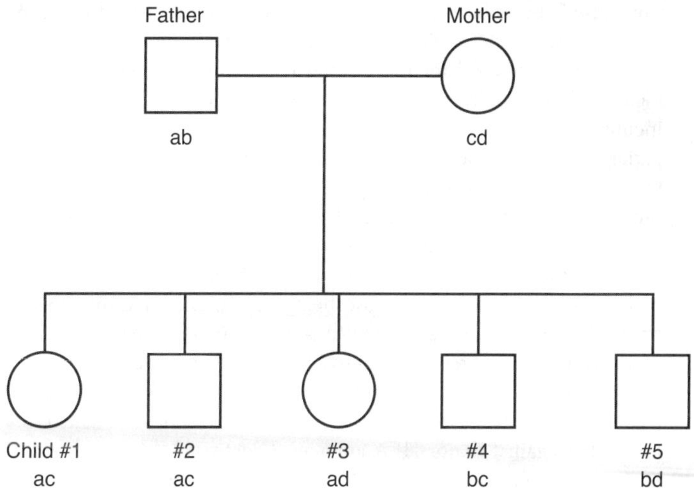

Code:	Haplotype:					
a	A1,	B8,	Cw1,	DR17,	DR52,	DQ2
b	A2,	B44,	Cw2,	DR11,	DR52,	DQ7
c	A3,	B7,	Cw3,	DR15,	DR51,	DQ6
d	A11,	B55,	Cw3,	DR4,	DR53,	DQ8

FIGURE 138–2. Pedigree representing inheritance of HLA antigens. Each of the four parental haplotypes is coded by a letter: *a* and *b* represent paternal haplotypes; *c* and *d* represent maternal haplotypes. Each child inherits one paternal and one maternal haplotype such that four combinations are possible.

Linkage Disequilibrium

Because the MHC is so highly polymorphic, the probability that any two unrelated individuals are HLA identical is extremely low. However, the system exhibits a phenomenon known as *linkage disequilibrium.* That is, HLA alleles are inherited together on the same chromosome more often than would be predicted if HLA loci were in equilibrium. At equilibrium, the frequency of an allele at one locus is independent of the frequencies of alleles at linked loci. For example, the gene frequency of HLA-A1 is 0.145 and that of HLA-B8 is 0.1 in North American whites. Given no preferential association between A1 and B8, then the haplotype frequency would be 0.0145 (0.145×0.1). However, population studies demonstrate that the actual frequency of the HLA-A1, B8 haplotype is 0.0726.[16] The degree of linkage disequilibrium is defined as the observed frequency minus its expected frequency, 0.0581 in this example. Although particular alleles found in linkage disequilibria differ for various racial groups, all racial groups display significant disequilibria. Different races and ethnic groups can vary greatly in the frequency with which HLA antigens are found.[17]

■ HUMAN LEUKOCYTE ANTIGEN TYPING

Tissue typing for HLA antigens can be performed by various methods using serologic, cellular, and molecular technologies. The most frequent procedures used in the clinical setting are serologic and molecular. Cellular assays such as the mixed lymphocyte reaction and the primed lymphocyte test were common prior to the widespread adoption of DNA methods. Compared to DNA techniques, cellular methods are labor-intensive and require the use of radioisotopes; they are mainly used in research laboratories.

Serology

The microlymphocytotoxicity complement-dependent cytotoxicity (CDC) test has been a fundamental procedure for defining HLA antigens for over 30 years.[18] In this assay, a suspension of lymphocytes is incubated with human alloantisera or monoclonal antibody in a microtiter tray.[19] Rabbit serum is added as a source of complement. Cell death is induced when antibody binds to antigen on the cell surface and the complement cascade activated. Death is visualized microscopically by the uptake of vital dye or by immunofluorescence. Panels used to determine a patient's HLA type consist of two to four antisera that recognize the same specificity, which requires approximately 150 different reagents for class I antigens and 80 to 150 for class II antigens. Antisera are usually obtained from multiparous women, multiply transfused patients, and from patients who have rejected allografts. Monoclonal antibodies are also commercially available for many HLA specificities. Serology for class II (DR and DQ) antigens requires enrichment for B lymphocytes, which can be accomplished with antibody or immunomagnetic bead reagents.

Molecular HLA Typing

The development of the polymerase chain reaction (PCR)[20] revolutionized the approach to HLA typing. Several DNA-based methods are commonly accepted for HLA typing. These include sequence-based typing, sequence-specific primer amplification (SSP)[21] and sequence-specific oligonucleotide (SSO) probe hybridization. All of these methods involve amplification of genomic DNA from selected portions of HLA genes with oligonucleotide primer pairs. Generally exons 2 and 3 of the class I and exon 2 of class II genes are amplified. These exons encode most of the polymorphisms of the classes I and II molecules. Molecular HLA typing is primarily of clinical interest in marrow/blood stem cell transplantation.

Detection of Antibodies to HLA Molecules

In addition to typing for HLA antigens, most laboratories also use technology to detect antibodies to HLA antigens. This is very important for solid-organ transplantation where the presence of anti-HLA antibodies can cause irreversible rejection upon transplantation. It is of less concern for marrow/stem cell transplantation where donors and recipients are generally matched for HLA antigens. The microcytotoxicity serologic test is a standard antibody detection method. However, instead of incubating an unknown patient cell with defined antisera for typing, a patient's serum is reacted with a panel of lymphocytes of defined HLA type. Analysis of the reaction patterns yields information about the breadth of alloimmunization, or PRA (percent reactive antibody), and the specificity of the reactions. Solid-phase assays have also become common methods for identifying anti-HLA antibody. These assays include enzyme-linked immunosorbent assay (ELISA) and microbead-based flow assays such as FlowPRA and Luminex® assays. The solid-phase assays are much more sensitive than the cytotoxic assays.

Prior to most solid-organ transplants, a donor-specific crossmatch is also performed to ensure that the recipient does not have anti-HLA antibodies against donor HLA antigens. Crossmatches are performed by microlymphocytotoxicity (CDC), flow cytometry, and by solid-phase (ELISA and microbead) assays.

CLINICAL APPLICATIONS

The HLA antigens coded by the MHC play a central role in transplantation, regulation of immune responses, and susceptibility to a variety of diseases. The most common application, however, is the field of transplantation. In renal and stem cell transplantation, allografts from HLA-identical sibling donors have significantly greater survival than grafts from nonmatched family or unrelated donors.

For solid-organ transplantation, a living donor is not always available or feasible (e.g., for heart transplantation). HLA typing for matching of kidneys and pancreas is performed at the HLA-A, HLA-B, and HLA-DR loci at low resolution (serologic or antigen level by DNA). In the early years of renal transplantation a high degree of match was sought between recipients and donors. However, as more potent immunotherapies have developed, the level and use of HLA matching has declined. HLA matching is not prospectively performed for hepatic or cardiac transplantation. Detection of alloantibody by screening techniques and the donor specific crossmatch is of prime importance for solid-organ transplants where its existence could cause a hyperacute rejection and graft failure.

Marrow or stem cell transplantation engenders problems other than allograft survival. In these cases an immunocompetent graft is transplanted to an immunocompromised/immunoablated host. The graft may recognize the host tissue as foreign and mount an immune response resulting graft-versus-host disease (GVHD). With HLA-identical sibling donors, disease-free survival of greater than 80 percent can be achieved for some hematopoietic malignancies.[22,23] However, fewer than 30 percent of individuals have an HLA-identical sibling. For these patients, alternative donors, such as phenotypically matched unrelated volunteers and partially matched family members, may be considered. However, the risks and incidence of graft failure and GVHD are higher than seen with HLA-identical siblings, and increase with the level of HLA disparity. HLA typing for stem cell transplants is generally performed by molecular methods. For those with a family donor, low-resolution typing may be sufficient to identify a match. However for unrelated or haplo-identical family donors, high-resolution (allele-level) typing for HLA-A, HLA-B, HLA-C, HLA-DR, and HLA-DQ should be performed, and is required by the national registry program (National Marrow Donor Program [NMDP]).[22]

Patients requiring platelet transfusions may be broadly sensitized to HLA-A, and -B (i.e., have high PRA) through prior transfusions (particularly nonleukoreduced) or pregnancies. HLA antibody screening to select nonreactive donors and/or HLA donor platelet matching may enable these refractory patients to achieve improved platelet transfusion count increments.

TABLE 138–2. Human Neutrophil Antigens

System	Alleles	Location of Antigens	Genes
HNA-1	HNA-1a, -1b, and -1c	FcγRIIIb	*FCGR3B*1*, *FCGR3B*2*, and *FCGR3B*3*
HNA-2	HNA-2a	NB1gp	*CD177*1*
HNA-3	HNA-3a	Unknown	Unknown
HNA-4	HNA-4a	α_M integrin, C3bi-receptor (CR3)	*CD11B*1*
HNA-5	HNA-5a	αL integrin, LFA-1	*CD11A*1*

HLA typing at one or a few antigens or alleles may also be performed to support diagnosis of diseases associated with specific HLA antigens. The most common of these is the association between HLA-B27 and ankylosing spondylitis[24] and HLA-DQ2's association with narcolepsy.[25] HLA typing may also be performed to determine eligibility for vaccine trials that utilize tumor peptides and HLA.[26,27] HLA antigens also are implicated in drug hypersensitivity. For example HLA-B*5701 is associated with hypersensitivity to the drug for treatment of the human immunodeficiency virus, abacavir.[28]

HLA tetramers may be used to monitor the efficacy of HLA-based peptide vaccines. Recombinant HLA molecules are loaded with the peptide vaccine and linked via a fluoresceinated streptavidin molecule. They are incubated with patient blood lymphocytes. Effector T cells specific for the peptide-HLA will be bound by the tetramer and monitored by flow cytometry.

NEUTROPHIL ANTIGENS AND ANTIBODIES

Clinically significant alloantigens expressed only or predominantly by neutrophils are known as human neutrophil antigens (HNAs).[29] In this nomenclature, the antigen systems are indicated by integers, and specific antigens within each system are designated alphabetically by date of publication (Table 138–2).

THE HNA-1 ANTIGEN SYSTEM

HNA-1 Antigens

The neutrophil-specific HNA-1 antigen system is made up of the three alleles, HNA-1a, -1b, and -1c (see Table 138–2).[30] HNA-1 antigens are located on the low-affinity Fcγ receptor IIIb (FcγRIIIb), CD16, and are expressed only on neutrophils.[31–34] FcγRIIIb and HNA-1 antigens are expressed on all segmented neutrophils, on approximately one-half of neutrophilic metamyelocytes, and on approximately 10 percent of neutrophilic myelocytes.[35] Soluble FcγRIIIb is present in plasma and has the same HNA-1 polymorphisms found on neutrophils.[36]

Molecular Biology

FcγRIIIb and the HNA-1 antigens are encoded by the *FCGR3B* gene located on chromosome 1q23–24. *FCGR3B* is highly homologous to *FCGR3A*, which encodes FcγRIIIa. In addition to the polymorphic FCGRB3B nucleotides only four others differ between *FCGR3B* and *FCGR3A*. The most important difference between the two genes is a

TABLE 138–3. Human Neutrophil Antigen Frequencies

		Antigen Frequencies			
System	Alleles	Europeans/ North Americans	Africans and African Americans	Asians	Brazilians/ Argentineans
HNA-1	HNA-1a	58%	59–67%	91%	68%
	HNA-1b	88%	71–88%	54%	76%
	HNA-1c	5%	25–38%	<1%	5–10%
HNA-2	HNA-2a	95–97%	95%	89–99%	NA
HNA-3	HNA-3a	89–92%	NA	NA	NA
HNA-4	HNA-4a	99%	NA	99%	97%
HNA-5	HNA-5a	85%	88%	81–96%	78–92%

NA, not available.

C-to-T change at 733 in *FCGR3B* that creates a stop codon. As a result, *FCGR3A* has 21 more amino acids than *FCGR3B* and *FCGR3B* is a glycosyl phosphatidylinositol (GPI)-anchored rather than a transmembrane glycoprotein.

The *FCGR3B*1* allele differs from *FCGR3B*2* by only five nucleotides in the coding region, at positions 141, 147, 227, 277, and 349.[31–34] Four of the nucleotide changes result in changes in amino acid sequence between the HNA-1a and HNA-1b forms of FcγRIIIb. The glycosylation pattern of FcγRIIIb differs between the two antigens because of two nucleotide changes at bases 227 and 277. The HNA-1b form of FcγRIIIb has six *N*-linked glycosylation sites and the HNA-1a form has four glycosylation sites.

The *FCGR3B*3* allele is identical to *FCGR3B*2* except for a C to A substitution at nucleotide 266 resulting in an alanine to aspartate change at amino acid 78 of FcγRIIIb.[30] In many cases, *FCGR3B*3* exists on the same chromosome with a second or duplicate *FCGR3B* gene.[37,38]

The antigen frequencies of the three alleles vary widely among different racial groups. Among whites, HNA-1b is the most common antigen (Table 138–3),[39–44] but in Japanese and Chinese populations HNA-1a is most common.[39,41–43,45] The frequency of the gene encoding HNA-1c antigen also varies among racial groups. HNA-1c is expressed by neutrophils in 4 percent to 5 percent of whites, 25 percent to 38 percent of African Americans, and 10 percent of Brazilians.[46,47]

Several other sequence variations in FCGR3B have been described.[41] Most of these chimeric alleles have single-base substitutions involving one of the five single nucleotide polymorphisms (SNPs) that distinguish *FCGR3B*1* and *FCGR3B*2*. *FCGR3B* alleles that most closely resembled *FCGR3B*2* were found more often in African Americans than in whites or Japanese.[41]

Genetic deficiencies of neutrophil FcγRIIIb and HNA-1 antigens have also been reported. Among whites the incidence of individuals homozygous for *FCGR3B* deletion is approximately 0.1 percent.[46,48,49] However, among Africans and African Americans the incidence is much higher. In one study, 3 of 126 Africans were found to be *FCGR3B* deficient,[42] and in another study, 1 of 53 were found to be *FCGR3B* deficient.[41]

Function of HNA-1 Antigens

Polymorphisms in FcγRIIIb have some effect on neutrophil function. Neutrophils that are homozygous for HNA-1b have a lower affinity for immunoglobulin (Ig) G_3 than those homozygous for HNA-1a.[50] Neutrophils from those who are homozygous for HNA-1b phagocytize erythrocytes sensitized with IgG_1 and IgG_3 anti-Rh monoclonal antibodies and bacteria opsonized with IgG_1 at a lower level than neutrophils homozygous for HNA-1a.[51,52]

THE HNA-2 ANTIGEN SYSTEM

The HNA-2a Antigen

The HNA-2 system has one well-described allele, HNA-2a. HNA-2a is expressed only on neutrophils, neutrophilic metamyelocytes, and myelocytes.[35,53] It's unique in that it is expressed on subpopulations of neutrophils. The mean size of the HNA-2a-positive subpopulation of neutrophils is 45 to 65 percent[54–56] and is dependent on gender. The size of the HNA-2a positive subpopulation of neutrophils from women is approximately 60 percent, compared with approximately 50 percent for men.[56,57] Neutrophil expression of HNA-2a is greater in pregnant women than in healthy female blood donors.[58]

HNA-2a Molecular Biology

The glycoprotein carrying HNA-2a, NB1 glycoprotein, is located on neutrophil plasma membranes and secondary granules[54,58] and is a GPI-anchored glycoprotein.[54] The gene encoding NB1 glycoprotein, *CD177*, is located on chromosome 19q13.31[59,60] and belongs to the *Ly-6* snake toxin superfamily. Other genes in this family include urokinase-type plasminogen activator receptor (CD87) and decay accelerating factor (CD59).

HNA-2a is expressed on neutrophils by approximately 95 to 97 percent of whites, 95 percent of African Americans, and 89 to 99 percent of Japanese.[56,61,62] SNPs have been identified in *CD177*. These SNPs have been associated with the size of the HNA-2a–positive population of neutrophils, but not the HNA-2a–negative phenotype.[63] The HNA-2a–negative neutrophil phenotype is the result of a *CD177* transcription defect.[64]

Role of NB1 Glycoprotein in Neutrophil Function

NB1 glycoprotein binds to platelet endothelial cell adhesion molecule-1 (PECAM-1, CD31) and functions as a cell adhesion molecule.[65] PECAM-1 is expressed on both neutrophils and endothelial cells and PECAM-1–PECAM-1 interactions are important in the migration of neutrophils through endothelial cells. Interactions between NB1 glycoprotein and PECAM-1 are also involved with neutrophil–endothelial cell interactions, and mediate neutrophil transendothelial cell migration.[65] However, women who produce HNA-2a specific alloantibodies and who lack NB1 glycoprotein are healthy.

CD177 messenger RNA (mRNA) is overexpressed by neutrophils from patients with polycythemia rubra vera and essential thrombocytosis, but the expression of HNA-2a is not.[66,67] The increased expression of CD177 mRNA in neutrophils from these patients may be secondary to the constitutive activation of Janus kinase 2 (JAK2) by JAK2 V617F.

THE HNA-3 ANTIGEN SYSTEM

The HNA-3 antigen system has one antigen, HNA-3a, that was previously known as 5b. HNA-3a is expressed by neutrophils, lymphocytes, platelets, endothelial cells, kidney, spleen, and placental cells. HNA-3a has an antigen frequency of 89 to 92 percent and is located on a 70- to 95-kDa neutrophil glycoprotein.[68] The gene encoding HNA-3a has not yet been cloned, and the nature and function of the 70- to 95-kDa glycoproteins is not known. Although a biologic role for this system has not been established, several cases of transfusion-related acute lung injury (TRALI) have been associated with transfusion of plasma containing anti–HNA-3a.[69–71]

■ THE HNA-4 AND HNA-5 ANTIGEN SYSTEMS

The HNA-4 and HNA-5 antigens are located on the β_2 integrins. Each antigen system contains only a single antigen, HNA-4a and HNA-5a, respectively. The HNA-4a antigen was previously known as Mart(a). HNA-4a was defined by an antibody in the sera of three nontransfused multiparous blood donors. This antigen has an autosomal dominant inheritance and an antigen frequency of 99 percent in whites[72] and Asians,[73] and 97 percent in Brazilians.[74] HNA-4a is located on the α_M chain (CD11b) of the C3bi receptor (CR3) and is caused by a single nucleotide substitution of G to A at position 302[75] that results in an Arg-to-His polymorphism at amino acid 61. The significance of the antibody is not known, and none of the infants of the three multiparous women with anti–HNA-4a showed evidence of neonatal alloimmune neutropenia.

A second polymorphism of the β_2 integrins, HNA-5a, was first described as Ond(a). A chronically transfused man with aplastic anemia became alloimmunized to HNA-5a. HNA-5a was found to be expressed on the α_L integrin unit, leukocyte function antigen-1 (CD11a), and is a result of a G to C single nucleotide substitution at position 2446 that results in a change of Arg to Thr at amino acid 766.[78] The antigen frequency of HNA-5a is 78 to 96 percent.[73,74,76]

■ ANTIBODIES TO NEUTROPHIL ANTIGENS

Alloimmune Neonatal Neutropenia

Neutrophil antibody tests are performed by agglutination or fluorescent techniques, and these are not widely available because clinical syndromes caused by these antibodies are uncommon. During pregnancy, mothers can become alloimmunized to fetal neutrophil antigens. Maternal IgG directed to neutrophils can cross the placenta and destroy the neonate's neutrophils. Maternal alloimmunization to neutrophil antigens can affect the first child. Most neonates experience isolated neutropenia, but the cytopenias are self-limiting and resolve as the antibody is cleared. Antibodies to neutrophil-specific antigens HNA-1a, HNA-1b, and HNA-2a most commonly cause neonatal alloimmune neutropenia.[68,77] Mothers with FcγRIIIb deficiency have also produced antibodies to FcγRIIIb, causing neonatal neutropenia.[49,68,77]

Most often the neutropenia is detected in the first week of life when the neonate becomes febrile or develops an infection and a neutrophil count is done. Typically, the counts are 0.100 to 0.200 × 10^9/L. White blood cell count, platelet count, and hemoglobin are usually normal, but eosinophilia or monocytosis may be present. The clinical course is quite variable. An occasional infant is asymptomatic, but almost all affected children have an infection. The duration of the neutropenia may be as short as a few days or as long as 28 weeks.[77] The mean duration of neutropenia is about 11 weeks.[77] Intravenous immunoglobulin (IVIg) and granulocyte colony-stimulating factor (G-CSF) have a limited role in the treatment of neonatal alloimmune neutropenia.[77]

Autoimmune Neutropenia of Childhood

Autoimmune neutropenia is well described in children.[78–81] Typically, the onset of the autoimmune neutropenia of children begins at 8 months of age, but children between 1 and 36 months of age can be affected. Most studies have found that neutrophil counts recover spontaneously by the age of 5 years, with a median duration of neutropenia of 13 to 20 months.[78–81] In most cases, children presented with severe neutropenia, having neutrophil counts less than 0.5 × 10^9/L. Monocytosis has been reported to occur in up to 38 percent of patients. Marrow biopsies in affected patients usually show normal to hypercellular marrow with a decreased number of mature neutrophils.

Antibodies to neutrophils can be detected in up to 98 percent of affected patients. If an antibody specificity is identified, the antibodies are almost always specific to epitopes located on FcγRIIIb. The antibodies are directed to HNA-1a in 10 to 46 percent of patients, to HNA-1b in 2 to 3 percent of patients, and rarely to FcγRIIIb epitopes expressed by neutrophils from all donors.[79,80] Autoimmune neutropenia has been treated with glucocorticoids, IVIg, and G-CSF.[79]

Transfusion Reactions

Antibodies to neutrophil and HLA antigens in transfused blood can cause febrile nonhemolytic reactions. Febrile nonhemolytic transfusion reactions occur within a few hours of a transfusion and can be associated with chills and rigors. These reactions are a result of neutrophil antibodies in the transfusion recipient binding to leukocytes in the transfused blood component. Febrile transfusion reactions can be prevented in recipients of platelet and red blood cell component transfusions by the use of leukocyte-reduced blood components.

A more serious type of neutrophil antibody-mediated transfusion reaction is TRALI. TRALI is often caused by the transfusion of neutrophil antibodies in the plasma portion of a blood component. TRALI occurs within 6 hours of a transfusion when hypoxia and noncardiogenic pulmonary edema occur, as measured by a fall in hemoglobin oxygen saturation to less than 90 percent or a partial pressure of arterial oxygen (PaO_2)-to-fraction of inspired oxygen (FIO_2) ratio (PaO_2:FIO_2) of less than 300 torr.[82]

Many case reports have associated TRALI with the inadvertent transfusion of neutrophil antibodies. Investigations of transfusion recipients of blood components from donors with neutrophil antibodies who have been implicated in cases of TRALI suggest that a large proportion of neutrophil antibodies can cause TRALI and less-severe pulmonary transfusion reactions.[70,83–85] Antibodies to HNA-2a and -3a have most frequently been implicated in lung injury. Animal models have also shown that the transfusion of anti–HNA-2a and –HNA-3a can cause acute lung injury.[86–88]

HUMAN PLATELET ANTIGENS

Platelets express a variety of immunogenic markers on the cell surface. Some of these antigens are shared with other cell types as in the case of human leukocyte or blood group (ABO) antigens, whereas others are specific to platelets. Some of these platelet-specific markers can be recognized by autoantibodies[89–92] or by antibodies induced by certain drugs,[93–95] and still others by antibodies made by pregnant women or recipients of blood transfusions.

■ PLATELET ALLOANTIGENS

Platelet alloantigens are associated with polymorphisms of platelet surface glycoproteins (GPs) and can induce production of alloantibodies when individuals lacking a particular polymorphism are exposed via pregnancy or transfusion.[96] Immune responses to platelet alloantigens are involved in the pathogenesis of several clinical syndromes, including neonatal alloimmune thrombocytopenia (NAIT), posttransfusion purpura (PTP), and occasionally in refractory unresponsiveness to platelet transfusion.[97] Alloimmune thrombocytopenia can also be an unusual complication of solid-organ transplantation in which donor lymphocytes make alloantibodies specific for the platelets produced by the recipient of an organ allograft.[98]

PLATELET ISOANTIGENS

A condition similar to alloimmune platelet destruction occurs in patients who lack part or all of a particular platelet glycoprotein (GP) because of defective alleles of the GP-encoding genes. Such patients can make *iso*antibodies against platelets of virtually all donors that bear the platelet GP. For example, patients with Bernard-Soulier syndrome, who lack platelet GPIb-V-IX, or patients with Glanzmann thrombasthenia, who lack expression of GPIIb (CD41) and GPIIIa (CD61), can be induced to make broadly reactive antiplatelet isoantibodies (see Chap. 121).[99–102]

Platelet GPIV (CD36) is expressed on various human cells including platelets, macrophages, capillary endothelium, erythroblasts, and adipocytes.[103,104] Some apparently normal individuals lack CD36 on their platelets (type II deficiency) or platelets and monocytes (type I deficiency).[105] CD36 deficiency is common in Asians (3–11%)[106] and Africans (3–6%),[107] but is extremely rare in white populations (0.1%).[107] CD36 deficiency may confer protection from malaria and has been shown to be a receptor for red cells infected with *Plasmodium falciparum*. However, one report suggests CD36 deficiency may actually *increase the risk* for more severe forms of malarial infection.[108] Type I CD36-deficient individuals can become immunized via transfusion or pregnancy and make isoantibodies against CD36 that have been implicated in cases of NAIT, PTP, and platelet transfusion refractoriness.[106,109,110]

TABLE 138–4. Human Platelet Alloantigens[112,*]

Alloantigens	Other Names	Phenotypic Frequency	Glycoprotein Location/Amino Acid Change Substitution	Nucleotide
HPA-1a (PlA1)	PlA, Zw	72% a/a	GPIIIa /Leu:Pro33	T:C 196
HPA-1b (PlA2)		26% a/b	GPIIIa/Leu:Val33	C:G 175
HPA-1c		2% b/b		
		< 1 % a/c		
HPA-2a (Kob)	Ko, Sib	85% a/a	GPIb/Thr:Met145	C:T 524
HPA-2b (Koa)		14% a/b		
		1% b/b		
HPA-3a (Baka)	Bak, Lek	37% a/a	GPIIb/Ile:Ser843	T:G 622
HPA-3b (Bakb)		48% a/b		
		15% b/b		
HPA-4a (Pena)	Pen, Yuk	>99.9% a/a	GPIIIa/Arg:Gln143	G:A 526
HPA-4b (Penb)		<0.1% a/b		
		<0.1% b/b		
HPA-5a (Brb)	Br, Hc, Zav	80% a/a	GPIa/Glu:Lys 505	G:A648
HPA-5b (Bra)		19% a/b		
		1% b/b		
HPA-6bw	Caa, Tu	<1%	GPIIIa/Arg:Gln489	A:G1564
HPA-7bw	Mob	<1%	GPIIa/Pro:Ala407	G:C1317
HPA-8bw	Sra	<0.1%	GPIIIa/Arg:Cys636	T:C2004
HPA-9bw	Maxa	<1%	GPIIb/Val:Met837	A:G 2603
HPA-10bw	Laa	1%	GPIIIa/Arg:Gln62	A:G 281
HPA-11bw	Groa	<0.5%	GPIIIa/Arg:His633	A:G 1996
HPA-12bw	Iya	1%	GPIbβ/Gly:Glu15	A:G 141
HPA-13bw	Sita	<1%	GPIa/Met:Thr799	T:C 2531
HPA-14bw	Oea	1%	GPIIIa/Del Lys611	AAG1929–31
HPA-15a (Gov†)	Gov	35% a/a	CD109/Tyr:Ser703	A:C2 108
HPA-15b (Gov*)		42% a/b		
		23% b/b		
HPA-16bw	Duva	<1%	GPIIIa/Thr:Ile140	C:T 517
HPA-17bw	Vaa	<1%	GPIIIa/Thr:Met195	C:T 622
NA†	Naka	99.8% (White)	CD36 (GPIV)	T:G1 264
		97% (African)		C:T 478
		96% (Asian)		

*Phenotypic frequencies for the antigens shown are for the white population only. Significant differences in gene frequencies may be found in African and Asian populations.

†Sensitization to CD36 (GPIV) is an example of isoimmunization. Anti-CD36 antibodies have been implicated in cases of NAIT and PTP and thus are included in the list of platelet alloantigens that are associated with these disorders.

PLATELET ANTIGENS: GENETICS AND STRUCTURE

Platelet-specific alloantigens result from genetic polymorphism in genes encoding platelet surface proteins.[111] These *allo*antigens were first defined by antiplatelet antibodies discovered in the sera of multiparous females who gave birth to thrombocytopenic infants (NAIT) or in patients who developed PTP. Many of these alloantibodies were subsequently found to recognize allotypic determinants of platelet-associated membrane GPs, such as GPIIb/IIIa (CD41/CD61). Almost all of these determinants are generated by single-amino-acid substitutions encoded by SNPs in the GP genes (Table 138–4).[112] In some cases, differential glycosylation may contribute to or influence the expression of certain human platelet antigen (HPA) epitopes, such as those associated with HPA-3.[113,114] In any case, these amino acid substitutions generally do not appear to affect platelet function *in vitro*. However, the genetic polymorphism in platelet GPs may be associated with more subtle differences in platelet physiology that can contribute to the relative risk for thrombosis and/or atherosclerosis.[115–118]

To date, 24 platelet-specific alloantigens have been described, including localization to platelet surface GPs, quantification of their density on the platelet surface, and determination of DNA polymorphisms in genes encoding for them (see Table 138–4).[96,112] Several others have been described serologically, but genetic polymorphisms underlying these have not yet been determined.

NOMENCLATURE

A nomenclature for human platelet alloantigens has been adopted to replace the old complex "classic" nomenclatures that previously were developed independently in laboratories throughout the world (see

Table 138–4). In most cases, an HPA site has two alleles, designated by the suffix *a* or *b*. These alleles are expressed by platelets codominantly. The *a* allele represents the more prevalent form of the protein, while the *b* allele represents the less common form. There is one example of a triallelic HPA system, HPA-1, with the *c* allele being least prevalent.[119] Allelic frequencies for some of the HPAs can vary among different racial groups. For example, HPA-lb is expressed on the platelets of approximately 15 percent of persons of European ancestry but of less than 1 percent of persons of Asian ancestry.

A number of HPA alleles, for example, HPA-6b, HPA-7b, HPA-8b, HPA-9b, and HPA-10b, are present at gene frequencies of less than 0.1 percent and were recognized in the sera of mothers of thrombocytopenic babies (NAIT) in a single or only a very few families. Their putative high-frequency alternative alleles or the *a* form of the HPAs have not yet been identified serologically, probably because of the extremely low frequency of individuals who are homozygous for the rare alleles and who could therefore be sensitized to the high-frequency alternative allele. When such low-frequency markers are detected in only one family, they are referred to as *private* alleles. When more than one family is discovered to have such low-frequency markers and the families are unrelated, the alleles are then designated as *rare*. Such extremely rare or private alleles are unlikely to be present in the blood donor population. For this reason, these markers are unlikely to account for cases of PTP, but can be found in isolated cases of NAIT in selected families. Alleles present at gene frequencies greater than 2 percent within the population are designated as *public* alleles. These alleles are more likely to encode alloantigens involved in PTP.

TESTING FOR PLATELET-SPECIFIC ANTIGENS AND ANTIBODIES

Three types of platelet antibody detection methods have been developed. The earliest were phase I assays that involved mixing of patient serum with normal platelets and used platelet function-dependent endpoints such as alpha granule release, aggregation, or agglutination. The serotonin release assay, used for the laboratory diagnosis of heparin-induced thrombocytopenia, and in which radiolabeled serotonin, a dense granule constituent, is measured, is the only major phase I assay remaining in wide use today.[120] Other phase I assays were largely succeeded by phase II tests that detect either surface or total platelet-associated immunoglobulin on patient platelets or on normal platelets after sensitization with patient serum. An example of a phase II assay in wide use today is the solid-phase red cell adherence test, used for platelet crossmatching.[121] Phase III assays have been developed in which the binding of antibodies to isolated platelet surface GPs is detected. These assays are used to detect alloantibodies in the evaluation of suspected NAIT and PTP cases as well as autoantibodies in some cases of idiopathic thrombocytopenic purpura.[122] Phase III assays have an advantage over both phase I and phase II tests in that they detect antibodies that bind to platelet GPs, and not to non–platelet-specific epitopes, such as class I HLA. Examples of phase III assays are the monoclonal antibody immobilization of platelet antigens assay[123] and the modified antigen capture ELISA.[124]

Although most of the platelet antibody detection methods can be employed to determine platelet alloantigen types, because of limited access to rare typing sera and the need to establish platelet typing in patients with very few platelets, they have been largely supplanted by molecular typing using methods based on the PCR. Molecular typing is now available for all of the platelet alloantigens that have been elucidated at the gene level. Several DNA-based HPA typing techniques, such as restriction fragment length polymorphism analysis, sequence-specific oligonucleotide hybridization, and PCR with SSPs have been developed.[125–128]

CLINICAL IMPORTANCE

Antibodies recognizing platelet-specific alloantigens have been discovered in three clinical situations, including mothers who give birth to infants with NAIT; patients who develop dramatic thrombocytopenia after blood transfusion (PTP); and patients who have received multiple transfusions. Chapter 119 discusses the clinical syndromes of NAIT and PTP.

Although antibodies to class I HLA antigens are the principal cause of immunologic platelet transfusion refractoriness (discussed in Chap. 141), occasionally patients receiving multiple platelet transfusions will develop antibodies to platelet specific alloantigens. Many of the best-documented platelet-specific antibodies detected in such patients are directed against platelet antigens whose phenotypic frequencies are less than 30 percent in the blood-donor population.[129–131] Therefore, it is difficult to attribute refractory responses in random-donor and/or HLA-matched platelet transfusions to these antibodies alone. Indeed, the majority of refractory patients with platelet-specific antibodies also have HLA antibodies. Alloimmunization to high-frequency platelet-specific antigens would be expected to present a major challenge in finding compatible platelets to support a patient requiring multiple platelet transfusions. Fortunately, these cases are extremely rare.[130,132] If platelet transfusion refractoriness does develop because of platelet-specific antibodies, compatible platelet products may be identified by using either platelet crossmatching or by accessing family member or other HPA-typed donors who are compatible with the patient's antibodies.[133] Although there are a few well-documented cases of transfusion failures attributable to platelet-specific antibodies,[134] platelet glycoprotein reactivity in transfusion recipients that lacks specificity usually does not influence transfusion responses.[129,135–137]

Antibodies against some HPA-allelic determinants can inhibit platelet function. Anti–HPA-1 alloantibodies, for example, can inhibit clot retraction and platelet aggregation, presumably because they block the binding of GPIIb/IIIa ($\alpha_{IIb}\beta_3$) (CD41/CD61) to fibrinogen. Moreover, anti–HPA-4 alloantibodies can completely inhibit aggregation of HPA-4 platelets that are homozygous for the allele recognized by the alloantibodies because the epitope is in close proximity to the RGD (arginine-glycine-aspartic acid peptide sequence)-binding domain of the $\alpha_{IIb}\beta_3$ integrin.[138,139] On the other hand, other anti–HPA-alloantibodies, such as alloantibodies specific for HPA-3, may not significantly interfere with platelet function but nonetheless can cause Fc-mediated platelet destruction and immune thrombocytopenia.[140]

REFERENCES

1. Breuning MH, van den Berg-Loonen EM, Bernini LF, et al: Localization of HLA on the short arm of chromosome 6. *Hum Genet* 37:131, 1977.
2. Complete sequence and gene map of a human major histocompatibility complex. The MHC sequencing consortium. *Nature* 401:921, 1999.
3. Berrih S, Arenzana-Seisdedos F, Cohen S, et al: Interferon-gamma modulates HLA class II antigen expression on cultured human thymic epithelial cells. *J Immunol* 135:1165, 1985.
4. Robinson J, Waller MJ, Parham P, et al: IMGT/HLA and IMGT/MHC: Sequence databases for the study of the major histocompatibility complex. *Nucleic Acids Res* 31:311, 2003.

4a. Holdsworth R, Hurley CK, Marsh SG, et al: The HLA dictionary 2008: A summary of HLA-A, -B, -C, DRB1/3/4/5, and DQB1 alleles and their association with serologically defined HLA-A, -B, -C, -DR, -DQ antigens. *Tissue Antigens* 73:95, 2009.

5. Horton R, Wilming L, Rand V, et al: Gene map of the extended human MHC. *Nat Rev Genet* 5:889, 2004.
6. Thorsby E: Structure and function of HLA molecules. *Transplant Proc* 19:29, 1987.
7. Le Bouteiller P: HLA class I chromosomal region, genes, and products: Facts and questions. *Crit Rev Immunol* 14:89, 1994.
8. Mueller-Eckhardt G, Hauck M, Kayser W, Mueller-Eckhardt C: HLA-C antigens on platelets. *Tissue Antigens* 16:91, 1980.
9. Bjorkman PJ, Saper MA, Samraoui B, et al: The foreign antigen binding site and T cell recognition regions of class I histocompatibility antigens. *Nature* 329:512, 1987.

10. Campbell RD, Trowsdale J: Map of the human MHC. *Immunol Today* 14:349, 1993.
11. Trowsdale J: Genetics and polymorphism: Class II antigens. *Br Med Bull* 43:15, 1987.
12. Germain RN, Margulies DH: The biochemistry and cell biology of antigen processing and presentation. *Annu Rev Immunol* 11:403, 1993.
13. Yewdell JW, Bennink JR: The binary logic of antigen processing and presentation to T cells. *Cell* 62:203, 1990.
14. Vyas JM, Van der Veen AG, Ploegh HL: The known unknowns of antigen processing and presentation. *Nat Rev Immunol* 8:607, 2008.
15. Boon T, Coulie PG, Van den Eynde BJ, van der Bruggen P: Human T cell responses against melanoma. *Annu Rev Immunol* 24:175, 2006.
16. Cao K, Hollenbach J, Shi X, et al: Analysis of the frequencies of HLA-A, B, and C alleles and haplotypes in the five major ethnic groups of the United States reveals high levels of diversity in these loci and contrasting distribution patterns in these populations. *Hum Immunol* 62:1009, 2001.
17. Maiers M, Gragert L, Klitz W: High-resolution HLA alleles and haplotypes in the United States population. *Hum Immunol* 68:779, 2007.
18. Terasaki PI, Park MS, Bernoco D, Iwaki Y: Serology of HLA. *Transplant Proc* 13:900, 1981.
19. Terasaki PI, McClelland JD: Microdroplet assay of human serum cytotoxins. *Nature* 204:998, 1964.
20. Saiki RK, Gelfand DH, Stoffel S, et al: Primer-directed enzymatic amplification of DNA with a thermostable DNA polymerase. *Science* 239:487, 1988.
21. Schaffer M, Olerup O: HLA-AB typing by polymerase-chain reaction with sequence-specific primers: More accurate, less errors, and increased resolution compared to serological typing. *Tissue Antigens* 58:299, 2001.
22. Flomenberg N, Baxter-Lowe LA, Confer D, et al: Impact of HLA class I and class II high-resolution matching on outcomes of unrelated donor bone marrow transplantation: HLA-C mismatching is associated with a strong adverse effect on transplantation outcome. *Blood* 104:1923, 2004.
23. Petersdorf EW, Gooley T, Malkki M, Horowitz M: Clinical significance of donor-recipient HLA matching on survival after myeloablative hematopoietic cell transplantation from unrelated donors. *Tissue Antigens* 69 Suppl 1:25, 2007.
24. Bowness P: HLA and the spondylarthropathies, in *HLA in Health and Disease*, Chap. 12, 2nd ed, edited by A Warrens, R Lechler, p 187. Academic Press, London, 2000.
25. Sollid L, Spurkland A, Thorsby T: HLA and gastrointestinal diseases, in *HLA in Health and Disease*, Chap. 17, 2nd Ed edited by A Warrens, R Lechler, p 249. Academic Press, London, 2000.
26. Riley JP, Rosenberg SA, Parkhurst MR: Identification of a new shared HLA-A2.1 restricted epitope from the melanoma antigen tyrosinase. *J Immunother* 24:212, 2001.
27. Rezvani K, Yong ASM, Mielke S, et al: Leukemia-associated antigen-specific T-cell responses following combined PR1 and WT1 peptide vaccination in patients with myeloid malignancies. *Blood* 111:236, 2008.
28. Abel S, Paturel L, Cabie A: Abacavir hypersensitivity. *N Engl J Med* 358:2515, 2008 (author reply 358:2515, 2008).
29. Bux J: Nomenclature of neutrophil alloantigens. ISBT Working Party on Platelet and Neutrophil Serology, Neutrophil Antigen Working Party. International Society of Blood Transfusion. *Transfusion* 39:662, 1999.
30. Bux J, Stein EL, Bierling P, et al: Characterization of a new alloantigen (SH) on the human neutrophil Fc gamma receptor IIIb. *Blood* 89:1027, 1997.
31. Trounstine ML, Peltz GA, Yssel H, et al: Reactivity of cloned, expressed human Fc gamma RIII isoforms with monoclonal antibodies which distinguish cell-type-specific and allelic forms of Fc gamma RIII. *Int Immunol* 2:303, 1990.
32. Ory PA, Clark MR, Kwoh EE, et al: Sequences of complementary DNAs that encode the NA1 and NA2 forms of Fc receptor III on human neutrophils. *J Clin Invest* 84:1688, 1989.
33. Ravetch JV, Perussia B: Alternative membrane forms of Fc gamma RIII(CD16) on human natural killer cells and neutrophils. Cell type-specific expression of two genes that differ in single nucleotide substitutions. *J Exp Med* 170:481, 1989.
34. Huizinga TW, Kleijer M, Tetteroo PA, et al: Biallelic neutrophil Na-antigen system is associated with a polymorphism on the phospho-inositol-linked Fc gamma receptor III (CD16). *Blood* 75:213, 1990.
35. Stroncek DF, Shankar R, Litz C, Clement L: The expression of the NB1 antigen on myeloid precursors and neutrophils from children and umbilical cords. *Transfus Med* 8:119, 1998.
36. Huizinga TW, de Haas M, Kleijer M, et al: Soluble Fc gamma receptor III in human plasma originates from release by neutrophils. *J Clin Invest* 86:416, 1990.
37. Koene HR, Kleijer M, Roos D, et al: Fc gamma RIIIB gene duplication: Evidence for presence and expression of three distinct Fc gamma RIIIB genes in NA(1+,2+)SH(+) individuals. *Blood* 91:673, 1998.
38. Steffensen R, Gulen T, Varming K, Jersild C: FcgammaRIIIB polymorphism: Evidence that NA1/NA2 and SH are located in two closely linked loci and that the SH allele is linked to the NA1 allele in the Danish population. *Transfusion* 39:593, 1999.
39. Hessner MJ, Curtis BR, Endean DJ, Aster RH: Determination of neutrophil antigen gene frequencies in five ethnic groups by polymerase chain reaction with sequence-specific primers. *Transfusion* 36:895, 1996.
40. Bux J, Stein EL, Santoso S, Mueller-Eckhardt C: NA gene frequencies in the German population, determined by polymerase chain reaction with sequence-specific primers. *Transfusion* 35:54, 1995.
41. Matsuo K, Procter J, Stroncek D: Variations in genes encoding neutrophil antigens NA1 and NA2. *Transfusion* 40:645, 2000.
42. Lin M, Chen CC, Wang CL, Lee HL: Frequencies of neutrophil-specific antigens among Chinese in Taiwan. *Vox Sang* 66:247, 1994.
43. Ohto H, Matsuo Y: Neutrophil-specific antigens and gene frequencies in Japanese. *Transfusion* 29:654, 1989.
44. de La Vega Elena CD, Nogues N, Fernandez MA, et al: HNA-1a, HNA-1b and HNA-1c gene frequencies in Argentineans. *Tissue Antigens* 71:475, 2008.
45. Abid S, Zili M, Bouzid L, et al: Gene frequencies of human neutrophil antigens in the Tunisian blood donors and Berbers. *Tissue Antigens* 58:90, 2001.
46. Kissel K, Hofmann C, Gittinger FS, et al: HNA-1a, HNA-1b, and HNA-1c (NA1, NA2, SH) frequencies in African and American Blacks and in Chinese. *Tissue Antigens* 56:143, 2000.
47. Kuwano ST, Bordin JO, Chiba AK, et al: Allelic polymorphisms of human Fcgamma receptor IIa and Fcgamma receptor IIIb among distinct groups in Brazil. *Transfusion* 40:1388, 2000.
48. Muniz-Diaz E, Madoz P, de la Calle MO, Puig L: The polymorphonuclear neutrophil Fc gamma RIIIb deficiency is more frequent than hitherto assumed. *Blood* 86:3999, 1995.
49. Fromont P, Bettaieb A, Skouri H, et al: Frequency of the polymorphonuclear neutrophil Fc gamma receptor III deficiency in the French population and its involvement in the development of neonatal alloimmune neutropenia. *Blood* 79:2131, 1992.
50. Nagarajan S, Chesla S, Cobern L, et al: Ligand binding and phagocytosis by CD16 (Fc gamma receptor III) isoforms. Phagocytic signaling by associated zeta and gamma subunits in Chinese hamster ovary cells. *J Biol Chem* 270:25762, 1995.
51. Salmon JE, Edberg JC, Kimberly RP: Fc gamma receptor III on human neutrophils. Allelic variants have functionally distinct capacities. *J Clin Invest* 85:1287, 1990.
52. Bredius RG, Fijen CA, de Haas M, et al: Role of neutrophil Fc gamma RIIa (CD32) and Fc gamma RIIIb (CD16) polymorphic forms in phagocytosis of human IgG1- and IgG3-opsonized bacteria and erythrocytes. *Immunology* 83:624, 1994.
53. Clement LT, Lehmeyer JE, Gartland GL: Identification of neutrophil subpopulations with monoclonal antibodies. *Blood* 61:326, 1983.
54. Goldschmeding R, van Dalen CM, Faber N, et al: Further characterization of the NB1 antigen as a variably expressed 56–62 kD GPI-linked glycoprotein of plasma membranes and specific granules of neutrophils. *Br J Haematol* 81:336, 1992.
55. Stroncek DF, Shankar RA, Noren PA, et al: Analysis of the expression of NB1 antigen using two monoclonal antibodies. *Transfusion* 36:168, 1996.
56. Matsuo K, Lin A, Procter JL, et al: Variations in the expression of neutrophil antigen NB1. *Transfusion* 40:654, 2000.
57. Caruccio L, Bettinotti M, Matsuo K, et al: Expression of human neutrophil antigen-2a (NB1) is increased in pregnancy. *Transfusion* 43:357, 2003.
58. Stroncek DF, Skubitz KM, McCullough JJ: Biochemical characterization of the neutrophil-specific antigen NB1. *Blood* 75:744, 1990.
59. Kissel K, Santoso S, Hofmann C, et al: Molecular basis of the neutrophil glycoprotein NB1 (CD177) involved in the pathogenesis of immune neutropenias and transfusion reactions. *Eur J Immunol* 31:1301, 2001.
60. Caruccio L, Bettinotti M, Director-Myska AE, et al: The gene overexpressed in polycythemia rubra vera, PRV-1, and the gene encoding a neutrophil alloantigen, NB1, are alleles of a single gene, CD177, in chromosome band 19q13.31. *Transfusion* 46:441, 2006.
61. Taniguchi K, Kobayashi M, Harada H, et al: Human neutrophil antigen-2a expression on neutrophils from healthy adults in western Japan. *Transfusion* 42:651, 2002.
62. Bierling P, Poulet E, Fromont P, et al: Neutrophil-specific antigen and gene frequencies in the French population. *Transfusion* 30:848, 1990.
63. Caruccio L, Walkovich K, Bettinotti M, et al: CD177 polymorphisms: Correlation between high-frequency single nucleotide polymorphisms and neutrophil surface protein expression. *Transfusion* 44:77, 2004.
64. Kissel K, Scheffler S, Kerowgan M, Bux J: Molecular basis of NB1 (HNA-2a, CD177) deficiency. *Blood* 99:4231, 2002.
65. Sachs UJ, Andrei-Selmer CL, Maniar A, et al: The neutrophil specific antigen CD177 is a counter-receptor for endothelial PECAM-1 (CD31). *J Biol Chem* 282:23603, 2007.
66. Temerinac S, Klippel S, Strunck E, et al: Cloning of PRV-1, a novel member of the uPAR receptor superfamily, which is overexpressed in polycythemia rubra vera. *Blood* 95:2569, 2000.
67. Klippel S, Strunck E, Busse CE, et al: Biochemical characterization of PRV-1, a novel hematopoietic cell surface receptor, which is overexpressed in polycythemia rubra vera. *Blood* 100:2441, 2002.
68. de Haas M, Muniz-Diaz E, Alonso LG, et al: Neutrophil antigen 5b is carried by a protein, migrating from 70 to 95 kDa, and may be involved in neonatal alloimmune neutropenia. *Transfusion* 40:222, 2000.
69. Nordhagen R, Conradi M, Dromtorp SM: Pulmonary reaction associated with transfusion of plasma containing anti-5b. *Vox Sang* 51:102, 1986.
70. Kopko PM, Marshall CS, MacKenzie MR, et al: Transfusion-related acute lung injury: Report of a clinical look-back investigation. *JAMA* 287:1968, 2002.
71. Reil A, Keller-Stanislawski B, Gunay S, Bux J: Specificities of leucocyte alloantibodies in transfusion-related acute lung injury and results of leucocyte antibody screening of blood donors. *Vox Sang* 95:313, 2008.
72. Clague HD, Fung YL, Minchinton RM: Human neutrophil antigen-4a gene frequencies in an Australian population, determined by a new polymerase chain reaction method using sequence-specific primers. *Transfus Med* 13:149, 2003.
73. Han TH, Han KS: Gene frequencies of human neutrophil antigens 4a and 5a in the Korean population. *Korean J Lab Med* 26:114, 2006.
74. Cardone JD, Bordin JO, Chiba AK, et al: Gene frequencies of the HNA-4a and -5a neutrophil antigens in Brazilian persons and a new polymerase chain reaction-

restriction fragment length polymorphism method for HNA-5a genotyping. *Transfusion* 46:1515, 2006.
75. Simsek S, van der Schoot CE, Daams M, et al: Molecular characterization of antigenic polymorphisms (Ond(a) and Mart(a)) of the beta 2 family recognized by human leukocyte alloantisera. *Blood* 88:1350, 1996.
76. Sachs UJ, Reil A, Bauer C, et al: Genotyping of human neutrophil antigen-5a (Ond). *Transfus Med* 15:115, 2005.
77. Bux J, Jung KD, Kauth T, Mueller-Eckhardt C: Serological and clinical aspects of neutrophil antibodies leading to alloimmune neonatal neutropenia. *Transfus Med* 2:143, 1992.
78. Bux J, Behrens G, Jaeger G, Welte K: Diagnosis and clinical course of autoimmune neutropenia in infancy: Analysis of 240 cases. *Blood* 91:181, 1998.
79. Bruin MC, dem Borne AE, Tamminga RY, et al: Neutrophil antibody specificity in different types of childhood autoimmune neutropenia. *Blood* 94:1797, 1999.
80. Lalezari P, Khorshidi M, Petrosova M: Autoimmune neutropenia of infancy. *J Pediatr* 109:764, 1986.
81. Conway LT, Clay ME, Kline WE, et al: Natural history of primary autoimmune neutropenia in infancy. *Pediatrics* 79:728, 1987.
82. Toy P, Popovsky MA, Abraham E, et al: Transfusion-related acute lung injury: Definition and review. *Crit Care Med* 33:721, 2005.
83. Davoren A, Curtis BR, Shulman IA, et al: TRALI due to neutrophil-agglutinating human neutrophil antigen-3a (5b) alloantibodies in donor plasma: A report of 2 fatalities. *Transfusion* 43:641, 2003.
84. Muniz M, Sheldon S, Schuller RM, et al: Patient-specific transfusion-related acute lung injury. *Vox Sang* 94:70, 2008.
85. Fadeyi EA, Los Angeles MM, Wayne AS, et al: The transfusion of neutrophil-specific antibodies causes leukopenia and a broad spectrum of pulmonary reactions. *Transfusion* 47:545, 2007.
86. Seeger W, Schneider U, Kreusler B, et al: Reproduction of transfusion-related acute lung injury in an ex vivo lung model. *Blood* 76:1438, 1990.
87. Sachs UJ, Hattar K, Weissmann N, et al: Antibody-induced neutrophil activation as a trigger for transfusion-related acute lung injury in an *ex vivo* rat lung model. *Blood* 107:1217, 2006.
88. Silliman CC, Curtis BR, Kopko PM, et al: Donor antibodies to HNA-3a implicated in TRALI reactions prime neutrophils and cause PMN-mediated damage to human pulmonary microvascular endothelial cells in a two-event in vitro model. *Blood* 109:1752, 2007.
89. McMillan R: The pathogenesis of chronic immune thrombocytopenic purpura. *Semin Hematol* 44(4 Suppl 5):S3, 2007.
90. McMillan R: Antiplatelet antibodies in chronic adult immune thrombocytopenic purpura: Assays and epitopes. *J Pediatr Hematol Oncol* 25 Suppl 1:S57, 2003.
91. Wadenvik H, Stockelberg D, Hou M: Platelet proteins as autoantibody targets in idiopathic thrombocytopenic purpura. *Acta Paediatr Suppl* 424:26, 1998.
92. Beardsley DS, Ertem M: Platelet autoantibodies in immune thrombocytopenic purpura. *Transfus Sci* 19:237, 1998.
93. Bougie DW, Wilker PR, Wuitschick ED, et al: Acute thrombocytopenia after treatment with tirofiban or eptifibatide is associated with antibodies specific for ligand-occupied GPIIb/IIIa [see comment]. *Blood* 100:2071, 2002.
94. Gentilini G, Curtis BR, Aster RH: An antibody from a patient with ranitidine-induced thrombocytopenia recognizes a site on glycoprotein IX that is a favored target for drug-induced antibodies. *Blood* 92:2359, 1998.
95. Peterson JA, Nyree CE, Newman PJ, Aster RH: A site involving the "hybrid" and PSI homology domains of GPIIIa (beta 3-integrin subunit) is a common target for antibodies associated with quinine-induced immune thrombocytopenia. *Blood* 101:937, 2003.
96. McFarland JG: Platelet and granulocyte antigens and antibodies, in *Technical Manual*, edited by JD Roback, p 525. American Association of Blood Banks, Bethesda, MD, 2008.
97. Warkentin TE, Smith JW: The alloimmune thrombocytopenic syndromes. *Transfus Med Rev* 11:296, 1997.
98. West KA, Anderson DR, McAlister VC et al: Alloimmune thrombocytopenia after organ transplantation. *N Engl J Med* 341:1504, 1999.
99. Li C, Pasquale DN, Roth GJ: Bernard-Soulier syndrome with severe bleeding: Absent platelet glycoprotein Ib alpha due to a homozygous one-base deletion. *Thromb Haemost* 76:670, 1996.
100. Conte R, Cirillo D, Ricci F et al: Platelet transfusion in a patient affected by Glanzmann's thrombasthenia with antibodies against GPIIb-IIIa. *Haematologica* 82:73, 1997.
101. Skouri H, Bettaieb A, Fromont P, et al: Platelet and granulocyte alloimmunisation in multitransfused Tunisian patients. *Eur J Haematol* 75:248, 2005.
102. Kashyap R, Kriplani A, Saxena R, et al: Pregnancy in a patient of Glanzmann's thrombasthenia with antiplatelet antibodies. *J Obstet Gynaecol Res* 23:247, 1997.
103. Greenwalt DE, Lipsky RH, Ockenhouse CF, et al: Membrane glycoprotein CD36: A review of its roles in adherence, signal transduction, and transfusion medicine. *Blood* 80:1105, 1992.
104. Yanai H, Chiba H, Morimoto M, et al: Human CD36 deficiency is associated with elevation in low-density lipoprotein cholesterol. *Am J Med Genet* 93:299, 2000.
105. Yanai H, Chiba H, Fujiwara H, et al: Phenotype-genotype correlation in CD36 deficiency types I and II. *Thromb Haemost* 84:436, 2000.
106. Ikeda H, Mitani T, Ohnuma M, et al: A new platelet-specific antigen, Naka, involved in the refractoriness of HLA-matched platelet transfusion. *Vox Sang* 57:213, 1989.
107. Curtis BR, Aster RH: Incidence of the Nak(a)-negative platelet phenotype in African Americans is similar to that of Asians. *Transfusion* 36:331, 1996.
108. Aitman TJ, Cooper LD, Norsworthy PJ, et al: Malaria susceptibility and CD36 mutation. *Nature* 405:1015, 2000.
109. Bierling P, Godeau B, Fromont P, et al: Posttransfusion purpura-like syndrome associated with CD36 (Naka) isoimmunization. *Transfusion* 35:777, 1995.
110. Kankirawatana S, Kupatawintu P, Juji T, et al: Neonatal alloimmune thrombocytopenia due to anti-Nak(a). *Transfusion* 41:375, 2001.
111. Newman PJ, Valentin N: Human platelet alloantigens: Recent findings, new perspectives. *Thromb Haemost* 74:234, 1995.
112. Santoso S: Human platelet alloantigens. *Transfus Apher Sci* 28:227, 2003.
113. Lyman S, Aster RH, Visentin GP, Newman PJ: Polymorphism of human platelet membrane glycoprotein IIb associated with the Baka/Bakb alloantigen system. *Blood* 75:2343, 1990.
114. Harrison CR, Curtis BR, McFarland JG, et al: Severe neonatal alloimmune thrombocytopenia caused by antibodies to human platelet antigen 3a (Baka) detectable only in whole platelet assays. *Transfusion* 43:1398, 2003.
115. Bray PF: Integrin polymorphisms as risk factors for thrombosis. *Thromb Haemost* 82:337, 1999.
116. Goldschmidt-Clermont PJ, Roos CM, Cooke GE: Platelet PlA2 polymorphism and thromboembolic events: From inherited risk to pharmacogenetics. *J Thromb Thrombolysis* 8:89, 1999.
117. Harris K, Nguyen P, Van Cott EM: Platelet PlA2 Polymorphism and the risk for thrombosis in heparin-induced thrombocytopenia. *Am J Clin Pathol* 129:282, 2008.
118. Ollikainen E, Mikkelsson J, Perola M, et al: Platelet membrane collagen receptor glycoprotein VI polymorphism is associated with coronary thrombosis and fatal myocardial infarction in middle-aged men. *Atherosclerosis* 176:95, 2004.
119. Santoso S, Kroll H, Andrei-Selmer CL, et al: A naturally occurring LeuVal mutation in beta3-integrin impairs the HPA-1a epitope: The third allele of HPA-1. *Transfusion* 46:790, 2006.
120. Sheridan D, Carter C, Kelton JG: A diagnostic test for heparin-induced thrombocytopenia. *Blood* 67:27, 1986.
121. Rachel JM, Summers TC, Sinor LT, Plapp FV: Use of a solid phase red blood cell adherence method for pretransfusion platelet compatibility testing. *Am J Clin Pathol* 90:63, 1988.
122. Davoren A, Bussel J, Curtis BR, et al: Prospective evaluation of a new platelet glycoprotein (GP)-specific assay (PakAuto) in the diagnosis of autoimmune thrombocytopenia (AITP). *Am J Hematol* 78:193, 2005.
123. Kiefel V, Santoso S, Weisheit M, Müeller-Eckhardt C: Monoclonal antibody-specific immobilization of platelet antigens (MAIPA): A new tool for the identification of platelet-reactive antibodies. *Blood* 70:1722, 1987.
124. Visentin GP, Wolfmeyer K, Newman PJ, Aster RH: Detection of drug-dependent, platelet-reactive antibodies by antigen-capture ELISA and flow cytometry. *Transfusion* 30:694, 1990.
125. McFarland JG, Aster RH, Bussel JB, et al: Prenatal diagnosis of neonatal alloimmune thrombocytopenia using allele-specific oligonucleotide probes. *Blood* 78:2276, 1991.
126. Simsek S, Faber NM, Bleeker PM, et al: Determination of human platelet antigen frequencies in the Dutch population by immunophenotyping and DNA (allele-specific restriction enzyme) analysis. *Blood* 81:835, 1993.
127. Panzer S: Report on the Tenth International Platelet Genotyping and Serology Workshop on behalf of the International Society of Blood Transfusion. *Vox Sang* 80:72, 2001.
128. Skogen B, Bellissimo DB, Hessner MJ, et al: Rapid determination of platelet alloantigen genotypes by polymerase chain reaction using allele-specific primers. *Transfusion* 34:955, 1994.
129. Leukocyte reduction and ultraviolet B irradiation of platelets to prevent alloimmunization and refractoriness to platelet transfusions. The Trial to Reduce Alloimmunization to Platelets Study Group. *N Engl J Med* 337:1861, 1997.
130. Taaning E, Simonsen AC, Hjelms E, et al: Platelet alloimmunization after transfusion. A prospective study in 117 heart surgery patients. *Vox Sang* 72:238, 1997.
131. Kiefel V, König C, Kroll H, Santoso S: Platelet alloantibodies in transfused patients. *Transfusion* 41:766, 2001.
132. Langenscheidt F, Kiefel V, Santoso S, Mueller-Eckhardt C: Platelet transfusion refractoriness associated with two rare platelet-specific alloantibodies (anti-Baka and anti-PlA2) and multiple HLA antibodies. *Transfusion* 28:597, 1988.
133. Kekomaki S, Volin L, Koistinen P, et al: Successful treatment of platelet transfusion refractoriness: The use of platelet transfusions matched for both human leucocyte antigens (HLA) and human platelet alloantigens (HPA) in alloimmunized patients with leukaemia. *Eur J Haematol* 60:112, 1998.
134. Murata M, Furihata K, Ishida F, et al: Genetic and structural characterization of an amino acid dimorphism in glycoprotein Ib alpha involved in platelet transfusion refractoriness. *Blood* 79:3086, 1992.
135. Godeau B, Fromont P, Seror T, et al: Platelet alloimmunization after multiple transfusions: A prospective study of 50 patients. *Br J Haematol* 81:395, 1992.
136. Novotny VM: Prevention and management of platelet transfusion refractoriness. *Vox Sang* 76:1, 1999.
137. Meenaghan M, Judson PA, Yousaf K, et al: Antibodies to platelet glycoprotein V in polytransfused patients with haematological disease. *Vox Sang* 64:167, 1993.
138. Wang R, Furihata K, McFarland JG, et al: An amino acid polymorphism within the RGD binding domain of platelet membrane glycoprotein IIIa is responsible for the formation of the Pena/Penb alloantigen system. *J Clin Invest* 90:2038, 1992.
139. Furihata K, Nugent DJ, Bissonette A, et al: On the association of the platelet-specific alloantigen, Pena, with glycoprotein IIIa. Evidence for heterogeneity of glycoprotein IIIa. *J Clin Invest* 80:1624, 1987.
140. Glade-Bender J, McFarland JG, Kaplan C, et al: Anti-HPA-3A induces severe neonatal alloimmune thrombocytopenia. *J Pediatr* 138:862, 2001.

CHAPTER 139

BLOOD PROCUREMENT AND SCREENING

Jeffrey McCullough

SUMMARY

Blood procurement is a vital national priority that is met in the United States by volunteer donors and a pluralistic blood collection program that includes the American Red Cross, independent community blood centers, and hospitals. More than 13 million units of whole blood are collected from approximately 10 million donors annually. Recruitment of donors is preceded by a medical history and limited physical examination. The donated blood is subjected to as many as 15 tests, which include determination of blood type, examination for red cell antibodies, and a series of studies for infectious agents that may be transmitted by blood transfusion. The process usually starts with donations from random, unrelated donors but may include autologous, patient-specific, or patient-directed donors in special circumstances. In some cases, collection of red cells, platelets, leukocytes, or plasma is achieved by hemapheresis. Plasma for the subsequent manufacture of derivatives such as albumin and intravenous immunoglobulin is obtained from paid donors by for-profit organizations different from those that collect whole blood and prepare blood components. The meticulous attention to donor risk characteristics and the use of sensitive assays to detect infectious agents that may be transmitted by blood have greatly improved the safety of blood as a therapeutic product in countries that apply these practices. Nevertheless, a risk of viral and bacterial infection, albeit small, remains. The introduction of nucleic acid amplification and bacterial detection techniques to detect microbial contaminants are the latest steps to further decrease the risk of acquiring an infection through transfusion.

OVERVIEW OF THE BLOOD BANKING SYSTEM

SYSTEM IN THE UNITED STATES

The United States has a pluralistic rather than the single national system of blood collection that exists in other developed countries.[1,2] In the United States during 2005, approximately 15,019,000 units of blood were available for use (Table 139–1). Approximately 94 percent of the blood was collected in regional blood centers and hospitals collected 6 percent.[3] Approximately 2 percent of the units donated in the United States were autologous donations and another 0.9 percent were directed donations—that is, blood given by family or friends for a specific patient. Both autologous and directed donations decreased from 2001.[3] Of red cells collected, 97.7 percent of allogeneic, 59 percent of autologous, and 100 percent of directed donor red cells were transfused.[3] Approximately 5,300,000 patients received a red cell transfusion for an average of 2.7 units per patient.[3] A single organization, the American Red Cross, collects approximately 45 percent of the blood through its network of 36 regional blood centers. Community blood centers and hospitals collect the remainder. Community blood centers are individual, locally operated, nonprofit organizations, whereas the American Red Cross is a single national corporation with a single FDA license and set of operating procedures for all its regional centers.

Acronyms and abbreviations that appear in this chapter include: AABB, American Association of Blood Banks; CPD, citrate, phosphate, dextrose; G-CSF, granulocyte colony-stimulating factor; U, units.

All whole blood for transfusion in the United States is donated by volunteers; however, costs are incurred in the collection, testing, production, and distribution of blood components. Blood banks are nonprofit organizations that pass on these costs to hospitals. In the past, patients possibly could partially reduce the cost of blood by arranging for replacement of the blood they used. This practice has generally been discontinued because of the demand it places on the patient or family during the difficult time of the illness. Instead, blood banks assume the responsibility of ensuring that the community's blood needs are met by developing public education and donor recruitment programs.

Some areas of the United States are able to provide more blood than is needed locally and other areas are unable to collect enough blood to meet their local needs. The misalignment of blood use and blood availability is a long-standing phenomenon. Several inventory-sharing systems are used to move blood around the United States so as to alleviate the shortages, but these systems are complex and fragile arrangements that are not always effective. As a result, blood shortages occasionally occur in some areas of the United States.

Blood is considered a drug and all aspects of the selection of donors, collection, processing, testing, preservation, and dispensing are regulated by the FDA as specified in the Code of Federal Regulations. The requirements in the code define the procedures, record-keeping, staff proficiency, specific testing, and donor medical requirements that blood banks must follow. Blood banks meet these requirements using the FDA-defined good manufacturing practices that are similar to those used by pharmaceutical manufacturers.[1,4] Additional standards are formulated by the American Association of Blood Banks (AABB), a voluntary organization that accredits blood banks.

INTERNATIONAL PRACTICES

Approximately 80 million units of blood are collected annually worldwide.[5] Considerable difference exists in the availability of blood and blood components throughout the world.[6–8] In general, this difference is related to the extent of development in the country and the country's healthcare system. The amount of blood collected in relation to the population ranges from 50 donations per 1000 population in industrialized countries to 5 to 15 per 1000 in developing countries and 1 to 5 per 1000 in the least-developed countries. Thus, industrialized countries utilize transfused blood products far more commonly.[5] In developed countries, especially Western Europe and parts of Asia, a governmental agency usually oversees the blood collection activities, although the extent to which the government sets requirements and monitors or inspects the blood collection system varies.[9] Where national blood programs have been developed, usually a national blood policy is established that includes definition of the organization(s) responsible for the program, source of funding, type of blood donation, and regulations ensuring blood safety.[2,6,9] In these countries, the basic processes of donor medical screening, blood collection, laboratory testing, and preparation of blood components are similar to the system found in the United States. In virtually all developed countries, blood is donated by volunteers and paid donors are arduously avoided, a system shown to reduce transfusion-associated complications by removing the fiscal benefit that could compromise the self-reporting of donor behaviors associated with blood-borne disease.[10,11] The blood may be collected by hospitals, community-based regional blood centers, or a combination of these facilities. The supply systems and sharing among hospitals and blood centers vary with the extent of development of the country's blood supply system. The basic blood components—red cells, platelets, plasma, and cryoprecipitate—

TABLE 139–1. U.S. Blood Supply System in 2004*

	Number	Percent
Total units whole blood	15,019,000	100
Blood centers	14,050,000	94
Hospitals	968,000	6
Red blood cell transfusions	14,182,000	100
Allogeneic	13,720,000	96.7
Autologous	270,000	1.9
Directed	132,000	0.9
Other	60,000	0.4
Discarded	503,000	3.3
Platelets	13,362,000	100
SDP collected	9,161,000	69
Platelet concentrates	4,202,000	31
Total platelets transfused*	9,875,000	
Fresh-frozen plasma	4,089,000	–
FFP transfused	4,089,000	–
Cryoprecipitate	1,164,000	
Cryo transfused	890,000	

SDP, single-donor platelet concentrate prepared by plateletpheresis. One SDP is equivalent to six platelet concentrates.

*Data from Whitaker BI, Sullivan M.[3]

usually are available, and apheresis instruments are used to collect platelets. Plasma derivatives such as albumin, coagulation factor VIII, and immune globulins are available. In many developed countries, these plasma derivatives are prepared from plasma collected from volunteer donors instead of the paid donor plasma used to prepare these derivatives in the United States.

However, in the developing world, "transfusion practice is fragmented and disorganized and it is difficult, if not impossible, to provide the five basic blood components . . . in an adequate supply."[5,8] These countries usually do not have an organized blood supply system. Patients may be required to arrange for the blood they need so donors may be friends or family members of patients or even individuals who have been paid by the patient's family to donate the blood needed. Considerable evidence exists that blood from paid donors is more likely to transmit disease.[12] Donor screening may not be as extensive, transmissible disease testing may be lacking, and equipment may be reused. These difficulties may be compounded by the presence of endemic transfusion-transmissible diseases for which screening is difficult or expensive and thus not performed as extensively as in more developed countries. Blood components, such as fresh-frozen plasma or platelets, are not available in most developing countries. Thus, the availability of blood and its components around the world varies widely, from inadequate supplies and uncertain safety to sophisticated supply systems and component availability equal to or surpassing those of the United States.

PROCUREMENT OF PLASMA DERIVATIVES

The plasma industry is separate from the blood banking system described above (see "Overview of the Blood Banking System" above). Plasma can be subjected to a fractionation process to produce several medically valuable products referred to as *plasma derivatives*. Examples are albumin, coagulation factor concentrates, immune serum globulins, and many others. Plasma fractionation is performed in manufacturing plants in batches of up to 10,000 L involving the pooling of plasma from as many as 50,000 donors. Plasma for manufacture or fractionation into derivatives can be obtained from units of whole blood, but this amount of plasma is inadequate to meet the needs for plasma derivatives. Consequently, large amounts of plasma are obtained by plasmapheresis in which only the plasma and not red cells or platelets are retained from the donor. Individuals can donate plasma up to two times per week and usually are paid because of the more extensive time commitment. This plasma collection system usually is operated by for-profit organizations and functions separately from the system for whole-blood donation.

Approximately 13 million L of plasma are collected annually in the United States from about 15 million donations.[13] Twenty-two plasma derivatives are approved for licensure by the FDA (Table 139–2). Some derivatives are produced by only one manufacturer; other derivatives are produced by several manufacturers. Thus, disruption in the sources of plasma or in one manufacturer's plant can have serious consequences and create shortages of certain derivatives.

The remainder of this chapter describes the blood collection system operated by voluntary community organizations to provide cellular and whole-blood–derived components.

RECRUITMENT OF BLOOD DONORS

Although most Americans will require a blood transfusion at some time in their lives, only about one-third of the United States population is eligible to donate blood,[14] and only a small portion of those actually donate. Blood donors are more likely than the general population to be male, age 30 to 50 years, white, employed, and have more education and higher income.[15] It is generally believed that the most effective way to get someone to donate blood is to ask him or her personally.[16] Factors such as the convenience of donation, peer pressure, receipt of blood by a family member, and perceived community needs are important factors that are superimposed onto the individual's basic social commitments.[16] Usually blood donors are asked to give to the general community supply. Some donors are asked to give for a specific patient, which is referred to as *directed donation*. Such donations may be easier to obtain and leave the donor with a stronger sense of satisfaction because of the personal nature of the donation.

The heightened concern about blood safety since the onset of the AIDS epidemic has resulted in expanded requirements for the suitability for blood donation. Thus, a larger proportion of the population of potential donors is being excluded and the most common reason is a low hemoglobin. The expanded requirements, along with the aging population, geographic and ethnic shifts in the population, and people's changing priorities, are causing a shrinking donor pool.[14] Deferrals that have little if any benefit to patient or donor safety are a serious problem for the blood supply because individuals who have been deferred from donation are unlikely to return.[17,18]

WHOLE-BLOOD DONOR SCREENING

The approach to the selection of blood donors is designed to (1) ensure the safety of the donor and (2) obtain a high-quality blood component that is as safe as possible for the recipient. Some specific steps that are taken to ensure that blood is as safe as possible are the use of only volunteer blood donors; questioning of donors about their general health before their donation is scheduled; obtaining a medical history, including

TABLE 139–2. Plasma Derivative Products and Their Uses

Blood Product	Purpose of Blood Product Use
Albumin	Restoration of plasma volume subsequent to shock, trauma, surgery, and burns
α_1-Proteinase inhibitor	Treatment of emphysema caused by a genetic deficiency
Activated prothrombin complex	Treatment of bleeding episodes in the presence of factor VIII and factor IX inhibitors
Antihemophilic factor	Treatment of prevention of bleeding in patients with hemophilia A
Antithrombin III	Treatment of bleeding episodes associated with liver disease, antithrombin III deficiency, and thromboembolism
Cytomegalovirus immune globulin	Passive immunization subsequent to exposure to cytomegalovirus
Factor IX complex	Prophylaxis and treatment of hemophilia B bleeding episodes and other bleeding disorders
Factor XIII	Treatment of bleeding and disorders of wound healing resulting from factor XIII deficiency
Fibrinogen	Treatment of hemorrhagic diathesis in hypofibrinogenemia, dysfibrinogenemia, and afibrinogenemia
Hepatitis B immune globulin	Passive immunization subsequent to exposure to hepatitis B
IgM-enriched immune globulin	Treatment and prevention of septicemia and septic shock resulting from toxin liberation in the course of antibiotic treatment
Immune globulin (intravenous and intramuscular)	Treatment of agammaglobulinemia and hypogammaglobulinemia; passive immunization for hepatitis A and measles
Plasma protein fraction	Restoration of plasma volume subsequent to shock, trauma, surgery, and burns
Rabies immune globulin	Passive immunization subsequent to exposure to rabies
Rho(D) immune globulin	Treatment and prevention of hemolytic disease of fetus and newborn resulting from Rh incompatibility and incompatible blood transfusions
Rubella immune globulin	Passive immunization subsequent to exposure to German measles
Serum cholinesterase	Treatment of prolonged apnea after administration of succinylcholine chloride
Tetanus immune globulin	Passive immunization subsequent to exposure to tetanus
Vaccinia immune globulin	Passive immunization subsequent to exposure to smallpox
Varicella-zoster immune globulin	Passive immunization subsequent to exposure to chicken pox

SOURCE: From information provided by the American Blood Resources Association.

specific risk factors, before donation; conducting a brief physical examination before donation; laboratory testing of donated blood; checking the donor's identity against a donor deferral registry[19]; and providing a method by which the donor can confidentially designate the unit as unsuitable for transfusion after the donation is completed.[15]

Health History

The health history is done by personal interview, although a computer-assisted self-interview is used increasingly and may provide more accurate information.[20,21] The questions designed to protect the safety of the donor include whether the donor is under the care of a physician or has a history of cardiovascular or lung disease, seizures, present or recent pregnancy, recent donation of blood or plasma, recent major illness or surgery, unexplained weight loss, unusual bleeding, or is taking medication(s). Questions designed to protect the safety of the recipient include those related to the donor's general health, history of receipt of growth hormone, and occurrence of or exposure to patients with hepatitis or other liver disease, or a previous diagnosis of AIDS (or symptoms of AIDS), Chagas disease, or babesiosis. A history also is obtained regarding the injection of drugs; receipt of coagulation factor concentrates; blood transfusion; tattoos; acupuncture; body piercing; receipt of an organ or tissue transplant; recent travel to areas endemic for malaria; recent immunizations; ingestion of medications (especially aspirin); presence of a major illness or surgery; and previous notice of a positive test for a transmissible disease. In addition, several questions are related to AIDS risk behavior, including whether the potential donor has had sex with anyone with AIDS, given or received money or drugs for sex, (for males) had sex with another male, or (for females) had sex with a male who has had sex with another male. This series of sex-related questions is highly specific although they seem to be acceptable to blood donors.

Situations may arise in which the donor's physician believes donation would be safe but the blood bank does not accept the donor. For instance, donors with a history of cancer, other than minor skin cancer or carcinoma *in situ* of the cervix, usually are rejected because the genesis of malignant disease is not known, although there is no convincing evidence that malignancy can be transmitted by blood transfusion. The donor is questioned about medications. Some medications may make the donor unsuitable because of the condition requiring the medication, whereas other medications may be potentially harmful to the recipient. Many other conditions must be evaluated individually by the blood bank physician and that physician's assessment of conformance with FDA regulations, which view blood as a pharmaceutical, may not always coincide with the personal physician's view of the health of the patient who is the potential blood donor.

Physical and Laboratory Examination of the Blood Donor and Collected Blood Products

The examination includes determination of the temperature, pulse, blood pressure, weight, and blood hemoglobin concentration. The FDA has mandated limits for each of these factors. In addition, the donor's general appearance is assessed for any signs of illness or the influence of drugs or alcohol. The skin at the venipuncture site is examined for signs of intravenous drug abuse, lesions suggestive of Kaposi sarcoma, and local lesions that would make disinfecting the skin difficult and thus lead to contamination of the blood unit during venipuncture.

■ COLLECTION OF WHOLE BLOOD

Blood Containers

Blood must be collected into single-use, sterile, FDA-licensed containers. The containers are made of plasticized material that is biocompatible with blood cells and allows diffusion of gases so as to provide optimal cell preservation. These blood containers are combinations of bags and integral tubing that allow separation of the whole blood into its components in a closed system, thus minimizing the chance of bacterial contamination while making storage of the components for days or weeks possible. Plasticizers from the bags accumulate in red cell components during storage and can be found in tissues of multitransfused patients. However, no evidence indicates that transfusion of this material causes clinical problems.[22]

Preparation of the Venipuncture Site

The blood should be drawn from an area free of skin lesions and the phlebotomy site should be properly decontaminated. The site is scrubbed with a soap solution, followed by the application of tincture of iodine or iodophor complex solution. The selection of the venipuncture site and its decontamination are important steps because bacterial contamination of blood can be a serious or even fatal complication of transfusion.[23–26]

Venipuncture and Blood Collection

The venipuncture is done with a needle that should be used only once in order to prevent contamination. The blood must flow freely and be mixed with anticoagulant frequently as the blood fills the container to prevent the development of small clots. The actual time for collection of 450 to 500 mL usually is approximately 7 minutes and almost always is less than 10 minutes. During blood donation, cardiac output falls slightly but heart rate changes little. A slight decrease in systolic pressure results with a rise in peripheral resistance and diastolic blood pressure.

Usually 450 mL (±10%) is collected, although many blood banks now collect 500 mL. Some blood centers use containers that divert the first few milliliters into a waste bag so that skin contaminants do not enter the container of transfusible blood.[27] The blood is mixed with 63 to 70 mL of anticoagulant composed of citrate, phosphate, and dextrose (CPD). The amount of blood withdrawn must be within prescribed limits so as to maintain the proper ratio with the anticoagulant; otherwise, the blood cells may be damaged and/or anticoagulation may be unsatisfactory. Although the red cells can be stored in the CPD-anticoagulant solution, customarily almost all the anticoagulated plasma is removed and the red cells resuspended in a solution that provides optimum red cell preservation.

Postdonation Observation and Adverse Reactions to Blood Donation

An untoward reaction occurs after approximately 2 to 5 percent of blood donations, but, fortunately, most of the reactions are not serious.[28–30] Donors who have reactions are more likely to be younger, unmarried, have a higher predonation heart rate and lower diastolic blood pressure, lower weight, female, and first-time or infrequent donors.[28,29] The interpersonal nature of the phlebotomist may affect the reactions,[31] and donors who experience a reaction are less likely to donate in the future.[18,32]

The most common reactions to blood donation are weakness, cool skin, and diaphoresis. More extensive, but still moderate, reactions are dizziness, pallor, hypertension, and bradycardia. Bradycardia usually is considered a sign of a vasovagal reaction rather than hypotensive or cardiovascular shock, where tachycardia would be expected. In a more severe form, this kind of reaction may progress to loss of consciousness, convulsions, and involuntary passage of urine or stool.[28,29,33,34] Other reactions include nausea and vomiting; hyperventilation, sometimes leading to twitching or muscle spasms; hematoma at the venipuncture site; convulsions; and serious cardiac difficulties. Such serious reactions are rare.[28,29,34,35] Injury of the brachial nerve and resulting pain and/or paresthesia may occur as a result of needle puncture of the nerve or compression from a hematoma.[36,37]

Donors are advised to drink extra fluids to replace lost blood volume and to avoid strenuous exercise for the remainder of the day of donation. The latter advice is given to prevent fainting and to minimize the possibility of hematoma development at the venipuncture site. Some donors are subject to lightheadedness or even fainting if they change position quickly. Therefore, donors are advised not to return to work for the remainder of the day if they have an occupation where fainting would be hazardous to themselves or others.

■ SPECIAL BLOOD DONATIONS

In several situations involving blood donation, the blood is not obtained from the community's general blood supply. Examples of such situations include autologous donation, directed donation, patient-specific donation, and therapeutic bleeding. In some of these situations, the FDA requirements for blood donation may not apply.

Autologous Donor Blood

Autologous blood donation is an old concept but was little used until the AIDS epidemic raised fears of blood transfusion among both patients and physicians. Individuals can donate blood for their own use if the need for blood can be anticipated and a donation plan developed. Most commonly this situation occurs with elective surgery.

Autologous blood for transfusion can be obtained by preoperative donation, acute normovolemic hemodilution, intraoperative salvage, and postoperative salvage, but only preoperative donation is discussed here. If patient candidates for autologous blood donation meet the usual FDA criteria for blood donation, their blood can be used for other patients if the original autologous donor has no need for the blood. However, this practice is not allowed by AABB standards and is usually not relevant because most patients do not meet the FDA donation criteria. If the autologous donor does not meet the FDA criteria for blood donation, the blood must be specially labeled, segregated during storage, and discarded if it is not used by that specific patient. Thus, the autologous blood donation should be collected only for procedures with a substantial likelihood that the blood will be used.[38] Without this type of planning, a very high rate of wastage of autologous blood is observed, estimated at 59 percent in 2004. Thus, the cost of autologous blood is high.[39]

No age or weight restrictions exist for autologous donation.[15] Pregnant women can donate, but this practice is not recommended routinely because these patients rarely require transfusion. The autologous donor's hemoglobin may be lower (11 g/dL) than that required for routine donors (12.5 g/dL), and autologous donors may donate as often as every 72 hours up to 72 hours prior to the planned surgery, although usually only 2 to 4 U of blood can be obtained before the hemoglobin falls below 11 g/dL. Autologous blood donors can be given erythropoietin and iron to increase the number of units of blood they can donate,[40] although the value of erythropoietin is dubious because this strategy has not been shown to reduce the need for allogeneic donor blood and only results in the ability to donate one additional unit of blood.[41,42] Contraindications for autologous blood donation include bacteremia, symptomatic angina, recent seizures, and symptomatic valvular heart lesions. The final decision on whether to withdraw blood from an autologous donor rests with the medical director of the blood bank. Often consultation between the donor's (patient's) physician and the blood bank physician is necessary to decide on a wise course of action. Reactions in autologous donors are similar to allogeneic donors and are related to first-time donation, female gender, lower age, and lower weight.[43]

Autologous blood must be typed for ABO and Rh antigens.[15] If the unit is to be shipped to another facility for transfusion, it must be tested for transmissible diseases similar to allogeneic blood.[15] If any of the transmissible disease tests are positive, the unit must be labeled with a biohazard label. This labeling sometimes is confusing or disconcerting to physicians but is required by the FDA to alert healthcare personnel to the hazard presented by the potentially infectious blood.

Directed Donor Blood

Directed donors are friends or relatives who wish to give blood for a specific patient because the patient hopes those donors will be safer than the regular blood supply. In general, the data do not indicate that directed donors have a lower incidence of transmissible disease markers[44,45] and thus do not support a realistic rationale for these donations. Moreover, when friends or relatives are asked to donate blood, they may be reluctant to disclose risk factors that would preclude them from voluntary donation, which may actually increase risk. Some blood banks refuse directed donations, but most accept them as a service to the patients. However, because the blood becomes part of the community's general blood supply if it is not used for the originally intended patient, directed donors must meet all the usual FDA requirements for routine blood donation.

Patient-Specific Donation

In a few situations, appropriate transfusion therapy involves collecting blood from a particular donor for a particular patient. Examples are donor-specific transfusions prior to kidney transplantation, maternal platelets for a fetus projected to have neonatal alloimmune thrombocytopenic purpura (NATP), or family members of a patient with a rare blood type. Usually, these donors must meet all the usual FDA requirements, except that they may donate as often as every 3 days so long as the hemoglobin remains above the normal donor minimum of 12.5 g/dL.[15] An exception is donation of maternal platelets for a neonate with NATP. Patient-specific donated units must undergo all routine laboratory testing.[15]

Therapeutic Bleeding

Blood can be collected as part of the therapy of diseases such as polycythemia vera or hemochromatosis. Often the patient or physician asks that the blood be used for transfusion as a way of comforting the patient. However, usually such blood is not used for transfusion because the donors do not meet the FDA standards for donor health. As the genetic basis of hemochromatosis has become better understood, blood removed from these patients appears to be safe[46] and has been proposed for transfusion, although this has not gained general acceptance,[47,48] in part because it is believed that the patient with hemochromatosis or polycythemia vera is fiscally advantaged by donation to the blood center rather than seeing his or her physician and being charged for the procedure. Red cells from patients with hemochromatosis are normal during blood bank storage,[49] and although a blood collection program can operate successfully,[50] this may not be an important contribution to the blood supply.[51]

COLLECTION AND PRODUCTION OF BLOOD COMPONENTS BY APHERESIS

Blood components can be obtained by apheresis rather than prepared from a standard unit of whole blood. In apheresis, the donor's anticoagulated whole blood is passed through an instrument in which the blood is separated into red cells, plasma, and a leukocyte/platelet fraction. Several semiautomated blood-cell-separator instruments are available for collection of platelets, granulocytes, blood stem cells, mononuclear cells, and plasma.[15,52] All of these instruments use centrifugation to separate the blood components.[52] Some apheresis procedures involve two venipunctures with continuous flow of blood from the donor through the blood cell separator; others can be accomplished with a single venipuncture and intermittent blood withdrawal and return. Apheresis has been used to collect 2 U of red cells[53–55] or various combinations of components.[56]

PLATELETPHERESIS

Platelet concentrates can be produced from whole blood, but use of plateletpheresis has been increasing. By 2004, approximately 69 percent, or 1,527,000 doses, of platelets produced in the United States were produced by plateletpheresis. Platelets prepared from 4,202,000 units of whole blood provided 700,333 doses.[3] The trend to produce platelets by apheresis instead of from whole blood is increasing.[3] Plateletpheresis requires approximately 90 minutes, during which approximately 4000 to 5000 mL of the donor's blood is processed through the blood cell separator. The process results in a platelet concentrate with a volume of approximately 200 mL and containing approximately 4.0×10^{11} platelets and less than 0.5 mL red cells. Currently manufactured blood cell separators produce a platelet concentrate that contains less than 5×10^6 leukocytes and thus can be considered leukocyte reduced. Following plateletpheresis, the donor's platelet count declines by approximately 30 percent and does not return to preplateletpheresis levels for approximately 4 days (see Chap. 141).[57]

COLLECTION OF RED CELLS BY APHERESIS

Chronic shortages of group O red cells stimulated interest in the use of apheresis for collecting the equivalent of 2 U of red cells from some donors, especially group O.[53–56] The collection procedure is similar to other apheresis procedures, except that red cells are retained rather than returned to the donor. The red cells usually have a very high hematocrit as they are removed from the instrument, but an additive solution is incorporated and the red cells can be stored for the usual 42 days. The red cell products obtained by apheresis have a more standard volume than do red cells prepared from whole blood, but otherwise red cells obtained by apheresis have the same characteristics as those produced from whole blood. Donors for 2-U red cell apheresis must meet weight and hemoglobin standards specified for each instrument. Because 2 U of red cells are removed, donors may donate only every 4 months. Double-unit red cell collection allows fewer donor visits, may increase red cell availability, and could reduce the patient's donor exposure if both donor units are given to the same patient, although this is rarely done because of logistical difficulties.

LEUKAPHERESIS

Leukapheresis has been used to produce a granulocyte concentrate for transfusion therapy of infections unresponsive to antibiotics.[15] In the past, leukapheresis provided only a marginally adequate dose of granulocytes for therapeutic benefit and its use had declined to very low levels. Leukapheresis usually is a more lengthy and complex procedure than plateletpheresis. Because the efficiency of granulocyte extraction from whole blood is less than for platelets, the leukapheresis procedure involves processing 6500 to 8000 mL of donor blood for approximately 3 hours.[52] To increase the separation of granulocytes from other blood components, hydroxyethyl starch is added to the blood-cell–separator flow system.[52] In addition, glucocorticoids have been administered to the donor to increase the blood granulocyte count and thus increase the yield. Granulocyte colony-stimulating factor (G-CSF) has been administered to granulocyte donors to achieve much larger increases in granulocyte count and a much greater granulocyte yield.[58–61] Transfusion of these high-yield granulocyte concentrates results in substantially increased granulocyte count and has led to renewed interest in granulocyte transfusions.[62,63]

PLASMAPHERESIS

Plasmapheresis is done using semiautomated instruments. The volume of plasma that can be collected depends on the size of the donor. Plasmapheresis usually can be performed in approximately 30 minutes and produces up to 750 mL of plasma. Because few red cells are removed, the procedure can be repeated up to two times per week, so theoretically a donor could provide up to approximately 50 L of plasma in 1 year. Because of the nature and possible frequency of plasma donation, special donor criteria apply.

SELECTION OF APHERESIS DONORS

The selection of donors for apheresis uses the same criteria as for whole-blood donation.[15] Because of the unique nature of apheresis, some additional donor requirements are necessary. Many apheresis procedures involve two venipunctures and continuous blood flow, so good venous access is important. No more than 15 percent of the donor's blood should be extracorporeal during apheresis; thus, the donor's size is considered when making decisions about specific apheresis procedures or instruments to be used. Following plateletpheresis, the donor's platelet count declines by approximately 30 percent and does not return to preplateletpheresis levels for approximately 4 days.[57] Donors may undergo plateletpheresis every 48 hours; however, if they are donating more often than every 8 weeks, a platelet count must be obtained to ensure that the count is at least 150,000/μL (150×10^9/L). Apheresis donors of 2-U red cells must wait 4 months before they may donate again. Following leukapheresis of G-CSF donors, the granulocyte count decreases slightly, the platelet count decreases by 20 to 25 percent, and the hematocrit decreases by approximately 1 percent.[59,60] Thus, the platelet count must be monitored in donors undergoing frequent leukaphereses. Because a plateletpheresis concentrate would be the sole source of platelets for the transfusion, the donor must not have taken aspirin for at least 3 days. For donors undergoing plasmapheresis more often than once every 8 weeks, the serum protein must be at least 6 g/dL. In addition, a protein electrophoresis or a quantitative immunoglobulins assay should be obtained every 4 months, and the results must be normal to allow further donation.[15] The amount of blood components removed from apheresis donors must be monitored. Not more than 200 mL of red cells per 2 months or approximately 1500 mL of plasma per week can be removed.[15] The laboratory testing of donors and apheresis components for transmissible diseases is the same as for whole-blood donation. Thus, the likelihood of disease transmission from apheresis components is the same as from whole blood.

REACTIONS IN APHERESIS DONORS

Apheresis donors can experience the same kind of reactions as whole-blood donors. In addition, apheresis donors experience a higher incidence of paresthesias, probably because of the infusion of citrate used to anticoagulate the donor's blood while it is in the cell separator.[64,65] This type of reaction is managed by slowing the blood flow rate through the instrument, which slows the rate of citrate infusion. The additional donor selection and monitoring requirements for apheresis prevent the development of reactions or complications resulting from excess removal of blood cells or plasma. In leukapheresis, donors can be given glucocorticoid and/or G-CSF to elevate the granulocyte count, and the sedimenting agent hydroxyethyl starch is used in the cell separator to improve the granulocyte yield (see Chap. 26). When G-CSF is used, approximately 60 percent of donors experience side effects, usually myalgia, arthralgia, headache, or flu-like symptoms.[58-61] This rate of side effects may be higher if the donors also receive glucocorticoids.[60] The major side effect of hydroxyethyl starch is blood volume expansion manifested by headache and/or hypertension.[15] Donor selection techniques are intended to minimize the likelihood of hypertension resulting from hydroxyethyl starch.

LABORATORY TESTING OF DONATED BLOOD

Each unit of whole blood or each apheresis component undergoes a standard battery of tests, including those for blood type, red cell antibodies (including ABO, Rh, minor antigens), and transmissible diseases (Table 139–3). Additional tests, such as those for cytomegalovirus (CMV) antibodies to aid in directed transfusions (i.e., for transfusions into CMV-negative, immunosuppressed recipients), may be done. The total number of test results for each unit of donated blood is approximately 15, depending on the specific methodology used. In addition, because each unit of whole blood is separated into several components and a donor history record and 2 or 3 tubes of blood for tests are available, each donation generates up to 30 different data elements. All data are amalgamated to ensure that the results are satisfactory for release of the blood into the transfusion inventory. Because busy blood collection centers deal with hundreds of donors each day, this amount of data has made essential the need for blood banks to operate sophisticated computer systems and, where possible, automated laboratory testing equipment. Thus, the modern blood center uses pharmaceutical-type manufacturing processes to ensure accuracy and cost effectiveness.[1,4,15]

SAFETY OF THE BLOOD SUPPLY

Ironically, the improvements in blood safety have occurred at a time of the public's increased fear of transfusion and the more cautious use of blood components by physicians. The steps in donor selection and laboratory testing described have resulted in the nation's blood supply being safer than ever.[66-73] Each step in the overall process of donor evaluation and testing adds to blood safety in important ways, and the medical history is important as illustrated by the 90 percent reduction in HIV infectivity from the use of donor-selection criteria identifying HIV risk behavior.[74] Tests for transmissible diseases further reduce the proportion of infectious donors. Donor deferral registries detect individuals who previously were deferred as blood donors but who for various reasons attempt to donate again. Currently, the risk of acquiring a

TABLE 139–3. Laboratory Tests for Transmissible Agents of Donated Blood

Agent	Disease
Treponema	Syphilis
Hepatitis B_s antigen	Hepatitis B
Hepatitis B_c antibody	Hepatitis B
	Hepatitis non-A, non-B
Hepatitis C antibody	Hepatitis C
Hepatitis C nucleic acids	Hepatitis C
HIV-1 and HIV-2 antibody	AIDS
West Nile virus nucleic acids	West Nile infection
HIV nucleic acids	AIDS
Bacteria*	Sepsis
HTLV-I antibody	Leukemia
	Lymphoma
	Tropical paresis
HTLV-II antibody	Disease unknown
CMV†	CMV disease

CMV, cytomegalovirus; HTLV, human T-cell lymphotropic virus.

*Only platelet concentrates tested.

†Of use for immunodeficient recipients.

TABLE 139–4. Incidence of Transfusion-Transmitted Diseases

	Data from Strong and Katz (2002)[75]	Data from Dodd, Notari, and Stramer (2002)[76]	Data from Tabor (2002)[77]	Total U.S. Cases*
Hepatitis C	1/1,200,000	1/1,935,000	1/625,000	8
Hepatitis B	1/150,000	–	1/150,000	80†
HTLV-I/HTLV-II	1/641,000	–	–	20†
HIV	1/1,400,000	1/2,135,000	1/769,230	7

HTLV, human T-cell lymphotropic virus.

*Calculated based on transfusion of 15,000,000 U of blood annually and Dodd[76] incidence figures.

†Calculations based on data from Strong and Katz.[75]

transfusion-transmitted disease ranges from 1 per 150,000 U for hepatitis B to 1 per 2,135,000 U for HIV (Table 139–4). Thus, although the blood supply is safer than ever,[66–73] transfusion is not risk free and should be undertaken only after careful consideration of the patient's clinical situation and specific blood component needs.

REFERENCES

1. McCullough J: The nation's changing blood supply system. *JAMA* 269:2239, 1993.
2. World Health Organization: National blood transfusion services [on the Internet]. www.who.int/bloodsafety/transfusion_services/en/. Accessed September 1, 2009.
3. Whitaker BI, Sullivan M: *2005 Nationwide Blood Collection and Utilization Survey Report*. United States Department of Health and Human Services, Rockville, MD, 2005. Available at www.aabb.org/apps/docs/05nbcusrpt.pdf. Accessed September 1, 2009.
4. Zuck TF: Current good manufacturing practices. *Transfusion* 35:95, 1995.
5. World Health Organization: Blood safety and donation [on the Internet]. Fact sheet No. 279, June 2008. www.who.int/mediacentre/factsheets/fs279/en/index.html. Accessed September 1, 2009.
6. Koistinen J: Organization of blood transfusion services in developing countries. *Vox Sang* 64:247, 1994.
7. Emanuel JC: Blood transfusion systems in economically restricted countries. *Vox Sang* 64:267, 1994.
8. Beal R: Transfusion science and practice in developing countries: A high frequency of empty shelves. *Transfusion* 33:276, 1993.
9. McCullough J: National blood programs in developed countries. *Transfusion* 36:1019, 1996.
10. Beal RW, van Aken WG: Gift or good? *Vox Sang* 63:1, 1992.
11. Barker LF, Westphal RG: Voluntary, nonremunerated blood donation: Still a world health goal? *Transfusion* 38:803, 1998.
12. Eastlund T: Monetary blood donation incentives and the risk of transfusion-transmitted infection. *Transfusion* 38:874, 1998.
13. Plasma Protein Therapeutics Association, 2009. Available at www.pptaglobal.org/faq/default.aspx.
14. Riley W, Schwei M, McCullough J: The United States' potential blood donor pool: Estimating the prevalence of donor exclusion factors on the pool of potential donors. *Transfusion* 47:1180, 2007.
15. McCullough J: *Transfusion Medicine*, 2nd ed. Elsevier, Philadelphia, 2005.
16. Piliavin JA, Callero PL (eds): *Giving Blood. The Development of an Altruistic Identity*. Johns Hopkins University, Baltimore, 1991.
17. Zou S, Musavi F, Notari E, et al: Donor deferral and resulting donor loss at the American Red Cross Blood Services, 2001–2006. *Transfusion* 48:2531, 2008.
18. Newman BH, Newman DT, Ahmad R, Roth AJ: The effect of whole-blood donor adverse events on blood donor return rates. *Transfusion* 46:1374, 2006.
19. Grossman BJ, Springer KM, Zuck TF: Blood donor deferral registries: Highlights of a conference. *Transfusion* 32:868, 1992.
20. Sanchez AM, Schreiber GV, Glynn SA, et al: Blood-donor perceptions of health history screening with a computer-assisted self-administered interview. *Transfusion* 43:165, 2003.
21. Katz LM, Cumming PD, Wallace EL: Computer-based blood donor screening: A status report. *Transfus Med Rev* 21:13, 2009.
22. Rubin RJ, Ness PM: What price progress? An update on vinyl plastic blood banks. *Transfusion* 29:3358, 1989.
23. Morduchowicz G, Pitlik SD, Huminer D, et al: Transfusion reactions due to bacterial contamination of blood and blood products. *Rev Infect Dis* 13:307, 1991.
24. Klein HG, Dodd RY, Ness PM, et al: Current status of microbial contamination of blood components: Summary of a conference. *Transfusion* 37:95, 1997.
25. Kuehnert MJ, Roth VR, Haley NR, et al: Transfusion-transmitted bacterial infection in the United States, 1998 through 2000. *Transfusion* 41:1492, 2001.
26. Benjamin RJ, Kline L, Dy BA, et al: Bacterial contamination of whole blood-derived platelets: The introduction of sample diversion and prestorage pooling with culture testing in the American Red Cross. *Transfusion* 48:2348, 2008.
27. Bruneau C, Perez P, Chassaigne M, et al: Efficacy of a new collection procedure for preventing bacterial contamination of whole-blood donations. *Transfusion* 41:74, 2001.
28. Eder AF, Hillyer CD, Dy BA, et al: Adverse reactions to allogeneic whole blood donation by 16- and 17-year-olds. *JAMA* 299:2279, 2008.
29. Eder AF, Dy BA, Kennedy JM, et al: The American Red Cross donor hemovigilance program: Complications of blood donation reported in 2006. *Transfusion* 48:1809, 2008.
30. Trouern-Trend JJ, Cable RG, Badon SJ, et al: A case-controlled multicenter study of vasovagal reactions in blood donors: Influence of sex, age, donation status, weight, blood pressure, and pulse. *Transfusion* 39:316, 2002.
31. Stewart KR, France CR, Rager AW, Stewart JC: Phlebotomist interpersonal skill predicts a reduction in reactions among volunteer blood donors. *Transfusion* 46:1394, 2006.
32. Rader AW, France CR, Carlson B: Donor retention as a function of donor reactions to whole-blood and automated double red cell collections. *Transfusion* 47:995, 2007.
33. Popovsky MA: Vasovagal donor reactions: An important issue with implications for the blood supply. *Transfusion* 42:1534, 2002.
34. Popovsky MA, Whitaker B, Arnold NL: Severe outcomes of allogeneic and autologous blood donation: Frequency and characterization. *Transfusion* 35:734, 1995.
35. Kasprisin DO, Glynn SH, Taylor F, Miller KA: Moderate and severe reactions in blood donors. *Transfusion* 32:23, 1992.
36. Newman BH, Waxman DA: Blood donation-related neurologic needle injury: Evaluation of 2 years' worth of data from a large blood center. *Transfusion* 36:213, 1996.
37. Berry PR, Wallis WE: Venipuncture nerve injuries. *Lancet* 1:1236, 1997.
38. Axelrod FB, Pepkowitz SH, Goldfinger D: Establishment of a schedule of optimal preoperative collection of autologous blood. *Transfusion* 29:677, 1989.
39. Birkmeyer JD, Goodnough LT, AuBuchon JP, et al: The cost-effectiveness of preoperative autologous blood donation for total hip and knee replacement. *Transfusion* 33:544, 1993.
40. Goodnough LT, Rednick S, Price TH, et al: Increased preoperative collection of autologous blood with recombinant human erythropoietin therapy. *N Engl J Med* 321:1163, 1989.
41. Spivak JL: Recombinant human erythropoietin and its role in transfusion medicine. *Transfusion* 34:1, 1994.
42. de Pree C, Mermillod B, Hoffmeyer P, Beris P: Recombinant human erythropoietin as adjuvant treatment for autologous blood donation in elective surgery with large blood needs (> or = 5 units): A randomized study. *Transfusion* 37:708, 2003.
43. McVay PA, Andrews A, Kaplan EB, et al: Donation reactions among autologous donors. *Transfusion* 30:249, 2003.
44. Starkey NM, MacPherson JL, Bolgiano DC, et al: Markers for transfusion-transmitted disease in different groups of blood donors. *JAMA* 262:3452, 1989.
45. Williams AE, Kleinman S, Gilcher RO, et al: The prevalence of infectious disease markers in directed versus homologous blood donations [abstract]. *Transfusion* 32:45S, 1992.
46. Sanchez AM, Schreiber GV, Bethel J, et al: Prevalence, donation practices, and risk assessment of blood donors with hemochromatosis. *JAMA* 286:1475, 2001.
47. Jeffrey G, Adams PC: Blood from patients with hereditary hemochromatosis—A wasted resource? *Transfusion* 39:549, 1999.
48. Sacher RA: Hemochromatosis and blood donors: A perspective. *Transfusion* 39:551, 1999.
49. Luten M, Roerdinkholder-Stoelwinder B, Rombout-Sestrienkova E, et al: Red cell concentrates of hemochromatosis patients comply with the storage guidelines for transfusion purposes. *Transfusion* 48:436, 2007.

50. Leitman SF, Browning JN, Ying Uau Y, et al: Hemochromatosis subjects as allogeneic blood donors: A prospective study. *Transfusion* 43:1538, 2003.
51. Newman B: Hemochromatosis blood donor programs: Marginal for the red blood cell supply but potentially good for patient care. *Transfusion* 44:1535, 2004.
52. McLeod BC, Price TH, Drew MI (eds): *Apheresis: Principles and Practice*, 2nd ed. AABB, Bethesda, MD, 2003.
53. Meyer D, Bolgiano DC, Sayers M, et al: Red cell collection by apheresis technology. *Transfusion* 33:819, 1993.
54. Shi PA, Ness PM: Two-unit red cell apheresis and its potential advantages over traditional whole-blood donation. *Transfusion* 39:219, 1999.
55. Snyder EL, Elfath MD, Taylor H, et al: Collection of two units of leukoreduced RBCs from a single donation with a portable multiple-component collection system. *Transfusion* 43:1695, 2003.
56. Smith JW, Gilcher RO: Red blood cells, plasma, and other new apheresis-derived blood products: Improving product quality and donor utilization. *Transfus Med Rev* 13:118, 1999.
57. Lasky L, Lin A, Kahn R, McCullough J: Donor platelet response and product quality assurance in plateletpheresis. *Transfusion* 21:247, 1981.
58. Bensinger WI, Price TH, Dale DC, et al: The effects of daily recombinant human granulocyte-colony-stimulating factor administration on normal granulocyte donors undergoing leukapheresis. *Blood* 81:1883, 1993.
59. McCullough J, Clay M, Herr G, et al: Effects of granulocyte colony stimulating factor (G-CSF) on potential normal granulocyte donors. *Transfusion* 39:1136, 1999.
60. Hester J, Dignani MC, Anaissie EJ, et al: Collection and transfusion of granulocyte concentrates from donors primed with granulocyte stimulating factor and response of myelosuppressed patients with established infection. *J Clin Apher* 10:188, 1995.
61. Liles WC, Huang JE, Llewellyn C, et al: A comparative trial of granulocyte-colony-stimulating factor and dexamethasone, separately and in combination, for the mobilization of neutrophils in the peripheral blood of normal volunteers. *Transfusion* 37:182, 1997.
62. Dale DC, Liles WC, Llewellyn C, et al: Neutrophil transfusions: Kinetics and functions of neutrophils mobilized with granulocyte colony-stimulating factor (G-CSF) and dexamethasone. *Transfusion* 38:713, 1998.
63. Strauss RG: Neutrophil (granulocyte) transfusions in the new millennium. *Transfusion* 38:710, 1998.
64. Olson PR, Cox C, McCullough J: Laboratory and clinical effects on the infusion of ACD solution during plateletpheresis. *Vox Sang* 33:79, 1977.
65. Bolan CD, Greer SE, Cecco SA, et al: Comprehensive analysis of citrate effects during plateletpheresis in normal donors. *Transfusion* 41:1165, 2001.
66. Busch MP, Bernard EE, Khayam-Bashi H, et al: Evaluation of screened blood donations from human immunodeficiency virus type 1 infection by culture and DNA amplification of pooled cells. *N Engl J Med* 325:1, 1991.
67. Donahue JG, Munoz A, Ness PM, et al: The declining risk of post-transfusion hepatitis C virus infection. *N Engl J Med* 327:369, 1992.
68. Dodd RY: The risk of transfusion-transmitted infection. *N Engl J Med* 327:419, 1992.
69. Kleinman S, Alter H, Busch M, et al: Increased detection of hepatitis C virus (HCV)-infected blood donors by a multiple-antigen HCV enzyme immunoassay. *Transfusion* 32:805, 1992.
70. Williams AE, Thomson RA, Schreiber GB, et al: Estimates of infectious disease risk factors in U.S. blood donors. *JAMA* 277:967, 1997.
71. Sloand EM, Pitt E, Klein HG: Safety of the blood supply. *JAMA* 274:1368, 1995.
72. Lackritz EM, Satten GA, Aberle-Grasse J, et al: Estimated risk of transmission of the human immunodeficiency virus by screened blood in the United States. *N Engl J Med* 333:1721, 1995.
73. Schreiber GB, Busch MP, Kleinman SH: The risk of transfusion-transmitted viral infections. *N Engl J Med* 334:1685, 1996.
74. Busch MP, Young MJ, Samson SM, et al: Risk of human immunodeficiency virus (HIV) transmission by blood transfusions before the implementation of HIV-1 antibody screening. *Transfusion* 31:4, 1991.
75. Strong DM, Katz L: Blood-bank testing for infectious diseases: How safe is blood transfusion? *Trends Mol Med* 8:355, 2002.
76. Dodd RY, Notari EP, Stramer SL: Current prevalence and incidence of infectious disease markers and estimated window-period risk in the American Red Cross blood donor population. *Transfusion* 42:975, 2002.
77. Tabor E, Epstein JS: NAT screening of blood and plasma donations: Evolution of technology and regulatory policy. *Transfusion* 42:1230, 2002.

CHAPTER 140
RED CELL TRANSFUSION

Norma B. Lerner, Majed A. Refaai, and Neil Blumberg

SUMMARY

Red cell transfusion is one of the oldest and most commonly employed therapies in medicine. The first successful stored red cell transfusions occurred fewer than 100 years ago. The special place of red cell transfusion in medical practice is the result of its lifesaving applications in exsanguinating hemorrhage and life-threatening anemia, for which transfusion remains today virtually the only effective therapy. Methods of red cell preservation have been improved, and the risks of hemolytic transfusion reactions and transmission of infectious diseases significantly reduced. Red cell transfusion is used both to prevent complications of anemia and to treat the symptoms and signs of hypoxia due to anemia. These signs generally do not develop unless hemoglobin level falls below 5 g/dL. Nonetheless, common clinical practice is to maintain hemoglobin levels above 7 g/dL in most patients, and above 8 g/dL in those patients with symptomatic coronary artery disease. In transfusion-dependent outpatients, transfusion to hemoglobins of 9 to 11 g/dL is considered to provide improved quality of life with modest risk, but scant data support the safety of this practice employing transfusion as opposed to erythropoietic agents. In patients with severe hereditary hemoglobinopathies, transfusion also serves to reduce the production of abnormal red cells, in some cases decreasing pathologic effects, as well as provide therapy of the anemia. Alternative strategies exist but cannot fully substitute for transfusion of donor red cells. Transfused stored red cells are not normal, having reduced or absent 2,3-biphosphoglycerate and nitric oxide, and abnormal biophysical properties. The exact importance of these changes to transfusion efficacy and safety is not known. Adverse effects of red cell transfusion related to immunologic incompatibility and disease transmission are uncommon to rare, especially in the era of modern serologic and microbial testing, and use of leukoreduced red cells, but uncommon mild allergic reactions can occur, and are prevented by saline washing or plasma removal of red cells. Acute lung injury is rare after red cell transfusion, but can be life-threatening. Circulatory overload as a result of too rapid or too high volume red cell transfusion is more frequent than lung injury, but less likely to be fatal, and more easily managed in most cases. The potential toxicity and questionable efficacy of stored red cells are now major foci of clinical concern and research. Immunomodulation leading to increases in infection, tumor recurrence, multiorgan failure, decreased organ allograft rejection, and similar phenomena is an important area of basic and clinical research. Preliminary findings raise the question of whether red cell transfusion may predispose to arterial and venous thrombosis. Storage duration of transfused red cells has become one issue in these associations with transfusion. Leukoreduction of red cell transfusions reduces alloimmunization to human leukocyte antigens, cytomegalovirus transmission, refractoriness to platelet transfusion, febrile transfusion reactions, and multiorgan failure after cardiac surgery. Leukoreduction has become standard practice throughout most of the developed world, but has not been adopted universally in the United States. Red cell transfusion remains a key therapy prescribed by physicians of all specialties, but there is little evidence base for current practices, nor is it clear what the indications for transfusion should be in many clinical settings. Furthermore, the degree to which red cells should be processed to remove contaminating white cells, platelets, and stored supernatant, is a matter of controversy and uncertainty. Finally, transfused red cells are metabolically and physically abnormal in many ways, and the degree to which correcting these abnormalities might improve transfusion efficacy and safety is unknown. As red cell transfusion begins its second century, new questions have arisen as to how best to benefit patients employing this powerful therapy and to assess its risks.

Acronyms and abbreviations that appear in this chapter include: ACD, acid, citrate, and dextrose; AHTR, acute hemolytic transfusion reaction; ATR, allergic transfusion reaction; BPG, bisphosphoglycerate; CMV, cytomegalovirus; CPD, citrate, phosphate, and dextrose; DAT, direct antiglobulin test; DHTR, delayed hemolytic transfusion reaction; FNHTR, febrile nonhemolytic transfusion reaction; HDN, hemolytic disease of newborn; HNA, human neutrophil antigen; ICU, intensive care unit; LDH, lactic dehydrogenase; PTP, posttransfusion purpura; SCD, sickle cell disease; TACO, transfusion-associated cardiac overload; TA-GVHD, transfusion-associated graft-versus-host disease; TNF, tumor necrosis factor; TRALI, transfusion-related lung injury; TRICC, transfusion requirement in critical care.

HISTORY AND OVERVIEW

Red cell transfusions are among the oldest therapeutics of the modern era of medical practice. Their lifesaving potential in catastrophic postpartum hemorrhage and massive bleeding following trauma or surgery, were realized more than a hundred years ago. Blood transfusion is the most commonly employed procedure among discharge codes recorded for hospital inpatients.[1] Estimates are that 3 to 4 million patients a year are transfused in the United States, and that most individuals will receive a transfusion at some point in their lives. Transfusions of red cells have rarely been subjected to modern assessments of efficacy and safety. Indeed, as in most clinical research, when randomized trials have been performed, surrogate endpoints of clinical benefit have been employed (e.g., hematocrit increments) rather than clinically more important outcomes (e.g., reduced morbidity and mortality from anemia).

Great advances in transfusion medicine have been achieved by pretransfusion testing for red cell compatibility, hepatitis viruses, HIV, and other pathogens. Red cells are not purified, and are usually contaminated with donor white cells, platelets, and plasma, all of which are modulated by storage-induced changes. Changes in red cell properties during storage have been known for decades, but the clinical significance of these changes is still largely uncertain.[2] The most abundant contaminating cells are donor platelets. Leukoreduction removes 99.9 percent of contaminating white cells and platelets, but approximately 20 percent of red cell transfusions in the United States are nonleukoreduced. Many of the associations between blood transfusion and adverse clinical outcomes likely are related to their effects on innate immunity and hemostasis. Examples include acute lung injury,[3] bacterial infection,[4,5] multiorgan failure,[6] myocardial infarction,[7] and other thrombotic conditions.[8,9] There are randomized trials demonstrating that leukoreduction mitigates some of these effects of red cell transfusions, particularly infection and multiorgan failure.[4–6,10] The supernatant of stored donor red blood cells also contributes to adverse events in recipients, presumably through interactions of cytokines with recipient white cells, platelets, and endothelial.[11–13]

TRANSFUSION THERAPY

Red cell transfusions are administered to improve tissue oxygenation in the context of anemia or acute blood loss. Adaptive responses to a declining hemoglobin concentration include increased cardiac output, augmented oxygen extraction, blood flow redistribution to the heart and brain, a right shift in the oxyhemoglobin dissociation curve, and increased red cell production by the marrow. These compensatory mechanisms help to ensure continued oxygen delivery.[14] There are no specific clinical signs or laboratory parameters that can consistently and reliably indicate the need of patients for transfusion. Physicians most often base their decision to transfuse red blood cells upon their clinical experience and the patient's hemoglobin concentration. The "critical" hemoglobin level is considered to be that at which adaptive mechanisms have been maximized and the prediction that further reduction would result in compromised function. The critical hemoglobin level in healthy adults is not known but is below 5 g/dL.[15] In sick patients, for whom compensatory responses may be compromised, the threshold hemoglobin level is likely higher.

In the past, the benefit of red cell transfusions was believed to outweigh related risks. Since the 1980s, however, hazards associated with red cell transfusion have been closely examined. This scrutiny was initially provoked by infectious concerns, but subsequently was prompted by other hazards such as induction of immunomodulation and red cell storage lesions. Leukoreduction, shorter storage times, and a decreased number of transfusions have been employed to reduce these complications.[16–21] There is consensus that whenever transfusion is deemed necessary, patients should be well informed about risks and benefits and consent should be obtained.[22]

CRITICALLY ILL ADULTS

Red cell transfusions are administered to approximately 40 percent of adults and 14 percent of children who are hospitalized in intensive care units (ICUs).[23,24] A large, randomized controlled study of transfusion requirements in critical care (TRICC) compared a standard "liberal" transfusion strategy with a more "restrictive" one.[19] The study documented a similar 30-day mortality using either strategy, and revealed lower mortality rates in less acutely ill and younger patients using the restrictive approach. It should be noted that the transfusions in this study were not leukoreduced. The authors concluded that adult ICU patients should receive red cell transfusions for a hemoglobin less than 7.0 g/dL and that the hemoglobin should be maintained between 7.0 and 9.0 g/dL. Possible exceptions to this recommendation were patients with active coronary ischemia.[19] A later multicenter observational study also found an association between transfusions and increased mortality and recorded diminished organ function in transfused patients.[25]

The approach to ill adults with cardiovascular disease has been less clear. A followup subgroup analysis of the TRICC data showed that a restrictive transfusion strategy was safe in such patients, with the possible exception of those with acute myocardial infarction or unstable angina.[26] Other studies suggest that anemia is less-well tolerated in patients with significant coronary disease.[7,27] Recent guidelines based on findings of adverse events when patients were transfused for a hematocrit greater than 25 percent, recommend transfusing patients with hematocrits less than 25 percent with non–ST-segment elevation acute coronary syndromes.[7,29] A more liberal transfusion strategy was proposed in older patients, and a more restrictive approach was suggested in younger patients with cardiac disease.[30] Table 140–1 shows current published ICU transfusion recommendations.[30]

TABLE 140–1. Recommendations for Transfusion in Patients in ICUs[30,*]

	Hemoglobin Level (g/dL)	
Critical Patient Variable	Trigger Value	Goal Value
No acute bleeding	7.0	7.0–9.0
Septic shock (>6 h)	7.0	7.0–9.0
Septic shock (<6 h)	8.0–10.0	10.0
Chronic cardiac disease	7.0	7.0–9.0
Acute cardiac disease	8.0–10.0	10.0

*One unit of red cells should be administered at a time, and hemoglobin level monitored closely.

CRITICALLY ILL CHILDREN

Liberal versus restrictive transfusion strategies were also compared in a large randomized trial involving stable critically ill children.[21] There were no significant between-group differences in the incidence of multiple organ dysfunction syndrome, 28-day death rates, or adverse events. The restrictive approach resulted in a substantial reduction in the number of patients transfused and in the number of transfusions. Unlike the TRICC study, all transfusions in this study were leukoreduced. Based upon their findings, the authors recommended a hemoglobin threshold of 7 g/dL for the transfusion of stable, pediatric ICU patients. Premature infants and children with severe hypoxemia, hemodynamic instability, active bleeding, or cyanotic heart disease were not included in this recommendation.[21]

Despite their frequent use, the impact of red cell transfusions in premature newborns is not well understood. While clinical factors such as poor weight gain, respiratory difficulties, and tachycardia have prompted transfusion in these patients, a beneficial effect of red cells for these indications has not been documented. Laboratory findings like blood lactate, erythropoietin level, and mixed venous oxygen saturation have also proved to have poor predictive value with regard to the need for transfusion. Two randomized controlled trials comparing liberal and restrictive leukoreduced transfusion strategies documented somewhat fewer red cell transfusions in the restrictive group without increased mortality or morbidity.[17,20] However, one of these studies showed that the restrictive group experienced more brain hemorrhage, periventricular leukomalacia, and apnea,[17] whereas the Premature Infants in Need of Transfusion study did not.[20] Differences in trial design and in the populations studied were likely responsible for the outcome disparities. A recent followup of subjects enrolled in the Premature Infants in Need of Transfusion study found that the difference in cognitive delay approached statistical significance and a *post hoc* analysis using a redefined definition of cognitive delay showed a significantly better outcome in the liberal transfusion group.[31] Because a liberal approach may be associated with better neuroprotection, most consensus-based guidelines continue to advise this strategy pending further study. Table 140–2 presents a reasonable approach to red cell transfusions in premature infants.[32]

MAJOR HEMORRHAGE

Massive hemorrhage has been defined as the loss of one blood volume within a 24-hour period, a 50 percent blood volume loss within 3 hours, or a rate of loss of 150 mL/min. Acute blood loss is initially treated by volume support and is only secondarily concerned with the loss of red cell mass. Volume support consists of rapid infusion of crystalloid or colloid solutions. Red cell transfusion is usually required after 30 to 40 percent of blood volume has been lost or when hemoglobin concentration has fallen to <6 g/dL. Transfusion when higher hemoglobin levels are present may be dictated by a perceived risk of complications from inadequate oxygenation. In this regard, it should be kept in mind that tissue ischemia may occur in the face of normal vital signs.[33]

TABLE 140-2. Suggested RBC Transfusion Guidelines for the Anemia of Prematurity[32,*]

Maintain >40–45% hematocrit (Hct) for *severe* cardiopulmonary disease
Maintain >30–35% Hct for *moderate* cardiopulmonary disease
Maintain >30–35% Hct for *major* surgery
Maintain >20–25% Hct for infants with *stable* anemia, especially if accompanied by:
Unexplained breathing disorder
Unexplained tachycardia
Unexplained poor growth

*Words in italics designate parameters that must be defined in each center. For example, *severe* pulmonary disease may be defined as requiring mechanical ventilation with >0.35 FiO_2 (fraction of inspired oxygen) and *moderate* as less-intensive ventilation.

GENERAL SURGERY

Although recommendations derived from the randomized ICU trials may have influenced perioperative practices, studies that specifically address general surgical patients are limited in number. In the recent past, transfusion in healthy patients with a hemoglobin <7 g/dL and the avoidance of transfusion in circumstances where the hemoglobin was ≥10 g/dL was recommended. There was general adherence to these guidelines in a retrospective study of patients undergoing surgery for hip fracture, wherein no reduction in mortality was found when red cell transfusions were administered at hemoglobin concentrations of ≥8 g/dL.[18]

CARDIAC SURGERY

Most perioperative investigations have been performed in the context of cardiac surgery. In a randomized trial involving patients undergoing coronary artery bypass grafting, there was no difference in morbidity or mortality when the group receiving postoperative transfusion for a hemoglobin <8 g/dL was compared with a control group receiving transfusions as dictated by clinical judgment and institutional guidelines (hemoglobin <9 g/dL).[34] Other cardiac surgery studies have found associations between red cell transfusions and important complications including infection, myocardial infarction, stroke, renal failure, as well as early and late mortality.[10,35–38] One of these investigations found no benefit from transfusions given at hematocrits as low as 21.[38] The authors suggested that this might represent a reasonable restrictive threshold for future randomized studies. Other reports have linked decreased survival in women undergoing cardiac surgery to their greater likelihood of being transfused.[39,40] In another study, both preoperative anemia and intraoperative blood transfusion were independent risk factors for adverse outcomes, and as the number of transfused red cell units increased, the number of adverse outcomes rose at comparable hemoglobin levels.[28] A retrospective cohort study found that preoperative anemia, independent of the effects of red cell transfusions, was associated with adverse outcomes.[41] Patients undergoing cardiac surgery have strikingly reduced mortality and multiorgan failure when only leukoreduced transfusions are used.[10]

EMERGENCY TRANSFUSIONS

Massive bleeding from the gastrointestinal tract or ruptured aneurysm and during surgery or following trauma may not allow the typing, selecting, and cross-matching of blood.[42] In such cases, uncross-matched blood, type O, Rh-negative blood is used for women of child-bearing age or younger, and type O, Rh-negative or Rh-positive blood is used in males or older females. The use of packed red blood cells is preferable because it reduces the quantity of anti-A or anti-B administered. If time permits, ABO group and Rh type-specific blood should be used. Because this can be available within 5 to 15 minutes, the first blood sample that should be sent in a massively bleeding patient should be sent to the blood bank. The advantage of using uncross-matched ABO group-specific blood is the prevention of hemolysis that may occur if a high-titered anti-A or anti-B group O blood is given to a non-O recipient. If 15 to 30 minutes are available, an abbreviated antibody screen can be carried out using low ionic strength conditions.[43] Group- and type-specific uncross-matched blood with a negative antibody screen provides compatibility for the recipient that is equivalent to that of cross-matched blood in essentially all cases.[44]

CHRONIC ANEMIA

Adaptive physiologic mechanisms allow most individuals to tolerate chronic anemia. Consequently, blood transfusion in most patients with chronic stable anemia is probably unjustifiable if the hemoglobin level is above 7 g/dL. Over this level, red cell transfusion is usually reserved for older patients, patients with symptoms that interfere with daily functioning, and patients with cardiac or pulmonary disease.

HEMOGLOBINOPATHIES

Sickle Cell Disease

For a detailed discussion of sickle cell disease, see Chap. 48.

Although transfusions are generally not needed in the context of baseline anemia and vasoocclusive crisis, they are a mainstay of therapy for certain complications of sickle cell disease (SCD).[45] Transfusion is often needed to treat the severe anemia associated with splenic sequestration crisis and parvovirus B19-related aplastic crisis. Acute sequestration should be considered an emergency as it has been associated with a mortality rate of close to 10 percent.[46] Red cells should be transfused promptly but cautiously. Transfusion may cause the spleen to unload sequestered cells that, when added to the allogeneic cells, may produce an unexpectedly high hemoglobin concentration. To avoid raising the hemoglobin above 10 to 12 g/dL and the resultant hyperviscosity, approximately half of the anticipated transfusion (5 mL/kg in children) should be given initially, following which the hemoglobin should be rechecked to determine if additional transfusion is needed.

Parvovirus B19 infection compromises erythropoiesis for 7 to 10 days. Because sickle cell disease is a hemolytic anemia associated with a significantly shortened erythrocyte life span and active compensatory reticulocytosis, marrow shut down and reticulocytopenia lead to severe symptomatic anemia in patients with this disorder. Anemia in aplastic crisis develops gradually and the associated expanded plasma volume may cause a red cell transfusion to precipitate pulmonary edema. Consequently, consideration should be given to diuretic administration halfway through the transfusion or, alternatively, partial exchange transfusion should be carried out.

Transfusion is also recommended in patients with sickle cell disease if the hemoglobin is less than 10 g/dL prior to surgery requiring general anesthesia.[47] It is also often useful in acute chest syndrome. For patients who fail to improve with a simple transfusion or those with a baseline high hemoglobin, exchange transfusion may be indicated.

In children with an acute ischemic stroke, an exchange transfusion with the goal of reducing the hemoglobin S level to less than 20 to 25 percent should be performed as soon as possible. The management of adults with acute stroke is less clear. A standard approach used in adults without SCD who experience ischemic stroke has been advocated.[48] One might question, however, the prudence of using antiplatelet agents or tissue plasminogen activator in a population prone to cerebral hemorrhage.

Chronic prophylactic transfusion therapy substantially reduces the incidence of recurrent stroke. Simple transfusion or manual exchange/erythrocytapheresis should be pursued with the intent of maintaining the hemoglobin S level at less than 30 percent.[45,46] After 3 years of neurologic stability, some hematologists believe the hemoglobin S cutoff can be increased to 50 percent. This approach, as well as exchange and erythrocytapheresis, is associated with decreased iron loading.[49,50] In most instances, continued transfusion is recommended, given the high incidence of recurrent stroke when it is curtailed. For secondary prophylaxis, a gradual transition from transfusion to hydroxyurea therapy has been investigated.[51] An ongoing study should provide answers to whether or not such an approach is effective.

Chronic transfusion therapy is also effective for the primary prevention of stroke. Transfusions decrease the incidence of stroke by 92 percent in children with SCD and abnormally high cerebral transcranial Doppler ultrasound velocity, a known risk factor for stroke.[52] Unfortunately, recent evidence supports continuing prophylactic transfusions indefinitely to prevent reversion to high transcranial Doppler ultrasound velocities and/or stroke.[53]

The combined use of leukoreduced red cells matched for ABO, minor Rh and K antigens decreases alloimmunization and hemolytic transfusion reactions in patients with SCD.[54] Many centers also test donor red cells for hemoglobin S trait when large volume or exchange transfusions are required, and when the hemoglobin S level in the recipient is targeted to be less than 30 percent. Most blood units, however, are negative for sickle cell trait.[55]

All patients receiving chronic transfusions ultimately will require iron-chelation therapy to avoid organ damage from iron overload. A new oral agent, deferasirox, has been effective and will likely improve compliance when compared with continuous infusion subcutaneous desferrioxamine (see Chaps. 47 and 48).[56]

β-Thalassemia

For a detailed discussion of *β*-thalassemia, see Chap. 48.

Patients with thalassemia major are dependent on red cell transfusions. Over the years, a variety of transfusion modalities have been tested with the goal of maximizing symptom control and minimizing iron loading. A successful approach has been to maintain a pretransfusion hemoglobin of 9 to 10 g/dL while targeting an average hemoglobin of 12 g/dL. At this level, endogenous erythropoiesis with the associated bone deformities is suppressed and poor growth and organomegaly are ameliorated.[57] This target hemoglobin is usually achieved with monthly transfusions. Chelation therapy is generally required after the first year of transfusions or when the serum ferritin is repeatedly greater than 1000 ng/mL.

The clinical picture in thalassemia intermedia can be quite variable and the age at presentation appears to be a good indicator of future need for transfusion. The decision to transfuse such patients is primarily clinical and based upon poor growth, skeletal deformities, splenic enlargement and well being. Once the decision to transfuse is made, guidelines used in thalassemia major are generally pursued.[57]

Autoimmune Hemolytic Anemia

For a detailed discussion of autoimmune hemolytic anemia, see Chap. 53.

Many patients with *de novo* or secondary autoimmune hemolytic anemia may require red cell transfusions to treat life-threatening anemia. Finding compatible blood for these individuals can be difficult because of the presence of autoantibodies that complicate compatibility testing. Ideally, donor blood should be selected so that it lacks major antigens corresponding to the antibodies in the recipient, but frequently, no autoantibody specificity can be established. Previously transfused or pregnant patients may also have clinically significant alloantibodies that are difficult to detect in the presence of an autoantibody. Transfusion of serologically incompatible red cells should be avoided but may sometimes be necessary.[58] In such cases there is a shortened life span of red cells but transfusion reactions are rare.

Hemolytic Disease of the Newborn

For a detailed discussion of hemolytic disease of the newborn, see Chap. 54.

In the not-so-distant past, hemolytic disease of the newborn (HDN) was predominately associated with Rh(D) alloimmunization which often necessitated multiple exchange transfusions. Postnatal prophylactic anti-D immunoglobulin greatly reduced its incidence. Other etiologies for HDN are ABO incompatibility, maternal alloantibodies, as well as red cell enzyme and membrane defects. In most instances, transfusion can be avoided using other interventions.[59] If exchange transfusion is needed in the context of ABO incompatibility, this may be performed with washed group O red cells suspended in AB plasma or saline/albumin, depending on the volume and frequency of exchange needed.

■ CONGENITAL AND ACQUIRED ANEMIAS

Patients with congenital anemias such as Diamond Blackfan and Fanconi anemia (Chap. 39) may need acute or chronic red cell transfusion support. Children with transient erythroblastopenia of childhood generally require transfusion pending marrow recovery (see Chap. 52). Strict guidelines are generally employed for patients with acquired severe aplastic anemia because sensitization reduces the chances of recovery. Transfusions are reserved for symptomatic anemia or bleeding and are generally not given unless the hemoglobin is <7 g/dL.

Controlled trials regarding a reasonable hemoglobin target level are lacking for patients with marrow suppression secondary to chemotherapy and/or radiation therapy for malignancies. Most centers maintain the hemoglobin level over 8 g/dL. Although low hemoglobin levels are associated with a poor quality of life in patients receiving chemotherapy, transfusions are associated with thrombosis and mortality.[9]

■ HEMATOPOIETIC STEM CELL TRANSPLANTATION

For a detailed discussion of hematopoietic stem cell transplantation, see Chap. 21.

Transplant recipients usually require special blood components including leukocyte-reduced and irradiated red cells and platelets. Leukoreduction reduces the risk of transfusion reactions, cytomegalovirus (CMV) transmission, and human leukocyte antigen (HLA) alloimmunization/platelet refractoriness. Some data suggest leukoreduction may reduce infectious complications, graft-versus-host disease, and other serious complications, including lung injury.[60,61] Family directed donations may be contraindicated because of concerns regarding sensitization to minor HLA antigens and consequent graft rejection. Transfusion guidelines generally follow those discussed for individuals with marrow suppression, namely maintaining the hemoglobin above 8 g/dL in healthy patients and somewhat higher in those with cardiac disease, although good evidence-based data are not available on the risks and benefits of this approach. Hematopoietic stem cell transplantation does not require the donor and recipient to be ABO identical, but transfusions should be ABO/Rh compatible.[62]

■ ORGAN TRANSPLANTATION

Kidney Transplant

Random donor blood transfusions can result in allogeneic immunization,[63] and in the early days of transplantation they were avoided so as to prevent the possibility of inducing anti-HLA antibodies in potential transplant recipients. However, a series of reports from 1973 to 1978 surprisingly demonstrated that kidney transplant patients who had received multiple blood transfusions before transplantation actually had better graft survival.[64] This provided the first evidence of the immunomodulatory effects of transfusions. Prior to the introduction of cyclosporine, the purposeful administration of random donor blood transfusions to reduce rejection became common. Current practice in kidney transplantation has been changed dramatically by three developments: the introduction of cyclosporine and erythropoietin and the increasing concern over the danger of exposure to random donor transfusions. Cyclosporine is a potent immunosuppressive drug that reduces the beneficial immunomodulatory effects of blood transfusions that might otherwise outweigh the risks of transfusion-induced HLA sensitization. The widespread use of erythropoietin has ended the routine practice of blood transfusions to treat the anemia of end-stage renal disease and transfusions are to be avoided in any potential renal transplant recipient.[65]

Liver Transplantation

For a detailed discussion of liver transplantation, see Chap. 129.

Large volumes of blood have frequently been used for liver transplantation[66] but are associated with increased morbidity and reduced survival.[67] The demand for blood is influenced by the underlying liver disease, the nature of the preoperative coagulation defect, and the intraoperative blood loss associated with surgery on a large vascular organ. Improved surgical and anesthetic practices to prevent blood loss have reduced the number of red cell transfusions, and currently almost 40 percent of liver transplantations are performed without transfusion.[67]

MODE OF ADMINISTRATION

Blood should always be transfused at the bedside through a filter (approximately 170 microns) to remove small clots and aggregates that may have accumulated during storage. These devices do not provide leukoreduction. Blood should not be warmed up before its use. The use of a blood warmer is recommended when unusually large amounts must be given (>3 L) at a rapid rate (>100 mL/min; in children, >15 mg/kg per hour), during exchange transfusions, and in patients with cold agglutinin disease. Blood should be administered slowly during the first 30 minutes to minimize the amount given if an untoward reaction occurs, but should be infused within 4 hours. It is usually safe to transfuse 1000 mL of blood (approximately 2–3 units) within a period of 2 to 3 hours to the average adult patient who has no cardiovascular disease. In children, a rate of approximately 2.5 mL/kg per hour will usually prevent circulatory overload. Vascular instability may warrant slower infusion rates and more rapid rates may be needed when there is major acute blood loss.

Drugs or medications should not be added to blood or blood components. Several intravenous solutions are incompatible with banked blood and should not be administered through the blood lines. Aqueous dextrose solutions cause agglomeration (clumping) and hemolysis of red blood cells, and calcium-containing solutions such as Ringer lactate may exceed the calcium-binding capacity of the citrate in the anticoagulated blood with formation of clots. Physiologic saline is compatible with all blood components.

Most transfusions are administered intravenously. A vein in the forearm or antecubital fossa is ordinarily used, although any accessible vein or a central venous line may be employed. Because of the hazards, transfusion into an artery should be reserved for patients who have failed to respond to rapid, large-volume intravenous transfusion.

Exchange transfusion is recommended to control severe anemia and/or hyperbilirubinemia in the neonate. It is also employed for various indications in patients with SCD (see "Hemoglobinopathies" above). Exchange transfusion can be manually performed or carried out by an automated approach (erythrocytapheresis). Most instruments require vascular access for draw and return which may be difficult to find in children. Exchange should only be undertaken by experienced individuals as the procedure has the potential to lead to serious adverse events if not performed properly (see Chap. 26).

Intrauterine transfusion may be indicated to reverse fetal anemia secondary to red cell alloimmunization, parvovirus infection, or other etiology. This procedure can be hazardous to the fetus and is only used when the fetus is hydropic or at high risk of becoming so before 34 to 35 weeks of gestation. A high degree of skill is required, and the procedure is carried out only at tertiary prenatal centers.

In infants and young children, small red cell volumes may be all that are needed at any one time. It is good practice to "split" units derived from a single donor to allow sequential transfusions to be given as required. Single-unit transfusions are often justifiable. Examples include elderly surgical patients with coronary heart disease, patients who have sustained an acute blood loss who can achieve circulatory stability by reaching an appropriate hematocrit, and patients whose bleeding during surgery or from the gastrointestinal tract is controlled after transfusion of the first unit.[68]

DECREASING THE NEED OF TRANSFUSION

Given the increasing evidence for potential harm, physicians now rely on a variety of strategies to decrease the need for allogeneic transfusion. Some approaches are described below.

Limiting Blood Loss

Frequent blood sampling for diagnostic purposes and followup is an important and often overlooked cause of blood loss.[16,23,25] Critical care patients have their blood drawn frequently, particularly when the process is simplified by the existence of an indwelling catheter. Catheters also require infusate-blood discards which substantially add to iatrogenic loss. Useful ways to reduce losses include careful consideration regarding what testing is actually necessary and eliminating those blood draws that are not. The use of small volume collection tubes (micro volumes in infants) has also proved useful, as has the elimination or reduction of discarded blood from catheters. Point-of-care testing may also reduce losses.[16]

Control of bleeding during surgery is of paramount importance and is primarily achieved with good surgical technique. In all settings, other interventions may be used to reduce blood loss. Blood products (platelets, fresh-frozen plasma/cryoprecipitate) often provide hemostatic support. Antifibrinolytic agents that decrease clot dissolution have been used effectively in the perioperative setting, reducing transfusions and reoperations without increasing morbidity.[16] Recent safety concerns have been raised with regard to one of these agents, aprotinin, and it is no longer readily available.[69] Desmopressin acetate has been used effectively in patients with specific bleeding disorders but is of unproven help for other patients. Although recombinant activated factor VII has been studied in a variety of settings, its prophylactic and therapeutic effectiveness in nonhemophiliacs has not been proven.[16]

Preventing Anemia

Erythropoietin receptor agonists, usually recombinant erythropoietin, have been used widely to reduce transfusions in patients with chronic renal failure and in cases where endogenous erythropoietin levels are low. The use of erythropoietin in cancer patients undergoing chemotherapy has been associated with a reduction in transfusion requirements, but there have been concerns regarding an associated increase in venous thrombosis and possibly more rapid tumor progression.[70]

Erythropoietin has been effectively employed to increase the red cell count prior to elective surgery. In a randomized study of critically ill patients treated or not by erythropoietin, there was no significant difference in the number of transfusions between the treated and placebo groups.[71] There was no overall difference in mortality, but a subgroup analysis of trauma patients found improved survival in the treated group. Notably, there was a significant increase in the incidence of deep vein thrombosis in the erythropoietin-treated group.[71]

Alternative Transfusion Strategies

Although transfusion of autologous blood may avert some problems associated with the use of donor blood, some of the risks remain.[14] Three variations of autologous blood transfusion have been used: preoperative blood collection, with storage for a variable time and retransfusion during surgery; normovolemic hemodilution (immediate preoperative phlebotomy and hemodilution, with postoperative return of the phlebotomized blood); and intraoperative salvage of shed blood with reinfusion during surgery. Preoperative autologous red cell donation is associated with a 40 percent reduction in the number of transfusions, as well as a 30 percent increase in the need for transfusion.[14] Because it can be frozen, predeposited autologous blood may be most useful for patients with rare blood types and for those with antibodies in numbers and combinations that make it nearly impossible to find compatible units of blood. Acute normovolemic hemodilution at the start of a surgical procedure with reinfusion on completion results in the same number of transfused patients, but fewer units of blood are used.[72] This approach may be most useful in the setting of expected major surgical blood loss. Overall, randomized trials have demonstrated that autologous transfusion techniques reduce morbidity in surgical patients, but these findings remain controversial.[73]

Some but not all cohort studies, retrospective and prospective, have demonstrated an association between prolonged red cell storage times and adverse outcomes, including mortality and organ failure.[74] Further research will be necessary to determine the true nature and magnitude of these effects, and in which patients they may be relevant. The negative impact of a "storage lesion" may be related to a decrease in red cell oxygen transport and delivery, impeded microvascular flow, and/or an associated heightened inflammatory response. Investigations have been limited by small sample size and confounding factors. A large retrospective study in patients undergoing cardiac surgery found that the transfusion of red cells stored for more than 2 weeks was associated with a significantly increased risk of postoperative complications and reduced survival.[74] Although prospective randomized controlled trials are needed to verify these findings, it is possible that in the future, rejuvenated, supernatant removed, and/or "fresher" red cells may prove to be a useful technique to decrease transfusion associated complications in selected patient populations. Universal use of "fresher blood," although attractive in principle, is not feasible with the current blood donation and storage system, thus modifications to the stored red cells seem the most likely avenue to reductions in the toxicity of transfusion.

■ EFFECTS OF STORAGE ON BLOOD

Red cells, as currently stored, do not acutely improve oxygen delivery to the tissues. This may be due, in part, to striking storage changes in important red cell regulatory molecules (see "Liquid Preservation of Red Cells" below). Decreased 2,3-bisphosphoglycerate, which aids oxygen unloading from hemoglobin, and severe deficiency of nitric oxide, that is needed for normal vasodilation in the microcirculation, have been described, along with rheologic and morphologic changes.[75,76] However, there are no human studies demonstrating that modifications of 2,3-bisphosphoglycerate or nitric oxide can improve clinical outcomes, nor are there modifications that improve red cell rheology. Complement activation may also occur in some stored blood products.[77]

Randomized controlled clinical trials have demonstrated that leukoreduction of stored red cells[5,10,78,79] and removal of supernatant by washing ameliorate inflammatory responses and reduce overall mortality.[11,80,81]

■ ADVERSE EFFECTS OF RED CELL TRANSFUSIONS

Blood transfusion therapy carries significant risks[82] and should be regarded as a temporary organ transplant. In the late 1980s, acute transfusion reactions were estimated to occur in 20 percent of total transfusions, with severe reactions observed in approximately 0.5 percent.[83] Subsequently, the rate has declined because of the introduction of leukoreduction.[60] The precise risk of adverse reactions is difficult to assess because many posttransfusion reactions may be wrongly attributed to the patient's underlying illness. Approximately half of all transfusions are given to anesthetized patients in the operating room where reactions may be blunted or more difficult to recognize.[84]

Adverse reactions may occur within minutes to hours as in acute hemolytic reactions or acute lung injury, or may be delayed by days to weeks as in delayed hemolytic reactions, multiorgan failure, thrombosis, tumor recurrence, and infections.[4–13,78–81] Most acute transfusion reactions are mild and manageable. Many of the reported transfusion-related fatalities are caused by human errors. In one study of 70 transfusion-related deaths, 75 percent resulted from administration of correctly cross-matched blood to the wrong patient.[85,86] The rate of a technical error was estimated to be 1:18,000 transfusions.[87]

■ IMMEDIATE TRANSFUSION REACTIONS

Immediate transfusion reactions include chills, fever, urticaria, tachycardia, dyspnea, nausea, vomiting, chest tightness, chest and back pain, hypotension, bronchospasm, angioneurotic edema, anaphylaxis, shock, pulmonary edema, and congestive heart failure. Immediate immunologic transfusion reactions in an anesthetized patient may manifest signs such as generalized oozing of blood from the operative site, hypotension, and shock. In general, immediate transfusion reactions are more dangerous than delayed reactions. Severe complications, including death, can, on rare occasions, develop within a few minutes of initiating transfusion. Close attention and early vital sign assessments are therefore recommended at the beginning and within 15 minutes of starting a transfusion. Once a reaction is suspected, transfusion should be discontinued immediately. Intravenous access should be maintained. Treating the patient's symptoms, ordering appropriate laboratory tests, and notifying the transfusion service for further investigation are typical procedures.

Acute Hemolytic Transfusion Reactions

Acute hemolytic transfusion reaction (AHTR) is typically caused by the immune-mediated destruction of ABO-incompatible transfused blood,[88,89] and rarely by other blood group incompatibilities, such as the Kidd blood group.

Incidence The incidence of ABO-incompatible transfusions is unknown but is estimated to occur in 1 in 38,000 to 1 in 70,000 red cell transfusions.[88,89] The severity of AHTR is extremely variable and usually depends on the rate and total volume of blood administered. Approximately 47 percent of the recipients of ABO-incompatible blood show no effects even after receiving a whole blood unit. Forty-one percent of recipients exhibit symptoms of AHTR (see below). The mortality rate is approximately 2 percent.[88,89]

Until recently, AHTR was the leading cause of transfusion-related mortality but this has changed because of better recognition of transfusion-related acute lung injury (TRALI), which is now the leading reported cause of death.[90]

Pathophysiology The severity of AHTR is thought to depend on the potency of the naturally occurring immunoglobulin (Ig) M antibodies (anti-A or anti-B) in the recipient's plasma. Anti-A and anti-B antibodies can activate the complement and coagulation systems. C3a and C5a can activate white blood cells to release inflammatory cytokines (interleukin [IL]-1, IL-6, IL-8 and tumor necrosis factor [TNF]-α) that cause fever, hypotension, wheezing, chest pain, nausea, and vomiting.[91] The presence of antigen–antibody complexes and activated complement on donor red cells may lead to generation of bradykinin. This can increase capillary permeability and arteriolar dilatation, causing a fall in systemic blood pressure. Activation of factor XII may initiate the coagulation cascade with formation of thrombin and lead to disseminated intravascular coagulation. Renal failure may also develop as a result of ischemia, hypotension, antigen–antibody complex deposition, and thrombosis.[92,93]

Clinical Features The most common presenting symptom is fever with or without chills or rigors. In mild cases, this may be accompanied with abdominal, chest, flank, or back pain, whereas dyspnea, hypotension, hemoglobinuria, and eventually shock can be seen in severe cases. Bleeding caused by the consumptive coagulopathy can also be seen in one-third to one-half of patients with intravascular hemolysis following an incompatible transfusion.[94] Hemoglobinuria can be the first sign of intravascular hemolysis, particularly in anesthetized or unconscious patients.

Laboratory Evaluation In all suspected acute transfusion reactions, the Blood Transfusion Service will immediately check for technical and identification errors, examine a posttransfusion specimen for hemolysis, and perform a direct antiglobulin test (DAT) to detect any incompatibility.[93] If AHTR is suspected, repeat ABO and Rh typing of the patient and the transfused blood should be carried out, along with repeat antibody screening and cross-matching. Additional laboratory findings consistent with intravascular hemolysis include decreased hemoglobin level, hemoglobinemia, hemoglobinuria, hyperbilirubinemia, low haptoglobin level, and elevated level of lactic dehydrogenase (LDH). A negative DAT occurs in rare cases when all transfused red cells are lysed.

Management Severe complications rarely occur with transfusion of less than 200 mL of red cells. Immediate discontinuation of transfusion should always be the first step in any transfusion reaction. Maintaining vascular access with slow infusion of normal saline, monitoring vital signs, and assessing urine output are key early steps. A blood specimen should be collected immediately for laboratory evaluation. The donor unit bag should be returned to the blood bank. If severe hemolysis has occurred, therapy focuses on management of hypotension, coagulation disorders, and renal function. A urine output of approximately 100 mL/h for 24 hours should be maintained in adults without contraindications. In simple cases, normal saline infusion may be sufficient; however, diuretics may be necessary in some cases. Intravenous administration of furosemide (40–80 mg) promotes diuresis and improves blood flow to the renal cortex. In severe cases of hypotension, dopamine, which dilates renal vasculature and increases cardiac output, can be used at a dosage of 1 mg/kg of body weight per hour. Expert renal consultation may be sought for patients with renal compromise. Patients with coagulopathy and active bleeding may require administration of platelets, fresh-frozen plasma, and cryoprecipitate.

Prevention The common causes of AHTR are errors in identifying the patient, labeling the pretransfusion sample, and identifying the correct red cell unit for the patient.[85–87] Identifying where an error occurred may help prevent future errors and accidents. It is recommended to use at least two patient identifiers whenever administering blood products or collecting blood samples.

Febrile Nonhemolytic Transfusion Reactions

A febrile nonhemolytic transfusion reaction (FNHTR) is defined, arbitrarily, as a temperature increase of 1°C (1.8°F) or more associated with transfusion in the absence of other identifiable causes for fever. This reaction may occur either during or within 1 to 2 hours following the transfusion. Chills and rigors without fever or a low fever are also defined as FNHTR. Symptoms can also include increases in respiratory rate, changes in blood pressure, anxiety, and more unusually, nausea or vomiting.

Incidence FNHTRs are commonly encountered transfusion reactions. The incidence varies with the clinical setting such as age, prior transfusion history, and underlying illness. FNHTRs occur in approximately 0.5 to 2.0 percent of units transfused and are more likely to occur following transfusion of platelets (1–38%) than following transfusion of red cells (0.01–6%).[95] Leukocyte reduction decreases the incidence of FNHTRs with both whole-blood-derived and apheresis platelets.[96] Universal leukoreduction of red cell and platelet transfusions has been adopted in most European nations, but not the United States. Individuals with a history of repeated transfusions and women with a history of multiple pregnancies are at higher risk of FNHTRs. [96]

Pathophysiology Fever is triggered by the action of cytokines (e.g., IL-1, IL-6, TNF-α) on the thermoregulatory center of the anterior hypothalamus inducing production of prostaglandin E_2. The generation of these cytokines after transfusion, speculatively, may be the result of activation of donor leukocytes by anti-HLA or other antibodies in the recipient, activation of recipient leukocyte and endothelial cells by transfused donor leukocytes or plasma constituents, or by the passive transfer of cytokines that have accumulated in the unit during storage. Stored platelets accumulate IL-1β, IL-6, IL-8, and TNF-α, and transfusion of supernatant can elicit FNHTRs.[96,97] Prestorage is more effective than poststorage leukocyte reduction in preventing reactions. Another mediator present in nonleukoreduced red cells and both leukoreduced and nonleukoreduced platelets, CD40 ligand (CD154), has been associated with febrile responses to platelet transfusions.[98]

Clinical Features Fever should not be solely attributed to FNHTR. Other potential life-threatening transfusion reactions, such as AHTR, bacterial contamination, acute lung injury, and other concomitant causes of fever (such as infection or drug reaction), have to be excluded. The temperature curve, hospital course, and the status of indwelling catheters should also be examined. The patient's current vital signs should be compared to the pretransfusion values and monitored until the fever and/or other symptoms resolve. Past transfusion reaction history should be reviewed to determine if additional measures should be undertaken for future transfusions.

Laboratory Evaluation As in almost all transfusion reactions, laboratory investigation should include (1) review of the accuracy of clerical transfusion records, (2) evaluation of hemolysis, and (3) comparison of the pre- and posttransfusion DATs. If any of these tests are positive, additional laboratory evaluation is required to rule out AHTR. If all results are negative and the patient's presentation is consistent with a mild FNHTR, no additional tests are required.

Management As mentioned above, the first step in the management of any transfusion reaction is to discontinue transfusion procedure immediately. FNHTRs are typically benign, and usually resolve completely within 1 to 2 hours after the transfusion is discontinued. The remainder of the transfused unit and a posttransfusion blood sample from the patient should be sent to the laboratory for investigation. Bacterial sepsis caused by contaminated red cell units is very rare and usually not considered in the differential diagnosis unless severe signs and symptoms are present, in which case Gram stain and culture of the transfusion bag may be indicated. Antipyretics may be administered to shorten the duration of the fever and provide analgesia. Acetaminophen 325 to 650 mg orally for adults or 10 to 15 mg/kg per dose orally for children is effective for ameliorating symptoms.

Prevention Approximately 10 to 15 percent of patients who experience a FNHTR will have a similar reaction to the next transfusion.[96] Administration of antipyretics (acetaminophen) 30 to 60 minutes before starting transfusion is often recommended for a patient who has had two or more FNHTRs. However, the evidence supporting this approach is limited. The routine use of premedication for all intended transfusion recipient is unnecessary, as is the routine use of antihistamines. FNHTRs to red cell transfusions are almost completely prevented by leukocyte reduction. In some cases, FNHTRs may recur despite premedication and/or leukoreduction saline-washed red cell transfusions invariably abrogate further reactions in such patients. The major disadvantage of washing red cells or platelets is a loss of 5 to 10 percent of red cells and 20 percent of platelets during preparation.[99–101]The single most important factor in preventing FNHTR from red cell transfusions is implementing universal leukoreduction of blood transfusions.[93,101]

Allergic Transfusion Reactions

Allergic transfusion reaction (ATR) is the most common adverse reaction to transfusion therapy. Depending on the severity of these reactions, different forms are recognized: mild, anaphylactoid, and anaphylaxis.

Incidence The mild form of ATR occur in 1 to 3 percent of transfusions of plasma or platelets and in 0.1 to 0.3 percent for red cells.[93] Severe anaphylactic reactions are estimated to occur in 1:20,000 to 1:50,000 transfusions.

Pathophysiology Mild ATRs are hypothesized to be caused by antibody response in recipients to soluble proteins present within the donor plasma.[100–102] This interaction between previously preformed antibodies and the alloantigen can activate mast cells. As a result, histamine, chemotactic factors, proteases, leukotrienes, prostaglandins, and platelet-activating factor are released and contribute to the development of this reaction. Severe anaphylactic reactions may occur after transfusion of blood products to IgA deficient patients with high titers of anti-IgA antibodies. The estimated incidence of IgA deficiency in whites is 1:900 individuals, and only 30 percent develop anti-IgA antibodies. Most patients with anti-IgA antibodies do not experience anaphylaxis with transfusion. Anaphylactoid reactions are similar to anaphylaxis but clinically less severe and caused by non–IgE-mediated activation of mast cells.[102]

Clinical Features ATRs usually begin during or within an hour of starting a transfusion but may not become evident until several hours later. Common findings include hives, rash, pruritus, and flushing. More severe reactions occur sooner and may include chest tightness, dyspnea, cyanosis, hoarseness, stridor, or wheezing. In addition, gastrointestinal symptoms such as abdominal pain, nausea, vomiting, and diarrhea may also occur. Unlike other acute transfusion reactions, fever is usually absent. The clinical evaluation of ATRs should include preexisting conditions such as atopy to drugs, food, and other allergens, as well as asthma. Classically anaphylaxis occurs immediately after starting the transfusion. Symptoms can include bronchospasm, respiratory distress, nausea, vomiting, abdominal cramps, diarrhea, shock, and loss of consciousness.

Laboratory Evaluation There is no need for laboratory investigation with simple urticaria. However, the incident should be reported to the blood bank to update the patient's record for any future transfusions. Generalized signs and symptoms are an indication for ruling out an AHTR. In anaphylactic reactions, it is recommended to test the patient for complete IgA deficiency and, if possible, for the presence of anti-IgA antibodies. However, life-threatening anaphylactic reactions mandate use of washed red cells and platelets and avoidance of fresh-frozen plasma and other plasma transfusions regardless of the results of these tests, so anti-IgA antibody testing is superfluous unless IgA deficiency is documented.

Management Most ATRs are mild, self-limited and respond well to discontinuation of transfusion and to administration of antihistaminic drugs such as diphenhydramine hydrochloride. In simple cases of urticaria and hives, resuming transfusion of the blood product may be possible 15 minutes after treatment with an antihistamine. Transfusion should never be resumed in patients with severe ATR especially in atopic patients. In acute anaphylaxis, fluid resuscitation may be needed to maintain blood pressure followed by administration of subcutaneous or intramuscular epinephrine (0.3 mL of 1:1000 dilution), as well as airway management and intensive care. For shock, a higher concentration of intravenous epinephrine (3–5 mL of a 1:10,000 dilution) can be administered.[102] Glucocorticoids are usually not helpful in acute crises.

Prevention Patients with a history of mild ATRs can be premedicated with an antihistaminic drug 30 to 60 minutes prior to transfusion. In case of repeated reactions, patients may be premedicated with a glucocorticoid several hours before transfusion. Plasma-depleted or saline-washed red cells may benefit patients with repeated ATRs. In IgA-deficient patients with a history of anaphylaxis to transfusion, plasma products from IgA-deficient donors sometimes can be provided. Extensively saline-washed red cells are an alternative for such patients.

Transfusion-Related Acute Lung Injury

TRALI is a syndrome of acute hypoxia as a result of noncardiogenic pulmonary edema that follows transfusion. All blood components have been implicated in TRALI, but most frequent are plasma-containing products,[3,90,103–108] which account for 50 to 63 percent of TRALI fatalities.[107]

Incidence The true incidence of TRALI is unknown because of the difficulty in making the diagnosis and because of underreporting. It is estimated to occur in 1:1300 to 1:5000 transfusions of plasma-containing products.[108] TRALI is the leading reported cause of death related to transfusion in the United States; more than 20 cases were reported per year from 2003 to 2005.[90]

Pathophysiology The precise mechanisms of the capillary leak syndrome in TRALI have not been fully determined, but two main hypotheses have been proposed. One involves white cell antibody-mediated TRALI and the other cytokine-mediated TRALI. The former suggests that TRALI is often a result of infusion of antibodies to HLA class I or class II or human neutrophil antigens (HNAs).[90,103,106] Following transfusion, these antibodies react with neutrophils in the pulmonary microvasculature. Activated neutrophils damage the endothelium. Vascular leakage into the alveolar space with pulmonary edema ensues. In 90 percent of reported cases, antibodies were present in the donor plasma; in 10 percent of the cases antibodies were present in the recipient plasma.[90] The second hypothesis suggests that neutrophils accumulate and are primed in the patient's pulmonary microvasculature as a result of preexisting systemic inflammation. Activation of these neutrophils by lipids[104] or other mediators, such as CD40L,[13] which accumulate in cellular blood components during storage, contributes to endothelial damage in susceptible patients, leading to vascular leaks and pulmonary edema.[104] Because 20 percent of blood components contain HLA antibodies yet TRALI is relatively uncommon, it is conceivable that additional factors play a role in the development of TRALI.

Clinical Features It is often impossible to distinguish TRALI from adult respiratory distress syndrome. The typical presentation of TRALI is the sudden development of dyspnea, severe hypoxemia (O_2 saturation <90% in room air),[90,106,108] hypotension, and fever that develop within 6 hours after transfusion and usually resolve with supportive care within 48 to 96 hours. Although hypotension is considered one of the important signs in diagnosing TRALI, hypertension can occur in some cases.

Laboratory Evaluation In addition to new or worsening oxygen desaturation, TRALI is characterized by chest radiographic findings of bilateral diffuse patchy pulmonary densities without cardiac enlargement.[90] TRALI can be ruled out as the sole cause of pulmonary failure by the presence of rales, jugular vein distention, and/or dilated pulmonary arteries on chest radiography; these are signs of congestive heart failure with or without transfusion-associated cardiac overload (TACO).[110] Transient leukopenia, which follows the onset of TRALI by a few hours, can also distinguish it from TACO.

Management Supportive care is the mainstay of therapy in TRALI. Oxygen supplementation is employed in all reported cases of TRALI and aggressive respiratory support is needed in 72 percent of patients.[108] Intravenous administration of fluids, as well as vasopressors, are essential for blood pressure support. Use of diuretics, which are indicated in TACO management, should be avoided in TRALI. Corticosteroids can be beneficial.[108,110]

Prevention Screening the entire blood supply for HLA and HNA antibodies is currently considered impractical. Several strategies have been implemented to minimize TRALI. In 2004, the American Association of Blood Banks recommended that blood collection centers minimize the preparation of high-plasma-volume components from donors who are at risk for leukocyte alloimmunization (i.e., females). Other approaches also may theoretically minimize TRALI; prestorage leukoreduction and washing of cellular components before transfusion will reduce the amount of TRALI mediators and TRALI inducers, respectively. Exclusion of female donors has been reported to decrease the incidence of, but not eliminate, TRALI.[109]

Transfusion-Associated Circulatory Overload

TACO is defined as an expansion in the intravascular volume when the infused blood components and/or other fluids volume exceed the cardiovascular ability to handle the additional workload.[110] A new hypothesis suggests that congestive heart failure is mediated in part by inflammation and this may be another mechanism underlying TACO.[111]

Incidence Adults older than 60 years of age, infants, patients with compromised myocardial function, and patients with hypervolemia caused by, for example, renal failure or congestive heart failure, are at risk of TACO. TACO is estimated to occur in 0.1 to 1 percent of transfusions. An incidence of 1 percent and 8 percent was reported in patients undergoing hip and knee replacement, respectively.[112]

Pathophysiology TACO occurs most often following infusion of large volumes of blood components. The increase in intravascular blood volume increases central venous pressure and can result in pulmonary edema. Patients with compensated chronic anemia may be more susceptible to TACO because their cardiac output may be close to maximal at the time of transfusion.

Clinical Features Nonspecific symptoms of TACO include dyspnea, chest tightness, dry cough, headache, and agitation. Signs such as rales, hypertension, and jugular vein distention provide strong evidence of TACO and distinguish it from TRALI.

Laboratory Evaluation Oxygen saturation may decrease along with PaO_2 (partial pressure of arterial oxygen). New bilateral infiltrates on chest radiography is characteristic for TACO as it is for TRALI.

Management Once TACO is suspected, intravenous fluids should be restricted and followed by the administration of oxygen and a diuretic if not contraindicated. Placing the patient in a sitting position can also be helpful. In severe cases, mechanical ventilation may be required. Phlebotomy with or without return of packed red cells may sometimes be effective.

Prevention If a patient is at risk for TACO and blood transfusion is imperative, blood should be administered slowly at a rate of 1 to 4 mL/kg per hour. Most blood banks can also reduce the transfusion volume by removing plasma from cellular transfusions or splitting the blood product into smaller volumes if the transfusion is going to last longer than 4 hours.

Transfusion-Related Sepsis

Red cells stored at 4°C (39.2°F) are very rarely contaminated by unusual cold-growing organisms (e.g., *Yersinia, Serratia, Pseudomonas*). Visual inspection of the blood unit may reveal clots or color change, and suggest the presence of bacterial contamination.[113]

Clinical Features The infusion of large numbers of Gram-negative microorganisms may lead to fever (>38.5°C [101°F]), rigors, marked hypotension, abdominal pain, vomiting, diarrhea, and the development of profound shock. Rapid diagnosis usually can be made via Gram stain of the residual donor blood.

Management Septic shock is a complex disorder, and expert consultation should be sought. Broad-spectrum antibiotics may be initiated but are often ineffective. The fatality rate from sepsis as a consequence of red cell transfusion is estimated to be 1:500,000 units.[82]

Reactions Associated with Massive Transfusions

Massive transfusion is defined as transfusion of more than 10 units of red cells or replacement of 1 blood volume in 24 hours. The use of large quantities of stored blood in massive transfusions may lead to a number of complications. Among these are dilutional coagulopathy, circulatory overload, hyperkalemia, hypoglycemia, hypothermia, and, rarely, citrate-induced hypocalcemia.[114]

Citrate Toxicity Sodium citrate is the anticoagulant in all blood components. In massive transfusion, citrate can produce a transient hypocalcemia and hypomagnesemia that may affect the cardiac rate and function. This is usually seen only in patients with liver failure and/or severe hypothermia where citrate metabolism is slowed. Treatment with calcium and, rarely, magnesium, is tailored to the clinical findings and ion levels.

Hyperkalemia During storage, red cell intracellular potassium leaks from red cells into the supernatant. Gamma irradiation of the blood unit accelerates this process. The total amount of potassium in transfused red cells is modest: less than 0.5 mEq in briefly stored red cells, and between 5 and 7 mEq in units at expiration. Thus, there is little concern for most settings. However, massive and rapid transfusions of red cells may lead to significant hyperkalemia in patients with renal failure. Hyperkalemia can be avoided by slow transfusion in renal failure patients. Washed or volume-depleted units are another alternative.

Coagulopathy In major trauma, a complex coagulopathy may develop as a result of multiple factors, including hypothermia, acidosis, shock, tissue damage, disseminated intravascular coagulation, and hemodilution of platelets and coagulation factors. The exact means of how to prevent and when to treat the coagulopathy of massive transfusion is uncertain.

■ DELAYED TRANSFUSION REACTIONS

Delayed Hemolytic Transfusion Reactions

Delayed hemolytic transfusion reaction (DHTR) occurs as a result of recall of secondary immune responses to donor red cell antigen(s) at more than 24 hours after transfusion. The red cell antibody screen is negative prior to transfusion, but hemolysis occurs nonetheless. A decline in hematocrit and evidence of hemolysis during a week following transfusion is typical.

Incidence DHTRs occur in 0.2 to 2.6 percent of patients. It is very rare in infants younger than 4 months of age, and more common in chronically transfused patients.[82,83] Children with hereditary hemoglobinopathies who begin transfusion therapy before the age of 10 years are less likely to become alloimmunized than are older children or adults despite greater numbers of exposure. This may be a result of the induction of immune tolerance in very young children.[115]

Pathophysiology When alloimmunization is *de novo*, hemolysis may occur several weeks after exposure. When alloimmunization has already occurred because of prior transfusions or pregnancy, hemolysis may occur within hours to few days following the reexposure to the same antigen. Thirty to 40 percent of alloantibodies become undetectable over periods ranging from months to years.[116] Antibodies in the Kidd system frequently exhibit this pattern. Hemolysis for DHTR is typically extravascular, without dramatic clinical symptoms and signs.

Clinical Features Decreasing hematocrit noted within several days to weeks of blood transfusion, along with unexplained fever are characteristic of DHTRs. DHTR may also present as an inadequate response to blood transfusion. Hemolysis in DHTRs is usually mild and gradual, and hemoglobinemia and hemoglobinuria are rare.

Laboratory Evaluation Failure to see the typical 1 g/dL rise in hemoglobin concentration following transfusion of 1 unit of red cells should raise the suspicion of DHTR and warrants investigation. Laboratory evidence of DHTR includes the appearance of spherocytes in blood film, reticulocytosis, and increased concentrations of unconjugated bilirubin and LDH. DAT and antibody screen should be repeated on a fresh blood sample in all suspected cases of DHTRs. The DAT may be negative if all the transfused red cells have been eliminated from the circulation.

Management No specific management is usually needed as these reactions are usually quite subtle. Once DHTRs is suspected, adequate hydration is required as well as monitoring of renal function particularly in acutely ill patients.

Posttransfusion Purpura

Posttransfusion purpura (PTP) is a rare immune-mediated disorder that occurs in patients who lack a specific platelet antigen, most commonly human platelet antigen-1a (HPA-1a), and who have a history of transfusion or pregnancy (see Chap. 141). Female-to-male ratio of affected patients is 5:1. PTP is rarely seen after red cell transfusion because almost all platelets are currently removed by leukoreduction.

Iron Overload

One of the most common complications of chronic red cell transfusion is iron overload (see Chaps. 47 and 48).

Transfusion-Associated Graft-Versus-Host Disease

Transfusion-associated graft-versus-host disease (TA-GVHD) is a very rare complication of transfusion that develops following the engraftment of allogeneic lymphocytes that attack the recipient's tissues.[117] TA-GVHD begins within 3 to 30 days after transfusion. It occurs when transfusions from close relatives or other genetically matched donors are administered to severely immunocompromised recipients; however, cases of TA-GVHD have also been reported in recipients with an intact immune system.[118,119] TA-GVHD is particularly uncommon in recipients of leukoreduced red cells according to United Kingdom national data.[61]

TA-GVHD may present as maculopapular rash, fever, watery diarrhea, liver dysfunction, and marrow failure. The mortality rate in patients with TA-GVHD is approximately 90 percent and the downhill course often rapid. Irradiation of the blood components prior to transfusion is very reliable in reducing the number of viable lymphocytes to a level that can prevent TA-GVHD.[117]

Transfusion-Associated Thrombosis and Immunomodulation/Inflammation

Patients transfused according to current standards of practice experience striking increases in morbidity and mortality compared with nontransfused patients, or patients receiving fewer transfusions.[120–122] For example, critical care patients receiving transfusions at hemoglobin levels of 7 to 8 g/dL rather than 9 to 10 g/dL had equivalent or better clinical outcomes.[19] However, this effect may not be generalizable to patients with cardiac disease.[26,125] Randomized trials of alternative strategies, such as conservative transfusion triggers,[19] and autologous[123] or leukoreduced[5,6,10,60,78,79] transfusions, have demonstrated reduced morbidity and mortality in some, but not all, settings.[124]

Transfusions are associated with an increased venous and arterial thrombosis.[8,9] Several groups have described mediators, such sCD40L (CD154),[98] IL-6,[97,98,126] and IL-8,[96–98,126] whose increased levels in stored blood units are associated with adverse outcomes such as fever,[96–98] acute lung injury,[13] and possibly thrombosis. In general, both downregulation of T-cell and natural killer immunity and inappropriate inflammatory responses have been documented *in vitro* and *in vivo* after red cell transfusions.[127] Although these results are not definitive, and much uncertainty remains, it is very likely that cells[5,6,10,60,78,79,128] and supernatant mediators[11,81,129–131] present in stored blood unfavorably affect clinical outcomes.

High levels of free hemoglobin as seen in the supernatant of red cell units have been implicated in vascular pathology, lung injury, and thrombosis in patients with SCD.[132] It is well known that intravascular hemolysis, as in paroxysmal nocturnal hemoglobinuria, is somehow associated with thrombotic complications,[133] and *in vitro* exposure to as little as 35 mg/dL of free hemoglobin activates normal platelets.[134]

Table 140–3 lists some major severe adverse effects of blood transfusions, both known and hypothesized.

STORAGE AND PRESERVATION OF RED CELLS

Red cells are preserved by either liquid storage at 4°C (39.2°F) or frozen storage with various cryoprotective agents at −80°C (−176°F). During

TABLE 140–3. Severe Adverse Effects of Transfusions

Multiorgan failure in surgery[10,19,35–40,74,78,121,124]
Increased postoperative infection[4,5,6,10,35–40,78,79,123,127]
Increased tumor recurrence[11,81,120,127,128,130]
Increased lung injury[3,13,90,103–110]
Increased severity of existing infections[127,131]
Increased incidence of thrombosis[7–9,19,35]
ABO-mismatched transfusions[82,83,85–87,107]
Transfusion reactions
Bacterial contamination of platelets[82]
Transmission of unconventional organisms (*Mycoplasma*, *Chlamydia*, etc.)

liquid storage, red blood cells undergo changes that lead to a loss in viability and a diminished capacity to offload oxygen. When stored red blood cells are reinfused, some perish within a few hours, but the remainder appear to return to an entirely normal state. The survival of those cells not removed within the first 24 hours is normal. The critical changes associated with loss of red cell viability have not been identified. One possible mechanism is related to multiple and complex changes in membrane structure that occur in stored red cells.[135] Following reinfusion, stored red blood cells need to function properly in delivering oxygen to the tissues. The loss of 2,3-bisphosphoglycerate (2,3-BPG) during storage results in increased oxygen affinity that may compromise the ability of the stored erythrocytes to deliver oxygen to the tissues (see Chap. 30). After reinfusion, the red cell 2,3-BPG level returns to half-normal level within 4 hours and to normal level within 24 hours.[136] Although the clinical significance of 2,3-BPG loss in stored blood is difficult to assess, there is general agreement that blood with near-normal oxygen affinity would, if logistically possible, be preferable for massive transfusions, particularly in infants, older patients, and patients with cardiovascular and pulmonary disease.[137]

■ LIQUID PRESERVATION OF RED CELLS

The preservative solutions used for the storage of whole blood or red blood cells contain glucose and a citrate buffer at an acid pH. The citrate ion chelates calcium and thus prevents coagulation of the blood, glucose sustains the metabolism of red blood cells during storage, and the acid pH counteracts the marked rise of pH that occurs when blood is cooled to 4°C (39.2°F). The two preservative solutions of this type in use until CPD-adenine was introduced in 1978, were acid, citrate, and dextrose (ACD) and citrate, phosphate, and dextrose (CPD; see below).

When whole blood or packed red blood cells are stored in either ACD or CPD, a series of well-defined biochemical changes, designated collectively as the storage lesion, take place in the erythrocytes. Erythrocytes stored at 4°C (39.2°F) also show a progressive increase in rigidity as measured by their rate of flow through filters. Blood collected in ACD or CPD will yield a 70 percent 24-hour survival of transfused red blood cells for up to 21 days of storage.

Major efforts have been directed toward development of preservative solutions that will maintain adequate erythrocyte levels of ATP and 2,3-BPG. Addition of adenine to give a final concentration of 0.25 to 0.75 mM at the beginning of storage helps to prevent the loss of ATP[138] because it can serve as a substrate for synthesis of adenine nucleotides.

The low 2,3-BPG content of stored blood can be restored to normal or supranormal levels[139] by incubating the erythrocytes with phosphate, inosine, and pyruvate (PIP). Both 2,3-BPG and ATP levels in outdated blood can be restored by incubation with PIP and adenine. The rejuvenated erythrocytes can be recovered by centrifugation and washing and either used for transfusion or frozen for future use.

■ ADDITIVE SOLUTIONS

The conversion of whole blood into components requires the removal of a significant fraction of both plasma and red cell preservative solution from the red blood cells. Red cell preservation, however, can be optimized if a nutrient solution is added to the isolated red blood cells.[140] The initial blood collection can be into CPD solution or half-strength CPD (0.5 CPD).[141] The nutrient solutions that have been developed generally contain glucose as a source of energy, adenine to help support ATP levels, and mannitol to prevent hemolysis. Several different additive solutions are now available in the United States. ATP levels are well maintained and good survival is obtained after 42 days storage with the use of additive solutions, but the 2,3-BPG level is reduced by 90 percent at 42 days.

■ FROZEN STORAGE OF RED CELLS

Uncontrolled freezing and thawing of erythrocytes results in hemolysis. Preservation of erythrocytes by freezing retards or arrests the deleterious biochemical changes that occur during liquid storage. Frozen cells are considered to have a storage time of at least 10 years but have maintained satisfactory viability for as long as 21 years.[142] Glycerol is the most commonly used cryoprotective agent for freeze preservation of erythrocytes. All methods of freeze preservation of erythrocytes involving the use of cryoprotective agents require the technical capability for introducing and removing high concentrations of the cryoprotective agent (glycerol) under sterile conditions. Under optimal conditions of processing, storage, and cell washing, greater than 80 percent of the freeze-preserved red blood cells from 1 U of blood will survive and function normally after transfusion. Such thawed and washed red blood cells must be used within 24 hours because processing breaks the closed system and introduces the possibility of bacterial contamination.

WHOLE BLOOD PREPARATIONS

Most clinical situations require the use of specific blood components, and the use of whole blood is quite rare in most developed nations, and usually restricted to autologous blood collections for surgical use.

FRESH BLOOD

For practical purposes, despite the desire to avoid the deterioration in red cell function and accumulation of potentially toxic changes, freshly collected red cells are only used for autologous transfusion or in military situations. Use of fresh blood is not logistically possible given the safety requirements, and no studies have demonstrated conclusively any benefits to this approach. Blood stored at 4°C (39.2°F) over 48 hours using ACD, CPD, or their adenine-containing derivatives is depleted of viable platelets. Factor V remains at adequate levels (>80% of baseline) for at least 5 days; factor VIII remains above 80 percent of its original level for 1 to 2 days; and factor XI activity declines to approximately 20 percent of its original level within the first week of storage. All other clotting factors appear to be stable during liquid storage.

RED CELL PREPARATIONS

Four types of red cell preparations are in common use: red cell concentrates, either with or without additive solutions, washed red cells, leukocyte-reduced red cells, and frozen red cells.

■ RED CELL CONCENTRATES

Red cells can be separated and recovered from ACD, CPD, or CPDA-1 whole blood by centrifugation and removal of plasma to give a hematocrit of 60 to 90 percent. Red cells packed to a hematocrit of less than 80 percent or sedimented red blood cells stored at 1 to 6°C (33.8–42.8°F) are suitable for transfusion for the full shelf-life of the preservative-anticoagulant solution (21–42 days).

■ LEUKOCYTE-REDUCED RED CELL CONCENTRATES

There are four widely accepted reasons for the use of leukocyte-reduced red cells: (1) to prevent or avoid nonhemolytic febrile reactions resulting from antibodies to white cells and platelets in recipients alloimmunized to platelets or white cells by previous transfusions or pregnancies; (2) to prevent or reduce allosensitization of patients to HLA antigens and subsequent risks of platelet transfusion refractoriness, acute lung injury, and multiorgan failure after cardiac surgery; (3) to minimize transmission of white cell-associated transfusion-transmitted viral diseases such as cytomegalovirus; and (4) to reduce the risks of postoperative infection, thrombosis, and multiorgan failure in some surgical settings, particularly cardiac surgery.[5,10,78,79] These benefits have led to widespread adoption of leukoreduction in most developed countries. In the United Kingdom, leukoreduction is associated, for the first time, with a significant decrease in reported cases of graft-versus-host disease and post-transfusion purpura.[61] Preliminary data suggest that leukoreduction also reduces the risks of TRALI and TACO.[111,143]

■ WASHED RED CELLS

Packed red cells collected by centrifugation can be washed with saline using either manual batch centrifugation or continuous-flow cell separators. Washed red cells must be used within 24 hours after processing because of the risk of bacterial contamination during preparation. Washed red cells are indicated in patients who have repeat nonhemolytic febrile or allergic reactions to leukoreduced red cell preparations. Other potential benefits to washed transfusions, such as removal of supernatant mediators, are under investigation.[11,81]

■ FROZEN RED CELLS

Frozen red cells have a very prolonged shelf-life (see "Frozen Storage of Red Cells" above), which simplifies the efficient management of blood inventories. Frozen red cells are well suited for autotransfusion when liquid storage is not practical, and are particularly important for maintaining an inventory of rare blood types.

■ ARTIFICIAL BLOOD SUBSTITUTES

Some functions of blood, such as maintaining circulating volume and oncotic pressure, can be replaced with various crystalloid and colloid macromolecules such as dextran and hydroxyethyl starch. These blood substitutes, however, do not provide oxygen transport. Materials with the potential for supporting oxygen transport, such as stroma-free hemoglobin solutions, liposome-encapsulated hemoglobin, and perfluorocarbons, have been under active investigation, but none have been applied for clinical use, in part because of concerns about efficacy and safety.[144]

REFERENCES

1. Health Care Cost and Utilization Project (HCUP) facts and figures, 2005, Exhibit 3.1. Most frequent procedures available at www.ahrq.gov/data/hcup/.
2. Schrier SL, Sohmer PR, Moore GL, et al: Red blood cell membrane abnormalities during storage: Correlation with *in vivo* survival. *Transfusion* 22:261, 1982.
3. Popovsky MA, Moore SB: Mechanism of transfusion-related acute lung injury. *Blood* 77:2299, 1991.
4. Tartter PI, Quintero S, Barron DM: Perioperative blood transfusion associated with infectious complications after colorectal cancer operations. *Am J Surg* 152:479, 1986.
5. Tartter PI, Mohandas K, Azar P, et al: Randomized trial comparing packed red cell blood transfusion with and without leukocyte depletion for gastrointestinal surgery. *Am J Surg* 176:462, 1998.
6. van Hilten JA, van de Watering LM, van Bockel JH, et al: Effects of transfusion with red cells filtered to remove leucocytes: Randomised controlled trial in patients undergoing major surgery. *BMJ* 328:1281, 2004.
7. Rao SV, Jollis JG, Harrington RA, et al: Relationship of blood transfusion and clinical outcomes in patients with acute coronary syndromes. *JAMA* 292:1555, 2004.
8. Nilsson KR, Berenholtz SM, Garrett-Mayer E, et al: Association between venous thromboembolism and perioperative allogeneic transfusion. *Arch Surg* 142:126, 2007.
9. Khorana AA, Francis CW, Blumberg N, et al: Blood transfusions, thrombosis, and mortality in hospitalized patients with cancer. *Arch Intern Med* 168:2377, 2008.
10. van de Watering LMG, Hermans J, Houbiers JGA, et al: Beneficial effects of leukocyte depletion of transfused blood on postoperative complications in patients undergoing cardiac surgery—A randomized clinical trial. *Circulation* 97:562, 1998.
11. Blumberg N, Heal JM, Liesveld JL, et al: Platelet transfusion and survival in adults with acute leukemia. *Leukemia* 22:631, 2008.
12. Blumberg N, Gettings KF, Turner C, et al: An association of soluble CD40 ligand (CD154) with adverse reactions to platelet transfusions. *Transfusion* 46:1813, 2006.
13. Khan SY, Kelher MR, Heal JM, et al: Soluble CD40 ligand accumulates in stored blood components, primes neutrophils through CD40, and is a potential cofactor in the development of transfusion-related acute lung injury. *Blood* 108:2455, 2006.
14. Klein HG, Spahn DR, Carson JL: Red blood cell transfusion in clinical practice. *Lancet* 370:415, 2007.
15. Viele MK, Weiskopf RB: What can we learn about the need for transfusion from patients who refuse blood? The experience with Jehovah's Witnesses. *Transfusion* 34:396, 1994.
16. Tinmouth AT, McIntyre LA, Fowler RA: Blood conservation strategies to reduce the need for red blood cell transfusion in critically ill patients. *CMAJ* 178:49, 2008.
17. Bell EF, Strauss RG, Widness JA, et al. Randomized trial of liberal versus restrictive guidelines for red blood cell transfusion in preterm infants. *Pediatrics* 115:1685, 2005.
18. Carson JL, Duff A, Berlin JA, et al: Perioperative blood transfusion and postoperative mortality. *JAMA* 279:199, 1998.
19. Hebert PC, Wells G, Blajchman MA, et al: A multicenter, randomized, controlled clinical trial of transfusion requirements in critical care. Transfusion requirements in critical care investigators, Canadian critical care trials group. *N Engl J Med* 340:409, 1999.
20. Kirpalani H, Whyte RK, Andersen C, et al: The Premature Infants in Need of Transfusion (PINT) study: A randomized, controlled trial of a restrictive (low) versus liberal (high) transfusion threshold for extremely low birth weight infants. *J Pediatr* 149:301, 2006.
21. Lacroix J, Hebert PC, Hutchison JS, et al: Transfusion strategies for patients in pediatric intensive care units. *N Engl J Med* 356:1609, 2007.
22. Widman FK: Informed consent for blood transfusion: Brief historical survey and summary of a conference. *Transfusion* 30:460, 1990.
23. Corwin HL, Gettinger A, Pearl RG, et al: The CRIT study: Anemia and blood transfusion in the critically ill—Current clinical practice in the United States. *Crit Care Med* 32:39, 2004.
24. Armano R, Gauvin F, Ducruet T, Lacroix J: Determinants of red blood cell transfusions in a pediatric critical care unit: A prospective, descriptive epidemiological study. *Crit Care Med* 33:2637, 2005.
25. Vincent JL, Baron JF, Reinhart K, et al: Anemia and blood transfusion in critically ill patients. *JAMA* 288:1499, 2002.
26. Hebert PC, Yetisir E, Martin C, et al: Is a low transfusion threshold safe in critically ill patients with cardiovascular diseases? *Crit Care Med* 29:227, 2001.
27. Wu WC, Rathore SS, Wang Y, et al: Blood transfusion in elderly patients with acute myocardial infarction. *N Engl J Med* 345:1230, 2001.
28. Kulier A, Levin J, Moser R, et al: Impact of preoperative anemia on outcome in patients undergoing coronary artery bypass graft surgery. *Circulation* 116:471, 2007.
29. Aronson D, Suleiman M, Agmon Y, et al: Changes in haemoglobin levels during hospital course and long-term outcome after acute myocardial infarction. *Eur Heart J* 28:1289, 2007.
30. Hebert PC, Tinmouth A, Corwin HL: Controversies in RBC transfusion in the critically ill. *Chest* 131:1583, 2007.
31. Whyte RK, Kirpalani H, Asztalos EV, et al: Neurodevelopmental outcome of extremely low birth weight infants randomly assigned to restrictive or liberal hemoglobin thresholds for blood transfusion. *Pediatrics* 123:207, 2009.
32. Strauss RG: How I transfuse red blood cells and platelets to infants with the anemia and thrombocytopenia of prematurity. *Transfusion* 48:209, 2008.
33. Stainsby D, MacLennan S, Thomas D, et al: Guidelines on the management of massive blood loss. *Br J Haematol* 135:634, 2006.
34. Bracey AW, Radovancevic R, Riggs SA, et al: Lowering the hemoglobin threshold for transfusion in coronary artery bypass procedures: Effect on patient outcomes. *Transfusion* 39:1070, 1999.
35. Engoren MC, Habib RH, Zacharias A, et al: Effect of blood transfusion on long-term survival after cardiac operation. *Ann Thorac Surg* 74:1180, 2002.
36. Koch CG, Li L, Duncan AI, et al: Morbidity and mortality risk associated with red blood cell and blood-component transfusion in isolated coronary artery bypass grafting. *Crit Care Med* 34:1608, 2006.
37. Koch CG, Li L, Duncan AI, et al: Transfusion in coronary artery bypass grafting is associated with reduced long-term survival. *Ann Thorac Surg* 81:1650, 2006.
38. Murphy GJ, Reeves BC, Rogers CA, et al: Increased mortality, postoperative morbidity, and cost after red blood cell transfusion in patients having cardiac surgery. *Circulation* 116:2544, 2007.
39. Rogers MA, Blumberg N, Heal JM, Hicks GL Jr: Increased risk of infection and mortality in women after cardiac surgery related to allogeneic blood transfusion. *J Womens Health* 16:1412, 2007.
40. Ranucci M, Pazzaglia A, Bianchini C, et al: Body size, gender, and transfusions as determinants of outcome after coronary operations. *Ann Thorac Surg* 85:481, 2008.
41. Karkouti K, Wijeysundera DN, Yau TM, et al: The influence of baseline hemoglobin concentration on tolerance of anemia in cardiac surgery. *Transfusion* 48:666, 2008.
42. Blumberg N, Bove JR: Uncrossed matched blood for emergency transfusion. One year's experience in a civilian setting. *JAMA* 240:2057, 1978.
43. Moore HC, Mollison PL: Use of a low-ionic-strength medium in manual tests for antibody detection. *Transfusion* 16:291, 1976.

44. Oberman HA, Barnes BA, Steiner EA: Role of the crossmatch in testing for serologic incompatibility. *Transfusion* 22:12, 1982.
45. Wahl S, Quirolo KC: Current issues in blood transfusion for sickle cell disease. *Curr Opin Pediatr* 21:15, 2009.
46. Josephson CD, Su LL, Hillyer KL, Hillyer CD: Transfusion in the patient with sickle cell disease: A critical review of the literature and transfusion guidelines. *Transfus Med Rev* 21:118, 2007.
47. Vichinsky EP, Haberkern CM, Neumayr L, et al: A comparison of conservative and aggressive transfusion regimens in the perioperative management of sickle cell disease. The Preoperative Transfusion in Sickle Cell Disease Study Group. *N Engl J Med* 333:206, 1995.
48. Atweh GF, DeSimone J, Saunthararajah Y, et al: Hemoglobinopathies. *Hematology Am Soc Hematol Educ Program* 2003: pp 14–39.
49. Cohen AR, Martin MB, Silber JH, et al: A modified transfusion program for prevention of stroke in sickle cell disease. *Blood* 79:1657, 1992.
50. Kim HC, Dugan NP, Silber JH, et al: Erythrocytapheresis therapy to reduce iron overload in chronically transfused patients with sickle cell disease. *Blood* 83:1136, 1994.
51. Ware RE, Zimmerman SA, Sylvestre PB, et al: Prevention of secondary stroke and resolution of transfusional iron overload in children with sickle cell anemia using hydroxyurea and phlebotomy. *J Pediatr* 145:346, 2004.
52. Adams RJ, McVie VC, Hsu L, et al: Prevention of a first stroke by transfusions in children with sickle cell anemia and abnormal results on transcranial Doppler ultrasonography. *N Engl J Med* 339:5, 1998.
53. Adams RJ, Brambilla D; for the Optimizing Primary Stroke Prevention in Sickle Cell Anemia (STOP 2) Trial Investigators: Discontinuing prophylactic transfusions used to prevent stroke in sickle cell disease. *N Engl J Med* 353:2769, 2005.
54. Vichinsky EP, Luban NL, Wright E, et al: Stroke Prevention Trail in Sickle Cell Anemia. Prospective RBC phenotype matching in a stroke-prevention trial in sickle cell anemia: A multicenter transfusion trial. *Transfusion* 41:1086, 2001.
55. Afenyi-Annan A, Willis MS, Konrad TR, Lottenberg R: Blood bank management of sickle cell patients at comprehensive sickle cell centers. *Transfusion* 47:2089, 2007.
56. Vichinsky E, Onyekwere O, Porter J, et al: A randomised comparison of deferasirox versus deferoxamine for the treatment of transfusional iron overload in sickle cell disease. *Br J Haematol* 136:501, 2007.
57. Borgna-Pignatti C: Modern treatment of thalassaemia intermedia. *Br J Haematol* 138:291, 2007.
58. Buetens OW, Ness PM: Red blood cell transfusion in autoimmune hemolytic anemia. *Curr Opin Hematol* 10:429, 2003.
59. Roberts IA: The changing face of haemolytic disease of the newborn. *Early Hum Dev* 84:515, 2008.
60. Blumberg N, Heal JM: Universal leukoreduction of blood transfusions. *Clin Infect Dis* 45:1014, 2007.
61. Williamson LM, Stainsby D, Jones H, et al: The impact of universal leukodepletion of the blood supply on hemovigilance reports of posttransfusion purpura and transfusion-associated graft-versus-host disease. *Transfusion* 47:1455, 2007.
62. Gajewski JL, Johnson VV, Sandler SG, et al: A review of transfusion practice before, during, and after hematopoietic progenitor cell transplantation. *Blood* 112:3036, 2008.
63. Brittingham TE, Chaplin H Jr: Febrile transfusion reactions caused by sensitivity to donor leukocytes and platelets. *JAMA* 165:819, 1957.
64. Opelz G, Terasaki PI: Improvement of kidney graft survival with increased number of transfusions. *N Engl J Med* 299:799, 1978.
65. Englesbe MJ, Pelletier SJ, Diehl KM, et al: Transfusions in surgical patients. *J Am Coll Surg* 200:249, 2005.
66. Owen CA, Rettke SR, Bowie EJW, et al: Hemostatic evaluation of patients undergoing liver transplantation. *Mayo Clin Proc* 62:761, 1987.
67. Boin IF, Leonardi MI, Luzo AC, et al: Intraoperative massive transfusion decreases survival after liver transplantation. *Transplant Proc* 40:789, 2008.
68. Cass RM, Blumberg N: Single-unit blood transfusion: Doubtful dogma defeated. *JAMA* 257:628, 1987.
69. Mangano DT, Tudor IC, Dietzel C: The risk associated with aprotinin in cardiac surgery. *N Engl J Med* 354:353, 2006.
70. Glaspy JA: Erythropoietin in Cancer Patients. *Annu Rev Med* 60:181, 2009.
71. Corwin HL, Gettinger A, Fabian TC, et al: Efficacy and safety of epoetin alfa in critically ill patients. *N Engl J Med* 357:965, 2007.
72. Segal JB, Blasco-Colmenares E, Norris EJ, Guallar E: Preoperative acute normovolemic hemodilution: A meta-analysis. *Transfusion* 44:632, 2004.
73. Vanderlinde E, Heal JM, Blumberg N: Autologous transfusion. *BMJ* 324:772, 2002.
74. Koch CG, Li L, Sessler DI, et al: Duration of red-cell storage and complications after cardiac surgery. *N Engl J Med* 358:1229, 2008.
75. Moroff G, Holme S, Keegan T, Heaton A: Storage of ADSOL-preserved red cells at 2.5 and 5.5 degrees C: Comparable retention of *in vitro* properties. *Vox Sang* 59:136, 1990.
76. Bonaventura J: Clinical implications of the loss of vasoactive nitric oxide during red blood cell storage. *Proc Natl Acad Sci U S A* 104:19165, 2007.
77. Yazdanbakhsh K: Controlling the complement system for prevention of red cell destruction. *Curr Opin Hematol* 12:117, 2005.
78. Bilgin YM, van de Watering LM, Eijsman L, et al: Double-blind, randomized controlled trial on the effect of leukocyte-depleted erythrocyte transfusions in cardiac valve surgery. *Circulation* 109:2755, 2004.
79. Blumberg N, Zhao H, Wang H, et al: The intention-to-treat principle in clinical trials and meta-analyses of leukoreduced blood transfusions in surgical patients. *Transfusion* 47:573, 2007.
80. Vo TD, Cowles J, Heal JM, Blumberg N: Platelet washing to prevent recurrent febrile reactions to leucocyte-reduced transfusions. *Transfus Med* 11:45, 2001.
81. Blumberg N, Heal JM, Rowe JM: A randomized trial of washed red blood cell and platelet transfusions in adult acute leukemia. *BMC Blood Disord* 4:6, 2004.
82. Goodnough LT: Risks of blood transfusion. *Crit Care Med* 31:S678, 2003.
83. Walker RH: Special report: Transfusion risks. *Am J Clin Pathol* 88:374, 1987.
84. Van Dijk PM, Kleine JW: The transfusion reaction in anesthesiological practice. *Acta Anaesthesiol Belg* 27:247, 1976.
85. Schmidt PJ: Transfusion mortality with special reference to surgical and intensive care facilities. *J Fla Med Assoc* 67:151, 1980.
86. Sazama K: Reports of 355 transfusion-associated deaths: 1976 through 1985. *Transfusion* 30:583, 1990.
87. Linden JV, Wagner K, Voytovich AE, Sheehan J: Transfusion errors in New York State: An analysis of 10 years' experience. *Transfusion* 40:1207, 2000.
88. Goldfinger D: Acute hemolytic transfusion reactions—A fresh look at pathogenesis and considerations regarding therapy. *Transfusion* 17:85, 1977.
89. Pineda AA, Brzica SM Jr, Taswell HF: Hemolytic transfusion reaction. Recent experience in a large blood bank. *Mayo Clin Proc* 53:378, 1978.
90. Kopko P, Popovsky MA: Transfusion reactions in *Transfusion-Related Acute Lung Injury*, 3rd ed, p 207. AABB Press, Bethesda, MD, 2007.
91. Davenport RD: The role of cytokines in hemolytic transfusion reactions. *Immunol Invest* 24:319, 1995.
92. Ingram GIC: The bleeding complications of blood transfusion. *Transfusion* 5:1, 1965.
93. *AABB Technical Manual*, 16th ed, edited by EM Brecher, and *AABB Standards for Blood Banks and Transfusion Services*, 25th ed, edited by EM Brecher. AABB Press, Bethesda, MD, 2008.
94. Bick RL, Schmalhorst WR, Fekete L: Disseminated intravascular coagulation and blood component therapy. *Transfusion* 16:361, 1976.
95. Miller JP, AuBuchon JP: Leukocyte-reduced and cytomegalovirus-reduced-risk blood components, in *Transfusion Therapy: Clinical Principles and Practice*, edited by EPD. Minz, p 313. AABB Press, Bethesda, MD, 1999.
96. Stack G, Judge JV, Snyder EL: Febrile and non-immune transfusion reactions, in *Principles of Transfusion Medicine*, 2nd ed, edited by TLS EC Rossi, G S Moss, SA Gould, p 773. Williams & Wilkins, Baltimore, MD, 1996.
97. Heddle NM, Klama L, Singer J, et al., The role of the plasma from platelet concentrates in transfusion reactions. *N Engl J Med* 331:625, 1994.
98. Phipps RP, Kaufman J, Blumberg N: Platelet derived CD154 (CD40 ligand) and febrile responses to transfusion. *Lancet* 357:2023, 2001.
99. Pineda AA, Zylstra VW, Clare DE, et al: Viability and functional integrity of washed platelets. *Transfusion* 29:524, 1989.
100. Sandler SG, Eckrich R, Malamut D, Mallory D: Hemagglutination assays for the diagnosis and prevention of IgA anaphylactic transfusion reactions. *Blood* 84:2031, 1994.
101. Davenport RD: Management of transfusion reactions, in *Transfusion Therapy: Clinical Principles and Practice*, edited by EPD Mintz. AABB Press, Bethesda, MD, 1999.
102. Davenport RD, Burnie KL, Barr RM: Transfusion management of patients with IgA deficiency and anti-IgA during liver transplantation. *Vox Sang* 63:247, 1992.
103. Popovsky MA, Chaplin HC Jr, Moore SB: Transfusion-related acute lung injury: A neglected, serious complication of hemotherapy. *Transfusion* 32:589, 1992.
104. Silliman CC, Boshkov LK, Mehdizadehkashi Z et al: Transfusion-related acute lung injury: Epidemiology and a prospective analysis of etiologic factors. *Blood* 101:454, 2003.
105. Fasano R, Luban NL: Blood component therapy. *Pediatr Clin North Am* 55:421, 2008.
106. Popovsky MA, Moore SB: Diagnostic and pathogenetic considerations in transfusion-related acute lung injury. *Transfusion* 25:573, 1985.
107. Eder AF, Chambers LA: Noninfectious complications of blood transfusion. *Arch Pathol Lab Med* 131:708, 2007.
108. Goldman M, Webert KE, Arnold DM, et al: Proceedings of a consensus conference: Towards an understanding of TRALI. *Transfus Med Rev* 19:2, 2005.
109. Insunza A, Romon I, Gonzalez-Ponte ML, et al: Implementation of a strategy to prevent TRALI in a regional blood centre. *Transfus Med* 14:157, 2004.
110. Popovsky MA: Transfusion and the lung: Circulatory overload and acute lung injury. *Vox Sang* 2:62, 2004.
111. Blumberg N, Heal J, Masel D, et al: Decreased TACO, TRALI and febrile but not allergic reactions after implementation of universal leukoreduction [abstract]. *Transfusion* 48 Suppl:202, 2008.
112. Popovsky MA, Audet AM, Andrzejewski C Jr: Transfusion-associated circulatory overload in orthopedic surgery patients: A multi-institutional study. *Immunohematol* 12:87, 1996.
113. Braude AI: Transfusion reactions from contaminated blood: Their recognition and treatment. *N Engl J Med* 258:1289, 1958.
114. Hardy JF, de Moerloose P, Samama CM: The coagulopathy of massive transfusion. *Vox Sang* 89:123, 2005.
115. Rosse WF, Gallagher D, Kinney TR et al: Transfusion and alloimmunization in sickle cell disease. The Cooperative Study of Sickle Cell Disease. *Blood* 76:1431, 1990.
116. Ramsey G, Larson P: Loss of red cell alloantibodies over time. *Transfusion* 28:162, 1988.
117. Anderson, K: Broadening the spectrum of patient groups at risk for transfusion-associated GVHD: Implications for universal irradiation of cellular blood components. *Transfusion* 43:1652, 2003.

118. Triulzi D, Duquesnoy R, Nichols L, et al: Fatal transfusion-associated graft-versus-host disease in an immunocompetent recipient of a volunteer unit of red cells. *Transfusion* 46:885, 2006.
119. Petz LD, Calhoun L, Yam P, et al: Transfusion-associated graft-versus-host disease in immunocompetent patients: Report of a fatal case associated with transfusion of blood from a second-degree relative, and a survey of predisposing factors. *Transfusion* 33:742, 1993.
120. Blumberg N: Deleterious clinical effects of transfusion immunomodulation: Proven beyond a reasonable doubt. *Transfusion* 45:33S, discussion 39S, 2005.
121. Tinmouth A, Fergusson D, Yee IC, Hebert PC: Clinical consequences of red cell storage in the critically ill. *Transfusion* 46:2014, 2006.
122. Gianotti L, Pyles T, Alexander JW, et al: Impact of blood transfusion and burn injury on microbial translocation and bacterial survival. *Transfusion* 32:312, 1992.
123. Heiss MM, Mempel W, Jauch KW, et al: Beneficial effect of autologous blood transfusion on infectious complications after colorectal cancer surgery. *Lancet* 342:1328, 1993.
124. Weinberg JA, McGwin G Jr, Griffin RL, et al: Age of transfused blood: An independent predictor of mortality despite universal leukoreduction. *J Trauma* 65:279, 2008.
125. Deans KJ, Minneci PC, Suffredini AF, et al: Randomization in clinical trials of titrated therapies: Unintended consequences of using fixed treatment protocols. *Crit Care Med* 35:1509, 2007.
126. Stack G, Snyder EL: Cytokine generation in stored platelet concentrates. *Transfusion* 34:20, 1994.
127. Blumberg N, Heal JM: Transfusion immunomodulation, in *Blood Banking and Transfusion Medicine*, 2nd ed, edited by CD Hillyer, LE Silberstein, PM Ness, KC Anderson, JD Roback, p 701. Churchill Livingstone Elsevier, Philadelphia, 2007.
128. Blajchman MA, Bardossy L, Carmen R, et al: Allogeneic blood transfusion-induced enhancement of tumor growth: Two animal models showing amelioration by leukodepletion and passive transfer using spleen cells. *Blood* 81:1880, 1993.
129. Davenport RD, Kunkel SL: Cytokine roles in hemolytic and nonhemolytic transfusion reactions. *Transfus Med Rev* 8:157, 1994.
130. Blumberg N, Heal JM, Murphy P, et al: Association between transfusion of whole blood and recurrence of cancer. *Br Med J* 293:530, 1986.
131. Blumberg N, Heal JM: Evidence for plasma-mediated immunomodulation: Transfusions of plasma-rich blood components are associated with a greater risk of acquired immunodeficiency syndrome than transfusions of red blood cells alone. *Transplant Proc* 20:1138, 1988.
132. Gladwin MT, Vichinsky E: Pulmonary complications of sickle cell disease. *N Engl J Med* 359:2254, 2008.
133. Parker CJ: Paroxysmal nocturnal hemoglobinuria: An historical overview. *Hematology Am Soc Hematol Educ Program* 2008: p 93.
134. Villagra J, Shiva S, Hunter LA, et al: Platelet activation in patients with sickle disease, hemolysis-associated pulmonary hypertension, and nitric oxide scavenging by cell-free hemoglobin. *Blood* 110:2166, 2007.
135. Wolfe LC: The membrane and the lesions of storage in preserved red cells. *Transfusion* 25:185, 1985.
136. Valeri CR, Hirsch NM: Restoration in vivo of erythrocyte adenosine triphosphate 2,3-diphosphoglycerate, potassium ion, and sodium ion concentrations following the transfusion of acid-citrate-dextrose-stored human red blood cells. *J Lab Clin Med* 73:722, 1969.
137. Beutler E: What is the clinical importance of alterations of the hemoglobin oxygen affinity in preserved blood–especially as produced by variations of red cell 2,3-DPG content? *Vox Sang* 34:113, 1978.
138. Simon ER: Adenine and purine nucleosides in human red cell preservation: A review. *Transfusion* 7:395, 1967.
139. Duhm J, Deuticke B, Gerlach E: Complete restoration of oxygen transport function and 2,3-diphosphoglycerate concentration in stored blood. *Transfusion* 11:147, 1971.
140. Beutler E, Wood LA: Preservation of red cell 2,3-DPG and viability in bicarbonate containing medium: The effect of blood-bag permeability. *J Lab Clin Med* 80:723, 1972.
141. Högman CF, Eriksson L, Gong J, et al: Half-strength citrate CPD combined with a new additive solution for improved storage of red blood cells suitable for clinical use. *Vox Sang* 65:271, 1993.
142. Valeri CR, Pivacek LE, Gray AD, et al: The safety and therapeutic effectiveness of human red cells stored at −80°C for as long as 21 years. *Transfusion* 29:429, 1989.
143. Plurad D, Belzberg H, Schulman I, et al: Leukoreduction is associated with a decreased incidence of late onset acute respiratory distress syndrome after injury. *Am Surg* 74:117, 2008.
144. Natanson C, Kern SJ, Lurie P, et al: Cell-free hemoglobin-based blood substitutes and risk of myocardial infarction and death: A meta-analysis. *JAMA* 299:2304, 2008.

CHAPTER 141
PRESERVATION AND CLINICAL USE OF PLATELETS

Mike Murphy and Ralph Vassallo*

SUMMARY

Increasingly aggressive medical and surgical treatment modalities spurred dramatic growth in the use of platelet transfusions in the United States in the 1980s. This growth slowed somewhat in the 1990s, based on evidence that the threshold for transfusion can be safely set at a lower level. Worldwide, many methods are used for the preparation of platelets for transfusion. In the United States, the "platelet-rich plasma" method is popular for the separation of platelets from whole-blood donations, whereas in Canada and Europe, the "buffy coat method" is more commonly used. In addition, platelets obtained from single donors and prepared by apheresis are gaining in popularity worldwide in order to limit the numbers of donors to whom recipients are exposed and to minimize the number of contaminating leukocytes in the preparations. Many institutions are making their platelet products universally leukoreduced at the time of their preparation based on evidence that such products have a reduced incidence of adverse events. After preparation, platelets are generally stored at 20 to 24°C (68–75.2°F) in containers that are permeable to oxygen. Optimally, these preparations should be agitated continuously. Storage at lower temperatures decreases *in vivo* survival after transfusion, and adequate access to oxygen and agitation are required to prevent deleterious declines in pH. Platelets stored in this fashion produce satisfactory clinical responses after storage for 5 to 7 days. Currently, storage is limited to 5 days because of concerns about overgrowth of bacteria that might have inadvertently contaminated the preparation.

The clinical response to platelet transfusion can be assessed by measuring the increment in platelet concentration achieved in the patient's blood. This measurement generally correlates directly with the dose of platelets infused and inversely with the patient's size. Using physiologic principles, one can calculate what this response should be. Although the ideal theoretical response is occasionally achieved, on average the response is approximately half the predicted value because of immunologic and nonimmunologic clinical factors that impact negatively on the response. No single correct dose of platelets exists for all patients. On average, both the initial increment and the time to next transfusion increase with increasing platelet dose. The appropriate dose varies with the clinical circumstances, the patient's size, and the individual response to transfusion. The traditional platelet concentration that should trigger a platelet transfusion had been 20,000/μL, but studies have shown that this level can safely be reduced to 10,000/μL in patients with production disorders that are stable. Raising the transfusion trigger above this level in response to a variety of clinical circumstances that increase the likelihood of bleeding is important. Although most platelet transfusions are given to patients with suppressed platelet production, platelet transfusion occasionally is indicated when the thrombocytopenia results from massive blood loss, cardiopulmonary bypass, splenomegaly, immune-mediated thrombocytopenia, and hereditary thrombocytopenia.

The complications of platelet transfusion most frequently result from contaminating leukocytes, red cells, plasma proteins, and microorganisms. The frequency of complications resulting from contaminating leukocytes can be reduced by prestorage leukoreduction of the platelet products. Alloimmunization to class I human leukocyte antigens can be managed by a variety of strategies using apheresis platelet concentrates that lack the antigens to which the patient has formed antibody.

Acronyms and abbreviations that appear in this chapter include: AABB, American Association of Blood Banks; ACE, angiotensin-converting enzyme; ATP, adenosine triphosphate; BSA, body surface area; CCI, corrected count increment; CMV, cytomegalovirus; CREG, cross-reactive group; DMSO, dimethyl sulfoxide; ELISA, enzyme-linked immunosorbent assay; FNHTR, febrile nonhemolytic transfusion reaction; GVHD, graft-versus-host disease; HLA, human leukocyte antigen; HPA, human platelet antigen; HTLV, human T-cell lymphotrophic virus; Ig, immunoglobulin; LCT, lymphocytotoxicity; PRA, percent reactive antibody; TTP, thrombotic thrombocytopenic purpura.

*Dr. Scott Murphy cowrote this chapter in the 7th edition and some of that material has been retained.

In the 1980s, the use of platelet transfusion increased rapidly in the United States, doubling between 1982 and 1989.[1,2] Overall, platelet use continued to grow, albeit at a somewhat slower rate of approximately 2.9 percent annually between 1989 and 2006 (Fig. 141–1).[2–9] In 2006, the percentage of platelets infused in the United States obtained by apheresis reached 87.5 percent.[9] The ongoing increase in platelet use correlates with increasingly aggressive myelosuppressive therapy for malignancies and increased availability of platelets, made possible by the development of cost-effective methods for storage of platelet concentrates.

TECHNIQUES FOR PLATELET PREPARATION

Platelet concentrates for transfusion can be obtained from donations of whole blood anticoagulated with citrate-based preservative solutions or by apheresis with a variety of apheresis devices that also use citrate as the anticoagulant. Two methods of preparing platelet concentrates from whole blood are used: the platelet-rich plasma method and the buffy coat method.

In addition to appropriate platelet content, attention is also focused on the level of contaminating leukocytes in these products. Problems produced by contaminating leukocytes are discussed in "Complications of Platelet Transfusion" below. In the United States, an apheresis platelet concentrate or a pool of six platelet-rich plasma platelet concentrates is considered leukoreduced if it contains less than 5×10^6 leukocytes. In Europe, the standard is 1×10^6 leukocytes. Because most apheresis instruments are capable of consistently producing products meeting the U.S. standard through in-process leukoreduction, this issue is mostly confined to whole-blood-derived platelets which must be leukoreduced by filtration. Platelet concentrates can be filtered during infusion at the bedside, but, for reasons to be discussed, accomplishing leukoreduction at the time of product preparation is preferable.

WHOLE-BLOOD-DERIVED PLATELET CONCENTRATES

Whole-blood-derived platelet concentrates often are termed *random-donor platelet concentrates.* This term was used to distinguish whole-blood-derived platelet concentrates from apheresis platelet concentrates collected from specific donors for specific refractory patients generally based on human leukocyte antigen (HLA) matching. Now, apheresis platelet concentrates commonly are given "randomly" to patients who do not require products from specific donors. Consequently, the term *whole-blood-derived platelet concentrates* is preferred.

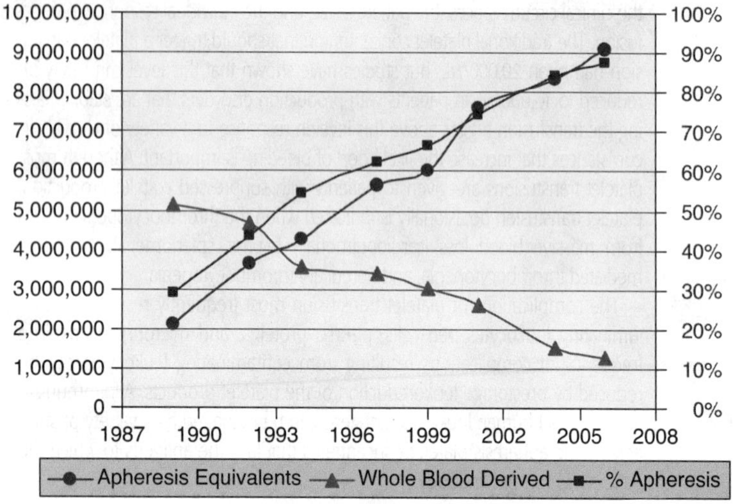

FIGURE 141–1. Trends in U.S. use of whole-blood-derived platelet concentrate equivalent units per year.[1–9] In 1994, for the first time, more than 50% of platelet transfusions were given as apheresis platelet concentrates (*red line*). For comparability, data use an older 6 whole-blood-derived units to 1 apheresis unit equivalency rather than the more recent 5:1 actual value.

Platelet-Rich Plasma Platelet Concentrates

The platelet-rich plasma method is the only method used in the United States for whole-blood-derived platelet concentrates. From 450 to 500 mL (1 U) of whole blood is held at room temperature for up to 8 hours, and platelet-rich plasma is separated from red cells and the buffy coat by low-speed centrifugation. After the platelet-rich plasma is transferred to another bag, the plasma is centrifuged rapidly to produce a platelet pellet. Most of the plasma is removed, and the platelet pellet is allowed to "rest" for 1 to 2 hours before it is resuspended in approximately 50 mL of autologous citrated plasma. The need for a rest period, originally designed to prevent irreversible clumping upon resuspension, has been called into question.[10] The separated red cells are used for transfusion, whereas the supernatant plasma is used for transfusion or sent for fractionation.

Over the past 20 years, technical improvements have doubled the number of platelets in each unit, resulting in an average content of 0.8 to 0.9×10^{11} platelets per unit. The range around this average, however, is high ($0.4–1.8 \times 10^{11}$), primarily related to the variability in donor platelet level.[11,12] One unit is adequate only for the transfusion of a small child who weighs less than 30 lb. Because of the wide range of platelet counts in individual units, at least 5 U must be pooled to be certain the pool contains at least 3×10^{11} platelets.[12] For transfusion of adults, 4 to 8 U must be pooled to provide a therapeutic dose (see "Platelet Dose" below).

Whole-blood-derived platelet pools of 4 to 8 U have a high level of leukocyte (primarily lymphocyte) contamination of 0.4 to 4.0×10^9, which is three orders of magnitude higher than the level found in a leukoreduced product. Collection sets are available with integrated leukocyte-reduction filters in various places between the primary blood bag and the platelet container.[13,14] These systems leukoreduce either whole blood or platelet-rich plasma to produce platelets with less than 5×10^6 leukocytes in more than 99 percent of products.[15]

In 2006, whole-blood-derived platelets constituted fewer than 18 percent of the platelet doses transfused in the United States.[9] This erosion of "market share" is likely because of blood center inconvenience (as platelet separation must occur within 8 hours of donation), physician-perceived advantages of apheresis platelets, and the additional effort required in hospital blood banks to pool and screen whole-blood-derived platelets for bacterial contamination (see "Relative Merits of Different Platelet Concentrates" below).

Buffy Coat Platelet Concentrates

The buffy coat method is used in Europe and Canada.[16,17] An initial hard centrifugation sediments all blood cells so that the plasma, buffy coat, and red cells can be collected in three separate containers. Segregating by density, the platelets at the top of the bag fall to the buffy coat between the red cells and plasma, while platelets at the bottom of the bag rise to the buffy coat. Platelet yields in the buffy coat are excellent. One can prepare platelet concentrates from individual buffy coats[18] or pool four to six buffy coats, add two to four volumes of one donor's plasma or an additive solution, centrifuge the pool at low speed to remove red cells and leukocytes, and push the supernatant through a leukoreduction filter to produce a therapeutic, leukoreduced dose of platelets for an adult.[19,20]

Each method has its advantages and disadvantages.[16,21–23] Each method produces platelets of high quality, and platelet yields are equivalent. In the buffy coat method, 20 to 25 mL of red cells are lost with the buffy coat, but an extra 70 to 80 mL of plasma can be collected. Despite Canada's initiation of conversion to the buffy coat method in 2004, it is not approved in the United States.

APHERESIS PLATELET CONCENTRATES

From 2.5 to 14×10^{11} platelets (equivalent to 3–18 U of whole-blood-derived platelet concentrates) can be obtained by apheresis of donors over 1 to 2 hours using a variety of devices,[24–27] with an extraordinarily high level of safety for the donors.[28] The number of platelets obtained during the procedure varies according to the platelet concentration in the blood of the donor, the duration of the donation, and the efficiency of the device. The efficiency of the newest devices is such that collection of at least 60 percent of the platelets that pass through the devices can be expected, and most donors become restless if the donation time exceeds more than 90 to 120 minutes. Therefore, the wide range of platelet concentrations in the blood of normal donors (150,000–500,000/μL) accounts for the wide range in platelet yields.[29] Reports of yield enhancement through administration of recombinant human thrombopoietin to enhance donor platelet concentrations have been abandoned because of the development of antibody-mediated thrombocytopenia in volunteer donors.[30] However, devices capable of maximizing donors' contributions by obtaining apheresis platelet concentrates and a unit of red cells and/or plasma from the same donor at a single sitting are available.[31]

The original goal of apheresis was to obtain a therapeutic dose of platelets for an adult from a single donor during one apheresis sitting. Current controversies concerning the appropriate dose for platelet transfusion are discussed in the section Platelet Dose below. Current FDA standards state only that 75 percent of apheresis platelet products must contain more than 3.0×10^{11} platelets. The AABB (the international association of blood banks, formerly known as the American Association of Blood Banks) has set a 90 percent target for this platelet content.[32] The goal of 3×10^{11} platelets probably reflects the capabilities of apheresis devices available at the time the standards were established rather than the needs of the wide variety of patients undergoing treatment. Although 2.5 to 3.5×10^{11} probably is a satisfactory dose for the prophylactic transfusion of a child or small adult, that number probably is unsatisfactory for a large adult who is bleeding or has other clinical features that interfere with an optimal response to platelet transfusion. On the other hand, administration of high-yield platelet products to small adults and children may be wasteful. Blood centers are considering the best way to handle the preparation process for apheresis platelets. Many centers divide high-yield products (i.e., >6.5–7 × 10^{11} platelets) to provide a therapeutic dose for two patients. Very-high-yield products (>10–11 × 10^{11} platelets) can be divided to treat three patients. Results from recent trials examining the impact of prophylactic platelet dose on bleeding risk appear to validate the practice of "splitting" and are discussed further in "Platelet Dose" below.[33,34]

RELATIVE MERITS OF DIFFERENT PLATELET CONCENTRATES

Table 141–1 lists the advantages of each platelet preparation method. Among the advantages of apheresis platelet products is their slightly lower infectious disease risk through exposure to fewer, often repeat, apheresis donors. Repeat donors have approximately half the risk of incident viral infections of first-time donors who more commonly donate whole blood.[35] The risk of bacterial infection in whole-blood-derived products increases with the number of units pooled (each requiring a separate venipuncture, the primary source of contamination).[36] Also, because the low volume of individual whole-blood-derived platelets disallows more sensitive culture-based bacterial detection methods, the risk of sepsis from whole-blood-derived platelets is significantly higher than for apheresis platelets.[37] Efficient in-process apheresis leukoreduction results in platelet products with fewer than 5 × 10^6 leukocytes over 99.9 percent of the time, in contrast to the one order of magnitude-higher leukoreduction failure rate with filtration.[24,25,38] Because apheresis products contain a bacterially tested transfusable platelet dose, there are no delays in blood bank issue necessitated by pooling and point-of-issue bacterial testing. Prestorage pooling of whole-blood-derived platelets does not reduce platelet increments compared to nonpooled platelets.[39] A recent meta-analysis indicated that platelet increments, corrected for platelet dose and recipient blood volume, are higher with apheresis platelets than whole-blood-derived platelets produced with the platelet-rich plasma method, but not the buffy coat method.[40] The clinical significance of this finding (bleeding and effect on transfusion intervals), however, is not yet known. Of note, apheresis platelets will continue to be the product of choice when special characteristics are required, such as HLA-matched, human platelet antigen (HPA)-matched, or immunoglobulin (Ig) A-deficient platelets.

Whole-blood-derived platelets also have a number of advantages. They afford superior dosing flexibility as the number of units in a pool can be altered to suit patient need. Unlike apheresis platelets that contain high volumes of plasma (up to 500 mL) from a single donor, whole-blood-derived platelets generally contain no more than 60 mL of single-donor's plasma. Transfusing lower volumes of substances which mediate transfusion-related acute lung injury (TRALI), recipient hemolysis from donor anti-A or anti-B, and allergic reactions may be beneficial. Because whole-blood-derived platelets are a by-product of whole-blood donation, they are also less expensive to procure. Prestorage pools of platelet-rich plasma whole-blood-derived platelets, available in the United States since 2005, take advantage of culture-based bacterial detection strategies and provide a pooled, issue-ready product. Buffy coat whole-blood-derived platelets are also prestorage pooled and appear to produce platelet increments not significantly different from apheresis platelets. Although not licensed in the United States, buffy coat platelet production also results in slightly higher volumes for transfusion in the plasma coproduct.

TABLE 141–1. Advantages of Different Platelet Products

Apheresis platelets
Exposure to fewer, repeatedly tested donors (slightly lower viral risk)
Acceptable product volume loss for more sensitive bacterial detection methods
Slightly more consistent leukoreduction and fewer contaminating red cells
Permit immediate release of a transfusable dose from the blood bank
Higher transfusion increments than platelet-rich plasma whole-blood-derived platelets
Products can be collected from special-attribute donors (HLA- or HPA matched and IgA deficient)
Platelet-rich plasma, whole-blood-derived platelets
Superior dosing flexibility
Reduced single-donor plasma exposure (may mitigate TRALI, ABO-hemolytic, and allergic reactions)
Public health benefit of lower procurement cost
Prestorage pools benefit from enhanced bacterial detection and elimination of pooling delays
Buffy coat, whole-blood-derived platelets
Shares benefits of prestorage pooled platelet-rich plasma whole-blood-derived platelets
Production spares plasma, providing higher volumes of transfusable plasma

HLA, human leukocyte antigen; HPA, human platelet antigen; IgA, immunoglobulin A; TRALI, transfusion-related acute lung injury.

STORAGE OF PLATELET CONCENTRATES

LIQUID STORAGE AT 20 TO 24°C (68–75.2°F)

Both whole-blood-derived and apheresis platelet concentrates can be stored for 5 days using the same principles: (1) the temperature must be 20 to 24°C (68–75.2°F)[41]; (2) the storage container must be constructed of a plastic material that allows adequate diffusion of oxygen to meet the cells' metabolic needs[42,43]; and (3) the platelet concentrates must be agitated during storage.[42,43]

Using radiolabeling of stored platelets (Fig. 141–2), *in vivo* survival after reinfusion is nearly normal if storage, even for several days, is performed at 20 to 24°C (68–75.2°F). However, at colder temperatures, the cells undergo irreversible disc-to-sphere transformation, and survival is dramatically shortened.[41] If oxygen influx is inadequate at 20 to 24°C (68–75.2°F), the cells increase their production of lactic acid in an effort to maintain adenosine triphosphate (ATP) levels, leading to depletion of bicarbonate buffer and a fall in pH.[42,43] If the pH drops to below 6.2, an irreversible disc-to-sphere transformation occurs, resulting in rapid clearance from the circulation after transfusion. A similar fall in pH occurs if the platelet concentrates are not agitated during storage. Data suggest that agitation can be discontinued for up to 24 hours of the 5-day storage interval without harm to the platelets.[44–46]

Synthetic media are used for storage of buffy coat platelet concentrates[19] and are expected to be available by the end of 2010 for storage of apheresis platelets in the United States.[47,48] Definition of the optimal solution is still in progress, but the solution appears to be relatively simple, relying upon 20 to 40 percent residual plasma and added acetate as an oxidative fuel for platelets.[48] Oxidation of an organic anion such as acetate utilizes a proton from the medium, thus providing an alkalinizing effect that spares bicarbonate, the major buffer during platelet concentrate storage.[49]

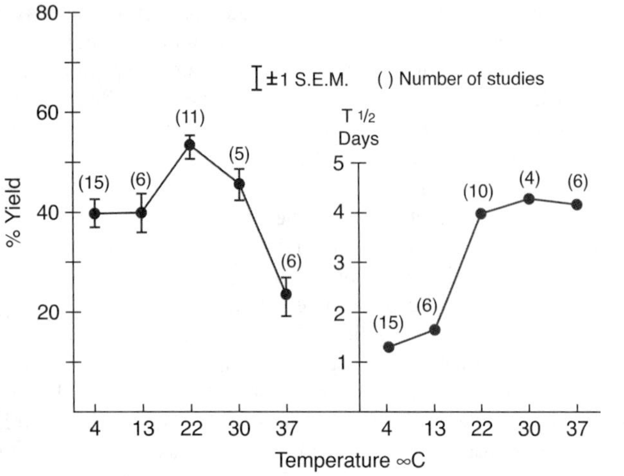

FIGURE 141–2. Relationship between storage temperature and platelet viability after transfusion. Platelet-rich plasma was obtained from normal volunteers and stored overnight at the indicated temperatures. Thereafter, the platelets were labeled with radioactive chromium and reinfused. Percent yield refers to the percent of platelets infused that circulate in the first 3 hours after infusion. The 50 to 60 percent yield at 22°C (71.6°F) is a result of physiologic pooling in the spleen (see Chap. 110, not cell damage. The combination of percent yield and subsequent *in vivo* survival ($T_{1/2}$) is optimal at 22°C (71.6°F).

Some investigators have been unable to find any practical difference in clinical response between fresh and stored platelets.[50,51] However, most investigators find reduced *in vivo* recovery for the latter, with survival reduced by approximately 20 to 25 percent after 5 days of storage as judged by radiolabeling studies in normal volunteers and by the increase in platelet concentrations in thrombocytopenic patients.[52] Furthermore, some authors have reported an even greater defect in stored platelets relative to fresh platelets in sick patients with fever, sepsis, splenomegaly, and disseminated intravascular coagulation.[53,54]

Several studies have shown that platelet recovery and survival are satisfactory after 7 days of storage (albeit with a 15–20% loss of efficacy over the last 2 days of storage).[55–57] However, when storage was extended from 5 to 7 days in 1984, bacterial overgrowth and clinical sepsis in recipients of stored platelets occurred with sufficient frequency to warrant returning the storage period to 5 days 2 years later.[58] If methods for bacterial decontamination[59] or reliable bacterial detection are developed,[60] prolonging storage beyond 5 days may again be possible.[61]

Platelet products deteriorate to some extent even during storage under optimal conditions. A number of *in vitro* abnormalities have been described after *ex vivo* storage, collectively termed the *platelet storage lesion*.[62–64] At present, *in vitro* research assay characteristics that correlate best with the capacity to circulate *in vivo* are retention of disc shape and good function in the hypotonic shock response.[65] With few exceptions, platelets with normal discoid morphology circulate normally after transfusion. Platelets that are damaged by cold, acidity, or bacterial contamination generally lose their discoid morphology and become spheres. Normal discoid morphology is reflected by the "swirling" or "shimmering" appearance of well-preserved platelet concentrates during gross, visual inspection.[66] Blood bank staff and clinical personnel are urged to check platelet concentrates for this phenomenon prior to transfusion (Fig. 141–3). Several additional characteristics of stored platelets—induction of markers of cellular apoptosis, microparticle release with platelet activation, and morphologic responses to temperature change—hold some promise as new strategies for monitoring the quality of platelet products.[67,68] As yet, however, no single *in vitro* parameter (or battery of tests) has been demonstrated to reliably reflect the *in vivo* survival of platelets once infused into recipients.

The activities of coagulation factors are well maintained in the suspending plasma of platelet concentrates during storage, except for modest decreases in the activity of factors V and VIII.[69] Thus, a pool of four to eight whole-blood-derived platelet concentrates or an apheresis platelet concentrate provides the equivalent of 1 to 2 U of fresh-frozen plasma.

FROZEN STORAGE

The most widely used method for frozen storage involves controlled rate freezing (1°C [1.8°F] per minute), 5 to 6 percent dimethyl sulfoxide (DMSO) as a cryoprotective agent, rapid thawing, graded reduction of the DMSO concentration, and washing prior to infusion. *In vivo* viability is approximately 40 to 50 percent relative to fresh platelets.[70] Thus, this technology is more complex, expensive, and less effective than liquid storage at 20 to 24°C (68–75.2°F).[71] However, these preparations can be effective clinically[72] and may be valuable for autologous transfusion of

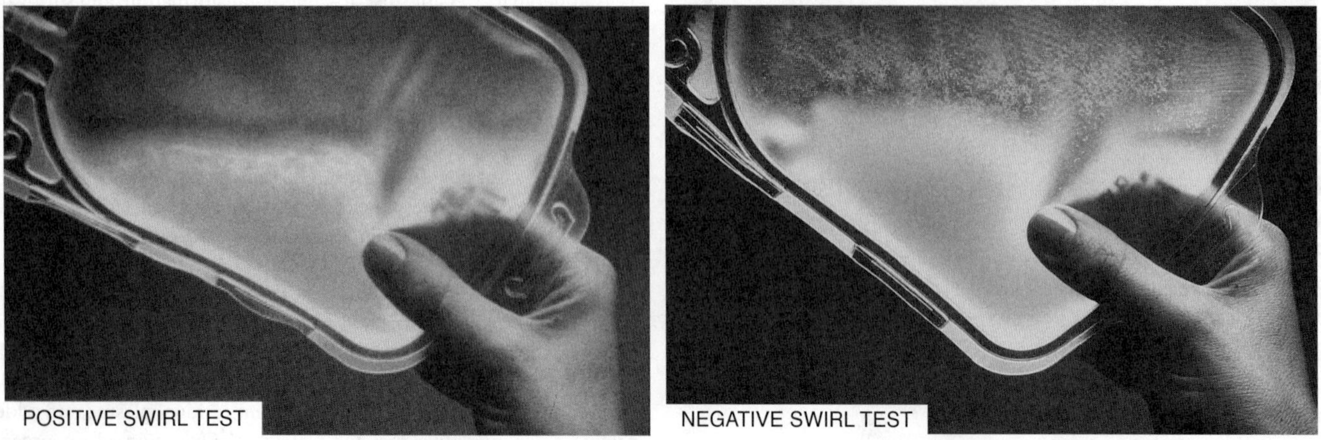

FIGURE 141–3. Swirling of platelet concentrates. Platelets in platelet concentrates that have been prepared and stored well retain their normal discoid configuration, which confers a swirling or shimmering appearance to the platelet concentrates (*left*). If the platelets are damaged by cold temperature, a fall in pH, or bacterial contamination, the discoid shape and swirling appearance are lost (*right*). Loss of swirling allows a transfusion technologist or clinician to identify potentially ineffective or dangerous platelet concentrates.

selected patients who do not respond well to allogeneic platelets. Platelets can be obtained before myelosuppressive therapy, then frozen and administered during subsequent periods of thrombocytopenia.[73] Newer approaches using a second-messenger effector-containing storage solution permit the use of lower concentrations of DMSO and correspondingly less cumbersome freezing and thawing protocols.[74] Despite reports of the effectiveness of human recombinant thrombopoietin-stimulated autologous high-yield platelet collections in supporting patients through intensive multicycle chemotherapy regimens, enthusiasm for thrombopoietin use has waned in light of reported antibody formation and severe thrombocytopenia with recombinant preparations.[75,76] It is not yet clear if thrombopoietin mimics (see Chaps. 113 and 119) will find use in this setting.

■ COLD LIQUID STORAGE

Room temperature storage of platelets limits their shelf-life by facilitating bacterial overgrowth.[77] Cold storage may allow the extension of shelf-life by reducing the risk of bacterial contamination and by further decreasing platelet metabolism below the 44 percent reduction in aging seen with 22°C (71.6°F) storage versus that seen at 37°C (98.6°F) *in vivo*.[78] As noted previously, however, platelet exposure to temperatures below 20°C (68°F) results in loss of discoid shape and marked shortening of posttransfusion survival.[41] Chilled platelets continue to function normally however, despite their markedly reduced circulation time.[79] Storage of murine platelets at 0°C (32°F) for 2 hours results in clustering of glycoprotein Ibα complexes and β-*N*-acetylglucosamine residue exposure. This neoantigen is recognized by complement type 3 receptors on hepatic macrophages, which rapidly clear the chilled platelets.[80] Galactosylation of glycoprotein Ibα neoantigens prevents the hepatic clearance of briefly cold-exposed murine platelets.[80,81] Unfortunately, reinfusion studies with galactosylated platelets exposed to 4°C (39.2°F) for longer periods (48 hours) in both humans and mice demonstrated rapid platelet clearance.[82] It appears that β-*N*-acetylglucosamine exposure is not the only mechanism of cold-exposed platelet clearance.[83] Other relevant mechanisms must be elucidated before cold platelet storage becomes a viable option.

LYOPHILIZED PLATELETS, PLATELET MEMBRANES, AND PLATELET SUBSTITUTES

Because of periodic supply shortages, having a safe and effective platelet substitute with a long shelf-life that simply could be rehydrated and infused into bleeding patients would be ideal. A great deal of research in this area is examining paraformaldehyde-treated lyophilized platelets, lyophilized platelet membrane microvesicles, fibrinogen-coated albumin microcapsules, platelet glycoprotein-containing liposomes, and other platelet substitutes.[84] This is an important area, but all of these developments await validation in appropriate clinical trials.

Nontransfusional agents, including the antifibrinolytic drugs ε-aminocaproic acid and tranexamic acid, may help stop bleeding in thrombocytopenic patients.[85] Antifibrinolytics have been effective in controlling mucosal and dental bleeding in thrombocytopenic patients without increasing the blood platelet concentration. Recombinant factor VIIa, in pharmacologic doses, enhances thrombin generation on activated platelets. A number of clinical reports describing bleeding time reduction and diminution or cessation of thrombocytopenic bleeding suggest a potential role for this agent in hemorrhage resulting from low platelet concentrations or platelet dysfunction.[86] However, further data from randomized controlled trials are needed to confirm its safety and effectiveness in different settings of major hemorrhage.[87,88]

CLINICAL RESPONSE

■ GENERAL PRINCIPLES IN PATIENTS WITH MARROW FAILURE

Assuming that one-third of infused platelets are pooled reversibly in a spleen of normal size (see Chap. 119) and that the recipient's blood volume is 2.5 L/m^2, infusion of 1 U of whole-blood-derived platelet concentrates containing 0.8×10^{11} platelets into a recipient with 1 m^2 of body surface area (BSA) should result in an increased platelet concentration of 21,000/μL. Of course, the response to 1 U is inversely proportional to the patient's size, expressed as the BSA. Thus, the response to a platelet transfusion can be evaluated by calculating the corrected count increment (CCI):[89]

$$\frac{\text{Measured increase in platelet concentration} \times \text{BSA (in m}^2\text{)}}{\text{No. of platelets infused } (\times 10^{11})}$$

The measurement of CCI has its critics,[90] but it is the most widely used method. Under optimal circumstances, the response should be 21,000/μL per square meter per whole-blood-derived unit infused or 26,000/μL per square meter per 10^{11} platelets infused.

In practice, in patients with thrombocytopenia secondary to marrow failure, the average CCI is approximately half the value expected: 10,000/μL per square meter per whole-blood-derived unit infused (Fig. 141–4).[89] Many studies have attempted to identify the factors responsible for this consistent but less than optimal response.[54,89,91–96] Alloimmunization has been incriminated, as have a variety of nonimmune factors such as platelet storage, bacterial sepsis, concomitant use of antibacterial antibiotics and amphotericin B, graft-versus-host disease, splenomegaly, disseminated intravascular coagulation, and even a recent allogeneic marrow transplantation. No one factor predominates in the majority of studies, suggesting that the crucial factors vary with the patient populations being studied. Often, none of these factors are present, but the response still is suboptimal. Other factors, as yet undefined, likely also are at work.

The initial CCI can be measured in 10 minutes[97] to a few hours after transfusion. The time until the platelet concentration returns to a level below the institution's threshold for prophylactic platelet transfusions

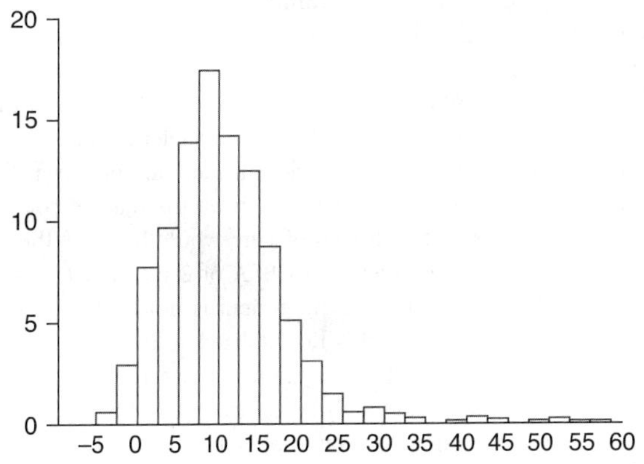

FIGURE 141–4. Rise in platelet concentration 1 hour after infusion in patients with acute leukemia. As described in the text, the increment in concentration for each unit infused has been corrected for body surface area. Without complicating factors, the concentration should be approximately 21,000/μL. The *vertical axis* refers to the percent of transfusions achieving the increments indicated. Marked heterogeneity in response is seen, with a median of approximately 10,000/μL, which is approximately half of the predicted amount. *(Redrawn with permission from Bishop JF, McGrath K, Wolf MM, et al.[89])*

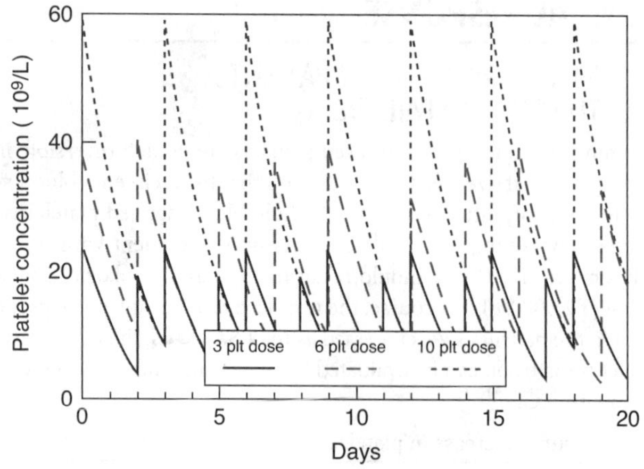

FIGURE 141–5. Response to varying doses of units of whole-blood-derived platelet concentrates during repetitive transfusion of patients who are thrombocytopenic because of marrow failure. Larger doses produce an initially higher increase in platelet concentration and a longer time to next transfusion. Fewer transfusion episodes are required over a 20-day transfusion period. *(Redrawn with permission from calculations in Hersh JK, Hom EG, Brecher ME,[99] and validated by empirical data in Norol F, Bierling P, Roudot-Thoraval F, et al.,[100] and Klumpp TR, Herman JH, Gaughan JP, et al.[101])*

(time to next transfusion) also varies with the immune and nonimmune factors affecting the initial CCI.[98] Time to next transfusion is also dependent upon the peak platelet count achieved by the transfusion and, therefore, the dose of platelets administered.[99–101] This finding follows from the fact that platelet survival is reduced in all patients with thrombocytopenia, regardless of the cause, with progressive reduction as the platelet concentration in the blood decreases (see Chap. 119).[102] Therefore, all other factors being equal, the larger the dose, the higher the platelet count achieved by transfusion and the longer the time to the next transfusion (Fig. 141–5).

■ PLATELET DOSE

If the average patient has an increase in platelet concentration of 10,000/μL per square meter per whole-blood-derived unit of platelets, the relationship between the dose administered and the platelet count achieved can be calculated. Furthermore, using calculations and data from references 99 to 101, the time to the next transfusion can be estimated. Table 141–2 gives these values for the transfusion of a myelosuppressed patient having a BSA of 2 m^2 and platelet count of 5000/μL. The results indicate that no standard dose fits all patients, regardless of size and clinical situation. For the doses given, the platelet concentrations achieved in a patient with BSA of 1 m^2 would be twice the values given in the table. In the patient with BSA of 2 m^2, 4 U (3.2×10^{11}) probably would be satisfactory if the patient is not bleeding, is being transfused prophylactically, and is hospitalized so that the patient can be transfused again 24 to 48 hours later, because raising the platelet concentration to 20,000 to 30,000/μL protects most thrombocytopenic patients against spontaneous, catastrophic bleeding. However, 10 U (8.0×10^{11}) is a better choice if the goal is to achieve a platelet concentration greater than 50,000/μL because the patient is bleeding or is being prepared for an invasive procedure.[103] Achieving this level of platelet concentration probably is most critical if the surgical field is highly vascular, as with inflammation or portal hypertension; if coexisting defects in plasma coagulation are present; if the procedure is "blind," as in needle biopsy of the liver; or when no opportunity to achieve hemostasis mechanically exists. If surgery is necessary in an area where even a small hemorrhage would be disastrous, as in the central nervous system, even higher doses may be required to increase the platelet concentration to greater than 100,000/μL.[104] A higher dose also might be chosen to facilitate transfusion in the outpatient setting where a longer transfusion interval would be preferable.

Patients vary dramatically in their responses. Therefore, the measurement of increments 1 and 24 hours after transfusion is a simple and cost-effective way to modify the dose and frequency of transfusion based on the pathophysiology of the individual patient.

Prophylactic use of platelets currently is the largest single indication in the United States, representing 52 to 74 percent of transfusions.[105,106] Large, randomized, controlled trials have compared different prophylactic dose strategies in patients with hypoproliferative thrombocytopenia (≤10,000/μL) in the setting of intensive chemotherapy or stem cell transplantation. The first of these, comparing standard-dose ($3–6 \times 10^{11}$ platelets/dose) versus half-dose prophylaxis was inconclusive because the study was terminated prematurely.[33] There was no overall difference in the primary endpoint of World Health Organization (WHO) grade 2 or greater bleeding (approximately 50% in both study arms). However, three patients (5.2%) in the half-dose arm had grade 4 bleeding, compared with none in the standard-dose arm of the study, triggering a prespecified stopping criterion and leaving the study underpowered with regards to its primary endpoint. Whether the difference in grade 4 bleeding was a result of chance or represented a real finding remains unknown. A larger trial of three dose strategies (standard [$2.2 \times 10^{11}/m^2$], half, and double dose) concluded that platelet doses ≥$1.1 \times 10^{11}/m^2$ given at a platelet count trigger ≤10,000/μL have no effect on the frequency of any bleeding grade.[34] Although low-dose prophylaxis consumed 9 percent fewer platelets than standard dose, the median number of transfusion events was 1.7 times greater. Consequently, the full economic benefits of lower-dose prophylaxis may only be applicable to whole-blood-derived platelet doses, assuming that savings from reductions in pool size are not offset by the cost of more frequent administration. Surprisingly, high-dose prophylaxis did not result in fewer transfusion events and there was no difference in the number of thrombocytopenic days in any arm. The latter finding suggests that the different dosing strategies did not significantly alter stimuli promoting spontaneous recovery of thrombopoiesis.

■ PLATELET TRANSFUSION TRIGGER

A thrombocytopenic patient who is actively bleeding requires platelet transfusion. The decision to transfuse platelets is more difficult if the platelet count is simply very low and the patient has no bleeding or relatively minor hemorrhage, such as petechiae or small cutaneous

TABLE 141–2. Relationship between Platelet Dose and Clinical Response in a Patient with a 2-m^2 Body Surface with a Platelet Count of 5000/μL, Prior to Transfusion

Dose $\times 10^{11}$	Dose Units*	Platelet Concentration Achieved, per μL	Transfusion Interval (Days)†
3.2	4	25,000	1.8
4.8	6	35,000	2.3
6.4	8	45,000	2.8
8.0	10	55,000	3.5

*Whole-blood-derived platelet concentrates.

†Time to return to 5000/μL.

ecchymoses. Clinical experience suggests that if the platelet count is low enough for long enough, there is a significant risk of "spontaneous" major hemorrhage, particularly into the central nervous system. Unfortunately, a number of studies have shown that the platelet count *per se* does not reliably predict the bleeding risk for thrombocytopenic patients.[107,108]

A classic study of patients with acute leukemia performed prior to the availability of platelet transfusion described the relationship between platelet concentration in the blood and clinical hemorrhage.[109] Minor and major hemorrhage began (i.e., >1% chance per day) when the platelet count fell below 50,000 and 20,000/μL, respectively. Major hemorrhage was observed in the range from 5000 to 20,000/μL but on only 3 percent of patient-days. The rate of major bleeding increased rapidly when the platelet concentration fell below 5000/μL and reached a frequency of 33 percent of patient-days as the platelet concentration approached zero. However, many of these children were receiving aspirin for pain and fever, and these bleeding rates may be overestimates.

Subsequently, the same group described the effect of prophylactic platelet transfusion administered whenever the platelet count fell below 20,000/μL.[110] Although major hemorrhage was strikingly reduced when the pretransfusion platelet count was below 5,000/μL, no substantial change was noted when the platelet count ranged from 5000 to 20,000/μL. Nonetheless, for many years, this experience was used to justify prophylactic platelet transfusion whenever the platelet concentration fell below 20,000/μL, although the data actually suggested 5000/μL was an appropriate trigger.

Prospective but uncontrolled studies by one group supported the safety and efficacy of a more restrictive policy using 5000/μL as the platelet transfusion trigger.[111,112] Subsequently, three prospective studies assigned patients to one of two groups receiving prophylactic platelet transfusion at either 10,000/μL or 20,000/μL.[113–115] Uniformly, no increase in bleeding risk was observed at the lower transfusion trigger, which has been adopted by most transfusion services.[116]

Clinical factors commonly are assumed to increase the risk of hemorrhage by accelerating platelet consumption. These factors include fever and sepsis, administration of drugs that interfere with platelet function, coexistent abnormalities of plasma coagulation factors, disseminated intravascular coagulation, and high leukocyte concentrations in the blood.[117] A retrospective analysis of the hospital course of almost 3000 thrombocytopenic adults showed no relationship between the first morning platelet count, or the lowest platelet count of the day, and the risk of hemorrhage.[107] This study identified several important patient-specific factors that appear to be associated with a greater risk for severe bleeding. These included a history of recent bleeding, uremia, marrow transplantation within 100 days, and hypoalbuminemia. Yet another study found no clear evidence for an association between the occurrence of major intracranial bleeding and absolute platelet count just prior to the event.[118] A recent study in experimental animals also suggests that the presence of inflammation, particularly during periods of severe thrombocytopenia, may be an important factor in the occurrence of life-threatening bleeding.[119] Thus, raising the transfusion trigger in complicated, clinically ill patients is common practice, although it is not (yet) supported by data from clinical trials.

Moderate to severe bleeding is observed in 11 to 23 percent of patients after marrow transplantation despite aggressive use of prophylactic platelet transfusion and maintenance of morning platelet counts above 20,000/μL.[120,121] Gastrointestinal and urinary bleeding are most common; pulmonary and intracranial bleeding are less common. Usually, an anatomic cause, such as gastrointestinal ulceration, hemorrhagic cystitis, or diffuse alveolar hemorrhage, can be identified. In effect, common practice in the myelosuppressed patient is to treat bleeding, not prevent it.

Interest in comparing the use of prophylactic versus therapeutic platelet transfusions is gaining ground. A preliminary report of a trial in autologous peripheral stem cell transplant patients found only one patient with major bleeding amongst 171 patients randomized to either prophylactic platelet transfusions or platelet transfusion only after nonminor bleeding, although there was an increase in minor bleeding in the therapeutic-only transfusion group (28.7% of patients versus 9.5%).[122] Reports from European trials underway may increase enthusiasm for this approach in the United States.[123]

THROMBOCYTOPENIA RESULTING FROM PLATELET LOSS, SEQUESTRATION, OR DESTRUCTION

MASSIVE TRANSFUSION

Dilutional thrombocytopenia occurs when massive blood loss is replaced with stored red cells lacking viable platelets. Following replacement of one blood volume (approximately 10 red cell units for adults), 35 to 40 percent of patients' platelets usually remain. Even when one to two blood volumes are replaced, the platelet count is usually not less than 50,000/μL, thrombocytopenic bleeding usually does not develop, and routine transfusion is not indicated simply because the platelet count is low.[124,125] Platelets have been traditionally given to patients who demonstrate abnormal bleeding associated with platelet counts less than 50,000/μL. Retrospective data from battlefield resuscitations have revived enthusiasm for massive transfusion protocols incorporating early aggressive plasma transfusion and empiric platelet dosing strategies.[126] The absence of prospective data, the lack of statistically significant contribution of early platelet use to possible improvements in mortality and the unclear applicability of military protocols in civilian settings collectively provide no compelling rationale for changes in platelet transfusion practice.[127,128]

CARDIOPULMONARY BYPASS

Immediately following and for several days after cardiac surgery, the platelet count commonly falls to subnormal levels, occasionally as low as 50,000/μL. An associated defect in platelet function is observed. Prospective studies have shown no benefit of prophylactic administration of platelet transfusions to such patients.[129] The platelet count following cardiac surgery gives no indication of functioning platelets and an appropriate platelet function test is lacking. Thromboelastography has been found to aid the decision-making process regarding platelet transfusion in some institutions. Transfusions should be reserved for the relatively rare patient who demonstrates clinically abnormal microvascular bleeding where a surgical cause has been excluded.

An increasing number of patients are referred for cardiac surgery while on treatment with antiplatelet drugs such as aspirin and clopidogrel. This treatment should be discontinued 5 to 7 days before surgery unless the procedure is urgent, as it increases the risk of bleeding and the requirements for red cell and platelet transfusions.[130]

Antifibrinolytic agents reduce bleeding and transfusion requirements in cardiac surgery patients, but aprotinin was associated with increased mortality compared to other agents such as tranexamic acid, prompting its withdrawal from the market.[131]

SPLENOMEGALY

Patients with massive splenomegaly have thrombocytopenia related predominantly to excessive sequestration in a splenic pool in continuous exchange with platelets in the circulation (see Chap. 119). In patients with splenomegaly resulting from hepatic cirrhosis and organ failure, thrombopoietin deficiency also contributes by reducing platelet production. The platelet count rarely falls below 30,000/μL as a result of splenomegaly alone, so platelet transfusion is rarely considered except in anticipation of invasive procedures such as surgery and needle biopsy of the liver. Under these circumstances, depending upon the degree of splenic enlargement, administration of 10 to 15 U of whole-blood-derived platelet concentrates per square meter BSA may be necessary to achieve a substantial increase in platelet count. In many patients with severe splenomegaly, achieving adequate platelet increments may not be possible, even with large numbers of platelet concentrates. If such patients require elective surgery, consideration should be given to splenectomy prior to the elective procedure.

IMMUNE (IDIOPATHIC) THROMBOCYTOPENIC PURPURA

In immune (idiopathic) thrombocytopenic purpura, platelet transfusion generally is not used because the bleeding tendency is less severe than in thrombocytopenia resulting from diminished production, and the response to medical therapy generally is satisfactory and rapid (see Chap. 119). Furthermore, the survival of transfused platelets is relatively brief, similar to that of the patient's own platelets. Nonetheless, when critical bleeding occurs or urgent surgery is needed, 3 to 6 U of whole-blood-derived platelet concentrates per square meter BSA generally raise the platelet count for 12 to 48 hours.[132] The same general principles apply to other diseases in which accelerated destruction of platelets occurs, such as disseminated intravascular coagulation.

NEONATAL ALLOIMMUNE THROMBOCYTOPENIA

In this syndrome, the mother produces an alloantibody against antigens on fetal platelets that have crossed the placenta (see Chap. 119). The antibody, in turn, crosses the placenta, causing fetal thrombocytopenia that may persist for weeks after delivery. The optimal postnatal management of neonatal alloimmune thrombocytopenia (NAIT) depends on its rapid recognition, and prompt correction by transfusion of platelet concentrates to neonates who are severely thrombocytopenic or bleeding. It is inappropriate to wait for laboratory confirmation of the diagnosis in suspected cases. Because maternal platelets are compatible, platelets harvested from the mother's blood by apheresis can produce an adequate increase in the infant's platelet count after infusion.[133] Ideally, such platelets should be concentrated in a small volume of plasma or washed so that additional antibody is not infused. Unfortunately, arranging for apheresis of the mother often is difficult.

Although there is debate about the use of randomly chosen apheresis platelet aliquots or a whole-blood-derived platelet unit in the immediate postnatal management of NAIT, several studies have shown that these are often effective.[134,135] However, compatible platelet concentrates, for example, from HPA-1a– and -5b–negative donors, give larger platelet count increments and have a longer half-life and should be used initially, if they are available, on the basis of the certainty of their effectiveness in the more than 90 percent of cases of NAIT that are caused by anti-HPA-1a or anti-HPA-5b.[136] Unfortunately, the routine availability of such HPA-1a– and -5b–negative platelets for immediate use in suspected cases of NAIT is limited. Strategies for antenatal treatment of NAIT include the use of serial intrauterine platelet transfusions, which, although effective, are invasive and associated with significant morbidity and mortality. Maternal therapy involving the administration of intravenous immunoglobulin and/or steroids is also effective and associated with fewer risks to the fetus.[137]

HEREDITARY THROMBOCYTOPENIA

These syndromes are rare and generally are not associated with severe bleeding.[138] Because the survival of allogeneic platelets is normal, platelet transfusion is effective and can be used for critical bleeding and surgery. However, like all cases in which repeated platelet transfusions are required, the risk for alloimmunization is high and should be considered when generating a long-term care plan.

QUALITATIVE PLATELET DISORDERS

Despite normal platelet counts, patients with qualitative platelet disorders have a clinical bleeding tendency associated with abnormal *in vitro* tests of platelet function and a prolonged bleeding time *in vivo*. The basis may be hereditary (see Chap. 121) or acquired (see Chap. 122). Platelet transfusion is generally not indicated when the cause is extrinsic to the platelet, as in uremia, von Willebrand disease, and hyperglobulinemia, because the transfused platelets will function no better than the patient's own platelets. Exceptions are certain types of von Willebrand disease in which normal platelets can be used to deliver von Willebrand factor to a bleeding site (see Chap. 127). Most inherited intrinsic platelet disorders are mild and do not require transfusions even for surgery if the procedure is carried out under direct vision, so hemostasis may be achieved mechanically. If the bleeding tendency is more severe, as in Glanzmann thrombasthenia or Bernard-Soulier syndrome, platelet transfusions may be necessary for bleeding. However, in this setting isoimmunization to the missing platelet glycoproteins may occur and result in platelet refractoriness, so every effort should be made to avoid prophylactic transfusion, if possible. The acquired defects, as in the myeloproliferative and myelodysplastic syndromes, generally do not require platelet transfusion except in cases of coexistent thrombocytopenia.

POSSIBLE CONTRAINDICATIONS TO PLATELET TRANSFUSION

Concern has been voiced that platelet transfusions should not be administered to patients with forms of thrombocytopenia associated with platelet activation and thrombosis, such as thrombotic thrombocytopenic purpura (TTP) or heparin-induced thrombocytopenia (see Chap. 133), because infusion of platelets might worsen the thrombotic tendency. Unfortunately, particularly in TTP, platelet transfusion is often requested prior to invasive procedures such as insertion of intravenous catheters for plasma exchange. While experience suggests that platelet transfusions are generally tolerated in this setting, a prudent approach avoids prophylactic administration.[139,140] Platelet transfusion should never be withheld when patients experience significant bleeding.

COMPLICATIONS OF PLATELET TRANSFUSION

Platelet transfusions are associated with many complications (Table 141–3). Paradoxically, most complications are not caused by the platelets themselves but rather the contaminating leukocytes, leukocyte-derived cytokines, red cells, plasma proteins, and microorganisms.

COMPLICATIONS RESULTING FROM CONTAMINATING LEUKOCYTES

Alloimmunization to Class I Human Leukocyte Antigens

HLAs are expressed on integral membrane glycoproteins. Almost all cells have class I antigens (platelets have abundant amounts of HLA-A and -B antigens), whereas only a few types of circulating leukocytes (dendritic cells, monocytes, subsets of B cells) have class II antigens. Primary alloimmunization to class I HLAs appears to require presentation of these antigens on cells that also express HLA class II antigens

TABLE 141–3. Complications of Platelet Transfusion

Because of contaminating leukocytes
Alloimmunization to class I HLA antigens
Refractoriness to platelet transfusion
FNHTR
Cytokine formation
FNHTR
Transmission of cytomegalovirus
Graft-versus-host disease
Because of contaminating red cells
Rh alloimmunization
Parasites—malaria, babesiosis
Because of plasma and its contents
Contaminating microorganisms
Bacteria
Viruses—e.g., HBV, HCV, HIV, HTLV
Parasites—e.g., Chagas disease
Plasma proteins
Minor and major allergic reactions
ABO antibody-mediated hemolysis
Transfusion-related acute lung injury
Because of the platelets themselves
FNHTR
Refractoriness to platelet transfusion
Posttransfusion purpura

FNHTR, febrile nonhemolytic transfusion reaction; HBV, hepatitis B virus; HCV, hepatitis C virus; HTLV, human T-cell lymphotropic virus.

and other costimulatory molecules.[141] Abundant evidence now indicates the incidence of HLA alloimmunization can be reduced by more than half with consistent use of leukoreduced blood products.[142–144] Transfused red cells also must be leukoreduced because leukocytes contained in the transfused red cells are capable of inducing HLA alloimmunization.[145]

Alloimmunization to HLA should be suspected clinically if two or more transfusions result in 1-hour CCIs of less than 7500/μL per square meter per 10^{11} platelets transfused.[146] Rapid confirmatory flow cytometry-based assays and enzyme-linked immunosorbent assays (ELISA) can screen for the presence of HLA antibodies and even define their specificity.[147,148] The presence of HLA antibodies has been a good predictor of poor response to platelets from randomly selected donors[149] and improved response when platelets are matched for HLA type.[150] In the future, it may be more economical to periodically screen transfused individuals and multiparous women for HLA antibody so that HLA alloimmunization is detected prior to the development of refractoriness rather than vice versa.[151] Before matched support is denied, one should ensure that HLA antibody screening was performed with the most sensitive technology available and that appropriate screening for the presence of antibodies to HPA was also carried out (see Role of ABO and Platelet-Specific Antibodies below).

The incidence of HLA alloimmunization should gradually decrease as the use of leukoreduced blood products becomes widespread.[144] Some patients do not develop HLA antibodies after many transfusions, whereas others do so after exposure to only two to four transfusions.[152,153] The pattern and breadth of alloimmunization vary greatly among patients, presumably because some have class I HLA molecules with epitopes present on a wide variety of other class I molecules, whereas others' are relatively restricted, mismatched epitopes on transfused white blood cells may be of high or low immunogenicity and the innate capacity for immune responsiveness varies by individual, by disease state and the immune effects of treatment.[154] HLA antibody panels can characterize the breadth of alloimmunization by the percentage of HLA antigens in the population against which the patient's serum reacts, that is, the percent reactive antibody (PRA). Patients may have PRA values between 1 and 100 percent. The precise identification of HLA allotypes to which recipients are immunized lends itself to the provision of so-called antigen-negative platelet transfusions, discussed further in "Management of Refratory Patients" below and in Chap. 138. HLA-C antigens are expressed on the platelet surface, but they are present in sufficiently low density that they play an insignificant role in the majority of patients with platelet refractoriness,[155] although some cases of HLA-C–mediated refractoriness have been reported.[156]

The majority of patients who become alloimmunized establish a specificity pattern and PRA plateau, which they maintain as they continue receiving transfusions. However, approximately 30 percent lose their antibodies over time despite continuing transfusion.[157] Thus, monitoring antibody PRA and specificity is helpful, because such patients may regain some measure of responsiveness having been previously refractory.

Cross-reactive groups (CREGs) of HLAs have been defined by serologic testing. Cross-reactivity among antigens in a CREG is based upon the sharing of one or more public epitopes by those antigens.[158] Patients commonly develop antibodies to one or more public epitopes in a CREG, but less frequently develop antibodies to private epitopes (those unique to a particular HLA allele).[159] Some patients even develop intra-CREG antibodies, that is, antibodies to antigens in the same CREG as their own antigens.[160] This unpredictability complicates attempts to provide HLA-selected products armed only with the patient's HLA type (i.e., without knowledge of precise antibody specificity available through ELISA, flow cytometry-based assays, and older technologies).

MANAGEMENT OF REFRACTORY PATIENTS

In 1969, studies showed that platelet transfusion-refractory patients respond to platelets from siblings who are identical for all four class I HLA-A and HLA-B antigens.[161] This simple clinical observation remains one of the most compelling pieces of evidence supporting the role of HLA alloimmunization in platelet refractoriness. Similarly, thrombocytopenic patients can be supported by platelets from unrelated donors who are HLA identical or closely matched. Because some patients do not make antibody to antigens within their own CREGs, it became popular to choose donors according to CREG classification, particularly BX matches, that is, donors whose antigens are identical to or within the same CREGs as those of the patient.[162] Table 141–4 lists the categorization of such matches.

Responses were better with directed matching than with random donor selection, but many BX matches failed and many C and D matches succeeded. Figure 141–6 suggests potential explanations for the relatively poor predictive capacity of this method. Some patients with relatively low PRAs have antibody to only one or two CREGs, so success with some C and D matches would be expected. On the other hand, failure of some BX matches would be expected in patients with intra-CREG antibody. Furthermore, this method does not quickly provide a good match. Finding an excellent match in a blood center's

TABLE 141–4. Classification of Donor/Recipient Pairs on the Basis of HLA Class I Matching

A	All 4 antigens in donor identical to those of recipient.
B1U	Only 3 antigens detected in donor (i.e., donor homozygous at one HLA-A or -B sublocus); all present in recipient.
B1X	Three donor antigens identical to recipient; fourth antigen cross-reactive* with recipient.
B2U	Only 2 antigens detected in donor; both present in recipient.
B2UX	Only 3 antigens detected in donor; 2 identical with recipient, third cross-reactive.
B2X	Two donor antigens identical to recipient; third and fourth antigens cross-reactive with recipient.
C	One antigen of donor not present in recipient and not cross-reactive with recipient.
D	Two antigens of donor not present in recipient and not cross-reactive with recipient.

*Antigen in a cross-reactive group (CREG) that contains one of the patient's antigens.

Revised with permission from Duquesnoy RJ, Filip DJ, Rodey GE, et al.[162]

inventory is uncommon, and days are required to recruit and apherese one or more well-matched donors from an HLA-typed donor file.

In the late 1980s and early 1990s, practical methods for platelet cross-matching became available.[163] Many centers found that they could simply cross-match the patient's serum with unselected apheresis platelet concentrates in inventory to find, within hours, a compatible product that would be successful *in vivo*.[91,164] However, in a highly immunized patient, one might cross-match with dozens of donors and not find a compatible product.[164] For many such patients, only the identification of an A or BU match (see Table 141–4) suffices.

One other approach to these patients has been proposed.[165] If the PRA in an HLA antibody panel is less than 100 percent, one should be able to identify the HLAs to which the patient has not formed antibody. The patient then can be supported with "antigen-negative" platelets, that is, platelets that lack the antigens to which the patient has formed antibody. If the results of an HLA antibody panel are known, one often can provide a product from inventory on an urgent basis using this approach.

No reason exists for choosing one of these approaches to the exclusion of the other two. If the PRA is reasonably low (<33%), successful support usually can be provided by any means. Crossmatching is most useful when HLA typing and antibody results are pending. When the PRA is relatively high (>67%), a strategy of selective recruitment of A and BU matches from an HLA-typed donor file and provision of "antigen-negative" units of the best mismatch grade when no identical matches are available appears to enjoy the most success.[151,166]

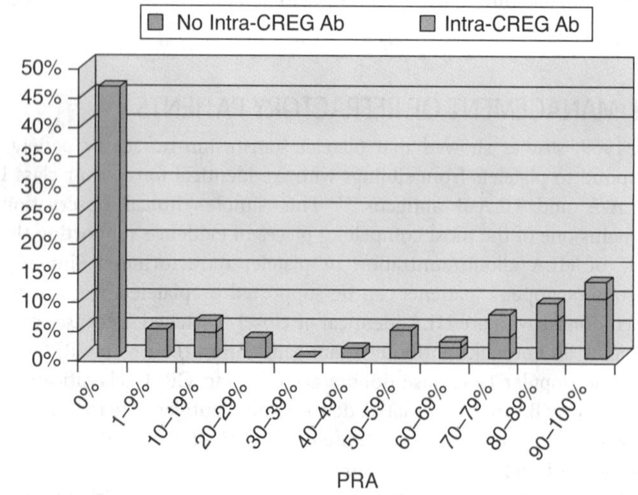

FIGURE 141–6. Percent reactive antibody (PRA) distribution by lymphocytotoxicity assay in serum samples from 108 thrombocytopenic patients referred to a regional blood center for matched platelet support during a 6-month period. Fifty patients showed no reactivity, whereas 58 patients showed PRAs that varied from 4 to 100 percent. The *shaded portions* of the bars indicate patients who had demonstrable antibody against antigens within their own cross-reactive groups, that is, intra–cross-reactive group antibody (CREG Ab). *(Data provided by Dr. Susan Hsu, American Red Cross Blood Services, Penn-Jersey Region. Redrawn from Murphy S,[219] with permission.)*

Role of ABO and Platelet-Specific Antibodies

ABO determinants are carried by platelet glycoproteins and glycolipids, as they are on erythrocytes.[167,168] Although ABO identity is not absolutely critical for successful platelet transfusion, transfused platelets incompatible with recipients' plasma antibodies (e.g., O recipient, A donor) predictably result in yields up to one-third less than ABO-identical transfusions.[169,170] Even ABO-compatible platelets in donor plasma with incompatible antibodies (e.g., A recipient, O donor) produce lower increments, possibly as a result of circulating immune complexes.[169,171] In addition, transfusion of incompatible plasma (especially O plasma to A recipients) can result in accelerated red cell destruction in the recipient, occasionally leading to acute hemolysis.[172,173] Furthermore, formation of immune complexes between A and B substance and corresponding antibodies has been proposed to have additional deleterious effects.[174] Thus, observing ABO compatibility whenever possible seems wise.

The platelet surface carries many platelet-specific antigens (HPAs; see Chap. 138), which are capable of eliciting a strong alloantibody response. A number of patients with such alloantibodies accounting for refractoriness to platelet transfusion have been described.[175–179] From 4 to 10 percent of heavily transfused patients in several series developed HPA antibodies, most often coexisting with HLA antibodies.[180–182] Fewer than 2 percent of patients developed HPA antibodies alone. However, faced with clinically refractory patients who do not demonstrate HLA antibody, investigation for HPA antibodies would be prudent. Similarly, the consistent failure of well HLA-matched platelet products mandates investigation for coexisting HPA antibodies. HPA antibody detection methods continue to evolve, but most commonly involve ELISA or monoclonal antibody immobilization of antigen techniques.[183,184] HPA genotyping has been helpful in predicting the potential for HPA antibody formation and confirming the results of antibody studies.[185]

FEBRILE NONHEMOLYTIC TRANSFUSION REACTIONS

Prior to the availability of methods for leukoreduction, approximately 20 percent of platelet transfusions were accompanied by febrile nonhemolytic transfusion reaction (FNHTR).[186] Some of these reactions undoubtedly were caused by antibodies in the patient directed against either leukocyte specific antigens or HLAs on leukocytes contaminating the platelet product. Leukocyte depletion by filtration during infusion reduced the frequency of these reactions, but many continued to occur.[186,187] Contaminating leukocytes now are known to produce inflammatory cytokines, such as interleukin-1, interleukin-6, interleukin-8, and tumor necrosis factor-alpha, during storage at 20 to 24°C (68–75.2°F), and these compounds are responsible for many FNHTRs given that they are not removed by bedside filtration.[188,189] Thus, febrile reactions occur more when platelets are transfused at the end of the storage interval.[190] These reactions provide a strong argument for routine, prestorage removal of leukocytes.

Nonetheless, FNHTRs occur in approximately 4.6 percent of platelet transfusions even with prestorage leukoreduction.[191] The cause of these reactions is not known. They may be related to plasma proteins or products produced during storage by the platelets themselves, such as CD154, a potent cyclooxygenase-2 inducer.[192] In the unusual case of distressing recurrent febrile reactions, platelets can be washed free of plasma prior to infusion.[193]

It is estimated that premedication with acetaminophen and diphenhydramine is used before 50 to 80 percent of transfusion episodes in the United States to prevent acute transfusion reactions, both febrile (nonhemolytic) and allergic reactions. A single-center study found no benefit from the routine administration of pretransfusion premedication, and there remains a need for a better understanding of the mechanisms involved in acute transfusion reactions and the means to prevent them.[194]

TRANSMISSION OF CYTOMEGALOVIRUS

In asymptomatic carriers, the cytomegalovirus (CMV) resides in the nuclei of subsets of leukocytes with little virus free in plasma. Use of leukoreduced blood components was shown to be essentially equivalent to use of components from CMV-negative donors in terms of risk of CMV transmission.[195] A later cohort study challenged this assertion but was unable to demonstrate increased CMV transmission resulting from use of leukoreduced platelet products, and no significant difference in the incidence of CMV disease was observed, possibly because of aggressive antigenic surveillance.[196] Because this infection is particularly dangerous for severely immunocompromised CMV-negative patients, such as recent allogeneic marrow transplant recipients, some clinicians continue to request leukoreduced, CMV-negative blood products in this select population.

GRAFT-VERSUS-HOST DISEASE

Immunosuppressed patients may develop graft-versus-host disease (GVHD) from T lymphocytes present in any cellular blood product, including platelets. Thus, standard practice is to treat platelet concentrates with γ-irradiation to inhibit proliferation of transfused T lymphocytes in cellular immune response suppressed recipients.[197] Transfusions from biologic relatives and HLA-matched or crossmatch-compatible platelets should also be irradiated. Exposure to 2500 cGy appears to have no deleterious effect on platelets.[198] Of importance to note is that current methods of leukoreduction do not remove enough T cells to prevent GVHD.

COMPLICATIONS OF FILTRATION OF PLATELET CONCENTRATES

Complications of platelet transfusion related to the removal of leukocytes by filtration of platelet concentrates at the bedside may occur. Severe hypotension has been reported,[199] predominantly when negatively charged leukocyte reduction filters are used in patients who are receiving angiotensin-converting enzyme (ACE) inhibitors.[200] In one proposed mechanism, high molecular weight kininogen is converted to bradykinin, a potent vasodilator, by exposure to a negatively charged surface. Bradykinin normally is metabolized by ACE in a few seconds but may circulate much longer in patients receiving ACE inhibitors.[201] Although there have been no reports of hypotensive reactions from prestorage leukoreduced platelet concentrates, warmed, microfiltered, prestorage, leukoreduced red cell products have caused such reactions.[202]

COMPLICATIONS RESULTING FROM CONTAMINATING RED CELLS

When transfusing platelet concentrates to Rh-negative women of childbearing potential, one must be concerned about sensitization by Rh-positive red cells contaminating infused platelets. Apheresis-derived platelets contain far fewer contaminating red cells than whole-blood-derived platelet concentrates, often below levels known to produce Rh-alloimmunization.[173] In practice, with either product, sensitization is uncommon in immunosuppressed patients.[203,204] However, where possible, platelets from Rh-negative donors should be administered. When this is not possible, Rh immune globulin, about 20 mcg per unit of whole-blood-derived platelets, can be administered so that the infused red cells will be cleared prior to sensitization. A full dose of 300 mcg is sufficient to suppress the immune response to 15 mL of Rh-positive red cells.

Enough red cells contaminate platelet concentrates (0.2–0.7 μL per apheresis unit, 0.3–0.5 mL per whole-blood-derived unit)[204] to transmit both malaria and babesiosis if the donor is parasitemic.

COMPLICATIONS RESULTING FROM PLASMA AND ITS CONTENTS

Contaminating Microorganisms

Storage of platelet concentrates at 20 to 24°C (68–75.2°F) allows proliferation to dangerous levels of bacteria that occasionally contaminate units of blood or apheresis platelet concentrates.[205] Contamination may occur because of asymptomatic bacteremia in the donor at the time of venipuncture, inadequate decontamination of the skin, or venipuncture through areas of the skin where bacterial colonization is deeper than can be reached by such decontamination.[206] Bacterial contamination that might not be clinically significant after 2 to 3 days of storage may become significant after 5 to 7 days.[207] For this reason, platelet concentrate storage is limited to 5 days.

The magnitude of this problem is commonly underestimated.[208] Estimates suggest contamination of 3 to 10 U per 10,000 whole-blood-derived platelet concentrates and 150 clinical episodes associated with severe morbidity and death in the United States per year.[209] These values equate to 1 episode of severe morbidity or mortality per 20,000 platelet units transfused, which is 50- to 250-fold higher than the risk of mortality from transmission by transfusion of human immunodeficiency virus (HIV), hepatitis B virus (HBV), or hepatitis C virus (HCV).

Several potential approaches to this important problem can be used. Apheresis, which involves only one donor and one venipuncture, is associated with less risk than pooled whole-blood-derived platelet concentrates.[36] The AABB, in recognition of the significant risk of platelet bacterial contamination, has instituted standards requiring implementation of methods that limit and detect bacteria in all platelet products.[32] Detection technology is evolving.[210] Methods for viral inactivation that also inactivate bacteria are under investigation. The methods of viral inactivation also may inactivate T lymphocytes and prevent GVHD.[59]

The plasma diluent of platelet concentrates can transmit viruses such as HBV and HCV, human T-cell lymphotrophic virus (HTLV) I/II, and HIV. Improved methods of donor screening and testing have reduced, but not eliminated, this risk. Methods for viral inactivation are being sought.[59] Transmission of the parasite *Trypanosoma cruzi*, which is responsible for Chagas disease, has occurred with platelet transfusion.[211]

Plasma Proteins

Many transfusion services attempt to transfuse ABO-identical platelet concentrates; however, such transfusion is not always possible. When anti-A or anti-B is transfused to a patient whose red cells carry A or B, a positive direct antiglobulin test may be observed in the laboratory, making red cell compatibility testing more difficult.[212] Actual accelerated destruction of the patient's red cells is rare.[213] However, very rare cases of frank acute hemolysis have been observed.[214]

As with any plasma infusion, urticaria or even anaphylactic shock in patients with specific protein deficiencies and circulating antibodies (e.g., anti-IgA, antihaptoglobin) can occur,[215] and transfusion-associated acute lung injury can be observed when a donor has HLA or human neutrophil antigen (HNA) antibodies that can react with antigens on the recipient's neutrophils.[216] Efforts underway to reduce the amount of these antibodies in platelet concentrates involve a shift away from multiparous female donors, donor testing for HLA/HNA antibodies, introduction of platelet additive solutions to replace donor plasma and use of whole-blood-derived concentrates that contain less plasma from a single donor.[216]

COMPLICATIONS RESULTING FROM PLATELETS THEMSELVES

In addition to the potential role of platelets in cytokine-mediated FNHTRs, alloimmunization to HPAs can result in recipient adverse reactions. As discussed above in Role of ABO and Platelet-Specific Antibodies, platelet refractoriness may uncommonly result from HPA antibody formation. Posttransfusion purpura, another uncommon reaction, results in severe acute thrombocytopenia in individuals previously sensitized to HPAs. It usually occurs an average of 9 days following transfusion of platelet antigen-containing blood products, usually red cells.[217] Through an as-yet-unknown mechanism, recipients' antigen-negative platelets are destroyed in the anamnestic alloimmune response, most often to HPA-1 system antigens. Following acute therapy with intravenous immunoglobulin, patients may preferentially respond to HPA-matched platelet products.[218] Efforts to prevent recurrence include prophylactic use of antigen-negative blood products and washed or frozen deglycerolized red cells (washed free of cellular antigens).

REFERENCES

1. Surgenor DM, Wallace EL, Hao SHS, et al: Collection and transfusion of blood in the United States, 1982–1988. *N Engl J Med* 322:1646, 1990.
2. Wallace EL, Surgenor DM, Hao HS, et al: Collection and transfusion of blood and blood components in the United States, 1989. *Transfusion* 33:139, 1993.
3. Wallace EL, Churchill WH, Surgenor DM, et al: Collection and transfusion of blood and blood components in the United States, 1992. *Transfusion* 35:802, 1995.
4. Wallace EL, Churchill WH, Surgenor DM, et al: Collection and transfusion of blood and blood components in the United States, 1994. *Transfusion* 38:625, 1998.
5. Sullivan MT, McCullough J, Schreiber GB, Wallace EL: Blood collection and transfusion in the United States in 1997. *Transfusion* 42:1253, 2002.
6. Sullivan MT, Wallace EL: Blood collection and transfusion in the United States in 1999. *Transfusion* 45:141, 2005.
7. Sullivan MT, Cotton R, Read EJ, Wallace EL: Blood collection and transfusion in the United States in 2001. *Transfusion* 47:385, 2007.
8. Whitaker BI, Sullivan M: *The 2005 Nationwide Blood Collection and Utilization Survey Report.* Department of Health & Human Services, Washington, DC, 2006.
9. Whitaker BI, Green J, King MR, et al: The 2007 Nationwide Blood Collection and Utilization Survey Report. Department of Health & Human Services, Washington, DC, 2008.
10. Moroff G, Kline L, Dabay M, et al: Reevaluation of the resting time period when preparing whole blood-derived platelet concentrates with the platelet-rich plasma method. *Transfusion* 46:572, 2006.
11. Kelley DL, Fegan RL, Ng AT, et al: High-yield platelet concentrates attainable by continuous quality improvement reduce platelet transfusion cost and donor exposure. *Transfusion* 37:482, 1997.
12. Hoeltge GA, Shah A, Miller JP: An optimized strategy for choosing the number of platelet concentrates to pool. *Arch Pathol Lab Med* 123:928, 1999.
13. Sweeney JD, Holme S, Heaton WA, et al: White cell-reduced platelet concentrates prepared by in-line filtration of platelet-rich plasma. *Transfusion* 35:131, 1995.
14. Lozano ML, Perez-Ceballos E, Rivera J, et al: Evaluation of a new whole-blood filter that allows preparation of platelet concentrates by platelet-rich plasma methods. *Transfusion* 43:1723, 2003.
15. Wilkinson SL, Lipton KS: Leukocyte reduction. *AABB Assoc Bull* 99–7, 1999.
16. Murphy S: Platelets from pooled buffy coats: An update. *Transfusion* 45:634, 2005.
17. Levin E, Culibrk B, Gyongyossy-Issa MI, et al: Implementation of buffy coat platelet component production: Comparison to platelet-rich plasma platelet production. *Transfusion* 48:2331, 2008.
18. Pietersz RN, Loos JA, Reesink HW: Platelet concentrates stored in plasma for 72 hours at 22°C prepared from buffy coats of citrate-phosphate-dextrose blood collected in a quadruple-bag saline-adenine-glucose-mannitol system. *Vox Sang* 49:81, 1985.
19. Bertolini F, Rebulla P, Riccardi D: Evaluation of platelet concentrates prepared from buffy coats and stored in a glucose-free crystalloid medium. *Transfusion* 29:605, 1989.
20. Bertolini F, Rebulla P, Marangoni F, et al: Platelet concentrates stored in synthetic medium after filtration. *Vox Sang* 62:82, 1992.
21. Heaton WAL, Rebulla P, Pappalettera M, Dzik WH: A comparative analysis of different methods for routine blood component preparation. *Transfus Med Rev* 11:116, 1997.
22. Van Delden CJ, de Wit HJC, Smit Sibinga CTH: Comparison of blood component preparation systems based on buffy coat removal: Component specifications, efficiency, and process costs. *Transfusion* 38:860, 1998.
23. Vassallo RR, Murphy S: A critical comparison of platelet preparation methods. *Curr Opin Hematol* 13:323, 2006.
24. Adams MR, Dumont LJ, McCall M, Heaton WA: Clinical trial and local process evaluation of an apheresis system for preparation of white cell-reduced platelet components. *Transfusion* 38:966, 1998.
25. Yockey C, Murphy S, Eggers L, et al: Evaluation of the Amicus separator in the collection of apheresis platelets. *Transfusion* 38:848, 1998.
26. Holme S, Andres M, Goermar N, Giordano GF: Improved removal of white cells with minimal platelet loss by filtration of apheresis platelets during collection. *Transfusion* 39:74, 1999.
27. Moog R, Valbonesi M, Carlier P: Collection of platelets and peripheral progenitor cells with Fresenius ASTEC 204 blood cell separator. *J Clin Apher* 12:126, 1997.
28. McLeod BC, Price TH, Owen H, et al: Frequency of immediate adverse effects associated with apheresis donation. *Transfusion* 38:938, 1998.
29. Goodnough LT, Ali S, Despotis G, et al: Economic impact of donor platelet count and platelet yield in apheresis products: Relevance for emerging issues in platelet transfusion therapy. *Vox Sang* 76:43, 1999.
30. Li J, Yang C, Xia Y, et al: Thrombocytopenia caused by the development of antibodies to thrombopoietin. *Blood* 98:3241, 2001.
31. Burgstaler EA: Blood component collection by apheresis. *J Clin Apher* 21:142, 2006.
32. AABB: Standards 5.7.5.19–20. *Standards for Blood Banks and Transfusion Services*, 25th ed. AABB Press, Bethesda, MD, 2008.
33. Heddle NM, Cook RJ, Tinmouth A, et al: A randomized controlled trial comparing standard- and low-dose strategies for transfusion of platelets (SToP) to patients with thrombocytopenia. *Blood* 113:1564, 2009.
34. Slichter SJ, Kaufman RM, Assmann SF, et al: Effects of prophylactic platelet (Plt) dose on transfusion (Tx) outcomes (PLADO trial) [abstract 285]. (ASH Annual Meeting Abstracts). *Blood* 2008.
35. Dodd RY, Notari IV EP, Stramer SL: Current prevalence and incidence of infectious disease markers and estimated window-period risk in the American Red Cross blood donor population. *Transfusion* 42:975, 2002.
36. Benjamin RJ, Kline L, Dy BA, et al: Bacterial contamination of whole blood-derived platelets: The introduction of sample diversion and pre-storage pooling with culture testing in the American Red Cross. *Transfusion* 48:2348, 2008.
37. Pietersz RN, Englefriet CP, Reesink HW, et al: Detection of bacterial contamination of platelet concentrates. *Vox Sang* 93:260, 2007.
38. Popovsky MA: Quality of blood components filtered before storage and at the bedside: Implications for transfusion practice. *Transfusion* 36:470, 1996.
39. Heddle NM, Cook RJ, Blajchman MA, et al: Assessing the effectiveness of whole blood-derived platelets stored as a pool: A randomized block noninferiority trial. *Transfusion* 45:896, 2005.
40. Heddle NM, Arnold DM, Boyle D, et al: Comparing the efficacy and safety of apheresis and whole blood-derived platelet transfusions: A systematic review. *Transfusion* 48:1447, 2008.
41. Murphy S, Gardner FH: Platelet preservation. Effect of storage temperature on maintenance of platelet viability—Deleterious effect of refrigerated storage. *N Engl J Med* 280:1094, 1969.
42. Murphy S: Platelet storage for transfusion. *Semin Hematol* 22:165, 1985.
43. Moroff G, Holme S: Concepts about current conditions for the preparation and storage of platelets. *Transfus Med Rev* 5:48, 1991.
44. Hunter S, Nixon J, Murphy S: The effect of the interruption of agitation on platelet quality during storage for transfusion. *Transfusion* 41:809, 2001.
45. van der Meer PF, Gulliksen H, Aubuchon JP, et al: Interruption of agitation of platelet concentrates: Effects on *in vitro* parameters. *Vox Sang* 88:227, 2005.
46. Wagner SJ, Vassallo R, Skripchenko A, et al: The influence of simulated shipping conditions (24- or 30-hr interruption of agitation) on the *in vitro* properties of apheresis platelets during 7-day storage. *Transfusion* 48:1072, 2008.
47. Gulliksen K: Platelet additive solutions: Current status. *Immunohematol* 23:14, 2007.
48. Ringwald J, Zimmermann R, Eckstein R: The new generation of platelet additive solution for storage at 22°C: Development and current experience. *Transfus Med Rev* 20:158, 2006.

49. Murphy S, Shimizu T, Miripol J: Platelet storage for transfusion in synthetic media: Further optimization of ingredients and definition of their roles. *Blood* 86:3951, 1995.
50. Shanwell A, Larsson S, Aschan J, et al: A randomized trial comparing the use of fresh and stored platelets in the treatment of bone marrow transplant recipients. *Eur J Haematol* 49:77, 1992.
51. Leach MR, AuBuchon JP: Effect of storage time on clinical efficacy of single-donor platelet units. *Transfusion* 33:661, 1993.
52. Murphy S, Kahn RA, Holme S, et al: Improved storage of platelets for transfusion in a new container. *Blood* 60:194, 1982.
53. Peter-Salonen K, Bucher UE, Nydegger UE: Comparison of post-transfusion recoveries achieved with either fresh or stored platelet concentrates. *Blut* 54:207, 1987.
54. Norol F, Kuentz M, Cordonnier C, et al: Influence of clinical status on the efficiency of stored platelet transfusion. *Br J Haematol* 86:125, 1994.
55. Rock G, Neurath D, Cober N, et al: Seven-day storage of random donor concentrates PLT. *Transfusion* 43:1374, 2003.
56. Dumont LJ, AuBuchon JP, Whitley P, et al: Seven-day storage of single-donor platelets: Recovery and survival in an autologous transfusion study. *Transfusion* 42:847, 2002.
57. AuBuchon JP, Taylor H, Holme S, Nelson E: *In vitro* and *in vivo* evaluation of leukoreduced platelets stored for 7 days in CLX containers. *Transfusion* 45:1356, 2005.
58. Food and Drug Administration: *Reduction of the Maximum Platelet Storage Period to 5 Days in an Approved Container*. CBER Office of Communication, Training and Manufacturers' Assistance, Rockville, MD, June 1986.
59. Webert KE, Cserti CM, Hannon J, et al: Proceedings of a consensus conference: Pathogen inactivation—Making decisions about new technologies. *Transfus Med Rev* 22:1, 2008.
60. Eder AF, Kennedy JM, Dy BA, et al: Bacterial screening of apheresis platelets and the residual risk of septic transfusion reactions: The American Red Cross experience (2004–2006). *Transfusion* 47:1134, 2007.
61. Blajchman MA, Goldman M, Baeza F: Improving the bacteriological safety of platelet transfusions. *Transfus Med Rev* 18:11, 2004.
62. Murphy S, Rebulla P, Bertolini F, et al: *In vitro* assessment of the quality of stored platelet concentrates. *Transfus Med Rev* 8:29, 1994.
63. Seghatchian J, Krailadsiri P: The platelet storage lesion. *Transfus Med Rev* 11:130, 1997.
64. Thon JN, Schubert P, Devine DV: Platelet storage lesion: A new understanding from a proteomic perspective. *Transfus Med Rev* 22:268, 2008.
65. Holme S, Moroff G, Murphy S: A multi-laboratory evaluation of *in vitro* platelet assays: The tests for extent of shape change and response to hypotonic shock. *Transfusion* 38:31, 1998.
66. Bertolini F, Murphy S: A multicenter evaluation of reproducibility of swirling in platelet concentrates. *Transfusion* 34:796, 1994.
67. Maurer-Spurej E, Chipperfield K: Past and future approaches to assess the quality of platelets for transfusion. *Transfus Med Rev* 21:295, 2007.
68. Albanyan AM, Harrison P, Murphy MF: Markers of platelet activation and apoptosis during storage of apheresis- and buffy coat-derived platelet concentrates for 7 days. *Transfusion* 49:108, 2009.
69. Ciavarella D, Lavallo E, Reiss RF: Coagulation factor activity in platelet concentrates stored up to 7 days: An *in vitro* and *in vivo* study. *Clin Lab Haematol* 8:233, 1986.
70. Murphy S, Sayar SN, Abdou NL, et al: Platelet preservation by freezing. Use of dimethylsulfoxide as cryoprotective agent. *Transfusion* 14:139, 1975.
71. Towell BL, Levine SP, Knight WA III, et al: A comparison of frozen and fresh platelet concentrates in the support of thrombocytopenic patients. *Transfusion* 26:525, 1986.
72. Lazarus HM, Kaniecki-Green EA, Warm SE, et al: Therapeutic effectiveness of frozen platelet concentrates for transfusion. *Blood* 57:243, 1981.
73. Schiffer CA, Aisner J, Wiernik PH: Frozen autologous platelet transfusion for patients with leukemia. *N Engl J Med* 299:7, 1978.
74. Currie LM, Livesey SA, Harper JR, Connor J: Cryopreservation of single-donor platelets with a reduced dimethyl sulfoxide concentration by the addition of second-messenger effectors: Enhanced retention of *in vitro* functional activity. *Transfusion* 38:160, 1998.
75. Vadhan-Raj S, Kavanagh JJ, Freedman RS, et al: Safety and efficacy of transfusions of autologous cryopreserved platelets derived from recombinant human thrombopoietin to support chemotherapy-associated severe thrombocytopenia: A randomized cross-over study. *Lancet* 359:2145, 2002.
76. Wautier JL: Safety and usefulness of autologous cryopreserved platelets. *Lancet* 360:1985, 2002.
77. Hillyer CD, Josephson CD, Blajchman MA, et al: Bacterial contamination of blood components: Risks, strategies, and regulation: Joint ASH and AABB educational session in transfusion medicine. *Hematology Am Soc Hematol Educ Program* 2003:575, 2003.
78. Holme S, Heaton A: *In vitro* platelet ageing at 22°C is reduced compared to *in vivo* ageing at 37°C. *Br J Haematol* 91:212, 1995.
79. Kaufman RM: Uncommon cold: Could 4 degrees C storage improve platelet function? *Transfusion* 45:1407, 2005.
80. Hoffmeister KM, Felbinger TW, Falet H, et al: The clearance mechanism of chilled blood platelets. *Cell* 112:1, 2003.
81. Hoffmeister KM, Josefsson EC, Isaac NA, et al: Glycosylation restores survival of chilled blood platelets. *Science* 301:1531, 2003.
82. Wandall HH, Hoffmeister KM, Sorenson AL, et al: Galactosylation does not prevent the rapid clearance of long-term, 4 degrees C-stored platelets. *Blood* 111:3249, 2008.
83. Sorenson AL, Hoffmeister KM, Wandall HH: Glycans and glycosylation of platelets: Current concepts and implications for transfusion. *Curr Opin Hematol* 15:606, 2008.
84. Blajchman MA: Substitutes and alternatives to platelet transfusions in thrombocytopenic patients. *J Thromb Haemost* 1:1637, 2003.
85. Mannucci PM: Hemostatic drugs. *N Engl J Med* 339:245, 1998.
86. Goodnough LT: Experiences with recombinant human factor VIIa in patients with thrombocytopenia. *Semin Hematol* 41(Suppl 1):25, 2004.
87. Birchall J, Stanworth SJ, Duffy MR, et al: Evidence for the use of recombinant factor VIIa in the prevention and treatment of bleeding in patients without hemophilia. *Transfus Med Rev* 22:177, 2008.
88. Levi M, Peters M, Büller HR: Efficacy and safety of recombinant factor VIIa for treatment of severe bleeding: A systematic review. *Crit Care Med* 33:883, 2005.
89. Bishop JF, McGrath K, Wolf MM, et al: Clinical factors influencing the efficacy of pooled platelet transfusions. *Blood* 71:383, 1988.
90. Davis KB, Slichter SJ, Corash L: Corrected count increment and percent platelet recovery as measures of posttransfusion platelet response: Problems and a solution. *Transfusion* 39:586, 1999.
91. Friedberg RC, Donnelly SF, Boyd JC, et al: Clinical and blood bank factors in the management of platelet refractoriness and alloimmunization. *Blood* 81:3428, 1993.
92. Klumpp TR, Herman J, Innis S, et al: Factors associated with response to platelet transfusion following hematopoietic stem cell transplantation. *Bone Marrow Transplant* 17:1035, 1996.
93. Doughty HA, Murphy MF, Metcalfe P, et al: Relative importance of immune and non-immune causes of platelet refractoriness. *Vox Sang* 66:200, 1994.
94. Alcorta I, Pereira A, Ordinas A: Clinical and laboratory factors associated with platelet transfusion refractoriness: A case-control study. *Br J Haematol* 93:220, 1996.
95. Bock M, Muggenthaler KH, Schmidt U, et al: Influence of antibiotics on posttransfusion platelet increment. *Transfusion* 36:952, 1996.
96. Slichter SJ, Davis K, Enright H, et al: Factors affecting posttransfusion platelet increments, platelet refractoriness, and platelet transfusion intervals in thrombocytopenic patients. *Blood* 105:4106, 2005.
97. O'Connell B, Lee EJ, Schiffer CA: The value of 10-minute posttransfusion platelet counts. *Transfusion* 28:66, 1988.
98. Bishop JF, Matthews JP, McGrath K, et al: Factors influencing 20-hour increments after platelet transfusion. *Transfusion* 31:392, 1991.
99. Hersh JK, Hom EG, Brecher ME: Mathematical modeling of platelet survival with implications of optimal transfusion practice in the chronically platelet transfusion-dependent patient. *Transfusion* 38:637, 1998.
100. Norol F, Bierling P, Roudot-Thoraval F, et al: Platelet transfusion: A dose-response study. *Blood* 92:1448, 1998.
101. Klumpp TR, Herman JH, Gaughan JP, et al: Clinical consequences of alterations in platelet transfusion dose: A prospective, randomized, double-blind trial. *Transfusion* 39:674, 1999.
102. Hanson SR, Slichter SJ: Platelet kinetics in patients with bone marrow hypoplasia: Evidence for a fixed platelet requirement. *Blood* 66:1105, 1985.
103. McVay PA, Toy PT: Lack of increased bleeding after liver biopsy in patients with mild hemostatic abnormalities. *Am J Clin Pathol* 94:747, 1990.
104. Anonymous: Practice parameter for use of fresh-frozen plasma, cryoprecipitate, and platelets. *JAMA* 271:777, 1994.
105. Tinmouth AT, Freedman J: Prophylactic platelet transfusions: Which dose is the best dose? A review of the literature. *Transfus Med Rev* 17:181, 2003.
106. Brecher ME: The platelet prophylactic transfusion trigger: When expectations meet reality. *Transfusion* 47:188, 2007.
107. Friedmann AM, Sengul H, Lehmann H, et al: Do basic laboratory tests or clinical observations predict bleeding in thrombocytopenic oncology patients? A reevaluation of prophylactic platelet transfusions. *Transfus Med Rev* 16:34, 2002.
108. Slichter SJ: Relationship between platelet count and bleeding risk in thrombocytopenic patients. *Transfus Med Rev* 18:152, 2004.
109. Gaydos LA, Freireich EJ, Mantel N: The quantitative relation between platelet count and hemorrhage in patients with acute leukemia. *N Engl J Med* 266:905, 1962.
110. Freireich EJ, Kliman A, Lawrence AG, et al: Response to repeated platelet transfusion from the same donor. *Ann Intern Med* 59:277, 1963.
111. Gmur J, Burger J, Schanz U, et al: Safety of stringent prophylactic platelet transfusion policy for patients with acute leukemia. *Lancet* 338:1223, 1991.
112. Sagmeister M, Oec L, Gmur J: A restrictive platelet transfusion policy allowing long-term support of outpatients with severe aplastic anemia. *Blood* 93:3124, 1999.
113. Heckman KD, Weiner GJ, Davis CS, et al: Randomized study of prophylactic platelet transfusion threshold during induction therapy for adult acute leukemia: 10,000/μL versus 20,000/μL *J Clin Oncol* 15:1143, 1997.
114. Rebulla P, Finazzi G, Marangoni F, et al: The threshold for prophylactic platelet transfusions in adults with acute myeloid leukemia. *N Engl J Med* 337:1870, 1997.
115. Wandt H, Frank M, Ehninger G, et al: Safety and cost effectiveness of a 10×10^9/L trigger for prophylactic platelet transfusion compared with the traditional 20×10^9/L trigger: A prospective comparative trial in 105 patients with acute myeloid leukemia. *Blood* 91:3601, 1998.
116. Contreras M: The appropriate use of platelets: An update from the Edinburgh Consensus Conference. *Br J Haematol* 101:10, 1998.
117. Schiffer CA, Anderson KC, Bennett CL, et al: Platelet transfusions for patients with cancer: Clinical practice guidelines of the American Society of Clinical Oncology. *J Clin Oncol* 19:1510, 2001.

118. Stanworth SJ, Hyde C, Brunskill S, et al: Platelet transfusion prophylaxis for patients with haematological malignancies: Where to now? *Br J Haematol* 131:588, 2005.
119. George T, Ho-Tin-Noe B, Carbo C, et al: Inflammation induces hemorrhage in thrombocytopenia. *Blood* 111:4958, 2008.
120. Nevo S, Swan V, Enger C, et al: Acute bleeding after bone marrow transplantation (BMT)—Incidence and effect on survival. A quantitative analysis in 1,402 patients. *Blood* 91:1469, 1998.
121. Bernstein SH, Nademanee AP, Vose JM, et al: A multicenter study of platelet recovery and utilization in patients after myeloablative therapy and hematopoietic stem cell transplantation. *Blood* 91:3509, 1998.
122. Wandt H, Wendelin K, Schaefer-Eckart K, et al: A therapeutic platelet transfusion strategy without routine prophylactic transfusion is feasible and safe and reduces platelet transfusion numbers significantly: Preliminary analysis of a randomized study in patients after high dose chemotherapy and autologous peripheral blood stem cell transplantation. *Blood* 112:286, 2008.
123. Blajchman MA, Slichter SJ, Heddle NM, Murphy MF: New strategies for the optimal use of platelet transfusions. *Hematology Am Soc Hematol Educ Program* 2008:198, 2008.
124. Reed RL, Ciavarella D, Heimbach DM, et al: Prophylactic platelet administration during massive transfusion. A prospective, randomized, double-blind clinical study. *Ann Surg* 203:40, 1986.
125. Hiippala ST, Myllyla GJ, Vahtera EM: Hemostatic factors and replacement of major blood loss with plasma-poor red cell concentrates. *Anesth Analg* 81:360, 1995.
126. Duchesne JC, Hunt JP, Wahl G, et al: Review of current blood transfusion strategies in a mature level I trauma center: Were we wrong for the last 60 years? *J Trauma* 65:272, 2008.
127. Gunter OL Jr, Au BK, Isbell JM, et al: Optimizing outcomes in damage control resuscitation: Identifying blood product ratios associated with improved survival. *J Trauma* 65:527, 2008.
128. Scalea TM, Bochiccio KM, Lumpkins K, et al: Early aggressive use of fresh frozen plasma does not improve outcome in critically injured trauma patients. *Ann Surg* 248:578, 2008.
129. Simon TL, Aki Bechara F, Murphy W: Controlled trial of routine administration of platelet concentrates in cardiopulmonary bypass surgery. *Ann Thorac Surg* 37:359, 1984.
130. Ferraris VA, Ferraris SP, Saha SP, et al: Perioperative blood transfusion and blood conservation in cardiac surgery: The Society of Thoracic Surgeons and the Society of Cardiovascular Anesthesiologists clinical practice guideline. *Ann Thorac Surg* 83:S27, 2007.
131. Fergusson DA, Hebert PC, Mazer CD, et al: A comparison of aprotinin and lysine analogues in high-risk cardiac surgery. *N Engl J Med* 258:2319, 2008.
132. Carr JM, Kruskall MS, Kaye JA, et al: Efficacy of platelet transfusions in immune thrombocytopenia. *Am J Med* 80:1051, 1986.
133. McIntoch S, O'Brien RT, Schwartz AD, et al: Neonatal isoimmune purpura: Response to platelet infusions. *J Pediatr* 82:1020, 1973.
134. Bussel JB, Zacharoulis S, Kramer K, et al: Clinical and diagnostic comparison of neonatal alloimmune thrombocytopenia to non-immune causes of thrombocytopenia. *Pediatr Blood Cancer* 45:176, 2005.
135. Kiefel V, Bassler D, Kroll H, et al: Antigen-positive platelet transfusion in neonatal alloimmune thrombocytopenia. *Blood* 107:3761, 2006.
136. Allen D, Verjee S, Rees S, et al: Platelet transfusion in neonatal alloimmune thrombocytopenia. *Blood* 109:388, 2007.
137. Murphy MF, Bussel JB: Advances in the management of alloimmune thrombocytopenia. *Br J Haematol* 136:366, 2007.
138. Murphy S: Hereditary thrombocytopenia, in *Clinics in Haematology*, edited by JR O'Brien Jr, p 359. WB Saunders, London, 1972.
139. Swisher KK, Terrell DR, Vesely SK, et al: Clinical outcomes after platelet transfusions in patients with thrombotic thrombocytopenic purpura. *Transfusion* 49:873, 2009.
140. Hopkins CK, Goldfinger D: Platelet transfusions in heparin-induced thrombocytopenia: A report of 4 cases and review of the literature. *Transfusion* 48:2128, 2008.
141. Kao KJ, del Rosario MLU: Role of class-II major histocompatibility complex (MHC)-antigen-positive donor leukocytes in transfusion-induced alloimmunization to donor class-I antigens MHC. *Blood* 92:690, 1998.
142. The Trial to Reduce Alloimmunization to Platelets Study Group: Leukocyte reduction and ultraviolet B irradiation of platelets to prevent alloimmunization and refractoriness to platelet transfusions. *N Engl J Med* 337:1861, 1997.
143. Vamvakas EC: Meta-analysis of randomized controlled trials of the efficacy of white cell reduction in preventing HLA-alloimmunization and refractoriness to random-donor platelet transfusions. *Transfus Med Rev* 12:258, 1998.
144. Seftel MD, Growe GH, Petraszko T, et al: Universal prestorage leuko-reduction in Canada decreases platelet alloimmunization and refractoriness. *Blood* 103:333, 2004.
145. Friedman DF, Lukas MB, Jawad A, et al: Alloimmunization to platelets in heavily transfused patients with sickle cell disease. *Blood* 88:3216, 1996.
146. Bishop JF, Matthews JP, Yuen K, et al: The definition of refractoriness to platelet transfusions. *Transfus Med* 2:35, 1992.
147. Worthington JE, Robson AJ, Sheldon S, et al: A comparison of enzyme-linked immunoabsorbent assays and flow cytometry techniques for the detection of HLA specific antibodies. *Hum Immunol* 62:1178, 2001.
148. Chesterton KA, Pretl K, Sholander JT, et al: Rapid and reliable detection of HLA-specific antibodies with the Luminexx platform. *Hum Immunol* 64(Suppl 10):S108, 2003.
149. Hogge DE, Dutcher JP, Aisner J, et al: Lymphocytotoxic antibody is a predictor of response to random donor platelet transfusion. *Am J Hematol* 14:363, 1983.
150. McFarland JG, Anderson AJ, Slichter SJ: Factors influencing the transfusion response to HLA-selected apheresis donor platelets in patients refractory to random platelet concentrates. *Br J Haematol* 73:380, 1989.
151. Vassallo RR Jr: New paradigms in the management of alloimmune refractoriness to platelet transfusions. *Curr Opin Hematol* 14:655, 2007.
152. Dutcher JP, Schiffer CA, Aisner J, et al: Long-term follow-up of patients with leukemia receiving platelet transfusions: Identification of a large group of patients who do not become alloimmunized. *Blood* 58:1007, 1981.
153. Dutcher JP, Schiffer CA, Aisner J, et al: Alloimmunization following platelet transfusion: The absence of a dose-response relationship. *Blood* 57:395, 1981.
154. Duquesnoy RJ, Claas FH: 14th International HLA and immunogenics workshop: Report on the structural basis of HLA compatibility. *Tissue Antigens* 69(Suppl 1):108, 2007.
155. Datema G, Stein S, Eijsink C, et al: HLA-C expression on platelets: Studies with an HLA-Cw1-specific human monoclonal antibody. *Vox Sang* 79:108, 2000.
156. Saito S, Ota S, Seshimo H, et al: Platelet transfusion refractoriness caused by a mismatch in HLA-antigens C. *Transfusion* 42:302, 2002.
157. Lee EJ, Schiffer CA: Serial measurement of lymphocytotoxic antibody and response to nonmatched platelet transfusion in alloimmunized patients. *Blood* 70:1727, 1987.
158. Rodey GE, Neylan JF, Whelchel JD, Revels KW: Epitope specificity of HLA class I alloantibodies: I. Frequency analysis of antibodies to private versus public specificities in potential transplant recipients. *Hum Immunol* 39:272, 1994.
159. Zimmermann R, Wittmann G, Zingsem J, et al: Antibodies to private and public HLA class I epitopes in platelet recipients. *Transfusion* 39:772, 1999.
160. MacPherson BR: HLA antibody formation within the HLA-A1 cross reactive group in multitransfused platelet recipients. *Am J Hematol* 30:228, 1989.
161. Yankee RA, Grumet FC, Rogentine GN: Platelet transfusion. The selection of compatible platelet donors for refractory patients by lymphocyte typing HLA. *N Engl J Med* 281:1208, 1969.
162. Duquesnoy RJ, Filip DJ, Rodey GE, et al: Successful transfusion of platelets "mismatched" for HLA antigens to alloimmunized thrombocytopenic patients. *Am J Hematol* 22:219, 1977.
163. von dem Borne AEG, Ouwehand WH, Kuijpers RW: Theoretic and practical aspects of platelet crossmatching. *Transfus Med Rev* 4:265, 1990.
164. Gelb AB, Leavitt AD: Crossmatch-compatible platelets improve corrected count increments in patients who are refractory to randomly selected platelets. *Transfusion* 37:624, 1997.
165. Petz LD, Garratty G, Calhoun C, et al: Selecting donors of platelets for refractory patients on the basis of HLA antibody specificity. *Transfusion* 40:1446, 2000.
166. Hod E, Schwartz, J: Platelet transfusion refractoriness. *Br J Haematol* 142:348, 2008.
167. Santoso S, Kiefel V, Mueller-Eckhardt C: Blood groups A and B determinants are expressed on platelet glycoproteins IIa, IIIa, Ib. *Thromb Haemost* 65:196, 1991.
168. Cooling L: ABO and platelet transfusion therapy. *Immunohematol* 23:20, 2007.
169. Heal JM, Blumberg N, Masel D: An evaluation of crossmatching, HLA and ABO matching for platelet transfusions to refractory patients. *Blood* 70:23, 1987.
170. Jimenez TM, Patel SB, Pineda AA, et al: Factors that influence platelet recovery after transfusion: Resolving donor quality from compatibility ABO. *Transfusion* 43:328, 2003.
171. Heal JM, Masel D, Rowe JM, Blumberg N: Circulating immune complexes involving the ABO system after platelet transfusion. *Br J Haematol* 85:566, 1993.
172. McManigal S, Sims KL: Intravascular hemolysis secondary to ABO incompatible platelet products. An under-recognized transfusion reaction. *Am J Clin Pathol* 111:202, 1999.
173. Lozano M, Cid J: The clinical implications of platelet transfusions associated with ABO or Rh(D) incompatibility. *Transfus Med Rev* 17:57, 2003.
174. Heal M, Blumberg N: The second century of ABO: And now for something completely different. *Transfusion* 39:1155, 1999.
175. Langenscheidt F, Kiefel V, Santoso S, et al: Platelet transfusion refractoriness associated with two rare platelet-specific alloantibodies (anti-Bak^{a} and anti-P1^{A2}) and multiple HLA antibodies. *Transfusion* 28:597, 1988.
176. Ikeda H, Mitani T, Ohnuma M, et al: A new platelet-specific antigen, Nak^{a}, involved in the refractoriness of HLA-matched platelet transfusion. *Vox Sang* 57:213, 1989.
177. Saji H, Maruya E, Fujii H, et al: New platelet antigen, Sib^{a}, involved in platelet transfusion refractoriness in a Japanese man. *Vox Sang* 56:283, 1989.
178. Kekomaki S, Volin L, Koistinen P, et al: Successful treatment of platelet transfusion refractoriness: The use of platelet transfusions matched for both human leucocyte antigens (HLA) and human platelet alloantigens (HPA) in alloimmunized patients with leukaemia. *Eur J Haematol* 60:112, 1998.
179. Pappalardo PA, Secord AR, Quitevis P, et al: Platelet transfusion refractoriness associated with HPA-1a (Pl^{A1}) alloantibody without coexistent HLA antibodies successfully treated with antigen-negative platelet transfusions. *Transfusion* 41:984, 2001.
180. Uhrynowska M, Zupanska B: Platelet-specific antibodies in transfused patients. *Eur J Haematol* 56:248, 1996.
181. Sanz C, Freire C, Alcorta I, et al: Platelet-specific antibodies in HLA immunized patients receiving chronic platelet support. *Transfusion* 41:762, 2001.
182. Kiefel V, Konig C, Kroll H, Santoso S: Platelet alloantibodies in transfused patients. *Transfusion* 41:766, 2001.
183. Lucas GF, Rogers SE: Evaluation of an enzyme-linked immunosorbent assay kit (GTI PakPlus) for the detection of antibodies against human platelet antigens. *Transfus Med* 9:63, 1999.

184. Allen D, Ouwehand WH, de Haas M, et al: Interlaboratory variation in the detection of HPA-specific alloantibodies and in molecular HPA typing. *Vox Sang* 93:316, 2007.
185. Curtis BR: Genotyping for human platelet alloantigen polymorphisms: Applications in the diagnosis of alloimmune platelet disorders. *Semin Thromb Hemost* 34:539, 2008.
186. Mangano MM, Chambers LA, Kruskall MS: Limited efficacy of leukopoor platelets for prevention of febrile transfusion reactions. *Am J Clin Pathol* 95:733, 1991.
187. Goodnough LT, Riddell J, Lazarus H, et al: Prevalence of platelet transfusion reactions before and after implementation of leukocyte depleted platelet concentrates by filtration. *Vox Sang* 65:103, 1993.
188. Heddle NM, Klama L, Singer J, et al: The role of the plasma from platelet concentrates in transfusion reactions. *N Engl J Med* 331:625, 1994.
189. Heddle NM, Klama L, Meyer R, et al: A randomized controlled trial comparing plasma removal with white cell reduction to prevent reactions to platelets. *Transfusion* 39:231, 1999.
190. Kelley DL, Mangini J, Lopez-Plaza I, Triulzi D: The utility of ≤3-day old whole-blood platelets in reducing the incidence of febrile nonhemolytic transfusion reactions. *Transfusion* 40:439, 2000.
191. Geiger TL, Howard SC: Acetaminophen and diphenhydramine premedication for allergic and febrile nonhemolytic transfusion reactions: Good prophylaxis or bad practice? *Transfus Med Rev* 21:1, 2007.
192. Phipps RP, Kaufman J, Blumberg N: Platelet derived CD154 (CD40 ligand) and febrile responses to transfusion. *Lancet* 357:2023, 2001.
193. Buck SA, Kickler TS, McGuire M, et al: The utility of platelet washing using an automated procedure for severe platelet allergic reactions. *Transfusion* 27:391, 1987.
194. Kennedy LD, Case LD, Hurd DD, et al. A prospective, randomized, double-blind controlled trial of acetaminophen and diphenhydramine pretransfusion medication versus placebo for the prevention of transfusion reactions. *Transfusion* 48:2285, 2008.
195. Bowden RA, Slichter SJ, Sayers M, et al: A comparison of filtered leukocyte-reduced and cytomegalovirus (CMV) seronegative blood products for the prevention of transfusion-associated CMV infection after marrow transplant. *Blood* 86:3598, 1995.
196. Nichols WG, Price TH, Gooley T, et al: Transfusion-transmitted cytomegalovirus infection after receipt of leukoreduced blood products. *Blood* 101:4195, 2003.
197. Leitman SF, Holland PV: Irradiation of blood products. Indications and guidelines. *Transfusion* 25:293, 1985.
198. Sweeney JD, Holme S, Moroff G: Storage of apheresis platelets after gamma irradiation. *Transfusion* 34:779, 1994.
199. Hume HA, Popovsky MA, Benson K, et al: Hypotensive reactions: A previously uncharacterized complication of platelet transfusion? *Transfusion* 36:904, 1996.
200. Mair B, Leparc GF: Hypotensive reactions associated with platelet transfusions and angiotensin-converting enzyme inhibitors. *Vox Sang* 74:27, 1998.
201. Cyr M, Eastlund T, Blais C Jr, et al: Bradykinin metabolism and hypotensive transfusion reactions. *Transfusion* 41:136, 2001.
202. Arnold DM, Molinaro G, Warkentin TE, et al: Hypotensive transfusion reactions can occur with blood products that are leukoreduced before storage. *Transfusion* 44:1361, 2004.
203. Goldfinger D, McGinniss MH: Rh-incompatible platelet transfusion—Risks and consequences of sensitizing immunosuppressed patients. *N Engl J Med* 284:942, 1971.
204. Menitove JL: Immunoprophylaxis for D− patients receiving transfusions from D+ donors. *Transfusion* 42:136, 2002.
205. Blajchman MA, Beckers EA, Dickmeiss E, et al: Bacterial detection of platelets: Current problems and possible resolutions. *Transfus Med Rev* 19:259, 2005.
206. Anderson KC, Lew MA, Gorgone BC, et al: Transfusion-related sepsis after prolonged platelet storage. *Am J Med* 81:405, 1986.
207. Heal JM, Singal S, Sardisco E, et al: Bacterial proliferation in platelet concentrates. *Transfusion* 26:388, 1993.
208. AuBuchon JP, Kruskall MS: Transfusion safety: Realigning efforts and risks. *Transfusion* 37:1211, 1997.
209. Svoboda R, Lipton KS: Bacterial contamination of blood components. *AABB Assoc Bull* 96–6, 1996.
210. Blajchman MA, Goldman M, Baeza F: Improving the bacteriological safety of platelet transfusions. *Transfus Med Rev* 18:11, 2004.
211. Leiby DA, Lenes BA, Tibbals MA, Tames-Olmedo MT: Prospective evaluation of a patient with *Trypanosoma cruzi* infection transmitted by transfusion. *N Engl J Med* 341:1237, 1999.
212. Garratty G: Problems associated with passively transfused blood group alloantibodies. *Am J Clin Pathol* 109:769, 1998.
213. Mair B, Benson K: Evaluation of changes in hemoglobin levels associated with ABO-incompatible plasma in apheresis platelets. *Transfusion* 38:51, 1998.
214. McManigal S, Sims KL: Intravascular hemolysis secondary to ABO incompatible platelet products. An under recognized transfusion reaction. *Am J Clin Pathol* 111:202, 1999.
215. Gilstad CW: Anaphylactic transfusion reactions. *Curr Opin Hematol* 10:419, 2003.
216. Mair DC, Hirschler N, Eastlund T: Blood donor and component management strategies to prevent transfusion-related acute lung injury (TRALI). *Crit Care Med* 34(5 Suppl):S137, 2006.
217. McFarland JG: Posttransfusion purpura, in *Transfusion Reactions*, 3rd ed, edited by MA Popovsky, p 275. AABB Press, Bethesda, MD, 2007.
218. Win N, Peterkin MA, Watson WH: The therapeutic value of HPA-1a-negative platelet transfusion in post-transfusion purpura complicated by life-threatening haemorrhage. *Vox Sang* 69:138, 1995.
219. Murphy S: Platelet transfusion therapy, in *Thrombosis and Hemorrhage*, 2nd ed, edited by J Loscalzo, AI Schafer, p 1119. Williams & Wilkins, Philadelphia, 1998.

INDEX

Page numbers in **boldface** *type indicate a major discussion. A "t" following a page number indicates tabular material, and an "f" following a page number indicates a figure.*

A

C

D

F

G

M

N

O

P

Q

R

T

U

W

X

Y

Z